MW00453751

The ASAM Principles of Addiction Medicine

Seventh Edition

Senior Editor

Shannon C. Miller, MD, DFASAM, DLFAPA

Dayton VA Medical Center
Clinical Professor of Psychiatry and Population and Public Health Sciences
Boonshoft School of Medicine
Wright State University
Founding Co-Editor
Journal of Addiction Medicine (2006-2016)
American Society of Addiction Medicine
Lieutenant Colonel, Retired
United States Air Force
Dayton/Cincinnati, Ohio

Associate Editors

Richard N. Rosenthal, MD, MA, DLFAPA, DFAAAP, FASAM

Professor of Psychiatry
Director of Addiction Psychiatry
Department of Psychiatry
Stony Brook University Medical Center
Stony Brook, New York

Sharon Levy, MD, MPH, FASAM, FAAP

Chief, Division of Addiction Medicine
Boston Children's Hospital
Professor of Pediatrics
Harvard Medical School
Boston, Massachusetts

Andrew J. Saxon, MD, FASAM

Professor
Department of Psychiatry and Behavioral Sciences
University of Washington School of Medicine
Seattle, Washington

Jeanette M. Tetrault, MD, FACP, FASAM

Professor of Medicine and Public Health
Vice Chief for Education
Section of General Internal Medicine
Program Director, Addiction Medicine Fellowship
Associate Director for Education and Training
Program in Addiction Medicine
Yale School of Medicine
New Haven, Connecticut

Sarah E. Wakeman, MD, FASAM

Medical Director for Substance Use Disorder at Mass General Brigham
Medical Director for the MGH Substance Use Disorder Initiative
Director of the Program for Substance Use and Addiction Services
MGH Division of General Internal Medicine
Boston, Massachusetts

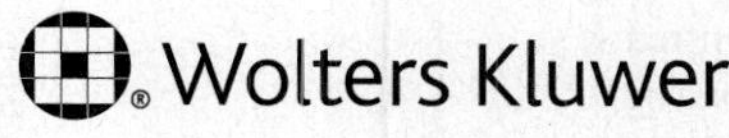

Philadelphia • Baltimore • New York • London
Buenos Aires • Hong Kong • Sydney • Tokyo

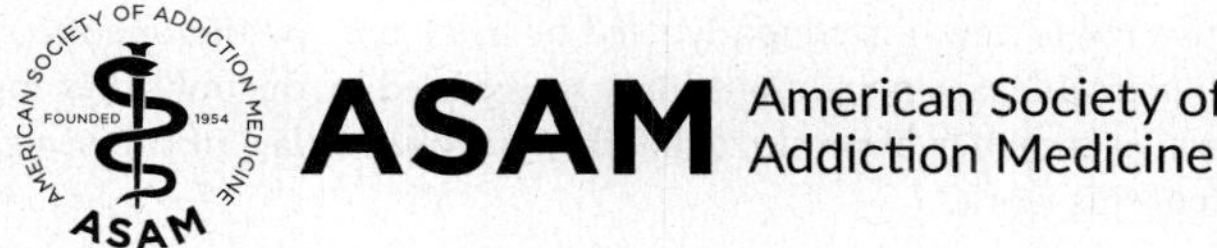

Acquisitions Editor: Chris Teja
Development Editor: Ariel S. Winter
Editorial Coordinator: Sean Hanrahan
Editorial Assistant: Jaida Lively
Marketing Manager: Kirsten Watrud
Production Project Manager: Bridgett Dougherty
Manager, Graphic Arts & Design: Stephen Druding
Manufacturing Coordinator: Lisa Bowling
Prepress Vendor: Straive

ASAM Staff
Director of Quality Improvement: Leigh Hause-Alvarado
Sr. Manager, Scientific Publications: Anne Luzier

Cover Photos Are Stock Photos. Posed by models.

7th Edition

9 8 7 6 5 4 3 2 1
Printed in Mexico

Cataloging-in-Publication Data available on request from the Publisher

ISBN: 978-1-9752-0156-2

This work is provided "as is," and the publisher disclaims any and all warranties, express or implied, including any warranties as to accuracy, comprehensiveness, or currency of the content of this work.

This work is no substitute for individual patient assessment based upon healthcare professionals' examination of each patient and consideration of, among other things, age, weight, gender, current or prior medical conditions, medication history, laboratory data and other factors unique to the patient. The publisher does not provide medical advice or guidance and this work is merely a reference tool. Healthcare professionals, and not the publisher, are solely responsible for the use of this work including all medical judgments and for any resulting diagnosis and treatments.

Given continuous, rapid advances in medical science and health information, independent professional verification of medical diagnoses, indications, appropriate pharmaceutical selections and dosages, and treatment options should be made and healthcare professionals should consult a variety of sources. When prescribing medication, healthcare professionals are advised to consult the product information sheet (the manufacturer's package insert) accompanying each drug to verify, among other things, conditions of use, warnings and side effects and identify any changes in dosage schedule or contraindications, particularly if the medication to be administered is new, infrequently used or has a narrow therapeutic range. To the maximum extent permitted under applicable law, no responsibility is assumed by the publisher for any injury and/or damage to persons or property, as a matter of products liability, negligence law or otherwise, or from any reference to or use by any person of this work.

shop.lww.com

QUADM0224

Dedicated to all people whose lives have been affected by addiction and related conditions and to those who care for them based on empathy, understanding, respect, and the best science available.

Section Editors

Anika Alvanzo, MD, MS, DFASAM, FACP
Eastern Region Medical Director for Pyramid Healthcare, Inc.
Physician Consultant to Behavioral Health Administration
Maryland Department of Health
Managing Partner of Uzima Consulting Group, LLC
Baltimore, Maryland

Sarah M. Bagley, MD
Assistant Professor of Medicine and Pediatrics
Boston University School of Medicine
Boston, Massachusetts

William C. Becker, MD
Associate Professor
Department of Internal Medicine
Yale School of Medicine
New Haven, Connecticut

J. Wesley Boyd, MD, PhD
Professor
Medical Ethics and Psychiatry
Baylor College of Medicine
Houston, Texas

Timothy K. Brennan, MD, MPH
Chief of Clinical Services–Addiction
Department of Psychiatry
Icahn School of Medicine at Mount Sinai
New York, New York

Deepa R. Camenga, MD, MHS
Associate Professor
Emergency Medicine and Pediatrics
Yale School of Medicine
New Haven, Connecticut

Martin D. Cheatle, PhD
Associate Professor
Department of Psychiatry and Anesthesiology
Perelman School of Medicine
University of Pennsylvania
Philadelphia, Pennsylvania

Wilson M. Compton, MD, MPE
Deputy Director
National Institute on Drug Abuse
National Institutes of Health
Bethesda, Maryland

Dennis C. Daley, PhD
Professor of Psychiatry (Adjunct)
Department of Psychiatry
University of Pittsburgh School of Medicine
Pittsburgh, Pennsylvania

Smita Das, MD, PhD, MPH
Clinical Associate Professor
Department of Psychiatry and Behavioral Sciences
Stanford School of Medicine
Stanford, California

Antoine Douaihy, MD
Professor of Psychiatry and Medicine
Department of Psychiatry
University of Pittsburgh School of Medicine
Pittsburgh, Pennsylvania

Robert L. DuPont, MD
President
Institute for Behavior and Health, Inc.
Rockville, Maryland

Babalola Faseru, MD, MPH
Professor, Family Medicine and Community Health
Director, KU Tobacco Treatment Education Program
Population Health
Consultant Medical Epidemiologist
Bureau of Health Promotion
Kansas Department of Health and Environment
Adjunct Faculty
School of Health Professions
University of Kansas Medical Center
Kansas City, Kansas

Deborah S. Finnell, PhD
Professor Emerita
School of Nursing
Johns Hopkins University
Baltimore, Maryland

Maria Gabriela Garcia Vassallo, MD
Assistant Professor of Psychiatry
Yale School of Medicine
New Haven, Connecticut

Eric L. Garland, PhD, LCSW
Distinguished Professor
College of Social Work
University of Utah
Salt Lake City, Utah

R. Jeffrey Goldsmith, MD, DLFAPA, FASAM
Self-employed
Biddeford Pool, Maine

Adam J. Gordon, MD, MPH, FACP, DFASAM
Elbert F. and Marie Christensen Endowed Research Professorship
Professor of Medicine and Psychiatry
Director, Program for Addiction Research, Clinical Care, Knowledge, and Advocacy
Codirector, Greater Intermountain Node of the NIH NIDA Clinical Trials Network
University of Utah School of Medicine
National Director, Medication Addiction Treatment in the VA
Initiative National Codirector
Coordinating Center of the Interprofessional Advanced Fellowship in Addiction Treatment Director (Emeritus)
Vulnerable Veteran Innovative Patient Aligned Care Team (VIP) Initiative
Salt Lake City, Utah

David A. Gorelick, MD, PhD
Professor
Department of Psychiatry
University of Maryland
Baltimore, Maryland

Jon E. Grant, MD
Professor
Department of Psychiatry and Behavioral Neuroscience
University of Chicago
Chicago, Illinois

Sion Kim Harris, PhD, RN
Associate Professor
Department of Pediatrics
Harvard Medical School
Boston, Massachusetts

Ana Holtey, DO, MS
Adjunct Assistant Professor
Department of Psychiatry
University of Utah
Salt Lake City, Utah

Michael A. Incze, MD, MSED
Associate Professor of Medicine
Division of General Internal Medicine
University of Utah Health
Salt Lake City, Utah

Amy J. Kennedy, MD, MS
Acting Assistant Professor of Medicine
Division of General Internal Medicine
VA Puget Sound Healthcare System
University of Washington School of Medicine
Seattle, Washington

Thomas R. Kosten, MD
Waggoner Professor
Department of Psychiatry, Neuroscience, Pharmacology
Baylor College of Medicine
Houston, Texas

Catalina Lopez-Quintero, PhD
Assistant Professor
Department of Epidemiology
University of Florida
Gainesville, Florida

Paula Lum, MD, MPH
Professor
School of Medicine
University of California, San Francisco
San Francisco, California

Lisa J. Merlo, PhD, MPE
Professor of Psychiatry
University of Florida
Gainesville, Florida

Edward V. Nunes, MD
Professor
Department of Psychiatry
Columbia University Irving Medical Center
New York, New York

Karran A. Phillips, MD, MSc
Deputy Director
Center for Substance Abuse Treatment
Substance Abuse and Mental Health Services Administration
Rockville, Maryland

Darius A. Rastegar, MD
Associate Professor of Medicine
Division of Addiction Medicine
Department of Medicine
Johns Hopkins University School of Medicine
Baltimore, Maryland

Richard K. Ries, MD
Professor of Psychiatry
Director Addictions Division
Department of Psychiatry and Behavioral Sciences
University of Washington School of Medicine
Seattle, Washington

Corrine L. Shea, MA
Executive Director
Institute for Behavior and Health, Inc.
Rockville, Maryland

Daryl Shorter, MD
Associate Professor
Menninger Department of Psychiatry and Behavioral Sciences
Baylor College of Medicine
Houston, Texas

Frank Vocci, PhD
President and Senior Research Scientist
Social Research Center
Friends Research Institute
Bethesda, Maryland

Emily C. Williams, PhD, MPH
Professor
Department of Health Systems and Population Health
University of Washington
Seattle, Washington

Sarah W. Yip, PhD, MSc
Associate Professor of Psychiatry
Yale School of Medicine
New Haven, Connecticut

Contributors

Hoover Adger, MD, MPH, MBA
Professor
Department of Pediatrics
Johns Hopkins University School of Medicine
Baltimore, Maryland

Majid Afshar, MD, MS
Assistant Professor
Department of Medicine
University of Wisconsin–Madison
Madison, Wisconsin

Nassima Ait-Daoud Tiouririne, MD
Professor of Psychiatry
Department of Psychiatry and Neurobehavioral Sciences
University of Virginia
Charlottesville, Virginia

Mona Al Banna, MB BCH, MSc (Res)
Neurologist
Cerebrovascular Institute
Cleveland Clinic
Cleveland, Ohio

Daniel P. Alford, MD, MPH, FACP, DFASAM
Professor of Medicine
General Internal Medicine
Boston University School of Medicine
Boston, Massachusetts

Rachel H. Alinsky, MD, MPH
Assistant Professor
Department of Pediatrics
Johns Hopkins University School of Medicine
Baltimore, Maryland

Steven Allen, MD
Addiction Psychiatrist
Los Angeles County Department of Mental Health
Los Angeles, California

Hamada Hamid Altalib, DO, MPH, FAES
Chief of Neurology
VA Connecticut Healthcare System
Associate Professor
Department of Neurology
Yale School of Medicine
New Haven, Connecticut

James C. Anthony, MSc, PhD
Professor
Department of Epidemiology and Biostatistics
Michigan State University College of Human Medicine
East Lansing, Michigan

Ayesha Appa, MD
Infectious Diseases and Addiction Medicine Physician
Department of Medicine
University of California, San Francisco
San Francisco, California

Nicholas Athanasiou, MD, MBA
Associate Clinical Professor, Health Sciences
Department of Psychiatry
UCLA–Olive View Medical Center
Los Angeles, California

Sanford Auerbach, MD
Director, Sleep Disorders Center
Department of Neurology
Boston Medical Center
Boston, Massachusetts

Nicole Avena, PhD
Associate Professor
Department of Neuroscience
Icahn School of Medicine at Mount Sinai
New York, New York

Thomas F. Babor, PhD, MPH
Emeritus Professor
Department of Public Health Sciences
University of Connecticut School of Medicine
Farmington, Connecticut

Sudie E. Back, PhD
Professor
Department of Psychiatry
Medical University of South Carolina
Mt. Pleasant, South Carolina

Ruben Baler, MsC, PhD
Health Scientist
National Institute on Drug Abuse
National Institutes of Health
Bethesda, Maryland

Robert L. Balster, PhD
Butler Professor
Department of Pharmacology and Toxicology
Virginia Commonwealth University
Richmond, Virginia

Declan T. Barry, PhD
Associate Professor
Psychiatry and Child Study Center
Yale School of Medicine
New Haven, Connecticut

Kristen J. Barry, PhD
Emeritus Research Professor
Department of Psychiatry
University of Michigan
Ann Arbor, Michigan

Andrea G. Barthwell, MD
President
Department of Medical
Encounter Medical Group, PC
Chicago, Illinois

Michael H. Baumann, PhD
Staff Scientist
Designer Drug Research Unit
Intramural Research Program
National Institute on Drug Abuse
Baltimore, Maryland

Louis E. Baxter Sr, MD
Executive Medical Director and CEO
Executive Office
Professional Assistance Program of New Jersey
Princeton, New Jersey

William C. Becker, MD
Associate Professor
Department of Internal Medicine
Yale School of Medicine
New Haven, Connecticut

Neal L. Benowitz, MD
Professor Emeritus
Department of Medicine
University of California, San Francisco
San Francisco, California

Lisa K. Berger, MSW, PhD
Professor
Social Work
University of Wisconsin–Milwaukee
Milwaukee, Wisconsin

Anya Bershad, MD, PhD
Resident Physician
Department of Psychiatry and Biobehavioral Sciences
University of California, Los Angeles
Los Angeles, California

Nicolas Bertholet, MD, MSc
Associate Professor
Department of Psychiatry
Lausanne University Hospital and University of Lausanne
Lausanne, Switzerland

Thomas J. R. Beveridge, MSc, PhD
Assistant Professor
Department of Physiology and Pharmacology
School of Medicine
Wake Forest University
Winston Salem, North Carolina

Manjit Bhandal, MD
Psychiatrist
Department of Psychiatry
University of California, Los Angeles
Los Angeles, California

Snehal Bhatt, MD
Associate Professor
Department of Psychiatry and Behavioral Sciences
University of New Mexico
Albuquerque, New Mexico

Richard D. Blondell, MD
Professor Emeritus
Department of Family Medicine
University at Buffalo
Buffalo, New York

Frederic C. Blow, PhD
Professor
Department of Psychiatry
University of Michigan
Ann Arbor, Michigan

Michael P. Bogenschutz, MD
Professor
Department of Psychiatry
New York University Grossman School of Medicine
New York, New York

Cassandra L. Boness, PhD
Research Assistant Professor
Center on Alcohol, Substance Use, and Addictions
University of New Mexico
Albuquerque, New Mexico

Gilbert J. Botvin, BA, MA, MPhil, PhD
Professor Emeritus of Psychology
Department of Population Health Sciences
Weill Cornell Medical College
New York, New York

J. Wesley Boyd, MD, PhD
Professor
Medical Ethics and Psychiatry
Baylor College of Medicine
Houston, Texas

Katharine A. Bradley, MD, MPH
Senior Investigator
Kaiser Permanente Washington Health Research Institute
Seattle, Washington

Kathleen T. Brady, MD, PhD
Distinguished University Professor
Department of Psychiatry
University of South Carolina
Charleston, South Carolina

Jeffrey Bratberg, PharmD
Clinical Professor
Department of Pharmacy Practice
University of Rhode Island
Kingston, Rhode Island

Hannan M. Braun, MD
Assistant Professor
Department of General Internal Medicine
Denver Health and Hospital Authority
Denver, Colorado

Alyssa Braxton, MD
Addiction Psychiatrist
Psychiatry
Ralph H Johnson VA/Medical University of South Carolina
Charleston, South Carolina

Timothy K. Brennan, MD, MPH
Chief of Clinical Services–Addiction
Department of Psychiatry
Icahn School of Medicine at Mount Sinai
New York, New York

Lawrence S. Brown Jr, MD, MPH, FACP, DFASAM
Clinical Associate Professor of Medicine
Public Health
Weill Cornell Medical College
New York, New York

Connor J. Buchholz, MPH, MS
Clinical Research Coordinator
Division of Adolescent and Young Adult Medicine
Massachusetts General Hospital
Boston, Massachusetts

Oscar Bukstein, MD, MPH
Professor of Psychiatry
Department of Psychiatry and Behavioral Sciences
Boston Children's Hospital
Boston, Massachusetts

Chris Bundy, MD, MPH
Executive Medical Director
Washington Physicians Health Program
Seattle, Washington

Gregory C. Bunt, MD
Clinical Assistant Professor
Department of Psychiatry
New York University Grossman School of Medicine
New York, New York

Megan E. Buresh, MD, DFASAM
Assistant Professor
Department of Medicine
Johns Hopkins University School of Medicine
Baltimore, Maryland

Jessica B. Calihan, MD, MS
Addiction Fellow
Department of Pediatrics
Boston Children's Hospital
Boston, Massachusetts

Randy L. Calisoff, MD
Physician
Physical Medicine and Rehabilitation
Lake Villa, Illinois

Deepa R. Camenga, MD, MHS
Associate Professor
Emergency Medicine and Pediatrics
Yale School of Medicine
New Haven, Connecticut

Kenneth M. Carpenter, PhD
Associate Professor of Clinical Psychology
Division on Substance Use Disorders
Department of Psychiatry
Columbia University Medical Center
New York, New York

Emily R. Casey, BS, PharmD
Pharmacist
Department of Pharmacy
Hospital of the University Of Pennsylvania
Philadelphia, Pennsylvania

Martin D. Cheatle, PhD
Associate Professor
Departments of Psychiatry and Anesthesiology
Perelman School of Medicine
University of Pennsylvania
Philadelphia, Pennsylvania

Ahyeon Cho, MD
Medical Student
Department of Medicine
Penn State College of Medicine
Hershey, Pennsylvania

H. Westley Clark, MD, JD, MPH
Consultant
Columbia, Maryland

Marianne Cloeren, MD, MPH
Associate Professor of Medicine
Division of Occupational and Environmental Medicine
University of Maryland School of Medicine
Baltimore, Maryland

Jeffrey S. Cluver, MD
Owner and Founder
Cluver Psychiatric Group
Charlestown, South Carolina

Peter R. Cohen, BA, MD
Child and Adolescent Psychiatrist
Research and Instruction
Institute for Research, Education and Training in Addictions
Pittsburgh, Pennsylvania

John J. Coleman, MS, MA, PhD
Assistant Administrator (Retired)
Operations
U.S. Drug Enforcement Administration
Arlington, Virginia

Jennifer A. Collins, PhD
VP Operations
Occupational Testing Services
Laboratory Corporation of America Holdings
Saint Paul, Minnesota

Peggy Compton, RN, PhD
Professor and van Ameringen Endowed Chair
School of Nursing
University of Pennsylvania
Philadelphia, Pennsylvania

Wilson M. Compton, MD, MPE
Deputy Director
National Institute on Drug Abuse
National Institutes of Health
Bethesda, Maryland

David J. Copenhaver, MD, MPH
Professor and Chief, Division of Pain Medicine
Director of Cancer Pain Management
Director of Pain Medicine Tele-Health
Department of Anesthesiology and Pain Medicine
UC Davis Medical Center
Sacramento, California

Edouard Coupet Jr, MD, MS
Assistant Professor
Department of Emergency Medicine
Yale School of Medicine
New Haven, Connecticut

Silvia L. Cruz, PhD
Professor
Department of Pharmacobiology
Cinvestav
Ciudad de Mexico, Mexico

K. Michael Cummings, PhD, MPH
Professor
Department of Psychiatry and Behavioral Sciences
Medical University of South Carolina
Charleston, South Carolina

Dennis C. Daley, PhD
Professor of Psychiatry (Adjunct)
Department of Psychiatry
University of Pittsburgh School of Medicine
Pittsburgh, Pennsylvania

John A. Dani, PhD
Professor and Chair
Department of Neuroscience
University of Pennsylvania
Philadelphia, Pennsylvania

Itai Danovitch, MD, MBA
Professor and Chair
Department of Psychiatry and Behavioral Neurosciences
Cedars-Sinai
Los Angeles, California

Smita Das, MD, PhD, MPH
Clinical Associate Professor
Department of Psychiatry and Behavioral Sciences
Stanford School of Medicine
Stanford, California

George De Leon, PhD
Science Director, Behavioral Science Training NIDA Grant
New York University Grossman School of Nursing
New York, New York

Adam Demner, MD
Director of Addiction Psychiatry
Department of Clinical Neurosciences
Charles E. Schmidt College of Medicine
Florida Atlantic University
Boca Raton, Florida

Nicholas Denomme, BS, MS
PhD Candidate
Department of Pharmacology
University of Michigan
Ann Arbor, Michigan

Eric T. Dobson, MD
Addiction Psychiatry Fellow
Department of Psychiatry and Behavioral Sciences
Medical University of South Carolina
Charleston, South Carolina

Coreen B. Domingo, DrPH, MPH, LMSW
Assistant Professor
Department of Psychiatry and Behavioral Sciences
Baylor College of Medicine
Houston, Texas

Gail D'Onofrio, MD, MS
Professor
Department of Emergency Medicine
Yale School of Medicine
New Haven, Connecticut

Dennis M. Donovan, BS, MA, PhD
Professor Emeritus
Department of Psychiatry and Behavioral Sciences
University of Washington School of Medicine
Seattle, Washington

Antoine Douaihy, MD
Professor of Psychiatry and Medicine
Department of Psychiatry
University of Pittsburgh School of Medicine
Pittsburgh, Pennsylvania

Mark H. Duncan, MD
Physician
Department of Psychiatry
University of Washington
Seattle, Washington

Robert L. DuPont, MD
President
Institute for Behavior and Health, Inc.
Rockville, Maryland

Paul H. Earley, MD
Medical Director
Georgia Professionals Health Program
Atlanta, Georgia

Steven J. Eickelberg, MD, DFASAM, FAPA
Senior Behavioral Health Medical Director
Arizona Complete Health
Tucson, Arizona

Mahmoud A. El-Sohly, PhD
Research Professor and Professor of Pharmaceutics and Drug Delivery
National Center for National Products Research
University of Mississippi
Oxford, Mississippi

Honora Englander, MD
Professor of Medicine
Division of Hospital Medicine
Oregon Health and Science University
Portland, Oregon

Tyler G. Erath, PhD
Postdoctoral Fellow
Vermont Center on Behavior and Health
University of Vermont
Burlington, Vermont

Norah Essali, MD
Acting Assistant Professor
Department of Psychiatry and Behavioral Sciences
University of Washington
Seattle, Washington

Xiaoduo Fan, MD, MPH
Psychiatrist
Department of Psychiatry
University of Massachusetts Chan Medical School
Worcester, Massachusetts

Luis C. Farhat, MD
Graduate Student
Department of Psychiatry
Faculdade de Medicina FMUSP
Universidade de Sao Paulo
Sao Paulo, Brazil

James L. Ferguson, DO
Medical Director
Recovery Management Solutions
FSS/Vault Health
Willow Grove, Pennsylvania

Sergi Ferré, MD, PhD
Senior Investigator
Integrative Neurobiology Section
National Institute on Drug Abuse Intramural Research Program
Baltimore, Maryland

James W. Finch, MD
Adjunct Professor
Department of Family Medicine
University of North Carolina
Durham, North Carolina

Brandi C. Fink, PhD
Associate Professor
Department of Psychiatry and Behavioral Science
University of Oklahoma Health Sciences Center
Oklahoma City, Oklahoma

Deborah S. Finnell, PhD
Professor Emerita
School of Nursing
Johns Hopkins University
Baltimore, Maryland

Marc Fishman, MD
Medical Director
Maryland Treatment Centers
Baltimore, Maryland

Scott M. Fishman, MD
Fullerton Endowed Chair in Pain Medicine
Professor of Anesthesiology and Pain Medicine
Professor of Psychiatry and Behavioral Sciences (Secondary)
Director, Center for Advancing Pain Relief
Executive Vice Chair, Department of Anesthesiology and Pain Medicine
University of California, Davis School of Medicine
Sacramento, California

Julianne C. Flanagan, PhD
Associate Professor
Department of Psychiatry and Behavioral Sciences
Medical University of South Carolina
Charleston, South Carolina

James H. Ford II, PhD
Assistant Professor
School of Pharmacy
University of Wisconsin Madison
Madison, Wisconsin

Laura Morgan Frankart, PharmD, MEd
Associate Professor
Director of Education and Assessment
Department of Pharmacotherapy and Outcomes Science
Virginia Commonwealth University
Richmond, Virginia

Shelby Franklin, BS
Research assistant
Department of Psychology
University of Minnesota, Twin Cities
Minneapolis, Minnesota

P. Joseph Frawley, MD
Physician
Private Practice
Medical Group Inc.
Santa Barbara, California

Jodi J. Frey, PhD, LCSW-C
Professor
School of Social Work
University of Maryland
Baltimore, Maryland

Peter D. Friedmann, MD, MPH, FACP, DFASAM
Associate Dean for Research
Office of Research
University of Massachusetts Medical School–Baystate
Springfield, Massachusetts

Marc Galanter, MD
Research Professor of Psychiatry
Department of Psychiatry
New York University Grossman School of Medicine
New York, New York

Nan Gallagher, JD
Managing Member
Healthcare Division
The Nan Gallagher Law Group
Morristown, New Jersey

Eric L. Garland, PhD, LCSW
Distinguished Professor
College of Social Work
University of Utah
Salt Lake City, Utah

David R. Gastfriend, MD, DFASAM
Chief Architect
ASAM CONTINUUM(R)
American Society of Addiction Medicine
Rockville, Maryland

Ashley N. Gearhardt, PhD
Associate Professor
Department of Psychology
University of Michigan
Ann Arbor, Michigan

Sarah Gilligan, MD, MS
Assistant Professor
Division of Nephrology
Department of Internal Medicine
University of Utah
Salt Lake City, Utah

Mark S. Gold, MD
Professor
Department of Psychiatry
Washington University in St. Louis
St Louis, Missouri

Paula Goldman, MD
Adolescent and Young Adult Medicine Fellow
Division of Adolescent and Young Adult Medicine
UPMC Children's Hospital of Pittsburgh
Pittsburgh, Pennsylvania

R. Jeffrey Goldsmith, MD, DLFAPA, FASAM
Self-employed
Biddeford Pool, Maine

Adam J. Gordon, MD, MPH, FACP, DFASAM
Elbert F. and Marie Christensen Endowed Research Professorship
Professor of Medicine and Psychiatry
Director, Program for Addiction Research, Clinical Care, Knowledge, and Advocacy
Codirector, Greater Intermountain Node of the NIH NIDA Clinical Trials Network
University of Utah School of Medicine
National Director, Medication Addiction Treatment in the VA
Initiative National Codirector
Coordinating Center of the Interprofessional Advanced Fellowship in Addiction Treatment Director (Emeritus)
Vulnerable Veteran Innovative Patient Aligned Care Team (VIP) Initiative
Salt Lake City, Utah

David A. Gorelick, MD, PhD
Professor
Department of Psychiatry
University of Maryland
Baltimore, Maryland

Jon E. Grant, MD
Professor
Department of Psychiatry and Behavioral Neuroscience
University of Chicago
Chicago, Illinois

Kenneth W. Griffin, PhD, MPH
Professor
Department of Global and Community Health
George Mason University
Fairfax, Virginia

Roland R. Griffiths, PhD
Professor
Department of Psychiatry and Behavioral Sciences
Johns Hopkins University School of Medicine
Baltimore, Maryland

Skylar Gross, MPH
Project Manager
Social Solutions and Services Research
Nathan Kline Institute
New York, New York

Joel W. Grube, PhD, MS, AB
Senior Research Scientist
Prevention Research Center
Pacific Institute for Research and Evaluation
Berkeley, California

Paul J. Gruenewald, PhD
Senior Research Scientist
Prevention Research Center
Pacific Institute for Research and Evaluation
Oakland, California

Kimberly Guy
Engagement Specialist
Recovery Mentor
Department of Psychiatry
Program for Recovery and Community Health
Yale School of Medicine
New Haven, Connecticut

Carolina L. Haass-Koffler, PharmD, PhD
Associate Professor
Department of Psychiatry and Human Behavior
Brown University
Providence, Rhode Island

Paul S. Haber, MD, FRACP, FAChAM
Clinical Director
Drug Health Service
Sydney Local Health District
Camperdown, Australia

Scott E. Hadland, MD, MPH, MS
Chief
Division of Adolescent and Young Adult Medicine
MassGeneral Hospital for Children/Harvard Medical School
Boston, Massachusetts

Timothy M. Hall, MD, PhD
Assistant Clinical Professor
Department of Family Medicine
University of California, Los Angeles
Los Angeles, California

Benjamin Han, MD
Associate Professor
Division of Geriatrics, Gerontology, and Palliative Care
Department of Medicine
University of California, San Diego
San Diego, California

Beth Han, MD, PhD, MPH
Epidemiologist
National Institute on Drug Abuse
National Institutes of Health
Bethesda, Maryland

Colleen A. Hanlon, PhD
Professor
Departments of Cancer Biology and Physiology and Pharmacology
School of Medicine
Wake Forest University
Winston Salem, North Carolina

Roxanne F. Harfmann, MA
Predoctoral Trainee
Vermont Center on Behavior and Health
University of Vermont
Burlington, Vermont

Sion Kim Harris, PhD, RN
Associate Professor
Department of Pediatrics
Harvard Medical School
Boston, Massachusetts

Karen J. Hartwell, MD
Associate Professor
Psychiatry and Behavioral Sciences
Ralph H Johnson VA Medical Center
Medical University of South Carolina
Charleston, South Carolina

Kathryn Hawk, MD, MHS
Associate Professor
Department of Emergency Medicine
Yale School of Medicine
New Haven, Connecticut

Sarah H. Heil, PhD
Professor
Department of Psychiatry and Psychological Science
University of Vermont
Burlington, Vermont

Amy A. Herrold, PhD
Research Associate Professor and Research Health Scientist
Department of Psychiatry and Behavioral Sciences
Feinberg School of Medicine and Edward Hines Jr., VA Hospital
Northwestern University
Chicago, Illinois

Stephen T. Higgins, PhD
Director
Vermont Center on Behavior and Health
University of Vermont
Burlington, Vermont

Omari Hodge, MD
Program Director
Family Medicine
Advent Health
Wesley Chapel, Florida

Kenneth Hoffman, MD, MPH
Colonel (Retired)
Medical Corps
U.S. Army
Rockville, Maryland

Kim A. Hoffman, PhD
Assistant Research Professor
Department of Internal Medicine
Oregon Health and Science University
Portland, Oregon

Mark Hrymoc, MD
Addiction Psychiatrist
Mental Health Center
Los Angeles, California

Martha J. Ignaszewski, MD, FRCPC
Physician
Psychiatry
BC Children's Hospital
Vancouver, British Columbia, Canada

Matthew Iles-Shih, MD, MPH
Assistant Professor
Department of Psychiatry and Behavioral Sciences
University of Washington
Seattle, Washington

Karen S. Ingersoll, PhD
Professor
Department of Psychiatry and Neurobehavioral Sciences
University of Virginia Health
Charlottesville, Virginia

Gwendolyne Anyanate Jack, MD, MPH
Assistant Professor of Medicine
Division of Endocrinology, Diabetes, and Metabolism
Department of Medicine
NewYork-Presbyterian/Weill Cornell Medicine
New York, New York

Steven L. Jaffe, MD
Professor Emeritus
Department of Psychiatry
Emory University School of Medicine
Atlanta, Georgia

Priya Jaisinghani, MD
Endocrinology Fellow
Department of Endocrinology
NewYork-Presbyterian/Weill Cornell Medicine
New York, New York

Oluwole O. Jegede, MD, MPH
Assistant Professor
Department of Psychiatry
Yale School of Medicine
New Haven, Connecticut

David H. Jernigan, PhD
Professor
Department of Health Law, Policy and Management
Boston University School of Public Health
Boston, Massachusetts

Indira G. Jetton, BS
Medical Student
School of Medicine
University of Maryland
Baltimore, Maryland

Kimberly Johnson, PhD, MBA, MSEd
Associate Professor
Department of Mental Health Law and Policy
University of South Florida
Tampa, Florida

Abenaa Jones, PhD
Assistant Professor
Human Development and Family Studies
Penn State: The Pennsylvania State University
State College, Pennsylvania

Christopher M. Jones, PharmD, DrPH, MPH
Acting Director
National Center for Injury Prevention and Control
Centers for Disease Control and Prevention
Atlanta, Georgia

Hendrée E. Jones, PhD
Professor, Executive and Division Director, UNC Horizons
Department of Obstetrics and Gynecology
School of Medicine
The University of North Carolina at Chapel Hill
Chapel Hill, North Carolina

Ayana Jordan, MD, PhD
Barbara Wilson Associate Professor of Psychiatry
Department of Psychiatry
New York University Grossman School of Medicine
New York, New York

Laura M. Juliano, PhD
Professor
Department of Psychology
American University
Washington, District of Columbia

David Kan, MD
Chief Medical Officer, Bright Heart Health
Department of Psychiatry
University of California, San Francisco
Walnut Creek, California

Lori D. Karan, MD, DFASAM, FACP
Professor of Internal Medicine and Preventive Medicine
Program Director, Addiction Medicine Fellowship
Loma Linda University and VA Loma Linda Healthcare System
Loma Linda, California

Jeffrey Katra, DO, MA, AB
Addiction Medicine Physician
Private Practice
University of Virginia
Office of Pain Management and Opioid Stewardship
Charlottesville, Virginia

John F. Kelly, PhD
Elizabeth R. Spallin Professor of Psychiatry in Addiction Medicine
Department of Psychiatry
Massachusetts General Hospital, Harvard Medical School
Boston, Massachusetts

Amy J. Kennedy, MD, MS
Acting Assistant Professor of Medicine
Division of General Internal Medicine
VA Puget Sound Healthcare System
University of Washington School of Medicine
Seattle, Washington

Jag H. Khalsa, MS, PhD
Adjunct Professor
Department of Microbiology, Immunology, and Tropical Diseases
School of Medicine and Health Sciences
The George Washington University
Washington, District of Columbia

Maliha Khan, MD
Physician
Department of Internal Medicine
University of California, Los Angeles
Los Angeles, California

Therese K. Killeen, PhD, APN
Professor
Addiction Science Division
Department of Psychiatry and Behavioral Sciences
Medical University of South Carolina
Charlestown, South Carolina

Jason R. Kilmer, PhD
Associate Professor
Department of Psychiatry and Behavioral Sciences
Adjunct Associate Professor
Department of Psychology
University of Washington
Seattle, Washington

Jungjin Kim, MD
Medical Director of Alcohol, Drug, and Addiction Inpatient Program
Division of Alcohol, Drugs and Addiction
McLean Hospital/Harvard Medical School
Belmont, Massachusetts

Simeon D. Kimmel, MD, MA
Assistant Professor of Medicine
Department of Medicine
Sections of General Internal Medicine and Infectious Diseases
Boston University School of Medicine and Boston Medical Center
Boston, Massachusetts

Kaitlin R. Kinney, MSc
PhD Candidate
Department of Physiology and Pharmacology
Wake Forest School of Medicine
Winston Salem, North Carolina

Barbara M. Kirrane, MD, MPH
Medical Toxicology Consultant
Department of Emergency Medicine
Cooperman Barnabas Medical Center
Livingston, New Jersey

John R. Knight, MD
Associate Professor (Ret.)
Department of Pediatrics
Harvard Medical School
Boston, Massachusetts

Brian B. Koo, MD
Associate Professor of Neurology
Yale School of Medicine
New Haven, Connecticut

George F. Koob, PhD
Director of the National Institute on Alcohol Abuse and Alcoholism
National Institutes of Health
Bethesda, Maryland

Nicholas C. Kortt, MBBS, BSc (Hons)
Advanced Trainee
Gastroenterology
Campbelltown Hospital
Sydney, Australia

Thomas R. Kosten, MD
Waggoner Professor
Departments of Psychiatry, Neuroscience, Pharmacology
Baylor College of Medicine
Houston, Texas

Shyam Kottilil, MD, PhD
Professor
Department of Medicine
Institute of Human Virology
University of Maryland School of Medicine
Baltimore, Maryland

Connor Kubeisy, BA
MPH Candidate
Department of Health Policy and Management
Harvard T.H. Chan School of Public Health
Cambridge, Massachusetts

Kevin Kunz, MD, MPH
ADM Physician
SUD Prevention and Treatment Team
West Hawaii Community Health Center
Kailua-Kona, Hawaii

Eugene Lambert, MD, MBA
Medical Director, Addiction Consult Team
Department of Medicine
Massachusetts General Hospital
Boston, Massachusetts

Mary E. Larimer, PhD
Professor
Departments of Psychiatry and Behavioral Sciences and Psychology
University of Washington
Seattle, Washington

Amanda Latimore, PhD
Director
Center for Addiction Research and Effective Solutions
American Institutes for Research
Center for Addiction Research and Effective Solutions
Rockville, Maryland

Bernard Le Foll, MD, PhD
Professor and Chair
Department of Family and Community Medicine
University of Toronto
Toronto, Canada

Janet H. Lenard, EdD
Counseling Psychology, MSSW, and Bachelors in Psychology/Sociology
Retired Department of the Army Civilian
Clinical Quality Program Manager
Headquarters, Installation Management Command
Army Substance Abuse Programs
San Antonio, Texas

Frank T. Leone, MD, MS
Director, Comprehensive Smoking Treatment Program
Pulmonary Medicine and Critical Care
University of Pennsylvania
Philadelphia, Pennsylvania

Annie Lévesque, MD, MSc
Assistant Professor
Department of Psychiatry
Icahn School of Medicine at Mount Sinai
New York, New York

Frances Rudnick Levin, MD
Kennedy-Leavy Professor of Psychiatry
Addiction Psychiatry
Division on Substance Use Disorders
New York State Psychiatric Institute/Columbia University Irving Medical Center
New York, New York

Sharon Levy, MD, MPH, FASAM, FAAP
Chief, Division of Addiction Medicine
Boston Children's Hospital
Professor of Pediatrics
Harvard Medical School
Boston, Massachusetts

Ty W. Lostutter, PhD
Associate Professor
Department of Psychiatry and Behavioral Sciences
University of Washington
Seattle, Washington

Eric Lott, MD, FASAM
Associate Program Director
HonorHealth Addiction Medicine Fellowship Program
Medical Director, Professional Medical Monitoring Program of Arizona
Department of Addiction Medicine
HonorHealth, Community Bridges Inc.
Scottsdale, Arizona

Scott E. Lukas, PhD
Director, McLean Imaging Center and Behavioral Psychopharmacology Research Lab
Department of Psychiatry
McLean Hospital/Harvard Medical School
Belmont, Massachusetts

Katrina Mark, MD
Associate Professor
Department of Obstetrics, Gynecology and Reproductive Sciences
University of Maryland School of Medicine
Baltimore, Maryland

Douglas B. Marlowe, JD, PhD
Senior Scientific Consultant
National Drug Court Institute
National Association of Drug Court Professionals
Alexandria, Virginia

Silvia S. Martins, MD, PhD
Professor
Department of Epidemiology
Columbia University
New York, New York

Megan E. Marziali, MPH, BSc
Doctoral Student
Department of Epidemiology
Columbia University
New York, New York

Suena H. Massey, MD
Associate Professor
Department of Psychiatry and Behavioral Sciences
Northwestern University Feinberg School of Medicine
Chicago, Illinois

David S. Mathai, MD
Postdoctoral Research Fellow
Department of Psychiatry
Johns Hopkins University School of Medicine
Baltimore, Maryland

Justin Matheson, PhD
Postdoctoral Research Fellow
Translational Addiction Research Laboratory
Centre for Addiction and Mental Health
Toronto, Ontario, Canada

Myra L. Mathis, MD
Assistant Professor
Department of Psychiatry
University of Rochester Medical Center
Rochester, New York

Pia M. Mauro, PhD
Assistant Professor
Department of Epidemiology
Columbia University Mailman School of Public Health
New York, New York

Elinore F. McCance-Katz, MD, PhD
Clinical Professor of Psychiatry and Behavioral Sciences
Alpert School of Medicine
Brown University
Providence, Rhode Island

Lauren McClain, MS
Graduate Student
Department of Psychology
University of Washington
Seattle, Washington

Emma E. Mcginty, PhD, MS
Professor
Department of Health Policy and Management
Johns Hopkins Bloomberg School of Public Health
Baltimore, Maryland

Mark McGovern, PhD
Professor
Department of Psychiatry and Behavioral Sciences and Medicine
Stanford University School of Medicine
Palo Alto, California

Jennifer McNeely, MD, MS
Associate Professor
Section on Tobacco, Alcohol and Drug Use
Department of Population Health
Division of General Internal Medicine and Clinical Innovation
Department of Medicine
New York University Grossman School of Medicine
New York, New York

John G. McNutt, MD
Fellow
Addiction Medicine
Loma Linda University
Loma Linda, California

Lisa J. Merlo, PhD, MPE
Professor of Psychiatry
University of Florida
Gainesville, Florida

Shannon C. Miller, MD, DFASAM, DLFAPA
Dayton VA Medical Center
Clinical Professor of Psychiatry and Population and Public Health Sciences
Boonshoft School of Medicine
Wright State University
Founding Co-Editor
Journal of Addiction Medicine (2006-2016)
American Society of Addiction Medicine
Lieutenant Colonel, Retired
United States Air Force
Dayton/Cincinnati, Ohio

Richard Montgomery, MD
Attending Psychiatrist
Schick Shadel Hospital
Seattle, Washington

Kenneth L. Morford, MD
Assistant Professor of Medicine
Department of Internal Medicine
Yale School of Medicine
New Haven, Connecticut

Hamilton Morris, BSc
Medicinal Chemist
Department of Pharmaceutical Sciences
Saint Joseph's University
Philadelphia, Pennsylvania

Angela M. Mueller, PhD
Postdoctoral Scholar
Department of Psychiatry
University of California, San Francisco
San Francisco, California

Hugh Myrick, MD
Director, Military Sciences Division
Department of Psychiatry
Medical University of South Carolina (MUSC)
Charleston, South Carolina

Edgar P. Nace, MD
Adjunct Professor of Psychiatry
Department of Psychiatry
University of Texas Southwestern Medical School
Dallas, Texas

Rohit Nalamasu, DO
Physician
Pain Management
The Permanente Medical Group
Oakland, California

Emily Nash, BAppSc (MRS), MBBS (Hons), MPH
Gastroenterology and Addiction Medicine Advanced Trainee
AW Morrow Gastroenterology and Liver Centre
Royal Prince Alfred Hospital
Camperdown, Australia

David E. Nichols, BSc, PhD
Distinguished Professor Emeritus
Department of Medicinal Chemistry and Molecular Pharmacology
Purdue University School of Pharmacy
West Lafayette, Indiana

Edward V. Nunes, MD
Professor
Department of Psychiatry
Columbia University Irving Medical Center
New York, New York

Patrick G. O'Connor, MD, MPH
Dan Adams and Amanda Adams Professor and Chief, General Internal Medicine
Department of Internal Medicine
Yale School of Medicine
New Haven, Connecticut

Brian L. Odlaug, PhD, MPH
Researcher
Department of Neurology
N. Bud Grossman Center
University of Minnesota
Minneapolis, Minnesota

Yngvild Olsen, MD, MPH
Director
Center for Substance Abuse Treatment
Substance Abuse and Mental Health Services Administration
Rockville, Maryland

Deirdre O'Sullivan, PhD
Associate Professor
Department of Educational Psychology, Counseling, and Special Education
Pennsylvania State University
University Park, Pennsylvania

Anna Parisi, PhD, MSW
Postdoctoral Research Associate
College of Social Work
University of Utah
Salt Lake City, Utah

Elyse R. Park, PhD, MPH
Professor
Psychiatry and Medicine
Massachusetts General Hospital
Boston, Massachusetts

Theodore V. Parran Jr, MD
Professor of Medical Education
Internal Medicine
School of Medicine
Case Western Reserve University
Cleveland, Ohio

Mallie J. Paschall, PhD
Senior Research Scientist
Prevention Research Center
Pacific Institute for Research and Evaluation
Berkeley, California

David L. Pennington, PhD
Associate Professor
Department of Psychiatry and Behavioral Sciences
University of California, San Francisco
San Francisco, California

India Perez-Urbano, BA
MD Candidate
School of Medicine
University of California, San Francisco
San Francisco, California

Alyssa F. Peterkin, MD
Assistant Professor
General Internal Medicine
Boston Medical Center
Boston, Massachusetts

Petros Petridis, MD, MS
Resident Physician
Department of Psychiatry
New York University
New York, New York

Steven E. Pfau, MD
Chief of Cardiology, West Haven VA Medical Center
Department of Internal Medicine
Yale School of Medicine
New Haven, Connecticut

Karran A. Phillips, MD, MSc
Deputy Director
Center for Substance Abuse Treatment
Substance Abuse and Mental Health Services Administration
Rockville, Maryland

Daniele Piomelli, PhD, MD
Distinguished Professor
Department of Anatomy and Neurobiology
University of California, Irvine
Irvine, California

Marc N. Potenza, MD, PhD
Professor
Departments of Psychiatry and Neuroscience and the Child Study Center
Yale School of Medicine
New Haven, Connecticut

Steven Prakken, MD
Chief Medical Pain Service
Psychiatry
Avance Health Care
Raleigh, North Carolina

Wesley R. Prickett, MD
Pain Physician
Anesthesiology/Extended Care and Rehabilitation
Department of Veterans Affairs
Omaha, Nebraska

James O. Prochaska, PhD
Professor Emeritus
Department of Psychology
University of Rhode Island
Kingston, Rhode Island

Janice M. Prochaska, PhD
Consultant
Prochaska Change Consultants
Mill Valley, California

Miranda P. Ramirez, BA
Graduate Student
Department of Psychology
University of Kentucky
Lexington, Kentucky

Lynsie Ranker, PhD, MPH
Postdoctoral Research Associate
Department of Community Health Sciences
Boston University School of Public Health
Boston, Massachusetts

Darius A. Rastegar, MD
Associate Professor of Medicine
Division of Addiction Medicine
Department of Medicine
Johns Hopkins University School of Medicine
Baltimore, Maryland

Naveen Rathi, MD
Resident Physician
Department of Internal Medicine
University of Cincinnati
Cincinnati, Ohio

Richard K. Ries, MD
Professor of Psychiatry
Director Addictions Division
Department of Psychiatry and Behavioral Sciences
University of Washington School of Medicine
Seattle, Washington

Daniel Roberts, MD, MSW
Resident Psychiatrist
Department of Psychiatry
New York University
New York, New York

Rachel L. Rosen, MS
Clinical Fellow
Department of Psychiatry
Massachusetts General Hospital
Boston, Massachusetts

Richard N. Rosenthal, MD, MA, DLFAPA, DFAAAP, FASAM
Professor of Psychiatry
Director of Addiction Psychiatry
Department of Psychiatry
Stony Brook University Medical Center
Stony Brook, New York

Stephen Ross, MD
Associate Director
NYU Langone Center for Psychedelic Medicine
Department of Psychiatry
New York University Grossman School of Medicine
New York, New York

Fred Rottnek, MD, MAHCM, FAAFP, FASAM
Director of Community Medicine
Program Director for Addiction Medicine Fellowship
Department of Family and Community Medicine
Saint Louis University
St. Louis, Missouri

Kevin A. Sabet, PhD, MS, BA
Fellow, ISPS
Yale School of Medicine
New Haven, Connecticut

Stanley Sacks, PhD
Senior Research Scientist, Emeritus
Center for the Integration of Research and Practice
National Development and Research Institutes
New York, New York

Corey Sadd, MD
Physician
Pulmonary and Critical Care
University of Wisconsin
Madison, Wisconsin

Michael E. Saladin, PhD
Professor
Health Sciences and Research
Medical University of South Carolina
Charlestown, South Carolina

Robert F. Saltz, BA, MA, PhD
Senior Scientist
Prevention Research Center
Pacific Institute for Research and Evaluation
Berkeley, California

Jeffrey H. Samet, MD, MA, MPH
John Noble, MD, Professor of Medicine
General Internal Medicine
Boston University School of Medicine
Boston, Massachusetts

Friedhelm Sandbrink, MD
Chief, Pain Medicine
Neurology
Washington DC Veterans Affairs Medical Center
Washington, District of Columbia

Tanya C. Saraiya, PhD
Assistant Professor
Center of Alcohol and Substance Use Studies
Rutgers University
New Brunswick, New Jersey
Adjunct Research Assistant Professor
Department of Psychiatry and Behavioral Sciences
Medical University of South Carolina
Charleston, South Carolina

David Saunders, MD, PhD
Assistant Professor of Psychiatry
Department of Psychiatry
Columbia University–New York State Psychiatric Institute
New York, New York

Andrew J. Saxon, MD, FASAM
Professor
Department of Psychiatry and Behavioral Sciences
University of Washington School of Medicine
Seattle, Washington

Emmanuelle A. D. Schindler, MD, PhD
Medical Director
Headache Center of Excellence
VA Connecticut Healthcare System
West Haven, Connecticut

Robert Schnoll, PhD
Professor
Department of Psychiatry
University of Pennsylvania
Philadelphia, Pennsylvania

Frank J. Schwebel, PhD
Research Assistant Professor
Center on Alcohol, Substance Use, and Addictions
University of New Mexico
Albuquerque, New Mexico

Ripal Shah, MD, MPH
Clinical Assistant Professor
Department of Psychiatry and Behavioral Sciences
Stanford University
Stanford, California

Samit M. Shah, MD, PhD
Assistant Professor
Department of Internal Medicine
Yale School of Medicine
New Haven, Connecticut

Andi Shahu, MD, MHS
Cardiology Fellow
Section of Cardiovascular Medicine
Yale School of Medicine
New Haven, Connecticut

Julia M. Shi, MD
Associate Clinical Professor
General Internal Medicine
Yale School of Medicine
New Haven, Connecticut

Steven Shoptaw, PhD
Professor
Department of Family Medicine
David Geffen School of Medicine at UCLA
Los Angeles, California

Daryl Shorter, MD
Associate Professor
Menninger Department of Psychiatry and Behavioral Sciences
Baylor College of Medicine
Houston, Texas

Lydia A. Shrier, MD, MPH
Research Director and Codirector of the Center for Adolescent Behavioral Research
Division of Adolescent/Young Adult Medicine
Boston Children's Hospital
Boston, Massachusetts

Jason J. Sico, MD, MHS
Associate Professor
Department of Neurology and Internal Medicine
Yale School of Medicine
New Haven, Connecticut

Marisa M. Silveri, MA, PhD
Neuroscientist
Associate Professor of Psychiatry
Department of Psychiatry
McLean Hospital
Harvard Medical School
Belmont, Massachusetts

Kevin M. Simon, MD
Chief Behavioral Health Officer
Boston Public Health Commission
Pediatric Psychiatrist
Department of Psychiatry & Behavioral Sciences
Boston Children's Hospital
Addiction Medicine Specialist
Division of Addiction Medicine
Boston Children's Hospital
Instructor of Psychiatry
Department of Psychiatry
Harvard Medical School
Boston, Massachusetts

Jennifer T. Sneider, PhD
Associate Neuroscientist
Department of Psychiatry
McLean Hospital
Belmont, Massachusetts

David Spiegel, MD
Jack, Lulu and Sam Wilson Professor and Associate Chair
Department of Psychiatry & Behavioral Sciences
Stanford University School of Medicine
Stanford, California

Gideon St.Helen, PhD
Associate Professor of Medicine
Department of Medicine
University of California, San Francisco
San Francisco, California

Andie Stallman, BS
Research Assistant
Neurodevelopmental Laboratory on Addictions and Mental Health
McLean Hospital
Belmont, Massachusetts

Sharon Stancliff, MD
Addiction Medicine Specialist
Primary Care
Project Renewal
New York, New York

Steven Stanos, DO
Executive Medical Director
Rehabilitation and Performance Medicine
Swedish Medical Group
Swedish Health System
Seattle, Washington

Tessa L. Steel, MD, MPH
Acting Assistant Professor
Department of Medicine
University of Washington
Seattle, Washington

Randy Stinchfield, PhD
Clinical Psychologist
Department of Psychiatry
University of Minnesota Medical School
Minneapolis, Minnesota

Kenneth B. Stoller, MD, DFAPA
Associate Professor
Department of Psychiatry and Behavioral Sciences
Johns Hopkins University School of Medicine
Baltimore, Maryland

Susan Storti, PhD, RN, NEA-BC, CARN-AP
President/CEO
The Substance Use and Mental Health Leadership Council of RI
Warwick, Rhode Island

Joanna M. Streck, PhD
Member of the Faculty and Staff Psychology
Department of Psychiatry
Massachusetts General Hospital/Harvard Medical School
Boston, Massachusetts

Kimberly Sue, MD, PhD
Assistant Professor
General Internal Medicine
Yale School of Medicine
New Haven, Connecticut

Carol A. Sulis, MD
Associate Professor of Medicine (Retired)
Department of Medicine
Boston University School of Medicine
Boston, Massachusetts

John W. Sullenbarger, MD
Associate Professor
Department of Psychiatry
Wright State University
Dayton, Ohio

Javier Ponce Terashima, MD
Psychiatry Fellow
Department of Psychiatry
Yale School of Medicine
New Haven, Connecticut

Jeanette M. Tetrault, MD, FACP, FASAM
Professor of Medicine and Public Health
Vice Chief for Education, Section of General Internal Medicine
Program Director, Addiction Medicine Fellowship
Associate Director for Education and Training, Program in Addiction Medicine
Yale School of Medicine
New Haven, Connecticut

Angela M. Tiberia, MPH
Research Area Specialist Lead
Department of Psychiatry
University of Michigan
Ann Arbor, Michigan

Hanne Tonnesen, MD, DMSc
Professor
WHO CC
Clinical Health Promotion Centre
The Parker Institute
Bispebjerg and Frederiksberg Hospital
Copenhagen, Denmark

Michael Torres, MD
Resident Physician
Department of Clinical Neurosciences
Charles E. Schmidt College of Medicine
Boca Raton, Florida

Sacha N. Uljon, MD, PhD
Medical Director, Core Laboratory
Department of Pathology
Massachusetts General Hospital
Boston, Massachusetts

Tanya J. Uritsky, PharmD
Opioid Stewardship Coordinator
Department of Pharmacy
Hospital of the University of Pennsylvania,
Penn Medicine
Philadelphia, Pennsylvania

Federico E. Vaca, MD, MPH
Professor and Vice Chair
Department of Emergency Medicine
Yale School of Medicine
New Haven, Connecticut

Ana Ventuneac, PhD
Vice President
Research and Evaluation
START Treatment and Recovery Centers, Inc.
Brooklyn, New York

Kenneth W. Verbos II, MD, MPH, MSc
Primary Care Research Fellow
Department of Family and Community Medicine
Penn State College of Medicine
Hershey, Pennsylvania

Frank Vocci, PhD
President and Senior Research Scientist
Social Research Center
Friends Research Institute
Baltimore, Maryland

Nora D. Volkow, MD
Principal Investigator
Institute Director
National Institute on Drug Abuse
National Institutes of Health
Bethesda, Maryland

Darren C. Volpe, MD
Associate Professor
Department of Neurology
Yale School of Medicine
New Haven, Connecticut

Sarah E. Wakeman, MD, FASAM
Medical Director for Substance Use Disorder at Mass General Brigham
Medical Director for the MGH Substance Use Disorder Initiative
Director of the Program for Substance Use and Addiction Services
MGH Division of General Internal Medicine
Boston, Massachusetts

Jason Wallach, PhD
Assistant Professor
Department of Pharmaceutical Sciences
University of the Sciences
Philadelphia, Pennsylvania

R. Corey Waller, MD, MS, FACEP, DFASAM
Managing Director
Institute of Addiction
Health Management Associates
Lansing, Michigan

Alexander Y. Walley, MD, MSc
Professor of Medicine
Department of Medicine
Boston University School of Medicine
Boston, Massachusetts

Angela Wangari Walter, PhD, MPH, MSW
Associate Professor
Department of Public Health
University of Massachusetts Lowell
Lowell, Massachusetts

Alan A. Wartenberg, MD, FACP, DFASAM
Affiliated Faculty
Center for Alcohol and Addiction Studies
Brown University
Providence, Rhode Island

Darian Weaver, BS
Clinical Psychology Doctoral Student/Graduate TA
Department of Psychology
American University
Washington, District of Columbia

Michael F. Weaver, MD, DFASAM
Professor and Medical Director
Department of Psychiatry
University of Texas Health Science Center at Houston
Houston, Texas

Julia Megan Webb, MD
Attending Physician
Interventional Spine and Pain Medicine Physical Medicine and Rehabilitation
Spaulding Rehabilitation Network/Mass General Bingham
Boston, Massachusetts

Zoe M. Weinstein, MD, MS
Assistant Professor
General Internal Medicine
Boston University School of Medicine
Boston, Massachusetts

Roger D. Weiss, MD
Chief
Division of Alcohol, Drugs, and Addiction
McLean Hospital
Belmont, Massachusetts
Professor of Psychiatry
Harvard Medical School
Boston, Massachusetts

Arthur F. Weissman, MD
Assistant Professor
Department of Family Medicine
Jacobs School of Medicine and Biomedical Sciences
State University of New York at Buffalo
Buffalo, New York

Justine Welsh, MD
Director, Addiction Services, Emory Healthcare
Department of Psychiatry and Behavioral Sciences
Emory University
Atlanta, Georgia

Michael J. Wesley, PhD
Assistant Professor
Department of Behavioral Science
University of Kentucky
Lexington, Kentucky

William L. White, MA
Emeritus Sr. Research Consultant
Lighthouse Institute
Chestnut Health Systems
Bloomington, Illinois

Ursula Whiteside, MS, PhD
Clinical Faculty
Department of Psychiatry and Behavioral Sciences
University of Washington
Seattle, Washington

Jeffery N. Wilkins, MD
Clinical Professor
UCLA Department of Psychiatry and Biobehavioral Sciences
David Geffen School of Medicine at UCLA
Los Angeles, California

Mark Willenbring, MD
Adjunct Full Professor
Department of Psychiatry
University of Minnesota
Minneapolis, Minnesota

Emily C. Williams, PhD, MPH
Professor
Department of Health Systems and Population Health
University of Washington
Seattle, Washington

Randi M. Williams, PhD, MPH
Assistant Professor
Oncology
Lombardi Comprehensive Cancer Center
Georgetown University Medical Center
Washington, District of Columbia

Jacqueline Deanna Wilson, MD, MPH
Assistant Professor of Medicine, Pediatrics, and Clinical and Translational Sciences
Department of Medicine
University of Pittsburgh
Pittsburgh, Pennsylvania

Ken C. Winters, PhD
Senior Scientist
Oregon Research Institute
Falcon Heights, Minnesota

John J. Woodward, BS, MS, PhD
Professor
Department of Neuroscience
Medical University of South Carolina
Charleston, South Carolina

Tara M. Wright, MD
ACOS, Mental Health Service Line
Mental Health
Ralph H Johnson VAMC
Charleston, South Carolina

Martha J. Wunsch, MD, FAAP, DFASAM
Director
Medication for Addiction Treatment Program
Alameda County Santa Rita Jail
Dublin, California

Stephen A. Wyatt, DO
Addiction Psychiatry Fellowship Director
Psychiatry
Mountain Area Health Education Center
Asheville, North Carolina

Ziming Xuan, ScD
Associate Professor
Department of Community Health Sciences
Boston University School of Public Health
Boston, Massachusetts

David B. Yaden, PhD
Assistant Professor
Department of Psychiatry and Behavioral Sciences
Johns Hopkins University School of Medicine
Baltimore, Maryland

Warren Yamashita, MD, MPH
Adjunct Instructor
Psych/General Psychiatry and Psychology
Stanford University
Palo Alto, California

Jih-Cheng Yeh, MPH
Doctoral Candidate
Department of Health Law, Policy and Management
Boston University School of Public Health
Boston, Massachusetts

Sarah W. Yip, PhD, MSc
Associate Professor of Psychiatry
Yale School of Medicine
New Haven, Connecticut

Richard Youins
Research Assistant
Psychiatry
Yale School of Medicine
New Haven, Connecticut

Amy M. Yule, MD
Director of Adolescent Addiction Psychiatry
Department of Psychiatry
Boston Medical Center
Boston University School of Medicine
Boston, Massachusetts

Anne Zajicek, MD, PharmD
Deputy Associate Director for Clinical Research
Office of Clinical Research
National Institutes of Health
Bethesda, Maryland

Aleksandra E. Zgierska, MD, PhD
Professor
Vice Chair of Research
Department of Family and Community Medicine
Penn State College of Medicine
Hershey, Pennsylvania

Alice Zhang, MD
Family Medicine Physician
Department of Family and Community Medicine
Penn State College of Medicine
Hershey, Pennsylvania

Douglas Ziedonis, MD, MPH
Executive Vice President, Health Sciences
CEO, UNM Health System
Department of Psychiatry
University of New Mexico
Albuquerque, New Mexico

Cara Zimmerman, MD, MBA
Addiction Medicine/Internal Medicine Physician
Addiction Medicine/Internal Medicine
Brown University
Providence, Rhode Island

Joan E. Zweben, PhD
Clinical Professor/Staff Psychologist
Department of Psychiatry
University of California, San Francisco/SF VA Medical Center
San Francisco, California

Preface

Welcome to the seventh edition of *The ASAM Principles of Addiction Medicine*. Our goal, as with previous editions of Principles, is to provide a reference text that reflects the state of the art in the science and practice of addiction medicine. This goal is supported through the textbook's link to the American Society of Addiction Medicine (ASAM), the world's largest addiction medicine professional association, and through the involvement of the world's leading researchers and experts in our field. This edition of Principles is being released after the COVID-19 Federal Public Health Emergency officially ended, the removal of DATA Waiver requirements and changed educational requirements, the extended relaxation of telehealth policies, and the relaxation of rules for take-home opioid use disorder treatment. Clinicians face challenging and ever changing legal and social landscapes that shape addiction medicine. The material in this book offers scientific research and evolving best practices to better equip clinicians and policymakers to prevent, recognize, and treat addiction-related disorders more efficiently.

The text is organized pyramidally under senior editor, associate editors, lead section editors, section editors, and authors. To accommodate the expansion of the seventh edition with 11 new chapters and 7 sidebars, and to replace the departure of David Fiellin, MD, and the passing of Rich Saitz, MD, four new associate editors have joined the editorial team: Sarah E. Wakeman, MD, Jeanette M. Tetrault, MD, Sharon Levy, MD, and Andy Saxon, MD.

Dr. Wakeman, provides her strength in internal medicine and addiction medicine, with a focus on the integration of substance use disorder care into general medical settings. Dr. Wakeman was the lead editor for ASAM's Pocket Addiction Medicine.

Dr. Tetrault, provides her strength in internal medicine, with a focus on care of patients with addiction and the medical conditions associated with substance use, in particular HIV and hepatitis C. She returns to the textbook after previous service as a section editor.

Dr. Levy, provides her strength in pediatrics, with a focus on prevention, screening, evaluation, and treatment of adolescents and young adults with substance use disorders, and the integration of substance use treatment into primary care pediatrics.

Dr. Saxon, provides his strength in addiction psychiatry, with a focus on substance use disorder treatment and education. He returns to the textbook after previous service as a section editor.

Dr. Rosenthal, returns as associate editor from the sixth edition and provides his strengths in addiction psychiatry and co-occurring psychiatric disorders, behavioral and 12-step approaches, technology-associated disorders, and collaborative team–based care for addiction-related disorders.

Both Richard Saitz, MD, and David Fiellin, MD, who served as associate editors for the fourth, fifth, and sixth editions, provided cornerstones to our links to patient-oriented research, screening and brief intervention, and the management of opioid use disorders, while sharing their wide-ranging expertise in internal medicine.

Shannon C. Miller, MD, returns from the fourth and fifth editions, where he served as an associate editor. He moved into the Senior Editor role for the sixth edition and has returned to lead this seventh edition of Principles. He provides strengths in psychiatry and neuroscience, military and veteran medical care, and his editorial strength as a founding coeditor of ASAM's peer-reviewed medical journal, *Journal of Addiction Medicine*.

The editors have updated, deleted, added, and reorganized chapters to provide coherent and compete information, including updates to all chapters and substantial revisions to most. Also, importantly, this edition expanded the frontiers of nonstigmatizing terminology by incorporating recently evolved terminology into all chapters. As well, most authors have provided a unique focus on how the topics of race, diversity, equity, inclusion, and justice relate to their chapter contents, especially in chapters dealing with the topics of genetics, epidemiology, assessment, and treatment. Work continued to ensure usage of DSM-5-TR language throughout its chapters, while attempting to preserve linkages to previous DSM editions. To maintain Principles as current and relevant to the medical community as our field rapidly expands in breadth and depth, a substantial number of new chapters have been added that are not traditionally covered in addiction related publications.

Frank Vocci, PhD, leads Section 1, Basic Science and Core Concepts. The opening chapter, Substance Use Disorders: The Neurobiology of Motivation Gone Awry, is written by Nora D. Volkow, MD, and George F. Koob, PhD, directors of the National Institute on Drug Abuse (NIDA) and the National Institute on Alcohol Abuse and Alcoholism (NIAAA), respectively. In addition to orienting the reader to basic principles in neurobiology and epidemiology of addiction, important chapter updates have been added on recommended use of terminology in the field of addiction medicine (Chapter 2), understanding research in addiction-related clinical trials (Chapter 4), and the addiction medicine physician as a change agent toward public health (Chapter 5). Three new chapters explore the important influence and impact industry has on tobacco, alcohol, and cannabis use disorders (Chapters 7, 8, and 9). As well, a novel chapter on the increasingly relevant intersection of addiction medicine and climate change is provided.

Thomas R. Kosten, MD, along with David A. Gorelick, MD, and Daryl Shorter, MD, lead Section 2, Pharmacology. This team has worked to better elucidate the clinical relevance of this section's content to readers. Expansion into increasingly important topics such as the rapidly evolving field of electronic drug delivery devices (Chapter 22), cannabinoids (Chapter 17), and hallucinogens and dissociatives (Chapters 18 and 19) have been incorporated, and the chapter on novel psychoactive substances has been enriched (Chapter 23).

Section 3 is a new section devoted to epidemiology and prevention. Led by a new trio of editors, Deepa R. Camenga, MD, Babalola Faseru, MD, and Catalina Lopez-Quintero, PhD, the section features new content on primary, secondary and tertiary prevention (24, SB1) and five substantially updated chapters focused on prevention for different populations, harm reduction, and public policy to address military personnel.

Section 4, Diagnosis, Assessment, and Early Intervention Treatment, led by Emily C. Williams, PhD and Lisa J. Merlo, PhD, features expanded material on screening and brief interventions in a variety of settings, laboratory testing, assessment, and community-based prevention. Three new sidebars have been added: Hospital-Based Addiction Care (33 SB1), Prevention and Early Treatment in the Workplace Setting (33, SB2), and an often neglected topic of Health Care Professional Wellness After Patient Overdose Death (34, SB1).

Wilson M. Compton, MD, Karran A. Phillips, MD, and Deborah S. Finnell, PhD, lead Section 5 on Overview of Addiction Treatment. The section includes 4 new chapters: Race, Ethnicity, Gender, and Social Determinants of Health, Disparities, and Access to Care; Treatment Considerations for LGBTQ Patients; Reducing Inequities of Care Through Changes in Practice (Chapters 38, 42, and 49); and Delivery of Addiction Medicine Care via Video or Phone—the evolution of which was greatly influenced by the COVID-19 pandemic, which began and ended during the production of this textbook.

Jon E. Grant, MD, and Sarah W. Yip, PhD, lead Section 6, devoted to Nonsubstance Addiction-Related Disorders and provide updates on Gambling Disorder, Compulsive Sexual Behaviors and the global concern for Disorders Associated With Technology and Social Media (Chapter 54).

Section 7, Management of Intoxication and Withdrawal, is led by Adam J. Gordon, MD, Mike A. Incze, MD, and Ana Holtey, DO, provides updates on the critical safety and patient engagement topic of management of substance withdrawal.

Section 8, Pharmacological Interventions and Other Somatic Therapies, led by Amy J. Kennedy, MD, Smita Das, MD, and Maria Gabriela Garcia Vassallo, MD, includes discussion of FDA-approved pharmacotherapies, off-label uses of pharmacotherapies, as well as complimentary and integrative interventions for addiction-related disorders. Medical Director Stewardship of Opioid Treatment Programs (OTPs) is a newly added sidebar (62, SB1). The management and pharmacologic treatment chapters in these sections have all been fully updated to include the most current information. A novel chapter on neuromodulation has also been expanded.

Antoine Douaihy, MD, and Eric L. Garland, PhD, lead Section 9 on Psychologically Based Interventions. The section incorporates the latest research on a wide variety of behavioral therapies and adds two new chapters on motivational interviewing and mindfulness-based treatments as well as updates on digital media as treatment platforms. Richard K. Ries, MD, leads Section 10 on Mutual Help: Twelve Step and Other Programs in Addiction Recovery and contributes a chapter on spirituality and recovery.

Section 11 has new leadership, Paula Lum, MD, Anika Alvanzo, MD, and Darius A. Rastegar, MD, and includes the latest research about medical disorders and complications of addiction. Arranged by body systems, this section includes important updates relating to hepatitis C and HIV, as well as approaches to the pregnant patient.

Section 12, led by Edward V. Nunes, MD, and R. Jeffrey Goldsmith, MD, includes updated chapters on co-occurring addiction and mood, anxiety, psychotic, personality, eating, and substance-induced disorders, as well as ADHD and PTSD.

Section 13 retains leadership from William C. Becker, MD, and Martin D. Cheatle, PhD, to review the biopsychosocial intersections between pain and addiction. Legal and regulatory issues in opioid prescribing are also addressed for the reader.

Sarah M. Bagley, MD, Sion Kim Harris, MD, and J. Wesley Boyd, MD, lead Section 14 on Children and Adolescents. This section has been interwoven with content in other sections relating to subject matter on addiction-related issues in children and adolescents. Relevant to today's policymaking climate, the impact of cannabis legalization and cannabis used as treatment on youth are presented (Sidebar to Chapter 116). Newly added is a chapter focusing on Biopsychosocial Determinants of Development of Addiction in Children and Adolescents, as well as a renewed focus on Treating SUD in justice involved youth (Sidebar to Chapter 116 and Chapters 118, respectively).

Timothy K. Brennan, MD, Robert L. DuPont, MD, and Corinne L. Shea, MA, lead Section 15, "Ethical, Legal, and Liability Issues in Addiction Practice." In addition to several chapters on each of these topics, this section provides a chapter on Therapeutic Effectiveness of Cannabis and Cannabinoids for medical (including psychiatric) conditions, Legal and Ethical Considerations for Clinicians Recommending Cannabis Used as Treatment to patients (Sidebar to Chapter 126). Attention is also given to chapters on drug testing, the MRO, and court-leveraged treatment as well as incarcerated populations.

Martha "Marty" Wunsch, MD, provided her strength in addition medicine as one of the founding editors of *Journal of Addiction Medicine*. Dr. Wunsch reviewed and updated the Appendices as we moved from Principles of Addiction Medicine sixth edition to the seventh edition.

As the first and only addiction textbook to fully embrace nonstigmatizing terminology throughout the entire textbook, this was an inspiring endeavor for which the editors and ASAM thank all of our contributors. We aim to retain and revitalize effective coverage of foundational issues in our field, while also constantly sharpening the blade relating to novel and emerging topics in addiction medicine. We hope you find this textbook useful in your education, research, policymaking, and most importantly in the care of patients whom we all serve.

Terminology

A Note on Terminology

The editors of *The ASAM Principles of Addiction Medicine* recognize that addiction is a medical condition with its own terminology used by not only clinicians and researchers but also patients, policy makers, the press, families, and other stakeholders. There are certain terms that can have several meanings and often unintended effects. Most importantly, such terms can further the stigma about people and patients with addiction-related conditions. The terms "alcoholic" and "addict" are examples of such terms—they can be used by health care workers in a pejorative manner to label a problem medical patient, by family to label a member's violent and irresponsible behavior, by persons with a substance use disorder attending 12-step meetings as a positive label defining themselves as actively participating in recovery, by the general public to define anybody "who drinks too much" or "is a drug user," and by addiction professionals to indicate a patient's substance use disorder. Pejorative terms can erode the motivation of people affected by these conditions to accept help from family, friends, or professionals. Medically inaccurate terms can cause confusion and lead to unclear research results, difficulty translating such results into practice, and inappropriate clinical care. Furthermore, inappropriate and imprecise terms can dehumanize patients as well as undermine and erode efforts toward scientifically informed and ethically appropriate public policy or legislation, including funding for research, treatment, or graduate medical education. This most current edition of the textbook maintains the importance of terminology and continues with a dedicated terminology chapter (Chapter 2) and encourages all clinicians to lead by example with the use of medically clear, accurate, and nonstigmatizing terminology.

For the seventh edition of the textbook, we expanded the frontiers of nonstigmatizing terminology by encouraging our authors and editors to consider how the topics of race, diversity, equity, inclusion, and justice relate to their chapter contents, especially in chapters dealing with the topics of genetics, epidemiology, assessment, and treatment. This has provided attention to these topics throughout the textbook. More specifically, we have also added three new chapters to bring deeper understanding and meaning within addiction medicine: Race, Ethnicity, Gender, and Social Determinants of Health, Disparities, and Access to Care; Treatment Considerations for LGBTQ Patients; and Reducing Inequities of Care Through Changes in Practice.

Addiction medicine is shaped by constantly evolving science and practical clinical experience. It is our sincere hope that this textbook will embody the best of what both of these can offer to clinicians as we work to serve our patients and society.

Acknowledgments

The editors wish to thank the American Society of Addiction Medicine (ASAM) for the opportunity to work on this textbook. Our section editors and authors generously lent their time and expertise, and we celebrate new authors and editors who have joined the team of experts in updating the seventh edition. All authors and editors have made a significant contribution to the field of addiction medicine.

Our publishing partners at Wolters Kluwer—Chris Teja, Ariel S. Winter, Sean Hanrahan, and Bridgett Dougherty—worked with authors and editors and behind the scenes to help lead this project to fruition. Anne Luzier, Sr. Manager, Scientific Publications, nurtured most every aspect of this textbook from beginning to end, under the sage stewardship and advocacy of ASAM Director of Quality Improvement, Leigh Hause-Alvarado, MEd, MBA.

Finally, with enduring respect and recognition, we wish to acknowledge the contributions and leadership of the editors of previous editions of *The ASAM Principles of Addiction Medicine*: Norman S. Miller, MD, Martin C. Doot, MD, Bonnie B. Wilford, MS, Allan W. Graham, MD, Terry K. Schultz, MD, Michael F. Mayo-Smith, MD, David A. Fiellin, MD, Richard K. Ries, MD, and Richard Saitz, MD.

Shannon C. Miller, MD, DFASAM, DLFAPA

Richard N. Rosenthal, MD, MA, DLFAPA, DFAAAP, FASAM

Sharon Levy, MD, MPH, FASAM, FAAP

Andrew J. Saxon, MD, FASAM

Jeanette M. Tetrault, MD, FACP, FASAM

Sarah E. Wakeman, MD, FASAM

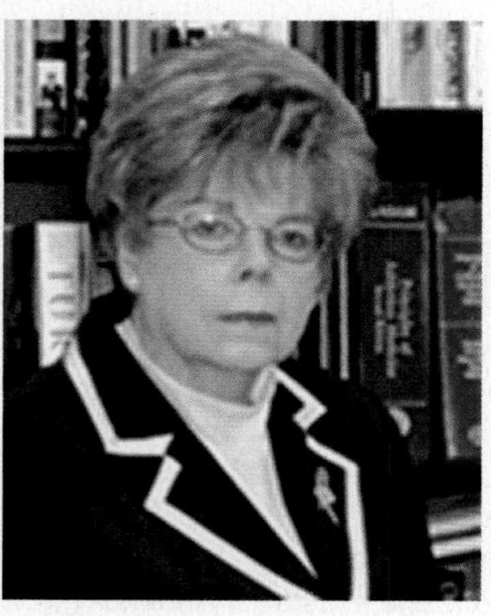

Bonnie Baird Wilford, MS (1944-2019)

An Icon and Paragon Devoted to ASAM, Advancing Addiction Medicine

As a consultant for ASAM for nearly three decades, Mrs. Wilford's knowledge and leadership were pivotal in helping ASAM to evolve into a mature specialty society. Her work not only raised the awareness of addiction as a medical issue but helped redefine addiction medicine through education and public policy—ultimately assisting ASAM to gain acceptance among the other well-established medical specialty organizations. Bonnie Wilford was central in helping ASAM leadership to understand that connecting medical education and U.S. federal public policy were critical to its mission. With her experience leading addiction-related education and outreach programs with the AMA, developing working relationships with NIH and other federal entities, and performing policy work with SAMSHA and ONDCP, Bonnie was a natural at networking federal policymakers with ASAM and its growing body of educators.

Mrs. Wilford's passion was education. She skillfully worked with ASAM to organize its first Review Course in 1986 and recognized the value the Review Course syllabus had in educating physicians in Addiction Medicine. Bonnie persuaded ASAM to compile and publish the syllabus making it available to anyone. This compilation of work later evolved into ASAM's first textbook: the first edition of the *ASAM Principles of Addiction Medicine* (1994). Bonnie led and was the heartbeat for the first four editions of this respected textbook. She served as the Managing Editor for the first four editions of the textbook and then worked to personally help identify and recruit its following editors. Bonnie served as the collaborating shepherd for ASAM's continued growth and influence resulting in publishing landmark books and educational programs and supporting documents, including the 1991, 1996, and 2001 editions of The ASAM Criteria. Her leadership and successes above carried over into the U.S. federal agencies that were becoming interested in and supportive of addiction medicine research and discovery.

She was the catalyst for ONCDP to sponsor three White House Conferences on medical education in addiction. Wanting to keep the momentum alive, she worked with leaders of the White House to form the Coalition on Physician Education in Substance Use Disorders (COPE) in 2002, along with several organizations. COPE's mission remains today to ensure all physicians are trained to identify, prevent, and provide specialty-appropriate interventions for patients with substance use disorders. A passion for the remainder of her career, Bonnie took on the volunteer role of Executive Director of COPE where she remained until the time of her passing in 2019.

We fondly remember Bonnie as kind, approachable, friendly, and inclusive. Bonnie was seen at most every ASAM-related educational event—always working her way through the masses to meet new attendees, identifying needed areas of talent in old and new members, and inspiring them to contribute their time and expertise to help ASAM evolve forward. Many did so on a volunteer basis and with Bonnie mentoring them along the way. Bonnie was warm, passionate, smart, and highly interpersonally skilled. These qualities made her successful in bringing people, organizations, and ideas together toward accepting of addiction as a true medical illness. Bonnie literally planted multiple ASAM pillars of education (medical conferences, textbooks, educational organizations, etc.) that today exponentially bear fruits year-upon-year, serving to motivate and equip clinicians, researchers, and policy makers to battle this deadly disease. ASAM is eternally grateful to Bonnie as a pioneer in our field and organization, as many of ASAM's educational and policy-related accomplishments today began with Bonnie's vision and collective efforts over the preceding decades.

It is in this spirit that we pay tribute to Bonnie B. Wilford in this seventh edition of this landmark publication.

Michael M. Miller, MD, DFASAM, DLFAPA
ASAM President, 2007-2009

Louis E. Baxter Sr, MD, DFASAM
ASAM President, 2007-2009

Shannon C. Miller, MD, DFASAM, DLFAPA
Sr. Editor, Principles of Addiction Medicine

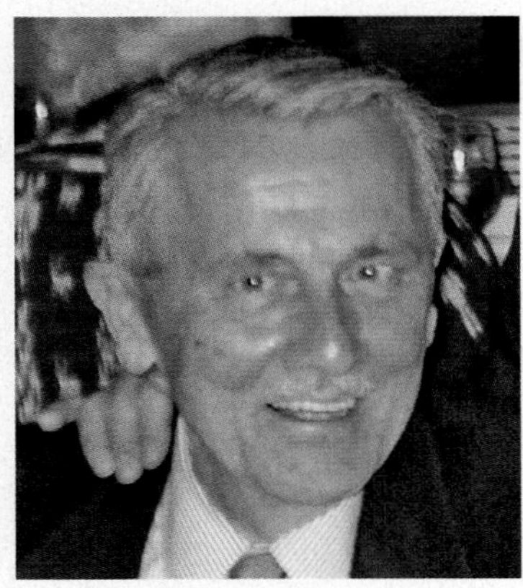

Terry K. Schultz, MD, FASAM (1938-2019)

Terry K. Schultz, MD, FASAM, and Allan Graham, MD, FASAM, met in 1994 in Washington, DC, while attending an ASAM conference. ASAM EVP/CEO James "Jim" Callahan knew that Graham and Schultz were interested in advancing the intellectual content of ASAM's meetings and publications. ASAM had just produced its first textbook in 1994 with Norman Miller, MD, as Editor and Martin "Marty" Doot, MD, (1948-2008) as Associate Editor. Callahan requested Schultz and Graham be coeditors for the second edition of *Principles of Addiction Medicine*. Both physicians understood that establishing the science of addiction medicine was critical to the American Board of Medical Specialties (ABMS) accepting the field as a medical specialty, so they accepted Callahan's request to update the textbook. They served as coeditors for the second edition (1994) along with Bonnie Wilford as Associate Editor and returned again as Senior Editors on the third edition (2003) along with Editors Richard "Rick" K. Ries and Michael F. Mayo-Smith and Bonnie Wilford as Associate Editor.

Both Graham and Schultz thought that ASAM needed a "booster shot" program of cutting-edge advances in the field. They thought ASAM was large enough to have an interested subgroup of physicians wanting new addiction research and established a biannual symposium for ASAM members called "The State of the Art of Addiction Medicine." They launched the first symposium in 1995, naturally in Washington, DC. The meeting was a great success, both in content and in attendance, and they were overjoyed. The State of the Art Course allowed ASAM to invite researchers to speak from the DC area (especially from the National Institute on Alcohol Abuse and Alcoholism [NIAAA] and the National Institute on Drug Abuse and policy experts from the Substance Abuse and Mental health Services Administration) to share their work and findings with clinicians who could take the lessons home and apply them. The conference also allowed Graham and Schultz to recruit authors for the third edition of *Principles of Addiction Medicine*.

Dr. Schultz had a unique interest and mastery of addiction neuroscience, far ahead of his time for the subject. He was a primary moving force for ASAM to embrace neuroscience in its conferences and publications. He loved to discuss anything related to the subject and was often the first to ask questions of conference presenters—stimulating academic discussion for all attendees. He was a gifted organizer and shepherd of authors. He served a full career in the U.S. Army, reaching the rank of Colonel. It was Terry Schultz who introduced George Koob, PhD, (ex-U.S. Navy, alcohol and addiction neuroscientist, and now Director of NIAAA) to Shannon Miller, MD, (a USAF reservist) at the time that Shannon Miller and Martha "Marty" Wunsch, MD, were founding ASAM's new Journal of Addiction Medicine. Shannon Miller invited Dr. Koob to apply for the position as Senior Editor of ASAM's new journal, and Koob was later selected as its first Senior Editor. Without Dr. Schultz, this would have never happened.

Graham and Schultz's textbooks were landmark publications and contributed to the prestige of ASAM and the field of addiction medicine. The texts successfully advanced the field by providing a reference textbook on addiction science and addiction medicine treatment, including new information on withdrawal management, addiction treatment outcome studies, and research into the genetic and neurobiological aspects of addiction. These remain important cornerstone foci for the textbook today.

David E. Smith, MD, DFASAM

Allan W. Graham, MD, DFASAM

Shannon C. Miller, MD, DFASAM, DLFAPA

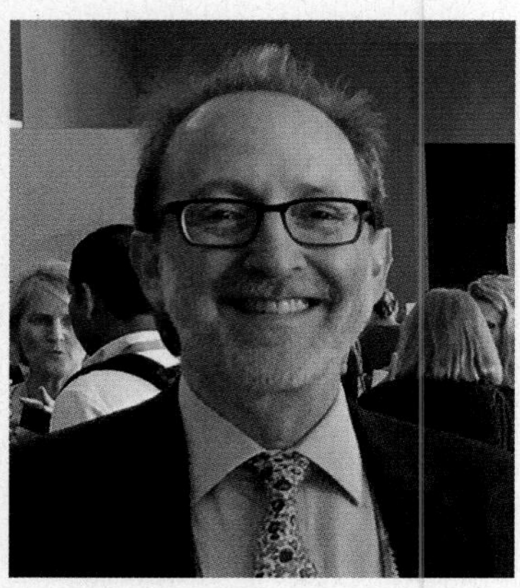

Richard Saitz, MD, MPH, FACP, DFASAM (1963-2022)

In 2022, we lost a brilliant, critical voice in the addiction medicine community. Dr. Rich Saitz left behind a 35-year legacy of research, critical insights, clinical innovations, editorial leadership, and research mentorship. As a physician trained in internal medicine and addiction and as Professor of Medicine and Professor and Chair of Community Health Sciences at Boston University Schools of Medicine and Public Health, he was a physician giant. Rich Saitz created a community of inspired practitioners and researchers who helped define how we approach patients with a spectrum of clinical problems from unhealthy alcohol use to alcohol withdrawal syndrome in varying settings, from the community to primary care to the hospital.

This tribute in the seventh edition of *The ASAM Principles of Addiction Medicine* is most appropriate given his commitment to advancing the editorial enterprise that ASAM supports. Dr. Saitz was Associate Editor for the fourth, fifth, sixth, and the early phase of the seventh edition of this landmark tome. In addition, he was appointed Editor-in-Chief to ASAM's *Journal of Addiction Medicine* in 2014, and under his leadership, ASAM's journal experienced remarkable growth.

I (Dr. Samet) will always remember Rich as that intern who stood out to me, his Chief Resident. His passion, humor, and intellect would accept critical input and revise and resubmit work that would ultimately shine. Over the years, as his mentor, colleague, and beneficiary of his wisdom, I saw these same wonderful talents yield great benefit providing medical care in the hospital and in the clinic, responding to highly critical grant reviews, advancing a complex research project, teaching motivational interviewing, demanding the evidence for science-based decisions, and supporting talented trainees.

My experience (Dr. Miller) working with Rich spanned the fourth through seventh editions of this textbook, as well as working with Rich on *Journal of Addiction Medicine* for several years on a no less than weekly basis. Rich was a very warm person who exuded a unique combination of academic brilliance balanced with humility. In particular, he significantly strengthened the textbook's approach on matters relating to screening and brief intervention. Rich was always available to help people, projects, and efforts aimed toward improving the experience of learners and patients in our field. His humor and spirit always managed to find the positive side of challenging situations, benefitting those who worked with him.

May the life work of Professor Rich Saitz be an inspiration for those of us who seek to provide compassionate, evidence-based high-quality care to individuals impacted by substance use.

Jeffrey H. Samet, MD, MA, MPH

Shannon C. Miller, MD, DFASAM, DLFAPA

Contents

Section Editors iv
Contributors vi
Preface xxiii
Acknowledgments xxv
Tributes xxvi

SECTION 1
BASIC SCIENCE AND CORE CONCEPTS 1

1 Substance Use Disorders: The Neurobiology of Motivation Gone Awry 2
Nora D. Volkow, George F. Koob, and Ruben Baler

2 Recommended Use of Terminology in Addiction Medicine 27
Shannon C. Miller, Richard N. Rosenthal, Jeanette M. Tetrault, Sarah E. Wakeman, Andrew J. Saxon, and Sharon Levy

3 The Anatomy of Addiction 34
Michael J. Wesley, Colleen A. Hanlon, and Thomas J. R. Beveridge

4 Clinical Trials in Substance-Using Populations 48
Frank Vocci

5 Addiction Medicine Physicians and Collaborative Care Clinicians as Change Agents for Prevention and Public Health 64
Warren Yamashita, Kevin Kunz, and Omari Hodge

6 Climate Change and Addiction Medicine 76
Shannon C. Miller and John W. Sullenbarger

7 The Cigarette Industry's Role in Promoting Tobacco Use Disorder 89
K. Michael Cummings

8 The Impact of the Alcohol Industry on Alcohol Use Disorder 105
Thomas F. Babor

9 The Impact of the Cannabis Industry on Cannabis Use Disorder 116
David H. Jernigan, Jih-Cheng Yeh, Connor Kubeisy, and Kevin A. Sabet

SECTION 2
PHARMACOLOGY 128

10 Pharmacokinetic, Pharmacodynamic, and Pharmacogenomic Principles 129
Lori D. Karan, John G. McNutt, and Anne Zajicek

11 The Pharmacology of Alcohol 148
John J. Woodward

12 The Pharmacology of Nonalcohol Sedative Hypnotics 165
Carolina L. Haass-Koffler and Elinore F. McCance-Katz

13 The Pharmacology of Opioids 178
Daryl Shorter, Coreen B. Domingo, and Thomas R. Kosten

14 The Pharmacology of Stimulants 191
David A. Gorelick and Michael H. Baumann

15 The Pharmacology of Caffeine 217
Laura M. Juliano, Sergi Ferré, Darian Weaver, and Roland R. Griffiths

16 The Pharmacology of Nicotine and Tobacco 230
John A. Dani, Thomas R. Kosten, and Neal L. Benowitz

17 The Pharmacology of Cannabinoids 248
Justin Matheson, Katrina Mark, Daniele Piomelli, David A. Gorelick, and Bernard Le Foll

18 The Pharmacology of Hallucinogens 269
David B. Yaden, David S. Mathai, Michael P. Bogenschutz, and David E. Nichols

19 The Pharmacology of Dissociatives 293
Nicholas Denomme, Hamilton Morris, Jason Wallach, and Shannon C. Miller

20 The Pharmacology of Inhalants 308
Robert L. Balster and Silvia L. Cruz

21 The Pharmacology of Anabolic-Androgenic Steroids 317
Scott E. Lukas

22 Electronic Drug Delivery Devices 337
Gideon St.Helen and Shannon C. Miller

23 Novel Psychoactive Substances 357
Kathryn Hawk, Barbara M. Kirrane, and Gail D'Onofrio

SECTION 3
EPIDEMIOLOGY AND PREVENTION 366

24 The Epidemiology of Substance Use Disorders 367
Silvia S. Martins, Megan E. Marziali, and Pia M. Mauro

Sidebar Primary, Secondary, and Tertiary Prevention 385
James C. Anthony

25 Preventing Substance Use Among Children and Adolescents 390
Kenneth W. Griffin and Gilbert J. Botvin

26 Environmental Approaches to Prevention: Communities and Contexts 399
Mallie J. Paschall, Joel W. Grube, Robert F. Saltz, and Paul J. Gruenewald

27 Prevention of Prescription Medication Misuse 408
Beth Han, Christopher M. Jones, and Wilson M. Compton

28 The Harm Reduction Approach to Caring for People Who Use Substances 423
Alexander Y. Walley, Sharon Stancliff, and India Perez-Urbano

29 College Student Drinking 437
Lauren McClain, Frank J. Schwebel, Ursula Whiteside, Jason R. Kilmer, Ty W. Lostutter, and Mary E. Larimer

30 Policy and Leadership: Impact on Primary, Secondary, and Tertiary Prevention of Substance Use Disorders in Military Personnel and Beyond 453
Kenneth Hoffman and Janet H. Lenard

Sidebar Challenges of Reintegration for Military Personnel and Their Families 464
Joan E. Zweben and Susan Storti

SECTION 4

DIAGNOSIS, ASSESSMENT, AND EARLY INTERVENTION TREATMENT 471

31 Screening and Brief Intervention 472
Kenneth W. Verbos II, Alice Zhang, Ahyeon Cho, Suena H. Massey, and Aleksandra E. Zgierska

Sidebar 1 Screening and Brief Intervention in Pregnancy 496
Nicolas Bertholet

Sidebar 2 Screening and Brief Intervention in Trauma Centers, Hospitals, and Emergency Departments 504
Arthur F. Weissman and Richard D. Blondell

Sidebar 3 Implementation of Screening and Brief Intervention in Clinical Settings Using Quality Improvement Principles 506
Emily C. Williams and Katharine A. Bradley

Sidebar 4 Screening for Unhealthy Alcohol and Drug Use in Older Adults 510
Jennifer McNeely and Benjamin Han

32 Laboratory Assessment 515
Sacha N. Uljon, Eugene Lambert, and Eric Lott

33 Assessment 526
Deirdre O'Sullivan and Abenaa Jones

Sidebar 1 Hospital-Based Addiction Care 535
Honora Englander, Jennifer McNeely, and Zoe M. Weinstein

Sidebar 2 Prevention and Early Treatment in the Workplace Setting 542
Marianne Cloeren, Jodi J. Frey, and Indira G. Jetton

34 Addiction Among Physicians and Physician Health Programs 551
Paul H. Earley and Chris Bundy

Sidebar Health care Professional Wellness After Patient Overdose Death 575
Amy M. Yule and Frances Rudnick Levin

SECTION 5

OVERVIEW OF ADDICTION TREATMENT 579

35 Addiction Medicine in America: Its Birth, Early History, and Current Status (1750-2022) 580
Kevin Kunz, Hoover Adger, William L. White, Timothy K. Brennan, Annie Lévesque, and Jacqueline Deanna Wilson

36 The Treatment of Substance Use Disorders: An Overview 594
Lawrence S. Brown Jr, Andrea G. Barthwell, and Ana Ventuneac

37 Identification and Treatment of High-Risk Alcohol Use and Alcohol Use Disorder: An Overview 609
Mark Willenbring

38 Race, Ethnicity, Gender, and Social Determinants of Health, Disparities, and Access to Care 621
Oluwole O. Jegede, Myra L. Mathis, Richard Youins, Kimberly Guy, Skylar Gross, and Ayana Jordan

39 Cultural Issues in Addiction Medicine 627
Andrea G. Barthwell

40 Substance Use and Co-occurring Conditions in Women 635
Joan E. Zweben

41 Treatment of Substance Use Disorders in Older Adults 653
Frederic C. Blow, Kristen J. Barry, and Angela M. Tiberia

42 Treatment Considerations for LGBTQ Patients 666
Timothy M. Hall, Maliha Khan, and Steven Shoptaw

43 Military Sexual Trauma 680
Joan E. Zweben

44 Traumatic Brain Injury and Substance Use Disorders 685
David L. Pennington, Amy A. Herrold, and Angela M. Mueller

45 Integrated Care for Substance Use Disorder 701
Emma E. McGinty, Rachel H. Alinsky, and Mark McGovern

46 Substance Use–Related Care—Interprofessional Collaborative Practice 713
Deborah S. Finnell, Jeffrey Bratberg, and Lisa K. Berger

47 *The ASAM Criteria* and Matching Patients to Treatment 725
David R. Gastfriend and R. Corey Waller

48 Linking Addiction Treatment With Other Medical and Psychiatric Treatment Systems 740
Alyssa F. Peterkin, Karran A. Phillips, Peter D. Friedmann, and Jeffrey H. Samet

49 Reducing Inequities of Care Through Changes in Practice 758
Kimberly Sue, Amanda Latimore, and India Perez-Urbano

50 Quality Improvement for Addiction Treatment 768
James H. Ford II, Kim A. Hoffman, Kimberly Johnson, and Javier Ponce Terashima

Sidebar Delivery of Addiction Medicine Care via Video or Phone 780
Christopher M. Jones and Yngvild Olsen

SECTION 6

NONSUBSTANCE ADDICTION-RELATED DISORDERS 787

51 Understanding Nonsubstance Addictions 788
Luis C. Farhat, Sarah W. Yip, and Marc N. Potenza

52 Gambling Disorder: Clinical Characteristics and Treatment 812
Jon E. Grant and Brian L. Odlaug

53 Compulsive Sexual Behaviors 826
Timothy M. Hall, Anya Bershad, and Steven Shoptaw

54 Disorders Associated With Technology and Social Media 842
Richard N. Rosenthal and Jon E. Grant

SECTION 7

MANAGEMENT OF INTOXICATION AND WITHDRAWAL 859

55 Management of Intoxication and Withdrawal: General Principles 860
Tara M. Wright, Jeffrey S. Cluver, and Hugh Myrick

56 Management of Alcohol Intoxication and Withdrawal 868
Alan A. Wartenberg, Hannan M. Braun, and Cara Zimmerman

57 Management of Sedative-Hypnotic Intoxication and Withdrawal 888
Steven J. Eickelberg and Adam J. Gordon

58 Management of Opioid Intoxication and Withdrawal 908
Kenneth L. Morford, Julia M. Shi, Patrick G. O'Connor, and Jeanette M. Tetrault

59 Management of Stimulant, Hallucinogen, Cannabis, Phencyclidine, and Other Drug Intoxication and Withdrawal 923
Jeffery N. Wilkins, David A. Gorelick, Itai Danovitch, Nicholas Athanasiou, and Steven Allen

SECTION 8

PHARMACOLOGICAL INTERVENTIONS AND OTHER SOMATIC THERAPIES 945

60 Pharmacological Interventions for Alcohol Use Disorder 946
Norah Essali, Hugh Myrick, and Andrew J. Saxon

61 Pharmacological Interventions for Sedative-Hypnotic Use Disorder 961
Alyssa Braxton, Jeffrey S. Cluver, Tara M. Wright, and Hugh Myrick

62 Pharmacological Treatment for Opioid Use Disorder 969
David Kan and Joan E. Zweben

Sidebar Medical Director Stewardship of Opioid Treatment Programs 994
Kenneth B. Stoller

63 Special Issues in Office-Based Opioid Treatment (OBOT) 999
Amy J. Kennedy and Andrew J. Saxon

64 Pharmacological Treatment of Stimulant Use Disorders 1014
David A. Gorelick and Jeffery N. Wilkins

65 Pharmacological Interventions for Nicotine and Tobacco Use 1030
Randi M. Williams, Frank T. Leone, and Robert Schnoll

66 Pharmacological Interventions for Other Substances and Multiple Substance Use Disorders 1045
Jeffery N. Wilkins, Mark Hrymoc, Manjit Bhandal, and David A. Gorelick

67 Complementary and Integrative Interventions for Substance Use Disorders 1052
Ripal Shah and David Spiegel

68 Neuromodulation for Substance Use Disorders 1064
Colleen A. Hanlon, Kaitlin R. Kinney, Miranda P. Ramirez, and Michael J. Wesley

SECTION 9

PSYCHOLOGICALLY BASED INTERVENTIONS 1073

69 Enhancing Motivation to Change 1074
James O. Prochaska and Janice M. Prochaska

70 Motivational Interviewing 1085
Cassandra L. Boness, Antoine Douaihy, and Karen S. Ingersoll

71 Group Therapies 1094
Dennis C. Daley, Antoine Douaihy, and Roger D. Weiss

72 Individual Treatment 1107
Edward V. Nunes and Kenneth M. Carpenter

73 Contingency Management and the Community Reinforcement Approach 1128
Sarah H. Heil, Tyler G. Erath, Roxanne F. Harfmann, and Stephen T. Higgins

74 Behavioral Interventions for Tobacco Use Disorder 1143
Joanna M. Streck, Angela Wangari Walter, Rachel L. Rosen, and Elyse R. Park

75 Network Therapy 1164
Marc Galanter

76 Therapeutic Communities and Modified Therapeutic Communities for Co-occurring Mental and Substance Use Disorders 1175
George De Leon and Stanley Sacks

77 Aversion Therapies 1189
Hanne Tonnesen, P. Joseph Frawley, and Richard Montgomery

78 Family Involvement in Addiction, Treatment, and Recovery 1198
Julianne C. Flanagan and Brandi C. Fink

79 Twelve-Step Facilitation Approaches 1213
Antoine Douaihy, Dennis M. Donovan, and Dennis C. Daley

80 Relapse Prevention: Clinical Models and Intervention Strategies 1219
Antoine Douaihy, Dennis C. Daley, and Dennis M. Donovan

81 Mindfulness-Based Treatment of Addiction 1236
Eric L. Garland and Anna Parisi

82 Digital Health Interventions for Substance Use Disorders: The State of the Science 1250
Smita Das

83 Medical Management Techniques and Collaborative Care: Integrating Behavioral With Pharmacological Interventions 1261
Richard N. Rosenthal, Richard K. Ries, and Joan E. Zweben

SECTION 10

MUTUAL HELP: TWELVE STEP AND OTHER PROGRAMS IN ADDICTION RECOVERY 1278

84 Twelve-Step and Other Programs in Addiction Recovery 1279
Edgar P. Nace

85 Recent Research Into Twelve-Step Programs 1289
John F. Kelly

86 Spirituality in the Recovery Process 1308
Marc Galanter

SECTION 11

MEDICAL DISORDERS AND COMPLICATIONS OF ADDICTION 1313

87 Medical Care of Patients With Unhealthy Substance Use 1314
Darius A. Rastegar

88 Cardiovascular Disorders Related to Substance Use 1335
Andi Shahu, Steven E. Pfau, and Samit M. Shah

89 Liver Disorders Related to Substance Use 1355
Paul S. Haber and Emily Nash

90 Renal and Metabolic Disorders Related to Substance Use 1376
Sarah Gilligan and Naveen Rathi

91 Gastrointestinal Disorders Related to Substance Use 1389
Paul S. Haber and Nicholas C. Kortt

92 Pulmonary Disorders Related to Substance Use 1402
Tessa L. Steel, Corey Sadd, and Majid Afshar

93 Neurological Disorders Related to Substance Use 1420
Emmanuelle A. D. Schindler, Mona Al Banna, Brian B. Koo, Darren C. Volpe, Hamada Hamid Altalib, and Jason J. Sico

94 Human Immunodeficiency Virus, Tuberculosis, and Other Infectious Diseases Related to Substance Use 1444
Carol A. Sulis, Ayesha Appa, and Simeon D. Kimmel

95 Sleep Disorders Related to Substance Use 1463
Sanford Auerbach

96 Traumatic Injuries Related to Alcohol and Other Drug Use 1482
Edouard Coupet Jr, Deepa R. Camenga, Gail D'Onofrio, and Federico E. Vaca

97 Endocrine and Reproductive Disorders Related to Substance Use 1490
Priya Jaisinghani and Gwendolyne Anyanate Jack

98 Substance Use During Pregnancy 1509
Michael F. Weaver, Hendrée E. Jones, and Martha J. Wunsch

99 Perioperative Management of Patients With Substance Use 1530
Zoe M. Weinstein, Megan E. Buresh, and Daniel P. Alford

SECTION 12
CO-OCCURRING ADDICTION AND OTHER PSYCHIATRIC DISORDERS 1544

100 Substance-Induced Mental Disorders 1545
Mark H. Duncan, R. Jeffrey Goldsmith, Matthew Iles-Shih, and Richard K. Ries

101 Co-occurring Mood Disorders and Substance Use Disorders 1559
Edward V. Nunes and Jungjin Kim

102 Co-occurring Substance Use, Anxiety Disorders, and Obsessive-Compulsive Disorders 1589
Alyssa Braxton, Eric T. Dobson, and Karen J. Hartwell

103 Co-occurring Psychosis and Substance Use Disorders 1601
Douglas Ziedonis, Xiaoduo Fan, Snehal Bhatt, and Stephen A. Wyatt

104 Co-occurring Attention Deficit Hyperactivity Disorder and Substance Use Disorders 1622
David Saunders and Frances Rudnick Levin

105 Co-occurring Personality Disorders and Substance Use Disorders 1643
Stephen Ross, Adam Demner, Daniel Roberts, Petros Petridis, and Michael Torres

106 Co-occurring Posttraumatic Stress Disorder and Substance Use Disorders 1658
Tanya C. Saraiya, Sudie E. Back, Michael E. Saladin, Therese K. Killeen, and Kathleen T. Brady

107 Co-occurring Eating Disorders and Substance Use Disorders 1678
Lisa J. Merlo, Nicole Avena, Ashley N. Gearhardt, and Mark S. Gold

SECTION 13
PAIN AND ADDICTION 1690

108 The Pathophysiology of Chronic Pain and Clinical Interfaces With Substance Use Disorder 1691
Laura Morgan Frankart and Michael F. Weaver

109 Psychological Issues in the Management of Pain 1708
Martin D. Cheatle

110 Assessing and Mitigating Risk of Suicide in Patients With Pain and Substance Use Disorders 1726
Martin D. Cheatle

111 Rehabilitation Approaches to Pain Management 1734
Steven Stanos and Randy L. Calisoff

112 Nonopioid Pharmacotherapy of Pain 1747
Emily R. Casey and Tanya J. Uritsky

113 Opioid Therapy of Pain 1761
Peggy Compton and Friedhelm Sandbrink

114 Co-occurring Pain and Substance Use Disorders 1791
William C. Becker and Declan T. Barry

115 Legal and Regulatory Considerations in Opioid Prescribing 1800
David J. Copenhaver, Rohit Nalamasu, Wesley R. Prickett, Julia Megan Webb, and Scott M. Fishman

SECTION 14
CHILDREN AND ADOLESCENTS 1810

116 Screening and Brief Intervention for Adolescents 1811
Jessica B. Calihan and Lydia A. Shrier

Sidebar 1 Neurobiological Determinants of Addiction in Children and Adolescents 1822
Marisa M. Silveri, Andie Stallman, and Jennifer T. Sneider

Sidebar 2 Governmental Policy on Cannabis Legalization and Use: Impact on Youth 1827
Ziming Xuan, Lynsie Ranker, and Sion Kim Harris

117 Assessing Adolescent Substance Use 1833
Ken C. Winters, Randy Stinchfield, and Shelby Franklin

118 Placement Criteria and Strategies for Adolescent Treatment Matching 1838
Marc Fishman

Sidebar 1 Confidentiality in Caring for Adolescents 1850
Connor J. Buchholz and Scott E. Hadland

Sidebar 2 Drug Testing Adolescents in School 1853
J. Wesley Boyd and John R. Knight

119 Treating Substance Use Disorders in Carceral-Involved Youth 1855
Kevin M. Simon

120 Treatment of Addiction-Related Disorders in Adolescents 1862
Steven L. Jaffe, Justine Welsh, and Peter R. Cohen

121 Pharmacotherapy for Adolescents With Substance Use Disorders 1871
Jacqueline Deanna Wilson and Paula Goldman

122 Co-occurring Psychiatric Disorders in Adolescents With Addiction-Related Issues 1883
Martha J. Ignaszewski and Oscar Bukstein

SECTION 15

ETHICAL, LEGAL, AND LIABILITY ISSUES IN ADDICTION PRACTICE 1895

123 Ethical Issues in Addiction Practice 1896
Timothy K. Brennan and H. Westley Clark

124 Consent and Confidentiality Issues in Addiction Practice 1904
Louis E. Baxter Sr and Nan Gallagher

125 Clinical, Ethical, and Legal Considerations in Prescribing Medications With Potential for Nonmedical Use and Addiction 1911
James W. Finch, Theodore V. Parran Jr, and Steven Prakken

Sidebar 1 Drug Control Policy: History and Future Directions 1927
John J. Coleman and Robert L. DuPont

Sidebar 2 Guidance on the Use of Opioids to Treat Chronic Pain 1933
Steven Prakken and James W. Finch

126 Therapeutic Effectiveness of Cannabis and Cannabinoids 1937
Jag H. Khalsa, Gregory C. Bunt, Marc Galanter, Mahmoud A. El-Sohly, and Shyam Kottilil

Sidebar Legal and Ethical Considerations for Clinicians Recommending Cannabis Used as Treatment 1954
Nassima Ait-Daoud Tiouririne and Jeffrey Katra

127 Practical Considerations in Drug Testing 1957
Jennifer A. Collins

Sidebar Workplace Drug Testing and the Role of the Medical Review Officer 1969
James L. Ferguson and Robert L. DuPont

128 Reducing Substance Use in Court-Leveraged Treatment 1975
Douglas B. Marlowe

Sidebar Reducing Disparities in Substance Use Services in Legal System Settings Among BIPOC and Minority Groups 1982
Fred Rottnek

Index 1989

APPENDICES (ONLINE ONLY)

Appendix 1: Changes to ASAM Criteria Levels of Care
Martha J. Wunsch

Appendix 2: Consolidated Appropriations Act of 2023 and Buprenorphine Prescribing Requirements
Martha J. Wunsch

Basic Science and Core Concepts

Associate Editor: Jeanette M. Tetrault
Lead Section Editor: Frank Vocci

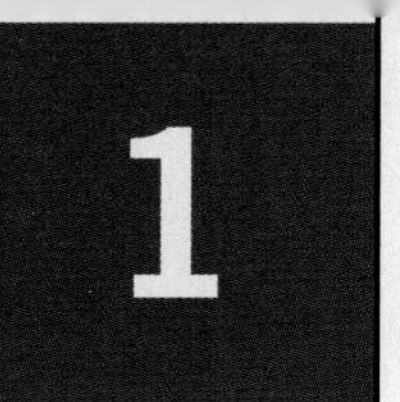

Substance Use Disorders: The Neurobiology of Motivation Gone Awry

Nora D. Volkow, George F. Koob, and Ruben Baler

CHAPTER OUTLINE

- Introduction
- Substance use disorder: a developmental disorder
- Neurobiology of addictive drugs: binge-intoxication stage
- Neurobiology of substance use disorders: withdrawal-negative affect stage
- Neurobiology of substance use disorders: preoccupation-anticipation ("craving") stage
- Vulnerability to substance use disorders
- Strategies to combat substance use disorders
- Challenges for society
- Summary

INTRODUCTION

Substance use disorders (SUD) are chronic relapsing disorders that, as they transition from mild to severe, manifest as an increasingly stronger compulsive drive to take a drug despite adverse consequences, loss of control over intake, and the emergence of a negative emotional state during abstinence. Substance Use Disorders or SUD is the terminology used by the *Diagnostic and Statistical Manual of Mental Disorders*, 5th ed. (DSM-5). In this dimensional nomenclature, the former diagnosis of addiction corresponds roughly to moderate to severe SUD. This maladaptive behavior has traditionally been viewed as a bad "choice" made voluntarily by the person with the disorder, a view that engendered the lingering stigma of addiction as a moral failure. However, addiction researchers have collected converging evidence showing that frequent substance use changes the brain in ways that can lead to the profound behavioral disruptions seen in individuals with SUD. This is because addictive substances impact many neuronal circuits, including those that are involved in processing responses to rewarding stimuli and motivating behavioral actions, negative emotions, interoception, decision-making, and cognitive control, turning substance use into a compulsive behavior. The fact that these changes are progressive and that, once developed, are long lasting, persisting even after years of substance use discontinuation, is what makes SUD a chronic and relapsing disorder but also one that offers unique opportunities for prevention. Growing knowledge about the vulnerability factors that increase the risk for substance use and SUD, including genetic, developmental, and social factors, and much better understanding of the effects of addictive substances in the brain has led to improved approaches to the prevention, diagnosis, and treatment of SUD.

Drugs, both legal (eg, alcohol, nicotine) and illegal (eg, cocaine, methamphetamine, heroin, etc.), and nonprescribed psychotherapeutics (opioid analgesics, stimulant medications, benzodiazepines, and barbiturates) can be used for various reasons, including to experience pleasure, alter mental states, improve performance, or self-medicate negative emotional states or a mental disorder. The repeated use of a psychoactive drug by vulnerable individuals can result in a SUD. In its more severe presentations the intense urge for the drug and the loss of control over drug taking increase the risk of catastrophic consequences (eg, death, incarceration, loss of child custody, loss of medical license, adverse health effects, homelessness).

It is important to emphasize the marked difference between a state of addiction and a state of physical dependence. Physical dependence results in strong withdrawal symptoms when drugs, such as alcohol, benzodiazepines, barbiturates and opioid drugs like heroin, are discontinued, but the adaptations that are responsible for these effects are relatively short lasting and distinct from those that underlie addiction, which are much longer lasting and are described in detail in this chapter. Partly because this distinction has often led to confusion, the DSM-5 eliminated the categories of "substance abuse" and "substance dependence" and uses instead the category of "SUD." The DSM-5 nomenclature identifies each drug in its own SUD category along with its severity (mild, moderate or severe), which captures better the dimensionality of the disorder and the complex progression of neural and behavioral impairments that afflict individuals with addiction. In this review the term addiction refers to moderate to severe SUD, which is often associated with most impairment to the individual. However, mild, moderate, and severe SUD are a single DSM diagnostic and clinical entity.

A growing body of basic research in animal models and imaging evidence in humans provides critical insights that help explain the maladaptive behavioral manifestations of SUD. The convergent results suggest that individuals with SUD undergo progressive structural and functional disruption in brain regions that underlie normal processes of reward and motivation, emotional regulation, inhibitory control, and self-awareness.[1,2] Drug addiction has been conceptualized as a cycle of three stages, each representing basic neurocircuitry linked to a functional domain and associated brain functional networks, while recognizing that brain networks interact with one

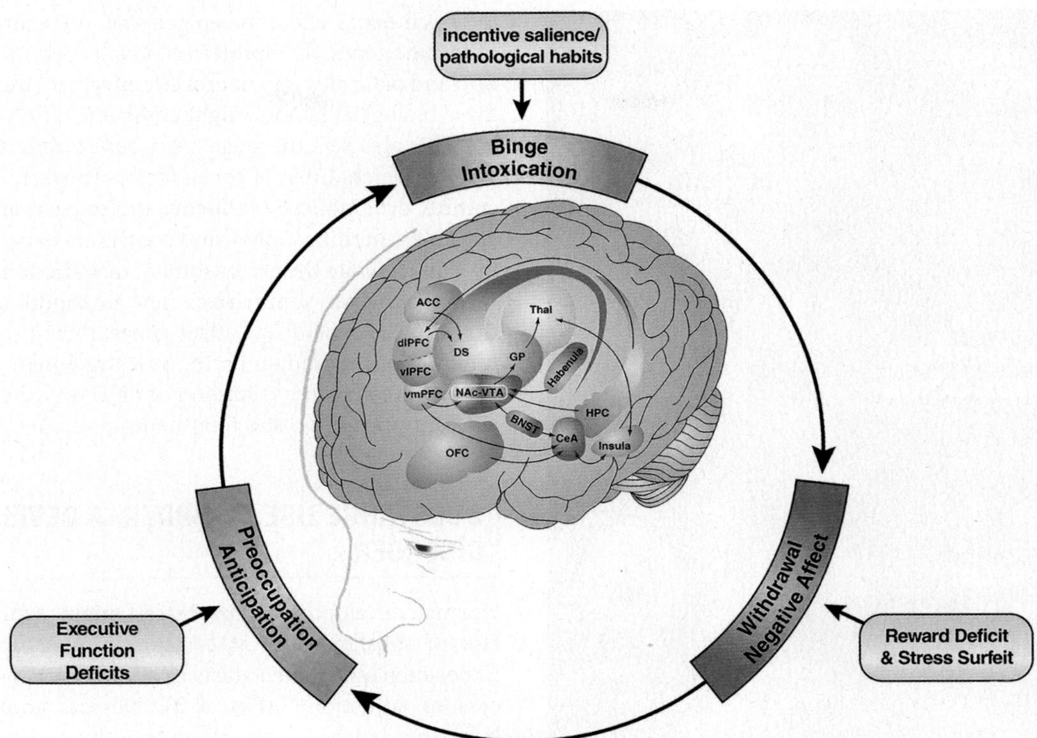

Figure 1-1. Conceptual framework for neurobiology of addiction. The three stages of the addiction cycle (see text) are linked to three domains of neurocircuitry, which mediate three domains of dysfunction: binge-intoxication (basal ganglia-incentive salience), withdrawal-negative affect (extended amygdala-negative emotional states), preoccupation-anticipation ("craving") (prefrontal cortex-executive dysfunction). In parallel, the disruption of the default mode network (DMN) necessary for interoceptive awareness makes it harder to ignore drug craving as well as the negative emotional states during the withdrawal-negative affect stage. (Modified from Koob GF. Drug addiction: hyperkatifeia/negative reinforcement as a framework for medications development. *Pharmacol Rev.* 2021;73(1):163-201.)

another (**Fig. 1-1**). The binge-intoxication stage via the neurocircuitry of the basal ganglia reflects the rewarding effects of drugs and the ways in which drugs impart motivational significance to associated cues and contexts in the environment, termed incentive salience, which is experienced as "well-being," "high," "euphoria," or "relief," depending on the degree of tolerance to the rewarding effects of the drug (see **Fig. 1-1**). In addition, the binge-intoxication stage with repeated drug use enables the development of pathological repetitive learned behaviors, which engage dorsal-striatal circuits involved in automatic and compulsive-like responding for drugs. The withdrawal-negative affect stage, via the extended amygdala and habenula, reflects the loss of reward and motivation and the enhanced sensitivity and recruitment of brain stress systems, resulting in a negative emotional state that is experienced as dysphoria, anhedonia, and irritability (see **Fig. 1-1**). The preoccupation-anticipation ("craving") stage via the neurocircuitry of the prefrontal cortex (PFC) reflects the impulsivity and loss of control over drug taking, described as impairment of executive control, and the input from the default mode network (DMN) including the insula that accounts for the enhanced interoceptive awareness of the desire for the drug, which is experienced as drug craving (see **Fig. 1-1**).[3]

This provides a compelling rationale for the argument that addiction is a chronic disorder of the brain (because the changes are long-lasting, persisting months or years after drug discontinuation) and that the associated maladaptive behaviors (such as those associated with nicotine, opioid, cocaine or alcohol use disorders [AUD]) are the result of impairments in brain functional networks that are necessary for everyday activities. As a result, SUD is conceptually not different from other medical disorders (ie, cardiac insufficiency is the result of impaired myocardial function that impairs the heart's circulation to the body)[4] (**Fig. 1-2**). Therefore, although initial drug experimentation and recreational use may be controllable in many cases, once addiction develops, behavioral control becomes markedly disrupted. Importantly, although imaging studies consistently show specific changes in the brain in individuals with addiction, not all people with addiction present with these changes, and the severity is not the same across all subjects with addiction. The dimensional and heterogeneous nature of this disorder has implications for its prevention and treatment and for public health policy, highlighting the need for further research to delineate the nature and diversity of the genetic, neurodevelopmental, and social factors that are involved in addiction.

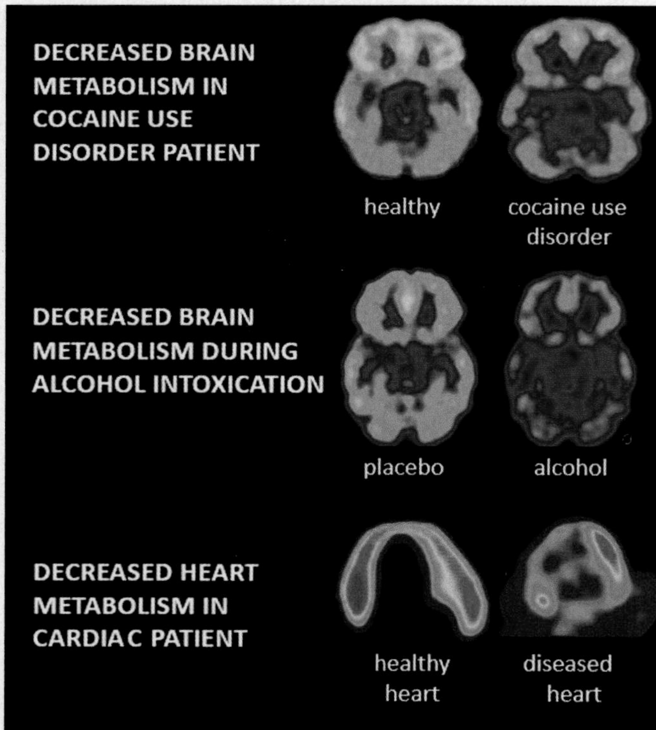

Figure 1-2. Substance use disorder as a disorder of the brain. Images of the brain in a healthy control and in an individual with addiction to cocaine **(top panel)** and in an individual acutely exposed to placebo or alcohol **(middle panel)** and parallel images of the heart in a healthy control and in an individual with a myocardial infarction **(bottom panel)**. The images were obtained with positron emission tomography (PET) and [^{18}F]fluoro-2-deoxyglucose (FDG-PET) to measure glucose metabolism, which is a sensitive indicator of damage to the tissue in the brain and the heart. Note the decreased glucose metabolism in the orbitofrontal cortex (OFC) of the person with addiction and the decreased metabolism in the myocardial tissue in the person with a myocardial infarct. Damage to the OFC will result in improper inhibitory control and compulsive behavior, and damage to the myocardium will result in improper blood circulation. Although abnormalities in the OFC are some of the most consistent findings in imaging studies of individuals with addiction (including alcohol addiction), they are not detected in all individuals with addiction. This implies that disruption of this frontal region is not the only mechanism that underlies the addictive process. (From Heart images courtesy of H. Schelbert, University of California at Los Angeles. Images of glucose metabolism during alcohol intoxication reprinted from Volkow ND, Kim SW, Wang G-J, et al. Acute alcohol intoxication decreases glucose metabolism but increases acetate uptake in the human brain. *Neuroimage.* 2013;64:277-283.)

The emergence of SUD involves complex interactions between biological and social factors.[5] This can help explain why some individuals develop addiction and why others do not, and why attempts to understand addiction as a purely biological or social disorder have been largely unsuccessful. Recently, important discoveries have provided a means of explaining this social/biological interaction via better knowledge of the ways in which drugs affect the epigenome, the expression patterns of specific genes, their protein products, neuronal communication and plasticity, and neural circuitry[6] and the ways in which these biological factors might conflate to affect human behavior. This also sets the stage for a better understanding of the ways in which different social factors (poverty, stress, income, culture, drug policies) influence molecular traits (eg, through epigenetic modifications)[7] and contribute to patterns of behavior that facilitate the establishment of addiction.

This chapter summarizes new methodologies that allow the study of how drugs affect genes, their products, and the function of the human brain; how these methodologies have yielded greater understanding of SUD and their implications for their prevention and treatment.

SUBSTANCE USE DISORDER: A DEVELOPMENTAL DISORDER

Normal developmental processes might result in a higher risk of substance use at certain times in life than others. Experimentation often starts in adolescence, as does the process of addiction[8,9] (**Fig. 1-3**). Normal adolescent-specific behaviors (such as risk-taking, novelty seeking, and heightened sensitivity to peer pressure) increase the likelihood of experimenting with legal and illegal drugs,[10,11] which likely reflects the incomplete development and connections between brain regions (eg, pruning of frontal cortical regions and myelination of projections that connect cortical and limbic brain regions)[12,13] that are involved in the processes of executive control and necessary for regulating emotions and desires. The frontal lobes and connections between the frontal lobes do not fully develop until well into the 20s.[12] This is relevant because drug experimentation emerges in adolescence, and the highest rates of drug use for most substances occur between 18 and 24 years of age, when the connectivity between functional networks is still developing. Preclinical studies with animal models and human imaging studies indicate that drug exposure during adolescence might result in different neuroadaptations from those that occur during adulthood. For example, adolescent rats that are exposed to nicotine exhibit significant changes in nicotinic acetylcholine receptors, with greater reinforcement value for nicotine later in life.[14] Lasting reductions of synaptic metabotropic glutamate receptor type 2 are also observed in the medial PFC, leading to attention deficits later in adulthood.[15] Similarly, recent studies in both humans and animals have demonstrated that the adolescent period is distinctly sensitive to long-term alterations by chronic alcohol and drug exposure[16-19] and may explain the greater vulnerability to ADU among individuals who start using alcohol and drugs, including cannabis, early in life.[18,20] For example, adolescents who had engaged in episodes of heavy drinking presented faster-declining volumes in lateral frontal and temporal cortex gray matter regions and smaller increases in regional white matter volumes relative to adolescents who do not drink.[21] Similarly, a recent Bayesian causal network (BCN)

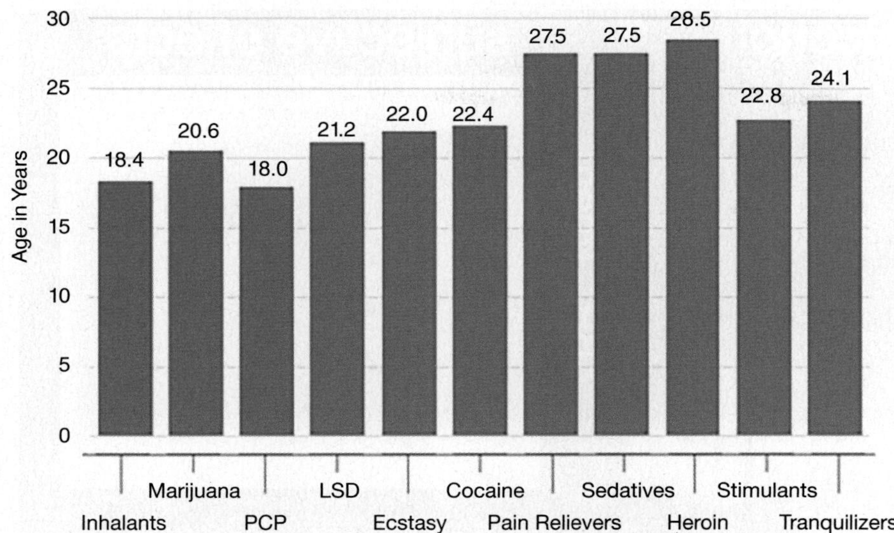

Figure 1-3. Past year initiation of substance use among persons 12 to 49 and mean age at first substance use among past year initiates aged 12 to 49, by gender: numbers and averages in thousands, 2018 and 2019. Mean age at first use for specific illicit drugs among past year initiates aged 12 to 49, in 2011. (Source: From SAMHSA, Center for Behavioral Health Statistics and Quality, *National Survey on Drug Use and Health, 2018 and 2019.*)

modeling study suggested that early cannabis use may be causally responsible for accelerating the prefrontal cortical thinning that occurs during brain development.[22]

NEUROBIOLOGY OF ADDICTIVE DRUGS: BINGE-INTOXICATION STAGE

During the binge-intoxication stage, large surges of dopamine (DA) and the release of opioid peptides have been consistently associated with the reinforcing effects of most addictive drugs. Addictive drugs induce large increases in extracellular DA concentrations in the basal ganglia, including the nucleus accumbens (NAc).[23,24] Specifically, the reinforcing effects of these drugs are seemingly attributable to their ability to surpass the magnitude and duration of the fast DA increases that occur in the NAc when triggered by natural reinforcers, such as food and sex, that are necessary to stimulate DA D_1 receptors and needed for reward-associative learning.[25] Stimulant drugs such as cocaine, amphetamine and methamphetamine as well as ecstasy increase DA in the synaptic space by inhibiting DA reuptake or by promoting the release of intravesicular DA into the cytoplasm.[26-28] Other drugs, such as nicotine, alcohol, opioids, and cannabis, work directly or indirectly to modulate DA cell firing through their effects on nicotinic, γ-aminobutyric acid (GABA), opioid, and cannabinoid receptors (predominantly CB_1), respectively.[29,30] For example, alcohol has prominent effects on DA and opioid peptide release in the basal ganglia[31,32] (**Figs. 1-4** and **1-5**), whereas heroin, via its metabolites morphine and monoacetyl morphine, directly stimulates μ opioid receptors (MORs), activating dopamine and brain reward regions.

It is common to describe the effects of DA in the NAc as one that signals "reward," but this traditional concept is an oversimplification.[33] Rather, DA is a versatile modifier of motivation; its firing patterns help predict the arrival of a reward and calculate any prediction errors. The effects of DA signaling depend on the receptor it activates (there are five different DA receptors). Psychopharmacological studies show that, depending on the magnitude and time course of DA-mediated neuronal activity, the system can encode different kinds of information to subcortical and cortical brain structures that convey different messages about stimulus–response, approach behavior, learning, and decision-making.[34-36] For example, abrupt and large increases in DA stimulate D_1 receptors and are related to reward-predictive stimuli, whereas slower and lower increases in DA stimulate D_2 receptors and are related to preparedness of the neuronal system to stimulation and are necessary for sustaining motivation, effort, and attention. Dopaminergic neurons also respond to aversive stimuli or the absence of an expected reward by decreasing DA release, thus influencing subsequent behaviors to avoid aversive stimuli or to avoid placing effort on nonrewarding stimuli. Interestingly, imaging studies with individuals who are diagnosed with cocaine addiction have shown the expected, drug-induced fast increases in DA in the striatum (including the NAc) associated with the drug's rewarding effect, but such increases are markedly blunted compared with controls[37] (see below). These same subjects with SUD, however, present significant increases in DA in the striatum in response to drug-conditioned cues that are associated with self-reports of drug craving, and these DA responses appear to have a greater magnitude than those produced by consumption of the drug itself. We postulate that the discrepancy between the expectation for the drug's effects (ie, conditioned responses) and the blunted pharmacological effects of the drug's consumption maintains drug taking in an attempt to obtain the expected reward (see Preoccupation-Anticipation Stage section). This explains the commonly reported experience of people with cocaine use disorder who continue to chase the original "high" achieved with initial use but without finding it again.

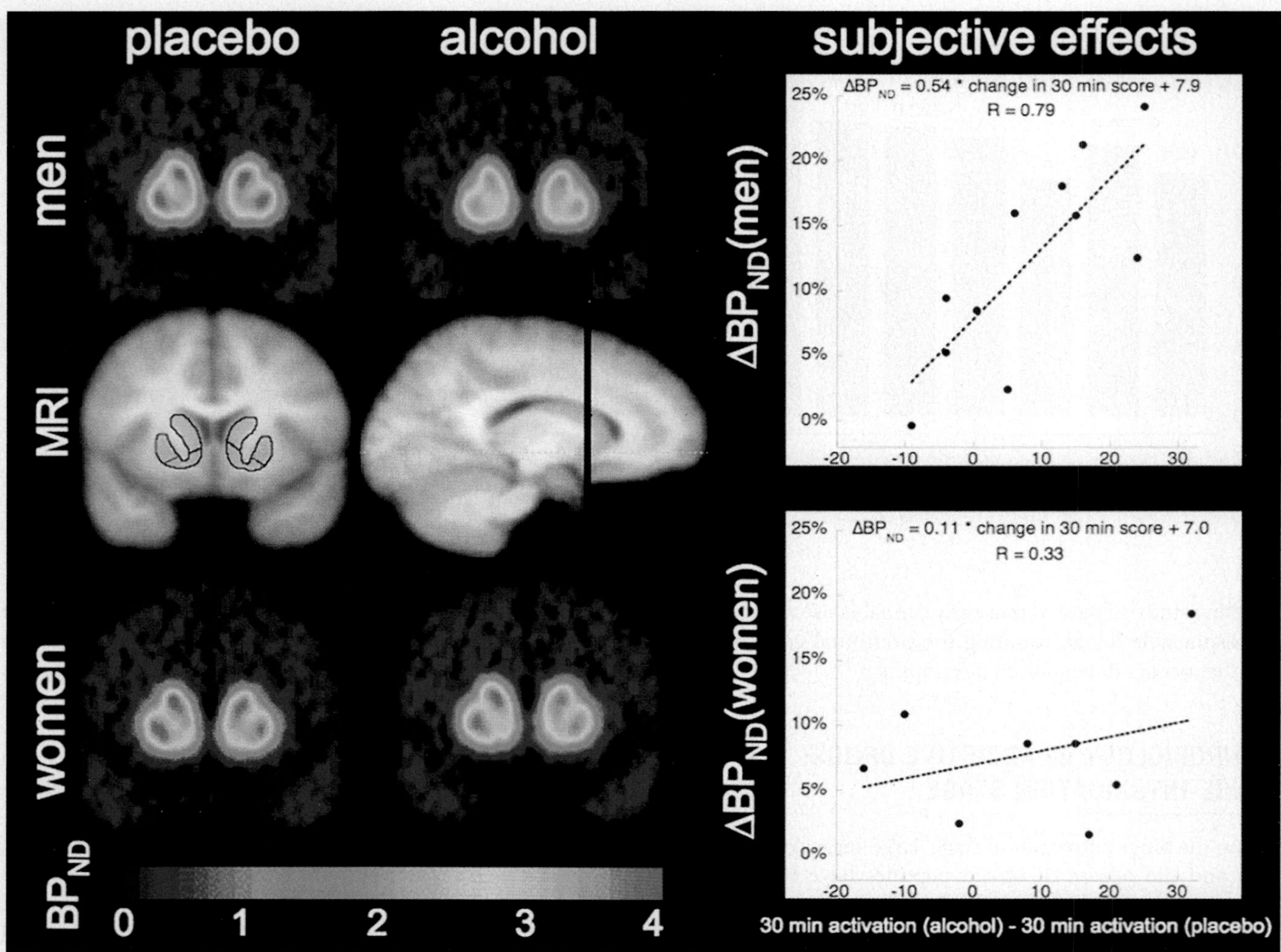

Figure 1-4. Neuroimaging of reward activation (binge-intoxication stage). Alcohol releases DA in the striatum in humans. *Left*, striatal change in [11C]raclopride nondisplaceable binding potential (BP_{ND}) maps and subjective activation in response to alcohol. The placebo consisted of cranberry juice and soda alone, while the alcohol drink in addition contained the equivalent of three standard drinks of 100 proof vodka designed to deliver an average of 0.75 g alcohol per kg body water. BAL peaked at 55 minutes after drink (1.15 ± 0.3 mg/mL in men and 1.02 ± 0.4 mg/mL in women). BP_{ND} maps averaged across men (*N* = 11, *top*) and women (*N* = 10, *bottom*) following placebo drink (*left*) and alcohol drink (*right*). The MRI images (*center*) are averaged across all 21 subjects. Images were all nonlinearly warped into MNI space in the SPM2 software environment. The ROIs on the coronal MRI image (*left*) are the preDCA, preDPU, and VST. The line through the sagittal MRI slice (*right*) shows the coronal slice level of the other images. The graphs on the right show the correlation between subjective activation at 30 minutes after drink (total score post alcohol minus total score post placebo, not adjusted for baseline) and absolute ΔBP_{ND} (reflecting changes in DA). The relationship is stronger for men (*top*). Note that the absolute value of ΔBP_{ND} is presented here. (Taken from Urban NB, Kegeles LS, Slifstein M, et al. Sex differences in striatal dopamine release in young adults after oral alcohol challenge: a positron emission tomography imaging study with [11C]raclopride. *Biol Psychiatry.* 2010;68:689-696, with permission.)

Another important question can be posed: If natural reinforcers increase DA, then why would they not lead to addiction? The difference might be attributable to qualitative and quantitative differences in the increases in DA that are induced by drugs, which are greater in magnitude (by at least 5- to 10-fold as measured by microdialysis) and duration than those that are induced by natural reinforcers.[25] Additionally, increases in DA that are produced by natural reinforcers in the NAc undergo satiation, whereas those that are induced by addictive drugs do not.[23] For natural reinforcers (but not for drugs) lower DA release in NAc is associated with satiety (highly rewarding food that is rich in fat and sugar is a special case that is discussed elsewhere in more detail).[38]

Finally, engagement of the dorsal striatum during addiction is thought to help solidify habitual behaviors that are associated with drug seeking and taking, leading to pathological, compulsive-like habits. Neuroadaptations in the dorsal striatum and NAc also involve changes in glutamate, GABA, and the endocannabinoid system.[39,40]

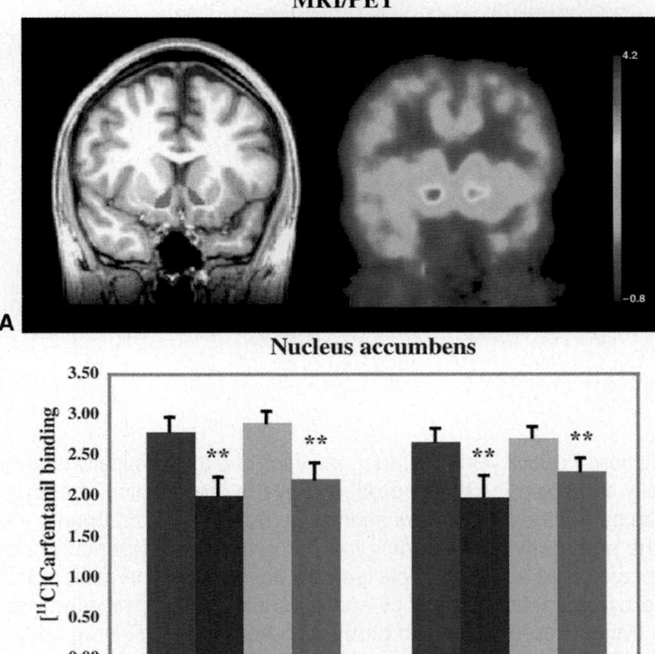

Figure 1-5. Neuroimaging of reward activation (binge-intoxication stage). Alcohol consumption induces opioids in the NAc in humans. Changes in MOR binding in ROIs following alcohol consumption. **A** (*Top*). Spatially coregistered coronal MRI (*left*) and PET (*right*) images from a single representative control subject indicating designation of individually drawn NAc ROIs. *Left*: Coronal section MRI with the NAc ROI in *orange*. *Right*: [11C]carfentanil binding potential, with highest binding potential in hot colors (see color scale) **B**. Binding potential (BP = Bmax/Kd − 1) for the NAc region $*p < 0.05$; $**p < 0.01$, paired *t* tests for heavy drinking ($N = 12$) and control subjects ($N = 13$) before and after alcohol consumption. Alcohol consumption of one standard drink in fruit juice resulted in blood alcohol levels of 0.04-0.05 g%. (Data from Mitchell JM, O'Neill JP, Janabi M, Marks SM, Jagust WJ, Fields HL. Alcohol consumption induces endogenous opioid release in the human orbitofrontal cortex and nucleus accumbens. *Sci Transl Med.* 2012;4:116ra6.)

NEUROBIOLOGY OF SUBSTANCE USE DISORDERS: WITHDRAWAL-NEGATIVE AFFECT STAGE

Substance use disorder has been conceptualized as a reward deficit disorder.[41] More specifically, a defining characteristic of SUD is the transition from impulsive drug intake to compulsive intake that is mediated by positive and negative reinforcement, respectively. Once a person transitions to compulsive drug use, negative reinforcement mechanisms play a substantial role in continued, escalated drug use. Negative reinforcement is a behavioral mechanism whereby greater drug taking is strengthened by the alleviation of a negative emotional state that is precipitated by absence of the drug. In recent years, attention has focused on understanding the neurobiological mechanisms, including specific neuroadaptations that underlie this negative emotional state that is produced by drug withdrawal and abstinence because of its central role in return to use. These mechanisms contribute to negative emotional state also referred to as hyperkatifeia during the withdrawal/negative affect stage of the addiction cycle[42] (**Fig. 1-6**).

Neuroadaptations in the brain reward/motivation, executive/self-regulation, stress/emotion and internal awareness/interoceptive systems are key drivers of the compulsion to continue drug intake despite adverse consequences. Decreases in DA and GABA in the ventral striatum (where the NAc is located) are coupled with the recruitment of brain stress systems in the extended amygdala and habenula, which in turn inhibit DA cell firing and DA release.[43] The extended amygdala is a composite structure that comprises the central nucleus of the amygdala (CeA), the bed nucleus of the stria terminalis (BNST), and a transition area in the medial and caudal portions of the NAc.[44] A key player in the brain stress systems is dysregulation of the hypothalamic-pituitary-adrenal (HPA) axis and the recruitment of extrahypothalamic corticotropin-releasing factor (CRF) in the extended amygdala.[45] In animal models, CRF receptor antagonists blocked alcohol self-administration in dependent rats during both acute withdrawal and protracted abstinence and also blunted compulsive-like responding for all major addictive drugs, and many of these effects have been localized to the extended amygdala.[45] Withdrawal from all addictive drugs that have been studied to date leads to an activated HPA stress response. However, repeated withdrawal and the repeated activation of glucocorticoids (effectors of the HPA axis) can lead to a blunted HPA stress response along with sensitization of the CRF-CRF_1 receptor systems of the extended amygdala, causally linking the neuroendocrine and extrahypothalamic CRF system stress responses in the development of a SUD.[45]

Consistent with a functional role for the HPA axis component of the opponent process, glucocorticoid receptor antagonists reduced the development and expression of excessive alcohol self-administration that resulted from repeated, intermittent alcohol intoxication[46] and alcohol seeking in a human laboratory study.[47]

The excessive release of DA and opioid peptides also produces the subsequent activation of dynorphin systems, which through their activation of κ opioid receptors decreases DA release. A decrease in DA release contributes to the dysphoria that is associated with addiction[48] and more generally to negative emotional states.[49] Indeed, κ opioid receptor antagonists block the depression-like, aversive responses to stress, and dysphoric-like responses during drug withdrawal and compulsive-like responding in animal models.[50] Additionally, there is evidence that norepinephrine, vasopressin, substance P, hypocretin (orexin), and inflammatory cytokines also contribute to negative emotional states of drug withdrawal, which are most prominent for alcohol and opioids.[51] Recruitment of the brain stress systems in the extended amygdala is also accompanied by compensatory mechanisms that oppose these effects. Such "buffer systems" include neuropeptide Y (NPY), nociceptin, and the endocannabinoid system, which act to

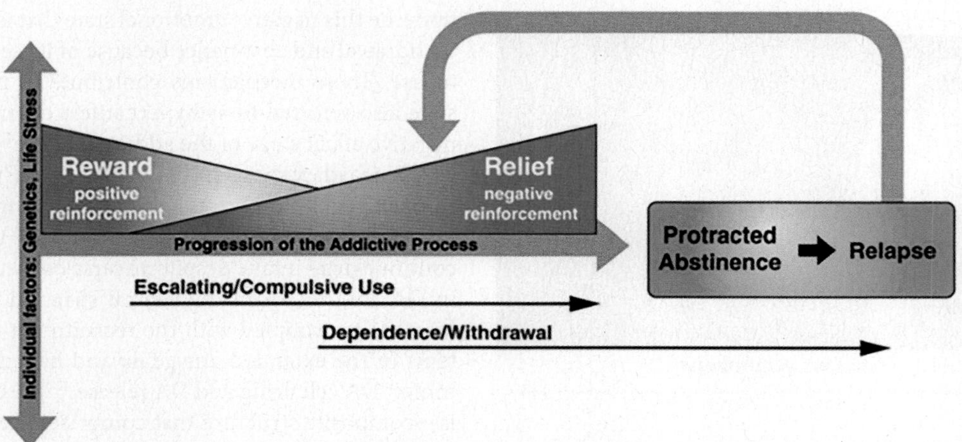

Figure 1-6. Conceptual framework of sources of reinforcement in addiction. Positive reinforcement, in which the drug typically engenders positive hedonic effects, is defined as an increase in the probability of responding that is produced by the presentation of a drug. Positive reinforcement is associated with the early stages of addiction as part of the binge/intoxication stage but persists throughout the addiction cycle. Negative reinforcement is defined as an increase in the probability of responding for a drug to relieve hyperkatifeia or stress, in which drug withdrawal during the withdrawal/negative affect stage of the addiction cycle typically engenders hyperkatifeia and stress. Both sources of reinforcement can coexist and be perpetuated by protracted abstinence and cue-, drug-, and stress-induced reinstatement in the preoccupation/anticipation stage of the addiction cycle. (Reproduced with permission from Koob GF. Drug addiction: hyperkatifeia/negative reinforcement as a framework for medications development. *Pharmacol Rev.* 2021;73(1):163-201.)

restore homeostasis to extended amygdala circuits and modulate stress responses.[52,53] Thus, one can envision stress system recruitment (the overactivation of CRF or dynorphin-κ opioid receptors) or buffer system failure (low activation of NPY, nociceptin, or endocannabinoids) that contributes to vulnerability, severity, and return to substance use in addiction under the conceptual framework that is conveyed by negative reinforcement. In human imaging studies, hyperactivity of the amygdala, thalamus, and hippocampus and a decrease in amygdala connectivity with the anterior cingulate gyrus were observed in response to angry and fearful facial expressions in people with a current cocaine use disorder compared with controls[54] (**Fig. 1-7**). Increases in amygdala activation were also independently associated with an earlier age of first cocaine use and longer exposure to cocaine.[55]

There is also evidence of impairments in ancillary circuits that are likely to contribute to compulsive-like behaviors that are seen in individuals with addiction. For example,

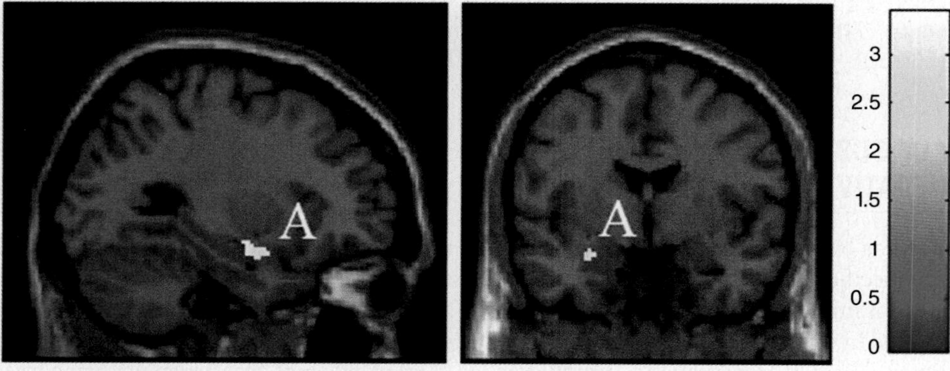

Figure 1-7. Neuroimaging showing sensitization of amygdala during fear responses (withdrawal-negative affect stage). Brain image of a patient with DSM-IV defined cocaine dependence showing significantly increased activation in the left amygdala in response to fearful and angry faces during an emotional face-matching task. Amygdala activity and amygdala connectivity during the emotional face-matching task, known to activate the amygdala (Morris et al.[54]) were assessed in 51 cocaine-using males and 32 non–drug-using healthy males using functional magnetic resonance imaging (fMRI). Male healthy non–drug-using controls and males who were currently using cocaine, 22 to 50 years old, were included when using at least 1 g of cocaine during at least two occasions per week for the last six consecutive months. (From Crunelle CL, Kaag AM, van den Munkhof HE, et al. Dysfunctional amygdala activation and connectivity with the prefrontal cortex in current cocaine users. *Hum Brain Mapp.* 2015;36:4222-4230.)

insular dysfunction can affect the ability to properly evaluate internal states,[56] and impairments in the lateral habenula can compromise the ability to properly process and learn from disappointments and might disrupt mood.[57] Finally, in addition to classic neurotransmitter systems, recent studies link neuroinflammatory signaling in the brain to substance use and SUD. For example, central immune signaling activation is associated with the use of alcohol, opioids, cocaine, and methamphetamine.[58] Alterations of neuroimmune signaling regulate alcohol drinking behavior and may contribute to negative affect and depression-like behaviors induced by alcohol[59,60] and opioids[61,62] and additionally contribute to the toxicity associated with alcohol[63,64] and other drugs, such as methamphetamine[65] and opioids.[66,67]

NEUROBIOLOGY OF SUBSTANCE USE DISORDERS: PREOCCUPATION-ANTICIPATION ("CRAVING") STAGE

A hallmark of SUD involves poor executive function, including impaired self-regulation, which is mediated by prefrontal cortical regions. Regions in the PFC are damaged by chronic intermittent drug (alcohol, cocaine, cannabis) use and result in poor decision making that can perpetuate the addiction cycle. Indeed, gray matter volume deficits in specific medial frontal and posterior parietal-occipital brain regions are predictive of risk for return to use, suggesting a significant role for gray matter atrophy in poor clinical outcomes in AUD[68] (see **Fig. 1-8**). Similar, although not identical, findings have been observed for opioid, cocaine, and cannabis use disorders.[69-72] Adaptations also appear to occur in regions that are innervated by mesolimbic DA circuits (including NAc, amygdala, hippocampus, and PFC), which may contribute to the greater salience value of the drug and drug stimuli and the lower sensitivity to natural reinforcers.[6] Whether tested during early or protracted withdrawal, individuals with addiction present lower levels of DA D_2 receptors in the striatum (including the NAc), which in turn are associated with decreases in the baseline activity of frontal brain regions that are implicated in salience attribution (orbitofrontal cortex [OFC]), inhibitory control, and error monitoring (anterior cingulate gyrus [ACC]). These results point to an imbalance between dopaminergic circuits that underlie reward and conditioning and those that underlie executive function (emotional control and decision-making). We postulate that this imbalance (and especially the disruptions it causes in OFC function, according to optogenetic studies in mice,[73] results in impulsivity and compulsivity.[74]

The impaired attribution of salience is a particularly consequential aspect of this imbalance. Salience refers to stimuli or environmental changes that are arousing or that elicit an attentional behavioral switch.[75] This salience, which applies not only to reward but also to aversive, new, or unexpected stimuli,

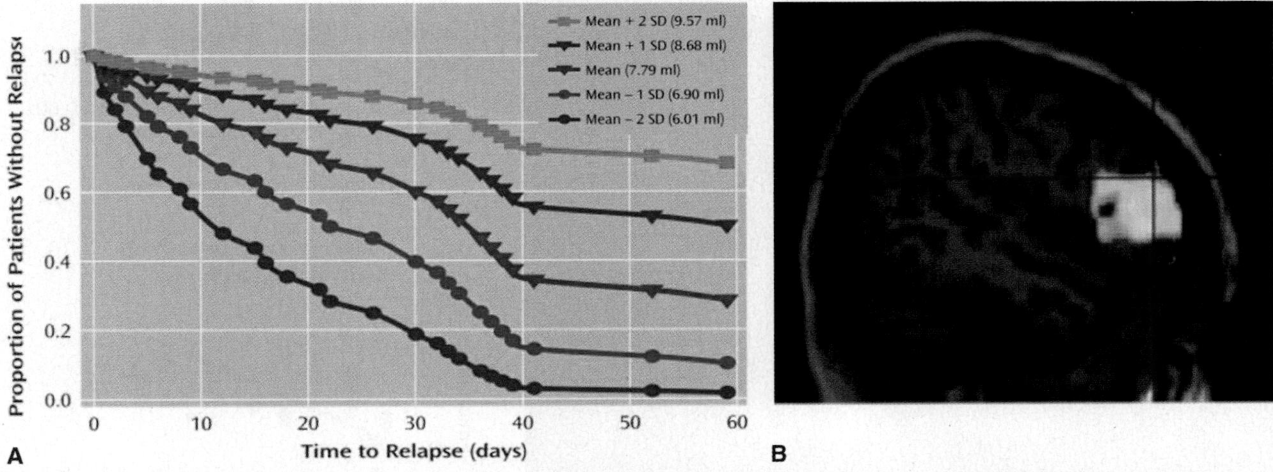

Figure 1-8. Neuroimaging showing decreased frontal activity correlated with return to use vulnerability (preoccupation-anticipation stage), with significant clusters of gray matter volume deficit in patients with alcohol dependence relative to healthy comparison subjects. **Panel A** presents estimated survival risk functions (with mean age, IQ, and baseline total amount of alcohol consumed held constant) for mean gray matter volumes as well as for volumes one and two standard deviations above and below the mean for the medial frontal cluster (cluster $\chi^2 = 6.7$, $p < 0.009$; hazard ratio = 0.52, 95% CI = 0.31-0.85). Although the survival function was a 90-day analysis, the graphs are cut off at day 60 because all patient with alcohol dependence with gray matter volumes two standard deviations below the mean for each of the two regions returned to use by day 60. For patients with volumes two standard deviations above the mean in the medial frontal cluster, the estimated survival function at day 60 spans a 0.68 (68%) proportion of surviving return to use, whereas for patients with volumes two standard deviations below the mean, the estimated survival function at day 60 for both regions spans only a 0.02% chance of surviving recurrence of substance use. **Panel B** shows the right lateral prefrontal cortex with crosshairs at Montreal Neurological Institute (MNI) coordinates $x = 51$, $y = 40$, $z = 19$ (Brodmann area 46; dorsolateral prefrontal cortex). (Adapted and reprinted with permission from the *American Journal of Psychiatry*, as content originally appeared in Issue 168:2, Figure 2 and Figure 3, pages 183-192 (Copyright © 2011). American Psychiatric Association. All Rights Reserved.)

affects the motivation to seek the anticipated reward and facilitates conditioned learning and engages DA D_1 receptors.[76,77] This provides a different perspective about drugs because it implies that drug-induced increases in DA will inherently motivate further procurement of more drug (regardless of whether the effects of the drug are consciously perceived to be pleasurable or not). Indeed, some individuals with addiction report that they seek the drug even though its effects are no longer pleasurable. Drug-induced increases in DA through D_1 receptor stimulation will also facilitate conditioned learning, in which previously neutral stimuli that are associated with the drug become salient. These previously neutral stimuli then increase DA by themselves and elicit the desire for the drug.[78] This may explain why a person with addiction is at risk of return to use when exposed to an environment where they previously administered the drug.

At the neurotransmitter level, addiction-related adaptations have been reported not only for DA but also for glutamate, GABA, opioids, serotonin, cannabinoids, and various neuropeptides.[79] These changes contribute to the abnormal function of brain circuits. The combined research of the last decade reveals that drug-induced impairments in areas of the PFC exert a twofold greater impact on addiction, first through its perturbed regulation of limbic reward regions and second through its involvement in higher-order executive function (eg, self-control, salience attribution, and awareness),[80] and third via dysregulation of the brain stress systems via disinhibition of medial prefrontal control over the extended amygdala[81,82] (**Fig. 1-9**). Note, that negative affect/stress during protracted withdrawal contributes significantly to return to use in AUD.[83] Therefore, abnormalities in these PFC regions could underlie both the compulsive nature of drug administration in individuals with addiction and their inability to control their urges to take the drug when they are exposed to it.[84,85] They are also likely to contribute to the impaired judgment and cognitive deficits that are seen in many people with addiction. Additionally, animal studies have shown that drug-related adaptations in these PFC regions result in greater activity of the glutamatergic pathway that regulates DA release in the NAc.[86] Adaptations in this pathway appear to play a role in the return to substance use that occurs after drug withdrawal in animals that are previously trained to self-administer a drug when they are again exposed to the drug, a drug-related stimulus, or stress.[86]

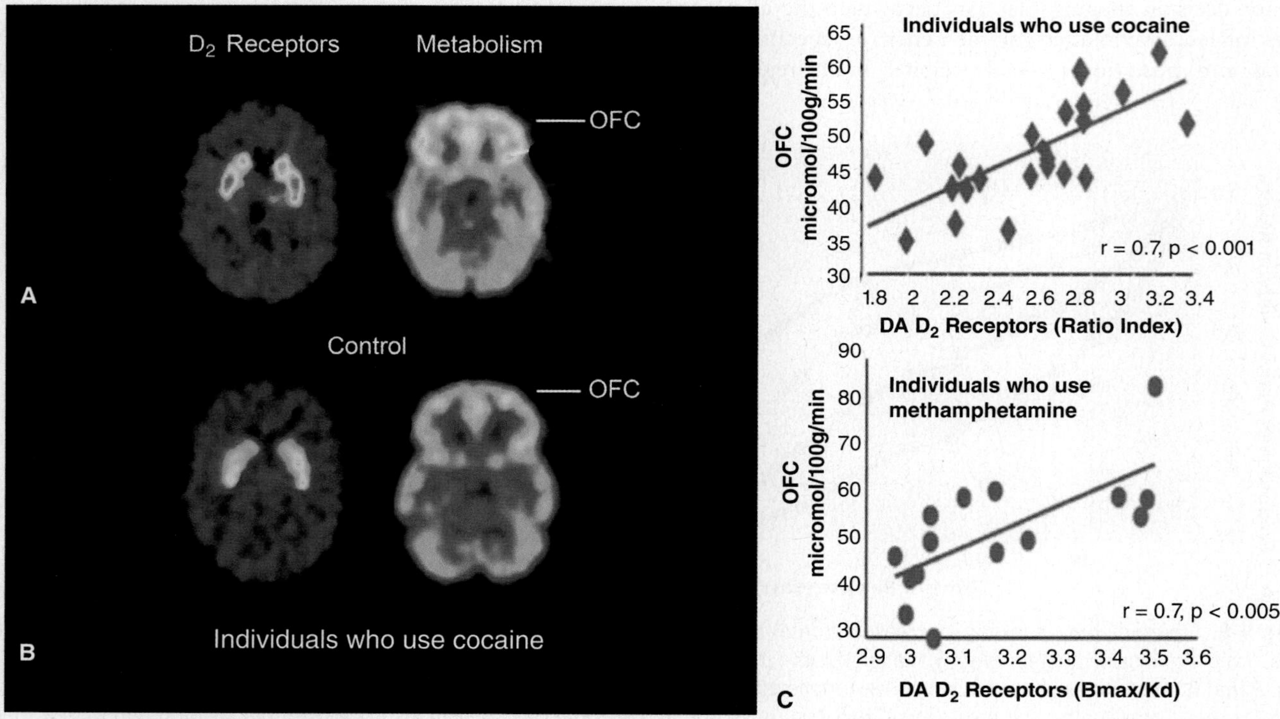

Figure 1-9. Dopamine D_2 receptors and glucose metabolism in addiction. **A, B**. Positron emission tomography (PET) images showing DA D_2 receptors and brain glucose metabolism in the OFC (orbitofrontal cortex) in controls **(A)** and in individuals who use cocaine **(B)**. Note that the individuals using cocaine have reductions in both D_2 receptors and in OFC metabolism. **C**. Correlation between measures of D_2 receptors and brain glucose metabolism in the OFC and anterior cingulate gyrus (CG) of both people who used cocaine and methamphetamine. The lower the D_2-receptor expression, the lower the metabolism in the OFC and CG. Decreased activity in the OFC, a brain region that is implicated in salience attribution and whose disruption results in compulsive behavior, could underlie the compulsive drug administration that occurs in addiction. Decreased activity in the CG, a brain region that is involved in inhibitory control, could underlie the inability to restrain from taking the drug when the person with addiction is exposed to it. (From Volkow ND, Fowler JS, Wang GJ, et al. Dopamine in drug abuse and addiction: results of imaging studies and treatment implications. *Arch Neurol.* 2007;64:1575-1579.)

Moreover, brain imaging studies have shown that the more individuals with a cocaine use disorder can engage the PFC, the more they can inhibit activation of the NAc that follows exposure to cocaine-related cues.[87]

At the molecular-cellular level, drugs have been reported to alter the expression of certain transcription factors (nuclear proteins that bind to regulatory regions of genes, thereby regulating their transcription into mRNA), and a wide variety of proteins that are involved in neurotransmission in several key brain regions. Growing evidence suggests that epigenetic mechanisms mediate many drug-induced changes in gene expression patterns that lead to structural, synaptic, and behavioral plasticity in the brain.[88] The dynamic and often long-lasting changes that occur in the transcription factors ΔFosB, cAMP-responsive element-binding protein (CREB), and nuclear factor κB after chronic drug administration are particularly interesting because they appear to modulate the synthesis of proteins that are involved in key aspects of the addiction phenotype, such as synaptic plasticity.[89-91]

Indeed, chronic drug exposure can alter the morphology of neurons in DA-regulated circuits. For example, in rodents, chronic cocaine, alcohol, or amphetamine administration alters neuronal dendritic branching and spine density in the NAc and PFC. This adaptation is thought to play a role in the greater incentive motivational value of the drug in addiction.[92-94] These molecular changes can influence all three stages of the addiction cycle, thereby loading the circuits that contribute to neuroadaptations in reward-motivation, stress-emotion, executive function, self-regulation, and interoceptive self-awareness networks in the brain whose dysfunctions coalesce to drive compulsive alcohol and drug intake.

VULNERABILITY TO SUBSTANCE USE DISORDERS

Genetic Factors

It is estimated that 40% to 60% of the vulnerability to SUD is attributable to genetic factors.[95] In animal studies, several genes have been identified that are involved in drug responses, and their experimental modifications markedly affect drug self-administration.[96] While acknowledging the intrinsic biases introduced by the "streetlight effect" and complexities engendered by the effect of gene-gene interactions,[97] animal studies have identified candidate genes and genetic loci for alcohol responses that overlap with genes and loci that are identified in human studies.[98,99] For example, genes on mouse chromosome 1 and human chromosome 1q are associated with alcohol withdrawal responses. Genome-wide association studies (GWASs), which interrogate all of the common genetic variants for correlations with alcohol phenotypes, have proven to be a useful approach to identify novel variants.[100] A GWAS of alcohol consumption identified the autism susceptibility candidate 2 (*AUTS2*) gene in a large population-based sample.[101] A family based GWAS of frontal theta oscillations, an endophenotype of AUD, found that the potassium channel gene *KCNJ6* was responsible for a significant amount of variations in that measure.[102] Progress in identifying candidate genes for alcoholism and alcohol-related responses continues at a rapid pace.[103] However, identifying the biological function of these new candidate genes will be a major challenge in the next decade. The hope is that a better understanding of the myriad interacting genetic factors and networks that influence addiction risk and trajectory will help increase the efficacy of SUD treatments and reduce the likelihood of recurrence of use.[104] A prime example of a successful move from gene identification to biological function is the association between drug-metabolizing genes and protection against AUD. Some of these polymorphisms interfere with drug metabolism, influencing the amount of time a drug circulates through the body. For example, specific alleles of the genes that encode alcohol dehydrogenases ADH1B and ALDH2 (enzymes that are involved in the metabolism of alcohol) are reportedly protective against alcoholism.[105] Similarly, polymorphisms in the gene that encodes cytochrome P-450 2A6 (an enzyme that is involved in nicotine metabolism) are reportedly protective against nicotine addiction.[106] Furthermore, genetic polymorphisms in the cytochrome P-450 2D6 gene (an enzyme that is involved in the conversion of codeine to morphine) appear to provide a degree of protection against the nonmedical use of codeine.[107] These polymorphisms of drug-metabolizing genes operate by modulating the accumulation of toxic metabolites that are aversive; therefore, if alcohol or drugs are consumed by individuals who carry variants that convert their substrate at high rates, then the accumulation of toxic metabolites serves as a negative stimulus to prevent further consumption.

Some polymorphisms of receptor genes that mediate effects of drug have also been associated with a higher risk of addiction. For example, a number of convergent results support a *CHRNA5/CHRNA3/CHRNB4* gene cluster association with nicotine addiction[108-111] and the risk of such smoking-related diseases as lung cancer and peripheral arterial disease.[112] Similarly, polymorphisms of the MOR gene have been associated with a higher risk for an opioid or AUD.[113,114] Associations have also been found between AUD and the genes that encode $GABA_A$ (*GABRG3*[115] and *GABRA2*[116]). Particularly interesting in this context are findings related to the association between *DRD4* variable number tandem repeat polymorphisms and attention-deficit/hyperactivity disorder (ADHD), personality traits that influence risk taking, addiction, and addiction-related phenotypes.[117] The likely involvement of *DRD4* in SUD trajectories is potentially very important in light of its alleged ability to moderate the impact of environments on behavior and health.[118] The replication of many of the genetic findings in SUDs is still pending, but such techniques as exome sequencing (where one sequences all of the protein-coding regions of the genome) is likely to identify variants that play some role in altering the function of the corresponding protein.

Social Factors

Social and cultural factors that have been consistently associated with a propensity to drug use include low income, poor education, social neglect, including poor parental support and discrimination, within-peer group deviancy, and drug availability, all of which contribute to stress, which may be a common feature of a wide variety of social factors that increase substance use risk. Disparities in addiction outcomes by race and ethnicity are deeply connected to social determinants of health. For example, non-Hispanic Black individuals in four U.S. states experienced a 38% increase in the rate of opioid overdose deaths from 2018 to 2019, while the rates for other race and ethnicity groups held steady or decreased.[119,120] These alarming data are consistent with previous research documenting a widening of disparities in overdose deaths in Black communities in recent years, largely driven by heroin and illicit fentanyl.[121] Making matters worse, the COVID pandemic has exposed (and accelerated) long standing disparities that can significantly impact an individual's general health and particularly his or her risk of substance use and SUD and their consequences.[122,123] These facts emphasize the need for expanding research that can lead to effective, equitable, sustainable data-driven, community-based interventions to address disparities relevant to diversity, equity, inclusion, and racial justice, particularly when dealing with topics of genetics, neurodevelopment, epidemiology, assessment, prevention and treatment.

The mechanisms that are responsible for stress-induced increases in vulnerability to substance use and recurrence in people with SUD are not yet well understood. However, there is strong evidence that dysregulation of stress-responsive CRF, vasopressin, dynorphin, hypocretin, norepinephrine, and neuroinflammatory systems may contribute to a variety of psychiatric disorders and SUDs,[124] likely through their effects on the HPA axis, extended amygdala, and other stress-responsive regions, such as the insula and habenula[125] (see Withdrawal-Negative Affect Stage section above). A recent study showed that social isolation during a critical period of adolescence increases the vulnerability to addiction.[126] Social isolation in adolescence also increases anxiety and alcohol intake.[127] On the other hand, social interaction offered as a nondrug reward, has been recently shown capable of sustaining voluntary abstinence in a rat model of opioid return to use.[128]

Imaging techniques now allow researchers to investigate the ways in which environmental factors affect the brain and the ways in which these affect behavioral responses to addictive drugs. For example, in nonhuman primates, social status affects DA D_2 receptor expression in the brain, which in turn affects the propensity for cocaine self-administration in males[129] but not females.[130] Animals (males and females) that achieve a dominant status in the group show greater numbers of DA D_2 receptor availability in the striatum and are reluctant to self-administer cocaine (males only), whereas animals that are subordinate have lesser DA D_2 receptor availability and readily administer cocaine. Because studies in male rodents have shown that increasing DA D_2 receptors in the NAc markedly decreases drug consumption (which has been shown for alcohol and cocaine),[131,132] this could provide a mechanism by which a social stressor can modify the propensity to self-administer drugs, at least for males. These results also highlight the need to understand potential gender differences in the neurobiological responses of the brain to stressors and their subsequent contribution to drug taking.

Long-lasting changes in gene expression that are induced by environmental events, such as drug or alcohol exposure, are now being studied as a means to identify the ways in which the environment can contribute to SUD. These long-lasting changes in gene expression are mediated by epigenetic mechanisms, including DNA methylation, histone modification, and microRNAs. For example, the acute anxiolytic effects of alcohol in rats were associated with a decrease in histone deacetylase (HDAC) activity and an increase in the acetylation of histones H3 and H4. CREB-binding protein (CBP) and NPY expression levels increased in the amygdala, a major brain region that is implicated in stress and anxiety.

Conversely, anxiety-like behaviors during withdrawal after chronic alcohol exposure were highly correlated with an increase in HDAC activity and decreases in the acetylation of H3 and H4 and levels of CBP and NPY in the amygdala.[92] Treatment with the HDAC inhibitor trichostatin A in rats reversed the deficits in H3, H4, and NPY expression and prevented the development of alcohol withdrawal-related anxiety in the elevated plus maze and light/dark box test. Based on the effect of trichostatin A, the authors suggested the possibility that neuroadaptations in the amygdala during chronic alcohol exposure may involve both histone acetyltransferases and HDACs in the dynamic process of chromatin remodeling.[133] Consistent with this prediction, a preclinical study recently showed that CRISPR/dCas9 mediated targeted epigenomic editing at the Synaptic Activity Response Element (SARE) of the Arc gene (one of the most affected genes displaying an altered synaptic gene network in the adult amygdala after adolescent alcohol exposure in rats) bidirectionally modulated the behavioral changes caused by adolescent alcohol exposure.[134]

An increasingly relevant example of an environmental factor that negatively impacts brains that are hardwired to respond and seek immediate rewards can be found in the ubiquitous availability of high calorie "junk" food, which can co-opt deeply entrenched (evolved) homeostatic mechanisms to easily override inhibitory controls in vulnerable individuals and facilitate behaviors that lead to obesity.[38] A similarly deleterious relationship between greater availability and negative impacts on health can also be found in the more widespread nonmedical use of stimulant (eg, ADHD) medications,[135,136] high rates of opioid analgesic prescriptions and overdose deaths,[137,138] and the steady increase in cannabis use among young people.[139]

Comorbidity With Mental Illness

The risk of a SUD in individuals with mental illness is significantly higher than for the general population.[140] The high comorbidity probably reflects, in part, overlapping social, genetic, and neurobiological factors that influence drug use and mental illness.[141-143]

Alcohol use disorder also often presents in combination with the use of other drugs and psychiatric disorders, including mood, anxiety, sleep, and psychotic disorders. Among individuals with AUD, nearly 40% have at least one lifetime psychiatric diagnosis and more than 20% have another SUD. Similarly, individuals with a mood disorder are at increased risk for an opioid use disorder, which in turn increases their risk for overdose fatalities and suicidality.[144] Almost 30% of people with psychiatric disorders present with a SUD, and 25% have an AUD and 15% have another drug use disorder. These comorbidities are problematic because they can complicate treatment and lead to synergistic negative effects on health that are worse than any of the disorders alone. For example, depression can deplete patients of the motivation that is required to maintain recovery from alcohol. Depressed individuals with AUD have 59% more severe suicidal symptoms compared with depressed individuals without AUD, and depression is predictive of return to use after AUD treatment.[145,146]

It is likely that different neurobiological factors are involved in comorbidity, depending on the temporal course of its development (ie, mental illness followed by substance use or vice versa). In some instances, the mental illness and the SUD appear to co-occur independently.[147] In others, there might be a sequential relationship. It has been proposed that comorbidity might be attributable to use of a drug to self-medicate the mental illness in cases in which the onset of mental illness is followed by the use of some types of drugs. When substance use is followed by mental illness, chronic excessive drug exposure could lead to neurobiological changes, which might explain the greater risk of mental illness.[148] For example, the high prevalence of smoking that is initiated after individuals experience depression could at least partially reflect the antidepressant effects of nicotine and the antidepressant effects of monoamine oxidase A and B inhibition by cigarette smoke.[149] The reported risk for depression with early substance use[150] could reflect neuroadaptations of the DA systems and the recruitment of brain stress systems that might make individuals more vulnerable to depression. Also in this category are the multiple observations that suggest that cannabis exposure may be a "component cause" that, in combination with other factors (eg, preexisting/genetic vulnerabilities), may increase risk for schizophrenia or other psychotic disorders.[151]

The higher risk of substance use in individuals with mental illness highlights the relevance of the early evaluation and treatment of mental disorders as an effective strategy to prevent a SUD that starts as self-medication.

STRATEGIES TO COMBAT SUBSTANCE USE DISORDERS

Knowledge of the neurobiology of drugs and the adaptive changes that occur with SUD is guiding new strategies for prevention and treatment and identifying areas in which further research is required.

Preventing SUD

The greater vulnerability of adolescents to experimentation with addictive drugs and to subsequent addiction underscores why the prevention of early exposure is such an important strategy to combat SUD. Epidemiological studies show that the prevalence of substance use in adolescents has changed significantly over the past 30 years, and some of the decreases appear to be related to education about the risks of drugs, but some of the increases may be related to changes in the perception of such risks. For example, for cannabis, the prevalence rates of use in the United States in 1979 were as high as 50%. In 1992, they were as low as 20%[152] (**Fig. 1-10**) but now have increased significantly among 18 to 25-year-olds, although these rates have remained stable among adolescents. Interestingly, in contrast to the stable levels of cannabis use among teenagers, the use of other drugs, both legal (alcohol and nicotine) and illegal (cocaine, methamphetamine, heroin, ecstasy, and inhalants), and prescription medications (stimulants, opioids, benzodiazepines) has continued to decrease[153] whereas vaping of nicotine and cannabis has increased dramatically in the United States.[154,155] Moreover, the historically strong relationship between perception of the risks associated with cannabis consumption and its use; such that when adolescents perceived cannabis to be risky, the use was low, whereas when they did not, the use was high, is no longer evident. Thus, despite significant decreases over the past 5 years in the perception of cannabis as risky, its use has not changed during this time period.[153] Some of the significant decreases in ecstasy use and cigarette smoking in adolescents[153] reflect effective prevention campaigns, which provide evidence that, despite the fact that adolescents are more likely to take risks, interventions that educate them about the harmful effects of drugs through age-appropriate messages can decrease the rate of substance use.[156-158] From 2006 to 2014, there is also evidence that there has been a steady decrease in underage alcohol use, and binge drinking,[153] though in the same time period emergency room visits linked to alcohol have increased, which may reflect increases in high-intensity drinking (10-15 drinks in a given setting).[159] This pattern of use is concerning for several reasons, including recent findings that the long-term sequelae for adolescents with more severe SUD symptoms are more deleterious than with no or low severity.[160,161] Also, it suggests that not all media campaigns and school-based educational programs have been successful in preventing hazardous or unhealthy substance use.[162,163] Tailored interventions that take into account socioeconomic, cultural, and age and gender characteristics of children and adolescents are more likely to improve their effectiveness.

Currently, prevention strategies include not only educational interventions that are based on comprehensive school-based programs and effective media campaigns and strategies that decrease access to drugs and alcohol but also strategies that provide supportive community activities that engage adolescents in productive and creative ways. However, as the neurobiological consequences that underlie the adverse environmental factors that increase the risks for substance use and SUD begin to be understood, it will be possible to develop

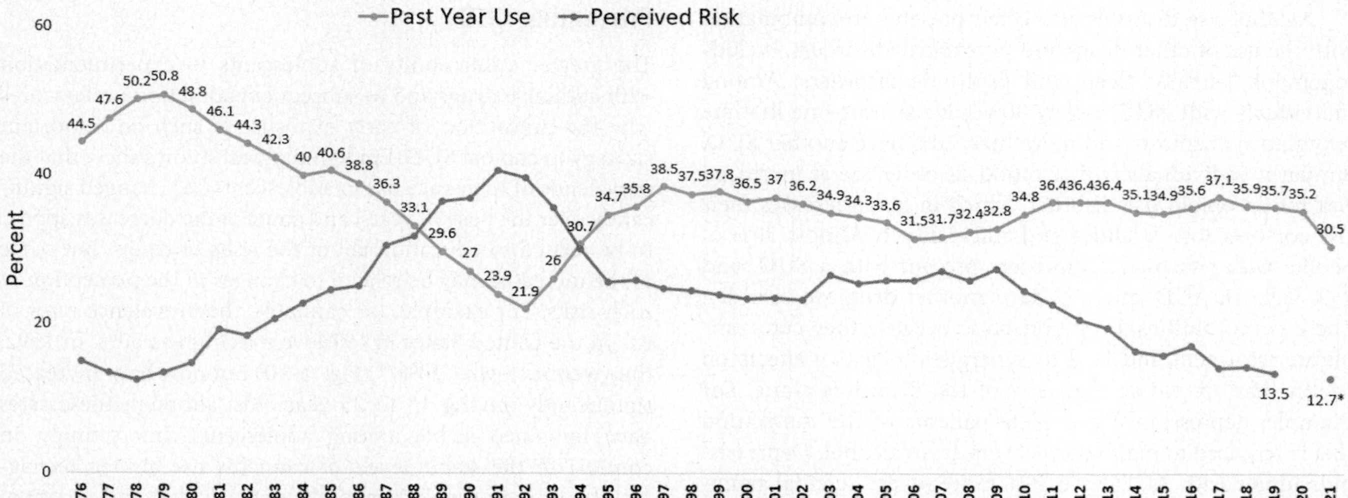

Figure 1-10. Use and risk perception of cannabis. The prevalence rate in perceived availability, perceived risk of regular use, and prevalence of use in past 30 days in 12th graders (18-19 years old) between 1975 and 2021. When teenagers perceived cannabis as dangerous, the prevalence of drug use was low and vice versa. (Modified from Miech R, Johnston L, O'Malley P, Bachman G, Schulenberg J, Patrick M. *Monitoring the Future National Survey Results on Drug Use.* 2021.)

interventions to counteract these changes. With increased knowledge of the ways in which different genes (and their encoded proteins) make a person more or less vulnerable to taking drugs and to SUD, more targets will be available to tailor interventions for those at higher risk.

Finally, there is likely to be a renewed focus, in the near future, on the research and development of interventions that increase general resilience that leads to universally better outcomes. Particularly promising in this context are the landmark results of a major longitudinal study that showed a dramatic positive influence of childhood self-control on a wide range of life outcomes, including substance use risk, overall health, and financial status.[164] Studies are needed to investigate whether there are other factors that also contribute to the significant reduction of the consumption of alcohol and other drugs among adolescents in the United States (ie, some [prosocial] forms of interactions among teenagers through social media rather than in physical venues that favor peer pressure for drug consumption, alternative sources of rewarding behaviors such as some video games).

To address this and other gaps in understanding of the causal connections between adverse social exposures, genetics, brain development, and SUD and health related outcomes, NIDA, NIAAA and other sister agencies launched the largest long-term studies of brain development and child health in the United States: The Adolescent Brain Cognitive Development (ABCD) study[165] has recruited close to 12,000 children ages 9 to 10 whose biological and behavioral development has been followed prospectively for the past 5 years and continue to do so as they transition into young adulthood. Using cutting-edge imaging and wireless technologies, scientists are determining how childhood experiences (such as sports, videogames, social media, unhealthy sleep patterns, and smoking) interact with each other and with a child's changing biology to affect brain development and social, behavioral, academic, health, and other outcomes. The results of the ABCD study have already begun to provide families, school superintendents, principals, teachers, health professionals, and policymakers with practical information to promote the health, well-being, and success of children. Last year NIDA, in partnership with other NIH institutes and the HEAL initiative, launched the HEALthy Brain and Child Development Study (HBCD),[166] which will recruit a large cohort of pregnant people from regions of the country significantly affected by the opioid crisis and follow them and their children through early childhood. This longitudinal study which aims to recruit 7,500 mother/infant pairs will collect information beginning prenatally and continuing through early childhood, including structural and functional brain imaging; anthropometrics; medical history; family history; biospecimens; and social, emotional, and cognitive development. Data obtained from HBCD will lead to better understanding of brain development beginning in the perinatal period and extending through early childhood, including variability in development and how it contributes to cognitive, behavioral, social, and emotional function. Knowledge of normative brain trajectories is critical to understanding how they may be affected by exposure to opioids and other substances (eg, alcohol, tobacco, cannabis), stressors, trauma, and other significant social and economic influences, including those that promote resilience.

Treating Substance Use Disorders

The adaptations in the brain that result from chronic drug exposure are long lasting which is why addiction is considered a chronic disorder.[52] This explains why long-term treatment is required for optimal outcomes, just as it is for other chronic disorders, like hypertension, diabetes, or asthma.[167]

By recognizing the likelihood of recurrence of use, this perspective radically modifies the expectations of addiction treatment outcomes, establishing the need for a more rational, continuous management model for addiction treatment.[168] The discontinuation of treatment, as for other chronic disorders, is likely to result in recurrence of use/disease. As for other chronic medical conditions, return to use should not be interpreted as a failure of treatment (as is the prevailing view for most people who are diagnosed with addiction), but instead as a temporary setback due to a lack of adherence or tolerance to an effective treatment.[167] It is rather telling that the rates of recurrence and recovery in the treatment of SUD are equivalent to those of other chronic medical disorders.[167]

The involvement of multiple brain circuits (reward, motivation, memory, learning, stress, emotion, interoception, inhibitory control, and executive function) and the associated behavioral disruptions point to the need for a multimodal approach to the treatment of addiction. Therefore, interventions should not be limited to inhibiting the rewarding effects of a drug—they should include strategies to enhance the salience of natural reinforcers (including social support), strengthen inhibitory control, decrease conditioned responses, improve mood, reduce stress, and strengthen executive function and decision-making.

Among the recommended multimodal approaches, the most obvious rely on the combination of pharmacological and behavioral interventions, which might target different underlying factors and thus have synergistic effects. Such combined treatments are strongly recommended because behavioral and pharmacological treatments are thought to operate through different yet complementary mechanisms that can have additive or even synergistic effects. Thus, it could be expected that addiction treatments that use behavioral interventions would be more effective when complemented with medications to help the patient remain drug-free. For example, behavioral approaches complement most tobacco addiction treatment programs. They can amplify the effects of medications by teaching people how to manage stress, recognize and avoid high-risk situations for return to smoking, and develop alternative coping strategies (eg, cigarette refusal skills, assertiveness, and time management skills) that they can practice in treatment, social, and work settings.[169,170]

Pharmacological Interventions

Pharmacological interventions can be grouped into two classes. First, there are those that interfere with the reinforcing effects of addictive drugs (ie, medications that interfere with binding to a target, drug-induced DA increase, postsynaptic responses, or the drug's delivery to the brain, like antidrug antibodies or medications that trigger aversive responses). Second, there are those that compensate for the adaptations that either preceded or developed after long-term use (ie, medications that decrease the prioritized motivational value of the drug, enhance the salience of natural reinforcers, or interfere with conditioned responses, stress-induced relapse, or motivational aspects of withdrawal). The usefulness of some addiction medications has been clearly validated; for others, the data are still preliminary. For these, most results are limited to promising preclinical findings. **Tables 1-1** and **1-2** and **Figures 1-11** to **1-13** summarize U.S. Food and Drug Administration (FDA) approved medications and medications for which there are preliminary clinical/preclinical data. Many of these promising new medications target different neurotransmitters (such as GABA, serotonin, or glutamate) relative to older drugs, offering a wider range of therapeutic options. Combining medications may increase their efficacy, as shown for a tobacco (nicotine) use disorder treatment.[171]

TABLE 1-1 FDA-Approved Medications for Treating Substance Use Disorders

Medication	Neurobiological target
FDA-approved medications for alcohol use disorder	
Disulfiram (Antabuse; Wyeth-Ayerst)	Aldehyde dehydrogenase (triggers aversion)
Naltrexone	MOR antagonist (interferes w/reinforcement)
Acamprosate	Glutamate related
FDA-approved medications for nicotine use disorder	
Nicotine replacement	Nicotine receptor (agonist with different pharmacokinetics)
Varenicline (Chantix; Pfizer)	Nicotine receptor (4α2β nicotine [partial agonist])
Bupropion	DA transporter blocker (amplified DA signals)
FDA-approved medications for opioid use disorder	
Naltrexone	MOR antagonist (interferes w/reinforcement)
Methadone	MOR (agonist with different pharmacokinetics)
Buprenorphine	MOR (partial agonist)

TABLE 1-2 Alcohol Use Disorder Medication Pipeline

Medication	Biological target
Oxytocin	Oxytocin
ASP8062	Positive GABA-B modulator
Ghrelin antagonist	Ghrelin receptor
Baclofen	GABAb receptor (antagonist)
Mifepristone	Glucocorticoid antagonist
Gabapentin	Calcium channel/GABA
Varenicline (Chantix, Pfizer)	4α2β nicotinic (partial agonist)
Doxazosin, prazosin	A1 adrenergic (antagonist)
LY686017	NK1 (antagonist)
Cannabidiol (CBD)	Endocannabinoid system
N-acetylcysteine	Glutamate modulating activity

Opioid Use Disorder medication pipeline					
Drug Discovery / Early Preclinical	Late Preclinical	Clinical Trials			New Formulation
		Phase I	Phase II	Phase III	
GPR151 antagonist *	Brexpiprazole *	Cannabidiol *	Cannabidiol *	Brivoligide *	Naltrexone 2-month injection [μ]
AT-121 *	Tezampanel *	Ketamine *	Guanfacine *		BICX104 Naltrexone 3-month implant [μ]
PTPRD inhibitor *	BTRX-246040 *	Lemborexant *	Pregabalin + Lofexidine *		Naltrexone 6-month implant [μ]
SBI-553 *	DCUKA/Kindolor *	Liraglutide/Semaglutide *			Naltrexone 6-month implant [μ]
5HT2R agonist *	EC5026 *	Suvorexant *			Naltrexone 1-year implant [μ]
HBS087/HBS093 *	KNX100 *	Lofexidine *			LAAM Oral [μ]
D24M [μ]	NYX-783 *	ASP8062 *			LYN-014-Long-acting methadone [μ]
NAN/NAQ [μ]	PF5190457 *	CVL-354 *			OPNT003 - Nasal Nalmefene [μ]
Opioid biased agonist [μ]	SBS-1000 *	CVL-936 *			Nalmefene implant [μ]
Carfentanyl mAb [B]	Biased MOR Agonist [μ]	INDV-2000 *			AP007 Extended-release Nalmefene [μ]
Fentanyl vaccine [B]	Methocinnamox [μ]	ST-2427 *			LYN-013 - BUP/NX Oral, long acting [μ]
Oxy/Fentanyl nano-vaccine [B]	Mitragynine analogs [μ]	AZD4041 *			Nanoparticle-based ADF [μ]
Fentanyl/heroin vaccine [B]	NRS-033 methadone prodrug [μ]	ITI-333 [μ]			Nafamostat/PF614 –Oxycodone [μ]
GDNF gene therapy [B]	PZM21 [μ]	Oxycodone vaccine [B]			Naloxone [μ]
	R-methadone prodrug [μ]				
	Heroin vaccine [B]				
	P1A4 Fentanyl mAb [B]				

KEY: **Black:** New Molecular Entity **Red:** New Indication **Blue:** New Formulation [μ] mu opioid receptor * Non-mu opioid receptor [B] Biological

Figure 1-11. Opioid use disorder medication pipeline.

Nicotine Use Disorder medication pipeline					
Early Preclinical	Late Preclinical (Initiated IND enabling)	Clinical Trials			
		Phase I	Phase Ib	Phase II	Phase III
	TriCoil-based nicotine vaccine	**SBI-0069330 (mGlu2 PAM)**	Suvorexant (orexin antagonist)	**High-dose bupropion in smokers with anhedonia**	
		Novel α3β4 partial agonist	Oral Cannabidiol	**Varenicline+Guanfacine**	
			Isradipine +VR Cue Exposure	**Varenicline+Naltrexone in heavy drinking people who smoke**	

KEY: **Black: New molecular entity,** Blue: Repurpose of FDA approved medication, Green: novel medication combination or dosing parameters, Red: Recent updates

Figure 1-12. Nicotine use disorder medication pipeline.

Stimulant (Cocaine/Amphetamine) Use Disorder medication pipeline					
Drug discovery/ Early Preclinical	Late Preclinical	Clinical Trials			
		Phase I	Phase Ib	Phase II	Phase III
cocaine hydrolase [C]	Methamphetamine conjugate vaccine [M]	Cocaine hydrolase gene therapy [C]	Cariprazine [C]	Bupropion [C]	
GLT-1 up-regulator [C]		dAdGNE [C]	Clavulanic acid [C]	Guanfacine [C]	
Peptidic KOR agonists [C]		h2E2 [C]	Duloxetine & Methylphenidate [M]	Ketamine [C]	
PTPRD ligands [CM]		IXT-m200 [M]	Mirtazapine [M]	Pioglitazone [C]	
VMAT-2 inhibitor [M]			Pomaglumetad methionil [M]	EMB-001 [C]	
CS-1103 [M]				IXT-m200 [M]	

KEY: **Black:** New Molecular Entity **Red:** New Indication **Blue:** Biological **Green:** Gene Therapy [C] cocaine [M] meth

Figure 1-13. Stimulant (cocaine and methamphetamine) use disorder medication pipeline.

The therapeutic potential of hallucinogenic drugs also deserves a brief mention in this context, given the renaissance this field has experienced in recent years,[172] fueled by a more permissive research environment and growing evidence suggesting psychedelics could have a legitimate place in an expanded psychiatric pharmacopeia. The reported associations between life-time use of some psychedelics and lower rates of DSM-defined nicotine dependence[173] and the historical accounts (from the 1950s to 1970s),[174] suggest that classic psychedelics (eg, psylocibin) might have potential as therapeutics for SUD and deserve further evaluation.

Behavioral Interventions

In a similar fashion, behavioral interventions can be classified according to their intended remedial function, such as to strengthen inhibitory control circuits, provide alternative reinforcers, reduce stress, improve mood, or strengthen executive function. Traditionally, behavioral therapy has focused on symptom-based targets rather than underlying causes of addiction. However, for other brain disorders, new views of brain plasticity that recognize the capacity of neurons in the adult brain to increase synaptic connections and in certain instances to regenerate[175] have resulted in more focused cognitive-behavioral interventions that are designed to increase the efficiency of dysfunctional brain circuits. This has been applied to attempts to improve reading in children with learning disabilities,[176] improve memory-related brain activity in patients with Alzheimer's disease,[177] strengthen voluntary cortical control in children with ADHD,[178] and facilitate motor and memory rehabilitation after brain injury.[95] It is now possible to see the first glimpses of this general approach as potentially applicable to the treatment of SUD. For example, a small positive relationship was found between cognitive-specific strategies, such as using positive self-talk and a better ability to cope with the urge to smoke.[179] Similarly, a recent imaging study of people who used cocaine showed that specific instructions to purposefully inhibit cue-induced craving were associated with inhibition in the (limbic) NAc, insula, and orbitofrontal and cingulate cortices and reduced cocaine craving.[87,180] Dual approaches that pair cognitive-behavioral strategies with medications to compensate for or counteract the neurobiological changes that are induced by chronic drug exposure are also a promising area of translational research that might, in the near future, provide more robust and longer-lasting treatments for SUD than when given in isolation.[181] A new and exciting area of research in this context is the emerging area of translational research that focuses on understanding how and why behavioral interventions work in terms of neurobiological function and structure.[182,183]

Neuromodulation

Recent advances in the use of brain stimulation technologies for the treatment of not only specific neurologic (eg, Parkinson disease[184] but potentially some psychiatric (eg, depression,[185] obsessive-compulsive[186] disorders, have inspired addiction researchers to consider electrical neuromodulation also for the treatment of SUD. These investigations involved studies of both invasive (ie, deep-brain stimulation [DBS]) as well as peripheral or noninvasive (ie, trans-cranial direct current stimulation [tDCS] and repetitive trans-magnetic stimulation [rTMS]) neuromodulation.

Initial clues regarding the potential of DBS for the treatment of SUD, came from early incidental clinical findings that appeared to link deep brain stimulation of the NAc with the facilitation of stopping smoking[187,188] and with remission from alcoholism.[189] These observations are consistent with almost two decades of animal studies showing that DBS targeting not only NAc[190] but also the insula,[191] lateral habenula,[192] and the subthalamic nucleus,[193] could reduce drug self-administration and seeking. Meanwhile, human studies have focused primarily on DBS stimulation during active drug use and, since the relevant clinical trials have been relatively small, most of the clinical data comes from case reports, reducing the weight of the available evidence. Even so, results have been generally positive,[194] particularly for the treatment of nicotine addiction.[195] The quality of the current evidence, combined with the nonnegligible risks of adverse consequences during DBS[196,197] make it premature to recommend DBS for the treatment of most cases of SUD at this point.[198]

On the other hand, although the effects of peripheral stimulation are typically transient and limited to the brain surface and its subjacent cortical areas, the clinical advantages of noninvasive approaches to modulate brain function, like tDCS or rTMS, are self-evident. Indeed, existing evidence suggests that tDCS and TMS may offer promising approaches for the treatment of SUD.[199-201] For example, preliminary evidence suggests that rTMS could help reduce heroin[202] and methamphetamine[203] craving.

Both invasive and noninvasive neuromodulation are promising approaches for the treatment of SUD. However, more research and larger clinical trials are needed to understand their mechanisms of action, calibrate the key therapeutic variables in different clinical situations, and evaluate their long-term effectiveness. This topic is reviewed further in Chapter 68, "Neuromodulation for Addiction-Related Disorders."

Treating Comorbidities

The use of multiple substances (eg, alcohol + nicotine or alcohol + cocaine) should be considered in the proper management of individuals with SUD. Similarly, comorbidities with other mental illnesses will require treatment for the mental illness concurrent with treatment for substance use. Because addictive drugs adversely affect many organs in the body (**Fig. 1-14**), they can contribute to the burden of many physical health disorders, including death from overdoses, cancer, cardiovascular and pulmonary diseases, HIV/AIDS, and hepatitis C, as well as to accidents and violence. Therefore, substance use treatment will help prevent or improve the

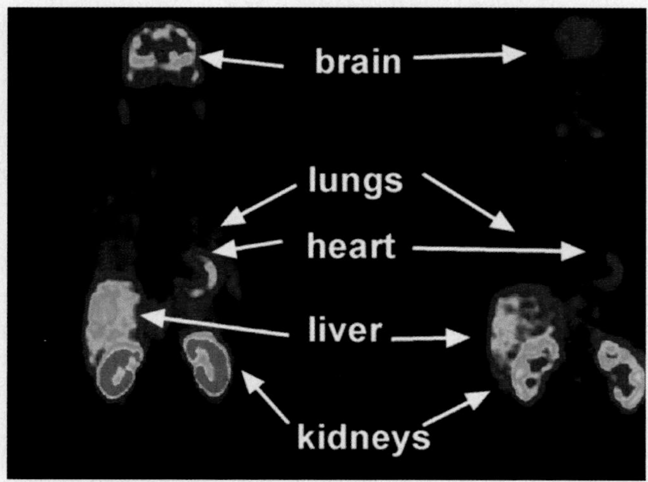

Figure 1-14. Monoamine oxidase B concentration and cigarette smoking. Positron emission tomography (PET) images of the concentration of the enzyme MAO-B (monoamine oxidase B) in the body of a healthy control (*left*) and of a person who smoked tobacco cigarettes (*right*). There are significant decreases in the concentration of the enzyme throughout the body of the person who smoked. (Reproduced from Fowler JS, Logan J, Wang GJ, Volkow ND. Monoamine oxidase and cigarette smoking. *Neurotoxicology.* 2003;24:75-82, with permission.)

outcome for many such diseases. The HIV/AIDS epidemic provides one of the best examples. Substance use and SUD have been fueling the global spread of HIV from the very beginning of the AIDS epidemic. This inextricable connection is predicated on at least three major threads: (1) the direct effects of contaminated injection drug use on infection rates, (2) the indirect impact of addictive drugs on high-risk sexual behaviors and treatment adherence, and (3) the drugs' ability to worsen neurological complications that stem from HIV infection. Fortunately, recent research has now shown conclusively that (1) HIV prevention among people who use drugs (which includes HIV treatment) is effective in reducing HIV prevalence and (2) treating SUDs (particularly with the aid of new and more effective medications) improves HIV treatment outcomes and should be parlayed into global instruments for severing those threads once and for all.[204,205] A particularly promising approach in this context has emerged in the form of the Seek, Test, Treat, and Retain paradigm that seeks out hard-to-reach/high-risk populations, including people who use drugs and those in the justice system, tests them for HIV, links those who test positive to HIV treatment and other services, and provides the necessary support to ensure these individuals remain in the care system.[204,205] Similarly, the treatment of SUD decreases the incidence of hepatitis C infection.[206]

A frequent comorbidity of SUD is that with pain, which is particularly challenging for patients with OUD who may have a legitimate need for opioid medication to manage a pain condition. The OUD pain co-morbidity is fueled in part by the overreliance on opioids for analgesia due in part to the limited therapeutic options (including the limited efficacy of opioid medications) for managing severe chronic pain.[207] Clinical management of patients with OUD and chronic pain is confounded by opioid-induced hyperalgesia that can lead to increases in the doses of opioid prescribed that further exacerbate pain.[208] Specific consideration for these patients is the use of buprenorphine or of methadone to treat both the pain and the OUD. Patients with severe pain that do not receive proper treatment may revert to the use of nonprescribed or illegal opioids for analgesia.

Harm Reduction

The opioid epidemic has shifted the way that public health officials and politicians view the potential of evidence-based harm-reduction approaches, which are steadily becoming part of a more comprehensive strategy to address addiction and the overdose epidemic. Indeed, the President's latest National Drug Control Strategy[209] is the first-ever to champion harm reduction to meet people where they are and engage them in care and services. It also calls for actions that will expand access to evidence-based treatments that have been shown to reduce overdose risk and mortality.

Harm reduction (HR) is a patient-centered component of the continuum of care consistent with the practice of all medical specialties. A fundamental goal of HR is to reduce the negative consequences of drug use by presenting a menu of options with a nonjudgmental, noncoercive approach. HR has long been explored in the treatment of AUD[210] and forms the basis for operational definitions of recovery that do not require abstinence.[211] HR seeks to keep patients safe and to engage, connect with, and empower patients in their care through various methods, including teaching sterile injection practices to avoid infections. Harm reduction is still controversial for some people in the United States who consider its principles as enabling, or contradictory to the goal of treating substance use disorders (SUDs). However, this is a false dichotomy for SUD treatment and reducing the harm of drug use should be a complementary goal as supported by a substantial amount of scientific evidence.[212-216] Indeed, outside the United States, harm reduction is often seen as a co-equal fourth category of drug-control interventions alongside law enforcement, treatment, and prevention.[213]

There is strong evidence of the efficacy of providing of sterile syringes as well as the provision of naloxone for overdose reversal. There is also evidence of the efficacy of overdose prevention centers but research is still very limited on the value of drug testing strips. More research is also needed to explore the clinical potential of phytocannabinoids (eg, THC and CBD) as opposed to cannabis used as treatment (so called "medical marijuana") in order to maximize therapeutic (or HR) index. More specifically, while CBD might have effects on heroin seeking[217,218] the cumulative evidence is rather weak, cannabis used as treatment use may result in rapid onset of cannabis use disorder.[219] Similarly, more research is needed to assess the value of electronic drug delivery devices to determine if long-term harms are indeed reduced. Note that in this vein,

NIAAA has recently developed an operational research definition of recovery that emphasizes reduction in heavy drinking and removal of criteria for an AUD.[211] Importantly, abstinence, per se, is not a criterion of recovery.

CHALLENGES FOR SOCIETY

SUDs can alienate individuals from both their families and communities, increasing isolation and interfering with treatment and recovery. Because both the family and the community provide integral aspects of effective treatment and recovery, this identifies an important challenge: to reduce the stigma of addiction that interferes with intervention and proper rehabilitation.

The effective treatment of SUD in many individuals requires the consideration of social policy, such as the treatment of people with addiction in the justice system, the role of unemployment in the vulnerability to substance use, and family dysfunctions that contribute to stress and that might block the efficacy of otherwise effective interventions. For example, studies have shown that providing SUD treatment to incarcerated individuals who had a SUD and continuing treatment after they leave prison dramatically reduced not only their rate of return to drug use but also their rate of reincarceration[220,221] and overdose.[222-224] Similarly, drug courts in the United States, which incorporate SUD treatment into the carceral system, have proved to be beneficial in decreasing drug use and arrests of individuals who break the law who are involved in drug taking.[225] However, despite these preliminary positive results, there are lingering challenges[226] and there are many unanswered questions that future research should address. For example, what are the active ingredients in the treatment of substance use in people under a criminal justice supervision? How does the system address the fact that few individuals with substance use in criminal legal settings stay in treatment long enough to receive the minimally required services? What are the implications of these findings for pretrial diversion laws, postprison reentry initiatives, and so on? There are also numerous emerging challenges with respect to specific substances. For example, there is a real possibility that the wave of cannabis legalization could be connected to recent spikes in the prevalence of cannabis use among college students,[227] which in turn, could negatively impact health outcomes.[228] Meanwhile, the steady emergence of new psychoactive drugs (NPS),[229] highly potent or toxic adulterants, like fentanyl and xylazine, and novel administration modalities, like vaping of nicotine[230] or THC[231] is increasingly hampering the ability to monitor trends and assess the health consequences of substance use and SUD.

The recognition of addiction as a chronic disorder that affects the brain is essential for large-scale prevention and treatment programs that require participation by the medical community. The understanding that SUD puts people at significantly higher risk of suffering the adverse effects of unrelated medical emergencies, like the recent COVID-19 pandemic is also essential.[232] The engagement of primary care physicians (internists, family physicians, pain specialists, obstetricians/gynecologists, and pediatricians) and emergency medicine and preventive medicine physicians will facilitate the early detection of drug use in childhood and adolescence. A prerequisite for these essential issues will be the implementation of adequate competencies and curricula in medical school education and postgraduate residency training in addiction medicine. These models should be replicated across all health professional training (nursing, physician assistants, dental, pharmacy).

Moreover, screening for drug use could help clinicians better manage medical disorders that are likely to be adversely affected by the concomitant use of drugs, such as cardiac and pulmonary disorders.[233] Unfortunately, physicians, nurses, psychologists, and social workers receive little training in the identification and management of SUD, despite being one of the most common chronic disorders, a situation that the National Institute on Drug Abuse and the National Institute on Alcohol Abuse and Alcoholism are trying to address through the development and deployment of such products as a Screening, Brief Intervention, and Referral to Treatment (SBIRT) service program,[234,235] as well as a Web-based tutorial to train health care providers who care for individuals who use substances. Such approaches for alcohol are well outlined in the NIAAA Healthcare Professional's Core Resource.[236]

Participation of the medical community in many countries, including the United States, is further curtailed by the lack of reimbursement by most private medical insurance policies for the evaluation or treatment of SUD. This lack of reimbursement limits the treatment infrastructure and the choices that the person with SUD has with respect to their treatment. It also sends a negative message to medical students who are interested in clinical practice, discouraging them from choosing a specialty for which the reimbursement of their services is limited by the lack of parity. But the tide may slowly be turning and as value-based payments (VBP) models are being adopted. Indeed, health care systems should identify ways to mitigate challenges and support SUD treatment providers where there are limited resources to address complex workforce, client, and infrastructure needs.[237]

Another considerable obstacle in the treatment of SUD is the limited involvement of the pharmaceutical industry in the development of new medications. Such issues as stigmatization, the lack of reimbursement for SUD treatment, and the perceived lack of a large market all contribute to the limited involvement of the pharmaceutical industry in the development of medications to treat SUD.[238] The importance of this issue had been identified by the Institute of Medicine of the United States, which recommended in 1995 a program to provide incentives to the pharmaceutical industry as a way of helping address this problem.[239]

The translation of scientific findings from substance use research into prevention and treatment initiatives clearly requires partnerships with federal agencies, such as the Substance Abuse and Mental Health Services Administration (which is responsible for U.S. programs to prevent and treat drug use) and the Office of National Drug Control Policy (which is responsible for U.S. programs to control availability and reduce demand for addictive drugs). A good example of progress in this area is the publication of the Surgeon General's Report: Facing Addiction: Alcohol Drugs and Health.[240] Furthermore, improvements in prevention and treatment programs could result from collaborations with other agencies and groups, such as the Department of Education (which can bring prevention interventions into the school environment), the Department of Justice (which can implement treatment strategies that will minimize the chances of recidivism and reincarceration of inmates with substance use problems), and state and local agencies (which can bring evidence-based and science-based treatments into the communities).

As the neurobiology of normal and pathological human behavior is better understood, a challenge for society will be to harness this knowledge to effectively guide public policy. For example, as understanding of the neurobiological underpinnings of voluntary actions increases, how will society define the boundaries of personal responsibility in those individuals who have impairments in these very same brain circuits? The answer to this and other questions will have implications not only for the management of people in legal settings who use substances but also for those with other diagnoses such as antisocial personality or conduct disorders. Critics of the medical model of addiction argue that this model removes the responsibility of the individual with addiction from his behavior. However, the value of the medical model of addiction as a public policy guide is not to excuse the behavior of the individual with a SUD but rather to provide a framework to understand it and to treat it more effectively.

SUMMARY

Remarkable scientific advances have been made in the neurobiology of SUD in the domains of genetics, molecular biology, behavioral neuropharmacology, and brain imaging that offer critical new insights into the ways in which the human brain engages in self-destructive compulsive drug seeking that characterizes addiction and the ways in which the human brain engages executive and motivational functional networks that allow individuals to optimize everyday decisions and plan for the future. Substance use disorders engage fundamental neurocircuits of motivation in three stages: the basal ganglia in the binge-intoxication stage to drive incentive salience and habits, the extended amygdala in the withdrawal-negative affect stage to drive stress and negative emotional states, and the PFC in the preoccupation-anticipation ("craving") stage to drive executive dysfunction, while at the same time enhancing the engagement of interoceptive brain networks that make it difficult to ignore the craving and negative emotional states that dominate the mental state of a person with addiction.

However, the field is at a crossroads where major advances in understanding the neurobiology of addiction have helped identify promising new medications and improve behavioral treatments but where the translation of these findings into clinical practice is limited by several factors, including the limited involvement of the medical community in the treatment of SUD, the restricted involvement of the pharmaceutical industry, the lack of reimbursement by private insurance policies, and the stigma associated with SUD. One of the main challenges for agencies like the National Institute on Drug Abuse and the National Institute on Alcohol Abuse and Alcoholism is to develop and disseminate knowledge that will help to overcome these obstacles.[240,241]

REFERENCES

1. Parvaz MA, Alia-Klein N, Woicik PA, Volkow ND, Goldstein RZ. Neuroimaging for drug addiction and related behaviors. *Rev Neurosci.* 2011;22:609-624.
2. Seo D, Lacadie CM, Tuit K, Hong K-I, Constable RT, Sinha R. Disrupted ventromedial prefrontal function, alcohol craving, and subsequent relapse risk. *JAMA Psychiatry.* 2013;70(7):727-739.
3. Koob GF, Volkow ND. Neurobiology of addiction: a neurocircuitry analysis. *Lancet Psychiatry.* 2016;3:760-773.
4. Leshner AI. Addiction is a brain disease, and it matters. *Science.* 1997;278:45-47.
5. Baler RD, Volkow ND. Addiction as a systems failure: focus on adolescence and smoking. *J Am Acad Child Adolesc Psychiatry.* 2011;50:329-339.
6. Koob GF, Volkow ND. Neurocircuitry of addiction. *Neuropsychopharmacology.* 2010;35:217-238.
7. Nielsen DA, Utrankar A, Reyes JA, Simons DD, Kosten TR. Epigenetics of drug abuse: predisposition or response. *Pharmacogenomics.* 2012; 13:1149-1160.
8. Chen CY, Storr CL, Anthony JC. Early-onset drug use and risk for drug dependence problems. *Addict Behav.* 2009;34:319-322.
9. Substance Abuse and Mental Health Services Administration. *Results from the 2011 National Survey on Drug Use and Health: Summary of National Findings and Detailed Tables.* SAMHSA, Office of Applied Studies; 2012.
10. Doremus-Fitzwater TL, Varlinskaya EI, Spear LP. Motivational systems in adolescence: possible implications for age differences in substance abuse and other risk-taking behaviors. *Brain Cogn.* 2009;72:114-123.
11. Spear LP. The adolescent brain and age-related behavioral manifestations. *Neurosci Biobehav Rev.* 2000;24:417-463.
12. Giedd JN, Blumenthal J, Jeffries NO, et al. Brain development during childhood and adolescence: a longitudinal MRI study. *Nat Neurosci.* 1999;2:861-863.
13. Sowell ER, Peterson BS, Thompson PM, Welcome SE, Henkenius AL, Toga AW. Mapping cortical change across the human life span. *Nat Neurosci.* 2003;6:309-315.
14. Adriani W, Spijker S, Deroche-Gamonet V, et al. Evidence for enhanced neurobehavioral vulnerability to nicotine during periadolescence in rats. *J Neurosci.* 2003;23:4712-4716.
15. Goriounova NA, Mansvelder HD. Nicotine exposure during adolescence leads to short- and long-term changes in spike timing-dependent plasticity in rat prefrontal cortex. *J Neurosci.* 2012;32:10484-10493.
16. Fleming RL, Acheson SK, Moore SD, Wilson WA, Swartzwelder HS. In the rat, chronic intermittent ethanol exposure during adolescence alters the ethanol sensitivity of tonic inhibition in adulthood. *Alcohol Clin Exp Res.* 2012;36:279-285.
17. Fleming RL, Li Q, Risher M-L, et al. Binge-pattern ethanol exposure during adolescence, but not adulthood, causes persistent changes in GABA(A) receptor-mediated tonic inhibition in dentate granule cells. *Alcohol Clin Exp Res.* 2013;37(7):1154-1160.
18. Hanson KL, Medina KL, Padula CB, Tapert SF, Brown SA. Impact of adolescent alcohol and drug use on neuropsychological functioning in young adulthood: 10-year outcomes. *J Child Adolesc Subst Abuse.* 2011;20:135-154.

19. Vargas WM, Bengston L, Gilpin NW, Whitcomb BW, Richardson HN. Alcohol binge drinking during adolescence or dependence during adulthood reduces prefrontal myelin in male rats. *J Neurosci.* 2014;34:14777-14782.
20. Grant BF, Stinson FS, Harford TC. Age at onset of alcohol use and DSM-IV alcohol abuse and dependence: a 12-year follow-up. *J Subst Abuse.* 2001;13:493-504.
21. Squeglia LM, Tapert SF, Sullivan EV, et al. Brain development in heavy-drinking adolescents. *Am J Psychiatry.* 2015;172:531-542.
22. Albaugh MD, Ottino-Gonzalez J, Sidwell A, et al. Cannabis use during adolescence is associated with neurodevelopment. *JAMA Psychiatry.* 2021;78:1031-1040.
23. Di Chiara G, Bassareo V, Fenu S, et al. Dopamine and drug addiction: the nucleus accumbens shell connection. *Neuropharmacology.* 2004; 47(Suppl 1):227-241.
24. Gupta S, Kulhara P. Cellular and molecular mechanisms of drug dependence: an overview and update. *Indian J Psychiatry.* 2007;49:85-90.
25. Wise RA. Brain reward circuitry: insights from unsensed incentives. *Neuron.* 2002;36:229-240.
26. Madras BK, Fahey MA, Bergman J, Canfield DR, Spealman RD. Effects of cocaine and related drugs in nonhuman primates. I. [3H] cocaine binding sites in caudate-putamen. *J Pharmacol Exp Ther.* 1989;251:131-141.
27. McFadden LM, Stout KA, Vieira-Brock PL, et al. Methamphetamine self-administration acutely decreases monoaminergic transporter function. *Synapse.* 2012;66:240-245.
28. Partilla JS, Dempsey AG, Nagpal AS, Blough BE, Baumann MH, Rothman RB. Interaction of amphetamines and related compounds at the vesicular monoamine transporter. *J Pharmacol Exp Ther.* 2006;319:237-246.
29. Kreek MJ, LaForge KS, Butelman E. Pharmacotherapy of addictions. *Nat Rev Drug Discov.* 2002;1:710-726.
30. Morikawa H, Morrisett RA. Ethanol action on dopaminergic neurons in the ventral tegmental area: interaction with intrinsic ion channels and neurotransmitter inputs. *Int Rev Neurobiol.* 2010;91:235-288.
31. Mitchell JM, O'Neill JP, Janabi M, Marks SM, Jagust WJ, Fields HL. Alcohol consumption induces endogenous opioid release in the human orbitofrontal cortex and nucleus accumbens. *Sci Transl Med.* 2012;4:116ra6.
32. Urban NB, Kegeles LS, Slifstein M, et al. Sex differences in striatal dopamine release in young adults after oral alcohol challenge: a positron emission tomography imaging study with [^{11}C]raclopride. *Biol Psychiatry.* 2010;68:689-696.
33. Salamone JD, Correa M. The mysterious motivational functions of mesolimbic dopamine. *Neuron.* 2012;76:470-485.
34. Cohen JY, Haesler S, Vong L, Lowell BB, Uchida N. Neuron-type-specific signals for reward and punishment in the ventral tegmental area. *Nature.* 2012;482:85-88.
35. Schultz W. Behavioral dopamine signals. *Trends Neurosci.* 2007; 30:203-210.
36. Schultz W, Tremblay L, Hollerman JR. Reward processing in primate orbitofrontal cortex and basal ganglia. *Cereb Cortex.* 2000;10:272-284.
37. Volkow ND, Wang GJ, Fowler JS, Tomasi D, Telang F. Addiction: beyond dopamine reward circuitry. *Proc Natl Acad Sci U S A.* 2011;108:15037-15042.
38. Volkow ND, Wang GJ, Tomasi D, Baler RD. The addictive dimensionality of obesity. *Biol Psychiatry.* 2013;73(9):811-818.
39. Bock R, Shin JH, Kaplan AR, et al. Strengthening the accumbal indirect pathway promotes resilience to compulsive cocaine use. *Nat Neurosci.* 2013;16:632-638.
40. Cuzon Carlson VC, Seabold GA, Helms CM, et al. Synaptic and morphological neuroadaptations in the putamen associated with long-term, relapsing alcohol drinking in primates. *Neuropsychopharmacology.* 2011;36:2513-2528.
41. Koob GF. Theoretical frameworks and mechanistic aspects of alcohol addiction: alcohol addiction as a reward deficit disorder. *Curr Top Behav Neurosci.* 2013;13:3-30.
42. Koob GF. Drug addiction: hyperkatifeia/negative reinforcement as a framework for medications development. *Pharmacol Rev.* 2021; 73(1):163-201.
43. Volkow ND, Morales M. The brain on drugs: from reward to addiction. *Cell.* 2015;162:712-725.
44. Alheid GF. Extended amygdala and basal forebrain. *Ann N Y Acad Sci.* 2003;985:185-205. doi:10.1111/j.1749-6632.2003.tb07082.x
45. Zorrilla EP, Logrip ML, Koob GF. Corticotropin releasing factor: a key role in the neurobiology of addiction. *Front Neuroendocrinol.* 2014;35:234-244.
46. Vendruscolo LF et al. Corticosteroid-dependent plasticity mediates compulsive alcohol drinking in rats. *J Neurosci.* 2012;32:7563-7571.
47. Vendruscolo LF, Estey T, Goodell V, et al. Glucocorticoid receptor antagonism decreases alcohol seeking in alcohol-dependent individuals. *J Clin Invest.* 2015;125:3193-3197.
48. Carlezon WA Jr, Nestler EJ, Neve RL. Herpes simplex virus-mediated gene transfer as a tool for neuropsychiatric research. *Crit Rev Neurobiol.* 2000;14:47-67.
49. Shippenberg TS, Zapata A, Chefer VI. Dynorphin and the pathophysiology of drug addiction. *Pharmacol Ther.* 2007;116:306-321.
50. Chavkin C, Koob GF. Dynorphin, dysphoria, and dependence: the stress of addiction. *Neuropsychopharmacology.* 2016;41:373-374.
51. Koob GF, Le Moal M. Review. Neurobiological mechanisms for opponent motivational processes in addiction. *Philos Trans R Soc Lond B Biol Sci.* 2008;363:3113-3123.
52. Volkow ND, Koob GF, McLellan AT. Neurobiologic Advances from the brain disease model of addiction. *N Engl J Med.* 2016;374:363-371.
53. Volkow ND, Hampson AJ, Baler R. Don't Worry, be happy: endocannabinoids and cannabis at the intersection of stress and reward. *Annu Rev Pharmacol Toxicol.* 2017;57:285-308. doi:10.1146/annurev-pharmtox-010716-104615
54. Morris JS, Friston KJ, Büchel C, et al. A neuromodulatory role for the human amygdala in processing emotional facial expressions. *Brain.* 1998;121(Pt 1):47-57.
55. Crunelle CL, Kaag AM, van den Munkhof H, et al. Dysfunctional amygdala activation and connectivity with the prefrontal cortex in current cocaine users. *Hum Brain Mapp.* 2015;36:4222-4230.
56. Naqvi NH, Bechara A. The insula and drug addiction: an interoceptive view of pleasure, urges, and decision-making. *Brain Struct Funct.* 2010;214:430-450.
57. Baldwin PR, Alanis R, Salas R. The role of the habenula in nicotine addiction. *J Addict Res Ther.* 2011;S1:2.
58. Namba MD, Leyrer-Jackson JM, Nagy EK, Olive MF, Neisewander JL. Neuroimmune mechanisms as novel treatment targets for substance use disorders and associated comorbidities. *Front. Neurosci.* 2021;15:650785.
59. Grantham EK, Warden AS, McCarthy GS. Role of toll-like receptor 7 (TLR7) in voluntary alcohol consumption. *Brain Behav Immun.* 2020;89:423-432.
60. Macht VA, Vetreno RP, Crews FT. Cholinergic and neuroimmune signaling interact to impact adult hippocampal neurogenesis and alcohol pathology across development. *Front Pharmacol.* 2022;13:849997.
61. Lacagnina MJ, Rivera PD, Bilbo SD. Glial and neuroimmune mechanisms as critical modulators of drug use and abuse. *Neuropsychopharmacology.* 2017;42:156-177.
62. Taylor AM, Castonguay A, Ghogha A, et al. Neuroimmune regulation of GABAergic neurons within the ventral tegmental area during withdrawal from chronic morphine. *Neuropsychopharmacology.* 2016;41:949-959. doi:10.1038/npp.2015.221
63. Crews FT, Sarkar DK, Qin L, Zou J, Boyadjieva N, Vetreno RP. Neuroimmune function and the consequences of alcohol exposure. *Alcohol Res.* 2015;37(2):331-341, 344-351.
64. Doremus-Fitzwater TL, Deak T. Adolescent neuroimmune function and its interaction with alcohol. *Int Rev Neurobiol.* 2022;161:167-208.
65. Wang X, Northcutt AL, Cochran TA, et al. Methamphetamine activates toll-like receptor 4 to induce central immune signaling within the ventral tegmental area and contributes to extracellular dopamine increase in the nucleus accumbens shell. *Chem Neurosci.* 2019;10(8):3622-3634.

66. Chastain LG, Sarkar DK. Role of microglia in regulation of ethanol neurotoxic action. *Int Rev Neurobiol.* 2014;118:81-103. doi:10.1016/B978-0-12-801284-0.00004-X
67. McConnell SE, O'Banion MK, Cory-Slechta DA, Olschowka JA, Opanashuk LA. Characterization of binge-dosed methamphetamine-induced neurotoxicity and neuroinflammation. *Neurotoxicology.* 2015;50:131-141. doi:10.1016/j.neuro.2015.08.006
68. Rando K, Hong KI, Bhagwagar Z, et al. Association of frontal and posterior cortical gray matter volume with time to alcohol relapse: a prospective study. *Am J Psychiatry.* 2011;168:183-192.
69. Hanlon CA, Dowdle LT, Jones JL. Biomarkers for success: using neuroimaging to predict relapse and develop brain stimulation treatments for cocaine-dependent individuals. *Int Rev Neurobiol.* 2016;129:125-156. doi:10.1016/bs.irn.2016.06.006
70. McHugh MJ, Demers CH, Braud J, Briggs R, Adinoff B, Stein EA. Striatal-insula circuits in cocaine addiction: implications for impulsivity and relapse risk. *Am J Drug Alcohol Abuse.* 2013;39:424-432. doi:10.3109/00952990.2013.847446
71. Wang A-L, Elman I, Lowen SB, et al. Neural correlates of adherence to extended-release naltrexone pharmacotherapy in heroin dependence. *Transl Psychiatry.* 2015;5:e531. doi:10.1038/tp.2015.20
72. Blair MA, Stewart JL, May AC, Reske M, Tapert SF, Paulus MP. Blunted frontostriatal blood oxygen level-dependent signals predict stimulant and marijuana use. *Biol Psychiatry Cogn Neurosci Neuroimaging.* 2018;pii: S2451-9022(18)30068-5. doi:10.1016/j.bpsc.2018.03.005
73. Pascoli V, Hiver A, Van Zessen R, et al. Stochastic synaptic plasticity underlying compulsion in a model of addiction. *Nature.* 2018;564(7736):366-371.
74. Volkow ND, Fowler JS. Addiction, a disease of compulsion and drive: involvement of the orbitofrontal cortex. *Cereb Cortex.* 2000;10:318-325.
75. Horvitz JC. Mesolimbocortical and nigrostriatal dopamine responses to salient non-reward events. *Neuroscience.* 2000;96:651-656.
76. McClure SM, Daw ND, Montague PR. A computational substrate for incentive salience. *Trends Neurosci.* 2003;26:423-428.
77. Schultz W. Reward signaling by dopamine neurons. *Neuroscientist.* 2001;7:293-302.
78. Ito R, Dalley JW, Howes SR, Robbins TW, Everitt BJ. Dissociation in conditioned dopamine release in the nucleus accumbens core and shell in response to cocaine cues and during cocaine-seeking behavior in rats. *J Neurosci.* 2000;20:7489-7495.
79. Cui C et al. New insights on neurobiological mechanisms underlying alcohol addiction. *Neuropharmacology.* 2012;67:223-232.
80. Goldstein RZ, Volkow ND. Dysfunction of the prefrontal cortex in addiction: neuroimaging findings and clinical implications. *Nat Rev Neurosci.* 2011;12:652-669.
81. Etkin A, Egner T, Kalisch R. Emotional processing in anterior cingulate and medial prefrontal cortex. *Trends Cogn Sci.* 2011;15(2):85-93.
82. Voon V, Grodin E, Mandali A, et al. Addictions NeuroImaging Assessment (ANIA): towards an integrative framework for alcohol use disorder. *Neurosci Biobehav Rev.* 2020;113:492-506.
83. Marlatt G, Gordon J. Determinants of relapse: implications for the maintenance of behavioral change. In: Davidson P, Davidson S, eds. *Behavioral Medicine: Changing Health Lifestyles.* Brunner/Mazel; 1980:410e52.
84. Volkow ND, Wang GJ, Tomasi D, Baler RD. Unbalanced neuronal circuits in addiction. *Curr Opin Neurobiol.* 2013;23(4):639-648.
85. Morie KP, DeVito EE, Potenza MN, Worhunsky PD. Longitudinal changes in network engagement during cognitive control in cocaine use disorder. *Drug Alcohol Depend.* 2021;229(Pt A):109151.
86. McFarland K, Davidge SB, Lapish CC, Kalivas PW. Limbic and motor circuitry underlying footshock-induced reinstatement of cocaine-seeking behavior. *J Neurosci.* 2004;24:1551-1560.
87. Volkow ND, Fowler JS, Wang G-J, et al. Cognitive control of drug craving inhibits brain reward regions in cocaine abusers. *Neuroimage.* 2010;49:2536-2543.
88. Cadet JL, McCoy MT, Jayanthi S. Epigenetics and addiction. *Clin Pharmacol Ther.* 2016;99:502-511. doi:10.1002/cpt.345
89. Bali P, Kelly P. Transcriptional mechanisms of drug addiction. *Dialogues Clin Neurosci.* 2019;21(4):379-387.
90. Teague CD, Nestler EJ. Key transcription factors mediating cocaine-induced plasticity in the nucleus accumbens. *Mol Psychiatry.* 2022;27(1):687-709.
91. Pandey SC, Kyzar EJ, Zhang H. Epigenetic basis of the dark side of alcohol addiction. *Neuropharmacology.* 2017;122:74-84.
92. Kroener S, Mulholland PJ, New NN, Gass JT, Becker HC, Chandler LJ. Chronic alcohol exposure alters behavioral and synaptic plasticity of the rodent prefrontal cortex. *PLoS One.* 2012;7:e37541.
93. Robinson TE, Gorny G, Mitton E, Kolb B. Cocaine self-administration alters the morphology of dendrites and dendritic spines in the nucleus accumbens and neocortex. *Synapse.* 2001;39:257-266.
94. Zhou FC, Anthony B, Dunn KW, Lindquist WB, Xu ZC, Deng P. Chronic alcohol drinking alters neuronal dendritic spines in the brain reward center nucleus accumbens. *Brain Res.* 2007;1134:148-161.
95. Uhl GR, Grow RW. The burden of complex genetics in brain disorders. *Arch Gen Psychiatry.* 2004;61:223-229.
96. Laakso A, Mohn AR, Gainetdinov RR, Caron MG. Experimental genetic approaches to addiction. *Neuron.* 2002;36(2):213-228.
97. Hall FS, Chen Y, Resendiz-Gutierrez F. The Streetlight Effect: reappraising the study of addiction in light of the findings of genome-wide association studies. *Brain Behav Evol.* 2020;95(5):230-246.
98. Ehlers CL, Walter NA, Dick DM, Buck KJ, Crabbe JC. A comparison of selected quantitative trait loci associated with alcohol use phenotypes in humans and mouse models. *Addict Biol.* 2010;15:185-199.
99. Patriquin MA, Bauer IE, Soares JC, Graham DP, Nielsen DA. Addiction pharmacogenetics: a systematic review of the genetic variation of the dopaminergic system. *Psychiatr Genet.* 2015;25:181-193. doi:10.1097/YPG.0000000000000095
100. Treutlein J, Rietschel M. Genome-wide association studies of alcohol dependence and substance use disorders. *Curr Psychiatry Rep.* 2011;13:147-155.
101. Schumann G, Coin LJ, Lourdusamy A, et al. Genome-wide association and genetic functional studies identify autism susceptibility candidate 2 gene (AUTS2) in the regulation of alcohol consumption. *Proc Natl Acad Sci U S A.* 2011;108:7119-7124.
102. Kang SJ, Rangaswamy M, Manz N, et al. Family-based genome-wide association study of frontal theta oscillations identifies potassium channel gene KCNJ6. *Genes Brain Behav.* 2012;11:712-719.
103. Kalsi G, Prescott CA, Kendler KS, Riley BP. Unraveling the molecular mechanisms of alcohol dependence. *Trends Genet.* 2009;25:49-55.
104. Kreek MJ, Levran O, Reed B, Schlussman SD, Zhou Y, Butelman ER. Opiate addiction and cocaine addiction: underlying molecular neurobiology and genetics. *J Clin Invest.* 2012;122:3387-3393.
105. Chen CC, Lu R-B, Chen Y-C, et al. Interaction between the functional polymorphisms of the alcohol-metabolism genes in protection against alcoholism. *Am J Hum Genet.* 1999;65:795-807.
106. Rao Y, Hoffmann E, Zia M, et al. Duplications and defects in the CYP2A6 gene: identification, genotyping, and in vivo effects on smoking. *Mol Pharmacol.* 2000;58(4):747-755.
107. Kathiramalainathan K, Kaplan HL, Romach MK, et al. Inhibition of cytochrome P450 2D6 modifies codeine abuse liability. *J Clin Psychopharmacol.* 2000;20(4):435-444.
108. Berrettini W, Yuan X, Tozzi F, et al. α-5/α-3 Nicotinic receptor subunit alleles increase risk for heavy smoking. *Mol Psychiatry.* 2008;13:368-373.
109. Bierut LJ, Madden P, Breslau N, et al. Novel genes identified in a high-density genome wide association study for nicotine dependence. *Hum Mol Genet.* 2007;16:24-25.
110. Saccone SF, Hinrichs AL, Saccone NL, et al. Cholinergic nicotinic receptor genes implicated in a nicotine dependence association study targeting 348 candidate genes with 3713 SNPs. *Hum Mol Genet.* 2007;16:136-149.
111. Schlaepfer IR, Hoft NR, Collins AC, et al. The CHRNA5/A3/B4 gene cluster variability as an important determinant of early alcohol and tobacco initiation in young adults. *Biol Psychiatry.* 2008;63:1039-1046.

112. Thorgeirsson TE, Geller F, Sulem P, et al. Variant associated with nicotine dependence, lung cancer and peripheral arterial disease. *Nature.* 2008;452:638-642.
113. Berrettini W. Alcohol addiction and the mu-opioid receptor. *Prog Neuropsychopharmacol Biol Psychiatry.* 2016;65:228-233. doi:10.1016/j.pnpbp.2015.07.011
114. Hancock DB, Levy JL, Gaddis NC, et al. Cis-expression quantitative trait loci mapping reveals replicable associations with heroin addiction in OPRM1. *Biol Psychiatry.* 2015;78:474-484. doi:10.1016/j.biopsych.2015.01.003
115. Dick DM, Edenberg HJ, Xiaoling X, et al. Association of GABRG3 with alcohol dependence. *Alcohol Clin Exp Res.* 2004;28(1):4-9.
116. Edenberg HJ, Dick DM, Xuei X, et al. Variations in GABRA2, encoding the alpha 2 subunit of the GABA(A) receptor, are associated with alcohol dependence and with brain oscillations. *Am J Hum Genet.* 2004;74:705-714.
117. McGeary J. The DRD4 exon 3 VNTR polymorphism and addiction-related phenotypes: a review. *Pharmacol Biochem Behav.* 2009;93:222-229.
118. Grady DL, Thanos PK, Corrada MM, et al. DRD4 genotype predicts longevity in mouse and human. *J Neurosci.* 2013;33:286-291.
119. Kariisa M, Davis NL, Kumar S, et al. Vital signs: drug overdose deaths, by selected sociodemographic and social determinants of health characteristics—25 States and the District of Columbia, 2019-2020. *MMWR Morb Mortal Wkly Rep.* 2022;71(29):940-947.
120. Larochelle MR, Slavova S, Root ED, et al. Disparities in opioid overdose death trends by race/ethnicity, 2018-2019, from the HEALing Communities Study. *Am J Public Health.* 2021;111(10):1851-1854.
121. Hoopsick R. Differences in opioid overdose mortality rates among middle-aged adults by race/ethnicity and sex, 1999-2018. *Public Health Rep.* 2021;136(2):192-200.
122. Skolnick P. Treatment of overdose in the synthetic opioid era. *Pharmacol Ther.* 2022;233:108019.
123. Chandler R, Villani J, Clarke T, McCance-Katz E, Volkow N. Addressing opioid overdose deaths: the vision for the HEALing communities study. *Drug Alcohol Depend.* 2020;217:108329.
124. Haass-Koffler CL, Bartlett SE. Stress and addiction: contribution of the corticotropin releasing factor (CRF) system in neuroplasticity. *Front Mol Neurosci.* 2012;5:91.
125. Koob GF. The role of CRF and CRF-related peptides in the dark side of addiction. *Brain Res.* 2010;1314:3-14.
126. Whitaker LR, Degoulet M, Morikawa H. Social deprivation enhances VTA synaptic plasticity and drug-induced contextual learning. *Neuron.* 2013;77:335-345.
127. Chappell AM, Carter E, McCool BA, Weiner JL. Adolescent rearing conditions influence the relationship between initial anxiety-like behavior and ethanol drinking in male Long Evans rats. *Alcohol Clin Exp Res.* 2012;37(Suppl 1):E394-E403.
128. Reiner DJ, Fredriksson I, Lofaro OM, Bossert JM, Shaham Y. Relapse to opioid seeking in rat models: behavior, pharmacology and circuits. *Neuropsychopharmacology.* 2019;44(3):465-477.
129. Morgan D, Grant KA, Gage HD, et al. Social dominance in monkeys: dopamine D2 receptors and cocaine self-administration. *Nat Neurosci.* 2002;5:169-174.
130. Nader MA, Nader SH, Czoty PW, et al. Social dominance in female monkeys: dopamine receptor function and cocaine reinforcement. *Biol Psychiatry.* 2012;72:414-421. doi:10.1016/j.biopsych.2012.03.002
131. Thanos PK, Volkow ND, Freimuth P, et al. Overexpression of dopamine D2 receptors reduces alcohol self-administration. *J Neurochem.* 2001; 78:1094-1103.
132. Thanos PK, Michaelides M, Umegaki H, Volkow ND. D2R DNA transfer into the nucleus accumbens attenuates cocaine self-administration in rats. *Synapse.* 2008;62:481-486.
133. Pandey SC, Ugale R, Zhang H, Tang L, Prakash A. Brain chromatin remodeling: a novel mechanism of alcoholism. *J Neurosci.* 2008; 28:3729-3737.
134. Bohnsack JP, Zhang H, Wandling GM, et al. Targeted epigenomic editing ameliorates adult anxiety and excessive drinking after adolescent alcohol exposure. *Sci Adv.* 2022;8(18).
135. Bogle KE, Smith BH. Illicit methylphenidate use: a review of prevalence, availability, pharmacology, and consequences. *Curr Drug Abuse Rev.* 2009;2:157-176.
136. Varga MD. Adderall abuse on college campuses: a comprehensive literature review. *J Evid Based Soc Work.* 2012;9:293-313.
137. Bohnert AS, Valenstein M, Bair MJ, et al. Association between opioid prescribing patterns and opioid overdose-related deaths. *JAMA.* 2011;305:1315-1321.
138. Compton WM, Volkow ND. Major increases in opioid analgesic abuse in the United States: concerns and strategies. *Drug Alcohol Depend.* 2006;81:103-107.
139. Thurstone C, Lieberman SA, Schmiege SJ. Medical marijuana diversion and associated problems in adolescent substance treatment. *Drug Alcohol Depend.* 2011;118:489-492.
140. Compton WM, Thomas YF, Stinson FS, Grant BF. Prevalence, correlates, disability, and comorbidity of DSM-IV drug abuse and dependence in the United States: results from the national epidemiologic survey on alcohol and related conditions. *Arch Gen Psychiatry.* 2007;64:566-576.
141. Brady KT, Sinha R. Co-occurring mental and substance use disorders: the neurobiological effects of chronic stress. *Am J Psychiatry.* 2005; 162:1483-1493.
142. Hassel S, Almeida JR, Frank E, et al. Prefrontal cortical and striatal activity to happy and fear faces in bipolar disorder is associated with comorbid substance abuse and eating disorder. *J Affect Disord.* 2009;118:19-27.
143. Moran LV, Sampath H, Stein EA, Hong LE. Insular and anterior cingulate circuits in smokers with schizophrenia. *Schizophr Res.* 2012;142:223-229.
144. Oquendo MA, Volkow ND. Suicide: a silent contributor to opioid-overdose deaths. *N Engl J Med.* 2018;378(17):1567-1569.
145. Pompili M, Serafini G, Innamorati M, et al. Suicidal behavior and alcohol abuse. *Int J Environ Res Public Health.* 2010;7(4):1392-1431.
146. Nguyen L-C, Durazzo TC, Dwyer CL, et al. Predicting relapse after alcohol use disorder treatment in a high-risk cohort: the roles of anhedonia and smoking. *J Psychiatr Res.* 2020;126:1-7.
147. Grant BF, Stinson FS, Dawson DA, et al. Prevalence and co-occurrence of substance use disorders and independent mood and anxiety disorders: results from the National Epidemiologic Survey on Alcohol and Related Conditions. *Arch Gen Psychiatry.* 2004;61:807-816.
148. Markou A, Kosten TR, Koob GF. Neurobiological similarities in depression and drug dependence: a self-medication hypothesis. *Neuropsychopharmacology.* 1998;18:135-174.
149. Fowler JS, Logan J, Wang GJ, Volkow ND. Monoamine oxidase and cigarette smoking. *Neurotoxicology.* 2003;24:75-82.
150. Brook DW, Brook JS, Zhang C, Cohen P, Whiteman M. Drug use and the risk of major depressive disorder, alcohol dependence, and substance use disorders. *Arch Gen Psychiatry.* 2002;59:1039-1044.
151. D'Souza D, DiForti M, Ganesh S, et al. Consensus paper of the WFSBP task force on cannabis, cannabinoids and psychosis. *World J Biol Psychiatry.* 2022;23(10):719-742.
152. Johnston LD, O'Malley PM, Bachman JG, Schulenberg JE. *Monitoring the Future National Survey Results on Drug Use 2012 Overview.* National Institutes of Health Publication No. 07-6205. National Institute on Drug Abuse National Institutes of Health U.S. Department of Health & Human Services; 2012.
153. Johnston LD, Miech R, O'Malley P, Bachman J, Schulenberg J, Patrick ME. *Monitoring the Future. National Survey Results on Drug Use, 1975-2021. Overview Key Findings on Adolescent Drug Use.* Accessed October 2023. https://deepblue.lib.umich.edu/bitstream/handle/2027.42/171751/mtf-overview2021.pdf?sequence=1&isAllowed=y
154. Harrell MB, Chen B, Clendennen SL, et al. Longitudinal trajectories of E-cigarette use among adolescents: a 5-year, multiple cohort study of vaping with and without marijuana. *Prev Med.* 2021;150:106670.
155. Cullen K. E-cigarette use among youth in the United States, 2019. *JAMA.* 2019;322(21):2095-2103.
156. Block LG, Morwitz VG, Putsis WP Jr, Sen SK. Assessing the impact of antidrug advertising on adolescent drug consumption: results from a behavioral economic model. *Am J Public Health.* 2002;92:1346-1351.

157. Carpenter CS, Pechmann C. Exposure to the above the influence antidrug advertisements and adolescent marijuana use in the United States, 2006-2008. *Am J Public Health.* 2011;101:948-954.
158. Terry-McElrath YM, Emery S, Szczypka G, Johnston LD. Potential exposure to anti-drug advertising and drug-related attitudes, beliefs, and behaviors among United States youth, 1995-2006. *Addict Behav.* 2011;36:116-124.
159. Agency for Healthcare Research and Quality. *Overview of the Nationwide Emergency Department Sample (NEDS).* Accessed August 29, 2023. http://www.hcup-us.ahrq.gov/nedsoverview.jsp
160. McCabe S, Schulenberg J, Schepis T, McCabe V, Veliz P. Longitudinal analysis of substance use disorder symptom severity at age 18 years and substance use disorder in adulthood. *JAMA Netw Open.* 2022;5(4):e225324.
161. Volkow N, Wargo E. Association of severity of adolescent substance use disorders and long-term outcomes. *JAMA Netw Open.* 2022; 5(4):e225656.
162. Clayton RR, Cattarello AM, Johnstone BM. The effectiveness of Drug Abuse Resistance Education (project DARE): 5-year follow-up results. *Prev Med.* 1996;25:307-318.
163. Gruber AJ, Pope HG Jr. Marijuana use among adolescents. *Pediatr Clin North Am.* 2002;49:389-413.
164. Moffitt TE, Arseneault L, Belsky D, et al. A gradient of childhood self-control predicts health, wealth, and public safety. *Proc Natl Acad Sci U S A.* 2011;108:2693-2698.
165. Adolescent Brain Cognitive Development Study. Accessed October 2023. https://abcdstudy.org/
166. National Institutes of Health. HEALthy Brain and Child Development Study (HBCD). Accessed August 31, 2022. https://heal.nih.gov/research/infants-and-children/healthy-brain
167. McLellan AT, Lewis DC, O'Brien CP, Kleber HD. Drug dependence, a chronic medical illness: implications for treatment, insurance, and outcomes evaluation. *JAMA.* 2000;284:1689-1695.
168. Saitz R, Larson MJ, Labelle C, Richardson J, Samet JH. The case for chronic disease management for addiction. *J Addict Med.* 2008;2:55-65.
169. Alterman AI, Gariti P, Mulvaney F. Short- and long-term smoking cessation for three levels of intensity of behavioral treatment. *Psychol Addict Behav.* 2001;15:261-264.
170. Hall SM, Humfleet GL, Muñoz RF, Reus VI, Prochaska JJ, Robbins JA. Using extended cognitive behavioral treatment and medication to treat dependent smokers. *Am J Public Health.* 2011;101:2349-2356.
171. Ebbert JO, Hatsukami DK, Croghan IT, et al. Combination varenicline and bupropion SR for tobacco-dependence treatment in cigarette smokers: a randomized trial. *JAMA.* 2014;311(2):155-163.
172. Heal D, Henningfield J, Smith S, Belouin S, Xi D. Eds. *Neuropharmacology.* Special Issue. Accessed August 31, 2022. https://www.sciencedirect.com/journal/neuropharmacology/special-issue/10TFVWPHZCS
173. Jones G, Lipson J, Nock M. Associations between classic psychedelics and nicotine dependence in a nationally representative sample. *Sci Rep.* 2022;12(1):10578.
174. Johnson M. Classic psychedelics in addiction treatment: the case for psilocybin in tobacco smoking cessation. *Curr Top Behav Neurosci.* 2022;56:213-227.
175. Schaffer DV, Gage FH. Neurogenesis and neuroadaptation. *Neuromolecular Med.* 2004;5:1-9.
176. Kujala T, Karma K, Ceponiene R, et al. Plastic neural changes and reading improvement caused by audiovisual training in reading-impaired children. *Proc Natl Acad Sci U S A.* 2001;98:10509-10514.
177. van Paasschen J, Clare L, Yuen KSL, et al. Cognitive rehabilitation changes memory-related brain activity in people with Alzheimer disease. *Neurorehabil Neural Repair.* 2013;27(5):448-459.
178. Liechti MD, Maurizio S, Heinrich H, et al. First clinical trial of tomographic neurofeedback in attention-deficit/hyperactivity disorder: evaluation of voluntary cortical control. *Clin Neurophysiol.* 2012; 123:1989-2005.
179. Merchant G, Pulvers K, Brooks RD, Edwards J. Coping with the urge to smoke: a real-time analysis. *Res Nurs Health.* 2013;36:3-15.
180. Ceceli AO, Parvaz MA, King S, et al. Altered prefrontal signaling during inhibitory control in a salient drug context in cocaine use disorder. *Cereb Cortex.* 2023;33(3):597-611.
181. Stead LF, Lancaster T. Behavioural interventions as adjuncts to pharmacotherapy for smoking cessation. *Cochrane Database Syst Rev.* 2013;12:CD009670.
182. Feldsten-Ewing S, Chung T. Neuroimaging mechanisms of change in psychotherapy for addictive behaviors: emerging translational approaches that bridge biology and behavior. *Psychol Addict Behav.* 2013;27(2):329-335.
183. Morgenstern J, Bechara A, Breiter HC. The contributions of cognitive neuroscience and neuroimaging to understanding mechanisms of behavior change in addiction. *Psychol Addict Behav.* 2013;27(2):336-350.
184. Brittain J, Cagnan H. Recent trends in the use of electrical neuromodulation in Parkinson's disease. *Review Curr Behav Neurosci Rep.* 2018;5(2):170-178.
185. Dell'osso B, Camuri G, Castellano F, et al. Meta-review of metanalytic studies with repetitive transcranial magnetic stimulation (rTMS) for the treatment of major depression. *Clin Pract Epidemiol Ment Health.* 2011;7:167-177.
186. Rehn S, Eslick G, Brakoulias V. A meta-analysis of the effectiveness of different cortical targets used in repetitive transcranial magnetic stimulation (rTMS) for the treatment of obsessive-compulsive disorder (OCD). *Psychiatr Q.* 2018;89(3):645-665.
187. Mariska Mantione M, de Brink W, Schuurman P, Denys D. Smoking cessation and weight loss after chronic deep brain stimulation of the nucleus accumbens: therapeutic and research implications: case report. *Neurosurgery.* 2010;66(1):E218.
188. Kuhn J, Bauer R, Pohl S, et al. Observations on unaided smoking cessation after deep brain stimulation of the nucleus accumbens. *Eur Addict Res.* 2009;15:196-201.
189. Kuhn J, Lenartz D, Huff W, et al. Remission of alcohol dependency following deep brain stimulation of the nucleus accumbens: valuable therapeutic implications? *J Neurol Neurosurg Psychiatry.* 2007;78:1152-1153.
190. Knapp CM, Tozier L, Pak A, Ciraulo DA, Kornetsky C. Deep brain stimulation of the nucleus accumbens reduces ethanol consumption in rats. *Pharmacol Biochem Behav.* 2009;92(3):474-479.
191. Ibrahim C, Rubin-Kahana DS, Pushparaj A, et al. The insula: a brain stimulation target for the treatment of addiction. *Front Pharmacol.* 2019;10:720.
192. Friedman A, Lax E, Dikshtein Y, et al. Electrical stimulation of the lateral habenula produces enduring inhibitory effect on cocaine seeking behavior. *Neuropharmacology.* 2010;59(6):452-459.
193. Rouaud T, Lardeux S, Panayotis N, Paleressompoulle D, Cador M, Baunez C. Reducing the desire for cocaine with subthalamic nucleus deep brain stimulation. *Proc Natl Acad Sci U S A.* 2010;107(3):1196-1200.
194. Wang T, Moosa S, Dallapiazza RF, Elias WJ, Lynch WJ. Deep brain stimulation for the treatment of drug addiction. *Neurosurg Focus.* 2018;45(2):E11.
195. Petit B, Dornier A, Meille V, Demina A, Trojak B. Non-invasive brain stimulation for smoking cessation: a systematic review and meta-analysis. *Addiction.* 2022;117(11):2768-2779. doi:10.1111/add.15889
196. Coley E, Farhadi R, Lewis S, Whittle IR. The incidence of seizures following Deep Brain Stimulating electrode implantation for movement disorders, pain and psychiatric conditions. *Br J Neurosurg.* 2009;23(2):179-183.
197. Wang X, Li N, Li J, et al. Optimized deep brain stimulation surgery to avoid vascular damage: a single-center retrospective analysis of path planning for various deep targets by MRI image fusion. *Brain Sci.* 2022;12(8):967.
198. Yuen J, Kouzani AZ, Berk M, et al. Deep brain stimulation for addictive disorders-where are we now? *Neurotherapeutics.* 2022;19(4):1193-1215. doi:10.1007/s13311-022-01229-4

199. Luigjes J, Segrave R, de Joode N, Figee M, Denys D. Efficacy of invasive and non-invasive brain modulation interventions for addiction. *Neuropsychol Rev.* 2019;29:116-138.
200. Mahoney JJ III, Hanlon CA, Marshalek PJ, Rezai AR, Krinke L. Transcranial magnetic stimulation, deep brain stimulation, and other forms of neuromodulation for substance use disorders: review of modalities and implications for treatment. *J Neurol Sci.* 2020;418: 117149.
201. Tseng PT, Jeng J-S, Zeng B-S, et al. Efficacy of non-invasive brain stimulation interventions in reducing smoking frequency in patients with nicotine dependence: a systematic review and network meta-analysis of randomized controlled trials. *Addiction.* 2022;117(7):1830-1842.
202. Shen Y, Cao X, Tan T, et al. 10-Hz repetitive transcranial magnetic stimulation of the left dorsolateral prefrontal cortex reduces heroin cue craving in long-term addicts. *Biol Psychiatry.* 2016;80(3):e13-e14.
203. Yuan J, Liu W, Liang Q, Cao X, Lucas MV, Yuan T-F. Effect of low-frequency repetitive transcranial magnetic stimulation on impulse inhibition in abstinent patients with methamphetamine addiction: a randomized clinical trial. *JAMA Netw Open.* 2020;3:e200910.
204. Volkow ND, Baler RD, Normand JL. The unrealized potential of addiction science in curbing the HIV epidemic. *Curr HIV Res.* 2011;9:393-395.
205. Volkow N, Montaner J. The urgency of providing comprehensive and integrated treatment for substance abusers with HIV. *Health Aff.* 2011;30(8):1411-1419.
206. Tsui JI, Evans JL, Lum PJ, Hahn JA, Page K. Association of opioid agonist therapy with lower incidence of hepatitis C virus infection in young adult injection drug users. *JAMA Intern Med.* 2014;174:1974-1981. doi:10.1001/jamainternmed.2014.5416
207. Rosenblum A, Marsch L, Joseph H, Portenoy R. Opioids and the treatment of chronic pain: controversies, current status, and future directions. *Exp Clin Psychopharmacol.* 2008;16(5):405-416.
208. Yi P, Pryzbylkowski P. Opioid induced hyperalgesia. *Pain Med.* 2015;16(suppl 1):S32-S36.
209. The White House. *Fact sheet: White House releases 2022 national drug control strategy that outlines comprehensive path forward to address addiction and the overdose epidemic.* Accessed August 31, 2022. https://www.whitehouse.gov/briefing-room/statements-releases/2022/04/21/fact-sheet-white-house-releases-2022-national-drug-control-strategy-that-outlines-comprehensive-path-forward-to-address-addiction-and-the-overdose-epidemic
210. Marlatt G, Witkiewitz K. Harm reduction approaches to alcohol use: health promotion, prevention, and treatment. *Addict Behav.* 2002;27:867-886.
211. Hagman BT, Falk D, Litten R, Koob GF. Defining recovery from alcohol use disorder: development of an NIAAA research definition. *Am J Psychiatry.* 2022;179(11):807-813.
212. Hawk M, Coulter RWS, Egan JE, et al. Harm reduction principles for healthcare settings. *Harm Reduct J.* 2017;14(1):70.
213. Caulkins J. *Cost-Benefit Analyses of Investments to Control Illicit Substance Abuse and Addiction.* Carnegie Mellon University; 2006.
214. Potier C, Laprevote V, Dubois-Arber F, Cottencin O, Rolland B. Supervised injection services: what has been demonstrated? A systematic literature review. *Drug Alcohol Depend.* 2014;145:48-68.
215. Masterman PW, Kelly AB. Reaching adolescents who drink harmfully: fitting intervention to developmental reality. *J Subst Abuse Treat.* 2003;24(4):347-355.
216. McBride N, Farringdon F, Midford R, Meuleners L, Phillips M. Harm minimization in school drug education: final results of the School Health and Alcohol Harm Reduction Project (SHAHRP). *Addiction.* 2004;99(3):278-291.
217. Ren Y, Whittard J, Higuera-Matas A, Morris CV, Hurd YL. Cannabidiol, a nonpsychotropic component of cannabis, inhibits cue-induced heroin seeking and normalizes discrete mesolimbic neuronal disturbances. *J Neurosci.* 2009;29(47):14764-14769.
218. Humphreys K, Saitz R. Should physicians recommend replacing opioids with cannabis? *JAMA.* 2019;321(7):639-640.
219. Gilman JM, Schuster RM, Potter KW, et al. Effect of medical marijuana card ownership on pain, insomnia, and affective disorder symptoms in adults. *JAMA Netw Open.* 2022;5(3):e222106.
220. Butzin CA, Martin SS, Inciardi JA. Evaluating component effects of a prison-based treatment continuum. *J Subst Abuse Treat.* 2002;22:63-69.
221. Hiller ML, Knight K, Simpson DD. Prison-based substance abuse treatment, residential aftercare and recidivism. *Addiction.* 1999; 94:833-842.
222. Lee JD, Friedmann PD, Kinlock TW, et al. Extended-release naltrexone to prevent opioid relapse in criminal justice offenders. *N Engl J Med.* 2016;374:1232-1242.
223. Wakeman SE, Bowman SE, McKenzie M, Jeronimo A, Rich JD. Preventing death among the recently incarcerated: an argument for naloxone prescription before release. *J Addict Dis.* 2009;28:124-129.
224. Brinkley-Rubinstein L, McKenzie M, Macmadu A, et al. A randomized, open label trial of methadone continuation versus forced withdrawal in a combined US prison and jail: findings at 12 months post-release. *Drug Alcohol Depend.* 2018;184:57-63. doi:10.1016/j.drugalcdep.2017.11.023
225. Mitchell O, Wilson DB, Eggers A, MacKenzie DL. Assessing the effectiveness of drug courts on recidivism: a meta-analytic review of traditional and non-traditional drug courts. *J Crim Just.* 2012;40:60-71.
226. Cropsey KL, Binswanger IA, Clark CB, Taxman FS. The unmet medical needs of correctional populations in the United States. *J Natl Med Assoc.* 2012;104:487-492.
227. Marijuana use at historic high among college-aged adults in 2020 Annual NIH-supported study reports changing substance use trends among college students and college-aged adults. Accessed October 2023. https://www.nih.gov/news-events/news-releases/marijuana-use-historic-high-among-college-aged-adults-2020
228. O'Grady M, Iverson MG, Suleiman AO, Rhee TG. Is legalization of recreational cannabis associated with levels of use and cannabis use disorder among youth in the United States? A rapid systematic review. *Eur Child Adolesc Psychiatry.* 2022 May 4; doi:10.1007/s00787-022-01994-9
229. Simão AY, Antunes M, Cabral E, et al. An update on the implications of new psychoactive substances in public health. *Int J Environ Res Public Health.* 2022;19(8):4869.
230. Virgili F. E-cigarettes and youth: an unresolved Public Health concern. *Ital J Pediatr.* 2022;48(1):97.
231. Harrell M, Clendennen SL, Sumbe A, Case KR, Mantey DS, Swan S. Cannabis vaping among youth and young adults: a scoping review. *Curr Addict Rep.* 2022;9(3):217-234.
232. Wang L, Wang Q, Davis PB, Volkow ND, Xu R. Increased risk for COVID-19 breakthrough infection in fully vaccinated patients with substance use disorders in the United States between December 2020 and August 2021. *World Psychiatry.* 2022;21(1):124-132.
233. National Institute of Drug Abuse. *Screening for Drug Use in General Medical Settings: Quick Reference Guide.* Accessed August 31, 2022. https://nida.nih.gov/sites/default/files/pdf/screening_qr.pdf
234. Madras BK, Compton WM, Avula D, Stegbauer T, Stein JB, Clark HW. Screening, brief interventions, referral to treatment (SBIRT) for illicit drug and alcohol use at multiple healthcare sites: comparison at intake and 6 months later. *Drug Alcohol Depend.* 2009;99:280-295.
235. Pilowsky DJ, Wu LT. Screening instruments for substance use and brief interventions targeting adolescents in primary care: a literature review. *Addict Behav.* 2013;38:2146-2153.
236. National Institute on Alcohol Abuse and Alcoholism. *The Healthcare Professional's Core Resource on Alcohol. Knowledge. Impacts. Strategies.* Accessed August 29, 2023. https://www.niaaa.nih.gov/health-professionals-communities/core-resource-on-alcohol?utm_source=niaaa-eblast&utm_medium=email&utm_campaign=directormessage-52022
237. O'Grady M, Lincourt P, Gilmer E, et al. How are substance use disorder treatment programs adjusting to value-based payment? A statewide qualitative study. *Subst Abuse.* 2020;14:1178221820924026.

238. Volkow ND, Skolnick P. New medications for substance use disorders: challenges and opportunities. *Neuropsychopharmacology.* 2012;37:290-292.
239. Fulco CE, Liverman CT, Earley LE. *Development of Medications for the Treatment of Opiate and Cocaine Addictions: Issues for the Government and Private Sector (Institute of Medicine).* National Academy Press; 1995.
240. Substance Abuse and Mental Health Services Administration (US); Office of the Surgeon General (US). *Facing Addiction in America. The Surgeon General's Report on Alcohol, Drugs, and Health.* US Department of Health and Human Services; 2016.
241. Volkow N, Gordon J, Koob G. Choosing appropriate language to reduce the stigma around mental illness and substance use disorders. *Neuropsychopharmacology.* 2021;46(13):2230-2232.

CHAPTER

2 Recommended Use of Terminology in Addiction Medicine

Shannon C. Miller, Richard N. Rosenthal, Jeanette M. Tetrault, Sarah E. Wakeman, Andrew J. Saxon, and Sharon Levy

CHAPTER OUTLINE

- Introduction
- Recommended concepts and terminology by construct
- Conclusions

INTRODUCTION

Addiction specialists are uniquely positioned to be change agents toward public health.[1] Each should lead by example with the use of medically clear, accurate, person-centered, and nonstigmatizing terminology. Words reflect and impact the way we think. Nowhere is this perhaps more evident than in the field of addiction medicine.[2] The terminology used in addiction medicine has appropriately evolved with a changing understanding of the condition and evolving attitudes. This evolution is less a reflection of political correctness than it is a response to a need for greater clarity and objectivity and a recognition of the harms of stigmatizing language. Terminology used by clinicians and researchers should be both scientifically accurate and nonstigmatizing. This chapter serves only to introduce and briefly discuss key issues in terminology, provide references for further exploration, and make recommendations. It is not exhaustive in its coverage of all possible terms related to addiction and its treatment.

In 2002,[3] the American Society of Addiction Medicine (ASAM) first laid a foundation to identify and remove potentially stigmatizing or imprecise terminology[4] from its conferences, textbooks, and medical journal. ASAM provided the first known major conference dealing with addiction where the problem of stigmatizing or inaccurate terminology was formally addressed.[5] While ASAM's textbook first dedicated space to this topic in its fourth edition[6]; ASAM's sixth edition provided the first major medical textbook on the subject of addiction wherein methods were used to remove stigmatizing or imprecise terminology throughout.[7] ASAM's *Journal of Addiction Medicine* and other leading journals have encouraged the use of precise, nonstigmatizing terminology.[8-11] Furthermore, the International Society of Addiction Journal Editors (ISAJE) published a recommendation statement against the use of stigmatizing terms.[12] In 2018, the *Associated Press Stylebook* was published to guide journalists not to use stigmatizing language. Unfortunately, even after this guide was published, a study found that 56% to 94% of articles by major news outlets still used stigmatizing language.[13] Stigmatizing language continues to be used in the medical literature including in clinical trials. For example, both a systematic search of the medical literature on alcohol use disorder[14] and a search of clinical trials relating to alcohol use from 2017 to 2021[15] found that roughly 80% of the publications were not adherent to person-centered language and/or continued to use stigmatizing terminology.

RECOMMENDED CONCEPTS AND TERMINOLOGY BY CONSTRUCT

Avoid Stigmatizing the Patient or the Condition, and Seek Medically Defined Terminology

Stigmatizing terms can negatively impact clinician judgment and quality of care.[16-18] For example, research demonstrates that when patients are described as having substance "abuse" instead of a "use disorder," clinicians are more likely to recommend punitive approaches to treatment.[16,17] While there may not be consensus on exactly which terms in and of themselves are stigmatizing versus which are not, clearly using terminology in a way that ignores the many human aspects of the patient beyond their substance use and defines them by their behavior or condition is potentially stigmatizing. Examples include the use of the terms "alcoholic," "abuser," "drunk," "user," "addict," or "junkie." While some may view the use of terms such as "alcoholic" and "addict" as acceptable in 12-step or other nonmedical settings, these terms should be replaced with more medically defined and less stigmatizing terms that incorporate person-first language (eg, patient with "alcohol use disorder" and not "alcoholic," "patient with OUD" and not "OUD patient," etc.). Our patients are people first, who secondarily have a disease or disorder; using proper terminology reinforces this concept to clinicians, families, patients, administrators, and politicians. This concept transcends addiction medicine and is not different from refraining from referring to "the sickler in bed 3," instead appropriately describing "the patient with sickle cell disease in bed 3."

The Spectrum of Use

Several terms[19] are preferred when discussing the spectrum of unhealthy alcohol and other substance use, as conceptually illustrated in **Figure 2-1**.

1. Lower-risk use
2. Unhealthy (alcohol, other substances) use
   a. Hazardous use[20,21] or at-risk use
   b. Harmful use (including addiction and substance use disorder)

1. **Lower risk use** refers to consumption of an amount of alcohol or other drugs below the amount *currently known* or *identified* as causally associated with future risk, or that has already caused present/past harm—physically and/or psychosocially. This amount could be any (even a small) amount and is empirically derived for each substance. Of course, use of any substance (or engagement in behaviors) known to carry risk for developing a substance use disorder, or addiction could thus carry some risk; albeit lower than risk as described below. The term "lower risk" may be preferred over "low" risk because the latter may be more susceptible to conflation with "no" risk, and the former emphasizes risk typically being relative when exposing the human body to substances.
2. **Unhealthy use** covers the entire spectrum of use related to health consequences including addiction. Unhealthy alcohol and other substance use is any use that increases the risk or likelihood for health consequences (hazardous use) or has already led to health consequences (harmful use). Unhealthy use is an umbrella term that encompasses all levels of use relevant to health, from at-risk use through addiction. Unhealthy use is a useful descriptive term referring to all the conditions or states that should be targets of preventive activities or interventions.
3. The exact threshold for unhealthy use is a clinical and/or public health decision based on epidemiological evidence for measurably increased risks for the occurrence of use-related injury, illness, or other health consequences. The term "unhealthy" (just as with the descriptors "unsafe" or "hazardous" or "harmful" or "misuse") does not imply the existence of "healthy" or "safe" or "nonhazardous" or "harmless" use or that there is a way to use the substances properly (ie, without "misuse").
   a. **Hazardous or at-risk use** is use that increases the risk for health consequences. These terms refer only to use that increases the risk or likelihood of health consequences. They do not include use that has already led to health consequences (this would be referred to as "harmful use"—see below). Thresholds are defined by the amount and frequency of use and/or by circumstances of use. Some of these thresholds are substance-specific and others are not. For example, use of a substance that impairs coordination, cognition, or reaction time while driving or operating heavy machinery is hazardous. Nonmedical use or use in doses more than what is prescribed for prescription drugs can be hazardous. Use of substances that interact (eg, two medications with sedative effects like benzodiazepines and opioids) is hazardous. Use of substances that may exacerbate underlying medical conditions is hazardous (eg, alcohol use and hepatitis C virus infection or alcohol use and postgastrectomy states). Any cocaine use can increase risk for myocardial infarction; one-time use of hydrocarbon inhalants can lead to sudden cardiac death; no known level of tobacco use is considered risk-free; any alcohol or nicotine use during pregnancy is hazardous; any use by young people is likely increases risk for later consequences; use of any potentially addictive substance is more hazardous for persons with a family history or genetic predisposition to addiction than it is to those at average risk in the general population. Alcohol is a known carcinogen, so there is likely no use that is completely risk-free. On the other hand, there are thresholds at which the risk increases for alcohol, and these hazardous or at-risk amounts have been specified.[19]

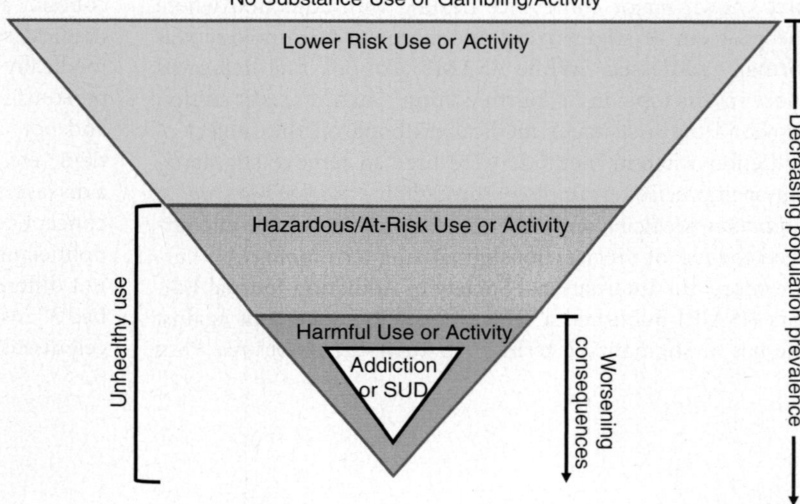

Figure 2-1. Diagram of terminology relating to substance use (or engagement in behaviors) known to carry risk for developing a substance use disorder or addiction. Concepts are not represented to exact scale.

Nicotine is a known cancer promoter, so tobacco and nontobacco nicotine use may be hazardous in the setting of cancer—known or unknown. The exact definitions may change with evolving epidemiological evidence and can also vary by preferences of those making clinical or public health decisions regarding thresholds. In addition, individual factors beyond age, sex, and other characteristics can affect risk (eg, weight), and thresholds are not individualized; although they are useful guides clinically, they cannot be thought of as absolute. For example, it is not the case that drinking just under the threshold is associated with no risk or that drinking just above the threshold confers a substantially greater risk.

b. **Harmful substance use** is the use that results in health consequences. The ICD-10 definition of harmful use can be summarized as repeated use that causes physical or mental damage.[22] Hazardous and harmful are mutually exclusive of each other. These terms apply also to prescription and nonprescription or over-the-counter medications. The terms could also apply to potentially addictive behaviors. **Addiction or substance use disorder** are a subset of harmful substance use and are further discussed in the section entitled "Addiction or Substance Use Disorder" below.

The WHO lexicon defines misuse as use for a purpose not consistent with legal or medical guidelines.[23] However, "misuse" is also a term used to describe not taking (nonaddictive or others) medication as directed or missing doses (eg, of an antihypertensive medication). The U.S. Department of Veterans Affairs has described misuse as the target of alcohol screening and intervention, including disorder and addiction. "Misuse" is not an appropriate descriptor for "addiction," or "substance use disorder" because it minimizes the seriousness of the disorder (to "misuse" the substance). "Misuse" also seems to have a value judgment at least potentially implied, as if it were an accident, mistake, or alternatively purposeful (a choice), neither of which would be appropriate for describing the varied states of unhealthy use. As such, "misuse" can be seen as pejorative or stigmatizing.

"Problem" use is not preferred because it is not well-defined and may be considered stigmatizing. It is used sometimes to refer to harmful use but other times to encompass the spectrum, and can lead to stigmatizing discussion (eg, "you have a problem" or "you are a problem"). "Inappropriate use" is not well-defined and carries a similar pejorative nuance. "Binge or binge drinking" can be useful for public health messaging but needs to be clearly defined as it is sometimes used to mean a heavy drinking (ie, quantity) episode but also used to mean a several day long (duration) episode of heavy drinking or other drug use (eg, cocaine). "Moderate" drinking (or use) is not preferred as a term because it implies safety, restraint, avoidance of excess, and, even, health. Since alcohol is a carcinogen and cancer risk appears at amounts lower than those generally defined as hazardous, and lower limit amounts harmful to the fetus are not well-defined, better terms for amounts lower than amounts defined as risky or hazardous include "lower-risk" alcohol use.

Addiction or Substance Use Disorder

When referring to the medical diagnosis, terms that have been defined and agreed upon should be used. This specificity is essential in allowing clinicians to communicate accurately with each other and researchers and policy makers to compare populations accurately. Examples of terms that typically indicate a medical disease and that are roughly synonymous include "addiction" and "substance use (or gambling) disorder." "Addiction" is a term long used by laypeople, patients, and health care providers. However, the term "addicted" can be problematic because it often incorrectly conflates addiction and physical dependence.

In past decades, the American Psychiatric Association (APA) and the World Health Organization International Classification of Diseases developed criteria to provide a consensus definition of this medical disease known commonly as addiction.[22-25] We provide some historical context here.

The APA's Diagnostic and Statistical Manual of Mental Disorders (DSM) Committee on Substance-Related Disorders had "good agreement among committee members as to the definition of the medical disease known as addiction, but there was disagreement as to the label that should be used."[26]

"Addiction" was a consideration; however, there was concern that labeling it as such could be pejorative and invite stigma. While there was agreement that the term "addiction" would "convey the appropriate meaning of the compulsive drug-taking condition and would distinguish it well from 'physical' dependence,"[26] the concern for stigma resulted in changing the term from "addiction" to (substance) "dependence." Thus, "addiction" and "substance dependence" (at least three DSM criteria met at that time) were considered as synonymous and describing the same clinical disease. In fact, a vote for (substance) "dependence" to be used and not "addiction" was won by only one committee member vote.

The term "addiction" however remained quite acceptable in other medical realms. The APA, ASAM, and the American Board of Medical Specialties retained the medical subspecialty designations of "Addiction Psychiatry" and "Addiction Medicine" throughout these deliberations, and over decades through to today—lending support to the utility of the term "addiction" as descriptive to the layperson, scientifically valuable, and nonstigmatizing.

Years later, the DSM-5 Substance-Related Disorders Committee Chair, Charles P. O'Brien, as well as the directors of the National Institute on Drug Abuse and National Institute on Alcohol Abuse and Alcoholism, published an editorial[26] recognizing that the use of "substance dependence" and not "addiction" as the label for this clinical disease was "a serious mistake," as "this has resulted in confusion among clinicians regarding the difference between 'dependence' in a DSM sense, which is really 'addiction,' and (physical) 'dependence' as a normal physiological adaptation to repeated dosing of a medication." As such, they urged the APA to adopt the word "addiction" for DSM-5.

With the publication of DSM-5 in 2013, the previous DSM terms "substance abuse" and "substance dependence" were made obsolete.[25] This was after consistent findings from studies of over 200,000 participants revealing that these two terms "abuse" and "dependence" were clinically and statistically recognized as representing a *single* disease with varying degrees of severity, renamed in DSM-5 as "substance use disorder" with mild, moderate, or severe severity ratings. Criteria for the disorder no longer included legal problems but did (newly) include craving. In addition, rather than have the threshold as one or more criteria (as in "substance abuse") or three or more criteria (as in "substance dependence"), the threshold was set at two or more criteria for "substance use disorder."[27] Again, the Committee on Substance-Related Disorders chose against using the term "addiction" to avoid possible stigma, even though feedback to the committee from the College on Problems of Drug Dependence in 2009 and the Research Society on Alcoholism (2010) supported the use of the term "addiction."[28]

"Substance use disorder" is well-defined,[25] and the features of "addiction" are described by ASAM. Each can be appropriately used if referenced. The terms overlap and have similar meaning. However, DSM-5 criteria do not define "addiction." The DSM-5 clarifies that "addiction" was not chosen as the label for substance use disorder, not only because of stigma but also because of a desire to avoid conflict with the varied ways the construct is used. While "addiction" is "in common usage in many countries to describe severe *problems*" (not necessarily DSM *criteria*) "related to compulsive and habitual use of substances," and "some clinicians will choose to use the word *addiction* to describe more extreme presentations,"[25] the DSM-5 does not state that addiction should only be used to represent a "severe" substance use disorder. The DSM-5 does not exclude addiction as present in a "moderate" or "mild" substance use disorder, nor does a diagnosis of addiction require that six (or more) criteria of a substance use disorder be present (O'Brien CP, Chair, DSM-5 Substance-Related Disorders Committee. Personal Communication with Miller SC. 2016).

With respect to "dependence," although this term is used as an ICD-10 disorder, given the transition from DSM-IV to DSM-5 as well as frequent confusion between addiction and physical dependence, which does not necessarily indicate any disorder and may simply reflect a pharmacological effect, avoiding the term dependence is recommended. Finally, with these concerns about the words "abuse" and "alcoholism," the Directors of the National Institute on Drug Abuse and the National Institute on Alcohol Abuse and Alcoholism have expressed openness to changing their institute names using less stigmatizing terms.[2]

Treatment

Medication (including opioid agonist) treatment of addiction has been mislabeled "drug," "medication-assisted," "substitution," or "replacement." These terms are inaccurate; their pejorative nature and their implicit communication that pharmacotherapy is in some way inferior to psychosocial or mutual help pathways to remission of substance use disorders may be partly responsible for the slow uptake of these efficacious treatments. These treatments do not substitute for, reproduce the effects of, or replace nonprescribed drugs. And medications do not "assist" treatment, they are treatments shown to be efficacious on their own, and studies often fail to show additional benefits of added psychosocial therapies.[29-33] More accurate alternatives would be medication treatment, treatment, opioid agonist treatment, or even psychosocially assisted pharmacotherapy.[34] The jarring nature of the sound of this last example (from a guide published by the World Health Organization [WHO] in 2009) demonstrates how important language and terminology are in shaping how patients and treatments are viewed. Describing patients as "using" medications, rather than "taking" medications, reflects an even subtler stigma that equates medically supervised receipt of medications with unsupervised drug use.

"Medical marijuana" is not a scientifically accurate term and is potentially stigmatizing. Thus, an alternative term should be used. "Medical" infers that (a) the ingredients are well-defined and measurable (yet, cannabis has over 125 ingredients, which vary), (b) ingredients should be consistent from one dose to the next, (c) indications for use should be reasonably evidence-based, (d) with well-established safe dosing ranges, and (e) have clinical warnings and precautions within the product labeling; and (f) are prescribed and clinically supervised throughout care by a medically trained professional with expertise in the condition for which the patient is seeking treatment. The cannabis plant is not FDA-approved or approved by any (medication) regulatory agency. The term "marijuana" has historical roots, which can be harmful to minoritized populations. An alternative to the term "medical marijuana," which is clear, accurate, nonpolitical, and nonstigmatizing is "cannabis used as treatment."

During substance use disorder treatment, testing is often performed for addictive substances. In these cases, results should be presented like other medical tests, as "positive" versus "negative" and "detected" versus "not detected" test results; not "dirty" versus "clean," which are then often used to describe people in a highly stigmatizing way ("I am clean," "your urine was dirty," "I tested you today and you were dirty.").[35] In addition, referring to patients in remission from substance use disorder as "clean" implies that those with active substance use are "dirty." Appropriate clinical terminology to refer to remission is preferred.

CONCLUSIONS

This chapter does not make recommendations regarding what terms people with substance use disorders should use to describe themselves or their experience. Some patients (eg, those succeeding in part with participation in social networks such as Alcoholics Anonymous) clearly find benefit to calling themselves an "alcoholic" or an "addict" even if it might reflect some internalized stigma. However, as patients frequently carry negative self-appraisals and shame about their substance use disorder, other patients have strong negative associations to being labeled a "drug addict" or "drunk," which impedes their treatment engagement. Furthermore, patient acceptance of such labels has not been shown to be necessary to achieve good clinical outcomes.

The purpose of this chapter is not to police language used or to call out those who use a term with good intentions. It takes time for language to change in society and even in clinical practice, including these last two decades of change highlighted above. Doing so now in clinical and scientific speaking and writing is part of an ongoing process and will ultimately lead to wider use of scientifically accurate, nonstigmatizing terms.[36] Thus, this chapter has made recommendations regarding terms that should be preferred versus those that should be avoided. In general, stigmatizing terms should be avoided, as should disease first constructions. Terms to be avoided by clinicians and scientists because they may be potentially stigmatizing or clinically unclear are outlined in **Table 2-1**; however, this table is not exhaustive. Scientific and medical terms that are clearly defined and nonstigmatizing are preferred over vague or inaccurate terms, terms that are difficult to define, and terms that are used to mean many different things. Better use of terminology can improve clear communication of addiction science and improve the quality of care for the patients we serve daily under the Hippocratic Oath.

TABLE 2-1 Recommendations for Nonstigmatizing, More Clinically Accurate Language

Avoid the Term	Preferred Term (and relevant discussion)
(substance) Abuse	(substance) Use (or specify lower-risk vs unhealthy use)
Addict, user, abuser, alcoholic, crack head, pot head, dope fiend, junkie	Person with (the disease of) addiction, a substance use disorder, or gambling disorder
Addicted baby	Baby experiencing substance withdrawal
Addictive disease	Person with alcohol use disorder, or person with addiction. The person is not addicted to a disease; rather, the person has the medical disease of addiction, or addiction to a substance, gambling, etc.
Alcoholic hepatitis/cirrhosis/pancreatitis	Alcohol-associated hepatitis/cirrhosis/pancreatitis, or alcohol-related
Binge	Heavy drinking episode
Detoxification	Withdrawal management, withdrawal
Dirty vs clean urine, failed a test	Positive or negative test result, substance was detected or not detected
Dropped out of treatment, treatment dropout	Discontinued participation. "Drop-out" is synonymous with leaving high school early and being viewed as having an inadequate education. Dropping out of treatment or a study might also not be fully their choice, but rather a consequence of barriers such as lack of transportation, need to work, loss of housing, lack of family support, etc.[15]
Drunk, smashed, bombed, messed up, strung out	Intoxicated
Fix	Dose, use
Medical marijuana	Cannabis used as treatment. "Medical" infers that (a) the ingredients are well-defined and measurable (yet, cannabis has over 125 ingredients, which vary), (b) ingredients should be consistent from one dose to the next, (c) indications for use should be reasonably evidence-based, (d) with well-established safe dosing ranges, and (e) have clinical warnings and precautions within the product labeling; and (f) are prescribed and clinically supervised throughout care by a medically trained professional with expertise in the condition for which the patient is seeking treatment. The marijuana plant is not FDA-approved or approved by any (medication) regulatory agency. The term "marijuana" has historical roots, which can be harmful to minoritized populations. An alternative and more medically clear, accurate, nonpolitical, and nonstigmatizing term recommended by the authors is "cannabis used as treatment."
Meth	Methamphetamine, methadone, methylphenidate, methcathinone, methanol
Misuse, problem use	Could be used if clearly defined and most useful for prescription drug (misuse) when the nature or severity of the condition is unknown. Avoid calling the person a problem or their use a problem. More accurate terms include nonmedical use, use not consistent with the prescription, vs at-risk use/hazardous use, vs harmful use.
Moderate drinking (or drug use)	Lower-risk use.
Noncompliant, unmotivated, resistant (11) patient	Patient not in agreement with the treatment plan, patient opted out of treatment, patient experiencing ambivalence about change, patient is in the precontemplative stage of change. These terms affirm a person's agency and preference.
Quit, quitter	"Quit" is imprecise (define the period of time, as there can be great variability). "Quitter" carries stigma, instead consider "patient in remission of use since (insert date/duration)" or other more precise and less-stigmatizing language.

(Continued)

TABLE 2-1 Recommendations for Nonstigmatizing, More Clinically Accurate Language *(Continued)*

Avoid the Term	Preferred Term (and relevant discussion)
Recidivism, Recidivist	Patient with recurrence of use, recurrence of SUD. The term "recidivism" is a term that originated in the criminal justice arena. It refers to a person's return to criminal behavior. The use of the term in a patient to refer to a re-activation of their disease or substance use inappropriately denotes clinical "relapse" as a criminal offense[11]
Relapse[37]	Use, return to use, recurrence of substance/gambling use, or of DSM criteria, or of SUD/Gambling Disorder, vs remission specifiers (early or sustained) as defined by the DSM. "Relapse" artificially creates a binary outcome whereby any return to use of a substance is considered a loss of all gains made thus far; this would be like telling a patient with diabetes in the ER that they have "relapsed" and/or "failed."[15] A systematic review found 25 different definitions of relapse in the alcohol literature alone[38]
Smoking cessation	Tobacco use disorder treatment, reduction or cessation of tobacco use.[39] This term is often mis-stated as "smoking sensation." A similar term is not typically used for other drugs with addiction liability. This term seems to place tobacco in a category different than other drugs, which may not be helpful considering its high addiction risk and high morbidity and mortality. More favored terms for "smoking" include "tobacco" (or "nicotine").
Substitution, replacement, medication-assisted treatment	Opioid agonist treatment, medication treatment, psychosocially-assisted pharmacological treatment, treatment

The original table for this work first appeared in Salsitz E, Miller SC, Wilford B. *Organizational Committee for the American Society of Addiction Medicine Review Course*. Accessed April 20, 2022. http://naabt.org/documents/ES-lettervoc.pdf. Published 2002. And also in Salsitz EA, Miller SC. Perspectives: the language of addiction. *American Society of Addiction Medicine News*. 2002, November/December 17;(6):13.

REFERENCES

1. Kunz K, Yamashita W. The addiction medicine physician as a change agent for prevention and public health. In: Miller SC, Levy S, Rosenthal RN, Saxon A, Tetrault J, Wakeman S, eds. *The ASAM Principles of Addiction Medicine*. 7th ed. Wolters Kluwer; 2023.
2. Volkow ND, Gordon JA, Koob GF. Choosing appropriate language to reduce the stigma around mental illness and substance use disorders. *Neuropsychopharmacology*. 2021;46:2230-2232.
3. Salsitz EA, Miller SC. Perspectives: the language of addiction. *American Society of Addiction Medicine News*. 2002 November/December 17;(6):13.
4. Miller SC; for the ASAM History Writing Committee. Combating stigma, changing conversations: The language of addiction medicine. In: Graham AW, Barthwell AG, Jara G, Miller MM, Smith DE, eds. *Treat Addiction—Saves Lives: The History of the American Society of Addiction Medicine*. The American Society of Addiction Medicine; 2022:196.
5. Salsitz E, Miller SC, Wilford B. *Organizational Committee for the American Society of Addiction Medicine Review Course*. Accessed April 20, 2022. http://naabt.org/documents/ES-lettervoc.pdf
6. Ries RK, Fiellin DA, Miller SC, Saitz R. *Principles of Addiction Medicine*. 4th ed. Lippincott, Williams, and Wilkins; 2009.
7. Miller SC, Fiellin DA, Rosenthal RN, Saitz R. *The ASAM Principles of Addiction Medicine*. 6th ed. Wolters Kluwer; 2019.
8. Saitz R. Things that work, things that don't work, and things that matter: including words. *J Addict Med*. 2015;9:429-430.
9. Language and terminology guidance for Journal of Addiction Medicine manuscripts. Accessed April 23, 2022. http://journals.lww.com/journaladdictionmedicine/Pages/Instructions-and-Guidelines.aspx#languageandterminologyguidance
10. Botticelli MP, Koh HK. Changing the language of addiction. *JAMA*. 2016;316(13):1361-1362.

Disclaimer: Dr Miller is employed by the Department of Veterans Affairs, Dayton VA Medical Center, Dayton, Ohio. The VA had no role in the design, literature review or analysis, writing, or in the decision to submit this chapter for publication. The contents do not necessarily represent the views of the Department of Veterans Affairs or the United States Government.

11. Broyles LM, Binswanger IA, Jenkins JA, et al. Confronting inadvertent stigma and pejorative language in addiction scholarship: a recognition and response. *Subst Abuse*. 2014;35:217-221.
12. Saitz R. International statement recommending against the use of terminology that can stigmatize people. *J Addict Med*. 2016;10(1):1-2.
13. Bessette LG, Hauc SC, Danckers H, Atayde A, Saitz R. The *associated press stylebook* changes and the use of addiction-related stigmatizing terms in news media. *Subst Abuse*. 2020;43(1):127-130.
14. Hartwell M, Naberhaus B, Arnhart C, et al. The use of person-centered language in scientific research articles focusing on alcohol use disorder. *Drug Alcohol Depend*. 2020;216:1-6.
15. Hartwell M, Lin V, Hester M, et al. Stigmatizing terminology for outcomes and processes (STOP) in alcohol research: A meta-epidemiologic assessment of language used in clinical trial publications. *J Addict Med*. 2022;16(5):527-533.
16. Kelly JF, Dow SJ, Westerhoff C. Does our choice of substance-related terms influence perceptions of treatment need? An empirical investigation with two commonly used terms. *J Drug Issues*. 2010;40:805-818.
17. Kelly JF, Westerhoff C. Does it matter how we refer to individuals with substance-related problems? A randomized study with two commonly used terms. *Int J Drug Policy*. 2010;21:202-207.
18. Van Boekel LC, Brouwers EP, van Weeghal J, Garretsen HF. Stigma among health professionals towards patients with substance use disorders and its consequences for healthcare delivery: a systematic review. *Drug Alcohol Depend*. 2013;131:23-35.
19. Saitz R. Unhealthy alcohol use. *N Engl J Med*. 2005;352:596-607.
20. Saunders JB, Lee NK. Hazardous alcohol use: Its delineation as a subthreshold disorder, and approaches to its diagnosis and management. *Compr Psychiatry*. 2000;41(2 suppl 1):95-103.
21. Saunders JB, Room R. Enhancing the ICD system in recording alcohol's involvement in disease and injury. *Alcohol*. 2012;47(3):216-218.
22. *The ICD-10 Classification of Mental and Behavioural Disorders: Clinical Descriptions and Diagnostic Guidelines*. World Health Organization; 1992.
23. Babor T, Campbell R, Room R, et al. *Lexicon of Alcohol and Drug Terms*. World Health Organization; 1994. Accessed April 23, 2022. https://apps.who.int/iris/bitstream/handle/10665/39461/9241544686_eng.pdf?sequence=1&isAllowed=y

24. American Psychiatric Association. *Diagnostic and Statistical Manual of Mental Disorders.* 4th ed., text rev. ed. APA; 2000.
25. American Psychiatric Association. *Diagnostic and Statistical Manual of Mental Disorders: DSM-5.* APA; 2013.
26. O'Brien CP, Volkow N, Li TK. What's in a word? Addiction versus dependence in DSM-V. *Am J Psychiatry.* 2006;163(5):764-765.
27. Hasin DS, Obrien CP, Auriacombe M, et al. DSM-5 criteria for substance use disorders: recommendations and rationale. *Am J Psychiatry.* 2013;170(8):834-851.
28. O'Brien CP. Addiction and dependence in DSM-V. *Addiction.* 2011;106(5):1-3.
29. Schwartz RP. When added to opioid agonist treatment, psychosocial interventions do not further reduce the use of illicit opioids: A comment on Dugosh et al. *J Addict Med.* 2016;10(4):283-285.
30. Friedmann PD, Schwartz RP. Just call it "treatment." *Addict Sci Clin Pract.* 2012;7:10.
31. Samet JH, Fiellin DA. Opioid substitution therapy-time to replace the term. *Lancet.* 2015;385(9977):1508-1509.
32. Wakeman SE. Medications for addiction treatment: changing language to improve care. *J Addict Med.* 2017;11(1):1-2.
33. Amato L, Minozzi S, Davoli M, Vecchi S. Psychosocial combined with agonist maintenance treatments versus agonist maintenance treatments alone for treatment of opioid dependence. *Cochrane Database Syst Rev.* 2011;(10):CD004147.
34. *Guidelines for the Psychosocially Assisted Pharmacological Treatment of Opioid Dependence.* World Health Organization; 2009.
35. Kelly JF, Wakeman SE, Saitz R. Stop talking 'dirty': clinicians, language, and quality of care for the leading cause of preventable death in the United States. *Am J Med.* 2015;128:8-9.
36. U.S. Department of Health and Human Services (HHS), Office of the Surgeon General. *Facing Addiction in America: The Surgeon General's Report on Alcohol, Drugs, and Health.* HHS; November 2016.
37. Miller WR. Retire the concept of relapse. *Subst Use Misuse.* 2015;50(8-9):976-977.
38. Maisto SA, Witkiewitz K, Moskal D, et al. Is the construct of relapse heuristic, and does it advance alcohol use disorder clinical practice? *J Stud Alcohol Drugs.* 2016;77(6):849-858.
39. Wolff F, Hughes JR, Woods SS. New terminology for the treatment of tobacco dependence: a proposal for debate. *J Smok Cessat.* 2013;8:71-75.

CHAPTER

3 The Anatomy of Addiction

Michael J. Wesley, Colleen A. Hanlon, and Thomas J. R. Beveridge

CHAPTER OUTLINE

- Introduction
- Primer on neuroanatomy
- Neuroanatomy of drug reinforcement
- Neuroanatomy of drug addiction
- Moving forward

INTRODUCTION

Dr Watson admiring Sherlock Holmes "But consider! Count the cost! Your brain may, as you say, be roused and excited, but it is a pathological and morbid process, which involves increased tissue change and may at least leave permanent weakness.... Why should you, for a mere passing pleasure, risk the loss of those great powers with which you have been endowed?"—*Sign of Four*, Sherlock Holmes (Arthur Conan Doyle, 1894).

This quote from Dr Watson comes as a plea to Sherlock Holmes who has started using cocaine in a "7% solution" when he is feeling bored. This may be one of the first suggestions that regular use of psychostimulants could change the structure of the brain—a fictional assertion from 221B Baker Street, which can now be supported by shelves of brain imaging journals in the nonfiction section of your local university. Over one hundred years later, we now know that chronic use of many commonly used addictive drugs (including but not limited to cocaine, alcohol, nicotine, and opioids) can lead to structural and functional pathology in the brain. This pathology is not restricted to a single brain region, a single cell type, or a single neurotransmitter system. Additionally, the topography of drug-associated neural changes evolves in a spatially progressive manner as the vulnerable individual progresses from a set of initially rewarding experiences to addiction. The temporal continuum of substance use disorder is recognized by the DSM-5, and we are consistently learning more about its neural correlates.

There are three primary goals of this chapter. They are (a) introducing the reader to a common set of neural regions, which appear to be critical to the acquisition and maintenance of substance use disorder, (b) discussing changes in these regions during the initial phases of reward-based learning, and (c) concluding with a discussion of functional and structural neuropathology associated with addiction. Whether we are observing young adults after a high school football game, or rodents in cages in a research laboratory, initial drug taking is nearly always a reinforced behavior. Consequently, in order to understand why certain individuals may be more vulnerable to eventual substance use disorder (SUD) or addiction, it is critical to understand the neural mechanisms that underlie basic drug reinforcement. Following a basic primer on the neuroanatomy of addiction, Part 2 (Neuroanatomy of Drug Reinforcement) focuses on the systems associated with the primary reinforcing effects of three specific classes of substances, namely, psychostimulants, opioids, and cannabinoids. We focus on the site of action, which defines the access points for a drug to influence a specific brain process and highlights the role of the limbic system. In Part 3 (Neuroanatomy of Drug Addiction), we will describe how an initial reinforcing drug action influences brain areas beyond the limbic system, which are involved in habit formation and maintenance of the initially reinforced behavior.

For the most part, the discussion of the anatomy of reinforcement and addiction maps onto structures associated with the limbic system and the basal ganglia.

PRIMER ON NEUROANATOMY

The brain is a complex organ with interconnected yet distinct anatomy. When attempting to understand how neuroanatomy relates to behavior in general, and addiction specifically, it is helpful to consider neuroanatomy at various spatial levels of analysis. For example, at the cellular level (on the order of nanometers and micrometers) drugs have direct physiological effects on specific molecular targets according to the topography of a given receptor system. Cellular receptor systems are often a part of pathways that span multiple brain structures. Zooming out several orders of magnitude (on the order of millimeters and centimeters), it is the concerted activity of diverse cellular physiology within a given location (which is not limited to the primary molecular effect of a single drug) that gives rise to the multiple functions of a specific brain structure. Thus, it is unlikely that there is a 1:1 relationship between a primary cellular drug effect and the multifaceted behaviors and symptoms of addiction. It is more likely that the coordinated neural network activity of several brain structures within a given neural system (which may be heavily influenced by a primary drug effect) is responsible for the many behaviors and symptoms of addiction. While there is still much to learn about the neuroanatomy of addiction, preclinical and clinical research has uncovered multiple cellular systems and brain structures involved in the addiction process.

The brain structures most often mentioned in the context of unhealthy substance use and addiction are closely associated with the limbic system, lateral hypothalamus, basal ganglia, and frontal cortical regions. Here we present a brief description of each of these systems. Readers interested in a more complete description of the anatomy of these regions are referred to the following reviews.[1-4]

Subcortical Limbic System

Research into the limbic system has a long and venerable history, but some scholars have suggested that the term may have outlived its usefulness. Nonetheless, a brief historic review of the term is a useful way of introducing some of the regions involved in drug addiction. The term *limbic* is derived from the Latin term *limbus*, meaning border, and was used to describe a ring of phylogenetically older cortex that separates the diencephalon and the neocortex. This limbic lobe consisted of the subcallosal area, cingulate, and parahippocampal gyri (**Fig. 3-1**). This purely anatomic distinction was expanded by MacLean[5] in 1952 to describe a functional unit that was proposed to be responsible for emotional expression. He made the distinction between the older, medial cortex and the more lateral neocortex, which is involved in cognitive functions.

MacLean's concept was that most human behavior is the result of cooperation between three systems of the brain. The cerebral cortex is responsible for higher-order reasoning and speech, whereas the limbic system was the source of emotions, aspects of personal identity, and fight-or-flight instincts. The third aspect of MacLean's system is the reptilian brain. Early work with primates showed that when various parts of the limbic system were electrically stimulated, a range of emotional responses was produced, such as rage, fear, and joy.[6] This phylogenetically older brain is responsible for the organism avoiding things that are "disagreeable" and approaching those that are "agreeable"—reactions that MacLean saw as having survival value. It is now clear that structures associated with the limbic system (such as the hypothalamus, hippocampus, and amygdala) are essential not only for learning and memory but also for the emotional context and the affective response to learned associations.

As is detailed, many addictive drugs have their sites of action within the limbic system, and the neurochemistry within these structures is altered during the addiction process. This may help explain why decisions surrounding drug seeking and drug taking seem to be driven more by emotion and instinct rather than by logic.

From an anatomic perspective, MacLean defined the limbic system as the original limbic lobe along with other structures sharing direct connections with them. These include the olfactory cortex, hippocampal formation, amygdala, septum, hypothalamus, habenula, anterior thalamic nuclei, and parts of the basal ganglia. With further anatomic research, more and more areas were shown to share direct connections with these structures and some of these began to be included in the limbic system. The result was that the boundaries of the limbic system became overly broad. Brodal[7] observed that the term *limbic system* was becoming less useful, and he argued that it should be discarded altogether; however, the concept of a phylogenetically older forebrain system responsible for emotional control is now firmly entrenched.

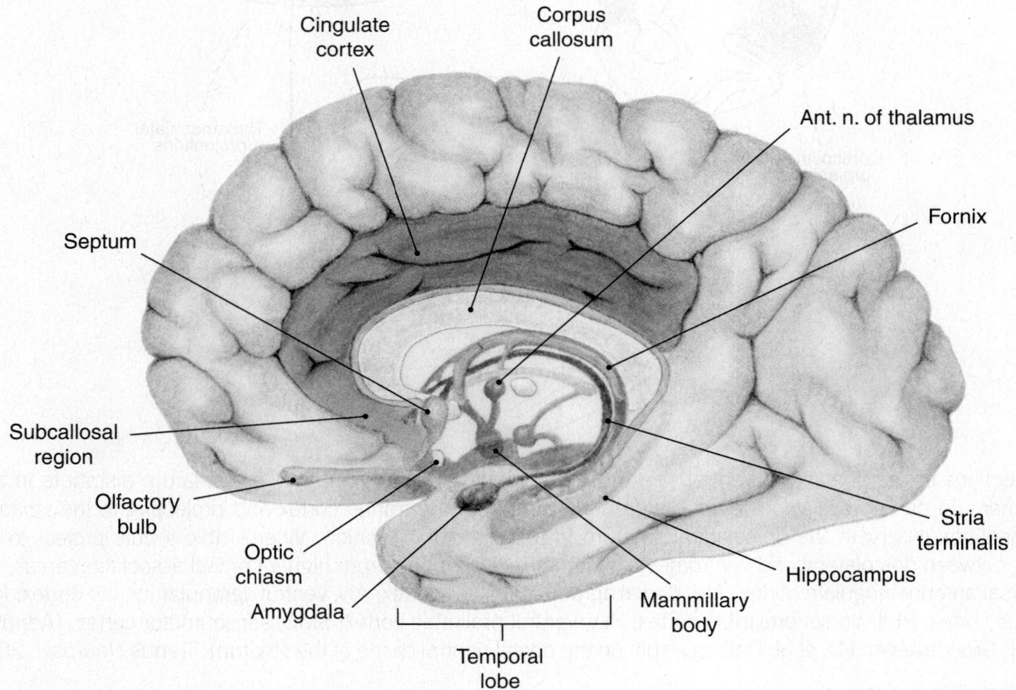

Figure 3-1. Regions of the human brain associated with the limbic system, which includes a loop of cortex extending from the subcallosal region through cingulate cortex to the parahippocampal gyrus. Also shown are the hippocampal formation, septum, amygdala, and mammillary bodies.

Swanson[8] has helped crystallize the anatomic definition by characterizing the limbic system as a network of highly interconnected regions that appear to form the only major route for information transfer between the neocortex and the hypothalamus. **Figure 3-1** illustrates these areas in the human brain.

The Dorsal and Ventral Striatum

The basal ganglia is traditionally thought of as a motor system; however, the idea that this system deals only with motor function while the limbic system deals with reinforcement and emotion is oversimplified and misleading. As later sections illustrate, there is reason to believe that parts of the basal ganglia, and connected striatal subdivisions, are very much involved in memory formation and a variety of cognitive tasks. For example, neuroimaging research in primates and humans has led to computational theories about the role of striatal and prefrontal cortical dopamine in behavioral control.[9] As more is learned about how the basal ganglia and limbic system communicate, it is becoming increasingly clear that the two systems are jointly involved in coordinating motivated behavior.

The largest mass associated with the basal ganglia is the striatum (caudate–putamen). The dorsal portion has long been considered part of the basal ganglia, whereas the ventral striatum is considered to be part of the limbic system.[10] This dorsal/ventral distinction is clearly important; however, more recent debate has focused on the idea that gradations rather than sharp boundaries mark the transition from the dorsolateral to ventromedial striatum. **Figure 3-2** shows the topographic organization of inputs to the striatum in the rat. Voorn et al.[11] make the point, as **Figure 3-2** illustrates, that no histological or immunohistochemical border exists that can be used to define or divide the region. Note that although the dorsolateral parts receive primarily motor inputs and the ventromedial striatal areas receive primarily limbic projections, it is a gradual topographic transition.

The accumbens forms the ventral portion of the striatum, thus accumbens and ventral striatum are used synonymously in the addiction literature. Famously, in 1993 Mogenson et al.[12] described the ventral striatum as the crossroad of the limbic and motor systems and "the place where motivation is translated into action." **Figure 3-2** also shows two regions identified as the nucleus accumbens (NAcc) core and shell. Extensive data suggests that these two regions are involved in behavioral and electrophysiological responses to drug reinforcement, however the functional specificity of these regions to different aspects of drug reinforcement is an area of debate.

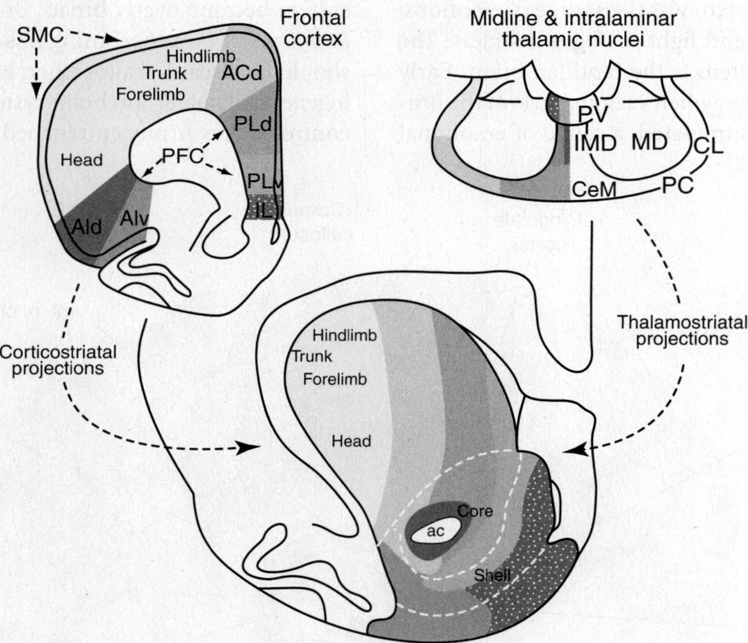

Figure 3-2. Connections of the dorsal and ventral striatum. Cortical and thalamic inputs to the striatum distribute in a dorsomedial-to-ventrolateral manner. To paraphrase Voorn et al.,[9] afferents arising from the frontal cortex and projecting to the striatum are depicted. Sensorimotor projections innervate the dorsolateral striatum in a somatotopic fashion. Vicerolimbic inputs project to the ventromedial striatum. Areas in between dorsolateral and ventromedial striatum receive inputs from higher cortical association areas: ac, anterior commissure; ACd, dorsal anterior cingulate cortex; AId, dorsal agranular insular cortex; AIv, ventral agranular insular cortex; IL, infralimbic cortex; PFC, prefrontal cortex; PLd, dorsal prelimbic cortex; PLv, ventral prelimbic cortex; SMC, sensorimotor cortex. (Adapted from Voorn P, Vanderschuren LJ, Groenewegen HJ, et al. Putting a spin on the dorsal-ventral divide of the striatum. Trends Neurosci. 2004;27:468-474.)

PV, paraventricular thalamic nucleus
IMD, intermediodorsal thalamic nucleus
MD, mediodorsal thalamic nucleus
CL, central lateral thalamic nucleus
CeM, central medial thalamic nucleus
PC, paracentral thalamic nucleus

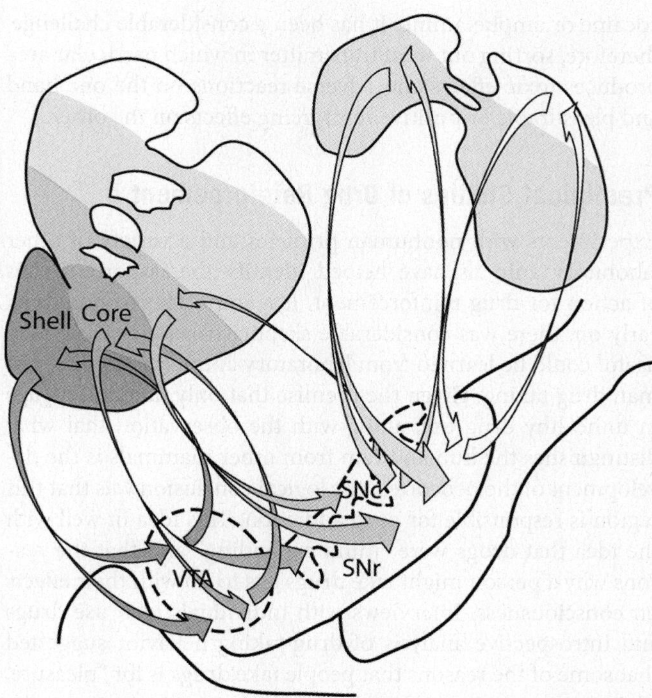

Figure 3-3. Striatonigrostriatal connections form a series of ascending spiraling loops. Projections from the NAcc shell terminate in both the VTA and ventromedial SNc. The VTA sends reciprocal projections back to the shell and neurons from the medial SN project forward to the NAcc core. The projections continue to go back and forth between the striatum and substantia nigra, spiraling upward, so that the shell influences the core, the core influences the central striatum, and so on. These striatonigrostriatal connections continue to occur even past the anterior commissure (*top right schematic*). These posterior portions of the caudate and putamen have reciprocal connections with the dorsal portions of the SN. VTA, ventral tegmental area; SNc, substantia nigra pars compacta; SNr, substantia nigra pars reticulate. (Adapted from Haber SN, Fudge JL, McFarland NR. Striatonigrostriatal pathways in primates form an ascending spiral from the shell to the dorsolateral striatum. *J Neurosci.* 2000;20:2369-2382.)

As one may expect, the topographical organization of these striatal connections is more complex in primates than rodents. Haber et al.[13] have elegantly described the topography of striatonigrostriatal circuitry, including reciprocal synaptic connections between the striatum and substantia nigra pars compacta/reticulate. This complex intrastriatal connectivity provides an iterative and redundant network for integration of various cortical inputs with thalamic outputs (**Fig. 3-3**). This circuitry has been described as a series of ascending spiraling connections between adjacent striatal regions via the ventral midbrain (substantia nigra). In this manner the accumbens shell influences the accumbens core, the core influences the central striatum, and the central striatum influences the dorsolateral striatum.

Executive Function and the Prefrontal Cortex

Executive function refers to multiple aspects of cognitive control (eg, decision making, future thinking, choice) which often provide a counterbalance to limbic activity (eg, arousal, drive, motivation). Some of these executive functions include the ability to differentiate conflicting thoughts, evaluate future consequences of current activities, planning goal-directed activities, and behavioral inhibition.

The prefrontal cortex (PFC) is thought to be the "hub" of executive function in the brain, and contains dense projections to the striatal areas listed previously. While modern human functional brain imaging studies often parcellate the frontal cortex into 15 or more subregions (eg, Automated Anatomical Labeling atlas), broadly there are three widely established functional parcellations: (a) the orbitofrontal and the ventromedial areas (often considered complements to the limbic system[14]; (b) the dorsolateral PFC (often considered a key hub in the executive control system)[15]; and (c) the cingulate cortex (involved in error monitoring, salience detection, and modulating the intensity of a stimulus-response).[16]

NEUROANATOMY OF DRUG REINFORCEMENT

"Site of action" is a concept that defines the access point for a drug to produce a specific response. If that response is defined behaviorally (eg, anorexic, convulsant, antidepressant effect), then the site of action may refer to the receptors (primary molecular component) or the brain regions responsible for that particular behavioral response. It is one thing to describe all possible sites where a drug can affect the brain; it is a more difficult matter to narrow down the possibilities to a particular binding site in a circumscribed region. Research into the site of action for the reinforcing effects of psychostimulant drugs, such as cocaine and amphetamine, offers a good example of how this investigative process occurs.

In vitro experiments have shown that cocaine binds to dopamine, noradrenaline, and serotonin (DA, NA, and 5-HT) transporters and blocks the reuptake of these neurotransmitters[17]; amphetamine acts additionally as a releasing agent. Both of these actions result in an increased concentration of monoamine neurotransmitters in the synapse. Therefore, psychostimulant drugs act as indirect agonists everywhere these transmitters are found.

An examination of the anatomic projections of the catecholamine systems shows that they have extensive and diffuse projections throughout the neural axis. The cell bodies of these transmitter systems are loosely organized in an anteroposterior fashion. Based on their histochemical mapping studies, Dahlstroem and Fuxe[18] proposed a nomenclature wherein cell clusters were numbered from posterior to anterior and given a letter prefix according to whether they were dopaminergic/noradrenergic (A) or serotoninergic (B). **Fig. 3-4A** shows the distribution of NA fibers. The locus coeruleus (LC) (A6) is located in the dorsal brain stem and sends ascending projections to terminal regions of the cortex, hippocampus, and cerebellum. More caudal and ventral NA cells groups (A1-A5) innervate the hypothalamus and brain stem. Dopaminergic innervations are more circumscribed (**Fig. 3-4B**). DA cell groups within the ventral tegmental area (VTA) and substantia nigra (A8, A9, and A10) project in a topographic manner to the striatum. The more medial group (A10) sends projections to the ventral striatum, whereas the more lateral groups form a nigrostriatal

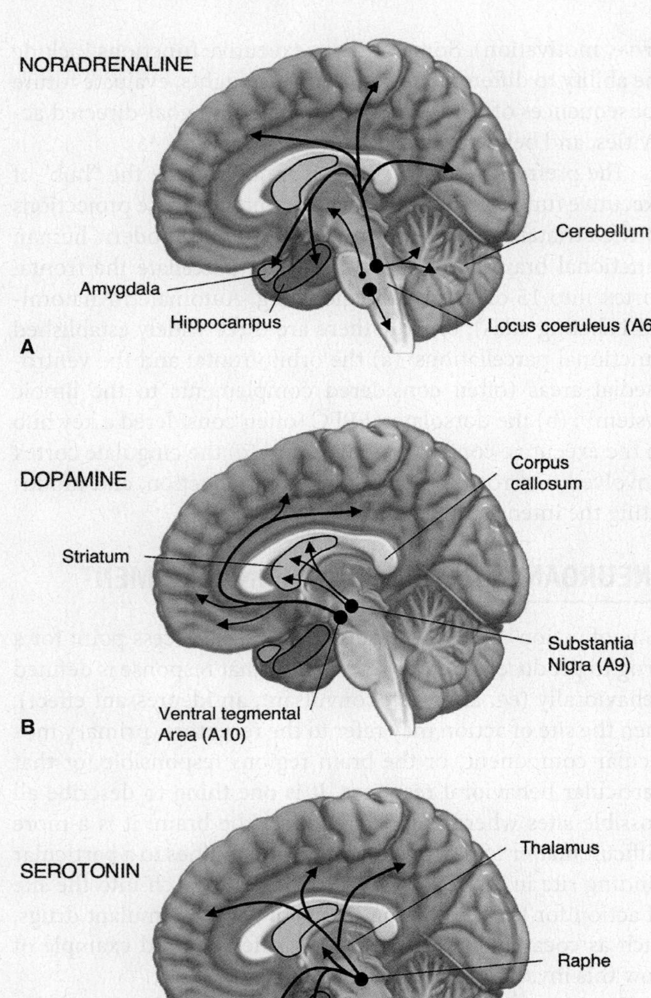

Figure 3-4. Schematic diagram illustrating the distribution of the main central neuronal pathways containing noradrenaline **(A)**, dopamine **(B)**, and serotonin **(C)**. The location of cell bodies of origin is indicated by *circles* with the projections indicated by *arrows*.

bundle that innervates the caudate–putamen. This latter projection is known to degenerate in Parkinson disease and is thus associated with motor function. An additional cluster of DA cells in the hypothalamus composes the tuberoinfundibular DA system, which innervates the external layer of the median eminence. Dahlstroem and Fuxe[19] also described 5-HT cell groups (B1-B9), which lie near the midline of the pons and upper brain stem. Later studies showed clusters of cells also in the caudal LC, area postrema, and interpeduncular nucleus.[14] Generally, the more caudal cell groups innervate the medulla and spinal cord, whereas the more anterior clusters project rostrally (**Fig. 3-4C**).

The main point to be taken from an examination of the areas innervated by DA, NA, and 5-HT is that there is hardly a region that is not innervated by at least two of the monoamines. Given that psychostimulants have an effect at the terminal regions of each of these systems, every area of the brain would be expected to be affected to some extent by an injection of cocaine or amphetamine. It has been a considerable challenge, therefore, sorting out what transmitter in which particular area produces toxic effects and adverse reactions on the one hand and pleasurable or positive reinforcing effects on the other.

Preclinical Studies of Drug Reinforcement

Experiments with nonhuman primates and a variety of other laboratory animals have helped identify the important sites of action for drug reinforcement. It is important to note that, early on, there was considerable skepticism whether anything useful could be learned from laboratory animals regarding human drug taking. Given the premise that only humans engage in unhealthy drug use, along with the observation that what distinguishes the human brain from other mammals is the development of the neocortex, the logical conclusion was that this region is responsible for drug addiction. This idea fit well with the idea that drugs were "mind expanding" and that the reasons why a person might take drugs has to do with their effects on consciousness. Interviews with individuals who use drugs and introspective analysis of drug-taking behavior suggested that some of the reasons that people take drugs is for "pleasure, curiosity, the desire to experiment, the sense of adventure, the search for self-knowledge, the relief of stress and tension, depression, the feeling of powerlessness, and the lack of belief in the future."[20] Although these observations are entirely appropriate for discussion at one level, they also serve to perpetuate the idea that human consciousness and reasoning are the bases for drug reinforcement. The demonstration that nonhuman primates and rodents will voluntarily self-administer drugs such as cocaine and heroin has prompted a consideration of concepts other than human consciousness to account for use of drugs, forcing an examination of brain regions other than the cortex.

There is an extremely high correlation between the addictive drugs that are used by humans and drugs that are self-administered by other mammalian species such as rat, dog, cat, rabbit, and nonhuman primate.[21,22] These data support the idea that addictive drugs have their reinforcing actions on brain structures that have been relatively conserved through the course of human evolution—that is, limbic and brainstem areas. This being the case, the development of self-administration techniques, through intravenous (IV),[23-25] intracranial,[26-28] and inhalation[29] routes, has provided a means to study brain structures responsible for drug reinforcement in animal models. Next, as opposed to providing a review of all drug classes, we expand on three specific drug classes commonly explored in reference to addiction. These classes are psychostimulants, opioids, and cannabinoids.

Psychostimulants

Pharmacological experiments were the first to narrow down the range of possible sites of action for the reinforcing effects of psychostimulant drugs.[30,31] In these studies, rats and monkeys were trained to self-administer cocaine and amphetamine until they showed a stable baseline level of responding (**Fig. 3-5**). They were then pretreated with a variety of agonists or

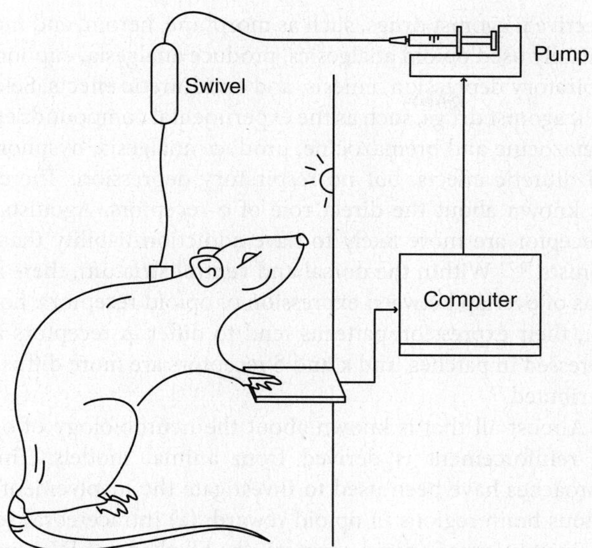

Figure 3-5. In self-administration studies, animals are implanted with permanent indwelling catheters and placed in an experimental chamber. The catheter is connected to a syringe pump through a fluid swivel that allows free movement throughout the chamber. A computer detects responses on a lever and controls the timing of drug delivery according to the schedule of reinforcement. For example, on a fixed-ratio one schedule (FR1), every response on the lever results in an infusion of drug.

antagonists in an effort to identify the specific transmitter systems that modulate reinforcing efficacy. Importantly, it was shown that pretreatment with DA receptor antagonists caused the animals to self-administer cocaine and amphetamine more frequently.[32-34] This is the same result one sees if the concentration of drug is diluted: The animals appear to compensate for the reduction in drug effect by increasing their intake. Note that pretreatment with NA or 5-HT antagonists did not have consistent effects on drug intake. These data prompted Wise[35,36] to champion the idea that stimulation of DA receptors must be essential for psychostimulant reinforcement.

Peripheral injections of DA antagonists narrowed the site of action to DA receptors, but it remained unclear which brain regions mediated this effect. Central manipulations were necessary to identify which brain regions were important. Neurotoxins specific to catecholamine and indolamine neurons provided a useful tool to examine whether the loss of a particular fiber system would affect drug self-administration. A considerable literature developed around the neurotoxin 6-hydroxydopamine (6-OH-DA) that, depending on the site of injection and other parameters, could be used to completely deplete various brain regions of either DA or NA. Early experiments showed that removing the noradrenergic innervation of the entire forebrain had almost no effect on cocaine self-administration. In contrast, removal of the DA innervation of the NAcc resulted in a substantial reduction in cocaine's reinforcing effects.[37-39] In fact, animals will no longer self-administer cocaine if DA levels in the NAcc are reduced by more than 80%. Destroying the DA neurons in the VTA also drastically reduced cocaine self-administration.[40] These data were the first to draw attention to the NAcc (more recently referred to as ventral striatum) as a site for action for psychostimulant reinforcement.

6-OH-DA lesions in other brain regions have had much less dramatic effects. Lesions of the dorsal striatum do not change the rate of cocaine intake, supporting the idea that the ventral striatum has a preferential involvement.[41] Additionally, destruction of DA terminals in the medial PFC or amygdala has only minor effects on the cocaine dose-response curve, which seems to reflect changes in the reinforcing threshold or a change in the anxiogenic effects of cocaine.[42,43]

Injections of DA antagonists directly into the brain have also been used to identify the important anatomic sites involved in cocaine action. The evidence consistently shows that the DA receptors in the ventral striatum are an important site of action. Blockade of D_2 receptors produce an apparent decrease in potency. That is, animals compensate by increasing their hourly drug intake and will "work" less hard for each injection. Injections of D_2 antagonists into the dorsal striatum and the medial PFC produce similar effects, albeit less strongly.[44,45]

In summary, the data presented are from a wide range of studies using neurotoxins, and specific pharmacological agents are consistent with the idea that the most important site of action for the reinforcing effects of cocaine and amphetamine is at DA terminals in the ventral striatum. It should be emphasized however that, although the ventral striatum is essential for the reinforcing effects of cocaine and amphetamine, other DA projection areas (such as the PFC, amygdala, and dorsal striatum) also contribute to some extent.

The site of action for the locomotor-activating effects of psychostimulant drugs seems to largely overlap with the regions responsible for drug reinforcement. Experiments using either lesion or intracerebral injections of DA drugs have shown that stimulation of the DA receptors in the ventral striatum produces behavioral activating effects (locomotion); stimulation of DA receptors in the dorsal striatum produces stereotypy,[46] which is characterized by repetitive sequences of movements, such as licking and grooming in rodents. 6-OH-DA–induced destruction of DA terminals in the ventral striatum almost completely abolishes the locomotor stimulant effects of cocaine, while lesions of the dorsal striatum abolish psychostimulant stereotypy. Similarly, direct injections of DA agonists into the ventral striatum produce locomotion, whereas injections into the dorsal striatum produce stereotypy.[47-49]

The stereotypic response elicited from the dorsal striatum may have relevance to addiction. In rats, stereotyped behavior is often measured on a categorical scale, which includes licking, chewing, and gnawing. These high-frequency movements have the appearance of being "hard-wired" responses that are elicited by the drug. It should be emphasized, however, that almost any behavior can become stereotyped. In their influential article, Randrup and Munkvad[50] described how the precise forms of stereotyped behavior differ across species and offer the example of a man who repeatedly rebuilt his car engine. They suggested that inhibition of drug-induced stereotypy might be useful in screening antipsychotics. We know now that this is true because of the relationship between the importance of DA in stimulating stereotypy and the action of neuroleptic drugs. To re-emphasize, anything can become stereotyped.

Behaviors that occur with high frequency have a high likelihood of becoming stereotyped (ie, they occur repetitively and ritualistically) if they occur in the presence of a drug.[51] Lyon and Robbins[52] argue that stereotypy is a process in which there is an increase in frequency in a diminishing number of response categories. The effect is that psychostimulant drugs narrow the behavioral repertoire such that only a few predominant behaviors remain. Put another way, the behavioral repertoire becomes focused around the things that occur most frequently. In the case of a person with addiction, the frequent behaviors associated with drug seeking and drug taking become repetitive and ritualistic.

In conclusion, strong evidence from studies using widely different strategies suggests that stimulation of DA receptors in the ventral striatum is associated with drug reinforcement. There is a wealth of evidence from a parallel literature showing that the mesolimbic DA system is also involved in reward from natural behaviors such as feeding,[53-55] drinking,[56,57] sexual behaviors,[58,59] and intracranial self-stimulation.[60-62] This enormous amount of literature has resulted in the mesolimbic DA system being called a *reward pathway*. Whether this term is accurate or biologically meaningful (we think it is not) lies outside the scope of this chapter. However, the immense interest in the mesolimbic DA pathway demands some discussion of its interconnections.

Data from electrophysiological studies show that VTA-DA neurons respond to primary reinforcing stimuli (eg, food) and to environmental cues that predict the presentation of rewards.[63,64] Although these neurons receive no direct input from visual, auditory, or somatosensory systems, this information is likely sent via thalamic relays.[65] In fact, the VTA is a part of a widespread collection of neurons that belong to the "isodendritic core."[66] This system is a network of neurons stretching from brainstem to telencephalon. The neurons within the network have similar morphology, send out long projections, and are themselves the target of a great number of contacts from distant sources.[67] This network serves an integrative function and responds to changes in the environment that are biologically significant. Although VTA-DA neurons respond differentially than others in the network when exposed to drug cues, they are likely responsive to salience rather than specific rewarding properties of a drug—a topic that is the center of a long debate.

Opioids

Opioid receptors are expressed throughout the brain, especially in limbic and limbic-related structures; they are found in the amygdala, insular cortex, caudate, anterior hypothalamus, cortex, parietal cortex, putamen, thalamus, and periaqueductal gray.[68] There are three different types of G protein–coupled opioid receptors: μ, κ, and δ, which are acted on by both endogenous and exogenously applied opioids.[69] Selective μ agonist drugs, such as morphine, heroin, and most clinically used opioid analgesics, produce analgesia, euphoria, respiratory depression, emesis, and antidiuretic effects. Selective κ agonist drugs, such as the experimental compounds ethylketazocine and bremazocine, produce analgesia, dysphoria, and diuretic effects, but no respiratory depression. There is less known about the direct role of δ receptors. Agonists at μ receptor are more likely to have addiction liability than κ agonists.[70-72] Within the dorsal and ventral striatum, there are areas of overlap between expression of opioid receptors; however, their expression patterns tend to differ. μ receptors are expressed in patches, and κ and δ receptors are more diffusely distributed.[73]

Almost all that is known about the neurobiology of opioid reinforcement is derived from animal models. Three approaches have been used to investigate the involvement of various brain regions in opioid reward: (a) intracerebral self-administration of opioid agonists, (b) blockade of IV heroin self-administration by intracerebral injections of opioid antagonists, and (c) disruption of IV heroin self-administration by lesions. Generally, the focus has been on areas associated with the mesolimbic DA system (ventral striatum and VTA), although other regions have also been implicated.

Self-administration of drugs directly into various brain regions would seem to be the most straightforward test of their involvement in reinforcement processes; however, the procedures have a number of technical problems that limit their appeal. Issues involving diffusion, osmolarity, and tissue damage demand thoughtful consideration (see Ref.[74] for review). Nonetheless, several papers have provided evidence that opioid-like compounds are self-administered into discrete brain regions. The early work focused on the lateral hypothalamus[26,75,76] because this area was intensely studied for its ability to support intracranial electrical self-stimulation.[77] Later, because of interest in the mesolimbic system, interest switched to the ventral striatum and the VTA. The role of the lateral hypothalamus has been challenged, and it is possible that the early results were due to diffusion of drug to other areas.[78] The ventral striatum appears to support intracranial self-administration of morphine[79] and methionine-enkephalin.[80] These data fit well with the demonstration that intra-NAcc opioids produce a conditioned place preference.[81] Techniques have also been developed to study intracerebral self-injection in mice by using a Y-maze. Selection of one arm of the maze results in a morphine injection, whereas the other arm results in a saline injection. Using this method, mice have been shown to self-inject morphine into the lateral septum[82] and the ventral striatum but not the dorsal striatum.[83]

By far the most sensitive site for intracerebral self-administration of opioids is the VTA. Both μ and δ opioids are self-administered into this region at doses that are not supported in other areas.[28,84-86] The idea that opioids have a significant impact on reinforcement mechanisms through an action in the VTA is supported by a variety of other techniques. For example, injections of opioid agonists into the VTA also produce a conditioned place preference,[87] facilitate brain stimulation reward,[88,89] and reinstate extinguished lever responding that was trained under IV heroin reward.[90]

It should be noted that there are a few reports of reinforcing effects produced by intracerebral injections of opioids into the hippocampus[91] and periaqueductal gray. The doses used in these studies are relatively high, and it remains unclear whether these are important but less sensitive sites or whether diffusion of the drug to other areas accounts for those observation.

When self-administering IV heroin, animals respond to a decrease in the unit injection dose by taking injections more frequently. A similar phenomenon can be observed when animals are treated with a systemic injection of naloxone (a μ antagonist), suggesting that animals compensate for a reduced drug effect by increasing their drug intake.[92] Several laboratories have used this compensatory response to evaluate the effects of opioid antagonists injected into various brain regions. Increases in IV heroin self-administration have been shown after injections of low doses of opioid antagonists into the NAcc,[93-95] periaqueductal gray,[94] stria terminalis,[96] and lateral hypothalamus, but not the PFC.[97] Surprisingly, injections of an opioid antagonist into the VTA have relatively little effect.[98] It remains unclear why many studies have shown that the VTA is one of the most sensitive brain sites for intracerebral self-administration of opioid agonists, whereas it is one of the least effective sites for disrupting IV heroin self-administration studies with an intracerebral injection of opioid antagonists.

Lesions offer a third method for identifying critical brain areas responsible for the reinforcing effects of opioids. Zito et al.[99] showed that the size of a kainic acid–induced lesion of the NAcc correlated with impaired heroin self-administration. This effect is site specific because lesions of other areas, such as the lateral hypothalamus, do not necessarily affect heroin self-administration.[100] More recent studies have attempted to define the relative contribution of subregions within the ventral striatum comparing acquisition of heroin self-administration after excitotoxic lesions of the NAcc core or shell. Rats with lesions of the NAcc core lesion group showed impairments in acquisition, whereas the group with lesions of the NAcc shell was similar to controls. This effect was found either with acquisition of low-dose heroin on a simple fixed-ratio schedule[101] or with acquisition of a second-order schedule with a high injection dose.[102] These data suggest a relatively greater role for the NAcc core in the acquisition of heroin-seeking behavior.

Martin et al.[103] examined regional differences in the ventral striatum by using beta-FNA. This drug is an irreversible antagonist at the μ-opioid receptor producing what amounts to a reversible lesion. Beta-FNA blocks the receptor rendering it unavailable for many days, until new receptor populations can be synthesized. Beta-FNA was found to produce site-specific effects, attenuating heroin self-administration when injected into the caudal but not rostral NAcc.

The hypothesis that the mesolimbic DA systems mediate the reinforcing effects of opioids has been proposed. Certainly, it is clear that psychostimulants and opioids have independent sites of action at the receptor level. DA antagonists potently affect cocaine but not heroin self-administration; conversely, opioid antagonists potently affect heroin but not cocaine self-administration.[104,105] However, it has been shown that opioids indirectly affect DA cell firing through inhibition of GABA interneurons in the VTA.[106] This disinhibition can result in enhanced DA release in the NAcc.[107] Heroin self-administration increases DA in the ventral striatum, and this has been argued to be the mechanisms of action for heroin reinforcement.[108]

Curiously, DA cell bodies in the VTA seem to be more important for heroin self-administration than the DA innervation of the ventral striatum. Bozarth and Wise[109] showed that 6-OH-DA lesions of the VTA impair the acquisition of IV heroin self-administration. By contrast, 6-OH-DA–induced depletion within of the NAcc has very little effect on heroin self-administration in spite of the fact that 6-OH-DA such lesions dramatically reduce or abolish cocaine self-administration.[110,111] It appears that some, but not all, of the reinforcing effects of opioids are mediated through an action on DA mechanisms.

Cannabinoids

The characterization of cannabinoid receptors in the brain has been an important first step in identifying the site of action for the reinforcing effects of cannabis. Two cannabinoid receptors (CB1 and CB2) have been identified to date. Both are G protein–coupled receptors and function to inhibit adenylate cyclase. They are acted on by endogenous cannabinoids and exogenous activators such as cannabis. **Figure 3-6** represents CB1 expression in the rat brain. As in humans, the CB1 receptor is highly expressed in the brain and found in the basal ganglia, hippocampus, cerebellum, cerebral cortex,

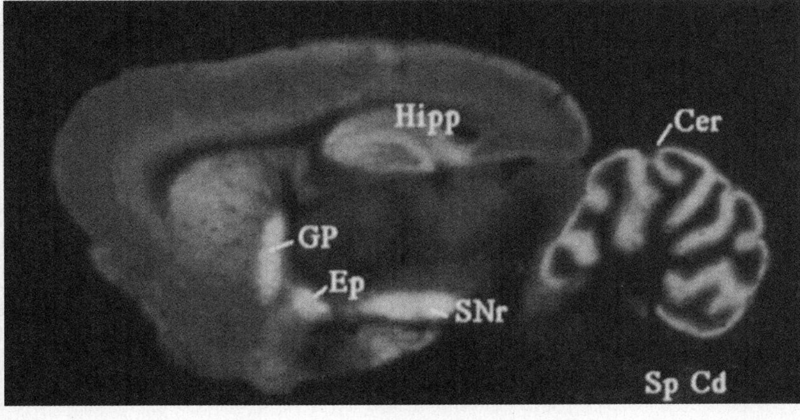

Figure 3-6. Cannabinoid receptor expression in the rat brain. Areas with brightest colors indicate a greater expression. Cannabinoid receptors are expressed in high numbers in the cerebellum (Cer), hippocampus (Hipp), globus pallidus (GP), external globus pallidus (Ep), and the substantia nigra pars reticulate (SNr). Sp Cd, spinal cord. (Courtesy of Dr Allyn Howlett.)

and striatum.[112] This expression may explain some of the behavioral effects of cannabis (motor, memory, or cognitive impairment).[113] The CB2 receptor was once thought to be only expressed in peripheral immune cells but has recently been identified in the brain at low levels.[114]

Progress in identifying the brain mechanisms associated with the reinforcing effects of cannabinoids has been hampered until recently by the lack of a good animal model. Route of administration is a major influence on the reinforcing effects of drugs, and smoking is the preferred route for cannabis use in humans. Smoking, of course, is not an option for studying cannabinoid use in rats, and there have been no reports of successfully training nonhuman primates to smoke cannabis. Instead, attempts have been made to demonstrate IV self-administration of Δ9-tetrahydrocannabinol (THC), the active ingredient in cannabis, and other cannabinoid receptor agonists. Despite a good deal of effort, early studies provided little evidence that rats would self-administer THC,[113] although self-administration of THC and anandamide analogs has been reported in squirrel monkeys.[115,116] More success has been achieved with the synthetic CB1 receptor agonist WIN 55,212-2, which has been shown to be self-administered by mice[117] and rats.[118,119]

The neurobiological investigation of cannabinoid self-administration is in the early stages although it appears that both opioid and DA mechanisms may interact with cannabinoid reinforcement.[120-122]

NEUROANATOMY OF DRUG ADDICTION

As discussed above, the acquisition and maintenance of substance use disorder involves multiple cortical and subcortical brain regions. It also occurs on a continuum where initial exposure may lead to increased and compulsive drug taking. This evolution of drug taking behavior (initial reward-based use leads to habit-based use) is accompanied by a parallel evolution in neural-network involvement (initial limbic ventral striatal involvement leads to more dorsal striatal governance). This process often occurs despite adverse consequences and at the expense of more socially or biologically important behaviors. Stress and anxiety (both of which are also fueled by the limbic system), in fact precipitate this process and render people who use drugs recreationally particularly vulnerable to risky drug use and substance use disorder.

To understand how the behavioral repertoire becomes subverted, it is necessary to consider the structures involved in decision-making and in generating motivated behavior. The research questions that can be addressed by using animal models are necessarily different than those that can be asked with human subjects. Animal studies have a number of advantages and are well suited for the investigation of the site of action of drug reinforcement through the use of receptor agonists, antagonists, and lesion techniques. Animal self-administration studies allow tight control over many variables that could possibly affect the addiction process including genetics, frequency of access, dosage, route of administration, and drug history. Understandably, this type of control is unattainable in the investigation of humans with addiction; however, human studies allow for the examination of aspects of addiction that are uniquely human. Addiction is a condition that expresses in the real world and thus encompasses many different facets, such as polydrug use, co-occurrence with other disorders, predisposition, drug use history, and environmental context. Thus, the literature on human unhealthy substance use and addiction offers quite different insights.

Imaging technology has been a key tool for identifying several subcortical and cortical brain regions important for addiction (see **Fig. 3-7** for highlights). The widely used types of functional imaging are positron emission tomography (PET) and functional magnetic resonance imaging (fMRI). These technologies have very different temporal resolutions and lend themselves to assessing distinct aspects of brain function. PET uses a radioisotope that is introduced into the body and binds to specific receptors, transporters, and enzymes. Specific ligands can be visualized, thereby offering insights into drug distribution and changes in receptor mechanism in vivo. fMRI offers much greater temporal and spatial resolution. Changes in the fMRI signal can be assessed on the order of seconds rather than minutes, making it possible to detect metabolic changes associated with transient cognitive demands or craving states.

Early imaging studies asked the questions, "Where does cocaine act in the brain, and how does it affect brain function?" One of the first imaging studies on individuals addicted to cocaine was conducted by Volkow et al.[123] in 1988. She found that individuals who chronically use cocaine have decreased relative cerebral blood flow (as measured by PET) in the PFC. Volkow later showed changes in metabolic activity (as measured by fluorodeoxyglucose), which depended on the time since the last drug experience. An overall increase in metabolic activity was observed in frontal brain regions during the first week of withdrawal,[124] whereas decreases in metabolic activity were found after several months.[125] PET has also been used to map the binding sites of cocaine in the human brain. Fowler et al.[126] conducted the first of these studies showing high cocaine binding in the corpus striatum in nondrug using human subjects.

More recent work with PET has shown that striatal dopamine D_2 receptor binding is reduced in those who use cocaine,[127] heroin,[128] and methamphetamine[129] and also in DSM-IV defined alcohol dependence.[130] This area of work is in good concordance with nonhuman primate PET studies showing decreased D_2 receptor availability in animals that are more susceptible to the reinforcing aspects of cocaine.[131,132]

fMRI studies have been used to examine transient drug states, such as drug craving and the "rush" feeling associated with drug use. Much of the work in this area has been done by giving cocaine-addicted subjects (because of ethical limitations on giving drug-naive people cocaine) infusions of cocaine and other stimulants while in the fMRI scanner.

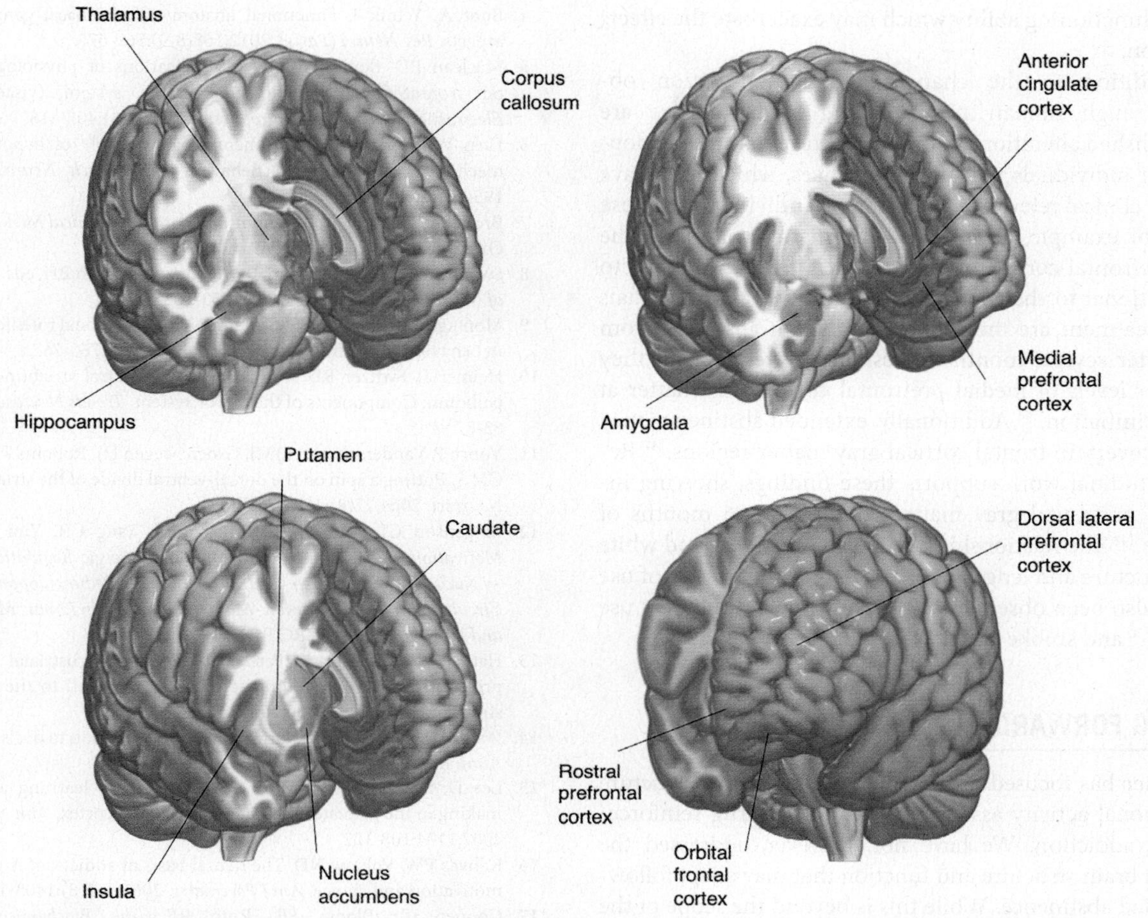

Figure 3-7. Diagram illustrating brain regions commonly identified as important for addiction in human neuroimaging studies. The *right* hemisphere (cutout side) images primarily highlight deeper and limbic brain areas. The *left* hemisphere (whole side) images primarily highlight prefrontal brain areas.

Breiter et al.[133] found that self-reports of craving for the upcoming infusion of cocaine corresponded to increases in activity in the NAcc and decreases in activity in the amygdala. He also observed increases in the ventral tegmentum (VTA and substantia nigra), pons, basal forebrain, caudate, and cingulate that correlated with self-reported feelings of rush. Further work into drug craving has shown that drug-addicted individuals have greater increases in brain activity in limbic areas and the PFC following the presentation of drug-associated cues (such as pictures of drugs and drug paraphernalia) when compared with nondrug-addicted people[134-136] and decreased responsiveness when presented with nondrug reinforcers (eg, sexually evocative cues).[137]

One brain area, the insula, has recently been recognized as having an essential role in the detection of interoceptive cues. These cues can also provoke powerful cravings for drugs and are a key component in the addiction process. Naqvi et al.[138] discovered that individuals with physiologic nicotine dependence with lesions to their insula reported disruption of smoking at a far greater frequency than did patients with lesions to other brain areas. Furthermore, those individuals who acquired insula damage were more likely to quit smoking easily and immediately and to remain abstinent. Remarkably, drug-associated cues can produce limbic activation in individuals who use cocaine even when these stimuli are not consciously perceived. Childress et al.[139] presented stimuli for only 33 ms. Although this short presentation was too brief for the image to be correctly identified, the drug-related stimuli nonetheless produced an increase in activity in the ventral pallidum and amygdala. The intensity of this response also predicted the magnitude of the subject's affective response when later shown visible versions of the same cues.[139] These data suggest that drug cues can stimulate drug craving even before there is conscious awareness. Childress et al.[139] speculate that "by the time the motivational state is experienced and labeled as conscious desire, the ancient limbic reward circuitry already has a running start." The imaging field now provides concrete evidence of limbic involvement in drug craving that fits well with the wealth of evidence for animal studies. Finally, activity of the medial and lateral prefrontal cortices has been linked to suboptimal performance on complex decision making and working memory tasks in people with chronic alcohol,[140] cannabis,[141] and cocaine[142] use disorders. These data suggest that long-term heavy drug use may result in compromised executive functioning ability which may exacerbate the effects of addiction.

In addition to the changes in brain function observed through human neuroimaging studies, there are well-established alterations in brain structure in multiple populations of individuals who use substances, which may have important clinical relevance to treatment. Individuals who use cocaine, for example, have lower gray matter volume in the medial prefrontal cortex than controls,[143,144] which appears to be proportional to their length of cocaine use.[145] Individuals seeking treatment are more likely to remain abstinent from cocaine after several months of residential treatment if they had higher levels of medial prefrontal cortex gray matter at treatment initiation.[146] Additionally, extended abstinence may lead to recovery in frontal cortical gray matter regions.[147] Recent longitudinal work supports these findings, showing increases in prefrontal gray matter volume over 6 months of abstinence.[148] The relationship between altered gray and white matter structure and length of use as well as recurrence of use rates has also been observed in people who compulsively use alcohol[149,150] and smoke tobacco.[151,152]

MOVING FORWARD

This chapter has focused on the alterations in brain structure and functional activity associated with initial drug reinforcement and addiction. We have not, however, addressed the changes in brain structure and function that may adapt following extended abstinence. While this is beyond the scope of the present chapter, there are many studies, which suggest that the limbic system is a critical biomarker for abstinence.[153-155] Additionally, as we attempt to bridge the neurobiological findings from clinical and preclinical studies of chronic drug use to abstinence, it will also be important to integrate the literature on behavioral patterns that predict successful recovery. Through the integration of these components, we will be much more likely to generate individually tailored therapies, both pharmacological and behavioral, for those that find themselves on the continuum of addiction, from vulnerable adolescents to treatment-seeking individuals that recurrently return to previous use.

ACKNOWLEDGEMENTS

This chapter represents an update and revision of previous chapters in this series, most recently by Dr David Roberts from the last edition. We are indebted to Dr Roberts for his work and retain much of his prose in this current edition.

REFERENCES

1. Zahm DS. The evolving theory of basal forebrain functional-anatomical 'macrosystems.' *Neurosci Biobehav Rev.* 2006;30(2):148-172.
2. Gerfen CR. The neostriatal mosaic: Multiple levels of compartmental organization in the basal ganglia. *Annu Rev Neurosci.* 1992;15:285-320.
3. Squire LR, Stark CE, Clark RE. The medial temporal lobe. *Annu Rev Neurosci.* 2004;27:279-306.
4. Buot A, Yelnik J. Functional anatomy of the basal ganglia: Limbic aspects. *Rev Neurol (Paris).* 2012;168(8-9):569-575.
5. Maclean PD. Some psychiatric implications of physiological studies on frontotemporal portion of limbic system (visceral brain). *Electroencephalogr Clin Neurophysiol.* 1952;4(4):407-418.
6. Hess WR, Akert K. Experimental data on role of hypothalamus in mechanism of emotional behavior. *AMA Arch Neurol Psychiatry.* 1955;73(2):127-129.
7. Brodal A. *Neurological Anatomy in Relation to Clinical Medicine.* 2nd ed. Oxford University Press; 1969.
8. Swanson LW. Limbic system. In: Adelman G, Smith BH, eds. *Encyclopedia of Neuroscience.* Elsevier; 1987:1053-1055.
9. Montague PR, Hyman SE, Cohen JD. Computational roles for dopamine in behavioural control. *Nature.* 2004;431(7010):760-767.
10. Heimer L, Switzer RD, Vanhoesen GW. Ventral striatum and ventral pallidum: Components of the motor system. *Trends Neurosci.* 1982;5(3): 83-87.
11. Voorn P, Vanderschuren LJMJ, Groenewegen HJ, Robbins TW, Pennartz CMA. Putting a spin on the dorsal-ventral divide of the striatum. *Trends Neurosci.* 2004;27(8):468-474.
12. Mogenson GJ, Brudzynski SM, Wu M, Yang CR, Yim CCY. *From Motivation to Action: A Review of Dopaminergic Regulation of Limbic → Nucleus Accumbens → Ventral Pallidum → Pedunculopontine Nucleus Circuitries Involved in Limbic-Motor Integration, in Limbic Motor Circuits and Neuropsychiatry.* CRC Press; 1993:193-236.
13. Haber SN, Fudge JL, McFarland NR. Striatonigrostriatal pathways in primates form an ascending spiral from the shell to the dorsolateral striatum. *J Neurosci.* 2000;20(6):2369-2382.
14. Wallis JD. Orbitofrontal cortex and its contribution to decision-making. *Annu Rev Neurosci.* 2007;30:31-56.
15. Lee D, Seo H. Mechanisms of reinforcement learning and decision making in the primate dorsolateral prefrontal cortex. *Ann N Y Acad Sci.* 2007;1104:108-122.
16. Kalivas PW, Volkow ND. The neural basis of addiction: A pathology of motivation and choice. *Am J Psychiatry.* 2005;162(8):1403-1413.
17. Cooper JR, Bloom FE, Roth RE. *The Biochemical Basis of Neuropharmacology.* 8th ed. Oxford University Press; 2003.
18. Dahlstroem A, Fuxe K. Evidence for the existence of monoamine-containing neurons in the central nervous system. I. Demonstration of monoamines in the cell bodies of brain stem neurons. *Acta Physiol Scand Suppl.* 1964;(Suppl. 232):1-55.
19. Dahlstroem A, Fuxe K. Evidence for the existence of monoamine neurons in the central nervous system. II. Experimentally induced changes in the intraneuronal amine levels of bulbospinal neuron systems. *Acta Physiol Scand Suppl.* 1965;(Suppl 247):1-36.
20. Le Dain G, Campbell IL, Lehmann HE, Stein JP, Bertrand MA. *The Final Report of the Canadian Government Commission of Inquiry into the Non-Medical Use of Drugs.* Information Canada; 1972.
21. Brady JV. Animal models for assessing drugs of abuse. *Neurosci Biobehav Rev.* 1991;15(1):35-43.
22. Schuster CR, Johanson CE. An analysis of drug-seeking behavior in animals. *Neurosci Biobehav Rev.* 1981;5(3):315-323.
23. Deneau G, Yanagita T, Seevers MH. Self-administration of psychoactive substances by the monkey. *Psychopharmacologia.* 1969;16(1):30-48.
24. Thompson T, Schuster CR. Morphine self-administration, food-reinforced, and avoidance behaviors in rhesus monkeys. *Psychopharmacologia.* 1964;5:87-94.
25. Weeks JR. Experimental morphine addiction: Method for automatic intravenous injections in unrestrained rats. *Science.* 1962;138 (3537):143-144.
26. Olds J, Yuwiler A, Olds ME, Yun C. Neurohumors in hypothalamic substrates of reward. *Am J Physiol.* 1964;207:242-254.
27. Phillips AG, Mora F, Rolls ET. Intracerebral self-administration of amphetamine by rhesus monkeys. *Neurosci Lett.* 1981;24(1):81-86.
28. Bozarth MA, Wise RA. Intracranial self-administration of morphine into the ventral tegmental area in rats. *Life Sci.* 1981;28(5): 551-555.

29. Comer SD, Turner DM, Carroll ME. Effects of food deprivation on cocaine base smoking in rhesus monkeys. *Psychopharmacology (Berl).* 1995;119(2):127-132.
30. Davis WM, Smith SG. Effect of haloperidol on (+)-amphetamine self-administration. *J Pharm Pharmacol.* 1975;27(7):540-542.
31. Wilson MC, Schuster CR. The effects of chlorpromazine on psychomotor stimulant self-administration in the rhesus monkey. *Psychopharmacologia.* 1972;26(2):115-126.
32. Yokel RA, Wise RA. Increased lever pressing for amphetamine after pimozide in rats: Implications for a dopamine theory of reward. *Science.* 1975;187(4176):547-549.
33. Yokel RA, Wise RA. Attenuation of intravenous amphetamine reinforcement by central dopamine blockade in rats. *Psychopharmacology (Berl).* 1976;48(3):311-318.
34. De Wit H, Wise RA. Blockade of cocaine reinforcement in rats with the dopamine receptor blocker pimozide, but not with the noradrenergic blockers phentolamine or phenoxybenzamine. *Can J Psychol.* 1977;31(4):195-203.
35. Wise RA. Catecholamine theories of reward: A critical review. *Brain Res.* 1978;152(2):215-247.
36. Wise RA, Bozarth MA. Brain substrates for reinforcement and drug self-administration. *Prog Neuropsychopharmacol.* 1981;5(5-6):467-474.
37. Roberts DC, Mason ST, Fibiger HC. 6-OHDA lesion to the dorsal noradrenergic bundle alters morphine-induced locomotor activity and catalepsy. *Eur J Pharmacol.* 1978;52(2):209-214.
38. Caine SB, Koob GF. Effects of mesolimbic dopamine depletion on responding maintained by cocaine and food. *J Exp Anal Behav.* 1994;61(2):213-221.
39. Lyness WH, Friedle NM, Moore KE. Destruction of dopaminergic nerve terminals in nucleus accumbens: Effect on d-amphetamine self-administration. *Pharmacol Biochem Behav.* 1979;11(5):553-556.
40. DCS R, Koob GF, Klonoff P, Fibiger HC. Extinction and recovery of cocaine self-administration following 6-hydroxydopamine lesions of the nucleus accumbens. *Pharmacol Biochem Behav.* 1980;12(5):781-787.
41. Roberts DCS, Corcoran ME, Fibiger HC. Recovery of cocaine self-administration after 6-OHDA lesion of the n.accumbens correlates with residual dopamine levels. In: Usdin E, Kopin IJ, Barchas J, eds. *Catecholamines: Basic and Clinical Frontiers*. Pergamon; 1979:1774-1776.
42. McGregor A, Baker G, Roberts DC. Effect of 6-hydroxydopamine lesions of the amygdala on intravenous cocaine self-administration under a progressive ratio schedule of reinforcement. *Brain Res.* 1994;646(2):273-278.
43. McGregor A, Baker G, Roberts DC. Effect of 6-hydroxydopamine lesions of the medial prefrontal cortex on intravenous cocaine self-administration under a progressive ratio schedule of reinforcement. *Pharmacol Biochem Behav.* 1996;53(1):5-9.
44. McGregor A, Roberts DC. Dopaminergic antagonism within the nucleus accumbens or the amygdala produces differential effects on intravenous cocaine self-administration under fixed and progressive ratio schedules of reinforcement. *Brain Res.* 1993;624(1-2):245-252.
45. McGregor A, Roberts DC. Effect of medial prefrontal cortex injections of SCH 23390 on intravenous cocaine self-administration under both a fixed and progressive ratio schedule of reinforcement. *Behav Brain Res.* 1995;67(1):75-80.
46. Kelly PH, Iversen SD. Selective 6OHDA-induced destruction of mesolimbic dopamine neurons: abolition of psychostimulant-induced locomotor activity in rats. *Eur J Pharmacol.* 1976;40(1):45-56.
47. Van Rossum JM. Mode of action of psychomotor stimulant drugs. *Int Rev Neurobiol.* 1970;12:307-383.
48. Pijnenburg AJ, van Rossum JM. Letter: Stimulation of locomotor activity following injection of dopamine into the nucleus accumbens. *J Pharm Pharmacol.* 1973;25(12):1003-1005.
49. Pijnenburg AJ, Honig WM, Van Rossum JM. Inhibition of d-amphetamine-induced locomotor activity by injection of haloperidol into the nucleus accumbens of the rat. *Psychopharmacologia.* 1975;41(2):87-95.
50. Randrup A, Munkvad I. Stereotyped behavior. *Pharmacol Ther B.* 1975;1(4):757-768.
51. Ellinwood EH Jr, Kilbey MM. Amphetamine stereotypy: the influence of environmental factors and prepotent behavioral patterns on its topography and development. *Biol Psychiatry.* 1975;10(1):3-16.
52. Lyon M, Robbins TW The action of central nervous system stimulant drugs: A general theory concerning amphetamine effects. *Curr Dev Psychopharmacology.* 1975;2:81-163.
53. Ahn S, Phillips AG. Modulation by central and basolateral amygdalar nuclei of dopaminergic correlates of feeding to satiety in the rat nucleus accumbens and medial prefrontal cortex. *J Neurosci.* 2002;22(24):10958-10965.
54. Ahn S, Phillips AG. Independent modulation of basal and feeding-evoked dopamine efflux in the nucleus accumbens and medial prefrontal cortex by the central and basolateral amygdalar nuclei in the rat. *Neuroscience.* 2003;116(1):295-305.
55. Phillips AG, Ahn S, Howland JG. Amygdalar control of the mesocorticolimbic dopamine system: Parallel pathways to motivated behavior. *Neurosci Biobehav Rev.* 2003;27(6):543-554.
56. Ågmo A, Galvan A, Talamantes B. Reward and reinforcement produced by drinking sucrose: 2 processes that may depend on different neurotransmitters. *Pharmacol Biochem Behav.* 1995;52(2):403-414.
57. Ågmo A, Federman I, Navarro V, Padua M, Velazquez G. Reward and reinforcement produced by drinking water: Role of opioids and dopamine receptor subtypes. *Pharmacol Biochem Behav.* 1993;46(1):183-194.
58. Fibiger HC, Nomikos GG, Pfaus JG, Damsma G. Sexual behavior, eating and mesolimbic dopamine. *Clin Neuropharmacol.* 1992;15(Suppl 1 Pt A):566A-567A.
59. Mitchell JB, Gratton A. Involvement of mesolimbic dopamine neurons in sexual behaviors: Implications for the neurobiology of motivation. *Rev Neurosci.* 1994;5(4):317-329.
60. Gratton A, Wise RA. Brain stimulation reward in the lateral hypothalamic medial forebrain bundle: Mapping of boundaries and homogeneity. *Brain Res.* 1983;274(1):25-30.
61. Tzschentke TM. The medial prefrontal cortex as a part of the brain reward system. *Amino Acids.* 2000;19(1):211-219.
62. Wise RA. Brain reward circuitry: Insights from unsensed incentives. *Neuron.* 2002;36(2):229-240.
63. White FJ. Synaptic regulation of mesocorticolimbic dopamine neurons. *Annu Rev Neurosci.* 1996;19:405-436.
64. Schultz W. Behavioral dopamine signals. *Trends Neurosci.* 2007;30(5):203-210.
65. Phillipson OT. A Golgi study of the ventral tegmental area of Tsai and interfascicular nucleus in the rat. *J Comp Neurol.* 1979;187(1):99-115.
66. Ramon-Moliner E, Nauta WJ. The isodendritic core of the brain stem. *J Comp Neurol.* 1966;126(3):311-335.
67. Geisler S, Zahm DS. Afferents of the ventral tegmental area in the rat-anatomical substratum for integrative functions. *J Comp Neurol.* 2005;490(3):270-294.
68. Martin M, Hurley RA, Taber KH. Is opiate addiction associated with longstanding neurobiological changes? *J Neuropsychiatry Clin Neurosci.* 2007;19(3):242-248.
69. Dykstra LA, Preston KL, Bigelow GE. Discriminative stimulus and subjective effects of opioids with mu and kappa activity: Data from laboratory animals and human subjects. *Psychopharmacology.* 1997;130(1):14-27.
70. Koob GF, Vaccarino FJ, Amalric M, Bloom FE. Neurochemical substrates for opiate reinforcement. *NIDA Res Monogr.* 1986;71:146-164.
71. Mucha RF, Herz A. Motivational properties of kappa and mu opioid receptor agonists studied with place and taste preference conditioning. *Psychopharmacology (Berl).* 1985;86(3):274-280.
72. Tang AH, Collins RJ. Behavioral effects of a novel kappa opioid analgesic, U-50488, in rats and rhesus monkeys. *Psychopharmacology (Berl).* 1985;85(3):309-314.
73. Mansour A, Khachaturian H, Lewis ME, Akil H, Watson SJ. Autoradiographic differentiation of mu, delta, and kappa opioid receptors in the rat forebrain and midbrain. *J Neurosci.* 1987;7(8):2445-2464.
74. Wise RA, Hoffman DC. Localization of drug reward mechanisms by intracranial injections. *Synapse.* 1992;10(3):247-263.

75. Olds ME. Hypothalamic substrate for the positive reinforcing properties of morphine in the rat. *Brain Res.* 1979;168(2):351-360.
76. Olds ME, Williams KN. Self-administration of D-Ala2-Met-enkephalinamide at hypothalamic self-stimulation sites. *Brain Res.* 1980;194(1):155-170.
77. Olds J, Milner P. Positive reinforcement produced by electrical stimulation of septal area and other regions of rat brain. *J Comp Physiol Psychol.* 1954;47(6):419-427.
78. Bozarth MA, Wise RA. Localization of the reward-relevant opiate receptors. *NIDA Res Monogr.* 1982;41:158-164.
79. Olds ME. Reinforcing effects of morphine in the nucleus accumbens. *Brain Res.* 1982;237(2):429-440.
80. Goeders NE, Lane JD, Smith JE. Self-administration of methionine enkephalin into the nucleus accumbens. *Pharmacol Biochem Behav.* 1984;20(3):451-455.
81. van der Kooy D, Mucha RF, O'Shaughnessy M, Bucenieks P. Reinforcing effects of brain microinjections of morphine revealed by conditioned place preference. *Brain Res.* 1982;243(1):107-117.
82. Le Merrer J, Gavello-Baudy S, Galey D, Cazala P. Morphine self-administration into the lateral septum depends on dopaminergic mechanisms: Evidence from pharmacology and Fos neuroimaging. *Behav Brain Res.* 2007;180(2):203-217.
83. David V, Cazala P. Anatomical and pharmacological specificity of the rewarding effect elicited by microinjections of morphine into the nucleus accumbens of mice. *Psychopharmacology.* 2000;150(1):24-34.
84. David V, Durkin TP, Cazala P. Differential effects of the dopamine D-2/D-3 receptor antagonist sulpiride on self-administration of morphine into the ventral tegmental area or the nucleus accumbens. *Psychopharmacology.* 2002;160(3):307-317.
85. Devine DP, Wise RA. Self-administration of morphine, DAMGO, and DPDPE into the ventral tegmental area of rats. *J Neurosci.* 1994;14(4):1978-1984.
86. Welzl H, Kuhn G, Huston JP. Self-administration of small amounts of morphine through glass micropipettes into the ventral tegmental area of the rat. *Neuropharmacology.* 1989;28(10):1017-1023.
87. Phillips AG, LePiane FG. Reinforcing effects of morphine microinjection into the ventral tegmental area. *Pharmacol Biochem Behav.* 1980;12(6):965-968.
88. Jenck F, Gratton A, Wise RA. Opioid receptor subtypes associated with ventral tegmental facilitation of lateral hypothalamic brain stimulation reward. *Brain Res.* 1987;423(1-2):34-38.
89. Broekkamp CL, Phillips AG. Facilitation of self-stimulation behavior following intracerebral microinjections of opioids into the ventral tegmental area. *Pharmacol Biochem Behav.* 1979;11(3):289-295.
90. Stewart J. Reinstatement of heroin and cocaine self-administration behavior in the rat by intracerebral application of morphine in the ventral tegmental area. *Pharmacol Biochem Behav.* 1984;20(6):917-923.
91. Corrigall WA, Linseman MA. Conditioned place preference produced by intra-hippocampal morphine. *Pharmacol Biochem Behav.* 1988;30(3):787-789.
92. Koob GF, Pettit HO, Ettenberg A, Bloom FE. Effects of opiate antagonists and their quaternary derivatives on heroin self-administration in the rat. *J Pharmacol Exp Ther.* 1984;229(2):481-486.
93. Britt MD, Wise RA. Ventral tegmental site of opiate reward: antagonism by a hydrophilic opiate receptor blocker. *Brain Res.* 1983;258(1):105-108.
94. Corrigall WA, Vaccarino FJ. Antagonist treatment in nucleus accumbens or periaqueductal grey affects heroin self-administration. *Pharmacol Biochem Behav.* 1988;30(2):443-450.
95. Vaccarino FJ, Bloom FE, Koob GF. Blockade of nucleus accumbens opiate receptors attenuates intravenous heroin reward in the rat. *Psychopharmacology.* 1985;86(1-2):37-42.
96. Walker JR, Ahmed SH, Gracy KN, Koob GF. Microinjections of an opiate receptor antagonist into the bed nucleus of the stria terminalis suppress heroin self-administration in dependent rats. *Brain Re.* 2000; 854(1-2):85-92.
97. Corrigall WA. Heroin self-administration: Effects of antagonist treatment in lateral hypothalamus. *Pharmacol Biochemand Behav.* 1987;27(4):693-700.
98. Vaccarino FJ, Pettit HO, Bloom FE, Koob GF. Effects of intracerebroventricular administration of methyl naloxonium chloride on heroin self-administration in the rat. *Pharmacol Biochem Behav.* 1985;23(3):495-498.
99. Zito KA, Vickers G, Roberts DCS. Disruption of cocaine and heroin self-administration following kainic acid lesions of the nucleus accumbens. *Pharmacol Biochem Behav.* 1985;23(6):1029-1036.
100. Britt MD, Wise RA. Opiate rewarding action: Independence of the cells of the lateral hypothalamus. *Brain Res.* 1981;222(1):213-217.
101. Alderson HL, Parkinson JA, Robbins TW, Everitt BJ. The effects of excitotoxic lesions of the nucleus accumbens core or shell regions on intravenous heroin self-administration in rats. *Psychopharmacology.* 2001;153(4):455-463.
102. Hutcheson DM, Parkinson JA, Robbins TW, Everitt BJ. The effects of nucleus accumbens core and shell lesions on intravenous heroin self-administration and the acquisition of drug-seeking behaviour under a second-order schedule of heroin reinforcement. *Psychopharmacology.* 2001;153(4):464-472.
103. Martin TJ, Kim SA, Lyupina Y, Smith JE. Differential involvement of mu-opioid receptors in the rostral versus caudal nucleus accumbens in the reinforcing effects of heroin in rats: Evidence from focal injections of beta-funaltrexamine. *Psychopharmacology.* 2002;161(2):152-159.
104. Ettenberg A, Pettit HO, Bloom FE, Koob GF. Heroin and cocaine intravenous self-administration in rats: Mediation by separate neural systems. *Psychopharmacology.* 1982;78(3):204-209.
105. Gerber GJ, Wise RA. Pharmacological regulation of intravenous cocaine and heroin self-administration in rats: A variable dose paradigm. *Pharmacol Biochem and Behav.* 1989;32(2):527-531.
106. Johnson SW, North RA. Opioids excite dopamine neurons by hyperpolarization of local interneurons. *J Neurosci.* 1992;12(2):483-488.
107. Hemby SE, Martin TJ, Co C, Dworkin SI, Smith JE. The effects of intravenous heroin administration on extracellular nucleus-accumbens dopamine concentrations as determined by in-vivo microdialysis. *J Pharmacol Exp Ther.* 1995;273(2):591-598.
108. Lecca D, Valentini V, Cacciapaglia F, Acquas E, Di Chiara G. Reciprocal effects of response contingent and noncontingent intravenous heroin on in vivo nucleus accumbens shell versus core dopamine in the rat: a repeated sampling microdialysis study. *Psychopharmacology.* 2007;194(1):103-116.
109. Bozarth MA, Wise RA. Involvement of the ventral tegmental dopamine system in opioid and psychomotor stimulant reinforcement. *NIDA Res Monogr.* 1986;67:190-196.
110. Pettit HO, Ettenberg A, Bloom FE, Koob GF. Destruction of dopamine in the nucleus accumbens selectively attenuates cocaine but not heroin self-administration in rats. *Psychopharmacology (Berl).* 1984;84(2):167-173.
111. Gerrits MAFM, VanRee JM. Effect of nucleus accumbens dopamine depletion on motivational aspects involved in initiation of cocaine and heroin self-administration in rats. *Brain Res.* 1996;713(1-2):114-124.
112. Herkenham M, Lynn AB, Little MD, et al. Cannabinoid receptor localization in brain. *Proc Natl Acad Sci USA.* 1990;87(5):1932-1936.
113. Abood ME, Martin BR. Neurobiology of marijuana abuse. *Trends Pharmacol Sci.* 1992;13(5):201-206.
114. Onaivi ES. Neuropsychobiological evidence for the functional presence and expression of cannabinoid CB2 receptors in the brain. *Neuropsychobiology.* 2006;54(4):231-246.
115. Justinova Z, Tanda G, Redhi GH, Goldberg SR. Self-administration of delta9-tetrahydrocannabinol (THC) by drug naive squirrel monkeys. *Psychopharmacology (Berl).* 2003;169(2):135-140.
116. Justinova Z, Solinas M, Tanda G, Redhi H, Goldberg SR. The endogenous cannabinoid anandamide and its synthetic analog R(+)-methanandamide are intravenously self-administered by squirrel monkeys. *J Neurosci.* 2005;25(23):5645-5650.
117. Martellotta MC, Cossu G, Fattore L, Gessa GL, Fratta W. Self-administration of the cannabinoid receptor agonist WIN 55,212-2 in drug-naive mice. *Neuroscience.* 1998;85(2):327-330.
118. Fattore L, Cossu G, Martellotta CM, Fratta W. Intravenous self-administration of the cannabinoid CB1 receptor agonist WIN 55,212-2 in rats. *Psychopharmacology (Berl).* 2001;156(4):410-416.

119. Fattore L, Spano MS, Altea S, Angius F, Fadda P, Fratta W. Cannabinoid self-administration in rats: Sex differences and the influence of ovarian function. *Br J Pharmacol.* 2007;152(5):795-804.
120. Justinova Z, Tanda G, Munzar P, Goldberg SR. The opioid antagonist naltrexone reduces the reinforcing effects of delta 9 tetrahydrocannabinol (THC) in squirrel monkeys. *Psychopharmacology (Berl).* 2004;173(1-2): 186-194.
121. Fadda P, Scherma M, Spano MS, et al. Cannabinoid self-administration increases dopamine release in the nucleus accumbens. *Neuroreport.* 2006;17(15):1629-1632.
122. Lecca D, Cacciapaglia F, Valentini V, Di Chiara G. Monitoring extracellular dopamine in the rat nucleus accumbens shell and core during acquisition and maintenance of intravenous WIN 55,212-2 self-administration. *Psychopharmacology (Berl).* 2006;188(1):63-74.
123. Volkow ND, Mullani N, Gould KL, Adler S, Krajewski K. Cerebral blood flow in chronic cocaine users: A study with positron emission tomography. *Br J Psychiatry.* 1988;152:641-648.
124. Volkow ND, Fowler JS, Wolf AP, et al. Changes in brain glucose metabolism in cocaine dependence and withdrawal. *Am J Psychiatry.* 1991;148(5):621-626.
125. Volkow ND, Hitzemann R, Wang GJ, et al. Long-term frontal brain metabolic changes in cocaine abusers. *Synapse.* 1992;11(3): 184-190.
126. Fowler JS, Volkow ND, Wolf AP, et al. Mapping cocaine binding sites in human and baboon brain in vivo. *Synapse.* 1989;4(4):371-377.
127. Volkow ND, Fowler JS, Wang GJ, et al. Decreased dopamine D2 receptor availability is associated with reduced frontal metabolism in cocaine abusers. *Synapse.* 1993;14(2):169-177.
128. Wang GJ, Volkow ND, Fowler JS, et al. Dopamine D2 receptor availability in opiate-dependent subjects before and after naloxone-precipitated withdrawal. *Neuropsychopharmacol.* 1997;16(2):174-182.
129. Volkow ND, Chang L, Wang GJ, et al. Low level of brain dopamine D2 receptors in methamphetamine abusers: Association with metabolism in the orbitofrontal cortex. *Am J Psychiatry.* 2001;158(12):2015-2021.
130. Volkow ND, Wang GJ, Fowler JS, et al. Decreases in dopamine receptors but not in dopamine transporters in alcoholics. *Alcohol Clin Exp Res.* 1996;20(9):1594-1598.
131. Morgan D, Grant KA, Gage HD, et al. Social dominance in monkeys: dopamine D2 receptors and cocaine self-administration. *Nat Neurosci.* 2002;5(2):169-174.
132. Nader MA, Morgan D, Gage HD, et al. PET imaging of dopamine D2 receptors during chronic cocaine self-administration in monkeys. *Nat Neurosci.* 2006;9(8):1050-1056.
133. Breiter HC, Gollub RL, Weisskoff RM, et al. Acute effects of cocaine on human brain activity and emotion. *Neuron.* 1997;19(3):591-611.
134. Garavan H, Pankiewicz J, Bloom A, et al. Cue-induced cocaine craving: neuroanatomical specificity for drug users and drug stimuli. *Am J Psychiatry.* 2000;157(11):1789-1798.
135. Maas LC, Lukas SE, Kaufman MJ, et al. Functional magnetic resonance imaging of human brain activation during cue-induced cocaine craving. *Am J Psychiatry.* 1998;155(1):124-126.
136. Wexler BE, Gottschalk CH, Fulbright RK, et al. Functional magnetic resonance imaging of cocaine craving. *Am J Psychiatry.* 2001;158(1): 86-95.
137. Garavan H, Pendergrass JC, Ross TJ, Stein EA, Risinger RC. Amygdala response to both positively and negatively valenced stimuli. *Neuroreport.* 2001;12(12):2779-2783.
138. Naqvi NH, Rudrauf D, Damasio H, Bechara A. Damage to the insula disrupts addiction to cigarette smoking. *Science.* 2007;315(5811): 531-534.
139. Childress AR, Ehrman RN, Wang Z, et al. Prelude to passion: limbic activation by "unseen" drug and sexual cues. *PLoS One.* 2008;3(1): e1506.
140. Wesley MJ, Lile JA, Fillmore MT, Porrino LJ. Neurophysiological capacity in a working memory task differentiates dependent from nondependent heavy drinkers and controls. *Drug Alcohol Depend.* 2017;175: 24-35.
141. Wesley MJ, Hanlon CA, Porrino LJ. Poor decision-making by chronic marijuana users is associated with decreased functional responsiveness to negative consequences. *Psychiatry Res.* 2011;191(1):51-59.
142. Wesley MJ, Lohrenz T, Koffarnus MN, et al. Choosing money over drugs: the neural underpinnings of difficult choice in chronic cocaine users. *J Addict.* 2014;2014:189853.
143. Ersche KD, Jones PS, Williams GB, Turton AJ, Robbins TW, Bullmore ET. Abnormal brain structure implicated in stimulant drug addiction. *Science.* 2012;335(6068):601-604.
144. Matochik JA, London ED, Eldreth DA, Cadet J-L, Bolla KI. Frontal cortical tissue composition in abstinent cocaine abusers: A magnetic resonance imaging study. *Neuroimage.* 2003;19(3):1095-1102.
145. Ide JS, Zhang S, Hu H, Sinha R, Mazure CM, Li C-SR. Cerebral gray matter volumes and low-frequency fluctuation of BOLD signals in cocaine dependence: duration of use and gender difference. *Drug Alcohol Depend.* 2014;134:51-62.
146. Hanlon CA, Dufault DL, Wesley MJ, Porrino LJ. Elevated gray and white matter densities in cocaine abstainers compared to current users. *Psychopharmacology (Berl).* 2011;218(4):681-692.
147. Connolly CG, Bell RP, Foxe JJ, Garavan H. Dissociated grey matter changes with prolonged addiction and extended abstinence in cocaine users. *PLoS One.* 2013;8(3):e59645.
148. Parvaz MA, Moeller SJ, d'Oleire Uquillas F, et al. Prefrontal gray matter volume recovery in treatment-seeking cocaine-addicted individuals: A longitudinal study. *Addict Biol.* 2017;22(5):1391-1401.
149. Infante MA, Eberson SC, Zhang Y, et al. Adolescent binge drinking is associated with accelerated decline of gray matter volume. *Cereb Cortex.* 2021;32(12):2611-2620.
150. McCalley DM, Hanlon CA. Regionally specific gray matter volume is lower in alcohol use disorder: implications for noninvasive brain stimulation treatment. *Alcohol Clin Exp Res.* 2021;45(8):1672-1683.
151. Hanlon CA, Owens MM, Joseph JE, et al. Lower subcortical gray matter volume in both younger smokers and established smokers relative to non-smokers. *Addict Biol.* 2016;21(1):185-195.
152. Pan P, Shi H, Zhong J, et al. Chronic smoking and brain gray matter changes: Evidence from meta-analysis of voxel-based morphometry studies. *Neurol Sci.* 2013;34(6):813-817.
153. Balodis IM, Kober H, Worhunsky PD, et al. Neurofunctional reward processing changes in cocaine dependence during recovery. *Neuropsychopharmacology.* 2016;41(8):2112-2121.
154. Camchong J, Macdonlad AW III, Mueller BA, et al. Changes in resting functional connectivity during abstinence in stimulant use disorder: a preliminary comparison of relapsers and abstainers. *Drug Alcohol Depend.* 2014;139:145-151.
155. Jia ZR, Worhunsky PD, Carroll KM, et al. An initial study of neural responses to monetary incentives as related to treatment outcome in cocaine dependence. *Biol Psych.* 2011;70(6):553-560.

4 Clinical Trials in Substance-Using Populations

Frank Vocci

CHAPTER OUTLINE

- Introduction
- Elements of a clinical trial
- Types of clinical trials
- Features of clinical trials
- The research question dictates various aspects of trial design
- Outcome metrics used in clinical trials
- Monitoring and quality control
- Reporting results in a journal article
- Conclusions

INTRODUCTION

Clinical trials play an important role in the evaluation of interventions designed to prevent, assess, treat, and educate in the field of addiction medicine. The U.S. National Institutes of Health (NIH) defines a clinical trial as "A research study in which one or more human subjects are prospectively assigned to one or more interventions (which may or may not include placebo or other control), to evaluate the effects of those interventions on health-related biomedical or behavioral outcomes." This chapter contains general information on human subjects in clinical trials as well as comments on behavioral and pharmacotherapy trials in populations of individuals who use substances. Reference will be made to the published literature of trials in populations of individuals who use substances as illustrative examples of the designs and outcomes being discussed. NIH trial requirements and Food and Drug Administration (FDA) regulations and guidance documents, especially with clinical trials involving pharmacological interventions, will be noted so the reader can develop an appreciation for trial designs, outcome measures, and clinical trial evidence needed to secure medication approval from the FDA.

ELEMENTS OF A CLINICAL TRIAL

Clinical trials are conducted within a legal-regulatory framework. A proposed clinical trial must be reviewed and approved by an institutional review board (IRB) prior to commencement (ie, http://www.fda.gov/RegulatoryInformation/Guidances/ucm126420.htm#IRBOrg).[1] The role of the IRB is to protect the rights and welfare of human subjects. A principal investigator and co-investigator will submit drafts of the following materials for review: a detailed protocol; surveys, questionnaires, and rating scales that will be used in the trial; an informed consent document; advertising material; qualifications of the investigators; evidence of certification of training in human research for the research staff; and financial disclosure forms for the determination of potential conflict of interest. In trials involving investigational or approved medications, the investigators will also submit evidence of investigational new drug (IND) approval from the FDA, FDA 1572 forms, the investigator's brochure or package insert, the data and safety monitoring plan, or the composition of the Data and Safety Monitoring Board (DSMB, if applicable).

The study protocol contains the following elements: the primary and secondary objectives of the study, inclusion/exclusion criteria, recruitment strategies and participant discontinuation criteria, information on the dosage form, administration schedule, and duration of pharmacotherapy in a medication trial or type, intensity, and duration of behavioral therapy in a behavioral intervention trial, concomitant medications or other treatments allowed (if any), the outcome measures, type and frequency of efficacy and safety assessments, procurement, handling, shipping, and assay of biospecimens, justification of the sample size to be recruited, the proposed statistical analyses, collection of adverse event data and reporting of safety issues to the IRB and other regulatory agencies, participant and trial stopping rules, interactions with the IRB and DSMB, the informed consent process, information on confidentiality of participant information, including certificates of confidentiality that are usually obtained when working with populations of individuals who use substances, data handling and data management procedures, and publication and data sharing intentions. A protocol is a "living document." Changes to a protocol may be made to enhance the safety of the trial participants, for example, lowering the maximum dose or duration of therapy due to adverse events observed in the trial. Changes may also be made to the statistical analysis plan prior to the opening of the trial data set. The NIH has developed a protocol template that they expect prospective grantees to use when filing grants to perform clinical trials.[2] The template outline meets the standards elucidated in the International Conference on Harmonization (ICH) Guidance for Industry, E6 Good Clinical Practice, and Consolidated Guidance (ICH-E6). Thus, the template is acceptable to the FDA for developing protocols to determine the safety and efficacy of medications, including those for treating substance use disorders (SUDs). Details regarding individual studies and the totality of studies necessary for approval by the FDA of a new medication are usually discussed in a series of meetings with the FDA along the medication development pathway.

The informed consent document, which in most instances is a written document, contains the following elements that are detailed in 45 Code of Federal Regulations 46.16[3]: a statement that the trial involves research, the purpose of the research and the expected duration of the participant's involvement, the procedures to be followed and identification of any procedures considered experimental, a description of the risks, a description of the potential benefits to the participants and possibly others, a disclosure of alternative treatments, a statement of the extent of confidentiality of the participant's records, an explanation as to whether any compensation or treatment is available if an injury occurs, an explanation as to whom to contact in the event of questions related to the research and the participant's research rights and contact information in the case of a research-related injury, and a statement that participation is voluntary and the participant can withdraw from the trial at any time without penalty or loss of benefits. Additionally, other elements may be added to the consent form, for example, a statement that the treatment may involve unforeseeable risks either to the participant or fetus, if the participant becomes pregnant, circumstances under which the investigator may discontinue the participants from the trial; additional costs that the participant may incur from trial participation; consequences of withdrawal and procedures for orderly termination; a statement that new findings that may affect the course of the research and participant's willingness to continue will be provided; and the number of expected trial participants to be enrolled. For example, a tapering regimen for a medication that should not be abruptly discontinued will be included in the consent form in the case of a participant's withdrawal from the trial.

The investigator or their co-investigators describe the consent form to the prospective participant and obtain their written consent. The consent form should be written at a 6th-8th grade reading level. The prospective participant must not be under the influence of alcohol or drugs at the time consent is obtained. A written quiz may be given to ensure that the participants understand the purpose of the study and their right to withdraw at any time without prejudice. A copy of the signed consent form is given to the trial participant.

The federal regulations cited above also note that special protections should be given to vulnerable populations, that is, pregnant women, human fetuses, neonates, children, adolescents, and prisoners. Individuals with SUDs are also considered vulnerable and actions must be taken to ensure a lack of coercion and that the participant understands their rights as a study participant. Lack of coercion is often operationalized as keeping payments to participants to be reasonable; for example, $25 per visit with additional fees given for urine testing or blood samples. Payments are made at the end of the study period in increments over several weeks or months. Participants are often asked to provide a drug-free urine sample as a contingent prerequisite to obtain a payment.

There are additional requirements for conducting research in prisoners (45 CFR 46.301 306); for example, the risks involved must not be greater than those that would be acceptable to volunteers without criminal legal history. The Secretary of Health and Human Services has delineated the types of research that can be carried out with individuals under supervision by the criminal legal system, for example, alcohol use disorder and drug use disorder, and, following IRB approval, must approve each study. The approval for studies of individuals under criminal justice supervision has been delegated to the Office of Human Research Protection in the Office of the Secretary of Health and Human Services.

TYPES OF CLINICAL TRIALS

There are three main types of clinical trials that evaluate the impact of an intervention in a clinical population: efficacy, effectiveness, and comparative effectiveness.[4] These trials are on a continuum of control in design and external validity or generalizability to the patient population who has the disorder, with efficacy trials being the most restrictive and controlled but least generalizable and effectiveness trials having high generalizability. Efficacy can be defined as the performance of an intervention under ideal and controlled circumstances, whereas effectiveness refers to its performance under real-world conditions. Each type of clinical trial will be discussed in turn.

Efficacy Trials

Efficacy trials (phase II) compare an intervention to another treatment in a rigorous, controlled design that is optimized for detection of an efficacy signal. For example, in the initial phase II trial evaluating efficacy of varenicline for treatment of alcohol use disorder (AUD),[5] the following inclusion/exclusion criteria usually found in phase II trials were noted: the participants met criteria for diagnosis of an AUD but do not have other SUDs, participants did not have co-occurring psychiatric or medical disorders, and concomitant medications affecting the central nervous system were not allowed. The following features typical of a phase II trial were noted: participants were randomized to the medication or control treatment (placebo), neither the investigators nor the participants knew the treatment assignment (double blinding), the investigators were highly trained in the delivery of the intervention, the doses of the medication were fixed after the initial titration, and the duration of treatment (8-12 weeks) was shorter than a full treatment course; behavioral treatment was minimized and consisted of participants viewing a computerized bibliotherapy platform derived from the Rethinking Drinking program of the National Institute on Alcohol Abuse and Alcoholism (NIAAA), the primary efficacy end point was defined as percent heavy drinking days measured weekly; secondary measures of drinking, craving for alcohol, consequences of drinking, cigarette use, and quality of life outcome measures were defined and assessed, and adverse events were ascertained at clinic visits and during telephone interviews. The advantages of such a design are that it has high internal validity, minimizes potential bias through the random assignment to treatment arms, has a homogenous study population, optimizes efficacy signal detection, and allows investigators to determine rating scales that are sensitive to the effect of the medication. The disadvantages are that it lacks external validity or generalizability to patients most likely to get the medication in clinical settings, and given the usually stringent exclusion criteria, it can underestimate the safety profile of the medication in the ultimate patient population for which it is intended.

Double-blind, placebo-controlled trials are also conducted in phase III efficacy trials with several differences noted between the two phases: in phase III trials a larger sample size is enrolled, there are fewer exclusion criteria so that the study population is more similar to patients seen in clinical practice, a longer duration of treatment is administered, sometimes exceeding 1 year of dosing, fixed dosing, flexible dosing regimens, and titration schemes can be evaluated; concomitant medications may be allowed, and behavioral treatments may mimic the standard of care so that placebo-treated participants are treated ethically. The larger sample size allows the assessment of benefit and risk in the population most likely to get the medication in the real world and improves the chances of discovering serious adverse events that occur at low frequency in the patient population. The FDA and other regulatory agencies usually request a study census of 300 to 600 participants in order to assess event rates that occur in the 0.5% to 5% range (ICH E1 guideline). Studies with 100 participants dosed at levels intended for clinical use for a minimum of 1 year are acceptable to the regulatory agencies to allow indefinite prescribing in the product label of the medication. The multicenter phase III trial of buprenorphine and buprenorphine/naloxone versus placebo serves as an illustration of a phase III trial.[6] The study was conducted in two parts: initially, 326 persons with opioid use disorder were enrolled at eight sites and randomized to fixed doses of buprenorphine tablets (16 mg), buprenorphine/naloxone tablets (16/4 mg), or placebo for 1 month. Participants came to an outpatient clinic Monday through Friday and received take-home doses for the weekend. Participants received HIV counseling and up to 1 hour of substance use counseling per week. After 1 month, the second part began with all remaining participants ($N = 279$) administered buprenorphine for 2 days up to a maximum of 12 mg and then switched to buprenorphine/naloxone in an open-label fashion for an additional 11 months. Four additional clinics admitted 193 new participants for 11 months of dosing. Thus, 472 participants received open-label buprenorphine/naloxone, up to 24/6 mg daily dose, for 11 months, resulting in 92,930 days of exposure to the medication. For the first 2 weeks, participants received their medication at the clinic in the same fashion as part one. Thereafter, they could get a 10-day take-home supply of medication with each clinic visit. Two hundred sixty-one (261) participants completed 6 months of dosing with buprenorphine/naloxone. This trial contained multiple elements of a phase III trial: a large sample size, collection of safety data during 1-year duration of dosing, fixed dosing and doses that are titrated, allowance for take-home medication, random collection of urine samples twice a month, results of the urine tests during part two of the trial were available to investigators, and multiple outpatient settings where the research was conducted.

In some circumstances, large sample, simple trials (LSSTs) are conducted in phase III. In these trials, participants are randomized to treatment groups and are focused on an adverse event of interest, for example, hepatotoxicity that is not resolved with the safety database that has been accumulated in the development of a medication.

Phase IV Trials

LSSTs can also be conducted in phase IV (postapproval) as part of a commitment to evaluate a lingering toxicity concern (FDA premarket safety assessment guidance). Such was the case with the approval of buprenorphine and buprenorphine/naloxone for the management of DSM-IV–defined opioid dependence. The FDA requested a postmarketing study of the hepatic effects of buprenorphine. The study was conducted by the Clinical Trials Network (CTN) of the National Institute on Drug Abuse (NIDA). Twelve hundred sixty-nine participants with DSM-IV defined opioid dependence were randomized to buprenorphine/naloxone or methadone; their serum transaminase levels were followed for 32 weeks.[7] Neither medication was associated with liver damage during the initial 6 months of the study.

Effectiveness Trials

Effectiveness trials assess the impact of an effective therapy in real-world settings. Effectiveness trials are usually conducted in phase IV by practicing clinicians in a heterogeneous population that often has multiple co-occurring disorders. The protocols are usually more flexible with regard to dosing, and concurrent treatment modalities may be permitted. Participants can be randomized to a treatment arm, but the comparison group is often a "treatment-as-usual" group as opposed to a placebo-controlled group.[4] Effectiveness trials evaluate factors at the level of patient, provider, and system that may influence the efficacy of a therapy. Contingency management reinforces a target behavior, either abstinence from substance use or clinic attendance. An example of a behavioral effectiveness study is the addition of contingency management, that is, voucher incentives for abstinence from cocaine or amphetamines added onto treatment as usual (TAU) versus TAU without incentives.[8] Participants randomized to the voucher incentive group remained in treatment longer, had fewer positive urines for stimulants and alcohol, and attended more counseling sessions than the TAU group (all $p = 0.02$). An example of an add-on behavioral therapy to pharmacotherapy trial is the addition of cognitive-behavioral therapy to physician management of 141 patients treated with buprenorphine/naloxone-treated in a primary care clinic.[9] Following randomization to baseline medical management or medical management plus cognitive-behavioral therapy, patients were followed for 24 weeks. The self-reported reduction in opioid use during the trial was similar between the two groups ($p = 0.96$). There was also no difference reported between the groups in terms of maximum consecutive weeks of abstinence ($p = 0.84$). Another example of an add-on pharmacotherapy is a multicenter effectiveness trial of extended-release naltrexone for treatment of opioid use disorder versus TAU. The trial was designed to evaluate whether extended-release naltrexone reduced the likelihood of a return to opioid use in a community-dwelling population with a history of legal system involvement and opioid use disorder.[10] Participants were randomized to extended-release naltrexone with TAU, consisting of brief counseling and referral to treatment programs, or TAU. The percentage of participants experiencing return to opioid use, defined as evidence of >10 days of opioid use in a 28-day period, was lower in the extended-release naltrexone group (43% versus 64%, $p = 0.001$).[11] Moreover, there were no overdose events in the extended-release naltrexone group, while seven overdose events were recorded in the TAU group ($p = 0.02$).

Comparative Effectiveness Studies

Comparative effectiveness studies are a subset of effectiveness studies and have been defined as "the generation of and synthesis of evidence that compares the benefits and harms of alternative methods to prevent, diagnose, treat, and monitor a clinical condition or to improve the delivery of care."[12] The purpose and setting are nearly identical to the purpose and setting of effectiveness studies although the comparator may be a different modality of treatment, for example, medical versus surgical management of coronary artery disease. Rawson et al.[13] compared the effects of 16 weeks of contingency management (CM), cognitive-behavioral therapy (CBT), and the combination of the two therapies (CM + CBT) in 171 individuals with DSM-IV–defined stimulant dependence. Retention was superior in the CM and CM + CBT groups compared to the CBT group, $p < 0.02$. The percentage of study participants achieving 3 weeks of continuous abstinence was also higher in the CM and CM+ CBT groups compared to the CBT group (60%, 69.5% versus 40%, respectively, p, 0.0001). None of the treatments were superior to the others at the week 26 and week 52 follow-up time points. Similar results were reported in a study of CM and CBT in treating patients with opioid use disorder taking methadone who were also using cocaine.[14] A pharmacotherapy example of a comparative effectiveness trial is the comparison of sublingual buprenorphine/naloxone versus extended-release naltrexone in the NIDA CTN (ClinicalTrials.gov # NCT02032433). The primary outcome measure was the estimated time to return to opioid use over 24 weeks. Return to use was defined as 4 consecutive weeks of nonstudy opioid use or 7 consecutive days of self-reported opioid use. Return to opioid use at 24 weeks was greater in the group treated with extended-release naltrexone group (65%) versus the group treated with buprenorphine/naloxone (57%) [hazard ratio = 1.36], primarily due to the higher percentage of participants randomized to naltrexone who failed to complete induction. Rates of return to opioid use between the groups were not significantly different in the participants who were successfully inducted.[15]

FEATURES OF CLINICAL TRIALS

Randomization

As described above, clinical trials often use a randomization scheme to assign participants to different treatment arms. The randomized clinical trial (RCT) is considered to be the gold standard trial design in the assessment of efficacy.[16] The purpose of randomization is to avoid selection bias. Randomization schemes used in SUD trials have been described.[17] Randomization can be as simple as assigning each participant to a treatment arm with equal probability, although this can lead to imbalances in treatment assignment. The most common randomization method used is the stratified permuted block, which allows for balancing of covariates across treatment arms.[16] Block sizes can be varied to minimize the possibility of the investigators deducing the randomization scheme. More complex randomization schemes such as urn randomization attempt to reduce differences in baseline characteristics by adjusting the probability of assignment to a treatment arm based on the degree of current treatment imbalance.[18] Irrespective of the type of randomization scheme used, differences in baseline characteristics of the groups may occur. The degree of influence of the baseline differences on treatment outcome may be estimated using propensity scoring.[19]

Blinding

Blinding refers to the process of concealment of the treatments or group assignments.[20] A single-blind protocol conceals the treatment assignment from the participant but not the investigator. The more common double-blind design masks treatment assignment from both the investigator and the study participant. In placebo-controlled, double-blind studies, the active medication and placebo should appear identical in appearance and taste. Since most medications are bitter, placebo capsules or tablets can match bitterness by adding denatonium benzoate.[21]

Some studies compare two completely different looking medications under blinded conditions. In this instance, participants receive the active medication of one treatment and a placebo treatment of the comparator drug in a balanced fashion. This type of blinding is called by the term "double dummy."

It is not possible to mask treatment assignment in trials comparing different psychosocial therapies. In these types of trials, a new psychosocial therapy is usually compared to an established therapy.

Sample Size, Power, and Effect Size

All clinical trials should have a sufficient sample size to detect treatment differences. The estimation of the sample size required for a clinical trial assessing superiority of a medication versus placebo is based on the characteristics of the population under study, whether there are data from clinical trials in this population suggesting a drug-placebo difference and how variable the difference is across studies and statistical considerations, that is, α, the probability of concluding a difference exists between groups when one does not (false-positive rate also known as type I error), usually set at 5%, whether the trial is one tailed or two tailed; β, the probability of concluding no difference between the groups when one exists (false-negative rate also known as type II error); and the desired power ($1-\beta$) to find a true difference if one exists between the treatments. Power is the ability to detect an effect, if, in fact, an effect actually exists; it is strongly influenced by sample size and projected differences between treatment groups. Sample sizes are usually projected to yield power of 80% or greater so that the false-negative rate is 20% or less. Small pilot trials are not considered useful in determining sample size as the confidence intervals are large.[22] A confidence interval, expressed as a percentage of probability such as 90%, 95%, or 99%, is an interval estimate in which a derived value such as a mean or median might lie. Thus, a large confidence interval suggests a less reliable estimate of the statistical parameter in question and may lead to an underestimation of the necessary sample size. Sample size estimates may utilize previously published response rates, when available. Suppose an investigator wanted to propose a trial of bupropion for the treatment of methamphetamine use disorder. Previous trials had reported end-of-treatment placebo response rates of 7%,[23] 14% (25), and 19% (26). Of note, Elkashef et al.[23] enrolled both individuals who used methamphetamines less-than-daily and those who used daily, while the higher placebo response rates reported by Heinzerling et al.[24] and Anderson et al.[25] were in those who used methamphetamines less-than-daily. Thus, use characteristics may be taken into account when selecting appropriate placebo response rates. The sample size can then be estimated using the placebo response rate and the proposed differential response in the treatment group. In the absence of literature denoting a drug-placebo difference or placebo response rates, the investigator must choose a difference thought to be clinically meaningful. The placebo response rate might be estimated from other clinical trials involving the population of individuals who use a particular substance. Once this is known, the estimated sample size can be calculated.[26] The larger the hypothesized difference between the two groups, the smaller the sample size estimate for the trial response rates in clinical trials can be. Trials in populations of individuals who use substances may have a higher dropout rate than trials in other disciplines. For example, dropout rates were >40% in those who used cocaine in 8-week randomized trials,[27] 47% in a 12-week trial of those who used methamphetamine,[28] 50% in those who smoked cigarettes in a 13-week pharmacotherapy trial,[29] 26% and 54% for patients receiving methadone or buprenorphine in a 24-week trial.[30] Trials with high dropout rates have missing data issues that can compromise the integrity of the findings, likely leading to type II errors. One way to reduce this possibility would be to increase sample sizes to correct for the high dropout rates.

Another form of missing data in clinical trials is data that is missing intermittently during a clinical trial. Three types of intermittent missing data have been characterized.[31,32] These are data missing completely at random (MCAR) defined as being completely unrelated to any constructs being studied, missing at random (MAR) defined as possibly related to observed values but completely unrelated to unobserved outcomes, and missing not at random (MNAR) defined as related to unobserved outcomes. Multiple imputation and full information maximum likelihood models are valid when used to analyze MCAR and MAR data,[33,34] whereas MNAR data should be subjected to sensitivity analyses.[35,36]

Statistical Analysis Plans

Statistical analysis plans should specify the proposed analyses for primary, secondary, and exploratory outcomes. The statistical analysis plan can be modified up to the breaking of the blind in a double-blind trial. The plan should define the intent-to-treat (all randomized participants whether they received the intervention or not and whether they may or may not have had data assessments), the modified intent-to-treat (usually randomized, received the intervention, and had at least one assessment), and the per protocol (usually the adherent population that completed the protocol with minimal or no missing data) populations, state the null hypothesis (no difference between groups) and the alternate hypothesis (there is a difference between groups) for a superiority trial, anticipate missing data and define how the missing data patterns will be analyzed, and describe the methods that could be used for missing data in the determination of efficacy. It should be noted that there is no universal set of recommendations from regulatory agencies as to how to handle missing data (ICH E9 Statistical Principles for Clinical Trials). The statistical analysis plan should describe the monitoring and reporting of adverse events, with particular emphasis on events of significance, that is, deaths, near-deaths, and other SAEs.

Statistical Significance and Effect Sizes

A statistically significant drug-placebo difference obtained in a superiority trial (usually $p < 0.05$) may be due to bias, chance, fraud, or a true effect. Given the possible causes of the statistically significant results, the significance of $p < 0.05$ is commonly but incorrectly interpreted to mean that there is a 5% probability that the null hypothesis is true. Thus, investigators may overestimate the veracity of the findings. To avoid overstating a statistically significant result, it has been recommended to report effect sizes in conjunction with p values.[37] An effect size is a measure of the magnitude of an effect. For example, Cohen's d, defined as the difference between two means divided by the pooled standard deviation, is a measure of effect size.[38] Cohen's d effect sizes are defined as small (0.2), medium (0.5), or large (0.8 or greater).

The reproducibility of the results and the effect size can be tested though replication studies, one of the foundational principles of the scientific method. Reproduction of study results by different investigators in a different set of patients with the disorder adds credence to the findings. In the case of data needed for drug approvals, the concept of "adequate and well-controlled studies" was entered into law in 1962 with the passage of the Kefauver-Harris amendments of the Federal Food, Drug, and Cosmetic Act. Thus, with rare exceptions that are spelled out in the Food and Drug Modernization Act of 1997, the FDA requires replication of study results for drug approvals.[39] NIH has also issued a guidance for investigators to enhance rigor and reproducibility of grant findings.[40] Thus, both the FDA and NIH encourage rigor in designs to enhance the possibility of replication of findings.

THE RESEARCH QUESTION DICTATES VARIOUS ASPECTS OF TRIAL DESIGN

Superiority Designs

In randomized, efficacy, and effectiveness trials, the outcome of interest is whether one intervention comparator produces a superior outcome versus the comparator. For instance, in a double-blind, placebo-controlled efficacy trial, the null hypothesis is that there are no differences between the active and placebo medication groups. If statistically significant differences are found, the null hypothesis is rejected and the alternate hypothesis (medication efficacy) is accepted. In the comparison of buprenorphine 16 mg, buprenorphine/naloxone 16/4 mg, and placebo, the proportion of urine samples negative for opioids in the first month of the trial was 17.8%, 20.7%, and 5.8%, respectively ($p < 0.001$ for both active medication groups).[6] Missing urines were categorized conservatively as "not negative." The reduction in opioid use at 4 weeks was considered to demonstrate efficacy of the buprenorphine and buprenorphine/naloxone tablet formulations over the placebo.

Another type of superiority design is a comparison of a test medication to an active control group. Johnson, Jaffe, and Fudala[41] randomized 162 individuals using heroin to daily doses of 8 mg of sublingual buprenorphine or 20 mg of oral methadone and 60 mg of oral methadone. A double-blind, double-dummy design was used to maintain the blind; that is, participants randomized to the buprenorphine treatment received placebo oral methadone and those randomized to one of the methadone groups received placebo sublingual buprenorphine. (Of note, the double-dummy design is employed to mask treatment assignment when disparate dosage forms are being compared.) Urine samples were collected three times weekly for the 17-week maintenance phase of the study and analyzed for the presence of opioids and cocaine. The buprenorphine, methadone 20 mg, and methadone 60-mg group participants submitted urines that were 53%, 29%, and 44% negative for opioids, respectively. The reductions of opioid use in the buprenorphine group and 60-mg methadone group were superior to the percentage noted in the 20-mg methadone group ($p < 0.001$ buprenorphine versus 20 mg methadone; $p = 0.04$ methadone 60 mg versus methadone 20-mg group). Thus, a superior response in comparison to a dose of an active control is considered to demonstrate efficacy. Moreover, assay sensitivity was demonstrated as a higher dose of methadone was superior to a lower dose of methadone.

Dose-response studies also fall under superiority designs. Since the field of addiction medicine is mostly dealing with patients with chronic conditions (such as SUDs), several doses of a medication should be tested in a parallel, fixed-dose group design. A statistically significant positive slope is considered to be evidence of efficacy of a medication (ICH-E4 dose-response information to support drug registration), although the lowest dose should also have evidence of efficacy from other studies. Multiple, ascending doses of sublingual buprenorphine (1, 4, 8, and 16 mg/d) were assessed for their ability to reduce opioid use in patients with DSM-III defined opioid-dependence.[42] Although the a priori comparison for determination of efficacy was the difference in urines negative for opioids between the 1- and 8-mg dose groups (the 8-mg group had more urines negative for opioids [$p < 0.0001$], and a higher percentage of patients with 13 consecutive negative urines [$p < 0.0001$]), the trial could also have been analyzed for a dose-response relationship. For example, there was a doubling and tripling of the percentage of participants in the 8- and 16-mg groups who achieved 13 consecutive negative urines, respectively, compared to the 1-mg dose group.

Superiority trials may sometimes add a third arm; an active control group. If the active control demonstrates efficacy versus the placebo group, the trial is said to demonstrate "assay sensitivity" as it aids in the interpretation of findings seen with the drug in question. For example, varenicline was tested against bupropion and placebo for efficacy in abstinence from tobacco. Bupropion was more effective than placebo, demonstrating assay sensitivity. Varenicline's efficacy was superior to both bupropion and the placebo groups in this study.[43] Conversely, if the active control fails to demonstrate efficacy versus placebo, it can be considered to be a failed trial rather than a failure to show efficacy if the effect seen with the drug in question also does not separate from placebo responses.

Dose-response relationships can also be studied in behavioral therapy trials. Some CM trials evaluate the "dose" or magnitude of a reinforcer given in response to adherence with the targeted behavior. Petry et al.[44] evaluated two different magnitudes of monetary reinforcement ($250 or $560) in 106 individuals who used cocaine. Both groups reduced their cocaine use relative to standard care. The higher magnitude monetary reinforcement group also had the longest duration of abstinence relative to standard care ($p < 0.05$).

The frequency of counseling given in medications for SUD is another example of assessment of dose-response relationships. One hundred sixty-six participants with DSM-IV–defined opioid-dependence were randomized to standard medical management (SMM) and either once weekly (group 1) or three times weekly medication dispensing (group 2) or enhanced medical management and three times weekly medication dispensing (group 3; Fiellin et al.[45]). The percent negative urine samples for opioids in groups 1, 2, and 3 were 44%, 40%, and 40%, respectively, $p = 0.82$. Enhanced medical management and three times per week dispensing did not increase the treatment response.

Noninferiority Designs

Noninferiority designs are clinical trials that compare two active treatments with the purpose of determining whether the efficacy or effectiveness of one treatment is not worse than the standard established behavioral or pharmacological therapy. Noninferiority trials, previously called equivalence trials, must be of high quality and rigorously conducted. A poorly conducted noninferiority trial could yield a result consistent with noninferiority when a difference between the two treatments could actually exist. Design considerations include the following: (a) what is the noninferiority margin? (b) what is the sample size and power to detect differences between the treatments? (c) how will the blind be maintained? (d) will the study population be similar to those in which the standard treatment was already established? (e) is the population being analyzed the "intent-to-treat" population, a modified "intent-to-treat" population, or a "per protocol" population that was fully compliant with the protocol? In an ITT population, none of the patients are excluded and the patients are analyzed according to the randomization scheme. In other words, for the purposes of ITT analysis, everyone who is randomized in the trial is considered to be part of the trial regardless of whether he or she is dosed or completes the trial; (f) what statistical analyses are being used? and (g) will sensitivity analyses be conducted to test the robustness of the results?

The noninferiority margin can be determined by the treatment effect noted in drug versus placebo superiority trials. Without such data, the noninferiority margin can be established by expert consensus as it was in the case described below. Noninferiority margins can be as high as 50%, but smaller margins in the 20% range certainly meet the FDA guidelines for a noninferiority margin choice.[46] If a 20% margin is chosen, noninferiority of the new treatment may be concluded if the lower bound of the 95% confidence interval (CI) of the difference between the treatments is within the lower bound of the 95% CI of the intent-to-treat population, that is, all randomized participants. The sample size needs to be justified in the protocol and the power should be 90% or greater. It should be appreciated that small sample sizes would bias toward a failure to find differences between the treatments due to a lack of power.

A noninferiority trial of buprenorphine implants versus sublingual buprenorphine is an example of a noninferiority trial in a population of individuals who use opioids.[47] The purpose of the study was to determine whether buprenorphine implants were capable of maintaining low opioid use or abstinence compared to daily sublingual buprenorphine therapy in currently stable patients with DSM-IV–defined opioid-dependence who are taking sublingual buprenorphine/naloxone dose of 8/2 mg or less. Stability was defined as being on a stable dose of buprenorphine/naloxone with abstinence from illicit opioid use for at least 90 days. To maintain the blind, participants were randomized in a 1:1 ratio to buprenorphine implants with placebo sublingual buprenorphine/naloxone tablets or sublingual buprenorphine/naloxone tablets with placebo implants. Further, since the buprenorphine implants were distinguishable from the placebo implants, the study employed two sets of physicians at each of the 21 sites: one group implanted study participants and the other group treated the participants during the 6-month study. Participants were assessed at week 1 and thereafter at 4-week intervals. A total of 10 urine samples were collected, at monthly visits and four times at random during the 6 months of treatment. Treatment response was defined as achieving 4 out of 6 months in which no illicit opioid use was detected, either by urine testing or self-report. Urine was analyzed for multiple opioids (codeine, fentanyl, hydrocodone, hydromorphone, methadone, morphine, oxycodone, and oxymorphone) by liquid chromatography-tandem mass spectrometry. A 20% penalty, that is, considering 20% of missing urines as positive for opioids, was imputed to missing urines only in the buprenorphine implant group, adding to the rigor of the trial. Participants could receive supplemental buprenorphine, if necessary. Opioid craving, withdrawal, and adverse events were also measured.

Power was estimated to be 87.3%, assuming each group had 75% responders. One hundred seventy-seven patients were admitted to the trial. The trial employed a modified intent-to-treat analysis, defined as those randomized to treatment, received implants and sublingual doses of buprenorphine/naloxone or placebo, and had at least one post-baseline assessment.

One hundred sixty-five participants completed the study. The buprenorphine implant and the sublingual buprenorphine groups have 96.4% and 87.6% responders, respectively. The lower bound of the 95% CI was within the lower bound of the study confidence interval, establishing noninferiority. Once noninferiority is established, the group difference can be tested for superiority. The response in the buprenorphine implant group was not only noninferior; it was superior to the response rate in the sublingual group ($p = 0.03$). Sensitivity analyses were conducted; the cumulative 6-month abstinence rate in the buprenorphine implant group (85.7%) was superior to the abstinence rate in the sublingual buprenorphine/naloxone group (71.9%) ($p = 0.03$).

Adaptive Designs

Clinical trials in which sequential assignments of participants to new treatments are made following predetermined decisions rules are called adaptive designs.[48] These designs can more closely replicate the type of care clinicians often provide to patients by allowing those patients to receive sequential treatments contingent upon their clinical response. Adaptive designs take into account the order of treatments and adherence to treatment and response of participants during the trial.[49-51] The Sequential Multiple Assignment Randomized trial (SMART) design has been proposed to address the types of issues facing clinicians in treating patients with SUDs in which multiple treatments, both behavioral and pharmacological, are available. In the simplest model, participants are randomized to a treatment group and are assessed for response/nonresponse at a decision point. Those patients who do not respond can then be assigned an alternate treatment assignment while responders may continue with their treatment. Study participants can also be randomized twice, initially to a treatment group and then following a decision point, to a second randomized assignment. Advantages of the SMART design are that it provides options for study participants who do not respond to one treatment type and it allows an assessment of the potential synergistic effects of a treatment sequence. An example of a SMART design in the substance use field is the treatment of patients with methamphetamine use disorder with injectable naltrexone plus oral bupropion or matching naltrexone and bupropion placebos, randomized 0.26:0.74 for 6 weeks. Treatment response was defined as a participant with at least 3 of 4 urines negative for methamphetamine at the end of the first or second stage. Individuals in the placebo group who did not respond at the end of the first stage were re-randomized to naltrexone plus bupropion or matching placebos for an additional 6 weeks and assessed for response to treatment. The naltrexone plus bupropion group had 13.6% responders versus 2.5 % on the placebo group when the responses for the two stages were combined.[52]

OUTCOME METRICS USED IN CLINICAL TRIALS

Abstinence and/or reduction of alcohol or other substance use are often primary outcome variables in clinical trials involving populations of individuals who use substances. The FDA has a guidance on the development of medications for the treatment of alcohol use disorder that illustrates the FDA's current thinking on outcome measures and trial designs.[53] The FDA advises that trials of treatments for alcohol use disorder should employ randomized, placebo-controlled, superiority designs of at least 6 months duration with a primary end point based on a responder analysis. A responder is either a participant who is abstinent for a significant period of time at the end of a trial, following a negotiated grace period, or a participant who has not experienced any heavy drinking days (defined as having more than four standard drinks for men or three standard drinks for women per drinking occasion). The requirement for the 6-month trial duration is based on literature that abstinence at 6 months predicts abstinence at 5 years,[54] with health benefits accruing to the individual who has achieved abstinence. The FDA's acceptance of the validity of the percent heavy drinking days end point as a surrogate for clinical benefit is based on studies examining alcohol consumption using a graduated frequencies measure from the National Alcohol Surveys,[55] the National Epidemiological Survey on Alcohol and Related Conditions,[56] an analysis of transitioning in and out of problem drinking (defined as at least two of the following: heavy episodic drinking, social consequences, or dependence symptoms according to DSM-IV) in a 7-year longitudinal study,[57] and a pooled analysis of three clinical trials involving people experiencing problems with alcohol.[58] Although an unofficial opinion, an FDA medical reviewer has opined that efficacy trials of medications for treatment of stimulant use should have similar durations and outcome measures.[59] The definition of response in these trials would include those participants exhibiting abstinence of a duration that predicts "ongoing abstinence and/or good psychosocial functioning and physical functioning" and those with less than full abstinence if the remaining level of use "can be considered nonharmful." This is in contrast to the recommendations of a group of research and treatment experts who opined that a 50% reduction in substance use was clinically meaningful.[60] An analysis of several continuous variables of cocaine use (percent days abstinent, percent negative urine samples, maximum days of cocaine abstinence) and one dichotomous variable (at least 3 weeks of abstinence), measured in multiple clinical trials, related these improvements to reduced cocaine use and improvement of functioning on the addiction severity index (ASI)[61] during a 12-month follow-up period.[62] Cocaine abstinence and reduced use of cocaine have also been shown to correlate with decreased levels of endothelin-1 (ET-1), a marker of endothelial dysfunction.[63] Moreover, the number of cocaine use days was correlated to the reduction in ET-1 levels.

Quantification of Substance Use

The measurement of alcohol or other substance use can be by biological assay, self-report, or a combination of the two measures.[64] Urine is the biological fluid most tested for the presence of substances, likely due in part to the noninvasive nature of collecting urine. Relating the measurement of alcohol or other substances in urine is more complex than originally thought. Detection times for alcohol and other substances are reported in **Table 4-1**. Alcohol and most other substances, with the exception of cannabis and PCP, have detection times in urine of 2 to 4 days. Thus, urine sampling once a week would not cover the potential days of use, possibly resulting in falsely concluding that a patient was abstinent. Increasing urine sampling to 3 days per week certainly covers the majority of the week but brings up the problem of frequent research visits and carryover, that is, consecutive semiquantitative urine positive samples in the absence of new use. Quantitative analysis of benzoylecgonine has been proposed as a method to correct carryover in assessment of cocaine.[72] Urine samples and self-reporting can be discrepant for identification of use. An algorithm integrating both quantitative urinalysis of benzoylecgonine and self-reporting of cocaine use has been developed.[64] Finally, clinical trials in populations of individuals who use substances often involve missing data, and urinalysis data are no exception. Missing urines can be imputed as positive, neutral, or negative, leading to different results in terms of percent days abstinent or consecutive days abstinent. The worst-case scenario can produce biased estimates in a

TABLE 4-1 Detection Times for Drugs and Alcohol in Urine Samples

	Detection time	Reference
Alcohol	Ethyl glucuronide median = 66 h, range = 30-110 h	65
Cannabis Single use 1.75% or 3.55% cigarette	THC carboxylate 33 ± 9.2 h or 88 ± 9.5 h	66
Cannabis Chronic use	THC carboxylate Mean excretion time = 46 d Range up to 77 d	67
Cocaine	Benzoylecgonine (150 mg/mL) 93 h	68
Methamphetamine	Methamphetamine (500 ng/mL cutoff) 66.9 ± 7.5 h	69
Heroin 12-mg IV dose	(2000 ng/mL cutoff) 12 h (300 ng/mL cutoff) 24-48 h	70
Oxycodone 20-mg dose	(50 ng/mL cutoff) Oxycodone 30 h Noroxycodone 40 h Oxymorphone 40 h	71

treatment effect. Missing data in the COMBINE study were subjected to five imputation methods: complete case analysis, last observation carried forward, missing = heavy drinking, multiple imputation (MI) method, and full information maximum likelihood (FIML). The MI and FIML produced the least biased estimates of the effect of naltrexone.[73]

Measuring Withdrawal Syndromes

Withdrawal syndromes associated with discontinuation of alcohol, caffeine, cannabis, opioid, sedative-hypnotics, stimulants, and nicotine/tobacco are described in DSM-5.[74] Management of withdrawal symptoms is recognized by the FDA as a potential indication for use of medications in alcohol and opioid withdrawal. Management of nicotine/tobacco withdrawal is considered to be a mechanism affecting efficacy of nicotine replacement therapies.[75] Management of withdrawal for other SUDs would be a potential indication if clinical benefit can be demonstrated; for example, reduction of withdrawal signs and symptoms is associated with concomitant ability to remain abstinent. There are multiple withdrawal scales to measure components of opioid withdrawal: the Short Opiate Withdrawal Scale,[76] the Subjective Opiate Withdrawal Scale and the Objective Opiate Withdrawal Scale,[77] and the Clinical Opiate Withdrawal Scale,[78] Alcohol withdrawal domains can be reliably measured using the Clinical Institute Withdrawal Assessment for Alcohol (CIWA-Ar).[79,80]

Measuring Drug Craving

There is no universal definition of craving. It is usually defined as a conscious awareness of a desire to use a drug.[81] Craving is included in the DSM-5 diagnostic criteria to consider for a SUD and in the ASAM definition of addiction. In the ASAM definition of addiction, craving is noted as a component of addiction whereby the individual has increased hunger for a substance or its rewarding experiences. Craving has a complex relationship with substance use. A full discussion of craving and the limitations of its measurement are beyond the scope of this chapter. Craving can be measured as a single-item construct, but this has been criticized as lacking the breadth to describe dimensional aspects of the experience.[82] Craving can also be measured as a multi-item construct like the questionnaire on smoking urges.[80] In clinical trials, craving is usually measured as a secondary outcome variable that often serves a role in the convergent validity of behavioral findings, that is, reduced craving associated with reduced use or abstinence. Craving can be measured in real time using ecological momentary assessment techniques through mobile devices where study participants are queried on craving and its relationship to drug intake or abstinence.[83]

Measuring Cognitive Function

Although not routinely measured in clinical trials, cognitive functioning may impact outcomes in trials and treatment. Individuals with cognitive deficits have higher discontinuation rates in substance use treatment,[84,85] and populations of individuals who use substances often have deficits in cognitive tests. For a full discussion of cognitive deficits in this population and their possible remediation, the reader is referred to Vocci.[86] A few examples will suffice. Those who use cocaine demonstrated cognitive inflexibility (perseverative responding) in the Wisconsin Card Sorting Test.[87,88] There is some evidence that medications may be able to affect set-shifting, improving cognitive flexibility. A 200-mg dose of modafinil corrected a set-shifting deficit in patients with schizophrenia,[89] suggesting that medications can affect perseverative responding. Attentional bias toward drugs may factor into treatment response. Poor performance on a drug-related Stroop test[90] and a conventional Stroop test by patients who use cocaine[91] predicted treatment discontinuation, although further research is needed to establish causality. A cognitive battery could be used during the screening process to evaluate cognitive deficits and balance groups with respect to cognitive dysfunction. Cognitive tests incorporated into clinical trials would need to show that improvement was not due to practice effects. Additionally, improvements in cognition would need to be accompanied by a clinical benefit to serve as an outcome measure for FDA approval of a medication.

Psychiatric Scales

There are multiple psychiatric scales used in clinical trials. The Structured Clinical Interview for DSM-5 (SCID-5) is used to systematically evaluate psychiatric diagnoses during screening. The SCID-5 has multiple versions, including a research version and a clinical trial version (SCID-5-CT) that can be customized to map onto the inclusion and exclusion criteria of a trial. Other psychiatric rating scales that measure mood disorders used in trials involving populations of individuals who use substances are the Beck Depression Inventory,[92] the Hamilton Depression Rating Scale,[93] and the Hamilton Anxiety Rating Scale.[94] These scales can be incorporated into screening procedures as ancillary inclusion or exclusion criteria, as stratification criteria, or as outcome measures.[95] A wide array of psychiatric scales have been developed for various clinical trials over the decades. For example, scales used in the DSM-5 field studies can be found at www.psychiatry.org/dsm5. A *Handbook of Psychiatric Measures* has also been published.[96]

Addiction-Focused Scales

The Addiction Severity Index (ASI) measures problems associated with addiction in several domains: alcohol and other substance use, medical and psychiatric issues, legal problems, family issues, and employment status.[61,97] Although originally designed to tailor treatment to address problems of patients entering treatment, it has been used in clinical trials to measure alcohol and substance use and associated functioning.[98] A fairly comprehensive and easily accessible resource for instruments used in NIDA studies can be found at https://datashare.nida.nih.gov/assessments.

Reduction of HIV Risk Scales

The Risk Assessment Battery measures behaviors associated with substance use and sexual behavior that are associated with HIV risk. It is one of the scales used in trials with populations of individuals who use substances that measures infectious disease risk. A computerized version exists.[99] Substance and sexual risk sub scores can be evaluated separately. It is usually measured at the beginning and at the end of a trial. The HIV Risk Behavior Scale is an 11-item questionnaire that is also used to quantify substance and sexual risk behaviors that may put the individual at risk of contracting or transmitting HIV.[100]

Quality of Life Measures

The Medical Outcome Study (MOS) 36-item short form health survey (SF-36) assesses eight domains of physical and emotional health.[101] It can be used to assess changes in health across time in a clinical trial and can be used to satisfy the FDA's request to demonstrate that changes in drug use produce medical benefit or improvements in well-being to an individual. Another quality-of-life scale that has gained wide usage is the EQ-5D.[102] This scale measures the domains of mobility, self-care, usual activities, pain/discomfort, and anxiety/depression. It has been translated into more than 60 languages, making it a good choice for measuring quality of life issues in international clinical trials where multiple languages would be used in data collection.

Patient-Reported Outcome Measures

The NIH has developed a standardized, validated Patient-Reported Outcome Measures Information System (PROMIS) to fill a gap in research on self-reported health measures (https://commonfund.nih.gov/promis/index). Approximately 70 domains of self-reported health can be evaluated using PROMIS. It has been translated into multiple languages and is available on paper, electronic, mobile, and Web-based platforms.

Pharmacokinetic Measures

The plasma pharmacokinetics of a medication can yield important information on dosing intervals and pharmacokinetic-pharmacodynamic correlations. For example, daily dosing of 8 mg sublingual and alternate daily dosing of 16 mg sublingual buprenorphine yielded trough plasma levels of 0.80 and 0.77 ng/mL, respectively.[103] There were no differences in withdrawal scores, suggesting plasma concentrations above 0.7 ng/mL would suppress withdrawal symptoms. Higher doses of buprenorphine yielding higher plasma concentration and higher mu receptor occupancy were associated with greater blockade of hydromorphone's effects.[104] Blockade of hydromorphone agonist effects required buprenorphine plasma concentrations ≥3 ng/mL.[105]

In vaccine trials, the antibody titer may be correlated to efficacy. Vaccines will produce a variable immune response, resulting in an array of antibody titers. In a cocaine vaccine trial, 21 participants with IgG levels ≥42 μg/mL had more cocaine-negative urines than placebo-dosed participants ($p < 0.03$).[106] The correlation to antibody titers can guide future vaccine development.

Health Care Service Utilization Measures

Health care service utilization can be measured from the standpoint of the patient or the provider/health care system.[107] Indicators of health care quality include accessibility to treatment, continuity of treatment, the range of services offered, and the integration of care.[108] These indicators appear to be more geared to evaluating an existing treatment system but could be incorporated into a clinical trial evaluating one or more of these indicators. For example, treatment accessibility has been studied in a trial where patients seeking methadone maintenance treatment were randomized to an interim methadone group that received methadone for up to 120 days or to a waiting list control.[109] To evaluate continuity of treatment and range of services, the Treatment Services Review (TSR) surveys treatment services addressing the seven domains of the ASI provided to patients receiving alcohol or substance use counseling.[110,111] Again, it is geared more toward addressing issues in the extant treatment system, but it could be used to evaluate the amount of services accessed by participants during a clinical trial.

Cost Analysis-Related Measures

Although rarely a primary outcome measure, economic data obtained during effectiveness trials can assess the economic value of an intervention.[112] An economist should be involved in the design of the trial if an economic analysis is contemplated.

The main types of analyses are cost-effectiveness analysis measuring benefits in terms of quantity or quality of life as a unitary construct, cost-utility analysis measuring quantity and quality of life across several aspects of health and well-being (eg, quality-adjusted life years or healthy years equivalent are estimates of the benefit of a health care intervention), and cost-benefit analysis addresses whether the benefits associated with an intervention exceed its costs. For example, a cost and cost-effectiveness analysis of the nine treatment groups comprising the COMBINE study was conducted in terms of percent days abstinent, the incremental cost per patient to avoid heavy drinking, and the incremental cost per patient of achieving a good clinical outcome.[113] Three intervention groups were noted to be cost-effective relative to the other treatment groups: medical management (MM) with placebo, MM with naltrexone, and MM with naltrexone and acamprosate. A benefit-cost analysis comparison of interim versus standard methadone treatment failed to reveal any significant monetary differences between the interventions although there was a net monetary benefit noted in the combined study sample.[114]

Treatment Adherence Measures

Adherence to therapy is an important variable to measure in both behavioral and medication trials. Behavioral therapy sessions can be recorded and assessed for fidelity to the therapy and the therapist's competence in delivering the therapy.[115] Adherence to medication regimens is an issue in clinical trials for all pharmacotherapy trials except those in which the administration of the therapeutic agent is directly observed. Medication adherence can be measured through multiple means: addition of riboflavin into oral medications for measurement in urine samples,[116] pill count and medication diaries,[117] medication event monitoring systems (MEMS) in which opening of a bottle containing medication is captured electronically,[118] self-report,[119] direct measurement of the medication in urine,[24,25] capsule photographs taken with cellular telephones,[120] and pharmacy fill-refill. The reliability and comparability of the various forms of adherence are another consideration in designing clinical trials. In a study of buspirone as a treatment for people with cannabis dependence, riboflavin (a water-soluble vitamin) was added to the dosage form to measure medication adherence. Both riboflavin and serum 6-OH buspirone levels in urine showed a declining adherence to medication, whereas pill counts and diaries overreported adherence,[117] calling into question the reliability of self-reporting.

The effect of medication adherence can be illustrated in clinical studies attempting to replicate the initial finding of the efficacy of bupropion to reduce methamphetamine use.[23] A NIDA-funded replication study of bupropion in individuals who used methamphetamines less than daily reported no difference in reduction of methamphetamine use at the end of the trial between the bupropion and placebo groups ($p = 0.32$).[25] Adherence, measured by urinary bupropion levels, was reported in 47% of the bupropion-treated group. Thus, this could be considered a failed trial rather than a failure to replicate. A second trial of bupropion in individuals who used methamphetamines less than daily found no significant difference in abstinence between the bupropion (29%) versus placebo (14%) groups in the intent-to-treat analysis ($p = 0.08$).[24] Medication adherence, measured by bupropion plasma levels, was low (32%). A post hoc analysis of participants who were medication-adherent (13/41) versus participants who were nonadherent to bupropion (28/41) reported end-of-treatment abstinence in 54% and 18%, respectively ($p = 0.018$). These positive and negative findings show the impact of adherence in the replication of bupropion's efficacy.

MONITORING AND QUALITY CONTROL

Data gathered in clinical trials are entered into a confidential database during the trial. The Public Health Service Act (301 (d), 42 U.S.C. 241 (d)) authorizes investigators performing trials involving populations of individuals who use substances to withhold information from civil, criminal, administrative, or legislative bodies unless the information is considered a reportable issue, that is, child abuse, elder abuse, or threats of violence toward self or others.[121] The privacy of research participants is ensured by the obtaining a Certificate of Confidentiality from the NIH or the FDA. Participants' data are coded to establish confidentiality. Confidentiality at the research site is maintained by keeping the linking file separate from the database, password protecting the database, and restricting access to individuals who need to input or review data. The informed consent document explains that certain outside entities may review case report forms and the database, that is, the FDA, industry monitors if the trial is industry sponsored, or NIH personnel if the trial is NIH funded. Industry-sponsored trial monitors visit a clinical site at least three times: before participants are enrolled, during the study, and at the end of the study. The privacy of the research participant is maintained since only coded data are reviewed.

Safety is monitored at the clinical site by the investigators and by the IRB, the DSMBs, the FDA, the pharmaceutical industry (if industry sponsored), and the NIH (if the study is NIH funded). The protocol contains the definition of serious adverse events (SAEs) and how, when, and to whom SAEs will be reported. The investigators have the primary role for participant safety and can discontinue a participant if they think it is in the participant's best interest to do so. The IRB reviews the protocol prior to study commencement and then periodically reviews enrollment and adverse events. Sometimes, a medical monitor (who is usually blinded with respect to treatment assignment) will review safety issues and advise investigators. In other cases, a DSMB, a collection of clinical trial experts and medical experts that advise the investigators on trial design features, study enrollment, and safety and efficacy issues, will be chartered. The DSMB, when appropriate, can recommend changes in the protocol, up to and including termination of the study. It is the investigator's responsibility to report DSMB recommendations to the IRB and other regulatory entities. The NIH requires DSMBs for multicenter trials funded by NIH[122] and encourages consideration of setting up a DSMB for trials involving randomized, blinded data.[2]

The public reporting and monitoring of national and international clinical trials are done through the ClinicalTrials.gov website. Section 801 of the FDA's Amendment Act mandates that applicable clinical trials, including NIH-funded trials, be reported on ClinicalTrials.gov. Although phase I studies are exempt from posting on the site, many phase I studies are posted.

REPORTING RESULTS IN A JOURNAL ARTICLE

There are over 65 journals in the addiction medicine field. An important consideration by investigators is selecting an appropriate journal. A list of well-managed addiction journals can be accessed by downloading chapter 3 of *Publishing Addiction Science* at https://www.ubiquitypress.com/site/books/10.5334/bbd/. The quality of a particular journal can be checked at the following address: https://libguides.rutgers.edu/c.php?g=644942&p=4519187. Once a journal has been selected, the authors should visit that journal's website to determine the formatting, word count, and other specific requirements, for example, reporting oversight/institutional review and informed consent procedures. Items to be included in a published clinical study to enhance trial utility, replicability, and transparency have recently been published.[123] The outcome measures and statistical methods used in a trial should be described in the methods section of the paper. The statistical methods used for imputation of missing data should be stated. Planned versus post hoc analyses should be clearly described as the former carries more weight with reviewers, editors, and the journal readership. It is recommended that effect sizes accompany the p values so that readers can judge the strength of the effects reported. The conclusions and recommendations to changes in practice should not go beyond what is supported by the results.

CONCLUSIONS

Clinical trials in populations of individuals who use substances must comply with all the requirements of performing investigations in human subjects. Additionally, there are unique challenges to performing and interpreting clinical trials in these populations. The determination of abstinence is not straightforward as carryover may be observed in urine samples, necessitating a correction algorithm. Moreover, there is no consensus as to what constitutes an adequate duration of abstinence or what level of improvement in psychosocial functioning or well-being would be acceptable in those who do not achieve full abstinence. More research is needed to engage the FDA in determining the issue of what constitutes an adequate response to a pharmacotherapy for cannabis, opioid, and stimulant disorders. Moreover, abstinence from substance use is not the only valid indication the FDA would accept. The NIAAA has worked with the FDA in determining the level of drinking reduction that is associated with a therapeutic response to a pharmacotherapy.[53] Additionally, high discontinuation rates and other missing data in clinical trials in populations of individuals who use substances may lead to type II errors and require sophisticated analyses to account for the missing data. Adherence to taking medication, although not unique to patients with SUDs, may be low to moderate in this patient population, another variable that could lead to a type II error. Clinical trial designs need to consider these issues in the design and analysis of future trials in patients with SUDs with the goals of preventing missing data, improving medication adherence, and increasing the reproducibility of results.

Acronyms Explained

Certificate of Confidentiality (CoC)

A Certificate of Confidentiality is a document obtained from either the NIH or the FDA that allows a researcher to refuse to disclose names or other identifying information about participants in a clinical trial in response to local, state, or federal subpoenas.

Data and Safety Monitoring Board (DSMB)

A DSMB is composed of medical and clinical trial experts who are charged with making recommendations regarding study design, enrollment, efficacy issues up to and including trial termination due to overwhelming efficacy, and protocol changes due to safety issues up to and including trial termination for safety reasons. DSMB functions and oversight are distinct from the requirement of study review and approval by an institutional review board. A DSMB is required for all NIH-funded multicenter trials and is encouraged in other situations.

Institutional Review Board (IRB)

An institutional review board is composed of a group of at least five individuals possessing professional competence to review research activities and able to ascertain the acceptability of proposed research in terms of institutional commitments and regulations, applicable laws, and standards of professional conduct and practice.

Investigational New Drug (IND) Application

A commercial IND is an exemption to the law that a pharmaceutical company must have an approved drug in order to ship across state lines. The investigational drug can then be shipped to investigators across the United States and internationally if the FDA approves the IND. Another type of IND is an investigator IND, obtained by clinical investigators to study already marketed drugs for indications other than those approved in the labeling.

New Drug Application (NDA)

An NDA is a compilation of relevant information regarding the chemistry, manufacturing control data, pharmacology, pharmacokinetics, toxicology, and clinical and statistical analyses of data on a drug product that a pharmaceutical company submits to the FDA in pursuit of marketing approval.

Clinical Trial Phases

Phase I studies are the initial studies of a drug in human subjects. Most phase I drug research is conducted in healthy volunteers in inpatient settings. The usual number of participants is 20 to 80 and the emphasis is on safety and pharmacokinetics of the drug. In the development of medications for substance use disorders, the FDA often requests an interaction study of a putative medication with a known drug, for example, cocaine, in cocaine-experienced nontreatment seeking volunteers before allowing outpatient studies to commence in persons with cocaine use disorder.

Phase II studies, usually conducted in 100 to 200 study participants, are the initial determination of a drug's efficacy and safety in the intended patient population.

Phase III studies are intended to replicate the efficacy of a drug in an expanded population and to explore the efficacy and safety of the proposed dose range, fixed versus flexible dosing strategies, duration of therapy, and interactions with concomitant medications. It is not uncommon to have 1,000 to 3,000 study participants in phase III studies in order to capture serious adverse events that occur at low incidence rates.

Phase IV studies, also known as postmarketing studies, are often performed to gather further safety data on specific clinical issues, for example, concerns about hepatotoxicity, under real-world conditions. Comparative effectiveness trials, also conducted in phase IV, compare different treatments using flexible protocols that allow clinician judgment with regard to dose changes, for example. The comparison group is often a "treatment-as-usual" group.

REFERENCES

1. FDA guidance. February 1, 2016. Accessed August 12, 2022. http://www.fda.gov/RegulatoryInformation/Guidances/ucm126420.htm#IRBOrg
2. *NIH Clinical Trial Template* [NIH website]. February 1, 2016. Accessed October 20, 2016. https://osp.od.nih.gov/sites/default/files/Protocol_Template_01Feb2016_shell_508_mh
3. OHRP guidance. Accessed August 12, 2022. https://www.hhs.gov/ohrp/regulations-and-policy/guidance/faq/45-cfr-46/index.html
4. Singal AG, Higgins PD, Waljee AK. A primer on effectiveness and efficacy trials. *Clin Transl Gastroenterol.* 2014;5:e45.
5. Litten RZ, Ryan ML, Fertig JB, et al. A double-blind, placebo-controlled trial assessing the efficacy of varenicline tartrate for alcohol dependence. *J Addict Med.* 2013;7(4):277-286.
6. Fudala PJ, Bridge TP, Herbert S, et al. Office-based treatment of opiate addiction with a sublingual-tablet formulation of buprenorphine and naloxone. *N Engl J Med.* 2003;349(10):949-958.
7. Saxon AJ, Ling W, Hillhouse M, et al. Buprenorphine/naloxone and methadone effects on laboratory indices of liver health: a randomized trial. *Drug Alcohol Depend.* 2013;128(1-2):71-76.
8. Petry NM, Peirce JM, Stitzer ML, et al. Effect of prize-based incentives on outcomes in stimulant abusers in outpatient psychosocial treatment programs: a national drug abuse treatment clinical trials network study. *Arch Gen Psychiatry.* 2005;62(10):1148-1156.
9. Fiellin DA, Barry DT, Sullivan LE, et al. A randomized trial of cognitive behavioral therapy in primary care-based buprenorphine. *Am J Med.* 2013;126(1):74.e11-74.e17.
10. Lee JD, Friedmann PD, Boney TY, et al. Extended-release naltrexone to prevent relapse among opioid dependent, criminal justice system involved adults: rationale and design of a randomized controlled effectiveness trial. *Contemp Clin Trials.* 2015;41:110-117.
11. Lee JD, Friedmann PD, Kinlock TW, et al. Extended-release naltrexone to prevent opioid relapse in criminal justice offenders. *N Engl J Med.* 2016;374(13):1232-1242.
12. Sox HC, Greenfield S. Comparative effectiveness research: a report from the Institute of Medicine. *Ann Intern Med.* 2009;151(3):203-205.
13. Rawson RA, McCann MJ, Flammino F, et al. A comparison of contingency management and cognitive-behavioral approaches for stimulant-dependent individuals. *Addiction.* 2006;101(2):267-274.
14. Rawson RA, Huber A, McCann M, et al. A comparison of contingency management and cognitive-behavioral approaches during methadone maintenance treatment for cocaine dependence. *Arch Gen Psychiatry.* 2002;59(9):817-824.
15. Lee JD, Nunes EV, Novo P, et al. Comparative effectiveness of extended-release naltrexone versus buprenorphine-naloxone for opioid relapse prevention (X-BOT): a multicentre, open-label, randomized controlled trial. *Lancet.* 2018;391(10118):309-318.
16. Witkiewitz K, Finney JW, Harris AH, Kivlahan DR, Kranzler HR. Recommendations for the design and analysis of treatment trials for alcohol use disorders. *Alcohol Clin Exp Res.* 2015;39(9):1557-1570.
17. Hedden SL, Woolson RF, Malcolm RJ. Randomization in substance abuse clinical trials. *Subst Abuse Treat Prev Policy.* 2006;1:6.
18. Wei LJ, Lachin JM. Properties of the urn randomization in clinical trials. *Control Clin Trials.* 1988;9(4):345-364. Erratum in: *Control Clin Trials.* 1989;10(1):following 126.
19. Berger VW. The reverse propensity score to detect selection bias and correct for baseline imbalances. *Stat Med.* 2005;24(18):2777-2787.
20. Karanicolas PJ, Farrokhyar F, Bhandari M. Practical tips for surgical research: blinding: who, what, when, why, how? *Can J Surg.* 2010;53(5):345-348.
21. Farr BM, Conner EM, Betts RF, Oleske J, Minnefor A, Gwaltney JM Jr. Two randomized controlled trials of zinc gluconate lozenge therapy of experimentally induced rhinovirus colds. *Antimicrob Agents Chemother.* 1987;31(8):1183-1187.
22. Kraemer HC, Mintz J, Noda A, Tinklenberg J, Yesavage JA. Caution regarding the use of pilot studies to guide power calculations for study proposals. *Arch Gen Psychiatry.* 2006;63(5):484-489.
23. Elkashef AM, Rawson RA, Anderson AL, et al. Bupropion for the treatment of methamphetamine dependence. *Neuropsychopharmacology.* 2008;33(5):1162-1170.
24. Heinzerling KG, Swanson AN, Hall TM, Yi Y, Wu Y, Shoptaw SJ. Randomized, placebo-controlled trial of bupropion in methamphetamine-dependent participants with less than daily methamphetamine use. *Addiction.* 2014;109(11):1878-1886.
25. Anderson AL, Li SH, Markova D, et al. Bupropion for the treatment of methamphetamine dependence in non-daily users: a randomized, double-blind, placebo-controlled trial. *Drug Alcohol Depend.* 2015;150:170-174.
26. Friedman L, Furberg C, DeMets D. Sample size. In: Friedman LM, Furberg C, DeMets DL, eds. *Fundamentals of Clinical Trials.* John Wright; 1982:165-200.
27. Elkashef A, Holmes TH, Bloch DA, et al. Retrospective analyses of pooled data from CREST I and CREST II trials for treatment of cocaine dependence. *Addiction.* 2005;100(Suppl 1):91-101.
28. Elkashef A, Rawson RA, Smith E, et al. The NIDA Methamphetamine Clinical Trials Group: a strategy to increase clinical trials research capacity. *Addiction.* 2007;102(Suppl 1):107-113.
29. Evins AE, Culhane MA, Alpert JE, et al. A controlled trial of bupropion added to nicotine patch and behavioral therapy for smoking cessation in adults with unipolar depressive disorders. *J Clin Psychopharmacol.* 2008;28(6):660-666.

30. Hser YI, Saxon AJ, Huang D, et al. Treatment retention among patients randomized to buprenorphine/naloxone compared to methadone in a multi-site trial. *Addiction.* 2014;109(1):79-87.
31. Little R, Rubin D. *Statistical Analysis with Missing Data.* 2nd ed. Wiley; 2002.
32. Rubin D. Inference and missing data. *Biometrika.* 1976;63:581-592.
33. Hedden SL, Woolson RF, Carter RE, Palesch Y, Upadhyaya HP, Malcolm RJ. The impact of loss to follow-up on hypothesis tests of the treatment effect for several statistical methods in substance abuse clinical trials. *J Subst Abuse Treat.* 2009;37(1):54-63.
34. Barnes SA, Larsen MD, Schroeder D, Hanson A, Decker PA. Missing data assumptions and methods in a smoking cessation study. *Addiction.* 2010;105(3):431-437.
35. National Research Council (U.S.) Panel on Handling Missing Data in Clinical Trials. *The Prevention and Treatment of Missing Data in Clinical Trials.* National Academies Press; 2010. Accessed November 11, 2016. https://nap.nationalacademies.org/catalog/12955/the-prevention-and-treatment-of-missing-data-in-clinical-trials
36. Enders CK. Missing not at random models for latent growth curve analyses. *Psychol Methods.* 2011;16(1):1-16.
37. Chavalarias D, Wallach JD, Li AH, Ioannidis JP. Evolution of reporting P values in the biomedical literature, 1990-2015. *JAMA.* 2016;315(11):1141-1148.
38. Cohen J. *Statistical Power Analysis for the Behavioral Sciences.* Routledge; 1988.
39. Katz R. FDA: evidentiary standards for drug development and approval. *NeuroRx.* 2004;1(3):307-316.
40. *NIH Guide on Rigor and Reproducibility.* [NIH website]. Accessed November 11, 2016. https://grants.nih.gov/reproducibility/index.htm#guidance
41. Johnson RE, Jaffe JH, Fudala PJ. A controlled trial of buprenorphine treatment for opioid dependence. *JAMA.* 1992;267(20):2750-2755.
42. Ling W, Charuvastra C, Collins JF, et al. Buprenorphine maintenance treatment of opiate dependence: a multicenter, randomized clinical trial. *Addiction.* 1998;93(4):475-486.
43. Gonzales D, Rennard SI, Nides M, et al. Varenicline, an alpha4beta2 nicotinic acetylcholine receptor partial agonist, vs sustained-release bupropion and placebo for smoking cessation: a randomized controlled trial. *JAMA.* 2006;296(1):47-55.
44. Petry NM, Barry D, Alessi SM, Rounsaville BJ, Carroll KM. A randomized trial adapting contingency management targets based on initial abstinence status of cocaine-dependent patients. *J Consult Clin Psychol.* 2012;80(2):276-285.
45. Fiellin DA, Pantalon MV, Chawarski MC, et al. Counseling plus buprenorphine-naloxone maintenance therapy for opioid dependence. *N Engl J Med.* 2006;355(4):365-374.
46. *Guidance for Industry: Non-Inferiority Clinical Trials.* [FDA website]. March 2010. Accessed May 9, 2012. https://www.fda.gov/media/78504/download.
47. Rosenthal RN, Lofwall MR, Kim S, et al. Effect of buprenorphine implants on illicit opioid use among abstinent adults with opioid dependence treated with sublingual buprenorphine: a randomized clinical trial. *JAMA.* 2016;316(3):282-290.
48. Almirall D, Compton SN, Gunlicks-Stoessel M, Duan N, Murphy SA. Designing a pilot sequential multiple assignment randomized trial for developing an adaptive treatment strategy. *Stat Med.* 2012;31(17):1887-1902.
49. Lavori PW, Dawson R. Dynamic treatment regimes: practical design considerations. *Clin Trials.* 2004;1(1):9-20.
50. Murphy SA, Lynch KG, Oslin D, McKay JR, TenHave T. Developing adaptive treatment strategies in substance abuse research. *Drug Alcohol Depend.* 2007;88(Suppl 2):S24-S30.
51. TenHave TR, Coyne J, Salzer M, Katz I. Research to improve the quality of care for depression: alternatives to the simple randomized clinical trial. *Gen Hosp Psychiatry.* 2003;25(2):115-123.
52. Trivedi MH, Walker R, Ling W, et al. Naltrexone and bupropion for methamphetamine use disorder. *N Engl J Med.* 2021;384(2):140-153.
53. Guidance for Industry: *Alcoholism: Developing Drugs for Treatment.* [FDA website]. February 9, 2015. Accessed May 9, 2023. https://www.fda.gov/media/91222/download
54. Weisner C, Ray GT, Mertens JR, Satre DD, Moore C. Short-term alcohol and drug treatment outcomes predict long-term outcome. *Drug Alcohol Depend.* 2003;71(3):281-294.
55. Greenfield TK. Ways of measuring drinking patterns and the difference they make: experience with graduated frequencies. *J Subst Abuse.* 2000;12(1-2):33-49.
56. Dawson DA, Goldstein RB, Grant BF. Rates and correlates of relapse among individuals in remission from DSM-IV alcohol dependence: a 3-year follow-up. *Alcohol Clin Exp Res.* 2007;31(12):2036-2045.
57. Delucchi KL, Weisner C. Transitioning into and out of problem drinking across seven years. *J Stud Alcohol Drugs.* 2010;71(2):210-218.
58. Sanchez-Craig M, Wilkinson DA, Davila R. Empirically based guidelines for moderate drinking: 1-year results from three studies with problem drinkers. *Am J Public Health.* 1995;85(6):823-828.
59. Winchell C, Rappaport BA, Roca R, Rosebraugh CJ. Reanalysis of methamphetamine dependence treatment trial. *CNS Neurosci Ther.* 2012;18(5):367-368.
60. Donovan DM, Bigelow GE, Brigham GS, et al. Primary outcome indices in illicit drug dependence treatment research: systematic approach to selection and measurement of drug use end-points in clinical trials. *Addiction.* 2012;107(4):694-708.
61. McLellan AT, Kushner H, Metzger D, et al. The fifth edition of the addiction severity index. *J Subst Abuse Treat.* 1992;9(3):199-213.
62. Carroll KM, Kiluk BD, Nich C, et al. Toward empirical identification of a clinically meaningful indicator of treatment outcome: features of candidate indicators and evaluation of sensitivity to treatment effects and relationship to one year follow up cocaine use outcomes. *Drug Alcohol Depend.* 2014;137:3-19.
63. Lai H, Stitzer M, Treisman G, et al. Cocaine abstinence and reduced use associated with lowered marker of endothelial dysfunction in African Americans: a preliminary study. *J Addict Med.* 2015;9(4):331-339.
64. Somoza E, Somoza P, Lewis D, et al. The SRPHK1 outcome measure for cocaine-dependence trials combines self-report, urine benzoylecgonine levels, and the concordance between the two to determine a cocaine-use status for each study day. *Drug Alcohol Depend.* 2008;93(1-2):132-140.
65. Helander A, Bottcher M, Fehr C, Dahmen N, Beck O. Detection times for urinary ethyl glucuronide and ethyl sulfate in heavy drinkers during alcohol detoxification. *Alcohol Alcohol.* 2009;44(1):55-61.
66. Huestis MA, Mitchell JM, Cone EJ. Urinary excretion profiles of 11-nor-9-carboxy-delta 9-tetrahydrocannabinol in humans after single smoked doses of marijuana. *J Anal Toxicol.* 1996;20(6):441-452.
67. Ellis GM Jr, Mann MA, Judson BA, Schramm NT, Tashchian A. Excretion patterns of cannabinoid metabolites after last use in a group of chronic users. *Clin Pharmacol Ther.* 1985;38(5):572-578.
68. Jufer R, Walsh SL, Cone EJ, Sampson-Cone A. Effect of repeated cocaine administration on detection times in oral fluid and urine. *J Anal Toxicol.* 2006;30:458-462.
69. Huestis MA, Cone EJ. Methamphetamine disposition in oral fluid, plasma, and urine. *Ann N Y Acad Sci.* 2007;1098:104-121.
70. Smith ML, Shimomura ET, Summers J, et al. Detection times and analytical performance of commercial urine opiate immunoassays following heroin administration. *J Anal Toxicol.* 2000;24(7):522-529.
71. Cone EJ, Heltsley R, Black DL, Mitchell JM, Lodico CP, Flegel RR. Prescription opioids. I. Metabolism and excretion patterns of oxycodone in urine following controlled single dose administration. *J Anal Toxicol.* 2013;37(5):255-264.
72. Preston KL, Silverman K, Schuster CR, Cone EJ. Assessment of cocaine use with quantitative urinalysis and estimation of new uses. *Addiction.* 1997;92(6):717-727.
73. Hallgren KA, Witkiewitz K. Missing data in alcohol clinical trials: a comparison of methods. *Alcohol Clin Exp Res.* 2013;37(12):2152-2160.
74. American Psychiatric Association. *Diagnostic and Statistical Manual of Mental Disorders.* 5th ed. American Psychiatric Association; 2013.

75. Register F. *78 FR 19718*; April 2, 2013:19718-19721.
76. Gossop M. The development of a Short Opiate Withdrawal Scale (SOWS). *Addict Behav.* 1990;15(5):487-490.
77. Handelsman L, Cochrane KJ, Aronson MJ, Ness R, Rubinstein KJ, Kanof PD. Two new rating scales for opiate withdrawal. *Am J Drug Alcohol Abuse.* 1987;13(3):293-308.
78. Wesson DR, Ling W. The Clinical Opiate Withdrawal Scale (COWS). *J Psychoactive Drugs.* 2003;35(2):253-259.
79. Substance Abuse and Mental Health Services Administration (SAMHSA), NIAA. *Medication for the Treatment of Alcohol Use Disorder: A Brief Guide.* HHS Publication; 2015.
80. Sullivan JT, Sykora K, Schneiderman J, Naranjo CA, Sellers EM. Assessment of alcohol withdrawal: the revised clinical institute withdrawal assessment for alcohol scale (CIWA-Ar). *Br J Addict.* 1989;84(11):1353-1357.
81. Sayette MA, Shiffman S, Tiffany ST, Niaura RS, Martin CS, Shadel WG. The measurement of drug craving. *Addiction.* 2000;95(Suppl 2): S189-S210.
82. Tiffany ST, Drobes DJ. The development and initial validation of a questionnaire on smoking urges. *Br J Addict.* 1991;86(11): 1467-1476.
83. Epstein DH, Willner-Reid J, Vahabzadeh M, Mezghanni M, Lin JL, Preston KL. Real-time electronic diary reports of cue exposure and mood in the hours before cocaine and heroin craving and use. *Arch Gen Psychiatry.* 2009;66(1):88-94.
84. Fals-Stewart W, Schafer J. The relationship between length of stay in drug-free therapeutic communities and neurocognitive functioning. *J Clin Psychol.* 1992;48(4):539-543.
85. Aharonovich E, Hasin DS, Brooks AC, Liu X, Bisaga A, Nunes EV. Cognitive deficits predict low treatment retention in cocaine dependent patients. *Drug Alcohol Depend.* 2006;81(3):313-322.
86. Vocci FJ. Cognitive remediation in the treatment of stimulant abuse disorders: a research agenda. *Exp Clin Psychopharmacol.* 2008;16(6): 484-497.
87. Rosselli M, Ardila A, Lubomski M, Murray S, King K. Personality profile and neuropsychological test performance in chronic cocaine-abusers. *Int J Neurosci.* 2001;110(1-2):55-72.
88. Ardila A, Rosselli M, Strumwasser S. Neuropsychological deficits in chronic cocaine abusers. *Int J Neurosci.* 1991;57(1-2):73-79.
89. Turner DC, Clark L, Pomarol-Clotet E, McKenna P, Robbins TW, Sahakian BJ. Modafinil improves cognition and attentional set shifting in patients with chronic schizophrenia. *Neuropsychopharmacology.* 2004;29(7):1363-1373.
90. Carpenter KM, Schreiber E, Church S, McDowell D. Drug Stroop performance: relationships with primary substance of use and treatment outcome in a drug-dependent outpatient sample. *Addict Behav.* 2006;31(1):174-181.
91. Streeter CC, Terhune DB, Whitfield TH, et al. Performance on the Stroop predicts treatment compliance in cocaine-dependent individuals. *Neuropsychopharmacology.* 2008;33(4):827-836.
92. Beck AT, Ward CH, Mendelson M, Mock J, Erbaugh J. An inventory for measuring depression. *Arch Gen Psychiatry.* 1961;4:561-571.
93. Hamilton M. A rating scale for depression. *J Neurol Neurosurg Psychiatry.* 1960;23:56-62.
94. Hamilton M. The assessment of anxiety states by rating. *Br J Med Psychol.* 1959;32(1):50-55.
95. Mason BJ, Kocsis JH, Ritvo EC, Cutler RB. A double-blind, placebo-controlled trial of desipramine for primary alcohol dependence stratified on the presence or absence of major depression. *JAMA.* 1996;275(10):761-767.
96. American Psychiatric Association. *Handbook of Psychiatric Measures.* 2nd ed. American Psychiatric Association; 2008.
97. McLellan AT, Luborsky L, Woody GE, O'Brien CP. An improved diagnostic evaluation instrument for substance abuse patients. The addiction severity index. *J Nerv Ment Dis.* 1980;168(1):26-33.
98. Kiluk BD, Nich C, Witkiewitz K, Babuscio TA, Carroll KM. What happens in treatment doesn't stay in treatment: cocaine abstinence during treatment is associated with fewer problems at follow-up. *J Consult Clin Psychol.* 2014;82(4):619-627.
99. Navaline HA, Snider EC, Petro CJ, et al. Preparations for AIDS vaccine trials. An automated version of the Risk Assessment Battery (RAB): enhancing the assessment of risk behaviors. *AIDS Res Hum Retroviruses.* 1994;10(Suppl 2):S281-S283.
100. Ward J, Darke S, Hall W; National Drug and Alcohol Research Centre. *The HIV Risk-Taking Behavior Scale (HRBS) Manual*; 1990.
101. Ware JE Jr, Sherbourne CD. The MOS 36-item short-form health survey (SF-36). I. Conceptual framework and item selection. *Med Care.* 1992;30(6):473-483.
102. EuroQol group. EuroQol—a new facility for measurement of health-related quality of life. *Health Policy.* 1990;161:99-208.
103. Kuhlman JJ Jr, Levine B, Johnson RE, Fudala PJ, Cone EJ. Relationship of plasma buprenorphine and norbuprenorphine to withdrawal symptoms during dose induction, maintenance and withdrawal from sublingual buprenorphine. *Addiction.* 1998;93(4):549-559.
104. Greenwald MK, Johanson CE, Moody DE, et al. Effects of buprenorphine maintenance dose on mu-opioid receptor availability, plasma concentrations, and antagonist blockade in heroin-dependent volunteers. *Neuropsychopharmacology.* 2003;28(11):2000-2009.
105. Greenwald MK, Comer SD, Fiellin DA. Buprenorphine maintenance and mu-opioid receptor availability in the treatment of opioid use disorder: implications for clinical use and policy. *Drug Alcohol Depend.* 2014;144:1-11.
106. Martell BA, Orson FM, Poling J, et al. Cocaine vaccine for the treatment of cocaine dependence in methadone-maintained patients: a randomized, double-blind, placebo-controlled efficacy trial. *Arch Gen Psychiatry.* 2009;66(10):1116-1123.
107. Da Silva RB, Contandriopoulos AP, Pineault R, Tousignant P. A global approach to evaluation of health services utilization: concepts and measures. *Health Policy.* 2011;6(4):e106-e117.
108. Starfield B. *Primary Care: Balancing Health Needs, Services and Technology*. Rev. ed. Oxford University Press; 1998.
109. Schwartz RP, Highfield DA, Jaffe JH, et al. A randomized controlled trial of interim methadone maintenance. *Arch Gen Psychiatry.* 2006;63(1): 102-109.
110. Cacciola JS, Alterman AI, Lynch KG, Martin JM, Beauchamp ML, McLellan AT. Initial reliability and validity studies of the revised Treatment Services Review (TSR-6). *Drug Alcohol Depend.* 2008;92(1-3):37-47.
111. McLellan AT, Alterman AI, Cacciola J, Metzger D, O'Brien CP. A new measure of substance abuse treatment. Initial studies of the treatment services review. *J Nerv Ment Dis.* 1992;180(2):101-110.
112. Ramsey S, Willke R, Briggs A, et al. Good research practices for cost-effectiveness analysis alongside clinical trials: the ISPOR RCT-CEA Task Force report. *Value Health.* 2005;8(5):521-533.
113. Zarkin GA, Bray JW, Aldridge A, et al. Cost and cost-effectiveness of the COMBINE study in alcohol-dependent patients. *Arch Gen Psychiatry.* 2008;65(10):1214-1221.
114. Schwartz RP, Alexandre PK, Kelly SM, O'Grady KE, Gryczynski J, Jaffe JH. Interim versus standard methadone treatment: a benefit-cost analysis. *J Subst Abuse Treat.* 2014;46(3):306-314.
115. Carroll KM, Nich C, Sifry RL, et al. A general system for evaluating therapist adherence and competence in psychotherapy research in the addictions. *Drug Alcohol Depend.* 2000;57(3):225-238.
116. Herron AJ, Mariani JJ, Pavlicova M, et al. Assessment of riboflavin as a tracer substance: comparison of a qualitative to a quantitative method of riboflavin measurement. *Drug Alcohol Depend.* 2013;128(1-2):77-82.
117. McRae-Clark AL, Baker NL, Sonne SC, DeVane CL, Wagner A, Norton J. Concordance of direct and indirect measures of medication adherence in a treatment trial for cannabis dependence. *J Subst Abuse Treat.* 2015;57:70-74.
118. Mooney ME, Sayre SL, Hokanson PS, Stotts AL, Schmitz JM. Adding MEMS feedback to behavioral smoking cessation therapy increases compliance with bupropion: a replication and extension study. *Addict Behav.* 2007;32(4):875-880.

119. Das M, Santos D, Matheson T, et al. Feasibility and acceptability of a phase II randomized pharmacologic intervention for methamphetamine dependence in high-risk men who have sex with men. *AIDS.* 2010;24(7):991-1000.
120. Galloway GP, Coyle JR, Guillen JE, Flower K, Mendelson JE. A simple, novel method for assessing medication adherence: capsule photographs taken with cellular telephones. *J Addict Med.* 2011;5(3):170-174.
121. Certificates of Confidentiality-Privacy Protection for Research Subjects: OHRP Guidance (2003). February 25, 2003. Accessed May 9, 2023. https://www.hhs.gov/ohrp/regulations-and-policy/guidance/certificates-of-confidentiality/index.html
122. NIH Policy for Data and Safety Monitoring. June 10, 1998. Accessed November 8, 2016. https://grants.nih.gov/grants/guide/notice-files/not98-084.html
123. Butcher NJ, Monsour A, Mew EJ, et al. Guidelines for reporting outcomes in trial reports The Consort-Outcomes 2022 Extension. *JAMA.* 2022;328(22):2252-2264. doi:10.1001/jama.2022.21022

5 Addiction Medicine Physicians and Collaborative Care Clinicians as Change Agents for Prevention and Public Health

Warren Yamashita, Kevin Kunz, and Omari Hodge

CHAPTER OUTLINE

- We are responsible for protecting the public's health
- The role of the addiction medicine physician and collaborative care clinicians
- Transformational change
- A proven approach to effecting change in health care and the community
- Summary

WE ARE RESPONSIBLE FOR PROTECTING THE PUBLIC'S HEALTH

"Everyone is really responsible to all [people] for all [people] and for everything." – Fyodor Dostoyevsky, *The Brothers Karamazov*

There is an urgent need to translate addiction science into everyday clinical practice, while also translating it into institutional and public policies that constructively impact health. While this textbook presents a vast array of effective evidence-based interventions, which can be applied in clinical and community settings, cultural and structural barriers continue to prevent these lifesaving practices from being adequately implemented in the real world. Unhealthy substance use is one of the world's largest and most costly health issues, accounting for the top causes of preventable death and disability on a global scale. In the United States, unhealthy substance use and addiction cause at least 22% of all deaths.[1-3] While tobacco and alcohol cause the largest number of these deaths, the current unrelenting opioid use and drug overdose crisis of the last four decades has not yet peaked, led by rising overdose rates of synthetic opioids such as fentanyl.[3] The annual increase on illicit drug overdose deaths has exponentially increased despite all medical, social and legal interventions[4] (**Fig. 5-1**). This disturbing trend has finally brought the field of medicine and American public to acknowledge the need to address unhealthy substance use in our country.

The American health care field may reasonably take pride in the technical application of science and discovery, yet the U.S. continues to rank among the lowest among high-income countries on global ratings of health care outcomes and equity.[5,6] This is most exemplified in disease and social dysfunction caused or exacerbated by unhealthy substance use. Unhealthy substance use and addiction are America's number one health problem, yet the health care system still primarily focuses on treating complications of substance use rather than on the prevention and treatment of substance use disorders (SUDs).[7,8,9] One fifth of annual deaths in the U.S. are attributable to unhealthy substance use and addiction. Fortunately SUDs are not only treatable conditions, but they are also responsive to well-coordinated prevention and public health initiatives.[10] This is true also for other conditions often referred to as "process" or "behavioral" addictions, such as gambling disorder, sexual "addiction," problematic internet use, etc.

The current U.S. epidemic of overdose deaths (primarily related to opioids), in which the medical field has been complicit, has compelled both individual clinicians as well as the health care system to urgently develop and deploy the field of addiction medicine. Clinicians and the American public have been sensitized by the opioid crisis rocking our national health and our collective consciousness. Concern and calls to action to combat the opioid crisis stand in stark contrast to the passivity expressed in relation to the high prevalence of nicotine addiction over the past 50 years and in relation to decades of unhealthy use of other substances.

Missing from the current approach of medicine today is the front end of the continuum of health care practice: attention to issues of public health and illness prevention. America's current acute care health system resulted from transformative change triggered by the 1910 Flexner report.[11] This report was the basis for a sweeping reform and renewal of American medical education and practice. Physician training was increased to a minimum of 6 years post-secondary education, medical research adhered to the protocols of the scientific method, physician training itself was restructured in a scientific manner, literally half of all medical schools were closed, and the state regulation of physician education and practice was instituted. These changes—substantial improvements at the time—were fundamental and have remained dominant and are accepted as unalterable. The need for a new shift from an acute care model to one that attends to the full continuum of care from prevention and early intervention to chronic disease management now demands a transformation of similar magnitude to that initiated by Flexner over a century ago.[12] Nowhere is this more obvious than with the prevention and treatment of unhealthy substance use. The acute care focus of American medicine has historically rewarded the short-term care of back-end medical complications of substance use, while

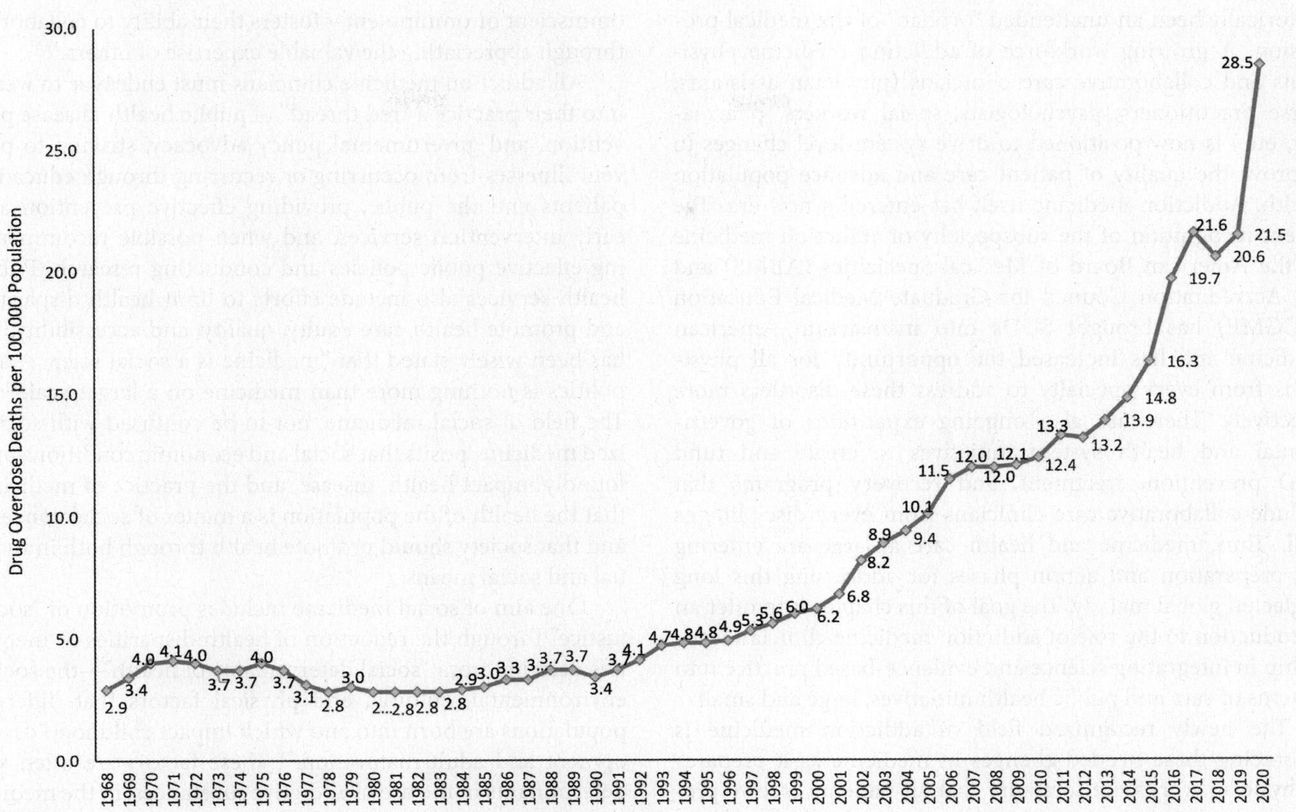

Figure 5-1. Drug overdose deaths per 100,000 population from 1968 to 2020. (From Compton WM, Einstein EB, Jones CM. Exponential increases in drug overdose: implications for epidemiology and research. *Int J Drug Policy.* 2022;104:103676. doi:10.1016/j.drugpo.2022.103676).

providing minimal reward for front-end and often more cost-effective prevention. There is sparse implementation of available evidence-based prevention and treatment strategies, while there are easily accessible advanced and costly treatment options for late-stage complications of addiction: trauma, organ damage, cancer, metabolic disorders, psychiatric complications, etc. As well, late stage "interventions" for social sequelae of substance use, such as incarceration, disability, and unemployment assistance, are usually more readily available than less costly and more effective prevention and public health initiatives. Addiction care is often sub-adequate because collaboration with other health professionals and the existence of multi-professional teams are generally absent. This entire situation is now being considered "upside down."

Feinberg suggests that there are other reasons why it is difficult to gain broad institutional support for prevention. These reasons include: success is invisible, lack of drama makes prevention less interesting, statistical lives have little emotional effect, there is usually a long delay before rewards appear, benefits for prevention often do not accrue to the payer, persistent behavioral change may be required, bias against errors of commission may deter action, avoidable harm is accepted as normal, there is a financial double standard in the evaluation of prevention as compared to treatment, commercial interests may conflict with disease prevention, advice is inconsistent or changes, and advice may conflict with personal or religious or cultural beliefs.[13] To address these and other concerns, the landscape of health care and health care training in this country must change to a more comprehensive and integrated approach. Thibault has noted that this requires addressing the full continuum of care from prevention and early intervention to chronic disease management, breaking down the silos of health professional education and practice, and assuring competency rather than curricular completion.[14,15] As our modern health care system begins to appreciate Dostoyevsky's wisdom in the saying "Everyone is really responsible to all [people] for all [people] and for everything," we will begin to imagine new ways for clinicians to become system leaders, communities to have their own voices integrated into the systems that provide them health care, and previously siloed disciplines to develop fully integrated and team-based models of care to lead a new era of transformational change required to turn the tide on this current overdose crisis.

THE ROLE OF THE ADDICTION MEDICINE PHYSICIAN AND COLLABORATIVE CARE CLINICIANS

It is the ethical responsibility of every clinician to provide competent medical care and to incorporate current scientific knowledge into their medical practice. Yet SUDs have historically been an unattended "orphan" of the medical profession. A growing workforce of addiction medicine physicians and collaborative care clinicians (physician assistants, nurse practitioners, psychologists, social workers, pharmacist, etc.) is now positioned to drive system-level changes to improve the quality of patient care and advance population health. Addiction medicine itself has entered a new era. The recent recognition of the subspecialty of addiction medicine by the American Board of Medical Specialties (ABMS) and the Accreditation Council for Graduate Medical Education (ACGME) has brought SUDs into mainstream American medicine and has increased the opportunity for all physicians from every specialty to address these disorders more effectively. There are also ongoing expansions of governmental and health system initiatives to create and fund SUD prevention, treatment, and recovery programs that include collaborative care clinicians from every discipline as well. Thus, medicine and health care at-large are entering the preparation and action phases for addressing this long neglected global malady. The goal of this chapter is to offer an introduction to the role of addiction medicine clinician leadership in integrating science and evidence-based practice into systems of care and public health initiatives, large and small.

The newly recognized field of addiction medicine is embracing these needed changes in medicine as it prepares a physician workforce to assure that all patients receive prevention and early intervention services and effective treatment and disease management for addiction and its many co-occurring disorders. Addiction medicine physicians play four essential roles in this process: providing clinical expertise in direct patient care and in consultation with other clinicians in multispecialty and interdisciplinary settings, serving as faculty and teachers to educate and train others, performing clinical and health policy research, and functioning as change agents to speed the evolution of needed reforms.[16] They can do this by serving as expert clinicians, teachers, faculty, researchers and community or governmental-level change agents. Within addiction medicine and focusing on the role of physicians as change agents, the ABMS and ACGME competencies of systems-based practice and professionalism are especially salient. Systems-based practice is the physician's ability to "demonstrate awareness of and responsibility to the larger context and systems of health care" and to "be able to call on system resources to provide optimal care."[17,18] The competency of professionalism includes accountability to society. Recognizing that cultural competencies often fail to consider the institutional, political, and economic forces that produce structural racism and persistent addiction stigmas, developing structural competencies have become particularly pertinent to the addiction medicine physician. They include the physician's ability to understand their patient's illness in the context of their socio-ecological environments, implement interventions for their patients that address social determinants of health, and maintain a posture of structural humility and patience with an openness to collaborate and learn from other disciplines and the community. Importantly, structural humility—the ability of physicians to recognize they are not omniscient or omnipotent—fosters their ability to collaborate through appreciating the valuable expertise of others.[19]

All addiction medicine clinicians must endeavor to weave into their practice a "red thread" of public health, disease prevention, and governmental policy advocacy, striving to prevent illnesses from occurring or recurring through educating patients and the public, providing effective prevention and early intervention services, and when possible recommending effective public policies and conducting research. Public health services also include efforts to limit health disparities and promote health care equity, quality, and accessibility.[20] It has been wisely stated that "medicine is a social science, and politics is nothing more than medicine on a larger scale."[21,22] The field of social medicine, not to be confused with socialized medicine, posits that social and economic conditions profoundly impact health, disease, and the practice of medicine; that the health of the population is a matter of social concern; and that society should promote health through both individual and social means.

One aim of social medicine includes promotion of "social justice" through the reduction of health disparities or inequities deriving from "social determinants of health"—the social, environmental, cultural, and physical factors that different populations are born into and which impact childhood development and adult maturation.[23] These factors are often key determinants in the use of addictive substances, in the medical and social consequences of their use, and in the opportunities for medical and social interventions available for prevention, treatment, and recovery. While the task ahead may seem insurmountable, it is important for each and every addiction medicine clinician to remember that as an agent of change in their communities and health systems, they have within them the possibility to ignite transformational change in the people around them and to keep our eyes on the goal, even when the days are long and hard.

TRANSFORMATIONAL CHANGE

The old adage that a "Band-Aid approach won't fix this problem" clearly applies to the unsuccessful efforts of medicine to attenuate the morbidity and mortality associated with unhealthy substance use and addiction. Health care systems, and key stakeholders are now being challenged to produce a thorough and dramatic change in the form, character, and appearance of the antiquated interventions, or complete lack thereof, necessary to address unhealthy substance use and addiction. As the 21st century proceeds, we are entering an era ripe for transformational change in the prevention and treatment of SUDs.

Transformational change derives from a radical divergence from the underlying consciousness, strategy, and processes that an organization or system has been using. It can be identified by a shift in the culture of an organization, field, or population that results in new expectations and new practices.[24] Examples include the near-total restriction of tobacco smoking in public places as well as more private venues, the removal of all tobacco products from major health and drug stores, and the acceptance of routine vaccinations. The U.S. is now witnessing the emergence of another transformative shift of consciousness: that addiction is a health condition and not a character, moral, or criminal problem. Addiction medicine physicians are challenged to lead, contribute to, and actualize strategies and processes driving system changes to reflect this new public and medical reality. Health care clinicians are the ultimate purveyors of messaging and action in this arena because SUDs are medical disorders impacted by genetics and environment, and these same medical disorders significantly impact human environment and society.

A key prerequisite for transformational change is its dependence on leadership that integrates and models the change being sought. If clinicians were still using tobacco in large numbers, how would that have impacted the public health campaign for reducing the prevalence of tobacco use and related disease? If clinicians seek to collaborate across traditional boundaries with other stakeholders, they can both model a winning strategy and improve the health of patients and our nation. In this, they can lead. In fact, the skills which seasoned clinicians use so well in the clinical care of patients to positively accentuate and promote the benefits of personal change are needed now to achieve advancement in structure and cooperation between interdependent elements in health care systems.

Finally, and most importantly, transformational change engages the heart. Science, economics, analysis, and critical thinking are necessary yet insufficient to produce lasting changes in behaviors and the collective consciousness. And just as the science of medicine is incomplete without the art of the sacred patient-physician relationship, so too are relationships key to driving positive changes in systems. Systems are driven by individuals who interact, cooperate, and collaborate with one another. We are not computers or robots. We are driven by our aspirations, by issues, and activities we deeply care about that give meaning to our lives.

To actualize system change, addiction medicine clinicians armed with the science of addiction and knowledge of best practices for reform have much to offer. The Institute of Healthcare Improvement has promoted and validated the well-known Plan-Do-Study-Act cycle, which breaks the change process into straightforward steps.[25] The detail of these steps is incorporated into the content below and illustrated with the case of Dr Brave.

A PROVEN APPROACH TO EFFECTING CHANGE IN HEALTH CARE AND THE COMMUNITY

1. Become a change agent.
2. Take a systems approach.
3. Put together a diverse, multispecialty, interdisciplinary team.
4. Develop a shared purpose and plan of action.
5. Act.
6. Set up a strategy for evaluation and improvement.

Become a Change Agent

As humanitarian physician Albert Schweitzer said, "my life is my argument." A physician leader first seeks to be the change they wish to see in their community. This grounding allows them to honor the past and hope for the future, while keeping a strong focus on the present moment with openness to new ideas, insights and barriers that may arise. To borrow a motivational interviewing phrase, they know how to "roll with resistance."

Albert Einstein had said, "problems cannot be solved by the same level of thinking that created them." Thus, a clinician-leader will sometimes need to think outside the box at the risk of criticism from their colleagues. In this frame, they assess the current situation, imagine new possibilities, and seek a process for improvement. The clinician-leader can participate in changing the system shortcomings or in creating a new system. There are several realities leaders can recognize early: leadership is an action, not a position; leadership is not victimhood—you cannot be a leader and a victim simultaneously; leaders define reality—with vision and data; leaders develop and test changes; leaders take risk and have courage, because complacent or threatened persons or organizations may react loudly and negatively to a proposed change; leaders must cross boundaries, stepping outside and letting go of defending their silo; and physician leaders seek and achieve new interactions with a diversity of stakeholders.[26]

The case of Dr Brave: Emergence as a Change Agent

A family medicine physician we will call Dr Brave is a fellowship-trained addiction medicine specialist. He returned home after his fellowship because he wanted to make an impact in the community in which he grew up. As a Black/African American physician, Dr Brave was aware of the persistent health disparities and structural racism within medicine from his lived experience, clinical practice, and medical literature. He had borrowed substantially to afford medical school and still carries exorbitant undergraduate and medical school loans. His younger brother was not as fortunate. He had experimented with cannabis through high school and suffered a sports injury in college, which then started the trajectory from prescription opioids to illegal opioids. Rather than being referred to treatment, he was expelled from college and was incarcerated for several years for possession. Dr Brave was well acquainted with the obstacles individuals of minoritized backgrounds must overcome.

Dr Brave landed his hometown dream job at a local Federally Qualified Health Center: he was brought on and assigned to start an integrated primary care addiction medicine program in the inner-city. After building a robust comprehensive addiction program, he became frustrated to see a continued lack of representation among his patient panel. Most of his patients were White, including those receiving buprenorphine, although the city's overdose rates were increasing most amongst the Black and Indigenous American/Alaskan Native communities.[27] During his practice, he had seen several barriers causing this discrepancy including social determinants of health in housing, transportation, food insecurity, child support, domestic violence, and inadequate legal services. He recognized that racial and ethnic minoritized communities had a greater distrust of the health care system. He was aware these communities have long suffered systemic racism in medicine and that this left a wound of mistrust that particularly discouraged individuals with SUDs from seeking addiction treatment.

He was particularly disturbed by how his clinic administration trumpeted his program's success amongst city officials with numbers and charts that avoided breaking down the disparities by race/ethnicity, income, and zip code. He experienced subtle microaggressions such as when a medical colleague told him he was "rocking the boat" too much in bringing up racial disparities at meetings, and suggested he be grateful for the impact they have already made. When he suggested hiring a Spanish-speaking, Latinx addiction medicine practitioner to help reach the Latinx community to attenuate its high rate of alcohol use disorder, he was asked, "Can't you just use the translation service to treat these patients yourself?" Although he valued and respected his team, he was increasingly discouraged by the implicit biases that persisted within his own clinic.

Unfortunately, these situations are not uncommon. They usually derive from addiction stigma, ignorance, persistent racial biases, and outmoded and inefficient health care systems. Dr Brave knew he could address one individual or service at a time to educate them about the disease of addiction, structural competencies to address racial biases, and the modern treatment of SUD. Yet he alone would still never be able to address all the systemic factors preventing people of color from accessing equitable addiction care. While his burden seemed insurmountable, Dr Brave held hope and remained open for a breakthrough that might morph a daunting obstacle into a creative opportunity. By applying a systems approach, he learned he could involve strategic and key stakeholders, which would be a better use of his time and energy toward long-term, integrated, and mutually appreciated solutions. As a physician, he could go to key community leaders, state his concern clearly, and propose a new collaborative approach that addresses everyone's goals and overcomes traditionally accepted barriers to improving care.

Desperate for a breakthrough, Dr Brave called his brother and asked if he could air his frustrations with his clinic. His brother by then had been attending a 12-step group at his church, which helped him get into and stay in recovery after incarceration. He was sponsoring and mentoring others and speaking with his church congregation and leadership about addiction prevention, treatment, and recovery. The conversation that ensued changed Dr Brave's perspective and life trajectory from a physician about to burn out to an impassioned change agent with renewed hope and fresh vision. What did they talk about? Read on.

Take a Systems Approach

A system is a set of interdependent elements interacting to achieve a common goal.[28] Physicians can learn the elements and processes of the systems in which they inhabit and can engage in interactions for improvement. Cooperation across traditional boundaries is not as daunting a barrier as often perceived. Medical specialties, other health professions, and system managers often operate in "silos of excellence." Administrators, financial stakeholders, policy makers, nonprofits, the public, and other interest groups also have their own world views, cultures, goals, and preferred practices. Although a physician entering this larger system may initially feel intimidation, most newcomers will find this can be a welcoming environment—"boots on the ground" physicians are rare visitors. In this milieu, physicians have a unique capacity to be accepted as participants and critical leaders in improving systems and advancing the quality of care for their patients and their community. Leaders holding the precept "do what is best for the patient," can bring quality of care into discussions where other outcomes and agendas have historically dominated. Health care professionals, and especially addiction medicine physicians, have been absent or scarce in deliberations at nearly every system level due to a limited workforce, overwhelming patient care considerations, or the assumption that someone else is already working on the issue. Key decisions in the care of patients thus have often excluded effective input from addiction medicine clinicians and defaulted to stakeholders with more provincial interests.

As addiction medicine professionals bring new perspective and leadership to their communities, they come to appreciate Aristotle's wisdom that "the whole is greater than the sum of its parts." Thus they learn to acknowledge the multi-layered complexity of the human systems they serve. To address the opioid crisis, for example, one must consider the individual, interpersonal, community and societal dimensions of the problem[29] (**Fig. 5-2**).

They must stay up to date with evidence-based practice as well as practice-based evidence by listening and learning from their community's lived experience. Addiction medicine leaders often adopt frameworks to help them maintain perspective and navigate these complex systems. The Strengths Model is one example of a proven framework.[30]

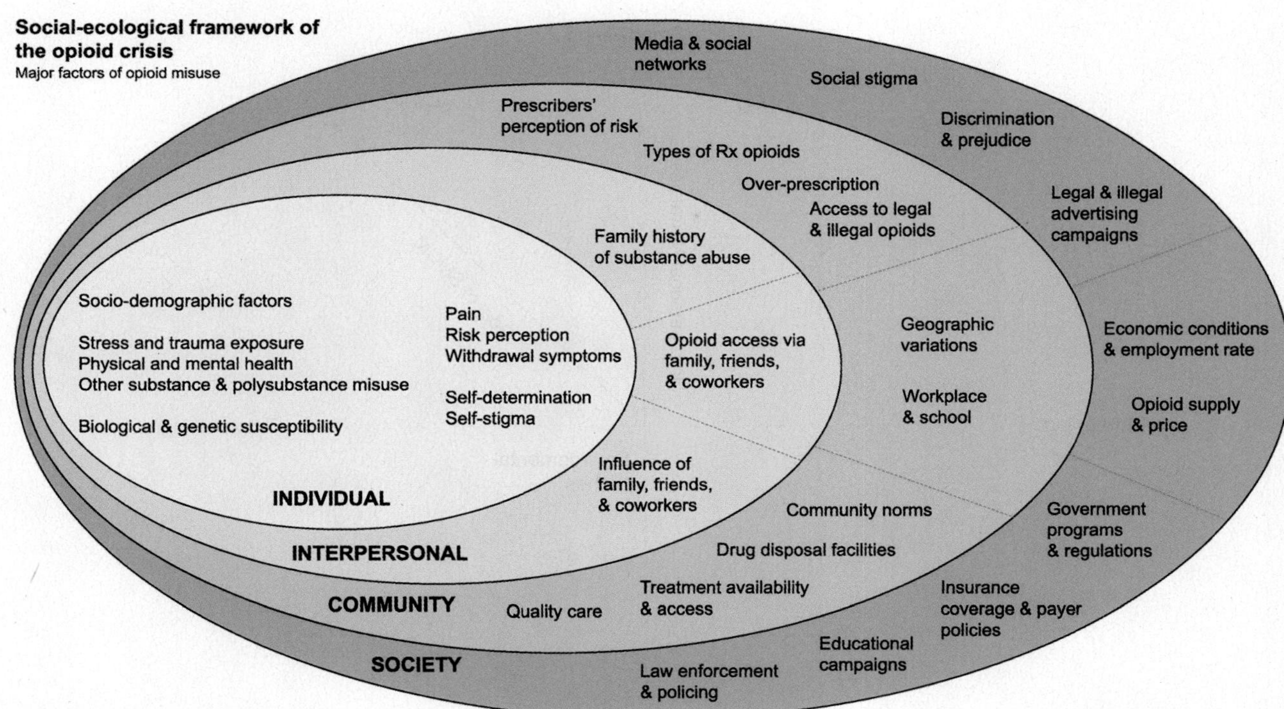

Figure 5-2. Social-ecological framework of the opioid crisis highlighting major factors contributing to opioid misuse. (From Jalali MS, Botticelli M, Hwang RC, Koh HK, McHugh RK. The opioid crisis: a contextual, social-ecological framework. *Health Res Policy Syst.* 2020;18(1):87. doi:10.1186/s12961-020-00596-8).

Dr Brave Moves Beyond the Four Walls of the Clinic

Dr Brave's brother commented how he could relate to Dr Brave's difficulties from "the other side." While Dr Brave's clinic wasn't reaching the Black community, his brother commented how there are no opioid treatment programs in the zip code where he lives. And his brother never had access to buprenorphine treatment before, during or after incarceration. Dr Brave's brother proposed they both partner with their church and recovery ministry. Dr Brave had never thought of partnering with churches or any nonprofit organization for that matter. He had only focused on medical-led interventions. Dr Brave also expressed that he had negative experiences with his church when his patients were told their medication treatment was a "crutch" or "just replacing one addiction for another." But his brother came ready with a story about the Imani Breakthrough Program's community-driven faith-based opioid recovery initiative that was specifically reaching Black and Latinx communities.[31] His brother said he and his pastor had wanted to do something like that with their church and asked Dr Brave what he thought about it. Intrigued, Dr Brave started looking up other community-focused initiatives, and was pleased to find similar models globally such as the Friendship Bench intervention in Zimbabwe that partnered with grandmothers to address a severe mental health crisis amid a mental health workforce shortage.[32] He began to imagine new possibilities.

Inspired to collaborate with the community outside of the four walls of the clinic, Dr Brave chose to use the Strengths Model to inform how he could partner with his brother's church which consisted of mostly African American families. He specifically liked how this model emphasized helping people make changes in two dimensions of their recovery: (1) moving from entrapping intrapersonal narratives to empowering ones; and (2) moving from entrapping environmental niches to empowering ones[33] (**Fig. 5-3**).

In the following months, Dr Brave and his brother's pastor met several times to brainstorm how their efforts might synergize. The pastor shared he never expected to be counseling families through addiction and overdose prevention when he started ministry. He was frustrated by repeatedly seeing families traumatized by their loved ones' drug use, overdoses and legal issues and was aware how the drug use was becoming more prevalent and the drugs more deadly. In the past year, the church had experienced emotional trauma with overdose death of one of their high school students. The pastor knew that other Black and Latinx churches in the area were facing similar problems and invited them into discussions. Several

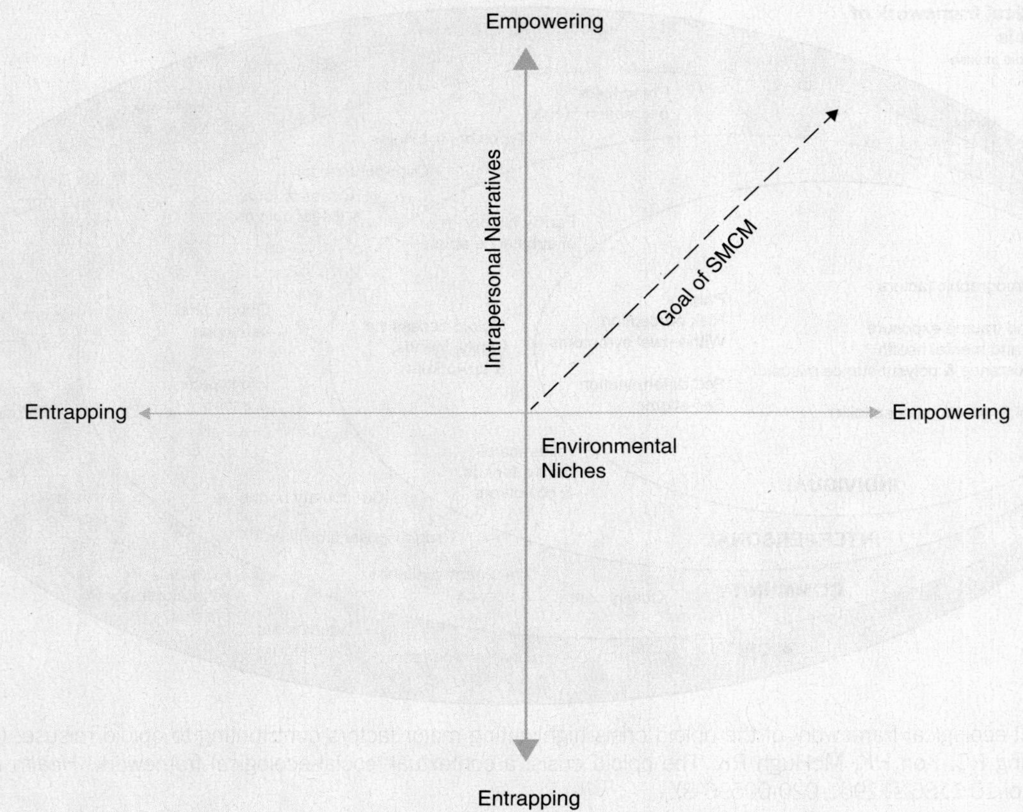

Figure 5-3. Strengths model for case management. (From Goscha, R. Strengths model case management: moving strengths from concept to action. In: Mendenhall AN, Carney MM, eds. In Rooted in Strengths: Celebrating the Strengths Perspective in Social Work; 2022:165-186).

months later, one Latinx and two Black churches asked to collaborate with Dr Brave to see how their partnership could make an impact in their community.

Dr Brave had found impassioned partners who understood the need to reach the Black and Latinx communities with addiction care; unexpected partners he discovered only through his critical conversation with his brother. As he continued this outreach, he developed effective communication and teaching skills to foster the engagement and education of the many diverse stakeholders he recruited. Dr Brave became both an advocate internally within the four walls of his clinic and externally in the community. He became an enduring champion for change. He learned that a single phone call or visit with one church leader or nonprofit board would not suffice. Instead of complaining about churches and residential programs that "don't get it," his approach to system change mimicked his approach with his patients: they deserve understanding, care for their ailments, optimization of their functioning, and attention to their ongoing well-being. Dr Brave let stakeholders know change is possible, he assisted them as an equal partner, and he collaborated and was accountable to them. Now with attention of key stakeholders and system lever pullers, he wondered what was next. Read on.

Put Together a Diverse, Multispecialty, and Interdisciplinary Team

Transformational change needs a broad set of participating diverse stakeholders: from medicine, nursing and other health disciplines; from financial, governmental, and policy players; from patients and the public. It truly takes a village. Health care affects all Americans. It is one of our highest national values and impacts all aspects of public and social health. It is central to the successes and failures of American society and culture. We all own it, and we must all participate in improving it. Every addiction medicine leader has a contribution they can make.

Diverse, multispecialty, interdisciplinary teams provide a breadth of perspective from varied and complimentary backgrounds that work together toward achieving common goals. Transformational change requires this revolutionary shift in understanding that these diverse teams are not just for outward display of solidarity, but essential to the process of transformation itself. We are all profoundly interconnected. Leadership can be defined as the ability to inspire and align others to successfully achieve common goals, with an emphasis on "others" and "common."[34] Physicians can assume the role of champion, but they do not always have to be the team leader; they can also model valuable listening skills, openness to change, willingness to make suggestions and continued participation on the team. Physicians should expect and encourage a diversity of styles—most health care professions have their own cultures and values, and the reality is physicians do not own the single standard—and they are usually newcomers to groups already networking or known to each other. Stakeholders who are involved in the process of change are more likely to be cooperative if they sense openness instead of resistance when offering a view. This collaborative systems approach requires physicians to desert their traditionalist top-down and authoritarian approaches of providing the ultimate answer and the final say. This is often a difficult pill for physicians to swallow. Embracing an egalitarian style with nonphysicians increases the pool for ideas and suggestions. The physician or group leader can then ask each person for his or her concerns and opinions and create a safe space for everyone to contribute. Inclusion of freely expressed ideas from a group of diverse stakeholders is essential for change from the heart that can lead to a change in systems of care. Externally motivated change is effervescent; change from the inside is nearly indelible.

Dr Brave Builds a Team on Common Ground

Dr Brave returned to his clinic with his hope and conviction restored that the status quo can be changed with the help of his new community partners. For several weeks, he slowly introduced the idea of collaborating with churches of color with his internal colleagues and "socialized" the idea of an interdepartmental health disparities meeting. He sought out sympathetic and at least open-minded staff to participate in opening a dialogue. To his surprise he found impassioned advocates in the clinic's warm-hearted Latinx pediatrician who was concerned about the trends in adolescent vaping and cannabis use and the Filipino American Licensed Clinical Social Worker (LCSW) who had previous experience with street medicine. He invited the administration and staff from each department to a 60-minute lunch meeting titled "Addressing the Health Disparities in Substance Use Disorder Care with Community Partnerships." After his welcome, he acknowledged and celebrated how far their program had come in helping hundreds of patients with SUDs. After acknowledging their strengths, he reviewed how their medical model of addiction treatment was not reaching communities of color, particularly those affected by alarming rises in overdose rates. He guided the group towards a holistic approach to addiction care that added prevention, harm reduction and recovery to their current treatment heavy model. Dr Brave also put his presentation in context of other successful programs that were partnering with communities to offer prevention education, naloxone distribution and to build community-based peer recovery programs. The pediatrician and LCSW also shared their view on how they saw Dr Brave's holistic approach elevating the care for all patients at the clinic while narrowing the existing disparities in addiction care. Dr Brave ended the lunch with a surprise appearance from his own brother who shared his recovery story and difficulty finding help in his community when he most needed it. His brother emphasized that real change wasn't going to be made without partnering with all segments of the community, using the slogan "Nothing about us without us." Dr Brave shared how he had met with local Black and Latinx pastors recently, and how they were open to partnering with the clinic to hold substance use prevention and education classes, harm reduction interventions such as naloxone distribution, and even integrate peer recovery coaches into their churches to support people with SUDs and increase referrals to addiction treatment programs. The clinic session was well attended. Although one colleague criticized Dr Brave for not "staying in his lane," everyone else was enthusiastic. Dr Brave's brother's story had silenced the room, and the message that community partnerships were needed sunk in. Dr Brave left the door open, and he and his brother reached out to the administration's leadership with an invitation to meet. A week later the Medical Director approached Dr Brave privately to apologize for not understanding him earlier and shared that his brother's story really helped her see the clinic's blind spots. She told him he had her full support and would talk to their CEO to grant permission to create a working group to draft a proposal.

Develop a Shared Purpose and Plan of Action

Human systems derive their identity from a shared, common purpose. The dialogue of change thus begins with the question, "What are we trying to accomplish?" And to engage the passion of the participants asks, "Why is this important to you?"

It is crucial to develop and gain consensus on the purpose and aim of the desired improvement, enlisting and aligning as many stakeholders as necessary or possible to consider alternatives to the status quo. State clearly the testable objective of the plan. The "aim" of the desired improvement should be time specific, measurable, and define the patients, populations, and system(s) to be involved. The Institute of Medicine has suggested that there are six broad categories for most desired improvements: safety, effectiveness, patient-centeredness, timeliness, efficiency, and equity.[35]

Detail the components of the plan, remembering you may be starting small, and develop quantitative measures, which can be used to monitor and track the outcome. With the outcome data, it can be determined whether the plan resulted in an improvement. As a physician leader, your own commitment and endurance are essential. Physicians who desire and work for change that will result in a system's improvement become knowledgeable and gain experience in making small improvements and always cooperate with others. They start with small goals and objectives and seek collaboration. Defined rules are a critical attribute of a cooperative environment.

This is a group process, since persons both within and outside of the departments or organization have varying experience on the system elements involved. No change effort will succeed without cooperation. Cooperative interactions may be ethical and altruistic, yet they are a prerequisite and pragmatic strategy for engineering change in interdependent systems.

Effective leaders learn, model, and teach expertise in basic dialogue and group communication. Basic negotiation attitudes and skills are requisite for success and can be acquired from reading or courses. Success is more likely when the decision process focuses on issues and not individuals and empowers ownership in the change process and results. The frequently expressed complaint that nothing will change until "that person moves on" is counterproductive. There are always issues that can be win-win for all parties. Change is dependent on new solutions, not lamenting current shortcomings.

Dr Brave and the Embrace Recovery Initiative

Dr Brave's Medical Director kept her promise and in the following weeks, the CEO asked him to officially create a working group around how they could close their clinic's racial disparities. The CEO asked their grant writer to support Dr Brave with identifying and applying for grants to support the work. At the next official work group meeting, the pediatrician and LCSW as well as staff from the front desk, medical assistant, pharmacy, psychiatry, and nursing met to brainstorm next steps. Dr Brave used the white board to draw out a Driver Diagram analysis[36] to start the conversation on how they could better serve the whole community and close the substance use disparities among people of color. The group continued to meet weekly for 7 weeks and self-named the group the "Embrace Recovery Initiative."

During four of those meetings, they invited community stakeholders from the churches to meet and help inform the initiatives they were developing. A stakeholder from one of the Black churches shared that: "Black communities need harm reduction because we are always under assault from drug use." A community recovery coach said "The key strength is that we [recovery coaches] understand addiction, we went through the same stuff…recovery coaches are there to support and give guidance. We connect them with [addiction treatment], help with job seeking, housing applications; if they relapse, recovery coaches are there to help you pick up there all the time… sometimes can spend four hours in a day with getting them to appointments and assisting transportation…we can sit with you three hours in a courtroom. How many professionals can do that?" The community input was critical, because it reinforced to the clinic staff that their addiction treatment program was necessary, yet insufficient to meet the structural needs of communities of color struggling with SUDs in their city. A more complex understanding of addiction was needed that took into context people's lived experience and socio-ecological environments. One stakeholder summarized this idea with a comment: "So much evidence that addiction is beyond the neuroreceptor level—it's the criminal justice system, daily life, the neighborhood—all have an impact on outcomes in addiction treatment…medication is essential but not a magic bullet for treating opioid use disorder, [you] need more to recover successfully…not a single med that sustains recovery on its own, especially for those living in toxic environments…rather, a comprehensive, holistic approach tailored to the community is required."[37,38]

At the end of the meetings, they identified five initiatives that they all agreed were attainable: (1) a 3-session workshop series on preventing and treating SUDs that their staff could give at churches in their community, (2) a routine screening, brief intervention and referral to treatment (SBIRT) for all their adolescent and adult primary care patients, (3) a naloxone distribution program for their clinic and church partners, (4) a peer recovery coaching program at their clinic that would facilitate a by-directional bridge to connect the clinic with its partners in the community, and (5) a community addiction treatment referral process with warm handoffs utilizing recovery coaches that the churches could easily utilize. The recovery coaches would connect patients to housing, transportation, as well as mutual support group recovery resources, but inversely, they were available to connect the churches' recovery ministries to addiction medicine referrals for church members with SUDs. The team produced a document with these targeted changes and a detailed plan for implementation and evaluating results. Team representatives brought their proposal to the administration, including the Medical Director and CEO, who were all impressed that personnel from various departments had worked together on the proposal that was so clearly detailed and measurable. They helped the team identify a grant and offered help in applying to acquire funding to implement the proposal.

Act

With a detailed plan in place and the assurance that the people, procedures, and processes needed to execute it are in place, and after all stakeholders—including patients if they are involved—are onboard, begin on a planned start date.

Dr Brave's Community Initiative Begins!

Honoring Dr Brave's brother's words "nothing about us without us," the first step the clinic took was hiring one Black and one Latinx recovery coach who were from the communities they intended to reach. With their recovery coaches' input, the interdisciplinary team spent several months designing the educational curricula, SBIRT workflows, peer recovery coaching program and community referral process. They decided to roll out the initiatives in phases. They held one last clinic-wide meeting where their team outlined the rationale and objectives for the initiatives with a detailed timeline, responsibilities, and evaluative methodology to track progress. The implementation start dates for each phase were announced at the meeting and subsequently through email and clinic huddle announcements.

Set Up a Strategy for Evaluation and Improvement

Monitor key aspects and measures for the plan, document problems and unexpected observations, and begin preliminary analysis of the data. Recall the saying "what gets measured gets done," and remember that there is no innovation without data. Take the time and engage the people and system elements that the cycle will involve or impact.

At appropriate and strategic intervals, analyze the emerging data. Compare them with your predictions and discuss with the team, reflecting on what was learned. Determine what modifications should be made and prepare a plan for next steps.

The Embrace Recovery Team Follows Through

Implementing the five initiatives of the plan had some early bumps and unexpected consequences. Modifications were made along the way. At the 3-month evaluation mark, the predetermined evaluative indices were reported: number of community education sessions held with pre/post surveys, SBIRT referrals, number of naloxone kits distributed and administrations for overdoses reported, patient evaluations of the recovery coach sessions, and community referrals through the church partnerships. Dr Brave also tracked the addiction program's panel and reported that the number of previously underserved, minoritized patients receiving treatment for SUDs increased by 15% at the 6-month mark. A survey of involved churches indicated that community stakeholders believed the community partnerships had reduced stigma of addiction and racial biases and overall reflected a high satisfaction with the program.

The Embrace Recovery Initiative Becomes a Movement! As the success of the Embrace Recovery Initiative spread throughout the community, the County's Opioid Task Force reached out to Dr Brave to invite him to present on their program. During the meeting, Dr Brave presented on the structural racism that caused the racial disparities in the addiction treatment setting. After the meeting, interested clinicians at nearby clinics and a hospital addiction medicine consult liaison service asked for follow-up to discuss helping them launch similar programs. They were encouraged that Dr Brave was forthright in bringing up the racial disparities in their field and were impressed that the clinic team was making an impact to reduce them. Over the following year, these clinicians and other new participants increased their engagement with community partners and soon recognized their need to better coordinate their care across agencies. For example, the hospital consult liaison service began utilizing recovery coaches to ensure smooth transitions from inpatient to outpatient. Recovery coaches acted as a bridge not only with the community but also between their hospital and clinics. In several years, this coordinated effort began to see the gap between addiction care racial disparities close by 50%. As Dr Brave saw the community partnership model replicated across the county with measurable outcomes to show progress, he regained the conviction that communities of color could someday receive equitable addiction care in the U.S. using this proven approach to effecting change in health care and the community.

SUMMARY

Unhealthy substance use impacts people we work with, live with, and those with whom we share community; persons we care about; and those we love. On some level, it is personal for all of us. Foremost, health care is much more than a calculated business venture; it is compassion and caring for all with whom we are connected. Every addiction medicine clinician is needed to bring prevention, high-quality treatment, recovery support and systems improvement into reality. Addiction medicine can lead and contribute to the well-being of communities and nations as well as to our patients and their families. Whether clinician contributions are made in assessing, planning, or acting on improvements in a small clinic, a large health care system, or at the level of governmental policy impacting public health, this is all within the mission and character of the field of addiction medicine. Addiction medicine clinicians are clinical experts, faculty and teachers, researchers, and change agents. This is our work and we can succeed.

REFERENCES

1. Centers for Disease Control and Prevention. *Alcohol-Attributable Deaths*. Accessed May 1, 2022. https://nccd.cdc.gov/DPH_ARDI/default/default.aspx
2. National Center for Chronic Disease Prevention and Health Promotion (U.S.) Office on Smoking and Health. *The Health Consequences of Smoking—50 Years of Progress: A Report of the Surgeon General*. Department of Health and Human Services, Centers for Disease Control and Prevention; 2014.
3. Centers for Disease Control and Prevention. *Provisional Drug Overdose Death Counts*. Accessed May 1, 2022. https://www.cdc.gov/nchs/nvss/vsrr/drug-overdose-data.htm
4. Compton WM, Einstein EB, Jones CM. Exponential increases in drug overdoses: Implications for epidemiology and research. *Int J Drug Policy*. 2022;104:103676.
5. STATISTA. *Health and health systems ranking of countries worldwide in 2021, by health index score*. Accessed May 1, 2022. https://www.statista.com/statistics/1290168/health-index-of-countries-worldwide-by-health-index-score/
6. The Commonwealth Fund. *Health Care in the U.S. Compared to Other High-Income Countries*. Accessed August 8, 2023. https://www.commonwealthfund.org/publications/fund-reports/2021/aug/mirror-mirror-2021-reflecting-poorly
7. *Adolescent Substance Use: America's #1 Public Health Problem*. The National Center on Addiction and Substance Abuse at Columbia University. June 2011. Accessed November 15, 2023. https://cdn-01.drugfree.org/web/prod/wp-content/uploads/2011/06/19202754/Adolescent-substance-use-americas-no-1-public-health-problem.pdf?_gl=1*gyfdn2*_ga*MTYxOTExMTI4Mi4xNzAwMDkyNDQ2*_ga_ECZGQ0GWSZ*MTcwMDA5MjQ0NS4xLjEuMTcwMDA5MjQ2OC4zNy4wLjA
8. Mokdad AH, Marks JS, Stroup DF, Gerberding JL. Actual causes of death in the United States, 2000. *JAMA*. 2004;291(10):1238-1245.
9. Marvasti FF, Stafford RS. From sick care to health care—reengineering prevention into the U.S. System. *N Engl J Med*. 2002;367(10):889-891.
10. Richter L, Kunz K, Foster SE. A public health approach to addiction: the health professional's role. In: Herron AJ, Brennan TK, eds. *Essentials of Addiction Medicine*. 2nd ed. American Society of Addiction Medicine/Wolters Kluwer; 2015.
11. Flexner A. *Medical Education in the United States and Canada: A Report to the Carnegie Foundation for the Advancement of Teaching, Bulletin No. 4. The Carnegie Foundation for the Advancement of Teaching*; 1910:346. OCLC 9795002. Accessed November 15, 2023. https://archive.org/details/medicaleducation00flexiala/mode/2up
12. Duffy TP. The Flexner Report—100 Years Later. *Yale J Biol Med*. 2011;84(3):269-276.
13. Feinberg HV. The paradox of disease prevention: celebrated in principle, resisted in practice. *JAMA*. 2013;310(1):85-90.
14. Thibault GE. Reforming health professions education will require culture change and closer ties between classroom and practice. *Health Aff (Millwood)*. 2013;32(11):1928-1932.
15. Thibault GE. The future of health professions education: emerging trends in the United States. *FASEB Bioadv*. 2020;2(12):685-694. doi:10.1096/fba.2020-00061
16. O'Connor PG, Sokol RJ, D'Onofrio G. Addiction medicine: the birth of a new discipline. *JAMA Intern Med*. 2014;174(11):1717-1718. doi:10.1001/jamainternmed.2014.4211
17. American Board of Medical Specialties. *A Trusted Credential*. Accessed on March 6, 2023. http://www.abms.org/board-certification/a-trusted-credential/based-on-core-competencies/
18. Association for Multidisciplinary Education and Research in Substance use and Addiction. Specific Disciplines Addressing Substance Use: AMERSA in the 21st Century - 2018 Update. Accessed on March 6, 2023. https://amersa.org/wp-content/uploads/AMERSA-Competencies-Final-31119.pdf
19. Hansen H, Braslow J, Rohrbaugh RM. From cultural to structural competency—training psychiatry residents to act on social determinants of health and institutional racism. *JAMA Psychiatry*. 2018;75(2):117-118. doi:10.1001/jamapsychiatry.2017.3894
20. CDC Foundation. *What is Public Health?* Accessed August 8, 2023. http://www.cdcfoundation.org/content/what-public-health
21. Der Virchow R. Armenarzt. *Die Medicinische Reform*. 1848;125-127.
22. Mackenbach JP. Politics is nothing but medicine on a larger scale: reflections on public health's biggest idea. *J Epidemiol Community Health*. 2009;63:181-184.
23. Healthypeople.gov. *Social Determinants of Health*. https://wayback.archive-it.org/5774/20220413203948/https://www.healthypeople.gov/2020/topics-objectives/topic/social-determinants-of-health
24. Gass R. What is Transformational Change? Accessed August 8, 2023. http://transform.transformativechange.org/2010/06/robertgass
25. Institute for Healthcare Improvement. Accessed 8 August, 2023. http://www.ihi.org
26. Reinertsen JL. Physicians as leaders in the improvement of health care systems. *Ann Intern Med*. 1998;128(10):834-838.
27. Han B, Einstein EB, Jones CM, Cotto J, Compton WM, Volkow ND. Racial and ethnic disparities in drug overdose deaths in the US during the COVID-19 pandemic. *JAMA Netw Open*. 2022;5(9):e2232314. doi:10.1001/jamanetworkopen.2022.32314
28. Nolan TW. Understanding medical systems. *Ann Intern Med*. 1998;128(4):293-298.
29. Jalali MS, Botticelli M, Hwang RC, Koh HK, RK MH. The opioid crisis: a contextual, social-ecological framework. *Health Res Policy Syst*. 2020;18(1):87. doi:10.1186/s12961-020-00596-8
30. Monsen KA, Vanderboom CE, Olson KS, Larson ME, Holland DE. Care coordination from a strengths perspective: a practice-based evidence evaluation of evidence-based practice. *Res Theory Nurs Pract*. 2017;31(1):39-55. doi:10.1891/1541-6577.31.1.39
31. Bellamy CD, Costa M, Wyatt J, et al. A collaborative culturally-centered and community-driven faith-based opioid recovery initiative: the Imani Breakthrough project. *Soc Work Ment Health*. 2021;19(6):558-567. doi:10.1080/15332985.2021.1930329
32. Chibanda D, Weiss HA, Verhey R, et al. Effect of a primary care–based psychological intervention on symptoms of common mental disorders in Zimbabwe: a randomized clinical trial. *JAMA*. 2016;316(24):2618-2626. doi:10.1001/jama.2016.19102
33. Strengths Model Case Management. California Institute for Behavioral Health Solutions. Accessed May 1, 2022. https://work.cibhs.org/strengths-model-case-management

34. Gass R. *What is Transformation? And How It Advances Social Change.* Accessed August 8, 2023. https://www.robertgass.com/_files/ugd/17ff8d_693caff6096b411b9dd0d0fdef122ec8.pdf
35. Agency for Healthcare Research and Quality. *Six Domains of Health Care Quality.* Accessed May 1, 2022. https://www.ahrq.gov/talkingquality/measures/six-domains.html
36. Institute for Healthcare Improvement. Tools: Driver Diagram. Accessed May 1, 2022. https://www.ihi.org/resources/Pages/Tools/Driver-Diagram.aspx
37. SAMHSA. *The Opioid Crisis and the Black/African American Population: An Urgent Issue.* Accessed August 8, 2023. https://store.samhsa.gov/sites/default/files/pep20-05-02-001.pdf
38. SAMHSA. *What are Peer Recovery Support Services?* Accessed August 8, 2023. https://www.samhsa.gov/sites/default/files/programs_campaigns/brss_tacs/peers-supporting-recovery-substance-use-disorders-2017.pdf

CHAPTER 6

Climate Change and Addiction Medicine

Shannon C. Miller and John W. Sullenbarger

CHAPTER OUTLINE

- Introduction
- Impacts of CC on mental health
- Vulnerable populations
- Impact of CC on populations with greater identification with the environment (eg, Indigenous and rural communities)
- Interactions between CC and substance use
- Contributions of substance use to CC and environmental degradation
- Approach to the patient impacted by CC
- Addiction medicine clinicians as change agents to slow CC
- Conclusions

INTRODUCTION

Climate change (CC) is "the single biggest health threat facing humanity"[1] and yet there is little attention to this topic in the field of addiction medicine. CC is defined as significant, long-term changes in climate *measures* (air temperature and quality, precipitation, humidity, ocean temperature and pH, wind patterns, sea level, sea ice, etc.) and how these changes affect life on Earth. Climate change drivers (also referred to as climate forcings or climate drivers) are actions that force a change in the climate set point subsequently creating abnormal climate measures and resulting in extreme weather or other CC related meteorological events.[2] Natural CC drivers include pattern shifts in the dynamics of our oceans and atmosphere (El Niño/La Niña, and the Pacific Decadal Oscillation), volcanic eruptions that emit various gasses and aerosols, long-term changes in the Earth's orbit around the sun, and variations in the amount of energy from the Sun that reaches Earth.[3] Examples of non-natural, human caused (or anthropogenic) CC drivers include greenhouse gas emissions (created from the burning of fossil fuels, which in turn create carbon dioxide/CO_2 and other heat-trapping gases and pollutants), and deforestation (which enables heat energy to more readily penetrate and heat the Earth, while also reducing air filtration and carbon sequestration), as well as a myriad of lesser but still significant anthropogenic CC drivers.

Since the industrial revolution of the mid-1800s, anthropogenic CC drivers have dominated Earth's climate forces resulting in a warming of the Earth and destabilization of climate measures, as well as extreme weather events.[4] The direct and indirect impacts of CC driver exposures are far reaching for human health, particularly mental health. For the purposes of this chapter, we will be focusing on the primary source of CC in the last two centuries (anthropogenic) and its relationships with mental health and addiction medicine.

IMPACTS OF CC ON MENTAL HEALTH

Anthropogenic CC has increased the average number of extreme weather events such as hurricanes, floods, heavy precipitation and other severe conditions; as well as heat waves, wildfires, droughts, air pollution, acidification of the oceans, rising ocean levels, and loss of biodiversity and habitats. CC can be visualized through a variety of online models, such as NASA's interactive climate time machine, which allows the visualization of four key climate measures over time: global temperature, sea ice, sea level, and carbon dioxide.[5]

CC negatively impacts human health including psychiatric and addiction medicine-related. A 2021 U.S. general population survey on CC-related concerns indicates that 70% of Americans were worried about global warming, with 35% of this group having great worry.[6] As for the younger generation, among 10,000 youth studied in 10 countries (Australia, Brazil, Finland, France, India, Nigeria, Philippines, Portugal, the United Kingdom, and the United States; 1,000 participants per country between May-June 2021), 84% reported at least moderate anxiety about CC and 45% of that majority reported a daily negative impact to their life and functioning; 75% said that they think the future is frightening, and 83% said that they think people have failed to take care of the planet.[7]

Among people with mental health disorders, CC is associated with increased distress, anxiety, depression, PTSD, cognitive impairment, substance use, psychiatric hospitalizations, suicide, and overall mortality.[8] In the last decade, this growing impact of CC on mental health has crystalized a novel lexicon to describe the expanding psychological responses to CC, overarchingly referred to as "psychoterratic syndromes."[9] "Ecoanxiety" is defined as anxiety regarding future/potential environmental degradation or loss due to CC, whereas "ecological grief" refers to those CC-related degradations and losses already experienced. For example, 20% to 41% of Europeans described ecoanxiety in 2016 over CC-related issues.[10] However, after the repeated heat waves, droughts, and other extreme events in the years following 2016 it is likely these numbers are higher. "Ecoparalysis" is defined as the inability to act on environmental degradation or CC due to a belief it is insurmountable. "Solastalgia"[11] is a term derived from the Latin word for "comfort" plus the Greek word for "pain" and is defined as pain/distress resulting from a loss of solace/comfort from a geographical area that has been environmentally degraded and no longer provides the comfort or meaning that it used to. These syndromes are not viewed as pathological,[12] but rather are expected and normal responses to abnormal events. These concepts are increasingly applied to substance use disorder (SUD)-related research and practice.

People with SUDs may be more vulnerable to CC-related events; either due to the direct interactions of their substance with the CC event (such as impaired thermoregulation from stimulant use during heat waves), or in relation to common co-occurring conditions such as homelessness. Further, certain substance-related behaviors or industries may contribute, albeit in smaller ways, to CC.

VULNERABLE POPULATIONS

CC negatively impacts disadvantaged people more often and disproportionally as a result of their greater geographic exposure to CC-related events, as well as impoverished resources and reserves to adapt and cope with CC effects. For instance, those struggling with homelessness, which influences and is influenced by substance use,[13] are at increased risk of experiencing detrimental outcomes from CC; such as heat stroke during heat waves, as well as greater exposure to air pollution impacting neurocognitive and cardiovascular functioning. In brief, CC can worsen the housing crisis further through damage to homes, disruption of resources, and financial pressures.[12] Youth and elderly populations, ethnic and racial minorities, those living in rural communities, and those who have close identities with the Earth are also all placed at higher risk for greater impact from CC due to neurobiological vulnerabilities, complex and historically racist policies, and emotional and geographical proximity to the effects of CC, amongst others.

IMPACT OF CC ON POPULATIONS WITH GREATER IDENTIFICATION WITH THE ENVIRONMENT (EG, INDIGENOUS AND RURAL COMMUNITIES)

Greater identification and connection to the Earth, such as in Indigenous and rural communities, creates a vulnerability for broader and more intense impacts from CC. Many of these communities are also located in areas more prone to experience CC-related extreme events, such as wildfires, derechos, drought, and flooding. The resultant identity disruption can confer greater risk for negative psychological effects and maladaptive coping mechanisms, such as through unhealthy substance use. Although complex in its etiology and largely owing to systematic oppression, those in Indigenous communities are at higher risk for SUDs compared to other cultural groups[14] and part of this risk can be inferred from environmental degradation as a result of a changing climate and environment.[8] Rural communities are also at higher risk due to their close economic and identifying relationship with the surrounding land that is experiencing CC through drought, severe heat, and extreme weather events. This is exemplified by elevated rates of suicide by farmers during droughts.[15,16] Direct and indirect impacts of CC, as well as the psychological effects of a changing environment, places a significant burden on the mental health of these populations, which likely confers a greater risk for reliance on substance use as a coping means. For example, solastalgia has impacted rural American mountain communities as evidenced in a quantitative study by Canu et al.[17] who examined Kentucky emergency department visits and found a greater risk of depression and SUDs in areas with mountain top removal mining, after controlling for other demographic factors.

INTERACTIONS BETWEEN CC AND SUBSTANCE USE

Heat Waves

It is unequivocal that human influence has warmed (global warming) the Earth's atmosphere, ocean, and land; and at a current rate of about 0.2 °C (0.36 °F) incrementally per decade, more rapidly than any period observed historically.[18] The rate of "hottest year ever recorded" has increased since 2005, compared to before the industrial revolution in America.[19] Global warming (a main indicator of CC) is occurring roughly ten times faster than the average rate of expected natural ice-age-recovery warming with some areas around the world experiencing greater rates of warming than others, such as the oceans, which absorb most of the temperature increase currently, as well as the greenhouse gas carbon dioxide which acidifies the oceans. Carbon dioxide from human activity is increasing more than 250 times faster than it did from natural sources after the last Ice Age.[20]

Excessive heat is associated with an increase of 1% in the suicide rate for every 1 °F of mean ambient temperature increase,[21] as well as a 3.9% increase in interpersonal violence and a 13.6% increase in inter-group violence per standard deviation increase in temperature.[22]

During heat waves, neurocognitive function is eroded resulting in reduced working memory, reaction time, and attention,[23] which may then erode impulse control resulting in greater risk for maladaptive substance or gambling use. Sleep quality is reduced during heat waves,[24] which may then increase risk for substance use in an attempt to self-medicate.

Bouchama et al.[25] conducted a meta-analysis of observational studies published between 1982 and 2005 on a broad array of risk and protective factors in heat wave-related deaths and found that being confined to bed (OR, 6.44; 95% confidence interval [CI], 4.5-9.2), not leaving home daily (OR, 3.35;

95% CI, 1.6-6.9), and being unable to care for oneself (OR, 2.97; 95% CI, 1.8-4.8) were associated with the highest risk of death during heat waves. Preexisting psychiatric illness tripled the risk of death, followed by cardiovascular and pulmonary illness. Access to home air-conditioning, visiting cool environments, and increasing social contact were strongly associated with better outcomes. Taking extra showers or baths and using fans were associated with a trend toward lower risk of death. Each of these factors can be applied to patient populations with SUDs during heat waves to assess or reduce risk.

A significantly higher heat-related mortality rate is seen in those with SUDs.[8] Alcohol and other substance use places people at higher risk for impaired thermoregulation during heat waves via disruption in serotonergic, adrenergic, cholinergic, GABAergic, and glutaminergic pathways, which all play roles in thermoregulation.[26,27] For instance, stimulant use increases the presence of catecholamine neurotransmitters, which increase peripheral vasoconstriction through alpha 1 and 2 signaling, diminishing the body's ability to release heat through conduction and radiation.[27] Smoked and vaped/aerosolized drugs compromise the cardiorespiratory system, which may be further negatively impacted during heat waves. Alcohol is a central nervous system depressant and causes diuresis and dehydration. Opioids may interfere with heat-induced vasculature responses. Sedative-hypnotics depress the central nervous system causing dehydration. There is an association between fatal cocaine overdoses and hot weather.[28]

Page et al. [29] assessed a large, well-validated, longitudinal primary care dataset to determine the risk of mortality in people with psychosis, dementia and unhealthy substance use during hot weather in England (1998-2007). Overall, a classic "hockey stick" plot was observed, whereby these populations showed an overall increase in risk of death of 4.9% (95% CI 2.0-7.8) per 1 °C (1.8 °F) increase in temperature above the 93rd percentile (in this case, 64.4 °F) of the annual temperature distribution (**Fig. 6-1**). Younger patients, those prescribed sedative-hypnotics or antipsychotics, and those with a primary diagnosis of unhealthy substance use demonstrated the greatest mortality risk. This effect is compared against that seen in general population samples using similar methodology, where an increased risk of around 2% per 1 °C increase is seen in England and Wales.

More generally, a study by Martin-Latry et al.[30] highlighted greater odds for hospitalization and heat-related deaths while on psychotropics as a result of the thermoregulatory disruption.

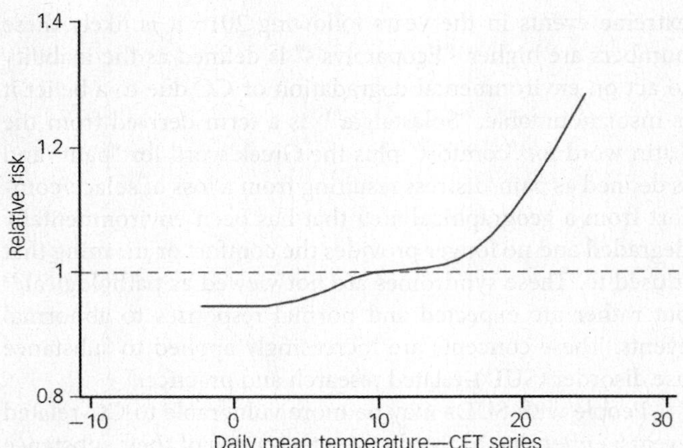

Figure 6-1. Seasonally adjusted relationship between risk of death and central England temperature (CET) series in patients with psychosis, dementia and unhealthy substance use. (From Page LA, Hajat S, Sari Kovats R, Howard LM. Temperature-related deaths in people with psychosis, dementia and substance misuse. *Br J Psychiatry.* 2012;200:485-490.)

Air Pollution and Wildfires

Air pollution negatively impacts at least 90% of the world's population causing 4.2 years of life lost per person globally on average.[31] CC-related air pollution includes products of fossil fuel burning, burning of other matter including during wildfires, products of industrialization, etc. This consists of increased ozone, dust, pollen, nitrogen dioxide and carbon dioxide and other heat trapping or toxic gases, and three sizes of particulate matter (PM).

Wildfires are occurring more frequently and with more severity. CC has doubled the forest fire area in the western United States between 1984 and 2016.[32] In addition to the biological impact of air pollution on mental health, the psychological impact is significant. For example, rates of depression and PTSD were high among those directly exposed to wildfires: 31% to 33% for depression and 24% to 37% for PTSD.[33]

Air pollutants, especially PM, can be carried throughout the body after entry via the respiratory and olfactory systems. Such exposure has been associated with cerebral oxidative distress and inflammation resulting in possible increased risk for various brain diseases. Prolonged exposure to PM of 2.5 μm diameter or smaller (equal to about 1/20th the diameter of a human hair, or smaller, and a size that can be inhaled very deeply into lung tissue) has been associated with increased risk for dementia, including Parkinson and Alzheimer diseases, as well as autism spectrum disorders.[34] PM has also been associated with increased risk for depression and suicide,[35] and disorders of the developing brain (behavioral, ADHD, reduced IQ, and developmental delay).[36] Additionally, risk for violence is increased; for every 10 μm^2 increase in PM 2.5 μm there is an associated 1.1% increased rate of violence, with a 0.6% increase on days with high ozone levels.[37]

Air pollution may further compromise the cardiorespiratory system in those who smoke or vape/aerosolize drugs, with higher rates of hospitalization, morbidity, and mortality for obstructive airway disease in areas and days with high air pollution levels, especially PM.[38]

Extreme Weather Events

People exposed to extreme weather events are 90% more likely to experience depression, anxiety, PTSD, hyperarousal, insomnia, reduced concentration, or increased substance use.[33]

Rohrbach et al.[39] examined relationships between exposure to Hurricane Rita, and posttraumatic stress (PTS) symptoms, and changes in adolescent substance use from 13-months predisaster to 7-months and 19-months postdisaster. Subjects involved 280 Louisiana high school students who participated in a substance use prevention intervention trial prior to the hurricane. Two-thirds were female and 68% were White. Students completed surveys at baseline (13 months prehurricane) and two follow-ups (7-months and 19-months posthurricane). Results indicated a positive bivariate relationship between PTS symptoms, assessed at 7-months post-hurricane, and increases in alcohol ($p < .05$) and cannabis use ($p < .10$) from baseline to the 7-month posthurricane follow-up. When these associations were examined collectively with other hurricane-related predictors in multivariate regression models, PTS symptoms did not predict increases in substance use. However, objective exposure to the hurricane predicted increases in cannabis use, and post-hurricane negative life events predicted increases in all three types of substance use (p's $< .10$), suggesting that increased adolescent substance use may result after hurricane exposure.

Flory et al.[40] studied 209 adult survivors of Hurricane Katrina interviewed in Columbia, South Carolina or New Orleans, Louisiana between October 2005 and May 2006. Results revealed that survivors were smoking cigarettes, drinking alcohol, and experiencing alcohol-related problems at a substantially higher rate than expected based on prehurricane prevalence data. Results also suggested that certain psychosocial factors were associated with participants' substance use and unhealthy use following the hurricane. Additional studies of the effects of Hurricane Katrina support these findings. For example, Kessler found a doubling of prevalence of any mental disorders (increasing from 15% to 31%) and in "serious" mental illness (increasing from 6.1% to 11.3%) following Hurricane Katrina.[41]

The MH-related consequences from CC may be long-lasting at times. Floods have impacted mental health for as long as 5 years,[42] and Hurricane Katrina victims from 2005 continued to need trauma-related care more than 10 years later.[43]

Drought

CC has resulted in higher average temperatures along with longer periods of time between precipitation. Droughts then result and are only worsened with human population growth and corresponding greater water use. Droughts are associated with depression, anxiety, domestic violence, as well as conflicts between spouses, peoples, and between communities.[15]

Those who reside on the land (such as farmers and Indigenous peoples) and rely upon it for their own sustenance and economic viability and identity are among those hit with significant mental health impacts. For example, drought conditions are associated with a 15% increased risk for suicide among rural middle-aged males in New South Wales, Australia, many of whom were farmers.[44,45] This is supported by a study from Carleton[16] who found that rising temperatures, and the related reduction in precipitation, can be attributed to an additional excess of 59,300 suicides from 1980 to 2017 in India, largely in farmers.

CONTRIBUTIONS OF SUBSTANCE USE TO CC AND ENVIRONMENTAL DEGRADATION

While the production and use of substances relating to SUDs can have a variety of impacts (however small) to CC, here we briefly focus on a few substances that have potential to increasingly impact CC over time due to their high prevalence of use, high amounts of new initiates, and the greatest prevalence of substance-specific SUD[46]; and for which significant studies exist (**Figs. 6-2** to **6-4**).

Nicotine and Tobacco

While the prevalence of tobacco smoking has been declining in developed countries,[47] the rate of traditional (nonelectronic) cigarette consumption has still been increasing globally due in a large part to increasing marketing to and consumption by youth and young adults in developing countries.[48] Annually, 6 trillion cigarettes are produced and 5.8 trillion are consumed.[49] Nicotine (including both tobacco-derived and synthetic) and tobacco leaf products are used by one-fifth of Americans over the age of 12 (**Fig. 6-5**).

While the health effects of smoking are increasingly known, the impact of the tobacco industry on the environment and CC is less understood. With support from the World Health Organization (WHO), Zafeiridou et al.[50] studied the impact of the traditional cigarette industry on the environment by quantifying the environmental footprint of traditional cigarettes (a major portion of the tobacco industry) across the global tobacco supply chain (cultivation, curing, primary processing and trading, manufacturing, distribution, use, and final disposal). A cumulative mass balance model was produced using material flow analysis (an established analytical method for quantifying flows and stocks of materials and substances), while the environmental footprint of cigarette smoking was captured from cradle-to-grave using life cycle assessment (a well-established and internationally standardized method for assessing the potential environmental and health impacts of goods and services) (**Figs. 6-6** and **6-7**). Despite detailed accounting, their efforts likely underestimated the environmental impacts.

The authors concluded that the cultivation of 32.4 megatons (Mt) of green tobacco used for the production of 6.48 Mt of dry tobacco in the 6 trillion cigarettes manufactured worldwide in 2014 were shown to contribute almost 84 Mt CO_2 equivalent emissions to CC—approximately 0.2% of the global total; including 490,000 tons of 1,4-dichlorobenzene equivalent to ecosystem ecotoxicity levels; over 22 billion m^3 equivalents of water consumption, and 21 Mt of oil equivalents to fossil fuel consumption. A typical single cigarette was shown to have a water footprint of 3.7 L, a CC contribution of 14 g of CO_2 equivalents, and a fossil fuel consumption of

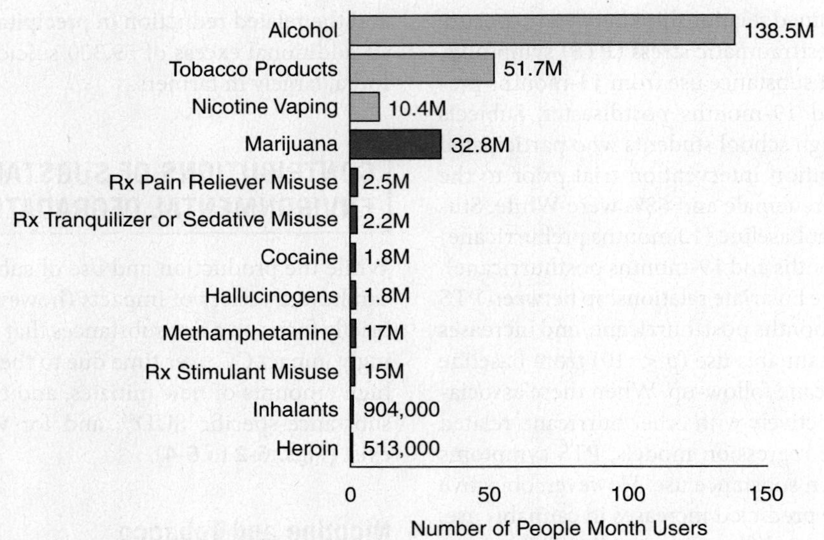

Figure 6-2. Past month general substance use and nicotine vaping: among people aged 12 or older, 2020. Rx = prescription. Note: General Substance Use includes any illicit drug, alcohol, and tobacco product use. Tobacco products are defined as cigarettes, smokeless tobacco, cigars, and pipe tobacco. Note: The estimated numbers of people who current use different substances are not mutually exclusive because people could have used more than one type of substance in the past month. (From SAMHSA. Key substance use and mental health indicators in the United States: Results from the 2020 National Survey on Drug Use and Health. *HHS Publication No. PEP21-07-01-003, NSDUH Series H-56.* Center for Behavioral Health Statistics and Quality, Substance Abuse and Mental Health Services Administration; 2021. Accessed July 9, 2022. https://www.samhsa.gov/data/)

3.5 g oil equivalents. They concluded that "Tobacco competes with (more) essential (consumer) commodities for resources and places significant pressures on the health of our planet and its most vulnerable inhabitants. Increased awareness, as well as better monitoring and assessment of the environmental issues associated with tobacco, should support the current efforts to reduce global tobacco use as an important element of sustainable development."

The authors[50] put this into perspective. Describing a typical person who smokes traditional cigarettes, the authors conclude that a person who smokes a pack a day over 50 years creates a carbon footprint that would require 132 tree saplings to be planted and grown for an entire decade to offset the carbon cost of manufacturing those cigarettes for that single person. The manufacture of that single person's supply of cigarettes costs an amount of water that could have otherwise been used

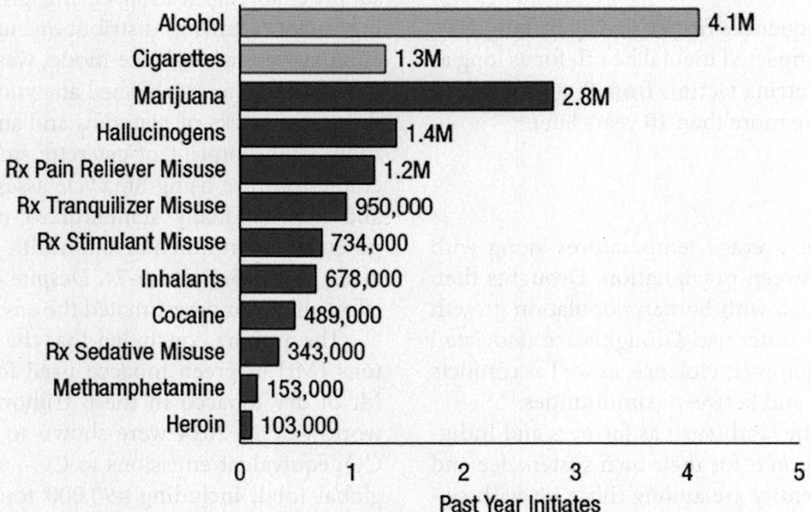

Figure 6-3. Past year initiates of substances among people aged 12 and older, 2020. Rx = prescription. Note: Estimates for prescription pain relievers, prescription tranquilizers, prescription stimulants, and prescription sedatives are for the initiation of misuse. (From SAMHSA. Key substance use and mental health indicators in the United States: Results from the 2020 National Survey on Drug Use and Health. *HHS Publication No. PEP21-07-01-003, NSDUH Series H-56.* Center for Behavioral Health Statistics and Quality, Substance Abuse and Mental Health Services Administration; 2021. Accessed July 9, 2022. https://www.samhsa.gov/data/)

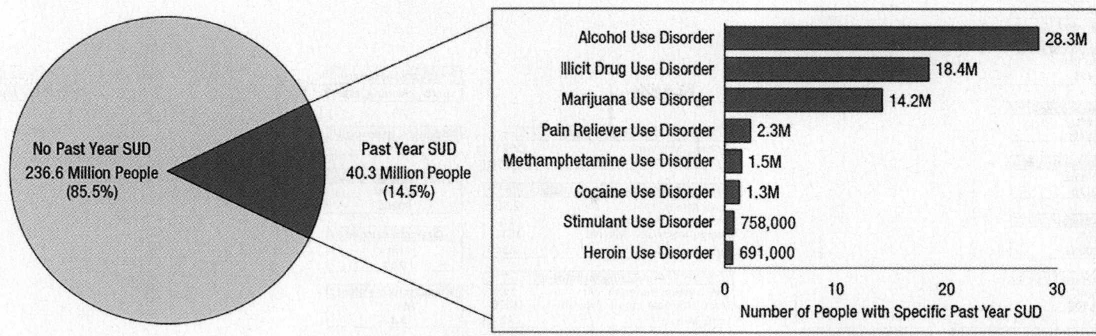

Figure 6-4. People aged 12 or older with a past year substance use disorder (SUD), 2020. Note: The estimated numbers of people who currently use different tobacco products or nicotine vaping are not mutually exclusive because people could have used more than one type of tobacco product or used tobacco products and vaped nicotine in the past month. (From SAMHSA. Key substance use and mental health indicators in the United States: Results from the 2020 National Survey on Drug Use and Health. *HHS Publication No. PEP21-07-01-003, NSDUH Series H-56.* Center for Behavioral Health Statistics and Quality, Substance Abuse and Mental Health Services Administration; 2021. Accessed July 9, 2022. https://www.samhsa.gov/data/)

to provide for three people's basic water-related hygiene and food needs for 62 years of life, and costs an amount of fossil fuel that could have otherwise been used to power the average electricity needs for a household in India for 15 years.

Given the broad and increasing prevalence of smoking globally, the impacts to CC are increasingly relevant. Smoking cigarettes kills roughly half of all people who smoke. Addiction medicine clinicians who help patients who smoke cigarettes to permanently stop smoking not only prolong the patient's lifespan, but may also erode the force of CC drivers on our planet.

The tobacco industry's contribution to metal depletion at 3.3 Mt iron equivalent is at least as high as that caused by 8% of the United States' annual iron mining. The cigarette industry's total annual contribution to CC at 84 Mt CO_2 equivalent makes up about 0.2% of the world's total greenhouse gas emissions; nearly as much as the greenhouse emissions of entire countries such as Israel and Peru. While the U.S. healthcare sector contributes as much as 10% of the country's carbon emissions,[51] one can argue that the benefits weigh significantly against this cost; especially as this industry works to lower its impact on CC.

Given that global traditional cigarette consumption is expected to continue to rapidly expand by 50% to 9 trillion by 2025,[52] the environmental impacts and contribution to CC will only expand as well. And since roughly 90% of tobacco leaf production and most of the traditional cigarette consumption is being done by developing countries, these countries are burdened with most of the environmental degradation and personal medical health risks from this addiction-related industry. Further, the developed countries that own these industries are literally burning through the resources of the less developed countries; thus, promoting disparities on a global scale.[50]

Traditional cigarettes contain more than 7,000 chemicals, and their combustion produces toxicants in mainstream smoke, sidestream smoke, secondhand smoke, thirdhand smoke, and discarded cigarette butts.[53] Incorrect disposal of cigarette butts is commonplace with up to two-thirds of all smoked cigarettes being discarded onto the ground. Cigarettes and their butts are causally linked to fires, which can contribute to CC. Moreover, these butts leave substantial amounts of toxins in the environment, including nicotine, arsenic, and heavy metals.[54]

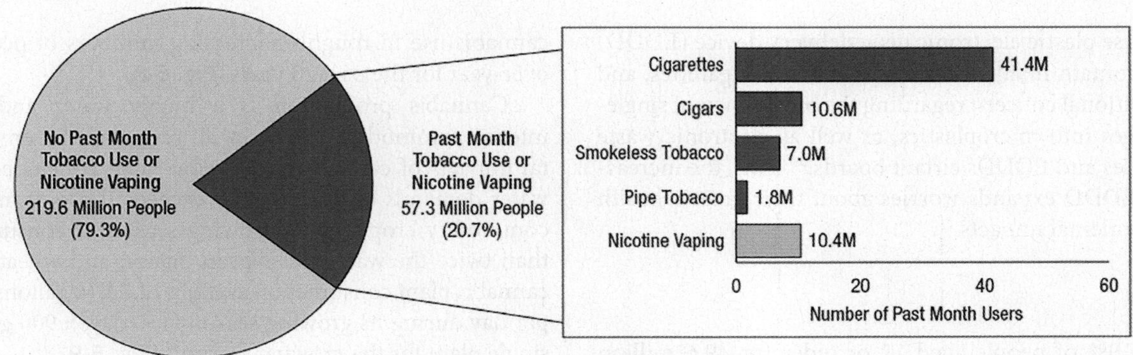

Figure 6-5. Past month tobacco use and nicotine vaping among people aged 12 or older, 2020. (From SAMHSA. Key substance use and mental health indicators in the United States: Results from the 2020 National Survey on Drug Use and Health. *HHS Publication No. PEP21-07-01-003, NSDUH Series H-56.* Center for Behavioral Health Statistics and Quality, Substance Abuse and Mental Health Services Administration; 2021. Accessed July 9, 2022. https://www.samhsa.gov/data/)

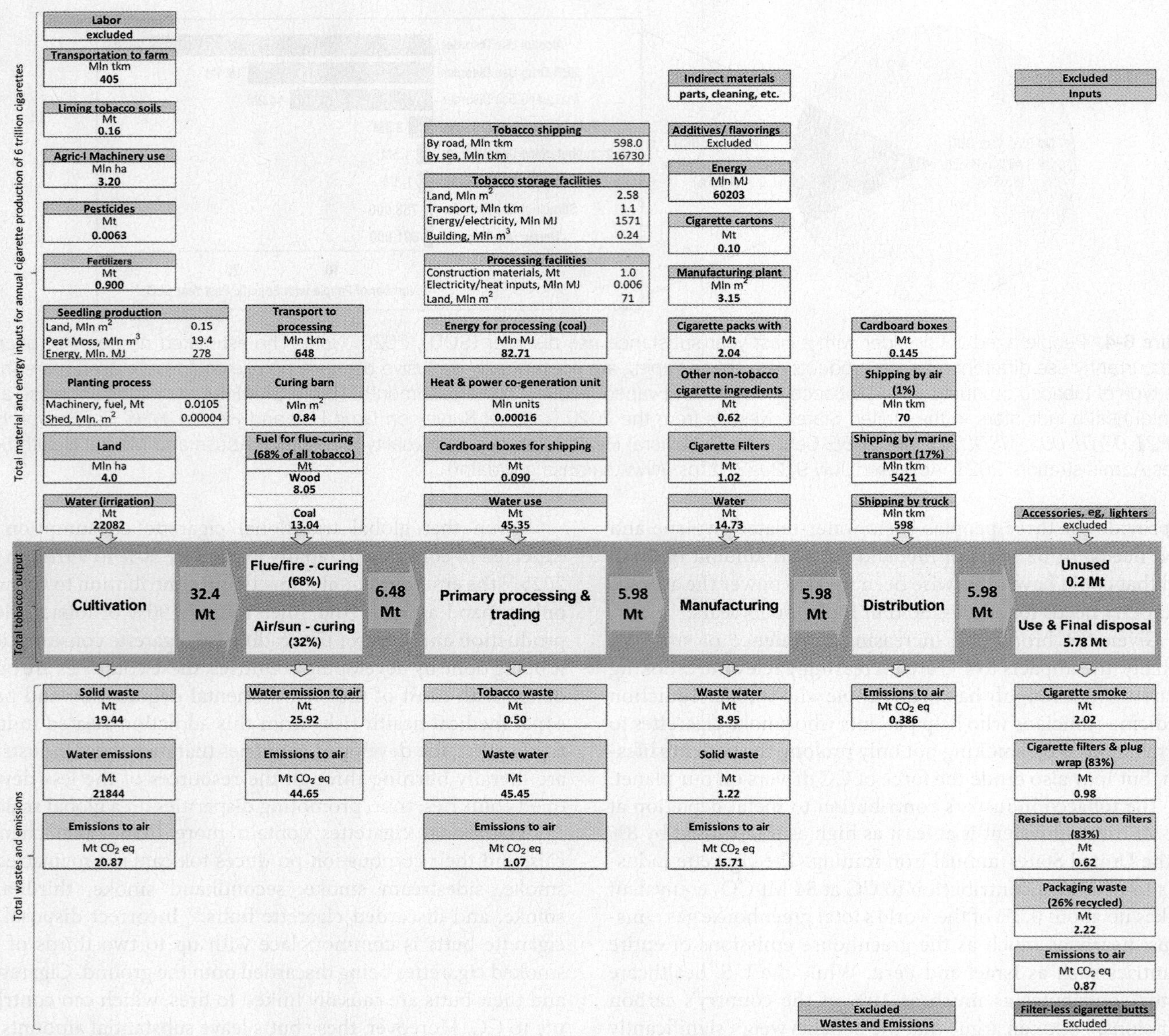

Figure 6-6. Total annual input, waste, and emission flows across the global tobacco supply chain. (From Zafeiridou M, Hopkinson NS, Voulvoulis N. Cigarette smoking: an assessment of tobacco's global environmental footprint across its entire supply chain. *Environ Sci Technol.* 2018;52(15):8087-8094)

Single-use plastic electronic drug delivery device (EDDD) cartridges contain many of the same toxins as cigarettes, and there is additional concern regarding the breakdown of single-use cartridges into microplastics, as well as electronic waste from batteries and EDDDs circuit boards.[55] Thus, the increasing use of EDDD expands worries about their greater health and environmental impacts.

Cannabis

In 2020, 17.9% of people aged 12 or older (or 49.6 million people) used cannabis in the past year,[46] and this number may increase significantly with the ongoing spread of cannabis legalization and cannabis used as treatment. For example, in nearly all age groups over 12 years old, Americans are initiating cannabis use in roughly increasing numbers of people year-over-year for the past 20 years (**Fig. 6-8**).

Cannabis production is a highly water and nutrient intense commodity. Zheng et al. reviewed the environmental impacts of cannabis production[56] and concluded that the water demands of this crop far exceeds those of many other commodity crops. In its growing season, it consumes more than twice the water as soybean, maize, and wheat. A single cannabis plant consumes on average 22.7 L (6 gallons) of water per day during its growing season (150 days); 900 gallons per single plant for the growing season[57] (**Fig. 6-9**).

Cannabis is grown both outdoors in crops and in indoor facilities as well. Outdoor growth may be having impacts on water supply, its quality, as well local biodiversity. Water diversion is the removal of water from one watershed source to

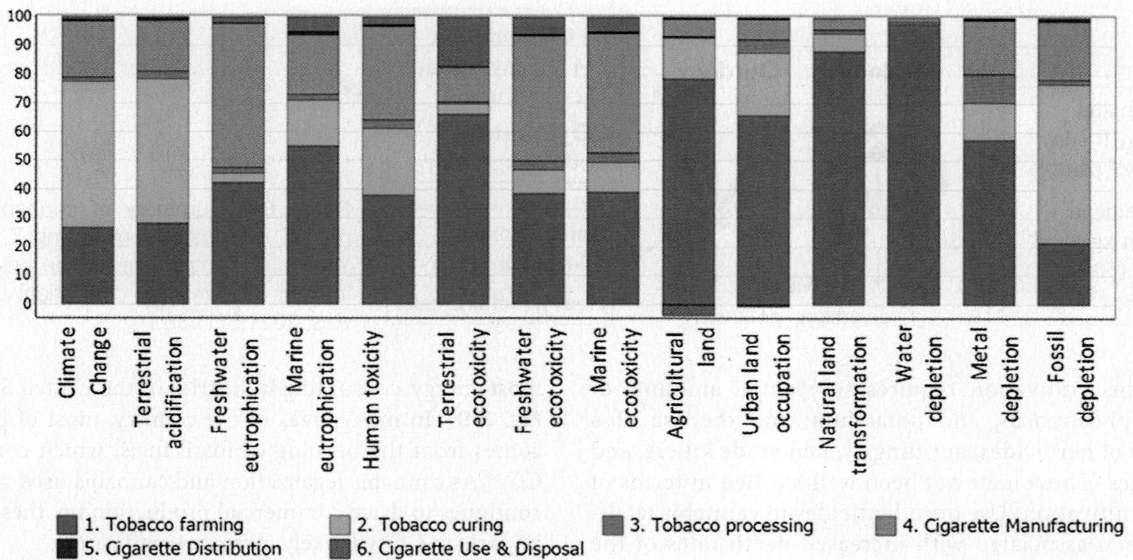

Figure 6-7. Environmental impacts and contribution of the global tobacco supply chain stages across the full life cycle of cigarette production and consumption. (From Zafeiridou M, Hopkinson NS, Voulvoulis N. Cigarette smoking: an assessment of tobacco's global environmental footprint across its entire supply chain. *Environ Sci Technol.* 2018;52(15):8087-8094.)

another to irrigate crops. A quantitative study of surface water diversions to support outdoor cannabis crops found reduced flows and dewatering of local streams.[58] This study chose 4 sites that were rural and less impacted by human activity. Cannabis cultivation in 3 of the 4 sites outstripped local stream flow during low flow periods, and the 7-day average low flow was reduced by roughly one-quarter among the least impacted watersheds.

Reduced streamflow has significant harmful impacts to biodiversity, especially on amphibians and salmonid fish in particular. Lower stream flows positively correlate with increased water temperatures, lower dissolved oxygen, lower growth rate, and increased risk for biodiversity to be preyed upon.[59] There has been an 80% to 116% increase in cannabis cultivation sites being located near high quality habitat sites for endangered or threatened salmonid fishes.[57] Because flow modification is one of the greatest threats to aquatic diversity, and loss of biodiversity is a significant negative outcome from CC, cannabis cultivation-related aquatic impacts require careful attention.

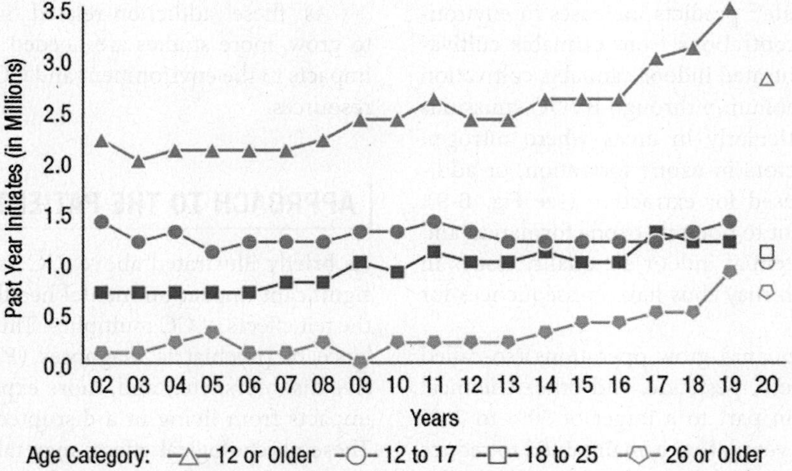

Figure 6-8. Past year cannabis initiates among people aged 12 or older, 2002-2020. Note: Estimates of less than 0.05 million round to 0.0 million when shown to the nearest tenth of a million. Note: There is no connecting line between 2019 and 2020 to indicate caution should be used when comparing estimates between 2020 and prior years because of methodological changes for 2020. Due to these changes, significance testing between 2020 and prior years was not performed. (From SAMHSA. Key substance use and mental health indicators in the United States: Results from the 2020 National Survey on Drug Use and Health. *HHS Publication No. PEP21-07-01-003, NSDUH Series H-56.* Center for Behavioral Health Statistics and Quality, Substance Abuse and Mental Health Services Administration; 2021. Accessed July 9, 2022. https://www.samhsa.gov/data/)

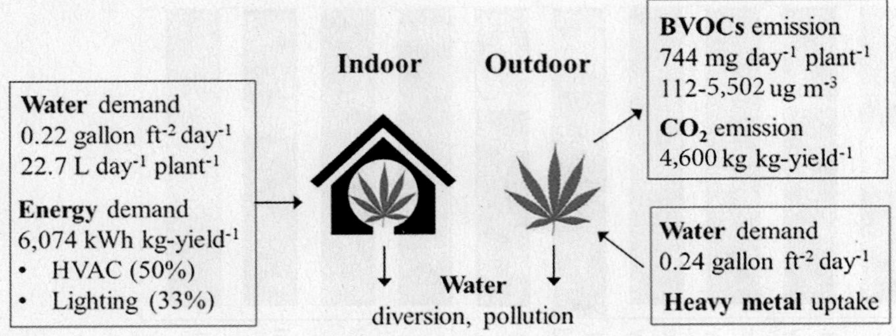

Figure 6-9. Summary of cannabis environmental impacts. (From Zheng Z, Fiddes K, Yang L. A narrative review on environmental impacts of cannabis cultivation. *J Cannabis Res.* 2021;3(1):35.)

Cannabis cultivation requires substantial amounts of nitrogen, phosphorus, and potassium; and the use of a wide array of herbicides, antifungals, nematode killers, and rodenticides. These have not been well-studied in terms of cannabis cultivation. Use of rodenticides in cannabis facilities has been associated with increased death rates of the northern spotted owl, a threatened species native to the northwest.[60]

The cannabis plant has also been found to absorb and store heavy metals, pulling them out of the soil and potentially into its flowers,[61] which can be beneficial to contaminated soil. However, this also may be achieved via simply growing cannabis hemp as opposed to recreational cannabis or cannabis used as treatment.

Not only does the cannabis plant consume significant amounts of water, but as part of its normal physiology it also emits volatile organic compounds. Volatile organic compounds contribute to the formation of ozone and PM, which then trap heat, contribute to global warming, and to air pollution. The cannabis plant contains significant numbers of biogenic volatile organic compounds (BVOCs) including various terpenes, terpenoids, methanol, and acetone. A recent review of the limited studies to date[62] predicts increases in environmental hourly ozone concentrations from cannabis cultivation, indicating that concentrated indoor cannabis cultivation may increase local ozone pollution through BVOC emissions (including terpenes), particularly in areas where nitrogen oxides are not limiting factors in ozone formation, or additionally where butane is used for extraction (see **Fig. 6-9**). These findings are important to not only ozone formation and CC, but also highlight potential indoor air quality issues in production facilities, which may thus have consequences for worker safety.

Indoor cannabis (marijuana) grow operations (so-called IMGOs) pose a risk of mold, pesticide, and other chemical exposure to workers due in part to a target of 50% to 70% humidity, and worse if low ventilation is maintained to reduce emittance of BVOCs or odors to the outside (especially in illegal IMGOs, to avoid detection).

By 2012, cannabis cultivation accounted for at least 1% of the total electricity expenditures in the United States.[63] By 2015, cannabis cultivation accounted for 3% of total electricity expenditures in California, and nationally it ranked among the most energy-consuming industries in the United States[64] (see **Fig. 6-9**). In many areas of the country, most of this energy comes from the burning of fossil fuels, which contribute to CC.[56] As cannabis legalization and cannabis used a treatment continues to drive commercial production up, these potential impacts to CC will likely increase significantly.

Carbon footprint refers to "a measure of the exclusive total amount of carbon dioxide emissions that is directly and indirectly caused by an activity or is accumulated over the life stages of a product."[65] In the context of cannabis cultivation, a carbon footprint can be defined as the total amount of greenhouse gases emitted during the production of cannabis.[56] Producing one kilogram of processed cannabis (roughly 1,000 joints) indoors is estimated to create 4,600 kg of CO_2 emissions to the atmosphere, equivalent to one average US passenger vehicle driven for one year (11,414 miles).[63]

From 2012 to 2016 the number of northern California cannabis farms increased 58% and the total expansion area increased 91%, with many in areas of environmental sensitivity.[66] As the demand grows, so will the number of farms and indoor growing facilities. Without careful regulation, the negative environmental impact will grow as well.

As these addiction-related industries above continue to grow, more studies are needed to better understand their impacts to the environment and CC amid increasingly limited resources.

APPROACH TO THE PATIENT IMPACTED BY CC

As briefly illustrated above, CC and its drivers are having a significant impact on mental health, which will only grow as the felt effects of CC multiplies. This includes increased prevalence of psychiatric diagnoses (PTSD, anxiety and depressive disorders, etc.) and, more expansively, the psychological impacts from living in a disrupted and destabilized climate. These psychological effects may take the form of "psychoterratic syndromes," such as solastalgia, ecoanxiety, ecological grief, existential distress, moral injury, and more.

Certainly, extreme weather events can acutely erode many systems of care. This is more so in those populations who are disadvantaged and stigmatized before such extreme weather events, and in particular in certain lifesaving addiction clinics where the patient is legally required to transport themselves physically to and from appointments to ensure the provision of urine specimen collection, provision of methadone or buprenorphine medication, etc., so as to maintain the basic flow of opioid agonist therapy.[67,68] Not only do such services need to have pre-rehearsed response plans to ensure service delivery during an extreme weather event, but also efforts must be made in advance to ensure adequate funding for these situations, along with creative bridge solutions—such as telehealth services or mobile clinics.

Similar to the clinician's role in educating the public and patients regarding the negative health impacts from maladaptive substance and gambling use, there is a responsibility for the clinician to be well versed on CC, its health impacts, and means to cope. This education should include the risks of climate drivers to health (air pollution exposure exacerbating obstructive lung disease, vulnerability to heat-related illnesses in those with addiction and on psychotropic medications, etc.) as well as possible interventions such as location of cooling centers during heat waves, air filtration, emergency preparation kits, and reducing or stopping their substance use, which may negatively interact with aspects of CC. Given the unique and interconnected impacts of CC, creative solutions are also needed to adapt to climate drivers; this may include expanding alert systems for climate drivers, such as providing advisories during heat waves to those that are most vulnerable (elderly, those experiencing houselessness, using substances, etc.) with guidelines on how to mitigate effects.

Strengthening the patient's capability to navigate the psychological pressure of the climate crisis will prove to be a growing area of importance within medicine. "Social prescriptions" may be helpful wherein the patient is advised to spend more time with nature—an activity with mounting evidence of benefits.[69] Other activities that patients may find empowering include participating locally in actions to combat CC or seeking involvement in activities relating to equity or conservation. Each of these can help build a sense of self-efficacy while addressing the potential development of isolation in the face of a felt existential issue like CC. Therapy, both individual and in groups, may also prove to be of some benefit. Existing groups, such as the Good Grief Network,[70] which is structured similarly to Alcoholic Anonymous 12-step groups, can assist with CC-related distress by finding healing and support in groups of similarly struggling individuals.[71]

Meanwhile, current therapeutic models (acceptance and commitment therapy, ecotherapy, and dialectic-behavioral therapy) can be flexibly applied to address current psychological responses to CC.[12] For instance, Lewis et al.[72] describe how stressors felt to be insurmountable can cause a collapse of dialectical thinking into extreme poles (eg, hope versus hopelessness), thus applying dialectical techniques can help reestablish simultaneous holding of dialectical poles and subsequent balance in psychological disposition.

ADDICTION MEDICINE CLINICIANS AS CHANGE AGENTS TO SLOW CC

Addiction medicine clinicians have potential to impact CC in a positive way. Roles include those of clinician, public health officer, addiction medicine advocate, activist, researcher, community leader, and policy advisor.[12]

Clinicians should inquire about the impact of CC on their patient's MH and substance use, encourage them to talk about it, and provide them resources to further explore and manage these impacts. Clinicians should educate patients regarding how their substance use may increase their risk for health problems in relation to CC events. Clinicians should be mindful about their medication prescribing practices, the carbon footprint of medications, and work to reduce unnecessary prescriptions (both in terms of numbers of different prescriptions the patient is taking, and the number dispensed per prescription). Further, clinicians may encounter patients who desire to learn more about how the production and consumption of their substance may contribute to CC.

Addiction medicine clinicians are well-positioned within their community to educate others about CC and its medical impacts; while also providing education to public officials and lawmakers about the unique needs of our patients in relation to CC. Finally, there is a growing interest in how certain substance use and addiction-related industries may be negatively impacting our environment, climate, and the world within which we live.

There are important lessons from nicotine/tobacco control policy that may be applied to climate policy (**Fig. 6-10**).[73] It took roughly half a century to move from general scientific agreement about the health harms of tobacco use[74,75] to then develop and implement global nicotine/tobacco health policy. This delay cost 100 million lives.[76]

Nicotine/tobacco control and CC have many similarities. Both cause significant damage to population health; both cause significant adverse social, economic, equity, and gender effects; both have long lag times between cause and effect—thus eroding political will for policy change. Both require long term policies and monitoring systems, and both cause major adverse impacts to low-income countries and the poor. Policy development in both are influenced by strong vested interests to maintain the momentum of the status quo, despite personal and societal harms. This includes the use of delaying tactics and "junk science" by opponents of change. The lesson from nicotine/tobacco policy for CC policy is that there is an urgent need for comprehensive and sustained action. Public policy intervention is required because the markets will not enact meaningful change on their own, and political will and strong leadership—including from clinicians—is required. Delays in policy agreement and implementation will cost lives.[73] The question for CC is just how many lives will be lost before policy agreement and implementation is a reality?

The principles and approach of motivational interviewing, created in relation to helping individual patients with tobacco/

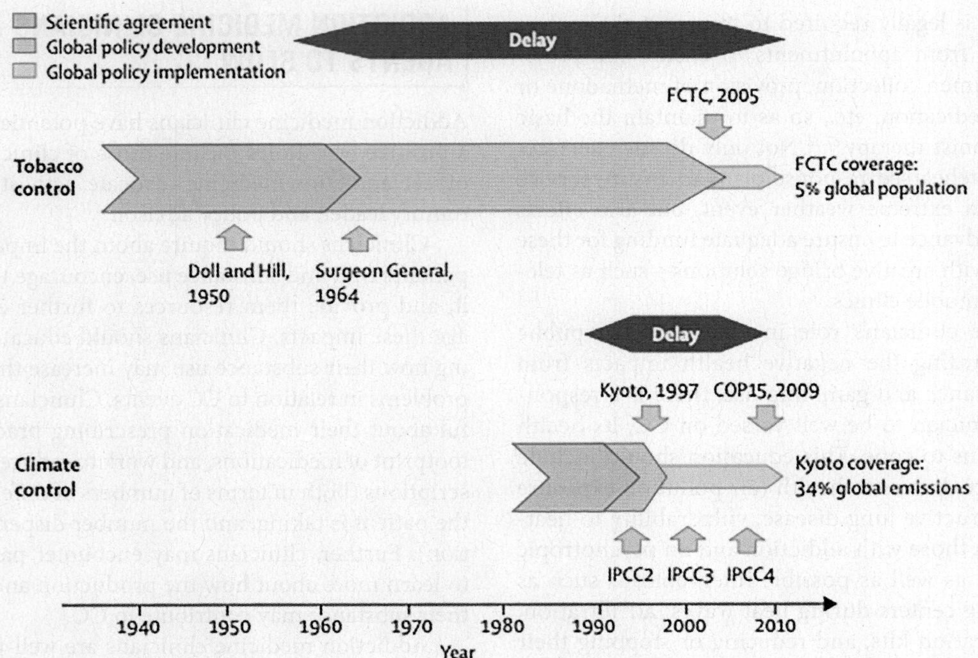

Figure 6-10. Time delays from science to policy: Tobacco and climate change. (From Nilsson M, Beaglehole R, Sauerborn R. Climate policy: lessons from tobacco control. *Lancet*. 2009;374:1955-1956.)

nicotine use disorder to mobilize their ambivalence to change, may also be useful on a population health level for approaching ambivalence about CC in the clinician's public community.

The American Psychiatric Association's Climate Psychiatry Alliance (www.climatepsychiatry.org) and other professional groups serve as resource sharing groups for this topic. The Climate Psychiatry alliance website provides free resources for clinicians, including topics such as "Coping with extreme heat," "Green your office," "Climate and health organizations," and a "Climate-aware therapist directory." The American Psychiatric Association Committee on Climate Change and Mental Health has published key curriculum components for graduate medical education on CC-related issues.[77] ASAM's lobbying resources[78] may also serve as an outlet for addressing CC.

CONCLUSIONS

Anthropogenic CC is an accepted scientific fact and an existential threat to modern human society and health. As reflected in the literature, mental health and substance use are progressively and negatively affected as a result, with amplified impacts within vulnerable populations. Meanwhile, substance use has a bidirectional relationship with CC given its production, distribution, and waste, which all worsen anthropogenic CC as well as other associated environmental degradations, while the effects of CC are known to exacerbate substance use. As such, addiction medicine clinicians have an obligation to increase their knowledge base regarding the issue, become involved in patient-centered and population-based interventions, and apply lessons learned from other international substance use issues to the climate crisis. It is our hope that this novel chapter will stimulate readers to close that gap.

REFERENCES

1. World Health Organization. *Climate Change and Health*. 2021. Accessed August 12, 2022. https://www.who.int/news-room/fact-sheets/detail/climate-change-and-health
2. Climate.gov. *Climate Forcing*. National Oceanic and Atmospheric Association; 2022. Accessed July 18, 2022. https//www.climate.gov/maps-data/climate-data-primer/predicting-climate/climate-forcing
3. NOAA. *What's the Difference Between Climate and Weather?* National Oceanic and Atmospheric Association; 2022. Accessed July 4, 2022. https://www.noaa.gov/explainers/what-s-difference-between-climate-and-weather
4. NOAA. *Global Climate Report*. National Centers for Environmental Information. National Oceanic and Atmospheric Administration; 2022. Accessed July 17, 2022. https://www.ncei.noaa.gov/access/monitoring/monthly-report/global/202113
5. NASA. *Climate Time Machine*. National Aeronautics and Space Administration; 2022. Accessed July 4, 2022. https://climate.nasa.gov/interactives/climate-time-machine
6. Leiserowitz A, Roser-Renouf C, Marlon J, et al. Global Warming's six Americas: a review and recommendations for climate change communication. *Curr Opin Behav Sci*. 2021;42:97-103.

Disclaimer: Dr Miller is employed by the Department of Veterans Affairs, Dayton VA Medical Center, Dayton, Ohio. The VA had no role in the design, literature review or analysis, writing, or in the decision to submit this chapter for publication. The contents do not necessarily represent the views of the Department of Veterans Affairs or the United States Government.

7. Hickman C, Marks E, Pihkala P, et al. Climate anxiety in children and young people and their beliefs about government responses to climate change: a global survey. *Lancet Planet Health*. 2021;5(12):e863-e873.
8. Charlson F, Ali S, Benmarhnia T, et al. Climate change and mental health: a scoping review. *Int J Environ*. 2021;18(9):4486.
9. Albrecht G. Chronic environmental change: Emerging 'psychoterratic' syndromes. In: Weisbecker I, ed. *Climate Change and Human Wellbeing*. Springer; 2011.
10. Steentjes K, Pidgeon N, Poortinga W, et al. *European Perceptions of Climate Change: Topline findings of a survey conducted in four European countries in 2016*. Cardiff University; 2017. Accessed August 13, 2022. https://orca.cardiff.ac.uk/id/eprint/98660/7/epcc.pdf
11. Albrecht G, Sartore GM, Connor L, et al. Solastalgia: The distress caused by environmental change. *Australas Psychiatry*. 2007;15(S1):S95-S98.
12. Sullenbarger J, Schutzenhofer E, Haase E. Climate Change: Implications for Mental Health. In: Sowers WE, HL MQ, Ranz JM, Feldman JM, Ranz JM, Runnels P, eds. *American Association for Community Psychiatry Textbook of Community Psychiatry*. 2nd ed. Springer Nature AG; 2022.
13. National Coalition for the Homeless. *Substance Abuse and Homelessness*. National Coalition for the Homeless; 2017. Accessed July 18, 2022. https://nationalhomeless.org/wp-content/uploads/2017/06/Substance-Abuse-and-Homelessness.pdf
14. SAMHSA. *National Survey on Drug Use and Health Detailed Tables*. Substance Abuse and Mental Health Services Administration; 2019. Accessed July 20, 2022. https://www.samhsa.gov/data/report/2018-nsduh-detailed-tables
15. Vins H, Bell J, Saha S, Hess JJ. The mental health outcomes of drought: A systematic review and causal process diagram. *Int J Environ*. 2015; 12(10):13251-13275.
16. Carleton T. Crop-damaging temperatures increase suicide rates in India. *PNAS*. 2017;114(33):8751.
17. Canu WH, Jameson JP, Steele EH, Denslow M. Mountain top removal coal mining and emergent cases of psychological disorder in Kentucky. *Community Ment Health J*. 2017;53(7):802-810.
18. NASA Global Warming vs Climate Change. National Aeronautical and Space Administration; 2022. Accessed 4 July, 2022. https://climate.nasa.gov/resources/global-warming-vs-climate-change/
19. Masson-Delmotte V, Zhai P, Pirani A, et al. Climate change 2021: The physical science basic. *Contribution of Working Group I to the Sixth Assessment Report of the Intergovernmental Panel on Climate Change*. IPCC; 2021. Accessed January 5, 2022. https://www.ipcc.ch/report/ar6/wg1/downloads/report/IPCC_AR6_WGI_Full_Report.pdf
20. NASA. *How Do We Know Climate Change Is Real?* National Aeronautical and Space Administration; 2022. Accessed July 4, 2022. https://climate.nasa.gov/evidence/
21. Dumont C, Haase E, Dolber T, et al. Climate change and risk of completed suicide. *J Nerv Ment Dis*. 2020;208(7):559-565.
22. Hsiang SM, Burke M, Miguel E. Quantifying the influence of climate on human conflict. *Science*. 2013;341:6151.
23. Schlader ZJ, Gagnon D, Adams A, et al. Cognitive and perceptual responses during passive heat stress in younger and older adults. *American J Physiol Regul Integr Comp Physiol*. 2015;308:847-854.
24. Obradovich N, Fowler JH. Climate change may alter human physical activity patterns. *Nat Hum Behav*. 2017;1(5):97.
25. Bouchama A, Dehbi M, Mohamed G, et al. Prognostic factors in heat wave related deaths: A meta-analysis. *Arch Intern Med*. 2007; 167(20):2170-2176.
26. Hayes K, Poland B, Cole D, Agic B. Psychosocial adaptation to climate change in High River, Alberta: implications for policy and practice. *Can J Public Health*. 2020;111(6):880-889.
27. Morrison SF, Nakamura K. Central mechanisms for thermoregulation. *Ann Rev Physiology*. 2019;81:285-308.
28. Marzuk PM, Tardiff K, Leon AC, et al. Ambient temperature and mortality from unintentional cocaine overdose. *JAMA*. 1998;279:795-800.
29. Page LA, Hajat S, Sari Kovats R, Howard LM. Temperature-related deaths in people with psychosis, dementia and substance misuse. *Br J Psychiatry*. 2012;200:485-490.
30. Martin-Latry K, Goumy MP, Latry P, et al. Psychotropic drugs use and risk of heat-related hospitalization. *Eur Psychiatry*. 2007;22(6):335-338.
31. Cohen AJ, Brauer M, Burnett R, et al. Estimates and 25-year trends of the global burden of disease attributable to ambient air pollution: An analysis of data from the Global Burden of Diseases Study 2015. *Lancet*. 2017;389(10082):1907-1918.
32. Abatzoglou JT, Williams AP. Impact of anthropogenic climate change on wildfire across western US forests. *PNAS*. 2016;113(42):11770-11775.
33. Chique C, Hynds P, Nyhan MM, et al. Psychological impairment and extreme weather event (EWE) exposure, 1980-2020: A global pooled analysis integrating mental health and well-being metrics. *Int J Hyg Environ Health*. 2021;238:113840.
34. Fu P, Guo X, Cheung FMH, Yung KKL. The association between PM2.5 exposure and neurological disorders: A systematic review and meta-analysis. *Sci Total Environ*. 2019;655:1240-1248.
35. Gu X, Liu Q, Deng F, et al. Association between particular matter air pollution and risk of depression and suicide: Systematic review and meta-analysis. *Br J Psychiatry*. 2019;215:456-467.
36. Perera FP. Multiple threats to child health from fossil fuel combustion: Impacts of air pollution and climate change. *Environ Health Perspect*. 2017;125(3):141-148.
37. Berman JD, Burkhardt J, Bayham J, et al. Acute air pollution exposure and the risk of violent behavior in the United States. *Epidemiology*. 2019;30(6):799-806.
38. Li X, Cao X, Guo M, et al. Trends and risk factors of mortality and disability adjusted life years for chronic respiratory diseases from 1990 to 2017: systematic analysis for the Global Burden of Disease Study 2017. *BMJ*. 2020;368(m237):1-10.
39. Rohrbach LA, Grana R, Vernberg E, et al. Impact of Hurricane Rita on substance use. *Psychiatry*. 2009;72(3):222-237.
40. Flory K, Hankin BL, Kloos B, Cheely C. Alcohol and cigarette use and misuse among Hurricane Katrina survivors: Psychosocial risk and protective factors. *Subst Use Misuse*. 2009;44(12):1711-1724.
41. Kessler RC, Galea S, Jones RT, Parker HA. Mental illness and suicidality after Hurricane Katrina. *Bull World Health Organ*. 2006;84:930-939.
42. Tunstall S, Tapsell S, Green C, et al. The health effects of flooding: social research results from England and Wales. *J Water Health*. 2006;4:365-380.
43. Hayes K, Blashki G, Wiseman J, et al. Climate change and mental health: risks, impacts and priority actions. *Int J Ment Health Syst*. 2018;12:28.
44. Hanigan IC, Butler CD, Kokic PN, Hutchinson MF. Suicide and drought in new South Wales, Australia, 1970–2007. *PNAS*. 2012; 109(35):13950-13955.
45. Parida Y, Dash DP, Bhardwaj P, Chowdhury JR. Effects of drought and flood on farmer suicides in Indian states: An empirical analysis. *Econ Dis Cli Cha*. 2018;2(2):159-180.
46. SAMHSA. *Key Substance Use and Mental Health Indicators in the United States: Results from the 2020 National Survey on Drug Use and Health (HHS Publication No. PEP21-07-01-003, NSDUH Series H-56)*. Center for Behavioral Health Statistics and Quality, Substance Abuse and Mental Health Services Administration; 2021. Accessed 9 July, 2022. https://www.samhsa.gov/data/
47. WHO Report on the Global Tobacco Epidemic. World Health Organization; 2015. Raising taxes on tobacco. Accessed June 12, 2017. https://www.who.int/publications/i/item/9789241509121
48. Leppan W, Lecours N, Buckles D. *Tobacco Control and Tobacco Farming: Separating Myth from Reality*. International Development Research Centre (IDRC); 2014.
49. Eriksen M, Mackay J, Schluger N, et al. Tobacco Companies. *The Tobacco Atlas [Online]*. American Cancer Society, Inc; 2015.
50. Zafeiridou M, Hopkinson NS, Voulvoulis N. Cigarette smoking: An assessment of tobacco's global environmental footprint across its entire supply chain. *Environ Sci Technol*. 2018;52(15):8087-8094.
51. Sherman JD, MacNeill A, Thiel C. Reducing pollution from the health care industry. *JAMA*. 2019;322(11):1043-1044.
52. Novotny TE, Lum K, Smith E, et al. Cigarette butts and the case for an environmental policy on hazardous cigarette waste. *Int J Environ Res Public Health*. 2009;6(5):1691-1705.

53. Soleimani F, Dobaradaran S, De-la-Torre GE, et al. Content of toxic components of cigarette, cigarette smoke vs cigarette butts: A comprehensive systematic review. *Sci Total Environ.* 2022;20(813):152667.
54. World Health Organization. *Tobacco and Its Environmental Impact: An Overview.* 2022. Accessed August 14, 2022. https://www.who.int/publications/i/item/9789241512497
55. Pourchez J, Mercier C, Forest V. From smoking to vaping: A new environmental threat? *Lancet Respir Med.* 2022;10(7):e63-e64.
56. Zheng Z, Fiddes K, Yang L. A narrative review on environmental impacts of cannabis cultivation. *J Cannabis Res.* 2021;3(1):35.
57. Butsic V, Brenner J. Cannabis (*Cannabis sativa* or *C. indica*) agriculture and the environment: A systematic, spatially-explicit survey and potential impacts. *Environ Res Lett.* 2016;11(4):044023.
58. Bauer S, Olson J, Cockrill A, et al. Impacts of surface water diversions for marijuana cultivation on aquatic habitat in four northwestern California watersheds. *PloS One.* 2015;10(3):e0120016. https://doi.org/10.1371/journal.pone.0120016
59. Marine KR, Cech JJ. Effects of high water temperature on growth, smoltification, and predator avoidance in juvenile Sacramento River chinook salmon. *North Am J Fisheries Manag.* 2004;24(1):198-210.
60. Franklin AB, Carlson PC, Rex A, et al. Grass is not always greener: Rodenticide exposure of a threatened species near marijuana growing operations. *BMC Res Notes.* 2018;11(1):94.
61. Seltenrich N. Cannabis contaminants: Regulating solvents, microbes, and metals in legal weed. *Environ Health Perspect.* 2019;127(8):082001.
62. Wartenberg AC, Holden PA, Bodwitch H, et al. Cannabis and the environment: What science tells us and what we still need to know. *Environ Sci Technol Lett.* 2021;8:98-107.
63. Mills E. The carbon footprint of indoor Cannabis production. *Energy Policy.* 2012;46:58-67.
64. Warren GS. Regulating pot to save the polar bear: Energy and climate impacts of the marijuana industry. *Colum J Envtl Lett.* 2015;40:385.
65. Wiedmann T, Minx J. A definition of "carbon footprint." *Ecolog Econ Res Trends.* 2008;1:1-11.
66. Butsic V, Carah JK, Baumann M, et al. The emergence of cannabis agriculture frontiers as environmental threats. *Environ Res Lett.* 2018;13(12):124017.
67. Bottner R, Weems J, Hill LG, et al. Commentary: addiction treatment networks cannot withstand acute crises: lessons from 2021 winter storm uri in Texas. *Natl Acad Med.* 2021; Accessed August 30, 2022. https://nam.edu/addiction-treatment-networks-cannot-withstand-acute-crises-lessons-from-2021-winter-storm-uri-in-texas/
68. Biegacki E. First opinion: Emergency response systems must not overlook people with substance use disorders. *Stat.* 2022; Accessed August 30, 2022. https://www.statnews.com/2022/03/16/emergency-response-systems-mustnt-overlook-people-substance-use-disorders/
69. Dean JH, Shanahan DF, Bush R, et al. Is nature relatedness associated with better mental and physical health? *Int J Environ.* 2018;15(7):1371.
70. Good Grief Network. *Steps to Personal Resilience & Empowerment in a Chaotic Climate.* Good Grief Network; 2022. Accessed August 13, 2022. https://www.goodgriefnetwork.org
71. Mark B, Lewis J. *Group Interventions for Climate Change Distress.* Psychiatric Times; 2020. Accessed July 26, 2022. https://www.psychiatrictimes.com/view/group-interventions-climate-change-distress
72. Lewis J, Haase E, Trope A. Climate dialectics in psychotherapy: Holding open the space between abyss and advance. *Psychodyn Psychiatry.* 2020;48(3): 271-294.
73. Nilsson M, Beaglehole R, Sauerborn R. Climate policy: Lessons from tobacco control. *Lancet.* 2009;(374):1955-1956.
74. Doll R, Hill AB. Smoking and carcinoma of the lung. *BMJ.* 1950;2:739-748.
75. Surgeon General's Advisory Committee on Smoking and Health. Smoking and Health; 1964. Accessed July 27, 2022. http://profiles.nlm.nih.gov/NN/B/B/M/Q
76. Frieden TR, Bloomberg MR. How to prevent 100 million deaths from tobacco. *Lancet.* 2007;369:1758-1761.
77. Pollack D, Haase E. What every psychiatrist should know about the climate crisis. *Psychiatr News.* 2022;40-41.
78. ASAM. *Advocacy.* American Society of Addiction Medicine. Accessed August 13, 2022. https://www.asam.org/advocacy

CHAPTER

7 The Cigarette Industry's Role in Promoting Tobacco Use Disorder

K. Michael Cummings

CHAPTER OUTLINE

- Introduction
- Tobacco product design
- Concealing the truth about nicotine addiction
- Mass marketing
- Interference with the provision of therapies for people who smoke
- Interference with policies that could reduce the harms caused by tobacco use
- Denying justice to those harmed by addiction to cigarettes
- The economic realities of the cigarette business
- Summary

INTRODUCTION

The main reason people use tobacco on a persistent daily basis for months, years and decades is addiction to nicotine.[1-8] This chapter focuses primarily on cigarettes and the role that cigarette companies have historically played in promoting tobacco use disorder.[1] Tobacco use disorder is defined as a problematic pattern of tobacco use leading to clinically significant impairment or distress, as manifest by at least two of 11 criteria, occurring in the individual who uses tobacco within a 12-month period.[1] This definition implies compulsive use of tobacco products that cause problems, typically harm to health. Commonly observed factors of tobacco use disorder in individuals who smoke cigarettes include smoking daily, frequency of smoking per day, smoking within 30 minutes of waking, and waking up at night to smoke.[1]

A common misconception about tobacco use is that the most dangerous component of the product is nicotine.[9-11] Most of the preventable morbidity and mortality is due to the long-term use of combusted tobacco smoking (mostly cigarettes), not to nicotine itself.[1-5] However, nicotine exposure alone does have health risks.[7] Nicotine can cause neuroadaptive changes in the brain that contribute to the risk of developing physiological dependence.[2-4,7,8] As one Philip Morris scientist observed, "No one has ever become a cigarette smoker by smoking cigarettes without nicotine."[12] At extremely high doses, higher than those experienced by the vast majority of nicotine and tobacco product users, nicotine can cause serious acute toxicity.[2,7] During pregnancy, nicotine can harm fetal development.[7] Nicotine exposure can increase catecholamines, alter hemodynamic function and may contribute to cardiovascular disease, although its impact is much less, compared to the use of smoked tobacco.[7] Nicotine is not known to cause cancer but is a cancer promoter.[3]

Nicotine exerts its effects by binding to receptors located in the brain, producing in the average person who smokes cigarettes on an established basis a sensation described as both stimulating and relaxing.[2-4,7,8] The mood altering effects are the result of the release of neurotransmitters such as dopamine and serotonin.[7,8] The response to nicotine varies widely in the population with some people exhibiting a strong affinity for nicotine and others very little or none at all.[13] The biological, likely hereditary, affinity to nicotine most likely explains in part why some people who try smoking don't need to smoke every day or at all, while others seem to crave nicotine and find it difficult to go more than a few hours without a cigarette and struggle to refrain from smoking in some cases even after experiencing serious health problems caused by smoking.[14]

Tobacco use disorder is common among individuals who use tobacco products daily, and significantly less common among those who do not use tobacco daily or use nicotine replacement therapies without tobacco or other nicotine sources.[1,15] Most people who evolve to smoking on a persistent daily basis as adults report having started smoking during their teenage years and end up struggling to stop smoking as adults.[16,17] Epidemiologic evidence shows that the younger a person is when they start smoking, the more likely they are to become strongly addicted to nicotine.[16,17]

The challenge to cigarette companies has always been how to recruit enough "replacement smokers" to make up for the adults who quit or die every year. As one cigarette industry executive observed "if younger people turn away from smoking the industry must decline, just as a population that does not give birth will eventually dwindle."[18] A 1973 business record from R.J. Reynolds discussed the importance and challenge of designing cigarettes to appeal to both the confirmed regular smoker and also to the starter end of the market as follows:

"The things which keep a confirmed smoker habituated and satisfied, i.e., nicotine and secondary physical and manipulative gratifications, are unknown and/or largely unexplained to the nonsmoker. The nonsmoker does not start smoking to obtain undefined physiological gratifications or reliefs, and certainly he does not start to smoke to satisfy a nonexistent craving for nicotine. Rather, the nonsmoker appears to start to smoke for purely psychological reasons such as to emulate a valued image, to conform, to experiment, to defy, to be daring, to have something to do with their hands, and the like. It is only after experiencing smoking for some period of time that the physiological satisfactions and habituation become apparent and needed. Indeed, the first smoking experiences are often unpleasant until a tolerance for nicotine has been developed."[19]

This chapter discusses the role that the cigarette industry has played in promoting tobacco use disorder through its design of products, efforts to downplay the role of nicotine and tobacco use disorder in smoking behavior, mass marketing, interference with the provision of therapies for people who smoke, interference with policies that that would accelerate a decline in smoking behavior, and by denying justice to those harmed by addiction to nicotine in commercially manufactured cigarettes. The chapter ends with a brief discussion of the economic realities of the cigarette business and how these realities define what can be done to change the trajectory of health harms caused by tobacco use disorder.

TOBACCO PRODUCT DESIGN

Tobacco use disorder can develop with use of all forms of nicotine containing tobacco products including cigarettes, cigars, pipe tobacco, chewing tobacco, moist snuff, snus, and electronic drug (nicotine) delivery devices (EDDDs), which include both e-cigarettes and heated tobacco products, and even with prescription or nonprescription nicotine-containing products (eg, nicotine gum, lozenges, and patches).[4] However, the way different tobacco products are designed can influence the bioavailability of nicotine and associated down-stream health problems people experience.[5,6] All commercially available cigarettes in the United States contain the drug nicotine. The vast majority of cigarette brands on the market today contain more than 8 milligrams (mg) of nicotine in the tobacco of which about 10% is absorbed when smoked, yielding an average delivery of 0.8 mgs or more of nicotine per cigarette.[5] Nicotine from cigarette smoke is rapidly absorbed in the lungs, and then quickly passes into the brain.[2-8] The speed of absorption is an important determinant of the addictiveness of a drug, and nicotine delivered in cigarette smoke is the most rapid method of nicotine delivery.[2-8] Commercially manufactured cigarettes and their variants, such as roll-your-own cigarettes, and mass produced cigars pose the highest risks for disease because the design of these products optimize nicotine delivery while also exposing the person to a toxic mixture of chemicals including more than 60 carcinogens in every puff.[2-8]

Most commercial manufactured cigarettes have a "filter"-tip (a device that, while alleged to remove toxins, may actually enable deeper inhalation of smoke and nicotine into the person's airways), include additives (eg, urea, ammonia compounds, glycerin, menthol) that facilitate smoke inhalation, and contain enough nicotine in the tobacco blend to induce and sustain physiologic nicotine addiction in those who smoke cigarettes.[2-8] A 1972 R.J. Reynolds document describes the cigarette business as a "specialized, highly ritualized and stylized segment of the pharmaceutical industry...whose products uniquely contain and deliver nicotine, a potent drug with a variety of physiological effects."[20] Commercial cigarettes are not merely a roll of tobacco wrapped in paper, but rather a highly engineered product to ensure efficient nicotine delivery.[2-6] As a 1963 document from Brown & Williamson Tobacco Company noted that the nicotine level of our cigarettes is not obtained by accident, "...we can regulate fairly precisely the nicotine and sugar levels to almost any desired level management might require."[21] While publicly downplaying the role of nicotine in cigarettes, cigarette companies have viewed nicotine as the *sine qua non* of product design.[22,23] **Table 7-1** provides excerpts of cigarette company business records illustrating the role of nicotine in cigarette design including research to define the threshold level of nicotine needed to create and sustain product use and methods to manipulate nicotine impact by altering smoke pH to change the form of nicotine from "bound" to "free."[24-38]

Today, about 80% percent of people who smoke cigarettes in the United States report smoking daily, while 20% report nondaily use, although some of the nondaily use reflects younger people who are still transitioning from experimental use to regular smoking.[39] Among people who smoke daily, the average cigarette intake is about 14 cigarettes per day, which represents a reduction from 20 per day (equal to one pack) in the early 1990s.[39,40] The reduction in daily cigarette use over the past three decades reflects less societal acceptance of smoking, higher cigarette prices, environmental restrictions on where smoking is permitted, combined with increasing access and use of other forms of tobacco products such as cigars, oral tobacco products, and most recently EDDDs.[4,40,41]

However, even among individuals who smoke daily, the numbers of cigarettes consumed per day does not tell the whole story of nicotine dosing since how different people smoke a cigarette can vary in terms of number of puffs per cigarette, volume of smoke per puff, length of cigarette smoked and so on. Smoking topography and biomarker studies show that people self-titrate to their needed level of nicotine delivery.[42,43] The unique design features of the cigarette such as the overall amount and blend of tobaccos used, length and circumference, the mixture of additives and how they are applied, which can influence smoke pH and inhalation, and the filter design (ie, material, density, ventilation holes on the filter tip) can interact in complex ways to impact how a person puffs on the cigarette and ultimately the deliveries of smoke constituents received.[32,44,45]

Cigarette manufacturers have long had the technical capability to control the nicotine content in cigarettes and to minimize product abuse liability.[24,46] From time to time, very low nicotine cigarettes were commercialized for sale, which also demonstrates the technical feasibility of controlling and reducing nicotine levels in tobacco. Methods for nicotine reduction date back over a hundred years and include things such as plant breeding and various nicotine extraction methods using solvents, steam, gases, and microbes.[46] Patents for extracting nicotine from tobacco date back to the 1920s and 1930s.[46-48]

TABLE 7-1 Examples of Company Records Discussing the Role of Nicotine in Cigarette Design

Date	Source	Quote and citation
December 9, 1935	ATC	It is quite possible to denicotinized a cigarette by chemical or thermal methods. The makers of Lucky Strike Cigarettes deliberately refrain from this because (1) such removal of nicotine cannot be secured without affecting adversely certain other desirable taste-constituents; and (2) such removal of nicotine produces an emasculated cigarette, shorn of those very qualities which give a cigarette character and appeal.[24]
September 22, 1959	PM	One of the main reasons people smoke is to experience the physiological effects of nicotine on the human system. Nicotine, to the best of present knowledge, does not produce cancer. Hence, in theory one could achieve the major advantage of smoking without the hazard of cancer.[25]
November 2, 1959	RJR	Regarding the extracted tobacco…the physiological requirements of the smoker with respect to nicotine can be met by the application of the optimum amount of nicotine to the extracted tobacco.[26]
February 13, 1962	BAT	As a result of these various research projects we now possess a knowledge of the effects of nicotine far more extensive than exists in public scientific literature.[27]
July 17, 1963	B&W	Moreover, nicotine is addictive. We are, then, in the business of selling nicotine, an addictive drug effective in the release of stress mechanisms.[28]
February 1, 1965	PM	Determine minimum nicotine drop to keep human smoker "hooked."[29]
November 26, 1969	PM	We are of the conviction, in view of the foregoing, that the ultimate explanation for the perpetuated cigarette habit resides in the pharmacological effect of smoke upon the body of the smoker, the effect being most rewarding to the individual under stress.[30]
May 24, 1971	RJR	Habituating level of nicotine (how low can we go?)[31]
October 25, 1972	PM	Think of the cigarette pack as a storage container for a day's supply of nicotine…think of the cigarette as a dispenser for a dose unit of nicotine…think of a puff of smoke as the vehicle of nicotine. Smoke is beyond question the most optimized vehicle of nicotine and the cigarette the most optimized dispenser of smoke.[12]
April 14, 1972	RJR	Our industry is then based upon design, manufacture and sale of attractive dosage forms of nicotine, and our Company's position in our industry is determined by our ability to produce dosage forms of nicotine which have more overall value, tangible or intangible, to the consumer than those of our competitors.[20]
September, 1973	RJR	Methods which may be used to increase smoke pH and/or nicotine "kick" include: (1) increasing the amount of (strong) burley in the blend, (2) reduction of casing sugar used on the burley and/or blend, (3) use of alkaline additives, usually ammonia compounds, to the blend, (4) addition of nicotine to the blend, (5) removal of acids from the blend, (6) special filter systems to remove acids from or add alkaline materials to the smoke, and (7) use of high air dilution filter systems. Methods 1-3, in combination, represent the Philip Morris approach and are under active investigation.[32]
October 19, 1977	PM	Without the chemical compound [nicotine] the cigarette market would collapse, PM would collapse, and we'd all lose our jobs and our consulting fees….our research effort can now be ground out: What is the lower delivery level limit [for nicotine] beyond which the smoking act is not reinforced?[33]
May 30, 1978	RJR	Winston filtered cigarettes using our basic burley blend (#300827) have an optimum "nicotine strength" rating in an area mean pH 6.2-6.3 and 0.12-0.13 mg/puff nicotine.[34]
February 13, 1980	LTC	Determine the minimum level of nicotine that will allow continued smoking.[35]
December 1, 1982	RJR	We cannot ever be comfortable selling a product which most of our customers would stop using if they could…if the exit gate from our market should suddenly open, we could be out of business almost overnight.[36]
January 18, 1982	PM	No statistically significant effects (ie, pattern reversal evoked potential) were obtained by the smoking of the three-low delivery (0.1 mg) cigarettes. This suggests that, with respect to the conditions of our experiment, a threshold exists somewhere between 0.1 and 0.3 mg of nicotine.[37]
July 29, 1987	PM	Any future reduction of tar levels will come into conflict with a twofold limit, as (1) a minimum amount of nicotine is needed for the smoker's satisfaction (~0.8 mg/cig) and (2) there exists a maximum concentration of nicotine in smoke to let the taste of the latter unaffected (less than 10%).[38]

Company abbreviations as follows: ATC, American Tobacco Company; BAT, British American Tobacco Company; B&W, Brown & Williamson Tobacco Company; LTC, Lorillard Tobacco Company; PM, Philip Morris Tobacco Company; RJR, R.J. Reynolds Tobacco Company.

More recently, genetic engineering methods have been used to control the level of nicotine in tobacco.[49]

Additional information about nicotine in cigarettes can be found in the Pharmacology section of this textbook.

CONCEALING THE TRUTH ABOUT NICOTINE ADDICTION

While internal cigarette company documents reveal the critical role of nicotine in product design dating back over a half a century ago (see **Table 7-1**), it was not until 1997, when the CEO of Liggett Group became the first cigarette company executive to publicly acknowledge that nicotine and cigarettes are addictive[50] (see **Fig. 7-1**). Once this admission was made by Liggett Group, the other cigarette manufacturers soon changed their public stance on nicotine, acknowledging that nicotine was an addictive drug and could cause physiological dependence in some people who use it. But, even today, as indicated by how cigarette makers defend themselves in lawsuits brought by those claiming personal injury from cigarettes, the role of nicotine in addiction to nicotine in cigarettes is downplayed along with the design of the cigarette, with arguments made that those individuals who fail to quit simply lack sufficient motivation to refrain from smoking and that continued smoking is a matter of choice[51] (see section Denying Justice to Those Harmed by Addiction to Nicotine in Cigarettes).

So why deny the obvious? The answer to this question relates to the way cigarette companies represented smoking and tobacco as "free choice," which of course would be negated if the person smoking was addicted. As a 1980 Tobacco Institute memo noted, "the entire matter of addiction is the most potent weapon a prosecuting attorney can have in a lung cancer/cigarette case. We can't defend continued smoking as "free choice" if the person was addicted."[52]

Cigarette manufacturers also worried that labelling smoking as addiction could open the door to product regulation, which is something they had worked to avoid for nearly a century. As a 1969 memo from a Philip Morris executive cautioned, "Do we really want to tout cigarette smoke as a drug? It is, of course, but there are dangerous FDA implications to having such conceptualization go beyond these walls."[53]

The Pure Food and Drug Act of 1906 was the first federal food and drug law in the United States. It defined a drug as including medicines and preparations recognized in the United States Pharmacopeia (USP).[54] Tobacco had been listed in the 1890 edition of the USP, but was deleted in the next edition, released in 1905 with rumors that the deletion of tobacco had been made in exchange for support of the law from tobacco state congressional members.[55] In 1914, the chief of the Bureau of Chemistry in the Department of Agriculture interpreted the 1906 Act to include tobacco only if there is a claim made that tobacco is used for the cure, mitigation, or prevention of disease; if no such claim is made, tobacco and its preparation would not be subject to the provisions of the Act.[54] In 1938 the 1906 Act was replaced by Federal Food, Drug, and Cosmetic Act which made no specific reference to tobacco.[54]

During the 20th century cigarette companies collectively denied that nicotine was addictive and instead referred to smoking of tobacco as a habit and not an addiction.[56-59] For example, in response to a 1976 consumer letter which asked the manufacturer of Vantage cigarette (ie, R.J. Reynolds Tobacco Company) if nicotine has any habit-forming properties, the response from the Tobacco Institute sent back to the customer was that "nicotine is not physically addictive"[60] (see **Fig. 7-2**). Instead, the response letter referred the consumer to an excerpt of the 1964 Surgeon General's Report

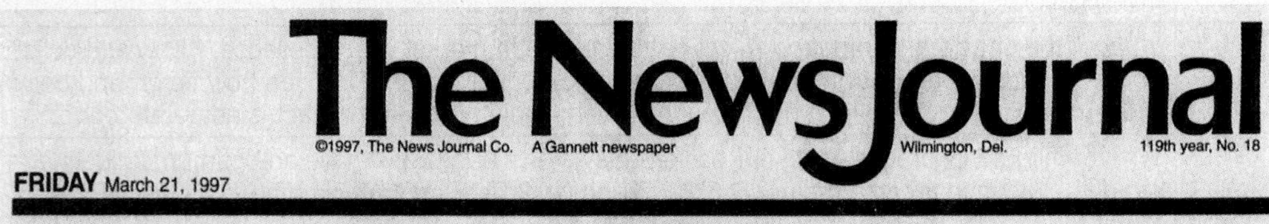

The News Journal

©1997, The News Journal Co. A Gannett newspaper Wilmington, Del. 119th year, No. 18

FRIDAY March 21, 1997

40¢ New Castle County stores, 50¢ all other stores
FINAL EDITION

Tobacco firm admits deceit, settles suits

Liggett will turn over documents

By LAURAN NEERGAARD
Associated Press

WASHINGTON — In a dramatic confession, the maker of Chesterfield cigarettes settled 22 state lawsuits Thursday by agreeing to warn on every pack that smoking is addictive and admitting the industry markets cigarettes to teen-agers.

▶Bigger firms won't yield. A10

"They know it and they will help us prove it," said Arizona Attorney General Grant Woods in announcing the settlement. He called the deal "the beginning of the end for this conspiracy of lies and deception perpetuated on the American public by the tobacco companies."

Liggett also provided thousands of documents that detail industry-wide discussions of tobacco dangers and marketing, and Woods said Liggett has begun transferring papers to the custody of state judges.

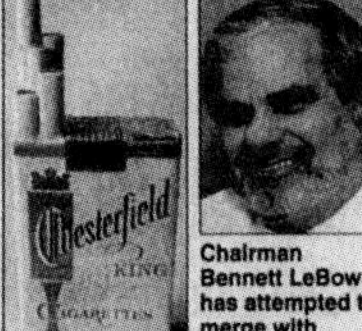

Chairman Bennett LeBow has attempted to merge with another company

"On the basis of these documents, tobacco company executives could go to jail," said Florida Attorney General Robert Butterworth.

But tobacco giant Philip Morris and three other Liggett competitors won a temporary restraining order Thursday to keep those documents secret for at least 10 more days.

And Philip Morris said in a statement it "will continue to defend vigorously against the meritless lawsuits."

Woods said the attorneys general will not attempt to see the disputed papers until judges decide whether they must remain confidential.

The 22 states will divide 25 percent of pretax profits over the next 25 years from Liggett, which has just 2 percent of the U.S. cigarette market. But if Liggett merges with another tobacco firm, which chief executive Bennett LeBow has attempted to do, it would immediately pay an additional $25 million to the states, Woods said.

The prosecutors emphasized they pursued Liggett not for money, but for evidence in the states' continuing lawsuits against the industry.

Settling the state lawsuits, which seek to recover Medicaid funds spent treating sick smokers, does not end litigation against Liggett's competitors.

Sheri L. Woodruff, a spokeswoman for Gov. Carper, said the administration has until this point stayed out of the tobacco litigation because it hasn't been clear that the state would collect more money than it would spend on investigating health problems related to smoking. Woodruff said the administration would review the Liggett development over the next few weeks to make sure that stance still makes sense.

Figure 7-1. 1997 newspaper clip cover Bennett LeBow of Liggett Group. (From Cummings KM, Brown A, Philipson B. History of the evolution of tobacco products. In: Hecht SS, Hatuskami DK, eds. *Tobacco and Cancer: The Science and the Story*. World Scientific Publishing Company; 2022.)

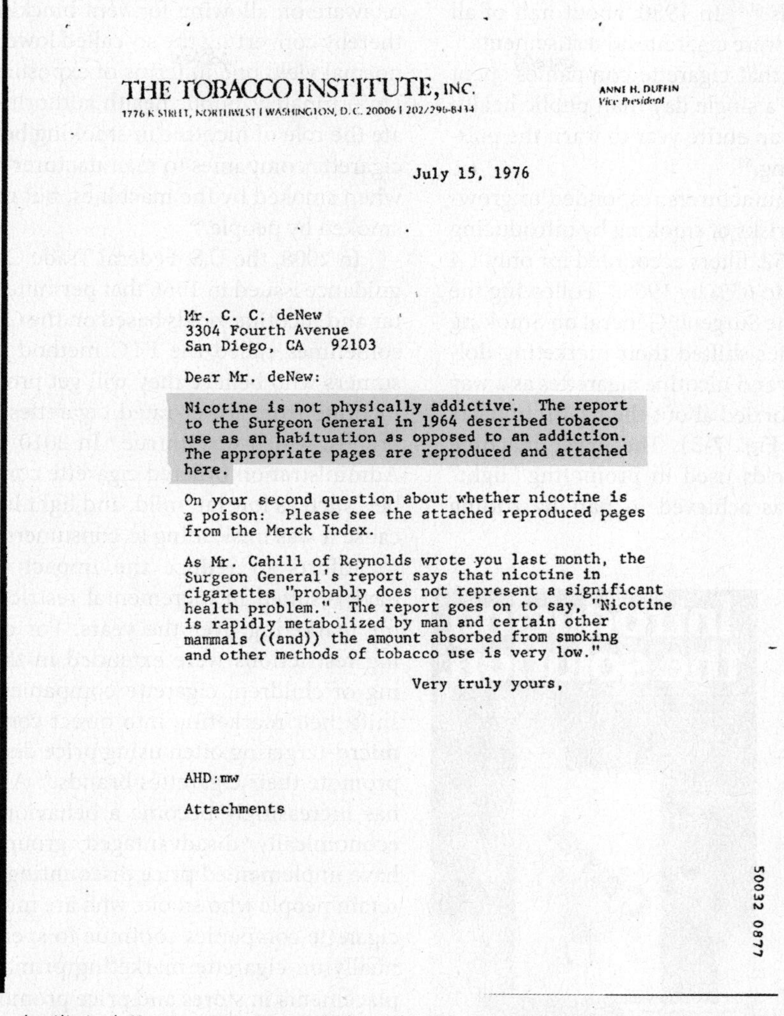

THE TOBACCO INSTITUTE, INC.
1776 K STREET, NORTHWEST | WASHINGTON, D.C. 20006 | 202/296-8434

ANNE H. DUFFIN
Vice President

July 15, 1976

Mr. C. C. deNew
3304 Fourth Avenue
San Diego, CA 92103

Dear Mr. deNew:

Nicotine is not physically addictive. The report to the Surgeon General in 1964 described tobacco use as an habituation as opposed to an addiction. The appropriate pages are reproduced and attached here.

On your second question about whether nicotine is a poison: Please see the attached reproduced pages from the Merck Index.

As Mr. Cahill of Reynolds wrote you last month, the Surgeon General's report says that nicotine in cigarettes "probably does not represent a significant health problem.". The report goes on to say, "Nicotine is rapidly metabolized by man and certain other mammals ((and)) the amount absorbed from smoking and other methods of tobacco use is very low."

Very truly yours,

AHD:mw

Attachments

50032 0877

Figure 7-2. 1976 Tobacco Institute letter to consumer stating nicotine is not physically addictive. (From Duffin AH. *Letter*. Tobacco Institute, July 15, 1976. Accessed August 9, 2023. https://www.industrydocuments.ucsf.edu/docs/hnmk0056)

that defined smoking as an habituation rather than an addiction. However, what was not revealed in the response letter was that the 1964 report used an outdated definition of drug addiction, which at the time required a drug to be intoxicating in order for the drug to be labelled addictive. In fact, using the outdated definition neither cocaine nor methamphetamine would have been classified as addictive.[2] Shortly, after the 1964 Surgeon General's report was issued, the World Health Organization modified its criteria for drug addiction dropping the intoxication requirement.[2]

MASS MARKETING

Cigarette makers have long recognized the importance of advertising in selling cigarettes as an acceptable lifestyle choice.[61,62] As one tobacco company executive noted, "The rise and fall of every brand of consequence has been traced in detail and their year to year success or failure shown to be the direct result of consumer advertising."[63] Between 1940 and 2004 cigarette companies collectively spent about $250 billion to advertise their cigarette brands, an amount that exceeds any other consumer product sold in America.[61] In the 1920s cigarette companies were among the first to sponsor radio shows linking their brands with popular celebrities of the era.[62] As movies became a popular form of entertainment, cigarette makers worked with Hollywood producers to create tie-ins, paying actors and studios for brand endorsements.[64]

As television viewing became commonplace in the 1950s, cigarette makers were also early and frequent sponsors of TV shows, sponsoring comedy sitcoms (eg, Beverly Hillbillies) RJR), variety shows (eg, Lucky Strike Hit Parade), sporting events (eg, NFL football), and dramas (eg, Twilight Zone). Public concern about cigarette advertising impacting children led Congress to eventually ban cigarette advertising on television and radio in 1971.[61] However, cigarette companies simply shifted their marketing dollars to newspapers, magazines, sports sponsorship (eg, NASCAR, Virginia Slims Tennis), concerts (eg, Kool Jazz Festival), brand placement in movies (eg, Superman), and billboards.[61,65] In 1980, about half of all billboards in the United States were cigarette advertisements.[65] A 1981 FTC report observed that cigarette companies spent more to advertise cigarettes in a single day than public health authorities spent combined in an entire year to warn the public about the dangers of smoking.[65]

In the 1950s, cigarette manufacturers responded to growing concerns about the health risks of smoking by introducing "filtered" cigarettes.[61,62,66] In 1952, filters accounted for only 1.4 percent of sales, but increased to 65% by 1965.[67] Following the release of the 1964 Report of the Surgeon General on Smoking and Health, cigarette companies shifted their marketing dollars to promote filtered low-tar and nicotine cigarettes as a way to recruit and retain people worried about the health impacts of cigarette smoking[61,66] (see **Fig. 7-3**). The lower machine measured tar and nicotine yields used in promoting "light" and "ultra-light" cigarettes was achieved in part by adding ventilation holes to the filter tip, which consumers were mostly unaware of, allowing for vent blocking with fingers and lips, thereby converting the so-called lower yield product back to a normal yield one in terms of exposure to tar and nicotine.[66,68] Unfortunately, public health authorities did not fully appreciate the role of nicotine in smoking behavior and the ability of cigarette companies to manufacturer products with low yields when smoked by the machines, but much higher yields when smoked by people.[66]

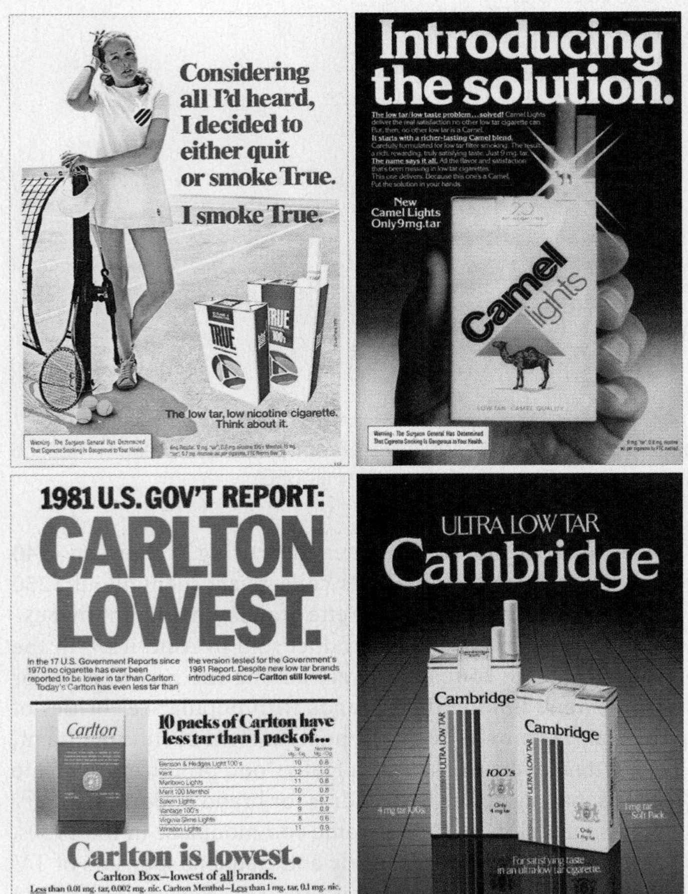

Figure 7-3. Collage of low tar and ultra-low tar cigarette brand advertising. (From The history of tobacco policy—exhibits. Accessed August 9, 2023. https://tobaccoexhibits.musc.edu/#. *The Evolving Cigarette*. Accessed August 9, 2023. https://tobaccoexhibits.musc.edu/wp-content/uploads/2016/12/Evolving-Cigarette-1-1.pdf)

In 2008, the U.S. Federal Trade Commission rescinded its guidance issued in 1966 that permitted statements concerning tar and nicotine yields based on the Cambridge Filter Method, sometimes called the FTC method because it mislead consumers who believe they will get proportionately less tar and nicotine from lower-rated cigarettes than from higher-rated brands, which was untrue.[4] In 2010, the U.S. Food and Drug Administration ordered cigarette companies to stop using labels such as low tar, mild, and light in cigarette marketing because it was misleading to consumers.[4,69]

Efforts to reduce the impact of cigarette advertising have resulted in incremental restrictions on different forms for marketing over the years. For example, when advertising restrictions were extended in the 1990s to limit targeting of children, cigarette companies had already started to shift their marketing into direct consumer advertising, with micro-targeting often using price discounts and incentives to promote their cigarettes brands.[61] Also, as cigarette smoking has increasingly become a behavior more prevalent among economically disadvantaged groups, cigarette companies have implemented price discounting strategies to induce and retain people who smoke who are more price sensitive. Today, cigarette companies continue to spend billions of dollars annually on cigarette marketing primarily supporting product placements in stores and price promotions.[67] Ironically, many tobacco products (ie, smokeless and EDDDs) sold in the United States today include a required warning about nicotine addiction on the package, the most addictive and dangerous form of tobacco product, cigarettes, still do not include a warning about the risk of nicotine addiction. Efforts by government regulators to update cigarette pack labeling with inclusion of a warning of the addictive nature of cigarettes has been opposed by cigarette manufacturers through litigation and lobbying.[54,70,71]

INTERFERENCE WITH THE PROVISION OF THERAPIES FOR PEOPLE WHO SMOKE

Recognizing tobacco use as an addiction is critical both for treating the individual who uses tobacco and for understanding why people continue to use tobacco despite known health risks.[1] As evidence of the neurobiology of addictive substances such as opiates and nicotine began to emerge in the 1970s, the cigarette companies began to worry about the implications that this line of research might have in redefining smoking as a physiological addiction and the potential this research might have in terms of leading to effective therapies to help people to stop smoking.[72,73] As one Philip Morris scientist observed when discussing some of the research it was funding on the neurobiology of addictive substances, "...it is my strong feeling that with the progress that has been claimed, we are in the process of digging our own grave."[74]

Cigarette companies also have a history of opposing efforts to promote abstinence from smoking. In 1973 when the National Cancer Institute budget included a line item for funding abstinence from smoking, cigarette companies opposed the plan arguing that such research was propaganda-oriented rather than scientific.[75] In 1976 when the American Psychiatric Association (APA) considered classifying smoking tobacco as an addiction, the tobacco industry organized a successful lobbying effort both within APA and outside to oppose the change in status, suggesting that classifying smoking tobacco as an addiction would increase the cost of drug treatment since smoking would need to be covered in the same way as other substance use disorder treatments[76,77] (see **Fig. 7-4**). In the 1980s when the American Cancer Society sponsored its annual national Great American Smoke Out event urging people who smoke to try to give up cigarettes for a day, Philip Morris launched its Great American Smoker's Campaign offering tips on how to avoid being nagged about smoking and while claiming to defend a person's right to smoke.[78,79]

Nicotine gum was introduced as a stop smoking treatment in the late 1970s, first registered as a drug for treating tobacco smoking addiction in Switzerland in 1978, and later approved in Canada in 1979, the United Kingdom in 1980, and in Sweden in 1981. It was not until 1984, after a 34-month review, that the U.S. Food and Drug Administration (FDA) approved nicotine gum as a prescription for stop-smoking treatment.[54] Nicotine gum was brought to the U.S. market by Merrell Dow, part of the Dow chemical company, ironically which was also a supplier of millions of dollars of chemicals used by Philip Morris in cigarette manufacturing.[80,81] Nicotine gum became a top selling prescription medication in the United States reflecting the high demand for an effective stop smoking treatment.[54] However, what was not known at the time was the effort made by Philip Morris to use its leverage with Dow to influence the marketing of nicotine gum. In 1984,

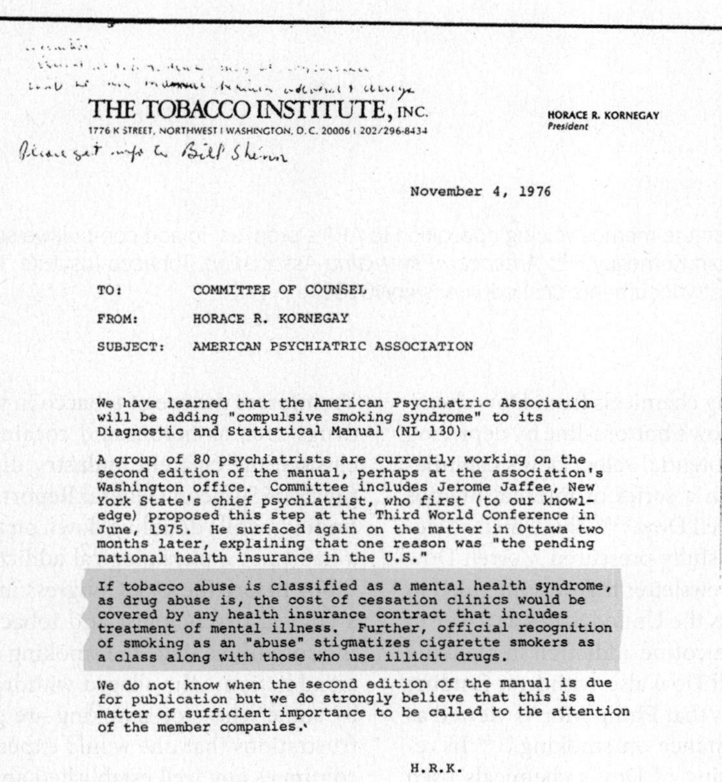
THE TOBACCO INSTITUTE, INC.
1776 K STREET, NORTHWEST | WASHINGTON, D.C. 20006 | 202/296-8434

HORACE R. KORNEGAY
President

Please get info to Bill Shinn

November 4, 1976

TO: COMMITTEE OF COUNSEL
FROM: HORACE R. KORNEGAY
SUBJECT: AMERICAN PSYCHIATRIC ASSOCIATION

We have learned that the American Psychiatric Association will be adding "compulsive smoking syndrome" to its Diagnostic and Statistical Manual (NL 130).

A group of 80 psychiatrists are currently working on the second edition of the manual, perhaps at the association's Washington office. Committee includes Jerome Jaffee, New York State's chief psychiatrist, who first (to our knowledge) proposed this step at the Third World Conference in June, 1975. He surfaced again on the matter in Ottawa two months later, explaining that one reason was "the pending national health insurance in the U.S."

If tobacco abuse is classified as a mental health syndrome, as drug abuse is, the cost of cessation clinics would be covered by any health insurance contract that includes treatment of mental illness. Further, official recognition of smoking as an "abuse" stigmatizes cigarette smokers as a class along with those who use illicit drugs.

We do not know when the second edition of the manual is due for publication but we do strongly believe that this is a matter of sufficient importance to be called to the attention of the member companies.

H.R.K.

50368 389

Figure 7-4. *(Continued)*

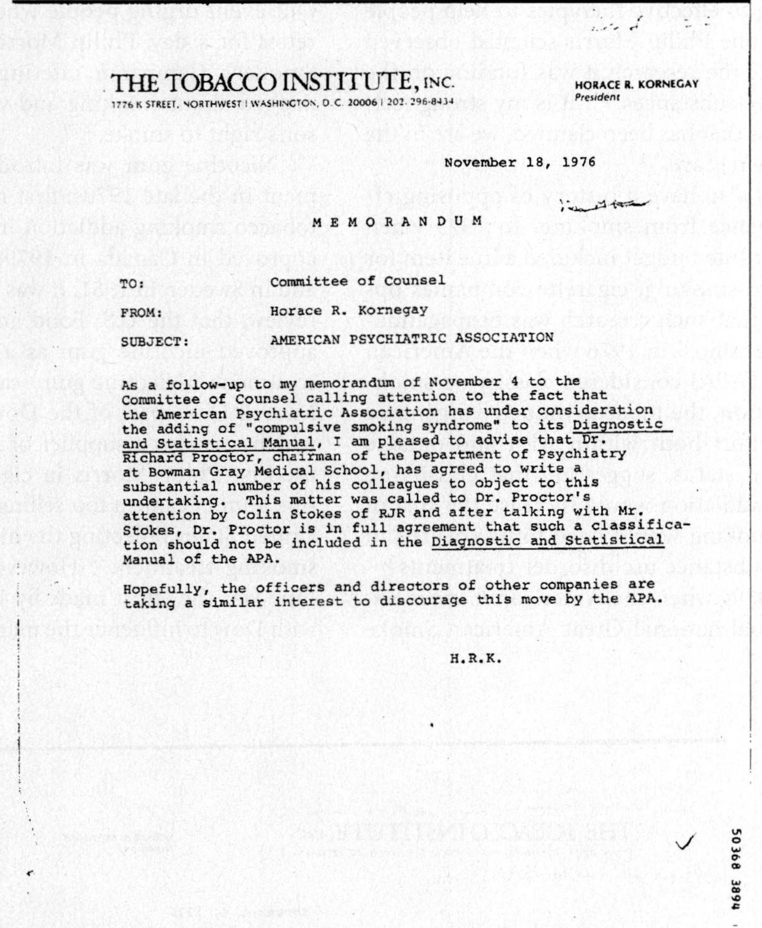

THE TOBACCO INSTITUTE, INC.
1776 K STREET, NORTHWEST | WASHINGTON, D.C. 20006 | 202-296-8434

HORACE R. KORNEGAY
President

November 18, 1976

M E M O R A N D U M

TO: Committee of Counsel

FROM: Horace R. Kornegay

SUBJECT: AMERICAN PSYCHIATRIC ASSOCIATION

As a follow-up to my memorandum of November 4 to the Committee of Counsel calling attention to the fact that the American Psychiatric Association has under consideration the adding of "compulsive smoking syndrome" to its Diagnostic and Statistical Manual, I am pleased to advise that Dr. Richard Proctor, chairman of the Department of Psychiatry at Bowman Gray Medical School, has agreed to write a substantial number of his colleagues to object to this undertaking. This matter was called to Dr. Proctor's attention by Colin Stokes of RJR and after talking with Mr. Stokes, Dr. Proctor is in full agreement that such a classification should not be included in the Diagnostic and Statistical Manual of the APA.

Hopefully, the officers and directors of other companies are taking a similar interest to discourage this move by the APA.

H.R.K.

50368 3894

Figure 7-4. Two 1976 Tobacco Institute memos voicing opposition to APA's proposal to add compulsive smoking syndrome to the Diagnostic and Statistical Manual. (From Kornegay HE. *American Psychiatric Association*. Tobacco Institute, November 4, 1976. Accessed August 9, 2023. https://www.industrydocuments.ucsf.edu/docs/gryv0101)

Philip Morris stopped purchasing chemicals from Dow chemical company, thereby hurting Dow's bottom-line by depriving them of millions of dollars of potential sales. Dow's capitulation then followed as detailed in a series of internal memos between Philip Morris and Merrell Dow.[80-86] These memos describe how Philip Morris successfully pressured Merrell Dow to discontinue a stop-smoking newsletter that was intended to be circulated to physicians across the United States as a way to educate them about the role of nicotine addiction in smoking behavior[80] (see **Fig. 7-5**). Merrell Dow also withdrew funding support of various health groups that Philip Morris viewed as objectionable because of their stance on smoking.[80-86] In return for the continued purchasing of Dow's chemicals used in cigarette manufacturing, Philip Morris was also given the opportunity to comment on proposed advertising and promotional activities associated with the marketing of nicotine gum.[83-86]

Public awareness about the role of nicotine in smoking behavior began to shift, after the 1988 Surgeon General Report concluded that nicotine is a psychoactive drug that Vreinforces the use of tobacco in ways that are similar to other drugs such as heroin and cocaine.[2] In response to this conclusion, the cigarette industry did what they had done with previous Surgeon General Reports, denying the validity of the findings while doubling down on their claim that smoking was a habit not a physiological addiction.[56] For example, in testimony before the U.S. Congress in 1988, Theodore Blau, PhD, a clinical psychologist and tobacco industry consultant told the committee that "the smoking of tobacco is a habit and not an addiction…the alleged withdrawal symptoms experienced by some who stop smoking are generally the same kinds of frustrations that one would expect to see when someone discontinues any well established and well liked habit."[87] Similar testimony was given by the CEOs of the major cigarette companies that appeared before another Congressional committee in April 1994 (see **Fig. 7-6**). When asked whether they believe nicotine is addictive, all seven company CEOs answered no. A few years later, James Morgan, President of Philip Morris was asked in a deposition if he thought that cigarettes were addictive to which he replied,

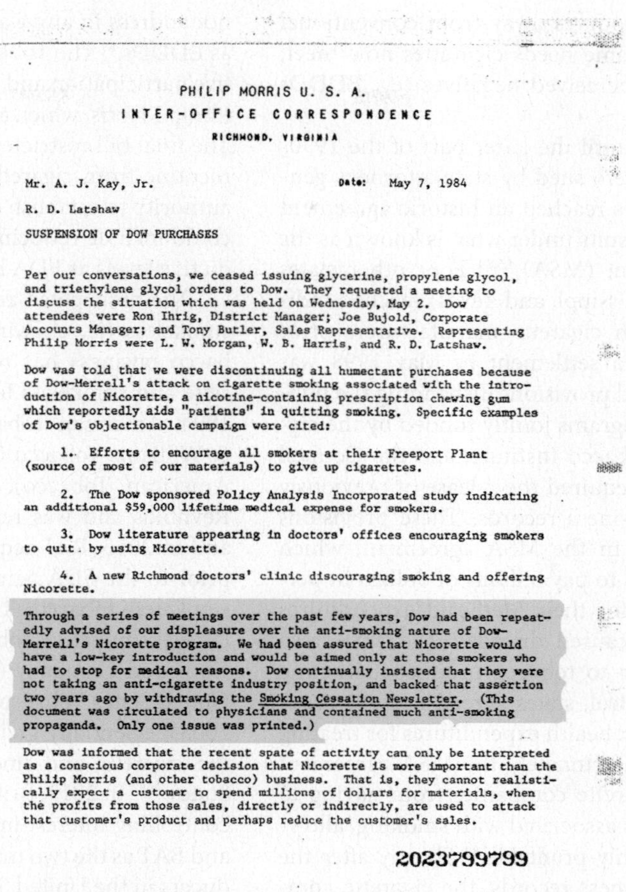

PHILIP MORRIS U. S. A.

INTER-OFFICE CORRESPONDENCE

RICHMOND, VIRGINIA

To: Mr. A. J. Kay, Jr. **Date:** May 7, 1984

From: R. D. Latshaw

Subject: SUSPENSION OF DOW PURCHASES

Per our conversations, we ceased issuing glycerine, propylene glycol, and triethylene glycol orders to Dow. They requested a meeting to discuss the situation which was held on Wednesday, May 2. Dow attendees were Ron Ihrig, District Manager; Joe Bujold, Corporate Accounts Manager; and Tony Butler, Sales Representative. Representing Philip Morris were L. W. Morgan, W. B. Harris, and R. D. Latshaw.

Dow was told that we were discontinuing all humectant purchases because of Dow-Merrell's attack on cigarette smoking associated with the introduction of Nicorette, a nicotine-containing prescription chewing gum which reportedly aids "patients" in quitting smoking. Specific examples of Dow's objectionable campaign were cited:

1. Efforts to encourage all smokers at their Freeport Plant (source of most of our materials) to give up cigarettes.

2. The Dow sponsored Policy Analysis Incorporated study indicating an additional $59,000 lifetime medical expense for smokers.

3. Dow literature appearing in doctors' offices encouraging smokers to quit by using Nicorette.

4. A new Richmond doctors' clinic discouraging smoking and offering Nicorette.

Through a series of meetings over the past few years, Dow had been repeatedly advised of our displeasure over the anti-smoking nature of Dow-Merrell's Nicorette program. We had been assured that Nicorette would have a low-key introduction and would be aimed only at those smokers who had to stop for medical reasons. Dow continually insisted that they were not taking an anti-cigarette industry position, and backed that assertion two years ago by withdrawing the Smoking Cessation Newsletter. (This document was circulated to physicians and contained much anti-smoking propaganda. Only one issue was printed.)

Dow was informed that the recent spate of activity can only be interpreted as a conscious corporate decision that Nicorette is more important than the Philip Morris (and other tobacco) business. That is, they cannot realistically expect a customer to spend millions of dollars for materials, when the profits from those sales, directly or indirectly, are used to attack that customer's product and perhaps reduce the customer's sales.

2023799799

Figure 7-5. 1984 Philip Morris memo suspending purchase of chemicals used in cigarette manufacturing because of Merrell Dow's marketing of nicotine gum. (From Latshaw RD. *Suspension of Dow Purchases*. Philip Morris Tobacco Company, May 7, 1984. Accessed August 9, 2023. https://www.industrydocuments.ucsf.edu/docs/pjhv0125)

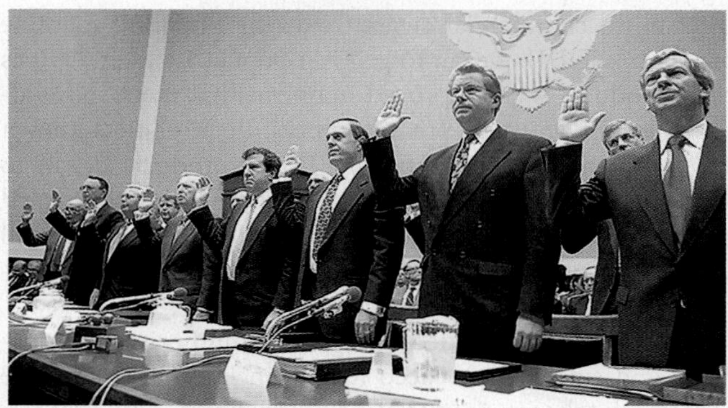

Figure 7-6. 1994 cigarette company executives testify before Congress that cigarettes are not addictive. (From The history of tobacco policy—exhibits. Accessed August 9, 2023. https://tobaccoexhibits.musc.edu/#, *The Evolving Cigarette*. Accessed August 9, 2023. https://tobaccoexhibits.musc.edu/wp-content/uploads/2016/12/Evolving-Cigarette-1-1.pdf)

"…if they [cigarettes] are behaviorally addictive or habit-forming, they are much more like caffeine, or in my case, gummy bears. I love gummy bears…and I want gummy bears, and I like gummy bears, and I eat gummy bears, and I don't like it when I don't eat my gummy bears, but I'm certainly not addicted to them."[88]

INTERFERENCE WITH POLICIES THAT COULD REDUCE THE HARMS CAUSED BY TOBACCO USE

Despite the public pronouncements from cigarette companies that cigarette and nicotine are not addictive, a 1982 R.J. Reynolds business record makes it clear that the company understood that most of their customers who have smoked for any significant time would like to stop smoking and that most were unable to do so.[36] This memo goes on to observe that in the early 1980s there was no universal, easy method for individuals to use to help them stop smoking but looking to the future the situation would likely change. The executive writing the memo observed that if the exit gate from the cigarette market (ie, people being able to stop smoking) was to open, then R.J. Reynolds and other cigarette companies could be out of business overnight (which he said was not an option). The author goes on to discuss strategies the company could employ to stay in business should the exit gate to the cigarette market begin to open. One option suggested was finding ways to eliminate the desire of people to stop smoking (eg, reassurance about the safety of smoking as the companies were already doing with the marketing of "light" and "ultra-light" cigarette brands). A second strategy was to consider offering consumers other products away from conventional cigarettes, which meet the same needs cigarettes now meet, but without the associated perceived negatives (eg, EDDDs and oral tobacco).[36]

Nothing really changed until the latter part of the 1990s when cigarette companies were sued by state attorneys general. In 1998 cigarette makers reached an historic agreement to settle the various state lawsuits under what is known as the Master Settlement Agreement (MSA).[4,5,89] Four other states (ie, Florida, Minnesota, Mississippi, and Texas) reached individual state settlements with cigarette manufacturers prior to the MSA. The Minnesota settlement in May 1998 was important because it included provisions disbanding the public relations and research programs jointly funded by the cigarette companies (ie, the Tobacco Institute, and the Council for Tobacco Research) and required the release of previously secret internal company business records. These provisions were adopted and updated in the MSA agreement, which required cigarette companies to pay billions of dollars in perpetuity to reimburse states for their Medicaid expenditures allocated to treat smoking-caused diseases. The MSA also required companies to agree to tobacco product marketing restrictions. As part of the deal, states agreed not to pursue future efforts to recoup public health expenditures for treating tobacco caused diseases. Unfortunately the MSA agreement also shielded the major cigarette companies from having to pay the full cost of the harms associated with smoking, allowing cigarettes to remain highly profitable.[89] Shortly after the release of their internal business records, the cigarette companies quietly adjusted their decades-long position that cigarettes were not harmful or addictive.[58,59]

Around the same time as the MSA was unfolding, the FDA attempted to exert its authority to regulate tobacco products as drug delivery systems for nicotine.[4] Cigarette manufacturers opposed this effort and filed suit in federal court arguing that the FDA had no such statutory authority.[90] In March 2000, the U.S. Supreme Court ruled that Congress never intended to give FDA the power to regulate tobacco products under the Federal Food, Drug and Cosmetic Act. After the Supreme Court decision, Congressional efforts to pass some form of legislation granting FDA authority over tobacco multiplied.[90] Around this time Philip Morris would be the first major cigarette company to break from the rest of the industry acknowledging that there needed to be FDA oversight of the industry, reasoning that regulation was likely going to be inevitable so they began to lobby Congress in support of regulatory structure that would allow cigarettes to continue to be sold in a way that would be favorable to them (Phillip Morris) as the market leader.[90]

However, it was not until 2009 when Congress finally passed the Family Smoking Prevention and Tobacco Control Act, that FDA was granted regulatory authority over cigarettes and smokeless tobacco.[4,5,89] The Tobacco Control Act was written in part to rein in the cigarette industry's decades of fraud, conspiracy and misrepresentation.[89] However, the statute, a long time in the making, was a political compromise and did not address in any way novel nicotine delivery products such as EDDDs.[89] The Tobacco Control Act was passed with the active participation and support of Altria, the parent company of Philip Morris, which at the time had half the cigarette market.[90] The final bill restricted FDA's authority to completely remove nicotine from cigarettes, although the law did give FDA the authority to establish science-based product standards, which could include reducing nicotine levels in cigarettes to nonaddictive levels as FDA has proposed.[4,5,89]

The anticipated regulatory oversight of the cigarette and smokeless (ie, chewing tobacco, moist snuff, snus, etc.) tobacco business has resulted in a consolidation of the cigarette and smokeless tobacco industry in the United States. In 1994, American Tobacco Company was acquired by Brown & Williams Tobacco Company (B&W) (affiliated with British American Tobacco), in 2004 B&W was acquired by R.J. Reynolds and was renamed Reynolds American, Inc (RAI), and in 2015, RAI acquired Lorillard Tobacco Company.[5] Just prior to the FDA gaining authority to regulate cigarettes and smokeless tobacco, RAI and Philip Morris acquired the two largest smokeless tobacco companies in the United States, Conwood Company (acquired by R.J. Reynolds in 2006) and United States Tobacco Company (acquired by Philip Morris in 2008), essentially giving them controlling interests over both the cigarette and smokeless tobacco markets in the United States.[91,92] In 2017, British American Tobacco (BAT) acquired a controlling interest in Reynolds American, Inc, leaving Altria and BAT as the two major cigarette and smokeless tobacco producers in the United States.[93]

However, the internet and EDDDs product innovations allowed for a growing spectrum of next generation nicotine delivery products, most of which were not manufactured by cigarette companies at that time, to reach consumers and threaten to commercial cigarettes as the preferred nicotine product.[89] EDDDs began to grow in popularity after 2010 as early products were improved upon making them more affordable and acceptable to consumers. Retail outlets known as "vape" shops specializing in EDDDs products began to appear in local communities offering competition to gas and convenient stores that cigarette companies have used to sell their tobacco products (ie, cigarettes, cigars, smokeless tobacco).[5,89]

In 2016, FDA extended its regulatory authority over cigarettes and smokeless tobacco to also include other nicotine containing tobacco products including cigars, pipe tobacco, and EDDDs. In July 2017, the FDA announced an innovative new framework for regulating tobacco products based on a recognition that there is a continuum of risk across different nicotine delivery products offering an opportunity to markedly improved population health by reducing the addictiveness of commercial cigarette tobacco products while at the same time increasing people's access to potentially less harmful nicotine products (ie, both consumer and medicinal nicotine products).[94,95] The guiding principle behind the strategy was finding a way to reduce the diseases and premature deaths caused by smokeable tobacco products, primarily cigarettes.

As the FDA's Center for Tobacco Products' press release noted: "Envisioning a world where cigarettes would no longer create or sustain addiction and where adults who need or want nicotine could get it from less harmful alternative sources, needs to be the cornerstone of our efforts—and we believe it's vital that we pursue common ground."[95]

The concept for reducing the addictiveness of cigarettes was initially proposed in 1994, when Benowitz and Henningfield suggested the idea of a federal regulation of the nicotine content of cigarettes to reduce nicotine addiction.[96] These authors suggested a potential maximum level of 0.5 mg of nicotine per gram of tobacco in a cigarette, which would yield 0.05 mg/cigarette available to the person who smokes. Access to previously secret cigarette company documents revealed that the companies had long known about consumer interest in a nonaddictive cigarette and the feasibility of creating such a cigarette (see **Table 7-1**). In the late 1950s and early 1960s, Philip Morris even had a research program to engineer very low nicotine cigarettes.[97-102] The research program was shut down in 1964 when the U.S. Surgeon General's Report labelled smoking as a habit rather than as a drug addiction[103] (see **Fig. 7-7**).

In March 2018, the FDA sought public comment on a proposed regulation to lower the absolute nicotine content of tobacco used in smoked tobacco products, not the amount of nicotine delivered in smoke, to nonaddictive levels, asking about the merits of maximum nicotine levels like 0.3, 0.4, and 0.5 mg nicotine/g of tobacco filler (ie, the amount of nicotine in the cigarette rod).[104] In the background section discussing the proposed rule, FDA references the extensive scientific evidence on the public health impact of establishing a very low nicotine standard for smoked tobacco products, including a population-based simulation modeling study that estimated that the policy if enacted could prevent 8.5 million deaths by the year 2100.[104,105] Cigarette manufacturers, in their comments to the FDA, were dubious on the very low nicotine product standard for smoked tobacco, warning the FDA that it could take decades to implement and would potentially create an illicit market for normal nicotine cigarettes.[106,107] The suggestion that an illicit market for normal nicotine products would flourish if the FDA product standard were to be implemented may be unlikely in the United States since cigarette manufacturers are already regulated by FDA and the market is highly concentrated, combined with the fact that most people

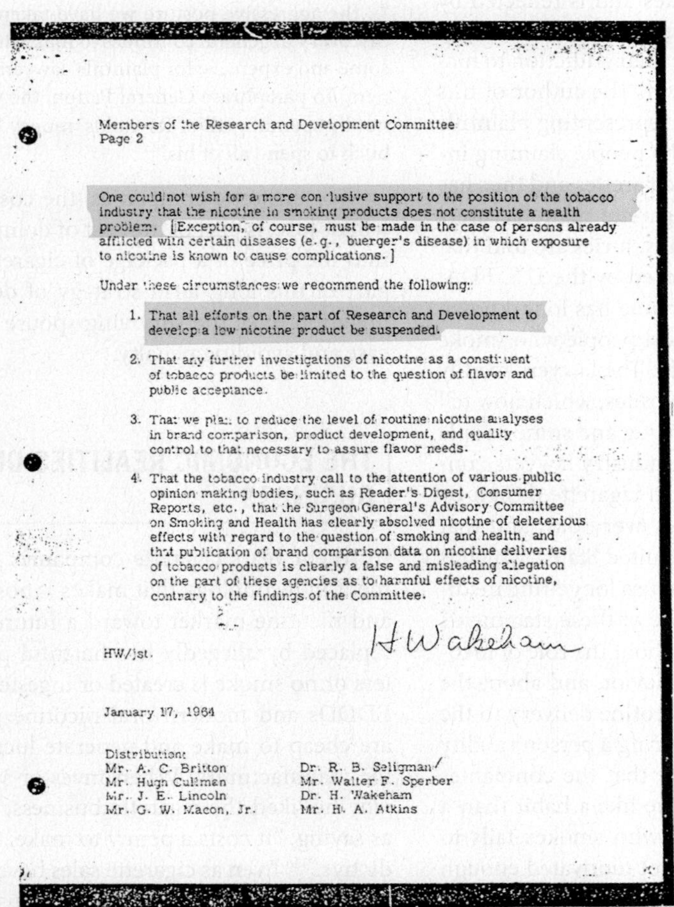

Members of the Research and Development Committee
Page 2

One could not wish for a more con·lusive support to the position of the tobacco industry that the nicotine in smoking products does not constitute a health problem. [Exception, of course, must be made in the case of persons already afflicted with certain diseases (e.g., buerger's disease) in which exposure to nicotine is known to cause complications.]

Under these circumstances we recommend the following:

1. That all efforts on the part of Research and Development to develop a low nicotine product be suspended.

2. That any further investigations of nicotine as a constituent of tobacco products be limited to the question of flavor and public acceptance.

3. That we plan to reduce the level of routine nicotine analyses in brand comparison, product development, and quality control to that necessary to assure flavor needs.

4. That the tobacco industry call to the attention of various public opinion making bodies, such as Reader's Digest, Consumer Reports, etc., that the Surgeon General's Advisory Committee on Smoking and Health has clearly absolved nicotine of deleterious effects with regard to the question of smoking and health, and that publication of brand comparison data on nicotine deliveries of tobacco products is clearly a false and misleading allegation on the part of these agencies as to harmful effects of nicotine, contrary to the findings of the Committee.

H Wakeham

HW/jst.

January 17, 1964

Distribution:

Mr. A. C. Britton	Dr. R. B. Seligman
Mr. Hugh Cullman	Mr. Walter F. Sperber
Mr. J. E. Lincoln	Dr. H. Wakeham
Mr. G. W. Macon, Jr.	Mr. H. A. Atkins

1001502929

Figure 7-7. 1964 Philip Morris memo announcing the suspension of their low nicotine research program. (From Wakeham H. *Nicotine.* Philip Morris Tobacco Company, January 17, 1964. Accessed August 9, 2023. https://www.industrydocuments.ucsf.edu/docs/pfyw0107)

who smoke want to stop smoking and are unlikely to be willing to pay a premium price to purchase illegal normal nicotine cigarettes.

As of 2023, the FDA had not formally issued a product standard to establish a very low nicotine threshold for smoked tobacco products, although recent news reports suggest a proposed guidance will be forthgoing.[108] At the same time, the health ministry in New Zealand has recently announced plans to move ahead with a policy similar to what the FDA had sought comment on in 2018.[109] In 2019, the FDA did approve a premarket tobacco application from a small plant biotechnology firm (ie, 22nd Century) to allow the sale of a very low nicotine product called VLN (very low nicotine).[110]

DENYING JUSTICE TO THOSE HARMED BY ADDICTION TO CIGARETTES

In recent years cigarette companies have told investors that they are working to diversify their business so that their profits are less dependent on selling commercial cigarettes.[111,112] However, the sincerity of cigarette manufacturers to transform out of the cigarette business is questionable given the enormous profits made from selling cigarettes and is reflected by how cigarette manufacturers defend themselves in court when challenged by customers who claim that their addiction to nicotine in cigarettes has caused them harm. The author of this chapter has served as an expert witness representing plaintiffs in many personal injury cases brought by people claiming injury from their addiction to nicotine in cigarettes and thus has had an opportunity to observe how cigarette manufacturers defend themselves in such cases. Typically, juries are told that cigarettes are a legal product and regulated by the U.S. FDA. Industry lawyers advise juries that everyone has long-known the health risks of smoking, and that most people who smoke recognize that it is hard to stop smoking. The lawyers readily acknowledge what is on the company websites, which now tell consumers that nicotine is an addictive drug and some people do get addicted to cigarettes. However, industry lawyers consistently downplay the role of nicotine in cigarette design by explaining that people do stop smoking every day, and that there are millions of ex-smokers in the United States, which is proof that nicotine addiction is not an excuse for getting medical diseases from smoking.[51] The purpose of these statements is to create doubt in the minds of jurors about the role of nicotine addiction in persistent smoking behavior, and about the engineering of cigarettes to maximize nicotine delivery to the human brain as a significant factor impairing a person's ability to stop smoking in much the same way that the companies argued decades ago that smoking is more like a habit than a serious drug addiction.[51] If the person who smokes fails to stop smoking, jurors are told they were not motivated enough to stop. If, on the other hand, the person does stop smoking, but too late to prevent the injury, industry lawyers tell jurors that the fact that the person has stopped smoking is evidence they were not seriously addicted to nicotine and could have stopped sooner to avoid injury in the first place. In either case, the industry lawyers attempt to shift blame from the cigarette industry who knowingly engineered and sold a product that is dangerous and addictive, and instead blame the individuals who smoke whose apparent failure to stop smoking in time to prevent their injuries reflects poor motivation and decision-making.[51]

Of course, in a legal context, companies have a right to defend themselves, but how cigarette companies do this is illustrative of their sincerity in moving their business away from cigarettes. It has been my observation that plaintiffs and their families are typically subjected to a long and arduous process that can take many years whereby highly skilled attorneys demand unreasonable evidence about reasons for starting and continuing to smoke while berating the sincerity of quit attempts.

Even if the plaintiff is able to convince a jury that the companies have some degree of responsibility for the injuries caused by smoking, these cases can be dragged on for years through various legal appeals. The entire process is costly and uncertain for the families involved, which is exactly what the companies hope to accomplish. As explained in a 1988 industry memo discussing plaintiff's cigarette cases

> "...the aggressive posture we have taken regarding depositions and discovery in general continues to make these cases extremely burdensome and expensive for plaintiffs' lawyers, particularly sole practitioners. To paraphrase General Patton, the way we won these cases was not by spending all of Reynolds' money but make the other son of a bitch to spend all of his."[113]

For cigarette companies, the cost of defending litigation, win or lose, is part of the cost of doing business and is factored into the price of a package of cigarettes. Also, it appears that part of this long-term strategy of defense may be to extend litigation until the surviving spouse dies, thus dissolving the case and avoiding penalty.

THE ECONOMIC REALITIES OF THE CIGARETTE BUSINESS

In recent years cigarette companies have touted their investment in technology that makes it possible to shift the tobacco and nicotine market toward a future in which cigarettes are replaced by allegedly less harmful products whereby ideally less or no smoke is created or ingested, such as is alleged with EDDDs and modern oral nicotine products.[114,115] Cigarettes are cheap to make and generate lucrative operating margins for manufacturers. When investor Warren Buffet was asked why he liked the cigarette business, he allegedly was quoted as saying, "It costs a penny to make. Sell it for a dollar, it's addictive."[116] Even as cigarette sales have declined, cigarette companies continue to report enormous operating margins that are two to three times higher compared to food and beverage companies, providing a strong economic incentive for cigarette makers to remain in the business as long as possible.[117]

However, as cigarette sales have fallen, cigarette manufacturers have started to market their own EDDD products. Much of the investment to date has involved acquiring (buying out, purchasing, assuming control of) popular EDDD brands allowing for greater control of the EDDDs market.[118-120] In 2019 Altria, the parent company of Philip Morris USA, acquired a 35% share of JUUL labs, which at the time was the best-selling EDDD brand in the United States.[120] In 2021, PMI acquired three companies, Fertin Pharma, OptiTopic, and Venture, all three of which have expertise in oral and intra-oral drug delivery systems.[116] In 2022, PMI acquired Swedish-Match one of the leading smokeless tobacco companies globally.[121] No doubt cigarette companies are attempting to position themselves for a future where normal nicotine cigarettes may not be as predominant in the marketplace as they are today. However, expecting cigarette manufacturers to voluntarily transition out of the cigarette business is unrealistic, which is why tobacco product regulations based on sound science that encourages and rewards new or existing manufacturers to invest in consumer acceptable but independently research-proven lower risk products to replace cigarettes needs to be encouraged.[119]

SUMMARY

This chapter discussed the role that cigarette companies have played in promoting tobacco use disorder (addiction) through its design of cigarettes, efforts to downplay the role of nicotine and physiological dependence in smoking behavior, mass marketing, interference with the provision of therapies for people who smoke, interference with policies that that would accelerate a decline in smoking behavior, and by denying justice to those harmed by smoking and nicotine addiction. The chapter concluded with a brief discussion of the economic realities of the cigarette business and what can be done to change the trajectory of health harms caused by tobacco use disorder.

REFERENCES

1. American Psychiatric Association. *Diagnostic and Statistical Manual of Mental Disorders.* 5th ed., Text Revision. American Psychiatric Association Publishing; 2022.
2. U.S. Department of Health and Human Services. Nicotine Addiction. *A Report of the Surgeon General.* U.S. Department of Health and Human Services, Public Health Service, Centers for Disease Control, Center for Health Promotion and Education, Office on Smoking and Health; 1988.
3. U.S. Department of Health and Human Services. *How Tobacco Smoke Causes Disease: The Biology and Behavioral Basis for Smoking-Attributable Disease: A Report of the Surgeon General.* U.S. Department of Health and Human Services, Centers for Disease Control and Prevention, National Center for Chronic Disease Prevention and Health Promotion, Office on Smoking and Health; 2010.
4. U.S. Department of Health and Human Services, Centers for Disease Control and Prevention, National Center for Chronic Disease Prevention and Health Promotion, Office on Smoking and Health. 2014.
5. Hecht SS, Hatsukami DK, eds. *Tobacco and Cancer: The Science and the Story.* World Scientific Publishing; 2022.
6. Slade J. Nicotine delivery devices. In: Orleans CT, Slade J, eds. *Nicotine Addiction: Principles and Management.* Oxford University Press; 1993:3-23.
7. Benowitz NL. *Nicotine Safety and Toxicity.* Oxford University Press; 1998.
8. Benowitz NL. Pharmacology of nicotine: addiction, smoking-induced disease, and therapeutics. *Annu Rev Pharmacol Toxicol.* 2009;49:57-71.
9. Cummings KM, Hyland A, Giovino GA, Hastrup JL, Bauer JE, Bansal MA. Are smokers adequately informed about the health risks of smoking and medicinal nicotine? *Nicotine Tob Res.* 2004;6(Suppl 3):S333-S340.
10. O'Brien EK, Nguyen AB, Persoskie A, Hoffman AC. U.S. adults' addiction and harm beliefs about nicotine and low nicotine cigarettes. *Prev Med.* 2017;96:94-100.
11. Steinberg MB, Bover-Manderski MT, Wackowski OA, Singh B, Strasser AA, Delnevo CD. Nicotine risk misperception among US physicians. *J Gen Intern Med.* 2021;36(12):3888-3890.
12. Dunn WL Jr. *Motives and incentives in cigarette smoking—paper approved for presentation at the CORESTA/TCRC Joint Conference, October 22-28, 1972, at Williamsburg, Virginia.* Philip Morris Tobacco Company; 1972. Accessed August 9, 2023. https://www.industrydocuments.ucsf.edu/docs/zhfg0117
13. Senkus M. *Smoking Satisfaction.* R.J. Reynolds; 1976. Accessed August 9, 2023. https://www.industrydocumentslibrary.ucsf.edu/tobacco/docs/lxfv0093
14. Liu M, Jiang Y, Wedow R, Li Y, et al. Association studies of up to 1.2 million individuals yield new insights into the genetic etiology of tobacco and alcohol use. *Nat Genet.* 2019;51(2):237-244.
15. Strong DR, Leas E, Noble M, et al. Predictive validity of the adult tobacco dependence index: findings from waves 1 and 2 of the Population Assessment of Tobacco and Health (PATH) study. *Drug Alcohol Depend.* 2020;214:108134.
16. Lynch BS, Bonnie RJ, eds. *Institute of Medicine Committee on Preventing Nicotine Addiction in Children and Youths.* National Academies Press; 1994.
17. U.S. Department of Health and Human Services. *Preventing Tobacco Use Among Youth and Young Adults: A Report of the Surgeon General.* U.S. Department of Health and Human Services, Centers for Disease Control and Prevention, National Center for Chronic Disease Prevention and Health Promotion, Office on Smoking and Health; 2012.
18. Burrows S. *Strategic Research Report. Younger Adult Smokers Strategies and Opportunities.* R.J. Reynolds; February 29, 1984. Accessed August 9, 2023. https://www.industrydocuments.ucsf.edu/docs/kqwv0001
19. Teague CE Jr. *Research Planning Memorandum on Some Thoughts About New Brands of Cigarettes for the Youth Market.* RJ Reynolds; February 2, 1973. Accessed August 9, 2023. https://www.industrydocuments.ucsf.edu/docs/ylnx0096
20. Teague CE Jr. *Research Planning Memorandum on the Future of the Tobacco Business and the Crucial Role of Nicotine Therein.* R.J. Reynolds Tobacco Company; April 14, 1972. Accessed August 9, 2023. https://www.industrydocumentslibrary.ucsf.edu/tobacco/docs/stdb0184
21. Griffith RB. *Letter to John Kirwan.* Brown & Williamson Tobacco Company; September 18, 1963. Accessed August 9, 2023. https://www.industrydocumentslibrary.ucsf.edu/tobacco/docs/jglw0200
22. McCue MJ. *Re: Future Consumer Reaction to Nicotine.* 1978 August 24; Philip Morris Records. Accessed August 9, 2023. https://www.industrydocuments.ucsf.edu/docs/ztdb0184
23. Teague CE Jr. *Proposal of a New, Consumer-Oriented Business Strategy for RJR Tobacco Company.* R.J. Reynolds Tobacco Company; September 19, 1969. Accessed August 9, 2023. https://www.industrydocuments.ucsf.edu/docs/hrpb0094
24. American Tobacco Company. *Improving the Taste and Character of Cigarette Tobacco With a View to Removing Irritants and Producing a Light Smoke.* American Tobacco Company; December 9, 1935. Accessed August 9, 2023. https://www.industrydocumentslibrary.ucsf.edu/tobacco/docs/sxwv0024
25. Wakeham H. *An Opinion on Cigarette Smoking and Cancer.* Philip Morris Tobacco Company; September 22, 1969. Accessed August 9, 2023. https://www.industrydocuments.ucsf.edu/docs/skbc0040
26. Rodgman AF. *The Optimum Composition of Tobacco and Its Smoke.* R.J. Reynolds Tobacco Company; November 2, 1959. Accessed August 9, 2023. https://www.industrydocumentslibrary.ucsf.edu/tobacco/docs/fxkp0034

27. Ellis C. *The Effects of Smoking: Proposal for Further Research Contracts With Battelle*. British American Tobacco Company; February 13, 1962. Accessed August 9, 2023. https://www.industrydocuments.ucsf.edu/docs/pjnc0200
28. Yeaman A. *Implications of Battelle Hippo I & II and The Griffith Filter*. Brown & Williamson Tobacco Company; July 17, 1963. Accessed August 9, 2023. https://www.industrydocumentslibrary.ucsf.edu/tobacco/docs/rhxp0042
29. Tamol RA. *Notes*. Philip Morris Tobacco Company; February 1, 1965. Accessed August 9, 2023. https://www.industrydocumentslibrary.ucsf.edu/tobacco/docs/qynn0226
30. Wakeham H. *Smoker Psychology Program*. Philip Morris Tobacco Company; November 26, 1969. Accessed August 9, 2023. https://www.industrydocuments.ucsf.edu/docs/gqpx0037
31. Laurene AH. *Possible IBT Projects*. R.J. Reynolds Tobacco Company; May 24, 1971. Accessed August 9, 2023. https://www.industrydocuments-library.ucsf.edu/tobacco/docs/tjvk0191
32. Teague CE Jr. *Implication and Activities Arising From Correlation of Smoke pH with Nicotine Impact, Other Smoke Qualities, and Cigarettes Sales*. R.J. Reynolds Tobacco Company; September 1973. Accessed August 9, 2023. https://www.industrydocuments.ucsf.edu/docs/xphv0094
33. Dunn WL, Osdene TS. *Smoker Psychology Program Review*. Philip Morris Tobacco Company. October 1977; Accessed August 9, 2023. https://www.industrydocuments.ucsf.edu/docs/ysmp0042
34. Neumann CL. *Formulation of Blends and Consumer Testing, Monthly Status Report*. R.J. Reynolds Tobacco Company; May 30, 1978. Accessed August 9, 2023. https://www.industrydocuments.ucsf.edu/docs/gkhp0042
35. Smith RE. *Memo*. Lorillard Tobacco Company; February 13, 1980. Accessed August 9, 2023. https://www.industrydocumentslibrary.ucsf.edu/tobacco/docs/kpmv0035
36. Teague CE Jr. *Nordine Study*. R.J. Reynolds Tobacco Company; December 1, 1982. Accessed August 9, 2023. https://www.industrydocuments.ucsf.edu/docs/jtjc0094
37. Gullotta FP, Shultz CJ. *Memo: Repetitive Smoking and the Pattern Reversal Evoked Potential*. Philip Morris Tobacco Company; January 18, 1982. Accessed August 9, 2023. https://www.industrydocumentslibrary.ucsf.edu/tobacco/docs/tnbx0108
38. Reif H. *New Tar Quality Pyrolysates to Distillates*. Philip Morris Tobacco Company; July 29, 1987. Accessed August 9, 2023. https://www.industrydocuments.ucsf.edu/docs/pxgg0111
39. Kasza KA, Ambrose NK, Conway KP, Borek N, et al. Tobacco-product use by adults and youths in the United States in 2013 and 2014. *N Engl J Med*. 2017;376(4):342-353.
40. O'Connor RJ, Giovino GA, Kozlowski LT, et al. Changes in nicotine intake and cigarette consumption over two nationally representative cross-sections of smokers. *Am J Epidemiol*. 2006;164(8):750-759.
41. Foundation for a Smokefree World. *Global Trends in Nicotine*. Accessed August 9, 2023. https://www.smokefreeworld.org/advancing-industry-transformation/global-trends-nicotine/
42. Ashton H, Stepney R, Thompson JW. Self-titration by cigarette smokers. *Br Med J*. 1979;2(6186):357-360.
43. Woodward M, Tunstall-Pedoe H. Self-titration of nicotine: evidence from the Scottish Heart Health Study. *Addiction*. 1993;88(6):821-830.
44. Hammond D, Fong GT, Cummings KM, Hyland A. Smoking topography, brand switching, and nicotine delivery: results from an in vivo study. *Cancer Epidemiol Biomarkers Prev*. 2005;14(6):1370-1375.
45. O'Connor RJ, Hammond D, McNeill A, et al. How do different cigarette design features influence the standard tar yields of popular cigarette brands sold in different countries? *Tob Control*. 2008;17(Suppl 1):i1-i5.
46. Havermans A, Pieper E, Henkler-Stephani F, Talhout R. Feasibility of manufacturing tobacco with very low nicotine levels. *Tob Regul Sci*. 2020;6(6):405-425.
47. Federman H. Removing nicotine from tobacco. US Patent 1,719,291. July 2, 1929.
48. Lippmann LM, Faitelowitz A. Method of denicotinizing tobacco. US Patent 2,000,855. May 7, 1935.
49. Conkling MA. Modifying nicotine and nitrosamine levels in tobacco. US Patent 6908776B2, June 21, 2005.
50. Lebow BS. *Videotaped Deposition*; July 18, 1997. Accessed August 9, 2023. https://www.industrydocuments.ucsf.edu/docs/fjvn0016
51. Patterson AM. *Shook, Hardy & Bacon Memo Regarding STIC File*. R.J. Reynolds Tobacco Company; June 25, 1985. Accessed August 9, 2023. https://www.industrydocuments.ucsf.edu/docs/nzfn0174
52. Knopick P. *Memo*. Tobacco Institute; September 9, 1980 Accessed August 9, 2023. https://www.industrydocuments.ucsf.edu/docs/ynmd0145
53. Dunn WL Jr. *Jet's Money Offer*. Philip Morris Tobacco Company, February 19, 1969. https://www.industrydocuments.ucsf.edu/docs/fnfm0061
54. U.S. Department of Health and Human Services. *Reducing the Health Consequences of Smoking: 25 Years of Progress. A Report of the Surgeon General*. U.S. Department of Health and Human Services, Public Health Service, Centers for Disease Control, Center for Chronic Disease Prevention and Health Promotion, Office on Smoking and Health. DHHS Publication No. (CDC) 89-8411; 1989.
55. Neuberger MB. *Smoke Screen: Tobacco and the Public Welfare*. Prentice-Hall; 1963.
56. Tobacco Institute. *Press Release*. Tobacco Institute; May 16, 1988. Accessed August 9, 2023. https://www.industrydocuments.ucsf.edu/docs/fpkp0141
57. Davis RM. The language of nicotine addiction: purging the word 'habit' from our lexicon. *Tob Control*. 1992;1(3):163-164.
58. Cummings KM, Brown A, Douglas CE. Consumer acceptable risk: how cigarette companies have responded to accusations that their products are defective. *Tob Control*. 2006;15(Suppl 4):iv84-iv89.
59. Cummings KM, Brown A, O'Connor R. The cigarette controversy. *Cancer Epidemiol Biomarkers Prev*. 2007;16(6):1070-1076.
60. Duffin AH. *Letter*. Tobacco Institute; July 15, 1976. Accessed August 9, 2023. https://www.industrydocuments.ucsf.edu/docs/hnmk0056
61. U.S. National Cancer Institute. *The Role of the Media in Promoting and Reducing Tobacco Use*. Tobacco Control Monograph No. 19. U.S. Department of Health and Human Services, National Institutes of Health, National Cancer Institute; 2008.
62. Proctor RN. *Golden Holocaust: Origins of the Cigarette Catastrophe and the Case for Abolition*. University of California Press; 2011.
63. Burgard JW. *A Study of Cigarette Advertising*. Lorillard Tobacco Company; 1953. Accessed August 9, 2023. https://www.industrydocuments.ucsf.edu/docs/qymm0104
64. Mekemson C, Glantz SA. How the tobacco industry built its relationship with Hollywood. *Tob Control*. 2002;11(Suppl 1):81-91.
65. U.S. Federal Trade Commission. *Staff Report on the Cigarette Advertising Investigation*. U.S. Federal Trade Commission; 1981.
66. US National Cancer Institute. *Risks Associated with Smoking Cigarettes with Low Machine-Measured Yields of Tar and Nicotine*. Smoking and Tobacco Control Monograph No. 13. Department of Health and Human Services, National Institutes of Health, National Cancer Institute; 2001.
67. Federal Trade Commission. *Cigarette Report for 2021*. Issued in 2023. Accessed August 9, 2023. https://www.ftc.gov/system/files/ftc_gov/pdf/p114508cigarettereport2021.pdf
68. Kozlowski LT, Goldberg ME, Yost BA, Ahern FM, Aronson KR, Sweeney CT. Smokers are unaware of the filter vents now on most cigarettes: results of a national survey. *Tob Control*. 1996;5(4):265-270.
69. Yong HH, Borland R, Cummings KM, et al. Impact of the removal of misleading terms on cigarette pack on smokers' beliefs about "light/mild" cigarettes: cross-country comparisons. *Addiction*. 2011;106(12):2204-2213.
70. Cummings KM, Gdanski J, Veatch N, Sebrié EM. Assumption of risk and the role of health warnings labels in the United States. *Nicotine Tob Res*. 2020;22(6):975-983.
71. Tobacco Reporter. *U.S. Health Warnings Date Pushed Back Again*. Accessed August 9, 2023. https://tobaccoreporter.com/2022/11/15/u-s-graphic-health-warnings-date-pushed-back-again/
72. Pepples E. *Future Problems*. Brown & Williamson Tobacco Company; February 14, 1973. Accessed August 9, 2023. https://www.industrydocuments.ucsf.edu/docs/mskb0172
73. Blackman LCF. *Notes of a Meeting of the Tobacco Company Research Directors*. British American Tobacco Company; February 16, 1983. Accessed August 9, 2023. https://www.industrydocuments.ucsf.edu/docs/ygnn0197

74. Osdene TS. *Some Comments About the CTR Program.* Philip Morris Tobacco Company; November 29, 1977. Accessed August 9, 2023. https://www.industrydocuments.ucsf.edu/docs/mzmd0119
75. Bryant D. *Meeting of Committee of Counsel of the Tobacco Institute with regards to Dr. Gio Gori and the Tobacco Working Group.* Brown & Williamson Tobacco Company; March 14, 1973. Accessed August 9, 2023. https://www.industrydocuments.ucsf.edu/docs/ghgn0050
76. Kornegay HE. *American Psychiatric Association.* Tobacco Institute; November 4, 1976. Accessed August 9, 2023. https://www.industrydocuments.ucsf.edu/docs/fxyg0001
77. Kornegay HE. American Psychiatric Association. Tobacco Institute, November 4, 1976. Accessed August 9, 2023. https://www.industrydocuments.ucsf.edu/docs/gryv0101
78. Los Angeles Herald Dispatch. *Freedom of Choice Urged: Philip Morris Counters Smokeout with "Great American Smoker's Kit."* Philip Morris Tobacco Company; November 20, 1986. Accessed August 9, 2023. https://www.industrydocuments.ucsf.edu/docs/yhwy0127
79. Whist A. *Great American Smoker Campaign.* Philip Morris Tobacco Company; November 21, 1986. Accessed August 9, 2023. https://www.industrydocuments.ucsf.edu/docs/xlbj0111
80. Osdene TS. *Merrell Dow Smoking Cessation Newsletter.* Philip Morris Tobacco Company; January 4, 1982. Accessed August 9, 2023. https://www.industrydocuments.ucsf.edu/docs/tqdy0111
81. Latshaw RD. *Merrell Dow Pharmaceutical Meeting—July 13, 1982.* Philip Morris Tobacco Company; July 21, 1982. Accessed August 9, 2023. https://www.industrydocuments.ucsf.edu/docs/tjwd0040
82. Latshaw RD. *Suspension of Dow Purchases.* Philip Morris Tobacco Company; May 7, 1984. Accessed August 9, 2023. https://www.industrydocuments.ucsf.edu/docs/pjhv0125
83. Latshaw RD. *Dow—Nicorette Meeting, October 23, 1984.* Philip Morris Tobacco Company; October 25, 1984. Accessed August 9, 2023. https://www.industrydocuments.ucsf.edu/docs/rjwd0040
84. Kay AJ Jr. *Letter.* Philip Morris Tobacco Company; December 17, 1984. Accessed August 9, 2023. https://www.industrydocuments.ucsf.edu/docs/yjhv0125
85. Kay AJ Jr. *Dow Nicorette. Philip Morris Tobacco Company.* September 6, 1985. Accessed August 9, 2023. https://www.industrydocuments.ucsf.edu/docs/hrmb0106
86. Kay AJ Jr. *Dow Nicorette. Philip Morris Tobacco Company.* 1985;December 16. Accessed August 9, 2023. https://www.industrydocuments.ucsf.edu/docs/lxdp0042
87. Blau TH. *Health consequences of smoking: nicotine addiction. Hearing before the subcommittee on Health and the Environment on Energy and Commerce, US House of Representatives, 100th Congress, 2nd session, 29 July 1988, Serial No. 100-168.* Government Printing Office; 1988:319-332.
88. Associated Press. *Smoking No More Addictive Than Gummy Bears.* Newspaper article, May 2, 1997. Accessed August 9, 2023. https://www.industrydocuments.ucsf.edu/docs/gsgw0070
89. Cummings KM, Ballin S, Sweanor D. The past is not the future in tobacco control. *Prev Med.* 2020;140:106183. doi:10.1016/j.ypmed.2020.106183
90. McDaniel PA, Malone RE. Understanding Philip Morris's pursuit of US government regulation of tobacco. *Tob Control.* 2005;14:193-200.
91. Baron M. Reynolds American to Acquire Conwood for $3.5 billion. MarketWatch, April 25, 2006. Accessed August 9, 2023. https://www.marketwatch.com/story/reynolds-american-to-acquire-smokeless-tobacco-co-for-35b
92. Unknown Altria buys maker of smokeless tobacco for $10 billion. *New York Times*, September 8, 2008. Accessed August 9, 2023. https://www.nytimes.com/2008/09/08/business/worldbusiness/08iht-08deal.15971153.html
93. BAT. Press release: *BAT completes acquisition of Reynolds.* July 25, 2017. Accessed August 9, 2023. https://www.bat.com/group/sites/UK__9D9KCY.nsf/vwPagesWebLive/DOAPKCXS#:~:text=the%20premium%20segment%20of%20the,time)%20on%2026%20July%202017
94. Gottlieb S, Zeller MA. Nicotine-focused framework for public health. *N Engl J Med.* 2017;377(12):1111-1114.
95. US Food and Drug Administration. *FDA Announces Comprehensive Regulatory Plan to Shift Trajectory Of Tobacco-Related Disease, Death.* Accessed August 9, 2023. https://www.fda.gov/news-events/press-announcements/fda-announces-comprehensive-regulatory-plan-shift-trajectory-tobacco-related-disease-death
96. Benowitz NL, Henningfield JE. Establishing a nicotine threshold for addiction. The implications for tobacco regulation. *N Engl J Med.* 1994;331(2):123-125.
97. Unknown. *Project 0302—Nicotine Control.* Philip Morris Tobacco Company; 1959. Accessed August 9, 2023. https://www.industrydocuments.ucsf.edu/docs/nnnh0119
98. Seligman RB. *Experimental Cigarette Samples—Controlled Nicotine Delivery.* Philip Morris Tobacco Company; September 13, 1960. Accessed August 9, 2023. https://www.industrydocuments.ucsf.edu/docs/gqbw0115
99. Seligman RB. *Consumer Test—Low Nicotine Parliament Cigarette.* Philip Morris Tobacco Company; June 20, 1961. Accessed August 9, 2023. https://www.industrydocuments.ucsf.edu/docs/lqbw0115
100. Seligman RB. *Nicotine Free Cigarette.* Philip Morris Tobacco Company; October 3, 1962. Accessed August 9, 2023. https://www.industrydocuments.ucsf.edu/docs/rqbw0115
101. Clarke AB. *Project 0302. Nicotine Control as Related to Cigarette Acceptability.* Philip Morris Tobacco Company; April 24, 1963. Accessed August 9, 2023. https://www.industrydocuments.ucsf.edu/docs/msbw0115
102. Dunn WL. *Project 0302: Field Testing of the Low Nicotine Blend Cigarette.* Philip Morris Tobacco Company; November 5, 1963. Accessed August 9, 2023. https://www.industrydocuments.ucsf.edu/docs/jtkw0119
103. Wakeham H. *Nicotine.* Philip Morris Tobacco Company; January 17, 1964. Accessed August 9, 2023. https://www.industrydocuments.ucsf.edu/docs/pfyw0107
104. U.S. Food and Drug Administration. *Advance Notice of Proposed Rulemaking: Tobacco Product Standard for Nicotine Level of Combusted Cigarettes.* Document number: 2018–05345. Federal Register; 2018:1-99.
105. Apelberg BJ, Feirman SP, Salazar E, et al. Potential public health effects of reducing nicotine levels in cigarettes in the United States. *N Engl J Med.* 2018;378(18):1725-1733.
106. Altria Client Services. Comment re: Docket FDA-2017-N-6189, Advance notice of proposed rulemaking on tobacco product standard for nicotine level of certain tobacco products. Comment ID: FDA-2017-N-6189-7074; 2018.
107. RAI Services Company. Comment re: Docket FDA-2017-N-6189, Advance notice of proposed rulemaking on tobacco product standard for nicotine level of certain tobacco products. Comment ID: FDA-2017-N-6189-6710; 2018.
108. Prater E. Tobacco companies will be forced to reduce nicotine in U.S. cigarettes until they're non-addictive, if the Biden administration has its way. *Fortune.* June 11, 2022. Accessed Auguts 9, 2023. https://fortune.com/2022/06/11/tobacco-companies-will-be-forced-to-reduce-nicotine-in-us-cigarettes-until-theyre-non-addictive-if-the-biden-administration-has-its-way-report/
109. McClure T. New Zealand to ban smoking for next generation in bid to outlaw habit by 2025. *The Guardian.* December 8, 2021. Accessed August 9, 2023. https://www.theguardian.com/world/2021/dec/09/new-zealand-to-ban-smoking-for-next-generation-in-bid-to-outlaw-habit-by-2025
110. US Food and Drug Administration. *FDA permits sale of two new reduced nicotine cigarettes through premarket tobacco product application pathway. Press release.* December 17, 2019. Accessed August 9, 2023. https://www.fda.gov/news-events/press-announcements/fda-permits-sale-two-new-reduced-nicotine-cigarettes-through-premarket-tobacco-product-application
111. Perrone M. Altria expands sales of heated-cigarette as revenue slides. *The Washington Post.* July 28, 2020. Accessed August 9, 2023. https://www.washingtonpost.com/business/altria-expands-sales-of-heated-cigarette-as-revenue-slides/2020/07/28/edc29878-d0db-11ea-826b-cc394d824e35_story.html
112. R.J. Reynolds. *Transforming Tobacco.* https://rjrt.com/transforming-tobacco/our-mission-and-vision/

113. Jordan M. John Robinson's California cases. *S&H Attorneys*. April 29, 1988. Accessed August 9, 2023. https://www.industrydocuments.ucsf.edu/docs/xfcj0005
114. Foundation for a Smokefree World. *Tobacco Transformation Index*. Accessed August 9, 2023. https://www.smokefreeworld.org/advancing-industry-transformation/tobacco-transformation-index/
115. Philip Morris International. *2021 ESG Highlights*. June 2022. Accessed August 9, 2023. https://pmidotcom3-prd.s3.amazonaws.com/docs/default-source/sustainability-reports-and-publications/2021-esg-highlights_final.pdf
116. Lubitz L. Investopedia. *Warren Buffett's Best Buys*. Accessed August 9, 2023. https://www.investopedia.com/articles/stocks/08/buffett-best-buys.asp#:~:text=Choosing%20Investments%20With%20Long%2DTerm,It's%20addictive
117. Barclays. *State of Global Tobacco and Cannabis, 1Q22*. April 24, 2022.
118. Sweanor D, Yach D. Looking for the next breakthrough in tobacco control and health. *S Afr Med J*. 2013;103(11):810-811.
119. Levy DT, Thirlway F, Sweanor D, Liber A, et al. Do tobacco companies have an incentive to promote "harm reduction" products?: the role of competition. *Nicotine Tob Res*. 2023;ntad014. doi:10.1093/ntr/ntad014
120. Levy DT, Douglas CE, Sanchez-Romero LM, Cummings KM, Sweanor DT. An analysis of the FTC's attempt to stop the Altria-Juul Labs deal. *Tob Regul Sci*. 2020;6(4):302-305.
121. Ringstrom A. Philip Morris bets on cigarette alternatives with $16 bln Swedish Match bid. *Reuters*. May 11, 2022. Accessed August 9, 2023. https://www.reuters.com/business/philip-morris-launches-16-bln-cash-offer-swedish-match-2022-05-11/

CHAPTER

8 The Impact of the Alcohol Industry on Alcohol Use Disorder

Thomas F. Babor

CHAPTER OUTLINE

- Introduction: The elephant in the room
- Alcohol as a commercial determinant of health
- Alcohol use disorders as a corporation-induced disorder: A heuristic model
- Level 1: Corporate power and the strategies formulated by corporate decision-makers
- Level 2: Corporate activities aimed at profits
- Levels 3 and 4: Impact on alcohol use disorders
- Implications for addiction medicine
- Conclusions

INTRODUCTION: THE ELEPHANT IN THE ROOM

Using terms of justification such as "corporate social responsibility" and "partnerships with the public health community," the alcoholic beverage industry supports a variety of activities designed to show how they can be "good corporate citizens" who contribute to the prevention of alcohol use disorders (AUDs) and other alcohol-related problems. Despite their apparent good intentions, there is growing evidence that some segments of the industry follow a broader strategy that at the same time contributes to the development and maintenance of AUDs. Although most research related to addiction medicine focuses on the etiology and management of AUDs, recently the industry itself has become the subject of scientific inquiry because of its harmful commercial activities, such as aggressive alcohol marketing and its corporate political activities, which are designed to maximize profits by increasing alcohol sales. This chapter describes research and theory relevant to the question of whether the alcohol industry can be considered an inducer of AUDs and other consequences of harmful drinking, especially at the population level where rates of alcohol-related problems vary tremendously over time and among countries.

For the purposes of this chapter, an AUD is an interrelated set of behavioral, cognitive and physiological symptoms used in addiction medicine primarily for assigning persons with alcohol-related problems to treatment and early intervention services.[1] Two important diagnostic systems used in addiction medicine to diagnose AUDs are the eleventh revision of the *International Classification of Diseases* (ICD-11) and the substance use disorder section of the fifth edition of the American Psychiatric Association's *Diagnostic and Statistical Manual* (DSM 5).[2] In ICD-11, dependence is defined in terms of three criteria: (1) impaired control over the amount and timing of alcohol ingestion; (2) the use of alcohol taking precedence over other major life interests; and (3) physiological tolerance to the effects of alcohol, withdrawal symptoms following abstinence or reduction in use of alcohol, and the repeated use of alcohol to alleviate withdrawal symptoms. In ICD-11, a second AUD category, harmful pattern of use, refers to the repeated use of alcohol in ways that cause damage to a person's physical or mental health, or regular use that has resulted in harm to the health of others. Harmful use typically precedes the development of alcohol dependence, but often occurs in the absence of dependence, especially when it results from occasional acute intoxication. The following diagnostic criteria are characteristic of AUDs in DSM 5: alcohol taken in larger amounts or over a longer period than intended; a great deal of time spent in activities necessary to obtain, use or recover from the effects of alcohol; a strong desire or urge to use alcohol; recurrent use resulting in a failure to fulfill major role obligations; continued use despite recurrent social or interpersonal problems caused or exacerbated by the effects of alcohol; important activities given up or reduced because of alcohol use; recurrent use in physically hazardous situations; continued use despite knowledge of having a physical or psychological problem caused or exacerbated by alcohol; tolerance to effects of alcohol; the characteristic withdrawal syndrome for alcohol or use of alcohol to relieve or avoid withdrawal symptoms. DSM 5 specifies three levels of severity: mild (2-3 symptoms), moderate (4 or 5 symptoms) and severe (6 or more). For the purposes of this chapter, dependence as defined in ICD-11 will be considered comparable to DSM 5 moderate and severe AUD.

Because the alcohol industry has been generally ignored as a potential contributor to AUD,[3] its presence in the field of addiction medicine fits the metaphor of the "elephant in the room," that is, a large and powerful entity that is obviously present but is avoided even as a subject for discussion because it is uncomfortable to deal with. This chapter will not only provide evidence that the industry is a major part of the global alcohol problem, but also consider how addiction medicine can become more effective in managing AUDs by counteracting the activities of the alcohol industry.

Alcohol has long been recognized by the World Health Organization as one of the main contributors to mortality and morbidity globally.[4] That recognition poses a direct threat to the industry's public image and its profits. For this reason, the friendly, albeit unobtrusive elephant has been throwing its weight around during the past decade to avoid the mistakes of the tobacco industry, which for many years was very adept at creating doubt about scientific evidence of tobacco's health harms in order to avoid regulation.[5] "Big Alcohol" has been following the same playbook. Research reviewed in this chapter will show how effective they have been in applying the same tactics.

ALCOHOL AS A COMMERCIAL DETERMINANT OF HEALTH

The alcohol industry is a multinational business complex that includes producers of beer, wine, and distilled spirits, as well as a large network of distributors, wholesalers, and related industries, such as hotels, restaurants, bars, and advertisers. Industry-sponsored social aspects and public relations organizations (SAPROs) and the large trade associations for beer, spirits and wine are also part of this complex. The "industry" is not monolithic but it often acts in concert in relation to regulatory policies, especially under the leadership of the large transnational producers that operate indirectly through their trade associations and SAPROs.

In recent years, the global alcohol market has become highly concentrated in terms of beer and spirits production, though the wine sector remains more fragmented.[6,7] This trend toward consolidation of hundreds of different brands into a small number of transnational corporations has made it possible for the alcohol industry to become an important part of the environment in which drinking patterns are learned and practiced—especially with the growth of modern industrial production, the proliferation of new products (eg, caffeinated alcohol "energy drinks") and the development of sophisticated marketing and promotional techniques. With increased concentration, the industry has adopted strategies and tactics, many borrowed by from the tobacco industry, that have been used effectively to influence the policy environment for their products.[8]

In its broad outlines, what has just been described positions alcohol as a "Commercial Determinant of Health (CDoH)," a concept that has been applied to other health conditions attributed to use of hazardous industrial products such as tobacco, processed food, guns, and gambling machines.[9-11] A modified version of the concept has been adapted to the alcohol industry in several theoretical articles and narrative reviews of research.[12-14] In this chapter the concept is extended into a heuristic model that explores its practical implications for addiction medicine.

ALCOHOL USE DISORDERS AS A CORPORATION-INDUCED DISORDER: A HEURISTIC MODEL

A heuristic model is a practical approach to problem solving and theoretical explanation that suggests how a problem can be understood and solved. The traditional public health model is one such heuristic. It proposes that many diseases, especially infectious diseases, result from the interaction of agent, host and environment. Although these elements are key parts of the Corporate-induced Disorder (CID) heuristic model for alcohol, the "agent" is more than an infectious microorganism or a toxic substance like alcohol, the host is more than just the person who drinks, and the environment consists of both policy environment and drinking environment that results from alcohol-related policies. Alcohol as an agent has complex cultural meanings that can either increase or decrease its likelihood of harming the host. Religious injunctions against alcohol, for example, render the Islamic countries among the most abstemious in the world, whereas the culture of heavy drinking on American college campuses can contribute to problem drinking. The causal "agents" in the CID model are complex and extend far beyond the agent, ethyl alcohol. They include the major alcohol producers, their conduits or influence extenders, as well as retailers and others in the distribution chain.

The "host" in the CID model refers to the person who drinks and who may develop an AUD. A variety of factors intrinsic to the host, sometimes called risk factors, can influence a person's exposure, susceptibility, and response to alcohol products. These can be genetic, psychological, and social. Almost all segments of the population, including children, can be considered the targets of corporate activities because of their roles as actual or potential consumers.

In the parlance of public health, an inducer is a causal mechanism that is neither an agent, nor a risk factor, nor a vector. Rather, it coordinates these different factors to maximize the exposure of susceptible hosts to a given agent. Transnational alcohol producers and their extenders in the alcohol industry can function as inducers when their commercial and political agendas serve to enhance alcohol consumption and heavy drinking.[15] As illustrated in the heuristic model shown in **Figure 8-1**, the alcohol industry functions as an inducer through an epidemiologic cascade of sequential causes and effects, which starts with the enormous economic and political power behind government-sanctioned corporate profit making and ends with individual-level consequences to health and social welfare. These consequences add up to population rates of alcohol-related morbidity, mortality, disability, AUDs and harm to others. The explained variable at one level is also the explanatory variable at the next lower level, establishing a causal chain that can be followed from the site of societal power (eg, corporate decisions affecting government policies) down to the exposure environment that induces AUDs in the susceptible host. As described in **Table 8-1**, each level of the model includes a set of actors, processes (ie, modes of transmission) and outcomes with public health implications.

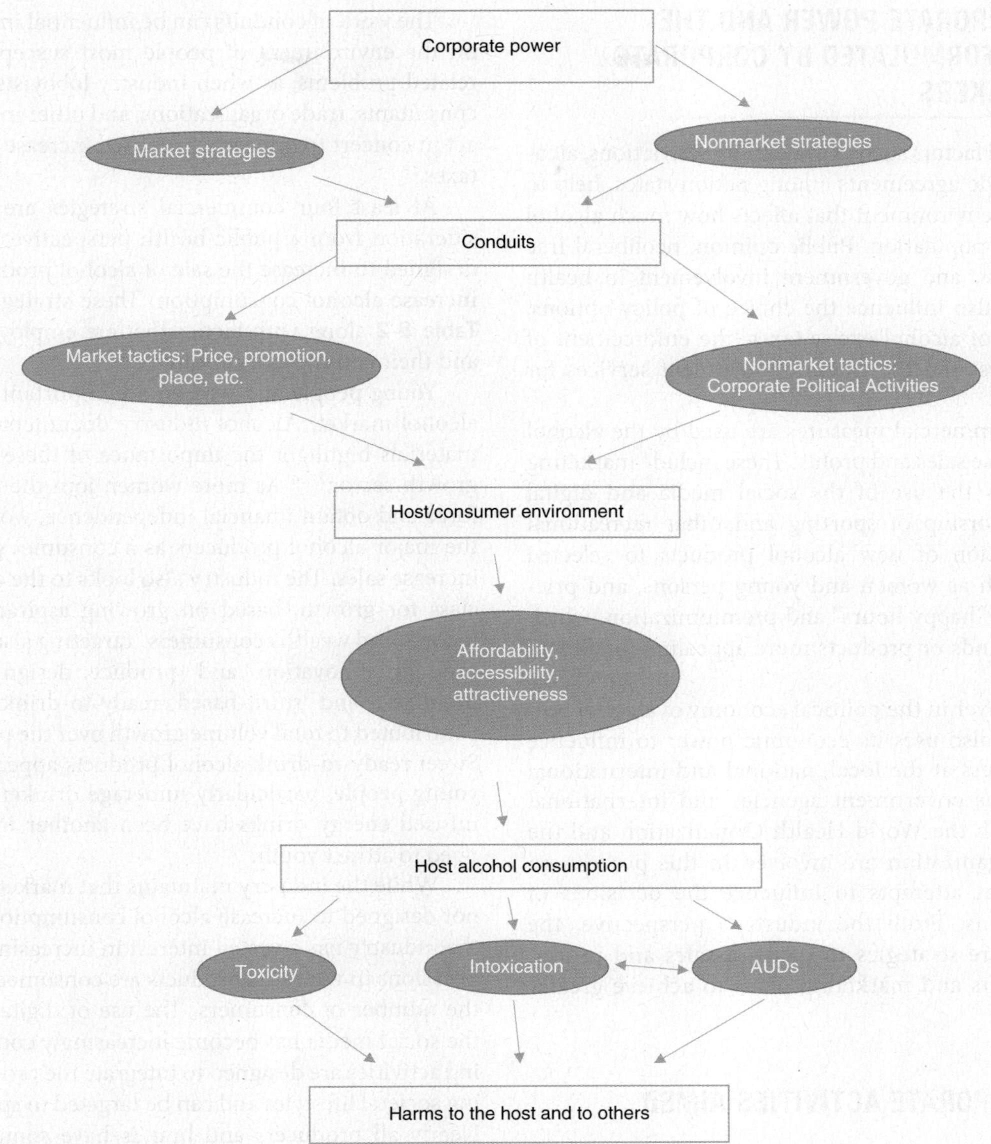

Figure 8-1. Heuristic model of corporate-induced alcohol use disorders.

TABLE 8-1 Actors, Processes and Outcomes for Heuristic Model of Corporate-Induced Alcohol Use Disorders

Level	Actors	Processes	Outcomes
Level 1: Corporate power and the aims and strategies of corporate decision-makers	Alcohol industry, especially transnational corporations, and their key decision-makers	Exercise of corporate power through commercial activities (product design, marketing) and corporate political activities; delegation of tasks to conduits	Strategies to increase sales and profits
Level 2: Conduits and their tactics to implement strategies	Conduits commissioned to implement strategies eg, lobbyists, trade associations, SAPROs, industry funded NGOs, marketing firms	Corporate social responsibility activities, corporate political activities	Changes in drinking environment and policies conducive to alcohol use; increased alcohol availability (physical, financial and psychosocial)
Level 3: Host alcohol consumption	Host (alcohol consumer)	Physical, financial and psychosocial availability of alcohol	Host alcohol consumption
Level 4: Host AUD and alcohol-related problems; harm to others	Host and those affected by the person who drinks	Intoxication, toxic effects, and AUD	Host alcohol-related problems; harm to others

LEVEL 1: CORPORATE POWER AND THE STRATEGIES FORMULATED BY CORPORATE DECISION-MAKERS

At level 1, political factors such as availability restrictions, alcohol taxes, and trade agreements among nation states, help to define the policy environment that affects how much alcohol is consumed in a population. Public opinion, neoliberal free market economics, and government involvement in health promotion, may also influence the choice of policy options, such as the level of alcohol excise taxes, the enforcement of drink-driving laws, and the extent of treatment services for AUDs.

Numerous commercial measures are used by the alcohol industry to increase sales and profits. These include marketing activities, such as the use of the social media and digital marketing, sponsorship of sporting and other recreational activities; promotion of new alcohol products to selected target groups such as women and young persons, and pricing measures like "happy hours" and premiumization, which makes certain brands or products more appealing to affluent consumers.

As a major player in the political economy of alcohol policy, the industry also uses its economic power to influence the political process at the local, national and international levels.[16] Numerous government agencies and international organizations such the World Health Organization and the World Trade Organization are involved in this process, so there are constant attempts to influence the decisions of these organizations. From the industry's perspective, the main outcomes are strategies to increase sales and profits, as well as products and marketing plans to achieve greater market share.

LEVEL 2: CORPORATE ACTIVITIES AIMED AT PROFITS

At level 2, the strategies of corporate decision-makers are implemented using market and nonmarket (political) tactics. Tasks are often passed on to corporate conduits, which are individuals or organizations acting in the interests of corporations. Advertising firms and social media platforms are examples of commercial conduits. SAPROs, law firms and trade associations are examples of political conduits. To the extent that scientific information is sometimes used to justify alcohol control policies, conduits can also include scientists recruited to conduct industry-favorable research or to question independent research that threatens industry interests. For example, in 2018 a group of five major alcohol producers and a SAPRO representing them pledged more than 60 million dollars to the U.S. National Institutes of Health to fund a 9-nation study that was designed to show the health benefits of moderate drinking. After an independent review, the study was discontinued because of a biased research design and potential conflicts of interest (COI) among the investigators.[17]

The work of conduits can be influential in putting pressure on the environment of people most susceptible to alcohol-related problems, as when industry lobbyists, paid economic consultants, trade organizations, and other industry groups all act in concert to oppose a proposed increase in alcohol excise taxes.[18]

At least four commercial strategies are worthy of consideration from a public health perspective because they are designed to increase the sale of alcohol products and thereby increase alcohol consumption. These strategies are shown in **Table 8-2** along with tactics that are employed by producers and their commercial conduits.

Young people and women are important segments of the alcohol market. Alcohol industry documents and marketing materials highlight the importance of these groups as a key growth sector.[19,20] As more women join the organized workforce and obtain financial independence, women are seen by the major alcohol producers as a consumer group that could increase sales. The industry also looks to the emerging middle class for growth, based on growing aspirations of middle-income and wealthy consumers. Targeting also occurs through product innovation and product design. High-strength premixes, and spirit-based ready-to-drink products have contributed to total volume growth over the past several years. Sweet ready-to-drink alcohol products appeal to women and young people, particularly underage drinkers,[21] and alcohol-infused energy drinks have been another innovation developed to attract youth.

While the industry maintains that marketing activities are not designed to increase alcohol consumption, it is clear that the industry has a vested interest in increasing the number of occasions in which its products are consumed, and increasing the number of consumers. The use of digital marketing and the social media has become increasingly common.[20] Marketing activities are designed to integrate the product into emerging societal lifestyles and can be targeted to specific audiences. Nearly all producers and brands have some type of online presence, with many using multiple social media channels

TABLE 8-2 Corporate Commercial Strategies and Tactics Used by the Alcohol Industry

Strategy	Tactics
Increase sales through pricing innovations	• Price discounts • Happy hours • Premiumization to attract more affluent segments
Introduce product innovations	• Integrated marketing campaigns • Advertising to new and traditional market segments
Appeal to new and traditional market segments	• Target segments with different marketing approaches • Integrated marketing campaigns
Increase physical availability	• Home delivery • Supermarket sales

TABLE 8-3 Corporate Political Strategies and Tactics Used by the Alcohol Industry

Strategy	Tactics
Political access/information control	• Campaign contributions • Direct and indirect lobbying (meetings and correspondence with policy makers) • Shaping the evidence base (eg, funding and dissemination of research, use of paid consultants, position papers, technical reports) • Partnerships/collaboration (eg, working with civil society groups and academia to provide technical support and advice)
Constituency building	• Forming alliances with trade associations, other industry sectors • Forming alliances with or mobilizing civil society organizations, consumers, employees, and/or the public • Creation of SAPROs • Corporate-image advertising[a] • Advocacy advertising[b] (press releases, publicity campaigns)
Policy substitution	• Develop/promote self-regulation • Develop/promote alternative regulatory policy, often under the guise of "modernization" of state regulatory regimes • Develop/promote voluntary activities
Financial incentives	• Contributions to political parties • Hiring, or offering future employment to people with political, regulatory, governmental or academic connections • Other financial enticement (travel, honoraria)
Legal actions	• Pre-emption, when a higher level of government restricts the authority of a lower level to impose alcohol control policies • Litigation (or threat of litigation) • Circumvention of existing alcohol control regulations and laws

[a]Corporate-image advertising seeks to build a favorable image and keep the company's name in the public eye.

[b]Advocacy advertising is defined as an advertisement or public communication that attempts to influence public opinion on a specific issue.

Adapted from Robaina K, Babor T, Pinksy I, Johns P. *The Alcohol Industry's Commercial and Political Activities in Latin America and the Caribbean: Implications for Public Health.* NCD Alliance, Global Alcohol Policy Alliance, Healthy Latin America Coalition, and Healthy Caribbean Coalition; 2020; Hillman AJ, Hitts MA. Corporate political strategy formulation: a model of approach, participation and strategy decision. *Acad Manag Rev.* 1999;24(4):825-842; Savell E, Gilmore AB, Fooks G. How does the tobacco industry attempt to influence marketing regulations? A systematic review. *PLoS One.* 2014;9(2):e87389.

(ie, Facebook, Instagram, X(previously known as Twitter), YouTube) that appeal especially to youth. Websites and social media are used to encourage personal interactions with a brand in various ways, including interactive games and sharing messages, images, videos, and links to other websites.

Table 8-3 describes the corporate political strategies and tactics that have been identified in research on the alcohol industry. According to the CID model, conduits for the alcohol industry producers and trade associations engage in corporate political activities (CPA) to create a favorable regulatory environment in which to increase sales and profits. Reviews of CPA used by the alcohol industry document five main political strategies: (1) a strategy to gain access to political decision makers, (2) a constituency-building strategy, (3) a substitution strategy to promote alternative policy or voluntary measures, (4) a financial incentive strategy to influence government policymakers to act in a certain way, and (5) a legal strategy employing pre-emption, litigation and circumvention, as well as measures to influence trade policy. **Box 8-1** provides examples of these various types of legal action. Each long-term strategy is implemented using a variety of tactics. Although conduits do not usually engage in direct interaction with the hosts (people who consume alcohol), their activities indirectly serve to modify the policy environment in ways that increase exposure to alcohol products.

Corporate strategies to deregulate alcohol marketing, oppose alcohol taxes, or increase access are often successful in changing the environment of the host. Examples of the latter include political pressure by industry groups to allow home delivery of alcohol during the COVID pandemic, and the relaxation of zoning regulations to promote more alcohol sales in late-night entertainment districts. In some U.S. states and in several countries (eg, Iceland, Sweden, Norway), government monopolies were created after national prohibition was repealed in the 1930s to remove the profit motive from alcohol sales and to impose strict controls on alcohol availability. Many of these state monopolies have been abolished under pressure from the alcohol industry, despite evidence of their public health benefits.[24] The modified local environment at Level 2 results not only in increased alcohol availability, it

BOX 8-1

LEGAL ACTIONS USED BY THE ALCOHOL INDUSTRY TO DELAY, PRE-EMPT OR CIRCUMVENT PUBLIC HEALTH MEASURES IN DIFFERENT COUNTRIES

When governments propose new regulations, industry conduits (eg, legal firms, trade associations) are sometimes used to threaten or initiate legal action against alcohol policies. There have also been cases where the industry circumvents existing laws, particularly regarding marketing restrictions. The following are examples of legal activities initiated by the alcohol industry in different countries.

Threat of legal action

- In Canada, industry representatives threatened legal action as a way to temporarily stop a program that was testing the effectiveness of warning labels advising consumers that alcohol is a cause of cancer.[22]
- In Brazil, a country with one of the highest rates of soccer-related violence, InBev's Budweiser pressured the government to suspend a national ban on serving alcoholic drinks in soccer stadiums, as a condition for its sponsorship of the 2014 FIFA World Cup games.[23]

Litigation

- The Scottish Whiskey Association brought suit against the Scottish government to prevent implementation of a law that imposed minimum unit prices on alcoholic beverages. The case involved six years of litigation within the European Union legal system before it was denied and the law was finally allowed to be implemented.

Circumvention of existing laws and regulations

- Despite a 2008 ban on alcohol sales in roadside businesses, AB InBev in 2014 launched "Pit Stop Skol kiosks", or alcohol vending machines, in an effort to improve brand penetration and increase sales in Brazil. Located in the parking lots of supermarkets and in large urban centers, consumers were able to purchase beer without getting out of their car.[21]
- Alcohol advertisements frequently violate marketing regulations and the industry's own self-regulation codes. In 2013, Ambev was fined by the Guatemalan Health Ministry for running soccer-related advertisements without government approval.[21]
- In Brazil, Ambev (now part of AB InBev) faced significant backlash for a Skol marketing campaign that appeared to be condoning rape. Following a counter-campaign and fierce criticism over social media, Ambev stopped the ads.[21]

Pre-emption

- The Trans-Pacific Partnership and other international trade agreements have at the urging of the alcohol industry included pre-emptive conventions that prevent countries from mandating health warnings on alcohol and other alcohol control measures.

These cases indicate that legal actions such as litigation (or threat of litigation), and circumvention of laws and regulations are effective industry tactics because local and municipal governments often do not have the financial resources to become involved in protracted litigation, even when the case is based on sound legal precedent.

can also lead to changes in public perceptions that alcohol is an ordinary commodity, one where drinking is considered normative and even necessary, and drunkenness acceptable. Alcohol availability has often been defined in terms of physical availability, which is strongly influenced by the arrangements made by governments that determine how convenient or difficult it is to obtain and consume alcoholic beverages. In a broader definition of the concept,[25,26] several other mechanisms have been introduced that either control or facilitate access to alcohol. These include economic, subjective and social types of availability. Economic availability refers to how price and disposable income affect the affordability of alcohol. Social availability refers to the degree of normative support for drinking provided by a person's key social groups, such as family, friends, and the neighborhood bar or restaurant, or local college, military base, or employer. Subjective, or psychological, availability refers to how acceptable alcohol is to them. This is often learned from alcohol marketing. To the extent that corporate activities influence these different types of alcohol availability, it should be possible to establish evidence for a causal chain that describes how alcohol problems develop as a function of corporate activities.

One additional process at this level that is related to both commercial and political activities is corporate social responsibility (CSR) initiatives. CSR activities take numerous forms, including partnerships with governments and civil society organizations, philanthropic donations, sponsorship of sporting events, responsible drinking campaigns, support for designated driver programs and contributions to scientific research. In 2012 the Global Producers announced that they had contributed 3,550 "Industry Actions" in support of the World Health Organization's Global Strategy to Reduce the Harmful Use of Alcohol. A content analysis of a sample of the Industry Actions from 2010 to 2012 found that only 3.2% of them could be considered as "evidence-based" activities likely to have a positive impact on drinking behavior or alcohol-related problems, 30% had the marketing potential to promote a brand or product and 10% had the potential to create harm.[15] For example, many industry organizations sponsored designated driver campaigns, safe rides programs, self-regulation codes for marketing and alcohol education programs in schools, all of which lack evidence of effectiveness.[16,27] In addition, the prominent association of brand names with these programs was considered to have a marketing potential, and programs that engaged young persons in wine-tasting parties and driver education programs where alcohol was given were considered potentially harmful.

Regarding industry involvement in scientific research, McCambridge and colleagues highlight the way in which the alcohol industry uses both industry-funded research and their relationships with researchers to demonstrate their credibility and good intentions.[28] For example, industry involvement in the funding of a $100 million trial of the cardiovascular benefits of moderate doses alcohol resulted in the choice of investigators who had been previously funded by industry organizations and the development of a biased research design.[17] This is consistent with the findings of an analysis of systematic reviews of research on alcohol and cardiovascular disease,[29] which found that reviews with industry funding connections were more likely to report positive outcomes for low-dose alcohol consumption than reviews conducted by authors with no history of industry funding.

LEVELS 3 AND 4: IMPACT ON ALCOHOL USE DISORDERS

What is likely to be the impact of the alcohol industry activities on alcohol use disorders? So far, we have shown how industry strategies and tactics are likely to influence the exposure environment that increases alcohol availability. This section describes research that supports the contention that industry activities have both a direct and indirect impact on AUDs, one that could influence the initiation, development, course, and consequences of AUDs, as well as recovery from more severe forms of AUD.

At Level 3, alcohol consumers are affected at the individual and population levels by the expanded amount of alcohol availability. The outcome (see **Fig. 8-1**) is increased host alcohol consumption. At Level 4, the impact of increased alcohol consumption is the increased likelihood of alcohol-related problems and harm to others.

Remarkable progress has been made in the scientific understanding of alcohol's harmful effects. As addiction scientists continue to uncover genetic, biological, social, and psychological explanations for humans' propensity to consume alcohol, it has now become apparent that the adverse effects of alcohol stem from three mechanisms of harm: intoxication, toxicity, and ICD-defined dependence, also called addiction. Each of these mechanisms is attributable in part to the influence of the alcohol industry on the exposure environment for alcohol consumption.

The drinking patterns in a particular society are in part created, if not reinforced, by industry marketing of alcohol as normative, enjoyable, and socially rewarding. Drinking patterns are characterized mainly by the frequency of drinking and the quantity consumed per occasion. Different patterns can lead to different types of problems. Sustained heavy drinking may not lead to evident intoxication, but frequent elevated blood alcohol levels can cause tissue damage and AUD. Daily drinking of even moderate amounts of wine or beer per occasion over a long period of time can lead to cirrhosis because of the cumulative effects of alcohol on the liver. In contrast, consumption of a high number of drinks per occasion, even if done infrequently, can lead, through the mechanism of acute intoxication, to a variety of medical and social problems, including harm to others, such as accidents, injuries, and interpersonal violence. Finally, sustained drinking may result in increasingly severe AUD, which, once established, can feed back to increase or sustain both the overall volume of drinking and the occurrence of heavy drinking occasions. This is why AUD is associated with numerous chronic medical problems, as well as acute and chronic social problems.

There is considerable evidence that alcohol is a toxic substance in terms of its direct and indirect effects on a wide range of body organs and organ systems. Some of alcohol's adverse health impacts result from acute intoxication or binge drinking, including alcohol poisoning, acute pancreatitis, and acute cardiac arrhythmias. Another type of harm is chronic disease resulting from long-term exposure to high doses of alcohol. There is clear evidence for a causal role of alcohol in various cancers, including cancer of the mouth, esophagus, larynx, and pharynx, as well as cirrhosis of the liver, diseases of the heart muscle, pancreatitis, and hypertension.[16,ch4] And heavy drinking by pregnant women can cause serious harm to the fetus.[30] In summary, alcoholic beverages are consumer products with toxic effects even when used "responsibly" as recommended in industry marketing messages. They have the potential to adversely affect nearly every organ and system of the body. Few, if any, other commodities legally sold for ingestion, has such wide-ranging physical effects.

In addition to its toxic effects, another cause of alcohol-related harm is alcohol intoxication. The major types of impairments are mostly dose-related, such as impaired driving ability. Alcohol intoxication and accompanying changes in behavior are conditioned by cultural and personal expectations and attitudes, as well as by the concentration of alcohol in the blood.

Intoxication, whether occasional or regular, is a key risk factor for many of the adverse consequences of drinking, especially social harms, such as a failure to fulfil major social obligations associated with family, job, and public demeanor. Social harms also affect the person's immediate social network (eg, co-workers, relatives, and friends) and have a collective effect on society in terms of lost productivity in the workplace, public disorder, interpersonal violence and driving after drinking. Intoxication, even when it occurs infrequently, can result in substantial injury and social harm.[31] These findings highlight the riskiness of intoxication for infrequent heavy drinkers and suggest that frequent heavy drinkers, while still at an elevated risk for injury, mitigate their risk through tolerance and avoiding risky activities while intoxicated.

A number of studies have examined the relationship between drinking patterns and ICD-10-defined alcohol dependence. The more a population engages in sustained or recurrent heavy alcohol consumption, the higher the rate of ICD-10-defined alcohol dependence.[32] The prevalence of alcohol dependence thus varies according to the level of drinking in the general population, a phenomenon that is driven in part by the marketing activities of the alcohol industry. Both the average volume of drinking and the pattern of drinking larger amounts on an occasion are related to the prevalence of DSM-IV-defined alcohol dependence.[33] The fact that some psychoactive substances have self-reinforcing potential is of fundamental importance to understanding how consumer products like alcohol and nicotine can have such devastating effects on population health. Although AUD has many different contributory causes, including genetic vulnerability, it is a condition that is developed by exposure to, and regular consumption of, alcohol. The heavier the drinking, the greater the risk. The challenge to addiction medicine is to identify policies that make it less likely that people who drink will develop AUDs, which, once established, is typically a chronic influence on drinking behavior, one likely to generate more and more problems over the individual's drinking trajectory. In this respect, heavy drinking becomes a major challenge for the alcohol industry because most of its revenues depend on providing alcohol to people who drink heavily with moderate to high levels of AUD.[34]

For illustrative purposes, three groups can be considered in terms of their susceptibility to alcohol-related harm and to the effects of industry activities that constitute the epidemiologic cascade from the corporate boardroom to the clinician's office and hospital emergency room: (1) children and adolescents, (2) adult population groups targeted by industry marketing campaigns (eg, women, males who drink heavily, ethnic/racial minorities), and (3) persons in recovery.

Initiation of Drinking During Childhood and Adolescence

Children and adolescents are particularly vulnerable to alcohol marketing and product design innovations (eg, sugar-sweetened alcoholic beverages, alcohol containing energy drinks). There is considerable evidence that these groups are not only exposed, but also initiate alcohol use and develop problems because of such exposure.[35] Some of this evidence derives from neurobiological research showing that as the human brain undergoes normal biological development during childhood and adolescence,[36] behavioral controls, judgment skills and the capacity to postpone gratification do not mature until after adolescence, thus rendering adolescents particularly prone to risky behavior such as binge drinking. Early onset of heavy drinking has been found to increase the likelihood of developing AUDs later in life, potentially due to lasting effects on brain function.[37]

Developmental research strongly suggests that young children may be more susceptible to media imagery because they do not have the ability to compensate for biases in advertising portrayals and glamorized media imagery.[38] The relationship between exposure to alcohol marketing and youth drinking, viewed in the context of criteria for causality, shows that the alcohol industry can be considered a major contributor to the early onset of youth drinking and an inducer of alcohol-related problems. A descriptive synthesis of findings[35] from 11 narrative and systematic reviews showed evidence of causality according to nine criteria typically used to establish scientific certainty. The reviews document that a substantial amount of empirical research leading to this conclusion has been conducted in a variety of countries using different but complementary research designs.

Adult Population Groups Targeted by the Industry

A variety of alcohol-related problems experienced by adults who drink, including those with AUDs, have been linked to the activities of the alcohol industry. These problems have been studied in relation to population groups often targeted by the alcohol industry in their marketing and other commercial activities such as women and people who drink heavily, including people in recovery.

There are two primary health concerns regarding alcohol use by women. First, women typically have increased vulnerability to alcohol-related harm because of lower body weight, smaller liver capacity to metabolize alcohol, and a higher proportion of body fat.[39] A meta-analysis that included 23 prospective studies concluded that women with moderate and heavy drinking have an increased risk of mortality from cardiovascular disease compared to men.[40] The risk of liver cirrhosis is higher among women compared to men with the same level of alcohol consumption.[41] Alcohol use is also a risk factor for breast cancer, with the risk beginning at 1 to 2 drinks per day.[42]

Second, women who drink alcohol while pregnant risk giving birth to a child with physical, cognitive, and behavioral problems, including fetal alcohol spectrum disorder (FASD).[43] Alcohol can disrupt fetal development at all stages of pregnancy, especially during the early stages before the individual may know they are pregnant.

Despite these health concerns, women are targeted by the alcohol industry through a number of strategies[44]: the creation of new products (eg, Jim Beam's new product campaign called Jane Beam), the use of lifestyle messages underpinned by gender stereotypes (eg, slimness/weight, pink, all-female friendships), and advertising messages of female empowerment and representations of women as sexually active.

Are people with AUD more susceptible to alcohol marketing? Exposure to marketing can affect drinking behavior through visual and auditory cues, such as a picture of an alcohol containing drink or the sound of music associated with a bar-room setting, which can trigger neurobiological responses that are perceived as alcohol craving. Marketing messages are processed differently by individuals with heavy drinking. The more someone drinks, the more likely they are to pay attention to alcohol cues, which in turn leads to increased cravings. Responsiveness to cues is also predictive of alcohol consumption and relapse after treatment in people with alcohol problems.[45] Research suggests that the risk of returning to previous levels of alcohol intake in persons with AUD is related to the person's severity of AUD and craving.[36] Craving and intentions to drink are influenced by the same kinds of "cues" used in alcohol advertising. People in treatment for AUD report increased desire to drink when exposed to alcohol ads,[45] and those trying to abstain describe difficulty with advertising themes suggesting that it is normal to drink alcohol and that a good time involves drinking.[46] Does the alcohol industry proactively target individuals with heavy drinking and persons in recovery? Digital platforms are designed to learn the preferences and vulnerabilities of consumers. These tools are used to disproportionately target people at risk for unhealthy drinking and those with an AUD. People in recovery in particular report feeling "bombarded" with alcohol ads on social media.[47] The integration of digital marketing with the opportunity to instantly purchase a product through a "click here to buy now" button presents an added risk to those in recovery.

IMPLICATIONS FOR ADDICTION MEDICINE

The addiction medicine community consists of a loose coalition of health practitioners, academics and government officials who deliver addiction services and study the causes and consequences of addiction. As discussed in this chapter, evidence and theory suggest that the alcohol industry can be considered an inducer of AUDs. This conclusion has important implications for clinical practice, research, training, policy development and ethical conduct in professional affairs.

There is a need for addiction medicine professionals to support effective, evidence-based practices in prevention, treatment and public policy, especially because these practices are often opposed by the alcohol industry. Children and adolescents, adults at risk for unhealthy drinking, and those with current or past history of unhealthy alcohol use (including those with AUD) need to be protected from alcohol industry practices that promote unhealthy use, including alcohol marketing. Current self-regulation codes, which rely on vague descriptions of nonpermissible content (eg, situations where people are drinking excessively), should be replaced by statutory regulations like those found in France's Loi Evin, which only permit product information instead of lifestyle advertising and images of social drinking that are likely to stimulate craving in persons with AUD. Targeting of individuals with heavy drinking (market segmentation) should be monitored and exposed. Evidence-based practices should be supported.

Public health policy derived from alcohol research has demonstrated the value of numerous policy options that can significantly reduce the burden of disease attributable to alcohol. The "Best Practices" demonstrated in a recent comprehensive review of the policy research literature[16] include measures that decrease the affordability of alcohol products, such as excise taxes, restrictions on the physical availability of alcohol, and total bans on alcohol marketing. In addition, a variety of "Good Practices" are recommended, including treatment services and drink-driving countermeasures. Other implications for policy can be inferred from the analysis of the four levels of the epidemiological cascade. To deal with the upstream causes of AUD at Levels 1 and 2 (government and industry), policies should address the source of the problems upstream (eg, availability, affordability, access, and promotion) and expose or limit the unethical activities of industry conduits in the host environment and political arena. At Level 4, improved access to effective individual-level interventions for unhealthy drinking are recommended.

Clinical, social and policy research is needed not only to conduct surveillance of industry activities that impact vulnerable groups, but also to provide better theoretical models. Research on the alcohol industry as an inducer of alcohol-related problems is needed to answer the following questions: Is the corporation-induced disease model a useful heuristic device? Does the model offer predictability, falsifiability and public verifiability? Is the epidemiological cascade a useful concept for studying mediators and moderators of alcohol-related problems and AUDs?

Beyond studies of the industry as an inducer, there is a need to improve the ethical training of scientists who are prone to become complicit in the industry's harmful activities by accepting funding from industry sources, or engaging in other activities that present potential COI, such as serving on industry-sponsored advisory committees or expert panels. The concept of corporate-induced disorders proposed in this chapter should be included in training programs for health professionals and in continuing education programs. The International Society of Addiction Journal Editors has published a review of useful prevention measures[48] that describe how to avoid COI and other threats to scientific integrity. The measures include online workshops on ethical decision-making, ethics-awareness exercises and COI guidelines developed by professional societies. The concept of corporate-induced disorders proposed in this chapter provides a clear rationale for the need to enhance ethical training programs for health professionals and scientific investigators that goes beyond the clinical ethics training that they are typically exposed to.

A considerable amount of marketing research is conducted for the alcohol industry by social scientists and contract research organizations. Scientists trained in or conversant with behavioral research methods have been involved in laboratory studies of taste and sensory preferences, public opinion surveys, marketing campaigns and program evaluations. In the case of tobacco, an analysis of previously secret internal industry documents revealed that research on sensory perception was used to inform product design for targeted segments of the cigarette market, including young adults.[49] There is evidence that the alcohol industry conducts similar research.[50] To the extent that this research requires the services of social and behavioral scientists, it may pose ethical problems because it could facilitate the marketing of products (eg, alcopops) that are misused by vulnerable populations. Acceptance of research funding from the alcohol industry not only has the potential for reputational damage, it may also affect the objectivity of independent scientists and contribute to the problems experienced by vulnerable populations.

For these reasons, professional associations have developed guidelines regarding the ethical behavior of acceptable funding bodies, competing or conflicting interests, and related issues. In one of the most thorough policy statements about competing interests, the International Network on Brief Interventions for Alcohol and Other Drugs (INEBRIA) issued a position statement that is summarized in **Box 8-2**.

BOX 8-2

SUMMARY OF THE INTERNATIONAL NETWORK ON BRIEF INTERVENTIONS FOR ALCOHOL AND OTHER DRUGS (INEBRIA) POSITION STATEMENT ON THE ALCOHOL INDUSTRY

1. The commercial activities of the alcohol industry pose a conflict-of-interest of such magnitude that any form of engagement may influence the independence, objectivity, integrity, and credibility of the person or organization involved with the alcohol industry.
2. All individuals wishing to present at an INEBRIA meeting are required to complete a conflict-of-interest declaration for the work being presented.
3. Members of the coordinating committee may not have worked with or received funding from the alcohol industry in the five years before their election date or during their term of office.

Adapted from International Network on Brief Interventions for Alcohol & Other Drugs (INEBRIA). *INEBRIA Position Statement on the Alcohol Industry.* n.d. https://inebria.net/wp-content/uploads/2016/02/position_statement_on_the_alcohol_industry.pdf

Addiction medicine professional organizations can best fulfill their public health responsibilities by avoiding direct partnerships with commercial or vested alcohol interest groups, and their representatives, especially in the development or implementation of alcohol policy. The addiction medicine community can also provide critical support for governments to implement evidence-based policies by avoiding funding from alcohol industry sources for prevention, research and information dissemination activities, refraining from any form of association with alcohol industry education programs and improving the dissemination of information for advocacy and policy development to combat the extensive lobbying power of the alcohol industry.

Finally, addiction scientists and addiction medicine professionals can become more active in public health advocacy through global health policy networks, which have been shown to be effective in addressing the global epidemic of tobacco-related disease through the WHO Framework Convention on Tobacco Control. Public health responses must be matched to alcohol's dual role as a commodity and as a drug. Population-level policies (universal interventions) should be considered, together with those directed at people with high-risk for unhealthy drinking (selective interventions) and those targeting individuals who have already developed alcohol-related dysfunction (targeted interventions). The responses need to reflect an improved understanding of the nature of an industry that can serve as an inducer of alcohol-related problems.

CONCLUSIONS

The major public health implications of the evidence reviewed in this chapter can be stated as follows. The dangers in alcohol use are multiple and varied in kind and degree; some, but not all, are dose-related; they may result directly from the effect of alcohol or through interaction with other factors; intoxication is often an important mediator of harm; and AUDs can significantly exacerbate the hazards and cause protracted exposure to danger. Alcohol's harm to others extends the damage caused by alcohol significantly beyond the harm done to the individual who consumes alcohol.

For these reasons, alcohol is not an ordinary commodity, even when it is used in moderation, because the risk of acute and chronic effects begins at low doses of alcohol. To focus on this level of the AUD problem (Level 4) is appropriate, but the upstream distal causes should not be ignored.

Global health is being threatened as never before by a coalition of transnational corporations capable of acting in concert to expand their operations into every corner of the world. Although the industry may appear to many as the friendly elephant always ready to promote "responsible drinking" and corporate philanthropy, their political strategies and business tactics suggest two less flattering animal analogies. One is the fox guarding the henhouse, as when the industry falsely claims its self-regulation guidelines are protecting young people from exposure to their sophisticated advertising. The other is the cash cow, ready to contribute to civil society organizations and health scientists to show they are good corporate citizens, even as they use their financial influence to undermine advocacy for effective policy and unbiased research.

REFERENCES

1. Saunders JB, Degenhardt L, Reed GM, Poznyak V. Alcohol use disorders in ICD-11: past, present, and future. *Alcohol Clin Exp Res.* 2019;43:1617-1631.
2. American Psychiatric Association. *Diagnostic and Statistical Manual of Mental Disorders.* 5th ed., text rev. ed. American Psychiatric Association Publishing; 2022.
3. PLoS Medicine Editors. Let's be straight up about the alcohol industry. *PLoS Med.* 2011;8(5):e1001041.
4. World Health Organization. *Global Status Report on Alcohol and Health 2018.* World Health Organization; 2018.
5. Oreskes N, Conway EM. *Merchants of Doubt: How a Handful of Scientists Obscured the Truth on Issues from Tobacco Smoke to Global Warming.* Bloomsbury Press; 2010.
6. Jernigan D, Ross C. The alcohol marketing landscape: alcohol industry size, structure, strategies, and public health responses. *J Stud Alcohol Drugs Suppl.* 2020;19(Suppl 19):13-25.
7. Jernigan DH, Babor TF. The concentration of the global alcohol industry and its penetration in the African region. *Addiction.* 2015;110(4):551-560. doi:10.1111/add.12468
8. Savell E, Gilmore AB, Fooks G. How does the tobacco industry attempt to influence marketing regulations? A systematic review. *PLoS One.* 2014;9(2):e87389.
9. Maani N, Petticrew M, Galea S, eds. *The Commercial Determinants of Health.* Oxford University Press; 2023.
10. Wood B, Baker P, Sacks G. Conceptualising the commercial determinants of health using a power lens: a review and synthesis of existing frameworks. *Int J Health Policy Manag.* 2022;11(8):1251-1261. doi:10.34172/ijhpm.2021.05
11. Kickbusch I. Addressing the interface of the political and commercial determinants of health. *Health Promot Int.* 2012;27(4):427-428. doi:10.1093/heapro/das057
12. Jahiel RI. Corporate-induced diseases, upstream epidemiologic surveillance, and urban health. *J Urban Health.* 2008;85(4):517-531.

13. Jahiel R, Babor TF. Industrial epidemics, public health advocacy and the alcohol industry: lessons from other fields. *Addiction.* 2007;102:1335-1339.
14. Babor TF, Robaina K. Public health, academic medicine, and the alcohol industry's corporate social responsibility activities. *Am J Public Health.* 2013;103:206-214.
15. Babor TF, Robaina K, Brown K, et al. Is the alcohol industry doing well by "doing good"? Findings from a content analysis of the Alcohol Industry's Actions to Reduce Harmful Drinking. *BMJ Open.* 2018;8:e024325. doi:10.1136/bmjopen-2018-024325
16. Babor T, Casswell S, Graham K, et al. *Alcohol: No Ordinary Commodity. Research and Public Policy*. 3rd ed. Oxford University Press; 2023.
17. Mitchell G, Lesch M, McCambridge J. Alcohol industry involvement in the moderate alcohol and cardiovascular health trial. *Am J Public Health.* 2020;110:485-488.
18. Babor, TF, Monteiro, M, Collin, J. Health taxes on unhealthy commodities: a political economy analysis. In: Lauer J, Sassi F, Soucat A, Vigo A, eds. *Health Taxes: A Policy and Practice Guide.* World Scientific Publishing; 2022:431-484.
19. Hastings G. "They'll drink bucket loads of the stuff": an analysis of internal alcohol industry advertising documents. *Alcohol and Education Research Council.* Accessed November 20, 2017. http://oro.open.ac.uk/22913/1/AERC_FinalReport_0060.pdf
20. Atkinson AM, Meadows BR, Emslie C, Lyons A, Sumnall HR. 'Pretty in Pink' and 'Girl Power': an analysis of the targeting and representation of women in alcohol brand marketing on Facebook and Instagram. *Int J Drug Policy.* 2021;101:103547.
21. Robaina K, Babor T, Pinksy I, Johns P. *The Alcohol Industry's Commercial and Political Activities in Latin America and the Caribbean: Implications for Public Health.* NCD Alliance, Global Alcohol Policy Alliance, Healthy Latin America Coalition, and Healthy Caribbean Coalition; 2020.
22. Stockwell T, Solomon R, O'Brien P, Vallance K, Hobin E. Cancer warning labels on alcohol containers: a consumer's right to know, a government's responsibility to inform, and an industry's power to thwart. *J Stud Alcohol Drugs.* 2020;81:284-292.
23. Noel JK, Babor TF, Robaina K, Feulner M, Vendrame A, Monteiro M. Alcohol marketing in the Americas and Spain during the 2014 FIFA World Cup Tournament. *Addiction.* 2017;112(Suppl 1):64-73. doi:10.1111/add.13487
24. Holder H. The state monopoly as a public policy approach to consumption and alcohol problems: a review of research evidence. *Contemporary Drug Problems.* 2003;293-322.
25. Abbey A, Scott RO, Smith MJ. Physical, subjective, and social availability: their relationship to alcohol consumption in rural and urban areas. *Addiction.* 1993;88:489-499.
26. Single E. The availability of alcohol: prior research and future directions. *Aust Drug Alcohol Rev.* 1988;7:273-284.
27. Babor TF, Robaina K, Noel J. *The Role of the Alcohol Industry in Policy Interventions for Alcohol-Impaired Driving. Appendix C in National Academies of Sciences, Engineering and Medicine. Getting to Zero Alcohol-Impaired Driving Fatalities. A Comprehensive Approach to a Persistent Problem. National Academies Press.* 2018;C1-C37.
28. McCambridge J, Hawkins B, Holden C. Industry use of evidence to influence alcohol policy: a case study of submissions to the 2008 Scottish government consultation. *PLoS Med.* 2013;10(4):e1001431.
29. Golder S, McCambridge J. Alcohol, cardiovascular disease and industry funding: a co-authorship network analysis of systematic reviews. *Soc Sci Med.* 2021;289:1144-1150.
30. Lange S, Probst C, Gmel G, Rehm J, Burd L, Popova S. Global prevalence of fetal alcohol spectrum disorder among children and youth: a systematic review and meta-analysis. *JAMA Pediatr.* 2017;171(10):948-956. doi:10.1001/jamapediatrics.2017.1919
31. Cherpitel CJ, Ye Y, Kerr WC. Risk of past year injury related to hours of exposure to an elevated Blood Alcohol Concentration and Average Monthly Alcohol Volume: Data from 4 National Alcohol Surveys (2000 to 2015). *Alcohol Clin Exp Res.* 2018;42(2):360-368.
32. Rehm J, Eschmann S. Global monitoring of average volume of alcohol consumption. *Soz Praventivmed.* 2020;47:48-58. doi:10.1007/BF01318406
33. Caetano R, Tam T, Greenfield T, Cherpitel C, Midanik L. DSM-IV alcohol dependence and drinking in the US population: a risk analysis. *Ann Epidemiol.* 1997;7:542-549.
34. Bhattacharya A, Angus C, Pryce R, Holmes J, Brennan A, Meier P. How dependent is the alcohol industry on heavy drinking in England? *Addiction.* 2018;113:2225-2232.
35. Sargent JD, Babor TF. The relationship between exposure to alcohol marketing and underage drinking is causal. *J Stud Alcohol Drugs Suppl.* 2020;(Suppl 19):113-124. doi:10.15288/jsads.2020.s19.113
36. Babor TF, Robaina K, Noel JK, Ritson EB. Vulnerability to alcohol-related problems: a policy brief with implications for the regulation of alcohol marketing. *Addiction.* 2017;112:94-101. doi:10.1111/add.13626
37. Bava S, Tapert SF. Adolescent brain development and the risk for alcohol and other drug problems. *Neuropsychol Rev.* 2010;20:398-413.
38. Institute of Medicine. *Food Marketing to Children and Youth: Threat or Opportunity?* The National Academies Press; 2004. Accessed August 9, 2023. https://www.nap.edu/catalog/11514/food-marketing-to-children-and-youth-threat-or-opportunity
39. Cannon MJ, Guo J, Denny CH, et al. Prevalence and characteristics of women at risk for an alcohol-exposed pregnancy (AEP) in the United States: estimates from the National Survey of Family Growth. *Matern Child Health J.* 2015;19(4):776-782.
40. Zheng YL, Lian F, Shi Q, et al. Alcohol intake and associated risk of major cardiovascular outcomes in women compared with men: a systematic review and meta-analysis of prospective observational studies. *BMC Public Health.* 2015;15:773.
41. Rehm J, Taylor B, Mohapatra S, et al. Alcohol as a risk factor for liver cirrhosis: a systematic review and meta-analysis. *Drug Alcohol Rev.* 2010;29:437-435.
42. Scoccianti C, Lauby-Secretan B, Bello PY, Chajes V, Romieu I. Female breast cancer and alcohol consumption: a review of the literature. *Am J Prevent Med.* 2014;46(3):S16-S25.
43. Zuccolo L, Lewis SJ, Smith GD, et al. Prenatal alcohol exposure and offspring cognition and school performance. A 'Mendelian randomization' natural experiment. *Int J Epidemiol.* 2013;42(5):1358-1370.
44. Atkinson AM, Sumnall H, Begley E, Jones L. *A Rapid Narrative Review of Literature on Gendered Alcohol Marketing and Its Effects: Exploring the Targeting and Representation of Women.* Public Health Institute, Liverpool John Moores University; 2019.
45. Litt MD, Cooney NL, Morse P. Reactivity to alcohol-related stimuli in the laboratory and in the field: predictors of craving in treated alcoholics. *Addiction.* 2000;95(6):889-900.
46. Thomson A, Bradley E, Casswell S. A qualitative investigation of the responses of in-treatment and recovering heavy drinkers to alcohol advertising on New Zealand television. *Contemp Drug Probl.* 1997;24(1):133-146.
47. Elvin S. Fears alcoholics are being 'bombarded' as they struggle to hide Instagram adverts. *Metro News.* Accessed August 9, 2023. https://metro.co.uk/2021/03/10/alcoholics-claim-they-are-struggling-to-hide-adverts-on-instagram-14208953/
48. Miller P, Babor TF, McGovern T, Obot I, Bühringer G. Relationships with the alcoholic-beverage industry, pharmaceutical companies, and other funding agencies: holy grail or poisoned chalice? In: Babor TF, Stenius K, Pates R, Miovský M, O'Reilly J, Candon P, eds. *Publishing Addiction Science: A Guide for the Perplexed.* Ubiquity Press; 2017:323-352.
49. Carpenter CM, Wayne GF, Connolly GN. Designing cigarettes for women: New findings from the tobacco industry documents. *Addiction.* 2005;100:837-851.
50. Babor TF. Alcohol research and the alcoholic beverage industry issues, concerns and conflicts of interest. *Addiction.* 2009;104:34-47.

CHAPTER

9

The Impact of the Cannabis Industry on Cannabis Use Disorder

David H. Jernigan, Jih-Cheng Yeh, Connor Kubeisy, and Kevin A. Sabet

CHAPTER OUTLINE

- Cannabis use and disorder trends in the United States
- Cannabis marketing and cannabis use

As of 2022, both cannabis use and the nature and structure of the cannabis industry are rapidly changing in the United States. This chapter will review current trends in cannabis use and cannabis use disorder (CUD), among both youth and adults, as a backdrop to a description of the U.S. cannabis market and industry, and an exploration of how the evolution of these two is affecting and is likely to affect CUD, through the vectors of product development and proliferation, advertising and marketing, pricing, physical availability, and the changing regulatory landscape at the state and federal levels. We will conclude by providing some specific recommendations for how to mitigate possible negative effects of these trends. Note: Throughout this chapter, we use the term "cannabis" to refer to the psychoactive components of the cannabis plant, specifically those above 0.3% THC (tetrahydrocannabinol) (ie, not hemp).

CANNABIS USE AND DISORDER TRENDS IN THE UNITED STATES

National

Between 2002 and 2012, the year Colorado became the first state to legalize cannabis for adult non–medical use, the number of individuals who used cannabis in the past year increased from approximately 25.75 to 31.53 million, a 22.4% increase.[1,2] By 2020, the number of individuals with past-year use had reached 49.63 million, a 57.4% increase since 2012 and a 92.7% increase since 2002.[2]

Beyond these numerical increases, those who use cannabis are now using the drug more frequently. According to the National Survey on Drug Use and Health (NSDUH), in 2002 there were 14.58 million individuals with past-month use, representing 56.6% of those with past-year use.[1] However, this increased to 32.78 million by 2020, accounting for 66.0% of those with past-year use.[3] This shift suggests that many individuals who use cannabis infrequently—such as those who might have used it once or twice each year at a party—now use it semiregularly throughout the year. Moreover, the use category increasing most quickly is daily use: in 2002, there were 4.76 million individuals with daily or almost daily use, accounting for approximately 18.5% of those with past-year use.[1] This number grew to 7.60 million in 2012, representing 24.1% of those with past-year use.[4] By 2020, 15.06 million individuals reported daily cannabis use, or 30.3% of those who used cannabis in the past year.[3]

Viewed in terms of percentages, in 2020, 45.7% of the U.S. population aged 12 and older reported having used cannabis in their lifetime (compared to 40.4% in 2002), 17.9% used it in the past year (up from 11.0% in 2002), 11.8% used in the past month (an increase from 6.2% in 2002), and 4.0% used it daily (up from 1.3% in 2002).[1,3,5] More people are using cannabis, and they are using it more frequently.

Figure 9-1 shows the distribution of past 30-day and daily consumption by age, according to the National Institute on Drug Abuse's Monitoring the Future (MTF) survey.[6] As the figure makes clear, use peaks in the young adult years, and declines significantly after age 30. Because earlier and heavier use has implications for the development of CUD, we will return to this below.

Young People

The rise in cannabis use seems to have been driven primarily by growth in numbers and frequency among those age 26 or older who use; in fact, use among 12- to 17-year-olds appears to have fallen slightly between 2017 and 2020, although a change in survey methods in 2020 precludes making more definitive statements.[5] Still, youth consumption is substantial. According to NSDUH, 16.9% of 12- to 20-year-olds used cannabis in 2020, varying from 1.3% of 12- to 13-year-olds to 30.5% of 18- to 20-year-olds—nearly one in three 18- to 20-year-olds used cannabis in the past year. Regarding past-month use, 0.4% of 12- to 13-year-olds fell into this category, compared to 19.9% of 18- to 20-year-olds.[3] Looking at the period from 2002 to 2020, it is apparent that older young people and young adults—specifically, 18- to 25-year-olds—are driving the increase in daily use among youth: while there has been little change in daily use among 12- to 17-year-olds or 12- to 20-year-olds during this period, daily or almost daily use among 18- to 25-year-olds nearly doubled, from 4.3% in 2002 to 7.8% in 2020.[3]

Young people are at the forefront of changes in the form of delivery of cannabis as a drug. An analysis of 3 years of data on use by young people from MTF from 2017 to 2019 concluded that vaping (ie, inhaling what is more accurately termed an aerosol) was increasingly the most popular form of cannabis delivery among young people, and that frequent use (six or more times per month) was rising faster than occasional use.[7] Young people can use vapes more discreetly, in locations such as school bathrooms, and vapes are often more potent than smoked cannabis. When MTF first asked

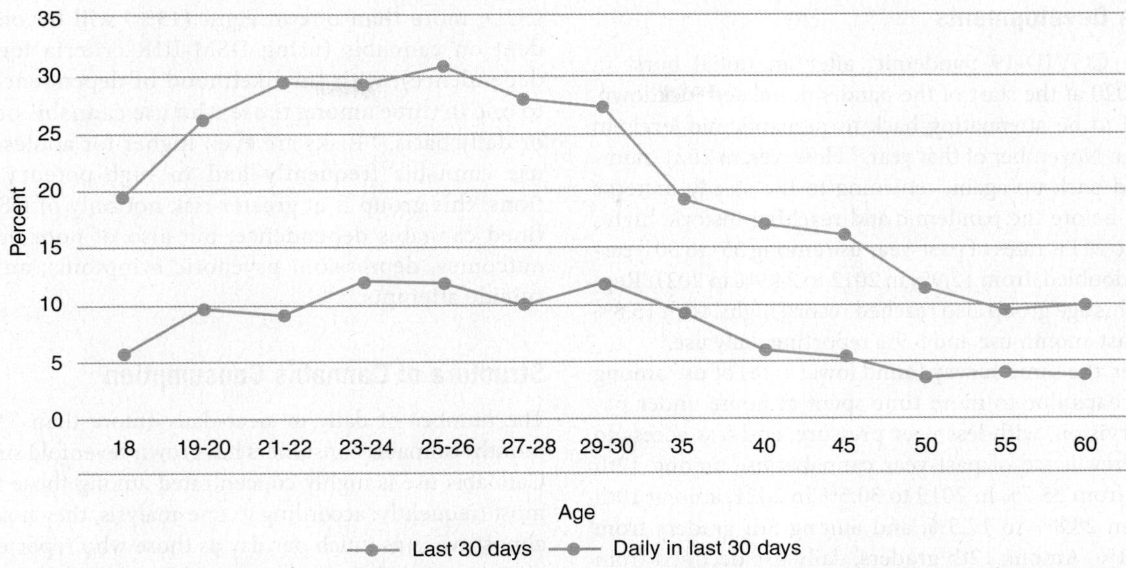

Figure 9-1. Cannabis use among 12- to 60-year-olds, 2021. (Adapted from Patrick ME, Schulenberg JE, Miech RA, Johnston LD, O'Malley PM, Bachman JG. *Monitoring the Future Panel Study Annual Report: National Data on Substance Use Among Adults Ages 19 to 60, 1976–2021*. University of Michigan Institute for Social Research; 2022.)

young people about their use of cannabis vapes in 2017, 9.5% of 12th graders indicated that they had used one in the past year. This number more than doubled to 20.8% in 2019 and 22.1% in 2020.[8] A 2021 meta-analysis of 17 studies about adolescent use of cannabis vapes published in *JAMA Pediatrics* found that lifetime prevalence doubled from 2013 to 2020 (6.1%-13.6%), use in the past year nearly doubled from 2017 to 2020 (7.2%-13.2%), and 30-day prevalence of cannabis vaping was five times as high in 2020 as in 2013 (1.6%-8.4%).[9]

Racial Differences

Rates of cannabis use are not equal across racial groups. In 2020, 6.7% of Native Hawaiian or Pacific Islanders (NHOPI), 7.5% of Asians, 15.3% of Hispanics or Latinx, 19.2% of Whites, 19.4% of Blacks, 26.3% of American Indians and Alaska Natives (AIAN), and 27.8% of people who are of two or more races used cannabis in the past year. Regarding past-month use, 4.0% of NHOPI, 4.0% of Asians, 9.6% of Hispanics or Latinx, 12.5% of Whites, 14.2% of Blacks, and 19.3% of people of two or more races reported this. As a study in *JAMA Network Open* concluded, "higher-frequency cannabis use is more common among young and racial minority populations, as well as respondents with low socioeconomic status."[10]

Gender

The same national surveys find that males are slightly more likely than females to use cannabis: as of 2020, 48.0% of males had used cannabis at some point in their lifetime, compared to 43.5% of females. In 2020, 19.9% of males reported use in the past year, compared to 16.0% of females, and 13.3% of males reported use in the past month, compared to 10.4% of females.[3] In general, males are more likely to use joints, vapes, and concentrates; females are more likely to use pipes and take the drug orally.[11] Males also tend to use products with higher potency.[12] As one study concluded, "Men and boys tend to have greater prevalence of cannabis use, initiate earlier and use cannabis more frequently; and being male has been identified as one of the greatest risk factors for developing CUD."[13]

Additional Groups

Rates of use among lesbian, gay, bisexual, transgender, queer, and/or questioning (LGBTQ+) individuals are well above the national average. In 2019, 43.6% of LGBTQ+ individuals over the age of 18 reported use in the past year, up from 37.6% in 2018 and more than twice the national average of 18.0% of the general population over the age of 18. Between 2016 and 2019, rates of past-month use among 18- to 25-year-old LGBTQ+ individuals grew from 30.5% to 35.6%. Over that same time period, among individuals older than 26, past-month rates of use increased from 17.8% to 29.7%. In 2019, 9.3% of LGBTQ+ individuals over the age of 18 had CUD, compared to 7.6% in 2016.[14]

There has also been an increase in the rates of use among pregnant people. In 2020, 8.0% of pregnant people reported past-month use of cannabis, up from 5.4% in 2019 and 4.7% in 2018.[15] In 2019, 9.1% of pregnant people used cannabis in the first trimester, compared to 4.4% in the second trimester and 3.3% in the third trimester. This is a concern because, as the Substance Abuse and Mental Health Services Administration (SAMHSA) has summarized findings of the available literature, "[cannabis] use during pregnancy can be harmful to a [fetus'] health and cause many serious problems, including stillbirth, preterm birth, and growth and development issues."[16]

COVID-Era Developments

During the COVID-19 pandemic, after an initial burst in March of 2020 at the start of the pandemic-related lockdown, use seemed to be attenuating back to prepandemic levels in June through November of that year.[17] However, in 2021, numbers jumped back up again, returning to the steady increase in evidence before the pandemic and reaching historic highs. According to MTF, rates of past-year use among 35- to 50-year-olds nearly doubled, from 12.9% in 2012 to 24.9% in 2021. Regular use in this age group also reached record highs, with 15.8% reporting past-month use and 5.9% reporting daily use.[6]

However, the same survey found lower rates of use among minors, perhaps due to more time spent at home under parental supervision, with less peer pressure, and less access to the drug. Prevalence of past-year cannabis use among 12th graders fell from 35.7% in 2019 to 30.5% in 2021, among 10th graders from 28.8% to 17.3%, and among 8th graders from 11.8% to 7.1%. Among 12th graders, daily use declined from 6.4% in 2019 to 5.8% in 2021; the analogous decline among 10th graders was from 4.8% to 3.2%, and from 1.3% to 0.6% among 8th graders.[8]

Trends in Prevalence of Cannabis Use Disorder

Critical to understanding the impact of this industry on CUD is comprehending current trends in the prevalence of CUD among youth and adults. The American Psychiatric Association (APA) defines CUD as a problematic pattern of cannabis use leading to clinically significant personal, social, physical, and/or psychological distress or impairment.

Based on the fifth edition of the *Diagnostic and Statistical Manual of Mental Disorders* (DSM-V), the 11 diagnostic criteria for CUD identified by the APA include taking cannabis in larger amounts or over a longer period than intended, having a persistent desire or unsuccessful efforts to cut down or control cannabis use, spending a great deal of time obtaining or using cannabis, or recovering from its effects, craving or having a strong desire or urge to use cannabis, repeatedly having cannabis use lead to failure in fulfilling major school, work or home obligations, continuing to use cannabis despite persistent or recurrent social or interpersonal problems caused or made worse by it, reducing important social, occupational or recreational activities because of cannabis use, repeatedly using cannabis in physically hazardous situations, continuing to use cannabis despite knowing that one has a physical or psychological problem related to cannabis use, tolerance, that is, needing more cannabis to become intoxicated, or getting less effect from continued use of the same amount of cannabis, and symptoms of withdrawal from cannabis. The greater the number of criteria met, the more severe the CUD.[18]

According to NSDUH, in 2020 14.2 million people met the criteria for CUD, including 1 million 12- to 17-year-olds and 4.9 million 18- to 25-year-olds.[3] More than one in five (22%) individuals who use cannabis will develop a CUD; more than one in eight (13%) will become dependent on cannabis (using DSM-IIIR criteria for cannabis dependence), with the likelihood of dependence growing to one in three among those who use cannabis on a weekly or daily basis.[19] Risks are even higher for adolescents who use cannabis frequently and in high-potency formulations: this group is at greater risk not only of DSM-IV defined cannabis dependence, but also of poor educational outcomes, depression, psychotic symptoms, anxiety, and suicide attempts.[20,21]

Structure of Cannabis Consumption

The number of daily or near-daily (more than 21 days per month) cannabis consumers has grown sevenfold since 1992.[22] Cannabis use is highly concentrated among those who use it most frequently: according to one analysis, they not only used almost twice as much per day as those who reported less frequent use, but they also accounted for 80% of all consumption and 71% of the days of use.[23] NSDUH reports this group as comprising 4% of the population. This suggests that cannabis consumption is even more concentrated in a small segment of the population than alcohol use, where the top-consuming 10% of the population accounts for 56.5% of the total alcohol consumed.[24]

Product Development and Vulnerability to CUD

The cannabis industry's role in CUD begins with catering to this group of individuals, their best customers. The industry has developed product offerings with higher potencies that place individuals who use at an increased risk of developing a CUD. Product offerings include dried cannabis flower (the type used in joints), edibles (drinks and foods), concentrates (vapes and oils), and infused non-edible products (like lotions and bath salts). Many individuals now favor stronger—and trendier—products: in 2014, in Colorado, flower accounted for 66.5% of sales in the recreational market. Edibles and concentrates accounted for 14.6% and 11.4%, respectively. By 2019, the market share of flower decreased to 46.8%, while the share for edibles more than doubled to 32.4% and concentrates rose to 13.2%.[25]

If these trends hold, the structure of consumption will continue to shift from flower toward edibles and concentrates, representing a shift from low- to high-potency products. As individuals who use cannabis move to more potent products, the products themselves are becoming more potent. Since 1995, there has been a consistent rise in the average THC potency of flower nationwide, quadrupling from 3.75% to more than 15%. The percentage of samples above 12% THC increased from 1.1% to 70.3%.[26] Between 2014 and 2020, the average potency of joints in Colorado increased from 14% to 19.2%. The potency of concentrates in Colorado increased from 46.4% to 67.8%.[25,27] In its report on THC concentration, Colorado's Department of Public Health & Environment concluded that "almost all retail [cannabis] products contain high THC concentration."[28]

In this case, the "market" drives even those who use casually to higher-potency products, use of which has in turn been associated with four times greater odds of developing use resulting in problems.[29]

The development of tolerance is a key factor driving this trend toward the development of ever-stronger products in mature markets. Individuals who use for the first time may find a 5% THC joint brings them a sufficient level of intoxication, but this may have a negligible effect among those who use cannabis for much of their lifetimes. To counteract their tolerance, the latter will look to use stronger products more frequently. Stronger products come in the form of vapes and concentrates, instead of traditional joints. A 2017 survey of 2,400 adults, evenly split between those who used cannabis and those who did not, incorporated discrete choice experiments to demonstrate that both groups preferred higher-potency products, specifically choosing 20% and 30% THC over 15% THC products.[30] Far from improving population health, the industry is in what one group of researchers described as "a race to sell higher-potency" products[31] to differentiate themselves from their numerous competitors.

Complement or Substitute for Other Drug Use?

While alcohol continues to be the most popular intoxicant among both adults and youth in the United States,[5] the future of cannabis use depends at least in part on whether it complements or substitutes for alcohol use. Supporters of legalization argued cannabis could be a risk-reducing alternative to alcohol, while opponents worried that cannabis use might lead to a progression of alcohol use. However, there have been mixed results. The legalization of recreational cannabis was associated with a 13% decrease in purchases of alcohol products in Colorado but a 24% increase in purchases of spirits in Washington, with researchers concluding "alcohol and cannabis are not clearly substitutes nor complements to one-another."[32] The most recent systematic review of 95 studies found multiple mechanisms that condition the relationship between cannabis and alcohol use, including individual patterns of co-use, the context in which co-use occurs, sequencing of use, the formulation of cannabis being used, and pharmacokinetic interactions, as well as particular characteristics of users themselves.[33] This question becomes ever more complex as the cannabis industry itself grows and innovates.

Similarly, some wondered how the legalization of cannabis would influence tobacco use, which has trended downward. Evidence that these two are complements is more conclusive, a relationship that can make the cessation of either product more difficult.[34] Researchers have found a six times higher prevalence of daily cannabis use among individuals who smoke tobacco daily, and a 3.5 times higher prevalence among those who do not smoke tobacco daily, compared to individuals who do not smoke tobacco at all.[35] Among young adults who smoked at least one cigarette in the past month, 53% also used cannabis in the last 30 days, and co-used on 45% of the days they used either substance.[36] Researchers have found that people who use both cannabis and tobacco are more likely to report heavier use of each, as well as higher numbers of problematic behaviors.[37]

Although few experts continue to subscribe to the idea that cannabis is a gateway drug—the view that using cannabis leads to the use of stronger, more lethal drugs—many agree that cannabis use is associated with the use of other drugs. According to the NSDUH, individuals who use cannabis daily were more than five times as likely to have misused opioids in the past year, compared to those who did not use cannabis (11.9% versus 2.1%).[38] Individuals with daily use were nearly five times as likely to have had "heavy alcohol use" in the past month, compared to those who did not use cannabis (17.8% versus 4.8%).[38] They were also 48 times as likely to have used cocaine (14.4% versus 0.3%) and 25 times as likely to have used methamphetamine in the past year (5.0% versus 0.2%).[38] Additionally, 48.9% of those who misused opioids in the past year used cannabis, compared to 16.8% who did not. Of those with past-month "heavy alcohol use," 47.6% also used cannabis, compared to 9.2% who did not. And 78.3% of individuals who used methamphetamines in the past year also used cannabis, compared to 17.4% who did not.[38]

Data from SAMHSA's Drug Abuse Warning Network, which tracks drug-related emergency department visits, further confirm the polysubstance use tendencies of cannabis consumers. In 2021, cannabis was the most common substance in polysubstance alcohol-related ED visits, in 30.60% of visits, and the second most common drug in polysubstance methamphetamine-related ED visits, in 23.94% of visits. It was also the second most common drug in polysubstance cocaine-related ED visits, in 28.62% of visits. Alcohol was in 52.74% of polysubstance cannabis-related ED visits; methamphetamine was in 31.04%; cocaine was in 25.08%; fentanyl was in 7.21%; and amphetamine was in 5.51%. Approximately 63.5% of the nearly 800,000 cannabis-related ED visits in 2021 involved additional substances.[39]

Cannabis Use and Mental Illness

The relationship between mental illness and substance use is bidirectional: substance use can lead to and worsen mental health outcomes, and mental illness can be a precursor to substance use.[40] According to NSDUH, individuals with past-year cannabis use over the age of 18 were more than twice as likely to have experienced a "major depressive episode" (18.0% versus 7.3%) and nearly three times as likely to have had a "serious mental illness" (12.0% versus 4.2%).[38] This phenomenon is sometimes referred to as "self-medication," but if so it is not only occurring without medical supervision, but also is extremely difficult to do with any accuracy given the rapidly changing potency of cannabis products and the resulting difficulties users experience in titrating dosages. This phenomenon also implies that the development of a CUD may be an indicator of other disorders related both to substance use and to mental health.

CANNABIS MARKETING AND CANNABIS USE

Clearly, cannabis use is rising in the United States, while the bulk of it remains concentrated in a small population at high risk of CUD. Key to understanding vulnerability to CUD is examining how the cannabis industry is responding to this current state of the cannabis market. The most important change in this market of course is legalization, but how legalization is structured can have important ramifications for the likelihood of increased prevalence of CUD. "Cannabis used as treatment" (CUAT) is the preferred (more precise, less stigmatizing) terminology over the term "medical marijuana" (see Chapter 2). While there are a range of options available to states in decriminalizing or legalizing the adult non–CUAT use of cannabis, from solely decriminalizing to cannabis social clubs (cooperatives with limited membership that produce solely for their own members, which is one of the options available to Uruguayans) to state monopolies as occur in some states regarding alcohol, to date, U.S. states have all chosen a single structure, a licensed private commercial industry.[41] In doing so, they have granted permission to the cannabis industry to market its products in ways that were not possible when the product was illegal. This entails using all the different tools of marketing—from pricing to product innovation to promotion and placement—to increase the consumption of their products.

Because these activities aim at increasing cannabis consumption, if cannabis use spreads in the population but continues to concentrate among those with the heaviest use, and if approximately one in five people who use cannabis will develop CUD, then increasing use will drive up the prevalence of CUD. Furthermore, if regulatory structures permit entry into the cannabis market of large corporations with deep pockets and long experience in consumer marketing, these structures will also facilitate greater expenditures on marketing. As is the case in alcohol, marketing spending and industry concentration are a positive feedback loop: the more the largest players can spend, the more their spending becomes a barrier to entry into the marketplace for newer and smaller firms, driving concentration of the industry into a smaller number of companies, which are then able to extract oligopoly "rents" from a less competitive marketplace, which in turn give them more money to spend on marketing.[42]

The Size and Structure of the Cannabis Market

This drive toward concentration appears already to be happening. Cannabis is a global industry, but most of the legal business is still in North America. The value of the total global legal and illicit cannabis market stood at $150 billion in 2019,[43] the last year for which we were able to obtain data, with legal (CUAT and non–CUAT) accounting only for a 10th of that ($14.9 billion). Of this, there were $12.4 billion in legal sales in the United States alone.[44] However, Euromonitor, our source for these figures and projections, anticipates that the share of the global market of legal cannabis will grow to 77% of total cannabis sales by 2025, or $166 billion, if the U.S. legalizes cannabis for adult non–medical use at the federal level.[43]

The United States is the largest market in the world, with Euromonitor estimating it will grow to $60 billion in 2025. While much of the growth of the legal cannabis market will come from the conversion of illicit sales to legal ones, there will also likely be new consumers, as well as new product types, as described above.[43]

Unlike alcohol in the United States, there are no limits on vertical integration in the legal cannabis industry, and thus different sectors in the cannabis market are interconnected and influence each other. These sectors range from small, home-based facilities to expansive, extended farms, to companies that provide unique equipment or specific extraction services, to versatile companies offering several different products, brands, and services. At the center of the industry are cannabis cultivation and production companies. Their operations require appropriate indoor facilities or space for outdoor growing, as well as related products such as watering or light supplies, nutrients, and other accessories needed for the cultivation and care of the cannabis plants. With the legalization of cannabis in Canada and in more states in the United States, the overall industry has evolved into a multi-billion-dollar market. Based on companies' revenue analysis, the global market for cannabis agriculture and cultivation was estimated to be worth approximately $1.5 billion in 2019. This sector is expected to triple to $4.5 billion by 2024.[45]

Table 9-1 shows the top 10 companies involved in the cultivation and growth of cannabis for recreational or medicinal purposes by market capitalization[46] as of 2019, the last year for which figures were available.

The market saw increasing consolidation in 2018-2019 with several mergers between cannabis producers, most notably Aurora's acquisition of MedReleaf and Tilray's acquisition of Natura Naturals, both aimed at increasing overall production capacity for their respective parent companies. **Table 9-2** lists the leading global cannabis producers by

TABLE 9-1 Leading Cannabis Production Companies by Market Cap (2019)

Company	Headquarters	Market cap (billions USD)
Trulieve Cannabis	USA	$4.33
Curaleaf	USA	$4.29
Green Thumb Industries	USA	$2.62
Tilray	Canada	$2.33
Verano Holdings	USA	$1.66
Canopy Growth	Canada	$1.58
Cronos Group	Canada	$1.19
Cresco Labs	USA	$1.03
Sundial Growers	Canada	$0.71
Columbia Care	USA	$0.65

TABLE 9-2 Leading Cannabis Producers by Estimated Production Capacity, 2018

Company	Headquarters	Production (kg)	Notes
Aurora Cannabis	Canada	150,000	GBO of CanniMed and MedReleaf. 17.6% stake in Green Organic Dutchman
Tilray	Canada	90,000	GBO of Natura Naturals (2019)
Canopy Growth Corp	Canada	>70,000[a]	Extraction, retail, online (Tweed), pet care (CannaPet), sleep aids. Constellation has 38% stake
Cronos Group	Canada	40,000	Medical, GBO of Peace Naturals, Original BC. Altria has 45% stake
OrganicGram	Canada	36,000	Financial services provider
Aphria	Canada	35,000	Extraction, GBO of Nuuvera
Hexo Corp	Canada	25,000	Hydropothecary = medical; HEXO = recreational
CannTrust	Canada	15,000	
Green Organic Dutchman	Canada	14,000	
Emerald Health	Canada	13,000[a]	Cannabis used as treatment

Note: All production figures estimated based on company information to January 2019, excludes funded capacity potential; market capitalization figures sourced January 2019.

[a]Minimum Canadian supply commitment.

GBO, Global Brand Owner (ie, ultimate owner of the brand).

From Euromonitor. *Cannabis Market Disruptor Handbook Part 1: An Introduction.* 2019.

estimated production capacity[43] in 2018. Note that Aphria merged with Tilray in 2021—this is not reflected in the table.

Other industries adept at marketing addictive and/or intoxicating products have also been increasing their activity regarding cannabis. Recent acquisitions include tobacco giant Altria's purchase of a 45% stake in Cronos; they are competing with alcohol companies such as U.S.-based Constellation Brands with its 38% share in Canadian cannabis producer Canopy Growth, and Heineken, which in 2015 acquired Lagunitas. That company has launched hops-flavored sparkling water Hi-Fi Hops in a cannabidiol (CBD)/THC combo and 10 mg THC-only version, as well as cannabis-infused beers. In summer 2018, Lagunitas introduced IPA SuperCritical (6.8% ABV) made with cannabis terpenes (by CannaCraft's AbsoluteXtracts) in tandem with SuperCritical vape oils, combining cannabis with hops. Terpenes (the essential oils in cannabis, shared also with hops) have also been used in spirits such as The Myrcene Hemp Gin by The CannaCo.

After the plant is grown, there is further distribution and retail of cannabis and cannabis-infused products into dispensaries. There is a specific sector in the cannabis industry that deals with the processing and packaging of the plant into related products. Dispensaries provide cannabis for recreational as well as treatment purposes. In addition, the cannabis plant can be processed to obtain extracts or concentrates that are further developed into other cannabis-containing products. This has created another sector in the cannabis industry that provides either equipment or extraction services. Since cannabis is consumed internally, its extracts and products need to be tested analytically to be compliant with the law. Therefore, the cannabis industry has a specific sector that provides analytical testing equipment or services.

Because there are no limits on vertical integration in the U.S. cannabis industry, some of the largest producers are also the largest sellers of cannabis. Curaleaf operates 101 dispensaries in 23 states. Truelieve has 80 dispensaries, and dominates its home market, Florida, with more than 50% of sales in that state coming from its stores. Green Thumb Industries controls RISE, a retail chain with 54 dispensaries spread from coast to coast.[47]

Impact of Advertising and Marketing

This integration among tiers of the industry creates economic efficiencies that further drive profitability, which in turn feeds the concentration of ownership in the market. As outlined above, marketing spending plays a key role in erecting and maintaining barriers to entry into the marketplace. Cannabis marketers are significant spenders. The website dashtwo.com quoted estimates from Kantar Media of $2.26 billion in cannabis marketing spending in the United States in 2019, including $719.4 million on newspapers, $370.2 million on internet display ads, $213.6 million on spot (local) television, $190.2 million on cable television, and $110 million on out-of-home ad placements (primarily billboards and bus shelters).[48]

What is the impact of all this marketing spending, in particular on the development of CUD? Most research on the effects of similar advertising, such as with tobacco or alcohol, focuses on young people. From the perspective of CUD, this population matters, since CUD appears to develop much more quickly among young people than among emerging adults,[49] putting teens who use cannabis at nearly four times the odds of having a CUD as older individuals with recent onset cannabis use between the ages 22 and 26.[50] Multiple systematic reviews of the effect of alcohol marketing on young people have found that, in longitudinal studies, advertising exposure is associated with a greater likelihood of drinking and progression to heavier drinking over time.[51,52] A recent review of this literature used the Bradford Hill criteria for causality to conclude that exposure to alcohol marketing played a causal role in subsequent youth drinking behavior.[53]

There have been similar findings for youth exposure to electronic drug delivery devices (EDDDs) (such as e-cigarettes) marketing: a systematic review of 124 studies concluded that EDDD marketing content was attractive to youth, and that adolescents and young adults exposed to the adverts were more likely to try EDDDs.[54] One study, of college students in Texas, connected EDDD advertising to a greater likelihood of using cannabis in those devices one year later.[55]

The impact of exposure to cannabis marketing on young people's likelihood of using cannabis and of developing CUD is a small but developing literature. Cross-sectional studies have consistently found associations between youth exposure to cannabis marketing and youth use.[56,57] One such study extended the analysis from use to development of CUD: in a survey in 2018 of 15- to 19-year-olds in states where cannabis had been legalized for adult non–CUAT use, 90% reported having been exposed to some kind of cannabis advert or promotion, and one-third had interacted with the marketing. This interaction was associated with a five times greater likelihood of having used cannabis in the past year, compared with young people who were not engaging, while those who reported having a favorite cannabis brand were eight times as likely to have used cannabis in the past year.[58] Exposure to particular types of advertising was also associated with the development of CUD: adolescents who reported exposure to billboards advertising cannabis had five times the odds of CUD even if that exposure was described as rarely or sometimes; with self-reported exposure most or all of the time, there was sixfold greater odds of CUD. Ownership of cannabis-branded merchandise was associated with three times the odds of CUD.[59]

However, cross-sectional studies cannot differentiate between whether individuals with heavier use were more likely to notice and engage with the marketing, or whether the marketing led to heavier use and/or CUD. Only one study has used a longitudinal design to assess the impact of youth exposure on cannabis use over time. Researchers interviewed middle school-age students from Southern California in 2010-2011, when only CUAT was legally allowed. Nearly a quarter of respondents at baseline (22%) and nearly a third of respondents at 1-year follow-up (30%) reported seeing a CUAT advertisement in the prior 3 months; those who had seen the ads were twice as likely at follow-up to say they intended to use cannabis during the next year.[60] Follow-up 6 years later revealed that students who reported above-average exposure to the CUAT ads in 2010-2011 were using cannabis. The researchers interviewed the students again in 2017 and found that those with higher-than-average exposure to CUAT ads in 2010-2011 reported more frequent cannabis use and more negative consequences, including trouble concentrating, or missing or getting in trouble at school, from use at follow-up.[61]

Impact of Exposure to Outlets/Dispensaries

Exposure to street-level cannabis marketing, through signage on dispensaries, was also associated cross-sectionally with increased past-month use and a four-to-six times larger effect on the number of times used during a day and positive expectancies about cannabis use, among 18- to 22-year-olds in Los Angeles County who lived near higher numbers of dispensaries for medical cannabis.[62] This exposure may be one mechanism that accounts for why research has found that higher percentages of young people living in areas with higher densities of cannabis outlets use cannabis, compared to their peers in neighborhoods with fewer outlets.[63] Higher density of outlets, whether licensed or unlicensed, within a four-mile radius of a young adult's home was associated with heavy cannabis use and CUD, according to a study in Los Angeles County that surveyed young adult use at two points in time that bracketed the opening of licensed recreational outlets in California.[64]

These findings have significant equity implications. Multiple studies have found that cannabis retail outlets are concentrated in communities of color and low-income neighborhoods. For instance, in the medical cannabis era in California, a statewide analysis found cannabis outlets clustered in block groups with greater cannabis demand but also higher poverty rates and numbers of alcohol outlets.[65] As cannabis laws evolved in California, Los Angeles attempted to limit the location and density of CUAT cannabis dispensaries. Analysis of dispensary locations before and after the enactment of these limits found the new restrictions left the total number of dispensaries unchanged, but the remaining dispensaries were more likely to be in areas with greater proportions of African American residents.[66] Mapping by a cannabis business site of retail cannabis stores in Seattle and Denver in 2017 found 40% of Seattle and 45% of Denver dispensaries were located in poor neighborhoods, that is, neighborhoods where average earnings were in the bottom 25th percentile.[67] This concentration of cannabis outlets in communities of color and low-income areas likely concentrates the health-related harms of use, which perpetuate preexisting health disparities. These communities often lack the resources to oppose the opening of dispensaries; the result, ironically, is a worsening of racial and economic inequities, which proponents of cannabis legalization often claim that legalization will ameliorate.[68]

Additionally, the industry is actively introducing initiatives to reach customers who do not live near a dispensary. For instance, companies now deliver purchased products to a customer's house. Kiosks are also being tested, which would allow cannabis products to be sold wherever vending machines can be placed. The industry is also working to open consumption lounges, which would allow individuals to smoke cannabis indoors, in settings comparable to hookah lounges.

Pricing

In the wake of legalization, product innovation, the decline of flower as the leading form of cannabis consumed, and the lack of meaningful government intervention are producing trends in the pricing of cannabis that are also putting individuals who use at greater risk of CUD. Prices postlegalization have tended to decline, and contrary to expectations, this decline has continued recently even as inflation has spiked and driven the prices of other quantities higher.[69] The rising dominance in the market of a variety of nonflower formulations such as concentrates and edibles permits more convenient ingestion of cannabis, facilitating more discrete as well as on-the-go consumption of products with significantly higher concentrations of THC. The industry offers these at prices "per dose" that are comparable to those of flower, particularly if, as in the case of edibles, price per dose is adjusted to account for the greater effectiveness in delivering THC compared to smoking or vaporization.[70]

The price of cannabis, often defined by the price per gram of cannabis or the price per dose, influences the consumption patterns of individuals who currently use or may potentially use cannabis. Assuming this is an ordinary commodity in an economic sense, as the price of cannabis declines, more individuals may be expected to use it and individuals with prior use may be expected to consume more, following the consumption patterns of other products. Conversely, as the price of cannabis increases, usage rates may be expected to decline. A 2014 research review of evidence regarding cannabis pricing concluded that a 10% drop in the price of cannabis would lead to a 3% to 5% increase in the number of young people who will use for the first time.[71] Analysis of cannabis use among Australian youth reached a similar conclusion, that is, that lower prices would be associated with a greater likelihood of initiating at younger ages.[72]

As the cannabis market has matured in states where it is legal, the industry has been able to take advantage of innovation, streamlining and economies of scale in production, driving prices down. In Colorado, for example, where data are readily available, the price per gram of flower decreased from slightly above $14 in 2014 to an average of $4.80 in 2020, and the price per gram of concentrate decreased from a high of approximately $47 in 2014 to $16.55 in 2020. Thus the price per dose of cannabis—defined by Colorado regulators as 57.1 mg of inhaled THC or 10.0 mg of ingested THC—has fallen substantially.[27]

Current pricing in the cannabis marketplace thus encourages individuals to use products that are more convenient and deliver THC in higher concentrations, putting those who use at greater risk of heavy use. The obvious government intervention to prevent this would be to tax cannabis products by potency, but as of 2020, just one state—Illinois—was doing this.[41]

Stakeholder Marketing (Lobbying)

Another form of industry marketing activity has played a critical role in the evolution of cannabis consumption: marketing to key stakeholders such as state and federal policymakers. After Colorado and Washington voted to legalize cannabis in 2012, the U.S. Department of Justice issued the "Cole Memorandum,"[73] which signaled that the federal government would not enforce federal prohibition laws against states that legalized cannabis. This effectively cleared the way for states to begin commercializing this Schedule 1 drug, as well as other state-level initiatives to liberalize additional Schedule 1 drugs.

In response to this sea change in the legal landscape, as regulators worked to play catch up, the cannabis industry invested heavily to convince legislators at the state and federal levels to continue to loosen restrictions on the drug. At the federal level, where cannabis remains illegal, cannabis interests employed 86 lobbyists as of 2022; from 2018 to 2022, the industry spent $18.2 million on federal lobbying.[74] Although their ultimate goal is likely full legalization and commercialization for adult non–CUAT use, industry-backed lobbyists have worked around the edges of the issue by trying to decriminalize the drug and increase banking access for cannabis companies. While thus far most of their federal efforts to legalize and legitimize the industry have fallen short, they have been able to increase funding for cannabis research on a bipartisan basis.

As is common in other industries, cannabis companies have hired former federal officials to advance their interests. For instance, former Speaker of the House John Boehner, a Republican, joined the board of Acreage Holdings in 2018.[75] In 2021, former Deputy Attorney James Cole and Senator Cory Gardner, a Republican from Colorado, joined the National Cannabis Roundtable.[76] Former Speaker of the House Nancy Pelosi's son Paul Pelosi Jr. is the board chair for Freedom Leaf, Inc., which uses the trademarked subtitle "The Marijuana Legalization Company."[77] And former Senator Thomas Daschle and former Congressman Greg Walden co-chair the Coalition for Cannabis Policy, Education, and Regulation, whose members include Altria, Constellation Brands, and Molson Coors, all of whom have invested in the cannabis industry.[78]

At the state level, the cannabis industry is also active. Producers and growers donated $15.4 million in the past 20 years to state legislators and spent an additional $24 million on state-level lobbying.[79] Prior to legalization, industry-funded lobbyists worked at the state level to pass CUAT legislation and liberalize related policies around hemp and CBD. The industry has also funded ballot initiatives: in California, for example, supporters of Proposition 64, the initiative to legalize adult non–CUAT use, outspent opponents 12-to-1, helping it pass with 57% of the vote in 2016.[80] In states that have legalized cannabis for adult non–CUAT use, companies have lobbied to accelerate the transition between the illicit market and a legal licensing system, to keep taxes low, and to remove restrictions on cannabis advertising.[81-83] According to news reports, in Arizona, social equity advocates charged the industry with lobbying against the distribution of "equity" licenses to entrepreneurs of color.[84]

In many states, after the passage of legalization, municipalities have considerable control over how the cannabis industry can operate within their borders, if at all. When given the choice to opt out of opening cannabis dispensaries, many cities and towns have done so. More than two-thirds of municipalities opted out of sales in California and New Jersey after legalization, for example. In response to this trend, other states like New Mexico have preemptively prohibited local jurisdictions from having a say in whether shops are allowed to open. Then, debates ensue about how and where shops may open. While some localities have required shops to open 1,000 ft from schools, others may set a buffer of only 500 ft. Some might allow only one license, while others might have no cap at all. Local jurisdictions have routinely zoned dispensaries and limited their hours of operation. These decisions are left to local officials, who then become another target of industry lobbyists.

Of note, the efforts of industry-backed lobbyists are countered by groups that oppose the liberalization of cannabis laws, which often represent the interests of public health and public safety groups. These organizations work to increase funding for cannabis research and to hold the cannabis industry accountable. Public health-focused groups often lobby for more stringent policies, such as potency caps and strict bans on advertising. However, they are heavily outspent by the industry, which looks forward to billions in profits from the legalization and sale of cannabis.

Impact of Legalization on CUD Prevalence

Because so much of the industry's efforts have been directed at achieving full legalization, the impact of legalization on CUD prevalence is highly relevant. A 2019 national study looking at the relationship between state legalization of cannabis for adult non–CUAT use and prevalence of CUD found that past-year CUD diagnoses among 12- to 17-year-olds increased 25% more (from 2.18% to 2.72%) in legalized states. The authors cautioned that unmeasured confounders may have been the explanation for the association among youth, but they had no such qualification for their finding that the prevalence of past-year CUD in those age 26 and older increased from 0.9% to 1.23%.[85]

CUAT cannabis laws have also been associated with higher adult treatment admissions for CUD,[86] particularly in states that have allowed dispensaries.[87,88] According to one study, between 1992 and 2012, an additional 500,000 cases of CUD among adults may have been attributable to the implementation of CUAT laws.[89] However, national surveys indicate that individuals who use CUAT represent less than 10% of those who used cannabis in the past year, making it difficult to credit effects of this size to CUAT laws alone.[90]

Canada legalized cannabis for adult non–CUAT use nationwide in late 2018, creating the possibility for a retrospective study of the impact of legalization on cannabis use and CUD. Examination of records for patients who visited a psychiatrist in the emergency unit of a major hospital both pre- ($n = 1,247$) and postlegalization ($n = 1,368$) revealed significant increases in cannabis use and in CUD, with postlegalization patients between the ages of 18 and 24, in particular, having 2.27 times the odds of presenting with CUD compared with prelegalization patients in the same age group.[91]

Where to From Here?

The close relationship between the legalization of cannabis and the rising prevalence of use and CUD, both generally and in vulnerable populations, may not be inevitable. Evidence, particularly from Uruguay, which has taken a much more restrictive approach to legalization, suggests that cannabis can be made more widely available without, for instance, inadvertently increasing young people's use of the drug. Proponents of cannabis legalization have touted this as support for their stance in the United States.[92] However, there are significant differences in how Uruguay accomplished legalization: it only permits the sale of flower (not vapes, edibles, or concentrates), it limits access to a small number of pharmacies (currently 16 for a national population of 3.5 million people), to home cultivators, or to members of cannabis social clubs of up to 45 people, and consumers may select only one of these routes of access. It also bans advertising, requires plain packaging with warning labels, and limits the strength of products to 9% THC.[93]

These restrictions essentially remove the possibility that a cannabis industry like what is developing in the United States can emerge in Uruguay. The United States has a robust and growing legal cannabis industry. An effort 5 years ago to assess the impact of cannabis legalization on the development of CUD laid out clear principles to be followed and directed policymakers to the large body of scientific literature that exists regarding pharmacologic, access and availability, and environmental factors that influence the development of substance use disorders.[94] There is little evidence that policymakers have done so in their structuring of legalization at the state level. At the same time, there is broad consensus in the public health field on what must be done to keep this industry in check from a public health standpoint. Use of state monopolies (which exist for alcohol in 17 states), restricting retail physical availability, setting restrictions on discounting such as minimum prices and minimum unit prices, using taxes at least as much for public health as for revenue-raising purposes, and emphasizing regulating business rather than consumer behavior were key recommendations of one consensus panel.[95] A recent publication from the American Public Health Association (APHA), as well as that organization's policy statement on regulating commercially legalized cannabis developed by APHA's Section on Alcohol, Tobacco and Other Drugs, echo these recommendations.

They also add to them the importance of regulating advertising and marketing as well as product potency, form, and characteristics, providing sufficient funds for enforcement, monitoring, and evaluation as well as for community-level prevention, education, and health promotion, developing better technology for detecting and preventing impaired driving, limiting the environmental effects of the larger cannabis industry, including regulating pesticide use, monitoring and mitigating effects of cultivation on water usage and climate change (see also Chapter 6) and limiting exposure to secondhand cannabis smoke, and addressing social justice issues by using cannabis revenues to promote general wealth development rather than more cannabis businesses in communities historically targeted by the War on Drugs.[41,96]

Without these steps, it is likely that the principal impact of the cannabis industry on CUD will be to drive the prevalence of CUD in the U.S. population steadily higher. Furthermore, this impact will likely manifest in ways that exacerbate current health disparities, with the effects most profoundly felt by young people and young adults, poor people, and communities of color. This outcome may be avoidable, but only if policymakers attend both to the lessons of the past, in terms of experiences with other legal drugs such as alcohol and nicotine, and to the emerging lessons of the present. Cannabis legalization is currently a vast national and natural experiment. It is incumbent upon the medical community to prevent this experiment from harming the human subjects involved, particularly populations and communities already struggling from histories of discrimination, disenfranchisement, and exploitation by profit-seeking entities such as many in the emerging cannabis industry.

REFERENCES

1. Substance Abuse and Mental Health Services Administration (SAMHSA). *Results From the National Survey on Drug Use and Health: National Findings*. Office of Applied Studies; 2002. Accessed September 18, 2022. https://files.eric.ed.gov/fulltext/ED479833.pdf
2. Statista. *Number of People in the U.S. Who Used Marijuana in The Past Year From 2009 to 2020*. 2022. Accessed September 17, 2022. https://www.statista.com/statistics/611714/marijuana-use-during-past-year-in-the-us/
3. Substance Abuse and Mental Health Services Administration. *Results From the 2020 National Survey on Drug Use and Health: Detailed Tables*. Substance Abuse and Mental Health Services Administration; 2021. Accessed May 2, 2022. https://www.samhsa.gov/data/report/2020-nsduh-detailed-tables
4. Substance Abuse and Mental Health Services Administration (SAMHSA). *Results From the 2012 National Survey on Drug Use and Health: Summary of National Findings*. Office of Applied Studies; 2013. Accessed February 6, 2014. http://www.samhsa.gov/data/NSDUH/2012SummNatFindDetTables/NationalFindings/NSDUHresults2012.htm#ch2.2
5. Substance Abuse and Mental Health Services Administration (SAMHSA). *2020 National Survey of Drug Use and Health (NSDUH) Releases*. Substance Abuse and Mental Health Services Administration (SAMHSA); 2021. Accessed December 2021. https://www.samhsa.gov/data/sites/default/files/reports/rpt35323/NSDUHDetailedTabs2020/NSDUHDetailedTabs2020/NSDUHDetTabsSect2pe2020.htm
6. Patrick ME, Schulenberg JE, Miech RA, Johnston LD, O'Malley PM, Bachman JG. *Monitoring the Future Panel Study Annual Report: National Data on Substance Use Among Adults Ages 19 to 60, 1976–2021*. University of Michigan Institute for Social Research; 2022. Accessed September 20, 2023. https://monitoringthefuture.org/wp-content/uploads/2022/09/mtfpanelreport2022.pdf
7. Keyes KM, Kreski NT, Ankrum H, et al. Frequency of adolescent cannabis smoking and vaping in the United States: trends, disparities and concurrent substance use, 2017-19. *Addiction*. 2022;117(8):2316-2324. doi:10.1111/add.15912
8. Miech RA, Johnston LD, O'Malley PM, Bachman JG, Schulenberg JE, Patrick ME. *Monitoring the Future National Survey Results on Drug Use, 1975–2021: Volume I, Secondary School Students*. Institute for Social Research, University of Michigan; 2022. Accessed September 17, 2022. https://monitoringthefuture.org/wp-content/uploads/2022/08/mtf-vol1_2020.pdf
9. Lim CCW, Sun T, Leung J, et al. Prevalence of adolescent cannabis vaping: a systematic review and meta-analysis of US and Canadian Studies. *JAMA Pediatr*. 2022;176(1):42-51. doi:10.1001/jamapediatrics.2021.4102
10. Jeffers AM, Glantz S, Byers A, Keyhani S. Sociodemographic characteristics associated with and prevalence and frequency of cannabis use among adults in the US. *JAMA Netw Open*. 2021;4(11):e2136571. doi:10.1001/jamanetworkopen.2021.36571
11. Cuttler C, Mischley LK, Sexton M. Sex differences in cannabis use and effects: a cross-sectional survey of cannabis users. *Cannabis Cannabinoid Res*. 2016;1(1):166-175. doi:10.1089/can.2016.0010
12. Daniulaityte R, Zatreh MY, Lamy FR, et al. A twitter-based survey on marijuana concentrate use. *Drug Alcohol Depend*. 2018;187:155-159. doi:10.1016/j.drugalcdep.2018.02.033
13. Greaves L, Hemsing N. Sex and gender interactions on the use and impact of recreational cannabis. *Int J Environ Health Res*. 2020;17(2): doi:10.3390/ijerph17020509
14. Substance Abuse and Mental Health Services Administration. *2019 National Survey on Drug Use and Health: Lesbian, Gay, & Bisexual (LGB) Adults*. Substance Abuse and Mental Health Services Agency; 2020. Accessed September 17, 2022. https://www.samhsa.gov/data/sites/default/files/reports/rpt31104/2019NSDUH-LGB/LGB%202019%20NSDUH.pdf
15. Substance Abuse and Mental Health Services Administration. *2019 National Survey on Drug Use and Health: Women*. Substance Abuse and Mental Health Services Agency; 2020. Accessed September 17, 2022. https://www.samhsa.gov/data/sites/default/files/reports/rpt31102/2019NSDUH-Women/Women%202019%20NSDUH.pdf
16. Substance Abuse and Mental Health Services Administration. *Marijuana and Pregnancy*. Substance Abuse and Mental Health Services Agency; 2022. Accessed September 17, 2022. https://www.samhsa.gov/marijuana/marijuana-pregnancy
17. Brenneke SG, Nordeck CD, Riehm KE, et al. Trends in cannabis use among U.S. adults amid the COVID-19 pandemic. *Int J Drug Policy*. 2022;100:103517. doi:10.1016/j.drugpo.2021.103517
18. American Psychiatric Association. *The Diagnostic and Statistical Manual of Mental Disorders*. 5th ed. American Psychiatric Association; 2013.
19. Leung J, Chan GCK, Hides L, Hall WD. What is the prevalence and risk of cannabis use disorders among people who use cannabis? A systematic review and meta-analysis. *Addict Behav*. 2020;109:106479. doi:10.1016/j.addbeh.2020.106479
20. Silins E, Horwood LJ, Patton GC, et al. Young adult sequelae of adolescent cannabis use: an integrative analysis. *Lancet Psychiatry*. 2014;1(4):286-293. doi:10.1016/S2215-0366(14)70307-4
21. Wilson J, Freeman TP, Mackie CJ. Effects of increasing cannabis potency on adolescent health. *Lancet Child Adolesc Health*. 2019;3(2):121-128. doi:10.1016/S2352-4642(18)30342-0
22. Davenport SS, Caulkins JP. Evolution of the United States marijuana market in the decade of liberalization before full legalization. Article. *J Drug Issues*. 2016;46(4):411-427. doi:10.1177/0022042616659759
23. Caulkins JP, Pardo B, Kilmer B. Intensity of cannabis use: findings from three online surveys. *Int J Drug Policy*. 2020;79:102740. doi:10.1016/j.drugpo.2020.102740
24. Greenfield T, Rogers JD. Who drinks most of the alcohol in the U.S.? The policy implications. *J Stud Alcohol*. 1999;60(1):78-89.

25. MPG Consulting, Leeds School of Business University of Colorado Boulder. *2019 Regulated Marijuana Market Update*. n.d. Accessed September 18, 2022. https://sbg.colorado.gov/sites/sbg/files/documents/2019%20Regulated%20Marijuana%20Market%20Update%20Report%20Final_0.pdf
26. University of Mississippi National Center for Natural Products Research. *Quarterly Report #139 From the Potency Monitoring Program*. School of Pharmacy. University of Mississippi; 2019. Accessed September 17, 2022. https://pharmacy.olemiss.edu/marijuana/wp-content/uploads/sites/30/2020/03/U-Miss-Marijuana-Potency-Monitoring-Program-Quarterly-Report-139-December-23-2018-March-22-2019.pdf
27. MPG Consulting, Leeds School of Business University of Colorado Boulder. *2020 Regulated Marijuana Market Update*. n.d. Accessed September 18, 2022. https://sbg.colorado.gov/sites/sbg/files/2020-Regulated-Marijuana-Market-Update-Final.pdf
28. Colorado Department of Public Health and Environment. *THC Concentrationi in Colorado Marijuana: Health Effects and Public Health Concerns*. Colorada Department of Public Health & Environment; 2020. Accessed September 18, 2022. https://adai.uw.edu/wordpress/wp-content/uploads/2020/11/THCinColorado2020.pdf
29. Hines LA, Freeman TP, Gage SH, et al. Association of high-potency cannabis use with mental health and substance use in adolescence. *JAMA Psychiatry*. 2020;77(10):1044-1051.
30. Shi Y, Cao Y, Shang C, Pacula RL. The impacts of potency, warning messages, and price on preferences for Cannabis flower products. *Int J Drug Policy*. 2019;74:1-10. doi:10.1016/j.drugpo.2019.07.037
31. Smart R, Caulkins JP, Kilmer B, Davenport S, Midgette G. Response to commentaries: new data sources for understanding cannabis markets. *Addiction*. 2017;112(12):2180-2181. doi:10.1111/add.14051
32. Calvert CM, Erickson D. Recreational cannabis legalization and alcohol purchasing: a difference-in-differences analysis. *J Cannabis Res*. 2021;3(1):27. doi:10.1186/s42238-021-00085-x
33. Gunn RL, Aston ER, Metrik J. Patterns of cannabis and alcohol co-use: substitution versus complementary effects. *Alcohol Res*. 2022;42(1):04. doi:10.35946/arcr.v42.1.04
34. Berg CJ, Payne J, Henriksen L, et al. Reasons for marijuana and tobacco co-use among young adults: a mixed methods scale development study. *Subst Use Misuse*. 2018;53(3):357-369. doi:10.1080/10826084.2017.1327978
35. Weinberger AH, Wyka K, Goodwin RD. Impact of cannabis legalization in the United States on trends in cannabis use and daily cannabis use among individuals who smoke cigarettes. *Drug Alcohol Depend*. 2022;238:109563. doi:10.1016/j.drugalcdep.2022.109563
36. Ramo DE, Prochaska JJ. Prevalence and co-use of marijuana among young adult cigarette smokers: an anonymous online national survey. *Addict Sci Clin Pract*. 2012;7(1):5. 10.1186/1940-0640-7-5
37. Tucker JS, Pedersen ER, Seelam R, Dunbar MS, Shih RA, D'Amico EJ. Types of cannabis and tobacco/nicotine co-use and associated outcomes in young adulthood. *Psychol Addict Behav*. 2019;33(4):401-411. doi:10.1037/adb0000464
38. Substance Abuse and Mental Health Services Administration. *Key Substance Use and Mental Health Indicators in the United States: Results From the 2020 National Survey on Drug Use and Health*. Substance Abuse and Mental Health Services Administration; 2021. https://www.samhsa.gov/data/sites/default/files/reports/rpt35325/NSDUHFFRPDFWHTMLFiles2020/2020NSDUHFFR1PDFW102121.pdf
39. Drug Abuse Warning Network. *Preliminary Findings from Drug-Related Emergency Department Visits*, 2021. https://store.samhsa.gov/sites/default/files/SAMHSA_Digital_Download/PEP22-07-03-001.pdf
40. Substance Abuse and Mental Health Services Administration. *2020 National Survey on Drug Use and Health: Lesbian, Gay, or Bisexual (LGB) Adults*. 2020. Accessed May 10, 2023. https://www.samhsa.gov/data/sites/default/files/reports/rpt37929/2020NSDUHLGBSlides072522.pdf
41. Jernigan DH, Ramirez RR, Castrucci B, Patterson C, Castillo G. *Cannabis: Moving Forward, Protecting Health*. American Public Health Association Press; 2021.
42. Jernigan D, Ross CS. The alcohol marketing landscape: alcohol industry size, structure, strategies, and public health responses. *J Stud Alcohol Drugs Suppl*. 2020;(Sup 19):13-25.
43. Euromonitor. *Cannabis Market Disruptor Handbook Part 1: An Introduction*. 2019.
44. Arcview Market Research. *The State of Legal Cannabis Markets*. 2020.
45. BCC Research. *Cannabis Market: Products, Technologies and Applications*. 2019.
46. Largest Cannabis Companies by Market Cap. Accessed May 10, 2023. https://companiesmarketcap.com/cannabis/largest-cannabis-companies-by-market-cap/
47. MediaJel. *Top 10 Cannabis Dispensary Chains in 2021*. MediaJel; 2021. Accessed October 1, 2022. https://www.mediajel.com/blogs/top-10-cannabis-dispensary-chains/
48. Sesto G. *60 Unbelievable Cannabis Marketing Statistics*. Dash Two; 2019. Accessed September 25, 2022. https://dashtwo.com/cannabis-marketing-statistics/
49. Han B, Compton WM, Blanco C, Jones CM. Time since first cannabis use and 12-month prevalence of cannabis use disorder among youth and emerging adults in the United States. *Addiction*. 2019;114(4):698-707. doi:10.1111/add.14511
50. Winters KC, Lee C-YS. Likelihood of developing an alcohol and cannabis use disorder during youth: association with recent use and age. *Drug Alcohol Depend*. 2008;92(1):239-247. doi:10.1016/j.drugalcdep.2007.08.005
51. Jernigan D, Noel J, Landon J, Thornton N, Lobstein T. Alcohol marketing and youth alcohol consumption: a systematic review of longitudinal studies published since 2008. *Addiction*. 2017;112:7-20. doi:10.1111/add.13591
52. Anderson P, De Bruijn A, Angus K, Gordon R, Hastings G. Impact of alcohol advertising and media exposure on adolescent alcohol use: a systematic review of longitudinal studies. *Alcohol Alcohol*. 2009;44(3):229-243.
53. Sargent JD, Babor TF. The relationship between exposure to alcohol marketing and underage drinking is causal. *J Stud Alcohol Drugs Suppl*. 2020;(Suppl 19):113-124. doi:10.15288/jsads.2020.s19.113
54. Collins L, Glasser AM, Abudayyeh H, Pearson JL, Villanti AC. E-cigarette marketing and communication: how E-cigarette companies market E-cigarettes and the public engages with E-cigarette information. *Nicotine Tob Res*. 2019;21(1):14-24. doi:10.1093/ntr/ntx284
55. Kreitzberg DS, Hinds JT, Pasch KE, Loukas A, Perry CL. Exposure to ENDS advertising and use of marijuana in ENDS among college students. *Addict Behav*. 2019;93:9-13. doi:10.1016/j.addbeh.2019.01.012
56. Cabrera-Nguyen EP, Cavazos-Rehg P, Krauss M, Bierut LJ, Moreno MA. Young adults' exposure to alcohol- and marijuana-related content on twitter. *J Stud Alcohol Drugs*. 2016;77(2):349-353. doi:10.15288/jsad.2016.77.349
57. Roditis ML, Delucchi K, Chang A, Halpern-Felsher B. Perceptions of social norms and exposure to pro-marijuana messages are associated with adolescent marijuana use. *Prev Med*. 2016;93:171-176. doi:10.1016/j.ypmed.2016.10.013
58. Trangenstein PJ, Whitehill JM, Jenkins MC, Jernigan DH, Moreno MA. Active cannabis marketing and adolescent past-year cannabis use. *Drug Alcohol Depend*. 2019;204:107548. doi:10.1016/j.drugalcdep.2019.107548
59. Trangenstein PJ, Whitehill JM, Jenkins MC, Jernigan DH, Moreno MA. Cannabis marketing and problematic cannabis use among adolescents. *J Stud Alcohol Drugs*. 2021;82(2):288-296.
60. D'Amico EJ, Miles JN, Tucker JS. Gateway to curiosity: medical marijuana ads and intention and use during middle school. *Psychol Addict Behav*. 2015;29(3):613-619. doi:10.1037/adb0000094
61. D'Amico EJ, Rodriguez A, Tucker JS, Pedersen ER, Shih RA. Planting the seed for marijuana use: changes in exposure to medical marijuana advertising and subsequent adolescent marijuana use, cognitions, and consequences over seven years. *Drug Alcohol Depend*. 2018;188:385-391. doi:10.1016/j.drugalcdep.2018.03.031
62. Shih RA, Rodriguez A, Parast L, et al. Associations between young adult marijuana outcomes and availability of medical marijuana dispensaries

and storefront signage. *Addiction*. 2019;114(12):2162-2170. doi:10.1111/add.14711

63. Everson EM, Dilley JA, Maher JE, Mack CE. Post-legalization opening of retail cannabis stores and adult cannabis use in Washington state, 2009–2016. *Am J Public Health*. 2019;109(9):1294-1301. doi:10.2105/AJPH.2019.305191
64. Pedersen ER, Firth CL, Rodriguez A, et al. Examining associations between licensed and unlicensed outlet density and cannabis outcomes from preopening to postopening of recreational cannabis outlets. *Am J Addict*. 2021;30(2):122-130. doi:10.1111/ajad.13132
65. Morrison C, Gruenewald PJ, Freisthler B, Ponicki WR, Remer LG. The economic geography of medical cannabis dispensaries in California. *Int J Drug Policy*. 2014;25(3):508-515. doi:10.1016/j.drugpo.2013.12.009
66. Thomas C, Freisthler B. Evaluating the change in medical marijuana dispensary locations in Los Angeles following the passage of local legislation. *J Prim Prev*. 2017;38(3):265-277. doi:10.1007/s10935-017-0473-8
67. MjBizDaily. *Chart: Recreational Marijuana Stores Are Clustered in Low-Income Areas of Denver*. 2017. Accessed May 10, 2023. https://mjbizdaily.com/chart-recreational-marijuana-stores-clustered-low-income-areas-denver-seattle/
68. Altieri E. *Marijuana Legalization and the Fight for Racial Justice*. NORML; 2020. Accessed May 10, 2023. https://norml.org/blog/2020/06/01/marijuana-legalization-and-the-fight-for-racial-justice/
69. Nguyen J, Blood M. *Declining Cannabis Prices*. EisnerAmper; 2022. Accessed May 10, 2023. https://www.eisneramper.com/declining-cannabis-prices-0722/
70. Davenport S. Price and product variation in Washington's recreational cannabis market. *Int J Drug Policy*. 2021;91:102547. doi:10.1016/j.drugpo.2019.08.004
71. Pacula RL, Lundberg R. Why changes in price matter when thinking about marijuana policy: a review of the literature on the elasticity of demand. *Public Health Rev*. 2014;35(2):1-18.
72. van Ours JC, Williams J. Cannabis prices and dynamics of cannabis use. *J Health Econ*. 2007;26(3):578-596. doi:10.1016/j.jhealeco.2006.10.001
73. Cole JM. *Memorandum for All United States Attorneys*. U.S. Department of Justice, Office of the Deputy Attorney General; 2013. Accessed October 3, 2022. https://www.justice.gov/iso/opa/resources/3052013829132756857467.pdf
74. Center for Responsive Politics. Industry Profile: Marijuana. 2022. Accessed October 3, 2022. https://www.opensecrets.org/industries/lobbying.php?cycle=2022&ind=G2860
75. Victor D. *John Boehner's Marijuana Reversal: 'My Thinking on Cannabis Has Evolved'*. The New York Times. https://www.nytimes.com/2018/04/11/us/politics/boehner-cannabis-marijuana.html
76. Jaeger K. *Former Justice Department Official and GOP Senator Join Marijuana Group as Legalization Advances in Congress*. Marijuana Moment. Accessed May 10, 2023. https://www.marijuanamoment.net/former-justice-department-official-and-gop-senator-join-marijuana-group-as-legalization-advances-in-congress/
77. Freedom Leaf Inc. *The Marijuana Legalization Company, Appoints Paul Pelosi Jr. as Chairman of the Board*. Global Newswire; 2017. Accessed March 3, 2023. https://www.globenewswire.com/news-release/2017/11/02/1246879/0/en/Freedom-Leaf-Inc-The-Marijuana-Legalization-Company-Appoints-Paul-Pelosi-Jr-as-Chairman-of-the-Board.html
78. Coalition for Cannabis Policy Education, and Regulation. *Who Are We?* 2022. https://www.cpear.org/who-we-are/
79. Open Secrets. *State-Level Lobbyist Spending by Marijuana Growers and Product Sales Spenders*. 2022. Accessed October 3, 2022. https://www.followthemoney.org/show-me?dt=3&lby-y=2022,2021,2020,2019,2018,2017,2016,2015,2014,2013,2012,2011,2010&lby-f-fc=2&lby-f-cci=151&lby-f-fc=2#[{1|gro=lby-y
80. California Secretary of State. November 8, 2016 General Election. 2016. Accessed May 10, 2023. https://elections.cdn.sos.ca.gov/sov/2016-general/sov/2016-complete-sov.pdf
81. Koseff A. California cuts cannabis taxes to heal ailing industry. *Cal Matters*. 2022. Accessed October 7, 2022. https://calmatters.org/politics/2022/07/california-cannabis-tax/
82. Inside Radio. *Effort to Allow Cannabis Ads on Local Radio and TV Clear House*. Inside Radio; 2022. Accessed October 7, 2022. https://www.insideradio.com/free/effort-to-allow-cannabis-ads-on-local-radio-and-tv-clears-house/article_47e122da-086f-11ed-b3c6-d7cd74fbc5c9.html
83. Molina T. *With License Delays Persisting and Illinois Legislative Session Ending, Situation Called 'dire' for Some Marijuana Entrepreneurs*. CBS News; 2022. Accessed October 7, 2022. https://www.cbsnews.com/chicago/news/with-license-delays-persisting-and-illinois-legislative-session-ending-situation-called-dire-for-some-marijuana-entrepreneurs/
84. Schroyer J. *Finger-Pointing in Arizona Over Marijuana Social Equity Hurdles*. MJ Biz Daily; 2022. Accessed October 7, 2022. https://mjbizdaily.com/who-is-to-blame-for-marijuana-social-equity-hurdles-in-arizona/
85. Cerda M, Mauro C, Hamilton A, et al. Association between recreational marijuana legalization in the united states and changes in marijuana use and cannabis use disorder from 2008 to 2016. *JAMA Psychiatry*. 2020;77(2):165-171. doi:10.1001/jamapsychiatry.2019.3254
86. Chu YW. The effects of medical marijuana laws on illegal marijuana use. *J Health Econ*. 2014;38:43-61. doi:10.1016/j.jhealeco.2014.07.003
87. Pacula RL, Powell D, Heaton P, Sevigny EL. Assessing the effects of medical marijuana laws on marijuana use: the devil is in the details. *J Policy Anal Manage*. 2015;34(1):7-31.
88. Wen H, Hockenberry JM, Cummings JR. The effect of medical marijuana laws on adolescent and adult use of marijuana, alcohol, and other substances. *J Health Econ*. 2015;42:64-80. doi:10.1016/j.jhealeco.2015.03.007
89. Hasin DS, Sarvet AL, Cerda M, et al. US adult illicit cannabis use, cannabis use disorder, and medical marijuana laws: 1991-1992 to 2012-2013. *JAMA Psychiatry*. 2017;74(6):579-588. doi:10.1001/jamapsychiatry.2017.0724
90. Smart R, Pacula RL. Early evidence of the impact of cannabis legalization on cannabis use, cannabis use disorder, and the use of other substances: findings from state policy evaluations. *Am J Drug Alcohol Abuse*. 2019;45(6):644-663 doi:10.1080/00952990.2019.1669626
91. Vignault C, Massé A, Gouron D, Quintin J, Asli KD, Semaan W. The potential impact of recreational cannabis legalization on the prevalence of cannabis use disorder and psychotic disorders: a retrospective observational study. *Can J Psychiatry*. 2021;66(12):1069-1076. doi:10.1177/0706743720984684
92. NORML. *Uruguay: No Sustained Changes in Young People's Cannabis Use Patterns Following Legalization*. NORML; 2022. Accessed October 4, 2022. https://norml.org/news/2022/05/05/uruguay-no-sustained-changes-in-young-peoples-cannabis-use-patterns-following-legalization/
93. Dilley JA. Commentary on Rivera-Aguirre et al: what are the effects of cannabis legalization on youth use? It may depend on what you mean by 'legalization'. *Addiction*. 2022;117(11):2878-2879. doi:10.1111/add.16006
94. Budney AJ, Borodovsky JT. The potential impact of cannabis legalization on the development of cannabis use disorders. *Prev Med*. 2017;104:31-36. doi:10.1016/j.ypmed.2017.06.034
95. Blanchette JG, Pacula RL, Smart R, et al. Rating the comparative efficacy of state-level cannabis policies on recreational cannabis markets in the United States. *Int J Drug Policy*. 2022;106:103744. doi:10.1016/j.drugpo.2022.103744
96. American Public Health Association. *A Public Health Approach to Regulating Commercially Legalized Cannabis*. 2020. Accessed January 4, 2021. https://www.apha.org/policies-and-advocacy/public-health-policy-statements/policy-database/2021/01/13/a-public-health-approach-to-regulating-commercially-legalized-cannabis

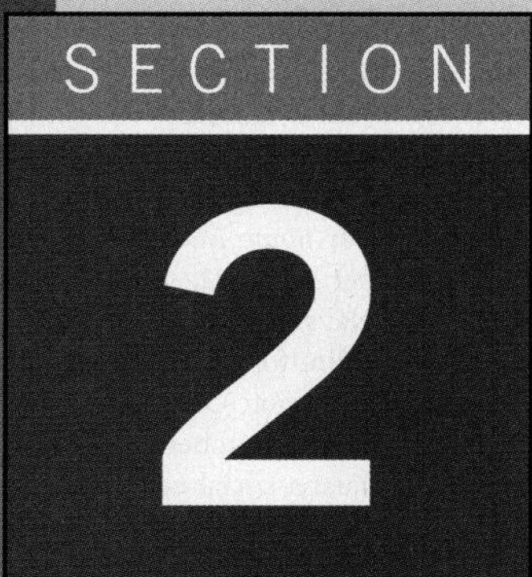

Pharmacology

Associate Editor: Shannon C. Miller
Lead Section Editor: Thomas R. Kosten
Section Editors: David A. Gorelick and Daryl Shorter

CHAPTER

10 Pharmacokinetic, Pharmacodynamic, and Pharmacogenomic Principles

Lori D. Karan, John G. McNutt, and Anne Zajicek

CHAPTER OUTLINE

- Introduction
- Pharmacokinetics
- Drug-drug interactions
- Pharmacokinetics and the brain
- Pharmacokinetics and pregnancy
- Pharmacodynamics
- Individual differences in drug response and addiction susceptibility
- Summary

INTRODUCTION

Addiction medicine requires an understanding of the application of pharmacologic principles to both the substances used and to the medications used to treat these disorders.

Pharmacokinetics describes how drugs are handled by the body. Drug concentrations are determined by their absorption, distribution, metabolism, and elimination (often referred to as ADME). These processes determine the time course of drug concentrations in the blood, tissues and organs, including the placenta and brain. The magnitude of a drug's pharmacological effect depends upon the free (unbound) drug concentration at its site of action.

Pharmacodynamics is the study of the effects of drugs on the body and the body's response to these drugs. Most drugs act on specific endogenous targets, or receptors, to modulate the rate and extent of the body's functions. Drug effects are also influenced by desensitization, tolerance, sensitization and withdrawal.

Pharmacogenomics is the study of how the genetic makeup of an individual affects drug pharmacokinetics and pharmacodynamics. Improved understanding of pharmacogenomics is the basis of precision medicine. Epigenetics refers to modifications in gene expression that are not due to changes in DNA (ie, the gene itself).

PHARMACOKINETICS

Pharmacokinetics describes the amounts and rates by which drugs enter the body, reach their site of action, and leave the body. This encompasses four phases: absorption, distribution, metabolism, and elimination (ADME). After absorption, a common measure of drug exposure is the area under the curve (AUC) of the plasma concentration of a drug as a function of time. Other useful measures are the time (T_{max}) of peak drug concentration (C_{max}), and the lowest (trough) drug concentration (C_{min}).

Absorption

Absorption is the process of drug movement from the site of drug delivery to the body's circulatory system. The "rate hypothesis" holds that the faster a drug reaches the brain and produces a psychoactive effect, the greater its reinforcing effects and unhealthy use and addiction liability.[1] The faster the rate of absorption, the shorter the time to maximum concentration. Intravenous and inhaled drugs have a more rapid absorption than transmucosal, intramuscular (IM), subcutaneous (SC), oral, and transdermal preparations. This explains why a given drug administered intravenously or by inhalation has more unhealthy use liability than that same drug given orally (eg, cocaine, opioids).

Potentially addictive prescription drugs are reformulated to reduce the rates of absorption in order to reduce the peak concentrations and reduce this reinforcing effect.[2] In animal studies, the rate of change in drug-induced synaptic dopamine concentration, rather than the dopamine concentration itself, correlates best with the unhealthy use liability of a drug.[3] Routes of administration and delivery systems that produce slower rates of dopamine transporter blockade and rates of dopamine increases have less unhealthy use liability than delivery systems that lead to faster dopamine changes. For instance, sustained-release methylphenidate has a slower peak dopamine transporter blockade in the striatum and cerebellum than does immediate-release methylphenidate.[4]

Inhaled (smoked or vaporized) substances have a fast rate of absorption because they have direct access to the bloodstream across the large, highly vascularized surface area of the lung alveoli. Absorption of an inhaled drug depends on the physical characteristics of the drug, including its volatility, and particle size. Upon inhalation, each drug proceeds directly from the pulmonary circulation to the heart and then to the arterial system. 12% to 20% of the cardiac output perfuses the brain.[5]

Intranasal, buccal, sublingual, and rectal drug administration rely on transmucosal absorption. Intranasal, buccal, and sublingual drug administration avoid first pass metabolism in the liver, whereas rectally administered drugs undergo about 50% first pass metabolism. This is because drugs absorbed in the upper rectum enter the superior rectal vein which drains through the mesenteric and portal veins into the liver. In contrast, drugs absorbed in the lower rectum enter the middle and inferior rectal veins which drain through the inferior vena cava directly into the systemic venous circulation.[6] Drugs have a more rapid onset of action when their absorption avoids first pass metabolism.

Examples of transmucosally administered drugs include sublingual buprenorphine, and sublingually and buccally absorbed nicotine polacrilex lozenges and gum. Limitations of transmucosal drug administration include a small volume of fluid for drug dissolution, relatively small surface area for effective drug absorption, and the presence of a mucus barrier. Penetrating the mucus barrier generally requires that drugs be small molecular weight substances, with high potency, and high lipophilicity.[6]

The nasal cavity is covered by a well-vascularized thin mucosa which allows ready absorption. Intranasally absorbed drugs flow to the cavernous sinus, pterygoid plexus and facial vein which drain the nose, and then to the heart and systemic circulation, bypassing first pass metabolism. Local anesthetics such as cocaine are vasoconstrictive and limit their own transmucosal absorption. The central nervous system activity of intranasal naloxone may be enhanced via absorption through the cribriform plate high in the nasal cavity as well as via the olfactory and trigeminal nerves.[7]

Transdermal drug administration produces a slow rate of absorption because it requires permeation of a drug across the lipophilic skin layers into the systemic circulation. Most drugs are not systemically absorbed through the skin, but can be made permeable by increasing their lipophilicity. Adding dimethyl sulfoxide (DMSO), for example, to impermeable compounds can dramatically increase topical permeability.[8]

Several factors affect the ability of drugs to cross biological membranes. Lipid-solubility and neutral electric charge enhance the ability of molecules to passively diffuse across membranes. For some drugs, transmembrane transporters promote active diffusion. Some drugs have diminished absorption because of a reverse transporter associated with P-glycoprotein. This reverse transporter actively pumps drugs out of the gut wall cells back into the gut lumen. A similar process occurs in the brain. Inhibiting P-glycoprotein increases drug absorption.

Multiple factors affect absorption for orally administered drugs, including pharmaceutical properties of the oral dosage form, gastric pH, rate of gastric emptying, presence of food, intestinal transit time, and integrity of the intestinal epithelium. Low gastric pH destroys some drug molecules. Faster gastric emptying provides more rapid delivery of drug to the small intestine. However, too rapid "dumping" into the small intestine may reduce absorption. For drugs absorbed in the small intestine, faster intestinal transit time lowers the rate of absorption. The presence of food can diminish the interaction time between the drug and the intestinal villi, reducing drug absorption.[9]

There are gender differences in absorption of orally administered drugs. Women have higher blood alcohol concentrations than men for the same amount of alcohol consumed. This is because women have a higher percentage of body fat (and less total body water), and they generally weigh less than men. Women also have less gastric alcohol dehydrogenase. Thus, women have a smaller volume of distribution and lower clearance of alcohol than men.

Surgery can affect absorption. As an example, gastric bypass surgery affects alcohol's absorption and pharmacokinetics, with less gastric alcohol dehydrogenase from the gastric pouch to break down alcohol. When alcohol bypasses the stomach and duodenum and is directly absorbed in the jejunum, blood alcohol concentrations peak sooner at approximately double the level of those who didn't have the surgery, unintentionally enhancing alcohol's rewarding effects.[10]

Orally administered drugs are exposed to hepatic drug metabolizing enzymes in the liver, via the portal vein, before reaching the rest of the body; this is termed first pass metabolism. Some first pass metabolism also takes place in the gut (eg, for benzylpenicillin and insulin). First-pass metabolism occurs most extensively for lipid-soluble drugs such as morphine, methylphenidate, and desipramine. Morphine, for example, requires nearly twice the dose when administered orally as compared to intravenously.

Bioavailability is the extent of absorption, defined as the fraction of unchanged drug that reaches the systemic circulation after administration by any route. The *bioavailability factor* (F) takes into account the portion of the administered dose that is able to enter the circulation unchanged. For intravenously administered drugs, F = 1.0 (100%). Bioavailability depends on a given drug's site-specific membrane permeability, activity of drug transporters, and its first-pass metabolism.

Some foods and drugs alter first-pass metabolism and absorption from the intestinal wall. For example, components of grapefruit juice and other foods either inhibit or induce intestinal wall CYP3A4 or P-glycoprotein, thereby altering bioavailability of drugs that are substrates for this cytochrome.[11,12]

Distribution

Once absorbed, a drug is distributed to the various organs and tissues of the body. Distribution is influenced by organ perfusion, organ size, binding of the drug within the blood and tissues, and the permeability of tissue membranes.[13]

Volume of distribution (V_d) relates the concentration of a drug in the plasma to the total amount of drug in the body. This volume is not an actual physical value, but describes the volume of plasma required to account for the total amount of the drug in the body. V_d can be thought of as the amount of drug in the body (D = dose) divided by the concentration of drug (C) in the plasma, or

$$V_d = \frac{D}{C}$$

Drugs with a small V_d are confined primarily to the intravascular space of approximately 5 L, and tend to be tightly bound to plasma proteins or have a high molecular weight. Drugs with large V_d values up to 50,000 L are highly bound to tissue sites or are lipophilic.

Protein binding affects free (active) drug concentration. Some drugs, such as caffeine, are not bound to plasma proteins, while other drugs are highly bound. Characteristics of binding proteins are capacity (amount of binding space) and affinity (tightness of binding interaction). Albumin is a high-capacity, low-affinity binding protein, whereas specific transport proteins such as transcortin are low capacity, high affinity. Acidic drugs commonly bind to albumin, the most abundant plasma protein; examples are barbiturates, benzodiazepines, and phenytoin. Basic drugs (alkaloids) such as methadone bind to alpha$_1$-acid glycoprotein, and others such as amitriptyline and nortriptyline bind to lipoproteins. Some binding sites are competitive, and a drug with a higher binding site affinity can displace a drug with a lower binding site affinity. Binding can also be stereospecific (specific for one stereoisomer of a compound). Drugs that are greater than 90% bound are considered highly protein bound; reduced protein binding for these highly protein-bound drugs can lead to large increases in free fraction of drug and therefore increased drug effect.

For volatile chemicals, distribution depends upon their solubility (and therefore vapor pressure), cardiac output, and the blood/gas partition coefficient. For example, a chemical highly soluble in blood will have a substantially greater volume of distribution and a slower onset of action because the "reservoir" of blood will dilute the agent at the site of action (brain).[14]

The rate of blood flow delivered to specific organs and tissues affects drug distribution. Well-perfused tissues can receive large quantities of drugs. In contrast, poorly perfused tissues, such as fat, receive and release drugs at a slow rate. This action explains why the concentration of drugs in fat can be maintained long after the concentration in plasma has begun to decrease. For example, FDA labeling for zolpidem was amended following reports of women having car accidents the morning after taking zolpidem, presumably because women were maintaining higher continuous zolpidem concentrations into the next morning. Women are to be prescribed half the dose of zolpidem as men.[15,16] The elderly have a higher proportion of body fat. With repeated dosing, lipophilic drugs, including many antidepressants and antipsychotics, can accumulate in fat and may be erratically released.

Metabolism

Drug metabolism is the process of chemical modification of drugs, generally into less active and more hydrophilic (renally excreted) compounds. Not all metabolites are inactive or nontoxic, and active metabolites need to be considered when assessing a drug's total activity. In some cases, the administered drug is intentionally designed to be a pharmacologically inactive prodrug that is converted in vivo to a pharmacologically active molecule. One example is lisdexamfetamine, a prodrug which is converted to active amphetamine in the body.

Drugs can be metabolized by phase 1 and/or phase 2 reactions. Phase 1 reactions are nonsynthetic reactions in which the drug is chemically oxidized, reduced or hydrolyzed by unmasking or inserting a polar functional group (eg, -OH, -SH, -NH_2) to make it more water soluble. Examples of phase 1 reactions include the oxidation of phenobarbital, amphetamine, meperidine, and codeine by liver microsomal enzymes. Phase 2 reactions are synthetic reactions in which the drug is conjugated with a polar moiety, such as glucuronide, acetate, or sulfate. Examples of synthetic reactions include the glucuronidation of morphine and meprobamate, the acetylation of clonazepam and mescaline, and the sulfation of dopamine and thyroid hormone. Phase 2 reactions produce compounds that are more polar than their parent chemicals in order to facilitate elimination. Substances may be metabolized by a combination of the above mechanisms. Ethanol, for example, is both oxidized (~90%) to acetaldehyde and conjugated (~1%) with glucuronic acid to form ethyl glucuronide and with sulfate to form ethyl sulfate. 3% to 10% ethanol is excreted unchanged in the breath, urine and sweat.[17]

Phase 1 Reactions

Enzymes are responsible for most drug metabolism. The CYP (pronounced "sip" for singular and "sips" for plural) enzymes are most commonly involved and exist in the gut, liver, and brain. The gut and liver enzymes are the best studied. Phase 1 reactions can take place by CYP-dependent and CYP-independent mechanisms. CYP-dependent reactions include aromatic (phenytoin, amphetamine) and aliphatic (pentobarbital, meprobamate) hydroxylation, epoxidation, and oxidative dealkylation (morphine, caffeine, codeine), deamination (amphetamine), desulfurization (thiopental), and dechlorination. CYP-independent reactions include dehydrogenations (ethanol); azo, nitro, and carbonyl reductions (methadone and naloxone); and ester and amide hydrolysis (cocaine).[18]

More than 50 individual CYPs have been identified in humans. The CYP family of enzymes is involved not only in the metabolism of dietary and environmental compounds and medications but also in the degradation of bile acids from cholesterol, the metabolism of retinoic and fatty acids including prostaglandins and eicosanoids, and the synthesis of steroids. A large number of specialized CYPs with specific substrate preferences are involved in these latter endogenous functions, in contrast to the relatively few CYPs that metabolize xenobiotics such as drugs. CYPs that metabolize medications not only have a tremendous capacity to oxidize a large number of structurally diverse compounds but also can metabolize a single compound at different positions on that molecule. Drug-metabolizing CYPs' large and fluid substrate-binding sites contribute to their slow catalytic rates. In part, this explains why the half-lives of drugs are much longer than the half-lives of most endogenous compounds.

Cytochromes P450 belong to the superfamily of proteins that are bound to the membrane in a cell ("cyto"), contain heme pigment as a cofactor ("chrome P"), and are often terminal oxidase enzymes in electron transfer chains. When the enzyme is in a reduced state and complexed with carbon monoxide, it has a 450-nm spectrophotometric absorption maximum.

CYPs are named with the root CYP followed by a number designating the family, a letter denoting the subfamily, and another number designating the CYP form. Thus, CYP2B6 is family 2, subfamily B, and gene number 6. Twelve CYPs (1A1, 1A2, 1B1, 2A6, 2B6, 2C8, 2C9, 2C19, 2D6, 2E1, 3A4, and 3A5) are known to metabolize xenobiotics in humans; CYP3A4 alone is responsible for metabolizing more than 50% of clinically prescribed drugs.

Substances that inhibit or induce CYPs may dramatically affect drug metabolism. Many commonly used medications induce or inhibit CYP3A4, creating clinically relevant changes in drug clearance and clinical response. For instance, ketoconazole, an antifungal, is an inhibitor of the CYP4-mediated metabolism of quetiapine, which can lead to increased risks of sedation, confusion and respiratory depression. Other factors also cause CYP inhibition or induction: the polycyclic aromatic hydrocarbons in cigarette smoke induce CYP3A4, 1A1, 1A2 and 2E1,[19] whereas grapefruit juice and several anti-retrovirals inhibit 3A4. Other significant drug interactions occur with antidepressants such as bupropion and fluoxetine, which inhibit CYP2D6.[20] An extensive list of clinically relevant inducers, inhibitors, and substrates of CYPs (originally developed by the late Dr David Flockhart) is available online.[21] Please see **Table 10-1** for an abbreviated version.

Phase 2 Synthetic Reactions

A phase 2 synthetic reaction adds a large hydrophilic group (most commonly a glucuronide or sulfate) to increase the water solubility of the metabolite to aid in elimination.[22] These reactions are catalysed by a large group of broad-specificity transferases. An example of a phase 2 synthetic reaction is the conjugation of a phosphatidyl group to ethanol. Phosphatidylethanol, or PEth, is polar and therefore hydrophilic thus facilitating renal excretion. PEth may be detected in blood for 2 to 4 weeks after abstinence from significant alcohol consumption.[23,24] PEth 16:0/18:1 concentrations above 20 ng/mL indicate "social drinking," while concentrations above 150 or 221 ng/mL (depending on the source) suggest chronic and excessive alcohol consumption.[25]

Uridine 5' diphospho-glucuronsyl transferase (UGTs) have genetic polymorphisms and some have differing activity during pregnancy.[26]

Elimination

Elimination refers to disappearance of the parent and/or active metabolite from the bloodstream or body, which can occur by metabolism and/or excretion.

The term *clearance* (Cl) represents the theoretical volume of plasma that is completely cleared of drug in a given period of time. The factors that determine hepatic clearance are hepatic blood flow, the fraction of drug that is unbound, and the drug's intrinsic clearance. If the *intrinsic clearance* of an unbound drug is very large, blood flow to the liver becomes rate limiting. If the intrinsic clearance of an unbound drug is very small, then this metabolic capacity (ie, intrinsic clearance) of the liver, rather than hepatic blood flow, becomes the major determinant of hepatic clearance. In this case, activity of hepatic enzymes determines drug clearance. Metabolic capacity determines drug clearance in most cases.

Most drugs display *first-order elimination* kinetics: the *fraction* or *percentage* of the total amount of drug present in the body removed over time is constant and *independent* of dose. Following administration of a drug with first-order kinetics, concentrations show an exponential decline over time. The slope of this decay line is the elimination rate constant (k_{eel}), which is the percent of drug cleared per unit time (eg, percent/hour).

The *half-life* ($t_{1/2}$) of a drug with first-order elimination kinetics is the amount of time it takes for a drug concentration to decrease by half. For example, if the concentration at 2 hours postdose is 100 µg/mL, and the concentration at 5 hours postdose is 50 µg/mL, the $t_{1/2}$ is 3 hours. One half-life represents a 50% change and 2, 3, 4, and 5 half-lives represent 75%, 87.5%, 93.7% and 96.8% change, respectively. For drugs with dose-independent (first-order) elimination, five half-lives is a reasonable estimate of the time to reach steady-state. The amount of drug in the body at steady-state depends upon the dose and frequency of drug administration.

There is only one terminal half-life but, in some cases, there are multiple distribution half-lives, describing distribution of drug into multiple body compartments, eg, well-perfused (circulating blood volume), then CNS, and then less well-perfused compartments.

Half-life is directly related to the volume of distribution and inversely related to clearance. Conditions which increase the volume of distribution, such as increases in body fat for lipid soluble drugs or increases in body water for water soluble drugs, will increase the half-life, and conditions which decrease drug clearance, such as renal or hepatic dysfunction, will also increase the half-life. Drug elimination is best described by an exponential process, that is, log linear decline.

For drugs with *zero-order elimination* kinetics, the *amount* of drug removed (rather than the fraction of drug removed) at any one time is constant and *dependent* on dose. The maximal rate of metabolism and/or elimination is generally due to saturation of a key enzyme. This zero-order process is described by the Michaelis-Menten equation. Because half-life is inversely related to clearance and clearance changes with drug concentration, the half-life is not constant. Therefore, half-life is not a useful descriptor for drugs with zero-order elimination.

For drugs with zero-order kinetics, a small increase in dose can cause a large increase in concentration. This is in contrast to drugs with first-order kinetics, where there is proportionality between dose and concentration. Aspirin, phenytoin, and ethanol are examples of drugs with zero-order elimination kinetics.[27] See **Figure 10-1** for a calculation of the decline in blood alcohol concentrations over time.

A clinically useful concept is the context-sensitive half time, defined as the time associated with a 50% decrease in

TABLE 10-1 Inhibitors, Inducers and Substrates of Cytochrome P450 Isozymes

Inhibitors	Inducers	Substrates		Inhibitors	Inducers	Substrates	
CYP1A2				**CYP3A4**			
cimetidine fluoroquinolones macrolides fluvoxamine isoniazid	barbiturates carbamazepine charcoal-broiled foods omeprazole phenytoin rifampin smoking	caffeine clozapine cyclobenzaprine mirtazapine olanzapine propranolol ropinirole R-warfarin Tricyclic antidepressants zileuton		amiodarone azole antifungals cyclosporine danazol delavirdine diltiazem efavirenz ethinylestradiol grapefruit juice indinavir macrolides nelfinavir quinine ritonavir saquinavir verapamil	barbiturates carbamazepine efavirenz ethosuximide griseofulvin modafinil nevirapine oxcarbazepine phenytoin rifamycins St John's wort	amlodipine amprenavir atorvastatin azole antifungals benzodiazepines buspirone carbamazepine citalopram clomipramine corticosteroids cyclosporine dapsone delavirdine diltiazem disopyramide dofetilide donepezil efavirenz ethinylestradiol felodipine fentanyl analogs finasteride imipramine indinavir isradipine lansoprazole loratadine losartan lovastatin macrolides methadone mirtazapine montelukast nefazodone nelfinavir nicardipine nifedipine nimodipine nisoldipine pimozide	quetiapine quinidine quinine repaglinide rifabutin ritonavir saquinavir sertraline sibutramine sildenafil simvastatin tacrolimus tamoxifen testosterone tolterodine verapamil R-warfarin zaleplon zileuton zolpidem zonisamide

(Continued)

TABLE 10-1 Inhibitors, Inducers and Substrates of Cytochrome P450 Isozymes (*Continued*)

Inhibitors	Inducers	Substrates		Inhibitors	Inducers	Substrates	
CYP2C9							
amiodarone cimetidine isoniazid metronidazole azole antifungals	barbiturates carbamazepine rifamycins St John's wort	carvedilol celecoxib diclofenac ibuprofen losartan montelukast naproxen phenytoin S-warfarin					
CYP2C19							
fluoxetine modafinil omeprazole oxcarbazepine	None	amitriptyline citalopram clomipramine diazepam imipramine lansoprazole phenytoin omeprazole R-warfarin					
CYP2D6							
amiodarone chloroquine cimetidine clomipramine diphenhydramine fluoxetine haloperidol paroxetine perphenazine quinacrine quinidine ritonavir sertraline terbinafine	None	amitriptyline carvedilol chlorpromazine clomipramine clozapine codeine desipramine dextromethorphan dihydrocodeine donepezil flecainide fluoxetine haloperidol hydrocodone imipramine loratadine methamphetamine	metoprolol mexiletine mirtazapine nortriptyline oxycodone paroxetine perphenazine propranolol risperidone ritonavir thioridazine timolol tolterodine tramadol trazodone venlafaxine				

Adapted from Flockhart DA, Thacker D, McDonald C, Desta Z. The Flockhart Cytochrome P450 Drug-Drug Interaction Table. Division of Clinical Pharmacology, Indiana University School of Medicine (Updated 2021). Accessed December 28, 2023. https://drug-interactions.medicine.iu.edu/.

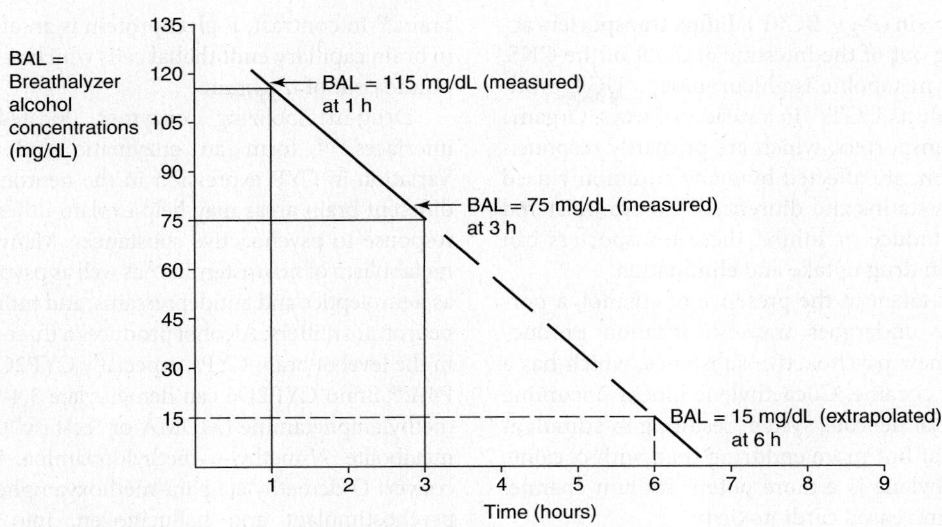

Figure 10-1. Extrapolating the decrease in blood alcohol concentration from two prior readings.

$$\text{Slope} = \frac{115\ \text{mg/dL} - 75\ \text{mg/dL}}{2\ \text{hours}}$$

$$= \frac{40\ \text{mg/dL}}{2\ \text{hours}} = 20\frac{\text{mg/dL}}{\text{hours}}$$

Expect at 4 hours, BAL to be 55 mg/dL; 5 hours, BAL to be 35 mg/dL; 6 hours, BAL to be 15 mg/dL; and 7 hours, BAL to have already reached 0.00 mg/dL.

drug concentration in a specific compartment of interest. For example, some drugs, such as midazolam, exert pharmacodynamic effects in the CNS but are inactive in other body compartments. As a result, consideration of the overall half-life alone may provide a misleading clinical picture.[28]

Excretion

Excretion is the process of removing a compound from the body without chemically changing that compound. Drugs can be excreted into the urine or feces, exhaled through the lungs (anesthetic gasses and volatile compounds), and secreted through the sweat and salivary glands.

Excretion of drugs by the kidney involves three main mechanisms: Glomerular filtration of the unbound drug, active secretion of both free and protein-bound drugs utilizing transporters (ie, ionized or conjugated compounds such as urate, choline, and glucuronide/sulfate), anions (ie, urate, penicillin, glucuronide, sulfate conjugates), or cations (ie, choline and histamine), and urinary concentration via a countercurrent multiplication process in the medullary interstitium, followed by osmotic equilibration of fluid in the collecting duct and passage out through the urine.[29]

Fecal excretion takes place when drugs enter the liver, are then excreted into the bile, which flows into the intestine and gets incorporated into feces, or move directly from the blood to the intestine and feces. Glandular excretion occurs through elimination of unchanged drug via sweat, saliva, and milk ducts.

DRUG-DRUG INTERACTIONS

Drug-drug interactions can occur by pharmacokinetic and pharmacodynamic mechanisms.

Pharmacokinetic drug interactions alter drug absorption, distribution, metabolism, or elimination. One drug either inhibits or induces (enhances) the activity of an enzyme metabolizing another drug, thereby altering the latter drug's pharmacokinetics (see **Table 10-1**). As an example, methadone is metabolized primarily by liver CYP3A4 and CYP2B6, with contributions from CYP2C19, CYP2D6, and CYP2C9.[30] Inhibitors of CYP3A4, including erythromycin, diltiazem, ketoconazole, and saquinavir, slow the metabolism of methadone and increase methadone concentrations. Inducers of CYP3A4, such as carbamazepine, phenobarbital, efavirenz, and St John's wort, increase the metabolism of methadone and decrease methadone concentrations.[31] Awareness of potential interactions, clinical observation, and tailoring medication regimens and dosages are needed to optimize therapy and minimize potential toxicities. Brain cytochromes, which metabolize endogenous and exogenous compounds, can also be altered by the exogenously administered drugs.[32]

Pharmacokinetic drug-drug interactions can also be caused by non–CYP enzymes and transporters, UDP-glucuronosyltransferases (UGTs), uptake transporters including organic anion transporters (OATs), organic anion transporting polypeptides (OATPs), organic cation transporters (OCTs), and efflux transporters P-glycoprotein and breast cancer resistance protein (*P-gp*, BCRP). Efflux transporters actively transport drug out of the intestine and out of the CNS. Morphine's primary metabolite is glucuronide, a UGT product. Cannabinoids affects UGTs[33] in a variety of ways. Organic anion and cation transporters, which are primarily responsible for renal secretion. are affected by many commonly used medications, such as statins and diuretics.[34] Co-administered medications which induce or inhibit these transporters can have a major effect on drug uptake and elimination.

When cocaine is taken in the presence of ethanol, a portion of the cocaine undergoes transesterification producing cocaethylene, a new psychoactive substance, which has a longer half-life than cocaine. Cocaethylene blocks dopamine reuptake in the central nervous system resulting in stimulant effects that are similar but more enduring than with cocaine. In the heart, cocaethylene is a more potent sodium channel blocker resulting in increased cardiotoxicity.[35,36]

Interactions can also occur by protein binding displacement of highly protein bound drugs (>90% bound)—increasing the free fraction of a drug increases the fraction of active drug. Warfarin, due to its high percentage of protein binding, narrow therapeutic index, and metabolism by CYP isoforms, is affected both by protein binding displacement and induction or inhibition of CYPs.[37]

pH changes caused by a medication can affect absorption and elimination. Proton pump inhibitors and H2 blockers raise gastic pH, reducing calcium and iron absorption.[38] Sodium bicarbonate increases urinary pH, increasing the urinary solubility of methotrexate (a weak acid).[39]

Pharmacodynamic drug interactions are either additive (total effect is the sum of individual drug effects), synergistic (total effect is greater than the sum of individual drug effects), or antagonistic (total effect is less than the sum of individual drug effects). These interactions are related to the action of the drugs. For example, opioids cause sedation; ingestion of other drugs causing sedation (eg, benzodiazepines) may cause increased sedation (additive or synergistic), albeit by different mechanisms of action. Cocaine administered with heroin, on the other hand, would provide an antagonistic effect between the stimulant (cocaine) and sedative (heroin) actions.[40]

PHARMACOKINETICS AND THE BRAIN

The blood-brain barrier hinders the ability of non–lipid-soluble drugs to reach brain tissue by passive diffusion from the bloodstream.[41] The endothelial cells lining brain capillaries have tight junctions which do not permit small (<25K daltons) molecules to pass through, unlike the fenestrated capillaries found outside the CNS. This blood-brain barrier is found throughout the brain and spinal cord central to the arachnoid membrane, except for the floor of the hypothalamus and the area postrema, including the chemoreceptor trigger zone (where direct-acting chemicals can provoke vomiting).

Active transport systems enable glucose, amino acids, amines, purines, nucleosides, and organic acids to access the brain.[42] In contrast, P-glycoprotein is an efflux carrier present in brain capillary endothelial cells which actively exports compounds out of the brain.

Drug-metabolizing enzymes located at blood-brain interfaces.[43,44] form an enzymatic and metabolic barrier. Variation in CYP expression in the neuronal and glial cells in different brain areas may help explain differences in individual response to psychoactive substances. Many CYPs catalyze the metabolism of neurosteroids[45] as well as psychoactive drugs such as neuroleptics and antidepressants, and influence the activity of neurotransmitters. Alcohol produces a three- to fivefold increase in the level of brain CYPs, especially CYP2C, CYP2E1, and CYP4A.[46] Brain CYP2D6 can demethylate 3,4-methylenedioxy-*N*-methylamphetamine (MDMA or "ecstasy") forming a harmful metabolite, *N*-methyl-α-methyldopamine. Brain CYP2D6 can convert *O*-demethylate para-methoxyamphetamine, a synthetic psychostimulant and hallucinogen, into 4-hydroxyamphetamine, which is also toxic.[47] Ethanol-induced brain CYP2E1 in rats contributes to increased formation of reactive oxygen species and ethanol-induced neurotoxicity.[48] People who smoke have higher levels of brain CYP2D6 in their basal ganglia, which by increasing the metabolism and elimination of neurotoxic substances might be neuroprotective for Parkinson disease.[48]

Novel brain CYPs, such as 5α-androstane-3β, 17β-diol hydroxylase, CYP7B, and CYP2D4, continue to be discovered.[49,50] Because the level of CYPs in the brain is approximately 0.5% to 2% of those in the liver and because brain CYP isoenzymes are of different types than those found in the liver, brain CYPs appear to be locally active but contribute little to overall pharmacokinetics of drugs in the body. The regulation of CYP isozyme expression in the brain and the demonstration of novel brain transporter pathways[51] are active areas of research.

PHARMACOKINETICS AND PREGNANCY

During pregnancy, the volume of distribution, protein binding and drug metabolism are significantly altered.[52] Pregnancy is associated with increased cardiac output, hepatic and portal vein blood flow, and increased unbound fraction of drugs, primarily due to hypoalbuminemia. During the third trimester of pregnancy, there is increased expression of CYP3A4 and UGT1A4. This leads to increased metabolism of buprenorphine, and contributes to the need for higher doses and increased frequency of buprenorphine dosing.[53,54] Increased CYP3A4 expression in the liver, intestine, and plasma also accelerates methadone metabolism. In a case report, the half-life of methadone fell from an average of 22 to 24 hours in nonpregnant women to 8.1 hours in a pregnant woman carrying twins.[55]

The placenta performs drug distribution and metabolic functions during pregnancy. Most transport from the maternal to fetal circulation occurs passively, so that protein binding, molecular weight, ionization, and lipophilicity affect transport. Lipid soluble opioids readily pass through the placenta to the fetus. Fentanyl is more lipophilic than morphine and so passes more readily. Nicotine is also transferred. The placenta has transporters, including the efflux transporter P-glycoprotein (Pgp), and the ability to metabolize compounds much like the liver. Placental metabolic enzymes become more mature as the pregnancy proceeds.[56,57]

Drug metabolizing enzymes in the fetal liver are much less active than in an adult. The fetal kidney is not an efficient route of elimination because excreted drug enters the amniotic fluid, which is swallowed by the fetus.[58] Fetal liver, kidney, and Pgp in the CNS become more mature as the fetus matures.

Since 1999, there has been a dramatic increase in the number of infants born to opioid-addicted mothers in the United States.[59,60] Many pregnant women use one or more other psychoactive substances, resulting in prenatal exposure of the fetus.[61] This prenatal exposure to a combination of addictive substances such as opioids, nicotine, alcohol, and benzodiazepines creates a complex withdrawal picture in the neonate.[62] Careful monitoring and treatment are necessary to avoid the cycle of recurrences of use alternating with an abstinence syndrome which are dangerous to the mother and fetus.[63] The literature on the preferred pharmacological management of neonatal withdrawal is evolving.[64]

PHARMACODYNAMICS

Pharmacodynamics refers to drug effects on the body and the body's homeostatic response. Most drugs act on specific endogenous targets, or receptors, to modulate the body's endogenous functions. Receptors and their associated effector and transducer proteins coordinate signals from multiple ligands with the metabolic activities of the cell to act as integrators of this information.

Potency, Efficacy, and Dose-Response

When the effect of a drug is plotted against the drug dose on a logarithmic scale, a sigmoidal curve often results (**Fig. 10-2**). The *efficacy* of a drug is the nature and strength of its effect when interacting with its receptor and associated effector system. *Potency* denotes the amount of drug needed to produce a given effect, often measured in terms of the concentration of drug needed to produce a 50% maximal effect (EC_{50}). Potency is primarily determined by the affinity of the drug for its receptor. Fentanyl illustrates the importance of potency. Even a small amount of street drug contamination with fentanyl can be fatal, as fentanyl is highly potent. In general, low potency is important only if it results in the medication having to be administered in undesirably large amounts. Because medication doses are readily adjusted, it is the maximal efficacy that is more often clinically relevant.

A similar sigmoidal curve is attained when the percentage of receptors that bind a drug is plotted against log drug concentration. The concentration at which 50% of the receptors are bound is denoted K_d, which is the dissociation rate at equilibrium. The maximum number of receptors bound is termed B_{max}. Both "dose-response" and "dose-receptor–bound" graphs have a linear or nearly linear middle segment, indicating a first-order process. As the concentration of a drug increases, a constant proportion of the drug binds to the receptor, causing a proportionate drug effect.

A system is said to have *spare receptors* when the activation of fewer than 50% of the receptors achieves 50% of maximal effect. This determination is made by comparing the EC_{50}, with K_d. If the EC_{50} is less than the K_d, spare receptors are present.[65] The presence of spare receptors does not alter the maximal biological response, but it does increase the sensitivity to the

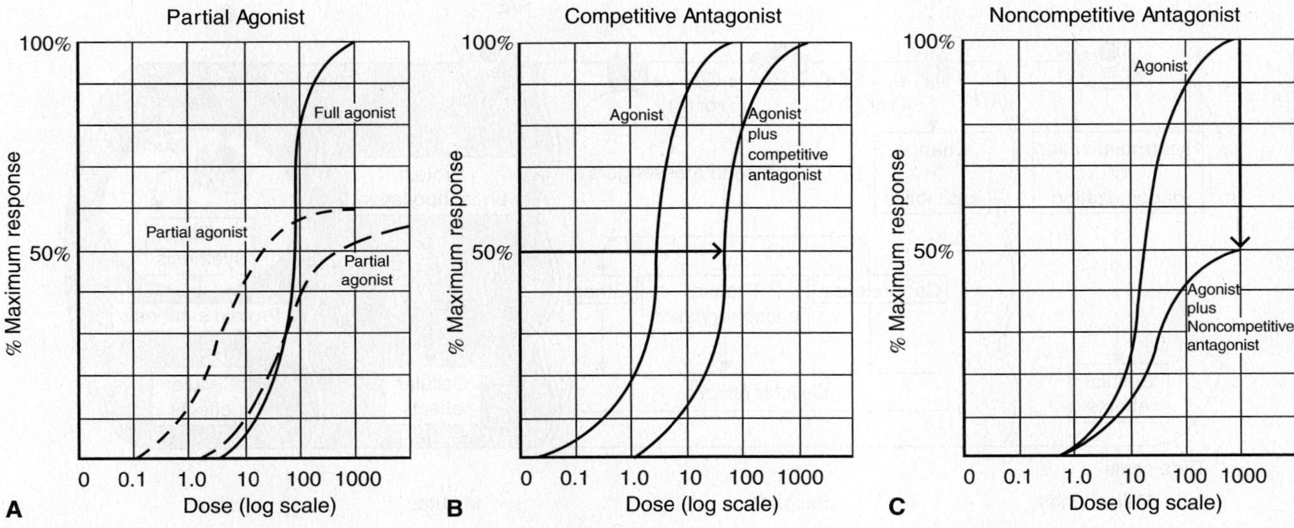

Figure 10-2. Full agonist, partial agonist, and competitive and noncompetitive antagonists. **A.** No matter how much the dose is increased, a partial agonist always will have a lower maximal efficiency (E_{max}). A partial agonist may be more potent, less potent, or equally potent as the agonist. In this example, both partial agonists decrease E_{max}. However, one partial agonist is more potent, and the other partial agonist is equipotent, when compared to the full agonist. **B.** If there are no spare receptors, competitive agonists increase the EC_{50} but do not alter the other E_{max}. **C.** Noncompetitive antagonists decrease the E_{max}. (Modified from Katzung BG, Masters SB. Pharmacodynamics. In: *Katzung and Trevor's Pharmacology Examination and Board Review*. Lange Medical Books/McGraw Hill; 2002:13.)

drug ligand. This relationship occurs because drug-receptor interactions are more likely when there are proportionately more available receptors.

A graded dose-response graph is attained when the response of a particular receptor-effector system is measured against increasing concentrations of drug. A quantal dose-response graph is achieved when the log dose of a drug is plotted against the cumulative percentage of a population that respond to it. The results of animal experiments can be plotted in this manner to discern the *median effective dose* (ED_{50}), *median toxic dose* (TD_{50}), and *median lethal dose* (LD_{50}). The *therapeutic index* is defined as the ratio of the TD_{50} to the ED_{50}. Because it is unethical to design experiments using a full range of drug doses to determine these indices in humans, the range of therapeutic drug concentrations and the margin of safety are estimated more broadly through extrapolation from animal studies, human drug trials, and clinical experience. In practice, both the risks and benefits of prescribing a medication are taken into account when making therapeutic decisions. Judgment about the clinically acceptable risk of toxicity often is influenced by the severity of the disease being treated.

Receptors

A *receptor* is an endogenous target to which a drug or other molecule (termed a ligand) binds. Receptors on membranes act as transducers for ligands, whether endogenous or exogenous. Ligand binding to a receptor triggers downstream effects.[66]

Receptors contain at least two functional domains: a ligand-binding site and an effector or message propagation (ie, signaling) site. Receptors can be grouped into four common types: (i) ligand-gated ion channels, (ii) G protein–coupled receptor signaling, (iii) receptors with intrinsic enzymatic activity, and (iv) receptors regulating nuclear transcription. Target cells integrate signals from multiple receptors to produce sequential, additive, synergistic, or inhibitory responses. (See **Fig. 10-3** for types of receptor-effector linkages and **Table 10-2** for a mechanistic classification of drugs involved in substance use disorders.)

Ligand-Gated Ion Channels

These receptors selectively gate the flow of ions into the cell through transmembrane channels. Each unit of these multi-subunit proteins spans the plasma membrane several times. The association of the subunits allows the formation of a wall or pore. Ligand binding to single or multiple subunits enables these subunits to rapidly and cooperatively control channel opening and closing. Excitatory neurotransmitters (eg, acetylcholine and glutamate) result in a net inward current of cations such as Na^+, Ca^{2+}, and K^+, which depolarize the cell and increase the generation of action potentials. In contrast, inhibitory neurotransmitters (eg, GABA and glycine) result in the net inward flux of anions, such as Cl^-, which hyperpolarize the cell and decrease the generation of action potentials.

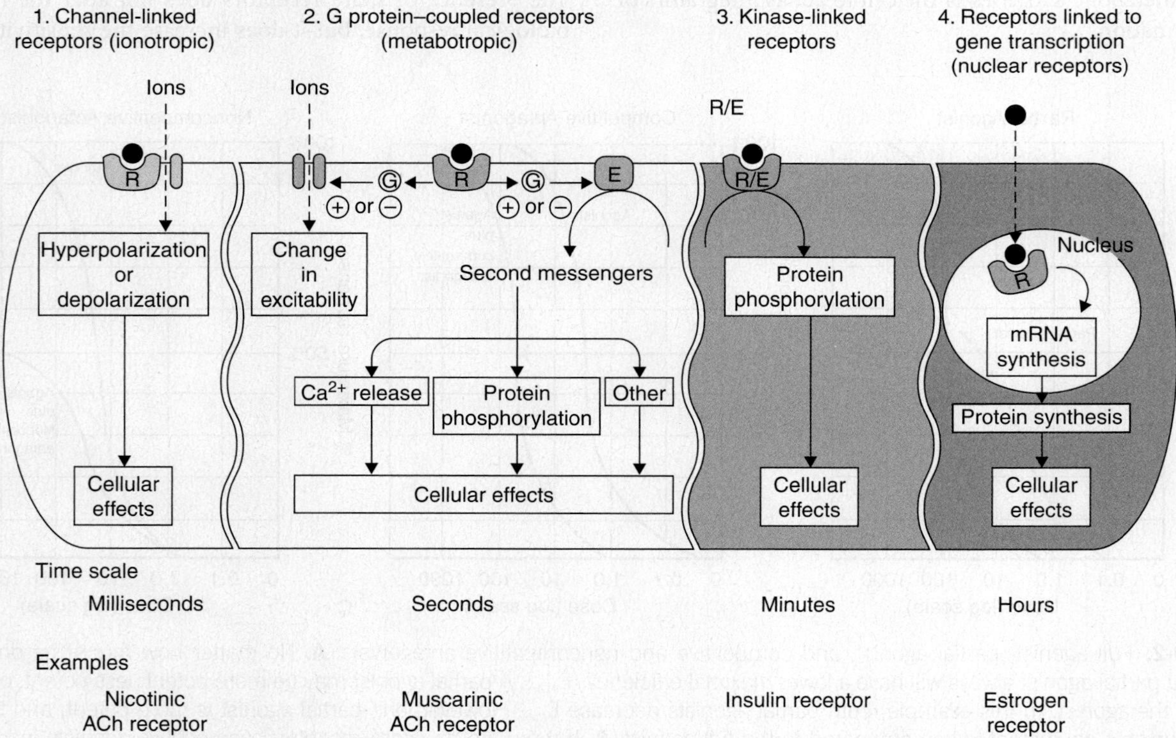

Figure 10-3. Types of receptor-effector linkage. (From Rang HP, Dale MM, Ritter JM, et al., eds. *Pharmacology*. 5th ed. Churchill Livingstone; 2003.)

TABLE 10-2 The Mechanistic Classification of Drugs Involved in Substance Use Disorders

Name	Main molecular target	Pharmacology	Effect on dopamine (DA) neurons
Drugs that bind to ionotropic receptors and ion channels			
Nicotine	nAChR	Agonist	Disinhibition
Alcohol	$GABA_AR$, $5\text{-}HT_3R$, nAChR, NMDAR, Kir3 channels	—	Disinhibition
Benzodiazepines	$GABA_AR$	Positive modulator	Disinhibition
Phencyclidine, ketamine, dextromethorphan	NMDAR	Antagonist	—
Drugs that activate G protein–coupled receptors			
Opioids	-OR (G_{io})	Agonist	Excitation, disinhibition (?)
Cannabinoids	CB1R (G_{io})	Agonist	Excitation, disinhibition (?)
γ-Hydroxybutyric acid	$GABA_BR$ (G_{io})	Weak agonist	Disinhibition
LSD, mescaline, psilocybin	$5\text{-}HT_{2A}R$ (G_q)	Partial agonist	—
Drugs that bind to transporters of biogenic amines			
Cocaine	DAT, SERT, NET	Inhibitor	Blocks DA uptake
Amphetamine	DAT, NET, SERT, VMAT	Reverses transport	Blocks DA uptake, synaptic depletion
Methylenedioxymethamphetamine	SERT > DAT, NET	Reverses transport	Blocks DA uptake, synaptic depletion

5-HTxR, serotonin receptor; CB1R, cannabinoid-1; DAT, dopamine transporter; GABA, gamma-aminobutyric acid; Kir3 channels, G protein–coupled inwardly rectifying potassium channels; LSD, lysergic acid diethylamide; -OR, -opioid receptor; nAChR, nicotinic acetylcholine receptor; NET, norepinephrine transporter; NMDAR, *N*-methyl-D-aspartate receptor; SERT, serotonin transporter; VMAT, vesicular monoamine transporter; ?, data not available.

Ligand-gated channels enable rapid transmission of information across synapses. They are involved in synaptic plasticity required for learning and memory.[67]

G Proteins and Second Messengers

"Serpentine" receptors coupled to G-proteins have an extracellular amino (N) terminal and an intracellular carboxyl (C) terminal and commonly transverse the plasma membrane seven times. Ligands bind to G-protein receptors at a site surrounded by the transmembrane regions. This triggers a change of conformation that is transmitted to the cytoplasmic loops of the receptor that in turn activates the appropriate intracellular G-protein.[68] Examples of G protein coupled receptors include muscarinic acetylcholine receptors, receptors for adrenergic amines, most serotonin receptors, and many peptide hormone receptors.

G proteins modify the activity of intracellular regulatory proteins and/or ion channels, which in turn alter the activity of intracellular second messengers that enable signal transduction and amplification. Cells of different tissues may have different G protein-dependent responses to the same initial ligand (eg, norepinephrine, acetylcholine, serotonin).[69]

Major second messenger systems include cyclic adenosine monophosphate (cAMP) (by means of G_s and G_i), cyclic guanosine monophosphate (cGMP), and phosphoinositides (by means of G_q).[68,70] β-adrenergic amines, glucagon, histamine, serotonin, and numerous other hormones act on G_s to increase adenylyl cyclase and in turn increase the second messenger, cAMP, whereas 2-adrenergic amines, acetylcholine acting on muscarinic cholinergic receptors, opioids, serotonin, and others act on G_{i1}, G_{i2}, and G_{i3} to decrease adenylyl cyclase and in turn decrease cAMP. cAMP stimulates distinct cAMP-dependent protein kinases that are differentially expressed in varying tissues. When cAMP binds to the regulatory dimer (D) of the kinase, two catalytic (C) chains are released, which diffuse through the cytoplasm and nucleus, transferring phosphate from ATP to other specific enzymes and substrate proteins. When the hormonal stimulation stops, a diverse group of specific and nonspecific phosphatases quickly reverse the cAMP-induced phosphorylation of enzyme substrates, and cAMP is degraded to 5′AMP by several cyclic nucleotide phosphodiesterases.

The cGMP-based signal transduction mechanism closely parallels the cAMP-mediated signaling mechanism, but its presence is limited to a few tissues, including intestinal mucosa and vascular smooth muscle. Whereas methylxanthines (eg, caffeine and theophylline) act by competitively inhibiting cAMP degradation, sildenafil produces vasodilation by inhibiting specific phosphodiesterases and inhibiting cGMP degradation.

Receptors for G_q, including muscarinic acetylcholine, bombesin, serotonin ($5\text{-}HT_{1c}$), and others, act through G proteins or tyrosine kinases to stimulate phospholipase C in the cell membrane that splits phosphatidylinositol-4,5-bisphosphate (PIP_2) into two second messengers, diacylglycerol (DAG) and inositol-1,4,5-triphosphate (IP_3 or $InsP_3$). Confined to the membrane, diacylglycerol activates a phospholipid- and calcium-sensitive protein kinase C, whereas water-soluble IP_3 diffuses through the cytoplasm, enabling the release of Ca^{2+}. This signaling pathway is inactivated when IP_3 is dephosphorylated, and DAG is either phosphorylated to phosphatidic acid and converted back into phospholipids or deacylated to arachidonic acid, and Ca^{2+} is actively removed by calcium pumps from the cytoplasm. The phosphoinositide signaling pathway is more complex than the cAMP pathway, owing to multiple second messengers and protein kinases. For instance, more than nine structurally distinct types of protein kinase C have been identified. In addition, protein kinases of different cell types may have general or specific substrate targets.

Receptors With Intrinsic Enzyme Activity

Polypeptide receptors typically consist of an extracellular growth factor or hormone-binding domain connected to a cytoplasmic enzyme domain by a hydrophobic segment that crosses the plasma membrane's lipid bilayer. The cytoplasmic enzyme domain may be a tyrosine kinase, a serine/threonine kinase, or a guanylate cyclase that, when activated, catalyzes the activity of substrate proteins followed by additional downstream signaling proteins. For instance, when epidermal growth factor binds to its receptor, it converts the receptor from its inactive monomeric state to an active dimeric state of two noncovalently bound receptor polypeptides. The enzymatic cytoplasmic domains become activated and catalyze the phosphorylation of substrate proteins. Drugs may target the agonist binding site and/or the enzymatic activity of the receptor.

Receptors Regulating Nuclear Transcription

Receptors that regulate nuclear transcription are soluble DNA-binding proteins that include an N-terminal variable domain, a DNA binding domain, a hinge region, and a C-terminal hormone binding domain. Type 1 nuclear receptors are bound to accessory heat shock proteins located in the cytoplasm of the cell. On activation, the heat shock protein dissociates and two steroid-receptor proteins dimerize and translocate to the nucleus. Type 2 nuclear receptors present in the nucleus are activated by the ligand entering through nuclear pores.[71] Once activated, both types of receptors bind to specific DNA sequences (called *response elements*) on the genome to activate or inhibit transcription of the nearby gene. Examples of Type 1 nuclear receptors include targets for sex hormones (androgen, estrogen, and progesterone receptors), glucocorticoid, and mineralocorticoid receptors. Examples of type 11 nuclear receptors include the thyroid/retinoid family consisting of thyroid hormone, vitamin D, and retinoic acid receptors. These hormone-mediated gene actions require time for synthesis of new proteins. They have a relatively slower onset and offset of action, which can take hours to days.

Ligand-Receptor Interactions

Affinity of a ligand refers to the tightness of its binding to the receptor, which is often measured in terms of the fraction of ligand that is bound at a particular concentration. The dissociation constant (K_d) reflects the inverse of binding strength, that is, the lower the K_d, the higher the affinity (strength of binding). *Intrinsic activity* refers to the ligands ability to evoke a response after binding to the receptor.

Receptors can exist in multiple conformational states: active, inactive, partially active, and selectively active and those that produce nonproductive signaling. If the inactive state predominates, there will be little or no downstream effect in the absence of a drug.

When drugs bind to receptors, the relative affinity of the drug for various conformations of the receptor will determine the extent to which the equilibrium is shifted toward the active state. A drug is considered an *agonist* or a *positive allosteric modulator* if binding to the receptor produces a biochemical response similar to that of an endogenous ligand. Agonists bind to the same site as the endogenous ligand, while allosteric modulators bind to a receptor site that is topographically distinct from the primary agonist binding site. The allosteric modulation can be either full or partial depending upon the degree of the elicited response. Even at saturating concentrations, *allosteric partial positive modulators (partial agonists)* will not produce a full response, sometimes termed a ceiling effect (see **Fig. 10-2**).

Buprenorphine is an example of a highly potent mu opioid receptor (MOR) partial agonist. The drug has a high affinity for MORs and, depending on the relative concentrations, may displace full agonists such as morphine and methadone from these receptors. At the receptor level, buprenorphine is competing with full mu agonists but is exerting only partial agonist effects, thereby potentially precipitating withdrawal in the opioid physically dependent individual. Because buprenorphine is a partial agonist, higher doses have a longer duration of action but not a stronger effect. This ceiling effect makes buprenorphine safer than full agonists such as methadone in that respiratory depression is less likely.

Biased agonism refers to the preferential activation of second messenger and downstream pathways after agonist-receptor binding (see **Fig. 10-4**). Preferential signaling may occur differently depending upon the specific receptor subtype.[69] For example, opioid receptors (mu, delta, and kappa) have two intracellular signaling pathways: G-protein and β-arrestin.[72] These pathways mediate different effects of opioids, for example, analgesia or nausea and respiratory depression, respectively. An unbiased agonist activates both pathways equally. Existing opioid mediations are unbiased agonists. Biased agonists activate one pathway more than the other.[69] Drug development aims to use biased agonism to develop more selective compounds that produce desired clinical effects with minimal side-effects.

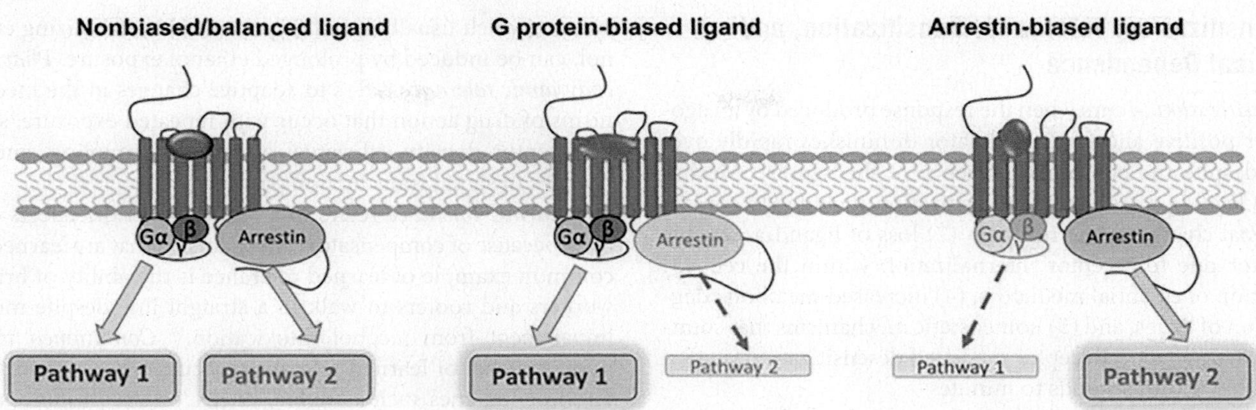

Figure 10-4. Signaling of biased agonists. In most cases agonists regarded as nonbiased can efficiently activate both G protein- and arrestin-dependent signaling. Relative to this, biased agonists preferentially activate either G protein- or arrestin-dependent signaling as shown in *bold arrows*. (From Conibear AE, Kelly E. A biased view of mu-opioid receptors. *Mol Pharm.* 2019;96(5):542-549. doi:10.1124/mol.119.115956.)

Attempts to develop a biased agonist at the MOR that produces analgesia without respiratory depression have not been successful to date.[73] The direct measurement of the degree of bias is difficult and may be dependent on the cellular assay.[74]

Neutral allosteric modulators or *antagonists* bind to a receptor but have no intrinsic activity, that is, they don't trigger a downstream response. Thus, their presence prevents a positive allosteric modulator or agonist from binding to the receptor and inducing a response.[75] Antagonists physically block access of the agonist to the receptor, whereas neutral allosteric modulators interact at a different site on the receptor to diminish the ability of the agonist to bind to its primary site. Competitive antagonists or neutral allosteric modulators are reversible by adding additional agonist or positive allosteric modulators. Naloxone is an example of a competitive neutral allosteric modulator at MOR. The effects of *noncompetitive antagonists* cannot be overcome by the addition of agonist or positive allosteric modulators because they cause a conformational change in the receptor. Ketamine is an example of a noncompetitive antagonist of the NMDA receptor. Ketamine binds to a site deep within an open NMDA ion channel and can remain in the channel when it closes, occluding the flow of ions through that channel.[76,77]

Negative allosteric modulators or *inverse agonists* bind the same receptor site as positive allosteric modulators or agonists but exert the opposite downstream effect. Inverse agonists have preferential affinity for inactive receptor conformations, rather than shifting equilibrium toward the active conformation, as would a positive allosteric modulator (agonist). If the basal equilibrium lies in the direction of the inactive receptor, there will be little change in activity, and it will be difficult to distinguish negative allosteric modulation from neutral allosteric modulation.[78] This concept gives rise to that of "constitutive activity" which implies ongoing receptor activity without a bound ligand. Receptors can be constitutively in an active conformation, or they can be activated by physiological events even in the absence of a positive allosteric modulator. If a drug were to block this tonic activity, it would perhaps be considered a negative allosteric modulator or an inverse agonist.[79] It would be considered a negative allosteric modulator if it blocked tonic activity by operating at a receptor site that was topographically distinct from the primary agonist binding site, or it would be considered an inverse agonist if it blocked tonic activity by operating at the same site as the endogenous ligand. Negative allosteric modulator medications may be clinically useful if they can selectively prevent the adverse aspects of receptor activation.[78]

Agents that act at $GABA_A$-gated chloride ion channels illustrate the spectrum of positive and neutral modulating allosteric (agonist and antagonist) activities. The endogenous agonist GABA acts at this receptor to produce inhibitory, hyperpolarizing postsynaptic potentials. This activity produces an assortment of sedative, anxiolytic, and anticonvulsant effects. Both barbiturates and benzodiazepines are exogenous positive allosteric modulators that act at the GABA receptor. Binding of each of these drugs to the GABA receptor complex occurs at distinct sites and facilitates the activity of GABA to open the chloride ion channel. Benzodiazepines increase the frequency of GABA-mediated chloride ion channel opening, whereas barbiturates increase the *duration* of this opening.[80] Bicuculline, a competitive antagonist of GABA, binds selectively to the GABA site, interfering with GABA binding to that site. In contrast, picrotoxin, a noncompetitive antagonist of GABA, binds to the barbiturate site on the receptor, blocking the channel directly. Beta-carboline is a negative allosteric modulator that reduces chloride ion conductance and increases excitability and irritability of the central nervous system. Flumazenil, a GABA neutral allosteric modulator has therapeutic utility in treating benzodiazepine overdose. Flumazenil does not antagonize the actions of ethanol or barbiturates. However, by removing the tonic chloride ion gated flow at the receptor, flumazenil may precipitate the onset of seizures if given in the clinical setting of chronic ethanol or barbiturate use.[81]

Desensitization, Tolerance, Sensitization, and Physical Dependence

Desensitization occurs when the response produced by an agonist or positive allosteric modulator diminishes rapidly over time despite the continued presence of the agonist. Mechanisms leading to receptor desensitization include (1) conformational change in the receptor, (2) loss of ligand-accessible receptor due to receptor internalization within the cell, (3) depletion of essential mediators, (4) increased metabolic degradation of drugs, and (5) homeostatic mechanisms that counteract drug effect.[82] Receptor mediated desensitization is often reversible within seconds to minutes.

Desensitization may be homologous or heterologous. Homologous desensitization indicates feedback directed to the specific receptor molecule, whereas heterologous desensitization (also known as cross desensitization) extends to the action of all receptors that share a common signaling pathway. Heterologous desensitization may also involve inhibition of one or more downstream proteins that participate in signaling from other receptors. For instance, desensitization of some G protein-coupled receptors involves phosphorylation of specific residues by G-protein receptor kinases (homologous desensitization) or PKA (heterologous desensitization) enzymes.[83]

Positive allosteric modulators (agonists) can induce endocytosis and membrane trafficking of receptors. For example, β-arrestin accelerates endocytosis of receptors from the plasma membrane by binding to endocytic structures in the plasma membrane called *coated pits*. This endocytosis can either result in the receptor's recycling through the plasma membrane with continued cellular responsiveness or cause receptor trafficking into lysosomes that degrade the receptor, causing downregulation and attenuated cellular responsiveness. Increased endocytosis and recycling of opioid receptors in the plasma membrane (created by a knock-in mouse expressing mutant MOR) is associated with continued morphine analgesia but reduced tolerance and physical dependence.[84,85] Changes at the MOR, including phosphorylation and internalization, are biochemical components of desensitization.[86]

Tolerance and sensitization reflect changes in response with repeated drug use. *Tolerance* is the reduction in response to a drug after its repeated administration. Tolerance shifts the dose-response curve to the right, requiring higher doses to achieve the same effect. *Sensitization* indicates an increase in drug response after its repeated administration. Sensitization shifts the dose-response curve to the left, so that repeated doses cause a greater effect than that seen with the initial dose. Both tolerance and sensitization can take days, weeks, and even longer for recovery.

Tolerance and sensitization develop more readily to some drug effects than to others. For example, tolerance to the opioid-induced "high" or euphoria develops more rapidly than tolerance to constipation and constricted pupils.[87]

Tolerance can occur by several mechanisms. *Pharmacokinetic tolerance* occurs as a consequence of increased metabolism of a drug, resulting in less drug being available at its site of action. For example, the microsomal ethanol-metabolizing system, which usually is not important in metabolizing ethanol, can be induced by prolonged ethanol exposure. *Pharmacodynamic tolerance* refers to adaptive changes in the mechanisms of drug action that occur with repeated exposure, such as receptor density, efficiency of receptor coupling, and/or changes in signal transduction pathways.[88]

Learned tolerance refers to a reduction in the effects of a drug because of compensatory mechanisms that are learned. A common example of learned tolerance is the ability of bridge workers and roofers to walk in a straight line despite motor impairment from alcohol intoxication.[89] *Conditioned tolerance*, a subset of learned tolerance, occurs when specific environmental cues such as sights, smells, or circumstances are paired with drug administration so that the drug response is altered by expectations when the drug is taken in the presence of the specific environmental cue. With expectation, the drug effect may be experienced before the drug is taken—and an adaptive response may be learned.[90]

Cross-tolerance occurs when tolerance to a specific drug generalizes to other drugs in that same structural or pharmacological category. Cross-tolerance can have therapeutic value, for example, cross-tolerance among alcohol, long-acting benzodiazepines, and barbiturates allows benzodiazepines (or barbiturates) to facilitate the smooth withdrawal of a patient with physical dependence on alcohol (see Section 7, "Management of Intoxication and Withdrawal").

Physical dependence or withdrawal develops as a result of physiological adaptation to repeated drug use. Withdrawal signs and symptoms occur in a physically dependent person when drug administration is stopped or substantially reduced. Tolerance and withdrawal are two of the 11 DSM-5-TR diagnostic criteria[91] for substance use disorder, but are neither necessary nor sufficient for making this diagnosis.

Patients who take prescribed medications for appropriate medical indications can show tolerance, physical dependence, and withdrawal if the medication is stopped abruptly or quickly tapered, even if they do not exhibit compulsive substance seeking and taking and other adverse consequences associated with a substance use disorder. Such tolerance or physical dependence to an appropriately taken prescribed medication is not considered a DSM-5-TR criterion for substance use disorder. For example, patients with chronic pain taking opioid analgesics may develop tolerance and physical dependence on their opioid analgesics, as evidenced by withdrawal signs and symptoms when the medication is quickly tapered or abruptly discontinued. Such patients do not fulfill the diagnostic criteria for an opioid use disorder[92] (see Section 13, "Pain and Addiction").

INDIVIDUAL DIFFERENCES IN DRUG RESPONSE AND ADDICTION SUSCEPTIBILITY

Pharmacogenomics

Pharmacogenetics refers to how variation in a single gene influences the pharmacology of a single drug. *Pharmacogenomics* encompasses how all of the genes (entire genome) can influence drug pharmacology. However, these terms are often used interchangeably.[93] Pharmacogenomic variants affect the probability of drug response or adverse drug reactions.[94]

Pharmacokinetic-related genetic polymorphisms lead to variations in the concentrations of drugs or their metabolites at the site of action. Pharmacodynamic-related genomic variations lead to variations in the physiological response to a drug, which is often measured at the whole-organism level. The genetic variations relating to the pharmacodynamics of drug response are less well described.[95]

The small percentage of the genome that differs among individuals can cause profound variation in phenotypes, including drug response. Genetic variability in drug-metabolizing enzymes can affect drug bioavailability and clearance.[96-99] Single nucleotide polymorphisms (SNPs), combinations of SNPs (haplotypes), insertions, deletions, and copy number variation may alter CYP activity.[96]

Genetically defined differences in drug metabolism may influence risk of addiction, with relative protection for persons who experience adverse drug reactions at lower drug doses. Both the ADH1B2-His47Arg allele of alcohol dehydrogenase 1B and the ALDH-Glu487Lys allele of aldehyde dehydrogenase 2 alone or together can lead to flushing, nausea, and headache after alcohol intake, owing to the accumulation of acetaldehyde.[100] Each of these alleles reduces the risk of alcohol use disorder, with an additive protective effect when both alleles are present. Persons of South Asian descent are likely to carry both alleles, whereas those with Jewish ancestry often carry the Arg47 allele. Heterozygous carriers of ALDH2 Lys487 have low concentrations of ALDH2 enzyme activity, whereas ALDH2 Lys487/Lys487 homozygotes are nearly completely protected from alcohol use disorder.[101] In addition, slow nicotine metabolism by CYP2D6 to cotinine appears to protect against nicotine addiction.[102]

Twin studies indicate approximately 50% of the risk for developing opioid use disorder is inherited.[103] Many alleles, each of small effect (odds ratio of <1.5) contribute to the genetic risk for opioid use disorder, including alleles in genes for potassium ion channel genes (KCNC1 and KCNG2), a glutamate receptor auxiliary protein (CNIH3), and the expression quantitative loci SNP, C allele of rs3778150, near the gene encoding the mu-opioid receptor (OPRM1) on chromosome 6.[104] Several genome-wide association studies have revealed variants (CYP2B6 and locus 300 kb 5' to the OPRM1 in African Americans) that impact methadone dose requirements.[104] Such findings may be used in the future to help clinicians select the optimum opioid agonist medication for individual patients.

Important genotypic influences on CYP2B6 enzyme function have been identified.[105] For instance, the *4 allele, which results in higher enzyme function than the wild type, has been associated with increased bupropion toxicity due to increased rates of conversion of bupropion to its active and longer-lasting metabolite, hydroxybupropion. Conversely, increasing the dose of bupropion (FDA-approved for for helping abstinence from tobacco) in poor metabolizers (PMs) improves tobacco abstinence rates.[106,107]

CYP2D6, which metabolizes codeine to morphine, is the best studied of the drug metabolic enzymes; over 100 alleles and numerous mutations have been identified.[108,109] Genotype and enzyme activity vary with genetic ancestry: from no gene/no enzyme activity (6% of those with European ancestry) to two copies of a fully active gene (33% of Ethiopians). Individuals can be characterized as PMs, intermediate metabolizers [IMs], extensive metabolizers [EMs], or ultra-rapid metabolizers [UMs]).[110] Those with PM phenotypes generally do not receive adequate analgesia from codeine due to limited conversion to the more potent morphine. UMs, on the other hand, metabolize codeine rapidly and extensively to morphine, producing life-threatening morphine intoxication.[111,112] Breast-feeding infants of mothers who are UMs may experience morphine overdoses when their mothers are prescribed codeine for postpartum pain relief.[113] After several case reports of excessive narcosis and unexpected postoperative death in children who were UMs of codeine, the FDA issued a black box warning regarding the administration of acetaminophen with codeine elixir in children following tonsillectomy.[114]

Tramadol is a prodrug that is metabolized, in part by CYP2D6, to the *O*-desmethyltramadol active metabolite, which has a 200-fold greater affinity for the MOR receptor than its parent compound. Similar to codeine, individuals who are CYP2D6 UMs should take lower than standard tramadol doses to avoid opioid side effects. Individuals who are CYP2D6 intermediate or poor metabolizers may experience reduced efficacy and inadequate analgesia at standard tramadol doses.[115]

Nonsteroidal anti-inflammatory drugs (NSAIDs) interfere with prostaglandin synthesis by reversibly inhibiting cyclooxygenase-1 (COX-1) and/or cyclooxygenase-2 (COX-2). Hepatic CYP2C9 enzyme contributes to the metabolism of many NSAIDs including ibuprofen, indomethacin, meloxicam, naproxen, piroxicam, celecoxib, and diclofenac. The CYP2C9 gene is highly polymorphic, with at least 61 variant alleles and multiple sub-alleles. Since CYP2C9 PMs have an increased risk of developing NSAID-induced gastrointestinal distress and bleeding, it is advised that CYP2C9 PMs begin with a starting NSAID dose of 25% to 50% the recommended maximum and that upward dose titration not be initiated until steady state has been achieved. It is also suggested that if NSAIDs are utilized, that meloxicam and piroxicam be substituted by NSAIDs with a shorter half-life.[115]

Another example of how genetic variations can predispose to adverse drug reactions is the interaction between several anticonvulsants, especially carbamazepine, and human leukocyte antigen (HLA) variant HLA-B*15:02. The human leukocyte antigen complex helps the immune system differentiate between its own proteins and foreign proteins. Individuals with HLA-B*15:02 are at increased risk of severe hypersensitivity reactions, including StevensJohnson syndrome and toxic epidermal necrolysis, from carbamazepine, oxcarbazepine, phenytoin, or lamotrigine (odds ratios of 80.7, 26.4, 5.65, and 2.4, respectively).[115] Therefore, testing for HLA-B*15:02 may be performed prior to initiating therapy. HLA-B*15:02 testing is particularly important in patients of Asian descent, and especially those from Hong Kong, Thailand, Malaysia, parts of the Philippines, Taiwan and India.[116]

Pharmacogenomic testing offers the possibility of more precise "personalized' therapeutics,[117,118] but it has been difficult to demonstrate clinical utility in large populations where drug response is influenced by complex multifactorial traits rather than a single genotype.[58] With many mental health disorders, there is only a modest correlation between a medication's plasma concentration and the patient's clinical response. Pharmacogenomic testing may afford a larger margin of safety in light of the narrow therapeutic window encountered with many psychotropic and pain medications.

The Pharmacogenomics Knowledgebase (PharmGKB; https://www.pharmgkb.org) collects, curates and disseminates knowledge about clinically actionable gene-drug associations and genotype-phenotype relationships.[119] Created in 2009 as a shared project between PharmGKB and NIH, the Clinical Pharmacogenetics Implementation Consortium (CPIC; www.cpicpgx.org) provides freely available, evidence-based, peer-reviewed, and updated pharmacogenetic clinical practice guidelines. The goal is to give clinical guidance on how to use genetic test results to adjust the use or dose of medications.[120,121] The recommendations for codeine, tramadol, carbamazepine, oxcarbazepine, phenytoin and lamotrigine mentioned above can be found on the CPIC website.

Epigenetics

Epigenetics are heritable and possibly reversible modifications in gene expression that occur without alterations in the DNA sequence.[122] Epigenetic factors such as DNA methylation and histone modifications may play a role in individual vulnerability to develop a substance use disorder, the response to substance use, and the response to pharmacotherapy.[123]

The development of epigenetic interventions to treat substance use disorders is made possible by the discovery of mechanisms that regulate DNA methylation and chromatin remodeling. Clinically useful epigenetic agents need to be directed to precise segments of DNA and targeted to specific brain regions.

Epigenomic editing can alter alcohol-seeking and anxiety behaviors in rats.[124] Adolescent alcohol exposure was associated with decreased activity-regulated cytoskeleton-associated protein (Arc), a key regulator of synaptic plasticity. Using the CRISPR-dCas9 system to increase histone acetylation at the Arc synaptic activity response element (SARE) normalized deficits in Arc expression. This attenuated adult anxiety and excessive alcohol drinking in rats who were exposed to alcohol during adolescence. In contrast, increased repressive histone methylation at the Arc SARE, decreased Arc expression, and produced anxiety and alcohol drinking in control rats who were not exposed to alcohol during adolescence. The CRISPR-dCas9 system functions by targeting a single gene. However, instead of modifying the DNA sequence, the CRISPR-dCas9 system modifies how tightly chromatin is condensed at a particular gene region by acetylating histones and other transcription-related proteins, changing the ease with which transcription-boosting activator proteins can access the genetic sequence.

SUMMARY

This chapter introduces the pharmacological principles that underlie the use of drugs for both therapeutic and nontherapeutic purposes. A key principle is the so-called rate hypothesis: the more rapid a drug is absorbed and reaches maximal concentration in the brain, that is, the more rapid the onset of action, the more reinforcing is that drug.

Pharmacokinetics, the processes of absorption, distribution, metabolism, and elimination, determine drug concentrations in the body. For example, effective opioid agonist treatment in pregnant women needs to take into consideration changes in the volume of distribution, metabolism and clearance of drugs that occur during pregnancy.

Orally administered drugs undergo first pass metabolism in the liver, whereas drugs administered intravenously, intranasally, buccally, transdermally, or by inhalation enter the systemic circulation directly, bypassing the liver. Drugs may undergo specific enzymatic and synthetic reactions prior to elimination. Pharmacokinetic drug-drug interactions occur when one drug induces or inhibits the metabolizing enzymes of another drug. Drug-drug interactions also can cause changes in free drug concentration through alterations in efflux transporters, protein binding, and pH. Pharmacodynamic drug-drug interactions can occur with addictive drugs, both purposeful (eg, to increase euphoria) and unintended (concomitant use of opiates and benzodiazepines resulting in increased respiratory depression and possible death).

Pharmacodynamics encompasses the mechanisms of drug action and response, including receptor physiology, as well as desensitization, tolerance/cross-tolerance, and the behavioral and environmental aspects of drug effects. Drug action can be understood in terms of positive (agonist), neutral (antagonist), and negative (inverse agonist) allosteric modulation of a receptor. Our advancing knowledge of intracellular signaling pathways and receptor desensitization and internalization may enable manipulation of downstream processes so that we can develop more targeted and effective medications, for example, more potent opioid analgesics with fewer side effects such as respiratory depression.

Pharmacogenomics, the relationship between genetic polymorphisms and drug pharmacokinetics and pharmacodynamics, can explain much of the individual variability in response to medications. Precision medicine aims to improve drug selection and dosing of medication based upon an individual's genetic make-up. Pharmacogenetic clinical practice guidelines are being developed to translate such research into practice.

Epigenetic changes in gene expression without alterations in the DNA sequence are being studied for their role in individual vulnerability to develop a substance use disorder, the response to substance use, and the response to pharmacotherapy. Understanding the mechanisms that regulate DNA methylation and chromatin remodeling has opened the door to epigenetic interventions.

The following chapters in this section describe the pharmacology of specific drug classes that contribute to substance use disorders.

REFERENCES

1. Nelson RA, Boyd SJ, Zieglestein RC, et al. Effect of rate of administration on subjective and physiological effects of intravenous cocaine in humans. *Drug Alcohol Depend.* 2006;82:19-24. doi:10.1016/j.drugalcdep.2005.08.004
2. Johnson F, Setnik B. Morphine sulfate and naltrexone hydrochloride extended-release capsules: Naltrexone release, pharmacodynamics, and tolerability. *Pain Physician.* 2011;14(4):391-406.
3. Volkow N. Stimulant medications: How to minimize their reinforcing effects? *Am J Psychiatry.* 2006;163(3):359-361. doi:10.1176/appi.ajp.163.3.359
4. Spencer TJ, Biederman J, Ciccone PE, et al. PET study examining pharmacokinetics, detection and likeability, and dopamine transporter receptor occupancy of short- and long-acting oral methylphenidate. *Am J Psychiatry.* 2006;163(3):387-395. doi:10.1176/appi.ajp.163.3.387
5. Xing CY, Tarumi T, Liu J, et al. Distribution of cardiac output to the brain across the adult lifespan. *J Cereb Blood Flow Metab.* 2017;37(8):2848-2856.
6. Lam JKW, Cheung CCK, Chow MYT, et al. Transmucosal drug administration as an alternative route in palliative and end-of-life care during the COVID-19 pandemic. *Adv Drug Deliv Rev.* 2020;160:234-243.
7. Chapman CD, Frey WH II, Craft S, et al. Intranasal treatment of central nervous system dysfunction in humans. *Pharm Res.* 2013;30(10):2475-2484. doi:10.1007/s11095-012-0915-1
8. Marren K. Dimethyl sulfoxide: An effective penetration enhancer for topical administration of NSAIDs. *Physician Sports Med.* 2011;39(3):75-82. doi:10.3810/psm.2011.09.1923
9. Stepensky D. Prediction of drug disposition on the basis of its chemical structure. *Clin Pharmacokinet.* 2013;52:415-431.
10. Klockhoff H, Näslund I, Jones AW. Faster absorption of ethanol and higher peak concentration in women after gastric bypass surgery. *Br J Clin Pharmacol.* 2002;54(6):587-591. doi:10.1046/j.1365-2125.2002.01698.x
11. Won CS, Oberlies NH, Paine MF. Mechanisms underlying food-drug interactions: Inhibition of intestinal metabolism and transport. *Pharmacol Ther.* 2012;136:186-201.
12. Hermann R, von Richter O. Clinical evidence of herbal drugs as perpetrators of pharmacokinetic drug interactions. *Planta Med.* 2012;78(13):1458-1477.
13. Rowland M, Tozer TN. *Clinical Pharmacokinetics: Concepts and Applications.* 3rd ed. Lippincott Williams & Wilkins; 1995.
14. Miller RD, Cohen NH, Eriksson LI, et al. *Miller's Anesthesia.* 8th ed. Saunders Elsevier; 2015.
15. FDA Drug Safety Communication: FDA Approves New Label Changes and Dosing for Zolpidem Products and A Recommendation to Avoid Driving the Day After Using Ambien CR. Accessed September 10, 2022. https://www.fda.gov/drugs/drug-safety-and-availability/fda-drug-safety-communication-fda-approves-new-label-changes-and-dosing-zolpidem-products-and
16. Greenblatt DJ, Harmatz JS, Roth T. Zolpidem and gender: Are women really at risk. *Psychopharmacology.* 2019;39(3):189-199. doi:10.1097/JCP.0000000000001026

Disclaimer: The views expressed in this chapter do not necessarily represent the views of the National Institutes of Health or the Department of Health and Human Services.

17. Jones AW. Pharmacokinetics of ethanol-issues of forensic importance. *Forensic Sci Rev.* 2011;23:91-136.
18. Ince I, Knibbe CA, Danhof M, et al. Developmental changes in the expression and function of cytochrome P450 3A isoforms: Evidence from in vitro and in vivo investigations. *Clin Pharmacokinet.* 2013;52(5):333-345.
19. Kumagai T, Suzuki H, Sasaki T, et al. Polycyclic aromatic hydrocarbons activate CYP3A4 gene transcription through human pregnane X receptor. *Drug Metab Pharmacokinet.* 2012;27(2):200-206.
20. Drug Interactions. Relevant Regulatory Guidance and Policy Documents. Accessed September 10, 2022. https://www.fda.gov/drugs/drug-interactions-labeling/drug-interactions-relevant-regulatory-guidance-and-policy-documents
21. Indiana University, School of Medicine. Drug interactions: Flockhart table. Accessed September 10, 2022. https://drug-interactions.medicine.iu.edu/MainTable.aspx
22. deLeon J. Glucuronidation enzymes, genes and psychiatry. *Int J Neuropsychopharmacol.* 2003;6:57-72. doi:10.1017/S1461145703003249
23. Neumann J, Olof B, Helander A, Boettcher M. Performance of PEth compared with other alcohol biomarkers in subjects presenting For occupational and pre-employment medical examination. *Alcohol Alcohol.* 2020;55(4):401-408.
24. Andresen-Strichert H, Beres Y, Weinmann W, et al. Improved detection of alcohol consumption using the novel marker phosphatidylethanol in the transplant setting: Results of a prospective study. *Transpl Int.* 2017;611-620. doi:10.1111/tri.12949
25. Hill-Kapturczak H, Dougherty DM, Roache JD, Karns-Wright TE, Lopez-Cruzan M, Javors MA. Chapter 58 – Phosphatidylethanol homologs in blood as biomarkers for the time frame and amount of recent alcohol consumption. In: Preedy VR, ed. *Neuroscience of Alcohol: Mechanisms and Treatment.* Academic Press; 2019:567-576. doi:10.1016/B978-0-12-813125-1.00058-1. Synopsis. Accessed September 11, 2022. https://www.sciencedirect.com/topics/neuroscience/phosphatidylethanol.
26. Khatri R, Fallon JK, Sykes C, et al. Pregnancy-related hormones increase UGT1A1-mediated labetalol metabolism in human hepatocytes. *Front Pharmacol.* 2021;12:655320. doi:10.3389/fphar.2021.655320
27. Atkinson AJ. Clinical pharmacokinetics. In: Atkinson AJ, Abernathy DR, Daniels CE, et al., eds. *Principles of Clinical Pharmacology.* Academic Press; 2007:9-20.
28. Bailey JM. Context-sensitive half-times. *Clin Pharmacokinet.* 2002;41:793-799. doi:10.2165/00003088-200241110-00001
29. Huang W, Isoherranen N. Development of a dynamic physiologically based mechanistic kidney model to predict renal clearance. *CPT Pharmacometrics Syst Pharmacol.* 2018;7(9):593-602. doi:10.1002/psp4.12321
30. Medsafe. Medicines interacting with methadone. *Prescriber Update.* 2018;39(2):20. Accessed August 11, 2022. https://www.medsafe.govt.nz/profs/PUArticles/June2018/Methadone.htm
31. Tian JN, Ho IK, Isou HH, et al. UCT2B7 genetic polymorphisms are associated with the withdrawal symptoms in methadone maintenance patients. *Pharmacogenomics.* 2012;13(8):879-888.
32. Daniel WA, Bromek E, Danek PJ, Haduch A. The mechanisms of interactions of psychotropic drugs with liver and brain cytochrome P450 and their significance for drug effect and drug-drug interactions. *Biochem Pharmacol.* 2022;199:115006.
33. Qian Y, Gurley BJ, Markowitz JS. The potential for pharmacokinetic interactions between cannabis products and conventional medications. *J Clin Psychopharmacol.* 2019;39(5):462-471. doi:10.1097/JCP.0000000000001089
34. Burckhardt G. Drug transport by organic anion transporters (OATs). *Pharmacol Ther.* 2012;136(1):106-130. doi:10.1016/j.pharmthera.2012.07.010
35. Jones AW. Forensic drug profile: cocaethylene. *J Anal Toxicol.* 2019;43(3):155-160. doi:10.1093/jat/bkz007
36. McCance-Katz EF, Sullivan LE, Nallani S. Drug interactions of clinical importance among the opioids, methadone and buprenorphine, and other frequently prescribed medications: a review. *Am J Addict.* 2010;19(1):4-16. doi:10.1111/j.1521-0391.2009.00005.x

37. Nadkarni A, Oldham MA, Howard M, Berenbaum I. Drug-drug interactions between warfarin and psychotropics: Updated review of the literature. *Pharmacotherapy.* 2012;32(10):932-942. doi:10.1002/j.1875-9114.2012.01119
38. Drost SA, Wentzell JR, Giguère P, et al. Outcomes associated with reducing the urine alkalinization threshold in patients receiving high-dose methotrexate. *Pharmacotherapy.* 2017;37(6):684-691. doi:10.1002/phar.1935
39. Urbas R, Huntington W, Napoleon LA, Wong P, Mullin JM. Malabsorption-related issues associated with chronic proton pump inhibitor usage. *Austin J Nutr Metab.* 2016;3(2):1041.
40. Leri F, Bruneau J, Stewart J. Understanding polydrug use: Review of heroin and cocaine co-use. *Addiction.* 2003;98(1):7-22. doi:10.1046/j.1360-0443.2003.00236.x
41. Shawahna R, Decleves X, Scherrmann JM. Hurdles with using in vitro models to predict human blood–brain barrier drug permeability: A special focus on transporters and metabolizing enzymes. *Curr Drug Metab.* 2013;14(1):120-136.
42. Geier EG, Schlessinger A, Fan H, et al. Structure-based ligand discovery for the large-neutral amino acid transporter 1, LAT-1. *Proc Natl Acad Sci USA.* 2013;110(14):5480-5485.
43. Ferguson CS, Tyndale RF. Cytochrome P450 enzymes in the brain: Emerging evidence of biological significance. *Trends Pharmacol Sci.* 2011;32(12):708-714.
44. Ghosh C, Hossain M, Solanki J, Dadas A, Marchi N, Janigro D. Pathophysiological implications of neurovascular P450 in brain disorders. *Drug Discov Today.* 2016;21(10):1609-1619.
45. Wojciech K, Władysława AD. Cytochrome P450 expression and regulation in the brain. *Drug Metab Rev.* 2021;53:1-29. doi:10.1080/03602532.2020.1858856
46. Hedlund E, Gustafsson JA, Warner M. Cytochrome P450 in the brain: A review. *Curr Drug Metab.* 2001;2(3):245-263.
47. Dutheil F, Beaune P, Loriot MA. Xenobiotic metabolizing enzymes in the central nervous system: contribution of cytochrome P450 enzymes in normal and pathological human brain. *Biochimie.* 2008;90(3):426-436.
48. Sheng Y, Yang H, Wu T, Shu L, Liu L, Liu X. Alterations of cytochrome P450s and UDP-glucuronosyltransferases in brain under diseases and their clinical significances. *Front Pharmacol.* 2021;12:650027. doi:10.3389/phar.2021.65027
49. Booth Depaz IM, Toselli F, Wilce PA, et al. Differential expression of human cytochrome P450 enzymes from the CYP3A subfamily in the brains of alcoholics and drug free controls. *Drug Metab Dispos.* 2013;41(6):1187-1194. doi:10.1124/dmd.113.051359
50. Ravindranath V, Strobel HW. Cytochrome P450-mediated metabolism in brain: Functional roles and their implications. *Expert Opin Drug Metab Toxicol.* 2013;9(5):551-558.
51. Eiden LE, Weihe E. VMAT2: a dynamic regulator of brain monoaminergic neuronal function interacting with drugs of abuse. *Ann N Y Acad Sci.* 2011;1216:86-98.
52. Feghali M, Venkataramanan R, Caritis S. Pharmacokinetics of drugs in pregnancy. *Semin Perinatol.* 2015;39(7):512-519. doi:10.1053/j.semperi.2015.08.003
53. Bastian JR, Chen H, Zhang H, et al. Dose-adjusted plasma concentrations of sublingual buprenorphine are lower during than after pregnancy. *Am J Obstet Gynecol.* 2017;216(1):64.e1-64.e7.
54. Caritis SN, Bastian JR, Zhang H, et al. An evidence-based recommendation to increase the dosing frequency of buprenorphine during pregnancy. *Am J Obstet Gynecol.* 2017;217(4):459.e1-459.e6.
55. Swift RM, Dudley M, DePetrillo P, Camara P, Griffiths W. Altered methadone pharmacokinetics in pregnancy: Implications for dosing. *J Subst Abuse.* 1989;1(4):453-460.
56. Griffiths SK, Campbell JP. Placental structure, function and drug transfer. *Contin Educ Anaesth Crit Care Pain.* 2015;15(2):84-89.
57. Syme MR, Paxton JW, Keelan JA. Drug transfer and metabolism by the human placenta. *Clin Pharmacokinet.* 2004;43(8):487-514.
58. Ritter JM, Flower R, Henderson G, Loke YK, MacEwan D, Rang HP. Chapter 12: Individual variation, pharmacogenomics and personalized medicine. In: Ritter JM, Flower R, Henderson G, Loke YK, MacEwan D, eds. *Rang & Dale's Pharmacology.* Elsevier; 2020:152-162.
59. Centers for Disease Control and Prevention. Data and Statistics About Opioid Use During Pregnancy. Accessed September 12, 2022. https://www.cdc.gov/pregnancy/opioids/data.html
60. Opioid use and opioid use disorder in pregnancy. Committee opinion no. 711. American college of obstetricians and gynecologists. *Obstet Gynecol.* 2017;130:e81-e94.
61. Use of psychoactive medication during pregnancy and possible effects on the fetus and newborn. Committee on drugs. American academy of pediatrics. *Pediatrics.* 2000;105(4 Pt 1):880-887. doi:10.1542/peds.105.4.880
62. Jansson LM, Patrick SW. Neonatal abstinence syndrome. *Pediatr Clin North Am.* 2019;66(2):353-367. doi:10.1016/j.pcl.2018.12.006
63. Jones HE, Kraft WK. Analgesia, opioids, and other drug use during pregnancy and neonatal abstinence syndrome. *Clin Perinatol.* 2019;25(2):346-366.
64. Jones HE, Heil SH, Baewert A, et al. Buprenorphine treatment of opioid-dependent pregnant women: a comprehensive review. *Addiction.* 2012;107(Suppl 1 (01)):5-27. doi:10.1111/j.1360-0443.2012.04035.x
65. Homer LD, Nielsen TB. Spare receptors, partial agonists, and ternary complex model of drug action. *Am J Physiol.* 1987;253(1 Pt 1):E114-E121. doi:10.1152/ajpendo.1987.253.1.E114
66. von Zastrow M. Chapter 2: Drug receptors & pharmacodynamics. *Access Medicine.* McGraw Hill; 2022:1-28. Accessed May 10, 2023. https://accessmedicine.mhmedical.com/content.aspx?bookId=2249§ionId=175215570
67. Abraham WC, Jones OD, Glanzman DL. Is plasticity of synapses the mechanism of long-term memory storage? *NPJ Sci Learn.* 2019;4:9. doi:10.1038/s41539-019-0048-y
68. Wen RT, Zhang FF, Zhang HT. Cyclic nucleotide phosphodiesterases: Potential therapeutic targets for alcohol use disorder. *Psychopharmacology (Berl).* 2018;235(6):1793-1805.
69. Ippolito M, Benovic JL. Biased agonism at beta-adrenergic receptors. *Cell Signal.* 2021;80:109905.
70. Wang Y, Yutuc E, Griffiths WJ. Neuro-oxysterols and neuro-sterols as ligands to nuclear receptors, GPCRs, ligand-gated ion channels and other protein receptors. *Br J Pharmacol.* 2021;178(16):3176-3193. doi:10.1111/bph.15191
71. Stevens CW. Pharmacodynamics or what the drug does to the body. In: Stevens CW, ed. *Brenner and Stevens' Pharmacology.* 6th ed. Elsevier, Inc; 2023:27-34. IBSN: 978-0-323-75898-7
72. Conibear AE, Kelly E. A biased view of mu- opioid receptors. *Mol Pharm.* 2019;96(5):542-549. doi:10.1124/mol.119.115956
73. Hill R, Disney A, Conibear A, et al. The novel u-opioid receptor agonist PZM21 depresses respiration and induces tolerance to antinociception. *Br J Pharmacol.* 2018;175(13):2653-2661. doi:10.1111/bph.14224
74. Schmid CL, Kennedy NM, Ross NC, et al. Bias factor and therapeutic window correlate to predict safer opioid analgesics. *Cell.* 2017;171(5):1165-1175.e13. doi:10.1016/j.cell.2017.10.035
75. Gilchrist A. Modulating G protein-coupled receptors: from traditional pharmacology to allosterics. *Trends Pharmacol Sci.* 2007;28(8):431-437.
76. Zorumski CF, Izumi Y, Mennerick S. Ketamine: NMDA receptors and beyond. *J Neurosci.* 2016;36(44):11158-11164.
77. Sleigh J, Harvey M, Voss L, Denny B. Ketamine-More mechanisms of action than just NMDA blockade. *Trends Anaesth Crit Care.* 2014;4:76-81. doi:10.1016/j.tacc.2014.03.002
78. Buxton ILO. Rethinking drug action in light of current models of receptor pharmacology. In: Brunton LL, Lazo JS, Parker KL, eds. *Goodman & Gilman's the Pharmacological Basis of Therapeutics [Supplement to Main Textbook].* 11th ed. McGraw Hill, Inc; 2005.
79. Milligan G. Constitutive activity and inverse agonists of G protein coupled receptors: a current perspective. *Mol Pharmacol.* 2003;64(6):1271-1276. doi:10.1124/mol.64.6.1271

80. Trevor AJ, Way WL. Sedative-hypnotic drugs. In: Katzung BG, ed. *Basic and Clinical Pharmacology*. 8th ed. Lange Medical Books/McGraw Hill; 2001:364-381.
81. Nelson LS. Alcohol withdrawal and flumazenil: Not for the faint of heart. *J Med Toxicol*. 2014;10(2):123-125.
82. Williams JT, Ingram SL, Henderson G, et al. Regulation of μ-opioid receptors: desensitization, phosphorylation, internalization, and tolerance. *Pharmacol Rev*. 2013;65:223-254.
83. Chandni D. *Mechanisms in Desensitization*. AuthorSTREAM. Accessed July 22, 2022. https://www.authorstream.com/Presentation/chandni.dave-1451948-desensitization-new/
84. Kim JA, Bartlett S, He L, et al. Morphine induced receptor endocytosis in a novel knockin mouse reduces tolerance and dependence. *Curr Biol*. 2008;18(2):129-135.
85. He L, Gooding SW, Lewis E, Felth LC, Gaur A, Whistler JL Pharmacological and genetic manipulations at the u-opioid receptor reveal arrestin-3 engagement limits analgesic tolerance and does not exacerbate respiratory depression in mice. *Neuropsychopharmacology*. 2021;46:2241-2249. doi:10.1038/s41386-021-01054-x
86. Gondin AB, Halls ML, Canals M. Briddon SJ FRK mediates U-opioid receptor plasma membrane reorganization. *Front Mol Neurosci*. 2019;2:104. doi:10.3389/fnmol.2019.00104
87. Kasai S, Ikeda K. Pharmacogenomics of the human u-opioid receptor. *Pharmacogenomics*. 2011;12(9):1305-1320.
88. Williams JT, Ingram SL, Henderson G, et al. Regulation of mu-opioid receptors: desensitization, phosphorylation, internalization, and tolerance. *Pharmacol Rev*. 2013;65(1):223-254.
89. O'Brien CP. Drug addiction and drug abuse. In: Hardman JG, Limbird LE, Gilman AG, eds. *Goodman and Gilman's The Pharmacologic Basis of Therapeutics*. 10th ed. McGraw Hill Inc; 2001:621-642.
90. Siegel S, Hinson RE, Krank MD, et al. Heroin "overdose" death: The contribution of drug-associated environmental cues. *Science*. 1982;216(4544):436-437.
91. American Psychiatric Association. *Diagnostic and Statistical Manual of Mental Disorders*. 5th ed., text rev. ed.; 2022. doi:10.1176/appi.books.9780890425787
92. Manhapra A, Sullivan MD, Ballantyne JC, MacLean RR, Becker WC. Complex persistent opioid dependence with long-term opioids: A gray area that needs definition, better understanding, treatment guidance, and policy changes. *J Gen Intern Med*. 2020;3535(Suppl3):964-971.
93. What is the Difference Between Pharmacogenetics and Pharmacogenomics? Accessed September 10, 2022. https://www.pharmgkb.org/page/faqs#what-is-the-difference-between-pharmacogenetics-and-pharmacogenomics
94. Guo X, Liu Z, Wang X, et al. Large-scale association analysis for drug addiction: Results from SNP to gene. *Scientific World Journal*. 2012;2012:939584.
95. Zdanowicz MM. *Concepts in Pharmacogenomics*. American Society of Health-System Pharmacists; 2010:414. ISBN: 978-1-58528-234-0
96. Daly AK. Genetic polymorphisms affecting drug metabolism: Recent advances and clinical aspects. *Adv Pharmacol*. 2012;63:137-167.
97. Meyer MR, Maurer HH. Absorption, distribution, metabolism and excretion pharmacogenomics of drugs of abuse. *Pharmacogenomics*. 2011;12(2):215-233.
98. Mroziewicz M, Tyndale RF. Pharmacogenetics: A tool for identifying genetic factors in drug dependence and response to treatment. *Addict Sci Clin Pract*. 2010;5(2):17-29.
99. Sturgess JE, George TP, Kennedy JL, et al. Pharmacogenetics of alcohol, nicotine and drug addiction treatments. *Addict Biol*. 2011;16(3):357-376.
100. Chen YC, Yang LF, Lai CL, Yin SJ. Acetaldehyde enhances alcohol sensitivity and protects against alcoholism: evidence from alcohol metabolism and in subjects with variant ALDH2*2 gene allele. *Biomolecules*. 2021;11(8):1183.
101. Shen Y-C, Fan J-H, Edenberg H, et al. Polymorphisms of ADH and ALDH genes among four ethnic groups in China and effects upon the risk for alcoholism. *Alcohol Clin Exp Res*. 1997;21(7):1272-1277. doi:10.1111/j.1530-0277.1997.tb04448.x
102. Chenoweth MJ, O'Loughlin J, Sylvestre MP, et al. CYP2A6 slow nicotine metabolism is associated with increased quitting by adolescent smokers. *Pharmacogenet Genomics*. 2013;23(4):232-235.
103. Kendler KS, Jacobson KC, Prescott CA, Neale MC. Specificity of genetic and environmental risk factors for use and abuse/dependence of cannabis, cocaine, hallucinogens, sedatives, stimulants, and opiates in male twins. *Am J Psychiatry*. 2003;160(4):687-695.
104. Berrettini W. A brief review of the genetics and pharmacogenetics of opioid use disorders. *Dialogues Clin Neurosci*. 2017;19(3):229-236. doi:10.31887/DCNS.2017.19.3/wberrettini
105. Zanger UM, Klein K, Saussele T, et al. Polymorphic CYP2B6: Molecular mechanisms and emerging clinical significance. *Pharmacogenomics*. 2007;8(7):743-759.
106. Zhu AZX, Cox LS, Nollen N, et al. CYP2B6 and bupropion's smoking-cessation pharmacology: The role of hydroxybupropion. *Clin Pharmacol Ther*. 2012;92(6):771-777.
107. Chenoweth MJ, Tyndale FR. Pharmacogenetic optimization of smoking cessation treatment. *Trends Pharmacol Sci*. 2017;38(1):55-66.
108. The Pharmacogene Variation (Pharm Var) Consortium. Accessed July 24, 2023. https://www.pharmvar.org/gene/CYP2D6
109. Del Tredici AL, Malhotra A, Dedek M, et al. Frequency of CYP2D6 alleles including structural variants in the United States. *Front Pharmacol*. 2018;9. doi:10.3389/fphar.2018.00305
110. Dean L, Kane M. Codeine therapy and CYP2D6 genotype. 2012 Sep 20 [Updated Mar 30 2021]. In: Pratt VM, Scott SA, Pirmohamed M, et al., eds. *Medical Genetics Summaries [Internet]*. National Center for Biotechnology Information; 2012. Accessed May 10, 2023.https://www.ncbi.nlm.nih.gov/books/NBK61999/
111. Kelly LE, Madadi P. Is there a role for therapeutic drug monitoring with codeine? *Ther Drug Monit*. 2012;34(3):249-256.
112. Crews KR, Monte AA, Huddart R, et al. Clinical pharmacogenetics implementation consortium guideline for CYP2D6, OPRM1, and COMT genotypes and select opioid therapy. *Clin Pharmacol Ther*. 2021;110(4):888-896. doi:10.1002/cpt.214918
113. Madadi P, Avard D, Koren G. Pharmacogenetics of opioids for the treatment of acute maternal pain during pregnancy and lactation. *Curr Drug Metab*. 2012;13(6):721-727.
114. Van Cleve WC. Pediatric posttonsillectomy analgesia before and after the black box warning against codeine use. *JAMA Otolaryngol Head Neck Surg*. 2017;143(10):1052-1054.
115. Hamann K, Daut RA, Gutierrez MA. Psychiatry and neurology pharmacogenomics. In: Lam JT, Gutierrez MA, Shah S, eds. *Pharmacogenomics: A Primer for Clinicians*. McGraw Hill; 2021:14.
116. Tegretol Label. Accessed September 10, 2022. https://www.accessdata.fda.gov/drugsatfda_docs/label/2007/016608s098lbl.pdf
117. Eap CB. Personalize prescribing: A new medical model for clinical implementation of psychotropic drugs. *Dialogues Clin Neurosci*. 2016;18(3):313-322.
118. Iosifescu DV. Pharmacogenomic testing for next-step antidepressant selection: Still a work in progress. *JAMA*. 2022;328(2):146-147.
119. PharmGKB. Accessed July 28, 2022. http://www.pharmgkb.org
120. Whirl-Carrillo M, Huddart R, Gong L, K., et al. An evidence-based framework for evaluating pharmacogenomics knowledge for personalized medicine. *Clin Pharmacol Ther*. 2021;110(3):563-572. doi:10.1002/cpt.2350
121. Relling MV, Klein TE, Gammal RS, Whirl-Carrillo M, Hoffman JM, Caudle KE. The clinical pharmacogenetics implementation consortium: 10 years later. *Clin Pharmacol Ther*. 2020;107(1):171-175. doi:10.1002/cpt.1651
122. Nielsen DA, Utrankar A, Reyes JA, Simons DD, Kosten TR. Epigenetics of drug abuse: Predisposition or response. *Pharmacogenomics*. 2012;13(10):1149-1169. doi:10.2217/pgs 12.94
123. Kaplan G, Xu H, Abreu K, Feng J. DNA epigenetics in addiction susceptibility. *Front Genet*. 2022;13:806685. doi:10.3389/gene.2022.806685
124. Bohnsack JP, Zhang H, Wandling GM, et al. Targeted epigenomic editing ameliorates adult anxiety and excessive drinking after adolescent alcohol exposure. *Sci Adv*. 2022;8(18): doi:10.1126/sciadv.abn2748

CHAPTER 11

The Pharmacology of Alcohol

John J. Woodward

CHAPTER OUTLINE

- Definition
- Substances included in this class
- Formulations and methods of use
- Clinical uses
- Brief historical features
- Epidemiology
- Pharmacokinetics
- Pharmacodynamics
- Drug-drug interactions
- Neurobiology (mechanisms of addiction)
- Addiction liability
- Conclusions/future research

DEFINITION

Alcohol is a chemical name for a group of related compounds that contain a hydroxyl group (-OH) bound to a carbon atom. The form of alcohol that is voluntarily consumed by humans is ethyl alcohol or ethanol and consists of two carbons and a single hydroxyl group (written as C_2H_5OH or C_2H_6O). Unless otherwise noted, the term *alcohol* will be used throughout this chapter to mean ethanol.

SUBSTANCES INCLUDED IN THIS CLASS

In terms of human consumption, all commercially available alcoholic beverages contain ethyl alcohol with concentrations depending upon the type of beverage. Beverages made by fermentation of sugar-containing fruits and grains include beer (3%-8% ethanol by volume), and wines (11%-13% ethanol by volume). Spirits or liquor are produced after distillation and generally contain at least 30% ethanol. Ethanol can be concentrated by simple distillation up to approximately 95%, while pure ethanol requires addition of benzene or related substances or desiccation using glycerol. Denatured alcohol contains additives or toxins to prevent human consumption. Rubbing alcohol is prepared from denatured alcohol or isopropyl alcohol and is used for topical purposes.

FORMULATIONS AND METHODS OF USE

A bewildering array of alcoholic beverages is available for consumption and these products contain a wide range of alcohol concentrations. In the United States and Canada, a standard alcoholic drink is defined as one that contains about 14 grams (approximately 0.6 fluid ounces or approximately 18 milliliters) of pure alcohol. This amount of alcohol is typically contained in 12 ounces of beer, 5 ounces of wine, or 1.5 ounces of distilled spirits (40% ethanol by volume); this can vary depending on the specific type of beverage (**Table 11-1**). Although most alcohol is consumed orally, there are isolated cases of individuals injecting ethanol intravenously[1] as well as other means of administration. For example, ethanol vapor is often used to induce physical dependence in rodent models of alcohol use disorder (AUD)[2,3] and machines called AWOL (alcohol without liquid) have been marketed as a novel means of self-administering alcohol. Various U.S. states have since banned the sale or use of these devices. Ethanol vapor may also be inhaled from e-cigarettes that often contain ethanol as part of the carrier fluid or following adulteration by the consumer.[4] The impact of this route of administration is not yet fully known but could contribute to higher blood alcohol levels when combined with drinking. Forms of powdered alcohol have also been developed including those using micro-encapsulation with a water-soluble carrier such as maltodextrin. Concerns over the safety of these products, particularly with regard to unauthorized use by children and adolescents, led to their ban by a majority of U.S. states.[5]

CLINICAL USES

Alcohol has several clinical indications, primarily as a topical antiseptic and for treatment of accidental or voluntary ingestion of methanol or ethylene glycol.[6] Ethanol has a higher affinity for alcohol dehydrogenase than methanol and thus reduces the formation of the toxic methanol metabolites formaldehyde and formic acid. However, hemodialysis is the recommended first line of treatment. Alcohol has also been used for treatment of various types of cysts (sclerotherapy) and was used historically for treatment of premature labor.[7] Safer and more effective medications have largely replaced these uses. Alcohol combined with dextrose given intravenously was previously used to increase caloric intake and for replenishing fluids but has since been withdrawn for safety reasons.[8] In addition, alcohol,

TABLE 11-1 Amount of Alcohol in Different Beverages and Relationship to a Standard Drink

Beverage	Volume (oz)	%Alcohol (v:v)	No. of Std Drinks
Beer			
Light beer	12	4.2%	approximately 1
Standard beer (U.S.)	12	5%	1
Pint/super	16-20	5%	1.3-1.5
Craft beer/malt liquor	12	7%-9%	1.5
Wine			
Table wine	5	12%-14%	1
Fortified (sherry)	3.5	17%	1
Brandy	1.5	35%-50%	1
Spirits/Liquors			
80 proof "shot"	1.5	40%	1
100 proof	1.5	50%	1.25
190 proof	1.5	95%	2.38

In the United States, a "standard drink" is one that contains approximately 0.6 fluid ounces (14 g) of pure alcohol.

either given orally or IV, was used in the past to treat alcohol withdrawal, particularly in a hospital setting[9] or in an austere or remote setting away from healthcare resources, but this use has been replaced by benzodiazepines or other pharmacotherapies.

BRIEF HISTORICAL FEATURES

Alcohol is one of the oldest used psychoactive substances. Consumption of alcohol-containing beverages predates recorded human history while written records of its use are found in Chinese and Middle Eastern texts as far back as 9,000 years ago. Alcoholic beverages have long been consumed as part of the daily diet and are also used for medicinal or symbolic effects. In modern times, alcohol is second only to caffeine in incidence of use, and its manufacture, distribution, and sale are of major economic importance across the world. Alcohol use worldwide is regulated by both societal and religious beliefs. In the United States, consumption of alcohol was legally restricted on the national level with passage of the Volstead Act and the Eighteenth Amendment to the U.S. Constitution in 1919.[10] Amid growing public outcry, prohibition was repealed in 1933 with the ratification of the twenty-first Amendment that gave states the right to regulate the purchase and sale of alcohol. Today, sales and consumption of alcohol are under control of a wide variety of local and state laws.

EPIDEMIOLOGY

Lifetime exposure to alcohol is high with nearly 86% of the U.S. population over 18 years old reporting using alcohol at least once in their lifetime.[11] In 2020, the 12-month prevalence for DSM-5 defined alcohol use disorder (AUD) was approximately 10%[11] while previous studies report a lifetime prevalence of approximately 29%.[12] Men show higher a rate than women and prevalence is higher among whites and Indigenous Americans[12] and the risk of developing alcohol dependence shows a strong inverse correlation with the age at which heavy drinking begins. In 2020, current self-reported alcohol use (defined as use in the past 30 days) by community-dwelling United States residents ranged from an estimated 8.2% among 12- to 17-year-olds to 59.6% for adults 26 to 49 and 50.2% for those 50 and older.[11] Rates of binge drinking (5 or more drinks within a few hours) within the past 30 days were estimated as 22.2% of persons aged 12 and older and was highest (38.5%) among those aged 21 to 25. Annual alcohol-related costs in the United States in terms of lost productivity and health care were last estimated in 2010 to be $249 billion.[13]

Initial studies of patients with alcohol-related problems resulted in binary classifications such as the Type I and II forms proposed by Cloninger and colleagues and the Type A and B forms proposed by Babor.[14] Subsequent studies expanded these to include additional typologies with three, four or five clusters of symptoms that reflected various personality traits as well as patterns and age of onset of drinking.[14] These criteria have been refined and expanded over time to accommodate a growing awareness of the heterogenous nature of AUD that is clinically diagnosed using eleven criteria outlined in the 5th edition of the *Diagnostic and Statistical Manual of Mental Disorders* (DSM-5).[15] Based on the number of criteria identified, AUD severity ranges from mild (2-3 symptoms) to moderate (4-5 symptoms) to severe (>6 symptoms).

Although the prevalence of AUD in the United States is relatively low (2020 current-year estimate was 10.2% for those 12 and older),[11] this is likely an underestimate as the annual National Survey on Drug Use and Health (NSDUH) interviews a nationally representative, community-based sample that excludes individuals residing in long-term care facilities, prisons, and other residential institutions. Factors that increase an individual's risk for developing AUD are complex and involve usage patterns, environmental and genetic factors such as a family history of AUD. Risk is also enhanced by heavy drinking during adolescence and younger ages of drinking onset,[16] co-occurring psychiatric conditions including depression and anxiety[17] and experiencing adverse and/or traumatic events especially during childhood.[18] Twin studies indicate that the heritability of AUD is approximately 50%[19] with risk spread among a large number of genes each generally having only a small (<1%) effect.[20] Of these, recent genome-wide association studies (GWAS) suggest that polymorphisms in genes coding for enzymes that metabolize ethanol including alcohol dehydrogenase (ADH) and aldehyde dehydrogenase (ALDH) significantly increase the probability of heavy drinking and AUD, while other polymorphisms convey protection.[21] Other genes associated with developing AUD include *GCKR*, a regulator of glucokinase, and *CRHR1*, which codes for the corticotrophin releasing hormone receptor 1. Genes that correlate with the amount of drinking, such as beta-klotho (*KLB*) and fibroblast growth factor 21 (*FGF21*), are not associated with the incidence of AUD,[13] illustrating the importance of distinguishing between drinking, per se, and AUD.

PHARMACOKINETICS

Absorption and Metabolism

Alcohol is a small, water-soluble molecule that is rapidly and efficiently absorbed into the bloodstream from the stomach, small intestine, and colon. The rate of absorption depends on the gastric emptying time and can be delayed by the presence of food in the small intestine. Once in the bloodstream, alcohol is rapidly distributed throughout the body and gains access to all tissues, including the fetus in pregnant women. Although the relationship between alcohol intake and blood levels is body weight-dependent, gender is also important. When body weights are equivalent, women show a 20% to 25% higher blood alcohol level than men following ingestion of the same amount of alcohol (Table 11-2). This appears to be due primarily to lower gastric metabolism of alcohol in women as blood levels are not significantly different when alcohol is administered intravenously.[22]

Alcohol is metabolized primarily by enzymatic pathways and only small amounts of alcohol are excreted through the lungs as vapor.[23] In the liver, alcohol is broken down by alcohol dehydrogenase (ADH) and to a lesser extent mixed function oxidases such as cytochrome P450IIE1 (CYP2E1).[23] Levels of CYP2E1 may be increased in people who drink chronically. ADH converts alcohol to acetaldehyde, which subsequently can be converted to acetate by the actions of acetaldehyde dehydrogenase (ALDH).

The rate of alcohol metabolism by ADH is relatively constant, as the enzyme is saturated at relatively low blood alcohol levels and thus exhibits zero order kinetics (constant amount oxidized per unit of time).[23] Alcohol metabolism is proportional to body weight (and probably liver weight) and averages approximately 1 ounce of pure alcohol (about two standard alcoholic beverages) per 3 hours in adults. Although stimulants are often used to mask the depressant effects of alcohol, there is no truly effective "alcohol antagonist" (amethystic agents) that can quickly reverse the intoxicating effects of alcohol (see Section 7, Management of Intoxication and Withdrawal).

PHARMACODYNAMICS

Central Nervous System

Alcohol acts acutely as a central nervous system (CNS) depressant. During the initial phase of drinking when blood alcohol concentrations are in the range from 10 to 50 mg/dL (0.01%-0.05%), there is a feeling of warmth as cutaneous blood flow is increased and this is accompanied by a reduction in core body temperature. Gastric secretions are usually increased, although the concentration of alcohol ingested affects this response, with high concentrations (>20%) inhibiting secretions.[24] These effects are accompanied by a period of disinhibition and the onset of common signs of behavioral arousal including relief of anxiety, increased talkativeness, feelings of confidence and euphoria and enhanced assertiveness. As drinking continues and blood concentrations exceed legal limits (United States and Canada, 80 mg/dL or 0.08%), DSM-5 defined signs and symptoms of intoxication develop including slurred speech, incoordination, unsteady gait, nystagmus, impairment in attention or memory, stupor or coma.[15] At higher concentrations, alcohol acts as a sedative and hypnotic, although the quality of sleep is reduced after alcohol intake. In patients with obstructive sleep apnea, alcohol increases the frequency and severity of apneic episodes and the resulting hypoxia.[25] Higher levels (150-200 mg%) produce marked ataxia and reduced reaction time. Some individuals may experience blackouts, postintoxication periods during

TABLE 11-2 Estimated Blood Alcohol Levels Following Drinking

Body Weight (lb)	120		140		160		180		200	
No. of Drinks	M	F	M	F	M	F	M	F	M	F
1	0.03	0.04	0.03	0.03	0.02	0.03	0.02	0.03	0.02	0.02
2	0.06	0.08	0.05	0.07	0.05	0.06	0.04	0.05	0.04	0.05
3	0.09	0.11	0.08	0.10	0.07	0.09	0.06	0.08	0.06	0.07
4	0.12	0.15	0.11	0.13	0.09	0.11	0.08	0.10	0.08	0.09
5	0.16	0.19	0.13	0.16	0.12	0.14	0.11	0.13	0.09	0.11
6	0.19	0.23	0.16	0.19	0.14	0.17	0.13	0.15	0.11	0.14
7	0.22	0.27	0.19	0.23	0.16	0.20	0.15	0.18	0.13	0.16
8	0.25	0.30	0.21	0.26	0.19	0.23	0.17	0.20	0.15	0.18

Data represent blood alcohol concentration (gram per 100 mL or gram %) for men (M) and women (F) following consumption of different number of drinks. Subtract 0.01 from each value for each hour of drinking to account for effects of metabolism. One drink represents 12 oz beer, 5 oz wine, or 1.5 oz liquor.

which the individual cannot recall events that occurred during intoxication. As concentrations reach and exceed 300 mg%, an anesthetic level is approached and individuals may show severe motor impairment and vomiting. Lethal doses of alcohol in nontolerant individuals are on the order of 400 to 500 mg% although this varies widely. Acute alcohol intoxication is not always associated with sedation or coma; indeed, some intoxicated individuals display violent behavior that requires administration of other sedative or antipsychotic agents. These agents must be used cautiously in a severely intoxicated individual to avoid precipitating respiratory failure.

DRUG-DRUG INTERACTIONS

Alcohol has depressant actions on the CNS similar to other centrally acting drugs, such as opioids, barbiturates, benzodiazepines, general anesthetics and solvents, and anticonvulsants and can potentiate the sedative-hypnotic properties of these substances. Alcohol also enhances the sedative effects of antihistamines that are commonly used in the treatment of nasal congestion. Combining these medications with alcohol can result in significant CNS depression and reduced ability to carry out normal functions safely, such as motor vehicle driving. Alcohol can also enhance the hepatotoxic effects of acetaminophen and the gastric irritating effects of nonsteroidal anti-inflammatory drugs, thus increasing the risk for development of gastritis and upper GI bleeding.[26] Alcohol has also been shown to alter the pharmacokinetic profile of certain medications including diazepam, chlordiazepoxide and erythromycin.[26]

NEUROBIOLOGY (MECHANISMS OF ADDICTION)

Addictive substances are considered to produce pleasurable effects that promote further drug-seeking and taking. This concept suggests that substances like alcohol produce, at least initially, some form of positive reinforcement that provides a strong incentive to re-experience the substance. As use proceeds, the degree of acute reinforcement may be attenuated and drinking is motivated less for pleasure (positive reinforcement) and more to relieve aversive symptoms that accompany withdrawal (negative reinforcement).[27] The repetitive nature of substance use also engages mechanisms of learning leading to entrained behaviors that may become highly ritualistic, habit-like or compulsive. These findings suggest that substance use disorders (SUDs) are a form of dysfunctional, maladaptive learning that, once established, is difficult to reverse.[28] Recent studies suggest that interactions between midbrain dopamine-based reward systems and cortical mechanisms of brain plasticity and learning that are mediated by the neurotransmitter glutamate underlie the development of SUDs.[29] As substance use transitions into more habitual and compulsive behaviors and aversive symptoms appear, brain stress systems such as the extended amygdala are recruited and modulators such as corticotrophin-releasing factor (CRF) and dynorphin may gain importance.

Alcohol affects reward pathways by enhancing the release of dopamine (DA) from midbrain dopaminergic projections onto neurons within limbic and cortical circuits that regulate motivated behavior. The DA neurons involved in this action reside in the midbrain ventral tegmental area (VTA) and project to discrete areas of the brain, including the nucleus accumbens (ventral striatum), olfactory tubercle, frontal cortex, amygdala, and the septal/hippocampal areas. This circuitry is thought to be involved in translating emotion and perception into action through the activation of motor pathways; thus, these dopamine-rich regions may be important in initiating and sustaining drug-seeking behavior. In studies with mice, repeated self-stimulation of midbrain dopamine neurons produces aversion-resistant behavior[30] while lesions or inactivation of brain areas innervated by these neurons can reduce both the acquisition of drug-seeking as well as its reinstatement following long periods of abstinence.[31,32]

The initial reinforcing actions of alcohol appear to involve excitation of VTA dopamine neurons. Alcohol acutely enhances the firing rate of midbrain DA neurons and animals will self-administer alcohol directly into the posterior but not anterior VTA.[33,34] Chronic exposure to alcohol reduces the excitability of these neurons producing hypoactive dopaminergic signaling, which may persist for significant periods of time after the exposure[35,36] and result in a negative affective state. Electrophysiological studies show enhanced efficiency of glutamatergic signaling in neurons following exposure to alcohol or other addictive substances.[37-39] These findings suggest that enhanced firing of VTA DA neurons during exposure to alcohol facilitates glutamatergic transmission in limbic, cortical, and striatal areas thus strengthening the association between behavioral action and outcome. Studies using in vivo microdialysis to monitor levels of dopamine in freely behaving animals report significant dose-dependent increases in extracellular dopamine concentration in the nucleus accumbens in rats self-administrating alcohol[40,41] Importantly, in rats genetically selected to consume large amounts of alcohol, significant increases in dopamine were also observed during the 15-minute waiting period that preceded alcohol self-administration.[42] This finding suggests that, in animals with drinking experience, the expected reward that ingestion of alcohol provides is itself sufficient to enhance activity in this pathway. The subsequent pharmacologically induced elevation of dopamine that occurs during drinking may further strengthen the motivation to consume alcohol in future sessions. Genetic differences in the responsiveness of this pathway may contribute to the motivational factors that drive greater alcohol-seeking behavior in certain individuals.

Studies with individuals with AUD have examined the neurobehavioral aspects of alcohol use using drug discrimination procedures similar to those used in animal studies. In these studies, subjects rate the effects produced by a variety of substances in terms of their similarity to alcohol. For example, ketamine, a dissociative anesthetic that blocks the ethanol-sensitive N-methyl-D-aspartate (NMDA) subtype of glutamate receptors, induces ethanol-like subjective effects in people who recently underwent withdrawal management.[43]

These effects were dose dependent: at low doses, they mimicked the effects of one to two standard drinks of alcohol, whereas higher doses produced effects similar to those of eight to nine drinks. The ethanol-like ketamine effects were associated with the descending phase of blood alcohol concentration that is associated with ethanol-induced sedation.

Human clinical studies using selective pharmacological agents have implicated neurotransmitters such as γ-aminobutyric acid (GABA), serotonin, and endorphin and enkephalin opioids in mediating the rewarding and craving aspects of alcohol action. Human imaging studies have identified differences in brain activation during exposure to alcohol or alcohol-related cues between control and DSM-IV defined alcohol-dependent subjects.[44,45] Such human studies are important for understanding the underlying causes of AUD because alcohol, unlike most drugs, interacts with a wide variety of molecular and cellular processes to produce its physiologic, and psychological effects.

Molecular Sites of Alcohol Action

Psychostimulants such as cocaine and amphetamine, or opiates like heroin and morphine, all produce their primary effect by binding to specific proteins expressed on brain neurons. In contrast, alcohol is rather promiscuous and interacts with a wide variety of targets including both lipids and proteins. Initial observations made by the German scientists Meyer and Overton over 100 years ago led to a lipid disordering hypothesis of alcohol and anesthetic action due to the high correlation between lipid solubility of a compound and its potency as an anesthetic. Support for this theory has waned over the years as contrary evidence has accumulated. For example, measurable changes in membrane fluidity usually require supra-physiological concentrations of alcohol, are relatively modest, and are less marked than the effects produced by small changes in temperature that are not associated with behavioral signs of intoxication.[46] These findings and the demonstration that some effects of ethanol persist in lipid-free systems have led to the idea that alcohol's acute actions are likely due to effects on ion channel proteins that regulate the excitability of neurons.[47] In most in vitro studies of alcohol action, the range of concentrations needed to cause significant effects is similar to that associated with the behavioral actions of alcohol. Blood alcohol concentrations in the range 40 to 400 mg% are equivalent to 8 to 88 mM in vitro and are associated with the full spectrum of alcohol intoxication. Thus, in vitro studies of alcohol's effect on ion channels are usually conducted at concentrations below 100 mM in order to approximate concentrations found in the brain during drinking.

Table 11-3 shows a variety of neuronally expressed ligand-gated and voltage-activated ion channels that are sensitive to behaviorally relevant concentrations of alcohol.

Alcohol's acute depressant action on neuronal excitability likely results from its ability to enhance the function of inhibitory ion channels while blocking the activity of excitatory receptors (**Fig. 11-1**).

$GABA_A$ and Glycine Receptors

As shown in **Table 11-3**, distinct families of subunits make up functional $GABA_A$ and glycine receptors. Each subunit class may have multiple members that differ slightly in their sequence and effect on channel function including sensitivity to pharmacologic agents such as alcohol. Alcohol generally enhances $GABA_A$ and glycine receptor function, although $GABA_A$ ρ receptors are inhibited by alcohol. Knockout mice

TABLE 11-3 Properties of Alcohol-Sensitive Ion Channels

Neurotransmitter Agonist or Activator	Channel Name	Channel Subunits	Common Brain Receptors	Major Permeant Ions	Alcohol Effect (Acute)
GABA	$GABA_A$	α,β,γ,δ,ρ	α1/β1/γ2, α4(6)βxδ	Cl^-	Enhance
Glycine	Glycine	α,β	α2/β1	Cl^-	Enhance
Acetylcholine	nAchR	α,β	α4β2, α7–9, α6β2*	Na^+	Enhance/inhibit
Serotonin	$5HT_3$	$5HT_{3a,b}$	$5HT_3$	Na^+	Enhance
ATP	$P2_X$	$P2X_{1-7}$	$P2X_3$, $P2X_4$	Na^+	Inhibit/enhance
Glutamate	NMDA	GluN1, GluN2A-D	GluN1/GluN2A, GluN1/GluN2B	Ca^{++}/Na^+	Inhibit
Glutamate	Non-NMDA	GluA1-4, GluK1-5	GluA1, GluA2/3	Na^+/Ca^{++}	Inhibit
Voltage-gated (potassium)	BK_{Ca},	α,β_{1-4}	α, α/β,	K^+	Enhance
Voltage-gated (potassium)	M-current	Kv7(KCNQ)	Kv7.2, Kv7.3	K^+	Inhibit
Voltage-gated (calcium)	L,P/Q,N,R,T	$Ca_v1,2,3\alpha,\alpha_2\delta,\beta,\gamma$	Multiple	Ca^{++}	Inhibit

Ion channels are listed according to their natural agonist or mode of activation. Subunit families represent those found in the brain or spinal cord. Brain subtypes are examples of subunit combinations commonly expressed by neurons (* indicates other subunits likely required). Alcohol effect indicates change in ion channel function by alcohol acutely administered to recombinant or native receptor preparations.

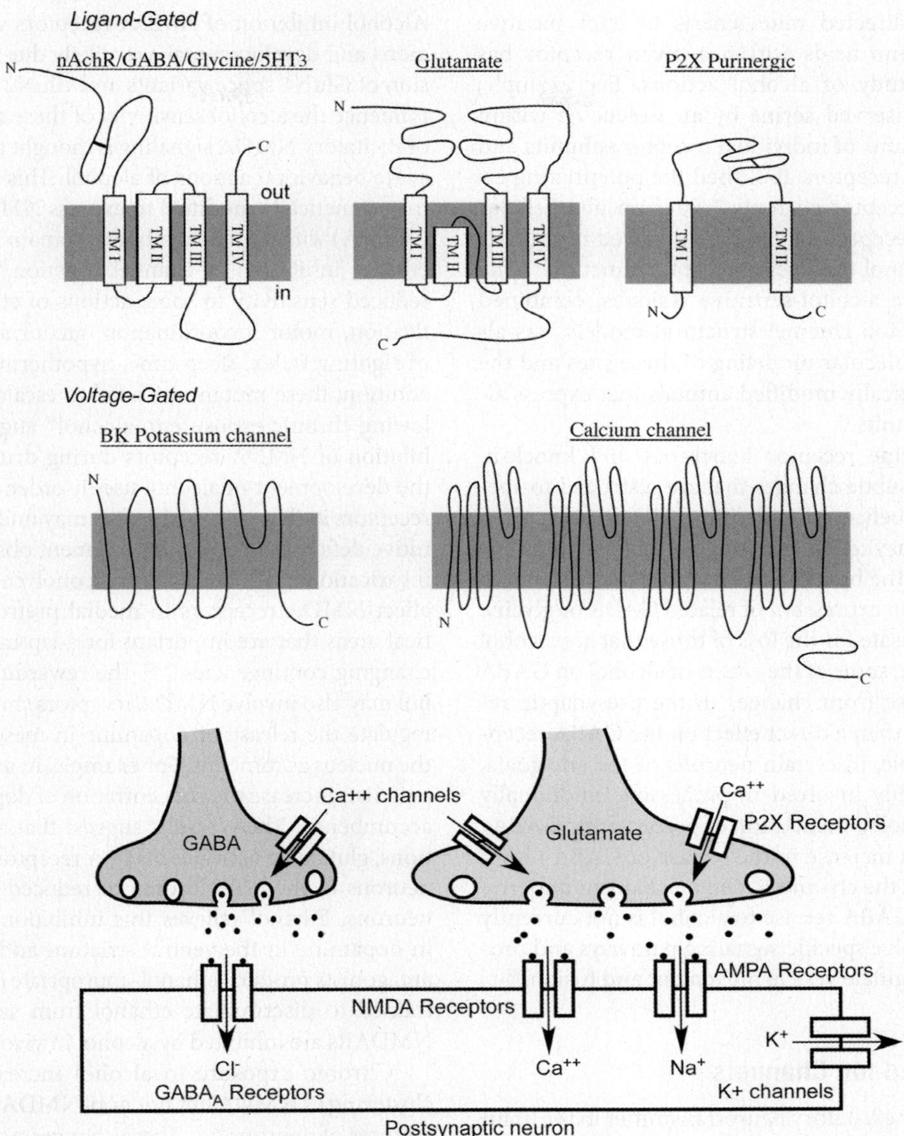

Figure 11-1. Structure and location of alcohol-sensitive ion channels in the neuronal synapse.

lacking the γ2L subunit, which contains an additional 8 amino acids, including a site for phosphorylation of the receptor by protein kinase C, show normal sensitivity to alcohol, although their responsiveness to benzodiazepines is enhanced.[48,49] The role of the γ2 subunit in mediating alcohol action on GABA$_A$ receptors may be phosphorylation dependent, as the alcohol sensitivity of GABA$_A$ α1β2γ2 receptors is markedly enhanced when the kinase PKCε is inhibited.[50] Mice lacking PKCε also show an enhanced response to ethanol suggesting that specific subtypes of GABA$_A$ receptors may show appreciable alcohol sensitivity under certain conditions.[51]

δ-containing GABA receptors are highly sensitive to relatively low concentrations of alcohol and may mediate some effects of alcohol. These receptors contain the α4(6), β and the δ subunit instead of the γ subunit and are affected by concentrations of ethanol (5-10 mM) achieved after only 1 standard drink[52] although not all studies have replicated this finding[53] suggesting that other mechanisms may underlie the effects of alcohol. For example, following restraint stress in rats, GABA$_A$ receptors in GABA interneurons in the VTA became depolarizing due to reduced function of the KCC2 chloride transporter.[54] This results in enhanced inhibition of VTA DA neurons, blunted ethanol-induced increases in nucleus accumbens DA and increased drinking in the stressed rats.

Glycine receptors also gate the flux of chloride and reduce neuronal excitability in both spinal cord and brain. As with GABA$_A$ receptors, ethanol can enhance glycine receptor currents although this depends on the subtypes of α and β subunits expressed.[55,56] Ethanol can also indirectly reduce excitability through release of glycine from astrocytes and activation of inhibitory glycine receptors on neighboring neurons[57,58] although this effect appears to be brain region dependent.

The use of site-directed mutagenesis to alter putative alcohol-sensitive amino acids within a given receptor has revolutionized the study of alcohol actions. For example, replacement of a conserved serine by an isoleucine within transmembrane domains of individual receptor subunits and in $GABA_A$ or glycine receptors abolished the potentiating effects of alcohol on receptor currents.[59] Sites on intracellular loops of the glycine receptor may also be involved in mediating the effects of ethanol on glycine receptor function.[55] The identification of these alcohol-sensitive residues, combined with development of ion channel structural models, has allowed for detailed molecular modeling of these sites and the development of genetically modified animals that express alcohol insensitive subunits.[60]

$GABA_A$ and glycine receptor knock-out and knock-in mice show relatively subtle changes that are restricted to specific alcohol-induced behaviors with little effect on other alcohol actions.[61-66] This may reflect the fact that there are multiple targets for alcohol in the brain and that in the case of knockout animals, changes in expression of related GABA or glycine subunits may compensate for the loss of those that are alcohol sensitive.[67] In addition, some of the effects of alcohol on GABA receptor function arise from changes in the presynaptic release of GABA rather than a direct effect on the GABA receptor itself.[68] For example, in certain neurons of the amygdala, a brain structure highly involved in processing emotionally relevant stimuli, alcohol's potentiation of postsynaptic $GABA_A$ responses is due to an increase in the release of GABA rather than a direct effect on the channel.[69] The mechanism underlying the sensitivity of GABA release to alcohol is not currently known but could involve specific signaling pathways and proteins that normally regulate vesicle movement and fusion.[70]

Glutamate Activated Ion Channels

Glutamate is the major excitatory neurotransmitter in the brain and activates three major subtypes of ion channels: AMPA, kainate, and NMDA receptors. These channels mediate most of the fast excitatory synaptic transmission in the brain and are critical for most forms of synaptic plasticity that underlie learning and memory. NMDA receptors are highly calcium-permeable and require both glutamate and glycine for activation while AMPA and kainate receptors only require glutamate for activation. NMDA receptors are inhibited by ethanol as well as other substances including nitrous oxide, dissociative anesthetics, and volatile solvents such as toluene.[71-73]

NMDA receptors show appreciable sensitivity to behaviorally relevant concentrations of alcohol while AMPA and kainate receptors show a more restricted pattern of ethanol sensitivity.[57,74,75] NMDA receptors expressed by most neurons are antagonized by alcohol at concentrations (10-100 mM) associated with intoxication and sedation although this varies by brain region.[57,75-79] As with $GABA_A$ and glycine receptors, alcohol inhibition of NMDA receptors may involve an interaction with specific residues within defined transmembrane domains of the receptor that control channel gating.[80-82] Alcohol inhibition of NMDA receptors varies across brain regions and developmental ages likely due to differential expression of GluN1 splice variants and GluN2 NMDA subunits that influence the alcohol sensitivity of these receptors.[83,84] Blunting of excitatory NMDA signaling is thought to mediate some of the acute behavioral actions of alcohol. This has been tested using mice genetically modified to express NMDA subunits (GluN1, GluN2A) with a transmembrane domain mutation that reduces ethanol inhibition of channel function.[85,86] These mice show reduced sensitivity to some actions of ethanol (locomotor activation, motor incoordination, anxiolysis) while others (loss of righting reflex, sleep time, hypothermia) are unaffected. In addition, these mutant mice fail to escalate their drinking following chronic exposure to alcohol[86] suggesting that acute inhibition of NMDA receptors during drinking is important in the development of alcohol use disorder. Inhibition of NMDA receptors in the prefrontal cortex may underlie some of the cognitive deficits and errors in judgment observed during alcohol intoxication.[75,87,88] Long-term alcohol consumption may also affect NMDA receptors in medial prefrontal and orbital cortical areas that are important for adapting behavior to rapidly changing contingencies.[89-92] The rewarding properties of alcohol may also involve NMDA receptors since these receptors can regulate the release of dopamine in mesolimbic areas such as the nucleus accumbens. For example, in awake rats, NMDA antagonists increase the concentration of dopamine in the nucleus accumbens.[93] These results suggest that, under normal conditions, glutamate activates NMDA receptors on inhibitory interneurons in the VTA leading to reduced activity of dopamine neurons. Ethanol relieves this inhibition leading to increases in dopamine in the ventral striatum and other areas. NMDA antagonists produce ethanol-appropriate lever responses in rats trained to discriminate ethanol from saline confirming that NMDARs are inhibited by alcohol in vivo.[94]

Chronic exposure to alcohol increases the density and clustering of NMDA but not non-NMDA receptors in primary cultures of neurons.[95-97] These changes occur specifically within the glutamatergic synapse as there is no change in NMDA receptors in extra-synaptic locations. These results suggest that NMDA receptors serve as alcohol sensors and that neurons compensate for the reduction in activity by trafficking more receptors to the synapse where they can be activated by glutamate. While adaptive, this response also increases the susceptibility of animals and humans to seizures that develop during withdrawal from alcohol. NMDA-induced seizure activity is elevated in mice made physically dependent on alcohol and NMDA antagonists reduce or prevent seizures during alcohol withdrawal.[98] Enhanced NMDA receptor function after chronic alcohol exposure involves changes in the expression of specific NMDA receptor subunits.[89,91,99-102]

Other Ethanol-Sensitive Ion Channels

$5HT_3$ Receptors

$5HT_3$ receptors are ion channels activated by serotonin and are permeable to monovalent cations, such as sodium and potassium. Low concentrations of alcohol potentiate ion flow through $5HT_3$ receptors[103,104] and in behavioral studies, $5HT_3$ receptor antagonists block an animal's ability to discriminate ethanol from saline.[105] Some human studies report that the $5HT_3$ antagonist ondansetron reduces alcohol drinking, especially in individuals with early-onset AUD, but this is not a consistent finding[106] (see Section 8, Chapter 60, "Pharmacologic Interventions for Alcohol Use Disorder").

Acetylcholine Nicotinic Receptors

Acetylcholine ligand-gated ion channels are expressed in brain neurons and are related to the nicotinic receptor expressed at the neuromuscular junction.[107] Heteromeric nicotinic receptors composed of αβ subunits are potentiated by ethanol, whereas homomeric receptors composed of just α subunits (α7, for example) are inhibited by ethanol.[108] Alcohol may also indirectly activate nicotinic receptors via increased firing of ACh-expressing cholinergic neurons that project to brain areas involved in reward.[47] Nicotinic receptors containing the α6 subunit are found on VTA dopamine and GABA neurons and are sensitive to low concentrations of ethanol.[109] These subunits are often co-expressed along with α4β2 subunits that are targeted by varenicline, a medication approved for nicotine/tobacco use disorder, and a partial agonist at the α4β2 nicotinic receptor. Varenicline reduces alcohol seeking in rodents without altering responding for sucrose.[110] Human trials have also supported the efficacy of varenicline in alcohol use disorder.[111-113]

ATP-gated Ion Channels

Adenosine triphosphate (ATP) is released into synapses where it activates ion channels of the P2X family.[114] Alcohol inhibits ATP-gated currents in some neurons[115] while the effect of alcohol on recombinant P2X receptors is subtype specific with P2X2 and P2X4 channel currents being inhibited,[115-117] while P2X3 currents are enhanced.[118] Subunit-dependent differences in a small number of amino acids at sites that control channel gating may underlie these differential effects.[119] The anthelminthic drug ivermectin is a positive allosteric modulator of P2X4 channels and blocks the ethanol inhibition of these channels. Ivermectin and some related analogs reduce ethanol consumption in rodent drinking models.[120]

Potassium and Calcium Selective Ion Channels

Potassium channels including those regulated by calcium (SK and BK channels) or G-proteins (GiRK) channels serve as a brake on excitatory glutamatergic transmission by hyperpolarizing the membrane potential. BK channel activity is acutely enhanced by alcohol, and this enhancement may contribute to the inhibition of vasopressin release from neurohypophysial terminals and the resulting diuresis that accompanies alcohol ingestion.[121] SK potassium channels are not directly inhibited by alcohol but are down-regulated in hippocampal and orbitofrontal cortex neurons following chronic alcohol exposure.[91,122] Reductions in SK channel expression may contribute to enhanced neuronal excitability observed during ethanol withdrawal. Alcohol-induced down regulation of SK channels in nucleus accumbens neurons may contribute to elevated drinking as enhancing SK activity in this area with an allosteric modulator (chlorzoxazone) reduced alcohol consumption in rats.[123] In contrast, inhibiting SK2 channels in the rat infralimbic prefrontal cortex enhanced the extinction of alcohol-seeking behavior.[124] While SK2 modulators may represent a novel means of treating individuals with AUD, their efficacy may vary depending on whether subjects are actively drinking or are abstinent. Most voltage-gated potassium and sodium channels are relatively insensitive to relevant concentrations of alcohol although there are exceptions. For example, recombinant Kv7 (in the KCNQ family) channels are inhibited by moderate concentrations of ethanol[125] and Kv7.2/Kv7.3 heteromers underlie the slow, noninactivating M-current that reduces neuronal excitability. In VTA DA neurons, M-current is inhibited by acute ethanol at concentrations that enhance DA neuron firing.[126] Ethanol inhibition of leak potassium channels such as KCNK13, which are important regulators of the resting membrane potential, also leads to enhanced VTA DA neuron firing.[127] Alcohol inhibits certain sub-types of voltage-gate calcium channels.[128] Genetically modified mice lacking the N-type calcium channel show reduced ethanol consumption compared to wild-type animals.[129] Altered expression of T-type calcium channels in thalamic neurons following chronic alcohol exposure may underlie disruptions in sleep commonly observed in individuals with AUD.[130]

Pharmacologic Studies Implicating Other Neurotransmitter Systems

Much of the working knowledge of alcohol's effects on neuronal function comes from animal studies examining the effects of neurotransmitter specific agents on alcohol drinking. A brief review of this literature is presented here and is summarized in **Table 11-4**.

Adenosine

Adenosine is a major inhibitory neurotransmitter in the brain and may serve as an endogenous anti-epileptic. Alcohol inhibits the function of the nucleoside transporter ENT1, leading to increased extracellular adenosine levels,[131] activation of A2 adenosine receptors and increases in cellular levels of cAMP that can activate PKA and stimulate cAMP-dependent changes in gene expression. A2 receptors can form heteromers with D2 dopamine receptors to regulate the activity of medium spiny neurons in the ventral and dorsal striatum. Adenosine analogs that target ENT1 and A2 receptors can reduce voluntary alcohol drinking in experimental animals.[132]

Dopamine

Increases in the activity of mesolimbic projecting dopamine neurons is a critical step mediating the reinforcing effects of substances, including alcohol.[133] Alcohol increases the firing of VTA dopamine-containing neurons leading to enhanced

TABLE 11-4 Alcohol Interactions With Brain Neurotransmitter Systems

Neurotransmitter or Modulator	Effect of Acute Alcohol	Effect of Chronic Alcohol	Role in Alcohol-Induced Behavior
$GABA_A$	Enhance channel activity	Reduced function, altered subunit expression	**Acute**: sedation, anxiolysis **Chronic**: withdrawal symptoms; increased anxiety
Acetylcholine	Enhance/inhibit channel activity	Decreased receptor expression	**Acute**: reward, arousal **Chronic**: maintain drinking; recurrence of use
Serotonin	Enhance channel activity	Variable effects on receptor expression	**Acute**: reward **Chronic**: modulate drinking
Endocannabinoids	Increase release	Reduced receptor expression	**Acute**: reward, euphoria **Chronic**: cognitive effects
Dopamine	Increase release	Blunted responsiveness	**Acute**: reward, euphoria **Chronic**: anhedonia
Glutamate	Inhibit channel activity	Increased receptor expression; function	**Acute**: intoxication, anxiolysis **Chronic**: tolerance, withdrawal excitability, seizures, craving, recurrence of use
Opioid peptides	Enhance release	Altered expression and coupling to signaling pathways	**Acute**: reward (mu) **Chronic**: craving, recurrence of use, dysphoria (kappa)
CRF/NPY	Mixed	Increased (CRF)/decreased (NPY) levels and receptors during withdrawal	**Acute**: stress indicators, increased appetite **Chronic**: increased anxiety, craving, elevated drinking

The table summarizes effects of acute and chronic alcohol on various brain ion channels and neurotransmitter signaling systems. Right column lists alcohol-related behaviors that each system/neurotransmitter may contribute to.

dopamine release in the nucleus accumbens and other areas.[34] This may involve a direct effect on potassium channels that regulate the excitability of VTA neurons[35,126,127] as well as indirectly via modulation of inputs into the VTA. The sensitivity of VTA neurons to alcohol-induced excitation is lower in mice that show a higher voluntary consumption of alcohol, suggesting that these animals may consume more alcohol to sufficiently activate a dopaminergic reward pathway.[34,134] In addition, VTA DA neurons that project to the nucleus accumbens but not those that project to the prefrontal cortex show enhanced glutamatergic plasticity following brief exposure to substances such as cocaine or toluene.[38,135]

Systemic administration of the long-acting dopamine agonists bromocriptine or apomorphine shifts a rat's preference from alcohol to water, especially in those strains of rats that show alcohol preference.[136] These results suggest that activating dopamine receptors with direct agonists reduces the need for alcohol's dopamine-enhancing activity, such that a "reward state" was achieved at lower alcohol levels. Human studies with these agents have not found significant effects on alcohol drinking or recurrence of use.[137]

Opioids and Other Neuropeptides

The involvement of endogenous opioids (endorphins, enkephalins, dynorphin) and other neuropeptides in AUD is suggested by several lines of research. Initial studies showed that acetaldehyde undergoes a metabolic reaction with monoamines to form compounds (tetrahydroquinolines or TIQs) structurally related to morphine.[138] TIQs elicit alcohol-drinking behavior and alcohol preference even after cessation of TIQ administration.[139] However, these findings remain controversial due to lack of reproducibility and the demonstration that TIQ formation in vivo may arise from dietary factors rather than direct effects of alcohol.[140] Alcohol increases the release of certain opioid peptides (such as β-endorphin) from rat pituitary glands, and increases blood levels of β-endorphins in humans.[141] Naloxone and naltrexone, two mu-opioid receptor antagonists, reduce alcohol intake in both animals and humans, and various formulations of naltrexone, including sustained-release and depot forms, are now approved for treating AUD (see Section 8, Chapter 60, "Pharmacological Interventions for Alcohol Use Disorder"). Antagonists of the kappa opioid receptor may also have clinical efficacy for reducing drinking. Kappa receptors are activated by the opioid peptide dynorphin that is involved in aspects of negative reinforcement that occurs during withdrawal from alcohol and other addictive substances.[27] Kappa receptor antagonists reduce alcohol self-administration in rodents, including that induced or augmented by stress.[142-144]

Other neuropeptides such as neuropeptide Y (NPY) and corticotropin releasing factor (CRF) are involved in mediating stress and anxiety and are important regulators of alcohol drinking. CRF is released following activation of the hypothalamic-pituitary-adrenal (HPA) axis leading to elevated levels of cortisol indicative of a stress response. Alcohol also induces CRF release and chronic alcohol use is associated with enhanced anxiety that can be blocked by CRF antagonists.[145]

CRF antagonists reduce the elevated drinking observed in alcohol-(physically) dependent rats without altering consumption in nondependent animals.[146] Mice lacking CRF1 receptors do not show enhanced drinking following chronic ethanol exposure again suggesting an important link between stress and alcohol drinking.[147] However, two different CRF1 antagonists (pexacerfont and verucerfont) failed to reduce cue-induced craving for alcohol in human clinical trials.[148,149] Injected NPY, a neuropeptide associated with the general regulation of feeding behavior and anxiety, reduces drinking in rodents while mice lacking NPY or the NPY Y1 receptor display enhanced ethanol intake.[150] The neuropeptide orexin (also called hypocretin) is synthesized by a small number of neurons in the lateral hypothalamus and axons from these neurons innervate a wide array of brain structures including those involved in reward and cognition.[151] In rodent models, orexin antagonists reduce drinking with greatest efficacy in alcohol-preferring animals.[152,153]

Serotonin

While alcohol enhances cation conductance through $5HT_3$ receptors,[103] serotonin also activates a large number of non-ion channel G-protein linked receptors coupled to various signal transduction pathways. 5HT and 5HT-metabolite concentrations are reduced in the cerebrospinal fluid of individuals with mild AUD, suggesting that reduced 5HT levels or a reduction in 5HT-mediated neurotransmission may predispose certain people to uncontrollable drinking behavior.[154] Similar deficiencies in 5HT neurotransmission may underlie the development of other disorders, including bulimia and obsessive-compulsive behavior, disorders that are characterized by a loss of behavioral control. Pharmacologic agents that enhance 5HT neurotransmission (eg, serotonin selective-uptake inhibitors such as fluoxetine, and sertraline) have no efficacy in treating AUD.[155,156] The 5HT1b receptor may be especially involved in regulating alcohol intake although the data are conflicting regarding whether receptor activity should be enhanced or blocked to reduce ethanol intake.[157-159] In addition, it is not clear whether these manipulations are selective for alcohol as 5HT plays a central role in feeding and drinking behaviors.

Metabotropic Glutamate Receptors

Metabotropic glutamate receptors (mGluR) are G-protein coupled glutamate receptors expressed at both pre- and postsynaptic sites where they influence excitability by reducing neurotransmitter release and regulating membrane excitability. The presynaptic mGluR2 subtype may be particularly important in regulating drinking as P rats previously generated by selective breeding for high alcohol consumption express a premature stop codon in the *Grm2* gene leading to a loss of expression and function of mGluR2 receptors.[160] Pharmacological blockade of mGluR2 receptors in control rats enhances alcohol consumption[160] and alcohol-(physically) dependent animals show a reduction in mGluR2 expression in certain areas of the prefrontal cortex that may regulate drinking.[161]

Endocannabinoids

Endocannabinoids (ECs) are endogenous lipid-derived molecules that activate cannabinoid receptors (CB1, CB2), which also bind Δ^9-tetrahydrocannabinol (THC), the primary psychoactive constituent of cannabis. ECs regulate both GABAergic and glutamatergic synaptic transmission and are synthesized during periods of intense neuronal depolarization. CB1 receptor agonists, including THC, enhance appetite. Animal studies show that CB1 antagonists such as rimonabant reduce ethanol preference in wild-type mice and that mice lacking CB1 receptors show reduced alcohol preference[162] and no alcohol-induced increase in nucleus accumbens dopamine.[163] This effect was also observed for cocaine and nicotine-induced increases in dopamine suggesting an important role of ECs in general drug-induced reward.

Neuroimmune Modulators

Mediators of immune function have recently been identified as important determinants of alcohol-induced neurodegeneration and may also influence brain systems that regulate ethanol intake. Of these, the family of Toll-like receptors (TLR) and the receptor for advanced glycation end products (RAGE) are involved in the brain's response to alcohol.[164] Genetically modified mice lacking the TLR4 receptor show reduced neurodegeneration following chronic exposure to ethanol and show blunted expression of neuroimmune genes.[165] In wild-type mice, repeated exposures to binge-like levels of alcohol induced the expression of TLR receptors including TL4 and activators of TLR signaling such as HMGB1.[166] Similar increases have been reported in postmortem brains from individuals with moderate-severe AUD.[166] These changes correlate with the age of onset of drinking and the lifetime consumption of alcohol with individuals who started drinking earlier and those who consumed the most ethanol showing highest expression.[166,167] Ethanol also induces HMGB1-TLR4 signaling in the gut with subsequent leakage into the circulation of bacterial products that are powerful stimulators of the innate immune system.[168] These mediators then cross the blood brain barrier where they induce pro-inflammatory responses in the brain. Ibudilast, a neuroimmune modulator that blocks TLR4 signaling, reduces alcohol drinking in various rodent models of AUD.[169] In nontreatment seeking individuals with AUD, ibudilast reduced heavy drinking and blunted alcohol cue-induced activation of the ventral striatum.[170]

ADDICTION LIABILITY

Although reward mechanisms are undoubtedly important in the development of heavy alcohol use, other processes and brain areas may be critical for maintaining continued drinking by generating anxiety or stress during withdrawal that is relieved by alcohol (negative reinforcement). In support of this idea, a variety of studies now implicate activation of brain areas such as the amygdala and associated structures ("extended amygdala") with returning to drinking precipitated by alcohol specific cues or stress.[171] In combination with brain stress systems and areas involved in decision-making (prefrontal cortex), these areas may be critically important in driving continued drinking in individuals with AUD.[172] Chronic use of alcohol produces several neuroadaptive changes that may be important in the development of AUD.

Sensitization

Sensitization is defined as an increase in the pharmacologic and physiologic response to a substance after repeated exposures. In mice, sensitization to the locomotor effects of alcohol is well demonstrated although the magnitude and duration of this effect vary depending on the background strain of the animal.[173] Sensitization also occurs for withdrawal as the severity and intensity of withdrawal signs increase after multiple episodes of alcohol intoxication and withdrawal.[174] This form of sensitization is similar to the kindling phenomena observed after repeated brain seizures and may share some of the same mechanisms.[173]

Tolerance and Physical Dependence

Tolerance is manifested as a reduced sensitivity to alcohol and can be of two forms: pharmacokinetic, that is, increased enzymatic capacity (eg, ADH, ALDH, cytochrome P450) to metabolize alcohol, or pharmacodynamic, that is, decreased cellular response to alcohol. A form of short-term acute functional tolerance to alcohol (termed the "Mellanby effect") is the difference in intensity of intoxication effects produced by the same blood concentration of alcohol achieved during the rising phase of the blood alcohol curve (with higher perceived level of intoxication) as compared to the falling phase (lower perceived level of intoxication) several hours later.[175] Tolerance development, in both humans and animal models, is strongly influenced by context and environment.[176] Individuals who regularly consume large amounts of alcohol can develop profound tolerance to the CNS depressant effects of alcohol. For example, the lethal dose 50 percent (LD50) in nontolerant humans is approximately 400 to 500 mg%, while even higher concentrations are often reported in highly tolerant individuals, such as some arrested for driving under the influence.[177] Physical dependence is defined by the occurrence of withdrawal signs and symptoms that appear after the abstinence from alcohol drinking. Typical alcohol withdrawal signs include disturbed sleep, tremor, convulsions; symptoms include anxiety, depression, and increased craving for alcohol. Tolerance and physical dependence also develop at the cellular level so that the acute effects of alcohol on ion channel or receptor function are diminished in animals chronically exposed to alcohol. For example, acute ethanol no longer inhibits action potential firing of OFC neurons in chronically drinking mice[178] or monkeys[179] or in mice made physically dependent on alcohol.[58] As mentioned earlier, this adaptation may involve changes in signaling pathways that regulate receptor subunit expression or the functional state of alcohol-sensitive ion channels as neurons adapt to the chronic presence of alcohol.[180,181]

AUD, like other substance use disorders, is a chronic, relapsing condition and a strong desire or craving for alcohol is one of the possible criteria for diagnosing AUD.[15] The risk of reuse declines logarithmically after abstinence from use but may occur even after long periods of abstinence. Such recurrence of use suggest that prolonged alcohol use induces long-lasting or permanent changes in brain circuitry and processes that mediate alcohol use. These include reduced function of prefrontal cortical areas involved in cognitive control of behavior and enhanced activity of stress-related areas such as the central nucleus of the amygdala.[172] Animal models of craving and recurrence of use involve measuring consumption in alcohol-trained animals following various periods of forced abstinence.[182,183] Animals display a robust increase in alcohol consumption when it is re-introduced, and this effect is characterized by not only higher rates of drinking but also increased preference for solutions containing higher alcohol concentrations. In addition, the alcohol deprivation effect in animals can persist for very long periods of abstinence (up to 9 months; about 1/3 the lifespan of a rat), suggesting long-lasting or even irreversible changes in mechanisms regulating drinking behavior in humans.

Medical Complications

Alcohol affects nearly all tissues and organ systems. People who drink heavily show skeletal fragility and damage to tissues such as brain, liver, and heart, as well as increased susceptibility to some cancers.[184-186] Long-term ingestion of high concentrations of alcohol can lead to a variety of pathologies associated with the gastrointestinal tract including esophageal varices and bleeding, erosive gastritis, and diarrhea and malabsorption of nutrients and vitamins.[24] Alcohol consumption is also associated with an increased risk of tumors in the GI system[184] as well as in other tissues including lung and breast.[185] Acute and chronic ingestion of alcohol generally decreases sexual performance in both men and women although sexual behavior may be enhanced due to loss of inhibitory control and judgment. Alcohol has manifold effects on the cardiovascular system. Drinking is associated with hypertension and increased risk for cardiac arrhythmia, heart attack and stroke.[187] The deleterious effect of alcohol on the heart and other organ systems may be countered by protective effects of small amounts of alcohol on cardiovascular tissue although this remains controversial.[187] For example, some previous studies suggested that low to moderate alcohol use (approximately 1-2 drinks per day) is associated with a reduced risk of coronary disease, possibly due to alcohol-induced changes in plasma lipoproteins and alterations in cell protection pathways. However, data from more recent studies suggest that these beneficial effects may have been overestimated and could have resulted from other factors including diet, genetic background and health issues among participants.[188] Chronic alcohol ingestion increases fat accumulation in the liver that can progress to liver enzyme elevation and fatty infiltration (nonalcoholic fatty liver disease), and eventually to cirrhosis.[186] Alcohol-induced liver damage is due in part to the production of acetaldehyde that readily reacts with proteins, lipids and other compounds leading to impaired mitochondrial function. Although moderate to heavy alcohol consumption leads to fatty liver in most individuals, only a small fraction (8%-20%) of people who drink develop cirrhosis suggesting that other factors are involved.[189] These include sex (women are at a higher risk of developing alcoholic liver disease; ALD), obesity, and viral hepatitis. Genetic factors are also important as suggested by increased risk of ALD in the second monozygotic twin if the first twin has ALD. Individual genes shown to be associated with risk of developing ALD include those involved in alcohol metabolism including variants of *ADH* (alcohol dehydrogenase), *ALDH* (acetaldehyde dehydrogenase) and *CYP450* (cytochrome P450).[189] Gene association studies indicate that ALD risk is enhanced in individuals with polymorphisms in genes involved in lipid metabolism (*PNPLA3, TM6SF2, MBOAT7*), oxidative stress (*SOD2*) and immune function (*TNF, ILB, CTLA4*). Changes in epigenetic modifiers including microRNAs, histone acetylation/deacetylation enzymes and DNA methylases have also been implicated in the development of ALD.[189]

Brain magnetic resonance imaging (MRI) studies show decreases in brain volume in adults with AUD with corresponding increases in cortical cerebrospinal fluid that can be distinguished from those found in other neuropsychiatric disorders such as schizophrenia and Alzheimer disease.[190,191] When corrected for age-related changes in these parameters, the frontal lobes and cerebellar gray matter are particularly sensitive to alcohol-induced shrinkage.[192] These studies also show that volume deficits are found in anterior but not poster hippocampus and that these deficits were more severe in patients who displayed symptoms of memory loss and possible Korsakoff syndrome (memory loss due to thiamine deficiency). Prenatal as well as postnatal exposure to alcohol disrupts and reduces the area of the corpus callosum.[193] Functional imaging techniques such as positron emission tomography (PET) show reduced brain glucose metabolism in cortical areas and reductions in striatal dopamine D2/3 receptors in individuals with AUD as compared to control subjects.[194,195] Changes in blood flow coupled with structural damage to frontal brain areas may underlie the deficits in cognitive and emotional behaviors observed in patients with AUD.[196,197]

In humans, chronic heavy drinking (>4 drinks per day, 8 per week for females; >5 drinks per day, 15 per week for males) produces substantial changes in brain neuron density.[198] Animal studies suggest that even brief episodes of heavy drinking, or binges, also cause neuron loss.[199] These findings are particularly relevant for critical periods of brain development that span from early adolescence through young adulthood as longitudinal imaging studies reveal accelerated loss of gray matter in frontal cortex[200] and cerebellum[201] of adolescent who drink compared to adolescents who don't.

The mechanisms underlying ethanol-induced neurotoxicity are not completely understood but may arise from overactivation of NMDA receptors during alcohol withdrawal. Chronic exposure of neurons to ethanol up-regulates the functional status of the NMDA receptor; these effects are revealed during withdrawal.[202,203] Enhanced receptor activation by glutamate may lead to above-normal production of cellular signals such as reactive oxygen species that contribute to cell death.

In other cases of ethanol-induced neurotoxicity, non–NMDA-mediated mechanisms are involved. In an acute binge model of alcohol intoxication, rats given large doses of alcohol over a 3- to 4-day period show pronounced loss of neurons in specific brain areas, including the entorhinal cortex and dentate gyrus. The toxic action of ethanol was not blocked by NMDA antagonists but was attenuated by the diuretic furosemide suggesting other pathways for ethanol-induced brain damage.[204] Chronic alcohol drinking may also induce activation of microglia and astrocytes in brain tissue and promote aberrant signaling of the neuroimmune system.[205] This may lead to over-expression of pro-inflammatory molecules such as cytokines, oxidases and proteases that contribute to dysfunctional frontal circuits observed in subjects with AUD.[206]

Alcohol use during pregnancy can lead to a variety of birth defects and alterations in normal growth and development of the newborn.[207] One in three infants born to mothers with AUD display symptoms of fetal alcohol spectrum disorder (FASD) that include, among others, CNS dysfunction such as low IQ and microcephaly, delayed growth, and facial abnormalities.[208] Current findings suggest that while binge drinking during pregnancy may be particularly damaging, even low levels of alcohol can have adverse effects. The U.S. Surgeon General and various medical societies in the United States, Canada and other countries recommend women abstain from alcohol during pregnancy.[209] Similar to findings with alcohol-induced liver damage, gene association studies suggest that alcohol metabolizing enzymes (ADH, ALDH) are important in determining the severity of FASD.[210] In addition, there is an association between prenatal alcohol exposure and epigenetic mechanisms including DNA methylation and histone acetylation of key genes involved in early development. Polymorphisms in these genes that affect their modulation by epigenetic processes may enhance the risk of FASD, although more studies are needed to confirm these findings.[210]

CONCLUSIONS/FUTURE RESEARCH

A great deal of progress has been made in recent years in understanding the sites and mechanisms of alcohol's effect on the brain. There is a growing appreciation that alcohol and other substances initially target brain circuits involved in reward and learning and with repeated use causes long-lasting changes in areas involved in habit and compulsion, stress, and cognitive control of behavior. A consensus has emerged that specific ligand-gated and voltage-gated ion channels represent the sites of action for many of the acute effects of alcohol on neuronal function, although exactly how alcohol produces these effects remains unclear. Homeostatic mechanisms of neuroplasticity are likely engaged during repeated episodes of alcohol drinking and withdrawal as neurons and brain circuits attempt to adapt to the periodic presence of alcohol. These effects may involve changes in the expression and distribution of ion channel subunits and their downstream signaling processes that are normally involved in allowing an organism to learn and adapt to its environment. Chronic use of alcohol may usurp these mechanisms and result in a near permanent altered neuropsychological state that promotes continued alcohol consumption even in the face of adverse consequences. More work is needed with transgenic or knock-in animals that express proteins with altered alcohol sensitivity to better understand the correlation between these targets and alcohol's behavioral effects. For example, if ion channels gated by glutamate, GABA, acetylcholine, ATP, and serotonin represent primary targets of alcohol action, how does perturbation of these channels lead to behaviors such as reward, craving, and reinforcement that appear to involve complex neurocircuitry and multiple neurotransmitters such as dopamine, opioids, and neuropeptides?

Other areas that need attention include elucidating the normal physiological processes that guide responses and seeking for food and other natural reinforcers, as well as what genetic and environmental factors contribute to an individual's risk for developing AUD. Better use of brain imaging techniques in conjunction with electrophysiological recording and network modeling would also improve our understanding of regional changes in brain function in individuals with AUD. More effort is needed to develop better treatments for AUD including using noninvasive brain stimulation techniques. Lastly, more emphasis and support for research into the causes and treatments of AUD is needed to enhance public awareness that AUD is a chronic relapsing disease that, like other chronic diseases, can be successfully treated.

REFERENCES

1. Mahdi AS, McBride AJ. Intravenous injection of alcohol by drug injectors: report of three cases. *Alcohol Alcohol.* 1999;34(6):918-919.
2. Becker HC, Lopez MF. An animal model of alcohol dependence to screen medications for treating alcoholism. *Int Rev Neurobiol.* 2016;126:157-177.
3. Vendruscolo LF, Roberts AJ. Operant alcohol self-administration in dependent rats: focus on the vapor model. *Alcohol.* 2014;48(3):277-286.
4. Valentine GW, Jatlow PI, Coffman M, Nadim H, Gueorguieva R, Sofuoglu M. The effects of alcohol-containing e-cigarettes on young adult smokers. *Drug Alcohol Depend.* 2016;159:272-276.
5. Garcia AM. U.S. state statutes banning powdered alcohol: exceptions and penalties. *Am J Public Health.* 2017;107(6):880-882.
6. Le Dare B, Gicquel T. Therapeutic applications of ethanol: a review. *J Pharm Pharm Sci.* 2019;22(1):525-535.
7. Haas DM, Morgan AM, Deans SJ, Schubert FP. Ethanol for preventing preterm birth in threatened preterm labor. *Cochrane Database Syst Rev.* 2015;(11):CD011445.
8. FDA. *Determination That Alcohol and Dextrose Injection, 5 Milliliters/100 Milliliters, 5 Grams/100 Milliliters; and 10 Milliliters/100 Milliliters, 5 Grams/100 Milliliters, Were Withdrawn From Sale for Reasons of Safety or Effectiveness. In. Vol FDA-2021-P-0375.* Federal Register: United States Government; 2021.
9. Rosenbaum M, McCarty T. Alcohol prescription by surgeons in the prevention and treatment of delirium tremens: historic and current practice. *Gen Hosp Psychiatry.* 2002;24(4):257-259.
10. Blocker JS Jr. Did prohibition really work? Alcohol prohibition as a public health innovation. *Am J Public Health.* 2006;96(2):233-243.
11. Substance Abuse and Mental Health Services Administration. *Key Substance Use and Mental Health Indicators in the United States: Results from the 2020 National Survey on Drug Use and Health (HHS Publication No. PEP21-07-01-003, NSDUH Series H-56).* Center for Behavioral Health Statistics and Quality, Substance Abuse and Mental Health Services Administration.
12. Grant BF, Goldstein RB, Saha TD, et al. Epidemiology of DSM-5 alcohol use disorder: results from the national epidemiologic survey on alcohol and related conditions III. *JAMA Psychiatry.* 2015;72(8):757-766.
13. Sacks JJ, Gonzales KR, Bouchery EE, Tomedi LE, Brewer RD. 2010 national and state costs of excessive alcohol consumption. *Am J Prev Med.* 2015;49(5):e73-e79.
14. Leggio L, Kenna GA, Fenton M, Bonenfant E, Swift RM. Typologies of alcohol dependence. From Jellinek to genetics and beyond. *Neuropsychol Rev.* 2009;19(1):115-129.
15. *Diagnostic and Statistical Manual of Mental Disorders: DSM-5-TR.* 5th ed. Text Revision DSM-5-TR ed. American Psychiatric Association; 2022.
16. Hingson RW, Heeren T, Winter MR. Age at drinking onset and alcohol dependence: age at onset, duration, and severity. *Arch Pediatr Adolesc Med.* 2006;160(7):739-746.
17. Kwako LE, Patterson J, Salloum IM, Trim RS. Alcohol use disorder and co-occurring mental health conditions. *Alcohol Res.* 2019;40(1):arcr.v40.1.00.
18. Hall OT, Phan KL, Gorka S. Childhood adversity and the association between stress sensitivity and problematic alcohol use in adults. *J Trauma Stress.* 2022;35(1):148-158.
19. Verhulst B, Neale MC, Kendler KS. The heritability of alcohol use disorders: a meta-analysis of twin and adoption studies. *Psychol Med.* 2015;45(5):1061-1072.
20. Edenberg HJ, Gelernter J, Agrawal A. Genetics of alcoholism. *Curr Psychiatry Rep.* 2019;21(4):26.
21. Sanchez-Roige S, Palmer AA, Clarke TK. Recent efforts to dissect the genetic basis of alcohol use and abuse. *Biol Psychiatry.* 2020;87(7):609-618.
22. Baraona E, Abittan CS, Dohmen K, et al. Gender differences in pharmacokinetics of alcohol. *Alcohol Clin Exp Res.* 2001;25(4):502-507.
23. Cederbaum AI. Alcohol metabolism. *Clin Liver Dis.* 2012;16(4):667-685.
24. Bujanda L. The effects of alcohol consumption upon the gastrointestinal tract. *Am J Gastroenterol.* 2000;95(12):3374-3382.
25. Burgos-Sanchez C, Jones NN, Avillion M, et al. Impact of alcohol consumption on snoring and sleep apnea: a systematic review and meta-analysis. *Otolaryngol Head Neck Surg.* 2020;163(6):1078-1086.
26. Chan LN, Anderson GD. Pharmacokinetic and pharmacodynamic drug interactions with ethanol (alcohol). *Clin Pharmacokinet.* 2014; 53(12):1115-1136.
27. Koob GF. Drug addiction: hyperkatifeia/negative reinforcement as a framework for medications development. *Pharmacol Rev.* 2021;73(1):163-201.
28. Everitt BJ, Robbins TW. Drug addiction: updating actions to habits to compulsions ten years on. *Annu Rev Psychol.* 2016;67:23-50.
29. Bellone C, Loureiro M, Luscher C. Drug-evoked synaptic plasticity of excitatory transmission in the ventral tegmental area. *Cold Spring Harb Perspect Med.* 2021;11(4):a039701.
30. Pascoli V, Hiver A, Van Zessen R, et al. Stochastic synaptic plasticity underlying compulsion in a model of addiction. *Nature.* 2018;564(7736):366-371.
31. Bobadilla AC, Heinsbroek JA, Gipson CD, et al. Corticostriatal plasticity, neuronal ensembles, and regulation of drug-seeking behavior. *Prog Brain Res.* 2017;235:93-112.
32. Stefanik MT, Moussawi K, Kupchik YM, et al. Optogenetic inhibition of cocaine seeking in rats. *Addict Biol.* 2013;18(1):50-53.
33. Ding ZM, Oster SM, Hauser SR, et al. Synergistic self-administration of ethanol and cocaine directly into the posterior ventral tegmental area: involvement of serotonin-3 receptors. *J Pharmacol Exp Ther.* 2012;340(1):202-209.

34. Brodie MS, Pesold C, Appel SB. Ethanol directly excites dopaminergic ventral tegmental area reward neurons. *Alcohol Clin Exp Res.* 1999;23(11):1848-1852.
35. Okamoto T, Harnett MT, Morikawa H. Hyperpolarization-activated cation current (Ih) is an ethanol target in midbrain dopamine neurons of mice. *J Neurophysiol.* 2006;95(2):619-626.
36. Hopf FW, Martin M, Chen BT, Bowers MS, Mohamedi MM, Bonci A. Withdrawal from intermittent ethanol exposure increases probability of burst firing in VTA neurons in vitro. *J Neurophysiol.* 2007;98(4):2297-2310.
37. Saal D, Dong Y, Bonci A, Malenka RC. Drugs of abuse and stress trigger a common synaptic adaptation in dopamine neurons. *Neuron.* 2003;37(4):577-582.
38. Beckley JT, Evins CE, Fedarovich H, Gilstrap MJ, Woodward JJ. Medial prefrontal cortex inversely regulates toluene-induced changes in markers of synaptic plasticity of mesolimbic dopamine neurons. *J Neurosci.* 2013;33(2):804-813.
39. Wang J, Lanfranco MF, Gibb SL, Yowell QV, Carnicella S, Ron D. Long-lasting adaptations of the NR2B-containing NMDA receptors in the dorsomedial striatum play a crucial role in alcohol consumption and relapse. *J Neurosci.* 2010;30(30):10187-10198.
40. Weiss F, Hurd YL, Ungerstedt U, Markou A, Plotsky PM, Koob GF. Neurochemical correlates of cocaine and ethanol self-administration. *Ann N Y Acad Sci.* 1992;654:220-241.
41. Doyon WM, York JL, Diaz LM, Samson HH, Czachowski CL, Gonzales RA. Dopamine activity in the nucleus accumbens during consummatory phases of oral ethanol self-administration. *Alcohol Clin Exp Res.* 2003;27(10):1573-1582.
42. Weiss F, Lorang MT, Bloom FE, Koob GF. Oral alcohol self-administration stimulates dopamine release in the rat nucleus accumbens: genetic and motivational determinants. *J Pharmacol Exp Ther.* 1993;267(1):250-258.
43. Krystal JH, Petrakis IL, Webb E, et al. Dose-related ethanol-like effects of the NMDA antagonist, ketamine, in recently detoxified alcoholics. *ArchGenPsychiatry.* 1998;55:354-360.
44. Sinha R, Li CS. Imaging stress- and cue-induced drug and alcohol craving: association with relapse and clinical implications. *Drug Alcohol Rev.* 2007;26(1):25-31.
45. Schacht JP, Yeongbin I, Hoffman M, Voronin KE, Book SW, Anton RF. Effects of pharmacological and genetic regulation of COMT activity in alcohol use disorder: a randomized, placebo-controlled trial of tolcapone. *Neuropsychopharmacology.* 2022;47:1953-1960.
46. Forman SA, Miller KW. Molecular sites of anesthetic action in postsynaptic nicotinic membranes. *Trends Pharmacol Sci.* 1989; 10(11):447-452.
47. Abrahao KP, Salinas AG, Lovinger DM. Alcohol and the brain: neuronal molecular targets, synapses, and circuits. *Neuron.* 2017;96(6):1223-1238.
48. Homanics GE, Harrison NL, Quinlan JJ, et al. Normal electrophysiological and behavioral responses to ethanol in mice lacking the long splice variant of the gamma2 subunit of the gamma-aminobutyrate type A receptor. *Neuropharmacology.* 1999;38(2):253-265.
49. Quinlan JJ, Firestone LL, Homanics GE. Mice lacking the long splice variant of the gamma 2 subunit of the GABA(A) receptor are more sensitive to benzodiazepines. *Pharmacol Biochem Behav.* 2000;66(2):371-374.
50. Qi ZH, Song M, Wallace MJ, et al. Protein Kinase C epsilon regulates $GABA_A$ receptor sensitivity to ethanol and benzodiazepines through phosphorylation of γ2 subunits. *J Biol Chem.* 2007;282(45):33052-33063.
51. Hodge CW, Mehmert KK, Kelley SP, et al. Supersensitivity to allosteric GABA(A) receptor modulators and alcohol in mice lacking PKCepsilon. *Nat Neurosci.* 1999;2(11):997-1002.
52. Wallner M, Hanchar HJ, Olsen RW. Ethanol enhances alpha 4 beta 3 delta and alpha 6 beta 3 delta gamma-aminobutyric acid type A receptors at low concentrations known to affect humans. *Proc Natl Acad Sci U S A.* 2003;100(25):15218-15223.
53. Borghese CM, Storustovu S, Ebert B, et al. The delta subunit of gamma-aminobutyric acid type A receptors does not confer sensitivity to low concentrations of ethanol. *J Pharmacol Exp Ther.* 2006;316(3):1360-1368.
54. Ostroumov A, Thomas AM, Kimmey BA, Karsch JS, Doyon WM, Dani JA. Stress increases ethanol self-administration via a shift toward excitatory GABA signaling in the ventral tegmental area. *Neuron.* 2016;92(2):493-504.
55. Burgos CF, Munoz B, Guzman L, Aguayo LG. Ethanol effects on glycinergic transmission: from molecular pharmacology to behavior responses. *Pharmacol Res.* 2015;101:18-29.
56. Munoz B, Mariqueo T, Murath P, et al. Modulatory actions of the glycine receptor beta subunit on the positive allosteric modulation of ethanol in alpha2 containing receptors. *Front Mol Neurosci.* 2021;14:763868.
57. Badanich KA, Mulholland PJ, Beckley JT, Trantham-Davidson H, Woodward JJ. Ethanol reduces neuronal excitability of lateral orbitofrontal cortex neurons via a glycine receptor dependent mechanism. *Neuropsychopharmacology.* 2013;38(7):1176-1188.
58. Nimitvilai-Roberts S, Gioia D, Zamudio PA, Woodward JJ. Ethanol inhibition of lateral orbitofrontal cortex neuron excitability is mediated via dopamine D1/D5 receptor-induced release of astrocytic glycine. *Neuropharmacology.* 2021;192:108600.
59. Mihic SJ, Ye Q, Wick MJ, et al. Sites of alcohol and volatile anaesthetic action on $GABA_A$ and glycine receptors. *Nature.* 1997;389:385-389.
60. Howard RJ, Slesinger PA, Davies DL, Das J, Trudell JR, Harris RA. Alcohol-binding sites in distinct brain proteins: the quest for atomic level resolution. *Alcohol Clin Exp Res.* 2011;35(9):1561-1573.
61. Werner DF, Blednov YA, Ariwodola OJ, et al. Knockin mice with ethanol-insensitive alpha1-containing gamma-aminobutyric acid type A receptors display selective alterations in behavioral responses to ethanol. *J Pharmacol Exp Ther.* 2006;319(1):219-227.
62. Mihalek RM, Bowers BJ, Wehner JM, et al. GABA(A)-receptor delta subunit knockout mice have multiple defects in behavioral responses to ethanol. *Alcohol Clin Exp Res.* 2001;25(12):1708-1718.
63. Blednov YA, Borghese CM, McCracken ML, et al. Loss of ethanol conditioned taste aversion and motor stimulation in knockin mice with ethanol-insensitive alpha2-containing GABA(A) receptors. *J Pharmacol Exp Ther.* 2011;336(1):145-154.
64. Blednov YA, Benavidez JM, Homanics GE, Harris RA. Behavioral characterization of knockin mice with mutations M287L and Q266I in the glycine receptor alpha1 subunit. *J Pharmacol Exp Ther.* 2012;340(2):317-329.
65. Aguayo LG, Castro P, Mariqueo T, et al. Altered sedative effects of ethanol in mice with α1 glycine receptor subunits that are insensitive to Gβγ modulation. *Neuropsychopharmacology.* 2014;39(11):2538-2548.
66. San Martin L, Gallegos S, Araya A, et al. Ethanol consumption and sedation are altered in mice lacking the glycine receptor alpha2 subunit. *Br J Pharmacol.* 2020;177(17):3941-3956.
67. Woodward JJ. GABAA alpha 4 receptor subunits and ethanol: a knockout punch? *Alcohol Clin Exp Res.* 2008;32(1):8-9.
68. Weiner JL, Valenzuela CF. Ethanol modulation of GABAergic transmission: the view from the slice. *Pharmacol Ther.* 2006;111(3): 533-554.
69. Roberto M, Madamba SG, Moore SD, Tallent MK, Siggins GR. Ethanol increases GABAergic transmission at both pre- and postsynaptic sites in rat central amygdala neurons. *Proc Natl Acad Sci U S A.* 2003;100(4):2053-2058.
70. Bajo M, Cruz MT, Siggins GR, Messing R, Roberto M. Protein kinase C epsilon mediation of CRF- and ethanol-induced GABA release in central amygdala. *Proc Natl Acad Sci U S A.* 2008;105(24):8410-8415.
71. Ogata J, Shiraishi M, Namba T, Smothers CT, Woodward JJ, Harris RA. Effects of anesthetics on mutant N-methyl-D-aspartate receptors expressed in Xenopus oocytes. *J Pharmacol Exp Ther.* 2006;318(1):434-443.
72. Cruz SL, Balster RL, Woodward JJ. Effects of volatile solvents on recombinant N-methyl-D-aspartate receptors expressed in Xenopus oocytes. *Br J Pharmacol.* 2000;131(7):1303-1308.
73. Beckley JT, Woodward JJ. The abused inhalant toluene differentially modulates excitatory and inhibitory synaptic transmission in deep-layer neurons of the medial prefrontal cortex. *Neuropsychopharmacology.* 2011;36(7):1531-1542.

74. Mameli M, Zamudio PA, Carta M, Valenzuela CF. Developmentally regulated actions of alcohol on hippocampal glutamatergic transmission. *J Neurosci*. 2005;25(35):8027-8036.
75. Weitlauf C, Woodward JJ. Ethanol selectively attenuates NMDAR-mediated synaptic transmission in the prefrontal cortex. *Alcohol Clin Exp Res*. 2008;32(4):690-698.
76. Lovinger DM, White G, Weight FF. Ethanol inhibits NMDA-activated ion current in hippocampal neurons. *Science*. 1989;243:1721-1724.
77. Hoffman PL, Moses F, Tabakoff B. Selective inhibition by ethanol of glutamate-stimulated cyclic GMP production in primary cultures of cerebellar granule cells. *Neuropharmacology*. 1989;28:1239-1243.
78. Woodward JJ, Gonzales RA. Ethanol inhibition of N-methyl-D-aspartate-stimulated endogenous dopamine release from rat striatal slices: reversal by glycine. *J Neurochem*. 1990;54(2):712-715.
79. Gonzales RA, Brown LM. Brain regional differences in glycine reversal of ethanol-induced inhibition of N-methyl-D-aspartate-stimulated neurotransmitter release. *Life Sci*. 1995;56:571-577.
80. Ronald KM, Mirshahi T, Woodward JJ. Ethanol inhibition of N-methyl-D-aspartate receptors is reduced by site-directed mutagenesis of a transmembrane domain phenylalanine residue. *J Biol Chem*. 2001; 276(48):44729-44735.
81. Honse Y, Ren H, Lipsky RH, Peoples RW. Sites in the fourth membrane-associated domain regulate alcohol sensitivity of the NMDA receptor. *Neuropharmacology*. 2004;46(5):647-654.
82. Xu M, Smothers CT, Trudell J, Woodward JJ. Ethanol inhibition of constitutively open N-methyl-D-aspartate receptors. *J Pharmacol Exp Ther*. 2012;340(1):218-226.
83. Jin C, Smothers CT, Woodward JJ. Enhanced ethanol inhibition of recombinant N-methyl-D-aspartate receptors by magnesium: role of NR3A subunits. *Alcohol Clin Exp Res*. 2008;32(6):1059-1066.
84. Jin C, Woodward JJ. Effects of 8 different NR1 splice variants on the ethanol inhibition of recombinant NMDA receptors. *Alcohol Clin Exp Res*. 2006;30(4):673-679.
85. den Hartog CR, Beckley JT, Smothers TC, et al. Alterations in ethanol-induced behaviors and consumption in knock-in mice expressing ethanol-resistant NMDA receptors. *PLoS One*. 2013;8(11):e80541.
86. Zamudio PA, Gioia DA, Lopez M, Homanics GE, Woodward JJ. The escalation in ethanol consumption following chronic intermittent ethanol exposure is blunted in mice expressing ethanol-resistant GluN1 or GluN2A NMDA receptor subunits. *Psychopharmacology (Berl)*. 2021;238(1):271-279.
87. Tu Y, Kroener S, Abernathy K, et al. Ethanol inhibits persistent activity in prefrontal cortical neurons. *J Neurosci*. 2007;27(17):4765-4775.
88. Abernathy K, Chandler LJ, Woodward JJ. Alcohol and the prefrontal cortex. *Int Rev Neurobiol*. 2010;91:289-320.
89. Kroener S, Mulholland PJ, New NN, Gass JT, Becker HC, Chandler LJ. Chronic alcohol exposure alters behavioral and synaptic plasticity of the rodent prefrontal cortex. *PLoS One*. 2012;7(5):e37541.
90. Badanich KA, Becker HC, Woodward JJ. Effects of chronic intermittent ethanol exposure on orbitofrontal and medial prefrontal cortex-dependent behaviors in mice. *Behav Neurosci*. 2011;125(6):879-891.
91. Nimitvilai S, Lopez MF, Mulholland PJ, Woodward JJ. Chronic intermittent ethanol exposure enhances the excitability and synaptic plasticity of lateral orbitofrontal cortex neurons and induces a tolerance to the acute inhibitory actions of ethanol. *Neuropsychopharmacology*. 2016;41(4):1112-1127.
92. Gioia DA, Woodward JJ. Altered activity of lateral orbitofrontal cortex neurons in mice following chronic intermittent ethanol exposure. *eNeuro*. 2021;8(2):ENEURO.0503-20.2021.
93. Jentsch JD, Tran A, Taylor JR, Roth RH. Prefrontal cortical involvement in phencyclidine-induced activation of the mesolimbic dopamine system: behavioral and neurochemical evidence. *Psychopharmacology (Berl)*. 1998;138(1):89-95.
94. Colombo G, Grant KA. NMDA receptor complex antagonists have ethanol-like discriminative stimulus effects. *Ann N Y Acad Sci*. 1992; 654:421-423.
95. Iorio KR, Reinlib L, Tabakoff B, Hoffman PL. Chronic exposure of cerebellar granule cells to ethanol results in increased N-methyl-D-aspartate receptor function. *Mol Pharmacol*. 1992;41:1142-1148.
96. Carpenter-Hyland EP, Woodward JJ, Chandler LJ. Chronic ethanol induces synaptic but not extrasynaptic targeting of NMDA receptors. *J Neurosci*. 2004;24(36):7859-7868.
97. Clapp P, Gibson ES, Dell'acqua ML, Hoffman PL. Phosphorylation regulates removal of synaptic N-methyl-D-aspartate receptors after withdrawal from chronic ethanol exposure. *J Pharmacol Exp Ther*. 2010;332(3):720-729.
98. Grant KA, Valverius P, Hudspith M, Tabakoff B. Ethanol withdrawal seizures and the NMDA receptor complex. *EurJPharmacol*. 1990; 176:289-296.
99. Blevins T, Mirshahi T, Chandler LJ, Woodward JJ. Effects of acute and chronic ethanol exposure on heteromeric N-methyl-D-aspartate receptors expressed in HEK 293 cells. *J Neurochem*. 1997;69(6):2345-2354.
100. Follesa P, Ticku MK. Chronic ethanol treatment differentially regulates NMDA receptor subunit mRNA expression in rat brain. *Mol Brain Res*. 1995;29:99-106.
101. Snell LD, Nunley KR, Lickteig RL, Browning MD, Tabakoff B, Hoffman PL. Regional and subunit specific changes in NMDA receptor mRNA and immunoreactivity in mouse brain following chronic ethanol ingestion. *Brain Res Mol Brain Res*. 1996;40(1):71-78.
102. Szumlinski KK, Ary AW, Lominac KD, Klugmann M, Kippin TE. Accumbens Homer2 overexpression facilitates alcohol-induced neuroplasticity in C57BL/6J mice. *Neuropsychopharmacology*. 2008;33(6):1365-1378.
103. Lovinger DM, White G. Ethanol potentiation of 5-hydroxytryptamine3 receptor-mediated ion current in neuroblastoma cells and isolated adult mammalian neurons. *Mol Pharmacol*. 1991;40:263-270.
104. Hu XQ, Hayrapetyan V, Gadhiya JJ, Rhubottom HE, Lovinger DM, Machu TK. Mutations of L293 in transmembrane two of the mouse 5-hydroxytryptamine3A receptor alter gating and alcohol modulatory actions. *Br J Pharmacol*. 2006;148(1):88-101.
105. Grant KA, Barrett JE. Blockade of the discriminative stimulus effects of ethanol with 5-HT3 receptor antagonists. *Psychopharmacology (Berl)*. 1991;104(4):451-456.
106. Johnson BA. Update on neuropharmacological treatments for alcoholism: scientific basis and clinical findings. *Biochem Pharmacol*. 2008;75(1):34-56.
107. Dani JA, Bertrand D. Nicotinic acetylcholine receptors and nicotinic cholinergic mechanisms of the central nervous system. *Annu Rev Pharmacol Toxicol*. 2007;47:699-729.
108. Cardoso RA, Brozowski SJ, Chavez-Noriega LE, Harpold M, Valenzuela CF, Harris RA. Effects of ethanol on recombinant human neuronal nicotinic acetylcholine receptors expressed in Xenopus oocytes. *J Pharmacol Exp Ther*. 1999;289(2):774-780.
109. Steffensen SC, Shin SI, Nelson AC, et al. alpha6 subunit-containing nicotinic receptors mediate low-dose ethanol effects on ventral tegmental area neurons and ethanol reward. *Addict Biol*. 2018;23(5):1079-1093.
110. Steensland P, Simms JA, Holgate J, Richards JK, Bartlett SE. Varenicline, an alpha4beta2 nicotinic acetylcholine receptor partial agonist, selectively decreases ethanol consumption and seeking. *Proc Natl Acad Sci U S A*. 2007;104(30):12518-12523.
111. Litten RZ, Ryan ML, Fertig JB, et al. A double-blind, placebo-controlled trial assessing the efficacy of varenicline tartrate for alcohol dependence. *J Addict Med*. 2013;7(4):277-286.
112. Falk DE, Castle IJ, Ryan M, Fertig J, Litten RZ. Moderators of varenicline treatment effects in a double-blind, placebo-controlled trial for alcohol dependence: an exploratory analysis. *J Addict Med*. 2015;9(4):296-303.
113. Verplaetse TL, Pittman BP, Shi JM, Tetrault JM, Coppola S, McKee SA. Effect of lowering the dose of varenicline on alcohol self-administration in drinkers with alcohol use disorders. *J Addict Med*. 2016;10(3):166-173.
114. Boue-Grabot E, Pankratov Y. Modulation of central synapses by astrocyte-released ATP and postsynaptic P2X receptors. *Neural Plast*. 2017;2017:9454275.
115. Li C, Aguayo L, Peoples RW, Weight FF. Ethanol inhibits a neuronal ATP-gated ion channel. *Mol Pharmacol*. 1993;44(4):871-875.
116. Xiong K, Li C, Weight FF. Inhibition by ethanol of rat P2X(4) receptors expressed in Xenopus oocytes. *Br J Pharmacol*. 2000;130(6):1394-1398.

117. Koles L, Wirkner K, Furst S, Wnendt S, Illes P. Trichloroethanol inhibits ATP-induced membrane currents in cultured HEK 293-hP2X3 cells. *Eur J Pharmacol.* 2000;409(3):R3-R5.
118. Davies DL, Kochegarov AA, Kuo ST, et al. Ethanol differentially affects ATP-gated P2X(3) and P2X(4) receptor subtypes expressed in Xenopus oocytes. *Neuropharmacology.* 2005;49(2):243-253.
119. Asatryan L, Popova M, Woodward JJ, King BF, Alkana RL, Davies DL. Roles of ectodomain and transmembrane regions in ethanol and agonist action in purinergic P2X2 and P2X3 receptors. *Neuropharmacology.* 2008;55(5):835-843.
120. Khoja S, Huynh N, Warnecke AMP, Asatryan L, Jakowec MW, Davies DL. Preclinical evaluation of avermectins as novel therapeutic agents for alcohol use disorders. *Psychopharmacology (Berl).* 2018;235(6): 1697-1709.
121. Cannady R, Rinker JA, Nimitvilai S, Woodward JJ, Mulholland PJ. Chronic alcohol, intrinsic excitability, and potassium channels: neuroadaptations and drinking behavior. *Handb Exp Pharmacol.* 2018;248:311-343.
122. Mulholland PJ, Becker HC, Woodward JJ, Chandler LJ. Small conductance calcium-activated potassium type 2 channels regulate alcohol-associated plasticity of glutamatergic synapses. *Biol Psychiatry.* 2010;69(7):625-632.
123. Hopf FW, Simms JA, Chang SJ, Seif T, Bartlett SE, Bonci A. Chlorzoxazone, an SK-type potassium channel activator used in humans, reduces excessive alcohol intake in rats. *Biol Psychiatry.* 2010;69(7):618-624.
124. Cannady R, McGonigal JT, Newsom RJ, Woodward JJ, Mulholland PJ, Gass JT. Prefrontal cortex KCa2 channels regulate mGlu5-dependent plasticity and extinction of alcohol-seeking behavior. *J Neurosci.* 2017;37(16):4359-4369.
125. Cavaliere S, Gillespie JM, Hodge JJ. KCNQ channels show conserved ethanol block and function in ethanol behaviour. *PLoS One.* 2012; 7(11):e50279.
126. Koyama S, Brodie MS, Appel SB. Ethanol inhibition of M-current and ethanol-induced direct excitation of ventral tegmental area dopamine neurons. *J Neurophysiol.* 2006;97(3):1977-1985.
127. You C, Savarese A, Vandegrift BJ, et al. Ethanol acts on KCNK13 potassium channels in the ventral tegmental area to increase firing rate and modulate binge-like drinking. *Neuropharmacology.* 2019;144:29-36.
128. Walter HJ, Messing RO. Regulation of neuronal voltage-gated calcium channels by ethanol. *Neurochem Int.* 1999;35(2):95-101.
129. Newton PM, Orr CJ, Wallace MJ, Kim C, Shin HS, Messing RO. Deletion of N-type calcium channels alters ethanol reward and reduces ethanol consumption in mice. *J Neurosci.* 2004;24(44):9862-9869.
130. Graef JD, Huitt TW, Nordskog BK, Hammarback JH, Godwin DW. Disrupted thalamic T-type Ca^{2+} channel expression and function during ethanol exposure and withdrawal. *J Neurophysiol.* 2011;105(2):528-540.
131. Choi DS, Cascini MG, Mailliard W, et al. The type 1 equilibrative nucleoside transporter regulates ethanol intoxication and preference. *Nat Neurosci.* 2004;7(8):855-861.
132. Hong SI, Peyton L, Chern Y, Choi DS. Novel adenosine analog, N6-(4-hydroxybenzyl)-adenosine, dampens alcohol drinking and seeking behaviors. *J Pharmacol Exp Ther.* 2019;371(2):260-267.
133. Luscher C, Malenka RC. Drug-evoked synaptic plasticity in addiction: from molecular changes to circuit remodeling. *Neuron.* 2011;69(4): 650-663.
134. Brodie MS, Appel SB. Dopaminergic neurons in the ventral tegmental area of C57BL/6J and DBA/2J mice differ in sensitivity to ethanol excitation. *Alcohol Clin Exp Res.* 2000;24(7):1120-1124.
135. Lammel S, Hetzel A, Hackel O, Jones I, Liss B, Roeper J. Unique properties of mesoprefrontal neurons within a dual mesocorticolimbic dopamine system. *Neuron.* 2008;57(5):760-773.
136. Weiss F, Mitchiner M, Bloom FE, Koob GF. Free-choice responding for ethanol versus water in alcohol preferring (P) and unselected Wistar rats is differentially modified by naloxone, bromocriptine, and methysergide. *Psychopharmacology (Berl).* 1990;101(2):178-186.
137. Burnette EM, Nieto SJ, Grodin EN, et al. Novel agents for the pharmacological treatment of alcohol use disorder. *Drugs.* 2022;82(3):251-274.
138. Davis VE, Walsh MJ. Alcohol, amines, and alkaloids: a possible biochemical basis for alcohol addiction. *Science.* 1970;167(920):1005-1007.
139. Myers RD. Isoquinolines, beta-carbolines and alcohol drinking: involvement of opioid and dopaminergic mechanisms. *Experientia.* 1989;45(5):436-443.
140. Collins MA. Acetaldehyde and its condensation products as markers in alcoholism. *Recent Dev Alcohol.* 1988;6:387-403.
141. Oswald LM, Wand GS. Opioids and alcoholism. *Physiol Behav.* 2004;81(2):339-358.
142. Walker BM, Koob GF. Pharmacological evidence for a motivational role of kappa-opioid systems in ethanol dependence. *Neuropsychopharmacology.* 2008;33(3):643-652.
143. Anderson RI, Lopez MF, Becker HC. Stress-induced enhancement of ethanol intake in C57BL/6J mice with a history of chronic ethanol exposure: involvement of kappa opioid receptors. *Front Cell Neurosci.* 2016;10:45.
144. Haun HL, Griffin WC, Lopez MF, Becker HC. Kappa opioid receptors in the bed nucleus of the stria terminalis regulate binge-like alcohol consumption in male and female mice. *Neuropharmacology.* 2020; 167:107984.
145. Valdez GR, Roberts AJ, Chan K, et al. Increased ethanol self-administration and anxiety-like behavior during acute ethanol withdrawal and protracted abstinence: regulation by corticotropin-releasing factor. *Alcohol Clin Exp Res.* 2002;26(10):1494-1501.
146. Funk CK, Zorrilla EP, Lee MJ, Rice KC, Koob GF. Corticotropin-releasing factor 1 antagonists selectively reduce ethanol self-administration in ethanol-dependent rats. *Biol Psychiatry.* 2007;61(1):78-86.
147. Zorrilla EP, Schulteis G, Ling N, Koob GF, De Souza EB. Performance-enhancing effects of CRF-BP ligand inhibitors. *Neuroreport.* 2001; 12(6):1231-1234.
148. Kwako LE, Spagnolo PA, Schwandt ML, et al. The corticotropin releasing hormone-1 (CRH1) receptor antagonist pexacerfont in alcohol dependence: a randomized controlled experimental medicine study. *Neuropsychopharmacology.* 2015;40(5):1053-1063.
149. Schwandt ML, Cortes CR, Kwako LE, et al. The CRF1 antagonist verucerfont in anxious alcohol-dependent women: translation of neuro-endocrine, but not of anti-craving effects. *Neuropsychopharmacology.* 2016;41(12):2818-2829.
150. Thiele TE, Koh MT, Pedrazzini T. Voluntary alcohol consumption is controlled via the neuropeptide Y Y1 receptor. *J Neurosci.* 2002;22(3): RC208.
151. Hopf FW. Recent perspectives on orexin/hypocretin promotion of addiction-related behaviors. *Neuropharmacology.* 2020;168:108013.
152. Moorman DE, Aston-Jones G. Orexin-1 receptor antagonism decreases ethanol consumption and preference selectively in high-ethanol–preferring Sprague–Dawley rats. *Alcohol.* 2009;43(5):379-386.
153. Lawrence AJ, Cowen MS, Yang HJ, Chen F, Oldfield B. The orexin system regulates alcohol-seeking in rats. *Br J Pharmacol.* 2006;148(6):752-759.
154. Sellers EM, Higgins GA, Sobell MB. 5-HT and alcohol abuse. *Trends Pharmacol Sci.* 1992;13:69-75.
155. Nunes EV, Levin FR. Treatment of depression in patients with alcohol or other drug dependence: a meta-analysis. *JAMA.* 2004;291(15):1887-1896.
156. Kranzler HR, Mueller T, Cornelius J, et al. Sertraline treatment of co-occurring alcohol dependence and major depression. *J Clin Psychopharmacol.* 2006;26(1):13-20.
157. Crabbe JC, Phillips TJ, Feller DJ, et al. Elevated alcohol consumption in null mutant mice lacking 5-HT1B serotonin receptors. *Nat Genet.* 1996;14:98-101.
158. Yan QS, Zheng SZ, Feng MJ, Yan SE. Involvement of 5-HT1B receptors within the ventral tegmental area in ethanol-induced increases in mesolimbic dopaminergic transmission. *Brain Res.* 2005;1060(1-2):126-137.
159. Hoplight BJ, Sandygren NA, Neumaier JF. Increased expression of 5-HT1B receptors in rat nucleus accumbens via virally mediated gene transfer increases voluntary alcohol consumption. *Alcohol.* 2006;38(2):73-79.
160. Zhou Z, Karlsson C, Liang T, et al. Loss of metabotropic glutamate receptor 2 escalates alcohol consumption. *Proc Natl Acad Sci U S A.* 2013;110(42):16963-16968.
161. Meinhardt MW, Hansson AC, Perreau-Lenz S, et al. Rescue of infralimbic mGluR2 deficit restores control over drug-seeking behavior in alcohol dependence. *J Neurosci.* 2013;33(7):2794-2806.

162. Kunos G. Interactions between alcohol and the endocannabinoid system. *Alcohol Clin Exp Res*. 2020;44(4):790-805.
163. Cheer JF, Wassum KM, Sombers LA, et al. Phasic dopamine release evoked by abused substances requires cannabinoid receptor activation. *J Neurosci*. 2007;27(4):791-795.
164. Liu J, Li JX, Wu R. Toll-like receptor 4: a novel target to tackle drug addiction? *Handb Exp Pharmacol*. 2022;276:275-290.
165. Alfonso-Loeches S, Guerri C. Molecular and behavioral aspects of the actions of alcohol on the adult and developing brain. *Crit Rev Clin Lab Sci*. 2011;48(1):19-47.
166. Crews FT, Qin L, Sheedy D, Vetreno RP, Zou J. High mobility group box 1/Toll-like receptor danger signaling increases brain neuroimmune activation in alcohol dependence. *Biol Psychiatry*. 2013;73(7):602-612.
167. Vetreno RP, Qin L, Crews FT. Increased receptor for advanced glycation end product expression in the human alcoholic prefrontal cortex is linked to adolescent drinking. *Neurobiol Dis*. 2013;59:52-62.
168. de Timary P, Starkel P, Delzenne NM, Leclercq S. A role for the peripheral immune system in the development of alcohol use disorders? *Neuropharmacology*. 2017;122:148-160.
169. Bell RL, Lopez MF, Cui C, et al. Ibudilast reduces alcohol drinking in multiple animal models of alcohol dependence. *Addict Biol*. 2015;20(1):38-42.
170. Grodin EN, Bujarski S, Towns B, et al. Ibudilast, a neuroimmune modulator, reduces heavy drinking and alcohol cue-elicited neural activation: a randomized trial. *Transl Psychiatry*. 2021;11(1):355.
171. Koob G, Kreek MJ. Stress, dysregulation of drug reward pathways, and the transition to drug dependence. *Am J Psychiatry*. 2007;164(8): 1149-1159.
172. Koob GF. Anhedonia, hyperkatifeia, and negative reinforcement in substance use disorders. *Curr Top Behav Neurosci*. 2022;58:147-165.
173. Nona CN, Hendershot CS, Le AD. Behavioural sensitization to alcohol: bridging the gap between preclinical research and human models. *Pharmacol Biochem Behav*. 2018;173:15-26.
174. Becker HC, Hale RL. Repeated episodes of ethanol withdrawal potentiate the severity of subsequent withdrawal seizures: an animal model of alcohol withdrawal "kindling". *Alcohol Clin Exp Res*. 1993;17(1):94-98.
175. Elvig SK, McGinn MA, Smith C, Arends MA, Koob GF, Vendruscolo LF. Tolerance to alcohol: a critical yet understudied factor in alcohol addiction. *Pharmacol Biochem Behav*. 2021;204:173155.
176. Haass-Koffler CL, Cannella N, Ciccocioppo R. Translational dynamics of alcohol tolerance of preclinical models and human laboratory studies. *Exp Clin Psychopharmacol*. 2020;28(4):417-425.
177. Jones AW. The drunkest drinking driver in Sweden: blood alcohol concentration 0.545% w/v. *J Stud Alcohol*. 1999;60(3):400-406.
178. Cannady R, Nimitvilai-Roberts S, Jennings SD, Woodward JJ, Mulholland PJ. Distinct region- and time-dependent functional cortical adaptations in C57BL/6J mice after short and prolonged alcohol drinking. *eNeuro*. 2020;7(3):ENEURO.0077-20.2020.
179. Nimitvilai S, Uys JD, Woodward JJ, et al. Orbitofrontal neuroadaptations and cross-species synaptic biomarkers in heavy-drinking macaques. *J Neurosci*. 2017;37(13):3646-3660.
180. Ron D, Messing RO. Signaling pathways mediating alcohol effects. *Curr Top Behav Neurosci*. 2013;13:87-126.
181. Wu PH, Coultrap S, Browning MD, Proctor WR. Correlated changes in NMDA receptor phosphorylation, functional activity, and sedation by chronic ethanol consumption. *J Neurochem*. 2010;115(5):1112-1122.
182. Schulteis G, Markou A, Cole M, Koob GF. Decreased brain reward produced by ethanol withdrawal. *Proc Natl Acad Sci U S A*. 1995; 92(13):5880-5884.
183. Goltseker K, Hopf FW, Barak S. Advances in behavioral animal models of alcohol use disorder. *Alcohol*. 2019;74:73-82.
184. Scherubl H. Alcohol use and gastrointestinal cancer risk. *Visc Med*. 2020;36(3):175-181.
185. Boffetta P, Hashibe M. Alcohol and cancer. *Lancet Oncol*. 2006;7(2): 149-156.
186. Neuman MG, Seitz HK, French SW, et al. Alcoholic-hepatitis, links to brain and microbiome: mechanisms, clinical and experimental research. *Biomedicines*. 2020;8(3):63.
187. Goel S, Sharma A, Garg A. Effect of alcohol consumption on cardiovascular health. *Curr Cardiol Rep*. 2018;20(4):19.
188. Rehm J, Roerecke M. Cardiovascular effects of alcohol consumption. *Trends Cardiovasc Med*. 2017;27(8):534-538.
189. Choudhary NS, Duseja A. Genetic and epigenetic disease modifiers: non-alcoholic fatty liver disease (NAFLD) and alcoholic liver disease (ALD). *Transl Gastroenterol Hepatol*. 2021;6:2.
190. Sullivan EV, Pfefferbaum A. Neurocircuitry in alcoholism: a substrate of disruption and repair. *Psychopharmacology (Berl)*. 2005;180(4): 583-594.
191. Harper C. The neurotoxicity of alcohol. *Hum Exp Toxicol*. 2007;26(3): 251-257.
192. Sullivan EV, Pfefferbaum A. Brain-behavior relations and effects of aging and common comorbidities in alcohol use disorder: a review. *Neuropsychology*. 2019;33(6):760-780.
193. Donald KA, Eastman E, Howells FM, et al. Neuroimaging effects of prenatal alcohol exposure on the developing human brain: a magnetic resonance imaging review. *Acta Neuropsychiatr*. 2015;27(5):251-269.
194. Martinez D, Kim JH, Krystal J, Abi-Dargham A. Imaging the neurochemistry of alcohol and substance abuse. *Neuroimaging Clin N Am*. 2007;17(4):539-555. x
195. Volkow ND, Wiers CE, Shokri-Kojori E, Tomasi D, Wang GJ, Baler R. Neurochemical and metabolic effects of acute and chronic alcohol in the human brain: studies with positron emission tomography. *Neuropharmacology*. 2017;122:175-188.
196. Fama R, Le Berre AP, Sassoon SA, et al. Memory impairment in alcohol use disorder is associated with regional frontal brain volumes. *Drug Alcohol Depend*. 2021;228:109058.
197. Sullivan EV, Zhao Q, Pohl KM, Zahr NM, Pfefferbaum A. Attenuated cerebral blood flow in frontolimbic and insular cortices in alcohol use disorder: relation to working memory. *J Psychiatr Res*. 2021;136: 140-148.
198. Morris LS, Dowell NG, Cercignani M, Harrison NA, Voon V. Binge drinking differentially affects cortical and subcortical microstructure. *Addict Biol*. 2018;23(1):403-411.
199. Obernier JA, White AM, Swartzwelder HS, Crews FT. Cognitive deficits and CNS damage after a 4-day binge ethanol exposure in rats. *Pharmacol Biochem Behav*. 2002;72(3):521-532.
200. Infante MA, Eberson SC, Zhang Y, et al. Adolescent binge drinking is associated with accelerated decline of gray matter volume. *Cereb Cortex*. 2022;32(12):2611-2620.
201. Sullivan EV, Brumback T, Tapert SF, et al. Disturbed cerebellar growth trajectories in adolescents who initiate alcohol drinking. *Biol Psychiatry*. 2020;87(7):632-644.
202. Chandler LJ, Newsom H, Sumners C, Crews F. Chronic ethanol exposure potentiates NMDA excitotoxicity in cerebral cortical neurons. *J Neurochem*. 1993;60:1578-1581.
203. Mulholland PJ, Chandler LJ. The thorny side of addiction: adaptive plasticity and dendritic spines. *Scientific World Journal*. 2007;7:9-21.
204. Collins MA, Zou JY, Neafsey EJ. Brain damage due to episodic alcohol exposure in vivo and in vitro: furosemide neuroprotection implicates edema-based mechanism. *Faseb J*. 1998;12(2):221-230.
205. Melbourne JK, Chandler CM, Van Doorn CE, et al. Primed for addiction: a critical review of the role of microglia in the neurodevelopmental consequences of adolescent alcohol drinking. *Alcohol Clin Exp Res*. 2021;45(10):1908-1926.
206. Agarwal K, Manza P, Chapman M, et al. Inflammatory markers in substance use and mood disorders: a neuroimaging perspective. *Front Psychiatry*. 2022;13:863734.
207. Spadoni AD, McGee CL, Fryer SL, Riley EP. Neuroimaging and fetal alcohol spectrum disorders. *Neurosci Biobehav Rev*. 2007;31(2):239-245.
208. Gomez DA, Abdul-Rahman OA. Fetal alcohol spectrum disorders: current state of diagnosis and treatment. *Curr Opin Pediatr*. 2021;33(6):570-575.
209. Dejong K, Olyaei A, Lo JO. Alcohol use in pregnancy. *Clin Obstet Gynecol*. 2019;62(1):142-155.
210. Kaminen-Ahola N. Fetal alcohol spectrum disorders: genetic and epigenetic mechanisms. *Prenat Diagn*. 2020;40(9):1185-1192.

12 The Pharmacology of Nonalcohol Sedative Hypnotics

Carolina L. Haass-Koffler and Elinore F. McCance-Katz

CHAPTER OUTLINE

- Introduction
- Formulations and chemical structure
- Brief historical features
- Pharmacodynamics
- Pharmacokinetics
- Pharmacogenomics
- Drug–drug interactions
- Special consideration of concominant use of benzodiazepines and opioids
- Mechanism of tolerance and withdrawal
- Liability for development of a substance use disorder
- Epidemiology of unhealthy use
- Toxicities
- Medical complications
- Conclusion

INTRODUCTION

Sedative hypnotic drugs represent a diverse group of chemical agents that depress the function of the central nervous system (CNS).[1] They are used in medicine as anxiolytics, sleep inducers, hypnotics, anticonvulsants, muscle relaxants, and anesthesia induction agents. Their calming (sedative) effects are dose-dependent and on *a continuum* with sleep-inducing (hypnotic) effects, unconsciousness and, for some agents, coma and death. Agents discussed in this chapter include benzodiazepines, nonbenzodiazepine hypnotics, and miscellaneous related compounds.

FORMULATIONS AND CHEMICAL STRUCTURE

The name benzodiazepine is derived from the chemical structure comprised by a benzene ring fused to a seven-membered diazepine ring (Fig. 12-1).[2] Modification in the ring system yields compounds with altered potency and efficacy.[3]

The more recent sedative hypnotic agents include the nonbenzodiazepines (ie, zopiclone, eszopiclone, zaleplon and zolpidem). While the chemical structure of these compounds is not similar to the benzodiazepines, their therapeutic effect is via the benzodiazepine binding site at the γ-aminobutyric acid ($GABA_A$) receptor; their actions are not identical to classic benzodiazepines. The clinically available formulations of benzodiazepines and nonbenzodiazepines, half-life ($t_{1/2}$), biotransformation and active metabolites are shown in Table 12-1.

BRIEF HISTORICAL FEATURES

Barbituric acid was synthesized in 1864 by the German chemist Adolf von Baeyer,[4] but it did not have any therapeutic use. Only later, its derivates have been used in medicine: barbital in 1903 and phenobarbital in 1912. In the 1950s, the synthesis of chlordiazepoxide with hypnotic, sedative, and muscle-relaxant effects opened the era of benzodiazepine use in the United States. In 1960, chlordiazepoxide was marketed as Librium, a safe and effective anxiolytic agent. The elimination of the basic nitrogen moiety from the original structure increased the potency of chlordiazepoxide by 3 to 10 fold and produced diazepam, which was marketed in 1963 as the popular drug Valium. The widespread clinical use of benzodiazepines as anxiety-relieving and sleep-inducing medications was well established by the end of the 1970s when benzodiazepines were

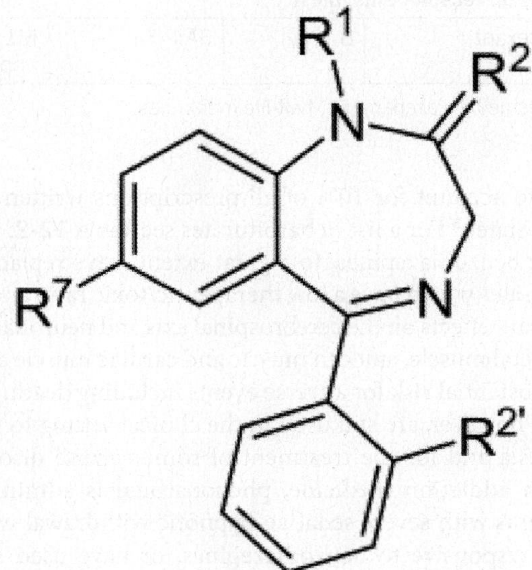

Figure 12-1. The core structure of benzodiazepines comprised by a benzene ring fused to a seven-membered diazepine ring. The "R" groups denote side chains of which yielded compounds with altered potency and efficacy.

TABLE 12-1 Elimination Half-Life ($t_{1/2}$), Cytochrome P450 Enzymes (CYP) that Mediate Metabolism and Production of Active Metabolites

Parent drug	$t_{1/2}$, (min)	CYP	Active metabolites ($t_{1/2}$, min)
Benzodiazepines			
alprazolam	10-14	3A4, 3A5	α-hydroxyalprazolam
clonazepam	17-56	3A5	7-aminoclonazepam → 7-acetamidoclonazepam
clorazepate			DMD (30-100) → oxazepam (5-20)
chlordiazepoxide	7-25		desmethylchlordiazepoxide (10-30) → demoxepam (14-95) → DMD (30-100) → oxazepam (5-20)
diazepam	28-54	2C19, 3A4	DMD (30-100) → oxazepam (5-20) temazepam (5-17)
estazolam	15-17		1-oxo-etazolam
flurazepam	2-3		hydroxyethylflurazepam → desalkylflurazepam (47-100) → 3-hydroxymetabolite ↓ desmethylchlordiazepoxide → demoxepam → DMD (30-100) → oxazepam (5-20)
halazepam			DMD (30-100) → oxazepam (5-20)
lorazepam	10-20		
midazolam	2-5	3A4, 3A5	α-hydroxymidazolam (1-4)
oxazepam	5-20		
prazepam	1-2		DMD (30-100) → oxazepam (5-20)
quazepam	36	2C19, 3A4	2-oxo-quazepam → 3-hydroxy-2-oxo-quazepam ↓ desalkylflurazepam → 3-hydroxymetabolite
temazepam	5-17		oxazepam (5-20)
triazolam	2-3	3A4	α-hydroxytriazolam → 4-hydroxytrazolam
Nonbenzodiazepines			
eszopiclone	6	2E1, 3A4	desmethylzopiclone
zaleplon	1-5	3A4	
zolpidem	1.5-3	3A4, 1A1, 2D6	
Dual orexin receptor antagonist			
daridorexant	8	3A4	M1, M3, and M10, but with lower affinity to OX1 and OX2 receptors and with no apparent pharmacological effect

DMD, desmethyldiazepam; $t_{1/2}$, half-life in minutes.

found to account for 10% of all prescriptions written in the United States.[5] For a list of barbiturates see **Table 12-2**.

The benzodiazepines, to a great extent, have replaced the barbiturates which have a low therapeutic/toxic ratio and exert depressant effects on the cerebrospinal axis and neuronal activity, skeletal muscle, smooth muscle and cardiac muscle activity with substantial risk for adverse events including death. Barbiturates, however, are still used in the clinical setting to induce anesthesia and for the treatment of some seizure disorders.[6] Also, in addiction medicine, phenobarbital is administered in patients with severe sedative-hypnotic withdrawal who are poorly responsive to benzodiazepines, or have used several different drugs of this class. For example, patients who have heavily misused analgesics formulated with butalbital (short to intermediate-acting barbiturate co-formulated with acetaminophen, aspirin, etc.) may require phenobarbital medical withdrawal, whereas individuals taking 10 or less tablets per day of Fiorinal (butalbital 50 mg, aspirin 325 mg, and caffeine 40 mg) can usually be weaned off the medication gradually.[7]

In addition, it is important to note that there are other less used sedative hypnotics which include paraldehyde (anticonvulsant), chloral hydrate (insomnia), ethchlorvynol (insomnia) and meprobamate (carisoprodol, muscle relaxant) that not only share risk for unhealthy use, but also have risk for a withdrawal syndrome upon abrupt discontinuation after chronic use. Phenobarbital withdrawal protocols are recommended for these agents.

Benzodiazepines are less toxic in overdose than other sedative-hypnotics, have less capacity to produce fatal CNS effects and are associated with fewer drug-drug interactions. Nonbenzodiazepine hypnotics have been the most recent addition to this group of drugs and these compounds are more potent than the benzodiazepines. They may offer an advantage of lower liability for unhealthy use, though clinical experience is insufficient to make definitive judgments.

TABLE 12-2 List of Barbiturates

Generic name	Duration of action	Therapeutic use
methohexital	ultrashort acting (15 min-3 h)	general anesthetic
thiopental		general anesthetic, emergency treatment of seizures
pentobarbital	short acting (3-6 h)	sedation, emergency treatment of seizures
secobarbital		sedation, emergency treatment of seizures
amobarbital	intermediate acting (6-12 h)	hypnotic, sedation, emergency treatment of seizures
butabarbital		hypnotic, sedative
butalbital		combination with headache therapies
phenobarbital	Long acting (12-24 h)	sedation, seizures, many combination products
mephobarbital		sedation, seizures

At the present time, benzodiazepines are widely utilized in the management of many medical and psychiatric conditions and are often used for long periods of times—sometimes years.

Conditions for which benzodiazepines are frequently used include acute relief of anxiety and insomnia, which may extend to long-term, chronic use. Benzodiazepines are often administered as adjuncts to anesthesia prior to surgery and as muscle relaxants in pain management; such as low back pain. Further, the United States Food and Drug Administration (FDA) has approved the use of benzodiazepine medications for the treatment of panic disorder and generalized anxiety disorder. Benzodiazepines also remain a frequently utilized approach to management of acute agitation in psychiatric syndromes, often in combination with antipsychotic medications. The multiple clinical uses for benzodiazepines and the chronic nature of their use has made benzodiazepines and nonbenzodiazepine hypnotics some of the most frequently prescribed medications in the United States.

Only recently (2022), daridorexant, a dual orexin receptor antagonist for treating insomnia in adults with limited GABA-receptor agonist side-effects was approved in the United States.[8,9] Daridorexant blocks binding of wake-promoting neuropeptides and has been shown in clinical trials to improve sleep latency and reduce waking. Its use is associated with improved daytime functioning relative to other benzodiazepines.[10] However, potentially serious side effects similar to that seen with other benzodiazepines and nonbenzodiazepines including sleep paralysis, hallucinations and amnesia for complex behaviors during sleep have been reported.[11] Daridorexant is a Schedule IV controlled substance under the Controlled Substance Act in the United States.

PHARMACODYNAMICS

Benzodiazepines and nonbenzodiazepines exert their clinical effects through allosteric modulation of the $GABA_A$ receptor.[12] As GABA is the major inhibitory neurotransmitter system in the brain, positive modulation of the receptor by benzodiazepines is responsible for sedative, anticonvulsant, hypnotic, and amnestic effects of these drugs. The $GABA_A$ receptor is a heteropentameric protein structure surrounding a central chloride channel.[13] The five subunits that are linked to form the chloride ion channel are classified into several subtypes: alpha ($\alpha_{1\text{-}6}$), beta ($\beta_{1\text{-}3}$), gamma ($\gamma_{1\text{-}3}$), delta (δ), epsilon (ε), rho (ρ), and pi (π), each of which has a unique sequence of amino acids and determines the pharmacological properties of the receptor.[13] In the human brain, the most common structure of the $GABA_A$ receptor consists of two α, two β, and one γ subunit.[13] Benzodiazepines bind at the interface of the γ_2 and α subunits.[12] $GABA_A$ receptors containing $\alpha_{1\text{-}3,5}$ subunits mediate effects of benzodiazepines. Binding at the α_1 subunit mediates sedative and amnestic effects, while binding at the α_2 subunit[14] and possibly the α_3 subunit[15,16] modulates anxiolytic and muscle relaxant effects. Anticonvulsant activity is modulated by $\alpha_{1\text{-}3}$ subunits.[17] The α_5 subunit is located extrasynaptically and regulates tonic GABAergic currents, while the other subunits are located predominately within the synapse and mediate the rapid phasic GABA currents.[18] In contrast, the presence of $\alpha 4$ or $\alpha 6$ subunits leads to a lack of sensitivity to benzodiazepines.

The $GABA_A$ receptors that contain α_1 have been implicated in playing a key role in the production of the ataxic effects of both benzodiazepines and zolpidem.[15,19] There is also evidence that the α_2 and α_3 subunits mediate the rewarding effects of diazepam.[20] In contrast, other research has implicated the $\alpha 1$ subunit in mediating the reinforcing effects of benzodiazepines.[21]

Barbiturates and benzodiazepines share some pharmacodynamic properties. At low concentrations, barbiturates act as positive modulators of the $GABA_A$ receptor via an allosteric mechanism[22]; however, at higher concentrations, barbiturates act as direct $GABA_A$ receptor agonists by prolonging the duration of the opening of the chloride channel. $GABA_A$ receptors that contain the β_2 or β_3 subunit show greater sensitivity to the effects of pentobarbital than receptors with the β_1 subunit.[23] Pentobarbital shows the greatest efficacy as a GABA receptor agonist in receptor complexes that contain the α_6 subunit, which is a benzodiazepine-insensitive subunit.[24] Barbiturates may reduce excitatory neurotransmission through inhibition of α-amino-3-hydroxy-5-methyl-4-isoxazolepropionic acid (AMPA) receptors and inhibit neurotransmitter release by blockade of voltage-sensitive calcium channels.[25,26]

Currently the FDA approved nonbenzodiazepines are zolpidem, zaleplon and eszopiclone (*S*-enantiomer of zopiclone, not available in the United States). Zolpidem is also formulated as an extended-release medication. This reduced dose formulation is marketed for middle-of-the-night insomnia to reduce next-day sedation. The nonbenzodiazepines may have less amnestic effects and are less likely to be associated with the development of tolerance compared to the classic benzodiazepines.[27]

Nonbenzodiazepines share many pharmacologic actions with benzodiazepines including sedative-hypnotic, anxiolytic, myorelaxant, and anticonvulsant effects, although their selectivity for these actions differs. For example, animal studies suggest that zolpidem is more selective in its sedative effects as compared to its anticonvulsant actions than are quazepam, zaleplon, or zopiclone.[28,29] Among the nonbenzodiazepines, eszopiclone has the strongest antianxiety effect in animal models, which is produced at nonhypnotic doses.[30,31]

Benzodiazepines and nonbenzodiazepines may act through overlapping binding sites between α and β subunits of the $GABA_A$ receptor.[32-34] Zolpidem, however, binds to additional sites on these subunits that are not crucial for benzodiazepine activity.[35-37]

Benzodiazepines have roughly similar affinities for $GABA_A$ subtype receptors that contain the $\alpha_{1-3,5}$ subunits. In contrast, zaleplon and zolpidem have more than 10-fold greater affinity for receptors with a $\alpha_1\beta_2\gamma_2$ composition than for those with a $\alpha_2\beta_2\gamma_2$ composition, whereas zopiclone has essentially equivalent affinity for these receptors. Zolpidem in contrast to the benzodiazepines and other nonbenzodiazepines has little affinity for α_5-containing $GABA_A$ receptors, and the presence of the γ_3 subunit produces insensitivity to zolpidem.[38] Therefore, it is possible that patients may respond differently and pharmacogenomics trials (precision/personalized medicine approaches) of these medications may be needed to determine the most effective and individualized treatment.[39]

Finally, daridorexant selectively binds equally to the orexin receptors (OX1 and OX2) with no effect on the GABA receptors.[40,41]

PHARMACOKINETICS

The effectiveness of a benzodiazepine as a hypnotic is based on its pharmacokinetic properties including development of acute tolerance, which will diminish CNS effects before the drug is eliminated, redistribution from the CNS to other peripheral tissues and finally, the rate of biotransformation and formation of active metabolites.

Many benzodiazepines, and daridorexant, undergo hepatic metabolism involving oxidative reactions mediated by cytochrome P450 (CYP450) enzymes. Oxidative metabolism reactions include N-dealkylation or aliphatic hydroxylation. The CYP3A4 enzyme mediates the oxidative metabolism of many of the benzodiazepines and also plays a role in the biotransformation of nonbenzodiazepine sedative-hypnotic agents. Several of the benzodiazepines are converted into active metabolites such as diazepam to desmethyldiazepam, which are then slowly cleared from the body. The final phase of metabolism for most benzodiazepines consists of conjugation of either the parent drug or their metabolites with glucuronide. Drugs or metabolites that undergo glucuronidation contain a hydroxyl group. Parent drugs, such as lorazepam and oxazepam, which undergo direct glucuronidation, are less subject to drug interactions or reduced clearance associated with impairment of hepatic function than are the other benzodiazepines.[42]

Distinct metabolic pathways mediate the biotransformation of the different nonbenzodiazepines. Zolpidem is extensively metabolized by CYP3A4, CYP2C9, and CYP2C19 to inactive hydroxylated metabolites.[43,44] Aldehyde dehydrogenase may play a major role in the metabolism of zaleplon, which involves the biotransformation of this drug into metabolites including 5-oxozaleplon that are excreted into the urine. Nearly 50% of zopiclone is transformed by esterase into a decarboxylated metabolite that is excreted through the lungs. This drug is also converted by CYP3A4 into the active metabolite zopiclone N-oxide and the inactive metabolite N-desmethylzopiclone.

Daridorexant metabolism is primarily via CYP3A4 oxidative transformation (89%) and it is excreted in the feces (57%) and urine (28%). There are three major metabolites (M1, M3, and M10) but they have lower affinity to OX1 and OX2 receptors compared to the parent drug with limited pharmacological effect.[45-47]

The relationship between the pharmacokinetic profile of benzodiazepines and unhealthy use liability is complex. It is generally believed that rapid onset of action is associated with euphoria.[48] Onset of action after oral administration relies on the formulation of the drug, the intrinsic activity of the drug, lipid solubility, protein binding, and rate of entry into the brain. Some animal data suggest that greater lipid solubility increases the rate of uptake by the brain, with diazepam having more rapid brain uptake as compared to lorazepam.[49] In clinical practice, pharmacokinetic factors do not always predict unhealthy use liability. For example, clorazepate, rarely cited as a benzodiazepine with a high unhealthy use potential, is rapidly decarboxylated in the stomach to desmethyldiazepam, which then reaches maximum plasma concentrations within 30 minutes or less and has a long half-life ($t_{1/2}$ = 40-50 hours).[50] Subjective ratings by individuals with substance use disorder (SUD) of the "high" induced by clorazepate, however, are lower than ratings for diazepam or lorazepam.[51] Also, even though alprazolam and oxazepam differ only slightly in lipid solubility,[52-54] intrinsic activity and rate of absorption are greater with alprazolam, which has higher unhealthy use potential than oxazepam.[55-60] Lower unhealthy use potential is more consistently predicted with prodrugs that require hepatic metabolism to form the active moiety, such as the formation of desmethyldiazepam from halazepam, which appears to have lower unhealthy use liability than diazepam.[61] Therefore, the rate of absorption and entry into the brain are factors that may influence unhealthy use liability.

PHARMACOGENOMICS

Pharmacogenomic investigation of benzodiazepines have focused on metabolizing enzymes.[62] The impact of polymorphisms in CYP3A4 and CYP3A5 on benzodiazepine metabolism is mixed. CYP3A4 and CYP3A5 genetic variations evaluated in healthy volunteers[63] and in vitro[64] did not contribute to large inter-individual variability in midazolam hydroxylation. On the other hand, one in vitro midazolam study indicated that CYP3A4*16 showed substrate-dependent altered kinetics compared with wild type.[65]

Unlike CYP3A4/5, polymorphisms of CYP2C19 have been reported to have more consistent impact on the metabolism of benzodiazepines. Poor metabolizers had significantly lower plasma clearance of both diazepam and desmethydiazepam[66,67] and longer elimination half-life[68] when compared to extensive metabolizers.

DRUG-DRUG INTERACTIONS

The most serious drug-drug interactions occur when sedative hypnotics are combined with drugs that depress CNS activity (ie, alcohol, opioids, muscle relaxants, etc.), potentially resulting in overdose and death. Benzodiazepines do not induce their own metabolism; however, those that are metabolized through CYP3A4 (Table 9-1) are subject to altered plasma levels by agents that inhibit this metabolic pathway. Common inhibitors are ketoconazole, itraconazole, macrolide antibiotics (erythromycin), fluoxetine, nefazodone, and cimetidine. Drugs that induce or inhibit CYP2C19 may also influence the metabolism of some benzodiazepines. For example, oral contraceptives containing estrogen and progesterone impair the metabolism of some substrates of CYP1A2, CYP3A4, and CYP2C19, although findings with benzodiazepines are inconsistent.[69] One study found inhibition of alprazolam metabolism in women taking low-dose estrogen oral contraceptives,[70] and another did not.[71] Similarly, lorazepam metabolism was unaffected by oral contraceptives in one study,[72] yet increased in another.[70] The latter study also found enhanced elimination of temazepam. Oxazepam kinetics are not affected by oral contraceptives.[72] The clearance of both chlordiazepoxide and diazepam are impaired in women taking oral contraceptives.[73-75]

Lorazepam and oxazepam are eliminated by glucuronidation and are not substrates of the CYP450 system. As such, lorazepam kinetics in women taking oral contraceptives was unaffected in one study,[72] however, in another study, lorazepam metabolism and elimination were enhanced.[70] Oxazepam kinetics are not affected by oral contraceptives.[72]

Inducers of CYP3A4 enzymes also may significantly reduce plasma concentrations of benzodiazepines and non-benzodiazepines as has been demonstrated with zaleplon, zolpidem, and zopiclone[43] and other benzodiazepines that are CYP3A4 substrates. In particular, rifampin, carbamazepine, and phenytoin have been shown to greatly decrease the maximum serum concentration (C_{max}) and area under the curve (*AUC*) of midazolam.[76,77] Similarly, repeated administration of the CYP3A4 inducer carbamazepine increases the clearance of zolpidem.[78]

Administration of the CYP3A4 enzyme inhibitors such as erythromycin or ketoconazole, in contrast, can decrease the clearance of zolpidem.[43] Compounds which inhibit CYP3A and CYP2C19 (eg, cimetidine, ketoconazole, fluvoxamine, fluoxetine, and omeprazole) may lead to increased and prolonged sedation with diazepam administration.[77]

The ability of benzodiazepines to inhibit CYP450 enzymes has not been extensively evaluated. One study found that flurazepam inhibits the organic cation transporter 2 (OCT2, SLC22A2) which plays an important role in renal drug elimination.[79] Barbiturates present a serious risk of CNS depression, coma, and death when taken in high doses or with ethanol or other sedative hypnotics. They induce their own metabolism (pharmacokinetic tolerance) and induce CYP2B6, CYP2C9, and CYP3A4, resulting in enhanced metabolism of drugs that are substrates of these cytochromes, reducing their therapeutic effects. Patients taking phenobarbital may experience decreased effects of anticoagulants, oral contraceptives, corticosteroids, some antibiotics, and other drugs.[80]

With the ongoing public health issue of unhealthy use of prescription drugs (specifically opioids), the interaction between opioid analgesics and sedative hypnotics is a significant concern. There is extensive evidence implicating benzodiazepines in both fatal and nonfatal cases of opioid overdose.[81] Pharmacodynamic interactions between benzodiazepines and opioids may lead to over-sedation and impaired motor function. The combination of oxycodone and alprazolam, for example, when co-administered at therapeutic doses produced greater impairment in psychomotor performance and increased difficulty in concentrating than was seen when these agents were administered alone.[82] High dose diazepam (40 mg) also enhanced psychomotor impairment and sedation when given concurrently with either buprenorphine or methadone.[83] CNS depression is also a risk associated with the use of daridorexant, therefore concomitant use of CYP3A inhibitors that may increase daridorexant exposure, which is a CYP3A4 substrate, should be avoided.[41]

SPECIAL CONSIDERATION OF CONCOMITANT USE OF BENZODIAZEPINES AND OPIOIDS

Benzodiazepines have been linked to adverse events and deaths when taken with opioids. From a historical perspective, in 2004 benzodiazepines were mentioned in 18% of opioid overdose deaths, which increased to 31% by 2011.[84] From 1999 to 2013, the rate of prescription opioid-related deaths quadrupled. The majority of these deaths involved the use of other drugs or alcohol with opioids, and benzodiazepines were the most frequent medication class associated with opioid overdose deaths.[85] In 2015, nearly 30% of opioid overdose deaths included benzodiazepines.[86] This trend continues with the Centers for Disease Control and Prevention (CDC) reporting increases in availability of illicit benzodiazepines and a substantial increase in benzodiazepine-associated deaths of which nearly 93% involved opioids.[87] In 2020, FDA required updated black box labeling on benzodiazepines to warn of unhealthy use liability and harm when mixed with opioids, alcohol, or other illicit drugs.[88]

One question that arises is why benzodiazepines are so frequently identified as a secondary drug in an opioid-associated adverse event or death. Although there is evidence of substantial nonmedical use of benzodiazepines as described below (see Epidemiology of Unhealthy Use), it is also the case that benzodiazepines are frequently prescribed in treatment of pain and so may be co-prescribed with opioid analgesics. However, the limited studies that have been conducted have shown little to no benefit of benzodiazepines in pain management.[89] In one older study of alprazolam 1.5 mg daily for pain management showed improvement in reported pain severity at 12 weeks.[90] However, other studies have shown no efficacy for benzodiazepines in treatment of acute lumbar disc prolapse with sciatica[91] or for low back pain.[92] Studies in rodents showed that concomitant use of benzodiazepines was associated with reduced morphine analgesia, which was blocked using the $GABA_A$ antagonist, flumazenil.[93] In humans administered diazepam preoperatively, postoperative administration of flumazenil, a benzodiazepine antagonist, was shown to reduce morphine analgesia requirements.[94,95] In a study that examined concurrent use of benzodiazepines in patients with chronic pain; it was reported that 38% of a sample of 114 individuals were taking more than one benzodiazepine medication, 46% had been using these medications for more than 2 years and the stated reason for use was all or in part to assist with sleep. Interestingly, there was no difference in reported sleep problems in those taking benzodiazepines as compared to those in the sample who were not. However, while there were no signs of excessive intake in those prescribed benzodiazepines, no individuals were willing to stop taking these medications despite their reported lack of effectiveness for insomnia.[96] In a study of 1, 220 patients receiving chronic opioid therapy, benzodiazepine use was examined. In this study, 33% of participants had used benzodiazepines in the past month and 17% were people who used daily. Benzodiazepine use was associated with a number of adverse effects including reports of greater pain severity, pain interference in life, and lower feelings of self-efficacy regarding pain. Those receiving benzodiazepines in the context of pain management were more likely to be prescribed higher risk opioid doses (> 200 mg morphine equivalents per day) and to be using antidepressant or antipsychotic medications. These patients were also more likely to have an alcohol use disorder (AUD), to use illicit substances and had greater mental health comorbidity. Further, those taking opioids concomitantly with benzodiazepines had greater past month use of emergency healthcare and were more likely to experience an overdose event.[89]

In summary, benzodiazepines are frequently utilized in pain management. Addiction to benzodiazepines used in pain management appears to be uncommon. However, evidence for benefit of benzodiazepines in acute pain management is small and there is no evidence for the benefit of benzodiazepines in pain management when used chronically. There is evidence for harm associated with benzodiazepine use in pain treatment[97] including drug-drug interactions particularly with opioid analgesics, impairment and accidents, and rebound anxiety related to withdrawal as chronicity of use increases. The weak evidence for benefit of benzodiazepines versus risk of serious adverse events in the setting of pain management should be carefully considered by prescribing clinicians.

MECHANISM OF TOLERANCE AND WITHDRAWAL

The pharmacodynamic mechanisms underlying the development of tolerance and withdrawal to sedative hypnotics have been extensively studied. Tolerance, as evidenced by decreased responsiveness of $GABA_A$ receptors to benzodiazepines, has been demonstrated using measures of both electrophysiologic activity[98,99] and GABA-mediated chloride flux.[100] The decreased ability of benzodiazepines to positively modulate $GABA_A$ receptors may result, in part, from the loss of interaction between benzodiazepine and GABA-binding sites within these receptors, referred to as "uncoupling."[101,102] Zolpidem may also produce uncoupling between these binding sites.[103] Another possible mechanism of tolerance may involve benzodiazepine-induced internalization of surface $GABA_A$ receptors into intraneuronal sequestration sites.[102] In vitro studies indicate that levels of the messenger RNAs (mRNAs) that are involved in the synthesis of the α_1 $GABA_A$ receptor subunit are reduced during prolonged exposure to benzodiazepines, whereas mRNAs for the benzodiazepine-insensitive α_4 subunit are increased soon after benzodiazepine withdrawal.[104] These changes in α_4 subunit expression correlate with decreased sensitivity to the effects of benzodiazepines on GABA-mediated chloride currents.[105] This loss of sensitivity can be prevented by blockade of the expression of α_4 subunits. These findings point to the possible role of increased α_4 subunit expression in early benzodiazepine withdrawal.

The glutamatergic (Glu) system may play a major role in the benzodiazepine withdrawal syndrome. In animal models, anxiety associated with benzodiazepine withdrawal may involve upregulation of hippocampal AMPA receptors as evidenced by increased AMPA receptor Glu receptor 1 (GluR) subunits and increased AMPA receptor binding.[106-109] Other studies have confirmed increased AMPA receptor binding in the hippocampus and thalamus using different experimental paradigms of withdrawal, but have not found corresponding alterations in levels of the GluR1 or GluR2 subunits in these brain regions.[110] AMPA mediated conductance in hippocampal neurons has been shown to be enhanced by abrupt withdrawal from benzodiazepines.[111] These changes occur in association with the presence of anxiety-related behaviors.

LIABILITY FOR DEVELOPMENT OF A SUBSTANCE USE DISORDER

The benzodiazepines occupy an intermediate position for addiction liability, with barbiturates and older sedative hypnotics (eg, methaqualone, ethchlorvynol) having greater risk of unhealthy use and nonbenzodiazepines have lower potential, although both classes of medications are controlled substances.

Benzodiazepines, depending on assessment of addiction liability, have been placed on Schedules IV and V (the lower the schedule number, the greater the unhealthy use liability of a medication) and nonbenzodiazepines have been placed on Schedule V. More controversial is the issue of relative addiction liability among the benzodiazepines themselves. Using the sole criterion of euphoric mood (positive reinforcement) effect in humans, benzodiazepines with the highest liability for addiction are flunitrazepam, diazepam, alprazolam, and possibly lorazepam. Those with the lowest positive reinforcing effects in humans are clonazepam, chlordiazepoxide, halazepam,[61] prazepam,[112] quazepam, and oxazepam. However, individuals at risk for sedative-hypnotic addiction (eg, those with an AUD disorder) may use any of the benzodiazepines, even those with relatively low potential for addiction. Benzodiazepines with the highest addiction potential are those that produce rapid onset of pleasant mood, a sense of well-being, relief of dysphoria and anxiety, and a general state of contentment.[113]

The relative addiction liability of nonbenzodiazepines, compared to benzodiazepines, is a matter of some controversy. While the nonbenzodiazepines were initially thought to have little addiction liability, human laboratory studies have shown that zolpidem administration increases subjective responses such as "Drug Liking" and "Good Effects" in both people who use drugs[114] and in healthy volunteers[115] indicating addiction potential. In other human laboratory studies that assessed addiction potential, these drugs produce euphoric effects at doses above their typical therapeutic ranges. For example, eszopiclone, at doses of 6 mg and 12 mg, produced euphoric effects comparable to diazepam 20-mg in people who previously used sedative-hypnotic. Studies examining the addiction liability of 25 mg, 50 mg, and 75 mg of zaleplon (doses above the approved therapeutic range) in subjects with a history of sedative-hypnotic addiction, indicated addiction potential similar to benzodiazepines and benzodiazepine-like hypnotics.

Daridorexant, in a large unhealthy use potential study, showed "Drug Liking" scores greater than placebo with similar effects at higher doses compared to supratherapeutic doses of suvorexant and zolpidem.[116] This new orexin receptor antagonist, recently approved for the treatment of insomnia, has been recommended for placement on Schedule IV. DEA has preliminarily placed this drug on Schedule IV and will finalize the schedule following public comment.[117]

EPIDEMIOLOGY OF UNHEALTHY USE

Benzodiazepines including alprazolam, clonazepam, and lorazepam remain some of the most commonly prescribed psychiatric medications. FDA reported that over 92 million prescriptions were written for benzodiazepines in 2019.[118] Sedative-hypnotic unhealthy use is reported in the National Survey on Drug Use and Health (NSDUH). After a decline in the number in 2016 from 2.6 million to 2.1 million in 2019, in 2020 unhealthy use increased to 4.8 million with highest rates in 18- to 25-year old at 3.3 percent or 1.1 million, followed by adults 26 and older (3.5 million).[119] These increases may be related to the restrictions and social isolation associated with coronavirus (COVID-19) pandemic mitigation strategies as a near doubling of SUD prevalence was reported for 2020. Sedative-hypnotic use disorders were present in 1.2 million people over age 12 and will contribute to greater need for SUD treatment and greater complexity of those treatments. A recent analysis of longitudinal data showed the relationship between adolescent binge alcohol, cigarette and cannabis use as risk factors for prescription drug unhealthy use in adulthood including sedative-hypnotic medications[120] underscoring the need to consider polysubstance use in the clinical approach to addressing SUD(s).

A recent literature review,[86] summarized findings regarding demographics of benzodiazepine unhealthy use (men and women have similar rates). Older studies have shown unhealthy use is more frequent in those who identify as non-Hispanic Whites. However, in recent years benzodiazepine unhealthy use has increased in racial/ethnic minority groups. Individuals with low education, unemployment, low income and who are unmarried are reported to have higher rates of benzodiazepine unhealthy use. Other epidemiological correlates include that subgroups of sexual minority groups may be at higher risk for benzodiazepine unhealthy use.

Other SUD are associated with benzodiazepine unhealthy use. For example, individuals with a history of AUD have higher rates of benzodiazepine-related problems according to NSDUH findings. In an analysis of data from 2008-2014, 7.6% of individuals with AUD were using benzodiazepines in an unhealthy manner; a rate more than 3 times that of the general public.[96] People with opioid use disorders (OUD) also have significant rates of benzodiazepine unhealthy use (up to 43%). Those in treatment for OUD also have substantial rates of benzodiazepine unhealthy use ranging from 7% to 73% of those queried and the majority of studies reporting upwards of 40% of those in treatment for OUD use benzodiazepines in an unhealthy manner.[86] Benzodiazepines may be used to manage anxiety and opioid withdrawal in this population and to enhance euphoria or "high" when ingested concomitantly with opioids increasing the risk of co-administration.[121] Benzodiazepine unhealthy use is common in those who use other illicit drugs including stimulants such as cocaine and methamphetamine. Further, benzodiazepine unhealthy use is associated with much greater risk for prescription drug use disorders.[122] Co-occurring mental illness is common in those with SUD. Benzodiazepine unhealthy use has been reported in association with mental disorders, particularly anxiety and affective disorders[123] underscoring the need to consider and address unhealthy benzodiazepine use in individuals with SUD and/or mental disorders. The frequent unhealthy use of benzodiazepines raises concern for risk of overdose particularly given increasing availability of illicit benzodiazepines that may contain fentanyl.[124]

TOXICITIES

It is well established that acute doses of benzodiazepines can be associated with adverse effects that include anterograde amnesia, difficulty acquiring new learning,[125] and sedation that may affect attention and concentration; however benzodiazepines provide a greater margin of safety than barbiturates and older agents. With continued use, tolerance develops to most of the cognitive effects, but not in everyone. Those who use intermittent doses (such as "as needed" dosing) of high-potency agents may not develop tolerance and continue to be at risk for impaired psychomotor and memory function, especially in the first few hours after taking a dose. Furthermore, studies[126] and clinical experience suggest that not all benzodiazepines produce the same type or severity of cognitive impairment. Although some studies have found no cognitive impairment associated with long-term benzodiazepine treatment,[127,128] others have reported persistent problems in psychomotor function, learning, concentration, and visuospatial skills.[129,130] In people whose use is chronic, greater impairment is seen in men, the elderly, and individuals taking the highest doses.[125] Long-term cognitive impairment was observed in concentration, general intelligence, problem-solving and psychomotor speed at three months following abstinence from use of benzodiazepines.[110] Further, these patients still perform worse than controls at 6 months after the medication is stopped.[131]

Benzodiazepines are widely prescribed in the elderly, despite the known risks in older people (eg, impaired cognition and mobility as well as increased risk of falls and associated injuries). An association between benzodiazepine use in older people and increased risk of Alzheimer disease has also been described,[132] though one study found the memory impairment in elderly taking benzodiazepines to be small.[133] Falls present a serious risk to the elderly. Classic benzodiazepines, nonbenzodiazepine hypnotics, selective serotonin reuptake inhibitors (SSRI) antidepressants, and antipsychotics have all been linked to falls and fractures in the elderly,[134-136] underscoring the need to consider the risk/benefit ratio of such medications in this population.

Zolpidem also produces anterograde amnesia and has been associated with somnambulism and complex nocturnal behaviors, such as eating, shopping, and driving. Similar problems may be seen with zaleplon, especially at high doses. It is not known whether all hypnotics are capable of producing such effects; however, the FDA has required a label change for benzodiazepine and nonbenzodiazepine hypnotics to include a warning describing these complex sleep-related behaviors.

Several surveys in different countries have found a higher incidence of motor vehicle accidents associated with benzodiazepine use.[137,138] It is not known whether this reflects acute psychomotor impairment, somnolence, or persistent visuospatial impairment. Zolpidem at a high (20 mg) dose when administered in the middle of the night can produce decrements in driving performance the following morning.[139]

The risks of benzodiazepines during pregnancy and lactation have been the subject of controversy. Data pooled from cohort studies have not demonstrated an increased risk of major malformations or cleft palate.[140] Conversely, when data from case control studies were pooled in the same meta-analysis, a small but statistically significant association was found between exposure to benzodiazepines and oral cleft abnormalities or other major malformations. The rate of cleft palate in the general population is estimated at 0.06%,[141] and case-control studies show that with benzodiazepines the risk may be approximately doubled at 0.12%.

Most recent studies have not found an association of in utero benzodiazepine exposure alone with major congenital anomalies.[142,143]

Two other clinically important problems may be encountered during pregnancy and are worth noting. Newborns who have been exposed to benzodiazepines in utero during the third trimester or during delivery may present with floppy baby syndrome. This condition is characterized by low Apgar scores, poor sucking, hypotonia, poor reflexes, and apnea.[144] Neonatal withdrawal syndromes have also been reported.[145]

Benzodiazepines administered to nursing mothers enter breast milk, but in such low concentrations that adverse effects in infants are generally not observed.[146-149] There are two important exceptions to this general rule: the risk to the infant is higher (1) if the benzodiazepine is given in high doses antepartum and continued postpartum, and (2) if infants have impaired hepatic function (eg, hyperbilirubinemia).[148] Despite their relative safety, breastfed infants whose mothers are taking benzodiazepines should be monitored for lethargy, weight loss, and signs of an abstinence syndrome.

The use of anticonvulsants, including phenobarbital, by pregnant women with epilepsy has been associated with reports of harm to the fetus, with inconsistent results.[150] The frequency of anticonvulsant embryopathy (ie, major malformations, growth retardation, and hypoplasia of the midface and fingers), is increased in infants exposed to phenobarbital alone or in combination with other anticonvulsants, compared to those whose mothers had a history of epilepsy but took no medications during pregnancy.[151]

In summary, benzodiazepines and nonbenzodiazepines can present a risk for significant adverse events associated with their use both acutely and chronically. These medications are widely prescribed for anxiety, insomnia, and in pain management. Tolerance rapidly develops over weeks to months for anxiolytic and sleep producing effects. Therefore, while acute or short-term administration of these medications can be useful, chronic use should generally be discouraged as a primary means of avoiding the toxicities that have been reported.

MEDICAL COMPLICATIONS

The principal medical complications with benzodiazepines are related to overdose and withdrawal syndromes. All sedative/hypnotics produce effects on a continuum from sedation to obtundation. Barbiturates have a greater risk for respiratory depression than do benzodiazepines. In overdose situations, sedative hypnotics are often combined with ethanol or other CNS depressants. When high doses of benzodiazepines are ingested, either as a therapeutic intervention or in an overdose, initial signs of toxicity are ataxia and impaired gag reflex as well as CNS depression. Respiratory depression may also occur in overdose and the medical approach to overdose treatment is supportive care. Rarely, medical complications of sedative hypnotic use can include disinhibition or paradoxical excitement.

A severe withdrawal syndrome after high-dose chronic administration of chlordiazepoxide or diazepam was demonstrated in the early 1960s[152,153] and, in its most severe form, can include grand mal seizures and psychosis. A characteristic abstinence syndrome may develop upon abrupt discontinuation of therapeutic doses of benzodiazepines that are administered for several weeks.[154] When administered for short periods and at therapeutic doses, the withdrawal syndrome is usually mild, consisting of anxiety, headache, insomnia, dysphoria, tremor, and muscle twitching. After long-term treatment with therapeutic doses, the syndrome increases in severity and may include autonomic dysfunction, nausea, vomiting, depersonalization, derealization, delirium, hallucinations, illusions, agitation, and grand mal seizures. The time course of the abstinence syndrome is related to the half-life of the agent, with patients taking short half-life agents (lorazepam, alprazolam, temazepam) developing symptoms within 24 hours of discontinuation, the severity of which peaks at 48 hours. With longer-half-life agents such as diazepam, symptoms may develop as much as a week after drug discontinuation and last for several weeks. This timeline should be used as a general guideline, because some patients on long-acting agents will develop symptoms earlier than predicted by the pharmacokinetics of the drug. In addition, some clinicians believe that there is a prolonged withdrawal syndrome that persists for several months, but it has not been clearly distinguished from return of original anxiety symptoms. Longer duration of treatment with benzodiazepines and/or the administration of higher doses of these agents increases the odds for the development of physical dependence and, potentially, development of a SUD.[155]

In general, longer treatment periods, higher doses, sudden drug discontinuation, and psychopathology increase the severity of the withdrawal syndrome. Clinical experience has shown that there is great variability in the sensitivity of patients to discontinuation of benzodiazepines. Benzodiazepines are most effective in short term (days to several weeks) use. Clinical evaluation of risks and benefits of long-term use should be an ongoing consideration.

The withdrawal syndrome upon abrupt discontinuation from barbiturates includes: apprehension, uneasiness, muscular weakness, coarse tremors, postural hypotension, anorexia, vomiting, and myoclonic jerks occurring within the first day following the last dose taken and lasting up to 2 weeks. Grand mal seizures may occur within 2 to 3 days of discontinuation and last as long as 8 days. Delirium was most likely to develop 3 to 8 days after drug discontinuation and lasted up to 2 weeks.[156] Management of the barbiturate withdrawal syndrome includes transition to an equivalent dose of phenobarbital, determined by either a challenge dose, or loading dose procedure and taper.[157]

CONCLUSION

Benzodiazepines are the most widely used of the sedative/hypnotic medications and lead other drugs in the sedative/hypnotic class in unhealthy use. In animal models and human laboratory studies, they occupy a lesser position of addiction liability relative to opioids and some stimulant medications as indicated by their placement in Schedules IV and V. In patients with anxiety and affective disorders, unhealthy use is less common though should be clinically monitored. Certain subgroups, such as individuals with AUD and those receiving opioid therapies for OUD are also at high risk for unhealthy use of these agents. Compared to the general population, higher rates of benzodiazepine use are found in the elderly and in those with chronic pain. Benzodiazepines can pose significant risks for adverse events and overdose deaths, particularly when used in combination with opioid medications and/or when unhealthy use of either is present. Risks associated with illicit benzodiazepines sold on the street include the presence via adulteration with fentanyl and other potent opioids that increase risk of overdose and death. The newer nonbenzodiazepine hypnotics may have a lower potential for tolerance or the development of a SUD, though they are not devoid of such risk. Newer medications for insomnia including orexin receptor antagonists also have unhealthy use liability and will be scheduled as the benzodiazepines.[117] The identification of $GABA_A$ receptor subtypes and clarification of their function provide optimism that drug development will lead to $GABA_A$ agonists and modulators that have fewer adverse effects, lower risk for addiction, and greater specificity of action.[158]

REFERENCES

1. Ciraulo D, Sarid-Segal O. *Sedative-, hypnotic-, or anxiolytic-related disorders*. In: Sadock B, Sadock B, eds. *Comprehensive Textbook of Psychiatry*. Lippincott Williams & Wilkens; 2004:1300-1318.
2. Greenblatt D, Shader R. *Benzodiazepines in Clinical Practice*. Raven Press; 1974.
3. Charney D, Mihic S, Harris R. *Hypnotics and Sedatives*. In: Hardman J, Limbird L, Gilman A, eds. *The Pharmacological Basis of Therapeutics*. McGraw Hill, Medical Publishing Edition; 2006.
4. Carter MK. *The story of barbituric acid*. *J Chem Educ*. 1951;28(10):524.
5. Lader M. History of benzodiazepine dependence. *J Subst Abuse Treat*. 1991;8(1):53-59.
6. Suddock JT, Cain MD. *Barbiturate Toxicity*. StatPearls Publishing; 2018.
7. Shader RI, Ciraulo DA. *Clinical Manual of Chemical Dependence*. American Psychiatric Press; 1991.
8. Herring WJ, Connor KM, Ivgy-May N, et al. Suvorexant in patients with insomnia: results from two 3-month randomized controlled clinical trials. *Biol Psychol*. 2016;79(2):136-148.
9. Rosenberg R, Murphy P, Zammit G, et al. Comparison of lemborexant with placebo and zolpidem tartrate extended release for the treatment of

older adults with insomnia disorder: a phase 3 randomized clinical trial. *JAMA Netw Open*. 2019;2(12):e1918254-e1918254.

10. Mignot E, Mayleben D, Fietze I, et al. Safety and efficacy of daridorexant in patients with insomnia disorder: results from two multicentre, randomised, double-blind, placebo-controlled, phase 3 trials. *Lancet Neurol*. 2022;21(2):125-139.
11. Markham A. Daridorexant: first approval. *Drugs*. 2022;82:601-607.
12. Jones-Davis DM, Song L, Gallagher MJ, Macdonald RL. Structural determinants of benzodiazepine allosteric regulation of GABA(A) receptor currents. *J Neurosci*. 2005;25(35):8056-8065.
13. Benarroch EE. $GABA_A$ receptor heterogeneity, function, and implications for epilepsy. *Neurology*. 2007;68(8):612-614.
14. Crestani F, Löw K, Keist R, Mandelli M, Möhler H, Rudolph U. Molecular targets for the myorelaxant action of diazepam. *Mol Pharmacol*. 2001;59(3):442-425.
15. Rowlett JK, Platt DM, Lelas S, Atack JR, Dawson GR. Different GABAA receptor subtypes mediate the anxiolytic, abuse-related, and motor effects of benzodiazepine-like drugs in primates. *Proc Natl Acad Sci U S A*. 2005;102(3):915-920.
16. Dias R, Sheppard WFA, Fradley RL, et al. Evidence for a significant role of alpha 3-containing $GABA_A$ receptors in mediating the anxiolytic effects of benzodiazepines. *J Neurosci*. 2005;25(46):10682-10688.
17. Rudolph U, Mohler H. Analysis of GABAA receptor function and dissection of the pharmacology of benzodiazepines and general anesthetics through mouse genetics. *Annu Rev Pharmacol Toxicol*. 2004;44:475-498.
18. Luscher B, Fuchs T, Kilpatrick CL. GABAA receptor trafficking-mediated plasticity of inhibitory synapses. *Neuron*. 2011;70(3):385-409.
19. Savic MM, Huang S, Furtmüller R, et al. Are GABAA receptors containing alpha5 subunits contributing to the sedative properties of benzodiazepine site agonists? *Neuropsychopharmacology*. 2008;33(2): 332-339.
20. Reynolds LM, Engin E, Tantillo G, et al. Differential roles of GABA(A) receptor subtypes in benzodiazepine-induced enhancement of brain-stimulation reward. *Neuropsychopharmacology*. 2012;37(11):2531-2540.
21. Tan KR, Brown M, Labouèbe G, et al. Neural bases for addictive properties of benzodiazepines. *Nature*. 2010;463(7282):769-774.
22. Thompson S, Whiting P, Wafford K. Barbiturate interactions at the human GABAA receptor: Dependence on receptor subunit combination. *Brit J Pharmacol*. 1996;117(3):521-527.
23. Dias R, et al. Evidence for a significant role of α3-containing GABAA receptors in mediating the anxiolytic effects of benzodiazepines. *J Neurosci*. 2005;25(46):10682-10688.
24. Drafts BC, Fisher JL. Identification of structures within GABAA receptor α subunits that regulate the agonist action of pentobarbital. *J Pharmacol Exp Ther*. 2006;318(3):1094-1101.
25. Taverna FA, Cameron BR, Hampson DL, Wang LY, Mac Donald JF. Sensitivity of AMPA receptors to pentobarbital. *Eur J Pharmacol*. 1994;267(3):R3-R5.
26. Zhan R, Fujiwara N, Yamakura T, Taga K, Fukuda S, Shimoji K. Differential inhibitory effects of thiopental, thiamylal and phenobarbital on both voltage-gated calcium channels and NMDA receptors in rat hippocampal slices. *Br J Anaesth*. 1998;81(6):932-939.
27. Drover DR. Comparative pharmacokinetics and pharmacodynamics of short-acting hypnosedatives: Zaleplon, zolpidem and zopiclone. *Clin Pharmacokinet*. 2004;43(4):227-238.
28. Sanger DJ. The pharmacology and mechanisms of action of new generation, non-benzodiazepine hypnotic agents. *CNS Drugs*. 2004;18(1):9-15. discussion 41, 43-5.
29. Sanger DJ, Morel E, Perrault G. Comparison of the pharmacological profiles of the hypnotic drugs, zaleplon and zolpidem. *Eur J Pharmacol*. 1996;313(1–2):35-42.
30. Carlson JN, Haskew R, Wacker J, Maisonneuve IM, Glick SD, Jerussi TP. Sedative and anxiolytic effects of zopiclone's enantiomers and metabolite. *Eur J Pharmacol*. 2001;415(2–3):181-189.
31. Griebel G, Perrault G, Sanger DJ. Limited anxiolytic-like effects of non-benzodiazepine hypnotics in rodents. *J Psychopharmacol*. 1998;12(4):356-365.
32. Sanna E, Busonero F, Talani G, et al. Comparison of the effects of zaleplon, zolpidem, and triazolam at various GABA(A) receptor subtypes. *Eur J Pharmacol*. 2002;451(2):103-110.
33. Noguchi H, Kitazumi K, Mori M, Shiba T. Binding and neuropharmacological profile of zaleplon, a novel nonbenzodiazepine sedative/hypnotic. *Eur J Pharmacol*. 2002;434(1–2):21-28.
34. Doble A, Canton T, Dreisler S, et al. RP 59037 and RP 60503: anxiolytic cyclopyrrolone derivatives with low sedative potential: Interaction with the gamma-aminobutyric acidA/benzodiazepine receptor complex and behavioral effects in the rodent. *J Pharmacol Exp Ther*. 1993;266(3):1213-1226.
35. Davies M, Newell JG, Derry JM, Martin IL, Dunn SM. Characterization of the interaction of zopiclone with gamma-aminobutyric acid type A receptors. *Mol Pharmacol*. 2000;58(4):756-762.
36. Hanson SM, Czajkowski C. Structural mechanisms underlying benzodiazepine modulation of the GABA(A) receptor. *J Neurosci*. 2008;28(13):3490-3499.
37. Sancar F, Ericksen SS, Kucken AM, Teissére JA, Czajkowski C. Structural determinants for high-affinity zolpidem binding to GABA-A receptors. *Mol Pharmacol*. 2007;71(1):38-46.
38. Dämgen K, Lüddens H. Zaleplon displays a selectivity to recombinant GABAA receptors different from zolipdem, zopiclone and benzodiazepines. *Neurosci Res Comm*. 1999;25(3):139-148.
39. McMahon FJ, Insel TR. Pharmacogenomics and personalized medicine in neuropsychiatry. *Neuron*. 2012;74(5):773-776.
40. Roch C, Bergamini G, Steiner MA, Clozel M. Nonclinical pharmacology of daridorexant: A new dual orexin receptor antagonist for the treatment of insomnia. *Psychopharmacology (Berl)*. 2021;238(10): 2693-2708.
41. US Food and Drug Administration. *Highlights of Prescribing Information*. 2022.
42. Monti JM, Monti D. Overview of currently available benzodiazepine and nonbenzodiazepine hypnotics. *Clinical Pharmacology of Sleep*. Springer; 2006:207-223.
43. Hesse LM, von Moltke LL, Greenblatt DJ. Clinically important drug interactions with zopiclone, zolpidem and zaleplon. *CNS Drugs*. 2003;17(7):513-532.
44. Mandrioli R, Mercolini L, Raggi MA. Metabolism of benzodiazepine and non-benzodiazepine anxiolytic-hypnotic drugs: an analytical point of view. *Curr Drug Metab*. 2010;11(9):815-829.
45. Muehlan C, Heuberger J, Juif P-E, Croft M, van Gerven J, Dingemanse J. Accelerated development of the dual orexin receptor antagonist ACT-541468: Integration of a microtracer in a first-in-human study. *Clin Pharmacol Ther*. 2018;104(5):1022-1029.
46. Boof M-L, Alatrach A, Ufer M, Dingemanse J. Interaction potential of the dual orexin receptor antagonist ACT-541468 with CYP3A4 and food: results from two interaction studies. *Eur J Clin Pharmacol*. 2019;75(2):195-205.
47. Muehlan C, Fischer H, Zimmer D, et al. Metabolism of the dual orexin receptor antagonist ACT-541468, Based on microtracer/accelerator mass spectrometry. *Curr Drug Metab*. 2019;20(4):254-265.
48. Greenblatt DJ, Arendt RM, Shader RI. Pharmacodynamics of benzodiazepines after single oral doses: Kinetic and physiochemical correlates. *Psychopharmacology Suppl*. 1984;1:92-97.
49. Greenblatt DJ, Sethy VH. Benzodiazepine concentrations in brain directly reflect receptor occupancy: studies of diazepam, lorazepam, and oxazepam. *Psychopharmacology (Berl)*. 1990;102(3):373-378.
50. Norman TR, Fulton A, Burrow GD, Maguire KP. Pharmacokinetics of N-desmethyldiazepam after a single oral dose of clorazepate: The effect of smoking. *Eur J Clin Pharmacol*. 1981;21(3):229-233.
51. O'Brien CP. Benzodiazepine use, abuse, and dependence. *J Clin Psychiatry*. 2005;66(Suppl 2):28-33.
52. Arendt RM, Greenblatt DJ, Leibisch DC, Luu MD, Paul SM. Determinants of benzodiazepine brain uptake: lipophilicity versus binding affinity. *Psychopharmacology (Berl)*. 1987;93(1):72-76.
53. Scavone JM, Friedman H, Greenblatt DJ, Shader RI. Effect of age, body composition, and lipid solubility on benzodiazepine tissue distribution in rats. *Arzneimittelforschung*. 1987;37(1):2-6.

54. Greenblatt DJ, Arendt RM, Abernethy DR, Giles HG, Sellers EM, Shader RI. In vitro quantitation of benzodiazepine lipophilicity: Relation to in vivo distribution. *Br J Anaesth*. 1983;55(10):985-989.
55. Ciraulo D, Barnhill JG, Ciraulo AM, et al. Alterations in pharmacodynamics of anxiolytics in abstinent alcoholic men: Subjective responses, abuse liability, and electroencephalographic effects of alprazolam, diazepam, and buspirone. *J Clin Pharmacol*. 1997;37(1):64-73.
56. Ciraulo D, Barnhill JG, Greenblatt DJ, et al. Abuse liability and clinical pharmacokinetics of alprazolam in alcoholic men. *J Clin Psychiatry*. 1988;49(9):333-337.
57. Griffiths RR, Bigelow G, Liebson I. Human drug self-administration: double-blind comparison of pentobarbital, diazepam, chlorpromazine and placebo. *J Pharmacol Exp Ther*. 1979;210(2):301-310.
58. Griffiths RR, Bigelow GE, Liebson I, Kaliszak JE. Drug preference in humans: Double-blind choice comparison of pentobarbital, diazepam and placebo. *J Pharmacol Exp Ther*. 1980;215(3):649-661.
59. Griffiths RR, McLeod DR, Bigelow GE, Liebson IA, Roache JD, Nowowieski P. Comparison of diazepam and oxazepam: Preference, liking and extent of abuse. *J Pharmacol Exp Ther*. 1984;229(2):501-508.
60. Griffiths RR, Wolf B. Relative abuse liability of different benzodiazepines in drug abusers. *J Clin Psychopharmacol*. 1990;10(4):237-243.
61. Jaffe JH, Ciraulo DA, Nies A, Dixon RB, Monroe LL. Abuse potential of halazepam and of diazepam in patients recently treated for acute alcohol withdrawal. *Clin Pharmacol Ther*. 1983;34(5):623-630.
62. Whirl-Carrillo M, McDonagh EM, Herbert JM, et al. Pharmacogenomics knowledge for personalized medicine. *Clin Pharmacol Ther*. 2012;92(4):414.
63. He P, Court MH, Greenblatt DJ, Von Moltke LL. Genotype-phenotype associations of cytochrome P450 3A4 and 3A5 polymorphism with midazolam clearance in vivo. *Clin Pharmacol Ther*. 2005;77(5):373-387.
64. He P, Court MH, Greenblatt DJ, Von Moltke LL. Factors influencing midazolam hydroxylation activity in human liver microsomes. *Drug Metab Dispos*. 2006;34(7):1198-1207.
65. Maekawa K, Yoshimura T, Saito Y, et al. Functional characterization of CYP3A4.16: Catalytic activities toward midazolam and carbamazepine. *Xenobiotica*. 2009;39(2):140-147.
66. Bertilsson L, Henthorn TK, Sanz E, Tybring G, Säwe J, Villén T. Importance of genetic factors in the regulation of diazepam metabolism: Relationship to S-mephenytoin, but not debrisoquin, hydroxylation phenotype. *Clin Pharmacol Ther*. 1989;45(4):348-355.
67. Sohn DR, Kusaka M, Ishizaki T, et al. Incidence of S-mephenytoin hydroxylation deficiency in a Korean population and the interphenotypic differences in diazepam pharmacokinetics. *Clin Pharmacol Ther*. 1992;52(2):160-169.
68. Zhang YA, Reviriego J, Lou YQ, Sjöqvist F, Bertilsson L. Diazepam metabolism in native Chinese poor and extensive hydroxylators of S-mephenytoin: Interethnic differences in comparison with white subjects. *Clin Pharmacol Ther*. 1990;48(5):496-502.
69. Granfors MT, Backman JT, Laitila J, Neuvonen PJ. Oral contraceptives containing ethinyl estradiol and gestodene markedly increase plasma concentrations and effects of tizanidine by inhibiting cytochrome P450 1A2. *Clin Pharmacol Ther*. 2005;78(4):400-411.
70. Stoehr GP, Kroboth PD, Juhl RP, Wender DB, Phillips JP, Smith RB. Effect of oral contraceptives on triazolam, temazepam, alprazolam, and lorazepam kinetics. *Clin Pharmacol Ther*. 1984;36(5):683-690.
71. Scavone JM, Greenblatt DJ, Locniskar A, Shader RI. Alprazolam pharmacokinetics in women on low-dose oral contraceptives. *J Clin Pharmacol*. 1988;28(5):454-457.
72. Abernethy D, Greenblatt DJ, Ochs HR, et al. Lorazepam and oxazepam kinetics in women on low-dose oral contraceptives. *Clin Pharmacol Ther*. 1983;33(5):628-632.
73. Abernethy D, Greenblatt DJ, Divoll M, Arendt R, Ochs HR, Shader RI. Impairment of diazepam metabolism by low-dose estrogen-containing oral-contraceptive steroids. *N Engl J Med*. 1982;306(13):791-792.
74. Roberts RK, Desmond PV, Wilkinson GR, Schenker S. Disposition of chlordiazepoxide: sex differences and effects of oral contraceptives. *Clin Pharmacol Ther*. 1979;25(6):826-831.
75. Patwardhan RV, Mitchell MC, Johnson RF, Schenker S. Differential effects of oral contraceptive steroids on the metabolism of benzodiazepines. *Hepatology*. 1983;3(2):248-253.
76. Backman, J. T., Olkkola, K. T., Ojala, M., Laaksovirta, H., & Neuvonen, P. J. Concentrations and effects of oral midazolam are greatly reduced in patients treated with carbamazepine or phenytoin. *Epilepsia*. 1996;37(3):253-257.
77. Backman, J. T., Olkkola, K. T., & Neuvonen, P. J. Rifampin drastically reduces plasma concentrations and effects of oral midazolam. *Clinical pharmacology & therapeutics*. 1996;59(1):7-13.
78. Vlase L, Popa A, Neag M, Muntean D, Bâldea I, Leucuța SE. Pharmacokinetic interaction between zolpidem and carbamazepine in healthy volunteers. *J Clin Pharmacol*. 2011;51(8):1233-1236.
79. Zolk O, Solbach TF, König J, Fromm MF. Functional characterization of the human organic cation transporter 2 variant p.270Ala>Ser. *Drug Metab Dispos*. 2009;37(6):1312-1318.
80. Ciraulo DA. *Drug Interactions in Psychiatry*. Lippincott Williams & Wilkins; 2006.
81. Jones JD, Mogali S, Comer SD. Polydrug abuse: A review of opioid and benzodiazepine combination use. *Drug Alcohol Depend*. 2012;125(1–2):8-18.
82. Zacny JP, Paice JA, Coalson DW. Separate and combined psychopharmacological effects of alprazolam and oxycodone in healthy volunteers. *Drug Alcohol Depend*. 2012;124(3):274-282.
83. Lintzeris N, Mitchell TB, Bond AJ, Nestor L, Strang J. Pharmacodynamics of diazepam co-administered with methadone or buprenorphine under high dose conditions in opioid dependent patients. *Drug Alcohol Depend*. 2007;91(2–3):187-194.
84. Jones CM, McAninch JK. Emergency department visits and overdose deaths from combined use of opioids and benzodiazepines. *Am J Prev Med*. 2015;49(4):493-501.
85. Substance Abuse and Mental Health Services Administration. *Mental Health Services Administration, Drug Abuse Warning Network, 2011: National Estimates of Drug-Related Emergency Department Visits. HHS Publication No.(SMA) 13-4760, DAWN Series D-39*. Substance Abuse and Mental Health Services Administration. Accessed May 12, 2023. https://www.samhsa.gov/data/sites/default/files/DAWN2k11ED/DAWN2k11ED/DAWN2k11ED.pdf
86. Votaw VR, Geyer R, Rieselbach MM, RK MH. The epidemiology of benzodiazepine misuse: A systematic review. *Drug Alcohol Depend*. 2019;200:95-114.
87. Liu S, O'Donnell J, Gladden RM, McGlone L, Chowdhury F. Trends in nonfatal and fatal overdoses involving benzodiazepines—38 states and the District of Columbia, 2019–2020. *Am J Transplant*. 2021;21(11):3794-3800.
88. US Food and Drug Administration. *FDA Drug Safety Communication: FDA Requiring Boxed Warning Updated to Improve Safe Use of Benzodiazepine Drug Class*. US FDA; 2020.
89. Nielsen S, Lintzeris N, Bruno R, et al. Benzodiazepine use among chronic pain patients prescribed opioids: Associations with pain, physical and mental health, and health service utilization. *Pain Med*. 2015;16(2):356-366.
90. Westbrook L, Cicala RS, Wright H. Effectiveness of alprazolam in the treatment of chronic pain: Results of a preliminary study. *The Clin J Pain*. 1990;6(1):32-36.
91. Brotz D, Maschke E, Burkard S, et al. Is there a role for benzodiazepines in the management of lumbar disc prolapse with acute sciatica? *Pain*. 2010;149(3):470-475.
92. Chou R, Huffman LH; American Pain Society, American College of Physicians. Medications for acute and chronic low back pain: A review of the evidence for an American Pain Society/American College of Physicians clinical practice guideline. *Ann Intern Med*. 2007;147(7):505-514.
93. Ito K, Yoshikawa M, Maeda M, et al. Midazolam attenuates the antinociception induced by d-serine or morphine at the supraspinal level in rats. *Eur J Pharmacol*. 2008;586(1–3):139-144.
94. Pakulska W, Czarnecka E. Effect of diazepam and midazolam on the antinociceptive effect of morphine, metamizol and indomethacin in mice. *Pharmazie*. 2001;56(1):89-91.

95. Gear RW, et al. Benzodiazepine mediated antagonism of opioid analgesia. *Pain*. 1997;71(1):25-29.
96. King SA, Strain JJ. Benzodiazepines and chronic pain. *Pain*. 1990;41(1):3-4.
97. Dowell D, Ragan KR, Jones CM, Baldwin GT, Chou R. CDC Clinical practice guideline for prescribing opioids for pain – United States, 2022. *MMWR Recomm Rep*. 2022;71(No. RR-3):1–95. doi: http://dx.doi.org/10.15585/mmwr.rr7103a1
98. Zeng XJ, Tietz EI. Role of bicarbonate ion in mediating decreased synaptic conductance in benzodiazepine tolerant hippocampal CA1 pyramidal neurons. *Brain Res*. 2000;868(2):202-214.
99. Zeng XJ, Tietz EI. Benzodiazepine tolerance at GABAergic synapses on hippocampal CA1 pyramidal cells. *Synapse*. 1999;31(4):263-277.
100. Yu O, Chiu TH, Rosenberg HC. Modulation of GABA-gated chloride ion flux in rat brain by acute and chronic benzodiazepine administration. *J Pharmacol Exp Ther*. 1988;246(1):107-113.
101. Li M, Szabo A, Rosenberg HC. Down-regulation of benzodiazepine binding to alpha 5 subunit-containing gamma-aminobutyric Acid(A) receptors in tolerant rat brain indicates particular involvement of the hippocampal CA1 region. *J Pharmacol Exp Ther*. 2000;295(2):689-696.
102. Ali NJ, Olsen RW. Chronic benzodiazepine treatment of cells expressing recombinant GABA(A) receptors uncouples allosteric binding: Studies on possible mechanisms. *J Neurochem*. 2001;79(5):1100-1108.
103. Vlainić J, Jembrek MJ, Strac DS, Pericić D. The effects of zolpidem treatment and withdrawal on the in vitro expression of recombinant alpha1beta2gamma2s GABA(A) receptors expressed in HEK 293 cells. *Naunyn Schmiedebergs Arch Pharmacol*. 2010;382(3):201-212.
104. Follesa P, Cagetti E, Mancuso L, et al. Increase in expression of the GABA(A) receptor alpha(4) subunit gene induced by withdrawal of, but not by long-term treatment with, benzodiazepine full or partial agonists. *Brain Res Mol Brain Res*. 2001;92(1-2):138-148.
105. Smith SS, Gong QH, Hsu FC, Markowitz RS, Ffrench-Mullen JM, Li X. GABA(A) receptor alpha4 subunit suppression prevents withdrawal properties of an endogenous steroid. *Nature*. 1998;392(6679):926-930.
106. Izzo E, Auta J, Impagnatiello F, Pesold C, Guidotti A, Costa E. Glutamic acid decarboxylase and glutamate receptor changes during tolerance and dependence to benzodiazepines. *Proc Natl Acad Sci U S A*. 2001;98(6):3483-3488.
107. Allison C, Pratt JA. Neuroadaptive processes in GABAergic and glutamatergic systems in benzodiazepine dependence. *Pharmacol Ther*. 2003;98(2):171-195.
108. Van Sickle BJ, Xiang K, Tietz EI. Transient plasticity of hippocampal CA1 neuron glutamate receptors contributes to benzodiazepine withdrawal-anxiety. *Neuropsychopharmacology*. 2004;29(11):1994-2006.
109. Das P, Lilly SM, Zerda R, Gunning WT, Alvarez FJ, Tietz EI. Increased AMPA receptor GluR1 subunit incorporation in rat hippocampal CA1 synapses during benzodiazepine withdrawal. *J Comp Neurol*. 2008;511(6):832-846.
110. Allison C, Pratt JA. Differential effects of two chronic diazepam treatment regimes on withdrawal anxiety and AMPA receptor characteristics. *Neuropsychopharmacology*. 2006;31(3):602-619.
111. Xiang K, Tietz EI. Benzodiazepine-induced hippocampal CA1 neuron alpha-amino-3-hydroxy-5-methylisoxasole-4-propionic acid (AMPA) receptor plasticity linked to severity of withdrawal anxiety: Differential role of voltage-gated calcium channels and N-methyl-D-aspartic acid receptors. *Behav Pharmacol*. 2007;18(5–6):447-460.
112. Orzack MH, Cole JO, Ionescu-Pioggia M, Beake BJ, Bird MP, Lobel M. A comparison of some subjective effects of prazepam, diazepam, and placebo. *NIDA Res Monogr*. 1982;41:309-317.
113. Ciraulo DA, Knapp CM, LoCastro J, Greenblatt DJ, Shader RI. A benzodiazepine mood effect scale: reliability and validity determined for alcohol-dependent subjects and adults with a parental history of alcoholism. *Am J Drug Alcohol Abuse*. 2001;27(2):339-347.
114. Rush CR, Baker RW, Wright K. Acute behavioral effects and abuse potential of trazodone, zolpidem and triazolam in humans. *Psychopharmacology (Berl)*. 1999;144(3):220-233.
115. Licata SC, Mashhoon Y, Maclean RR, Lukas SE. Modest abuse-related subjective effects of zolpidem in drug-naive volunteers. *Behav Pharmacol*. 2011;22(2):160-166.
116. Ufer M, Kelsh D, Schoedel KA, Dingemanse J. Abuse potential assessment of the new dual orexin receptor antagonist daridorexant in recreational sedative drug users as compared to suvorexant and zolpidem. *Sleep*. 2022;45(3): zsab224.
117. Milgram A. *Schedules of Controlled Substances: Placement of Daridorexant in Schedule IV*; 2022. Accessed May 12, 2023. https://www.regulations.gov/document/DEA-2022-0025-0001
118. Brooks M. *FDA Orders Stronger Warnings on Benzodiazepines*; 2020. Accessed May 12, 2023. https://www.medscape.com/viewarticle/937997?ecd=ppc_google_rlsa-traf_mscp_news-perspectives_t1-psych_us
119. Substance Abuse and Mental Health Services Administration. Key substance use and mental health indicators in the United States: Results from the 2019 National Survey on Drug Use and Health (HHS Publication No. PEP20-07-01-001, NSDUH Series H-55). Rockville, MD: Center for Behavioral Health Statistics and Quality, Substance Abuse and Mental Health Services Administration. 2020. Retrieved from https://www.samhsa.gov/data/
120. McCabe SE, Schulenberg JE, Schepis TS, et al. Trajectories of prescription drug misuse among US adults from ages 18 to 50 years. *JAMA Netw Open*. 2022;5(1):e2141995-e2141995.
121. Stein MD, Kanabar M, Anderson BJ, Lembke A, Bailey GL. Reasons for benzodiazepine use among persons seeking opioid detoxification. *J Subst Abuse Treat*. 2016;68:57-61.
122. Jones CM, McCance-Katz EF. Co-occurring substance use and mental disorders among adults with opioid use disorder. *Drug Alcohol Depend*. 2019;197:78-82.
123. Schepis TS, Hakes JK. Non-medical prescription use increases the risk for the onset and recurrence of psychopathology: Results from the national epidemiological survey on alcohol and related conditions. *Addiction*. 2011;106(12):2146-2155.
124. Sutter ME, Gerona RR, Davis MT, et al. Fatal fentanyl: One pill can kill. *Acad Emerg Med*. 2017;24(1):106-113.
125. Stewart SA. The effects of benzodiazepines on cognition. *J Clin Psychiatry*. 2005;66(Suppl 2):9-13.
126. Curran HV, Gorenstein C. Differential effects of lorazepam and oxazepam on priming. *Int Clin Psychopharmacol*. 1993;8(1):37-42.
127. Lucki I, Rickels K, Geller AM. Chronic use of benzodiazepines and psychomotor and cognitive test performance. *Psychopharmacology (Berl)*. 1986;88(4):426-433.
128. Buffett-Jerrott SE, Stewart SH. Cognitive and sedative effects of benzodiazepine use. *Curr Pharm Des*. 2002;8(1):45-58.
129. Barker MJ, Greenwood KM, Jackson M, Crowe SF. Cognitive effects of long-term benzodiazepine use: a meta-analysis. *CNS Drugs*. 2004;18(1):37-48.
130. Golombok S, Moodley, Lader M. Cognitive impairment in long-term benzodiazepine users. *Psychol Med*. 1988;18(2):365-374.
131. Barker MJ, Greenwood KM, Jackson M, Crowe S. Persistence of cognitive effects after withdrawal from long-term benzodiazepine use: A meta-analysis. *Arch Clin Neuropsychol*. 2004;19(3):437-454.
132. Olfson M, King M, Schoenbaum M. Benzodiazepine use in the United States. *JAMA Psychiatry*. 2015;72(2):136-142.
133. Bierman EJ, Comijs HC, Gundy CM, Sonnenberg C, Jonker C, Beekman ATF. The effect of chronic benzodiazepine use on cognitive functioning in older persons: Good, bad or indifferent? *Int J Geriatr Psychiatry*. 2007;22(12):1194-1200.
134. Vestergaard P, Rejnmark L, Mosekilde L. Anxiolytics, sedatives, antidepressants, neuroleptics and the risk of fracture. *Osteoporos Int*. 2006;17(6):807-816.
135. Hartikainen S, Lonnroos E, Louhivuori K. Medication as a risk factor for falls: critical systematic review. *J Gerontol A Biol Sci Med Sci*. 2007;62(10):1172-1181.
136. Pariente A, Dartigues J-F, Benichou J, Letenneur L, Moore N, Fourrier-Réglat A. Benzodiazepines and injurious falls in community dwelling elders. *Drugs Aging*. 2008;25(1):61-70.
137. Hebert C, Delaney JAC, Hemmelgarn B, Lévesque E, Suissa S. Benzodiazepines and elderly drivers: A comparison of pharmacoepidemiological study designs. *Pharmacoepidemiol Drug Saf*. 2007;16(8):845-849.

138. Engeland A, Skurtveit S, Morland J. Risk of road traffic accidents associated with the prescription of drugs: A registry-based cohort study. *Ann Epidemiol.* 2007;17(8):597-602.
139. Verster JC, Volkerts ER, Schreuder AHCML, et al. Residual effects of middle-of-the-night administration of zaleplon and zolpidem on driving ability, memory functions, and psychomotor performance. *J Clin Psychopharmacol.* 2002;22(6):576-583.
140. Dolovich LR, Addis A, Vaillancourt JM, Power JD, Koren G, Einarson TR. Benzodiazepine use in pregnancy and major malformations of oral cleft: meta-analysis of cohort and case-control studies. *BMJ.* 1998;317(7162):839-843.
141. Addis A, Dolovitch LR, Einarson TR, Koren G. Can we use anxiolytics during pregnancy without anxiety? *Can Fam Physician.* 2000;46:549-551.
142. Czeizel AE, Rockenbauer M, Sørensen HT, Olsen J. A population-based case-control study of oral chlordiazepoxide use during pregnancy and risk of congenital abnormalities. *Neurotoxicol Teratol.* 2004;26(4):593-598.
143. Lin AE, Peller AJ, Westgate M-N, Houde K, Franz A, Holmes LB. Clonazepam use in pregnancy and the risk of malformations. *Clin Mol Teratol.* 2004;70:534-536.
144. Gillberg C. "Floppy infant syndrome" and maternal diazepam. *Lancet.* 1977;2(8031):244.
145. Iqbal MM, Sobhan T, Ryals T. Effects of commonly used benzodiazepines on the fetus, the neonate, and the nursing infant. *Psychiatr Serv.* 2002;53(1):39-49.
146. Burt VK, Suri R, Altshuler L, Stowe Z, Hendrick VC, Muntean E. The use of psychotropic medications during breast-feeding. *Am J Psychiatry.* 2001;158(7):1001-1009.
147. Menon SJ. Psychotropic medication during pregnancy and lactation. *Arch Gynecol Obstet.* 2008;277(1):1-13.
148. Birnbaum CS, Cohen LS, Bailey JW, Grush LR, Roberston LM, Stowe ZN. Serum concentrations of antidepressants and benzodiazepines in nursing infants: A case series. *Pediatrics.* 1999;104(1):e11.
149. McElhatton PR. The effects of benzodiazepine use during pregnancy and lactation. *Reprod Toxicol.* 1994;8(6):461-475.
150. Bertollini R, Källen B, Mastroiacovo P, Robert E. Anticonvulsant drugs in monotherapy. Effect on the fetus. *Eur J Epidemiol.* 1987;3(2): 164-171.
151. Holmes L. The teratogenicity of anticonvulsant drugs: A progress report. *J Med Genet.* 2002;39(4):245-247.
152. Hollister LE, Motzenbecker FP, Degan RO. Withdrawal reactions from chlordiazepoxide ("Librium"). *Psychopharmacologia.* 1961;2:63-68.
153. Hollister LE, Bennett JL, Kimbell I Jr, Savage C, Overall JE. Diazepam in newly admitted schizophrenics. *Dis Nerv Syst.* 1963;24:746-750.
154. American Psychiatric Association. *Benzodiazepine Dependence, Toxicity, and Abuse.* APA; 1990.
155. Kan CC, Hilberink SR, Breteler MH. Determination of the main risk factors for benzodiazepine dependence using a multivariate and multidimensional approach. *Compr Psychiatry.* 2004;45(2):88-94.
156. Wikler A. Diagnosis and treatment of drug dependence of the barbiturate type. *Am J Psychiatry.* 1968;125(6):758-765.
157. Kranzler HR, Ciraulo DA, Zindel L. *Clinical Manual of Addiction Psychopharmacology.* American Psychiatric Publishing, Inc.; 2005.
158. Korpi ER, Sinkkonen ST. GABA(A) receptor subtypes as targets for neuropsychiatric drug development. *Pharmacol Ther.* 2006;109(1–2): 12-32.

13 The Pharmacology of Opioids

Daryl Shorter, Coreen B. Domingo, and Thomas R. Kosten

CHAPTER OUTLINE

- Definition of drugs and substances included in the class
- Epidemiology of opioids and use disorder
- Pharmacokinetics of specific drugs
- Pharmacodynamics
- Tolerance development
- Toxicity states and their medical management
- Drug-drug interactions
- Conclusions and future research directions

DEFINITION OF DRUGS AND SUBSTANCES INCLUDED IN THE CLASS

The three distinct types of opioid drugs can be classified as plant-derived, semisynthetic, and synthetic. Opium is a plant-derived, naturally occurring mixture directly derived from the juice of the opium poppy (*Papaver somniferum*). Opioid analgesic medications are agonists at MOP-r (mu opioid receptors). Morphine (the prototypical MOP-r agonist) is the main active alkaloid in opium and constitutes roughly 10% (by weight), while codeine and thebaine are also present, but in much lower concentrations. Codeine is used medicinally as an analgesic and antitussive, whereas thebaine can be used as a starting point for producing semisynthetic MOP-r ligands. Several synthetic and semi-synthetic opioids also are significant for opioid use disorder: heroin, oxycodone, hydromorphone, and hydrocodone, as well as meperidine, pentazocine, methadone, levo-alpha-acetylmethadol (LAAM), and buprenorphine.

Opium was first cultivated around 3400 BCE along the banks of the Tigris and Euphrates River in lower Mesopotamia. Unearthed Sumerian clay tablets (3000 BCE) referred to the opium poppy as "hul gil" ("joy plant"). The ancient Egyptians also cultivated poppies. "Thebaine" is derived from the name for the Egyptian city Thebes. "Opium" may be a Greek-derived word ("opion" = poppy juice). Opium is also featured prominently in Greek mythology and was found in the writings of Hippocrates' (460-377 BCE) who wrote of its usefulness as a narcotic and analgesic in the treatment of pain. The ancient Roman philosopher Pliny the Elder (23-79 CE) warned of the dangers of compulsive use of opium. In 1804, a young German pharmacist, Friedrich Sertürner, isolated morphine (which he named after Morpheus, the Greek god of dreams) from the raw opium seed. A major development in the delivery of opioids, the hypodermic needle, was perfected in 1853. This allowed for rapid analgesia, but also greater morbidity and mortality when misused. Diacetylmorphine, a derivative of morphine, was first synthesized as a semisynthetic analog in the 1870s by the Bayer company and marketed under the name "heroin." The American experience with opiate addiction has been historically documented in the literature and is particularly well evidenced in the book, *Dark Paradise* by David Courtwright.[1]

Plant-Derived Agents

Opium and Morphine

Opium refers to the extract of the opium poppy plant, *P somniferum.* Morphine is the major analgesic found in opium and is the prototypical plant-derived agent. It is the basis for comparison to other opioids, which are commonly referenced in terms of morphine equivalents using tools such as the CDC Opioid Conversion Guide (https://www.cdc.gov/drugoverdose/training/dosing/accessible/index.html). Codeine is also found in opium but in very small amounts. Codeine used clinically is a semisynthetic product of morphine (see below).

Semisynthetic Agents

Semisynthetic opioids include heroin, codeine, oxycodone, hydrocodone, hydromorphone, and oxymorphone.

Heroin

Heroin is derived from morphine, and its rapid onset of action and short half-life make it preferred over morphine among people who engage in unhealthy opioid use. Heroin is classified as a Schedule I drug (ie, not available for any therapeutic use in the United States), although a few countries (eg, Switzerland, the Netherlands, Spain, Germany, Canada, and the United Kingdom) use it as a medication for treatment of intravenous heroin use disorder. In these countries heroin is used only in patients who have not responded to methadone or buprenorphine maintenance treatment or residential rehabilitation.[2,3] A prodrug that is not itself active, heroin is rapidly deacetylated to 6-monoacetyl morphine (6-MAM) and morphine, both of which are active at the MOP-r. It is most effective intravenously but increasingly is used intranasally and smoked, which is possible with high-purity heroin, and reduces the risk of human immunodeficiency virus (HIV-1) transmission and overdose.[4]

Codeine

Codeine is methylmorphine and is one of the plant-derived products from the poppy plant, but its low concentration makes its production more efficient as a semisynthetic derivative of morphine. It crosses the blood-brain barrier faster and has less first-pass metabolism in the liver for greater oral bioavailability than morphine. It also is metabolized to morphine via cytochrome 2D6.

Oxycodone

Although oxycodone is structurally similar to codeine, it is pharmacodynamically comparable to morphine with 50% greater potency than morphine.[5] It is combined with aspirin or acetaminophen for treating moderate pain and is available orally without a co-analgesic for severe pain. By the mid-2000s, oxycodone had become one of the most widely nonmedically used and diverted opioids in the United States, particularly in the controlled-release (CR) formulation, since it could be easily crushed and self-administered (intranasally or IV) for a potentially toxic, rapid "high."[6,7] Subsequently, in 2010, the medication was reformulated and released in a tamper-resistant, unhealthy use-deterrent form characterized by reduced euphoria, nasal irritation with insufflation, and difficulty with extraction of the active compound.[8] Following reformulation, oxycodone nonmedical use dropped, but heroin use rose.

Hydromorphone

First synthesized in the 1920s, hydromorphone is a more potent opioid analgesic than morphine. It is used for the treatment of moderate to severe pain and is excreted, along with its metabolites, by the kidneys. It can be given intravenously, by infusion, orally, and per rectum, with low oral bioavailability. On a milligram basis, it is five times more potent than morphine when given orally and 8.5 times as potent when given intravenously.[9]

Hydrocodone

Hydrocodone is a prescription medication for relatively minor pain, such as oral/dental or osteoarthritis. Hydrocodone undergoes hepatic metabolism entirely by the *CYP2D6* system to its active metabolite, hydromorphone, which is then further converted by phase 2 glucuronidation. When used in combination with acetaminophen, there can be an increased risk of hepatotoxicity when used in unhealthy ways.

The amount of hydrocodone used in the United States dropped substantially since October 2014, when the Drug Enforcement Administration (DEA) rescheduled hydrocodone from Schedule III to Schedule II, in large part due to its high potential for unhealthy use. In the year following the change, hydrocodone prescriptions decreased by 22%, from approximately 120 to 93.5 million. These numbers have continued to steadily decline; as of 2018, only 5.5 million individuals in the United States were prescribed hydrocodone.[10]

Synthetic Agents

Thebaine and Synthetic Compounds

Thebaine is not used clinically or recreationally, but is a potent convulsant and the chemical basis for several semisynthetic and synthetic opioids. Modifications of thebaine result in semisynthetics as reviewed above including hydrocodone (Vicodin), oxycodone (OxyContin), hydromorphone (Dilaudid), and heroin. Synthetic modifications also include antagonists such as naloxone (Narcan), naltrexone (Trexan or ReVia or Vivitrol), and nalmefene (Revex), as well as partial agonists such as buprenorphine alone (Subutex) or, when combined with naloxone, (Suboxone, Zubsolv). Other unrelated synthetics include methadone, fentanyl and tramadol.

Meperidine

Meperidine is a phenylpiperidine with limited potency and a short duration of action. Clinically, meperidine is used primarily for the management of acute, postoperative pain in the central nervous system (CNS) and gastrointestinal and genitourinary systems, and prophylactic use of meperidine has been shown to reduce postoperative shivering, particularly for patients undergoing spinal anesthesia.[11] Meperidine is no longer used for treatment of chronic pain owing largely to concerns regarding toxicity of its major metabolite, normeperidine, which can produce seizures and CNS excitation, for example, disorientation, drowsiness, vertigo, or urinary retention. While meperidine is metabolized primarily by the liver, normeperidine is renally excreted, has a substantially longer half-life (15-30 hours), and carries a risk of accumulation in those with renal disease and the elderly.[12] Meperidine should not be used for more than 48 hours or at doses greater than 600 mg/d. Because it has serotonergic activity, it can produce a serotonin syndrome (ie, clonus, hyperreflexia, hyperthermia, and agitation) when combined with monoamine oxidase inhibitors.[13] Additionally, meperidine use has been associated with electrocardiogram (ECG) changes, such as QT_c prolongation, which can lead to torsade de pointes, a potentially fatal arrhythmia.[14]

Pentazocine

Pentazocine was first approved for use in the United States in 1967 for treatment of mild-to-moderate pain but is now rarely used. Pentazocine is a weak antagonist or partial agonist (ie, it has a "ceiling effect," plateau in maximal effect, contrasted with a full agonist) at the mu opioid receptor. It is also a kappa opioid receptor partial agonist and displays activity at the delta opioid receptor as well as the sigma receptor. Pentazocine shows differences in CNS effect and degree of analgesia depending on the medication dose. In addition, pentazocine has two enantiomers with different pharmacological profiles, and the prescribed formulation, (±)-pentazocine, provides pain reduction and is rewarding. In rats, (−)-pentazocine is rewarding through mu and delta opioid receptors, while

(+)-pentazocine is not rewarding through agonism of the selective sigma-1 receptor, which also underlies its hallucinogenic and psychotomimetic properties.[15] In 1983, as a deterrent to unhealthy use, pentazocine was manufactured in combination with naloxone (Talwin NX). Thus, if injected, this formulation would actually precipitate withdrawal in those with physiological dependence. After this change, unhealthy use of pentazocine in the United States declined. Currently, it is only available in tablet form in fixed combinations (50 mg) with either acetaminophen (Talacen and generics) or naloxone (Talwin Nx and generics).[16]

Methadone

Methadone is a synthetic, long-acting, full mu opioid agonist, active by parenteral and oral routes. It was first synthesized as a potential analgesic in Germany in the late 1930s and first studied for human use in the 1950s in the United States. It has been used primarily as a maintenance treatment for heroin use disorder since the first research done in 1964, and it was approved by the U.S. Food and Drug Administration (FDA) in 1972. Methadone is also effective in the treatment of chronic pain; however, it should be used with caution in opioid-naive patients due to the risk of accumulation and respiratory depression. Methadone has a diphenylheptylamine chemical structure and consists of a racemic mixture of D(*S*)- and L(*R*)-methadone.[17] The L(*R*)-methadone enantiomer has up to 50 times more analgesic activity and the potential to produce more respiratory depression than the D(*S*)-enantiomer. Both enantiomers have modest *N*-methyl-D-aspartate (NMDA) receptor antagonism, which is thought to be the underlying neurobiological mechanism for the limited development of tolerance observed with this medication.[18,19]

Levo-alpha-acetylmethadol

LAAM is a synthetic, longer-acting (48-hour) congener of methadone that is also orally administered. LAAM was first studied in the 1970s for the treatment of heroin use disorder and approved in 1993 by the FDA after a large multicenter safety trial. A black box warning was added to the product label due to postmarketing reports of prolonged QT_c interval on ECG that were associated with treatment with LAAM.[20] Although LAAM remains approved for human use in the United States, no pharmaceutical company is manufacturing the medication currently. As the new drug application for LAAM has not been withdrawn, LAAM could once again be made available in the United States.

Buprenorphine

Buprenorphine, alone and in combination with opioid antagonist, naloxone, was approved in 2002 by the FDA as an office-based treatment for heroin and opioid use disorder[21]; at the same time, buprenorphine was reclassified by the Drug Enforcement Administration from a Schedule V to a Schedule III drug. Buprenorphine is primarily a MOP-r–directed partial agonist, but also acts as a kappa partial agonist. The structure of buprenorphine is that of an oripavine with a C7 side chain, which contains a tert-butyl group. Norbuprenorphine is a major metabolite of buprenorphine in humans, with activity at the MOP-r as well.[22]

The SAMHSA DATA 2000 (Drug Addiction Treatment Act 2000) established eligibility requirements for physicians to use buprenorphine in the office-based treatment of opioid use disorders.[23] Although these requirements were loosened in 2016 by increasing the number of patients who could be prescribed buprenorphine for opioid use disorder under a waiver, and by expanding the variety of qualified practitioners who could prescribe it as such, by 2023 they were removed such that a DATA 2000 waiver is no longer required to prescribe buprenorphine for opioid use disorder if permitted by applicable state law.

The formulations of specific opioids are shown in **Table 13-1**.

Formulations to Deter Unhealthy Use

Formulations are being developed for many opioids to deter unhealthy use, as defined in section 1 of this textbook "Recommended Use of Terminology in Addiction Medicine." The addition of an opioid antagonist, such as naloxone or naltrexone, to the parent opioid compound is a common

TABLE 13-1 Formulations of Opioids and Their Routes of Administrations

Drug	Formulation	Routes of administration
Heroin	Powder Free base	IV, intranasal, smoked, SC
Morphine	Oral, injectable solution	Oral, SC, IV
Oxycodone	Tablet: can be With aspirin With acetaminophen (potentially hepatotoxic)	Oral, crushed and then snorted or injected IV, SC
Codeine	Tablet	
Pentazocine	Tablet Also combined with naloxone	Oral, SC, IV
Hydromorphone	Oral	Oral (low bioavailability), IV, PR
Hydrocodone	Tablet With acetaminophen	Oral
Methadone	Tablet, liquid	Oral, IV
LAAM	Tablet	Oral
Buprenorphine	Tablet With naloxone Film (SL)	SL, IV, SC

SC, subcutaneous; IV, intravenous; PR, per rectum; SL, sublingual.

pharmacological strategy, employed with medications including pentazocine/naloxone (Talwin NX) and buprenorphine/naloxone. Other formulations are designed with physical deterrents to intranasal or parenteral use and include adding capsaicin or a gelling polymer to make dissolved pills unpleasant to use due to nasal irritation or difficult to crush or dissolve due to structurally resistant, tamper-proof outside coatings.[24]

Clinical Uses

Clinically used opioids (ie, MOP-r agonists) are indicated primarily for treatment of acute and chronic pain conditions. For minor pain, such as postdental procedures, opioids such as hydrocodone are used. For moderate to severe, postsurgical, or chronic pain, opioids such as morphine may be prescribed. Neuropathic or regional pain syndromes can sometimes be relieved by opioids, though their prolonged use in these conditions remains an area of continued investigation. Opioids have been well established as cough suppressants; however, only codeine is typically used for this indication. Low-dose opioids, particularly buprenorphine, have been used as relatively rapidly acting antidepressants,[25] although they are not FDA-approved for this indication.

The opioid agonists methadone and buprenorphine are employed as treatment for opioid use disorder; either as withdrawal management to reduce withdrawal symptoms or as maintenance therapy (to reduce craving and re-establish physiological homeostasis). All opioid medications carry the risk for development of substance use disorder and diversion, and as a result, they must be dispensed cautiously. This caution, however, must be carefully balanced against the risk of undermedicating pain for each individual patient. Depot naltrexone (Vivitrol) was approved in 2010 as a monthly IM injection for prevention of recurrence of use following withdrawal management from opioid use disorder. An implantable version of buprenorphine, Probuphine, is also FDA approved as of 2016 as well as two other depot forms of buprenorphine, Sublocade and Brixadi, approved in 2017 and 2018 for monthly and weekly or monthly use, respectively.[26,27]

Nonmedical Use of Prescription Medications (NUPM)

Recreational or illicit use of opioids may initiate from a desire to experience the euphorigenic effects of these agents. There are also those who favor use of prescription medications because they are not associated with the societal stigma of heroin or the negative consequences of IV drug use. Additionally, some patients are prescribed opioids for pain treatment and go on to develop unhealthy opioid use. Heroin is not available for medical indications in the United States. Methadone and buprenorphine are sometimes diverted by those for whom it is prescribed, generally not for euphoria-inducing effects, but rather to prevent the onset of opioid withdrawal symptoms.[28]

The medical implications of unhealthy opioid use and diversion are quite significant. Family members and friends are the most common source of nonmedically used opioids; however, family members and friends most commonly receive those medications directly from physicians. Prescribing practices related to opioids are not the sole clinical concern. Benzodiazepines and opioid pain medications are commonly used in combination, and recent guidelines from the CDC clarify the dangers of concomitant use and caution against it, given the elevated risk of respiratory depression, coma, and death.

EPIDEMIOLOGY OF OPIOIDS AND USE DISORDER

After a steady increase in the overall national opioid dispensing rate starting in 2006, within a short 6-year span, the total number of prescriptions dispensed peaked in 2012 to an all-time high of more than 255 million; the equivalent of 81.3 prescriptions per 100 persons. Eight years later, in 2020, the dispensing rate had fallen almost 50% to 43.3 prescriptions per 100 persons, the equivalent of a total of 142 million prescriptions dispensed. This was the lowest recorded rate over the past 15 years. Despite this significant overall drop however, also in 2020, a small segment of U.S. counties (3.6%) had opioid dispensing rates that were nine times higher than that experienced across the United States; the equivalent of almost 400 prescriptions per 100 persons.[29] Such regional variation clearly indicates that we have not solved the over-supply of opioids, as shown in the 2020 National Survey on Drug Use and Health (NSDUH).[30]

The NSDUH 2020 report estimated that of the 9.5 million community-dwelling U.S. residents aged 12 and over who nonmedically used opioids in the past year, 8.6 million were people who nonmedically used prescription pain relievers (representing 90.5% of the total overall) and 902,000 people were people who used heroin (representing 9.5% of people who used opioids nonmedically overall.[30] An estimated 2.7 million persons (aged 12 or older) met putative *Diagnostic and Statistical Manual of Mental Disorders*, 5th edition (DSM-5) criteria for current (past-year) opioid use disorder, with 2.3 million having prescription pain reliever use disorder and 691,000 people having heroin use disorder. In 2020, an estimated 3.7% of persons aged 12 to 17 years old were currently using nonmedical opioid pain relievers. This estimate for adolescent use differs from adults, whose use has remained stable. This near-continuous decline over the last several years in adolescents is supported by other epidemiological studies, including Monitoring the Future, which found that use of "narcotics other than heroin" in 12th graders over the previous 12 months peaked at 8.5% of respondents in 2004, but had declined to a rate of 1.0% in 2020.[31,32]

Other epidemiological databases about opioid use include TEDS, DAWN, NFLIS, and NCHS. According to the Substance Abuse and Mental Health Services Administration (SAMHSA) Treatment Episode Data Set (TEDS), annual admissions to substance use disorder treatment for primary opioid use disorder increased from 2014 to 2017 in publicly funded U.S. treatment programs and has continued to remain high throughout the COVID-19 pandemic. Importantly, the ethnic and age distributions have altered substantially. Among White individuals, the mean number of admissions per 3-year groupings increased since 2000 and the age distribution remained centered around ages 21 to 34 years. Among Black individuals, however, admissions decreased from 2000 to 2014 and the age distribution shifted to older ages with a mean of 45 years[33]; a trend that has stabilized during the past 7 years. Starting in 2005, methadone maintenance treatment programs (MMTP) admitted individuals abusing oral prescription opioids like oxycodone and hydrocodone much more commonly than heroin, and since 2017 fentanyl has been displacing oxycodone as the most commonly nonmedically used opioid.[34] The Drug Abuse Warning Network (DAWN) is a nationwide public health surveillance system that captures data on emergency department (ED) visits related to recent drug use.[35] Opioids, at 14%, were the second most common drug class involved in drug-related ED visits in 2021, following alcohol at 39%. Fentanyl-related ED visits rose throughout 2021, peaking in the fourth quarter. Heroin-related ED visits rose from the first through the third quarter, and declined in the fourth quarter. Methamphetamine was the most common additional drug involved in heroin- and fentanyl-related polysubstance ED visits. National Forensic Laboratory Information System (NFLIS), a program of the Drug Enforcement Administration (DEA), finds fentanyl detection rates in submitted forensic samples growing more than 10-fold, while oxycodone rates have dropped more than 60%, from 2015 to 2020.[36] The National Center for Health Statistics (*NCHS*), a part of the Centers for Disease Control and Prevention (CDC), carefully tracks opioid overdose rates and estimated 100,306 drug overdose deaths in the United States during the 12-month period ending in April 2021, an increase of 28.5% from the 78,056 deaths during the same period the year before.[37]

Interesting racial/ethnic group differences occur in the nonmedical use of prescription opioids. For example, a study of 18- to 23-year-old emerging adults who used opioids nonmedically but did not meet DSM-IV-TR criteria for opioid dependence found an ethnic difference: a higher proportion of White adults than non-White adults used opioids for its euphoric effects by oral ingestion or by snorting, while non-White adults tended to use opioids to self-medicate health problems via oral ingestion.[38] These findings were confirmed by a separate study in college students, where researchers found recreational use was more prevalent among white people who use opioids, while self-treatment of pain was more prevalent among African Americans. Recent studies examining racial bias in pain assessment and treatment further suggest that the undermedication of pain among certain groups is related to false beliefs and misperceptions about physiological differences between whites and people of color regarding pain tolerance.[39] Altogether, these factors may contribute to the differing manifestations of nonmedical use of prescription opioids among diverse populations and represents an important area of future study, particularly as it is related to potential opportunities for targeted intervention.

Additionally, opioid-related overdoses have become an area of significant concern, particularly since fentanyl and now counterfeit stimulants that look like Adderall (mixed amphetamine salts) but contain fentanyl have flooded the illicit market and may contribute significantly to toxicity. According to the National Center for Health Statistics, the number of deaths involving fentanyl increased from 730 deaths in 1999 to 107,000 deaths in 2021.[40] The "fourth phase" of the lethal opioid epidemic, which started with prescription opioids such as oxycodone in late 1990, involves the combination of stimulants (cocaine and methamphetamine) with fentanyl with a steep rise in this combination starting in 2016 and particularly impacting Black communities.[41] Of note, benzodiazepines continue to contribute to lethal overdoses since their peak involvement in 31% of opioid analgesic deaths in 2011.[42]

Although concerns regarding access to treatment persist, some improvement is evident. According to August 2022 SAMHSA data (before the Drug Addiction Treatment Act 2000 restrictions were changed), there were approximately 130,671 U.S. prescribers eligible to prescribe buprenorphine as office-based treatment to patients for treatment of opioid use disorder. Most prescribers (92,563) are certified to treat up to 30 patients, 28,970 are certified to treat up to 100 patients, and 9,138 can treat up to 250 patients.[43]

Neurobiology, Mechanisms of Action, Genetics and Relationship to Addiction liability

Three types of opioid receptors are found in the nervous system: mu, kappa, and delta. These opioid receptors are G-protein–coupled, 7-transmembrane receptors. The endogenous opioid neuropeptide agonists include the endorphins, enkephalins, and dynorphins as well as the more recently characterized endomorphins.[44] The endorphins are cleavage products of the protein, pro-opiomelanocortin (POMC), which is produced primarily in the anterior pituitary of humans by the *POMC* gene. The major endorphin agonist produced from POMC is beta-endorphin, while the shorter products, alpha-endorphin and gamma-endorphin, are less biologically active peptides. Beta-endorphin stimulates mu opioid receptors (MOP-r) in mediating both the analgesic and rewarding effects of opioids. The enkephalins and dynorphins are opioid peptides with affinity for MOP-r as well, but enkephalins are primarily active at delta opioid receptors, while dynorphins exert their activity primarily through kappa opioid receptors. The endomorphins, endomorphin-1 and endomorphin-2, are opioid tetrapeptides with high affinity and selectivity for MOP-r. Although the parent gene and precursor protein of the endomorphins are still yet to be characterized, these agents may represent an important advance in development of opioid medications due to their potent antinociception and reduced adverse effects in rodent models.[45]

Opioids have primarily agonist effects at the MOP-r (encoded by the MOP-r gene [*OPRM1*]). MOP-r are members of the G-protein–coupled 7-transmembrane domain superfamily; they are coupled to G_i and G_o proteins. Thus, MOP-r agonists typically acutely result in the downstream inhibition of adenylyl cyclase with a consequent reduction in the production of cyclic AMP (cAMP), the opening of potassium channels, the inhibition of calcium channels, and the activation of mitogen-activated protein kinase (MAPK).[46]

Distribution in CNS and Mediation of Different Functions

MOP-r are widely distributed in both the CNS and peripheral nervous system (PNS), with the constellation of their psychological and analgesic effects being mediated primarily in the CNS.[47] Therapeutically desirable analgesic effects can be mediated in areas including dorsal spinal cord and thalamus, whereas undesirable effects are thought to be mediated elsewhere. Respiratory depression, for example, is thought to be mediated primarily by activity in the brain stem,[48] while gastrointestinal effects, such as constipation (experienced by as many as 40% of those prescribed opioids), are thought to be mediated through CNS activity as well as activation of MOP-r in the gastrointestinal tract: submucosa, ileal mucosa, stomach, and proximal colon.[49] The classic rewarding effects of MOP-r agonists are likely mediated to a substantial degree in ventral and dorsal striatal areas and can depend (although not exclusively) on downstream activation of the dopaminergic mesocorticolimbic and nigrostriatal systems. Symptoms of physiological dependence and withdrawal from MOP-r agonists, such as autonomic instability (eg, blood pressure and heart rate elevation), diaphoresis, and anxiety, are thought to stem from increased noradrenergic activity within the locus coeruleus and related centers.[50,51]

Genetics of Opioid Effects Including Opioid Use Disorder

Understanding the genetics of MOP-r function remains in an early stage. There are five single nucleotide polymorphisms (SNPs) in the coding region of the human *OPRM1* gene.[52] Three of these 5 SNPs lead to amino acid changes, and one (the A118G and the C17T variants) has a high allelic frequency of more than 40% in some ethnic groups. The C17T variant may have some association with opioid use disorder and contribute to inter-subject variability in response to opioid ligands or especially the opioid antagonists.[53]

MOP-r Signaling Properties and Addiction Liability

A major underlying concept in the addiction liability of MOP-r agonists is their pharmacodynamic efficacy (ie, their relative ability to stimulate downstream second messenger systems). In general, compounds with progressively greater efficacy (eg, morphine or fentanyl-like compounds) have greater analgesic effects but also have greater potential for unhealthy use, including addiction, than partial agonists such as buprenorphine. Furthermore, other downstream effects of MOP-r agonist exposure are now postulated to be of relevance to the relative balance of therapeutic and undesirable effects of MOP-r agonists, including propensity to cause tolerance or potential for unhealthy use. Major mechanisms of current interest are the relative propensity of compounds to cause MOP-r desensitization and internalization, potentially related to their ability to stimulate the β-arrestin signaling pathways.[54,55] For example, the main active heroin metabolite, morphine, results in lesser desensitization and internalization of receptors, compared to the endogenous neuropeptide ligands or methadone.[56] Thus, methadone maintenance can be used effectively for extended periods without the development of further tolerance (or progressively greater methadone dose requirements). By contrast, heroin (through its primary metabolite, morphine), or prescription opioids, may result in progressive cycles of physical dependence and tolerance, secondary to a lesser recruitment of endogenous MOP-r desensitization/internalization mechanisms.[57]

PHARMACOKINETICS OF SPECIFIC DRUGS

It is beyond the scope of this chapter to provide a comprehensive table of dosing equivalents and the procedures for conversion from one opioid to another. There are a number of excellent web-based applications for this purpose. One such example is located at: https://www.oregonpainguidance.org/opioidmedcalculator/.

Morphine Pharmacokinetics

Morphine is largely selective for MOP-r and most physicians consider it the drug of choice for the treatment of moderate to severe cancer pain.[58] The pharmacokinetics of morphine and its metabolites vary, depending on the route of administration. Its favorable safety profile is due in large part to its pharmacokinetic profile. The oral bioavailability varies, from 35% to 75%, with a plasma half-life ranging from 2 to 3.5 hours. The half-life is less than the time course of analgesia, which is 4 to 6 hours, thus reducing accumulation.

Morphine is biotransformed mainly by hepatic glucuronidation to the major but inactive metabolite morphine-3-glucuronide (M3G) and the biologically active M6G compound,[59] with prolonged clearance because of enterohepatic cycling with oral dosing. In the setting of chronic liver disease, morphine oxidation is more affected than is glucuronidation. Use of lower doses or longer dosing intervals is recommended to minimize the risk of accumulation of morphine when chronic liver disease is present, particularly with repeated dosing. At 24 hours, more than 90% of morphine has been excreted in urine. M6G elimination seems to be closely tied to renal function, so accumulation of metabolites can occur. With renal compromise, less than 10% of morphine and its metabolites are excreted in feces; therefore, morphine should be used with great caution in patients with renal disease.[60,61]

Codeine Pharmacokinetics

Codeine has a high oral-parenteral effect, owing to low first-pass metabolism in the liver. Metabolites are mostly inactive and excreted in the urine, with about 10% demethylated via CYP2D6 to morphine, which may be primarily responsible for the analgesic effect of codeine, as codeine itself has very low affinity for opioid receptors. Codeine (~ 80%) is mostly conjugated with glucuronic acid to form codeine-6-glucuronide, which is also believed to contribute somewhat to the analgesic properties of the medication.[62] Genetic variations in 2D6 impact the effects of codeine, with poor metabolizers experiencing less analgesia due to reduced conversion to morphine and potentially reduced addiction liability, while ultrarapid metabolizers (ie, those carrying a CYP2D6 gene duplication) may have increased side effects, such as sedation.[63] The allelic variants have different frequency in different ethnic groups and can affect the depth of analgesia. Repeated doses of codeine may result in the accumulation of the active metabolite M6G in patients with renal disease.

Heroin (Diacetylmorphine) Pharmacokinetics

Heroin is an efficient prodrug with greater water solubility and potency than morphine.[64] It is synthesized from morphine by acetylation at both the 3 and 6 positions and metabolized in humans to active opioid compounds first by deacetylation to the active 6-monoacetylmorphine (6-MAM, also known as 6-acetylmorphine [6-AM]) and then by further deacetylation to morphine. Well-designed studies of heroin pharmacokinetics in humans have shown that it has an average half-life in blood of 3 minutes after intravenous administration; the half-life of 6-AM in humans appears to be 30 minutes.

The use of intranasal, intramuscular, and subcutaneous heroin produces peak blood levels of heroin or 6-AM within 5 minutes; however, intranasal use has about half the relative potency of parenteral routes. Most of the enzymes involved in the metabolism of opioids are part of the P450 microsomal enzyme system, though heroin and morphine are also biotransformed outside this system.

Oxycodone Pharmacokinetics

The onset of action of oxycodone begins 1 hour following oral administration. Although the immediate-release (IR) formulation of oxycodone has a plasma half-life of 3 to 4 hours, the controlled-release (CR) formulation lasts for approximately 12 hours. Stable plasma levels are achieved within 24 hours. Oral bioavailability ranges from 60% to 87%, with 45% protein bound. Oxycodone is mostly metabolized in the liver, with the remainder as well as the metabolites metabolized in the kidneys. The two main metabolites are oxymorphone, which is also a potent analgesic, and the weaker analgesic noroxycodone, which is its major metabolite.[65] Its protein binding and lipophilicity is like morphine, but it has a slightly longer half-life and greater bioavailability. The cytochrome enzyme CYP2D6 mostly metabolizes oxycodone, while morphine in humans is primarily glucuronidated.[66]

Meperidine Pharmacokinetics

Onset of analgesia begins with the oral route after 15 minutes, with peak in 1 to 2 hours, which is close to peak level in plasma, with duration of about 1.5 to 3 hours. It is absorbed by all routes, but intramuscular administration results in a less reliable peak plasma level after 45 minutes, with wide range of plasma concentrations. After oral administration, about 50% of meperidine enters circulation without first-pass metabolism, with peak at 1 to 2 hours. Meperidine is mostly metabolized in the liver, with half-life of about 3 hours. Cirrhosis leads to increased bioavailability and half-life of both meperidine and normeperidine. Sixty percent of meperidine is protein bound and little is excreted unmetabolized.[13]

Pentazocine Pharmacokinetics

Pentazocine is a mixed agonist–antagonist with intermediate activity at both MOP-r and KOP-r (kappa opioid receptors) that can be given intramuscularly or orally, but it is not currently available in the oral formulation. It can cause psychotomimetic effects (likely due to its KOP-r actions) and therefore has a very limited role in the treatment of chronic pain. Its peak effect is at 0.5 to 1 hour when given intramuscularly and 1 to 2 hours when given orally, and the overall duration of action is 3 to 6 hours. The drug half-life is 2 to 3 hours. Sixty percent of the drug is bound to protein. Pentazocine is metabolized by the liver via oxidative and glucuronide conjugation with an extensive first-pass effect. When administered orally, the bioavailability of pentazocine is about 10%, except in patients with cirrhosis, which increases bioavailability to 60% to 70%. Small amounts of unchanged pentazocine are excreted with urine. It is also a sigma-1 receptor antagonist that blocks the toxic effects of glutamate in the brain.[67]

Hydromorphone Pharmacokinetics

Hydromorphone is shorter acting than morphine. It is derived from morphine, although it may also be produced in the body in small amounts by N-demethylation of hydrocodone. It has an oral bioavailability of 30% to 40%, with an analgesic onset after 10 to 20 minutes, which peaks at about 30 to 60 minutes and persists for about 3 to 5 hours. The oral–parenteral ratio is about 5:1, with an equivalency of 1.5 mg of hydrocodone to 10 mg morphine.[68]

Hydrocodone Pharmacokinetics

The pharmacokinetics of hydrocodone depends on formulation since there are commercially available immediate-release (IR) and extended-release (ER) compounds available. Of note, hydrocodone ER has been reformulated with unhealthy use-deterrent technology, which limits the release of the active ingredient in cases of unhealthy use (ie, crushing, snorting) or in combination with alcohol.[69] Hydrocodone IR has a peak effect at 0.5 to 1 hour and duration of action of 3 to 4 hours. The half-life of hydrocodone IR is approximately 3 hours (range: 2-4 hours).[70] Hydrocodone ER has a peak plasma level at roughly 14 hours (range: 6-30 hours) and analgesic duration of action of approximately 12 hours, allowing for twice-daily dosing. The half-life of hydrocodone ER, in comparison, is 6 hours. Hydrocodone is converted by cytochrome P450 2D6 to its active metabolite, hydromorphone, and via cytochrome 3A4 to inactive metabolite, norhydrocodone. Codeine may show up as trace quantities of hydrocodone in urine testing as up to 11% of codeine is metabolized to hydrocodone, which could be misinterpreted as unhealthy hydrocodone use.

Methadone Pharmacokinetics

Methadone, as used in the United States, is a racemic compound; the L(*R*)-enantiomer is the active component, while the other D(*S*)-enantiomer is inactive. Both enantiomers are weak NMDA receptor antagonists; racemic methadone retards and attenuates the development of opioid tolerance.[71] Methadone meets two important criteria for a medication used in the treatment of an opioid use disorder: high systemic bioavailability (>90%) with oral administration and long apparent half-life with long-term administration in humans.

Oral methadone has a rapid absorption but delayed onset of action, with peak plasma levels achieved by 2 to 4 hours and sustained over a 24-hour dosing period.[72] Moreover, the mean plasma apparent terminal half-life of racemic D,L-methadone in human subjects is around 24 hours. The L-enantiomer has a half-life of 36 hours.[71] Biotransformation of methadone is accelerated in the third trimester; therefore, methadone dose may need to be increased in the final stages of pregnancy.

When taken on a chronic basis, methadone is stored and accumulated mostly in the liver. Methadone plasma levels are relatively constant because of the slow release of unmetabolized methadone into the blood, which extends the apparent terminal half-life. Methadone is more than 90% plasma protein bound both to albumin and globulins. These properties help explain why methadone maintenance treatment is effective as a once-daily, orally administered pharmacotherapy for opioid use disorder. Methadone is biotransformed in the liver by the cytochrome P450–related enzymes (primarily by the CYP3A4 and, to a lesser extent, the CYP2B6, CYP2D6, and CYP1A2 systems) to two N-demethylated biologically inactive metabolites, which undergo additional oxidative metabolism.[72] Methadone and its metabolites are excreted in nearly equal amounts in urine and in feces. In patients with renal disease, methadone can be cleared almost entirely by the GI tract, reducing potential toxicity by preventing accumulation. Methadone disposition is relatively normal in patients with mild to moderate liver impairment.[73] Patients with severe long-standing liver disease have decreased methadone metabolism and thus slower metabolic clearance of methadone, yet lower than expected plasma methadone levels due to lower hepatic reservoirs of methadone because of reduced liver size. Interestingly, due to genetic differences, select patients may require higher doses of methadone due to "rapid metabolism" of the medication.

Levo-Alpha-Acetylmethadol Pharmacokinetics

LAAM, a congener of methadone, shares with methadone the properties of long duration of effect (48 versus 24 hours for methadone, in part owing to its active metabolites norLAAM and dinorLAAM, as well as its steady-state perfusion of MOP-rs), oral effectiveness, and function as a pure opioid agonist, active mostly at the MOP-r.[74] NorLAAM and dinorLAAM accumulate with chronic administration. In addition, LAAM and its metabolites bind to tissue proteins.

The clearance of norLAAM and LAAM is similar, whereas the clearance of dinorLAAM is more prolonged than that of its parent compound. The peak pharmacological effect of LAAM as measured by amount of pupillary constriction occurred at 8 hours and then diminished at a rate like that of norLAAM metabolism.

Because of the metabolism of LAAM by the cytochrome P450 3A4 system-related microsomal enzymes to norLAAM and dinorLAAM, drug interactions can occur (eg, rifampin and long-term unhealthy alcohol use tend to induce this enzyme system). In their presence, increased biotransformation of LAAM could accelerate the production of norLAAM and dinorLAAM. LAAM metabolism theoretically could be retarded if hepatic drug metabolism is diminished, as occurs in the presence of very large quantities of either ethanol, perhaps with large doses of benzodiazepines, or with intake of cimetidine.

Buprenorphine Pharmacokinetics

Buprenorphine undergoes extensive first pass metabolism in the liver; thus, it is administered sublingually with 50% to 60% bioavailability. Buprenorphine is metabolized to norbuprenorphine through dealkylation in the cytochrome P450–related enzyme 3A4 system, of which buprenorphine itself is a weak inhibitor. Buprenorphine has a long duration of action (24-48 hours) when administered on a chronic basis, not because of its pharmacokinetic profile, but because of its very slow dissociation from MOP-r. Given intravenously, buprenorphine has an apparent beta-terminal plasma half-life of about 3 to 5 hours. When given orally, it is relatively ineffective because of its first-pass metabolism, that is, rapid biotransformation, probably by the intestinal mucosa and, especially, by the liver.

Sublingual preparations of buprenorphine can be film or tablet, both of which require about 120 minutes for time to peak. However, peak plasma concentrations of the sublingual tablet and film and mean area under the plasma concentration time curve are lower than that of the liquid at equivalent doses.[75-79]

PHARMACODYNAMICS

The pharmacodynamics of the clinically important MOP-r agonists are wide ranging, with the most pronounced effects produced in the CNS and GI tract.

The mechanism of action for all of the clinically relevant opioids described here is at the MOP-r, in which they act preferentially as agonists, except for pentazocine and buprenorphine, which are partial mu opioid agonists and low efficacy ligands (antagonists) at kappa receptors.[80] The euphorigenic effects of any opioid agonists are mediated in part by the ventral tegmentum, where opioid agonist–mediated inhibition of GABAergic neurons results in disinhibition and thus activation of dopamine neurons extending to the nucleus accumbens.

Opioids in general affect heat regulation mechanisms in the hypothalamus. Body temperature decreases slightly, except with chronic high doses where temperature may be increased. Opioids also act in the hypothalamus to inhibit the release of gonadotropin-releasing hormone (GNRH) and corticotropin-releasing hormone (CRH), producing a reduction in luteinizing hormone (LH), follicle-stimulating hormone (FSH), adrenocorticotropin hormone (ACTH), and beta-endorphin.[81] With decrease in these hormones, plasma concentrations of testosterone and cortisol are lowered. Mu agonists increase the amount of prolactin in plasma by decreasing dopaminergic inhibition. Given chronically, there is tolerance to the effects of morphine on the neuroendocrine system. Mu opioid agonists also tend to have antidiuretic effects[81] and can cause constriction of the pupil. Additionally, opioids can cause seizures at doses much higher than those used clinically, and these overdoses can be managed with opioid antagonist medications, such as naloxone. Of note, naloxone is less potent in antagonizing seizures due to meperidine in comparison to other opioids such as morphine or methadone, likely due to its proconvulsant metabolite, normeperidine. Because of the increased risk of seizure with long-term use of meperidine, it is no longer used for chronic pain; when used for treatment of acute pain, meperidine should not be used for greater than 48 hours or at doses greater than 600 mg/d.

All opioids must be used cautiously in patients with impaired respiratory function. Opioids have the potential to elevate intracranial pressure (eg, in the setting of head injury, they can produce an exaggerated respiratory depression, as well as mental status changes that can confuse the clinical picture). Typical side effects of all opioids include drowsiness, nausea, and constipation, while vomiting, pruritus, and dizziness are less common; all of these lessen in intensity over time.

Codeine is commonly used to suppress cough at doses lower than those used for analgesia (starting with 10-20 mg given orally); higher doses are used for chronic (lower airway) cough. Codeine reduces cough via a central mechanism by stimulation of MOP-r on different neurons than those involved in analgesia or addiction, with doses greater than 65 mg not indicated, owing to little increased therapeutic effect but increasing side effects.

Pentazocine, as a mixed agonist-antagonist, has a "ceiling effect," like buprenorphine, which limits the degree of analgesia. Pentazocine can produce psychotomimetic side effects, not reversible with naloxone, suggesting these may not be mediated through MOP-r. Pentazocine also has affinity for kappa opioid receptors. Pentazocine can precipitate withdrawal in opioid-tolerant patients currently taking opioids, due to its weak antagonist effects.

Methadone, like all MOP-r agonists, affects multiple organ systems, with tolerance developing at different rates to each effect. In the treatment of either opioid use disorder or chronic pain, proper dosing (titrated to the tolerance of the individual patient) is essential to avoid CNS depression. The precise neuronal and molecular mechanisms of physical tolerance have not been fully elucidated. Studies of the D(R)-enantiomer of methadone (which is relatively inactive at the MOP-r) show that this isomer has modest NMDA antagonist activity, which attenuates the development of morphine tolerance in rodents, but does not affect physical dependence.[16]

Buprenorphine's pharmacodynamics include two important properties: (1) its apparent lower severity of withdrawal signs and symptoms on cessation, compared with heroin and other opioids, and (2) its reduced potential to produce lethal overdose when used alone in opioid-naive or nontolerant persons, because of its partial agonist properties. Acute buprenorphine intoxication with buprenorphine alone is associated with mild mental status changes, mild to minimal respiratory effects, small but not pinpoint pupils, and essentially stable vital signs. In some situations, naloxone apparently can improve the respiratory depression but with limited effect on the other symptoms. Nevertheless, patients should be observed for 24 to 48 hours after an episode of intoxication. While generally safe when used alone, deaths have occurred when buprenorphine is combined with large doses of benzodiazepines.[75] There also have been many reports of the intravenous use of the sublingual preparation of buprenorphine in many countries, which is the main reason that naloxone is added for deterrence against unhealthy use. A second formulation of sublingual buprenorphine (combined with naloxone) was developed in 1984 and is now increasingly used in the United States and worldwide. In this formulation, naloxone will not precipitate withdrawal when taken sublingually because of its limited oral bioavailability; however, it may block the initial euphoric effects of buprenorphine if used by the intravenous route and can also precipitate acute opioid withdrawal.[76]

Initially developed as an analgesic, buprenorphine is as effective as morphine in many situations. In addition to its activity in the MOP-r system, buprenorphine has kappa opioid receptor (KOP-r) antagonist activity. Owing to its ceiling effect, increasing buprenorphine doses in humans beyond 32 mg sublingually using the film version has no greater MOP-r agonist effect and at 16 mg appears to occupy all the available mu opiate receptors.[80]

Chronic administration of opioids can lead to the gradual development of tolerance to the effects on hypothalamic-releasing factors, with return to normal levels and activity of anterior pituitary-derived ACTH and beta-endorphin and normal ACTH stimulation in approximately 3 months and resumption of normal menses and return of plasma levels of testosterone to normal within 1 year.[81] In humans, prolactin release is under tonic inhibition by tuberoinfundibular dopaminergic tone. With the use of short-acting opioids, there is a prompt increase in the release of prolactin resulting from abrupt lowering of dopamine levels in the tuberoinfundibular dopaminergic system. With heroin use, thyroid levels may be elevated because of raised thyroid-binding globulin, while function remains normal. The hypothalamic and pituitary effects of opioids can produce antidiuretic effects by the release of vasopressin.

Short-acting opioids can cause many effects in the cardiovascular system, including peripheral vasodilatation, decreased peripheral resistance, reduced baroreceptor reflexes, histamine release, and decreased reflex vasoconstriction caused by raised PCO_2. In the stomach, hydrochloric acid secretion may be inhibited, and somatostatin release from the pancreas may be elevated. Acetylcholine release from the GI tract is inhibited, resulting in slowed motility and reductions in the absorption of many drugs. The presence of increased appetite has also been noted. Biliary, pancreatic, and intestinal secretions may be reduced and digestion in the small intestine slowed. In the large intestine, there is reduced propulsion and higher tone. Tolerance to each of these effects develops with chronic administration.

TOLERANCE DEVELOPMENT

Tolerance is a reduced effect after repeated use, leading to the need for higher doses to get the equivalent effect.[82] All opioid medications lead to tolerance and physical dependence, but rates of development vary by medication, different effects, and individuals. Development of tolerance to opioids does not involve changes in drug disposition and metabolism (ie, pharmacokinetic), but changes at the cellular and neuronal system levels. Methadone has modest NMDA antagonism that may attenuate tolerance.[18] The GI and neuroendocrine side effects of short-acting opioids tend not to develop tolerance.

TOXICITY STATES AND THEIR MEDICAL MANAGEMENT

Acute opioid overdose is characterized by the triad of altered mental status (ie, stupor, coma), respiratory depression, and "pinpoint" pupils, and is extensively covered in later chapters. Mydriasis or normal pupils may be observed in patients with an overdose of meperidine, propoxyphene, dextromethorphan, pentazocine, and diphenoxylate with atropine (ie, Lomotil). A full opioid overdose can be effectively treated with an opioid antagonist. However, repeated naloxone administration is usually needed, or the overdose may be only transiently reversed, and the patient may lapse back into coma. Importantly for the current fentanyl overdose epidemic, larger doses of naloxone may be needed for reversal of overdoses with fentanyl and its derivatives compared to other opioids.[83] This larger dose may be the result of the much greater potency of fentanyl compared to other opioids and the direct activation of beta-arrestin rather than the cyclic AMP system when fentanyl binds to the mu opioid receptor.[84] Another option under development for fentanyl overdose is nalmefene, which is a longer acting and more potent opioid antagonist than naloxone.[85]

Medical Complications of Opioids

The two main effects of opioid overdose on the CNS are depression of the mental status and depression of respiratory activity. A suppressed gag reflex predisposes the patient to aspiration of gastric contents into the lungs. A few opioids may cause generalized seizures (eg, high-dose meperidine). Respiratory depression is the most frequent cause of death.

Chronic opioid use has complications that can be milder versions of these overdose effects, as well as three serious risks.[86] The first risk is prolongation of QT_c interval and torsades de pointes. Because a QT_c interval greater than 500 ms is a risk factor for sudden death, this needs to be monitored during methadone maintenance.[87,88] Second, opioid-induced spasm of the sphincter of Oddi can produce biliary colic and lead to unnecessary gall bladder surgery. Third, chronic constipation needs to be prevented; if left unaddressed, it can produce a toxic megacolon, which, if burst, will result in sepsis and possible death.

Patients with chronic opioid use show atypical responses to stress and stressors, as demonstrated by changes in HPA axis function. During cycles of physical dependence, abstinence, and recurrence of use, there is a flattened circadian rhythm of glucocorticoid levels, with increased levels during opioid withdrawal. Other hormonal systems altered by chronic opioid use include elevated prolactin and suppression of luteinizing and follicle stimulating hormones and testosterone.

Besides these direct effects of opioids, intravenous opioid use can lead to bacterial endocarditis; venous thrombosis; septic pulmonary emboli; emboli of cornstarch and talc (additives) to the retina, lungs, kidney, and liver; pseudoaneurysms; and mycotic aneurysms. Heroin, morphine, and pentazocine may cause rhabdomyolysis and nephropathy when used intravenously, leading to glomerulonephritis. Centrally mediated muscle rigidity of the chest and abdominal wall can occur, and intravenously used opioids may also cause osteomyelitis, septic arthritis, polymyositis, and fibrous myopathy. Injection routes (intravenous, subcutaneous) of opioids can transmit HIV-1 infection, hepatitis B, hepatitis C, and bacteria causing cellulitis, skin and neck abscesses, endocarditis, and botulism.

DRUG-DRUG INTERACTIONS

Other drugs can interact with opioids because of their additive pharmacodynamic effects, as well as pharmacokinetically via their hepatic enzyme effects on the cytochrome P450–related enzyme system. The pharmacodynamic interactions occur primarily with other brain depressants such as alcohol, sedatives including benzodiazepines (see buprenorphine interaction above) and therapeutic agents at normal doses that induce sedation and respiratory suppression. The pharmacokinetic drug-drug interactions with opioids based on hepatic enzyme variations are complex and must be considered on a case-by-case basis in individual patients. The major categories of drugs potentially interacting with opioids include both inducers and inhibitors of CYP3A4, as well as inhibitors of CYP2D6, such as paroxetine. CYP3A4 inducers typically have minimal clinical effects but include rifampin, rifabutin, carbamazepine, phenytoin, and phenobarbital; given the ability of these medications to increase the rate of metabolism of opioids, there is a chance that use of these medications in combination with opioids may induce withdrawal symptoms. CYP3A4 inhibitors, which include fluconazole, fluvoxamine, fluoxetine, paroxetine, and possibly erythromycin and ketoconazole, have shown few clinically significant drug interactions. A number of studies have examined specific antiretroviral medications used in the treatment of HIV-1 and their interaction with methadone. The reported pharmacokinetic interactions, usually through the CYP3A4 system, affect either methadone or the antiretroviral medication, which sometimes have clinical manifestations.[89,90] Finally, methadone levels are significantly increased by the regular consumption of more than four alcoholic drinks per day.

CONCLUSIONS AND FUTURE RESEARCH DIRECTIONS

The most pressing opioid-related clinical issue over the past 15 years has been the expanding opioid overdose epidemic, which has moved into a fourth phase of evolution. While the initial phase involved opioid over-prescription, particularly of extended-release oxycodone, the subsequent phases involved heroin, then illicit fentanyl-related drugs, and now stimulants in combination with fentanyl derivatives. Because fentanyl has a different binding site on the MOP-r than other opioids and naloxone, and very high potency, the usual naloxone doses are insufficient for reversal of overdoses. Higher naloxone doses can be effective, but new agents are needed. Nalmefene, an opioid antagonist medication similar in structure and activity to naltrexone, is a leading candidate due to its higher potency and longer duration of action than naloxone.

The most pressing opioid basic science issue is the neuronal and molecular basis of opioid tolerance and physical dependence, which appears to differ for different effects (eg, analgesia versus respiratory depression versus mediation of reward). Two specific areas for investigation are the genetics of MOP-r function and relating stress responsivity to opioid function with the partial agonists such as buprenorphine and the synthetic fentanyl related agonists. The effects of MOP-r partial agonists such as buprenorphine on specific indices of neuroendocrine function have not been extensively studied and warrant attention based on the persistent changes observed with chronic full opioid agonists. Overall, the molecular mechanisms for partial opioid agonism, with low doses producing agonist and high doses producing antagonist responses, would benefit from a comprehensive theory as well as data to support that theory, as new opioids are developed. These contributions may also significantly improve our therapeutic options for analgesia and treatment of addiction.

REFERENCES

1. Courtwright DT. *Dark Paradise: A History of Opiate Addiction in America*. Harvard University Press; 2001.
2. Blanken P, Hendriks VM, van Ree JM, et al. Outcome of long-term heroin-assisted treatment offered to chronic, treatment-resistant heroin addicts in The Netherlands. *Addiction*. 2010;105:300-308.
3. Strang J, Groshkova T, Uchtenhagen A, et al. Heroin on trial: Systematic review and meta-analysis of randomised trials of diamorphine-prescribing as treatment for refractory heroin addiction. *Br J Psychiatry*. 2015;207(1):5-14.
4. Stöver HJ, Schäffer D. SMOKE IT! Promoting a change of opiate consumption pattern—from injecting to inhaling. *Harm Reduct J*. 2014;11:18.
5. Ordonez Gallego A, Gonzalez Baron M, Espinosa AE. Oxycodone: A pharmacological and clinical review. *Clin Transl Oncol*. 2007;9:298-307.
6. Comer S, Ashworth J. The growth of prescription opioid abuse. In: Smith H, Passik S, eds. *Pain and Chemical Dependence*. Oxford University Press; 2008:19-23.
7. Van Zee A. Promotion and marketing of OxyContin: Commercial triumph, public health tragedy. *Am J Public Health*. 2009;99(2):221-227.
8. Perrino PJ, Colucci SV, Apseloff G, Harris SC. Pharmacokinetics, tolerability, and safety of intranasal administration of reformulated OxyContin® tablets compared with original OxyContin® tablets in healthy adults. *Clin Drug Investig*. 2013;33:441-449.
9. Sarhill N, Walsh D, Nelson KA. Hydromorphone: pharmacology and clinical applications in cancer patients. *Support Care Cancer*. 2001;9:84-96.
10. Drug Enforcement Agency (DEA). *Hydrocodone, 2019*. Accessed September 9, 2022. https://www.deadiversion.usdoj.gov/drug_chem_info/hydrocodone.pdf
11. Sohlpour A, Jafari A, Hashemi M, et al. A comparison of prophylactic use of meperidine, meperidine plus dexamethasone, and ketamine plus midazolam for preventing of shivering during spinal anesthesia: A randomized, double-blind, placebo-controlled study. *J Clin Anesth*. 2016;34:128-135.
12. Friesen KJ, Falk J, Bugden S. The safety of meperidine prescribing in older adults: A longitudinal population-based study. *BMC Geriatr*. 2016;16:100.
13. Latta KS, Ginsberg B, Barkin RL. Meperidine: A critical review. *Am J Ther*. 2002;9:53-68.
14. Keller GA et al. Meperidine-induced QTc-interval prolongation: Prevalence, risk factors, and correlation to plasma drug and metabolite concentrations. *Int J Clin Pharmacol Ther*. 2017;55(3):275-285.

15. Mori T, Itoh T, Yoshizawa K, et al. Involvement of μ- and δ-opioid receptor function in the rewarding effect of (±)-pentazocine. *Addict Biol.* 2015;20:724-732.
16. *LiverTox: Clinical and Research Information on Drug-Induced Liver Injury* [Internet]. National Institute of Diabetes and Digestive and Kidney Diseases; 2012. Pentazocine. [Updated 2020 Nov 24]. Accessed August 11, 2022. https://www.ncbi.nlm.nih.gov/books/NBK548498/
17. Ferrari A, Coccia CP, Bertolini A, et al. Methadone—metabolism, pharmacokinetics and interactions. *Pharmacol Res.* 2004;50:551-559.
18. Davis AM, Inturrisi CE. D-Methadone blocks morphine tolerance and N-methyl-D-aspartate-induced hyperalgesia. *J Pharmacol Exp Ther.* 1999;289:1048-1053.
19. Mendez IA, Trujillo KA. NMDA receptor antagonists inhibit opiate antinociceptive tolerance and locomotor sensitization in rats. *Psychopharmacology (Berl).* 2008;196:497-509.
20. Kang J, Chen XL, Wang H, et al. Interactions of the narcotic L-alpha-acetylmethadol with human cardiac K+ channels. *Eur J Pharmacol.* 2003;458:25-29.
21. Vocci F, Ling W. Medications development: Successes and challenges. *Pharmacol Ther.* 2005;108:94-108.
22. Huang P, Kehner GB, Cowan A, et al. Comparison of pharmacological activities of buprenorphine and norbuprenorphine: norbuprenorphine is a potent opioid agonist. *J Pharmacol Exp Ther.* 2001;297:688-695.
23. SAMHSA. *Become a Buprenorphine Waivered Practitioner*. Accessed September 9, 2022. https://www.samhsa.gov/medication-assisted-treatment/become-buprenorphine-waivered-practitioner
24. Li X, Shorter D, Kosten TR. Prescription opioid misuse: Effective methods for reducing the epidemic. *Curr Treat Options Psychiatry.* 2015;2:122.
25. Serafini G, Adavastro G, Canepa G, et al. The efficacy of buprenorphine in major depression, treatment-resistant depression and suicidal behavior: a systematic review. *Int J Mol Sci.* 2018;19(8):2410.
26. Voelker R. Implant for opioid dependence. *JAMA.* 2016;316:24.
27. Ling W, Shoptaw S, Goodman-Meza D. Depot buprenorphine injection in the management of opioid use disorder: From development to implementation. *Subst Abuse Rehabil.* 2019;10:69-78. doi:10.2147/SAR.S155843. Correction appears in *Subst Abuse Rehabil.* 2020;11:19-20.
28. Mitchell SG, Kelly SM, Brown BS, et al. Uses of diverted methadone and buprenorphine by opioid-addicted individuals in Baltimore, Maryland. *Am J Addict.* 2009;18:346-355.
29. Centers for Disease Control & Prevention (CDC). *U.S. Opioid Dispensing Rate Maps.* Accessed September 11, 2022. https://www.cdc.gov/drugoverdose/rxrate-maps/index.html#:~:text=After%20a%20steady%20increase%20in,81.3%20prescriptions%20per%20100%20persons
30. Substance Abuse and Mental Health Services Administration. *Key substance use and mental health indicators in the United States: Results from the 2020 National Survey on Drug Use and Health* (HHS Publication No. PEP21-07-01-003, NSDUH Series H-56). Center for Behavioral Health Statistics and Quality, Substance Abuse and Mental Health Services Administration; 2021. Accessed May 13, 2023. 2021 https://www.samhsa.gov/data/sites/default/files/reports/rpt35325/NSDUHFFRPDFWHTMLFiles2020/2020NSDUHFFR1PDFW102121.pdf
31. Michigan News, University of Michigan. 2016. Teen use of any illicit drug other than marijuana at new low, same true for alcohol. Accessed September 11, 2022. https://news.umich.edu/teen-use-of-any-illicit-drug-other-than-marijuana-at-new-low-same-true-for-alcohol/. http://www.monitoringthefuture.org/pubs/monographs/mtf-overview2021.pdf
32. Warren EC, Kolodny A. Trends in heroin treatment admissions in the United States by race, sex, and age. *JAMA Netw Open.* 2021;4(2):e2036640. doi:10.1001/jamanetworkopen.2020.36640
33. Rosenblum A, Parrino M, Schnoll SH, et al. Prescription opioid abuse among enrollees into methadone maintenance treatment. *Drug Alcohol Depend.* 2007;90:64-71.
34. Carlson RG, Nahhas RW, Daniulaityte R, Martins SS, Li L, Falck R. Latent class analysis of non-opioid dependent illegal pharmaceutical opioid users in Ohio. *Drug Alcohol Depend.* 2014;134:259-266.
35. Substance Abuse and Mental Health Services Administration. *Preliminary Findings from Drug-Related Emergency Department Visits, 2021; Drug Abuse Warning Network (HHS Publication No. PEP22-07-03-001).* Center for Behavioral Health Statistics and Quality; 2022. Accessed August 22, 2022. https://store.samhsa.gov/sites/default/files/SAMHSA_Digital_Download/PEP22-07-03-001.pdf
36. US Drug Enforcement Administration. *Diversion Control Division. National Forensic Laboratory Information System: NFLIS-Drug2020 Midyear Report.* U.S. Drug Enforcement Administration; 2021. Accessed May 13, 2023. https://www.nflis.deadiversion.usdoj.gov/nflisdata/docs/13915NFLISdrugMidYear2020.pdf
37. Ahmad FB, Cisewski JA, Rossen LM, Sutton P. *Drug Overdose Death Counts.* National Center for Health Statistics; 2022. Accessed August 10, 2022. https://www.cdc.gov/nchs/nvss/vsrr/drug-overdose-data.htm
38. Conn BM, Marks AK. Ethnic/racial differences in peer and parent influence on adolescent prescription drug misuse. *J Dev Behav Pediatr.* 2014;35(4):257-265.
39. Hoffman KM, Trawalter S, Axt JR, Oliver MN. Racial bias in pain assessment and treatment recommendations, and false beliefs about biological differences between Blacks and Whites. *Proc Natl Acad Sci U S A.* 2016;113:4296-4301.
40. Centers for Disease Control and Prevention, National Vital Statistics System. *Mortality Multiple Cause of Death.* Accessed July 4, 2022. https://www.cdc.gov/nchs/nvss/mortality_public_use_data.htm.
41. NYU Langone Health News Hub. Overdose Deaths Caused by Opioids in Combination with Stimulants Hit Black Communities Hardest. Research, Press Release, Feb 08, 2022. Accessed July 4, 2022. https://nyulangone.org/news/overdose-deaths-caused-opioids-combination-stimulants-hit-black-communities-hardest
42. Chen LJ, Hedegaard H, Warner M. *Drug-Poisoning Deaths Involving Opioid Analgesics: United States, 1999–2011.* NCHS data brief, no. 166. National Center for Health Statistics; 2014. Accessed September 10, 2022. https://www.cdc.gov/nchs/products/databriefs/db166.htm
43. Substance Abuse and Mental Health Services Administration. Practitioner and Program Data, Updated Aug 19, 2022. Accessed September 10, 2022. https://www.samhsa.gov/medication-assisted-treatment/practitioner-resources/data-program-data
44. Varamini P, Blanchfield JT, Toth I. Endomorphin derivatives with improved pharmacological properties. *Curr Med Chem.* 2013;20:2741-2758.
45. Zhao J, Xin X, Xie G-X, Palmer PP, Huang Y-G. Molecular and cellular mechanisms of the age-dependency of opioid analgesia and tolerance. *Mol Pain.* 2012;8:38.
46. Kling MA, Carson RE, Borg L, et al. Opioid receptor imaging with positron emission tomography and [(18)F]cyclofoxy in long-term, methadone-treated former heroin addicts. *J Pharmacol Exp Ther.* 2000;295:1070-1076.
47. Zubieta JK, Dannals RF, Frost JJ. Gender and age influences on human brain mu-opioid receptor binding measured by pet. *Am J Psychiatry.* 1999;156:842-848.
48. Pattinson KT. Opioids and the control of respiration. *Br J Anaesth.* 2008;100:747-758.
49. Camilleri M. Opioid-induced constipation: Challenges and therapeutic opportunities. *Am J Gastroenterol.* 2011;106(5):835-842.
50. McClung CA, Nestler EJ, Zachariou V. Regulation of gene expression by chronic morphine and morphine withdrawal in the locus ceruleus and ventral tegmental area. *J Neurosci.* 2005;25:6005-6015.
51. Han MH, Bolanos CA, Green TA, et al. Role of camp response element-binding protein in the rat locus ceruleus: regulation of neuronal activity and opiate withdrawal behaviors. *J Neurosci.* 2006;26:4624-4629.
52. Bart G, Heilig M, LaForge KS, et al. Substantial attributable risk related to a functional mu-opioid receptor gene polymorphism in association with heroin addiction in central Sweden. *Mol Psychiatry.* 2004;9:547-549.
53. Bart G, Kreek MJ, Ott J, et al. Increased attributable risk related to a functional mu-opioid receptor gene polymorphism in association with alcohol dependence in central Sweden. *Neuropsychopharmacology.* 2005;30:417-422.

54. Alvarez VA, Arttamangkul S, Dang V, et al. Mu-opioid receptors: Ligand-dependent activation of potassium conductance, desensitization, and internalization. *J Neurosci.* 2002;22:5769-5776.
55. Raehal KM, Bohn LM. The role of beta-arrestin2 in the severity of antinociceptive tolerance and physical dependence induced by different opioid pain therapeutics. *Neuropharmacology.* 2011;60:58-65.
56. Quillinan N, Lau EK, Virk M, et al. Recovery from mu-opioid receptor desensitization after chronic treatment with morphine and methadone. *J Neurosci.* 2011;31:4434-4443.
57. Arttamangkul S, Quillinan N, Low MJ, et al. Differential activation and trafficking of micro-opioid receptors in brain slices. *Mol Pharmacol.* 2008;74:972-979.
58. Caraceni A, Hanks G, Kaasa S, et al. Use of opioid analgesics in the treatment of cancer pain: Evidence-based recommendations from the EAPC. *Lancet Oncol.* 2012;13:e58-e68.
59. Inturrisi CE. Clinical pharmacology of opioids for pain. *Clin J Pain.* 2002;18:S3-S13.
60. Lugo RA, Kern SE. Clinical pharmacokinetics of morphine. *J Pain Palliat Care Pharmacother.* 2002;16:5-18.
61. Wilder-Smith OH. Opioid use in the elderly. *Eur J Pain.* 2005;9:137-140.
62. Vree TB, van Dongen RT, Koopman-Kimenai PM. Codeine analgesia is due to codeine-6-glucuronide, not morphine. *Int J Clin Pract.* 2000; 54(6):395-398.
63. Kirchheiner J, Schmidt H, Tzvetkov M, et al. Pharmacokinetics of codeine and its metabolite morphine in ultrarapid metabolizers due to CYP2D6 duplication. *Pharmacogenomics J.* 2007;7:257-265.
64. Knapp CM, Ciraulo DA, Jaffe J. Opiates: clinical aspects. In: Lowinson JH, Ruiz P, Millman RB, eds. *Substance Abuse: A Comprehensive Textbook.* 4th ed. Lippincott Williams & Wilkins; 2005:180-195.
65. Lugo RA, Kern SE. The pharmacokinetics of oxycodone. *J Pain Palliat Care Pharmacother.* 2004;18:17-30.
66. Davis MP, Varga J, Dickerson D, et al. Normal-release and controlled-release oxycodone: Pharmacokinetics, pharmacodynamics, and controversy. *Support Care Cancer.* 2003;11:84-92.
67. Colabufo NA, Contino M, Inglese C, et al. In vitro and ex vivo characterization of sigma-1 and sigma-2 receptors: agonists and antagonists in biological assays. *Cent Nerv Syst Agents Med Chem.* 2009;9(3):161-171.
68. Bao YJ, Hou W, Kong XY, et al. Hydromorphone for cancer pain. *Cochrane Database Syst Rev.* 2016;10:CD011108.
69. Darwish M, Yang R, Tracewell W, Robertson P Jr, Bond M. Single- and multiple-dose pharmacokinetics of a hydrocodone bitartrate extended-release tablet formulated with abuse-deterrence technology in healthy, naltrexone-blocked volunteers. *Clin Ther.* 2015;37:390-401.
70. Robinson CY, Rubino CM, Farr SJ. A pharmacokinetic evaluation of single and multiple doses of extended-release hydrocodone bitartrate in subjects experiencing surgical or osteoarthritic pain. *J Opioid Manag.* 2015;11:405-415.
71. Lugo RA, Satterfield KL, Kern SE. Pharmacokinetics of methadone. *J Pain Palliat Care Pharmacother.* 2005;19:13-24.
72. Eap CB, Buclin T, Baumann P. Interindividual variability of the clinical pharmacokinetics of methadone: Implications for the treatment of opioid dependence. *Clin Pharmacokinet.* 2002;41:1153-1193.
73. Begre S, von Bardeleben U, Ladewig D, et al. Paroxetine increases steady-state concentrations of (R)-methadone in Cyp2d6 extensive but not poor metabolizers. *J Clin Psychopharmacol.* 2002;22:211-215.
74. Stotts AL, Dodrill CL, Kosten TR. Opioid dependence treatment: options in pharmacotherapy. *Expert Opin Pharmacother.* 2009;10(11): 1727-1740.
75. Lintzeris N, Mitchell TB, Bond AJ, et al. Pharmacodynamics of diazepam co-administered with methadone or buprenorphine under high dose conditions in opioid dependent patients. *Drug Alcohol Depend.* 2007;91:187-194.
76. Sporer KA. Buprenorphine: A primer for emergency physicians. *Ann Emerg Med.* 2004;43:580-584.
77. Ciraulo DA, Hitzemann RJ, Somoza E, et al. Pharmacokinetics and pharmacodynamics of multiple sublingual buprenorphine tablets in dose-escalation trials. *J Clin Pharmacol.* 2006;46:179-192.
78. Strain EC, Moody DE, Stoller KB, et al. Relative bioavailability of different buprenorphine formulations under chronic dosing conditions. *Drug Alcohol Depend.* 2004;74:37-43.
79. Compton P, Ling W, Moody D, et al. Pharmacokinetics, bioavailability and opioid effects of liquid versus tablet buprenorphine. *Drug Alcohol Depend.* 2006;82:25-31.
80. Greenwald MK, Johanson CE, Moody DE, et al. Effects of buprenorphine maintenance dose on mu-opioid receptor availability, plasma concentrations, and antagonist blockade in heroin-dependent volunteers. *Neuropsychopharmacology.* 2003;28:2000-2009.
81. Kreek MJ, Borg L, Zhou Y. Relationships between endocrine functions and substance abuse syndromes: Heroin and related short-acting opiates in addiction contrasted with methadone and other long-acting opioid agonists used in pharmacotherapy of addiction. In: Pfaff D, ed. *Hormones, Brain and Behavior*. Academic Press; 2002:781-830.
82. Bailey CP, Connor M. Opioids: Cellular mechanisms of tolerance and physical dependence. *Curr Opin Pharmacol.* 2005;5:60-68.
83. Moss RB, Carlo DJ. Higher doses of naloxone are needed in the synthetic opioid era. *Subst Abuse Treat Prev Policy.* 2019;14(1):6. doi:10.1186/s13011-019-0195-4
84. Kosten TR, Graham DP, Nielsen DA. Neurobiology of opioid use disorder and comorbid traumatic brain injury. *JAMA Psychiatry.* 2018;75(6):642-648. doi:10.1001/jamapsychiatry.2018.0101
85. Krieter P, Gyaw S, Crystal R, Skolnick P. Fighting fire with fire: Development of intranasal nalmefene to treat synthetic opioid overdose. *J Pharmacol Exp Ther.* 2019;371(2):409-415. doi:10.1124/jpet.118.256115
86. McHugh PF, Kreek MJ. The medical consequences of opiate abuse and addiction and methadone pharmacotherapy. In: Brick J, ed. *Handbook of the Medical Consequences of Alcohol and Drug Abuse.* 2nd ed. The Haworth Press; 2008:303-339.
87. Martell BA, Arnsten JH, Ray B, et al. The impact of methadone induction on cardiac conduction in opiate users. *Ann Intern Med.* 2003;139:154-155.
88. Krantz MJ, Lowery CM, Martell BA, et al. Effects of methadone on Qt-interval dispersion. *Pharmacotherapy.* 2005;25:1523-1529.
89. McCance-Katz EF. Treatment of opioid dependence and coinfection with HIV and hepatitis C virus in opioid-dependent patients: The importance of drug interactions between opioids and antiretroviral agents. *Clin Infect Dis.* 2005;41(suppl 1):S89-S95.
90. Bruce RD, Altice FL, Gourevitch MN, et al. Pharmacokinetic drug interactions between opioid agonist therapy and antiretroviral medications: Implications and management for clinical practice. *J Acquir Immune Defic Syndr.* 2006;41:563-572.

CHAPTER 14

The Pharmacology of Stimulants

David A. Gorelick and Michael H. Baumann

CHAPTER OUTLINE

- Definition
- Substances included
- Formulations and methods of use
- Historical features
- Epidemiology
- Pharmacokinetics
- Drug-drug interactions
- Pharmacodynamic actions
- Neurobiology
- Future research directions

DEFINITION

Stimulants are a class of drugs that enhance activity in the central and sympathetic peripheral nervous systems, chiefly by augmenting neurotransmission at catecholaminergic synapses. Most stimulants exert their effects by binding to presynaptic plasma membrane monoamine reuptake transporters. By disrupting the function of norepinephrine, dopamine, and serotonin transporters, stimulant drugs inhibit the presynaptic reuptake process, thereby increasing extracellular concentrations of these neurotransmitters and amplifying associated receptor signaling and neuron-to-neuron transmission.

SUBSTANCES INCLUDED

Stimulants include both naturally occurring plant alkaloids, such as cocaine (**Fig. 14-1**), ephedra, and khat, and more than a dozen synthetic compounds, including amphetamine-type stimulants (ATS) (ie, amphetamine, methamphetamine, and methylphenidate), synthetic cathinones, and modafinil. Most of these compounds are variants of the basic phenethylamine chemical structure, which is shared by the endogenous catecholamine neurotransmitters norepinephrine and dopamine (**Fig. 14-2**). The wakefulness-promoting agents modafinil and its (*R*)-isomer, armodafinil, have a mechanism of action similar to that of stimulants, but a different chemical structure and reduced propensity for addiction.[1]

All stimulants share the same range of psychological and physiologic effects, while differing in potency and pharmacokinetic characteristics. Caffeine, the most widely used stimulant, is considered separately in Chapter 15, "The Pharmacology of Caffeine." 3,4-Methylenedioxymethamphetamine (MDMA, "ecstasy"), a structural analogue of methamphetamine with both stimulant and hallucinogenic characteristics, is considered separately in Chapter 18, "The Pharmacology of Hallucinogens."

FORMULATIONS AND METHODS OF USE

Plant-Derived Stimulants

Several stimulant-containing plants are available for oral use by indigenous populations. These include coca (containing cocaine) in South America, ephedra (containing ephedrine) in North America and East Asia, and khat (containing cathinone) in East Africa and the Arabian Peninsula. Oral use often is culturally sanctioned and may not be associated with a substance use disorder. Use of more potent formulations or more rapidly acting routes of administration has significant addiction potential and is illegal even where oral formulations are allowed.

Cocaine

Cocaine is an alkaloid with a tropane ester chemical structure (see **Fig. 14-1**). It occurs in leaves of several *Erythroxylum* species (coca bush), especially *Erythroxylum coca* and *Erythroxylum novogranatense*, which grow in the Andean region of South America.[2] Cocaine exists as two stereoisomers: naturally occurring (−)-cocaine and (+)-cocaine. The (−) isomer of cocaine is responsible for pharmacological activity, as the (+) isomer has substantially less affinity for the dopamine transporter and is rapidly metabolized in the periphery.[3]

The coca bush is cultivated primarily in Bolivia, Colombia, and Peru. Local indigenous use of oral (coca tea) or buccal transmucosal (coca leaves) cocaine is legal in these countries.[2] Coca leaves typically are "chewed" by placing crushed leaf between the buccal mucosa and teeth. An alkaline environment is created with lime or plant ash to enhance absorption. Cocaine is legally available (schedule II of the Controlled Substances Act [CSA]) in the United States only as a 4% solution for use as a topical anesthetic on mucous membranes. Legal cocaine preparations rarely are diverted for misuse.

Illicit cocaine is smuggled into the United States specifically for recreational (ie, nonmedical) purposes from its countries of origin. The coca leaves are crushed and heated in an organic solvent (often kerosene) to extract the cocaine.[4] The extraction and filtering process is usually repeated several

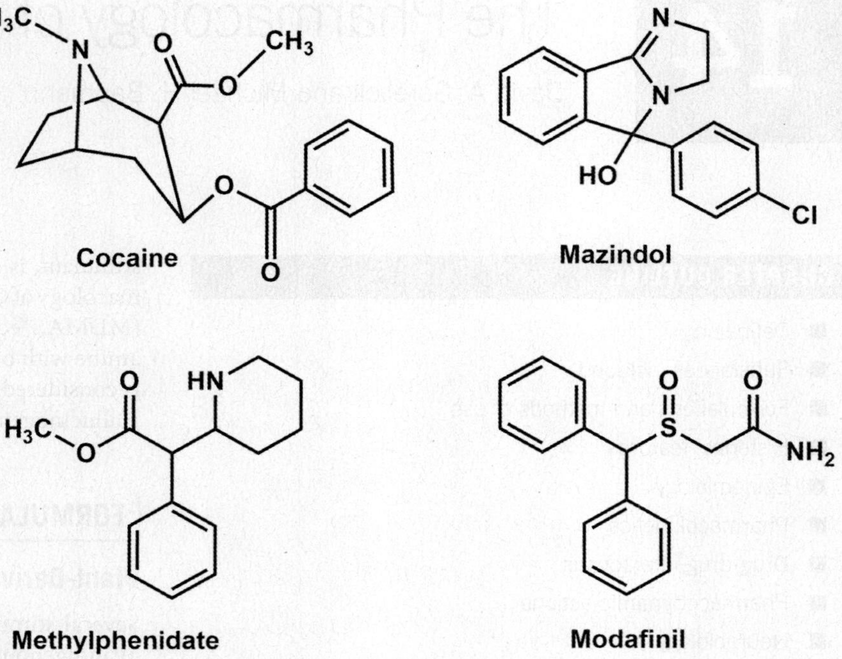

Figure 14-1. Chemical structures of cocaine, mazindol, methylphenidate, and modafinil.

times to achieve 80% to 90% cocaine content. This coca paste can be heated in an organic solvent (often ether or acetone) with concentrated acid to convert it to salt form. The salt is readily converted back to the base by heating in an organic solvent at basic pH. This process of heating the salt form is known as "freebasing" and was practiced by people who used cocaine during the 1980s, before cocaine base (or "freebase") was widely available on the retail illicit market. "Crack" as a street name for base cocaine reportedly derives from the crackling sound made during this heating process.

Cocaine is available for illicit use in two forms: base and salt.[4] These forms have different physical properties, which favor different routes of administration. The base has a relatively low melting point (98 °C) and vaporizes before substantial pyrolytic destruction has occurred. This allows cocaine base to be smoked (eg, in a pipe) or vaporized without burning for inhalation via electronic drug delivery devices (EDDDs, including "e-cigarettes") (see Chapter 22 for more information about EDDDS). The majority of smoked cocaine is probably inhaled in the form of small particles (<5 μm) that reach the alveoli, rather than true cocaine vapor.[5] Cocaine base is insoluble in water (alcohol to water solubility ratio of 100:1), making it difficult to dissolve for injection purposes. In contrast, cocaine salt does not melt below 195 °C, so heating it for smoking results in destruction of most of the cocaine. Cocaine salt is highly water soluble (alcohol to water solubility ratio of 1:8), making it easy to dissolve for injection purposes or be absorbed across mucus membranes, for example, in the nose (insufflation or "snorting"). Regardless of the chemical form or route of administration, the cocaine molecule exerts the same actions once it reaches the brain or other target organ.[4]

Adulterants are added (ie, the cocaine is "cut") to enhance dealer profits. Adulterants include both inert fillers that look like cocaine (eg, dextrose, lactose, mannitol, starch) and active chemicals that either mimic the local anesthetic effect of cocaine (eg, benzocaine, lidocaine, procaine) or provide some psychoactive effect (eg, ephedrine, amphetamine, caffeine, phenacetin, phencyclidine [PCP]).[6] The veterinary antihelminthic agent levamisole is increasingly common as a cocaine adulterant, found in up to three-quarters of analyzed street cocaine samples in the United States.[7] Cocaine adulterated with levamisole is associated with serious side effects, including agranulocytosis, leukopenia, purpura, and cutaneous vasculitis. Street cocaine may also contain contaminants from the preparation process (such as benzene, acetone, or sodium bicarbonate).

Ephedra

Ephedrine and pseudoephedrine are naturally occurring alkaloids with a phenethylamine chemical structure (see **Fig. 14-2**) that are found in several *Ephedra* species.[8] Ephedra is a preparation of dried plant material, typically containing 1% to 3% ephedrine. This may be converted into a capsule, tincture, liquid extract, or tea. Ephedra products are widely used in East Asia and North America.

Ephedra products often are advertised as legal alternatives to more strictly regulated manufactured stimulants. They appeal to consumers as safer than synthetic stimulants because they are "natural" or "herbal." Synthetic ephedrine and pseudoephedrine are available as tablets or capsules (see below). Ephedra alkaloids have the same range of psychological and physiological effects as do cocaine and ATS. There is limited evidence of their efficacy for weight loss in obese individuals.[8] Ephedra products were banned from the U.S. market in 2006 due to severe cardiovascular and central nervous system (CNS) adverse effects.[8]

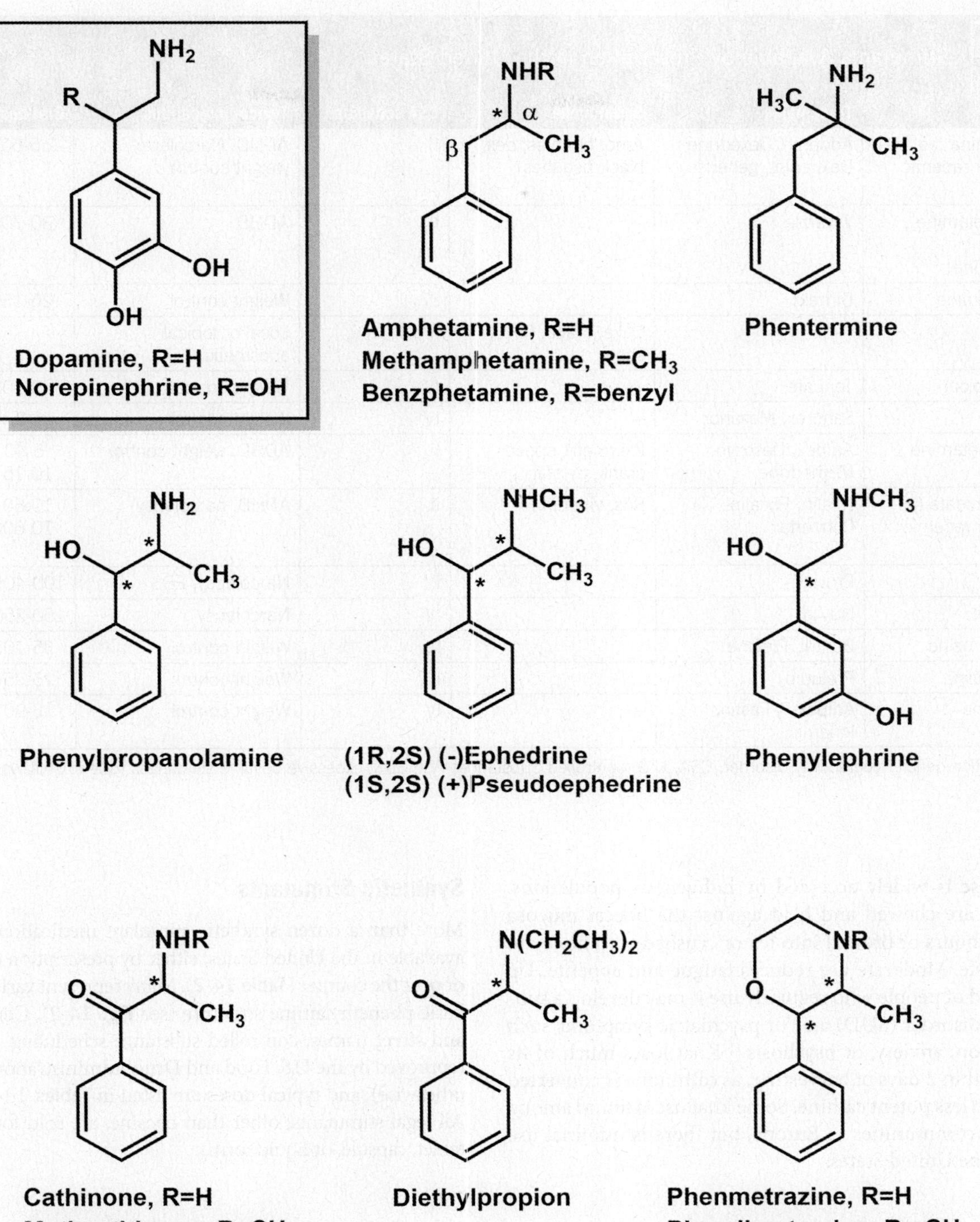

Figure 14-2. Chemical structures of endogenous catecholamine neurotransmitters (dopamine, norepinephrine) and phenethylamine stimulant drugs. Asterisks (*) denote chiral centers associated with stereoisomers; the α and β carbon positions are shown.

Khat

Khat is the common term for preparations of the *Catha edulis* plant, which is native to East Africa (Sudan to Madagascar) and the southwestern Arabian Peninsula (Yemen).[9,10] Fresh khat leaves contain at least two stimulant alkaloids with phenethylamine chemical structures: cathinone (present at 1%-3%) (see **Fig. 14-2**) and cathine (norpseudoephedrine).

Cathinone is a Schedule I controlled substance; cathine is in Schedule IV. Cathinone displays neuropharmacological potency similar to ATS.[8] Recreational use of potent synthetic methcathinone congeners such as mephedrone, methylone, and 3,4-methylenedioxypyrovalerone (MDPV), often marketed as "bath salts," has increased markedly around the world in the past decade (see "Synthetic Stimulants" below).

TABLE 14-1 Stimulants Available by Prescription in the United States

Drug	Trade name	Street name	CSA schedule	Typical indications	Oral dose (mg/d)
Amphetamine (as D-isomer or racemic mixture)	Adderall, Dexedrine, Dextrostat, generic	Amp, bennies, dex, black beauties	II	ADHD, Narcolepsy, weight control	2.5-60
Lisdexamfetamine (L-lysine-D-amphetamine)	Vyvanse	—	II	ADHD	30-70
Benzphetamine	Didrex	—	III	Weight control	25-150
Cocaine		Coke, crack, flake, snow	II	Local or topical anesthetic	—
Diethylpropion	Tenuate	—	IV	Weight control	75-100
Mazindol	Sanorex, Mazanor	—	IV	Weight control	1-3
Methamphetamine	Adipex, Desoxyn, Methedrine	Ice, meth, speed, crank, crystal	II	ADHD, weight control	5-40 10-15
Methylphenidate (as D-isomer or racemic mixture)	Ritalin, Focalin, Concerta	Rits, vitamin R	II	ADHD, narcolepsy	10-60 10-60
Modafinil	Provigil		IV	Narcolepsy, EDS	100-400
R-Modafinil	Nuvigil		IV	Narcolepsy	150-250
Phendimetrazine	Bontril, Plegine		III	Weight control	35-105
Phenmetrazine	Preludin		II	Weight control	25-75
Phentermine	Adipex-P, Fastin, Ionamin	—	IV	Weight control	15-90

ADHD, attention deficit/hyperactivity disorder; CSA, U.S. Controlled Substances Act; EDS, excessive daytime sleepiness (due to shift-work, obstructive sleep apnea).

Khat use is widely accepted by indigenous populations. The leaves are chewed and held against the buccal mucosa for several hours or brewed into tea or crushed with honey to make a paste. Moderate use reduces fatigue and appetite. Up to one-third of people who regularly use it may develop a substance use disorder (SUD) and/or psychiatric symptoms such as depression, anxiety, or psychosis.[11] Khat loses much of its potency within 2 days of harvesting, as cathinone is converted to the much less potent cathine. Some khat use is found among immigrant communities in Europe, but there is minimal use of khat in the United States.

Synthetic Stimulants

More than a dozen synthetic stimulant medications are legally available in the United States, either by prescription (**Table 14-1**) or over the counter (**Table 14-2**). Many represent variations on the basic phenethylamine structure (see **Fig. 14-2**). Common trade and street names, controlled substance scheduling, clinical uses (approved by the U.S. Food and Drug Administration [FDA] and otherwise), and typical doses are listed in **Tables 14-1** and **14-2**. All legal stimulants, other than cocaine, are sold for oral use in tablet, capsule, or liquid form.

TABLE 14-2 Stimulants Available as Over-the-Counter Preparations in the United States

Drug	Trade name	Indications	Typical oral dose (mg/d)
Caffeine	(Various)	Weight control, alertness	50-250
Ephedrine	Marax, Quadrinal	Decongestant, bronchodilation	50-100
Phenylephrine	Comhist, Dristan, Neo-Synephrine	Decongestant	40-60
Pseudoephedrine	Sudafed, Sine-Aid	Decongestant	90-240
Propylhexedrine	Benzedrex, Dristan, Obesin	Decongestant, weight control	50-150

Several stimulants are available in extended or sustained-release formulations,[12] chiefly prescribed for treatment of attention deficit/hyperactivity disorder (ADHD). Methylphenidate and amphetamine are also available as a transdermal patch.[12] Amphetamine is available as a prodrug, lisdexamfetamine, consisting of d-amphetamine coupled to the amino acid L-lysine.[13] The active drug is formed as the inactive lysine is hydrolyzed by enzymes in the intestines and liver. All slow release formulations have two theoretical advantages over conventional immediate release formulations: (1) improved patient compliance and effectiveness because of longer duration of action, and (2) reduced recreational use and addiction liability because of slower onset of action and weaker peak subjective effects.[14]

Some over-the-counter (OTC) stimulants are available in aerosolized formulations for nasal inhalation for use as decongestants. Phenylephrine is available as a sterile solution for parenteral administration to treat hypotension.

Prescription synthetic stimulants are often misused (ie, used for nonmedical purposes, rather than as prescribed), especially by adolescents and young adults.[15] Amphetamines, especially highly pure crystallized methamphetamine ("ice"), may be used intranasally or smoked, as is cocaine. The stimulants may be obtained via a physician's prescription, diverted from a relative or friend who has a prescription, or purchased illegally.[16] If oral administration is not intended, the original tablet or capsule may be crushed or opened to allow the drug to be taken intranasally or mixed with water for injection. Amphetamines, especially methamphetamine, are often synthesized in clandestine laboratories directly for illicit use. The synthesis can be done with standard chemical reactions applied to legally available precursors. For example, methamphetamine (desoxyephedrine) can be made by reducing ephedrine or pseudoephedrine. For this reason, retail purchases of products containing ephedrine or pseudoephedrine in the United States are limited to 3.6 g/day and 9 g/month.

Stimulants with a phenylisopropylamine structure (such as amphetamine and methamphetamine) have a chiral center at the alpha-carbon atom (see **Fig. 14-2**) and exist in two stereoisomeric forms that differ in pharmacodynamic and pharmacokinetic properties.[17,18] The D- or *S*-(+) isomer generally has three to five times greater CNS activity and about one-third the half-life of the L- or *R*-(−) isomer. The L-isomers usually have more peripheral alpha-adrenergic activity. For example, D-methamphetamine is a potent CNS stimulant, whereas L-methamphetamine (L-desoxyephedrine) is used as a decongestant (as in the Vicks nasal inhaler). Methylphenidate has two chiral centers so exists in four stereoisomeric forms, of which the D-threo enantiomer is the active one.[19]

The recreational use of synthetic stimulants unrelated to prescription medications has increased substantially in recent years. These compounds are typically synthetic analogues of cathinone and are now classified in Schedule I of the CSA. Products containing synthetic cathinones are purchased over the Internet or from street dealers and marketed with innocuous names (eg, "bath salts," "research chemicals") as "legal" alternatives to cocaine and methamphetamine.[20] Synthetic cathinones fall into two broad structural categories: pyrrolidine-containing compounds like MDPV and ring-substituted cathinones like methylone. MDPV is a common constituent of bath salts products, whereas methylone is often found in counterfeit MDMA ("ecstasy") tablets. Synthetic cathinones exert potent ATS effects and can cause serious cardiovascular and neurological side effects requiring emergency medical care.[21] See Chapter 23 for more information about synthetic cathinones.

Clinical Uses

Cocaine (4% solution) is FDA-approved (CSA schedule II) for clinical use as a topical anesthetic for the nasal mucosa and is used off-label for other ear, nose, and throat procedures.[22] Such use is now uncommon in the United States,[23] but more common in the United Kingdom.[24] Other prescription stimulants generally are used for one of several FDA-approved indications: ADHD in both children[12] and adults,[25] narcolepsy and excessive daytime sleepiness,[26,27] or appetite suppression to promote weight loss in exogenous obesity[28] (see **Table 14-1**). Stimulants prescribed for ADHD are misused by about 10% of patients for whom they are prescribed.[29]

OTC stimulants generally are used for decongestion[30] and bronchodilation in the treatment of asthma, upper respiratory infections, allergic rhinitis, sinusitis, or bronchitis, and for appetite suppression to promote weight loss in exogenous obesity (all of which are FDA-approved indications) (see **Table 14-2**). Parenteral phenylephrine is approved by the FDA as an adjunct to prolong the duration of spinal anesthesia, to terminate paroxysmal supraventricular tachycardia, and for immediate, short-term treatment of hypotension.

In addition to their FDA-approved indications, oral stimulants have a long history of accepted, off-label clinical use for other indications.[31] Amphetamines and methylphenidate are used as adjunctive or augmentation treatment for treatment-resistant major (unipolar)[32] or bipolar depression[33] and as quick acting (2- to 3-day), short-term antidepressants in persons who are elderly, medically ill, or HIV-infected, or those with neurological conditions such as stroke or traumatic brain injury, especially those who cannot tolerate the side effects of standard antidepressants.[34] Such patients may exhibit apathy, fatigue, and psychomotor retardation, rather than a full-blown classic depressive syndrome. It is often unclear whether the beneficial effect of stimulants in such patients is due to activating effects of the drug or true antidepressant actions. Stimulants are used to improve functional recovery after stroke and traumatic brain injury[35,36] and to reduce fatigue in palliative care,[37] but their efficacy is limited. ATS and mazindol have been used to potentiate opiate analgesia and to counteract opiate-induced sedation and respiratory suppression, thus allowing larger doses of opioids to be used. Cocaine is used for this purpose as part of Brompton's cocktail (with alcohol and an opioid) in the treatment of cancer pain. Ephedrine and phenylephrine are used parenterally to counteract hypotension associated with spinal anesthesia, especially in obstetrical and urological surgery. Most other clinical uses of stimulants for their pressor effect have been superseded by more selective agents.

There is little evidence that medical use of stimulants at therapeutic doses in appropriately diagnosed and monitored patients leads to a stimulant use disorder (StUD) or increases the risk of serious adverse events, although there are little data from long-term, controlled trials.[38] Prospective, longitudinal studies of children receiving stimulant treatment for ADHD find no increased risk of developing a SUD.[39]

Nonmedical Use and Addiction

Oral stimulants (both prescription and OTC) are widely used in work, school, military, and sports settings, often without medical supervision, for their alerting, antifatigue, sleep-suppressing, and performance-enhancing properties.[40,41] Among individuals reporting nonmedical use of prescription stimulants, about two-thirds use stimulants to improve alertness, concentration, or studying or to stay awake.[42]

The antifatigue and sleep-suppression effects of stimulants are well demonstrated in laboratory and field studies. Enhancement of cognitive and psychomotor performance is more difficult to demonstrate in controlled studies and occurs more robustly in persons who already are fatigued or sleep deprived.[43] Low-quality evidence suggests that stimulants mildly improve athletic performance, especially in endurance sports, such as cycling, which require anaerobic exercise.[44,45] Stimulants of all types (illicit, prescription, and OTC) are banned by the World Anti-Doping Agency and most other sports organizations.[45]

All stimulants have a potential for misuse and addiction, varying only in their potency. Cocaine, amphetamine, and methamphetamine have high addiction potential, as reflected in their placement in Schedule II of the CSA. Nationally representative, community-based, cross-sectional surveys suggest that about one-sixth of individuals currently using cocaine will develop a cocaine use disorder in the same year[46]; about half of individuals currently using methamphetamine have a methamphetamine use disorder.[47] Frequency and quantity, but not duration, of cocaine use are positively associated with risk of developing a cocaine use disorder.[48] Individuals engaged in daily or weekly cocaine use have 12.1 and 8.8 times greater risk, respectively, of developing cocaine use disorder when compared to those engaged in low-frequency use (once or twice a year). Individuals using very high (2 g or more daily) or high (1-2 g daily) quantities of cocaine have 4.8 and 2.7 times the risk, respectively, of developing cocaine use disorder when compared to those using lower quantities (0.2 g or less daily). Individuals who smoke cocaine are at higher risk of developing cocaine use disorder than individuals using other routes of administration,[48] probably due to the quicker onset of action with the smoked route.[49] Even lower potency stimulants in Schedule IV, such as pemoline and phentermine, or OTC stimulants, such as ephedrine, pseudoephedrine, and phenylpropanolamine, have been misused and result in a StUD.[50]

Family, twin, and adoption studies suggest that genes contribute about 40% of the variability in development of cocaine use disorder,[51] that is, cocaine use disorder has a heritability of about 40%. About 90% of this genetic influence appears to be from common factors that similarly influence other SUDs. Genome-wide association studies (GWAS) have identified several candidate genes and genetic variants associated with cocaine use disorder, but none has been consistently identified in high-quality studies.[51] There are no good-quality studies on the heritability of methamphetamine use disorder.[52]

Stimulants are used in a variety of patterns.[53,54] "Binge" use involves short periods of heavy use (eg, on weekends or payday), separated by longer periods of little or no use.[54] Others use daily for an extended period until their finances are exhausted or their access to drug is interrupted. A majority of people who use it take low doses and/or use infrequently without escalation of dose over time. Typical cocaine doses are 12 to 15 g orally (coca leaf chewing), 20 to 100 mg intranasally, 10 to 50 mg intravenously, and 50 to 200 mg smoked.

Stimulant intoxication is weakly associated with agitation and aggression in human laboratory studies.[55] Community surveys suggest a strong association between stimulant use and violence.[56] This association may be more due to witnessing or experiencing violence than to perpetrating it.[57]

Unintended use of cocaine may occur in persons who swallow the drug in their possession to avoid arrest or prosecution (ie, "body stuffers") or who swallow large quantities to transport it without detection by law enforcement authorities (ie, "body packers," "mules").[58] The drug may be wrapped in plastic bags, balloons, condoms, paper, or aluminum foil. If the wrapper fails, the carrier may be exposed suddenly to large doses of cocaine in the gastrointestinal tract, resulting in severe acute cocaine intoxication.

Stimulants often are used in combination with other drugs, especially alcohol, cannabis, and opioids.[59,60] Such use may be concurrent (at the same time, often termed "co-use") or sequential. Concurrent use of CNS depressants is believed to enhance the subjective experience and temper unpleasant effects of intoxication. Concurrent intravenous use of cocaine plus heroin is termed speedballing[61]; concurrent use of methamphetamine and heroin is termed goofballing.[62] Sequential use may relieve symptoms of stimulant withdrawal. The recent rise in stimulant overdose deaths in the United States is related to concurrent use (either intentional or unintentional due to adulteration) with opioids, particularly illicitly manufactured fentanyl.[63] (See Chapter 59 for more information about stimulant overdose.)

HISTORICAL FEATURES

Naturally occurring plant alkaloids have been used for their CNS stimulant properties for thousands of years. Chinese medicine has used the herbal preparation ma-huang (ephedra) for at least 5,000 years.[64] Chewing of coca leaves and drinking of coca tea have been prevalent in the Andean regions of South America for at least 2,000 years.[2]

Coca received little attention in Europe until Albert Niemann isolated cocaine as the active ingredient of coca leaf in 1850.[2,65] This discovery generated the popularity of cocaine-containing products throughout Europe and North America. A nonalcoholic beverage (containing 4.5 mg of cocaine per 6 oz) was introduced in 1886 and quickly became one of the world's most popular soft drinks: Coca-Cola. A fluid extract of coca for medical use (containing 0.5 mg of cocaine per mL) appeared in the *U.S. Pharmacopeia* in 1882. The first specific use of cocaine in medicine came in 1884, when the German ophthalmologist Koller discovered its efficacy as a local anesthetic during surgery. In the same year, Sigmund Freud published his monograph, *Uber Coca*, describing the first systematic study of cocaine's psychological effects (albeit with a sample of one, himself) and suggesting its use as a treatment for morphine addiction.

With widespread use of cocaine came increasing reports of adverse effects. By 1903, cocaine had been removed from Coca-Cola. In 1914, the Harrison Narcotic Act banned cocaine from OTC medications, beverages, and foods in the United States. For the next 50 years, cocaine remained largely out of public view and medical attention, except for limited use as a local anesthetic.

Synthetic stimulants first appeared with the synthesis of amphetamine in 1887 and of methamphetamine in 1919.[66] These stimulants attracted little attention until amphetamine became popular as an OTC bronchodilator (Benzedrine inhaler) in the early 1930s. By 1933, the CNS stimulant properties of amphetamine were recognized, leading to its use for weight loss, narcolepsy, depression, and childhood hyperactivity. The increasing medical use of amphetamine during the 1930s led to a concomitant increase in StUD. This growing abuse pattern led to a switch in 1937 from OTC to prescription-only status. During World War II, amphetamine was widely used by both Allied and Axis countries to enhance the performance of troops and factory workers. After the war, widespread use in Japan and Sweden led to tight restrictions on amphetamine manufacture and dispensing. In response to increasing rates of intravenous misuse of amphetamine extracted from Benzedrine inhalers, the FDA banned the inhalers in 1959. With passage of the CSA in 1970, cocaine, amphetamine, and methamphetamine were placed in Schedule II because they have high potential for misuse and accepted medical use only with severe restrictions.

EPIDEMIOLOGY

Stimulant Use

There are substantial geographic and sociodemographic differences in the epidemiology of stimulant use.[67] Cocaine is the predominant stimulant in the Western Hemisphere, Western Europe, coastal West Africa, and Australia, while ATS are predominant in Central and Eastern Europe, Scandinavia, Middle East, North Africa, and Asia. About three-quarters (73%) of people who use cocaine are men, as are slightly more than half (55%) of people who use ATS and prescription stimulants. In 2020, there were an estimated 20 million people using cocaine worldwide, representing 0.4% of the 15- to 64-year-old population. This represented a leveling of the steady increase seen over the 2010-2019 decade. The highest prevalence of cocaine use was in Oceania (2.7%, 0.73 million current users), followed by North America (1.9%, 6.35 million), South America (1.6%, 4.34 million), Western and Central Europe (1.4%, 4.55 million), and Central America (0.9%, 0.31 million). Lowest prevalence of cocaine use was in Asia (0.1%, 2.0 million) and Africa (0.25%, 2.0 million). In 2020, there were an estimated 34 million (0.6% prevalence) people globally who used ATS nonmedically, representing a slight increase over the past decade. Such use is most prevalent in North America (3.8%, 12.48 million), Oceania (1.3%, 0.33 million), Central America (1.0%, 0.31 million), and South America (0.6%, 2.3 million). Lowest prevalence of ATS use was in Africa (0.4%, 2.72 million), Asia (0.5%, 12.73 million), and Western and Central Europe (0.5%, 2.33 million).

Oral use of cocaine is legal in Bolivia and Peru.[68] Purified cocaine, suitable for intravenous, smoked, or intranasal administration, is illegal in all Andean countries. The lifetime prevalence of such cocaine use is similar to that reported in North America.

The 2020 National Survey on Drug Use and Health (NSDUH), which interviewed a nationally representative sample of 36,284 community-dwelling U.S. residents 12 years and older, provides a detailed view of stimulant epidemiology in the United States[69] (see **Table 14-3**).

With regard to current use (ie, in the past month), cocaine was the most commonly used stimulant (1.83 million people), followed by methamphetamine (1.72 million), prescription stimulants (1.49 million), and synthetic cathinones ("bath salts," flakka) (51,000). In 2020, there were an estimated 489,000 new people using cocaine (more than two-thirds [69.7%] 18 to 25 years old), 153,000 new people using methamphetamine (almost two-thirds [63.3%] older than 25 years), and 734,000 who began misuse of prescription stimulants (more than two-fifths [44.1%] older than 25 years). Cocaine use occurs in all segments of U.S. society but is significantly more prevalent in young adult men with low income who live in urban areas.[46]

Cocaine use is highly associated with alcohol and tobacco use,[70] and with psychiatric syndromes.[71] Those who smoke cigarettes or drink alcohol heavily are significantly more likely to use cocaine than are those who do not smoke or who drink moderately (nonbinge). People who currently use cocaine are twice as likely to have symptoms of depressive or anxiety disorders than are those that do not.

Stimulant Use Disorder

An analysis of publicly available data from 195 countries (Global Burden of Disease Study [GBDS]) estimated that 5.84 million individuals (68.4% men) worldwide had a cocaine use

TABLE 14-3 Epidemiology of Stimulant Use in the United States, 2020

Stimulant	Lifetime use Number in thousands (% prevalence)	Past-year use Number in thousands (% prevalence)	Past-month use Number in thousands (% prevalence)
Cocaine	39,261 (14.2%)	5,172 (1.9%)	1,831 (0.7%)
"Crack" cocaine	9,356 (3.4%)	637 (0.2%)	335 (0.1%)
Methamphetamine	15,397 (5.6%)	2,550 (0.9%)	1,722 (0.6%)
Misuse of prescription stimulants	nr	5,092 (1.8%)	1,493 (0.5%)
CNS stimulants	nr	10,306 (3.7%)	4,483 (1.6%)

Data from the 2020 National Survey on Drug Use and Health, a nationally representative, cross-sectional survey of 36,284 community-dwelling U.S. residents 12 years of age or older.

CNS, central nervous system; nr, not reported due to measurement issues; CNS stimulant, use or misuse (for prescription stimulants) of one or more of cocaine, methamphetamine, or prescription stimulant; "crack," cocaine base in chunk or rock form; misuse, use other than as prescribed for that individual.

Source: From Center for Behavioral Health Statistics and Quality. *Results From 2020 National Survey on Drug Use and Health: Detailed Tables*. Substance Abuse and Mental Health Services Administration; 2021. Accessed January 21, 2022. https://www.samhsa.gov/data/

disorder in 2016 and 4.96 million individuals (66.7% men) had an ATS use disorder.[72]

In 2020, an estimated 1.28 million U.S. residents 12 years or older met putative psychiatric diagnostic criteria (*Diagnostic and Statistical Manual for Mental Disorders*—5th edition [DSM-5])[73] for cocaine use disorder in the past year (four-fifths [79.6%] older than 25 years), 1.54 million for methamphetamine use disorder (almost all [92.4%] older than 25 years), and 758,000 for prescription stimulant use disorder (three-quarters [75.7%] older than 25 years).[69]

Only a minority of individuals with StUD receive treatment. In 2020, an estimated 492,000 people received some form of past-year treatment for their cocaine use disorder (slightly more than one-third [38.4%] the number of those with current cocaine use disorder), 562,000 received treatment for methamphetamine use disorder (about one-third [36.4%] of those with methamphetamine use disorder), and 118,000 received treatment for their prescription stimulant use disorder (about one-sixth [15.6%] of those with prescription stimulant use disorder).[69]

PHARMACOKINETICS

Absorption and Distribution

Route of administration has a major effect on the pharmacokinetic characteristics of stimulants.[65,74] Smoked stimulants are rapidly absorbed through the lungs and reach the brain in 6 to 8 seconds. The peak effect occurs within minutes of administration. As the stimulant redistributes from the brain, there is a rapid decline in effect. Intravenous administration produces peak brain uptake in 4 to 7 minutes, based on positron emission tomography (PET) studies.[75] Greatest cocaine uptake occurs in the striatum (caudate, putamen, and nucleus accumbens) and least uptake in the orbital cortex and cerebellum. Clearance to half-peak brain levels requires 17 to 30 minutes. The rapid offset of drug effects is often experienced as a "crash" by people who use smoked or intravenous stimulants.

Intranasal and oral stimulants have a slower absorption and onset of effect (30-45 minutes), a longer peak effect, and a more gradual decline from peak.[65,74] The peak intensity of effect is weaker than with smoked or intravenous administration because less active drug reaches its site of action in the brain. Coca leaf chewing produces less than half the peak cocaine plasma concentrations of an equivalent dose of intranasal cocaine.[2] However, even a single oral dose of cocaine (such as 2 mg in a cup of coca tea) may yield detectable urine concentrations of cocaine metabolites for at least 24 hours.[2] Pharmacokinetic parameters for oral stimulants are given in **Table 14-4**.

Cocaine and amphetamines are well absorbed through mucus membranes of the nose, mouth, vagina, and rectum[76] and are absorbed through intact skin or by passive (second-hand) inhalation of smoked drug.[77,78] Passive exposure from second-hand smoke, aerosolized particles, or contact with contaminated environmental surfaces (third-hand exposure)[5] can result in detectable urine concentrations of cocaine metabolites in medical and laboratory personnel. These concentrations are often too low to trigger a positive result on routine urine toxicology testing.

Stimulants distribute into most tissues of the body. Cocaine is rapidly taken up into the heart, kidney, adrenal glands, and liver.[76] In addition to blood and urine,[79] stimulants and their metabolites appear in hair,[80] sweat,[81] oral fluid (saliva),[81] nails,[82] and breast milk,[81] and cross the placenta to appear in umbilical cord blood, amniotic fluid, and meconium.[83] Analysis of these biological matrices is used for drug detection in workplace,[84] legal, and clinical settings.[85] Stimulants can also be detected postmortem in body fluids and tissues.[86]

TABLE 14-4 Pharmacokinetic Parameters of Oral Stimulants

Drug	T_{max} (h)	$T_{1/2}$ (h)	V_d (L/kg)	pK_a	F_b
Amphetamine	2-4	7-34[a]	3.2-5.6	9.9	0.16
Benzphetamine	—	—	—	6.6	—
Chlorphentermine	4	35-44	3.0	9.6	—
Cocaine	1	0.75-1.5	1.6-2.7	8.6	0.92
Diethylpropion		2.5			
Ephedrine	1	4-10	2.6-3.1	9.6	—
Mazindol	1	12-36	—	8.6	—
Methamphetamine	1-3	6-15[a]	3-7	9.9	0.1-0.2
Methylphenidate	1-3	1.4-4.2	11-33	8.8	0.15
Modafinil	2-3	14-16	0.9	8.8	—
Phendimetrazine	1	—		7.6	
Phenmetrazine	2	8	—	8.5	—
Phentermine	4	19-24	3-4	10.1	—
Phenylephrine	1	2-3	5	8.8	—
Propylhexedrine		—	—	10.4	—
Pseudoephedrine	2-3	3-16[a]	2-3	9.4	0.2

[a]Urine pH dependent: lower pH yields shorter half-life.

T_{max}, time of maximum plasma concentration (in hours); $T_{1/2}$, half-life (in hours); V_d, apparent volume of distribution (in L/kg of body weight); pK_a, acid dissociation constant (pH at which drug is 50% ionized); F_b, fraction of bound drug.

Source: From Drake LR, Scott PJH. DARK classics in chemical neuroscience: cocaine. *ACS Chem Neurosci.* 2018;9:2358-2372; Markowitz JS, Melchert PW. The pharmacokinetics and pharmacogenomics of psychostimulants. *Child Adolesc Psychiatr Clin N Am.* 2022;31(3):393-416.

Metabolism

In humans and other primates, 95% of cocaine is metabolized by hydrolysis of ester bonds to form benzoylecgonine (the primary urinary metabolite) and ecgonine methyl ester by the action of carboxylesterases in the liver and butyrylcholinesterase in the liver, plasma, brain, lung, and other tissues.[4,76] The remaining 5% of cocaine is *N*-demethylated by the CYP3A4 isozyme of the liver cytochrome P450 microsomal enzyme system to form norcocaine. The cytochrome P450 system is the predominant metabolic pathway in rodents.

Norcocaine has some pharmacological actions similar to those of cocaine and is hepatotoxic.[4,76] This may account for the significant hepatotoxicity of cocaine in rodents, which is not found in primates. Cocaine's hydrolytic metabolites are much less active pharmacologically, though this has not been well studied.

Amphetamines are metabolized in the liver via three different pathways: deamination to inactive metabolites, oxidation to norephedrine and other active metabolites, and para-position ring hydroxylation to active metabolites.[74,87] Amphetamine itself is the initial *N*-demethylated metabolite of methamphetamine.

When cocaine is smoked, a pyrolysis product is formed (methylecgonidine or anhydroecgonine methyl ester), the presence of which allows identification of the smoked route of administration.[4,76]

Elimination

Stimulants and their metabolites are largely eliminated in the urine.[74,76] Benzoylecgonine is the cocaine metabolite found in highest concentration in urine for several days after cocaine use. It is benzoylecgonine, rather than cocaine, that is measured in routine urine drug tests for cocaine. GI absorption and urinary elimination of amphetamines is highly pH dependent. Because amphetamines are weak bases (pK_a around 9.9),[74] acidification of the GI tract or urine substantially decreases absorption and increases excretion.[88] Conversely, alkalinization of the GI tract or urine can increase GI absorption and reduce excretion to negligible levels. This fact motivates people to take large doses of sodium bicarbonate to prolong the action of amphetamines and reduce the amount present in the urine for detection by drug tests.

DRUG-DRUG INTERACTIONS

Stimulants have adverse drug interactions by both pharmacokinetic and pharmacodynamic mechanisms.[89,90] The primary pharmacokinetic mechanism is altered activity of liver cytochrome P-450 drug-metabolizing enzymes. A lesser pharmacokinetic mechanism is altered activity of the P-glycoprotein drug transporter. For example, cocaine use is associated with reduced plasma concentrations of buprenorphine and methadone and increased concentrations of phenytoin. Methylphenidate is associated with enhanced cardiovascular effects of MDMA ("ecstasy"). Stimulants do not have clinically significant interactions with antiviral medications.[91,92] The primary pharmacodynamic drug interaction of clinical concern is with other stimulants or medications that enhance catecholamine activity. Such interactions risk overstimulation of the sympathetic nervous system, with possible severe cardiovascular effects and death. The greatest risk is presented by monoamine oxidase inhibitors (MAOIs) such as phenelzine and selegiline, which are used as antidepressants. MAOIs inhibit the enzymatic breakdown of catecholamines. Prescription stimulants should not be used within 2 weeks of MAOI use because the simultaneous blockade of catecholamine uptake and inhibition of catecholamine breakdown could result in dangerously high levels of catecholamine activity.

Alcohol used in conjunction with cocaine often results in enhanced or prolonged effects of cocaine, in part because of formation of a new pharmacologically active compound, cocaethylene.[93] Cocaethylene has actions similar to, but less potent than, those of cocaine, with a longer half-life. Human laboratory studies of the cocaine/alcohol/cocaethylene interaction have yielded inconsistent results.

PHARMACODYNAMIC ACTIONS

Adverse Health Effects

Chronic stimulant use generates a significant health and public health burden, although substantially less than that generated by alcohol, tobacco, or opioids. The GBDS estimated that in 2016 cocaine use was directly responsible for 8,800 deaths, 357,000 years of life lost, and 798,000 years lived with disability.[72] Amphetamine use was responsible for 5,200 deaths, 224,000 years of life lost, and 657,000 years lived with disability. Separate meta-analyses of cohort studies found regular or problematic cocaine or amphetamine use associated with a sixfold increased risk of death compared with age- and sex-matched peers.[94,95] The leading causes of death were suicide, unintended injury, homicide, and AIDS-related conditions for cocaine[94] and acute intoxication, cardiovascular disease, suicide, unintended injury, and homicide for amphetamine.[95] Cocaine- and methamphetamine-related cases were involved in an estimated 1.13 million visits to U.S. emergency departments in 2021, representing 15.7% of all substance-related visits.[96] For comparison, alcohol accounted for more than one-third (39.3%) of such visits and opioids for 14.1%. An estimated 65% of cocaine-related visits also involved at least one other psychoactive substance (chiefly alcohol, cannabis, and methamphetamine), as did about half (48.7%) of methamphetamine related visits (chiefly alcohol, cannabis, and heroin).

Central Nervous System

Intoxication

All stimulants produce a similar range of psychological, behavioral, and physical effects, with the intensity and duration depending on potency, dose, route of administration, and duration of use. The initial effects—usually desired—include increased energy, alertness, and sociability; elation or euphoria; and decreased fatigue, decreased need for sleep, and decreased appetite.[62,76,97] These effects may occur after 5 to 20 mg of oral amphetamine, methamphetamine, or methylphenidate; 100 to 200 mg of oral cocaine; 40 to 100 mg of intranasal cocaine; or 15 to 25 mg of IV or smoked cocaine. Such single oral doses of stimulants improve cognitive and psychomotor performance in subjects whose performance has been impaired by fatigue, sleep deprivation, or alcohol, especially in tasks that require focused and sustained attention (vigilance).[43]

There is less consistent evidence that stimulants are of any benefit in subjects who are fully alert and attentive or engaged in tasks involving learning, memory, or problem solving. With increasing potency, dose, duration of use, or a more efficient route of administration, stimulant effects often progress to include dysphoric effects such as anxiety, irritability, panic attacks, interpersonal sensitivity, hypervigilance, suspiciousness, paranoia, grandiosity, impaired judgment, and psychotic symptoms such as delusions and hallucinations.[62,76] Stimulant use is often associated with insomnia (delayed sleep onset, shortened total sleep time)[98,99] and weight loss (due to appetite suppression and metabolic changes).[100] Up to 50% of individuals using stimulants experience psychotic symptoms such as severe paranoia and/or hallucinations.[101,102] The proportion of people who use stimulants experiencing paranoia or psychotic symptoms varies with intensity and duration of use and severity of StUD.

Patients with stimulant psychosis may closely resemble those with acute schizophrenia.[103,104] Stimulant-induced psychosis differs in having more frequent visual hallucinations and fewer negative symptoms such as alogia and inattention. Stimulant-induced hallucinations may be of any sensory modality, but tactile hallucinations are especially typical. These include the sensation of something (eg, insects) crawling under the skin ("formication," "cocaine bugs").[105]

Parallel behavioral effects include restlessness, agitation, tremor (resembling essential tremor),[106] tics, dyskinesia, and repetitive or stereotyped behaviors such as picking at the skin or foraging for drug ("punding," "hung-up activity").[107,108] Associated physiological effects include tachycardia, pupil dilation, diaphoresis, and nausea, reflecting stimulation of the sympathetic nervous system. Treatment of acute stimulant intoxication is reviewed in Chapter 59. Cocaine and the more potent synthetic stimulants (such as amphetamines) produce these adverse effects at readily available doses by any route of administration. Less potent oral stimulants require chronic, high-dose use or diversion to intravenous use to cause adverse effects. Even OTC stimulants have been associated with severe psychological effects, misuse, and addiction.

There is wide individual variability in the response to stimulants.[97] The reasons for variable sensitivity are poorly understood but presumably are related to differences in genetics, psychological characteristics (including personality traits), previous drug experience, the setting in which the drug is taken, and the existence of psychiatric or medical comorbidities. Identical twins are highly concordant in their response to single doses of stimulants, suggesting an important genetic component. In animals, response to stimulants appears to be under polygenic control, with independent genetic influences on responses to cocaine or amphetamine.[109] In rats, behavioral response to cocaine shows a negative correlation with baseline brain dopamine concentrations, and a positive correlation with the increase in dopamine concentration elicited by a cocaine challenge.[110]

Individual differences in tolerance and sensitization to stimulants (see Neuroadaptation below) may account for the poor correlation between stimulant plasma concentrations and toxic effects.[111,112]

Chronic Effects

Chronic cocaine or ATS use is associated with cognitive impairment that varies with intensity and duration of use, and at least partially recovers after several months of abstinence.[113,114]

Chronic cocaine use is associated with decreased gray matter volume in some brain regions, including the frontal cortex and insula,[115] enlarged basal ganglia, and lower concentrations of *N*-acetyl aspartate (a magnetic resonance spectroscopy marker for normal neuronal function) and higher concentrations of creatine and myoinositol (markers of glial cell activity and inflammation).[116]

Long-term use of ATS by any route of administration is associated with a psychotic syndrome including paranoia, delusions, and hallucinations; negative symptoms are less common.[117,118] Methamphetamine-associated psychosis may persist for years after the last drug use, even in persons with no personal or family history of psychiatric disorder. Risk increases with longer duration and heavier intensity of use and past history of psychiatric disorder, especially psychotic symptoms.[119] Psychotic flashbacks have been reported in people who use ATS years after their last drug use and often are precipitated by threatening experiences.[120] A persisting psychosis after long-term cocaine use is apparently rare. Prescription ATS taken as medically directed are rarely associated with psychosis.[121]

Withdrawal

Cessation of heavy and/or chronic stimulant use results in a withdrawal syndrome that usually does not have prominent physical features and is rarely medically serious.[122] Stimulant withdrawal symptoms are thought to be mediated by decreased brain dopaminergic activity due to down-regulation from chronic stimulant exposure.[123] Withdrawal symptoms generally are the opposite of those associated with stimulant intoxication and include depressed mood, irritability, anhedonia (ie, inability to experience pleasure), fatigue, difficulty concentrating, increased appetite, increased stimulant craving, hypersomnolence, and increased dreaming[122] (due to increased rapid eye movement sleep[124]). Symptoms typically peak in 2 to 3 days (commonly termed the "crash") and resolve within 1 to 2 weeks without treatment. Some individuals experience more protracted withdrawal, with mild depression and cognitive impairment lasting a month or more. This is commoner with ATS than with cocaine withdrawal, possibly because of the longer half-life of the former.

Treatment of stimulant withdrawal is reviewed in Chapter 59.

Behavioral Pharmacology

Cocaine, ATS, cathinone, ephedrine, and most other stimulants tested in animals consistently produce increased motor activity, repetitive stereotyped behavior, drug discrimination, and evidence of reinforcing effects (such as drug self-administration and conditioned place preference).[125] Animals allowed free access to stimulants often self-administer in a "binge-abstinence" pattern: periods of high levels of drug intake (producing stereotyped behavior, hyperactivity, decreased eating, and little sleep), alternating with periods of abstinence, during which behavior returns to normal. Animals given unlimited access to stimulants may self-administer to the point of death during a binge period. The rewarding effects of stimulants in animals are influenced by the same factors as are other drug and natural reinforcers. The dose of drug available, schedule of reinforcement, past history of drug exposure, current environment, and current condition of the animal can all influence rewarding effects of stimulants. Stimulant self-administration is reduced by increased work requirements, availability of an alternative potent reinforcer, or the concurrent presence of punishment (as by electric shock). Stimulant self-administration is increased by food deprivation or stress.

Animals undergoing forced abstinence after a period of stimulant self-administration initially increase their responding in an apparent attempt to obtain drug but eventually extinguish their drug-seeking behavior.[110] However, they will promptly resume drug-seeking behavior if given a single "priming" dose of the drug or exposed to drug-associated stimuli or stress (such as electric foot shock).[126] This reinstatement of drug-seeking behavior has been considered an animal model of relapse to drug use after treatment.

Stimulants produce a distinctive set of subjective psychological effects (including euphoria, drug liking, increased energy, and increased alertness) in humans under controlled double-blind experimental conditions.[97] D-Amphetamine, benzphetamine, cocaine, ephedrine, mazindol, methylphenidate, phenmetrazine, and phenylpropanolamine are readily distinguished from placebo or sedative drugs but often are not distinguished from each other when equipotent doses are given.

Other Central Nervous System Effects

Acute stimulant administration is associated with transient increases in electroencephalographic (EEG) alpha, beta, and theta activity, which correlate with the acute psychological effects.[127] Case series suggest that stimulant use by any route of administration can cause seizures (usually single, generalized tonic-clonic), even in persons without a preexisting seizure disorder.[128] Most cocaine-associated seizures occur within 90 minutes of drug use, during the time of peak plasma concentration. However, a systematic review of 22 cross-sectional and 1 case-control study did not find cocaine use a significant risk factor for seizures.[129]

Long-term stimulant use is associated with cerebral vasoconstriction, cerebrovascular atherosclerosis, cerebrovascular disease, and ischemic stroke.[130-132] A population-based, 4-year longitudinal study of 617,863 adults living in British Columbia, Canada found that those with a stimulant use disorder had a more than twofold greater risk of having an ischemic stroke than those with no SUD (adjusted OR 2.54, 95% CI 1.14-5.68), after adjusting for age, sex, tobacco use disorder, benzodiazepine use, psychiatric comorbidity, medical comorbidity (eg, diabetes, chronic obstructive lung disease), and socioeconomic status.[133] There was no increased risk for hemorrhagic stroke. A population-based case-control study involving 2,244 subjects found past-24-hour cocaine use significantly associated with stroke (adjusted odds ratio 5.7).[134] An underlying cerebrovascular abnormality, such as arterial aneurysm or arteriovenous malformation, probably increases the risk of cocaine-associated stroke, but the majority of such stroke patients do not have any identified cerebrovascular risk factors. The OTC stimulant phenylpropanolamine, marketed as a decongestant and appetite suppressant, was associated with a significant risk of hemorrhagic stroke, even at recommended doses.[135] Such findings led the FDA to remove phenylpropanolamine from the U.S. market in October 2000.

Stimulant use is associated with a variety of movement disorders, presumably as the result of increased dopamine activity in the basal ganglia and other brain areas that control movement.[136] Such disorders include repetitive stereotyped behaviors (such as repeated dismantling of objects, cleaning, doodling, searching for imaginary objects), acute dystonic reactions, choreoathetosis and akathisia (so-called "crack dancers"), buccolingual dyskinesias ("twisted mouth" or "boca torcida"), and exacerbation of Tourette syndrome and tardive dyskinesia. People who use cocaine are at increased risk of extrapyramidal symptoms (but not akathisia) when taking antipsychotic medications.[137]

Cardiovascular System

Stimulants act acutely on the cardiovascular system both directly (by increasing adrenergic activity at sympathetic nerve terminals) and indirectly via the CNS to increase heart rate, blood pressure, and systemic vascular resistance.[138,139] Stimulant-induced increases in heart rate and blood pressure are significantly correlated with increases in plasma norepinephrine and epinephrine concentrations,[140,141] suggesting mediation by increased activity of the sympathetic nervous system. The mechanism may be prolonged blockade of norepinephrine transporters in the heart, amplifying the action of endogenous norepinephrine.

Cocaine-induced tachycardia increases myocardial oxygen demand and may be accompanied by decreased coronary blood flow (from vasospasm and vasoconstriction). This mismatch between oxygen demand and supply may cause acute myocardial infarction, even in young persons without atherosclerosis. This process may be promoted by cocaine-induced increases in circulating activated platelets, platelet aggregation, and thromboxane synthesis. Cocaine use is a factor in about one-fourth of nonfatal heart attacks in persons younger than 45 years.[142] People who frequently use cocaine are up to seven times more likely to have a nonfatal heart attack than those who do not use cocaine.[142]

Cocaine use is associated with cardiac arrhythmias (such as ventricular tachycardia or fibrillation) and sudden death.[138,143] The mechanisms underlying arrhythmias include blockade of myocyte sodium channels (resulting in impaired cardiac conduction and areas of localized conduction block) and increased concentration of plasma norepinephrine (which sensitizes the myocardium).

Long-term use of stimulants is associated with several cardiovascular conditions, including heart failure, ischemic heart disease, and arrhythmia.[132] Chronic cocaine or amphetamine use is associated with cardiomyopathy and myocarditis.[144-146] Case series of asymptomatic persons with cocaine use disorder find up to half with echocardiographic abnormalities such as left ventricular hypertrophy and abnormal segmental wall motion. Cocaine-associated cases of dilated cardiomyopathy and myocardial fibrosis may be due to direct toxic effects of high concentrations of circulating norepinephrine. Cocaine-associated myocarditis (whose acute symptoms may mimic myocardial infarction) may be a direct toxic effect of cocaine or a hypersensitivity effect. Autopsy series of people who used cocaine have found myocarditis in up to 20%.

Other Organ Systems

No large surveys or prospective studies have comprehensively evaluated the natural history of stimulant use or the frequency of adverse effects. Existing knowledge derives largely from case reports or case series of persons who come to medical attention. In the absence of experimental data, it may be difficult to determine the extent to which an observed adverse effect is the result of a direct action on the affected organ or tissue, an indirect action, an effect of street drug contaminants, or secondary to other factors that are part of a drug-using lifestyle, such as infection, malnutrition, and use of other substances. The most relevant indirect action of cocaine in producing adverse effects in many organs and tissues is ischemia and infarction. These effects result from several mechanisms, including vasoconstriction, vasospasm, damage to vascular endothelium, and increased clotting as the result of increased number of circulating activated platelets, enhanced platelet aggregation, and increased thromboxane synthesis. These mechanisms often reinforce one another. For example, vasospasm may damage endothelium, endothelial damage increases thromboxane synthesis, and thromboxane causes platelet aggregation and vasoconstriction.

Adverse effects of stimulant use on particular organ systems often depend on the route of administration. For example, smoked stimulants produce lung toxicity not found with other routes, injection use is associated with infectious diseases such as AIDS and hepatitis C, and intranasal use is associated with damage to the nasal septum.

Pulmonary

Smoked cocaine produces both acute and chronic pulmonary toxicity.[147-149] Acute respiratory symptoms develop in up to half of people using cocaine within minutes to several hours after smoking. Symptoms include productive cough, shortness of breath, wheezing, chest pain, hemoptysis, and exacerbation of asthma. More severe, and rarer, acute effects include pulmonary edema, pulmonary hemorrhage, pneumothorax, pneumomediastinum, and thermal airway injury. Pulmonary edema has been reported after intravenous cocaine use. Chronic cocaine smoking is associated in case reports with pulmonary and peripheral eosinophilia, interstitial pneumonitis, and bronchiolitis obliterans. The pathophysiology of these adverse effects is not definitively understood but presumably involves a combination of direct damage by cocaine or inhaled microparticles to the alveolar capillary membrane, vasoconstriction, and damage to the pulmonary vascular bed, and/or interstitial disease.

The long-term effect of cocaine smoking on pulmonary function remains unclear.[149] Standard pulmonary function tests (spirometry) are normal in most studies. Some studies find increased alveolar epithelial permeability and moderately decreased (up to 20%) pulmonary diffusion capacity among people who smoke cocaine without acute symptoms, although other studies have found normal function. The attribution of these abnormalities to cocaine use is confounded by the fact that the vast majority of people who smoke cocaine also smoke tobacco and/or cannabis.

Renal

Stimulants have little direct toxic effect on the kidneys. Acute renal failure can occur as a result of renal ischemia or infarction, malignant hypertension, or rhabdomyolysis[150,151] (see Musculoskeletal below). Release of myoglobin during rhabdomyolysis may cause renal tubular obstruction or direct myoglobin damage to renal tubules. Intrarenal arterial constriction with resulting renal medullary ischemia also may contribute to renal tubular damage.

Gastrointestinal

Cocaine reduces gastric motility and delays gastric emptying, in part by affecting medullary centers that regulate these functions. The major gastrointestinal effects of cocaine use are due to vasoconstriction and ischemia: gastroduodenal ulceration and perforation, intestinal infarction and perforation, and ischemic colitis.[152,153] The distribution of cocaine-associated ulcers is primarily in the greater curvature and prepyloric region of the stomach, pyloric canal, and first portion of the duodenum, whereas peptic ulcers occur primarily in the duodenal bulb. Concealing cocaine by swallowing large packets ("body packing") may result in severe acute toxicity if the wrapping deteriorates and allows cocaine into the gastrointestinal tract.[58]

Liver

Cocaine is hepatotoxic in rodents, presumably because of oxidative metabolism to norcocaine by the cytochrome P450 microsomal enzyme system in the liver, with further transformation to reactive hepatotoxic compounds such as *N*-hydroxy-norcocaine.[154] This cytochrome P450 system is a very minor metabolic pathway in humans (see Metabolism above). There is no direct evidence that cocaine is hepatotoxic in humans. Liver abnormalities reported in case series of people who use cocaine are likely due to viral hepatitis from injection drug use, liver disease because of alcohol use, rhabdomyolysis, or other consequences of a drug-using lifestyle.[155]

Endocrine

Acute cocaine and ATS use activates the hypothalamic-pituitary-adrenal (HPA) axis, stimulating secretion of epinephrine, corticotropin-releasing hormone (CRH), ACTH, and cortisol and reducing plasma prolactin concentrations,[156,157] presumably because of increased dopamine activity (dopamine inhibits prolactin release from the pituitary). Stimulants increase blood glucose concentration; their use is associated with increased risk of diabetic ketoacidosis.[158]

Musculoskeletal

Stimulants may cause rhabdomyolysis by several different mechanisms: a direct toxic effect causing myofibrillar degeneration (probably rare except at very high doses), indirectly by vasoconstriction of intramuscular arteries resulting in ischemia, and secondary to stimulant-induced hyperthermia or seizures.[152,159] Up to one-third of patients with rhabdomyolysis will develop acute renal failure, sometimes accompanied by disseminated intravascular coagulation and liver damage. This syndrome often is fatal.

Head and Neck

Common head and neck complications of stimulant use depend on the route of administration. Intranasal cocaine use ("snorting") is associated with chronic rhinitis, erosion or perforation of the nasal septum or palate, oropharyngeal ulcers, and osteolytic sinusitis, presumably due to vasoconstriction and resulting ischemic necrosis.[160] Changes in the senses of smell and taste are rare,[161] except in severe cases. Smoked cocaine ("crack") or amphetamines may cause corneal ulcers due to exposure to aerosolized drug.[162] Use of cocaine or amphetamines by any route of administration reduces salivary secretions (xerostomia) and causes bruxism.[163] Chronic use is associated with several dental problems, including caries, cracking of tooth enamel, and loss of teeth ("meth mouth"). Because oral health problems are pervasive among people who use stimulants, dental professionals serve an important role in identifying these individuals and getting them into treatment.

Immune System

Cocaine use is associated with a variety of vasculitic syndromes primarily affecting the skin and muscle.[164] These may mimic rheumatological conditions such as Henoch-Schönlein purpura, Steven-Johnson syndrome, or Raynaud phenomenon. Cocaine-associated midline destructive lesions may resemble Wegener granulomatosis.[165] In experimental studies, cocaine impairs innate immune mechanisms (eg, the response of monocytes to bacterial lipopolysaccharide).[166]

Sexual Function

Stimulants are commonly regarded as aphrodisiacs, but chronic use usually reduces libido and impairs sexual function.[167-169] Men may experience erectile dysfunction or delayed or inhibited ejaculation. Priapism is rare. Women may develop irregular menses. Cocaine has been applied to the penis or clitoris to use its local anesthetic effect to delay orgasm.[167]

Reproductive, Fetal, and Neonatal Health

Prescription stimulants, including cocaine and amphetamines, are classified by the FDA in pregnancy category C, meaning that risk cannot be ruled out because human studies are lacking. One exception is diethylpropion, which is category B (no evidence of risk in humans). Men who use cocaine chronically have reduced sperm count and motility.[168]

Prenatal (in utero) exposure to cocaine or ATS is associated with vaginal bleeding, abruptio placenta, placenta previa, and premature rupture of membranes in the mother, whereas newborns display decreased head circumference, low birth weight, tremulousness, irritability, poor feeding, and autonomic instability.[170] It is usually difficult in prenatal exposure studies to distinguish a direct effect of the stimulant from the effects of concomitant factors frequently present in people who use drugs, such as other substance use (including alcohol, nicotine, and opioids), poor nutrition, and lack of prenatal care. Long-term studies suggest that prenatal cocaine exposure is associated with small but statistically significant impairments in sustained attention and behavioral self-regulation among preschool- and school-aged children[171] and in language and memory among adolescents.[172] These effects appear modifiable by environmental factors such as prenatal care and the care-giving environment. Their causal mechanisms remain unknown. Cocaine, amphetamines, phentermine, ephedrine, and pseudoephedrine appear in breast milk. Cocaine and amphetamines may cause irritability, sleep disturbance, and tremors in the infant. Medical use by the mother of other prescription and OTC stimulants in appropriate doses usually does not have clinically significant adverse effects on nursing infants.

NEUROBIOLOGY

Mechanisms of Action

Molecular Mechanisms

All stimulant drugs enhance extracellular concentrations of monoamine neurotransmitters in the central and peripheral nervous systems. Stimulants achieve this effect by disrupting the function of plasma membrane transporter proteins expressed on neurons that synthesize and release these neurotransmitters[173] (**Fig. 14-3**). Under normal circumstances, monoamine transporters mediate the reuptake of previously released neurotransmitter molecules from the extracellular space back into nerve cells, thus terminating neurotransmitter action. Because transporters are not confined to nerve endings (ie, synapses), being also found on cells bodies, dendrites, and axons, they are critically involved with controlling extrasynaptic volume transmission of monoamines.[174]

Stimulant drugs can be divided into two classes based on their molecular mechanism of action: transporter blockers (see **Fig. 14-3A**) and transporter substrates (see **Fig. 14-3B**; **Table 14-5**). Transporter blockers, like cocaine and methylphenidate, bind to the extracellular face of transporters and inhibit the reuptake of previously released monoamine neurotransmitters. Thus, transporter blockers are often called *uptake* or *reuptake blockers*. Transporter substrates, like amphetamine and phentermine, have a more complex mechanism of action.[175] These drugs bind to transporters, are transported into the neuronal cytoplasm along with sodium ions, and trigger release of intracellular monoamines by reversing the normal direction of transporter flux. Once inside the neuronal cytoplasm, transporter substrates interact with vesicular monoamine transporters (VMATs) to disrupt monoamine storage, thereby greatly increasing cytoplasmic concentrations of amines available for release. Because transporter substrates elicit transmitter efflux by reverse transport, they are often termed *releasers*.

Potent stimulants like cocaine and amphetamine are active at dopamine and norepinephrine transporters, whereas weaker stimulants like (−)-ephedrine and its isomers preferentially target norepinephrine transporters.[176] Higher affinity binding to the dopamine transporter in vitro is associated with stronger stimulant effects in vivo in animal models. Drugs that selectively interact with serotonin transporters are generally not perceived as stimulant-like and have little or no recreational or SUD liability (eg, serotonin selective reuptake inhibitors, SSRIs).

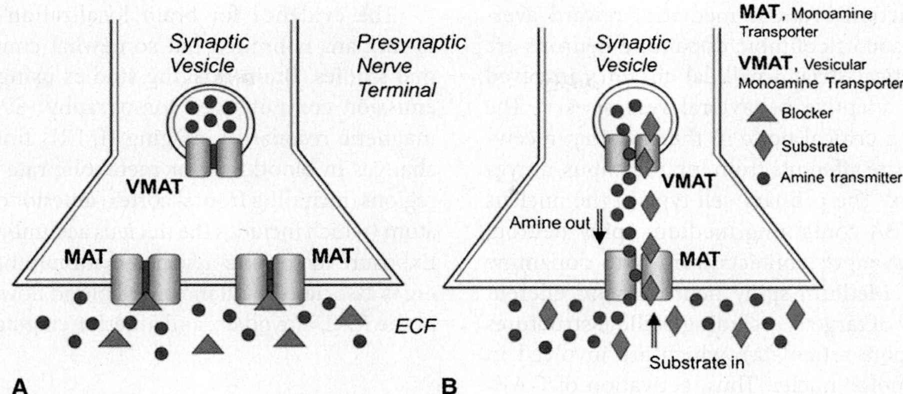

Figure 14-3. Mechanism of action of stimulants acting as monoamine transporter blockers **(A)** or substrates (releasers) **(B)**. Drugs that act as monoamine transporter (MAT) blockers increase the concentration of amine neurotransmitters (ie, dopamine, norepinephrine, and serotonin) in the extracellular fluid (ECF) by blocking reuptake of previously released neurotransmitter molecules. Drugs that act as MAT substrates increase concentrations of amine transmitters in the ECF by a two-pronged mechanism: (1) they promote nonexocytotic release of cytoplasmic amine transmitters by entering neurons and reversing the normal direction of transporter flux (ie, reverse transport), and (2) they disrupt storage of transmitters in vesicles by interacting with vesicular monoamine transporters (VMATs). The disruption of transmitter storage increases cytoplasmic concentration of transmitter molecules available for transporter-mediated release.

Some stimulant drugs have nontransporter sites of action that contribute to their pharmacological effects (see **Table 14-5**). Cocaine blocks plasma membrane voltage-gated sodium ion channels. This action accounts for its local anesthetic effect and may contribute to cardiac arrhythmias. Amphetamines and phentermine are competitive, reversible inhibitors of monoamine oxidase, although this action probably is not significant at the drug concentrations achieved with typical therapeutic or recreational doses.[177] Ephedrine, pseudoephedrine, phenylephrine, and phenylpropanolamine are weak agonists at alpha-adrenergic receptors, which mediate vasoconstriction (hence their use as decongestants and antihypotensive agents). Ephedrine also has some action at beta-adrenergic receptors, which mediate bronchodilation.

Neural Circuits and Systems

Animal studies demonstrate that rewarding effects of stimulants and other addictive substances are mediated by activation of the mesocorticolimbic dopamine system.[178] In the rat, this pathway consists of cells bodies in the ventral tegmental area (VTA) that send axonal projections to the prefrontal cortex (PFC), nucleus accumbens, and amygdala. Distinct subpopulations of VTA dopamine neurons are associated with

TABLE 14-5 Neuropharmacological Actions of Selected Stimulants

	Catecholamine		Serotonin			
	Transporter blocker	Transporter substrate (releaser)	Transporter blocker	Transporter substrate (releaser)	MAO inhibition	Na channel blocker
Amphetamine	++	+++	0	+	+	0
Cocaine	+++	0	++	0	0	+++
Ephedrine[a]	+	++	0	0	0	0
Mazindol	+++	0	+	0	0	0
Methamphetamine	++	+++	+	++	+	0
Methylphenidate	+++	0	+	0	0	0
Modafinil	+++	0	0	0	0	0
Phentermine	+	++	0	0	+	0

[a]Also direct agonist at adrenergic (norepinephrine) receptors.

MAO, monoamine oxidase; 0, no effect; +, marginal effect; ++, substantial effect; +++, predominant effect.

Source: From Docherty JR, Alsufanyi HA. Pharmacology of drugs used as stimulants. *J Clin Pharmacol.* 2021;61(S2):S53-S69; Reyes-Parada M, et al. Amphetamine derivatives as monoamine oxidase inhibitors. *Front Pharmacol.* 2020;10:1590.

projection-specific functional roles in mediating reward, aversion, and stress.[179] Mesocorticolimbic dopamine neurons are part of a complex cortical-striatal-pallidal circuitry involved with the selection of adaptive behavioral responses.[180] The nucleus accumbens is a critical node in the circuitry, receiving stimulatory glutamate afferents from hippocampus, amygdala, and frontal cortex. The primary cell type in the nucleus accumbens is the GABA-containing medium spiny neuron, which receives direct synaptic contacts from both dopamine and glutamate inputs. Medium spiny neurons send efferent projections to a variety of targets, including pallidal structures (eg, substantia nigra pars reticulata), which are involved in tonic suppression of motor nuclei. Thus, activation of GABAergic medium spiny neurons can recruit motor behaviors by inhibiting pallidal output (ie, via disinhibition).

Medium spiny neurons can be divided into two types based on phenotype: neurons expressing low-affinity D_1 dopamine receptors and those expressing high-affinity dopamine D_2 receptors.[181] Medium spiny neurons require glutamate stimulation to drive their activity; dopamine receptors differentially modulate responsiveness to glutamate input. In general, activation of D_1 receptors increases excitability of medium spiny neurons (so-called up state), making them more receptive to glutamate stimulation, whereas activation of D_2 receptors has the opposite effect. Under basal resting conditions, when extracellular dopamine levels are low, high-affinity D_2 receptors inhibit activity of spiny neurons, and behavior is suppressed. When dopamine levels are increased, activation of low-affinity D_1 receptors facilitates excitation of spiny neurons and behavior is executed. Natural rewards induce transient, localized changes in extracellular dopamine in nucleus accumbens (via VTA cell firing) that are capable of modulating stimulatory drive in discrete populations of medium spiny neurons. By contrast, stimulant drugs induce sustained supraphysiological elevations in extracellular dopamine that cause widespread excitation of medium spiny neurons, and repeated drug exposure changes circuit function.

The nucleus accumbens and PFC are the key sites for stimulant reward.[110] In rodents, selective dopamine lesions or administration of dopamine receptor blockers in the nucleus accumbens, but not in other sites, abolish the rewarding effects of cocaine or amphetamine. Rodents will self-administer amphetamine directly into the nucleus accumbens or PFC and cocaine directly into the PFC, but not into other brain sites. Cocaine administration into the PFC increases dopamine turnover in the nucleus accumbens. The relationship between cocaine self-administration and extracellular dopamine concentration in the nucleus accumbens also suggests a key role for this site.[110] A period of cocaine self-administration increases tonic concentrations of extracellular dopamine, with each individual dose producing a time-locked phasic increase. The subsequent decline in dopamine concentration predicts the self-administration of the next dose. Overall, the animal appears to be titrating extracellular dopamine concentration in the nucleus accumbens to maintain an increase above baseline concentration.

The evidence for brain localization of stimulant effects in humans is limited but somewhat consistent with the animal studies. Brain imaging studies using PET, single-photon emission computerized tomography (SPECT), or functional magnetic resonance imaging (fMRI) find stimulant-induced changes in blood flow or metabolic rate in a variety of brain regions, including frontal cortex, anterior cingulate, ventral striatum (which includes the nucleus accumbens), and amygdala.[182] Exposure to cocaine-associated stimuli that elicit cocaine craving is associated with increased blood flow or metabolic activity in the PFC, amygdala, and anterior cingulate gyrus.

Dopamine

Cocaine, ATS, and modafinil enhance dopamine transmission by acting at dopamine transporters, as described earlier (see **Table 14-5**). The cocaine-binding site on the dopamine transporter overlaps with the binding sites for dopamine and amphetamine.[183] Acute administration of cocaine or amphetamine transiently increases brain extracellular dopamine concentrations in animals and humans, especially in the striatum (which includes the nucleus accumbens).[184] Repeated administration of cocaine or amphetamine increases D_1 receptor sensitivity in the nucleus accumbens but has variable effects on other dopamine receptor measures.[185]

Several lines of evidence from animal studies show that increased synaptic dopamine activity in the mesocorticolimbic reward circuit mediates the behavioral effects of stimulants.[178] In rats, the magnitude of locomotor activation produced by methamphetamine and other stimulants is positively correlated with extracellular concentrations of dopamine in the nucleus accumbens.[186] Fluctuations in extracellular dopamine and neuronal firing in the nucleus accumbens parallel cocaine self-administration.[187] The potency of cocaine analogues and other stimulants for being self-administered or producing cocaine-like discriminative stimuli is highly correlated with their affinity for and speed of binding to the dopamine transporter,[188] but not with their binding to other monoamine transporters or receptors.[189] Conversely, lesions of dopamine neurons in the reward circuit (but not other brain regions) reduce cocaine self-administration.[190] Mice genetically engineered to express functional dopamine transporters without a cocaine-binding site do not show reinforcing or other behavioral effects of cocaine.[191-194]

Dopamine D_1 and D_2/D_3 receptors play reciprocal roles in the behavioral effects of stimulants.[185] Blockade of D_1 receptors in regions of the brain reward circuit (eg, the shell of the nucleus accumbens or VTA) reduces the rewarding effects of cocaine or amphetamine in the rat, as does stimulation of D_3 receptors.[195,196] Knockout mice that lack the D_1 receptor do not self-administer cocaine,[197] whereas D_3 knockout mice show enhanced responses to cocaine or amphetamine.[198] In vivo calcium imaging studies, carried out in transgenic mice expressing fluorescent proteins to label defined cell types, show that psychomotor stimulant effects of cocaine are accompanied by rapid activation of D_1 receptors on striatal medium spiny neurons, followed by slower more persistent deactivation of D_2 receptors in the same region.[199]

Evidence from human brain imaging studies using PET or SPECT is largely consistent with an important role for dopamine in the acute psychological effects of stimulants. The acute positive psychological response (euphoria or "high") to cocaine or methylphenidate correlates in time course and intensity with drug concentration in the brain, with dopamine transporter occupancy (in the case of cocaine),[189] and with extracellular dopamine release in the striatum (as measured by ligand displacement from dopamine receptors).[183,184] Exposure to cocaine-associated cues is also associated with dopamine release in the striatum; the degree of release is correlated with intensity of cocaine craving.[184] Blockade of more than half the dopamine receptors is needed to reduce cocaine self-administration in animals[189] or reduce the subjective effects in humans.

Some clinical evidence does not support an important role for dopamine activity in stimulant effects. For example, patients with schizophrenia taking first-generation antipsychotics (which are potent dopamine D_2 receptor antagonists) at doses that control their psychotic symptoms still experience the psychoactive effects of cocaine and frequently use it recreationally.[200] In human laboratory studies, acute pretreatment with dopamine receptor antagonists does not reduce the rewarding effects of cocaine.[201]

Brain imaging studies (PET) in individuals who used stimulants chronically suggest down-regulation of dopamine function in the striatum and frontal cortex, with some differences between cocaine and ATS.[202,203] Postmortem brain studies are largely consistent with these findings. **Table 14-6** presents the pattern of findings. In vivo human studies using PET show that people who use cocaine have decreased dopamine D_2 receptor binding in striatum and frontal cortex, which may persist for months of abstinence, but normal levels of dopamine transporter binding.[184,204,205] Individuals with cocaine use disorder display blunted dopamine release in response to amphetamine challenge, suggesting a presynaptic dopamine deficiency.[205] In contrast, individuals who use methamphetamine have increased D_1 receptors in the nucleus accumbens and decreased dopamine transporter density in nucleus accumbens, striatum, and PFC.[202]

TABLE 14-6 Brain Dopamine Function in People Who Use Stimulants

Dopamine measure	In vivo studies (PET)		Postmortem studies	
	Cocaine	ATS	Cocaine	ATS
D_1 receptor binding	No Δ	No Δ		
D_1 receptor number			No Δ	↑
D_2/D_3 receptor availability	↓	↓		
D_3 receptor binding			↑	
DA synthesis	No Δ	No Δ		
DA release striatum	↓	↓		
DAT availability	↑	↓	↑	↓
VMAT	No Δ	No Δ		

Data show differences from healthy controls with no known history of stimulant use. Blank cells indicate no data available.

ATS, amphetamine, methamphetamine; DA, dopamine; DAT, dopamine transporter; PET, positron emission tomography; VMAT, vesicular monoamine transporter.

Source: From Kohno M, et al. Dopamine dysfunction in stimulant use disorders: mechanistic comparisons and implications for treatment. *Mol Psychiatry.* 2022;27:220-229; Proebstl L, et al. Effects of stimulant drug use on the dopaminergic system: a systematic review and meta-analysis of in vivo neuroimaging studies. *Eur Psychiatry.* 2019;59:15-24.

Norepinephrine

Cocaine, ATS, phentermine, and ephedrine enhance norepinephrine neurotransmission by acting at norepinephrine transporters (see **Table 14-5**), but the importance of norepinephrine in mediating behavioral effects of cocaine is not well understood. Intravenous cocaine increases plasma norepinephrine and epinephrine concentrations within minutes of injection, probably due to blockade of norepinephrine transporters on peripheral sympathetic nerve terminals.[140] There is a significant positive correlation between potency of norepinephrine release (measured in vitro) and the oral stimulant dose that produces stimulant like subjective effects in humans, suggesting a role for norepinephrine in the psychological effects of stimulants.[206] Chronic cocaine exposure increases norepinephrine transporter function in monkey and human brain.[190,207]

Evidence supports a modulatory role for specific norepinephrine receptor subtypes in the effects of cocaine and other stimulants. Blockade of α_1 adrenergic receptors attenuates locomotor effects of stimulants in rats[208] and blunts the subjective effects in individuals who use cocaine.[209] Activation of α_2 adrenergic receptors with clonidine reduces stress-induced reinstatement of extinguished cocaine seeking in rats[210] and drug craving in abstinent individuals with cocaine use disorder.[211] The therapeutic effects of α_2 adrenergic agonists in cocaine use disorder are most likely related to activation of presynaptic auto-receptors on norepinephrine cells, which serve to dampen norepinephrine cell firing and transmitter release.

Serotonin

Most stimulant drugs exhibit lower potency at serotonin transporters than at catecholamine transporters (see **Table 14-5**). Cocaine is an exception, as it blocks uptake at transporters for serotonin, dopamine, and norepinephrine with comparable potency. Acute cocaine administration increases extracellular serotonin concentrations in the nucleus accumbens and VTA and reduces firing of serotonin neurons in the dorsal raphe. The latter action probably is mediated by negative feedback from stimulation of 5-HT_{1A} auto-receptors.[212]

The role of serotonin in stimulant reward in animals is unclear. Knockout mice lacking the serotonin transporter show increased cocaine reward, possibly via a glutamatergic mechanism.[213] Double knockout mice lacking both the dopamine and serotonin transporters do not find cocaine rewarding;

Mice lacking both the norepinephrine and serotonin transporters show increased cocaine reward.[214] These findings suggest a permissive, but not obligatory, role for the serotonin transporter in cocaine reward.

Determining the importance of serotonin receptors in mediating effects of cocaine is complicated by the presence of more than a dozen receptor subtypes, which can differentially influence cocaine-induced behavior.[215] Activation of 5-HT_{1A}, 5-HT_{1B}, 5-HT_{2A}, or 5-HT_3 receptors enhances the locomotor and rewarding actions of cocaine, whereas activation of 5-HT_{2C} receptors reduces the effects of cocaine and other stimulants. 5-HT_{2A} antagonists and 5-HT_{2C} agonists exert similar inhibitory modulation of cocaine's effects. The 5-HT_{2A} antagonist M100907 and 5-HT_{2C} agonist Ro60-0175 attenuate reinstatement of extinguished cocaine-seeking behavior produced by priming injections of cocaine or cue exposure.[216] These same drugs inhibit the premature responding produced by cocaine and amphetamine in the five-choice serial reaction test, a measure of impulsive behavior.[217] Microinjection studies reveal that 5-HT_{2A} receptors in VTA and 5-HT_{2C} receptors in the PFC could be involved with the effects of serotonergic receptor drugs on cocaine-induced behaviors.[218]

Human studies using nonselective serotonin manipulations provide an inconsistent picture of the influence of serotonin on cocaine reward. Enhancement of synaptic serotonin activity with selective serotonin reuptake inhibitors, activation of serotonin receptors with a partial agonist, or depletion of serotonin levels (via a tryptophan-free diet) all reduce the acute subjective effects ("high," craving) of cocaine in humans.[219] Neuroendocrine challenge studies in individuals with cocaine use disorder show that hormonal responses to serotonin releasers (fenfluramine) and serotonin receptor agonists (mCPP) are blunted during withdrawal.[220,221] These findings suggest that chronic cocaine use engenders deficits in serotonergic transmission.[222] The clinical availability of receptor-selective agonists and antagonists will aid in determining the role of serotonin in stimulant reward.

Endogenous Opioids

Stimulants do not directly interact with opioid receptors but do influence endogenous opioid (endorphin, enkephalin) systems in the brain. In rats, single doses of cocaine or amphetamine increase extracellular endorphin levels in the nucleus accumbens and enkephalin and dynorphin mRNA levels in striatum.[223,224] The mechanism is indirect, via other neurotransmitters, especially dopamine, that influence endogenous opioid release.

Repeated cocaine administration increases brain mu and delta opioid receptor expression in rodents, with no change in kappa opioid receptors.[225] Human subjects who use cocaine show increased mu opioid receptor binding in some brain regions with PET scanning, and this increased binding correlates with self-reported cocaine craving.[226] Postmortem brains from fatal cocaine overdose victims show increased kappa opioid receptor binding in limbic areas, although rodent studies show no consistent effect of kappa opioid receptor ligands on cocaine reward.[224]

Glutamate

The acute administration of cocaine or ATS increases glutamate release in the VTA, nucleus accumbens, dorsal striatum, ventral pallidum, septum, and cerebellum.[227,228] Low doses of cocaine enhance glutamate-evoked neuronal firing and have variable effects on the different subtypes of glutamate receptors. Several glutamate receptor subtypes play an important role in cocaine reinforcement. Blockade of *N*-methyl-D-aspartate receptors in the nucleus accumbens reduces cocaine reinforcement, as does reduction of mGluR5 receptor activity. Indirect reduction of glutamate activity by stimulating presynaptic mGluR2 receptors also reduces cocaine reinforcement, whereas inhibiting mGluR2 activity enhances reinforcement.

Rat studies suggest that chronic treatment with noncontingent or self-administered cocaine changes nucleus accumbens glutamate transmission, which persists for weeks after abstinence from cocaine exposure.[228] For instance, chronic cocaine treatment is accompanied by a marked decrease in nonsynaptic extracellular glutamate levels, due to a reduction in cysteine-glutamate exchange. Cocaine-induced decreases in nucleus accumbens glutamate levels may be involved in drug-seeking behavior because treatment with the prodrug *N*-acetylcysteine restores extracellular glutamate to normal levels and attenuates reinstatement of extinguished cocaine-seeking behavior. Withdrawal from chronic cocaine decreases membrane excitability in GABA-containing medium spiny neurons, which in turn induces a persistent up-regulation of AMPA-type glutamate receptors on these cells. Up-regulation of AMPA receptors renders medium spiny neurons more receptive to glutamate inputs from the cortex and other regions. Enhanced glutamate responsiveness in mesolimbic circuits could underlie stronger responding to drug-associated cues.

γ-Amino-Butyric Acid

γ-Amino-butyric acid (GABA) is the major inhibitory neurotransmitter in the CNS; GABA-ergic neurons in the nucleus accumbens play a key role in the mesocorticolimbic reward circuit[229] (see Neural Circuits and Systems above). In rats, acute administration of cocaine or methamphetamine indirectly reduces activity at VTA $GABA_B$ receptors, which disinhibits dopamine neurons.[229] At the same time, the stimulant is increasing extracellular dopamine concentration, thereby increasing dopamine D_1 receptor activity, which stimulates $GABA_B$ receptor (inhibitory) activity. Chronic administration of cocaine or methamphetamine also decreases $GABA_B$ receptor activity in several brain regions, including VTA and medial PFC.[229] Rodents in withdrawal from self-administering cocaine show large decreases in $GABA_B$ receptor binding in several regions of the mesocorticolimbic reward circuit, including the VTA, nucleus accumbens, and medial PFC.[229]

Acetylcholine

Both muscarinic and nicotinic cholinergic receptors are expressed in regions of the brain reward circuit.[230] Cocaine and ATS block neuronal nicotinic acetylcholine (ACh) receptors[231-233]; cocaine also blocks muscarinic ACh receptors in the brain.[231] Cocaine, amphetamine, and methamphetamine release ACh in several brain regions, including the striatum, nucleus accumbens, medial thalamus, and interpeduncular nucleus.[230,231,234] Chronic cocaine or methamphetamine exposure down-regulates brain cholinergic systems, reflected in decreased muscarinic receptors[230,231] and decreased choline acetyltransferase activity,[235] although findings vary depending on dose and duration of treatment.

Signal Transduction

When monoamine neurotransmitters such as dopamine activate their membrane receptors on the nerve cell surface, they trigger a cascade of intracellular chemical events.[236] The neurotransmitter receptors are coupled to G-proteins, which regulate adenylyl cyclase activity to alter levels of cyclic 3′,5′-adenosine monophosphate (cAMP), an intracellular "second messenger." Cyclic AMP, in turn, regulates the activity of protein kinases, phospholipases, and other intracellular enzymes. These enzymes regulate various intracellular processes, including the activity of transcription factors that regulate gene transcription, by binding to specific DNA sequences in the regulatory regions of genes (see Gene Expression below). Stimulants activate several signaling pathways in neurons of the brain reward circuit, including cAMP, extracellular signal-regulated kinase, mitogen-activated protein kinase, and phosphoinositide 3-kinase, as well as altering expression of proteins that regulate G protein signaling. Direct manipulation of steps in these pathways can modify stimulant-induced behavior.[237,238] Changes to these pathways from chronic exposure to stimulants may mediate tolerance and sensitization (see Neuroadaptation below).

Gene Expression

Acute administration of stimulants (such as cocaine, amphetamine, and methylphenidate) to rodents promptly activates several "immediate early" genes in the brain, such as cAMP response element-binding protein (CREB), c-*fos*, *zif268*, and c-*jun*, probably via activation of dopamine receptors.[239] The protein products of these genes are nuclear transcription factors that regulate gene expression. Repeated administration of stimulants results in a long-lasting blunting of the gene activation effect in many brain regions. Chronic stimulant administration leads to accumulation of some transcription factors, which may mediate the development of sensitization (see Neuroadaptation below).

In animal studies, acute or chronic stimulant administration results in changes in expression of a variety of genes in many brain regions related to SUD, including genes involved in neuronal growth, cytoskeletal structure, synaptic plasticity, and receptors and signal transduction.[51] Human postmortem studies of individuals who used cocaine chronically do not always find the same changes. Genes significantly up-regulated in human studies include cocaine- and amphetamine-related transcript, CREB, and several glutamate receptor subunits, whereas several myelin-related genes were down-regulated.

Neuroadaptation

Repeated exposure to stimulants can result in two distinct neuroadaptations: sensitization (increased drug response)[240] and tolerance (decreased drug response).[241] Development of these neuroadaptations depends on pharmacological, genetic,[242] and environmental factors.

Behavioral sensitization has two temporally distinct phases: *initiation* or *induction* and *expression*.[240] A combination of pharmacological and environmental factors influences both phases. Sensitization is promoted by intermittent stimulant exposure and rapid stimulant administration, while tolerance is more likely to occur with continuous, high-dose exposure.[243] Sensitization is more likely to occur when the stimulant is taken in the same environment (so-called "context-specific" or "conditioned" sensitization).[244] In utero exposure to stimulants in rodents leads to long-term stimulant sensitization in the offspring.[245] Behavioral sensitization to stimulants is mediated, in part, by changes in glutamatergic and GABAergic activity in the PFC, which in turn promote increased dopaminergic activity in the nucleus accumbens and VTA.[246] There can be cross-sensitization between cocaine and amphetamines.[247]

Behavioral sensitization to stimulants has been suggested as a mechanism for drug craving and relapse[248] and for stimulant-induced psychosis.[249] Neither has been directly demonstrated in humans. Several retrospective evaluations of patients presenting with stimulant-induced psychosis found that psychotic symptoms were more severe than during prior episodes of use or were elicited at lower doses that previously had not caused such symptoms.[249] This pattern is consistent with sensitization (ie, an enhanced response to the drug after prior exposure).

Attempts to demonstrate sensitization prospectively in humans have yielded inconsistent results.[250] Studies using intravenous, intranasal, or oral cocaine in people experienced with using cocaine failed to show sensitization after one to several prior cocaine doses. One study using oral cocaine did find significant sensitization to cocaine's cardiovascular effects but not to its psychological effects.[251] Studies using oral amphetamines in subjects with little or no prior stimulant exposure have shown sensitization to psychological and physiological (eye blink rate) responses after one to three prior oral amphetamine doses. This sensitized response was still present 1 year after the last amphetamine dose and included increased dopamine release in the ventral striatum (measured by PET scanning).[252] The failure to show sensitization in other studies may have been due to the substantial prior stimulant exposure of most subjects, resulting in sensitization already having occurred (ie, a "ceiling" effect).

Tolerance to the behavioral (eg, hyperactivity, reinforcement, euphoria) and physiological (tachycardia) effects of stimulants has been demonstrated in animals and humans.[241,248,253] Tolerance to different stimulant effects may develop at different rates[107] and can sometimes develop after just a few exposures.[253,254] There is significant cross-tolerance among various stimulants.

Stimulant tolerance is pharmacodynamic (ie, due to adaptive changes in the brain) rather than pharmacokinetic; chronic stimulant exposure does not change stimulant pharmacokinetics.[253,254] Development of tolerance is associated with attenuation of the dopamine response to stimulants.[241]

In clinical use, tolerance to stimulants develops differentially to various effects. Patients typically become tolerant to the appetite-suppressing effects within several weeks of daily use, whereas the beneficial effects in narcolepsy or ADHD often remain over months of treatment.[254]

Neurotoxicity

Long-term use of stimulants (cocaine, ATS, cathinones) is associated with neurotoxicity in animals.[255,256] ATS appear more neurotoxic than cocaine, with methamphetamine being the most neurotoxic, especially to serotonergic neurons. Neurotoxicity appears in both gray matter (neurons and glia) and white matter (axons).[257,258] Several mechanisms are involved, including increased oxidative stress from generation of oxygen free radicals and disruption of mitochondrial function, resulting in cell death (apoptosis).[259] Tissue hypoxia from vasoconstriction may contribute to cocaine-associated neurotoxicity.[255]

Neurotoxicity has not been as conclusively demonstrated in people who use stimulants long-term. Such individuals have reduced density of dopamine transporters in the brain (measured by PET scanning), with only partial recovery after long-term abstinence.[256] It remains unclear whether this loss of transporters represents a reversible physiological response (down-regulation) to chronic stimulant exposure or a true loss of dopamine nerve endings. People who use cocaine or methamphetamine chronically show significant abnormalities of white matter microstructure on MRI, suggesting abnormalities in myelination and axon structure.[257,258] A postmortem brain study of individuals with methamphetamine use disorder found increased neuronal degeneration and cell death in the prefrontal cortex.[260]

Use of cocaine, ATS, and cathinones is associated with genotoxicity in in vitro and in vivo animal studies, including DNA damage and abnormal DNA methylation, as well as with fetal malformations.[261-265] Exposure to smoked cocaine is especially damaging, possibly because of the presence of pyrolytic compounds.[264-266] Individuals who smoke cocaine have genetic damage in cells of peripheral blood and oral mucosa.[264]

The clinical relevance of data from preclinical toxicity studies remains unclear. Earlier studies finding cocaine- and methamphetamine-associated teratogenesis had small samples sizes and often failed to adequately control for known confounds such as use of other substances, exposure to environmental toxins, and poor diet.[267] Recent more rigorous studies do not find a significant association between stimulant use and increased risk of fetal malformation.[267,268]

FUTURE RESEARCH DIRECTIONS

Future research at both preclinical and clinical levels is needed to increase understanding of the mechanisms of stimulant addiction and to develop more effective prevention and treatment approaches. Productive areas for preclinical research include the neurochemical mechanisms that underlie stimulant sensitization and tolerance, the role of nondopamine neurotransmitter systems (eg, glutamate, neuropeptides, trace amino acids[269]) in modulating the dopamine reward circuit, the molecular mechanisms underlying stimulant interactions with transporter proteins, and the role of various genes and gene transcription factors in stimulant action.

Productive areas for clinical research include the genetic, hormonal, psychological, and environmental factors that influence response to stimulants and the progression to stimulant use disorder and the development of effective treatments for stimulant use disorder and its adverse consequences.

REFERENCES

1. Hashemian SM, Farhadi T. A review on modafinil: the characteristics, function, and use in critical care. *J Drug Assess*. 2020;9(1):82-86.
2. Bauer I. Travel medicine, coca, and cocaine: demystifying and rehabilitating *Erythroxylum*—a comprehensive review. *Tropical Dis Travel Med Vaccine*. 2019;5:20.
3. Fowler JS, Volkow ND, Wang GJ, et al. [11]Cocaine: PET studies of cocaine pharmacokinetics, dopamine transporter availability and dopamine transporter occupancy. *Nucl Med Biol*. 2001;28(5):407-416.
4. Dinis-Oliveira RS. Metabolomics of cocaine: implications in toxicity. *Toxicol Mech Methods*. 2015;25(6):494-500.
5. Yeh K, Li L, Wania F, et al. Thirdhand smoke from tobacco, e-cigarettes, cannabis, methamphetamine, and cocaine: Partitioning, reactive fate, and human exposure in indoor environments. *Environ Int*. 2022;160:107063.
6. Broseus J, Gentile N, Esseiva P. The cutting of cocaine and heroin: a critical review. *Forensic Sci Int*. 2016;262:73-83.
7. Midthun KM, Nelson LS, Logan BK. Levamisole—a toxic adulterant in illicit drug preparations: a review. *Ther Drug Monit*. 2021;43:221-228.
8. Costa VM, Grando LGR, Milandri E, et al. Natural sympathomimetic drugs: from pharmacology to toxicology. *Biomolecules*. 2022;12:1793.
9. Patel NB. Khat (Catha edulis Forsk)—and now there are three. *Brain Res Bull*. 2019;145:92-96.
10. Silva B, Soares J, Rocha-Pereira C, Mladenka P, Remião F. Khat, a cultural chewing drug: a toxicokinetic and toxicodynamic summary. *Toxins*. 2022;14:71.
11. Edwards B, Atkins N. Exploring the association between khat use and psychiatric symptoms: a systematic review. *BMJ Open*. 2022;12:e061865.
12. Steingard R, Taskiran S, Connor DF, et al. New formulations of stimulants: an update for clinicians. *J Child Adolesc Psychopharmacol*. 2019;29(5):324-339.
13. Carton L, Icick R, Weibel S, et al. What is the potential for abuse of lisdexamfetamine in adults? A preclinical and clinical literature review and expert opinion. *Expert Rev Clin Pharmacol*. 2022;15(8):921-925.

14. Gorelick DA. The rate hypothesis and agonist substitution approaches to cocaine abuse treatment. *Adv Pharmacol.* 1998;42:995-997.
15. Robitaille C, Collin J. Prescription psychostimulant use among young adults: a narrative review of qualitative studies. *Subst Use Misuse.* 2016;51(3):357-369.
16. Chen LY, Crum RM, Strain EC, Alexander GC, Kaufmann C, Mojtabai R. Prescriptions, nonmedical use, and emergency department visits involving prescription stimulants. *J Clin Psychiatry.* 2016;77(3):e297-e304.
17. Jacobs DS, Blough BE, Kohut SJ. Reinforcing and stimulant-like effects of methamphetamine isomers in Rhesus macaques. *J Pharmacol Exp Ther.* 2021;378:124-132.
18. Heal DJ, Smith SL, Gosden J, et al. Amphetamine, past and present—a pharmacological and clinical perspective. *J Psychopharmacol.* 2013; 27(6):479-496.
19. Combs CC, Hankins EL, Copeland CL, et al. Quantitative determination of D- and L-threo enantiomers of methylphenidate in brain tissue by liquid chromatography—mass spectrometry. *Biomed Chromatogr.* 2013; 27:1587-1589.
20. Baumann MH, Walters HM, Niello M, Sitte HH. Neuropharmacology of synthetic cathinones. *Handb Exp Pharmacol.* 2018;252:113-142.
21. Soares J, Costa VM, Bastos ML, Carvalho F, Capela JP. An updated review on synthetic cathinones. *Arch Toxicol.* 2021;95(9):2895-2940.
22. Said AM, Farboud A, Delfosse E, et al. Assessing the safety and efficacy of drugs used in preparing the nose for diagnostic and therapeutic procedures: a systematic review. *Clin Otolaryngol.* 2016;41:546-563.
23. Armbuster YC, Banas BN, Feikert KD, et al. Decline and pronounced regional disparities in medical cocaine usage in the United States. *J Pharmacy Technol.* 2021;37(6):278-285.
24. Murdoch I, Surda P, Nguyen-Lu N. Anaesthesia for rhinological surgery. *BJA Educ.* 2021;21(6):225-231.
25. Stuhec M, Lukic P, Locatelli I. Efficacy, acceptability, and tolerability of lisdexamfetamine, mixed amphetamine salts, methylphenidate, and modafinil in the treatment of attention-deficit hyperactivity disorder in adults: a systematic review and meta-analysis. *Ann Pharmacotherapy.* 2019;53(2):121-133.
26. Gandhi KD, Mansukhani MP, Silber MH, et al. Excessive daytime sleepiness: a clinical review. *Mayo Clin Proc.* 2021;96(5):1288-1301.
27. Ono T, Takenoshita S, Nishino S. Pharmacologic management of excessive daytime sleepiness. *Sleep Med Clin.* 2022;17(3):485-503.
28. Ahmad NN, Robinson S, Kennedy-Martin T, Poon JL, Kan H. Clinical outcomes associated with anti-obesity medications in real-world practice: a systematic literature review. *Obes Rev.* 2021;22(11):e13326.
29. Clemow DB, Walker DJ. The potential for misuse and abuse of medications in ADHD: a review. *Postgrad Med.* 2014;126(5):64-81.
30. Deckx L, De Sutter AI, Guo L, Mir NA, van Driel ML. Nasal decongestants in monotherapy for the common cold. *Cochrane Database Syst Rev.* 2016;(10):CD009612.
31. Sinita E, Coghill D. The use of stimulant medications for non-core aspects of ADHD and in other disorders. *Neuropharmacology.* 2014;87:161-172.
32. Bahji A, Mesbah-Oskui L. Comparative efficacy and safety of stimulant-type medications for depression: a systematic review and network meta-analysis. *J Affect Disord.* 2021;292:416-423.
33. Perugi G, Vannucchi G, Bedani F, Favaretto E. Use of stimulants in bipolar disorder. *Curr Psychiatry Rep.* 2017;19(1):7.
34. Malhi GS, Byrow Y, Bassett D, et al. Stimulants for depression: on the up and up? *Aust N Z J Psychiatry.* 2016;50(3):203-207.
35. Huang CH, Huang CC, Sun CK, Lin GH, Hou WH. Methylphenidate on cognitive improvement in patients with traumatic brain injury: a meta-analysis. *Curr Neuropharmacol.* 2016;14(3):272-281.
36. Walker-Batson D, Mehta J, Smith P, Johnson M. Amphetamine and other pharmacological agents in human and animal studies of recovery from stroke. *Prog Neuropsychopharmacol Biol Psychiatry.* 2016;64:225-230.
37. Mucke M, Mochamat, Cuhls H, et al. Pharmacological treatments for fatigue associated with palliative care: executive summary of a Cochrane Collaboration systematic review. *J Cachexia Sarcopenia Muscle.* 2016;7(1):23-27.
38. Martinez-Raga J, Knecht C, Szerman N, Martinez MI. Risk of serious cardiovascular problems with medications for attention-deficit hyperactivity disorder. *CNS Drugs.* 2013;27(1):15-30.
39. Humphreys KL, Eng T, Lee SS. Stimulant medication and substance use outcomes: a meta-analysis. *JAMA Psychiat.* 2013;70(7):740-749.
40. Bagot KS, Kaminer Y. Efficacy of stimulants for cognitive enhancement in non-attention deficit hyperactivity disorder youth: a systematic review. *Addiction.* 2014;109(4):547-557.
41. Franke AG, Bagusat C, Rust S, Engel A, Lieb K. Substances used and prevalence rates of pharmacological cognitive enhancement among healthy subjects. *Eur Arch Psychiatry Clin Neurosci.* 2014;264(Suppl 1): S83-S90.
42. Vosburg SK, Robbins RS, Antshel KM, et al. Characterizing prescription stimulant nonmedical use (NMU) among adults recruited from Reddit. *Addict Behav Rep.* 2021;14:100376.
43. Schifano F, Catalani V, Sharif S, et al. Benefits and harms of 'smart' drugs (nootropics) in healthy individuals. *Drugs.* 2022;82:633-647.
44. Berezanskaya J, Cade W, Best TM, et al. ADHD prescription medications and their effect on athletic performance: a systematic review and meta-analysis. *Sports Med Open.* 2022;8:5.
45. Heuberger JAAC, Cohen JF. Review of WADA prohibited substances: limited evidence for performance-enhancing effects. *Sports Med.* 2019;49:525-539.
46. Mustaquim D, Jones CM, Compton WM. Trends and correlates of cocaine use among adults in the United States, 2006-2019. *Addict Behav.* 2021;120:106950.
47. Jones CM, Houry D, Han B, et al. Methamphetamine use in the United States: epidemiological update and implications for prevention, treatment, and harm reduction. *Ann NY Acad Sci.* 2022;508:3-22.
48. Liu Y, Cheong JW, Vaddiparti K, et al. The association between quantity, frequency, and duration of cocaine use during heaviest use period and risk of DSM-5 cocaine use disorder. *Drug Alcohol Depend.* 2020;213:108114.
49. Allain F, Minogianis EA, Roberts DC, et al. How fast and how often: the pharmacokinetics of drug use are decisive in addiction. *Neurosci Biobehav Rev.* 2015;82(1):166-179.
50. Le VT, Turner AN, McDaniel A, et al. Nonmedical use of over-the-counter medications is significantly associated with nonmedical use of prescription drugs among university students. *J Am College Health.* 2018;61(1):1-8.
51. Fernandez-Castillo N, Cabana-Dominguez J, Corominas R, et al. Molecular genetics of cocaine use disorder in humans. *Molec Psychiatry.* 2022;27:624-639.
52. Guerin AA, Nestler EJ, Berk M, et al. Genetics of methamphetamine use disorder: a systematic review and meta-analyses of gene association studies. *Neurosci Biobehav Rev.* 2021;120:48-74.
53. Liu Y, Vaddiparti K, Cheong JW, et al. Identification of typologies of cocaine use based on quantity, frequency, and duration of use: a latent profile analysis. *J Addict Med.* 2021;15:211-218.
54. Roy E, Arruda N, Jutras-Aswad D, et al. Examining the link between cocaine binging and individual, social, and behavioral factors among street-based cocaine users. *Addict Behav.* 2017;68:66-72.
55. Kuypers KPC, Verkes RJ, van den Brink W, et al. Intoxicated aggression: do alcohol and stimulants cause dose-related aggression? A review. *Eur Neuropsychopharmacol.* 2020;30:114-147.
56. Zhong S, Yu R, Fazel S. Drug use disorders and violence: associations with individual drug categories. *Epidemiol Rev.* 2020;42:103-116.
57. Butler AJ, Rehm J, Fischer B. Health outcomes associated with crack-cocaine use: systematic review and meta-analyses. *Drug Alcohol Depend.* 2017;180:401-416.
58. Cappelletti S, Piacentino D, Sani G, et al. Systematic review of the toxicological and radiological features of body packing. *Int J Legal Med.* 2016;130:693-709.
59. Liu Y, Williamson V, Setlow B, et al. The importance of considering polysubstance abuse: lessons from cocaine research. *Drug Alcohol Depend.* 2018;192:16-28.

60. Leeman RF, Sun Q, Bogart D, et al. Comparison of cocaine-only, opioid-only, and users of both substances in the National Epidemiological Survey of Alcohol and Related Conditions (NESARC). *Substance Use Misuse.* 2016;51(5):553-564.
61. Goodwin RD, Moeller SJ, Zhu J, et al. The potential role of cocaine and heroin co-use in the opioid epidemic in the United States. *Addict Behav.* 2021;113:106680.
62. Ciccarone D, Shoptaw S. Understanding stimulant use and use disorders in a new era. *Med Clin N Am.* 2022;106:81-97.
63. Ciccarone D. The rise of illicit fentanyls, stimulants and the fourth wave of the opioid overdose crisis. *Curr Opin Psychiatry.* 2021;34(4):344-350.
64. Shuang-Man M, Qi Z, Xiao-Bao B, et al. A review of the phytochemistry and pharmacological activities *Ephedra* herb. *Chinese J Nat Med.* 2020;18(5):321-344.
65. Drake LR, Scott PJH. DARK classics in chemical neuroscience: cocaine. *ACS Chem Neurosci.* 2018;9:2358-2372.
66. Morelli M, Tognotti E. Brief history of the medical and non-medical use of amphetamine-type stimulants. *Exp Neurol.* 2021;342:113754.
67. United Nations Office on Drugs and Crime. *World Drug Report 2022.* United Nations Publication; 2022.
68. Molina-Avila I, Rojas AA, Gilligan G, et al. Oral squamous cell carcinoma in coca chewers from a north region of Argentina: a case series and review of literature. *J Oral Maxillofac Pathol.* 2022;26:S124-S128.
69. Center for Behavioral Health Statistics and Quality. *Results From 2020 National Survey on Drug Use and Health: Detailed Tables.* Substance Abuse and Mental Health Services Administration; 2021. Accessed January 21, 2022. https://www.samhsa.gov/data/
70. Crummy EA, O'Neal TJ, Baskin BM, et al. One is not enough: understanding and modeling polysubstance use. *Front Neurosci.* 2020;14:569.
71. Jegede O, Rhee TG, Stefanovics EA, et al. Rates and correlates of dual diagnosis among adults with psychiatric and substance use disorders in a nationally representative US sample. *Psychiatry Res.* 2022;315:114720.
72. GBD 2016 Alcohol and Drug Use Collaborators. The global burden of disease attributable to alcohol and drug use in 195 countries and territories, 1990–2016: a systematic analysis for the Global Burden of Disease Study 2016. *Lancet Psychiatry.* 2018;5:987-1012.
73. American Psychiatric Association. *Diagnostic and Statistical Manual of Mental Disorders, Fifth Edition (DSM-5).* American Psychiatric Association; 2013.
74. Markowitz JS, Melchert PW. The pharmacokinetics and pharmacogenomics of psychostimulants. *Child Adolesc Psychiatr Clin N Am.* 2022;31(3):393-416.
75. Fowler JS, Volkow ND, Logan J. Fast uptake and long-lasting binding of methamphetamine in the human brain: comparison with cocaine. *NeuroImage.* 2008;43:756-763.
76. Roque Bravo R, Faria AC, Brito-da-Costa AM, et al. Cocaine: an updated review on chemistry, detection, biokinetics, and pharmacotoxicological aspects including abuse patterns. *Toxins.* 2022;14:278.
77. Gelhausen JM, Klette JL, Stout PR. Occupational cocaine exposure of crime laboratory personnel preparing training aids for a military working dog program. *J Anal Toxicol.* 2003;27:453-458.
78. Stout PR, Horn CK, Klette KL, et al. Occupational exposure to methamphetamine in workers preparing training aids for drug detection dogs. *J Anal Toxicol.* 2006;30:551-553.
79. Verstraete AG. Detection times of drugs of abuse in blood, urine, and oral fluid. *Ther Drug Monit.* 2004;26(2):200-205.
80. Cuypers E, Flanagan RJ. The interpretation of hair analysis for drugs and drug metabolites. *Clin Toxicol.* 2018;56(2):90-100.
81. de Campos EG, da Costa BRB, dos Santos FS, et al. Alternative matrices in forensic toxicology: a critical review. *Forensic Toxicol.* 2022;40:1-18.
82. Solimini R, Minutillo A, Kyriakou C, et al. Nails in forensic toxicology: an update. *Curr Pharm Des.* 2017;23(36):5468-5479.
83. Wabuyele SL, Colby JM, McMillan GA. Detection of drug-exposed newborns. *Ther Drug Monit.* 2018;40(2):166-185.
84. Morse AK, Askovic M, Sercombe J, et al. A systematic review of efficacy, effectiveness, and cost-effectiveness of workplace-based interventions for the prevention and treatment of problematic substance use. *Front Public Health.* 2022;10:1051119.
85. Jarvis M, Williams J, Hurford M, et al. Appropriate use of drug testing in clinical addiction medicine. *J Addict Med.* 2017;11:163-173.
86. Drummer OH. Postmortem toxicology of drugs of abuse. *Forensic Sci Int.* 2004;142(2-3):101-113.
87. Abbruscato TJ, Trippier PC. DARK classics in chemical neuroscience: methamphetamine. *ACS Chem Neurosci.* 2018;9:2373-2378.
88. Huang W, Czuba LC, Isoherranen N. Mechanistic PBPK modeling of urine pH effect on renal and systemic disposition of methamphetamine and amphetamine. *J Pharmacol Exp Ther.* 2020;373:488-501.
89. Abbott KL, Flannery PC, Gill KS, et al. Adverse pharmacokinetic interactions between illicit substances and clinical drugs. *Drug Metab Rev.* 2020;52(1):44-65.
90. Schoretsanitis G, de Leon J, Eap CB, et al. Clinically significant drug–drug interactions with agents for attention-deficit/hyperactivity disorder. *CNS Drugs.* 2019;33:1201-1222.
91. Lorenzini KI, Girardin F. Direct-acting antiviral interactions with opioids, alcohol or illicit drugs of abuse in HCV-infected patients. *Liver Int.* 2020;40:32-44.
92. Desai N, Burns L, Gong Y, et al. An update on drug-drug interactions between anti-retroviral therapies and drugs of abuse in HIV systems. *Expert Opin Drug Metab Toxicol.* 2020;16(11):1005-1018.
93. Pergolizzi J, Breve F, Magnusson P, et al. Cocaethylene: when cocaine and alcohol are taken together. *Cureus.* 2022;14(2):e22498.
94. Peacock A, Tran LT, Larney S, et al. All-cause and cause-specific mortality among people with regular or problematic cocaine use: a systematic review and meta-analysis. *Addiction.* 2020;116:725-742.
95. Stockings E, Tran LT, Santo T Jr, et al. Mortality among people with regular or problematic use of amphetamines: a systematic review and meta-analysis. *Addiction.* 2019;114:1738-1750.
96. Substance Abuse and Mental Health Services Administration. *Preliminary Findings From Drug-Related Emergency Department Visits, 2021.* Drug Abuse Warning Network (HHS Publication No. PEP22-07-03-001). Center for Behavioral Health Statistics and Quality, Substance Abuse and Mental Health Services Administration; 2022. Accessed June 1, 2022. https://www.samhsa.gov/data/
97. Strzelecki A, Weafer J, Stoops WW. Human behavioral pharmacology of stimulant drugs: an update and narrative review. *Adv Pharmacol.* 2022;23:77-103.
98. Ogeil RP, Phillips JG, Savic M, et al. Sleep- and wake-promoting drugs: where are they being sourced, and what is their impact? *Subst Use Misuse.* 2019;54(12):1916-1928.
99. Angarita GA, Emadi N, Hodges S, et al. Sleep abnormalities associated with alcohol, cannabis, cocaine, and opiate use: a comprehensive review. *Addict Sci Clin Pract.* 2016;11:9.
100. Maboub N, Rizk R, Karaveetian M, et al. Nutritional status and eating habits of people who use drugs and/or are undergoing treatment for recovery: a narrative review. *Nutr Rev.* 2020;79(6):627-635.
101. Sabe M, Zhao N, Kaiser S. A systematic review and meta-analysis of the prevalence of cocaine-induced psychosis in cocaine users. *Progr Neuropsychopharmacol Biol Psychiatry.* 2021;109:110263.
102. Bramness JG, Rognli EB. Psychosis induced by amphetamines. *Curr Opin Psychiatry.* 2016;29(4):236-241.
103. Vergara-Moragues E, Mestre-Pinto JI, Gomez PA, et al. Can symptoms help in differential diagnosis between substance-induced vs independent psychosis in adults with a lifetime diagnosis of cocaine use disorder? *Psychiatry Res.* 2016;242:94-100.
104. Waters F, Fernyhough C. Hallucinations: a systematic review of points of similarity and difference across diagnostic classes. *Schiz Bull.* 2017;43(1):32-43.
105. Juan Juan C, de la Hoya S, Zamácola P. Prickling or formication after the use of cocaine. *Rev Esp Sanid Penit.* 2018;20:70-72.
106. Baizabal-Carvallo JF, Morgan JC. Drug-induced tremor, clinical features, diagnostic approach and management. *J Neurol Sci.* 2022;435:120192.
107. Vorspan F, Icick R, Mekdad N, et al. Translational study of the whole transcriptome in rats and genetic polymorphisms in humans identifies

LRP1B and VPS13A as key genes involved in tolerance to cocaine-induced motor disturbances. *Transl Psychiatry*. 2020;10:381.

108. Nam S-H, Lim MH, Park TW. Stimulant induced movement disorders in attention deficit hyperactivity disorder. *J Korean Acad Child Adolesc Psychiatry*. 2022;33(2):27-34.
109. Elmer GI, Miner LL, Pickens RW. The contribution of genetic factors in cocaine and other drug abuse. In: Higgins ST, Katz JL, eds. *Cocaine Abuse: Behavior, Pharmacology, and Clinical Applications*. Academic Press; 1998:289-311.
110. O'Brien CP, Gardner E. Critical assessment of how to study addiction and its treatment: human and non-human animal models. *Pharmacol Ther*. 2005;108(1):18-58.
111. Heard K, Palmer R, Zahniser NR. Mechanisms of acute cocaine toxicity. *Open Pharmacol J*. 2008;2:70-78.
112. Stephens BG, Jentzen JM, Karch S, Mash DC, Wetli CV. Criteria for the interpretation of cocaine levels in human biological samples and their relation to the cause of death. *Am J Forensic Med Pathol*. 2004;25(1):1-10.
113. Hirsiger S, Hanggi J, Germann J, et al. Longitudinal changes in cocaine intake and cognition are linked to cortical thickness adaptations in cocaine users. *NeuroImage Clin*. 2019;21:101652.
114. Paulus MP, Stewart JL. Neurobiology, clinical presentation, and treatment of methamphetamine use disorder: a review. *JAMA Psychiatry*. 2020;77(9):959-966.
115. Dang J, Tao Q, Niu X, et al. Meta-analysis of structural and functional brain abnormalities in cocaine addiction. *Front Psychiatry*. 2022;13:927075.
116. Magalhaes AC. Functional magnetic resonance and spectroscopy in drug and substance abuse. *Top Magn Reson Imaging*. 2005;16(3):247-251.
117. Chiang M, Lombardi D, Du J, et al. Methamphetamine-associated psychosis: clinical presentation, biological basis, and treatment options. *Hum Psychopharmacol Clin Exp*. 2019;34:e2710.
118. Voce A, Calabria B, Burns R, et al. A systematic review of the symptom profile and course of methamphetamine-associated psychosis. *Subst Use Misuse*. 2019;54(4):549-559.
119. Arunogiri S, Foulds JA, McKetin R, et al. A systematic review of risk factors for methamphetamine-associated psychosis. *Austral New Zealand J Psychiatry*. 2018;52(6):514-529.
120. Yui K, Goto K, Ikemoto S. The role of noradrenergic and dopaminergic hyperactivity in the development of spontaneous recurrence of methamphetamine psychosis and susceptibility to episode recurrence. *Ann NY Acad Sci*. 2004;1025:296-306.
121. Gallagher KE, Funaro MC, Woods SW. Prescription stimulants and the risk of psychosis: a systematic review of observational studies. *J Clin Psychopharmacol*. 2022;42:308-314.
122. Li MJ, Shoptaw SJ. Clinical management of psychostimulant withdrawal: review of the evidence. *Addiction*. 2023;118(4):750-762.
123. Solinas M, Belujon P, Fernagut PO, et al. Dopamine and addiction: what have we learned from 40 years of research. *J Neural Transm (Vienna)*. 2019;126(4):481-516.
124. Garcia AN, Salloum IM. Polysomnographic sleep disturbances in nicotine, caffeine, alcohol, cocaine, opioid, and cannabis use: a focused review. *Am J Addict*. 2015;24(7):590-598.
125. Huskinson SL, Naylor JE, Rowlett JK, et al. Predicting abuse potential of stimulants and other dopaminergic drugs: overview and recommendations. *Neuropharmacology*. 2014;87:66-80.
126. Bossert JM, Ghitza UE, Lu L, Epstein DH, Shaham Y. Neurobiology of relapse to heroin and cocaine seeking: an update and clinical implications. *Eur J Pharmacol*. 2005;526(1-3):36-50.
127. Reid MS, Flammino F, Howard B, Nilsen D, Prichep LS. Topographic imaging of quantitative EEG in response to smoked cocaine self-administration in humans. *Neuropsychopharmacology*. 2006;31(4):872-884.
128. Brust JC. Neurologic complications of illicit drug abuse. *Continuum (Minneap, Minn)*. 2014;20(3 Neurology of Systemic Disease):642-656.
129. Sordo L, Indave BI, Degenhardt L, et al. A systematic review of evidence on the association between cocaine use and seizures. *Drug Alcohol Depend*. 2013;133(3):795-804.
130. Harro J. Neuropsychiatric adverse effects of amphetamine and methamphetamine. *Int Rev Neurobiol*. 2015;120:179-204.
131. Sanchez-Ramos J. Neurologic complications of psychomotor stimulant abuse. *Int Rev Neurobiol*. 2015;120:131-160.
132. Gan WQ, Buxton JA, Scheuermeyer FX, et al. Risk of cardiovascular diseases in relation to substance use disorders. *Drug Alcohol Depend*. 2021;229:109132.
133. Sordo L, Indave BI, Barrio G, Degenhardt L, de la Fuente L, Bravo MJ. Cocaine use and risk of stroke: a systematic review. *Drug Alcohol Depend*. 2014;142:1-13.
134. Cheng YC, Ryan KA, Qadwai SA, et al. Cocaine use and risk of ischemic stroke in young adults. *Stroke*. 2016;47(4):918-922.
135. Blankfield RP, Iftikhar IH. Food and Drug Administration regulation of drugs that raise blood pressure. *J Cardiovasc Pharmacol Ther*. 2015;20(1):5-8.
136. Asser A, Taba P. Psychostimulants and movement disorders. *Front Neurol*. 2015;6:75.
137. Zhornitsky S, Stip E, Pampoulova T, et al. Extrapyramidal symptoms in substance abusers with and without schizophrenia and in nonabusing patients with schizophrenia. *Mov Disord*. 2010;25(13):2188-2194.
138. Phillips K, Luk A, Soor GS, Abraham JR, Leong S, Butany J. Cocaine cardiotoxicity: a review of the pathophysiology, pathology, and treatment options. *Am J Cardiovasc Drugs*. 2009;9(3):177-196.
139. Paratz ED, Cunningham NJ, MacIsaac AI. The cardiac complications of methamphetamines. *Heart Lung Circ*. 2016;25(4):325-332.
140. Sofuoglu M, Nelson D, Babb DA, Hatsukami DK. Intravenous cocaine increases plasma epinephrine and norepinephrine in humans. *Pharmacol Biochem Behav*. 2001;68(3):455-459.
141. Volkow ND, Wang GJ, Fowler JS, et al. Cardiovascular effects of methylphenidate in humans are associated with increases of dopamine in brain and of epinephrine in plasma. *Psychopharmacology (Berl)*. 2003;166(3):264-270.
142. Qureshi AI, Suri MF, Guterman LR, Hopkins LN. Cocaine use and the likelihood of nonfatal myocardial infarction and stroke: data from the Third National Health and Nutrition Examination Survey. *Circulation*. 2001;103(4):502-506.
143. Ramirez FD, Femenia F, Simpson CS, Redfearn DP, Michael KA, Baranchuk A. Electrocardiographic findings associated with cocaine use in humans: a systematic review. *Expert Rev Cardiovasc Ther*. 2012;10(1):105-127.
144. Schwartz BG, Rezkalla S, Kloner RA. Cardiovascular effects of cocaine. *Circulation*. 2010;122(24):2558-2569.
145. Maceira AM, Ripoll C, Cosin-Sales J, et al. Long term effects of cocaine on the heart assessed by cardiovascular magnetic resonance at 3T. *J Cardiovasc Magn Reson*. 2014;16:26.
146. Jafari Giv M. Exposure to amphetamines leads to development of amphetamine type stimulants associated cardiomyopathy (ATSAC). *Cardiovasc Toxicol*. 2017;17(1):13-24.
147. Megarbane B, Chevillard L. The large spectrum of pulmonary complications following illicit drug use: features and mechanisms. *Chem Biol Interact*. 2013;206(3):444-451.
148. Almeida RR, Zanetti G, Souza AS, et al. Cocaine-induced pulmonary changes: HRCT findings. *J Bras Pneumol*. 2015;41(4):323-330.
149. Tseng W, Sutter ME, Albertson TE. Stimulants and the lung: review of literature. *Clin Rev Allergy Immunol*. 2014;46(1):82-100.
150. Goel N, Pullman JM, Coco M. Cocaine and kidney injury: a kaleidoscope of pathology. *Clin Kidney J*. 2014;7(6):513-517.
151. Pendergraft WF III, Herlitz LC, Thornley-Brown D, Rosner M, Niles JL. Nephrotoxic effects of common and emerging drugs of abuse. *Clin J Am Soc Nephrol*. 2014;9(11):1996-2005.
152. Glauser J, Queen JR. An overview of non-cardiac cocaine toxicity. *J Emerg Med*. 2007;32(2):181-186.
153. Hagan IG, Burney K. Radiology of recreational drug abuse. *Radiographics*. 2007;27(4):919-940.
154. Graziani M, Antonilli L, Togna AR, Grassi MC, Badiani A, Saso L. Cardiovascular and hepatic toxicity of cocaine: potential beneficial effects of modulators of oxidative stress. *Oxid Med Cell Longev*. 2016;2016:8408479.
155. Guollo F, Narciso-Schiavon JL, Barotto AM, Zannin M, Schiavon LL. Significance of alanine aminotransferase levels in patients admitted for cocaine intoxication. *J Clin Gastroenterol*. 2015;49(3):250-255.

156. Manetti L, Cavagnini F, Martino E, et al. Effects of cocaine on the hypothalamic–pituitary–adrenal axis. *J Endocrinol Invest.* 2014;37:701-708.
157. Zatelli MC, Cavagnini F, Ambrosio MR. Pituitary side effects of old and new drugs. *J Endocrinol Invest.* 2014;37:917-923.
158. Malinovska J, Urbanova J, Lustigova M, et al. Diabetes mellitus a nelegální drogy. *Vnitř Lék.* 2020;66(2):e16-e19.
159. Doctora JS, Williams CW, Bennett CR, Howlett BK. Rhabdomyolysis in the acutely cocaine-intoxicated patient sustaining maxillofacial trauma: report of a case and review of the literature. *J Oral Maxillofac Surg.* 2003;61(8):964-967.
160. Di Cosola M, Ambrosino M, Limongelli L, et al. Cocaine-induced midline destructive lesions (CIMDL): a real challenge in diagnosis. *Int J Environ Res Public Health.* 2021;18:7831.
161. Kao HH, Chen HH, Chiang KW, et al. Illicit drug use and smell and taste dysfunction: a National Health and Nutrition Examination Survey 2013-2014. *Healthcare.* 2022;10:909.
162. Heer JS, Heavey S, Quesada D, et al. Keratolysis associated with methamphetamine use—incidental diagnosis of corneal melt in a patient with acute methamphetamine intoxication. *Clin Pract Cases Emerg Med.* 2020;4(3):472-473.
163. Fratto G, Manzon L. Use of psychotropic drugs and associated dental diseases. *Int J Psychiatry Med.* 2014;48(3):185-197.
164. Graf J. Rheumatic manifestations of cocaine use. *Curr Opin Rheumatol.* 2013;25(1):50-55.
165. Peikert T, Finkielman JD, Hummel AM, et al. Functional characterization of antineutrophil cytoplasmic antibodies in patients with cocaine-induced midline destructive lesions. *Arthritis Rheum.* 2008;58(5):1546-1551.
166. Irwin MR, Olmos L, Wang M, et al. Cocaine dependence and acute cocaine induce decreases of monocyte proinflammatory cytokine expression across the diurnal period: autonomic mechanisms. *J Pharmacol Exp Ther.* 2007;320(2):507-515.
167. Palha AP, Esteves M. Drugs of abuse and sexual functioning. *Adv Psychosom Med.* 2008;29:131-149.
168. Fronczak CM, Kim ED, Barqawi AB. The insults of illicit drug use on male fertility. *J Androl.* 2012;33(4):515-528.
169. Chou NH, Huang YJ, Jiann BP. The impact of illicit use of amphetamine on male sexual functions. *J Sex Med.* 2015;12(8):1694-1702.
170. Cain MA, Bornick P, Whiteman V. The maternal, fetal, and neonatal effects of cocaine exposure in pregnancy. *Clin Obstet Gynecol.* 2013;56(1):124-132.
171. Behnke M, Smith VC. Prenatal substance abuse: short- and long-term effects on the exposed fetus. *Pediatrics.* 2013;131(3):e1009-e1024.
172. Buckingham-Howes S, Berger SS, Scaletti LA, Black MM. Systematic review of prenatal cocaine exposure and adolescent development. *Pediatrics.* 2013;131(6):e1917-e1936.
173. Docherty JR, Alsufanyi HA. Pharmacology of drugs used as stimulants. *J Clin Pharmacol.* 2021;61(S2):S53-S69.
174. Vizi ES, Fekete A, Karoly R, Mike A. Non-synaptic receptors and transporters involved in brain functions and targets of drug treatment. *Br J Pharmacol.* 2010;160(4):785-809.
175. Sitte HH, Freissmuth M. Amphetamines, new psychoactive drugs and the monoamine transporter cycle. *Trends Pharmacol Sci.* 2015;36(1):41-50.
176. Niello M, Sideromenos S, Gradisch R, et al. Persistent binding at dopamine transporters determines sustained psychostimulant effects. *Proc Natl Acad Sci USA.* 2023;120(6):e2114204120.
177. Reyes-Parada M, Iturriaga-Vasquez P, Cassels BK. Amphetamine derivatives as monoamine oxidase inhibitors. *Front Pharmacol.* 2020;10:1590.
178. Volkow ND, Morales M. The brain on drugs: from reward to addiction. *Cell.* 2015;162(4):712-725.
179. Juarez B, Han MH. Diversity of dopaminergic neural circuits in response to drug exposure. *Neuropsychopharmacology.* 2016;41(10):2424-2446.
180. Sesack SR, Grace AA. Cortico-basal ganglia reward network: microcircuitry. *Neuropsychopharmacology.* 2010;35(1):27-47.
181. Gerfen CR, Surmeier DJ. Modulation of striatal projection systems by dopamine. *Annu Rev Neurosci.* 2011;34:441-466.
182. Buttner A. Neuropathological alterations in cocaine abuse. *Curr Med Chem.* 2012;19(33):5597-5600.
183. Beuming T, Kniazeff J, Bergmann ML, et al. The binding sites for cocaine and dopamine in the dopamine transporter overlap. *Nat Neurosci.* 2008;11(7):780-789.
184. Volkow ND, Fowler JS, Wang GJ, Baler R, Telang F. Imaging dopamine's role in drug abuse and addiction. *Neuropharmacology.* 2009;56 (Suppl 1):3-8.
185. Goodman A. Neurobiology of addiction. An integrative review. *Biochem Pharmacol.* 2008;75(1):266-322.
186. Zolkowska D, Jain R, Rothman RB, et al. Evidence for the involvement of dopamine transporters in behavioral stimulant effects of modafinil. *J Pharmacol Exp Ther.* 2009;329(2):738-746.
187. Anderson SM, Pierce RC. Cocaine-induced alterations in dopamine receptor signaling: implications for reinforcement and reinstatement. *Pharmacol Ther.* 2005;106(3):389-403.
188. Wee S, Carroll FI, Woolverton WL. A reduced rate of in vivo dopamine transporter binding is associated with lower relative reinforcing efficacy of stimulants. *Neuropsychopharmacology.* 2006;31(2):351-362.
189. Kimmel HL, O'Connor JA, Carroll FI, Howell LL. Faster onset and dopamine transporter selectivity predict stimulant and reinforcing effects of cocaine analogs in squirrel monkeys. *Pharmacol Biochem Behav.* 2007;86(1):45-54.
190. Weinshenker D, Schroeder JP. There and back again: a tale of norepinephrine and drug addiction. *Neuropsychopharmacology.* 2007;32(7):1433-1451.
191. Chen R, Tilley MR, Wei H, et al. Abolished cocaine reward in mice with a cocaine-insensitive dopamine transporter. *Proc Natl Acad Sci U S A.* 2006;103(24):9333-9338.
192. Tilley MR, Cagniard B, Zhuang X, Han DD, Tiao N, Gu HH. Cocaine reward and locomotion stimulation in mice with reduced dopamine transporter expression. *BMC Neurosci.* 2007;8:42.
193. Tilley MR, Gu HH. Dopamine transporter inhibition is required for cocaine-induced stereotypy. *Neuroreport.* 2008;19(11):1137-1140.
194. Thomsen M, Han DD, Gu HH, Caine SB. Lack of cocaine self-administration in mice expressing a cocaine-insensitive dopamine transporter. *J Pharmacol Exp Ther.* 2009;331(1):204-211.
195. Kim ES, Lattal KM. Context-dependent and context-independent effects of D1 receptor antagonism in the basolateral and central amygdala during cocaine self-administration. *eNeuro.* 2019;6(4).
196. Galaj E, Ewing S, Ranaldi R. Dopamine D1 and D3 receptor polypharmacology as a potential treatment approach for substance use disorder. *Neurosci Biobehav Rev.* 2018;89:13-28.
197. Caine SB, Thomsen M, Gabriel KI, et al. Lack of self-administration of cocaine in dopamine D1 receptor knock-out mice. *J Neurosci.* 2007;27(48):13140-13150.
198. Zhang J, Xu M. Toward a molecular understanding of psychostimulant actions using genetically engineered dopamine receptor knockout mice as model systems. *J Addict Dis.* 2001;20(3):7-18.
199. Luo Z, Volkow ND, Heintz N, Pan Y, Du C. Acute cocaine induces fast activation of D1 receptor and progressive deactivation of D2 receptor striatal neurons: in vivo optical microprobe [Ca2+]i imaging. *J Neurosci.* 2011;31(37):13180-13190.
200. Hartz SM, Pato CN, Medeiros H, et al. Comorbidity of severe psychotic disorders with measures of substance use. *JAMA Psychiat.* 2014;71(3):248-254.
201. Regnier SD, Lile JA, Rush CR, et al. Clinical neuropharmacology of cocaine reinforcement: a narrative review of human laboratory self-administration studies. *J Exp Anal Behav.* 2022;117:420-441.
202. Kohno M, Dennis LE, McCready H, et al. Dopamine dysfunction in stimulant use disorders: mechanistic comparisons and implications for treatment. *Mol Psychiatry.* 2022;27:220-229.
203. Proebstl L, Kamp F, Manz K, et al. Effects of stimulant drug use on the dopaminergic system: a systematic review and meta-analysis of in vivo neuroimaging studies. *Eur Psychiatry.* 2019;59:15-24.

204. Martinez D, Kim JH, Krystal J, Abi-Dargham A. Imaging the neurochemistry of alcohol and substance abuse. *Neuroimaging Clin N Am*. 2007;17(4):539-555.
205. Martinez D, Narendran R, Foltin RW, et al. Amphetamine-induced dopamine release: markedly blunted in cocaine dependence and predictive of the choice to self-administer cocaine. *Am J Psychiatry*. 2007;164(4):622-629.
206. Rothman RB, Baumann MH, Dersch CM, et al. Amphetamine-type central nervous system stimulants release norepinephrine more potently than they release dopamine and serotonin. *Synapse*. 2001;39(1):32-41.
207. Mash DC, Ouyang Q, Qin Y, Pablo J. Norepinephrine transporter immunoblotting and radioligand binding in cocaine abusers. *J Neurosci Methods*. 2005;143(1):79-85.
208. Drouin C, Blanc G, Villegier AS, Glowinski J, Tassin JP. Critical role of alpha1-adrenergic receptors in acute and sensitized locomotor effects of D-amphetamine, cocaine, and GBR 12783: influence of preexposure conditions and pharmacological characteristics. *Synapse*. 2002;43(1):51-61.
209. Newton TF, De La Garza R II, Brown G, Kosten TR, Mahoney JJ III, Haile CN. Noradrenergic alpha(1) receptor antagonist treatment attenuates positive subjective effects of cocaine in humans: a randomized trial. *PLoS One*. 2012;7(2):e30854.
210. Erb S, Hitchcott PK, Rajabi H, Mueller D, Shaham Y, Stewart J. Alpha-2 adrenergic receptor agonists block stress-induced reinstatement of cocaine seeking. *Neuropsychopharmacology*. 2000;23(2):138-150.
211. Jobes ML, Ghitza UE, Epstein DH, Phillips KA, Heishman SJ, Preston KL. Clonidine blocks stress-induced craving in cocaine users. *Psychopharmacology (Berl)*. 2011;218(1):83-88.
212. Muller CP, Carey RJ, Huston JP, De Souza Silva MA. Serotonin and psychostimulant addiction: focus on 5-HT1A-receptors. *Prog Neurobiol*. 2007;81(3):133-178.
213. Caffino L, Mottarlini F, Targa G, et al. Responsivity of serotonin transporter knockout rats to short and long access to cocaine: modulation of the glutamate signaling in the nucleus accumbens shell. *Br J Pharmacol*. 2022;179:3727-3739.
214. Hall FS, Li XF, Randall-Thompson J, et al. Cocaine-conditioned locomotion in dopamine transporter, norepinephrine transporter and 5-HT transporter knockout mice. *Neuroscience*. 2009;162(4):870-880.
215. Muller CP, Huston JP. Determining the region-specific contributions of 5-HT receptors to the psychostimulant effects of cocaine. *Trends Pharmacol Sci*. 2006;27(2):105-112.
216. Filip M, Alenina N, Bader M, Przegalinski E. Behavioral evidence for the significance of serotoninergic (5-HT) receptors in cocaine addiction. *Addict Biol*. 2010;15(3):227-249.
217. Fletcher PJ, Rizos Z, Noble K, Higgins GA. Impulsive action induced by amphetamine, cocaine and MK801 is reduced by 5-HT(2C) receptor stimulation and 5-HT(2A) receptor blockade. *Neuropharmacology*. 2011;61(3):468-477.
218. Bubar MJ, Cunningham KA. Prospects for serotonin 5-HT2R pharmacotherapy in psychostimulant abuse. *Prog Brain Res*. 2008;172:319-346.
219. Nonkes LJP, van Bussel IGP, Verheij MMM, et al. The interplay between brain 5-hydroxytryptamine levels and cocaine addiction. *Behav Pharmacol*. 2011;22(8):723-738.
220. Haney M, Ward AS, Gerra G, Foltin RW. Neuroendocrine effects of D-fenfluramine and bromocriptine following repeated smoked cocaine in humans. *Drug Alcohol Depend*. 2001;64(1):63-73.
221. Patkar AA, Mannelli P, Hill KP, Peindl K, Pae CU, Lee TH. Relationship of prolactin response to meta-chlorophenylpiperazine with severity of drug use in cocaine dependence. *Hum Psychopharmacol*. 2006;21(6):367-375.
222. Rothman RB, Blough BE, Baumann MH. Dual dopamine-5-HT releasers: potential treatment agents for cocaine addiction. *Trends Pharmacol Sci*. 2006;27(12):612-618.
223. Yoo JH, Kitchen I, Bailey A. The endogenous opioid system in cocaine addiction: what lessons have opioid peptide and receptor knockout mice taught us? *Br J Pharmacol*. 2012;166(7):1993-2014.
224. Wee S, Koob GF. The role of the dynorphin-kappa opioid system in the reinforcing effects of drugs of abuse. *Psychopharmacology (Berl)*. 2010;210(2):121-135.
225. Sun H, Luessen DJ, Kind KO, et al. Cocaine self-administration regulates transcription of opioid peptide precursors and opioid receptors in rat caudate putamen and prefrontal cortex. *Neurosci*. 2020;443:131-139.
226. Gorelick DA, Kim YK, Bencherif B, et al. Imaging brain mu-opioid receptors in abstinent cocaine users: time course and relation to cocaine craving. *Biol Psychiatry*. 2005;57(12):1573-1582.
227. Niedzielska-Andres E, Pomierny-Chamiolo L, Andres M, et al. Cocaine use disorder: a look at metabotropic glutamate receptors and glutamate transporters. *Pharmacol Ther*. 2021;221:107797.
228. Fischer KD, Knackstedt LA, Rosenberg PA. Glutamate homeostasis and dopamine signaling: Implications for psychostimulant addiction behavior. *Neurochem Int*. 2021;144:104896.
229. Li X, Slesinger PA. $GABA_B$ receptors and drug addiction: psychostimulants and other drugs of abuse. *Curr Top Behav Neurosci*. 2022;52:119-155.
230. Walker LC, Lawrence AJ. Allosteric modulation of muscarinic receptors in alcohol and substance use disorders. *Adv Pharmacol*. 2020;88:233-375.
231. Williams MJ, Adinoff B. The role of acetylcholine in cocaine addiction. *Neuropsychopharmacology*. 2008;33(8):1779-1797.
232. Ma Z, Jiang N, Huang Y, et al. Cocaine potently blocks $\alpha 3\beta 4$ nicotinic acetylcholine receptors in SH-SY5Y cells. *Acta Pharmacol Sin*. 2020;41:163-172.
233. Garton DR, Ross SG, Maldonado-Hernandez R, et al. Amphetamine enantiomers inhibit homomeric $\alpha 7$ nicotinic receptor through a competitive mechanism and within the intoxication levels in humans. *Neuropharmacology*. 2019;144:172-183.
234. Ferrucci M, Limanaqi F, Ryskalin L, et al. The effects of amphetamine and methamphetamine on the release of norepinephrine, dopamine and acetylcholine from the brainstem reticular formation. *Front Neuroanat*. 2019;13:48.
235. Farar V, Valuskova P, Sevcikova M, et al. Mapping of the prenatal and postnatal methamphetamine effects on D_1-like dopamine, M_1 and M_2 muscarinic receptors in rat central nervous system. *Brain Res Bull*. 2018;137:17-22.
236. McGinty JF, Shi XD, Schwendt M, Saylor A, Toda S. Regulation of psychostimulant-induced signaling and gene expression in the striatum. *J Neurochem*. 2008;104(6):1440-1449.
237. Lu L, Koya E, Zhai H, Hope BT, Shaham Y. Role of ERK in cocaine addiction. *Trends Neurosci*. 2006;29(12):695-703.
238. Stipanovich A, Valjent E, Matamales M, et al. A phosphatase cascade by which rewarding stimuli control nucleosomal response. *Nature*. 2008;453(7197):879-884.
239. Bisagno V, Cadet JL. Histone deacetylases and immediate early genes: key players in psychostimulant-induced neuronal plasticity. *Neurotox Res*. 2021;39:2134-2140.
240. Wearne TA, Cornish JL. Inhibitory regulation of the prefrontal cortex following behavioral sensitization to amphetamine and/or methamphetamine psychostimulants: a review of GABAergic mechanisms. *Prog Neuropsychopharmacol Biol Psychiatry*. 2019;95:109681.
241. Calipari ES, Ferris MJ, Jones SR. Extended access of cocaine self-administration results in tolerance to the dopamine-elevating and locomotor-stimulating effects of cocaine. *J Neurochem*. 2014;128:224-232.
242. Bailey LS, Bagley JR, Wherry JD, et al. Repeated dosing with cocaine produces strain-dependent effects on responding for conditioned reinforcement in Collaborative Cross mice. *Psychopharmacology*. 2023;240(3):561-573.
243. Allain F, Delignat-Lavaud B, Beaudoin MP, et al. Amphetamine maintenance therapy during intermittent cocaine self-administration in rats attenuates psychomotor and dopamine sensitization and reduces addiction-like behavior. *Neuropsychopharmacology*. 2021;46:305-315.
244. Post RM, Kalivas P. Bipolar disorder and substance misuse: pathological and therapeutic implications of their comorbidity and cross-sensitisation. *Br J Psychiatry*. 2013;202:172-176.
245. Slamberova R. Review of long-term consequences of maternal methamphetamine exposure. *Physiol Res*. 2019;68(Suppl. 3):S219-S231.
246. Marie N, Canestrelli C, Noble F. Role of pharmacokinetic and pharmacodynamic parameters in neuroadaptations induced by drugs of

abuse, with a focus on opioids and psychostimulants. *Neurosci Biobehav Rev*. 2019;106:217-226.

247. Carr CC, Ferrario CR, Robinson TE. Intermittent access cocaine self-administration produces psychomotor sensitization: effects of withdrawal, sex and cross-sensitization. *Psychopharmacology (Berl)*. 2020;237:1795-1812.

248. Small AC, Kampman KM, Plebani J, et al. Tolerance and sensitization to the effects of cocaine use in humans: a retrospective study of long-term cocaine users in Philadelphia. *Subst Use Misuse*. 2009;44:1888-1898.

249. Ujike H, Sato M. Clinical features of sensitization to methamphetamine observed in patients with methamphetamine dependence and psychosis. *Ann N Y Acad Sci*. 2004;1025:279-287.

250. Leyton M. Conditioned and sensitized responses to stimulant drugs in humans. *Prog Neuropsychopharmacol Biol Psychiatry*. 2007;31(8):1601-1613.

251. Kollins SH, Rush CR. Sensitization to the cardiovascular but not subject-rated effects of oral cocaine in humans. *Biol Psychiatry*. 2002;51(2):143-150.

252. Boileau I, Dagher A, Leyton M, et al. Modeling sensitization to stimulants in humans: an [11C]raclopride/positron emission tomography study in healthy men. *Arch Gen Psychiatry*. 2006;63(12):1386-1395.

253. Foltin FW, Haney M. Intranasal cocaine in humans: acute tolerance, cardiovascular and subjective effects. *Pharmacol Biochem Behav*. 2004;78:93-101.

254. Handelman K, Suriya F. Tolerance to stimulant medication for attention deficit hyperactivity disorder: literature review and case report. *Brain Sci*. 2022;12(8):959.

255. Jitca G, Osz BE, Tero-Vescan A, et al. Psychoactive drugs—from chemical structure to oxidative stress related to dopaminergic neurotransmission. a review. *Antioxidants*. 2021;10:381.

256. Moratalla R, Khairnar A, Simola N, et al. Amphetamine-related drugs neurotoxicity in humans and in experimental animals: main mechanisms. *Prog Neurobiol*. 2017;155:149-170.

257. Gaudreault PO, King SG, Malaker P, et al. Whole-brain white matter abnormalities in human cocaine and heroin use disorders: association with craving, recency, and cumulative use. *Mol Psychiatry*. 2023;28:780-791.

258. Ottino-Gonzalez J, Uhlmann A, Hahn S, et al. White matter microstructure differences in individuals with dependence on cocaine, methamphetamine, and nicotine: findings from the ENIGMA-Addiction working group. *Drug Alcohol Depend*. 2022;230:109105.

259. Wen S, Aki T, Funakoshi T, et al. Role of mitochondrial dynamics in cocaine's neurotoxicity. *Int J Mol Sci*. 2022;23:5418.

260. Koshsirat S, Khoramgah MS, Mahmoudiasl GR, et al. LC3 and ATG5 overexpression and neuronal cell death in the prefrontal cortex of postmortem chronic methamphetamine users. *J Chem Neuroanat*. 2020;107:101802.

261. Al-Serori H, Ferk F, Angerer V, et al. Investigations of the genotoxic properties of two synthetic cathinones (3-MMC, 4-MEC) which are used as psychoactive drugs. *Toxicol Res*. 2016;5:1410-1420.

262. Mahna D, Puri S, Sharma S. DNA methylation signatures: biomarkers of drug and alcohol abuse. *Mutat Res Rev Mutat Res*. 2018;777:19-28.

263. Ropek N, Al-Serori H, Misik M, et al. Methamphetamine ("crystal meth") causes induction of DNA damage and chromosomal aberrations in human derived cells. *Food Chem Toxicol*. 2019;128:1-7.

264. Yujra VQ, Moretti EG, Claudio SR, et al. Genotoxicity and mutagenicity induced by acute crack cocaine exposure in mice. *Drug Chem Toxicol*. 2016;39(4):388-391.

265. Malacarne IT, De Souza DV, Rosario BDA, et al. Genotoxicity, oxidative stress, and inflammatory response induced by crack-cocaine: relevance to carcinogenesis. *Environ Sci Pollut Res*. 2021;28:14285-14292.

266. Souza-Silva EM, Alves RB, Simon KA, et al. Crack cocaine smoke on pregnant rats: maternal evaluation and teratogenic effect. *Human Exp Toxicol*. 2020;39(4):411-422.

267. Smith LM, Santos LS. Prenatal exposure: the effects of prenatal cocaine and methamphetamine exposure on the developing child. *Birth Defects Res C Embryo Today*. 2016;108:142-146.

268. Garey JD, Lusskin SI, Schialli AR. Teratogen update: amphetamines. *Birth Defects Res*. 2020;112:1161-1182.

269. Liu J, Wu R, Li J-X. TAAR1 and psychostimulant addiction. *Cell Mol Neurobiol*. 2020;40(2):229-238.

CHAPTER

15

The Pharmacology of Caffeine

Laura M. Juliano, Sergi Ferré, Darian Weaver, and Roland R. Griffiths

CHAPTER OUTLINE

- Introduction
- Drugs in the class
- History
- Epidemiology
- Sources of caffeine
- Therapeutic uses
- Neurobiology
- Pharmacokinetics
- Physiological effects
- Subjective effects
- Performance effects
- Reinforcing effects
- Caffeine tolerance
- Caffeine intoxication
- Caffeine withdrawal
- Caffeine use disorder
- Genetics
- Effects on physical health
- Drug-drug interactions

INTRODUCTION

Caffeine, a mild central nervous system (CNS) stimulant, is the most widely used mood-altering drug in the world.[1] It's primary mechanism of action is antagonism of A_1 and A_{2A} adenosine receptors. Adenosine serves an important modulatory role in many brain processes and functions including but not limited to sleep, arousal, and dilation of blood vessels. Moderate caffeine consumption is not generally associated with negative health effects. Moreover, caffeine has valuable therapeutic effects and may offer protective effects from some diseases. However, caffeine can produce clinically significant negative physiologic and psychological effects, tolerance, withdrawal, and psychiatric disorders. Furthermore, its interactions with recreational and psychotherapeutic drugs can have important clinical implications. The widespread use of caffeine and its integration into daily customs and routines can make the recognition and treatment of caffeine-associated problems particularly challenging.

DRUGS IN THE CLASS

Caffeine is the common name for 1,3,7-trimethylxanthine (**Fig. 15-1**). Caffeine is found in more than 60 types of plants, including coffee, tea, cola, guarana, cacao, and yerba maté. Caffeine is a member of the methylxanthine class of alkaloids, which includes the structurally related dimethylxanthines, theophylline, and theobromine. In its free base form caffeine is a bitter white powder that is moderately soluble in water (21.7 mg/mL).[2] Pharmaceutical preparations of caffeine include caffeine anhydrous, caffeine sodium benzoate, and caffeine citrate.

HISTORY

Caffeine was first isolated from coffee and tea in the early 1800s, and its chemical structure was identified in 1875. The use of tea, coffee beans, and cacao pod for psychoactive effects may predate recorded history.[3] The development of worldwide trade in the 17th and 18th centuries propagated global use of caffeinated foods and beverages.[4] In America, the protest of a British tax on tea became a symbolic focal point for revolution, resulting in the famous "Boston tea party" in 1773. After the Continental Congress passed a resolution against tea consumption, coffee became America's caffeinated drink of choice.[3] Presently, coffee, cocoa, and tea products represent major imports of the United States. In 2020, the total value of coffee, cocoa, and tea product imports were $5.7 billion, $5.18 billion, and $473 million, respectively. Caffeinated soft drinks (eg, Coca-Cola), introduced at the end of the 19th century, and caffeinated energy drinks (eg, Red Bull), introduced at the end of the 20th century, now represent multibillion dollar markets with hundreds of different brands available to consumers worldwide. Regulation of energy drinks in the United States has been heretofore quite lax relative to other countries,[5] but increasing incidences of adverse events after consumption of energy have led to public scrutiny and an ongoing FDA investigation on the safety of energy drinks and other caffeine-containing foods (eg, caffeine-containing gum, candy).[6] Caffeinated alcoholic beverages became available to consumers in the early 2000s. However, in 2010 these products were removed from the market by manufacturers as the US Food and Drug Administration (FDA) deemed that caffeine added to alcoholic malt beverages was an "unsafe food additive."[7]

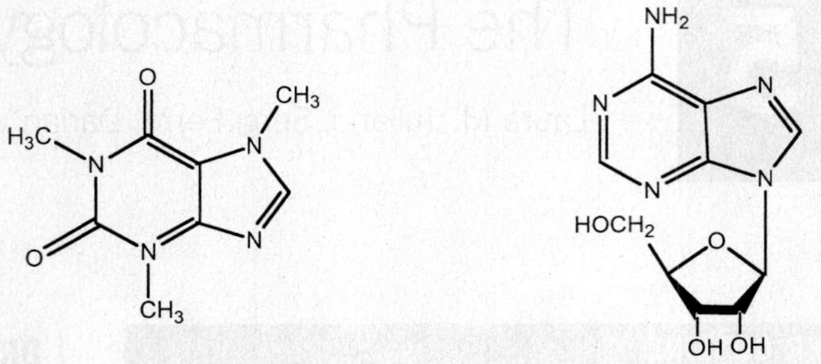

CAFFEINE
(an adenosine receptor antagonist)

ADENOSINE
(an endogenous neuromodulator)

Figure 15-1. The chemical structure of caffeine. The chemical structure of caffeine (1,3,7-trimethylxanthine) and adenosine. Adenosine is an endogenous neuromodulator that has structural similarities to caffeine. Most of the physiological effects of caffeine, including the central nervous system stimulant effects, are likely mediated through adenosine receptor antagonism.

EPIDEMIOLOGY

Population-based epidemiological data on caffeine use are derived from two main sources. The National Health and Nutrition Examination Survey (NHANES) is administered each year to a representative sample of children and adults in the United States and collects information on all foods, beverages, and supplements consumed in a 24-hour period. The Kantar World Beverage Consumption Panel includes a representative sample of the US population that complete 7-day diaries of beverage consumption. These surveys consistently find a high rate of regular caffeine use among children and adults with ~85% of the population age 2 years and older[8] and 89% of adults[9] consuming at least one caffeinated beverage per day. Daily caffeine exposure rates are estimated to be 43%-63% among 2- to 5-year-olds,[8,10] 75% among older children and adolescents,[10] 86% to 90% among teenagers and young adults.[11]

More than 95% of all caffeine ingestion comes from beverages. Among adults, the primary source of caffeine is coffee followed by soft drinks and tea.[8,9] The 2022 National Coffee Data Trends report found that 66% of individuals in the US drink coffee each day and consume an average of about 3.3 cups per day. This is a marked increase in prevalence from recent prior years.[12] A review of 2003-2016 NHANES data from more than 33,000 respondents ages 12 to 59 found that the prevalence of energy drink consumption increased over time across all age groups and per capita consumption increased among young adults.[13] The report also concluded that energy drinks were a major source of caffeine among those who consume them. A nationally representative survey of adolescents conducted in 2014 found that nearly two-thirds had reported ever trying energy drinks and 41% had used energy drinks in the prior three months.[14] In the absence of current large scale epidemiological data on energy drink usage it is notable that sales of energy drinks quadrupled from 2015 to 2020[15] and are projected to increase.

Determining the absolute level of caffeine exposure in the general population is challenging and estimates tend to vary widely depending on the study sample and methodology. There also tends to be a considerable lag in the time from data collection to publication of data summaries. A report was commissioned by the US Food and Drug Administration (FDA) that summarized the US population's consumption of caffeine between 2003 and 2008. The mean daily caffeine intake among adults (over age 22) was estimated to be 300 mg.[16] Among coffee drinkers, the mean daily caffeine intake was estimated to be 375 mg. Another study based on NHANES data from 2001 to 2010 estimated average daily caffeine intake among consumers to be 211 mg, with 14% consuming more than 400 mg caffeine per day.[9]

Across various studies, men tend to consume more caffeine than women.[9] Non-Hispanic White individuals tend to consume more caffeine than non-Hispanic Black individuals, with Hispanic individuals falling in between.[17,18]

SOURCES OF CAFFEINE

As shown in **Table 15-1**, sources of caffeine include beverages, foods, dietary supplements, and over-the-counter and prescription medications. Estimating caffeine exposure can be difficult because of the wide variety of products that contain caffeine, large differences in serving sizes, variability in caffeine content across products of the same type, and undisclosed caffeine amounts in some products. For example, a 12-oz cup of coffee may contain anywhere from 107 to 420 mg of caffeine. Energy drinks can vary more than 10-fold in caffeine content across brands. Presently, there is widespread marketing of highly caffeinated dietary supplements and energy shots (eg, 5-hour ENERGY), and caffeine is added to various food products (eg, gum, jelly beans).

THERAPEUTIC USES

Caffeine is often taken to increase energy and alertness and prevent sleepiness. Some over-the-counter and prescription analgesics contain caffeine because of its analgesic-enhancing

TABLE 15-1 Caffeine Content of Common Foods and Medications

Product	Serving size (volume or weight)	Typical caffeine content (mg)	Range (mg)
Beverages			
Brewed drip coffee	12 oz	200	107-420
Instant coffee	12 oz	140	40-260
Espresso	1 oz	70	60-95
Decaffeinated coffee	12 oz	8	0-20
Starbucks bottled frappuccino	13.7 oz	110	45-130
Brewed tea	6 oz	40	30-90
Instant tea	6 oz	30	10-35
Canned or bottled tea	12 oz	20	8-32
Chocolate milk	6 oz	4	2-7
Cocoa/hot chocolate	6 oz	7	2-10
Soft drinks typical amount	12 oz	varies	0-69
Pepsi Zero Sugar	12 oz	69	
Mountain Dew/Diet Mountain Dew	12 oz	54	
Coca-Cola Classic/Diet Coke	12 oz	34/46	
Dr. Pepper/Diet Dr. Pepper	12 oz	42/41	
Pepsi/Diet Pepsi	12 oz	38/35	
Barq's Root Beer/Diet Root Beer	12 oz	22/0	
Energy drinks/shots typical amount	Varies	Varies	25-400
Hyde Extreme Preworkout	12 oz	400	
Celsius Energy Drink	12 oz	200	
5-hour ENERGY	1.93 oz	200	
Rockstar	16 oz	160	
Monster	16 oz	160	
Red Bull	8.46 oz	80	
Kill Cliff	12 oz	25	
Foods			
Military Energy Gum	1 stick	100	
Jelly Belly Extreme Sport Beans	1 oz	50	
Jolt caffeinated gum	1 stick	45	
Dannon coffee yogurt	5.3 oz	32	
Hershey's special dark	1.45 oz	20	
Hershey's chocolate bar	1.5 oz	9	
Medications/dietary supplements/weight loss products			
Vivarin/NoDoz	1 tablet	200	
Excedrin Extra Strength	2 tablets	130	
BC Original	1 powder packet	65	
Diurex Ultra Water Pills	2 tablets	200	
Midol Complete	2 caplets	120	
Cafergot	2 tablets	200	
Fiorinal	2 capsules	80	
Swarm Extreme Energizer	1 capsule	300	
Hydroxycut Hardcore	2 capsules	270	
Stacker 3	1 capsule	250	
Dexatrim Max Daytime	1 capsule	200	
Dexatrim Max Complex	2 capsules	110	

Caffeine values for name brand items were obtained directly from product labels, the manufacturer's website, customer service department, or www.caffeineinformer.com.

effects.[19] Caffeine withdrawal symptoms and postoperative headache can be treated with caffeine.[20] As a respiratory stimulant, caffeine is used to treat apnea in neonates and infants.[21] Because of its lipolytic and thermogenic effects,[22,23] caffeine is commonly added to weight loss preparations and nutritional supplements. Caffeine and other xanthines have also been used to treat postprandial hypotension.[24]

NEUROBIOLOGY

Psychostimulant Pharmacological Profile of Caffeine

Caffeine is a psychostimulant with milder psychomotor and reinforcing effects than classical psychostimulants,[25] such as amphetamine or cocaine, and it does not directly target dopaminergic neurotransmission. Caffeine is a nonselective adenosine receptor antagonist with similar in vitro affinities for A_1, A_{2A}, and A_{2B} receptors and with lower affinity for A_3 receptors.[1] A_1 and A_{2A} receptors are the preferential targets for caffeine in the CNS because physiological extracellular levels of adenosine are sufficient to occupy and, therefore, activate A_1 and A_{2A} receptors. On the other hand, adenosine only binds and activates A_{2B} receptors at high pathological extracellular concentrations.[1] A_1 receptors are widely expressed in the CNS, including the spinal cord,[1,26] whereas A_{2A} receptors are particularly concentrated in the striatum, in the GABAergic striatal efferent neuron.[1,25,27] Striatal adenosine receptors have been associated with the psychomotor and reinforcing effects of caffeine. On the other hand, adenosine receptors localized in the brainstem, basal forebrain, and hypothalamus, in the loci of origin of ascending arousal systems, have been suggested to be involved in caffeine-induced hyperarousal. Generally, it can be concluded that striatal A_{2A} and extrastriatal A_1 receptors are preferentially involved in the psychomotor-reinforcing effects and hyperarousal induced by caffeine, respectively.[25,28]

Adenosine A_{2A}-Dopamine D_2 Receptor Heteromers as Main Targets for the Psychomotor and Reinforcing Effects of Caffeine

The enigmatic psychomotor activating effects of caffeine provided one of the main findings that would lead to the field of G protein–coupled receptor (GPCR) heteromers.[29,30] More specifically, it led to the discovery of adenosine-dopamine receptor heteromers and, even more specifically, to the establishment of A_{2A}-D_2 receptor heteromers as mainly responsible for the psychomotor-reinforcing effects of caffeine.[25,31] A GPCR heteromer is defined as a macromolecular complex composed of at least two different GPCR units with biochemical properties that are demonstrably different from those of its individual components.[29,30] Simultaneous allosteric interactions between caffeine and endogenous adenosine and dopamine within the A_{2A}-D_2 receptor heteromer determine the ability of caffeine to increase D_2 receptor–mediated signaling in the GABAergic striatopallidal neurons.[31,32] Accumulated knowledge about the function of the A_{2A}-D_2 receptor heteromer indicates that it is a main target for the psychomotor activating and also reinforcing effects of caffeine.[25] However, this is still an incomplete picture and caffeine also increases dopamine neurotransmission by additional mechanisms related to blockade of presynaptic striatal A_1 receptors localized in dopaminergic terminals and also in glutamatergic terminals, where they form heteromers with A_{2A} receptors, and which exert an inhibitory modulation of glutamate and dopamine release,[33,34] and postsynaptic A_1 receptors that form heteromers with D_1 receptors in the GABAergic striatonigral neuron.[25] In addition, recent evidence indicates that A_1-D_1 receptor heteromers expressed by the spinal motor neuron also govern the effect of caffeine at the spinal level, where it potentiates a spinal-generated locomotor activation.[26]

Adenosine A_1 Receptors as Main Targets for the Arousal Effects of Caffeine

Adenosine is a main mediator of sleepiness following prolonged wakefulness, when it accumulates in the extracellular space of basal forebrain, cortex, and hypothalamus.[28,35] This accumulation leads to A_1 receptor–mediated inhibition of the cells of origin of the corticopetal basal forebrain system,[28,35] inhibition of corticofugal neurons from the prefrontal cortex that target the origin of pontine ascending arousal systems, also mediated by A_1 receptor[36]; and inhibition of hypothalamic histaminergic and orexinergic ascending arousal systems, with both A_1 and A_{2A} receptors being involved.[28,35,36] Several studies indicate that the A_1 receptor is a marker of homeostatic sleep responses and the need for recovery of lost sleep, which involves rebound sleepiness upon acute sleep deprivation and cumulative sleepiness upon chronic sleep deprivation.[37,38] In fact, both acute and chronic sleep deprivation lead to an increase of A_1 receptor density in the brain.[38-40] Chronic caffeine consumption also leads to up-regulation of A_1 receptors, which therefore seems to play an important role in the sleepiness, marked fatigue, and drowsiness of caffeine withdrawal.[25,40] Therefore, an important component of the improvement in attention, performance, and wakefulness by caffeine could be explained by relieving these A_1 receptor–mediated withdrawal symptoms.[25,41] The very prevalent consumption of caffeine may therefore depend largely on A_{2A} receptor blockade–mediated reinforcing effects and A_1 receptor blockade–mediated and reversal withdrawal-related arousing effects.[25]

PHARMACOKINETICS

Absorption and Distribution

Caffeine is rapidly and completely absorbed after oral administration, with peak levels reached in 30 to 45 minutes.[42] It is readily distributed throughout the body, with concentrations in blood correlating with those in saliva, breast milk, amniotic fluid, fetal tissue, semen, and the brain.[43] Binding to plasma proteins is estimated to range between 10% and 35%.[44] Saliva caffeine concentrations, which often exceed 75% of plasma concentrations, are used as a noninvasive alternative to serum monitoring.

Metabolism

Caffeine metabolism is complex, with more than 25 metabolites identified in humans.[45] Caffeine is metabolized by the cytochrome P-450 liver enzyme system. In particular the CYP1A2 isoenzyme demethylates caffeine to three biologically active dimethylxanthines: paraxanthine, theobromine, and theophylline, accounting for approximately 84%, 12%, and 4% of caffeine metabolism, respectively.[46]

Elimination

On average, caffeine half-life is 4 to 6 hours, but there are wide individual differences, which are due in large part to CPY1A2 genetic variation.[46] Drugs or conditions that affect the cytochrome P-450 liver enzyme system significantly alter caffeine elimination.[47] Caffeine's half-life is prolonged with liver disease,[44] presumably because of lower CYP1A2 activity.[48] Caffeine half-life is markedly increased in infants whose liver enzyme capacity is not completely developed until about 6 months of age.[49] Cigarette smoking, which induces liver enzymes, decreases caffeine half-life by as much as 50%.[47] Numerous compounds inhibit caffeine metabolism including oral contraceptives, cimetidine, some antibiotics (eg, ciprofloxacin, pipemidic acid, enoxacin), and the antidepressant fluvoxamine.[46,47] A more complete list of drugs that affect caffeine pharmacokinetics can be found elsewhere.[46,47] Caffeine half-life increases markedly during the last trimester of pregnancy,[50] which could increase the risk of caffeine toxicity among women who maintain high levels of caffeine use during pregnancy.[51]

PHYSIOLOGICAL EFFECTS

At moderate dietary dose levels, caffeine increases systolic and diastolic blood pressure,[52] constricts blood vessels in the head and neck, increases urine volume,[53] stimulates gastric acid secretions, and is a colonic stimulant.[54] As a diuretic, caffeine also increases detrusor pressure on the bladder of patients with complaints of urinary urgency and confirmed detrusor instability.[55] Caffeine is a respiratory stimulant[56] and a bronchodilator at high doses.[57] Caffeine increases plasma epinephrine, norepinephrine, renin, and free fatty acids, particularly in nontolerant individuals.[58-60] It also increases adrenocorticotropic hormone and cortisol.[61,62] Caffeine increases insulin levels in healthy subjects[63] and impairs postprandial glucose responses.[64,65]

SUBJECTIVE EFFECTS

Low to moderate doses of caffeine (eg, 20-200 mg) typically produce positive subjective effects, including increased well-being, happiness, energy, arousal, alertness, and sociability, with greater positive effects observed among people who regularly use caffeine.[66,67] Negative subjective effects are more likely to be reported after ingestion of higher acute doses (eg, >400 mg) and include anxiety, nervousness, jitteriness, negative mood, upset stomach, sleeplessness, and "bad effects."[66,67] Individual differences in use, sensitivity, and tolerance play an important role in the likelihood and severity of negative subjective effects and some individuals may report adverse effects at lower doses (eg, 200 mg)[68] such as those prone to anxiety.[69] High acute doses of caffeine can trigger panic.[70] The DSM-5-TR recognizes Caffeine-Induced Anxiety Disorder, which is defined as anxiety symptoms or an anxiety disorder (eg, Generalized Anxiety Disorder) caused by caffeine use.[71]

PERFORMANCE EFFECTS

Cognitive Performance

Caffeine has been shown to improve performance especially when it has been degraded by sleep deprivation, fatigue, prolonged vigilance, or caffeine abstinence.[72] Compared with placebo, caffeine reliably improves reaction time, tapping speed, and sustained attention.[73] The effects of caffeine on various memory tasks, higher-order executive functioning, and decision-making have also been investigated, but results tend to be less consistent.[73]

Physical Performance

Caffeine is ergogenic across a variety of exercise situations. Relative to placebo, caffeine enhances performance during long-term (30-60 minutes) aerobic exercise, reduces ratings of perceived exhaustion, and improves power output or speed. Some studies have also shown caffeine-related enhancement during short-term, high-intensity exercise, resistance training, and other sport specific actions.[74-76] According to a recent review, the most reliable and potent effects are observed during aerobic exercise when caffeine (3-6 mg/kg) is consumed approximately 60 minutes prior. High doses of caffeine (eg, 9 mg/kg) produce no additional benefit and can result in negative side effects.[76]

Withdrawal Reversal

A problem in interpreting the effects of caffeine on performance is that most studies have compared the effects of caffeine and placebo on the performance of people who use caffeine habitually who have been required to abstain from caffeine, usually overnight. Thus, improvements in performance after caffeine relative to placebo may simply reflect a reversal of withdrawal effects or restoration to baseline performance.[77,78] However, some studies have shown caffeine-related performance enhancements among light nondependent caffeine consumers and nonconsumers,[79,80] nonwithdrawn caffeine consumers,[81] as well as caffeine consumers after a protracted period of abstinence.[82] Based on the preclinical literature, which clearly documents the behavioral stimulant effects of caffeine, it seems quite likely that caffeine enhances human performance on some types of tasks (eg, vigilance), especially among nontolerant individuals. Among habitual caffeine consumers, performance enhancements above and beyond withdrawal reversal effects are perhaps modest at best.[78,83]

REINFORCING EFFECTS

Given that caffeine is the most widely self-administered mood-altering drug in the world, the circumstantial evidence for caffeine functioning as a reinforcer is compelling. Carefully controlled research studies provide unequivocal evidence for the reinforcing effects of caffeine. Caffeine reinforcement has been demonstrated with various participant populations, using a variety of methodological approaches (eg, choice procedures, ad libitum self-administration), and across different caffeine vehicles (eg, coffee, soft drinks, capsules). The average incidence of caffeine reinforcement across studies in people who use caffeine normally is approximately 40%, with higher rates observed (ie, 82%-100%) among certain subsamples such as heavy caffeine consumers, those with histories of substance use disorders (SUD), in studies involving repeated exposure to caffeine and placebo test conditions before reinforcement testing, and in the context of having to perform a vigilance task after drug administration. Doses as low as 25 mg per cup of coffee and 33 mg per serving of soft drink function as reinforcers.[84,85] Doses greater than 50 or 100 mg tend to decrease choice or self-administration, with relatively high doses of caffeine (eg, 400 or 600 mg) sometimes producing significant caffeine avoidance.[66] Positive subjective effects of caffeine predict the subsequent choice of caffeine relative to placebo, and negative subjective effects predict the subsequent choice of placebo relative to caffeine.[86] There is good evidence to suggest avoidance of caffeine withdrawal symptoms increases the reinforcing effects of caffeine among regular caffeine consumers. For instance, people who use caffeine who report negative effects of placebo (ie, withdrawal symptoms) tend to choose caffeine over placebo, and when physical dependence is manipulated, subjects chose caffeine more than twice as often when they were physically dependent than when they were not physically dependent.[87]

CAFFEINE TOLERANCE

The degree of tolerance development to caffeine depends on the caffeine dose, the dose frequency, the number of doses, and individual differences.[88] Complete tolerance does not occur at typical daily dietary doses and tolerance develops for some pathways and not others.[46] At the peripheral level, tolerance develops to blood pressure, heart rate, diuresis, plasma adrenaline and noradrenaline levels, and renin activity.[46] However, it has been argued that tolerance to caffeine induced increases in blood pressure is incomplete enough to be clinically significant.[52] Partial tolerance has also been observed for sleep disruption, subjective effects, and performance effects.[46,83]

CAFFEINE INTOXICATION

Caffeine intoxication is a diagnosis in DSM-5-TR[71] and in the ICD-11.[89] Caffeine intoxication is defined by the DSM-5-TR as the emergence of five or more of the following symptoms after excess ingestion of caffeine: restlessness, nervousness, excitement, insomnia, flushed face, diuresis, gastrointestinal disturbance, muscle twitching, rambling flow of thought and speech, tachycardia or cardiac arrhythmia, inexhaustibility, and psychomotor agitation.[71]

Among adults, negative effects are not usually observed at acute doses less than 250 mg, and caffeine intoxication is typically associated with higher acute doses (eg, >500 mg). Individual differences in sensitivity (eg, metabolic differences) and tolerance likely influence dose effects.

Caffeine intoxication typically resolves within a day (consistent with caffeine's half-life of 4-6 hours) and often with no long-lasting consequences. However, medical treatment and monitoring are necessary when significant caffeine overdose occurs. Caffeine can be lethal after ingestion of very high doses (ie, about 5-10 g), and there is documentation of accidental death and suicide by caffeine ingestion.[90,91]

It has been suggested that the lack of regulation and availability of highly caffeinated energy drinks/shots in recent years may be increasing the incidence of caffeine intoxication, especially among young people. A recent comprehensive review of adverse effects of energy drinks among children and adults found reports of symptoms consistent with caffeine intoxication with tachycardia, slurred speech, rapid speech, stress, jitteriness, insomnia, decreased coordination, weakness all reported at relatively high frequencies.[92]

A report by the Drug Abuse Warning Network found that the number of emergency department visits involving energy drinks doubled from 2007 to 2011 with most of the 20,783 energy drink-related visits involving males and individuals between the ages of 18 and 25.[93] A review of the National Poison Data System from 2008 to 2015 revealed that the large majority of energy drink cases involved young children and adolescents.[94] Claims that energy drinks have contributed to sudden deaths have led to public scrutiny and an FDA investigation on the safety of energy drinks.[6,7]

CAFFEINE WITHDRAWAL

The caffeine withdrawal syndrome is well characterized. A 2004 comprehensive review of carefully controlled caffeine withdrawal research provided a strong empirical basis for 13 symptoms (**Table 15-2**). The symptoms were conceptually grouped into the following five categories and later validated

TABLE 15-2 Empirically Validated Signs and Symptoms Resulting From Caffeine Abstinence

Headache
Tiredness/fatigue
Drowsiness/sleepiness
Decreased energy/activeness
Decreased alertness/attentiveness
Decreased contentedness/well-being
Irritability
Depressed mood
Difficulty concentrating
Muggy/foggy/not clearheaded
Flu-like symptoms
Nausea/vomiting
Muscle pain/stiffness

Reprinted by permission from Springer. Juliano LM, Griffiths RR. A critical review of caffeine withdrawal: Empirical validation of symptoms and signs, incidence, severity, and associated features. *Psychopharmacology.* 2004;176(1):1-29.

by a factor analysis[95,96]: (a) headache, (b) fatigue or drowsiness, (c) dysphoric mood, depressed mood, or irritability, (d) difficulty concentrating, and (e) flu-like somatic symptoms—nausea, vomiting, and muscle pain/stiffness. The caffeine withdrawal syndrome is defined by the DSM-5-TR as the presence of at least three symptoms within 24 hours of abrupt caffeine reduction or abstinence.[71] Symptoms must cause clinically significant distress or impairment in social, occupational, or other important areas of functioning (eg, unable to care for children, unable to work). Headache is a hallmark feature of caffeine withdrawal with approximately 50% of people who use caffeine regularly reporting headache by the end of the first day of abstinence.[96] Caffeine withdrawal headaches have been described as gradual in development, diffuse, throbbing, and sensitive to movement. Caffeine abstinence produces rebound cerebral vasodilatation and increased cerebral blood flow, and such vascular changes are the likely mechanism underlying caffeine withdrawal headache.[97,98]

Caffeine withdrawal usually begins 12 to 24 hours after terminating daily caffeine intake, although onset as early as 6 hours and as late as 43 hours has been documented. Peak withdrawal intensity generally occurs 20 to 51 hours after abstinence. The duration of withdrawal ranges from 2 to 9 days, with headache possibly persisting for 3 weeks.[96]

Although there is wide variability across individuals, the incidence and severity of caffeine withdrawal appears to be positively correlated with daily caffeine dose.[99] Nevertheless, caffeine withdrawal has been observed after repeated dosing as low as 100 mg/d,[99,100] and after relatively short-term exposure to daily caffeine (eg, 3 consecutive days of 300 mg/d), with greater severity after 7 and 14 consecutive days.[99] Low doses of caffeine can suppress caffeine withdrawal. Among individuals maintained on 300 mg caffeine/day and tested with a range of lower doses, a substantial reduction in caffeine dose (to <100 mg/d) was necessary for caffeine withdrawal to manifest.[99]

Individuals who abstain from caffeine during religious holidays and in preparation for certain medical procedures (eg, blood tests, colonoscopies) and surgeries may be at risk for caffeine withdrawal.[20] Caffeine withdrawal symptoms can sometimes be misattributed to other ailments among those who are not aware of their physical dependence on caffeine.

It has been suggested that expectancy may play a role in caffeine withdrawal,[101] although these conclusions were in the absence of controlled research.[102] More recent experimental studies have found that the belief that caffeine has been consumed among withdrawn caffeine consumers results in transient reductions in withdrawal and craving[102,103]; however, there is no evidence that expectancy has an effect after more protracted abstinence.[102]

CAFFEINE USE DISORDER

Caffeine Use Disorder is included in the DSM-5-TR as a condition for further study.[71] The research diagnosis requires that individuals meet a more restrictive criteria than that of the generic DSM-5-TR SUD criteria. Individuals must show a problematic pattern of caffeine use leading to clinically significant impairment or distress, as manifested by *all* three of the following characteristics occurring within a 12-month period: (1) difficulty cutting down or controlling caffeine use, (2) caffeine use despite physical or psychological problems that are made worse by caffeine, and (3) caffeine withdrawal or the use of caffeine to avoid withdrawal. The DSM-5-TR SUD diagnosis that applies to other drugs requires meeting two of eleven potential criteria. A stricter set of criteria are being tested for caffeine to avoid potential overdiagnosis. Of the eight additional criteria that define SUDs per the DSM-5-TR, six may also apply to caffeine including tolerance and craving.

Studies that have identified individuals with problematic caffeine use find that such individuals show a wide range of daily caffeine intake, consume various types of caffeinated products, are more likely to experience caffeine reinforcement and severe withdrawal, and are more likely to have a history of DSM-defined alcohol use or dependence.[104,105] Among a representative sample of 1,006 US adults, approximately 8% met criteria for the Caffeine Use Disorder research criteria, which was significantly associated with overall caffeine-related distress, sleep problems, and psychological distress.[106] A convenience survey of more than 2,000 adults in New Zealand found that 20% endorsed proposed criteria for Caffeine Use Disorder, rates were higher among women and people who smoke cigarette, and that 50% would be interested in a self-help program for caffeine reduction.[107] Controlled studies have shown that gradual caffeine reduction, self-monitoring, and cognitive behavioral coping strategies are effective for problematic caffeine use.[108,109] Additional research is warranted in order to better understand the features and prevalence of Caffeine Use Disorder, its clinical significance, prognosis, and effective treatment strategies.[110]

GENETICS

Genetic factors account for some of the variability in the use of and effects of caffeine.[46] Relative to dizygotic twins, monozygotic twins have higher concordance rates for total caffeine consumption, heavy caffeine consumption, coffee and tea intake, caffeine intoxication, caffeine withdrawal, caffeine tolerance, and caffeine-related sleep disturbances with heritability ranging between 30% and 77%.[111] There is evidence that a common genetic factor (polysubstance use) underlies the use of caffeine, cigarette, and alcohol use, with 28% to 41% of the heritable effects of caffeine use (or heavy use) shared with alcohol and smoking.[112] Additional research shows DSM-defined caffeine and nicotine dependence to be associated with genetic factors unique to these licit drugs[113] and distinct from illicit drugs.[114] Twin studies have also concluded that caffeine use shares genetic factors with some psychiatric disorders.[115]

There have been numerous studies examining associations between candidate genes and caffeine-related effects and caffeine use. Most research has focused on polymorphisms in the adenosine A2A receptor gene (*ADORA2A*), the CYP12A enzyme gene (the primary enzyme responsible for caffeine metabolism), and the aryl hydrocarbon receptor gene (ACH), which influences the transcription of CYP12A. Polymorphisms in these genes have been shown to be associated with caffeine consumption, the acute effects of caffeine, and some health outcomes.[46,116] Polymorphisms in the CYP1A2 and ACH receptor genes are most reliably associated with variability in caffeine consumption.[116] Various studies have also shown associations between ADORA2A polymorphisms and anxiety.[116] Associations between the "fast metabolizer" CYP1A2 variant and enhanced performance outcomes have been observed but are unreliable across studies.[116,117]

EFFECTS ON PHYSICAL HEALTH

The relationship between caffeine consumption and physical health has been the focus of several scholarly books and reviews.[118-121] Although caffeine is not associated with any life-threatening illnesses, there are some medical conditions that may be adversely affected by caffeine or coffee consumption. Epidemiological research has also provided evidence that caffeine or coffee consumption may have some protective effects against specific diseases, most notably Parkinson disease.[122]

Dietary Guidelines

The 2020-2025 Dietary Guidelines of the U.S. Department of Agriculture suggest that up to 400 mg/d of caffeine from coffee may be part of a healthy diet.[123] The Dietary Guidelines are consistent with a scholarly review of the effects of caffeine on health, which suggested limits of 300 mg/d for reproductive aged women, 400 mg/d for healthy adults, and 2.5 mg/kg/d for children.[49] For pregnant women, the American College of Obstetricians and Gynecologists concluded that consuming less than 200 mg of caffeine per day is unlikely to cause miscarriage or preterm birth.[124] The American Academy of Pediatrics advises against energy drink consumption among children and adolescents.[125] Caffeine-related consumption guidelines for 81 countries can be found elsewhere.[126]

Adverse Health Effects

Caffeine can increase blood pressure, influence heart rate variability, and increase arterial stiffness, but whether such effects represent clinically significant cardiovascular risk factors is debated.[43,127,128] Both caffeinated and decaffeinated coffees contain lipids that raise total and low-density lipoprotein cholesterol with higher levels obtained from unfiltered brewing methods (eg, French press, boiled). Coffee has been shown to exacerbate gastroesophageal reflux[129]; however, it is not clear if it is due to caffeine or other coffee constituents.[130,131] Caffeine is a general risk factor for urinary incontinence in women[132] and men,[133] and reducing caffeine intake has been shown to decrease urinary incontinence.[134] Caffeine consumption increases urinary calcium excretion and has been linked to bone loss and fractures, but it has been suggested that the effects of caffeine on calcium loss may be offset by relatively small intake of milk.[135] There is no evidence that caffeine consumption increases the risk of cancer development.[136] There is also no clear association between caffeine use and peptic or duodenal ulcers.[137]

Evidence from large-scale prospective studies and meta-analyses suggests caffeine consumption prepregnancy and during pregnancy may dose-dependently increase the rate of spontaneous abortion (miscarriage), still birth, low birth weight, and infants that are small for gestational age.[124,138,139] Caffeine use is not reliably associated with decreased fecundity.[140]

Caffeine can also have negative effects on planned sleep. Caffeine delays sleep onset, reduces total sleep time and efficiency, alters the normal stages of sleep, and decreases the reported quality of sleep.[141] Even caffeine taken early in the day can disrupt nighttime sleep.[142] Genetic differences may account for some of the variability in caffeine related sleep disruption and effects may worsen as people age.[141] Caffeine-Induced Sleep Disorder is a diagnosis recognized by DSM-5-TR characterized by a prominent sleep disturbance etiologically related to caffeine use.[71]

Health Protective Effects

There is an inverse association between coffee, tea, and caffeine consumption and risk of Parkinson disease,[143,144] and caffeine-derived compounds have been suggested as potential therapeutic agents for the treatment of Parkinson disease.[145] There is some evidence suggesting protective effects of caffeine consumption against other forms of dementia and depression, but the data are more ambiguous.[146,147] Systematic review of studies examining the effects of coffee on liver health outcomes suggest that increased coffee drinking is associated with reduced progression to cirrhosis for individuals with chronic liver disease, decreased mortality in individuals with cirrhosis, decreased rate of liver cancer, improved response to antiviral treatment in individuals with hepatitis C, and decreased steatohepatitis in individuals with nonalcoholic fatty liver disease.[148] The potential mechanisms of coffee's hepatoprotective effects are many, and some are unrelated to caffeine.[148] Preclinical research and systematic review provide evidence that antioxidant coffee constituents improve glucose metabolism and insulin sensitivity and consequently offer a protective effect of coffee drinking against type 2 diabetes mellitus, with similar effects for caffeinated and decaffeinated coffee.[149,150]

DRUG-DRUG INTERACTIONS

Nicotine and Cigarette Smoking

People who smoke cigarettes consume more caffeine than those who do not smoke cigarettes,[151] and twin studies suggest a high genetic correlation between caffeine use and smoking.[113] Coffee drinking and cigarette smoking tend to temporally covary. Caffeine can increase the reinforcing and stimulant subjective effects of nicotine.[152,153] However, caffeine administration has not been shown to reliably increase cigarette or nicotine self-administration,[154,155] suggesting that the coffee–smoking interaction is not controlled by the pharmacological effects of caffeine alone.

Alcohol

Heavy alcohol use is associated with greater caffeine use.[156,157] One study reported substantial increases in caffeine consumption after alcohol withdrawal management in patients with alcoholism.[158] A study of individuals fulfilling DSM-IV diagnostic criteria for substance dependence as applied to caffeine found that almost 60% had a past diagnosis of DSM-defined alcohol use or dependence.[159]

Alcohol and Energy Drinks

There is some evidence that the co-ingestion of alcohol and caffeinated energy drinks (AEDs) may be associated with increased harm relative to alcohol consumed alone.[160,161] Alcohol consumers who consume AEDs tend to drink more than those who do not.[161,162] Associations have been shown between AEDs and increased stimulation, decreased fatigue, risky sexual behavior, the urge to keep drinking, and drinking and driving.[160,161] Some of these associations may be explained in part by individual differences in risk-seeking that precede alcohol and energy drink consumption. However, self-reported motivations for AED use and evidence from controlled laboratory studies suggest that caffeine decreases the sedative effects of alcohol and increases stimulant effects, prolongs drinking, and thus may result in a greater risk of alcohol-related harms.[161,163]

Studies have also found that young adults who have a higher frequency of energy drink consumption drink more heavily,[164] drive while drunk more frequently,[165] and are at greater risk for DSM-defined alcohol dependence,[166] psychological issues,[167] and other substance use.[168,169] More research is needed regarding the risks associated with energy drink use both alone and in combination with alcohol, including their possible roles in the development of substance use problems.

Other Drug Interactions

Across animal and human studies, caffeine may potentiate the discriminative stimulus effects of cocaine.[170] Caffeine and ephedrine have been shown to mutually potentiate each other's discriminative stimulus effects.[171] Various drugs or conditions that affect the cytochrome P-450 liver enzyme system significantly alter the pharmacokinetics of caffeine.[46,47] There is also preclinical evidence to suggest that caffeine may increase the toxic effects of other stimulant drugs such as d-amphetamine, cocaine, and MDMA.[172-174] Both animal and human studies suggest a mutually antagonistic relationship between caffeine and benzodiazepines.[175]

Caffeine inhibits the metabolism of the antipsychotic clozapine to an extent that might be clinically significant.[176] Because caffeine and theophylline mutually inhibit each other's metabolism, caffeine consumption during theophylline therapy should be monitored. Lithium toxicity may occur after caffeine withdrawal because of decreased renal clearance of lithium.[45]

REFERENCES

1. Fredholm BB, Bättig K, Holmén J, Nehlig A, Zvartau EE. Actions of caffeine in the brain with special reference to factors that contribute to its widespread use. *Pharmacol Rev.* 1999;51(1):83-133.
2. Budavari S, O'Neil M, Smith A. *The Merck Index*. Merck and Co. Published online; 1996.
3. Weinberg BA, Bealer BK. *The World of Caffeine: The Science and Culture of the World's Most Popular Drug*. Routledge; 2004.
4. Fredholm B. Notes on the history of caffeine use. *Handb Exp Pharmacol.* 2011;200:1-9.
5. Reissig CJ, Strain EC, Griffiths RR. Caffeinated energy drinks—a growing problem. *Drug Alcohol Depend.* 2009;99(1-3):1-10.
6. Beauchamp G, Amaducci A, Cook M. Caffeine toxicity: A brief review and update. *Clin Pediat Emerg Med.* 2017;18(3):197-202. doi:10.1016/j.cpem.2017.07.002
7. Institute of Medicine. *Caffeine in Food and Dietary Supplements: Examining Safety—Workshop Summary*. The National Academies Press; 2014.
8. Mitchell DC, Knight CA, Hockenberry J, Teplansky R, Hartman TJ. Beverage caffeine intakes in the US. *Food Chem Toxicol.* 2014;63:136-142.
9. Fulgoni VL III, Keast DR, Lieberman HR. Trends in intake and sources of caffeine in the diets of US adults: 2001-2010. *Am J Clin Nutr.* 2015;101(5):1081-1087.
10. Ahluwalia N, Herrick K. Caffeine intake from food and beverage sources and trends among children and adolescents in the United States: Review of national quantitative studies from 1999 to 2011. *Adv Nutr.* 2015;6(1):102-111.
11. Tran N, Barraj L, Bi X, Jack M. Trends and patterns of caffeine consumption among US teenagers and young adults, NHANES 2003-2012. *Food Chem Toxicol.* 2016;94:227-242.
12. *National Coffee Drinking Trends*. National Coffee Association; 2022.
13. Vercammen KA, Koma JW, Bleich SN. Trends in energy drink consumption among US adolescents and adults, 2003-2016. *Am J Prev Med.* 2019;56(6):827-833.
14. Miller KE, Dermen KH, Lucke JF. Caffeinated energy drink use by US adolescents aged 13-17: A national profile. *Psychol Addic Behav.* 2018;32(6):647.

15. Jagim AR, Harty PS, Barakat AR, et al. Prevalence and amounts of common ingredients found in energy drinks and shots. *Nutrients.* 2022;14(2):314. doi:10.3390/nu14020314
16. Somogyi LP. *Caffeine Intake by the US Population*. Prepared for the Food and Drug Administration and Oakridge National Laboratory. Published online; 2010:475-485.
17. Lieberman HR, Agarwal S, Fulgoni VL. Daily patterns of caffeine intake and the association of intake with multiple sociodemographic and lifestyle factors in US adults based on the NHANES 2007-2012 surveys. *J Acad Nutr Diet.* 2019;119(1):106-114. doi:10.1016/j.jand.2018.08.152
18. Rehm CD, Ratliff JC, Riedt CS, Drewnowski A. Coffee consumption among adults in the United States by demographic variables and purchase location: Analyses of NHANES 2011-2016 data. *Nutrients.* 2020;12(8):2463.
19. Weiser TW. Caffeine as analgesic adjuvant. In: Rajendram R, Patel VB, Preedy VR, Martin CR, eds. *Treatments, Mechanisms, and Adverse Reactions of Anesthetics and Analgesics*. Academic Press; 2022:63-72. doi:10.1016/B978-0-12-820237-1.00007-7
20. Agritelley MS, Goldberger JJ. Caffeine supplementation in the hospital: Potential role for the treatment of caffeine withdrawal. *Food Chem Toxicol.* 2021;153:112228.
21. Chen J, Jin L, Chen X. Efficacy and safety of different maintenance doses of caffeine citrate for treatment of apnea in premature infants: A systematic review and meta-analysis. Muraskas J, ed. *BioMed Res Int.* 2018;2018:9061234. doi:10.1155/2018/9061234
22. Astrup A, Toubro S, Cannon S, Hein P, Breum L, Madsen J. Caffeine: a double-blind, placebo-controlled study of its thermogenic, metabolic, and cardiovascular effects in healthy volunteers. *Am J Clin Nutr.* 1990;51(5):759-767. doi:10.1093/ajcn/51.5.759
23. Kim TW, Shin YO, Lee JB, Min YK, Yang HM. Effect of caffeine on the metabolic responses of lipolysis and activated sweat gland density in human during physical activity. *Food Sci Biotechnol.* 2010;19(4):1077-1081. doi:10.1007/s10068-010-0151-6
24. Ong AC, Myint PK, Potter JF. Pharmacological treatment of postprandial reductions in blood pressure: A systematic review. *J Am Geriatr Soc.* 2014;62(4):649-661.
25. Ferré S. Mechanisms of the psychostimulant effects of caffeine: Implications for substance use disorders. *Psychopharmacology.* 2016;233(10):1963-1979.
26. Rivera-Oliver M, Moreno E, Álvarez-Bagnarol Y, et al. Adenosine A1-dopamine D1 receptor heteromers control the excitability of the spinal motoneuron. *Mol Neurobiol.* 2019;56(2):797-811.
27. Schiffmann SN, Fisone G, Moresco R, Cunha RA, Ferré S. Adenosine A2A receptors and basal ganglia physiology. *Prog Neurobiol.* 2007;83(5):277-292.
28. Ferré S. Role of the central ascending neurotransmitter systems in the psychostimulant effects of caffeine. *J Alzheimers Dis.* 2010;20(s1):S35-S49.
29. Ferré S, Baler R, Bouvier M, et al. Building a new conceptual framework for receptor heteromers. *Nat Chem Biol.* 2009;5(3):131-134.
30. Ferré S, Casadó V, Devi LA, et al. G protein-coupled receptor oligomerization revisited: Functional and pharmacological perspectives. *Pharmacol Rev.* 2014;66(2):413-434.
31. Bonaventura J, Navarro G, Casadó-Anguera V, et al. Allosteric interactions between agonists and antagonists within the adenosine A2A receptor-dopamine D2 receptor heterotetramer. *Proc Natl Acad Sci U S A.* 2015;112(27):E3609-E3618.
32. Ferré S, Bonaventura J, Zhu W, et al. Essential control of the function of the striatopallidal neuron by pre-coupled complexes of adenosine A2A-dopamine D2 receptor heterotetramers and adenylyl cyclase. *Front Pharmacol.* 2018;9:243.
33. Borycz J, Pereira MF, Melani A, et al. Differential glutamate-dependent and glutamate-independent adenosine A1 receptor-mediated modulation of dopamine release in different striatal compartments. *J Neurochem.* 2007;101(2):355-363.
34. Ciruela F, Casadó V, Rodrigues RJ, et al. Presynaptic control of striatal glutamatergic neurotransmission by adenosine A1-A2A receptor heteromers. *J Neurosci.* 2006;26(7):2080-2087.
35. McCarley RW. Neurobiology of REM and NREM sleep. *Sleep Med.* 2007;8(4):302-330.
36. Van Dort CJ, Baghdoyan HA, Lydic R. Adenosine A1 and A2A receptors in mouse prefrontal cortex modulate acetylcholine release and behavioral arousal. *J Neurosci.* 2009;29(3):871-881.
37. Bjorness TE, Kelly CL, Gao T, Poffenberger V, Greene RW. Control and function of the homeostatic sleep response by adenosine A1 receptors. *J Neurosci.* 2009;29(5):1267-1276.
38. Kim Y, Bolortuya Y, Chen L, Basheer R, McCarley RW, Strecker RE. Decoupling of sleepiness from sleep time and intensity during chronic sleep restriction: Evidence for a role of the adenosine system. *Sleep.* 2012;35(6):861-869.
39. Elmenhorst D, Meyer PT, Winz OH, et al. Sleep deprivation increases A1 adenosine receptor binding in the human brain: A positron emission tomography study. *J Neurosci.* 2007;27(9):2410-2415.
40. Jacobson KA, von Lubitz DK, Daly JW, Fredholm BB. Adenosine receptor ligands: differences with acute versus chronic treatment. *Trends Pharmacol Sci.* 1996;17(3):108-113.
41. James JE, Keane MA. Caffeine, sleep and wakefulness: Implications of new understanding about withdrawal reversal. *Hum Psychopharmacol Clin Exp.* 2007;22(8):549-558.
42. Mumford G, Benowitz N, Evans S, et al. Absorption rate of methylxanthines following capsules, cola and chocolate. *Eur J Clin Pharmacol.* 1996;51(3):319-325.
43. James JE. *Understanding Caffeine: A Biobehavioral Analysis.* Sage Publications, Inc; 1997.
44. Denaro CP, Benowitz NL. Caffeine metabolism. *Liver Pathology and Alcohol.* Springer; 1991:513-539.
45. Carrillo JA, Benitez J. Clinically significant pharmacokinetic interactions between dietary caffeine and medications. *Clin Pharmacokinet.* 2000;39(2):127-153.
46. Nehlig A. Interindividual differences in caffeine metabolism and factors driving caffeine consumption. *Pharmacol Rev.* 2018;70(2):384-411.
47. Grzegorzewski J, Bartsch F, Köller A, König M. Pharmacokinetics of caffeine: a systematic analysis of reported data for application in metabolic phenotyping and liver function testing. *Front Pharmacol.* 2022;12:752826-752826. doi:10.3389/fphar.2021.752826
48. Frye RF, Zgheib NK, Matzke GR, et al. Liver disease selectively modulates cytochrome P450-mediated metabolism. *Clini Pharmacol Ther.* 2006;80(3):235-245.
49. Nawrot P, Jordan S, Eastwood J, Rotstein J, Hugenholtz A, Feeley M. Effects of caffeine on human health. *Food Addit Contam.* 2003;20(1):1-30.
50. Yu T, Campbell SC, Stockmann C, et al. Pregnancy-induced changes in the pharmacokinetics of caffeine and its metabolites. *J Clin Pharmacol.* 2016;56(5):590-596.
51. Anderson BL, Juliano LM, Schulkin J. Caffeine's implications for women's health and survey of obstetrician-gynecologists' caffeine knowledge and assessment practices. *J Women's Health.* 2009;18(9):1457-1466.
52. James JE. Critical review of dietary caffeine and blood pressure: A relationship that should be taken more seriously. *Psychosom Med.* 2004;66(1):63-71.
53. Wemple R, Lamb D, McKeever K. Caffeine vs caffeine-free sports drinks: Effects on urine production at rest and during prolonged exercise. *Int J Sports Med.* 1997;18(01):40-46.
54. Rao S, Welcher K, Zimmerman B, Stumbo P. Is coffee a colonic stimulant? *Eur J Gastroenterol Hepatol.* 1998;10(2):113-118.
55. Creighton SM, Stanton S. Caffeine: Does it affect your bladder? *Br J Urol.* 1990;66(6):613-614.
56. Pianosi P, Grondin D, Desmond K, Coates AL, Aranda JV. Effect of caffeine on the ventilatory response to inhaled carbon dioxide. *Respir Physiol.* 1994;95(3):311-320.
57. Becker AB, Simons KJ, Gillespie CA, Simons FER. The bronchodilator effects and pharmacokinetics of caffeine in asthma. *N Engl J Med.* 1984;310(12):743-746.
58. Benowitz NL, Jacob P III, Mayan H, Denaro C. Sympathomimetic effects of paraxanthine and caffeine in humans. *Clin Pharmacol Ther.* 1995;58(6):684-691.

59. Patwardhan RV, Desmond PV, Johnson RF, et al. Effects of caffeine on plasma free fatty acids, urinary catecholamines, and drug binding. *Clin Pharmacol Ther.* 1980;28(3):398-403.
60. Robertson D, Wade D, Workman R, Woosley RL, Oates J. Tolerance to the humoral and hemodynamic effects of caffeine in man. *J Clin Invest.* 1981;67(4):1111-1117.
61. Al'Absi M, Lovallo WR, McKey B, Sung BH, Whitsett TL, Wilson MF. Hypothalamic-pituitary-adrenocortical responses to psychological stress and caffeine in men at high and low risk for hypertension. *Psychosom Med.* 1998;60(4):521-527.
62. Lovallo WR, Farag NH, Vincent AS, Thomas TL, Wilson MF. Cortisol responses to mental stress, exercise, and meals following caffeine intake in men and women. *Pharmacol Biochem Behav.* 2006;83(3):441-447.
63. MacKenzie T, Comi R, Sluss P, et al. Metabolic and hormonal effects of caffeine: randomized, double-blind, placebo-controlled crossover trial. *Metabolism.* 2007;56(12):1694-1698.
64. Lane JD, Feinglos MN, Surwit RS. Caffeine increases ambulatory glucose and postprandial responses in coffee drinkers with type 2 diabetes. *Diabetes Care.* 2008;31(2):221-222.
65. Robertson TM, Clifford MN, Penson S, Chope G, Robertson MD. A single serving of caffeinated coffee impairs postprandial glucose metabolism in overweight men. *Br J Nutr.* 2015;114(8):1218-1225. doi:10.1017/S0007114515002640
66. Griffiths RR, Woodson PP. Reinforcing effects of caffeine in humans. *J Pharmacol Exp Ther.* 1988;246(1):21.
67. Stern KN, Chait LD, Johanson CE. Reinforcing and subjective effects of caffeine in normal human volunteers. *Psychopharmacology.* 1989; 98(1):81-88. doi:10.1007/BF00442010
68. Rogers PJ, Heatherley SV, Mullings EL, Smith JE. Faster but not smarter: effects of caffeine and caffeine withdrawal on alertness and performance. *Psychopharmacology.* 2013;226(2):229-240.
69. Lara DR. Caffeine, mental health, and psychiatric disorders. *J Alzheimers Dis.* 2010;20(s1):S239-S248.
70. Vilarim MM, Rocha Araujo DM, Nardi AE. Caffeine challenge test and panic disorder: a systematic literature review. *Expert Rev Neurother.* 2011;11(8):1185-1195.
71. American Psychiatric Association. *Diagnostic and Statistical Manual of Mental Disorders* (DSM-5-Text Revision (TR)). Published online; 2022.
72. Irwin C, Khalesi S, Desbrow B, McCartney D. Effects of acute caffeine consumption following sleep loss on cognitive, physical, occupational and driving performance: A systematic review and meta-analysis. *Neurosci Biobehav Rev.* 2020;108:877-888.
73. McLellan TM, Caldwell JA, Lieberman HR. A review of caffeine's effects on cognitive, physical and occupational performance. *Neurosci Biobehav Rev.* 2016;71:294-312.
74. Grgic J, Grgic I, Pickering C, Schoenfeld BJ, Bishop DJ, Pedisic Z. Wake up and smell the coffee: Caffeine supplementation and exercise performance—an umbrella review of 21 published meta-analyses. *Br J Sports Med.* 2020;54(11):681-688.
75. Grgic J, Del Coso J. Ergogenic effects of acute caffeine intake on muscular endurance and muscular strength in women: A meta-analysis. *Int J Environ Res Public Health.* 2021;18(11):5773.
76. Guest NS, VanDusseldorp TA, Nelson MT, et al. International society of sports nutrition position stand: Caffeine and exercise performance. *J Int Soc Sports Nutr.* 2021;18(1):1-37.
77. James JE. Caffeine and cognitive performance: Persistent methodological challenges in caffeine research. *Pharmacol Biochem Behav.* 2014;124:117-122. doi:10.1016/j.pbb.2014.05.019
78. James JE, Rogers PJ. Effects of caffeine on performance and mood: Withdrawal reversal is the most plausible explanation. *Psychopharmacology.* 2005;182(1):1-8.
79. Childs E, de Wit H. Subjective, behavioral, and physiological effects of acute caffeine in light, nondependent caffeine users. *Psychopharmacology.* 2006;185(4):514-523.
80. Haskell CF, Kennedy DO, Wesnes KA, Scholey AB. Cognitive and mood improvements of caffeine in habitual consumers and habitual non-consumers of caffeine. *Psychopharmacology.* 2005;179(4):813-825.
81. Addicott MA, Laurienti PJ. A comparison of the effects of caffeine following abstinence and normal caffeine use. *Psychopharmacology.* 2009;207(3):423-431.
82. Smith AP, Christopher G, Sutherland D. Acute effects of caffeine on attention: A comparison of non-consumers and withdrawn consumers. *J Psychopharmacol.* 2013;27(1):77-83.
83. Beaumont R, Cordery P, Funnell M, Mears S, James L, Watson P. Chronic ingestion of a low dose of caffeine induces tolerance to the performance benefits of caffeine. *J Sports Sci.* 2017;35(19):1920-1927. doi:10.1080/02640414.2016.1241421
84. Hughes JR, Oliveto AH, Bickel WK, Higgins ST, Badger GJ. The ability of low doses of caffeine to serve as reinforcers in humans: A replication. *Exp Clin Psychopharmacol.* 1995;3(4):358.
85. Liguori A, Hughes JR. Caffeine self-administration in humans: 2. A within-subjects comparison of coffee and cola vehicles. *Exp Clin Psychopharmacol.* 1997;5(3):295.
86. Sigmon SC, Griffiths RR. Caffeine choice prospectively predicts positive subjective effects of caffeine and d-amphetamine. *Drug Alcohol Depend.* 2011;118(2-3):341-348.
87. Garrett BE, Griffiths RR. Physical dependence increases the relative reinforcing effects of caffeine versus placebo. *Psychopharmacology.* 1998;139(3):195-202. doi:10.1007/s002130050704
88. Shi J, Benowitz NL, Denaro CP, Sheiner LB. Pharmacokinetic-pharmacodynamic modeling of caffeine: Tolerance to pressor effects. *Clin Pharmacol Ther.* 1993;53(1):6-14.
89. World Health Organization. *International Classification of Diseases* (11th Revision); 2019.
90. Cappelletti S, Piacentino D, Fineschi V, Frati P, Cipolloni L, Aromatario M. Caffeine-related deaths: Manner of deaths and categories at risk. *Nutrients.* 2018;10(5):611. doi:10.3390/nu10050611
91. Jabbar SB, Hanly MG. Fatal caffeine overdose: A case report and review of literature. *Am J Forensic Med Pathol.* 2013;34(4):321-324. Accessed June 16, 2023. https://journals.lww.com/amjforensicmedicine/Fulltext/2013/12000/Fatal_Caffeine_Overdose__A_Case_Report_and_Review.8.aspx
92. Nadeem IM, Shanmugaraj A, Sakha S, Horner NS, Ayeni OR, Khan M. Energy drinks and their adverse health effects: A systematic review and meta-analysis. *Sports Health.* 2021;13(3):265-277.
93. Substance Abuse and Mental Health Services Administration. *The DAWN Report: Update on Emergency Department Visits Involving Energy Drinks: A Continuing Public Health Concern.* 2013.
94. Markon AO, Jones OE, Punzalan CM, Lurie P, Wolpert B. Caffeinated energy drinks: adverse event reports to the US Food and Drug Administration and the National Poison Data System, 2008 to 2015. *Public Health Nutr.* 2019;22(14):2531-2542. doi:10.1017/S1368980019001605
95. Juliano LM, Huntley ED, Harrell PT, Westerman AT. Development of the caffeine withdrawal symptom questionnaire: Caffeine withdrawal symptoms cluster into 7 factors. *Drug Alcohol Depend.* 2012;124(3):229-234.
96. Juliano LM, Griffiths RR. A critical review of caffeine withdrawal: Empirical validation of symptoms and signs, incidence, severity, and associated features. *Psychopharmacology.* 2004;176(1):1-29.
97. Jones HE, Herning RI, Cadet JL, Griffiths RR. Caffeine withdrawal increases cerebral blood flow velocity and alters quantitative electroencephalography (EEG) activity. *Psychopharmacology.* 2000; 147(4):371-377.
98. Sigmon SC, Herning RI, Better W, Cadet JL, Griffiths RR. Caffeine withdrawal, acute effects, tolerance, and absence of net beneficial effects of chronic administration: cerebral blood flow velocity, quantitative EEG, and subjective effects. *Psychopharmacology.* 2009;204(4):573-585.
99. Evans SM, Griffiths RR. Caffeine withdrawal: a parametric analysis of caffeine dosing conditions. *J Pharmacol Exp Ther.* 1999;289(1):285-294.
100. Griffiths R, Evans S, Heishman S, et al. Low-dose caffeine physical dependence in humans. *J Pharmacol Exp Ther.* 1990;255(3):1123-1132.
101. Dews PB, Curtis GL, Hanford KJ, O'Brien CP. The frequency of caffeine withdrawal in a population-based survey and in a controlled, blinded pilot experiment. *J Clin Pharmacol.* 1999;39(12):1221-1232.

102. Juliano LM, Kardel PG, Harrell PT, Muench C, Edwards KC. Investigating the role of expectancy in caffeine withdrawal using the balanced placebo design. *Human Psychopharmacol Clin Exp.* 2019;34(2):e2692.
103. Shephard A, Barrett SP. The impacts of caffeine administration, expectancies, and related stimuli on coffee craving, withdrawal, and self-administration. *J Psychopharmacol.* 2022;36(3):378-386.
104. Juliano LM, Evatt DP, Richards BD, Griffiths RR. Characterization of individuals seeking treatment for caffeine dependence. *Psychol Addict Behav.* 2012;26(4):948-954. doi:10.1037/a0027246
105. Meredith SE, Juliano LM, Hughes JR, Griffiths RR. Caffeine use disorder: a comprehensive review and research agenda. *J Caffeine Res.* 2013;3(3):114-130.
106. Sweeney MM, Weaver DC, Vincent KB, Arria AM, Griffiths RR. Prevalence and correlates of caffeine use disorder symptoms among a United States Sample. *J Caffeine Adenosine Res.* 2020;10(1):4-11. doi:10.1089/caff.2019.0020
107. Booth N, Saxton J, Rodda S. Estimates of caffeine use disorder, caffeine withdrawal, harm and help-seeking in New Zealand: A cross-sectional survey. *Addict Behav.* 2020;109:106470.
108. Evatt DP, Juliano LM, Griffiths RR. A brief manualized treatment for problematic caffeine use: a randomized control trial. *J Consult Clin Psychol.* 2016;84(2):113.
109. Sweeney MM, Meredith SE, Juliano LM, Evatt DP, Griffiths RR. A randomized controlled trial of a manual-only treatment for reduction and cessation of problematic caffeine use. *Drug Alcohol Depend.* 2019;195: 45-51.
110. Hasin DS, O'Brien CP, Auriacombe M, et al. DSM-5 criteria for substance use disorders: recommendations and rationale. *AJP.* 2013;170(8):834-851. doi:10.1176/appi.ajp.2013.12060782
111. Yang A, Palmer AA, de Wit H. Genetics of caffeine consumption and responses to caffeine. *Psychopharmacology.* 2010;211(3):245-257.
112. Hettema JM, Corey LA, Kendler KS. A multivariate genetic analysis of the use of tobacco, alcohol, and caffeine in a population based sample of male and female twins. *Drug Alcohol Depend.* 1999;57(1):69-78.
113. Treur JL, Taylor AE, Ware JJ, et al. Smoking and caffeine consumption: a genetic analysis of their association. *Addict Biol.* 2017;22(4):1090-1102.
114. Kendler KS, Chen X, Dick D, et al. Recent advances in the genetic epidemiology and molecular genetics of substance use disorders. *Nat Neurosci.* 2012;15(2):181-189.
115. Bergin JE, Kendler KS. Common psychiatric disorders and caffeine use, tolerance, and withdrawal: An examination of shared genetic and environmental effects. *Twin Res Hum Genet.* 2012;15(4):473-482.
116. Fulton JL, Dinas PC, Carrillo AE, Edsall JR, Ryan EJ, Ryan EJ. Impact of genetic variability on physiological responses to caffeine in humans: A systematic review. *Nutrients.* 2018;10(10):1373.
117. Grgic J, Pickering C, Del Coso J, Schoenfeld BJ, Mikulic P. CYP1A2 genotype and acute ergogenic effects of caffeine intake on exercise performance: A systematic review. *Eur J Nutr.* 2021;60(3):1181-1195.
118. Cornelis MC. The impact of caffeine and coffee on human health. *Nutrients.* 2019;11(2):416.
119. Higdon JV, Frei B. Coffee and health: A review of recent human research. *Crit Rev Food Sci Nutr.* 2006;46(2):101-123.
120. James J. *Caffeine and Health.* Academic Press; 1991.
121. van Dam RM, Hu FB. Caffeine consumption and cardiovascular health. *Nat Rev Cardiol.* 2022;19(7):429-430.
122. Hong CT, Chan L, Bai CH. The effect of caffeine on the risk and progression of Parkinson's disease: a meta-analysis. *Nutrients.* 2020;12(6):1860.
123. U.S. Department of Agriculture and U.S. Department of Health and Human Services. *Dietary Guidelines for Americans, 2020-2025.* 9th ed.
124. James JE. Maternal caffeine consumption and pregnancy outcomes: A narrative review with implications for advice to mothers and mothers-to-be. *BMJ Evid Based Med.* 2021;26(3):114-115.
125. Schneider MB, Benjamin HJ. Sports drinks and energy drinks for children and adolescents: Are they appropriate? *Pediatrics.* 2011;127(6):1182-1189.
126. Reyes CM, Cornelis MC. Caffeine in the diet: country-level consumption and guidelines. *Nutrients.* 2018;10(11):1772.
127. De Giuseppe R, Di Napoli I, Granata F, Mottolese A, Cena H. Caffeine and blood pressure: a critical review perspective. *Nutr Res Rev.* 2019; 32(2):169-175.
128. Lim D, Chang J, Ahn J, Kim J. Conflicting effects of coffee consumption on cardiovascular diseases: Does coffee consumption aggravate pre-existing risk factors? *Processes.* 2020;8(4):438.
129. Boekema PJ, Samsom M, van Berge Henegouwen GP, Smout AJ. Coffee and gastrointestinal function: facts and fiction: A review. *Scand J Gastroenterol.* 1999;34(230):35-39.
130. Mehta RS, Song M, Staller K, Chan AT. Association between beverage intake and incidence of gastroesophageal reflux symptoms. *Clin Gastroenterol Hepatol.* 2020;18(10):2226-2233.e4. doi:10.1016/j.cgh.2019.11.040
131. Pehl C, Pfeiffer A, Wendl B, Kaess H. The effect of decaffeination of coffee on gastro-oesophageal reflux in patients with reflux disease. *Aliment Pharmacol Ther.* 1997;11(3):483-486.
132. Balalau DO, Olaru OG, Bacalbasa N, Paunica S, Balan DG, Stanescu AD. The analysis of risk factors associated with women's urinary incontinence; literature review. *J Mind Med Sci.* 2021;8(1):53-59.
133. Davis NJ, Vaughan CP, Johnson TM II, et al. Caffeine intake and its association with urinary incontinence in United States men: Results from National Health and Nutrition Examination Surveys 2005-2006 and 2007-2008. *J Urol.* 2013;189(6):2170-2174.
134. Bryant CM, Dowell CJ, Fairbrother G. Caffeine reduction education to improve urinary symptoms. *Br J Nurs.* 2002;11(8):560-565.
135. O'Keefe JH, Bhatti SK, Patil HR, DiNicolantonio JJ, Lucan SC, Lavie CJ. Effects of habitual coffee consumption on cardiometabolic disease, cardiovascular health, and all-cause mortality. *J Am Coll Cardiol.* 2013;62(12):1043-1051.
136. van Dam RM, Hu FB, Willett WC. Coffee, caffeine, and health. *N Engl J Med.* 2020;383(4):369-378.
137. Aldoori WH, Giovannucci EL, Rimm EB, Wing AL, Trichopoulos DV, Willett WC. A prospective study of alcohol, smoking, caffeine, and the risk of symptomatic diverticular disease in men. *Ann Epidemiol.* 1995;5(3):221-228.
138. Gaskins AJ, Rich-Edwards JW, Williams PL, Toth TL, Missmer SA, Chavarro JE. Pre-pregnancy caffeine and caffeinated beverage intake and risk of spontaneous abortion. *Eur J Nutr.* 2018;57(1):107-117.
139. Greenwood DC, Thatcher NJ, Ye J, et al. Caffeine intake during pregnancy and adverse birth outcomes: A systematic review and dose-response meta-analysis. *Eur J Epidemiol.* 2014;29(10):725-734.
140. Lyngsø J, Ramlau-Hansen CH, Bay B, Ingerslev HJ, Hulman A, Kesmodel US. Association between coffee or caffeine consumption and fecundity and fertility: A systematic review and dose-response meta-analysis. *Clin Epidemiol.* 2017;9:699-719. doi:10.2147/CLEP.S146496
141. Clark I, Landolt HP. Coffee, caffeine, and sleep: A systematic review of epidemiological studies and randomized controlled trials. *Sleep Med Rev.* 2017;31:70-78.
142. Landolt HP, Werth E, Borbély AA, Dijk DJ. Caffeine intake (200 mg) in the morning affects human sleep and EEG power spectra at night. *Brain Res.* 1995;675(1-2):67-74.
143. Costa J, Lunet N, Santos C, Santos J, Vaz-Carneiro A. Caffeine exposure and the risk of Parkinson's disease: A systematic review and meta-analysis of observational studies. *J Alzheimers Dis.* 2010;20(s1):S221-S238. doi:10.3233/JAD-2010-091525
144. Qi H, Li S. Dose-response meta-analysis on coffee, tea and caffeine consumption with risk of Parkinson's disease. *Geriatr Gerontol Int.* 2014;14(2):430-439.
145. Roshan MHK, Tambo A, Pace NP. Potential role of caffeine in the treatment of Parkinson's disease. *Open Neurol J.* 2016;10:42-58. doi:10.2174/1874205X01610010042
146. Carman A, Dacks P, Lane R, Shineman D, Fillit H. Current evidence for the use of coffee and caffeine to prevent age-related cognitive decline and Alzheimer's disease. *J Nutr Health Aging.* 2014;18(4):383-392.
147. Grosso G, Micek A, Castellano S, Pajak A, Galvano F. Coffee, tea, caffeine and risk of depression: a systematic review and dose-response meta-analysis of observational studies. *Mol Nutr Food Res.* 2016;60(1):223-234.

148. Saab S, Mallam D, Cox GA, Tong MJ. Impact of coffee on liver diseases: A systematic review. *Liver Int.* 2014;34(4):495-504.
149. Carlström M, Larsson SC. Coffee consumption and reduced risk of developing type 2 diabetes: A systematic review with meta-analysis. *Nutrition Rev.* 2018;76(6):395-417. doi:10.1093/nutrit/nuy014
150. Jiang X, Zhang D, Jiang W. Coffee and caffeine intake and incidence of type 2 diabetes mellitus: a meta-analysis of prospective studies. *Eur J Nutr.* 2014;53(1):25-38. doi:10.1007/s00394-013-0603-x
151. Swanson JA, Lee JW, Hopp JW. Caffeine and nicotine: A review of their joint use and possible interactive effects in tobacco withdrawal. *Addict Behav.* 1994;19(3):229-256.
152. Jones HE, Griffiths RR. Oral caffeine maintenance potentiates the reinforcing and stimulant subjective effects of intravenous nicotine in cigarette smokers. *Psychopharmacology.* 2003;165(3):280-290.
153. Tanda G, Goldberg SR. Alteration of the behavioral effects of nicotine by chronic caffeine exposure. *Pharmacol Biochem Behav.* 2000;66(1):47-64.
154. Chait LD, Griffiths RR. Effects of caffeine on cigarette smoking and subjective response. *Clin Pharmacol Ther.* 1983;34(5):612-622.
155. Perkins KA, Fonte C, Stolinski A, Blakesley-Ball R, Wilson AS. The influence of caffeine on nicotine's discriminative stimulus, subjective, and reinforcing effects. *Exp Clin Psychopharmacol.* 2005;13(4):275.
156. Istvan J, Matarazzo JD. Tobacco, alcohol, and caffeine use: A review of their interrelationships. *Psychol Bull.* 1984;95(2):301.
157. Kozlowski L, Henningfield JE, Keenan R, et al. Patterns of alcohol, cigarette, and caffeine and other drug use in two drug abusing populations. *J Subst Abuse Treat.* 1993;10(2):171-179.
158. Aubin H, Laureaux C, Tilikete S, Barrucand D. Changes in cigarette smoking and coffee drinking after alcohol detoxification in alcoholics. *Addiction.* 1999;94(3):411-416.
159. Strain EC, Mumford GK, Silverman K, Griffiths RR. Caffeine dependence syndrome: Evidence from case histories and experimental evaluations. *JAMA.* 1994;272(13):1043-1048.
160. Marczinski CA, Fillmore MT. Energy drinks mixed with alcohol: What are the risks? *Nutr Rev.* 2014;72(suppl. 1):98-107.
161. McKetin R, Coen A, Kaye S. A comprehensive review of the effects of mixing caffeinated energy drinks with alcohol. *Drug Alcohol Depend.* 2015;151:15-30.
162. Verster JC, Benson S, Johnson SJ, Alford C, Godefroy SB, Scholey A. Alcohol mixed with energy drink (AMED): A critical review and meta-analysis. *Human Psychopharmacol Clin Exp.* 2018;33(2):e2650.
163. Sweeney MM, Meredith SE, Evatt DP, Griffiths RR. Effects of caffeine on alcohol reinforcement: beverage choice, self-administration, and subjective ratings. *Psychopharmacology.* 2017;234(5):877-888.
164. Brache K, Stockwell T. Drinking patterns and risk behaviors associated with combined alcohol and energy drink consumption in college drinkers. *Addict Behav.* 2011;36(12):1133-1140.
165. Arria AM, Caldeira KM, Bugbee BA, Vincent KB, O'Grady KE. Energy drink use patterns among young adults: associations with drunk driving. *Alcohol Clin Exp Res.* 2016;40(11):2456-2466.
166. Arria AM, Caldeira KM, Kasperski SJ, Vincent KB, Griffiths RR, O'Grady KE. Energy drink consumption and increased risk for alcohol dependence. *Alcohol Clin Exp Res.* 2011;35(2):365-375.
167. Dawodu A, Cleaver K. Behavioural correlates of energy drink consumption among adolescents: A review of the literature. *J Child Health Care.* 2017;21(4):446-462. doi:10.1177/1367493517731948
168. Galimov A, Hanewinkel R, Hansen J, Unger JB, Sussman S, Morgenstern M. Association of energy drink consumption with substance-use initiation among adolescents: A 12-month longitudinal study. *J Psychopharmacol.* 2020;34(2):221-228. doi:10.1177/0269881119895545
169. Yasuma N, Imamura K, Watanabe K, Nishi D, Kawakami N, Takano A. Association between energy drink consumption and substance use in adolescence: A systematic review of prospective cohort studies. *Drug Alcohol Depend.* 2021;219:108470. doi:10.1016/j.drugalcdep.2020.108470
170. Oliveto A, McCance-Katz E, Singha A, Hameedi F, Kosten T. Effects of d-amphetamine and caffeine in humans under a cocaine discrimination procedure. *Behav Pharmacol.* 1998;9(3):207-217.
171. Young R, Gabryszuk M, Glennon RA. Ephedrine and caffeine mutually potentiate one another's amphetamine-like stimulus effects. *Pharmacol Biochem Behav.* 1998;61(2):169-173.
172. Derlet RW, Tseng JC, Albertson TE. Potentiation of cocaine and d-amphetamine toxicity with caffeine. *Am J Emerg Med.* 1992;10(3):211-216.
173. McNamara R, Kerans A, O'Neill B, Harkin A. Caffeine promotes hyperthermia and serotonergic loss following co-administration of the substituted amphetamines, MDMA ("Ecstasy") and MDA ("Love"). *Neuropharmacology.* 2006;50(1):69-80.
174. McNamara R, Maginn M, Harkin A. Caffeine induces a profound and persistent tachycardia in response to MDMA ("Ecstasy") administration. *Eur J Pharmacol.* 2007;555(2-3):194-198.
175. White JM. Behavioral effects of caffeine coadministered with nicotine, benzodiazepines, and alcohol. *Caffeine and Behavior.* CRC Press; 1999:75-86.
176. Hägg S, Spigset O, Mjörndal T, Dahlqvist R. Effect of caffeine on clozapine pharmacokinetics in healthy volunteers. *Br J Clin Pharmacol.* 2000;49(1):59-63.

16 The Pharmacology of Nicotine and Tobacco

John A. Dani, Thomas R. Kosten, and Neal L. Benowitz

CHAPTER OUTLINE

- Introduction and nicotine chemistry
- Methods of use
- Epidemiology and historical features
- Pharmacokinetics
- Pharmacological actions
- Clinical manifestations
- Neurobiological mechanisms of action
- Systemic toxicity

INTRODUCTION AND NICOTINE CHEMISTRY

Tobacco use and tobacco (nicotine) use disorder are worldwide health challenges not only because of this addiction disorder, but also because smoke contains more than 7,000 chemicals, including over 70 known carcinogens.[1] While multiple constituents may contribute to the reinforcing properties of tobacco[2] including nornicotine, anabasine and acetaldehyde, nicotine is the main addictive component. Therefore, understanding the pharmacology of nicotine is important in devising effective treatments for this substance use disorder.

Nicotine is the only drug in this class of substances. It is a naturally occurring alkaloid that serves as an insecticide in many plants. Chemically, nicotine is a tertiary amine that consists of a pyridine and a pyrrolidine ring. There are two stereoisomers of nicotine. The (S)-nicotine form (**Fig. 16-1**) found in tobacco is the active isomer that binds to diverse nicotinic acetylcholine receptor (nAChR) subtypes throughout the central nervous system (CNS). The (R)-nicotine form is a weak agonist at cholinergic receptors, but has similar efficacy on transient receptor potential A1 (TRPA1) receptors which are involved in sensory response to nicotine.[3] Also, it is reported that the increase in nicotine receptor binding sites with chronic nicotine administration in rats is increased similarly by (S)- and (R)-nicotine, which may be important in the pathophysiology of DSM-defined nicotine dependence.[4] During smoking, some racemization takes place, and small quantities of (R)-nicotine are found in cigarette smoke. The pharmacology of (R)-nicotine is particularly relevant now because a number of electronic cigarette brands as well as oral nicotine products are being marketed with synthetic nicotine, which is often racemic.[5] Because nicotine is a tertiary amine, it can exist in a charged and uncharged form. In the charged form, nicotine cannot cross cell membranes unaided, and it binds to nAChRs.[6] In the uncharged form, nicotine is membrane permeable. Therefore, nicotine can influence intracellular processes indirectly via nAChRs and directly by entering the cytoplasm.[7]

METHODS OF USE

Multiple routes of administration are used for nicotine, and include inhalation through smoke or aerosol, transmucosal by intranasal or buccal (snus), oral, and transdermal. The delivery devices and formulations for these various methods of use involve both nonmedical and therapeutic aims. Overall, nicotine and the reinforcing sensory stimulation associated with tobacco use are responsible for the compulsive use of tobacco in the form of cigarettes, bidis, cigars, pipes, water pipes, snuff, and chewing tobacco.[7-9] Nicotine replacement medications that are used to stabilize the nicotine withdrawal syndrome include nicotine polacrilex gum, transdermal patches, nasal spray and inhalers. Other delivery mechanisms include e-cigarettes and heated tobacco products, collectively referred to as electronic drug delivery devices [EDDDs] (for additional detail, please see Chapter 22 "Electronic Drug Delivery Devices") that have become widely available. They heat a nicotine solution to generate a nicotine-containing aerosol that is inhaled. In contrast to regular cigarettes, EDDD aerosol is generated by heating, but combustion of plant material is debatable as some evidence of combustion has recently been demonstrated in some so-called heat-not-burn EDDD products. Edds have been marketed for use as a recreational product, or in settings where one cannot smoke regular cigarettes, and/or to cut down or quit combustible cigarette use; however, their effectiveness for the latter purpose on a population level is debated[10] and remains uncertain.[11] In this chapter we will use the term "vaping" which is commonly used by the EDDD industry, the lay public, and our patients; however, a more correct and medically precise term is "aerosol/aerosolizing." A Cochrane review of 34 clinical trials found moderate evidence that EDDDs increased cessation of tobacco use.[12] In population studies, regular and frequent use of e-cigarettes is associated with (but not necessarily causally linked with) increased quitting, but occasional use of e-cigarettes may be associated with a lower quit rate, possibly because e-cigarettes provide a source of nicotine where smoking is prohibited.[13,14] Vaping among young people who do not smoke has been a concern as a potential cause of incident nicotine/tobacco use disorder, possibly via socially renormalizing

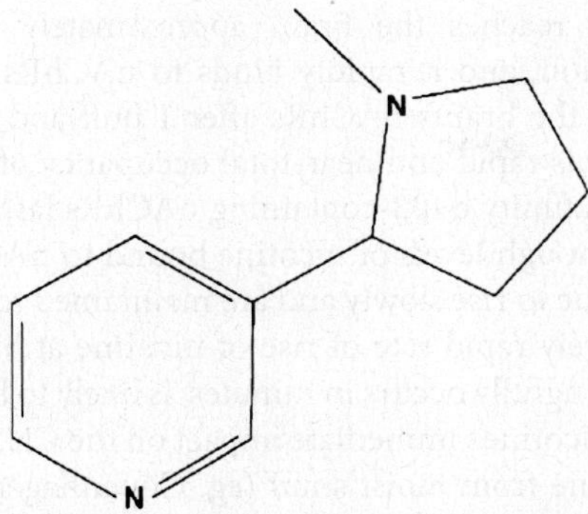

Figure 16-1. The chemical structure of nicotine. The chemical IUPAC name is 3-(1-methylpyrrolidin-2-yl)pyridine and the chemical formula is $C_{10}H_{14}N_2$.

smoking and/or by having adverse effects on the adolescent brain.[10] However, despite an increase in vaping, smoking rates among adolescents have been declining since 1997. Importantly, vaping is prevalent in U.S. middle and high schoolers, and when used without traditional cigarette exposures can lead to nicotine use disorder which may have similar adverse effects on the developing brain (which continues to mature biologically into age early 20s).

While switching 100% from traditional smoking to EDDDs may reduce exposure to many toxic compounds generated by combustion of tobacco, EDDDs may still provide smaller exposures to some toxicants (with long term consequences being uncertain) and does introduce other new toxicants—all while still maintaining exposure to inhaled nicotine, which may have its own long-term harms. Nicotinic AChRs are involved in critical brain maturation processes, and there is some concern that nicotine exposure from EDDDs may induce epigenetic changes that sensitize the brain to other drugs and prime it for future substance use.[15,16] Nicotine may contribute to acute cardiovascular events in people with underlying cardiovascular disease, and may promote tumor development, but it is not a tumor initiator in carcinogenesis.[17] Thus, completely substituting tobacco cigarettes with EDDDs may reduce exposure to selected tobacco-specific toxicants, but EDDDs are not safe.[9,18] Further, dual-use of both combustible tobacco and EDDDs is not uncommon; thus causing overlapping of unique EDDD-specific toxicant exposures alongside combustion-related toxicants. Dual toxicant exposure from dual use (in parallel or in series, or both) over a significant lifespan of use to enable assessment for adverse outcomes has not been well-studied. Like most addictive drugs, the method of administration modifies the addictive influence. Nicotine is much more addictive during rapid administration, as obtained by smoking tobacco or as increasingly obtained by subsequent generations of EDDD development (vaping); whereas the nicotine patch provides slow administration. The potential harms of EDDDs, as well as their use to possibly stop traditional tobacco use, is covered in more detail in Chapter 22 "Electronic Drug Delivery Devices".

EPIDEMIOLOGY AND HISTORICAL FEATURES

Indigenous American tribes cultivated and used tobacco for many ceremonies and religious customs for thousands of years before the arrival of Europeans. Tobacco was first commercially grown for the European market at the first permanent English settlement in America, Jamestown, which was founded in 1607. Tobacco became an important economic influence in the British American colonies and the early United States. Tobacco over the past three centuries has remained an important economic influence in the United States and world-wide, and gone from a ceremonial symbol to a broadly used substance requiring clinical attention.

The World Health Organization and Global Burden of Disease research has found that over the past 30 years, smoking prevalence—the percent of people who smoke in a population —has decreased, but the number of people smoking cigarettes worldwide has increased because of population growth. Overall, one-third of the global adult population smokes tobacco. In the United States, 12.5% of adults (30.8 million) smoked regularly in 2020.[19-22] This level of smoking is a decrease from 21% of adults smoking in 2005, but this level is likely to be more difficult to decrease further because of the co-occurrence of psychiatric disorders in the core group of people who still smoke.[21,23] Greece has the highest proportion of people smoking in the European Union at around 42% in 2020, and more broadly cigarette smoking prevalence is linked to lower income levels worldwide. The association of high smoking rates in poorer areas of the world has been attributed to tobacco companies targeting these communities, and to the stresses of living in poverty and sometimes hopelessness also leading people to turn to cigarettes. In most countries, men are more likely to smoke than women and 90% of people who smoke began smoking by the age of 25.[23] The age of smoking onset is often in adolescence, and about 23.6% of high school students reported in 2020 that they had used any tobacco product including cigarettes in the past 30 days—a decrease from 31.2% in 2019. After increasing between 2017 and 2019, current (past 30 day) use of e-cigarettes also went down among middle and high school students from 2019 to 2020. About 1 of every 5 high school students (19.6%) reported in 2020 that they used electronic cigarettes in the past 30 days—a decrease from 27.5% in 2019. However, these reporting windows overlap with the early wave of the COVID pandemic wherein socialization and access to goods and transportation fell sharply, while concern for respiratory health increased sharply.

A more severe condition than simply any smoking is tobacco use disorder as defined in DSM-5. This disorder is present in approximately 80% of people who smoke, with higher rates among those with co-occurring psychiatric disorders. For example, rates of DSM-5 defined tobacco use disorder are substantially higher among adults with ADHD (40%) than in the general population (about 12.5%). Among adults who smoke, the presence of ADHD is associated with early initiation of regular cigarette smoking, even after controlling for confounding variables such as socioeconomic status, IQ, and psychiatric disorders. A similar high rate of co-occurrence occurs with depression. The lifetime prevalence of depression is 59% among subjects who had ever smoked, compared with 17% in the general population. The prevalence of smoking in individuals with major depression is twice that observed in the general population.[24] Nicotine use has even higher prevalence among patients with bipolar disorder (60%-70% rates) and schizophrenia (70%-80% rates) and has a strong association with suicide among these patients. A history of mood disorder or schizophrenia may speed the progression from tobacco use to tobacco use disorder. Twin studies support a model with common risk factors for both depression and cigarette smoking. The genetic correlation between major depression and smoking behavior is relatively high and driven by additive genetic effects ($r_G = 0.249$).

PHARMACOKINETICS

Absorption, Distribution, Metabolism, and Elimination

The absorption of nicotine depends on its pH. Below pH 6, tobacco smoke contains less than 1% unprotonated (free or free base) nicotine. As the pH rises, so does the proportion of unprotonated nicotine. At pH 7.26, 15% of the nicotine is unprotonated, increasing to 50% at pH 8. Unprotonated nicotine is present mainly in the gas phase of the aerosol of smoke, whereas protonated nicotine is contained primarily within semisolid particles in the smoke aerosol. Unprotonated (free base) nicotine is readily absorbed through the mucous membranes of the oral and nasal cavities. Tobacco products such as large cigars, many pipe tobaccos, snuffs, and chewing tobaccos present nicotine either as predominantly unionized (unprotonated), aerosolized component of smoke or as an alkaline solution of nicotine. Tobacco smoke with pH levels above 6.2 contains increasing amounts of free ammonia, nitrates that are partially reduced to ammonia during smoking, and other volatile basic components.

Because alkaline smoke is irritating to the pharynx, it is harsh and difficult to inhale, and particular strains of tobacco and curing processes can reduce this alkaline pH to reduce the irritation (ie, "smoother" or "smoothing" the tobacco, respectively) and thus enable deeper inhalation. The ionized nicotine in such smoke is largely dissolved in the aerosol droplets. After small droplets of tar and nicotine are inhaled and deposited in small airways and alveoli, the protonated nicotine is buffered to a physiological pH and absorbed. Inhaled nicotine avoids first-pass hepatic metabolism. It is quickly delivered from the large surface area of the alveoli and circulation in the lung to the arterial bloodstream and then to the brain and other tissues. Thus, various combinations of tobacco species, curing processes, additives, and other measures are involved to deliver a wide array of tobacco products.

Nicotine reaches the brain approximately 20 seconds after inhalation, and it rapidly binds to nAChRs (occupying one-third of the brain's nAChRs after 1 puff and 88% after 1 cigarette). This rapid and near-total occupancy of the human brain's high-affinity $\alpha4\beta2$-containing nAChRs lasts more than 3 hours. Although levels of nicotine bound to nAChRs in the brain continue to rise slowly and are maintained for hours, the initial relatively rapid rate of rise of nicotine at brain targets, which meaningfully occurs in minutes, is likely to be the determinant for nicotine's immediate impact on the CNS. The delivery of nicotine from moist snuff (eg, Copenhagen) is slower, with the plasma concentration of nicotine continuing to rise throughout a 30-minute period of use and relieving subjective nicotine craving for a longer time than from smoked tobacco.

The relatively rapid delivery of nicotine to the brain in the smoking process allows precise dose titration so that the person who smokes can obtain the desired effects. People who smoke can control nicotine intake by altering their puff volume, the number of puffs they take, the frequency of puffing, and the depth to which they inhale. They also can increase smoke/nicotine intake by blocking the ventilation holes on the cigarette filter with their fingers or their lips, thereby reducing the amount of outside air drawn in to mix with the smoke being pulled in from the burning end of the cigarette into the person's mouth. Because of the complexity of smoking, the dose of nicotine taken in by a person cannot be accurately predicted from the nicotine content of the tobacco or a cigarette's machine-rated yield. Individuals smoke to obtain desired levels of nicotine from cigarettes and they will largely compensate for the engineering features, such as blocking the filter ventilation holes as described above. Importantly, the term filter is generally a misnomer, as filters do not protect the person smoking; instead they work to make the smoke particles inhaled through the cigarette smaller, thus increasing drug delivery into the person.

Nicotine is poorly absorbed from the stomach because of the acidity of the gastric fluid, but it is well absorbed in the small intestine, which has an alkaline pH as well as a large surface area. When nicotine is administered in capsules, peak concentrations are reached in just over an hour. Nicotine undergoes first-pass metabolism; its oral bioavailability is approximately 45%.

Nicotine obtained from smoking tobacco or vaping nicotine reaches high initial concentrations in the arterial blood and lungs. After nicotine is absorbed into the bloodstream, it has a volume of distribution of about 180 L, with less than 5% binding to plasma proteins. Subsequently, nicotine distributes into the brain and is stored in adipose and muscle tissue. Arterial blood levels of nicotine are two- to sixfold higher than venous blood levels. The average steady-state concentration of nicotine in the body tissues is 2.6 times the average steady-state concentration of nicotine in the blood. Nicotine crosses the placenta freely and has been found in the amniotic fluid and in the umbilical cord blood of neonates. Nicotine also is found in breast milk at concentrations approximately twice those found in the mother's blood.

Based on a half-life of 2 to 3 hours, nicotine accumulates during a day of regular smoking (3-4 half-lives) and persists for 6 to 8 hours after smoking ceases. Steady-state plasma nicotine levels, which plateau in the early afternoon (for typical smoking patterns of starting upon awakening in the morning) typically range between 10 and 50 ng/mL. The increment in blood nicotine concentration after smoking one cigarette ranges from 5 to 30 ng/mL, depending on how the cigarette is smoked. Peak blood concentrations of nicotine are similar for people who use cigars, snuff, chewing tobacco, and those who smoke cigarettes. The rate of rise of nicotine concentrations is slower with use of snuff and chewing tobacco, with peak nicotine levels occurring at 20 to 30 minutes. People who smoke seem to manipulate their nicotine intake to maintain a consistent level of nicotine from day to day. Based on positron emission tomography imaging, the distribution of nicotine onto brain nAChRs is slower than the rise in the bloodstream.

Smoking represents a multiple-dosing situation throughout the day, with considerable accumulation of nicotine in the body tissues (including the brain). Nicotine persists in the body around the clock. Peaks and troughs in blood nicotine concentrations follow each cigarette (**Fig. 16-2**), but those variations are smoothed out within the brain. As the day progresses for the person who regularly smokes, the overall level of nicotine accumulates and rises, and the potential influence of each dose becomes less important. Rapid tolerance occurs, so that the effects of individual cigarettes tend to lessen throughout the day. Overnight abstinence results in low nicotine levels overnight and upon awakening, which then causes considerable re-sensitization of nicotinic receptors to nondesensitized states (**Fig. 16-2**), and nicotine withdrawal. For these reasons, the first smoke in the morning is often described as the most rewarding (a result of both positive reinforcement from the rapid rise of nicotine from its low overnight trough levels, and negative reinforcement from the rapid relief of withdrawal symptoms such as irritability, poor concentration, etc.). The populations of nAChR subtypes begin to change as other molecular mechanisms involving neuroadaptations come into play after days and weeks of tobacco use.[6,25]

Nicotine is extensively metabolized primarily in the liver and to a lesser extent in the lung and in the brain with the metabolite cotinine having the highest blood concentration but little pharmacological effect compared to nicotine. On average, 80% of nicotine is metabolized to cotinine, with smaller fractions metabolized to nicotine *N*-oxide and nicotine glucuronide. Cotinine is further metabolized to trans-3'-hydroxycotinine, the major nicotine metabolite found in the urine, as well as cotinine glucuronide, cotinine methonium ion, 5'-hydroxycotinine, and cotinine-*N*-oxide and trans 3'-hydroxycotinine glucuronide. About 17% of cotinine is excreted unchanged in the urine. CYP2A6 is primarily responsible both for the C-oxidation of nicotine to cotinine and for the oxidation of cotinine to trans-3'-hydroxycotinine. The ratio of trans-3'-hydroxycotinine to cotinine, which can be measured in blood, saliva, or urine of people who use tobacco, is a relatively stable biomarker of CYP2A6 activity and the rate of metabolism of nicotine. Allelic differences in CYP2A6 alter the rate of its activity and, thus, alter the rate and pathways of nicotine metabolism.[26] Slower nicotine metabolism usually results in less nicotine taken in per day by the person who smokes, achieving the same levels of nicotine in the body as faster metabolizers who inhale more nicotine. The rate of nicotine metabolism is an important determinant of the level of nicotine addiction and response to nicotine/tobacco use disorder treatments.[27] Renal clearance accounts for 2% to 35% (averaging 10%) of total nicotine clearance depending on the urine pH.

Although differences in the *CYP2A6* gene contribute to the widely differing rates of nicotine metabolism among people who smoke, differences in metabolism are present even among those with similar *CYP2A6* genotype.[28] Rapid metabolizers smoke more cigarettes per day than slower metabolizers, presumably to maintain desired levels of nicotine. Studies using the ratio of the nicotine metabolites trans-3'-hydroxycotinine/cotinine (known as the nicotine metabolite ratio or NMR) have shown that slow metabolizers are more likely to quit smoking than normal metabolizers.[29] The mechanism of this effect is not definitely known, but it may be that fast metabolizers eliminate nicotine faster from the blood and so have more severe withdrawal symptoms between cigarettes, making smoking more of a negative reinforcer.[30] In addition, more rapid elimination of nicotine from the brain in faster metabolizers could reduce the extent of tolerance such that the next cigarette is more rewarding, making smoking more

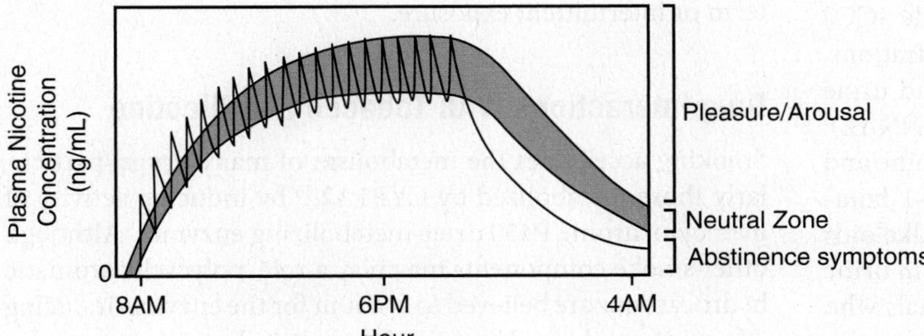

Figure 16-2. A simulation of the plasma nicotine concentration throughout the day in relation to continued cigarette smoking until later in the evening.

of a positive reinforcer. The rate of nicotine metabolism is being evaluated as a way to personalize tobacco use disorder treatment. A prospective clinical trial demonstrated that slow metabolizers undergoing treatment had similar quit rates when treated with nicotine patch or varenicline, while normal metabolizers had much higher quit rates with varenicline compared to nicotine patch.[31]

Gender and ancestry also influence nicotine metabolism.[28] Women metabolize nicotine faster than men, and women who take estrogen-containing oral contraceptives metabolize nicotine faster than women who do not. The metabolism of nicotine during pregnancy is even faster, consistent with a dose effect of estrogen on CYP2A6 activity. Blacks (individuals of African ancestry) obtain on average 30% more nicotine per cigarette, and they clear nicotine and cotinine more slowly than do Whites. The slower nicotine clearance is due to the less rapid oxidative metabolism of nicotine to cotinine, related at least in part to a higher prevalence of *CYP2A6* gene variants associated with reduced activity in Blacks.[32] Blacks also exhibit population polymorphism in the rate of nicotine *N*-glucuronidation, with a subpopulation of slow metabolizers, due to UGT2B10 gene variants, not found in Whites.[32] Black men also have a higher incidence of mortality from lung cancer than do White men, particularly at lower levels of cigarette consumption. Individuals of Chinese ancestry living in the United States have both a lower nicotine intake per cigarette and smoke fewer cigarettes per day than do Whites. Individuals of Chinese ancestry metabolize nicotine and cotinine more slowly than do Whites. Slower metabolism in Americans of Chinese ancestry is consistent with the higher prevalence of *CYP2A6* alleles associated with slow metabolism among Asians. Because nicotine intake per cigarette is a marker for tobacco smoke exposure per cigarette, these findings suggest why Chinese American people who smoke have lower rates of lung cancer than either Blacks or Whites. Ethnic variations in nicotine intake per cigarette, the number of cigarettes smoked, and the metabolism of nicotine may form the basis for population-based differences in the incidence and prevalence of progression from nicotine use to use disorder, as well as the associated risk of tobacco-related disease.

Biochemical Assessment of Exposure to Nicotine and Tobacco

Blood, salivary, and plasma cotinine are most commonly used as biochemical markers of nicotine intake. Other measures of smoking include expired breath carbon monoxide (CO) concentrations, blood carboxyhemoglobin concentrations, and plasma or salivary thiocyanate concentrations and urine 4-(methylnitrosamino)-1-(3) pyridyl-1-butanol (NNAL). NNAL is a metabolite of the tobacco-specific nitrosamine and lung carcinogen 4-(methylnitrosamino)-1-(3)pyridyl-1-butanone (NNK).[32] Measurement of the minor tobacco alkaloids anabasine, anatabine, and nicotelline as well as NNAL in urine can be used as a biomarker of tobacco use in individuals who are using nicotine medications.[33]

The 16-hour half-life of cotinine makes it useful as a plasma and salivary marker of nicotine intake. Salivary cotinine concentrations correlate well with blood cotinine concentrations (r = 0.82-0.90). The cotinine level produced by a single cigarette is 8 to 10 ng/mL. It takes several hours for the cotinine to peak after a cigarette is smoked. A cotinine value greater than 5 ng/mL typically indicates smoking.[34] A person who smokes and has a plasma cotinine concentration of 100 ng/mL would have an estimated intake of 8 mg nicotine per day, which corresponds to smoking approximately a half pack of cigarettes per day. Cotinine blood levels average about 250 to 300 ng/mL in people who smoke daily but range from 10 to 900 ng/mL. Because of individual variability in the fractional conversion of nicotine to cotinine and in the rate of elimination of cotinine itself, blood levels of cotinine are not perfect quantitative markers of nicotine intake in individuals who smoke but are useful in studying populations. Detectable cotinine levels may persist for up to 7 days after beginning abstinence from tobacco. The gold standard for estimating daily nicotine intake from tobacco use is the sum of nicotine and its metabolites in urine.

Breath measurements of expired air that contain more than 10 parts/million of CO usually indicate tobacco or cannabis smoking within the past 8 to 12 hours.[34] Elevated CO levels in the absence of smoking may be the result of exposure to environmental pollutants, such as faulty gas boilers, car exhausts, and smog. Persons who are lactose intolerant exhale hydrogen after ingesting milk. Several monitors misinterpret this exhaled hydrogen as CO.[35]

Hydrogen cyanide is inhaled (10-400 μg per cigarette) from tobacco smoke and is a combustion product of nitrogen-containing compounds. Thiocyanate results from the body metabolizing hydrogen cyanide and thiosulfate into thiocyanate, which can be detected in the blood and saliva as an indirect measure of smoking. Thiocyanate levels also may be affected by consumption of common foods (such as almonds, tapioca, cabbage, broccoli, and cauliflower). In addition, hydrogen cyanide is produced when burning other plant materials, in building fires, and car exhaust fumes. Assays of thiocyanate are insensitive to low amounts of smoking, and thiocyanate levels can remain elevated for weeks after smoking has ceased. CO and cotinine levels generally are preferred to thiocyanate levels in the assessment of smoking.

Unique to tobacco is the nicotine-derived nitrosamine NNK, which is metabolized in the body to NNAL, which in turn is excreted in urine. The half-life of NNAL is much longer than cotinine (10-16 days) and is a better biomarker of long-term or intermittent exposure.

Drug Interactions With Tobacco and Nicotine

Smoking accelerates the metabolism of many drugs, particularly those metabolized by CYP1A2,[36] by inducing activity of liver cytochrome P450 drug-metabolizing enzymes. Although other smoke components may play a role, polycyclic aromatic hydrocarbons are believed to account for the enzyme-inducing effects of smoking. Nicotine does not induce most enzymes but may increase CYP2E1 and inhibit CYP2A6 enzymatic activity. Cigarette smoking induces the metabolism of theophylline, propranolol, flecainide, tacrine, caffeine, olanzapine, clozapine, imipramine, haloperidol, pentazocine, estradiol, and other drugs. When people stop smoking, as often occurs during hospitalization for an acute illness, the doses of these medications may need to be lowered to avoid toxicity.

Several pharmacodynamic interactions arise between cigarette smoking and other drugs. Cigarette smoking results in faster clearance of heparin, possibly because of smoking-related activation of thrombosis, with enhanced heparin binding to antithrombin III. Cigarette smoking and oral contraceptives interact synergistically to increase the risk of stroke and premature myocardial infarction in women. Cigarettes appear to enhance the procoagulant effect of estrogens. For this reason, oral contraceptives are relatively contraindicated in women who smoke cigarettes. The stimulant actions of nicotine inhibit reductions in blood pressure and heart rate from beta-adrenergic blockers. Smoking results in less sedation from benzodiazepines and less analgesia from some opioids. Smoking also impairs the therapeutic effects of histamine H_2-receptor antagonists used in treating peptic ulcers. Cutaneous vasoconstriction by nicotine can slow the rate of absorption of subcutaneously administered insulin.

PHARMACOLOGICAL ACTIONS

Central Nervous System

Nicotine has a complex dose-response relationship.[37] At lower doses (such as those achieved by smoking a cigarette), nicotine acts on the sympathetic nervous system to acutely increase blood pressure, heart rate, and cardiac output and to cause cutaneous vasoconstriction. At higher doses, nicotine produces ganglionic stimulation and the release of adrenal catecholamines. At extremely high doses, nicotine causes hypotension and slowing of the heart rate, possibly via peripheral ganglionic blockade or vagal afferent nerve stimulation. Although blood pressure throughout the day while smoking is higher than when that person is not smoking, chronic nicotine exposure in and of itself does not cause hypertension because of the development of tolerance to nicotine's cardiovascular effects. Nicotine also causes muscle relaxation by stimulating discharge of the spinal cord's inhibitory Renshaw cells on the alpha motor neurons of the diaphragm and chest muscles or pulmonary afferent nerves to inhibit the activity of motor neurons that contract the diaphragm muscles for expanding the lungs during breathing. nAChRs are centrally involved in learning and memory functions within the human brain. As such, nicotine use disorder is increasingly understood as a learning disorder, and this expectation is especially applicable in relation to the effect of nicotine on the adolescent brain. Secondhand smoke exposure to the developing brain has been associated with attention deficit hyperactivity disorder (ADHD), but social-economic issues may confound this finding.[38]

Psychoactive Effects

The primary CNS effects of nicotine in people who smoke are arousal, relaxation (particularly in stressful situations), and enhancement of mood, attention, and reaction time, with improvement in performance of some behavioral tasks. Some of this improvement results from the relief of withdrawal symptoms in people addicted to nicotine, rather than as a direct enhancing effect.[39] It is important for patients and clinicians to realize that nicotine/smoking more often acts by reversing some effects of acute withdrawal, rather than directly relieving stress and improving cognition. In a comparison of self-rated feelings of stress, arousal, pleasure, and evaluations of cognitive function in 75 people (25 who smoke cigarettes regularly, 25 who temporarily abstained, and 25 who were historically nonsmoking), those who abstained reported significantly worse psychological states on every assessment measure than did the other two groups, who did not differ from each other. Thus, people who smoke may need regular doses of nicotine to feel normal rather than to enhance their capabilities.

The psychoactive effects of nicotine are determined not only by the route and speed of drug administration and the pharmacokinetic parameters that determine the concentration at receptor sites over time but also by a variety of host and environmental factors. The magnitude of nicotine's subjective effects may depend on the predrug subjective state, level of activity, genetic predisposition, history or current intake of other drugs, expectancy of the individual, and other situational factors.[40-42] Nicotine's effects are dependent on the initial conditions. For example, low-activity rats become more active on exposure to nicotine, whereas the reverse occurs in high-activity rats. Similarly, nicotine has stimulant-like effects on human electroencephalograms during quiet ambient conditions but minimal effects during high-noise ambient conditions.

In people who smoke daily, nicotine's ability to cause stimulation when smoked at a low level of arousal (such as fatigue) and to affect relaxation when smoked at a high level of arousal (such as anxiety) underlies its reinforcing effects under a range of conditions. People who smoke increase their smoking under both low- and high-arousal conditions. People who use nicotine to adjust their subjective state at a given time may think subtle stimulation or relaxation effects from smoking are beneficial. However, many of these effects are more a result of relief of withdrawal symptoms (negative reinforcement) as opposed to gains in brain function above that of a nonsmoking person.

In summary, for humans, nicotine is a psychostimulant and mood modulator. Like other psychostimulants, nicotine may temporarily improve alertness, mood, and produce positive reinforcement. However, the onset of negative reinforcement is perhaps faster than most drugs (within a day), resulting in self-administration based more to relieve withdrawal symptoms (including irritability, anxiety, poor concentration, depressed mood, etc., as outlined below).

Gender differences appear to affect nicotine responsiveness. Women have less sensitivity to changes in nicotine dose during nicotine discrimination experiments, and they may not benefit as much as men from nicotine replacement therapy during tobacco use disorder treatment. Women may be influenced more by nonnicotine stimuli, such as the olfactory and taste attributes of cigarette smoke, indicating greater conditioned reinforcement.

Genetic Predisposition

Genetics mediate differences in the development of nicotine/tobacco use disorder. Different mice strains react differently to nicotine, self-administer nicotine to different extents, differ in the ability to develop tolerance, and have different numbers of nicotine receptor binding sites. In humans, monozygotic twins are more similar than dizygotic twins with respect to smoking behavior; the heritability of DSM-IV-defined nicotine dependence is 0.59 in males who smoke and 0.46 in females who smoke. Heritability estimates for smoking initiation in male twins range from 46% to 84% and estimates of the genetic contribution to long-term persistent smoking range from 58% to 74%. Thus, genetics contributes approximatively half of the variability in risk of developing nicotine dependence. Twin studies also demonstrate a genetic influence on nicotine withdrawal symptoms.

Family linkage studies and candidate gene association studies suggest a number of loci or particular genes that are associated with smoking behavior, but the smoking phenotypes vary considerably from study to study.[40] Although candidate genes coding for various receptors and neurotransmitter systems have been suggested, genome-wide association studies have most compellingly identified single nucleotide polymorphisms in the genes encoding nicotinic acetylcholine receptor subunits.[41,42] The *CHRNA5–CHRNA3–CHRNB4* nAChR subunit cluster on chromosome 15q25 is associated with the number of cigarettes smoked per day and serum cotinine levels, as well as with risk for lung cancer, peripheral arterial disease, and chronic lung disease.[40,41] SNP rs16969968 in *CHRNA5*, leading to an amino acid change in the α5 nAChR subunit protein, produced a slight loss of function of the α5-containing nAChRs and was compellingly linked to increased cigarette usage.[43] Also, the *CHRNB3–CHRNA6* gene cluster on chromosome 8 was implicated from both genome-wide association studies and candidate gene-based association studies.[42] Two distinct loci within this region were implicated: one upstream of the *CHRNB3* gene and the other, rs4952, a coding SNP in that gene. Functional studies by genetic manipulation in animal models also have indicated the importance of the nAChR α6 subunit, which is highly expressed within the midbrain dopamine (DA) system where it influences nicotine self-administration.[6]

The other gene that clearly affects smoking behavior and cancer risk is the *CYP2A6* gene, which codes for the primary enzyme responsible for the oxidation of nicotine and cotinine.[40] *CYP2A6* affects cigarette smoking behavior and cancer risk. This gene is polymorphic, and reduced function variants of the gene are associated with smoking fewer cigarettes per day and a lower risk of lung cancer.[44,45] Other genome-wide association studies point to several other genes as potential genetic determinants of DSM-defined nicotine dependence, including *neurexin 1*, *VPS13A* (vacuolar sorting protein), *KCNJ6* (a potassium channel), and the *GABA A4* receptor genes. Some of these genes, such as the *neurexin 1* gene, are related to cell communication. Other genome-wide association studies have identified a number of genes affecting cell adhesion and extracellular matrix molecules that are common among various substance use disorders, consistent with the idea that neural plasticity and learning are key determinants of individual differences in vulnerability to substance use disorders. Studies with sample sizes up to 1.2 million individuals indicated 566 genetic variants in 406 loci associated with tobacco usage (ie, initiation, abstinence, and heaviness of use).[46,47]

Nicotine Discrimination and Self-administration

Squirrel monkeys and rodents can distinguish the subjective effects of nicotine and nicotine analogues from drugs of other classes.[48] This effect is attenuated by pretreatment with mecamylamine, a centrally acting nicotinic receptor antagonist, but not with hexamethonium, a peripheral antagonist that does not enter the brain. Animals will self-administer nicotine, but the environment, dose, and timing of the reinforcement schedule are more critical with nicotine than with, for example, cocaine. Likewise, human volunteers will self-administer intravenous nicotine. They describe the experience as pleasurable and similar to cocaine effects. People who smoke also regulate the nicotine levels that they self-administer. People who smoke regularly and then are pretreated with mecamylamine smoke more to overcome the blocking effects of this antagonist.

People who smoke get "secondary reinforcement" from the irritant effects of nicotine on the tissues of the mouth and throat. Those with significant experience with smoking can use the tissue-irritant effects to assess how much nicotine they are receiving when smoking. A short-term reduction in cigarette craving is seen when the sensory input from tobacco smoke is simulated with ascorbic acid or black pepper extract.[49] Products that replicate the taste, flavor, throat, and chest sensations of cigarette smoking or the sensorimotor handling of a cigarette may reduce craving and some of the symptoms of nicotine withdrawal. Some of these products are being developed as treatments for tobacco use disorder.

CLINICAL MANIFESTATIONS

Addiction Liability and Tobacco Use Disorder

Cigarette smoking typically starts at age 15 to 16, and 90% of adults who smoke cigarettes daily first try smoking before age 18. Nicotine obtained through chewing tobacco and cigarettes often precedes the use of other drugs.[50] In general, the earlier the age at which use begins, the more difficult it is for the person with addiction to quit. Many persons have been exposed to nicotine in utero as a result of smoking by their mothers. Nicotine exposure alters nicotinic receptor numbers and influences their function both in utero and after birth. In people who progress to chronic cigarette use, tolerance develops rapidly to the headache, dizziness, nausea, and dysphoria associated with the first cigarette. However, tolerance is incomplete; the intake of as little as 50% more than the usual dose can result in symptoms of toxicity. Chronic use is associated with the regular intake of quantities far larger than those used initially, even though consumption levels typically remain steady for many years after addiction has been established.

Conditioned cues (arising from drug-associated memories) become established during the fine-tuned dosing of nicotine. Chronic nicotine exposure increases brain nAChR numbers significantly, including in areas critical to storage and retrieval of memories. As a result of conditioning and the direct effects of nicotine on these brain areas, desiring a cigarette becomes associated with everyday events such as driving a car, finishing a meal, talking on the telephone, waking from sleep, and taking a break. People who smoke link the need to modulate their moods with smoking. The imagery promoted by cigarette advertising adds to this expectation. Thus, a person who begins smoking a pack of cigarettes per day at age 17 would experience thousands of finely tuned doses of nicotine-conditioned internal emotional states and external cues by their mid-20s. The quantity and power of this conditioning are unique to cigarette smoking, and it is a reason that permanently quitting smoking is so difficult. The regular use of tobacco commonly leads to its compulsive use. Factors such as the duration of smoking, nicotine yield of cigarettes, puff frequency, puff duration, and inhalation volume only weakly correlate with biochemical measures of nicotine intake and do not predict the intensity and extent of nicotine withdrawal symptoms. The Fagerstrom Test for Nicotine Dependence (FTND) is one of the most widely accepted measures of the severity of nicotine physical dependence. Many studies show a relationship between the FTND and the ability to achieve abstinence from tobacco. The two items in the FTND that convey the most predictive information are number of cigarettes smoked per day and time from waking to first cigarette of the day. These two items have been combined into the Heaviness of Smoking Index.

There is a high rate of recurrence of use among individuals who try to quit smoking.[9] Population surveys consistently find more than 80% of people who smoke attempt to quit at some time. About 55% actually try to stop each year, but only about 7% have recently quit.[51] Among persons who experience myocardial infarctions, laryngectomies, chronic obstructive pulmonary disease, and other medical sequelae of smoking, more than 50% revert to cigarette use within days or weeks after leaving the hospital.

Withdrawal

Tobacco use is sustained, in part, by the need to prevent the symptoms of nicotine withdrawal, that is, negative reinforcement.[39] The symptoms of withdrawal vary in severity from person to person, but the common symptoms include craving for nicotine, irritability and frustration or anger, anxiety, depression, difficulty concentrating, restlessness, and increased appetite. Performance measures such as reaction time and attention are impaired during withdrawal. Although these symptoms often are distressing and can be disruptive to interpersonal functioning, they are not in themselves life threatening. Most acute withdrawal symptoms reach maximum intensity 24 to 48 hours after abstinence from tobacco begins and then gradually diminish over a few weeks.[52] Some (including dysphoria, mild depression, and anhedonia) may persist for months. The extinction of tobacco-associated conditioned cues requires months to years. That nicotine itself is responsible for the withdrawal symptoms is supported by the appearance of similar symptoms with sudden withdrawal from the use of chewing tobacco, snuff, or nicotine gum and relief of those symptoms provided by nicotine replacement. Another motivating factor to resume smoking for some people is an average weight gain of 3 to 4 kg during the first year after stopping smoking.[53]

There is evidence that activation of the extra-hypothalamic corticotropin-releasing factor (CRF)-CRF1 receptor system contributes to negative affect during nicotine withdrawal. During precipitated nicotine withdrawal in rats, which is associated with anxiety-like behavior, CRF is released in the central nucleus of the amygdala. CRF activation produces anxiety behavior; pharmacological blockade of CRF1 receptors inhibits the anxiogenic effects of nicotine withdrawal. Withdrawal from other drugs such as alcohol, cocaine, opioids, and cannabinoids is also associated with activation of the extra-hypothalamic CRF system, suggesting that this is a common mechanism of affective manifestations of drug withdrawal. Both the hypoactivity of the dopaminergic system and the activation of the CRF system appear to mediate nicotine withdrawal symptoms that often precipitate recurrence of use.

Co-Occurring Psychiatric Conditions

Tobacco use is most highly prevalent and more intense among psychiatric patients and among those who use other drugs. Among those with mental illness, 36% currently smoke, compared to 12.5% among adults with no mental illness.[54] Individuals with schizophrenia, depression, and attention deficit/hyperactivity disorder (ADHD) have a higher prevalence of cigarette smoking than the general population. These groups of patients have more difficulty in quitting compared with people who smoke and are without mental illness, often experiencing greater depression after stopping smoking.

Among those with schizophrenia, 70% to 88% currently smoke. People with schizophrenia have diminished sensory gating to repeated stimuli, an abnormality that is reversed for tens of minutes by nicotine and clozapine, but not haloperidol. Nicotine also reverses some haloperidol dose-related impairments on a variety of cognitive tasks and relieves some of the negative symptoms (such as blunted affect, emotional withdrawal, and lack of spontaneity and flow of speech) that occur with schizophrenia. Genetic linkage in families with schizophrenia supports a role for the nAChR α7 subunit, with potential linkage at the α7 locus on chromosome 15. These data suggest there may be a shared underlying neurobiology for both nicotine/tobacco use and schizophrenia. People who smoke experience fewer side effects from antipsychotic drugs, presumably from the stimulating effects of nicotine, which also may contribute to a higher prevalence of smoking among people with schizophrenia.

Depression sensitizes people who smoke to the influence of stress, making the individual more susceptible to drug reward. Depression and anxiety often accompany nicotine withdrawal, particularly for people with psychiatric illness who also smoke. Relief from specific aspects of those symptoms motivates a return to smoking. Thus, people who smoke become conditioned to expect nicotine to provide partial relief from stress and depression, as smoking does from the symptoms of withdrawal. People with a history of depression and co-occurring tobacco use disorder who stop smoking are at risk of developing more severe nicotine withdrawal symptoms, have poorer outcomes including suicide, and are more likely to experience a depressive episode, especially during the first 3 months after stopping smoking.

NEUROBIOLOGICAL MECHANISMS OF ACTION

Nicotinic Acetylcholine Receptors

Nicotinic acetylcholine receptors (nAChRs) belong to a superfamily of ligand-gated ion channels that includes GABA, glycine, and 5-hydroxytryptamine (serotonin) receptors.[37] The basic conformational states of a nAChR channel are the closed state at rest, the open state, and the desensitized state. After binding the endogenous agonist, acetylcholine (ACh), or an exogenous agonist, nicotine, the nAChR ion channel enters the open-pore conformation for several milliseconds. While open, nAChRs conduct cations across the cellular member that cause a local depolarization of the neuron's transmembrane potential, and the entering cations produce an intracellular ionic signal. Although sodium and potassium ions carry most of the net inward current through open nAChR channels, calcium also can make a small but significant contribution. The open pore of the receptor/channel complex then closes to a resting state or to a desensitized state that is unresponsive to ACh or other agonists for varying lengths of time, usually in the milliseconds to seconds time range.

The kinetic rate at which the nicotinic receptor proceeds through the various conformational states and the selectivity with which it conducts cations in the open state depend on many factors, including the receptor-channel's subunit composition. The nAChR consists of five polypeptide subunits assembled like staves of a barrel around a central water-filled pore.[41] Various subunit combinations produce many different nAChR types. Three broad functional classes of nAChRs are recognized: muscle nAChRs (not discussed here), neuronal nAChRs formed from alpha and beta subunit combinations (α2-α6 and β2-β4), and neuronal nAChRs formed only of alpha subunits (α7-α9 or α10 with α9). Some evidence suggests that subunits of the separate classes are capable of combining to form nAChRs, but such combinations seem to be less common. Therefore, the extensive nAChR subunit-combinatorial diversity has the potential to produce many different responses to endogenous or exogenous agonists. The intensity of the membrane depolarization, the kinetics of gating activation, the rates of desensitization and recovery from desensitization, the size of the ionic signal, the pharmacology, and the regulatory controls of the ACh response all depend on the subunit composition of the nAChRs. In addition, the local environmental and regulatory factors influence the function of nAChRs. These influences include peptide transmitters, various protein kinases, the cytoskeleton, and calcium.

To add further complexity, the three basic conformational states (rest, open, and desensitized) do not account for the actual kinetic properties of nicotinic receptors. Rather, there are multiple conformations involved in the gating.[56] Desensitization, in particular, encompasses many time constants. Thus, there may be short- and long-lived states of desensitization. Long exposures to low concentrations of agonist will favor deeper levels of desensitization for some nAChR subtypes, and this situation is often the case for people who smoke, who maintain low concentrations of nicotine throughout the day.[6]

Genetic and neurophysiological studies in mice indicate the α4β2* nAChRs (where * indicates the potential presence of other nAChR subunits), often in combination with the α6 subunit, are primarily responsible for the initiation of nicotine addiction.[6] In β2-subunit knockout mice, nicotine is less able to release DA in the brain, and these animals do not self-administer nicotine. Genetic manipulation of the α4 subunit alters sensitivity to the effects of nicotine. The expression of somatic withdrawal symptoms mainly depends upon the α5, α2, and β4 nicotinic subunits.[6]

CNS Cholinergic Systems

Cholinergic neurons release the neurotransmitter ACh, which is the endogenous agonist for nAChRs. Cholinergic neurons project throughout the CNS, providing diffuse, sparse innervation to practically all of the brain. Cholinergic cell bodies are positioned along a loosely contiguous axis running from the cranial nerve nuclei of the brainstem to the medullary tegmentum and pontomesencephalic tegmentum, continuing rostrally through the diencephalon to the telencephalon. These systems include the following: (a) the pedunculopontine and lateral dorsal tegmental nuclei, providing widespread innervation to the thalamus and midbrain dopaminergic areas and also descending innervation to the caudal pons and brainstem, (b) various basal forebrain nuclei that make broad projections throughout the neocortex, hippocampus, thalamus, and amygdala. Another subsystem arises from a collection of cholinergic interneurons located in the striatum.[57,58] Unlike many broadly projecting cholinergic neurons throughout the brain, these cholinergic interneurons make up approximately 2% of the striatal neurons, and they provide very rich local innervation throughout the striatum and the olfactory tubercle.[57,58]

Cholinergic systems have significant complexity beyond nicotinic signaling, but acting via nAChRs, nicotine or nicotinic cholinergic innervation can increase arousal, heighten attention, influence stages of sleep, produce states of euphoria, decrease fatigue, decrease anxiety, act centrally as an analgesic, and influence cognitive function.[57-59] Cholinergic systems affect discriminatory processes by increasing the signal-to-noise ratio and by helping to evaluate the significance and relevance (salience) of stimuli.[60] These normal brain cholinergic functions are usurped by nicotine addiction and are believed unique and central to why nicotine addiction has perhaps the highest rate of recurrence among addictive drugs.

Nicotinic Mechanisms in the CNS

The most widely observed synaptic role of nAChRs in the mammalian CNS is to influence neurotransmitter release. Presynaptic nAChRs initiate a direct and indirect calcium signal that boosts the release of neurotransmitters. Exogenous application of nicotinic agonists enhances, and nicotinic antagonists often diminish, the release of ACh, dopamine, norepinephrine, serotonin, GABA, and glutamate. In many cases, the α7* nAChRs, which are highly calcium permeable, mediate the increased release of neurotransmitter, but in other cases, different nAChR subtypes are involved.

Nicotinic AChRs also have roles in neuronal development and plasticity. The density of nAChRs varies during the course of development, and nAChRs can contribute to activity-dependent calcium signals. Nicotinic regulatory, plasticity, and developmental influences may be important in the etiology of disease. Biological changes that inappropriately alter nicotinic mechanisms could immediately influence the release of many neurotransmitters and alter circuit excitability. Moreover, nicotinic dysfunction could have long-term developmental consequences that are expressed later in life.

The tremendous diversity of nAChRs provides the flexibility necessary for them to play multiple, varied roles.[61] Broad, sparse cholinergic projections ensure that nicotinic mechanisms modulate the neuronal excitability of relatively wide circuits. Although fast nicotinic transmission (as seen at the neuromuscular junction) is not the predominant mechanism in the CNS, it can contribute excitatory input to many synapses at one time. Nicotinic receptors located on presynaptic terminals or located on axons before the presynaptic terminals (ie, preterminal) modulate the release of many neurotransmitters. The activity of nAChRs at those locations induces a local depolarization that may initiate a local action potential, or the activity may directly or indirectly induce a calcium signal. Both the local action potential and calcium signal influence neurotransmitter release if the effects invade active release sites that are most commonly located in presynaptic terminals. In addition, ACh also diffuses from release sites depending on the local density of acetylcholinesterase (AChE), which is the enzyme that breaks down (ie, hydrolyzes) ACh. Although AChE is widely distributed in the CNS, evidence indicates that the density and location of AChE does not always match the location of ACh release sites. Consequently, ACh diffuses and acts at lower concentrations substantial distances away from the release site in a process called volume transmission. Owing to volume transmission, nAChRs influence broad circuit excitability owing to nAChR effects occurring well outside of the synaptic sites.

Nicotine Influences on Dopaminergic Neurons

While nicotine is not the only compound contributing to the addictive influence of tobacco, it is the primary addictive component.[6] Although many areas of the brain participate, the mesocorticolimbic DA system serves a vital role in the acquisition of behaviors that are reinforced by addictive drugs. An important dopaminergic pathway originates in the ventral tegmental area (VTA) of the midbrain and projects to the prefrontal cortex, as well as to limbic and striatal structures, including the nucleus accumbens. Blocking DA release in the nucleus accumbens with antagonists or lesions reduces nicotine self-administration in rodents.

Nicotine Activates and Desensitizes nAChRs on Mesocorticolimbic Neurons

In rat brain slices, nicotine, at concentrations comparable to those seen in people who use tobacco, activates and desensitizes nAChRs on VTA dopamine (DA) neurons and thereby potently modulates the firing of VTA neurons.[6,37] Nicotine reaches nAChRs at every brain location, including those at presynaptic, postsynaptic, and nonsynaptic (including somal) locations. On the DA neuron's cell bodies and postsynaptically, the majority of nAChRs contain α4β2 subunits, and those nAChRs have a high affinity for nicotine. The α4 and β2 subunits are often in combination with α5 or α6. α4β2-containing (α4β2*) nAChRs also predominate on inhibitory GABAergic neurons innervating this area. The DA neurons from the posterior VTA that provide the main projection to the nucleus accumbens commonly express α6 and β3 with the α4 and β2 subunits.[61,62] At the low concentrations of nicotine achieved by smoking, the presence of the α6 subunit, particularly in α6α4β2* nAChRs, slows the rate and degree of desensitization seen with the higher-affinity α4β2 nAChRs.[63] Therefore, those α6-containing receptors are important to maintain the more prolonged activation of DA neurons caused by nicotine from tobacco.[61] In addition, α4β2* nAChRs containing the α6 subunit regulate DA release in target areas such as the nucleus accumbens. The α7* nAChRs, which have a much lower affinity for nicotine, are at lower density in the midbrain; they are more commonly located on the presynaptic terminals of excitatory glutamatergic afferents into this midbrain area (in rodent studies). This arrangement of nAChRs is hypothesized to underlie their enhancement of excitatory synaptic potentiation.

When nicotine first arrives in the midbrain DA area, it excites nAChRs, particularly the high-affinity α4β2* nAChRs and related nAChR subtypes and, to a lesser degree, the lower-affinity α7* nAChRs. Activation of the presynaptic nAChRs enhances the release of glutamate. The postsynaptic (and somal) α4β2* nAChRs, including those containing α6, contribute to the depolarization of DA neurons, helping *N*-methyl-D-aspartate (NMDA) receptors to participate in glutamatergic synaptic potentiation.[6] After the initial exposure to nicotine and potentiation of glutamatergic afferents, there is significant, but incomplete, desensitization of the high-affinity α4β2* nAChR subtypes. Particularly owing to the presence of the α6 subunit in many α4β2* nAChRs as well as rarer α7* nAChRs, many nAChR subtypes are not strongly desensitized. Some of the inhibitory GABA transmission decreases because the α4β2 nAChR subtype is significantly desensitized, and the GABAergic inhibition of the DA neurons decreases because any afferent cholinergic activity that normally boosted GABA release no longer can act on all the α4β2* receptor subtypes. Further complicating the GABAergic signaling is the recent finding that nicotine (as well as stress) can increase GABA signaling onto DA neurons.[64-66] The blunted dopamine signaling results from a nicotine-induced excitation of GABA neurons in the VTA. Excitation of GABA neurons was mediated by $GABA_A$ receptor activation and involved stress- or nicotine-induced functional downregulation of the K^+,Cl- cotransporter, KCC2. The functional downregulation of KCC2 alters the Cl- gradient in midbrain GABA neurons, thereby shifting $GABA_A$ receptor signaling toward excitation of some downstream GABA neurons that, in turn, project to inhibit DA neurons. Overall, the direct and indirect modulation of midbrain GABAergic signaling and consequent impact on the immediate and long-term DA signaling has influence over the initiation of the nicotine addiction process.

Glutamatergic excitation of the DA neurons remains elevated after nicotine exposure because the synaptic potentiation that was initiated by nAChR activity persists for longer time periods (known as long-term synaptic potentiation). In addition, the presynaptic α7* nAChRs on glutamatergic afferents are much less desensitized by the low concentrations of nicotine that are present. Therefore, α7* nAChRs continue to enhance glutamate release, particularly at the potentiated synapses that provide ongoing excitation of DA neurons.[6] Thus, while a patient may have stopped smoking and is no longer self-administering nicotine, the effects of nicotine remain in the form of glutamate-mediated release of DA for as long as 2 months due to long-term potentiation. This glutamate excitation results in a higher risk for recurrence of use, and is one hallmark of nicotine's usurpation of free will—and lasting well beyond the last time nicotine was self-administered.

Distinct nAChRs subtypes contribute to the manifestations of the nicotine withdrawal syndrome. The withdrawal syndrome is not mediated by the same mechanisms or neural circuits that initiate nicotine/tobacco use disorder. The epithalamic habenular complex and its targets appear to be critical for the withdrawal syndrome. The medial habenula (MHb) and one of its primary targets, the interpeduncular nucleus (IPN), richly express β4 and α5 nAChR subunits (and α2 only in the IPN) that are necessary for the neuroadaptations that lead to somatic withdrawal symptoms during nicotine abstinence.[6] In mouse models, the absence of α5 or β4 nearly eliminates the somatic signs of withdrawal. This phenotype is in sharp contrast with that of β2-lacking mice, which display normal somatic signs of withdrawal.[6] Another nicotinic subunit that contributes to the somatic signs of withdrawal is the α2 subunit, which is selectively expressed in the IPN and the olfactory bulb of rodents. The α7 subunit plays a smaller role.

The α5, α3, α2, and β4 subunits are highly expressed in MHb and/or IPN.[6] Microinjection of the nAChR antagonist mecamylamine into the Hb and IPN precipitates nicotine withdrawal symptoms in mice chronically treated with nicotine. When the α2, α5 or β4 subunits of the nAChR are genetically knocked-out, the mice do not show somatic signs of withdrawal. On the other hand, mice with the most broadly expressed subunit in the brain, β2, knocked-out show less anxiety during withdrawal. The somatic signs of withdrawal are not influenced by β2 knockout.[66] Furthermore, mice lacking α5 in the MHb self-administer nicotine at doses that elicit strong aversion in wild-type mice. This result suggests that α5-containing nAChRs in the MHb control the amounts of nicotine self-administered. Taken together, these data suggest a prominent role of the MHb/IPN axis in mediating nicotine's aversive effects and the somatic symptoms of withdrawal.[6]

The single nucleotide polymorphism (SNP) rs16969968 within the *CHRNA5* gene correlates with nicotine addiction risk, heavy smoking, and the pleasurable sensation produced by a cigarette. Some people with that SNP may smoke more and become addicted at a younger age because of less functional activity by α5* nAChRs in the MHb/IPN axis. The presence of fewer aversive effects (even at higher nicotine doses) during the initial contact with nicotine would promote the hedonic drive, thereby promoting the transition from use to tobacco use disorder.

Hypotheses to Extrapolate the Cellular Results to People Who Smoke

The development and maintenance of nicotine use disorder results from a combination of positive reinforcements, including enhancement of mood, and avoidance of negative factors related to withdrawal symptoms[6] (**Fig. 16-3**). In addition, there is drug use associated learning that creates smoking-related cues that spur reinforced behaviors for continued use. That is, nicotine-induced cellular changes in the brain arise from the drug commandeering normal learning mechanisms that associate environmental input (in this case, smoking context and cigarettes) with behavioral repertoire (in this case, getting and smoking a cigarette).

Cellular studies of nAChR activation and desensitization suggest the process by which smoking a cigarette, each of which delivers about 20 to 100 nanoMolar nicotine (or about 12 ng/ml) to the brain[6] drives development of a use disorder. Initially, the brain is free of nicotine and nAChRs respond normally to cholinergic synaptic activity. When nicotine first arrives, the especially high-affinity α4β2* nAChRs are activated, causing the neurons to depolarize and fire action potentials. This process has multiple consequences throughout the brain[6,40] (Fig. 13-3). DA neurons are activated, contributing to the increase in DA that is broadcast throughout the brain via the mesocorticolimbic projections. Present theories hold that these neuronal events reinforce the behaviors (tobacco use and associated cues and events) that produce the DA release.[6,67] For example, the DA signal reaching the memory center of the hippocampus increases the likelihood for synaptic change as a mechanism for associating the environmental events (eg, the smoking place and context) with the behavior (eg, smoking a cigarette) that produced the DA signal.[67,68] Thus, smoking and associated behaviors, whether incidental or meaningful, are reinforced (in a type of learning process). As the nicotine from the cigarette lingers, desensitization of especially high-affinity subtypes of nAChRs begins. This process decreases the reinforcing effect obtained by smoking multiple cigarettes in a row. However, the desensitization process is not complete; there is considerable variability in desensitization of the various nAChR subtypes, and lower-affinity nAChRs, such as those containing α6 or α7, may show little desensitization from the low levels of nicotine.

Nicotinic receptor desensitization has other effects.[6] When nicotine is present, the high-affinity nicotine sites (including α4β2* nAChRs) are more likely to desensitize. At cholinergic synapses, nAChRs experience repeated exposures to synaptic ACh and are exposed to nicotine from the cigarette. The combination of agonist exposures increases the probability that these nAChRs at active cholinergic synapses will desensitize. Thus, smoking will turn down the gain for information arriving via nicotinic cholinergic synapses because fewer nAChRs will be able to respond to the released ACh. In summary, nicotine not only sends inappropriate information through the nicotinic and mesocorticolimbic DA systems, but it also decreases the amplitude for normal nicotinic information processing at cholinergic synapses.

Long-term nicotine exposure leads to neuroadaptations; the most well-known is an increase in the number of mainly high-affinity nAChR subtypes.[7] After long periods (weeks, months, or years) of smoking, nAChRs dramatically increase the number of nicotine-instigated mechanisms. For example, a coat protein complex I (COPI)-mediated process contributes to up-regulation of α6* or α4* nAChRs.[69] Nicotine exploits a COPI-dependent process to chaperone high-affinity nAChRs, leading to increased expression in the cell membrane. In addition, the regulation of nAChR numbers is complex, involving the ubiquitin-proteasome system that regulates the stability of neuronal nAChRs. Nicotine reduces proteasomal activity, which also contributes to the up-regulation of nAChRs and other synaptic proteins.

When nicotine is removed from the brain during abstinence, some of the excess nAChRs recover from desensitization, resulting in an excess excitability of the nicotinic cholinergic systems of people who stop smoking. This hyperexcitability, where nAChRs have been up-regulated, could contribute to the unrest and agitation (nicotine withdrawal) that contribute to the newly abstinent person's motivation (ie, negative reinforcement) for the next cigarette, which "medicates" the person by desensitizing the excess number of nAChRs back toward a more normal level.

These receptor changes may underlie the most common pattern of cigarette smoking. Most people who smoke report that the first cigarette of the day is the most pleasurable.[6] After a night of abstinence, nicotine concentrations in the brain are at their lowest level. Thus, smoking the first cigarette most strongly activates nAChRs, possibly causing the largest activity of the midbrain DA areas and contributing to the most reinforcing effects (**Fig. 16-3**, Step 1). After a few cigarettes, there is significant (albeit incomplete) desensitization, causing some acute tolerance and less effect from additional cigarettes (**Fig. 16-3**, Step 2). The process of activation and desensitization affects different nAChR types differently and influences synaptic plasticity, contributing to the long-term changes associated with addiction. When smoking continues for long periods, the nicotinic system undergoes various neuroadaptations, including an increase in the number of high-affinity nAChRs (**Fig. 16-3**, Step 3). Cigarettes are smoked throughout the day, in part, driven by smaller variable rewards and by the agitation (nicotine withdrawal) arising from the excess nAChRs and hyperexcitability at cholinergic synapses experienced during abstinence (**Fig. 16-3**, Step 4).

Episodes of cigarette smoking are often separated by hours of abstinence. During that time, nicotine levels drop, and some nAChRs recover from desensitization. People who smoke often report that cigarettes smoked during the day help them to focus and relax so that they can work more efficiently. As an individual smokes several times during the course of a day, the background level of nicotine slowly increases. Therefore, the person experiences some exposure to nicotine throughout the day, ensuring that some subtypes of nAChRs achieve states of desensitization. These episodes of nAChR desensitization ensure that the number of nAChRs becomes and remains elevated (owing to mechanisms of neuroadaptation). If nicotine is avoided for a few weeks, the number of nAChRs begins to return to the lower value seen in nonsmoking people. Although this readjustment suggests that disease remission may be underway, the nicotine-associated learning and memory are not extinguished. Thus, indelible smoking-associated conditioned cues can continue to produce cravings and to motivate tobacco use for long periods beyond this stage.

The design of various products (combustible tobacco cigarettes, snuff, snus, pipes, etc.) that deliver nicotine to the human brain has evolved from decades of industry research and careful engineering to enhance addiction liability. These involve additives and ingredients with chemosensory effects that act synergistically with nicotine to increase the probability and strength of the conditioned associations mentioned above as important for development of nicotine use disorder. Specifically these additions increase product appeal, improve product initiation, discourage abstinence from tobacco, and promote recurrence of use.[70,71] These include, but are not limited to, camouflaging the odor of smoke, adding menthol and ammonia, and adding flavorings. Similar approaches are being recycled and improved from the traditional cigarette industry and applied to encourage the use of electronic cigarettes.

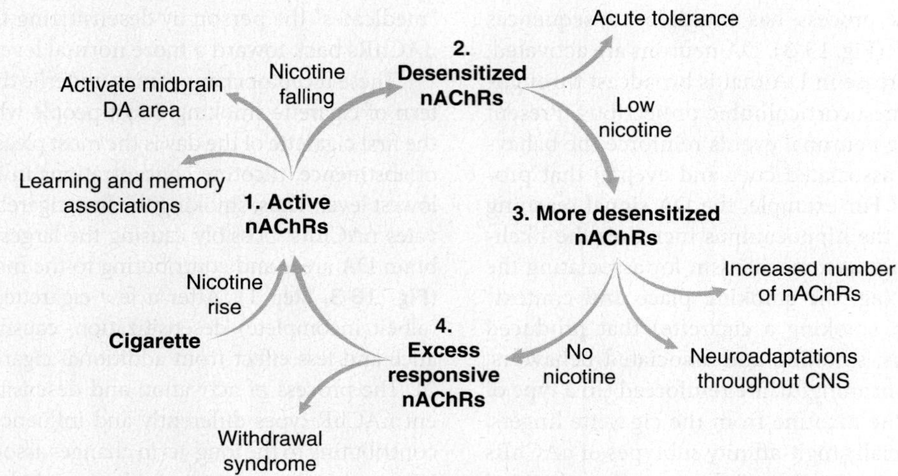

Figure 16-3. A simplified cycle for continued tobacco use, based on nicotine's cellular actions. The nicotinic acetylcholine receptors (nAChRs) are initially and transiently activated when nicotine first arrives. The incomplete desensitization of some nAChR subtypes follows as the concentration of nicotine is maintained during the day, and then slowly decreases overnight. The increased number of nAChRs and other neuroadaptations develop after chronic use of nicotine. The learned associations occur over the course of chronic tobacco use as nicotine causes reinforcements of behavior via the mesocorticolimbic systems. (Adapted from Dani JA, Heinemann S. Molecular and cellular aspects of nicotine abuse. *Neuron.* 1996;16:905-908.)

Fewer than 1 in 10 adults who smoke cigarettes succeed in quitting each year. Four out of every nine adults who smoke cigarettes and saw a health professional during the past year do not receive advice to quit (which is perhaps the most minimal of interventions). In fact, most people who smoke return to smoking within the first 10 days after cessation, which is before the weeks to months that it takes for the effects of nicotine on human brain nAChRs and glutamate-mediated DA release to approach normalization. Over years of smoking, long-term synaptic changes result in learned associations, including associations with the events, people, and context in which smoking takes place. Because these behaviors are repeatedly and variably reinforced by nicotine and its associated cues (people, places, and things such as cigarettes, lighters, e-cigarettes, advertising, etc.), these associations become conditioned cues that motivate tobacco usage. Thus, the desire for cigarettes extinguishes slowly and sometimes incompletely. Nicotine leaves an "indelible imprint," and the desire for cigarettes may be experienced even years after having quit, cued by learned associations.[6]

Monoamine Oxidase and Tobacco Use Disorder

Cigarette smoking is associated with reduced activity of the enzymes monoamine oxidase A (MAO-A) and monoamine oxidase B (MAO-B), as demonstrated by positron emission tomography scanning of the human brain using MAO substrates. Inhibition of MAO is produced not by nicotine, but by condensation products of acetaldehyde with biogenic amines, such as benzoquinones, 2-naphthylamine, harmon, and other chemicals. The acetaldehyde is produced from combustion, and from a wide range of normal metabolic processes, as well as the metabolism of alcohol, which is often a co-occurring problem with smoking. The main function of MAO is to metabolize catecholamines, including DA. Inhibition of MAO should result in higher brain levels of DA after exposure to nicotine. Studies in rats show that pretreatment with drugs that inhibit MAO make nicotine more rewarding and increase the likelihood and rate of acquisition of nicotine self-administration. Therefore, MAO inhibition may contribute to the addictiveness of smoking tobacco products. In addition, because MAO inhibitors have antidepressant action, smoking-induced inhibition of monoamine oxidase might contribute to the perceived benefit of smoking by some depressed patients.

SYSTEMIC TOXICITY

The Global Burden of Disease Study 2019[23] has estimated the health burden of smoking tobacco using mortality and disability adjusted life years (DALY), which represents the loss of the equivalent of 1 year of good health without any disability. Globally in 2019, smoking tobacco use accounted for 7.69 million (7.16-8.20) deaths and 200 million (185-214) disability-adjusted life-years, and was the leading risk factor for death among males (20.2% [19.3-21.1] of male deaths). 6.68 million (86.9%) of 7.69 million deaths attributable to smoking tobacco use were among people currently smoking. The economic cost of smoking in the United States is approximately $380 billion a year, including nearly $225 billion in direct medical costs and $155 billion in lost productivity.[21,72] The causes of this human morbidity and mortality are found in tobacco smoke, which is composed of volatile (gaseous) and particulate phases that contain many substances in addition to nicotine. The volatile phase contains many gaseous compounds, including nitrogen, CO, carbon dioxide, ammonia, hydrogen cyanide, acrolein, butadiene, and benzene. There are about 3,500 different compounds in the particulate phase, including the pharmacologically active alkaloids nornicotine, anabasine, anatabine, myosmine, nicotyrine, and nicotine. Assays for some of these alkaloids are used as biomarkers of tobacco use (see above). The "tar" in a cigarette is composed of the particulate matter minus its alkaloid and water content. Tar contains many carcinogens, including polynuclear aromatic hydrocarbons, *N*-nitrosamines, and aromatic amines. The health consequences of smoking have been reviewed in a recent U.S. Surgeon General's report emphasizing that permanently stopping smoking is beneficial at any age, that doing so improves health status and enhances quality of life, and that it reduces the risk of premature death and can add as much as a decade to life expectancy.[8]

Cardiovascular, Pulmonary, and Oncological Toxicities

People who smoke are exposed to more than 7,000 different chemicals, including at least 50 known carcinogens. The threefold increased risk of cardiovascular disease among people who smoke cigarette likely is related to exposure to oxidant chemicals, particulates, and CO, as well as acrolein, hydrogen cyanide, carbon disulfide, cadmium, and zinc.[73] Although CO reduces oxygen delivery to the heart, oxidant chemicals are primarily responsible for endothelial dysfunction, platelet activation, thrombosis, and coronary vasoconstriction.

Cigarette smoking has significant detrimental effects on both the structure and function of the lung. Cigarette smoking causes an imbalance between proteolytic and antiproteolytic forces in the lung and heightens airway responsiveness. Chronic obstructive lung diseases are linked with exposure to tar, nitrogen oxides, hydrogen cyanide, and volatile aldehydes, enhanced by inducers of superoxide and H_2O_2.[74]

The agents contributing most significantly to the 15 to 30 times greater likelihood of getting lung cancer are thought to be the carcinogenic polynuclear aromatic hydrocarbons and the tobacco-specific *N*-nitrosamines, followed by polonium-210 and volatile aldehydes. Catechol, the weakly acidic agents, volatile aldehydes, and nitrogen oxides that can serve as precursors in the exogenous and endogenous formation of *N*-nitrosamines enhance tobacco smoke-induced tumorigenesis. People actively smoking and who have elevated levels of DNA damage from polynuclear aromatic hydrocarbons in their white blood cells (DNA adducts) are three times more likely to be diagnosed with lung cancer 1 to 13 years later than are those with lower adduct concentrations (odds ratio, 2.98; 95% confidence interval, 1.05-8.42; $p = .04$). As with other tobacco-related diseases, the risk of cancer of the mouth, larynx, esophagus, lung, stomach, pancreas, kidney, urinary bladder, and uterine cervix as well as leukemia is directly related to the intensity and duration of exposure to cigarette smoke and to nicotine, which is itself a tumor promoter.

Other Physiological Effects and Toxicities

Cigarette smoking is associated with skin changes, including yellow staining of fingers, vasospasm and obliteration of small skin vessels, precancerous and squamous cell carcinomas on the lips and oral mucosa, and enhanced facial skin wrinkling. Tobacco smoke and exposure to ultraviolet A radiation each cause wrinkle formation. When excessive sun exposure (>2 hours per day) and heavy smoking (>35 pack years) occur together, the risk of developing wrinkles is 11.4 times higher than that of those who have not smoked and those with less sun exposure at the same age. The induction of matrix metalloproteinase-1, mediated by reactive oxygen species (especially in people with low glutathione content fibroblasts), is thought to be an important mechanism underlying premature skin aging caused by cigarette smoking and exposure to ultraviolet A radiation.

People who smoke 20 or more cigarettes per day have significant eye pathology, including statistically significant increases in nuclear sclerosis and posterior subcapsular cataracts compared with individuals who never smoked. After adjusting for age and average number of cigarettes smoked per day, people who had quit smoking 25 or more years previously have a 20% lower risk of cataracts, but still higher than among subjects who never smoked.[75] People who smoke more than 20 cigarettes per day also have an increased risk of age-related macular degeneration.

Cigarette smoking in women is associated with lower levels of estrogen, earlier menopause, and a 37% increased risk of osteoporosis. The alkaloids in tobacco smoke diminish estrogen formation by inhibiting an aromatase enzyme in granulosa cells or placental tissue.

In men, smoking may impair penile erection, primarily in those with underlying vascular disease, through the impairment of endothelium-dependent smooth muscle relaxation. Smoking 20 cigarettes daily doubles the likelihood of moderate or complete erectile dysfunction associated with other risk factors, such as coronary artery disease and hypertension. The prevalence of erectile dysfunction in people who quit smoking for 5 years is no different from that in individuals who never smoked.

Nicotine both suppresses appetite and increases metabolic rate.[76] People who smoke weigh an average 2.7 to 4.5 kg (6-10 lb) less than people who don't. After stopping smoking, individuals typically crave sweets. Individuals who stop smoking typically gain weight to approximately the levels of those who never smoked in the 6 to 12 months after stopping smoking.

Through release of catecholamines, nicotine increases lipolysis and releases free fatty acids, which are taken up by the liver. This could contribute to the increase in very low-density lipoprotein and low-density lipoprotein and the decrease in high-density lipoprotein seen in people who smoke.

Cigarette smoking is associated with the occurrence and delayed healing of peptic ulcers. Mechanisms include decreases in the mucous bicarbonate barrier in the stomach, reduction in the production of endogenous prostaglandins in the gastric mucosa, and increased proliferation of *Helicobacter pylori*.

Tobacco and Pregnancy

Smoking during pregnancy and lactation has been associated with a variety of untoward child health outcomes, including preterm birth, fetal growth restriction, low birth weight, sudden infant death syndrome, neurodevelopmental and behavioral problems, obesity, hypertension, type 2 diabetes, impaired lung function, asthma, and wheezing.[77,78] Nicotine itself has been implicated as at least partially causative for a number of these adverse outcomes from maternally derived exposures to smoking. Smoking during pregnancy nearly doubles the relative risk of having a low-birth-weight infant; and increases by about one-third the relative risks of spontaneous abortion and perinatal and neonatal mortality. The components of tobacco smoke responsible for obstetric and fetal problems have not been definitively identified. CO clearly is detrimental because it markedly reduces the oxygen-carrying capacity of fetal hemoglobin. The use of smokeless tobacco, which delivers nicotine but not combustion products, during pregnancy is associated with an increased risk of pre-eclampsia, while smoking during pregnancy is protective against pre-eclampsia. It is hypothesized that CO in cigarette smoke acts as a vasodilator to counter the vasoconstrictor effects of nicotine, while in smokeless tobacco and perhaps people who use electronic cigarette the nicotine effects are unopposed, leading to arteriolar vasoconstriction and hypertension, as seen in pre-eclampsia.

The effect of smoking in lowering birth weight interacts with the metabolic genes *CYP1A1* and *GSTT1*. Infants born to mothers who smoke and who had genetic variants associated with reduced *CYP1A1* activity—Aa and aa (heterozygous and homozygous variant types)—and reduced or absent *GSTT1* activity had greater reductions in birth weight than did infants born to mothers who smoked and had the normal metabolic activity genes *CYP1A1* AA (homozygous wild type) or *GSTT1* genotype. The CYP1A1 and GSTT1 enzymes have roles in metabolizing and excreting some toxic chemicals in cigarette smoke.

In the developing fetus, nicotine can arrest neuronal replication and differentiation and after birth this neuronal arrest can contribute to sudden infant death syndrome. Nicotine activates nicotinic cholinergic receptors in the fetal brain, resulting in abnormalities of cell proliferation and differentiation that lead to shortfalls in cell numbers and eventually to altered synaptic activity. Comparable alterations occur in peripheral autonomic pathways and are hypothesized to lead to increased susceptibility to hypoxia-induced brain damage, perinatal mortality, and sudden infant death.

Secondhand and Thirdhand Smoke

Secondhand smoke (SHS) is the complex mixture formed by the escaping smoke of a burning tobacco product, as well as smoke that is exhaled by a person who smokes. It can be detected using biological markers.[79] Side-stream smoke contains higher concentrations of some toxins than does mainstream smoke. SHS characteristics change as it combines with other constituents in the ambient air and ages. Exposure to SHS by people who don't smoke is causally associated with acute and chronic coronary heart disease, lung cancer, nasal sinus cancer, and eye and nasal irritation in adults and with asthma, chronic respiratory symptoms, acute lower respiratory tract infections such as bronchitis and pneumonia in children, and potentially certain psychiatric disorders. SHS is also causally associated with low birth weight and sudden infant death syndrome in infants. Young children's exposure to tobacco smoke comes mainly from people who smoke in the home, especially parents. Maternal smoking has the greatest effect on children's measured cotinine levels. Additional contributors include paternal smoking, smoking by other household members, and smoking by child-care personnel.

An average salivary fluid cotinine level of 0.4 ng/mL corresponds to an increased lifetime mortality risk of 1/1,000 for lung cancer and 1/100 for heart disease. Assuming a prevalence of 28% for unrestricted smoking in the workplace, passive smoking would yield 4,000 heart disease deaths and 400 lung cancer deaths annually in the United States. More than 95% of SHS-exposed office workers exceeded the significant risk level for heart disease mortality, and more than 60% exceeded the significant risk level for lung cancer mortality established by the Occupational Safety and Health Administration.

More recent concerns are thirdhand smoke, which is residual—nicotine, tobacco-derived nitrosamines, and other chemicals that remain on environmental surfaces such as clothing and furniture after someone smokes in the area. Dangerous residue from tobacco smoke sticks to carpets, walls and other surfaces after the smoke clears; and can re-enter the air. Thirdhand smoke poses a potential health hazard to people who do not smoke especially children. Homes of people who formerly smoked remain polluted with thirdhand smoke for up to 6 months after the residents quit smoking,[80] perhaps even years depending on if/how remediation attempts were made.

Morbidity and Mortality

The cumulative result of these health effects is that each pack of cigarettes sold in the United States costs the nation an estimated $7.18 in medical care expenditures and lost productivity. Tobacco use is a leading cause of death in the United States, causing more than 480,000 deaths per year,[19-22] which is about one in every five deaths.[8] This includes 148,605 deaths (36.9%) from cardiovascular causes, 155,761 deaths (38.7%) from cancer, and 98,008 deaths (24.3%) from nonmalignant pulmonary disease. Cigarette smoking also increases the risk of developing and increases the severity of respiratory tract infections, including influenza, pneumococcal pneumonia, and tuberculosis.[81] On average, adult men and women who smoke lost 13.2 and 14.5 years of life, respectively, due to smoking. In contrast, the annual mortality attributable to passive smoking between 1995 and 1999 was estimated at 39,060 deaths, including 35,053 from cardiovascular diseases, 3,000 from lung cancer, and 1,007 from perinatal conditions.

Nicotine and Other Addictions

There is a strong association between tobacco smoking and alcohol use disorder[82] some of which might be related to genetic factors.[83] People who are more severely addicted to alcohol smoke more and are less likely to quit. Tobacco also synergizes with alcohol in causing many medical complications. Smoking and heavy drinking, in combination, are associated with substantially increased rates of oral and esophageal cancers. Because lit cigarettes smolder when they fall onto upholstered furniture, alcohol use combines with smoking to cause household fires that claim more than 1,000 lives per year among children and adults. Nicotine and cannabis are often used together, and one appears to augment compulsive use with the other.[84-87] Also, smoking is more common in individuals with opioid and stimulant use disorders. Furthermore, people recovering from other substance use disorders often die from tobacco-related illnesses. In a landmark population-based retrospective cohort study, death certificates were examined for 214 of 854 persons who were admitted between 1972 and 1983 to an inpatient program for the treatment of alcoholism and other nonnicotine potentially addicting substances. Of the deaths reported, 50.9% were caused by tobacco use, whereas 34.1% were attributable to alcohol use. The cumulative 20-year mortality was 48.1% versus an expected 18.5% for a demographically matched control population ($p < .001$).

Adolescent cigarette smoking is a "gateway" to pathological drinking later in life.[65] Studies in mice showed that adolescent, but not adult, nicotine exposure altered GABA signaling within the VTA and led to a long-lasting enhancement of alcohol self-administration. Alterations in GABA signaling were dependent on glucocorticoid receptor activation and were associated with attenuated dopaminergic neuron responses to alcohol in the lateral VTA. In this case, the DA signal is still induced by alcohol, but the signal is depressed, suggesting that the animals self-administer more alcohol to recover more DA signaling.

Benefits of Stopping Smoking

Most people (70%) who smoke want to quit, and approximately 40% attempt to quit each year. However, without assistance, only about 2% to 5% of the attempts are successful.[9] The good news is that stopping smoking has benefits at any age by which abstinence is achieved. The immediately decreased risk of cardiovascular death in those who stop smoking may reflect a decrease in blood coagulability, improved tissue oxygenation, and reduced predisposition to cardiac arrhythmias. Among people who stopped smoking, the reduced risk of death compared with those who continue smoking begins shortly after quitting and continues for at least 10 to 15 years. After 10 to 15 years' abstinence, the risk of all-cause mortality returns nearly to that of persons who never smoked.[88]

REFERENCES

1. American Cancer Society. *Carcinogens in Tobacco Products.* American Cancer Society; 2015. Accessed 16 May, 2023. http://www.cancer.org/cancer/cancercauses/tobaccocancer/carcinogens-found-in-tobacco-products
2. Brennan KA, Crowther A, Putt F, Roper V, Waterhouse U, Truman P. Tobacco particulate matter self-administration in rats: Differential effects of tobacco type. *Addict Biol.* 2015;20:227-235.
3. Schreiner BS, Lehmann R, Thiel U, et al. Direct action and modulating effect of (+)- and (-)-nicotine on ion channels expressed in trigeminal sensory neurons. *Eur J Pharmacol.* 2014;5(728):48-58. doi:10.1016/j.ejphar.2014.01.060
4. Zhang X, Gong ZH, Nordberg A. Effects of chronic treatment with (+)- and (-)-nicotine on nicotinic acetylcholine receptors and N-methyl-D-aspartate receptors in rat brain. *Brain Res.* 1994;644(1):32-39. doi:10.1016/0006-8993(94)90343-3
5. Cwalina SN, McConnell R, Benowitz NL, Barrington-Trimis JL. Tobacco-free nicotine—new name, same scheme? *N Engl J Med.* 2021;385(26):2406-2408. doi:10.1056/NEJMp2111159
6. De Biasi M, Dani JA. Reward, addiction, withdrawal to nicotine. *Annu Rev Neurosci.* 2011;34:105-130.
7. Henderson BJ, Lester HA. Inside-out neuropharmacology of nicotinic drugs. *Neuropharmacology.* 2015;96:178-193.
8. Surgeon General Report 2020. Accessed 16 May, 2023. https://www.hhs.gov/surgeongeneral/reports-and-publications/tobacco/2020-cessation-sgr-factsheet-key-findings/index.html
9. Prochaska JJ, Benowitz NL. The past, present, and future of nicotine addiction therapy. *Annu Rev Med.* 2016;67:467-486.
10. Balfour DJK, Benowitz NL, Colby SM, et al. Balancing consideration of the risks and benefits of e-cigarettes. *Am J Public Health.* 2021;111(9):1661-1672. doi:10.2105/AJPH.2021.306416
11. Warren GW, Singh AK. Nicotine and lung cancer. *J Carcinog.* 2013;12:1.
12. Hartmann-Boyce J, McRobbie H, Butler AR, et al. Electronic cigarettes for smoking cessation. *Cochrane Database Syst Rev.* 2021;9(9):CD010216. doi:10.1002/14651858.CD010216.pub6
13. Levy DT, Yuan Z, Luo Y, Abrams DB. The relationship of E-cigarette use to cigarette quit attempts and cessation: insights from a large, nationally representative U.S. survey. *Nicotine Tob Res.* 2018;20(8):931-939. doi:10.1093/ntr/ntx166
14. Wang RJ, Bhadriraju S, Glantz SA. E-cigarette use and adult cigarette smoking cessation: a meta-analysis. *Am J Public Health.* 2021;111(2):230-246. doi:10.2105/AJPH.2020.305999
15. Grana R, Benowitz N, Glantz SA. E-cigarettes: A scientific review. *Circulation.* 2014;129:1972-1986.
16. Yuan M, Cross SJ, Loughlin SE, Leslie FM. Nicotine and the adolescent brain. *J Physiol.* 2015;593:3397-3412.
17. Benowitz NL, St Helen G, Dempsey DA, Jacob P III, Tyndale RF. Disposition kinetics and metabolism of nicotine and cotinine in African American smokers: impact of CYP2A6 genetic variation and enzymatic activity. *Pharmacogenet Genomics.* 2016;26:340-350.
18. Goniewicz ML, KnysakJ GM, et al. Levels of selected carcinogens and toxicants in vapour from electronic cigarettes. *Tob Control.* 2014;23:133-139.
19. Hu SS, Neff L, Agaku IT, et al. Tobacco product use among adults—United States, 2013–2014. *MMWR Morb Mortal Wkly Rep.* 2016;65:685-691.
20. U.S. Department of Health and Human Services. *The Health Consequences of Smoking—50 Years of Progress: A Report of the Surgeon General.* U.S. Department of Health and Human Services, Centers for Disease Control and Prevention, National Center for Chronic Disease Prevention and Health Promotion, Office on Smoking and Health; 2014. Accessed January 30, 2022.
21. Cornelius ME, Loretan CG, Wang TW, Jamal A, Homa DM. Tobacco product use among adults—United States, 2020. *MMWR Morb Mortal Wkly Rep.* 2022;71:397-405.
22. CDC. Current Cigarette Smoking Among Adults in the United States. 2020. Accessed May 16, 2023. https://www.cdc.gov/tobacco/data_statistics/fact_sheets/adult_data/cig_smoking/index.htm#:~:text=In%202020%2C%20nearly%2013%20of,with%20a%20smoking%2Drelated%20disease
23. GBD 2019 Tobacco Collaborators. Spatial, temporal, and demographic patterns in prevalence of smoking tobacco use and attributable disease burden in 204 countries and territories, 1990-2019: a systematic analysis from the Global Burden of Disease Study 2019. *Lancet.* 2021;397(10292):2337-2360. doi:10.1016/S0140-6736(21)01169-7
24. Mendelsohn C. Smoking and depression—a review. *Aust Fam Physician.* 2012;41:304-307.

25. Baker LK, Mao D, Chi H, et al. Intermittent nicotine exposure upregulates nAChRs in VTA dopamine neurons and sensitises locomotor responding to the drug. *Eur J Neurosci.* 2013;37:1004-1011.
26. Bergen AW, Michel M, Nishita D, et al. Drug metabolizing enzyme and transporter gene variation, nicotine metabolism, prospective abstinence, and cigarette consumption. *PLoS ONE.* 2015;10:e0126113.
27. Allenby CE, Boylan KA, Lerman C, Falcone M. Precision medicine for tobacco dependence: Development and validation of the nicotine metabolite ratio. *J Neuroimmune Pharmacol.* 2016;11:471-483.
28. Ross KC, Gubner NR, Tyndale RF, et al. Racial differences in the relationship between rate of nicotine metabolism and nicotine intake from cigarette smoking. *Pharmacol Biochem Behav.* 2016;148:1-7.
29. West O, Hajek P, McRobbie H. Systematic review of the relationship between the 3-hydroxycotinine/cotinine ratio and cigarette dependence. *Psychopharmacology (Berl).* 2011;218:313-322.
30. Liakoni E, Edwards KC, St Helen G, et al. Effects of nicotine metabolic rate on withdrawal symptoms and response to cigarette smoking after abstinence. *Clin Pharmacol Ther.* 2019;105(3):641-651. doi:10.1002/cpt.1238
31. Lerman C, Schnoll RA, Hawk LW Jr, et al. Use of the nicotine metabolite ratio as a genetically informed biomarker of response to nicotine patch or varenicline for smoking cessation: A randomised, double-blind placebo-controlled trial. *Lancet Respir Med.* 2015;3:131-138.
32. Benowitz NL, Dains KM, Hall SM, et al. Smoking behavior and exposure to tobacco toxicants during 6 months of smoking progressively reduced nicotine content cigarettes. *Cancer Epidemiol Biomarkers Prev.* 2012;21:761-769.
33. Jacob P III, Goniewicz ML, Havel CM, Schick SF, Benowitz NL. Nicotelline: a proposed biomarker and environmental tracer for particulate matter derived from tobacco smoke. *Chem Res Toxicol.* 2013;26(11):1615-1631. doi:10.1021/tx400094y.
34. Benowitz NL, Bernert JT, Foulds J, et al. Biochemical verification of tobacco use and abstinence: 2019 update. *Nicotine Tob Res.* 2020;22(7):1086-1097. doi:10.1093/ntr/ntz132
35. Ryter SW, Choi AM. Carbon monoxide in exhaled breath testing and therapeutics. *J Breath Res.* 2013;7:017111.
36. Anderson GD, Chan LN. Pharmacokinetic drug interactions with tobacco, cannabinoids and smoking cessation products. *Clin Pharmacokinet.* 2016;55:1353-1368.
37. Dani JA. Neuronal nicotinic acetylcholine receptor structure and function and response to nicotine. *Int Rev Neurobiol.* 2015;124:3-19.
38. Joo H, Lim M-H, Ha M, et al. Secondhand smoke exposure and low blood lead levels in association with attention-deficit hyperactivity disorder and its symptom domain in children: A community-based case-control study. *Nicotine Tob Res.* 2017;19:94-101.
39. McLaughlin I, Dani JA, De Biasi M. Nicotine withdrawal. *Curr Top Behav Neurosci.* 2015;24:99-123.
40. Loukola A, Wedenoja J, Keskitalo-Vuokko K, et al. Genome-wide association study on detailed profiles of smoking behavior and nicotine dependence in a twin sample. *Mol Psychiatry.* 2014;19:615-624.
41. Wen L, Jiang K, Yuan W, Cui W, Li MD. Contribution of variants in CHRNA5/A3/B4 gene cluster on chromosome 15 to tobacco smoking: From genetic association to mechanism. *Mol Neurobiol.* 2016;53:472-484.
42. Wen L, Yang Z, Cui W, Li MD. Crucial roles of the CHRNB3-CHRNA6 gene cluster on chromosome 8 in nicotine dependence: Update and subjects for future research. *Transl Psychiatry.* 2016;6:e843.
43. Bierut LJ. Genetic vulnerability and susceptibility to substance dependence. *Neuron.* 2011;69:618-627.
44. Tanner JA, Prasad B, Claw KG, et al. Predictors of variation in CYP2A6 mRNA, protein, and enzyme activity in a human liver bank: Influence of genetic and nongenetic factors. *J Pharmacol Exp Ther.* 2017;360:129-139.
45. Wassenaar CA, Dong Q, Wei Q, Amos CI, Spitz MR, Tyndale RF. Relationship between CYP2A6 and CHRNA5-CHRNA3-CHRNB4 variation and smoking behaviors and lung cancer risk. *J Natl Cancer Inst.* 2011;103:1342-1346.
46. Quach BC, Bray MJ, Gaddis NC, et al. Expanding the genetic architecture of nicotine dependence and its shared genetics with multiple traits. *Nat Commun.* 2020 Nov 3;11(1):5562. doi:10.1038/s41467-020-19265-z
47. Liu M, Jiang Y, Wedow R, et al. Association studies of up to 1.2 million individuals yield new insights into the genetic etiology of tobacco and alcohol use. *Nat Genet.* 2019;51(2):237-244. doi:10.1038/s41588-018-0307-5
48. Goodwin AK, Hiranita T, Paule MG. The reinforcing effects of nicotine in humans and nonhuman primates: A review of intravenous self-administration evidence and future directions for research. *Nicotine Tob Res.* 2015;17:1297-1310.
49. Cordell B, Buckle J. The effects of aromatherapy on nicotine craving on a U.S. campus: A small comparison study. *J Altern Complement Med.* 2013;19(8):709-713. doi:10.1089/acm.2012.0537
50. Doyon WM, Dong Y, Ostroumov A, Thomas AM, Zhang TA, Dani JA. Nicotine decreases ethanol-induced dopamine signaling and increases self-administration via stress hormones. *Neuron.* 2013;79:530-540.
51. Babb S, Malarcher A, Schauer G, Asman K, Jamal A. Quitting smoking among adults—United States, 2000–2015. *MMWR Morb Mortal Wkly Rep.* 2017;65(52):1457-1464. doi:10.15585/mmwr.mm6552a1
52. Zhang L, Dong Y, Doyon WM, Dani JA. Withdrawal from chronic nicotine exposure alters dopamine signaling dynamics in the nucleus accumbens. *Biol Psychiatry.* 2012;71:184-191.
53. Sahle BW, Chen W, Rawal LB, Renzaho AMN. Weight gain after smoking cessation and risk of major chronic diseases and mortality. *JAMA Netw Open.* 2021;4(4):e217044. doi:10.1001/jamanetworkopen.2021.7044
54. CDC. Vital signs: current cigarette smoking among adults aged ≥18 years with mental illness—United States, 2009–2011. *MMWR Morb Mortal Wkly Rep.* 2013;62:81-87.
55. American Psychiatric Association. *Diagnostic and Statistical Manual of Mental Disorders.* 5th ed., text rev. 2022. doi:10.1176/appi.books.9780890425787
56. Auerbach A. Agonist activation of a nicotinic acetylcholine receptor. *Neuropharmacology.* 2015;96:150-156.
57. Gonzales KK, Smith Y. Cholinergic interneurons in the dorsal and ventral striatum: Anatomical and functional considerations in normal and diseased conditions. *Ann N Y Acad Sci.* 2015;1349:1-45.
58. Lim SA, Kang UJ, McGehee DS. Striatal cholinergic interneuron regulation and circuit effects. *Front Synaptic Neurosci.* 2014;6:22.
59. Ballinger EC, Ananth M, Talmage DA, Role LW. Basal forebrain cholinergic circuits and signaling in cognition and cognitive decline. *Neuron.* 2016;91:1199-1218.
60. Minces V, Pinto L, Dan Y, Chiba AA. Cholinergic shaping of neural correlations. *Proc Natl Acad Sci U S A.* 2017;114(22):5725-5730. doi:10.1073/pnas.1621493114
61. Leslie FM, Mojica CY, Reynaga DD. Nicotinic receptors in addiction pathways. *Mol Pharmacol.* 2013;83:753-758.
62. Zhao-Shea R, Liu L, Soll LG, et al. Nicotine-mediated activation of dopaminergic neurons in distinct regions of the ventral tegmental area. *Neuropsychopharmacology.* 2011;36:1021-1032.
63. Liu L, Zhao-Shea R, McIntosh JM, Gardner PD, Tapper AR. Nicotine persistently activates ventral tegmental area dopaminergic neurons via nicotinic acetylcholine receptors containing alpha4 and alpha6 subunits. *Mol Pharmacol.* 2012;81:541-548.
64. Ostroumov A, Thomas AM, Kimmey BA, Karsch JS, Doyon WM, Dani JA. Stress increases ethanol self-administration via a shift toward excitatory GABA signaling in the ventral tegmental area. *Neuron.* 2016;92(2):493-504.
65. Thomas AM, Ostroumov A, Kimmey BA, et al. Adolescent nicotine exposure alters GABAA receptor signaling in the ventral tegmental area and increases adult ethanol self-administration. *Cell Rep.* 2018;23(1):68-77.
66. Ostroumov A, Wittenberg RE, Kimmey BA, et al. Acute nicotine exposure alters ventral tegmental area inhibitory transmission and promotes diazepam consumption. *eNeuro.* 2020;7(2). doi:10.1523/ENEURO.0348-19.2020 ENEURO.0348-19.2020
67. Broussard JI, Yang K, Levine AT, et al. Dopamine regulates aversive contextual learning and associated in vivo synaptic plasticity in the hippocampus. *Cell Rep.* 2016;14:1930-1939.
68. Tsetsenis T, Badyna JK, Wilson JA, et al. Midbrain dopaminergic innervation of the hippocampus is sufficient to modulate formation of aversive memories. *Proc Nat Acad Sci.* 2021;118(40):e2111069118. doi:10.1073/pnas.2111069118

69. Henderson BJ, Srinivasan R, Nichols WA, et al. Nicotine exploits a COPI-mediated process for chaperone-mediated up-regulation of its receptors. *J Gen Physiol.* 2014;143:51-66.
70. Alpert HR, Agaku IT, Connolly GN. A study of pyrazines in cigarettes and how additives might be used to enhance tobacco addiction. *Tob Control.* 2016;25:444-450.
71. Land T, Keithly L, Kane K, et al. Recent increases in efficiency in cigarette nicotine delivery: Implications for tobacco control. *Nicotine Tob Res.* 2014;16:753-758.
72. CDC. Fast Facts, Smoking and Tobacco Use. 2021. Accessed May 17, 2023. https://www.cdc.gov/tobacco/data_statistics/fact_sheets/fast_facts/index.htm#
73. Benowitz NL, Liakoni E. Tobacco use disorder and cardiovascular health. *Addiction.* 2022;117(4):1128-1138. doi:10.1111/add.15703
74. Decramer M, Janssens W, Miravitlles M. Chronic obstructive pulmonary disease. *Lancet.* 2012;379:1341-1351.
75. Weintraub JM, Willett WC, Rosner B, Colditz GA, Seddon JM, Hankinson SE. Smoking cessation and risk of cataract extraction among US women and men. *Am J Epidemiol.* 2002;155:72-79.
76. Audrain-McGovern J, Benowitz NL. Cigarette smoking, nicotine, and body weight. *Clin Pharmacol Ther.* 2011;90:164-168.
77. Banderali G, Martelli A, Moretti F, et al. Short and long term health effects of parental tobacco smoking during pregnancy and lactation: A descriptive review. *J Transl Med.* 2015;13:327.
78. Holz NE, Boeker R, Baumeister S, et al. Effect of prenatal exposure to tobacco smoke on inhibitory control: Neuroimaging results from a 25-year prospective study. *JAMA Psychiat.* 2014;71:786-796.
79. Avila-Tang E, Al-Delaimy WK, Ashley DL, et al. Assessing secondhand smoke using biological markers. *Tob Control.* 2013;22:164-171.
80. Jacob P III, Benowitz NL, Destaillats H, et al. Thirdhand smoke: New evidence, challenges, and future directions. *Chem Res Toxicol.* 2017;30(1):270-294. doi:10.1021/acs.chemrestox.6b00343
81. Huttunen R, Heikkinen T, Syrjanen J. Smoking and the outcome of infection. *J Intern Med.* 2011;269:258-269.
82. Weinberger AH, Platt J, Jiang B, Goodwin RD. Cigarette smoking and risk of alcohol use relapse among adults in recovery from alcohol use disorders. *Alcohol Clin Exp Res.* 2015;39(10):1989-1996. doi: 10.1111/acer.12840.
83. Sinkus ML, Graw S, Freedman R, Ross RG, Lester LA, Leonard S. The human CHRNA7 and CHRFAM7A genes: A review of the genetics, regulation, and function. *Neuropharmacology.* 2015;96:274-288.
84. Weinberger AH, Platt J, Zhu J, Levin J, Ganz O, Goodwin RD. Cigarette use and cannabis use disorder onset, persistence, and relapse: Longitudinal data from a representative sample of US adults. *J Clin Psychiatry.* 2021;82(4): 20m13713
85. Schauer GL, Rosenberry ZR, Peters EN. Marijuana and tobacco co-administration in blunts, spliffs, and mulled cigarettes: A systematic literature review. *Addict Behav.* 2017;64:200.
86. Hindocha C, Freeman TP, Ferris J, Chan A, et al. No smoke without tobacco: A global overview of cannabis and tobacco routes of administration and their association with intention to quit. *Front Psychiatry.* 2016;7:104.
87. McClure EA, Tomko RL, Salazar CA, et al. Tobacco and cannabis co-use: drug substitution, quit interest, and cessation preferences. *Exp Clin Psychopharmacol.* 2019;27:265.
88. Toll BA, Rogewski AM, Duncan LR, et al. "Quitting smoking will benefit your health": The evolution of clinician messaging to encourage tobacco cessation. *Clin Cancer Res.* 2014;20:301-309.

17 The Pharmacology of Cannabinoids

Justin Matheson, Katrina Mark, Daniele Piomelli, David A. Gorelick, and Bernard Le Foll

CHAPTER OUTLINE

- Introduction
- History, epidemiological, and legal status
- Substances included
- Cannabinoid pharmacokinetics
- The endocannabinoid system
- Clinical uses of cannabinoids
- Addiction liability
- Clinical manifestations of cannabis use
- Psychiatric adverse effects of cannabinoids
- Additional medical adverse effects of cannabinoids
- Effects of cannabis use during pregnancy
- Future developments
- Conclusion

INTRODUCTION

Cannabis has historically been, and continues to be, one of the most commonly used psychoactive drugs worldwide. The most recent data from the United Nations Office on Drugs and Crime (UNODC) estimate that 209 million people used cannabis in 2020.[1] Cannabis remains an illegal drug under international drug control treaties (eg, the 1961 United Nations (UN) Single Convention on Narcotic Drugs). However, the legal status of cannabis has been controversial since the late 1930s, and the past two decades have seen dramatic changes in individual state- and country-level regulation of cannabis worldwide.[2]

The story of cannabinoid pharmacology, which will be covered in more detail in the next section, began in the late nineteenth century and reached its first "peak" in the 1940s and 1960s with the isolation and synthesis of cannabis constituents (cannabinoids), such as Δ^9-tetrahydrocannabinol (Δ^9-THC), which mediate its pharmacological effects. Subsequent research from the 1980s to the present identified the endogenous cannabinoid (endocannabinoid) system, an important target of exogenous cannabinoids and an evolutionarily conserved lipid signaling system with ubiquitous presence throughout the body, not just the central nervous system. This chapter will present an overview of what is currently known and end with some ideas of where the field might be headed. The reader may also refer to other cannabis-related chapters in this textbook, including Chapter 9: Impact of the Cannabis Industry on Cannabis Use Disorder, Chapter 126: Therapeutic Effectiveness of Cannabis and Cannabinoid, and Sidebar to Chapter 126: Legal and Ethical Considerations When Choosing Whether to Recommend Dispensation of "Medical" Marijuana to Patients.

HISTORY, EPIDEMIOLOGICAL, AND LEGAL STATUS

History and Legal Status

The cannabis plant (*Cannabis sativa*) originated in Central Asia and has been used by humans for at least ten thousand years for three purposes: as a source of food and fiber, as a medication, and to create an altered state of consciousness (for both spiritual and recreational purposes).[3,4] Hemp was grown in Asia and Europe at least since the Bronze age.[5] Written records of cannabis use in China and South Asia date back four thousand years; it was also used by the Greeks and Romans.

Cannabis used as treatment was introduced to Europe and North America in the first half of the 19th century by European physicians, especially Jacques-Joseph Moreau de Tours, a French psychiatrist, and William O'Shaughnessy, a British Army surgeon. The successful use of cannabis used as treatment of Queen Victoria of the United Kingdom and Empress Elizabeth of Austria helped popularize its use as treatment, which was rapidly incorporated into practice along with other plant-based medications. Cannabis was added to the United States Pharmacopeia in 1850.

Attitudes toward cannabis changed in the early 20th century, for socio-political rather than scientific or medical reasons. Cannabis ("hashish" or "Indian hemp") was placed under strict international control by the 1925 International Opium Convention, which continued with the 1961 UN Single Convention on Narcotic Drugs and its 1972 amendments.[6] Cannabis and its extracts and tinctures were classified in Schedule I (use limited to medical or scientific purposes only under government licensing or ownership); cannabis was also classified in Schedule IV (which allows countries to impose complete prohibition if they consider it appropriate). Cannabis was made explicitly illegal in Canada in 1923 and functionally illegal in the United States through heavy taxation in 1937 (Marihuana Tax Act) and removed from the U.S. Pharmacopeia in 1942. Cannabis was made explicitly illegal in the United States in 1970 under the Controlled Substances Act (CSA). Against the advice of a scientific panel, cannabis and all cannabinoids were placed in Schedule I, meaning they were considered to have "high potential for abuse" and "no currently accepted medical use."

Attitudes toward cannabis changed again starting in the last decade of the 20th century. By 2021, 64 countries (32 in Europe) had legalized cannabis for treatment purposes several also legalized it for recreational or so-called "adult use," including Uruguay (2013), Canada (2018), South Africa (2018), and Mexico (2021).[1] In December 2020, the UN Commission on Narcotic Drugs narrowly voted (27-25) to remove cannabis from Schedule IV of the 1961 Single Convention. Cannabis remains illegal for any purpose in the United States at the national level. However, there is a growing movement at the U.S. state level to legalize cannabis for both recreational and nonrecreational (ie, cannabis used as treatment, CUAT) purposes, starting with California in 1996 (CUAT) and Colorado and Washington in 2012 (recreational). As of October 2022, 37 U.S. states, the District of Columbia, and three U.S. territories (Guam, Puerto Rico, and the U.S. Virgin Islands) had legalized CUAT; 19 states, the District of Columbia, and Guam had also legalized recreational cannabis.[7] One U.S. territory (Northern Mariana Islands) legalized recreational cannabis but has no CUAT program. Ten additional states had legalized cannabis with high cannabidiol (CBD)/low Δ^9-THC content for treatment of childhood seizures. Thus, only three U.S. states and one territory (American Samoa) have no type of legalized cannabis.

Hemp (defined as cannabis with a very low concentration of Δ^9-THC) remains an important commercial crop worldwide. The U.S. Farm Act of 2018 explicitly made hemp (defined as cannabis with no more than 0.3% Δ^9-THC by dry weight) legal by removing it from the jurisdiction of the CSA.

Epidemiology

Cannabis Use

In 2020, cannabis was used by an estimated 209.2 million people (95% CI 149.5-265.0 million) worldwide, 4.2% (95% CI 2.9%-5.2%) of the global population age 15 to 64 years.[1] This is an 8% increase in prevalence and 23% increase in number of people using it since 2010. Adolescents 15 to 16 years old had the highest use prevalence at 5.8%. About two-thirds of people using it were men, but this gender gap is smaller in high-income countries. Cannabis use was most prevalent in North America (16.6% [95% CI 16.4-16.8], 54.1 million), Australia and New Zealand (12.1% [95% CI 12.1-12.1], 2.4 million), and West and Central Africa (9.7% [95% CI 5.2-10.8], 28.5 million). Cannabis use was least prevalent in East and Southeast Asia (1.2% [95% CI 0.5-1.5], 19.4 million), Eastern and Southeastern Europe (2.0% [95% CI 1.5-2.8], 4.6 million), and Central Asia and Transcaucasia (2.6% [95% CI 0.8-4.3], 1.5 million).

An estimated 126.5 (standard error [se] 1.4) million U.S. residents reported lifetime use of cannabis in 2020, based on interviews with a nationally representative sample of 36,284 community-dwelling residents (National Survey on Drug Use and Health [NSDUH]).[8] The prevalence of lifetime cannabis use in this population group was 45.7 (se 0.50)%. An estimated 49.6 (se 1.0) million U.S. residents used cannabis in the prior year (17.9 [se 0.37]% prevalence) and 32.8 (se 0.83) million used in the past month (11.8 [se 0.30]% prevalence). These represent increases since 2002 of 13.1%, 62.7%, and 90.3% in lifetime, past-year, and past-month prevalence, respectively. However, cannabis use prevalence has decreased among adolescents (12-17 years old) by about one-third since 2002—39.8% lifetime, 36.1% past-year, and 28.0% past-month.

While cannabis use is present in all demographic groups and geographic areas, prevalence of use varies across groups and locations.[8] Prevalence of past-month use (in 2020) was highest in late adolescents/young adults (18-25 years old)—23.1 (se 0.83)% and lowest in adolescents (12-17 years old)—5.9 (se 0.45)% and the elderly (>65 years old)—3.7 (se 0.46)%. Men are significantly more likely than women to use cannabis (14.9 [se 0.73]% versus 12.1 [se 0.67]%). Cannabis use is significantly lower in the South of the United States (9.3 [0.44]%) than in other regions and in rural counties (5.6 [se 1.23]%) than in metropolitan and urbanized counties (11.9-12.3 [se 0.43-1.29]%). Cannabis use prevalence is significantly higher among non-Hispanics than Hispanics (14.0 [se 0.53]% versus 11.0 [se 1.25]%) but does not vary significantly across (self-identified) racial groups.

Cannabis use also varies across socioeconomic groups,[8] although these differences do not imply a causal relationship between cannabis use and these characteristics. There is an inverse association between household annual income and prevalence of cannabis use: below the federally defined poverty level—16.1 (se 0.85)%, 100% to 199% of poverty level—12.7 (se 0.67)%, at least 200% of poverty level—10.6 (se 0.35)%. Adults who are high school graduates (13.3 [se 1.13]%) or have some college (15.1 [se 0.90]%) have a significantly higher prevalence of cannabis use than those with other levels of education. Adults who are unemployed (22.0 [se 2.25]%) or work part-time (15.5 [se 1.27]%) have a significantly higher prevalence of cannabis use than those who work full-time (10.9 [se 0.74]%) or are not in the workforce (9.4 [se 0.94]%). Adults who self-identify as lesbian, gay, or bisexual have a substantially higher prevalence of cannabis use than the general population (29.8% versus 12.4%).

An estimated 2.84 (se 0.18) million individuals initiated cannabis use in 2020, representing 1.9 (se 0.12)% of the population not already using cannabis.[8] The mean age of those starting cannabis use was 20.2 (se 0.51) years (similar for males and females), more than half (57.6%) were female, more than one-third (36.2%) adolescents (12 to 17 years old), and two-fifths (40.4%) young adults (18 to 25 years old).

In Canada, where cannabis has been legal since 2018, prevalence of lifetime use in 2019 was 41.7% (95% CI 40.3-43.1), with 31.0 million people who used it in their lifetime, based on interviews with a nationally representative sample of 10,293 Canadian residents at least 15 years old (Canada Alcohol and Drugs Survey [CADS]).[9] Prevalence of past-year use was 20.7% (19.4-22.0) and of past 30-day use 13.9% (12.8-15.0). Males had a slightly higher use prevalence than females over all three time periods. Nova Scotia and New Brunswick had the highest prevalence over all three time periods, while Ontario and Quebec had the lowest. The mean age at initiation of cannabis use was 19.3 (19.0-19.5) years and was similar for males and females.

Cannabis Use Disorder

An estimated 22.1 million (95% uncertainty interval 19.0-25.9) individuals globally had cannabis use disorder (CUD) in 2016 (harmful use or cannabis dependence in ICD-10 terminology[10]), based on publicly available data from 195 countries.[11] This was a 25.6% increase from 1990. The estimated age-adjusted prevalence was 0.29% (0.25-0.34), a 7.1% decrease from 1990. Both absolute prevalence and age-adjusted prevalence were about twofold greater in men than in women. The estimated world-wide modal age of onset of cannabis use disorder, based on a systematic review of published studies, is 19.5 years, median (25th, 75th percentile) 22 years (19, 29).[12] More than one-sixth (17.5%) of cases have onset by 18 years; only 3.2% by 14 years.

In the United States, an estimated 14.2 million (se 0.49) individuals at least 12 years old had cannabis use disorder (DSM-5 criteria[10]) in 2020, an estimated 12-month prevalence of 5.1 (se 0.18)%.[8] Prevalence is greatest among young adults (18-25 years old)—13.5 (se 0.19)% and lowest among adolescents (12-17 years old)—4.1 (se 0.38)% and those 26 years and older—4.0 (se 0.19)%. Males had a higher prevalence of cannabis use disorder than did females.

SUBSTANCES INCLUDED

Complexity of *Cannabis sativa*

The taxonomy and nomenclature of cannabis has been a subject of debate since the Swedish naturalist Carl Linnaeus first identified and named one species he called *Cannabis sativa* in 1753.[13] A second species of cannabis that grew in India called *Cannabis indica* was proposed by Jean-Baptiste Lamarck in 1785, followed nearly two centuries later by a third proposed species, *Cannabis ruderalis*, identified in Russia.[13] Recently, some scientists have suggested that the taxonomic genus *Cannabis* contains a single species, *Cannabis sativa* L., with the three variants *sativa*, *indica*, and *ruderalis*,[13-15] though the dispute has not been fully resolved,[16] and alternative nomenclatures have been proposed based on the morphology and chemical characteristics of the plant.[17] The issue of classification has been further complicated by decades of intentional interbreeding to satisfy the rapidly evolving recreational cannabis and CUAT markets that have emerged in response to the changing legal status of cannabis, resulting in hundreds (or possibly thousands) of different cannabis varieties.[15,17] Thus, for the purposes of this chapter, "cannabis" will mean all varieties of the genus *Cannabis*, unless otherwise stated.

Regardless of taxonomic classification, from a pharmacological perspective, the key feature of cannabis is the presence of epidermal glandular structures called trichomes that line the leaves, bracts/flowers, and stems of the plant and produce a number of secondary metabolites.[16] Over 500 different compounds have been identified in cannabis, including flavonoids (eg, quercetin, luteolin, and orientin), terpenoids (eg, limonene, myrcene, and pinene) that give cannabis its aroma, and, most importantly, the phytocannabinoids.[16,18] The term "cannabinoid" refers to three classes of molecules[14]:

1. **Phytocannabinoids**: compounds isolated from the cannabis plant with the characteristic C_{21} terpenophenolic structure along with their derivatives and transformation products. There are at least 125 distinct phytocannabinoid compounds that are typically grouped together according to common structural elements.[19,20] In addition to Δ^9-THC and CBD, other phytocannabinoids that have been well characterized include tetrahydrocannabivarin (THCV), cannabinol (CBN), cannabigerol (CBG), and cannabichromene (CBC).[20]
2. **Endocannabinoids**: endogenous lipid signaling molecules that interact with cannabinoid receptors. The endocannabinoids are phospholipid derivatives containing a poly-unsaturated fatty acid moiety (arachidonate, which contains four cis double bonds, though endocannabinoids with different numbers of double bonds have been reported) and a polar head group, either ethanolamine in the case of anandamide or glycerol in the case of 2-AG.[21]
3. **Synthetic cannabinoids**: synthetic analogues not derived from the cannabis plant.

Cannabinoids have a range of pharmacological actions, both within the endocannabinoid system (ECS) and other signaling systems. Their most important target is the cannabinoid receptor type-1 (CB_1 receptor), whose activation by cannabinoids mediates the psychotropic (ie, intoxicating) effects of cannabis, as selective antagonism of CB_1 blocks behavioral effects of Δ^9-THC in laboratory animals and attenuates the subjective and physiological effects of smoked cannabis in humans.[22] Thus, cannabinoids are often distinguished by their pharmacological activity at CB_1 receptors: partial agonists (compounds that bind to the receptor but do not evoke a maximal response), full agonists, antagonists, and inverse agonists (compounds whose binding to the receptor suppresses spontaneous signaling).

Partial CB_1 Agonists

Among the phytocannabinoids, Δ^9-THC is by far the most studied; synthetic Δ^9-THC is FDA-approved (under the international nonproprietary name [INN] of dronabinol) for the treatment of chemotherapy-induced nausea and vomiting. Based on seminal work conducted in the 1940s,[23] Δ^9-THC was firmly identified as the primary intoxicating component of cannabis in the 1960s.[24,25] Δ^9-THC can fully displace CB_1 receptor ligands from receptor binding sites, yet its affinity is significantly lower than that of many synthetic cannabinoid agonists such as CP-55,940.[26] The maximal effect sizes

(E_{max} values) of CB_1-receptor-mediated effects produced by Δ^9-THC are significantly lower than those of full receptor agonists, indicating that Δ^9-THC is a partial agonist.[26] Other important partial agonists at the CB_1 receptor include the synthetic analogue, nabilone, and the less-studied phytocannabinoid Δ^8-THC.[27]

Full CB_1 Agonists

Most (if not all) of the full CB_1 receptor agonists are synthetic cannabinoid compounds that were initially developed to probe the ECS. These include the cyclohexylphenols (CPs), such as CP55,940; HU-210, a dibenzopyran that is structurally similar to Δ^9-THC developed by Raphael Mechoulam at Hebrew University (HU); and aminoalkylindoles such as WIN55,212.[28] In the early 2000s, illicit laboratories began to synthesize these cannabinoids, spray them directly on to dried plant materials, and market them as legal cannabis alternatives.[28] These designer drugs were first identified by brand names such as "Spice" and "K2," though newer brand names have continued to appear.

CB_1 Antagonists

The discovery of the cannabinoid receptors led to the development of numerous synthetic probe compounds to modulate CB receptor activity, including the CB_1 receptor antagonist/inverse agonist rimonabant. Studies administering rimonabant in rodent models[26] and human laboratory paradigms[29,30] have demonstrated that the CB_1 receptor mediates most of the acute effects of cannabis. Rimonabant initially showed promise as therapeutic agent to treat obesity[31] and substance use disorders,[32] though it was ultimately withdrawn from the market due to serious psychiatric adverse effects.[33,34]

Cannabidiol

Unlike Δ^9-THC, CBD does not act primarily through activating the ECS. While it does seem to act as a negative allosteric modulator at CB_1[35] and a partial agonist at CB_2,[36] CBD signaling is much more complex and involves a wide range of molecular targets. Important among them are the serotonin receptors $5HT_{1A}$ and $5HT_{3A}$, the dopamine D_2 receptor, the GABAa receptor, the glycine receptor, nuclear receptors such as the peroxisome proliferator-activated receptor gamma (PPAR-γ), the transient receptor potential (TRP) channels TRPV1 and TRPA1, as well as the orphan G-protein coupled receptors (GPCRs) GPR3/6 and GPR5.[37,38] Also unlike Δ^9-THC, CBD is generally considered to be nonintoxicating and lacking euphoria and addiction liability, although there is some evidence that CBD may be more likely to produce subjective effects when it is inhaled instead of taken orally (though it should be noted these subjective effects are not indicative of reward or reinforcement, rather just subjective perception of psychological effects).[39]

Combination Products

Sativex (nabiximols) is a phytocannabinoid extract and oromucosal spray containing a 1:1 ratio of Δ^9-THC to CBD. Sativex was created by GW Pharmaceuticals (acquired by Jazz Pharmaceuticals in 2021); it is produced from two cannabis chemovars containing high Δ^9-THC and CBD concentrations using a standardized process.[40] In 2010, Sativex became the first cannabis-based product to be approved in the United Kingdom, for treatment of spasticity due to multiple sclerosis.[40]

Other Phytocannabinoids

The phytocannabinoids have been classified into 11 sub-classes, including CBC, CBD, cannabielsoin (CBE), CBG, cannabicyclol (CBL), CBN, cannabinodiol (CBND), cannabitriol (CBT), Δ^8-THC, Δ^9-THC, and miscellaneous-type cannabinoids.[20]

Other Cannabis Constituents

In addition to the cannabinoids, other pharmacologically active compounds are present in the cannabis plant, such as terpenes. Terpenes are odorous compounds that give cannabis its characteristic smell, although growing evidence suggests that terpenes may also have clinically relevant pharmacological actions.[41,42] At least 120 terpenes have been identified in cannabis,[20] but the number varies widely (12-66) across individual chemovars.[41] The most common terpenes present across different cannabis chemovars include myrcene, β-caryophyllene, α-humulene, α-pinene, limonene, and linalool.[41] Cannabis also contains flavonoids (eg, the cannflavins, which are currently being investigated for therapeutic uses due to their anti-inflammatory properties[43]), as well as numerous other noncannabinoid phenols.[20]

Cannabis Potency

Cannabis potency is typically quantified as the concentration of Δ^9-THC or the Δ^9-THC to CBD ratio in a cannabis product. The average Δ^9-THC content in cannabis products has been increasing for decades, based largely on assays of samples seized by law enforcement; for example, in the United States it increased from 8.9% in 2008 to 17.1% in 2017, while the Δ^9-THC:CBD ratio increased dramatically from 23 in 2008 to 104 in 2017, largely because CBD content remained stable.[44] Similar increases in Δ^9-THC content and Δ^9-THC:CBD ratio have occurred in Europe.[45] The emergence of cannabis products with 50% or more Δ^9-THC content presents a serious public health concern, given the association between high Δ^9-THC content and risk for adverse psychological effects such as psychosis and cannabis use disorder.[45,46]

Diversity of Cannabis Formulations and Routes of Administration

Cannabis products are available in a variety of formulations that can be taken by several routes of administration. In the United States, smoking dried cannabis flower has historically been the most common method of cannabis use, either rolled in cigarette paper ("joint") or tobacco leaf ("blunt") or smoked in a pipe or water pipe ("bong"). However, as new legal cannabis markets have emerged, there has been a dramatic diversification in the range of cannabis product types and routes of administration available to consumers.[47] Cannabis can be taken orally when plant material is placed in capsules or pressed into tablets or when the plant material has been cooked into an oil and/or baked into a cookie, pastry, or other dessert. These so-called edibles are increasing in popularity.[48,49] Newer oral products have emerged, such as cannabis- or Δ9-THC-infused drinks or other foodstuffs such as gummy bears. Cannabis concentrates with up to 90% Δ9-THC content (eg, "waxes," "dabs," or "shatter") can be flash vaporized on a hot surface for inhalation. Δ9-THC can be inhaled ("vaped") via pen-like electronic drug delivery devices ("e-cigarettes" or EDDD) (see Chapter 22). Cannabinoids (chiefly, CBD) are available for topical administration in the form of lotions, creams, balms, and gels. Also available, but less common, are tongue strips, sublingual sprays, and rectal suppositories.[48,50] Administration by injection is extremely rare.

CANNABINOID PHARMACOKINETICS

There are hundreds of pharmacologically active compounds in the cannabis plant, but few have been studied pharmacokinetically other than Δ9-THC (the primary psychoactive component) and CBD (psychoactive but not euphorigenic). Thus, the focus here will be on Δ9-THC and CBD, with some mention of other phytocannabinoids. Δ9-THC and other phytocannabinoids are present in cannabis as inactive acids which must be decarboxylated. Decarboxylation occurs slowly at room temperature, whereas heating of the plant material produces rapid and efficient decarboxylation and is typically required to liberate enough of the pharmacologically active Δ9-THC to have psychotropic effects.[51] This is a primary reason why the most common routes of administration of cannabis have historically involved heating—either inhalational, by combusting the dried plant material (eg, in a cannabis cigarette or "joint") or by vaporizing it, or orally after preparation involving heating, for example, infusing oils with Δ9-THC at hot temperatures and baking foodstuffs with the resulting oils.[48]

Understanding the complex pharmacokinetics of Δ9-THC (see below) is essential to understanding the onset, duration, and magnitude of cannabinoid effects. For example, the strong lipophilicity of Δ9-THC results in its rapid redistribution after administration into brain and adipose tissue, which build up large stores of Δ9-THC with chronic use. This stored Δ9-THC is gradually released back into the circulation during periods of no use. These pharmacokinetic factors lead to detectable Δ9-THC in urine in individuals who have not used cannabis for several weeks and a poor association between blood Δ9-THC concentrations and cannabis effects. These phenomena have critical implications for drug testing for cannabis, especially in the forensic and workplace context.

Absorption

When cannabis is smoked or vaporized, Δ9-THC is detectable in blood within seconds and peak blood concentrations occur typically within 5 to 10 minutes.[51] Rapid absorption of Δ9-THC into the systemic circulation, which is paralleled by the onset of subjective drug effects within minutes, likely contributes to the addiction liability of smoked cannabis (though it should be noted that oral Δ9-THC has addiction liability as well).[52] When smoking a typical cannabis cigarette, an estimated 30 to 50% of Δ9-THC is lost through pyrolysis and sidestream smoke.[51,53] The observed bioavailability of Δ9-THC when cannabis is smoked is extremely variable (estimates range from 2% to 56%) due to smoking-related factors such as depth of inhalation, puff duration and frequency, and breath hold duration.[51,52] The observed bioavailability of CBD from smoked cannabis products is similar in range (ie, 11%-45%).[54] In general, people who are more experienced using cannabis have more efficient smoking practices and thus will inhale more Δ9-THC for a given quantity of cannabis, resulting in a greater observed bioavailability.[52] While people describe "vaping" cannabis products, a more accurate term is that this is not a vapor but an aerosol. Cannabis aerosols may lead to slightly higher blood Δ9-THC concentrations than smoking,[55] though the evidence remains limited.

In contrast to inhalation, oral administration of Δ9-THC leads to much slower onset of effects, more variability in peak concentrations, and lower bioavailability.[54] Peak plasma concentrations of Δ9-THC after oral absorption may not occur until 2 to 6 hours after ingestion, compared to just minutes after smoking.[52] Further, there may be two peaks observed with oral administration of Δ9-THC, which is thought to be due to enterohepatic recirculation.[52] The time to peak concentration of CBD after oral ingestion is similarly variable and estimated to be between 1 and 6 hours based on the few available studies.[56] The bioavailability, peak concentration, and half-life of CBD are dependent on co-ingestion with food, with studies finding greater CBD concentrations after co-ingestion with a high-fat meal.[56]

Distribution

Δ9-THC has a large volume of distribution (estimated to be 4 to 14 L/kg) and is highly bound to plasma lipoproteins (estimated at 95%-99%) in the systemic circulation,[51,54] with approximately only 3% of Δ9-THC present in plasma in the free-state.[57] Δ9-THC disappears rapidly from the blood as it passes through highly vascularized tissues such as lung, heart, and liver.[51] Due to its high lipophilicity, Δ9-THC eventually accumulates in the adipose organ (white and brown adipose tissues), possibly also as fatty acid conjugates.[51] Δ9-THC conjugates can be redistributed from adipose depots to the circulation and can be detectable even during periods of abstinence from cannabis.[52] Distribution of Δ9-THC into the brain is important for understanding and predicting the behavioral effects of cannabis. Studies in rodent models have found that less than 1% of the total dose of Δ^9-THC administered reaches the brain.[52] In human postmortem samples, Δ^9-THC can be detected in brain while undetectable in blood.[58] This likely contributes to the poor correlation between blood Δ^9-THC concentrations and acute effects,[52] which presents a challenge for roadside enforcement of cannabis-involving driving legislation.[59]

Metabolism

The primary site of Δ^9-THC metabolism is in the liver. The cytochrome P_{450} (CYP) enzymes CYP2C9, CYP2C19, and CYP3A4 are the most important enzymes involved in Δ^9-THC metabolism.[52] Over 100 metabolites of Δ^9-THC have been identified in humans, most involving oxidation of Δ^9-THC at the carbon-11 position to form the psychoactive metabolite 11-OH-THC, followed by further hydroxylation at this position to form the inactive metabolite 11-COOH-THC.[52,57] 11-OH-THC is about as potent as Δ^9-THC in humans, is better able to cross the blood-brain barrier, and is thought to contribute to the overall psychoactivity of Δ^9-THC, especially when Δ^9-THC is consumed orally.[57] As a result of significant first-pass hepatic metabolism, 11-OH-THC is detectable in higher concentrations after consumption of oral Δ^9-THC compared to smoked cannabis.[52] Aside from 11-OH-THC, other common oxidation products of Δ^9-THC include 8β-OH-THC and 8α-OH-THC.[52] 11-COOH-THC often undergoes glucuronidation by uridine 5'-diphosphoglucuronosyltransferase 1A9 (UGT1A9) and 1A10 (UGT1A10) to increase water solubility.[57] Extrahepatic metabolism of Δ^9-THC has also been observed, for example, in the brain, intestines, and lung.[52] The metabolism of CBD is similar to that of Δ^9-THC, though additional CYP enzymes such as CYP1A1, CYP1A2, and CYP2D6 may play more of a role.[60] Hydroxylation of CBD to 7-OH-CBD seems to be the primary initial metabolic pathway for CBD.[60]

Elimination

Approximately 20% to 35% of Δ^9-THC is excreted (either as the parent compound or a metabolite) in the urine, while the remaining 65% to 80% is excreted in the feces.[51,52] Renal clearance of lipophilic Δ^9-THC itself is quite low due to extensive tubular reabsorption in the nephron.[51] The glucuronide conjugate of 11-COOH-THC is the major metabolite excreted in the urine; concentrations of free 11-COOH-THC in the urine are insignificant.[51] The predominance of excretion in the feces is largely a result of significant enterohepatic recirculation of metabolites and high protein binding of cannabinoids.[51] Metabolites in the feces are present only in their nonconjugated forms.[51]

The detection window of 11-COOH-THC in urine is commonly used in drug treatment programs, criminal justice, and employee assistance testing programs as an indication of cannabis use, as it is well known that the elimination of 11-COOH-THC is much slower than the parent compound.[51] For example, the detection window of 11-COOH-THC in urine has been observed to be as long as 67 days following sustained abstinence.[61] Due to the slow redistribution of Δ^9-THC from the adipose tissue to the systemic circulation, and the subsequent metabolism of Δ^9-THC to 11-COOH-THC, urine samples may fluctuate between positive and negative as urinary 11-COOH-THC concentrations rise and fall.[52]

THE ENDOCANNABINOID SYSTEM

The endocannabinoid system (ECS) is a lipid signaling system found in all vertebrate animals and many invertebrates.[62] Widespread and versatile, the ECS plays a role in a vast range of physiological processes, including energy homeostasis, neural development, synaptic plasticity, and the processing of stress, pain, emotion, and reward.[63-66] With such a wide range of functions, it is unsurprising that endocannabinoid signaling is complex and tissue- and region-specific.

The two cannabinoid receptors, type-1 (CB_1) and type-2 (CB_2), are 7-transmembrane-domain G-protein coupled receptors (GPCRs) regarded as the most abundant GPCRs in the mammalian brain.[64] CB_1 is encoded by the *CNR1* gene and alternative splicing of this gene leads to three variants: a canonical long form and two additional isoforms with a shorter N-terminus.[67,68] The CB_2 receptor is encoded by the *CNR2* gene, which shares only 44% protein sequence homology with CB_1 and has two isoforms in humans.[69] The functional significance of the cannabinoid receptor isoforms remains unclear.[69] In addition to CB_1 and CB_2 receptors, several orphan receptors have been proposed as putative cannabinoid receptors, including G-protein-coupled receptor 55 (GPR55).[70] Other receptors that play a role in endocannabinoid-related signaling include the peroxisome proliferator activated receptors (PPARs) and transient receptor potential (TRP) channels.[65]

Early autoradiography studies revealed a wide expression of CB_1 receptors in the brain, especially in the cortex, basal ganglia, hippocampus, and cerebellum.[71] This binding pattern paralleled the known effects of cannabinoids; for example, high receptor expression in the basal ganglia and cerebellum was consistent with the characteristic motor effects of Δ^9-THC, while low or absent binding in the brainstem was consistent with the observation of low lethality from cannabinoid overdose.[71] Later in situ hybridization and immunohistochemistry studies confirmed these early observations and provided further evidence that CB_1 is expressed primarily presynaptically.[64] In the cortex, CB_1 receptors are widely distributed throughout the cingulate gyrus, the frontal cortex, the secondary somatosensory cortex, the motor cortex, several olfactory cortical areas, the hippocampus, and the cortical amygdala nuclei.[72] The highest expression of cortical CB_1 receptors is in large GABAergic cholecystokinin (CCK)-containing interneurons, with lower (but functionally relevant) expression on glutamatergic neurons.[72] In the striatum, CB_1 receptors are densely expressed on GABAergic medium spiny neurons in the dorsal and ventral striatum, with lower expression in the nucleus accumbens.[72] Finally, in the cerebellum, CB_1 receptors are most densely expressed on GABAergic and glutamatergic axon terminals of the climbing and parallel fibers and on the basket cells.[72] Non-neuronal expression of CB_1 receptors has also been observed, for example in immune cells, adipocytes, hepatocytes, and cells of the reproductive organs.[64,73]

The majority of CB_2 receptor expression is found in cells of the immune system,[64] with additional expression in bone, the gastrointestinal and reproductive systems, and in many other non-neuronal tissues.[74] Evidence indicates that CB_2 receptors are also expressed in microglia, vascular elements of the CNS, and certain neuron populations.[72] CB_2 receptors are highly inducible in the CNS, with up to 100-fold increases in neuronal expression after tissue injury or inflammation.[65] Their expression has been documented in the cerebellum, brainstem, hippocampus, thalamus, hypothalamus, and striatum, though generally at low levels.[74]

Endogenous agonists (the endocannabinoids) are phospholipid derivatives containing a poly-unsaturated fatty acid moiety (eg, arachidonate) and a polar head group, either ethanolamine in the case of arachidonoylethanolamide (anandamide) or glycerol in the case of 2-arachidonoylglycerol (2-AG).[21] Anandamide is a high-affinity partial (low-efficacy) agonist for the CB_1 receptor with very little activity at the CB_2 receptor, while 2-AG is a low-affinity, high-efficacy agonist for both receptors.[65] Although anandamide was the first to be identified, 2-AG is actually the more abundant endocannabinoid in the CNS, with nearly 1,000-fold greater basal levels.[69] A key characteristic of the endocannabinoid system that differentiates it from other classical neurotransmitter systems is that the endocannabinoids are not stored in cells, but are instead produced and released upon demand, normally in response to increased intracellular calcium concentrations or postsynaptic metabotropic receptor activation.[21,65]

Anandamide formation starts with the transfer of an arachidonate group from phosphatidylcholine to phosphatidylethanolamine (PE), which generates the anandamide precursor *N*-arachidonoyl-PE.[75,76] This reaction occurs predominantly upon demand—for example, *via* activation of transmitter or hormone receptors[77,78]—and is catalyzed by the enzyme cytosolic type-epsilon phospholipase A_2 (encoded by *PLA2G4E*).[79] Cleavage of *N*-arachidonoyl-PE by a unique phospholipase D (*NAPEPLD*)[80,81] releases anandamide, which diffuses out of the cell and into the external milieu.[77,82] Like anandamide, 2-AG is also generated upon demand. The membrane phospholipid that serves as its immediate precursor, phosphatidylinositol-4,5-bisphosphate (PIP_2), is hydrolyzed by a receptor-operated phospholipase C (*PLC*), probably PLCβ and/or PLCε, to produce 1,2-diacylglycerol (DAG), which is then cleaved by the α or β isoform of diacylglycerol lipase (*DGL*) to generate 2-AG.[83,84] In glutamate-sensitive neurons of the brain, PLC and DGL-α are physically linked to type-5 metabotropic glutamate receptors in a multimolecular complex (the "endocannabinoid signalosome") that enables efficient retrograde signaling from the postsynaptic spine (which houses the signalosome) to the axon terminal (where the majority of central CB_1 receptors are localized).[85]

Membrane trafficking followed by intracellular degradation of the endocannabinoids is responsible for signal termination. The mechanism of endocannabinoid uptake across the plasma membrane remains controversial,[66,69] whereas endocannabinoid hydrolysis is generally well characterized. The enzyme fatty acid amide hydrolase (FAAH) is responsible for anandamide degradation, a reaction that produces arachidonic acid and ethanolamine.[21] FAAH is also able to metabolize 2-AG in vitro, but the physiological pathway is hydrolysis of 2-AG by monoglyceride lipase (MGL) to form arachidonic acid and glycerol.[21,65] Oxidation of endocannabinoids by cyclooxygenases (COX), lipoxygenases (LOX), and the cytochrome P_{450} enzymes has also been observed.[21]

Endocannabinoid signaling is complex and varies in a ligand-, cell-type-, and region-dependent fashion. Early experiments in Allyn Howlett's laboratory clearly demonstrated that cannabinoid signaling was sensitive to inhibition by pertussis toxin, implicating the $G_{i/o}$ family of G proteins.[86] Indeed, a common feature of both cannabinoid receptors is that agonist activation leads to $G_{i/o}$-mediated inhibition of adenylyl cyclase, subsequent reduction in the production of cyclic AMP (cAMP), and dampening of protein kinase A (PKA) activity.[64] A reduction in PKA phosphorylation can in turn activate A-type potassium currents and inhibit voltage-gated L-, N-, P-, and Q-type calcium channels.[64] Often, this pathway tends to suppress neuronal excitability and inhibit presynaptic neurotransmitter release,[21,64] which can have either a net excitatory or inhibitory effect as CB_1 receptors are widely expressed on both inhibitory and excitatory synapses. There is evidence that CB_1 receptors can also signal through G_s proteins in certain cell types, leading to a stimulation of cAMP production.[73] Other common pathways involve the $G_{i/o}\beta\gamma$ subunit, which mediates the stimulation of intracellular calcium transients and the activation of phosphatidylinositol 3-kinase (PI3K), resulting in tyrosine phosphorylation, activation of Raf-1, and phosphorylation of mitogen-activated protein kinase (MAPK) to ultimately influence cell death/survival decisions.[64] Finally, an important G-protein-independent pathway is the association of the CB_1 receptor with β-arrestins,[69] which results in internalization of the receptor, is thought to underlie desensitization of the CB_1 receptor, and is at least partially responsible for tolerance to the effects of repeated cannabinoid agonist administration.[63,69]

An important role of 2-AG, which is not apparently shared by anandamide, is that of retrograde synaptic messenger. Three basic forms of retrograde endocannabinoid-mediated synaptic plasticity have been described, including depolarization-induced suppression of inhibition (DSI) and excitation (DSE), metabotropic-induced suppression of inhibition (MSI) and excitation (MSE), and long-term depression (LTD).[65] In most cases, these types of retrograde signaling begin with the production of 2-AG in response to either increases in postsynaptic intracellular calcium concentrations (in the case of DSI/DSE) or activation of postsynaptic $G_{q/11}$-coupled receptors (in the case of MSI/MSE).[65,69] 2-AG is then released into the synaptic cleft, travels across the synapse, and activates the CB_1 receptor, which in turn suppresses calcium influx into the neuron by inhibiting voltage-gated calcium channels.[65] The result is suppression of either inhibitory or excitatory neurotransmitter release (usually GABA or glutamate), dampening subsequent activity at the synapse for a brief duration. LTD, in contrast, is a longer-lasting form of synaptic dampening that involves additional CB_1-dependent and -independent signaling pathways, though is still heavily dependent on adenylyl cyclase activity.[69]

CLINICAL USES OF CANNABINOIDS

Approved Indications

Cannabis has been used for a wide variety of treatment purposes over the centuries, but only in a few cases have cannabinoid-based agents been approved by a national regulatory authority, that is, have adequate scientific evidence supporting efficacy and safety, usually in the form of well designed, replicated phase 3 controlled clinical trials.

The U.S. Food & Drug Administration (FDA) has approved four cannabinoid products (representing three distinct compounds). Synthetic Δ^9-THC (dronabinol), marketed in capsule (Marinol) and liquid (Syndros) formulations, is approved for treatment of nausea and vomiting associated with cancer chemotherapy and anorexia and weight loss associated with HIV/AIDS. The synthetic Δ^9-THC analogue nabilone is also approved for the treatment of nausea and vomiting associated with cancer chemotherapy. CBD derived from cannabis plant extract is approved for the treatment of several intractable childhood seizure syndromes such as Lennox-Gastaut syndrome, Dravet syndrome, or tuberous sclerosis complex.

In Canada and parts of Europe, nabilone (generic forms) is approved for severe chemotherapy-induced nausea and vomiting. In addition, nabiximols, a cannabis plant extract containing a 1:1 ratio of Δ^9-THC:CBD, is approved for the treatment of spasticity and neuropathic pain in adult patients with multiple sclerosis and for moderate to severe pain in adult patients with advanced cancer despite treatment with opioid analgesics.

Unapproved Indications

Cannabis has been used for treatment purposes for thousands of years often, albeit not only, as an analgesic and sedative.[3,4] Over the past several decades, a growing number of clinical studies of varying degrees of rigor have evaluated cannabis products and specific cannabinoids in the treatment of various medical conditions, including psychiatric. However, this research has been limited by two major factors: the illegal status of cannabis in most of the world, which limits funding and granting of regulatory permission for clinical studies, and the complex pharmacology of cannabis, as the plant contains hundreds of chemicals, most of which have not been adequately studied. Complicating interpretation of study findings is the substantial variation in cannabis formulations (plant-derived versus synthetic, whole plant versus specific cannabinoid(s)), doses, and routes of administration (smoked, vaporized, oral).[87] Listing in a U.S. state law as an approved indication for receiving legal CUAT is no guarantee that there is scientific evidence supporting that listing. Of the 42 different medical and psychiatric conditions listed in U.S. state CUAT laws, half have no published clinical studies showing efficacy; 9% have evidence of causing harm.[87]

Clinical trials and reviews on the subject of CUAT have been increasing over the years.[87-92] For additional information on cannabis used as treatment (CUAT), please see Chapter 2 "Recommended Use of Terminology in Addiction Medicine" for a brief discussion of the term "medical" marijuana and Chapter 126 "Therapeutic Effectiveness of Cannabis and Cannabinoids" and its side-bar "Legal and Ethical Considerations for Clinicians Recommending Cannabis Used as Treatment."

ADDICTION LIABILITY

Animal Addiction Liability

Various animal models are able to capture different facets of drug addiction.[93] For example, drug discrimination procedures allow studying subjective effects induced by psychoactive drugs. Conditioned place preference (CPP) and intra-cranial self-stimulation procedures allow to measure impact on reward system. Intravenous drug self-administration procedures allow studying reinforcing properties. Withdrawal states can be induced by administering a substance chronically and withdrawing its administration or by blocking its effects with an antagonist administration.

Drug discrimination studies have shown that animals can learn to discriminate effects induced by Δ^9-THC administration[32,93] and that those effects are mediated by cannabinoid CB_1 receptors.[94,95] Results with the CPP paradigm have been more complex to interpret. Indeed, the majority of studies performed in rodents have indicated that Δ^9-THC produced aversive effects.[96] It should be noted that some studies using low Δ^9-THC doses revealed some place preference,[96] suggesting that maybe most of studies were done using unit doses of Δ^9-THC that were too high. Typically, drugs that induce reward in the CPP paradigm are prone to produce self-administration. The drug self-administration paradigm is considered the best model to study reinforcing effects of drugs and to predict addiction liability potential in humans. It has been very difficult for investigators to establish intravenous self-administration (IVSA) of Δ^9-THC in rodents, while the full CB_1/CB_2 agonist, WIN 55,212-2 was able to support IVSA.[97,98] However, it should be noted that those experiments observed self-administration under very restricted conditions (eg, severe food restriction, animal immobilization and tail administrations). In addition, the fact that Δ^9-THC did not substitute to WIN 55,212-2 in a rodent study suggest also that models using full CB_1 ligand may not reflect the addictive potential of Δ^9-THC.[99]

The only preclinical model that reliably obtained Δ^9-THC IVSA has been developed in squirrel monkeys.[100] Δ^9-THC IVSA was self-administered at high rates in this species with animals first trained to self-administer psychostimulants[100] or drug naive animals only exposed to Δ^9-THC.[101] It has been possible also to produce reinstatement of drug seeking behavior after a phase of extinction in those animals. It should be noted that the doses used in those studies using squirrel monkeys were similar to those in cannabis smoke inhaled by humans. In squirrel monkeys, the Δ^9-THC IVSA was blocked by the cannabinoid CB_1 receptor antagonist/inverse agonist rimonabant[100] and by the neutral CB_1 antagonist AM4113.[102] Those two CB_1 blockers also prevented reinstatement of Δ^9-THC seeking.[102]

Recently, there has been an interest at developing animal models that would use aerosolized ("vaped") cannabis extracts instead of the IVSA route.[103] In this model, Sprague-Dawley rats have been trained to nose-poke in operant chambers to obtain puffs containing aerosol cannabis extracts in daily sessions. Interestingly, these animals were able to discriminate between active and inactive operanda. The aerosolized cannabis extracts maintained higher response rates under fixed ratio schedules and higher break points under progressive ratio schedule of reinforcements, although the intake levels were relatively low and the rates of responding much lower than typically observed with addictive drugs. Interestingly, removal of the reinforcer produced extinction and cue-induced reinstatement was observed in those animals.[103] Those promising findings suggest that such preclinical models may better reflect the inhalation of cannabis smoke performed by human participants and would accelerate preclinical research in this area in the future.

Human Addiction Liability

One metric of addiction liability is the proportion of people who use drugs who develop a substance use disorder. A recent meta-analysis of 21 published studies (both cross-sectional and longitudinal) found that 22% (95% CI 18%-26%) of people who use cannabis developed a cannabis use disorder.[104] Rates were similar in longitudinal and cross-sectional studies, but higher for lifetime use (27% [25%-28%]) than for recent (past-year or past-month) use (22% [20%-24%]) in longitudinal studies. Rates also vary substantially depending on cannabis use patterns and individual characteristics.

Risk Factors for Cannabis Use Disorder

There is a substantial positive association between frequency[105-107] and duration[108,109] of cannabis use and risk for developing cannabis use disorder. Quantity (amount) of use is presumably also an important risk factor but has not been adequately studied because of the difficulty in accurately measuring amounts and potency of an illegal substance. A nationally representative cross-sectional survey of U.S. adults found a 30% rate of past-year DSM-IV defined cannabis dependence among respondents using cannabis daily, a 22% rate among those using at least weekly, and a 9% rate among those using less than weekly.[105] Other nationally representative cross-sectional U.S. surveys found a significant positive association between lifetime duration of cannabis use and prevalence of past-year cannabis use disorder among adolescents (12-17 years old) or young adults (18-25 years old).[109] Among adolescents, prevalence of past-year cannabis use disorder increased from 11% (95% CI 9.3%-12.3%) among those using up to 1 year to 15% (95% CI 13.2%-16.2%) among those using 1 to 2 years, 17% (95% CI 15%-18.8%) using 2 to 3 years, and 20% (95% CI 18%-22.3%) among those using more than 3 years.

Family, twin and population-based studies (eg, genome-wide association studies [GWAS]) suggest that genetic factors account for one-quarter to one-third of the variability in initiation of cannabis use[110,111] and age at first cannabis use[112] and two-thirds to three-quarters of the variability in frequency of cannabis use[113] and development of cannabis use disorder in people who use cannabis.[110,113,114] A substantial proportion of this genetic influence is not specific to cannabis, but is shared with other psychoactive substances.[115-117] No gene or single nucleotide polymorphism (SNP) has been consistently associated with these traits,[115,116] suggesting that the genetic influence arises from many different genes each exerting a very small influence. There is also some evidence of genetic influence on the subjective effects of cannabis, such as cannabis craving[118,119] or other euphoric-related subjective effects as measured in human laboratory studies.[120,121]

Several clinical and sociodemographic factors are associated with increased risk of developing cannabis use disorder, based on several large population-based cross-sectional surveys and a few small longitudinal surveys.[122-126] However, these significant associations do not necessarily reflect direct causal influence. Use of alcohol, tobacco, or other psychoactive substances is associated with greater risk of cannabis use, daily use of cannabis, and developing cannabis use disorder. Adverse childhood experiences (such as physical, emotional, or sexual abuse),[127] pre-existing psychiatric disorder or conduct problems as a child or adolescent,[128] depressed mood, anxiety, or abnormal negative mood regulation, stressful life events (such as unemployment, financial difficulties,[123,127,129] and parental cannabis use[130,131]) are associated with increased risk of developing cannabis use disorder.

Several sociodemographic factors may be protective, that is, they are associated with lower risk of developing cannabis use disorder. These include personal attendance at religious services[132] and close parental monitoring of adolescent behavior.[133]

CLINICAL MANIFESTATIONS OF CANNABIS USE

Intoxication

Cannabis produces a variety of acute psychological and physiological effects,[134,135] which vary by dose, route of administration, and degree of tolerance in the people who use, among other factors.[136] Low to moderate doses produce euphoria ("high"), reduction of anxiety, and sedation, the effects desired by people who use recreationally. Other psychological effects include increased appetite ("munchies") and sociability and impaired short-term memory and concentration. Some people may experience anxiety, panic attacks, or paranoia, especially at higher doses. Less common are psychotomimetic symptoms such as perceptual alterations (eg, altered time sense, visual illusions), delusions, and hallucinations. These effects can be induced in healthy research volunteers with high doses or intravenous administration of Δ^9-THC.[137] Acute physical effects include poor motor coordination (ataxia), slurred speech, dry mouth, conjunctival injection ("red eye"), tachycardia, orthostatic hypotension, and horizontal nystagmus.

The onset and duration of acute cannabis intoxication varies with the route of administration, reflecting the pharmacokinetics of absorption and distribution. With inhalational (smoked or vaporized/aerosolized) administration, intoxication begins within a few minutes and lasts 3 to 4 hours. With oral administration, intoxication begins in 30 to 180 minutes and lasts 8 to 12 hours. The intensity and duration of intoxication is positively correlated with the dose of Δ^9-THC taken and negatively correlated with the individual's degree of tolerance. People who are cannabis-naive and those who use occasionally typically experience intoxication with Δ^9-THC doses of 2 to 3 mg inhaled or 5 to 10 mg oral.[135]

Most episodes of cannabis intoxication are mild, self-limited, and resolve without treatment. Many cases never come to medical attention. More severe cases may warrant a diagnosis of cannabis intoxication, for example, the individual has difficulty communicating or cooperating with others or taking adequate care of themselves. Examples include severe anxiety or panic attack, paranoia, inability to walk unaided, prominent hallucinations, or psychosis. The latter experiences may require inpatient psychiatric hospitalization, and the psychosis may be prolonged in some cases. Children who inadvertently ingest cannabis orally may require hospitalization due to coma, convulsions, or cardiopulmonary instability.[138] Treatment of cannabis intoxication is reviewed in Chapter 59.

Withdrawal

Cannabis withdrawal is a cluster of self-limiting signs and symptoms that occur within 1 week of substantial reduction in or abstinence of use of cannabis use by individuals who use it heavily or long-term.[139,140] The probability and severity of cannabis withdrawal are positively correlated with the intensity (quantity, frequency) and duration of cannabis use. A recent meta-analysis that included 23 published studies found a current (past-year) prevalence of cannabis withdrawal syndrome of 46% (95% CI 41%-52%) in those who used it daily and 23% (15.7%-33.4%) in those who used it regularly but less than daily.[141] Co-occurring psychiatric, alcohol, tobacco or other substance use disorders did not influence the prevalence of cannabis withdrawal syndrome. A population-based, nationally representative, cross-sectional survey of U.S. adults (2012-2013) found a 12.1% (standard error 1.13) prevalence of cannabis withdrawal syndrome (DSM-5 diagnostic criteria) among people who used it regularly (at least thrice weekly) in the past 12 months.[142] Using cannabis daily did not significantly increase the odds of having cannabis withdrawal syndrome, while smoking more than 6 joints daily was associated with a threefold increase in the odds. There was no association of withdrawal prevalence with age, gender, or other substance use disorders.

Common symptoms of cannabis withdrawal include depression, anxiety, irritability or aggression, restlessness, decreased appetite, and sleep disturbance (including vivid dreams).[139,140,142] Physical signs are less common and include abdominal cramps, muscle aches or tremor, headache, sweating or chills, and weight loss. Symptoms tend to begin within 1 to 2 days of abstinence or reduction of use and peak within 2 to 6 days, with symptoms lasting 2 to 3 weeks or longer in individuals with a long-term, heavy use.[140] These signs and symptoms greatly overlap with those of tobacco withdrawal, making the two withdrawal syndromes often difficult to distinguish in individuals who use both cannabis and tobacco.

Most cases of cannabis withdrawal resolve without treatment and do not come to medical attention. However, signs and symptoms can last for several weeks and cause discomfort. Therefore, cannabis withdrawal can serve as negative reinforcement for continuation or resumption of cannabis use, which may account for the threefold greater prevalence among patients in treatment than among the general population.[141] Treatment of cannabis withdrawal is reviewed in Chapter 59.

Tolerance

Repeated exposure to phyto-, synthetic, or endogenous cannabinoids in animals generates substantial tolerance to most behavioral and physiological effects.[143,144] This tolerance is accompanied by down-regulation or desensitization of cannabinoid receptors (ie, pharmacodynamic) rather than by significant increase in cannabinoid metabolism (pharmacokinetic).

Information about human tolerance to cannabis comes largely from self-reporting by people who use it long term and comparing the response to single doses of cannabis among individuals who use it regularly versus occasionally, rather than from controlled administration of cannabis at known doses over extended time periods.[144,145] Human studies show that repeated cannabis use, either inhaled or oral, generates substantial or complete tolerance to psychological effects such as cognitive and psychomotor impairment and partial tolerance to subjective effects such as euphoria ("high") and anxiety and cardiovascular effects such as tachycardia and orthostatic hypotension. Controlled cannabis administration studies show more consistent tolerance development than do other studies. In such experimental studies, tolerance to cognitive, psychomotor, and subjective effects develops within 4 to 6 days of multiple daily dosing. We are not aware of any studies evaluating the influence of cannabis dose on tolerance development or on the time course of tolerance dissipation.

Cannabis tolerance in humans is likely pharmacodynamic, as regular cannabis use is associated with down-regulation of brain CB_1 receptors.[144,145] There is no evidence of a pharmacokinetic mechanism, as the pharmacokinetic parameters of Δ^9-THC are similar whether it is used occasionally or regularly. Several studies suggest that laboratory animals can develop behavioral or learned tolerance to cannabis behavioral effects.[144] Human studies suggest that people with experience using cannabis can compensate for some expected acute effects of cannabis, thereby appearing to show tolerance. Such tolerance is limited and seen chiefly in studies of motor vehicle driving. In such studies, participants believing they received cannabis tend to drive more slowly and carefully.

PSYCHIATRIC ADVERSE EFFECTS OF CANNABINOIDS

Acute Effects

Transient adverse psychological symptoms are common acute effects of cannabis intoxication. Cannabis-related mental health adverse effects such as anxiety, suicidal thoughts, and psychotic symptoms such as paranoia and hallucinations are common reasons that individuals seek emergency medical services.[146] In human laboratory studies, administration of cannabis causes transient, dose-dependent psychotomimetic symptoms, including positive (hallucinations, delusions, etc.), negative (blunted affect, emotional withdrawal, and psychomotor retardation), and cognitive symptoms associated with psychotic illness.[147] Cannabis also causes acute dose-dependent, time-limited impairment of several cognitive and psychomotor functions, including episodic and working memory, attention (especially divided attention), concentration, executive functions (especially response inhibition), associative learning, reaction time, and visual-motor coordination that usually wear off within several hours.[136,148,149] These impairments contribute to the increased risk of motor vehicle collisions or other unintended injury associated with cannabis use.[59] Tolerance tends to develop to most of the acute effects of cannabis, including cognitive effects, where individuals who use more frequently or heavily may be less likely to experience cognitive impairment under the influence of cannabis.[145] Mounting evidence has suggested that increases in the diversity and Δ^9-THC potency of cannabis products has increased risk of acute cannabis-related harms and may be driving an increase in cannabis-attributable emergency department (ED) visits, especially among cannabis-naive individuals.[47]

Long-Term Effects

The long-term psychiatric adverse effects of cannabis use include cannabis use disorder, chronic impairment in cognitive performance, increased risk of psychosis-spectrum disorders, and increased risk of mood and anxiety symptoms.[150,151]

Cognition

Long-term use of cannabis is associated with chronic impairment in multiple domains of cognition, especially verbal episodic and working memory, attention, and certain executive functions.[152-155] Unlike acute cognitive effects of cannabis, which can be measured in placebo-controlled laboratory studies, chronic cognitive effects of cannabis are assessed in observational studies, either cross-sectionally, by comparing a sample of participants who use cannabis regularly to a sample of participants who use little or no cannabis, or longitudinally, where cohorts of cannabis-using and nonusing individuals have their cognitive performance measured at multiple time points. Both types of observational studies are potentially confounded by numerous factors, including group differences in cannabis use patterns, age, sex/gender, co-occurring disorders, and use of other psychoactive drugs.[150,156] One salient issue is distinguishing between residual or sub-acute effects of cannabis in individuals who use cannabis frequently from actual long-term effects. For example, in a recent meta-analysis, significant between-groups differences were observed in verbal recall performance only when cannabis-using groups were tested after fewer than 7 days of abstinence, suggesting that cognitive impairment may resolve after 7 days of abstinence.[153] The literature is mixed on the extent to which cognitive function can return to baseline (precannabis-using) levels and the duration of abstinence required for recovery of function.[156] Some recovery of verbal recall performance can be observed following 3 days of sustained abstinence from cannabis.[153] Duration of regular cannabis use is positively associated with greater impairment in verbal recall performance.[153]

Psychosis

Several converging lines of evidence strongly suggest a causal role of cannabis use in increasing the risk of psychosis, though the exact nature of the relationship remains under debate.[157] At least a dozen prospective longitudinal studies have documented an association between cannabis use and increased risk of subsequent psychotic symptoms or illness.[158] Cross-sectional studies suggest that people who use cannabis have a two- to threefold increased prevalence of schizophrenia and schizophrenia spectrum disorders than do those who do not use cannabis.[159] The association is stronger with earlier age of initiating cannabis use, more intense cannabis use, and use of cannabis with high Δ^9-THC content and high Δ^9-THC:CBD ratio.[160,161] A retrospective longitudinal study based on Danish national health registries found a fourfold increased risk of schizophrenia among those with cannabis use disorder, compared to with those without cannabis use disorder, after controlling for potential confounds such as age, sex, other psychiatric diagnoses (including other substance use disorders), and parents' education level, and psychiatric history.[162] The population-attributable risk fraction of schizophrenia due to cannabis use disorder increased from 2 in 1992 to 6 to 8 in 2010 to 2016, paralleling the increasing incidence of cannabis use disorder from 0.02% in 1992 to 0.18% in 2016. A third line of evidence is that genetic liability to cannabis use disorder is strongly associated with schizophrenia.[163] In addition, having an episode of cannabis-induced psychosis is a very strong risk factor for later development of schizophrenia. A meta-analysis of six studies found that 34% of individuals with cannabis-induced psychosis eventually transitioned to schizophrenia.[164] A longitudinal study based on Danish national health registries found that 41% of individuals with a diagnosis of cannabis-induced psychosis developed schizophrenia over the subsequent 20 years; half of those who converted to schizophrenia converted within 4 years.[165] Clinical studies have suggested that people who use cannabis who develop a psychotic disorder present for treatment at a significantly younger age than those who do not use cannabis and that there may be a dose-response relationship between the potency of cannabis and younger age of experiencing first psychotic symptoms.[157] A recent systematic review confirmed this association; compared to use of low-potency cannabis, use of high-potency cannabis was associated with an increased risk of psychosis (which was higher in individuals using cannabis daily), an earlier onset of psychosis, more symptoms of psychosis, and increase risk of recurrence of psychosis.[46] Of note, however, a 2021 analysis of two cohorts of twins found no evidence of a differential effect of cannabis on psychoticism.[166] Cannabis use also has adverse effects on individuals with pre-existing schizophrenia. A meta-analysis of 24 published longitudinal studies found that those who used cannabis had increased risk of recurrence of illness and rehospitalization, more severe positive symptoms, and poorer level of functioning and treatment adherence than those who never used or discontinued cannabis use.[167] In individuals with first episode of psychosis, cannabis use is associated with an increased risk of psychotic experiences[168] and of illness recurrence and re-hospitalization.[169]

Mood and Anxiety

The relationship between regular cannabis use and mood and anxiety disorders remains unclear.[150] A systematic review found that individuals reporting cannabis use were more likely to develop depression than controls, with a stronger relationship in individuals using cannabis more heavily.[170] Another systematic review found that cannabis use was associated with worsening of depressive symptoms in individuals with major depressive disorder and of both depressive and manic symptoms in bipolar disorder.[171] Other systematic reviews have found less consistent evidence for an association between cannabis use and depressive symptoms in healthy individuals[172] and limited evidence for an association between increasing cannabis potency and depression.[46] Systematic reviews suggest a significant association between cannabis use and increased odds of developing any anxiety disorder,[173] as well as an association between cannabis use and subclinical anxiety symptoms in healthy individuals[172] and increased potency associated with increased risk of anxiety.[46] Cannabis use disorder is often co-occurring with mood and anxiety disorders,[174] and some evidence suggests that mood and anxiety symptoms may increase the risk of conversion from cannabis use to CUD.[150] One of the biggest issues in the field is determining whether cannabis use itself is a risk factor for mood and anxiety disorders, or whether the co-occurrence between CUD and other psychiatric problems is the result of shared etiology.[174] Further complexity comes from the fact that while alleviation of anxiety and depression is a common motive for using cannabis,[175] cannabis can cause symptoms of anxiety and depression in human laboratory studies.[150]

Brain Structure and Function

Long-term cannabis use is associated with changes in brain structure and function as assessed with structural and functional magnetic resonance imaging (MRI). For example, a systematic review of 56 published studies in adults who used cannabis found consistent evidence of reduced hippocampal volume and lower hippocampal gray matter density in people who used cannabis relative to those who did not use cannabis, with no evidence for changes in whole brain volume and inconsistent or inconclusive evidence for changes in other brain regions.[176] A cross-sectional study involving 243 adults found that the 129 people who used cannabis had significantly smaller volume of the orbitofrontal cortex and cerebellar white matter than the 114 healthy people who did not use cannabis, after controlling for age, intelligence quotient, intracranial volume, and alcohol and tobacco use.[177] A prospective longitudinal study of 799 adolescents followed from before initiation of cannabis use (age 14 years) to age 19 years found a significant dose-dependent association between frequency of cannabis use and thinning of the frontal cortex bilaterally, after controlling for age, sex, handedness, total brain volume, and alcohol intake.[178]

Functional MRI studies find that adults who use cannabis have decreased neuronal activity in anterior cingulate cortex and right dorsolateral prefrontal cortex relative to adults that do not use cannabis, as well as increased functional connectivity across brain regions.[176] Abnormalities of neuronal activity were observed even when cognitive task performance was normal, suggesting that people who use cannabis may need to engage increased levels of neuronal activation to achieve normal cognitive performance.

ADDITIONAL MEDICAL ADVERSE EFFECTS OF CANNABINOIDS

It remains unclear whether cannabis use per se is associated with increased all-cause mortality.[179] A population-based, retrospective, longitudinal cohort study of all individuals born in Sweden between 1955 and 1980 found that those identified as having cannabis use disorder had a higher mortality rate than the general population (hazard ratio 10.93, 95% CI 11.36-12.03).[180] The major adverse health consequences with the strongest evidence of being caused by cannabis use are motor vehicle accidents (40% increased risk[181]), suicide, and cardiovascular and pulmonary disease.[182,183] Most other cannabis-associated morbidity and mortality is due to co-occurring psychiatric disorders and substance use (especially alcohol and tobacco), rather than to cannabis itself.[184]

Cannabis use disorder represents only a minor portion of the global disease burden.[11] In 2016, cannabis use disorder accounted for a negligible proportion of the estimated 144,000 deaths globally attributed to substance use disorders (not including alcohol or tobacco use disorders). By comparison, opioids accounted for 60.0%, cocaine 13.0%, and amphetamines 3.6%. Cannabis use disorder was associated with only 6.4% of the more than 6.1 million disability-adjusted life years attributed to substance use disorders (excluding tobacco) in the United States and Canada in 2016.[11]

Cannabis is not a major driver of visits to U.S. emergency departments (EDs), especially compared to other psychoactive substances. Cannabis use was associated with an estimated 788,000 visits to U.S. EDs in 2021, based on data from a representative sample of 53 hospitals (Drug Abuse Warning Network [DAWN]), where it ranked as the fourth commonest driver of ED visits, behind alcohol, opioids, and methamphetamine.[185] Cannabis-attributable ED visits represent about 10% of all substance-related visits. By comparison, alcohol accounted for more than one-third (39.3%) of such visits and opioids for 14.1%. Almost two-thirds (63.6%) of cannabis-related visits also involved another substance, primarily alcohol or stimulants (amphetamines, cocaine).

Cardiovascular Effects

The acute cardiovascular effects of cannabis smoking include tachycardia, vasodilation, increased myocardial oxygen demand, and reduced myocardial oxygen supply.[186,187] These changes provide plausible pathophysiological mechanisms for producing adverse cardiovascular outcomes such as cardiac arrhythmia, acute myocardial infarction (MI), and stroke.[188-190] However, the existing evidence supporting such associations is weak due to methodological limitations in many studies, including recall bias, inadequate assessment of cannabis exposure, failure to include participants with heavy or long-term cannabis use, and failure to control for many confounding factors, such as use of alcohol, tobacco, or other psychoactive substances.

A significant positive association between frequent cannabis use (>10 days per month) and risk of lifetime MI or coronary artery disease was found in a cross-sectional survey of a nationally representative sample of U.S. adults.[191] All participants had no lifetime cigarette use, ruling out confounding by tobacco use, a known risk factor for coronary artery disease. Another study found a fourfold increased risk of acute MI in the first hour after smoking cannabis.[192]

A modest but significant association between lifetime cannabis use and stroke, especially ischemic stroke, was found among young adults (18-49 years old) in a retrospective medical record review of U.S. hospitalization between 2007 and 2014.[193]

While cardiac arrhythmias, except sinus tachycardia, are rare among adolescent and young adults using cannabis,[193,194] some case series and case-control studies suggest a possible association between cannabis use and atrial fibrillation and ventricular tachycardia in this age group.[195] A significant association between current cannabis use disorder and cardiac arrhythmia in hospitalized adolescents and young adults (15 to 34 years old) was found in a retrospective medical record review covering 2010 to 2014, even after controlling for potential confounding factors such as race, sex, alcohol and tobacco use disorders, obesity, and medical comorbidities.[196] The most common arrhythmia among patients with cannabis use disorder was atrial fibrillation (42%).

Pulmonary Effects

Smoking cannabis causes acute respiratory symptoms (cough, wheezing, dyspnea, sputum production)[197] and acutely exacerbates asthma.[197] However, there is no clear association between chronic cannabis use and impaired pulmonary function or lung diseases such as chronic obstructive pulmonary disease (COPD).[197,198] The adverse effects of cannabis smoke, compared with tobacco smoke, may be moderated by the absence of nicotine and the presence of cannabinoids with anti-inflammatory action.[199,200]

Cancer

Cannabis use for more than 10 years is associated with an increased risk for only one type of cancer—testicular nonseminoma.[201] There is no clear evidence that cannabis use is associated with any other type of cancer, including lung cancer.[201] This may be due, in part, to the fact that people who smoke cannabis have less exposure to inhaled carcinogens than do those who smoke tobacco, either with or without tobacco.[202,203] Case-control, cohort, and cross-sectional studies have inconsistent results regarding an association between cannabis smoking and lung cancer. Most studies had high risk of bias.[201] A pooled analysis including 5,144 participants from six large, good-quality case control studies found no association between "habitual" cannabis use (at least one joint-year) and lung cancer when compared with nonhabitual or never use (odds ratio 0.96, 95% CI 0.66-1.38).[204] However, a large Mendelian randomization study including 85,716 individuals found a significant association between genetic liability for lifetime cannabis use (but not for cannabis use disorder) and squamous cell carcinoma of lung (odds ratio 1.22, 95% CI 1.07-1.39).[198] There was no such significant association with other forms of lung cancer. Meta-analyses have found no association between ever using cannabis and head and neck or oral cancer.[201]

Cannabis Hyperemesis Syndrome

Cannabis (or cannabinoid) hyperemesis syndrome (CHS) is a form of cyclical vomiting, often accompanied by abdominal pain, occurring in the context of heavy, frequent (often daily) cannabis use.[205] CHS may be impossible to distinguish from cyclical vomiting syndrome unless the history of heavy frequent cannabis use is elicited. Another distinctive feature is relief by heat; patients often take hot baths or showers. As cannabis itself can relieve nausea and vomiting (synthetic Δ^9-THC is FDA-approved for this condition), patients often unintentionally worsen their condition by "self-medicating" with more cannabis and are reluctant to accept the diagnosis. CHS is confirmed when abstinence from cannabis use results in cessation of vomiting.[205] The pathophysiology of CHS is unclear, but likely involves disruption of endocannabinoid system function, which leads to dysregulation of stress responses, thermoregulation, and various neurotransmitter systems, involved in pain perception.[206] While traditional antiemetics are typically ineffective in treating CHS, benzodiazepines, haloperidol, and topical capsaicin have shown some promise for managing symptoms.[205]

Sexual and Reproductive Function

Cannabis use was not associated with impairment of male or female sexual function in healthy individuals[207-209] in several large, cross-sectional surveys nor with delay in the time to pregnancy in healthy couples trying to conceive.[210] There is no good-quality evidence associating cannabis use with male erectile dysfunction,[211] as most published studies do not control for potential confounds such as other substance use or co-occurring psychiatric disorders. Cannabis use is associated with reduced spermatogenesis and impaired sperm function in most,[212,213] but not all,[214] studies.

At least some cannabinoids (Δ^9-THC, CBD) appear in the breast milk of lactating women who use cannabis.[215,216] The concentration of Δ^9-THC in breast milk is two- to sixfold higher than its concentration in plasma and is detectable in breast milk for several weeks after the mother stops cannabis use. The effects of cannabinoids in breast milk on the nursing infant are uncertain.

Other Organ System Effects

Cannabis use is not associated with acute hepatotoxicity[217] or nephrotoxicity[218,219] in healthy individuals or with adverse outcomes after kidney transplantation,[218] but may accelerate decline in kidney function in men with hypertensive kidney disease.[220] Cannabis use is associated with worsening progression of hepatic fibrosis[221] and increased risk of hepatic encephalopathy[222] in patients with chronic viral hepatitis C.

Cannabis use is not associated with obesity[223] or the development of type II diabetes; in fact, it is protective against diabetes in some studies[224-226] and epidemiological studies have found that people who use cannabis regularly are less likely to be obese.[227] Cannabis use is associated with poorer glycemic control and increased risk of diabetic ketoacidosis in adults with type I or type II diabetes.[228,229]

Cannabis causes several acute ocular effects, including decreased intraocular pressure, increased photosensitivity, reduced tear production ("dry eyes"), and conjunctival injection ("red eye").[230,231] Chronic cannabis use is not associated with increased risk of developing glaucoma, but may be associated with earlier age at onset of glaucoma.[232]

Chronic cannabis use is associated in cross-sectional studies with several adverse oral health effects, including xerostomia ("dry mouth"), leukoplakia, and periodontitis.[233] However, most studies did not rule out confounding by other substance use and poor oral hygiene.

EFFECTS OF CANNABIS USE DURING PREGNANCY

Many studies have attempted to evaluate the effects on the fetus of in utero cannabis exposure. To date, there is no evidence of direct teratogenicity resulting in birth defects or congenital anomalies.[234] Although randomized, controlled trials are not able to be performed given the Schedule I status of cannabis in the United States, animal studies and observational human studies have raised concerns regarding birth outcomes and long-term neurologic effects.[235]

Of all birth outcomes that have been evaluated, lower mean birth weight in infants with gestational cannabis exposure has the strongest evidence.[234,236,237] A systematic review and meta-analysis showed an OR of 1.77 for low birth weight and a mean difference of 109 g less in infants exposed to cannabis in utero.[234] Low birthweight, preterm birth, admission to the Neonatal Intensive Care Unit, low APGAR score and smaller head circumference have all been found to be associated with in utero cannabis exposure.[235] Although no causal link between adverse birth outcomes and exposure has been established, biologic plausibility exists. Given the endocannabinoid system involvement in embryonic implantation and placentation, it is feasible that exposure during early developmental stages decrease blood flow and placental changes.[238-241] Additionally, the Generation R study found that continued exposure throughout pregnancy resulted in the greatest negative impact on birthweight.[242]

Several large, prospective cohort studies attempted to evaluate the long-term neurodevelopmental effects of in utero cannabis exposure.[243-245] All of the studies found some outcomes that met statistical difference including measures of attention, memory and aggression.[237] However, the findings have been met with criticism given the inevitable confounders, the vast number of outcomes that were measured and the inconsistency of the findings.[246] Other studies have also found an association between in utero cannabis exposure and long-term behavioral and mental health disorders.[247,248] However, given the complexity of evaluating these neurodevelopmental outcomes and inability to account for all possible confounding factors, a causal link between exposure and outcome has not been established. On a molecular level, human studies have shown effects of in utero cannabis exposure on dopamine receptor development in the fetal brain, again supporting the biologic plausibility for concern.[249,250]

With the changing legal and social climate surrounding cannabis in the United States, rates of cannabis use in pregnancy have increased. Although precise numbers are difficult to obtain, many pregnant people report their reasons for use as symptomatic relief or CUAT purposes.[251,252] Given the concerns regarding in utero exposure, recreational use of cannabis in pregnancy is not recommended. For pregnant people who are considering CUAT, a thorough discussion of risks and benefits of cannabis compared to alternative treatments or untreated disease is recommended.[253]

FUTURE DEVELOPMENTS

As nonmedical use of cannabis becomes increasingly legal and more accessible on a global scale, there is an urgent need to monitor changes in cannabis potency, product availability, and related harms. The legal cannabis markets in the United States and Canada need time to mature and it will likely be many years before their effects on CUD and other cannabis-attributable harms are known.[254] Two concerns of note are (1) the marketing of high-potency cannabis products to young or cannabis-naive individuals who may be at increased risk of cannabis-related harms[47] and (2) the legal cannabis industry targeting individuals who use regularly to encourage escalation of use.[254] Another challenge in monitoring harms associated with cannabis use is the lack of standardized measures of cannabis consumption.[254] More work is needed to develop better metrics to assess the complex patterns of cannabis use that often include multiple product types.

Current pharmacological treatments for CUD are lacking, and the existing research is less developed than for other psychoactive drugs. Agonist substitution therapy with dronabinol (Δ^9-THC), nabilone, or nabiximols (oromucosal Δ^9-THC/CBD) seems to be a promising approach.[255] Other promising pharmacological treatments include FAAH inhibitors, CBD, the opioid receptor antagonist naltrexone, anticonvulsants such as topiramate and gabapentin, C-acetylcysteine, oxytocin, and varenicline.[254] Further refinement of animal models of CUD will help to better screen these medications, and translational clinical trials will be needed to evaluate their clinical potential and utility. Neuromodulation, such as repetitive transcranial magnetic stimulation (rTMS), has emerged as a new potential therapeutic strategy for treatment of CUD, but needs validation.[256] Neuroimaging studies have begun to examine brain alterations that occur with CUD, for example decreased CB_1 receptor binding in individuals with CUD,[257] but more work is needed to characterize these changes.

There is also a need to better understand relationships between cannabis use and mental health. Alleviation of anxiety and mood symptoms is a common motive for endorsing cannabis use,[175] and yet chronic cannabis use and CUD are both associated with worsening of mental health, though these relationships are complex.[258,259] More work is needed to characterize which patterns of cannabis use, cannabis product types, and individual-level factors such as age, sex, and gender may influence relationships between cannabis use and mental health.

CONCLUSION

The use of cannabis for myriad reasons dates back to at least 4,000 BCE, yet the isolation and synthesis of the primary psychoactive component of cannabis was a mere 80 years ago and discovery of the endocannabinoid system is even more recent. Thus, research in cannabinoid pharmacology is essentially in its infancy, with many outstanding questions regarding potential therapeutic applications and harms of cannabinoids. Adding to this complexity, the worldwide increase in legal access to recreational and CUAT use has created a multi-billion-dollar cannabis industry that is still in its infancy, yet has already created an unprecedented diversity of cannabis products, dramatically increased cannabis potency, and targeted young people and individuals who use cannabis regularly to increase sales. Further information on this subject can be found in Chapter 9 "Impact of the Cannabis Industry on Cannabis Use Disorder."

REFERENCES

1. UNODC. *World Drug Report 2022.* United Nations Office on Drugs and Crime. Accessed September 23, 2022. https://www.unodc.org/unodc/en/data-and-analysis/world-drug-report-2022.html
2. Hall W, Stjepanovic D, Caulkins J, et al. Public health implications of legalising the production and sale of cannabis for medicinal and recreational use. *Lancet.* 2019;394(10208):1580-1590.
3. Charitos IA, Gagliano-Candela R, Santacroce L, Bottalico L. The cannabis spread throughout the continents and its therapeutic use in history. *Endocr Metab Immune Disord Drug Targets.* 2021;21(3):407-417.
4. Crocq MA. History of cannabis and the endocannabinoid system. *Dialogues Clin Neurosci.* 2020;22(3):223-228.
5. Long T, Wagner M, Demske D, Leipe C, Tarasov PE. Cannabis in Eurasia: origin of human use and Bronze age trans-continental connections. *Veg Hist Archaeobotany.* 2017;26(2):245-258.
6. Collins J. A brief history of cannabis and the drug conventions. *AJIL Unbound.* 2020;114:279-284.
7. National Conference of State Legislatures. *State Medical Marijuana Laws.* Accessed October 7, 2022. http://www.ncsl.org/research/health/state-medical-marijuana-laws.aspx
8. Center for Behavioral Health Statistics and Quality. *Results from the 2020 National Survey on Drug Use and Health: Detailed Tables.* Accessed January 21, 2022. https://www.samhsa.gov/data
9. Statistics Canada. *Canadian Alcohol and Drugs Survey (CADS): 2019 Detailed Tables.* Accessed 19 May 2022. https://www.canada.ca/en/health-canada/services/canadian-alcohol-drugs-survey/2019-summary/detailed-tables.html#t5
10. Proctor SL, Williams DC, Kopak AM, Voluse AC, Connolly KM, Hoffmann NG. Diagnostic concordance between DSM-5 and ICD-10 Cannabis use disorders. *Addict Behav.* 2016;58:117-122.
11. GBD 2016 Alcohol and Drug Use Collaborators. The global burden of disease attributable to alcohol and drug use in 195 countries and territories, 1990-2016: a systematic analysis for the Global Burden of Disease Study 2016. *Lancet Psychiatry.* 2018;5(12):987-1012.
12. Solmi M, Radua J, Olivola M, et al. Age at onset of mental disorders worldwide: large-scale meta-analysis of 192 epidemiological studies. *Mol Psychiatry.* 2022;27(1):281-295.

13. Watts G. Cannabis confusions. *BMJ.* 2006;332(7534):175-176.
14. ElSohly MA, Radwan MM, Gul W, Chandra S, Galal A. Phytochemistry of *Cannabis sativa* L. *Prog Chem Org Nat Prod.* 2017;103:1-36.
15. de Meijer E. The chemical phenotypes (chemotypes) of cannabis. In: *Handbook of Cannabis.* Oxford University Press; 2014.
16. Bonini SA, Premoli M, Tambaro S, et al. *Cannabis sativa*: a comprehensive ethnopharmacological review of a medicinal plant with a long history. *J Ethnopharmacol.* 2018;227:300-315.
17. Pollio A. The name of cannabis: a short guide for nonbotanists. *Cannabis Cannabinoid Res.* 2016;1(1):234-238.
18. Russo EB. Taming THC: potential cannabis synergy and phytocannabinoid-terpenoid entourage effects. *Br J Pharmacol.* 2011;163(7):1344-1364.
19. Hanuš LO, Meyer SM, Muñoz E, Taglialatela-Scafati O, Appendino G. Phytocannabinoids: a unified critical inventory. *Nat Prod Rep.* 2016;33(12):1357-1392.
20. Radwan MM, Chandra S, Gul S, MA ES. Cannabinoids, phenolics, terpenes and alkaloids of cannabis. *Molecules.* 2021;26(9):2774.
21. Pamplona FA, Takahashi RN. Psychopharmacology of the endocannabinoids: far beyond anandamide. *J Psychopharmacol.* 2012;26(1):7-22.
22. Huestis MA, Gorelick DA, Heishman SJ, et al. Blockade of effects of smoked marijuana by the CB1-selective cannabinoid receptor antagonist SR141716. *Arch Gen Psychiatry.* 2001;58(4):322-328.
23. Adams R, Baker BR, Wearn RB. Structure of cannabinol. III. Synthesis of cannabinol, 1-hydroxy-3-n-amyl-6,6,9-trimethyl-6-dibenzopyran1. *J Am Chem Soc.* 1940;62(8):2204-2207.
24. Gaoni Y, Mechoulam R. Isolation, structure, and partial synthesis of an active constituent of hashish. *J Am Chem Soc.* 1964;86(8):1646-1647.
25. Mechoulam R, Gaoni Y. The absolute configuration of delta-1-tetrahydrocannabinol, the major active constituent of hashish. *Tetrahedron Lett.* 1967;12:1109-1111.
26. Pertwee RG, Cascio MG. Known pharmacological actions of delta-9-tetrahydrocannabinol and of four other chemical constituents of cannabis that activate cannabinoid receptors. In: Pertwee R, ed. *Handbook of Cannabis.* Oxford University Press; 2014.
27. Rock EM, Parker LA. Constituents of *Cannabis sativa. Adv Exp Med Biol.* 2021;1264:1-13.
28. Castaneto MS, Gorelick DA, Desrosiers NA, Hartman RL, Pirard S, Huestis MA. Synthetic cannabinoids: epidemiology, pharmacodynamics, and clinical implications. *Drug Alcohol Depend.* 2014;144:12-41.
29. Gorelick DA, Heishman SJ, Preston KL, Nelson RA, Moolchan ET, Huestis MA. The cannabinoid CB1 receptor antagonist rimonabant attenuates the hypotensive effect of smoked marijuana in male smokers. *Am Heart J.* 2006;151(3):754.e751-754.e755.
30. Huestis MA, Boyd SJ, Heishman SJ, et al. Single and multiple doses of rimonabant antagonize acute effects of smoked cannabis in male cannabis users. *Psychopharmacology (Berl).* 2007;194(4):505-515.
31. Christensen R, Kristensen PK, Bartels EM, Bliddal H, Astrup A. Efficacy and safety of the weight-loss drug rimonabant: a meta-analysis of randomised trials. *Lancet.* 2007;370(9600):1706-1713.
32. Le Foll B, Goldberg SR. Cannabinoid CB1 receptor antagonists as promising new medications for drug dependence. *J Pharmacol Exp Ther.* 2005;312(3):875-883.
33. Moreira FA, Crippa JA. The psychiatric side-effects of rimonabant. *Braz J Psychiatry.* 2009;31(2):145-153.
34. Le Foll B, Gorelick DA, Goldberg SR. The future of endocannabinoid-oriented clinical research after CB1 antagonists. *Psychopharmacology (Berl).* 2009;205(1):171-174.
35. Laprairie RB, Bagher AM, Kelly ME, Denovan-Wright EM. Cannabidiol is a negative allosteric modulator of the cannabinoid CB1 receptor. *Br J Pharmacol.* 2015;172(20):4790-4805.
36. Tham M, Yilmaz O, Alaverdashvili M, Kelly MEM, Denovan-Wright EM, Laprairie RB. Allosteric and orthosteric pharmacology of cannabidiol and cannabidiol-dimethylheptyl at the type 1 and type 2 cannabinoid receptors. *Br J Pharmacol.* 2019;176(10):1455-1469.
37. Vitale RM, Iannotti FA, Amodeo P. The (poly)pharmacology of cannabidiol in neurological and neuropsychiatric disorders: molecular mechanisms and targets. *Int J Mol Sci.* 2021;22(9).
38. Pisanti S, Malfitano AM, Ciaglia E, et al. Cannabidiol: state of the art and new challenges for therapeutic applications. *Pharmacol Ther.* 2017;175:133-150.
39. Kirkland AE, Fadus MC, Gruber SA, Gray KM, Wilens TE, Squeglia LM. A scoping review of the use of cannabidiol in psychiatric disorders. *Psychiatry Res.* 2022;308:114347.
40. Potter DJ. A review of the cultivation and processing of cannabis (*Cannabis sativa* L.) for production of prescription medicines in the UK. *Drug Test Anal.* 2014;6(1-2):31-38.
41. Booth JK, Bohlmann J. Terpenes in *Cannabis sativa*—from plant genome to humans. *Plant Sci.* 2019;284:67-72.
42. Weston-Green K, Clunas H, Jimenez NC. A review of the potential use of pinene and linalool as terpene-based medicines for brain health: discovering novel therapeutics in the flavours and fragrances of Cannabis. *Front Psych.* 2021;12:583211.
43. Erridge S, Mangal N, Salazar O, Pacchetti B, Sodergren MH. Cannflavins—from plant to patient: a scoping review. *Fitoterapia.* 2020;146:104712.
44. Chandra S, Radwan MM, Majumdar CG, Church JC, Freeman TP, ElSohly MA. New trends in cannabis potency in USA and Europe during the last decade (2008-2017). *Eur Arch Psychiatry Clin Neurosci.* 2019;269(1):5-15.
45. Freeman TP, Craft S, Wilson J, et al. Changes in delta-9-tetrahydrocannabinol (THC) and cannabidiol (CBD) concentrations in cannabis over time: systematic review and meta-analysis. *Addiction.* 2021;116(5):1000-1010.
46. Petrilli K, Ofori S, Hines L, Taylor G, Adams S, Freeman TP. Association of cannabis potency with mental ill health and addiction: a systematic review. *Lancet Psychiatry.* 2022;9(9):736-750.
47. Matheson J, Le Foll B. Cannabis legalization and acute harm from high potency cannabis products: a narrative review and recommendations for public health. *Front Psych.* 2020;11:591979.
48. Spindle TR, Bonn-Miller MO, Vandrey R. Changing landscape of cannabis: novel products, formulations, and methods of administration. *Curr Opin Psychol.* 2019;30:98-102.
49. Barrus DG, Capogrossi KL, Cates SC, et al. Tasty THC: promises and challenges of cannabis edibles. *Methods Rep RTI Press.* 2016:2016.
50. ElSohly MA, Gul W, Walker LA. Pharmacokinetics and tolerability of Δ9-THC-hemisuccinate in a suppository formulation as an alternative to capsules for the systemic delivery of Δ9-THC. *Med Cannabis Cannabinoids.* 2018;1(1):44-53.
51. Grotenhermen F. Pharmacokinetics and pharmacodynamics of cannabinoids. *Clin Pharmacokinet.* 2003;42(4):327-360.
52. Huestis MA. Human cannabinoid pharmacokinetics. *Chem Biodivers.* 2007;4(8):1770-1804.
53. Ashton CH. Pharmacology and effects of cannabis: a brief review. *Br J Psychiatry.* 2001;178:101-106.
54. Foster BC, Abramovici H, Harris CS. Cannabis and cannabinoids: kinetics and interactions. *Am J Med.* 2019;132(11):1266-1270.
55. Spindle TR, Cone EJ, Schlienz NJ, et al. Acute pharmacokinetic profile of smoked and vaporized cannabis in human blood and oral fluid. *J Anal Toxicol.* 2019;43(4):233-258.
56. Britch SC, Babalonis S, Walsh SL. Cannabidiol: pharmacology and therapeutic targets. *Psychopharmacology (Berl).* 2021;238(1):9-28.
57. Dinis-Oliveira RJ. Metabolomics of delta(9)-tetrahydrocannabinol: implications in toxicity. *Drug Metab Rev.* 2016;48(1):80-87.
58. Mura P, Kintz P, Dumestre V, Raul S, Hauet T. THC can be detected in brain while absent in blood. *J Anal Toxicol.* 2005;29(8):842-843.
59. Hartman RL, Huestis MA. Cannabis effects on driving skills. *Clin Chem.* 2013;59(3):478-492.
60. Lucas CJ, Galettis P, Schneider J. The pharmacokinetics and the pharmacodynamics of cannabinoids. *Br J Clin Pharmacol.* 2018;84(11):2477-2482.

61. Ellis GM Jr, Mann MA, Judson BA, Schramm NT, Tashchian A. Excretion patterns of cannabinoid metabolites after last use in a group of chronic users. *Clin Pharmacol Ther*. 1985;38(5):572-578.
62. Elphick MR, Egertova M. The phylogenetic distribution and evolutionary origins of endocannabinoid signalling. *Handb Exp Pharmacol*. 2005;168:283-297.
63. Ronan PJ, Wongngamnit N, Beresford TP. Molecular mechanisms of cannabis signaling in the brain. *Prog Mol Biol Transl Sci*. 2016;137:123-147.
64. Howlett AC, Barth F, Bonner TI, et al. International union of pharmacology. XXVII. Classification of cannabinoid receptors. *Pharmacol Rev*. 2002;54(2):161-202.
65. Lu HC, Mackie K. An introduction to the endogenous cannabinoid system. *Biol Psychiatry*. 2016;79(7):516-525.
66. Ligresti A, De Petrocellis L, Di Marzo V. From phytocannabinoids to cannabinoid receptors and endocannabinoids: pleiotropic physiological and pathological roles through complex pharmacology. *Physiol Rev*. 2016;96(4):1593-1659.
67. Rinaldi-Carmona M, Calandra B, Shire D, et al. Characterization of two cloned human CB1 cannabinoid receptor isoforms. *J Pharmacol Exp Ther*. 1996;278(2):871-878.
68. Ryberg E, Vu HK, Larsson N, et al. Identification and characterisation of a novel splice variant of the human CB1 receptor. *FEBS Lett*. 2005;579(1):259-264.
69. Zou S, Kumar U. Cannabinoid receptors and the endocannabinoid system: signaling and function in the central nervous system. *Int J Mol Sci*. 2018;19(3).
70. Morales P, Reggio PH. An update on non-CB1, non-CB2 cannabinoid related G-protein-coupled receptors. *Cannabis Cannabinoid Res*. 2017;2(1):265-273.
71. Herkenham M, Lynn AB, Little MD, et al. Cannabinoid receptor localization in brain. *Proc Natl Acad Sci U S A*. 1990;87(5):1932-1936.
72. Hu SS-J, Mackie K. Distribution of the endocannabinoid system in the central nervous system. In: Pertwee RG, ed. *Endocannabinoids*. Springer International Publishing; 2015:59-93.
73. Howlett AC, Blume LC, Dalton GD. CB(1) cannabinoid receptors and their associated proteins. *Curr Med Chem*. 2010;17(14):1382-1393.
74. Atwood BK, Mackie K. CB2: a cannabinoid receptor with an identity crisis. *Br J Pharmacol*. 2010;160(3):467-479.
75. Di Marzo V, Fontana A, Cadas H, et al. Formation and inactivation of endogenous cannabinoid anandamide in central neurons. *Nature*. 1994;372(6507):686-691.
76. Cadas H, di Tomaso E, Piomelli D. Occurrence and biosynthesis of endogenous cannabinoid precursor, N-arachidonoyl phosphatidylethanolamine, in rat brain. *J Neurosci*. 1997;17(4):1226-1242.
77. Giuffrida A, Parsons LH, Kerr TM, Rodríguez de Fonseca F, Navarro M, Piomelli D. Dopamine activation of endogenous cannabinoid signaling in dorsal striatum. *Nat Neurosci*. 1999;2(4):358-363.
78. Wei D, Lee D, Cox CD, et al. Endocannabinoid signaling mediates oxytocin-driven social reward. *Proc Natl Acad Sci U S A*. 2015;112(45): 14084-14089.
79. Ogura Y, Parsons WH, Kamat SS, Cravatt BF. A calcium-dependent acyltransferase that produces N-acyl phosphatidylethanolamines. *Nat Chem Biol*. 2016;12(9):669-671.
80. Okamoto Y, Morishita J, Tsuboi K, Tonai T, Ueda N. Molecular characterization of a phospholipase D generating anandamide and its congeners. *J Biol Chem*. 2004;279(7):5298-5305.
81. Tsuboi K, Ikematsu N, Uyama T, Deutsch DG, Tokumura A, Ueda N. Biosynthetic pathways of bioactive N-acylethanolamines in brain. *CNS Neurol Disord Drug Targets*. 2013;12(1):7-16.
82. Serrano A, Pavon FJ, Buczynski MW, et al. Deficient endocannabinoid signaling in the central amygdala contributes to alcohol dependence-related anxiety-like behavior and excessive alcohol intake. *Neuropsychopharmacology*. 2018;43(9):1840-1850.
83. Stella N, Schweitzer P, Piomelli D. A second endogenous cannabinoid that modulates long-term potentiation. *Nature*. 1997;388(6644):773-778.
84. Bisogno T, Howell F, Williams G, et al. Cloning of the first sn1-DAG lipases points to the spatial and temporal regulation of endocannabinoid signaling in the brain. *J Cell Biol*. 2003;163(3):463-468.
85. Jung KM, Sepers M, Henstridge CM, et al. Uncoupling of the endocannabinoid signalling complex in a mouse model of fragile X syndrome. *Nat Commun*. 2012;3:1080.
86. Howlett AC, Qualy JM, Khachatrian LL. Involvement of Gi in the inhibition of adenylate cyclase by cannabimimetic drugs. *Mol Pharmacol*. 1986;29(3):307-313.
87. Burnett GM, Gorelick DA, Hill KP. Policy ahead of the science: medical cannabis laws versus scientific evidence. *Psychiatr Clin North Am*. 2022;45(3):347-373.
88. Inglet S, Winter B, Yost SE, et al. Clinical data for the use of cannabis-based treatments: a comprehensive review of the literature. *Ann Pharmacother*. 2020;54(11):1109-1143.
89. Lim K, See YM, Lee J. A systematic review of the effectiveness of medical cannabis for psychiatric, movement and neurodegenerative disorders. *Clin Psychopharmacol Neurosci*. 2017;15(4):301-312.
90. McKee KA, Hmidan A, Crocker CE, et al. Potential therapeutic benefits of cannabinoid products in adult psychiatric disorders: a systematic review and meta-analysis of randomised controlled trials. *J Psychiatr Res*. 2021;140:267-281.
91. Montero-Oleas N, Arevalo-Rodriguez I, Nuñez-González S, Viteri-García A, Simancas-Racines D. Therapeutic use of cannabis and cannabinoids: an evidence mapping and appraisal of systematic reviews. *BMC Complement Med Ther*. 2020;20(1):12.
92. National Academies of Sciences Engineering, Medicine, Health, et al. The national academies collection: reports funded by national institutes of health. In: *The Health Effects of Cannabis and Cannabinoids: The Current State of Evidence and Recommendations for Research*. National Academies Press (US); 2017.
93. Panlilio LV, Justinova Z, Trigo JM, Le Foll B. Screening medications for the treatment of cannabis use disorder. *Int Rev Neurobiol*. 2016;126:87-120.
94. Järbe TU, Henriksson BG. Discriminative response control produced with hashish, tetrahydrocannabinols (delta 8-THC and delta 9-THC), and other drugs. *Psychopharmacologia*. 1974;40(1):1-16.
95. Kubena RK, Barry H III. Stimulus characteristics of marihuana components. *Nature*. 1972;235(5338):397-398.
96. Kubilius RA, Kaplick PM, Wotjak CT. Highway to hell or magic smoke? The dose-dependence of Δ(9)-THC in place conditioning paradigms. *Learn Mem*. 2018;25(9):446-454.
97. Fadda P, Scherma M, Spano MS, et al. Cannabinoid self-administration increases dopamine release in the nucleus accumbens. *Neuroreport*. 2006;17(15):1629-1632.
98. Lecca D, Cacciapaglia F, Valentini V, Di Chiara G. Monitoring extracellular dopamine in the rat nucleus accumbens shell and core during acquisition and maintenance of intravenous WIN 55,212-2 self-administration. *Psychopharmacology (Berl)*. 2006;188(1):63-74.
99. Lefever TW, Marusich JA, Antonazzo KR, Wiley JL. Evaluation of WIN 55,212-2 self-administration in rats as a potential cannabinoid abuse liability model. *Pharmacol Biochem Behav*. 2014;118:30-35.
100. Tanda G, Munzar P, Goldberg SR. Self-administration behavior is maintained by the psychoactive ingredient of marijuana in squirrel monkeys. *Nat Neurosci*. 2000;3(11):1073-1074.
101. Justinova Z, Tanda G, Redhi GH, Goldberg SR. Self-administration of delta9-tetrahydrocannabinol (THC) by drug naive squirrel monkeys. *Psychopharmacology (Berl)*. 2003;169(2):135-140.
102. Schindler CW, Redhi GH, Vemuri K, et al. Blockade of nicotine and cannabinoid reinforcement and relapse by a cannabinoid CB1-receptor neutral antagonist AM4113 and inverse agonist rimonabant in squirrel monkeys. *Neuropsychopharmacology*. 2016;41(9):2283-2293.
103. Freels TG, Baxter-Potter LN, Lugo JM, et al. Vaporized cannabis extracts have reinforcing properties and support conditioned drug-seeking behavior in rats. *J Neurosci*. 2020;40(9):1897-1908.
104. Leung J, Chan GCK, Hides L, Hall WD. What is the prevalence and risk of cannabis use disorders among people who use cannabis? A systematic review and meta-analysis. *Addict Behav*. 2020;109:106479.
105. Cougle JR, Hakes JK, Macatee RJ, Zvolensky MJ, Chavarria J. Probability and correlates of dependence among regular users of alcohol, nicotine, cannabis, and cocaine: concurrent and prospective analyses of the

national epidemiologic survey on alcohol and related conditions. *J Clin Psychiatry*. 2016;77(4):e444-e450.
106. Richter L, Pugh BS, Ball SA. Assessing the risk of marijuana use disorder among adolescents and adults who use marijuana. *Am J Drug Alcohol Abuse*. 2017;43(3):247-260.
107. Compton WM, Han B, Jones CM, Blanco C. Cannabis use disorders among adults in the United States during a time of increasing use of cannabis. *Drug Alcohol Depend*. 2019;204:107468.
108. Han B, Compton WM, Blanco C, Jones CM. Time since first cannabis use and 12-month prevalence of cannabis use disorder among youth and emerging adults in the United States. *Addiction*. 2019;114(4):698-707.
109. Volkow ND, Han B, Einstein EB, Compton WM. Prevalence of substance use disorders by time since first substance use among young people in the US. *JAMA Pediatr*. 2021;175(6):640-643.
110. Kendler KS, Jacobson KC, Prescott CA, Neale MC. Specificity of genetic and environmental risk factors for use and abuse/dependence of cannabis, cocaine, hallucinogens, sedatives, stimulants, and opiates in male twins. *Am J Psychiatry*. 2003;160(4):687-695.
111. Minică CC, Dolan CV, Hottenga JJ, et al. Heritability, SNP- and gene-based analyses of cannabis use initiation and age at onset. *Behav Genet*. 2015;45(5):503-513.
112. Minică CC, Verweij KJH, van der Most PJ, et al. Genome-wide association meta-analysis of age at first cannabis use. *Addiction*. 2018;113(11):2073-2086.
113. Hines LA, Morley KI, Rijsdijk F, et al. Overlap of heritable influences between cannabis use disorder, frequency of use and opportunity to use cannabis: trivariate twin modelling and implications for genetic design. *Psychol Med*. 2018;48(16):2786-2793.
114. Kendler KS, Ohlsson H, Maes HH, Sundquist K, Lichtenstein P, Sundquist J. A population-based Swedish Twin and Sibling Study of cannabis, stimulant and sedative abuse in men. *Drug Alcohol Depend*. 2015;149:49-54.
115. Prom-Wormley EC, Ebejer J, Dick DM, Bowers MS. The genetic epidemiology of substance use disorder: a review. *Drug Alcohol Depend*. 2017;180:241-259.
116. Lopez-Leon S, González-Giraldo Y, Wegman-Ostrosky T, Forero DA. Molecular genetics of substance use disorders: an umbrella review. *Neurosci Biobehav Rev*. 2021;124:358-369.
117. Vink JM, Veul L, Abdellaoui A, Hottenga JJ, Boomsma DI, Verweij KJH. Illicit drug use and the genetic overlap with Cannabis use. *Drug Alcohol Depend*. 2020;213:108102.
118. Agrawal A, Madden PA, Bucholz KK, Heath AC, Lynskey MT. Initial reactions to tobacco and cannabis smoking: a twin study. *Addiction*. 2014;109(4):663-671.
119. Hindocha C, Freeman TP, Schafer G, et al. Acute effects of cannabinoids on addiction endophenotypes are moderated by genes encoding the CB1 receptor and FAAH enzyme. *Addict Biol*. 2020;25(3):e12762.
120. Bourgault Z, Matheson J, Mann RE, et al. Mu opioid receptor gene variant modulates subjective response to smoked cannabis. *Am J Transl Res*. 2022;14(1):623-632.
121. Murphy T, Matheson J, Mann RE, et al. Influence of cannabinoid receptor 1 genetic variants on the subjective effects of smoked cannabis. *Int J Mol Sci*. 2021;22(14).
122. Dugas EN, Sylvestre MP, Ewusi-Boisvert E, Chaiton M, Montreuil A, O'Loughlin J. Early risk factors for daily cannabis use in young adults. *Can J Psychiatry*. 2019;64(5):329-337.
123. Blanco C, Rafful C, Wall MM, Ridenour TA, Wang S, Kendler KS. Towards a comprehensive developmental model of cannabis use disorders. *Addiction*. 2014;109(2):284-294.
124. Courtney KE, Mejia MH, Jacobus J. Longitudinal studies on the etiology of cannabis use disorder: a review. *Curr Addict Rep*. 2017;4(2):43-52.
125. Crane NA, Langenecker SA, Mermelstein RJ. Risk factors for alcohol, marijuana, and cigarette polysubstance use during adolescence and young adulthood: a 7-year longitudinal study of youth at high risk for smoking escalation. *Addict Behav*. 2021;119:106944.
126. Solmi M, Dragioti E, Croatto G, et al. Risk and protective factors for cannabis, cocaine, and opioid use disorders: an umbrella review of meta-analyses of observational studies. *Neurosci Biobehav Rev*. 2021;126:243-251.
127. Myers B, McLaughlin KA, Wang S, Blanco C, Stein DJ. Associations between childhood adversity, adult stressful life events, and past-year drug use disorders in the National Epidemiological Study of Alcohol and Related Conditions (NESARC). *Psychol Addict Behav*. 2014;28(4):1117-1126.
128. Bevilacqua L, Hale D, Barker ED, Viner R. Conduct problems trajectories and psychosocial outcomes: a systematic review and meta-analysis. *Eur Child Adolesc Psychiatry*. 2018;27(10):1239-1260.
129. van der Pol P, Liebregts N, de Graaf R, Korf DJ, van den Brink W, van Laar M. Predicting the transition from frequent cannabis use to cannabis dependence: a three-year prospective study. *Drug Alcohol Depend*. 2013;133(2):352-359.
130. Madras BK, Han B, Compton WM, Jones CM, Lopez EI, McCance-Katz EF. Associations of parental marijuana use with offspring marijuana, tobacco, and alcohol use and opioid misuse. *JAMA Netw Open*. 2019;2(11):e1916015.
131. O'Loughlin JL, Dugas EN, O'Loughlin EK, et al. Parental cannabis use is associated with cannabis initiation and use in offspring. *J Pediatr*. 2019;206:142-147.e141
132. Livne O, Wengrower T, Feingold D, Shmulewitz D, Hasin DS, Lev-Ran S. Religiosity and substance use in U.S. adults: findings from a large-scale national survey. *Drug Alcohol Depend*. 2021;225:108796.
133. Lobato Concha ME, Sanderman R, Pizarro E, Hagedoorn M. Parental protective and risk factors regarding cannabis use in adolescence: a national sample from the Chilean school population. *Am J Drug Alcohol Abuse*. 2020;46(5):642-650.
134. Noble MJ, Hedberg K, Hendrickson RG. Acute cannabis toxicity. *Clin Toxicol*. 2019;57(8):735-742.
135. Wong KU, Baum CR. Acute cannabis toxicity. *Pediatr Emerg Care*. 2019;35(11):799-804.
136. Ramaekers JG, Mason NL, Kloft L, Theunissen EL. The why behind the high: determinants of neurocognition during acute cannabis exposure. *Nat Rev Neurosci*. 2021;22(7):439-454.
137. Hindley G, Beck K, Borgan F, et al. Psychiatric symptoms caused by cannabis constituents: a systematic review and meta-analysis. *Lancet Psychiatry*. 2020;7(4):344-353.
138. Chartier C, Penouil F, Blanc-Brisset I, Pion C, Descatha A, Deguigne M. Pediatric cannabis poisonings in France: more and more frequent and severe. *Clin Toxicol*. 2021;59(4):326-333.
139. Bonnet U, Preuss UW. The cannabis withdrawal syndrome: current insights. *Subst Abuse Rehabil*. 2017;8:9-37.
140. Connor JP, Stjepanović D, Budney AJ, Le Foll B, Hall WD. Clinical management of cannabis withdrawal. *Addiction*. 2022;117(7):2075-2095.
141. Bahji A, Gorelick DA. Factors associated with past-year and lifetime prevalence of cannabis withdrawal: an updated systematic review and meta-analysis. *Can J Addict*. 2022;13(3):14-25.
142. Livne O, Shmulewitz D, Lev-Ran S, Hasin DS. DSM-5 cannabis withdrawal syndrome: demographic and clinical correlates in U.S. adults. *Drug Alcohol Depend*. 2019;195:170-177.
143. González S, Cebeira M, Fernández-Ruiz J. Cannabinoid tolerance and dependence: a review of studies in laboratory animals. *Pharmacol Biochem Behav*. 2005;81(2):300-318.
144. Ramaekers JG, Mason NL, Theunissen EL. Blunted highs: pharmacodynamic and behavioral models of cannabis tolerance. *Eur Neuropsychopharmacol*. 2020;36:191-205.
145. Colizzi M, Bhattacharyya S. Cannabis use and the development of tolerance: a systematic review of human evidence. *Neurosci Biobehav Rev*. 2018;93:1-25.
146. Crocker CE, Carter AJE, Emsley JG, Magee K, Atkinson P, Tibbo PG. When cannabis use goes wrong: mental health side effects of cannabis use that present to emergency services. *Front Psych*. 2021;12: 640222.
147. Sherif M, Radhakrishnan R, D'Souza DC, Ranganathan M. Human laboratory studies on cannabinoids and psychosis. *Biol Psychiatry*. 2016;79(7):526-538.

148. McCartney D, Arkell TR, Irwin C, McGregor IS. Determining the magnitude and duration of acute Δ(9)-tetrahydrocannabinol (Δ(9)-THC)-induced driving and cognitive impairment: a systematic and meta-analytic review. *Neurosci Biobehav Rev*. 2021;126:175-193.
149. Dellazizzo L, Potvin S, Giguère S, Dumais A. Evidence on the acute and residual neurocognitive effects of cannabis use in adolescents and adults: a systematic meta-review of meta-analyses. *Addiction*. 2022;117(7):1857-1870.
150. Curran HV, Freeman TP, Mokrysz C, Lewis DA, Morgan CJ, Parsons LH. Keep off the grass? Cannabis, cognition and addiction. *Nat Rev Neurosci*. 2016;17(5):293-306.
151. Hall W, Lynskey M. Assessing the public health impacts of legalizing recreational cannabis use: the US experience. *World Psychiatry*. 2020;19(2):179-186.
152. Figueiredo PR, Tolomeo S, Steele JD, Baldacchino A. Neurocognitive consequences of chronic cannabis use: a systematic review and meta-analysis. *Neurosci Biobehav Rev*. 2020;108:358-369.
153. Krzyzanowski DJ, Purdon SE. Duration of abstinence from cannabis is positively associated with verbal learning performance: a systematic review and meta-analysis. *Neuropsychology*. 2020;34(3):359-372.
154. Lovell ME, Akhurst J, Padgett C, Garry MI, Matthews A. Cognitive outcomes associated with long-term, regular, recreational cannabis use in adults: a meta-analysis. *Exp Clin Psychopharmacol*. 2020;28(4):471-494.
155. Scott JC, Slomiak ST, Jones JD, Rosen AFG, Moore TM, Gur RC. Association of cannabis with cognitive functioning in adolescents and young adults: a systematic review and meta-analysis. *JAMA Psychiatry*. 2018;75(6):585-595.
156. Broyd SJ, van Hell HH, Beale C, Yucel M, Solowij N. Acute and chronic effects of cannabinoids on human cognition—a systematic review. *Biol Psychiatry* 2016;79(7):557-567.
157. Murray RM, Di Forti M. Cannabis and psychosis: what degree of proof do we require? *Biol Psychiatry*. 2016;79(7):514-515.
158. Murray RM, Englund A, Abi-Dargham A, et al. Cannabis-associated psychosis: neural substrate and clinical impact. *Neuropharmacology*. 2017;124:89-104.
159. Gage SH, Hickman M, Zammit S. Association between cannabis and psychosis: epidemiologic evidence. *Biol Psychiatry*. 2016;79(7):549-556.
160. van Winkel R, Kuepper R. Epidemiological, neurobiological, and genetic clues to the mechanisms linking cannabis use to risk for nonaffective psychosis. *Annu Rev Clin Psychol*. 2014;10:767-791.
161. Di Forti M, Quattrone D, Freeman TP, et al. The contribution of cannabis use to variation in the incidence of psychotic disorder across Europe (EU-GEI): a multicentre case-control study. *Lancet Psychiatry*. 2019;6(5):427-436.
162. Hjorthøj C, Posselt CM, Nordentoft M. Development over time of the population-attributable risk fraction for cannabis use disorder in schizophrenia in Denmark. *JAMA Psychiatry*. 2021;78(9):1013-1019.
163. Johnson EC, Hatoum AS, Deak JD, et al. The relationship between cannabis and schizophrenia: a genetically informed perspective. *Addiction*. 2021;116(11):3227-3234.
164. Murrie B, Lappin J, Large M, Sara G. Transition of substance-induced, brief, and atypical psychoses to schizophrenia: a systematic review and meta-analysis. *Schizophr Bull*. 2020;46(3):505-516.
165. Starzer MSK, Nordentoft M, Hjorthøj C. Rates and predictors of conversion to schizophrenia or bipolar disorder following substance-induced psychosis. *Am J Psychiatry*. 2018;175(4):343-350.
166. Schaefer JD, Jang SK, Vrieze S, Iacono WG, McGue M, Wilson S. Adolescent cannabis use and adult psychoticism: a longitudinal co-twin control analysis using data from two cohorts. *J Abnorm Psychol*. 2021;130(7):691-701.
167. Schoeler T, Monk A, Sami MB, et al. Continued versus discontinued cannabis use in patients with psychosis: a systematic review and meta-analysis. *Lancet Psychiatry*. 2016;3(3):215-225.
168. Sami M, Quattrone D, Ferraro L, et al. Association of extent of cannabis use and psychotic like intoxication experiences in a multi-national sample of first episode psychosis patients and controls. *Psychol Med*. 2021;51(12):2074-2082.
169. Schoeler T, Petros N, Di Forti M, et al. Association between continued cannabis use and risk of relapse in first-episode psychosis: a quasi-experimental investigation within an observational study. *JAMA Psychiatry*. 2016;73(11):1173-1179.
170. Lev-Ran S, Roerecke M, Le Foll B, George TP, McKenzie K, Rehm J. The association between cannabis use and depression: a systematic review and meta-analysis of longitudinal studies. *Psychol Med*. 2014;44(4):797-810.
171. Tourjman SV, Buck G, Jutras-Aswad D, et al. Canadian network for mood and anxiety treatments (CANMAT) task force report: a systematic review and recommendations of cannabis use in bipolar disorder and major depressive disorder. *Can J Psychiatry*. 2023;68(5):299-311.
172. Sorkhou M, Bedder RH, George TP. The behavioral sequelae of cannabis use in healthy people: a systematic review. *Front Psych*. 2021;12:630247.
173. Xue S, Husain MI, Zhao H, Ravindran AV. Cannabis use and prospective long-term association with anxiety: a systematic review and meta-analysis of longitudinal studies: Usage du cannabis et association prospective à long terme avec l'anxiété: une revue systématique et une méta-analyse d'études longitudinales. *Can J Psychiatry*. 2021;66(2):126-138.
174. Hasin DS. US epidemiology of cannabis use and associated problems. *Neuropsychopharmacology*. 2018;43(1):195-212.
175. Wycoff AM, Metrik J, Trull TJ. Affect and cannabis use in daily life: a review and recommendations for future research. *Drug Alcohol Depend*. 2018;191:223-233.
176. Nader DA, Sanchez ZM. Effects of regular cannabis use on neurocognition, brain structure, and function: a systematic review of findings in adults. *Am J Drug Alcohol Abuse*. 2018;44(1):4-18.
177. Rossetti MG, Mackey S, Patalay P, et al. Sex and dependence related neuroanatomical differences in regular cannabis users: findings from the ENIGMA Addiction Working Group. *Transl Psychiatry*. 2021;11(1):272.
178. Albaugh MD, Ottino-Gonzalez J, Sidwell A, et al. Association of cannabis use during adolescence with neurodevelopment. *JAMA Psychiatry*. 2021;78(9):1-11.
179. Calabria B, Degenhardt L, Hall W, Lynskey M. Does cannabis use increase the risk of death? Systematic review of epidemiological evidence on adverse effects of cannabis use. *Drug Alcohol Rev*. 2010;29(3):318-330.
180. Kendler KS, Ohlsson H, Sundquist K, Sundquist J. Drug abuse-associated mortality across the lifespan: a population-based longitudinal cohort and co-relative analysis. *Soc Psychiatry Psychiatr Epidemiol*. 2017;52(7):877-886.
181. Arkell TR, McCartney D, McGregor IS. Medical cannabis and driving. *Aust J Gen Pract*. 2021;50(6):357-362.
182. Drummer OH, Gerostamoulos D, Woodford NW. Cannabis as a cause of death: a review. *Forensic Sci Int*. 2019;298:298-306.
183. Zahra E, Darke S, Degenhardt L, Campbell G. Rates, characteristics and manner of cannabis-related deaths in Australia 2000-2018. *Drug Alcohol Depend*. 2020;212:108028.
184. Weye N, Santomauro DF, Agerbo E, et al. Register-based metrics of years lived with disability associated with mental and substance use disorders: a register-based cohort study in Denmark. *Lancet Psychiatry*. 2021;8(4):310-319.
185. Substance Abuse and Mental Health Services Administration. *Preliminary Findings From Drug-Related Emergency Department Visits, 2021*. Accessed June 1, 2022. https://www.samhsa.gov/data/
186. Thomas G, Kloner RA, Rezkalla S. Adverse cardiovascular, cerebrovascular, and peripheral vascular effects of marijuana inhalation: what cardiologists need to know. *Am J Cardiol*. 2014;113(1):187-190.
187. Pacher P, Steffens S, Haskó G, Schindler TH, Kunos G. Cardiovascular effects of marijuana and synthetic cannabinoids: the good, the bad, and the ugly. *Nat Rev Cardiol*. 2018;15(3):151-166.
188. Ravi D, Ghasemiesfe M, Korenstein D, Cascino T, Keyhani S. Associations between marijuana use and cardiovascular risk factors and outcomes: a systematic review. *Ann Intern Med*. 2018;168(3):187-194.
189. Yang PK, Odom EC, Patel R, Loustalot F, Coleman KS. Nonmedical marijuana use and cardiovascular events: a systematic review. *Public Health Rep*. 2022;137(1):62-71.

190. Latif Z, Garg N. The impact of marijuana on the cardiovascular system: a review of the most common cardiovascular events associated with marijuana use. *J Clin Med*. 2020;9(6).
191. Shah S, Patel S, Paulraj S, Chaudhuri D. Association of marijuana use and cardiovascular disease: a behavioral risk factor surveillance system data analysis of 133,706 US adults. *Am J Med*. 2021;134(5):614-620.e611.
192. Mittleman MA, Lewis RA, Maclure M, Sherwood JB, Muller JE. Triggering myocardial infarction by marijuana. *Circulation*. 2001;103(23):2805-2809.
193. Desai R, Singh S, Patel K, et al. Stroke in young cannabis users (18-49 years): national trends in hospitalizations and outcomes. *Int J Stroke*. 2020;15(5):535-539.
194. Ramphul K, Joynauth J. Cardiac arrhythmias among teenagers using cannabis in the United States. *Am J Cardiol*. 2019;124(12):1966.
195. Richards JR, Blohm E, Toles KA, Jarman AF, Ely DF, Elder JW. The association of cannabis use and cardiac dysrhythmias: a systematic review. *Clin Toxicol*. 2020;58(9):861-869.
196. Patel RS, Gonzalez MD, Ajibawo T, Baweja R. Cannabis use disorder and increased risk of arrhythmia-related hospitalization in young adults. *Am J Addict*. 2021;30(6):578-584.
197. Ghasemiesfe M, Ravi D, Vali M, et al. Marijuana use, respiratory symptoms, and pulmonary function: a systematic review and meta-analysis. *Ann Intern Med*. 2018;169(2):106-115.
198. Baumeister SE, Baurecht H, Nolde M, et al. Cannabis use, pulmonary function, and lung cancer susceptibility: a mendelian randomization study. *J Thorac Oncol*. 2021;16(7):1127-1135.
199. Tashkin DP, Roth MD. Pulmonary effects of inhaled cannabis smoke. *Am J Drug Alcohol Abuse*. 2019;45(6):596-609.
200. Gracie K, Hancox RJ. Cannabis use disorder and the lungs. *Addiction*. 2021;116(1):182-190.
201. Ghasemiesfe M, Barrow B, Leonard S, Keyhani S, Korenstein D. Association between marijuana use and risk of cancer: a systematic review and meta-analysis. *JAMA Netw Open*. 2019;2(11):e1916318.
202. Meier E, Tessier KM, Luo X, et al. Cigarette smokers versus cannabis smokers versus co-users of cigarettes and cannabis: a pilot study examining exposure to toxicants. *Nicotine Tob Res*. 2022;24(1):125-129.
203. Meier E, Vandrey R, Rubin N, et al. Cigarette smokers versus cousers of cannabis and cigarettes: exposure to toxicants. *Nicotine Tob Res*. 2020;22(8):1383-1389.
204. Zhang LR, Morgenstern H, Greenland S, et al. Cannabis smoking and lung cancer risk: pooled analysis in the international lung cancer consortium. *Int J Cancer*. 2015;136(4):894-903.
205. Gajendran M, Sifuentes J, Bashashati M, McCallum R. Cannabinoid hyperemesis syndrome: definition, pathophysiology, clinical spectrum, insights into acute and long-term management. *J Invest Med*. 2020;68(8):1309.
206. DeVuono MV, Parker LA. Cannabinoid hyperemesis syndrome: a review of potential mechanisms. *Cannabis Cannabinoid Res*. 2020;5(2):132-144.
207. Sun AJ, Eisenberg ML. Association between marijuana use and sexual frequency in the united states: a population-based study. *J Sex Med*. 2017;14(11):1342-1347.
208. Lynn B, Gee A, Zhang L, Pfaus JG. Effects of cannabinoids on female sexual function. *Sex Med Rev*. 2020;8(1):18-27.
209. Shiff B, Blankstein U, Hussaen J, et al. The impact of cannabis use on male sexual function: a 10-year, single-center experience. *Can Urol Assoc J*. 2021;15(12):E652-e657.
210. Kasman AM, Thoma ME, McLain AC, Eisenberg ML. Association between use of marijuana and time to pregnancy in men and women: findings from the National Survey of Family Growth. *Fertil Steril*. 2018;109(5):866-871.
211. Pizzol D, Demurtas J, Stubbs B, et al. Relationship between cannabis use and erectile dysfunction: a systematic review and meta-analysis. *Am J Mens Health*. 2019;13(6):1557988319892464.
212. Rajanahally S, Raheem O, Rogers M, et al. The relationship between cannabis and male infertility, sexual health, and neoplasm: a systematic review. *Andrology*. 2019;7(2):139-147.
213. Gundersen TD, Jørgensen N, Andersson AM, et al. Association between use of marijuana and male reproductive hormones and semen quality: a study among 1,215 healthy young men. *Am J Epidemiol*. 2015;182(6):473-481.
214. Nassan FL, Arvizu M, Mínguez-Alarcón L, et al. Marijuana smoking and markers of testicular function among men from a fertility centre. *Hum Reprod*. 2019;34(4):715-723.
215. Wymore EM, Palmer C, Wang GS, et al. Persistence of Δ-9-tetrahydrocannabinol in human breast milk. *JAMA Pediatr*. 2021;175(6):632-634.
216. Moss MJ, Bushlin I, Kazmierczak S, et al. Cannabis use and measurement of cannabinoids in plasma and breast milk of breastfeeding mothers. *Pediatr Res*. 2021;90(4):861-868.
217. Goyal H, Rahman MR, Perisetti A, Shah N, Chhabra R. Cannabis in liver disorders: a friend or a foe? *Eur J Gastroenterol Hepatol*. 2018;30(11):1283-1290.
218. Rein JL. The nephrologist's guide to cannabis and cannabinoids. *Curr Opin Nephrol Hypertens*. 2020;29(2):248-257.
219. Wang T, Collet JP, Shapiro S, Ware MA. Adverse effects of medical cannabinoids: a systematic review. *CMAJ*. 2008;178(13):1669-1678.
220. Vupputuri S, Batuman V, Muntner P, et al. The risk for mild kidney function decline associated with illicit drug use among hypertensive men. *Am J Kidney Dis*. 2004;43(4):629-635.
221. Wijarnpreecha K, Panjawatanan P, Ungprasert P. Use of cannabis and risk of advanced liver fibrosis in patients with chronic hepatitis C virus infection: a systematic review and meta-analysis. *J Evid Based Med*. 2018;11(4):272-277.
222. Rashid W, Patel V, Ravat V, et al. Problematic cannabis use and risk of complications in patients with chronic hepatitis C. *Cureus*. 2019;11(8):e5373.
223. Alayash Z, Nolde M, Meisinger C, Baurecht H, Baumeister SE. Cannabis use and obesity-traits: a Mendelian randomization study. *Drug Alcohol Depend*. 2021;226:108863.
224. Sidney S. Marijuana use and type 2 diabetes mellitus: a review. *Curr Diab Rep*. 2016;16(11):117.
225. Danielsson AK, Lundin A, Yaregal A, Östenson CG, Allebeck P, Agardh EE. Cannabis use as risk or protection for type 2 diabetes: a longitudinal study of 18000 Swedish men and women. *J Diabetes Res*. 2016;2016:6278709.
226. Baumeister SE, Nolde M, Alayash Z, Leitzmann M, Baurecht H, Meisinger C. Cannabis use does not impact on type 2 diabetes: a two-sample Mendelian randomization study. *Addict Biol*. 2021;26(6):e13020.
227. Murphy T, Le Foll B. Targeting the endocannabinoid CB1 receptor to treat body weight disorders: a preclinical and clinical review of the therapeutic potential of past and present CB1 drugs. *Biomolecules*. 2020;10(6).
228. Porr CJ, Rios P, Bajaj HS, et al. The effects of recreational cannabis use on glycemic outcomes and self-management behaviours in people with type 1 and type 2 diabetes: a rapid review. *Syst Rev*. 2020;9(1):187.
229. Kinney GL, Akturk HK, Taylor DD, Foster NC, Shah VN. Cannabis use is associated with increased risk for diabetic ketoacidosis in adults with type 1 diabetes: findings from the T1D exchange clinic registry. *Diabetes Care*. 2020;43(1):247-249.
230. Peragallo J, Biousse V, Newman NJ. Ocular manifestations of drug and alcohol abuse. *Curr Opin Ophthalmol*. 2013;24(6):566-573.
231. Thayer A, Murataeva N, Delcroix V, Wager-Miller J, Makarenkova HP, Straiker A. THC regulates tearing via cannabinoid CB1 receptors. *Invest Ophthalmol Vis Sci*. 2020;61(10):48.
232. Lehrer S, Rheinstein PH. Cannabis smoking and glaucoma in the UK Biobank cohort. *J Fr Ophtalmol*. 2022;45(4):423-429.
233. Keboa MT, Enriquez N, Martel M, Nicolau B, Macdonald ME. Oral health implications of cannabis smoking: a rapid evidence review. *J Can Dent Assoc*. 2020;86:k2.
234. Gunn JK, Rosales CB, Center KE, et al. Prenatal exposure to cannabis and maternal and child health outcomes: a systematic review and meta-analysis. *BMJ Open*. 2016;6(4):e009986.

235. Marchand G, Masoud AT, Govindan M, et al. Birth outcomes of neonates exposed to marijuana in utero: a systematic review and meta-analysis. *JAMA Netw Open*. 2022;5(1):e2145653.
236. Conner SN, Bedell V, Lipsey K, Macones GA, Cahill AG, Tuuli MG. Maternal marijuana use and adverse neonatal outcomes: a systematic review and meta-analysis. *Obstet Gynecol*. 2016;128(4):713-723.
237. Metz TD, Borgelt LM. Marijuana use in pregnancy and while breastfeeding. *Obstet Gynecol*. 2018;132(5):1198-1210.
238. Correa F, Wolfson ML, Valchi P, Aisemberg J, Franchi AM. Endocannabinoid system and pregnancy. *Reproduction*. 2016;152(6):R191-R200.
239. Chang X, Li H, Li Y, et al. RhoA/MLC signaling pathway is involved in Delta(9)-tetrahydrocannabinol-impaired placental angiogenesis. *Toxicol Lett*. 2018;285:148-155.
240. Walker OS, Ragos R, Gurm H, Lapierre M, May LL, Raha S. Delta-9-tetrahydrocannabinol disrupts mitochondrial function and attenuates syncytialization in human placental BeWo cells. *Physiol Rep*. 2020;8(13):e14476.
241. Banerjee S, Deacon A, Suter MA, Aagaard KM. Understanding the placental biology of tobacco smoke, nicotine, and marijuana (THC) exposures during pregnancy. *Clin Obstet Gynecol*. 2022;65(2):347-359.
242. El Marroun H, Tiemeier H, Steegers EA, et al. Intrauterine cannabis exposure affects fetal growth trajectories: the Generation R Study. *J Am Acad Child Adolesc Psychiatry*. 2009;48(12):1173-1181.
243. Fried PA, Watkinson B, Gray R. Differential effects on cognitive functioning in 9- to 12-year olds prenatally exposed to cigarettes and marihuana. *Neurotoxicol Teratol*. 1998;20(3):293-306.
244. Huizink AC. Prenatal cannabis exposure and infant outcomes: overview of studies. *Prog Neuropsychopharmacol Biol Psychiatry*. 2014;52:45-52.
245. El Marroun H, Bolhuis K, Franken IHA, et al. Preconception and prenatal cannabis use and the risk of behavioural and emotional problems in the offspring; a multi-informant prospective longitudinal study. *Int J Epidemiol*. 2019;48(1):287-296.
246. Torres CA, Medina-Kirchner C, O'Malley KY, Hart CL. Totality of the evidence suggests prenatal cannabis exposure does not lead to cognitive impairments: a systematic and critical review. *Front Psychol*. 2020;11:816.
247. Paul SE, Hatoum AS, Fine JD, et al. Associations between prenatal cannabis exposure and childhood outcomes: results from the ABCD study. *JAMA Psychiatry*. 2021;78(1):64-76.
248. Corsi DJ, Donelle J, Sucha E, et al. Maternal cannabis use in pregnancy and child neurodevelopmental outcomes. *Nat Med*. 2020;26(10):1536-1540.
249. DiNieri JA, Wang X, Szutorisz H, et al. Maternal cannabis use alters ventral striatal dopamine D2 gene regulation in the offspring. *Biol Psychiatry*. 2011;70(8):763-769.
250. Wang X, Dow-Edwards D, Anderson V, Minkoff H, Hurd YL. In utero marijuana exposure associated with abnormal amygdala dopamine D2 gene expression in the human fetus. *Biol Psychiatry*. 2004;56(12):909-915.
251. Vanstone M, Taneja S, Popoola A, et al. Reasons for cannabis use during pregnancy and lactation: a qualitative study. *CMAJ*. 2021;193(50):E1906-E1914.
252. Mark K, Gryczynski J, Axenfeld E, Schwartz RP, Terplan M. Pregnant women's current and intended cannabis use in relation to their views toward legalization and knowledge of potential harm. *J Addict Med*. 2017;11(3):211-216.
253. Committee Opinion No. 722. Marijuana use during pregnancy and lactation. *Obstet Gynecol*. 2017;130(4):e205-e209.
254. Connor JP, Stjepanović D, Le Foll B, Hoch E, Budney AJ, Hall WD. Cannabis use and cannabis use disorder. *Nat Rev Dis Primers*. 2021;7(1):16.
255. Nielsen S, Gowing L, Sabioni P, Le Foll B. Pharmacotherapies for cannabis dependence. *Cochrane Database Syst Rev*. 2019;1:CD008940.
256. Kearney-Ramos T, Haney M. Repetitive transcranial magnetic stimulation as a potential treatment approach for cannabis use disorder. *Prog Neuropsychopharmacol Biol Psychiatry*. 2021;109:110290.
257. Sloan ME, Grant CW, Gowin JL, Ramchandani VA, Le Foll B. Endocannabinoid signaling in psychiatric disorders: a review of positron emission tomography studies. *Acta Pharmacol Sin*. 2019;40(3):342-350.
258. Botsford SL, Yang S, George TP. Cannabis and cannabinoids in mood and anxiety disorders: impact on illness onset and course, and assessment of therapeutic potential. *Am J Addict*. 2020;29(1):9-26.
259. Lowe DJE, Sasiadek JD, Coles AS, George TP. Cannabis and mental illness: a review. *Eur Arch Psychiatry Clin Neurosci*. 2019;269(1):107-120.

18 The Pharmacology of Hallucinogens

David B. Yaden, David S. Mathai, Michael P. Bogenschutz, and David E. Nichols

CHAPTER OUTLINE

- Definition
- Substances included
- Features of clinical use, nonmedical use, and addiction
- Historical features
- Epidemiology
- Neurobiology
- Pharmacokinetics and pharmacodynamics
- Drug-drug interactions
- Conclusions and future research

DEFINITION

The hallucinogens constitute several highly diverse classes of compounds. In this chapter, we will use the term to refer to substances whose most prominent subjective effects include dramatic alterations in perception, cognition, affect, sense of meaning, and/or sense of self, lasting (depending on the substance and dose) from several minutes to many hours. *The Diagnostic and Statistical Manual of Mental Disorders*, 5th edition[1] (DSM-5) classifies Phencyclidine (PCP) and related arylcyclohexylamines (such as ketamine which are also termed dissociatives or dissociative anesthetics) as hallucinogen-related substances, but this textbook reviews these substances in a separate chapter within this section. Anticholinergic deliriants, such as atropine, hyoscyamine, and scopolamine can cause true hallucinations, but are not typically considered to be hallucinogens and we do not cover them in in this chapter.

Many researchers consider the term "hallucinogen" a misnomer because most of the commonly used hallucinogens rarely cause true hallucinations. Some believe "hallucinogen" is often used as a somewhat pejorative term to emphasize the potential for harm from this class of substances, rather than their beneficial or therapeutic potential. Many other terms have been proposed. The word "psychotomimetic" has been used to stress the similarity between hallucinogen intoxication and psychotic illness. Despite the possibility of overlap between these states,[2] hallucinogens have many effects that are not typical of psychosis.[3] The term "psychedelic" (loosely meaning "mind manifesting") was coined by psychiatrist Humphrey Osmond to emphasize an aspect of the acute subjective effects, which are often referred to as a kind of "altered state of consciousness," produced by classic serotonergic hallucinogens such as lysergic acid diethylamide (LSD) and psilocybin.[4] The terms "entactogen" and less commonly "empathogen," have been proposed for 3,4-methylenedioxymethamphetamine (MDMA) and related compounds whose effects are dominated by feelings of emotional openness and interpersonal connection. For some users, the term "entheogen" has been used for hallucinogens when spiritual or religious aspects of the experience are of primary importance. Over the past decade, "psychedelic" has become the preferred name for this overall class of substances, although its use appears to be increasingly more specifically applied to the classic serotonergic hallucinogens (eg, psilocybin and LSD).

SUBSTANCES INCLUDED

Basic information about representative hallucinogens is summarized in **Table 18-1**, and chemical structures are shown in **Figure 18-1**. The serotonergic hallucinogens include what are called the classic hallucinogens—which are now generally referred to as psychedelics (as well as classic psychedelics or serotonergic psychedelics)—such as mescaline, psilocybin, LSD, *N,N*-dimethyltryptamine (DMT), and a large number of substituted phenylethylamines, such as 2,5-dimethoxy-4-bromoamphetamine (DOB) and 2,5-dimethoxy-4-bromophenethylamine (2C-B). Psychedelics, or classic hallucinogens, possess an arylethylamine skeleton, either as an indole ethylamine or as a β-phenethylamine. Agents from this class all bind to serotonin 5-HT_2 family receptors and are agonists or partial agonists at the 5-HT_{2A} receptor. Indole ethylamine hallucinogens include LSD, DMT, and psilocybin and many structurally related compounds. Hallucinogenic phenethylamines include mescaline, DOB, 2C-B, and a large number of 2,5-dimethoxyphenethylamines with various substituents at the aryl-4-position, such as small halogen, alkoxy, small unbranched alkyl, and alkylthio moieties. Synthesis and preliminary human psychopharmacology have been catalogued for many of these compounds.[5,6]

Another small group of phenethylamines is similar in structure, but whose pharmacology differs from the classic hallucinogens, have been named entactogens.[7] The prototype of this group is MDMA, and it also includes 3,4-methylenedioxyethylamphetamine (MDE), 3,4-methylenedioxy-*N*-methyl-α-ethylphenylethylamine (MBDB), and the (+)-enantiomer of methylenedioxyamphetamine [(+)-MDA]. The term entactogen is derived from the roots "en" (Greek, within), "tactus"

TABLE 18-1 Representative Hallucinogens

Class	Chemical name	Common or street name	Source	Typical dosage	Route	Duration of action	Major neurobiologic target	Notes
Ergoline (indolealkylamine)	LSD	LSD, acid, blotter	Semisynthetic	50-200 μg	PO	8-14 h	5-HT_{2A} partial agonist	Distributed on small squares of blotter paper, in gel caps, in small tablets, or in liquid solution
Indole ethylamine	Psilocybin	Magic mushrooms, "shrooms"	Numerous species of *Psilocybe* mushrooms	10-30 mg; 1-5 g of dried mushrooms, depending on species	PO	4-6 h	5-HT_{2A} partial agonist	Psilocybin is the phosphate ester of psilocin, which is cleaved in vivo to give psilocin, the active molecule. Long and continuing shamanic use in Mesoamerica. Mushrooms will turn blue when bruised
	N,N-Dimethyltryptamine	DMT, yopo, cohoba, "businessman's trip"	Synthesis; *Psychotria viridis, Mimosa hostilis*, many other plant species	5-75 mg	Smoked, insufflated, snuff	6-20 min	5-HT_{2A} partial agonist	Amazonian shamanic use; as a religious sacrament in teas containing beta-carbolines (ayahuasca)
	5-Methoxy-*N,N*-dimethyltryptamine	5-MeO-DMT	Synthesis; Colorado River toad (*Incilius alvarius*) venom, also known as the Sonoran Desert toad	5-15 mg	Smoked, insufflated, snuff	5-20 min	5-HT_{2A} partial agonist; 5-HT_{1A} agonist	A minor component of yopo snuff
	5-Methoxy-*N,N*-diallyltryptamine	5-MeO-DALT	Synthesis	12-20 mg	PO	2-4 h	Near-full agonist at all 5-HT_2 family receptors	Recent appearance as a "research chemical" often mixed with other psychoactive compounds

Phenethy-lamine	3,4,5-Trimethoxy-phenethylamine	Mescaline, peyote	Synthesis; *Lophophora williamsii*, several species of *Trichocereus* cacti	200-500 mg of the sulfate salt; 10-20 g of dried peyote buttons	PO	8-12 h	Near-full agonist at the 5-HT_{2A} receptors	The prototype of the phenethylamine-type hallucinogens
	2,5-Dimethoxy-4-methylamphetamine	DOM, STP	Synthesis	3-10 mg	PO	14-20 h	Partial agonist at 5-HT_{2A} receptor	First phenethylamine to appear as a street drug in the late 1960s
	2,5-Dimethoxy-4-bromophenethylamine	2C-B, Nexus	Synthesis	12-24 mg	PO	4-8 h	Partial agonist at 5-HT_{2A} receptor	More of a sensory amplifier, with less actual hallucinogenic effect
	N-(2-Methoxybenzyl)-2,5-dimethoxy-4-iodophenethylamine	25I-NBOMe	Synthesis	0.2-0.5 mg	Sublingual	6-10 h	Agonist at 5-HT_{2A} receptor	Extremely potent and often distributed on blotter paper. The 4-bromo and 4-chloro compounds are also very potent. Fatalities have occurred with the NBOMe compounds
	3,4-Methylenedioxyam-phetamine	MDA, love drug	Synthesis	80-160 mg	PO	8-12 h	Release of endogenous monoamines; weak agonist activity at 5-HT_{2A}R	Pronounced effect on emotion, increased affect; hallucinogenic effect at high doses
	3,4-Methylenedioxy-*N*-methylamphetamine	MDMA, ecstasy, Adam, X, XTC, Molly	Synthesis	80-1-50 mg	PO	4-6 h	Release of endogenous monoamines, esp. serotonin	Continuing widespread use at dance parties (raves); successfully used to treat PTSD in phase 2/3 clinical trials
Bicyclic diterpenoid (not an alkaloid)	Salvinorin A	Salvia	*Salvia divinorum*	200-500 µg	Smoked	10-30 min	Agonist at the kappa opioid receptor	Different from classic hallucinogens; strong dissociative effects; can be very disorienting

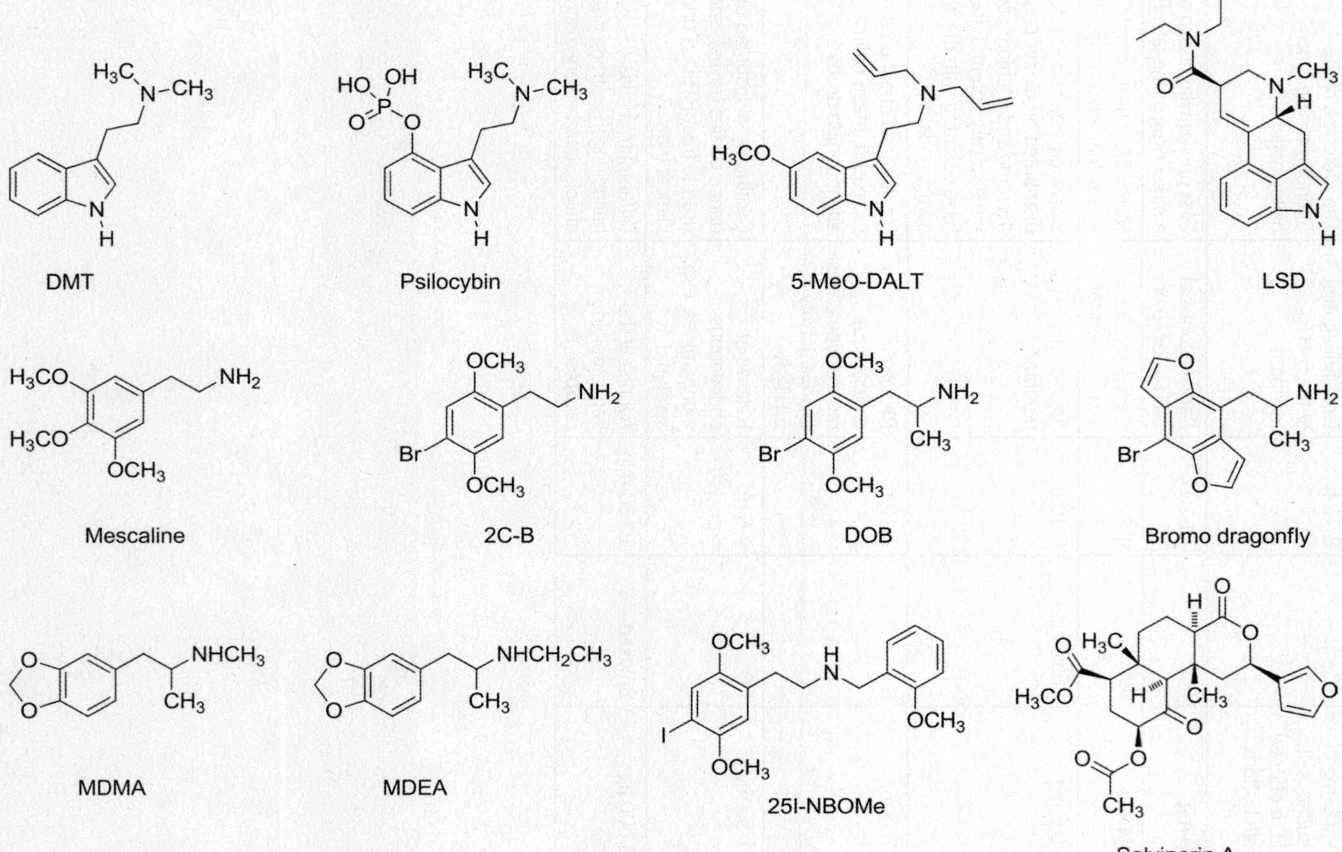

Figure 18-1. Chemical structures or representative hallucinogens of each class. Structural diagrams are taken from the PubChem Compound database. (Reprinted from Annual Reports in Computational Chemistry, Volume 4, Bolton E, Wang Y, Thiessen PA, Bryant SH, PubChem: integrated platform of small molecules and biological activities. Chapter 12. In: *Annual Reports in Computational Chemistry*, 2008, with permission from Elsevier.)

(Latin, *touch*), and "gen" (Greek, *produce*) connoting substances that "produce a touching within."[8] Entactogens have a mechanism of action and subjective effects distinct from the classic hallucinogens.[7] Although these substances affect emotion and promote social interaction, they do not produce the major alterations in sensory perceptions that are typical of the classic hallucinogens.[9] At the clinical level, MDMA is considered to have both hallucinatory and stimulant properties.[9] MDMA has significant stimulant discriminant stimulus properties in rodents, but MBDB, considered by some to be the prototypical drug of this class, does not.[9] Their ability to decrease anxiety and increase trust, self-acceptance, and openness has led to research on their use in treating patients suffering from post-traumatic stress disorder (PTSD).[10]

Another hallucinogen unrelated to those described above is Salvinorin A, which increased in popularity as a "legal high" during the last decade.[9] Salvinorin A is a potent nonnitrogenous (ie, nonalkaloid) substance obtained from a species of mint, *Salvia divinorum*. Although Salvinorin A has hallucinogenic-type effects, it is a specific kappa opioid agonist rather than a serotonergic agonist, differentiating it from the classic serotonergic hallucinogens/classic psychedelics (eg, LSD, psilocybin).

FEATURES OF CLINICAL USE, NONMEDICAL USE, AND ADDICTION

Compared to other recreational drug classes, classic psychedelics are unique for possessing relatively low addiction potential in addition to a long history of cultural use in healing and therapeutic contexts.[11,12] For people who use psychedelics, the experience is often about enhancing and expanding perception, and offering a new way to see the world.[13] Jaffe has opined "...the feature that distinguishes psychedelic agents from other classes of drugs is their capacity reliably to induce or compel states of altered perception, thought, and feeling that are not (or cannot be) experienced otherwise except in dreams or at times of religious exaltation."[14] Indeed, many persons who use these substances consider them to be "entheogens" (or substances that reveal the "god within"). This definition reflects the type of mystical or numinous experience often induced in people who use classic psychedelics.[13-15]

Clinical Uses

The history of classic psychedelics involved a period of intensive research interest for about a decade, a pause for several decades due to regulatory challenges, followed by a resurgence of interest in the past decade. More than 10,000 subjects received hallucinogens, mostly LSD, from 1950 to the mid-1960s in research settings.[16] Initial promotion of LSD by Sandoz Laboratories, where the drug was discovered in 1943, focused on the belief that LSD could induce a model psychosis (ie, was psychotomimetic) that could then be experienced by therapists of various kinds to better understand the psychoses of their patients by experiencing it themselves; or to improve their sense of empathy. The depth of self-reflection and introspection induced by LSD, however, led it to be tested in a variety of psychiatric conditions. In addition, hallucinogens engendered mystical and spiritual experiences.[17-19] Early research on clinical use of hallucinogens focused on investigation of their effects in the treatment of substance use disorders (SUD), particularly alcohol use disorder (AUD),[20,21] as well as the treatment of pain and end-of-life anxiety and depression.[22,23] A meta-analysis of the six randomized controlled trials of LSD-assisted treatment of AUD conducted in the 1960s found consistent, persistent (up to 6 months), and clinically meaningful benefits of LSD, administered at a high dose on a single occasion, over control treatments (although control groups varied in terms of active and inactive controls across studies).[24] Despite the promise that some of these approaches appeared to offer, all clinical work essentially ended with the criminalization of these substances in 1970.[25]

There is now renewed interest in psilocybin and LSD for their use in the treatment of SUD and other disorders, but no classic psychedelic has regulatory approval for clinical use.[26,27] Randomized placebo-controlled trials have demonstrated that psilocybin with psychotherapy can improve mood and anxiety symptoms in persons with a life-threatening cancer diagnosis.[28-30] Pilot studies have suggested large and clinically meaningful decreases in alcohol use and tobacco smoking following psilocybin-assisted treatment of AUD[31] and nicotine/tobacco use disorder (NUD),[32,33] respectively. Another pilot study demonstrated large persisting decreases in depressive symptoms in patients with chronic major depression following two administrations of psilocybin.[34] A very recent randomized, waiting-list controlled study observed significant decreases from baseline in scores on a standardized depression rating scale (GRID-HAMD) at 1-, 3-, 6-, and 12-month follow-up (Cohen d = 2.3, 2.0, 2.6, and 2.4, respectively).[35] Treatment response (>50% reduction in GRID-HAMD score from baseline) and remission were 75% and 58%, respectively, at 12 months.[36] However, there are some risks to classic psychedelic use in clinical settings, which are substantially increased in recreational settings (reviewed in detail below).

Recent studies of the psychotherapeutic utility of MDMA report significant clinical improvement in double-blind, placebo-controlled trials of MDMA-assisted psychotherapy for patients with PTSD.[37] Mitchell et al. report the findings of a recent randomized, double-blind, placebo-controlled, multisite phase 3 clinical trial in 90 participants to test the efficacy and safety of MDMA-assisted therapy for the treatment of patients with severe PTSD.[38] The Clinician-Administered PTSD Scale for DSM-5 (CAPS-5, the primary endpoint), and functional impairment, measured with the Sheehan Disability Scale (SDS, the secondary endpoint) were assessed at baseline and at 2 months after the last experimental session. MDMA significantly and robustly attenuated CAPS-5 score compared with placebo ($p < 0.0001$, $d = 0.91$) and significantly decreased the SDS total score ($p = 0.0116$, $d = 0.43$). All of these trials included a significant amount of psychotherapy (typically with two therapists present) prior to and after administration of the substance and carefully control the physical and psychological environment in which the drug is administered.

Nonmedical Use and Addiction

Nonmedical use of hallucinogens became widespread during the 1960s and was associated with the social turmoil that was occurring, most notably focused around protests against U.S. involvement in the Vietnam War. The extremely high potency and relative ease of synthesis of LSD led to its ready availability throughout the Western World. Careless experimentation with these drugs, along with inexperience among people who used them, led to a wave of complications, helping to establish a new image of hallucinogens as dangerous drugs.[39-41] These complications included physical injuries resulting from accidents[42] as well as psychological emergencies that resulted in emergency department visits.[43,44] However, according to the 2019 to 2020 U.S. National Survey on Drug Use and Health (NSDUH), the overall rates of hallucinogen use disorders (HUD) among community-dwelling U.S. residents 12 years and older are low compared to other substances (around 0.1% of the population in the past year),[45] although those who begin using hallucinogens at an early age are at increased risk for developing such a disorder.[46]

Diagnosis of HUD is based on 10 of the 11 substance use disorder criteria included in the DSM-5 nosology. These criteria are grouped separately into four clusters: impaired control, social impairment, risky use, and pharmacological criteria (including tolerance but not withdrawal). Withdrawal is not included as a criterion for hallucinogen use disorder because there is no established withdrawal syndrome for hallucinogens. The disorder severity is classified as mild (2 to 3 criteria), moderate (4 to 5 criteria), or severe (6 or more criteria). Frequent use of hallucinogens leads to a very rapid development of tolerance known as tachyphylaxis, where daily doses lead to rapidly diminishing effects until after about 4 days the drug no longer elicits any effect.[47] Comparisons of the harms to self and others from various psychoactive substances used recreationally tend to place psychedelics among the relatively safer of such substances.[48]

HISTORICAL FEATURES

Hallucinogens have been used ritualistically for centuries or possibly millennia in a number of cultures.[49] Some speculative and circumstantial evidence suggests that the *Soma* of the 3500-year-old Hindu Aryan Rig Veda and the *Kykeon* of the ancient Greek Eleusinian Mysteries were hallucinogens derived from plant sources.[50,51] Hallucinogens also played a prominent role in the cultures of Mesoamerican peoples. For example, mushrooms of the genus *Psilocybe*, known as *teonanácatl*, or flesh of the gods, were employed ritually by certain native tribes of Mexico such as the Aztecs. The seeds of *Rivea corymbosa*, a species of morning glory, also were used by the Aztec shaman and contain lysergamides.[52] Many native people of Latin America used DMT-containing plants for spiritual purposes.[53] For example, DMT is an active component of a powdered snuff from the seeds of *Anadenanthera peregrina* and the bark of *Virola* sp. trees. Ayahuasca is an orally active DMT-containing plant concoction prepared by boiling pounded *Banisteriopsis caapi* vines with leaves from *Psychotria*, the latter of which contain DMT.[54] Although DMT is not orally active, *Banisteriopsis* contains beta-carboline alkaloids (ie, harmine and harmaline) that inhibit the liver monoamine oxidase (MAO) that would normally break down orally ingested DMT. Ayahuasca remains an important spiritual medicine of many native people of the Amazon Basin as well as being a sacrament of the União do Vegetal (UDV) and Santo Daime churches.[55]

The peyote cactus (*Lophophora williamsii*) contains the hallucinogen mescaline. It has been venerated for possibly more than 3000 years by the Huichol and Tarahumara tribes of Northern Mexico and also is the sacrament of the Native American Church (NAC) in the United States and Canada.[55] The 1994 Amendment to the American Indian Religious Freedom Act provided legal protection for the use of peyote in the context of NAC ceremonies. Salvinorin A is a diterpene found in the mint *S. divinorum*, a plant originally cultivated in Oaxaca, Mexico, where it has been used for spiritual and divinatory purposes.[56]

Lysergic acid *N,N*-diethylamide (LSD; LSD-25; lysergide) was first synthesized in 1938, but its extremely potent psychoactive effects were not discovered until 1943, when Swiss natural products chemist Albert Hofmann accidentally ingested a minute amount.[57] Following the discovery of its psychoactive effects, it became a focus of intense interest in psychiatric research. At that time, it was believed that serotonin could be found only in the gut and blood, but when it was detected in the brain about a decade later,[58] it was recognized that LSD incorporated a tryptamine template, as did serotonin. That was the point at which it was first hypothesized that serotonin might be an important neurochemical in brain circuits that mediate behavior.[59,60]

By the early 1950s, psychedelics were hailed as a breakthrough for psychiatric research. Studies of hallucinogens, primarily LSD, resulted in more than 1,000 publications, describing results from about 40,000 subjects.[17] It was used during the 1950s and 1960s as an experimental drug in psychiatric research for producing a so-called experimental psychosis and in psychotherapeutic procedures ("psycholytic" and "psychedelic" therapy). Although adverse effects in laboratory and clinical settings were seldom seen, their recreational use was accompanied by a variety of adverse events.[43] Beginning in about the mid-1960s, hallucinogens "escaped" from the laboratory and became popular recreational drugs consumed on a broad scale, particularly in the United States. They became associated with youthful rebellion, particularly among young people who protested the war in Vietnam.[61] A number of social and political factors, as well as media exaggerations, ultimately led to severe restrictions on access to hallucinogens.[42] The classic hallucinogens were included as Schedule I substances under the Controlled Substances Act of 1970, meaning that they were considered to have high potential for unhealthy use, no accepted medical use, and no accepted safety under medical supervision. By the early 1970s, clinical research with hallucinogens had effectively stopped completely.

The history of 3,4-methylenedioxymethamphetamine (MDMA, commonly known as "ecstasy" or "Molly") is largely separated from that of the classic hallucinogens. It was first synthesized in Germany no later than 1912.[62] Alexander Shulgin became impressed with the psychotherapeutic potential of MDMA in the late 1970s and began synthesizing it and making it available to psychotherapists.[63] By the early 1980s, MDMA was becoming a popular street drug, and MDMA was listed as a Schedule I drug in 1985.[64]

Beginning in the early 1990s, after a hiatus of two decades, renewed interest developed in the potential therapeutic effects of these substances. The last decade has seen rapid growth in research on clinical uses of hallucinogens (summarized above in the section on clinical uses). In contrast to the chronic treatment required for efficacy with conventional pharmacotherapies (eg, selective serotonin reuptake inhibitors [SSRIs]), these short-term interventions using psychedelics, especially psilocybin, represent a new potential paradigm.[65]

EPIDEMIOLOGY

The best available data on rates of hallucinogen use and HUD in the United States are from the NSDUH and Monitoring the Future (MTF) surveys. Data from the 2020 NSDUH and 2020 MTF surveys[66] are summarized below, with further summary data presented in **Table 18-2**. 15.9% of the U.S. population aged 12 and over have used hallucinogens at least once. Rates of past-year and past-month use are highest in the 18- to 25-year-old age group, and lowest in the 12- to 17-year-old age group. The past-year peak is at age 21 to 25 (7.7%) and the past-month peak is at age 18 to 20 (2.2%). Rates of any hallucinogen use among 12- to 17-year-olds in the NSDUH study are marginally lower than those reported for high schoolers in the MTF survey (2.3, 1.5, and 0.3% vs 5, 3.4%, and 1.3% respectively for lifetime, annual, and monthly use). Rates of past-year and past-month use trend downward after age 25. On average, the age at first use was 22.3 years among individuals under age 50 reporting past-year initiation of hallucinogen use in 2020.

Data from the 2011 Drug Abuse Warning Network (DAWN) indicate that MDMA, LSD, and miscellaneous hallucinogens represented 1.8%, 0.4%, and 0.6% of all U.S. emergency department visits related to illicit drugs in 2011,

TABLE 18-2 Prevalence (%) of Hallucinogen Use and Hallucinogen Use Disorder in the United States in 2020

	NSDUH 2020[a]					MTF 2020[b]			
Substance	**Age group**	**Use lifetime**	**Use past year**	**Use past month**	**SUD past year[c]**	**Grade**	**Use lifetime**	**Use past year**	**Use past month**
Any hallucinogen[d]	**12+**	15.9	2.6	0.6	0.1	**8**	3.0	1.7	0.9
	12-17	2.3	1.5	0.3	0.3	**10**	4.8	3.4	1.4
	18-25	15.7	7.3	1.9	0.4	**12**	7.5	5.3	1.8
	>25	17.5	2.0	0.5	0.1				
LSD	**12+**	10.2	1.0	0.2		**8**	2.1	1.1	0.6
	12-17	1.3	0.9	0.1		**10**	3.8	2.5	1.0
	18-25	9.8	3.7	0.8		**12**	5.9	3.9	1.4
	>25	11.2	0.5	0.2					
MDMA	**12+**	7.4	0.9	0.2		**8**	1.7	0.8	0.3
	12-17	0.7	0.3	0.1		**10**	2.6	1.2	0.5
	18-25	8.8	2.5	0.6		**12**	3.6	1.8	0.8
	>25	7.9	0.8	0.2					

All numbers represent adjusted percentages of the surveyed sample: NSDUH = nationally representative sample of community-dwelling U.S. residents 12 years and older; MTF = nationally representative sample of U.S. school students. SUD, substance use disorder; LSD, lysergic acid diethylamide; MDMA, 3,4-methylenedioxymethamphetamine. MTF, Monitoring the Future; NSDUH, National Survey on Drug Use and Health.

[a]Data from Center for Behavioral Health Statistics and Quality. (2021). *Results from the 2020 National Survey on Drug Use and Health: Detailed Tables.* Substance Abuse and Mental Health Services Administration. https://www.samhsa.gov/data/

[b]Johnston LD, Miech RA, O'Malley PM, Bachman JG, Schulenberg JE, Patrick ME. *Monitoring the Future National Survey Results on Drug Use 1975-2020: Overview, Key Findings on Adolescent Drug Use.* Institute for Social Research, University of Michigan; 2021.

[c]DSM-5 criteria.

[d]Includes LSD, PCP, peyote, mescaline, psilocybin, MDMA, ketamine, dimethyltryptamine (DMT), alpha-methyltryptamine (AMT), 5-methoxy-diisopropyltryptamine (5-MeO-DIPT), *Salvia divinorum,* and others not listed.

respectively.[67] Hallucinogens were not among the top 10 drugs found in the 2021 DAWN report.[68] National data from the 2009 to 2019 Treatment Episode Data Set (TEDS) show that hallucinogens (including LSD, DMT, STP, mescaline, psilocybin, peyote, etc.) were reported as the primary substance of abuse by 0.1% of individuals 12 years or older admitted to publicly funded U.S. treatment programs.[69] In 2019, individuals aged 12 to 17 years comprised 5.7% of all primary hallucinogen admissions; the average age at admission was 32 years. These data represent a shift from 2015, when individuals aged 12 to 17 years comprised 13.9% of primary hallucinogen admissions, and the average age at admission was 28 years.[70]

Overall rates of hallucinogen use increased between 2015 and 2020, although rates vary across specific age and racial groups and geographic regions.[66-69] Increases over this period can be attributed to increased hallucinogen use in those age 18 or older, as rates of lifetime, annual, and monthly use in 12- to 17-year-olds are trending downward. Use of hallucinogens has most consistently increased in those age 26 or older. Between 2019 and 2020, most indices of hallucinogen use stayed the same or decreased, except for increased annual use in those 18 or older (7.2% to 7.3% for ages 18 to 25; 1.5% to 2% for ages 26 or older). Since 2006, significant increases have been seen in use of DMT, alpha-methyltryptamine (AMT), 5-methoxy-diisopropyltryptamine (5-MeO-DIPT), and *S. divinorum*. In the United States, rates of hallucinogen use are highest in the Western geographic region and lowest in the South and in urban counties. Higher socioeconomic status is positively associated with rate of lifetime use of hallucinogens but negatively associated with past year or past month use. Rates of hallucinogen use are highest in American Indian and Alaska natives (AIAN), Whites, and those declaring multiple races. Males are also more likely to report lifetime, annual, and monthly use of hallucinogens.

Epidemiologic surveys have not collected data on SUD criteria for specific classes of hallucinogens, so little is known about rates of HUD for most of the individual hallucinogens. Overall, HUDs are uncommon. Rates of past-year HUD are low in all age groups in the United States, with an overall rate of 0.1% for any DSM-5 HUD.[65] HUDs are most common in people under 25, with a peak in the 18 to 25 age group (0.4%). Among people who used hallucinogens in the past year, 3.7% of adults and 20% of adolescents met criteria for past-year HUD.

The 2015 NSDUH survey examined characteristics of people who used MDMA in the past year in contrast to those who used other hallucinogens in a similar time period (including LSD, PCP, mescaline, peyote, and psilocybin).[69,71] 1.4% of the adult sample had used one or more hallucinogens in the past year, and the overall prevalence of HUD was 0.11%. Both groups were approximately two-thirds male and aged 25 or younger. People who used other hallucinogens were more likely to be white than were people who used MDMA. The mean age of first use was 18 to 19 in both groups. 56% of people who used MDMA and 72% of people who used other hallucinogens had used less than 6 times in the past year, with 34% of people who used MDMA and 22% of people who used other hallucinogens having 12 or more occasions of use in the past year. Among people who used in the past-year, 4.9% of both groups met DSM-IV criteria for hallucinogen abuse, but 3.6% of the MDMA users versus 2.2% of people who used other hallucinogens met criteria for dependence.[72] In a parallel analysis of adolescents who used hallucinogens, MDMA use was similarly associated with a greater risk of hallucinogen dependence (adjusted odds ratio = 2.2).[73] These findings suggest that MDMA confers somewhat greater risk of DSM-IV hallucinogen dependence than does use of other hallucinogens.

NEUROBIOLOGY

Mechanisms of Action

Serotonergic hallucinogens (classic psychedelics) produce effects on central serotonergic systems. Although classic molecules such as LSD, psilocybin, and mescaline have affinity and agonist or partial agonist activity at the serotonin 5-HT_2 family of receptors (5-HT_{2A}, 5-HT_{2B}, 5-HT_{2C}), the 5-HT_{2A} subtype is now thought to be the primary target for all these molecules.[11,74,75] Glennon et al.[76,77] first proposed the central role of 5-HT_2–type receptors for the actions of hallucinogens in animal models, and Vollenweider et al.[78] later demonstrated that the selective 5-HT_{2A} receptor antagonist ketanserin could block the effects of psilocybin in humans, providing strong proof for the mediating role of the 5-HT_{2A} receptor in the effects of hallucinogens in humans. Quednow et al.[79] using [^{18}F]altanserin positron emitting tomography (PET) found that the intensity of psilocybin-induced subjective effects correlated positively with the level of 5-HT_{2A} receptor occupation by psilocin in the anterior cingulate and medial prefrontal cortices. Psilocin is the product of in vivo psilocybin dephosphorylation and is pharmacologically active, whereas psilocybin itself is a prodrug and is inactive as a hallucinogen.

Animal models further validate the conclusion that 5-HT_{2A} receptors function as the primary mediator of hallucinogen effect. For example, the head-twitch in mice is a behavior elicited by hallucinogens, but 5-HT_{2A} receptor knockout eliminates this behavior, whereas specific expression of the 5-HT_{2A} receptor in forebrain rescues the head-twitch.[80] Microinjection of LSD into the anterior cingulate in rats substituted for systemic LSD in drug discrimination assays, an effect mediated predominantly by 5-HT_{2A} receptors, and further suggesting an important role for this brain region in hallucinogen mechanism of action.[81] Some evidence suggests that some of the potentially therapeutic effects may be at least partly independent of 5-HT_{2A} activation.[82]

The 5-HT_{2A} receptor is highly expressed throughout the cortex, most notably on apical dendrites of cortical cells in Layer 5. Highest 5-HT_{2A} receptor density in the brain is found in the claustrum,[83,84] but high expression also is seen in the amygdala, the locus coeruleus, ventral tegmental area, reticular nucleus of the thalamus, the striatum, and several other important regions.[47,83,85,86] Widespread changes in neuronal excitability resulting from activation of 5-HT_{2A} receptors in these key brain regions would be expected to have marked effects on cognition.

The 5-HT_{2A} receptor is a family A type G protein–coupled receptor (GPCR). Canonical signaling at the 5-HT_{2A} receptor occurs through coupling to Gαq, activating phospholipase C, resulting in phosphoinositide hydrolysis, formation of diacylglycerol, and mobilization of intracellular calcium.[87] Activation of 5-HT_{2A} receptors on glutamatergic neurons within the brain causes cell depolarization that lowers the threshold for action potential firing, but generally does not actually generate action potentials (ie, the cells simply become more excitable). In addition, brain stem dorsal raphe cell firing is suppressed by psychedelics, either directly (LSD and similar compounds) or indirectly (by phenethylamine hallucinogens), an effect that also leads to excitation of the majority of cortical cells.[88]

Martin and Nichols,[89] using an improved fluorescence-activated cell sorting (FACS) method to purify hallucinogen-activated neurons from rat brain, demonstrated that a small subset of 5-HT_{2A}–expressing excitatory neurons (<5% of the total brain neuronal population) in key brain regions, including the prefrontal cortex (PFC) and the claustrum, is directly activated by the hallucinogenic phenethylamine 2,5-dimethoxy-4-iodoamphetamine (DOI). They also found that other cell types, including inhibitory somatostatin and parvalbumin GABAergic interneurons, as well as glia and astrocytes, are subsequently recruited. The neurons activated by hallucinogens expressed significantly higher levels of the gene for the 5-HT_{2A} receptor and are therefore more sensitive to the presence of hallucinogens than other neurons. Martin and Nichols hypothesize that the small population of directly responding neurons may represent a "trigger population" and that activation of these neurons initiates the cellular events leading to recurrent activity, cortical network destabilization, and the host of perceptual and cognitive behaviors associated with hallucinogens.

Although the 5-HT_{2A} receptor appears to be the key target for all the chemotypes of serotonergic hallucinogens, LSD and tryptamines such as *N,N*-dimethyltryptamine (DMT) or 5-methoxy-*N,N*-dimethyltryptamine (5-MeO-DMT) also are potent agonists at the serotonin 5-HT_{1A} receptor, which contributes to their behavioral effects in animal models.[74]

All of the serotonergic hallucinogens have agonist activity at the 5-HT_{2C} receptor that is nearly comparable to that observed at the 5-HT_{2A} receptor.[88] There is no evidence that 5-HT_{2C} receptor activation has a significant role in the behavioral effects of psychedelics, but agonist action at that receptor can functionally antagonize 5-HT_{2A} receptor activation in an animal model.[89-91] LSD is a potent agonist at the dopamine D_2 family of receptors.[92,93] It remains unknown whether that action is important to the effects of LSD in humans, but animal models indicate that dopaminergic effects may be important in the later temporal effects of LSD.[93,94] Early clinical studies of LSD, described the effects of LSD as occurring in two temporal phases: an early peak phase, followed by a later post peak phase 4 to 6 hours after LSD administration, and at times out to 10 hours.[95]

Except for LSD, none of the other serotonergic hallucinogens has been demonstrated to act directly through dopamine receptors. Nonetheless, it has been shown using [^{11}C]raclopride PET that psilocybin indirectly increases dopamine in the basal ganglia.[96] Thus, it seems possible that activation of dopaminergic systems may be a component of the overall psychopharmacology of hallucinogens.

Repeated administration of hallucinogens to rodents leads to a very rapid development of tolerance known as tachyphylaxis. Daily administration of LSD leads essentially to complete loss of sensitivity to the effects of the drug by day four.[97,98] Likewise, daily administration to humans of the hallucinogenic amphetamine 2,5-dimethoxy-4-methylamphetamine (DOM) also led, by day three, to significant tolerance to the drug effect.[99] In humans, cross-tolerance occurs between mescaline and LSD[100] and between psilocybin and LSD.[101] Tolerance and cross-tolerance to hallucinogens also develop in animal models.[102-109] Cross-tolerance between the various chemotypes of hallucinogens supports the notion that the classic serotonergic hallucinogens have a similar, if not identical, mechanism of action.

Rapid tolerance to hallucinogens correlates with downregulation of 5-HT$_{2A}$ receptors. For example, daily LSD administration selectively decreased 5-HT$_2$ receptor density in rat brain.[108-111] Not only LSD, but also the hallucinogenic amphetamines DOB and DOI produced 5-HT$_2$ receptor downregulation after repeated dosing in rats.[112] McKenna et al.[113] reported that chronic treatment of rats with DOI led to downregulation of brain 5-HT$_2$ receptors. In vitro agonist-induced receptor internalization has been observed previously for the 5-HT$_{2A}$ receptor,[114,115] and this phenomenon is also observed in vivo in rats.[89]

Brief 5-HT$_{2A}$ agonist treatment (eg, DOI) leads to desensitization of 5-HT$_{2A}$ receptor–mediated phosphoinositide hydrolysis in transfected cell lines.[116-118] Although the canonical signaling pathway for the 5-HT$_{2A}$ receptor is Gαq coupling and activation of phospholipase C (PLC), several other signaling pathways can be activated through this receptor. The relative activation of these different signaling pathways is ligand dependent, has most often been referred to as "functional selectivity" (and also as ligand bias),[119] and has been recently reviewed (eg,[120,121]).

Glutamate

Hallucinogens enhance glutamatergic transmission in the cortex at the neuronal level and also in behavioral responses. Aghajanian and Marek[122] reported that serotonin induced a calcium-dependent rapid and dramatic increase in frequency and amplitude of spontaneous (nonelectrically evoked) glutamatergic excitatory postsynaptic potentials/currents (EPSPs/EPSCs) in cortical pyramidal cells of layer V in rat brain slices. The effect was most robust in the medial PFC and other frontal areas with a high expression of 5-HT$_{2A}$ receptors in pyramidal apical dendrites. The specific 5-HT$_{2A}$ antagonist M100907 completely blocked the effect, as did the AMPA antagonist LY293558. Reverse dialysis of LSD for 30 minutes into rat PFC, followed by 45 minutes perfusion with drug-free solution, led to a significant increase of glutamate that remained elevated for at least 45 minutes after the LSD perfusion was ended.[123] The hallucinogenic amphetamine DOM (0.6 mg/kg, given intraperitoneally) similarly increased extracellular glutamate measured in rat PFC.

There is strong evidence for the interaction of glutamate systems with serotonin 5-HT$_{2A}$ receptor-mediated behaviors. For example, intracerebroventricular (ICV) administration of both competitive and noncompetitive *N*-methyl-d-aspartate (NMDA) antagonists potentiated the head-twitch response (HTR) produced in mice by a subsequent ICV injection of serotonin, providing evidence of glutamatergic modulation of serotonergic function in living mice.[124] Competitive and noncompetitive NMDA receptor antagonists also markedly enhanced the 5-HT–induced HTR in mice that had been treated with *p*-chlorophenylalanine (PCPA) to deplete endogenous serotonin.[125]

Group II metabotropic glutamate (mGlu2) receptor agonists can counteract the effects of hallucinogenic 5-HT$_{2A}$ agonists. For example, pretreatment of rats with either competitive or noncompetitive NMDA antagonists enhanced DOI-induced head shakes mediated by 5-HT$_{2A}$ receptor activation.[126] Pretreatment of rats with LY354740, a mGlu2/3 receptor agonist, attenuated the frequency of DOI-induced head shakes, whereas the selective mGlu2/3 antagonist LY341495 potentiated DOI-induced head shakes.[127] DOI-induced head twitches in mice were inhibited in a dose-dependent manner by the selective mGlu2/3 agonists LY354740 and LY379268.[128] The presynaptic location of mGlu2/3 receptors suggests that this effect occurs as a result of a presynaptic suppression of glutamate release, whereas antagonists block the presynaptic autoreceptor agonist effect of endogenously released glutamate.[129]

In rat drug discrimination studies, the effects of phenethylamine hallucinogens are potentiated by pretreatment with noncompetitive NMDA antagonists, such as PCP, dizocilpine, or ketamine.[130] Additionally, pretreatment with either the mGlu2/3 antagonist LY341495 or PCP enhanced the stimulus effect of LSD, whereas the mGlu2/3 agonist LY379268 significantly but incompletely blocked stimulus control by LSD. The 5-HT$_{2A}$ antagonists pirenperone and M100907 completely antagonized stimulus control by LSD.[131]

An in vivo functional interaction between 5-HT$_{2A}$ receptors and mGlu2 receptors has become widely accepted.[132] The 5-HT$_{2A}$ receptor forms a heterodimer with the mGlu2 receptor, creating a receptor complex that serves as a possible site of action for hallucinogenic drugs. 5-HT$_{2A}$ and mGlu2 receptors directly interact in recombinant cell lines and are present in the same neuronal cells in culture, and studies suggest this heterodimeric complex enhances $G\alpha_i$ activation by hallucinogenic 5-HT_{2A} agonists, a signaling event proposed to be involved in hallucinogen-specific signaling.[80,133]

GABA

GABA interneurons also play an important role. Administration of DOI through a microdialysis perfusion probe in rat medial PFC led to a significant dose-dependent increase in extracellular GABA.[134] Double-labeling immunohistochemical examination of cortical cells following systemic administration of DOI showed a significant increase in the number of interneurons expressing both glutamic acid decarboxylase (GAD) and *fos*-like immunoreactivity.[135] These findings suggest that 5-HT regulates cortical GABA interneurons, an effect similar to that seen in piriform cortex interneurons. 5-HT enhanced spontaneous inhibitory postsynaptic potentials (IPSPs) in rat frontal cortex pyramidal cells through activation of 5-HT_{2A} receptors located on GABAergic interneurons.[136] Neurons activated by DOI recruit small subpopulations (<10%) of inhibitory somatostatin and parvalbumin GABAergic interneurons.[89] Thus, activation of 5-HT_{2A} receptors in the cortex can produce both excitation and a feed-forward inhibition of cortical pyramidal cells.

Effects on Brain Functional Activity

Evidence from animal and human studies suggests that hallucinogens disrupt information processing in cortico-striato-thalamo-cortical (CSTC) feedback loops implicated in sensory and sensorimotor gating of internal and external information to the cortex.[137-139] The thalamocortical system is critical for conscious activity[140] and thalamocortical interactions play a role in the integration of distributed neural activity across wide cortical regions and in the generation of conscious experience,[141] although the term conscious experience refers here to certain kinds of conscious awareness and not the generation of phenomenal consciousness itself.[142] The CSTC model proposes that the thalamus plays a key role within CSTC feedback loops for gating external and internal information to the cortex and therefore is crucially involved in the regulation of the level of awareness and attention.[137,139,141]

This view may be consistent with the information integration theory of consciousness,[141-143] which proposes that the thalamus and thalamocortical system play a crucial role in integrating information related to conscious awareness. Hallucinogen stimulation of 5-HT_{2A} receptors located in several key components of the CSTC loops may alter thalamocortical transmission.[137,143] This interpretation is consistent with neuroimaging studies showing that oral administration of psilocybin, mescaline, or DMT alters neuronal activity during their peak effects in the frontomedial and frontolateral cortices, basal ganglia, and thalamus,[144-147] variously correlating with different dimensions of psychedelic states.[138]

The claustrum is the brain area with the highest expression of 5-HT_{2A} receptors.[83,84] This region was highly activated by DOI.[89] The claustrum is ideally positioned as a modulator that could desynchronize or terminate correlated activation of default mode network (DMN)-related brain regions.[148] The connectivity and anatomy of the claustrum would allow it to control temporal structure of network activity over component cortical areas of the salience network.[149] The claustrum has the highest density of fiber connections per unit volume of all brain regions examined and (1) the claustrum is a primary contributor to global brain network architecture and (2) significant connectivity exists between the claustrum, frontal lobe, and cingulate regions.[150] A study using functional magnetic resonance imaging (fMRI) found that in humans, psilocybin alters claustrum connectivity with networks that support cognition.[151] The subjective effects of psilocybin, and measures of the subjective quality of ineffability in particular, were associated with measures of claustrum activity. These findings support the notion that the claustrum may be involved at a circuit-level to exert psilocybin-induced disruptions in both the DMN and task-positive networks. The cortico-claustro-cortical (CCC) model places the claustrum at the center of 5-HT_{2A}-mediated disruptions.[152]

Blood oxygen level–dependent (BOLD) fMRI and magnetoencephalography (MEG) have been used to study human brain activity following administration of psilocybin or LSD. Carhart-Harris et al.[153] published the first study of resting state functional connectivity (RSFC) in 15 healthy humans after they received 2 mg of psilocybin IV. Using arterial spin labeling (ASL) perfusion and BOLD fMRI, the study revealed decreased cerebral blood flow and BOLD signal that were maximal in hub regions such as the thalamus and anterior and posterior cingulate cortex (PCC). Independent components and seed-based FC analyses revealed increased default mode network–task-positive network functional connectivity (DMN-TPN FC) and decreased DMN-TPN orthogonality after psilocybin.[154] They hypothesize that increased DMN-TPN coupling in the presence of preserved thalamocortical connectivity is related to a state in which arousal is preserved, but the distinction between inner thought and external focus becomes blurred.

Broadband (1-100 Hz) neural activity using MEG was recorded in 15 healthy volunteers with prior hallucinogen experience who were given 2 mg psilocybin IV.[155] The investigators observed decreased oscillatory power after psilocybin across a broad frequency range, localized primarily to association cortices, with marked decreases in areas of the DMN such as the PCC. They found post-psilocybin decreases in oscillatory power in 7 of 11 brain functional networks.

Muthukumaraswamy et al.[155] observed broadband desynchronization of cortical oscillatory rhythms after psilocybin infusion and decreased brain network integrity. They propose that there may be a general collapse of the normal rhythmic structure of cortical activity, consistent with the suggestion that psychedelics disorganize spontaneous brain activity.[153] The MEG source localizations included the PCC, precuneus, superior and middle frontal gyri, anterior cingulate, and supramarginal and precentral gyri, hub areas of the association cortex, consistent with previous fMRI results.[153] The PCC in particular showed marked effects that correlated with the subjective effects of the drug.

Carhart-Harris et al.[156] used ASL, BOLD, and MEG to image brain activity in 20 healthy human subjects administered 90 µg of IV LSD. They found visual cortex desynchronization and expanded functional connectivity in primary visual cortex area V1 to be correlated with visual hallucinations. Dysregulation of high-level regions and networks correlated with profound changes in consciousness. Decreased resting state functional connectivity in the parahippocampus correlated with ego-dissolution and altered meaning. Their results revealed that resting-state BOLD FC and MEG measures possess considerable power to predict the psychological effects of LSD. The effects of LSD on the visual system were pronounced, yet surprisingly did not correlate with its effects on self-reported qualities of the acute subjective effects. Consistent with their previous research with psilocybin, a significant relationship was found between decreased PCC alpha (and delta) power and ego-dissolution. Taken together with results from their earlier studies, it appears that psychedelics destabilize and disintegrate normally well-established brain networks and reduce the degree of segregation between them.

Relative Addiction Liability

The use of hallucinogens can lead to harmful patterns of compulsive use, and this appears to be more common with MDMA than with classic hallucinogens.[72,73] The 2009 to 2019 TEDS dataset indicates that hallucinogens were reported as the primary substance of use by 0.1% of substance-related treatment admissions aged 12 and older, with predominantly oral (49.7%) and smoking (33.9%) routes of administration.[69] Among individuals admitted primarily for hallucinogens, 40.6% reported no use in the past month, 30.2% reported some monthly use, and 29.2 % reported daily use—consistent with other data suggesting a varying typology of hallucinogen use.[157]

When considering the general population and not just those requiring substance use treatment, the proportion of people who used hallucinogens within the past year and also met criteria for HUD is substantially lower than that found for most other addictive substances (eg, past year cocaine users also meeting criteria for cocaine use disorder). For example, this ratio is 66.7% for heroin, 28.5% for cannabis, 26.3% for cocaine, and 3.8% for hallucinogens, based on a 2020 cross-sectional survey (NSDUH).[66] While the absolute values vary across studies, the relative differences among the substances show that hallucinogen use has a lower risk of developing into a SUD. Hallucinogens to varying degrees lack two important characteristics that contribute to the addiction liability of most drugs, namely, robust positive reinforcement, and negative reinforcement due to relief of withdrawal. With the exception of MDMA and similarly acting drugs, the hallucinogens discussed in this chapter are not consistently reinforcing in observational studies in humans or in animal self-administration models of addiction.[12,66] The rapid development of tolerance to the effects of most hallucinogens also limits whatever rewarding effects that they have.[11] MDMA is reinforcing, though less so than methamphetamine or cocaine.[157-159] However, moderate doses of MDMA do not appear to cause behavioral stimulant effects or significantly affect extracellular dopamine levels in nonhuman primates.[160] Although hallucinogen withdrawal is not recognized in DSM-5, some people who use MDMA experience a pronounced "crash" after using MDMA, which in 1% of such people meets DSM-IV diagnostic criteria for withdrawal.[161,162]

PHARMACOKINETICS AND PHARMACODYNAMICS

Because of the large number of compounds in the hallucinogen class, this section focuses on the hallucinogens whose effects are well characterized (LSD, psilocybin, DMT, mescaline, MDMA, and salvinorin A).

LSD

LSD was originally derived from ergot alkaloids produced by the ergot fungus *Claviceps purpurea*. Basic hydrolysis of ergot alkaloids yields lysergic acid, the precursor for LSD. LSD contains an indolealkylamine structure within a tetracyclic molecule (Fig. 15-1). LSD is often considered the prototypical classic hallucinogen (also referred to as a classic psychedelic, serotonergic psychedelic, or just psychedelic), and its effects are generally similar to those of the other classic hallucinogens.

Pharmacokinetics

LSD can be administered through a variety of routes (eg, IV, topical) but is typically taken orally. It is psychoactive in doses as low as 20 µg; 100 µg would be considered a moderate dose.[163] Street doses of LSD are extremely variable; some street samples contain no LSD. Following oral administration of 200 µg of LSD, plasma concentrations peak approximately 1.5 hours after administration, remain detectable for at least 12 hours, and are correlated with the intensity of sympathomimetic and subjective effects.[164] Concentrations of LSD decrease following first-order kinetics with an initial half-life of 3.6±0.9 hours and a terminal half-life of 8.9±5.9 hours. The distribution of LSD across tissue and organ systems has not been quantified in humans, but studies in rats and cats indicate that it readily crosses the blood–brain barrier.[165] Tolerance to autonomic and psychological effects of LSD occurs in humans after a few moderate daily doses, probably due to 5-HT_{2A} receptor downregulation or cellular internalization.[47] LSD is not tested for on standard drug screening tests.

Pharmacodynamics

Physiologic Effects

LSD induces physiologic effects including mydriasis, slight increases in blood pressure and heart rate, vasoconstriction, nausea and vomiting, minimal increase in core body temperature and blood glucose levels, sweat and saliva production, and tremor.[166-170] Other than mydriasis, these effects occur inconsistently and are generally not clinically significant. Cardiovascular effects peak about 2.5 hours after oral administration and last for several hours[171]; bradycardia and hypotension are rare.[172] In a recent double-blind, placebo-controlled human laboratory study, LSD (200 μg orally) significantly increased blood pressure, heart rate, body temperature, pupil size, prolactin, oxytocin, and epinephrine and decreased prepulse inhibition of acoustic startle response.[173] Plasma corticosteroids were increased between 2 and 6 hours after oral LSD administration.[174]

Psychological and Subjective Effects

The acute subjective and psychological effects of LSD are unpredictable and vary widely from person to person and within the same individual assessed on different occasions or even at different times during the same occasion.[47] Psychometric self-report measures are beginning to converge on several subjective qualities (outlined below) that commonly occur during psychedelic experiences.[173] Psychological effects of LSD begin 30 to 60 minutes after administration, peak within 2 to 4 hours, and last between 5 and 10 hours, depending on the dose.[47,166,175]

Commonly observed LSD effects include visual distortions and illusions, altered perception of time (time speeding up or slowing down), depersonalization and/or derealization, and rapid and sometimes extreme changes in mood, anxiety, weakness, dizziness, unusual bodily sensations, and synesthesias.[165] Insight is usually preserved so that people do not believe these experiences to be accurate representations of the objective world. However, people may have unusual thoughts or feelings about themselves or the world, including transient magical thinking or even delusional ideas.[176] Recent human laboratory studies with intravenous LSD have demonstrated acute enhancement of mood and increase in psychosislike symptoms.[176] Two weeks after dosing, no increase in delusional thinking, but increased optimism and trait openness were observed. At relatively high doses of LSD and other classic hallucinogens, people may experience a complete loss of bodily awareness, and/or a transcendent or mystical experience.[47,173,176] Psychedelic doses of LSD impair performance on working memory tasks such as digit span and word recall[177] and have significant effects on psychomotor speed and figure reconstruction.[178] LSD increases creative or unusual responses in word association tasks.[179] There is no evidence for persisting cognitive impairment after LSD intake.[180]

Toxicity/Adverse Effects

The oral lethal dose of LSD in humans is estimated as 100 mg,[181] but there have been no documented human deaths attributable to toxicity of LSD even after very large recreational doses. Slight unsteadiness or ataxia may be observed[172]; respiratory drive is unaffected.[173] There is no evidence for changes in liver and renal function, electrolytes, or blood cell counts with chronic use.[165] However, impaired judgment in an unsupervised situation can have dangerous and occasionally fatal consequences, such as walking onto a busy street or driving a car. Psychiatric complications including psychotic episodes can occur in the context of illicit use[43] but are extremely rare when LSD is administered in the context of a highly controlled clinical research environment.[182] Challenging experiences ("bad trips") can in some cases have long-lasting effects, including mood and anxiety symptoms and, more rarely, flashback phenomena.[43,183-187] It is important to distinguish between flash-back phenomena, which are common shortly after an experience (at least with LSD) and generally harmless; and hallucinogen persisting perception disorder (HPPD), which is very rare but can be disturbing.[187] HPPD is characterized by re-experiencing of perceptual symptoms of hallucinogen intoxication long after use which cause significant distress or impairment (DSM-5 criteria).[1] The number of emergency room visits related to LSD is relatively low, accounting for just 4,819 visits in 2011 (0.2% of all visits related to substance use).[188] This may be an underestimate, as LSD is not identified by readily available drug screening methods. Medical treatment of LSD intoxication is typically not necessary, but distressed patients should be managed with calm reassurance and environmental destimulation[182] (see Chapter 59).

Psilocybin and Psilocin

Psilocybin (4-phosphoryloxy-*N*,*N*-DMT) and psilocin (4-hydroxy-*N*,*N*-DMT) are substituted indolealkylamines found in many species of mushrooms.[47] The most commonly used psilocybin-containing mushroom, *Psilocybe cubensis*, contains 0.5% to 1.1% psilocybin when dried.[189] Fresh mushrooms may contain significant amounts of psilocin, but psilocin is relatively unstable, whereas psilocybin is very stable at room temperature in dry conditions.[189]

Pharmacokinetics

In rats, approximately 50% of orally administered C^{14}-labeled psilocybin is absorbed via gastrointestinal tract.[190] After oral ingestion in humans, 40% to 75% of the dose enters the systemic circulation as psilocin.[191] The vast majority of psilocybin is dephosphorylated to psilocin by phosphatases in the gut. Psilocin is thought to be the molecule that is primarily active in the brain.[192] In humans, psilocybin and psilocin are detectable in plasma within 20 to 40 minutes of ingestion. Within the first 30 minutes, psilocin concentration in the brain on average is comparable to concentrations in other organs.[193] Plasma psilocin concentrations peak at about 80 minutes, with substantial individual variation in the time course of plasma concentration.[192] The half-life of oral psilocybin is 163.3 ± 63.5 minutes, and the mean half-life of psilocin is 50 minutes. Psilocybin has four known metabolites: psilocin, 4-hydroxyindole-3-yl-acetaldehyde, 4-hydroxyindole-3-yl-acetic-acid, and 4-hydroxytryptophol.[192] Glucuronidated metabolites are excreted by the kidneys. Psilocybin is not tested for on standard drug screening tests.

Pharmacodynamics

Physiologic Effects

Physiologic effects of psilocybin within the usual dose range (10-30 mg orally) include mydriasis, slight acceleration in heart and breathing rate, increased blood pressure, and hyperreflexia.[192,194] Psilocybin and *Psilocybe* mushrooms can cause nausea and vomiting at or above the usual dose range. Mild, transient headaches are common, with onset occurring near the end of the intoxication state and usually ending within 24 hours.[195]

Psychological and Subjective Effects

The effects of oral psilocybin last about 6 hours. The onset of effect from psilocybin taken orally (usually taken in doses ranging from 10-30 mg) is typically between 30 and 60 minutes, and peak effects are observed between 90 and 180 minutes.[196] The psychological effects of psilocybin are very similar to those of LSD (see above; see also[15]). Oral psilocybin dose dependently alters the state of consciousness, marked by perceptual changes, intensified emotion, and alterations of thought, time sense, body sense, and sense of reality and self.[194,195] At higher doses, mystical-type experiences and significant anxiety become more common.[194]

Toxicity and Adverse Effects

The predicted human lethal dose of psilocybin is 6,000 mg,[181] which is approximately 500 times larger than the typical dose. There are few, if any, confirmed reports in the scientific literature of death directly caused by psilocybin. Electrolyte levels and blood sugar, liver enzyme, cortisol, prolactin, and growth hormone levels are unaffected.[192] Daily consumption of psilocybin results in acute tolerance, but such frequent use is virtually unknown.[197] As with other classic hallucinogens, physical dependence and withdrawal symptoms do not occur.[43] There is no evidence of mutagenic or teratogenic effects.[169] Severe anxiety and paranoia can occur even in highly controlled clinical research settings, but persisting adverse effects are very rare in clinical studies with psilocybin.[181] Many research participants report their experiences are highly meaningful and result in lasting psychological and behavioral benefits.[198] This may be due, at least in part, to the use of 1 or 2 well-trained therapists who carefully monitor and adjust the psychological set and setting of the experience.

DMT

N,N-dimethyltryptamine (DMT) is derived from various plant sources and animal venoms. It is also produced endogenously in humans in miniscule amounts,[199] although it is not known whether that has functional significance. In addition to its serotonergic actions, DMT binds to the sigma-1 receptor, which mediates some behavioral effects in mice.[200]

DMT alone is inactive when taken orally because it is almost completely oxidized by monoamine oxidase (MAO) in the liver before it can enter the systemic circulation.[201] Therefore, it is administered by smoking the free base form, insufflation, intravenous injection of the salt form, or orally in combination with an MAO inhibitor. Ayahuasca is the name given to various plant extracts containing DMT and β-carboline alkaloids such as harmine, harmaline, and tetrahydroharmine, which act as MAO inhibitors.[202] In the typical ayahuasca brew, leaves of the shrub *Psychotria viridis* (containing DMT) and the vine *B. caapi* (containing β-carbolines) are boiled together in water for several hours in order to extract the psychoactive constituents. After removing the spent plant material, portions of the dark aqueous solution are drunk. The use of ayahuasca has spread over the last 50 years from the Amazon rainforest into urban settings areas of Brazil and parts of Europe, Japan, Canada, and the United States.

Pharmacokinetics

Pharmacokinetics of DMT vary by route of administration. Peak plasma levels are reached 2 minutes after IV administration and 1.5 to 2 hours after oral intake of ayahuasca.[203,204] Once it reaches systemic circulation, DMT is quickly distributed throughout the body and the brain.[205,206] DMT is metabolized primarily by oxidative deamination (by MAO) and by N-oxidation to indole-3-acetic acid and dimethyltryptamine-*N*-oxide (DMT-NO), respectively.[201,207,208] DMT and its metabolites are eliminated through the kidneys. DMT is not tested for on standard drug screening tests.

Pharmacodynamics

Physiologic effects

The acute effects of DMT have been studied in dosages up to 0.4 mg/kg IV,[208] 25.4 mg smoked,[198] and 1.76 mg/kg orally as a component of ayahuasca.[209] After IV administration or smoking of freebase, the effects of DMT begin within 1 minute, peak within 3 minutes, and resolve within 30 minutes.[210-212] When it is ingested orally as a constituent of ayahuasca, the onset of effects begins after 30 to 60 minutes, peaks within 1 to 2 hours, and lasts for about 4 hours.[206]

Nausea and vomiting are common with ayahuasca and can occur with oral as well as with other routes of administration. Intravenous DMT significantly increases blood pressure (+15-30 mm Hg), heart rate (+10 bpm), and causes mydriasis.[203] Cardiovascular effects are less pronounced when DMT is ingested as ayahuasca.[213] IV DMT increases serum levels of prolactin, growth hormone, ACTH, cortisol, corticotropin, and β-endorphin.[207] Unlike other classic hallucinogens such as LSD, psilocybin, or mescaline, tolerance to DMT does not appear to develop rapidly in humans.[212,214]

Psychological and Subjective Effects

DMT produces alterations in sensation, perception, emotion, sense of self, and attribution of meaning comparable to those of other classic hallucinogens.[201,203,206,215] Psychoactive effects of DMT are often very intense, especially when they appear very rapidly, as with smoking or IV administration. With orally ingested ayahuasca, the psychological effects of DMT are much more gradual in onset than with other routes of administration, resembling those of LSD and psilocybin (see Table 15-2).

Toxicity and Adverse Effects

DMT has been associated with a loss of awareness of the physical environment and body. Medical and persisting psychiatric sequelae from such phenomena are rare.[212-214] DMT can cause seizures at high doses; however, there are no known reported cases of death due to DMT alone or ayahuasca brews not containing admixtures such as nicotine, belladonna alkaloids, or 5-methoxy DMT. In mice, the LD50 of DMT is 32 mg/kg IV.[214]

Mescaline

Mescaline (β-3,4,5-trimethoxyphenethylamine) occurs naturally in many species of cacti including peyote (*L. williamsii*) (up to 4.8% mescaline by dry weight)[216] and many species of the *Trichocereus* genus (up to 4.7% mescaline by dry weight).[217] Peyote is used as a sacrament by the Native American Church.[218]

Pharmacokinetics

Typical human oral doses are 200 to 400 mg of mescaline sulfate or 175 to 350 mg of mescaline hydrochloride.[5] Mescaline is rapidly absorbed in the gastrointestinal tract and readily crosses the blood–brain barrier.[219] Plasma concentrations of mescaline and metabolites peak after 2 hours and approach zero by 12 hours. The half-life of ingested mescaline in humans is about 6 hours.[220] Mescaline is excreted in the urine largely unchanged (55%-60%) and as metabolites including 3,4,5-trimethoxyphenylacetic acid (27%-30%), *N*-acetyl-β-(3,4,dimethoxy-5-hydroxyphenyl) ethylamine (5%), and *N*-acetylmescaline (<0.1%).[219] Mescaline is not tested for on standard drug screening tests.

Pharmacodynamics

Physiologic Effects

Physiologic research on mescaline is quite limited. The duration of action for mescaline is somewhat longer than that of LSD. Onset of effects is typically 30 to 45 minutes after ingestion, and peak effects occur within 2 to 3 hours, gradually resolving over the subsequent 4 to 8 hours.[221] Physiologic effects include increased blood pressure and heart rate, mydriasis, nausea and vomiting, diarrhea, abdominal cramps, headache, warm and cold sensations, dizziness, and tremor.[221] Plasma prolactin and growth hormone concentrations increase, with peak increases between 1.5 and 2 hours after administration.[222] Tolerance develops after a few days of daily usage and resolves after a few days of abstinence.[221]

Subjective Effects in Humans

The effects of mescaline are similar to those of LSD and psilocybin. There may be some qualitative and psychometrically quantifiable differences between mescaline, LSD, and psilocybin, such as lower ratings on mystical experience and ego-dissolution measures (though this may be due to lower doses taken as well as the lower overall potency of mescaline).[223] However, the limited comparative studies that have been conducted have not demonstrated significant differences between mescaline and these other hallucinogens across several primary dimensions, such as low addiction liability and self-reported beneficial effects.[221,224]

Toxicity and Adverse Effects

Medical emergencies due to mescaline are very rare.[188] There is no evidence in the scientific literature of physical complications from peyote or mescaline. No serious physiologic side effects or fatalities from mescaline have been reported in the scientific literature. Based on animal data, the human oral LD50 of mescaline is estimated to be 6000 mg.[182] There is no evidence of adverse cognitive or neuropsychiatric effects among Native American Church members who use peyote regularly in their religious ceremonies.[225]

MDMA

MDMA used recreationally is usually taken orally in tablet or powder form. The content of material sold as MDMA is highly variable, as it may contain no MDMA at all, or may include other ingredients such as amphetamines, various synthetic cathinones,[226] or unrelated compounds such as ketamine.[227] One common pattern of use is to ingest MDMA in the context of all-night dance parties or electronic dance music festivals (sometimes termed "raves," involving hours of dancing), often combined with other drugs.[227] People who use MDMA recreationally frequently take multiple doses over the course of an evening.[227] For these reasons, it is difficult to draw conclusions about the pharmacologic properties of MDMA from recreational experience, and it is difficult to extrapolate findings from human laboratory studies (controlled dosage of pure MDMA ingested in a standardized setting with healthy participants) to illicit use of MDMA.

The effects of MDMA have been studied primarily within a dose range of 80 to 150 mg orally. Although this range is considered typical, doses taken by people who use recreationally may be highly variable due to differences in potency and content in products sold as MDMA.[228] People who use MDMA frequently take additional "booster" doses after the first, to extend or heighten the effects of the initial dose.[227]

Pharmacokinetics

After a typical oral dose of MDMA (1.6 mg/kg), plasma concentrations peak around 1.5 to 2.5 hours after ingestion and decline gradually over the following 10 hours.[229] In this dose range (125 mg), the half-life is 8.6 hours.[228] Excretion is essentially complete within 24 hours.

MDMA is metabolized primarily by CYP2D6, CYP3A4, and catechol-*O*-methyltransferase.[230] MDMA itself inhibits CYP2D6, resulting in nonlinear kinetics, with elevated concentrations and longer half-life with higher doses or multiple consecutive doses.[231]

MDMA metabolites include 4-hydroxy-3-methoxymethamphetamine, 4-hydroxy-3-methoxyamphetamine, 3,4-dihydroxyamphetamine, and *N*-hydroxy-3,4-methylenedioxyamphetamine, and the active metabolite MDA.[232,233] MDMA is tested for by select organizations and drug test panels, typically as part of the amphetamine screening assays, with a detection window of typically up to 48 hours after dosing.[234]

Pharmacodynamics

Physiologic Effects

Typical somatic effects of MDMA include anorexia, diaphoresis, mydriasis, blurred vision, and bruxism.[235-237] Blood pressure increases in a dose-dependent manner with an increase of 20 to 35 mm Hg systolic and 10 to 20 mm Hg diastolic in clinically administered doses of 100 to 125 mg.[229,233] At doses up to 150 mg, heart rate increases by 10 to 20 bpm and body temperature by about 0.4 °C. Higher doses cause further increases in temperature, thought to be mediated by norepinephrine release, increased heat generation, and cutaneous vasoconstriction.[238] MDMA causes acute dose-dependent increases in plasma cortisol, prolactin, vasopressin, growth hormone, and oxytocin concentrations.[228,235-241] Acute immunologic effects include reduced CD4 T-cell count, increased NK cell count, and decreased lymphocyte proliferation.[242,243]

Subjective and Psychological Effects

When MDMA is taken orally, the onset of effect is around 30 minutes after ingestion.[244] With a single oral dose, peak effects occur at around 1.5 to 2 hours after ingestion and effects subside over the next 3 to 4 hours.[244] Women are more sensitive to the effects of MDMA than are men.[244-246]

Compared to the classic hallucinogens, MDMA produces mild sensory effects, as it is only a weak 5-HT_{2A} agonist, but produces feelings of emotional openness and closeness to others,[10] thought to be mediated primarily by the release of serotonin and inhibition of its uptake, as well as euphoria and other stimulantlike effects mediated primarily by release or reuptake inhibition of dopamine and noradrenaline.[245]

Moderate doses (75-150mg) of MDMA administered to MDMA-naive adult research volunteers produce effects including elevated mood, increased sense of physical well-being, vague symptoms of derealization and depersonalization, impaired thinking, and occasionally anxiety.[235-237] Subjects described a greater attention to feelings, a higher degree of openness, and increased sense of closeness to others. In a survey of 500 White American college students who reported taking MDMA at least once,[247] the most commonly reported effects were euphoria (97%), increased energy (91%), sexual arousal (83%), and feelings (not quantified) of "'love,' 'happiness,' 'peace,' and 'connection.'" Paranoia (20%), anxiety (16%), and depression (12%) were less commonly reported. After acute effects subside, "hangover" symptoms may emerge, including dysphoria, fatigue, headache, sore muscles, and insomnia, lasting for a few hours up to 1 to 2 days. Studies have demonstrated acute impairment[248] of sexual drive and functioning during intoxication, possibly due to prolactin release.[249] Some degree of tolerance to the desired effects may occur with chronic use.[250]

In moderate doses, MDMA has relatively modest effects on neuropsychological performance.[251] MDMA adversely affects driving performance, although it may also moderate aspects of driving impairment due to alcohol.[252-255]

Toxicity and Adverse Effects

The oral LD50 of MDMA in humans is estimated to be 1875 mg.[182] MDMA appears to be quite safe when moderate doses are administered to screened participants in the context of clinical research. No significant medical or psychiatric complications have been reported under such conditions.[38,228,236] MDMA ingested recreationally poses significant risks to those who use it, particularly when high doses are taken in the context of overexertion and elevated body temperature, for example, at all-night dance events ("raves")[256] (see Chapter 59).

MDMA is toxic to serotonergic neurons in animal models, although it is difficult to translate these findings into humans.[257] People with extensive histories of MDMA use have decreased serotonin transporter density and cognitive deficits.[258] However, these findings are difficult to interpret due to inconsistencies across studies and confounds such as other substance use, unknown MDMA content of the substance that was ingested, and characteristics predating MDMA use.[259] The mechanism for the serotonergic neurotoxicity of MDMA still remains enigmatic. Sprague et al.[260] suggested that MDMA-induced release of neuronal serotonin results in high levels of extracellular dopamine taken up into serotonin-depleted terminals by the serotonin uptake carrier (SERT). The absence of neuroprotective mechanisms within serotonergic terminals, which are present in dopaminergic neurons, allows breakdown of the intraneuronal dopamine, leading to formation of oxygen free radicals that subsequently damage the neurons. Saldaña and Barker[261] showed that the cloned human SERT expressed in HEK cells prefers dopamine over serotonin as a substrate as temperature increases from 37 °C to 40 °C. MDMA increases body temperature, which would enhance uptake of dopamine into serotonin terminals.

MDMA toxicity appears to be mediated by MDMA's metabolites, rather than MDMA itself, and to be potentiated by hyperthermia,[260-262] although evidence is mixed on this point. Low CYP2D6 activity due to genetics or the presence of enzyme inhibitors diminishes the neurotoxic effects of MDMA, presumably by decreasing the accumulation of toxic metabolites.[262] Behavioral toxicity has also been reported, and MDMA use can precipitate anxiety and/or depression[247] and, rarely, psychosis,[263-265] which in some cases may persist for days or weeks.

Other Serotonergic Hallucinogens

Hundreds of serotonergic hallucinogens have been characterized and new ones are synthesized every year (see Chapter 23). Many of these "research chemicals" find their way to people who use them in unhealthy, nonmedical ways; and they are not always accurately labeled. Most of these drugs have not been studied scientifically in humans. 2C-B and related compounds (eg, 2C-E, 2C-I) appear, based on self-reports by people who use them, to have effects that combine aspects of classic hallucinogen (or classic psychedelic) and entactogen agents.[266] Other drugs have unique effects that have not been characterized adequately. Recently, a number of highly potent hallucinogens with novel structures have been marketed, which feature strong LSD-like effects and considerably greater toxicity. For example, 1-(8-bromobenzo[1,2-b:4,5-b′]difuranyl-4-yl)-2-aminopropane (Bromo-DragonFLY), an agonist at 5-HT_{2A}, 5-HT_{2B}, and 5-HT_{2C} receptors, is active in doses under 1 mg and has effects that can last for several days.[267] 25I-NBOMe is a highly potent full agonist at the 5-HT_{2A} receptor (LSD is a partial agonist) and psychoactive in doses of under 1 mg.[268] These drugs are much more toxic than classic hallucinogens/classic psychedelics[269-271] and have caused a number of overdose fatalities.[272,273]

Salvinorin A

Salvinorin A occurs naturally in leaves of *S. divinorum*, a plant of the mint family. *S. divinorum* is used in ritual context by the Mazatec tribe of Mexico by chewing the leaves or drinking a decoction of the fresh leaves.[274] Salvinorin A is more commonly used recreationally in the United States by smoking the dried leaves or concentrated leaf extracts of *S. divinorum*.[275]

Pharmacokinetics

Salvinorin A has poor oral bioavailability, as most is degraded in the gastrointestinal tract.[274,275] When inhaled in vaporized form, blood levels peak at 2 minutes and then decrease rapidly.[276] When given intravenously to rhesus monkeys, the average elimination half-life was 56.6 minutes and was significantly longer in females than in males.[277] The principal metabolite is Salvinorin B, which is not psychoactive.[278] Salvinorin A is not tested for on standard drug screening tests.

Pharmacodynamics

Salvinorin A is a very potent, selective kappa opioid receptor agonist.[279] Salvinorin A produces conditioned place preference in rats at 0.1 to 40 μg/kg, associated with enhanced dopamine levels in the nucleus accumbens shell. It is aversive at higher doses.[280] Rewarding effects in rats are attenuated by rimonabant, indicating a role of the cannabinoid CB1 receptor in mediating reward.[281]

Physiologic Effects

Salvinorin A does not have significant cardiovascular effects, and no serious physiologic symptoms have been observed in human laboratory studies at doses up to 1.0 mg vaporized and inhaled.[281,282] Salvinorin A increased plasma concentrations of prolactin and (less robustly) cortisol.[276,282]

Subjective and Psychological Effects

The psychological effects of oral salvinorin A come on gradually over 5 to 10 minutes, plateau for about an hour, and subside over another hour.[274] When smoked or vaporized, the effects from leaves or extracts containing Salvinorin A can be extremely intense, peak after 2 minutes, and largely resolve within 20 minutes.[281] The subjective effects somewhat overlap with those of classic hallucinogens/classic psychedelics, with some distinctive characteristics including prominent dissociative and interoceptive effects.[281-283] Although the effects of high doses are somewhat comparable to those produced by intravenous DMT, salvinorin A users report that their perceptual world is perhaps even more strangely altered[283-285] Salvinorin A is not reliably euphorigenic[281,282] and can cause pronounced dysphoria and fear.[285]

Toxicity and Adverse Effects

There are no published reports of severe physiologic toxicity or deaths from overdose of salvinorin A. At high doses (1.0 mg vaporized), people who use it may become completely dissociated and disoriented,[286] which can lead to harmful behavior or apparent loss of consciousness. Harmful physical effects have not been observed in human laboratory studies. There is little evidence of *S. divinorum* causing addiction, and persisting adverse effects appear uncommon[287,288]; persistent psychosis following *S. divinorum* is rare.[289,290]

DRUG-DRUG INTERACTIONS

There are few known interactions between the classic hallucinogens/classic psychedelics and psychiatric medications, although serotonin syndrome is a theoretical concern when serotonergic hallucinogens are used when taking serotonergic medications. Based on limited retrospective self-reports, tricyclic antidepressants, lithium, and bupropion may increase sensitivity to LSD, whereas SSRIs and MAO inhibitors decrease its effects.[291] Retrospective analysis of online drug experience reports suggests that classic psychedelic coadministration with lithium is associated with seizures.[292] Because ayahuasca contains MAO inhibitors, serotonin syndrome is a concern if it is combined with serotonin reuptake inhibitors[293] or other serotonergic medications, although few such cases have been reported.

Several significant drug-drug interactions involving MDMA have been reported, mostly involving antidepressant medications. Serious complications from combinations of MDMA with antiretroviral agents have been reported.[294] Citalopram attenuates the psychological and cardiovascular effects of MDMA, presumably through interaction with the serotonin transporter.[295,296] Because MDMA is metabolized primarily by CYP2D6, medications that inhibit this enzyme can slow metabolism and increase levels of MDMA.[297-299] Alcohol, cannabis, and stimulants are commonly used together with MDMA.[300] Coingestion of stimulants (including caffeine) can worsen side effects and neurotoxicity of MDMA.[300,301] Coadministration of alcohol prolongs the euphoric effects of MDMA and modestly increases MDMA levels.[302] Alcohol decreases MDMA-induced fluid retention and possibly attenuates temperature increase but does not moderate heart rate or blood pressure effects.[303]

CONCLUSIONS AND FUTURE RESEARCH

The hallucinogens (or psychedelics, as they are increasingly being called) are an extremely diverse group (or groups) of substances, so few general conclusions can be drawn about them. The terminology is in flux, as the term "psychedelic" appears to be quickly replacing "hallucinogen" overall. The term psychedelic is also often used to specifically describe the classic hallucinogens, such as LSD and psilocybin (also increasingly further specified as "classic psychedelics" or "serotonergic psychedelics"). What these substances have in common is that their most obvious effects include marked alterations in perception, cognition, and affect in a manner that is sometimes referred to as a substantially "altered state of consciousness." The classic hallucinogens (or psychedelics), including LSD, mescaline, psilocybin, and DMT, are not reliably reinforcing, do not produce withdrawal, and rarely produce a SUD, although they can cause significant problems, particularly if used frequently or carelessly. MDMA, although sometimes classified as a hallucinogen or psychedelic, is more commonly called an entactogen (or empathogen). MDMA has very different effects from those of classic hallucinogens, including stimulant (amphetaminelike) effects, and poses enhanced risks and addiction liability, although it appears to be safe in a clinical research context. New hallucinogens with higher potency are being synthesized each year, most of which reach the black market before their effects have been studied. As a result, many of these compounds represent a significant danger, particularly in comparison to the well-known classic hallucinogens/classic psychedelics.

After many years of neglect, there is now renewed interest in the potential therapeutic effects of classic hallucinogens/classic psychedelics including psilocybin, DMT (or ayahuasca), and LSD in addition to the entactogen MDMA. This has largely been driven by the aforementioned clinical trial results with psilocybin[27-37] and MDMA.[38,259] However, there are a number of opportunities and challenges in terms of making hallucinogens/psychedelics available as safe and effective therapeutic agents,[304] including methodologic issues to overcome.[305] It is important that science communications about hallucinogens/psychedelics remain grounded in the available evidence and avoid both the overly negative extreme statements of decades past as well as the overly positive statements about therapeutic potential that have emerged in some quarters in recent years.[41,306] The hallucinogens/psychedelics are a fascinating class of substances that deserve study.

REFERENCES

1. *Diagnostic and Statistical Manual of Mental Disorders: DSM-5-TR*. 5th ed., text revision. ed. American Psychiatric Association Publishing; 2022.
2. Starzer MSK, Nordentoft M, Hjorthøj C. Rates and predictors of conversion to schizophrenia or bipolar disorder following substance-induced psychosis. *Am J Psychiatry*. 175(4):343-350.
3. Rucker JJ, Iliff J, Nutt DJ. Psychiatry & the psychedelic drugs. Past, present & future. *Neuropharmacology*. 2018;142:200-218.
4. Osmond H. A review of the clinical effects of psychotomimetic agents. *Ann N Y Acad Sci*. 1957;66(3):418-434.
5. Shulgin A, Shulgin A. *PIHKAL A Chemical Love Story*. Transform Press; 1991.
6. Shulgin AT, Shulgin A. *TIHKAL. The Continuation*. Transform Press; 1997.
7. Nichols DE. Differences between the mechanism of action of MDMA, MBDB, and the classic hallucinogens. Identification of a new therapeutic class: entactogens. *J Psychoactive Drugs*. 1986;18(4):305-313.
8. Nichols DE. Entactogens: how the name for a novel class of psychoactive agents originated. *Front Psych*. 2022;13:863088.
9. Nichols DE, Oberlender R. Structure-activity relationships of MDMA and related compounds: a new class of psychoactive drugs? *Ann N Y Acad Sci*. 1990;600:613-623. discussion 623-625.
10. Mithoefer MC, Wagner MT, Mithoefer AT, Jerome L, Doblin R. The safety and efficacy of {+/-}3,4-methylenedioxymethamphetamine-assisted psychotherapy in subjects with chronic, treatment-resistant posttraumatic stress disorder: the first randomized controlled pilot study. *J Psychopharmacol*. 2011;25(4):439-452.
11. Nichols DE. Psychedelics. *Pharmacol Rev*. 2016;68(2):264-355.
12. Schlag AK, Aday J, Salam I, Neill JC, Nutt DJ. Adverse effects of psychedelics: from anecdotes and misinformation to systematic science. *J Pharmacol*. 2022;36(3):258-272.
13. Griffiths RR, Hurwitz ES, Davis AK, Johnson MW, Jesse R. Survey of subjective "God encounter experiences": comparisons among naturally occurring experiences and those occasioned by the classic psychedelics psilocybin, LSD, ayahuasca, or DMT. *PLoS One*. 2019;14(4):e0214377.
14. Yaden DB, Le Nguyen KD, Kern ML, et al. Of roots and fruits: a comparison of psychedelic and nonpsychedelic mystical experiences. *J Humanist Psychol*. 2017;57(4):338-353.
15. Yaden DB, Griffiths RR. The subjective effects of psychedelics are necessary for their enduring therapeutic effects. *ACS Pharmacol Transl Sci*. 2020;4(2):568-572.
16. Grinspoon L, Bakalar JB. *Psychedelic Drugs Reconsidered*. Basic Books; 1979
17. Jaffe JH. Drug addiction and drug abuse. In: Gilman AG, et al., eds. *Goodman and Gilman's the Pharmacological Basis of Therapeutics*. Macmillan Publishing Co; 1985:532-581.
18. Pahnke WN. Drugs and mysticism. *An Analysis of the Relationship Between Psychedelic Drugs and the Mystical Consciousness*. Harvard University; 1963.

19. Pahnke WN, Richards WA. *Implications of LSD and experimental mysticism.* In: Tart CT, ed. *Altered States of Consciousness.* John Wiley & Sons, Inc; 1969:399-428.
20. Abramson HA. LSD in psychotherapy and alcoholism. *Am J Psychother.* 1966;20(3):415-438.
21. Bogenschutz MP, Johnson MW. Classic hallucinogens in the treatment of addictions. *Prog Neuropsychopharmacol Biol Psychiatry.* 2016;64:250-258.
22. Yaden DB, Nayak SM, Gukasyan N, Anderson BT, Griffiths RR. The potential of psychedelics for end of life and palliative care. *Curr Top Behav Neurosci.* 2022;56:169-184.
23. Grinspoon L, Balakar JB. *Psychedelic Drugs Reconsidered.* The Lindesmith Center; 1997.
24. Krebs TS, Johansen PO. Lysergic acid diethylamide (LSD) for alcoholism: meta-analysis of randomized controlled trials. *J Psychopharmacol.* 2012;26(7):994-1002.
25. Nutt D. Psychedelic drugs—a new era in psychiatry? *Dialogues Clin Neurosci.* 2019;21:139-147.
26. Vollenweider FX, Kometer M. The neurobiology of psychedelic drugs: implications for the treatment of mood disorders. *Nat Rev Neurosci.* 2010;11(9):642-651.
27. Kraehenmann R, Schmidt A, Friston K, Preller KH, Seifritz E, Vollenweider FX. The mixed serotonin receptor agonist psilocybin reduces threat-induced modulation of amygdala connectivity. *Neuroimage Clin.* 2016;11:53-60.
28. Grob CS, Danforth AL, Chopra GS, et al. Pilot study of psilocybin treatment for anxiety in patients with advanced-stage cancer. *Arch Gen Psychiatry.* 2011;68(1):71-78.
29. Griffiths RR, Johnson MW, Carducci MA, et al. Psilocybin produces substantial and sustained decreases in depression and anxiety in patients with life-threatening cancer: a randomized double-blind trial. *J Psychopharmacol.* 2016;30(12):1181-1197.
30. Ross S, Bossis A, Guss J, et al. Rapid and sustained symptom reduction following psilocybin treatment for anxiety and depression in patients with life-threatening cancer: a randomized controlled trial. *J Psychopharmacol.* 2016;30(12):1165-1180.
31. Bogenschutz MP, Forcehimes AA, Pommy JA, Wilcox CE, Barbosa PCR, Strassman RJ. Psilocybin-assisted treatment for alcohol dependence: a proof-of-concept study. *J Psychopharmacol.* 2015;29(3):289-299.
32. Garcia-Romeu A, Griffiths RR, Johnson MW. Psilocybin-occasioned mystical experiences in the treatment of tobacco addiction. *Curr Drug Abuse Rev.* 2014;7(3):157-164.
33. Johnson MW, Garcia-Romeu A, Cosimano MP, Griffiths RR. Pilot study of the 5-HT2AR agonist psilocybin in the treatment of tobacco addiction. *J Psychopharmacol.* 2014;28(11):983-992.
34. Carhart-Harris RL, Bolstridge M, Rucker J, et al. Psilocybin with psychological support for treatment-resistant depression: an open-label feasibility study. *Lancet.* 2016;3(7):619-627.
35. Davis AK, Barrett FS, May DG, et al. Effects of psilocybin-assisted therapy on major depressive disorder: a randomized clinical trial. *JAMA Psychiatry.* 2021;78(5):481-489.
36. Gukasyan N, Davis AK, Barrett FS, et al. Efficacy and safety of psilocybin-assisted treatment for major depressive disorder: prospective 12-month follow-up. *J Psychopharmacol.* 2022;36(2):151-158.
37. Mithoefer MC, Grob CS, Brewerton TD. Novel psychopharmacological therapies for psychiatric disorders: psilocybin and MDMA. *Lancet.* 2016;3(5):481-488.
38. Mitchell JM, Bogenschutz M, Lilienstein A, et al. MDMA-assisted therapy for severe PTSD: a randomized, double-blind, placebo-controlled phase 3 study. *Nat Med.* 2021;27(6):1025-1033.
39. Dyck E. Flashback: psychiatric experimentation with LSD in historical perspective. *Can J Psychiatry.* 2005;50(7):381-388.
40. Grob CS. Psychiatric research with hallucinogens: what have we learned? In: Ratsch C, Baker JR, eds. *Year Book for Ethnomedicine and the Study of Consciousness.* Verlag für Wissenschaft und Bildung; 1994:91-112.
41. Yaden DB, Yaden ME, Griffiths RR. Psychedelics in psychiatry—keeping the renaissance from going off the rails. *JAMA Psychiatry.* 2021;78(5):469-470.
42. Salas-Wright CP, Cano M, Hodges J, Oh S, Hai H, Vaughn MG. Driving while under the influence of hallucinogens: prevalence, correlates, and risk profiles. *Drug Alcohol Depend.* 2021;228(1):109055.
43. Strassman RJ. Adverse reactions to psychedelic drugs. A review of the literature. *J Nerv Ment Dis.* 1984;172(10):577-595.
44. Schwartz RH. LSD. Its rise, fall, and renewed popularity among high school students. *Pediatr Clin North Am.* 1995;42(2):403-413.
45. Center for Behavioral Health Statistics and Quality. *Results From the 2020 National Survey on Drug Use and Health: Detailed tables.* Substance Abuse and Mental Health Services Administration; 2021. Accessed 17 May, 2023. https://www.samhsa.gov/data/
46. Stone AL, O'Brien MS, De La Torre A, Anthony JC. Who is becoming hallucinogen dependent soon after hallucinogen use starts? *Drug Alcohol Depend.* 2007;87(2-3):153-163.
47. Nichols DE. Hallucinogens. *Pharmacol Ther.* 2004;101(2):131-181.
48. Nutt DJ, King LA, Phillips LD. Drug harms in the UK: a multicriteria decision analysis. *Lancet.* 2010;376(9752):1558-1565.
49. Schultes RE. Hallucinogens of plant origin: interdisciplinary studies of plants sacred in primitive cultures yield results of academic and practical interest. *Science.* 1969;163(3864):245-254.
50. Schultes RE, Hofmann A. *Plants of the Gods: Their Sacred, Healing, and Hallucinogenic Powers.* Healing Arts Press: Distributed to the book trade in the U.S by American International Distribution Corp; 1992.
51. Leonti M, Casu L. Soma, food of the immortals according to the Bower Manuscript (Kashmir, 6th century A.D.). *J Ethnopharmacol.* 2014;155(1):373-386.
52. Schultes RE. *A Contribution to our Knowledge of Rivea corymbosa: The Narcotic Ololiuqui of the Aztecs.* Botanical Museum of Harvard University; 1941.
53. Miller M. Chemical hints of ayahuasca use in pre-Columbian shamanic rituals. *Proc Natl Acad Sci U S A.* 2019;116(23):11079-11081.
54. Dobkin DR. Ayahuasca—the healing vine. *Int J Soc Psychiatry.* 1971;17(4):256-269.
55. Dinis-Oliveira RJ, Pereira CL, da Silva DD. Pharmacokinetic and pharmacodynamic aspects of peyote and mescaline: clinical and forensic repercussions. *Curr Mol Pharmacol.* 2019;12(3):184.
56. Schultes RE, Hofmann A. *Plants of the Gods. Origins of Hallucinogenic Use.* Alfred van der Marck ed.; 1979.
57. Hofmann A. *LSD My Problem Child.* McGraw Hill; 1980.
58. Twarog BM, Page IH. Serotonin content of some mammalian tissues and urine and a method for its determination. *Am J Physiol.* 1953;175(1):157-161.
59. Gaddum JH, Hameed KA. Drugs which antagonize 5-hydroxytryptamine. *Br J Pharmacol Chemother.* 1954;9(2):240-248.
60. Woolley DW, Shaw E. A biochemical and pharmacological suggestion about certain mental disorders. *Proc Natl Acad Sci U S A.* 1954;40(4):228-231.
61. Baumeister RF, Placidi KS. A social history and analysis of the LSD controversy. *J Humanist Psychol.* 1983;23(4):25-58.
62. Bernschneider-Reif S, Oxler F, Freudenmann RW. The origin of MDMA ("ecstasy")—separating the facts from the myth. *Pharmazie.* 2006;61(11):966-972.
63. Benzenhofer U, Passie T. Rediscovering MDMA (ecstasy): the role of the American chemist Alexander T Shulgin. *Addiction.* 2010;105(8):1355-1361.
64. Pentney AR. An exploration of the history and controversies surrounding MDMA and MDA. *J Psychoactive Drugs.* 2001;33(3):213-221.
65. Nutt D, Erritzoe D, Carhart-Harris R. Psychedelic psychiatry's brave new world. *Cell.* 2020;181(1):24-28.
66. Center for Behavioral Health Statistics and Quality. *Results From the 2020 National Survey on Drug Use and Health: Detailed Tables.* Substance Abuse and Mental Health Administration; 2021.
67. *2011: National Estimates of Drug-Related Emergency Department Visits.* Substance Abuse and Mental Health Services Administration; 2014.
68. Substance Abuse and Mental Health Services Administration. *Preliminary Findings From Drug-Related Emergency Department Visits, 2021*; Drug Abuse Warning Network Publication PEP22-07-03-001. Center for Behavioral Health Statistics and Quality, Substance Abuse

and Mental Health Services Administration; 2022. Accessed 17 May, 2023. https://www.samhsa.gov/data

69. Substance Abuse and Mental Health Services Administration Center for Behavioral Health Services and Quality. *Treatment Episode Data Set (TEDS): 2019, Admissions to and Discharges From Publically Funded Substance Abuse Treatment.* Substance Abuse and Mental Health Services Administration; 2021.
70. Substance Abuse and Mental Health Services Administration. *Center for Behavioral Health Statistics and Quality. Treatment Episode Data Set (TEDS): 2005-2015.* National Admissions to Substance Abuse Treatment Services. BHSIS Series S-91, HHS Publication No. (SMA) 17-5037. Substance Abuse and Mental Health Services Administration; 2017.
71. Center for Behavioral Health Statistics and Quality. *Results From the 2015 National Survey on Drug Use and Health: Detailed Tables.* Substance Abuse and Mental Health Services Administration; 2016.
72. Wu LT, Ringwalt CL, Mannelli P, Patkar AA. Hallucinogen use disorders among adult users of MDMA and other hallucinogens. *Am J Addict.* 2008;17(5):354-363.
73. Wu LT, Ringwalt CL, Weiss RD, Blazer DG. Hallucinogen-related disorders in a national sample of adolescents: the influence of ecstasy/MDMA use. *Drug Alcohol Depend.* 2009;104(1-2):156-166.
74. Halberstadt AL, Geyer MA. Multiple receptors contribute to the behavioral effects of indoleamine hallucinogens. *Neuropharmacology.* 2011;61(3):364-381.
75. Halberstadt AL. Recent advances in the neuropsychopharmacology of serotonergic hallucinogens. *Behav Brain Res.* 2015;277:99-120.
76. Glennon RA, Titeler M, McKenney JD. Evidence for 5-HT2 involvement in the mechanism of action of hallucinogenic agents. *Life Sci.* 1984;35(25):2505-2511.
77. Glennon RA, Young R, Rosecrans JA. Antagonism of the effects of the hallucinogen DOM and the purported 5-HT agonist quipazine by 5-HT2 antagonists. *Eur J Pharmacol.* 1983;91(2-3):189-196.
78. Vollenweider FX, Vollenweider-Scherpenhuyzen MF, Bäbler A, Vogel H, Hell D. Psilocybin induces schizophrenia-like psychosis in humans via a serotonin-2 agonist action. *Neuroreport.* 1998;9(17):3897-3902.
79. Quednow BB, Geyer MA, Halberstadt AL. Serotonin and schizophrenia. In: Muller CP, Jacobs B, eds. *Handbook of the Behavioral Neurobiology of Serotonin.* Academic Press; 2010:585-620.
80. Gonzalez-Maeso J, Weisstaub NV, Zhou M, et al. Hallucinogens recruit specific cortical 5-HT(2A) receptor-mediated signaling pathways to affect behavior. *Neuron.* 2007;53(3):439-452.
81. Gresch PJ, Barrett RJ, Sanders-Bush E, Smith RL. 5-Hydroxytryptamine (serotonin)2A receptors in rat anterior cingulate cortex mediate the discriminative stimulus properties of d-lysergic acid diethylamide. *J Pharmacol Exp Ther.* 2007;320(2):662-669.
82. Hesselgrave N, Troppoli TA, Wulff AB, Cole AB, Thompson SM. Harnessing psilocybin: antidepressant-like behavioral and synaptic actions of psilocybin are independent of 5-HT2R activation in mice. *Proc Natl Acad Sci U S A.* 2021;118(17).
83. Pazos A, Cortes R, Palacios JM. Quantitative autoradiographic mapping of serotonin receptors in the rat brain. II. Serotonin-2 receptors. *Brain Res.* 1985;346(2):231-249.
84. McKenna DJ, Saavedra JM. Autoradiography of LSD and 2,5-dimethoxyphenylisopropylamine psychotomimetics demonstrates regional, specific cross-displacement in the rat brain. *Eur J Pharmacol.* 1987;142(2):313-315.
85. Pasqualetti M, Nardi I, Ladinsky H, Marazziti D, Cassano GB. Comparative anatomical distribution of serotonin 1A, 1D alpha and 2A receptor mRNAs in human brain postmortem. *Brain Res Mol Brain Res.* 1996;39(1–2):223-233.
86. Weber ET, Andrade R. Htr2a gene and 5-HT2A receptor expression in the cerebral cortex studied using genetically modified mice. *Front Neurosci.* 2010;4:36.
87. Nichols DE, Nichols CD. Serotonin receptors. *Chem Rev.* 2008;108(5):1614-1641.
88. Puig MV, Artigas F, Celada P. Modulation of the activity of pyramidal neurons in rat prefrontal cortex by raphe stimulation in vivo: involvement of serotonin and GABA. *Cereb Cortex.* 2005;15(1):1-14.
89. Martin DA, Nichols CD. Psychedelics recruit multiple cellular types and produce complex transcriptional responses within the brain. *EBioMedicine.* 2016;11:262-277.
90. Sanders-Bush E, Breeding M. Choroid plexus epithelial cells in primary culture: a model of 5HT1C receptor activation by hallucinogenic drugs. *Psychopharmacology (Berl).* 1991;105(3):340-346.
91. Halberstadt AL, van der Heijden I, Ruderman MA, et al. 5-HT(2A) and 5-HT(2C) receptors exert opposing effects on locomotor activity in mice. *Neuropsychopharmacology.* 2009;34(8):1958-1967.
92. Giacomelli S, Palmery M, Romanelli L, Cheng CY, Silvestrini B. Lysergic acid diethylamide (LSD) is a partial agonist of D2 dopaminergic receptors and it potentiates dopamine-mediated prolactin secretion in lactotrophs in vitro. *Life Sci.* 1998;63(3):215-222.
93. Marona-Lewicka D, Thisted RA, Nichols DE. Distinct temporal phases in the behavioral pharmacology of LSD: dopamine D2 receptor-mediated effects in the rat and implications for psychosis. *Psychopharmacology (Berl).* 2005;180(3):427-435.
94. Marona-Lewicka D, Nichols DE. Further evidence that the delayed temporal dopaminergic effects of LSD are mediated by a mechanism different than the first temporal phase of action. *Pharmacol Biochem Behav.* 2007;87(4):453-461.
95. Freedman DX. LSD: the bridge from human to animal. In: Jacobs BL, ed. *Hallucinogens: Neurochemical, Behavioral, and Clinical Perspectives.* Raven Press; 1984:203-226.
96. Vollenweider FX, Vontobel P, Hell D, Leenders KL. 5-HT modulation of dopamine release in basal ganglia in psilocybin-induced psychosis in man—a PET study with [11C]raclopride. *Neuropsychopharmacology.* 1999;20(5):424-433.
97. Cholden LS, Kurland A, Savage C. Clinical reactions and tolerance to LSD in chronic schizophrenia. *J Nerv Ment Dis.* 1955;122:211-221.
98. Isbell H, Fraser HF, Isbell H, Logan CR, Wikler A. Studies on lysergic acid diethylamide (LSD-25). I. Effects in former morphine addicts and development of tolerance during chronic intoxication. *Arch Neurol Psychiatry.* 1956;76:468-478.
99. Angrist B, Rotrosen J, Gershon S. Assessment of tolerance to the hallucinogenic effects of DOM. *Psychopharmacologia.* 1974;36(3):203-207.
100. Balestrieri A, Fontanari D. Acquired and cross tolerance to mescaline, LSD-25, and BOL-148. *Arch Gen Psychiatry.* 1959;1:279-282.
101. Isbell H, Wolbach AB, Wikler A, Miner EJ. Cross tolerance between LSD and psilocybin. *Psychopharmacologia.* 1961;2:147-159.
102. Appel JB, Freedman DX. Tolerance and cross-tolerance among psychotomimetic drugs. *Psychopharmacologia.* 1968;13(3):267-274.
103. Commissaris RL, Lyness WH, Cordon JJ, Moore KE, rech RH. Behavioral tolerance to the effects of LSD in the rat. *Subst Alcohol Actions Misuse.* 1980;1(2):203-207.
104. Freedman DX, Aghajanian GK, Ornitz EM. Patterns of tolerance to lysergic acid diethylamide and mescaline in rats. *Science.* 1958;127:1173-1174.
105. Freedman DX, Boggan WO. Brain serotonin metabolism after tolerance dosage of LSD. *Adv Biochem Psychopharmacol.* 1974;10:151-157.
106. Smythies JR, Sykes EA, Lord CP. Structure-activity relationship studies on mescaline. II. Tolerance and cross-tolerance between mescaline and its analogues in the rat. *Psychopharmacologia.* 1966;9(5):434-446.
107. Trulson ME, Ross CA, Jacobs BL. Lack of tolerance to the depression of raphe unit activity by lysergic acid diethylamide. *Neuropharmacology.* 1977;16(11):771-774.
108. Wallach MB, Hine B, Gershon S. Cross tolerance or tachyphylaxis among various psychotomimetic agents on cats. *Eur J Pharmacol.* 1974;29(1):89-92.
109. Winter JC. Tolerance to a behavioral effect of lysergic acid diethylamide and cross-tolerance to mescaline in the rat: absence of a metabolic component. *J Pharmacol Exp Ther.* 1971;178(3):625-630.
110. Buckholtz NS, Freedman DX, Middaugh LD. Daily LSD administration selectively decreases serotonin2 receptor binding in rat brain. *Eur J Pharmacol.* 1985;109(3):421-425.
111. Buckholtz NS, Zhou DF, Freedman DX, Potter WZ. Lysergic acid diethylamide (LSD) administration selectively downregulates serotonin2 receptors in rat brain. *Neuropsychopharmacology.* 1990;3(2):137-148.

112. Buckholtz NS, Zhou DF, Freedman DX. Serotonin2 agonist administration down-regulates rat brain serotonin2 receptors. *Life Sci.* 1988;42(24):2439-2445.
113. McKenna DJ, Nazarali AJ, Himeno A, Saavedra JM. Chronic treatment with (+/−)DOI, a psychotomimetic 5-HT2 agonist, downregulates 5-HT2 receptors in rat brain. *Neuropsychopharmacology.* 1989;2(1):81-87.
114. Karaki S, Becamel C, Murat S, et al. Quantitative phosphoproteomics unravels biased phosphorylation of serotonin 2A receptor at Ser280 by hallucinogenic versus nonhallucinogenic agonists. *Mol Cell Proteomics.* 2014;13(5):1273-1285.
115. Berry SA, Shah MC, Khan N, Roth BL. Rapid agonist-induced internalization of the 5-hydroxytryptamine2A receptor occurs via the endosome pathway in vitro. *Mol Pharmacol.* 1996;50(2):306-313.
116. Gray JA, Roth BL. Paradoxical trafficking and regulation of 5-HT(2A) receptors by agonists and antagonists. *Brain Res Bull.* 2001;56(5):441-451.
117. Ivins KJ, Molinoff PB. Desensitization and down-regulation of 5-HT2 receptors in P11 cells. *J Pharmacol Exp Ther.* 1991;259(1):423-429.
118. Roth BL, Palvimaki EP, Berry S, et al. 5-Hydroxytryptamine2A (5-HT2A) receptor desensitization can occur without down-regulation. *J Pharmacol Exp Ther.* 1995;275(3):1638-1646.
119. Urban JD, Clarke WP, von Zastrow M, et al. Functional selectivity and classical concepts of quantitative pharmacology. *J Pharmacol Exp Ther.* 2007;320(1):1-13.
120. Seifert R. Functional selectivity of G-protein-coupled receptors: from recombinant systems to native human cells. *Biochem Pharmacol.* 2013;86(7):853-861.
121. Zhou L, Bohn LM. Functional selectivity of GPCR signaling in animals. *Curr Opin Cell Biol.* 2014;27:102-108.
122. Aghajanian GK, Marek GJ. Serotonin induces excitatory postsynaptic potentials in apical dendrites of neocortical pyramidal cells. *Neuropharmacology.* 1997;36(4-5):589-599.
123. Muschamp JW, Regina MJ, Hull EM, Winter JC, Rabin RA. Lysergic acid diethylamide and [−]-2,5-dimethoxy-4-methylamphetamine increase extracellular glutamate in rat prefrontal cortex. *Brain Res.* 2004;1023(1):134-140.
124. Kim HS, Park IS, Park WK. NMDA receptor antagonists enhance 5-HT2 receptor-mediated behavior, head-twitch response, in mice. *Life Sci.* 1998;63(26):2305-2311.
125. Kim HS, Park IS, Lim HK, Choi HS. NMDA receptor antagonists enhance 5-HT2 receptor-mediated behavior, head-twitch response, in PCPA-treated mice. *Arch Pharm Res.* 1999;22(2):113-118.
126. Dall'Olio R, Gaggi R, Bonfante V, Gandolfi O. The non-competitive NMDA receptor blocker dizocilpine potentiates serotonergic function. *Behav Pharmacol.* 1999;10(1):63-71.
127. Gewirtz JC, Marek GJ. Behavioral evidence for interactions between a hallucinogenic drug and group II metabotropic glutamate receptors. *Neuropsychopharmacology.* 2000;23(5):569-576.
128. Klodzinska A, Bijak M, Tokarski K, Pilc A. Group II mGlu receptor agonists inhibit behavioural and electrophysiological effects of DOI in mice. *Pharmacol Biochem Behav.* 2002;73(2):327-332.
129. Conn PJ, Pin JP. Pharmacology and functions of metabotropic glutamate receptors. *Annu Rev Pharmacol Toxicol.* 1997;37:205-237.
130. Winter JC, Doat M, Rabin RA. Potentiation of DOM-induced stimulus control by non-competitive NMDA antagonists: a link between the glutamatergic and serotonergic hypotheses of schizophrenia. *Life Sci.* 2000;68(3):337-344.
131. Winter JC, Eckler JR, Rabin RA. Serotonergic/glutamatergic interactions: the effects of mGlu2/3 receptor ligands in rats trained with LSD and PCP as discriminative stimuli. *Psychopharmacology (Berl).* 2004;172(2):233-240.
132. Gonzalez-Maeso J, Ang RL, Yuen T, et al. Identification of a serotonin/glutamate receptor complex implicated in psychosis. *Nature.* 2008;452(7183):93-97.
133. Fribourg M, Moreno JL, Holloway T, et al. Decoding the signaling of a GPCR heteromeric complex reveals a unifying mechanism of action of antipsychotic drugs. *Cell.* 2011;147(5):1011-1023.
134. Abi-Saab WM, Bubser M, Roth RH, Deutch AY. 5-HT2 receptor regulation of extracellular GABA levels in the prefrontal cortex. *Neuropsychopharmacology.* 1999;20(1):92-96.
135. Marek GJ, Aghajanian GK. Excitation of interneurons in piriform cortex by 5-hydroxytryptamine: blockade by MDL 100,907, a highly selective 5-HT2A receptor antagonist. *Eur J Pharmacol.* 1994;259(2):137-141.
136. Zhou FM, Hablitz JJ. Activation of serotonin receptors modulates synaptic transmission in rat cerebral cortex. *J Neurophysiol.* 1999;82(6):2989-2999.
137. Geyer MA, Vollenweider FX. Serotonin research: contributions to understanding psychoses. *Trends Pharmacol Sci.* 2008;29(9):445-453.
138. Vollenweider FX, Geyer MA. A systems model of altered consciousness: integrating natural and drug-induced psychoses. *Brain Res Bull.* 2001;56(5):495-507.
139. Vollenweider FX, Preller KH. Psychedelic drugs: neurobiology and potential for treatment of psychiatric disorders. *Nat Rev Neurosci.* 2020;21(11):611-624.
140. Edelman GM. Naturalizing consciousness: a theoretical framework. *Proc Natl Acad Sci U S A.* 2003;100(9):5520-5524.
141. Tononi G, Edelman GM. Consciousness and the integration of information in the brain. *Adv Neurol.* 1998;77:245-279.
142. Yaden DB, Johnson MW, Griffiths RR, et al. Psychedelics and consciousness: distinctions, demarcations, and opportunities. *Int J Neuropsychopharmacol.* 2021;24(8):615-623.
143. Vollenweider FX, Csomor PA, Knappe B, Geyer MA, Quednow BB. The effects of the preferential 5-HT2A agonist psilocybin on prepulse inhibition of startle in healthy human volunteers depend on interstimulus interval. *Neuropsychopharmacology.* 2007;32(9):1876-1887.
144. Gouzoulis-Mayfrank E, Schrekenberger M, Sabri O, et al. Neurometabolic effects of psilocybin, 3,4-methylenedioxyethylamphetamine (MDE) and d-methamphetamine in healthy volunteers. A double-blind, placebo-controlled PET study with [18F]FDG. *Neuropsychopharmacology.* 1999;20(6):565-581.
145. Hermle L, Füngeld M, Oepen G, et al. Mescaline-induced psychopathological, neuropsychological, and neurometabolic effects in normal subjects: experimental psychosis as a tool for psychiatric research. *Biol Psychiatry.* 1992;32(11):976-991.
146. Hermle L, Gouzoulis-Mayfrank E, Spitzer M. Blood flow and cerebral laterality in the mescaline model of psychosis. *Pharmacopsychiatry.* 1998;31(suppl 2):85-91.
147. Riba J, Romero S, Grasa E, Mena E, Carrió I, Barbanoj MJ. Increased frontal and paralimbic activation following ayahuasca, the pan-Amazonian inebriant. *Psychopharmacology (Berl).* 2006;186(1):93-98.
148. Reser DH, Richardson KE, Montibeller MO, et al. Claustrum projections to prefrontal cortex in the capuchin monkey (*Cebus apella*). *Front Syst Neurosci.* 2014;8:123.
149. Seeley WW, Menon V, Schatzberg AF, et al. Dissociable intrinsic connectivity networks for salience processing and executive control. *J Neurosci.* 2007;27(9):2349-2356.
150. Torgerson CM, Irimia A, Goh SYM, Van Horn JD. The DTI connectivity of the human claustrum. *Hum Brain Mapp.* 2015;36(3):827-838.
151. Barrett FS, Doss MK, Sepeda ND, Pekar JJ, Griffiths RR. Emotions and brain function are altered up to one month after a single high dose of psilocybin. *Sci Rep.* 2020;10(1):2214.
152. Doss MK, Madden MB, Gaddis A, et al. Models of psychedelic drug action: modulation of cortical-subcortical circuits. *Brain.* 2022;145(2):441-456.
153. Carhart-Harris RL, Erritzoe D, Williams T, et al. Neural correlates of the psychedelic state as determined by fMRI studies with psilocybin. *Proc Natl Acad Sci U S A.* 2012;109(6):2138-2143.
154. Carhart-Harris RL, Leech R, Erritzoe D, et al. Functional connectivity measures after psilocybin inform a novel hypothesis of early psychosis. *Schizophr Bull.* 2013;39(6):1343-1351.
155. Muthukumaraswamy SD, Carhart-Harris RL, Moran RJ, et al. Broadband cortical desynchronization underlies the human psychedelic state. *J Neurosci.* 2013;33(38):15171-15183.

156. Carhart-Harris RL, Muthukumaraswamy SD, Roseman L, et al. Neural correlates of the LSD experience revealed by multimodal neuroimaging. *Proc Natl Acad Sci U S A*. 2016;113(17):4853-4858.
157. Salas-Wright CP, Hodges JC, Hang Hai A, Alsolami A, Vaughn MG. Toward a typology of hallucinogen users in the United States. *Drug Alcohol Depend*. 2021;229(B1):109139.
158. Wang Z, Woolverton WL. Estimating the relative reinforcing strength of (+/−)-3,4-methylenedioxymethamphetamine (MDMA) and its isomers in rhesus monkeys: comparison to (+)-methamphetamine. *Psychopharmacology (Berl)*. 2007;189(4):483-488.
159. Lile JA, Ross JT, Nader MA. A comparison of the reinforcing efficacy of 3,4-methylenedioxymethamphetamine (MDMA, "ecstasy") with cocaine in rhesus monkeys. *Drug Alcohol Depend*. 2005;78(2):135-140.
160. Fantegrossi WE, Bauzo RM, Manvich DM, et al. Role of dopamine transporters in the behavioral effects of 3,4-methylenedioxymethamphetamine (MDMA) in nonhuman primates. *Psychopharmacology (Berl)*. 2009;205(2):337-347.
161. McKetin R, Copeland J, Norberg MM, Bruno R, Hides L, Khawar L. The effect of the ecstasy 'come-down' on the diagnosis of ecstasy dependence. *Drug Alcohol Depend*. 2014;139:26-32.
162. Degenhardt L, Bruno R, Topp L. Is ecstasy a drug of dependence? *Drug Alcohol Depend*. 2010;107(1):1-10.
163. Greiner T, Burch NR, Edelberg R. Psychopathology and psychophysiology of minimal LSD-25 dosage; a preliminary dosage-response spectrum. *AMA Arch Neurol Psychiatry*. 1958;79(2):208-210.
164. Dolder PC, Schmid Y, Haschke M, Rentsch KM, Liechti ME. Pharmacokinetics and concentration-effect relationship of oral LSD in humans. *Int J Neuropsychopharmacol*. 2015;19(1):pyv072.
165. Passie T, Halpern JH, Stichtenoth DO, Emrich HM, Hintzen A. The pharmacology of lysergic acid diethylamide: a review. *CNS Neurosci Ther*. 2008;14(4):295-314.
166. Cohen S. Psychotomimetic agents. *Annu Rev Pharmacol*. 1967;7:301-318.
167. Hollister LE, Sjoberg BM. Clinical syndromes and biochemical alterations following mescaline, lysergic acid diethylamide, psilocybin and a combination of the three psychotomimetic drugs. *Compr Psychiatry*. 1964;5:170-178.
168. Hollister LE, Hartman AM. Mescaline, lysergic acid diethylamide and psilocybin comparison of clinical syndromes, effects on color perception and biochemical measures. *Compr Psychiatry*. 1962;3:235-242.
169. Isbell H. Comparison of the reactions induced by psilocybin and LSD-25 in man. *Psychopharmacologia*. 1959;1:29-38.
170. Glennon RA. Pharmacology of classical hallucinogens and related designer drugs. In: Ries RK, Fiellin DA, Miller SC, Saitz R, eds. *Principles of Addiction Medicine*. 4th ed. Lippincott, Williams, and Wilkins; 2009:215-230.
171. Dimascio A, Greenblatt M, Hyde RW. A study of the effects of L.S.D.: physiologic and psychological changes and their interrelations. *Am J Psychiatry*. 1957;114(4):309-317.
172. Belleville RE, Fraser HF, Isbell H, Logan CR, Wikler A. Studies on lysergic acid diethylamide (LSD-25). I. Effects in former morphine addicts and development of tolerance during chronic intoxication. *AMA Arch Neurol Psychiatry*. 1956;76(5):468-478.
173. Schmid Y, Enzler F, Grasser P, et al. Acute effects of lysergic acid diethylamide in healthy subjects. *Biol Psychiatry*. 2015;78(8):544-553.
174. Strajhar P, Schmid Y, Liakoni E, et al. Acute effects of lysergic acid diethylamide on circulating steroid levels in healthy subjects. *J Neuroendocrinol*. 2016;28(3):12374.
175. Katz MM, Waskow IE, Olsson J. Characterizing the psychological state produced by LSD. *J Abnorm Psychol*. 1968;73(1):1-14.
176. Carhart-Harris RL, Kaelen M, Bolstridge M, et al. The paradoxical psychological effects of lysergic acid diethylamide (LSD). *Psychol Med*. 2016;46(7):1379-1390.
177. Jarvik ME, Abramson HA, Hirsch MW. Comparative subjective effects of seven drugs including lysergic acid diethylamide (LSD-25). *J Abnorm Psychol*. 1955;51(3):657-662.
178. Barendregt JT. Performance on some objective tests under LSD-25. *Fortschr Psychosom Med*. 1960;1:217-219.
179. Zegans LS, Pollard JC, Brown D. The effects of LSD-25 on creativity and tolerance to regression. *Arch Gen Psychiatry*. 1967;16(6):740-749.
180. Halpern JH, Pope HG Jr. Do hallucinogens cause residual neuropsychological toxicity? *Drug Alcohol Depend*. 1999;53(3):247-256.
181. Gable RS. Comparison of acute lethal toxicity of commonly abused psychoactive substances. *Addiction*. 2004;99(6):686-696.
182. Johnson M, Richards W, Griffiths R. Human hallucinogen research: guidelines for safety. *J Psychopharmacol*. 2008;22(6):603-620.
183. Carbonaro TM, Bradstreet MP, Barrett FS, et al. Survey study of challenging experiences after ingesting psilocybin mushrooms: acute and enduring positive and negative consequences. *J Psychopharmacol*. 2016;30(12):1268-1278.
184. Halpern JH, Pope HG Jr. Hallucinogen persisting perception disorder: what do we know after 50 years? *Drug Alcohol Depend*. 2003;69(2):109-119.
185. Halpern JH, Lerner AG, Passie T. A review of hallucinogen persisting perception disorder (HPPD) and an exploratory study of subjects claiming symptoms of HPPD. *Curr Top Behav Neurosci*. 2018;36:333-360.
186. Litjens RP, Brunt TM, Alderliefste G-J, Wetserink RHS. Hallucinogen persisting perception disorder and the serotonergic system: a comprehensive review including new MDMA-related clinical cases. *Eur Neuropsychopharmacol*. 2014;24(8):1309-1323.
187. Müller F, Kraus E, Holze F, et al. Flashback phenomena after administration of LSD and psilocybin in controlled studies with healthy participants. *Psychopharmacology (Berl)*. 2022;25:1-1.
188. Substance Abuse and Mental Health Services Administration, Drug Abuse Warning Network. 2011. *National Estimates of Drug-Related Emergency Department Visits, D.S.D.—HHS Publication No.* (SMA) 13-4760. Substance Abuse and Mental Health Services Administration; 2013.
189. Stamets P. *Psilocybin Mushrooms of the World*. Ten Speed Press; 1996.
190. Kalberer F, Kreis W, Rutschmann J. The fate of psilocin in the rat. *Biochem Pharmacol*. 1962;11:9.
191. Hasler F, Bourquin D, Brenneisen R, Bär T, Vollenweider FX. Determination of psilocin and 4-hydroxyindole-3-acetic acid in plasma by HPLC-ECD and pharmacokinetic profiles of oral and intravenous psilocybin in man. *Pharm Acta Helv*. 1997;72(3):175-184.
192. Passie T, Siefert J, Schneider U, Emrich HM. The pharmacology of psilocybin. *Addict Biol*. 2002;7(4):357-364.
193. Hopf A, Eckert H. Distribution patterns of 14-C-Psilocin in brains of various animals. *Act Nerv Super*. 1974;16(1):3.
194. Griffiths RR, Johnson MW, Richards WA, Richards BD, McCann U, Jesse R. Psilocybin occasioned mystical-type experiences: immediate and persisting dose-related effects. *Psychopharmacology (Berl)*. 2011;218(4):649-665.
195. Johnson MW, Andrew Sewell R, Griffiths RR. Psilocybin dose-dependently causes delayed, transient headaches in healthy volunteers. *Drug Alcohol Depend*. 2012;123(1-3):132-140.
196. Studerus E, Kometer M, Hasler F, Vollenweider FX. Acute, subacute and long-term subjective effects of psilocybin in healthy humans: a pooled analysis of experimental studies. *J Psychopharmacol*. 2011;25(11):1434-1452.
197. Riley SC, Blackman G. Between prohibitions: patterns and meanings of magic mushroom use in the UK. *Subst Use Misuse*. 2008;43(1):55-71.
198. Griffiths R, Richards W, Johnson M, McCann U, Jesse R. Mystical-type experiences occasioned by psilocybin mediate the attribution of personal meaning and spiritual significance 14 months later. *J Psychopharmacol*. 2008;22(6):621-632.
199. Barker SA, McIlhenny EH, Strassman R. A critical review of reports of endogenous psychedelic *N,N*-dimethyltryptamines in humans: 1955-2010. *Drug Test Anal*. 2012;4(7-8):617-635.
200. Fontanilla D, Johannessen M, Hajipour AR, Cozzi NV, Jackson MB, RuohoAE. The hallucinogen *N,N*-dimethyltryptamine (DMT) is an endogenous sigma-1 receptor regulator. *Science*. 2009;323(5916):934-937.
201. Riba J, McIlhenny EH, Bouso JC, Barker SA. Metabolism and urinary disposition of *N,N*-dimethyltryptamine after oral and smoked administration: a comparative study. *Drug Test Anal*. 2015;7(5):401-406.

202. McKenna DJ, Towers GH, Abbott F. Monoamine oxidase inhibitors in South American hallucinogenic plants: tryptamine and beta-carboline constituents of ayahuasca. *J Ethnopharmacol.* 1984;10(2):195-223.
203. Strassman RJ, Qualls CR. Dose-response study of *N,N*-dimethyltryptamine in humans. I. Neuroendocrine, autonomic, and cardiovascular effects. *Arch Gen Psychiatry.* 1994;51(2):85-97.
204. Callaway JC, McKenna DJ, Grob CS, et al. Pharmacokinetics of Hoasca alkaloids in healthy humans. *J Ethnopharmacol.* 1999;65(3):243-256.
205. Cohen I, Vogel WH. Determination and physiological disposition of dimethyltryptamine and diethyltryptamine in rat brain, liver and plasma. *Biochem Pharmacol.* 1972;21(8):1214-1216.
206. Barker SA, Littlefield-Chabaud MA, David C. Distribution of the hallucinogens *N,N*-dimethyltryptamine and 5-methoxy-*N,N*-dimethyltryptamine in rat brain following intraperitoneal injection: application of a new solid-phase extraction LC-APcI-MS-MS-isotope dilution method. *J Chromatogr B Biomed Sci Appl.* 2001;751(1):37-47.
207. Riba J, McIlhenny EH, Valle M, Bouso JC, Barker SA. Metabolism and disposition of *N,N*-dimethyltryptamine and harmala alkaloids after oral administration of ayahuasca. *Drug Test Anal.* 2012;4(7-8):610-616.
208. Osorio Fde L, Sanches RF, Macedo LR, et al. Antidepressant effects of a single dose of ayahuasca in patients with recurrent depression: a preliminary report. *Braz J Psychiatry.* 2015;37(1):13-20.
209. Riba J, Valle M, Urbano G, Yritia M, Moret A, Barbanoj MJ. Human pharmacology of ayahuasca: subjective and cardiovascular effects, monoamine metabolite excretion, and pharmacokinetics. *J Pharmacol Exp Ther.* 2003;306(1):73-83.
210. Cakic V, Potkonyak J, Marshall A. Dimethyltryptamine (DMT): subjective effects and patterns of use among Australian recreational users. *Drug Alcohol Depend.* 2010;111(1-2):30-37.
211. Strassman RJ, Qualls CR, Uhlenhuth EH, Kellner R. Dose-response study of *N,N*-dimethyltryptamine in humans. II. Subjective effects and preliminary results of a new rating scale. *Arch Gen Psychiatry.* 1994;51(2):98-108.
212. Strassman RJ, Qualls CR, Berg LM. Differential tolerance to biological and subjective effects of four closely spaced doses of *N, N*-dimethyltryptamine in humans. *Biol Psychiatry.* 1996;39(9):784-795.
213. Araujo AM, Carvalho F, de Lourdes Bastos M, de Pinho PG, Carvalho M. The hallucinogenic world of tryptamines: an updated review. *Arch Toxicol.* 2015;89(8):1151-1173.
214. Gable RS. Risk assessment of ritual use of oral dimethyltryptamine (DMT) and harmala alkaloids. *Addiction.* 2007;102(1):24-34.
215. Davis AK, Clifton JM, Weaver EG, Hurwitz ES, Johnson MW, Griffiths RR. Survey of entity encounter experiences occasioned by inhaled N, N-dimethyltryptamine: phenomenology, interpretation, and enduring effects. *J Psychopharmacol.* 2020;9:1008-1020.
216. Aragane M, Sasaki Y, Nakajima J, et al. Peyote identification on the basis of differences in morphology, mescaline content, and trnL/trnF sequence between *Lophophora williamsii* and *L. diffusa*. *J Nat Med.* 2011;65(1):103-110.
217. Ogunbodede O, McCombs D, Trout K, Daley P, Terry M. New mescaline concentrations from 14 taxa/cultivars of Echinopsis spp. (Cactaceae) ("San Pedro") and their relevance to shamanic practice. *J Ethnopharmacol.* 2010;131(2):356-362.
218. Stewart O. *The Peyote Religion: A History*. University of Oklahoma Press; 1987.
219. Charalampous KD, Walker KE, Kinross-Wright J. Metabolic fate of mescaline in man. *Psychopharmacologia.* 1966;9(1):48-63.
220. Seiler N, Demish L. Oxidative metabolism of mescaline in the central nervous system—III: side chain degradation of mescaline and formation of 3,4,5,-trimethoxy-benzoic acid in vivo. *Biochem Pharmacol.* 1974;23(2):259-271.
221. Wolbach AB Jr, Isbell H, Miner EJ. Cross tolerance between mescaline and LSD-25, with a comparison of the mescaline and LSD reactions. *Psychopharmacologia.* 1962;3:1-14.
222. Demisch L, Neubauer M. Stimulation of human prolactin secretion by mescaline. *Psychopharmacology (Berl).* 1979;64(3):361-363.
223. Uthaug MV, Davis AK, Haas TF, et al. The epidemiology of mescaline use: pattern of use, motivations for consumption, and perceived consequences, benefits, and acute and enduring subjective effects. *J Psychopharmacol.* 2022;36(3):309-320.
224. Wolbach AB Jr, Miner EJ, Isbell H. Comparison of psilocin with psilocybin, mescaline and LSD-25. *Psychopharmacologia.* 1962;3:219-223.
225. Halpern JH, Sherwood AR, Passie T, Blackwell KC, Ruttenber AJ. Evidence of health and safety in American members of a religion who use a hallucinogenic sacrament. *Med Sci Monit.* 2008;14(8):SR15-SR22.
226. Palamar JJ, Salomone A, Vincenti M, Cleland CM. Detection of "bath salts" and other novel psychoactive substances in hair samples of ecstasy/MDMA/"Molly" users. *Drug Alcohol Depend.* 2016;161:200-205.
227. Palamar JJ. There's something about molly: the under-researched yet popular powder form of ecstasy in the United States. *Subst Abus.* 2017;38(1):15-17.
228. Kolbrich EA, Goodwin RS, Gorelick DA, Hayes RJ, Stein EA, Huestis MA. Plasma pharmacokinetics of 3,4-methylenedioxymethamphetamine after controlled oral administration to young adults. *Ther Drug Monit.* 2008;30(3):320-332.
229. Mas M, Farré M, de la Torre R, et al. Cardiovascular and neuroendocrine effects and pharmacokinetics of 3,4-methylenedioxymethamphetamine in humans. *J Pharmacol Exp Ther.* 1999;290(1):136-145.
230. de la Torre R, Farré M, Ortuño J, et al. Non-linear pharmacokinetics of MDMA ('ecstasy') in humans. *Br J Clin Pharmacol* 2000;49(2):104-109.
231. Peiro AM, Farré M, Roset PN, et al. Human pharmacology of 3,4-methylenedioxymethamphetamine (MDMA, ecstasy) after repeated doses taken 2 h apart. *Psychopharmacology (Berl).* 2013;225(4):883-893.
232. Kraemer T, Maurer HH. Toxicokinetics of amphetamines: metabolism and toxicokinetic data of designer drugs, amphetamine, methamphetamine, and their N-alkyl derivatives. *Ther Drug Monit.* 2002;24(2):277-289.
233. Shima N, Katagi M, Zaitsu K, et al. Urinary excretion of the main metabolites of 3,4-methylenedioxymethamphetamine (MDMA), including the sulfate and glucuronide of 4-hydroxy-3-methoxymethamphetamine (HMMA), in humans and rats. *Xenobiotica.* 2008;38(3):314-324.
234. Abraham TT, Barnes AJ, Lowe RH, et al. Urinary MDMA, MDA, HMMA, and HMA excretion following controlled MDMA administration to humans. *J Anal Toxicol.* 2009;33(8):439-446.
235. Liechti ME, Vollenweider FX. Acute psychological and physiological effects of MDMA ("Ecstasy") after haloperidol pretreatment in healthy humans. *Eur Neuropsychopharmacol.* 2000;10(4):289-295.
236. Vollenweider FX, Gamma A, Leichti M, Huber T. Psychological and cardiovascular effects and short-term sequelae of MDMA ("ecstasy") in MDMA-naive healthy volunteers. *Neuropsychopharmacology.* 1998;19(4):241-251.
237. Greer G, Tolbert R. Subjective reports of the effects of MDMA in a clinical setting. *J Psychoactive Drugs.* 1986;18(4):319-327.
238. Liechti ME. Effects of MDMA on body temperature in humans. *Temperature (Austin).* 2014;1(3):192-200.
239. Harris DS, Baggott M, Mendelson JH, Mendelson JE, Jones RT. Subjective and hormonal effects of 3,4-methylenedioxymethamphetamine (MDMA) in humans. *Psychopharmacology (Berl).* 2002;162(4):396-405.
240. Henry JA, Fallon JK, Kicman AT, Hutt HJ, Cowan DA, Forsling M. Low-dose MDMA ("ecstasy") induces vasopressin secretion. *Lancet.* 1998;351(9118):1784.
241. Parrott AC. Oxytocin, cortisol and 3,4-methylenedioxymethamphetamine: neurohormonal aspects of recreational "ecstasy". *Behav Pharmacol.* 2016;27(8):649-658.
242. Pacifici R, Zuccaro P, Farré M, et al. Immunomodulating activity of MDMA. *Ann N Y Acad Sci.* 2000;914:215-224.
243. Pacifici R, Zuccaro P, Farré M, et al. Effects of repeated doses of MDMA ("ecstasy") on cell-mediated immune response in humans. *Life Sci.* 2001;69(24):2931-2941.
244. Holze F, Vizeli P, Müller F, et al. Distinct acute effects of LSD, MDMA, and D-amphetamine in healthy subjects. *Neuropsychopharmacology.* 2020;45(3):462-471.
245. Pardo-Lozano R, Farré M, Yubero-Lahoz S, et al. Clinical pharmacology of 3,4-methylenedioxymethamphetamine (MDMA, "ecstasy"): the influence of gender and genetics (CYP2D6, COMT, 5-HTT). *PLoS One.* 2012;7(10):e47599.

246. Liechti ME, Gamma A, Vollenweider FX. Gender differences in the subjective effects of MDMA. *Psychopharmacology (Berl)*. 2001;154(2):161-168.
247. Cohen RS. Subjective reports on the effects of the MDMA ('ecstasy') experience in humans. *Prog Neuropsychopharmacol Biol Psychiatry*. 1995;19(7):1137-1145.
248. Lamers CT, Ramaekers JG, Muntjewerff ND, et al. Dissociable effects of a single dose of ecstasy (MDMA) on psychomotor skills and attentional performance. *J Psychopharmacol*. 2003;17(4):379-387.
249. Passie T, Hartmann U, Schneider U, Emrich HM, Krüger THC. Ecstasy (MDMA) mimics the post-orgasmic state: impairment of sexual drive and function during acute MDMA-effects may be due to increased prolactin secretion. *Med Hypotheses*. 2005;64(5):899-903.
250. Karlsen SN, Spigset O, Slordal L. The dark side of ecstasy: neuropsychiatric symptoms after exposure to 3,4-methylenedioxymethamphetamine. *Basic Clin Pharmacol Toxicol*. 2008;102(1):15-24.
251. Cami J, Farré M, Mas M, et al. Human pharmacology of 3,4-methylenedioxymethamphetamine ("ecstasy"): psychomotor performance and subjective effects. *J Clin Psychopharmacol*. 2000; 20(4):455-466.
252. Stough C, Downey LA, King R, Papafotiou K, Swann P, Ogden E. The acute effects of 3,4-methylenedioxymethamphetamine and methamphetamine on driving: a simulator study. *Accid Anal Prev*. 2012;45:493-497.
253. Kuypers KP, Samyn N, Ramaekers JG. MDMA and alcohol effects, combined and alone, on objective and subjective measures of actual driving performance and psychomotor function. *Psychopharmacology (Berl)*. 2006;187(4):467-475.
254. Brookhuis KA, de Waard D, Samyn N. Effects of MDMA (ecstasy), and multiple drugs use on (simulated) driving performance and traffic safety. *Psychopharmacology (Berl)* 2004;173(3-4):440-445.
255. Veldstra JL, Brookhuis KA, de Waard D, et al. Effects of alcohol (BAC 0.5 per thousand) and ecstasy (MDMA 100 mg) on simulated driving performance and traffic safety. *Psychopharmacology (Berl)* 2012;222(3):377-390.
256. Kiyatkin EA, Sharma HS. Environmental conditions modulate neurotoxic effects of psychomotor stimulant drugs of abuse. *Int Rev Neurobiol*. 2012;102:147-171.
257. Green AR, King MV, Shortall SE, Fone KCF. Lost in translation: preclinical studies on 3,4-methylenedioxymethamphetamine provide information on mechanisms of action, but do not allow accurate prediction of adverse events in humans. *Br J Pharmacol*. 2012;166(5):1523-1536.
258. Parrott AC. MDMA, serotonergic neurotoxicity, and the diverse functional deficits of recreational 'Ecstasy' users. *Neurosci Biobehav Rev*. 2013;37(8):1466-1484.
259. Doblin R, Greer G, Holland J, Jerome L, Mithoefer MC, Sessa B. A reconsideration and response to Parrott AC (2013) "Human psychobiology of MDMA or 'Ecstasy': an overview of 25 years of empirical research". *Hum Psychopharmacol*. 2014;29(2): 105-108.
260. Sprague JE, Everman SL, Nichols DE. An integrated hypothesis for the serotonergic axonal loss induced by 3,4-methylenediosy-methamphetamine. *Neurotoxicology*. 1998;19(3):427-441.
261. Saldaña SN, Barker EL. Temperature and 3,4-methylenedioxymetham-phetamine alter human serotonin transporter-mediated dopamine uptake. *Neurosci Lett*. 2004;354(3):209-212.
262. Barbosa DJ, Capela JP, Silva R, et al. "Ecstasy"-induced toxicity in SH-SY5Y differentiated cells: role of hyperthermia and metabolites. *Arch Toxicol*. 2014;88(2):515-531.
263. Vallersnes OM, Dines AM, Wood DM, et al. Psychosis associated with acute recreational drug toxicity: a European case series. *BMC Psychiatry*. 2016;16:293.
264. Patel A, Moreland T, Haq F, et al. Persistent psychosis after a single ingestion of "Ecstasy" (MDMA). *Prim Care Companion CNS Disord*. 2011;13(6):
265. Vaiva G, Bos V, Bailly D, Lestavel P, Goudemand M. An "accidental" acute psychosis with ecstasy use. *J Psychoactive Drugs*. 2001;33(1):95-98.
266. Villalobos CA, Bull P, Sáez P, Cassels BK, Huidobro-Toro JP. 4-Bromo-2,5-dimethoxyphenethylamine (2C-B) and structurally related phenylethylamines are potent 5-HT2A receptor antagonists in Xenopus laevis oocytes. *Br J Pharmacol*. 2004;141(7):1167-1174.
267. Corazza O, Schifano F, Farré M, et al. Designer drugs on the internet: a phenomenon out-of-control? The emergence of hallucinogenic drug Bromo-Dragonfly. *Curr Clin Pharmacol*. 2011;6(2):125-129.
268. Bersani FS, Corraza O, Albano G, et al. 25C-NBOMe: preliminary data on pharmacology, psychoactive effects, and toxicity of a new potent and dangerous hallucinogenic drug. *Biomed Res Int*. 2014;2014:734749.
269. Hill SL, Dorsi T, Gurung S, et al. Severe clinical toxicity associated with analytically confirmed recreational use of 25I-NBOMe: case series. *Clin Toxicol (Phila)*. 2013;51(6):487-492.
270. Nielsen VT, Hogberg LC, Behrens JK. Bromo-Dragonfly poisoning of 18-year-old male. *Ugeskr Laeger*. 2010;172(19):1461-1462.
271. Wood DM, Looker JJ, Shaikh L, et al. Delayed onset of seizures and toxicity associated with recreational use of Bromo-dragonFLY. *J Med Toxicol*. 2009;5(4):226-229.
272. Walterscheid JP, Phillips GT, Lopez AE, Gonsoulin ML, Chen H-H. Pathological findings in 2 cases of fatal 25I-NBOMe toxicity. *Am J Forensic Med Pathol*. 2014;35(1):20-25.
273. Andreasen MF, Telving R, Birkler RID, Schmacher B, Johannsen M. A fatal poisoning involving Bromo-Dragonfly. *Forensic Sci Int*. 2009;183(1-3): 91-96.
274. Siebert DJ. *Salvia divinorum* and salvinorin A: new pharmacologic findings. *J Ethnopharmacol*. 1994;43(1):53-56.
275. Zawilska JB, Wojcieszak J. *Salvia divinorum*: from Mazatec medicinal and hallucinogenic plant to emerging recreational drug. *Hum Psychopharmacol*. 2013;28(5):403-412.
276. Johnson MW, MacLean KA, Caspers MJ, Prisinzano TE, Griffiths RR. Time course of pharmacokinetic and hormonal effects of inhaled high-dose salvinorin A in humans. *J Psychopharmacol*. 2016;30(4):323-329.
277. Schmidt MD, Schmidt MS, Butelman ER, et al. Pharmacokinetics of the plant-derived kappa-opioid hallucinogen salvinorin A in nonhuman primates. *Synapse*. 2005;58(3):208-210.
278. Schmidt MS, Prisinzano TE, Tidgewell K, et al. Determination of Salvinorin A in body fluids by high performance liquid chromatography-atmospheric pressure chemical ionization. *J Chromatogr B Analyt Technol Biomed Life Sci*. 2005;818(2):221-225.
279. Butelman ER, Kreek MJ. Salvinorin A, a kappa-opioid receptor agonist hallucinogen: pharmacology and potential template for novel pharmacotherapeutic agents in neuropsychiatric disorders. *Front Pharmacol*. 2015;6:190.
280. Braida D, Limonta V, Capurro V, et al. Involvement of kappa-opioid and endocannabinoid system on Salvinorin A-induced reward. *Biol Psychiatry*. 2008;63(3):286-292.
281. Johnson MW, MacLean KA, Reissig CJ, Prisinzano TE, Griffiths RR. Human psychopharmacology and dose-effects of salvinorin A, a kappa opioid agonist hallucinogen present in the plant *Salvia divinorum*. *Drug Alcohol Depend*. 2011;115(1-2):150-155.
282. Ranganathan M, Ashley Schnakenberg A, Skosnik PD, et al. Dose-related behavioral, subjective, endocrine, and psychophysiological effects of the kappa opioid agonist salvinorin A in humans. *Biol Psychiatry*. 2012;72(10):871-879.
283. Doss MK, May DG, Johnson MW, et al. The acute effects of the atypical dissociative hallucinogen salvinorin A on functional connectivity in the human brain. *Sci Rep*. 2020;10(1):1-2.
284. González D, Riba J, Bouso JC, Gómez-Jarabo G, Barbanoj MJ. Pattern of use and subjective effects of *Salvia divinorum* among recreational users. *Drug Alcohol Depend*. 2006;85(2):157-162.
285. Hutton F, Kivell B, Boyle O. "Quite a profoundly strange experience": an analysis of the experiences of *salvia divinorum* users. *J Psychoactive Drugs*. 2016;48(3):206-213.
286. Maqueda AE, Valle M, Addy PH, et al. Salvinorin-A induces intense dissociative effects, blocking external sensory perception and modulating interoception and sense of body ownership in humans. *Int J Neuropsychopharmacol*. 2015;18(12).
287. Baggott MJ, Erowid E, Erowid F, Galloway GP, Mendelson J. Use patterns and self-reported effects of *Salvia divinorum*: an internet-based survey. *Drug Alcohol Depend*. 2010;111(3):250-256.

288. Sumnall HR, Measham F, Brandt SD, Cole JC. *Salvia divinorum* use and phenomenology: results from an online survey. *J Psychopharmacol.* 2011;25(11):1496-1507.
289. Przekop P, Lee T. Persistent psychosis associated with *Salvia divinorum* use. *Am J Psychiatry.* 2009;166(7):832.
290. Meyer EG, Writer BW. *Salvia divinorum. Psychosomatics.* 2012;53(3):277-279.
291. Bonson KR, Murphy DL. Alterations in responses to LSD in humans associated with chronic administration of tricyclic antidepressants, monoamine oxidase inhibitors or lithium. *Behav Brain Res.* 1996;73(1-2): 229-233.
292. Nayak SM, Gukasyan N, Barrett FS, Erowid E, Griffiths RR. Classic psychedelic coadministration with lithium, but not lamotrigine, is associated with seizures: an analysis of online psychedelic experience reports. *Pharmacopsychiatry.* 2021;54(05):240-245.
293. Callaway JC, Grob CS. Ayahuasca preparations and serotonin reuptake inhibitors: a potential combination for severe adverse interactions. *J Psychoactive Drugs.* 1998;30(4):367-369.
294. Stolbach A, Paziana K, Heverling H, Pham P. A review of the toxicity of HIV medications II: interactions with drugs and complementary and alternative medicine products. *J Med Toxicol.* 2015;11(3):326-341.
295. Liechti ME, Baumann C, Gamma A, Vollenweider FX. Acute psychological effects of 3,4-methylenedioxymethamphetamine (MDMA, "Ecstasy") are attenuated by the serotonin uptake inhibitor citalopram. *Neuropsychopharmacology.* 2000;22(5):513-521.
296. Liechti ME, Vollenweider FX. The serotonin uptake inhibitor citalopram reduces acute cardiovascular and vegetative effects of 3,4-methylenedioxymethamphetamine ('Ecstasy') in healthy volunteers. *J Psychopharmacol.* 2000;14(3):269-274.
297. Farré M, Abanades S, Roset PN, et al. Pharmacological interaction between 3,4-methylenedioxymethamphetamine (ecstasy) and paroxetine: pharmacological effects and pharmacokinetics. *J Pharmacol Exp Ther.* 2007;323(3):954-962.
298. Hysek CM, Simmler LD, Nicola VG, et al. Duloxetine inhibits effects of MDMA ("ecstasy") in vitro and in humans in a randomized placebo-controlled laboratory study. *PLoS One.* 2012;7(5):e36476.
299. Schmid Y, Rickli A, Schaffner A, et al. Interactions between bupropion and 3,4-methylenedioxymethamphetamine in healthy subjects. *J Pharmacol Exp Ther.* 2015;353(1):102-111.
300. Gouzoulis-Mayfrank E, Daumann J. The confounding problem of polydrug use in recreational ecstasy/MDMA users: a brief overview. *J Psychopharmacol.* 2006;20(2):188-193.
301. Vanattou-Saifoudine N, McNamara R, Harkin A. Caffeine provokes adverse interactions with 3,4-methylenedioxymethamphetamine (MDMA, 'ecstasy') and related psychostimulants: mechanisms and mediators. *Br J Pharmacol.* 2012;167(5):946-959.
302. Hernández-López C, Farré M, Roset PN, et al. 3,4-Methylenedioxymethamphetamine (ecstasy) and alcohol interactions in humans: psychomotor performance, subjective effects, and pharmacokinetics. *J Pharmacol Exp Ther.* 2002;300(1):236-244.
303. Dumont GJ, Kramers C, Sweep FCGJ, et al. Ethanol co-administration moderates 3,4-methylenedioxymethamphetamine effects on human physiology. *J Psychopharmacol.* 2010;24(2):165-174.
304. Yaden DB, Earp D, Graziosi M, Friedman-Wheeler D, Luoma JB, Johnson MW. Psychedelics and psychotherapy: cognitive-behavioral approaches as default. *Front Psychol.* 2022;13:873279.
305. Aday JS, Heifets BD, Pratscher SD, Bradley E, Rosen R, Woolley JD. Great expectations: recommendations for improving the methodological rigor of psychedelic clinical trials. *Psychopharmacology (Berl).* 2022;1-22.
306. Yaden DB, Potash JB, Griffiths RR. Preparing for the bursting of the psychedelic hype bubble. *JAMA Psychiatry.* 2022;79(10): 943-944.

19 The Pharmacology of Dissociatives

Nicholas Denomme, Hamilton Morris, Jason Wallach, and Shannon C. Miller

CHAPTER OUTLINE

- Definition (drugs in this class)
- Substances included in this class
- Formulations, methods of use
- Historical features
- Epidemiology
- Pharmacokinetics
- Pharmacodynamics
- Drug-drug interactions
- Neurobiology

DEFINITION (DRUGS IN THIS CLASS)

Dissociatives are a structurally heterogeneous class of antagonists of the *N*-methyl-D-aspartate (NMDA) receptor subtype of the brain's primary excitatory neurotransmitter, glutamate. Termed dissociatives, these substances can be distinguished pharmacologically and clinically from classical hallucinogens like LSD and psilocybin. Although there are similarities in the subjective and toxicological actions of these substances, there are also differences. Classical hallucinogens are associated with a different 5-HT_{2A}-associated clinical syndrome of intoxication (whereby dissociation or impaired reality testing is less typically involved and visual hallucinations are more commonly involved). Dissociatives include various arylcyclohexylamines (of which phencyclidine [PCP] and ketamine are best known), dizocilpine (MK-801), and dextromethorphan (DXM). Many of these drugs have accepted medical uses. For example, DXM is used clinically as an antitussive and is present in more than 100 over-the-counter cough preparations in the United States. Ketamine and nitrous oxide are used clinically in humans and other animals, as general anesthetics. Nitrous oxide or "laughing gas" is not typically classified as a dissociative (more commonly considered an inhalant); however, given its NMDA antagonist and dissociative-like clinical effect, it merits inclusion in this chapter. The anesthetic noble gas, xenon, also targets NMDA receptors and displays dissociative-like clinical properties but will not be discussed.

The late Dr. Edward F. Domino (1924-2021)—who coined the term dissociative anesthesia along with Antoinette Domino—pioneered the clinical use of ketamine and was a longstanding author of previous editions of this chapter. In pursuit of a better understanding of dissociative pharmacology including unhealthy use and its management, we stand on the shoulders of Ed Domino's lifelong unparalleled contributions to the scientific and clinical understanding of dissociatives.

While many dissociatives cause anesthetic effects at high doses, most of the known dissociatives are used recreationally in subanesthetic doses/concentrations. Subanesthetic dissociative effects are complex but include euphoria, derealization, depersonalization, sensory hallucinations and altered thought and mood. Subanesthetic doses of PCP and ketamine induce distortions in consciousness that may mimic some of the clinical symptoms of schizophrenia.[1] The pharmacology of classical hallucinogens and other drugs capable of producing psychosis is discussed in their respective chapters in this section. The specific treatment of dissociative intoxication and withdrawal states is discussed in Chapter 59 of this book.

SUBSTANCES INCLUDED IN THIS CLASS

The chemical structures of the major dissociatives are shown in **Figure 19-1**. PCP, ketamine, and DXM are the best known illicit dissociatives. Other members of this class that are less commonly used include the pre-2000s street arylcyclohexylamines PCE (*N*-ethyl-1-phenylcyclohexylamine, CI, 400), TCP (1-(1-2-thienylcyclohexyl)-piperidine), and PCPy (1-(1-phenylcyclohexyl)-pyrrolidine). More recently a number of legal highs or "research chemical" dissociatives have been sold, largely over the internet. These include arylcyclohexylamines including 3-MeO-PCP, 3-Me-PCPy and 4-MeO-PCP, beta-keto-arylcyclohexylamines such as methoxetamine (MXE), deschloroketamine (DCK, 2-oxo-PCMe) and 2-fluorodeschloroketamine (FDCK)[2-4] and 1,2-diarylethylamines including diphenidine and ephenidine.

FORMULATIONS, METHODS OF USE

U.S. Food and Drug Administration-Approved Formulations

Ketamine hydrochloride (Ketalar) is available as a sterile solution for use in general anesthesia in humans and other animals. Ketamine is a U.S. Controlled Substances Act (CSA) Schedule III substance. It has also been used for prehospital analgesia and anesthesia[5] and conscious sedation.[6] As an anesthetic,

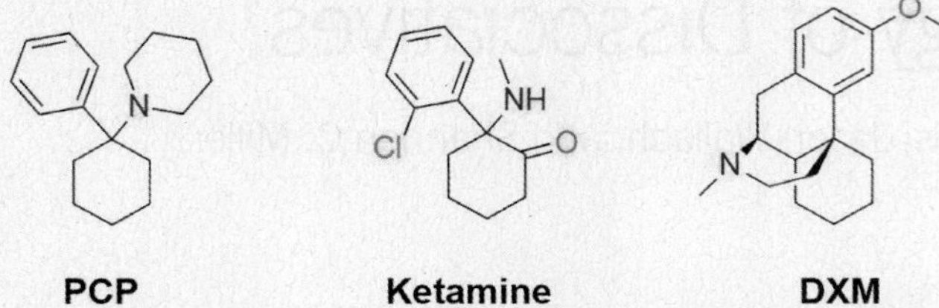

Figure 19-1. Chemical structures of the major dissociative drugs phencyclidine (PCP), ketamine, and dextromethorphan (DXM).

ketamine is used more often in children, who appear less susceptible than adults to emergent delirium.[7] Nonmedical ketamine use can be accomplished by various routes (including oral, smoked, insufflated, injection) in different doses; however, it is typically insufflated or injected intramuscularly. Ketamine is a racemic mixture of *S*- and *R*-enantiomers (explained further in pharmacology section of this chapter) and carries box warnings for hemodynamic instability, emergence reactions (vivid dreams, hallucinations, or delirium), respiratory depression, and drug-induced liver injury, among others.[8] Although ketamine is not approved by the U.S. Food and Drug Administration (FDA) for the treatment of any psychiatric disorder, one of its isomers known as *S*-ketamine (esketamine) is (Spravato). Spravato is FDA-approved (2019, Schedule III) as a nasal spray for treatment-resistant depression (TRD) in adults in conjunction with an oral antidepressant, and for depressive symptoms in adults with major depressive disorder with acute suicidal ideation or behavior. In addition to boxed warnings for sedation, dissociation, and unhealthy use[9] Spravato is subject to strict safety controls on dispensing and administration under a safety program called a Risk Evaluation and Mitigation Strategy (REMS). The Spravato REMS program requires Spravato (esketamine or S-ketamine) to be dispensed and administered in health care settings certified in the REMS. Patients must be monitored inside this health care setting for a minimum of 2 hours after administration until patients are deemed safe to leave. FDA has expressed concern that some pharmacies are compounding racemic ketamine either alone or in combination with other ingredients, enabling substitution of racemic ketamine as a nasal spray for FDA-approved Spravato/esketamine, and also enabling home use outside the REMS. The FDA Adverse Event Reporting System (FAERS) database and the medical literature from April 2011 through January 2022 provide five cases of psychiatric events such as delusion, dissociation, visual hallucination, and panic attack as well as unhealthy use following the use of compounded ketamine nasal spray. Compounded ketamine typically occurs as a nasal spray or sublingual troches and is typically used at different doses and a higher frequency of dosing than FDA-approved Spravato (esketamine). The use of compounded ketamine for home use carries additional risks given it is occurring outside a supervised setting. Appropriate safety measures are thus warranted to ensure safe use and continued access.

While PCP was used as a general anesthetic in humans and other animals, it is not currently available as a medical commercial preparation approved by the FDA. It is available in many illicit preparations in various forms and is used in a wide range of doses, which under a lack of regulation are uncontrolled. PCP has many of the pharmacological effects of ketamine but is more potent (~10-fold) and longer acting. It is encountered in various illicit forms: powder, tablets, and liquid solutions (eg, salt form in water, free base in ether). The solutions are typically soaked onto plant leaves such as tobacco, ginger, cannabis, mint, oregano, or parsley and then smoked. PCP is a CSA Schedule II substance although some of its congeners are Schedule I substances (eg, PCPy and TCP). Certain chemical intermediates to PCP, such as piperidinocyclohexanecarbonitrile (PCC) are also CSA Schedule I substances; this does little to deter illicit production but negatively impacts legitimate scientific investigation. PCC is also a common contaminant in illicit PCP and may contribute to adverse reactions.

Medical DXM preparations are typically administered orally. The salt forms usually encountered are DXM hydrobromide and less commonly DXM polistirex. Capsules, tablets, lozenges, or solutions of DXM are available alone or in combination with many other substances as cough, cold, and flu relief preparations. The usual antitussive dosage for adults is 10 to 20 mg every 4 hours or 30 mg every 6 to 8 hours, not to exceed 120 mg daily. Extended-release forms are given as 60 mg twice daily. Larger doses of DXM are used for psychoactive dissociative effects. DXM has a low toxicity and high therapeutic index.[10] Death is unlikely even at very high doses but has been reported.[11] The additional ingredients in over-the-counter preparations make for exacerbated hazards with high dose use including death[12]: decongestant/pseudoephedrine (causing cardiac toxicity), antihistamine/chlorpheniramine (antihistamine toxicity), pain/acetaminophen (liver toxicity), and bromides (bromide toxicity). While use may not be preventable, such adverse drug interactions are largely preventable with proper harm reduction strategies and education.

HISTORICAL FEATURES

The discovery of PCP in 1956 has been well documented by those involved with its therapeutic development.[2,13] PCP was initially developed under the trade name Sernyl as an intravenous general anesthetic, however the unique anesthesia it produced was complicated by a prolonged emergence delirium. This quickly led to its demise as a clinically useful agent. PCP is associated with symptoms that model both the positive (delusions, hallucinations) and negative (blunted affect, ambivalence, asociality, autistic-like effects) symptoms of schizophrenia, making for perhaps one of the more useful pharmacological models of schizophrenia.[14-16] Illicit PCP use began in the late 1960s and quickly spread throughout the United States.[2]

The desirable anesthetic properties of PCP were retained in the short-acting arylcyclohexylamine derivative ketamine, which produced a briefer emergence delirium due to a shorter elimination half-life. The term dissociative anesthetic was coined to emphasize that the anesthetized patient was psychologically "disconnected" from their environment. Ketamine subsequently was discovered by the recreational drug using community, where it is also known as "K," "super K," "special K," and "cat Valium," among other terms.

Illicit PCP use occurs primarily in large metropolitan areas. Because PCP is potent and relatively easy and inexpensive to synthesize, it is an inexpensive intoxicant. In the past it was not uncommon for PCP to be sold as another psychoactive substance like THC, LSD or mescaline.[2]

In contrast to the arylcyclohexylamines, MK-801 (dizocilpine) was developed as an anticonvulsant[17] and subsequently explored as a neuroprotective agent; however, its development was discontinued following observations of a specific type of neurotoxicity called Olney's lesions.[18] Clinical trials of MK-801 have been extremely limited, and the results are not easily available. Very little is known of its properties in humans. To date, it has been impossible to obtain from FDA all of their files on MK-801 via the Freedom of Information Act.

The history of DXM begins with the synthesis of racemethorphan (deoxydihydrothebaiodine) or methorphan (Dromoran) and was patented by Hoffmann-La Roche in 1954 as an opioid analgesic. After the D- and L-isomers were isolated, it was discovered that the D-isomer was antitussive and had much less analgesic and narcotic-like properties. DXM is nearly equal to codeine as an antitussive. However, unlike codeine, DXM is fairly devoid of other opioid effects such as analgesia, central nervous system depression, and respiratory depression. DXM is metabolized to dextrorphan (DXO), also an NMDAR antagonist. DXM's mechanism of action as an antitussive is unknown and more basic studies are needed. In doses of 300 to 1,800 mg (20-120 times the recommended dose), DXM produces PCP-like mental effects.[19,20] However, larger doses (237 times the recommended dose) are sometimes used recreationally.[21] Nonmedical DXM use has been a concern since at least the 1960s. An over-the-counter tablet form of DXM, Romilar, was replaced by a cough syrup in 1973 in an attempt to reduce its recreational use. In 1990, the FDA Drug Abuse Advisory Committee assessed DXM use by teenagers and recommended against placing the drug on the Controlled Drug Schedule but requested more study of the problem.[22] Although widespread recreational use of DXM began with the liquid cough syrup (claimed to hamper the use of large doses of DXM because of the distasteful nature of cough syrup), more convenient consumer products have since been developed, including high-dose (30 mg) tablets as well as high-dose gel capsules, and concentrated liquid solutions which are preferred by those who use DXM recreationally. While more conducive to use as an intoxicant, such products may actually reduce risk of adverse reactions as they typically only contain DXM as the active ingredient. Acid-base extraction techniques have been developed to isolate DXM as a powder.[23] DXM has become popular, particularly among adolescents, likely due to ease of access relative to other intoxicants and perceived safety as an approved drug as well as difficulty detecting in urinalysis drug testing.[24] Over the last decade or so, many states have enacted laws to restrict purchase of DXM to those over 18, which has likely helped reduce the frequency of adolescent misuse,[25] though more research is needed. Slang terms for the cough medicine preparations are "dex," "robo," "skittles" (owing to some tablets appearing similar to red Skittles candies), "tussin," and "triple Cs." Recreational use of DXM is sometimes described as "dexing," "roboing," and "robotripping" (referring to the popular DXM cough syrup Robitussin). Recently, a combination drug product containing DXM and quinidine was approved in the United States by the FDA for treatment of pseudobulbar affect. Additional indications for this combination are also being explored.

Nitrous oxide has been known for more than 225 years. It is widely used today in anesthesia. In addition, its recreational use as "laughing gas" has been well described since it first was discovered. Nitrous oxide is widely used today as part of the mixture of anesthetics used to achieve "balanced anesthesia."

Two other NMDAR antagonists are worth mentioning: amantadine and memantine. Amantadine is used in influenza and Parkinson disease. Memantine is FDA approved for moderate to severe Alzheimer disease. Memantine is an NMDAR antagonist with comparable potency to ketamine.[2,4] While there is some nonapproved medical use of these substances (especially memantine), it is largely for "self-medication" or claimed nootropic (cognitive enhancing effects) rather than for any intoxicating effect.[26] Memantine will cause clear dissociative effects even at low doses and can cause potent dissociative and hallucinogenic effects at higher doses (eg, 100 mg). The reason for the unpopularity of memantine and amantadine for their intoxicating properties is unknown though the long duration of action (over 24 hours) may be one factor. Though other explanations are likely. Both agents should be explored as potential replacement therapies for those with severe dissociative use disorder. Likewise further research on the underlying differences could provide valuable insight for future drug development of NMDAR antagonists with reduced misuse liability.

EPIDEMIOLOGY

Unhealthy or recreational PCP use may be more a problem in large cities than in the rest of the United States.[27] Ketamine is often used alone as well as with other drugs[28,29] and its nonmedical use is popular all over the world, particularly in Asian countries.[30]

DXM is considered one of the most common recreationally used over-the-counter medications in the United States and was first included in the Monitoring the Future epidemiological surveys in 2006. The proportion of U.S. students who reported in 2006 having used DXM during the prior year for the expressed purpose of "getting high" was 4%, 5%, and 7% in grades 8, 10, and 12, respectively.[31] Rates in 2011 were similar, at 3%, 6%, and 5%, respectively.[32] In 2015 rates dropped slightly (2%, 3%, 5%).[33] Poison Control Center data from the first half of the 2000 to 2010 decade reflected increasing recreational DXM use, particularly among adolescents.[34] For example, cases of DXM use reported to the California Poison Control System[35] increased 10-fold in all age groups and 15-fold in adolescents between 1999 and 2004. Similar trends were seen in national databases. Approximately 75% of California cases were aged 9 to 17 years. The highest frequency of use was in 15- to 16-year-olds. The most commonly used DXM product was Coricidin HBP Cough & Cold Tablets. The extent of DXM recreational use is likely far greater than what has been reported, because only the most severe cases are reported to poison control databases, and nearly all routine drug screening kits still do not screen or test for DXM or DXO. Studies of DXM in blood samples of suspected impaired drivers in the state of Wisconsin between 1999 and 2005 also supported an increasing prevalence of DXM-positive drivers, with a mean concentration of 207 ng/mL, compared with an expected therapeutic concentration range of 0.5 to 5.9 ng/mL (the highest concentrations being in males aged 16-20 years).[36] Intentional use of Coricidin products reported to the Illinois Poison Center occurred primarily among adolescents and was associated with significant short-term clinical effects and $353,314 in-hospital charges annually (2001-2006).[37] A 2004-2013 observational study of another national poison control database supports that cough medicines remain the most commonly reported drug class for intentional unhealthy drug ingestion among all years and regions for adolescents.[38]

The annual rate of single-substance DXM use calls peaked in 2006 and then decreased 56.3% from 2006 to 2015 among adolescents 14 to 17 years from 143.8 to 80.9 calls per million population.[25] This is likely in part due to a trend of many U.S. states implementing age restrictions on purchasing of DXM products and illustrates the potential for rational drug regulation policies to have a positive impact on adolescent drug use.

PHARMACOKINETICS

PCP is a lipophilic (logP = 5.1) weak base (pKa = 8.5) that readily crosses the blood-brain barrier.[3] Blood PCP concentrations ranging from 10 to 180 ng/mL (mean = 73.3 ng/mL) were found in 50 persons believed to be driving under the influence.[39] The plasma half-life (t½) of PCP has been reported to vary from 7 to 46 hours, suggesting the influence of dose and/or multiphase elimination processes.[3] A terminal PCP elimination phase (gamma) t½ of 1 to 4 days has been reported in cases of severe PCP poisoning.[10] PCP is biotransformed in the liver to several metabolites excreted in the urine as both free and glucuronide conjugates.[4] Acidification of the urine increases its renal clearance as PCP is a weak base. However, this intervention is no longer recommended clinically because of the risk of increasing urinary myoglobin precipitation.[39]

Ketamine is a moderately lipophilic (logP: 2.18) weak base (pKa: 7.5)[4] which readily crosses the blood-brain barrier. Bioavailability varies by route of administration (see **Table 19-1**). It is important to point out that bioavailability and potency,

TABLE 19-1 Bioavailability of Ketamine in Humans by Route of Administration

Route of administration	% Bioavailability (relative to IV)
Intravenous (IV)	100%
Intramuscular (IM)	93%[40]
Subcutaneous (SC)	75%-95%[41]
Oral (PO)	20%[40]
Intranasal (IN)	50%[40] 48% (esketamine) (Spravato)
Sublingual (SL)	30%[40] 29%[42]
Rectal (PR)	25%[43]
Transdermal	~0% (systemic absorption)[44] *likely to depend on vehicle

while often related, can differ. For example, potency of a drug effect will also be influenced by the rate of absorption which affects PK parameters like C_{max} (max plasma concentration) and T_{max} (time to max plasma concentration). Ketamine follows a three-phase plasma pharmacokinetic model when given intravenously.[10,45] There is a brief initial (alpha) phase with t½ of about 7 minutes because of rapid distribution, followed by a longer elimination (beta) phase. The elimination t½ of ketamine has been reported from 79.8 to 186 minutes.[43,46-48]

As used in general anesthesia, an intravenous dose of 2.0 mg/kg produces rapid induction. This dose produces an onset in 30 seconds, with the loss of consciousness lasting for 8 to 10 minutes. The intramuscular injection of ketamine has a latency of 3 to 5 minutes and a duration of 20 minutes or more, depending on the dose administered.

Ketamine is extensively metabolized producing a large number of phase I and II metabolites. The cytochrome P450 enzymes CYP3A4, CYP2B6 and CYP2C9 are especially relevant.[43] Potential for drug-drug or drug-food (eg, grapefruit) interactions involving ketamine through CYP metabolism exists.[49,50] There may also be genetic variability in ketamine metabolism due to CYP variants.[51] Research has shown ketamine interacts, albeit weakly, with various biological transporters which may influence its bioavailability.[52] Relevant metabolites include norketamine, dehydronorketamine, and various hydroxynorketamine metabolites.[4] Differences in the metabolism of *R*- and *S*-ketamine are known.[4] Excretion of ketamine is largely through urinary excretion of metabolites.[4]

The pharmacokinetics of DXM and its metabolites has recently been reviewed.[53] DXM is readily absorbed from the gut following oral ingestion. Peak serum levels are reached at 2 to 3 hours for immediate release and 6 hours for sustained release oral preparations. The major metabolite from *O*-demethylation, DXO, shows peak levels at 1.5 to 3 hours.[53] Metabolism is largely due to CYP2D6 and a lesser extent CYP3A4.[54] Humans have a genetic polymorphism for the biotransformation of DXM.[6] Rapid metabolizers have a plasma elimination t½ of about 3.4 hours, and slow metabolizers may have t½ exceeding 24 hours. Slow metabolizers of DXM represent about 10% to 15% of the population. Both *O*- and *N*-demethylation of DXM occur, with the *N*-demethylated version also having antitussive effects. Subsequent biotransformation results in various less potent compounds with respect to known pharmacological effects. Phenotypic "slow" metabolizers of DXM report fewer intoxication effects than normal subjects.[55]

A combination drug product containing DXM and quinidine (Nuedexta) is FDA approved for pseudobulbar affect. The rationale for the addition of quinidine is that quinidine inhibits CYP2D6 metabolism of DXM, elevating bioavailability, plasma levels (up to 20-fold) and extending the t½.[53] A similar product Auvelity, containing DXM and CYP2D6 inhibitor bupropion was recently approved by the FDA for major depressive disorder (MDD) in adults.

PHARMACODYNAMICS

A number of studies have explored ketamine's receptor pharmacology. While sometimes ketamine is called a "dirty drug" this is misleading. In fact, several studies have consistently found that ketamine is quite selective (at least 2 orders of magnitude) at physiologically relevant concentrations for NMDARs.[56-59]

NMDARs are ionotropic glutamate channels implicated in learning, memory, synaptic signaling and processing, synaptic plasticity, and more.[2-4] Structurally NMDARs are tetramers; composed of four protein subunits. These subunits come from three separate families called NR1, NR2, and NR3. There are various ways in which these may be combined, giving rise to distinct NMDARs; each seemingly with unique physiological properties and distributions.[60] Ketamine inhibits NMDARs by binding to a site inside the channel pore called the PCP binding site; by doing so it physically blocks the channel pore of the active-open NMDAR channel, in a manner referred to as uncompetitive inhibition.[4] Recently, structures of ketamine bound to the PCP site of different NMDAR subtypes were solved using cryo-EM.[61] Interestingly ketamine and some other channel blockers, have shown selectivity in inhibiting NR2C containing NMDARs, and to a lesser extent NR2D containing NMDARs.[62] Inhibition of NR2C containing NMDARs are hypothesized to underlie some of the acute psychoactive effects of ketamine.[63]

There is strong evidence to support the role of NMDARs in mediating the classical dissociative and hallucinogenic actions of ketamine and related dissociatives.[2-4,64]

At higher concentrations of ketamine (typically >10 μM), additional interactions will occur including binding to opioid receptors, monoamine transporters and sigma receptors.[4,59] Given these interactions only seem to reach significant degrees with high μM concentrations of ketamine, it is unclear the extent to which direct interactions have clinical significance in humans at the standard doses of ketamine used.[4,65]

Unfortunately, data on ketamine CSF levels in humans could not be readily found. However, extensive evidence on blood/plasma levels exist allowing some predictions. Plasma levels of ketamine can reach fairly high μM concentrations within the first minute following IV administration of anesthetic doses, however these levels quickly drop and stabilize, following distribution, to 10 μM or less.[45,46,66] Studies have shown patients start to recover consciousness from anesthesia between 1 and 4 μM.[45,46,67,68] The estimated plasma concentration of ketamine required for approximately 50% NMDAR occupancy in humans, was 1.42 μM.[69] Brain concentrations of *S*-ketamine at antidepressant doses were estimated to be around 0.4 μM.[65] Thus it seems likely that direct interactions with NMDARs are the major contributor to the actions of ketamine, with the exceptions of a brief time period following high anesthetic doses.

Despite this selectivity for NMDARs, there is evidence that NMDAR inhibition by ketamine leads to complex systemic effects throughout the CNS affecting the activity of countless other neurotransmitters and signaling molecules. Such complex effects will of course be species and dose dependent as well as show variance in location and through time. One must also consider the impact of the environment (past and present) on the state of CNS at the time of administration and measurement. To illustrate the complexity of this issue, ketamine has been reported to alter levels of virtually every neurotransmitter and hormonal system people have looked at. This includes glutamate,[70,71] GABA,[72] serotonin,[73] norepinephrine,[73,74] dopamine,[75-77] acetylcholine,[78] adenosine,[79] BDNF,[80] histamine,[81] nitric oxide,[82] and cortisol.[76]

Making sense of this complex information is challenging and is likely one reason new yet questionable hypotheses on ketamine's mechanism of action are reported regularly. There is strong evidence that elevations in glutamate are particularly relevant to the acute psychoactive effects of dissociative drugs,[71,83-85] and possibly antidepressant actions of ketamine.[86] With the leading hypothesis on ketamine's mechanism of action in both cases resulting from inhibition of GABAergic interneurons (via inhibiting NR2C containing NMDARs) which leads to disinhibition of excitatory glutamatergic neurons, especially pyramidal neurons, in various subcortical and cortical regions.[87] Consistent with elevated glutamatergic output, ketamine has been observed to enhance gamma band electroencephalography power, which may be related to cortical disinhibition.[88,89] In depression, it is hypothesized that this elevated glutamate signaling activates AMPA glutamate receptors, leading to BDNF release and activation of various signaling pathways (eg, mTOR) leading to synaptogenesis and neuritogenesis, countering deficits in depression.[90] However, many other drugs (eg, cocaine) have similar actions in this respect, seemingly without the same antidepressant effects[91] and it must be pointed out that countless other hypotheses exist.[92-94] In fact, virtually everything ketamine is observed to do seems to be hypothesized to mediate its antidepressant effects. Interestingly a clinical study in which subjects were pretreated with the mTOR inhibitor rapamycin prior to antidepressant doses of ketamine found potentiation of the antidepressant response rather than attenuation.[95] In preclinical models rapamycin attenuates the synaptogenesis and behavioral response in rodent models of depression.[90] The reason for this discrepancy is unclear and more research is required.

Ketamine contains a chiral carbon, which means that it can exist in two mirror image stereoisomer forms; called *R*-ketamine and *S*-ketamine (based on the spatial arrangement of the molecule). These forms are referred to as enantiomers.[96] Unless specified the term ketamine usually refers to the racemic form which is a 50:50 mixture of *R*- and *S*-ketamine. Ketamine (racemic) is approved as a general anesthetic in the United States and is the form most encountered in illicit markets. More recently *S*-ketamine, was approved in the United States and Europe for treatment resistant depression and major depression disorder (MDD) associated with suicidality.[97-99] *S*-ketamine is also an approved general anesthetic in Europe. Racemic and *S*-ketamine appear to exhibit comparable clinical profiles including treatment outcomes in depression.[100] In a recent phase 2a trial in TRD, *R*-ketamine failed to distinguish from placebo at the primary endpoint.

S-ketamine is about 2 to 5 times more potent than *R*-ketamine as an NMDAR antagonist.[74,101,102] Consistent with the higher NMDAR affinity, *S*-ketamine is a more potent dissociative in animals including humans than *R*-ketamine or racemic ketamine.[59,103-105] While claims have been made that *R*-ketamine lacks the same pharmacological effects as *S*- or racemic ketamine, especially with respect to *R*-ketamine lacking dissociative effects and risk for recreational use,[59,106] when doses used are equipotent for NMDAR antagonism there appears to be little difference across humans and other species including dissociative effects as well as behavioral models predictive of nonmedical use liability.[4,65,105,107]

When considering the pharmacological action of ketamine, its metabolites must be considered. Over 20 phase-I metabolites of ketamine are known.[108] The major metabolite that is likely of clinical relevance, given the plasma levels observed and known pharmacology, is norketamine, resulting from *N*-demethylaton.[4] Norketamine is a less potent NMDAR antagonist relative to ketamine.[109] Like ketamine it appears to be largely selective for NMDARs over other common CNS binding sites.[58] As with ketamine, *S*-norketamine is the more potent enantiomer as an NMDAR antagonist.[109] Other metabolites of interest are dehydronorketamine (DHNK) and a number of hydroxynorketamine (HNK) isomers, which may have activities independent of NMDAR antagonism.[92,109]

Clinical Pharmacology

Depending on dose and the specific arylcyclohexylamine ingested, patients who have taken a dissociative like PCP or ketamine present with widely different neurological and psychiatric signs and symptoms. These signs and symptoms can be generally subdivided into three major clinical pictures: (1) confusion, delirium, and psychosis; (2) semicoma and coma; and (3) coma with seizures. Patients may become progressively more obtunded and eventually comatose, or the reverse, with the patient emerging from coma and exhibiting emergence delirium. **Table 19-2** lists the various signs and symptoms of PCP intoxication at different intravenous doses. Common clinical presentations with ketamine intoxication include hallucinations, altered mental status, mydriasis, nystagmus, tachycardia and hypertension.[4] **Figure 19-2** shows the predicted molecular target sites with doses, concentrations, and clinical effects.[110] Most people who use dissociatives like PCP and ketamine do not grossly overdose themselves to the point of semicoma and coma. Hence, most patients intoxicated with dissociatives leading to medical intervention show a clinical picture of confusion, delirium, and psychosis. Rats show marked behavioral sensitization to both PCP and MK-801, with asymmetric cross-sensitization.[111-113] The significance of this phenomenon for humans is unknown. Whether individuals who use PCP or ketamine show enhanced psychotomimetic effects over time is also unknown. Tolerance occurs with PCP and to a greater degree with continuous dosing.[114] Animal models show severe withdrawal symptoms after cessation of repeated PCP exposure: vocalizations, bruxism, oculomotor hyperactivity, diarrhea, piloerection, somnolence, tremor, and seizures.[115] However, human dissociative withdrawal is not formally recognized by the Diagnostic and Statistical Manual, and human evidence remains limited.[116,117]

Ketamine induces a general anesthetic state in a dose-dependent manner. A minimum of 0.5 mg/kg intravenously is necessary to induce loss of consciousness for approximately 1.5 minutes. A dose of 1.0 mg/kg induces loss of consciousness for approximately 5.8 minutes, whereas a dose of 2.0 mg/kg induces a loss of consciousness for approximately 10 minutes.

During and after slow intravenous administration of 2.0 mg/kg ketamine, the following sequence of eye signs is observed: blinking, staring, closure of lids, nystagmus, strabismus, and loss of lid reflex. Initially, when the patient falls into a dissociative or cataleptic state, the eyelids are widely open and horizontal or vertical nystagmus is seen. Later, the eyeballs become centrally fixed in a gaze. During this stage, both somatosensory and visual stimulation elicit evoked potentials in the cortex. This finding supports the contention that the patient's brain cannot interpret the afferent impulses because of the disruption of the normal connections of the sensory cortex with association areas. The persistence of open eyes distinguishes ketamine-induced anesthesia from that caused by other intravenous and inhalational anesthetics or coma-producing substances. This dissociation between eye signs and anesthetic or coma depth is one of the major disadvantages of ketamine as an anesthetic agent because eye signs cannot be used to gauge the depth of anesthesia.

Adverse long-term chronic psychological effects include dysphoria, impaired memory and cognition, apathy, and irritability,[118] as well as distortion in the subjective experience of time.[119] Such adverse effects are dependent on dosages and the frequency of use. Physical dependence and discontinuation syndromes have been described with ketamine[120-122] but this needs further study. Ketamine associated deaths, while rare, have been reported however in general have involved behavioral toxicity or polydrug use.[4]

TABLE 19-2 Dose-Related Effects of PCP in Healthy Subjects

Total dose by intravenous infusion	1 mg	2 mg	7 mg	7-10 mg	14 mg	17.5 mg	35 mg	70 mg
mg/70kg	0.014	0.03	0.1		0.2	0.25	0.5	1
Subjective effects	+	+						
Nystagmus			+					
Gait ataxia			+					
Increased blood pressure			+					
Confusional state			+					
Theta slowing (EEG)			±	±				
Anesthesia-analgesia (loss of consciousness, no response to painful or auditory stimuli)					–	+		
Amnesia						+		
Purposeless movements (state of agitation)							+	
Muscle rigidity and extensor posturing (severe rigidity and catatonia)								+
Seizure activity								+
Respiration depression								–

Data summarized by Burns RS, Lerner SE. Chapter 21: The effects of phencyclidine in man: a review. In: Domino EF, ed. *Phencyclidine: Historical and Current Perspectives*. NPP Books; 1981:450. (From Ries RK, Fiellin DA, Miller SC, Saitz R, eds. *Principles of Addiction Medicine*. 5th ed. Lippincott Williams & Wilkins; 2014. Table 15-1.)

In the past several decades a large number of so-called "legal high" or "research chemical" dissociatives have been encountered.[2-4] Many of these compounds are β-keto-arylcyclohexylamines that are structurally similar to ketamine (eg, deschloroketamine or DCK, 2-oxo-PCE, and 2-fluorodeschloroketamine or FDCK), or arylcyclohexylamines and structurally similar to PCP (eg, 3-MeO-PCP, 4-MeO-PCP, 3-MeO-PCE, 3-Cl-PCP, 3,4-MD-PCP, 3-MeO-PCMo and 3-Me-PCPy). Another common structural class are the 1,2-diarylethylamines represented by diphenidine and ephenidine. All these compounds exhibit similar pharmacodynamics being NMDAR antagonists, and in general exert classic dissociative effects as well as similar clinical presentations in humans. Although specific compounds do have unique pharmacological aspects that may be clinically relevant.[3,4]

Dextromethorphan

The history of nonmedical use of DXM, beginning in the 1960s, has been reviewed.[2] The pharmacodynamics of DXM and its metabolites has been recently reviewed.[53] DXM and its active metabolite DXO are moderate potency NMDAR antagonists.[53] This pharmacology along with reported subjective effects are consistent with the classification of DXM as a dissociative drug. Interestingly, DXO is a more potent NMDA receptor antagonist than DXM,[53] though exhibits reduced BBB penetration.[123] Like DXM, DXO is relatively inactive at the mu, kappa, and delta opioid receptors; thus, it is essentially devoid of the more conventional opiate properties, although respiratory depression has been reported with massive ingestion.[124]

In addition, DXM has significant serotonergic properties, including increasing the synthesis and release of serotonin, as well as inhibiting the reuptake of serotonin from the synaptic cleft.[53] DXM in clinical therapeutic doses is well tolerated and produces relatively few side effects. These

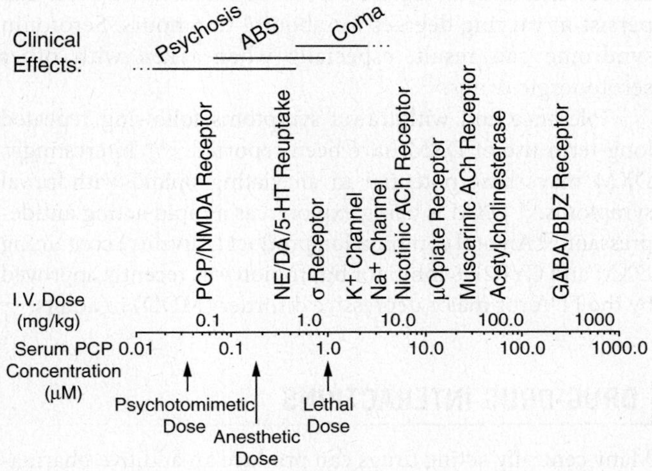

Figure 19-2. PCP doses, serum concentrations, molecular target sites, and clinical effects.

TABLE 19-3 Characteristics of the DXM Intoxication Syndrome

Psychotomimetic	Neurological	General
Auditory hallucinations	Slurred speech	Nausea
Visual hallucinations	Ataxia	Vomiting
Tactile hallucinations	Mydriasis	Diaphoresis
Hyperexcitability	Blurry vision	Hypertension
Pressure of thought	Bidirectional nystagmus	Respiratory suppression[a]
Lethargy	Hypertonia	Coma[a]
Nervousness	Choreoathetoid movements	Fatality[a]
Euphoria	Dystonic movements	
Confusion/disorientation	Dyskinesia	
Altered time perception	Restlessness	
Paranoia	Tremor	
Feeling of "floating"	Hyperreflexia	
Heightened perceptual awareness	Seizures[a]	

[a]Condition occurs only rarely.

From Bobo WV, Miller SC, Martin BD. The abuse liability of dextromethorphan among adolescents: a review. *J Child Adolesc Subst Abuse* 2005;14(4):55-75. (From Ries RK, Fiellin DA, Miller SC, Saitz R, eds. *Principles of Addiction Medicine*. 5th ed. Lippincott Williams & Wilkins; 2014. Table 15-2.)

include body rash, itching, nausea, and vomiting and are most likely when DXM is combined with the other ingredients in cough preparations. Depending on dose, the drug can cause drowsiness, dizziness, altered vision, cardiovascular, and significant central nervous system effects that may resemble PCP intoxication. Dissociative effects including euphoria and hallucinations can occur within 15 to 30 minutes of ingestion of intoxicating doses, with peak effects experienced after roughly 2.5 hours. Clinical effects of DXM are summarized in **Table 19-3**.[11] The intoxication state can persist in varying degrees for about 3 to 6 hours. Serotonin syndrome can result, especially when taken with other serotonergic drugs.[125]

Tolerance and withdrawal symptoms following repeated long-term use of DXM have been reported.[21,126] Interestingly, DXM may show potential in alleviating opioid withdrawal symptoms.[127] DXM is being explored as a rapid acting antidepressant.[128] An oral combination product (Auvelity) containing DXM and CYP2D6 inhibitor bupropion was recently approved by the FDA for major depressive disorder (MDD) in adults.

DRUG-DRUG INTERACTIONS

Many centrally acting drugs can produce an additive pharmacodynamic interaction with all of the agents described herein. Therapeutic combinations of ketamine with benzodiazepines reduce its emergence delirium with anesthetic use. Clonidine and related alpha-adrenergic agonists such as dexmedetomidine have also been given clinically with ketamine to reduce its dissociative effects.

As mentioned, DXM can induce a serotonin syndrome when taken with monoamine oxidase inhibitors, selective serotonin reuptake inhibitors, or other serotonergically active substances. Genetic polymorphism in the biotransformation of DXM via CYP2D6 may enhance the toxicity of the former by inhibitors of the latter. These include many drugs such as chlorpromazine, delavirdine, fluoxetine, miconazole, paroxetine, pergolide, quinidine, quinine, ritonavir, and ropinirole, as well as acute ingestion of large amounts of alcohol. Many DXM preparations contain other additives, and this can lead to adverse interactions if taken at higher doses.

NEUROBIOLOGY

The action of arylcyclohexylamines on NMDARs was first described by Anis et al.[129] NMDAR antagonism has come to be the leading hypothesis to explain the subjective and clinical action of dissociative drugs.[3,4,64] Alternative mechanisms involving biogenic amines and sigma-binding sites were suggested but have been largely disproven.[4,64,130-132] This important discovery stimulated interest in the role of glutamate in schizophrenia and related psychotic disorders.[133-135] Krystal et al.[136-140] were especially active in studying ketamine and glutamatergic antagonists in human volunteers, which ultimately led to the serendipitous discovery of ketamine's antidepressant properties.[1]

Imaging data (SPECT) show that ketamine-induced antagonism of the NMDARs is directly correlated with negative symptoms of schizophrenia (assessed with the Brief Psychiatric Rating Scale [BPRS] negative subscale), suggesting that dissociatives induce negative symptoms via NMDAR antagonism.[141] It has also been hypothesized that dissociatives induce positive symptoms via enhancing glutamate release. As discussed by Deakin et al.,[84] Olney and Farber[142] previously suggested that NMDAR antagonists block excitation of gamma aminobutyric acid (GABA) interneurons,[143] resulting in disinhibition of cholinergic, serotonergic, and glutamatergic afferents to the posterior retrosplenial cingulate cortex. Subsequent studies using in vivo microdialysis confirmed that the administration of NMDA antagonists increased glutamate release in the frontal cortex. Moreover, mGluR2 (metabotropic glutamate 2/3 receptor) agonists, acting presynaptically to decrease the release of glutamate, reverse the behavioral effects of PCP in rats.[70] Lamotrigine and nimodipine both attenuate dissociative effects of ketamine in humans, likely through blockade of glutamate release.[83,144]

Subanesthetic ketamine administration induces a rapid, focal decrease in ventromedial frontal cortex regional blood oxygenation level–dependent (BOLD) fMRI signals that strongly correlate with its dissociative effects. Ketamine also significantly increased BOLD activity in the mid-posterior cingulate, thalamus, and temporal cortical regions—increases correlated with BPRS psychosis scores.[84] Pretreatment with lamotrigine (a sodium channel blocker that decreases glutamate release) prevented many of the BOLD changes and increases in BPRS psychosis scores. Thus, dissociatives may induce certain subjective effects that have similarities to positive symptoms via enhancing glutamate release.[84] In humans, subanesthetic doses of ketamine show prominent alterations of consciousness that correlate with suppressed EEG alpha power that is source-localized to the precuneus and temporal-parietal junction. Given the involvement of temporal-parietal loci in multisensory integration and body representation, this region is a candidate for generating the tactile hallucinations as well as an "out-of-body" experience induced by ketamine and other dissociatives.[145] Moreover, a recent study identified a low frequency (1- to 3-Hz) oscillation in the deep posteromedial cortex (analogous to the mouse retrosplenial cortex) induced by ketamine, PCP, and MK-801 in mice that was claimed to underlie states of dissociation though this may be more of a measure of general sedation and more research is needed.[146]

Ketamine is widely used for depression in clinical settings, where potential adverse effects are mild, but include intoxication, hypertension, nausea, and tachycardia.[147] A precise unifying mechanism for the rapid antidepressant action of ketamine remains elusive, partly due to the complexity of the central nervous system and limitations of currently used "animal models" of depression. Ketamine's high affinity for NMDARs directed much of the early mechanistic focus, however a number of other NMDAR antagonists failed to show promise in clinical development.[92,148-152] However, it is notable that in all cases, nondissociative doses were used, whereas ketamine only shows efficacy in depression at doses that induce a clear dissociative intoxication comparable in intensity to several alcoholic beverages. Thus, it is likely that inadequate target engagement of NMDARs occurred in these other studies. Alternative mechanisms involving mTOR signaling, monoamines, opioids, cannabinoids, as well as sigma, acetylcholine and AMPA receptors, and calcium and hyperpolarization-activated cyclic nucleotide-gated (HCN) ion channels have been proposed—in fact almost everything ketamine has been observed to do pharmacologically has been proposed to mediate its antidepressant effects creating much confusion.[153-155] Ketamine-mediated blockade of NMDA receptors at rest, resulting in release of BDNF has gained much attention[156] though most psychoactive drugs are known to affect BDNF release in similar ways to ketamine; this is not surprising given it is a ubiquitous neurotrophin regulating neuronal connectivity.[157]

The action of nitrous oxide as an NMDAR antagonist is another major advance in our knowledge[158-160] that may have clinical applications for psychiatry.[161-163] Whether NMDAR antagonism plays a primary role in the action of nitrous oxide at recreational or "subanesthetic" concentrations remains controversial.[164-166] Nitrous oxide interacts with a wide range of molecular targets, weakly inhibiting numerous ion channels, and weakly potentiating glycine and GABA-A receptors.[167] Nitrous oxide is often used nonmedically for its euphoric and anxiolytic effects.[168] Nitrous oxide may exert some of its action through opioid receptors either via release of endogenous opioid peptides or through direct action as a partial agonist at the opioid receptors.[169-171]

Substance Use Disorder Liability

In addition to euphoria, dissociatives can induce an experience of floating in space, dissociation, sensory isolation, tactile and visual hallucinations and altered thought patterns. Dissociatives are self-administered by animals. Rhesus monkeys self-administer PCP, and social stimulation among monkeys in adjoining cages enhances the reinforcing strength of PCP.[172] A recent study in rats observed that with comparable doses, *S*-ketamine was more strongly self-administered than *R*-ketamine (likely a dose effect); interestingly animals showed rapid extinction of self-administration suggesting differences in the reinforcing actions relative to other commonly used drugs like opioids and psychostimulants.[59] Rodent and primate animal studies of DXM support reinforcement by DXO, akin to PCP. DXM is self-administered by animals.[173] DXM dissociative use disorder and risk of recurrence has been studied[174] though more research is needed. A variety of mechanisms have been proposed but not confirmed for its ability to cause a dissociative use disorder, and further research is needed.

Very little work has been done to develop medications to treat dissociative use disorder.[175] As mentioned previously memantine and amantadine should be explored further for potential utility here. Furthermore, harm reduction strategies and education can reduce some of the negative consequences around dissociative use (including overdose and fatal drug-drug interactions), while also reducing the stigma for those seeking treatment.

Toxicity/Adverse Effects

Since the 1970s, when Olney described the neurotoxic effects of glutamate, reducing its excess has been a target for brain-protective agents. NMDAR antagonists have remarkable effects on brain neurons under some experimental conditions,[176] including toxicity,[177] that can be reduced or prevented.[178] For example, these agents induce significant vesicular changes (termed Olney lesions) in rat brain posterior cingulate retrosplenial neurons. Interestingly not all species of animals show these changes and the relationship of such neurotoxicity to humans, especially those who engage in high dose use of dissociatives remains unclear. Such neurotoxic changes observed experimentally are reduced by pretreatment with benzodiazepines, supporting the mechanism of NMDA antagonists blocking GABA interneuron activity, leading to disinhibition of cholinergic, serotonergic, and glutamatergic afferents—resulting in excitotoxicity. However, Olney lesions are not evident following DXM administration in rats.[179] Repeated high-dose administration of DXM during adolescence in rats may induce permanent deficits in cognitive function; increased expression of NMDAR NR1 subunits in the prefrontal cortex and hippocampus may play a role in

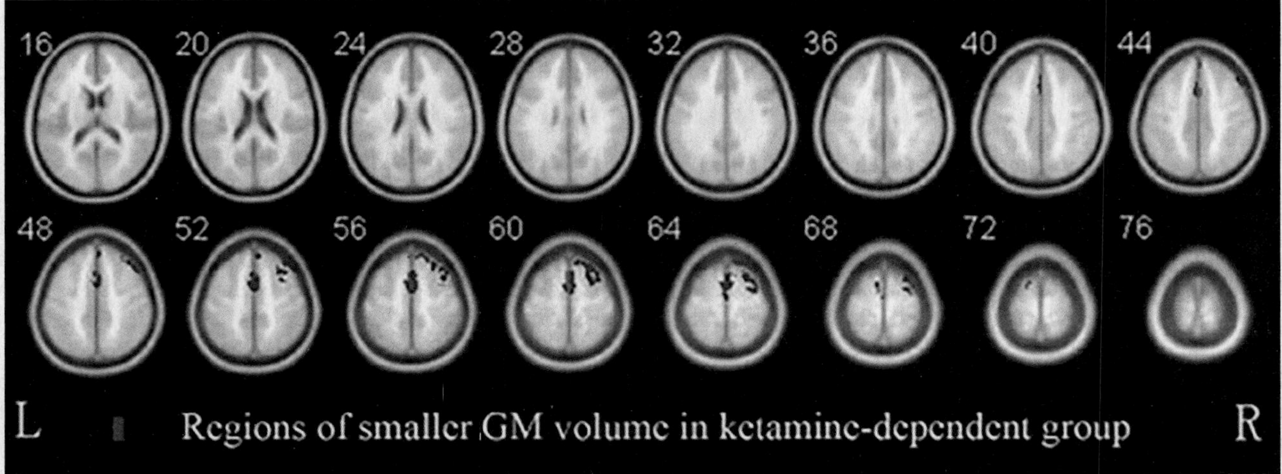

Figure 19-3. Brain maps of representative axial slices showing the differences of gray matter (GM) volume between the ketamine-use group and control group. Voxels of reduced GM volume in bilateral frontal cortex, including left superior frontal. (From Liao Y, et al. Reduced dorsal prefrontal gray matter after chronic ketamine use. *Biol Psychiatry.* 2011;69(1):42-48.)

DXM-induced memory deficits.[180] The significance of this in humans is however unclear. In addition to experimental challenges to translatability of experimental models, such research is highly politically and socially charged making reliable conclusions difficult.

High dose and frequent dissociative use do appear to lead to cognitive complications which are likely reversible. For example, studies in humans have shown impairments in working and episodic memory, among other cognitive problems, correlating with ketamine exposure levels.[181] Further supporting problems with working memory and other cognitive issues, people who use ketamine chronically, compared to controls, show less bilateral dorsal prefrontal gray matter, with duration of use negatively correlating with gray matter volume and estimated total lifetime consumption of ketamine negatively correlating with gray matter volume in the left superior frontal gyrus[182] (see **Fig. 19-3**). This same research group found white matter abnormalities in bilateral frontal and left temporoparietal cortices, with anisotropy values negatively correlating with the total lifetime ketamine consumption, suggesting pathology of the white matter/axons in these brain regions[183] (see **Fig. 19-4**) however cause and effect cannot be determined easily.

Nitrous oxide displays neuroprotective effects at physiological concentrations and neurotoxic effects at higher concentrations. Heavy use of nitrous oxide can deplete vitamin B_{12}[184,185] and the resulting deficiency may lead to neuropathy.[186,187] The mechanisms and long-term neurological sequelae of nitrous oxide-induced vitamin B_{12} deficiency deserve further investigation.

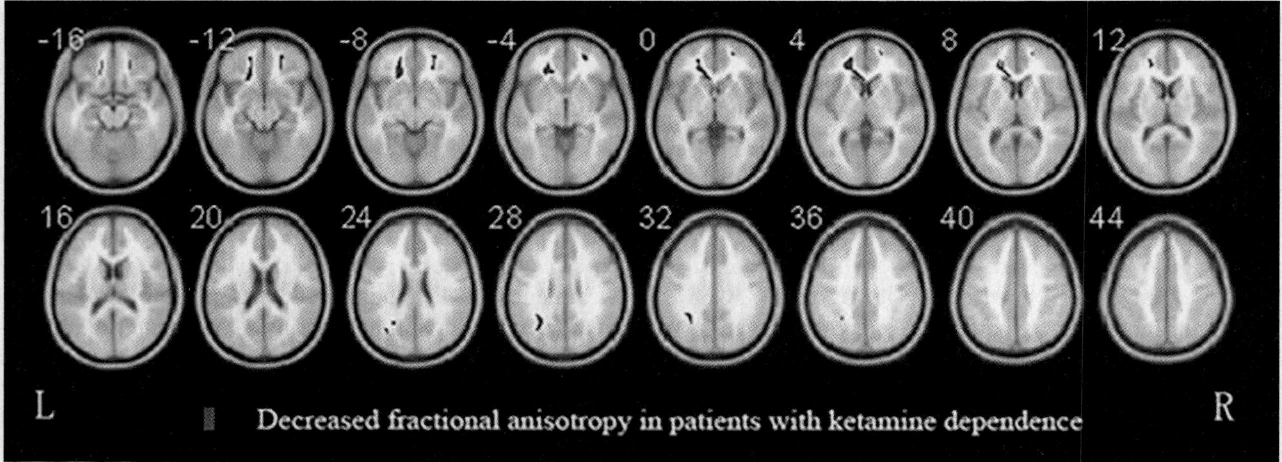

Figure 19-4. Brain maps of representative axial slices showing regions of abnormal fractional anisotropy in patients with ketamine use in relation to healthy comparison subjects. (From Liao Y, et al. Frontal white matter abnormalities following chronic ketamine use: a diffusion tensor imaging study. *Brain.* 2010;133(7):2115-2122.)

Intoxication and Overdose

Intoxication is discussed in greater detail in Section 7 of this book. Although a preliminary diagnosis of arylcyclohexylamine intoxication can be made on the basis of history, clinical signs, and symptoms, confirmation of exposure via a drug-positive blood or urine specimen is helpful. Most clinically used drug screening panels include PCP and/or ketamine but not most of the other agents discussed herein; thus, a request may be required for specialized testing. A large variety of different chemical assays are available, but gas chromatography-mass spectrometry is often ideal for confirmation.[188] The prevalence of novel psychoactive substance (NPS) dissociatives fueled by prohibition, greatly complicates the job of those identifying these substances in patients. Such knowledge is timely and can be lifesaving. It is worth noting that a number of commercial immunoassays show cross reactivity to certain dissociative NPS, suggesting value in such screenings as a preliminary approach. Likewise, development of more ubiquitous immunoassays for drug classes could have clinical value.

Cases of intoxication with PCP, ketamine, and various dissociative NPS have been described.[3,4] Serum skeletal creatinine phosphokinase levels are often increased, and the urine can contain myoglobin because of rhabdomyolysis. End-organ kidney damage may result.

The first step in the differential diagnosis of arylcyclohexylamine intoxication is identifying whether the patient is in coma with or without seizures, emerging from coma, descending into coma, or in a psychotic state. The patient in coma—with or without seizures—has a differential diagnosis that includes all other causes of coma and seizures. The history and laboratory analysis are crucial. This is further discussed in Section 7 of this book.

Psychotic manifestations of arylcyclohexylamine poisoning can be confused with catatonic schizophrenia, an acute toxic psychosis induced by other hallucinogens, and various acute organic brain syndromes. Dissociative intoxication can induce an organic brain syndrome, as well as cardiovascular (often tachycardia and hypertension) and renal complications that are seldom, if ever, seen with other psychiatric syndromes. With heavy ketamine use, lower urinary tract symptoms may exist, including severe pain, frequency, hematuria, dysuria and cystitis.[189] Distortions in body representation such as a floating feeling also can suggest dissociative use. DXM is associated with psychosis at doses greater than 300 to 600 mg or in fast metabolizers.[21] Psychosis-like signs and symptoms may occur at lower doses when DXM is combined with other drugs such as alcohol. Folate deficiency may also be associated with unhealthy DXM use.[190] Unhealthy DXM use may result in brain damage, seizure, loss of consciousness, irregular heart beat,[191] serotonin syndrome and death especially if taken with other drugs. Respiratory depression from DXM may be reversed with naloxone.[192] An evidence-based consensus guideline for out-of-hospital management of DXM toxicity is available,[193] as are other sources.[194]

Dissociatives include an array of compounds sharing antagonist activity at the NMDA receptors (among other actions on the human brain) and resulting in a clinical syndrome involving dissociation or disconnection of the brain from its external sensory input and altered internal processes. Such a disconnect is one of the many effects described by people who use dissociatives as the desired end state; however, it is not uncommon for people to exceed the dosing required for these effects, especially without adequate education or from use of impure or mislabeled unregulated chemicals resulting in serious untoward psychiatric and medical effects. It is often only then that such patients present for medical assistance. Antidotes or other effective treatments do not yet exist for these compounds, making supportive care the only treatment modality. The potential for developing substance use disorders with dissociatives and long-term consequences of high dose use requires further exploration, particularly in light of FDA-approval for certain more severe types of depression and suicidal ideation, increasing off-label use of the racemic compound including home use by patients with less prescriber supervision than outlined in the FDA REMS program, and increasing off-label use for certain psychiatric and neurological disorders. However, it is important that a rational and evidence based approach is taken, rather than the highly biased approach to this question of the past decades. The evaluation of this drug class for therapeutic qualities will likely prove increasingly fruitful. This is exemplified with the recent discovery of the rapid antidepressant qualities of ketamine and esketamine providing new treatments for depression. Interest in the potential of other NMDAR antagonists like DXM[195] and other dissociatives is growing. Finally, the prevalence and significance of unhealthy DXM use is concerning, particularly for the concentrated involvement of young people who appear largely unaware of its potential risks and may be at elevated risk of lasting consequences from chronic use.

REFERENCES

1. Krystal JH, Perry EB Jr, Gueorguieva R, et al. Comparative and interactive human psychopharmacologic effects of ketamine and amphetamine: implications for glutamatergic and dopaminergic model psychoses and cognitive function. *Arch Gen Psychiatry*. 2005;62(9):985-994.
2. Morris H, Wallach J. From PCP to MXE: a comprehensive review of the non-medical use of dissociative drugs. *Drug Test Anal.* 2014;6(7-8): 614-632.
3. Wallach J, Brandt SD. Phencyclidine-based new psychoactive substances. *New Psychoactive Substances*. Springer; 2018:261-303.
4. Wallach J, Brandt SD. 1, 2-Diarylethylamine- and ketamine-based new psychoactive substances. In: Maurer HH, Brandt SD, eds. *New Psychoactive Substances*. Springer; 2018:305-352.
5. Svenson JE, Abernathy MK. Ketamine for prehospital use: new look at an old drug. *Am J Emerg Med.* 2007;25(8):977-980.
6. Mikhael MS, Wray S, Robb ND. Intravenous conscious sedation in children for outpatient dentistry. *Br Dent J.* 2007;203(6):323-331.
7. Bhutta AT. Ketamine: a controversial drug for neonates. *Semin Perinatol.* 2007;31(5):303-308.

Disclaimer: Dr Miller is employed by the Department of Veterans Affairs, Dayton VA Medical Center, Dayton, Ohio. The VA had no role in the design, literature review or analysis, writing, or in the decision to submit this chapter for publication. The contents do not necessarily represent the views of the Department of Veterans Affairs or the United States Government.

8. Ketalar (ketamine hydrochloride) [package insert]. US Food and Drug Administration website. Accessed May 20, 2022. https://www.accessdata.fda.gov/drugsatfda_docs/label/2020/016812s046lbl.pdf
9. Spravato (esketamine) [package insert]. US Food and Drug Administration website. Accessed May 20, 2022. https://www.accessdata.fda.gov/drugsatfda_docs/label/2019/211243lbl.pdf
10. Baselt RC. *Disposition of Toxic Drugs and Chemicals in Man*. Biomedical Publications; 2011.
11. Bobo WV, Miller SC, Martin BD. The abuse liability of dextromethorphan among adolescents: a review. *J Child Adolesc Subst Abuse*. 2005;14(4):55-75.
12. Ontiveros S, Cantrell L. Fatal cold medication poisoning in an adolescent. *Am J Emerg Med*. 2022;52:269-e1.
13. Domino EF. *PCP (Phencyclidine). Historical and Current Perspectives*. NPP Books; 1981.
14. Ernst A, Ma D, Garcia-Perez I, et al. Molecular validation of the acute phencyclidine rat model for schizophrenia: identification of translational changes in energy metabolism and neurotransmission. *J Proteome Res*. 2012;11(7):3704-3714.
15. Domino EF, Luby ED. Phencyclidine/schizophrenia: one view toward the past, the other to the future. *Schizophr Bull*. 2012;38(5):914-919.
16. Domino E. From Sernyl to angel dust: the return of PCP. *Univ Mich Med Cent J*. 1981;XLVII:1-5.
17. Troupin AS, Mendius JR, Cheng F, et al. MK-801. In: Meldrum BS, Porter RJ, eds. *New Anticonvulsant Drugs*. Libbey; 1986:191-201.
18. Piercey M, Hoffmann W, Kaczkofsky P. Functional evidence for PCP-like effects of the anti-stroke candidate MK-801. *Psychopharmacology (Berl)*. 1988;96(4):561-562.
19. McFee RB, Mofenson HC, Caraccio TR. Dextromethorphan: another "ecstasy"? *Arch Fam Med*. 2000;9(2):123.
20. Nordt S. "DXM": a new drug of abuse? *Ann Emerg Med*. 1998;31(6):794.
21. Miller S. Dextromethorphan psychosis, dependence and physical withdrawal. *Addict Biol*. 2005;10(4):325-327.
22. US Food and Drug Administration. *Drug Abuse Advisory Committee, Open Session*. Vol. 1. Public Health Service; 1990.
23. Hendrickson RG, Cloutier RL. "Crystal Dex:" free-base dextromethorphan. *J Emerg Med*. 2007;32(4):393-396.
24. Bates MS, Trujillo KA. Use and abuse of dissociative and psychedelic drugs in adolescence. *Pharmacol Biochem Behav*. 2021;203:173129.
25. Karami S, Major JM, Calderon S, McAninch JK. Trends in dextromethorphan cough and cold products: 2000–2015 National Poison Data System intentional abuse exposure calls. *Clin Toxicol*. 2018;56(7):656-663.
26. Natter J, Michel B. Memantine misuse and social networks: a content analysis of internet self-reports. *Pharmacoepidemiol Drug Saf*. 2020;29(9):1189-1193.
27. Proceedings of the Community Epidemiology Working Group, National Institute of Drug Abuse. *Epidemiologic Trends in Drug Abuse: Highlights and Executive Summary*. Vol. 1. National Institutes of Health; 2011.
28. Bobo WV, Miller SC. Ketamine as a preferred substance of abuse. *Am J Addict*. 2002;11(4):332-334.
29. Lankenau SE, Clatts MC. Patterns of polydrug use among ketamine injectors in New York City. *Subst Use Misuse*. 2005;40(9-10):1381-1397.
30. Yew DT, ed. *Ketamine Use and Abuse*. CRC Press; 2015.
31. Johnston LD, O'Malley P, Bachman JG, et al. *Teen Drug Use Continues Down in 2006, Particularly Among Older Teens; But Use of Prescription-type Drugs Remains High*. University of Michigan News and Information Services. Accessed May 18, 2023. www.monitoringthefuture.org
32. Johnston LD, O'Malley P, Bachman JG, et al. *Monitoring the Future National Survey Results on Drug Use. 1975–2011, Volume 1, Secondary School Students*. Institute for Social Research, The University of Michigan. Accessed May 18, 2023. http://www.monitoringthefuture.org/results/publications/monographs/
33. Johnston LD, O'Malley PM, Miech RA, et al. *Monitoring the Future National Survey Results on Drug Use. 1975–2015: Overview, Key Findings on Adolescent Drug Use*. Institute for Social Research, The University of Michigan. Accessed May 18, 2023. http://www.monitoringthefuture.org/results/publications/monographs/
34. Wilson MD, Ferguson RW, Mazer ME, Litovitz TL. Monitoring trends in dextromethorphan abuse using the National Poison Data System: 2000–2010. *Clin Toxicol*. 2011;49(5):409-415.
35. Bryner JK, Wang UK, Hui JW, Bedodo M, MacDougall C, Anderson IB. Dextromethorphan abuse in adolescence: an increasing trend: 1999–2004. *Arch Pediatr Adolesc Med*. 2006;160(12):1217.
36. Cochems A, Harding P, Liddicoat L. Dextromethorphan in Wisconsin drivers. *J Anal Toxicol*. 2007;31(4):227-232.
37. Yin S, Wahl M. Intentional Coricidin product exposures among Illinois adolescents. *Am J Drug Alcohol Abuse*. 2011;37(6):509-514.
38. Sheridan DC, Hendrickson RG, Beauchamp G, Laurie A, Fu R, Horowitz BZ. Adolescent intentional abuse ingestions: overall 10-year trends and regional variation. *Pediatr Emerg Care*. 2019;35(3):176-179. doi:10.1097/PEC.0000000000000866
39. Stone CK, Humphries RL. *Current Diagnosis and Treatment Emergency Medicine*. 6th ed. McGraw Hill; 2011.
40. Fourcade EW, Lapidus KA. The basic and clinical pharmacology of ketamine. In: Mathew SJ, Zarate CA, eds. *Ketamine for Treatment-Resistant Depression*. Adis; 2016:13-29.
41. Cohen SP, Bhatia A, Buvanendran A, et al. Consensus guidelines on the use of intravenous ketamine infusions for chronic pain From the American Society of Regional Anesthesia and Pain Medicine, the American Academy of Pain Medicine, and the American Society of Anesthesiologists. *Reg Anesth Pain Med*. 2018;43(5):521-546.
42. Rolan P, Lim S, Sunderland V, Liu Y, Molnar V. The absolute bioavailability of racemic ketamine from a novel sublingual formulation. *Br J Clin Pharmacol*. 2014;77(6):1011-1016.
43. Dinis-Oliveira RJ. Metabolism and metabolomics of ketamine: a toxicological approach. *Forensic Sci Res*. 2017;2(1):2-10.
44. Lynch ME, Clark AJ, Sawynok J, Sullivan MJ. Topical 2% amitriptyline and 1% ketamine in neuropathic pain syndromes: a randomized, double-blind, placebo-controlled trial. *Anesthesiology*. 2005;103(1):140-146.
45. Idvall J, Ahlgren I, Aronsen KF, Stenberg P. Ketamine infusions: pharmacokinetics and clinical effects. *Br J Anaesth*. 1979;51(12):1167-1173.
46. Domino EF, Zsigmond EK, Domino LE, Domino KE, Kothary SP, Domino SE. Plasma levels of ketamine and two of its metabolites in surgical patients using a gas chromatographic mass fragmentographic assay. *Anesth Analg*. 1982;61(2):87-92.
47. Domino EF, Domino SE, Smith RE, et al. Ketamine kinetics in unmedicated and diazepam-premedicated subjects. *Clin Pharmacol Ther*. 1984;36(5):645-653.
48. Clements JA, Nimmo WS. Pharmacokinetics and analgesic effect of ketamine in man. *Br J Anaesth*. 1981;53(1):27-30.
49. Peltoniemi MA, Saari TI, Hagelberg NM, et al. Exposure to oral S-ketamine is unaffected by itraconazole but greatly increased by ticlopidine. *Clin Pharmacol Ther*. 2011;90(2):296-302.
50. Peltoniemi MA, Saari TI, Hagelberg NM, Laine K, Neuvonen PJ, Olkkola KT. S-ketamine concentrations are greatly increased by grapefruit juice. *Eur J Clin Pharmacol*. 2012;68(6):979-986.
51. Li Y, Jackson KA, Slon B, et al. CYP2B6* 6 allele and age substantially reduce steady-state ketamine clearance in chronic pain patients: impact on adverse effects. *Br J Clin Pharmacol*. 2015;80(2):276-284.
52. Keiser M, Hasan M, Oswald S. Affinity of ketamine to clinically relevant transporters. *Mol Pharm*. 2017;15(1):326-331.
53. Silva AR, Dinis-Oliveira RJ. Pharmacokinetics and pharmacodynamics of dextromethorphan: clinical and forensic aspects. *Drug Metab Rev*. 2020;52(2):258-282.
54. Yu A, Haining RL. Comparative contribution to dextromethorphan metabolism by cytochrome P450 isoforms in vitro: can dextromethorphan be used as a dual probe for both CYP2D6 and CYP3A activities? *Drug Metab Dispos*. 2001;29(11):1514-1520.
55. Zawertailo LA, Kaplan HL, Busto UE, Tyndale RF, Sellers EM. Psychotropic effects of dextromethorphan are altered by the CYP2D6 polymorphism: a pilot study. *J Clin Psychopharmacol*. 1998;18(4):332-337.
56. Roth BL, Gibbons S, Arunotayanun W, et al. The ketamine analogue methoxetamine and 3- and 4-methoxy analogues of phencyclidine are high affinity and selective ligands for the glutamate NMDA receptor. *PLoS One*. 2013;8:e59334.

57. Roth BL, Gibbons S, Arunotayanun W, et al. Correction: the ketamine analogue methoxetamine and 3- and 4-methoxy analogues of phencyclidine are high affinity and selective ligands for the glutamate NMDA receptor. *PLoS One.* 2018;13:E0194984.
58. Salat K, Siwek A, Starowicz G, et al. Antidepressant-like effects of ketamine, norketamine and dehydronorketamine in forced swim test: role of activity at NMDA receptor. *Neuropharmacology.* 2015;99:301-307.
59. Bonaventura J, Lam S, Carlton M, et al. Pharmacological and behavioral divergence of ketamine enantiomers: implications for abuse liability. *Mol Psychiatry.* 2021;26(11):6704-6722.
60. Paoletti P, Bellone C, Zhou Q. NMDA receptor subunit diversity: impact on receptor properties, synaptic plasticity and disease. *Nat Rev Neurosci.* 2013;14(6):383-400. doi:10.1038/nrn3504
61. Zhang Y, Ye F, Zhang T, et al. Structural basis of ketamine action on human NMDA receptors. *Nature.* 2021;596(7871):301-305.
62. Kotermanski SE, Johnson JW. Mg2+ imparts NMDA receptor subtype selectivity to the Alzheimer's drug memantine. *J Neurosci.* 2009;29(9):2774-2779.
63. Khlestova E, Johnson JW, Krystal JH, Lisman J. The role of GluN2C-containing NMDA receptors in ketamine's psychotogenic action and in Schizophrenia models. *J Neurosci.* 2016;36(44):11151-11157.
64. Lodge D, Mercier MS. Ketamine and phencyclidine: the good, the bad and the unexpected. *Br J Pharmacol.* 2015;172(17):4254-4276. doi:10.1111/bph.13222
65. Chen G, Mannens G, De Boeck M, et al. Comments to pharmacological and behavioral divergence of ketamine enantiomers by Jordi Bonaventura et al. *Mol Psychiatry.* 2022;27(4):1860-1896.
66. Geisslinger G, Hering W, Thomann P, Knoll R, Kamp HD, Brune K. Pharmacokinetics and pharmacodynamics of ketamine enantiomers in surgical patients using a stereoselective analytical method. *Br J Anaesth.* 1993;70(6):666-671.
67. White PF, Schüttler J, Shafer A, Stanski DR, Horai Y, Trevor AJ. Comparative pharmacology of the ketamine isomers: studies in volunteers. *Br J Anaesth.* 1985;57(2):197-203.
68. Little B, Chang T, Chucot L, et al. Study of ketamine as an obstetric anesthetic agent. *Am J Obstet Gynecol.* 1972;113(2):247-260.
69. Shaffer CL, Osgood SM, Smith DL, Liu J, Trapa PE. Enhancing ketamine translational pharmacology via receptor occupancy normalization. *Neuropharmacology.* 2014;86:174-180.
70. Moghaddam B, Adams BW. Reversal of phencyclidine effects by a group II metabotropic glutamate receptor agonist in rats. *Science.* 1988;281(5381):1349-1352.
71. Abdallah CG, De Feyter HM, Averill LA, et al. The effects of ketamine on prefrontal glutamate neurotransmission in healthy and depressed subjects. *Neuropsychopharmacology.* 2018;43(10):2154-2160.
72. Milak MS, Proper CJ, Mulhern ST, et al. A pilot in vivo proton magnetic resonance spectroscopy study of amino acid neurotransmitter response to ketamine treatment of major depressive disorder. *Mol Psychiatry.* 2016;21(3):320-327.
73. Kari HP, Davidson PP, Kohl HH, Kochhar MM. Effects of ketamine on brain monoamine levels in rats. *Res Commun Chem Pathol Pharmacol.* 1978;20(3):475-488.
74. Hirota K. Lambert DG Ketamine: its mechanism(s) of action and unusual clinical uses. *Br J Anaesth.* 1996;77:441-444.
75. Lindefors N, Barati S, O'Connor WT. Differential effects of single and repeated ketamine administration on dopamine, serotonin and GABA transmission in rat medial prefrontal cortex. *Brain Res.* 1997;759(2):205-212.
76. Smith GS, Schloesser R, Brodie JD. Glutamate modulation of dopamine measured in vivo with positron emission tomography (PET) and 11 C-raclopride in normal human subjects. *Neuropsychopharmacology.* 1998;18(1):18.
77. Vollenweider FX, Vontobel P, Øye I, Hell D, Leenders KL. Effects of (S)-ketamine on striatal dopamine: a [11C] raclopride PET study of a model psychosis in humans. *J Psychiatr Res.* 2000;34(1):35-43.
78. Hirota K. Special cases: ketamine, nitrous oxide and xenon. *Best Pract Res Clin Anaesthesiol.* 2006;20(1):69-79.
79. Mazar J, Rogachev B, Shaked G, et al. Involvement of adenosine in the antiinflammatory action of ketamine. *Anesthesiology.* 2005;102(6):1174-1181.
80. Haile CN, Murrough JW, Iosifescu DV, et al. Plasma brain derived neurotrophic factor (BDNF) and response to ketamine in treatment-resistant depression. *Int J Neuropsychopharmacol.* 2014;17(2):331-336.
81. Marone G, Stellato C, Mastronardi P, Mazzarella B. Mechanisms of activation of human mast cells and basophils by general anaesthetic drugs. *Ann Fr Anesth Reanim.* 1993;12(2):116-125.
82. Romero TR, Galdino GS, Silva GC, et al. Ketamine activates the L-arginine/nitric oxide/cyclic guanosine monophosphate pathway to induce peripheral antinociception in rats. *Anesth Analg.* 2011;113(5):1254-1259.
83. Anand A, Charney DS, Oren DA, et al. Attenuation of the neuropsychiatric effects of ketamine with lamotrigine: support for hyperglutamatergic effects of N-methyl-D-aspartate receptor antagonists. *Arch Gen Psychiatry.* 2000;57(3):270-276.
84. Deakin J, Lees J, McKie S, Hallak JEC, Williams SR, Dursun SM. Glutamate and the neural basis of the subjective effects of ketamine: a pharmaco-magnetic resonance imaging study. *Arch Gen Psychiatry.* 2008;65(2):154.
85. Stone JM, Dietrich C, Edden R, et al. Ketamine effects on brain GABA and glutamate levels with 1H-MRS: relationship to ketamine-induced psychopathology. *Mol Psychiatry.* 2012;17(7):664.
86. Abdallah CG, Sanacora G, Duman RS, Krystal JH. The neurobiology of depression, ketamine and rapid-acting antidepressants: is it glutamate inhibition or activation? *Pharmacol Ther.* 2018;190:148-158.
87. Zhang B, Yang X, Ye L, et al. Ketamine activated glutamatergic neurotransmission by GABAergic disinhibition in the medial prefrontal cortex. *Neuropharmacology.* 2021;194:108382.
88. Pinault D. N-methyl d-aspartate receptor antagonists ketamine and MK-801 induce wake-related aberrant γ oscillations in the rat neocortex. *Biol Psychiatry.* 2008;63(8):730-735.
89. Hong LE, Summerfelt A, Buchanan RW, et al. Gamma and delta neural oscillations and association with clinical symptoms under subanesthetic ketamine. *Neuropsychopharmacology.* 2010;35(3):632-640.
90. Aleksandrova LR, Phillips AG, Wang YT. Antidepressant effects of ketamine and the roles of AMPA glutamate receptors and other mechanisms beyond NMDA receptor antagonism. *J Psychiatry Neurosci.* 2017;42(4):222.
91. Dong Y, Nestler EJ. The neural rejuvenation hypothesis of cocaine addiction. *Trends Pharmacol Sci.* 2014;35(8):374-383.
92. Zanos P, Moaddel R, Morris PJ, et al. NMDAR inhibition-independent antidepressant actions of ketamine metabolites. *Nature.* 2016;533(7604):481. doi:10.1038/nature17998
93. Du Jardin KG, Liebenberg N, Cajina M, et al. S-ketamine mediates its acute and sustained antidepressant-like activity through a 5-HT1B receptor dependent mechanism in a genetic rat model of depression. *Front Pharmacol.* 2018;8:978.
94. Getachew B, Aubee JI, Schottenfeld RS, Csoka AB, Thompson KM, Tizabi Y. Ketamine interactions with gut-microbiota in rats: relevance to its antidepressant and anti-inflammatory properties. *BMC Microbiol.* 2018;18(1):1-10.
95. Abdallah CG, Averill LA, Gueorguieva R, et al. Modulation of the antidepressant effects of ketamine by the mTORC1 inhibitor rapamycin. *Neuropsychopharmacology.* 2020;45(6):990-997.
96. Abelian A, Dybek M, Wallach J, Gaye B, Adejare A. Pharmaceutical chemistry. In: Adejare A, ed. *Remington: The Science and Practice of Pharmacy.* 23rd ed. Academic Press; 2021:105-128.
97. Canady VA. FDA approves esketamine treatment for MDD, suicidal ideation. *Mental Health Weekly.* 2020;30(31):6-7.
98. Mahase E. Esketamine is approved in Europe for treating resistant major depressive disorder. *BMJ.* 2019;367:l7069.
99. Sanders B, Brula AQ. Intranasal esketamine: from origins to future implications in treatment-resistant depression. *J Psychiatr Res.* 2021;137:29-35.
100. Bahji A, Zarate CA, Vazquez GH. Efficacy and safety of racemic ketamine and esketamine for depression: a systematic review and meta-analysis. *Expert Opin Drug Saf.* 2022;21(6):853-866.

101. Ebert B, Mikkelsen S, Thorkildsen C, Borgbjerg FM. Norketamine, the main metabolite of ketamine, is a non-competitive NMDA receptor antagonist in the rat cortex and spinal cord. *Eur J Pharmacol.* 1997;333:99-104.
102. Oye I, Hustveit O, Maurset A, Ratti Moberg E, Paulsen O, Skoglund LA. The chiral forms of ketamine as probes for NMDA receptor functions in humans. In: Kameyama T, Nabeshima T, Domino EF, eds. *NMDA Receptor Related Agents: Biochemistry, Pharmacology and Behavior*. NPP Books; 1991:381-389.
103. Oye I, Paulsen O, Maurset A. Effects of ketamine on sensory perception: evidence for a role of N-methyl-D-aspartate receptors. *J Pharmacol Exp Ther*. 1992;260:1209-1213.
104. Vollenweider FX, Leenders KL, Øye I, Hell D, Angst J. Differential psychopathology and patterns of cerebral glucose utilisation produced by (S)- and (R)-ketamine in healthy volunteers using positron emission tomography (PET). *Eur Neuropsychopharmacol.* 1997;7:25-38.
105. Halberstadt AL, Slepak N, Hyun J, Buell MR, Powell SB. The novel ketamine analog methoxetamine produces dissociative-like behavioral effects in rodents. *Psychopharmacology (Berl)*. 2016;233:1215-1225.
106. Yang C, Shirayama Y, Zhang JC, et al. R-ketamine: a rapid-onset and sustained antidepressant without psychotomimetic side effects. *Transl Psychiatry*. 2015;5(9):e632-e632.
107. Klepstad P, Maurset A, Moberg ER, Øye I. Evidence of a role for NMDA receptors in pain perception. *Eur J Pharmacol.* 1990;187(3):513-518.
108. Desta Z, Moaddel R, Ogburn ET, et al. Stereoselective and regiospecific hydroxylation of ketamine and norketamine. *Xenobiotica*. 2012; 42(11):1076-1087.
109. Moaddel R, Abdrakhmanova G, Kozak J, et al. Sub-anesthetic concentrations of (R, S)-ketamine metabolites inhibit acetylcholine-evoked currents in α7 nicotinic acetylcholine receptors. *Eur J Pharmacol.* 2013;698(1-3):228-234.
110. Javitt DC, Zukin SR. Recent advances in the phencyclidine model of schizophrenia. *Am J Psychiatry*. 1991;148(10):1301-1308.
111. Xu X, Domino EF. Phencyclidine-induced behavioral sensitization. *Pharmacol Biochem Behav*. 1994;47(3):603-608.
112. Xu X, Domino EF. Asymmetric cross-sensitization to the locomotor stimulant effects of phencyclidine and MK-801. *Neurochem Int.* 1994;25(2):155-159.
113. Xu X, Domino EF. A further study on asymmetric cross-sensitization between MK-801 and phencyclidine-induced ambulatory activity. *Pharmacol Biochem Behav*. 1999;63(3):413-416.
114. Balster RL. Clinical implications of behavioral pharmacology research on phencyclidine. *NIDA Res Monogr*. 1986;64:148-162.
115. Balster RL, Woolverton WL. Continuous-access phencyclidine self-administration by rhesus monkeys leading to physical dependence. *Psychopharmacology (Berl)*. 1980;70(1):5-10.
116. American Psychiatric Association. *Diagnostic and Statistical Manual of Mental Disorders*. 5th ed. American Psychiatric Association; 2013.
117. Rawson RA, Tennant FS Jr, McCann MA. Characteristics of 68 chronic phencyclidine abusers who sought treatment. *Drug Alcohol Depend*. 1981;8(3):223-227.
118. White JM, Ryan CF. Pharmacological properties of ketamine. *Drug Alcohol Rev*. 1996;15(2):145-155.
119. Coull JT, Morgan H, Cambridge VC, et al. Ketamine perturbs perception of the flow of time in healthy volunteers. *Psychopharmacology (Berl)*. 2011;218(3):543-556.
120. Pal HR, Berry N, Kumar R, Ray R. Ketamine dependence. *Anaesth Intensive Care*. 2022;30:382-384.
121. Lim DK. Ketamine associated psychedelic effects and dependence. *Singapore Med J*. 2003;44:31-34.
122. Critchlow DG. A case of ketamine dependence with discontinuation symptoms. *Addiction*. 2006;101:1212-1213.
123. Scholz O, Otter S, Welters A, et al. Peripherally active dextromethorphan derivatives lower blood glucose levels by targeting pancreatic islets. *Cell Chem Biol*. 2021;28(10):1474-1488.
124. Paterson JW, Lulich KM. Antiallergic drugs and antitussives. In: Dukes NG, ed. *Meyler's Side Effects of Drugs: An Encyclopedia of Adverse Reactions and Interactions*. Elsevier; 1996.
125. Monte AA, Chuang R, Bodmer M. Dextromethorphan, chlorphenamine and serotonin toxicity: case report and systematic literature review. *Br J Clin Pharmacol*. 2010;70(6):794-798.
126. Olives TD, Boley SP, LeRoy JM, Stellpflug SJ. Ten years of robotripping: evidence of tolerance to dextromethorphan hydrobromide in a long-term user. *J Med Toxicol*. 2019;15(3):192-197.
127. Malek A, Amiri S, Habibi AB. The therapeutic effect of adding dextromethorphan to clonidine for reducing symptoms of opioid withdrawal: a randomized clinical trial. *ISRN. Psychiatry*. 2013;546030.
128. Majeed A, Xiong J, Teopiz KM, et al. Efficacy of dextromethorphan for the treatment of depression: a systematic review of preclinical and clinical trials. *Expert Opin Emerg Drugs*. 2021;26(1):63-74.
129. Anis NA, Berry SC, Burton NR, Lodge D. The dissociative anaesthetics, ketamine and phencyclidine, selectively reduce excitation of central mammalian neurones by N-methyl-aspartate. *Br J Pharmacol.* 1983;79(2):565-575.
130. Rao TS, Kim HS, Lehmann J, Martin LL, Wood PL. Differential effects of phencyclidine (PCP) and ketamine on mesocortical and mesostriatal dopamine release in vivo. *Life Sci*. 1989;45(12):1065-1072.
131. Rao TS, Kim HS, Lehmann J, et al. Interactions of phencyclidine receptor agonist MK-801 with dopaminergic system: regional studies in the rat. *J Neurochem*. 1990;54(4):1157-1162.
132. Rabin RA, Doat M, Winter JC. Role of serotonergic 5-HT2A receptors in the psychotomimetic actions of phencyclidine. *Int J Neuropsychopharmacol*. 2000;3(04):333-338.
133. Abi-Saab W, D'Souza DC, Moghaddam B, Krystal JH. The NMDA antagonist model for schizophrenia: promise and pitfalls. *Pharmacopsychiatry*. 1998;31(2):104-109.
134. Loh M, Rolls ET, Deco G. A dynamical systems hypothesis of schizophrenia. *PLoS Comput Biol*. 2007;3(11):e228.
135. Javitt DC. Glycine transport inhibitors and the treatment of schizophrenia. *Biol Psychiatry*. 2008;63(1):6-8.
136. Krystal JH, Karper LA, Seibyl JP, et al. Subanesthetic effects of the noncompetitive NMDA antagonist, ketamine, in humans: psychotomimetic, perceptual, cognitive, and neuroendocrine responses. *Arch Gen Psychiatry*. 1994;51(3):199.
137. Krystal JH, Karper LP, Bennett A, et al. Interactive effects of subanesthetic ketamine and subhypnotic lorazepam in humans. *Psychopharmacology (Berl)*. 1998;135(3):213-229.
138. Krystal JH, Petrakis IL, Webb E, et al. Dose-related ethanol-like effects of the NMDA antagonist, ketamine, in recently detoxified alcoholics. *Arch Gen Psychiatry*. 1998;55(4):354.
139. Krystal JH, D'Souza DC, Karper LP, et al. Interactive effects of subanesthetic ketamine and haloperidol in healthy humans. *Psychopharmacology (Berl)*. 1999;145(2):193-204.
140. Krystal JH, Bennett A, Abi-Saab D, et al. Dissociation of ketamine effects on rule acquisition and rule implementation: possible relevance to NMDA receptor contributions to executive cognitive functions. *Biol Psychiatry*. 2000;47(2):137-143.
141. Stone JM, Erlandsson K, Arstad E, et al. Relationship between ketamine-induced psychotic symptoms and NMDA receptor occupancy: a [123 I] CNS-1261 SPET study. *Psychopharmacology (Berl)*. 2008;197(3):401-408.
142. Olney JW, Farber NB. Glutamate receptor dysfunction and schizophrenia. *Arch Gen Psychiatry*. 1995;52:998-1007.
143. Drejer J, Honore T. Phencyclidine analogues inhibit NMDA-stimulated [3H] GABA release from cultured cortex neurons. *Eur J Pharmacol.* 1987;143(2):287-290.
144. Krupitsky EM, Burakov AM, Romanova TN, et al. Attenuation of ketamine effects by nimodipine pretreatment in recovering ethanol dependent men: psychopharmacologic implications of the interaction of NMDA and L-type calcium channel antagonists. *Neuropsychopharmacology*. 2001;25(6):936-947.
145. Vlisides PE, Bel-Bahar T, Nelson A, et al. Subanaesthetic ketamine and altered states of consciousness in humans. *Br J Anaesth*. 2018;121(1):249-259.
146. Vesuna S, Kauvar IV, Richman E, et al. Deep posteromedial cortical rhythm in dissociation. *Nature*. 2020;586(7827):87. doi:10.1038/s41586-020-2731-9

147. Yavi M, Lee H, Henter ID, Park LT, Zarate CA Jr. Ketamine treatment for depression: a review. *Discov Ment Health*. 2022;2(1):9.
148. Zarate CA Jr, Singh JB, Carlson PJ, et al. A randomized trial of an N-methyl-D-aspartate antagonist in treatment-resistant major depression. *Arch Gen Psychiatry*. 2006;63(8):856-864. doi:10.1001/archpsyc.63.8.856
149. Maeng S, Zarate CA Jr, Du J, et al. Cellular mechanisms underlying the antidepressant effects of ketamine: role of alpha-amino-3-hydroxy-5-methylisoxazole-4-propionic acid receptors. *Biol Psychiatry*. 2008;63(4):349-352. doi:10.1016/j.biopsych.2007.05.028
150. Autry AE, Adachi M, Nosyreva E, et al. NMDA receptor blockade at rest triggers rapid behavioural antidepressant responses. *Nature*. 2011;475(7354):91-95. doi:10.1038/nature10130
151. Kishi T, Matsunaga S, Iwata N. A meta-analysis of memantine for depression. *J Alzheimers Dis*. 2017;57(1):113-121. doi:10.3233/jad-161251
152. Gould TD, Zarate CA Jr, Thompson SM. Molecular pharmacology and neurobiology of rapid-acting antidepressants. *Annu Rev Pharmacol Toxicol*. 2019;59:213-236. doi:10.1146/annurev-pharmtox-010617-052811
153. Zanos P, Gould TD. Mechanisms of ketamine action as an antidepressant. *Mol Psychiatry*. 2018;23(4):801-811. doi:10.1038/mp.2017.255
154. Lavender E, Hirasawa-Fujita M, Domino EF. Ketamine's dose related multiple mechanisms of actions: dissociative anesthetic to rapid antidepressant. *Behav Brain Res*. 2020;390112631. doi:10.1016/j.bbr.2020. 112631
155. Riggs LM, Gould TD. Ketamine and the future of rapid-acting antidepressants. *Annu Rev Clin Psychol*. 2021;17:207-231. doi:10.1146/annurev-clinpsy-072120-014126
156. Kavalali ET, Monteggia LM. Synaptic mechanisms underlying rapid antidepressant action of ketamine. *Am J Psychiatry*. 2012;169(11):1150-1156.
157. Autry AE, Monteggia LM. Brain-derived neurotrophic factor and neuropsychiatric disorders. *Pharmacol Rev*. 2012;64(2):238-258.
158. De Lima J, Hatch D, Torsney C. Nitrous oxide analgesia—a 'sting in the tail'. *Anaesthesia*. 2000;55(9):932-933.
159. Franks NP, Lieb WR. A serious target for laughing gas. *Nat Med*. 1998;4(4):383-384.
160. Maze M, Fujinaga M. Recent advances in understanding the actions and toxicity of nitrous oxide. *Anaesthesia*. 2001;55(4):311-314.
161. Nagele P, Duma A, Kopec M, et al. Nitrous oxide for treatment-resistant major depression: a proof-of-concept trial. *Biol Psychiatry*. 2015;78(1):10-18. doi:10.1016/j.biopsych.2014.11.016
162. Nagele P, Palanca BJ, Gott B, et al. A phase 2 trial of inhaled nitrous oxide for treatment-resistant major depression. *Sci Transl Med*. 2021;13(597):eabe1376. doi:10.1126/scitranslmed.abe1376
163. Nagele P, Zorumski CF, Conway C. Exploring nitrous oxide as treatment of mood disorders: basic concepts. *J Clin Psychopharmacol*. 2018;38(2):144-148. doi:10.1097/jcp.0000000000000837
164. Jevtovic-Todorovic V, Todorovic SM, Mennerick S, et al. Nitrous oxide (laughing gas) is an NMDA antagonist, neuroprotectant and neurotoxin. *Nat Med*. 1998;4(4):460-463. doi:10.1038/nm0498-460
165. Gillman MA. Mini-review: a brief history of nitrous oxide (N2O) use in neuropsychiatry. *Curr Drug Res Rev*. 2019;11(1):12-20. doi:10.2174/187447371166181008163107
166. Gillman MA. Opioid properties of nitrous oxide and ketamine contribute to their antidepressant actions. *Int J Neuropsychopharmacol*. 2021;24(11):892-893. doi:10.1093/ijnp/pyab045
167. Zarate CA Jr, Machado-Vieira R. Potential pathways involved in the rapid antidepressant effects of nitrous oxide. *Biol Psychiatry*. 2015;78(1):2-4. doi:10.1016/j.biopsych.2015.04.007
168. Block RI, Ghoneim MM, Kumar V, Pathak D. Psychedelic effects of a subanesthetic concentration of nitrous oxide. *Anesth Prog*. 1990;37(6):271-276.
169. Gillman MA. Analgesic (sub anesthetic) nitrous oxide interacts with the endogenous opioid system: a review of the evidence. *Life Sci*. 1986;39(14):1209-1221. doi:10.1016/0024-3205(86)90181-5
170. Gillman MA, Lichtigfeld FJ. Pharmacology of psychotropic analgesic nitrous oxide as a multipotent opioid agonist. *Int J Neurosci*. 1994;76(1-2):5-12. doi:10.3109/00207459408985986
171. Emmanouil DE, Quock RM. Advances in understanding the actions of nitrous oxide. *Anesth Prog*. 2007;54(1):9-18.
172. Newman JL, Perry JL, Carroll ME. Social stimuli enhance phencyclidine (PCP) self-administration in rhesus monkeys. *Pharmacol Biochem Behav*. 2007;87(2):280-288.
173. Nicholson KL, Hayes BA, Balster RL. Evaluation of the reinforcing properties and phencyclidine-like discriminative stimulus effects of dextromethorphan and dextrorphan in rats and rhesus monkeys. *Psychopharmacology (Berl)*. 1999;146(1):49-59.
174. Xu J, Ou H, Sun P, Qin S, Yuan TF. Brief report: predictors of relapse for patients with dextromethorphan dependence. *Am J Addict*. 2021;30(2):192-194.
175. Miller SC. Treatment of dextromethorphan dependence with naltrexone. *Addict Disord Ther Treat*. 2005;4(4):145-148.
176. Bleakman D, Alt A, Lodge A, Monaghan DT, Jane DE, Nisenbaum ES. Chapter 10: Ionotropic glutamate receptors. In: Sibley DR, Hanin I, Kuhar M, Skolnick P, eds. *Handbook of Contemporary Neuropharmacology*. John Wiley & Sons, Inc; 2007.
177. Allen H, Iversen L. Phencyclidine, dizocilpine, and cerebrocortical neurons. *Science*. 1990;247:221.
178. Olney J, Labruyere J, Wang G, Wozniak DF, Price MT, Sesma MA. NMDA antagonist neurotoxicity: mechanism and prevention. *Science*. 1991;254(5037):1515.
179. Carliss R, Radovsky A, Chengelis CP, O'Neill TP, Shuey DL. Oral administration of dextromethorphan does not produce neuronal vacuolation in the rat brain. *Neurotoxicology*. 2007;28(4):813-818.
180. Zhang TY, Cho HJ, Lee S, et al. Impairments in water maze learning of aged rats that received dextromethorphan repeatedly during adolescent period. *Psychopharmacology (Berl)*. 2007;191(1):171-179.
181. Morgan CJA, Muetzelfeldt L, Curran HV. Ketamine use, cognition and psychological wellbeing: a comparison of frequent, infrequent and ex-users with polydrug and non-using controls. *Addiction*. 2008;104(1):77-87.
182. Liao Y, Tang J, Corlett PR, et al. Reduced dorsal prefrontal gray matter after chronic ketamine use. *Biol Psychiatry*. 2011;69(1):42-48.
183. Liao Y, Tang J, Ma M, et al. Frontal white matter abnormalities following chronic ketamine use: a diffusion tensor imaging study. *Brain*. 2010;133(7):2115-2122.
184. Massey TH, Pickersgill TT, Peall JK. Nitrous oxide misuse and vitamin B12 deficiency. *BMJ Case Rep*. 2016; doi:10.1136/bcr-2016-215728
185. Egan W, Steinberg E, Rose J. Vitamin B-12 deficiency-induced neuropathy secondary to prolonged recreational use of nitrous oxide. *Am J Emerg Med*. 2018;36(9):1717.e1. doi:10.1016/j.ajem.2018.05.029
186. Hathout L, El-Saden S. Nitrous oxide-induced B_{12} deficiency myelopathy: perspectives on the clinical biochemistry of vitamin B_{12}. *J Neurol Sci*. 2011;301(1-2):1-8.
187. Garakani A, Jaffe RJ, Savla D, et al. Neurologic, psychiatric, and other medical manifestations of nitrous oxide abuse: a systematic review of the case literature. *Am J Addict*. 2016;25:358-369.
188. Lau SS, Domino EF. Gas chromatography mass spectrometry assay for ketamine and its metabolites in plasma. *Biol Mass Spectrom*. 1977;4(5):317-321.
189. Winstock AR, Mitcheson L, Gillatt DA, Cottrell AM. The prevalence and natural history of urinary symptoms among recreational ketamine users. *BJU Int*. 2012;110(11):1762-1766.
190. Au W, Tsang J, Cheng TS, et al. Cough mixture abuse as a novel cause of megaloblastic anaemia and peripheral neuropathy. *Br J Haematol*. 2003;123(5):956-958.
191. FDA. FDA Talk Paper. FDA Warns Against Abuse of Dextromethorphan (DXM); 2005.
192. Schneider SM, Michelson EA, Boucek CD. Dextromethorphan narcosis reversed by naloxone. *Vet Hum Toxicol*. 1986;31:376.
193. Chyka PA, Erdman AR, Manoguerra AS, et al. Dextromethorphan poisoning: an evidence-based consensus guideline for out-of-hospital management. *Clin Toxicol*. 2007;45(6):662-677.
194. Journey JD, Agrawal S, Stern E. *Dextromethorphan Toxicity*. StatPearls Publishing; 2022. Accessed May 18, 2023. https://www.ncbi.nlm.nih.gov/books/NBK538502/
195. Lauterbach EC. Dextromethorphan as a potential rapid-acting antidepressant. *Med Hypotheses*. 2011;76(5):717-719.

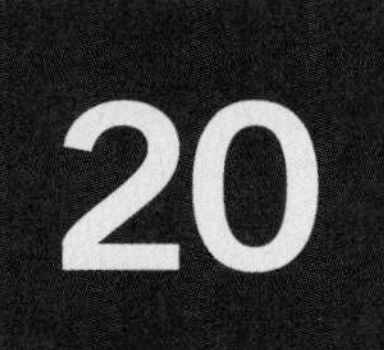

20 The Pharmacology of Inhalants

Robert L. Balster and Silvia L. Cruz

CHAPTER OUTLINE

- Definition
- Substances included in this class
- Historical features
- Epidemiology
- Pharmacokinetics
- Pharmacodynamics
- Addiction liability
- Toxicity, diagnosis, and intoxication management
- Future research directions

DEFINITION

Inhalants are breathable chemicals that are volatile at room temperature and can be self-administered as gases or vapors. There are historical examples of volatile liquids inhaled and consumed orally (eg, ether), but inhalants, by definition, are inhaled and do not need to be heated.[1]

SUBSTANCES INCLUDED IN THIS CLASS

It is useful for addiction medicine to classify the substances primarily based on shared mechanisms of action or pharmacologic effects rather than by chemical structure, source, or form. However, the toxicologic effects of inhalants differ, and these differences do not necessarily follow classifications based on acute adverse pharmacologic effects. Nonetheless, three broad pharmacologic subdivisions of inhalants are recognized: (1) volatile alkyl nitrites, (2) nitrous oxide, and (3) solvents, fuels, and anesthetics (**Table 20-1**). The rationale for this subclassification has been presented elsewhere[1] and is summarized below.

Volatile Alkyl Nitrites

The prototypic alkyl nitrite is amyl nitrite, used medically as a vasodilator for treatment of angina. Amyl nitrite is available as a volatile liquid in glass ampoules that are broken open and the vapor inhaled. At one time, the ampules were available over the counter, and people would "pop" them open—hence the street name "poppers." In 1968, when amyl nitrite was brought under prescription control in the United States, retailers made room for odorizer products from other alkyl nitrites, mainly isoamyl-, butyl-, isobutyl-, and cyclohexyl nitrites, with names such as "Locker Room" (nitrites smell like a locker room), "Rush," "Hardware," and "Climax." Very little is known about the safety of these products. Dietary supplements and other concoctions without nitrites are now being sold as performance enhancers using the brand names used previously for volatile nitrites.

Relatively little research has been done on volatile nitrites. In animal studies, they do not produce acute intoxication like those of solvents. Instead, they produce syncope secondary to venous pooling in the periphery, tumescence, and smooth muscle relaxation, making them popular as aids to sexual activity.[2]

Nitrous Oxide

Nitrous oxide is a low potency anesthetic gas at room temperature and pressure often diverted for illegitimate use. The tanks can be used to fill balloons for ready sale at concerts or parties. Nitrous oxide can also be obtained from whipped cream dispensers, and adapter paraphernalia is available to facilitate self-administration of the gas from the pressurized cans. The acute pharmacologic effects of subanesthetic concentrations of nitrous oxide are poorly understood. It can produce euphoria ("laughing gas") and feelings of intoxication,[3] but the qualitative nature of this intoxication appears to be different from that produced by anesthetic vapors such as isoflurane and sevoflurane.[4] Nitrous oxide requires concentrations of about 15% to 20% to produce intoxication. Many people who use it breathe almost 100% nitrous oxide (eg, from a balloon). This action can lead to anoxia and, as with nitrite-produced syncope, has acute psychological effects.

Volatile Solvents, Fuels, and Anesthetics

This category includes a large collection of chemicals, which cannot be further subclassified with current knowledge. Among the prototypic chemicals for this class are toluene and other alkyl benzenes, butane and other alkanes, R134a (1,1,1,2-tetrafluoroethane) and R152a (1,1-difluoroethane) and other haloalkanes, and various ketones, alcohols, and ethers (see **Table 20-1**). Many of these commercial chemicals share acute effects with subanesthetic concentrations of volatile anesthetics such as halothane, sevoflurane, and isoflurane.[5,6] These anesthetics offer a safer research alternative to the study of toluene and similar chemicals in humans, and they have been directly compared in many animal studies.[5,6]

TABLE 20-1 Pharmacologic Classification of Inhalants

Class	Examples	Sources
Volatile alkyl nitrites	Amyl nitrite*	Antianginal medication ampules
	Cyclohexyl nitrite	Room odorizers, video head cleaners
Nitrous oxide*		Whipped cream dispenser chargers, cylinders for anesthesia
Solvents, fuels, and anesthetics	Toluene	Adhesives, paint removers and thinners (toluol), inks, nail polish and remover, industrial solvents, and degreasers
	Xylene	Adhesives and printing inks, paints and varnishes, pesticides
	Difluoroethane (R152), tetrafluoroethane (R134a), dichlorodifluoromethane	Compressed "air" dusters for computers, refrigerants, and other uses
	Trichloroethane	This compound has almost entirely been removed from commercial use and not available for unhealthy use, but much of the research in this class has used it as a prototype
	Chloroethane (ethyl chloride)	Topical anesthetic/freezing spray, also sold on the internet as "popper-like" products
	Methylene chloride	A solvent in water repellants, automotive cleaners, primers and paints, adhesives and silicone lubricants, correction fluids, spray paints and paint removers, rust and spot removers, and other cleaning products
	Tetrachloroethylene	A solvent in water repellants, brake and carburetor cleaners, paints, adhesives and silicone lubricants, correction fluids, paint removers
	Butane, isopropane	Cigarette lighter fuel, aerosol propellant, bottled gas
	Ether, isoflurane	Anesthetics
	Ketones (MBK, MEK)	Solvents, adhesives

*Approved for clinical use by the FDA.

Comparatively, beverage alcohol (ethanol) is much less volatile and potent than other solvents for acute central nervous system (CNS) effects, discouraging use by inhalation.[7] Alcohol shares some pharmacologic effects with CNS depressant drugs such as barbiturates, nonbarbiturate sedatives, and benzodiazepines, all of which are positive $GABA_A$ allosteric modulators (see Pharmacodynamics). The acute depressant-like intoxication and presentation of overdose is similar among all these compounds.

HISTORICAL FEATURES

History

The use of anesthetics for purposes of intoxication began with their discovery more than 200 years ago.[8] The euphoriant effects of nitrous oxide were noted by Sir Humphrey Davy, who synthesized the substance in 1798 and called it "laughing gas." Laughing gas subsequently was used as part of comedic traveling shows at the beginning of the 19th century. The early vapor anesthetics, including ether and chloroform, were used recreationally and as "nerve tonics," both by inhalation and drinking. It may seem odd to drink an anesthetic, but one must remember that alcohol is a highly volatile liquid with irritant properties, yet its oral consumption surprises no one. Amyl nitrite was used for angina pectoris treatment in 1867, and first reports of recreational use are from the 1960s.[9]

Today, inhalants differ widely in their availability. Some, such as nitrous oxide and amyl nitrite, are under FDA control as prescription medications, although other forms of nitrous oxide are available commercially. Commercial sales of volatile alkyl nitrites are regulated in the United States by the Consumer Product Safety Commission. This step reduced the availability and unhealthy use of most of these substances; however, nitrites can be bought on internet sites. Many other types of inhalants used in unhealthy ways can be found in homes or workplaces or purchased at retail establishments. Gasoline, a very complex mixture of volatile compounds, is available everywhere, and butane lighter fluid is easy to obtain. Although inhalants are not regulated under the Controlled Substances Act or by international treaty, several states have restricted the sale and distribution of certain products commonly used as inhalants to minors. Some states have introduced fines, incarceration, or mandatory treatment for the sale, distribution, use, and/or possession of inhalant chemicals. Strategies to prevent access to inhalants, such as changing their labeling or reformulating products to limit their potential for unhealthy use, need a careful case-by-case analysis to the desired effect and not result in people seeking potentially more toxic products that almost certainly cannot be restricted (eg, gasoline).[10,11]

EPIDEMIOLOGY

U.S. national surveys suggest that the past-year prevalence of inhalant use is greatest among 12- to 17-year-olds compared to other age groups. The school-based Monitoring the Future (MTF) national survey of 8th, 10th, and 12th graders[12] estimated that rates of inhalant use in 2021 show a steady decline from their peak in the mid-1990s yet remain high (**Fig. 20-1**). The MTF no longer includes alkyl nitrites in its estimates because their use among high school students is currently very low. Inhalants are fourth behind alcohol, tobacco, and cannabis in this age range. One important difference from other substances is that the lifetime prevalence of inhalant use decreases from 8th to 12th grade. The 2020 U.S. National Survey on Drug Use and Health estimated the lifetime, past year, and past month prevalence for cannabis, inhalants, and cocaine in the United States.[13] About 1 in 20 youths used inhalants sometime in their life, and 1% used them in the past year (**Fig. 20-2**). Among older youth and adults, the prevalence of inhalant use falls considerably below that of cannabis, cocaine, and heroin. However, those engaged in unhealthy inhalant use remain a significant minority of all people who use substances. It is particularly prevalent among juvenile–justice-involved youth.[14] A study conducted in 2015 to 2017 found that 30% of gay men in the United States reported using nitrites in the previous 12 months.[15] Although many inhalant users quit as they reach young adulthood, it is incorrect to characterize this problem as a passing fad in youth. For about half of people who use currently, duration of use exceeds 1 to 2 years, with about 10% using inhalants for 6 years or more.[16]

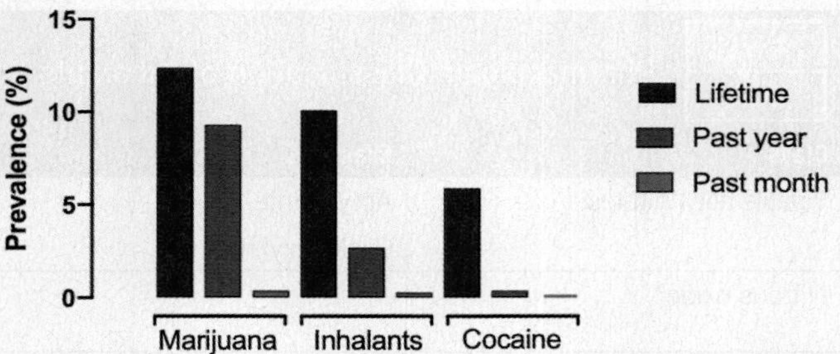

Figure 20-2. Lifetime, past-year, and past-month prevalence estimates for marijuana, inhalant, and cocaine use in 2020 for youth aging 12 to 17 in the United States. Based on data from the National Household Survey on Drug Use and Health. (From Center for Behavioral Health Statistics and Quality. *National Survey on Drug Use and Health: Detailed Tables.* 2020.)

Unhealthy use of inhalants is a significant problem throughout the world. The most recent report on Drug Use in the Americas (2019) estimated a past-year use of inhalants among secondary school students between 2% and 10%.[17] The European School Study Project on Alcohol and Other Drugs (2019) gathered data from 35 countries and found a 7.2% average for lifetime use among students aged 15 and 16 years.[18] Canada is an interesting case because it has a nationwide specialized program to treat youths that use inhalants. Data from the Ontario Student Drug Use and Health Survey (OSDUHS) indicate a decrease in past-year inhalant use among 7th and 12th graders from 8.9% in 1999 to 3.1% in 2019. The most recent data show that the prevalence is higher in females (3.6%) than in males (2.7%).[19] The past-year prevalence of inhalant

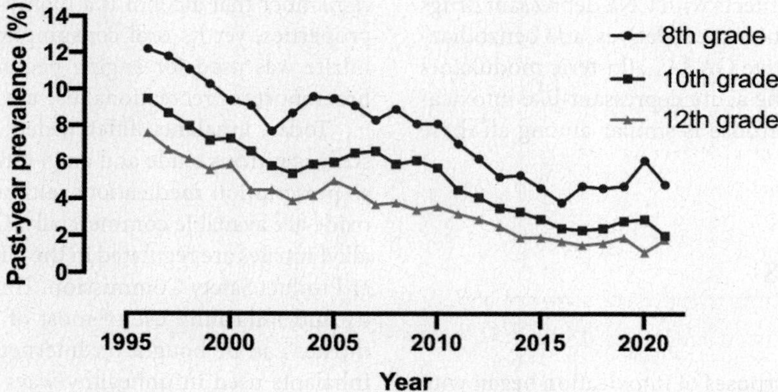

Figure 20-1. Trends in the annual prevalence of the use of inhalants for 8th, 10th, and 12th graders in the United States. Shown here is the estimated use in the past year during each of the reporting years from 1996 to 2021. (Modified from Johnston L, Miech R, O'Malley P, Bachman J, Schulenberg J, Patrick M. *Monitoring the Future National Results on Adolescent Drug Use 1975-2021: Overview, Key Findings on Adolescent Drug Use 1975-2021: Overview, Key Findings on Adolescent Drug Use.* Institute for Social Research, University of Michigan; 2022. Accessed May 18, 2023. https://monitoringthefuture.org/wp-content/uploads/2022/08/mtf-overview2021.pdf)

use in Australia increased from 0.4 % in 2001 to 1.4% in 2019 among people aged 14 years and over. The most used inhalants in 2019 were not solvents, but nitrous oxide and nitrites, which were reported by 6 out of 10 users who tried them in the previous 12 months.[20] These data highlight the importance of considering variations of the inhalants used among countries.

People who use inhalants can develop inhalant use disorders.[21] In addition, several studies have shown a clear progression from early inhalant use to later use of drugs such as cocaine and heroin. There is also evidence that people who use both inhalants and cannabis are at especially greater risk of using other substances.[22] For example, among adolescents who had used both, 35% had a 1-year prevalence of DSM-defined alcohol use disorder and 39% had another substance use disorder (SUD).[23]

PHARMACOKINETICS

Inhalants can be self-administered as gases, vapors and aerosols (ie, fine liquid droplets or solid particles suspended in the air). These three forms have somewhat different absorption characteristics and require different methods of use (eg, balloons for gases and bags or rags for volatile liquids). The likely "active ingredient" in aerosols (such as hair spray) is the propellant (eg, butane) that exists in the aerosol can under pressure; however, other materials in the cans (eg, pigments) also can be absorbed.

Gases and vapors rapidly penetrate deep into the lung and, because of their high lipophilicity, are rapidly absorbed and distributed into arterial blood. What distinguishes unhealthy inhalant use from clinical anesthetic use is that the partial pressure of the inhalant vapor inhaled generally is very high and quite variable over time, as people intermittently sniff from balloons, rags, or bags saturated with liquid. Once inhaled, solvents rapidly enter the brain and distribute to lipid-containing membranes within the CNS, placing them in proximity to key functional components, including the cellular sites responsible for their recreational effects. Because physical activity increases cardiac output, inhalant distribution to the brain in someone active will likely be greater than in someone at rest. Inhalants easily cross the placenta and expose the fetus, with consequences that will be discussed later.[11,24]

The situation with aerosols is somewhat different. When inhaled, the rapidity and efficiency of absorption are determined by particle size. Both the propellant and the aerosolized content may have behavioral effects. Gases, vapors, and aerosols have an almost immediate onset of action. Thus, it is common for people who use inhalants to stumble or fall, posing a risk to themselves and others.

For many use situations with inhalants, the concentrations in inspired air likely exceed concentrations that would be lethal if the person were exposed continuously. Lethal concentrations could occur, for example, if a person became unconscious while still exposed to the inhalant. This situation is probably the most common form of acute overdose. It happens when someone using a rag or a bag laden with solvent falls in such a way as to continue breathing the solvent. Some people have devised methods for exposing themselves to inhalants without having to use their hands, such as for sexual situations, and become vulnerable to overdose while using the devices.

Elimination of inhalants is very rapid once the source is removed from the inspired air. For most of these chemicals, expired air is the major route of elimination. Those that are relatively insoluble in the blood and brain are eliminated more quickly than those with greater solubility in these reservoirs (eg, toluene).

Most inhalants are metabolized to some extent, but this metabolism probably plays a greater role in determining their hepatic toxicity than their CNS effects. An important factor affecting recovery is the duration of the use episode. Someone who has been inhaling for a few hours might achieve considerable accumulation in the muscle, skin, and fat. For obese individuals, recovery can be a bit more prolonged, as the chemicals are more slowly relocated from adipose tissue to blood.

Intoxication with inhalants lasts less than with most other recreational substances. Unless comatose, such people typically are not brought to emergency departments because they will have recovered or died before they get there. Law enforcement personnel occasionally encounter inhalant intoxication if they arrive while the person is actively still using an inhalant. However, there is little they can do, even in cases of driving under the influence, because of the rapid recovery time. This lack of direct experience with intoxication and the difficulty of obtaining confirming toxicology (see Diagnosis and Intoxication Management sections) have contributed to an underappreciation of the adverse public health effects of this form of substance use.

PHARMACODYNAMICS

Solvents have effects at several ligand-gated and other ion channel receptors, including those for gamma-aminobutyric acid ($GABA_A$), glutamate, and acetylcholine.[5] Acute solvent intoxication has been associated with enhancement of $GABA_A$ and noncompetitive antagonism at the *N*-methyl-D-aspartate (NMDA) receptors.[25-27] These effects can be very selective for different structural subtypes of these heteromeric proteins, with different chemicals having somewhat different profiles of selectivity. Published descriptions include a much wider array of potential subjective and pharmacologic effects for inhalants than for alcohol and other typical CNS depressant substances, including hallucinations, tremor, and seizures.[28] GABAergic or NMDA antagonist effects have also been proposed as mechanisms for various effects of nitrous oxide,[29,30] and there is some evidence for opioid receptor involvement in its analgesic effects.[29] Alkyl nitrites produce hypotension because they are nitric oxide

(NO) donors, which cause blood vessel relaxation. Nitrites are also potent oxidizing agents and the high affinity of nitric oxide for the heme group can produce methemoglobinemia with chronic nitrite use. Some vapors can have excitatory effects in animals (such as flurothyl), and animal studies provide evidence that even aromatic hydrocarbons like benzene or isoparaffins can produce a different profile of acute effects than the prototypic depressant solvents such as toluene.[7] Considering that many commercial products contain complex mixtures, it should not be surprising that people who use inhalants experience a diverse array of acute effects, depending on the product used.

ADDICTION LIABILITY

All of the vapors that have been tested produce clear, reversible effects common to other used drugs. Self-administration studies in rodents[31] and humans[5] have shown toluene and nitrous oxide to have reinforcing properties. Toluene also produces a conditioned place preference in rats and mice.[32] When given repeatedly to animals, many drugs with addiction liability produce sensitization to their locomotor stimulant effects, a phenomenon thought to reflect the engagement of addiction-related processes in the brain. Trichloroethane produces locomotor sensitization in mice,[33] and repeated toluene exposure in rats produces cross-sensitization to cocaine and increased cocaine-produced dopamine release.[34] Toluene itself enhances dopamine release in various portions of the brain reward system,[35,36] suggesting that there may be a common neural basis for unhealthy use of inhalants and other substances with addiction liability.

Tolerance and Dependence

Little is known about the development of tolerance and physical dependence on inhalants, but they do not appear to be prominent features. With continuous exposure (such as that achieved with mice in inhalation exposure chambers), a mild withdrawal syndrome can be observed with TCE and toluene[37]; other vapors have not been systematically studied. The withdrawal effects appear within hours after discontinuation of exposure and can be considered excitatory in nature. Ethanol and barbiturates can suppress these withdrawal signs, suggesting a cross-dependence between inhalants and CNS depressants.

Unhealthy inhalant use typically is episodic and thus generally would not occur with sufficient frequency and intensity to maintain a constant exposure throughout a day, weeks, or months that it might take for physical dependence to develop. Nonetheless, several studies find that people who use inhalants report withdrawal signs associated with inhalant use.[38] A characteristic withdrawal syndrome is included in ICD-11[39] but not in DSM-5.[21] However, people who regularly use inhalants clearly can develop a pattern of uncontrolled use, investing considerable time and effort in obtaining and using inhalants that are characteristic of SUD.

TOXICITY, DIAGNOSIS, AND INTOXICATION MANAGEMENT

The toxicity of inhalants differs depending on the array of chemicals used and is reviewed in detail elsewhere.[40-43] A brief overview of the information is provided here. The known side effects of organic nitrites used clinically for smooth muscle relaxation are relevant to the nonmedical use of these compounds, but a systematic study of the health consequences in people with nitrite use disorder has not been done.

Acute Effects

Deaths related to the acute effects of inhalants are well documented.[41,44] There are two primary sources: behavioral toxicity and overdose. Because the solvent class of inhalants can produce profound intoxication and even anesthetic-like effects at high concentrations, accidents and injuries related to behavioral toxicity occur. The rapid onset of intoxication enhances vulnerability to these events. Additive effects are expected when inhalants are combined with alcohol or other CNS depressant drugs. An overdose occurs when people lose consciousness while being continually exposed to the inhalant, allowing lethal concentrations to accumulate in the brain. As with anesthetic vapors, the concentration-effect curves for inhalants are very steep, with toxic exposures achieved easily, especially in poorly ventilated indoor spaces.

The proximate cause of most inhalant overdose deaths is CNS depression, leading to respiratory problems or suffocation. Some inhalants can produce acute cardiotoxicity, even in otherwise healthy young people.[11,45] The mechanism may be increased sensitivity of the myocardium to circulating catecholamines, which may occur when an intoxicated individual engages in strenuous activity. This phenomenon has been termed "sudden sniffing death" and has been associated particularly with the use of aerosols containing chlorofluorocarbon and butane propellants and refrigerants that contain them. Inhalation of toluene-containing products can also be fatal due to cardiac arrhythmias, probably related to blockade of cardiac sodium channels[11] and low potassium levels. A high toluene concentration can cause hypokalemia and acid-basic changes, producing EKG alterations, weakness, cramps in the arms and legs, immobility, and diarrhea.[46] The contribution of hypoxia to the acute toxicity of inhalants should be considered, especially with the use of nitrous oxide, in which 100% concentrations are lethal only because of the lack of oxygen in the inhaled gas.

Chronic Toxicity

It is difficult to summarize chronic toxicity because of the complex composition of many commercial products and the fact that few people who regularly use inhalants confine themselves to a single product or a single chemical agent, making it difficult to ascertain the specific etiology of any adverse health effects. Some of them may be secondary to inhalant exposure or reflect lifestyles. These may include such known predictors of poor health as homelessness, inadequate diet, and other substance use. Thus, data from case reports in inhalant use situations should always be viewed cautiously. Careful epidemiologic work that controls for key covariables in this population has yet to be done. Despite this, many people who use inhalants chronically manifest adverse health effects, some of which can be used in diagnosing inhalant use disorder. A recent meta-analysis showed that inhalant use during adolescence is associated with growth impairments in both humans and rodents.[47] Common target organs are the nose and mouth area, lungs, brain, liver, and kidney. There also are physical dangers, such as the risk of burns[48] in using highly inflammable and explosive chemicals.

Most animal studies of inhalant toxicity simulate the long duration, low-concentration exposures experienced in home or workplace settings. Few animal studies model the periodic or occasional high-concentration exposure typical of people who use inhalants recreationally.

Neurotoxicity

Many, if not all, inhalants can be neurotoxic, and some components of these products are well-characterized neurotoxicants. Among these are hexane and methyl-n-butyl ketone, which produce axonopathies. Demyelination can also occur with nitrous oxide, and there are a few case reports of Guillain-Barré syndrome in chronic users.[43,49] Most information on the neurotoxicity of inhalants comes from case reports or small series of patients. It is not known what percentage of people have detectable brain damage nor whether the inhalants alone were responsible for the observed effects. Brain scanning, neurologic and neuropsychological assessment, or autopsy reports of people who use inhalants show many types of neuropathologies, including loss of white matter, brain atrophy, and damage to specific neural pathways.[50,51] Of particular concern are the effects of inhalants on the developing nervous system. Rodent studies show evidence for developmental delays[52] and reversible changes in white matter maturation,[53] suggesting that the prenatal period through adolescence may be particularly vulnerable periods for damage from inhalant exposure.

Psychiatric Disorders

Early inhalant use is associated with an increased risk of many SUDs. A 2001 to 2002 community-based, cross-sectional survey representative of the U.S. population estimated that 70% of people who use inhalants met DSM-IV criteria for at least one lifetime mood, anxiety, or personality disorder, and 38% experienced a mood or anxiety disorder in the past year.[54] Females were more likely than males to have multiple comorbid psychiatric illnesses. Suicidality has also been described among solvent users.[55] Conduct disorder, mood disorders, and suicidality are common among adolescents who use inhalants.[56,57] Nitrous oxide chronic use is associated with a high prevalence of psychotic symptoms and violent behavior.[58]

Effects on Major Organ Systems

With chronic use, inflammation of the lungs can result in coughing and may compromise respiration, and bone mass toxicity has been reported. Toluene and other hydrocarbon solvents may have ototoxic effects.[59] Chronic nitrite use can produce maculopathy.[60]

The liver is an important target in chronic exposure to many solvents, particularly those that undergo some hepatic metabolism.[61,62] Of particular concern are some of the halogenated hydrocarbons, such as carbon tetrachloride, and some gases used as propellants for computer dusters (eg, 1,1-difluoroethane). Persons with preexisting liver disease, such as hepatitis or alcohol-related liver disease, might be particularly vulnerable. Kidney damage also has been reported, in the form of glomerulonephritis and kidney stones. There have been reports of renal tubular acidosis in acute toluene intoxication.[63] Benzene and vinyl chloride are known carcinogens.[64] Alkyl nitrites can produce methemoglobinemia due to vitamin B_{12} deficiency.[65]

Fetal Solvent Syndrome

Decreased fertility and spontaneous abortions in some women may be related to inhalant use. Adverse effects in the offspring of mothers who use solvents include low birth weight, facial and other physical abnormalities, microcephaly, and delayed neurologic and physical maturation. Because certain features seen in these children resemble the fetal alcohol syndrome, a "fetal solvent syndrome" has been proposed. Whether these features result from direct teratologic effects of the chemicals, or some lifestyle variables associated with solvent use is unknown at this time. Confirmation of direct adverse effects of prenatal solvent exposure has been obtained in animal studies.[52] Thus, clinicians should be alert to this possibility in patients who use inhalants during pregnancy.

Diagnosis

Inhalants are not included in standard screening panels for recreational substances. Few, if any, clinical facilities routinely conduct tests for the presence of inhalants; such tests can be ordered through special services provided by commercial laboratories. Typically, these tests are performed using blood or urine and are available mainly for solvents such as toluene, benzene, and methyl ethyl ketone. Because inhalants are eliminated so rapidly after acute exposure, such tests have a high probability of producing false negatives. Problems associated with postmortem detection of volatile solvents have also been described.[66] Many people who use solvents chronically develop irritation of the eyes, nose, and mouth and exhibit rhinitis, nose bleeding, conjunctivitis, and a localized skin rash.[67] When these signs are accompanied by the odor of solvents on the breath or in clothing; by paint, adhesive, or other similar stains on clothing; or by possession of products in unusual circumstances or amounts, inhalant use should be suspected. Urinary phenol has been proposed as a marker for benzene use, and urinary hippuric acid, and o-cresol as a marker for the use of toluene.[68,69] A variety of potential biomarkers for nitrous oxide use have been proposed, including vitamin B_{12}, methionine, methylmalonate, and homocysteine, among others.[70]

Intoxication Management

Very little is known about effective treatment strategies for inhalant use disorder. A 2010 Cochrane review concluded that no data exist to form a recommendation.[71] Since most people who use inhalants are adolescents, they are usually treated within the context of general adolescent SUD treatment programs, often those targeting conduct disorder problems. However, in the last decade, there have been significant advances in inhalant intoxication management,[72] some of which are shown in **Table 20-2**.

FUTURE RESEARCH DIRECTIONS

Compared to other substances, there has been little research on inhalant use,[11] generally because of mistaken beliefs that exist within the scientific community. These beliefs include the ideas that (1) inhalant use is a transient phenomenon of adolescence that has relatively little associated morbidity and mortality, (2) inhalants have "nonspecific effects" on the brain and behavior that do not lend themselves to the study with modern scientific technologies in behavioral and molecular neurobiology, (3) laboratory studies of vapors and gases are very difficult to perform, and (4) there are too many chemicals to successfully sort out the similarities and differences in terms of their addiction potential and toxicity.

Our understanding should improve with the increasing information available from animal models.[11] However, there are some unique problems inherent in the study of inhalant use. The most significant is that it will be difficult to conduct laboratory-based human exposure studies of many of these compounds at behaviorally active concentrations. One approach to overcoming this problem may be to draw lessons about the effects of chemicals of this type by studying the medical use of general anesthetics. This approach has been used successfully in studying nitrous oxide.[4] Animal studies of inhalants will continue to be especially important because there are fewer limitations on the exposure conditions.

We need a lot more information on the phenomenology and adverse health and social consequences of acute inhalant intoxication, some of which could be obtained from prospective longitudinal studies of inhalant use.[73] Epidemiologic studies are made difficult by the numerous types of products and chemicals subject to inhalant use and by the fact that subclassifications have differed from study to study. There has been an increased appreciation that alkyl nitrite use differs from the rest, and this difference is reflected in separate analyses of prevalence data in many reports. The U.S. National Survey on Drug Use and Health now contains a breakdown of specific subtypes of inhalant products which should be useful for future analyses. Such progress should lead to a better understanding of inhalant use and improved treatment and prevention strategies.

Although chronic use of inhalants can cause damage to the brain and other organs, much more information is needed about the patterns of use that produce such effects and recovery programs. Considering the large number of persons who have experimented with inhalants, it seems likely that only a fraction of these experience organ damage. Much more data are needed on the etiologic factors in observed cases of organ toxicity from inhalant use, and more general population studies with appropriate control groups are needed to assess the incidence of these effects.

TABLE 20-2 Clinical Manifestations of Acute Inhalant Intoxication

Inhalants	Signs and symptoms	Cause	Management
Volatile alkyl nitrites	• Hypotension and tachycardia • Cyanosis and fatigue	• Blood vessels dilation • Methemoglobinemia	• Blood pressure stabilization • Methylene blue (1-2 mg/kg, IV over 5-10 min)
Nitrous oxide	Numbness in hands and feet in a stocking and glove distribution	Vitamin B_{12} inactivation	B_{12} supplementation
Toluene or toluene-containing products	Weakness, cramps in extremities, breathing difficulties, diarrhea, EKG alterations	Electrolyte imbalance and acid-basic disturbances	IV potassium replenishment HCO_3 supplementation, if needed

Adapted from Cámara-Lemarroy CR, Gónzalez-Moreno EI, Rodriguez-Gutierrez R, González-González JG. Clinical presentation and management in acute toluene intoxication: a case series. *Inhal Toxicol.* 2012;24(7):434-438; Cruz SL. Inhalant misuse management. The experience in Mexico and a literature review. *J Subst Use.* 2018;23(5):485-491.

CASE FOR CONSIDERATION

The parents of a 14-year-old boy report that they are concerned about behavioral changes they see taking place in their child. The boy often spends several hours a day after school in the garage, sometimes with friends and sometimes alone. He and his friends have stacked up boxes to sit on, but no obvious recreational activities are available in the garage. He does not spend as much time with the family, sleeps more, eats less, and has been more argumentative and more irritated. His school performance had deteriorated. Although the boy sometimes returned from the garage slightly intoxicated, a search of the garage and his room revealed no evidence of alcohol or other drug paraphernalia. The boy denied drinking alcohol or smoking cannabis. The mother becomes especially concerned when she noticed that her son had red eyes and sores around his mouth. The parents were advised to bring their son to their family physician for assessment. They make an appointment, but before the date for the physician visit, they found their son comatose in the garage. He had fallen with his face into a paint rag that had obviously been soaked with the fluid from an open can of paint thinner that was stored in the garage. The garage had a strong chemical smell. They opened the garage door, moved the boy outside, and called 911, but before the emergency response vehicle arrived, the boy recovered consciousness, displaying slurred speech and signs similar to alcohol intoxication. After a discussion with the family physician, the family arranged for their son to see a psychologist experienced in adolescent conduct disorder and SUDs.

REFERENCES

1. Balster RL, Cruz SL, Howard MO, Dell CA, Cottler LB. Classification of abused inhalants. *Addiction*. 2009;104(6):878-882.
2. Giorgetti R, Tagliabracci A, Schifano F, Zaami S, Marinelli E, Busardò FP. When "Chems" meet sex: a rising phenomenon called "ChemSex." *Curr Neuropharmacol*. 2017;15(5):762-770.
3. Xiang Y, Li L, Ma X, et al. Recreational nitrous oxide abuse: prevalence, neurotoxicity, and treatment. *Neurotox Res*. 2021;39(3):975-985.
4. Zacny JP, Janiszewski D, Sadeghi P, Black ML. Reinforcing, subjective, and psychomotor effects of sevoflurane and nitrous oxide in moderate-drinking healthy volunteers. *Addiction*. 1999;94(12):1817-1828.
5. Bowen SE, Batis JC, Paez-Martinez N, Cruz SL. The last decade of solvent research in animal models of abuse: mechanistic and behavioral studies. *Neurotoxicol Teratol*. 2006;28(6):636-647.
6. Shelton KL, Nicholson KL. Pharmacological classification of the abuse-related discriminative stimulus effects of trichloroethylene vapor. *J Drug Alcohol Res*. 2014;3:1-10.
7. Cruz S, Balster R. Neuropharmacology of inhalants. In: Miller PM, ed. *Biological Research on Addiction*. 2013:637-645.
8. Zandberg A. "Villages … reek of ether vapours": ether drinking in Silesia before 1939. *Med Hist*. 2010;54(3):387-396.
9. Haverkos HW, Kopstein AN, Wilson H, Drotman P. Nitrite inhalants: history, epidemiology, and possible links to AIDS. *Environ Health Perspect*. 1994;102(10):858-861.
10. d'Abbs P, MacLean S. *Volatile Substance Misuse: A Review of Interventions [Internet]*. Australian Government. 2008. Accessed May 18, 2023. https://vsu.mhc.wa.gov.au/media/1301/dha-2.pdf
11. Cruz SL, Bowen SE. The last two decades on preclinical and clinical research on inhalant effects. *Neurotoxicol Teratol*. 2021;87:106999.
12. Johnston L, Miech R, O´Malley P, Bachman J, Schulenberg J, Patrick M. *Monitoring the Future National Results on Adolescent Drug Use 1975-2021: Overview, Key Findings on Adolescent Drug Use 1975-2021: Overview, Key Findings on Adolescent Drug Use*. Institute for Social Research, University of Michigan; 2022. Accessed May 18, 2023. https://monitoringthefuture.org/wp-content/uploads/2022/08/mtf-overview2021.pdf
13. Center for Behavioral Health Statistics and Quality. *National Survey on Drug Use and Health: Detailed Tables*. 2020.
14. Snyder SM, Howard MO. Patterns of inhalant use among incarcerated youth. *PloS One*. 2015;10(9):e0135303.
15. Le A, Yockey A, Palamar JJ. Use of "Poppers" among adults in the United States, 2015-2017. *J Psychoactive Drugs*. 2020;52(5):433-439.
16. Dell CA, Gust SW, MacLean S. Global issues in volatile substance misuse. *Subst Use Misuse*. 2011;46(suppl 1):1-7.
17. Inter-American Drug Abuse Control Commission (CICAD) Secretariat for Multidimensional Security (SMS) Organization of American States (OAS). Report on Drug Use in the Americas; 2019. Accessed May 18, 2023. http://www.cicad.oas.org/main/pubs/Report%20on%20Drug%20Use%20in%20the%20Americas%202019.pdf
18. ESPAD Group. *ESPAD Report 2019: Results From the European School Survey Project on Alcohol and Other Drugs*. EMCDDA Joint Publications, Publications Office of the European Union; 2020. Accessed May 18, 2023. http://www.espad.org/espad-report-2019
19. Boak A, Elton-Marshall T, Mann R, Hamilton H. *Drug Use Among Ontario Students 1977-2019: Detailed Findings From the Ontario Student Drug Use and Health Survey (OSDUHS)*. Centre for Addiction and Mental Health. Accessed May 18, 2023. https://www.camh.ca/-/media/files/pdf---osduhs/drugusereport_2019osduhs-pdf.pdf
20. Australian Institute of Health and Welfare (AIHW). *National Drug Strategy Household Survey 2019. Drug Statistics Series no. 32. PHE 270*. Canberra AIHW; 2020. Accessed May 18, 2023. https://www.aihw.gov.au/reports/illicit-use-of-drugs/national-drug-strategy-household-survey-2019/contents/summary
21. American Psychiatric Association. Inhalant-Related Disorders. *Diagnostic and Statistical Manual of Mental Disorders*. 5th ed. 2022:601-668.
22. Wu LT, Howard MO. Is inhalant use a risk factor for heroin and injection drug use among adolescents in the United States? *Addict Behav*. 2007;32(2):265-281.
23. Wu LT, Pilowsky DJ, Schlenger WE. High prevalence of substance use disorders among adolescents who use marijuana and inhalants. *Drug Alcohol Depend*. 2005;78(1):23-32.
24. Bowen SE. Two serious and challenging medical complications associated with volatile substance misuse: sudden sniffing death and fetal solvent syndrome. *Subst Use Misuse*. 2011;46(suppl 1):68-72.
25. Cruz SL, Balster RL, Woodward JJ. Effects of volatile solvents on recombinant *N*-methyl-d-aspartate receptors expressed in *Xenopus* oocytes. *Br J Pharmacol*. 2000;131(7):1303-1308.
26. Shelton KL. Discriminative stimulus effects of abused inhalants. In: Porter JH, Prus AJ, eds. *The Behavioral Neuroscience of Drug Discrimination*. Springer Nature; 2018:113-140.
27. Mihic SJ, Ye Q, Wick MJ, et al. Sites of alcohol and volatile anaesthetic action on GABAA and glycine receptors. *Nature*. 1997;389(6649):385-389.
28. Cruz SL, Domínguez M. Misusing volatile substances for their hallucinatory effects: a qualitative pilot study with Mexican teenagers and a pharmacological discussion of their hallucinations. *Subst Use Misuse*. 2011;46(suppl 1):84-94.
29. Emmanouil DE, Quock RM. Advances in understanding the actions of nitrous oxide. *Anesth Prog*. 2007;54(1):9-18.
30. Richardson KJ, Shelton KL. *N*-methyl-d-aspartate receptor channel blocker–like discriminative stimulus effects of nitrous oxide gas. *J Pharmacol Exp Ther*. 2015;352(1):156-165.
31. Blokhina EA, Dravolina OA, Bespalov AY, Balster RL, Zvartau EE. Intravenous self-administration of abused solvents and anesthetics in mice. *Eur J Pharmacol*. 2004;485(1-3):211-218.

32. Gerasimov MR, Collier L, Ferrieri A, et al. Toluene inhalation produces a conditioned place preference in rats. *Eur J Pharmacol.* 2003;477(1):45-52.
33. Bowen SE, Balster RL. Tolerance and sensitization to inhaled 1,1,1-trichloroethane in mice: results from open-field behavior and a functional observational battery. *Psychopharmacology (Berl).* 2006;185(4):405-415.
34. Beyer CE, Stafford D, LeSage MG, Glowa JR, Steketee JD. Repeated exposure to inhaled toluene induces behavioral and neurochemical cross-sensitization to cocaine in rats. *Psychopharmacology (Berl).* 2001;154(2):198-204.
35. Gerasimov MR, Schiffer WK, Marstellar D, Ferrieri R, Alexoff D, Dewey SL. Toluene inhalation produces regionally specific changes in extracellular dopamine. *Drug Alcohol Depend.* 2002;65(3):243-251.
36. Riegel AC, Zapata A, Shippenberg TS, French ED. The abused inhalant toluene increases dopamine release in the nucleus accumbens by directly stimulating ventral tegmental area neurons. *Neuropsychopharmacology.* 2007;32(7):1558-1569.
37. Bowen SE, Hannigan JH, Davidson CJ, Callan SP. Abstinence following toluene exposure increases anxiety-like behavior in mice. *Neurotoxicol Teratol.* 2018;65:42-50.
38. Perron B, Glass JE, Ahmedani B, Vaughn MG, Roberts DE, Wu LT. The prevalence and clinical significance of inhalant withdrawal symptoms among a national sample. *Subst Abuse Rehabil.* 2011;2011(2):69-76.
39. ICD-11 for Mortality and Morbidity Statistics (Version: 02/2022)—6C4B.4 Volatile Inhalant Withdrawal. Accessed May 18, 2023. https://icd.who.int/browse11/l-m/en#/http://id.who.int/icd/entity/1317171068
40. Romanelli F, Smith KM, Thornton AC, Pomeroy C. Poppers: epidemiology and clinical management of inhaled nitrite abuse. *Pharmacotherapy.* 2004;24(1):69-78.
41. Tormoehlen LM, Tekulve KJ, Nañagas KA. Hydrocarbon toxicity: a review. *Clin Toxicol.* 2014;52(5):479-489.
42. Oussalah A, Julien M, Levy J, et al. Global burden related to nitrous oxide exposure in medical and recreational settings: a systematic review and individual patient data meta-analysis. *J Clin Med.* 2019;8(4):551.
43. Evans EB, Evans MR. Nangs, balloons and crackers: recreational nitrous oxide neurotoxicity. *Aust J Gen Pract.* 2021;50(11):834-838.
44. Maxwell JC. Deaths related to the inhalation of volatile substances in Texas: 1988-1998. *Am J Drug Alcohol Abuse.* 2001;27(4):689-697.
45. Cieślik-Guerra UI, Rechciński T, Trzos E, et al. Cardiotoxic effect due to accidental ingestion of an organic solvent. *Int J Occup Med Environ Health.* 2015;28:174-179.
46. Camara-Lemarroy CR, Rodríguez-Gutiérrez R, Monreal-Robles R, González-González JG. Acute toluene intoxication—clinical presentation, management and prognosis: a prospective observational study. *BMC Emerg Med.* 2015;15(1):19.
47. Crossin R, Lawrence A, Andrews Z, Churilov L, Duncan J. Growth changes after inhalant abuse and toluene exposure: a systematic review and meta-analysis of human and animal studies. *Hum Exp Toxicol.* 2019;38(2):157-172.
48. Kahn SA, Bierman TV, Larson KJ, Blache AL. Killing brain cells and skin cells simultaneously with inhalant abuse: pearls from the national burn repository. *J Burn Care Res.* 2019;40(3):347-348.
49. Dong X, Ba F, Wang R, Zheng D. Imaging appearance of myelopathy secondary to nitrous oxide abuse: a case report and review of the literature. *Int J Neurosci.* 2019;129(3):225-229.
50. Filley CM, Halliday W, Kleinschmidt-Demasters BK. The effects of toluene on the central nervous system. *J Neuropathol Exp Neurol.* 2004;63(1):1-12.
51. Borne J, Riascos R, Cuellar H, Vargas D, Rojas R. Neuroimaging in drug and substance abuse part II. *Top Magn Reson Imaging.* 2005;16(3):239-245.
52. Hannigan JH, Bowen SE. Reproductive toxicology and teratology of abused toluene. *Syst Biol Reprod Med.* 2010;56(2):184-200.
53. Duncan JR, Dick ALW, Egan G, et al. Adolescent toluene inhalation in rats affects white matter maturation with the potential for recovery following abstinence. *PloS One.* 2012;7(9):e44790.
54. Wu LT, Howard MO. Psychiatric disorders in inhalant users: results from the national epidemiologic survey on alcohol and related conditions. *Drug Alcohol Depend.* 2007;88(2-3):146-155.
55. Terán-Pérez G, Arana Y, Paredes L, Atilano-Barbosa D, Velázquez-Moctezuma J, Mercadillo RE. Diverse sleep patterns, psychiatric disorders, and perceived stress in inhalants users living on the streets of Mexico City. *Sleep Health.* 2020;6(2):192-196.
56. Sakai JT, Mikulich-Gilbertson SK, Crowley TJ. Adolescent inhalant use among male patients in treatment for substance and behavior problems: two-year outcome. *Am J Drug Alcohol Abuse.* 2006;32(1):29-40.
57. Howard MO, Perron BE, Sacco P, et al. Suicide ideation and attempts among inhalant users: results from the national epidemiologic survey on alcohol and related conditions. *Suicide Life Threat Behav.* 2010;40(3):276-286.
58. Chien WH, Huang MC, Chen LY. Psychiatric and other medical manifestations of nitrous oxide abuse. *J Clin Psychopharmacol.* 2020;40(1):80-83.
59. Gagnaire F, Langlais C. Relative ototoxicity of 21 aromatic solvents. *Arch Toxicol.* 2005;79(6):346-354.
60. Davies AJ, Borschmann R, Kelly SP, Ramsey J, Ferris J, Winstock AR. The prevalence of visual symptoms in poppers users: a global survey. *BMJ Open Ophthalmol.* 2017;1(1):1-1.
61. Tas U, Ogeturk M, Meydan S, et al. Hepatotoxic activity of toluene inhalation and protective role of melatonin. *Toxicol Ind Health.* 2011;27(5):465-473.
62. Yurtseven A, Türksoylu M, Yazıcı P, Karapınar B, Saz EU. A 'glue sniffer' teenager with anuric renal failure and hepatitis. *Turk J Pediatr.* 2018;60(2):206.
63. Cámara-Lemarroy CR, Gónzalez-Moreno EI, Rodriguez-Gutierrez R, González-González JG. Clinical presentation and management in acute toluene intoxication: a case series. *Inhal Toxicol.* 2012;24(7):434-438.
64. Yang M. A current global view of environmental and occupational cancers. *J Environ Sci Health C.* 2011;29(3):223-249.
65. Tello DM, Doodnauth AV, Patel KH, Gutierrez D, Dubey GR. Poppers-induced methemoglobinemia: a curious case of the blues. *Cureus.* 2021;13(5):e15276.
66. Wille SMR, Lambert WEE. Volatile substance abuse—post-mortem diagnosis. *Forensic Sci Int.* 2004;142(2-3):135-156.
67. Ford JB, Sutter ME, Owen KP, Albertson TE. Volatile substance misuse: an updated review of toxicity and treatment. *Clin Rev Allergy Immunol.* 2014;46(1):19-33.
68. Hubková B, Rácz O, Bódy G, Frišman E, Mareková M. Toluene abuse markers in marginalized populations. *Interdiscip Toxicol.* 2018;11(1):22-26.
69. Jain R, Verma A. Laboratory approach for diagnosis of toluene-based inhalant abuse in a clinical setting. *J Pharm Bioallied Sci.* 2016;8(1):18.
70. Joncquel Chevalier-Curt M, Grzych G, Tard C, et al. Nitrous oxide abuse in the emergency practice, and Review of toxicity mechanisms and potential markers. *Food Chem Toxicol.* 2022;162:112894.
71. Konghom S, Verachai V, Srisurapanont M, et al. Treatment for inhalant dependence and abuse. *Cochrane Database Syst Rev.* 2010;12:CD007537.
72. Cruz SL. Inhalant misuse management. The experience in Mexico and a literature review. *J Subst Use.* 2018;23(5):485-491.
73. Howard MO, Garland EL. Volatile substance misuse: toward a research agenda. *Am J Drug Alcohol Abuse.* 2013;39(1):3-7.

SUGGESTED READINGS

Balster RL, Cruz SL, Howard MO, et al. Classification of abused inhalants. *Addiction.* 2009;104:878-882.

Cruz SL, Bowen SE. The last two decades on preclinical and clinical research on inhalant effects. *Neurotoxicol Teratol.* 2021;87:106999.

Dell CA, Gust SW, MacLean S. Global issues in volatile substance misuse. *Subst Use Misuse.* 2011;46(suppl 1):1-7. (Note: the entire issue of this journal is devoted to international inhalant abuse research.)

Nguyen J, O'Brien C, Schapp S. Adolescent inhalant use prevention, assessment, and treatment: a literature synthesis. *Int J Drug Policy.* 2016;31:15-24.

21 The Pharmacology of Anabolic-Androgenic Steroids

Scott E. Lukas

CHAPTER OUTLINE

- Introduction
- Drugs in the class
- Therapeutic use and unhealthy use
- Adverse effects
- Addiction liability
- Absorption and metabolism
- Mechanisms of action
- Future vistas

INTRODUCTION

Within the addiction field, the term *steroids* defines those compounds that possess anabolic or tissue-building effects, but because most also have some androgenic properties, they are more appropriately called anabolic–androgenic steroids (AAS). This profile of effects distinguishes them from the corticosteroids and the female gonadotrophic hormones, neither of which is typically subject to unhealthy use. There are many AAS that have been produced for both human and veterinary use and the major source of illicit steroids is diversion from licit manufacture and distribution, as clandestine laboratory synthesis of these products is rare. The major distinction between use and unhealthy use is that the latter typically takes supraphysiological doses of these compounds to increase muscle growth and enhance performance. It is the consequence of these extremely high doses that results in serious and not always reversible, psychiatric and medical side effects.

DRUGS IN THE CLASS

The prototypic hormone, testosterone, is the standard to which all synthetic products are compared, and it is one of four structurally distinct groups of AAS. The other three groups are 17α-alkylated derivatives of testosterone, 17β-esterified derivatives of testosterone, and modified ring structure analogues[1] The history of how testosterone and its effects on male sexual development and tissue building were discovered is well detailed by Kochakian[2] Although hormonal involvement in male sexual development was known in 1849, it was not until 1930 when androsterone (a metabolite of testosterone) was isolated from human urine. In the 1940s, after chemists had succeeded in synthesizing testosterone, their efforts were directed toward separating its anabolic from its androgenic effects and to make a formulation that could be taken orally. The androgenic component of these synthetics has never been completely separated from the anabolic effects; only the relative percentage of the two has been manipulated. Commercially prepared products were used briefly during World War II to promote wound healing. In 1939, Boje[3] postulated that AAS might not only increase muscle mass but improve physical performance as well. Hartgens and Kuipers[4] provide a comprehensive review of the pharmacology and toxicity of AAS in athletes.

The introduction of AAS to the United States has been traced to the 1954 World Weightlifting Championships in Vienna, when the Soviet Union's coach informed the U.S. coach that his team members were taking testosterone[5] In the ensuing years, use of AAS by elite weightlifters, power lifters, and bodybuilders increased. Over the years, their use spread to many professional sports, especially those in which strength and body weight were important for success (eg, football). Testosterone was the drug of choice in the 1950s, which was replaced by more elegant synthetic compounds over the next three decades, primarily because of their slightly higher percent of anabolic versus androgenic effects and their relative resistance to detection by current laboratory tests. Use spread to collegiate and amateur athletes as evidenced by the 50% positive tests obtained by the International Olympic Committee during unannounced urine screens in 1984 and 1985.[6] The 1990s saw a return to the use of testosterone, which is thought to be due to improved gas chromatographic methods of detecting the synthetic compounds and the continued difficulty of accurately detecting exogenously administered testosterone.[7] However, another trend toward using other types of performance-enhancing aids has evolved in the wake of pure unhealthy AAS use.

It often is difficult to determine whether the attraction of the drugs is related to any beneficial effect on the individual's performance, because the drugs rarely are taken in the absence of a training program that includes exercise and sound nutrition.[8] This concept punctuates the second aspect of AAS unhealthy use among athletes—it usually occurs during training periods, which typically can begin weeks and even months before a competitive event or season. The need for these drugs by most athletes decreases during actual competition, and so the active use can decline. However, with the advent of mandatory urine testing at major athletic events, the risk of being caught also curtails use. Positive urine screens that are collected during the actual competitive event are usually due to the high sensitivity of the analytic methods to detect small amounts of metabolites that have persisted long since use of the AAS has ceased. Once a gas chromatographic test for hair samples had been validated, the ability to detect AAS among athletes increased,[9] and with more recent advances in mass spectrometry and bioassays,[10] the levels of detectability have decreased even to the picogram range, which could even pick up passive exposure.[11] Despite the enhanced methods of detecting these complex compounds, controversial use of AAS has tainted many sporting events including Major League Baseball, track and field, and professional cycling—some of these have led to congressional investigations, and elite athletes continue to be stripped of their titles because of discovered use. And in one case where such use was found to be so widespread—as in the Tour de France—no winner was declared for many years.

New-Generation "Performance Enhancers"

With the availability of more sophisticated urine testing procedures, the likelihood that an athlete can avoid being caught using AAS is decreasing somewhat, and the advent of detecting drugs like erythropoietin has contributed to the identification of a widespread use of this performance enhancer in professional cycling. Nevertheless, the desire for new-generation performance-enhancing drugs and nutritional supplements continues to grow. Moreover, many of these agents have been extremely difficult to detect using standard laboratory procedures, not because the technology is limited but because these substances are found naturally in the body,[12] and so carbon isotope mass spectrometry is needed.[13] Some of these challenging drugs include other hormones such as human growth hormone (somatotropin), dehydroepiandrosterone, erythropoietin, and thyroxine. Cadaver pituitary growth hormone has been replaced by recombinant human growth hormone, and the latter has been found to increase strength and peak power output and fat-free mass index decreased after only a short course of the recombinant hormone.[14]

Drugs belonging to other pharmacological classes continue to be popular as potential agents to "boost" performance. These include the mixed agonist/antagonist opioids such as butorphanol and nalbuphine; the beta-adrenergic agonist clenbuterol; "hormone helpers" such as gamma hydroxybutyrate, clonidine, and human chorionic gonadotropin; and testosterone stimulants such as clomiphene and human chorionic gonadotropin. In addition, a variety of diuretics (acetazolamide, furosemide, spironolactone, and triamterene) are used to help clear the AAS and their metabolites from the urine before drug testing. Knowledge of these drugs, where to get them, doses of use, and even recipes for adding them to training programs can be found in many "underground" guides as well as from a variety of websites. In fact, a growing concern is that many individuals have now turned to the internet as a major source for purchasing these agents, and it appears that there are hundreds of thousands of sites offering underground information on how to use them[15] and even offering to sell AAS outright[16]; clinicians are well advised to be aware of these practices because the sites are often very "pro" drug use and question the knowledge or authority of those in the medical field. The accuracy of many of the claims on these sites is dubious at best (**Table 21-1**).

It is not just the novel drugs that are of interest, but individuals with a substance use disorder (SUD) seek veterinary or animal husbandry products. For example, trenbolone is an AAS that is often used to increase muscle growth/meat production in cattle[17] and is usually implanted into the cow's ear. In their paper on web-based AAS information, Brennan et al.[15] noted that there were many sites that described how to remove the estrogens from this formulation, rendering it more suitable for human bodybuilding purposes.

At-Risk Populations

It is now well established that athletes are not the only individuals to use AAS in unhealthy ways. Unhealthy use has now appeared in adult nonathletes and even in young boys who may be using them to simply improve their appearance.[18] Women are also using these drugs, but all estimates indicate that the percentage remains much lower than in males. These factors encouraged the U.S. Congress to enact the Anabolic Steroids Control Act, which effectively placed all these compounds, including testosterone and its many analogues, into Schedule III of the federal Controlled Substances Act. States still have the option of scheduling these drugs even more restrictively under state law. Schedule III includes opioids such as nalorphine, stimulants such as benzphetamine, and depressants such as butabarbital and thiopental.

The 1990s was rife with surveys demonstrating that the incidence of AAS use and unhealthy use by adults and adolescents was lower than that of other drugs.[19,20] The data suggested that AAS were used by less than 2% of the adolescents surveyed and less than 1% of older respondents. During the ensuing 5 to 6 years, new data revealed some concerning trends in AAS use, particularly among the youth. Use among boys in general was reported to be more than 3%,[21] and in certain populations of 15- to 19-year-old boys, nearly 10% reported using AAS.[22] In a cross-sectional assessment using the 2003 Centers for Disease Control and Prevention National School-Based Youth Risk Behavior Survey database,[23] Elliot et al.[24] reported that 5.3% of the 7,544 females in grades 9 to 12 used AAS. In addition, these young women also engaged in a number of other unhealthy life choices including using tobacco, cannabis, and diet pills, carrying weapons, and having sexual relations before the age of 13. These authors also noted that AAS-using females were *less* likely to participate in team sports; this fuels the belief that children and adolescents have poor body images.[25] This rate of AAS use among females punctuates the twofold to fourfold increase in AAS use that was reported by Yesalis et al.[26] in the 1990s. However, steroid use appears to decline with age, and desire to weigh more was a strong predictor of AAS use by males, but females who use AAS were more likely to have higher body mass indices and a poorer knowledge of nutrition.[27] Another complicating factor in obtaining accurate information about AAS use in teenage

TABLE 21-1 List of Trade Names, Chemical Names, and Brief Summary of the Use of the More Common AAS Compounds

Popular/trade name	Chemical name	Description of uses/actions
Anabolic–Androgenic steroids (for human use)		
Anabolicum vister		Well tolerated but very weak androgen that has low side effect profile
Anadrol-50	Oxymetholone	One of the most powerful anabolic and androgenic steroids; used to treat anemia
Anavar	Oxandrolone	Primarily prescribed for weight gain
Androderm	Testosterone patch	Slow-release formulation of testosterone generally used for replacement therapy
Androgel	Testosterone topical gel	Topical ointment formulation of testosterone
Danocrine	Danazol	Used to treat pelvic pain and infertility secondary to uterine disorders and breast pain secondary to fibrocystic breast disease
Deca Durabolin	Nandrolone decanoate	Used to treat anemia, wasting syndrome, breast cancer and osteoporosis
Durabolin	Phenpropionate	Very popular injectable with high anabolic and low androgenic profile
Delatestryl	Testosterone enanthate	Moderately powerful androgen in an injectable oil preparation given every 1-4 weeks
Depo-Testosterone	Testosterone cypionate	Moderately powerful anabolic effects and androgen in an injectable oil preparation; its effects are relatively short-lived and water retention is a problem
Dianabol	Methandrostenolone	Popular oral preparation that has a rapid onset of effects; moderate androgenic effects limit its use
Halotestin	Fluoxymesterone	Powerful androgen with less anabolic effects, used to treat hypogonadism in males and metastastic breast cancer in females
Metandren, Testred	Methyltestosterone	Oral testosterone that is not very popular today but still taken because of its prominent anabolic effects
Android	Methyltestosterone	Synthetic derivative of testosterone used to treat hypogonadism
Oxandrin	Oxandrolone	Mild anabolic agent that increases strength without concomitant increase in mass; believed to be relatively safe although liver toxicity is possible
Primobolan	Methenolone	Mild, but relatively safe, anabolic agent with little androgenic effects and is available as an oral, buccal, and injectable depot formulation; used by athletes
Proviron	Mesterolone	Less effective anabolic as it is quickly metabolized to the diol metabolite and so may not reach receptors
Stenox	Halotestin	Strong oral androgen and mild anabolic but rather toxic; weight gain is minimal
Sustanon	Testosterone	Oil-based injectable preparation of four salts of testosterone, propionate, phenylpropionate, isocaproate, and decanoate, that are timed to release active testosterone from 1 to 30 days; pronounced anabolic and androgenic effects and has less water retention
Winstrol	Stanozolol	Oral preparation that has modest anabolic effects and weak androgenic effects and so is often stacked with other steroids; many counterfeits are available
Anabolic–Androgenic steroids/growth promoters (veterinary products)		
Cheque Drops	Mibolerone	No longer popular as is one of the most toxic of androgenic steroids available; it does increase mass and aggression
Equipoise	Boldenone	Strong anabolic with milder androgenic effects; often stacked with other steroids
Finiject	Bolasterone	Popular injectable but no longer available; strong anabolic and androgenic effects
Finaplix-H	Trenbolone	Implantable potent androgen that is no longer available
Implus	Testosterone	Implantable combination of testosterone and estradiol used to build muscle in cattle; also used by body builders
Nadrobolin	Nandrolone	Injectable long-acting version of Deca Durabolin; relatively inexpensive
Ralgro	Zeranol	Implantable agent that increases weight in cattle but efficacy in humans is unproven
Revalor	Trenbolone/estradiol	Implantable combination product of trenbolone and estradiol that will increase strength but little water retention; often used with dimethyl sulfoxide (DMSO) to promote skin absorption; renal toxicity is a common side effect
Synovex-H	Testosterone/estradiol	Implantable combination of testosterone and estradiol with similar profile as Revalor
Winstrol-V	Stanozolol	Both oral and injectable preparation that has modest anabolic effects and weak androgenic effects and so is often stacked with other steroids; many counterfeits exist for this preparation

(Continued)

TABLE 21-1 List of Trade Names, Chemical Names, and Brief Summary of the Use of the More Common AAS Compounds (*Continued*)

Popular/trade name	Chemical name	Description of uses/actions
Supplements, minerals, and other products (efficacy of these products for body building purposes have not been well characterized)		
Aldactazide	Aldactone/thiazide	Combination of the diuretics aldactone and thiazide used to lose excess water
Catapres	Clonidine	Antihypertensive taken to reduce steroid-induced elevated blood pressure
Clomid	Clomiphene	Increases FSH, which then increases testosterone; typically used to avoid crash after stopping steroids
Cynomel and others	Cytomel	Synthetic thyroid hormone (T3) used to increase basal metabolic rate by increasing synthesis of protein, carbohydrates, and fats; may work synergistically with steroids
Cytadren	Aminoglutethimide	Used to treat Cushing syndrome, it inhibits production of androgens, estrogens, and cortisone
EPO	Erythropoietin	Injectable protein hormone that stimulates red blood cell production in the bone marrow; dangerous elevations in hematocrit have accounted for some deaths
GHB	Gamma hydroxybutyrate	CNS depressant that increases growth hormone secretion, has a protein-sparing effect, improves sleep quality; dangerous when combined with other CNS depressants
Glucophage, Mellitron	Metformin	Oral hypoglycemic that mimics insulin; it is less toxic than phenformin
Humulin R	Insulin	Natural pancreatic hormone that regulates glucose and helps glycogen and other nutrients enter muscles; it is typically used right after a workout but is very dangerous
Fenformin	Phenformin	Oral hypoglycemic agent that can produce lactic acidosis, so it is not used as often as Glucophage
IGF-1		Insulin-like growth factor that is a structural analog of insulin; very short acting and so it is combined with IGFBP-3 to extend its half-life
Kyno-H	Kynoselen	A mixture of potassium, selenium, magnesium, vitamin B_{12}, and AMP that is promoted to inhibit protein breakdown; the claims have not been substantiated
Lasix	Furosemide	Strong diuretic that is used before competitions to remove excess subcutaneous water; can induce electrolyte imbalance if used improperly
Levothroid	L-thyroxine	Synthetic thyroid hormone (T4) that is used to increase the metabolism of carbohydrates, proteins, and fats; less popular than Cytomel
Naprosyn, Naxen	Naproxen	Potent oral nonsteroidal agent that reduces inflammation, stiffness, and pain; can result in stomach ulcers
Nubain	Nalbuphine	Opiate mixed agonist/antagonist pain killer that can be addictive
Pregnyl	Human chorionic gonadotropin (hCG)	Natural protein hormone that mimics luteinizing hormone's effects to stimulate release of testosterone; used to counter negative feedback effects of exogenous steroids. Also used to induce ovulation
Protropin	Growth hormone (GH)	Synthetic version of human growth hormone that is widely popular but may not be meeting expectations of protein buildup and breakdown of fat as an energy source; increases IGF-1 levels; cannot be detected by current testing procedures
Pump N Pose	Synthol	Fatty acid that is actually injected into specific muscles to increase their size via encapsulation within the muscle fibers; gains are reported to be permanent, but this is unlikely as it probably breaks down after a few years
Slow-K	Potassium chloride	Slow-release formulation used to prevent potassium depletion secondary to the use of strong diuretics
Spiropent	Clenbuterol	Bronchodilator used to treat asthma; as a $beta_2$ agonist, it burns fat but its anabolic effects are limited to livestock, not humans
Thiomucase		Dispersing agent that is included along with the injectable steroid to help it get into the system more quickly; also used by itself to reduce fatty spots (cellulite) on the body
Trisoralen	Trioxsalen	Oral medication that enhances pigmentation and thus promotes tanning to improve looks just before competition; not widely available

girls is that surveys may contain imprecise language so that the term *steroid* is misinterpreted,[28] leading to an inflated estimate of AAS use.

The incidence of drug use among 8th to 12th graders has been tracked by the Monitoring the Future National Survey for years and the recent 2021 report revealed some interesting trends in AAS use.[29] Use of androgenic steroids by 8th to 12th graders peaked between 2001 and 2005 with 12-month rates ranging 1.7%, 2.1%, and 2.5% for 8th, 10th and 12th graders, respectively. A slow but consistent decline followed until use flattened out in 2016 (0.4%-0.9%). A small increase ensued until 2020 where use peaked between 0.8 and 1.1%. Then in 2021, AAS use by all groups plummeted to less than 0.5%. This decrease was not restricted to AAS as the report noted that there was a decline in nearly all drug use in 2021. The Monitoring the Future Study[29] also collected data on perceived risk, disapproval rates, and perceived availability. It is counterintuitive, but the decline in use since 2001 to 2005 was paralleled by a decline in perceived risk, and no change in disapproval rates. Disapproval rates dropped dramatically in the past year, mimicking the fall in use. Some have attributed the decline in AAS use by adolescents as being related to this class of drugs being placed on Schedule III of the Control Substances Act. However, use by all three groups actually *increased* after they were scheduled in 1991 and it was not until 2007 that adolescents started to report a reduction in availability. The COVID pandemic contributed to a decrease in alcohol use but an increase in nicotine vaping and prescription drugs among 10- to 14-year-olds enrolled in the Adolescent Brain Cognitive Development (ABCD) study[30] with a dramatic increase in opiate overdoses in past years.[31] It is unknown whether the significant drop in AAS use among high school students is related to the COVID pandemic, but the combination of gradual reduced availability and the social isolation imposed by COVID restrictions could have made it more difficult for high school students to gain access to AAS drugs. What remains unclear is why use has declined even though the perceived risk of using these drugs continued downward.

While use among the lay public remains low, the incidence of use among individuals engaged in resistance training in gyms is closer to 17% for men and 6.5% for women.[32] The incidence of use among power sports and/or weightlifting can be 20% to more than 50%.[33,34] A recent meta-analysis[35] revealed that body builders were more likely to use AAS (36.3%) compared to other athletes (30.9%). Furthermore, there is a clear impact of the media, peer pressure, and teasing/comments from parents as factors that predict or at least facilitate AAS use among young boys. Many studies[36-38] reported that gaming, magazines, and the media and its portrayal of sports and image about male physical characteristics increase drive for muscularity. Indeed, in a internet-based survey of 500 people who use AAS, 78% were noncompetitive bodybuilders and not otherwise engaged in athletic events.[39]. However, very recent data suggest that depressive symptoms and victimization are two unexpected pathways to AAS use among adolescent boys because these factors enhance the impact of self-perceived underweight body image[40] but that there is also a significant risk factor for boys who perceive themselves to be either overweight or underweight.[41] Furthermore, a 2017 report revealed that sexual orientation and race/ethnicity may play a role in the misuse of AAS with a greater impact on Black and Hispanic adolescent boys.[42] Lifetime use of AAS has been difficult to track, but an analysis of multiple surveys revealed that AAS use begins later than most other drugs with only 22% starting before the age of 20.[43] After applying an age of onset analysis, these authors estimated that among 13- to 50-year-olds, between 2.9 and 4 million Americans have used AAS and roughly 1 million may have experienced pre-DSM-5-defined steroid dependence, which is surprisingly high.

Internet-based surveys have another role as revealing potential indicators of future AAS use, based on current drug use patterns. Dunn et al.[44] reported that 80% of respondents to the survey said that they used sports supplements such as vitamins and protein supplements. The authors suggest that the widespread use of sports supplements may in some way remove "barriers" for the future use of AAS. The sample also reported a high incidence (52%) of illicit drugs, which challenges the preconceived notion that people who use AAS are a health-conscious group as a whole and rarely engaged in other drug use. This is apparently not the case as it has been shown that AAS use is positively correlated with the use of other licit and illicit drugs such as alcohol, cocaine, licit painkillers, methylphenidate, ketamine, and legal performance-enhancing agents.[45] As might be expected, the use of the two smoked drugs, tobacco, and cannabis, was not consistently reported in these studies. The fact that people who use AAS are engaging in polypharmacy practices has only complicated efforts to define and implement safe and effective treatments. In fact, a recent meta-analysis of 50 studies published between 1985 and 2014 concluded that people who use AAS frequently used other substances with alcohol and cannabis leading the list, followed by cocaine, growth hormone, human chorionic gonadotropin (hCG), amphetamine/methamphetamine, clenbuterol, ephedrine, insulin, and thyroxine.[46]

A recent trend has been to use synthetic androgens or even "designer steroids" to achieve the same gains in strength, size, and performance but within legal measures.[47] A large number of these agents were originally developed for use in equine sports.[48] Many of these over-the-counter preparations having names like "prohormones," "natural steroids," testosterone booster" are sold over the internet and labeled as dietary supplements,[49,50] and because the chemical structures differ from the controlled AAS, they are not illegal. There is concern that these synthetic androgens induce a specific form of neurotoxicity resulting in neurodegenerative disease that is secondary to oxidative stress and apoptosis.[51] As a result, the use of nutritional supplements by adolescent athletes has increased dramatically (eg, testosterone precursors such as androstenedione, dehydroepiandrosterone, and androstenediol).[52-55] It is theoretically possible that these agents should increase lean muscle mass by being converted to testosterone. While many studies have failed to reliably demonstrate such effects[56-59] androstenedione will increase the testosterone to epitestosterone ratio—a marker used to indicate illegal use of testosterone in athletic competition and as such the FDA has ruled that it cannot be marketed as a dietary supplement.[60]

Although androstenedione is banned by the World Anti-Doping Agency, it is still sold as an oral supplement in many countries (but is under Schedule control in the U.S.). Theoretically, consuming large amounts of androstenedione should result in an increase in circulating testosterone concentrations and cause a net increase in body mass, reduced fat and increase RBC production. But does it really work as advertised? It is not regulated by the FDA and some healthcare professionals recommend its use to counteract the effects of age-related muscle loss (sarcopenia) to improve lifespan as well as quality of life in older people.[61] It is important to remember that the over-the-counter supplements that contain the word "andro" or claim to boost testosterone, do not in fact contain androstenedione. Androstenedione's ability to increase testosterone concentrations appears to be a function of dose. Testosterone concentrations were significantly increased in healthy 20- to 40-year-old men when given 300 mg/day for 7 days, but not when the dose was 100 mg/day.[62] However, an earlier randomized clinical trial failed to find significant increases in testosterone or enhance skeletal muscle adaptations to resistance training.[63] Thus, like most aspects of pharmacology, the key is the dose of the drug. But in the case of AAS, dose alone may not fully explain their efficacy or why they work for some and not for others. Improved performance from AAS and supplements like androstenedione are dependent on many other factors such as training intensity, training duration, diet, and genetics.

The chapter by McGinnis[64] demonstrated the remarkably close relationships between the effects of AAS in humans and a variety of animal models. One such model, the Syrian hamster, has been used to document that when adolescent animals are exposed to AAS, they appear to be far more sensitive to the effects of AAS than their adult counterparts. This model relates to the clinical condition as it is suspected that the neural "rewiring" that occurs in males during puberty sets the tone for future aggressive and violent tendencies and that exposure to AAS during this critical time can increase the likelihood that aggressive acts result in violent behavior. It would appear that the rewiring that normally occurs during puberty is affected by the exposure to higher concentrations of AAS and that this contributes to the changes in behavior later in life. The link between testosterone and aggressive behavior was made 2 years later by van Bokhoven et al.[65] who reported that 16-year-old boys who had criminal records had elevated testosterone concentrations compared to their peers and concluded that there was a positive relationship between testosterone and proactive and reactive aggression and self-reported delinquent behavior. This relationship was duplicated 9 years later in the hamster model and showed that exposure to AAS during adolescence results in increased aggressive responses during AAS exposure and enhanced anxiety-like responses during AAS withdrawal.[66] Exposure to AAS as adults failed to alter the behavior of the hamsters, which would suggest that the aggressive and anxiety-related responses to AAS are modulated by unique elements that appear during developmental stages.

Figure 21-1 depicts some of the more commonly identified effects and side effects of AAS use in adolescents. High-dose AAS use during adolescence has the potential of causing significantly more problems when adulthood is reached.[67] Some of the effects are easier to identify than others, so the challenge to the clinician in detecting AAS use in his or her patients is to know the risk factors, be able to identify the constellation of signs and symptoms of use and ask the correct questions when exploring use patterns.[68] The clinician may need to be vigilant

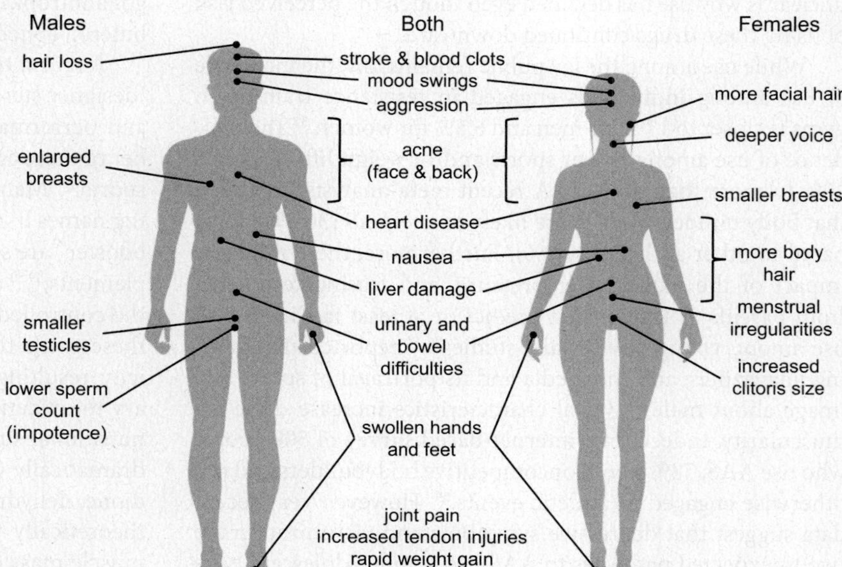

Figure 21-1. Side effect profiles of AAS in male and female persons with substance use disorder.

when presented with requests to treat moderate to severe acne, especially in 18- to 26-year-old males, because the incidence of acne is 50% in people who use AAS and thus may be a clinical indicator of unhealthy use.[69] As always, the clinician must be well informed of the facts about these drugs and be able to present themselves as a credible source of information.

THERAPEUTIC USE AND UNHEALTHY USE

Therapeutic Use

Although one might think that the therapeutic uses of AAS are of less concern to the addiction medicine specialist, most physicians are asked to give prescriptions for these drugs far more often than they are asked to help treat someone who is addicted to the drugs. Thus, knowledge of these medical situations might help in discussions with a person with a potential SUD because these individuals are likely to be aware of the medical reasons for their prescription and may use such information in their initial attempts to obtain legal medications to support their training or alter their appearance.

Males may receive AAS for replacement therapy when the testicles fail to function, because of either congenital or traumatic factors, or when puberty is delayed, and short stature would result. The doses that are prescribed, however, are much lower than those used by bodybuilders. The equivalent of 75 to 100 mg per week of testosterone suffices as replacement, but weightlifters and bodybuilders have reportedly used weekly doses of 1,000 to 2,100 mg of methandienone.[70,71] Women are occasionally treated with androgens when metastatic breast cancer has spread to the bone. Methyltestosterone is combined with estrogen to help alleviate some of the signs and symptoms of menopause. Nandrolone has been used in combination with exercise to increase lean body mass in patients who are on dialysis.[72]

Both males and females might receive the more anabolic agents during treatment of a rare form of hereditary angioedema. Acquired aplastic anemia and myelofibrosis both result in deficiencies of red blood cell production, which is combated with drugs that have equal amounts of anabolic and androgenic effects. Sometimes, these drugs can be useful in treating the trauma associated with burns and AIDS. Finally, just as was done in post-World War II, steroids with more anabolic activity are useful in treating muscle wasting that is secondary to starvation.

Unhealthy Use

AAS are used by three distinct populations: (1) athletes who use them to improve performance, (2) aesthetes who use them solely to improve appearance and perhaps gain some weight, and (3) the fighting elites who use them to enhance aggression and fighting skills. The "typology" of users has been suggested based on use patterns that include the "expert" on the pharmacology of AAS; the "you only live once" type who demonstrate little or no caution; the "athlete" type who only uses for competition, and the "wellbeing" type who is interested only in improving their physical appearance.[73] Identifying to which of these three populations a patient belongs to is the first step to understanding the pattern of use and determining the best treatment plan to follow.

Athletes

Athletes use AAS for one reason: to improve their performance. Perhaps one of the greatest mistakes a clinician makes in dealing with an athlete is attempting to dissuade their use because the drugs cannot improve performance. In fact, this is not true. The older research studies that purported to show that the effects of AAS were no different than placebo suffered from numerous methodological problems, did not control for motivation, and failed to document the amount of physical training. In addition, ethical considerations prevented the investigators from administering extremely high doses, which are considered necessary to achieve the muscle-building effect. Negative findings also have been attributed to the use of only one drug at a time in the research studies, whereas athletes in training typically use multiple drugs in combination. The continued use of these drugs is based on the belief that they increase muscle capacity, reduce body fat, increase strength and endurance, and hasten recovery from injury.[74] Many athletes also believe that AAS-assisted training allows the person to increase both the frequency and the intensity of workouts—factors that contribute to any direct benefits of the drugs.[75] An internet-based survey conducted in 2005 revealed that bodybuilders and weightlifters use on average 3.1 drugs, engage in cycles that last 5 to 10 weeks in length, and use doses that are 5 to 29 times greater than physiological replacement doses.[76] Rates of use among individuals in fitness centers are also much higher (approximately 12.5%) than the general population.[77]

In the world of professional weightlifting and bodybuilding, AAS are used in three basic patterns: "stacking," "pyramiding," and "cycling."[78] *Stacking* is the practice of using multiple products at the same time. Persons who use AAS believe that the beneficial effects of one drug will complement those of another and that they will only achieve real benefits through a specific combination. There are now animal data to support the notion that stacking AAS can result in an altered pharmacologic response. Wesson and McGinnis administered numerous combinations of testosterone, stanozolol, and nandrolone to adolescent male rats and found that behavioral and endocrine effects were altered. Furthermore, this simulated "stacking" procedure revealed that the level of androgen receptor occupation did not directly correlate with the effects of the combined agents.[79] A *pyramid* plan involves starting with a low dose and then gradually increasing the dose until peak levels are achieved a number of weeks before competition. The individual then slowly decreases or tapers the drug dose down, and because the beneficial effects of AAS persist long after their use has been discontinued, the athlete will be primed for the competitive event. *Cycling* refers to the practice of using different combinations over a period to avoid the development of tolerance or loss of effectiveness. Thus, different combinations of drugs are used over a 6- to 12-week period, after which another drug or combination is substituted.

A rather poignant example of how extensive the use pattern can be is provided in Table 4 of the review by Graham et al.[13] This table details a 16-week profile of stacking, pyramiding, and cycling of 19 different drugs from a half-dozen different pharmacological classes by a current UK bodybuilding champion. The breadth of combinations, patterns, and huge doses is quite extensive, and while this pattern appears to be on one end of the spectrum, this practice is widespread, and the clinician will find it necessary to become familiar with a number of different drugs (like diuretics, thyroid hormone, and insulin) as a reminder that few individuals engage in unhealthy use of a single agent and that other medications are used to either "boost" or facilitate the elimination of target drugs.

When prescriptions for AAS cannot be obtained, individuals may sometimes turn to veterinary products. It is an interesting paradox when young bodybuilders profess to be on strict diets and use only the purest of vitamin and dietary supplements, yet they will self-administer drugs for which use in humans has not been approved. Products that are not approved for use in the United States typically are obtained by mail order from abroad. Because the testing of these products in some other countries is not as stringent as that in the United States, patients should be cautioned about using such products. Finally, there is an extensive illegal market of AAS that supports a large percentage of inactive products that are falsely advertised as containing anabolic steroids.

Aesthetes

Another group of people who use AAS is composed of young boys and girls who use these drugs primarily to increase their weight or to improve their physical appearance.[73,80,81] This desire for weight gain among a group of adolescent boys who are not yet taking AAS may place them at risk for initiating use.[80] This trend is disturbing because these authors noted that a significant number of the boys were unaware of the most dangerous risks associated with AAS use. A recent study of the prevalence of AAS use among 6th to 12th grade Canadians revealed that 2.8% of the respondents had used these drugs over the past year.[82] A disturbing trend was that 29.4% of these students reported that they injected the drugs and 29.2% of these reported that they shared needles with friends. Young AAS users are also likely to use other drugs such as cannabis, smokeless tobacco, and cocaine.[83] These authors also reported a high percentage of needle-sharing behavior among adolescents.

In general, the doses used by adolescents and others who want to improve their appearance are substantially lower than those used by adult athletes.[84] Further, the pattern of lower doses and intermittent cycles of use is likely to obviate the development of major side effects. However, because young boys are often still in transition because of hormonal changes associated with puberty, these drugs can have other significant effects. For example, the epiphyseal plate of the femur can close prematurely and stunt a boy's growth,[85] which is contrary to what a significant number of adolescents believe. More importantly, these young people who use AAS may be particularly sensitive to the increased aggressive effects resulting from their use.[84]

Apparently, a substantial proportion of these adolescents are also unaware of the side effects of AAS. Although educational programs have been slow to incorporate these drugs in the lesson plans, the real reason that the public is so unaware of the risks is that these drugs are probably not a severe health hazard when taken intermittently and in low to moderate doses.[84] Because programs that simply emphasize the negative aspects of drugs are ineffectual at curtailing use,[86] the health professional should balance the discussion about unhealthy AAS use with the straight facts and not try to overstate the degree of harm. Such actions will only alienate the patient. Unfortunately, these young people know that only a small percentage of people who use AAS will experience very serious and deadly outcomes and that it will not happen to them. For the others, the side effects (except for some effects in women) are largely reversible.

Fighting Elite

Very little is known about this population of AAS users. This profile was originally described by Brower[87] and includes individuals who seek to increase their strength in order to perform their job. Another desired effect is the increase in aggressiveness that may also help them with their jobs. Thus, bouncers at bars, security personnel, and even law enforcement officers[88,89] have been reported to take these drugs.

Personality Profiles

A study of the personalities of people who use AAS by Cooper et al.[90] identified a high rate of abnormal personality traits in a sample of 12 bodybuilders who used AAS compared with a matched group who did not. Along with being heavier than the controls, the people who use AAS were more likely to score higher on measures of paranoia, schizoid, antisocial, borderline, histrionic, narcissistic, and passive–aggressive personality profiles. Further, the incidence of abnormal personality traits before AAS use began was not different from the control group, suggesting that such disturbances are secondary to their use. People who use AAS also reported that they believe that AAS not only enhance physical strength and athletic ability but increase confidence, assertiveness, feelings of sexuality, and optimism.[91] There appears to be both a pathological perception of body image and a very narrow (stereotypic) view of what a male body should look like among AAS users.[92] The term *reverse anorexia nervosa* has been coined by this group to describe symptoms association with muscle dysmorphia or a pathological preoccupation with muscularity (eg, not willing to let their bodies be seen in public). This form of body dysmorphic disorder may be associated with psychopathology as evidenced by a greater incidence of suicide attempts, higher frequency of unhealthy substance use, and poorer quality of life.[93] Indeed, a recent cross-sectional survey revealed that AAS users exhibited significantly more suicidal tendencies and mental health issues than matched people who do not use.[94]

ADVERSE EFFECTS

Pope et al.[95] have pointed out that the common belief that performance-enhancing drugs are fundamentally safe has led to their continued use, especially among the nonathlete weightlifter community. The dangers of supraphysiological doses of these drugs preclude the conduct of randomized controlled studies with humans, and so observational studies have remained the major source of knowledge. This review[95] provides a comprehensive overview of the adverse effects that have been associated with a number of different agents. As a result of the many observational studies, a great deal is known about the side effect and toxic profile of these drugs, and in the last few years, an even better appreciation for the risks of using these drugs has occurred. Much of the recent literature has focused on the short-term toxicity of these agents, particularly on cardiovascular and hepatic function. However, since people who use AAS rarely seek treatment for their unhealthy use of these drugs, they will present with just the side effects and may not reveal their history of high-dose AAS use. One important consequence to consider is that as AAS users age, their use may subside, but potentially long-lasting organ damage may have occurred that may accelerate the deterioration that occurs during the normal aging process. As unhealthy AAS use peaked in the 1980s, there is likely a generation of older men who may begin to experience the consequences of their past use. This issue has recently been addressed in a cross-sectional survey[96] showing that AAS users were more likely to report concomitant alcohol use (binge drinking) and report a higher incidence of anxiety disorders. There is also new evidence that AAS use among male weightlifters can result in ADHD-like symptoms that also affect cognitive function.[97]

Side effects are generally reversible, but more serious medical consequences and even toxic reactions appear to involve primarily blood chemistry, endocrine function, the liver, the cardiovascular system, and the nervous system. Reports that excessive amounts of these drugs lead to certain types of malignant cancers have not been substantiated. Overall, even the more serious side effects have disappeared within 3 months of discontinuing their use yet benefits such as increases in lean body mass and increased diameter of muscle fibers remain.[98] Although the side effect profile of AAS has been well documented in adults, less is known about how chronic use of high doses of AAS will affect adolescents.

Administration of the 17-alkylated androgens can cause a dramatic reduction in high-density lipoprotein (HDL) cholesterol, but there is no net change in total cholesterol levels.[99] Other agents such as nandrolone and testosterone esters fail to produce this profile.[99,100] Although the long-term detrimental effects of altered HDL/LDL ratios are known to predispose humans to atherosclerosis, documented morbidity, and mortality because of AAS use have been rare.[101,102] The lack of direct correlations may also be due to different steroids have varied effects on lipid dynamics.[100] Thus, although people who use AAS stack different drugs to improve the beneficial effects, this practice may afford some protection against these side effects. Further, the relative paucity of coronary vascular disease in athletes who use these drugs may also be due to other risk factors (eg, diet, exercise, low body fat) that may compensate for any negative contribution afforded by the HDL/LDL profile. Such protection, however, may not be present in individuals who use AAS just to improve their appearance and do not engage in athletic activity. Platelet aggregation[103] and increased red blood cell production and slight increases in systolic blood pressure have been suggested to be important factors that increase an individual's risk for thromboembolic disorders.[1,104]

Because testosterone exerts an inhibitory action on the hypothalamic–pituitary axis, administration of natural or synthetic analogues of testosterone decreases testicular size and sperm count.[105] Residual amounts of active metabolites may keep the levels of follicle-stimulating hormone and luteinizing hormone low and coupled with the relatively long cycle to produce sperm, the recovery is likely to be slow but often is complete. Aromatization is the process by which steroid hormones are interconverted. For example, testosterone is converted to estradiol and estrone, and high-dose male AAS users can have circulating estrogen levels of normally cycling women.[1] These circulating estrogens exert the usual feminizing effects, such as gynecomastia. Compounds that resist aromatization (eg, fluoxymesterone, mesterolone, stanozolol) may not result in the feminizing effects.[106]

Although a wide variety of medical disorders (and even exercise) can increase the amount of liver enzymes in the blood, this response is primarily limited to the use of oral, 17-alkylated AAS. The relationship between these drugs and elevated enzyme levels exists because these orally effective drugs are metabolized by the liver, the first-pass effect delivers an exceptionally large percentage of the dose to the liver, and people who use AAS typically take excessive doses that further stress liver function. This profile often results in cholecystic jaundice,[107] but because inflammation and necrosis are not present, the symptoms are limited to an accumulation of bile, which spills over into the blood. Interestingly, many bodybuilders use this side effect as a metric of their dosing regimen and titrate themselves to levels that just precipitate jaundice.[108]

Peliosis hepatitis is a disorder characterized by blood-filled cysts scattered throughout the liver; a detailed description of the history of this disorder and its relationship to unhealthy AAS use is presented elsewhere.[109] It has been associated with the 17-alkylated androgens, rarely results in symptoms, and likely resolves with discontinuation.[110]

The evidence linking 17-alkylated androgens with hepatic tumors is well established. Except for the fact that the androgen-related adenomas are typically larger, the profile resembles that of women who take birth control pills. The risk for developing hepatocellular adenomas ranges from 1% to 3% of people who use AAS,[99] and as with peliosis hepatitis, these adenomas rarely result in symptoms and are often not documented until a routine autopsy is performed.

A better appreciation for the mechanism of hepatic toxicity is now apparent as prolonged AAS use appears to increase lysosomal hydrolase activity and decrease some components of the microsomal drug-metabolizing system.[111] These macroscopic changes may very well lead to the inflammatory or degenerative lesions in centrilobular hepatocytes, ultrastructural alterations in canaliculi, and degenerative changes in mitochondria and lysosomes. Stanozolol, along with the other orally administered AAS, is known to induce these effects. Moreover, chronic AAS use may negatively impact immune function by over activating immune cell function while dampening immunological responses.[112] Testosterone, at higher concentrations, reduces extra- and intracellular superoxide and increases phagocytosis, indicating that the oxidative capacity of neutrophils has decreased.

AAS affect the cardiovascular system via their effects on HDL/LDL ratios and other blood products. However, there are reports that these drugs can directly affect myocardial tissue. Much of the evidence comes from animal studies in which high doses of methandrostenolone result in myocyte necrosis, cellular edema, and mitochondrial swelling.[113,114] Because these changes cannot be duplicated by exercise alone, it is likely that these effects were responsible for the clinical case report of an AAS user who suddenly died of cardiac arrest.[115] Recent preclinical studies suggest that the combination of vigorous exercise along with AAS use may precipitate myocardial injury that is manifested by myocardial disarray, contraction band necrosis, interstitial fibrosis, and apoptosis.[116] These direct cardiotoxic effects can result in hypertrophy, electrical and structural remodeling, and contractile dysfunction that can lead to increased risk of ventricular arrhythmias and sudden cardiac death.[117] A 2013 clinical report supports the notion that AAS use (possibly in combination with cannabis) can contribute to ischemic stroke in adolescents,[118] and a recent review of the extant clinical literature revealed a high incidence of cardiac toxicity associated with chronic use.[119] Angell et al,[120] present two case studies (a 25-year-old bodybuilder and a 27-year-old professional skater) that highlight the impact that performance-enhancing drugs have on cardiovascular function, especially in athletes. Frati et al,[121] have performed a review of the literature and have identified 19 AAS-related fatal cases that were not cardiac related.

An adverse effect of AAS use during high-intensity training periods that is not well documented is the incidence of injury that may occur as a direct result of their use. Cross-sectional cohort study revealed that ruptured tendons (especially upper body) occurred in 22% of the AAS users with a hazard ratio for first incident being 9.0, which was highly significant.[122] Although it might seem that the fact that people who use AAS can train with these drugs well beyond what they would be able to tolerate without the drugs is responsible for injuries of this type, it is possible that the growth of muscle mass is not paralleled by an increase in ligament support, which can result in such failures. Support for this contention was supplied by Turillazzi et al,[123] who posit that AAS-induced tolerance to exercise places muscles at risk for overload that may shield the fibers from damage and improve recovery but that this protective action breaks down when exercise programs are excessive.

Controversy remains over the degree and extent of the severity of AAS-induced extreme psychiatric effects often referred to as "roid rage." These eruptions of frenzied violent behavior during a cycle of high-dose AAS have been described in a few case reports, but no laboratory studies verifying such reactions have been published. More frequently, cases during which psychiatric effects appear associated with drug use have been reported.[124-126] The constellation of symptoms closely resembles those of hypomania or mania. The energized user of AAS talks faster, has more energy, sleeps less, and acts more impulsively, even to the extent of purchasing expensive cars.[126] At the far end of the spectrum, mania may lead to delusions and even hallucinations. Interestingly, many individuals with body dysmorphic disorder present with delusions as well.[127] Two studies[128,129] attempted to standardize the collection of these data and found that using structured interviews, the incidence of a full affective syndrome was present in 22% of a population of 41 bodybuilders.[129] Another 12% displayed psychotic symptoms that clearly emerged during AAS use. The cohort of 20 weightlifters who used AAS experienced more somatic, depressive, anxious, hostile, and paranoid complaints than those who did not use these drugs.[128] A 2012 survey[130] revealed that, compared to people who did not use AAS, those with pre-DSM-5 AAS dependence had a 25.9% incidence of any psychiatric illness, with the majority having anxiety disorder (16.1%) and major depression (15.2%), which were statistically elevated. The variables that contribute to these findings are now better understood to be related to an earlier onset of use (as in adolescence) because these individuals experience poorer performance on cognitive tasks and had worse impulse control while on cycle.[131] These cognitive deficits appear to be selective for certain elements such as visuospatial memory, while leaving response speed, sustained attention, and verbal memory intact.[132] A brain imaging study[133] revealed that long-term AAS users had enlarged right amygdala with reduced connectivity that paralleled brain chemistry changes that reflected a reduced turnover of glutamate. As the amygdala plays a role in cognitive control and spatial memory, these changes may reflect the neurobiological mechanisms of the psychiatric disturbances and cognitive difficulties[132] observed in people who used AAS chronically.

A recent survey has confirmed what the growing body of evidence has shown—that AAS use is associated with increased psychopathology that is expressed as anger and risk-taking.[134] Empirical evidence of drug effects on aggressive behavior has been obtained using the Karolinska Scales of Personality[135] and a human laboratory model of aggression, the Point Subtraction Aggression Paradigm.[136] More recently, psychiatric side effects after supraphysiological doses of combinations of

AAS were reported to correlate with severity of use.[136] Results from the personality scale indicate that a cohort of AAS users exhibits significantly more verbal aggression, impulsiveness, and indirect aggression. Yates et al.[137] reported that three measures of the Buss-Durkee Hostility Inventory,[138] assault, indirect aggression, and verbal aggression, were elevated in a group of people who currently or recently used AAS. The Point Subtraction Aggression Paradigm directly measures the amount of provoked aggressive behavior in the laboratory by ostensibly taking away points (that are worth money) from an individual who believes he is playing against another person. In reality, the subject plays against a computer program, and the experimenter actually controls the rate of provocation. Both aggressive and nonaggressive behaviors are recorded, so the effects of various drugs on responding per se can be viewed independent from aggressive responding. Using this model, moderately high doses of testosterone cypionate (600 mg, intramuscularly, once per week) can increase aggressive responding in individuals who had not used steroids before.[139] As weightlifters and bodybuilders have reportedly used weekly doses that exceed three times that used in research studies, it is reasonable to suspect that aggressive behavior can result from these training programs.

Collectively, it appears that AAS use can result in hypomania and even psychotic symptoms, whereas depression may ensue during withdrawal. The lack of well-controlled prospective studies has prevented a more definitive association between AAS use and psychiatric disorders. It is unlikely that such data will become available soon because ethical constraints will preclude the conduct of any double-blind assessments of supraphysiological doses of these drugs.

ADDICTION LIABILITY

Unhealthy AAS use includes a variety of social and psychological components that are not easy to imitate either in animal models or in currently validated methods of assessing addiction liability in human volunteers. The concepts of perception, motivation, and expectation play a pivotal role in the initial use and subsequent unhealthy use of these compounds. Because the anabolic effects of AAS can be profound but slow to develop, it has been difficult to separate these "desired" muscle-building effects from direct reinforcement. Demonstrating tolerance and physical dependence on these agents has also proved to be elusive because there are limitations in the doses that can be given to human subjects.

Reward

Although the anabolic steroid addiction hypothesis was proposed nearly 20 years ago,[140] few empirical studies have been conducted to test it. This has been primarily because it is often difficult to separate the direct rewarding effects of AAS from the ancillary positive effects on performance, weight gain, and physical strength, which are the primary reasons that these drugs are used.[141] Therefore, animal models of conditioned place preference and self-administration have been employed to test these relationships, and evidence is mounting that AAS may possess some reinforcing effects that are not related to athletic performance. There is mounting evidence that AAS have a direct impact on the mesolimbic reward system[141] and several animal studies have demonstrated that testosterone is reinforcing in both male rat and hamster animal models using intracerebroventricular (icv), intravenous, or oral self-administration.[142-144]

Ballard and Wood[145] showed that hamsters preferred to self-administer the injectable androgens nandrolone or drostanolone and failed to self-administer orally active androgens oxymetholone or stanozolol. However, self-administration of AAS drugs is modest compared to drugs like cocaine and heroin and, as such, does not appear to be directly related to dopamine.[146] This would suggest that the AAS reward circuitry is not directly tied to this neurotransmitter, much like that of alcohol and the benzodiazepines, even though their use can have a modulatory role on dopamine.

Perhaps the most important concept to understand about unhealthy AAS use is that these drugs are not used in the typical patterns that are observed with traditional drugs such as cocaine, heroin, alcohol, nicotine, and cannabis. Indeed, AAS are often taken or injected once per week as part of an exercise program. It is well known that if the subjective effects of a psychoactive drug are sufficiently delayed after self-administration, then the drug's reinforcing efficacy decreases, and drug-seeking behavior is reduced.[147] Although there are a few scattered anecdotal reports that high doses of AAS can elevate mood, no controlled studies have demonstrated that these drugs produce immediate positive mood effects or euphoria. AAS can act within minutes to hours on cell membrane receptor sites, but the real beneficial effects of such action (eg, protein synthesis) take more time. So, because of the difficulties of conducting such studies with humans, animal models have been proven to be the most valuable in discerning the nature of the reinforcing effects of these compounds. In one clinical study by Su et al.,[148] healthy non-AAS users described feeling euphoric, being full of energy, and having increased sexual arousal after an acute dose of methyltestosterone. Although the magnitude of the response was modest, the results were consistent but have not been replicated.

The rewarding effects of testosterone using conditioned place preference were described[149] but appeared to be dependent on the environmental cues as conditioned stimuli. A recent study in male rats demonstrated that these drugs may alter the sensitivity of brain reward systems.[150] In that study, a 2-week treatment with methandrostenolone alone had no effect on brain reward systems, but a 15-week treatment with a cocktail of three different AAS resulted in a shift in the response patterns to brain electrical reward and amphetamine. In a related study, dopamine receptor density in nucleus accumbens was altered by supraphysiological doses of testosterone in male rats, suggesting that dopamine levels are increased after AAS.[151] This action was verified using positron-emission tomography and found that chronic AAS treatment caused an up-regulation of the binding potential of dopamine in rat striatum.[152]

Another potential link to potentially addictive substances is that AAS share brain sites of action and neurotransmitter systems with opioids. In humans, unhealthy AAS use is often associated with prescription opioid use, and in animals, AAS overdose produces symptoms resembling opioid overdose.[153] This study also demonstrated that AAS modifies the activity of the endogenous opioid system. A review by Mhillaj et al.[154] summarizes the data suggesting that pre-DSM-5 AAS dependence may arise due to an enhancement of endogenous opioids,[140] which would explain the rather large number of studies demonstrating that AAS users are also prone to high rates of pre-DSM-5-defined opioid abuse and dependence,[155,156] and that use of both classes of drugs developed at about the same time.[32]

The absence of a well-defined pattern of self-administration in animals is confirmed by the finding that humans cannot tell whether they have been given an active AAS or placebo.[157] Marginal discriminations were made in two studies but only after a period of extended testing had been employed.[71,158] However, it is likely that it was the side effects of these drugs that were detected, rather than any positive reinforcing effects. Because the latter are thought to regulate drug-taking behavior in both humans and animals, the question that remains is "why do humans engage in unhealthy AAS use?"

Collectively, these data from animal models suggest that AAS may very well be reinforcing, but the magnitude and strength of the direct rewarding effects of these agents are modest at best and do not appear to approach that of the more classic drugs such as heroin, cocaine, or nicotine. Because of testosterone's role in many socially labile situations, it may be that it intensifies the rewarding aspects of these other behaviors and that is what contributes to the persistent use by a small fraction of the population.

Tolerance

The evidence supporting tolerance development is not strong, although there is a belief among people who use AAS that cycling is a necessary practice to avoid its development. Twenty percent of a sample of weightlifters believes that tolerance develops, but more than 80% believe that pre-DSM-5 substance dependence develops. Nevertheless, such concerns over lost efficacy with time appear to be without hard empirical evidence. As such, it must be assumed that the escalating doses that elite athletes use are not taken because tolerance develops to their effects, but because it increases the magnitude of the desired effects. The doses are increased slowly to minimize the side effects or to allow time to acclimate to them. When presented with this fact, some people who use AAS are likely to confuse their behavior with tolerance.

Substance Use Disorder

Although evidence of physical dependence on AAS has not been widespread, there are a few detailed reports of clear signs of withdrawal when their use was abruptly stopped.[159-161] Using DSM criteria in a study of 49 male weightlifters,[161] 84% reported experiencing withdrawal effects, and the most frequently reported symptoms were craving for more steroids (52%), fatigue (43%), depressed mood state (41%), restlessness (29%), anorexia (24%), insomnia (20%), decreased libido (20%), and headaches (20%). Interestingly, 42% of these subjects were dissatisfied with their body image during withdrawal as well. Those who reported being addicted to AAS generally took higher doses, completed more cycles of use, and reported more aggressive symptoms than those who did not report being addicted. However, the extent of addiction on AAS in the larger population of people who use AAS may be considerably smaller as there have been no reported cases of withdrawal effects in female athletes or among patients who have been prescribed with high doses for legitimate medical purposes.

AAS in fact can increase muscle mass and body weight, especially when used along with a regular training program. However, many of the illegal market AAS preparations sold during the late 1980s were devoid of any active ingredients, including AAS. In spite of the spread of these counterfeit drugs, people who use AAS claimed to have experienced improvements in their performance. Herein lies the real difficulty in assessing the addiction liability of these compounds. They are not expected to have immediate beneficial effects, and so the delay in any improvement does not raise suspicion that the preparation may be inert. Nevertheless, whether these drugs really do increase muscle mass, improve performance, or increase endurance is not the question that confronts the addiction medicine specialist. The fact that AAS-seeking behavior exists and that extremely high doses are used over relatively long periods suggests that there is a steroid use disorder and should trigger further inquiry and subsequent treatment.

Physical dependence on AAS may be more insidious than with other drugs. It is quite likely that the initial involvement with AAS is related to the anticipated increased physical strength and body mass. Brower proposed a two-stage model of AAS physical dependence that incorporated the anabolic benefits early on, but that physical dependence ensues after prolonged use of extremely high doses.[162]

Thus, although steroid use disorder with AAS may be rarer than substance use disorders (SUDs) for other drugs, the prudent clinician will be ever vigilant to identify the constellation of signs and symptoms that may signify steroid use disorder. Attempts to label the withdrawal signs and symptoms as opiate-like or ethanol-like may complicate the issue only because such an effort may conceal a real SUD with other drugs. Thus, when obvious signs of distress are observed during periods of forced abstinence, it is worthwhile to consider the possibility that the individual may, in fact, have a SUD with other drugs. There have been a few reports of pre-DSM-5-defined opioid dependence in bodybuilders,[155,163] and these individuals clearly met the criteria for substance dependence on both drug classes. Thus, the possibility of polydrug use should always be considered when dealing with people who use AAS.

Treatment Considerations

AAS users rarely seek treatment for their unhealthy use. Treating individuals who have an AAS use disorder has remained challenging for many of the reasons identified early in this chapter. While there is now evidence for a role of basic reward mechanisms in the effects of AAS, the impact is modest when compared to other drugs, and so conventional agonist or antagonist pharmacotherapies are not useful. Furthermore, a great deal of the "rewarding" aspects of AAS is their effects on body shape, size, weight, and image—all of which take time to develop and so the temporal relationship between use and desired effect is not solidified, making the choice to seek treatment difficult. Coupled with the attendant desire to perform at a higher level (and the financial rewards that can follow), treating AAS use disorder is a multifaceted endeavor.

Few empirical studies have been conducted, and current knowledge has relied on case reports from a handful of clinicians who have treated patients undergoing acute AAS withdrawal. We now have a better understanding of the constellation of issues that are present; current recommendations for treatment include a three-pronged approach[164]: (1) address the body image disorder, (2) address the depression due to the hypogonadism during withdrawal, and (3) address the hedonic effects via pharmacological and psychosocial treatments. Pharmacotherapy is targeted at restoring the effects of hormonal imbalance because hypogonadal symptoms can persist for years after cessation[165,166] and using antidepressants to treat the residual depression that emerges during withdrawal. Clinical management consists of supportive therapy and pharmacotherapy aimed at restoring normal endocrine function of the HPG axis.[167] Other medications for symptomatic relief include antidepressants (SSRI), nonsteroidal anti-inflammatory drugs and clonidine. Unfortunately, little gain has been made in developing a comprehensive, evidence treatment plan for AAS users as most publications are case reports with little or no empirical evidence for changing behavior, treating SUD or managing withdrawal.[168] As is the case with other forms of SUD, prevention is a valuable tool to avoid the need for treatment plans. A 2016 report[169] found that community-based prevention programs that target local gyms may be the best solution as this strategy will focus on not only where many AAS users congregate but where most illicit AAS are distributed.

Diagnostic Classifications

While AAS abuse and dependence were acknowledged in the American Psychiatric Association's *Diagnostic and Statistical Manual of Mental Disorders,* 4th ed. (DSM-IV),[170] it is no longer a specified diagnosis in DSM-5[171] and instead is now coded as "other substance use 305.90" and would be defined as mild, moderate, or severe anabolic steroid use disorder depending on the number of symptoms that is present. More specific AAS criteria for classifying a use disorder were proposed to be included in DSM-5[172] that have been validated in the laboratory,[173] but these were not included. The classification of mild would occur if 2 to 3 symptoms are present, while moderate and severe ratings would occur if the patient had 4 to 5 or more than 6 symptoms, respectively. The symptoms list is similar to that used in DSM-IV with items like taking larger amounts of AAS over a longer period of time, persistent desire or unsuccessful attempts to reduce use, spending a large amount of time to obtain AAS, experiencing craving or strong desire for AAS, use having negative impact on work, school, or home, having social or interpersonal problems with continued use, recurrent use in situations in which it is physically hazardous to use, continued use despite knowing that its use is causing problems, tolerance as defined by a need to increase the AAS dose or a noticeable diminished effect with continued use of the same dose. DSM-5 also includes craving for the substance as a criterion option.

There is another factor that must be considered when attempting to diagnose AAS use disorder. In a study of 108 bodybuilders, Pope et al.[174] noted a rather high percentage of anorexia nervosa and uncovered a body image disorder that they labeled *reverse anorexia.* This condition shares many signs and symptoms of body dysmorphic syndrome.[175] The profile of the former is that they view themselves as being too small and weak, when they are quite large and strong. The incidence of this disorder was 8% among people who used AAS and was not observed in any of those who did not. The authors postulate that these body image disorders may have some influence on an individual's decision to use AAS. Because the perceived size, shape, and attractiveness of one's body are likely tied to self-esteem[176] and, in general, men want to be 3-lb heavier, be taller, and have wider shoulders,[177] AAS use may be viewed as a way of speeding up the process to attain physical attractiveness. This similarity in profiles between body image disorders and drug use might suggest that those who present with a profile of body image disturbance may respond to the same treatments that have been used for body dysmorphic syndrome. Serotonin reuptake blockers have been marginally successful in treating body dysmorphic disorder,[178] and although there have been no published studies to this effect with people who use AAS, fluoxetine has been marginally successful in a small sample of bodybuilders who presented with depression during withdrawal from AAS use.[179]

A meta-analysis of 44 studies conducted in 11 countries revealed some very interesting consistent patterns in the etiology and trajectory of the initiation of AAS use.[180] Most of the individuals who use AAS reported that they began using before the age of 30, participated primarily in power-related sports, possessed a negative body image, and typically reported that feelings of depression preceded their use of AAS. These data confirm the results of other studies showing that psychosocial factors play a significant role in the decision to begin to use AAS, at least among males.

ABSORPTION AND METABOLISM

Historically, AAS have been taken either orally or injected deep into the muscle as there are no intravenous formulations or smoked products. More recently, testosterone gel and patches for topical administration have been released on the market and offer another route to consider. By far the greatest influence on subsequent development of toxic side effects is the route of administration. About half of an oral dose of testosterone is metabolized via the first-pass effect, so very large doses are needed. Some 17α-alkylated analogues of testosterone such as methyltestosterone resist such metabolism and so can be given orally in smaller doses. The oral route gives rise to many 17-alkylated metabolites, which are formed in the liver. This overload, not only of the metabolizing enzymes but also of the parent drug, because the doses taken are so high, causes significant stress on the liver.

Testosterone is metabolized to 5α-dihydrotestosterone in certain tissues such as prostate gland, seminal vesicles, and pubic skin. Because 5α-dihydrotestosterone has two to three times the affinity for the androgen receptor as the parent hormone, the effects of testosterone are enhanced in these tissues. One of the more interesting aspects of testosterone's metabolic pathways is that it is converted to estradiol in tissues that contain an aromatase enzyme.[181] The biological significance of circulating estrogens in males is unknown, but they may be involved with sex hormone–binding globulin and lipoproteins. Further, the estrogen that results from this metabolic process may interact with estrogen receptors to produce an anabolic effect.[182] The 17α-alkylated analogues discussed above are not metabolized to either 5α-dihydrotestosterone or estrogen. Instead, they interact with the androgen receptor.[1,183] Thus, the overall profile of relative anabolic to androgenic effects is not only due to the parent compound but to the profile of metabolites that result. With the advent of widespread use of these drugs during athletic competition, several analytic laboratories have been set up to detect either the parent drug or its metabolites.[184,185] In addition to providing quantitative analyses of the various synthetic analogues, most labs measure the testosterone/epitestosterone ratio (T/E ratio) as a metric of exogenous testosterone administration.[186] The ratio is normally 1:1 but United States and World Anti-Doping Agencies have now set the "passing" threshold at 4:1, lowering it from 6:1 as had been accepted in the past. This strategy of testing both the parent hormone testosterone and its major metabolite has provided a more reliable method of detecting illicit use of a hormone that is normally found in the body.

Another important advancement in detecting illicit testosterone use capitalizes on the natural abundance of ^{13}C and its dissociation from the abundance of ^{12}C in biological systems,[187] and the $^{13}C/^{12}C$ ratio should reflect that of the ingested carbon sources. Pharmaceutical grade testosterone is made from soya bean stigmasterol, which by its nature has a lower ^{13}C content. Using GC combustion isotope ratio mass spectrometry, these differences can be detected and used to identify the "source" of the testosterone that is present in a biological sample.

MECHANISMS OF ACTION

About 95% of the testosterone in males is synthesized in the testes, whereas the remaining 5% comes from the adrenals. The cholesterol used in the synthetic pathway comes from acetate that is stored in the testes and not from circulating blood levels. AAS have long been thought to exert their effects in the periphery, primarily by increasing the rate of RNA transcription.[7,188] About half of the circulating testosterone is tightly bound to sex hormone–binding globulin, and the other half is lightly bound to albumin, from which it freely dissociates and from whence it can diffuse passively into target cells. This process is thought to occur by intracellular metabolism and by altering the topology of the androgen receptor leading to changes in transcription.[189] After attaching to a steroid receptor in the cytoplasm, the hormone receptor complex moves into the nucleus where it binds to sites on the chromatin, resulting in the formation of new mRNA. If the target tissue is skeletal muscle, then new myofilaments are formed, which causes myofibrils to divide.[1,190] This mechanism is remotely supportive of the "muscle memory" hypothesis that may persist even after AAS use has stopped. It is unknown if myonuclei remain elevated and a recent cross-sectional longitudinal study failed to detect increased myonuclei or fiber, but the authors noted that the AAS doses used by the participants in their study were relatively low.[191] Because it is not completely understood whether this activity occurs at the supraphysiological doses typically taken by people who use AAS, another mechanism was sought.

The pharmacological profile of the AAS is thought to be due to androgen binding to intracellular androgen receptors. This process takes about 30 minutes and ultimately alters gene expression, but it is now believed that AAS possess a nongenomic action that can be mobilized in seconds or minutes.[192] There have been some advances in the understanding of how testosterone metabolites interact with the γ-aminobutyric acid ($GABA_A$)/benzodiazepine receptor complex or dopaminergic neurons in nucleus accumbens to mediate testosterone's hedonic effects.[193]

It has been suggested that high doses of AAS cross-react with glucocorticoid receptors that control the catabolic rates of protein.[1,194,195] This has led to the belief that AAS exert an anticatabolic effect via inhibition of glucocorticoids such as cortisol[189] that ultimately prevents the breakdown of muscle protein. It is also possible that the stress of strenuous workouts is not felt by athletes taking AAS because the stress-induced increase in cortisol is blocked. This action would also permit the workouts last longer and be more vigorous, which would further improve performance.

It is possible that the physical changes attributed to a direct effect of AAS on protein synthesis may be mediated via a direct effect on the central nervous system. Such effects might result in increased motivation and intensity of training to a degree that performance is improved. Increased aggressive behavior may also play a role in the training process. It is likely that the use of supraphysiological doses of these drugs can have both a direct effect on muscle tissue and an indirect effect by altering emotions such as motivation and drive such that the training periods are longer and more productive, resulting in improved performance.

Additional insight into the effects of AAS on skeletal muscle has been gleaned using an androgen receptor (AR) knockout mouse model.[196] These authors demonstrated that AR-regulated genes are responsible for the increases in muscle mass by maintaining myoblasts in a proliferation state and that, in addition, the AR also suppresses pathways that break down muscle. There have been some recent advances in the understanding of how testosterone metabolites interact with the $GABA_A$/benzodiazepine receptor complex or dopaminergic neurons in nucleus accumbens to mediate testosterone's hedonic effects.[193] The concept that AAS interact directly with peripheral benzodiazepine receptors in rat brain has been explored.[197] These receptors are mitochondrial proteins that are involved with regulating steroid synthesis and transport, so it seems plausible that their activation via exogenous AAS could have an impact on behavior that is mediated by these receptors.

The increase in body weight, especially during the first weeks of use, is almost certainly attributed to the stimulation of mineralocorticoid receptors, resulting in sodium and, ultimately, water retention as well as increasing amounts of circulating estrogen that has been aromatized from testosterone. This effect gives the muscles, particularly the deltoid, a "puffy" appearance. The increase in red blood cell production is probably the major reason that long-distance runners may use these drugs because endurance, rather than bulk muscle mass, is an asset in this sport. Blood volume probably increases as a result of erythropoietin synthesis. This effect is due to direct action on the bone marrow and easily leads to a rise in hematocrit.[198]

FUTURE VISTAS

Anabolic–androgenic steroids continue to be used in unhealthy ways by individuals for a wide range of reasons. Further, as people who previously used heavy amounts of AAS enter middle age, it remains to be seen whether there are psychiatric of other medical consequences of this form of unhealthy drug use,[199] an issue that the clinician may need to address when presented with organ diseases in individuals who, upon initial presentation, exercised regularly, ate balanced meals, and did not smoke for the past 30 years. The addiction liability of AAS may have a central nervous system mechanism that complements the anabolic effects. As quantitative methods for detecting AAS have become more sophisticated and specific, individuals have switched to using nutritional supplements, endogenous peptides such as growth hormone and erythropoietin. Attempts to determine reference ranges for urinary steroid "profiles"[200] represent a movement that may help to better define when illicit use has occurred. Although the anabolic effects of many oral supplements are not well documented, they are marketed and used as if they are. Selective androgen receptor modulators, capable of increasing muscle mass with little androgenic effects (and have already been banned from the Olympics), will join the ranks of the designer AAS like tetrahydrogestrinone and desoxymethyltestosterone as the performance-enhancing substances of the future. Indeed, selective androgen receptor modulators have already been explored and shown to possess tissue-selective anabolic effects on bone mineral content in female rats, without concomitant side effects.[201] While the designer drugs and novel peptides can now be detected, the way has been paved for an emerging biotechnique that implements recombinant DNA such that manipulated genes can be inserted into mammalian cells. This practice, called gene doping or performance-enhancing genetics, has been defined by the World Anti-Doping Agency as "the non-therapeutic use of genes, genetic elements and/or cells that have the capacity to enhance athletic performance."[202] This commission is unique in that human gene doping has not yet occurred, but the World Anti-Doping Agency has taken the initiative to set standards for future events. Conceptually, gene doping would involve using scientific techniques to manipulate DNA in a manner that would improve athletic performance.[203,204]

While there is a legitimate medical rationale for pursuing the development of selective androgen modulators because as AAS medications have been useful in treating a variety of medical conditions (eg, short stature, burns, wasting syndrome, anemia, and bone disorders), they tend to lack selectivity.[205] The drugs have the potential to target androgen receptors on specific end organs and, as such, are likely to have a safer profile. More recently, a new trend by AAS users is to take a mixture of aromatase inhibitors and selective estrogen receptor modulators.[206] These drugs are used secretly to either "revive" the hypothalamohypophyseal axis or combat androgen aromatization, both of which can impair the efficacy of AAS use. Most of the information on these drugs, doses and treatment plan are published on so-called cyber-forums as the trend is just emerging.

Finally, the medical community needs to appreciate the fact that few people who use AAS will seek drug addiction treatment, but as they age, the medical consequences of years of using excessive doses of these agents will take its toll on body organs and may present the clinician with conditions that will not have an obvious cause. To address this issue, one of the more exciting areas has been the development of molecular biomarkers that are selective for specific diseases or disorders. MicroRNA (miRNA) technologies are now being applied to identify the miRNA signature that identifies organ damage due to AAS use.[207] The approach will offer essentially noninvasive methods to detect these circulating miRNA biomarkers and thus identify AAS use.

REFERENCES

1. Wilson JD. Androgen abuse by athletes. *Endocr Rev.* 1988;9:181-199.
2. Kochakian CD. History of anabolic-androgenic steroids. In: Lin GC, Erinoff L, eds. *Anabolic Steroid Abuse (NIDA Research Monograph 102).* National Institute on Drug Abuse; 1990:29-59.
3. Boje O. Doping. *Bull Health Org League Nations.* 1939;8:439-469.
4. Hartgens F, Kuipers H. Effects of androgenic-anabolic steroids in athletes. *Sports Med.* 2004;34:513-554.
5. Todd T. Anabolic steroids: the gremlins of sport. *J Sport Hist.* 1987;14:87-107.

6. Yesalis C, Anderson W, Buckley W, et al. Incidence of the nonmedical use of anabolic-androgenic steroids. In: Lin GC, Erinoff L, eds. *Anabolic Steroid Abuse*. National Institute on Drug Abuse; 1990.
7. Lukas SE. Current perspectives on anabolic-androgenic steroid abuse. *Trends Pharmacol Sci.* 1993;14:61-68.
8. Bahrke MS, Yesalis CE III. Weight training: a potential confounding factor in examining the psychological and behavioural effects of anabolic-androgenic steroids. *Sports Med.* 1994;18(5):309-318.
9. Gambelunghe C, Sommavilla M, Ferranti C, et al. Analysis of anabolic steroids in hair by GC/MS/MS. *Biomed Chromatogr.* 2007;21(4):369-375.
10. Abushareeda W, Fragkaki A, Vonaparti A, et al. Advances in the detection of designer steroids in anti-doping. *Bioanalysis.* 2014;6(6):881-896.
11. Tsitsimpikou C, Tsarouhas K, Spandidos DA, Tsatsakis AM. Detection of stanozolol in the urine of athletes at a pg level: the possibility of passive exposure. *Biomed Rep.* 2016;5(6):665-666.
12. McHugh CM, Park RT, Sönksen PH, et al. Challenges in detecting the abuse of growth hormone in sport. *Clin Chem.* 2005;51:1587-1593.
13. Graham MR, Davies B, Grace FM, et al. Anabolic steroid use: patterns of use and detection of doping. *Sports Med.* 2008;38:505-525.
14. Graham MR, Baker JS, Evans P, et al. Physical effects of short-term recombinant human growth hormone administration in abstinent steroid dependency. *Horm Res.* 2008;69:343-354.
15. Brennan BP, Kanayama G, Pope HG Jr. Performance-enhancing drugs on the web: a growing public-health issue. *Am J Addict.* 2013;22(2):158-161. doi:10.1111/j.1521-0391.2013.00311.x
16. Cordaro FG, Lombardo S, Cosentino M. Selling androgenic anabolic steroids by the pound: identification and analysis of popular websites on the Internet. *Scand J Med Sci Sports.* 2011;21:247-259.
17. ZoBell D, Chapman C, Heaton K, et al. *Beef Cattle Implants (Revised from University of Nebraska publication number G97-1324A by Dee Griffin and Terry Mader)*. Utah State University Extension Electronic Publishing; 2000:1-9.
18. Yesalis CE, Kennedy NJ, Kopstein AN, et al. Anabolic-androgenic steroid use in the United States. *JAMA.* 1993;270(10):1217-1221.
19. Substance Abuse and Mental Health Services Administration. *National Household Survey on Drug Abuse: Main Findings 1994 (DHHS Publication No. [SMA] 96–3085)*. U.S. Government Printing Office; 1996.
20. National Institute on Drug Abuse. *National Survey Results on Drug Use from the Monitoring The Future Study, 1975–1994 (NIH Publication No. 96–4139)*. Vol. vol. II National Institutes of Health; 1996.
21. Irving LM, Wall M, Neumark-Sztainer D, et al. Steroid use among adolescents: findings from Project EAT. *J Adolesc Health.* 2002;4:243-252.
22. Cafri G, Thompson JK, Ricciardelli L. Pursuit of the muscular ideal: physical and psychological consequences and putative risk factors. *Clin Psychol Rev.* 2005;25:215-239.
23. National Center for Chronic Disease Prevention and Health Promotion. Youth risk behavior surveillance system. *Healthy Youth! National Data Files and Documentation: 1991–2005*. Accessed May 18, 2023.http://www.cdc.gov/HealthyYouth/yrbs/index.htm
24. Elliot DL, Cheong J, Moe EL, et al. Cross-sectional study of female students reporting anabolic steroid use. *Arch Pediatr Adolesc Med.* 2007;161(6):572-577.
25. Smolak L. Body image in children and adolescents: where do we go from here? *Body Image.* 2004;1:15-28.
26. Yesalis CE, Barsukiewicz CK, Koopstein AN, et al. Trends in anabolic-androgenic steroid use among adolescents. *Arch Pediatr Adolesc Med.* 1997;151:1197-1206.
27. vandenBerg P, Neumark-Sztainer D, Cafri G, et al. Steroid use among adolescents: longitudinal findings from Project EAT. *Pediatrics.* 2007;119:476-486.
28. Kanayama G, Boynes M, Hudson JI, et al. Anabolic steroid abuse among teenage girls: an illusory problem? *Drug Alcohol Depend.* 2007;88:156-162.
29. Johnston LD, Miech RA, O'Malley PM, Bachman JG, Schulenberg JE, Patrick ME. *Monitoring the Future National Survey Results on Drug Use 1975-2021: Overview, Key Findings on Adolescent Drug Use.* Institute for Social Research, University of Michigan; 2022.
30. Pelham WE, Tapert SF, Gonzalez MR, et al. Early adolescent substance use before and during the COVID-19 Pandemic: a longitudinal survey in the ABCD study cohort. *J Adoles Health.* 2021;69:390-397.
31. CDC National Center for Health Statistics: Vital Statistics Rapid Release. Accessed May 18, 2023. https://www.cdc.gov/nchs/nvss/vsrr/drug-overdose-data.htm
32. Pereira E, Moyses SJ, Ignacio SA, et al. Prevalence and profile of users and nonusers of anabolic steroids among resistance training practitioners. *BMC Public Health.* 2019;19:1650.
33. Beel A, Maycock B, McClean N. Current perspectives on anabolic steroids. *Drug Alcohol Rev.* 1998;17:87-103.
34. Kanayama G, Hudson JI, Pope HG. Features of men with anabolic androgenic steroid dependence: a comparison with nondependent AAS users and with AAS nonusers. *Drug Alcohol Depend.* 2009;102:130-137.
35. Selk-Ghaffari M, Shab-Bidar S, Halabchi F. The prevalence of anabolic-androgenic steroid misuse in Iranian athletes: a systematic review and meta-analysis. *Iran J Public Health.* 2021;50:1120-1134.
36. Cramblitt B, Pritchard M. Media's influence on the drive for muscularity in undergraduates. *Eat Behav.* 2013;14(4):441-446.
37. Slater A, Tiggemann M. Media matters for boys too! The role of specific magazine types and television programs in the drive for thinness and muscularity in adolescent boys. *Eat Behav.* 2014;15(4):679-682.
38. Harrison K, Bond BJ. Gaming magazines and the drive for muscularity in preadolescent boys: a longitudinal examination. *Body Image.* 2007;4(3):269-277.
39. Parkinson AB, Evans NA. Anabolic androgenic steroids: a survey of 500 users. *Med Sci Sports Exerc.* 2006;38:644-651.
40. Blashill AJ. A dual pathway model of steroid use among adolescent boys: results from a nationally representative sample. *Psychol Men Masc.* 2014;15(2):229-233.
41. Jampel JD, Murray SB, Griffiths S, Blashill AJ. Self-perceived weight and anabolic steroid misuse among US adolescent boys. *J Adolesc Health.* 2016;58(4):397-402.
42. Blashill AJ, Calzo JP, Griffiths S, Murray SB. Anabolic steroid misuse among US adolescent boys: disparities by sexual orientation and race/ethnicity. *Am J Public Health.* 2017;107(2):319-321.
43. Pope HG Jr, Kanayama G, Athey A, Ryan E, Hudson JI, Baggish A. The lifetime prevalence of anabolic-androgenic steroid use and dependence in Americans: current best estimates. *Am J Addict.* 2014;23(4):371-377.
44. Dunn M, Mazanov J, Sitharthan G. Predicting future anabolic-androgenic steroid use intentions with current substance use: findings from an internet-based survey. *Clin J Sport Med.* 2009;19(3):222-227. doi:10.1097/JSM.0b013e31819d65ad
45. Dodge T, Hoagland MF. The use of anabolic androgenic steroids and polypharmacy: a review of the literature. *Drug Alcohol Depend.* 2011;114(2–3):100-109. doi:10.1016/j.drugalcdep.2010.11.011
46. Sagoe D, McVeigh J, Bjørnebekk A, Essilfie MS, Andreassen CS, Pallesen S. Polypharmacy among anabolic-androgenic steroid users: a descriptive metasynthesis. *Subst Abuse Treat Prev Policy.* 2015;10:12.
47. Kaziauskas R. Designer steroids. *Handb Exp Pharmacol.* 2010;195:155-185.
48. Waller CC, McLeod MD. A review of designer anabolic steroids in equine sports. *Drug Test Anal.* 2016;9:1304-1319.
49. Rahnema CD, Crosnoe LE, Kim ED. Designer steroids—over-the-counter supplements and their androgenic component: review of an increasing problem. *Andrology.* 2015;3(2):150-155.
50. Joseph JF, Parr MK. Synthetic androgens as designer supplements. *Curr Neuropharmacol.* 2015;13(1):89-100.
51. Pomara C, Neri M, Bello S, Fiore C, Riezzo I, Turillazzi E. Neurotoxicity by synthetic androgen steroids: oxidative stress, apoptosis, and neuropathology: a review. *Curr Neuropharmacol.* 2015;13:132-145.
52. Laos C, Metzl JD. Performance-enhancing drug use in young athletes. *Adolesc Med Clin.* 2006;17(3):719-731.
53. Castillo EM, Comstock RD. Prevalence of use of performance-enhancing substances among United States adolescents. *Pediatr Clin North Am.* 2007;54:663-675.

54. Smurawa TM, Congeni JA. Testosterone precursors: use and abuse in pediatric athletes. *Pediatr Clin North Am.* 2007;54:787-796.
55. Hoffman JR, Faigenbaum AD, Ratamess NA, et al. Nutritional supplementation and anabolic steroid use in adolescents. *Med Sci Sports Exerc.* 2008;40:15-24.
56. Broeder CE, Quindry J, Brittingham K, et al. The andro project: physiological and hormonal influences of androstenedione supplementation in men 35 to 65 years old participating in a high-intensity resistance training program. *Arch Intern Med.* 2000;160:3093-3104.
57. Brown GA, Vukovich MD, Reifenrath TA, et al. Effects of anabolic precursors on serum testosterone concentrations and adaptations to resistance training in young men. *Int J Sport Nutr Exerc Metab.* 2000;10:340-359.
58. Foster ZJ, Housner JA. Anabolic-androgenic steroids and testosterone precursors: ergogenic aids and sport. *Curr Sports Med Rep.* 2004;3:234-241.
59. Bahrke MS, Yesalis CE. Abuse of anabolic androgenic steroids and related substances in sport and exercise. *Curr Opin Pharmacol.* 2004;4:614-620.
60. Badaway MT, Sobeh M, Xiao J, Farag MA. Androstenedione (a natural steroid and a drug supplement): a comprehensive review of its consumption, metabolism, health effects, and toxicity with sex differences. *Molecules.* 2021;26:6210.
61. Brown GA, Vukovich MD, Martini ER, et al. Endocrine responses to chronic androstenedione intake in 30- to 56-year-old men. *J Clin Endocrinol Metab.* 2000;85:4074-4080.
62. Leder BZ, Longcope C, Catlin DH, et al. Oral androstenedione administration and serum testosterone concentrations in young men. *JAMA.* 2000;283:779-782.
63. King DS, Sharp RL, Vukovich MD, et al. Effect of oral androstenedione on serum testosterone and adaptations to resistance training in young men: a randomized controlled trial. *JAMA.* 1999;2020-2028.
64. McGinnis MY. Anabolic androgenic steroids and aggression: studies using animal models. In: Devine J, Gilligan J, Miczek KA, et al., eds. *Youth Violence: Scientific Approaches to Prevention.* New York Academy of Sciences; 2004:399-409.
65. van Bokhoven I, van Goozen SH, van Engeland H, et al. Salivary testosterone and aggression, delinquency, and social dominance in a population-based longitudinal study of adolescent males. *Horm Behav.* 2006;50:118-125.
66. Morrison TR, Ricci LA, Melloni RH Jr. Anabolic/androgenic steroid administration during adolescence and adulthood differentially modulates aggression and anxiety. *Horm Behav.* 2015;69:132-138.
67. Sato SM, Schulz KM, Sisk CL, et al. Adolescents and androgens, receptors and rewards. *Horm Behav.* 2008;53:647-658.
68. Holland-Hall C. Performance-enhancing substances: is your adolescent patient using? *Pediatr Clin North Am.* 2007;54:651-662.
69. Melnik B, Jansen T, Grabbe S. Abuse of anabolic-androgenic steroids and bodybuilding acne: an underestimated health problem. *J Dtsch Dermatol Ges.* 2007;5(2):110-117.
70. Yesalis CE, Herrick RT, Buckley WE, et al. Self-reported use of anabolic androgenic steroids by elite powerlifters. *Phys Sportsmed.* 1988;16:91-100.
71. Freed DLJ, Banks AJ, Longson D, et al. Anabolic steroids in athletics: crossover double-blind trial on weightlifters. *Br Med J.* 1975;2: 471-473.
72. Johansen KL, Painter PL, Sakkas GK, et al. Effects of resistance training and nandrolone decanoate on body composition and muscle function among patients who receive hemodialysis: a randomized, controlled trial. *J Am Soc Nephrol.* 2006;17:2307-2314.
73. Ding JB, Ng MZ, Huang SS, et al. Anabolic-androgenic steroid misuse: mechanisms, patterns of misuse, user typology, and adverse effects. *J Sports Med.* 2021;7497346. doi:10.1155/2021/7497346
74. Haupt HA, Rovere GB. Anabolic steroids: a review of the literature. *Am J Sports Med.* 1984;12:469-484.
75. Anderson W, McKeag B. *The Substance Use and Abuse Habits of College Student Athletes, Research paper no. 2.* National Collegiate Athletic Association; 1985
76. Perry PJ, Lund BC, Deninger MJ, et al. Anabolic steroid use in weightlifters and bodybuilders: an internet survey of drug utilization. *Clin J Sport Med.* 2005;15:326-330.
77. Perikles S, Striegel H, Aust F, et al. Doping in fitness sports: estimated number of unreported cases and individual probability of doping. *Addiction.* 2006;101:1640-1644.
78. NIDA. 2018. Anabolic Steroids Drug Facts. Accessed May 18, 2023. https://nida.nih.gov/publications/drugfacts/anabolic-steroids
79. Wesson DW, McGinnis MY. Stacking anabolic androgenic steroids (AAS) during puberty in rats: a neuroendocrine and behavioral assessment. *Pharmacol Biochem Behav.* 2006;83:410-419.
80. Wang MQ, Fitzhugh EC, Yesalis CE, et al. Desire for weight gain and potential risk of adolescent males using anabolic steroids. *Percept Mot Skills.* 1994;78:267-274.
81. Tanner SM, Miller DW, Alongi C. Anabolic steroid use by adolescents: prevalence, motives, and knowledge of risks. *Clin J Sport Med.* 1995;5:108-115.
82. Melia P, Pipe A, Greenberg L. The use of anabolic-androgenic steroids by Canadian students. *Clin J Sport Med.* 1996;6(1):9-14.
83. Durant RH, Rickert VI, Ashworth CS, et al. Use of multiple drugs among adolescents who use anabolic steroids. *N Engl J Med.* 1993;328:922-926.
84. Rogol AD, Yesalis CE III. Anabolic-androgenic steroids and the adolescent. *Pediatr Ann.* 1992;21(3):175-188.
85. Moore WB. Anabolic steroid use in adolescents. *JAMA.* 1988;260:3484-3486.
86. Goldberg L, Bents R, Bosworth E, et al. Anabolic steroid education and adolescents: do scare tactics work? *Pediatrics.* 1991;87:283-286.
87. Brower KJ. Rehabilitation for anabolic-androgenic steroid dependence. *Clin Sports Med.* 1989;1:171-181.
88. Dart R. Drugs in the workplace: anabolic steroid abuse among law enforcement officers. *Police Ctef.* 1991;58(7):18.
89. Swanson C, Gaines L, Gore B. Abuse of anabolic steroids. *FBI Law Enforce Bull.* 1991;60(8):19-23.
90. Cooper CJ, Noakes TD, Dunne T, et al. A high prevalence of abnormal personality traits in chronic users of anabolic-androgenic steroids. *Br J Sports Med.* 1996;30(3):246-250.
91. Schwerin MJ, Corcoran KJ. Beliefs about steroids: user versus non-user comparisons. *Drug Alcohol Depend.* 1996;40(3):221-225.
92. Kanayama G, Barry S, Hudson JI, et al. Body image and attitudes toward male roles in anabolic-androgenic steroid users. *Am J Psychiatry.* 2006;163:697-703.
93. Pope CG, Pope HG, Menard W, et al. Clinical features of muscle dysmorphia among males with body dysmorphic disorder. *Body Image.* 2005;2(4):395-400.
94. Hussain B, Khalily MT, Khalily MA. Suicidal tendencies and psychiatric symptoms as consequence of anabolic androgenic steroid usage among athletes in District Rawalpindi. *J Pak Med Assoc.* 2022;72:616-619.
95. Pope HG Jr, Wood RI, Rogol A, Nyberg F, Bowers L, Bhasin S. Adverse health consequences of performance-enhancing drugs: an Endocrine Society scientific statement. *Endocr Rev.* 2014;35(3):341-375.
96. Ip EJ, Trinh K, Tenerowicz MJ, Pal J, Lindfelt TA, Perry PJ. Characteristics and behaviors of older male anabolic steroid users. *J Pharm Pract.* 2015;28:450-456.
97. Kildal E, Hassell B, Bjørnebekk A. ADHD symptoms and use of anabolic androgenic steroids among male weightlifters. *Sci Rep.* 2022;12:9479. doi:10.1038/s41598-022-12977-w
98. Hartgens F, Kuipers H, Wijnen JAG, et al. Body composition, cardiovascular risk factors and liver function in long term androgenic-anabolic steroids using body builders three months after drug withdrawal. *Int J Sports Med.* 1996;17:429-433.
99. Friedl KE. Reappraisal of the health risks associated with high doses of oral and injectable androgenic steroids. In: Lin GC, Erinoff L, eds. *Anabolic Steroid Abuse (NIDA Research Monograph 102).* National Institute on Drug Abuse; 1990:142-177.
100. Thompson PB, Curinane AN, Sady SP, et al. Contrasting effects of testosterone and stanozolol on serum lipoprotein levels. *JAMA.* 1989;261:1165-1168.

101. McNutt RA, Ferenchick GF, Kirlin PC, et al. Acute myocardial infarction in a 22 year old, world-class weightlifter using anabolic steroids. *Am J Cardiol.* 1988;62:164.
102. Bowman S. Anabolic steroids and infarction. *Br Med J.* 1990;300:750.
103. Ferenchick BS. Are androgenic steroids thrombogenic? *N Engl J Med.* 1990;322:476.
104. Lenders JWM, Demacker PN, Vos JA, et al. Deleterious effects of anabolic steroids on serum lipoproteins, blood pressure and liver function in amateur bodybuilders. *Int J Sports Med.* 1988;9:19-23.
105. Osta RE, Almont T, Diligent C, et al. Anabolic steroids abuse and male infertility. *Basic Clin Andrology.* 2016;26:2. doi:10.1186/s12610-016-0029-4
106. Kashkin KB. Anabolic steroids. In: Lowinson JH, Ruiz P, Millman RB, et al., eds. *Substance Abuse: A Comprehensive Textbook.* 2nd ed. Lippincott Williams & Wilkins; 1992:380-395.
107. Pecking A, Lejolly JM, Najean Y. Hepatic toxicity of androgen therapy in aplastic anemia. *Nouvelle Revue Francaise D Hematologie.* 1980;22:257-265.
108. Lukas SE. *Steroids.* Enslow Publishers; 1994
109. Karch SB. Anabolic steroids. *Karch's Pathology of Drug Abuse.* 3rd ed. CRC Press; 2002:481-499.
110. Westaby B, Ogle SJ, Paridians FJ, et al. Liver damage from long-term methyltestosterone. *Lancet.* 1977;1(8032):261-263.
111. Neri M, Bello S, Bonsignore A, et al. Anabolic androgenic steroids abuse and liver toxicity. *Mini Rev Med Chem.* 2011;11(5):430-437.
112. Brenu EW, McNaughton L, Marshall-Gradisnik SM. Is there a potential immune dysfunction with anabolic androgenic steroid use? A review. *Mini Rev Med Chem.* 2011;11(5):438-445.
113. Appell H, Heller-Umpfenbach B, Feraudi M, et al. Ultra-structural and morphometric investigations on the effects of training and administration of anabolic steroids on the myocardium of guinea pigs. *Int J Sports Med.* 1983;4:268-274.
114. Behrendt H, Boffin H. Myocardial cell lesions caused by an anabolic hormone. *Cell Tissue Res.* 1977;181:423-426.
115. Luke J, Farb A, Virmani R, et al. Sudden cardiac death during exercise in a weight lifter using anabolic androgenic steroids: pathological and toxicological findings. *J Forensic Sci.* 1991;35(6):1441-1447.
116. Riezzo I, De Carlo D, Neri M, et al. Heart disease induced by AAS abuse, using experimental mice/rats models and the role of exercise-induced cardiotoxicity. *Mini Rev Med Chem.* 2011;11(5):409-424.
117. Nascimento JH, Medei E. Cardiac effects of anabolic steroids: hypertrophy, ischemia and electrical remodelling as potential triggers of sudden death. *Mini Rev Med Chem.* 2011;11(5):425-429.
118. El Scheich T, Weber AA, Klee D, et al. Adolescent ischemic stroke associated with anabolic steroid and cannabis abuse. *J Pediatr Endocrinol Metab.* 2013;26(1-2):161-165.
119. Higgins JP, Heshmat A, Higgins CL. Androgen abuse and increased cardiac risk. *South Med J.* 2012;105:670-674.
120. Angell PJ, Chester N, Sculthorpe N, et al. Performance enhancing drug abuse and cardiovascular risk in athletes: implications for the clinician. *Br J Sports Med.* 2012;46(Suppl 1):i78-i84.
121. Frati P, Busardò FP, Cipolloni L, Dominicis ED, Fineschi V. Anabolic Androgenic Steroid (AAS) related deaths: autoptic, histopathological and toxicological findings. *Curr Neuropharmacol.* 2015;13:146-159.
122. Kanayama G, DeLuca J, Meehan WP III, et al. Ruptured tendons in anabolic-androgenic steroid users: a cross-sectional cohort study. *Am J Sports Med.* 2015;43(11):2638-2644.
123. Turillazzi E, Perilli G, Di Paolo M, Neri M, Riezzo I, Fineschi V. Side effects of AAS abuse: an overview. *Mini Rev Med Chem.* 2011;11(5):374-389.
124. Freinhar JP, Alvarez W. Androgen-induced hypomania. *J Clin Psychiatry.* 1985;46:354-355.
125. Conacher GN, Workman DG. Violent crime possibly associated with anabolic steroid use. *Am J Psychiatry.* 1989;146:679.
126. Pope HG Jr, Katz DL. Body-builder's psychosis. *Lancet.* 1987;1:863.
127. Phillips KA, McElroy SL, Keck PE Jr, et al. A comparison of delusional and nondelusional body dysmorphic disorder in 100 cases. *Psychopharmacol Bull.* 1994;30(2):179-186.
128. Perry PJ, Yates WR, Anderson KH. Psychiatric effects of anabolic steroids: a controlled retrospective study. *Ann Clin Psychiatry.* 1990;2:11-17.
129. Pope HG Jr, Katz DL. Affective and psychotic symptoms associated with anabolic steroid use. *Am J Psychiatry.* 1988;45(4):487-490.
130. Ip EJ, Lu DH, Barnett MJ, et al. Psychological and physical impact of anabolic-androgenic steroid dependence. *Pharmacotherapy.* 2012;32(10):910-919.
131. Hildebrandt T, Langenbucher JW, Flores A, Harty S, Berlin HA. The influence of age of onset and acute anabolic steroid exposure on cognitive performance, impulsivity, and aggression in men. *Psychol Addict Behav.* 2014;28(4):1096-1104.
132. Kanayama G, Kean J, Hudson JI, Pope HG Jr. Cognitive deficits in long-term anabolic-androgenic steroid users. *Drug Alcohol Depend.* 2013;130(1-3):208-214.
133. Kaufman MJ, Janes AC, Hudson JI, et al. Brain and cognition abnormalities in long-term anabolic-androgenic steroid users. *Drug Alcohol Depend.* 2015;152:47-56.
134. Nelson BS, Hildebrandt T, Wallisch P. Anabolic–androgenic steroid use is associated with psychopathy, risk-taking, anger, and physical problems. *Sci Rep.* 2022;12:9133. doi:10.1038/s41598-022-13048-w
135. Galligani N, Renck A, Hansen S. Personality profile of men using anabolic androgenic steroids. *Horm Behav.* 1996;30(2):170-175.
136. Cherek DR. Effects of smoking different doses of nicotine on human aggressive behavior. *Psychopharmacology (Berl).* 1981;75:339-345.
137. Yates WR, Perry P, Murray S. Aggression and hostility in anabolic steroid users. *Biol Psychiatry.* 1992;31:1232-1234.
138. Buss AH, Durkee A. An inventory for assessing different kinds of hostility. *J Consult Psychol.* 1957;21:343-349.
139. Kouri EM, Lukas SE, Pope HG Jr, et al. Increased aggressive responding in male volunteers following the administration of gradually increasing doses of testosterone cypionate. *Drug Alcohol Depend.* 1995;40:73-79.
140. Kashkin KB, Kleber HD. Hooked on hormones? An anabolic steroid addiction hypothesis. *JAMA.* 1989;262(22):3166-3170.
141. Grönbladh A, Nylander E, Hallberg M. The neurobiology and addiction potential of anabolic androgenic steroids and the effects of growth hormone. *Brain Res Bull.* 2016;126:127-137.
142. Johnson LR, Wood RI. Oral testosterone self-administration in male hamsters. *Neuroendocrinology.* 2001;73(4):285-292.
143. Wood RI. Oral testosterone self-administration in male hamsters: dose-response, voluntary exercise, and individual differences. *Horm Behav.* 2002;41:247-258.
144. Wood RI, Johnson LR, Chu L, Schad C, Self DW. Testosterone reinforcement: intravenous and intracerebroventricular self-administration in male rats and hamsters. *Psychopharmacology (Berl).* 2004;171(3):298-305.
145. Ballard CL, Wood RI. Intracerebroventricular self-administration of commonly abused anabolic-androgenic steroids in male hamsters (*Mesocricetus auratus*): nandrolone, drostanolone, oxymetholone, and stanozolol. *Behav Neurosci.* 2005;119:752-758.
146. Triemstra JL, Sato SM, Wood RI. Testosterone and nucleus accumbens dopamine in the male Syrian hamster. *Psychoneuroendocrinology.* 2008;33:386-394.
147. Balster RL, Schuster CR. Fixed-interval schedule of cocaine reinforcement: effect of dose and infusion duration. *J Exp Anal Behav.* 1973;20(1):119-129.
148. Su TP, Pagliaro M, Schmidt PJ, et al. Neuropsychiatric effects of anabolic steroids in male normal volunteers. *JAMA.* 1993;269:2760-2764.
149. Arnedo MT, Salvador A, Martinez-Sanchis S, et al. Rewarding properties of testosterone in intact male mice: a pilot study. *Pharmacol Biochem Behav.* 2000;65:327-332.
150. Clark AS, Lindenfeld RC, Gibbons CH. Anabolic-androgenic steroids and brain reward. *Pharmacol Biochem Behav.* 1996;53(3):741-745.
151. Kindlundh AM, Lindblom J, Bergström L, et al. The anabolic-androgenic steroid nandrolone decanoate affects the density of dopamine receptors in the male rat brain. *Eur J Neurosci.* 2001;13:291-296.
152. Kindlundh AM, Bergström M, Monazzam A, et al. Dopaminergic effects after chronic treatment with nandrolone visualized in rat brain

by positron emission tomography. *Prog Neuropsychopharmacol Biol Psychiatry.* 2002;26:1303-1308.

153. Peters KD, Wood RI. Androgen dependence in hamsters: overdose, tolerance, and potential opioidergic mechanisms. *Neuroscience.* 2005;130:971-981.
154. Mhillaj E, Morgese MG, Tucci P, Bove M, Schiavone S, Trabace L. Effects of anabolic-androgens on brain reward function. *Front Neurosci.* 2015;9:1-13.
155. McBride AJ, Williamson K, Petersen T. Three cases of nalbuphine hydrochloride dependence associated with anabolic steroid use. *Br J Sports Med.* 1996;30:69-70.
156. Wines JD Jr, Gruber AJ, Pope HG Jr, Lukas SE. Nalbuphine hydrochloride dependence in anabolic steroid users. *Am J Addict.* 1999;8:161-164.
157. Ariel G, Saville W. The physiological effects of placebos. *Med Sci Sports.* 1972;4:124.
158. Crist DM, Stackpole PJ, Peake GT. Effects of androgenic-anabolic steroids on neuromuscular power and body composition. *J Appl Physiol.* 1983;54:366-370.
159. Brower KJ, Eliopulos GA, Blow FC, et al. Evidence for physical and psychological dependence on anabolic-androgenic steroids in eight weightlifters. *Am J Psychiatry.* 1990;147:510-512.
160. Brower KJ. Anabolic steroids: addictive, psychiatric, and medical consequences. *Am J Addict.* 1992;1(2):100-114.
161. Brower KJ, Blow FC, Young JP, et al. Symptoms and correlates of anabolic-androgenic steroid dependence. *Br J Addict.* 1991;86:759-768.
162. Brower KJ. Anabolic steroid abuse and dependence. *Curr Psychiatry Rep.* 2002;4:377-387.
163. vans WS, Bowen JN, Giordano FL, et al. A case of Stadol dependence (letter). *JAMA.* 1985;253(15):2191-2192.
164. Kanayama G, Brower KJ, Wood RI, et al. Treatment of anabolic-androgenic steroid dependence: emerging evidence and its implications. *Drug Alcohol Depend.* 2010;109(1–3):6-13.
165. Rasmussen JJ, Selmer C, Østergren PB, et al. Former abusers of anabolic androgenic steroids exhibit decreased testosterone levels and hypogonadal symptoms years after cessation: a case-control study. *PLoS One.* 2016;11(8):e0161208.
166. Kanayama G, Hudson JI, DeLuca J. Prolonged hypogonadism in males following withdrawal from anabolic-androgenic steroids: an underrecognized problem. *Addiction.* 2015;110(5):823-831.
167. Medraś M, Tworowska U. Treatment strategies of withdrawal from long-term use of anabolic-androgenic steroids. *Polski Merkur Lekarski.* 2001;11:535-538.
168. Bates G, Van Hout M-C, Teck JTW, McVeigh J. Treatments for people who use anabolic androgenic steroids: a scoping review. *Harm Reduct J.* 2019;16:75.
169. Molero Y, Gripenberg J, Bakshi A-S. Effectiveness and implementation of a community-based prevention programme targeting anabolic androgenic steroid use in gyms: study protocol of a quasi-experimental control group study. *BMC Sports Sci Med Rehabil.* 2016;8:36.
170. American Psychiatric Association. *Diagnostic and Statistical Manual of Mental Disorders.* 4th ed. American Psychiatric Association; 1994.
171. American Psychiatric Association. *Diagnostic and Statistical Manual of Mental Disorders.* 5th ed. American Psychiatric Publishing; 2013.
172. Kanayama G, Brower KJ, Wood RI, et al. Issues for DSM-5: clarifying the diagnostic criteria for anabolic-androgenic steroid dependence. *Am J Psychiatry.* 2009;166(6):642-645.
173. Pope HG, Kean J, Nash A, et al. A diagnostic interview module for anabolic-androgenic steroid dependence: preliminary evidence of reliability and validity. *Exp Clin Psychopharmacol.* 2010;18(3):203-213.
174. Pope HG Jr, Katz DL, Hudson JI. Anorexia nervosa and "reverse anorexia" among 108 male bodybuilders. *Compr Psychiatry.* 1993;34(6):406-409.
175. Phillips KA. Body dysmorphic disorder: diagnosis and treatment of imagined ugliness. *J Clin Psychiatry.* 1996;57(Suppl 8):61-65.
176. Lombardo JA. Anabolic-androgenic steroids. In: Lin GC, Erinoff L, eds. *Anabolic Steroid Abuse (NIDA Research Monograph 102).* National Institute on Drug Abuse; 1992:60-73.
177. Wroblewski AM. Androgenic-anabolic steroids and body dysmorphia in young men. *J Psychosom Res.* 1997;42(3):225-234.
178. Hollander E, Liebowitz MR, Winchel R, et al. Treatment of body-dysmorphic disorder with serotonin reuptake blockers. *Am J Psychiatry.* 1989;146(6):768-770.
179. Malone DA Jr, Dimeff RJ. The use of fluoxetine in depression associated with anabolic steroid withdrawal: a case series. *J Clin Psychiatry.* 1992;53(4):130-132.
180. Sagoe D, Andreassen CS, Pallesen S. The aetiology and trajectory of anabolic-androgenic steroid use initiation: a systematic review and synthesis of qualitative research. *Subst Abuse Treat Prev Policy.* 2014;9:27.
181. Martini L. The 5-alpha-reduction of testosterone in the neuroendocrine structures: biochemical and physiological implications. *Endocr Rev.* 1982;3:1-25.
182. Bardin CW, Catterall JF, Janne OA. The androgen-induced phenotype. In: Lin GC, Erinoff L, eds. *Anabolic Steroid Abuse (NIDA Research Monograph 102).* National Institute on Drug Abuse; 1990:131-141.
183. Winters SJ. Androgens: endocrine physiology and pharmacology. In: Lin GC, Erinoff L, eds. *Anabolic Steroid Abuse (NIDA Research Monograph 102).* National Institute on Drug Abuse; 1990:113-130.
184. Schanzer W. Metabolism of anabolic androgenic steroids. *Clin Chem.* 1996;42(7):1001-1020.
185. Catlin DH. Detection of drug use by athletes. In: Strauss RH, ed. *Drugs and Performance in Sports.* WB Saunders; 1987:103-120.
186. Donike M, Barwald KR, Klosterman K, et al. Detection of exogenous testosterone. In: Heck H, Hollman W, Liesen H, et al., eds. *Sport: Leistung und Gesundheit Kongressbd Dtsch Sportarztekongress.* Deutscher Artze-Verlag; 1983:293-298.
187. Trout GJ, Kazlauskas R. Sports drug testing: an analysts perspective. *Chem Soc Rev.* 2004;33:1-13.
188. Lukas SE. CNS effects and abuse liability of anabolic-androgenic steroids. *Annu Rev Pharmacol Toxicol.* 1996;36:333-357.
189. Kicman AT. Pharmacology of anabolic steroids. *Br J Pharmacol.* 2008;154:502-521.
190. Rogivkin BA. The role of low molecular weight compounds in the regulation of skeletal muscle genome activity during exercise. *Med Sci Sports.* 1976;8:1-4.
191. Lima G, Kolliari-Turner A, Wang G, et al. The MMAAS Project: an observational human study investigating the effect of anabolic androgenic steroid use on gene expression and the molecular mechanism of muscle memory. *Clin J Sport Med.* 2022; doi:10.1097/JSM.0000000000001037
192. Michels G, Hoppe UC. Rapid action of androgens. *Front Neuroendocrinol.* 2008;29:182-198.
193. Frye CA. Some rewarding effects of androgens may be mediated by actions of its 5alpha-reduced metabolite 3alpha-androstanediol. *Pharmacol Biochem Behav.* 2007;86:354-367.
194. Mayer M, Rosen F. Interaction of glucocorticoids and androgens with skeletal muscle. *Metabolism.* 1977;27:937-962.
195. Raaka BM, Finnerty M, Samuels HH. The glucocorticoid antagonist 17 alpha-methyltestosterone binds to the 10S glucocorticoid receptor and blocks agonist-mediated disassociation of the 10S oligomer to the 4S deoxyribonucleic acid-binding subunit. *Mol Endocrinol.* 1989;3:322-341.
196. Rana K, Lee NK, Zajac JD, MacLean HE. Expression of androgen receptor target genes in skeletal muscle. *Asian J Androl.* 2014;16:675-683.
197. Masonis AE, McCarthy MP. Direct interactions of androgenic/anabolic steroids with the peripheral benzodiazepine receptor in rat brain: implications for the psychological and physiological manifestations of androgenic/anabolic steroid abuse. *J Steroid Biochem Mol Biol.* 1996;58:551-555.
198. Narducci WA, Wagner JC, Hendrickson TP, et al. Anabolic steroids—a review of the clinical toxicology and diagnostic screening. *Clin Toxicol.* 1990;28:287-310.
199. Kanayama G, Hudson JI, Pope HG. Long-term psychiatric and medical consequences of anabolic-androgenic steroid abuse: a looming public health concern? *Drug Alcohol Depend.* 2008;98:1-12.
200. Martínez-Brito D, Correa Vidal MT, de la Torre X, et al. Reference ranges for the urinary steroid profile in a Latin-American population. *Drug Test Anal.* 2013;5(8):619-626.

201. Furuya K, Yamamoto N, Ohyabu Y, et al. Mechanism of the tissue-specific action of the selective androgen receptor modulator S-101479. *Biol Pharm Bull.* 2013;36(3):442-451.
202. World anti-doping agency. *The 2007 Prohibited List: International Standard.* WADA; 2006.
203. Unal M, Unal DO. Gene doping in sports. *Sports Med.* 2004;34(6):357-362.
204. Azzazy HM, Mansour MM, Christenson RH. Doping in the recombinant era: strategies and counterstrategies. *Clin Biochem.* 2005;38:959-965.
205. Choi SM, Lee BM. Comparative safety evaluation of selective androgen receptor modulators and anabolic androgenic steroids. *Expert Opin Drug Saf.* 2015;14(11):1773-1785.
206. Rochov M, Danel A, Chazard E, et al. Doping with aromatase inhibitors and oestrogen receptor modulators in steroid users: analysis of a forum to identify dosages, durations and adverse drug reactions. *Therapie.* 2022;77(6):683-691.
207. Sessal F, Salerno M, Di Mizio G, et al. Anabolic androgenic steroids: searching new molecular biomarkers. *Front Pharmacol.* 2018; doi:10.3389/fphar.2018.01321

CHAPTER

22 Electronic Drug Delivery Devices

Gideon St.Helen and Shannon C. Miller

CHAPTER OUTLINE

- Electronic drug delivery devices, the product
- Constituents of EDDDs and their aerosols
- Nicotine delivery and addiction potential
- Secondhand and thirdhand exposure
- Epidemiology of EDDD use with nicotine
- EDDDs and their connection to traditional cigarettes
- Toxicant exposures and adverse health consequences of EDDDs
- EDDD use and stopping smoking
- What to tell patients
- Variation in EDDD design
- Other nonnicotine substance use with EDDDs
- Epidemiology of cannabis use via EDDDs
- U.S. regulation of EDDDs
- Conclusions

ELECTRONIC DRUG DELIVERY DEVICES, THE PRODUCT

Electronic drug delivery devices (EDDDs) are electrically-powered (typically battery) devices used to deliver a psychoactive substance in an aerosol produced from the heating of substances. Electronic cigarettes, a subset of EDDDs, typically contain a battery, a heating element called an atomizer, and a substance-containing solution (typically with vegetable glycerin [VG] and/or propylene glycol [PG] mixed with nicotine), oil, or plant material; and typically various other chemicals or additives—sometimes unknown—used to add flavoring, alter the taste sensation (such as menthol substitutes), or increase the likability of the product.

The invention of the modern e-cigarette is attributed to a Chinese pharmacist, Hon Lik, in the early 2000s, whose U.S. patent application describes the e-cigarette as "an electronic atomization cigarette that functions as substitutes [sic] for quitting smoking and cigarette substitutes" (Patent No. 8,490,628 B2).[1] Before Hon Lik, Philip Morris, a tobacco company, and its affiliates had been developing a nicotine aerosol device like the modern e-cigarette in the 1990s to complement traditional cigarettes (TCs).[2]

There is wide variability in the design of EDDDs and product engineering continues to evolve (**Fig. 22-1**). Initially, EDDDs were grouped into three main types: cig-a-likes, pen-style tank EDDDs, and advanced personal vaporizers (APVs); 1st generation, 2nd generation, and 3rd generation are used interchangeably with these three types, respectively (see **Fig. 22-1**). Cig-a-likes (1st generation) are cigarette-shaped devices, which consist of a low-capacity battery (~75-150 mAh) and cartridge containing an atomizer. Cig-a-likes can be disposable or rechargeable, containing rechargeable batteries and allowing cartridge replacement. Most cig-a-likes are puff-activated. These included brands of cig-a-likes such as Halo Cigs, Blu E-cigs, NJOY, and V2 Cigs.

Pen-style tank EDDDs (2nd generation) are larger than TCs or cig-a-likes, have higher-capacity batteries (450-1,100 mAh), and may contain a prefilled cartridge or refillable tank. The atomizer is usually a prebuilt coil made from high-resistance metals/alloys such as nichrome or kanthal, through which a wick is wound in a tank. Most pen-style EDDDs are activated by a manual switch. These included brands such as KangerTech's Protank and EVOD, Aspire ET, and Innokin iClear.

APV (3rd generation) EDDDs come in multiple shapes (see **Fig. 22-1**) and are typically larger than pen-shaped e-cigarettes. These devices contain high-capacity batteries (3,000-3,500 mAh). APVs come in two types: mechanical mods (modular) and regulated mods. Mechanical mods contain no circuitry and consist of a battery compartment, a button to activate the device, and a connector to attach to a tank. Regulated mods are more complex in design, include electrical circuit boards with built-in features to control voltage and/or power output (variable voltage/variable wattage) but are more user-friendly than mechanical mods. Mods are compatible with most standard tanks, including those used in pen-shaped e-cigarettes. Some APVs include automatic temperature control devices.

The most recent iteration of EDDDs is referred to as pods, pod-mods or 4th generation e-cigarettes. Pods have become the most popular type of EDDDs on the U.S. market, especially among youth and young adults.[3] These devices vary in shape and size, including those that resemble a USB flash drive (eg, JUUL and Puff Bar), box shaped but smaller than

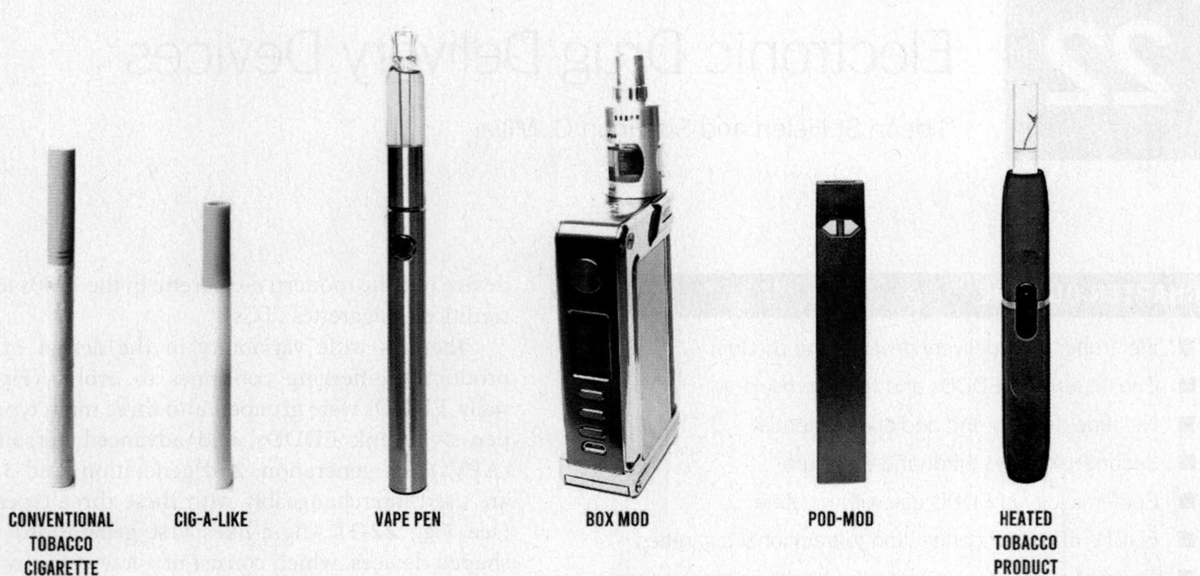

Figure 22-1. Types of EDDD products. From right to left, a combustible cigarette; a cig-a-like or 1st-generation e-cigarette; a vape pen-style or 2nd-generation e-cigarette; a large-size tank or box mod, also referred to as APVs or 3rd generation e-cigarette; a pod, pod-mod or 4th generation e-cigarette; and a heated tobacco product or heat-not-burn tobacco product. (From Benowitz NL, St. Helen G, Liakoni E. Clinical Pharmacology of Electronic Nicotine Delivery Systems (ENDS): implications for benefits and risks in the promotion of the combusted tobacco endgame. *J Clin Pharmacol.* 2021;61:S18-S36.)

3rd generation mods (eg, Lost Vape Ursa Baby), and even tear drop shaped (eg, Suorin Drop). The ease of use and concealment, along with their sleek, modern design and their packaging make pod EDDDs appealing to youth and easier to conceal them from parents, school staff, employers, and others who may raise concern about their use.[4]

CONSTITUENTS OF EDDDs AND THEIR AEROSOLS

Propylene Glycol and Vegetable Glycerin

In general, while the EDDD industry has promulgated the term "vapor," "vape," or "vaping" to describe what is released from EDDDs; rather than releasing a water vapor, EDDDs release an aerosol. These aerosols include liquids and gases suspended in air which can themselves carry various chemicals and semi-solid particulates, which may alter the likability of the product, introduce harm to the person using it, or both; or have no or other effects. Thus, "aerosol" is the more medically precise term than "vapor."

Humectant

For those EDDDs containing a humectant, the liquid refill, referred to as "e-liquid" or "e-juice," used in EDDDs contains PG and/or VG, nicotine, and flavorants. Propylene glycol (PG, 1,2-dihydroxypropane) is an odorless, colorless, and tasteless synthetic liquid. PG, a constituent of theatrical smoke and fog, produces the "smokiness" of the e-cigarette aerosol. PG also produces the sensory response in the upper airways colloquially referred to as the "throat hit."[5] VG, or propane-1,2,3-triol, is an odorless, colorless, and sweet-tasting viscous liquid. The ratios of VG to PG in e-liquids vary according to the desired smokiness of the aerosol, sweetness, viscosity, and throat hit. The concentration of VG and PG in e-cigarette aerosol depends on their concentration in the e-liquid.[6] While both PG and VG are generally recognized as safe (GRAS, "generally recognized as safe") for use in food and oral consumption by the Food and Drug Administration (FDA), there is no such safety assessment or rating for heated, aerosolized and inhaled formulations of VG/PG that enter the respiratory system. Heating of PG and VG in high-temperature conditions can lead to the production of toxic (including possibly cancerous) by-products such as acrolein, formaldehyde, and benzene.[7,8]

Nicotine

Nicotine levels in EDDDs or e-liquids range from low (eg, 3 mg/mL) to high (eg, 100 mg/mL). Some brands of e-liquids market zero-nicotine options,[9] presumably for nicotine-free vaping or for mixing with other nicotine-containing e-liquids. Due in part to lack of external regulation of this industry, there is poor concordance of labeled and actual nicotine content of some cig-a-like and refill e-liquid brands[6,10-12]; moreover, the nicotine content in the e-liquid is not necessarily predictive of nicotine exposure. The amount of nicotine delivered per puff is highly dependent on the actual (not labeled) amount of nicotine, the power applied to the EDDD atomizer, and the resultant temperature of the coil.[13] For instance, people who use high-powered APVs frequently use low nicotine concentration e-liquids because of the large amount of aerosol produced by these devices, resulting in nicotine intake comparable to or exceeding that from conventional cigarettes.[14]

As a weak organic base with a pKa of 8.0, 50% of nicotine is protonated and 50% unprotonated (also called freebase nicotine) at a pH of 8.0. Changes to the pH of the aerosol changes the proportion of protonated and freebase nicotine emitted. Freebase nicotine is more volatile than protonated nicotine. Given its higher volatility, a higher proportion of freebase nicotine is deposited in the upper airways than protonated nicotine, making the aerosol harsher and more difficult to inhale due to the impact of high concentrations of freebase nicotine on oropharyngeal and tracheal nicotinic cholinergic sensory receptors.[15] Compared to freebase nicotine, a lower proportion of protonated nicotine is deposited in the upper airways and a higher proportion is deposited in the lower airways (alveolar region) where absorption into the circulation is rapid, regardless of what form nicotine is in (protonated or freebase). Once in the alveoli, nicotine leaves the smoke or aerosol and, at the physiological pH of the lung, is absorbed quickly through the pulmonary capillaries and into the systemic circulation.[16] Importantly, protonated nicotine does not activate the trigeminal nerve, making it less harsh and easier to inhale than freebase nicotine.[17]

Traditional cigarette (TC) smoke typically has a pH of around 5.5 to 6.5 (ie, it has higher levels of protonated nicotine than freebase nicotine), which makes the smoke less harsh and easier to inhale. TCs have high addiction liability due to the rapidity with which inhaled nicotine enters the circulation and into the brain. Earlier iterations of EDDDs used e-liquids with higher pH (ie, no acid added). The aerosols with higher fractions of freebase nicotine produced harsher throat hits. To enhance the palatability of EDDDs aerosols, manufacturers added acids such as benzoic acid and lactic acid to the e-liquids, which reduces the pH of the e-liquids and increases the fraction of protonated nicotine in the aerosol. EDDDs with acid added (forms nicotine salts) such as JUUL, Puff Bar and other pod-mods, produce aerosols that are easier to inhale, and since a higher proportion of protonated nicotine is deposited in the lower airways, e-liquids with nicotine salts facilitate more rapid uptake of nicotine.

Given the lower electrical power (similar to 1st generation devices) of pod EDDDs and temperature regulation of some devices such as JUUL, the small volume of aerosol generated, and more tolerable aerosols, the nicotine content of e-liquids used in pod e-cigarettes is typically higher than that used in EDDDs from the first three generations. The higher nicotine content and rapid delivery to the brain may increase risk for nicotine use disorder, and may also pose higher risk for toxicity if the liquid is ingested (such as by toddlers, pets, etc.).

A recent evolution in EDDD product manufacture is the use of synthetic nicotine (nicotine not derived from tobacco). Previously, synthetic nicotine was presumed by scientists and regulators to be too expensive to be made and used in EDDDs, and thus was not a concern. This provided a loophole for EDDD expansion without regulatory oversight. The FDA's regulatory authority has since been clarified to include synthetic nicotine. Natural nicotine in the tobacco leaf is predominantly (S)-nicotine, with only 0.1% to 0.6% (R)-nicotine. Tobacco smoke may contain up to 10% (R)-nicotine, presumably due to formation (R)-nicotine during combustion. Pharmaceutical nicotine products contain 0.1% to 1.2% (R)-nicotine. Most synthetic nicotine products had contained approximately equal amounts of (S)- and (R)-nicotine; but more recently, they are more stereoselective.[18,19] These chemical differences are important because the pharmacology of (S)- and (R)-nicotine differ substantially. The (S) isomer has much higher affinity for most nicotinic cholinergic receptors (nAchR) compared to (R)-nicotine; and animal and cellular studies indicate that (S)-nicotine is more potent than (R)-nicotine for most nicotinic cholinergic receptor-mediated pharmacological effects.[20-24] However, the pharmacology of a racemic mixture (ie, containing equal fractions of (S)- and (R)-nicotine) or increasingly higher fractions of (S)-nicotine in EDDDs is currently unknown. Currently, most currently marketed synthetic nicotine EDDD products are predominantly (S)-nicotine. EDDD companies sometimes market their EDDDs that use synthetic nicotine as "tobacco-free"[25] EDDDs, which has been shown to reduce fears of tobacco-related harms (although nicotine may cause harm in youth) and increase product appeal.

Flavorants (Flavorings)

Flavorants are an important feature of EDDDs. In 2014, over 7,700 different e-liquid flavors were identified in the U.S. marketplace, including tobacco, fruit and beverage flavors, sweet flavors, menthol, and combinations.[9,26] Several flavorants used in EDDDs are toxic and could be harmful to people who use EDDDs. Diacetyl and 2,3-pentanedione, both of which give a buttery flavor and are known causes of bronchiolitis obliterans in humans with high-level exposure in occupational settings,[27,28] were previously used in EDDD liquids. Other flavorants such as cinnamaldehyde, 2-methoxycinnamaldehyde, vanillin, and 2,5-dimethypyrazine (chocolate flavoring), which have various toxic effects in vitro[29-31] are used in e-liquids today. The safety of these chemicals has not been evaluated in humans at the concentrations commonly found in EDDD aerosols. Some flavorants thermally decompose when heated in EDDDs, resulting in toxic and carcinogenic aldehydes, and generating concentrations that exceed safety limits.[32]

Recently, restrictions have been placed on the sale of flavored EDDDs in various jurisdictions. In January 2020, the FDA announced a policy prioritizing enforcement against sale of flavored cartridge-based EDDDs; tobacco flavor or menthol flavored EDDDs were exempted from this enforcement policy.[33] An analysis by Truth Initiative, a nonprofit tobacco control organization, found that by the end of March 2022, 361 localities and three Indigenous American tribes had restrictions on flavored tobacco products (including EDDDs); of those, 108 have fully comprehensive policies that prohibit sales of all types of flavors across all products at all retailers.[34] Nevertheless, disposable EDDDs were exempt from this FDA policy, and soon after disposables became the dominant EDDD sold. In July 2020, FDA ordered companies to remove unauthorized flavored disposable products from the market. Flavors and menthol/cooling agents significantly improve the palatability of inhaled EDDD aerosol—particularly important for attracting youth and those using EDDDs for the first time. As some municipalities have begun to ban flavors, the EDDD industry responded by switching from flavors to "blends" of flavors and "concepts" in an effort to both retain flavors and avoid regulation by making it more difficult for enforcement agencies to determine whether a product meets the legal definition of a flavored tobacco product.[35] For example, in 2021, the popular disposable e-cigarette brand BIDI Stick (founded in 2019) unveiled nearly a dozen new concept names as direct translations from its previous flavors.[36] Their marketing stated that this was done "to strengthen our advocacy against underage vaping through responsible marketing." In another example, San Francisco California eliminated flavored tobacco, including menthol cigarettes, and soon after R.J. Reynolds released two new cigarette brands, Camel Crisp and Newport EXP, marketing them as "nonmenthol" even though they still have synthetic cooling agents.[35] The use of fruit, sweet, menthol/mint or similar effects remain problematic toward attracting youth to EDDDs, while reducing the harshness and irritation from inhaled nicotine so as to enhance sales.

Contaminants

Contaminants in some e-liquids and EDDD aerosols include known human carcinogens such as tobacco-specific nitrosamines (eg, 4-(methylnitrosamino)-1-(3-pyridyl)-1-butanone, NNK),[37] polycyclic aromatic hydrocarbons (PAHs) (eg, pyrene),[38] heavy metals (eg, cadmium, lead, and copper)[37,39] and minor tobacco alkaloids (eg, nornicotine and myosmine).[10,12] Levels of NNK, PAHs, and minor tobacco alkaloids in e-liquids or EDDDs today are very low or not present.[37,40] The concentrations of these contaminants depend in part on the quality of the purification process when nicotine is extracted from tobacco. The metal coils of the atomizer and soldering in EDDDs are sources of heavy metal exposure such as chromium (likely in the trivalent state, chromium III), nickel, and tin.[39] While hexavalent chromium (chromium VI) is a known human carcinogen, there is no evidence that it is emitted from EDDDs.[41] When present, many contaminants in e-liquids and aerosols are found at much lower levels (9-450 times lower) compared to TCs and TC smoke.[37] Some are found in higher levels. Lower levels would suggest that the carcinogenic risk is lower for EDDDs compared to TCs.[42] Health implications of lower contaminant levels in EDDD aerosol for respiratory and cardiovascular disease risks are still uncertain given the presence of reactive aldehydes and toxic volatile organic compounds in EDDD aerosols. Long term exposure studies are critically needed, including not only health risks from exposures to those who use them, but also health risks from those exposed to second- and thirdhand sources (see below). Cadmium and lead, as well as drugs (such as amino-tadalafil and rimonabant) have also been detected in EDDDs.[43] In another study, other metals and silicates such as silver, iron, and aluminum were found; with nine of eleven elements in the EDDD aerosol being found in levels equal to or higher than in the corresponding TC smoke.[39]

Volatile Organic Compounds

Volatile organic compounds (VOCs) are a class of compounds produced from incomplete combustion of organic materials. Because of their abundance in TC smoke and their inherent carcinogenicity and/or toxicity, VOCs account for the majority of cancer, cardiovascular, and respiratory disease risks of tobacco smoke.[44,45] Although EDDDs do not burn (pyrolyze) the e-liquid, the heat applied by the atomizer can cause temperature-dependent thermal decomposition of e-liquid constituents to form toxic VOCs.[46] Under certain conditions (high power and dry puffs), VOCs such as formaldehyde, acetaldehyde, and acrolein are emitted in EDDD aerosol at pharmacologically significant concentrations, and also within the range of that achieved from smoking TCs.[37,46-49]

VG and PG both degrade to toxic aldehydes when heated.[7,8] One study reported that formaldehyde is generated from EDDDs at levels five times higher compared to TCs.[47] Another study suggested that flavoring compounds can also be substantial sources of aldehydes.[32] Whether people who use EDDDs use their devices under conditions that generate high levels of aldehydes has been questioned because the resultant aerosol would be harsh and unpleasant tasting.[48]

Acrolein, a cardiopulmonary toxicant, is estimated to account for as much as 88.5% of the noncancer risk index of traditional tobacco smoking.[45] Urinary biomarkers of acrolein exposure in people who use EDDDs are at much lower levels than those who smoke TCs and similar to levels in nonsmoking people, suggesting that actual levels of exposure and health risks from acrolein are low.[50-54] One of the major health risks from smoking TCs is cardiovascular disease.[55] Because cardiovascular disease risk has a nonlinear association with TC consumption, smoking just a few cigarettes per day imparts a majority of the cardiovascular disease risk. Thus, if VOCs such as acrolein are delivered in significant amounts from EDDDs, these compounds could contribute to cardiovascular disease risk. An inpatient study of healthy people who dually used both EDDDs and TCs found no evidence of elevated acrolein exposure from two days of EDDD use alone. However, the same study found increased levels of biomarkers of benzene and acrylamide after EDDD use, suggesting that toxic and carcinogenic VOCs are being emitted in EDDD aerosol, albeit at levels lower than that of TCs.[54] It is unknown if this lower level results in less risk of cardiovascular disease. Importantly, lower levels do not necessarily translate to lower risk, especially when the relationship between exposure and risk is nonlinear, as is seen with VOC exposure from TCs and heart disease risk.

Further discussion about cardiovascular risks from EDDDs can be found in the Chapter 88, "Cardiovascular Disorders Related to Substance Use."

Particles

Epidemiological studies have long associated exposure to particles in ambient air, particularly fine particles (those <2.5 μm in aerodynamic diameter) and ultrafine particles (those <0.1 μm), to increased risk of various cancers, cardiovascular, and respiratory diseases.[56-58] Both traditional tobacco smoke and EDDD emissions are best described as aerosols, that is, solid and/or liquid particles suspended in air. Particle size is an important factor in predicting the deposition fraction of the inhaled particles in various regions of the respiratory tract,[59] which in turn predicts the extent of nicotine absorption. Mainstream tobacco smoke (smoke directly inhaled) has a median particle size range of 180 to 340 nm.[60]

Initial studies reported that EDDDs have similar particle size compared to mainstream tobacco cigarette smoke,[61] including some particles in the nanoparticle range.[62,63] Aerosol characteristics likely vary significantly according to the power of the EDDDs and PG/VG ratio. One study reported that EDDD aerosol is bimodal, with median particle diameter at the modes of 11 to 25 nm and 96 to 175 nm.[64] This study found comparable particle concentrations in each mode and only nanoparticles present during "dry puffs." Dry puffs occur when insufficient e-liquid is drawn into the atomizer chamber during puffing and the wicking material (eg, cotton) overheats and burns. The aerosol or smoke given off produces what is described as an unpleasant sensory response in the throat. "Dripping" is another method of use that may result in this outcome, whereby e-liquid is dripped directly onto the heating element and then inhaled. Some EDDD products include versions and/or or instructions for dripping.

The composition of EDDD particles is quite different from that of particles in TC smoke. TC smoke particles are much more complex, include solid carbonaceous materials, and persist in the environment much longer than EDDD particles. The larger EDDD particles are liquid, comprised mostly of PG and VG, and such particles would be expected to dissolve and be absorbed quickly in the lung. Although constituents of EDDD nanoparticles have not been fully characterized, metals such as tin, chromium, and nickel have been detected.[39] There is also concern about the health consequences of exposure to EDDD-related nanoparticles because these particles can penetrate more deeply into the lungs (where particle clearance is slower[65]) than particles from TCs, leading to longer exposure times to toxicants (including carcinogens) associated with the particles as compared to those from TC. The specific hazards posed by particles generated by EDDDs are unknown, but remain of significant concern warranting more research.

NICOTINE DELIVERY AND ADDICTION POTENTIAL

Early studies in 2013 to 2014 estimating nicotine delivery from EDDDs were based on modified International Organization for Standardization (ISO) smoking machine tests or from the volume of e-liquid consumed. These studies showed that EDDDs delivered less nicotine than TCs.[11,66,67] The average nicotine yield for TCs is between 0.5 to 1.5 mg per cigarette.[68] Early pharmacokinetic studies of cig-a-like–type e-cigarettes reported very low plasma nicotine levels, indicative of low nicotine delivery and/or absorption.[69,70]

Later pharmacokinetic studies reported higher plasma nicotine concentrations among people experienced with EDDDs[71-74] although the average maximum plasma nicotine concentrations (C_{max}) from single use sessions were lower than previously reported levels from smoking TCs. Plasma nicotine C_{max} from smoking TCs vary but typical concentrations range between approximately 15 to 30 ng/mL.[68] Second- and third-generation EDDDs (tank-style and mods) produced greater levels of plasma nicotine than first generation (cig-a-likes).[73-75] Recent pharmacokinetic studies show EDDDs delivering similar levels of nicotine as do TCs. One study of EDDD use among people experienced with using them reported that EDDDs delivered an average of 1.3 mg (range 0.4-2.6 mg) of nicotine from 15 puffs, similar to TCs; several people who used EDDDs achieved TC-like plasma nicotine levels.[6] Another study among people experienced with EDDD use reported that those who used high-powered APVs were able to mimic the nicotine pharmacokinetic profile of TCs.[14] One study found similar maximum plasma nicotine levels from use of JUUL compared to TCs while another study showed lower nicotine intake from EDDDs compared to TCs among people who used both EDDDs and TCs.[74,76]

Pharmacokinetic parameters such as plasma nicotine C_{max} and time to maximum concentration (T_{max}) are important determinants of tobacco product addiction liability. Nicotine concentration peaks in blood within two to five minutes after the last puff of an EDDD,[6,71] similar to TCs.[68] Based on the type of EDDD, the maximum blood nicotine concentrations can be comparable to those from TC smoking. The basic shape of the plasma nicotine concentration-time curve after single administration (eg, 10-15 puffs) of nicotine from EDDDs is also comparable to TCs, that is, rapid increase in blood nicotine levels followed by quick decline. This indicates that EDDDs have the potential to initiate and sustain nicotine addiction. Further supporting risk for creating nicotine addiction, EDDDs reduce the urge to smoke and alleviate nicotine withdrawal symptoms (negative reinforcement) and are rated as satisfying by people who use them (positive reinforcement).[70,72,77,78] In addition to nicotine pharmacological effects, oral and tactile sensations may also contribute to the subjective effects of EDDDs and their addictiveness.[70] A review of the literature concluded that EDDD use results in symptoms of addiction and nicotine use disorder, but the risk and severity were subjectively rated as lower for EDDDs (manufactured and distributed at that time) than for TCs. As EDDD design rapidly evolves, addiction liability may also evolve as well.[79]

Nicotine intake and vaping behavior during ad libitum access to EDDDs should be considered when assessing the addictiveness of EDDDs. Blood nicotine concentrations during ad libitum access rise gradually to a maximum, in contrast to the rapid increase in blood nicotine concentrations that is characteristic of tobacco smoking and controlled EDDD use.[14,71,80] People who use EDDDs sustain their blood nicotine concentrations by vaping intermittently, often in single or groups of 2 to 5 puffs.[80] Given that a rapid rise in plasma nicotine concentration is associated with greater addiction liability of tobacco products, and given that EDDDs can deliver nicotine in a near-bolus dose, nicotine intake and the addictiveness of EDDDs likely depend on the manner in which they are used (as well as device characteristics).[79]

The relative level of DSM-IV defined nicotine dependence among adults who use EDDDs compared to TCs was examined in the Population Assessment of Tobacco and Health (PATH) study using the PATH nicotine dependence survey.[81] The PATH study is a nationally representative longitudinal study of tobacco use in the United States. Using baseline data collected in 2013 and 2014, aspects of addiction were compared in people who exclusively used EDDDs and those who exclusively smoked TCs. Based on a number of addiction-related criteria (DSM-5 equivalent criteria for tobacco use disorder in parenthesis) including time to first use after waking (an indicator of physical dependence, possibly withdrawal or craving), considering oneself addicted (continuing to use despite tobacco/nicotine causing problems to their mental health), strong cravings (experiencing intense cravings or urges to use tobacco/nicotine), difficulty in refraining from use in places where it is prohibited (loss of control), and feeling like they really needed the product (experiencing urges to use the substance), the people who used EDDDs self-reported lower scores than those who smoked TCs. 77% of people who used EDDDs (versus 94% of those who smoked TCs) still considered themselves addicted to EDDDs. The reason for higher self-reported addiction to TCs may relate to differences in nicotine delivery and pharmacokinetics and to user characteristics. The latter may include societal perceptions of lower addiction risk from EDDDs compared to TCs, younger age of the person using EDDDs, shorter lifetime use of EDDDs (EDDDs have been available for use for a very small fraction of the time as compared to TCs), or more social stigma from smoking TCs versus vaping. Importantly, at the time of the study, smoking was prohibited in most public places, whereas use of EDDDs was hardly if at all prohibited, likely causing under self-reporting in all but the first of the criteria discussed above. EDDDs have evolved significantly since this study a decade ago.

A survey study analyzed the cross-sectional National Youth Tobacco Surveys from 2014 to 2021 administered to national probability samples of roughly 150,000 U.S. students in grades 6 to 12.[82] Between 2014 and 2021, the age at initiation of EDDD use decreased, and intensity of use and addiction increased. By 2017, EDDDs became the most common first product used (77.0%). In contrast, for non-EDDD tobacco product use over this time period, age at initiation of use did not change, and changes in intensity of use were minimal. By 2019, more EDDD using youth were using their first product within 5 minutes of awakening (a marker of addiction to nicotine) than for TCs and all other products combined. Median EDDD use also increased from 3 to 5 days/month in between 2014 to 2018, to 6 to 9 days/month from 2019 to 2020, and further to 10 to 19 days/month in 2021. Thus, several markers for addiction to nicotine in EDDDs have been increasing significantly among 6th to 12th graders.

Further, some people modify the EDDD to increase the "hit" by various means to increase nicotine delivery. An example of this is "dripping," where the nicotine refill liquid is dripped directly onto the coil. One-quarter of adolescents who use e-cigarettes have engaged in "dripping" in a recent survey, and manufacturers are reportedly making their coils more accessible to enable this practice.[83] Since pod EDDDs, which are not designed to facilitate "dripping," are now the most popular EDDDs among adolescents, "dripping" may not be as widely practiced among adolescent e-cigarette users. However, a 2021 report (survey) that found 43.7% of young adults who ever used EDDDs (lifetime) reported dripping.[84]

Unknown and Undisclosed Chemicals

Tehrani et al. applied a chemical fingerprinting technique used to detect chemicals in food and wastewater, and applied it in a novel fashion to a variety of EDDDs.[85] Nearly two thousand unknown chemicals and substances (including those not disclosed by EDDD manufacturers) were detected in the e-liquid and even more in the aerosol, including industrial chemicals (such as tributylphosphine oxide), caffeine, and a pesticide. As well, they detected condensed hydrocarbon-like compounds previously associated with combustion. Other studies have found undisclosed substances in EDDDs as well.[86]

SECONDHAND AND THIRDHAND EXPOSURE

Unlike TCs, EDDDs do not generate side-stream emissions (from the burning tip of the cigarette), but bystanders can be exposed to constituents in the aerosol exhaled by the person using them, which is referred to as secondhand aerosol exposure. Thirdhand aerosol exposure, discussed below, results from the absorption of EDDD aerosol constituents onto environmental surfaces such as walls, carpets, draperies, furniture, clothing, car interiors, and toys after the use of the EDDD ends, followed by either touching these surfaces or inhaling their later release into the ambient air.

More than half of middle and high school students reported secondhand EDDD aerosol exposure in 2017.[87,88] One study measured nicotine in indoor air of the homes of nonsmoking volunteers who lived with people who use TCs, with people who use EDDDs, or in control homes where tobacco or EDDDs were not used. They measured cotinine in saliva and urine of the nonsmoking volunteers as a biomarker of exposure to secondhand smoke or to nicotine-containing EDDD aerosol. Air nicotine concentration was higher in the EDDD homes compared to the smoke-free homes, but lower than in the TC. Saliva and urine cotinine were 2 and 1.4 times higher, respectively, in people who did not smoke in the TC homes compared to the EDDD homes.[89] This study suggests that people who do not use EDDDs who live in homes where EDDDs are used are exposed to nicotine derived from the exhaled aerosol, but at lower levels than people exposed to secondhand TC smoke. Secondhand aerosol exposure is also expected to vary across devices. Mod users, given the large volume of aerosol generated, exhale a significant fraction of the inhaled aerosols; pods produce smaller volumes of aerosols for inhalation and the person exhales relatively lower amounts. Thus, device type is expected to have a notable effect on how much nicotine enters the environment.

A study of people who never smoked exposed to three conditions—(control session without smoking/vaping or passive exposure, passive TC tobacco smoke exposure session, and passive EDDD aerosol exposure)—found that there was no significant difference in serum cotinine concentrations between passive exposure to traditional tobacco smoke and passive exposure to EDDDs aerosol after one hour of exposure.[90] Changes in lung function (the ratio of forced expiratory volume in one second [FEV_1] to forced vital capacity [FVC], FEV_1/FVC) were smaller after passive exposure to EDDD aerosol than after passive exposure to TC smoke. Another study reported elevated levels of fine particulate matter ($PM_{2.5}$), 1,2-propanediol, glycerin, and nicotine in indoor air and increased concentrations of nitric oxide (FeNO) release in nonusing volunteers after two hours of secondhand EDDD exposure.[91] Other studies have also measured increased levels of $PM_{2.5}$ in indoor air following EDDD use, with similar findings.[92]

The contribution of EDDD emissions to thirdhand aerosol exposure and its potential health effects remain unknown. Thirdhand tobacco smoke is the result of physical and chemical transformations of smoke constituents in indoor and outdoor environments over time, which result in the creation of secondary pollutants.[93] Nicotine reacts with nitrous acid, a ubiquitous environmental contaminant, to form the potent lung carcinogen 4-(methylnitrosamino)-1-(3-pyridyl)-1-butanone (NNK).[94] Nicotine has been measured in the indoor environment after EDDD use (especially on the floor and glass windows) and is therefore a potential source of thirdhand aerosol exposure.[91,95-98] A study of indoor surfaces in five vape shops found surface nicotine concentrations comparable or higher than the reported surface nicotine levels induced by active TC smoking, though lower than those on casino surfaces.[99] The NNA and NNK levels observed in this study are of particular concern as they were higher than levels observed in the home of someone actively smoking TCs. Animal and in vitro studies show that thirdhand smoke exposure has toxic effects on several organs, including the liver and lungs, and is genotoxic.[100,101]

EPIDEMIOLOGY OF EDDD USE WITH NICOTINE

U.S. national data on EDDD use among adults aged 18 and over are derived from the 2019 National Health Interview Survey (NHIS).[102] Overall, 4.5% (estimated 10.9 million) of adults were currently using EDDDs, that is, they reported using EDDDs at least once during their lifetime and now used EDDDs "every day" or "some days." A greater proportion of adult men (5.5%) currently used EDDDs than did women (3.5%) and use was highest among 18 to 24 year olds (9.3%) and 25 to 44 years olds (6.4%) compared to adults aged 45 to 64 (3.0%) and those 65 years and older (0.8%). EDDD use also differed across race/ethnicity, with rates of current use as follows: non-Hispanic White (5.1%); non-Hispanic Black (3.4%); non-Hispanic Asian (2.7%); and Hispanic or Latinx (2.8%).

Past month EDDD use among adults differs by cigarette smoking status. Among current people who smoked TCs in 2018, 49.4% had ever-used an EDDD while 9.7% were currently using EDDDs.[103] Among people who formerly smoked cigarettes who had quit within the past year, 57.3% had ever-used EDDDs and 25.2% were currently using EDDDs. Rates of EDDD use decreased as time since quitting TCs increased. Prevalence of ever-use and current use of EDDDs were 48.6% and 17.3%, respectively, among people who formerly smoked TCs who quit 1 to 4 years ago and 9.0% and 1.7%, respectively, among people who formerly smoked who quit 5 or more years ago. Among people who had never smoked cigarettes, 6.5% and 1.1% had ever-used and currently used EDDDs.

A 2021 survey of a representative sample of U.S. middle and high school students (National Youth Tobacco Survey [NYTS]) estimated that 7.6% of U.S. youth (2.06 million) were currently (past 30-day) using EDDDs , including 2.8% of middle school students (320,000) and 11.3% high school students (1.72 million).[104] Current EDDD use among youth increased in 2022. The same survey estimated that, in 2022, 9.4% (2.55 million), including 3.3% (380,000) of middle school students and 14.1% (2.14 million) of high school students were currently using EDDDs.[105] In an FDA and CDC review of 2022 data, EDDDs were the most common tobacco product used by middle schoolers and high schoolers.[106]

The prevalence of youth who vape nicotine frequently (ie, on 20 or more days in past 30 days) is also increasing, suggesting increased addiction to nicotine in EDDDs. In 2021, 60.6% of youth currently using EDDDs did so on 1 to 19 days per month, 39.4% used on 20 to 30 days; and 24.6% used daily.[107] Among middle school students, 82.8% used EDDDs on 1 to 19 days, 17.2% used on 20 to 30 days; 8.3% used daily. Among high school students, 56.4% used on 1 to 19 days, 43.6% used on 20 to 30 days; 27.6% used daily. In contrast, in 2022, 57.7% of youth who used EDDDs did so on 1 to 19 days per month while 42.3% used on 20 to 30 days and 27.6% used daily.[105] Among middle school students, 79.3% used on 1 to 19 days while 20.8% used on 20 to 30 days and 11.7% used daily. For high school students, 54.0% used on 1 to 19 days while 46.0% used on 20 to 30 days and 30.1% used daily.

A majority of youth who currently use EDDDs use disposable EDDDs (55.3%) in 2022, compared to prefilled or refillable pods or cartridges (25.2%) and tanks or mod systems (6.7%); 12.8% of respondents did not know.[105] For middle and high school students, 45.8% and 57.2%, respectively, used disposables, compared to 21.6% and 25.7% who used prefilled or refillable pods or cartridges, and 9.8% and 5.9% who used tanks or mod systems; 22.8% and 11.2% of middle and high school students, respectively, did not know. The most popular brands among youth users were Puff Bar (overall, 29.7%; middle school, 30.9%; high school, 29.3%) followed by Vuse (overall, 23.6%; middle school, 20.9%; high school, 23.8%), JUUL (overall, 22.0%; middle school, 23.8%; high school, 21.2%), and SMOK (including NOVO) (overall, 13.5%; middle school, 7.8%; high school, 14.3%), among others.

In 2022, flavored EDDDs were the predominant choice of middle and high school-aged youth currently (past-30 days) using EDDDs: 84.9% (2.11 million) used flavored e-cigarettes while 9.3% (230,000) used unflavored e-cigarettes, and 5.7% (140,000) did not know.[105] The most frequently used flavors were fruit (69.1%, 1.45 million), candy, desserts, or other sweets (38.3%, 800,000), mint (29.4%, 610,000), menthol (26.6%, 550,000), alcoholic drink (7.6%, 150,000), chocolate (4.3%, 80,000), and clove or spice (2.9%, 60,000).

EDDDs AND THEIR CONNECTION TO TRADITIONAL CIGARETTES

Under the assumption that future TC use is a reasonable proxy for addiction, several observations are cause for concern. For example, the PATH study—a large representative sample of the U.S. population ages 12 to 24 with annual follow-up assessments—suggested that youth who first used EDDDs e-cigarettes had a three fold increased risk of TC use later in life. There is substantial evidence that EDDD use increases the risk of ever using TCs, moderate evidence that EDDD use increases the frequency and intensity of subsequent TC smoking, and limited evidence that EDDD use increases, in the near term, the duration of subsequent TC smoking among youth and young adults.[79]

Several prospective, longitudinal studies of nonsmoking people found that youth and young adults who had used EDDDs were two to eight times more likely to initiate TC use than those who had never used EDDDs.[108-112] Use of EDDDs among youth is also associated with use of other tobacco products. For example, the 2015 NYTS found that 58.8% of high school students who smoked TCs and those who smoked other traditional tobacco products, as well as 77% of those who used all traditional tobacco products (cigarettes, pipe, chew, snus, etc.), also used EDDDs in the past 30 days.[113] One study found that the association between EDDD use and TC initiation was stronger (odds ratio = 9.69, 95% CI, 4.02-23.4) for youth who were not originally susceptible to TC smoking (defined as those with a firm commitment not to smoke) compared to those who were susceptible, suggesting EDDD use may expand the pool of adolescents who will eventually smoke TC.[111]

Conversely, TC use among U.S. middle and high school students was 6.3% and 19.8%, respectively in 2006, the year before EDDDs entered the U.S. market, but dropped to 1.0% and 1.9% by 2021.[114] Concurrent with this time period were significant cost increases of TCs, increased public prohibitions and public health messaging against adolescent TC use, removal of smoking (and EDDD use) from public and commercial spaces, while EDDDs have been made more appealing in design, cost, and marketing to youth. A survey study found that between 2014 and 2021, the age of initiation among adolescents who ever used EDDDs continued to decrease (a poor prognostic variable for nicotine use disorder), while the intensity of use and level of addiction (use within the first 5 minutes after awakening—a strong indicator of physical dependence to nicotine) among adolescents who currently use EDDDs increased.[82]

Compared with older adults, the brain of youth and young adults is more vulnerable to the negative consequences of nicotine exposure. The effects in animals (not well-studied in humans) include addiction, priming for use of other addictive substances, reduced impulse control, deficits in attention and cognition, and mood disorders.[113] One mechanism for the gateway effect might be nicotine-induced delayed maturation of the adolescent brain (especially prefrontal cortex), as demonstrated in rodents,[115,116] or interference with myelination. This can result in impaired executive function and greater impulsiveness. Whether this occurs with nicotine exposure experienced by human adolescents is unclear. In a national cohort study of 17,073 children with neuroimaging outcomes, a significant association was found of early-age initiation of tobacco use with lower crystalized cognition composite score and impaired brain development in total cortical area and volume.[117] Region of interest analysis also revealed smaller cortical area and volume across frontal, parietal, and temporal lobes. Nicotine exposure during adolescence, a critical window for brain development, may have lasting adverse consequences for brain development and cognition.[113]

A survey study found that between 2014 and 2021, the age of initiation among adolescents who ever used EDDDs continued to decrease (a poor prognostic variable for nicotine use disorder), while the intensity of use and level of addiction (use within the first 5 minutes after awakening—a strong indicator of physical dependence to nicotine) among adolescents who currently use EDDDs increased.[82] The authors opined that these findings during this time interval may be due in part to the evolution of EDDDs to deliver protonated nicotine

TOXICANT EXPOSURES AND ADVERSE HEALTH CONSEQUENCES OF EDDDs

The potential adverse health effects of EDDDs among people who are exposed to them is of concern whether the exposure is secondhand or thirdhand, as discussed above, or is by primary exposure (using the product directly). Adverse health effects begin with an assessment of toxicant exposures, and end with the more important question of whether those exposures result in adverse health consequences. Toxicant exposure may not result in adverse health consequences, but on the other hand lower toxicant exposure does not necessarily result in lower risk for an adverse health consequence. Varying thresholds of exposures are needed to impart clinical risk, and some are known and some are unknown. Below, we summarize toxicant exposures and adverse health consequences relating to EDDDs.

Additional discussion of adverse health consequences from EDDDs may be found within the chapters of Section 11 of this textbook, and elsewhere.[118,119] As well, the toxicant exposures and potential health consequences of EDDDs versus TCs have been reviewed elsewhere.[118,119]

Understanding the toxicant exposures from EDDDs is not only important toward assessing whether they are safe to use in the absence of past or current TC smoking, but also whether they may be safer to use when the person is either still smoking TCs ("dual use"), or has permanently stopped TC use and replaced it with EDDD use. The latter two questions are an important consideration in determining the population-level benefit versus risk of EDDD use among those currently smoking TCs. As well, whether EDDDs significantly improve the rate by which people are able to permanently quit smoking is a separate question (discussed later), but one of obvious importance toward population health as well.

While a considerable amount of research on shorter term EDDD exposure has been conducted on vaping machines and studies with biomarkers in humans, exploration of long term exposure and its impact on later health and disease remains nascent. Importantly, many people who use EDDDs also smoke or have smoked TCs, thus confounding findings relating to toxicant exposures and possible health consequences from EDDDs. The landscape of people who are using EDDDs is changing, and may provide more opportunity for useful research. The most common first nicotine-related product used by youth is now EDDDs (with no smoking history), and EDDDs have now been in existence for more than 15 years.

EDDDs generally expose people who use them to some of the same toxic constituents of TC smoke, including nicotine, benzene metabolites, ethylene oxide, acrylonitrile, acrolein, acrylamide, aldehydes, ultrafine particles and metals; although often in much lower levels than those found in TC smoke.[79,118] These same exposures are still at higher levels than in people who neither smoked nor used EDDDs. For example, urinary biomarker levels of toxicants are significantly higher in those who only used EDDDs versus those who neither smoked nor used EDDDs, reaching levels up to twice as high in one study (including metabolites of acrylonitrile, acrolein, propylene oxide, acrylamide, and crotonaldehyde).[120]

EDDD use adds novel toxicant exposures not present in TCs, including potential carcinogenic or harmful substances either directly or indirectly present (through heating or other processes), including those from humectant, unique flavorings, unique aerosol components, and EDDD hardware device materials (wires, plastics, silicates, metals and other soldering components, fiberglass wicks, atomizer, etc.). EDDDs do not expose people who use them to carbon monoxide, which is a known cardiovascular and reproductive toxin. Levels of carcinogenic tobacco-specific nitrosamines are undetectable or much lower than levels seen in TC smoke.[37,121] No level of carcinogen is considered safe by regulatory bodies.

EDDDs are free of the combustion products (with possible exception, discussed later) in tobacco smoke that are the main chemical mediators of the cardiovascular toxicity of smoking TC tobacco, although nicotine itself may also contribute.[122,123] The major cardiovascular effect of EDDDs reflects the sympathetic nervous system stimulating effect of nicotine. EDDDs and cardiopulmonary health have been reviewed elsewhere.[119] EDDD use increases heart rate and blood pressure, increases arterial stiffness, and reduces heart rate variability, all actions related to sympathetic stimulation.[124,125] Acute EDDD use causes endothelial dysfunction, which could be mediated by nicotine and/or by oxidants or particulates in EDDD emissions.[126] Thrombosis is a central mechanism of acute cardiovascular events caused by smoking, but nicotine does not activate platelets in people. In vitro platelet activation with exposure to EDDD aerosol and oxidation of blood lipids in people who use EDDDs has been observed.[124,127] Increased platelet aggregation and activation (CD40L and P-selectin) in humans using EDDDs has been observed, and even more so in those who smoke.[128] Inflammatory effects of EDDD aerosol exposure are seen in human airway epithelial cells and human neutrophils in vitro[129] and in blood sampled from people after using an EDDD. While EDDD use acutely increases blood pressure, studies of people who smoke TCs and who also have hypertension showed a very slight (~3 mm Hg) reduction in blood pressure after they switched to EDDDs compared to baseline.[130,131]

Because EDDD use exposes people to nicotine at levels comparable to that of TCs, data on the cardiovascular safety of nicotine in people who use noncombusted tobacco may be relevant. A large proportion of Swedish men who use smokeless tobacco (snus) do not smoke TCs, thereby exposing themselves to nicotine for many years without the combustion products from TCs. Unlike cigarette smoking, snus use does not activate platelets or accelerate atherogenesis (based on carotid intima thickness, a noninvasive measure of atherosclerosis). The overall incidence of acute myocardial infarction (MI) and stroke in people who use snus is comparable to people who do not use tobacco products, but there is a small but significant increase in fatal MI or stroke. One retrospective study of acute MI in people who use snus found that mortality in the subsequent 2 years was higher in those who continued to use snus compared to those who quit. Thus, nicotine use per se may pose cardiovascular hazard, particularly in people with underlying cardiovascular disease. The same is likely to apply to people who use EDDDs.

Findings on the cardiovascular risk of EDDD use, primarily derived from cross-sectional studies, have methodological problems and have been conflicting.[132-135] A recent study used five waves of PATH data (2013-2019) to examine the risk of cardiovascular disease with EDDD.[136] Incident cardiovascular disease was defined as any self-reported past 12-month diagnosis of MI or cardiac bypass surgery, heart failure, other heart condition, or stroke. The study found no significant difference in the cardiovascular risk of exclusive EDDD use compared with nonuse of TCs and EDDDs. However, dual use of TCs and EDDDs was associated with a significantly increased risk of cardiovascular disease compared with nonuse, consistent with other studies.[134,135] Limitations included an EDDD-using population generally much younger than when cardiovascular complications arise. In vitro and animal studies find that EDDD liquids and aerosol can cause cytotoxicity, oxidant stress, inflammation, and impaired host defenses (including reduced cilia function), the latter resulting in reduced capacity to fight viral or bacterial lung infections.[137-141] As short as 1 hour exposure of cells to EDDD aerosol induced proteostasis/autophagy impairment and aggregation of misfolded proteins (aggresome), indicating that EDDD exposure may increase the risk of emphysema/chronic obstructive pulmonary disease (COPD).[142] Laboratory-based human studies report reduced pulmonary compliance and reduced expired nitric oxide, consistent with pulmonary irritation and oxidant stress.[143] EDDD use among youth may be associated with greater prevalence and exacerbation of asthma.[144-146] However, people who smoke TCs who have asthma or COPD demonstrated improved symptoms and improved pulmonary function tests when they used EDDDs while stopping or reduced TC consumption, suggesting pulmonary disease harm reduction.[147-149] This pattern of findings suggests the EDDD use may promote harm reduction if substituted completely for TC use but cause some harm themselves compared to nonuse. It may take 20 or more years for exposure to a carcinogen to result in cancer consequences, and EDDDs have only existed for roughly 15 years. Scant data are available on EDDD use and cancer risk in humans. Nicotine promotes cancer (via reduced apoptosis, increased cell proliferation, increased tumor vascularization, reduced removal of damaged DNA, etc.) in some animal studies[150,151] but not in others.[152-154] Epidemiological data from people who use snus in Sweden do not demonstrate an increased incidence of cancer (other than nitrosamine-related esophageal and pancreatic cancer). Long-term use (years) of nicotine replacement therapy (NRT) is not associated with increased risk of cancer.[155] Cancer risks from nicotine exposure are reviewed elsewhere.[154] Perhaps more relevant is that other chemicals in EDDD liquid and/or aerosol may be genotoxic and potentially cause DNA damage, which can initiate carcinogenesis.[156,157] Multiple EDDDs studies demonstrate cytotoxicity, oxidative stress, increased inflammatory markers, and human carcinogen and potential carcinogen exposures from EDDDs.[118] Some researchers have opined that "it is sensible to conclude that there is a high probability of (EDDD) aerosol being a human carcinogen."[158] The American Association of Cancer Research and the American Society of Clinical Oncology conclude that while EDDDs emit fewer carcinogens than TCs, preliminary evidence nonetheless links EDDDs use to DNA damage and inflammation, key steps in cancer development.[159] For example, a first-in-kind study of healthy people who never smoked but use EDDDs found quantified levels of DNA damage in oral epithelial cells that was the same (mean) compared to people who smoked but did not use EDDDs, with both groups being significantly higher than never smoking or vaping controls.[160] Further, pods showed more damage than mods, and sweet, mint, menthol, and fruit flavorings respectively had higher amounts of DNA damage. Because EDDDs have evolved to precisely these configurations, cancer risk from EDDDs deserves additional study.

Reproductive toxicity is related, at least in part, to nicotine exposure during fetal development and the use of EDDDs may pose similar risk.[161] Three studies of EDDD use in pregnant women found conflicting results. One study reported reduced birth weight and gestational age of babies prenatally exposed to EDDD use compared to nonsmoking women; another also found small for gestational age and more miscarriages, the other showed no difference.[162-164]

Nicotine itself in high doses can be toxic or even fatal. Nicotine toxicity, including some fatalities, has been reported in children who ingested EDDD liquids.[165,166] From September 2010 to February 2014, U.S. poison centers reported 2,405 EDDD exposure calls about possible EDDD liquid toxicity[167]; A more recent study reported 265 total cases of EDDD-related toxicity, including 193 children and 72 adults.[166] Both studies showed that exposure to EDDD liquids causes mild symptoms and systemic nicotine toxicity was rare.[166,168] Child-resistant packaging reduces toxicant exposures in children and associated mortality and should be mandated for all e-liquid solutions.[169] A number of cases of exploding EDDD batteries have been reported, some associated with serious burns.[170] Risk of nicotine poisoning is lower for disposable pod e-cigarettes since these devices are considered to be closed systems with ready-filled e-liquids rather than open systems which require manual refilling of EDDD tanks or pods.

EDDDs pose risk for cardiovascular and pulmonary disease, particularly for people with underlying cardiopulmonary disease (more commonly found in TC-using people). The available evidence base supports that EDDD use provides lower toxicant exposures for many but not all toxicants, but we do not as yet have studies to assess if they result in fewer adverse health effects or less harm. EDDD devices vary markedly in emissions and volume of aerosol generated, which could result in different cardiopulmonary risk for different products.

EDDD USE AND STOPPING SMOKING

EDDDs in Clinical Practice

People who smoke TCs report using EDDDs for several reasons, including for curiosity, from the belief they are less harmful than TCs, to help quit or reduce smoking, to inhale nicotine in places where smoking is forbidden, and for lifestyle reasons related to peer influences, marketing, social influences, etc. An assessment of the risks versus benefit of EDDDs in the general population is strongly influenced by the net effect of EDDD use on the prevalence of TC smoking. The use of EDDDs to aid stopping smoking has been studied in a growing number of clinical trials and population studies. These are summarized in **Table 22-1**. One concern has been that the performance of NRT in some of these studies has been lower than in previous NRT trials, raising questions about NRT versus EDDD study design.

EDDD Use and Stopping Smoking at the Population Level

Because most people who use EDDDs to stop smoking do so on their own and without professional assistance, it is important to assess population-based studies on this topic. In these studies, people who smoked reported their EDDD and TC use at baseline and then smoking status again at a later time point to assess for association (but not necessarily causation) between the use of EDDDs and quitting smoking. An analysis of repeated cross-sectional data from five waves of a large,

TABLE 22-1 Findings From e-Cigarette Smoking Cessation Studies

Design, location, year	Sample size/patient population	Device generation	Findings
Meta-analysis, 2020[49]	50 studies representing 12,430 patients; 26/50 were randomized clinical trials	NA	Use of electronic cigarettes with nicotine improves smoking cessation rates compared with electronic cigarettes without nicotine (RR, 1.71 [95% CI, 1.00–2.92]) and NRTs (RR, 1.69 [95% CI, 1.25–2.27])
Meta-analysis, 2016[56]	20 studies representing 40,815 individuals; 2/20 were randomized clinical trials with 757 patients combined	NA	The odds of quitting cigarettes were 28% lower (OR, 0.72 [95% CI, 0.57–0.91]) in those who used e-cigarettes compared with those who did not; data were driven by observational studies, as the two clinical trials collectively showed no change in abstinence rates
Meta-analysis, 2017[55]	12 studies representing 14,122 individuals; 3/12 were randomized clinical trials with 1,007 patients combined	NA	The odds of quitting cigarettes were 26% lower (OR, 0.74 [95% CI, 0.55–1.0]) in those who used e-cigarettes compared with those who did not; results were of low certainty on the basis of the Grading of Recommendations Assessment, Development and Evaluation approach
Randomized clinical trial, United Kingdom, 2019[51]	886 patients from UK stop-smoking services; largely middle-aged smokers, median age 41 years	2nd	1-year smoking abstinence rates were significantly higher (18%) for the e-cigarette group compared with 9.9% in the NRT group (RR, 1.83 [95% CI, 1.30–2.58]); patients in the e-cigarette group were more likely to still be using e-cigarettes (80%) than subjects who were treated with NRT (9%) after one year; 25% of participants in the e-cigarette group became dual users
Randomized clinical trial, Canada, 2020[53]	376 patients with a moderate to strong desire to attempt to quit; mean age 52 years	2nd	12-week smoking abstinence rates were significantly higher for the nicotine e-cigarette group with counseling (21.9%) versus counseling alone (9.1%); abstinence rates for the nicotine-free e-cigarette group with counseling were not significantly higher (17.3%) than counseling alone
Randomized intervention trial, United States, 2018[57]	6,006 smokers from 54 U.S. companies; median age 44 years	Unclear	6-month smoking abstinence rates were not significantly different in the e-cigarette group (1.0%) with standard care (free motivational text messaging and information about the benefits of abstinence) versus the NRT group (0.5%) with standard care or standard care alone (0.1%)

NRT, nicotine replacement therapy; OR, odds ratio; RR, risk ratio.

From Neczypor EW, Mears MJ, Ghosh A, et al. E-cigarettes and cardiopulmonary health: review for clinicians. *Circulation*. 2022;145(3):219-232. https://www.ahajournals.org/doi/10.1161/CIRCULATIONAHA.121.056777#T2

nationally representative survey in the United States (U.S. Current Population Survey-Tobacco Use Supplement [CPS-TUS]) found significantly higher population stopped smoking rates in 2014 to 2015 compared to 2010 to 2011 (5.6% versus 4.5%).[171] People who used EDDDs were more likely than people who did not to attempt to quit (65.1% versus 40.1%) and were more likely to succeed in quitting (8.2% versus 4.8%).

Population-based studies in the United Kingdom in people who self-selected EDDD use found substantially higher TC quit rates with use of EDDDs compared to use of other over-the-counter NRT.[172-174] EDDDs were most effective when more advanced devices were used and when EDDDs were used daily.[175] A longitudinal cohort study in the United Kingdom found that EDDD use at 1 year was associated with increased smoking quit attempts but not cessation.[176] A longitudinal cohort study in the United States found no overall effect of EDDD use on stopping smoking, but people who used EDDDs daily for at least 1 month were six times more likely to quit smoking (abstinent for a month) than those who used EDDDs at most once or twice in their lifetime).[177] Other studies in which people who smoke reported EDDD use at baseline and smoking status at a later time found that abstinence rates were lower in people who had used EDDDs in the past.[178] A potential bias in these studies is that people who used EDDDs who quit smoking using EDDDs at baseline would have been excluded from the analysis. Other limitations include no information available on the reason for EDDD use (eg, intent to quit may have been present or absent) or on the type and frequency of EDDD use, all of which may influence stopping smoking. Another factor that may influence the impact of EDDD use is the policy environment. Self-reported stopping smoking with EDDD use is higher in countries with less restrictive EDDD policies compared to countries with more restrictive policies.[179]

In sum, EDDD clinical trials suggest that EDDDs work as well as or better than NRT to help people stop using TCs, but have not been studied against bupropion, and are inferior to varenicline without therapy. In these trials, the NRT arms at times performed worse than has been seen in non-EDDD studies, raising some questions (some EDDD studies suffered from lack of compliance with consensus-based approaches with NRT, eg, which would place EDDDs at an artificial advantage). The available evidence supports that all of these comparators are likely safer than EDDDs in terms of toxicant exposures and potential for later adverse health consequences. However, for people using TCs who are unwilling to try approved stop smoking pharmacotherapies, EDDDs may offer an alternative to stop smoking.

On the other hand, some population-based analyses (of EDDD use without controlled settings or evidence-based approaches) indicate reduced odds of stopping smoking, which then prevents the reduction of toxin exposure, health consequences, and nicotine use disorder/addiction.[178,180] The available evidence regarding EDDD use to aid stopping smoking is notable for people who smoke and are intending to use EDDDs to quit TCs and have no interest in or who have failed FDA-approved treatments, but requires more study. Given that EDDD use is not harmless, any use of them to help stop smoking TC should be viewed as a strategy with continued efforts to help the person to eventually also quit the EDDD use. At present, controlled clinical trials of EDDDs for tobacco treatment cannot be conducted in the United States because an investigational new drug approval from the FDA is required, which has not been possible due to lack of the required toxicology testing. Clinical trials are ongoing elsewhere in the world.

See Chapter 65 for more information on pharmacological treatment of tobacco (nicotine) use disorder.

WHAT TO TELL PATIENTS

The most important action a person who smokes TCs can take to improve health is to stop smoking. Clinicians should support a person's attempt to quit and try to ensure that advice given does not undermine the motivation to quit. The safest and proven pharmacological aids for tobacco treatment are nicotine replacement products, varenicline, and bupropion, as well as off-label medications (nortriptyline, etc.).

There are conflicting opinions about how clinicians should respond when people who smoke ask about the use of EDDDs to help them quit smoking.[181] Acknowledging the controversy, we offer the following recommendations, which are supported by the American Heart Association.[182] If treatments (FDA-approved and evidence-based) have failed to provide encouraging results toward stopping smoking, or the patient has been intolerant of or refuses to use FDA-approved medications and/or psychotherapies and wishes to use EDDDS to aid quitting, that attempt should be supported, but not recommended. People who smoke should be informed that EDDDs are unregulated, deliver toxic chemicals and particles including some not in TCs, their long-term health effects are unknown, and the benefit of EDDDs for quitting smoking has not been proven by controlled clinical trials, the standard used for regulatory approval. People who use EDDDs to help quit smoking should be encouraged to quit smoking completely as soon as possible, as smoking, even at reduced levels, is still harmful to health. Motivational interviewing and other evidence-based techniques should be used by primary care and other frontline clinicians to help patients accept more proven modalities to stop smoking. Finally, we recommend that people who have quit smoking using EDDDs be urged to set a quit date for the EDDD use itself (especially if they have preexisting diseases such as cardiovascular disease), while continuing to see their tobacco/nicotine-related clinicians for ongoing care and support toward this goal.

VARIATION IN EDDD DESIGN

The tobacco industry is developing and marketing newer EDDDs such as so-called heat-not-burn (HNB) tobacco products. An example is Philip Morris' (PM)' product, IQOS (see https://www.ncbi.nlm.nih.gov/pmc/articles/PMC7572488/), which heats a modified tobacco cigarette without (allegedly, see below) combustion. By the end of 2021, IQOS was sold in over 60 countries with over 17 million consumers and had the largest market share globally among heated tobacco products.[183] Studies by the company found that IQOS substantially reduced yields of hazardous and potentially hazardous constituents (HPHCs) compared to 3R4F Kentucky reference TCs,[184,185] although they emit a host of other chemicals of unknown toxicology.[186] On switching from TCs to IQOS, the tobacco company alleges that biomarkers of toxicants fell 90%.[187] In July 2020, the U.S. FDA authorized the marketing of IQOS Tobacco Heating System as modified risk tobacco products (MRTPs). The product was the first to receive "exposure modification" orders, which "permits the marketing of a product as containing a reduced level of or presenting a reduced exposure to a substance or as being free of a substance when the issuance of the order is expected to benefit the health of the population."[188] Importantly, the FDA states that EDDDs are not a safe product, and that the FDA does not approve of or recommend their use. In the United States as of 2019, IQOS was sold in Georgia, Virginia, North Carolina, and South Carolina, but U.S. sales stopped in November 2021 due to a patent lawsuit.[183]

Since so-called HNB products are marketed as heating but not combusting tobacco, there are concerns that these products will be used to evade smoke-free air laws. Toxic substances can be generated at lower temperatures than required for combustion (including incomplete combustion/pyrolysis and thermogenic degradation). The first study of HNB toxicants independent of the tobacco industry quantified eight VOCs in IQOS emissions. Acrolein, benzaldehyde, formaldehyde, and isovaleraldehyde were at levels of 41% to 82% of levels released by TCs.[189] Carbon monoxide was also released but at lower levels than TCs (328 units, versus over 2,000 units in TCs). It is unknown if these lower exposure levels result in less frequent or intense adverse health consequences compared to smoking. Nicotine levels were 84% of those from TCs. IQOS also released 13 PAHs (almost all of which were vastly lower in amount compared to TCs—but unknown if low enough to avoid harm); however, acenaphthene (a PAH found in TC smoke) was released at levels 295% of those found in TC smoke. This compound is not known to be a carcinogen and implications for health are not known. The presence of PAHs in IQOS emissions suggests some degree of pyrolysis/combustion, contrary to tobacco industry claims that these are "heat-not-burn/HNB" products, thus bringing industry transparency (see Chapter 7, "The Cigarette Industry's Role in Promoting Tobacco Use Disorder") once again into question. A comparison of PM-affiliated research versus independent research on IQOS emissions showed agreement on nicotine yield and reductions in some IQOS emissions compared with TCs, but, importantly, independent studies, compared to PMI's data, showed increases in other emissions from and beyond the FDA's list of harmful and potentially harmful constituents (HPHCs).[190] Another study of HNB IQOS also found evidence of charring due to pyrolysis (a form of organic matter thermochemical decomposition) observed in the tobacco plug after use.[191] When the manufacturer's cleaning instructions were followed, both charring of the tobacco plug and melting of the polymer/plastic-film filter increased. Headspace analysis of the plastic-film filter revealed the release of formaldehyde cyanohydrin at 90°C, which is well below the maximum temperature reached during normal usage. Charring is increased when the device is not cleaned between heatsticks, and charring is likely far more common in routine consumer use. Release of formaldehyde cyanohydrin is a concern as it is highly toxic even at very low concentrations.

NONNICOTINE SUBSTANCE USE WITH EDDDs

The emergence and pervasiveness of nicotine EDDDs led to heightened concerns about the use of nicotine EDDDs to inhale other substances such as cannabis.[192] For example, EDDDs designed for use with nicotine refill e-liquids can be modified with cannabinoids for use in tank EDDDs. However, due to the poor solubility of tetrahydrocannabinol (THC) extracts and butane hashish oil in commercial e-liquid refills, especially those high in glycerin content, people who use EDDDs may find it challenging to aerosolize cannabis in tank EDDDs designed for use with nicotine e-liquids.[193] The viscous formulation does not flow readily into the atomizer where it can be vaporized. Until a modification is found, "dabbing" wax infused with THC directly onto the heating coils of rebuildable dripping atomizers is a well-known method of use and may be a more effective method of using cannabis via EDDDs. Dabbing has been linked with higher production of aldehydes/carcinogens.

While EDDD design is not optimized for delivery of drugs such as cannabis, reports confirm that EDDDs designed for nicotine use are being used for cannabis. An anonymous survey of high school students in Connecticut revealed that 26.5% of high schoolers who used EDDDs and cannabis had used EDDDs to inhale cannabis.[194] Young adults who use EDDDs are also inhaling cannabis using EDDDs. About 7% of undergraduates at a Midwestern U.S. university reported using an EDDD to aerosolize and inhale a substance other than nicotine.[195] Of those who used other substances with EDDDs, 78% used cannabis products (eg, butane hash oil, hashish, dabs, wax, THC); 2% reported use of other illegal substances. Other illegal drugs can also be delivered via EDDDs, including a designer drug "flakka" (a synthetic amphetamine-like cathinone),[196] amphetamine/methamphetamine, heroin, other opiates, and "crack" cocaine. EDDDs have been used to deliver gamma butyrolactone among club patrons.[197] Inhalation of a variety of other drugs, such as *Salvia*, has also been reported via EDDDs.

EPIDEMIOLOGY OF CANNABIS USE VIA EDDDs

"Vaporizers" that heat cannabis, such as commercially available tabletop devices (eg, Volcano) and portable, pocket devices (Pax by Ploom), were used for cannabis inhalation even before the popularization of nicotine EDDDs. The rapid expansion of legalized recreational cannabis and cannabis as used as treatment has remarkably increased access to cannabis-based substances for use in EDDDs. Recent data on cannabis EDDD use among young and older adults are derived from the 2021 Monitoring the Future survey.[198] Prevalence of 12-month cannabis EDDD use was 18.7% among adults aged 19 to 30 years and 2.9% among those aged 35 to 50 years. Prevalence of past 30-day cannabis EDDD use was 12.4% among those aged 19 to 30 years and 0.9% among those aged 35 to 50 years. Prevalence of cannabis EDDD use was similar for college and noncollege young adults. Among people who were 1 to 4 years beyond high school, 30-day prevalence of cannabis EDDD use was 11.8% among full-time college students compared to 15.3% among noncollege young adults.

Cannabis EDDD use is not the most popular form of cannabis use but its prevalence is increasing. The prevalence of cannabis EDDD use in the past 30 days increased among young adults aged 19 to 30 years from 10.8% in 2020 to 12.4% in 2021.[198] Data from 12 states in the 2016 Behavioral Risk Factor Surveillance System (BRFSS) found that 9.1% of adults (18 and older) used cannabis in the past month (current use).[199] Of those who were currently using cannabis, 19.4% reported any cannabis EDDD use and 2.1% reported cannabis EDDD use only. In contrast, 90.1% smoked cannabis, 58.3% reported cannabis smoking only, 24.5% reported any edible cannabis use, and 4.5% reported edible cannabis use only. Another analysis of adults (18 and older) in BRFSS from all 50 states and DC showed increasing cannabis EDDD use from 2017 to 2019.[200] The prevalence of past 30-day cannabis use increased from 10.0% in 2017 to 13.4% in 2019. The proportion of people currently using cannabis who smoke cannabis as their primary method of use decreased from 76.6% in 2017 to 66.3% in 2019 while the proportion of those who use cannabis via EDDD as their primary method of use increased from 9.9% to 14.9% over the same period. The prevalence of past 30-day cannabis EDDD use increased from 1.0% in 2017 to 2.0% in 2019. The prevalence of cannabis EDDD use was highest among people who used nicotine EDDDs, with a prevalence of 0.9% currently using cannabis EDDDs among those who never used nicotine EDDDs, 3.5% among those who formerly used EDDDs, and 6.5% among those currently using EDDDs in 2018.

Cannabis EDDD use is increasingly popular among adolescents. A metanalysis found that across all school grades of adolescents (18 years old and younger), the pooled prevalence of cannabis EDDD use increased for lifetime use (6.1% in 2013-2016 to 13.6% in 2019-2020), past 12-month use (7.2% in 2017-2018 to 13.2% in 2019-2020), and past 30-day use (1.6% in 2013-2016 to 8.4% in 2019-2020).[201] In the 2021 MTF survey, the portion of adolescents in grades 12, 10, and 8 who had ever tried cannabis EDDDs was 25.7%, 16.5%, and 6.5%, respectively.[202] In comparison, ever-use of any cannabis was 38.6%, 22.0%, and 10.2%, respectively. Past 30-day cannabis EDDD use prevalence among grades 12, 10, and 8 was 12.4%, 8.4%, and 2.9%, respectively. In comparison, 30-day prevalence of nicotine EDDD use was 19.6%, 13.1%, and 7.6%, respectively.

U.S. REGULATION OF EDDDs

The Family Smoking Prevention and Tobacco Control Act of 2009 gave the U.S. FDA authority over tobacco products. In May 2016, the FDA Deeming Rule extended its authority to e-cigarettes (EDDDs), cigars, hookah tobacco, and pipe tobacco[203]; e-cigarettes were considered tobacco products and subject to FDA regulation, including e-liquids, atomizers, batteries, delivery devices, and software. The rule required that manufacturers of all regulated products apply for marketing authorization, unless the product was on the market as of February 15, 2007. Thus, the vast majority of e-cigarettes/EDDDs require such authorization. There has been considerable controversy about this rule; it has been alleged that for most EDDD manufacturers, it would be financially difficult or impossible to submit the necessary product information to gain a modified tobacco product approval. It has been argued that such a rule favors large tobacco companies, which have the financial resources to develop and test EDDD products, while smaller EDDD manufacturers and sellers, some of whom advocate for stopping smoking of TCs, would be forced out of business. On the other hand, the allowance of products to be sold and marketed despite known toxins and risks posed to the consumer requires some degree of regulatory oversight.

EDDDs that were on the market as of August 8, 2016 were required to submit a premarket tobacco product application to the FDA by September 9, 2020.[204] Manufacturers of EDDDs containing synthetic nicotine which are on the market as of April 14, 2022 were required to submit a premarket tobacco product application (PMTA) by May 14, 2022. Some companies had changed from tobacco-sourced nicotine to synthetically sourced nicotine (a significantly more expensive option), which might then evade regulation. While not initially under FDA regulation, a 2022 amendment to the Federal Food, Drug, and Cosmetic Act now allows the FDA to regulate tobacco products containing nicotine from any source (including synthetic).[205]

Given the known and potential health risks associated with EDDDs, including uptake by youth, we recommend the following policy approach to EDDDs[1,182]:

- Include EDDDs in smoke-free air laws; prohibit use of EDDDs in any location where smoking of TCs is prohibited.
- Prohibit the sale of EDDDs to minors or anyone who cannot legally purchase cigarettes.
- Prohibit co-branding EDDDs with TCs in ways that promote dual use.
- Ensure that EDDDs are subjected to the same level of restrictions that apply to TCs, such as no television or radio advertising.
- Prohibit marketing claims that EDDDs are effective tobacco/nicotine treatment aids until the manufacturer and neutral third-party confirmation expert consensus provides sufficient evidence of efficacy and safety.
- Federal monitoring should be established to monitor and publicly report on the use of EDDDs for delivering drugs

other than nicotine. It is important that the relevant government agency, such as the FDA in the United States, monitor whether EDDDs are used to deliver potentially addictive or harmful drugs other than nicotine. All health claims associated with the EDDD products should be reviewed and approved by regulatory agencies applying scientific and regulatory standards.

- Product ingredients, components, and functioning should be labeled and regulated for safety concerns.
- All product ingredients, including externally verified nicotine concentration, tobacco-derived versus synthetic nicotine, humectants including PG/VG ratio, acid used for nicotine salts, all known or potential toxins, and flavorants should be listed on labels.
- Health warnings should be easily visible on the exterior packaging. Pregnancy warnings should be included.
- Use of flavors and concepts should be reviewed for toxicant risk and addiction risk, and consideration for banning.
- Eliminate sales of EDDDs in convenience stores and gas stations, on all online venues, and sell only in tobacco specialty shops where age limits can be enforced and monitored by third-party government entities.[206]
- Monitoring and enforcement of all age requirements should be implemented at least as soundly as is done for all tobacco products.
- EDDDs should not be modifiable, or vulnerable to be adapted for use with other addictive substances.
- EDDDs should be recyclable as much as possible to reduce environmental harm (plastics, metals), especially disposables.

Updated venues are available for consideration of regulations globally (such as http://globaltobaccocontrol.org/en/policy-scan/e-cigarettes).

CONCLUSIONS

EDDDs such as e-cigarettes, cannabis vaporizers, and heated tobacco products may deliver drugs without combustion although recent evidence suggests some may have physical and chemical evidence of thermal decomposition and possibly combustion. More importantly, toxicant exposures are increasingly recognized and being quantified as are potential adverse health consequences of solo use and dual use with TCs. EDDDs continue to evolve in design and popularity. In 2023, the most popular EDDDs in the U.S. were disposable pod devices. EDDD use continues to be widespread and increasing among adolescents and adults, with increasing use of pod design and those with flavorings (both of which require further study for added toxicant risk). EDDDs on the U.S. market are packaged in increasingly colorful external designs and with widening options of flavors or "concepts," which may then increase their appeal to youth, or reduce concern for any possible harm among all who consider using them.[207]

The FDA is now taking action against some products as a result, including some that are shaped to look like everyday objects, such as soft drink bottles, travel water bottles, children's toys, cell phones, etc.[208]

Cannabis EDDD use is less popular than nicotine EDDD use among adults and adolescents and is not as common as cannabis smoking, but prevalence of cannabis EDDD use is increasing, particularly among adolescents and young adults, which may in part relate to state-level legalization of recreational cannabis or cannabis used as treatment. Available evidence indicates that use of EDDDs leads to significant reduction in exposure to combustion-related toxicants compared to TCs or cannabis, but it is unknown if these reductions impart clinically meaningful reductions in disease risk or medical harm.

Still, known exposures remain to other toxicants derived from thermal breakdown of e-liquid or oil constituents, toxic flavor constituents, metals and other compounds (many unique to EDDDs) compared to TCs. Dual exposure (the most common form of EDDD use in adults) to both TC smoke and EDDD aerosol in the person using them or to those passively exposed likely expands the range of toxicant exposure types compared to smoking without EDDD use; additive, or even synergistic long term health risks have not been well investigated. The long-term effect of EDDD use is not understood; available evidence on health risks of cannabis and other substance-related aerosol use is even more sparse than that of nicotine aerosol. Cross-sectional studies indicate increased risk of cardiopulmonary disease from use of EDDDs. More robust study designs are needed to understand whether use of EDDDs causes cardiopulmonary diseases. Studies are also needed to understand the carcinogenic potential of EDDDs, particularly that of additives and chemicals contained in EDDD aerosol, as well as robust longitudinal studies on association between EDDD use and cancer risk. There is evidence supporting the opinion that EDDDs serve as a harm reduction tool, providing short term evidence of lowered toxin exposure compared to TCs. Others argue caution, because this assumes no dual use, EDDDs may introduce toxicants not in TCs, and because it is unknown if lower toxicant exposure impacts clinically meaningful reduction in disease risk or medical harm (harm reduction). Finally, medicolegal liability when recommending or providing EDDDs to patients is largely unknown.

Disclaimer: The content is solely the responsibility of the authors and does not necessarily represent the official views of the National Institutes of Health (NIH), the Department of Veterans Affairs, or the FDA.

REFERENCES

1. Grana R, Benowitz N, Glantz SA. E-cigarettes a scientific review. *Circulation.* 2014;129(19):1972-1986.
2. Dutra LM, Grana R, Glantz SA. Philip Morris research on precursors to the modern e-cigarette since 1990. *Tob Control.* 2017;26(e2):e97-e105.
3. Fadus MC, Smith TT, Squeglia LM. The rise of e-cigarettes, pod mod devices, and JUUL among youth: factors influencing use, health implications, and downstream effects. *Drug Alcohol Depend.* 2019;201:85-93.

4. Keamy-Minor E, McQuoid J, Ling PM. Young adult perceptions of JUUL and other pod electronic cigarette devices in California: a qualitative study. *BMJ Open.* 2019;9(4):e026306.
5. Bourke L, Bauld L, Bullen C, et al. E-cigarettes and urologic health: a collaborative review of toxicology, epidemiology, and potential risks. *Eur Urol.* 2017;71(6):915-923.
6. St. Helen G, Havel C, Dempsey DA, Jacob P III, Benowitz NL. Nicotine delivery, retention and pharmacokinetics from various electronic cigarettes. *Addiction.* 2016;111(3):535-544.
7. Pankow JF, Kim K, McWhirter KJ, et al. Benzene formation in electronic cigarettes. *PLoS One.* 2017;12(3):e0173055.
8. Jensen RP, Strongin RM, Peyton DH. Solvent chemistry in the electronic cigarette reaction vessel. *Sci Rep.* 2017;7:42549.
9. Zhu S-H, Sun JY, Bonnevie E, et al. Four hundred and sixty brands of e-cigarettes and counting: implications for product regulation. *Tob Control.* 2014;23(Suppl 3):iii3-iii9.
10. Trehy ML, Ye W, Hadwiger ME, et al. Analysis of electronic cigarette cartridges, refill solutions, and smoke for nicotine and nicotine related impurities. *J Liq Chromatogr Relat Technol.* 2011;34(14):1442-1458.
11. Goniewicz ML, Kuma T, Gawron M, Knysak J, Kosmider L. Nicotine levels in electronic cigarettes. *Nicotine Tob Res.* 2013;15(1):158-166.
12. Lisko JG, Tran H, Stanfill SB, Blount BC, Watson CH. Chemical composition and evaluation of nicotine, tobacco alkaloids, pH, and selected flavors in e-cigarette cartridges and refill solutions. *Nicotine Tob Res.* 2015;17(10):1270-1278.
13. Talih S, Balhas Z, Eissenberg T, et al. Effects of user puff topography, device voltage, and liquid nicotine concentration on electronic cigarette nicotine yield: measurements and model predictions. *Nicotine Tob Res.* 2015;17(2):150-157.
14. Wagener TL, Floyd EL, Stepanov I, et al. Have combustible cigarettes met their match? The nicotine delivery profiles and harmful constituent exposures of second-generation and third-generation electronic cigarette users. *Tob Control.* 2017;26(e1):e23-e28.
15. Henningfield JE, Pankow JF, Garrett BE. Ammonia and other chemical base tobacco additives and cigarette nicotine delivery: issues and research needs. *Nicotine Tob Res.* 2004;6(2):199-205.
16. Pankow JF. A consideration of the role of gas/particle partitioning in the deposition of nicotine and other tobacco smoke compounds in the respiratory tract. *Chem Res Toxicol.* 2001;14(11):1465-1481.
17. Mettam JJ, McCrohan CR, Sneddon LU. Characterisation of chemosensory trigeminal receptors in the rainbow trout, *Oncorhynchus mykiss*: responses to chemical irritants and carbon dioxide. *J Exp Biol.* 2012;215(4):685-693.
18. Hellinghausen G, Lee JT, Weatherly CA, Lopez DA, Armstrong DW. Evaluation of nicotine in tobacco-free-nicotine commercial products. *Drug Test Anal.* 2017;9(6):944-948. doi: 10.1002/dta.2145
19. Armstrong DW, Wang X, Ercal N. Enantiomeric composition of nicotine in smokeless tobacco, medicinal products, and commercial reagents. *Chirality.* 1998;10:587-591.
20. Aceto MD, Martin BR, Uwaydah IM, et al. Optically pure (+)-nicotine from (+/-)-nicotine and biological comparisons with (-)-nicotine. *J Med Chem.* 1979;22(2):174-177. doi: 10.1021/jm00188a009
21. Ikushima S, Muramatsu I, Sakakibara Y, Yokotani K, Fujiwara M. The effects of d-nicotine and l-isomer on nicotinic receptors. *J Pharmacol Exp Ther.* 1982;222(2):463-470.
22. Martin BR, Tripathi HL, Aceto MD, May EL. Relationship of the biodisposition of the stereoisomers of nicotine in the central nervous system to their pharmacological actions. *J Pharmacol Exp Ther.* 1983;226(1):157-163.
23. Risner ME, Cone EJ, Benowitz NL, Jacob P III. Effects of the stereoisomers of nicotine and nornicotine on schedule-controlled responding and physiological parameters of dogs. *J Pharmacol Exp Ther.* 1988;244(3):807-813.
24. Saareks V, Mucha I, Sievi E, Vapaatalo H, Riutta A. Nicotine stereoisomers and cotinine stimulate prostaglandin E2 but inhibit thromboxane B2 and leukotriene E4 synthesis in whole blood. *Eur J Pharmacol.* 1998;353(1):87-92. doi: 10.1016/s0014-2999(98)00384-7
25. Truth Initiative. *What is "tobacco-free" nicotine?* Accessed August 30, 2023. https://truthinitiative.org/research-resources/emerging-tobacco-products/what-tobacco-free-nicotine?utm_source=Truth+Initiative+Mailing+List&utm_campaign=d258730ff8-Newsletter_2023_05_11&utm_medium=email&utm_term=0_-d258730ff8-%5BLIST_EMAIL_ID%5D
26. Krishnan-Sarin S, Morean ME, Camenga DR, Cavallo DA, Kong G. E-cigarette use among high school and middle school adolescents in Connecticut. *Nicotine Tob Res.* 2015;17(7):810-818.
27. van Rooy FG, Rooyackers JM, Prokop M, Houba R, Smit LA, Heederik DJ. Bronchiolitis obliterans syndrome in chemical workers producing diacetyl for food flavorings. *Am J Respir Crit Care Med.* 2007;176(5):498-504.
28. Kreiss K, Gomaa A, Kullman G, Fedan K, Simoes EJ, Enright PL. Clinical bronchiolitis obliterans in workers at a microwave-popcorn plant. *N Engl J Med.* 2002;347(5):330-338.
29. Behar R, Davis B, Wang Y, Bahl V, Lin S, Talbot P. Identification of toxicants in cinnamon-flavored electronic cigarette refill fluids. *Toxicol In Vitro.* 2014;28(2):198-208.
30. Sherwood CL, Boitano S. Airway epithelial cell exposure to distinct e-cigarette liquid flavorings reveals toxicity thresholds and activation of CFTR by the chocolate flavoring 2, 5-dimethypyrazine. *Respir Res.* 2016;17(1):57.
31. Bahl V, Lin S, Xu N, Davis B, Wang Y-H, Talbot P. Comparison of electronic cigarette refill fluid cytotoxicity using embryonic and adult models. *Reprod Toxicol.* 2012;34(4):529-537.
32. Khlystov A, Samburova V. Flavoring compounds dominate toxic aldehyde production during E-cigarette vaping. *Environ Sci Technol.* 2016;50(23):13080-13085.
33. U.S. Food and Drug Administration. *FDA finalizes enforcement policy on unauthorized flavored cartridge-based e-cigarettes that appeal to children, including fruit and mint.* Accessed August 30, 2023. https://www.fda.gov/news-events/press-announcements/fda-finalizes-enforcement-policy-unauthorized-flavored-cartridge-based-e-cigarettes-appeal-children
34. Truth Initiative. *Local restrictions on flavored tobacco and e-cigarette products.* Accessed August 30, 2023. https://truthinitiative.org/research-resources/emerging-tobacco-products/local-restrictions-flavored-tobacco-and-e-cigarette
35. Truth Initiative. *Young e-cigarette users report widespread use of flavor blends and "concept" flavors like Iced Mango, Blue Dream, and OMG.* Accessed August 30, 2023. https://truthinitiative.org/research-resources/emerging-tobacco-products/young-e-cigarette-users-report-widespread-use-flavor
36. Kostygina G, Kreslake JM, Borowiecki M, et al. Industry tactics in anticipation of strengthened regulation: BIDI Vapor unveils non-characterising BIDI Stick flavours on digital media platforms. *Tob Control.* 2023;32:121-123.
37. Goniewicz ML, Knysak J, Gawron M, et al. Levels of selected carcinogens and toxicants in vapour from electronic cigarettes. *Tob Control.* 2014;23(2):133-139.
38. Laugesen M. Second safety report on the Ruyan® e-cigarette. *Cell.* 2008;27(488):4375.
39. Williams M, Villarreal A, Bozhilov K, Lin S, Talbot P. Metal and silicate particles including nanoparticles are present in electronic cigarette cartomizer fluid and aerosol. *PLoS One.* 2013;8(3):e57987.
40. Jacob P, Chan L, Cheung P, et al. Minor tobacco alkaloids as biomarkers to distinguish combusted tobacco use from electronic nicotine delivery systems (ENDS) use. Two new analytical methods. *Front Chem.* 2022;10:749089.
41. Farsalinos KE, Voudris V, Poulas K. Are metals emitted from electronic cigarettes a reason for health concern? A risk-assessment analysis of currently available literature. *Int J Environ Res Public Health.* 2015;12(5):5215-5232.
42. Stephens WE. Comparing the cancer potencies of emissions from vapourised nicotine products including e-cigarettes with those of tobacco smoke. *Tob Control.* 2018;27(1):10-17.
43. Cheng T. Chemical evaluation of electronic cigarettes. *Tob Control.* 2014;23:ii11-ii17. doi: 10.1136/tobaccocontrol-2013-051482
44. Fowles J, Dybing E. Application of toxicological risk assessment principles to the chemical constituents of cigarette smoke. *Tob Control.* 2003;12(4):424-430.

45. Haussmann H-J. Use of hazard indices for a theoretical evaluation of cigarette smoke composition. *Chem Res Toxicol.* 2012;25(4):794-810.
46. Sleiman M, Logue JM, Montesinos VN, et al. Emissions from electronic cigarettes: key parameters affecting the release of harmful chemicals. *Environ Sci Technol.* 2016;50(17):9644-9651.
47. Jensen RP, Luo W, Pankow JF, Strongin RM, Peyton DH. Hidden formaldehyde in e-cigarette aerosols. *N Engl J Med.* 2015;372(4):392-394.
48. Farsalinos KE, Voudris V, Poulas K. E-cigarettes generate high levels of aldehydes only in 'dry puff' conditions. *Addiction.* 2015;110(8):1352-1356.
49. Havel CM, Benowitz NL, Jacob P, St. Helen G. An electronic cigarette vaping machine for the characterization of aerosol delivery and composition. *Nicotine Tob Res.* 2017;19(10):1224-1231.
50. Goniewicz ML, Gawron M, Smith DM, Peng M, Jacob P III, Benowitz NL. Exposure to nicotine and selected toxicants in cigarette smokers who switched to electronic cigarettes: a longitudinal within-subjects observational study. *Nicotine Tob Res.* 2017;19(2):160-167.
51. Hecht SS, Carmella SG, Kotandeniya D, et al. Evaluation of toxicant and carcinogen metabolites in the urine of e-cigarette users versus cigarette smokers. *Nicotine Tob Res.* 2015;17(6):704-709.
52. McRobbie H, Phillips A, Goniewicz ML, et al. Effects of switching to electronic cigarettes with and without concurrent smoking on exposure to nicotine, carbon monoxide, and acrolein. *Cancer Prev Res (Phila).* 2015;8(9):873-878.
53. Shahab L, Goniewicz ML, Blount BC, et al. Nicotine, carcinogen, and toxin exposure in long-term E-cigarette and nicotine replacement therapy users: a cross-sectional study. *Ann Intern Med.* 2017;166(6):390-400.
54. St Helen G, Liakoni E, Nardone N, Addo N, Jacob P, Benowitz NL. Comparison of systemic exposure to toxic and/or carcinogenic volatile organic compounds (VOC) during vaping, smoking, and abstention. *Cancer Prev Res (Phila).* 2020;13(2):153-162.
55. USDHHS, Centers for Disease Control and Prevention, National Center for Chronic Disease Prevention and Health Promotion—Office on Smoking and Health. *The Health Consequences of Smoking—50 Years of Progress.* A Report of the Surgeon General. USDHHS; 2014.
56. Pope CA III, Burnett RT, Thun MJ, et al. Lung cancer, cardiopulmonary mortality, and long-term exposure to fine particulate air pollution. *JAMA.* 2002;287(9):1132-1141.
57. Peters A, Wichmann HE, Tuch T, Heinrich J, Heyder J. Respiratory effects are associated with the number of ultrafine particles. *Am J Respir Crit Care Med.* 1997;155(4):1376-1383.
58. Pope CA, Burnett RT, Krewski D, et al. Cardiovascular mortality and exposure to airborne fine particulate matter and cigarette smoke shape of the exposure-response relationship. *Circulation.* 2009;120(11):941-948.
59. Chang P-T, Peters LK, Ueno Y. Particle size distribution of mainstream cigarette smoke undergoing dilution. *Aerosol Sci Technol.* 1985;4(2): 191-207.
60. Bernstein DM. A review of the influence of particle size, puff volume, and inhalation pattern on the deposition of cigarette smoke particles in the respiratory tract. *Inhal Toxicol.* 2004;16(10):675-689.
61. Ingebrethsen BJ, Cole SK, Alderman SL. Electronic cigarette aerosol particle size distribution measurements. *Inhal Toxicol.* 2012;24(14): 976-984.
62. Fuoco F, Buonanno G, Stabile L, Vigo P. Influential parameters on particle concentration and size distribution in the mainstream of e-cigarettes. *Environ Pollut.* 2014;184:523-529.
63. Schripp T, Markewitz D, Uhde E, Salthammer T. Does e-cigarette consumption cause passive vaping? *Indoor Air.* 2013;23(1):25-31.
64. Mikheev VB, Brinkman MC, Granville CA, Gordon SM, Clark PI. Real-time measurement of electronic cigarette aerosol size distribution and metals content analysis. *Nicotine Tob Res.* 2016;18(9):1895-1902.
65. Asgharian B, Hofmann W, Miller F. Mucociliary clearance of insoluble particles from the tracheobronchial airways of the human lung. *J Aerosol Sci.* 2001;32(6):817-832.
66. Farsalinos KE, Romagna G, Tsiapras D, Kyrzopoulos S, Voudris V. Evaluation of electronic cigarette use (vaping) topography and estimation of liquid consumption: implications for research protocol standards definition and for public health authorities' regulation. *Int J Environ Res Public Health.* 2013;10(6):2500-2514.
67. Schroeder MJ, Hoffman AC. Electronic cigarettes and nicotine clinical pharmacology. *Tob Control.* 2014;23(Suppl 2):ii30-ii35.
68. Hukkanen J, Jacob P III, Benowitz NL. Metabolism and disposition kinetics of nicotine. *Pharmacol Rev.* 2005;57(1):79-115.
69. Vansickel AR, Cobb CO, Weaver MF, Eissenberg TE. A clinical laboratory model for evaluating the acute effects of electronic "cigarettes": nicotine delivery profile and cardiovascular and subjective effects. *Cancer Epidemiol Biomarkers Prev.* 2010;19(8):1945-1953.
70. Bullen C, McRobbie H, Thornley S, Glover M, Lin R, Laugesen M. Effect of an electronic nicotine delivery device (e cigarette) on desire to smoke and withdrawal, user preferences and nicotine delivery: randomised cross-over trial. *Tob Control.* 2010;19(2):98-103.
71. Vansickel AR, Weaver MF, Eissenberg T. Clinical laboratory assessment of the abuse liability of an electronic cigarette. *Addiction.* 2012;107(8):1493-1500.
72. Dawkins L, Corcoran O. Acute electronic cigarette use: nicotine delivery and subjective effects in regular users. *Psychopharmacology (Berl).* 2014;231(2):401-407.
73. Farsalinos KE, Spyrou A, Tsimopoulou K, Stefopoulos C, Romagna G, Voudris V. Nicotine absorption from electronic cigarette use: comparison between first and new-generation devices. *Sci Rep.* 2014;4(4133):1-7.
74. St. Helen G, Nardone N, Addo N, et al. Differences in nicotine intake and effects from electronic and combustible cigarettes among dual users. *Addiction.* 2020;115(4):757-767.
75. Hajek P, Przulj D, Phillips A, Anderson R, McRobbie H. Nicotine delivery to users from cigarettes and from different types of e-cigarettes. *Psychopharmacology (Berl).* 2017;234(5):773-779.
76. Hajek P, Pittaccio K, Pesola F, Myers Smith K, Phillips-Waller A, Przulj D. Nicotine delivery and users' reactions to Juul compared with cigarettes and other e-cigarette products. *Addiction.* 2020;115(6):1141-1148.
77. Vansickel AR, Eissenberg T. Electronic cigarettes: effective nicotine delivery after acute administration. *Nicotine Tob Res.* 2013;15(1):267-270.
78. Etter J-F. Explaining the effects of electronic cigarettes on craving for tobacco in recent quitters. *Drug Alcohol Depend.* 2015;148:102-108.
79. National Academies of Sciences Engineering and Medicine. *Public Health Consequences of E-cigarettes.* National Academies Press; 2018.
80. St. Helen G, Ross K, Dempsey D, Havel C, Jacob P III, Benowitz N. Nicotine delivery and vaping behavior during ad libitum e-cigarette access. *Tob Regul Sci.* 2016;2(3):363-376.
81. Liu G, Wasserman E, Kong L, Foulds J. A comparison of nicotine dependence among exclusive E-cigarette and cigarette users in the PATH study. *Prev Med.* 2017;104:86-91.
82. Glantz S, Jeffers A, Winickoff JP. Nicotine addiction and intensity of e-cigarette use by adolescents in the US, 2014 to 2021. *JAMA Netw Open.* 2022;5(11):e2240671.
83. Krishnan-Sarin S, Morean M, Kong G, et al. E-cigarettes and "dripping" among high-school youth. *Pediatrics.* 2017;139(3):e20163224.
84. Massey ZB, Brockenberry LO, Murray TE, Harrell PT. Dripping technology use among young adult e-cigarette users. *Tobacco Use Insights.* 2021;14:1179173X211035448. doi: 10.1177/1179173X211035448
85. Tehrani MW, Newmeyer MN, Rule AM, Prasse C. Characterizing the chemical landscape in commercial e-cigarette liquids and aerosols by liquid chromatography–high-resolution mass spectrometry. *Chem Res Toxicol.* 2021;34(10):2216-2226. doi: 10.1021/acs.chemrestox.1c00253
86. Larcombe A, Allard S, Pringle P, Mead-Hunter R, Anderson N, Mullins B. Chemical analysis of fresh and aged Australian e-cigarette liquids. *Med J Aust.* 2022;216(1):27-32.
87. Wang TW, Marynak KL, Agaku IT, King BA. Secondhand exposure to electronic cigarette aerosol among US youths. *JAMA Pediatr.* 2017;171(5):490-492.
88. Gentzke AS, Wang TW, Marynak KL, Trivers KF, King BA. Exposure to secondhand smoke and secondhand e-cigarette aerosol among middle and high school students. *Prev Chronic Dis.* 2019;16:180531. doi: 10.5888/pcd16.180531

89. Ballbè M, Martínez-Sánchez JM, Sureda X, et al. Cigarettes vs. e-cigarettes: Passive exposure at home measured by means of airborne marker and biomarkers. *Environ Res.* 2014;135:76-80.
90. Flouris AD, Chorti MS, Poulianiti KP, et al. Acute impact of active and passive electronic cigarette smoking on serum cotinine and lung function. *Inhal Toxicol.* 2013;25(2):91-101.
91. Schober W, Szendrei K, Matzen W, et al. Use of electronic cigarettes (e-cigarettes) impairs indoor air quality and increases FeNO levels of e-cigarette consumers. *Int J Hyg Environ Health.* 2014;217(6):628-637.
92. Soule EK, Maloney SF, Spindle TR, Rudy AK, Hiler MM, Cobb CO. Electronic cigarette use and indoor air quality in a natural setting. *Tob Control.* 2017;26(1):109-112.
93. Jacob P III, Benowitz NL, Destaillats H, et al. Thirdhand smoke: new evidence, challenges, and future directions. *Chem Res Toxicol.* 2016;30(1):270-294.
94. Sleiman M, Gundel LA, Pankow JF, Jacob P, Singer BC, Destaillats H. Formation of carcinogens indoors by surface-mediated reactions of nicotine with nitrous acid, leading to potential thirdhand smoke hazards. *Proc Natl Acad Sci.* 2010;107(15):6576-6581.
95. Goniewicz ML, Lee L. Electronic cigarettes are a source of thirdhand exposure to nicotine. *Nicotine Tob Res.* 2015;17(2):256-258.
96. Marcham CL, Floyd EL, Wood BL, Arnold S, Johnson DL. E-cigarette nicotine deposition and persistence on glass and cotton surfaces. *J Occup Environ Hyg.* 2019;16(5):349-354.
97. Marcham CL, Springston JP. Electronic cigarettes in the indoor environment. *Rev Environ Health.* 2019;34(2):105-124.
98. Melstrom P, Koszowski B, Hill Thanner M, et al. Measuring PM2.5, ultrafine particles, nicotine air and wipe samples following the use of electronic cigarettes. *Nicotine Tob Res.* 2017;19(9):1055-1061.
99. Son Y, Giovenco DP, Delnevo C, Khlystov A, Samburova V, Meng Q. Indoor air quality and passive e-cigarette aerosol exposures in vape-shops. *Nicotine Tob Res.* 2020;22(10):1772-1779. doi: 10.1093/ntr/ntaa094
100. Martins-Green M, Adhami N, Frankos M, et al. Cigarette smoke toxins deposited on surfaces: implications for human health. *PLoS One.* 2014;9(1):e86391.
101. Hang B, Sarker AH, Havel C, et al. Thirdhand smoke causes DNA damage in human cells. *Mutagenesis.* 2013;28(4):381-391.
102. Cornelius ME, Wang TW, Jamal A, Loretan CG, Neff LJ. Tobacco product use among adults - United States, 2019. *MMWR Morb Mortal Wkly Rep.* 2020;69(46):1736-1742. doi: 10.15585/mmwr.mm6946a4
103. Villarroel MA, Cha AE, Vahratian A. *Electronic cigarette use among U.S. adults, 2018.* NCHS Data Brief, no 365. Vol. 2020. National Center for Health Statistics.
104. Park-Lee E, Ren C, Sawdey MD, et al. Notes from the field: e-cigarette use among middle and high school students—National Youth Tobacco Survey, United States, 2021. *MMWR Morb Mortal Wkly Rep.* 2021;70(39):1387-1389.
105. Cooper M, Park-Lee E, Ren C, Cornelius M, Jamal A, Cullen KA. Notes from the field: e-cigarette use among middle and high school students — United States, 2022. *MMWR Morb Mortal Wkly Rep.* 2022;71:1283-1285. doi: 10.15585/mmwr.mm7140a3
106. Park-Lee E, Ren C, Cooper M, Cornelius M, Jamal A, Cullen KA. Tobacco product use among middle and high school students — United States, 2022. *MMWR Morb Mortal Wkly Rep.* 2022;71(45):1429-1435.
107. Gentzke AS, Wang TW, Cornelius M, et al. Tobacco Product Use and Associated Factors Among Middle and High School Students — National Youth Tobacco Survey, United States, 2021. *MMWR Surveill Summ.* 2022;71(SS-5):1-29. doi: 10.15585/mmwr.ss7105a1
108. Leventhal AM, Strong DR, Kirkpatrick MG, et al. Association of electronic cigarette use with initiation of combustible tobacco product smoking in early adolescence. *JAMA.* 2015;314(7):700-707.
109. Primack BA, Soneji S, Stoolmiller M, Fine MJ, Sargent JD. Progression to traditional cigarette smoking after electronic cigarette use among US adolescents and young adults. *JAMA Pediatr.* 2015;169(11):1018-1023.
110. Wills TA, Knight R, Sargent JD, Gibbons FX, Pagano I, Williams RJ. Longitudinal study of e-cigarette use and onset of cigarette smoking among high school students in Hawaii. *Tob Control.* 2016;26(1):34-39.
111. Barrington-Trimis JL, Urman R, et al. E-cigarettes and future cigarette use. *Pediatrics.* 2016;138(1):e20160379.
112. Unger JB, Soto DW, Leventhal A. E-cigarette use and subsequent cigarette and marijuana use among Hispanic young adults. *Drug Alcohol Depend.* 2016;163:261-264.
113. U.S. Department of Health and Human Services, Centers for Disease Control and Prevention, National Center for Chronic Disease Prevention and Health Promotion, Office on Smoking and Health. *E-Cigarette Use Among Youth and Young Adults. A Report of the Surgeon General.* USDHHS; 2016.
114. Johnston LD, O'Malley PM, Miech RA, Bachman JG, Schulenberg JE. *Monitoring the Future National Survey Results on Drug Use, 1975-2015: Overview, Key Findings on Adolescent Drug Use.* Institute for Social Research, The University of Michigan; 2016.
115. Dwyer JB, McQuown SC, Leslie FM. The dynamic effects of nicotine on the developing brain. *Pharmacol Ther.* 2009;122(2):125-139.
116. Slotkin TA, Orband-Miller L, Queen K, Whitmore W, Seidler F. Effects of prenatal nicotine exposure on biochemical development of rat brain regions: maternal drug infusions via osmotic minipumps. *J Pharmacol Exp Ther.* 1987;240(2):602-611.
117. Dai HD, Doucet GE, Wang Y, et al. Longitudinal assessments of neurocognitive performance and brain structure associated with initiation of tobacco use in children, 2016 to 2021. *JAMA Netw Open.* 2022;5(8):e2225991. doi: 10.1001/jamanetworkopen.2022.25991
118. Marques P, Piqueras L, Sanz MJ. An updated overview of e-cigarette impact on human health. *Respir Res.* 2021;22(1):151. doi: 10.1186/s12931-021-01737-5
119. Neczypor EW, Mears MJ, Ghosh A, et al. E-Cigarettes and cardiopulmonary health: review for clinicians. *Circulation.* 2022;145(3):219-232. doi: 10.1161/circulationaha.121.056777
120. Rubinstein ML, Delucci K, Benowitz NL, Ramo DE. Adolescent exposure to toxic volatile organic chemicals from e-cigarettes. *Pediatrics.* 2018;141(4):e20173557.
121. Goniewicz ML, Smith DM, Edwards KC, et al. Comparison of nicotine and toxicant exposure in users of electronic cigarettes and combustible cigarettes. *JAMA Netw Open.* 2018;1(8):e185937.
122. Benowitz NL, Burbank AD. Cardiovascular toxicity of nicotine: implications for electronic cigarette use. *Trends Cardiovasc Med.* 2016;26(6):515-523.
123. Benowitz NL, Fraiman JB. Cardiovascular effects of electronic cigarettes. *Nat Rev Cardiol.* 2017;14(8):447-456.
124. Moheimani RS, Bhetraratana M, Yin F, et al. Increased cardiac sympathetic activity and oxidative stress in habitual electronic cigarette users: implications for cardiovascular risk. *JAMA Cardiol.* 2017;2(3):278-284.
125. Vlachopoulos C, Ioakeimidis N, Abdelrasoul M, et al. Electronic cigarette smoking increases aortic stiffness and blood pressure in young smokers. *J Am Coll Cardiol.* 2016;67(23):2802-2803.
126. Carnevale R, Sciarretta S, Violi F, et al. Acute impact of tobacco versus electronic cigarette smoking on oxidative stress and vascular function. *Chest.* 2016;150(3):606-612.
127. Hom S, Chen L, Wang T, Ghebrehiwet B, Yin W, Rubenstein DA. Platelet activation, adhesion, inflammation, and aggregation potential are altered in the presence of electronic cigarette extracts of variable nicotine concentrations. *Platelets.* 2016;27(7):694-702.
128. Nocella C, Biondi-Zoccai G, Sciarretta S, et al. Impact of tobacco versus electronic cigarette smoking on platelet function. *Am J Cardiol.* 2018;122(9):1477-1481.
129. Higham A, Rattray NJ, Dewhurst JA, et al. Electronic cigarette exposure triggers neutrophil inflammatory responses. *Respir Res.* 2016;17(1):56.
130. Farsalinos K, Cibella F, Caponnetto P, et al. Effect of continuous smoking reduction and abstinence on blood pressure and heart rate in smokers switching to electronic cigarettes. *Intern Emerg Med.* 2016;11(1):85-94.
131. Polosa R, Morjaria JB, Caponnetto P, et al. Blood pressure control in smokers with arterial hypertension who switched to electronic cigarettes. *Int J Environ Res Public Health.* 2016;13(11): pii: E1123.
132. Alzahrani T, Pena I, Temesgen N, Glantz SA. Association between electronic cigarette use and myocardial infarction. *Am J Prev Med.* 2018;55(4):455-461.

133. Farsalinos KE, Polosa R, Cibella F, Niaura R. Is e-cigarette use associated with coronary heart disease and myocardial infarction? Insights from the 2016 and 2017 National Health Interview Surveys. *Ther Adv Chronic Dis.* 2019;10:2040622319877741.
134. Osei AD, Mirbolouk M, Orimoloye OA, et al. Association between e-cigarette use and cardiovascular disease among never and current combustible-cigarette smokers. *Am J Med.* 2019;132(8):949-954.e2.
135. Parekh T, Pemmasani S, Desai R. Risk of stroke with e-cigarette and combustible cigarette use in young adults. *Am J Prev Med.* 2020;58(3):446-452.
136. Berlowitz JB, Xie W, Harlow AF, et al. E-cigarette use and risk of cardiovascular disease: a longitudinal analysis of the PATH study (2013–2019). *Circulation.* 2022;145(20):1557-1559.
137. Lerner CA, Sundar IK, Yao H, et al. Vapors produced by electronic cigarettes and e-juices with flavorings induce toxicity, oxidative stress, and inflammatory response in lung epithelial cells and in mouse lung. *PLoS One.* 2015;10(2):e0116732.
138. Hiemstra PS, Bals R. Basic science of electronic cigarettes: assessment in cell culture and in vivo models. *Respir Res.* 2016;17(1):127.
139. Schweitzer KS, Chen SX, Law S, et al. Endothelial disruptive proinflammatory effects of nicotine and e-cigarette vapor exposures. *Am J Physiol Lung Cell Mol Physiol.* 2015;309(2):L175-L187.
140. Sussan TE, Gajghate S, Thimmulappa RK, et al. Exposure to electronic cigarettes impairs pulmonary anti-bacterial and anti-viral defenses in a mouse model. *PLoS One.* 2015;10(2):e0116861.
141. Park H-R, O'Sullivan M, Vallarino J, et al. Transcriptomic response of primary human airway epithelial cells to flavoring chemicals in electronic cigarettes. *Sci Rep.* 2019;9:1400.
142. Shivalingappa PC, Hole R, Van Westphal C, Vij N. Airway exposure to e-cigarette vapors impairs autophagy and induces aggresome formation. *Antioxid Redox Signal.* 2016;24(4):186-204.
143. Vardavas CI, Anagnostopoulos N, Kougias M, Evangelopoulou V, Connolly GN, Behrakis PK. Short-term pulmonary effects of using an electronic cigarette: impact on respiratory flow resistance, impedance, and exhaled nitric oxide. *Chest.* 2012;141(6):1400-1406.
144. Cho JH, Paik SY. Association between electronic cigarette use and asthma among high school students in South Korea. *Plos One.* 2016;11(3):e0151022.
145. Choi K, Bernat D. E-cigarette use among florida youth with and without asthma. *Am J Prev Med.* 2016;51(4):446-453.
146. Kim SY, Sim S, Choi HG. Active, passive, and electronic cigarette smoking is associated with asthma in adolescents. *Sci Rep.* 2017;7(1):1-8.
147. Cibella F, Campagna D, Caponnetto P, et al. Lung function and respiratory symptoms in a randomized smoking cessation trial of electronic cigarettes. *Clin Sci (Lond).* 2016;130(21):1929-1937.
148. Polosa R, Morjaria J, Caponnetto P, et al. Effect of smoking abstinence and reduction in asthmatic smokers switching to electronic cigarettes: evidence for harm reversal. *Int J Environ Res Public Health.* 2014;11(5):4965-4977.
149. Polosa R, Morjaria JB, Caponnetto P, et al. Evidence for harm reduction in COPD smokers who switch to electronic cigarettes. *Respir Res.* 2016;17(1):166.
150. Iskandar AR, Liu C, Smith DE, et al. β-Cryptoxanthin restores nicotine-reduced lung SIRT1 to normal levels and inhibits nicotine-promoted lung tumorigenesis and emphysema in A/J mice. *Cancer Prev Res.* 2013;6(4):309-320.
151. Hao J, Shi F-D, Abdelwahab M, et al. Nicotinic receptor β2 determines NK cell-dependent metastasis in a murine model of metastatic lung cancer. *PLoS One.* 2013;8(2):e57495.
152. Murphy SE, von Weymarn LB, Schutten MM, Kassie F, Modiano JF. Chronic nicotine consumption does not influence 4-(methylnitrosamino)-1-(3-pyridyl)-1-butanone–induced lung tumorigenesis. *Cancer Prev Res.* 2011;4(11):1752-1760.
153. Maier CR, Hollander MC, Hobbs EA, Dogan I, Linnoila RI, Dennis PA. Nicotine does not enhance tumorigenesis in mutant K-ras–driven mouse models of lung cancer. *Cancer Prev Res.* 2011;4(11):1743-1751.
154. Mishra A, Chaturvedi P, Datta S, Sinukumar S, Joshi P, Garg A. Harmful effects of nicotine. *Indian J Med Paediatr Oncol.* 2015;36:24-31.
155. Murray RP, Connett JE, Zapawa LM. Does nicotine replacement therapy cause cancer? Evidence from the Lung Health Study. *Nicotine Tob Res.* 2009;11(9):1076-1082.
156. Kadimisetty K, Malla S, Rusling JF. Automated 3-D printed arrays to evaluate genotoxic chemistry: e-cigarettes and water samples. *ACS Sens.* 2017;2(5):670-678.
157. Yu V, Rahimy M, Korrapati A, et al. Electronic cigarettes induce DNA strand breaks and cell death independently of nicotine in cell lines. *Oral Oncol.* 2016;52:58-65.
158. Tang M-S, Tang Y-L. Can electronic-cigarette vaping cause cancer? *Cancer Biol.* 2021;2(3):68-70. doi: 10.46439/cancerbiology.2.027
159. American Association of Cancer Research. *AACR and ASCO release joint policy statement on electronic nicotine delivery systems.* Accessed August 30, 2023. https://www.aacr.org/about-the-aacr/newsroom/news-releases/aacr-and-asco-release-joint-policy-statement-on-electronic-nicotine-delivery-systems
160. Tommasi S, Blumenfeld H, Besaratinia A. Vaping dose, device type, and e-liquid flavor are determinants of DNA damage in electronic cigarette users. *Nicotine Tob Res.* 2023;25(6):1145-1154.
161. Wong MK, Barra NG, Alfaidy N, Hardy DB, Holloway AC. Adverse effects of perinatal nicotine exposure on reproductive outcomes. *Reproduction.* 2015;150(6):R185-R193.
162. Hawkins SS, Wylie BJ, Hacker MR. Associations between electronic nicotine delivery systems and birth outcomes. *J Matern Fetal Neonatal Med.* 2022;35(25):6868-6875.
163. Nanninga EK, Weiland S, Berger MY, et al. Adverse maternal and infant outcomes of women who differ in smoking status: e-cigarette and tobacco cigarette users. *Int J Environ Res Public Health.* 2023;20:2632.
164. McDonnell BP, Dicker P, Regan CL. Electronic cigarettes and obstetric outcomes: a prospective observational study. *BJOG.* 2020;127(6):750-756.
165. Kim JW, Baum CR. Liquid nicotine toxicity. *Pediatr Emerg Care.* 2015;31(7):517-521. quiz 522-514.
166. Hughes A, Hendrickson RG. An epidemiologic and clinical description of e-cigarette toxicity. *Clin Toxicol.* 2019;57(4):287-293.
167. Chatham-Stephens K, Law R, Taylor E, et al. Notes from the field: calls to poison centers for exposures to electronic cigarettes—United States, September 2010–February 2014. *MMWR Morb Mortal Wkly Rep.* 2014;63(13):292-293.
168. Vakkalanka JP, Hardison LS Jr, Holstege CP. Epidemiological trends in electronic cigarette exposures reported to U.S. Poison Centers. *Clin Toxicol (Phila).* 2014;52(5):542-548.
169. Jo CL, Ambs A, Dresler CM, Backinger CL. Child-resistant and tamper-resistant packaging: a systematic review to inform tobacco packaging regulation. *Prev Med.* 2017;95:89-95.
170. Jiwani AZ, Williams JF, Rizzo JA, Chung KK, King BT, Cancio LC. Thermal injury patterns associated with electronic cigarettes. *Int J Burns Trauma.* 2017;7(1):1-5.
171. Zhu S-H, Zhuang Y-L, Wong S, Cummins SE, Tedeschi GJ. E-cigarette use and associated changes in population smoking cessation: evidence from US current population surveys. *BMJ.* 2017;358:j3262.
172. Beard E, West R, Michie S, Brown J. Association between electronic cigarette use and changes in quit attempts, success of quit attempts, use of smoking cessation pharmacotherapy, and use of stop smoking services in England: time series analysis of population trends. *BMJ.* 2016;354:i4645.
173. Brown J, Beard E, Kotz D, Michie S, West R. Real-world effectiveness of e-cigarettes when used to aid smoking cessation: a cross-sectional population study. *Addiction.* 2014;109(9):1531-1540.
174. West R, Shahab L, Brown J. Estimating the population impact of e-cigarettes on smoking cessation in England. *Addiction.* 2016;111(6):1118-1119.
175. Hitchman SC, Brose LS, Brown J, Robson D, McNeill A. Associations between E-cigarette type, frequency of use, and quitting smoking: findings from a longitudinal online panel survey in Great Britain. *Nicotine Tob Res.* 2015;17(10):1187-1194.
176. Brose LS, Hitchman SC, Brown J, West R, McNeill A. Is the use of electronic cigarettes while smoking associated with smoking cessation

attempts, cessation and reduced cigarette consumption? A survey with a 1-year follow-up. *Addiction.* 2015;110(7):1160-1168.

177. Biener L, Hargraves JL. A longitudinal study of electronic cigarette use among a population-based sample of adult smokers: association with smoking cessation and motivation to quit. *Nicotine Tob Res.* 2015;17(2):127-133.
178. Kalkhoran S, Glantz SA. E-cigarettes and smoking cessation in real-world and clinical settings: a systematic review and meta-analysis. *Lancet Respir Med.* 2016;4(2):116-128.
179. Yong HH, Hitchman SC, Cummings KM, et al. Does the regulatory environment for e-cigarettes influence the effectiveness of e-cigarettes for smoking cessation?: Longitudinal findings from the ITC Four Country Survey. *Nicotine Tob Res.* 2017;19(11):1268-1276.
180. Glantz SA. The evidence of electronic cigarette risks is catching up with public perception. *JAMA Netw Open.* 2019;2(3):e191032. doi: 10.1001/jamanetworkopen.2019.1032
181. Nickels AS, Warner DO, Jenkins SM, Tilburt J, Hays JT. Beliefs, practices, and self-efficacy of US physicians regarding smoking cessation and electronic cigarettes: a National Survey. *Nicotine Tob Res.* 2017;19(2):197-207.
182. Bhatnagar A, Whitsel LP, Ribisl KM, et al. Electronic cigarettes: a policy statement from the American Heart Association. *Circulation.* 2014;130(16):1418-1436.
183. Abroms L, Levine H, Romm K, et al. Anticipating IQOS market expansion in the United States. *Tob Prev Cessat.* 2022;8:04.
184. Mitova MI, Campelos PB, Goujon-Ginglinger CG, et al. Comparison of the impact of the Tobacco Heating System 2.2 and a cigarette on indoor air quality. *Regul Toxicol Pharmacol.* 2016;80:91-101.
185. Schaller JP, Keller D, Poget L, et al. Evaluation of the Tobacco Heating System 2.2. Part 2: Chemical composition, genotoxicity, cytotoxicity, and physical properties of the aerosol. *Regul Toxicol Pharmacol.* 2016;81(Suppl 2):S27-S47.
186. St. Helen G, Jacob P, Nardone N, Benowitz NL. IQOS: examination of Philip Morris International's claim of reduced exposure. *Tob Control.* 2018;27(Suppl 1):s30-s36.
187. Smith M, Haziza C, Hoeng J, et al. *The Science behind the Tobacco Heating System: A Summary of Published Scientific Articles.* Philip Morris International; 2016.
188. U.S. Food and Drug Administration. *FDA Authorizes Marketing of IQOS Tobacco Heating System With 'Reduced Exposure' Information.* Accessed August 30, 2023. https://www.fda.gov/news-events/press-announcements/fda-authorizes-marketing-iqos-tobacco-heating-system-reduced-exposure-information
189. Auer R, Concha-Lozano N, Jacot-Sadowski I, Cornuz J, Berthet A. Heat-not- burn tobacco cigarettes: smoke by any other name. *JAMA Intern Med.* 2017;177(7):1050-1052.
190. El-Kaassamani M, Yen M, Talih S, El-Hellani A. Analysis of mainstream emissions, secondhand emissions and the environmental impact of IQOS waste: a systematic review on IQOS that accounts for data source. *Tob Control.* 2022; tobaccocontrol-2021-056986.
191. Davis B, Williams M, Talbot P. iQOS: Evidence of pyrolysis and release of a toxicant from plastic. *Tob Control.* 2019;28:24-41.
192. Giroud C, de Cesare M, Berthet A, Varlet V, Concha-Lozano N, Favrat B. E-cigarettes: a review of new trends in cannabis use. *Int J Environ Res Public Health.* 2015;12(8):9988-10008.
193. Varlet V, Concha-Lozano N, Berthet A, et al. Drug vaping applied to cannabis: is "Cannavaping" a therapeutic alternative to marijuana? *Sci Rep.* 2016;6:25599.
194. Morean ME, Kong G, Camenga DR, Cavallo DA, Krishnan-Sarin S. High school students' use of electronic cigarettes to vaporize cannabis. *Pediatrics.* 2015;136(4):611-616.
195. Kenne DR, Fischbein RL, Tan AS, Banks M. The use of substances other than nicotine in electronic cigarettes among college students. *Subst Abuse.* 2017;11:1178221817733736.
196. Katselou M, Papoutsis I, Nikolaou P, Spiliopoulou C, Athanaselis S. α-PVP ("flakka"): a new synthetic cathinone invades the drug arena. *Forensic Toxicol.* 2016;34(1):41-50.
197. Thurtle N, Abouchedid R, Archer JR, et al. Prevalence of use of electronic nicotine delivery systems (ENDS) to vape recreational drugs by club patrons in South London. *J Med Toxicol.* 2017;13(1):61-65.
198. Patrick ME, Schulenberg JE, Miech RA, Johnston LD, O'Malley PM, Bachman JG. *Monitoring the Future Panel Study annual report: National data on substance use among adults ages 19 to 60, 1976-2021.* Monitoring the Future Monograph Series. University of Michigan Institute for Social Research; 2022. doi: 10.7826/ISRUM.06.585140.002.07.0001.2022
199. Schauer GL, Njai R, Grant-Lenzy AM. Modes of marijuana use–smoking, vaping, eating, and dabbing: Results from the 2016 BRFSS in 12 States. *Drug Alcohol Depend.* 2020;209:107900.
200. Boakye E, Obisesan OH, Uddin SI, et al. Cannabis vaping among adults in the United States: Prevalence, trends, and association with high-risk behaviors and adverse respiratory conditions. *Prev Med.* 2021;153:106800.
201. Lim CC, Sun T, Leung J, et al. Prevalence of adolescent cannabis vaping: a systematic review and meta-analysis of US and Canadian studies. *JAMA Pediatr.* 2022;176(1):42-51.
202. Miech RA, Johnston LD, O'Malley PM, Bachman JG, Schulenberg JE, Patrick ME. *Monitoring the Future National Survey Results on Drug Use, 1975–2021: Volume I, Secondary School Students.* Institute for Social Research, The University of Michigan; 2022.
203. U.S. Food and Drug Administration. Deeming tobacco products to be subject to the federal food, drug, and cosmetic act, as amended by the family smoking prevention and tobacco control act; restrictions on the sale and distribution of tobacco products and required warning statements for tobacco products. Final rule. *Fed Regist.* 2016;81(90):28973-29106.
204. U.S. Food and Drug Administration. *Submit Tobacco Product Applications for Deemed Tobacco Products.* Accessed August 30, 2023. https://www.fda.gov/tobacco-products/manufacturing/submit-tobacco-product-applications-deemed-tobacco-products
205. U.S. Food and Drug Administration. *Reminder: Electronic Submission of Premarket Applications for Non-tobacco Nicotine Products due May 14.* Accessed August 30, 2023. https://www.fda.gov/tobacco-products/ctp-newsroom/reminder-electronic-submission-premarket-applications-non-tobacco-nicotine-products-due-may-14
206. Public Health Law Center at Mitchell Hamline School of Law. *Online Sales of E-cigarettes and Other Tobacco Products.* Accessed August 30, 2023. https://www.publichealthlawcenter.org/sites/default/files/resources/Online-Sales-E-Cigarettes-Other-Tobacco-Products.pdf
207. Truth Initiative. *Elf Bar, Hyde, and Breeze – What You Need to Know About the Rise in Disposable e-Cigarettes.* Retrieved December 29, 2023. https://truthinitiative.org/research-resources/emerging-tobacco-products/high-nicotine-e-cigarettes-dominate-market-sales
208. U.S. Food and Drug Administration. *FDA Warns Retailers to Stop Selling Illegal Youth-Appealing E-Cigarettes Disguised as Everyday Items: Products Look Like Toys and Drink Containers That Can be Easily Concealed by Youth. CTP Newsroom.* Retrieved December 29, 2023. https://www.fda.gov/tobacco-products/ctp-newsroom/fda-warns-retailers-stop-selling-illegal-youth-appealing-e-cigarettes-disguised-everyday-items

23 Novel Psychoactive Substances

Kathryn Hawk, Barbara M. Kirrane, and Gail D'Onofrio

CHAPTER OUTLINE

- Introduction
- Recognition and diagnosis
- Treatment
- Specific examples of NPS
- Identifying and accessing information on newly emerging and novel psychoactive substances

INTRODUCTION

Novel psychoactive substances (NPS), especially synthetics, have appeared at an alarming rate over the past several years. While classic illicit substances such as cocaine and heroin were traditionally agents of concern and regulation, the development of NPS or designer drugs created in clandestine laboratories has been on the rise since the late 1970s, adding a whole new layer of complexity to detection and treatment. Typically, these drugs are designed to mimic already existing substances such as cannabis, amphetamines, or opioids, and are manufactured specifically to circumvent laws related to the sale and trafficking of controlled substances.[1] For example, the arylcyclohexylamine methoxetamine, shares clinical characteristics with ketamine, but has a much longer half-life owing to the presence of an additional *N*-ethyl group.[2] The NPS designation includes synthetic cannabimimetics, synthetic cathinones, phenylethylamines, piperazines, ketamine- and phencyclidine-type substances, tryptamines, benzofurans, and synthetic opioids, in addition to others. Two of the better understood novel drug categories include synthetic cathinones or "bath salts," which are derivatives of cathinone, a naturally occurring amphetamine analogue found in the leaves of the *Catha edulis* plant, and synthetic cannabinoids, marketed initially as Spice and K-2, that bind to cannabinoid receptors.[1,3,4] Another category of NPS includes nonpharmaceutical synthetic opioids such as acetyl fentanyl, acrylfentanyl,3-methyl fentanyl ("China white"), butyrfentanyl, U-47700, carfentanil, and the newly recognized isotonitazene, which bind μ-receptors and has been reported to be 500 times more potent than morphine.[5-11]

Little is known about the mechanisms of action, pharmacological effects, and toxicological profile for many other NPS, although specific details for "kratom" and newer sedative–hypnotics and cathinones are presented later in this chapter and resources with information on NPS are constantly being updated (**Table 23-1**).[12,13] More than 50 new substances were reported to the European Union Early Warning System in 2021, bringing the total of new NPS monitored by the European Monitoring Centre for Drugs and Drug Addiction (EMCDDA) to more than 884 substances. Synthetic cannabinoids represent the largest category, followed by synthetic cathinones.[12,14]

Some types of NPS are promoted as "legal highs" and are easily accessible in gas stations, convenience stores, "head shops," and the internet. These substances are a particular concern for teenagers and young adults, as they are easily available and affordable, often packaged in colorful wrappers that do not appear dangerous, sold as "herbal highs," "bath salts," "plant food," "insect repellent," "research chemicals," and "air fresheners," with disclaimers that they are "not for human consumption" or "for research purposes only" to circumvent regulation.[1,15] NPS use is often unintentional, as designer drugs, including high-potency fentanyl and analogues or other novel synthetic opioids such as U-47700 ("Pink"), are often detected in counterfeit black market prescription opioids and other traditional illicitly used drugs such as heroin and cocaine.[16-18]

Designer drugs are typically created when clandestine chemists modify the structure of an existing drug, for example, adding a methyl group to the compound, thereby creating an analog drug with similar properties, but not necessarily subject to regulation.[19] Legislative attempts both within and outside of the United States to regulate the sale and use of specific substances, have had limited impact given the targeted development of novel compounds specifically designed to skirt controlled substance regulations.[15,20-23]

RECOGNITION AND DIAGNOSIS

Acute clinical care for patients with toxicity related to NPS ingestion can be challenging for several reasons: wide variety of toxicological effects, batch to batch variability in potency, chemical composition, adulterants, limitations of patient-reported substance use history (in part due to unintended use), and lack of widely available, inexpensive screening assays. Toxicologists and emergency medicine physicians have traditionally focused on treating the poisoned or intoxicated patient based on the clinical presentation and characteristics (ie, toxidrome) rather than on the specific poison or drug.[24] NPS are largely undetectable using traditional methods for drug screening, which may be a perceived benefit for individuals who anticipate being monitored for illicit substance use.

TABLE 23-1 Online Resources for Information on Emerging Novel Psychoactive Substances

U.S. National Institutes of Health	www.drugabuse.gov
U.S. Drug Enforcement Administration	www.dea.gov
Monitoring the Future (University of Michigan)	www.monitoringthefuture.org
American Association of Poison Control Centers	www.aapcc.org
European Monitoring Centre for Drugs and Drug Addiction	www.emcdda.europa.eu
U.S. Substance Abuse and Mental Health Services Administration	www.samhsa.gov/data/
National Forensic Laboratory Information System	www.nflis.deadiversion.usdoj.gov

The different chemical structures of NPS ultimately mean different physiological effects, and with no oversight or regulation in the production of these substances, the resulting clinical picture can show wide variation across doses and individuals even when individuals use the same amount of product with the same label.[19,25] Acute intoxication with synthetic cathinones and synthetic cannabinoids predominantly presents clinically with a sympathomimetic toxidrome, which often includes tachycardia, hypertension, tachypnea, hyperthermia, agitation, tremors, and/or seizures.[21,24,26,27] Synthetic cannabinoids have been associated with nephrotoxicity, rhabdomyolysis, acute psychosis, and cardiac arrest. Synthetic cathinones have been associated with acute psychosis, hallucinations, paranoia, suicidality, and respiratory depression.[21,26,28-31] Daily use of synthetic cannabinoids has been associated with the development of a profound withdrawal syndrome, which can include seizures, tachycardia, chest pain, palpitations, anxiety, insomnia, diaphoresis, and anorexia; this is best managed by the administration of benzodiazepines and second-generation antipsychotics.

TREATMENT

Some people may be falsely reassured by the legal status of a number of these NPS, not realizing that they have been linked to a variety of life-threatening adverse events and have been implicated as the cause of numerous violent acts.[32-36] Based on the clinical presentation, including toxidrome and the best available history, emergency care frequently includes supportive care, including intravenous fluids; electrolyte repletion; evaluation for end-organ damage to the kidneys, lungs, heart, and brain; treatment with benzodiazepines and antipsychotics as needed; and observation. Naloxone administration should be considered for patients presenting with the opioid toxidrome of miosis, respiratory depression, and depressed mental status, even if a history of opioid use is not obtained, and high-dose naloxone should be considered if clinically indicated or if there is a suspicion for fentanyl or high-potency fentanyl analogues.[17] In the United States, poison control centers provide 24 hours per day, 7 days per week toll-free telephone access (800-222-1222) to trained toxicologists who are available to answer questions and provide consultations for clinical management .

SPECIFIC EXAMPLES OF NPS

See Chapters 17, 14, 18 and 13 for more information about synthetic cannabinoids, cathinones and other stimulants, hallucinogens and opioids, respectively.

Nonpharmaceutical Fentanyl Analogues

History

Fentanyl is a short-acting opioid with 50 to 100 times the potency of morphine. It was synthesized in 1960 by Janssen Pharmaceutica as part of an effort to identify anesthetics with a more favorable safety profile than what was currently available.[37] The synthesis of multiple analogues for clinical use, including sufentanil, carfentanil and alfentanil, soon followed. Although nonmedical use of pharmaceutical fentanyl and fentanyl analogues (fentanyls) has been reported, surveillance data suggest that increases in fentanyl-involved fatalities are related to illicitly manufactured fentanyls produced by clandestine laboratories primarily in China and other non-U.S. countries.[38-40] A U.S. Centers for Disease Control and Prevention (CDC) analysis of 27 states with consistent death certificate reporting of substances involved in opioid overdoses found a high degree of correlation ($r = 0.95$) between synthetic opioid-related deaths and increased fentanyl seizures reported to the National Forensic Laboratory Information System (NFLIS).[41] No changes in legal fentanyl prescribing rates were observed.[41] The Drug Enforcement Administration (DEA) reported an 18-fold increase in fentanyl-related submissions to the NFLIS from 5,541 in 2014 to 100,378 in 2019.[42]

Multiple fentanyl analogs have been associated with regional outbreaks of fatal overdose, including α-methyl fentanyl, 3-methyl fentanyl, acetyl fentanyl, carfentanil, butyrylfentanyl, ocfentanil, and furanylfentanyl.[10,17,24,43-45] New fentanyl analogues are identified yearly but the number has significantly decreased since 2019 due to restrictive Chinese legislation[22] and U.S. DEA restructuring.[23] A new generation of non-fentanyl-related synthetic opioids has appeared in counterfeit tablets or sold in bags/bundles similar to heroin. It is difficult to keep up with their identification and produce timely public health messaging, as the life cycle from initial synthesis to widespread distribution may be as short as 3-6 months. Over the past few years, isotonitazene and recently brorphine have dominated the U.S. market. Isotonitazine ("iso" or "toni") was identified in summer of 2019 and sold under the name "etonitazene," 1000 times more potent as an analgesic than morphine.[46] It was relatively underreported, as there were no laboratory readily available screening assay and it was not listed in the DEA Emerging Threat Report until late 2020. Subsequently brorphine, street name "purple heroin," emerged and is replacing isotonitazene. The DEA placed brorphine in Schedule I of the U.S. Controlled Substances Act (CSA) in March 2021. A recent case series from the ongoing national Toxicology Consortium Fentalog Study Group (October 2020-October 2021) found that 6 of 412 (1.5%) individuals with overdose had a New Age Opioid (NAO; brorphine, isotonitazene, or metonitazene) detected in their urine sample along with other opioids.[46] As these NPS will rapidly change, it is essential that there be a timely response from Early Warning Systems, laboratories and policy makers.

Epidemiology

The rapid increase in opioid-associated deaths has been largely attributed to non-pharmaceutical fentanyl analogues, although the true rate of synthetic opioid use has not been fully characterized. This is in part due to the frequent contamination of other substances with synthetic opioids and the frequent uncertainty of whether fentanyl use was intentional or unintentional. The CDC reported a 56% increase in synthetic opioid-related U.S. deaths between 2019 and 2020, with significant increases noted in 40 of 50 states.[47] The European Monitoring Centre for Drugs and Drug Addiction reports an ongoing shift away from fentanyl derivatives and towards benzimidazole opioids in 2020 and 2021. The presence of highly potent synthetic opioids, including isotonitazene and fentanyl analogues, as contaminants to the heroin supply and as components of fake opioid analgesic and benzodiazepine pills represents an ongoing risk.[48]

Pharmacology

Fentanyl is a synthetic mu-opioid receptor agonist, with a potency 50 to 100 times greater than morphine and 30 to 50 times greater than heroin.[39] Fentanyl analogues range in potency from acetyl fentanyl, 15 times more potent than morphine, to carfentanil, 10,000 times more potent than morphine.[10,44] Fentanyl is well absorbed transdermally and transmucosally, accounting for the lozenge, lollipop and transdermal pharmaceutical delivery systems.[24] In 2015, the DEA issued warnings to law enforcement and first responders about the possibility of fentanyl being absorbed through the skin and accidental inhalation of airborne powder.[39] The American College of Medical Toxicology and American Academy of Clinical Toxicology acknowledged the possibility of weaponized aerosolized fentanyl toxicity but concluded that incidental dermal absorption or inhalation is unlikely to cause opioid toxicity to first responders and law enforcement officers exposed during routine duties.[49] Clinical reports from responding physicians created a high suspicion that the gas used to subdue Chechen rebels holding 800 hostages at a Moscow Theater in 2002 contained aerosolized carfentanil or other high-potency fentanyl analogs.[50]

Clinical Implications

Fentanyl is used clinically in general and regional anesthesia and in the management of chronic and postoperative pain. Recreationally, fentanyls are used for their euphoric effects and to avoid opioid withdrawal. Fentanyls cause a typical opioid toxidrome with respiratory depression, miosis (constricted pupils), drowsiness and euphoria, and, at high doses, respiratory arrest and pulmonary edema.[44] The most common side effects include nausea, dizziness, vomiting, fatigue, headache, and constipation; repeated use leads to tolerance and physical dependence. Opioid overdose, manifested as decreased respiratory rate, decreased mental status, and miosis, can be reversed with the mu-opioid receptor antagonist naloxone, which can be administered via intranasal, intramuscular, or intravenous routes. Fentanyl is not included in many hospital urine toxicology screens, so exposure is often undetected. Like many exposures, source identification may be delayed or never occur, so clinical presentation and patient toxidrome should guide acute management.

Legal Status

Fentanyl, alfentanil, sufentanil, remifentanil, and carfentanil are Schedule II substances, while 3-methylfentanyl, α-methyl fentanyl, acetyl fentanyl, furanylfentanyl and brophine are categorized as Schedule I.[13,51]

Kratom

History

Kratom is a plant product derived from *Mitragyna speciosa* Korth, a leafy tree that is a member of the coffee family and native to Southeast Asia, although it is now cultivated elsewhere. Kratom was used in Thailand and Malaysia as early as the 1800s by manual laborers for euphoria, stimulation, and analgesia and to prevent withdrawal from opium.[52] Traditionally, the kratom leaves are chewed or brewed into a tea; they are rarely smoked. Today, kratom is widely available on the internet and specialty stores and can be found as capsules, tablets, gum, dried leaf, or powder. Kratom has become increasingly popular in the United States over the past several years, due to its wide availability in stores and on the internet along with its current legal status as an unscheduled substance. It has several slang names such as thang, kakuam, thom, ketum, and biak.[13] Kratom is commonly used today to self-treat chronic pain, prevent opioid withdrawal, and for its hallucinogenic effects, though other reported beneficial effects include antipyretic, antihypertensive, antidiarrheal, anti-inflammatory, and prolonging sexual intercourse.[34,53]

Epidemiology

The 2020 U.S. National Survey on Drug Use and Health (NSDUH) estimated that 2.1 million (0.8%) U.S. residents reported use of kratom during the past year and 1 million during the past month.[54] The 2016 Thailand national household survey estimated a 15.1% lifetime prevalence of kratom leaf usage, 2.1% past year prevalence and 1.4 past month prevalence.[55]

Pharmacology

Although more than 40 different alkaloids have been isolated from kratom, the primary psychoactive one is the indole alkaloid mitragynine.[13] The mitragynine metabolite 7-hydroxmitragynine is found in much lower concentration, but is more potent.[52] Mitragynine is an agonist of multiple receptors, including the opioid mu and delta receptors, as well as postsynaptic alpha-adrenergic receptors, dopamine and serotonin receptors.[34,56] Mitragynine is reported to have a mu-opioid receptor potency approximately 10 times that of morphine, a key reason why kratom is used to prevent opioid withdrawal. An analysis of multiple commercial kratom products found a substantially higher concentration of 7-hydroxymitragynine than found in natural *M. speciosa* leaves, suggesting the intentional adulteration of these products to increase opioid activity.[57]

Clinical Implications

Kratom has dual properties that result in both stimulation and analgesia, depending on the dose. At low doses, kratom acts primarily as a stimulant, producing a sympathomimetic toxidrome; at higher doses, effects are predominantly consistent with an opioid toxidrome.[58]

Kratom is used to increase pain tolerance, promote feelings of euphoria or alertness, or to treat opioid withdrawal symptoms.[52] Symptoms of acute intoxication reported to poison centers include tachycardia, agitation, drowsiness, nausea.[59] Published case reports have associated kratom exposure with psychosis, seizures, coma, and death, but the causal association with kratom is unclear, as many cases involve ingestion of multiple substances.[52,60,61] A withdrawal syndrome has been reported in individuals with kratom use disorder, including signs and symptoms such as nausea, vomiting, diarrhea, insomnia, hot flashes, and abdominal pain.[62] Treatment for acute kratom intoxication is primarily supportive, although naloxone, a mu-opioid receptor antagonist, is sometimes helpful. Buprenorphine, a partial mu-opioid receptor agonist, has been successful in treatment of kratom withdrawal and kratom use disorder.[52]

Legal Status

Kratom is currently unscheduled by the DEA, and so is legal to cultivate, buy, possess and sell. It was previously under consideration for a Schedule I classification and is currently listed as a "drug and chemical of concern."[13] Kratom is illegal in 6 states and several cities.

Sedative Hypnotics

Phenibut

History

Phenibut (beta phenyl-gamma aminobutyric acid) is a sedative hypnotic that was developed in Russia in the 1960s for treatment of insomnia, anxiety, and alcohol withdrawal.[63] Though it has never been approved by the U.S. Food and Drug Administration (FDA) for prescription use, it can been found in over-the-counter dietary supplements and through internet sales.[63,64] Participants in online drug discussion forums cite the disappearance of social anxiety and a sense of euphoria as commonly sought effects of phenibut.[65] The commonest reported route of use is oral; however rectal administration, nasal insufflation, and injection have been described.[63,65]

Pharmacology

Phenibut is structurally similar to the inhibitory neurotransmitter gamma-aminobutyric acid (GABA). It acts primarily by agonism at the GABA-B receptor. It also stimulates the GABA-A and dopamine receptors and antagonizes the phenethylamine receptor. Onset of symptoms occurs 2 to 4 hours after oral ingestion, peaking within 4 to 6 hours and may last up to 24 hours.[65]

Clinical Implications

A wide spectrum of clinical effects is reported with phenibut exposure, likely attributable to the multiple receptors affected by the drug, as well as differences in individual metabolism, dosing, purity of the substance and co-ingestants.[66,67] Commonly reported signs and symptoms include tachycardia, mental status changes ranging from lethargy to severe agitation, and respiratory depression that may require intubation.[66] Treatment should be targeted toward providing sedation for psychomotor agitation and ensuring adequate ventilation. There is no antidote available. Tolerance has been described after 1 to 2 weeks of consistent use.[66] As with other GABA agonists, abrupt cessation of phenibut may precipitate an acute, life-threatening withdrawal syndrome.[68]

Legal status

Phenibut is not a controlled substance in the U.S. In 2019, the FDA issued an advisory and warning letter clarifying that phenibut is not a legal supplement ingredient.[64]

Flualprazolam/Etizolam

History

"Designer benzodiazepines" refers to a class of illicit substances structurally related to benzodiazepines (BDZs) but have no approved clinical use in the U.S. This class of chemicals comprises both medications not legal in the U.S. but available in other countries and novel substances which have not been formally studied prior to sale and consumption.[69] First recognized in Western Europe in the 2000s, the use of novel BDZs is expected to continue to rise. Designer BDZs are sold as pills, tablets, capsules, pellets, powders, blotters and liquids.[70]

Examples of this class include flualprazolam, an analog of alprazolam which was never marketed for use and etizolam, a short acting thienodiazepine derivative not legal in the U.S.

though available by prescription in Italy, India, and Japan as an anxiolytic.[71,72]

Pharmacology

Benzodiazepines bind to the GABA-A receptor, resulting in enhanced chloride permeability in postsynaptic neurons in the central nervous system that leads to hyperpolarization.[67] The onset of action for flualprazolam is estimated to be 10 to 30 min after ingestion, with a duration of action ranging from 6 to 14 hours.[70] Etizolam has a half-life of 5 to 7 hours and it metabolized to an active metabolite alpha-hydroxyetizolam, which has a longer half-life than the parent drug.[67]

Clinical

Signs and symptoms described in case reports and case series are similar to those described with pharmaceutical BDZs and include somnolence, slurred speech, ataxia, slowed reaction time, impaired memory and respiratory depression.[67,69] Treatment is largely supportive. The BZD antagonist flumazenil (0.01mg/kg IV with a maximum dose of 0.2 mg) may be considered, with careful consideration given to the risk of precipitating life-threatening BZD withdrawal.[67] Chronic use results in the development of tolerance and abrupt cessation may lead to withdrawal.[70]

Legal Status

Flualprazolam and etizolam are not currently controlled in the U.S. under the CSA.

Xylazine

History

Originally developed in the 1960s as an antihypertensive agent, further development of xylazine was quickly stopped when it was discovered to have significant effects on the central nervous system.[73] Xylazine is structurally similar to clonidine, phenothiazines and imidazolines. Though not approved by the US FDA for human use, it is available as a veterinary medication for sedation and analgesia.[74] In recent years, xylazine has become an intended drug of use and is increasingly found as an adulterant in illicit drugs such as fentanyl, heroin and cocaine.[73,75,76] Xylazine has been detected in substantial numbers in postmortem toxicology reports of fatal drug overdoses, with a predominance in the northeastern U.S.[74,76-78] This suggests that xylazine adulteration of illicit drugs is far more prevalent than currently recognized. Recreational use of xylazine is most commonly via injection; oral ingestion and nasal insufflation are also described.[79]

Pharmacology

Xylazine is a presynaptic alpha-2-adrenergic agonist which acts to inhibit the release of norepinephrine and dopamine from nerve terminals in the CNS.

Clinical

Clinical effects in humans are mostly derived from published case report and case series. Commonly reported signs and symptoms include drowsiness, bradycardia, hypotension, hypertension, and loss of consciousness.[73] When mixed with opioids, xylazine may potentiate sedation and respiratory depression, increasing the risk of mortality.[74] Treatment is primarily supportive. Pure xylazine poisonings may clinically mimic opioid overdoses; but they will not respond to low-dose naloxone (less than 2 mg in adults).[73] Higher dose naloxone (10 mg in adults or 0.1 mg/kg in pediatrics), may be considered, based on recommendations for clonidine poisoning.[73]

Legal Status

Xylazine is not currently controlled under the U.S. CSA.

Cathinones

History

The plant *Catha edulis*, commonly known as khat, was historically used as a stimulant in the Middle East and East Africa. Khat leaves contain multiple compounds including alkaloids, flavonoids, and tannins, but cathinone ((2*S*)-2-amino-1-phenylpropan-1-one) is the primary psychoactive compound.[4,63] Examples of synthetic cathinones that have recently dominated the NPS market include methcathinone, initially used as an anti-depressant in Russia in the 1930s and 1940s, mephedrone, and methylone, which has potent psychostimulant action similar to MDMA.[4] Bupropion, a synthetic cathinone FDA approved for the treatment of depression, seasonal affective disorder and nicotine/tobacco use disorder, is one of the few synthetic cathinones currently approved for clinical use.[4]

Synthetic cathinones, often sold in gas stations, convenience stores or on the internet labeled as "bath salts," "flakka," "plant food," or "research chemicals," are marketed as legal alternatives to more regulated drugs, such as amphetamine and cocaine, and often labeled as "not for human consumption" to circumvent regulation. Over the past decade, cathinones have emerged as the second largest class of novel psychoactive substances, with 162 different compounds being monitored by the EMDCCA as of December 2021.[48] Several factors are associated with their proliferation and increased use, including affordability, ease of access, a public perception of increased safety given their legal status, and their inability to be detected using rapid drug screening technology.

Epidemiology

Data on synthetic cathinone use remains limited. Cathinones were the largest category of NPS seized in the European Union (EU) in 2020, suggesting increasing use. In 2020, seizures of synthetic cathinones in Europe increased to 3.3 tonnes, far surpassing its prior peak of 1.9 tonnes in 2016.[48] Few national population surveys of substance use include cathinones or synthetic stimulants; those that do estimate a prevalence rate of 1% or less.[80] In 2020, a question about synthetic stimulants (ie, "bath salts" or "flakka") was added to the U.S. NSDUH. That survey estimated a 0.1% of past-year prevalence of synthetic stimulant use, with similar prevalence across adolescents, young adults, and adults aged 26 and older.[54]

Pharmacology

Cathinone and its synthetic derivatives are CNS stimulants, exerting their effect by increasing the levels of brain monoamines, such as noradrenaline, serotonin, and dopamine.[81] Similar to phenethylamines such as MDMA, the psychoactive effects of synthetic cathinones may be caused by both their amphetamine-like properties and the ability to modulate serotonin. See Chapter 14 for more information.

Clinical Implications

Acute intoxication with synthetic cathinones predominantly presents clinically with a sympathomimetic toxidrome, which often includes tachycardia, hypertension, tachypnea, hyperthermia, agitation, tremors, and/or seizures.[21,24,26] Synthetic cathinones have amphetamine and cocaine-like psychostimulant effects and are associated with euphoria, empathy, increased openness and sociability, and increased libido.[4]

Legal Status

Khat is currently not under international control, but methcathinone is classified in Schedule I of the 1971 United Nations (UN) Convention on Psychotropic Substances.[4] The Synthetic Drug Abuse Prevention Act of 2012 classified two synthetic cathinone compounds (mephedrone and MDPV) as Schedule I and moved 10 additional synthetic cathinones from temporary to permanent DEA control.[82] In 2013, methylone was classified as Schedule I.[4] In 2015, China increased restrictions on a number of synthetic cathinones, including 3-MMC and 3-CMC. In 2022, the European Commission adopted a proposal to control these substances.[4]

Hallucinogens

History

Novel psychedelics (also termed hallucinogens) are defined by regulatory authorities as substances with similar effects to a scheduled compound, but are not listed in the 1961 United Nations Single Convention on Narcotic Drugs or the 1971 United Nations Convention on Psychotropic Substances.[83]

Psychedelics, both novel and classical (discussed in Chapter 18) generally fall into three structural families: tryptamines such as 4-AcO-DMT, lysergamides such as LSD and LDS analogues, or phenethylamines such as mescaline and 2C-B.[83] Common phenethylamines include N-2-methoxybenzyl phenethylamines, sometimes called N-Bomb, as well as the 2C-B-Fly and the more potent 2C-B-Dragonfly.[83] *Salvia divinorum,* a member of the mint family and endemic to a limited area of the highlands of the Mexican Oaxaca state, contains Salvinorin A, a potent psychedelic that was historically used by the indigenous population for medicinal and ceremonial purposes.[84,85] Since the late 1990s, salvia has had a surge in popularity due to its reputation as a "legal high," its wide availability on the internet and in head shops, lack of detection on drug screens, and perceived safety.[85]

Epidemiology

In 2020, an estimated 2.6% of U.S. residents aged 12 or older (7.1 million people) reported hallucinogen use in the past year on the U.S. NSDUH, with the highest prevalence among adults aged 18 to 25 (7.3 percent or 2.4 million people).[54] An anonymous online survey of 1180 predominantly North American (50.7%) and European (45.3%) respondents who use novel psychedelics found that phenethylamines had the highest prevalence of use (61.5%), followed by tryptamines (43.8%) and lysergamides (42.9%).[83]

Pharmacology

Although hallucinogenic effects have been attributed to serotonin 5-HT_{2A} agonism, a role for other pathways, including dopaminergic, glutamatergic, and 5HT_{2C} and 5HT_{1A} receptors, has been suggested.[83] In contrast to other hallucinogens, Salvinorin A does not demonstrate any binding affinity for the serotonin 5-HT_{2A} receptor, and is believed to cause vivid hallucinations as a highly selective agonist of the kappa opioid receptor[84,85].

Clinical Implications

Clinical symptoms associated with synthetic psychedelics can be variable, but consist mostly of hallucinations, euphoria, tachycardia and hypertension.[63] In addition, psychosis, agitation, seizures, hyperthermia, kidney injury, serotonin toxicity (serotonin syndrome) and death have been reported.[63] Treatment is largely supportive, including benzodiazepines, antipsychotics and intravenous fluid, as is generally the case for other etiologies for agitation and psychosis. Clinicians should have a low threshold for consulting poison control when clinical presentation suggests serotonin toxicity, including seizures, extreme hyperthermia, and agitation.

Legal Status

The Synthetic Drug Abuse Prevention Act of 2012 classified nine synthetic hallucinogens known as the 2C family as Schedule I. Neither *Salvia divinorum* nor salvinorin A is currently controlled under the CSA, although several states have regulated their use.

IDENTIFYING AND ACCESSING INFORMATION ON NEWLY EMERGING AND NOVEL PSYCHOACTIVE SUBSTANCES

A variety of organizations conduct surveillance and collate information to inform the public and clinicians and the development of public health and law enforcement policy. In the United States, poison control centers collect national surveillance data on drug exposures and provide toxicology support 24 hours per day, 7 days per week for lay people and clinicians (1-800-222-1222). The DEA enforces the controlled substance laws and regulations of the United States, collaborates with local law enforcement and health professionals regarding seizures and poisonings, and maintains the National Forensic Laboratory Information System (NFLIS) to collect, analyze, and disseminate information on analysis of substance-containing forensic samples.[86] EMCDDA conducts similar data collection, registration and analysis of both licit and illicit substances in the European Union, including wastewater and seized material chemical analysis, and analysis of global market and trade patterns. The U.S. Substance Abuse and Mental Health Services Administration (SAMHSA) and the National Institutes of Health fund periodic large-scale, population-based epidemiological studies (eg, NSDUH, Monitoring the Future (students)) that collect self-reported data on substance use that are available to the public. Local and state health departments, local law enforcement agencies, and medical examiners may also be a source of information.

REFERENCES

1. Baumann MH, Solis E, Watterson LR, Marusich JA, Fantegrossi WE, Wiley JL. Baths salts, spice, and related designer drugs: the science behind the headlines. *J Neurosci.* 2014;34(46):15150-15158. doi:10.1523/JNEUROSCI.3223-14.2014.
2. Corazza O, Schifano F, Simonato P, et al. Phenomenon of new drugs on the Internet: the case of ketamine derivative methoxetamine. *Hum Psychopharmacol.* 2012;27(2):145-149. doi:10.1002/HUP.1242
3. Alves VL, Gonçalves JL, Aguiar J, Teixeira HM, Câmara JS. The synthetic cannabinoids phenomenon: from structure to toxicological properties. A review. *Crit Rev Toxicol.* 2020;50(5):359-382. doi:10.1080/10408444.2020.1762539
4. Soares J, Costa VM, Bastos MDL, Carvalho F, Capela JP. An updated review on synthetic cathinones. *Arch Toxicol.* 2021;95(9):2895-2940. doi:10.1007/S00204-021-03083-3
5. Ayres WA, Starsiak MJ, Sokolay P. The bogus drug: three methyl & alpha methyl fentanyl sold as "China White". *J Psychoactive Drugs.* 1981;13(1):91-93. doi:10.1080/02791072.1981.10471455
6. Bäckberg M, Beck O, Jönsson KH, Helander A. Opioid intoxications involving butyrfentanyl, 4-fluorobutyrfentanyl, and fentanyl from the Swedish STRIDA project. *Clin Toxicol.* 2015;53(7):609-617. doi:10.3109/15563650.2015.1054505
7. Nonpharmaceutical Fentanyl-Related Deaths. Multiple States, April 2005--March 2007. *MMWR Weekly.* 2008;57(29): Accessed October 6, 2022. https://www.cdc.gov/mmwr/preview/mmwrhtml/mm5729a1.htm
8. European Monitoring Centre for Drugs and Drug Addiction. Fentanyl Drug Profile. Accessed October 17, 2022. http://www.emcdda.europa.eu/publications/drug-profiles/fentanyl
9. Fleming SW, Cooley JC, Johnson L, et al. Analysis of U-47700, a novel synthetic opioid, in human urine by LC–MS–MS and LC–QToF. *J Anal Toxicol.* 2016;37:334-341. doi:10.1093/jat/bkw131
10. Lozier MJ, Boyd M, Stanley C, et al. Acetyl fentanyl, a novel fentanyl analog, causes 14 overdose deaths in rhode Island, March-May 2013. *J Med Toxicol.* 2015;11(2):208-217. doi:10.1007/s13181-015-0477-9
11. Vandeputte MM, Krotulski AJ, Papsun DM, Logan BK, Stove CP. The rise and fall of isotonitazene and brorphine: two recent stars in the synthetic opioid firmament. *J Anal Toxicol* Published online July 8, 2021. doi:10.1093/jat/bkab082
12. European Monitoring Centre for Drugs and Drug Addiction, Evans-Brown M, Gallegos A, Christie R, et al. An update from the EU Early Warning System New psychoactive substances: 25 years of early warning and response in Europe. Published online 2022. doi:10.2810/882318
13. Department of Justice, Drug Enforcement Agency. *Drugs of Abuse, A DEA Resource Guide.* 2020th ed. Published online 2020. Accessed May 19, 2023. https://www.dea.gov/sites/default/files/2020-04/Drugs%20of%20Abuse%202020-Web%20Version-508%20compliant-4-24-20_0.pdf
14. European Monitoring Centre for Drugs and Drug Addiction. *European Drug Report 2022: Trends and Developments*; 2022 doi:10.2810/715044
15. Zawilska JB, Andrzejczak D. Next generation of novel psychoactive substances on the horizon—A complex problem to face. *Drug Alcohol Depend.* 2015;157:1-17. doi:10.1016/j.drugalcdep.2015.09.030
16. Vo KT, van Wijk XMR, Lynch KL, Wu AHB, Smollin CG. Counterfeit Norco Poisoning Outbreak—San Francisco Bay Area, California, March 25–April 5, 2016. *MMWR Morb Mortal Wkly Rep* 2016;65(16):420-423. doi:10.15585/mmwr.mm6516e1
17. Tomassoni AJ, Hawk KF, Jubanyik K, et al. Multiple fentanyl overdoses—New Haven, Connecticut, June 23, 2016. *Morb Mortal Wkly Rep.* 2017;66(4): doi:10.15585/mm6604a4
18. Emerging Trends and Alerts. National Institute on Drug Abuse (NIDA). Accessed October 17, 2022. https://www.drugabuse.gov/drugs-abuse/emerging-trends-alerts
19. Carroll FI, Lewin AH, Mascarella SW, Seltzman HH, Reddy PA. Designer drugs: a medicinal chemistry perspective. *Ann N Y Acad Sci.* 2012;1248(1):18-38. doi:10.1111/j.1749-6632.2011.06199.x
20. European Monitoring Centre for Drugs and Drug Addiction, Europol. *EU Drug Markets Report: Strategic Overview 2016.* Accessed October 18, 2022. https://www.emcdda.europa.eu/publications/joint-publications/eu-drug-markets/2016/strategic-overview_en
21. Cooper ZD. Adverse effects of synthetic cannabinoids: management of acute toxicity and withdrawal. *Curr Psychiatry Rep.* 2016;18(5):52. doi:10.1007/s11920-016-0694-1
22. Bao Y, Meng S, Shi J, Lu L. Control of fentanyl-related substances in China. *Lancet Psychiatry.* 2019;6(7):e15. doi:10.1016/S2215-0366(19)30218-4
23. Federal Register. Schedules of Controlled Substances: Temporary Placement of Fentanyl-Related Substances in Schedule I; Correction. Accessed May 19, 2023. https://www.federalregister.gov/documents/2020/04/10/2020-06984/schedules-of-controlled-substances-temporary-placement-of-fentanyl-related-substances-in-schedule-i
24. Hoffman RS, Howland MA, Lewin NA, Nelson LS, Goldfrank LR. *Goldfrank's Toxicologic Emergencies|Access Emergency Medicine.* 10th ed. McGraw Hill Medical Accessed January 29, 2017. http://accessemergencymedicine.mhmedical.com/book.aspx?bookid=1163
25. Slomski A. A trip on "bath salts" is cheaper than meth or cocaine but much more dangerous. *JAMA.* 2012;308(23):2445. doi:10.1001/jama.2012.34423
26. Banks ML, Worst TJ, Rusyniak DE, Sprague JE. Synthetic cathinones ("bath salts"). *J Emerg Med.* 2014;46(5):632-642. doi:10.1016/j.jemermed.2013.11.104
27. Spyres M, Jang D. Amphetamines. In: Nelson LS, Howland M, Lewin NA, Smith SW, Goldfrank LR, Hoffman RS, eds. *Goldfrank's Toxicologic Emergencies.* 11e ed. McGraw Hill Medical; 2019 Accessed October 20, 2022. https://accessemergencymedicine.mhmedical.com/content.aspx?sectionid=210259500&bookid=2569#1163017880

28. Kasper AM, Ridpath AD, Arnold JK, et al. Severe illness associated with reported use of synthetic cannabinoids—Mississippi, April 2015. *MMWR Morb Mortal Wkly Rep*. 2015;64(39):1121-1122. doi:10.15585/mmwr.mm6439a7
29. Hermanns-Clausen M, Kneisel S, Szabo B, Auwärter V. Acute toxicity due to the confirmed consumption of synthetic cannabinoids: clinical and laboratory findings. *Addiction*. 2013;108(3):534-544. doi:10.1111/j.1360-0443.2012.04078.x
30. Davis C, Boddington D. Teenage cardiac arrest following abuse of synthetic cannabis. *Heart Lung Circ*. 2015;24(10):e162-e163. doi:10.1016/j.hlc.2015.04.176
31. Miotto K, Striebel J, Cho AK, Wang C. Clinical and pharmacological aspects of bath salt use: a review of the literature and case reports. *Drug Alcohol Depend*. 2013;132(1–2):1-12. doi:10.1016/j.drugalcdep.2013.06.016
32. Harris CR, Brown A. Synthetic cannabinoid intoxication: a case series and review. *J Emerg Med*. 2013;44(2):360-366. doi:10.1016/j.jemermed.2012.07.061
33. Centers for Disease Control and Prevention (CDC). Acute kidney injury associated with synthetic cannabinoid use—multiple states, 2012. *MMWR Morb Mortal Wkly Rep*. 2013;62(6):93-98.
34. Rosenbaum CD, Carreiro SP, Babu KM. Here today, gone tomorrow … and back again? A review of herbal marijuana alternatives (K2, Spice), synthetic cathinones (bath salts), kratom, Salvia divinorum, methoxetamine, and piperazines. *J Med Toxicol*. 2012;8(1):15-32. doi:10.1007/s13181-011-0202-2
35. Levine M, Levitan R, Skolnik A. Compartment syndrome after "bath salts" use: a case series. *Ann Emerg Med*. 2013;61(4):480-483. doi:10.1016/j.annemergmed.2012.11.021
36. Suzuki J, Poklis JL, Poklis A. *"My Friend Said it was Good LSD": A Suicide Attempt Following Analytically Confirmed 25I-NBOMe Ingestion*. doi:10.1080/02791072.2014.960111
37. Stanley TH. The history and development of the fentanyl series. *J Pain Symptom Manage*. 1992;7(3):S3-S7. doi:10.1016/0885-3924(92)90047-L
38. Booth JV, Grossman D, Moore J, et al. Substance abuse among physicians: a survey of academic anesthesiology programs. *Anesth Analg*. 2002;95(4):1024-1030.
39. DEA Administrator Testifies on the Illicit Fentanyl Threat. February 15, 2023. URL: https://www.youtube.com/watch?v=oqCZrYL2nrM
40. Ciccarone D. The rise of illicit fentanyls, stimulants and the fourth wave of the opioid overdose crisis. *Curr Opin Psychiatry*. 2021;34(4):344-350. doi:10.1097/YCO.0000000000000717
41. Gladden RM, Martinez P, Seth P, et al. *MMWR Morb Mortal Wkly Rep*. 2016;65(33):837-843. doi:10.15585/mmwr.mm6533a2
42. Enforcement Administration D. 2020 National Drug Threat Assessment (NDTA). Published online 2020. Accessed May 19, 2023. https://deagovtest.dea.gov/documents/2021/03/02/2020-national-drug-threat-assessment#:~:text=The%202020%20National%20Drug%20Threat%20Assessment%20%28NDTA%29%20is,laundering%20of%20proceeds%20generated%20through%20illicit%20drug%20sales.
43. Somerville NJ, O'Donnell J, Gladden RM, et al. Characteristics of fentanyl overdose—Massachusetts, 2014–2016. *MMWR Morb Mortal Wkly Rep*. 2017;66(14):382-386. doi:10.15585/mmwr.mm6614a2
44. Zawilska JB. An expanding world of novel psychoactive substances: opioids. *Front Psych*. 2017;8:110. doi:10.3389/fpsyt.2017.00110
45. Swanson DM, Hair LS, Strauch Rivers SR, et al. Fatalities involving carfentanil and furanyl fentanyl: two case reports. *J Anal Toxicol*. 2017;41(6):498-502. doi:10.1093/jat/bkx037
46. Amaducci AM, Aldy K, Campleman SM, et al. Brorphine, isotonitazene and metonitazene emerge as new age opioids. ACMT annual scientific meeting abstract #40. *J Med Toxicol*. 2022;18:75-125.
47. Centers for Disease Control and Prevention. 2023. Synthetic Opioid Overdose Data | Drug Overdose | CDC Injury Center. Accessed October 18, 2022. https://www.cdc.gov/drugoverdose/deaths/synthetic/index.html
48. European Monitoring Centre for Drugs and Drug Addiction. New Psychoactive Substances: 25 Years of Early Warning and Response in Europe—An Update From the EU Early Warning System. Published 2022. Accessed October 18, 2022. https://www.emcdda.europa.eu/publications/rapid-communication/update-eu-early-warning-system-2022_en
49. Moss MJ, Warrick BJ, Nelson LS, et al. ACMT and AACT position statement: preventing occupational fentanyl and fentanyl analog exposure to emergency responders. *J Med Toxicol*. 2017;13(4):347-351. doi:10.1007/s13181-017-0628-2
50. Wax PM, Becker CE, Curry SC. Unexpected "gas" casualties in Moscow: a medical toxicology perspective. *Ann Emerg Med*. 2003;41(5):700-705. doi:10.1067/mem.2003.148
51. Federal Register. Temporary Placement of Brorphine in Schedule I. Accessed May 19, 2023. https://www.federalregister.gov/documents/2021/03/01/2021-04242/schedules-of-controlled-substances-temporary-placement-of-brorphine-in-schedule-i
52. Gorelick DA. Kratom: substance of abuse or therapeutic plant? *Psychiatr Clin North Am*. 2022;45(3):415-430. doi:10.1016/J.PSC.2022.04.002
53. Nelson ME, Bryant SM, Aks SE. Emerging drugs of abuse. *Emerg Med Clin North Am*. 2014;32(1):1-28. doi:10.1016/j.emc.2013.09.001
54. Center for Behavioral Health Statistics S. Key Substance Use and Mental Health Indicators in the United States: Results From the 2020 National Survey on Drug Use and Health; 2021. Accessed January 15, 2022. https://www.samhsa.gov/data/sites/default/files/reports/rpt35325/NSDUHFFRPDFWHTMLFiles2020/2020NSDUHFFR1PDFW102121.pdf
55. Angkurawaranon C, Jiraporncharoen W, Likhitsathian S, et al. Trends in the use of illicit substances in Thailand: results from national household surveys. *Drug Alcohol Rev*. 2018;37(5):658-663. doi:10.1111/DAR.12689
56. Nelsen JL, Lapoint J, Hodgman MJ, Aldous KM. Seizure and coma following Kratom (*Mitragynina speciosa* Korth) exposure. *J Med Toxicol*. 2010;6(4):424-426. doi:10.1007/s13181-010-0079-5
57. Lydecker AG, Sharma A, McCurdy CR, Avery BA, Babu KM, Boyer EW. Suspected adulteration of commercial kratom products with 7-hydroxymitragynine. *J Med Toxicol*. 2016;12(4):341-349. doi:10.1007/s13181-016-0588-y
58. Babu KM, McCurdy CR, Boyer EW. Opioid receptors and legal highs: *Salvia divinorum* and Kratom. *Clin Toxicol (Phila)*. 2008;46(2):146-152. doi:10.1080/15563650701241795
59. Anwar M, Law R, Schier J. Notes from the field: Kratom (*Mitragyna speciosa*) Exposures Reported to Poison Centers—United States, 2010–2015. *MMWR Morb Mortal Wkly Rep*. 2016;65(29):748-749. doi:10.15585/mmwr.mm6529a4
60. Post S, Spiller HA, Chounthirath T, Smith GA. Kratom exposures reported to United States poison control centers: 2011–2017. *Clin Toxicol*. 2019;57(10):847-854. doi:10.1080/15563650.2019.1569236
61. Cumpston KL, Carter M, Wills BK. Clinical outcomes after Kratom exposures: a poison center case series. *Am J Emerg Med*. 2018;36(1):166-168. doi:10.1016/J.AJEM.2017.07.051
62. Singh D, Müller CP, Vicknasingam BK. Kratom (Mitragyna speciosa) dependence, withdrawal symptoms and craving in regular users. *Drug Alcohol Depend*. 2014;139:132-137. doi:10.1016/j.drugalcdep.2014.03.017
63. Sam Wang G, Hoyte C. Novel drugs of abuse. *Pediatr Rev*. 2019;40(2):71-78. doi:10.1542/PIR.2018-0050
64. Cohen PA, Ellison RR, Travis JC, Gaufberg S, v., Gerona R. Quantity of phenibut in dietary supplements before and after FDA warnings. *Clin Toxicol*. 2022;60(4):486-488. doi:10.1080/15563650.2021.1973020
65. Owen DR, Wood DM, Archer JRH, Dargan PI. Phenibut (4-amino-3-phenyl-butyric acid): availability, prevalence of use, desired effects and acute toxicity. *Drug Alcohol Rev*. 2016;35(5):591-596. doi:10.1111/DAR.12356
66. McCabe DJ, Bangh SA, Arens AM, Cole JB. Phenibut exposures and clinical effects reported to a regional poison center. *Am J Emerg Med*. 2019;37(11):2066-2071. doi:10.1016/J.AJEM.2019.02.044
67. Levine M, Lovecchio F. New designer drugs. *Emerg Med Clin North Am*. 2021;39(3):677-687. doi:10.1016/J.EMC.2021.04.013
68. VanDreese B, Holland A, Murray A. Chronic phenibut use: symptoms, severe withdrawal, and recovery. *WMJ* 2022;12(1). Accessed August 20, 2022. https://wmjonline.org/wp-content/uploads/2022/121/1/E1.pdf
69. Greenblatt HK, Greenblatt DJ. Designer benzodiazepines: a review of published data and public health significance. *Clin Pharmacol Drug Dev*. 2019;8(3):266-269. doi:10.1002/CPDD.667

70. Zawilska JB, Wojcieszak J. An expanding world of new psychoactive substances—designer benzodiazepines. *Neurotoxicology*. 2019;73:8-16. doi:10.1016/J.NEURO.2019.02.015
71. Nielsen S, McAuley A. Etizolam: a rapid review on pharmacology, non-medical use and harms. *Drug Alcohol Rev*. 2020;39(4):330-336. doi:10.1111/DAR.13052
72. Blumenberg A, Hughes A, Reckers A, Ellison R, Gerona R. Flualprazolam: report of an outbreak of a new psychoactive substance in adolescents. *Pediatrics*. 2020;146(1): doi:10.1542/PEDS.2019-2953/37049
73. Ball NS, Knable BM, Relich TA, et al. Xylazine poisoning: a systematic review. *Clin Toxicol (Phila)*. 2020;60(8):892-901. doi:10.1080/15563650.2022.2063135
74. Kariisa M, Patel P, Smith H, Bitting J. Notes from the field: xylazine detection and involvement in drug overdose deaths—United States, 2019. *MMWR Morb Mortal Wkly Rep*. 2021;70(37):1300-1302. doi:10.15585/MMWR.MM7037A4
75. Bowles JM, McDonald K, Maghsoudi N, et al. Xylazine detected in unregulated opioids and drug administration equipment in Toronto, Canada: clinical and social implications. *Harm Reduct J*. 2021;18(1):1-6. doi:10.1186/S12954-021-00546-9/TABLES/2
76. Alexander RS, Canver BR, Sue KL, Morford KL. Xylazine and overdoses: trends, concerns, and recommendations. *Am J Public Health*. 2022;112(8):1212-1216. doi:10.2105/AJPH.2022.306881
77. Nunez J, DeJoseph ME, Gill JR. Xylazine, a veterinary tranquilizer, detected in 42 accidental fentanyl intoxication deaths. *Am J Forensic Med Pathol*. 2021;42(1):9-11. doi:10.1097/PAF.0000000000000622
78. Johnson J, Pizzicato L, Johnson C, Viner K. Increasing presence of xylazine in heroin and/or fentanyl deaths, Philadelphia, Pennsylvania, 2010–2019. *Inj Prev*. 2021;27(4):395-398. doi:10.1136/INJURYPREV-2020-043968
79. Thangada S, Clinton HA, Ali S, et al. Notes from the field: xylazine, a veterinary tranquilizer, identified as an emerging novel substance in drug overdose deaths—Connecticut, 2019–2020. *Morb Mortal Wkly Rep*. 2021;70(37):1303-1304. doi:10.1093/jat/bkw051
80. Karila L, Megarbane B, Cottencin O, Lejoyeux M. Synthetic cathinones: a new public health problem. *Curr Neuropharmacol*. 2015;13(1):12-20. doi:10.2174/1570159X13666141210224137
81. Pieprzyca E, Skowronek R, Nižnanský Ľ, Czekaj P. Synthetic cathinones—From natural plant stimulant to new drug of abuse. *Eur J Pharmacol*. 2020;875:173012. doi:10.1016/J.EJPHAR.2020.173012
82. Drug Enforcement Administration. 2020 "Bath Salts Drug Fact Sheet" URL: https://www.dea.gov/sites/default/files/2020-06/Bath%20Salts-2020.pdf
83. Mallaroni P, Mason NL, Vinckenbosch FRJ, Ramaekers JG. The use patterns of novel psychedelics: experiential fingerprints of substituted phenethylamines, tryptamines and lysergamides. *Psychopharmacology (Berl)*. 2022;239(6):1783-1796. doi:10.1007/s00213-022-06142-4
84. Brito-Da-costa AM, Dias-Da-silva D, Gomes NGM, Dinis-Oliveira RJ, Madureira-Carvalho Á. Pharmacokinetics and pharmacodynamics of Salvinorin A and *Salvia divinorum*: clinical and forensic aspects. *Pharmaceuticals (Basel)*. 2021;14(2):1-36. doi:10.3390/PH14020116
85. Coffeen U, Pellicer F. *Salvia divinorum*: from recreational hallucinogenic use to analgesic and anti-inflammatory action. *J Pain Res*. 2019;12:1069-1076. doi:10.2147/JPR.S188619
86. Underwood E. A new drug war. *Science*. 2015;347(6221):469-473. doi:10.1126/science.347.6221.469

SECTION

3

Epidemiology and Prevention

Associate Editor: Sharon Levy

Lead Section Editor: Babalola Faseru

Section Editors: Deepa R. Camenga and Catalina Lopez-Quintero

CHAPTER

24 The Epidemiology of Substance Use Disorders

Silvia S. Martins, Megan E. Marziali, and Pia M. Mauro

CHAPTER OUTLINE

- Epidemiological principles
- Alcohol use disorders
- Nicotine dependence and tobacco use disorders
- Cannabis use disorders
- Other drug use disorders and co-occurring issues
- Social determinants of health, socio-demographic, and structural factors associated with substance use disorders
- Substance use disorder remission and treatment
- Conclusions

EPIDEMIOLOGICAL PRINCIPLES

Epidemiology is the study of how diseases are distributed in populations as well as the study of the determinants of health.[1-3] Some basic terms used in epidemiology deserve attention in this chapter, to help understand the literature and studies reported here. *Prevalence* is taken to represent the ratio of the total number of cases of a particular disease divided by the total number of individuals in a particular population at a specific time. Prevalence considers both the incidence and duration of a disease because it depends not only on the rate of newly developed cases over time, but also on the length of time the disease exists in the population. In turn, the duration of the disorder is affected by the degree of recovery and death from the disease. *Incidence* is taken to represent the risk of disease, whereas *prevalence* is an indicator of the public health burden the disease imposes on the community.[4] More specifically, *incidence* refers to the occurrence of new cases of a disease divided by the total number at risk for the disorder during a specified period.[4] We refer to both the *cumulative incidence* and the *incidence rate*. *Cumulative incidence* is the proportion of new cases of a disease of interest within a population during a specified period.[5] *Incidence rate* is the proportion of new cases of a disease within *person-time* (ie, time contributed until becoming a case) of observation.[5] The key difference between cumulative incidence and incidence rates is the denominator, as the numerator remains the same.

In some instances we present *conditional probabilities*, which can take the form of the likelihood of disease (D) given the occurrence of exposure (E), often presented as P(D|E).[6] For example, a conditional probability in the context of substance use disorders (SUD) could be the likelihood of diagnosis among people who use psychoactive substances. (P(Substance use disorder) | (Use of substances)). The *relative risk* represents the strength of association between a particular characteristic or factor and the development of disease. The relative risk (sometimes called the *risk ratio*) measures the incidence of disease among those exposed to a particular characteristic (such as family history of alcohol use disorder), divided by the incidence of disease among those without exposure to that characteristic. The *odds ratio* is also a measure of the strength of association between a characteristic or exposure and disease or other outcomes. If there is no difference in the incidence among people with and without the characteristic or exposure, the relative risk or odds ratio is equal to 1. A relative risk or odds ratio of more than 1 indicates a positive association of disease with a given characteristic. A relative risk or odds ratio less than 1 signifies a negative association, which may indicate a protective effect associated with the characteristic. Because these are ratios, both relative risk and odds ratio have a lower bound of zero, meaning that negative associations will be between 0 and 1, but positive associations have no upper bound. When an outcome is rare, the odds ratio approximates the relative risk. Excellent detailed discussions of epidemiologic study designs can be found elsewhere.[1,2,4,7]

For the purposes of this chapter, observational epidemiologic studies can be divided into two types: (1) descriptive and (2) analytic. Observational studies may include case reports, case series, ecological, cross-sectional, case–control, and cohort studies. In cross-sectional studies or surveys, participant characteristics, risk factors, and disease occurrence or other outcomes are evaluated (eg, by interview or physical examination) at the same point in time.[4] In all observational studies, the investigator observes the study participants and gathers information for analysis.[4] Descriptive studies generate hypotheses to answer the questions: what, who, where and when. These include aggregate level studies (ecological studies) and individual level studies (case report, case series and cross-sectional studies). Descriptive studies do not include comparison groups. Analytic studies generally test a hypothesis (why and how?) of a suspected association between a particular exposure (risk factor) and a disease or other health related outcomes. Analytic studies include experimental studies (intervention studies eg, randomized controlled trials) and observational studies such as case–control (retrospective), and cohort (longitudinal, prospective, or retrospective). Cross-sectional and ecological studies could be categorized as analytical if they include comparison groups.

To describe SUD over the life-course, studies may report age, period, and cohort effects. *Age effects* refer to changes incurred developmentally by moving through the life-course independent of the time period (ie, physiological changes and accumulation of social effects).[8-10] *Period effects* are defined by experiences or changes (ie, historical or social events, such as war or policy changes) that impact an entire population at a specific time point, regardless of a person's age.[8-10] *Cohort effects* arise from a period effect impacting birth cohorts (which make up different age groups at a specific time) differently, or through which age groups have different susceptibility to the same exposure.[11] Cohort effect, therefore, can be conceptualized using both age and period effects. Modeling strategies to disentangle and differentiate age, period, and cohort effects for a specific outcome of interest can be used to better understand time-varying effects.[11] In this chapter, we will explore age–period–cohort effects related to SUD.

This chapter reviews the literature regarding prevalence and incidence concerning SUD, including alcohol, cannabis, nicotine, and other SUDs. We discuss social determinants of health, or social factors that influence health outcomes across populations encompassing "*environments in which people are born, live, learn, work, play, worship, and age that affect a wide range of health, functioning, and quality-of-life outcomes and risks*"[12] and key structural factors associated with increased risk for SUD. These can include *socioeconomic position* (eg, education, income, employment, etc.) and other living and working conditions.[13,14] Finally, we discuss treatment and remission of SUD.

A Note on Language

Prior to expanding on the substantive material, we want to draw attention to some terminology used throughout this chapter. We opt to use the term illegal rather than illicit when referring to substances not allowed for consumption within the current legal environment. This is because the term illicit refers to unlawful actions, but also to immorality and behaviors forbidden by social norms. To avoid the implication that substance use is an issue of morality, we use the term illegal, which strictly refers to being forbidden by law. When referencing illegal drugs, we are not including cannabis in this category; while federally illegal at this time in the United States, cannabis is legal for medical use (ie, cannabis used as treatment) or recreational consumption in many states.[15] We choose to use the term *cannabis* as opposed to *marijuana*, as the latter term is rooted in racism.[16] We also use person-centered, nonstigmatizing language throughout the chapter.[17] Lastly, we follow standards outlined by Flanagin et al., regarding the reporting of race and ethnicity.[18]

Epidemiological Surveys of Substance Use Disorders in the United States

Surveys in the United States and other nations assess the prevalence of SUD. Some surveys use structured interviews with standardized and universally recognized diagnostic criteria. These include the *Diagnostic and Statistical Manual of Mental Disorders*, most recently in its fifth edition (DSM-5),[19] and the 10th revision of the *International Classification of Diseases*.[20]

One of the earliest surveys to assess the epidemiology of SUDs in the United States using a structured psychiatric interview was the National Institute of Mental Health's Epidemiologic Catchment Area (ECA) study,[21-23] conducted between 1980 and 1984 with a 1-year follow-up. At the baseline interview, collaborators in the ECA assessed a probability sample of more than 20,000 adult participants (ages 18+) in five metropolitan areas of the United States. The National Comorbidity Survey (NCS) is another major survey providing information on SUD in the United States, first administered between 1990 and 1992.[24] The NCS included a 10-year follow-up of a subsample of the original survey with adults 18 years and older who screened positive for any disorder assessed in the first survey.[25,26] Below, we describe relevant nationally representative studies in the U.S. that we will refer to throughout this chapter.

The National Epidemiologic Survey on Alcohol and Related Conditions (NESARC), sponsored by the National Institute on Alcohol Abuse and Alcoholism, was first conducted in 2001 to 2002, with a prospective follow-up in 2003 to 2005.[27] The NESARC provided lifetime and 12-month estimates of SUD among adults ages 18 and older based on DSM-IV criteria[27,28] using the Alcohol Use Disorder and Associated Disabilities Interview Schedule.[29,30] The NESARC III, completed in 2012 to 2013, is an independent cross-sectional sampling of the U.S. adult population, based on DSM-5 criteria; importantly, NESARC III is not a longitudinal follow-up of wave 2.[31,32] To date, it is likely the largest nationally representative survey in the United States that provides 12-month as well as lifetime prevalence of DSM-5 SUD.

The National Survey on Drug Use and Health (NSDUH),[33] sponsored by the Substance Abuse and Mental Health Services Administration (SAMHSA), collects information in all 50 states and the District of Columbia on aspects related to drug use and SUD among the civilian, noninstitutionalized population ages 12 years and older.[34] The NSDUH is a cross-sectional survey conducted annually since 1971; however, substantial survey redesign limits some comparability of estimates over time,[34] such as providing incentives for participation starting in 2002 as well as changes in assessment of nonmedical prescription drug use in 2015.[35] Methodological changes to the 2020 NSDUH, necessary during the COVID-19 pandemic, require attention. In-person data collection was paused from mid-March 2020 until October 2020, leading to web-based data collection being implemented for the first time.[36,37] Survey questions also changed in 2020, including categorizing SUD using DSM-5 criteria, therefore affecting SUD population-level estimates.[36,37] The combination of methodological changes in data collection and survey redesign constrains comparability of the 2020 data to prior years. For this reason, we will be focusing mostly on data from the 2019 NSDUH survey with the inclusion of 2020 data for brief discussion on differences in estimates obtained across surveys.

The Population Assessment of Tobacco and Health (PATH) study is a longitudinal survey monitoring tobacco use and other substance use within the United States among the civilian, noninstitutionalized population ages 12 years and older.[38,39] The first wave of this study began in 2013 to 2015; data collection is ongoing, with the latest wave being completed in 2021.[38,39] As this study is longitudinal, respondents are asked to complete the study at each wave. Youth who turn 18 years old by the time the new wave of data is being collected are considered to have aged into the Adult Interview. Similarly, youth under the age of 12 (9-11 years) are sampled and referred to as "shadow youth"; once they turn 12 years old, they are then enrolled into the study cohorts with parental consent.[38] Another nationally representative study monitoring the use of tobacco and other substance use and nicotine dependence is the *National Youth Tobacco Study* (NYTS). The NYTS is a cross-sectional study conducted annually since 2011 (and periodically from 1999-2009), which samples middle through high school students (grades 6-12).[40,41]

The *Monitoring the Future* (MTF) study is a population-based, prospective study of drug use behaviors and related attitudes, with independent samples of 12th graders recruited annually and subsamples followed longitudinally into adulthood. MTF has thirteen waves of measurement from ages 18 to 60.[42] MTF conducts annual, in-school surveys of 12th-grade students, which are administered in classrooms to nationally representative samples of approximately 15,000 students from about 130 schools each year. Schools are selected using a multi-stage random sampling design with replacement and participate for 2 years, and participating schools are provided with a monetary incentive. Since 1976, participation by either an original or a replacement school has been obtained in 95% to 99% of sample units. Student response rates have averaged 83% (range = 77%-86%) and no systematic trend over time (most all non-response is due to student being absent during data collection, with only about 1% declining to participate). MTF also includes longitudinal follow-up of 12th graders, wherein sub-samples of approximately 2,400 respondents from each 12th-grade cohort complete follow-up mail surveys. These surveys oversample people who use substances at a ratio of 3 to 1. Across MTF cohorts, 40% to 75% of the originally targeted students complete the first follow-up; 42% to 67% complete follow-ups to age 45. The retention rate in MTF is similar to other commonly used longitudinal datasets in health research. Response rates in all studies have declined in the past several decades,[43-46] and differential attrition with respect to substance use is true of virtually all longitudinal studies.[47-51]

Comparing Across Studies: Methodological Reasons for Estimate Differences

Comparing estimates across studies is difficult at times because they employ different measures and definitions of SUD, different study populations, or have distinct data collection procedures.

Differences in estimates across surveys may be due to variations in the diagnostic instrumentation, such as the version of the DSM that was used at the time the survey was completed. In earlier versions of the DSM (eg, DSM-IV), SUD were conceptualized as a categorical variable, distinguishing past-year substance abuse (1 or more out of 4 criteria) and substance dependence (3 or more out of 7 criteria). In the DSM-5, these separate diagnostic categories were reconceptualized into one continuous construct distinguished by severity. Criteria used combined substance abuse and substance dependence indicators,[52] removed "having legal problems as a result of substance use" as a criterion, and instead added experiencing craving for the substance. SUD severity in the DSM-5 is defined based on the total number of criteria met: 2 to 3 criteria indicate mild disorder, 4 to 5 criteria indicate moderate disorder, and 6 or more criteria indicate severe disorder.[19] Throughout the text, when we use the term *substance use disorder*, we are referring to a combined substance abuse and/or dependence using DSM-IV or earlier diagnostic criteria. Additionally, some estimates for substance dependence are measured via survey scales; for example, nicotine dependence can be measured from the Nicotine Dependence Scale or the Wisconsin Inventory of Smoking Dependence Motives (WISDM), both of which are used to assess nicotine dependence in the Population Assessment of Tobacco and Health (PATH) dataset.[53]

Other differences in estimates can arise from different study populations in terms of person, place, and time. This includes the size of the survey sample, and the locale of the survey participants (nationally representative samples versus individual communities), as well as specific characteristics of the populations surveyed, including the age range of study participants. For example, the NCS included a relatively younger population (persons ages 15-54 years) than some other surveys,[54] and the NSDUH includes individuals from age 12 years and older,[55] whereas the ECA and NESARC surveys gathered information for participants age 18 years of age and above.[21-23,27,32] Lastly, through its nature of being a school-based sample, MTF does not include students who are not enrolled in school; these adolescents tend to have higher rates of SUD than their counterparts attending school.[56]

In addition, specific methods used during data gathering (eg, self-administered computerized versus face-to-face interviews, use of identifiers for follow-up assessment versus anonymity),[57] or a focus on clinically significance criteria[58] may relate to differences in survey findings. Differences in survey findings also may occur from use of "gated" procedures.[59] For example, to maximize efficiency, in some prior surveys, only people who screened positive for "substance abuse" (using DSM-IV criteria) were subsequently assessed for DSM-IV defined substance dependence. This approach was evaluated in several analyses that reported relatively small differences in estimated prevalence for some types of DSM-IV substance dependence (ie, cannabis, cocaine) when "gated" as compared with "ungated" protocols were in place,[59,60] but possibly more appreciable differences in assessment for other substances (ie, alcohol).[60] As a consequence, some people with DSM-IV defined substance dependence may not be identified among population-based surveys using gated procedures.[60,61] In some assessments, these cases appeared to be less likely to have received treatment and therefore less likely to be clinically apparent cases but more likely to have occurred among specific subgroups of the population.[61,62]

ALCOHOL USE DISORDERS

Almost a third of the population meets the criteria for DSM-5 alcohol use disorder (AUD) at some point in their lifetime: NESARC III data suggests that overall lifetime prevalence is 29.1%, with 8.6% having mild, 6.6% moderate, and 13.9% severe lifetime AUD. The overall prevalence of DSM-5 12-month AUD among adults, using NESARC III data, is 13.9%, which includes 7.3% mild, 3.2% moderate, and 3.4% severe AUD.[32] Data from the NESARC and NESARC III show that the prevalence of past-year DSM-IV AUD increased by 49.4%, from 8.5% in 2001 to 2002 to 12.6% in 2012 to 2013 among adults.[63]

Consistent with other surveys, data from the NESARC III also show that AUD is higher among males (17.6% 12-month and 36.0% lifetime prevalence) than among females (10.4% 12-month and 22.7% lifetime prevalence).[32] Most studies found that the prevalence of AUD is highest among young adults. For example, prevalence of 12-month AUD was highest among the 18- to 29-year-old age group in the NESARC III, and prevalence decreased among older age groups.[32] In the 2019 NSDUH, 5.3% of people ages 12 and older, including 10.1% of people ages 18 to 25, met criteria for an AUD in the past year using DSM-IV criteria.[64]

Incidence of Alcohol Use Disorders

Data from the 1-year follow-up of the ECA found that, among men, the estimated annual incidence of AUD in the 1-year follow-up of the ECA was 3.7 per 100 person years, and for women, the overall incidence was lower, 0.6 per 100 person years.[65] The peak incidence for both men and women was among those in late adolescence and young adulthood, 18 to 29 years of age. Analyses using the extended follow-up from the Baltimore site of the ECA (mean 12.6 years of follow-up, between 1981 and 1996) show similar trends for the development of alcohol dependence.[66] The most recent prospective data from the NESARC have provided annual incidence rates for DSM-IV AUD (1.66 per 100 person years) and also indicate that the greatest risk for AUD occurs during young adulthood.[67]

NICOTINE DEPENDENCE AND TOBACCO USE DISORDERS

Data from the NESARC III indicate that 20.0% of the adult population met the DSM-5 criteria for nicotine/tobacco use disorder in the prior year and 27.9% have a history of nicotine/tobacco use disorder during their lifetime.[68] The National Youth Tobacco Survey (NYTS) indicates that, in 2021, 27.2% of students from middle through high school that had used a tobacco product experienced cravings for tobacco in the previous 30 days and 19.5% wanted to use a tobacco product within 30 minutes of waking—both of which are indicators of tobacco dependence.[41] The PATH dataset includes measures validated for assessing tobacco dependence among people who smoke both traditional cigarettes and Electronic Drug Delivery Devices (EDDD), also known as e-cigarettes.[53,69,70] In studies using PATH, people who smoke traditional cigarettes are more likely to have higher dependence and consider themselves to have a tobacco/nicotine use disorder in comparison to people who use EDDDs[71,72]; it is possible this perception among people using EDDDs is related to the promotion of these products as an alternative to traditional cigarettes for harm reduction purposes.[73] Higher severity of tobacco dependence are also found to be associated with initiating or continuing co-use of traditional cigarettes and EDDDs.[74]

CANNABIS USE DISORDERS

Data from the NESARC (2001-2002) and the NESARC III (2012-2013) demonstrate that an approximation of DSM-5 cannabis use disorder (CUD) increased from 1.5% in 2001-2002 to 2.9% in 2012 to 2013 among adults ages 18+. However, CUD decreased among people ages 18+ who use cannabis during this same period (35.6% to 30.6%).[75] We should note that the NESARC III allows for the estimation of DSM-5-defined CUD, while only the DSM-IV definition is available in the earlier NESARC. The aforementioned study operationalizes CUD using the DSM-IV definition available in the NESARC III to allow for comparisons with NESARC data; other studies utilize the DSM-5 definition.[76,77] Recent data from the NSDUH indicate that the proportion of participants ages 12 and older with the approximation of CUD in 2002 was similar to the proportion in 2019 (1.8%), with some variation among years.[78] NSDUH data collected from 2002 to 2017 indicate the prevalence of CUD remained unchanged among adults 18 years and older during this period, at approximately 1.4% to 1.5%.[79] The prevalence of CUD decreased during this period among: adults who use cannabis (14.8% to 9.3%); adults who use cannabis daily or nearly daily (33.4% to 19.5%); adults who initiated cannabis use in the past year (7.4% to 2.4%); and, adults who did not initiate cannabis use in the past year (15.1% to 9.6%).[79] This study also approximated DSM-5 CUD diagnoses by examining criteria that overlap between DSM-IV and DSM-5 definitions (of which only the former was available in the NSDUH during this period). It is important to note that this study did not assess DSM-5 criteria for cannabis craving and withdrawal symptoms, since that information was not available in NSDUH data; thus, those earlier data likely underdiagnosed/under-represented the true amounts of cannabis use disorder present in pre-2013 NESARC data. While approximate DSM-5 CUD increased from 2.1% to 2.6% during this period among adults, prevalence decreased among adults who use cannabis and adults who use cannabis daily or almost daily.[79] Prevalence of CUD by age group differs notably, which will be further explored in the Social Determinants of Health, Socio-demographic, and Structural Factors Associated with Substance Use Disorders section.

Incidence of Cannabis Use Disorder

Few studies have explored CUD incidence in the United States. One study in Netherlands studied 199 young adults (18-30 years old) who used cannabis either daily or almost daily over the course of 3 years (2010-2012), and found 36.7% of people developed CUD during the study period.[80] Predictors of CUD incidence included cannabis use during the daytime, continual smoking and coping-related motives for using cannabis.[80] Among people who used cannabis at least five times in the 2007 Australian National Survey of Mental Health and Wellbeing , the cumulative incidence of CUD was 33.3% for all respondents (37% for male and 26.9% for female respondents).[81] The highest rate of onset of CUD was within the first year of cannabis use, with younger age at initiation associated with higher increased risk of transitioning to CUD.[81]

OTHER DRUG USE DISORDERS AND CO-OCCURRING ISSUES

The NESARC III survey has provided data on the prevalence of 12-month and lifetime DSM-5 drug use disorders (DUDs), the most recent edition of the *Diagnostic and Statistical Manual of Mental Disorders*.[19] The NESARC III also assessed the prevalence of DUD involving: sedatives (tranquilizer), opioids, stimulants, hallucinogens, club drugs (such as ecstasy, ketamine, and 3,4-methylenedioxymethamphetamine (MDMA)), and solvents (inhalants).[82] In the 2012 to 2013 NESARC III, 12-month prevalence of DSM-5 DUD was 3.9%, with 1.9% mild and 2.0% moderate to severe. Lifetime prevalence of DSM-5 DUD is 9.9%, with 3.4% mild and 6.6% moderate to severe.[82] Using data from the 2019 NSDUH, 12-month prevalence of any DUD (excluding cannabis, but including cocaine, heroin, hallucinogens, inhalants, methamphetamine, psychotherapeutics, and opioids) based on DSM-IV was 1.5% among participants 12 years of age and older.[64] The following sections will provide a more comprehensive overview of specific DUD that are of particular clinical relevance.

Opioid Use Disorder

People are classified as having an opioid use disorder (OUD) within the 2019 NSDUH if they meet the DSM-IV criteria for either heroin use disorder, prescription pain reliever disorder indicating the nonmedical use of prescription pain relievers, or both.[55] Of participants 12 years and older in the 2019 NSDUH, 0.6% had a past-year OUD, which is a decline from the proportion in 2015 (0.9%).[78] The NSDUH also reports heroin use disorder and prescription pain reliever (eg, hydrocodone, oxycodone, tramadol, oxymorphone, etc.) disorder separately.[55] Among people 12 and older, 0.2% reported a heroin use disorder and 0.5% reported a prescription pain reliever disorder in the 2019 NSDUH;[78] notably, neither measure specifically capture dependence on synthetic opioids, such as fentanyl.

Cocaine, Methamphetamine, and Stimulant Use Disorder

The 2019 NSDUH collects information on different types of stimulants, including cocaine, methamphetamine, and stimulant use disorder. In this survey, 0.4% of participants reported cocaine use disorder, which is a decrease from the percentage with cocaine use disorder in 2002 (0.6%).[78] As of 2015, the NSDUH inquired specifically about methamphetamine use disorder.[55] Methamphetamine use disorder was identified among 0.4% of participants in 2019, which was largely stable between 2015 through 2019.[78] Stimulant use disorder refers specifically to the use of prescription stimulants, including the misuse of prescription amphetamines (eg, Adderall®, Vyvanse®), methylphenidates (eg, Ritalin®) and other prescribed stimulants.[55] 0.2% of 2019 NSDUH participants had a prescription stimulant use disorder in the past year, a proportion which has remained approximately stable since 2015.[78]

Incidence of Drug Use Disorders

There is a relative paucity of information regarding the incidence of DUD overall, with less information available for specific substances. Early findings from the one-year prospective ECA data showed that the incidence of DUD was 1.09 per 100 person years of risk.[65] Analyses of the 3-year prospective NESARC data provided more recent estimates for the rate of development of DUD: annual incidence of DUD was reported to be 0.31 per 100 person years.[67] In both prospective studies, men developed a DUD at a higher rate than women, with the highest rates found for young adults. Incidence rates dropped sharply after young adulthood, and were particularly low or zero among the oldest participants, who are 65 years or older.[65,67]

Co-occurring Psychiatric Disorders

SUD commonly co-occur with psychiatric psychopathology[32,82-87] and are associated with other medical problems and risk for mortality.[88-93] In this section, we focus on co-occurrence between SUD and psychiatric conditions. Early data from the NCS show that most people with a lifetime AUD had at least one other substance use or psychiatric disorder in their lifetime.[24] The prevalence of AUD with another SUD is high. For example, the 12-month prevalence of AUD among those with an SUD in the prior 12 months was more than 50% for most substances assessed in the NESARC.[94] Analyses of the NESARC found positive associations between most SUDs with mood, anxiety, and personality disorders.[32,82] For example, DSM-IV alcohol and drug dependence were associated with all the independent mood and anxiety disorders assessed (those occurring independent from symptoms of withdrawal and intoxication with the substances involved) including major depression, dysthymia, mania, hypomania, social and specific phobia, panic, and generalized anxiety disorders.[95] A large proportion of individuals with personality disorders also have a co-occurring SUD.[32,96] Personality disorders also appear to be associated with the persistence of DUDs.[97] The temporal ordering of co-occurring psychiatric conditions with AUD appears to be bidirectional, although AUD is more commonly the primary condition.[98,99] In addition, some types of comorbidities differ by sex[100-102] and may differ by racial and ethnic group.[103]

The prevalence of psychiatric disorders among individuals in alcohol and drug treatment programs, or drug use among mental health patients in clinical facilities, is higher than in community samples; wide prevalence estimate ranges may depend on the assessment methods, population characteristics, specific diagnoses, and treatment setting.[104-107] Clinical outcomes tend to be worse for individuals with co-occurring psychiatric and SUDs than for those without the comorbid condition (eg, poorer psychological adjustment, worse psychiatric symptoms, reduced treatment effectiveness, greater risk for recurrence of substance use, risky behaviors, homelessness, emergency room visits, rehospitalization, and co-occurrence of medical problems).[108-118] Assessments of long-term outcomes highlight the impact that co-occurring conditions can have on the level of functioning, clinical status, and attainment in areas of educational level, occupation, and social relationships.[118-121] As more information becomes available from longitudinal studies, it will be possible to better assess these temporal relationships. In addition, future investigations into the progression of symptoms will improve our understanding of possible etiological relationships and should provide valuable information of potential clinical and treatment applications.

SOCIAL DETERMINANTS OF HEALTH, SOCIODEMOGRAPHIC, AND STRUCTURAL FACTORS ASSOCIATED WITH SUBSTANCE USE DISORDERS

Studies have examined social determinants of health and structural factors (eg, state-level drug policies) which increase the risk for SUD, including both AUD and DUD. We note that these factors often interact, which we have illustrated where possible, and are common across SUD. This section is restricted to a subset of individual characteristics found to be associated with alcohol and SUD and is by no means exhaustive. Social determinants and structural factors impacting the development and/or persistence of SUD are largely understudied. Our understanding of these issues will grow with future knowledge gained from investment in citizen science, epidemiological research, life course approaches, and advancements in neuroscience.

Age

Age correlates with the occurrence of SUDs. Data from the NESARC III demonstrates that AUD peaks in the twenties, with a prevalence of 32% for men at age 25 and 24% for women at age 22, with a gradual decrease in prevalence with age.[122] Similarly, incidence of AUD generally declines with age.[66,67] The hazard rate for DSM-IV alcohol abuse and dependence was reported to be highest at approximately age 19, and a steady reduction in hazard with increasing age was found.[27] The highest prevalence and incidence rates for DUDs are found among individuals in late adolescence and young adulthood.[65,67,82] NESARC III data indicates that the prevalence of CUD peaked at around age 18, with a prevalence of 13% for men and 7% for women, which subsequently declined with age.[122] Similarly, prevalence of OUD largely decreases with age after young adulthood; however, gender differences appear in prevalence by age, with women having a higher prevalence than men in older age.[122] Onset of DUD is the highest at approximately age 19, with sharp declines thereafter, so that hazard rates after age 25 are relatively low.[123] In addition, early onset of drug use is associated with elevated risk for subsequent DUD.[124-128] As with AUD, incidence of DUD decreases with age.[66,67]

Lower prevalence of AUD among older adults than younger age groups[27,32,129] may occur for several reasons. Because the measure of prevalence depends on the incidence as well as the duration of the disease,[1,2,4] AUD may be less prevalent among the elderly because the incidence decreases over the life span, the duration of the disorder is reduced, or some combination of the two factors is in effect. In terms of the duration of disorder being reduced, it may be a result of an increase in remission with age or a reduction in survival. In other words, with age, prevalence may be reduced because fewer individuals develop the disorder, because the substance-related problems have resolved, or because of premature mortality among people with SUD, or a combination of these factors. Explanations for a decreased prevalence with age also may include a reduced tolerance to alcohol with age,[130] poorer recall among older adults, or a cohort effect.[131] Further, AUD measurement in young adults may not generalize to older populations,[132-136] leading to unhealthy alcohol use and disorder being underrecognized in older adults.[134,136,137] Problems related to alcohol use among the elderly may occur at lower levels of consumption than in younger adults, and older adults with AUD may be at greater risk for co-occurring problems.[138-140] Surveys that include only household participants may miss people with AUD who reside in nursing homes. Although incidence is low among older adults, and survival may be decreased for individuals with SUD as they age, other factors, such as age–period–cohort effects, may be involved.

As described in the Epidemiological Principles section, age–period–cohort effects can explain differences in prevalence and incidence of SUDs. When analyzing data from a population, age–period–cohort effects can be obscured[141]; disentangling changes by age, period, and cohort can give researchers a better understanding of the landscape of SUDs. Some studies show that patterns of SUDs have changed and show a greater prevalence among cohorts born since World War II, starting with Baby Boomers.[49,142] For example, the risk of nicotine dependence has been reported to be greatest among people in the more recent birth cohorts who smoked tobacco.[143] Data from the *Monitoring the Future* study following U.S. adults who reached the age of 45 from 2003 to 2016 found that the prevalence of AUD symptoms decreased between ages 35 to 45; the rate of decrease slowed across cohorts, lending evidence to cohort effects.[144] Earlier age of onset of alcohol use among women observed in more recent birth cohorts has also been thought to be a possible explanation for the rise in prevalence of AUD among women,[145] early initiation is associated with greater with risk for subsequent AUD.[146] Further evidence examining birth cohort associations with initiation of use for specific substances also indicates that more recent birth cohorts are more likely to initiate drug use in childhood and early adolescence, particularly for cannabis, cocaine, and nonmedical use of drugs,[147] including nonmedical use of analgesics.[148,149] These patterns are also reported in other global areas (eg, U.S., Europe, South Africa, Australia).[49,150-152] However, in some analyses, there is evidence of a broader period effect across all age cohorts, which may explain the recent rise of cannabis use in the United States.[153] Researchers identified age–period–cohort effects in relation to nonmedical prescription OUDs using data from several nationally representative studies, with findings demonstrating higher rates of prescription OUD in each successive birth cohort.[141,149]

Self-identified Racial and Ethnic Group Membership

Information on the relationship between SUDs and racial and ethnic group membership is complex and sometimes conflicting. Racial and ethnic group membership is socially constructed and related to the types of racism and differential treatment that minoritized groups experience.[154-158] Some of the inconsistent findings result from the relative paucity of data involving distinct ethnic and racial subgroups, different classifications used to group ethnic minoritized groups leading to measurement error, variations in the social acceptability of drinking and drug use patterns within cultural groups, and the relationship of socioeconomic status and the availability of health care to racial and ethnic minority populations.

AUD is associated with immigration status, acculturation, discrimination, and ethnic identity.[159-161] Prevalence of lifetime AUD among Black adults is lower relative to White adults.[32,162,163] Although the odds of AUD tend to be lower for Black people compared with White people; Black people tend to experience more medical and social consequences from drinking, including injuries, higher mortality, and psychiatric comorbidity.[103,164-168] This may relate to differences in socioeconomic status, access to health care, health service utilization, and drinking trajectories over the life span as well as social and cultural environments and structural racism.[103,158,166,169-173] For example, neighborhood poverty may have a greater effect on problems related to unhealthy alcohol use among Black men relative to White or Hispanic men.[171] When socioeconomic factors are taken into account, differences due to race and ethnicity can be attenuated.[174-176]

In many reports, prevalence of AUD is lower for Hispanic people relative to White individuals.[32,64] Yet, alcohol-related mortality is higher for Hispanic men relative to non-Hispanic White men, and deaths from liver cirrhosis differ by race as well as ethnicity.[165,177,178] Drinking trajectories, prevalence, and incidence of alcohol-related problems and use disorders vary among people from different Hispanic subgroups in the United States,[169,178-184] and variations may reflect factors such as social and cultural environment, degree of acculturation, country of national origin, generational status, and time since immigration.[179,185-189] In some studies, acculturation has been found to relate to binge drinking and AUD in addition to characteristics that may relate to drinking such as suicide attempts and self-reported health status;[186-190] associations may differ by gender.[178]

Asian American people generally have the lowest prevalence of AUD in the United States.[32,64] Data from the 2019 NSDUH indicate that the lowest prevalence of AUD among people 12 and older is reported by people who identify as Asian (3.3%); people with AUD who identify as two or more races have the highest prevalence (6.5%).[64] However, as with Hispanic American people, the Asian American population is largely heterogeneous and composed of many subgroups with different backgrounds and cultural drinking patterns.[191,192] Distinguishing subgroups of Asian Americans (eg, Indian American or Korean Americans) could further elucidate SUD-related burdens in the U.S.

Indigenous American individuals historically,[32,64,193] and individuals from two or more racial groups more recently, have the highest prevalence of AUD in the United States (6.4% and 6.5%, respectively, according to the 2019 NSDUH).[64] Indigenous American people also have the highest drinking-related death rates.[166,194,195] However, these findings are not consistent across all studies,[196] and it is not accurate to generalize findings to all Indigenous American populations. Notably, drinking practices vary across groups[197-199] and cultural factors as well as socioeconomic characteristics and psychiatric symptoms may play a role in substance-related burden.[193,200,201]

Prevalence of DUDs vary by race and ethnicity,[64,202] gender and number of substances used—with those with polysubstance use being more likely to have persistent conditions.[203,204] Reports using data from the 2019 NSDUH indicate that the occurrence of past year DUD (including both CUD and other DUDs like cocaine or heroin) among individuals 12 years of age and older was highest among Indigenous Indian and Alaska Native people, and among those indicating two or more races, and lowest for Asian American people.[64] Similar relationships were documented in analyses of 12-month prevalence using the NESARC III, although there was no documentation for those from two or more racial subgroups.[82] However, there is limited evidence for differences in incidence of DUD by race and ethnicity as assessed with the prospective NESARC data.[67] In assessments of specific nonmedical prescription drug use and disorders (sedative, tranquilizer, opioid, and stimulants), relative to White people, people who identify as Black, Asian, and Hispanic were less likely and Indigenous American people were more likely to report lifetime SUD.[205,206] As with AUD, DUDs also vary by immigration status, country of origin, acculturation, discrimination, and socioeconomic status.[159,207-214] Patterns of comorbidity, and drug-related correlates and consequences, such as arrest risk, also vary by race and ethnicity.[215-219] Furthermore, there are racial and ethnic differences in service utilization as well as disparities in treatment of SUDs.[220-225] Addressing socioeconomic disparities and barriers to treatment, as well as cultural competency in treatment settings, could improve treatment outcomes across racial and ethnic groups.[226-230]

Sex and Gender

AUD, and SUDs broadly, are more common among males than among females. This finding has been shown in a number of cross-sectional surveys,[24,27,32,54,64] as well as in prospective studies.[65,67,231] In the 2019 NSDUH, the occurrence of past year AUD was slightly less than twofold greater for males (7.0% and 3.9% for males and females, respectively), with evidence from two national surveys finding that men progressed to alcohol dependence at a greater rate than women.[43] However, different age groups demonstrate sex and gender differences in AUDs; among people ages 12 to 17, the proportion of AUDs are higher among females then males (2.1% and 1.3%).[64] Studies in the United States[49] and other countries[232-234] over the past couple of decades provide evidence that the gender gap for prevalence of AUD is narrowing with declines in AUD being slower among women,[144] perhaps as the result of changes in drinking patterns.[49,232-236] Further, the increasing trends regarding AUD observed in nationally representative data have largely been concentrated among women.[63] Changes in AUD diagnoses among women are posited to be a result of shifting social norms or related to changes brought about by the increased number of women in the labor force, as well as the combined input of home and work environments.[237,238] Compounding stressors related to employment combined with more permissive drinking cultures could be pushing more women to engage in risky drinking.[63] While this pertains to alcohol use and not AUD, increases in binge-drinking among women are largely concentrated among women employed in careers with occupational prestige,[239] with higher incomes, and who are highly educated.[240,241] This could lend insight into changes in AUD diagnoses. Further, changes in social norms including gender, religion and family attitudes are important mediators of the cohort effects on gendered differences in alcohol consumption.[242] Many characteristics (eg, marital status, children in the home, full-time employment, ethnicity, age, occupation, educational level), as well as the occurrence of life events, and the presence of other psychopathology (such as depression) may play a role in gender variability with respect to alcohol consumption and the development of AUD.[243,244] There may be associations between physical or sexual violence and the occurrence of AUD.[245] Additionally, a potential predictor of women's risk for alcohol and SUD is a history of childhood maltreatment.[246,247]

There are sex and gender differences with respect to DUDs, as well. Boys and men generally have a higher prevalence[64,82,122] and incidence[67] of DUD than women. The 2019 NSDUH indicates that the prevalence of past year DUD and CUD was approximately 1.5 times higher for males (3.7%) than females (2.4%).[64] In the NCS Replication, males had a higher risk of progression from first use to cannabis dependence than females, but there were relatively small sex differences in progression risk for alcohol and cocaine.[248] NESARC III data indicate that while prevalence of SUDs are largely higher among men than women, the prevalence of OUD is higher among women than among men at older ages.[122]

Sexual Orientation and Identity

The prevalence of SUD differs by sexual orientation. Adults who identify as lesbian, gay, bisexual, those who are unsure about their sexual identity, or who report being attracted to same-sex people and/or report current same-sex sexual partners, have higher rates of DSM-5 AUD compared to adults who self-identify as heterosexual and report only opposite sex attraction or sexual partners.[249] Findings from the NESARC III suggest that while the prevalence for AUD is approximately 17% among heterosexual adults, the prevalence is about 30% (31.5% for males and 29.3% for females) among adults who are gay, lesbian, or bisexual.[250] This difference, with lesbian, gay, and bisexual adults having a higher prevalence of AUD than heterosexual adults, persists across ages 18 to 55.[250] Gay and bisexual men have the highest prevalence of AUD between the ages of 18 to 45, whereas lesbian, gay, and bisexual women have the highest prevalence of AUD between the ages of 45 to 55.[250] People who identify as bisexual, or who report being unsure of their sexual identity, have the highest likelihood of endorsing criteria for DSM-5 AUD.[249]

Similar to AUD, prevalence of DUD differs among people who identify as lesbian, gay, and bisexual.[251-253] Data from the NESARC III suggests that past-year DSM-5 tobacco use disorder is more prevalent among lesbian, gay, and bisexual adults in comparison to heterosexual adults.[251,254] One study found that women who identify as bisexual, gay/lesbian, or were unsure of their sexual orientation had a higher prevalence of past-year DUD (excluding alcohol and nicotine) in comparison to heterosexual women; this was not observed for men who identify as gay, bisexual, or unsure of their sexual orientation.[252] Similarly, one study found women who identify as lesbian, gay, or bisexual to have higher proportions of cannabis and tobacco use disorders, while only men who identify as bisexual have higher proportions of tobacco use disorder (and not CUD) in comparison to heterosexuals.[254] Data from the 2015 and 2016 NSDUH indicate that bisexual females have higher odds of SUD across all ages in comparison to heterosexuals; while lesbian or gay females and gay or bisexual males had higher odds of SUD than their heterosexual peers at certain ages, bisexual females were the only subgroup to consistently have higher odds across the lifespan.[253] More recent data (pooled 2015-2019 NSDUH data) indicates that gay, lesbian, and bisexual adults all have higher odds of CUD in comparison to heterosexual adults.[255]

The greater burden of SUDs among lesbian, gay, and bisexual adults is posited to be a result of discrimination and stigma. People reporting higher levels of discrimination as a result of sexual orientation also reporting higher levels of AUD severity.[249] Data from the NESARC III suggest that associations between discrimination and AUD is indicated among men (strongest in the mid-twenties through the late-forties and early fifties) and women.[250] Prior work exploring stress and discrimination found that, among men and women, people in lesbian, gay, and bisexual subgroups reported more stressful life events than heterosexual people; more stressful life events were associated with higher rates of SUDs (ie, alcohol, cannabis, and tobacco).[254]

Social Factors

Employment, Occupation, and Income

Most of the evidence presented in this section is derived from nationally representative cross-sectional studies, which lack temporality. Unless temporal relationships can be established,[256] we cannot rule out *reverse causality*. It is often not possible to determine whether lack of employment led to SUD via financial strain or whether SUD resulted in job loss, inability to obtain work, or selection into a specific occupation. Additionally, limitations of household surveys (such as the NSDUH) include selection bias resulting from non-response and measurement issues. It is possible that the exposure of interest, namely, employment or income, could be associated with non-response. Future research is needed with longitudinal data to further disentangle the role of employment, occupation, and income on SUDs. Nevertheless, insightful research suggests associations between finances and SUDs, which will be further explored in this section.

Financial positioning and issues causing financial concern, such as unemployment, job loss, or other financial stressors, can be intertwined with SUDs. Generally, in the U.S., perceptions of financial strain increase risk of SUDs.[257] Similar to the patterns as described for employment, people with the lowest income (ranging from \$0-\$19,999) have the highest prevalence of CUDs (5.4%) using NESARC III data; people with the highest income (≥\$70,000) have the lowest prevalence of CUD (1.5%).[75] People with CUD, AUD or both (ie, co-occurring CUD and AUD), all had higher odds of experiencing financial problems in comparison to people with no disorder, which included job loss, unemployment, homelessness, and unrepayable debt.[258] People with co-occurring CUD and AUD had a higher likelihood of reporting unemployment and unrepayable debt in comparison to people with only AUD.[258]

Employment status is related to the prevalence of AUD,[259-261] though associations with employment status may differ by specific substance type. Data from the 2019 NSDUH show that, among people 18 years of age and older, people working full-time or part-time have a lower prevalence of AUD (6.7% and 5.7%, respectively) in comparison to people who are unemployed (9.5%).[64] In the 2019 NSDUH, a higher proportion of DUDs (including cannabis and other DUDs) were reported among individuals who were unemployed (9.0%) in comparison to those employed part-time (3.5%) and full-time (2.7%) among people 18 years and older.[64]

The prevalence of AUD as well as alcohol-related morbidity and mortality differs by type of occupation,[259,261,262] which is also related to income. People in occupations involving manual labor report a higher prevalence of AUD and higher mortality from disease or injuries related to alcohol.[261-263] However, some find that employment in high occupational strata or in nonlabor jobs is associated with alcohol-related outcomes.[262,264] Findings from analyses of the NCS indicate that high occupational strata are associated with DUDs.[264] Further, as with AUD, there appear to be differences in the prevalence of DUDs and associated with specific occupations.[265]

Educational Level

Educational level often is included as part of broader socioeconomic or social class characteristics,[266] and studies of the relationship between educational level and drinking patterns as well as the development of AUD may yield conflicting results. Data from the 2019 NSDUH suggest that people who have completed some college have the highest prevalence of AUD (6.2%), followed closely however by both people with less than a high school education (5.4%) and with a college degree (5.4%).[64] However, data from the NESARC illustrates that people without a college degree have a higher risk of alcohol dependence relative to those with a college degree or more.[267] In a Swedish cohort, higher school achievement during adolescence and young adulthood was associated with reduced incidence of AUD.[268] Moreover, dropping out of high school or leaving college early is associated with an increased risk of AUD in adulthood.[175] These associations are bidirectional in that AUDs are associated with the level of subsequent educational achievement.[269] It should also be noted that the relationship between educational attainment and AUD may differ by race and ethnicity; for example, results from the NESERC show no relationship between educational attainment and alcohol dependence among people who identify as Hispanic.[267,270]

Lifetime prevalence of DUDs also vary by educational level. Data from the 2019 NSDUH indicate that the proportion of people with prior year DUD (including cannabis and other illegal DUDs) is lowest for college graduates (1.7%) in comparison to people with less than high school, high school, or some college education (3.3%, 3.5%, 3.7%, respectively).[64] Specifically in reference to CUD, studies using NESARC and NESARC III data found statistically significant increases in DSM-IV CUD across education levels; people who reported completing some college (the highest level of education attainment) had lower prevalence of CUD (2.5%), compared to people who completed less than high school (3.3%) or high school (3.7%).[75]

Marital Status

Marital status has been found to be related to the occurrence of AUD, but as discussed regarding employment status, understanding the temporal relationships may be difficult.[271,272] SUD may predate marital status changes, and problems associated with drinking and drug use may be causally related with marital status. Analyses of the NESARC indicate that individuals who never married or are separated, divorced, or widowed are more likely than are married or cohabiting couples to have prevalent or incident AUD.[32,67] Persons in stable marriages or cohabiting had the lowest 12-month prevalence of AUD (10.4%), as opposed to adults who had never married (25.0%) or who were widowed, divorced, or separated (11.4%).[32] Marriage has been shown to relate to decreases in subsequent risk for AUD for both men and women, and this potentially protective association was found to be strongest for those with a positive family history of AUD.[271] Divorce and widowhood appear to increase risk for AUD; subsequent remarriage, among those previously divorced, is associated with reduction in risk.[273]

Prevalence of DUD also varies by marital status. In the NESARC, adults who never married (and were not cohabiting with a partner) have the highest prevalence of DUD.[82] Adults who report being unmarried in the NESARC had the highest prevalence of CUD (7.3%), while married adults had the lowest prevalence (1.4%).[75] Lack of marital stability and the periods of transition to and from marriage or divorce have also been associated with substance use, treatment outcomes, and drug-related mortality.[274-279]

Structural Factors

Many structural and systemic factors have an impact on SUD. In this section, we detail state-level drug use policies, specifically. However, it is important to note that stigma and discrimination, and the stress incurred from encounters of discrimination, can impact SUDs and other substance use-related health outcomes.[280-283]

State-Level Drug Use Policies

Several empirical studies clearly demonstrate SUD arise in the context of complex socio-ecological systems, including risks at the individual-level, proximal family-level (ie, household composition), and community-levels (ie, neighborhood and school environment).[284-291] However, aside from some notable exceptions, few studies consider potential causes at the structural level.[292-294] In particular, most structural-level studies focused on drug use policies, mainly opioid and cannabis state-level policies, and few of them focus on SUD as an outcome.[295-303] For example, one study conducted with state-level NSDUH data on cannabis use as treatment (CUAT), also referred to as medical use, do not observe any significant increases in past-year CUD prevalence for any age or gender group after CUAT law enactment.[304] The broader state policy context may also modify the effects of CUAT laws on cannabis use and CUD. One study examined the association between state-level policy liberalism and past-year CUD for individuals aged 12 to 17, 18 to 25, and 26+. CUD among those using cannabis was lower in liberal states compared to conservative states for ages 12 to 17 (-2.87 percentage points; $p = 0.045$) and ages 26+ (-2.45 percentage points; $p = 0.05$).[305] Additional research is needed as effects of policy changes could impact rates of SUDs further into the future. Another example of structural policies, statewide cannabis decriminalization and legalization policies, disproportionately impact racial and ethnic groups. For example, a case-control study examining the impact of implementing cannabis decriminalization or legalization found differential policy effects among race-based arrests; states not implementing any policy change had no significant increases in arrests for White people, but increased arrest rates for Black people, emphasizing the persistence of racial disparities in cannabis-related arrests.[306]

SUBSTANCE USE DISORDER REMISSION AND TREATMENT

Remission from SUD in community samples varies by individual characteristics[307,308] and subtype of disorder based on age of onset, family history, specific disorder criteria, and concurrent conditions including other substance use and psychiatric disorders.[309-312] Maintaining remission is also dependent on consumption patterns while in remission. Data from the NESARC indicates maintenance of successful recovery from DSM-IV alcohol dependence was greatest for people who abstained from alcohol as compared with other groups in remission that continued to drink.[313]

Only a minority of individuals with SUD report using treatment services (including self-help groups, employee assistance programs, inpatient and outpatient facilities, rehabilitation centers, crisis centers, healthcare professionals, halfway houses, and withdrawal management units).[27,32,51,82,123,314-317] Based on the data from the NESARC III, Grant et al. found that only 13.5% of those with 12-month and 24.6% of individuals with lifetime DUD reported receiving treatment.[82] Among those with AUD, the proportion receiving treatment was even lower (7.7% among those with 12-month AUD and 19.8% of those with lifetime AUD).[32] A greater proportion of individuals with moderate or severe SUD enter treatment,[32,82] and in some reports, treatment is positively associated with having a co-occurring psychiatric disorder.[123] The relationship between co-occurring psychiatric disorders and treatment is complex; some psychiatric disorders (eg, bipolar disorder, avoidant and schizoid personality disorders) increase probability of seeking treatment for SUDs, while others (eg, specific phobias, narcissistic personality disorder) decrease probability of seeking treatment.[318] A more recent report using 2019 NSDUH data finds that only 27.8% of people who need treatment for OUD received medication for OUD in the past year, the gold standard to treat OUD.[319] Treatment use, and specifically medication, among people needing treatment was particularly low for certain age groups: no adolescents and only 13.2% of adults over the age of 50 reported past-year medication for OUD in 2019.[319]

CONCLUSIONS

This chapter summarized a sampling of major findings in epidemiological studies of SUDs. The ultimate goals for the study of SUD epidemiology are to improve our understanding of causal mechanisms, identify targets for prevention and intervention, and reduce the prevalence of SUD. For the epidemiology of SUDs to advance as a field, we need to pay particular attention to measurement of SUD and the role of social determinants of health as well as of structural factors to truly uncover mechanisms of action and trajectories of SUDs.

REFERENCES

1. Gordis L. *Epidemiology E-Book*. Elsevier Health Sciences; 2013.
2. Lilienfeld DE, Lilienfeld AM, Stolley PD. *Foundations of Epidemiology*. USA: Oxford University Press; 1994.
3. Porta M. *A Dictionary of Epidemiology*. Oxford University Press; 2014.
4. Mausner JS, Bahn AK. *Epidemiology: An Introductory Text*. 1974.
5. Aschengrau A, Seage GR. *Essentials of Epidemiology in Public Health*. Jones & Bartlett Learning; 2013.
6. Shafer G. Conditional probability. *Int Stat Rev Rev Int Stat*. 1985;53(3):261-275.
7. Rothman KJ, Greenland S, Lash TL. *Modern Epidemiology*. Vol. 3 Wolters Kluwer Health/Lippincott Williams & Wilkins; 2008.
8. Altman CE. Age, period, and cohort effects. Bean FD, Brown SK, eds. *Encyclopedia of Migration*. Springer; 2014:1-4.
9. Yang Y, Land KC. Age–period–cohort analysis of repeated cross-section surveys: fixed or random effects? *Soc Method Res*. 2008;36(3):297-326.
10. Blanchard RD, Bunker JB, Wachs M. Distinguishing aging, period and cohort effects in longitudinal studies of elderly populations. *Socio-Econ Plan Sci*. 1977;11(3):137-146.
11. Keyes KM, Utz RL, Robinson W, Li G. What is a cohort effect? Comparison of three statistical methods for modeling cohort effects in obesity prevalence in the United States, 1971-2006. *Soc Sci Med*. 2010;70(7):1100-1108.
12. Office of Disease Prevention and Health Promotion. *Healthy People 2030: Social Determinants of Health*. U.S. Department of Health and Human Services Accessed October 26, 2022. https://health.gov/healthypeople/priority-areas/social-determinants-health
13. Braveman P, Egerter S, Williams DR. The social determinants of health: coming of age. *Annu Rev Public Health*. 2011;32(1):381-398.
14. Braveman P, Gottlieb L. The social determinants of health: it's time to consider the causes of the causes. *Public Health Rep*. 2014;129(1 Suppl 2): 19-31.
15. Britannica ProCon.org. State-by-State Recreational Marijuana Laws. Accessed July 15, 2022. https://marijuana.procon.org/legal-recreational-marijuana-states-and-dc/
16. Solomon R. Racism and its effect on Cannabis research. *Cannabis Cannabinoid Res*. 2020;5(1):2-5.
17. Gonçalves PD, Gutkind S, Segura LE, Castaldelli-Maia JM, Martins SS, Mauro PM. Simultaneous alcohol/Cannabis use and driving under the influence in the U.S. *Am J Prev Med*. 2022;62(5):661-669.
18. Flanagin A, Frey T, Christiansen SL, Bauchner H. The reporting of race and ethnicity in medical and science journals: comments invited. *JAMA*. 2021;325(11):1049-1052.
19. American Psychiatric Association. *Diagnostic and statistical manual of mental disorders: DSM-5™*. 5th ed. American Psychiatric Publishing, Inc; 2013.
20. World Health Organization. *The ICD-10 Classification of Mental and Behavioural Disorders: Clinical Descriptions and Diagnostic Guidelines*. World Health Organization; 1992.
21. Eaton WW, Kessler LG. *Epidemiologic Field Methods in Psychiatry: The NIMH Epidemiologic Catchment Area Program*. Academic Press; 2012.
22. Eaton WW, Kramer M, Anthony JC, Chee EML, Shapiro S. Conceptual and methodological problems in estimation of the incidence of mental disorders from field survey data. In: Cooper B, Helgason T, eds. *Epidemiology and the Prevention of Mental Disorders*. Taylor & Frances; 1989:108-127.
23. Robins LN, Regier DA. *Psychiatric Disorders in America: The Epidemiologic Catchment Area Study*. The Free Press/MacMillan, Inc; 1991.
24. Kessler RC, Crum RM, Warner LA, Nelson CB, Schulenberg J, Anthony JC. Lifetime co-occurrence of DSM-III-R alcohol abuse and dependence with other psychiatric disorders in the National Comorbidity Survey. *Arch Gen Psychiatry*. 1997;54(4):313-321.
25. Kessler RC, Little RJ, Groves RM. Advances in strategies for minimizing and adjusting for survey nonresponse. *Epidemiol Rev*. 1995;17(1): 192-204.
26. Kessler RC, McGonagle KA, Nelson CB, Hughes M, Swartz M, Blazer DG. Sex and depression in the National Comorbidity Survey. II: Cohort effects. *J Affect Disord*. 1994;30(1):15-26.
27. Hasin DS, Stinson FS, Ogburn E, Grant BF. Prevalence, correlates, disability, and comorbidity of DSM-IV alcohol abuse and dependence in the United States: results from the National Epidemiologic Survey on Alcohol and Related Conditions. *Arch Gen Psychiatry*. 2007;64(7): 830-842.
28. Guze SB. Diagnostic and statistical manual of mental disorders, 4th ed. (DSM-IV). *Am J Psychiatry*. 1995;152(8):1228-1228.
29. Ruan WJ, Goldstein RB, Chou SP, et al. The alcohol use disorder and associated disabilities interview schedule-IV (AUDADIS-IV): reliability of new psychiatric diagnostic modules and risk factors in a general population sample. *Drug Alcohol Depend*. 2008;92(1–3):27-36.
30. Grant BF, Harford TC, Dawson DA, Chou PS, Pickering RP. The alcohol use disorder and associated disabilities interview schedule (AUDADIS): reliability of alcohol and drug modules in a general population sample. *Drug Alcohol Depend*. 1995;39(1):37-44.
31. Dawson DA, Goldstein RB, Saha TD, Grant BF. Changes in alcohol consumption: United States, 2001-2002 to 2012-2013. *Drug Alcohol Depend*. 2015;148:56-61.
32. Grant BF, Goldstein RB, Saha TD, et al. Epidemiology of DSM-5 alcohol use disorder: results from the National Epidemiologic Survey on Alcohol and Related Conditions III. *JAMA Psychiatry*. 2015;72(8):757-766.
33. Center for Behavioral Health Statistics and Quality. *National Survey on Drug Use and Health: 2014 and 2015 Redesign Changes*. Substance Abuse and Mental Health Services Administration; 2015.
34. RTI International. National Survey on Drug Use and Health (NSDUH): About the Survey. Accessed July 12, 2022. https://nsduhweb.rti.org/respweb/about_nsduh.html
35. Substance Abuse and Mental Health Services Administration (SAMHSA). 2002 National Survey on Drug Use and Health (NSDUH):

Population Data. Accessed August 3, 2022. https://www.datafiles.samhsa.gov/dataset/national-survey-drug-use-and-health-2002-nsduh-2002-ds0001

36. Substance Abuse and Mental Health Services Administration (SAMHSA). 2020 National Survey of Drug Use and Health (NSDUH) Releases. Accessed July 12, 2022. https://www.samhsa.gov/data/release/2020-national-survey-drug-use-and-health-nsduh-releases
37. Substance Abuse and Mental Health Services Administration (SAMHSA). *2020 National Survey on Drug Use and Health (NSDUH): Methodological Summary and Definitions*. Substance Abuse and Mental Health Services Administration; 2021.
38. Hyland A, Ambrose BK, Conway KP, et al. Design and methods of the Population Assessment of Tobacco and Health (PATH) Study. *Tobacco Control*. 2017;26(4):371-378.
39. United States Department of Health Human Services, National Institutes of Health, National Institute on Drug Abuse, United States Department of Health Human Services, Food Drug Administration, Center for Tobacco Products. Population Assessment of Tobacco and Health (PATH) Study [United States] Restricted-Use Files. *Inter-University Consortium for Political and Social Research [Distributor]*; 2022.
40. Office on Smoking and Health. *National Youth Tobacco Survey: Methodology Report*. Atlanta, GA: U.S. Department of Health and Human Services, Centers for Disease Control and Prevention, National Center for Chronic Disease Prevention and Health Promotion, Office on Smoking and Health; 2021.
41. Gentzke AS, Wang TW, Cornelius M, et al. Tobacco product use and associated factors among middle and high school students—National Youth Tobacco Survey, United States, 2021. *MMWR Surveill Summ*. 2022;71(5):1-29.
42. Schulenberg JE, Johnston LD, O'Malley PM, Bachman JG, Miech RA, Patrick ME. *Monitoring the Future National Survey Results on Drug Use, 1975-2019. Volume II, College Students & Adults Ages 19-60*. Institute for Social Research, University of Michigan; 2020.
43. Keyes KM, Martins SS, Blanco C, Hasin DS. Telescoping and gender differences in alcohol dependence: new evidence from two national surveys. *Am J Psychiatry*. 2010;167(8):969-976.
44. Keyes KM, Miech R. Age, period, and cohort effects in heavy episodic drinking in the US from 1985 to 2009. *Drug Alcohol Depend*. 2013; 132(1-2):140-148.
45. Keyes KM, Rutherford C, Hamilton A, Palamar JJ. Age, period, and cohort effects in synthetic cannabinoid use among US adolescents, 2011–2015. *Drug Alcohol Depend*. 2016;166:159-167.
46. Martins SS, Santaella J, Pacek LR, et al. Are medical marijuana users different than recreational marijuana users? *Drug Alcohol Depend*. 2015;156:e141.
47. Cerdá M, Sarvet AL, Wall M, et al. Medical marijuana laws and adolescent use of marijuana and other substances: alcohol, cigarettes, prescription drugs, and other illicit drugs. *Drug Alcohol Depend*. 2018;183:62-68.
48. Sarvet AL, Wall MM, Fink DS, et al. Medical marijuana laws and adolescent marijuana use in the United States: a systematic review and meta-analysis. *Addiction*. 2018;113(6):1003-1016.
49. Keyes KM, Li G, Hasin DS. Birth cohort effects and gender differences in alcohol epidemiology: a review and synthesis. *Alcohol Clin Exp Res*. 2011;35(12):2101-2112.
50. Huang X, Keyes KM, Li G. Increasing prescription opioid and heroin overdose mortality in the United States, 1999-2014: an age-period-cohort analysis. *Am J Public Health*. 2018;108(1):131-136.
51. Askari MS, Keyes KM, Mauro PM. Cannabis use disorder treatment use and perceived treatment need in the United States: time trends and age differences between 2002 and 2019. *Drug Alcohol Depend*. 2021; 229(Pt A):109154.
52. National Institute on Alcohol Abuse and Alcoholism (NIAAA). Alcohol Use Disorder: A Comparison Between DSM–IV and DSM–5. National Institutes of Health (NIH). Accessed July 28, 2022. https://www.niaaa.nih.gov/publications/brochures-and-fact-sheets/alcohol-use-disorder-comparison-between-dsm
53. Strong DR, Pearson J, Ehlke S, et al. Indicators of dependence for different types of tobacco product users: Descriptive findings from Wave 1 (2013-2014) of the Population Assessment of Tobacco and Health (PATH) study. *Drug Alcohol Depend*. 2017;178:257-266.
54. Kessler RC, McGonagle KA, Zhao S, et al. Lifetime and 12-month prevalence of DSM-III-R psychiatric disorders in the United States. Results from the National Comorbidity Survey. *Arch Gen Psychiatry*. 1994;51(1):8-19.
55. Substance Abuse and Mental Health Services Administration (SAMHSA). 2019 National Survey on Drug Use and Health (NSDUH): Methodological Summary and Definitions. Accessed July 12, 2022. https://www.samhsa.gov/data/sites/default/files/reports/rpt29395/2019NSDUHMethodsSummDefs/2019NSDUHMethodsSummDefs082120.pdf
56. Townsend L, Flisher AJ, King G. A systematic review of the relationship between high school dropout and substance use. *Clin Child Family Psychol Rev*. 2007;10(4):295-317.
57. Grucza RA, Abbacchi AM, Przybeck TR, Gfroerer JC. Discrepancies in estimates of prevalence and correlates of substance use and disorders between two national surveys. *Addiction*. 2007;102(4):623-629.
58. Narrow WE, Rae DS, Robins LN, Regier DA. Revised prevalence estimates of mental disorders in the United States: using a clinical significance criterion to reconcile 2 surveys' estimates. *Arch Gen Psychiatry*. 2002;59(2):115-123.
59. Degenhardt L, Bohnert KM, Anthony JC. Assessment of cocaine and other drug dependence in the general population: "gated" versus "ungated" approaches. *Drug Alcohol Depend*. 2008;93(3):227-232.
60. Degenhardt L, Bohnert KM, Anthony JC. Case ascertainment of alcohol dependence in general population surveys: 'gated' versus 'ungated' approaches. *Int J Methods Psychiatr Res*. 2007;16(3):111-123.
61. Hasin DS, Grant BF. The co-occurrence of DSM-IV alcohol abuse in DSM-IV alcohol dependence: results of the National Epidemiologic Survey on Alcohol and Related Conditions on heterogeneity that differ by population subgroup. *Arch Gen Psychiatry*. 2004;61(9):891-896.
62. Hasin DS, Hatzenbueler M, Smith S, Grant BF. Co-occurring DSM-IV drug abuse in DSM-IV drug dependence: results from the National Epidemiologic Survey on Alcohol and Related Conditions. *Drug Alcohol Depend*. 2005;80(1):117-123.
63. Grant BF, Chou SP, Saha TD, et al. Prevalence of 12-month alcohol use, high-risk drinking, and DSM-IV alcohol use disorder in the United States, 2001-2002 to 2012-2013: results from the national epidemiologic survey on alcohol and related conditions. *JAMA Psychiatry*. 2017;74(9):911-923.
64. Substance Abuse and Mental Health Services Administration (SAMHSA). 2019 National Survey of Drug Use and Health (NSDUH) Releases. Accessed July 12, 2022. https://www.samhsa.gov/data/release/2019-national-survey-drug-use-and-health-nsduh-releases
65. Eaton WW, Kramer M, Anthony JC, Dryman A, Shapiro S, Locke BZ. The incidence of specific DIS/DSM-III mental disorders: data from the NIMH Epidemiologic Catchment Area Program. *Acta Psychiatr Scand*. 1989;79(2):163-178.
66. Crum RM, Chan YF, Chen LS, Storr CL, Anthony JC. Incidence rates for alcohol dependence among adults: prospective data from the Baltimore Epidemiologic Catchment Area Follow-Up Survey, 1981-1996. *J Stud Alcohol*. 2005;66(6):795-805.
67. Grant BF, Goldstein RB, Chou SP, et al. Sociodemographic and psychopathologic predictors of first incidence of DSM-IV substance use, mood and anxiety disorders: results from the Wave 2 National Epidemiologic Survey on Alcohol and Related Conditions. *Mol Psychiatry*. 2009;14(11):1051-1066.
68. Chou SP, Goldstein RB, Smith SM, et al. The epidemiology of DSM-5 nicotine use disorder: results from the national epidemiologic survey on alcohol and related conditions-III. *J Clin Psychiatry*. 2016;77(10):1404-1412.
69. Strong DR, Leas E, Noble M, et al. Predictive validity of the adult tobacco dependence index: findings from waves 1 and 2 of the population assessment of tobacco and health (PATH) study. *Drug Alcohol Depend*. 2020;214:108134.
70. Piper ME, Baker TB, Benowitz NL, Smith SS, Jorenby DE. E-cigarette dependence measures in dual users: reliability and relations with

dependence criteria and E-cigarette cessation. *Nicotine Tob Res.* 2020;22(5):756-763.

71. Shiffman S, Sembower MA. Dependence on e-cigarettes and cigarettes in a cross-sectional study of US adults. *Addiction.* 2020;115(10):1924-1931.
72. Liu G, Wasserman E, Kong L, Foulds J. A comparison of nicotine dependence among exclusive E-cigarette and cigarette users in the PATH study. *Prev Med.* 2017;104:86-91.
73. National Academies of Sciences Engineering, and Medicine, Health and Medicine Division, Board on Population Health and Public Health Practice, Committee on the Review of the Health Effects of Electronic Nicotine Delivery Systems. Public health consequences of E-cigarettes. In: Eaton DL, Kwan LY, Stratton K, eds. *Harm Reduction.* Washington, DC National Academies Press; 2018.
74. Snell LM, Barnes AJ, Nicksic NE. A longitudinal analysis of nicotine dependence and transitions from dual use of cigarettes and electronic cigarettes: evidence from waves 1-3 of the PATH study. *J Stud Alcohol Drugs.* 2020;81(5):595-603.
75. Hasin DS, Saha TD, Kerridge BT, et al. Prevalence of marijuana use disorders in the United States between 2001-2002 and 2012-2013. *JAMA Psychiatry.* 2015;72(12):1235-1242.
76. Boyd CJ, Veliz PT, McCabe SE. Severity of DSM-5 cannabis use disorders in a nationally representative sample of sexual minorities. *Subst Abus.* 2020;41(2):191-195.
77. Feingold D, Livne O, Rehm J, Lev-Ran S. Probability and correlates of transition from cannabis use to DSM-5 cannabis use disorder: Results from a large-scale nationally representative study. *Drug Alcohol Rev.* 2020;39(2):142-151.
78. Substance Abuse and Mental Health Services Administration (SAMHSA). *Key substance use and mental health indicators in the United States: Results from the 2019 National Survey on Drug Use and Health (HHS Publication No. PEP20-07-01-001, NSDUH Series H-55).* Substance Abuse and Mental Health Services; 2020.
79. Compton WM, Han B, Jones CM, Blanco C. Cannabis use disorders among adults in the United States during a time of increasing use of cannabis. *Drug Alcohol Depend.* 2019;204:107468.
80. van der Pol P, Liebregts N, de Graaf R, Korf DJ, van den Brink W, van Laar M. Predicting the transition from frequent cannabis use to cannabis dependence: a three-year prospective study. *Drug Alcohol Depend* 2013;133(2):352-359.
81. Butterworth P, Slade T, Degenhardt L. Factors associated with the timing and onset of cannabis use and cannabis use disorder: results from the 2007 Australian National Survey of Mental Health and Well-Being. *Drug Alcohol Rev.* 2014;33(5):555-564.
82. Grant BF, Saha TD, Ruan WJ, et al. Epidemiology of DSM-5 drug use disorder: results from the national epidemiologic survey on alcohol and related conditions-III. *JAMA Psychiatry.* 2016;73(1):39-47.
83. Martins SS, Fenton MC, Keyes KM, Blanco C, Zhu H, Storr CL. Mood and anxiety disorders and their association with non-medical prescription opioid use and prescription opioid-use disorder: longitudinal evidence from the National Epidemiologic Study on Alcohol and Related Conditions. *Psychol Med.* 2012;42(6):1261-1272.
84. Regier DA, Farmer ME, Rae DS, et al. Comorbidity of mental disorders with alcohol and other drug abuse. Results from the Epidemiologic Catchment Area (ECA) Study. *JAMA.* 1990;264(19):2511-2518.
85. Farrell M, Howes S, Bebbington P, et al. Nicotine, alcohol and drug dependence and psychiatric comorbidity. Results of a national household survey. *Br J Psychiatry.* 2001;179:432-437.
86. Ross HE. DSM-III-R alcohol abuse and dependence and psychiatric comorbidity in Ontario: results from the Mental Health Supplement to the Ontario Health Survey. *Drug Alcohol Depend.* 1995;39(2):111-128.
87. Lai HM, Sitharthan T, Huang QR. Exploration of the comorbidity of alcohol use disorders and mental health disorders among inpatients presenting to all hospitals in New South Wales, Australia. *Subst Abus.* 2012;33(2):138-145.
88. Udo T, Vásquez E, Shaw BA. A lifetime history of alcohol use disorder increases risk for chronic medical conditions after stable remission. *Drug Alcohol Depend.* 2015;157:68-74.
89. Schoepf D, Heun R. Alcohol dependence and physical comorbidity: increased prevalence but reduced relevance of individual comorbidities for hospital-based mortality during a 12.5-year observation period in general hospital admissions in urban North-West England. *Eur Psychiatry.* 2015;30(4):459-468.
90. Disney E, Kidorf M, Kolodner K, et al. Psychiatric comorbidity is associated with drug use and HIV risk in syringe exchange participants. *J Nerv Ment Dis.* 2006;194(8):577-583.
91. Naji L, Dennis BB, Bawor M, et al. The association between age of onset of opioid use and comorbidity among opioid dependent patients receiving methadone maintenance therapy. *Addict Sci Clin Pract.* 2017;12(1):9.
92. Feng J, Iser JP, Yang W. Medical encounters for opioid-related intoxications in Southern Nevada: sociodemographic and clinical correlates. *BMC Health Serv Res.* 2016;16(1):438.
93. Schulte MT, Hser YI. Substance use and associated health conditions throughout the lifespan. *Public Health Rev.* 2014;35(2):
94. Stinson FS, Grant BF, Dawson DA, Ruan WJ, Huang B, Saha T. Comorbidity between DSM-IV alcohol and specific drug use disorders in the United States: results from the National Epidemiologic Survey on Alcohol and Related Conditions. *Drug Alcohol Depend.* 2005;80(1):105-116.
95. Grant BF, Stinson FS, Dawson DA, et al. Prevalence and co-occurrence of substance use disorders and independent mood and anxiety disorders: results from the National Epidemiologic Survey on Alcohol and Related Conditions. *Arch Gen Psychiatry.* 2004;61(8):807-816.
96. Trull TJ, Jahng S, Tomko RL, Wood PK, Sher KJ. Revised NESARC personality disorder diagnoses: gender, prevalence, and comorbidity with substance dependence disorders. *J Pers Disord.* 2010;24(4): 412-426.
97. Fenton MC, Keyes K, Geier T, et al. Psychiatric comorbidity and the persistence of drug use disorders in the United States. *Addiction.* 2012;107(3):599-609.
98. Flensborg-Madsen T, Mortensen EL, Knop J, Becker U, Sher L, Grønbaek M. Comorbidity and temporal ordering of alcohol use disorders and other psychiatric disorders: results from a Danish register-based study. *Compr Psychiatry.* 2009;50(4):307-314.
99. Fergusson DM, Boden JM, Horwood LJ. Tests of causal links between alcohol abuse or dependence and major depression. *Arch Gen Psychiatry.* 2009;66(3):260-266.
100. Dawson DA, Goldstein RB, Moss HB, Li TK, Grant BF. Gender differences in the relationship of internalizing and externalizing psychopathology to alcohol dependence: likelihood, expression and course. *Drug Alcohol Depend.* 2010;112(1-2):9-17.
101. Goldstein RB, Dawson DA, Chou SP, Grant BF. Sex differences in prevalence and comorbidity of alcohol and drug use disorders: results from wave 2 of the National Epidemiologic Survey on Alcohol and Related Conditions. *J Stud Alcohol Drugs.* 2012;73(6):938-950.
102. Husky MM, Mazure CM, Paliwal P, McKee SA. Gender differences in the comorbidity of smoking behavior and major depression. *Drug Alcohol Depend.* 2008;93(1-2):176-179.
103. Hesselbrock MN, Hesselbrock VM, Segal B, Schuckit MA, Bucholz K. Ethnicity and psychiatric comorbidity among alcohol-dependent persons who receive inpatient treatment: African Americans, Alaska Natives, Caucasians, and Hispanics. *Alcohol Clin Exp Res.* 2003;27(8):1368-1373.
104. Weaver T, Madden P, Charles V, et al. Comorbidity of substance misuse and mental illness in community mental health and substance misuse services. *Br J Psychiatry.* 2003;183:304-313.
105. Caton CL, Drake RE, Hasin DS, et al. Differences between early-phase primary psychotic disorders with concurrent substance use and substance-induced psychoses. *Arch Gen Psychiatry.* 2005;62(2): 137-145.
106. Sakai JT, Hall SK, Mikulich-Gilbertson SK, Crowley TJ. Inhalant use, abuse, and dependence among adolescent patients: commonly comorbid problems. *J Am Acad Child Adolesc Psychiatry.* 2004;43(9):1080-1088.
107. Johnson ME, Brems C, Mills ME, Fisher DG. Psychiatric symptomatology among individuals in alcohol detoxification treatment. *Addict Behav.* 2007;32(8):1745-1752.

108. Rosic T, Naji L, Bawor M, et al. The impact of comorbid psychiatric disorders on methadone maintenance treatment in opioid use disorder: a prospective cohort study. *Neuropsychiatr Dis Treat*. 2017;13:1399-1408.
109. Tross S, Feaster DJ, Thorens G, et al. Substance use, depression and sociodemographic determinants of HIV sexual risk behavior in outpatient substance abuse treatment patients. *J Addict Med*. 2015;9(6):457-463.
110. van Emmerik-van Oortmerssen K, van de Glind G, Koeter MW, et al. Psychiatric comorbidity in treatment-seeking substance use disorder patients with and without attention deficit hyperactivity disorder: results of the IASP study. *Addiction* 2014;109(2):262-272.
111. Willinger U, Lenzinger E, Hornik K, et al. Anxiety as a predictor of relapse in detoxified alcohol-dependent patients. *Alcohol Alcohol*. 2002;37(6):609-612.
112. Upadhyaya HP, Deas D, Brady KT, Kruesi M. Cigarette smoking and psychiatric comorbidity in children and adolescents. *J Am Acad Child Adolesc Psychiatry*. 2002;41(11):1294-1305.
113. Salloum IM, Cornelius JR, Douaihy A, Kirisci L, Daley DC, Kelly TM. Patient characteristics and treatment implications of marijuana abuse among bipolar alcoholics: results from a double blind, placebo-controlled study. *Addict Behav*. 2005;30(9):1702-1708.
114. Weisner C, Matzger H, Kaskutas LA. How important is treatment? One-year outcomes of treated and untreated alcohol-dependent individuals. *Addiction*. 2003;98(7):901-911.
115. Batki SL, Meszaros ZS, Strutynski K, et al. Medical comorbidity in patients with schizophrenia and alcohol dependence. *Schizophr Res*. 2009;107(2-3):139-146.
116. Curran GM, Sullivan G, Williams K, Han X, Allee E, Kotrla KJ. The association of psychiatric comorbidity and use of the emergency department among persons with substance use disorders: an observational cohort study. *BMC Emerg Med*. 2008;8:17.
117. Davis LL, Wisniewski SR, Howland RH, et al. Does comorbid substance use disorder impair recovery from major depression with SSRI treatment? An analysis of the STAR*D level one treatment outcomes. *Drug Alcohol Depend*. 2010;107(2-3):161-170.
118. Cardoso TA, Jansen K, Zeni CP, Quevedo J, Zunta-Soares G, Soares JC. Clinical outcomes in children and adolescents with bipolar disorder and substance use disorder comorbidity. *J Clin Psychiatry*. 2017;78(3): e230-e233.
119. Crawford TN, Cohen P, First MB, Skodol AE, Johnson JG, Kasen S. Comorbid axis I and axis II disorders in early adolescence: outcomes 20 years later. *Arch Gen Psychiatry*. 2008;65(6):641-648.
120. Wilton G, Stewart LA. Outcomes of offenders with co-occurring substance use disorders and mental disorders. *Psychiatr Serv*. 2017;68(7):704-709.
121. McHugo GJ, Drake RE, Xie H, Bond GR. A 10-year study of steady employment and non-vocational outcomes among people with serious mental illness and co-occurring substance use disorders. *Schizophr Res* 2012;138(2-3):233-239.
122. Vasilenko SA, Evans-Polce RJ, Lanza ST. Age trends in rates of substance use disorders across ages 18–90: differences by gender and race/ethnicity. *Drug Alcohol Depend*. 2017;180:260-264.
123. Compton WM, Thomas YF, Stinson FS, Grant BF. Prevalence, correlates, disability, and comorbidity of DSM-IV drug abuse and dependence in the United States: results from the national epidemiologic survey on alcohol and related conditions. *Arch Gen Psychiatry*. 2007;64(5):566-576.
124. Grant BF, Dawson DA. Age of onset of drug use and its association with DSM-IV drug abuse and dependence: results from the National Longitudinal Alcohol Epidemiologic Survey. *J Subst Abuse*. 1998;10(2):163-173.
125. Ehlers CL, Gizer IR, Vieten C, et al. Cannabis dependence in the San Francisco family study: age of onset of use, DSM-IV symptoms, withdrawal, and heritability. *Addict Behav*. 2010;35(2):102-110.
126. Chen CY, Storr CL, Anthony JC. Early-onset drug use and risk for drug dependence problems. *Addict Behav*. 2009;34(3):319-322.
127. McCabe SE, West BT, Morales M, Cranford JA, Boyd CJ. Does early onset of non-medical use of prescription drugs predict subsequent prescription drug abuse and dependence? Results from a national study. *Addiction*. 2007;102(12):1920-1930.
128. Le Strat Y, Dubertret C, Le Foll B. Impact of age at onset of cannabis use on cannabis dependence and driving under the influence in the United States. *Accid Anal Prev*. 2015;76:1-5.
129. Kandel D, Chen K, Warner LA, Kessler RC, Grant B. Prevalence and demographic correlates of symptoms of last year dependence on alcohol, nicotine, marijuana and cocaine in the U.S. population. *Drug Alcohol Depend*. 1997;44(1):11-29.
130. Meier P, Seitz HK. Age, alcohol metabolism and liver disease. *Curr Opin Clin Nutr Metab Care*. 2008;11(1):21-26.
131. Helzer JE, Burnam A, McEvoy LT. Alcohol abuse and dependence. In: Robins LE, Regier DA, eds. *Psychiatric Disorders in America*. The Free Press; 1991:81-115.
132. Conigliaro J, Kraemer K, McNeil M. Screening and identification of older adults with alcohol problems in primary care. *J Geriatr Psychiatry Neurol*. 2000;13(3):106-114.
133. O'Connell H, Chin AV, Hamilton F, et al. A systematic review of the utility of self-report alcohol screening instruments in the elderly. *Int J Geriatr Psychiatry*. 2004;19(11):1074-1086.
134. Berks J, McCormick R. Screening for alcohol misuse in elderly primary care patients: a systematic literature review. *Int Psychogeriatr*. 2008;20(6):1090-1103.
135. Pabst A, Kraus L, Piontek D, Baumeister SE. Age differences in diagnostic criteria of DSM-IV alcohol dependence among adults with similar drinking behaviour. *Addiction*. 2012;107(2):331-338.
136. Castro-Costa E, Ferri CP, Lima-Costa MF, et al. Alcohol consumption in late-life—the first Brazilian National Alcohol Survey (BNAS). *Addict Behav*. 2008;33(12):1598-1601.
137. Blow FC. Treatment of older women with alcohol problems: meeting the challenge for a special population. *Alcohol Clin Exp Res*. 2000;24(8): 1257-1266.
138. Shin MH, Kweon SS, Choi JS, et al. Average volume of alcohol consumed, drinking patterns, and metabolic syndrome in older Korean adults. *J Epidemiol*. 2013;23(2):122-131.
139. Caputo F, Vignoli T, Leggio L, Addolorato G, Zoli G, Bernardi M. Alcohol use disorders in the elderly: a brief overview from epidemiology to treatment options. *Exp Gerontol*. 2012;47(6):411-416.
140. Wakabayashi I, Araki Y. Influences of gender and age on relationships between alcohol drinking and atherosclerotic risk factors. *Alcohol Clin Exp Res*. 2010;34(Suppl 1):S54-S60.
141. Hu MC, Griesler P, Wall M, Kandel DB. Age-related patterns in nonmedical prescription opioid use and disorder in the US population at ages 12-34 from 2002 to 2014. *Drug Alcohol Depend*. 2017;177:237-243.
142. Warner LA, Kessler RC, Hughes M, Anthony JC, Nelson CB. Prevalence and correlates of drug use and dependence in the United States. Results from the National Comorbidity Survey. *Arch Gen Psychiatry*. 1995;52(3):219-229.
143. Breslau N, Johnson EO, Hiripi E, Kessler R. Nicotine dependence in the United States: prevalence, trends, and smoking persistence. *Arch Gen Psychiatry*. 2001;58(9):810-816.
144. Jager J, Keyes KM, Son D, Kloska D, Patrick ME, Schulenberg JE. Cohort and age trends in age 35–45 prevalence of alcohol use disorder symptomology, by severity, sex, race, and education. *Drug Alcohol Depend*. 2021;226:108820.
145. Grucza RA, Norberg K, Bucholz KK, Bierut LJ. Correspondence between secular changes in alcohol dependence and age of drinking onset among women in the United States. *Alcohol Clin Exp Res*. 2008;32(8):1493-1501.
146. Grant BF, Stinson FS, Harford TC. Age at onset of alcohol use and DSM-IV alcohol abuse and dependence: a 12-year follow-up. *J Subst Abuse*. 2001;13(4):493-504.
147. Chapman C, Slade T, Swift W, Keyes K, Tonks Z, Teesson M. Evidence for sex convergence in prevalence of Cannabis use: a systematic review and meta-regression. *J Stud Alcohol Drugs*. 2017;78(3):344-352.
148. Miech R, Bohnert A, Heard K, Boardman J. Increasing use of nonmedical analgesics among younger cohorts in the United States: a birth cohort effect. *J Adolesc Health*. 2013;52(1):35-41.

149. Martins SS, Keyes KM, Storr CL, Zhu H, Grucza RA. Birth-cohort trends in lifetime and past-year prescription opioid-use disorder resulting from nonmedical use: results from two national surveys. *J Stud Alcohol Drugs.* 2010;71(4):480-487.
150. Colell E, Sánchez-Niubò A, Domingo-Salvany A. Sex differences in the cumulative incidence of substance use by birth cohort. *Int J Drug Policy.* 2013;24(4):319-325.
151. Geels LM, Bartels M, van Beijsterveldt TC, et al. Trends in adolescent alcohol use: effects of age, sex and cohort on prevalence and heritability. *Addiction* 2012;107(3):518-527.
152. van Heerden MS, Grimsrud AT, Seedat S, Myer L, Williams DR, Stein DJ. Patterns of substance use in South Africa: results from the South African stress and Health study. *S Afr Med J.* 2009;99(5 Pt 2):358-366.
153. Miech R, Koester S. Trends in U.S., past-year marijuana use from 1985 to 2009: an age-period-cohort analysis. *Drug Alcohol Depend.* 2012;124(3):259-267.
154. Bailey ZD, Krieger N, Agénor M, Graves J, Linos N, Bassett MT. Structural racism and health inequities in the USA: evidence and interventions. *Lancet.* 2017;389(10077):1453-1463.
155. Krieger N. Discrimination and health inequities. *Int J Health Serv.* 2014;44(4):643-710.
156. Hardeman RR, Medina EM, Kozhimannil KB. Structural racism and supporting black lives—the role of health professionals. *N Engl J Med.* 2016;375(22):2113-2115.
157. Adkins-Jackson PB, Chantarat T, Bailey ZD, Ponce NA. Measuring structural racism: a guide for epidemiologists and other health researchers. *Am J Epidemiol.* 2022;191(4):539-547.
158. Castle B, Wendel M, Kerr J, Brooms D, Rollins A. Public health's approach to systemic racism: a systematic literature review. *J Racial Ethn Health Disparities.* 2019;6(1):27-36.
159. Savage JE, Mezuk B. Psychosocial and contextual determinants of alcohol and drug use disorders in the National Latino and Asian American Study. *Drug Alcohol Depend.* 2014;139:71-78.
160. Breslau J, Chang DF. Psychiatric disorders among foreign-born and US-born Asian-Americans in a US national survey. *Soc Psychiatry Psychiatr Epidemiol.* 2006;41(12):943-950.
161. Chae DH, Takeuchi DT, Barbeau EM, et al. Alcohol disorders among Asian Americans: associations with unfair treatment, racial/ethnic discrimination, and ethnic identification (the national Latino and Asian Americans study, 2002-2003). *J Epidemiol Community Health.* 2008;62(11):973-979.
162. Gibbs TA, Okuda M, Oquendo MA, et al. Mental health of African Americans and Caribbean blacks in the United States: results from the National Epidemiological Survey on Alcohol and Related Conditions. *Am J Public Health.* 2013;103(2):330-338.
163. Breslau J, Aguilar-Gaxiola S, Kendler KS, Su M, Williams D, Kessler RC. Specifying race-ethnic differences in risk for psychiatric disorder in a USA national sample. *Psychol Med.* 2006;36(1):57-68.
164. Polednak AP. Secular trend in U.S. black-white disparities in selected alcohol-related cancer incidence rates. *Alcohol Alcohol.* 2007;42(2): 125-130.
165. Stinson FS, Grant BF, Dufour MC. The critical dimension of ethnicity in liver cirrhosis mortality statistics. *Alcohol Clin Exp Res.* 2001;25(8): 1181-1187.
166. Shield KD, Gmel G, Kehoe-Chan T, Dawson DA, Grant BF, Rehm J. Mortality and potential years of life lost attributable to alcohol consumption by race and sex in the United States in 2005. *PLoS One.* 2013;8(1):e51923.
167. Witbrodt J, Mulia N, Zemore SE, Kerr WC. Racial/ethnic disparities in alcohol-related problems: differences by gender and level of heavy drinking. *Alcohol Clin Exp Res.* 2014;38(6):1662-1670.
168. Mulia N, Ye Y, Greenfield TK, Zemore SE. Disparities in alcohol-related problems among white, black, and hispanic Americans. *Alcohol Clin Exp Res.* 2009;33(4):654-662.
169. Vaeth PA, Wang-Schweig M, Drinking CR. Alcohol use disorder, and treatment access and utilization among U.S. racial/ethnic groups. *Alcohol Clin Exp Res.* 2017;41(1):6-19.
170. Zemore SE, Ye Y, Mulia N, Martinez P, Jones-Webb R, Karriker-Jaffe K. Poor, persecuted, young, and alone: toward explaining the elevated risk of alcohol problems among Black and Latino men who drink. *Drug Alcohol Depend.* 2016;163:31-39.
171. Jones-Webb R, Snowden L, Herd D, Short B, Hannan P. Alcohol-related problems among black, hispanic and white men: the contribution of neighborhood poverty. *J Stud Alcohol.* 1997;58(5):539-545.
172. Mulia N, Karriker-Jaffe KJ, Witbrodt J, Bond J, Williams E, Zemore SE. Racial/ethnic differences in 30-year trajectories of heavy drinking in a nationally representative U.S. sample. *Drug Alcohol Depend.* 2017;170:133-141.
173. Shih RA, Miles JN, Tucker JS, Zhou AJ, D'Amico EJ. Racial/ethnic differences in the influence of cultural values, alcohol resistance self-efficacy, and alcohol expectancies on risk for alcohol initiation. *Psychol Addict Behav.* 2012;26(3):460-470.
174. Lillie-Blanton M, Anthony JC, Schuster CR. Probing the meaning of racial/ethnic group comparisons in crack cocaine smoking. *JAMA.* 1993;269(8):993-997.
175. Crum RM, Helzer JE, Anthony JC. Level of education and alcohol abuse and dependence in adulthood: a further inquiry. *Am J Public Health.* 1993;83(6):830-837.
176. Fesahazion RG, Thorpe RJ Jr, Bell CN, LaVeist TA. Disparities in alcohol use: does race matter as much as place? *Prev Med.* 2012;55(5):482-484.
177. Mejia de Grubb MC, Salemi JL, Gonzalez SJ, Zoorob RJ, Levine RS. Trends and correlates of disparities in alcohol-related mortality between hispanics and non-hispanic whites in the United States, 1999 to 2014. *Alcohol Clin Exp Res.* 2016;40(10):2169-2179.
178. Yoon YH, Yi HY, Thomson PC. Alcohol-related and viral hepatitis C-related cirrhosis mortality among Hispanic subgroups in the United States, 2000-2004. *Alcohol Clin Exp Res.* 2011;35(2):240-249.
179. Vaeth PA, Caetano R, Rodriguez LA. The Hispanic Americans Baseline Alcohol Survey (HABLAS): the association between acculturation, birthplace and alcohol consumption across Hispanic national groups. *Addict Behav.* 2012;37(9):1029-1037.
180. Vaeth PA, Caetano R, Ramisetty-Mikler S, Rodriguez LA. Hispanic Americans Baseline Alcohol Survey (HABLAS): alcohol-related problems across Hispanic national groups. *J Stud Alcohol Drugs.* 2009;70(6):991-999.
181. Jetelina KK, Reingle Gonzalez JM, Vaeth PA, Mills BA, Caetano R. An investigation of the relationship between alcohol use and major depressive disorder across hispanic national groups. *Alcohol Clin Exp Res.* 2016;40(3):536-542.
182. Ríos-Bedoya CF, Freile-Salinas D. Incidence of alcohol use disorders among Hispanic subgroups in the USA. *Alcohol Alcohol.* 2014;49(5):549-556.
183. Caetano R, Mills BA, Vaeth PA, Reingle J. Age at first drink, drinking, binge drinking, and DSM-5 alcohol use disorder among Hispanic national groups in the United States. *Alcohol Clin Exp Res.* 2014;38(5):1381-1389.
184. Niño MD, Cai T, Mota-Back X, Comeau J. Gender differences in trajectories of alcohol use from ages 13 to 33 across latina/o ethnic groups. *Drug Alcohol Depend.* 2017;180:113-120.
185. Strunin L, Edwards EM, Godette DC, Heeren T. Country of origin, age of drinking onset, and drinking patterns among Mexican American young adults. *Drug Alcohol Depend.* 2007;91(2-3):134-140.
186. Lipsky S, Kernic MA, Qiu Q, Hasin DS. Posttraumatic stress disorder and alcohol misuse among women: effects of ethnic minority stressors. *Soc Psychiatry Psychiatr Epidemiol.* 2016;51(3):407-419.
187. Finch BK, Vega WA. Acculturation stress, social support, and self-rated health among Latinos in California. *J Immigr Health.* 2003;5(3): 109-117.
188. Wahl AM, Eitle TM. Gender, acculturation and alcohol use among Latina/o adolescents: a multi-ethnic comparison. *J Immigr Minor Health.* 2010;12(2):153-165.
189. Castro FG, Stein JA, Bentler PM. Ethnic pride, traditional family values, and acculturation in early cigarette and alcohol use among Latino adolescents. *J Prim Prev.* 2009;30(3-4):265-292.

190. Perez-Rodriguez MM, Baca-Garcia E, Oquendo MA, et al. Relationship between acculturation, discrimination, and suicidal ideation and attempts among US Hispanics in the National Epidemiologic Survey of Alcohol and Related Conditions. *J Clin Psychiatry*. 2014;75(4):399-407.
191. Iwamoto D, Takamatsu S, Castellanos J. Binge drinking and alcohol-related problems among U.S.-born Asian Americans. *Cultur Divers Ethnic Minor Psychol*. 2012;18(3):219-227.
192. Park SY, Shibusawa T, Yoon SM, Son H. Characteristics of Chinese and Korean Americans in outpatient treatment for alcohol use disorders: examining heterogeneity among Asian American subgroups. *J Ethn Subst Abuse*. 2010;9(2):128-142.
193. Spicer P, Beals J, Croy CD, et al. The prevalence of DSM-III-R alcohol dependence in two American Indian populations. *Alcohol Clin Exp Res*. 2003;27(11):1785-1797.
194. Landen M, Roeber J, Naimi T, Nielsen L, Sewell M. Alcohol-attributable mortality among American Indians and Alaska Natives in the United States, 1999-2009. *Am J Public Health*. 2014;104 Suppl 3:S343-S349.
195. Centers for Disease Control and Prevention (CDC). Alcohol-attributable deaths and years of potential life lost among American Indians and Alaska Natives—United States, 2001–2005. *MMWR Morb Mortal Wkly Rep*. 2008;57(34):938-941.
196. Cunningham JK, Solomon TA, Muramoto ML. Alcohol use among Native Americans compared to whites: Examining the veracity of the 'Native American elevated alcohol consumption' belief. *Drug Alcohol Depend*. 2016;160:65-75.
197. O'Connell JM, Novins DK, Beals J, Spicer P. Disparities in patterns of alcohol use among reservation-based and geographically dispersed American Indian populations. *Alcohol Clin Exp Res*. 2005;29(1):107-116.
198. Koss MP, Yuan NP, Dightman D, et al. Adverse childhood exposures and alcohol dependence among seven Native American tribes. *Am J Prev Med*. 2003;25(3):238-244.
199. Beals J, Novins DK, Whitesell NR, Spicer P, Mitchell CM, Manson SM. Prevalence of mental disorders and utilization of mental health services in two American Indian reservation populations: mental health disparities in a national context. *Am J Psychiatry*. 2005;162(9):1723-1732.
200. Les Whitbeck B, Chen X, Hoyt DR, Adams GW. Discrimination, historical loss and enculturation: culturally specific risk and resiliency factors for alcohol abuse among American Indians. *J Stud Alcohol*. 2004;65(4):409-418.
201. Emerson MA, Moore RS, Caetano R. Association between lifetime posttraumatic stress disorder and past year alcohol use disorder among American Indians/Alaska natives and non-hispanic whites. *Alcohol Clin Exp Res*. 2017;41(3):576-584.
202. Wu LT, Woody GE, Yang C, Pan JJ, Blazer DG. Racial/ethnic variations in substance-related disorders among adolescents in the United States. *Arch Gen Psychiatry*. 2011;68(11):1176-1185.
203. Evans EA, Grella CE, Washington DL, Upchurch DM. Gender and race/ethnic differences in the persistence of alcohol, drug, and poly-substance use disorders. *Drug Alcohol Depend*. 2017;174:128-136.
204. McCabe SE, West BT. The 3-year course of multiple substance use disorders in the United States: a national longitudinal study. *J Clin Psychiatry*. 2017;78(5):e537-e544.
205. Huang B, Dawson DA, Stinson FS, et al. Prevalence, correlates, and comorbidity of nonmedical prescription drug use and drug use disorders in the United States: results of the national epidemiologic survey on alcohol and related conditions. *J Clin Psychiatry*. 2006;67(7):1062-1073.
206. Saha TD, Kerridge BT, Goldstein RB, et al. Nonmedical prescription opioid use and DSM-5 nonmedical prescription opioid use disorder in the United States. *J Clin Psychiatry*. 2016;77(6):772-780.
207. Alegria M, Canino G, Stinson FS, Grant BF. Nativity and DSM-IV psychiatric disorders among Puerto Ricans, Cuban Americans, and non-Latino Whites in the United States: results from the national epidemiologic survey on alcohol and related conditions. *J Clin Psychiatry*. 2006;67(1):56-65.
208. Grant BF, Stinson FS, Hasin DS, Dawson DA, Chou SP, Anderson K. Immigration and lifetime prevalence of DSM-IV psychiatric disorders among Mexican Americans and non-Hispanic whites in the United States: results from the National Epidemiologic Survey on Alcohol and Related Conditions. *Arch Gen Psychiatry*. 2004;61(12):1226-1233.
209. Mercado A, Ramirez M, Sharma R, Popan J, Avalos Latorre ML. Acculturation and substance use in a Mexican American college student sample. *J Ethn Subst Abuse*. 2017;16(3):276-292.
210. Blanco C, Morcillo C, Alegría M, et al. Acculturation and drug use disorders among Hispanics in the U.S. *J Psychiatr Res*. 2013;47(2):226-232.
211. Borges G, Cherpitel CJ, Orozco R, et al. Substance use and cumulative exposure to American society: findings from both sides of the US-Mexico border region. *Am J Public Health*. 2016;106(1):119-127.
212. Carliner H, Delker E, Fink DS, Keyes KM, Hasin DS. Racial discrimination, socioeconomic position, and illicit drug use among US Blacks. *Soc Psychiatry Psychiatr Epidemiol*. 2016;51(4):551-560.
213. Le TN, Goebert D, Wallen J. Acculturation factors and substance use among Asian American youth. *J Prim Prev*. 2009;30(3-4):453-473.
214. Di Cosmo C, Milfont TL, Robinson E, et al. Immigrant status and acculturation influence substance use among New Zealand youth. *Aust NZ J Public Health*. 2011;35(5):434-441.
215. Smith SM, Stinson FS, Dawson DA, Goldstein R, Huang B, Grant BF. Race/ethnic differences in the prevalence and co-occurrence of substance use disorders and independent mood and anxiety disorders: results from the National Epidemiologic Survey on Alcohol and Related Conditions. *Psychol Med*. 2006;36(7):987-998.
216. Mericle AA, Ta Park VM, Holck P, Arria AM. Prevalence, patterns, and correlates of co-occurring substance use and mental disorders in the United States: variations by race/ethnicity. *Compr Psychiatry*. 2012;53(6):657-665.
217. Ramchand R, Pacula RL, Iguchi MY. Racial differences in marijuana-users' risk of arrest in the United States. *Drug Alcohol Depend*. 2006;84(3):264-272.
218. Harrell ZA, Broman CL. Racial/ethnic differences in correlates of prescription drug misuse among young adults. *Drug Alcohol Depend*. 2009;104(3):268-271.
219. Spillane NS, Weyandt L, Oster D, Treloar H. Social contextual risk factors for stimulant use among adolescent American Indians. *Drug Alcohol Depend*. 2017;179:167-173.
220. Cook BL, Alegría M. Racial-ethnic disparities in substance abuse treatment: the role of criminal history and socioeconomic status. *Psychiatr Serv*. 2011;62(11):1273-1281.
221. Delphin-Rittmon M, Andres-Hyman R, Flanagan EH, Ortiz J, Amer MM, Davidson L. Racial-ethnic differences in referral source, diagnosis, and length of stay in inpatient substance abuse treatment. *Psychiatr Serv*. 2012;63(6):612-615.
222. Cummings JR, Wen H, Druss BG. Racial/ethnic differences in treatment for substance use disorders among U.S. adolescents. *J Am Acad Child Adolesc Psychiatry*. 2011;50(12):1265-1274.
223. Nowotny KM. Race/ethnic disparities in the utilization of treatment for drug dependent inmates in U.S. state correctional facilities. *Addict Behav*. 2015;40:148-153.
224. Guerrero EG, Marsh JC, Cao D, Shin HC, Andrews C. Gender disparities in utilization and outcome of comprehensive substance abuse treatment among racial/ethnic groups. *J Subst Abuse Treat*. 2014;46(5):584-591.
225. Hatzenbuehler ML, Keyes KM, Narrow WE, Grant BF, Hasin DS. Racial/ethnic disparities in service utilization for individuals with co-occurring mental health and substance use disorders in the general population: results from the national epidemiologic survey on alcohol and related conditions. *J Clin Psychiatry*. 2008;69(7):1112-1121.
226. Sheffer CE, Stitzer M, Landes R, Brackman SL, Munn T, Moore P. Socioeconomic disparities in community-based treatment of tobacco dependence. *Am J Public Health*. 2012;102(3):e8-e16.
227. Saloner B, Cook BL. Blacks and hispanics are less likely than whites to complete addiction treatment, largely due to socioeconomic factors. *Health Affairs*. 2013;32(1):135-145.
228. Reid JL, Hammond D, Boudreau C, Fong GT, Siahpush M. Socioeconomic disparities in quit intentions, quit attempts, and smoking abstinence among smokers in four western countries: findings from the

International Tobacco Control Four Country Survey. *Nicotine Tob Res.* 2010;12(Suppl 1):S20-S33.

229. Campbell CI, Weisner C, Sterling S. Adolescents entering chemical dependency treatment in private managed care: ethnic differences in treatment initiation and retention. *J Adolesc Health.* 2006;38(4):343-350.
230. Quintero GA, Lilliott E, Willging C. Substance abuse treatment provider views of "culture": implications for behavioral health care in rural settings. *Qual Health Res.* 2007;17(9):1256-1267.
231. De Graaf R, Bijl RV, Ravelli A, Smit F, Vollebergh WA. Predictors of first incidence of DSM-III-R psychiatric disorders in the general population: findings from the Netherlands Mental Health Survey and Incidence Study. *Acta Psychiatr Scand.* 2002;106(4):303-313.
232. Bratberg GH, Sharon C. Wilsnack, Wilsnack R, et al. Gender differences and gender convergence in alcohol use over the past three decades (1984–2008), The HUNT Study, Norway, *BMC Public Health.* 2016;16(1):723.
233. Steingrímsson S, Carlsen HK, Sigfússon S, Magnússon A. The changing gender gap in substance use disorder: a total population-based study of psychiatric in-patients. *Addiction.* 2012;107(11):1957-1962.
234. Slade T, Chapman C, Swift W, Keyes K, Tonks Z, Teesson M. Birth cohort trends in the global epidemiology of alcohol use and alcohol-related harms in men and women: systematic review and metaregression. *BMJ Open.* 2016;6(10):e011827.
235. Keyes KM, Grant BF, Hasin DS. Evidence for a closing gender gap in alcohol use, abuse, and dependence in the United States population. *Drug Alcohol Depend.* 2008;93(1-2):21-29.
236. Grucza RA, Bucholz KK, Rice JP, Bierut LJ. Secular trends in the lifetime prevalence of alcohol dependence in the United States: a re-evaluation. *Alcohol Clin Exp Res.* 2008;32(5):763-770.
237. Parker DA, Harford TC. Gender-role attitudes, job competition and alcohol consumption among women and men. *Alcohol Clin Exp Res.* 1992;16(2):159-165.
238. Hall EM. Double exposure: the combined impact of the home and work environments on psychosomatic strain in Swedish women and men. *Int J Health Serv.* 1992;22(2):239-260.
239. McKetta S, Prins SJ, Bates LM, Platt JM, Keyes KM. US trends in binge drinking by gender, occupation, prestige, and work structure among adults in the midlife, 2006-2018. *Ann Epidemiol.* 2021;62:22-29.
240. Keyes KM. Age, period, and cohort effects in alcohol use in the United States in the 20th and 21st centuries: implications for the coming decades. *Alcohol Res.* 2022;42(1):02.
241. McKetta SC, Keyes KM. Trends in U.S. women's binge drinking in middle adulthood by socioeconomic status, 2006-2018. *Drug Alcohol Depend.* 2020;212:108026.
242. Keyes KM, Platt J, Rutherford C, et al. Cohort effects on gender differences in alcohol use in the United States: how much is explained by changing attitudes towards women and gendered roles? *SSM Popul Health.* 2021;15:100919.
243. Schulte MT, Ramo D, Brown SA. Gender differences in factors influencing alcohol use and drinking progression among adolescents. *Clin Psychol Rev.* 2009;29(6):535-547.
244. Thundal KL, Allebeck P. Abuse of and dependence on alcohol in Swedish women: role of education, occupation and family structure. *Soc Psychiatry Psychiatr Epidemiol.* 1998;33(9):445-450.
245. Lown AE, Vega WA. Alcohol abuse or dependence among Mexican American women who report violence. *Alcohol Clin Exp Res.* 2001;25(10):1479-1486.
246. Wilsnack SC, Vogeltanz ND, Klassen AD, Harris TR. Childhood sexual abuse and women's substance abuse: national survey findings. *J Stud Alcohol.* 1997;58(3):264-271.
247. Meng X, D'Arcy C. Gender moderates the relationship between childhood abuse and internalizing and substance use disorders later in life: a cross-sectional analysis. *BMC Psychiatry.* 2016;16(1):401.
248. Wagner FA, Anthony JC. Male-female differences in the risk of progression from first use to dependence upon cannabis, cocaine, and alcohol. *Drug Alcohol Depend.* 2007;86(2-3):191-198.
249. McCabe SE, Hughes TL, West BT, Veliz P, Boyd CJ. DSM-5 alcohol use disorder severity as a function of sexual orientation discrimination: a national study. *Alcohol Clin Exp Res.* 2019;43(3):497-508.
250. Fish JN, Exten C. Sexual orientation differences in alcohol use disorder across the adult life course. *Am J Prev Med.* 2020;59(3):428-436.
251. McCabe SE, Matthews AK, Lee JGL, Veliz P, Hughes TL, Boyd CJ. Tobacco use and sexual orientation in a national cross-sectional study: age, race/ethnicity, and sexual identity-attraction differences. *Am J Prev Med.* 2018;54(6):736-745.
252. Kerridge BT, Pickering RP, Saha TD, et al. Prevalence, sociodemographic correlates and DSM-5 substance use disorders and other psychiatric disorders among sexual minorities in the United States. *Drug Alcohol Depend.* 2017;170:82-92.
253. Schuler MS, Rice CE, Evans-Polce RJ, Collins RL. Disparities in substance use behaviors and disorders among adult sexual minorities by age, gender, and sexual identity. *Drug Alcohol Depend.* 2018;189:139-146.
254. Krueger EA, Fish JN, Upchurch DM. Sexual orientation disparities in substance use: investigating social stress mechanisms in a national sample. *Am J Prev Med.* 2020;58(1):59-68.
255. Mauro PM, Philbin MM, Greene ER, Diaz JE, Askari MS, Martins SS. Daily cannabis use, cannabis use disorder, and any medical cannabis use among US adults: associations within racial, ethnic, and sexual minoritized identities in a changing policy context. *Prev Med Rep.* 2022;28:101822.
256. Swendsen J, Conway KP, Degenhardt L, et al. Socio-demographic risk factors for alcohol and drug dependence: the 10-year follow-up of the national comorbidity survey. *Addiction.* 2009;104(8):1346-1355.
257. Maclean JC, Webber D, French MT. Workplace problems, mental health and substance use. *Appl Econ.* 2015;47(9):883-905.
258. Gutkind S, Fink DS, Shmulewitz D, Stohl M, Hasin D. Psychosocial and health problems associated with alcohol use disorder and cannabis use disorder in U.S. adults. *Drug Alcohol Depend.* 2021;229:109137.
259. Marchand A. Alcohol use and misuse: what are the contributions of occupation and work organization conditions? *BMC Public Health.* 2008;8(1):333.
260. Marchand A, Blanc ME. Occupation, work organization conditions, and alcohol misuse in Canada: an 8-year longitudinal study. *Subst Use Misuse.* 2011;46(8):1003-1014.
261. Cheng WJ, Cheng Y, Huang MC, Chen CJ. Alcohol dependence, consumption of alcoholic energy drinks and associated work characteristics in the Taiwan working population. *Alcohol Alcohol.* 2012;47(4):372-379.
262. Kaila-Kangas L, Koskinen A, Pensola T, Mäkelä P, Leino-Arjas P. Alcohol-induced morbidity and mortality by occupation: a population-based follow-up study of working Finns. *Eur J Public Health.* 2016;26(1):116-122.
263. Coggon D, Harris EC, Brown T, Rice S, Palmer KT. Occupation and mortality related to alcohol, drugs and sexual habits. *Occup Med (Lond).* 2010;60(5):348-353.
264. Diala CC, Muntaner C, Walrath C. Gender, occupational, and socioeconomic correlates of alcohol and drug abuse among U.S. rural, metropolitan, and urban residents. *Am J Drug Alcohol Abuse.* 2004;30(2):409-428.
265. Anthony JC, Eaton WW, Mandell W, Garrison R. Psychoactive drug dependence and abuse: more common in some occupations than others. *J Employee Assistance Res.* 1992;1(1):148-186.
266. McLaughlin KA, Breslau J, Green JG, et al. Childhood socio-economic status and the onset, persistence, and severity of DSM-IV mental disorders in a US national sample. *Soc Sci Med.* 2011;73(7):1088-1096.
267. Gilman SE, Breslau J, Conron KJ, Koenen KC, Subramanian SV, Zaslavsky AM. Education and race-ethnicity differences in the lifetime risk of alcohol dependence. *J Epidemiol Community Health.* 2008; 62(3):224-230.
268. Kendler KS, Ohlsson H, Sundquist J, Sundquist K. School achievement, IQ, and risk of alcohol use disorder: a prospective, co-relative analysis in a Swedish National Cohort. *J Stud Alcohol Drugs.* 2017;78(2): 186-194.
269. Grant JD, Scherrer JF, Lynskey MT, et al. Associations of alcohol, nicotine, cannabis, and drug use/dependence with educational attainment: evidence from cotwin-control analyses. *Alcohol Clin Exp Res.* 2012;36(8):1412-1420.

270. Sloan FA, Grossman DS. Alcohol consumption in early adulthood and schooling completed and labor market outcomes at midlife by race and gender. *Am J Public Health*. 2011;101(11):2093-2101.
271. Kendler KS, Lönn SL, Salvatore J, Sundquist J, Sundquist K. Effect of marriage on risk for onset of alcohol use disorder: a longitudinal and co-relative analysis in a Swedish national sample. *Am J Psychiatry*. 2016;173(9):911-918.
272. Power C, Rodgers B, Hope S. Heavy alcohol consumption and marital status: disentangling the relationship in a national study of young adults. *Addiction*. 1999;94(10):1477-1487.
273. Kendler KS, Lönn SL, Salvatore J, Sundquist J, Sundquist K. Divorce and the onset of alcohol use disorder: a Swedish population-based longitudinal cohort and co-relative study. *Am J Psychiatry*. 2017;174(5):451-458.
274. Fu H, Goldman N. The association between health-related behaviours and the risk of divorce in the USA. *J Biosoc Sci*. 2000;32(1):63-88.
275. Scott KM, Wells JE, Angermeyer M, et al. Gender and the relationship between marital status and first onset of mood, anxiety and substance use disorders. *Psychol Med*. 2010;40(9):1495-1505.
276. Hartmann DJ, Sullivan WP, Wolk JL. A state-wide assessment: marital stability and client outcomes. *Drug Alcohol Depend*. 1991;29(1):27-38.
277. Westhuis DJ, Gwaltney L, Hayashi R. Outpatient cocaine abuse treatment: predictors of success. *J Drug Educ*. 2001;31(2):171-183.
278. Kallan JE. Drug abuse-related mortality in the United States: patterns and correlates. *Am J Drug Alcohol Abuse*. 1998;24(1):103-117.
279. Homish GG, Leonard KE, Cornelius JR. Predictors of marijuana use among married couples: the influence of one's spouse. *Drug Alcohol Depend*. 2007;91(2-3):121-128.
280. Yang LH, Wong LY, Grivel MM, Hasin DS. Stigma and substance use disorders: an international phenomenon. *Curr Opin Psychiatry*. 2017;30(5):378-388.
281. Hunte HER, Barry AE. Perceived discrimination and DSM-IV-based alcohol and illicit drug use disorders. *Am J Public Health*. 2012;102(12):e111-e117.
282. McCabe SE, Bostwick WB, Hughes TL, West BT, Boyd CJ. The relationship between discrimination and substance use disorders among lesbian, gay, and bisexual adults in the United States. *Am J Public Health*. 2010;100(10):1946-1952.
283. Berger M, Sarnyai Z. More than skin deep: stress neurobiology and mental health consequences of racial discrimination. *Stress*. 2015;18(1):1-10.
284. Keyes KM, Cerda M, Brady JE, Havens JR, Galea S. Understanding the rural-urban differences in nonmedical prescription opioid use and abuse in the United States. *Am J Public Health*. 2014;104(2): e52-e59.
285. Compton WM, Jones CM, Baldwin GT. Relationship between nonmedical prescription-opioid use and heroin use. *N Engl J Med*. 2016;374(2):154-163.
286. Feder KA, Mojtabai R, Musci RJ, Letourneau EJ. U.S. adults with opioid use disorder living with children: treatment use and barriers to care. *J Subst Abuse Treat*. 2018;93:31-37.
287. Montiel Ishino FA, McNab PR, Gilreath T, Salmeron B, Williams F. A comprehensive multivariate model of biopsychosocial factors associated with opioid misuse and use disorder in a 2017-2018 United States national survey. *BMC Public Health*. 2020;20(1):1740.
288. Flores MW, Cook BL, Mullin B, et al. Associations between neighborhood-level factors and opioid-related mortality: a multi-level analysis using death certificate data. *Addiction*. 2020;115(10): 1878-1889.
289. McCabe SE, Schulenberg J, McCabe VV, Veliz PT. Medical use and misuse of prescription opioids in US 12th-grade youth: school-level correlates. *Pediatrics*. 2020;146(4):
290. Sara G, Burgess P, Harris M, Malhi GS, Whiteford H, Hall W. Stimulant use disorders: characteristics and comorbidity in an Australian population sample. *Aust NZ J Psychiatry*. 2012;46(12):1173-1181.
291. Martins SS, Segura LE, Santaella-Tenorio J, et al. Prescription opioid use disorder and heroin use among 12-34 year-olds in the United States from 2002 to 2014. *Addict Behav*. 2017;65:236-241.
292. Volkow ND. Collision of the COVID-19 and addiction epidemics. *Ann Intern Med*. 2020;173(1):61-62.
293. Alexander GC, Stoller KB, Haffajee RL, Saloner B. An epidemic in the midst of a pandemic: opioid use disorder and COVID-19. *Ann Intern Med*. 2020;173(1):57-58.
294. Volkow ND, Collins FS. The role of science in the opioid crisis. *N Engl J Med*. 2017;377(18):1798.
295. Martins SS, Ponicki W, Smith N, et al. Prescription drug monitoring programs operational characteristics and fatal heroin poisoning. *Int J Drug Policy*. 2019;74:174-180.
296. Cerda M, Ponicki W, Smith N, et al. Measuring relationships between proactive reporting state-level prescription drug monitoring programs and county-level fatal prescription opioid overdoses. *Epidemiology*. 2020;31(1):32-42.
297. Haffajee RL. Prescription drug monitoring programs—friend or folly in addressing the opioid-overdose crisis? *N Engl J Med*. 2019;381(8):699-701.
298. Smith N, Martins SS, Kim J, et al. A typology of prescription drug monitoring programs: a latent transition analysis of the evolution of programs from 1999 to 2016. *Addiction*. 2019;114(2):248-258.
299. Segura LE, Mauro CM, Levy NS, et al. Association of US medical marijuana laws with nonmedical prescription opioid use and prescription opioid use disorder. *JAMA Netw Open*. 2019;2(7):e197216.
300. Martins SS, Bruzelius E, Stingone JA, et al. Prescription opioid laws and opioid dispensing in US counties: identifying salient law provisions with machine learning. *Epidemiology*. 2021;32(6):868-876.
301. Kim JH, Martins SS, Shmulewitz D, Hasin D. Association between fatal opioid overdose and state medical cannabis laws in US national survey data, 2000-2011. *Int J Drug Policy*. 2021;99:103449.
302. Cerdá M, Wheeler-Martin K, Bruzelius E, et al. Spatiotemporal analysis of the association between pain management clinic laws and opioid prescribing and overdose deaths. *Am J Epidemiol*. 2021;190(12):2592-2603.
303. Castillo-Carniglia A, Ponicki WR, Gaidus AGP, et al. Prescription drug monitoring programs and opioid overdose: exploring sources of heterogeneity. *Am J Public Health*. 2019;30(2):212-220.
304. Mauro CM, Newswanger P, Santaella-Tenorio J, Mauro PM, Carliner H, Martins SS. Impact of medical marijuana laws on state-level marijuana use by age and gender, 2004-2013. *Prev Sci*. 2019;20(2):205-214.
305. Philbin MM, Mauro PM, SantaellaTenorio J, et al. Associations between state-level policy liberalism, cannabis use, and cannabis use disorder from 2004 to 2012: looking beyond medical cannabis law status. *Int J Drug Policy*. 2019;65:97-103.
306. Sheehan BE, Grucza RA, Plunk AD. Association of racial disparity of cannabis possession arrests among adults and youths with statewide cannabis decriminalization and legalization. *JAMA Health Forum*. 2021;2(10):e213435.
307. Gilder DA, Lau P, Corey L, Ehlers CL. Factors associated with remission from alcohol dependence in an American Indian community group. *Am J Psychiatry*. 2008;165(9):1172-1178.
308. Dawson DA, Goldstein RB, Ruan WJ, Grant BF. Correlates of recovery from alcohol dependence: a prospective study over a 3-year follow-up interval. *Alcohol Clin Exp Res*. 2012;36(7):1268-1277.
309. Moss HB, Chen CM, Yi HY. Prospective follow-up of empirically derived Alcohol Dependence subtypes in wave 2 of the National Epidemiologic Survey on Alcohol And Related Conditions (NESARC): recovery status, alcohol use disorders and diagnostic criteria, alcohol consumption behavior, health status, and treatment seeking. *Alcohol Clin Exp Res*. 2010;34(6):1073-1083.
310. McCutcheon VV, Schuckit MA, Kramer JR, et al. Familial association of abstinent remission from alcohol use disorder in first-degree relatives of alcohol-dependent treatment-seeking probands. *Addiction*. 2017;112(11):1909-1917.

311. Hufnagel A, Frick U, Ridinger M, Wodarz N. Recovery from alcohol dependence: do smoking indicators predict abstinence? *Am J Addict.* 2017;26(4):366-373.
312. McCabe SE, Cranford JA, Boyd CJ. Stressful events and other predictors of remission from drug dependence in the United States: longitudinal results from a national survey. *J Subst Abuse Treat.* 2016;71:41-47.
313. Dawson DA, Goldstein RB, Grant BF. Rates and correlates of relapse among individuals in remission from DSM-IV alcohol dependence: a 3-year follow-up. *Alcohol Clin Exp Res.* 2007;31(12):2036-2045.
314. Krasnova A, Diaz JE, Philbin MM, Mauro PM. Disparities in substance use disorder treatment use and perceived need by sexual identity and gender among adults in the United States. *Drug Alcohol Depend.* 2021;226:108828.
315. Mauro PM, Samples H, Klein KS, Martins SS. Discussing drug use with health care providers is associated with perceived need and receipt of drug treatment among adults in the United States: we need to talk. *Med Care.* 2020;58(7):617-624.
316. Cohen E, Feinn R, Arias A, Kranzler HR. Alcohol treatment utilization: findings from the national epidemiologic survey on alcohol and related conditions. *Drug Alcohol Depend.* 2007;86(2-3):214-221.
317. Alvanzo AA, Storr CL, Mojtabai R, et al. Gender and race/ethnicity differences for initiation of alcohol-related service use among persons with alcohol dependence. *Drug Alcohol Depend.* 2014;140: 48-55.
318. Blanco C, Iza M, Rodríguez-Fernández JM, Baca-García E, Wang S, Olfson M. Probability and predictors of treatment-seeking for substance use disorders in the U.S. *Drug Alcohol Depend.* 2015;149:136-144.
319. Mauro PM, Gutkind S, Annunziato EM, Samples H. Use of medication for opioid use disorder among US adolescents and adults with need for opioid treatment, 2019. *JAMA Netw Open.* 2022;5(3):e223821.

Sidebar

Primary, Secondary, and Tertiary Prevention

James C. Anthony

CONTEXT AND MEANING OF PRIMARY, SECONDARY, AND TERTIARY PREVENTION

When students in our field master the epidemiology of a specific disease, syndrome, or other disturbance of health and well-being, they can organize the evidence, estimates, and subject matter according to the five main rubrics and associated research questions shown in **Table 24-1**.

As Anthony and Van Etten described, for our work under Rubric #1, we often ask about the disturbance's incidence or mortality rate in the population designated for study.[1] The incidence rate estimate might involve an implicit passage of time when quantified as an attack rate. The estimated attack rate might refer to experiences during an interval of random but constrained length after a traumatic event or exposure to a toxic agent. If that interval is the entire life history of individuals in the population as of a specified date (eg, the date of a census or survey assessment), the attack rate can be expressed as a "cumulative incidence proportion."

Some incidence rates and mortality rates count up explicit units of person-time in the denominator of the rate, with units such as person-years, person-months, person-weeks, or even person-days, and person-hours. This formulation of the rate brings the estimates into closer alignment with concepts of "survival analysis" such as "the instantaneous hazard rate."

There is a bit of subtlety here when the condition is not immediately fatal, and even more subtlety when the condition involves recurrences. Take as an example the fact that a nonfatal drug overdose or suicide attempt might occur more than one time during the specified interval of time (eg, multiple nonfatal suicide attempts during one person-year in the life of an individual affected by bipolar disorder or borderline personality disorder). As is the case when a communicable disease (eg, influenza, gonorrhea) might occur more than once during the interval of time, it is important to draw a distinction

TABLE 24-1 The Five Main Rubrics of Epidemiology

1. Quantity: "In the population, as time passes, how many are becoming affected?"
2. Location: "Within the population, where are cases more or less likely to be found?" (in relation to place, time, person dimensions)
3. Causes: "What accounts for some population members becoming affected as cases while others are spared?"
4. Mechanisms: "What linkages of circumstances, conditions, states, and processes unfold as we study the earliest origins of the disturbance through its end-stages?"
5. Prevention & Control: "What can we do to reduce the numbers of newly incident cases, shorten duration, ameliorate, or otherwise reduce the suffering?"

From Anthony JC, Van Etten ML. Epidemiology and its rubrics. In: Bellack A, Hersen M, eds. *Comprehensive Clinical Psychology.* Elsevier; 1998:355-390. Courtesy of James C. Anthony.

between the "newly incident" occurrences versus the "recurrences." For public health officials trying to plan for how many person-days of effort are needed to do contact tracing for a communicable condition, there is a need to place the sum of the newly incidence occurrences plus the recurrences in the numerator of the rates. For calculation of a "first admission rate" to specialty psychiatric care, the recurrences are ignored, and it is the newly incident occurrences that are counted in the numerator of the rate.

Of course, for each condition that is not immediately fatal, with or without recurrences, we also ask about the population prevalence, specified as a proportion at some point in time or during an interval (eg, one year). For nonfatal conditions that leave residual disability, the Disability-Adjusted Life Years parameter has become popular because it quantifies the years of life lost due to premature deaths caused by the disease plus the years of disablement caused by the condition.

Working under Rubric #2, we focus on variations in the values of the estimated mortality or incidence rates and the other epidemiological parameters that hold for the population designated for study. Here, the term "location" encompasses more than geography and geopolitical boundaries. "Location" also refers to variations across time (eg, seasonal or other time trends) and across characteristics of the population members (eg, sex, age, ethnic self-identification).

In global health research, the variations might be region by region or country by country, considering the age pyramid, the female-male ratio, and other demographically crucial subgroups. The evidence might highlight the special needs of subgroups of inhabitants characterized by individual or sociocultural characteristics within a specific country or jurisdiction, such as a small public health district. The earliest epidemiological surveys generally produced estimates for dwellers in urban versus rural areas, native-born versus immigrant subgroups, religious affiliation, and occupation types. In the most recent epidemiological field studies that produce estimates under this rubric, the "locational" characteristics encompass subgroups defined by behavior (eg, men who have sex with men).

An epidemiologist's work under the third rubric builds from Rubric #2 estimates. Generally, it seeks increasingly definitive evidence needed to draw cause-effect inferences and to become increasingly precise about specific causal agents or processes. Nevertheless, the task has occasionally involved no new gathering of data or experimentation beyond what had been gathered under Rubric #2. Instead, the epidemiologist has organized available estimates and other evidence into a chain of inference sturdy enough to motivate prevention and control tactics. A classic example in epidemiology is John Snow's 19th-century inference that cholera epidemics ought to be prevented by improvements in the sanitary water supply decades before bacteriologist Robert Koch identified *Vibrio cholerae* as that disease's specific causal agent.

Our work under Rubric #4 shifts attention to mechanisms, sometimes studied as sequences of states and processes that lead toward and beyond a disease-state or other health disturbance; longitudinal research designs are often employed but are not required. The discovery of mechanisms helps to inspire new ideas about prevention and control. Occasionally, a prevention experiment sheds light on how a preventive intervention can reduce the incidence or prevalence of a condition. In an analysis of longitudinal data from their prevention trial of the Iowa Strengthening Families Program (ISFP), Spoth and colleagues studied shielding from drug exposure opportunities.[2] They concluded that ISFP shielding was an intermediate mechanism of later observed ISFP-associated reductions in the cumulative incidence of using glue or internationally regulated drugs such as cannabis.[2] Holmes and colleagues identified a potential mechanism of interest to neuroscientists in a suggestion that parenting behaviors might function to improve a multivariate array of health behaviors. The suggested mechanism involved changes in functional magnetic resonance imaging of resting-state functional connectivity within nodes of the anterior salience networks.[3]

The fifth rubric reflects epidemiology's explicit orientation to preventing and controlling diseases and other health disturbances. Here, the concept of "prevention and control" encompasses public health and clinical tactics that can reduce incidence or mortality rates or otherwise affect prevalence proportions by shortening a condition's duration. When the disturbance cannot be prevented or shortened, we can try to reduce the Disability-Adjusted Life Years or seek to relieve the associated pain, suffering, and economic hardship.

Condition by condition, we can map the definitions of primary, secondary, and tertiary prevention according to whether we see the effect of public health or clinical tactics in reduced incidence rates. If using the ISFP to shield youths from drug exposure opportunities prevents drug use before it occurs, we have reduced the incidence of drug use in the act of "primary" prevention. Effective use of an opioid antagonist such as naloxone to prevent a fatal outcome during overdose will reduce the drug overdose mortality rate—that is, "primary" prevention of overdose death.

When we have not prevented the use of alcohol, nicotine, or one of the internationally regulated drugs, each individual who starts using drugs counts toward an increase in the drug use prevalence proportion. If we cannot reduce the prevalence proportion by lowering the incidence rate, then the only other way to reduce prevalence is to shorten the duration of drug use. Public health and clinical tactics to shorten the duration of drug use might involve screening for active drug use, outreach to individuals who start using drugs, early intervention, and treatment services designed to be curative. These tactics qualify as "secondary" prevention when a "cure" occurs and shortens drug use duration. Thereby, the prevalence proportion drops.

Sometimes drug use per se can account for a residual disability without a diagnosable disease state. To illustrate, Takakuwa and Schears provide case reports of the EVALI syndrome (e-cigarette or vaping product use-associated lung injury), with residual consequences after vaping a vitamin E acetate-contaminated product.[4] Removal of the vitamin E acetate-contaminated products from the market represents a "tertiary prevention" tactic with respect to drug use because this tactic will influence neither incidence of drug use nor its duration, nor will it be curative with respect to the persistence of the vaping behavior. When we think about removal of the contamination with "drug use" as the specified target condition, it is a "tertiary prevention" tactic—a crucial ingredient in public health strategies designed to prevent and control such harmful effects of drug use in the form of disablement. When we think the "EVALI" syndrome as the specified target condition, removal of the contaminant would be a "primary prevention" tactic that should reduce incidence of the EVALI syndrome.

This example provides an illustration of the importance of specifying one's target condition before sorting tactics into the "primary," "secondary," and "tertiary" prevention subtypes. A tactic can be a "tertiary prevention" tactic for one specified target condition (eg, target = drug use; outcome = reduced occurrence of residual disability due to drug use) and that same tactic can be a "primary prevention" tactic for a different but related specified target condition (eg, target = EVALI syndrome; outcome = reduced incidence of the EVALI syndrome when vaping occurs).

Nolte characterized tertiary prevention as an attempt to reduce residual effects of "established disease by eliminating or reducing disability, minimizing suffering, and maximizing potential years of quality life." These tactics of treatment and rehabilitation seek to reduce the number and impact of complications, with an intended decline in the number of DALYs, as defined in the prior section.[5]

In this monograph, other target conditions for prevention and control are the drug dependence syndromes defined for the International Classification of Diseases (ICD) and the fourth edition of the *American Psychiatric Association's Diagnostic and Statistical Manual* (DSM-IV) or a related DSM-5 drug use disorder. The "secondary" prevention tactics described for "drug use" qualify as "primary" prevention tactics for these drug syndromes and disorders. Shortening drug use duration can reduce the incidence of drug dependence or a use disorder when there are "persistent use" and duration specifications in the ICD and DSM diagnostic criteria.

"Secondary" prevention of drug dependence or a related DSM-5 drug use disorder sometimes can encompass tactics that disrupt the progression from drug use onset to a diagnosable syndrome or disorder. These tactics might involve screening after initial drug exposure and some intervention designed to disrupt forward progress toward the syndrome or disorder.

Celentano, Szklo, and Gordis characterized one form of secondary prevention tactic as identifying people for whom a disease process has started but who have not yet qualified for the disease and might not even have signs or symptoms of any related illness. This form of "secondary" prevention intends to detect a pathological process earlier than it might have been detected otherwise.[6]

This characterization makes it possible to think that early screening for incipient use disorder for alcohol, nicotine, or other drugs might qualify as "secondary" prevention even though the intended effect of early screening is to reduce the disorder's incidence rate. The traditional specification for "primary" prevention encompasses tactics that reduce a disorder's incidence. The traditional specification for "secondary" prevention encompasses tactics that reduce prevalence proportions by shortening duration or being curative once the pathological process yields a case of the disorder. Logically, it would seem that early screening qualifies as "primary" prevention if the early screening makes it possible to prevent the occurrence of a condition that otherwise would have occurred.

JOHN D. SWISHER'S CONSTRUCTS OF PRIMARY, SECONDARY, AND TERTIARY PREVENTION

John D. Swisher might have been the first scientist to study alcohol, nicotine, cannabis, and other internationally regulated drugs, to master the concepts of primary, secondary, and tertiary prevention, and then apply these concepts to drug-related harms.[7] A summary of Swisher's ideas appears in **Table 24-2**.

ORIGINS OF THE CONCEPTS OF PRIMARY, SECONDARY, AND TERTIARY PREVENTION

Swisher attributed the concepts of primary, secondary, and tertiary prevention to Gerald Caplan.[8] Swisher neglected earlier work by psychiatric epidemiologist Ernest M. Gruenberg.[9] Perhaps inspired by Hilleboe,[10] Gruenberg organized his article into sections on "Demonstrated Primary Prevention" and "Presumptive Primary Prevention," as well as "Secondary Prevention" and the prevention of disability. Swisher also did not cite an important article by Lester Breslow nor the later publication of Volume 1 in a series of reports issued by the U.S. Commission on Chronic Illness.[11,12] The CCI often has been designated as the origin of these differentiated concepts of primary, secondary, and tertiary prevention; Gruenberg's article in 1953 covered all of these topics.

TABLE 24-2 John D. Swisher's Conceptualization of Primary, Secondary, and Tertiary Prevention of Unhealthy Drug Use

Timing	Activities	Terminology
During later states of use	Treatment Institutionalization maintenance Withdrawal management	Tertiary prevention
During early stages of use	Crises intervention Early diagnosis Crises monitoring Referral	Secondary prevention
Before use	Education Information Alternatives Personal and social growth	Primary prevention

From Swisher JD. Prevention issues. In: Dupont RL, Goldstein A, O'Donnell J, eds. *Handbook on Drug Abuse*. United States Government Printing Office; 1979:424.

BEYOND THE CONCEPTS OF PRIMARY, SECONDARY, AND TERTIARY PREVENTION

At present, any article on primary, secondary, and tertiary prevention should mention differentiated concepts for prevention research. Almost 30 years ago, Mrazek and Haggerty described the three-part prevention conceptualization and offered an embellishment as depicted in **Figure 24-1**.[13]

On the left side of the spectrum, we can see "universal" prevention tactics intended for all persons in a population. Then, "selective" prevention tactics are designed to benefit population members or subgroups with an excess risk of becoming cases. The concept of "indicated" prevention tactics refers to what we might do to prevent the onset of a diagnosable condition after a diagnostic workup. The workup might show (1) "minimal but detectable signs or symptoms" forming in a pathological process that foreshadows impending disorder onset or (2) biological markers that indicate an elevated predisposition to become a case.

SELECTED READINGS

Several contributions not cited in prior sections should interest the true scholars in this field of study. During graduate school, when studying poliovirus epidemiology, I learned an interesting prevention concept of "autarcesis," as described by Aycock.[14] Later, Aycock advocated "autarceology" as the study of host resistance characteristics of potential importance without the involvement of specific antibodies or generic mechanisms of immunity. The intact epidermis was described as an autarceologic shield against infection by agents that might cause disease via a skin lesion. Our research group later adapted this concept and explained how "behavioral autarcesis" might help shield young people from initial chances to try drugs. We suspected that a nonspecific protective process might dampen the probability of transitioning from that first chance to try the drug onward toward the onset of newly incident drug use. Chen and colleagues, in 2004, speculated that youths engaged in regular religious activities might benefit from "behavioral autarcesis" as a primary prevention mechanism with a protective influence against new drug use. Plus, there might be a dampening influence on the persistence and duration of drug use.[15,16] Spoth and colleagues recognized and exploited Aycock's concept of autarcesis as they tried to understand the mechanisms of protective influence conferred by exposure to their universal preventive intervention.[2]

Considering how parents, teachers, and others might shield their children from risks associated with early-onset alcohol, nicotine, or other drug use, we might pay more attention to Aycock's concept of autarcesis. The result might guide us to think more thoroughly about the modes of spread of drug use and the fact that most young people starting to use these drugs are introduced to drug-using behaviors by supposedly friendly peers. This way of thinking about the modes of spread of drug use prompts a consideration of epidemiological parameters such as the "reproduction number" recently made prominent in reports about the SARS-CoV-19 and COVID-19 pandemic. We have no definitive estimates for the "reproduction number" when studying the spread of drug use in youthful populations. The result is a gap in evidence that might help us in future preventive interventions. Without mentioning the reproduction number, Swedish epidemiologist Nils Bejerot advocated early identification of individuals who use drugs and a primary prevention tactic of sending them to the remote forests of Scandinavia so that they would not introduce other young people to drug-use behaviors. His ideas helped to shape Scandinavian policies in response to methamphetamine outbreak/epidemic conditions faced during the 1960s. Bejerot offered an alternative to the more draconian policy responses crafted in China, now resurgent within the United States.[17]

A question might be asked about the relationship between "resilience" and "autarcesis." The distinction involves the nature of the challenge that might give rise to a pathological process. Autarcesis is a phenomenon that can be observed even when there is no challenge, as in the case of an intact epidermis protecting the human organism from ambient microbes on the surface of the skin. The protection is there even if there never is an epidermal lesion followed by effective contact of the microbe with the human "host." In contrast, "resilience" as a concept is specified as a phenomenon that is observed only when there is a challenge. In the examples provided in this sidebar, there can be autarcesis traced to effective parenting behavior or levels of regular religious activity involvement

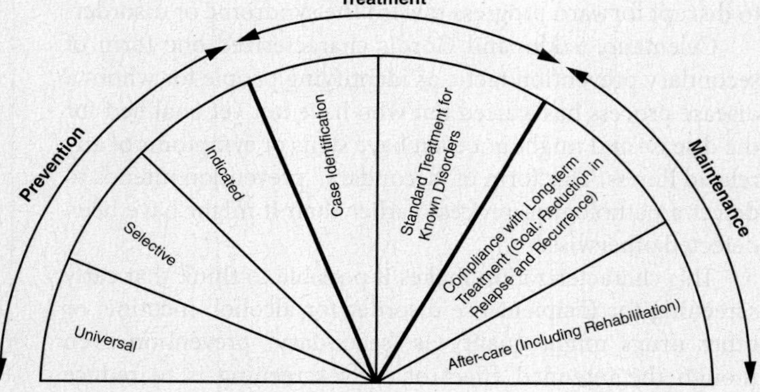

Figure 24-1. The mental health spectrum for mental disorders. (From Institute of Medicine (U.S.) Committee on Prevention of Mental Disorders, Mrazek PJ, Haggerty RJ, eds. *Reducing Risks for Mental Disorders: Frontiers for Preventive Intervention Research.* National Academies Press (U.S.); 1994:605 pages. Accessed May 22, 2023. https://www.ncbi.nlm.nih.gov/books/NBK236318/)

(eg, shielding young people from chances to try drugs), even when the young people never come into contact with someone who is a spreader of these exposure opportunities. In contrast, if there is a prevention program to build up "resilience," and the intent is to evaluate the efficacy or effectiveness of that prevention program, then the outcome to be studied should be the conditional occurrence of actually trying the drug for the first time, once the challenge of an exposure opportunity has occurred. Otherwise, any between-group variation in the unconditional occurrence of trying the drug for the first time might be due to the program's effect on whether and how often drug exposure opportunities occur, with no mechanism of "resilience" in play.

In addition to these drug-specific readings, interested readers might wish to read and understand the concepts and principles described in an American Public Health Association (APHA) monograph entitled *Mental Disorders: A Guide to Control Methods*.[18] It is fair to ask why anyone should look back and read a 1962 monograph that now is out of date and out of print (but available in online internet archives). This sidebar mentions the 1962 monograph because that monograph was intended to be a complement to the APHA *Control of Communicable Diseases manual* (CCDM). First published more than 100 years ago and updated regularly so that it now is in its 21st edition,[19] the CCDM is in the top rank of authoritative guides to what practitioners in the field of public health and medicine can do when they seek to prevent the occurrence of any communicable disease (or infection or other condition) in a population and to control the public health impact of the condition if it has not been prevented. Infection by infection, disease by disease, the CCDM summarizes the most up-to-date epidemiological and clinical evidence on best practices. This characteristic makes it an exceptionally useful manual for prevention scientists and other public health workers, as well as for practitioners who encounter a patient with what might be a challenging screening, diagnosis, or intervention-meriting condition. The 1962 monograph was intended as a complement to CCDM with deliberate coverage of neuropsychiatric conditions, including addictive behaviors and processes. Alas, it has not been updated since 1962, and there is no corresponding manual being regularly published with updated evidence and information for prevention specialists, other public health workers, or addiction medicine specialists. By mentioning it in this sidebar, I hope to encourage a collaborative venture of multiple organizations, including the American Society of Addiction Medicine and the American Public Health Association's Sections on Alcohol, Tobacco, and Other Drugs as well as Mental Health, in an initiative to update the 1962 manual and to foster the editing and publication of regularly issued updates of the manual during the rest of the 21st century and beyond.

REFERENCES

1. Anthony JC, Van Etten ML. Epidemiology and its rubrics. In: Bellack A, Hersen M, eds. *Comprehensive Clinical Psychology.* Vol. 1. Elsevier; 1998:355-390.
2. Spoth R, Guyll M, Shin C. Universal intervention as a protective shield against exposure to substance use: long-term outcomes and public health significance. *Am J Public Health.* 2009;99(11):2026-2033. doi:10.2105/AJPH.2007.133298
3. Holmes CJ, Barton AW, MacKillop J, et al. Parenting and salience network connectivity among African Americans: a protective pathway for health-risk behaviors. *Biol Psychiatry.* 2018;84(5):365-371. https://doi.org/10.1016/j.biopsych.2018.03.003
4. Takakuwa KM, Schears RM. The emergency department care of the cannabis and synthetic cannabinoid patient: a narrative review. *Int J Emerg Med.* 2021;14(1):10. doi:10.1186/s12245-021-00330-3
5. Nolte E. Disease prevention. In: Heggenhougen K, Quah S, eds. *International Encyclopedia of Public Health.* Elsevier; 2008:222-234.
6. Celentano DD, Szklo M. *Gordis Epidemiology.* 6th ed. Elsevier 2019:420 pages.
7. Swisher JD. Prevention issues. In: Dupont RL, Goldstein A, O'Donnell J, eds. *Handbook on Drug Abuse.* United States Government Printing Office; 1977:423-438.
8. Caplan G. *Support Systems and Community Mental Health.* Behavioral Publications; 1974:267 pages.
9. Gruenberg EM. The prevention of mental disease. *Ann Am Acad Pol Soc Sci.* 1953;286(1):158-166. doi:10.1177/000271625328600119
10. Hilleboe HE. Public health and medicine at the crossroads. *Public Health Rep (1896–1970).* 1952;67(8):767-771. doi:10.2307/4588196
11. Breslow L. Prevention of chronic illness. *Am J Public Health Nations Health.* 1956;46(12):1540-1542. doi:10.2105/ajph.46.12.1540
12. Commission on Chronic Illness. *Chronic Illness in the United States.* Vol. 1. Harvard University Press; 1957.
13. Institute of Medicine (U.S.) Committee on Prevention of Mental Disorders, Mrazek PJ, Haggerty RJ, eds. *Reducing Risks for Mental Disorders: Frontiers for Preventive Intervention Research.* National Academies Press (U.S.); 1994.
14. Aycock WL. A study of the significance of geographic and seasonal variations in the incidence of poliomyelitis. *J Prev Med.* 1929;3(3):245-278.
15. Chen CY, Dormitzer CM, Bejarano J, Anthony JC. Religiosity and the earliest stages of adolescent drug involvement in seven countries of Latin America. *Am J Epidemiol.* 2004;159(12):1180-1188. doi:10.1093/aje/kwh151
16. Chen CY, Dormitzer CM, Gutiérrez U, Vittetoe K, González GB, Anthony JC. The adolescent behavioral repertoire as a context for drug exposure: behavioral autarcesis at play. *Addiction.* 2004;99(7):897-906. doi:10.1111/j.1360-0443.2004.00774.x
17. Bejerot N. *Addiction and Society.* Charles C. Thomas; 1970.
18. American Public Health Association; Program Area Committee on Mental Health. *Mental Disorders: A Guide to Control Methods.* APHA; 1962.
19. Heymann DL. *Control of Communicable Diseases Manual 21st Edition: An Official Report of the American Public Health Association.* APHA Press. Accessed May 22, 2023. https://ccdm.aphapublications.org/doi/book/10.2105/CCDM.2745

CHAPTER

25 Preventing Substance Use Among Children and Adolescents

Kenneth W. Griffin and Gilbert J. Botvin

CHAPTER OUTLINE

- Introduction
- Prevalence rates and progression of use
- Etiology and implications for prevention
- Types of preventive interventions
- Summary and conclusions

INTRODUCTION

Substance use and substance use disorders (SUDs) are important public health problems that contribute significantly to morbidity and mortality in the United States and throughout the world. Over the past several decades, there have been significant advances in our understanding of the epidemiology and etiology of substance use and the development and testing of prevention and treatment approaches. Epidemiological research shows that, from a population perspective, the onset of substance use typically begins during the adolescent years. Many adolescents who use substances initiate with alcohol and "vaping," and research demonstrates that this typically begins in a social context with one's peer group. National and international data sets show that the prevalence of alcohol, tobacco, and other drug use increases rapidly from early to late adolescence, peaking during the years of young adulthood. Furthermore, a large body of research has shown that early initiation of substance use is associated with higher levels of use later in life, increased risk of addiction and negative outcomes including violent and delinquent behavior, poor physical health, and mental health problems.[1]

Given the well-established pattern of onset and developmental progression of substance use, a variety of prevention initiatives for children and adolescents have been developed. Relatively few prevention efforts have focused on adults because it is rare for adults to develop SUDs without a history of substance use during adolescence. Initiatives to prevent youth substance use include educational and skills training programs for young people in school settings, programs that teach parents ways to monitor their children and all family members the skills needed to communicate effectively, and community-based programs that combine school and family components with additional educational, mass media, or public policy components (eg, restricting access to alcohol and tobacco though enforcement of minimum purchasing age requirements; see Chapter 26. Environmental Approaches to Prevention). A goal of many prevention initiatives is to prevent early-stage substance use or delay the onset of use. Most aim to prevent alcohol, tobacco/nicotine, and cannabis use because these are widely used substances in our society and pose a great risk to individual and public health. Most prevention programs target middle or junior high school-age youth to prevent substance use initiation or delay the typical age of onset. The large body of research examining the efficacy and effectiveness of prevention programs for adolescent alcohol, tobacco, and other drug use demonstrates that the most effective approaches target salient risk and protective factors at the individual, family, and/or community levels and are guided by relevant psychosocial theories regarding the etiology of substance use.[2]

PREVALENCE RATES AND PROGRESSION OF USE

In the United States, the prevalence rates of substance use among adolescents peaked in the late 1970s and early 1980s, fell through much of the remainder of the 1980s, and began to increase again during the 1990s. Over the past two decades, prevalence rates of use for most substances have gradually declined among adolescents but remain problematic. The 2021 Monitoring the Future (MTF) study[3] found that among high school seniors, 54% of students reported lifetime alcohol use and 39% reported ever being drunk. The use of electronic drug delivery systems (including e-cigarettes) was reported by 41% of high school seniors, higher than the lifetime prevalence of cigarette smoking (18%). Findings showed that 41% of 12th graders reported ever using any illegal drug, and most of this was accounted for by cannabis use (39%). Lifetime prevalence rates were about 5% for LSD, hallucinogens other than LSD, and inhalants. Lifetime prevalence rates were in the range of 1% to 3% for ecstasy (MDMA), heroin, cocaine or crack cocaine, methamphetamine, and crystal methamphetamine. The misuse of any prescription drug (taking a medication "without a doctor telling you to use them") was reported by 9% of high school seniors, and this included the misuse of amphetamines (5%), narcotics other than heroin (2%), tranquilizers (3%), or sedatives/barbiturates (4%).

An analysis of demographic subgroup findings from the MTF study[4] revealed several differences in illegal drug use according to gender, race/ethnicity, and average education level of parents (a proxy for socioeconomic status). Annual prevalence rates of any illegal drug historically been higher among male relative to female high school seniors. However, in 2021, 33.4% of females reported illegal drug use in the past year compared to 29.5% of males. Illegal substance use rates have historically been highest among White high school seniors, though in 2021, 36.6% of Black high school seniors reported illegal drug use in the past year compared to 33.5% of Whites and 30.2% of Hispanics. Among 8th and 10th grade students, those whose parents have the lowest educational attainment have consistently reported higher rates of past year illegal drug use than students whose parents have higher educational attainment, but this pattern does not describe high school seniors. Studies have shown that adolescent substance use is associated with disadvantaged socioeconomic context and lower family income, and that these factors interact with family and peer risk and protective factors in complex ways.[5]

The MTF study and other national surveys revealed a decline in substance use rates among teens during 2020 and 2021 due to the Covid-19 pandemic. These declines can be understood in the context of the highly social nature of adolescent substance use. Due to school closings, stay-at-home and social distancing orders, and restricted opportunities for spending time with friends during the peak of the pandemic, teens spent considerably less time in the social environments where substance use often occurs, leading to reduced rates. On the other hand, pandemic-related disruptions in daily life led to increased reports of stress, isolation, boredom, anxiety, and depression among many teens—all of which are risk factors for adolescent substance use.[6] Rates of use for alcohol and cannabis use appeared to have increased during the pandemic among the relatively small proportion of mostly older adolescents who engage in solitary substance use to cope with negative affect.[6] Pandemic-related substance use trends should be interpreted with caution because data collection procedures changed due to the pandemic (eg, surveys completed at home rather than school) and the effects of these changes are unknown.

While the long-term effect of the pandemic on adolescent substance use is unknown, some level of substance use has and will continue to be commonplace among youth in contemporary American society. During early adolescence, substance use occurs largely in a social context and typically involves substances that are readily available from peers such as alcohol, tobacco/nicotine in all forms, and inhalants. Eventually, some youth may engage in more regular patterns of use and/or progress to cannabis, hallucinogens, and other illegal drugs in a predictable pattern.[7] A subset eventually develops patterns of use associated with problems or decrements in functioning. The likelihood of progressing to more serious levels of substance use and disorder is best understood in probabilistic terms. An individual's risk of greater substance use involvement increases at each additional step in the developmental progression. Furthermore, the initial social motivations for substance use typically yield to those driven increasingly by pharmacological, genetic, and psychological factors.[8] Knowledge of the typical patterns and progression of substance use has important implications for the focus and timing of preventive interventions. Prevention programs that effectively target risk factors for alcohol and tobacco/nicotine use may not only prevent the use of these substances but also may reduce or eliminate the risk of using other substances further along the progression.

ETIOLOGY AND IMPLICATIONS FOR PREVENTION

The predictable epidemiological patterns of substance use onset and progression during adolescence, combined with observations that substance use is frequently linked to important developmental goals and transitions of adolescence, support the notion that substance use can be thought of as fulfilling normal developmental drives to participate in risky and neurologically rewarding activities during adolescence. The degree of substance use involvement of any teenager is often a function of the negative prodrug social influences in their environment combined with their individual psychosocial vulnerabilities to these influences.

Developmental Aspects

A developmental perspective on the etiology of substance use is informative in understanding how best to prevent early experimentation with alcohol, tobacco/nicotine, and other drugs. Adolescence is a key period for experimentation not only with substances but with a wide range of behaviors and activities. Indeed, a great number of changes occur during adolescence, and experimenting with new behavior occurs as part of a natural process of separating from parents, gaining acceptance and popularity with peers, developing a sense of autonomy and independence, establishing a personal identity and self-image, seeking fun and adventure, and/or rebelling against authority. However, many of these same developmental goals can increase an adolescent's risk of smoking, drinking, or using drugs. Unfortunately, from the point of view of an adolescent, engaging in alcohol, tobacco, and other drug use may be a functional way of achieving independence, maturity, or popularity.

The Importance of Social Influences

Research has shown that social influences are among the most powerful factors promoting experimentation or initiation of alcohol, tobacco, and other drug use among young people. Important types of problematic social influence include the modeling of substance use behavior by significant others (eg, parents, older siblings, and especially peers) and exposure to positive attitudes and expectations regarding substance use.[9] The positive portrayal of substance use by celebrities in movies, television, and music videos is also a powerful and problematic social influence.[10] Advertisements that communicate positive messages about alcohol and tobacco use are likely to promote pro-substance use attitudes, expectancies, and perceived positive consequences of use that can translate into increases in substance use among young people.[11]

Risk and Protective Factors

Risk factors that contribute to the initiation, maintenance, and escalation of alcohol, tobacco, and illegal drug use—along with protective factors that offset the effects of risk—occur at the level of the individual, family, school, and community.

Individual Level

Individual-level factors include cognitive, attitudinal, social, personality, pharmacological, biological, and developmental factors.[12] Cognitive risk factors for substance use include lack of knowledge about the risks of substance use and exaggerated perceived norms regarding the prevalence and social acceptability of substance use. Affect regulation is another important factor in the etiology of substance use and SUDs, and psychiatric symptoms or disorders related to mood, anxiety, and attention can place youth at higher risk.[13] Psychological characteristics such as poor self-esteem, low assertiveness, and poor behavioral self-control are associated with substance use. As an individual's substance use increases in frequency and quantity, pharmacological risk factors become increasingly important. Drugs such as cocaine, amphetamine, morphine, as well as nicotine and alcohol have different molecular mechanisms of action but affect the brain in a similar way by increasing strength at excitatory synapses on midbrain dopamine neurons.[14] There are likely to be important individual differences in neurochemical reactivity to these drugs that place some individuals at a higher risk. Further, as a key developmental transition, a vast variety of neurobiological changes occur in the adolescent brain during the teen years. Complex brain maturation processes require an interdisciplinary approach to understand how the brain, behavior, and social contexts interact and are linked to substance use and other risk-taking behaviors.[15]

Family Level

In addition to the direct modeling of substance use behaviors and positive attitudes regarding use, factors within the family can contribute directly to increased substance use or indirectly by affecting established precursors of substance use such as aggressive behavior and other conduct problems. These family factors include harsh disciplinary practices, poor parental monitoring, low levels of family bonding, and high levels of family conflict. On the other hand, parenting practices characterized by firm and consistent limit setting, careful monitoring, nurturing, and open communication patterns with children are protective against substance use and other negative outcomes.[16]

School and Community Level

Characteristics of schools have been found to be associated with levels of substance use among students.[17] When large numbers of students feel unsafe or disengaged from school, fail academically, or do not have good relationships with teachers, this has been found to be associated with greater substance use prevalence. Similarly, feeling unsafe or disengaged from communities or neighborhoods is also associated with greater substance use.[18]

TYPES OF PREVENTIVE INTERVENTIONS

The terminology used to describe prevention efforts has evolved over time, moving away from primary, secondary, and tertiary prevention. More contemporary terminology for prevention by the Institute of Medicine[19] presented a new framework for classifying interventions along a continuum of care that includes prevention, treatment, and maintenance. In this framework, prevention refers only to interventions that occur prior to the onset of a disorder. Prevention is further divided into three types: universal, selective, and indicated interventions. Universal prevention programs focus on the general population and aim to deter or delay the onset of a condition. Selective prevention programs target selected high-risk groups or subsets of the general population believed to be at high risk due to membership in a particular group (eg, pregnant women or children of people who use drugs). Indicated prevention programs are designed for those already engaging in the behavior or those showing early danger signs or engaging in related high-risk behaviors. Thus, where recruitment and participation in a selective intervention are based on subgroup membership, recruitment and participation in an indicated intervention are based on early warning signs demonstrated by an individual.

There have been significant advances in the effectiveness of both drug treatment and prevention programs.[8] However, treatment remains expensive and labor intensive and suffers from high rates of recurrence. Prevention is therefore a key component in addressing the problem of substance use, especially given the increasing availability of effective programs. The first major breakthrough in prevention came at the end of the 1970s in the area of school-based smoking prevention. That work stimulated a great deal of prevention research and led to the development of several promising prevention approaches, including those designed to prevent the use of multiple substances. During the 1980s and up to the present, mounting empirical evidence from a growing number of methodologically sophisticated studies indicates that prevention can be highly effective. In the next several sections of this chapter, we describe contemporary approaches to drug prevention for children and adolescents at the school, family, and community levels.

School-Based Prevention Approaches

Schools are the most common implementation sites for universal prevention programs targeting children and adolescents. School settings are desirable because they provide access to large numbers of young people, and student substance use interferes with the education mission. Three types of contemporary approaches to school-based prevention of substance use are (1) social resistance skills training, (2) normative education, and (3) competence enhancement skills training. One or more of these approaches or components may be combined within a single preventive intervention.

Social Resistance Skills

These interventions are designed to increase the adolescent's awareness of the various social influences to engage in substance use and teach young people specific skills for effectively resisting both peer and media pressures to use substances. Resistance skills training programs teach adolescents how to recognize situations in which they are likely to experience peer pressure to smoke, drink, vape or use drugs along with ways to avoid or otherwise effectively deal with these high-risk situations. Participants are taught ways of handling pressure to engage in substance use, including what to say (ie, the specific content of a refusal message) and how to deliver it in the most effective way possible. Resistance skills programs also typically include content to increase students' awareness of the techniques used by advertisers to promote the sale of tobacco/nicotine products or alcoholic beverages and teach techniques for formulating counterarguments to the messages used by advertisers.

Normative Education

Because adolescents tend to overestimate the prevalence of smoking, drinking, and the use of certain drugs, normative education approaches include content and activities to correct inaccurate perceptions regarding the high prevalence of substance use. This can be done by providing feedback from survey data showing actual prevalence rates collected locally in the classroom, school, or community or by showing the relatively low prevalence rates in national survey data for young teens. Normative education also attempts to undermine popular but inaccurate beliefs that substance use is considered acceptable and not particularly dangerous. This can be done by highlighting evidence from national studies showing strong antidrug social norms and generally high perceived risks of drug use in the population. Material on normative education is often included in social resistance programs.

Competence Enhancement

These programs recognize that social learning processes are important in the development of adolescent drug use. However, they also recognize that youths with poor personal and social skills are more susceptible to influences that promote drug use, and these youths may be more motivated to use drugs as an alternative to more adaptive coping strategies.[20] Competence enhancement approaches typically teach some combination of the following life skills: general problem-solving and decision-making skills, general cognitive skills for resisting interpersonal or media influences, skills for increasing self-control and self-esteem, adaptive coping strategies for relieving stress and anxiety using cognitive coping skills or behavioral relaxation techniques, general social skills, and general assertive skills. In contrast to the more focused drug resistance skills training approaches, competence enhancement programs are designed to teach generic skills that will have a relatively broad application. The most effective personal and social skills training programs emphasize the application of general skills to situations directly related to substance use and demonstrate that these same skills can be used for dealing with many challenges confronting adolescents in their everyday lives.

Effectiveness of School-Based Prevention

There have been several published meta-analyses and systematic reviews of the prevention literature for school-based programs focused on preventing smoking, alcohol use, and illicit drug use among children and adolescents.[21-30]

Programs Focused on Preventing Smoking/e-Cigarette Use

A Cochrane review included randomized controlled trials (RCTs) of school-based interventions to prevent tobacco/nicotine smoking onset among children and adolescents aged 5 to 18.[21] Included were programs or curricula that focused on information only, social resistance skills only, social resistance plus competence enhancement skills, and multimodal curricula that included school-based programming with parent, community, or policy components. The main outcome variable in the meta-analysis was prevalence of nonsmoking at follow-up among those students not smoking at the baseline assessment. The analysis included 50 randomized controlled smoking prevention trials, of which 26 were conducted in the United States. Findings indicated that combined social resistance/social competence curricula was the only type that showed significant effects on smoking onset in both the short term (1 year or less) and longer term (more than a year).

A second meta-analysis of school-based smoking prevention examined 65 adolescent psychosocial smoking prevention programs among students in grades 6 to 12 published between 1978 and 1997 in the United States.[22] Programs were categorized into three prevention approaches (social resistance, social resistance + cognitive skills, and social resistance + cognitive + affective skills) and two delivery settings (school, school + community). Findings from the meta-analysis revealed that program effects on knowledge had the highest effect sizes in the short term (≤1 year) but rapidly decreased over time. Importantly, behavioral effects were observed and persisted over a 3-year period, with the strongest effects on smoking observed with programs that included social resistance combined with cognitive and/or affective skills training activities and/or programs that included both schools and community components in their implementation.

There is currently a research gap with regards to systematic reviews of school-based prevention programs aimed at e-Cigarette use, although one study is in progress.[23]

Programs Focused on Preventing Alcohol Use

A Cochrane review of universal alcohol prevention programs identified 53 school-based randomized trials that were designed to prevent alcohol use.[24] These were prevention trials conducted with children up to age 18 that met specific minimum criteria regarding the rigor of the research design. The prevention trials included educational interventions that focused primarily on raising awareness of the potential dangers of alcohol use and changing normative beliefs as well as more comprehensive psychosocial prevention programs that developed psychological and social skills in young people (eg, peer resistance, problem-solving and decision-making skills) to reduce alcohol use. Some of the studies included in the review (N = 11) focused on alcohol use as the sole outcome, and a second group of studies (N = 39) was more focused on generic prevention approaches that targeted alcohol use, smoking, illegal drug use, and/or antisocial behavior. Of the 11 alcohol-specific preventive interventions examined, 6 produced statistically significant reductions in alcohol use relative to controls. Of the 39 generic preventive interventions examined, 15 reported significant positive effects on alcohol use. Most of the programs were designed to discourage or prevent any alcohol use among youth. However, among the studies reporting significant prevention effects, the most observed beneficial effects were for heavier levels of alcohol use (eg, drunkenness and binge drinking).

A second meta-analysis of school-based prevention programs for adolescent alcohol use identified 28 RCTs published between 1990 and 2014.[25] Twelve of the studies reported continuous alcohol use outcomes (eg, frequency and quantity) and 16 reported categorical outcomes (eg, proportion of students who drank alcohol). Findings from the meta-analysis revealed a small but significant protective effect of the interventions on continuous alcohol use outcome variables. There were, however, no overall corresponding effects observed among the studies that reported categorical outcomes (eg, any alcohol use). These findings support the notion that alcohol prevention programs may be more effective in reducing frequency and quantity of use rather than onset of use. Moderator analyses revealed that there were no differences in effectiveness by school level (junior high versus high school) nor intervention duration (number of hours) on alcohol use outcomes.

Programs Focused on Preventing Illegal Drug Use

In recent years, there have been several meta-analytic reviews of the literature that have specifically examined the effectiveness of prevention programs on illegal substance use. A Cochrane review on school-based programs for preventing illegal drug use[26] examined 51 RCTs evaluating school-based interventions designed to prevent illegal substance use. The review focused on illicit drug use and did not include studies that looked at smoking or alcohol use prevention only. The authors classified the interventions as primarily focused on knowledge, social influence, or a combination of social influence and social competence skills. Most of the studies were conducted in the United States, and most interventions targeted 6th and 7th grade students. Findings from the meta-analysis indicated that programs based on a combination of social competence and social influence approaches had better results than the other categories, both in terms of preventing cannabis use and in preventing any drug use.

An additional meta-analysis examined the impact of school-based prevention programs on reducing cannabis use among youth from age 12 to 19.[27] Fifteen randomized prevention trials were included in the meta-analysis, and findings indicated that these programs had an overall positive effect on cannabis use compared to controls, with an average effect size of $d = 0.58$ (CI: 0.55, 0.62). Programs that focused on multiple hypothesized mediators (eg, social resistance skills, perceived norms, and competence skills) were more effective than those programs that focused solely on resistance skills. The more effective programs had 15 or more classroom sessions, were interactive in nature, and were facilitated by providers other than classroom teachers. The finding that comprehensive multisession programs are the most effective is consistent with the broader literature on school-based drug use prevention. However, programs that require a great deal of classroom time may be less feasible and require greater resources than more time-limited programs, potentially limiting their widespread adoption.

In summary, several meta-analyses and systematic reviews have examined the effectiveness of school-based programs to prevent alcohol, tobacco, and other forms of substance use. Overall, these studies have found that school-based prevention is effective in reducing smoking and other forms of substance use. Although the methodological rigor and theoretical bases of prevention programs included in these reviews varied considerably, findings have been useful in identifying characteristics of programs that are most effective. The most effective school-based prevention programs are interactive in nature, focus on building skills in drug resistance and general competence skills, and are implemented over multiple years. School-based programs that have a substantive community component that includes mass media or parental involvement also tend to be more effective than school-only programs. However, several major challenges remain in disseminating evidence-based prevention programs and adequately preparing prevention providers. Only about 27% of all schools in the United States use one of the ten most effective prevention curricula available,[28] and less than 1 in 5 providers use effective delivery of prevention program content.[29]

To address the challenges of facilitator-led classroom sessions, there is a growing body of research on using the internet, smartphones, or computers for alcohol and drug prevention programs delivered in schools. A recent systematic review of digital health interventions to prevent adolescent substance use found that of the seven programs with available data, six produced reductions in alcohol, cannabis, or tobacco use at post intervention and/or follow-up.[30] A second review identified 12 studies of digital health interventions designed to prevent adolescent substance use and found that a majority of studies supported the efficacy of such interventions for reducing substance use.[31] These findings suggest that digital health interventions offer a promising delivery method for school-based prevention, although more research is needed to identify best practices, barriers to implementation, and long-term effects of these programs on substance use behavior among students.

Family-Based Prevention Approaches

Family-based prevention programs include training in parenting skills, often provided to parents without children present. The specific parenting skills that are taught vary somewhat with the age of the target child or adolescent but may focus on ways to nurture, bond, and communicate with children, and how to help children develop prosocial skills and social resistance skills, training on rule setting and techniques for monitoring activities, and ways to help children reduce aggressive or antisocial behaviors. Prevention programs focusing on family skills often include sessions with the parents and children together (with or without additional parent-only training) that aim to improve family functioning, communication, and practice in developing, discussing, and enforcing family policies on substance use.[16]

Effectiveness of Family-Based Prevention

Parenting Programs

A recent systematic review evaluated parenting programs to prevent alcohol, tobacco, or drug use in children under 18 years of age.[32] Twenty controlled studies were reviewed, although the rigor of the studies and nature of the interventions varied considerably. Findings indicated statistically significant reductions in alcohol use in 6 of 14 studies, reduction in drug use in 5 of 9 studies, and reduction in tobacco use in 9 out of 13 studies. However, three interventions produced mixed findings, with increases in some alcohol, tobacco, or drug use measures among subgroups of youth. The authors concluded that parenting programs can be effective in reducing or preventing substance use and that the most effective programs were those emphasizing both active parental involvement and skills development in the areas of parenting, social competence, and self-regulation skills. Little is known about the long-term effectiveness of such interventions or the change mechanisms involved. In addition to improvements in parenting behaviors and other psychosocial mediating mechanisms, a future focus of research should explore neurological and biological mechanisms underlying effective programs, given the growing number of etiology studies demonstrating the important and complex links between parenting behaviors and youth outcomes.[33]

Family Programs

In a Cochrane review of family-based programs for preventing smoking, the authors identified RCTs designed to deter the use of tobacco among children (aged 5 to 12) or adolescents (aged 13 to 18) and other family members.[34] The authors identified 27 trials; 23 were conducted in the United States and one each in Australia, India, the Netherlands, and Norway. All studies focused on smoking prevention but several also focused on alcohol, cannabis, or substance use prevention in general. Eight studies could not be included in the analysis because there was insufficient data provided for the purposes of pooling results. The authors concluded that family intervention might reduce uptake or experimentation with smoking by between 16% and 32%, although these findings should be interpreted cautiously because effect estimates could not include data from all studies.

In a Cochrane review of family-based prevention programs for alcohol use in young people, the authors identified RCTs testing psychosocial or educational interventions that included the parents of school-aged children, and the studies included 27 universal, 12 selective, and 7 indicated interventions.[35] Overall, the authors found no impact of family intervention when compared to no intervention/standard care on alcohol use prevalence or frequency, and a small effect on volume of alcohol consumption. Subgroup analyses of universal, selective, and indicated prevention programs showed no differences for separate types of programs. The authors did not draw any conclusions about the potential benefits of family-based prevention programs for alcohol use among young people due to the relatively low quality of the evidence base and the variation and heterogeneity of studies included.

A meta-analysis focused on family-based approaches to preventing adolescent illegal drug use identified 22 RCTs.[36] Findings indicated that universal family interventions targeting parent–child dyads appear to be effective in preventing (OR 0.72; 95% CI 0.56, 0.94) and reducing adolescent cannabis use, but not in preventing other illicit drugs (OR 0.90; 95% CI 0.60, 1.34). The authors highlighted the need to strengthen the evidence base with more trials, especially among at-risk populations.

A systematic review of parent-based programs in preventing or reducing substance use (ie, alcohol, tobacco and cannabis) among 10- to 18-year-olds identified 39 publications that tested 13 programs.[37] Results revealed that the programs produced positive effects on parenting measures such as rule-setting, monitoring, and parent–child communication. There was also some evidence in terms of preventing or reducing adolescent substance use. Programs that improved parent–child communication and monitoring and reinforced strict rules against underage substance use were most effective, helping to curb adolescent substance use. Programs with multiple sessions over the course of several weeks, and those where the parenting skills best matched the developmental needs of young people, were most effective. The authors concluded that it is important to include parents in programs aiming to impede initiation of substance use or curb or reduce already existing substance use among adolescents. In summary, a variety of parenting skills and family-based drug prevention programs have been studied. Those that focus on both parenting skills and family bonding appear to be the most effective in reducing or preventing substance use. An important limitation of family-based prevention is the difficulty in getting parents to participate; families most at risk for drug use are least likely to participate in prevention programs.[38]

Community-Based Prevention Approaches

Community-based drug prevention programs typically have multiple components, including some combination of school-based programs, family or parenting components, mass media campaigns, public policy components such as restricting youth access to alcohol and tobacco, and other types of community organization and activities. The multiple components of a community-based intervention may be managed by a coalition of stakeholders including parents, educators, and key leaders in the community.

Effectiveness of Community-Based Prevention

A Cochrane review examined community-based programs to prevent smoking initiation in children and adolescents.[39] This qualitative narrative synthesis included RCTs and studies using quasi-experimental designs including a control or comparison group in which the effectiveness of multicomponent interventions was compared to no intervention, to a school-only program, or to another single-component intervention. Seventeen studies were included. Among the 13 studies that compared community interventions to no intervention controls, two programs produced lower smoking prevalence in the intervention versus control groups. One of two studies that compared a community intervention to school-only program found behavioral effects on smoking. Two studies found behavioral effects on smoking for multicomponent community interventions compared to mass media-only campaigns. The authors concluded that there is some limited support for the effectiveness of coordinated multicomponent community prevention programs in reducing smoking among young people and that programs with multiple components prevent smoking behavior more effectively than programs with a single component.

The importance of multicomponent community prevention programs can also be seen in the reviews of interventions that include mass media components. A Cochrane review examined the effectiveness of mass media campaigns in reducing illegal drug consumption and the intentions among youth under the age of 26.[40] The pooled analyses of eight mass-media interventions provided no evidence of an effect on illegal drug use or intentions. While four interventions provided some evidence of beneficial effects on behaviors and intentions, two showed possible iatrogenic effects. The review found significant heterogeneity in the types of mass media interventions reported in the literature, variability in the methods used to evaluate them, and inconsistent findings. Based on the review, the authors did not draw any general conclusions about the effectiveness of mass media interventions in preventing the use of illegal drugs among young people. A Cochrane review examining the effectiveness of mass media campaigns in preventing smoking in young people drew mixed results.[41] The majority of studies identified producing no effect on youth smoking, although those that included a school-based component in addition to a mass media component were more effective than stand-alone mass media campaigns. In summary, multicomponent community-based prevention programs can be effective in preventing adolescent substance use, particularly when the different components focus on a coordinated, comprehensive message. A limitation of community-based programs is the expense and high degree of coordination needed to implement and evaluate the type of comprehensive program most likely to be effective.

SUMMARY AND CONCLUSIONS

Substance use remains an important public health problem. The prevalence of alcohol, tobacco/nicotine, and other drug use increases rapidly from early to late adolescence, peaking during the transition to young adulthood. A variety of prevention initiatives for children and adolescents have been developed for schools, families, and communities. The most effective approaches target salient risk and protective factors and are guided by relevant psychosocial theories regarding the etiology of substance use and substance use disorder. The degree of substance use involvement of any teenager is often a function of the negative prodrug social influences in his or her environment combined with his or her individual vulnerabilities to these influences.

Contemporary school-based prevention programs focus on skills building in the areas of drug resistance and life skills and/or correcting inaccurate beliefs about the high prevalence of substance use. Reviews of the school-based prevention literature have found that overall, theory-based programs can reduce smoking and other forms of substance use. There has been some debate on the long-term effectiveness of prevention programs in general, but an increasing number of programs have shown clear evidence of long-term behavioral effects. A limitation of the meta-analytic approach is that by including all studies—including interventions that have no theoretical foundation and/or those with inadequate research designs—the overall meta-analytic findings can mask the impact of the most effective programs and obscure findings for specific population subgroups (eg, racial and ethnic minorities, low income, and rural youth). Despite these limitations, several conclusions can be made based on the available evidence. The most effective school-based prevention programs are interactive, focus on building skills in drug resistance and general competence skills, and are implemented over multiple years. School-based programs that include a substantive community component tend to be more effective than school-only programs. Family-based prevention programs include training in parenting skills and/or group interventions for the entire family that focus on improving family functioning, communication, and family policies on substance use. Family interventions that combine parenting skills and family bonding appear to be the most effective. Community-based drug prevention programs typically include some combination of school, family, mass media, public policy, and community organization components. The most effective community programs present a coordinated, comprehensive message across multiple delivery components. Several online resources are helpful in identifying exemplary evidence-based prevention programs, including Blueprints for Healthy Youth Development[42] and the Coalition for Evidence-Based Policy.[43]

Despite the progress that has been made in the field of drug prevention for children and adolescents, there are several factors that reduce the public health impact of effective school, family, and community prevention programs. Most schools still use non–evidence-based prevention programs, effective family programs often do not reach the families in greatest need, and community programs require substantial financial and human resources. In addition to refining our understanding of the risk and protective factors for substance use and translating this knowledge into improved interventions, future research is needed to find ways to effectively disseminate the most promising prevention programs into our schools, families, and communities.

REFERENCES

1. Newcomb MD, Locke T. Health, social, and psychological consequences of drug use and abuse. In: Sloboda Z, ed. *Epidemiology of Drug Abuse*. Springer; 2005:45-59.
2. Scheier LM. *Handbook of Adolescent Drug Use Prevention: Research, Intervention Strategies, and Practice*. American Psychological Association; 2015.
3. Johnston LD, Miech RA, O'Malley PM, Bachman JG, Schulenberg JE, Patrick ME. *Monitoring the Future National Survey Results on Drug Use 1975-2021: Overview, Key Findings on Adolescent Drug Use*. Institute for Social Research, University of Michigan; 2022.
4. Johnston LD, Miech RA, O'Malley PM, Bachman JG, Schulenberg JE, Patrick ME. *Demographic subgroup trends among adolescents in the use of various licit and illicit drugs. 1975–2021 (Monitoring the Future Occasional Paper No. 97)*. Institute for Social Research, The University of Michigan; 2022.
5. Cambron C, Kosterman R, Catalano RF, Guttmannova K, Hawkins JD. Neighborhood, family, and peer factors associated with early adolescent smoking and alcohol use. *J Youth Adolesc*. 2018;47:369-382.
6. Lundahl LH, Cannoy C. COVID-19 and Substance Use in Adolescents. *Pediatr Clin North Am*. 2021;68(5):977-990. doi:10.1016/j.pcl.2021.05.005
7. Kandel D, Kandel E. The gateway hypothesis of substance abuse: developmental, biological and societal perspectives. *Acta Paediatr*. 2015;104(2):130-137.
8. Hartel CR, Glantz MD. *Drug Abuse: Origins and Interventions*. American Psychological Association; 1997.
9. Branstetter SA, Low S, Furman W. The influence of parents and friends on adolescent substance use: a multidimensional approach. *J Subst Use*. 2011;16(2):150-160.
10. McCool JP, Cameron LD, Petrie KJ. Adolescent perceptions of smoking imagery in film. *Soc Sci Med*. 2001;52:1577-1587.
11. Jernigan DH. The extent of global alcohol marketing and its impact on youth. *Contemp Drug Probl*. 2010;37(1):57-89.
12. Swadi H. Individual risk factors for adolescent substance use. *Drug Alcohol Depend*. 1999;55:209-224.
13. Armstrong TD, Costello EJ. Community studies on adolescent substance use, abuse, or dependence and psychiatric comorbidity. *J Consult Clin Psychol*. 2002;70(6):1224-1239.
14. Saal D, Dong Y, Bonci A, et al. Drugs of abuse and stress trigger a common synaptic adaptation in dopamine neurons. *Neuron*. 2003;37:577-582.
15. Dahl RE. Adolescent brain development: a period of vulnerabilities and opportunities. Keynote address. *Ann N Y Acad Sci*. 2004;1021:1-22.
16. Lochman JE, van den Steenhoven A. Family-based approaches to substance abuse prevention. *J Prim Prev* 2002;23:49-114.
17. Fletcher A, Bonell C, Hargreaves J. School effects on young people's drug use: a systematic review of intervention and observational studies. *J Adolesc Health*. 2008;42:209-220.
18. Hays SP, Hays CE, Mulhall PF. Community risk and protective factors and adolescent substance use. *J Prim Prev*. 2003;24:125-142.
19. Institute of Medicine. *Preventing Mental, Emotional, and Behavioral Disorders Among Young People: Progress and Possibilities*. National Academy Press; 2009.
20. Botvin GJ. Preventing drug abuse in schools: social and competence enhancement approaches targeting individual-level etiological factors. *Addict Behav*. 2000;25:887-897.
21. Thomas RE, McLellan J, Perera R. Effectiveness of school-based smoking prevention curricula: systematic review and meta-analysis. *BMJ Open*. 2015;5(3):e006976.
22. Hwang MS, Yeagley KL, Petosa R. A meta-analysis of adolescent psychosocial smoking prevention programs published between 1978 and 1997 in the United States. *Health Educ Behav*. 2004;31:702-719.
23. Gardner LA, Rowe AL, Newton NC, et al. School-based preventive interventions targeting e-cigarette use among adolescents: a systematic review protocol. *BMJ Open*. 2022;12(9):e065509. doi:10.1136/bmjopen-2022-065509
24. Foxcroft DR, Tsertsvadze A. Universal school-based prevention programs for alcohol misuse in young people. *Cochrane Database Syst Rev*. 2011;5:CD009113:CD009113. doi:10.1002/14651858
25. Strøm HK, Adolfsen F, Fossum S, Kaiser S, Martinussen M. Effectiveness of school-based preventive interventions on adolescent alcohol use: a meta-analysis of randomized controlled trials. *Subst Abuse Treat Prev Policy*. 2014;9(1):48.
26. Faggiano F, Minozzi S, Versino E, Buscemi D. Universal school-based prevention for illicit drug use. *Cochrane Database Syst Rev*. 2014;12:CD003020. doi:10.1002/14651858.CD003020.pub3
27. Porath-Waller AJ, Beasley E, Beirness DJ. A meta-analytic review of school-based prevention for cannabis use. *Health Educ Behav*. 2010;37:709-723. doi:10.1177/1090198110361315
28. Ringwalt CL, Ennett S, Vincus A, et al. The prevalence of effective substance use prevention curricula in US middle schools. *Prev Sci*. 2002;3:257-265.
29. Ennett ST, Ringwalt CL, Thorne J, et al. A comparison of current practice in school-based substance use prevention programs with meta-analysis findings. *Prev Sci*. 2003;4:1-14.
30. Champion KE, Newton NC, Barrett EL, Teesson M. A systematic review of school-based alcohol and other drug prevention programs facilitated by computers or the Internet. *Drug Alcohol Rev*. 2013;32(2):115-123.
31. Kazemi DM, Borsari B, Levine MJ, Li S, Lamberson KA, Matta LA. A systematic review of the mHealth interventions to prevent alcohol and substance abuse. *J Health Commun*. 2017;22(5):413-432.
32. Petrie J, Bunn F, Byrne G. Parenting programmes for preventing tobacco, alcohol or drugs misuse in children <18: a systematic review. *Health Educ Res*. 2007;22:177-191.
33. Beach SR, Lei MK, Brody GH, Dogan MV, Philibert RA. Higher levels of protective parenting are associated with better young adult health: exploration of mediation through epigenetic influences on pro-inflammatory processes. *Front Psychol*. 2015;6:676.
34. Thomas RE, Baker PR, Thomas BC, Lorenzetti DL. Family-based programmes for preventing smoking by children and adolescents. *Cochrane Database Syst Rev*. 2015;(2):CD004493.

35. Gilligan C, Wolfenden L, Foxcroft DR, et al. Family-based prevention programmes for alcohol use in young people. *Cochrane Database Syst Rev*. 2019;3(3):CD012287.
36. Vermeulen-Smit E, Verdurmen JE, Engels RC. The effectiveness of family interventions in preventing adolescent illicit drug use: a systematic review and meta-analysis of randomized controlled trials. *Clin Child Fam Psychol Rev*. 2015;18(3):218-239.
37. Kuntsche S, Kuntsche E. Parent-based interventions for preventing or reducing adolescent substance use—A systematic literature review. *Clin Psychol Rev*. 2016;45:89-101.
38. Díaz S, Secades-Villa R, Pérez JE, et al. Family predictors of parent participation in an adolescent drug abuse prevention program. *Drug Alcohol Rev*. 2006;25:327-331.
39. Sowden A, Stead L. Community interventions for preventing smoking in young people. *Cochrane Database Syst Rev*. 2003;1:CD001291. doi:10.1002/14651858.CD001291
40. Allara E, Ferri M, Bo A, et al. Are mass-media campaigns effective in preventing drug use? A Cochrane systematic review and meta-analysis. *BMJ Open*. 2015;5:e007449. doi:10.1136/bmjopen-2014-007449
41. Carson-Chahhoud KV, Ameer F, Sayehmiri K, Hnin K, et al. Mass media interventions for preventing smoking in young people. *Cochrane Database Syst Rev*. 2017;6(6):CD001006.
42. Blueprints for Healthy Youth Development. Accessed July 18, 2023. http://www.blueprintsprograms.com
43. Coalition for Evidence-Based Policy. Accessed July 18, 2023. http://evidencebasedprograms.org

CHAPTER

26

Environmental Approaches to Prevention: Communities and Contexts

Mallie J. Paschall, Joel W. Grube, Robert F. Saltz, and Paul J. Gruenewald

CHAPTER OUTLINE

- Introduction
- Scope of the problem
- Environmental versus individual approaches to prevention
- Domains of environmental prevention
- Efficacy trials
- Environmental prevention and the social ecology of alcohol use
- Environmental prevention and implementation science
- Environmental prevention and the role of the medical professionals

INTRODUCTION

Environmental contexts around alcohol and other drug use are often governed with laws and regulations for the production, distribution, sale, and use of substances. These laws and regulations are importantly linked with the prevalence of substance use on a population level. For example, at the conclusion of prohibition in 1933, the 21st amendment to the United States Constitution broadly delegated control over production and sales of alcoholic beverages to the states, territories, and possessions of the United States (U.S. Constitution, Amend. XXI, Sec. 2). Since then, states progressively deregulated alcohol sales, allowed use in more contexts, lowered beverage taxes and prices, increased numbers of outlets, and, with the exception of the minimum legal drinking age and driving under the influence [DUI]) and zero tolerance laws, lowered legal restrictions on use. With the creation of large and profitable alcohol markets, continued deregulation is actively pursued as a goal by the alcohol beverage and social hosting industries to expand the times and places in which alcohol can be sold and consumed.[1] Although illegal production and distribution of alcohol have been essentially eliminated, this deregulation has led to an increase in alcohol-related public health problems which are acutely felt at local community and neighborhood levels.[2-4]

In this chapter, we outline effective environmental approaches to preventing substance use and related consequences with a focus on preventing harmful alcohol use in community settings. After a statement of the scope of the consequences of alcohol use, we distinguish environmental approaches from other approaches to prevention. We review the growing scientific bases for environmental prevention efforts. We then summarize current knowledge and best practices for community prevention efforts aimed at reducing alcohol-related harms.

SCOPE OF THE PROBLEM

Over 93,000 alcohol-attributable deaths occur in the U.S. each year (approximately 66,000 males and approximately 27,000 females), making alcohol use the third leading preventable cause of death.[5] About 55% of these deaths are caused by chronic conditions (eg, alcohol liver disease), while about 45% are due to acute conditions (eg, alcohol-related motor vehicle crashes).[5] This corresponds to 2.7 million years of potential life lost, the cost of which was estimated to be $249 billion in 2010.[6,7] Although women traditionally have consumed less alcohol and experienced fewer problems than men, rates of alcohol use and alcohol use disorder among women have been converging with those of men over the past decade.[8] Furthermore, excessive drinking among underage youth is responsible for at least 3,500 deaths and 210,000 years of potential life lost each year[9] and cost the U.S. $24 billion in 2010.[6] The costs associated with alcohol problems substantially exceed those resulting from illicit drug use and vary widely across communities, reflecting important differences in local alcohol environments.[10,11]

Alcohol-related motor vehicle crashes account for many acute deaths due to alcohol use. National Highway Traffic Safety Administration data indicate that 28% of traffic crashes in 2019 involved alcohol impairment and, despite declines in traffic fatalities, 10,142 people died in alcohol-involved traffic crashes that year.[12] The economic costs of alcohol-related motor vehicle crashes and fatalities were estimated to be $59 billion and $44 billion in 2014, respectively.[13] In 2019, 7% of people aged 16 and older reported driving while under the influence of alcohol at least once in the past year, corresponding to 19.9 million people in the U.S.[14]

Alcohol-related deaths are also attributable to a variety of other risks. Depending upon the body weight, gender, and drinking experience of people who are currently drinking, alcohol use alters motor skills, reaction time, and judgment[15,16] and increases risk of injury to the person and to others.[17] Alcohol use is involved in a substantial percentage of injuries caused by falls (32%), drownings (34%), and fires (42%).[9] Some researchers have concluded that there is no safe level of consumption in relation to injury risk.[18]

Alcohol also has been estimated to be involved in between 28% and 43% of violent injuries,[19] 24% of suicides, and 47% of homicides.[9] Much of the violence associated with drinking takes place among young people between the ages of 15 and 29 and this includes high rates of both interpersonal violence and suicide.[9,20,21] It has been found that alcohol is involved in 27% of hospital discharges recording the survival of a suicide attempt[21] and that 24% of suicides involve alcohol intoxication in excess of 0.08% Blood Alcohol Content (BAC).[20]

Medical care costs associated with excessive drinking are conservatively estimated to be $27.4 billion dollars per year.[6] Lost productivity related to drinking accounts for almost five times this amount ($179.3 billion per year).[6] Costs for law enforcement and criminal justice proceedings related to alcohol-related crimes are $25 billion per year.[6] Crimes attributable to alcohol have been estimated to cost $84 billion a year,[11] more than 2 times the estimated $38 billion attributable to illegal drugs. Alcohol-related injuries were estimated to cost employers $28.6 billion a year in 1998 to 2000.[22]

ENVIRONMENTAL VERSUS INDIVIDUAL APPROACHES TO PREVENTION

Both prevention and treatment are needed to reduce alcohol consequences and costs in community settings, the former to reduce use and prevent unhealthy use and consequences before they begin, and the latter to treat alcohol use disorder once established. Although important, treatment alone cannot effectively reduce use and consequences related to alcohol. A portion of people who drink alcohol progress to alcohol use disorder or addiction, but only a small proportion seek or enter treatment, and rates of return to use after treatment are high.[23,24] The consequence of these dynamics is that treatment would have to be nearly universally applied and very effective to substantially reduce alcohol use disorder in drinking populations.[25] A greater concern, however, is that most alcohol-related consequences, and the majority of healthcare and social costs related to alcohol use, arise among people who drink alcohol but do not meet criteria for formal treatment, meaning they neither drink heavily nor have an alcohol use disorder.[18] Therefore, prevention efforts are essential to reduce risky alcohol use before an alcohol use disorder is established.[26]

Individual approaches to prevention have largely focused on educational interventions that inform people about the effects and consequences of alcohol use, encourage people to abstain from use, or encourage the development of social norms that discourage risky use. Given their narrow focus on education, incomplete conceptual models of program effects, and poor program design, implementation, and evaluation, early educational prevention programs demonstrated limited success.[27-30] More recently, some newer preventive interventions have been shown to reduce or delay alcohol use among young people by focusing on correcting misperceptions about alcohol use norms.[31-33] Nonetheless, critical reviews continue to conclude that there is little evidence that educational programs alone are sufficient for long-term reductions in alcohol use or harms,[34-37] especially when people are immersed in an environment in which alcohol is readily available and heavily marketed.[38]

Environmental approaches to prevention recognize that alcohol consequences result from interactions among individuals in diverse social, economic, and community environments[39-41] and that some features of these environments can be changed to the benefit of community members.[42,43] Environmental approaches have been developed to complement educational approaches and have been shaped into programs that communities can implement without direct intervention with specific individuals.[44-47] While differing in detail, these programs share a common heritage of policy, regulatory, and enforcement interventions that attempt to reduce consequences of substance use by changing the economic, physical, or social environments in which alcohol or drugs are obtained or used.[48,49] They primarily focus on community systems within the geographic levels of neighborhoods and cities to influence alcohol use and consequences.[39,50] Community systems, such as families, schools, friends and neighbors, markets for alcohol and other drugs, enforcement agencies, treatment systems, and medical care are formal and informal political and social institutions in a community that can prevent alcohol consequences.

Environmental approaches contrast with educational approaches in at least five respects: First, they seek to change components of community systems that make the occurrence of substance use consequences more likely. These may include changes in functions of formal institutions (eg, reducing hours and days of alcohol sales)[51] and changes in informal systems (eg, making social hosts legally responsible for providing alcohol to underage youths).[52] Educational and other individualized approaches may encourage individual resistance to or desistance from use, but do not attempt to alter the formal or informal structures that enable use. Second, media environmental prevention approaches use media to motivate gatekeepers to pursue activities that are extensions of their normal efforts (eg, law enforcement) or increase public awareness of consequences (eg, underage drinking; DUI); and prevention efforts (eg, compliance checks to prevent alcohol sales to minors) to mobilize support for structural and system change as opposed to changing the behavior of individuals. In contrast, traditional educational approaches use media to target individual risk factors to elicit individual belief and behavior change through persuasion (eg, Just Say No; This Is your Brain on Drugs). Third, rather than targeting at-risk individuals, environmental approaches target broader environments and affect populations of people who use and do not use alcohol or other drugs. Thus, a workplace intervention may alter policies toward alcohol to reduce use in the workplace and thus provide greater safety for all employees.[53] Since people who do not use substances often suffer collateral damage from alcohol and other drug use by others,[54,55] everyone benefits and can be affected by the program. Fourth, many environmental approaches focus on the supply side of substance use, whereas individual educational approaches attempt to reduce the individual demand for drugs. Environmental efforts may include enforcement activities to reduce the ability of youths to purchase alcohol,[56] interdiction efforts to reduce availability of illicit drugs,[57] efforts to target risks related to sales or service of alcohol (eg, responsible beverage service [RBS] programs),[58] harm reduction efforts (eg, needle exchange programs),[49] and efforts to change drug distribution to ameliorate problem hot spots.[59] Fifth, as a final distinction, environmental approaches often focus on acute rather than chronic consequences related to use. Such consequences include motor vehicle crashes, injuries, and violence rather than alcohol use per se. Many medical conditions related to use, such as liver cirrhosis, are the outcome of rather long periods of heavy consumption. In contrast, consequences that are proximal to alcohol or illegal drug markets, such as alcohol-related motor vehicle crashes or drug-related crime,[60] are affected by acute use and can be prevented without necessarily affecting overall consumption. Thus, an RBS program may reduce sales to intoxicated patrons in bars and subsequently reduce driving while intoxicated[58] but need not have an overall effect on drinking to be effective.

An underappreciated aspect of environmental prevention strategies is that they can have a large impact on whole populations via small changes in individual behavior whereas individual approaches seek larger changes at the individual level. This is especially relevant to alcohol consumption, where risk of harm begins with any amount and thus translating small shifts in consumption into large population effects.[61]

Environmental prevention strategies are relevant and effective for demographically and geographically diverse communities as they place constraints on the availability of alcohol and other legal substances including nicotine/tobacco, cannabis, and potentially addictive prescription medications. Thus, implementation of evidence-based environmental interventions (eg, limits on the concentration of alcohol and cannabis outlets in economically disadvantaged neighborhoods) can help to reduce disparities in harmful use of alcohol and other substances, and related health, social and legal problems.

DOMAINS OF ENVIRONMENTAL PREVENTION

Environmental prevention programs act in four domains: physical, social, economic, and legal. Prevention programs may alter physical access by affecting proximity to sources of alcohol, tobacco, and other drugs. College dormitories may prohibit alcohol in dorm rooms, workplace administrators may eliminate tobacco vending machines, cities may limit the number and locations of legal retail cannabis outlets, and illicit markets for drugs may be disrupted by enforcement programs.[48] Environmental prevention programs may alter social access by affecting the social networks that encourage and enable informal distribution of alcohol and other substances. Thus, they may reduce social access to alcohol by restricting social activities at which alcohol is served (eg, during on-campus celebrations), reduce social access to tobacco through smoke-free policies, or moderate social access to illegal drugs by establishing and enforcing drug-free zones in a community. Environmental prevention interventions may alter economic access by increasing the price and opportunity costs (real costs) associated with obtaining and using alcohol, nicotine/tobacco, and other drugs through taxation, minimum pricing, regulating hours of sale, or changing the economic geography of availability (eg, restricting outlet density). Increased enforcement of minimum drinking age laws may increase the opportunity costs to youth for obtaining alcohol. Reducing the legal BAC for driving may increase the likelihood of incurring personal and monetary costs associated with drinking and driving.

The four domains of environmental influence interact in producing alcohol and other drug consequences. The physical, social, economic, and legal availabilities of alcohol (represented by outlets, use by others, beverage prices, and the laws regulating such) intersect at places where alcohol consequences may occur. The presence of other people who are drinking at bars exposes patrons to social influences for drinking and greater risks of violence.[61] Alcoholic beverages are more expensive at bars than at liquor or grocery stores, changing both the nature of drinking at bars and its relationship to consequences, such as driving while intoxicated and alcohol-related crashes.[62] The purchasing and over-consumption patterns of some patrons at these establishments can influence the behaviors of others by encouraging greater levels of intoxication.[63] Parallel arguments can be constructed for illegal drugs. Concentrated use of illegal drugs (eg, in and around crack houses) is associated with substantial degrees of crime and disease.[48,64] Prices of illegal drugs may be influenced by drug interdiction efforts (modestly), but certainly affect quantities of drug purchases.[65] Favored drug use changes as social access is restructured by enforcement efforts or changes in informal social systems that support drug distribution.[66] As a counterpoint, environmental harm reduction strategies (eg, increased availability of naloxone; needle exchange programs) do not directly target reductions in use, but may decrease mortality and morbidity and thus the societal costs associated with alcohol, nicotine/tobacco, and other drug use.[67,68]

EFFICACY TRIALS

The past three decades have seen the intensive development of community-based environmental prevention intervention programs to address unhealthy alcohol use and consequences. Community-based environmental prevention research has moved from trying to establish that environmental prevention programs can work to asking questions about what works, for whom, and why. Using a variety of case-comparison research methods, early studies demonstrated that:

1. The Communities Mobilizing for Change Project (CMCP) found that alcohol sales to underage youth, underage purchases and use of alcohol, and drinking and DUI could be reduced through community organization to monitor

sales to youth, increased underage sales decoy operations at alcohol outlets, keg registration, shortened hours of sale for alcohol, implementation of RBS training programs, sponsorship of alcohol-free events for youth, and educational programs for youth and adults.[69]

2. The "Community Trials (CT)" project found that media mobilization, RBS programs, reductions in sales to underage youth, increased enforcement of drinking and DUI laws, and reduced access to alcohol could together lead to reductions in alcohol involved motor vehicle crashes, injuries due to assaults, drinking and DUI, and heavy drinking among adults.[42] Clearly, communities can act to reduce alcohol consequences by modifying community environments. But each community requires some program adaptation in the different domains of environmental prevention to respond to their different environmental structures, needs, problems, and concerns. The current challenge is how to develop and field an adaptive framework that applies the logic of environmental prevention to the needs of different communities. This process may be illustrated by considering more recent studies.
3. The Sacramento Neighborhood Alcohol Prevention Project (SNAPP) implemented and evaluated neighborhood-level interventions intended to reduce youth and young adult access to alcohol, risky drinking, and associated consequences, particularly in low-income ethnically diverse neighborhoods. SNAPP posed three basic questions: Could an environmental approach be tailored to the unique needs of economically and ethnically diverse populations? Could environmental strategies address the problem of intentional injuries (ie, assaultive violence) in economically and ethnically diverse settings? Finally, could more specifically tailored interventions be implemented at the neighborhood level? To address these questions, SNAPP implemented five interventions focusing on individuals between ages 15 and 29: (1) community mobilization to support the overall project, (2) community awareness, (3) responsible beverage-service (RBS), (4) enforcement of underage-access laws, and (5) enforcement of service to intoxicated patrons laws. These interventions led to an estimated reduction of 3.9% in police calls related to assaults and a significant 33.4% reduction in emergency medical system (eg, ambulance) responses related to motor vehicle crashes in the initial intervention site relative to a subsequent intervention site. Subsequently, the project found significant estimated reductions of 36.5% in police calls related to assaults and 37.4% in emergency medical system responses related to assaults in the second intervention site relative to preintervention levels.[70]
4. The Stockholm Prevents Alcohol and Drug Problems (STAD) program was developed in 1996 as a project of the Stockholm, Sweden, City Council and the Karolinska Institute. The focus of STAD was on preventing risky alcohol use in restaurants, bars, and nightclubs. The program implemented a combination of strategies, including community mobilization, RBS training and practices to prevent overservice, and enforcement. The program increased service refusal rates to apparently intoxicated patrons from 5% prior to the program to 70% 5 years later.[71] Importantly, there was a 29% decrease in violent crimes reported to the police in the intervention area compared with the control area.[72] The program also significantly increased the likelihood that club doormen would refuse entrance to apparently impaired patrons.[73] Even after taking implementation costs into account, it has been estimated that the STAD program saved as much as €31 million over 10 years through reductions in judicial system costs, lost productivity, healthcare costs, and costs associated with other damage.[74]
5. The Safer California Universities Project aimed to determine whether environmental prevention strategies targeting specific off-campus settings would reduce the incidence of student intoxication on college campuses. Fourteen large public universities were recruited to participate in the project, campuses were matched on campus and community characteristics, and one member of each pair randomly assigned to the intervention condition. The intervention campuses implemented five environmental interventions: (1) nuisance party enforcement operations to reduce problems related to off-campus parties, (2) minor decoy operations at on- and off-premises outlets to reduce underage sales and sales to intoxicated persons, (3) police roadside checkpoints testing for intoxicated drivers, (4) development of local ordinances to discourage nuisance parties or provision of alcohol to people who are underage in social gatherings, and (5) the use of campus and local media to increase the visibility of all these environmental strategies. Significant reductions in the incidence and likelihood of intoxication at off-campus parties and bars/restaurants were observed among intervention campuses compared to controls. A lower likelihood of intoxication was also observed among intervention campuses for the last time students drank at an off-campus party, a bar or restaurant, or another setting. No increase in intoxication appeared in any setting, a sign that heavy drinking and intoxication were not displaced to other drinking contexts. Finally, stronger intervention effects were observed at those intervention campuses with the highest intensity of implementation.[75]
6. The Oregon Reducing Youth Access to Alcohol Project was a cluster randomized trial that incorporated a mix of law enforcement and other community-based activities to address underage drinking. The project involved 36 communities and was initiated as a collaborative effort involving researchers, local community members, the Oregon Liquor Control Commission, and the Addictions and Mental Health Division of Oregon's Department of Health and Human Services. The five program components were (1) community mobilization, (2) a reward and reminder program, (3) media advocacy, (4) enforcement, and (5) coordination and community outreach. The reward and reminder program educated alcohol merchants about

effective practices for identifying underage youth and conducted mystery shops with youthful shoppers after which clerks, managers, and owners were reinforced for using proper age checking procedures and given constructive feedback when proper procedures were not followed. This effort was combined with media advocacy focusing on topics such as county-specific costs of underage drinking, underage drinking during prom and graduation, dangers of underage drinking at home, social host liability, and highlighting law enforcement activities. Enforcement activities included compliance checks, which were completed once per year for 2 years in each of the off-premises alcohol outlets in the communities, along with shoulder tap operations, third-party purchase surveillance, enforcement of minor in-possession laws, DUI enforcement, and controlled party dispersal. The project demonstrated significant reductions in underage sales across intervention communities and reductions in drinking outcomes in communities with the highest levels of implementation.[76]

7. The Study to Prevent Alcohol-Related Consequences (SPARC) was a comprehensive intervention using a community organizing approach to implement environmental strategies in and around college campuses to reduce high-risk drinking and alcohol-related consequences among college students.[77] Eight public and two private universities in North Carolina were randomized to an intervention or comparison condition. Although each campus developed its own prevention plan, they were required to choose three of four strategy domains: (1) reduce alcohol availability, (2) address price and marketing of alcoholic beverages, (3) improve social norms, and (4) minimize harm related to alcohol. The interventions were expected to be comprehensive, including policy, enforcement, and awareness. Specific components included restricting alcohol at campus events and enforcing laws prohibiting sales to minors. These interventions led to approximately 228 fewer severe consequences per month on each campus and 107 fewer injuries caused to others per month. Higher levels of implementation were associated with reductions in negative consequences resulting from others' drinking and in alcohol-related injuries caused to others.
8. The California 24 cities project was a randomized trial focused on community interventions to reduce excessive drinking and alcohol-related vehicle crashes among adolescents and young adults.[78] The interventions consisted of enhanced enforcement of alcohol-impaired driving laws (roadside sobriety checkpoints, DUI saturation patrols), improving retail serving practices (RBS and enforcement of over-service laws), and reducing social and retail availability of alcohol to minors (social host ordinances, compliance checks, reward and reminder). These interventions were reinforced by activities to increase visibility of the program, including publicity through various media targeting adults and adolescents, periodic police visits to bars, and letters to retailers. The program resulted in a 17% reduction in alcohol-involved crashes among drivers aged 15 to 30 years in the intervention communities relative to control communities, which translated to about 310 fewer crashes over the 3 years of the program. A cost–benefit analysis estimated that the program saved the communities $27 dollars for every dollar spent.
9. The Southwest California Indians Project was a collaborative effort between clinicians, prevention scientists, and tribal leaders to prevent underage drinking in nine contiguous rural California Indigenous American reservations. The project included both individual- and community-level prevention strategies. The individual-level strategy consisted of brief motivational interviewing and psychoeducation for youth. The community-level strategies targeted the sale of alcohol to minors through a reward and reminder program in stores bordering the reservations, together with extensive outreach efforts to raise awareness of alcohol problems and mobilize support for project goals. The project showed significant reductions in sales of alcohol to youth,[79] and in 30-day frequency of drinking and heavy episodic drinking (5+ drinks in a row) among youth in the participating reservations compared with youth in nonparticipating reservations.[80]
10. A collaborative effort between the Cherokee Nation and researchers evaluated the effectiveness of environmental and individual strategies to reduce underage drinking and associated harms among youth living in rural communities within the Cherokee Nation. The interventions included evidence-based strategies adapted from Communities Mobilizing for Change on Alcohol (CMCA), a community-organizing approach designed to reduce alcohol access, and CONNECT, a screening and brief intervention (SBI) program implemented in schools. A significant reduction in sales of alcohol to minors and in overall availability of alcohol to youth was observed in the intervention communities.[81] Students in the intervention communities also showed significant reductions in the prevalence of 30-day alcohol use and heavy episodic drinking compared with students in control communities.[82]

ENVIRONMENTAL PREVENTION AND THE SOCIAL ECOLOGY OF ALCOHOL USE

Overall, these studies demonstrate the effectiveness of interventions targeting physical, economic, social, and legal aspects of the alcohol environment on drinking and related consequences across diverse community settings and populations. However, important questions remain about *how* environmental interventions affect alcohol use and related problems, since they are being implemented in complex and dynamic systems operating at macro and micro levels. There is still much to learn about how individuals or groups may adapt to constraints on alcohol availability in economic, physical, legal, and social domains, and how such adaptations may affect alcohol and other drug use and consequences in different contexts.

Figure 26-1 illustrates formal and informal systems through which state- and community-level environmental

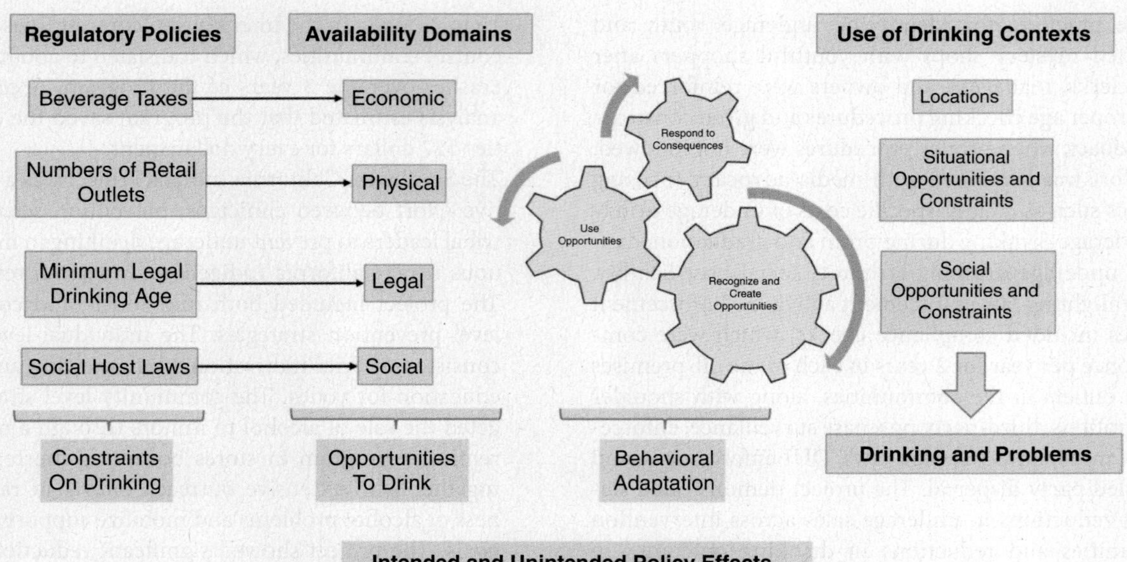

Figure 26-1. Conceptual framework for environmental prevention and the social ecology of alcohol use.

interventions (eg, beverage taxation, social host laws) can shape opportunities and constraints for alcohol use in the four domains. Individuals or groups may adapt to opportunities and constraints by shifting the way they obtain alcohol and where they drink (ie, drinking contexts). Behavioral adaptation may also be influenced by locational, situational, and social characteristics of drinking contexts and individuals' propensity for alcohol use, including how they respond to drinking consequences. Thus, formal and informal systems operating at macro and micro levels create opportunity structures that can influence when, where, and how much people drink and related risks for harms.

This conceptual framework sets the stage for future research on the effects of different environmental prevention strategies on harms related to alcohol and other substance use, including both intended and unintended consequences. By investigating effects of alcohol regulatory policies and related enforcement activities at state and local levels, and locational, situational, and social characteristics of specific drinking contexts that may lead to heavy drinking and consequences, we can better understand the social–ecological interactions in which we can intervene to reduce adverse outcomes. A better understanding of the social ecology of drinking and consequences and the dynamic human-to-human and human-to-environment interactions that lead to harm, can then help focus prevention efforts and even suggest novel interventions as well.

Two examples will help clarify how we can proceed. First, it has long been known that the availability of alcohol in the home, among peers, and through some alcohol outlets can affect youth access to and use of alcohol,[83] but locations where alcohol may be obtained (in the home, others' homes, a store) and then used (at home, at a park) vary a great deal by environmental circumstances (eg, local enforcement of underage alcohol sales laws and social host liability laws) and change with age.[84] Specific contexts are associated with greater risks for unhealthy alcohol use and related consequences,[85] and specific forms of social or parental control in those contexts can moderate alcohol use in adolescents.[86] Second, it has also long been known that numbers of bars and bar densities are related to assaults among adults.[87] But recently, it has become evident that people who drink heavily appear to self-select into these drinking environments[88] and that malleable characteristics both outside (eg, physical disorder, low-income neighborhoods) and inside (eg, crowding) these environments are related to greater likelihoods of assault.[89] Specific recommendations can be made to moderate heavy drinking among youth and adults with research efforts helping to direct prevention practitioners address the question, "What works in specific community contexts?" This research frontier of environmental approaches to prevention provides the working link between regulatory practices and individual behaviors in risky drinking and substance use environments.[90,91]

It is also the case that environmental interventions that are successful in one community may not work as effectively in others. For example, although the STAD program led to substantial reductions in alcohol-related violence in Stockholm, a replication in other communities in Sweden produced smaller effects that varied depending on community size.[92] A replication in Norway showed no significant change in alcohol-related consequences.[93,94] Although these discrepancies may reflect differences in the quality of implementation, they also may result from social and structural differences across communities. Understanding *why* environmental interventions work better in some communities than in others is a central issue that needs to be addressed.

ENVIRONMENTAL PREVENTION AND IMPLEMENTATION SCIENCE

As the number of effective environmental prevention strategies continues to grow, we are faced with the awareness that translational research into the most efficient ways to implement those strategies in community settings is sorely lacking.[95] Conventional approaches to dissemination of environmental interventions rely upon common understandings of means and goals that are often lacking among community members. These activities are, for this reason, often very slow and labor intensive, subject to distraction and entropy. Conventional practice provides materials and menus of environmental intervention options to community groups with little guidance for tying them into a synergistic whole.

In a review of implementation research, Fixsen and colleagues identified a need for interventions to have a "driver" to achieve success.[96] In their domain of education, this was likely a person with authority who could "champion" the needed organizational change. In community prevention, some similar person or small group may serve this function, but the concept of a "driver" may extend to other implementation strategies as well. One approach to facilitate implementation has evolved from experience with Holder's Community Trials project,[42] the SNAPP,[70] the Safer California Universities Project,[75] and the California 24 Cities projects[78] described earlier. Here, researchers used diagrams that merged a theory of change with elements found in logic models to provide a holistic view of the intervention objectives, measures, and expected outcomes. Evidence-based interventions can be laid over the diagram to show how they work to reduce adverse outcomes. Thus, this logic model is not simply a codification of the inputs and outputs of a program or intervention (as logic models are usually defined), but is instead of synthesis of research, a theory of change, and (eventually) an action plan, all built on the same simple platform. Furthermore, unlike community mobilization approaches, which advocate that a large group of stakeholders should be recruited as a first step, logic model approaches encourage recruitment of other community actors to support and implement specific components of the intervention, without the need to attend regular meetings or discussions irrelevant to their own area of responsibility. Examples of this approach include the Safer California Universities and California 24 cities projects described above.

In summation, this version of logic models clarifies the partnership between researchers and community members by drawing attention to what research recommends be done and what local expertise recommends about how to accomplish it. It leads communities to focus more on objectives than process, moves the community quickly through assessment and planning so members can be engaged in the action phase sooner, and, finally, keeps everyone focused on community-level outcomes.

The development of preventive interventions would be accelerated by greater support for implementation research. The use of rigorous designs to identify which elements of a promising preventive intervention are fundamental in achieving good outcomes, versus those that must be adapted to different populations or settings, is a necessary stage in creating practical programs and policies to reduce alcohol-related harm.

ENVIRONMENTAL PREVENTION AND THE ROLE OF THE MEDICAL PROFESSIONALS

Medical professionals, particularly physicians, can play an important role in advocating for effective environmental approaches to prevent alcohol, nicotine/tobacco, and other unhealthy drug use at multiple levels.[97] For example, physicians can collectively advocate for national, state, and local regulatory policies and enforcement activities that can reduce both acute and chronic harms of substance use through organizations such as the American Medical Association, American Academy of Pediatrics, and American Public Health Association. Physicians and other medical professionals can routinely implement substance use screening and brief interventions (SBI) in their practices, and discuss health issues related to alcohol, nicotine/tobacco and other drug use with parents and children to promote a healthy home environment. We note that SBI may only have modest, short-term effects on alcohol or other substance use,[98] indicating the need for effective individually-focused preventive interventions and effective population-level approaches to prevention. Additionally, they can work with local schools to improve school policies and programs aimed at promoting a healthy lifestyle and preventing substance use. To that end, medical professionals should receive appropriate undergraduate- and graduate-level education and training in advocacy work related to alcohol, nicotine/tobacco and other drug use to promote effective environmental prevention strategies.[97]

REFERENCES

1. Heffernan T. Last call. *Washington Monthly*. Accessed June 4, 2022. https://washingtonmonthly.com/2012/11/11/last-call/
2. Babor T, Caetano R, Casswell S, et al. *Alcohol No Ordinary Commodity: Research and Public Policy*. 2nd ed. Oxford University Press; 2010.
3. Cook P. *Paying the Tab: The Costs and Benefits of Alcohol Control*. Princeton University Press; 2008.
4. Gruenewald PJ. Regulating availability: how access to alcohol affects drinking and problems in youth and adults. *Alcohol Res Health*. 2011;34(2):248-256.
5. Esser MB, Sherk A, Liu Y, et al. Deaths and years of potential life lost from excessive alcohol use—United States, 2011-2015. *MMWR*. 2020;69:981-987. doi:10.15585/mmwr.mm6930a1
6. Sacks JJ, Gonzales KR, Bouchery EE, Tomedi LE, Brewer RD. 2010 National and state costs of excessive alcohol consumption. *Am J Prev Med*. 2015;49:e73-e79. doi:10.1016/j.amepre.2015.05.031
7. Stahre M, Roeber J, Kanny D, Brewer RD, Zhang X. Contribution of excessive alcohol consumption to deaths and years of potential life lost in the United States. *Prev Chronic Dis*. 2014;11:130293. Accessed May 22, 2023. https://www.cdc.gov/pcd/issues/2014/13_0293.htm
8. White AM. Gender differences in the epidemiology of alcohol use and related harms in the United States. *Alcohol Res: Curr Rev*. 2020;40:01.
9. Centers for Disease Control and Prevention. *Alcohol-Related Disease Impact (ARDI) Application*. Centers for Disease Control and Prevention,

National Center for Chronic Disease Prevention and Health Promotion, Division of Population Health; 2019.

10. Miller TR, Nygaard P, Gaidus A, et al. Heterogeneous costs of alcohol and drug problems across cities and counties in California. *Alcohol Clin Exp Res*. 2017;41:758-768. doi:10.1111/acer.13337
11. Miller TR, Levy DT, Cohen MA, Cox KL. The costs of alcohol and drug-involved crime. *Prev Sci*. 2006;7:333-342.
12. National Highway Traffic Safety Administration. *Traffic Safety Facts: Overview of Motor Vehicle Crashes in 2019*. National Highway Traffic Safety Administration; 2020.
13. Blincoe LJ, Miller TR, Zaloshnja E, Lawrence BA. *The Economic and Societal Impact of Motor Vehicle Crashes, 2010 (Revised)*. (Report No. DOT HS 812 013). National Highway Traffic Safety Administration; 2015.
14. Substance Abuse and Mental Health Services Administration. *National Survey on Drug Use and Health, 2019. Substance Abuse and Mental Health Data Archive*. Substance Abuse and Mental Health Services Administration; 2020.
15. Friedman TW, Robinson SR, Yelland GW. Impaired perceptual judgment at low blood alcohol concentrations. *Alcohol*. 2011;45:711-718.
16. Maylor EA, Rabbit PMA. Alcohol, reaction time and memory: a meta-analysis. *Br J Psychol*. 1993;84:301-317.
17. Cherpitel CJ. Alcohol and casualties: comparison of county-wide emergency room data with the county general population. *Addiction*. 1995;90:343-350.
18. Cherpitel CJ, Ye Y. Alcohol-attributable fraction for injury in the U.S. general population: data from the 2005 National Alcohol Survey. *J Stud Alcohol Drugs*. 2008;69:535-538.
19. Cherpitel CJ, Ye Y, Bond J. Attributable risk of injury associated with alcohol use: cross-national data from the Emergency Room Collaborative Alcohol Analysis Project. *Am J Public Health*. 2005;95:266-272.
20. Crosby AE, Espitia-Hardeman V, Hill HA, Ortega L, Clavel-Arcas C. Alcohol and suicide among racial/ethnic populations—17 states, 2005-2006. *MMWR*. 2009;58:637-641.
21. Miller TR, Teti LO, Lawrence BA, Weiss HB. Alcohol involvement in hospital-admitted nonfatal suicide acts. *Suicide Life Threat Behav*. 2010;40:492-499.
22. Zaloshnja E, Miller TR, Hendrie D, Galvin D. Employer costs of alcohol involved injuries. *Am J Ind Med*. 2007;50:136-142.
23. Durazzo TC, Meyerhoff DJ. Psychiatric, demographic, and brain morphological predictors of relapse after treatment for an alcohol use disorder. *Alcohol Clin Exp Res*. 2017;41:107-116.
24. Substance Abuse and Mental Health Services Administration. *Facing Addiction in America: The Surgeon General's Report on Alcohol, Drugs, and Health*. US Department of Health and Human Services; 2016.
25. Sánchez F, Wang X, Castillo-Chávez C, Gorman DM, Gruenewald PJ. Drinking as an epidemic—a simple mathematical model with recovery and relapse. In: Witkiewitz KA, Marlatt GA, eds. *Therapist's Guide to Evidence-Based Relapse Prevention*. Academic Press; 2007:351-366.
26. Stockwell T, Gruenewald PJ, Toumbourou JW, Loxley W. *Preventing Harmful Substance Use: The Evidence Base for Policy and Practice*. Wiley; 2005.
27. Gorman DM. Do school-based social skills training programs prevent alcohol use among young people? *Addict Res*. 1996;4:191-210.
28. Gorman DM. The failure of drug education. *Public Interest*. 1997;129:50-60.
29. Gorman DM. The irrelevance of evidence in the development of school-based drug prevention policy, 1986-1996. *Eval Rev*. 1998;22:118-146.
30. Holder HD, Flay B, Howard J, et al. Phases of alcohol problem prevention research. *Alcohol Clin Exp Res*. 23(1):183-194.
31. McNeal RG Jr, Hansen WB, Harrington NG, Giles SM. How all stars works: an examination of program effects on mediating variables. *Health Educ Behav*. 2004;31:165-178.
32. Paschall MJ, Antin TMJ, Ringwalt CL, Saltz RF. Evaluation of an Internet-based alcohol misuse prevention course for college freshmen: findings of a randomized multi-campus trial. *Am J Prev Med*. 2011;41:300-308.
33. Paschall MJ, Ringwalt CL, Wyatt T, DeJong W. Effects of an online alcohol education course among college freshmen: an investigation of potential mediators. *J Health Commun*. 2014;19:392-412.
34. Elder RW, Nichols JL, Shults RA, et al. Effectiveness of school-based programs for reducing drinking and driving and riding with drinking drivers: a systematic review. *Am J Prev Med*. 2005;28(Suppl):288-304.
35. Foxcroft DR, Ireland E, Lister-Sharp DJ, Lowe G, Breen R. Longer-term primary prevention for alcohol misuse in young people: a systematic review. *Addiction*. 2003;98:397-411.
36. Foxcroft DR, Moreira M, Almeida Santimano NML, Smith LA. Social norms information for alcohol misuse in university and college students. *Cochrane Database Syst Rev*. 2015;12:CD006748.
37. Foxcroft DR, Tsertsvadze A. Universal school-based prevention programs for alcohol misuse in young people. *Cochrane Database Syst Rev*. 2011;5:CD009113.
38. Grube JW. Environmental approaches to preventing adolescent drinking. In: Scheier L, ed. *Handboook of Drug Use Etiology: Theory, Methods and Empirical Findings*. American Psychological Association; 2009:493-509.
39. Holder HD. *Alcohol and the Community: A Systems Approach to Prevention*. Cambridge University Press; 1998.
40. Hawkins JD, Catalano RF, Miller JY. Risk and protective factors for alcohol and other drug problems in adolescence and early adulthood: implications for substance abuse prevention. *Psychol Bull*. 1992;112(1): 64-105.
41. Ammerman RT, Ott PJ, Tarter RE. *Prevention and Societal Impact of Drug and Alcohol Abuse*. Lawrence Erlbaum; 1999.
42. Holder HD, Gruenewald PJ, Ponicki WR, et al. Effect of community-based interventions on high risk drinking and alcohol-related injuries. *JAMA*. 2000;284:2341-2347.
43. Gruenewald PJ, Treno AJ, Holder HD, LaScala EA. Community-based approaches to the prevention of substance use related problems. In: Kenneth JS, ed. *Oxford Handbook of Substance Use Disorders*. Oxford University Press; 2016
44. Howard J. Community organizing, public policy and the prevention of alcohol problems. *Alcohol Clin Exp Res*. 1996;20(8 Suppl):265A-269A.
45. Holder HD, Grube JW, Gruenewald PJ, et al. Community approaches to prevention of alcohol-related accidents. In: Watson RR, ed. *Drug and Alcohol Abuse Reviews, Vol. 7: Alcohol, Cocaine, and Accidents*. Humana Press, Inc; 1995:175-194.
46. Pentz MA. Institutionalizing community-based prevention through policy change. *J Community Psychol*. 2000;28:257-270.
47. Wagenaar AC, Perry CL. Community strategies for the reduction of youth drinking: theory and application. *J Res Adolesc*. 1994;4:319-345.
48. Caulkins JP. Measurement and analysis of drug problems and drug control efforts. In: Duffee D, ed. *Measurement and Analysis of Crime and Justice, Vol. 4, Criminal Justice 2000*. National Institute of Justice (NIJ 182411); 2000:391-449.
49. Hingson R, Howland J. Alcohol, injury, and legal controls: some complex interactions. *Law Med Health Care*. 1989;17:58-68.
50. Holder HD, Reynolds RI. Application of local policy to prevent alcohol problems: experiences from a community trial. *Addiction*. 1997;92:285-292.
51. Stockwell T, Chikritzhs T. Do relaxed trading hours for bars and clubs mean more relaxed drinking? A review of international research on the impacts of changes to permitted hours of drinking. *Crime Prev Community Saf*. 2009;11:153-170.
52. Paschall MJ, Lipperman-Kreda S, Grube JW, Thomas S. Relationships between social host laws and underage drinking: findings from a study of 50 California cities. *J Stud Alcohol Drugs*. 2014;75(6):901-907.
53. McCrady BS, Zucker RA, Brooke SG, et al. Social environmental influences on the development and resolution of alcohol problems. *Alcohol Clin Exp Res*. 2006;30:688-699.
54. Wechsler H, Moeykens B, Davenport A, et al. The adverse impact of heavy episodic drinkers on other college students. *J Stud Alcohol*. 1995;56:628-634.

55. Gruenewald PJ, Millar AB, Treno AJ, et al. The geography of availability and driving after drinking. *Addiction*. 1996;91:967-983.
56. Grube JW. Preventing sales of alcohol to minors: results from a community trial. *Addiction*. 1997;92:S251-S260.
57. Reuter P. Quantity illusions and paradoxes of drug interdiction: federal intervention into vice policy. *Law Contemp Probl*. 1988;51:233-252.
58. Saltz RF, Stanghetta P. A community-wide responsible beverage service program in three communities: early findings. *Addiction*. 1997;92:S237-S249.
59. Gruenewald PJ, Treno AJ. Local and global alcohol supply: economic and geographic models of community systems. *Addiction*. 2000;95:S537-S545.
60. White HR, Gorman DM. Dynamics of the drug-crime relationship. In: LaFree G, ed. *Criminal Justice 2000, Vol. 1: The Nature of Crime: Continuity and Change*; 2000:151-218.
61. Rose G. Sick individuals and sick populations. *Int J Epidemiol*. 2001;30:427-432.
62. Homel R. *Policing for Prevention: Reducing Crime, Public Intoxication and Injury*. Criminal Justice Press; 1997.
63. Gruenewald PJ, Johnson FW, Millar A, et al. Drinking and driving: explaining beverage specific risks. *J Stud Alcohol*. 2000;61:515-523.
64. Hennessy M, Saltz RF. Modeling social influences on public drinking. *J Stud Alcohol*. 1993;54:139-145.
65. Reuter P, Caulkins JP. Redefining the goals of drug policy: report of a working group. *Am J Public Health*. 1995;85:1059-1063.
66. Gruenewald PJ. Geospatial analyses of alcohol and drug problems: empirical needs and theoretical foundations. *GeoJournal*. 2013;78(3):443-450. doi:10.1007/s10708-011-9427-5
67. Taylor M, Pradhan A, Ogando YM, Shaya F. Impact of the naloxone standing order on trends in opioid fatal overdose: an ecological analysis. *Am J Drug Alcohol Abuse*. 2022;48:338-346.
68. Khair S, Eastwood CA, Lu M, Jackson J. Supervised consumption site enables cost savings by avoiding emergency services: a cost analysis study. *Harm Reduct J*. 2022;19:32.
69. Wagenaar AC, Murray DM, Gehan JP, et al. Communities mobilizing for change on alcohol: outcomes from a randomized community trial. *J Stud Alcohol*. 2000;61:85-94.
70. Treno AJ, Gruenewald PJ, Lee JP, et al. The Sacramento Neighborhood Alcohol Prevention Project: outcomes from a community prevention trial. *J Stud Alcohol Drugs*. 2007;68(2):197-207.
71. Wallin E, Gripenberg J, Andréasson S. Overserving at licensed premises in Stockholm: effects of a community action program. *J Stud Alcohol*. 2005;66:806-814.
72. Wallin E, Norström T, Andréasson S. Alcohol prevention targeting licensed premises: a study of effects on violence. *J Stud Alcohol*. 2003;64:270-277.
73. Gripenberg J, Wallin E, Andréasson S. Effects of a community-based drug use prevention program targeting licensed premises. *Subst Use Misuse*. 2007;42:1883-1898.
74. Månsdotter AM, Rydberg MK, Wallin E, Lindholm LA, Andréasson S. A cost-effectiveness analysis of alcohol prevention targeting licensed premises. *Eur J Public Health*. 2007;17:618-623.
75. Saltz RF, Paschall MJ, McGaffigan RM, Nygaard PM. Alcohol risk management in college settings: the Safer California Universities Randomized Trial. *Am J Prev Med*. 2010;39:491-499.
76. Flewelling RL, Grube JG, Paschall MJ, et al. Reducing youth access to alcohol: findings from a community-based randomized trial. *Am J Community Psychol*. 2013;51:264-277.
77. Wolfson M, Champion H, McCoy TP, et al. Impact of a randomized campus/community trial to prevent high-risk drinking among college students. *Alcohol Clin Exp Res*. 2012;36:1767-1778.
78. Saltz RF, Paschall MJ, O'Hara SE. Effects of a community-Level intervention on alcohol-related motor vehicle crashes in California cities: a randomized trial. *Am J Prev Med*. 2021;60:38-46.
79. Moore RS, Roberts J, McGaffigan R, et al. Implementing a reward and reminder underage drinking prevention program in convenience stores near Southern California American Indian reservations. *Am J Drug Alcohol Abuse*. 2012;38:456-460.
80. Moore RS, Gilder DA, Grube JW, et al. Prevention of underage drinking on California Indian reservations using individual- and community-level approaches. *Am J Public Health*. 2018;108:1035-1041.
81. Wagenaar AC, Livingston MD, Pettigrew DW, Kominsky TK, Komro KA. Communities mobilizing for change on alcohol (CMCA): secondary analyses of a randomized controlled trial showing effects of community organizing on alcohol acquisition by youth in the Cherokee nation. *Addiction*. 2018;113:647-655.
82. Komro KA, Livingston MD, Wagenaar AC, Kominsky TK, Pettigrew DW, Garrett BA; Cherokee Nation Prevention Trial Team. Multilevel prevention trial of alcohol use among American Indian and White High School students in the Cherokee Nation. *Am J Public Health*. 2017;107:453-459.
83. Chen M-J, Grube JW, Gruenewald PJ. Community alcohol outlet density and underage drinking. *Addiction*. 2010;105:270-278.
84. Lipperman-Kreda S, Mair CF, Bersamin M, Grube GPJ, JW. Who drinks where: youth selection of drinking contexts. *Alcohol Clin Exp Res*. 2015;39:716-723.
85. Mair C, Lipperman-Kreda S, Gruenewald PJ, Bersamin M, Grube JW. Adolescent drinking risks associated with specific drinking contexts. *Alcohol Clin Exp Res*. 2015;39:1705-1711.
86. Bersamin M, Lipperman-Kreda S, Mair C, Gruenewald GJW, PJ. Identifying strategies to limit youth drinking in the home. *J Stud Alcohol Drugs*. 2016;77:943-949.
87. Mair C, Gruenewald PJ, Ponicki WR, Remer L. Varying impacts of alcohol outlet densities on violent assaults: explaining differences across neighborhoods. *J Stud Alcohol Drugs*. 2013;74:50-58.
88. Gruenewald PJ, Remer L, LaScala EA. Testing a social ecological model of alcohol use: the California 50-city study. *Addiction*. 2014;109:736-745.
89. Morrison C, Mair CF, Lee JP, Gruenewald PJ. Are barroom and neighborhood characteristics independently related to local-area assaults? *Alcohol Clin Exp Res*. 2015;39:2463-2470.
90. Gruenewald PJ. The spatial ecology of alcohol problems: niche theory and assortative drinking. *Addiction*. 2007;102:870-878.
91. Gruenewald PJ, Treno AJ, Ponicki WR, Huckle T, Yeh L-C, Casswell S. Impacts of New Zealand's lowered minimum purchase age on context-specific drinking and related risks. *Addiction*. 2015;110:1757-1766.
92. Trolldal B, Brännström L, Paschall MJ, Leifman H. Effects of a multi-component responsible beverage service programme on violent assaults in Sweden. *Addiction*. 2013;108:89-96.
93. Skardhamar T, Fekjær SB, Pedersen W. If it works there, will it work here? The effect of a multi-component responsible beverage service (RBS) programme on violence in Oslo. *Drug Alcohol Depend*. 2016;169:128-133.
94. Rossow I, Baklien B. Effectiveness of responsible beverage service: the Norwegian experiences. *Contemp Drug Probl*. 2010;2010(37):91-107.
95. Nygaard P, Saltz RF. Communication between researchers and practitioners: findings from a qualitative evaluation of a large-scale college intervention. *Subst Use Misuse*. 2010;45:77-97.
96. Fixsen DL, Naoom SF, Blase KA, Friedman RM, Wallace F. *Implementation Research: A Synthesis of the Literature*. University of South Florida; 2005.
97. Earnest MA, Wong SL, Frederico SG. Physician advocacy: what is it and how do we do it? *Acad Med*. 2010;85:63-67.
98. Tanner-Smith EE, Parr NJ, Schweer-Collins M, Saitz R. Effects of brief substance use interventions delivered in general medical settings: a systematic review and meta-analysis. *Addiction*. 2022;117:877-889.

CHAPTER 27

Prevention of Prescription Medication Misuse

Beth Han, Christopher M. Jones, and Wilson M. Compton

CHAPTER OUTLINE

- Introduction
- Historical perspective on the scheduling of prescription drugs in the United States
- Epidemiology of misuse of prescription medications
- The major classes of misused prescription medications
- Evidence-based prevention and harm-reduction and policy approaches
- Evidence-based treatment for prescription drug use disorders
- Ongoing research
- Summary/conclusions

INTRODUCTION

Prescription medication misuse has been a problem as long as such products have existed, and the current patterns in the United States represent the newest iteration.[1,2] The list of prescription medications that are misused is lengthy, but the primary categories of clinical importance are opioids, stimulants, and sedatives/tranquilizers. Misuse is often defined as using a psychotherapeutic medication without a prescription; in greater amounts, more often, or longer than prescribed; or for a reason other than as directed by a doctor.[3] A prescription drug use disorder (PDUD) as defined by the *Diagnostic and Statistical Manual of Mental Disorders,* 5th ed (DSM-5) is a medical illness that occurs when ongoing misuse of prescription drugs leads to clinically and functionally significant impairment, with endorsement of 2 or more of the 11 specific DSM-5 criteria (excluding tolerance and withdrawal if medications are taken solely under medical supervisions).

In 2020, approximately 16.1 million Americans ages 12 and older misused prescription opioids (assessed in the National Survey on Drug Use and Health as "prescription pain relievers," which are Predominantly opioids[4] and referred to as "prescription opioids" elsewhere in this chapter), prescription stimulants, or prescription sedatives/tranquilizers in the past year (**Fig. 27-1**), and among them, 3.6 million Americans had a past-year PDUP based on the DSM-5 diagnostic criteria.[5] In 2020, prescription opioid misuse was the most common form of prescription drug misuse, with 9.3 million people reporting misusing opioids in the past year and 2.3 million having a past-year prescription opioid use disorder.[5]

The most serious consequences of all substance use disorders (SUD) are deaths from drug use, and prescription medications have been associated with many deaths, particularly overdose deaths. In the United States, overall overdose deaths involving prescription opioids increased nearly five times from 3,442 in 1999 to 16,416 in 2020 (**Fig. 27-2**).[6] Deaths involving prescription opioids without the involvement of any other opioids (eg, heroin or synthetic opioids such as illicitly manufactured fentanyl) increased from 2,604 in 1999 to a peak of 13,226 in 2011, then declined to 7,114 in 2020. In contrast, overdose deaths involving prescription opioids in combination with other opioids increased modestly from 838 in 1999 to 1,712 in 2010 and then accelerated to 9,302 in 2020, driven by deaths involving prescription opioids in combination with illicit synthetic opioids such as illicitly manufactured fentanyl and fentanyl analogs during the late 2010s and during the COVID-19 pandemic. In particular, prescription opioids in combination with these synthetic opioids were almost nonexistent in 1999 and have increased markedly in recent years, and the number was higher than the number of deaths involving prescription opioids without any other opioids in 2020 (8,626 versus 7,114 deaths).[6a]

Misuse of prescription medications is linked to medical practice in ways quite different from alcohol, tobacco, and other illicit drugs. It presents unusual difficulties for clinicians for two reasons. First, the medical system is the origin of the substances in most cases. Prescription drugs are "legal" compounds, manufactured by pharmaceutical companies and distributed by the medical system before their diversion. Second, boundaries between therapeutic use, nonmedical use, and addiction can be quite vague. Overall, prescribers are in a unique situation of having to optimize medication dosage to minimize symptoms of the disease being treated while also monitoring their prescribing practices in order to reduce the risk of nonmedical use and addiction in their patients as well as diversion to the larger community. But ultimately, prescribers can only control what they prescribe, not how a prescription drug is taken.

In this chapter, several issues are covered: (1) historical perspectives on the scheduling of prescription medications, (2) epidemiology of prescription drug misuse, (3) review of the major classes of misused prescription medications (including a brief review of the pharmacology and neurobiological effects of each category as well as the particular harms associated

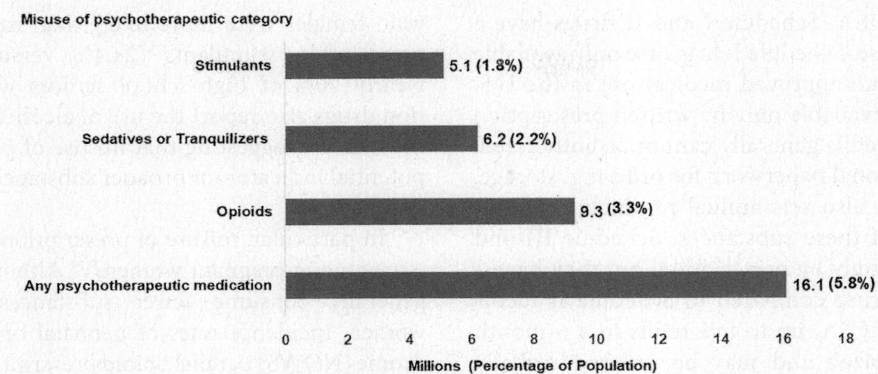

Figure 27-1. Past-year misuse of prescription psychotherapeutics among U.S. persons aged 12 and older, 2021. (From Center for Behavioral Health Statistics and Quality. *2020 National Survey on Drug Use and Health: Detailed Tables*. Substance Abuse and Mental Health Services Administration; 2021.)

with the category), (4) evidence-based prevention and harm-reduction approaches (including policy approaches), (5) evidence-based treatment for prescription drug use disorders, and (6) ongoing research.

HISTORICAL PERSPECTIVE ON THE SCHEDULING OF PRESCRIPTION DRUGS IN THE UNITED STATES

Use of opioids to obtain euphoria dates to antiquity. In the late 19th century, many Civil War veterans developed addiction to opioids ("the soldier's disease"), which began with exposure to injectable morphine for the treatment of pain from their war-related injuries. Simultaneously, the patent medicine industry was liberally promoting opioids and cocaine to treat a variety of conditions. In response, the U.S. Harrison Narcotics Act was enacted in 1914 in order to regulate and tax the production, importation, and distribution of opiates and coca products.

In 1970, the Controlled Substances Act (CSA) was enacted to regulate the manufacture, importation, possession, and distribution of drugs with misuse liability and their precursor compounds. The CSA created drug Schedules (classifications), based on whether a compound has an accepted medical use and on its potential for misuse. This legislation also created the Drug Enforcement Administration (DEA) within the Department of Justice, as the agency responsible for enforcing the CSA and its implementation.

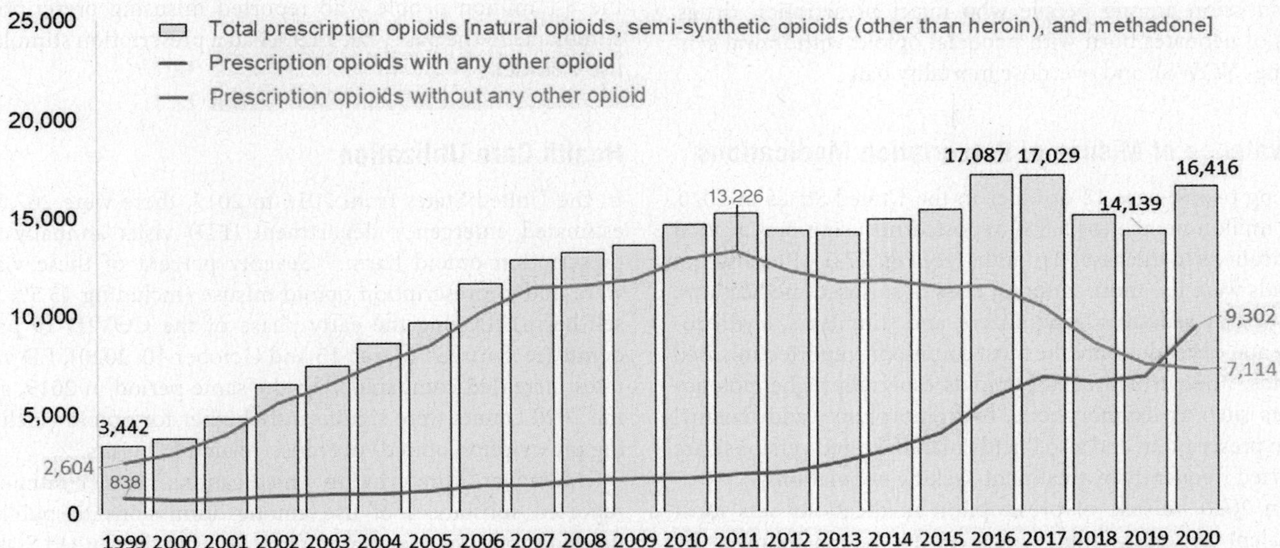

Figure 27-2. National overdose deaths involving prescription opioids, number among all ages, 1999-2020. Among deaths with drug overdose as the underlying cause, the prescription opioid subcategory does not include fentanyl (because it has not been possible to distinguish prescription-type fentanyl from illicit fentanyl based on the ICD codes) and was determined by **T40.2 or T40.3** for natural opioids, semi-synthetic opioids (other than heroin), and methadone. (Source: From Centers for Disease Control and Prevention, National Center for Health Statistics. *Multiple Cause of Death 1999-2020* on CDC WONDER Online Database.)

According to the DEA, Schedule I and II drugs have a high potential for misuse. Schedule I drugs are only available for research and have no approved medical use in the U.S. Schedule II drugs are available only by written prescription (paper or electronic); refills generally cannot be authorized, and they require additional paperwork for ordering, storage, and transfer. The DEA also sets annual production quotas for the manufacture of these substances. Schedule III and IV drugs are available only by prescription, but they have a lower potential for misuse compared to Schedule II medications and, under the CSA, up to five refills in a 6-month period may be authorized and may be ordered verbally (though state laws may be more stringent). Schedule V drugs have lower potential for misuse than Schedule IV medications and some are available over the counter (dependent upon state law). Scheduling is one mechanism that has been used to reduce diversion of prescription drugs. For example, hydrocodone combination products (eg, Vicodin and others) are the most commonly prescribed and misused[2] opioids, and their rescheduling from Schedule III to II in 2014 led to a 22% reduction in hydrocodone prescribing over the subsequent year.[7]

EPIDEMIOLOGY OF MISUSE OF PRESCRIPTION MEDICATIONS

Misuse of prescription medications is associated with a diverse range of potential health harms. Available epidemiological data include data from general populations reflecting the overall scope of nonmedical use, emergency department data demonstrating acute health harms, substance use disorder treatment data, data estimating rates of infectious disease transmission among people who inject prescription drugs, rates of neonates born with neonatal opioid withdrawal syndrome (NOWS), and overdose mortality data.

Prevalence of Misuse of Prescription Medications

Among people ages 12 or older in the United States in 2020, 16.1 million people (or 5.8%) reported misusing prescription medications in the past 12 months (see **Fig. 27-1**). Prescription opioids were the most common class of misused medications, followed by sedatives/tranquilizers, and stimulants. Hydrocodone and oxycodone are the most commonly reported misused opioids,[3-5] but virtually all the opioids, especially higher potency agents such as oxymorphone, hydromorphone, and fentanyl (both prescription and also illicitly manufactured versions), are reported frequently by treatment-seeking populations.

In 2020, misuse of prescription medications was most prevalent in young adults (ages 18-25: 9.5%), followed by adults (ages 26 or older: 5.6%) and adolescents (ages 12-17: 2.8%). In general, males had slightly higher misuse prevalence, with an important exception that among adolescents ages 12 to 17 who used prescription stimulants in the past year, females were more likely than males to have misused prescription stimulants (24.4% versus 14.0% in 2020).[5] Nearly 70% of high-school seniors who misuse prescription drugs also report the use of alcohol, cannabis, and other substances, suggesting that misuse of prescription drugs is a potential indicator for broader substance use problems in this population.[8]

In particular, misuse of prescription drugs is a significant issue among pregnant women.[9,10] Although pregnant women generally consume fewer substances than nonpregnant women, incidence rates of neonatal opioid withdrawal syndrome (NOWS) parallel opioid prescription rates, highlighting the need for adopting safe and appropriate opioid prescribing practices to help address this specific component of the opioid crisis. Of note, increases in maternal opioid use and NOWS have been even more pronounced in rural areas than in urban.[11,12] Treatment of women with opioid use disorder is covered in the chapters specific to pregnant and postpartum women.

Prevalence of Prescription Drug Use Disorders

In 2020, over 3.6 million Americans ages 12 or older met the DSM-5 diagnostic criteria for a past-year SUD related to misuse of prescription drugs—including 2.3 million with a prescription opioid use disorder, 1.2 million with a prescription sedative/tranquilizer use disorder, and 758,000 with a prescription stimulant use disorder.[5] Thus, in 2020, among the 9.3 million people who reported misusing prescription opioids in the past year, 25.2% had a prescription opioid use disorder; among the 6.2 million people who reported misusing prescription sedatives/tranquilizers in the past year, 18.6% had a prescription sedative/tranquilizer use disorder; and among the 5.1 million people who reported misusing prescription stimulants in the past year, 14.9% had a prescription stimulant use disorder.

Health Care Utilization

In the United States from 2016 to 2017, there were 267,020 estimated emergency department (ED) visits annually for prescription opioid harm.[13] Seventy percent of these visits were due to prescription opioid misuse (including 13.5% for self-harm). During the early phase of the COVID-19 pandemic (ie, between March 15 and October 10, 2020), ED visit rates increased compared with the same period in 2019, and the 2020 counts were significantly higher for opioid (including prescription opioid) overdose-related ED visits.[14]

Moreover, prescription medications are commonly reported substances of use among admissions to publicly funded substance use treatment facilities in the United States. In 2019, for example, 27,027 admissions were related to oxycodone (OxyContin, Percocet), 4,171 were due to hydrocodone (Vicodin), 29,739 were because of alprazolam (Xanax), and 7,070 were related to amphetamines.[15]

Overdose Deaths

Overdose deaths involving prescription medications also increased markedly throughout the United States between 1999 and 2020 (**Figs. 27-2** and **27-3**).[6] As mentioned above, overall overdose deaths involving prescription opioids increased 377% from 3,442 in 1999 to 16,416 in 2020, and deaths involving prescription opioids in combination with other opioids increased from 838 in 1999 to 9,302 in 2020, driven by prescription opioids in combination with illicit synthetic opioids such as illicitly manufactured fentanyl and fentanyl analogs in the late 2010s and during the COVID-19 pandemic. Although the number of prescription opioid-involved overdose deaths in 2020 (16,416) was lower than its peak in 2016 (17,087), it was higher than those in 2018 to 2019 (see **Fig. 27-2**). Factors that have contributed to the increase in prescription opioid overdose deaths,[16,17] include the prescribing of high-potency opioids, high dosages of opioids, or for longer durations, the co-prescribing of benzodiazepines, as well as the combined use of or exposure to highly potent illicitly-manufactured fentanyl (or related analogs) in the illicit drug supply, including in counterfeit pills designed to look like commonly misused prescription opioids or other prescription medications such as benzodiazepines and stimulants.[5] Overdose deaths involving benzodiazepines increased nearly 11 times from 1,135 in 1999 to 12,290 in 2020. In 2020, among the 12,290 benzodiazepine-involved overdose deaths, 10,771 deaths (or 87.6%) also involved an opioid; specifically, 4,425 deaths (or 36.0%) involved prescription opioids; 7,983 deaths (or 65.0%) involved synthetic opioids other than methadone; and 1,519 deaths (12.4%) did not involve any opioid.[6] Recent studies have also raised the possibility that interactions between opioids and some antidepressant medications—specifically selective serotonin reuptake inhibitors (SSRIs)—may increase the risk for overdose by increasing the risk for serotonin syndrome.[18]

Co-occurrence With Other Substance and Psychiatric Disorders

In general, there is a high rate of co-occurrence between addictive disorders and psychiatric disorders.[19,20] A PDUD defined by DSM-5 is highly predictive of a clinically significant SUD related to another prescription drug, an illicit drug, and/or alcohol.[9,10,21] Prescription opioid use disorders, specifically, have been shown to overlap considerably with other SUDs.[9,10,22]

Less is known, however, about the timing of the onset of co-occurring disorders. In one study, a prominent pathway from depression-related disorders to misuse of prescription opioids was reported.[23] In addition, recent work is showing that misuse of prescription drugs is generally part of a polydrug-use phenotype rather than a solitary condition.[24] Overall, common mental health disorders and illicit drug use are associated with misuse of prescription drugs, even though causality often cannot be determined. Clinicians need to carefully assess for co-occurring mental health and SUDs whenever misuse of prescription drugs is found.

THE MAJOR CLASSES OF MISUSED PRESCRIPTION MEDICATIONS

The division of drugs into classes is based on the pharmacological activity of the drug. Although anticholinergics, laxatives, neuroleptics, antidepressants, and other drug classes can be misused, this chapter is limited primarily to prescription opioids, stimulants, and sedatives-tranquilizers, each of which shares chemistry and physiological effects with illicit compounds in the same class. Strategies for withdrawal management and treatment can be found in the chapters specific to those drug classes. Nevertheless, diagnosis and management of PDUDs may have unique features, such as co-occurrence

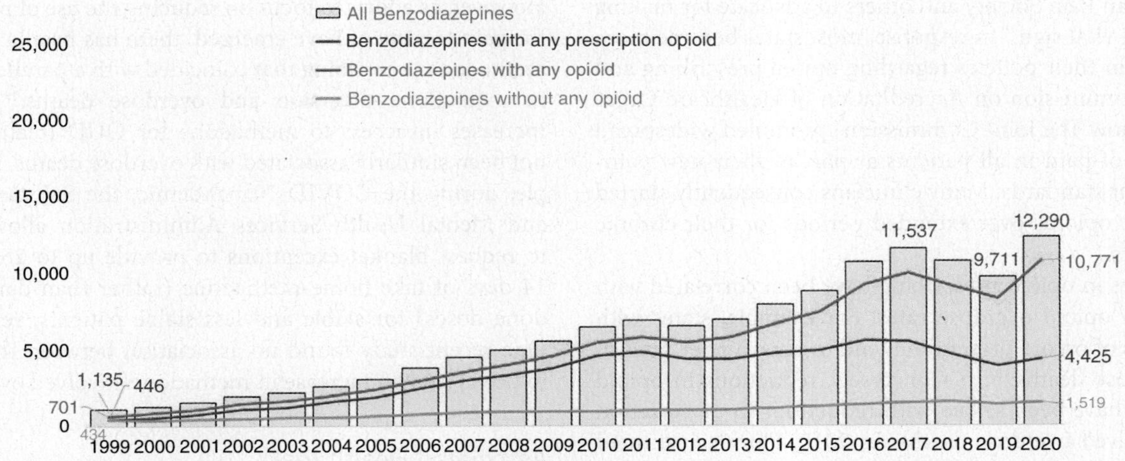

Figure 27-3. National Drug Overdose Deaths Involving Benzodiazepines,* by Opioid Involvement, Number Among All Ages, 1999-2020.*Among deaths with drug overdose as the underlying cause, the benzodiazepine category was determined by the T42.4 ICD-10 multiple cause-of-death code. (Source: From Centers for Disease Control and Prevention, National Center for Health Statistics. Multiple Cause of Death 1999-2020 on CDC WONDER Online Database.)

of a condition (eg, pain, anxiety, mood, or sleep disorders) for which the drug may have originally been prescribed.

Another issue of growing importance is how to conceptualize cannabis used as treatment (so-called "medical marijuana" or cannabis used a treatment). The U.S. Food and Drug Administration (FDA) has not approved the use of cannabis as a treatment for any medical condition. Several FDA-approved medications contain natural or synthetic cannabinoids, though these are distinct from cannabis used as treatment which typically consists of nonstandardized and nonpharmacologically produced preparations. As of July 2022, 38 states had taken legislative action to legalize cannabis used as treatment despite the lack of medical consensus around such use, and 18 states plus the District of Columbia had legalized its nonmedical use by adults. So far, data suggest that there is significant overlap in the demographic factors that cannabis used as treatment and the nonmedical use of cannabis[25]; and in states with permissive regulations for the former, it is not clear that the medical distinctions are meaningful. Thus, cannabis used as treatment is not included in this chapter and is covered Section 15, Ethical, Legal, and Liability Issues in Addiction Practice.

Prescription Opioids

In the United States,[26] prescription opioids are a common treatment for chronic pain despite longstanding recognition that not all pain syndromes are responsive to opioid therapy and addiction can arise from such use.[3,27-30] Following a period in which physicians had shied away from using opioids due to this risk, a confluence of events converged to reverse this trend in the 1990s. In 1996, Purdue Pharma released a new extended-release formulation of oxycodone, OxyContin, and launched an aggressive marketing campaign promoting its use and convincing prescribers that the risk for addiction was "less than one percent." Meanwhile, increasing recognition among the medical community of the under-treatment of pain led the American Pain Society and others to advocate for making pain a "fifth vital sign." In response, most states became more permissive in their policies regarding opioid prescribing and the Joint Commission on Accreditation of Healthcare Organizations (now The Joint Commission) promoted widespread assessment of pain in all patients as part of their new pain-management standards. Many clinicians consequently started to prescribe opioids over extended periods for their chronic pain patients.

Increases in opioid prescribing have been correlated with increases in opioid overdose rates. For example, states with higher rates of opioid prescribing tend to have higher rates of drug overdose deaths.[18,31,32] Conversely, reductions in opioid prescribing have been linked with reductions in prescription opioid-involved overdose deaths. In 2010, Florida instituted a series of major policy changes to reduce the inappropriate prescribing of prescription opioids, including cracking down on "pill mills," resulting in a curtailment of prescriptions and dispensing of opioids and a 27% reduction in overdose deaths related to prescription opioids between 2010 and 2012.[33]

Interestingly, despite the well-established efficacy of opioids for treating certain types of acute pain, there remains a dearth of evidence on the efficacy of opioids for treating chronic pain, even though chronic pain is highly prevalent in the United States.[26,34] Research suggests that opioids may cause hyperalgesia and exacerbate some chronic pain conditions. And while it was once thought that the use of prescription opioids for physiological pain treatment was not associated with a significant risk for misuse or addiction, this is now recognized to be incorrect; patients prescribed opioids to treat physiological pain are among those becoming addicted to these medications. The intersection of pain and addiction is covered in more detail in Section 13, Pain and Addiction, and is also summarized below.

Some studies have estimated the prevalence of misuse of prescription opioids among patients with chronic pain to be as high as 25%,[35] and another study found that appropriate medical use of opioids before the end of high school was independently associated with future misuse of opioids.[36] Among people ages 12 or older in 2020, relieving physical pain was the most commonly reported motivation for their most recent prescription opioid misuse (64.6%).[5] Prescription opioid misuse and use disorders were most commonly reported in adults who were uninsured, were unemployed, had low income, or had behavioral health problems.[3] Further adding to the complexity of these issues, patients with severe debilitating pain may be under-treated due to concerns about addiction.[37,38] The difficulty of treating pain while minimizing the risk of addiction clearly presents particular complexities for clinicians.

Methadone prescribed for pain management has also received considerable attention as a contributor to the rise in prescription opioid overdose deaths.[39] Methadone has a long half-life with significant variability across patients (ranging from 8 to 59 hours), substantially longer than the duration of its analgesic effects (4-8 hours). This has resulted in disproportionate involvement in overdose mortality in some states.[39] However, as efforts to focus on reducing the use of methadone for pain treatment have emerged, there has been a decline in methadone prescribing that coincided with a parallel decrease in methadone diversion and overdose deaths.[39] Of note, increases in access to methadone for OUD treatment have not been similarly associated with overdose deaths. For example, during the COVID-19 pandemic, the Substance Abuse and Mental Health Services Administration allowed states to request blanket exceptions to provide up to 28 days and 14 days of take-home-methadone (rather than daily methadone doses) for stable and less stable patients, respectively. One recent study found no association between this change in policy and an increase in methadone-involved overdoses.[40]

Associated Health Risks

Misuse of prescription opioids has been associated with the initiation of heroin use.[2] While prior research has documented that the majority of people who currently use heroin report misuse of prescription opioids before heroin initiation, heroin use among people who misuse prescription opioids is relatively rare, with heroin onset at a rate of about 1% to 3% per year.[41] As has been documented extensively, heroin initiation is predicted by more frequent nonmedical use of prescription opioids, presence of a prescription opioid use disorder, injection of prescription drugs, and polysubstance use.[2] Furthermore, adolescents who reported prescription opioid misuse were more likely to report the subsequent onset of heroin use than those without prescription opioid misuse.[42,43] The transition from prescription opioid misuse to heroin use appears to be part of the progression of addiction in a subset of individuals with nonmedical use of prescription opioids driven in part by the availability of high purity, low cost heroin. As individuals' tolerance outstrips the dose of opioids that they are able to obtain from their providers, they may turn to the illicit market for pills or heroin.

Misuse of prescription opioids has also been associated with increased transmission of infectious diseases including hepatitis C (HCV) and HIV due to sharing of needles, syringes, and drug injection preparation equipment by people who inject drugs, especially among young people who inject drugs in suburban and rural areas.[44-47] The risk of HCV transmission between people who inject drugs is roughly ten times higher than HIV transmission, partly because HCV lives longer outside of the body. The estimated annual incidence of HCV infection among young adults who inject drugs is between 8% and 25%, and currently over 200,000 may be infected. Regional rates of HCV are correlated with the severity of the opioid overdose epidemic[48] and prescription opioid injection in rural areas.[49] Data suggest that prescription opioid injection which is associated with higher-injection frequency may be a stronger risk factor for HCV infection than heroin or other drug injection.[47] HIV and HCV co-infection is also common. For example, during the 2015 outbreak of HIV in Scott County Indiana, wherein 181 patients who injected the prescription opioid oxymorphone were newly diagnosed with HIV, over 92% were co-infected with HCV.[44]

Heightening the sense of urgency for addressing prescription opioid misuse is the recent increase in the availability of and use of illicitly-manufactured fentanyl—a synthetic prescription opioid 50 to 100 times more potent than morphine, manufactured in clandestine labs and commonly mixed with heroin or sold alone in powder form or as counterfeit tablets. Epidemiological data indicate the population of individuals using fentanyl is similar in characteristics to those using heroin.[50,51] Fundamentally, prescription opioids, heroin, and illicit synthetic opioids such as fentanyl are elements of a larger epidemic of opioid-related morbidity and mortality. Viewing them from a unified perspective taking into account the interrelated factors that contribute to their use and the natural history of the transition from misuse of prescription opioids to heroin and fentanyl use is essential to improving public health.[2]

Prescription Stimulants

Prescription stimulants are primarily prescribed for attention deficit hyperactivity disorder (ADHD). Youth in the United States are treated with stimulants for ADHD more frequently than in Western European countries,[52] and the number of prescriptions for children and adults being treated for ADHD has increased markedly since 1990.[53] The recent increases in national prescription stimulant dispensing have been driven by significant increases in stimulant dispensing rates among women and adults aged 20 or older.[53] Unsurprisingly, among people aged 12 to 64 in the United States, the adjusted prevalence of prescription stimulant misuse has increased as well.[54] However, prescription stimulant misuse may be more common among friends/peers of youth prescribed these medications rather than the individuals with the prescription themselves.[55-57] Adolescent ADHD patients show lower rates of stimulant misuse than other young people, however, these same patients are often part of a sharing/diversion pathway for friends and classmates.

Among people aged 12 or older in the United States in 2020, 5.1 million (or 1.8%) reported misusing prescription stimulants in the past 12 months (see **Fig. 27-1**),[5] among them, 758,000 people (or 14.9%) had a prescription stimulant use disorder based on the diagnostic criteria specified in the DSM-5.[5] Misuse of amphetamines (and other pharmaceutical stimulants) has been relatively highly prevalent among young people for many years.[58] Preference for Adderall has been reported by both college and high school students.[59] National data show that stimulants are among the only substances used more by college students than by their non-college-attending same-age peers.[60] The motivations for misusing stimulant medication in college are varied and include weight loss, improving attention, partying, reducing hyperactivity, and improving grades (and sometimes a combination of the three—staying up to party and then using again to stay up to cram).[61]

Among U.S. adults, the most commonly reported motivations for misuse were to help be alert or concentrate.[62] The most likely source of misused prescription stimulants was by obtaining them free from friends or relatives, but more frequent prescription stimulant misuse and use disorder were associated with an increased likelihood of obtaining medications from physicians or from drug dealers or strangers and less likelihood of obtaining them from friends or relatives.[62]

Among U.S. adults with past-year prescription stimulant misuse, those with past-year prescription stimulant use disorders did not differ from those with misuse without use disorders in any of the examined sociodemographic characteristics and in many of the examined substance use problems.[62] These results suggest that these two groups may be related, and prescription stimulant misuse without use disorder may be an early expression of a trajectory toward prescription stimulant use disorder, highlighting the importance of judicious prescribing and screening for stimulant misuse and use disorder in patients for whom they prescribe stimulants.

Associated Health Risks

When used as directed, the side effects of prescription stimulants are typically mild and include headaches, decreased appetite, weight loss, and insomnia. However, misuse (which typically includes use at higher dosages) increases the risks for significant health effects including addiction, psychosis, cardiac events, seizures, and sudden death.

Prescription Sedative-Tranquilizers

The category of prescription sedatives-tranquilizers is often divided into separate classes of drugs based on their intended primary purpose—either relief from anxiety or insomnia. For example, benzodiazepines are a subcategory of drugs that may be prescribed either as tranquilizers for the relief of anxiety or as sedatives for the relief of insomnia. This division is not based on the pharmacological properties of the medication but often only on the dose administered or the time of administration (ie, at bedtime or not), and for that reason, we discuss them as one class.

Prescription sedatives-tranquilizers have been misused for decades, whether it was the earlier agents, such as the barbiturates and chloral hydrate, or the benzodiazepines available since the 1960s. Some have proven to be highly problematic and addictive (eg, methaqualone and the short-acting barbiturates) and are no longer accepted as standards of care except in limited circumstances—such as in hospitalized patients and in some cases of sedative withdrawal management—but all have significant misuse liability. Even the newest hypnotic agents, such as zolpidem and zopiclone, while shown to have lower potential to be misused than many earlier agents, have nonetheless been associated with such use.[63] Similar to the opioid and stimulant drugs classes, there has been an increase in the prescribing of benzodiazepines, which could account for increases in the misuse of these drugs.[64]

Among people ages 12 or older in the United States in 2020, 4.8 million (or 1.7%) reported misusing benzodiazepines in the past 12 months.[5] Among past-year adults that use benzodiazepine in the United States, 17.1% reported misusing benzodiazepines, and 1.5% had benzodiazepine use disorders.[5] Moreover, less than 20% of adults with past-year benzodiazepine misuse reported that their main motivation for their most recent misuse was to experiment, get high, or modify the effect of other drugs; by contrast, more than two-thirds reported that their main reason for misuse was to help sleep or relieve tension. Thus, better management of insomnia or anxiety symptoms could have a marked impact on reducing benzodiazepine misuse.[65]

Benzodiazepine misuse without use disorder was associated with younger age, male sex, being Black, poor educational attainment, being uninsured and unemployed, being single, having a family income below $50,000, and having suicidal ideation and other specific substance use problems.[65] Importantly, correlates of benzodiazepine use disorders were similar to the above, yet most correlates were more strongly associated with benzodiazepine use disorders.[65]

Although benzodiazepines alone do not typically result in overdose deaths, they have been linked to a growing number of overdoses and fatalities involving other drugs.[12] Between 1999 and 2020, the number of benzodiazepine overdose deaths increased almost 11 times from 1,135 to 12,290 (see **Fig. 27-3**). The number of overdose deaths involving benzodiazepine with any prescription opioid increased from 446 in 1999 to 4,425 in 2020, and the number of overdose deaths involving benzodiazepine with any opioid increased from 701 in 1999 to 10,771 in 2020; by contrast, the number of overdose deaths involving benzodiazepine without any opioid was much lower but did increase from 434 in 1999 to 1,519 in 2020.[6] In particular, a report from the Centers for Disease Control and Prevention (CDC) identified three concerning trends during 2019 to 2020:

1. Increases in both nonfatal and fatal overdoses involving benzodiazepines and opioids.
2. Marked increases in illicit benzodiazepine deaths, although overdose deaths involving prescription benzodiazepines still far outnumber those involving illicit benzodiazepines.
3. Increases in nonfatal benzodiazepine overdoses not involving opioids.[66]

Among patients who had a nonfatal opioid overdose, active daily benzodiazepine dispensing was also associated with an increased risk for repeated overdose.[67] An additional concern with sedatives is that withdrawal from these medications can pose significant health risks, including seizures. Thus, discontinuation of sedatives should be gradual and medically monitored. A hyperbolic reduction in dosage has been particularly recommended to reduce the risk of significant withdrawal and symptom recurrence.[68,69]

EVIDENCE-BASED PREVENTION AND HARM-REDUCTION AND POLICY APPROACHES

Prevention Programs

There are many evidence-based strategies to prevent or reduce misuse of prescription drugs and to reduce associated harms. Broad-based prevention approaches, including universal family-based interventions such as the *Strengthening Families Program: For Parents and Youth 10–14*, a family-based program for younger adolescents, and *PROmoting School-community-university Partnerships to Enhance Resilience* (PROSPER), a system for delivering evidence-based interventions during grades 6 and 7, have been demonstrated to reduce misuse of prescription drugs.[70] These approaches target families as key agents to address a range of adolescent-onset risk behaviors. The 2017 Surgeon General's *Report on Alcohol, Drugs, and Health* highlights the need to increase the implementation of evidence-based prevention practices both in the community and throughout health care systems.[71]

Prescription Take-Back Programs

Many persons who use prescription drugs nonmedically do not obtain them directly from physicians. For example, data from the *National Survey on Drug Use and Health* (**Fig. 27-4**)

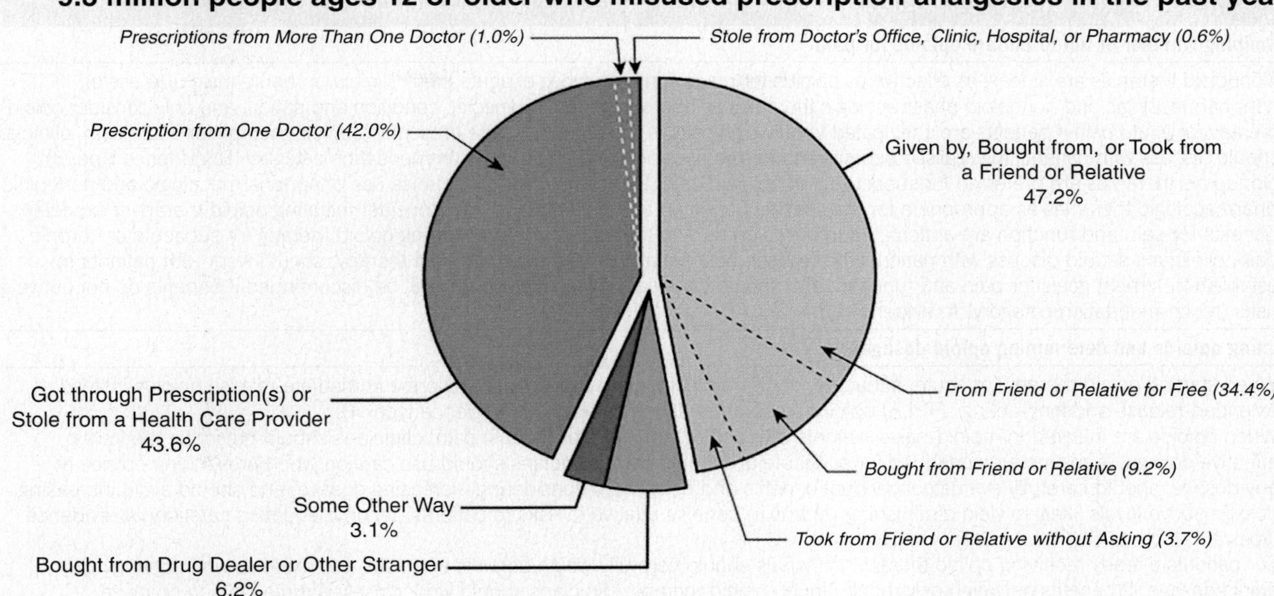

Figure 27-4. Source where pain relievers were obtained for most recent misuse: among people aged 12 or older who misused pain relievers in the past year; 2020. (Data Source: The 2020 National Survey on Drug Use and Health, SAMHSA.)

document that the major sources of misused prescription opioids are family and friends who have their own prescriptions. Notably, persons who frequently misused prescription opioids and those who are in treatment for opioid use disorders are more likely to obtain opioids from drug dealers and from personal prescriptions.[3,72,73] In response, efforts are underway to make it easier for patients to discard partially used prescriptions. While little empirical data addresses the effectiveness of take-back programs in reducing the rates of nonmedical prescription drug use or in reducing the harms from such use, these programs show promise in removing unwanted, commonly nonmedically used medications from people's medicine cabinets,[74] where they not only remain available for nonmedical use by the intended recipient but may also be found and taken by family members and friends. They also serve as an opportunity to amplify public messages about the appropriate use, storage, and disposal of medications.

Prescriber Education

The ongoing opioid overdose epidemic has highlighted the need to improve provider education and equip providers with the tools they need to improve prescribing practices. In 2016, the CDC released a *Guideline for Prescribing Opioids for Chronic Pain* to be used as a clinical tool to improve the safe and appropriate prescribing of opioids.[75] In 2022, the CDC updated and replaced the 2016 Guideline with the *CDC Clinical Practice Guideline for Prescribing Opioids for Pain*. This new guideline provides evidence-based recommendations for clinicians who are providing pain care, including those prescribing opioids, for outpatients aged 18 years or over with acute pain (duration <1 month), subacute (duration of 1-3 months) pain, or chronic (duration of >3 months) pain outside of sickle cell disease-related pain management, cancer-related pain treatment, palliative care, and end-of-life care (see **Table 27-1** for a summary of recommendations).[76]

Being aware of and adhering to evidence-based guidelines for pain management and advancing training in pain management and expanding access to and coverage of multiple pain care modalities are the responsibility of health care systems and clinicians. Alternate approaches to prescription opioid analgesics exist and often should be tried before prescription opioids are considered for many acute, subacute, and chronic pain conditions; they include psychosocial approaches (eg, cognitive behavioral therapy) and nonopioid medications (eg, nonsteroidal anti-inflammatory drugs [NSAIDs], antidepressants, and anticonvulsants), TENS units, acupuncture, exercise therapy, and among others. Routine review of prescription drug monitoring program (PDMP) data prior to writing prescriptions for controlled substances can also become standard practice among clinicians to inform individualized, patient-centered care. And given potential liability issues (eg, potential lawsuits for under-prescribing, and prosecution for overprescribing), well-written medical records and documented consultations are now an essential part of pain management. Good clinical practice includes meticulous medical records that document the logic for dosages (especially increases) and tapers or discontinuations, with particular caution against abrupt discontinuation of opioids or rapid dosage reductions, and if a patient is not responding to standard treatment or requires dosage increases, written consultation may be warranted. Finally, just as attention to PDMP data is recommended, clinicians should document and respond to clinical signals of inappropriate medication usage such as

TABLE 27-1 Summary of the CDC Clinical Practice Guideline for Prescribing Opioids for Pain—United States, 2022 Recommendations for Prescribing Opioids for Outpatients With Pain, Excluding Pain Management Related to Sickle Cell Disease, Cancer-Related Pain Treatment, Palliative Care, and End-of-Life Care; Recommendation Categories and Evidence Types

Determining whether or not to initiate opioids for pain

1. Nonopioid therapies are at least as effective as opioids for many common types of acute pain. Clinicians should maximize use of nonpharmacologic and nonopioid pharmacologic therapies as appropriate for the specific condition and patient and only consider opioid therapy for acute pain if benefits are anticipated to outweigh risks to the patient. Before prescribing opioid therapy for acute pain, clinicians should discuss with patients the realistic benefits and known risks of opioid therapy (recommendation category: B, evidence type: 3).
2. Nonopioid therapies are preferred for subacute and chronic pain. Clinicians should maximize use of nonpharmacologic and nonopioid pharmacologic therapies as appropriate for the specific condition and patients and only consider initiating opioid therapy if expected benefits for pain and function are anticipated to outweigh risks to the patient. Before starting opioid therapy for subacute or chronic pain, clinicians should discuss with patients the realistic benefits and known risks of opioid therapy, should work with patients to establish treatment goals for pain and function, and should consider how opioid therapy will be discontinued if benefits do not outweigh risks (recommendation category: A, evidence type: 2).

Selecting opioids and determining opioid dosages

3. When starting opioid therapy for acute, subacute, or chronic pain, clinicians should prescribe immediate-release opioids instead of extended-release and long-acting (ER/LA) opioids (recommendation category: A, evidence type: 4).
4. When opioids are initiated for opioid-naive patients with acute, subacute, or chronic pain, clinicians should prescribe the lowest effective dosage. If opioids are continued for subacute or chronic pain, clinicians should use caution when prescribing opioids at any dosage, should carefully evaluate individual benefits and risks when considering increasing dosage, and should avoid increasing dosage above levels likely to yield diminishing returns in benefits relative to risks to patients (recommendation category: A, evidence type: 3).
5. For patients already receiving opioid therapy, clinicians should carefully weigh benefits and risks and exercise when changing opioid dosage. If benefits outweigh risks of continued opioid therapy, clinicians should work closely with patients to optimize nonopioid therapies while continuing opioid therapy. If benefits do not outweigh risks of continued opioid therapy, clinicians should optimize other therapies and work closely with patients to gradually taper to lower dosages or, if warranted based on the individual clinical circumstances of the patient, appropriately taper and discontinue opioids. Unless there are indications of a life-threatening issue such as warning signs of impending overdose (eg, confusion, sedation, or slurred speech), opioid therapy should not be discontinued abruptly, and clinicians should not rapidly reduce opioid dosages from higher dosages (recommendation category: B, evidence type: 4).

Deciding duration of initial opioid prescription and conducting follow-up

6. When opioids are needed for acute pain, clinicians should prescribe no greater quantity than needed for the expected duration of pain severe enough to require opioids (recommendation category: A, evidence type: 4).
7. Clinicians should evaluate benefits and risks with patients within 1-4 weeks of starting opioid therapy for subacute or chronic pain or of dose escalation. Clinicians should regularly reevaluate benefits and risks of continued opioid therapy with patients (recommendation category: B, evidence type: 4).

Assessing risk and addressing potential harms of opioid use

8. Before starting and periodically during continuation of opioid therapy, clinicians should evaluate risk for opioid-related harms and discuss risk with patients. Clinicians should work with patients to incorporate into the management plan strategies to mitigate risk, including offering naloxone (recommendation category: A, evidence type: 4).
9. When prescribing initial opioid therapy for acute, subacute, or chronic pain, and periodically during opioid therapy for chronic pain, clinicians should review the patient's history of controlled substance prescriptions using state prescription drug monitoring program (PDMP) data to determine whether the patient is receiving opioid dosages or combinations that put the patient at high risk for overdose (recommendation category: B, evidence type: 4).
10. When prescribing opioids for subacute or chronic pain, clinicians should consider the benefits and risks of toxicology testing to assess for prescribed medications as well as other prescribed and nonprescribed controlled substances (recommendation category: B, evidence type: 4).
11. Clinicians should use particular caution when prescribing opioid pain medication and benzodiazepines concurrently and consider whether benefits outweigh risks of concurrent prescribing of opioids and other central nervous system depressants (recommendation category: B, evidence type: 3).
12. Clinicians should offer or arrange treatment with evidence-based medications to treat patients with opioid use disorder. Withdrawal management on its own, without medications for opioid use disorder, is not recommended for opioid use disorder because of increased risks for resuming drug use, overdose, and overdose death (recommendation category: A, evidence type: 1).

Recommendation categories:

- **Category A recommendation**: Applies to all persons; most patients should receive the recommended course of action.
- **Category B recommendation**: Individual decision-making needed; different choices will be appropriate for different patients. Clinicians help patients arrive at a decision consistent with patient values and preferences and specific clinical situations.

Evidence types:

- **Type 1 evidence**: Randomized clinical trials or overwhelming evidence from observational studies.
- **Type 2 evidence**: Randomized clinical trials with important limitations, or exceptionally strong evidence from observational studies.
- **Type 3 evidence**: Observational studies or randomized clinical trials with notable limitations.
- **Type 4 evidence**: Clinical experience and observations, observational studies with important limitations, or randomized clinical trials with several major limitations.

Source: From Dowell D, Ragan KR, Jones CM, Baldwin GT, Chou R. CDC Clinical Practice Guideline for Prescribing Opioids for Pain—United States, 2022. *MMWR Recomm Rep.* 2022;71(3):1-95.

repeated early refills, lost prescriptions, and lack of compliance with recommendations and work with patients to make shared decisions on how to proceed with treatment.

One recent cohort study examined whether trends in initial prescribing to patients who were opioid naive departed from preguideline trends after the 2016 CDC guideline release, and the results showed that both initial prescribing duration and dosage were significantly lower after the CDC guideline release than would be expected by extrapolating the preguideline trend.[77] Thus, nonmandatory, evidence-based guidelines from trusted sources may affect how clinicians prescribe opioids. However, reports of applying the 2016 CDC Guideline to patient populations not included in the 2016 CDC Guideline (eg, treatment of cancer pain) or in ways not intended (eg, abruptly discontinuing opioids among patients on long-term opioid therapy) have been identified and have resulted in significant harms to patients.[78] Thus, the 2022 CDC Clinical Practice explicitly states that the Guideline provides recommendations to clinicians and patients; it is not a law, regulation, or policy; does not require mandatory compliance and is intended to be flexible to support, not replace, clinical judgment and individualized, patient-centered decision-making.

Prescription Drug Monitoring Programs

Another strategy for improving prescribing practices for substances with liability for misuse is increasing the use of Prescription Drug Monitoring Programs (PDMPs), which have been implemented in almost every state in the United States since April 2017 and typically track prescribing of all controlled substances in Schedules II to V. The central aim of a PDMP is to reduce the misuse and diversion of controlled substances, like prescription opioids, by providing clinicians with information on past prescription histories that can be used to inform prescribing decisions. Widespread use of these programs could impact prescribing, such as limiting the degree to which patients can obtain multiple overlapping prescriptions. PDMPs are designed to identify risky prescribing patterns and alert prescribers, pharmacists, and (in some states) law enforcement officials to potential problems with the prescribing and use of controlled substances. Enabling prescribers to access PDMP data in a rapid, automated manner can inform clinicians about other controlled substances that may have been prescribed to their patients. Such information can change prescribing practices and has been shown to be effective when implemented fully.[79] Yet, prescriber enrollment and utilization continue to be rate-limiting factors in some locations due to variations in state requirements for use, technology maturity, and interoperability with electronic health records.[79] A number of jurisdictions around the country have passed laws requiring prescribers to check the PDMP before prescribing controlled substances, and recent research found that states with PDMPs that monitored all drug schedules (II-IV) and update data at least weekly had lower opioid-related overdose death rates, compared to other states with less robust PDMPs.[79]

Use-Deterrent Formulations

Another strategy for reducing inappropriate use of prescription drugs is the development of tamper-resistant drug formulations. These pharmaceutical approaches include efforts to reduce the administration of prescription drugs through unintended routes, via formulations that are designed to make it more difficult to inject, insufflate, crush, or dissolve.[80] While some evidence suggests that implementation of a tamper-resistant formulation of OxyContin can reduce nonmedical use of that specific agent,[80,81] other research suggests that high-risk groups of individuals who use opioids continue to report nonmedical use of OxyContin after the reformulation.[82] In addition, the outbreak of HIV detected in Indiana in 2015 was primarily among persons who injected extended-release oxymorphone, which had been reformulated to deter nonoral routes of misuse in 2012.[44] This formulation has also been implicated in an outbreak of thrombotic thrombocytopenic purpura.[83] Overall these data suggest caution in anticipating the impact of reformulated opioids purportedly designed to reduce harms.[84]

Harm-Reduction Policies

Other evidence-based strategies can be used to reduce the health harms associated with misuse of prescription drugs, including increasing access to the opioid-overdose-reversal drug naloxone as well as providing people who inject drugs with comprehensive services such as access to sterile syringes and other injection equipment and testing, prevention, and treatment services for HIV and HCV. Moreover, fentanyl test strips are valuable as a harm reduction tool to address increases in overdose deaths involving fentanyl and analogs.[85] However, the strips are no panacea for overdose since certain fentanyl analogs and other emerging synthetic opioids that do not share chemical structures with fentanyl are not detected. For a full discussion of the concepts of harm reduction, controversies surrounding them, and how they apply to addiction issues more broadly, readers are encouraged to consult Chapter 28 on harm reduction.

Naloxone

Direct approaches to reducing overdose mortality include widespread dissemination of opioid overdose education and naloxone distribution (OOEND), with naloxone being a safe and effective medication for the acute treatment of opioid overdose.[86,87] Its use is standard practice in emergency settings, where it can safely and quickly reverse an opioid-induced coma or respiratory depression because of its rapid action as a μ opioid receptor antagonist. Increasing ready access to naloxone for opioid overdose reversal demonstrates benefit in reducing overdose mortality among individuals who use opioids and in communities hard hit by overdoses.[87,88] In addition, co-prescribing of naloxone to persons receiving high-dose opioids for chronic pain is associated with a reduced risk of emergency department treatment for opioid complications.

This is particularly important, as early evidence suggests that patients on opioids for chronic pain have significant numbers of opioid overdose risk factors, have both witnessed or personally experienced overdoses in significant numbers, and yet perceive their own personal risk for overdose as lower than the general population.[89,90]

Naloxone has been approved in injectable form for about 50 years, whereas auto-injector and nasal spray formulations were approved by the FDA in 2014 and 2015, respectively, as a way to facilitate use by people without medical training. In April 2021, the FDA approved a higher-dose naloxone hydrochloride nasal spray product to treat opioid overdose. The newly approved product delivers 8 mg of naloxone into the nasal cavity. The FDA had previously approved 2 mg and 4 mg naloxone nasal spray products.

Despite its potential to save lives, the public health impact of naloxone has not yet reached its full potential.[88,91] Furthermore, with the dramatic increases in overdose deaths involving prescription opioids in combination with synthetic opioids other than methadone (primarily illicitly manufactured fentanyl) over time, the need for additional naloxone in communities has never been greater.[91] Despite increases in naloxone dispensing across all states, dispensing rates remain low, with substantial variation and increasing disparities over time at the state level.[92] The extent of naloxone distribution, especially through community-based programs and pharmacy-initiated access points, warrants substantial expansion in nearly every U.S. state.[91]

As the rate of synthetic opioid-involved overdoses rapidly increases, it should be recognized that multiple doses may be needed to revive someone experiencing an overdose. It is also important for first responders to know that, while fentanyl has a short duration of action (30-90 minutes), it can stay in fat deposits for hours, and patients should be monitored for up to 12 hours after resuscitation. In addition to expanding access to naloxone to the full populations who could benefit, a key next step includes determining the best ways to link persons who have been reversed with naloxone to substance use treatment and other support services (ie, transforming the rescue into a longer-term intervention opportunity).

Syringe Services Programs

Sharing injection equipment poses significant risks for the transmission of infectious diseases. One policy that has repeatedly been proven effective for reducing the spread of infectious diseases is access to sterile syringes and other injection equipment. Syringe exchange was implemented in Indiana in response to the prescription opioid-driven HIV outbreak and played a significant role in containing the outbreak.[93] In addition to reducing infectious disease transmission, these programs also offer counseling services, HIV testing, and referral to SUD treatment services as well as safe disposal of injection equipment, linkage to naloxone and overdose prevention education, and distribution of fentanyl test strips.

HIV Prevention and Treatment

The seek, test, treat, and retain model of care (STTR), also known as the HIV Care Continuum, involves reaching out to high-risk, hard-to-reach populations who use substances who have not been recently tested for HIV, engaging them in HIV testing, initiating, monitoring, and maintaining combined antiretroviral therapy (cART) for those testing positive, and retaining patients in care. Research has shown that the implementation of STTR has the potential to decrease the rate of HIV transmission by more than half.[94,95] Multiple interrelated mechanisms may account for this, including dramatic decreases in viral load from antiretroviral medications and significant increases in related medical care (including access to SUD treatment).

EVIDENCE-BASED TREATMENT FOR PRESCRIPTION DRUG USE DISORDERS

The class of medication being used (opioid, stimulant, or sedative-tranquilizer) determines the appropriate type of care for an individual with a PDUD. Treatment for individuals with opioid use disorder will generally be the same, whether the person uses prescription opioids or heroin. The opioid-agonist medication methadone and the opioid-partial-agonist medication buprenorphine are effective for the treatment of all opioid use disorders and have been shown to decrease opioid use, opioid overdose deaths, infectious disease transmission, and criminal justice involvement, while increasing social functioning and retention in treatment.[96,97] Yet, despite their well-documented benefits, methadone, and buprenorphine remained substantially underused due to multiple provider, system, and patient-level barriers.

To support greater provider uptake of buprenorphine treatment, in April 2021, the U.S. Department of Health and Human Services released *Practice Guidelines for the Administration of Buprenorphine for Treating Opioid Use Disorder*, aiming to increase treatment, primarily by allowing a limited waiver for prescribing buprenorphine without the specialized training requirement. The exemption allows licensed practitioners to (1) treat up to 30 patients with opioid use disorder using buprenorphine without having to make certain training-related certifications and (2) treat patients with buprenorphine without certifying their capacity to provide counseling and ancillary services. Although buprenorphine treatment is complicated by concerns about misuse, a study found that in 2019, nearly three-fourths of U.S. adults reporting past-year buprenorphine use did not misuse their prescribed buprenorphine, and most who misused reported using prescription opioids without having their own prescriptions.[98]

The opioid-antagonist medication naltrexone has also demonstrated efficacy in reducing illicit opioid use, but compliance and retention in treatment hinder this drug's utility; the extended-release version may be an appropriate treatment for some individuals, especially those who are highly motivated.[99] Just as for heroin use disorder, tapers and drug-free approaches for prescription opioid use disorder show a significant risk of returning to opioid use.[96]

No medications to treat stimulant use disorders or sedative/tranquilizer use disorders are currently FDA-approved. Treatments for these use disorders are via the same behavioral therapies as other substance use disorders such as cognitive behavioral therapy and contingency management approaches.

The treatment for prescription drug withdrawal depends on the drug class. Of course, the pharmacokinetics of the particular agent will influence acute care, and readers are encouraged to consult other relevant sections of this book for details. As mentioned above, a hyperbolic reduction in dosage has been particularly recommended to reduce the risk of significant withdrawal and symptom recurrence when tapering benzodiazepines.[68,69] It is also the case that a person with a PDUD may have co-occurring disorders for which they may have originally been prescribed the drug (eg, pain in the case of an opioid use disorder), and such comorbidities must be addressed as part of treatment.

ONGOING RESEARCH

Although studies show that current best practices can be effective in reducing misuse of prescription drugs and its adverse consequences, there is much room for improvement. In the shorter term, research is underway to test and improve prescribing approaches based on current knowledge about minimizing risk for diversion, misuse, and harm; to develop tamper-resistant formulations to minimize intranasal and injection use of all prescription medications; and to maximize the uptake of effective approaches for reducing and treating prescription drug misuse and use disorders (ie, implementation research).

Over the longer term, research aims to develop new treatments for pain, ADHD, anxiety, and insomnia (ie, the main indications for prescription opioids, stimulants, and sedatives-tranquilizers, respectively) with reduced potential for misuse, SUD, and/or overdose; and to better understand the neurobiology of SUDs as a foundation for developing better prevention and treatment approaches (ie, basic science research).

SUMMARY/CONCLUSIONS

Prescription drug misuse is associated with numerous health harms, including increased risk of developing a PDUD, contracting HIV/HCV, overdose, and death. Opioids have a role to play in the management of certain types of pain, but prescription opioid overdose deaths escalated in conjunction with increasing numbers of prescriptions from 1999 until at least 2012. In response, several strategies have been implemented both nationally and at the state, local, and organizational levels to reduce the supply of controlled prescription drugs available for misuse and diversion. These include prescription drug monitoring programs and related policies to promote their use, law enforcement efforts to shut down pill mills, moving problematic opioids to Schedule II, prescriber education including the issuance of prescriber guidelines, public education and prescription take-back events, and evidence-based drug-use prevention programs.

When it comes to misuse of prescription drugs, physicians find themselves on the horns of a dilemma. They are the principal "supply" of these substances while also being the first line of defense against their diversion and misuse. These complexities require the exercise of caution in addition to compassion. To accomplish this, physicians need to be knowledgeable about the conditions addressed by these medications (pain, anxiety, ADHD, etc.) as well as the potential of these medications that leads to SUDs both in their patients and in the wider community. This requires physicians to keep up to date with the latest prescribing guidelines and with evidence-based strategies to prevent and treat addiction.

Overall, physicians should receive better training to detect prescription drug misuse (and other substance use) through screening and to treat patients' SUDs. Those in addiction treatment settings or otherwise able to prescribe medications for opioid use disorders (methadone, buprenorphine, and extended-release naltrexone) should fully embrace these life-saving treatment modalities. Low adoption of these treatments due to infrastructure impediments and lingering stigma must, in the light of the evidence, be seen as systematically problematic and a contributor to the current scope of the drug overdose crisis. Effective utilization of medications for opioid use disorders means prescribing them at the recommended dose and for a sufficient duration (which may be indefinitely). Improving access to these treatments will also depend on better integration of SUD treatment or skills within general health care.

Harm-reduction strategies like syringe services programs and naloxone distribution are also essential to reducing significant health consequences of prescription drug misuse. Syringe services programs can reduce the spread of HIV and HCV as well as link people who use drugs to treatment, provide naloxone and overdose prevention education, and distribute fentanyl test strips. Providing naloxone in an easy-to-administer formulation to those at risk of opioid overdose (eg, people with opioid use disorders and those receiving high dosages of opioids or with other overdose risk factors) and potential bystanders can save lives; and reversing an overdose with naloxone can be a critical opportunity for engaging patients in SUD treatment, as has been shown for emergency department patients.[100] Despite studies showing that syringe services programs and naloxone distribution do not increase drug use in communities that implement them, longstanding attitudinal barriers to harm reduction impede their adoption.[101,102]

Disclaimers: The findings and conclusions of this study are those of the authors and do not necessarily reflect the views of the National Institute on Drug Abuse of the National Institutes of Health, the Centers for Diseases Control and Prevention, and the U.S. Department of Health and Human Services.

REFERENCES

1. Compton WM, Volkow ND. Abuse of prescription drugs and the risk of addiction. *Drug Alcohol Depend*. 2006;83(Suppl 1):S4-S7.
2. Compton WM, Jones CM, Baldwin GT. Relationship between nonmedical prescription opioid use and heroin abuse. *N Engl J Med*. 2016;374(2):154-163. doi:10.1056/NEJMra1508490
3. Han B, Compton WM, Blanco C, Crane E, Lee J, Jones CM. Prescription opioid use, misuse, and use disorders in U.S. adults: 2015 National Survey on Drug Use and Health. *Ann Intern Med*. 2017;167(5):293-301. doi:10.7326/M17-0865
4. Han B, Compton WM, Blanco C, Jones CM. Prescription opioid use, misuse, and use disorders in U.S. adults. *Ann Intern Med*. 2018; 168(5):383-384.
5. Center for Behavioral Health Statistics and Quality. *2020 National Survey on Drug Use and Health: Detailed Tables*. Substance Abuse and Mental Health Services Administration; 2021.
6. Centers for Disease Control and Prevention, National Center for Health Statistics. National Vital Statistics System, Mortality 1999-2020 on CDC WONDER Online Database, released in 2021. Accessed May 21, 2022. http://wonder.cdc.gov/mcd-icd10.html

6a. Kuehn B. Opioid prescriptions soar: increases in legitimate use as well as abuse. *JAMA*. 2007;297:249-251.

7. Jones CM, Lurie PG, Throckmorton DC. Effect of US Drug Enforcement Administration's rescheduling of hydrocodone combination analgesic products on opioid analgesic prescribing. *JAMA Intern Med*. 2016; 176(3):399-402.
8. McCabe SE, West BT, Teter CJ, et al. Co-ingestion of prescription opioids and other drugs among high school seniors: results from a national study. *Drug Alcohol Depend*. 2012;126:65-70.
9. Han B, Compton WM, Jones CM, et al. Nonmedical prescription opioid use and use disorders among adults aged 18 through 64 years in the United States, 2003-2013. *JAMA*. 2015;314(14):1468-1478. doi:10.1001/jama.2015.11859
10. Huang BD, Dawson DA, Stinson FS, et al. Prevalence, correlates, and comorbidity of nonmedical prescription drug use and drug use disorders in the United States: results of the National Epidemiologic Survey on Alcohol and Related Conditions. *J Clin Psychiatry*. 2006;67(7): 1062-1073.
11. Villapiano NLG, Winkelman TNA, Kozhimannil KB, et al. Rural and urban differences in neonatal abstinence syndrome and maternal opioid use, 2004 to 2013. *JAMA Pediatr*. 2017;1(2):194-196. doi:10.1001/jamapediatrics.2016.3750
12. Bagley SM, Wachman EM, Holland E, et al. Review of the assessment and management of neonatal abstinence syndrome. *Addict Sci Clin Pract*. 2014;9(1):19. doi:10.1186/1940-0640-9-19
13. Lovegrove MC, Dowell D, Geller AI, et al. US emergency department visits for acute harms from prescription opioid use, 2016-2017. *Am J Public Health*. 2019;109(5):784-791.
14. Holland KM, Jones C, Vivolo-Kantor AM, et al. Trends in US Emergency Department visits for mental health, overdose, and violence outcomes before and during the COVID-19 pandemic. *JAMA Psychiat*. 2021;78(4):372-379.
15. Substance Abuse and Mental Health Services Administration, Center for Behavioral Health Statistics and Quality. *Treatment Episode Data Set (TEDS): 2019. Admissions to and Discharges from Publicly Funded Substance Use Treatment*. Substance Abuse and Mental Health Services Administration; 2021.
16. Hall AJ, Logan JE, Toblin RL, et al. Patterns of abuse among unintentional pharmaceutical overdose fatalities. *JAMA*. 2008;300:2613-2620. doi:10.1001/jama.2008.802
17. Dunn KM, Saunders KW, Rutter CM, et al. Opioid prescriptions for chronic pain and overdose: a cohort study. *Ann Intern Med*. 2010; 152:85-92. doi:10.7326/0003-4819-152-2-201001190-00006
18. Jones CM, Mack KA, Paulozzi LJ. Pharmaceutical overdose deaths, United States, 2010. *JAMA*. 2013;309:657-659.
19. Compton WM, Thomas YT, Stinson FS, et al. Prevalence, correlates, disability, and comorbidity of DSM-IV drug abuse and dependence in the United States. *Arch Gen Psychiatry*. 2007;64:566-576.
20. Grant BF, Stinson FS, Dawson DA, et al. Prevalence and co-occurrence of substance use disorders and independent mood and anxiety disorders: results from the National Epidemiologic Survey on Alcohol and Related Conditions. *Arch Gen Psychiatry*. 2004;61(8):807-816.
21. McCabe SE, Cranford JA, Boyd CJ. The relationship between past-year drinking behaviors and nonmedical use of prescription drugs: prevalence of co-occurrence in a national sample. *Drug Alcohol Depend*. 2006;84(3):281-288. doi:10.1016/j.drugalcdep.2006.03.006
22. Jones CM. The paradox of decreasing nonmedical opioid analgesic use and increasing abuse or dependence—an assessment of demographic and substance use trends, United States, 2003-2014. *Addict Behav*. 2017;65:229-235. doi:10.1016/j.addbeh.2016.08.027
23. Sullivan MD, Edlund MJ, Zhang L, et al. Association between mental health disorders, problem drug use, and regular prescription opioid use. *Arch Intern Med*. 2006;166(19):2087-2093.
24. Sweeney CT, Sembower MA, Ertischek MD, et al. Nonmedical use of prescription ADHD stimulants and preexisting patterns of drug abuse. *J Addict Dis*. 2013;32(1):1-10. doi:10.1080/10550887.2012.759858
25. Compton WM, Han B, Hughes A, Blanco C, et al. Use of marijuana for medical purposes among adults in the United States. *JAMA*. 2017; 317(2):209-211.
26. Institute of Medicine. *Relieving Pain in America: A Blueprint for Transforming Prevention, Care, Education, and Research*. The National Academies Press; 2011.
27. Himmelsbach CK. Addiction liability of codeine. *JAMA*. 1934; 103(19):1420-1421. doi:10.1001/jama.1934.02750450004002
28. Joranson DE, Ryan KA, Gilson AM, et al. Trends in medical use and abuse of opioid analgesics. *JAMA*. 2000;283(13):1710-1714. doi:10.1001/jama.283.13.1710
29. Weppner RS, Wells KS, McBride DC, et al. Effects of criminal justice and medical definitions of a social problem upon the delivery of treatment: the case of drug abuse. *J Health Soc Behav*. 1976;17:170-177.
30. Wilford BB. Abuse of prescription drugs. *West J Med*. 1990;152(5): 609-612.
31. Manchikanti L, Helm S II, Fellows B, et al. Opioid epidemic in the United States. *Pain Physician*. 2012;15(3 Suppl):ES9-ES38.
32. Paulozzi LJ. Prescription drug overdoses: a review. *J Safety Res*. 2012; 43(4):283-289.
33. Johnson H, Paulozzi L, Porucznik C, Mack K, et al. Decline in drug overdose deaths after state policy change—Florida, 2010-2012. *Morb Mortal Wkly Rep*. 2014;63(26):569-574.
34. Chou R, Hartung D, Turner J, et al. *Opioid Treatments for Chronic Pain*. Comparative Effectiveness Review No. 229. (Prepared by the Pacific Northwest Evidence-based Practice Center under Contract No. 290-2015-00009-I.) AHRQ Publication No. 20-EHC011. Agency for Healthcare Research and Quality; 2020.
35. Boscarino JA, Rukstalis M, Hoffman SN, et al. Risk factors for drug dependence among out-patients on opioid therapy in a large US health-care system. *Addiction*. 2010;105(10):1776-1782. doi:10.1111/j.1360-0443.2010.03052.x
36. Miech R, Johnston L, O'Malley PM, Keyes KM, Heard K. Prescription opioids in adolescence and future opioid misuse. *Pediatrics*. 2015; 136(5):e1169-e1177.
37. Portenoy RK. Opioid therapy for chronic nonmalignant pain: a review of the critical issues. *J Pain Symptom Manage*. 1996;11(4): 203-217.
38. Zenz M, Sorge J. Is the therapeutic use of opioids adversely affected by prejudice and law (abstract). *Recent Results Cancer Res*. 1991;121:43-50. doi:10.1007/978-3-642-84138-5_6
39. Jones CM, Baldwin GT, Manocchio T, et al. Trends in methadone distribution for pain treatment, methadone diversion, and overdose deaths—United States, 2002-2014. *Morbid Mortal Wkly Rep*. 2016; 65(26):667-671. doi:10.15585/mmwr.mm6526a2
40. Jones CM, Compton WM, Han B, Baldwin G, Volkow ND. Methadone-involved overdose deaths before and after federal policy changes expanding take-home methadone doses from opioid treatment programs. *JAMA Psychiatry*. 2022;79(9):932-934.
41. Carlson RG, Nahhas RW, Martins SS, Daniulaityte R. Predictors of transition to heroin use among initially non-opioid dependent illicit

pharmaceutical opioid users: a natural history study. *Drug Alcohol Depend.* 2016;160:127-134. doi:10.1016/j.drugalcdep.2015.12.026

42. McCabe SE, Boyd CJ, Evans-Polce RJ, McCabe VV, Schulenberg JE, Veliz PT. Pills to powder: a 17-year transition from prescription opioids to heroin among US adolescents followed into adulthood. *Journal Addict Med.* 2021;15(3):241.
43. Kelley-Quon LI, Cho J, Strong DR, et al. Association of nonmedical prescription opioid use with subsequent heroin use initiation in adolescents. *JAMA Pediatr.* 2019;173(9):e191750. doi:10.1001/jamapediatrics.2019.1750
44. Peters PJ, Pontones P, Hoover KW, et al. HIV infection linked to injection use of oxymorphone in Indiana, 2014-2015. *N Engl J Med.* 2016;375(3):229-239. doi:10.1056/NEJMoa1515195
45. Zibbell JE, Iqbal K, Patel RC, et al. Increases in Hepatitis C virus infection related to injection drug use among persons aged ≤30 years—Kentucky, Tennessee, Virginia, and West Virginia, 2006–2012. *Morbid Mortal Wkly Rep.* 2015;64(17):453-458.
46. Ball LJ, Puka K, Speechley M, et al. Sharing of injection drug preparation equipment is associated with HIV infection: a cross-sectional study. *J Acquir Immune Defic Syndr.* 2019;81(4):e99-e103.
47. Zibbell JE, Hart-Mallow R, Barry J, et al. Risk factors for HCV infection among young adults in rural New York who inject prescription opioid analgesics. *Am J Public Health.* 2014;104(11):2226-2232.
48. Van Handel MM, Rose CE, Hallisey EJ, et al. County-level vulnerability assessment for rapid dissemination of HIV or HCV infections among persons who inject drugs, United States. *J Acquir Immune Defic Syndr.* 2016;73(3):323-331. doi:10.1097/QAI.0000000000001098
49. Lerner AM, Fauci AS. Opioid injection in rural areas of the United States: a potential obstacle to ending the HIV epidemic. *JAMA.* 2019; 322(11):1041-1042.
50. Peterson AB, Gladden RM, Delcher C, et al. Increases in fentanyl-related overdose deaths—Florida and Ohio, 2013–2015. *Morbid Mortal Wkly Rep.* 2016;65:844-849. doi:10.15585/mmwr.mm6533a3
51. Spies E, Peterson A, Garcia-Williams A, et al. *Undetermined Risk Factors for Fentanyl-Related Overdose Deaths—Ohio, 2015 (EpiAid 2016-003).* National Center for Injury Prevention and Control Centers for Disease Control and Prevention (CDC); 2016. Accessed March 17, 2017. http://www.healthy.ohio.gov/-/media/ODH/ASSETS/Files/health/injury-prevention/Ohio-PDO-EpiAid-Trip-Report_Final-Draft_3_18_2016.pdf?la=en
52. Goldman LS, Genel M, Bezman RJ, Slanetz PJ. Diagnosis and treatment of attention-deficit/hyperactivity disorder in children and adolescents. Council on Scientific Affairs, American Medical Association. *JAMA.* 1998;279(14):1100-1107.
53. Board AR, Guy G, Jones CM, Hoots B. Trends in stimulant dispensing by age, sex, state of residence, and prescriber specialty—United States, 2014-2019. *Drug Alcohol Depend.* 2020;217:108297. doi:10.1016/j.drugalcdep.2020.108297
54. Han B, Jones CM, Blanco C, Compton WM. National trends in and correlates of nonmedical use of prescription stimulants, nonmedical use frequency, and use disorders. *J Clin Psychiatry.* 2017;78(9):e1250-e1258. doi:10.4088/JCP.17m11760
55. Garcia C, Valencia B, Diaz Roldan K, et al. Prescription stimulant misuse and diversion events among college students: a qualitative study. *J Prev.* 2022;43(1):49-66.
56. Compton WM, Volkow ND. Major increases in opioid analgesic abuse in the United States: concerns and strategies. *Drug Alcohol Depend.* 2006;81(2):103-107.
57. Volkow ND, Swanson JM. Variables that affect the clinical use and abuse of methylphenidate in the treatment of ADHD. *Am J Psychiatry.* 2003;160:1909-1918.
58. Johnston LD, O'Malley PM, Bachman JG, et al. *Monitoring the Future National Results on Adolescent Drug Use: Overview of Key Findings.* The University of Michigan: Institute for Social Research; 2015. http://monitoringthefuture.org/pubs.html
59. Teter E, McCabe SE, LaGrange T, et al. Illicit use of specific prescription stimulants among college students: prevalence, motives, and routes of administration. *Pharmacotherapy.* 2006;26(10):1501-1510.
60. Johnston LD, O'Malley PM, Bachman JG, Schulenberg JE, Miech RA. Monitoring the Future National Survey Results on Drug Use, 1975-2015. *College Students and Adults Ages 19-55.* Vol. II. Institute for Social Research, The University of Michigan. Accessed May 22, 2023. https://monitoringthefuture.org/wp-content/uploads/2022/08/mtf-vol2_2015.pdf
61. Arria AM, Caldeira KM, Vincent KB, et al. Do college students improve their grades by using prescription stimulants nonmedically? *Addict Behav.* 2017;65:245-249.
62. Compton WM, Han B, Blanco C, Johnson K, Jones CM. Prevalence of prescription stimulant use, misuse, and use disorders and motivations for misuse in the U.S. *Am J Psychiatry.* 2018;175(8):741-755.
63. Hajak G, Muller WE, Wittchen HU, et al. Abuse and dependence potential for the non-benzodiazepine hypnotics zolpidem and zopiclone: a review of case reports and epidemiologic evidence. *Addiction.* 2003;98(10):1371-1378.
64. Hwang CS, Kang EM, Kornegay CJ, et al. Trends in the concomitant prescribing of opioids and benzodiazepines, 2002-2014. *Am J Prev Med.* 2016;51(2):151-160.
65. Blanco C, Han B, Jones CM, Johnson K, Compton WM. Prevalence and correlates of benzodiazepine use, misuse, and use disorders among in the U.S. *J Clin Psychiatry.* 2018;79(6):18m12174.
66. Liu S, O'Donnell J, Gladden RM, McGlone L, Chowdhury F. Trends in nonfatal and fatal overdoses involving benzodiazepines—38 States and the District of Columbia, 2019–2020. *Morbid Mortal Wkly Rep.* 2021;70:1136-1141.
67. Larochelle MR, Liebschutz JM, Zhang F, et al. Opioid prescribing after nonfatal overdose and association with repeated overdose: a cohort study. *Ann Intern Med.* 2016;164(1):1-9. doi:10.7326/M15-0038
68. Silvernail CM, Wright SL. Surviving benzodiazepines: a patient's and clinician's perspectives. *Adv Ther.* 2022;39(5):1871-1880.
69. Horowitz MA, Taylor D. How to reduce and stop psychiatric medication. *Eur Neuropsychopharmacol.* 2022;55:4-7.
70. Spoth R, Trudeau L, Shin C, et al. Longitudinal effects of universal preventive intervention on prescription drug misuse: three randomized controlled trials with late adolescents and young adults. *Am J Public Health.* 2013;103(4):665-672.
71. U.S. Department of Health and Human Services (HHS). *Office of the Surgeon General, Facing Addiction in America: The Surgeon General's Report on Alcohol, Drugs, and Health.* HHS; 2016.
72. Jones CM, Paulozzi LJ, Mack KA. Sources of prescription opioid pain relievers by frequency of past-year nonmedical use, United States, 2008-2011. *JAMA Intern Med.* 2014;174(5):802-803.
73. Rosenblum A, Parrino M, Schnoll SH, et al. Prescription opioid abuse among enrollees into methadone maintenance treatment. *Drug Alcohol Depend.* 2007;90(1):64-71.
74. Kaye L, Crittenden J, Gressitt S, et al. *Reducing Prescription Drug Misuse Through the Use of a Citizen Mail-Back Program in Maine: Safe Medicine Disposal Handbook and Summary Report.* University of Maine; 2010. Accessed July 11, 2023. https://digitalcommons.library.umaine.edu/moca_service/1/
75. Dowell D, Haegerich TM, Chou R. CDC Guideline for Prescribing Opioids for Chronic Pain—United States, 2016. *JAMA.* 2016;315(15):1624-1645. doi:10.1001/jama.2016.1464
76. Dowell D, Ragan KR, Jones CM, Baldwin GT, Chou R. CDC Clinical Practice Guideline for Prescribing Opioids for Pain—United States, 2022. *MMWR Recomm Rep.* 2022;713:1-95. doi:10.15585/mmwr.rr7103a1
77. Goldstick JE, Guy GP, Losby JL, Baldwin G, Myers M, Bohnert ASB. Changes in initial opioid prescribing practices after the 2016 release of the CDC Guideline for Prescribing Opioids for Chronic Pain. *JAMA Netw Open.* 2021;4(7):e2116860.
78. Dowell D, Haegerich T, Chou R. No shortcuts to safer opioid prescribing. *N Engl J Med.* 2019;380(24):2285-2287.
79. Bao Y, Pan Y, Taylor A, et al. Prescription Drug Monitoring Programs are associated with sustained reductions in opioid prescribing by physicians. *Health Affairs.* 2016;35(6):1045-1051.
80. Cicero TJ, Ellis MS, Surratt HL. Effects of abuse-deterrent formulation of OxyContin. *N Engl J Med.* 2012;367:187-189.

81. Dart RC, Surratt HL, Cicero TJ, et al. Trends in opioid analgesic abuse and mortality in the United States. *N Engl J Med.* 2015;372:241-248.
82. Jones CM, Muhuri PK, Lurie PG. Trends in the nonmedical use of OxyContin, United States, 2006-2013. *Clin J Pain.* 2016;33(5): 452-461.
83. Marder E, Kirschke D, Robbins D, et al. Thrombotic thrombocytopenic purpura (TTP)-like illness associated with intravenous Opana ER abuse—Tennessee, 2012. *Morbid Mortal Wkly Rep.* 2013;62(1):1-4.
84. U.S. Food and Drug Administration. *Data and Methods for Evaluating the Impact of Opioid Formulations With Properties Designed to Deter Abuse in the Postmarket Setting: A Scientific Discussion of Present and Future Capabilities.* Accessed May 22, 2023. https://www.fda.gov/Drugs/NewsEvents/ucm540845.htm
85. Bergh MS, Øiestad ÅML, Baumann MH, Bogen IL. Selectivity and sensitivity of urine fentanyl test strips to detect fentanyl analogues in illicit drugs. *Int J Drug Policy.* 2021;90:103065.
86. Boyer EW. Management of opioid analgesic overdose. *N Engl J Med.* 2012;367:146-155.
87. Coffin PO, Sullivan SD. Cost-effectiveness of distributing naloxone to heroin users for lay overdose reversal. *Ann Intern Med.* 2013;158:1-30.
88. Compton WM, Volkow ND, Throckmorton DC, et al. Access to opioid overdose intervention: research, practice, and policy needs. *Ann Intern Med.* 2013;168:65-66.
89. Wilder CM, Miller SC, Tiffany E, et al. Risk factors for opioid overdose and awareness of overdose risk among veterans prescribed chronic opioids for addiction or pain. *J Addict Dis.* 2016;35(1):42-51.
90. Tiffany E, Wilder CM, Miller SC, Winhusen T. Knowledge of and interest in opioid overdose education and naloxone distribution among US veterans on chronic opioids for addiction or pain. *Drugs Educ Prev Policy.* 2016;23(4):322-327.
91. Irvine MA, Oller D, Boggis J, et al. Estimating naloxone need in the USA across fentanyl, heroin, and prescription opioid epidemics: a modelling study. *Lancet Public Health.* 2022;7(3):e210-e218.
92. Guy GP Jr, Khushalani JS, Jackson H, Sims RSC, Arifkhanova A. Trends in state-level pharmacy-based naloxone dispensing rates, 2012-2019. *Am J Prev Med.* 2021;61(6):e289-e295.
93. Rich JD, Adashi EY. Ideological anachronism involving needle and syringe exchange programs: lessons from the Indiana HIV outbreak. *JAMA.* 2015;314(1):23-24.
94. Normand J, Montaner J, Fang CT, et al. HIV: seek, test, treat, and retain. *J Food Drug Anal.* 2013;21(4):S4-S6. doi:10.1016/j.jfda.2013.09.020
95. Johnson K, Jones C, Compton W, et al. Federal response to the opioid crisis. *Curr HIV/AIDs Rep.* 2018;15(4):293-301.
96. Fiellin DA, Schottenfeld RS, Cutter CJ, Moore BA, Barry DT, O'Connor PG. Primary care-based buprenorphine taper vs maintenance therapy for prescription opioid dependence: a randomized clinical trial. *JAMA Intern Med.* 2014;174(12):1947-1954.
97. Weiss RD, Potter JS, Fiellin DA, et al. Adjunctive counseling during brief and extended buprenorphine-naloxone treatment for prescription opioid dependence: a 2-phase randomized controlled trial. *Arch Gen Psychiatry.* 2011;69:1104-1112.
98. Han B, Jones CM, Einstein EB, Compton WM. Trends in and characteristics of buprenorphine misuse among adults in the US. *JAMA Netw Open.* 2021;4(10):e2129409.
99. Lee JD, Friedmann PD, Kinlock TW, et al. Extended-release naltrexone to prevent opioid relapse in criminal justice offenders. *N Engl J Med.* 2016;374:1232-1242.
100. D'Onofrio G, O'Connor PG, Pantalon MV, et al. Emergency department initiates buprenorphine/naloxone treatment for opioid dependence. *JAMA.* 2015;313(16):1636-1644.
101. Institute of Medicine. *Preventing HIV Infection Among Injecting Drug Users in High-Risk Countries. An Assessment of the Evidence.* National Academies Press; 2006.
102. Bazazi AR, Zaller ND, Fu JJ, et al. Preventing opiate overdose deaths: Examining objections to take-home naloxone. *J Health Care Poor Underserved.* 2010;21(4):1108-1113.

CHAPTER

28 The Harm Reduction Approach to Caring for People Who Use Substances

Alexander Y. Walley, Sharon Stancliff, and India Perez-Urbano

CHAPTER OUTLINE

- Introduction to harm reduction
- Interventions that reduce the harms of substance use
- Conclusion

INTRODUCTION TO HARM REDUCTION

Harm Reduction Definition and Principles

Harm reduction is a public health approach that seeks to reduce the harm of substance use via practical and evidence-based interventions, without a primary focus on altering the quantity or frequency of ongoing substance use or requiring abstinence.[1] Harm reduction is a practice in person-centered care that calls for care providers to "meet people where they are at" and assist them in developing their own substance use goals. Harm reduction recognizes the strengths of people who use substances and acknowledges that abstinence or reducing substance use may not be feasible, desired, or the best way to minimize the harms of substance use. Fundamentally, harm reduction approaches are built for, and by, people who use substances and emphasize de-stigmatization and their human rights.

Harm reduction also seeks to resist and reverse the systematic discrimination of all people who use substances and recognizes that additional efforts are needed for those groups of people that have been specifically targeted by drug criminalization. From the 1970s through the 2000s, national U.S. drug control policy has focused on efforts to reduce drug supply by trying to keep illegal drugs out of the country and punishing people who use drugs to discourage demand. This "War on Drugs"—which at its core criminalizes drug use, stigmatizes people who use drugs and onerously restricts access to high quality, evidence-based drug treatment—has been the primary driver of the mass incarceration of Black, Hispanic, and Indigenous people in the United States.[2,3] Mitigating the pervasive, racist harms to people who use drugs from the War on Drugs' systems, laws, and policies is fundamental to harm reduction. Studies have found consistently disproportionate access to harm reduction services based on race and ethnicity. Increasing the role of racially and ethnically minoritized people in designing and leading both harm reduction and treatment services is crucial to closing gaps in racial equity[4] and confronting the harms of drug criminalization and mass incarceration.

Harm reduction strategies and policies can be delivered across a diversity of settings and share the common goal of improving health and functioning. **Table 28-1** includes examples of tangible harm reduction strategies, many of which will be discussed throughout this chapter. Many of the adverse health consequences of substance use are not due directly to the substance itself, but to other factors that can be ameliorated—for example, the transmission of blood-borne infections from sharing injection equipment. Thus, harm reduction emphasizes the measurement of health, social, and economic outcomes, over the measurement of substance consumption. Overall, harm reduction can be integrated into the continuum of substance use prevention and treatment to reduce the harms associated with substance use that may occur before, after, and during treatment.

History of Harm Reduction

The evolution of what is now termed "harm reduction" may be traced back to the establishment of the first Syringe Service Program (SSP) in Amsterdam. In 1984, a group of individuals who used drugs (called the "Junky Union" [Junkiebund]), in collaboration with public health officials, developed an SSP to prevent the spread of Hepatitis B. SSPs were subsequently adopted across Europe and Australia to reduce the spread of HIV and have been credited in averting an HIV epidemic.[5] In the United Kingdom, the Mersey Harm Reduction Model responded to the threat of HIV through a collaboration between health educators and methadone treatment providers who included syringe–needle distribution among the services.[6] The first legally sanctioned SSP in the United States was established in Tacoma, Washington, in 1988. However, expansion was hindered in the United States by drug war policies that focused on punishing people who use drugs, especially Black, Hispanic, and Indigenous people, and specific laws that banned the use of federal funds for the provision of syringes and research of these programs.[7]

Despite these barriers, SSPs evolved into multiservice organizations serving people who use substances. Inspired by these programs and the harm reduction approach, other interventions have been innovated including take-home naloxone rescue kits for overdose prevention, supervised drug consumption venues, injectable opioid agonist treatment, pre- and postexposure HIV prophylaxis, Housing First, managed alcohol programs, and drug-checking.[8] For the first time ever, the 2022 United States National Drug Control Strategy prioritized the promotion of evidence-based harm reduction

TABLE 28-1 Interventions That Reduce the Harms to People Who Use Substances

	Reduce the acute harms of use (eg, overdose)	Reduce the complications of use (eg, infection, trauma)	Reduce harm by reducing use	Reduce harm by engaging in care
Overdose risk education and naloxone rescue kits	x			
Safe substance use materials: Syringe-service programs and safer smoking and sniffing supplies	x	x		x
Observation to keep people safe while using substances				
Overdose prevention sites (supervised injection facilities and drug consumption venues)	x	x		x
Postsubstance use observation sites: chill out rooms	x			
Virtual spotting	x			x
Medications				
Medication for opioid use disorder	x	x	x	x
Medication for stimulant use disorders	x	x	x	x
Target use of opioid antagonists for alcohol use disorder	x	x	x	
Preexposure and post-HIV prophylaxis (PEP and PrEP)		x		
Safer drug supply interventions				
Drug-checking at dance parties	x			
Fentanyl test strips				
Portable high specificity drug checking	x	x		x
Injectable opioid agonist treatment programs and prescribed safe supply				
Managed alcohol programs	x	x	x	x
Housing First		x		x
Designated driving		x		

programming and advancement of racial equity.[2] Many of the harm reduction interventions in the national strategy are also highlighted in this chapter, including integrating harm reduction into addiction treatment, naloxone rescue, syringe access services, buprenorphine through harm reduction programs, safer supply through drug checking, and increasing access to housing through harm reduction services.

The Integration of Harm Reduction and Addiction Treatment

The principles of harm reduction can be integrated into addiction treatment programs by acknowledging that return to use may occur and that when it does harm reduction strategies can keep people safer. Some abstinence-only focused addiction treatment programs silo themselves from harm reduction by not offering or referring to harm reduction services or stigmatizing medications to treat substance use disorders (SUDs).[9] People committed to abstinence may hesitate to engage with harm reduction programs because they do not want to acknowledge the possibility of returning to use and how to reduce the risks of using. Similarly, people who use substances and who are not willing or able to stop using may be less likely to seek out or learn about addiction treatment options. Yet, integrating harm reduction and SUD treatment benefits both people focused on abstinence and people not willing or able to discontinue use.[10]

People with severe SUDs, even when they are committed to abstinence, may return to use.[11] Returning to use despite the intention not to use a substance is one of the eleven DSM-5 criteria to be considered to diagnose a SUD.[12] Thus, return to use is common, despite the efforts of the person, the patient, or treatment providers and support networks. Treatment programs can improve the safety of their patients who return to use by incorporating harm reduction strategies, even if the program is designed for people committed to abstinence. Collaboration between, and integration of, harm reduction and addiction treatment programs is complimentary. Integration

BOX 28-1 Harm Reduction Online Resources

Website	Resource
prescribetoprevent.org	Information on naloxone rescue kits for prescribers and pharmacists, including patient materials, continuing education courses, and research reviews
pdaps.org—Prescription Drug Abuse Policy System	Interactive map of United States' overdose prevention naloxone and Good Samaritan laws
https://store.samhsa.gov/sites/default/files/d7/priv/sma18-4742.pdf	Substance Abuse Mental Health Services Administration overdose prevention toolkit for health care providers, first responders, treatment providers, and those recovering from opioid overdose
harmreduction.org	Harm Reduction Coalition resources including guide to developing and managing overdose prevention programs
harmreductionhelp.cdc.gov/s	The National Harm Reduction Technical Assistance Center (NHRTAC) provides free help to anyone in the country providing (or planning to provide) harm reduction services to their community. This may include syringe services programs, health departments, programs providing treatment for substance use disorder, as well as prevention and recovery programs
nasen.org	North America Syringe Exchange Network operates a directory of syringe service programs in the United States and Buyers Club for syringe service programs

has the potential to enhance the accessibility of effective treatment and harm reduction interventions to the broad continuum of people who use substances.

In addition, integration of harm reduction and addiction treatment may decrease stigma and increase acceptability of treatment services. Increased engagement in addiction treatment has been well documented at drug consumption programs and syringe service programs co-located with residential and medication treatment programs.[13,14] Examples of integrating harm reduction and addiction treatment include distributing naloxone to patients at opioid treatment programs[15] and offering medication for opioid use disorder at a syringe service program.[14] Engagement efforts built on harm reduction that also offer people addiction treatment, may further empower people to improve their own drug use safety. By facilitating access to treatment through harm reduction programs, people can access health promoting services earlier, including addiction treatment. Regardless of whether a person is committed to or interested in abstinence, what substances they use and how they use them evolves over time. Substance use treatment strategies, including medications, counseling, and residential care can help people who intend to continue using control their use.

Harm reduction integration may be particularly important for groups historically excluded from addiction treatment, including racially, ethnically, and gender minoritized people and Women.[16-21] Through drug courts and other forms of leveraged, involuntary, and mandated treatment, addiction treatment programs have partnered with legal systems that have arrested, convicted, and incarcerated these groups at disproportionately higher rates for drug-related crimes than cisgendered White men.[22,23] Integrating harm reduction principles into addiction treatment programming may be an important component of addressing historical trauma, destigmatizing and increasing the inclusivity of addiction treatment.[24]

The shared goals and principles of harm reduction programs and high-quality addiction treatment programs can help foster collaboration between these programs (**Box 28-1**).[25] These goals and principles include culturally-responsive, nonjudgmental care that respects individual dignity. Programs also need to provide care that addresses the socioeconomic and physical consequences of substance use. For example, integrating trauma-informed practices minimizes retraumatization. Outreach strategies can engage and motivate people who use substances. Adhering to these principles means that addiction treatment providers can emphasize the rewards and benefits of treatment, without shaming or stigmatizing return to use after abstinence. People who use substances already face damaging daily shame and stigma. Additionally, access to all medical, psychiatric, or addiction treatment regardless of current or previous medication treatment is recommended (eg, medical and residential addiction treatment settings can be accessible to people treated with methadone, but not require it). Finally, recognizing that collaboration between service programs makes the continuum of care stronger is important.

INTERVENTIONS THAT REDUCE THE HARMS OF SUBSTANCE USE

Overdose Risk Education and Naloxone Rescue Kits to Prevent Opioid Overdose

Unintentional overdose, primarily related to opioids, is a major cause of death in North America, Europe, Asia, and Australia. In the United States, the annual rate of unintentional drug-poisoning deaths more than doubled from 6.1 per 100,000 in 1999 to 13.1 per 100,000 in 2012.[26] In 2013, the overdose death rate further accelerated, doubling in 7 years from 13.8 per 100,000 to 28.3 in 2020. This acceleration of overdose deaths is driven by illicitly manufactured fentanyl (a synthetic opioid 50-100 times stronger than morphine), as well as, cocaine and psychostimulants (ie, methamphetamine).[27-29] In 2021, the number of overdose deaths in the United States was higher than ever at more than 107,000 deaths with over 71,000 involving fentanyl.[30] Since 2013, and especially during the COVID pandemic, studies from multiple states demonstrated surges in overdose deaths disproportionately among Black people.[31-33] Between 2019 and 2020, the overdose death rate among Black individuals was 36.8 per 100,000, 16.3% higher than White people (31.8 per 100,000). Indigenous American or Alaskan Natives had the highest rate at 41.4 per 100,000. Rates remain lower among Latinos (17.3 per 100,000) but also increased by 40.1% in 2020.[34]

Naloxone is an opioid antagonist that reverses the effects of opioid overdose by displacing opioid agonists (ie, heroin, fentanyl, oxycodone) from opioid receptors. Naloxone has minimal to no adverse effects aside from causing opioid withdrawal in physically dependent individuals and it is the standard overdose treatment used in the medical setting, including by emergency medical personnel. Distribution of naloxone rescue "kits"—which typically contain two doses of naloxone and instructions—alongside overdose reversal and prevention education, has become integral to community harm reduction programs. The U.S. Surgeon General, Centers for Disease Control and Prevention, the American Medical Association, and the American Society of Addiction Medicine each recommend prescribing of naloxone rescue kits to people at risk for overdose and their friends and family.[35-38] Laypersons with potential of being bystanders to an overdose (ie, people who use drugs, their friends and family, people recently released from jail and prison) are a primary target of these programs as they are most likely to witness an overdose and may fear calling 911 because of the criminalization of drug use or delays in arrival. Because most heroin overdoses evolve over minutes and occur in homes or residences removed from medical care, community programs train laypersons to respond to an overdose. Unfortunately, fentanyl overdoses can evolve to respiratory arrest more rapidly than those involving less potent opioids,[28] further underscoring the need for naloxone in the hands of those most at risk of witnessing an overdose. Overdose responder training often includes how to recognize signs of overdose, seek help, rescue breathe and/or provide chest compressions, administer naloxone, and stay with the person who is overdosing. Studies have found no evidence of compensatory drug use behavior among individuals who use heroin after being trained in overdose response and given a take-home naloxone rescue kit.[39]

In the United States, educating people who use opioids about overdose prevention and response and equipping them with take-home naloxone rescue kits started at an SSP, the Chicago Recovery Alliance in the 1990s.[40] Naloxone distribution programs have been established in many venues, including syringe service programs, HIV prevention outreach programs, methadone maintenance clinics, inpatient withdrawal management programs, emergency department settings, mail order services and community meetings.[15,41] Naloxone is available in retail pharmacies without a patient-specific prescription in all states but one.[42] To incentivize individuals to seek medical attention for an overdose, or after naloxone administration, "Good Samaritan" laws have been introduced in 47 U.S. states and the District of Columbia to provide legal protection to both the individual who administered naloxone and the individual who overdosed.[43] Good Samaritan laws are designed to grant immunity from arrest or prosecution if in possession of drug paraphernalia or certain amounts of controlled substances. Since 2010 in the United States, many police, fire, and emergency medicine first responders have been carrying and using naloxone, becoming enthusiastic advocates for widening access to life-saving antagonist; however, access to naloxone among Black and Latino populations lags as we continue to see increases in death in these populations.[44,45]

Studies of naloxone programs have demonstrated feasibility, increased knowledge and skills, and significant reduction in fatal overdoses after initiation of community naloxone rescue programs. In an interrupted-time series analysis of overdose education and nasal naloxone implementation in Massachusetts, compared to communities with no naloxone distribution, overdose deaths rates were 47% lower among communities with high naloxone distribution and 27% lower among those with low naloxone distribution.[46] A study on co-prescribing naloxone to patients being prescribed opioids, or otherwise at risk of overdose, found a 63% reduction in opioid-related emergency department visits compared to those not receiving a prescription.[47] A cohort study of naloxone training and distribution at an Opioid Treatment Program found that naloxone was administered 114 times by 395 participants over the course of a year, illustrating the crucial role of naloxone provision in opioid treatment programs.[48] The distribution of naloxone rescue kits has also been found to be cost-effective with estimated incremental cost per quality-adjusted life-years gained ranging from $438 to $14,000 in a conservative model.[49] While naloxone rescue kits are effective and cost-effective, fentanyl overdoses have surged. Naloxone does reverse overdose from fentanyl, yet the time to intervene is much shorter than with other opioids. Modeling studies have shown that while naloxone distribution has averted many deaths in the midst of the fentanyl surge, few communities are fully saturated with naloxone and have the opportunity to distribute more.[50,51]

Safer Drug Use Materials to Reduce HIV, HCV, and Other Infections

Syringe Service Programs

Syringe service programs (SSPs) are community-based prevention programs that distribute sterile syringe-needles, safer drug use supplies, drug safety education, and a range of other health and social services. In 2022, there were 402 SSPs operating in the United States.[52] Seven states (Alabama, Delaware, Kansas, Mississippi, Nebraska, South Dakota, and Wyoming) do not report any SSPs to the North American Syringe Exchange Network (NASEN). Reductions in HIV and hepatitis C incidence have been shown in several countries where access to new injecting equipment has been implemented on a large scale.[53] A study of 81 cities with HIV seroprevalence data found that cities with SSPs had a 5.8% decrease in HIV prevalence per year, whereas cities without SSPs had 5.9% increase in HIV prevalence per year.[5] In communities where they have been implemented, SSPs have reduced HIV incidence by reducing the sharing and reuse of hypodermic needles. Beyond syringe-needle access, many SSPs provide HIV, viral hepatitis, and tuberculosis screening, viral hepatitis vaccination, safe sex supplies and education, and on-site referral to substance use treatment to people who are often otherwise disconnected from medical services. Thus, secondary benefits have included increased enrollment in SUD treatment,[54,55] prevention of blood-borne and sexually transmitted infections, increased retention in HIV treatment among People Who Inject Drugs (PWID), increased proper disposal of syringe-needle, and reduced needle stick injuries among first responders.[56]

SSPs make use of different service delivery models: fixed site, mobile sites, vending machines, peer-delivered, street outreach, pharmacies, or a combination of such. Some deploy an "exchange" model where the number of syringe-needles that are distributed is limited by the number of used syringe-needles that a client brings into the program.[57] However, less restrictive distribution of injecting equipment has been associated with safer injection practices and lower HIV incidence compared to more conservative exchange schemes.[58]

Programs that involve people with lived experience using drugs ("peers") to staff and lead SSPs can improve the reach and impact of SSPs, particularly for those who are isolated and at especially high risk for the harms of injection drug use, including HIV infection and overdose. An evaluation of a peer-run outreach-based SSP in Vancouver, Canada found that a peer-run service was successful in engaging people who were not accessing SSPs elsewhere and that contact with them was associated with reduce frequency of re-using syringes.[59] Thus, peer-delivered syringe-needle exchange and peer outreach have become explicit elements to many SSPs.[59,60]

In many places, syringe-needles are available for purchase in pharmacies without a prescription.[61,62] Because pharmacies are broadly distributed across communities, pharmacy access to safer injection equipment has the potential to dramatically increase access. In many countries and communities where pharmacy access has been pursued and supported as an HIV and hepatitis C prevention policy, pharmacies have successfully distributed syringe-needles to PWID. Barriers have also been recognized including pharmacy staff attitudes, financial costs to PWID, mandated training, and requirements to show identification.

Laws regulating the possession and prescription of syringe-needles differ from state to state. A legal analysis in 2020[63] reported that syringe prescription was legal in all states except Delaware and Kansas, Puerto Rico and the District of Columbia; thus, physician-prescribed syringes is an option in communities where pharmacies require a prescription to purchase syringes.[64] This approach was implemented successfully

BOX 28-2 Discussing Safer Injection With People Who Inject Drugs

Educating patients on safer injection techniques can reduce the risks of injection and improve the patient-provider relationship.

Key techniques

Equipment:
- Use a sterile needle/syringe: a new needle/syringe with each injection.
- Use your own, clean cooker or spoon.
- Use sterile or clean water.
- Use a clean cotton filter. Ideally, a prepilled dental filter, rather than cotton pulled off a q-tip. Avoid lint or cigarette filters.
- Avoid sharing equipment.
- Keep used needle/syringes in a sturdy container until disposed in a biohazard box.

Hygiene:
- Wash your hands with soap and water or hand sanitizer.
- Use alcohol wipes to clean the injection site.
- Use clean surfaces for preparation.

Injection site:
- Veins on the arms and hands are safest. Avoid injecting into the groin or neck.

A video by Canadian organization CATIE demonstrates safer injection techniques. https://www.catie.ca/safer-substance-use-video-series
Six Moments of Infection Prevention in Injection Drug Use[67]
https://academic.oup.com/ofid/article/9/2/ofab631/6499355

in Providence, Rhode Island, in 1999 and demonstrated feasibility, acceptability, and enhanced communication between PWID and health care providers.[65] Prescribers offered syringe-needle prescriptions as part of general medical care, typically prescribing 100 syringes at a time. This is complimented by access to a portable disposal container and discussions on safer injection techniques (**Box 28-2**), how to recognize infections, and safe disposal of used equipment. A national survey of a representative sample of U.S. physicians with a 20% response rate found that most respondents were unaware of the laws in their state around syringe access. Almost half of the responding prescribers reported they would consider prescribing syringes to prevent transmission of infections yet only 3.4% reported that they had prescribed to PWID for this purpose.[66]

Sterile injection equipment can also be distributed via public syringe-dispensing vending machines (SDMs) 24 hours a day, 7 days a week, with reduced fixed overhead and staffing costs and with increased anonymity for participants. SDMs have been shown to attract PWID who would otherwise not go to SSPs or pharmacies: people who are younger, people who recently started injecting, and people with no contact with addiction service providers. In 2017, the first SDM was introduced to the United States (Las Vegas, Nevada)[68] but SDMs have been in operation for decades in more than 100 cities in Europe, Australia, and New Zealand.[69]

Despite the extensive evidence for SSPs, they have been politically controversial in the United States due to concerns that they would encourage injection drug use. A ban on federal funding for SSPs was initiated in 1988 and continued until it was lifted in 2009. The ban was reinstated in 2011 and then partially lifted in early 2016; specifically, the ban on using federal funds for the purchase of injection equipment remains, but federal funds may be used for other components of SSPs, based on evidence of demonstrated need due to an increase in HIV or hepatitis C infections.[70] Of note, after an outbreak of HIV and HCV infections among people using injection prescription opioids in Scott County, Indiana, was described in 2015,[71] the state government lifted restrictions and implemented a SSP through the public health department, along with increasing access to HIV and addiction treatment, resulting in the control of new HIV and HCV infections. In 2022 for the first time ever, the National Drug Control Strategy prioritized the promotion of harm reduction programming, including specific goals and support for the expansion of SSPs.[2]

Safer Smoking and Sniffing Supply Programs

Harm reduction programs often distribute inhalation and insufflation supplies to reduce health risks associated with smoking and sniffing drugs, as well as to support alternatives to injection. Smoking and sniffing drugs may be a safer alternative to injecting due to less risk of HIV transmission and potentially lower risk of overdose; however, more research is needed to understand the relative overdose risk of inhaling and snorting versus injecting different drugs. Some individuals who smoke and/or snort may also concurrently inject drugs, particularly in the context of polysubstance use. Some may use smoking or snorting as a reprieve from injection when they lack access to sterile injection supplies, wish to rest or heal their veins from the demands of injection, or aim to reduce their drug use risk or drug consumption.

Smoking substances such as heroin, fentanyl, methamphetamine or crack-cocaine involves heating the drug, usually with a flame, and inhaling the vapors through a pipe. These methods of inhalation can result in oral sores and burns that can pose infection risk to the person smoking substances, especially if pipes and/or mouthpieces are shared. In the absence of proper equipment, people often resort to makeshift equipment—such as plastic bottles or light bulbs—that either lacks proper protective measures, is prone to breaking and further causing cuts, and/or exposes people to unwanted chemicals and contaminants. Safer pipes distributed by harm reduction programs include glass stem-pipes with aluminum foil for heroin or fentanyl, glass stem-pipes with metal filters for crack cocaine, and glass bubble-pipes for methamphetamine. Safer smoking kits improve the safety of smoking by providing the following materials: rubber mouthpieces to prevent cuts, glass stems or bowl-pipes (depending on local drug paraphernalia laws), alcohol wipes to disinfect stems and mouthpieces, copper mesh (ie, ChoreBoy) or copper screens to serve as a filter in the stem, aluminum foil as a surface to heat and vaporize heroin or fentanyl, vitamin C to assist in dissolving substances, and vitamin E and/or lip balm to help lip cuts, sores, or burns.[72,73]

Similarly, insufflation of substances such as cocaine can result in irritant injury to the nasal septum; thus, exposing people to infection risk, that can be exacerbated by the use of makeshift equipment (eg, rolled up dollar bills). Safer sniffing kits will often supply the following materials: paper straws for snorting (sometimes multicolored to easily identify one's straw in the context of using in a group), spoons for snorting, sterile razor for cutting substances, and a flat surface (eg, plastic card) to prepare the substances on.

Observation to Keep People Safe While Using Substances to Reduce Overdose

Overdose Prevention Sites

Supervised Injection Facilities (SIFs), also called Drug Consumption Venues (DCVs) or Overdose Prevention Sites (OPS), are facilities where people may go to consume drugs obtained elsewhere under trained supervision in a hygienic environment, with appropriate equipment, and without fear of arrest. A primary goal of OPS are to improve the health status of people who use substances while reducing public drug use (ie, use of drugs in parks, empty lots, public restrooms).[74,75] The first SIF opened in Switzerland in 1986; today, there are more than 100 legally sanctioned sites in at least eight countries. In the United States, there were at least three facilities operating in 2022. One opened in 2014 in an undisclosed location and has reported reduced injection risk behaviors among participants.[76] Two more sites opened in New York City in well publicized locations[77]; these are constructed to allow not only supervised injection but also a safer site for other drug consumption such as smoking. SIFs are similar to other harm reduction interventions in that they are designed to reduce the risk of disease transmission and other infections, intervene in evolving overdoses and provide a point of entry into other services. These facilities serve marginalized populations with high rates of housing insecurity, HIV, and HCV. In 2021 an ASAM public policy recommended the development of pilot OPS.[78]

OPS are strongly associated with reductions in overdose fatalities in the vicinity of the facility, with no reported overdose deaths within the facilities.[79] They have not been associated with increases in drug use or drug crimes,[80] but rather cessation of drug injection, increased addiction treatment uptake, and reduced time to entry into addiction treatment.[81] They reduce isolated and public drug use, including public injection and public syringe disposal.[82] They have also been found to reduce risk behaviors for blood-borne infections such as reusing and sharing injection equipment, while increasing access to drug treatment and timely access to health care.[83] A number of modeling studies have found that SIFs are likely to reduce HIV and HCV infections and would be cost-effective and potentially cost-saving.[84] Related innovative programs that seek to create safer venues for people who use injection drugs, but do not offer fully supervised injection, include monitored spaces for people who are over-sedated from polysubstance use and monitored washrooms at agencies serving PWID in recognition of the reality that they may be used to inject.[85]

Postsubstance Use Observation Sites: Chill Out Rooms

Postsubstance use observation programs have been developed in communities where opioid overdose risk is high due to regular use of fentanyl, typically mixed with other sedating substances. These venues offer a comfortable, welcoming place for people who are over-sedated, where they can be monitored for overdose and kept safe. Boston's Healthcare for the Homeless Program developed such a program in 2016 that included a drop-in facility (that is open daily) with available medical care from a nurse and physician. The programs' overall goal is to avoid unnecessary emergency department visits, respond to potential overdoses, and provide individuals a gateway to other harm reductions services and substance use treatment. The core staff includes a harm reduction staff specialist with lived experience focused on engaging participants in services.[85]

Virtual Spotting

"Virtual spotting" includes efforts to observe people who are using drugs virtually or remotely so that, if the person overdoses or is otherwise at risk for harm while or after using, the harm can be recognized and addressed without having another person present or directly observing.[86] Overdose prevention programs advise people not to use substances alone as demonstrated by key overdose prevention messages such as "never use alone" and "take turns." Notwithstanding these messages, some people will use alone due to stigma, personal preference, or inability to use in the presence of trusted others. The further surge of overdose deaths after the onset of the COVID-19 pandemic in 2020 raised concerns that people may have increasingly isolated and used alone in efforts to reduce the spread of the COVID-19 virus.[83] Examples of virtual spotting interventions include contacting a person who can monitor for overdose or other harm by phone or via the internet, using a free call service such as neverusealone.com, or using a smartphone based application that can sound an alarm and notify a designated responder, such as Be Safe or Canary.[87] Reverse motion detectors have been deployed in public restrooms where overdoses have occurred to monitor if someone in the bathroom becomes motionless.[88-90] Naloxone auto-injectors with motion or hypoxia sensors are also under development.[91]

Medications That Reduce Overdose, Alcohol Intoxication, and HIV Infection Harms

A harm reduction-oriented approach to medications for substance use disorders prioritizes the reduction of risk behaviors associated with morbidity and mortality without requiring or emphasizing abstinence. This approach is supported by the American Society of Addiction Medicine's guidelines on the use of medications in the treatment of addiction involving opioids which recommend that "The use of cannabis, stimulants, or other addictive drugs should not be a reason to suspend OUD treatment."[92]

Targeted Use of Opioid Antagonists for Alcohol Use Disorder to Reduce Alcohol Use and the Side Effects of a Daily Medication

The strategy of targeted or "as-needed" use for Alcohol Use Disorder, meaning taking the medication at times when a person is more likely to drink alcohol, is a strategy that can be used to reduce the harms of alcohol use. The effectiveness of daily medications for alcohol use disorder, such as naltrexone, nalmefene, acamprosate and disulfiram, has been limited by poor adherence in many real-world populations. One study demonstrated greater reductions in alcohol use from a targeted naltrexone strategy than a daily naltrexone strategy.[93] Like daily medication use, targeted medication use can reduce episodes of alcohol intoxication and the consequences that follow and additionally reduce the risks of side effects of daily medication use (eg, hepatotoxicity).[94] Although the effect sizes were small, three randomized trials of targeted nalmefene use in Europe have demonstrated improvement in multiple alcohol-related outcomes over placebo. Prescribing these oral opioid antagonists, without an abstinence requirement, so that a person with an alcohol use disorder can decide which days to take the medication and which days to go without, is a patient-centered approach that tries to minimize the inconvenience of taking a medication daily and is consistent with a harm reduction approach.[94]

Pre- and Post-HIV Exposure Prophylaxis Medication to Reduce HIV Infection

HIV transmission risk can be reduced by taking anti-HIV medication within 24 hours before an unsafe exposure (pre-exposure prophylaxis [PrEP]) or within 72 hours after an unsafe exposure (postexposure prophylaxis [PEP]). People who use alcohol and drugs are at risk of transmission of HIV through high-risk sexual practices and the sharing of drug supplies. High sexual risk includes having a recent bacterial sexually transmitted infection (STI), multiple sexual partners, inconsistent or no condom use, and/or commercial sex work. A randomized controlled trial of PrEP among PWID in Thailand reported a 49% reduction in overall HIV infection risk and a 74% reduction in HIV risk among those who had the PrEP medication detectable in their blood.[95] Since 2014, the Centers for Disease Control and Prevention (CDC) has recommended that PrEP be considered for any adult who does not have HIV infection and who has injected drugs within the past 6 months, additionally, individuals who currently share injection equipment, are enrolled in addiction treatment, or are at an increased risk for sexual transmission.[96] Cost-effectiveness modeling has demonstrated a role for PrEP for PWIDs, along with opioid agonist treatment and antiretroviral treatment, in controlling HIV transmission in communities with HIV epidemics driven by injection use.[97]

PEP is indicated for anyone with a high-risk HIV exposure including sexual assault, unprotected sex, and needle-sharing incidents. PEP involves an assessment of the risk of the exposure, baseline testing, and prescription of a three-medication regime to be continued for 28 days. Treatment is best initiated as soon as possible, preferably within 2 hours of exposure, and is no longer indicated 72 hours after the exposure. Patients treated with PEP due to sexual- or injection-related exposure should be subsequently offered PrEP. Individuals with ongoing high-risk sexual or injection-related exposures should be initiated on PEP and then transitioned to PrEP.[98] In addition to CDC guidelines for PEP and PrEP[96,99] there is a national hotline for immediate consultation.[100]

Safer Substance Supply Interventions to Reduce Overdose and Other Harms From Contaminated Substance Supply

The economic principle called the Iron Law of Prohibition claims that the more drugs are prohibited or criminalized, the more potent and erratic they become.[101,102] The widespread advent of illegally manufactured fentanyl within the heroin supply as well as in other criminalized drugs demonstrates this principle, leading to a dynamic, unpredictable and increasingly toxic drug supply. In response, harm reduction providers are developing supply-focused tools to increase the safety of substance use, including drug-checking strategies that makes the content of drug samples known to people who use drugs and prescribed alternatives to criminalized drugs accessible for the purpose of a safer supply.[103]

Drug-Checking at Dance Parties to Reduce the Risks of Drug Contamination and Overdose

Drug-checking mitigates the harms of an increasingly potent and unpredictable drug supply by providing people who use drugs with more accurate information about the drugs they are using, so they can estimate the level of risk and adjust their drug use behavior to minimize their risk for harm. Drug-checking was first implemented by harm reduction organizations in the 1990s at raves and late-night dance scenes.[104] In these environments, stimulant and hallucinogen use (eg, ecstasy or MDMA, powder cocaine, lysergic acid diethylamide/LSD, ketamine) is prevalent and the risk of adulteration with unintended psychoactive agents (eg, synthetic cathinone or "bath salts") is high. Drug-checking can be conducted on-site or via self-testing kits sold online and can take the form of a range of methods such as colorimetric reagent testing, thin layer chromatography, mass spectrometry, and fentanyl test strips (FTS). Studies have shown adulteration detection rates to be 11% to 55% among dance festival attendees and detection results have shown to influence behavior change.[105] One study in the United Kingdom found that 19.5% of the samples tested at a dance festival contained unintended substances and 66.7% of participants disposed of their drugs upon learning that adulteration was detected.[106] Additional efforts are often taken to encourage a "healthy settings approach" by modifying nightlife venues to improve ventilation, promote hydration, arrange "chill-out" spots, distribute safe sex supplies, and have first aid teams on site.[107]

Fentanyl Test Strips to Reduce the Risks of Drug Contamination and Overdose

Between 2013 and 2020, the rate of opioid-related overdose deaths involving synthetic opioids other than methadone (eg, fentanyl and its chemic analogues) rose 18-fold (1.0-17.8 per 100,000 persons, age-adjusted) and accounted for more than half (51.5%) of all drug overdose deaths in 2019.[29,108,109] Since 2013, fentanyl has infiltrated all areas of the illicit drug supply market, including counterfeit prescription medications and nonopioid substances. Due to this ubiquity, many individuals are at risk of using fentanyl unintentionally; still, others may use fentanyl intentionally for its potency and affordability. Urine fentanyl test strips (FTS) have been reappropriated by the harm reduction community as a response to growing fentanyl adulteration. Testing a drug batch for fentanyl prior to use is an effective safety planning strategy that allows individuals to adjust their drug use behaviors to reduce risk of fatal overdose (eg, administer a smaller dose, use a different route of administration, prepare naloxone).

Most FTS are competitive lateral flow immunoassays on simple paper-based devices; they are easy-to-use, affordable, and provide quick results.[110] FTS sensitivity varies based on the brand and not all brands can identify all fentanyl analogues. Importantly, FTS only identify the presence of fentanyl or fentanyl analogues, not the concentration, and can be sensitive to minimal concentrations of fentanyl and its analogues. Thus, inform people who use FTS about the limits of FTS in their interpretation of results.

An FTS pilot program in San Francisco between 2017 and 2018 found that 68% to 79% of drug batches tested positive and 59% of clients shared the results of their FTS with their social network. Positive FTS results have been shown to promote risk reduction and overdose prevention behaviors among people who use substances. A study in Rhode Island found that, in response to a positive FTS, 45% of the people who use drugs reported using smaller amount of their drug batch, 42% went slower when using, 39% used with someone else, and 36% did a tester dose.[111] This same study demonstrated strong evidence for FTS acceptability (95% of participants wanted to continue using FTS) and feasibility (98% reported confidence in their ability to use FTS, 93% reported it would be easy to continue using FTS). In sum, FTS can be an essential component of the overdose prevention toolkit.[112]

Portable High Specificity Drug Checking to Reduce the Risks of Drug Contamination and Overdose

Portable high specificity drug-checking with mass spectrometry technology can provide precise information on drug supply components and the relative potency of each component. Several harm reduction programs have developed the capacity to test drug samples at this specificity, including residue from drug materials, like baggies, cookers, syringes, or pipes. The technology is especially useful in communities where fentanyl is ubiquitous in the opioid supply and FTS may provide little new knowledge. High specificity drug-checking is more responsive than FTS (which only indicates the presence of fentanyl) to the continually changing drug supply wherein multiple psychoactive components are being introduced. Initial efforts to incorporate high specificity drug-checking into harm reduction programs have demonstrated validity and utility in providing more precise and reliable information about the drug supply landscape and high levels of interest among staff and program participants, all consistent with the harm reduction principles of educating people who use drugs to promote their autonomy and safety.[113] However, challenges remain including the cost of the equipment, the technical expertise and experience required to collect, test and interpret samples using these machines, the ongoing need for expensive and delayed confirmatory testing, the legal ambiguity of such drug-checking services, and potentially disruptive or oppositional law enforcement activity.

Injectable Opioid Agonist Treatment Programs and Prescribed Safe Supply to Reduce the Risks of Participating in the Illegal Drug Economy and the Risks of Drug Contamination, Including Overdose

Injectable heroin was prescribed to patients for the treatment of opioid use disorder by physicians in the United States until the US Supreme Court ruled in the 1919 decision of *Webb v United States* that under the Harrison Narcotics Tax Act of 1914 that chronically prescribing opioids (including heroin) for opioid use disorder had no legitimate medical purpose. Heroin was placed on Schedule I under the 1970 Controlled Substances Act which further criminalized its use. Heroin was not similarly restricted or criminalized in the United Kingdom and continues to be prescribed for pain and for treatment of opioid use disorder, though due to some additional licensing requirements, its use is limited. Multiple randomized controlled trials comparing injectable heroin treatment to oral methadone treatment, conducted among people who have not responded to methadone treatment, have demonstrated reduced street opioid use, reduced criminal activity, and improved mental and physical health in United Kingdom,[114] Switzerland,[115] Netherlands,[116,117] Spain,[118] Germany,[119] Canada,[120] and Belgium.[121,122] These studies were conducted in supervised clinical settings where patients come to clinic multiple times a day and have their dose prepared by nurses who then supervise them while they inject themselves. A 2016 randomized clinical trial in Vancouver compared injectable heroin to injectable hydromorphone and found no significant differences in the decrease of street heroin use, but found increased rates of seizures and overdose in the heroin group.[123] Since the results of this trial, injectable hydromorphone clinics have opened in several Canadian cities.[124,125]

The toxicity of the illicit fentanyl supply has driven the surge in overdose deaths, even in places with strong underlying harm reduction and substance use treatment infrastructure like Vancouver, British Columbia. In 2019, in response to surging overdose deaths and inspired by the positive outcomes from the injectable hydromorphone study, the first prescription hydromorphone safe supply program was established at supervised consumption site, offering on-site use of pharmaceutical hydromorphone tablets. Qualitative evaluation from this pilot program reported acceptability, feasibility, reductions in illicit drug use, and improvements in quality of life.[126] At the same time, an injectable opioid agonist clinic in Vancouver is being piloted that offers prescribed dextroamphetamine to patients using stimulants as a safe supply option.[127] With the onset of COVID-19, such safe supply approaches were expanded to additional venues and there was a release of clinical guidance for providers to offer prescription opioids, stimulants, and benzodiazepines to people using similar substances illicitly in order to mitigate the risk of withdrawal and overdose in the setting of social isolation and an erratic illicit drug supply.[128,129] A qualitative study of 40 people who use drugs during this time in Vancouver found that people accessing the prescribed safe supply hydromorphone, dextroamphetamine, and benzodiazepines were able to relieve their withdrawal and cravings consistently with much lower risk of overdose and less need to raise money through crime.[130] Supplementing the prescribed safe supply with street drugs was common due to guideline limitations that made it so the safe supply pharmaceuticals were weaker and less likely to produce euphoria. A prescribed safe supply program set up in a COVID isolation hotel for unhoused people in Halifax, Nova Scotia, reported that among 62 residents receiving prescribed safe supply or managed alcohol, 60 completed a 14-day isolation and none overdosed.[131]

Managed Alcohol Programs to Reduce Lack of Housing, Acute Hospitalizations, the Consequences of Severe Intoxication and the Use of Nonbeverage Alcohol

People with severe alcohol use disorder who are actively drinking and unhoused are commonly restricted from housing due to eligibility guidelines that prohibit ongoing alcohol use. Housing First programs are designed to remove this barrier to housing (see next section). Managed alcohol programs further attempt to reduce the harms of daily heavy alcohol use among people who are unhoused by providing alcohol of known quality in order to stabilize alcohol use with the goals of improving health and well-being; as well as, reducing acute care hospitalizations, recurrent withdrawal management services, and hazardous alcohol use patterns (ie, severe intoxication and more dangerous nonbeverage alcohol, such as methanol and isopropyl alcohol). Longitudinal observational evaluations of managed alcohol programs have reported fewer emergency department visits, fewer police contacts, reduced alcohol consumption within the program over time,[132] less nonbeverage alcohol use, reductions in tests of liver inflammation,[133] and improved perception of quality of life and housing stability.[134] Peer-reviewed, published descriptions and evaluations of managed alcohol programs have mostly come from Canada.[131,135] However, during the COVID-19 pandemic, managed alcohol programs were developed and successfully implemented in three isolation units in Northern California and Anchorage, Alaska without any deaths or serious adverse events.[136,137]

Housing First to Reduce Barriers to Housing Among People Who Use Substances

In many communities in the United States, housing assistance is only accessible to people on the condition that they commit to abstinence and engage in addiction treatment, making housing contingent on abstinence. These policies structurally and directly discriminate against people who use substances, with a disproportionate effect on racially and ethnically minoritized individuals. This stigmatizing contingency couples entrenched substance use with entrenched lack of housing, undermining the health and wellness of people who use substances. Housing First programs house people who are unhoused without requiring abstinence from substances.[138,139] These programs seek to reduce health harms and costs by removing ongoing substance use as a barrier to providing stable housing. Typically, housing is combined with enhanced support services that both reduce the harms of ongoing substance use and increase the likelihood of engaging in treatment. A 2015 meta-analysis of Housing First programs found that shelter and emergency department costs are reduced, though overall costs may be increased.[140] A 2020 review that compared Housing First programs to treatment-contingent programs found improved housing stability.[139]

During the COVID-19 pandemic, those experiencing housing instability became particularly vulnerable to the downstream effects of the pandemic, notably exacerbations of SUDs, increased overdose risk, increased infection risk related to drug use, lapses in mental health treatment, and disruptions to drug supply. Concurrently, rates of housing instability spiked as individuals faced eviction and under-/unemployment at unprecedented rates. In some cities, programs emerged that provided people experiencing housing instability with temporary housing to fulfill shelter-in-place or quarantine requirements—some programs were created with the objective to serve as pathways to permanent housing.[141]

Designated Driving to Reduce Motor Vehicle Crash Injuries and Deaths

In the United States, the legal blood alcohol concentration limit is less than 80 mg/dL (0.08%), but drinking alcohol worsens driving performance at most any level in a dose-dependent fashion. A 2005 systematic review of two types of interventions to address alcohol-impaired driving found little evidence of effectiveness. The first intervention type was a population-level information campaign that conducted a study with a pre-post design. This study showed a 13% increase in designation of a driver who was not impaired, but no change in self-reported alcohol-impaired driving or riding with an alcohol-impaired driver. The second intervention type was the use of incentives at drinking venues to encourage designated driving. Among seven studies, the number of designated drivers per venue per night increased by a mean 0.9.[142] A 2020 systematic review found that some alternative transportation programs, such as designated drivers, produced reductions in some outcomes, such as impaired driving, crashes, driving under the influence arrests, and traffic crashes in general.[143] Others were not shown to be effective. More research with more rigorous designs and innovation is warranted to determine how best to implement designated driving as a harm reduction measure.

CONCLUSION

Harm reduction, as an approach to improve the lives of people who use substances, emerged amid widespread stigmatization and criminalization of substance use. People who use substances have developed innovative interventions to reducing the structural and health-related harms associated with substance use, including syringe access services and naloxone distribution. Their perspectives are invaluable, and their role should be core to the public health strategy to address the complications of substance use. These interventions advance public health and arise from a movement for social justice that is built on a belief in, and respect for, the rights and dignity of people who use drugs. Effective harm reduction efforts will require ongoing innovation and adaptation in collaboration with the people most impacted by substance use itself and the policies related to it.

REFERENCES

1. Stancliff S, Phillips BW, Maghsoudi N, Joseph H. Harm reduction: front line public health. *J Addict Dis.* 2015;34(2-3):206-219. doi:10.1080/10550887.2015.1059651
2. White House National Drug Control Strategy. Published online 2022. https://www.whitehouse.gov/wp-content/uploads/2022/04/National-Drug-Control-2022Strategy.pdf
3. Alexander M. *The New Jim Crow: Mass Incarceration in the Age of Colourblindness.* Penguin Books; 2019.
4. Hughes M, Suhail-Sindhu S, Namirembe S, et al. The crucial role of black, Latinx, and indigenous leadership in harm reduction and addiction treatment. *Am J Public Health.* 2022;112(S2):S136-S139. doi:10.2105/AJPH.2022.306807

5. Hurley SF, Jolley DJ, Kaldor JM. Effectiveness of needle-exchange programmes for prevention of HIV infection. *Lancet Lond Engl.* 1997;349(9068):1797-1800. doi:10.1016/S0140-6736(96)11380-5
6. O'Hare P. Merseyside, the first harm reduction conferences, and the early history of harm reduction. *Int J Drug Policy.* 2007;18(2):141-144. doi:10.1016/j.drugpo.2007.01.003
7. Lurie P, Reingold AL. *The Public Health Impact of Needle Exchange Programs in the United States and Abroad: Summary, Conclusions and Recommendations*; 1993. Accessed May 21, 2022. https://prevention.ucsf.edu/sites/prevention.ucsf.edu/files/uploads/pubs/reports/pdf/NEPReportSummary1993.pdf
8. Lopez AM, Thomann M, Dhatt Z, et al. Understanding racial inequities in the implementation of harm reduction initiatives. *Am J Public Health.* 2022;112(S2):S173-S181. doi:10.2105/AJPH.2022.306767
9. Abraham AJ, Andrews CM, Harris SJ, Friedmann PD. Availability of medications for the treatment of alcohol and opioid use disorder in the USA. *Neurother J Am Soc Exp Neurother.* 2020;17(1):55-69. doi:10.1007/s13311-019-00814-4
10. Denning P. Strategies for implementation of harm reduction in treatment settings. *J Psychoactive Drugs.* 2001;33(1):23-26. doi:10.1080/02791072.2001.10400464
11. Kellogg SH. On "Gradualism" and the building of the harm reduction-abstinence continuum. *J Subst Abuse Treat.* 2003;25(4):241-247. doi:10.1016/s0740-5472(03)00068-0
12. American Psychiatric Association. *Diagnostic and Statistical Manual of Mental Disorders (DSM).* 5th ed. American Psychiatric Publishing, Inc; 2013.
13. Gaddis A, Kennedy MC, Nosova E, et al. Use of on-site detoxification services co-located with a supervised injection facility. *J Subst Abuse Treat.* 2017;82:1-6. doi:10.1016/j.jsat.2017.08.003
14. Jakubowski A, Norton BL, Hayes BT, et al. Low-threshold buprenorphine treatment in a syringe services program: program description and outcomes. *J Addict Med.* 2022;16(4):447-453. doi:10.1097/ADM.0000000000000934
15. Walley AY, Doe-Simkins M, Quinn E, Pierce C, Xuan Z, Ozonoff A. Opioid overdose prevention with intranasal naloxone among people who take methadone. *J Subst Abuse Treat.* 2013;44(2):241-247. doi:10.1016/j.jsat.2012.07.004
16. Pinedo M. A current re-examination of racial/ethnic disparities in the use of substance abuse treatment: do disparities persist? *Drug Alcohol Depend.* 2019;202:162-167. doi:10.1016/j.drugalcdep.2019.05.017
17. Lagisetty PA, Ross R, Bohnert A, Clay M, Maust DT. Buprenorphine treatment divide by race/ethnicity and payment. *JAMA Psychiatry.* 2019;76(9):979. doi:10.1001/jamapsychiatry.2019.0876
18. Mays VM, Jones AL, Delany-Brumsey A, Coles C, Cochran SD. Perceived discrimination in health care and mental health/substance abuse treatment among blacks, latinos, and whites. *Med Care.* 2017;55(2):173-181. doi:10.1097/MLR.0000000000000638
19. Nuttbrock LA. Culturally competent substance abuse treatment with transgender persons. *J Addict Dis.* 2012;31(3):236-241. doi:10.1080/10550887.2012.694600
20. Kidd JD, Paschen-Wolff MM, Mericle AA, Caceres BA, Drabble LA, Hughes TL. A scoping review of alcohol, tobacco, and other drug use treatment interventions for sexual and gender minority populations. *J Subst Abuse Treat.* 2022;133:108539. doi:10.1016/j.jsat.2021.108539
21. Harris MTH, Laks J, Stahl N, Bagley SM, Saia K, Wechsberg WM. Gender dynamics in substance use and treatment: a women's focused approach. *Med Clin North Am.* 2022;106(1):219-234. doi:10.1016/j.mcna.2021.08.007
22. Ferrer B, Connolly JM. Racial inequities in drug arrests: treatment in Lieu of and after incarceration. *Am J Public Health.* 2018;108(8):968-969. doi:10.2105/AJPH.2018.304575
23. Nicosia N, Macdonald JM, Arkes J. Disparities in criminal court referrals to drug treatment and prison for minority men. *Am J Public Health.* 2013;103(6):e77-e84. doi:10.2105/AJPH.2013.301222
24. Komaromy M, Mendez-Escobar E, Madden E. Addressing racial trauma in the treatment of substance use disorders. *Pediatrics.* 2021;147(Suppl 2):S268-S270. doi:10.1542/peds.2020-023523L
25. Marlatt GA, Blume AW, Parks GA. Integrating harm reduction therapy and traditional substance abuse treatment. *J Psychoactive Drugs.* 2001;33(1):13-21. doi:10.1080/02791072.2001.10400463
26. Rudd RA, Aleshire N, Zibbell JE, Gladden RM. Increases in drug and opioid overdose deaths—United States, 2000-2014. *Morb Mortal Wkly Rep.* 2016;64(50-51):1378-1382. doi:10.15585/mmwr.mm6450a3
27. Gladden RM, Martinez P, Seth P. Fentanyl law enforcement submissions and increases in synthetic opioid-involved overdose deaths—27 states, 2013-2014. *Morb Mortal Wkly Rep.* 2016;65(33):837-843. doi:10.15585/mmwr.mm6533a2
28. Somerville NJ, O'Donnell J, Gladden RM, et al. Characteristics of fentanyl overdose—Massachusetts, 2014-2016. *Morb Mortal Wkly Rep.* 2017;66(14):382-386. doi:10.15585/mmwr.mm6614a2
29. Hedegaard H, Miniño A, Spencer MR, Warner M. *Drug Overdose Deaths in the United States, 1999–2020.* National Center for Health Statistics (U.S.); 2021. doi:10.15620/cdc:112340
30. Ahmad F, Cisewski J, Rossen L, Sutton P. *Provisional Drug Overdose Death Counts.* 2022. Accessed July 16, 2023. https://www.cdc.gov/nchs/nvss/vsrr/drug-overdose-data.htm
31. Larochelle MR, Slavova S, Root ED, et al. Disparities in opioid overdose death trends by race/ethnicity, 2018–2019, from the HEALing communities study. *Am J Public Health.* 2021;111(10):1851-1854. doi:10.2105/AJPH.2021.306431
32. Laurencin CT, Wu ZH, McClinton A, Grady JJ, Walker JM. Excess deaths among blacks and latinx compared to whites during Covid-19. *J Racial Ethn Health Disparities.* 2021;8(3):783-789. doi:10.1007/s40615-021-01010-x
33. Althoff KN, Leifheit KM, Park JN, Chandran A, Sherman SG. Opioid-related overdose mortality in the era of fentanyl: monitoring a shifting epidemic by person, place, and time. *Drug Alcohol Depend.* 2020;216:108321. doi:10.1016/j.drugalcdep.2020.108321
34. Friedman JR, Hansen H. Evaluation of increases in drug overdose mortality rates in the US by race and ethnicity before and during the COVID-19 pandemic. *JAMA Psychiatry.* 2022;79(4):379. doi:10.1001/jamapsychiatry.2022.0004
35. Adams JM. Increasing naloxone awareness and use: the role of health care practitioners. *JAMA.* 2018;319(20):2073-2074. doi:10.1001/jama.2018.4867
36. American Medical Association. *Help Save Lives: Co-prescribe Naloxone to Patients at Risk of Overdose.* Accessed May 22, 2023. American Medical Association; 2023. https://www.end-opioid-epidemic.org/wp-content/uploads/2017/08/AMA-Opioid-Task-Force-naloxone-one-pager-updated-August-2017-FINAL-1.pdf
37. HHS. *SAMHSA Opioid Overdose Prevention Toolkit.* 2023. Accessed May 22, 2023. https://store.samhsa.gov/sites/default/files/d7/priv/sma18-4742.pdf
38. ASAM. *Use of Naloxone for the Prevention of Opioid Overdose Deaths.* American Society of Addiction Medicine. Accessed May 22, 2023. https://www.asam.org/advocacy/public-policy-statements/details/public-policy-statements/2021/08/09/use-of-naloxone-for-the-prevention-of-drug-overdose-deaths
39. Jones JD, Campbell A, Metz VE, Comer SD. No evidence of compensatory drug use risk behavior among heroin users after receiving take-home naloxone. *Addict Behav.* 2017;71:104-106. doi:10.1016/j.addbeh.2017.03.008
40. Maxwell S, Bigg D, Stanczykiewicz K, Carlberg-Racich S. Prescribing naloxone to actively injecting heroin users: a program to reduce heroin overdose deaths. *J Addict Dis.* 2006;25(3):89-96. doi:10.1300/J069v25n03_11
41. Bennett AS, Elliott L. Naloxone's role in the national opioid crisis-past struggles, current efforts, and future opportunities. *Transl Res J Lab Clin Med.* 2021;234:43-57. doi:10.1016/j.trsl.2021.03.001
42. Laws Regulating Administration. *Naloxone Overdose Prevention Laws.* 2022. Published online January 1, 2022. Accessed July 1, 2022. https://pdaps.org/datasets/laws-regulating-administration-of-naloxone-1501695139

43. LAPPA. *Drug Overdose Immunity and Good Samaritan Laws. National Conference of State Legislatures.* Legislative Analysis and Public Policy Association; 2022. Accessed May 21, 2022. https://www.ncsl.org/research/civil-and-criminal-justice/drug-overdose-immunity-good-samaritan-laws.aspx
44. Oliva EM, Christopher MLD, Wells D, et al. Opioid overdose education and naloxone distribution: development of the Veterans Health Administration's national program. *J Am Pharm Assoc.* 2017;57(2S):S168-S179. doi:10.1016/j.japh.2017.01.022
45. Kinnard EN, Bluthenthal RN, Kral AH, Wenger LD, Lambdin BH. The naloxone delivery cascade: identifying disparities in access to naloxone among people who inject drugs in Los Angeles and San Francisco, CA. *Drug Alcohol Depend.* 2021;225:108759. doi:10.1016/j.drugalcdep.2021.108759
46. Walley AY, Xuan Z, Hackman HH, et al. Opioid overdose rates and implementation of overdose education and nasal naloxone distribution in Massachusetts: interrupted time series analysis. *BMJ.* 2013;346:f174. doi:10.1136/bmj.f174
47. Coffin PO, Behar E, Rowe C, et al. Nonrandomized intervention study of naloxone coprescription for primary care patients receiving long-term opioid therapy for pain. *Ann Intern Med.* 2016;165(4):245-252. doi:10.7326/M15-2771
48. Katzman JG, Takeda MY, Bhatt SR, et al. An innovative model for naloxone use within an OTP setting: a prospective cohort study. *J Addict Med.* 2018;12(2):113-118. doi:10.1097/ADM.0000000000000374
49. Coffin PO, Sullivan SD. Cost-effectiveness of distributing naloxone to heroin users for lay overdose reversal. *Ann Intern Med.* 2013;158(1):1-9. doi:10.7326/0003-4819-158-1-201301010-00003
50. Irvine MA, Oller D, Boggis J, et al. Estimating naloxone need in the USA across fentanyl, heroin, and prescription opioid epidemics: a modelling study. *Lancet Public Health.* 2022;7(3):e210-e218. doi:10.1016/S2468-2667(21)00304-2
51. Coffin PO, Maya S, Kahn JG. Modeling of overdose and naloxone distribution in the setting of fentanyl compared to heroin. *Drug Alcohol Depend.* 2022;236:109478. doi:10.1016/j.drugalcdep.2022.109478
52. KFF. *Sterile Syringe Exchange Programs.* KFF; 2022. Published January 24, 2022. Accessed June 30, 2022. https://www.kff.org/hivaids/state-indicator/syringe-exchange-programs/
53. Aspinall EJ, Nambiar D, Goldberg DJ, et al. Are needle and syringe programmes associated with a reduction in HIV transmission among people who inject drugs: a systematic review and meta-analysis. *Int J Epidemiol.* 2014;43(1):235-248. doi:10.1093/ije/dyt243
54. Hagan H, McGough JP, Thiede H, Hopkins S, Duchin J, Alexander ER. Reduced injection frequency and increased entry and retention in drug treatment associated with needle-exchange participation in Seattle drug injectors. *J Subst Abuse Treat.* 2000;19(3):247-252. doi:10.1016/s0740-5472(00)00104-5
55. Strathdee SA, Ricketts EP, Huettner S, et al. Facilitating entry into drug treatment among injection drug users referred from a needle exchange program: results from a community-based behavioral intervention trial. *Drug Alcohol Depend.* 2006;83(3):225-232. doi:10.1016/j.drugalcdep.2005.11.015
56. Groseclose SL, Weinstein B, Jones TS, Valleroy LA, Fehrs LJ, Kassler WJ. Impact of increased legal access to needles and syringes on practices of injecting-drug users and police officers—Connecticut, 1992-1993. *J Acquir Immune Defic Syndr Hum Retrovirol.* 1995;10(1):82-89.
57. Sherman SG, Patel SA, Ramachandran DV, et al. Consequences of a restrictive syringe exchange policy on utilisation patterns of a syringe exchange program in Baltimore, Maryland: implications for HIV risk. *Drug Alcohol Rev.* 2015;34(6):637-644. doi:10.1111/dar.12276
58. Bluthenthal RN, Ridgeway G, Schell T, Anderson R, Flynn NM, Kral AH. Examination of the association between syringe exchange program (SEP) dispensation policy and SEP client-level syringe coverage among injection drug users. *Addiction.* 2007;102(4):638-646. doi:10.1111/j.1360-0443.2006.01741.x
59. Hayashi K, Wood E, Wiebe L, Qi J, Kerr T. An external evaluation of a peer-run outreach-based syringe exchange in Vancouver, Canada. *Int J Drug Policy.* 2010;21(5):418-421. doi:10.1016/j.drugpo.2010.03.002
60. Brener L, Bryant J, Cama E, Pepolin L, Harrod ME. Patterns of peer distribution of injecting equipment at an authorized distribution site in Sydney, Australia. *Subst Use Misuse.* 2018;53(14):2405-2412. doi:10.1080/10826084.2018.1480039
61. Crawford ND, Amesty S, Rivera AV, Harripersaud K, Turner A, Fuller CM. Randomized, community-based pharmacy intervention to expand services beyond sale of sterile syringes to injection drug users in pharmacies in New York City. *Am J Public Health.* 2013;103(9):1579-1582. doi:10.2105/AJPH.2012.301178
62. Reich W, Compton WM, Horton JC, et al. Injection drug users report good access to pharmacy sale of syringes. *J Am Pharm Assoc Wash DC 1996.* 2002;42(6 Suppl 2):S68-S72. doi:10.1331/1086-5802.42.0.s68.reich
63. Lieberman A, Davis CS. *Harm Reduction and Overdose Prevention 50-State Survey.* Accessed May 22, 2023. https://www.networkforphl.org/wp-content/uploads/2020/12/50-State-Survey-Harm-Reduction-Laws-in-the-United-States-final.pdf
64. Burris S. Physician prescribing of sterile injection equipment to prevent HIV infection: time for action. *Ann Intern Med.* 2000;133(3):218. doi:10.7326/0003-4819-133-3-200008010-00015
65. Rich JD, McKenzie M, Macalino GE, et al. A syringe prescription program to prevent infectious disease and improve health of injection drug users. *J Urban Health Bull N Y Acad Med.* 2004;81(1):122-134. doi:10.1093/jurban/jth092
66. Macalino GE, Sachdev DD, Rich JD, et al. A national physician survey on prescribing syringes as an HIV prevention measure. *Subst Abuse Treat Prev Policy.* 2009;4:13. doi:10.1186/1747-597X-4-13
67. Harvey L, Boudreau J, Sliwinski SK, et al. Six moments of infection prevention in injection drug use: an educational toolkit for clinicians. *Open Forum Infect Dis.* 2022;9(2):ofab631. doi:10.1093/ofid/ofab631
68. Potera C. An innovative syringe exchange program. *Am J Nurs.* 2017;117(7):17. doi:10.1097/01.NAJ.0000520934.96160.36
69. Duplessy C, Reynaud EG. Long-term survey of a syringe-dispensing machine needle exchange program: answering public concerns. *Harm Reduct J.* 2014;11:16. doi:10.1186/1477-7517-11-16
70. CDC. *Federal Funding for Syringe Services Programs.* 2022. Accessed June 23, 2022. https://www.cdc.gov/ssp/ssp-funding.html
71. Peters PJ, Pontones P, Hoover KW, et al. HIV infection linked to injection use of oxymorphone in Indiana, 2014-2015. *N Engl J Med.* 2016;375(3):229-239. doi:10.1056/NEJMoa1515195
72. Imtiaz S, Strike C, Elton-Marshall T, Rehm J. Safer smoking kits for methamphetamine consumption. *Addiction.* 2020;115(6):1189-1190. doi:10.1111/add.14914
73. Prangnell A, Dong H, Daly P, Milloy MJ, Kerr T, Hayashi K. Declining rates of health problems associated with crack smoking during the expansion of crack pipe distribution in Vancouver, Canada. *BMC Public Health.* 2017;17(1):163. doi:10.1186/s12889-017-4099-9
74. Potier C, Laprévote V, Dubois-Arber F, Cottencin O, Rolland B. Supervised injection services: what has been demonstrated? A systematic literature review. *Drug Alcohol Depend.* 2014;145:48-68. doi:10.1016/j.drugalcdep.2014.10.012
75. Wolfson-Stofko B, Bennett AS, Elliott L, Curtis R. Drug use in business bathrooms: an exploratory study of manager encounters in New York City. *Int J Drug Policy.* 2017;39:69-77. doi:10.1016/j.drugpo.2016.08.014
76. Suen LW, Davidson PJ, Browne EN, Lambdin BH, Wenger LD, Kral AH. Effect of an unsanctioned safe consumption site in the United States on syringe sharing, rushed injections, and isolated injection drug use: a longitudinal cohort analysis. *J Acquir Immune Defic Syndr.* 2022;89(2):172-177. doi:10.1097/QAI.0000000000002849
77. Finke J, Chan J. The case for supervised injection sites in the United States. *Am Fam Physician.* 2022;105(5):454-455.
78. ASAM. *Overdose Prevention Sites.* 2023. Accessed May 22, 2023. https://www.asam.org/advocacy/public-policy-statements/details/public-policy-statements/2021/08/09/overdose-prevention-sites#

79. Marshall BDL, Milloy MJ, Wood E, Montaner JSG, Kerr T. Reduction in overdose mortality after the opening of North America's first medically supervised safer injecting facility: a retrospective population-based study. *Lancet Lond Engl.* 2011;377(9775):1429-1437. doi:10.1016/S0140-6736(10)62353-7
80. Freeman K, Jones CGA, Weatherburn DJ, Rutter S, Spooner CJ, Donnelly N. The impact of the Sydney Medically Supervised Injecting Centre (MSIC) on crime. *Drug Alcohol Rev.* 2005;24(2):173-184. doi:10.1080/09595230500167460
81. DeBeck K, Kerr T, Bird L, et al. Injection drug use cessation and use of North America's first medically supervised safer injecting facility. *Drug Alcohol Depend.* 2011;113(2-3):172-176. doi:10.1016/j.drugalcdep.2010.07.023
82. Wood E, Kerr T, Small W, et al. Changes in public order after the opening of a medically supervised safer injecting facility for illicit injection drug users. *CMAJ.* 2004;171(7):731-734. doi:10.1503/cmaj.1040774
83. Lloyd-Smith E, Wood E, Zhang R, et al. Determinants of hospitalization for a cutaneous injection-related infection among injection drug users: a cohort study. *BMC Public Health.* 2010;10:327. doi:10.1186/1471-2458-10-327
84. Irwin A, Jozaghi E, Bluthenthal RN, Kral AH. A cost-benefit analysis of a potential supervised injection facility in San Francisco, California, USA. *J Drug Issues.* 2017;47(2):164-184. doi:10.1177/0022042616679829
85. Providing a safe space and medical monitoring to prevent overdose deaths. *Health Affairs Forefront.* Accessed May 21, 2022. https://www.healthaffairs.org/do/10.1377/forefront.20160831.056280/full/
86. Perri M, Kaminski N, Bonn M, et al. A qualitative study on overdose response in the era of COVID-19 and beyond: how to spot someone so they never have to use alone. *Harm Reduct J.* 2021;18(1):85. doi:10.1186/s12954-021-00530-3
87. German K. *Canary—Prevent Overdose.* App Store; 2022. Accessed June 30, 2022. https://apps.apple.com/us/app/canary-prevent-overdose/id1396426874
88. Buchheit BM, Crable EL, Lipson SK, Drainoni ML, Walley AY. "Opening the door to somebody who has a chance."—The experiences and perceptions of public safety personnel towards a public restroom overdose prevention alarm system. *Int J Drug Policy.* 2021;88:103038. doi:10.1016/j.drugpo.2020.103038
89. Gaeta JM. A pitiful sanctuary. *JAMA.* 2019;321(24):2407. doi:10.1001/jama.2019.7998
90. Fozouni L, Buchheit B, Walley AY, Testa M, Chatterjee A. Public restrooms and the opioid epidemic. *Subst Abus.* 2020;41(4):432-436. doi:10.1080/08897077.2019.1640834
91. Chan J, Iyer V, Wang A, et al. Closed-loop wearable naloxone injector system. *Sci Rep.* 2021;11(1):22663. doi:10.1038/s41598-021-01990-0
92. Kampman K, Jarvis M. American Society of Addiction Medicine (ASAM) National Practice Guideline for the use of medications in the treatment of addiction involving opioid use. *J Addict Med.* 2015;9(5):358-367. doi:10.1097/ADM.0000000000000166
93. Hernandez-Avila CA, Song C, Kuo L, Tennen H, Armeli S, Kranzler HR. Targeted versus daily naltrexone: secondary analysis of effects on average daily drinking. *Alcohol Clin Exp Res.* 2006;30(5):860-865. doi:10.1111/j.1530-0277.2006.00101.x
94. Niciu MJ, Arias AJ. Targeted opioid receptor antagonists in the treatment of alcohol use disorders. *CNS Drugs.* 2013;27(10):777-787. doi:10.1007/s40263-013-0096-4
95. Martin M, Vanichseni S, Suntharasamai P, et al. Risk behaviors and risk factors for HIV infection among participants in the Bangkok tenofovir study, an HIV pre-exposure prophylaxis trial among people who inject drugs. *PloS One.* 2014;9(3):e92809. doi:10.1371/journal.pone.0092809
96. US Public Health Service. *Preexposure Prophylaxis for the Prevention of HIV Infection in the United States—2021 Update: A Clinical Practice Guideline.* Centers for Disease Control and Prevention; 2021. Accessed May 21, 2022. https://www.cdc.gov/hiv/pdf/risk/prep/cdc-hiv-prep-guidelines-2021.pdf
97. Bernard CL, Brandeau ML, Humphreys K, et al. Cost-effectiveness of HIV preexposure prophylaxis for people who inject drugs in the United States. *Ann Intern Med.* 2016;165(1):10-19. doi:10.7326/M15-2634
98. Taylor JL, Walley AY, Bazzi AR. Stuck in the window with you: HIV exposure prophylaxis in the highest risk people who inject drugs. *Subst Abus.* 2019;40(4):441-443. doi:10.1080/08897077.2019.1675118
99. CDC. *Updated Guidelines for Antiretroviral Postexposure Prophylaxis After Sexual, Injection Drug Use, or Other Nonoccupational Exposure to HIV—United States, 2016.* Centers for Disease Control and Prevention; 2022. Accessed June 30, 2022. https://stacks.cdc.gov/view/cdc/38856
100. NCCC. *PrEP: Pre-Exposure Prophylaxis.* National Clinician Consultation Center; 2022. Accessed May 21, 2022. https://nccc.ucsf.edu/clinician-consultation/prep-pre-exposure-prophylaxis/
101. Thornton M. The potency of illegal drugs. *J Drug Issues.* 1998;28(3):725-740. doi:10.1177/002204269802800309
102. Beletsky L, Davis CS. Today's fentanyl crisis: prohibition's iron law, revisited. *Int J Drug Policy.* 2017;46:156-159. doi:10.1016/j.drugpo.2017.05.050
103. Stringfellow EJ, Lim TY, Humphreys K, et al. Reducing opioid use disorder and overdose deaths in the United States: a dynamic modeling analysis. *Sci Adv.* 2022;8(25):eabm8147. doi:10.1126/sciadv.abm8147
104. NDARC. *Bulletin No. 24: Global Review of Drug Checking Services Operating in 2017.* NDARC—National Drug and Alcohol Research Centre; 2022. Accessed June 30, 2022. https://ndarc.med.unsw.edu.au/resource/bulletin-no-24-global-review-drug-checking-services-operating-2017
105. Palamar JJ, Fitzgerald ND, Keyes KM, Cottler LB. Drug checking at dance festivals: a review with recommendations to increase generalizability of findings. *Exp Clin Psychopharmacol.* 2021;29(3):229-235. doi:10.1037/pha0000452
106. Measham FC. Drug safety testing, disposals and dealing in an English field: exploring the operational and behavioural outcomes of the UK's first onsite 'drug checking' service. *Int J Drug Policy.* 2019;67:102-107. doi:10.1016/j.drugpo.2018.11.001
107. Bellis MA, Hughes K, Lowey H. Healthy nightclubs and recreational substance use. From a harm minimisation to a healthy settings approach. *Addict Behav.* 2002;27(6):1025-1035. doi:10.1016/s0306-4603(02)00271-x
108. Mattson CL, Tanz LJ, Quinn K, Kariisa M, Patel P, Davis NL. Trends and geographic patterns in drug and synthetic opioid overdose deaths—United States, 2013–2019. *Morb Mortal Wkly Rep.* 2021;70(6):202-207. doi:10.15585/mmwr.mm7006a4
109. CDC. *DOSE Dashboard: Nonfatal Overdose Data | Drug Overdose.* CDC Injury Center; 2022. Published May 23, 2022. Accessed June 30, 2022. https://www.cdc.gov/drugoverdose/nonfatal/dashboard/index.html
110. Bergh MSS, Øiestad ÅML, Baumann MH, Bogen IL. Selectivity and sensitivity of urine fentanyl test strips to detect fentanyl analogues in illicit drugs. *Int J Drug Policy.* 2021;90:103065. doi:10.1016/j.drugpo.2020.103065
111. Krieger MS, Goedel WC, Buxton JA, et al. Use of rapid fentanyl test strips among young adults who use drugs. *Int J Drug Policy.* 2018;61:52-58. doi:10.1016/j.drugpo.2018.09.009
112. NHRC. *Fentanyl Test Strip Pilot.* National Harm Reduction Coalition; 2022. Accessed June 30, 2022. https://harmreduction.org/issues/fentanyl/fentanyl-test-strip-pilot/
113. Carroll JJ, Mackin S, Schmidt C, McKenzie M, Green TC. The Bronze age of drug checking: barriers and facilitators to implementing advanced drug checking amidst police violence and COVID-19. *Harm Reduct J.* 2022;19(1):9. doi:10.1186/s12954-022-00590-z
114. Hartnoll RL. Evaluation of heroin maintenance in controlled trial. *Arch Gen Psychiatry.* 1980;37(8):877. doi:10.1001/archpsyc.1980.01780210035003
115. Perneger TV, Giner F, del Rio M, Mino A. Randomised trial of heroin maintenance programme for addicts who fail in conventional drug treatments. *BMJ* 1998;317(7150):13-18. doi:10.1136/bmj.317.7150.13

116. Blanken P, Hendriks VM, van Ree JM, van den Brink W. Outcome of long-term heroin-assisted treatment offered to chronic, treatment-resistant heroin addicts in the Netherlands. *Addiction*. 2010;105(2): 300-308. doi:10.1111/j.1360-0443.2009.02754.x
117. van den Brink W. Medical prescription of heroin to treatment resistant heroin addicts: two randomised controlled trials. *BMJ*. 2003;327(7410):310-0. doi:10.1136/bmj.327.7410.310
118. Oviedo-Joekes E, March JC, Romero M, Perea-Milla E. The Andalusian trial on heroin-assisted treatment: a 2 year follow-up. *Drug Alcohol Rev*. 2010;29(1):75-80. doi:10.1111/j.1465-3362.2009.00100.x
119. Haasen C, Verthein U, Degkwitz P, Berger J, Krausz M, Naber D. Heroin-assisted treatment for opioid dependence: randomised controlled trial. *Br J Psychiatry*. 2007;191(1):55-62. doi:10.1192/bjp.bp.106.026112
120. Oviedo-Joekes E, Brissette S, Marsh DC, et al. Diacetylmorphine versus methadone for the treatment of opioid addiction. *N Engl J Med*. 2009;361(8):777-786. doi:10.1056/NEJMoa0810635
121. Demaret I, Quertemont E, Litran G, et al. Efficacy of heroin-assisted treatment in Belgium: a randomised controlled trial. *Eur Addict Res*. 2015;21(4):179-187. doi:10.1159/000369337
122. Kilmer B, Taylor J, Caulkins J, et al. *Considering Heroin-Assisted Treatment and Supervised Drug Consumption Sites in the United States*. RAND Corporation; 2018. doi:10.7249/RR2693
123. Oviedo-Joekes E, Guh D, Brissette S, et al. Hydromorphone compared with diacetylmorphine for long-term opioid dependence: a randomized clinical trial. *JAMA Psychiatry*. 2016;73(5):447-455. doi:10.1001/jamapsychiatry.2016.0109
124. Eydt E, Glegg S, Sutherland C, et al. Service delivery models for injectable opioid agonist treatment in Canada: 2 sequential environmental scans. *CMAJ Open*. 2021;9(1):E115-E124. doi:10.9778/cmajo.20200021
125. Harris MT, Seliga RK, Fairbairn N, et al. Outcomes of Ottawa, Canada's Managed Opioid Program (MOP) where supervised injectable hydromorphone was paired with assisted housing. *Int J Drug Policy*. 2021;98:103400. doi:10.1016/j.drugpo.2021.103400
126. Ivsins A, Boyd J, Mayer S, et al. "It's helped me a lot, just like to stay alive": a qualitative analysis of outcomes of a novel hydromorphone tablet distribution program in Vancouver, Canada. *J Urban Health*. 2021;98(1):59-69. doi:10.1007/s11524-020-00489-9
127. Palis H, MacDonald S, Jun J, Oviedo-Joekes E. Use of sustained release dextroamphetamine for the treatment of stimulant use disorder in the setting of injectable opioid agonist treatment in Canada: a case report. *Harm Reduct J*. 2021;18(1):57. doi:10.1186/s12954-021-00500-9
128. British Columbia Centre on Substance Use. *Risk Mitigation in the Context of Dual Public Health Emergencies*. British Columbia Centre on Substance Use; 2022. Accessed July 16, 2023. https://www.bccsu.ca/wp-content/uploads/2022/02/Risk-Mitigation-Guidance-Update-February-2022.pdf
129. British Columbia Ministry of Mental Health and Addictions and Ministry of Health. Access to prescribed safer supply in British Columbia: policy direction. 2021. Published online July 15, 2021.
130. McNeil R, Fleming T, Mayer S, et al. Implementation of safe supply alternatives during intersecting COVID-19 and overdose health emergencies in British Columbia, Canada, 2021. *Am J Public Health*. 2022;112(S2):S151-S158. doi:10.2105/AJPH.2021.306692
131. Brothers TD, Leaman M, Bonn M, et al. Evaluation of an emergency safe supply drugs and managed alcohol program in COVID-19 isolation hotel shelters for people experiencing homelessness. *Drug Alcohol Depend*. 2022;235:109440. doi:10.1016/j.drugalcdep.2022.109440
132. Podymow T, Turnbull J, Coyle D, Yetisir E, Wells G. Shelter-based managed alcohol administration to chronically homeless people addicted to alcohol. *CMAJ*. 2006;174(1):45-49. doi:10.1503/cmaj.1041350
133. Vallance K, Stockwell T, Pauly B, et al. Do managed alcohol programs change patterns of alcohol consumption and reduce related harm? A pilot study. *Harm Reduct J*. 2016;13(1):13. doi:10.1186/s12954-016-0103-4
134. Pauly BB, Gray E, Perkin K, et al. Finding safety: a pilot study of managed alcohol program participants' perceptions of housing and quality of life. *Harm Reduct J*. 2016;13(1):15. doi:10.1186/s12954-016-0102-5
135. Pauly B, Brown M, Evans J, et al. "There is a Place": impacts of managed alcohol programs for people experiencing severe alcohol dependence and homelessness. *Harm Reduct J*. 2019;16(1):70. doi:10.1186/s12954-019-0332-4
136. Ristau J, Mehtani N, Gomez S, et al. Successful implementation of managed alcohol programs in the San Francisco Bay Area during the COVID-19 crisis. *Subst Abus*. 2021;42(2):140-147. doi:10.1080/08897077.2021.1892012
137. Brocious H, Trawver K, Demientieff LX. Managed alcohol: one community's innovative response to risk management during COVID-19. *Harm Reduct J*. 2021;18(1):125. doi:10.1186/s12954-021-00574-5
138. Collins SE, Malone DK, Clifasefi SL, et al. Project-based Housing First for chronically homeless individuals with alcohol problems: within-subjects analyses of 2-year alcohol trajectories. *Am J Public Health*. 2012;102(3):511-519. doi:10.2105/AJPH.2011.300403
139. Peng Y, Hahn RA, Finnie RKC, et al. Permanent supportive housing with housing first to reduce homelessness and promote health among homeless populations with disability: a community guide systematic review. *J Public Health Manag Pract*. 2020;26(5):404-411. doi:10.1097/PHH.0000000000001219
140. Ly A, Latimer E. Housing first impact on costs and associated cost offsets: a review of the literature. *Can J Psychiatry*. 2015;60(11):475-487. doi:10.1177/070674371506001103
141. Mejia-Lancheros C, Alfayumi-Zeadna S, Lachaud J, et al. Differential impacts of COVID-19 and associated responses on the health, social well-being and food security of users of supportive social and health programs during the COVID-19 pandemic: a qualitative study. *Health Soc Care Community*. 2022;30(6):e4332-e4344. doi:10.1111/hsc.13826
142. Ditter SM, Elder RW, Shults RA, Sleet DA, Compton R, Nichols JL. Effectiveness of designated driver programs for reducing alcohol-impaired driving: a systematic review. *Am J Prev Med*. 2005;28(5 Suppl):280-287. doi:10.1016/j.amepre.2005.02.013
143. Fell JC, Scolese J, Achoki T, Burks C, Goldberg A, DeJong W. The effectiveness of alternative transportation programs in reducing impaired driving: a literature review and synthesis. *J Safety Res*. 2020;75:128-139. doi:10.1016/j.jsr.2020.09.001

CHAPTER

29 College Student Drinking

Lauren McClain, Frank J. Schwebel, Ursula Whiteside, Jason R. Kilmer, Ty W. Lostutter, and Mary E. Larimer

CHAPTER OUTLINE

- Prevalence and consequences
- Prevention strategies and interventions
- Conclusions and future directions
- Acknowledgment

PREVALENCE AND CONSEQUENCES

Heavy drinking and significant alcohol-related problems impact college students nationwide.[1] An estimated 1707 college student deaths between 1998 and 2014 involved alcohol.[2] Heavy episodic (or binge) drinking and the resulting detrimental consequences have led the U.S. Department of Health and Human Services and the Surgeon General to classify college student binge drinking as a major public health problem. Though extensive research and administrative efforts have been aimed at decreasing college student binge drinking, problems and consequences such as driving under the influence, academic and relationship consequences, and student deaths due to alcohol-related injuries and suicide continue to occur at relatively high rates.[2] What follows is a review of the research on college student drinking including prevalence rates and consequences, risk factors for college drinking, and a discussion of empirically supported interventions and treatment practices.

Drinking Rates and Disorders Among College Students

Approximately four out of five (80%) college students have consumed alcohol in the past year and 65% have been drunk at least once in their lives.[3] When examining only the past month, 28% reported having been drunk and 2% reported drinking daily, while 24% have engaged in heavy episodic drinking (defined by the National Institute on Alcohol Abuse and Alcoholism [NIAAA] as reaching a blood alcohol level of 0.08 or higher, usually by consuming five or more drinks for men or four or more for women, over a 2-hour period) in the past 2 weeks.[1,3] These rates are comparable to young adults who are not in college. The estimated prevalence of alcohol use disorders (AUDs) among college students using DSM-5 criteria is about 33%.[4,5] Rates increased further during the COVID-19 pandemic.[5] While many students mature out of problematic alcohol use over time, an estimated 43% of students diagnosed with an AUD during early college continue to meet criteria for AUD after college.[6]

Alcohol-Related Problems and Consequences

The NIAAA Task Force on College Drinking categorized college student drinking consequences as damage to self, others, or the institution.[7] A wide variety of problems and consequences occur in relation to drinking by college students, such as death, injury, assault, sexual assault, unsafe sex, health problems, suicide, drunk driving, academic problems, vandalism, property damage, and police involvement.

Damage to Self

Nausea, vomiting, and hangovers are among the most reported negative physical effects produced by alcohol.[7] Structural changes to the brain, which may be less noticeable to the individual, can occur until 22 years old.[8] Beginning to drink during adolescence or young adulthood places individuals at risk of slower development of cognitive processing skills and intellectual functioning.[8] This may contribute to negative academic consequences due to drinking, including missing or falling behind in class, doing poorly on exams or papers, and receiving lower grades[9] as reported by about 25% of college students. Higher levels of drinking are associated with poorer academic performance, as indicated by grade point average.[10,11] College students risk legal consequences (in addition to injury or death) by driving under the influence (16%)[2] and/or may be involved with local or campus police because of drinking (5%).[12] Neurodevelopmental delays and immaturity of cognitive capacities with an inability to effectively inhibit behavioral responses[8] may exacerbate misbehavior in individuals who began drinking before college.

Damage to Others

In addition to direct harm to self, motor vehicle accidents, vandalism, litter, noise, fighting, public urination, vomiting, and problematic encounters with drunken individuals are all harms to others associated with college drinking. For example, among students who live on campus and drink either lightly or not at all, 60% experienced interrupted study or sleep due to other students' drinking, 48% took care of a drunk student, and almost 20% had a serious argument or experienced an unwanted sexual overture (for females) where alcohol was involved.[12] It is estimated that approximately half a million college students annually are unintentionally injured because of drinking; 646,000 experience physical assault by an intoxicated student. It is estimated that 50% to 80% of violence occurring on campuses is alcohol related.[13] Approximately 97,000 college students experience alcohol-related sexual assault annually.[14] Increased awareness of sexual assault and rape on campus has prompted research to further investigate the impact of alcohol on campus sexual assault.[15] Findings include that sexual assaults tend to occur at colleges with high rates of binge drinking and that three of four students who reported a sexual assault were under the influence of alcohol during the assault.[15,16] Sexual assault perpetration is also significantly associated with alcohol use.[17]

Damage to Institution

College administrators, staff, and campus police often have to deal with the consequences of student alcohol use. Associated problems, such as violence, vandalism, and property damage, are relatively common. More than one-fourth of colleges with low rates of drinking, and more than half of those with high rates of drinking, report moderate to major problems with alcohol-related vandalism and property damage.[18] Approximately 11% of students have damaged property while under the influence of alcohol.[12] Further, individuals who engaged in binge drinking sporadically or frequently were four and ten times more likely, respectively, to report having damaged property than were those who did not.[19] Furthermore, university reputation can be negatively impacted by alcohol-related incidents being publicized, leading to a popular perception of an institution as a "party school."[20]

Risk Factors for College Student Drinking

Identified risk factors for heavy drinking among college students include demographic and environmental influences, cognitive and motivational factors (eg, perceptions of the normative nature of drinking, expectations of positive outcomes from drinking), and affective factors (mood or anxiety problems, a desire to avoid negative emotions or enhance positive ones).[21] Parental drinking is a risk factor for AUD that acts through both behavioral modeling and genetic predisposition to problematic alcohol use. While these factors are at play across developmental stages, college student drinking is predominantly considered a contextually limited pattern of use characterized by high rates of alcohol use that often does not persist past students' transition to post-college roles. The tendency for college students to moderate or "mature out of" high rates of drinking is often attributed to their adopting a more conventional lifestyle toward the end of college.[13,19,20] However, a family history of AUD makes it less likely that an individual will experience maturation effects with respect to alcohol use.[19] Severity of use appears to impact maturation effects as well—approximately half of students who meet criteria for an AUD at 19 still meet criteria at 25,[6,22] and heavier involvement with alcohol early in college predicts meeting criteria for an AUD after graduation.[23] More recent nationally representative surveys indicate that this "maturing out" phenomenon may be decreasing, a worrying finding.[24]

Demographics

Sex and Ethnicity

On average, college men drink more often, consume larger quantities of alcohol, and are more likely to engage in heavy episodic drinking than are college women.[3,25] College men are also more likely to meet criteria for an AUD and experience more alcohol-related problems.[26-28] However, it has been hypothesized that current measures of alcohol-related problems emphasize externalizing behavior problems and neglect internalizing problems (eg, drinking related to the management of anxiety and depression), which may be more prevalent in females, suggesting that current estimates may be underrepresenting negative consequences of alcohol use for women.[29] Though the majority of research continues to suggest that men drink more and more often than do women, there is some evidence for an epidemiological shift toward reduced gender differences in alcohol use patterns and alcohol disorders.[30-34] There is also recent evidence to indicate that nonbinary college students drink less frequently than their cisgender peers and are less likely to engage in binge drinking.[35]

Research on both the national and local levels has found that White college students are the most likely to engage in heavy episodic drinking, as well as drinking games.[36] White college students and Indigenous American/Alaskan Native students tend to experience more problems related to drinking than other groups.[18,37] In contrast, African American students are least likely to engage in heavy drinking and are less likely to experience alcohol-related problems, possibly because of more negative alcohol outcome expectancies.[38] Asian American students have rates in between Black and White students.[25] Based on a review of national studies of adolescents and young adults, O'Malley and Johnston estimated that 40% to 50% of non-Hispanic White students engage in heavy episodic drinking, in comparison to 30% to 40% of Hispanic/Latinx and 10% to 20% of African American students.[25] African American female college students drink proportionally less than do African American male students, while the gender difference is less pronounced among Hispanic/Latinx and White students.

While it is true that in general non-Hispanic White students drink at higher rates than their peers of other racial and ethnic backgrounds, this fails to capture circumstances where minority students may be at increased risk for alcohol use as a result of stressors related to their identity. Experiences of discrimination may confer such risks for Black,[39-41] Asian[42] and Latinx,[43,44] students, and should not be ignored as environmental risk factors for negative alcohol-related outcomes in college students.

Sexual Minority Status

College students who are members of the LGBTQ+ community have higher rates of alcohol use[45-47] and binge drinking[48] than their heterosexual peers. These students are at increased risk for alcohol use associated with experiences of minority stressors such as identity-based harassment[49] and discrimination and stigma.[50,51] Little research has investigated how students with multiple minority identities may experience increased risk for alcohol use and alcohol-related consequences as a result of combined minority stressors (eg, both racism and homophobia) and future research is needed to investigate such possible interactions.

Athletics

For both males and females, involvement in athletics at the high school or college level is associated with more frequent drinking, including heavy episodic drinking and other risk behaviors.[52-55] Drinking rates vary from in-season to off-season, resulting in significantly reduced use and/or consequences during the competitive season and increased use and/or consequences when the season ends.[56-59] Students in team sports tend to report higher drinking and binge drinking rates than do students in individual sports.[53,60,61] Expectancies, particularly positive outcome expectancies for alcohol consumption, are associated with heavier drinking by student athletes,[62-66] even though many of these expectancies are placebo effects rather than pharmacological effects of alcohol.[62,63] Increased levels of athletic participation, for example, from nonparticipation to team participation to team captain, is positively associated with increased alcohol use and increased frequency of binge drinking.[52]

One need not be a team member to be at high risk for alcohol-related problems—across 140 colleges, students (team and nonteam members) who rated athletics as important to them (including fans, club sport athletes, and intramural competitors) had higher rates of heavy drinking.[12]

Membership in the Fraternity/Sorority (Greek) System

Fraternity and sorority organizations are environments in which heavy drinking may be considered normative and also seen as a sexuality, friendship, and socialization enhancer.[67,68] Members of the Greek system consume alcohol at greater frequencies and quantities than do their non-Greek peers.[18,69,70] Caudill et al.[69] surveyed more than 3,400 members of a single national fraternity across 32 states and found 97% drank alcohol, 86% reported heavy episodic drinking, and 64% reported frequent heavy episodic drinking (five or more drinks per occasion on three or more occasions in the past 2 weeks). Greek membership has consistently been shown to be a risk factor for heavy episodic drinking, especially among males,[18,68,69,71,72] and both *selection* (heavier drinking students choose to join the Greek system) and *socialization* (peer influence and drinking culture impact the drinking behavior of members after they join) have been found to influence drinking by fraternity and sorority members.[68,70,71] Additionally, membership in the Greek system may confer additional risk for alcohol-related emergency room visits,[73] and for meeting criteria for AUDs later in life.[74] However, there can be a great deal of variability in drinking rates and use of protective behavioral strategies related to drinking within fraternities or sororities,[75] and not all Greek organization members drink heavily or at all.[68]

Veterans and Military Service Members

The U.S. Post-9/11 Veterans Educational Assistance Act of 2008 (*the Post-9/11 GI Bill*) provides over 2 million U.S. veterans who served in either Afghanistan (Operation Enduring Freedom, OEF) or Iraq (Operation Iraqi Freedom, OIF) with the opportunity to attend college full time.[76] Although the Post-9/11 GI Bill gives OEF/OIF veterans access to educational benefits, many veterans return from deployment with physical and psychological challenges that may impede their academic success.[77,78] In particular, research suggests that OEF/OIF veterans have high rates of alcohol use and psychiatric disorders that can interfere with class attendance, decrease grades, and tests scores and lead to withdrawal/dropout from college.[79] High prevalence of PTSD among student veterans confers risk for problematic alcohol use, with severity of PTSD symptoms predicting increased alcohol use[80] and binge drinking.[81,82] Further, the transition from the battlefield to the classroom can be filled with unique stressors that veterans may not be prepared to handle.[83] Despite the potentially negative effects of alcohol use and psychiatric symptoms on academic success among OEF/OIF veterans, relatively little research has examined this relationship. A recent small study ($N = 27$) at a 4-year state university found that 73% of veteran college students who participated reported experiencing a difficult transition from military to college life, 62% felt academically unprepared for college, 21.4% reported a diagnosis of posttraumatic stress disorder (PTSD), and 14.3% reported a diagnosis of depression.[82,83] Other research has shown that veteran college students' past year alcohol use was higher than that of students in general (87.3% versus 82.5%, respectively), but veteran students engage in heavy episodic drinking rate like other students (39.1% versus 36.8%, respectively).[84] Collectively, these data suggest that returning veteran students are at risk for psychiatric symptoms and heavy alcohol consumption, both of which could interfere with their academic success. Please also read Chapter 30 and accompanying sidebar relating to military substance use that directly follow this chapter.

Individual and Environmental Risk Factors

Drinking Expectancies and Motives

Alcohol outcome expectancies refer to the set of beliefs one carries about the positive and negative effects of alcohol consumption and have been shown to predict both current and future alcohol use.[85-90] Drinking expectancies begin to form as early as the third grade.[85] The anticipated valued effects of alcohol consumption (eg, positive expectancies) are stronger predictors of drinking than are possible negative effects (eg, negative expectancies).[86] Positive expectancies have been shown to predict drinking[87] and to differentiate between problem and nonproblem college student drinking[86] and are associated with higher rates of lifetime alcohol use.[85,91] At the daily level, on days with higher alcohol expectancies, students have a higher likelihood of drinking and increased alcohol quantity.[92] Furthermore, positive expectancies have been found to explain a large degree of variance in the relationship between early experiences with alcohol (eg, parental, peer, and media modeling) and subsequent problem drinking in adolescence and in college.[85,93] Positive expectancies for specific drinking events are also associated with less use of alcohol-related protective behavioral strategies, leading to increased likelihood of intoxication and consequences.[94]

Expectancies measured with both explicit (eg, assessing conscious attitudes) and implicit (eg, assessing attitudes that are out of our awareness) measures predict alcohol consumption.[95] Recent evidence indicates that implicit measures predict additional unique variance over explicit measures of alcohol expectancies.[96] Furthermore, expectancies can be primed out of conscious awareness. Friedman et al.[96] presented participants with either an alcohol cue word (eg, drunk, vodka, keg) or a control cue word (eg, cup, tea, ice) for 40 milliseconds during what participants believed to be a lexical decision task. Participants with higher expectancies that alcohol increased sexual desire and who were primed with an alcohol cue word reported increased rating of sexual attraction to pictures presented. This indicates that expectancies influence alcohol use and can operate outside of awareness. Although expectancies are associated with both the onset and maintenance of alcohol use, studies evaluating interventions that challenge expectancies have demonstrated some efficacy, but results have been mixed; therapeutic effects, when present, are not maintained after a short period (ie, 4 weeks).[97]

Expectancies likely develop into motives, or a person's stated reason for drinking or not drinking, over time. Drinking motives are based on anticipated positive or negative reinforcement and predict alcohol use behaviors.[98-102] The most cited drinking motives are conformity—drinking to avoid social costs or rejection, enhancement—drinking to enhance positive mood, social—drinking to obtain positive social rewards, and coping—drinking to regulate negative affect.[98] Of these, social and enhancement motives, or anticipation of positive reinforcements (eg, drinking to induce a positive mood), are most commonly endorsed by college students,[100-102] followed by coping (eg, coping with feelings of depression or anxiety) or negative reinforcement.[103,104] This pattern of motives is consistent across cultures,[105] though college students from individualistic cultures tend to endorse social and enhancement motives more strongly than students from collectivistic cultures.[106]

Different motives are associated with differing patterns of use. In a review of the drinking motive literature for individuals aged 10 to 25, Kuntsche et al.[100] noted that social motives are more typically associated with light, infrequent, nonproblematic use of alcohol and have been shown to be negatively related to heavy drinking and negative consequences. Alternatively, enhancement and coping motives are most strongly associated with heavy alcohol use, and coping motives are further associated with more alcohol-related problems. The well-documented relationship between coping motives (eg, drinking to cope with depressed mood or anxiety) and problematic alcohol use is thought to represent a type of self-medication of emotional distress.[107,108] Although the lack of a strong association between social motives and alcohol-related problems is a reasonably robust finding, recent evidence suggests that this association may differ by gender. LaBrie et al.[101] demonstrated that for women college students, social drinking motives not only predicted quantity of alcohol consumption but also were directly associated with alcohol-related consequences, calling for more study of women's unique reasons for alcohol use and consequences.

Beyond a direct relationship to alcohol use behaviors, drinking motives have been found to mediate the relationship between a range of genetic, environmental, and individual difference factors and alcohol use[109-117] as well as mood states and alcohol-related consequences.[118-120] LaBrie et al.[121] examined the role of college adjustment and found that poor adjustment mediated the relationship between coping motives and drinking consequences, highlighting the importance of interventions to help students decrease stress and develop good coping skills. Drinking motives also appear to change with age and developmental stage. Littlefield et al.[122] prospectively assessed individuals over a 16-year period, beginning at the first year of college. They found that enhancement motives decreased from age 18 to 35, as did alcohol-related problems.

Social Norms and Misperceptions

One of the major forms of human learning is facilitated by the process of modeling—whereby one individual or group displays a behavior that others imitate. One consistent finding is that college students overestimate the rates at which other college students drink,[68] the amount they consume when drinking,[123] and the extent to which other students support heavy drinking[29] and risky drinking.[124] The degree to which students overestimate other students' drinking predicts their own increased consumption,[125,126] an overestimation that is among the strongest predictors of college student drinking when controlling for a variety of other individual risk factors.[127] Overestimation of other students' approval of heavy drinking likewise predicts increased alcohol consumption.[121,128] Identification with a specific reference group (eg, same sex, same race, same sexual orientation, same Greek status) within a larger reference group (college students) is a moderator of the relationship between perceived group drinking norms and own drinking levels such that the greater the identification with the group the more similar the individual drinking levels.[128,129]

Environmental Risk and Protective Factors

Environmental factors can also influence alcohol consumption, and college students have been found to seek out environments that facilitate binge drinking.[130-132] Presley and colleagues noted that the cost of alcohol in and surrounding the campus environment is related to alcohol use such that as the total cost to drink increases, consumption decreases.[25,133] This has significant implications for colleges surrounded by bars frequently offering drink specials or "happy hour" promotions in which the cost of a drink is dramatically reduced for a limited amount of time (which hastens the rate of consumption).[25] The authors also note that when multiple drinking venues exist, long-term and short-term drinking problems increase. Clapp and Shillington[134] found that, among other predictors, students who were in a setting where many people were intoxicated were almost 13 times more likely to report consumption of five or more drinks.

Events associated with high rates of drinking are generally well known (eg, New Year's eve, St. Patrick's Day, spring break, Halloween, and high-profile sporting events) or may be personal (eg, 21st birthdays, graduations, or celebrating major accomplishments).[135,136] Consuming alcohol prior to departing for one's intended social activity or eventual destination is referred to as "prepartying," "pregaming," "front loading," "preloading," or "prefunking."[137] Increased blood alcohol concentrations and a higher incidence of consequences are associated with prepartying."[138-140] particularly for women.[141] One-third of students who violate their campus alcohol policy prepartied on the night the violation occurred.[142] For those who preparty at least once per month, the type of alcohol consumed varies by gender[143] and, up to 50% of the time, involves the playing of "drinking games." Drinking games can be as simple as having everyone drink when a word or phrase is uttered during a movie, can be time-focused (eg, one sip per minute), can be team sport-focused such that losers of a game must drink (eg, "beer pong"), or could be quite complicated with a range of rules surrounding gambling, card games, motor skills, or verbal skills.[142] Drinking games have been identified as a risk factor for "problematic" drinking[21] and have been associated with heavy drinking episodes[134] and alcohol-related consequences.[144] In some places, there is a birthday tradition of downing one shot of hard liquor for every year of age. This behavior increases risks for frank alcohol poisoning and/or aspiration of vomitus.

Involvement in athletics is associated with risk for higher rates of drinking and for consequences associated with alcohol consumption,[21,145] and drinking-game participation can be associated with risky drinking for those involved in athletics.[146-148] Yet, the culture surrounding collegiate sporting events seems to also influence and be influenced by alcohol with many students and alumni participating in "tailgating," significant sporting events being associated with increased drinking, a high frequency of alcohol advertising aired during televised sports, and the general association of alcohol with celebration.[135,145,149]

Environmental variables can serve as protective factors against high-risk drinking. Many colleges have seen the emergence of designated substance-free housing options and 12-step recovery groups on campus. Students may self-select into various living options (eg, Greek systems, residence halls, and substance-free housing). Research suggests that living in a designated substance-free housing environment, even for those who drink, is a protective factor for negative consequences (eg, heavy episodic drinking) and is associated with increased use of preventive behaviors (eg, decreasing drinking-game involvement and increasing use of strategies for altering one's approach to drinking).[150] Clapp and Shillington[134] found that the only protective variable associated with lower risk of heavy episodic drinking was whether the event in which drinking occurred was a date. In attempting to explain this finding, the authors speculate that students who are dating may be less likely to use alcohol as a "social lubricant" and suggest that additional research is needed to further examine this apparent protective factor.

PREVENTION STRATEGIES AND INTERVENTIONS

College Drinking Prevention Strategies

Considerable research has focused on development of prevention and intervention approaches for the college student population. The NIAAA's influential 2002 report of the Task Force on College Drinking[151] represented the joint efforts of researchers and college presidents to address the harms of and solutions to college drinking. The Task Force report designated four tiers of prevention strategies:

- Tier I interventions have documented and replicated evidence of efficacy in college populations. Interventions may be delivered in an individual or group setting with a facilitator.
- Tier II interventions have documented evidence of efficacy in general populations and could be adapted for college students.
- Tier III interventions show logical and theoretical promise but need more research.
- Tier IV interventions show no evidence of effectiveness.

The Task Force report was accompanied by increased college drinking prevention research supported by the NIAAA, the Department of Education, and the Substance Abuse and Mental Health Services Administration (SAMHSA). In addition, several comprehensive reviews of the prevention literature have been conducted after the Task Force report,[152-160] and the report was updated in 2007 to reflect these findings.[161]

In 2015, the NIAAA created the College Alcohol Intervention Matrix (CollegeAIM) to help college administrators review findings regarding the cost and effectiveness of college drinking interventions and choose the optimal mix of strategies for their campuses[161] and this resource continues to be updated to reflect the most recent research. Thus, there has been considerable progress and a growing consensus to find what works in college drinking prevention. It is also important that the interventions that colleges select for their students be suitable for the populations of students they serve. Thus, where available, data are included here on the effectiveness of these interventions for student subpopulations by demographic and other relevant characteristics. Some of this information is relatively limited in nature, and it is to be hoped that future research will lead to additional information on the validity and effectiveness of these interventions with populations of students who have historically been minoritized.

Individually Focused Interventions

Each intervention listed in Tier I (having documented empirical evidence of efficacy) of the NIAAA Task Force report on College Drinking[151] has an individually focused intervention component. Research supporting the efficacy of these approaches has typically evaluated their use with students mandated to treatment (eg, sanctioned to complete a program after a policy violation), first-year students with high risk drinking, students within the Greek system, individuals who screen positive for AUDs in either a health or a counseling center setting, as well as other groups of students on campus. Additionally, studies have examined peer versus professional delivery and the efficacy and benefits of web-based delivery of interventions.

Multicomponent Skills-Based Interventions

Multicomponent skills-based interventions (eg, the Alcohol Skills Training Program—ASTP) typically combine cognitive-behavioral skills training (eg, identifying and planning for or avoiding risky situations; using protective behavioral strategies such as drink spacing, counting drinks, and setting limits to reduce intoxication during drinking events; discussing myths about alcohol's effects; and communicating assertively about drinking decisions) with norm clarification (eg, correcting misperceptions about drinking norms, exploring assumptions that everybody drinks), using a motivational interviewing (MI) style to reduce resistance and promote change.[162] The CollegeAIM[161] reviewed 32 studies including a multicomponent skills intervention and found that 20 of 32 produced statistically significant reductions in alcohol use, harmful consequences due to drinking, or both. Methodologically, stronger studies (eg, larger samples, longer follow-up, appropriate control groups) were the most likely to report statistically significant effects of the multicomponent skills approach. Culturally informed translations of skills-based interventions have shown equivalent effectiveness with Latino college students.[163]

Expectancy Challenge Interventions

The second Tier I cognitive-behavioral intervention is expectancy challenge interventions, which are aimed at changing students' positive expectations for alcohol intoxication and are delivered by two methods. The first method is experiential, and this intervention is classified as "moderate effectiveness" by the current iteration of CollegeAIM. Participants are informed that they will either be receiving alcohol or a placebo, and the alcohol placebo effect is directly applied to demonstrate how one's expectations about drinking influence their experience. As part of the intervention, students are told they are drinking alcohol but actually receive a nonalcoholic drink (ie, a placebo). These students still show the social or interpersonal effects associated with drinking for them (eg, they become more social, talkative). Alternatively, students are told they are not drinking alcohol when their beverage is actually alcoholic. These students do not exhibit the expected social effects of alcohol; instead, they feel some of the physical effects of drinking (eg, feel sleepy, flushed) but attribute these feelings to factors other than alcohol.

The second method is didactic, wherein students are educated about these phenomena (eg, discussion of alcohol myths, such as "I cannot be outgoing at a party without alcohol," and placebo effects). Initial reviews suggested that demonstrations of the placebo effect were associated with reduced alcohol use at short-term follow-up for college males.[155,164] Education about the placebo effect alone did not show the same effect in reducing drinking. More recent reviews found that 6 of 13 studies using experiential demonstrations of the alcohol placebo effect produced short-term reductions in alcohol use.[161] Again, these results were more consistent for men than women.[165] A recent review of expectancy challenge interventions (both experiential and didactic) found decreases in alcohol consumption in 12 of 18 studies.[166] Although one study[167] suggested that education about the placebo effect may have harmful effects (increased drinking postintervention) for women, two more recent studies[168,169] found that demonstrating the placebo effect was associated with reductions in alcohol use for both men and women.

Overall, results regarding the efficacy of expectancy challenge interventions are encouraging but mixed and suggest that implementation of expectancy challenges in single-gender groups may be more effective than mixed-gender challenges, especially for women[165] and that experiential expectancy challenge interventions are superior. Practical issues regarding the demonstration of the placebo effect (eg, administering alcohol to college students as part of the intervention) may limit wider application of this approach, though there has been a recent trend towards web-based versions of this intervention, to deliver the content in a more scalable, less resource intensive way.[170]

Brief Motivational Interventions

Motivational Intervention (MI), based on the work of Miller and Rollnick[162] is a nonjudgmental, nonconfrontational approach that emphasizes meeting people where they are regarding their readiness to change. For example, when people are ambivalent about changing a behavior (eg, problematic alcohol use), MI can be used to explore and resolve that ambivalence, and when people have not yet considered change, MI strategies can be used to prompt thinking about change. There is strong evidence and growing consensus that brief, in-person motivational feedback interventions (typically incorporating assessment and feedback regarding alcohol use, norms, and consequences) or brief motivational interventions (BMIs) are effective in reducing and preventing excessive alcohol use and related harm in college populations.[153,154,158-160,170-174] Brief motivational interventions for college student drinking are classified as either "higher effectiveness" for individual interventions or "moderate effectiveness" for group interventions—though group interventions have a much greater reach with equivalent facilitation resources.

Listed in the Task Force report as a Tier I intervention, Brief Alcohol Screening and Intervention for College Students (BASICS) developed by Marlatt et al.[175-177] includes a comprehensive assessment followed by a 1-hour personalized feedback interview. The interview is delivered in MI style, using specific strategies such as open questions, reflective listening, summarizing key observations or points, and supporting and affirming the student. The approach is designed to elicit personally relevant reasons for change (eg, change talk) and the adoption of cognitive-behavioral strategies to implement the desired changes. The interview is structured around a review of graphic feedback generated from the assessment (**Table 29-1**).

Larimer and Cronce reviewed 40 BMI studies of college drinking, most involving BASICS or similar interventions, and found that 36 of 40 were associated with reductions in alcohol use, consequences, or both, across follow-up periods up to 4 years.[153,154,159,160] Alcohol-related consequences and amount or pattern of alcohol use (rather than abstinence from alcohol) are the typical outcomes assessed in BMI studies of college students. Recent research has also suggested that personalized BMI content is more effective at reducing alcohol use and related problems than nonpersonalized BMI content (which can often vary between studies).[178-180] A meta-analysis[180] indicated that effect sizes for these interventions were generally in the small-to-medium range, with effects on alcohol use emerging within 1 month and effects on consequences emerging 6 months or more after intervention. Some research, though not all, suggests that effects weaken or decay by a 12-month follow-up.

A diagnosis of AUD during adolescence/young adulthood is relatively unstable compared to later in life. The natural trajectory of alcohol use in college and young adulthood is for a reduction in use over time even without intervention or within the control group.[6,175,180,181] Thus, brief motivational interventions may work to hasten the natural developmental progression out of high-risk drinking. In contrast, some research suggests that BMI effects persist or emerge over longer follow-up periods, up to 4 years post intervention.[182,183] Studies have successfully employed BMI approaches in both group[184] and individual formats,[168,185] with men,[185] women,[184] mixed genders,[168] and high-risk volunteers,[175] as well as mandated or judicially referred students.[183,186,187]

BASICS and similar interventions have been adapted and tested in a variety of subpopulations of students. Examples include students with ADHD,[188] and depression.[189] Further, this strategy has been successfully implemented in a variety of settings, including campus health clinics[190,191] and fraternities.[185] A majority of BMI studies focused on efficacy of this technique; however, newer studies have looked at effectiveness.[192] Thus, this type of intervention appears to be flexible

TABLE 29-1 Clinical Example of Brief Motivational Intervention (BASICS)

In the clinical case excerpt example below, "Tiffany," a college student, and a BASICS facilitator, as part of the feedback session, review the student's peak blood alcohol level (BAL) in the past month, an episode where she reported having consumed 14 drinks in 2 hours with a corresponding estimated BAL of 0.39. As is common in BASICS sessions, the facilitator noted that the student had been saying two, almost opposite, things during the earlier part of the session. On the one hand, she repeatedly reported that alcohol was not causing any serious problems in her life, while on the other hand, Tiffany reported notable negative consequences (eg, missing school, getting into fights, neglecting responsibilities) and concerns about her drinking habits. It was the facilitator's goal to hold both of these perspectives in mind and to reflect this disparity.

- Facilitator: "So, what do you make of that?"
- Student: "I don't know. That's kind of scary, but I don't know."
- Facilitator: "It's a little bit surprising."
- Student: "Yeah. I didn't think it would be that high."
- Facilitator: "Cause, like you said, you felt like you were safe [even though] you experienced a blackout."
- Student: "Yeah. I would never drink that much again though."

This last statement is a clear example of what is called *change talk.* Eliciting change talk is a key component of motivational approaches as the presence of change talk is associated with later reductions in alcohol use and improved outcomes.

The full BASICS intervention had a positive impact on Tiffany's alcohol use. Compared to her baseline consumption of 28 drinks per week, 3 months later, Tiffany was averaging 11 drinks per week. Her drinking reduced from 4 to 2 drinks per week and was associated with fewer alcohol-related problems. Her frequency of engaging in high-risk binge drinking, like the episode discussed above, had reduced from eight to three times per month. In addition, Tiffany reported key modifications to her pattern of drinking. For example, she increased the amount of time over which her drinks were consumed resulting in lower BACs.

and robust, reliably producing drinking reductions in a wide segment of the campus population in efficacy studies. BASICS has also been adapted for Latino students and is equally effective when delivered in English and Spanish.[193] Adaptations for use with Indigenous students attending tribal colleges and universities are still in progress.[194] Recent developments in BMIs include web-based delivery to reduce resources, and results of these adaptations are promising.[195]

Though BASICS and related motivational interventions have substantial evidence of efficacy and have been successfully utilized in a variety of settings, there are barriers to the more widespread utilization of this approach. Specifically, the approach requires the availability of trained providers and the resources and time to meet individually or in small groups with students. Some of these barriers can be reduced through the use of trained peers to provide the intervention[185,196] rather than professional providers and/or the integration of brief interventions into health or mental health settings through training of existing providers.[190]

Nonetheless, most campuses do not have the resources to extend in-person BASICS to all students who would benefit from intervention, nor do all students who would benefit want to attend an in-person session. As a result, researchers and practitioners have begun to evaluate more cost-effective methods for reaching a broader audience of students, using minimal intervention strategies such as provision of written, mailed, or internet-based motivational feedback.

Feedback-Only Interventions

As MI-based interventions are resource intensive, studies have evaluated the extent to which in-person intervention improves efficacy in comparison to feedback alone. Results of this research are encouraging.

The CollegeAIM reviewed 31 interventions involving an assessment component and a mailed, computerized, or written motivational feedback component.[161] Twenty-six of 31 interventions were associated with reductions in alcohol use after intervention. A mailed feedback and tips intervention was found to both prevent initiation of drinking among abstainers and reduce likelihood of heavy drinking among heavy episodic consumers at a 1-year follow-up.[197]

Two studies found no differences between in-person and mailed or written feedback, though neither study included an assessment-only control condition.[186,197] A meta-analysis by Carey et al.[180] found that effect sizes were largest for in-person, individual motivational feedback interventions as compared to mailed/computerized interventions. Nevertheless, they found that feedback alone was associated with significant reductions in drinking. A meta-analysis identified nine studies that evaluated the effects of computerized and Web-based normative feedback in reducing drinking and drinking-related harms.[198] These interventions provide simple information comparing the participant's own use to his or her perceptions of the typical college student's drinking pattern and the actual norm for college students.[199] All nine studies found reductions in alcohol use over follow-up periods ranging from 1 to 6 months.

Evidence suggests that gender-specific information (ie, comparison to typical same-sex college student) improves outcomes for both men and women as compared to gender-neutral information with larger effects for women who identified strongly with typical college females.[200] Recent studies indicate that these interventions may be effective only for students who are motivated to participate.[201] Taken together, these findings suggest that minimal interventions involving mailed or computerized feedback may be an important addition to the overall college drinking prevention toolbox, though BMIs may be a superior choice for students whose motivation to change behaviors needs enhancement.

An even simpler behavioral approach has shown efficacy in several recent studies of college drinking prevention. Specifically, Larimer and Cronce reviewed five studies of self-monitoring or self-assessment of alcohol use and/or consequences in the absence of other intervention strategies.[153,154,159,160] Four of five studies reported significant reductions in alcohol use and/or consequences. For example, Carey et al.[202] found that adding a timeline followback interview (a method for assessing drinking in detail daily over the past 3 months) to a standard assessment[203] resulted in reductions in peak and typical quantity as well as frequency of heavy consumption at a 1-month follow-up. This beneficial effect of recalling and reporting one's drinking levels to others may also contribute to increased self-awareness of harmful drinking patterns and to the overall efficacy of approaches utilizing screening and brief intervention methods.[13,155]

Pharmacotherapy

There is a lack of research on the use of pharmacotherapy (disulfiram, naltrexone, acamprosate) with college students for the treatment of AUD. This may in part be caused by the lack of college students who self-refer for treatment. A large proportion of college students receiving treatment may be under mandatory requirements, and they might not be informed about or inclined towards using medication. They might also be reluctant to use a medication that may lead to discomfort such as nausea when consumed alongside alcohol. One study examined the effects of naltrexone on alcohol drinking, urge to drink alcohol, and alcohol-induced sensations and mood in individuals near college age (participant age range, 21-32 years old).[204] The double-blind, placebo-controlled study found that individuals using naltrexone drank relatively less alcohol and drank alcohol more slowly. There was no significant difference found in urge to drink. These findings suggest that medication may be helpful in decreasing amount of drinking. However, the challenge remains in motivating college students to seek pharmacotherapy for AUD.

Structural Interventions

With data clearly supporting the use of brief interventions with high-risk or at-risk college students, optimism surrounds efforts to decrease harm and risk among college students who choose to drink alcohol. An important factor in the success of these efforts, however, is addressing the context in which alcohol use is occurring. Therefore, efforts to intervene at the level of environment are considered key. Recognizing the importance of context, the NIAAA Task Force on College Drinking[151] and their CollegeAIM[161] outlined several environmentally focused approaches.

With the amount of empirical data varying across approaches, these environmental strategies correspondingly vary between Tier II (strategies with demonstrated effectiveness with general populations) and Tier III (promising approaches that need further study). The report encouraged colleges to consider implementing these approaches as part of their overall strategic plan and to assist in evaluating strategies with less of an established evidence base to add to the field's understanding of "what works." Such approaches[151,161] include the following:

- Increased enforcement of minimum drinking age laws (Tier II). Despite interest in lowering the drinking age (eg, the "Amethyst Initiative" introduced in 2008), most studies have indicated that higher legal drinking ages are associated with reduced alcohol consumption, and over half demonstrate that higher legal drinking ages are associated with decreased rates of traffic crashes.[151,161] Despite conventional wisdom that lower drinking ages in European countries are associated with more moderate consumption patterns and reduced harm, cross-cultural research with college students indicates that young adult college students in countries with lower drinking ages drink more and have more alcohol-related consequences than U.S. students.[205]
- Increased publicity about and enforcement of underage drinking laws on campus and eliminating "mixed messages" (Tier III).[151,161]
- Restrictions on alcohol retail outlet density (Tier II). Research shows that higher outlet density, particularly around college campuses, is associated with increased binge drinking.[151,161]
- Consistently enforcing disciplinary actions associated with policy violations (Tier III). The NIAAA noted that failure to do so may suggest that "rules were made to be broken (p. 22)."[151]
- Informing new students and their parents about alcohol policies and penalties before arrival and during orientation periods.[151]

The list above represents only a sample of the various approaches listed by the NIAAA; any one strategy implemented on a college campus must be part of an overall strategic plan that may need multiple components to enhance success.

DeJong and Langford[206] recommend a college-focused prevention typology that identifies environmental change as one of the four areas of intervention. They outline five subcategories of strategic interventions within their environmental change category:

i. Promoting alcohol-free options (eg, creating or promoting alcohol-free events, publicizing volunteer opportunities, expanding hours for alcohol-free settings, promoting consumption of nonalcoholic beverages at events).
ii. Creating an environment that supports health-promoting norms (eg, modifying the academic schedule, offering substance-free residence halls, increasing faculty–student contact, creating programs to correct student misperceptions of drinking norms).
iii. Limiting alcohol availability on- and off-campus (eg, banning or restricting use of alcohol on campus, instituting responsible server training programs, limiting number and concentration of alcohol outlets near campus).
iv. Restricting alcohol promotion and marketing on- and off-campus (eg, banning or restricting alcohol advertising on campus, banning alcohol promotions with special appeal to underage people who drink, instituting cooperative agreements to limit special drink promotions).
v. Developing and enforcing policies and laws surrounding alcohol consumption (eg, revising campus policy as needed, increasing checks of identification at on-campus functions, increasing disciplinary sanctions for violation of campus policies).

In a discussion of specific high-risk events associated with problematic college drinking, Neighbors et al.[135] provide a number of recommendations involving environmental-level interventions for spring break, a notably high-risk situation with both heightened frequency of consumption and negative consequences (eg, sexual assault, legal involvement, lethal intoxication). Recommendations include inviting parents to visit campus during spring break, providing alternative activities (eg, community service trips), advertising lower-risk activities early before students plan spring break trips, and encouraging faculty to schedule major papers or exams the week after spring break. Similarly, when considering prevention of risky drinking games, another activity associated with increased alcohol consumption and negative consequences, Borsari[207] noted the importance of providing social alternatives to drinking games and taking steps to ensure students are aware of non-drinking-related activities as part of an environmental strategy.

Steps can be taken to promote an environment that may increase the effectiveness of minimum drinking age laws.[208] Keeling[209] found that laws restricting underage drinking and governing the volume of sales are associated with lower levels of drinking. Because inconsistent and ineffective enforcement of drinking laws is often a problem, Kypri et al.[210] stress the importance of effective communication surrounding laws, including clear definitions of key terms in increasing the impact of alcohol-focused regulations. For example, there is no clear definition of *intoxication*. It may refer to visible signs of inebriation or that an individual has consumed alcohol and it is affecting behavior (even if it is not obvious). More clarity could aid in enforcement.

As recognized by the NIAAA Task Force,[101] community-based interventions have demonstrated efficacy in reducing alcohol use and related consequences.[2,211,212] Although only a subset of these interventions has been specifically developed for use with younger people who drink, all programs included major targets related to alcohol use in teenagers and young adults and are relevant to college drinking issues. Programs have differed widely on key factors (eg, selection and makeup of targeted communities, intervention strategies, outcomes assessed), and currently, little is known about comparative efficacy. These factors aside, community-based interventions demonstrated significant reduction in alcohol sales to minors, alcohol consumption, self-reported drinking and driving, automotive crashes involving alcohol, and alcohol-related fatal crashes.[212] When the community and college or university campus both stand to benefit from efforts aiming to reduce consumption or related consequences, use of a campus-community coalition has been encouraged.[206]

A campus-community coalition typically assembles key stakeholders from both settings who can collaborate in efforts to reduce alcohol use problems on campus and in the surrounding area. Stakeholders generally include faculty, student leaders, administrators, staff (residence life, counseling center, health center, etc.), police, bar or restaurant owners, or landlords near campus. Clapp and Stanger[213] detail four examples in which a coalition (eg, the Collegiate-Community Alcohol Prevention Partnership) successfully worked with bars frequented by students to provide responsible beverage service training and to take steps toward modifying advertising practices, took steps to halt a bus provided by a bar in a Mexican border town that was unsafely transporting students, provided students with tips on hosting a safe party, and worked to remove paraphernalia associated with the promotion of heavy drinking from campus stores.

Since the original NIAAA Task Force report,[151] community-based interventions such as these have been applied specifically to college campuses.[208] As research efforts have begun to generate a small body of literature, studies have increasingly used more rigorous designs (eg, control/comparison campus). Like community-based programs, college community programs differ in intervention strategies and other key variables.[214] As outlined by Saltz,[214] results of studies are promising with interventions providing reductions in target alcohol-related behaviors. However, it is not known what combination of strategies will have the greatest impact, what is the most efficient manner to implement the strategies, and what is needed for universities to adopt these strategies.

CONCLUSIONS AND FUTURE DIRECTIONS

Alcohol use on college campuses is an important health, safety, liability, and risk management issue. Advances have been made in identifying effective strategies to reduce alcohol consumption and associated consequences. Increasingly, colleges and universities are recognizing the need for a strategic plan with multiple components, targets, and delivery strategies as they seek to reduce the harm associated with college student drinking.

Alcohol use does not occur in a vacuum, and attention should be paid to the context of college student alcohol use. In addition to reported alcohol use, 46% of college students also report the use of an illicit drug in the past year, 44% of students report past-year use of cannabis, and 16% of students report past-year use of any illicit drug other than cannabis.[3] In addition, a recent trend is for individuals to combine alcohol use with increasingly available and popular over-the-counter caffeinated energy drinks. This combination is uniquely problematic as the stimulant properties of these drinks can mask the depressant effects of alcohol, leading to the subjective impression that a person is less impaired.[215] The resulting lack of objective awareness may interfere with judgment regarding continued alcohol intake or engagement in activities where high levels of intoxication are increasingly dangerous. Efforts to prevent or intervene in unhealthy alcohol use in college students will need to consider these related behaviors. Future research efforts will need to more consistently measure the impact on other drug use when alcohol is the focus of prevention or intervention efforts and identify effective strategies for working with college students who use multiple substances. Prevention efforts targeted towards simultaneous alcohol and cannabis use may be increasingly important as cannabis continues to be legalized across the United States.

Also related to the context of student alcohol use are co-occurring mental health problems. In a national survey of counseling center directors conducted in 2014, 94% of directors felt that psychological problems were becoming more severe.[216] Schwartz[217] documented a more than fivefold increase in students prescribed a psychotropic medication on college campuses between 1992 and 2002. More recent surveys indicate that these trends towards increased mental health diagnoses among college students are continuing.[218,219] A number of explanations have been suggested for the perceived increase in the severity of mental health disorders on college campuses, including increased management of depression, anxiety, and behavioral/learning issues with psychotropic medications (allowing attendance of more severely ill students that otherwise would not have attended college), students using alcohol and drugs while on medication (resulting in an accentuation of depressant effects), or students stopping use of medication when entering college because, among other possible reasons, they want to use alcohol or other drugs instead.[220] Given success with brief interventions focused on depression[221] and alcohol,[154] future research must consider strategies to address the overlap of mental health issues and substance use.

Research to date indicates that BMIs utilizing assessment and individualized, in-person feedback are consistently efficacious in reducing alcohol use across college student settings and effectiveness trials on college campuses have supported these findings. In addition, cognitive-behavioral skills-based interventions have clear evidence of efficacy. Given the difficulties with engaging students in in-person interventions on college campuses, integration of these resources into existing points of contact (including academic courses, residence halls, Greek social organizations, student services, and campus health and mental health settings) holds promise for reaching students in need of services.

Although it may seem intuitive to screen for alcohol problems in a campus health setting, the data suggest that this is not a widespread practice. Although approximately one-third of health centers at 4-year colleges or universities routinely screen for alcohol problems, only 17% of these used standardized instruments as part of their screening.[222] Thus, in addition to integrating services into points of contact, reliable and valid screening strategies should be used.[223]

There is also reason for promise as various delivery strategies are considered. Given the success of mailed and computerized feedback,[199,215,224] the widespread implementation of online screening and brief feedback interventions is now feasible on college campuses. Several commercially available computerized screening and intervention products have emerged, and many are reviewed in the NIAAA CollegeAIM[161] resources.

In considering prevention and intervention strategies for college student alcohol use, future research is needed to assess efficacy and effectiveness of current best practices and interventions for minoritized college student communities.[225] Culturally informed adaptations of current interventions may be indicated to serve these college student subpopulations more effectively.[226]

Although there are documented barriers to dissemination, adoption, implementation, and maintenance of empirically tested approaches, fortunately, these barriers are surmountable.[227] College student alcohol use and associated consequences are not unique problems on any one campus. Rather, there are shared challenges across campuses and increasingly shared successes. As colleges and universities move toward developing campus–community coalitions and involvement in cooperative statewide coalitions, efforts to impact college student health move beyond the responsibility of the individual campus, allowing for shared knowledge and resources. With ever-changing and ever-growing student populations and venues for higher education, the challenge is not only to meet current needs but also to adapt to needs as they shift with demographic changes as well as structural ones.

ACKNOWLEDGMENT

This chapter represents an update and revision of previous chapters in this series, most recently by Dr Joyce N. Bittinger from the last edition. We are indebted to Dr Bittinger for her work and retain much of her prose in this current edition.

REFERENCES

1. National Institute on Alcohol Abuse and Alcoholism. *What Colleges Need to Know: An Update on College Drinking Research.* U.S. Department of Health and Human Services, Public Health Service, National Institutes of Health; 2007.
2. Hingson R, Zha W, Smyth D. Magnitude and trends in heavy episodic drinking, alcohol-impaired driving, and alcohol-related mortality and overdose hospitalizations among emerging adults of college ages 18–24 in the United States, 1998–2014. *J Stud Alcohol Drugs.* 2017;78(4):540-548.
3. Schulenberg JE, Patrick ME, Johnston LD, O'Malley PM, Bachman JG, Miech RA. Monitoring the Future National Survey Results on Drug Use, 1975-2020. *College Students & Adults Ages 19-60.* Volume II Institute for Social Research; 2021.
4. Arterberry BJ, Brooke J, Boyd CJ, West BT, Schepis TS, McCabe SE. DSM-5 substance use disorders among college-age young adults in the United States: prevalence, remission and treatment. *J Am Coll Health.* 2020;68(6):650-657.
5. Kim H, Rackoff GN, Fitzsimmons-Craft EE, et al. College mental health before and during the COVID-19 pandemic: results from a nationwide survey. *Cognit Ther Res.* 2022;46(1):1-10.
6. Sher KJ, Gotham HJ. Pathological alcohol involvement: a developmental disorder of young adulthood. *Dev Psychopathol.* 1999;11:933-956.
7. National Institute on Alcohol Abuse and Alcoholism. *High-Risk Drinking in College: What We Know and What We Need to Learn: Final Report of the Panel on Contexts and Consequences: Epidemiology of Alcohol Use Among College Students.* U.S. Department of Health and Human Services, Public Health Service, National Institutes of Health; 2002.
8. Silveri MM. Adolescent brain development and underage drinking in the United States: identifying risks of alcohol use in college populations. *Harv Rev Psychiatry.* 2012;20(4):189-200.
9. Wechsler H, Dowdall GW, Maenner G, et al. Changes in binge drinking and related problems among American college students between 1993 and 1997: results of the Harvard School of Public Health College Alcohol Study. *J Am Coll Health.* 1998;47(2):57-68.
10. Singleton RA. Collegiate alcohol consumption and academic performance. *J Stud Alcohol Drugs.* 2007;68:548-555.
11. Piazza-Gardner AK, Barry AE, Merianos AL. Assessing drinking and academic performance among a nationally representative sample of college students. *J Drug Issues.* 2016;46(4):347-353.
12. Wechsler H, Lee JE, Kuo M, et al. Trends in college binge drinking during a period of increased prevention efforts: findings from 4 Harvard School of Public Health College Alcohol Study surveys: 1993–2001. *J Am Coll Health.* 2002;50:203-217.
13. Roark ML. Conceptualizing campus violence: definitions, underlying factors, and effects. *J Coll Stud Psychother.* 1993;8:1-27.
14. Hingson RW, Zha W, Weitzman ER. Magnitude of and trends in alcohol-related mortality and morbidity among U.S. college students ages 18–24, 1998–2005. *J Stud Alcohol Drugs Suppl.* 2009;(16):12-20.
15. Wechsler H, Nelson TF. What we have learned from the Harvard School of Public Health College Alcohol Study: focusing attention on college student alcohol consumption and the environmental conditions that promote it. *J Stud Alcohol.* 2008;69(4):481-490.
16. Mohler-Kuo M, Dowdall GW, Koss MP, et al. Correlates of rape while intoxicated in a national sample of college women. *J Stud Alcohol.* 2004;65:37-45.
17. Reed E, Amaro H, Matsumoto A, Kaysen D. The relation between interpersonal violence and substance use among a sample of university students: examination of the role of victim and perpetrator substance use. *Addict Behav.* 2009;34(3):316-318.
18. Wechsler H, Dowdall GW, Davenport A, et al. Correlates of college student binge drinking. *Am J Public Health.* 1995;85(7):921-926.
19. Wechsler H, Lee JE, Kuo M, et al. College binge drinking in the 1990s: a continuing problem. Results of the Harvard School of Public Health 1999 College Alcohol Study. *J Am Coll Health.* 2000;48:199-210.
20. Milo KJ, McEuen VS. *Negative Publicity: Its Effect on Institutional Reputation and Student College Choice.* Accessed May 23, 2023. https://files.eric.ed.gov/fulltext/ED320181.pdf
21. Ham LS, Hope DA. College students and problematic drinking: a review of the literature. *Clin Psychol Rev.* 2003;23(5):719-759.
22. Rohde P, Lewinsohn PM, Kahler CW, Seeley JR, Brown RA. Natural course of alcohol use disorders from adolescence to young adulthood. *J Am Acad Child Adolesc Psychiatry.* 2001;40(1):83-90.
23. Prince MA, Read JP, Colder CR. Trajectories of college alcohol involvement and their associations with later alcohol use disorder symptoms. *Prev Sci.* 2019;20(5):741-752.
24. Lee MR, Sher KJ. "Maturing out" of binge and problem drinking. *Alcohol Res.* 2018;39(1):31.

25. Presley CA, Meilman PW, Leichliter JS. College factors that influence drinking. *J Stud Alcohol Suppl.* 2002;14:82-90.
26. Clements R. Prevalence of alcohol-use disorders and alcohol-related problems in a college student sample. *J Am Coll Health.* 1999;48(3):111-118.
27. Hill EM, Chow K. Life-history theory and risky drinking. *Addiction.* 2002;97(4):401-413.
28. Read JP, Wood MD, Davidoff OJ, et al. Making the transition from high school to college: the role of alcohol-related social influence factors in students' drinking. *Subst Abus.* 2002;23(1):53-65.
29. Perkins HW. Surveying the damage: a review of research on consequences of alcohol misuse in college populations. *J Stud Alcohol Suppl.* 2002;(14):91-100.
30. Keyes KM, Grant BF, Hasin DS. Evidence for a closing gender gap in alcohol use, abuse, and dependence in the United States population. *Drug Alcohol Depend.* 2008;93(1–2):21-29.
31. Holdcraft LC, Iacono WG. Cohort effects on gender differences in alcohol dependence. *Addiction.* 2002;97:1025-1036.
32. Rice JP, Neuman RJ, Saccone NL, et al. Age and birth cohort effects on rates of alcohol dependence. *Alcohol Clin Exp Res.* 2003;27:93-99.
33. Kuntsche E, Kuntsche S, Knibbe R, et al. Cultural and gender convergence in adolescent drunkenness: evidence from 23 European and North American countries. *Arch Pediatr Adolesc Med.* 2011;165(2):152-158.
34. White AM. Gender differences in the epidemiology of alcohol use and related harms in the United States. *Alcohol Res.* 2020;40(2):01.
35. Dinger MK, Brittain DR, Patten L, et al. Gender identity and health-related outcomes in a national sample of college students. *Am J Health Educ.* 2020;51(6):383-394.
36. Wegner R, Roy AR, DaCova A, Gorman KR. Similarities and differences in general drinking game behavior, game-specific behavior, and peer influence factors across race/ethnicity. *Am J Orthopsychiatry.* 2019;89(5):616.
37. O'Malley PM, Johnston LD. Epidemiology of alcohol and other drug use among American college students. *J Stud Alcohol Suppl.* 2002;(14):23-39.
38. Thorpe S, Tanner AE, Ware S, Guastaferro K, Milroy JJ, Wyrick DL. Black first-year college students' alcohol outcome expectancies. *Am J Health Educ.* 2020;51(2):78-86.
39. Pittman DM, Brooks JJ, Kaur P, Obasi EM. The cost of minority stress: risky alcohol use and coping-motivated drinking behavior in African American college students. *J Ethn Subst Abuse.* 2019;18(2):257-278.
40. Desalu JM, Goodhines PA, Park A. Racial discrimination and alcohol use and negative drinking consequences among Black Americans: a meta-analytical review. *Addiction.* 2019;114(6):957-967.
41. Metzger IW, Salami T, Carter S, et al. African American emerging adults' experiences with racial discrimination and drinking habits: the moderating roles of perceived stress. *Cultur Divers Ethnic Minor Psychol.* 2018;24(4):489.
42. Le TP, Iwamoto DK. A longitudinal investigation of racial discrimination, drinking to cope, and alcohol-related problems among underage Asian American college students. *Psychol Addict Behav.* 2019;33(6):520.
43. Cano MÁ, de Dios MA, Castro Y, et al. Alcohol use severity and depressive symptoms among late adolescent Hispanics: testing associations of acculturation and enculturation in a bicultural transaction model. *Addict Behav.* 2015;49:78-82.
44. Piña-Watson B, Cox K, Neduvelil A. Mexican descent college student risky sexual behaviors and alcohol use: the role of general and cultural based coping with discrimination. *J Am Coll Health.* 2021;69(1):82-89.
45. Schauer GL, Berg CJ, Bryant LO. Sex differences in psychosocial correlates of concurrent substance use among heterosexual, homosexual and bisexual college students. *Am J Drug Alcohol Abuse.* 2013;39(4):252-258.
46. Kerr D, Ding K, Burke A, Ott-Walter K. An alcohol, tobacco, and other drug use comparison of lesbian, bisexual, and heterosexual undergraduate women. *Subst Use Misuse.* 2015;50(3):340-349.
47. Coulter RW, Marzell M, Saltz R, Stall R, Mair C. Sexual-orientation differences in drinking patterns and use of drinking contexts among college students. *Drug Alcohol Depend.* 2016;160:197-204.
48. Haardörfer R, Windle M, Fairman RT, Berg CJ. Longitudinal changes in alcohol use and binge-drinking among young-adult college students: analyses of predictors across system levels. *Addict Behav.* 2021;112:106619.
49. Woodford MR, Kulick A, Atteberry B. Protective factors, campus climate, and health outcomes among sexual minority college students. *J Divers High Educ.* 2015;8(2):73.
50. Kidd JD, Jackman KB, Wolff M, Veldhuis CB, Hughes TL. Risk and protective factors for substance use among sexual and gender minority youth: a scoping review. *Curr Addict Rep.* 2018;5(2):158-173.
51. Reed E, Prado G, Matsumoto A, Amaro H. Alcohol and drug use and related consequences among gay, lesbian and bisexual college students: role of experiencing violence, feeling safe on campus, and perceived stress. *Addict Behav.* 2010;35(2):168-171.
52. Leichliter JS, Meilman PW, Presley CA. Alcohol use and related consequences among students with varying levels of involvement in college athletics. *J Am Coll Health.* 1998;46:257-262.
53. Ford JA. Alcohol use among college students: a comparison of athletes and nonathletes. *Subst Use Misuse.* 2007;42:1367-1377.
54. Nelson TF, Wechsler H. Alcohol and college athletes. *Med Sci Sports Exerc.* 2001;33:43-47.
55. Cimini MD, Monserrat JM, Sokolowski KL, et al. Reducing high-risk drinking among student-athletes: the effects of a targeted athlete-specific brief intervention. *J Am Coll Health.* 2015;63(6):343-352.
56. Yusko DA, Buckman JF, White HR, et al. Alcohol, tobacco, illicit drugs, and performance enhancers: a comparison of use by college student athletes and nonathletes. *J Am Coll Health.* 2008;57(3):281-290.
57. Bower BL, Martin M. African American female basketball players: an examination of alcohol and drug behaviors. *J Am Coll Health.* 1999;48(3):129-133.
58. Martens MP, Dams-O'Connor K, Duffy-Paiement C. Comparing off-season with in-season alcohol consumption among intercollegiate athletes. *J Sport Exerc Psychol.* 2006;28:502-510.
59. Thombs DL. A test of the perceived norms model to explain drinking patterns among university student athletes. *J Am Coll Health.* 2000;49(2):75-83.
60. Brenner J, Swanik K. High-risk drinking characteristics in collegiate athletes. *J Am Coll Health.* 2007;56(3):267-272.
61. Martens MP, Watson JC, Beck NC. Sport-type differences in alcohol use among intercollegiate athletes. *J Appl Sport Psychol.* 2006;18:136-150.
62. Yusko DA, Buckman JF, White HR, et al. Risk for excessive alcohol use and drinking-related problems in college student athletes. *Addict Behav.* 2008;33(12):1546-1556.
63. Martens MP, Pedersen ER, Smith AE, et al. Predictors of alcohol-related outcomes in college athletes: the roles of trait urgency and drinking motives. *Addict Behav.* 2011;36(5):456-464.
64. Zamboanga BL, Ham LS. Alcohol expectancies and context-specific drinking behaviors among female college athletes. *Behav Ther.* 2008;39(2):162-170.
65. Zamboanga BL, Horton NJ, Leitkowski LK, et al. Do good things come to those who drink? A longitudinal investigation of drinking expectancies and hazardous alcohol use in female college athletes. *J Adolesc Health.* 2006;39(2):229-236.
66. Pitts M, Chow GM, Donohue B. Relationship between general and sport-related drinking motives and athlete alcohol use and problems. *Subst Use Misuse.* 2019;54(1):146-155.
67. Baer JS. Effects of college residence on perceived norms for alcohol consumption: an examination of the first year in college. *Psychol Addict Behav.* 1994;8(1):43-50.
68. Bosari B. Alcohol use in the Greek system, 1999–2009: a decade of progress. *Curr Drug Abuse Rev.* 2009;2:216-255.
69. Caudill BD, Crosse SB, Campbell B, et al. High-risk drinking among college fraternity members: a national perspective. *J Am Coll Health.* 2006;55(3):141-155.
70. Larimer ME, Anderson BK, Baer JS, et al. An individual in context: predictors of alcohol use and drinking problems among Greek and residence hall students. *J Subst Abuse.* 2000;11(1):53-68.

71. McCabe SE, Schulenberg JE, Johnston LD, et al. Selection and socialization effects of fraternities and sororities on U.S. college student substance use: a multi-cohort national longitudinal study. *Addiction.* 2005;100(4):512-524.
72. Mallett KA, Varvil-Weld L, Borsari B, et al. An update of research examining college student alcohol-related consequences: new perspectives and implications for interventions. *Alcohol Clin Exp Res.* 2013;37(5):709-716.
73. Ngo DA, Ait-Daoud N, Rege SV, et al. Differentials and trends in emergency department visits due to alcohol intoxication and co-occurring conditions among students in a U.S. public university. *Drug Alcohol Depend.* 2018;183:89-95.
74. McCabe SE, Veliz P, Schulenberg JE. How collegiate fraternity and sorority involvement relates to substance use during young adulthood and substance use disorders in early midlife: a national longitudinal study. *J Adolesc Health.* 2018;62(3):S35-S43.
75. Myers JL, Sasso PA. Differences in informal alcohol protective behavior strategies between fraternity & sorority members. *J Sorority Fraternity Life.* 2022;16(02):17-36.
76. Radford AW; MPR Associates, Inc. *Military Service Members and Veterans in Higher Education: What the New GI Bill May Mean for Postsecondary Institutions.* American Council on Education; 2009.
77. Ackerman R, Diramio D, Mitchell RLG. Transitions: combat veterans as college students. *New Dir Stud Serv.* 2009;5-14.
78. Lostutter TW, Neighbors CR, Simpson T, Larimer ME. The relationship of college student and veteran identities to mental health symptoms and alcohol use among veteran and nonveteran students. *Mil Behav Health.* 2020;8(1):33-41.
79. Grossbard JR, Widome R, Lust K, et al. High-risk drinking and academic performance among college student veterans. *J Alcohol Drug Educ.* 2014;58(3):28-47.
80. Banducci AN, McCaughey VK, Gradus JL, Street AE. The associations between deployment experiences, PTSD, and alcohol use among male and female veterans. *Addict Behav.* 2019;98:106032.
81. Messerschmitt-Coen S. Considerations for counseling student veterans. *J College Stud Psychother.* 2021;35(2):181-200.
82. Cate CA, Gerber MM, Holmes DL. Prevalence of mental health disorders and service utilization among student veterans: a pilot study, 2010. *Paper presented at International Society for Traumatic Stress Studies (ISTSS).* University of California; 2009:2010.
83. Cate CA, Gerber MM, Holmes DL. Student veteran stressors in higher education: a pilot study, 2010. *Paper presented at International Society for Traumatic Stress Studies (ISTSS).* University of California; 2009:2010.
84. Widome R, Laska MN, Gulden A, et al. Health risk behaviors of Afghanistan and Iraq war veterans attending college. *Am J Health Promot.* 2011;26(2):101-108.
85. Dunn ME, Goldman MS. Age and drinking-related differences in the memory organization of alcohol expectancies in 3rd-, 6th-, 9th-, and 12th-grade children. *J Consult Clin Psychol.* 1998;66(3):579-585.
86. Young RM, Connor JP, Ricciardelli LA, et al. The role of alcohol expectancy and drinking refusal self-efficacy beliefs in university student drinking. *Alcohol Alcohol.* 2006;41(1):70-75.
87. Greenbaum PE, Del Boca FK, Darkes J, et al. Variation in the drinking trajectories of freshmen college students. *J Consult Clin Psychol.* 2005;73(2):229-238.
88. Jones BT, Corbin W, Fromme K. A review of expectancy theory and alcohol consumption. *Addiction.* 2001;96(1):57-72.
89. A Call to Action: Changing the Culture of Drinking at U.S. Colleges. 2002. www.collegedrinkingprevention.gov/Reports/TaskForce/Task-Force
90. Stacy AW, Widaman KF, Marlatt GA. Expectancy models of alcohol use. *J Pers Soc Psychol.* 1990;58(5):918-928.
91. Patrick ME, Wray-Lake L, Finlay AK, et al. The long arm of expectancies: adolescent alcohol expectancies predict adult alcohol use. *Alcohol Alcohol.* 2010;45(1):17-24.
92. Ramirez JJ, Rhew IC, Patrick ME, Larimer ME, Lee CM. A daily-level analysis of moderators of the association between alcohol expectancies and alcohol use among college student drinkers. *Subst Use Misuse.* 2020;55(6):973-982.
93. Leeman RF, Toll BA, Taylor LA, et al. Alcohol-induced disinhibition expectancies and impaired control as prospective predictors of problem drinking in undergraduates. *Psychol Addict Behav.* 2009;23(4):553-563.
94. Madden DR, Clapp JD. The event-level impact of one's typical alcohol expectancies, drinking motivations, and use of protective behavioral strategies. *Drug Alcohol Depend.* 2019;194:112-120.
95. Reich RR, Below MC, Goldman MS. Explicit and implicit measures of expectancy and related alcohol cognitions: a meta-analytic comparison. *Psychol Addict Behav.* 2010;24(1):13-25.
96. Friedman RS, McCarthy DM, Forster J, et al. Automatic effects of alcohol cues on sexual attraction. *Addiction.* 2005;100(5):672-681.
97. Scott-Sheldon LA, Terry DL, Carey KB, et al. Efficacy of expectancy challenge interventions to reduce college student drinking: a meta-analytic review. *Psychol Addict Behav.* 2012;26(3):393-405.
98. Cooper ML. Motivations for alcohol use among adolescents: development and validation of a four-factor model. *Psychol Assess.* 1994;6(2):117-128.
99. Cooper ML, Russell M, Skinner JB, et al. Stress and alcohol use: moderating effects of gender, coping, and alcohol expectancies. *J Abnorm Psychol.* 1992;101(1):139-152.
100. Kuntsche E, Knibbe R, Gmel G, et al. Why do young people drink? A review of drinking motives. *Clin Psychol Rev.* 2005;25(7):841-861.
101. LaBrie JW, Hummer JF, Pedersen ER. Reasons for drinking in the college student context: the differential role and risk of the social motivator. *J Stud Alcohol Drugs.* 2007;68(3):393-398.
102. Lewis MA, Phillippi J, Neighbors C. Morally based self-esteem, drinking motives, and alcohol use among college students. *Psychol Addict Behav.* 2007;21(3):398-403.
103. Brennan AF, Walfish S, AuBuchon P. Alcohol use and abuse in college students. I. A review of individual and personality correlates. *Int J Addict.* 1986;21(4–5):449-474.
104. Neighbors C. Feeling controlled and drinking motives among college students: contingent self-esteem as a mediator. *Self Identity.* 2004;3:207-224.
105. Wicki M, Kuntsche E, Gmel G. Drinking at European universities? A review of students' alcohol use. *Addict Behav.* 2010;35(11):913-924.
106. Mackinnon SP, Couture ME, Cooper ML, Kuntsche E, O'Connor RM, Stewart SH; DRINC Team. Cross-cultural comparisons of drinking motives in 10 countries: data from the DRINC project. *Drug Alcohol Rev.* 2017;36(6):721-730.
107. Greeley J, Oei T. Alcohol and tension reduction. In: Leonard KE, Blane HT, eds. *Psychological Theories of Drinking and Alcoholism.* 2nd ed. Guilford Press; 2002:14-53.
108. Khantzian EJ. The self-medication hypothesis of addictive disorders: focus on heroin and cocaine dependence. *Am J Psychiatry.* 1985;142(11):1259-1264.
109. Cooper ML, Agocha VB, Sheldon MS. A motivational perspective on risky behaviors: the role of personality and affect regulatory processes. *J Pers.* 2000;68(6):1059-1088.
110. Kuntsche E, Wiers RW, Janssen T, et al. Same wording, distinct concepts? Testing differences between expectancies and motives in a mediation model of alcohol outcomes. *Exp Clin Psychopharmacol.* 2010;18(5):436-444.
111. Magid V, Maclean MG, Colder CR. Differentiating between sensation seeking and impulsivity through their mediated relations with alcohol use and problems. *Addict Behav.* 2007;32(10):2046-2061.
112. Read JP, Wood MD, Kahler CW, et al. Examining the role of drinking motives in college student alcohol use and problems. *Psychol Addict Behav.* 2003;17(1):13-23.
113. Yurasek AM, Murphy JG, Dennhardt AA, et al. Drinking motives mediate the relationship between reinforcing efficacy and alcohol consumption and problems. *J Stud Alcohol Drugs.* 2011;72(6):991-999.
114. Lindgren KP, Neighbors C, Blayney JA, et al. Do drinking motives mediate the association between sexual assault and problem drinking? *Addict Behav.* 2012;37(3):323-326.

115. Goldstein AL, Flett GL, Wekerle C. Child maltreatment, alcohol use and drinking consequences among male and female college students: an examination of drinking motives as mediators. *Addict Behav.* 2010;35(6):636-639.
116. Grayson CE, Nolen-Hoeksema S. Motives to drink as mediators between childhood sexual assault and alcohol problems in adult women. *J Trauma Stress.* 2005;18(2):137-145.
117. Miranda R Jr, Meyerson LA, Long PJ, et al. Sexual assault and alcohol use: exploring the self-medication hypothesis. *Violence Vict.* 2002;17(2):205-217.
118. Bravo AJ, Pilatti A, Pearson MR, Mezquita L, Ibáñez MI, Ortet G. Depressive symptoms, ruminative thinking, drinking motives, and alcohol outcomes: a multiple mediation model among college students in three countries. *Addict Behav.* 2018;76:319-327.
119. Kenney SR, Anderson BJ, Stein MD. Drinking to cope mediates the relationship between depression and alcohol risk: different pathways for college and non-college young adults. *Addict Behav.* 2018;80:116-123.
120. Stevenson BL, Dvorak RD, Kramer MP, et al. Within- and between-person associations from mood to alcohol consequences: the mediating role of enhancement and coping drinking motives. *J Abnorm Psychol.* 2019;128(8):813.
121. LaBrie JW, Hummer JF, Neighbors C, et al. Whose opinion matters? The relationship between injunctive norms and alcohol consequences in college students. *Addict Behav.* 2012;35(4):343-349.
122. Littlefield AK, Sher KJ, Wood PK. Do changes in drinking motives mediate the relation between personality change and "maturing out" of problem drinking? *J Abnorm Psychol.* 2010;119(1):93-105.
123. Baer JS, Stacy A, Larimer M. Biases in the perception of drinking norms among college students. *J Stud Alcohol.* 1991;52(6):580-586.
124. Ward RM, Guo Y. Examining the relationship between social norms, alcohol-induced blackouts, and intentions to blackout among college students. *Alcohol.* 2020;86:35-41.
125. Clapp JD. The relationship of perceptions of alcohol promotion and peer drinking norms to alcohol problems reported by college students. *J Coll Stud Dev.* 2002;41:19-26.
126. Dumas TM, Davis JP, Neighbors C. How much does your peer group really drink? Examining the relative impact of overestimation, actual group drinking and perceived campus norms on university students' heavy alcohol use. *Addict Behav.* 2019;90:409-414.
127. Neighbors C, Lee CM, Lewis MA, et al. Are social norms the best predictor of outcomes among heavy-drinking college students? *J Stud Alcohol Drugs.* 2007;68(4):556-565.
128. Litt DM, Lewis MA, Rhew IC, Hodge KA, Kaysen DL. Reciprocal relationships over time between descriptive norms and alcohol use in young adult sexual minority women. *Psychol Addict Behav.* 2015;29(4):885.
129. Neighbors C, LaBrie JW, Hummer MA, et al. Group identification as a moderator of the relationship between perceived social norms and alcohol consumption. *Psychol Addict Behav.* 2010;24(3):522-528.
130. Courtney KE, Polich J. Binge drinking in young adults: data, definitions, and determinants. *Psychol Bull.* 2009;135(1):142-156.
131. Clapp JD, Lange J, Min JW, et al. Two studies examining environmental predictors of heavy drinking by college students. *Prev Sci.* 2003;4:99-108.
132. Lange JE, Voas RB. Youth escaping limits on drinking: binging in Mexico. *Addiction.* 2000;95:521-528.
133. Morrell MN, Reed DD, Martinetti MP. The behavioral economics of the bottomless cup: the effects of alcohol cup price on consumption in college students. *Exp Clin Psychopharmacol.* 2021;29(1):36.
134. Clapp JD, Shillington AM. Environmental predictors of heavy episodic drinking. *Am J Drug Alcohol Abuse.* 2001;27(2):301-313.
135. Neighbors C, Walters ST, Lee CM, et al. Event-specific prevention: addressing college student drinking during known windows of risk. *Addict Behav.* 2007;32(11):2667-2680.
136. Garcia TA, Hultgren BA, Canning JR, Gilson MS, Larimer ME. "On a night like this": a mixed-methods approach to understanding high-risk drinking events in college students. *Alcohol Clin Exp Res.* 2022;46(6):1121-1132.
137. Pedersen ER, LaBrie JW, Kilmer JR. Before you slip into the night, you'll want something to drink: exploring the reasons for prepartying behavior among college student drinkers. *Issues Ment Health Nurs.* 2009;30(6):354-363.
138. Chaney BH, Martin RJ, Barry AE, Lee JG, Cremeens-Matthews J, Stellefson ML. Pregaming: a field-based investigation of alcohol quantities consumed prior to visiting a bar and restaurant district. *Subst Use Misuse.* 2019;54(6):1017-1023.
139. Calhoun BH, Linden-Carmichael AN. Pre-game drinking among young adults and its association with positive and negative alcohol consequences. *Addict Behav.* 2022;124:107120.
140. Santos MG, Sanchez ZM, Hughes K, Gee I, Quigg Z. Pre-drinking, alcohol consumption and related harms amongst Brazilian and British university students. *PloS One.* 2022;17(3):e0264842.
141. LaBrie JW, Pedersen ER. Prepartying promotes heightened risk in the college environment: an event-level report. *Addict Behav.* 2008;33(7):955-959.
142. Bosari B, Boyle KE, Hustad JT, et al. Drinking before drinking: pregaming and drinking games in mandated students. *Addict Behav.* 2007;32:2694-2705.
143. Pedersen ER, Labrie J. Partying before the party: examining prepartying behavior among college students. *J Am Coll Health.* 2007;56(3):237-245.
144. Zamboanga BL, Newins AR, Cook MA. A meta-analysis of drinking game participation and alcohol-related outcomes. *Psychol Addict Behav.* 2021;35(3):263-273.
145. Martens MP, Dams-O'Connor K, Beck NC. A systematic review of college student-athlete drinking: prevalence rates, sport-related factors, and interventions. *J Subst Abuse Treat.* 2006;31(3):305-316.
146. Grossbard J, Geisner IM, Neighbors C, et al. Are drinking games sports? College athlete participation in drinking games and alcohol-related problems. *J Stud Alcohol Drugs.* 2007;68(1):97-105.
147. Zamboanga BL, Rodriguez L, Horton NJ. Athletic involvement and its relevance to hazardous alcohol use and drinking game participation in female college athletes: a preliminary investigation. *J Am Coll Health.* 2008;56(6):651-656.
148. Williams CM, Reynolds LM, Mastroleo NR. Comparison of pregaming alcohol use and consequences by season status and sex in college student athletes. *J Drug Educ.* 2020;49(3–4):71-86.
149. Neal DJ, Fromme K. Hook 'em horns and heavy drinking: alcohol use and collegiate sports. *Addict Behav.* 2007;32(11):2681-2693.
150. Boyd CJ, McCabe SE, d'Arcy H. Collegiate living environments: a predictor of binge drinking, negative consequences, and risk-reducing behaviors. *J Addict Nurs.* 2004;15:111-118.
151. National Institute on Alcohol Abuse and Alcoholism. *A Call to Action: Changing the Culture of Drinking at U.S. Colleges.* U.S. Department of Health and Human Services, Public Health Service, National Institutes of Health; 2002.
152. Barnett NP, Read JP. Mandatory alcohol intervention for alcohol-abusing college students: a systematic review. *J Subst Abuse Treat.* 2005;29(2):147-158.
153. Larimer ME, Cronce JM. Identification, prevention and treatment: a review of individual-focused strategies to reduce problematic alcohol consumption by college students. *J Stud Alcohol Suppl.* 2002;14:148-163.
154. Larimer ME, Cronce JM. Identification, prevention, and treatment revisited: individual-focused college drinking prevention strategies 1999–2006. *Addict Behav.* 2007;32(11):2439-2468.
155. Larimer ME, Neighbors C, Kilmer JR, et al. Brief interventions for college freshmen: direct comparison of group, individual, and web alcohol prevention formats. *Alcohol Clin Exp Res.* 2005;29:244D.
156. Walters ST, Miller E, Chiauzzi E. Wired for wellness: e-interventions for addressing college drinking. *J Subst Abuse Treat.* 2005;29(2):139-145.
157. Walters ST, Neighbors C. Feedback interventions for college alcohol misuse: what, why and for whom? *Addict Behav.* 2005;30(6):1168-1182.
158. White HR. Reduction of alcohol-related harm on United States, college campuses: the use of personal feedback interventions. *Int J Drug Policy.* 2006;17:310-319.

159. Cronce JM, Larimer ME. Individual-focused approaches to the prevention of college student drinking. *Alcohol Res Health*. 2011;34(2):210-221.
160. Cronce JM, Larimer ME. Individual-focused approaches to prevention of college student drinking. In: White H, Rabiner D, eds. *College Drinking and Drug Use*. Guilford Press; 2012.
161. National Institute on Alcohol Abuse and Alcoholism. *Planning Alcohol Interventions Using NIAAA's College AIM Alcohol Intervention Matrix*. U.S. Department of Health and Human Services, Public Health Service, National Institutes of Health; 2015.
162. Miller WR, Rollnick S. *Motivational Interviewing: Preparing People to Change Addictive Behavior*. Guilford Press; 2002.
163. Hernandez DV, Skewes MC, Resor MR, Villanueva MR, Hanson BS, Blume AW. A pilot test of an alcohol skills training programme for Mexican-American college students. *Int J Drug Policy*. 2006;17(4):320-328.
164. Darkes J, Goldman MS. Expectancy challenge and drinking reduction: experimental evidence for a mediational process. *J Consult Clin Psychol*. 1993;61(2):344-353.
165. Labbe AK, Maisto SA. Alcohol expectancy challenges for college students: a narrative review. *Clin Psychol Rev*. 2011;31(4):673-683.
166. Gesualdo C, Pinquart M. Expectancy challenge interventions to reduce alcohol consumption among high school and college students: a meta-analysis. *Psychol Addict Behav*. 2021;35(7):817-828.
167. Corbin WR, McNair LD, Carter JA. Evaluation of a treatment-appropriate cognitive intervention for challenging alcohol outcome expectancies. *Addict Behav*. 2001;26(4):475-488.
168. Wood MD, Capone C, Laforge R, et al. Brief motivational intervention and alcohol expectancy challenge with heavy drinking college students: a randomized factorial study. *Addict Behav*. 2007;32(11):2509-2528.
169. Lau-Barraco C, Dunn ME. Evaluation of a single-session expectancy challenge intervention to reduce alcohol use among college students. *Psychol Addict Behav*. 2008;22(2):168-175.
170. Dunn ME, Schreiner AM, Flori JN, et al. Effective prevention programming for reducing alcohol-related harms experienced by first year college students: evaluation of the expectancy challenge alcohol literacy curriculum (ECALC). *Addict Behav*. 2022;131:107338.
171. Carey KB, Merrill JE, Walsh JL, Lust SA, Kalichman SC, Carey MP. Predictors of short-term change after a brief alcohol intervention for mandated college drinkers. *Addict Behav*. 2018;77:152-159.
172. Dunn ME, Fried-Somerstein A, Flori JN, Hall TV, Dvorak RD. Reducing alcohol use in mandated college students: a comparison of a Brief Motivational Intervention (BMI) and the Expectancy Challenge Alcohol Literacy Curriculum (ECALC). *Exp Clin Psychopharmacol*. 2020;28(1):87.
173. Acuff SF, Voss AT, Dennhardt AA, Borsari B, Martens MP, Murphy JG. Brief motivational interventions are associated with reductions in alcohol-induced blackouts among heavy drinking college students. *Alcohol Clin Exp Res*. 2019;43(5):988-996.
174. Murphy JG, Dennhardt AA, Martens MP, Borsari B, Witkiewitz K, Meshesha LZ. A randomized clinical trial evaluating the efficacy of a brief alcohol intervention supplemented with a substance-free activity session or relaxation training. *J Consult Clin Psychol*. 2019;87(7):657.
175. Marlatt GA, Baer JS, Kivlahan DR, et al. Screening and brief intervention for high-risk college student drinkers: results from a 2-year follow-up assessment. *J Consult Clin Psychol*. 1998;66(4):604-615.
176. Dimeff LA, Baer JS, Kivlahan DR, et al. *Brief Alcohol Screening and Intervention for College Students (BASICS)*. The Guilford Press; 1999.
177. Larimer ME, Kilmer JR, Cronce JM, Hultgren BA, Gilson MS, Lee CM. Thirty years of BASICS: dissemination and implementation progress and challenges. *Psychol Addict Behav*. 2021;36(6):664-677.
178. Ray AE, Kim SY, White HR, et al. When less is more and more is less in brief motivational interventions: characteristics of intervention content and their associations with drinking outcomes. *Psychol Addict Behav*. 2014;28(4):1026-1040.
179. Yurasek AM, Borsari B, Magill M, et al. Descriptive norms and expectancies as mediators of a brief motivational intervention for mandated college students receiving stepped care for alcohol use. *Psychol Addict Behav*. 2015;29(4):1003-1011.
180. Carey KB, Scott-Sheldon LA, Carey MP, et al. Individual-level interventions to reduce college student drinking: a meta-analytic review. *Addict Behav*. 2007;32(11):2469-2494.
181. Jackson KM, Sher KJ, Gotham HJ, et al. Transitioning into and out of large-effect drinking in young adulthood. *J Abnorm Psychol*. 2001;110(3):378-391.
182. Baer JS, Kivlahan DR, Blume AW, et al. Brief intervention for heavy-drinking college students: 4-year follow-up and natural history. *Am J Public Health*. 2001;91(8):1310-1316.
183. White HR, Mun EY, Pugh L, et al. Long-term effects of brief substance use interventions for mandated college students: sleeper effects of an in-person personal feedback intervention. *Alcohol Clin Exp Res*. 2007;31(8):1380-1391.
184. JW LB, Thompson AD, Huchting K, et al. A group motivational interviewing intervention reduces drinking and alcohol-related negative consequences in adjudicated college women. *Addict Behav*. 2007;32(11):2549-2562.
185. Larimer ME, Turner AP, Anderson BK, et al. Evaluating a brief alcohol intervention with fraternities. *J Stud Alcohol*. 2001;62(3):370-380.
186. White HR, Morgan TJ, Pugh LA, et al. Evaluating two brief substance-use interventions for mandated college students. *J Stud Alcohol*. 2006;67(2):309-317.
187. Amaro H, Ahl M, Matsumoto A, et al. Trial of the university assistance program for alcohol use among mandated students. *J Stud Alcohol Drugs Suppl*. 2009;(16):45-56.
188. Oddo LE, Meinzer MC, Tang A, et al. Enhanced brief motivational intervention for college student drinkers with ADHD: goal-directed activation as a mechanism of change. *Behav Ther*. 2021;52(5):1198-1212.
189. Pedrelli P, Borsari B, Merrill JE, et al. Evaluating the combination of a Brief Motivational Intervention plus Cognitive Behavioral Therapy for Depression and heavy episodic drinking in college students. *Psychol Addict Behav*. 2020;34(2):308.
190. Martens MP, Cimini MD, Barr AR, et al. Implementing a screening and brief intervention for high-risk drinking in university-based health and mental health care settings: reductions in alcohol use and correlates of success. *Addict Behav*. 2007;32(11):2563-2572.
191. Schaus JF, Sole ML, McCoy TP, Mullett N, O'Brien MC. et al. Alcohol screening and brief intervention in a college student health center: a randomized controlled trial. *J Stud Alcohol Drugs Suppl*. 2009;(16):131-141.
192. Turrisi R, Larimer ME, Mallett KA, et al. A randomized clinical trial evaluating a combined alcohol intervention for high-risk college students. *J Stud Alcohol Drugs*. 2009;70:555-567.
193. Tomaka J, Palacios R, Morales-Monks S, Davis SE. An evaluation of the BASICS alcohol risk reduction model among predominantly Hispanic college students. *Subst Use Misuse*. 2012;47(12):1260-1270.
194. Blue Bird Jernigan V, D'Amico EJ, Duran B, Buchwald D. Multilevel and community-level interventions with Native Americans: challenges and opportunities. *Prev Sci*. 2020;21(1):65-73.
195. Shell DF, Newman IM. Effects of a web-based pre-enrollment alcohol brief motivational intervention on college student retention and alcohol-related violations. *J Am Coll Health*. 2019;67(3):263-274.
196. Fromme K, Corbin W. Prevention of heavy drinking and associated negative consequences among mandated and voluntary college students. *J Consult Clin Psychol*. 2004;72(6):1038-1049.
197. Larimer ME, Lee CM, Kilmer JR, et al. Personalized mailed feedback for college drinking prevention: a randomized clinical trial. *J Consult Clin Psychol*. 2007;75(2):285-293.
198. Dotson KB, Dunn ME, Bowers CA. Stand-alone personalized normative feedback for college student drinkers: a meta-analytic review, 2004 to 2014. *PloS One*. 2015;10(10):e0139518.
199. Neighbors C, Larimer ME, Lewis MA. Targeting misperceptions of descriptive drinking norms: efficacy of a computer-delivered personalized normative feedback intervention. *J Consult Clin Psychol*. 2004;72(3):434-447.
200. Lewis MA, Neighbors C. Who is the typical college student? Implications for personalized normative feedback interventions. *Addict Behav*. 2006;31(11):2120-2126.

201. Bedendo A, Ferri CP, de Souza AA, Andrade AL, Noto AR. Pragmatic randomized controlled trial of a web-based intervention for alcohol use among Brazilian college students: motivation as a moderating effect. *Drug Alcohol Depend.* 2019;199:92-100.
202. Carey KB, Carey MP, Maisto SA, et al. Brief motivational interventions for heavy college drinkers: a randomized controlled trial. *J Consult Clin Psychol.* 2006;74(5):943-954.
203. Sobell LC, Sobell MB. *Timeline Followback User's Guide: A Calendar Method for Assessing Alcohol and Drug Use.* Addiction Research Foundation; 1996.
204. Davidson D, Swift R, Fitz E. Naltrexone increases the latency to drink alcohol in social drinkers. *Alcohol Clin Exp Res.* 1996;20(4):732-739.
205. Hingson RW, Assailly JP, Williams AF. Underage drinking: frequency, consequences, and interventions. *Traffic Inj Prev.* 2004;5(3):228-236.
206. DeJong W, Langford LM. A typology for campus-based alcohol prevention: moving toward environmental management strategies. *J Stud Alcohol Suppl.* 2002;14:140-147.
207. Borsari B. Drinking games in the college environment: a review. *J Alcohol Drug Educ.* 2004;48:29-51.
208. Toomey TL, Lenk KM, Wagenaar AC. Environmental policies to reduce college drinking: an update of research findings. *J Stud Alcohol Drugs.* 2007;68:208-219.
209. Keeling RP. Binge drinking and the college environment. *J Am Coll Health.* 2002;50(5):197-201.
210. Kypri K, Saunders JB, Gallagher SJ. Acceptability of various brief intervention approaches for hazardous drinking among university students. *Alcohol Alcohol.* 2003;38(6):626-628.
211. Hingson RW, Howland J. Comprehensive community interventions to promote health: implications for college-age drinking problems. *J Stud Alcohol Suppl.* 2002;14:226-240.
212. Toomey TL, Lenk KM. A review of environmental-based community interventions. *Alcohol Res Health.* 2011;34(2):163-166.
213. Clapp JD, Stanger L. Changing the college AOD environment for primary prevention. *J Prim Prev.* 2003;23:515-523.
214. Saltz RF. Environmental approaches to prevention in college settings. *Alcohol Res Health.* 2011;34:204-209.
215. Ferreira SE, de Mello MT, Pompéia S, et al. Effects of energy drink ingestion on alcohol intoxication. *Alcohol Clin Exp Res.* 2006;30(4):598-605.
216. Gallagher RP. *National Survey of Counseling Center Directors.* The International Association of Counseling Services, Inc; 2014.
217. Schwartz AJ. Are college students more disturbed today? Stability in the acuity and qualitative character of psychopathology of college counseling center clients: 1992–1993 through 2001–2002. *J Am Coll Health.* 2002;54:327-337.
218. Oswalt SB, Lederer AM, Chestnut-Steich K, Day C, Halbritter A, Ortiz D. Trends in college students' mental health diagnoses and utilization of services, 2009–2015. *J Am Coll Health.* 2020;68(1):41-51.
219. Lipson SK, Lattie EG, Eisenberg D. Increased rates of mental health service utilization by U.S. college students: 10-year population-level trends (2007–2017). *Psychiatr Serv.* 2019;70(1):60-63.
220. The National Center on Addiction and Substance Abuse at Columbia University. *Depression, Substance Abuse and College Student Engagement: A Review of the Literature.* 2003.
221. Geisner IM, Neighbors C, Larimer ME. A randomized clinical trial of a brief, mailed intervention for symptoms of depression. *J Consult Clin Psychol.* 2006;74(2):393-399.
222. Foote J, Wilkens C, Vavagiakis P. A national survey of alcohol screening and referral in college health centers. *J Am Coll Health.* 2004;52(4):149-157.
223. Murphy JG, Benson TA, Vuchinich RE, et al. A comparison of personalized feedback for college student drinkers delivered with and without a motivational interview. *J Stud Alcohol.* 2004;65(2):200-203.
224. Kypri K, Saunders JB, Williams SM, et al. Web-based screening and brief intervention for hazardous drinking: a double-blind randomized controlled trial. *Addiction.* 2004;99(11):1410-1417.
225. Zemore SE, Karriker-Jaffe KJ, Mulia N, et al. The future of research on alcohol-related disparities across U.S. racial/ethnic groups: a plan of attack. *J Stud Alcohol Drugs.* 2018;79(1):7-21.
226. Barrera M Jr, Castro FG. A heuristic framework for the cultural adaptation of interventions. *Clin Psychol.* 2006;13(4):311-316.
227. Larimer ME, Kilmer JR, Lee CM. College student drug prevention: a review of individually oriented prevention strategies. *J Drug Issues.* 2005;35:431-456.

CHAPTER

30

Policy and Leadership: Impact on Primary, Secondary, and Tertiary Prevention of Substance Use Disorders in Military Personnel and Beyond

Kenneth Hoffman and Janet H. Lenard

CHAPTER OUTLINE

- Introduction
- Historical perspectives on policy and leadership leading to the military SUD prevention, early intervention, and treatment programs
- Development and implementation of drug testing as a deterrent: A drug-free workplace
- Policy and leadership: A different approach to alcohol, other drug use and tobacco
- Impact on prevalence and trends of alcohol and substance use in the military
- Learning from history: Connecting alcohol and other drug detection to early intervention, treatment, relapse prevention, and health promotion
- Impact for the nation
- Conclusions

INTRODUCTION

This chapter reviews the history and impact of military leadership and policy initiatives on the development of effective prevention and treatment of substance use disorders (SUDs). It highlights the development of the military's command and medical infrastructure, which focuses on developing and maintaining a "fit and ready" force through "zero tolerance" for illicit drug use, deglamorizing alcohol use, health promotion, and early identification of SUDs, followed by referral to treatment. Related to these initiatives are a series of comprehensive Department of Defense (DoD) Cross-sectional Surveys of Health-Related Behaviors Among Military Personnel, which assessed the prevalence of alcohol and drug use and trends over time.[1-3]

Noteworthy, is the fact that Substance Use Disorder Clinical Care (SUDCC) for the military is now realigned within the Behavioral Health System of Care (BHSOC) under the Surgeon General of the United States Army having primary responsibility. Military personnel identified or appearing at risk for SUDs are referred to SUDCC for a comprehensive assessment and treatment when indicated.[4] This includes an Impaired Healthcare Personnel Program (IHCPP) to identify and address multidisciplinary needs of its military and civilian health care personnel known or suspected to have physical, emotional, or psychiatric conditions, including SUDs.[4,5]

Treatment resources for early intervention and treatment are available to personnel, family members, and civilians through the Department of Veterans Affairs, TRICARE, Military One Source, and service-specific medical commands with staff and support SUD specialty providers located within military treatment facilities under behavioral health.[6,7]

Figure 30-1 highlights the prevention continuum of care with interventions that are possible within each level. Although this chapter will not directly address treatment of military personnel within any specific military or TRICARE treatment facility, the focus is to connect treatment with a continuum of preventive services and interventions. Prevention and early detection have a critical role in the continuum of care. Best patient placement and relapse prevention is dependent on the individual's recovery environment. Prevention activities within that environment impact treatment outcomes and relapse potential. The dimension "Recovery Environment" is nonmedical by nature and addresses social determinants of health, such as housing, finances, education, legal problems, transportation, family concerns, occupational concerns, and social network. This chapter focuses on prevention and early detection within the environment in which military personnel and their families live, and the impact that may have on personnel in treatment.

HISTORICAL PERSPECTIVES ON POLICY AND LEADERSHIP LEADING TO THE MILITARY SUD PREVENTION, EARLY INTERVENTION, AND TREATMENT PROGRAMS

Much can be learned from the nation's response to the opioid use epidemic in the 1960s, as well as the military's response during and following the Vietnam war, which conceptually relates to the Surgeon General's 2016 report.[8]

DoD Task Force

In 1967, DoD convened a task force to investigate the problem of drug use in the military. Congress ordered that hazardous alcohol use be accorded the same level of attention as did illicit

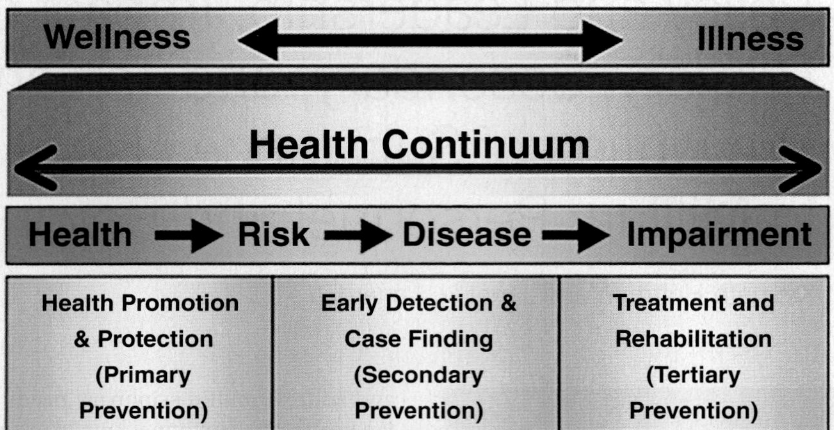

Figure 30-1. The relationship between the health continuum, intervention points, and primary, secondary, and tertiary prevention strategies. (From DoD TRICARE Management Activity, *Population Health Improvement Plan and Guide and Guide and Guide*. TRICARE Management Activity, Government Printing Office; 2001:10, figure 5.)

drug use, and this became part of the charge to the task force. Based on their recommendations, a policy directive set forth in 1970 came to guide military efforts to confront drug and alcohol use disorders (AUDs) over the ensuing decade.[9]

The 1970 DoD policy emphasized prevention of SUDs through education and enforcement procedures that focused on detection and early intervention. The policy also called for treatment of risky use of alcohol and nonmedical use of drugs, with an emphasis on helping those engaged in such use to return to service.

In 1971, President Richard Nixon delivered a special message to Congress on "Drug Abuse Prevention and Control," in which he said, "America has the largest number of heroin addicts of any nation in the world [and] an especially disheartening aspect of that problem involves those of our men in Vietnam who have used drugs. Peer pressures combine with easy availability to foster drug use. We are taking steps to end the availability of drugs in South Vietnam but, in addition, the nature of drug addiction and the peculiar aspects of the present problem as it involves veterans, make it imperative that rehabilitation procedures be undertaken immediately."[10]

Around the same time, the Secretary of Defense issued a memorandum to all commands, encouraging military personnel to submit themselves voluntarily for treatment and rehabilitation under the Drug Identification and Treatment Program of the Department of Defense.[11] This led to Public Law 92–129 §501(a), enacted in 1971 and titled "Identification and Treatment of Drug and Alcohol Dependent Persons in the Armed Forces"—a mandate to identify and provide treatment that continues today under Title 10 US Code §1090.[12]

Individual service branches were tasked with implementing programs that were consistent with the overall policy, but which also met the needs of personnel in their branch of the military.[9] Several new directives issued in the early 1970s clarified how treatment and prevention initiatives were to be set in motion.[13] Decades later, the Veterans Health Administration/Department of Defense Clinical Practice Guidelines for the Management of Substance Use Disorders in the Primary Care Setting in 2001 were created.[14] These guidelines have been regularly updated over the years to the current 2021 version. This is consistent with the Institute of Medicine's 2013 recommendations to the DoD for prevention, diagnosis, treatment, and management of SUDs throughout military medical and mental health care systems; and an outgrowth from first concerns of unhealthy substance use.[15]

The Vietnam Experience

The military's policy toward SUDs developed in response to concerns about illicit drug use among American service personnel returning from Vietnam. A study of 451 Army enlisted men who had returned from duty in Vietnam found that, before their deployment, half had used alcohol regularly and one in four had problems related to drinking, currently defined as problems that negatively impact ability to perform military duties or conduct appropriate for active duty personnel.[16] Once in Vietnam, the prevalence of risky drinking in this group declined, but their nonmedical use of opioids rose sharply: half reported that they had tried opioids, and 20% said they had become physically dependent or people who use.[17]

When these personnel returned to the United States, their use of opioids declined sharply (with only 2% reporting physical dependence or usage), while their rate of hazardous alcohol use increased.[18]

Drug Amnesty and Rehabilitation

In the Vietnam theater, the fourth Infantry Division piloted a Drug Amnesty and Rehabilitation Program for Soldiers who, although not otherwise identified as using or involved with illicit drugs, had voluntarily presented themselves as persons with a SUD to their chaplain, unit surgeon, or commander. Without punishment or adverse personnel actions, these soldiers were provided with (1) rapid medical assessment, (2) individual counseling and group therapy, and (3) assignment of a "buddy" who could deliver positive reinforcement for abstinence. Throughout treatment, soldiers were expected to continue full duty. The results were very positive, and the success of this approach became the model for an Army-wide program implemented 2 years later.[19]

DEVELOPMENT AND IMPLEMENTATION OF DRUG TESTING AS A DETERRENT: A DRUG-FREE WORKPLACE

Drug testing has been a key component of the military's response to the 1971 Presidential directive, which led to the establishment of a urine screening program that grew almost immediately to include service members returning from Vietnam, many of whom were people who used heroin. The program initially tested for opioids, barbiturates, and amphetamines and was a massive undertaking. It consisted of mandatory testing of all service members leaving Southeast Asia, as well as mandatory random testing of U.S. forces worldwide.[20] This approach later became a model for the creation of civilian employee workplace drug-testing programs in the United States.

The mid-1970s proved a difficult time for the fledgling urine screening program. In June 1974, the program was challenged in the courts on the grounds that it violated Fifth Amendment protections against self-incrimination. The court ruled that because general discharge had a potentially adverse effect on an individual's status, service members could refuse to submit a urine sample for testing.[21]

As a result, DoD issued new drug-testing guidelines in 1975. These stipulated that, although drug testing was mandatory, the results could be used only to support entry into a drug treatment program. The new guidelines also affirmed that personnel identified through urine drug testing could be given only an honorable discharge.[22]

In 1976, Congress discouraged the use of large-scale random drug testing as not cost-effective. Consequently, from 1976 until 1981, the testing program went dormant. By 1977, however, there were widespread reports—particularly in the Federal Republic of Germany—of increased drug use among military personnel. In response, the House Select Committee on Narcotics Abuse and Control ordered a series of observational surveys that supported reports of increased drug use. The overwhelming drug of choice appeared to be cannabis.[23]

The crash of a jet on the flight deck of the aircraft carrier Nimitz in 1981 riveted public attention on drug use in the military.[24] Autopsies of 14 Navy personnel found evidence of cannabis use among 6 of the 13 sailors killed in the crash, as well as nonprescription antihistamine use by the pilot, leading to the conclusion that illicit drug use may have been a contributing factor. Based on these results, Congress demanded action by the Secretary of Defense. In response, DoD announced a 10-point program to control nonmedical drug use that called for increased drug testing, discharge of military members who had recurrent problems, improved rehabilitation programs, and a massive education effort.[25]

In the summer of 1981, a major scientific breakthrough provided an important impetus for DoD's antidrug efforts. Scientists at the Armed Forces Institute of Pathology (AFIP) developed procedures that employed gas chromatography to confirm the presence of tetrahydrocannabinol (THC), the active ingredient in cannabis.[26] In December 1981, the Deputy Secretary of Defense issued a major change in DoD policy on evidentiary use of drug testing.[27] The new policy stated that test results could be used as evidence if they were properly obtained and if a strict chain of custody was maintained (ie, processes were followed that ensured that the urine sample was properly identified at the time it was obtained and processed, and not confused with that of another individual).

Concurrent with the policy change, in December 1981, the Department of the Navy launched its "War on Drugs,"[28] an aggressive program that involved extensive use of urinalysis to test for use of cannabis, widespread use of portable drug-testing equipment, unit-wide "sweep testing," and testing of all recruits during accession. The Navy also launched an intensive program of drug education, which featured an unequivocal message that drug use would not be tolerated. The Navy's program thus marked the beginning of DoD's zero tolerance emphasis, and the other services soon announced similar programs. Although help was offered to personnel who sought treatment for SUDs, the message was clear that those who did not follow the zero-tolerance policy would be discharged.

Forensic Testing Sufficient for Adverse Personnel Action

DoD has developed a series of directives and instructions (DoDIs) for use in developing and implementing regulations that meet the 1981 "War on Drugs." Current policies address prevention and management of "Problematic Substance Use by DoD Personnel"[29] and include the "DoD Civilian Employee Drug-Free Workplace Program,"[30] which outlines specific policies and technical procedures to be used in implementing the "Military Personnel Drug Abuse Testing Program."[31] The DoDIs deterrence testing focuses on three key areas: (1) deterrence testing for common and easily detected illicit drugs, (2) education to prevent harmful use of alcohol and/or to intervene early when harmful use is detected, and (3) quickly initiating treatment whenever an SUD is diagnosed.[32] In addition, DoD Forensic Drug Testing Labs can conduct additional tests such as differentiating the synthetic THC of dronabinol and the THC in cannabis.[33]

Since the initiation of the military forensic drug testing program, military service members' urine specimens are collected under direct observation, with strict chain-of-custody documentation and secure processing of specimens for shipment to the supporting drug testing laboratory. A two-step testing procedure provides legally sufficient information to commanders about personnel who have violated drug use policy. Defined cut-off values are used to identify service members with positive urine screens. A medical officer, functioning as a medical review officer (MRO), reviews the results and determines if a test-positive urine could be attributable to a prescribed medication. Commanders who receive urine test-positive results then have evidence sufficient to support administrative or legal action against the service member.[34]

Clinical Testing and Limited Use

In response to the mandate to treat, the military has created a path for active-duty service-members to self-identify as having a drug use problem or concerned about having a drug-positive urine: in all cases, individuals may seek treatment before being command-directed for a urine test. Seeking treatment proactively and voluntarily bypasses the punitive side.

Under limited use, or "safe harbor" policy, as part of the evaluation, a treatment provider can request a urine drug test, with any positive drug test protected from potential adverse personnel or command action. This is a one-time exemption from adverse personnel action.[35] Future forensic urine samples can be required on a regular basis, with a positive test sufficient cause for adverse administrative or legal action. Adverse actions can include suspension of any favorable personnel actions like awards, promotions, or attendance at schools or more drastic measures such as a dishonorable discharge or legal charges. Whether to take adverse administrative or legal action is a command decision without need for further medical input[36] (eg, UCMJ article 112a).

POLICY AND LEADERSHIP: A DIFFERENT APPROACH TO ALCOHOL, OTHER DRUG USE AND TOBACCO

Alcohol

Historically, alcohol use in the military is accepted if not interfering with military duties nor rising to the level of adverse legal problems within the military or civilian community and in keeping with military tradition.[37,38] Consequently, use of alcohol is common and generally accepted by the community. An innovative intervention/treatment program was initiated by a Medical Corps Major in the United States Air Force (USAF) in 1953. In that year, 50 pilots diagnosed with AUD who otherwise would have been discharged were instead provided with brief but effective interventions that included participation in Alcoholics Anonymous (AA) and use of AUD pharmacotherapy. Of this group, 25 were able to continue active duty, thereby salvaging their careers and saving the Air Force an estimated $1 million.[39] A comprehensive review of military alcohol treatment programs between 1964 and 1974 found that the military had developed effective alcohol treatment programs but had difficulty in identifying personnel with AUDs and getting them into treatment.[40]

Attitudes toward alcohol use and AUD in the military have changed remarkably little in the decades since that study. For example, a 1971 study found that the Army had spent $300,000 on 100 persons with AUD, mostly for court-martials, while only about 5% of that sum had been spent on treatment.[41] At the same time, the Army had implemented an effective intervention program that used a systems approach to ensure comprehensive and continuous care. The rationale for that program acknowledged that the military appeared to have a larger drinking problem than the civilian population, and that more than 20% of hospital admissions to one Army hospital were related to AUDs.[42]

Developing and conducting effective treatment (and prevention) programs requires an understanding of the perceptions, norms, and other factors that influence alcohol use. Using observations and interviews with soldiers, Ingraham[43] examined junior enlisted life in the barracks in the 1970s. He found that to "fit in," soldiers had to abide by the norms of barracks living and that, on post, there were sanctioned and unsanctioned drinking occasions. *Sanctioned* occasions included drinking during company or battalion "organization days" to ease interpersonal tensions (such as when a unit returned from a field exercise, or during a medical center picnic where the military serves alcohol), during athletic events, or in the barracks during off-duty time. *Unsanctioned* occasions involved drinking on duty, drinking that was related to vandalism or fighting, or drinking "hard liquor" in the barracks. A third occasion for drinking occurred off post.

Ingraham concluded that these drinking patterns reflected the local social structure and values, drawing members closer to each other through shared drinking experiences.[43] Participation required little in the way of social skills except the ability to drink without becoming ill or dysfunctional. As part of barracks life, young soldiers drank heavily but generally did not overtly demonstrate problems because of their alcohol use. This is consistent with reports from several clinical treatment studies that younger patients had more difficulty in perceiving themselves as having either unhealthy alcohol use or an AUD than did their older peers.[44]

Since the mid-1990s, the military health care system has become increasingly integrated with national civilian health care systems and standard health insurance practices. The command-medical linkages transitioned to military-civilian linkages and the military health care system was augmented with the TRICARE military insurance plan. Treatment of SUDs is included as an insurance benefit. Recommended care follows VA/DoD clinical practice guidelines for SUDs.[45]

In 2004, Warren Air Force Base operationalized the concept of "responsible drinking" after a base-wide survey found that the average airman thought "unsafe drinking" began with eight or more drinks. Based upon a 2002 NIAAA Call to action to reduce binge drinking in college students, the base command led a coalition of base agencies, leadership, and personnel to develop a "0-0-1-3" unhealthy alcohol use tool, defined as: "0" = Zero drinks if under 21 years old, "0" = Zero DUIs, "1" = One drink per hour, and "3" = no more than three drinks per outing or evening. One drink per hour was selected because 60 minutes is roughly the amount of time it takes to metabolize the alcohol from one drink. "Binge drinking" was defined as more than 3 drinks in an outing for both males and females. A three-pronged approach was used: (1) all personnel were screened for binge drinking using a standardized instrument, with referral for early intervention or treatment as determined by medical personnel, and all personnel with an alcohol-related event were referred for evaluation and treatment; (2) prevention activities included education on social norms, low-risk drinking and hazards of binge drinking, development of activities and events without alcohol use, for the 18- to 25-year old population; and (3) involvement of law enforcement, chambers of commerce and colleges in the surrounding community, to promote responsible sales, service, and use. Within the first year, alcohol-related incidents were reduced by 74%, underage drinking incidents reduced by 81%, and DUI cases reduced 45%.[46,47]

Current VA/DoD clinical practice guidelines no longer require abstinence as the sole successful outcome and are more tolerant of returning to use. IOM recommendations are being integrated into the TRICARE policy manual, and there is growing recognition of the need for more TRICARE network physicians who are educated, trained, and skilled in the practice of addiction medicine.

Potential Legal Issues

There is "zero tolerance" for use of Schedule I—which includes cannabis—or nonprescribed Schedule II drugs. A positive random or for-cause forensic urine test is sufficient grounds for adverse personnel or legal action, including separation from service, where treatment might be provided either within TRICARE or the Veterans Administration. However, there is a limited use or "safe harbor" policy that allows an individual to self-refer and seek treatment for a substance use problem. As well, a positive urine test collected when entering treatment does not subject the individual to adverse personnel or legal action. However, after treatment entry, the individual is expected to maintain abstinence, and any urine sample collected for forensic testing later can result in adverse action.[48,49]

Individuals using illicit drugs, and alcohol use with adverse consequences, are subject to punishment under the Uniformed Code of Military Justice (UCMJ).[50] Three articles under UCMJ specifically related to alcohol and controlled substances: Article 111—"Drunken or reckless operation of vehicle, aircraft, or vessel";[51] Article 112—"Drunk on duty";[52] and Article 112a—"Wrongful use, possession, etc., of controlled substances."[36]

Tobacco

Tobacco use has been addressed independently from alcohol and other drugs, with policies supporting tobacco cessation, tobacco-free living, and tobacco-free worksites.[53,54]

Smoking cigarettes as part of the military culture dates to World War I. Supported by congressional appropriations, tobacco products could be sold through commissaries and were in some instances included free of charge in deployed rations and settings. This resulted in lowest cost and tax-free cigarettes that could be found most anywhere the military member was serving around the globe.[55] By the 1980s, there were growing concerns about the negative impact of tobacco on health of DoD personnel and increasing awareness of the inverse relationship between price and smoking rates. With a strong tobacco industry and lobby, with Congressional interest, there has been long-standing interest that tobacco products continue to be made readily available on DoD installations for easy access and low-cost consumption. However, a compromise was reached that supported continued sales while increasing the price and have allowed continuing health promotion efforts for tobacco cessation. Tobacco sales were moved from the commissary system to the exchange system that operated on nonappropriated funds and where the system was required to break even financially. Although still tax-free, pricing could be increased to break even. This resulted in prices that were still low compared to the community, but marginally over wholesale and still within Congressional appropriation language.

Efforts to reduce tobacco use in the 1980s had become a key component of military health promotion programs. At that time, the Army's community health nurses engaged in health promotion using a computer-mediated survey: the Army Health Risk Appraisal (HRA) that was based on the Rhode Island Wellness Check. Compatible with computing capability at the time, answers were handwritten and then scanned with an interpretation, including smoking status, printed at the time of encounter. Using a prudent advice model, a "wellness score" was generated based upon modifiable risk factors such as tobacco use, alcohol use, nutrition, weight, depression, exercise pattern, and suicidal ideation. The HRA was designed to allow immediate and brief intervention with a community health nurse. It also allowed deidentified aggregate data for command reports and gave a demographic breakdown of risk profiles. This helped in designing targeted health promotion programs.

In 1991, the Army funded the Center for Training and Education in Addiction Medicine at the Uniformed Services University that in 1994, conducted a tobacco cessation demonstration project. In more than 3,500 surveys completed, 30% of soldiers who smoked were precontemplative, 19% were contemplative, 20% were in the preparation stage, 5% were in the action stage, and 6% had achieved maintenance. Younger soldiers who smoked were more likely to be in precontemplation, and older people who smoke were more likely to be in maintenance.

Soldiers in the precontemplative stage were more likely to believe that smoking improved concentration than soldiers in the contemplative stage and less likely to use seatbelts than other soldiers who smoked. They were also less likely to believe that smoking impaired their physical performance or that their friends would discourage them from smoking. From these findings, interventions were designed to move people who smoked from precontemplation to contemplation with greater awareness of the immediate impact of smoking on physical performance and to perceive greater social support for nonsmoking. Most soldiers who had successfully quit agreed with the statement: "I tell myself that if I try hard enough, I can keep from smoking." This suggested an intervention that soldiers who quit smoking should be trained to encourage themselves to maintain their success (Internal status report of The U.S. Army Smoking Cessation Demonstration Project, 1996). Soldiers who quit smoking were more likely to report problems with alcohol than were soldiers who were still smoking (Internal status report, 1996).[56]

Through the 1990s, within each of the service-specific health programs, tobacco cessation became part of an overall integrated health promotion and disease prevention program.

Today, health promotion includes targeted priorities on (1) tobacco-free living, (2) preventing drug use disorder and excessive alcohol use, (3) healthy eating, (4) active living, (5) injury and violence-free living, (6) reproductive and sexual health, and (7) mental and emotional well-being.[54,57] Within each uniformed service, there are specific wellness and health promotion programs. To support these programs, a DoD Center of Excellence, the Consortium for Health and Military Performance (CHAMP) was established at the Uniformed Services University. Its mission is to translate research into practice to improve the resilience and performance of service members and their families. Programs take a holistic approach that involves leadership, community engagement, and specific tools and guidelines for clinical providers. Resources and approaches for early and brief interventions related to tobacco, alcohol, and controlled substance use are available on the website.[58]

In the most current VA/DoD clinical practice guideline for SUDs, the focus is on treatment of SUDs but also affords some flexibility on nondysfunctional substance use for beneficiaries entitled for care within TRICARE or the VA health care system. A separate practice guideline now exists for tobacco use and follows U.S. preventive task force recommendations and updated clinical practice guidelines from the Agency for Healthcare Research and Quality.[59-61]

Figure 30-2 highlights seven steps for population and individual health improvement that links health care to the

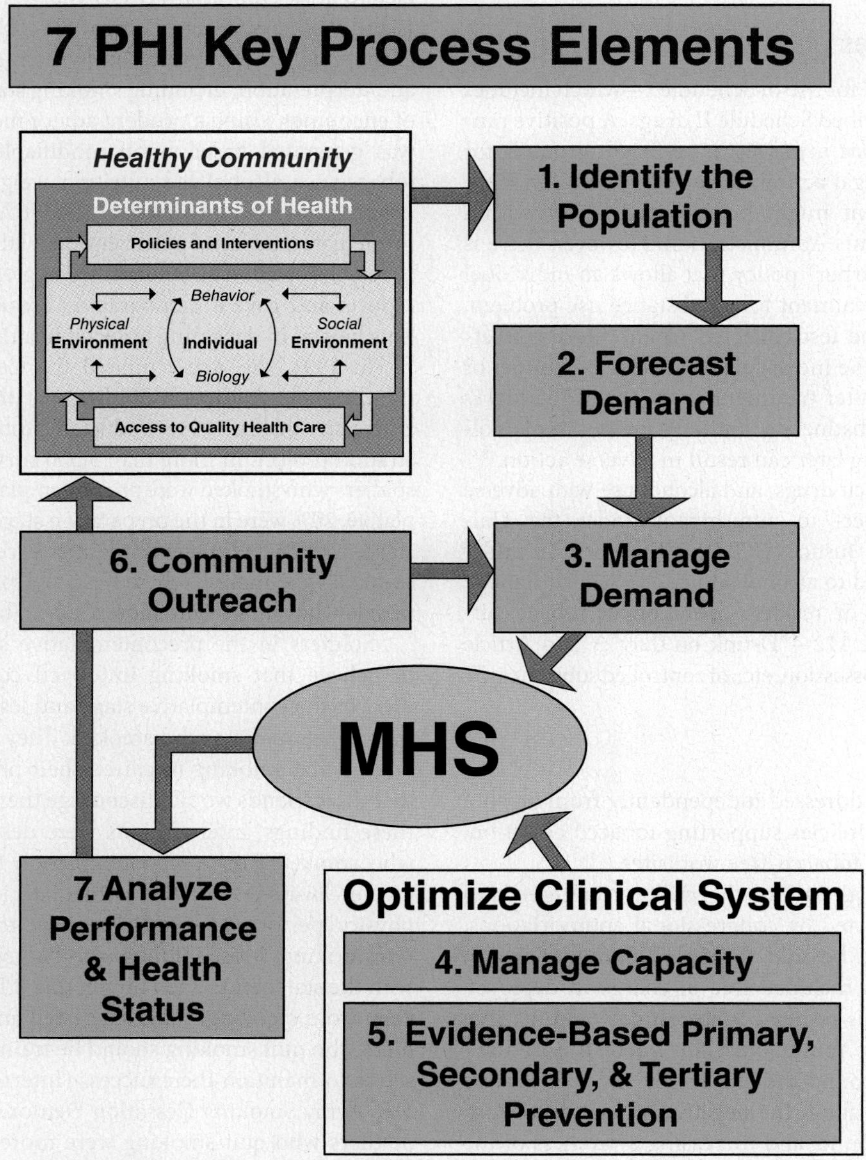

Figure 30-2. Seven population health improvement key process elements. (From *DoD TRICARE Management Activity. Population Health Improvement Plan and Guide and Guide and Guide*; 2001:33, figure 10.)

community. This model was consistent with the early alcohol, drug, and prevention treatment program. Cross-sectional surveys and HRAs could be used to determine health and problems in the community, opportunities for interventions in at-risk populations, and earlier interventions with individuals having identified SUDs. Decreasing the community prevalence of unhealthy alcohol use and other drug use was central. Primary prevention was focused on education and "deglamorization" of alcohol use throughout military commands and communities. Secondary prevention focused on identifying at-risk populations for early interventions through health promotion programs. Tertiary prevention involved ensuring treatment was available for those active-duty members clinically diagnosed with a SUD and was designed so that the individual patient had a high likelihood of achieving full sustained remission. Since patients treated at a residential treatment facility (ASAM Level III) would be returning to the referring provider and command, higher level treatment was seamlessly linked to at least 1-year aftercare by outpatient programs located at the home base. At that time, some residential programs were also running concurrent family programs where family members could receive a week of psychoeducation—that could include individual and family therapy—related to the impact of SUDs within the family and actions that the family might take.

IMPACT ON PREVALENCE AND TRENDS OF ALCOHOL AND SUBSTANCE USE IN THE MILITARY

To better understand and monitor substance use in the active-duty military, DoD initiated a series of comprehensive large, representative, anonymous personnel surveys that are administered every 3-4 years. A weighted sampling strategy is used to ensure sufficient representation of women, services and paygrades with lower numbers of active-duty personnel. Approximately 200,000 active-duty personnel were invited to participate between 1980 and 2008, with just over 17,000 providing usable surveys. The Health Risk Behavior Survey (HRBS), funded by the Department of Defense, is the primary cross-sectional survey for understanding the health and well-being of service members.

Sociodemographic Characteristics of Active-Duty Personnel

In 1980, military personnel were predominantly male, White, had some college education or a college degree, relatively young (almost half were aged 25 or younger), and married.[1-3]

This has changed over time with an increasing proportion of women, Hispanic and other racial/ethnic groups, more who are college-educated, and personnel aged 35 years and older increased significantly.[1-3,62] Significant sociodemographic differences between the branches of the military with implications related to diversity and equity are covered in other chapters.[63]

Trends in Substance Use and SUDs

From 1980 through 2018, the percentage of active-duty military personnel who engaged in heavy alcohol use defined as 5 or more drinks on one occasion, or illicit drug use during the 30 days prior to the survey was higher than the general population, and more than one in four of all service members agree that the military culture is supportive of drinking. In the last survey, 2018, an estimated 34% of military personnel reported binge drinking in the prior 30 days with 10% reporting current heavy drinking (1-2 days/week). Drinking behavior was more common in the junior enlisted ranks, among men, and within the Marine Corps and Navy.[64] Higher levels of drinking were associated with higher rates of alcohol-related problems, with people who drank "heavily" reporting nearly three times the rate of serious consequences and more than twice the rate of productivity loss compared to those who drank "moderate to heavy."[1,3] Such problems compromise the ability of military personnel to execute their mission and can lead to reduced readiness and lowered total force fitness.[65] In 2018, nearly 40% of service members reported the use of tobacco/nicotine with use of e-cigarettes increasing similarly to the civilian population.

Between 2015 and 2018, rates of binge drinking, heavy drinking, current cigarette/e-cigarette/pipe/hookah use all increased.[63] In 2018, rates of binge drinking, current cigarette smoking, current cigar smoking, and current smokeless tobacco use continued to significantly exceed the lower rates of Healthy People 2020 goals, in contrast to illicit drug use where rates were consistently significantly lower than Healthy People 2020 goals.[64]

In the 2015 HRBS survey, fewer than 1% of respondents reported past year drug use across all military branches between officers and enlisted service members, much lower than civilian populations across five categories: cannabis, synthetic cannabis, inhalants to get high, synthetic stimulants, and other illegal drugs.[66]

LEARNING FROM HISTORY: CONNECTING ALCOHOL AND OTHER DRUG DETECTION TO EARLY INTERVENTION, TREATMENT, RELAPSE PREVENTION, AND HEALTH PROMOTION

SUDS and Barriers to Treatment

There are significant benefits for the military community when engaging in SUD treatment. The accessibility of medical care through military benefits has been connected to decreased racial disparities in time to seeking treatment.[67] However, engagement with services are low both among active-duty personnel and veterans.[68] Recent research has been looking at the barriers to utilization of the military health care system, identifying major themes that include social norms and stigma, financial and other logistical barriers, lack of confidence in the providers/system, navigating through the services, and privacy and security concerns.[69] Additional disparities are shown to exist in screening and referrals to care in the military health care system.[70-72]

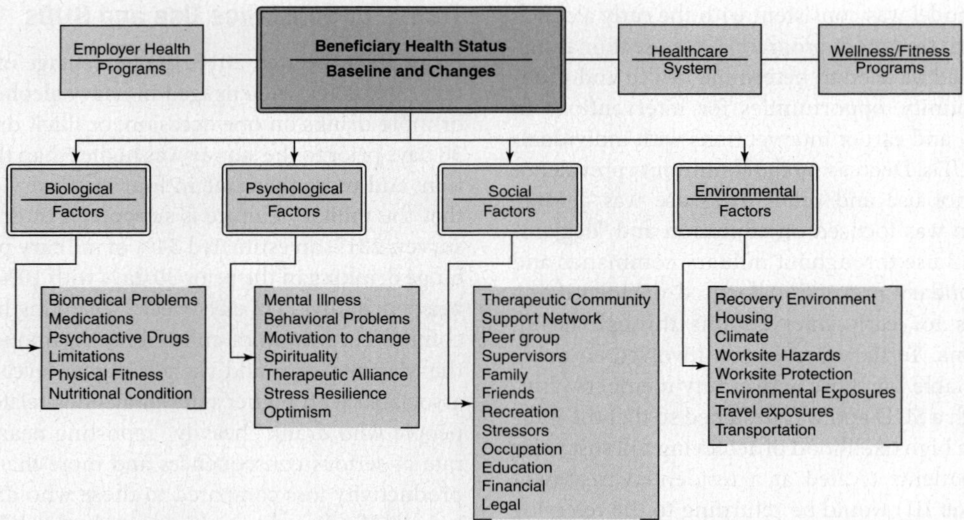

Figure 30-3. A comprehensive multidimensional framework for assessment and intervention for optimized individual and population health improvement. A multidimensional approach to individual and population health improvement: Measuring baseline multidimensional health status and changes through population-based and individual interventions. (From Hoffman KJ. Demystifying mental health information needs through Integrated Definition (IDEF) activity and data modeling. *Proc AMIA Annual Fall Symp.* 1997:111-116; Hoffman, KJ, Neven T. *The Alcohol and Drug Prevention and Control Program (ADAPCP) Clinical Information System (ACIS): User Manual for the ADAPCP Prototype Electronic Patient Record.* Center for Training and Education in Addiction Medicine, USUHS/Henry M Jackson Foundation; 1995.)

Efforts to address SUDs among military veterans has been integrating both SUD treatment and treatment of one or more of the most common co-occurring conditions (eg, PTSD, military sexual trauma).[73-76] These innovations hold significant promise both through addressing interrelated issues simultaneously, and through patient buy-in.[77] There is limited research available on racial, ethnic minorities, women, sexual, and gender minorities regarding the outcomes of military health care–based SUD treatment for communities experiencing disparities.

ASAM developed a six-dimensional model for patient placement and continuum of care, within the same time frame DoD had developed an optimized model for person-centric care in a more global model for prevention and treatment. If able to change the current healthcare focus from facility-centric patient care to person-centric care, specific problems and strengths assessed in both a bio-psycho-social assessment and ASAM criteria could guide culturally and ethnically sensitive interventions at each level of prevention.

Figure 30-3, initially developed within the Army's alcohol and drug treatment program, highlights specific components that were part of a comprehensive biopsychosocial assessment that was used to develop individualized comprehensive treatment plan; it is also applicable to interventions that might occur in the community, at the worksite, and in health promoting settings.

IMPACT FOR THE NATION

Original concepts that led to DoD's prevention and treatment programs were implemented by leadership who saw the continuum between prevention and treatment, and the continuum of treatment that connected residential treatment programs to 1-year follow-up in the community. The recursive relationship between military communities and medical treatment providers have been modeled in nonmilitary settings nationally and globally.

Policy and Leadership: A Healthy Alcohol-Drug-Free Living Environment for Relapse Prevention and Health Improvement: The Oxford House Model

The Oxford House (OH) model, which was extensively studied by Center for Community Research at DePaul University and recognized as an evidence-based program, emphasizes a supportive home environment and social network for individuals.[78] OH strives to create an environment where individuals can reestablish healthy behaviors, connect with others, and function as a healthy family member and good neighbor. An OH is not a treatment facility. They do not provide medical care, but provides an optimal recovery environment for relapse prevention.

The DoD conducted a pilot study of the OH model for TRICARE beneficiaries in 2001 to evaluate feasibility, effectiveness, and cost-efficiency.[78] Key findings from the study included the following:

1. In none of the five regions studied was there a designated "alcohol-free" living environment within barracks, and active-duty service members living in OH were fearful that their careers would be terminated should anyone connected to the base discover they had chosen to live in an OH.

2. At the time of the study, from a network of approximately 1,000 Oxford Houses, approximately one-third of Oxford House residents within the five study regions were veterans. Oxford House had connections to sections of the Veterans Administration working with homeless veterans. However, only a total of 105 OH residents identified themselves as TRICARE beneficiaries. Most were retirees, junior, midcareer, and senior enlisted pay grades from all services, with only a few self-identified as being active duty. All had remained abstinent and found living in OH very helpful and would recommend it to others.
3. The report recommended DoD Health Affairs reestablish a full-time senior officer as a dedicated program manager for SUD prevention and treatment intervention programs, which would include alcohol, illicit drugs, and nicotine. Working with community support networks and healthy recovery environments was considered essential to enhance the likelihood that patients treated for SUDs achieved sustained full remission. Most residents appear to have found their way into Oxford House independently of any systematic medical referral process.[78]

Impact Following Other Prevention Recommendations: COVID-19 Experience

With the COVID-19 pandemic, OH leadership quickly implemented recommendations to adhere to CDC guidelines in keeping with the OH model for recovery. Significantly lower rates of infection and mortality were found for residents of recovery homes, and their COVID-19 mortality rates were extremely low. Throughout the pandemic, among the approximately 45,000 people who had lived in an OH, and approximately 26,000 recovery beds across approximately 3,200 houses in 47 states, there were 1,423 positive COVID-19 cases and 3 confirmed deaths. These findings demonstrate the capability and outcomes when OH residents followed CDC guidelines consistent with the home's OH charter and leadership recommendations.

Global Health: Integrating the Continuum of Prevention and Treatment in a PEPFAR-Funded DoD-Supported Program in Tanzania

DoD has had an important role supporting national initiatives, such as the President's Emergency Plan for AIDS Relief (PEPFAR), with an established international presence in Mbeya, Tanzania, including collaboration with its Ministry of Health and Drug Commission and Enforcement Authority and with local community organizational support and the Regional Zonal Hospital in Mbeya.[79,80]

Because of the relationship between intravenous (IV) drug use and HIV infection, in 2017, PEPFAR, DoD, HJF, the Tanzania Ministry of Health, and the Zonal Hospital supported establishing an opioid treatment program at the hospital. Modeled on optimal clinical practices, an integrated biopsychosocial model was used to evaluate and treat patients, with an integrated team of physicians, nurses, social workers, psychologists, and pharmacists to medically manage opioid withdrawal and stabilize the patient on methadone for maintenance therapy while providing other medical treatment and counseling services. In 2017, there were an estimated 450 people who used drugs and could benefit from services of this new opioid treatment program (OTP). As of June 2021, a total of 383 people had benefited from opioid treatment services, and as of July 2021, there were 173 current patients receiving methadone. Directly Observed Treatment is used to administer methadone, with no opioid-related deaths.[81]

A unique feature of this program has been the connection with patients to a community support organization at the time an individual comes into the clinic for evaluation and treatment. This new patient is also connected at the first opportunity to a peer-support individual, who may already be an established patient at the clinic.

Transportation was identified as a major treatment barrier as the clinic grew. A second clinic was established at a border town, Tunduma, in its Health Centre, where patients would be able to reengage in care. This was also in a region where there was a known problem with illicit drug use across the border and had greatest need for a clinic.

Providers and hospital saw the potential to treat patients with other chronic conditions within the OTP, including HIV and tuberculosis. Additionally, consistent with the opioid agonist therapy (OAT) treatment model, patients received enhanced adherence counseling, with group and individual peer support. For the patients who initially had high HIV titers, at the end of 3 months, all had achieved viral suppression. For patients who initially had active tuberculosis infection, after 6 months of observed treatment, all had negative sputum tests.

Figure 30-4 schematically diagrams the components of care provided by the Mbeya OAT clinic. In this model, the clinic has worked with the surrounding community and health care providers to assure patients coming in for assessment already have the support of one of the community-service organizations and includes peer support for treatment adherence and relapse prevention. This combined approach includes close connections to community support organizations, law enforcement, group and patient peer support are models for collaborative patient-centered integrated health care within the United States.

CONCLUSIONS

Implicit within the military command and health care system has been the concept of prevention and treatment of addiction, which includes the following:

- Periodic worldwide surveys estimating the prevalence of alcohol, drug, and tobacco use/unhealthy use/adverse consequences of use within DoD.

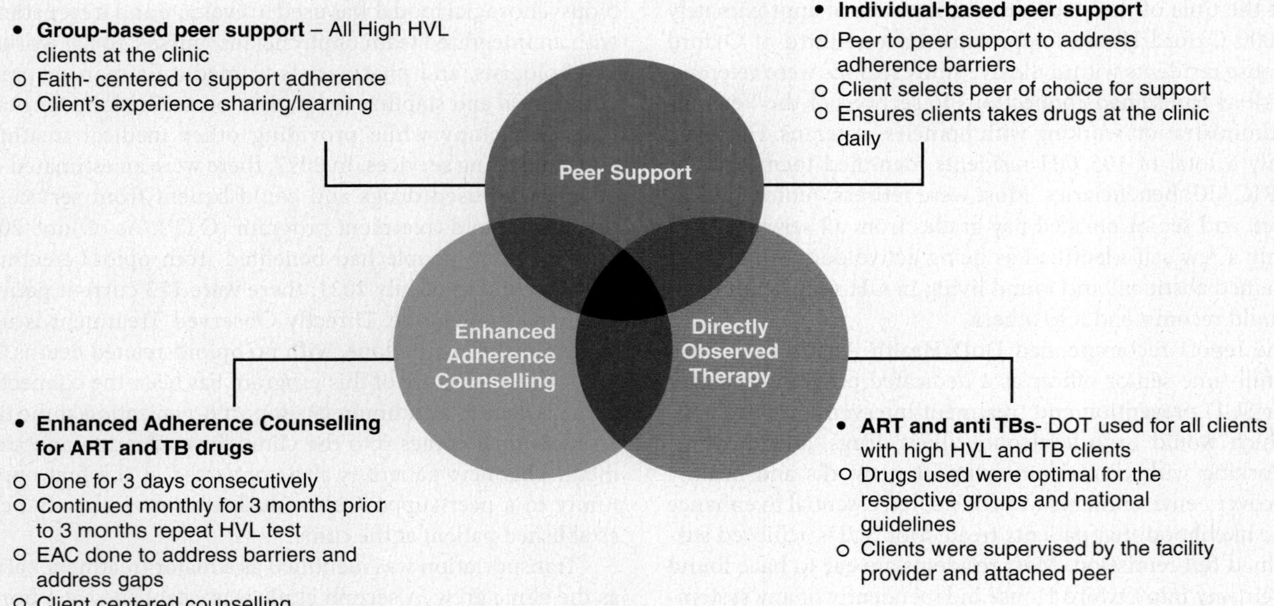

Figure 30-4. Opioid treatment program model for adherence. A combined approach of opioid agonist therapy (OAT), HIV/tuberculosis (HIV/TB), directly observed therapy (DOT), and enhanced adherence counseling (EAC) with psychosocial and community support results in optimal HIV and TB treatment outcomes for people who use drugs (PWUDs).

- Since nondysfunctional alcohol use has been supported throughout history within DoD, abstinence following treatment is not specifically required as long as there is no recurrence of dysfunctional behaviors.
- "Zero tolerance" for illicit use and full responsibility for behavior and actions taken under the influence of alcohol or drugs has been a central theme.
- A "safe harbor" for anyone who volunteers for or requests treatment for a SUD.
- Treatment consistent with IOM 2013 recommendations and VA/DoD practice guidelines.
- Treatment of tobacco use disorder following AHRQ and USPTF recommendations.
- The importance of a healthy living environment and alcohol-drug-free housing has a proven positive impact on the recovery environment.
- The ASAM multidimensional model for assessment and treatment of patients with SUD and co-occurring conditions have been successfully deployed with DoD assistance into international, nonmilitary settings hard hit by HIV and SUDs.

REFERENCES

1. Bray RM, Pemberton MR, Hourani LL, et al. *2008 Department of Defense Survey of Health-Related Behaviors Among Active-Duty Military Personnel.* Report prepared for TRICARE Management Activity, Office of the Assistant Secretary of Defense (Health Affairs) and U.S. Coast Guard. RTI International; 2009.
2. Bray RM, Pemberton MR, Lane ME, et al. Substance use and mental health trends among U.S. military active duty personnel: key findings from the 2008 DoD Health Behavior Survey. *Mil Med.* 2010(175):390-399.
3. Bray RM, Hourani LL, Williams J, et al. *Understanding Military Workforce Productivity: Effects of Substance Abuse, Health, and Mental Health.* Springer; 2014.
4. *Army Regulation 600-85: The Army Substance Abuse Program.* Department of the Army. Accessed June 21, 2022. https://armypubs.army.mil/epubs/DR_pubs/DR_a/ARN38035-AR_600-85-002-WEB-5.pdf
5. *Army Regulation 40-68: Clinical Quality Management.* Department of the Army. Accessed June 21, 2022. https://armypubs.army.mil/epubs/DR_pubs/DR_a/pdf/web/r40_68.pdf
6. Teeter JB, Lancaster CL, Brown DG, Back SE. Substance use disorders in military veterans: prevalence and treatment challenges. *Subst Abuse Rehabil.* 2017;8:69-77. https://www.ncbi.nlm.nih.gov/pmc/articles/PMC5587184/
7. Sirratt D, Ozanian A, Traenkner B. Epidemiology and prevention of substance use disorders in the military. *Mil Med.* 2012;177(8 Suppl):21-28.
8. Surgeon General of the United States. *Facing Addiction in America: The Surgeon General's Report on Alcohol, Drugs, and Health.* Office of the Surgeon General. U.S. Department of Health and Human Services; 2016.
9. Committee on Prevention, Diagnosis, Treatment, and Management of Substance Use Disorders in the U.S. Armed Forces; Board on the Health of Select Populations; Institute of Medicine; O'Brien CP, Oster M, Morden E, eds. Chapter 2, Understanding Substance Use Disorders in the Military. *Substance Use Disorders in the U.S. Armed Forces.* National Academies Press (US); 2013. Accessed October 2, 2023. https://www.ncbi.nlm.nih.gov/books/NBK207276/
10. Nixon RM. *Special Message to the Congress on Drug Abuse Prevention and Control, June 17, 1971.* The American Presidency Project;2017.
11. Office of the Under Secretary for Personnel and Readiness. *Military Drug Program Historical Timeline 1960's to 2008.* Accessed October 2, 2023. https://prhome.defense.gov/Portals/52/Documents/RFM/Readiness/DDRP/docs/72208/DoD%20Drug%20Policy%20History.pdf
12. United States Code. *Identifying and Treating Drug and Alcohol Dependent Persons in the Armed Forces (Public Law 92–129, Title 10 US Code §1090), 2006 Edition, Supplement 4, Title 10.* Armed Forces; 1971.

13. Bray RM, Marsden ME, Herbold JR, et al. Progress toward eliminating drug and alcohol use among U.S. military personnel. In: Stanley J, Blair JD, eds. *Challenges in Military Health Care: Perspectives on Health Status and the Provision of Care.* Transaction Publishers; 1993.
14. Kivlahan D, Miller SC, McNicholas LF, Willenbring M, Susskind, Eds. *Veterans Health Administration and Department of Defense Clinical Practice Guideline for the Management of Substance Use Disorders in the Primary Care Setting.* VHA and DoD; 2001.
15. Institute of Medicine (IOM), Committee on Prevention, Diagnosis, Treatment, and Management of Substance Use Disorders in the U.S. Armed Forces. *Substance Use Disorders in the U.S. Armed Forces.* National Academies Press; 2013:247-268.
16. Goodwin DW, Davis DH, Robins LN. Drinking amid abundant illicit drugs: the Vietnam case. *Arch Gen Psychiatry.* 1975;32:230-233.
17. Robins LN, Davis DH, Goodwin DW. Drug use by U.S. Army enlisted men in Vietnam: a follow-up on their return home. *Am J Epidemiol.* 1974;99(4):235-249.
18. Robins LN, Helzer JE, Davis DH. Narcotic use in southeast Asia and afterward. An interview study of 898 Vietnam returnees. *Arch Gen Psychiatry.* 1975;32(8):955-961.
19. Camp NM. *U.S. Army Psychiatry in the Vietnam War: New Challenges in Extended Counterinsurgency Warfare.* U.S. Government Printing Office; 2015.
20. U.S. Department of Defense (DoD). *Problematic Substance Use by DoD Personnel (Number 1010.04).* DoD; 2014. http://www.esd.whs.mil/Portals/54/Documents/DD/issuances/dodi/101004p.pdf
21. U.S. Department of Defense (DoD). *DoD Civilian Employee Drug-Free Workplace Program (1010.09).* DoD; 2012. Accessed October 2, 2023. https://www.esd.whs.mil/Portals/54/Documents/DD/issuances/dodi/101009p.pdf
22. U.S. Department of Defense. *Military Personnel Drug Abuse Testing Program (MPDATP) (Number 1010.01).* U.S. Department of Defense; 2012. Accessed October 2, 2023. https://www.esd.whs.mil/Portals/54/Documents/DD/issuances/dodi/101001p.pdf
23. DuPont RL. Personal communication, February 9, 2017.
24. Wilson GC. Jet crashes on Carrier Nimitz, Kills 14. *Washington Post.* Published May 28, 1981.
25. Office of the Under Secretary for Personnel and Readiness. *Military Drug Program Historical Timeline.* U.S. Department of Defense. https://prhome.defense.gov/ForceResiliency/DDRP/Timeline/
26. Debruyne D, Moulin M, Bigot MC, et al. Identification and differentiation of resinous cannabis and textile cannabis: combined use of HPLC and high-resolution GLC. *Bull Narc.* 1981;33(2):49-58.
27. Ammerman RT, Ott PJ, Tarter RE, eds. *Prevention and Societal Impact of Drug and Alcohol Abuse.* Lawrence Erlbaum Associates, Publishers; 1999.
28. Reinhold R. Congressman says most killed in Nimitz crash showed traces of drugs. New York Times; 1981.
29. US Department of Defense (DoD). *Problematic Substance Use by DoD Personnel, DOD Instruction 1010.04.* Accessed May 23, 2023. http://www.esd.whs.mil/Portals/54/Documents/DD/issuances/dodi/101004p.pdf
30. *DoD Civilian Employee Drug-Free Workplace Program. DOD Instruction 1010.09.* Accessed May 23, 2023. http://www.esd.whs.mil/Portals/54/Documents/DD/issuances/dodi/101009p.pdf?ver=2018-06-28-074214-763
31. *US Department of Defense (DoD) Military Personnel Drug Abuse Testing Program DOD Instruction 1010.01.* Accessed May 23, 2023. http://www.esd.whs.mil/Portals/54/Documents/DD/issuances/dodi/101001p.pdf
32. U.S. Department of Defense (DoD), Office of the Under Secretary for Personnel and Readiness. *Military Drug Program Historical Timeline 1960's to 2008.* Accessed October 2, 2023. https://prhome.defense.gov/Portals/52/Documents/RFM/Readiness/DDRP/docs/72208/DoD%20Drug%20Policy%20History.pdf
33. Department of Defense. *Instruction 1010.16: Technical Procedures for the Military Personnel Drug Abuse Testing Program.* Issued June 15, 2020. Accessed May 23, 2023. https://www.esd.whs.mil/Portals/54/Documents/DD/issuances/dodi/101016p.pdf
34. Ferdinando L. DoD implements expanded drug testing for military applicants. *DoD News.* March 9, 2017. Accessed May 23, 2023. https://www.defense.gov/News/Article/Article/1108009/dod-implements-expanded-drug-testing-for-military-applicants/
35. Tripp J. *Legal News for Soldiers: Taking Prescribed Medications That Include Synthetic THC.* US Army Soldier Legal Services; October 17, 2019. Accessed May 23, 2023. https://www.jbsa.mil/News/News/Article/1990902/legal-news-for-soldiers-taking-prescribed-medications-that-include-synthetic-thc/
36. United States Code. *10 US Code 912a – Article 112a. Wrongful Use, Possession, etc., of Controlled Substances.* Issued 1983. Accessed May 23, 2023.https://ucmj.us/912a-article-112a-wrongful-use-possession-etc-of-controlled-substances/
37. Howard MR. Red jackets and red noses: alcohol and the British Napoleonic soldier. *J R Soc Med.* 2000;93(1):38-41.
38. Powlson M. Red jackets and red noses. *J R Soc Med.* 2000;93(4):214.
39. West LJ, Swegan WH. An approach to alcoholism in the military service. *Am J Psychiatry.* 1956;112(12):1004-1009.
40. Long JR, Hewitt LE, Lane HC. Alcohol abuse in the armed services: a review. I. Policies and programs. *Mil Med.* 1976;141(12):844-850.
41. Conroy RW, Friedberg B. A community plan for military alcoholics. *Am J Psychiatry.* 1971;128(6):130-133.
42. Fiman BG, Connor DR, Segal AC. A comprehensive alcoholism program in the Army. *Am J Psychiatry.* 1973;130(5):532-535.
43. Ingraham LH. *The Boys in the Barracks: Observations on American Military Life.* Institute for the Study of Human Behavior; 1984.
44. Skuja AT, Wood D, Bucky SF. Reported drinking among post-treatment alcohol abusers: a preliminary report. *Am J Drug Alcohol Abuse.* 1976;3(3):473-483.
45. US Department of Veterans Affairs. *VA/DoD Clinical Practice Guidelines: Management of Substance Use Disorder (SUD) (2021).* Accessed May 23, 2023. https://www.healthquality.va.gov/guidelines/MH/sud/index.asp
46. Cameron BA. "0-0-1-3" A different approach to responsible drinking, Army article, 12/1/2011. Accessed May 23, 2023. https://www.army.mil/article/70190/0_0_1_3_a_different_approach_to_responsible_drinking#:~:text=It%20can%20also%20affect%20a%20military%20person%27s%20career,is%20not%20an%20excuse%20to%20drink%20every%20day
47. Task Force of the National Advisory Council on Alcohol Abuse and Alcoholism: Call to Action, Changing the Culture of Drinking at U.S. Colleges. *A Call to Action: Changing the Culture of Drinking at U.S. Colleges.* NIH Publication no. 02-5010, April 2002. Accessed May 23, 2023. https://www.collegedrinkingprevention.gov/media/TaskForceReport.pdf
48. Department of Defense. *Instruction Number 1010.04: Problematic Substance Use by DoD Personnel.* Issued February 20, 2014, updated May 6, 2020. Accessed May 23, 2023. https://www.esd.whs.mil/Portals/54/Documents/DD/issuances/dodi/101004p.pdf
49. Department of Defense. *Instruction Number 1010.09: DoD Civilian Employee Drug-Free Workplace Program.* Issued June 22, 2012, updated June 28, 2018.
50. United States Code. *Chapter 47: Uniform Code of Military Justice.* https://ucmj.us/
51. United States Code. *10 US Code 911—Article 111. Drunken or Reckless Driving.* Accessed May 23, 2023. https://ucmj.us/911-article-111-drunken-or-reckless-driving/
52. United States Code. *10 US Code 912—Article 112. Drunk on Duty.* Accessed May 23, 2023. https://ucmj.us/912-article-112-drunk-on-duty/
53. Institute of Medicine (IOM). *Combating Tobacco Use in Military and Veteran Populations.* The National Academies Press; 2009. doi:10/17226/12632.
54. Department of Defense. *Instruction Number 1010.10: Health Promotion and Disease Prevention.* Issued April 28, 2014, updated May 16, 2022. Accessed May 23, 2023. https://www.esd.whs.mil/Portals/54/Documents/DD/issuances/dodi/101010p.pdf
55. Brandt A. Chapter 2. Tobacco as much as bullets. *The Cigarette Century, the Rise, Fall, and Deadly Persistence of the Product That Defined America.* Basic Books; 2009:45-68.
56. Ahmad A, Singh J. Influence of processes of change on stages of change for smoking cessation. *J Appl Soc Sci.* 2022;16(1):209-222. doi:10.1177/19367244211036994

57. Defense Health Agency. *TRICARE*. Accessed May 23, 2023. https://www.tricare.mil/
58. Uniformed Services University. *Consortium for Health and Military Performance*. Accessed May 23, 2023. https://champ.usuhs.edu/
59. Agency for Healthcare Research and Quality. *For Clinicians: Treating Tobacco Use and Dependence: 2008 Update—Clinical Practice Guide*. Accessed May 23, 2023. https://www.ahrq.gov/prevention/guidelines/tobacco/clinicians/index.html
60. US Preventive Services Task Force. *Final Recommendation Statement: Tobacco Smoking Cessation in Adults, Including Pregnant Persons: Interventions*. Accessed May 23, 2023. https://www.uspreventiveservicestaskforce.org/uspstf/index.php/recommendation/tobacco-use-in-adults-and-pregnant-women-counseling-and-interventions
61. *VA/DoD Clinical Practice Guideline for the Management of Tobacco Use*. Department of Veterans Affairs and Department of Defense, Update Version 2.0a; June 2004. Accessed May 23, 2023. https://www.healthquality.va.gov/tuc/tuc_fulltext.pdf
62. Burt MR. Prevalence and consequences of alcohol use among U.S. military personnel, 1980. *J Stud Alcohol*. 1982;43(11):1097-1107.
63. Meadows SO, Engel CC, Collins RL, et al. *2018 Department of Defense Health Related Behaviors Survey (HRBS): Results for the Active Component*. RAND Corporation; 2021. Accessed May 23, 2023. https://www.rand.org/pubs/research_reports/RR4222.html
64. Meadows SO, Engel CC, Collins RL, et al. 2018 *Department of Defense Health Related Behaviors Survey (HRBS): Results for the Active Component*. RAND Corporation; 2021. Accessed May 23, 2023. https://www.rand.org/pubs/research_reports/RR4222.html. Chapter 5, p. 85-102 tables 5.1-5. 3030 Appendix D p. 298-308, tables D.21-D.40
65. Department of the Army. *The Army Substance Abuse Program, Army Regulation 600–85*. U.S. Department of Defense; 2012:54.
66. National Institute on Drug Abuse (NIDA). *Methamphetamine Research Report*. Accessed May 23, 2023. https://nida.nih.gov/publications/research-reports/methamphetamine/overview
67. Goldberg SB, Fortney JC, Chen JA, Young BA, Lehavot K, Simpson TL. Military service and military health care coverage are associated with reduced racial disparities in time to mental health treatment initiation. *Adm Policy Ment Health*. 2020;47(4):555-568.
68. Adams RS, Garnick DW, Harris AHS, et al. Assessing the postdeployment quality of treatment for substance use disorders among Army enlisted soldiers in the Military Health System. *J Subst Abuse Treat*. 2020;114:108026.
69. Cheney AM, Koenig CJ, Miller CJ, et al. Veteran-centered barriers to VA mental healthcare services use. *BMC Health Serv Res*. 2018;18(1):591.
70. Pugatch M, Chang G, Garnick D, et al. Rates and predictors of brief intervention for women veterans returning from recent wars: examining gaps in service delivery for unhealthy alcohol use. *J Subst Abuse Treat*. 2021;123:108257.
71. McDaniel JT, Albright DL, Laha-Walsh K, Henson H, McIntosh S. Alcohol screening and brief intervention among military service members and veterans: rural-urban disparities. *BMJ Mil Health*. 2022;168(3):186-191.
72. Wooten NR, Mohr BA, Lundgren LM, et al. Gender differences in substance use treatment utilization in the year prior to deployment in Army service members. *J Subst Abuse Treat*. 2013;45(3):257-265.
73. Back SE, Killeen T, Badour CL, et al. Concurrent treatment of substance use disorders and PTSD using prolonged exposure: a randomized clinical trial in military veterans. *Addict Behav*. 2019;90:369-377.
74. Brown DG, Flanagan JC, Jarnecke A, Killeen TK, Back SE. Ethnoracial differences in treatment-seeking veterans with substance use disorders and co-occurring PTSD: presenting characteristics and response to integrated exposure-based treatment. *J Ethn Subst Abuse*. 2022;21(3):1141-1164.
75. Beckman KL, Williams EC, Hebert PL, et al. Associations among military sexual trauma, opioid use disorder, and gender. *Am J Prev Med*. 2022;62(3):377-386.
76. Matthews M, Farris C, Tankard M, Dunbar MS. Needs of male sexual assault victims in the U.S. armed forces. *Rand Health Q*. 2018;8(2):7.
77. Back SE, Killeen TK, Teer AP, et al. Substance use disorders and PTSD: an exploratory study of treatment preferences among military veterans. *Addict Behav*. 2014;39(2):369-373.
78. Hoffman K, Barrett-Ballinger C. *Department of Defense Oxford House Feasibility Study Final Report*. Accessed May 23, 2023. https://www.oxfordhouse.org/doc/2004_Hoffman_Report.pdf
79. US President's Emergency Plan For AIDS Relief. *Guiding Principles for the Next Phase of PEPFAR*. Accessed May 23, 2023. https://www.state.gov/wp-content/uploads/2020/12/Guiding-Principles-for-the-Next-Phase-of-PEPFAR.pdf
80. Chai, C, Wazee H, et al. *Opioid Agonist Therapy Improves Outcomes*. 53rd ASAM Annual Conference, 1 April 2022, Poster 48.
81. Reddon H et al. Methadone maintenance therapy decreases the rate of antiretroviral therapy discontinuation among HIV-positive illicit drug users. *AIDS Behav*. 2014;18(4):740-746.

Sidebar

Challenges of Reintegration for Military Personnel and Their Families

Joan E. Zweben and Susan Storti

Military families often are overlooked as a cultural group that has its own constellation of stressors and issues. Such families tend to have a "must function" ethos, which often discourages them from seeking help with problems that put them at risk for both substance use and other mental disorders. When military members, veterans, and family members do seek help, community clinicians may not be attuned to the unique features of military culture that affect willingness to seek help and engage in treatment. The clinicians also may lack the preparation and experience necessary to provide care for service-related conditions.

RECOGNIZING THE NEEDS OF MILITARY MEMBERS AND FAMILIES

While the landscape of military deployment has changed over the past 10 years, deployments (being sent to foreign countries, often to a combat zone, in defense of national interests; or to domestic or nondomestic areas of the world often in response to a natural disaster or similar challenge) continue to carry the substantial risk of exposure to events and experiences that may physically and mentally impair those directly engaged in combat or in support functions. The number of deployed military personnel returning home since December 2017 has heightened the importance of community health care clinicians being aware of their special issues. It is especially important that primary care clinicians are alert to the needs and vulnerabilities of these patients because those providers are in an excellent position to identify behavioral issues in a population that is generally resistant to seeking care. Familiarity with the key issues confronting military members and their families strengthens the process of assessment and treatment planning and promotes more effective care.

At the height of the U.S. Operation Enduring Freedom (OEF), Operation Iraqi Freedom (OIF), and Operation New Dawn (OND), more than 2.7 million U.S. forces had been deployed to Iraq, Afghanistan, and beyond. The majority (60.7%) were in the 18- to 30-year age range. More than half (51%) were married, and 42.1% had children.[1] (The military defines family narrowly as "heterosexual marriages and parents with dependent children who live with them at least part of the time,"[2] so these studies do not reflect the true diversity of affected families.) This is particularly true of families of those serving with the national guard or reserve. In some cases, both parents are deployed simultaneously, leaving grandparents or guardians responsible for the care of children.

Over the past several years, the number of deployed military members have decreased. As of March 31, 2020, over 2.3 million military members have been and are deployed in various regions throughout the world with 42.6% representing members of the national guard and reserve. It is important to note that these numbers do not include countries in which U.S. military are engaged in active combat operations.[3]

Nearly one in three military members are married with children and more than 8% are single parents. Across the active duty population, about half are married and nearly a third are married with children, many of whom (41.4%) are below the age of 5 years.[4]

The terrorist attacks of September 11, 2001, caused a paradigm shift in tempo of military deployment operations, and predeployment readiness. In a study released by The Pew Research Center in 2019,[5] approximately 77% of post 9/11 veterans were deployed at least once, and many experienced longer deployments and shorter times between deployments than in the past. There has been an increase in the deployment of women, parents of young children, and reserve and national guard troops. Although many readjust to civilian life without great difficulty, significant numbers have trouble resuming their family life, education, and employment. Many military personnel and their families feel that other Americans are oblivious to their situation.

MAJOR STRESSORS WHILE IN THEATER

While deployed, the military member may live in difficult conditions, characterized by poor food, lack of privacy, harsh climates, and extreme physical exertion. Periods of intense violence are followed by inactivity, but always accompanied by a need to sustain a high degree of vigilance. There are long hours, multiple demands, and sleep deprivation. Military members often witness death and suffering, while constantly under the threat of injury or death. Simple decisions take on a life-and-death significance. Military personnel experience ethical dilemmas over what they would consider "right" and "wrong" under normal conditions versus what they must do to fulfill their mission and survive.

During the stress of deployment, military members are separated from family and friends and often have concerns about what is happening at home. They may say little about their hardships to avoid worrying family members, and the family may be reluctant to share difficulties in order to avoid burdening the absent member. Communication can become strained, superficial, and emotionally unsatisfying, setting the stage for a difficult reentry. Alcohol and tobacco use often becomes a coping strategy, and for many segments of the military, heavy drinking is the prevailing custom.

FAMILY MEMBERS COPING WITH WARTIME DEPLOYMENT

Family members may have only a vague understanding of life on active duty and must deal with their own series of stressors. It is common for them to withdraw emotionally and become detached as the time of departure nears. Initially, there can be intense fear and worry, followed by an adjustment period that includes loneliness, sadness, and fear of the unknown. Although the internet offers important new ways to stay in touch, military security may require that communication be limited for extended periods of time, and media portrayals of the conflict add to family members' anxiety.

Family structure often changes significantly in response to new challenges. Spouses at home are faced with managing unfamiliar tasks. The definition of family may be expanded to include friends and extended family. Younger families may move to be near parents who can provide help and support. Concerns about being away from the family are paramount for women and mothers who are deployed, as well as single parents and often men/husbands as well, many of whom experience great guilt, particularly if they are not comfortable with the arrangements at home. Families that are flexible regarding roles and responsibilities usually are better able to adapt. Although there are online and community support groups for partners and spouses of military members, not everyone uses them. A study involving more than 250,000 wives of active-duty service members found that spouses of deployed soldiers received significantly more mental health diagnoses and that the risk increased with the length of deployment.[6] The most common diagnoses were depression, sleep disorders, anxiety, acute stress reaction, and adjustment disorder. Many women had more than one disorder.

Children's reactions vary with their age, developmental stage, and preexisting problems.[7] Young children may experience separation anxiety, temper tantrums, and changes in eating habits. School-age children may show a decline in academic performance, mood changes, and physical complaints.[8] Adolescents may more readily express anger and act out or may show signs of apathy and withdraw.[9] Those who can use diverse, active coping behaviors frequently show enhanced resilience.[10]

It is very important that families develop skills in talking with children about a parent going to war, before as well as during deployment. Such discussions should include sharing feelings as well as coping strategies to deal with practical problems. Maintaining familiar family traditions is comforting, and monitoring children's exposure to TV coverage of war is recommended when possible. Conflict-avoidance usually exacerbates problems; frustration and other emotions can be turned against each other in unproductive ways. Family conflict resolution skills are very useful.

Case 1: The Impact of Deployment on Children of Military Personnel

Nathan, a second grader, had increasingly strong reactions to his father's multiple deployments to Iraq and struggled hard to adjust as he grew older. One day in class, he drew battle scenes involving tanks and other military armaments. His drawing was confiscated, and he was sent to the principal's office for possessing "dangerous contraband."

Nathan was attempting to manage his emotions and bring his father closer by depicting his father's situation in Iraq in his drawing. The drawings could have opened an opportunity for a child life expert to engage Nathan in conversations that would validate his feelings and help him learn to manage and express his emotions. The reaction from school personnel demonstrates the need for greater training among teachers and other professionals.

HOMECOMING AFTER DEPLOYMENT

Although the military member's return home is often eagerly anticipated by both the military member and the family, it is filled with challenges. Responses that are adaptive while on active duty become problems during the transition phase. For example, the "fight-or-flight" response is a survival asset in the war zone, but hyperarousal at home leads to jumpiness, poor sleep, and difficulty concentrating. These greatly elevate the risk for SUDs.

Military members usually feel that much has changed at home since they were deployed, which can lead them to feel out of place. National guard members and reservists may feel particularly alone because they do not return to a full time job as part of an active duty unit, but rather to their civilian job, negating the opportunity for continued bonding and destressing from deployment. Because active-duty personnel are accustomed to a high level of arousal, civilian life can seem insignificant. Free time is a burden, especially if the military member is unemployed and having difficulty finding work.

Family roles usually have shifted, and new roles established.[11] Couples have learned to live apart and to be independent, and return of the military member requires creation of a new relationship. Spouses and partners may enjoy learning and exercising newly acquired skills and thus be reluctant to give up some responsibilities. The returning parent may be keenly aware that he or she has missed important developmental milestones in his or her child's life and may be uncertain as to when to "jump in" with parenting or discipline. The returning partner may simultaneously feel overwhelmed by responsibility for the family while bored with the mundane aspects of civilian life.

Family members may encounter their own reintegration challenges. They may feel emotionally disconnected and alone, especially when trying to assist a loved one who has sustained a serious injury or other medical condition. Family members struggle with not knowing what will trigger anger or upset in their loved one and, if triggered, how they will react and when it is time for to ask for help.

Significant others often do not understand why, after being away for a long period of time, their veteran chooses to be with other members of his or her military unit rather than at home. Some male partners may experience resentment toward a returning woman veteran, contributing to relationship difficulties. Parents of returning military members, especially those serving in the national guard or reserve, face similar challenges. They often are uncertain as to how to deal with their child's struggles and, as a result, may experience emotional, physical, or psychological symptoms.

Case 2: Living With the Unknown—The Stress of War on Relationships

Angelina was often asked: "When did you begin to see changes in John?" She described that following John's return home from his second deployment, she saw subtle differences, but all of them were easily explained as reactions to his experiences during the preceding 12 months.

The changes became more evident shortly after his return from Iraq; his third deployment. The man who left for that deployment was kind, gentle, compassionate, and fun-loving; the man who returned was a shell. When Angelina looked into his eyes, it was as though his soul was missing. John would say, "I can't feel anything" and "You don't understand—leave me alone." He was distant, irritable, argumentative, and easily angered.

John never slept for more than short periods of time. He often woke screaming. His need to protect himself led him to keep a loaded gun as his constant companion, even at night while in bed. He would tie fishing line across the stairs and leave newspapers at the inside of doors so that he could hear anyone entering the house. There was a constant sense of uncertainty for family members—they never knew when a comment, a smell, or a sound would trigger John's anger. There also was constant worry for his safety and the safety of others.

John now spent the majority of his time chasing the "adrenaline train." He was fixated on doing things that would keep him moving and, more important than anything, that would test his strength or courage. When Angelina raised safety concerns, he would say: "Don't worry, if I didn't get killed there, I won't here."

John's belief that he was invincible culminated when he bought a motorcycle. About two weeks later Angelina received a call from a local police department reporting that John had been in an accident and was being transported to the hospital. Within hours, he was in surgery to repair his injuries.

During and following his recuperation, John's behavior continued to escalate. The number of angry outbursts and arguments increased, as did his drinking and gambling. This added more stress to his relationship with Angelina, which already was on the brink of collapse.

While this was happening externally, Angelina was experiencing internal turmoil. She knew and understood what was happening but was unable to stop it. She found herself living in a new reality, in which she could offer hope, guidance, and support to others but could not find the right words or actions to help John or save their relationship.

Even more difficult were the questions Angelina posed to herself. Could she walk away from a man she loved and admired? At what point would she be willing to accept the potential consequences of ending the relationship? Adding to Angelina's confusion were occasional glimpses of the man she fell in love with—a smile or act of kindness shown to a child or animal or the selfless effort to do something kind.

John continued to fight to be "normal." He believed he could "handle it on his own." Angelina was finally able to convince him to go for help. Although he went, he was not engaged in the process. His anger, irritation, nightmares, and anxiety continued to worsen.

One weekend in early fall, during another one of their heated arguments, both Angelina and John realized that they could not allow their current situation to continue. The strain of war had proved destructive. It was at that moment—with mixed emotions and heavy hearts—that they decided to let go of their relationship.

John moved into his own apartment. The downward spiral continued, leading him to question his will to live. With the support of friends and family that he returned to treatment. The healing had finally begun.

This account describes the actual experience of a national guard troop who was deployed three times in 4 years. It exemplifies the need for clinicians to understand how the mental health of the returning service member affects relationships as well as family functioning. Therefore, it is important that the needs of the entire family are considered when assisting military members returning from deployment.

Special Considerations With National Guard and Reservists

National guard members and reservists experience many of the same issues as other military personnel, but there are some important differences. Members of the Guard and Reserve are "weekend warriors"—civilians who suddenly are called to active duty for periods of up to 12 months. Although the law requires that their employer hold a job for them, there is no guarantee that they can return to the position they left; they may be offered a different or lower-level position upon return. This creates considerable economic hardship and other stressors for the returning service members and their families.

When they return to the United States, they do return to their unit, which typically operates out of a base, but unlike the active duty members they do not return to that base or unit for daily work; but instead scatter to their home community and civilian employer. If they elected to serve in a unit composed of individuals in a different geographic location, they will not enjoy the camaraderie that easy access allows. This may compound feelings of isolation. Reserve personnel require more mental health treatment than active-duty personnel upon returning home.[12] Reservists whose deployment involves combat exposure are significantly more likely to experience new-onset heavy drinking, binge drinking—defined by the National Institute on Alcohol Abuse and Alcoholism as a pattern of consuming 5 or more drinks (male), or 4 or more drinks (female), in about 2 hours, and alcohol-related problems, with the youngest service members at highest risk for alcohol-related problems.[13]

There is emerging evidence of the effects of reserve duty on the family. Issues that may present a challenge include emotional or mental health, health care, civilian employment, the spouse/partner relationship, financial or legal matters, child well-being, and education. Some problems may present soon after the service member returns home, while others emerge later.[14,15]

Medical and Psychological Issues That Affect Reintegration

Modern technology has dramatically improved survival rates, so that large numbers of seriously wounded soldiers return home. While all military members are eligible for health care, many are hesitant to access services for fear that information will be shared with commanding officers, which may erode their ability to remain in military service (by revealing physical and mental health problems that may erode their ability to deploy in the future, their ability to pilot aircraft, their ability to work with nuclear material, etc.). Instead, they may choose to seek health care from nonmilitary clinicians to keep their potentially disqualifying conditions from military awareness. Contrary to the troops' concerns above, there are many cases where such medical issues are repairable, or the troop is retainable by cross training into another area—and thus seeking medical care may not result in impairing their ability to serve.

Service members from minoritized communities experience disparities consistent with civilians however, patterns vary. For example, non-Hispanic Black and Asian service members are more likely than non-Hispanic Whites to report a suicide attempt, and military women exhibit greater prevalence of mental health conditions, but lower prevalence of substance use relative to military men.[16]

Common service-related injuries among U.S. military veterans in 2020 included musculoskeletal/joint injuries, posttraumatic stress disorder (PTSD), tinnitus, anxiety, depression, hearing loss, traumatic brain injury, pulmonary issues, burns/scarring, vision loss, paralysis, loss of limb among others.[17] Joint and other musculoskeletal ailments are the most common diagnoses among service members. Pain is a significant cause of disability, particularly among veterans of OEF, OIF, and OND.[18] About 15% of OEF/OIF/OND veterans have been prescribed opioid medications, and 25% to 35% of this group report being addicted to prescription or illegal opioids. The growing prevalence of illicit and synthetic opioids such as fentanyl in the drug supply led to a 65% increase in rates of opioid-related deaths among veterans between 2010 and 2016.[19] Polypharmacy, defined as the concurrent use of four or more prescription medications, of which at least one is a psychotropic drug or a controlled substance[20] is becoming more common. The appropriate emphasis on adequate pain management has resulted in unintended consequence of significant quantities of opioid medications in many homes, elevating the risk for SUDs in veterans and their family members.

In 2020, 65% of veterans with a service-related injury had PTSD and 56% had depression,[17] which may become more severe in the postdeployment period and have a profound effect on family functioning. Many of the wounded are young and require frequent and costly medical care for the rest of their lives.

Many caregivers, whether family members and/or other health care professionals assist with activities of daily living (ADLs), such as bathing, dressing, getting in and out of bed and chairs, as well as administering medications and injections, and coordinating medical and rehabilitation appointments.[21] Caring for someone with traumatic brain injury or PTSD can be enormously stressful for the caregiver. It can present in a variety of ways including but not limited to, grief, fear and anxiety, isolation and loneliness, guilt, and remorse and/or anger and resentment.

Alcohol and tobacco are commonly used substances among veterans,[22] followed by prescription opioids. Illicit drug use is less common among veterans than the general population, though still problematic. Stimulants may be used to lessen fatigue or to help cope with boredom or the panic of battle situations. Cannabis is often used to relieve tension and for recreational purposes.[23]

Veterans have high rates of co-occurring SUDs and mental health disorders. Estimates of co-occurring PTSD and depression range from 48% to 60% across studies of military and veteran populations, and rates of PTSD and SUD co-occurrence range from 34% to 88%. Alcohol use disorder (other than perhaps tobacco/nicotine) is the most common SUD that co-occurs with both PTSD and depression. The presence of co-occurring problems has important implications for treatment, as the mix of symptoms can exacerbate the consequences and treatment of each.[23]

Service members returning from combat have high rates of intimate partner violence, especially if they have PTSD or traumatic brain injury.[24] The high prevalence of military sexual trauma (MST) has a major impact on returning veterans, who often feel betrayed by the military if they report the assault.[25,26] According to the 2019-2020 National Health and Resilience in Veterans Study, 44.2% of female veterans and 3.5% of male veterans reported MST.[27] These conditions place great burdens on family members and are associated with elevated rates of separation and divorce.

Case 3

David is a male veteran of OEF, in his late 40s, married and the father of three children. His unit was hit by a sandstorm and the members were running for cover when David struck his head on the top of a doorway into a concrete bunker. He lost consciousness. When he regained it, he was dazed, disoriented, and confused. David was taken to a Mobile Army Surgical Hospital unit, where he remained overnight. He was given medications for pain and sleep, in addition to a week of restricted duty. He had no memory of what happened to him.

On his return to the United States, David sought treatment for persistent symptoms, including suicidal thoughts, depression, racing thoughts, military sexual trauma (MST), and drug use. During his assessment other problems were identified, including dizziness, loss of balance, poor coordination, severe headaches, nausea, sensitivity to light and noise, numbness/tingling in his extremities, appetite changes, poor concentration and memory, problems making decisions, slowed thinking and difficulties in completing organizational tasks, fatigue, poor quality sleep, nightmares, anxiety, depression, irritability, and little tolerance for frustration.

David's wife makes his medical appointments, organizes their lives, and takes care of all household responsibilities. David lost his job because of memory loss and problems functioning. He spends his days drinking at home, while his wife considers whether she should move him out of their home because of his angry outbursts.

Cases as complex as David's require access to multiple resources for the veteran and family members over an extended period. Substance use is one of many complex problems and can undermine the success of other efforts. Effective care for patients like David requires a high level of expertise and teamwork, as well as the resources needed to sustain them over time.

Community providers are ill-equipped by virtue of training or access to military-informed, evidence-based services for PTSD and similar disorders.[28] However, strength-based, family-centered interventions that are now emerging have demonstrated effectiveness in reducing symptoms of psychological problems and improving the resilience of military families.[29-31]

CONCLUSIONS

Reintegration after military deployment presents a number of unique stressors and challenges. Family members are an essential support to military service members, playing an important role in their readiness and effective functioning while deployed, as well as support and care when they return home. However, family members have their own set of stressors and problems. Helping them meet their challenges is essential to the well-being of the service member on active duty as well as those who return.

Spouses, children, and other family members more broadly defined than the military's current definition need sensitive care attuned to their unique needs. Specialized interventions to strengthen families have begun to emerge and hopefully will be disseminated and implemented more widely. Examples include Parent Management Training-Oregon model, a family of interventions that improves parenting practices and child adjustment in highly stressed families[32]; FOCUS (Families OverComing Under Stress), a family-centered, resilience-enhancing program,[33] behavioral health homes, and structure resiliency and parent training.[34]

The resources provided by the military for active duty and returning personnel are inadequate in some locations. Community providers can make a major contribution if they are prepared to meet the needs of this important population.

Understanding military culture, the experiences of deployment and reintegration, and learning of available resources to care for service members, veterans and their families within the Veterans Administration hospital system as well as within the community is imperative to the long-term care of individuals and their families.

REFERENCES

1. *Obergefell v Hodges*, 135 S. Ct. 2071, 576 US 644, 191 L. Ed. 2d 953 - Supreme Court, 2015.
2. Encyclopedia Britannica. *Obergefell v Hodges*. Encyclopedia Britannica. Accessed May 23, 2023. https://www.britannica.com/event/Obergefell-v-Hodges
3. Bledsoe E. (2023). *The Soldiers Project—What Percentages of Americans Have Served in the Military?* Accessed September 1, 2023. https://www.thesoldiersproject.org/what-percentage-of-americans-have-served-in-the-military/
4. Department of Defense. *2020 Demographics—Profile of the Military Community*. Department of Defense; 2020:222.
5. Parker K, Igielnick R, Barroso A, Cilluffo A. *The American Veteran Experience and the Post-9/11 Generation*. Pew Research Center; 2019.
6. Mansfield AJ, Kaufman JS, Marshall SW. Deployment and the use of mental health services among U.S. Army wives. *N Engl J Med*. 2010;362(2):101-109.
7. Huebner CR. Health and mental health needs of children in U.S. Military families. *Pediatrics*. 2019;143(1):e20183258. doi:10.1542/peds.2018-3258
8. Ormeno MD, Roh Y, Heller M, et al. Special concerns in military families. *Curr Psychiatry Rep*. 2020;22(12):82. doi:10.1007/s11920-020-01207-7
9. American Psychological Association (APA) Presidential Task Force on Military Deployment Services for Youth. *Families and Their Families: A Preliminary Report [Executive Summary]*. APA; 2007. Accessed August 22, 2022. www.apa.org/pubs/reports/military-deployment-summary.pdf
10. Okafor E, Lucier-Greer M, Mancini JA. Social stressors, coping behaviors, and depressive symptoms: a latent profile analysis of adolescents in military families. *J Adolesc*. 2016;51:133-143.
11. Armstrong K, Best S, Domenici P. *Courage After Fire: Coping Strategies for Troops Returning From Iraq and Afghanistan and Their Families*. Ulysses Press; 2006.
12. Milliken CS, Auchterlonie JL, Hoge CW. Longitudinal assessment of mental health problems among Active and Reserve Component soldiers returning from Iraq war. *JAMA*. 2007;298:2141-2148.
13. Jacobson IG, Ryan MAK, Hooper TI, et al. Alcohol use and alcohol-related problems before and after military combat deployment. *JAMA*. 2008;300(6):663-675.
14. Jones CE. *Staying Health After Deployment*. 2022. Accessed July 8, 2022. https://www.military.com/deployment/staying-healthy-after-deployment.html
15. Werber L, Gereben Schaefer A, Chan OK, et al. *Reintegration After Deployment: Supporting Citizen Warriors and Their Families*. RAND Corporation; 2013.
16. Wong EC, Meadows SO, Schell TL, et al. *The Behavioral Health of Minority Active Duty Members*. Rand Corporation; 2021.
17. Elflien, J. *Distribution of Injuries Among U.S. Military Veterans With Service-Related Injuries in the U.S. in 2021*. Accessed May 23, 2023. https://www.statista.com/statistics/779730/injires-services-related-in-us-veterans/
18. Nahin RL. Severe pain in Veterans: the impact of age and sex, and comparisons to the general population. *J Pain*. 2017;18(3):247-254.
19. Lin L, Peltzman T, McCarthy JF, Oliva EM, Trafton JA, Bohnert ASB. Changing trends in opioid overdose deaths and prescription opioid receipt among Veterans. *Am J Prev Med*. 2019;1:106-110.
20. Department of the Army. *Army 2020: Generating Health and Discipline in the Force Ahead of the Strategic Reset*. U.S. Department of Defense; 2012.
21. Institute of Medicine (IOM). Committee on the assessment of readjustment needs of military personnel and their families. *Returning Home From Iraq and Afghanistan: Assessment of Readjustment Needs of Veterans, Service Members, and Their Families*. National Academies Press; 2013.
22. Odani S, Agaku IT, Graffunder CM, et al. Tobacco product use among military veterans—United States, 2010-2015. *Morb Mortal Wkly Rep*. 2018;67:7-12. doi:10.15585/mmwr.mm6701a2
23. Pedersen ER, Bouskill KE, Holliday SB, et al. *Improving Substance Use Care: Addressing Barriers to Expanding Integrated Treatment Options for Post-9/11 Veterans*. RAND Corporation; 2020.
24. Committee on the Assessment of Readjustment Needs of Military Personnel, Veterans, and Their Families, Institute of Medicine. *Returning Home From Iraq and Afghanistan: Assessment of Readjustment Needs of Veterans, Service Members, and Their Families*. The National Academies Press; 2013.
25. Wilson LC. The prevalence of military sexual trauma: a meta-analysis. *Trauma Violence Abuse*. 2018;19(5):584-597. doi:10.1177/1524838016683459
26. Gibson CJ, Maguen S, Xia F, Barnes DE, Peltz CB, Yaffe K. Military sexual trauma in older women veterans: prevalence and comorbidities. *J Gen Intern Med*. 2020;35(1):207-213. doi:10.1007/s11606-019-05342-7

27. Nichter B, Holliday R, Monteith LL, et al. Military sexual trauma in the United States: results from a population-based study. *J Affect Disord*. 2022;306:19-27. doi:10.1016/j.jad.2022.03.016
28. Richards LK, Bui E, Charney M, et al. Treating veterans and military families: evidence based practices and training needs among community clinicians. *Community Ment Health J*. 2017;53:215-223.
29. Flittner O'Grady A, Burton ET, Chawla N, Topp D, MacDermid WS. Evaluation of a multimedia intervention for children and families facing multiple military deployments. *J Prim Prev*. 2016;37(1):53-70.
30. Lester P, Liang L-J, Milburn N, et al. Evaluation of a family-centered preventive intervention for military families: parent and child longitudinal outcomes. *J Am Acad Child Adolesc Psychiatry*. 2016;55(1):14-24.
31. Moriarty H, Winter L, Robinson K, et al. A randomized controlled trial to evaluate the Veterans' in-home program for military veterans with traumatic brain injury and their families: report on impact for family members. *PM R*. 2016;8(6):495-509.
32. Gewirtz AH, Erbes CR, Polusny MA, Forgatch MS, DeGarmo DS. Helping military families through the deployment process: strategies to support parenting. *Prof Psychol Res Pract*. 2011;42(1):56-62.
33. Saltzman WR, Lester P, Beardslee WR, Layne CM, Woodward K, Nash WP. Mechanisms of risk and resilience in military families: theoretical and empirical basis of a family-focused resilience enhancement program. *Clin Child Fam Psychol Rev*. 2011;14:213-230.
34. Murphy RA, Fairbank JA. Implementation and dissemination of military informed and evidence-based interventions for community dwelling military families. *Clin Child Fam Psychol Rev*. 2013;16(4):348-364.

SECTION

4

Diagnosis, Assessment, and Early Intervention Treatment

Associate Editor: Sarah E. Wakeman
Lead Section Editor: Emily C. Williams
Section Editor: Lisa J. Merlo

CHAPTER

31 Screening and Brief Intervention

Kenneth W. Verbos II, Alice Zhang, Ahyeon Cho, Suena H. Massey, and Aleksandra E. Zgierska

CHAPTER OUTLINE

- Introduction
- National recommendations on the implementation of unhealthy substance use screening and treatment in medical care settings
- Screening and brief intervention: clinical guidelines
- Current evidence on screening and brief intervention: a brief summary
- Systematic reviews and meta-analyses of screening and brief interventions for unhealthy alcohol use
- Individual studies of SBI for unhealthy alcohol use
- Studies of SBI for unhealthy drug use
- SBI: special settings
- Summary
- Ackowledgments

INTRODUCTION

In 2020, a nationally representative epidemiologic survey in the United States estimated that 40.3 million or 14.5% of individuals aged 12 years or older met the *Diagnostic and Statistical Manual of Mental Disorders*, 5th edition's (DSM-5) criteria for substance use disorder (SUD). Of those with SUD, 28.3 million individuals met criteria for alcohol use disorder (AUD), 18.4 million for drug use disorder (DUD), and 6.5 million for both AUD and DUD.[1] While estimated rates of SUD had remained stable from 2015 to 2019, the rate increased by 97.5% from 2019 to 2020. Rates of AUD are considerably higher among individuals with mental health problems and those presenting with trauma in emergency settings.[1] Furthermore, unhealthy alcohol use is fairly common in the United States—in 2016, 26% of adults and 4.9% of adolescents reported heavy episodic drinking (≥5 drinks during the same occasion on ≥1 day in the previous month, formerly referred to as "binge" drinking, a term that is now thought to be pejorative and stigmatizing) and 6.6% of adults reported episodic heavy drinking (≥5 drinks in the same occasion on ≥5 days).[2] In 2020, the prevalence of past-year drug use disorder in those aged 12 years or older was estimated at 6.6%,[1] with unhealthy prescription opioid use cited as a "national epidemic."[3] Additionally, in 2018, 11.7% of U.S. residents 12 years or older were currently using illegal drugs; with estimated of 10.1% using cannabis and 2.0% using nonmedical prescription psychotherapeutic drugs.[4] Thus, a sizeable proportion of individuals within our communities and patients presenting to primary care or hospital settings have problems with alcohol or drugs. On any given day, physicians are likely to provide medical care to patients with unhealthy alcohol or drug use, particularly since substance use has been linked to medical symptoms or conditions, including liver disease, cardiovascular problems, obesity, glucose intolerance, memory loss, and a variety of mental health conditions. Adding to the complexity of the problem is the challenge of engaging patients, and also their clinicians, in systematic evidence-based solutions. Research suggests that patients prefer to address their alcohol use with their own clinician rather than seeking help from Alcoholics Anonymous (AA) or specialty addiction treatment programs.[2]

Over the past six decades, research has demonstrated the potential benefits of screening and brief interventions (SBIs) as a brief behavioral therapy for tobacco and unhealthy alcohol use in a variety of public health and clinical settings. A unique aspect of SBI is its harm reduction paradigm, which emphasizes reduction in substance use to reduce negative consequences rather than the goal of abstinence that may not be accepted by or important to some patients. SBIs can be effective at least for those with unhealthy substance use at lower severity levels, especially since SBIs were developed specifically for implementation in primary care settings and have documented effectiveness in reducing tobacco use among those with tobacco use disorder and alcohol use among those with unhealthy alcohol use (but not without additional intervention among those with AUD). The U.S. Preventive Services Task Force (USPSTF) recommends routine SBI to reduce "unhealthy alcohol use" among adults, including pregnant people, in primary care settings (grade B).[4] It also strongly recommends that clinicians screen all adults, including pregnant people, for tobacco use, and provide tobacco abstinence interventions for people who use tobacco (grade A).[5] SBI for drug use has less robust evidence supporting its efficacy, and, in the case of cannabis, needs to take into consideration discrepancies in cannabis legalization status across the states. In 2020, the USPSTF issued recommendations to screen for unhealthy drug use in adults, including pregnant persons and postpartum people (grade B).[6] The USPSTF also found evidence to support pharmacotherapy and psychosocial interventions as effective treatments for improving substance use-related outcomes in adults. Although the USPSTF recommends SBI in adults, it did not find sufficient evidence to recommend for or against routine SBI for alcohol, tobacco or drugs among children and adolescents.[6]

Based on the available evidence and the USPSTF recommendations, recent years have witnessed structured efforts to disseminate SBI, especially for alcohol and tobacco, into clinical practice. However, plans for widespread implementation of SBI and its acceptability by clinicians have room for improvement, leading in part to investigations on SBI delivered by in different settings or platforms, such as smartphones and online approaches.[7]

NATIONAL RECOMMENDATIONS ON THE IMPLEMENTATION OF UNHEALTHY SUBSTANCE USE SCREENING AND TREATMENT IN MEDICAL CARE SETTINGS

A number of professional medical organizations have adopted policies calling on their members to be knowledgeable, trained, and involved in all phases of prevention (including SBI) for tobacco and unhealthy alcohol use. For example, the American College of Surgeons (ACS) Committee on Trauma requires screening of all level I and level II trauma patients for unhealthy alcohol use as well as providing BI for those who screen positive in level I trauma centers.[8] These recommendations have also been endorsed by the National Institute on Alcohol Abuse and Alcoholism (NIAAA), the National Institute on Drug Abuse (NIDA), the Substance Abuse and Mental Health Services Administration (SAMHSA), and the National Quality Forum (NQF) (for alcohol), a voluntary consensus evidence-based standard-setting organization. While many professional organizations recommend screening for alcohol and tobacco use in adults and adolescents, the specific age of onset of such services is less well defined. The NQF recommends alcohol and tobacco SBI services for patients 10 years of age or older during new patient encounters, then at least annually.[9] The NIAAA recommends alcohol screening starting at age nine and provides a clear algorithm for youth SBI in its *Guide for Youth*.[10] NIDA tools have been developed for drug SBI in adults.[11] Less unified recommendations regarding SBI for cannabis likely reflect an evolving view of cannabis use that varies by state—advocacy for improving safety and advancing research on the effects of recreational cannabis use is essentially universal.[12]

Validated standard assessments for SUD are important; however, their implementation into routine care has been subpar, and few have been validated that are brief enough for many clinical settings. With the adoption of billing codes by the AMA and the Centers for Medicare and Medicaid Services for tobacco as well as alcohol/other drug use structured SBI services has represented a step toward this goal.[13] For example, Medicare waives coinsurance, copayment, or deductible for the preventive services graded as A or B by the USPSTF; SBI for unhealthy use of alcohol (grade B), tobacco (grade A) and drugs (grade B) for adults and pregnant persons in primary care fall into this category. Medicare also has specific regulations about the settings of SBI delivery. It covers tobacco SBI for both outpatient and inpatient beneficiaries. It also covers annual screening for unhealthy alcohol use and for those who screen positive and are diagnosed with unhealthy use but not AUD—up to four face-to-face BIs in a 12-month period. Each intervention should be consistent with the Five A's approach (Ask, Advise, Assess, Assist, Arrange) and provided by a qualified physician (general practice, family medicine, geriatrics, pediatrics, internal medicine, or OB/GYN) or other recognized clinician in primary care settings, which, of note, excludes emergency departments and skilled nursing facilities. Medicare does not identify specific tools to screen for or diagnose unhealthy alcohol use; they can be chosen, as appropriate, by the clinician.[14]

SCREENING AND BRIEF INTERVENTION: CLINICAL GUIDELINES

"If you aren't already doing so, we encourage you to incorporate alcohol screening and intervention into your practice. You're in a prime position to make a difference."

These first lines of the booklet *Helping Patients Who Drink Too Much: A Clinician's Guide* summarize the current NIAAA guidelines on alcohol SBI in primary care and mental health settings.[15] While this guide provides an algorithm for a step-by-step approach to alcohol SBI for adults, another guide recently released by the NIAAA addresses nuances of alcohol SBI delivery in youth.[16] Both guides are available in extended (yet concise) and pocket (one small booklet) sizes. NIDA's guide incorporates SBI for alcohol, tobacco, and other drugs in one document.[11]

Clinical Approach to SBI Services in Primary Care Settings

Though screening tools and content of BIs vary in use and effectiveness, a commonly recommended framework for delivery of SBI, particularly for tobacco use, is the Five A's (Ask, Advise, Assess, Assist, Arrange):

- *Ask* refers to *screening and assessment* of the risk level: "Screen, then intervene." *Intervention* may then include all remaining "A's" and is tailored to the screening results and determined risk level. This step should optimally be conducted using validated screening tools.
- *Advise* means providing direct, personal advice to the patient about their substance use. The goal of the clinician's advice is for the patients to hear clearly that a change in their behavior is recommended as based on medical concerns (review results with the patient), and to learn about their

personal substance use and its effects on health (provide advice). Presentation of the facts in an objective, nonjudgmental way, using strong and personalized language, by a knowledgeable and trusted professional, has been shown to facilitate change.

- *Assess* refers to evaluating the severity of the patient's problem and the patient's willingness ("readiness") to change the unhealthy behavior (reduction of use or quitting), after hearing the clinician's advice. Assessment of severity should also be conducted using structured and/or validated instruments. These validated instruments include tools such as the Alcohol Use Disorders Identification Test (AUDIT) or AUDIT-C which assesses symptoms, severity, consequences of use, and likelihood of AUD or more structured DSM-5 assessments such as the recently validated SUD symptom checklist, which may help prompt a more patient centered discussion about the consequences of alcohol use, as well as guiding diagnosis, treatment, and management. If the patient is not currently interested in changing their substance use, the clinician should restate the substance use-related health concerns, reaffirm a willingness to help when the patient is ready, and encourage the patient to reflect about perceived "benefits" of continued use versus decreasing or stopping use and barriers to change. Assessment may also include the evaluation of other experiences, which may influence unhealthy substance use, including co-occurring physical or mental health problems, HIV and sexually transmitted disease risk, and social determinants of health.[17]
- *Assist* involves helping the patient who is interested in change to develop goals and to put in place a plan, which can help meet these goals. Using behavior change techniques (eg, motivational interviewing [MI]), the clinician should aid the patient in achieving their own goals, and acquiring the appropriate skills, confidence, and social/environmental support. It is helpful if the plan describes in concrete terms the specific steps the patient elects to take to reduce/quit drinking, for example, the maximum number of drinks per day or week and how to prevent and manage high-risk situations or establish a support network. Starting with "small steps" while working toward a larger goal (abstinence or safe use) may be most reasonable and achievable for many patients. Experts recommend a shared decision-making approach during this step.[18]

Following a shared decision-making approach, clinicians should offer a range of treatment options (pharmacological and behavioral), including consideration of whether the patient would benefit from a medical treatment for SUD, such as withdrawal management or pharmacotherapy, as well as consideration of the patient's whole health and lived experiences that may influence substance use. All sexually active patients with unhealthy alcohol or drug use—a risk factor for "risky behaviors"—should be counseled to practice safe sex and offered HIV and other sexually transmitted disease testing and prevention (eg, preexposure prophylaxis). Patients reporting any injection drug use should be encouraged to undergo HIV and hepatitis B/C testing (if they have not had it *twice* over a 6-month period following the last injection) and connect with appropriate follow-up care.

- Finally, *Arrange* refers to the consideration of a follow-up visit and specialty referrals. A follow-up appointment should be arranged for all patients who screened positive to provide ongoing assistance and adjust the treatment plan as needed. Optimally, all patients should also receive educational materials to take home.

All patients with a SUD should be encouraged to see an addiction specialist or other clinician who can provide it, including their primary care clinician, to consider treatment options, including the appropriateness of pharmacotherapy. While many patients may decline, especially during the initial meeting, and/or not be able to successfully seek such services (particularly persons experiencing multigenerational effects of structural racism and other lived experiences of societal marginalization) due to too few treatment options, clinician with such skills not available, distance to the nearest center, incompatibility of treatment schedule with work hours, or inadequate insurance coverage, clinicians should work to link patients with services and/or directly provide pharmacological treatment, which now show promise across many SUDs.[19] Though special training used to be required prior to the COVID-19 pandemic to prescribe buprenorphine for OUD, since 2021 prescribers can now prescribe buprenorphine without any special licensing or training. As well, COVID-related expansions of telehealth and other virtual health approaches can serve to bridge gaps in access to care (see the sidebar of Chapter 50, "Delivery of Addiction Medicine Care via Video or Phone").

SAMHSA's Treatment Facility Locator (https://www.samhsa.gov/find-treatment) and NIDA's National Drug Abuse Treatment Clinical Trials Network List of Associated Community Treatment Programs (https://nida.nih.gov/about-nida/organization/cctn/clinical-trials-network-ctn/resources) can help find addiction treatment programs around the country. Although not professional treatment, mutual self-help groups, such as AA, Narcotics Anonymous (NA) or SMART Recovery, are free-of-charge, available across locations, times, and in-person and remote meeting options, and can serve as a recovery-supportive social network. Engagement in mutual self-help groups has been shown to improve outcomes in people with addiction.

Follow-up visits allow clinicians to offer continued support and care for the patient. With patients who adhere to the set goals, clinicians should reinforce progress; renegotiate treatment goals, if indicated; and encourage regular follow-up. At each follow-up, patient progress should be documented ("Did the patient meet and sustain his goals?"), with re-screening and assessment, if needed, completed annually. Those who screen positive and/or have an existing diagnosis of SUD should be reassessed at the next appointment and re-offered interventions. Patient-centered care is essential for the delivery of high-quality SUD management and clinicians should acknowledge that change is difficult; reemphasize willingness to help; readdress the impact of continued substance use; reevaluate the diagnosis, treatment goals, and plan; consider engaging significant others; and schedule close follow-up.

SBI for Unhealthy Substance Use (Alcohol, Drugs, Nicotine/Tobacco): Approaches

Unhealthy Substance Use Screening

In the context of guidelines discussed previously, a variety of tools of varying length exist for screening for unhealthy substance use in clinical practice. Smith and colleagues showed that a single question, "How many times in the past year have you used an illegal drug or used a prescription medication for nonmedical reasons?" accurately identified unhealthy drug use in primary care patients, with a response of at least "one time" constituting a positive screen. In 2022, NIDA recommended the TAPS (Tobacco, Alcohol, Prescription medication, and other Substance use) tool, which is a brief substance-specific questionnaire for screening and assessing substance use severity (**Table 31-1**) (https://nida.nih.gov/taps2/). An adaptation from the NIDA quick screen and NM-ASSIST, TAPS consists of two parts. TAPS-1, is a 4-item screen for tobacco, alcohol, and illicit and nonmedical prescription-based drug use; and TAPS-2, which should be initiated for individuals who screened positive on TAPS-1. TAPS-1 has been found to be highly accurate and may be particularly useful for triage of unhealthy substance use in primary care due to the simple and brief nature of this tool.[20] Additionally, TAPS-1 is validated for both interviewer- and self-administration, with participants shown to disclose higher rates of substance use on the self-administered version for all substances except tobacco.

Regardless of the exact methods used, it is important for clinicians to screen for substance use routinely and repeatedly, and, when appropriate, assess consequences of substance use to avail opportunities for intervention and prevention.

Drug SBI

Assessment of Severity: At-Risk Use, or Disorder

Those with a positive screen for unhealthy drug use ("yes" to any use) should complete the NIDA-Modified ASSIST questionnaire,[21] called NM-ASSIST, available as an interactive Web-based (www.drugabuse.gov/nmassist) or "full text" survey (www.drugabuse.gov/sites/default/files/pdf/nmassist.pdf); the NIDA approach favors NM-ASSIST, but screening for, and severity assessment of, unhealthy drug use can be accomplished using other tools, such as the DAST-10. The eight-question NM-ASSIST inquires about the type of drugs, frequency of their use, and symptoms suggestive of a disorder. Its total score, the so-called *substance involvement score*, determines the level of risk associated with illicit or nonmedical prescription-based drug use (0-3 points: lower risk; 4-26 points: moderate risk; and 27 or more points: high risk, consistent with moderate to severe disorder). If the use of more than one drug is reported, the patient receives a score for *each* substance endorsed (the NM-ASSIST questions are "repeated" for each reported drug), rather than a single cumulative score. Therefore, the patient's risk level may differ from substance to substance. In addition to its "scored" questions, the NM-ASSIST also includes a question about injection substance use.

While the NM-ASSIST is one of the recommended screening tools, it may not be optimal for busy primary care settings.[20] Austin et al. conducted formative evaluation

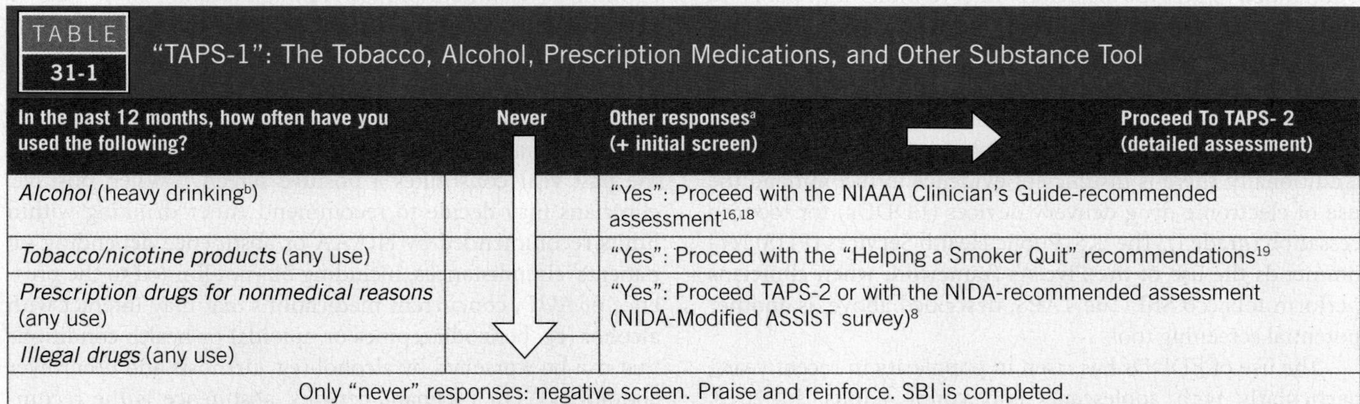
TABLE 31-1 "TAPS-1": The Tobacco, Alcohol, Prescription Medications, and Other Substance Tool

In the past 12 months, how often have you used the following?	Never	Other responses[a] (+ initial screen) → Proceed To TAPS-2 (detailed assessment)
Alcohol (heavy drinking[b])	↓	"Yes": Proceed with the NIAAA Clinician's Guide-recommended assessment[16,18]
Tobacco/nicotine products (any use)	↓	"Yes": Proceed with the "Helping a Smoker Quit" recommendations[19]
Prescription drugs for nonmedical reasons (any use)	↓	"Yes": Proceed TAPS-2 or with the NIDA-recommended assessment (NIDA-Modified ASSIST survey)[8]
Illegal drugs (any use)	↓	
Only "never" responses: negative screen. Praise and reinforce. SBI is completed.		

[a]Possible responses: "never," "less than monthly," "monthly," "weekly," or "daily or almost daily."

[b]Heavy drinking: five or more (for men) or four or more (for women) drinks in a day.

Based on National Institute on Drug Abuse Clinical Trials Network. The Tobacco, alcohol, prescription medication, and other substance (TAPS) use tool; 2017. https://nida.nih.gov/taps2/

during a multisite randomized controlled trial in 10 geographically distinct primary clinics engaged in implementing and a 12-question NM-ASSIST for OUD screening. They found that clinic staff viewed the NM-ASSIST as overly complicated and challenging to administer, corroborating prior research, which suggested that screening tools for SUD should be brief and easy to administer and interpret.[22] As of 2022, NIDA recommends using TAPS tool as described above, to assess substance use severity over the NM-ASSIST.

Clinicians should screen for unhealthy drug use and deliver interventions when determined appropriate as recommended in the updated 2020 USPSTF guidelines. Screening is only one indicator of a patient's potential drug use risk. In case of an elevated "risk level" identified for more than one drug, a decision about which substance to address first also needs to be clinically driven; in general, focusing intervention on the substance with the "highest risk" or the patient's expressed greatest "motivation to change" may produce best results, though an approach to addressing all substances simultaneously can also be appropriate. A shared decision-making with the patient is recommended. Similarly, a cautious, clinically-driven approach relates to the urine toxicology results, which represent only one of the multiple pieces of the clinical puzzle; the NIDA guide has a separate appendix with the tips on biologic sample testing. Addition of biomarker testing, such as toxicology testing (see Section 4 for more information on this topic), may be beneficial in selected patients, particularly for follow-up monitoring.[23]

Tobacco/Nicotine SBI

Tobacco/Nicotine Use Screening

USPSTF recommends screening all adults, including pregnant persons, as well as school-aged children and adolescents who have not started using tobacco and advising those who use tobacco to stop tobacco use (grade A). Furthermore, it is recommended to provide behavioral interventions and U.S. Food and Drug Administration (FDA) approved pharmacotherapy for abstinence to nonpregnant adults who use tobacco (grade A). In pregnant persons and school-aged children and adolescents there is currently insufficient evidence to recommend pharmacological intervention for tobacco cessation (grade I). Additionally, there is insufficient evidence to recommend the use of electronic drug delivery devices (EDDDs) for tobacco cessation (grade I). The U.S. Public Health Services (PHS) recommends the use of the Five A's framework when clinicians perform tobacco SBI. The TAPS, described above, is another potential screening tool.

The use of EDDDs has risen in popularity in recent years, particularly with adolescents and young adults. In 2018, approximately three million high school and 0.5 million middle school students used nicotine via EDDDs,[24] representing a dramatic increase from the past trends and threatening the gains achieved through the decades of prevention efforts. While screening for tobacco use in the form of cigarettes or chewable tobacco is rather common, clinicians often overlook screening for nicotine EDDDs and vaping of other substances. It is not well documented whether currently available tools, are sensitive enough to accurately screen for EDDDs use.[25,26]

There is currently moderate to high certainty evidence that a variety of behavioral support and counseling and the seven FDA approved medications for stopping nicotine/tobacco use, and combination therapy of pharmacotherapy and psychosocial interventions, can significantly increase rates of stopping smoking among adults.[24] Further work is needed regarding the comparative effectiveness of the FDA approved pharmacotherapies for tobacco/nicotine use and in special populations (pregnant persons, persons with mental illness, persons with HIV, and people who smoke nondaily/intermittently).[27] Evidence is limited on the use of EDDDs as an intervention for stopping smoking, mostly due to the limited number of robust RCTs. Further information on EDDDs can be found in Section 2 of this textbook.

Alcohol SBI for Adults

Adult Alcohol Screening

Consistent with the NIDA algorithm (described above), the NIAAA recommends a single question (see Table 28-1) about the presence of heavy drinking as an initial screen: "How many times in the past year have you had five or more (for men) or four or more (for women) drinks in a day?"[15,16] This single question is sensitive and specific for detecting unhealthy alcohol use in primary care[13,28] and, to a lesser degree, inpatient settings.[29] The NIAAA suggests an optional *prescreening question* about *any* alcohol use ("Do you sometimes drink beer, wine, or other alcoholic beverages?") that can help "ease" the patient into the more detailed screening for those who answered "yes." During this conversation, it is important to discuss with the patient what constitutes a single or "standard" drink (**Table 31-2**); presenting the patient with a chart of "standard drinks"—as the one available in the NIAAA's Clinician's Guide or online (www.RethinkingDrinking.niaaa.nih.gov)—can be very useful. This latter site can additionally help the patients screen themselves for unhealthy alcohol use.

With the endorsement of not drinking any alcohol or not engaging in any heavy drinking in the past year, the screen is considered *negative* and completed. *Any* heavy drinking in the past year constitutes a positive screen.[11] When positive, clinicians may decide to recommend either drinking within limits recommended by NIAAA or abstinence depending on patients' circumstances, including but not limited to the presence of AUD, concurrent medications that may interact with alcohol (eg, benzodiazepines or opioids) or health conditions that can be worsened by alcohol (eg, cirrhosis and other liver conditions). For pregnant persons, abstinence is the recommended healthiest choice. In all populations recent research suggests that any amount of alcohol used is unsafe and should be avoided. A systemic review by the Global Burden of Disease Collaborative (2018) found that increasing levels of consumed alcohol led to increased risk of all-cause mortality, and that there was no safe level of alcohol consumption.[30]

TABLE 31-2 Maximum (Low-Risk) Drinking Limits for Adults

	Daily[a]	Weekly[b]
Healthy men ≤65 years old	≤4 drinks	≤14 drinks
Healthy women and men >65 years old	≤3 drinks	≤7 drinks

One standard drink is equivalent to 12 oz of beer, 5 oz of wine, or 1.5 oz of 80-proof spirits.

[a]Exceeded daily limit: heavy drinking.

[b]Exceeded daily or weekly limit: at-risk drinking.

Data from National Institute on Alcohol Abuse and Alcoholism. (n.d.). Rethinking Drinking. https://www.rethinkingdrinking.niaaa.nih.gov/

A *positive screen* (indicating heavy drinking or drinking above the clinician-recommended limits in the past year) also warrants further inquiry about the alcohol use pattern and impact. At this point, clinicians should determine the patient's usual weekly alcohol consumption by asking questions about frequency and quantity ("On average, how many days a week do you have an alcoholic drink?" and "On a typical drinking day, how many drinks do you have?"). These two questions enable estimation of the number of drinks per week, which, if it exceeds the recommended weekly limits (see **Table 31-2**), increases the level of concern for unhealthy alcohol use. All the gathered information should be recorded in the patient's chart; it can be used later for targeted counseling and to help monitor treatment progress.

A notable alternative approach to the single screening question is administration of the three questions about alcohol consumption from the Alcohol Use Disorders Identification Test (AUDIT) developed by the World Health Organization,[31] or the AUDIT-C.[32] Answers to these questions have been associated with high predictive validity for screening for unhealthy alcohol use in veterans[33] also non-Veteran primary care patients[32] and college students.[34] The AUDIT-C (for "consumption") reflects the first three questions of the AUDIT: "How often did you have a drink containing alcohol in the past year?" "How many drinks containing alcohol did you have on a typical day when you were drinking in the past year?" "How often did you have six or more drinks on one occasion in the past year?" Generally, a score of 4 or more is considered positive for men, and a score of 3 or more is considered positive in women as a screen for unhealthy alcohol use. However, the cut-off score for the AUDIT-C has varied across clinical settings and in different populations, with some opting to choose a higher cut-off score ranging from 5 to 8 to decrease the number of false positives. AUDIT-C scores have also been shown to correlate well with consumption and increasing number of AUD symptoms, as well as risk for multiple health outcomes, including mortality risk, the latter particularly among men.[35,36] More specifically, higher AUDIT-C scores were associated with an increased risk of alcohol-related medical complications and death. AUDIT-C score of 5 or greater has been shown to be associated with medication noncompliance, fractures, and gastrointestinal illnesses.[37,38] Additionally, the study by Rubinsky et al. found that AUDIT-C scores could help estimate mean daily alcohol consumption level, AUD severity, and the probability of AUD.[39] A systematic review and meta-analysis of 36 studies conducted by Lange et al. suggested that AUDIT-C performs less well in identifying at-risk women. In addition, higher false-positive rates were noted in countries with a lower prevalence of AUD compared to countries with a higher AUD prevalence.[40]

Assessment of Severity in Adults: At-Risk Drinking Versus AUD

The Alcohol Symptom Checklist is one tool that clinicians can use to both identify individuals with undiagnosed AUD and to assess the AUD severity. The Checklist is an 11-item questionnaire based on DSM-5 criteria and previously validated within primary care settings. An individual scoring positively for at least two of the criteria would prompt the clinician to evaluate for AUD, with severity based upon the total number of positive criteria (ie, 2-3 criteria for mild, 4-5 criteria for moderate, and 6-11 criteria for severe).[41]

Another tool to assess AUD severity is the NIAAA's Clinician's Guide. While the NIAAA's Clinician's Guide and its associated materials use DSM-IV terminology of alcohol "abuse and dependence," it remains an easily accessible and easy-to-use method for discerning the level of risk and appropriate treatment tailored to routine day-to-day clinical practice. Specifically, patients who exceed recommended drinking limits or the questionnaire cutoffs but do not meet the criteria for AUD are categorized as engaging in "at-risk drinking," a risk factor for the development of AUD and other negative health consequences. Distinguishing between "at-risk drinking" and AUD is clinically relevant because it helps formulate appropriate clinical recommendations. Existing evidence indicates that those who are classified as having "at-risk drinking" but do not meet criteria for AUD are most likely to benefit from BI alone, while patients with AUD are less likely to do well without an additional, more-intensive intervention and/or behavioral or pharmacologic treatment.

Alcohol Brief Intervention in Adults

A brief intervention is appropriate for patients meeting criteria for unhealthy drinking. With the patient's agreement, the clinician should provide, in an empathic and nonconfrontational manner, an objective assessment of drinking and its consequences (information about personal health harms, and possible benefits of cutting down or quitting) as well as clear, specific, and personalized behavior change *advice*: "You're drinking more than what is medically safe. I strongly recommend that you cut down on your drinking." "I believe that your drinking is a serious risk to your health and I strongly recommend that you quit drinking." "As your physician, I want to partner with you to help you reduce or quit drinking."

Abstinence can produce better treatment outcomes than drinking reduction in people with AUD, especially those with advanced disease. Abstinence may also be recommended as a primary treatment goal for patients with specific comorbid medical or psychiatric conditions. However, for many people who should, but may not be willing to abstain, drinking reduction may be more acceptable or feasible. Even modest reductions in drinking can result in decreased alcohol-related harms. For example, cutting down from daily drinking to three days a week may be appropriate for some patients; for college students, cutting down from 12 to 15 drinks to 5 to 6 drinks on a weekend night may reduce the risk of significant harm and convince the student to begin the longer-term process of cutting back even further to lower the risk level.

SBI for Youth

Substance Use in Youth: General Considerations

In spite of the fact that the legal drinking age is 21 years in the United States, many youth start drinking earlier in life. In 2021, The Monitoring the Future national survey found 7% of 8th graders and 26% of 12th graders reported drinking alcohol in the past 30 days.[36] Drinking contributes to the top three causes of death among adolescents: unintentional injury (eg, motor vehicle accidents), homicide, and suicide.[42] Evidence shows that drinking at a younger age increases the risk of developing addiction and alcohol-related harms, which include serious consequences such as death, injuries, motor vehicle crashes, and high-risk behaviors, as well as mental and physical health problems. Mental health problems most likely to co-occur with AUD include depression and suicide, anxiety, attention deficit hyperactivity, conduct, schizophrenia, and eating disorders. Associated physical health conditions include trauma and its sequelae, sleep, gastrointestinal problems, liver disease, sexually transmitted infections (STIs) or unintended pregnancy. Patterns of substance use in the community have influence on the youth's substance use. Permissive parental attitudes toward substance use and having friends or family members who use alcohol, tobacco, or drugs are strong predictors of substance use by youth. Parental monitoring and presence of clear household rules about substance use are protecting factors against the youth's substance use.[43]

Although the guidelines by the USPSTF state the existing evidence is insufficient to recommend routine screening for unhealthy substance use in youth, new research lends support for effectiveness of SBI for adolescents,[44] and most professional organizations, including the American Academy of Pediatrics (AAP), the AAFP, the NIAAA, the NIDA, and the NQF, recommend implementing SBI in youth. In 2011, the NIAAA, in collaboration with the AAP, released a guide for practitioners describing the rationale for and an approach to alcohol SBI for youth.[45] According to this guide, *all children and youth between ages 9 and 18 years should be screened for alcohol use at least annually*, with more frequent screening considered for those who can be at higher risk for alcohol use and use disorders, such as youth who use tobacco/nicotine, have mental health problems known to co-occur with SUDs, have physical health conditions that might be alcohol related, or engage in high-risk behaviors (eg, as manifested by presence of an STI or pregnancy), or substantial negative behaviors. In its updated 2016 policy statement, the AAP continues to emphasize the importance of screening of adolescents for alcohol use and integrating SBI into the medical home.[45]

Confidentiality and Parental Involvement

Screening minors for substance use and related disorders inevitably brings to light the issue of confidentiality and parental involvement. Setting the stage in advance for the scope and extent of confidentiality is very helpful. Optimally, clinicians would share with the patient and the parents all the details about confidentiality policies and disclosure provisions in advance, ideally starting at 7- or 8-year-old well-child visits, or at least prior to the screening. With all adolescents who use substances, the clinician should inquire about parental awareness, and seek the patient's permission to speak to the parents (or guardians) or, at least, encourage the patient to discuss substance use with the parents.

In general, the discussion about and treatment for the minor's substance use can usually be kept confidential if the minor wishes to do so; preserving confidentiality may help strengthen the trust and treatment alliance between the clinician and the minor. Although most medical organizations and laws support the ability of clinicians to provide confidential care for minors in relation to substance use, it is important to be aware of specific laws governing each state. Information about minor consent laws can be obtained from the state medical societies or the Center for Adolescent Health and the Law (www.cahl.org).

There are circumstances, though, when a clinician should consider breaking confidentiality and engage the parents to ensure safety, for example, the presence of "acute danger signs" (see below in Assessment of Severity in Youth), a need for referral for further treatment, or negative health consequences related to substance use. The NIAAA guide also suggests engaging parents, even against the minor's wishes, for *any* alcohol use by elementary school kids, alcohol-related (even mild) problems in middle school, or significant problems in high school students. In general, the clinicians should apply their best medical judgment, together with the state's laws, to decide whether breaking confidentiality is warranted. Confidentiality can be unintentionally compromised if, for example, the substance use-related diagnostic codes are included in "explanation of benefits" sent to parents by the insurance company or when a follow-up visit is scheduled for "substance use" and may reveal the nature of the adolescent's problems; these aspects of care require consideration in advance (eg, a follow-up visit may be labeled as for immunizations or acne follow-up).

Alcohol Screening in Youth

Practitioners should strive to establish good rapport with adolescent patients and encourage honest answers. Building in alone time (without parents) during the visit and explaining confidentiality policies (see above) can facilitate it. Explaining the purpose of asking about sensitive issues can further promote a trusting relationship and alleviate the youth's perception of being singled out ("My goal is to help my patients be healthy and that's why I talk to all my patients about alcohol use and other health risks").

The NIAAA guide recommends using two screening questions about the *past year* alcohol use to facilitate stratification of the child's drinking behavior into a lowest-, moderate-, or highest-risk category. The choice of initial questions depends on the child's school level and age (**Table 31-3**). For elementary and middle school kids, the recommended first screening question is about their *friends' alcohol use (any use)*, with the second question about the patient's personal alcohol use. For high school students, the first screening question is about the patient's personal alcohol use frequency in the past year, and the second question asks about *friends' binge drinking*. Presence of friends who drink among younger kids or friends who have episodic heavy drinking among high school students has been shown to increase the patient's risk of unhealthy substance use and should trigger additional probing questions.

Assessment of Severity in Youth: At-Risk Drinking and AUD

Youth who do not drink (negative screen) should be affirmed and counseled on the continuation of their healthy behaviors. It is helpful to elicit and affirm their reasons for not drinking and educate about risks associated with drinking. Jointly with the clinician, they should also explore plans on how to continue staying alcohol free when their friends drink and be advised never to ride in a car with a driver who used alcohol or drugs. Nondrinkers with nondrinking friends should be rescreened at least yearly. However, those with drinking friends should be rescreened more frequently, ideally during the next visit.

All drinking youth should be evaluated in more depth to assess and stratify risk (**Table 31-4**). *Any* past year drinking places an elementary school student in a high risk category and a child 12 to 15 years old (middle or early high school) in a moderate-risk category. Moderate- and high-risk patients should be additionally evaluated for the presence of AUD. Additional questionnaires, asking in more detail about alcohol consumption and related problems, can assist this process.

Substance Use Assessment Questionnaires for Youth

For drinking youth, several brief questionnaires are available to help more in-depth assessment and gauging of risk of the adolescent's substance use. They can identify negative consequences, which can then be discussed during MI and BI. Although the AUDIT can be used in drinking adolescents, lower thresholds are used to identify unhealthy alcohol use than in adults.[44] The CRAFFT (Car, Relax, Alone, Forget, Friends, Trouble), on the other hand, is an easy-to-use, validated, and reliable six-question survey, inquiring about both alcohol and drug use in several contexts. It is endorsed by the NIDA and the AAP and can discriminate between substance use, at-risk use, and disorder in adolescents.[46] It can be prefaced with the phrase "in the past year" and administered in verbal, electronic, or paper-pencil format. Positive responses to two or three of the CRAFFT questions raise suspicion for substance use condition that warrants further inquiry, while four or more "yes" responses suggests DSM-IV–defined substance dependence (diagnostically similar to a moderate to severe SUD). In addition, the Problem Oriented Screening Instrument for Teenagers (POSIT)'s 17-item substance use/use disorder subscale has been validated for screening adolescents and adults in primary care for substance use and substance use

TABLE 31-3 Two-Question Initial Screen: Ask About Personal Alcohol Use and Friends' Drinking

	First question	Second question
Elementary school (9-11 years old)	Do you have any friends who drank beer, wine, or any drink containing alcohol in the past year?	How about you—have you ever had more than a few sips of any drink containing alcohol?
Middle school (11-14 years old)		How about you—in the past year, on how many days have you had more than a few sips of any drink containing alcohol?
High school (14-18 years old)	How about you—in the past year, on how many days have you had more than a few sips of any drink containing alcohol?	If your friends drink, how many drinks do they usually drink on an occasion?* *Binge drinking: • Girls: 3+ drinks • Boys: 9-13 years old: 3+ drinks 14-15 years old: 4+ drinks 16+ years old: 5+ drinks

Adapted from National Institute on Alcohol Abuse and Alcoholism. *Alcohol screening and brief intervention for youth: A practitioner's guide.* https://www.niaaa.nih.gov/sites/default/files/publications/NIAAA_AlcoholScreening_Youth_Guide.pdf

TABLE 31-4 Adolescents Who Report Drinking in the Past Year: Risk Stratification by Age and the Number of Past Year Drinking Days

Risk	9-11 years old	12-14 years old	15 years old	16 years old	17 years old	18 years old
Lowest	—	—	—	≤5 days	≤5 days	≤11 days
Moderate	—	1+ day	1+ day	6+ days	6+ days	12+ days
Highest	1+ day	6+ days	6+ days	12+ days	24+ days	52+ days

Elementary school, 9-11 years old; middle school, 11-14 years old; high school, 14-18 years old.

Data from National Institute on Alcohol Abuse and Alcoholism. *Alcohol screening and brief intervention for youth: A practitioner's guide.* https://www.niaaa.nih.gov/sites/default/files/publications/NIAAA_AlcoholScreening_Youth_Guide.pdf

disorder.[47] Although reliable, the POSIT's subscale is lengthy compared to AUDIT and AUDIT-C tools, which have good psychometric properties.

Brief tools have also shown promise as initial screening tools for unhealthy alcohol or cannabis use among young people (12-21 years old) in the emergency department (ED).[48] Positive screen results identify youth at risk for having an alcohol or cannabis use disorder who should receive a more detailed assessment, most likely on an outpatient basis. A two-question instrument may provide a "quick screen" in the ED to detect a probable AUD ("In the past year, have you sometimes been under the influence of alcohol in situations where you could have caused an accident or gotten hurt?" and "Have there often been times when you had a lot more to drink than you intended to have?").[49,50] Youth answering "yes" to one or both of these screening questions have an eight times higher risk of having an AUD. Youth who report cannabis use more than two times over the previous year on a one-question screen for unhealthy cannabis use (Diagnostic Interview Schedule for Children, DISC)[51,52] have an almost sevenfold risk of having a cannabis use disorder compared to those who used cannabis less frequently ("In the past year, how often have you used cannabis [0 to 1 time; >2 times]?"). In general, it is worth noting that many available screening instruments aim at identifying SUD; for most (if not all) youth, *any use*, and especially at-risk use, should be inquired about and approached seriously.

Just as with adults, it is important to clarify what a "single" drink means while inquiring about alcohol quantity. Charts defining "standard" drink equivalents are very useful. Incorporating "what else I know" about the patient into the risk assessment and then intervention can strengthen and personalize treatment; for example, family history of SUDs, permissive environment at home toward substance use, or low parental involvement would heighten concern about the degree of risk.

Alcohol Brief Intervention in Youth

All drinking youth should receive BI, with BI principles similar to those as for adults. Lowest- and moderate-risk patients without an AUD should be advised to stop (or at least reduce) drinking and receive counseling similar to that described above for the nondrinking youth, though adjusted appropriately. Referral to addiction treatment should always be considered for the highest-risk patients and those with an AUD. In addition, adolescents who display "acute danger signs" will need *immediate* intervention and, likely, parental or guardian involvement that may require breaking of the minor's confidentiality. The most common and potentially lethal *acute danger signs* include driving under the influence of alcohol or drugs; high-amount intake (eg, prior poisoning or overdose); combining alcohol with drugs, especially sedatives; engaging in high-risk behaviors in relation to substance use (eg, unprotected sex, injuries due to risks taken); signs of AUD; or injection drug use.[50,52]

Follow-up is crucial for the success of attaining treatment goals by both adults and youth.[52] Negotiating the timing of follow-up with the patient as well as scheduling it for additional reasons (eg, acne care) may increase the likelihood that the patient keeps that appointment. As with adults, the starting point of the follow-up evaluation is to ask the patient if they were able to meet and sustain goals, prior to the reassessment and risk re-stratification. Treatment goals and plans should be revised as appropriate, and as based on the newly obtained information and the patient's preferences.

CURRENT EVIDENCE ON SCREENING AND BRIEF INTERVENTION: A BRIEF SUMMARY

Screening and Brief Intervention for Unhealthy Alcohol Use

With the caveat that randomized controlled trials of SBI generally rely on patients' reports of drinking, which may be subject to bias (reporting what the participant believes the interviewer, who has recommended less use, wants to hear), a meta-analysis of studies on screening and counseling interventions for unhealthy alcohol use found that such interventions could lead to a 14% improvement in individuals abiding by the recommended drinking limits.[53]

Moderate-quality evidence also indicates that SBI delivered in ED settings can lead to reductions in alcohol use, drinking-related negative consequences (eg, injury), and repeated ED visits among children 12 years of age or older, and adults engaging in unhealthy drinking. Although the health impact of alcohol SBI has been compared to that of other cost-effective preventive services, such as screening for colorectal cancer, hypertension, visual acuity (for adults over 64 years of age), or immunizations for influenza and pneumococcal infections, SBI for unhealthy alcohol use continues to be delivered at much lower rates than these other commonly performed preventive services.[54] A nationally representative internet-based survey of over 2,500 adult primary care patients in 2013 showed that just under one in four patients received alcohol screening in the past year, with men and women being screened at similar rates. Individuals with less than a college degree and non-Hispanic Black patients were significantly less likely to be screened relative to college-educated non-Hispanic White patients.[55] A number of barriers can impede SBI implementation in the clinical setting, including inadequate resources and staff training, or societal-level stigma resulting in an unintentionally stigmatizing or stereotyping approach to the identification of those at risk, all critical factors to facilitating delivery of SBI in primary care setting.[56] The Committee on Trauma of the American College of Surgeons has recommended that all level I and II trauma centers be equipped with alcohol screening tools and that level I centers offer a BI when necessary.[57,58] In trauma settings, SBI may reduce drinking, drinking-related harms, and recurrence of injuries requiring ED care or hospital admissions among people with injury and at-risk drinking.[59-62] However, the overall evidence is not as strong as for a primary care setting—a recent meta-analysis on 28 separate randomized controlled trials of SBI in ED settings including 14,456 patients revealed very small effect sizes of SBI on subsequent drinking and ED visits.[63]

Indeed, evidence from individual studies in the ED settings is mixed; some suggest SBI can reduce drinking and result in fewer future ED visits among people with at-risk drinking,[62-64] while other studies with high quality methodology have yielded null results.[65-70]

In general inpatient medical settings, evidence on the effectiveness of opportunistic alcohol SBI is inconclusive and suggests that SBI may be overall beneficial[68,69,71] yet does not work as well as in primary care. One potential key issue in the inpatient setting is, based on findings from a single RCT in an urban hospital, that the vast majority of general medical inpatients, identified as "positive" by screening, may have DSM-IV–defined alcohol dependence.[68]

Limited evidence suggests that SBI can reduce morbidity and mortality.[70] SBI appears to reduce drinking in adults, including young adults ages 18 to 25[28] and older adults ages 65 and older,[72,73] college students,[74-76] pregnant and childbearing age persons,[77,78] though in the latter, the evidence is not as strong. According to the USPSTF guidelines, there is still insufficient evidence on the efficacy of alcohol SBI in adolescents; however, the growing evidence is encouraging, and main professional organizations and expert panels advise conducting SBI in youth at least annually, starting at age 9 years.[11,43-45,79]

Although a single, short 5- to 15-minute intervention may be helpful, a multiple-contact BI, usually including one to three booster sessions, has been shown to reduce self-reported drinking and is recommended.[80,81] The optimal interval for SBI is unknown, although routine annual screening may be a reasonable interval. Patients with past alcohol-related consequences, young adults, and other higher-risk groups (eg, people who use tobacco) may benefit from frequent screening and, if indicated, BI.[80] The counseling style of effective BI is based on MI and commonly includes elements such as empathy, feedback, advice with an emphasis on patient responsibility and self-efficacy, and a treatment plan with a menu of options. The BI studies with the largest effect sizes utilized primary care clinicians to deliver the intervention.[81]

Electronic SBI (e-SBI) such as computerized approaches for alcohol use have shown promise in a variety of contexts, including trauma and other medical settings,[82-86] college students,[87,88] people with at-risk drinking,[89-93] and pregnant and postpartum persons.[94-97] Technology may facilitate the process of identifying and initially addressing alcohol (and drug) use due to the perception of privacy by the user, and nearly unlimited moment-to-moment access, particularly as it pertains to smartphone-based tools (ie, apps). However, the effect sizes of e-SBI noted in systematic reviews of randomized controlled trials have been very small.

Screening and Brief Intervention for Unhealthy Drug Use

Recent years have seen an increase in the number of randomized controlled trials of SBI for unhealthy drug use in primary care[89,98-101] and ED[102,103] settings, paralleling the growing national recognition of morbidity and mortality associated with drug use in the United States, especially in relation to opioid use, and increasing acceptability and legalization of cannabis use.[104] Based on the growing evidence, now including thousands of patients in several settings, the USPSTF updated its 2008 guidance in 2020 to recommend screening for unhealthy drug use among adults 18 years old or older (grade B), with screening referring to asking questions or using validated questionnaires about unhealthy drug use, rather than testing of biological specimens.[6]

SBI for Nonmedical Opioid Use

SBI for opioid use disorder (OUD), including among those treated with long-term opioid therapy, may help reduce the nonmedical use of opioids (eg, heroin, fentanyl, and/or prescribed medications) and associated harms, and identify those with OUD. In 2020, an estimated 9.5 million persons aged 12 years or older reported using prescription opioids nonmedically.[1] The first wave of the current overdose crisis involved rising rates of nonmedical prescription opioid use, with the second and third waves of the overdose crisis being driven by heroin and illicitly manufactured fentanyl respectively. ED visits linked to opioid use increased between 2005 and 2017 from 89 to 249 visits per 100,000 people, and admissions to addiction treatment programs for OUD involving opioids more than quadrupled between 2002 and 2012.[105,106] The number of deaths involving prescription opioids rose from 3,442 in 1999 to 17,029 in 2017.[107] Moreover, overdose death rates continued to increase by 17% from 2019 to 2020.[108] Even more alarming is the expanding availability of powerful illicitly manufactured synthetic opioids, which may have emerged in response to increasing demands for illicit opioids. From 2019 to 2020, the age-adjusted rate of death involving natural and semisynthetic opioids increased by 11%, while mortality due to synthetic opioids other than methadone (eg, fentanyl) increased by 56%. During the same time, the age-adjusted rate of death involving heroin decreased by 6.8%.[106] The sharp increase in deaths involving synthetic opioids has been driven by contamination of the drug supply with illicitly manufactured fentanyl and its analogs. In 2021, the provisional number of drug-related overdose deaths in the United States reached 100,306, representing the highest number ever recorded, and a 28.5% increase from the previous year.[109,110]

Research designed to develop screening methods for the detection of unhealthy opioid use and use disorder has been growing in response to the opioid-related addiction and overdose crisis. Most studies have focused on survey-based screening and/or toxicology screens. Four specific behaviors among people prescribed chronic opioid therapy have been strongly associated with DSM-IV–defined opioid dependence; these included early refills, self-reports of feeling intoxicated, self-increasing dose, and over-sedating oneself.[111] One screening tool commonly used in ambulatory settings is the Screener and Opioid Assessment for Patients with Pain-Revised (SOAPP-R).[112] This questionnaire, validated in patients treated with opioids in a specialty pain clinic, has been widely used in both pain and primary care practices, and can help determine which patients may require additional monitoring while being treated with opioids long-term. When initiating opioid therapy for individuals with chronic pain, opioid risk tool (ORT) has been a popular screening tool to assess the risk of future unhealthy opioid use, although it has not been validated in populations without pain.[113] NIDA recommends the NIDA-Modified ASSIST questionnaire (described above) for unhealthy prescription drug use screening, though this can be a challenging instrument to integrate in primary care.

Despite the multiple questionnaire-based screening instruments available, unfortunately, no tool has been validated for universal screening in primary care for unhealthy opioid use. There is also limited literature to support the efficacy of SBI for unhealthy opioid use or use disorder. However, strong evidence for the benefits of OUD treatment, particularly medication for OUD, which reduce both all-cause and overdose specific mortality. This evidence emphasizes the need for early diagnosis and initiation of treatment among individuals with OUD, including in nontraditional addiction treatment settings, such as the EDs. The RCT by D'Onofrio et al. evaluated the efficacy of ED-initiated buprenorphine on addiction treatment engagement. among 329 ED patients with OUD, and found that those randomized to receive SBIRT along with ED-initiated buprenorphine had a higher rate of treatment engagement at 30 days than those who received SBIRT only or screening and referral to treatment only (78% versus 45% versus 37% of engaged individuals, respectively). These findings indicated that SBIRT combined with ED-initiated buprenorphine can be more effective in facilitating addiction treatment engagement among those with OUD than the more traditional SBIRT (ie, without ED initiation of buprenorphine therapy).[114] Additional tools that may assist clinicians in screening for unhealthy prescription opioid use include the Prescription Drug Monitoring Programs (PDMPs), which are in place in the majority of the U.S. states. The PDMPs are online databases, implemented on a state-by-state basis, that record details of prescribed opioids after they are dispensed by a pharmacy, including the date, type and quantity of dispensed opioid (and other controlled substance) medications, the name of the prescriber(s), and the pharmacies utilized.[115-117] Some include data on state-authorized cannabis used as treatment. The PDMP-based information can help identify patients who obtain prescriptions for opioids from multiple sources or request a medication refill too early. While mandatory PDMP use has been associated with decreased opioid prescribing, it may have the unintended effect of increasing overdose mortality due to illegal opioids.

Finally, while there is limited information on the sensitivity and specificity of routine toxicology drug screening to identify unhealthy opioid use in patients with opioid-treated chronic pain, this has become a routine practice in many regions to detect substances not prescribed and confirm use of the prescribed medications. Yet, this does not represent SBI; rather, such testing is indicated to monitor the use of prescription medications and to assess for illegal drug use in this subset of patients at higher risk for unhealthy opioid use.

SYSTEMATIC REVIEWS AND META-ANALYSES OF SCREENING AND BRIEF INTERVENTIONS FOR UNHEALTHY ALCOHOL USE

The following studies, among others, were used to support the summary statements in the previous sections. What follows is a brief overview of SBI-related research for unhealthy alcohol use or use disorder.

O'Connor et al. conducted a systematic review of the literature on the effectiveness and harm of SBI for unhealthy alcohol use.[118] This review included 113 studies of alcohol SBI among adolescents and adults. Its findings documented that screening instruments available for use in the primary care setting can effectively identify adults with unhealthy alcohol use, and BIs can help safely reduce unhealthy alcohol use.

A meta-analysis of randomized controlled trials by Kaner et al. provided an overall evaluation of the effects of SBI[119] for unhealthy alcohol consumption in general practice or ED settings. This review evaluated 69 studies with a total of 33,642 participants who received either BI or a minimal/no intervention. The results indicated that BI was effective in reducing unhealthy alcohol consumption compared to minimal or no intervention, and that longer BI duration (>15 minutes) had little additional effect.

A systematic review by Jonas et al. included 23 trials and evaluated the benefits and harms of SBI for unhealthy drinking among adolescents, pregnant persons, and adults with "nondependent" (based on DSM-IV criteria) drinking.[53] The best evidence for efficacy was found for brief (10 to 15 minute) multi-contact BIs. This review found a moderate strength of evidence supporting SBI efficacy for self-reported drinking reduction among adults with nondependent unhealthy alcohol use as well as young adults or college students who engage in at-risk drinking. Compared to controls, adults with unhealthy drinking reduced their consumption by 3.6 drinks per week (10 trials, 4,332 participants), with 12% fewer adults reporting heavy drinking (7 trials, 2,737 participants) and 11% more adults reporting drinking below the recommended limit (9 trials, 5,973 participants) over 12 months. Among young adults and college students, SBI also resulted in decreased alcohol use by 1.7 fewer drinks per week (3 trials, 1,421 participants) and heavy drinking by 0.9 fewer heavy drinking days per month (3 trials, 1,448 participants). The review did not find sufficient evidence to draw conclusions about SBI efficacy for pregnant persons, adolescents, or for the reduction in injuries, accidents, or alcohol-related liver problems among adult "unhealthy drinkers." In general, little-to-no evidence of SBI harm was found, though consequences of confidentiality breaches were not specifically studied.

Solberg et al. conducted a meta-analysis of primary care studies and evaluated the clinically preventable burden (CPB) and cost-effectiveness of SBI implementation, and compared these values across other recommended preventive services.[120] The CPB was calculated as the product of effectiveness times the alcohol-attributable fraction of both mortality and morbidity (measured in quality-adjusted life years or QALYs). Cost-effectiveness from both the societal perspective and the health system perspective was estimated. Randomized controlled trials (RCTs; $N = 10$) and cost-effectiveness studies ($N = 5$) were included. The mean percentage of SBI effectiveness for unhealthy drinking in primary care was found to be 17.4% (range: 9.8% to 30.1%), reflecting behavior change at 6 months to 2 years after intervention. The calculated CPB was 176,000 QALYs saved over the lifetime of a birth cohort of 4,000,000 people. From both the societal and health system perspectives, SBI was estimated to be cost effective and may be cost saving, assuming that the self-report outcomes were accurate. This meta-analysis suggested SBI as one of the highest-ranking preventive services among the 25 effective services evaluated using standardized methods. As current levels of delivery are the lowest of comparably ranked services, SBI deserves special attention by clinicians and care delivery systems for improvement.

A meta-analysis, conducted by the Cochrane Group led by Kaner et al., evaluated the effectiveness of SBI to reduce alcohol consumption among nontreatment-seeking patients in primary care settings and EDs.[121] The meta-analysis included 21 RCTs ($N = 7{,}286$ participants) and showed robust results that participants receiving SBI significantly reduced their self-reported alcohol consumption as compared to the control group (mean difference: 41 g of alcohol per week), yet with substantial heterogeneity of findings noted between trials. The percentage of adults reporting heavy drinking or binge drinking was also significantly reduced in the SBI as compared to the control group. When broken down by gender, the analysis noted the primary benefit of SBI in men rather than women. When compared with brief BIs, extended BIs were likely associated with a greater reduction in alcohol consumption and an increased reduction in alcohol use of 1.1 g/week for each extra minute of BI exposure ($p = 0.06$). Reduction of drinking was also observed in some of the control groups. The overall loss to follow-up rate was 27%, with the SBI group having a 3% higher attrition than the control groups. The results of this meta-analysis are broadly similar to previous findings in primary care samples and showed that SBI consistently produced modest reductions in self-reported alcohol consumption. The effect was clearer in men at one year of follow-up, but unproven in women. Of important note, given self-reported outcomes, there was no effect found of BI on biologic measures of alcohol consumption.

The systematic review by Saitz et al. evaluated efficacy of alcohol SBI in primary care, with the main focus on effects for those with very heavy alcohol use or DSM-IV–defined dependence. The review identified 16 RCTs ($N = 6{,}839$).[122] However, only two of these RCTs did not exclude participants based on very heavy drinking or dependence. One of these studies, in which 35% of 175 Mexican American patients (mostly men) had alcohol dependence, found no difference in drinks per week or severity scores between groups, and the other, in which 58% of 24 women with dependence, showed no difference in alcohol consumption between groups. Findings of this review highlight the absence of evidence and the need for further research on SBI efficacy in primary care patients with AUDs or very heavy drinking.

A systematic review and meta-analysis by Beich et al. evaluated the effectiveness of screening, as a part of an SBI program, for excessive alcohol use in general practice. The eight included studies used health questionnaires for screening, and the BIs included feedback, information, and advice.[90] Of 1,000 screened individuals, 90 screened positive and required further assessment, after which 25 qualified for BI. After 1 year, the pooled effect was 2.6 patients per 1,000 screened reporting that they drank less than the maximum recommended level. Although SBI can reduce self-reported excessive drinking, universal screening in general practice may be inefficient as a precursor to BIs targeting excessive alcohol use. This meta-analysis raised questions about the feasibility of screening in general practice for excessive alcohol use.

A systematic review by the Cochrane Group, led by Dinh-Zarr, assessed the effect of interventions intended to reduce alcohol consumption, or prevent injuries or their antecedents among "problem drinkers" in diverse settings.[91] Seventeen RCTs were included. Among those, seven evaluated BIs in the clinical setting. BIs were associated with a significant reduction of injury-related deaths (relative risk, RR = 0.65) and showed beneficial effects on diverse nonfatal injury-related outcomes. Overall, interventions, including BIs, for problem drinking appeared to reduce injuries and their antecedents. One should use caution in applying these results to SBI, however, since these were studies of BI, not universal screening and SBI in primary care settings.

INDIVIDUAL STUDIES OF SBI FOR UNHEALTHY ALCOHOL USE

Primary Care Settings

SBI is efficacious for unhealthy alcohol use (that has not yet developed into an AUD) and recommended in primary care settings. Implementation of SBI in primary care settings can allow for a better integration of medical care and SUD prevention and treatment. Such an integrated approach may benefit individuals with substance use-related medical conditions and be cost effective compared to a "treatment-as-usual model," in which primary care and SUD services are provided separately.[123]

Project TrEAT and Project Health are examples of the positive SBI trials in primary care. Project TrEAT was the first U.S. study to evaluate long-term efficacy and cost-benefit of SBI among 774 at-risk drinkers in primary care.[72] After two short BI sessions delivered by a clinician, each followed by a phone call, adults drinking at-risk amounts who received BI significantly decreased alcohol use, health resource utilization, and alcohol-related costs compared to controls. These effects were observed at 6 months and maintained during a 48-month follow-up. In Project Health, after a very short BI, delivered by a clinician as part of a routine primary care visit, participants significantly reduced self-reported drinking and were less likely to report return to at-risk drinking than controls at 6 and 12 months.[124,125]

Only one study evaluated efficacy of SBI over a period more than 4 years.[126] After up to three sessions of BI, delivered over a 6-month period, 554 adults with at-risk or harmful drinking in the BI group significantly reduced their self-reported drinking at 9 months compared to "no-treatment" controls. Although these between-group differences dissipated over a decade-long follow-up, at 10 years, both the BI and control groups tended to drink less by self-report than at baseline or at 9 months, which suggests "assessment effects" or a favorable natural history of unhealthy alcohol use.

Hilbink et al. conducted an RCT evaluating effects of a multifaceted BI in primary care aimed at the reduction of unhealthy drinking. Physician practices in the Netherlands were randomized to control condition (unhealthy drinkers were mailed the guidelines and information letters about unhealthy drinking) or the "improvement intervention." The intervention included the entire clinical practice team who received short training in SBI, thus facilitating changes on the organizational, and staff awareness and skill level, with emphasis on educating clinicians; people with unhealthy drinking in the BI practices received a personalized feedback letter with a suggestion to discuss drinking further with their clinician. Among 6,318 screened, 712 patients from 70 practices scored positive for unhealthy drinking (AUDIT score 8-19) without meeting criteria for the DSM-IV–based alcohol dependence. Over the course of 2 years, a sizable proportion (41.6%) of patients reduced their unhealthy drinking to a low-risk level; however, a significantly larger reduction was demonstrated in the control (47%) than in the intervention (35.5%) group. Certain patient characteristics (eg, older age, female sex, attitudes toward drinking), but not characteristics of the practices, were associated with drinking reduction. The authors drew conclusions that "the intervention has been counterproductive," and hypothesized that these unexpected results or, rather, lack of favorable results of the clinic-based BI may be related to the overall low level of engagement of the participating clinicians. At the very least, this study raised the possibility that SBI done poorly could yield subpar results.[127]

One study supports the low engagement of primary care clinicians by examining the levels of documentation as a proxy for communication about alcohol and drug screening.[128] Health educators in this study assessed patients for unhealthy alcohol consumption prior to patients seeing their primary care clinician. If warranted, health educators provided a BI to patients with a "positive screen." Health educators then completed a "provider education form" to convey these results but did not enter this information into the patient's electronic medical record. Of the 347 primary care patients who screened positive for unhealthy alcohol use, 97% (338/347) had risky substance use, and the remaining 3% (9/347) AUD. When examining medical records, only 58% of patients with identified substance use had documentation that matched the type of substance and rate of use. All patients with AUD had appropriate documentation, but only 64% of those with risky alcohol use did. In addition, documentation of the BI only existed for 25% of patients, although all patients were provided with some type of intervention. Such subpar documentation practices make it challenging for clinicians to properly follow-up with their patients about substance use, and introduces the risk of potential mishandling of risky situations that patients may be experiencing. It is impossible to test the efficacy of BIs in a real-world setting if clinicians are unwilling or unable to properly document their efforts.

Adolescents and Young Adults

Research on SBI efficacy for adolescent unhealthy drinking is limited, but its results are encouraging. Rates of adolescent alcohol use range from 5% among general ED admissions to nearly 50% among trauma admissions, and alcohol use by adolescents is associated with increases in severity of injury and cost of medical treatment.[104]

A 2013 review article examined 15 randomized controlled trials of SBI in adolescents aged 14 through 17 years. Among the included studies, one found that structured approach to screening produced higher rates of detection of unhealthy substance use than routine screening traditionally used by primary care physicians. Other studies highlighted the need to consider all youths, including in settings such as community outreach centers, as at risk for unhealthy substance use. Screening of adolescents must account for the context of the screening; it is important to remember that adolescents may not always tell the truth on self-report screening measures. In addition, research is limited on confirmatory measures, such as blood alcohol testing, due to the limits on the logistics, and cost of collecting data and extrapolating to long-term patterns of use. BIs for adolescents range from short conversations with a physician to lengthier and repeated exposures in a school setting. MI has repeatedly been found to be an effective tool for promoting change in adolescents with unhealthy alcohol use. Despite these positive findings, overall evidence on the effectiveness of SBI in adolescents is limited by the small number of studies, and heterogeneous nature of the participants and interventions used.

A systematic review by Yuma-Guerrero et al. focused on the efficacy of alcohol SBI in adolescents in acute care settings.[44] The review identified seven RCTs evaluating SBI effects on alcohol consumption and/or consequences among 3,309 individuals with at-risk alcohol use, aged 12 to 24 years, all patients in the EDs of the level I trauma centers. All but one study used MI-based interventions. These studies produced overall promising but inconsistent results. The authors concluded that the evidence is not sufficient at this point to provide an unambiguous support for the SBI efficacy for adolescent ED patients who engage in risky drinking. The Yuma-Guerrero et al.'s review included several RCTs conducted in the ED settings. The RCT by Monti et al. evaluated adolescents aged 18 to 19 years ($N = 94$) who either self-reported alcohol use or had a positive blood alcohol level. Although both the intervention and control groups reduced their drinking at 3 and 6 months, no significant differences between the groups were found in alcohol consumption.[129] Compared to controls, the intervention group was less likely to report negative consequences of drinking at 6 months ($p < 0.05$) though. Johnston et al.[130] examined effects of SBI among 12- to 20-year-old adolescents ($N = 631$) receiving ED care for injury. At 3- and 6-month follow-up assessments, both the intervention and the control groups reduced prevalence of risky behaviors, but there were no significant differences between the groups on alcohol-related outcomes (driving after drinking, riding with an impaired driver, or binge drinking). Spirito et al. evaluated outcomes of a single BI session in the ED setting among 13- to 17-year-old adolescents ($N = 152$) admitted for an alcohol-related injury.[131] Over 12 months, both intervention and control groups significantly reduced number of drinks per occasion; the groups did not differ on alcohol-related outcomes. However, the subgroup of adolescents with "problematic" alcohol use (almost 50% of the sample) reported significantly more reduced frequency of drinking and high-volume drinking if they received intervention ($p < 0.01$), indicating that BIs had some efficacy at least on self-reports, particularly for adolescents engaging in the riskiest drinking behavior. Maio et al. compared effects of an interactive computer program–based intervention versus standard of care among 14- to 18-year-old ED patients ($N = 655$). There were no statistically significant differences between the groups on main outcomes. Both groups showed a reduction in unhealthy alcohol use and "binge" drinking at 3 months, but these levels returned to baseline at 12 months. Interestingly, within the subgroups of adolescents, who reported either riding with an intoxicated driver or "drinking and driving" at baseline, those in the intervention group showed greater improvement in unhealthy alcohol use compared to controls.[132]

A meta-analytic review by Jensen et al. assessed effectiveness of MI-based BI for adolescent substance use.[50] Among 21 identified controlled trials of BIs, including 5,471 adolescents aged 12 to 23 years recruited primarily from the community settings, most addressed alcohol ($N = 12$) and cannabis ($N = 12$), then multiple substances ($N = 9$), tobacco ($N = 7$), and various nonprescribed drugs ($N = 6$). Meta-analysis revealed statistically homogeneous sample of effect sizes, with an overall small but significant mean posttreatment effect size of the MI interventions on self-reported outcomes that was retained over time. The MI interventions appeared effective across a variety of self-reported substance use behaviors, varying BI session lengths, and different settings, thus providing a strong support for the effectiveness of MI interventions for adolescent self-report of substance use behavior change.

A review by Tevyaw and Monti presented the use and efficacy of motivational enhancement and other brief interventions for substance use, particularly drinking, in adolescents and young adults.[79] This review found that positive results demonstrated in clinical trials using motivational enhancement interventions with adolescents and college students primarily stem from reductions in alcohol-related problems and, to a lesser extent, from reductions in drinking. Although most young people do mature out of hazardous drinking patterns, motivational enhancement-based interventions may help accelerate that maturation process in high-risk individuals. The review concluded that motivational enhancement-based BIs can decrease alcohol-related negative consequences, reduce alcohol use, and increase treatment engagement among adolescents and young adults. Grossberg et al. examined 226 primary care patients aged 18 to 30 years with at-risk drinking.[28] Young adults who received the BI significantly reduced self-reported drinking, had fewer ED visits, motor vehicle crashes and events, and fewer alcohol or drug use related arrests over the 4-year follow-up.[74] SBIs seem feasible and accepted by young adults.[129]

College Students

The 2019 National Survey on Drug Use and Health (NSDUH) reported that 53% of full-time college students drank alcohol in the past month, with 33% of them reporting episodic heavy drinking and 8% reporting heavy drinking.[133] Additionally, the 2019 NSDUH survey estimated that 104,000 of 18-year-old and 231,000 of 21-year-old college students met the DSM-5 criteria for AUD.[133] College students appear to be receptive to alcohol SBIs.[74,75] In addition, alcohol SBIs have been found effective for reducing unhealthy drinking among college students in general[74] as well as mandated college students,[134] and those admitted to the ED.[135-137]

While there are a limited number of SBI studies conducted in health care settings, one study, conducted by Campbell and Maisto, assessed the validity of the AUDIT-C for detecting at-risk alcohol use among college students utilizing the on-campus primary care clinic. This study found that the AUDIT-C scores correlated with alcohol consumption and negative drinking-related consequences, and can be used as a valid screen for detecting at-risk alcohol use among college students utilizing the on-campus primary care clinic.[138]

A robust set of studies evaluated BIs delivered outside of health care settings. In a study of 461 college freshmen, identified as engaging in at-risk drinking or a "normative control" group during their final high school year, the at-risk drinking students were randomized into the "no-treatment" control arm or the BI arm, with BI consisting of one to two BI sessions, delivered by psychologists, along with a personalized feedback letter.[74] Over 4 years of follow-up, although at-risk students in both the BI and the no-treatment control groups reported significantly reduced drinking and alcohol-related harms, the observed magnitude of changes favored the BI group; these long-term benefits occurred even in the context of maturational, natural trends, observed in the "normative control" group.[75]

A review of counselor-delivered BI by Larimer et al. summarized the results of 16 studies evaluating effects of alcohol SBIs in college settings and concluded that research provides strong support for the efficacy of SBIs.[76] The strongest evidence exists brief, personalized, individual, motivational feedback-based BIs. There also is emerging support for the efficacy of mailed or computerized feedback alone in producing at least short-term reductions in students' reported alcohol consumption. A systematic review by Zisserson et al. reviewed evidence for the utility of SBIs delivered without direct, real-time contact to college students engaging in at-risk drinking.[139] The results suggested that "no-contact" interventions (eg, printed materials or computer-based modalities) are feasible and may have efficacy in this population. The "no-contact" interventions may be helpful with broader dissemination of SBIs to college students.

A meta-analysis of SBI among college students, conducted by Fachini et al., included 18 trials that varied in sample sizes from 54 to 1,275 students, and found modest reduction in self-reported alcohol use and related harms over a 12-month period.[135]

In addition to the traditional counselor-delivered BI, there is an emerging literature with BI being conducted by primary care clinicians in student health centers. Fleming et al., in an RCT conducted across five student health centers in the United States and Canada, randomly assigned 986 students to usual care or BI delivered by 15 physicians and three nurse practitioners. They found significant modest reductions in self-reported alcohol use and related harm in the BI group compared to the usual care group.[140] Schaus and colleagues also reported positive findings from their study of BI delivered by physicians in the context of routine care in a student health clinic.[141]

A recent systematic review and meta-analysis by Samson et al. reviewed 73 studies and found that brief single-session alcohol BIs modestly reduced alcohol consumption among college students with unhealthy drinking. Additionally, BIs relying on motivational enhancement therapy or MI may be more effective.[142]

Another recent meta-analysis by Mun et al. of 15 RCTs involving a total of 6,801 college students revealed that alcohol BIs containing MI with personalized feedback and group MI reduced the risk of driving after heavy drinking among college students.[143]

When looking at specific alcohol BIs for college students, a meta-analysis by Henessy et al. of 52 trials assessed the effectiveness of different manualized BIs, such as the Brief Alcohol Screening Intervention for College Students (BASICS) (https://crimesolutions.ojp.gov/ratedprograms/138), the Electronic Checkup to Go (e-Chug) (https://www.echeckuptogo.com), and the Tertiary Health Research Intervention Via Email (THRIVE) (https://beacon.anu.edu.au/service/website/view/188/23#:~:text=Description%3A,information%20on%20available%20support%20services). The BASICS is delivered as two 50-minute counseling sessions, where MI is used to motivate and provide students with skills to change drinking behaviors. The e-Chug is a 15- to 30-minute online intervention, which consists of educational content, personal assessment (demographics, drinking behaviors, and consequences), and customized feedback about students' drinking. The THRIVE intervention is a 5-minute computer survey, which generates and delivers immediate, customized feedback on drinking behaviors, risks, as well as strategies and resources for reducing alcohol consumption. Findings from this study showed that several types of BIs appeared to be particularly effective. While all BIs examined showed some efficacy depending on the different measures of alcohol consumption, BASICS was consistently the most effective in reducing problematic alcohol use, yet resource intensive and possibly better suited for higher risk students, while THRIVE and e-Chug were found to be less resource intensive and, as such, potentially better suited for broader, universal prevention efforts.[144]

Older Adults

SBIs seem to be effective for older adults.[72] Project GOAL, conducted in parallel to Project TrEAT and based on similar methodology, showed that SBI can decrease self-reported alcohol use over a 2-year follow-up among primary care patients aged 65 years or older who engaged in unhealthy drinking.[145] The Florida BRITE (Brief Interventions and Treatment for Elders) project was created to provide and promote alcohol, tobacco, and drug SBI services for older adults aged 55 years or older, and was implemented at 75 health care and non–health care sites across 18 Florida counties.[146] The Florida Department of Children and Families visited each site and provided a 2-day staff training covering program competencies, such as prescreening, screening tools, MI, BI, and data entry. Following a positive substance use prescreen, the ASSIST tool was administered to determine substance use-related risk. Those with a moderate-to-higher risk based on the ASSIST score received BI, and individuals at highest risk received referral to treatment. Over the 5-year project (2006-2011), 85,001 individuals were screened for substance use, with 9.6% ($N = 8,165$) screening positive for moderate- to higher-risk substance use. A total of 5,035 individuals received BI. At the 6-month follow-up, significant reduction in substance use was noted, suggesting that SBI can be delivered in both health care and non–health care settings that serve people 65 years old or older.

STUDIES OF SBI FOR UNHEALTHY DRUG USE

In 2018, around 11.7% of the U.S. residents 12 years or older were identified as using illicit drugs, including cannabis and nonmedical prescription psychotherapeutics. Based on a systematic review of 99 studies, the USPSTF updated in 2020 its recommendations for screening for drug use in adolescents and adults. Additionally, the USPSTF found that pharmacotherapy and psychosocial interventions are effective at improving drug use outcomes.[147] Computerized interventions might be more effective for the use of some substances than others. Pregnant and postpartum persons have reported high acceptability of computer-based BIs.[94-97]

Brief interventions can be effective in reducing drug use outcomes among treatment seeking adults and those with less severe patterns of drug use. Chou et al. conducted a systematic review of psychosocial intervention trials for persons using substances (opioid, stimulant, cannabis, and polysubstance use). The included 52 trials used cognitive-behavioral or MI-based interventions, which showed effectiveness for increasing abstinence from drug use at 3- to 4-month follow-up (15 trials, RR = 1.60 [95% CI: 1.24, 2.13]; number needed to treat, NNT = 11) as well as at 6- to 12-month follow-up (14 trials; RR = 1.25 [95% CI: 1.11, 1.52]; NNT = 17). Additionally, the interventions included were associated with decreased number of drug-use days and drug use severity at the 3- to 4-month follow-up, but not at the 6- to 12-month follow-up. While the results support BI as effective in reducing drug use, most of the evidence was derived from trials conducted among treatment-seeking adults; therefore, their generalizability and applicability to SBI in primary care settings remains uncertain.[148]

Gelberg and colleagues found a reduction in reported days using individuals' self-identified "highest scoring drug" 3 months following BI relative to usual care.[98] Participants in this study were 334 adult primary care patients (171 intervention; 163 controls) with risky psychoactive drug use scores on the World Health Organization (WHO) Alcohol, Smoking, and Substance Involvement Screening Test (ASSIST). The BIs consisted of 3 to 4 minutes of clinician advice to quit/reduce drug use, reinforced by a video-based doctor message, a health education booklet, and up to two 20- to 30-minute follow-up telephone coaching sessions. Patients in the BI group reported using their "highest scoring drug" on 3.5 fewer days in the previous month relative to controls. Moreover, no compensatory increases in use of other substances were found. The results were not confirmed by biologic testing, and, surprisingly, the effects seemed to be strongest in a subgroup of patients engaged in more frequent drug use; if valid, these findings could be explained by having the BI delivered by the patient's own clinician, a video doctor, and a rather lengthy follow-up contact, the latter two components rarely appearing in typical SBI approaches.

Blow et al. conducted a RCT to examine the efficacy of drug BIs among adults presenting to the ED. The study included 780 ED patients (44% male) who completed the ASSIST tool and scored at least 4 points, and provided a urine sample for urine drug screen. These assessments were completed at baseline as well as at 3-, 6-, and 12-month follow-up. Initially, participants were randomized to (1) 30-minute computer BI, an interactive computer-delivered program guided by a virtual health counselor; (2) 30-minute therapist BI, delivered in person by a Master's-level therapist; or (3) enhanced usual care. After the 3-month assessment, participants were further randomized to either adapted motivational enhancement therapy booster or enhanced usual care booster to determine the effectiveness of booster BI sessions. The study results showed that, compared to the enhanced usual care, both the computer BI and the therapist BI reduced drug use at 6 and 12 months. Interestingly, the receipt of a booster session did not appear to offer added benefit.[149]

Krupski et al. conducted a prospective observation study of a statewide SBIRT program in Washington state known as WASBIRT. The program placed SUD clinicians in nine EDs across the state to carry out the SBIRT services, with the goal to investigate whether the SBIRT at an ED visit would lead to a better addiction treatment engagement. Study participants with elevated DAST-10 or AUDIT scores received a BI consisting of feedback about the screening tools and the individuals' scores, as well as exploration of the individuals' feeling about substance use, and provision of options for changing behaviors. A matched comparison group consisted of individuals who had a high likelihood of having an alcohol/drug use disorders based on their medical or arrest records, and were not screened for substance use as part of their visit in one of the nine participating EDs. The study included 2,493 individuals who received BI and 2,493 individuals in the matched comparison group. The authors found that those without prior addiction treatment who received BI were 1.90 (95% CI: 1.61, 2.23) times more likely than the comparison group to subsequently initiate addiction treatment following the SBIRT. The effect of BI was strongest 1 month after the BI; individuals in the BI group who did not have prior addiction treatment were 2.17 times more likely than the comparison group to engage in treatment at 1 month; this dropped to 1.64 times at 6 months after receiving the BI. Overall, these results suggest that that drug SBIRT delivered in the ED settings by highly-trained professionals could play an important role in helping patients engage in addiction treatment.[150]

Bertholet et al. conducted a RCT to determine the efficacy of BIs in those with lower-risk drug use versus no BI in the primary care setting. Individuals identified by ASSIST with drug specific scores of 2 to 3 were randomly assigned to the BI with brief negotiated interview (BNI, $N = 23$), BI with MI (MOTIV, $N = 19$), or no BI (control, $N = 19$). BNI consisted of a single 10 to 15 minute structured interview conducted by specially trained health educators discussing "pros and cons" of drug use and ways to change current behaviors. MOTIV consisted of a 30 to 45-minute session of MI about negative consequences of drug use-related health concerns, as well as providing opportunities for change. Cannabis was the most common drug used (70% of participants), followed by cocaine (15%), prescription opioid (10%), and 5% other substances, with average days of substance use of 3.4 days in the past 30 days at baseline. Follow up was conducted at 6 months and found that mean days of use was decreased in both the BNI and MOTIVE groups when compared to the control group. Although limited by a small sample size, BI in this study reduced substance use in those with less severe drug use in the primary care setting.[151]

Several earlier studies, such as those by Humeniuk et al.,[152] Saitz et al.,[101] Roy-Byrne et al.,[153] Woodruff et al.,[100] and Bogenschutz et al.,[103] did not show benefit of SBI for reducing unhealthy drug use.

Humeniuk et al.'s multinational study evaluated SBI's efficacy for illicit drug use (cannabis, cocaine, amphetamine-type stimulants, and opioids) among 731 primary care patients, aged 16 to 62 years, in four countries: Australia, Brazil, India, and the United States. Screening was conducted using the ASSIST questionnaire.[152] Enrolled participants were randomly assigned to receive usual care or a motivational BI, which took on average 13.8 minutes to deliver, and targeted the drug receiving the highest ASSIST score. At 3 months, those who received BI reported a reduction in total illicit substance involvement scores compared to controls; however, the differences were very small. Country-specific analyses indicated that profile of substance use changes varied by country. Compared to controls, the BI group reported improved (1) total substance use-related scores in Australia, Brazil, and India; (2) cannabis scores in Brazil and India; (3) stimulant scores in Brazil and Australia; and (4) opioid scores in India; in the United States, BI did not show efficacy for any substance.

Saitz and colleagues conducted a 3-group randomized trial involving 528 adult primary care patients with unhealthy drug use (ASSIST substance-specific scores of ≥4) to test the efficacy of two BIs, BNI and MOTIV, compared with no BI control.[101] The BNI was a 10- to 15-minute structured interview conducted by health educators; the MOTIV was a 30- to 45-minute BI based on MI, with a 20- to 30-minute booster conducted by master's level counselors. At baseline, 63% of participants reported cannabis as their main drug, followed by 19% reporting cocaine, and 17% reporting opioids. At 6 months, the mean adjusted number of days using the main drug was 12 for no BI group versus 11 for the BNI (incidence rate ratio [IRR], 0.97; 95% CI, 0.77-1.22) and 12 for the MOTIV (IRR, 1.05; 95% CI, 0.84-1.32) groups, without significant effects of BNI or MOTIV on other outcomes of interest, including drug use measures according to hair sample-based toxicology testing.

Roy-Byrne et al.'s RCT did not demonstrate efficacy of BI in the primary care setting in improving drug use-related outcomes compared with enhanced care.[153] Participants recruited from seven safety-net primary care clinics received a single BI involving MI, a handout and list of treatment/recovery resources, and an attempted 10-minute telephone booster within 2 weeks ($N = 435$), or enhanced care as usual, which included a handout and a list of treatment/recovery resources ($N = 433$). During the 12-month postintervention follow-up, no significant differences were found between the BI and enhanced usual care groups in self-reported drug use days, Addiction Severity Index-Lite drug use composite scores, ED and hospital admissions, arrests, mortality, or human immunodeficiency virus risk behaviors.

Woodruff and colleagues' RCT involving 700 ED patients also did not find a significant change in self-reported past 30-day abstinence at 6 months following a BI for illicit drug use relative to an attention-placebo control intervention.[100] Similarly, a multisite RCT by Bogenschutz et al. of 1,285 ED patients randomized to BI with telephone boosters (BI-B), screening, assessment, and referral to treatment (SAR), versus minimal screening only (MSO) found no significant differences at 3-, 6-, and 12-month follow-up in self-reported drug and alcohol use related outcomes or drug use based on hair sample toxicology.[103]

SBI: SPECIAL SETTINGS

Technology-Based SBI

There are many challenges to widespread implementation of SBI including time, training, and commitment. The COVID-19 pandemic added additional barriers to providing SBI through the shifting of health care resources toward helping fight the pandemic, stay at home orders, closures of health care facilities, travel restrictions, and infection control methods, among others.[154] The use of technology can help address these implementation challenges. The use of technological innovations, including electronic SBI (e-SBI), has been accelerated by and during the pandemic, providing the opportunity of delivering SBIs at lower cost, and more efficiently reaching those in need who may otherwise not have sought evaluation and/or treatment.

Substantial evidence exists regarding the use of technology-based (computerized, internet, text-messaging, or smartphone based) interventions in addressing unhealthy alcohol[85] and tobacco/nicotine use.[86] The e-SBI encompasses at minimum a screening process and personalized feedback BI, which have demonstrated benefits in raising awareness and reducing unhealthy alcohol use among college students.[155] Tansil et al.

conducted a systematic review on the effectiveness of brief e-SBI across different settings for excessive alcohol consumption and related harms, with e-SBI defined as at least screening and personalized feedback BI. Most of the included 31 studies reported that e-SBI reduced excessive alcohol consumption, with some of the studies noting a median reduction in binge drinking intensity (maximum number of drinks/binge episode) by 23.9% and frequency by 16.5%, sustained at 12 months. These findings suggested e-SBIs can be effective for reducing unhealthy alcohol use and may complement population-level strategies for reducing excessive drinking and related harms.[156] Although the implementation of e-SBI in primary care has been limited, this approach may be more feasible and acceptable than the traditional SBI models.[94]

While promising, the existing research on technology-based drug SBIs is still limited. Stand-alone, computer-and mobile text-messaging based tobacco e-SBI can be effective among college students.[157] Technology-based approaches for cannabis use have also been studied, confronting the barriers toward in-person SBI such as stigma associated with use.[158,159] According to a meta-analysis of 10 studies involving 4,125 participants, the frequency of cannabis use decreased following internet- and/or computer-based interventions in diverse target populations.[157] High attrition rates due to a lack of in-person guidance and accountability with a coach or therapist have been suggested as potential challenges to be considered when implementing drug e-SBIs.[160]

Other Provider/Setting-Based SBI

Although physician-driven SBI in clinical settings has documented efficacy, barriers to successful, wider implementation of SBI in real-life practice have shifted attention to the evaluation of the effects of SBI when delivered by other health care and other professionals across different settings.

Pharmacy-Based SBI

Pharmacist- and pharmacy staff-delivered SBI appears to be acceptable to consumers and feasible within the settings of retail pharmacy. Hattingh et al. recruited five pharmacies to receive training in alcohol SBI. To facilitate alcohol SBI among pharmacy customers who might be at increased risk for unhealthy alcohol use (eg, those requesting help with hang-over symptoms, heartburn, or sleep problems; filling prescriptions associated with certain chronic conditions or contraindicated with alcohol) were approached by pharmacist to participate. Fifty individuals, aged 25 to 55 years, were screened for unhealthy alcohol use with the AUDIT tool. Their AUDIT scores ranged from 0 to 39 points, with 11 individuals categorized as "hazardous" (AUDIT score 8-15), four as "harmful" (AUDIT score 16-19), and eight as "probably dependent" (AUDIT score 20+) alcohol use. Individuals with AUDIT scores 8 to 19 received BI consisting of discussion of their score and MI to facilitate behavioral change. Those with AUDIT scores of 20+ received the BI along with recommendations to seek help from their clinician regarding their alcohol consumption. Eleven of twenty-three individuals (47.8%) with a positive screen for unhealthy drinking agreed to follow up at 3 months; at that time, 54.4% had their AUDIT score in "low-risk," 9.1% had their score in "hazardous," and 36.4% had their score in "probably dependent" drinking categories. Those in the low-risk category at baseline remained low-risk, and three of the five individuals with the highest AUDIT scores had reduced their risk level at 3 months.[161]

Shonesy et al. recruited adults to determine the feasibility of performing SBI, using the NIDA Quick Screen, NIDA Modified ASSIST, and AUDIT, in a retail pharmacy setting by pharmacy staff. Participants were drawn from a convenience sample of adults who presented to the pharmacy and agreed to participate in the study. Among 24 study participants who were screened, 20.8% were at low to moderate risk for SUD, 16.7% screened 4 or more on AUDIT-C, and 37.5% were using one or more tobacco product. Furthermore, 50% of subjects required BI consisting of education about substance use. Overall, although more research is needed before solid conclusions can be drawn, the existing studies suggest feasibility, acceptability and effectiveness of SBIs in pharmacy settings.[162]

Nursing-Based SBI

In a study by Bachhuber et al., nursing staff delivered SBI for unhealthy drinking among adult primary care patients of federally qualified health centers in Bronx, NY. Over the span of one year, 9,119 patients were seen at the clinic and 46.5% of them were screened for unhealthy alcohol use using AUDIT-C. Of those screened, 255 (5.3%) screened positive, and 122 received a BI, suggesting that integrating SBI into routine primary care with the assistance of nursing staff can help improve SBI implementation in primary care.[163]

Vipond and Mennengaconducted a systematic review of literature from 2010 to 2018 to evaluate the feasibility (5 studies) and effectiveness (4 studies) of alcohol SBI when delivered by nurses in the ED settings. This review indicated that SBI delivered by nurses in the ED is feasible and can be effective for reducing drinking and related outcomes, such as lower future risk assessment screening scores, and decreased number of maximum drinks per single occasion, and number of drinking days per week. More research is needed to confirm these results due to the small sample sizes of the studies included in the review.[164]

Non-physician Provider and Medical Assistant-Based SBI

Mertens et al. conducted an implementation RCT, called ADVISe or Alcohol Drinking as a Vital Sign. In this study, 54 primary care clinics were randomly selected to one of three study arms: primary care physician (PCP), nonphysician provider/medical assistant (NPP/MA), or usual care (control). To facilitate system-wide SBI delivery, the NIAAA-recommended screening questions were built into the electronic health record and available to all study arms; additionally, clinicians/staff in the PCP and NPP/MA study arms received a 2-hour training in alcohol SBI at baseline as well as a 30-minute booster 6 months into the study. The average screening rates were highest in the NPP/MA arm (50.9%), followed by 9.2% in the PCP arm, and, finally, 3.5% in the usual care control arm. However, when looking at the rates of BI delivery, the PCP arm had higher rates (44.0%) versus 3.4% in the NPP/MA arm and 2.7% in the control arm. Within 12 months after the SBI training, screening increased in the NPP/MA arm, but remained stable in the PCP arm. Overall, these results suggest that while NPPs/MAs are well positioned to provide alcohol screening, primary care physicians and their teams can be more effective at implementing BIs to those with a positive screen.[165]

Dental-Based SBI

The efficacy of SBI in dental clinics is receiving increased attention.[166] In a cluster randomized trial study by Neff et al., 13 dental practices were randomized to either the intervention or control groups. In the intervention group practices, dental hygienists were trained to screen patients by phone prior to their scheduled visit and then deliver a brief 3 to 5 minute alcohol BI in person during the dental visit for those with a positive screen for unhealthy alcohol use. Among 1,039 individuals screened, 103 screened positive for unhealthy drinking. In that group, 50 individuals received the BI, consisting of information personalized to each individual's drinking pattern and impact, and 53 individuals in the control group did not receive the BI. By 6 months, those who received BI decreased their drinking by an average of eight drinks a week, compared to those in the control group who decreased their drinking by an average of four drinks per week. Despite the study limitations, these results point to the dental care setting as an additional potential venue for SBI for unhealthy alcohol use.

Peer-Based SBI

A study by Winn et al. evaluated the feasibility of SBI among moderate-risk youth when delivered by individuals with lived experience of addiction and recovery, leveraging the unique role and experience that recovery peers or mentors have. The SBI was implemented by 30 peers/mentors in three schools and three health clinics with 71 practitioners (physicians, nurses, social workers, counselors). During the study, 1,192 adolescents were screened for substance use using the CRAFFT tool. Of those screened, 139 (12%) met eligibility criteria (13-17 years old, had moderate risk for substance use based on the CRAFFT tool score), yet only 51 agreed to enroll in the study, and 28 completed the intervention. Five of the six sites were able to conduct Project Amp successfully, suggesting that the peer/mentor-led SBI was feasible but operational barriers related to recruitment, readiness, and sustainability presented challenges to implementation.[167]

Bernstein et al. conducted an RCT to assess the impact of BI delivered by peer-educators among those who used cocaine or heroin in the past 30 days and sought routine non-acute care at clinics associated with Boston Medical Center. Among 23,669 patients screened for cocaine or heroin use, 1,232 screened positive (DAST score ≥3) and were eligible for the study, and 1,175 enrolled into the study. Biochemical hair testing was used as an additional assessment of substance use among the study participants. Participants were then randomized to either an intervention group, which received motivational interview by peer-educators, active referral, the written handout (treatment resources), and a 10-day follow-up phone call; or a control group only receiving the handout. Follow-up was conducted at 6-months including biochemical hair testing. The results indicated that participants in the peer-delivered BI group, compared to those in the control group, were more likely to abstain from cocaine (22.3% versus 16.9%, respectively, p = 0.045) and heroin (40.2% versus 30.6%, respectively, p = 0.05). Nonsignificant results were observed and both cocaine and heroin (17.4% versus 12.8%, respectively, p = 0.052). Overall, these findings suggest that the involvement of peers may play an important role in expanding SBI delivery.[168]

SUMMARY

As commonly observed in medicine, the implementation and dissemination of novel clinical approaches rarely follows the pace of scientific advances.[169] Alcohol SBI in primary care settings shows efficacy for reducing self-reported use for people who engage in unhealthy drinking but do not have an AUD, findings consistent across decades of research. The challenge remains to confirm that it can affect any meaningful health outcomes consistently and retain effectiveness in real clinical practice. In general, this evidence has led to clear preventive recommendations because SBI is thought to have minimal harm and cost, patients should be informed about risky drinking regardless, and if the self-report findings translate to effects on significant consequences as some studies suggest, it could be a very effective public health prevention effort. Tobacco SBI is effective and has been implemented widely. Growing evidence supports drug SBI, however more research is needed to identify the patient population that is most likely to benefit from drug SBI as previous research focuses on treatment seeking adults. Additionally, the setting, in which the drug SBI takes place, may impact effectiveness; for example, in comparison with alcohol SBI where these services may be less effective in the hospital or trauma settings compared to primary care. It is also worth noting there are other reasons besides screening, to advise patients with the goal of reducing harms, and to identify and address substance use. For example, in order to diagnose any symptom (eg, sleep problem, high blood pressure, heartburn) or prescribe any medication (particularly those with an addictive potential, such as opioids), clinicians need to know if their patients are using substances.

The evidence for the use of SBI for adolescents in general clinical settings has strengthened over time, and currently, the major professional organizations recommend the SBI services for youth, starting as early as 9 years old. Identification and treatment of illicit drug use and prescription drug misuse in primary care and specialized clinical nonaddiction care settings is a relatively new area of work. Although evidence behind the utility of SBI for these risks and conditions is not as strong as for alcohol or tobacco, the growing problem of unhealthy drug use, especially misuse of prescription drugs, has led to the endorsement of SBI for drugs by multiple professional organizations, and, based on the growing evidence, by the USPSTF. More research is needed on the use of SBI for hospitalized patients, a sizable proportion of whom have severe AUD, and on the impact of SBI on morbidity and mortality. The use of SBI in psychiatric or co-occurring/settings remains an understudied area.

Since SBI is not simple or cheap to implement on a system level, it is critical to base practice on high-quality evidence and sound implementation science principles. The study of SBI in all clinical settings has become a high priority for federal funding initiatives. From clinical, evidence, and policy perspectives, much work still needs to be done. Implementation science, especially for SUD-related treatment, remains in its infancy, with a rather limited number of scientists working in this area. Electronic medical record systems offer an excellent opportunity to move SBI into point of care and routine clinical practice. Even with the foregoing areas that need further study, SBI has come a long way since the first large study reported by Wallace et al. in 1988 demonstrated evidence for alcohol SBI efficacy in the primary care settings.[170]

ACKNOWLEDGMENTS

The authors would like to acknowledge Dr Michael Fleming, MD, MPH and the late Dr Richard Saitz, MD, MPH, FACP, DFASAM for their contributions to the earlier versions of this chapter and the field of screening and brief interventions in addiction medicine.

REFERENCES

1. Substance Abuse and Mental Health Services Administration. *Key substance use and mental health indicators in the United States: Results from the 2020 National Survey on Drug Use and Health (HHS Publication No. PEP21-07-01-003, NSDUH Series H-56).* Center for Behavioral Health Statistics and Quality, SAMHSA; 2021.
2. Lieberman DZ, Massey SH, Collantes RS, Moore BB. Treatment preferences among problem drinkers in primary care. *Int J Psychiatry Med.* 2014;3:231-240.
3. Nelson LS, Juurlink DN, Perrone J. Addressing the opioid epidemic. *JAMA.* 2015;314:1453-1454.
4. Curry SJ, Krist AH, Owens DK, et al. Screening and behavioral counseling interventions to reduce unhealthy alcohol use in adolescents and adults: US Preventive Services Task Force Recommendation Statement. *JAMA.* 2018;320(18):1899-1909. doi:10.1001/jama.2018.16789
5. Krist AH, Davidson KW, Mangione CM, et al. Interventions for tobacco smoking cessation in adults, including pregnant persons: US Preventive Services Task Force Recommendation Statement. *JAMA.* 2021;325(3):265-279. doi:10.1001/jama.2020.25019
6. Krist AH, Davidson KW, Mangione CM, et al. Screening for unhealthy drug use: US Preventive Services Task Force Recommendation Statement. *JAMA.* 2020;323(22):2301-2309. doi:10.1001/jama.2020.8020
7. Agerwala SM, McCance-Katz EF. Integrating screening, brief intervention, and referral to treatment (SBIRT) into clinical practice settings: a brief review. *J Psychoactive Drugs.* 2012;44:307-317.
8. Gentilello LM. Alcohol and injury: American College of Surgeons Committee on trauma requirements for trauma center intervention. *J Trauma Acute Care Surg.* 2007;62:S44-S45.
9. National Quality Forum. *National Voluntary Consensus Standards for the Treatment of Substance Use Conditions: Evidence-Based Treatment Practices.* National Quality Forum; 2007. Accessed August 9, 2023. http://www.policyarchive.org/handle/10207/21566
10. Moyer VA. Screening and behavioral counseling interventions in primary care to reduce alcohol misuse: US preventive services task force recommendation statement. *Ann Intern Med.* 2013;159:210-218.
11. United States Department of Health and Human Services. NIDA. Screening for Drug Use in General Medical Settings: Resource Guide. Accessed August 9, 2023. https://nida.nih.gov/sites/default/files/pdf/screening_qr.pdf
12. Volkow ND, Baler RD, Compton WM, Weiss SR. Adverse health effects of marijuana use. *N Engl J Med.* 2014;370:2219-2227.
13. Fleming MF, Mundt MP, French MT, Manwell LB, Stauffacher EA, Barry KL. Brief physician advice for problem drinkers: long-term efficacy and benefit-cost analysis. *Alcohol Clin Exp Res.* 2002;26:36-43.
14. U.S. Department of Health and Human Services. *Medicare Learning Network: Screening and Behavioral Counseling Interventions in Primary Care to Reduce Alcohol Misuse in MLN Matters Information for Medicare Fee-for-Service Health Care Professionals* (Item No.:MM76332011). Accessed September 5, 2017. https://www.cms.gov/medicare-coverage-database/view/ncd.aspx?NCDId=347
15. U.S. Department of Health and Human Services. National Institute on Alcohol Abuse and Alcoholism: Helping Patients Who Drink Too Much: A Clinician's Guide. Accessed August 9, 2023. https://www.samhsa.gov/resource/ebp/helping-patients-who-drink-too-much-clinicians-guide
16. U.S. Department of Health and Human Services. National Institute on Alcohol Abuse and Alcoholism: Alcohol Screening and Brief Intervention for Youth: A Practitioner's Guide. National Institute on Alcohol Abuse and Alcoholism (NIAAA); 2011. Accessed August 9, 2023. https://www.niaaa.nih.gov/sites/default/files/publications/NIAAA_AlcoholScreening_Youth_Guide.pdf
17. Fletcher OV, Chen JA, van Draanen J, et al. Prevalence of social and economic stressors among transgender veterans with alcohol and other drug use disorders. *SSM Popul Health.* 2022;19:101153.
18. Bradley KA, Kivlahan DR. Bringing patient-centered care to patients with alcohol use disorders. *JAMA.* 2014;311(18):1861-1862.
19. Miller SC, Fiellin DA, Rosenthal RN, Saitz R; American Society of Addiction Medicine. *The ASAM Principles of Addiction Medicine.* 6th ed. Wolters Kluwer; 2019.
20. Gryczynski J, McNeely J, Wu LT, et al. Validation of the TAPS-1: a four-item screening tool to identify unhealthy substance use in primary care. *J Gen Intern Med.* 2017;32(9):990-996.
21. World Health Organization. The alcohol, smoking and substance involvement screening test (ASSIST): development, reliability, and feasibility. *Addiction.* 2002;97:1183-1194.

Disclaimer: The contents are those of the author(s) and do not necessarily represent the official views of, nor an endorsement, by HRSA, HHS, or the U.S. Government. For more information, please visit HRSA.gov.

22. Austin EJ, Briggs ES, Ferro L, et al. Integrating routine screening for opioid use disorder into primary care settings: experiences from a national cohort of clinics. *J Gen Intern Med.* 2023;38(2):332-340.
23. Kapoor A, Kraemer KL, Smith KJ, Roberts MS, Saitz R. Cost-effectiveness of screening for unhealthy alcohol use with % carbohydrate deficient transferrin: results from a literature-based decision analytic computer model. *Alcohol Clin Exp Res.* 2009;33:1440-1449.
24. Department of Health and Human Services. *Smoking Cessation. A Report of the Surgeon General.* U.S. Department of Health and Human Services, Centers for Disease Control and Prevention, National Center for Chronic Disease Prevention and Health Promotion, Office on Smoking and Health; 2020. Accessed July 15, 2020. https://www.cdc.gov/tobacco/sgr/2020-smoking-cessation/index.html
25. Cano Rodriguez Z, Chen Y, Siegel JH, Rousseau-Pierre T. Vaping: impact of improving screening questioning in adolescent population: a quality improvement initiative. *Pediatr Qual Saf.* 2021;6(1):e370. doi:10.1097/pq9.0000000000000370
26. Liu J, Halpern-Felsher B, Harris SK. Does tobacco screening in youth primary care identify youth vaping? *J Adolesc Health.* 2021;69(3):519-522. doi:10.1016/j.jadohealth.2021.01.017
27. Shahrir S, Crothers K, McGinnis KA, et al. Receipt and predictors of smoking cessation pharmacotherapy among veterans with and without HIV. *Prog Cardiovasc Dis.* 2020;63(2):118-124.
28. Grossberg PM, Brown DD, Fleming MF. Brief physician advice for high-risk drinking among young adults. *Ann Fam Med.* 2004;2:474-480.
29. Massey SH, Norris L, Lausin M, Nwaneri C, Lieberman DZ. Identifying harmful drinking using a single screening question in a psychiatric consultation-liaison population. *Psychosomatics.* 2011;52:362-366.
30. GBD 2016 Alcohol Collaborators. Alcohol use and burden for 195 countries and territories, 1990-2016: a systematic analysis for the Global Burden of Disease Study 2016. *Lancet.* 2018;392(10152):1015-1035.
31. Babor TF, Higgins-Biddle JC, Saunders JB, Monteiro MG. *World Health Organization. AUDIT: The Alcohol Use Disorders Identification Test: Guidelines for Use in Primary Health Care.* 2nd ed. World Health Organization; 2001.
32. Bradley KA, DeBenedetti AF, Volk RJ, Williams EC, Frank D, Kivlahan DR. AUDIT-C as a brief screen for alcohol misuse in primary care. *Alcohol Clin Exp Res.* 2007;31:1208-1217.
33. Bradley KA, Rubinsky AD, Lapham GT, et al. Predictive validity of clinical AUDIT-C alcohol screening scores and changes in scores for three objective alcohol-related outcomes in a Veterans Affairs population. *Addiction.* 2016;111:1975-1984.
34. Wahesh E, Lewis TF. Psychosocial correlates of AUDIT-C hazardous drinking risk status: implications for screening and brief intervention in college settings. *J Drug Educ.* 2015;45:17-36.
35. Kuitunen-Paul S, Roerecke M. Alcohol Use Disorders Identification Test (AUDIT) and mortality risk: a systematic review and meta-analysis. *J Epidemiol Community Health.* 2018;72(9):856-863. doi:10.1136/jech-2017-210078
36. Johnston LD, Miech RA, O'Malley PM, Bachman JG, Schulenberg JE, Patrick ME. *Monitoring the Future national survey results on drug use, 1975-2021: Overview, key findings on adolescent drug use.* Institute for Social Research, The University of Michigan; 2022.
37. Bryson CL, Au DH, Sun H, Williams EC, Kivlahan DR, Bradley KA. Alcohol screening scores and medication nonadherence. *Ann Intern Med.* 2008;149(11):795-804.
38. Harris AH, Bryson CL, Sun H, Blough D, Bradley KA. Alcohol screening scores predict risk of subsequent fractures. *Subst Use Misuse.* 2009;44(8):1055-1069.
39. Rubinsky AD, Dawson DA, Williams EC, Kivlahan DR, Bradley KA. AUDIT-C scores as a scaled marker of mean daily drinking, alcohol use disorder severity, and probability of alcohol dependence in a U.S. general population sample of drinkers. *Alcohol Clin Exp Res.* 2013;37(8):1380-1390.
40. Lange S, Shield K, Monteiro M, Rehm J. Facilitating screening and brief interventions in primary care: a systematic review and meta-analysis of the AUDIT as an indicator of alcohol use disorders. *Alcohol Clin Exp Res.* 2019;43(10):2028-2037. doi:10.1111/acer.14171
41. Hallgren KA, Matson TE, Oliver M, et al. Practical assessment of alcohol use disorder in routine primary care: performance of an alcohol symptom checklist. *J Gen Intern Med.* 2022;37(8):1885-1893.
42. Centers for Disease Control and Prevention. QuickStats: percentage of deaths from leading causes among teens aged 15–19 years—National Vital Statistics System (US); 2005. *MMWR Morb Mortal Wkly Rep.* 2008;57:1234.
43. Committee on Substance Abuse. Alcohol use by youth and adolescents: a pediatric concern. *Pediatrics.* 2010;125:1078-1087.
44. Yuma-Guerrero PJ, Lawson KA, Velasquez MM, von Sternberg K, Maxson T, Garcia N. Screening, brief intervention, and referral for alcohol use in adolescents: a systematic review. *Pediatrics.* 2012;130:115-122.
45. Levy SJ, Williams JF. Substance use screening, brief intervention, and referral to treatment. *Pediatrics.* 2016;138(1):e20161211.
46. Newton AS, Gokiert R, Mabood N, et al. Instruments to detect alcohol and other drug misuse in the emergency department: a systematic review. *Pediatrics.* 2010;128:1-10.
47. Kelly SM, O'Grady KE, Gryczynski J, Mitchell SG, Kirk A, Schwartz RP. The concurrent validity of the Problem Oriented Screening Instrument for Teenagers (POSIT) substance use/abuse subscale in adolescent patients in an urban federally qualified health center. *Subst Abus.* 2017;38(4):382-388. doi:10.1080/08897077.2017.1351413
48. Knight JR, Sherritt L, Harris SK, Gates EC, Chang G. Validity of brief alcohol screening tests among adolescents: a comparison of the AUDIT, POSIT, CAGE, and CRAFFT. *Alcohol Clin Exp Res.* 2003;27:67-73.
49. Vinson DC, Kruse RL, Seale JP. Simplifying alcohol assessment: two questions to identify alcohol use disorders. *Alcohol Clin Exp Res.* 2007;31:1392-1398.
50. Jensen CD, Cushing CC, Aylward BS, Craig JT, Sorell DM, Steele RG. Effectiveness of motivational interviewing interventions for adolescent substance use behavior change: a meta-analytic review. *J Consult Clin Psychol.* 2011;79:433-440.
51. Shaffer D, Fisher P, Dulcan MK, et al. The NIMH Diagnostic Interview Schedule for Children Version 2.3 (DISC-2.3): description, acceptability, prevalence rates, and performance in the MECA study. *J Am Acad Child Adolesc Psychiatry.* 1996;35:865-877.
52. Tripodi SJ, Bender K, Litschge C, Vaughn MG. Interventions for reducing adolescent alcohol abuse: a meta-analytic review. *Arch Pediatr Adolesc Med.* 2010;164:85-91.
53. Jonas DE, Garbutt JC, Amick HR, et al. Behavioral counseling after screening for alcohol misuse in primary care: a systematic review and meta-analysis for the U.S. Preventive Services Task Force. *Ann Intern Med.* 2012;157:645-654.
54. Glass JE, Hamilton AM, Powell BJ, Perron BE, Brown RT, Ilgen MA. Specialty substance use disorder services following brief alcohol intervention: a meta-analysis of randomized controlled trials. *Addiction.* 2015;110:1404-1415.
55. Denny CH, Hungerford DW, McKnight-Eily LR, et al. Self-reported prevalence of alcohol screening among U.S. adults. *Am J Prev Med.* 2016;50:380-383.
56. Johnson M, Jackson R, Guillaume L, Meier P, Goyder E. Barriers and facilitators to implementing screening and brief intervention for alcohol misuse: a systematic review of qualitative evidence. *J Public Health.* 2010;33:412-421.
57. D'Onofrio G, Degutis LC. Preventive care in the emergency department: screening and brief intervention for alcohol problems in the emergency department: a systematic review. *Acad Emerg Med.* 2002;9:627-638.
58. Blow FC, Barry KL, Walton MA, et al. The efficacy of two brief intervention strategies among injured, at-risk drinkers in the emergency department: impact of tailored messaging and brief advice. *J Stud Alcohol.* 2006;67:568-578.
59. Soderstrom CA, DiClemente CC, Dischinger PC, et al. A controlled trial of brief intervention versus brief advice for at-risk drinking trauma center patients. *J Trauma Acute Care Surg.* 2007;62:1102-1112.
60. Crawford MJ, Patton R, Touquet R, et al. Screening and referral for brief intervention of alcohol-misusing patients in an emergency

department: a pragmatic randomised controlled trial. *Lancet.* 2004;364:1334-1339.

61. Academic ED SBIRT Research Collaborative. The impact of screening, brief intervention, and referral for treatment on emergency department patients' alcohol use. *Ann Emerg Med.* 2007;50:699-710.
62. Schmidt CS, Schulte B, Seo HN, et al. Meta-analysis on the effectiveness of alcohol screening with brief interventions for patients in emergency care settings. *Addiction.* 2016;111:783-794.
63. Jouriles NJ, Chaney WC, Jones CA, et al., eds. *Advancing Emergency Care: Policy Compendium.* American College of Emergency Physicians; 2007. Accessed September 5, 2017. https://www.acep.org/siteassets/new-pdfs/policy-statements/policy-compendium.pdf
64. D'Onofrio G, Pantalon MV, Degutis LC, et al. Brief intervention for hazardous and harmful drinkers in the emergency department. *Ann Emerg Med.* 2008;51:742-750.
65. Daeppen JB, Gaume J, Bady P, et al. Brief alcohol intervention and alcohol assessment do not influence alcohol use in injured patients treated in the emergency department: a randomized controlled clinical trial. *Addiction.* 2007;102:1224-1233.
66. Drummond C, Deluca P, Coulton S, et al. The effectiveness of alcohol screening and brief intervention in emergency departments: a multicentre pragmatic cluster randomized controlled trial. *PLoS One.* 2014;9:e99463.
67. Duroy D, Boutron I, Baron G, Ravaud P, Estellat C, Lejoyeux M. Impact of a computer-assisted screening, Brief Intervention and Referral to Treatment on reducing alcohol consumption among patients with hazardous drinking disorder in hospital emergency departments. The randomized BREVALCO trial. *Drug Alcohol Depend.* 2016;165:236-244.
68. Saitz R, Palfai TP, Cheng DM, et al. Brief intervention for medical inpatients with unhealthy alcohol use: a randomized, controlled trial. *Ann Intern Med.* 2007;146:167-176.
69. McQueen J, Howe TE, Allan L, Mains D, Hardy V. Brief interventions for heavy alcohol users admitted to general hospital wards. *Cochrane Database Syst Rev.* 2011;8:CD005191.
70. Cuijpers P, Riper H, Lemmers L. The effects on mortality of brief interventions for problem drinking: a meta-analysis. *Addiction.* 2004;99(7):839-845. doi:10.1111/j.1360-0443.2004.00778.x
71. Emmen MJ, Schippers GM, Bleijenberg G, Wollersheim H. Effectiveness of opportunistic brief interventions for problem drinking in a general hospital setting: systematic review. *BMJ.* 2004;328:318.
72. Fleming MF, Manwell LB, Barry KL, Adams W, Stauffacher EA. Brief physician advice for alcohol problems in older adults: a randomized community-based trial. *J Fam Pract.* 1999;48:378-386.
73. Mundt MP, French MT, Roebuck MC, Manwell LB, Barry KL. Brief physician advice for problem drinking among older adults: an economic analysis of costs and benefits. *J Stud Alcohol.* 2005;66:389-394.
74. Marlatt GA, Baer JS, Kivlahan DR, et al. Screening and brief intervention for high-risk college student drinkers: results from a 2-year follow-up assessment. *J Consult Clin Psychol.* 1998;66:604.
75. Baer JS, Kivlahan DR, Blume AW, McKnight P, Marlatt GA. Brief intervention for heavy-drinking college students: 4-year follow-up and natural history. *Am J Public Health.* 2001;91:1310-1316.
76. Larimer ME, Cronce JM, Lee CM, Kilmer JR. Brief intervention in college settings. *Alcohol Res Health.* 2004;28:94.
77. Manwell LB, Fleming MF, Mundt MP, Stauffacher EA, Barry KL. Treatment of problem alcohol use in women of childbearing age: results of a brief intervention trial. *Alcohol Clin Exp Res.* 2000;24:1517-1524.
78. Floyd RL, Sobell M, Velasquez MM, et al. Preventing alcohol-exposed pregnancies: a randomized controlled trial. *Am J Prev Med.* 2007;32:1-10.
79. Tevyaw TOL, Monti PM. Motivational enhancement and other brief interventions for adolescent substance abuse: foundations, applications and evaluations. *Addiction.* 2004;99:63-75.
80. U.S. Preventative Services Task Force. *Recommendations for Primary Care Practice Published Recommendations. Alcohol Misuse: Screening and Behavioral Counseling Interventions in Primary Care.* USPSTF; 2016.
81. Vasilaki EI, Hosier SG, Cox WM. The efficacy of motivational interviewing as a brief intervention for excessive drinking: a meta-analytic review. *Alcohol Alcohol.* 2006;41:328-335.
82. Rooke S, Thorsteinsson E, Karpin A, Copeland J, Allsop D. Computer-delivered interventions for alcohol and tobacco use: a meta-analysis. *Addiction.* 2010;105:1381-1390.
83. White A, Kavanagh D, Stallman H, et al. Online alcohol interventions: a systematic review. *J Med Internet Res.* 2010;12:e62.
84. Cunningham JA, Khadjesari Z, Bewick BM, Riper H. Internet-based interventions for problem drinkers: from efficacy trials to implementation. *Drug Alcohol Rev.* 2010;29:617-622.
85. Lotfipour S, Howard J, Roumani S, et al. Increased detection of alcohol consumption and at-risk drinking with computerized alcohol screening. *J Emerg Med.* 2013;44:861-866.
86. Harris SK, Knight JR. Putting the screen in screening: technology-based alcohol screening and brief interventions in medical settings. *Alcohol Res.* 2014;36:63.
87. Kypri K, Vater T, Bowe SJ, et al. Web-based alcohol screening and brief intervention for university students: a randomized trial. *JAMA.* 2014;311:1218-1224.
88. Strohman AS, Braje SE, Alhassoon OM, Shuttleworth S, Van Slyke J, Gandy S. Randomized controlled trial of computerized alcohol intervention for college students: role of class level. *Am J Drug Alcohol Abuse.* 2016;42:15-24.
89. Saitz R, Alford DP, Bernstein J, Cheng DM, Samet J, Palfai T. Screening and brief intervention for unhealthy drug use in primary care settings: randomized clinical trials are needed. *J Addict Med.* 2010;4:123.
90. Beich A, Thorsen T, Rollnick S. Screening in brief intervention trials targeting excessive drinkers in general practice: systematic review and meta-analysis. *BMJ.* 2003;327:536-542.
91. Dinh-Zarr TB, Goss CW, Heitman E, Roberts IG, DiGuiseppi C. Interventions for preventing injuries in problem drinkers. *Cochrane Database Syst Rev.* 2004;3:CD001857.
92. Mullen J, Ryan SR, Mathias CW, Dougherty DM. Feasibility of a computer-assisted alcohol screening, brief intervention and referral to treatment program for DWI offenders. *Addict Sci Clin Pract.* 2015;10:25.
93. Bertholet N, Cunningham JA, Faouzi M, et al. Internet-based brief intervention for young men with unhealthy alcohol use: a randomized controlled trial in a general population sample. *Addiction.* 2015;110:1735-1743.
94. Nayak MB, Korcha RA, Kaskustas LA, Avalos LA. Feasibility and acceptability of a novel, computerized screening and brief intervention (SBI) for alcohol and sweetened beverage use in pregnancy. *BMC Pregnancy Childbirth.* 2014;14:379.
95. Ondersma SJ, Beatty JR, Svikis DS, et al. Computer-delivered screening and brief intervention for alcohol use in pregnancy: a pilot randomized trial. *Alcohol Clin Exp Res.* 2015;39:1219-1226.
96. Ondersma SJ, Chase SK, Svikis DS, Schuster CR. Computer-based brief motivational intervention for perinatal drug use. *J Subst Abuse Treat.* 2005;28:305-312.
97. Ondersma SJ, Svikis DS, Schuster CR. Computer-based brief intervention: a randomized trial with postpartum women. *Am J Prev Med.* 2007;32:231-238.
98. Gelberg L, Andersen RM, Afifi AA, et al. Project QUIT (Quit Using Drugs Intervention Trial): a randomized controlled trial of a primary care-based multi-component brief intervention to reduce risky drug use. *Addiction.* 2015;110:1777-1790.
99. Gryczynski J, Mitchell SG, Gonzales A, et al. A randomized trial of computerized vs. in-person brief intervention for illicit drug use in primary care: outcomes through 12 months. *J Subst Abuse Treat.* 2015;50:3-10.
100. Woodruff SI, Clapp JD, Eisenberg K, et al. Randomized clinical trial of the effects of screening and brief intervention for illicit drug use: the life shift/shift gears study. *Addict Sci Clin Pract.* 2014;9:8.
101. Saitz R, Palfai TP, Cheng DM, et al. Screening and brief intervention for drug use in primary care: the ASPIRE randomized clinical trial. *JAMA.* 2014;312:502-513.
102. Bonar EE, Walton MA, Cunningham RM, et al. Computer-enhanced interventions for drug use and HIV risk in the emergency room: preliminary results on psychological precursors of behavior change. *J Subst Abuse Treat.* 2014;46:5-14.

103. Bogenschutz MP, Donovan DM, Mandler RN, et al. Brief intervention for patients with problematic drug use presenting in emergency departments: a randomized clinical trial. *JAMA Intern Med.* 2014;174:1736-1745.
104. Berg CJ, Stratton E, Schauer GL, et al. Perceived harm, addictiveness, and social acceptability of tobacco products and marijuana among young adults: marijuana, hookah, and electronic cigarettes win. *Subst Use Misuse.* 2015;50:79-89.
105. Agency for Healthcare Research and Quality. National Healthcare Quality and Disparities Report: Introduction and Methods. Publication No. 20(21)-0045-EF. AHRQ; 2020.
106. Rudd RA, Aleshire N, Zibbell JE, Matthew GR. Increases in drug and opioid overdose deaths—United States, 2000–2014. *Am J Transplant.* 2016;16:1323-1327.
107. Centers for Disease Control and Prevention, National Center for Health Statistics. Multiple Cause of Death 1999-2020. CDC WONDER Online Database. Accessed August 9, 2023. https://www.cdc.gov/nchs/data/databriefs/db428.pdf
108. Hedegaard H, Miniño AM, Spencer MR, Warner M. *Drug Overdose Deaths in the United States, 1999–2020. NCHS Data Brief, no 428.* National Center for Health Statistics; 2021. doi:10.15620/cdc:112340
109. Ahmad FB, Cisewski JA, Rossen LM, Sutton P. *Provisional Drug Overdose Death Counts.* National Center for Health Statistics; 2022.
110. National Center for Injury Prevention and Control. *Understanding the Opioid Overdose Epidemic.* Centers for Disease Control and Prevention; 2022. Accessed August 9, 2023. https://stacks.cdc.gov/view/cdc/119116
111. Turk DC, Swanson KS, Gatchel RJ. Predicting opioid misuse by chronic pain patients: a systematic review and literature synthesis. *Clin J Pain.* 2008;24:497-508.
112. Butler SF, Fernandez K, Benoit C, Budman SH, Jamison RN. Validation of the revised Screener and Opioid Assessment for Patients with Pain (SOAPP-R). *J Pain.* 2008;9:360-372.
113. Webster, L. R., & Webster, R. M. (2005). Predicting aberrant behaviors in opioid-treated patients: preliminary validation of the Opioid Risk Tool. *Pain Med.* 2005;6(6):432-442.
114. D'Onofrio G, O'Connor PG, Pantalon MV, et al. Emergency department-initiated buprenorphine/naloxone treatment for opioid dependence: a randomized clinical trial. *JAMA.* 2015;313(16):1636-1644. doi:10.1001/jama.2015.3474
115. Gugelmann HM, Perrone J. Can prescription drug monitoring programs help limit opioid abuse? *JAMA.* 2011;306:2258-2259.
116. Weiner SG, Griggs CA, Mitchell PM, et al. Clinician impression versus prescription drug monitoring program criteria in the assessment of drug-seeking behavior in the emergency department. *Ann Emerg Med.* 2013;62:281-289.
117. Perrone J, Nelson LS. Medication reconciliation for controlled substances—an "ideal" prescription-drug monitoring program. *N Engl J Med.* 2012;366:2341-2343.
118. O'Connor EA, Perdue LA, Senger CA, et al. Screening and behavioral counseling interventions to reduce unhealthy alcohol use in adolescents and adults: updated evidence report and systematic review for the US Preventive Services Task Force. *JAMA.* 2018;320(18):1910-1928. doi:10.1001/jama.2018.12086
119. EFS K, Beyer FR, Muirhead C, et al. Effectiveness of brief alcohol interventions in primary care populations. *Cochrane Database Syst Rev.* 2018;2(2):CD004148. doi:10.1002/14651858.CD004148.pub4
120. Solberg LI, Maciosek MV, Edwards NM. Primary care intervention to reduce alcohol misuse: ranking its health impact and cost effectiveness. *Am J Prev Med.* 2008;34:143-152.
121. Kaner EF, Dickinson HO, Beyer FR, et al. Effectiveness of brief alcohol interventions in primary care populations. *Cochrane Database Syst Rev.* 2007;2:CD004148.
122. Saitz R. Alcohol screening and brief intervention in primary care: absence of evidence for efficacy in people with dependence or very heavy drinking. *Drug Alcohol Rev.* 2010;29:631-640.
123. Weisner C, Mertens J, Parthasarathy S, Moore C, Lu Y. Integrating primary medical care with addiction treatment: a randomized controlled trial. *JAMA.* 2001;286:1715-1723.
124. Okene J, Adams A, Hurley T, Wheeler E, Hebert J. Brief physician-and nurse practitioner-delivered counseling for high-risk drinkers. *Arch Intern Med.* 1999;159:2198-2205.
125. Reiff-Hekking S, Ockene JK, Hurley TG, Reed GW. Brief physician and nurse practitioner–delivered counseling for high-risk drinking. *J Gen Intern Med.* 2005;20:7-13.
126. Wutzke SE, Conigrave KM, Saunders JB, Hall WD. The long-term effectiveness of brief interventions for unsafe alcohol consumption: a 10-year follow-up. *Addiction.* 2002;97:665-675.
127. Hilbink M, Voerman G, van Beurden I, Penninx B, Laurant M. A randomized controlled trial of a tailored primary care program to reverse excessive alcohol consumption. *J Am Board Fam Med.* 2012;25:712-722.
128. Kim TW, Saitz R, Kretsch N, et al. Screening for unhealthy alcohol and other drug use by health educators: do primary care clinicians document screening results? *J Addict Med.* 2013;7:204-209.
129. Monti PM, Tevyaw T, Borsari B. Drinking among young adults. Screening, brief intervention, and outcome. *Alcohol Res Health.* 2005;28:236-244.
130. Johnston BD, Rivara FP, Droesch RM, Dunn C, Copass MK. Behavior change counseling in the emergency department to reduce injury risk: a randomized, controlled trial. *Pediatrics.* 2002;110(2 Pt 1):267-274.
131. Spirito A, Monti PM, Barnett NP, et al. A randomized clinical trial of a brief motivational intervention for alcohol-positive adolescents treated in an emergency department. *J Pediatr.* 2004;145:396-402.
132. Maio RF, Shope JT, Blow FC, et al. A randomized controlled trial of an emergency department–based interactive computer program to prevent alcohol misuse among injured adolescents. *Ann Emerg Med.* 2005;45:420-429.
133. Substance Abuse and Mental Health Services Administration. *Key substance use and mental health indicators in the United States: Results from the 2019 National Survey on Drug Use and Health (HHS Publication No. PEP20-07-01-001, NSDUH Series H-55).* Center for Behavioral Health Statistics and Quality, SAMHSA; 2020.
134. Doumas DM, Workman CR, Navarro A, Smith D. Evaluation of web-based and counselor-delivered feedback interventions for mandated college students. *J Addict Offend Counsel.* 2011;32:16-28.
135. Fachini A, Aliane PP, Martinez EZ, Furtado EF. Efficacy of brief alcohol screening intervention for college students (BASICS): a meta-analysis of randomized controlled trials. *Subst Abuse Treat Prev Policy.* 2012;7:40.
136. Helmkamp JC, Hungerford DW, Williams JM, et al. Screening and brief intervention for alcohol problems among college students treated in a university hospital emergency department. *J Am Coll Health.* 2003;52:7-16.
137. Hungerford DW, Williams JM, Furbee PM, et al. Feasibility of screening and intervention for alcohol problems among young adults in the ED. *Am J Emerg Med.* 2003;21:14-22.
138. Campbell CE, Maisto SA. Validity of the AUDIT-C screen for at-risk drinking among students utilizing university primary care. *J Am Coll Health.* 2018;66(8):774-782. doi:10.1080/07448481.2018.1453514
139. Zisserson RN, Palfai TP, Saitz R. "No-contact" interventions for unhealthy college drinking: efficacy of alternatives to person-delivered intervention approaches. *Subst Abuse.* 2007;28:119-131.
140. Fleming MF, Balousek SL, Grossberg PM, et al. Brief physician advice for heavy drinking college students: a randomized controlled trial in college health clinics. *J Stud Alcohol Drugs.* 2010;71:23-31.
141. Schaus JF, Sole ML, McCoy TP, Mullett N, O'Brien MC. Alcohol screening and brief intervention in a college student health center: a randomized controlled trial. *J Stud Alcohol Drugs Suppl.* 2009;16:131-142.
142. Samson JE, Tanner-Smith EE. Single-session alcohol interventions for heavy drinking college students: a systematic review and meta-analysis. *J Stud Alcohol Drugs.* 2015;76(4):530-543. doi:10.15288/jsad.2015.76.530
143. Mun EY, Li X, Lineberry S, et al. Do brief alcohol interventions reduce driving after drinking among college students? A two-step meta-analysis of individual participant data. *Alcohol Alcohol.* 2022;57(1):125-135. doi:10.1093/alcalc/agaa146
144. Hennessy EA, Tanner-Smith EE, Mavridis D, Grant SP. Comparative effectiveness of brief alcohol interventions for college students:

results from a network meta-analysis. *Prev Sci.* 2019;20(5):715-740. doi:10.1007/s11121-018-0960-z

145. Sorocco KH, Ferrell SW. Alcohol use among older adults. *J Gen Psychol.* 2006;133:453-467.
146. Schonfeld L, Hazlett RW, Hedgecock DK, Duchene DM, Burns LV, Gum AM. Screening, brief intervention, and referral to treatment for older adults with substance misuse. *Am J Public Health.* 2015;105(1):205-211. doi:10.2105/AJPH.2013.301859
147. Patnode CD, Perdue LA, Rushkin M, et al. Screening for unhealthy drug use: updated evidence report and systematic review for the US Preventive Services Task Force. *JAMA.* 2020;323(22):2310-2328. doi:10.1001/jama.2019.21381
148. Chou R, Dana T, Blazina I, et al. *Interventions for unhealthy drug use—supplemental report: a systematic review for the U.S. Preventive Services Task Force. Evidence Synthesis, No. 187.* Agency for Healthcare Research and Quality; 2020. Accessed August 9, 2023. https://www.ncbi.nlm.nih.gov/books/NBK558205/
149. Blow FC, Walton MA, Bohnert ASB, et al. A randomized controlled trial of brief interventions to reduce drug use among adults in a low-income urban emergency department: the HealthiER You study. *Addiction.* 2017;112(8):1395-1405. doi:10.1111/add.13773
150. Krupski A, Sears JM, Joesch JM, et al. Impact of brief interventions and brief treatment on admissions to chemical dependency treatment. *Drug Alcohol Depend.* 2010;110(1-2):126-136.
151. Bertholet N, Meli S, Palfai TP, et al. Screening and brief intervention for lower-risk drug use in primary care: a pilot randomized trial. *Drug Alcohol Depend.* 2020;213:108001.
152. Humeniuk R, Ali R, Babor T, et al. A randomized controlled trial of a brief intervention for illicit drugs linked to the Alcohol, Smoking and Substance Involvement Screening Test (ASSIST) in clients recruited from primary health-care settings in four countries. *Addiction.* 2012;107:957-966.
153. Roy-Byrne P, Bumgardner K, Krupski A, et al. Brief intervention for problem drug use in safety-net primary care settings: a randomized clinical trial. *JAMA.* 2014;312:492-501.
154. Ghosh A, Sharma K. Screening and brief intervention for substance use disorders in times of COVID-19: potential opportunities, adaptations, and challenges. *Am J Drug Alcohol Abuse.* 2021;47(2):154-159. doi:10.1080/00952990.2020.1865996
155. Ganz T, Braun M, Laging M, Schermelleh-Engel K, Michalak J, Heidenreich T. Effects of a stand-alone web-based electronic screening and brief intervention targeting alcohol use in university students of legal drinking age: a randomized controlled trial. *Addict Behav.* 2018;77:81-88. doi:10.1016/j.addbeh.2017.09.017
156. Tansil KA, Esser MB, Sandhu P, et al. Alcohol electronic screening and brief intervention: a Community Guide systematic review. *Am J Prev Med.* 2016;51:801-811.
157. Crocamo C, Carretta D, Ferri M, Dias S, Bartoli F, Carrá G. Web and text-based interventions for smoking cessation: meta-analysis and meta-regression. *Drugs Educ Prev Policy.* 2018;25:207-216.
158. Lee CM, Neighbors C, Kilmer JR, Larimer ME. A brief, web-based personalized feedback selective intervention for college student marijuana use: a randomized clinical trial. *Psychol Addict Behav.* 2010; 24:265.
159. Tait RJ, Spijkerman R, Riper H. Internet and computer based interventions for cannabis use: a meta-analysis. *Drug Alcohol Depend.* 2013;133:295-304.
160. MIA O, Blankers M, van Laar MW, Goudriaan AE. ICan, an Internet-based intervention to reduce cannabis use: study protocol for a randomized controlled trial. *Trials.* 2021;22(1):28. doi:10.1186/s13063-020-04962-3
161. Hattingh HL, Hallett J, Tait RJ. Making the invisible visible' through alcohol screening and brief intervention in community pharmacies: an Australian feasibility study. *BMC Public Health.* 2016;16(1):1141. doi:10.1186/s12889-016-3805-3
162. Shonesy BC, Williams D, Simmons D, Dorval E, Gitlow S, Gustin RM. Screening, brief intervention, and referral to treatment in a retail pharmacy setting: the pharmacist's role in identifying and addressing risk of substance use disorder. *J Addict Med.* 2019;13(5):403-407. doi:10.1097/ADM.0000000000000525
163. Bachhuber MA, O'Grady MA, Chung H, et al. Delivery of screening and brief intervention for unhealthy alcohol use in an urban academic Federally Qualified Health Center. *Addict Sci Clin Pract.* 2017;12(1):33. doi:10.1186/s13722-017-0100-2
164. Vipond J, Mennenga HA. Screening, brief intervention, and referral to treatment by emergency nurses: a review of the literature. *J Emerg Nurs.* 2019;45(2):178-184. doi:10.1016/j.jen.2018.10.004
165. Mertens JR, Chi FW, Weisner CM, et al. Physician versus non-physician delivery of alcohol screening, brief intervention and referral to treatment in adult primary care: the ADVISe cluster randomized controlled implementation trial. *Addict Sci Clin Pract.* 2015;10(1):26. doi:10.1186/s13722-015-0047-0
166. Neff JA, Kelley ML, Walters ST, et al. Effectiveness of a Screening and Brief Intervention protocol for heavy drinkers in dental practice: a cluster-randomized trial. *J Health Psychol.* 2015;20(12):1534-1548. doi:10.1177/1359105313516660
167. Winn LAP W, Paquette KL, LRW D, Wilkey CM, Ferreira KN. Enhancing adolescent SBIRT with a peer-delivered intervention: an implementation study. *J Subst Abuse Treat.* 2019;103:14-22. doi:10.1016/j.jsat.2019.05.009
168. Bernstein J, Bernstein E, Tassiopoulos K, Heeren T, Levenson S, Hingson R. Brief motivational intervention at a clinic visit reduces cocaine and heroin use. *Drug Alcohol Depend.* 2005;77:49-59.
169. Tabak RG, Padek MM, Kerner JF, et al. Dissemination and implementation science training needs: insights from practitioners and researchers. *Am J Prev Med.* 2017;52:S322-S329.
170. Wallace P, Cutler S, Haines A. Randomised controlled trial of general practitioner intervention in patients with excessive alcohol consumption. *BMJ.* 1988;297:663-668.

Sidebar 1

Screening and Brief Intervention in Pregnancy

Nicolas Bertholet

SUBSTANCE USE AND PREGNANCY

Introduction

Alcohol

Alcohol can have a harmful effect on the fetus, can be responsible for lifelong consequences such as the fetal alcohol syndrome (FAS; see Chapter 98 "Substance Use During Pregnancy" for additional information), and is completely preventable (by not drinking), making screening an important clinical priority.[1-3] Alcohol is teratogenic and, because of the absence of a developed blood filtration system, the fetus is unprotected from alcohol. In addition to FAS, alcohol can have detrimental effects on child development, with developmental problems such as moderate intellectual and behavioral deficits associated with even low levels of alcohol exposure (including at levels less than daily).[4] These "fetal alcohol effects" are similar to FAS but less severe and much more common.[5-7] Alcohol exposure during the first trimester of pregnancy is associated with low birth weight, decreased birth length and head circumference, minor physical abnormalities, and alcohol-related neurodevelopmental disorders.[8] Second- and third-trimester exposure can lead to developmental delay.[5] Though minimal alcohol consumption (eg, one drink every 10 days or less) might be very low risk during pregnancy, no definitive threshold level of safe alcohol consumption has been identified, mostly because of differences in fetal vulnerability to the toxic effects of alcohol.[9] Research suggests a linear association between prenatal alcohol exposure and birth defects and growth deficiencies, without evidence of a threshold.[10-14] Effective prevention of alcohol use by pregnant persons is an important public health measure with direct impact on infant outcomes.

Other Drugs

Drug use can also be associated with medical complications for women and people with other gender identities who are pregnant (eg, placental abruption, chorioamnionitis, placental insufficiency, spontaneous abortion, maternal hypertension, vasoconstriction, postpartum hemorrhage, and preeclampsia).[15] In addition, drug use can have negative impacts on the fetus, especially when combined with alcohol (see Chapter 98).[16] Rates of unhealthy prescription drug use in pregnancy increased in the early 2000s, and the incidence of neonatal abstinence syndrome increased threefold between 2000 and 2009.[17] Increasing prevalence of cannabis use has also made screening and intervention for perinatal drug use important, as cannabis can have negative effects on fetal outcomes (eg, impaired fetal growth).[18,19] Increasing rates of opioid use in pregnancy and prevalence of neonatal abstinence or neonatal opioid withdrawal syndrome emphasize the importance of ensuring access to effective and nonpunitive screening, diagnosis, and treatment initiation is available for pregnant people.[20,21] Opioid agonist treatment (ie, prescription of an opioid agonist such as methadone or partial agonist such as buprenorphine to prevent withdrawal, reduce cravings, reduce harms and provide opioid blockade) is the first-line indicated treatment for pregnant persons with an opioid use disorder.[22]

SCREENING

Universal screening with a validated set of questions for substance use is currently recommended by numerous professional organizations including the American College of Obstetricians and Gynecologists (ACOG), the American Academy of Pediatrics, the American Medical Association, and the Centers for Disease Control. Screening and brief interventions for unhealthy alcohol use are recommended by the U.S. Preventive Services Task Force (USPSTF),[23] and, for drug use, USPSTF recommends screening in "settings and populations for which services for accurate diagnosis, effective treatment, and appropriate care can be offered or referred."[24] The World Health Organization also recommends universal screening for alcohol and other drug use during antenatal visits. In 2008, the Committee on Ethics of the ACOG, based on an ethical rationale, recommends universal screening and brief intervention for alcohol and illicit drug use.[25] Systematic screening and brief intervention for alcohol and drugs is also recommended by Wright et al.[26] Nonetheless, screening for substance use other than alcohol has been less studied among pregnant persons.[27,28] Toxicology testing is not recommended for screening.

Screening for Unhealthy Alcohol Use

The goal of screening is to identify women and people with other gender identities who are pregnant or considering/planning pregnancy that are using any alcohol, and to advise them to abstain (or remain abstinent). In the early stages of pregnancy, before pregnancy recognition, alcohol consumption is commonly reported.[29] In addition, alcohol use and specifically heavy episodic drinking (defined by the World Health Organization as drinking 60 or more grams of ethanol during a single occasion) are associated with higher rates of unintended pregnancies.[30] The evaluation of prenatal alcohol use is complex as many pregnant persons will reduce their alcohol use as soon as they are aware of their pregnancy.[31] Assessing alcohol use during the pregnancy will therefore not be an accurate evaluation of what the alcohol consumption was at the time of conception. Day et al. have demonstrated that asking about alcohol consumption before pregnancy was a more accurate measure of drinking during the first trimester.[32] Even though many people will stop drinking during pregnancy, a significant proportion will continue to drink (from low amounts to heavy drinking episodes).[29] Nonetheless, pregnancy is a powerful motivational factor in stopping using substances.[33]

Because of fear and stigma associated with alcohol use during pregnancy, pregnant persons may under report their alcohol consumption.[34] In addition, despite the widespread effort to inform the population about the harmful effects of alcohol use on the fetus (eg, via warning labels on containers), many individuals believe that the consumption of small amounts will not have harmful consequences. Studies failing to find effects of alcohol on the fetus and child can erroneously prop up these beliefs, when more accurate reporting would clarify that failure to detect an effect is not the same as safe, or no effect. Furthermore, individual studies often examine only one outcome domain, and thus could only be reassuring in that regard, and not for all possible alcohol harms.[35]

Screening instruments developed for general populations may perform less well during pregnancy or the prenatal period.[9] Consequently, instruments have been developed specifically to ascertain drinking in pregnancy. The T-ACE, based on the "CAGE"[36] (each letter stands for one key word in each of the items), is a four-question instrument.[37] T-ACE stands for T (*Tolerance*): How many drinks does it take to make you feel high? A: Have people *annoyed* you by criticizing your drinking? C: Have you ever felt you ought to *cut down* on your drinking? E (*Eye-opener*): Have you ever had a drink first thing in the morning to steady your nerves or get rid of a hangover? Affirmative answers to questions A, C, or E are 1 point each. Reporting tolerance to more than two drinks (T question) is scored 2 points. A score of 2 or more is considered positive. The TWEAK, also derived from the CAGE, is a five-question instrument.[38] TWEAK stands for T (*Tolerance*): How many drinks can you hold? (positive if ≥6 drinks) *Or* How many drinks does it take before you begin to feel the first effects of alcohol? (positive if ≥3 drinks) W: Have close friends or relatives *worried* or complained about your drinking in the past year? E (*Eye-opener*): Do you sometimes take a drink in the morning when you first get up? A (*Amnesia*): Has a friend or a family member ever told you about things you said or did while you were drinking that you could not remember? K: Do you sometimes feel the need to *cut down* on your drinking? Affirmative answers to question E, A, K are 1 point each. Affirmative answers to question W and T are 2 points each. The cutoff score is 2. The NET is a three-question instrument. It shares two questions with the T-ACE (Eye-opener and Tolerance) and one with the Michigan Alcohol Screening Test (MAST) (Do you feel you are a normal drinker?). The tolerance question scores 2 points, the two other questions score 1 point each, and ≥2 is considered positive.

Tested in routine gynecology and obstetrics services, the T-ACE questionnaire showed better sensitivity compared to the Alcohol Use Disorders Identification Test (AUDIT) and the Short MAST (SMAST) for a lifetime diagnosis of an alcohol use disorder, risky drinking, and current alcohol use in pregnant women.[37,39] It outperformed obstetrics staff assessment of any alcohol use,[39] and its brevity makes it useful for routine practice.[40] Russell et al. demonstrated that the TWEAK and the T-ACE were sensitive for periconceptional risky drinking[41] and outperformed the CAGE and the MAST. At a cutoff of 2, the NET appears to be less sensitive than the T-ACE, the TWEAK, and the MAST.[38] In conclusion, the T-ACE and the TWEAK are two brief questionnaires with satisfactory performance during pregnancy (and during the periconception stage). These two questionnaires have similar sensitivities (69%-88% for the T-ACE, 71%-91% for the TWEAK) and specificities (71%-89%; 73%-83%).[42] Although not specifically developed to screen during pregnancy, the Alcohol Use Disorders Identification Test-Consumption (AUDIT-C),[43] with a cutoff of 3 or more, could also be used to screen for at-risk drinking (sensitivity: 95%; specificity: 85%) and alcohol use disorders (sensitivity: 96%; specificity: 71%).[42] The National Institute on Alcohol Abuse and Alcoholism (NIAAA) single screening question has not been tested specifically during pregnancy. According to a recent systematic review conducted on the performances of seven instruments (T-ACE, TWEAK, CAGE, NET, AUDIT, AUDIT-C, and SMAST), the three instruments with the best performances in patients receiving prenatal care are the T-ACE, the TWEAK, and the AUDIT-C.[42]

Screening for Unhealthy Other Drug Use

Unlike those for testing alcohol use, drug use screening tools to address use during pregnancy have not been extensively studied.[28] In its *Guidelines for the identification and management of substance use and substance use disorders in pregnancy*, the WHO gives a strong recommendation to screen all pregnant people, while acknowledging a low quality of evidence. In the same guidelines are listed the screening tests with reported performances in screening pregnant persons: the Substance Use Risk Profile-Pregnancy (SURP-P) scale, the 4Ps Plus©, and the NIDA quick screen and modified ASSIST.[44] Other available screening questionnaires tested in pregnancy include the CRAFFT, the 5Ps (an adaptation of the 4Ps©: parents, peers, partner, pregnancy, past), and the Wayne Indirect Drug Use Screener (WIDUS).

Chasnoff et al. demonstrated that the 4Ps Plus© was a reliable measure with good sensitivity and specificity for substance use (alcohol, cannabis, heroin, cocaine, and methamphetamines) during pregnancy.[45] This proprietary questionnaire (positive if questions about use during or before pregnancy are affirmative) asks about *P*ast substance use, use during *P*regnancy, and use by *P*arents and *P*artners. The questions are: Did either of your parents ever have a problem with alcohol or drugs? Does your partner have a problem with alcohol or drugs? Have you ever drunk beer, wine, or liquor? In the month before you knew you were pregnant, how many cigarettes did you smoke? In the month before you knew you were pregnant, how many beers/how much wine/how much liquor did you drink?

The SURP-P is a three-item questionnaire. The questions are: Have you ever smoked cannabis? In the months before you were pregnant, how many beers, how much wine, or how much liquor did you drink (classified as none compared with any). Have you ever felt that you needed to cut down on your drug or alcohol use? Each affirmative item scores 1. A score of 0 indicates a low risk, 1 moderate, and 2-3 high risk of substance use.[46] In the SURP-P validation study, for populations at low risk of substance use, the sensitivity was 91% and specificity 67%.[47]

The NIDA quick screen is a two-part instrument with a four question prescreen and a follow-up modified ASSIST with tobacco and alcohol use items removed (National Institute on Drug Abuse. Resource guide: screening for drug use in general medical settings. Available at https://nida.nih.gov/sites/default/files/resource_guide.pdf). The four-question prescreen asks about the use of alcohol, tobacco, prescription drugs for nonmedical reasons, and illegal drugs. In case of a positive answer, ASSIST questions are asked and a substance involvement score is computed.

The WIDUS consists of six true-false items. The items are not directly focused on drug use but on correlates of drug use (such as "I get mad easily and feel a need to blow off some steam"). Answers are summed to create an index of risk ranging from 0 to 6. In the screener development study, conducted among 400 postpartum women, a score of 2 had a 88% sensitivity and 42% specificity to detect drug use (compared to toxicology reports).[48]

The CRAFFT is a five-item screener (car, relax, alone, forget, friends, trouble) initially developed to screen adolescents for alcohol and other drug use. It has been evaluated among pregnant women for alcohol and cannabis use.[49]

In a study comparing the performances of the SURP-P, the 4Ps Plus© and the NIDA quick screen in prenatal care to detect substance use (compared to biological testing in urine and hair), the 4P's Plus© had a sensitivity = 90.2% and specificity = 29.6%, the NIDA Quick Screen-ASSIST had sensitivity = 79.7% and specificity = 82.8% and the SURP-P had sensitivity = 92.4% and specificity = 21.8%. Another study compared the performances of five instruments to identify illicit drug (including opioids) use: the SURP-P, the CRAFFT, 5Ps, WIDUS, and NIDA quick screen. No single instrument emerged as the most effective, and performances were limited.[50] The best two instruments, CRAFFT and SURP-P, showed only modest accuracy. Thus, currently available screening instruments have limited performances among pregnant people. In its 2019 report, the USPSTF also indicated that instruments are less accurate in detecting unhealthy drug use than unhealthy alcohol use in pregnancy.[51]

BRIEF INTERVENTIONS

Alcohol

Various studies of brief intervention included but did not specifically report on women of childbearing age. One of the largest studies conducted in primary care, a randomized controlled trial (Trial for Early Alcohol Treatment, project TrEAT),[52] reported results of a subgroup analysis of 205 women aged 18 to 40. Brief intervention decreased the self-reported number of drinks consumed in the past 7 days and the number of heavy drinking episodes in the past month by about 20% to 25%.[53] This study included women who drank more than 11 drinks per week, more than four standard drinks per occasion, or had positive CAGE screening tests (2+) but excluded those with DSM-IV alcohol dependence. The brief intervention consisted of two 15-minute visits with a physician, 1 month apart, and supportive phone calls by a nurse 2 weeks after each clinician visit. These results support the hypothesis that brief interventions conducted in primary care among women of childbearing age with unhealthy alcohol use are effective in reducing alcohol consumption and heavy drinking episodes.

Recent systematic reviews focusing on efficacy of screening and brief interventions for pregnant women conclude that brief interventions may result in increased abstinence from alcohol, but evidence is scarce. A 2009 Cochrane review identified 4 randomized controlled trials (not including trials of pregnant patients participating in treatment programs for alcohol use disorder).[54] These included a total of 715 pregnant women. Chang et al. randomly assigned 250 pregnant women identified using the T-ACE questionnaire (score ≥2) as they attended prenatal care.[55] Women with gestational age greater than 28 weeks and without alcohol consumption in the 6 months preceding study participation were excluded. Participants were randomly assigned to a comprehensive assessment only or to a comprehensive assessment and a 45-minute brief intervention. Brief intervention included review of the subject's health and pregnancy, review of lifestyle changes made since pregnancy, articulation of drinking goals while pregnant and reasons for these goals, recommendation of abstinence as the most prudent drinking goal, and identification of high-risk situations for drinking and alternatives to drinking. There was a similar decrease in alcohol consumption during pregnancy in the control and intervention groups (0.4 versus 0.3 drinks per drinking day, respectively). The groups did not differ on the number of drinking episodes either (1.0 versus 0.7 episodes, respectively). There was an effect of brief intervention on the subgroup of women (n = 142) who were abstinent at study entry, with significantly more maintenance of abstinence in the intervention group (86% versus control group 72%), relative risk (RR) = 1.20 (95% confidence interval [CI] 1.01-1.42). Unpublished data from Chang et al. are reported in the Cochrane review, showing no difference in abstinence from alcohol between the intervention and the control groups (69% and 62% abstinence, respectively).[55] Two studies reported positive significant intervention effects on abstinence.[56,57] O'Connor and Whaley compared brief intervention versus advice to stop drinking only, among 345 pregnant currently drinking women.[57] Brief interventions were delivered by trained nutritionists as part of an individual nutrition education program and included education, feedback, goal setting, cognitive-behavioral procedures, and a contract. There was a substantial decrease in alcohol use in both groups, and authors reported a significant effect of the intervention on abstinence by the third trimester: Participants in the intervention group were five times more likely to abstain than were participants in the control group (OR 5.39 [95% CI, 1.59-18.25]). Brief intervention also improved birth weight and reduced fetal death (from 2.9% to 0.9%), though it is unclear that brief intervention impact on abstinence could have plausibly accounted for effects of this size on these secondary outcomes. Handmaker et al.[56] compared a 1-hour motivational interviewing intervention to a written letter in a pilot study with 42 pregnant women. Results showed no impact of the intervention except on a subgroup of those with the highest drinking levels at study enrollment.

The fourth identified study, by Reynolds et al., compared a cognitive-behavioral self-help intervention (including a 10-minute educational session with a self-help manual to be completed over 9 days) to usual care. The study recruited low-income pregnant women attending public health clinics in an urban setting. Results suggest an intervention effect on abstinence, although the difference between groups was not significant (RR 1.25 [95% CI, 0.97-1.61]). There were no differences between treatment groups on number of drinks per week (mean difference -0.78 [-1.58; 0.02]). In subgroup analyses, there was a significant effect of the intervention on abstinence among African American women.[58]

Gilinsky et al. identified randomized and nonrandomized trials.[59] Two additional randomized trials not included in the Cochrane review were identified.[60,61] Reading et al. compared real-time ultrasound with verbal and visual feedback to ultrasound without feedback and showed no difference between groups.[61] Chang et al. compared a 25-minute brief intervention that could involve a partner to a no-intervention control condition. All participants completed a diagnostic interview on alcohol use.[60] The partner could be a spouse, father of the child, or any other supportive adult, and was chosen by the pregnant woman. Participants were enrolled as they initiated prenatal care in obstetric practices and included if they scored 2 or more on the T-ACE, reported any alcohol consumption while pregnant, reported consumption of at least one drink per day in the 6 months before study enrollment, or drank during a previous pregnancy. Exclusion criteria were receiving treatment for a substance use disorder, physical dependence to alcohol requiring medically supervised withdrawal management, use of cocaine, opioids, or other illicit drugs. The brief intervention included knowledge assessment with feedback on drinking and pregnancy, goal setting, and behavioral modification (identification of high-risk situations, alternative behaviors, support from the partner). Both the intervention and control groups showed similar reductions in alcohol consumption. In exploring the absence of intervention effect, the authors reported a significant interaction between participation in the brief intervention and prenatal alcohol use. Specifically, they indicated that the brief intervention was more effective among participants who drank more upon study enrollment. Similarly, in a subgroup analysis examining the impact of the partner's participation, the authors reported a significant impact of the brief intervention on alcohol consumption only when a partner participated.

Thus, research findings regarding the efficacy of alcohol screening and brief intervention in pregnancy are largely null with perhaps one exception[57] and some hypothesis-generating subgroup analyses, which suggested avenues for further research and confirmation. Furthermore, it should be noted that the Cochrane review concludes that the complexity of interventions limits the determination of which type of intervention would be most effective for which populations, and that there is a lack of information on possible intervention effects on the health of the babies.[54]

Another study, not included in the Cochrane review, offers some additional information: 300 women drinking more than three drinks per week during conception were randomly assigned postpartum to receive or not receive a brief intervention aimed at reducing prenatal alcohol use during the next pregnancy, and were followed up to 5 years. The intervention consisted of 5 sessions based on a cognitive behavioral approach with booster session over the 5-year follow-up period. Of the 300 participants, 96 delivered one or more infants during the follow-up period. The intervention decreased alcohol use and improved infant outcomes (low birth weight, fewer premature deliveries).[62]

In its 2018 evaluation of the evidence, the USPSTF noted that interventions increased the proportion abstinence in pregnancy (OR 1.92) compared to control group but that the between group difference in abstinence was significant in only two trials[57,58] (evidence synthesis 171).

Similar to the development of information technology-based brief interventions for other populations, the use of electronic interventions is developing for pregnant people and appears acceptable.[63,64] A pilot study tested the acceptability and efficacy of an electronic intervention (20-minute electronic interactive session compared to a 20-minute intervention on infant nutrition). Participants had to screen positive on the T-ACE and report drinking weekly or more in the past month or having at least 4 drinks at least monthly in the 12 months before becoming pregnant. Participants were recruited among pregnant patients seeking services at prenatal care clinics in Detroit. The intervention was favorably rated by users ($n = 48$). The study showed medium-size, but not significant, intervention effects on 90-day period prevalence (odds ratio [OR] = 3.4, $p = 0.19$), and on a combined pregnancy outcome variable (live birth, normal birthweight, no neonatal intensive care; OR = 3.3, $p = 0.09$).[65] This study was followed by a multisite study comparing electronic brief intervention to assessment-only among 123 postpartum low-income women reporting 4 or more drinks per occasion twice a month or scoring 2 or more on the T-ACE. Results did not show a significant difference between groups.[66]

Another intervention strategy consists of targeting the risk of alcohol-exposed pregnancy by reducing drinking and/or increasing contraception when alcohol use may occur. Floyd et al. randomly assigned 830 nonpregnant women aged 18 to 44 years and currently at risk for alcohol-exposed pregnancies (drinking more than five drinks any day or more than eight drinks per week and having unprotected sex) to receive information or information and a brief motivational alcohol intervention (four sessions) and one contraception consultation.[67] For up to 9 months, participants in the intervention group were significantly less likely to be at risk for an alcohol-exposed pregnancy (related to drinking risky amounts and/or not using effective contraception), confirming results from a previous report.[68] The same approach has been shown successful among college student heavy drinkers: Ceperich and Ingersoll published the results of a randomized trial comparing motivational interviewing (lasting 60-75 minutes) and a feedback intervention to a minimal control condition consisting of a brochure.[69] Study participants were female students aged 18 to 24 ($n = 280$) who were at risk for alcohol-exposed pregnancy (defined as having had sexual intercourse that could lead to a pregnancy in the past 90 days, ineffective contraception, and consumption of more than 4 standard drinks per occasion at least once in the past 90 days or consumption of more than 7 drinks per week on average). At 4-month follow-up, alcohol-exposed pregnancy risk was lower in the intervention group (20%) compared to the control group (35%). Control group assignment was associated with a doubling of the risk (OR = 2.2). Considering that around half of pregnancies can be unintended,[70] and that alcohol use is associated with sexual risk-taking,[30] this double approach is promising in reducing the risk of alcohol-exposed pregnancies. A methodological concern that applies to all of these studies is that outcomes rely on unbiased self-report—which may not be possible from persons who were advised to avoid alcohol use during pregnancy.

Expert Recommendations on Screening and Brief Intervention

In 2010, Carson et al. published consensus guidelines on alcohol use and pregnancy.[71] They recommend universal screening for all pregnant persons and persons of child-bearing age, emphasizing that:

- At-risk drinking should be identified before pregnancy to allow for behavior change
- Health care providers should create a safe environment to allow for the reporting of alcohol consumption
- The public should be informed that alcohol screening and support for persons at risk is part of usual care
- Brief interventions should be delivered by health care providers for persons with at-risk drinking
- Health care providers should be aware of the risk factors associated with at-risk drinking
- Harm reduction and treatment strategies should be encouraged for persons continuing to use alcohol during their pregnancy
- Pregnant persons should be given priority access to withdrawal management and treatment
- Providers should advise pregnant persons that low level consumption of alcohol in early pregnancy is not an indication for termination of pregnancy

In 2016, Wright et al. reported on conclusions from a 2012 expert meeting. Recommendations are to screen universally for at-risk drinking, at the first prenatal visit and repeated at least every trimester for those who screened positive, to provide brief advice to those who report abstinence from drinking, to provide brief intervention to those screening positive, and referral to treatment for persons in high-risk categories.[26]

The U.S. Surgeon General states that no level of alcohol consumption by pregnant persons can be considered safe and that persons who are, may be, or are considering becoming pregnant should abstain from alcohol. The Center for Disease Control and Prevention also recommends that persons who are pregnant or might be pregnant not drink alcohol at all (http://www.cdc.gov/vitalsigns/fasd/). Although it is possible that very low amounts of alcohol may not have adverse fetal effects in some subgroups of pregnant persons, these recommendations are supported by: (1) the linear dose response consequences of alcohol exposure, (2) its potentially irreversible and catastrophic effects, (3) the limited ability of research to prove the null, and (4) the absence of a compelling reason/need to drink alcohol during pregnancy.

Other Drugs

Screening and brief interventions are usually delivered with protection of confidentiality, notably to enhance accuracy of screening and establish trust in the clinician-patient relationship. This confidentiality may be challenged in states where the law requires physicians to report illicit drug use by pregnant persons, and where laws define this use as criminal behavior. Physicians should also be aware of their state's laws regarding the reporting of substance use during pregnancy. If thought to present legal risk, patients could be screened and advised anonymously, for example, via the internet or other self-administered materials, though few have been tested in pregnant persons.

While the USPSTF recommends screening in primary care for drug use among pregnant persons, available research findings show no clear benefits. Five studies were identified in the evidence review, but no significant impact on drug abstinence rates was found (RR 1.24 [0.99; 1.89]).[51] And, because screening is recommended conditional on the possibility of offering or referring to effective treatment,[24] implementation of systematic screening will depend on how health care is organized and whether adequate care, beyond brief interventions, is available. Specifically, availability and access to opioid agonist treatment will be key for those identified with opioid use disorder, and referral to specialized addiction treatment will allow for close monitoring of the potential development of a neonatal abstinence syndrome in the newborn. As noted by Saitz in his editorial published alongside the USPSTF recommendation, "Screening for drug use is reasonable to consider in clinical practice, but it is not evidence-based for improving health."[72]

Studies of information technology-based interventions for unhealthy drug use in pregnant people suggest brief intervention may have efficacy in this circumstance. However, research findings are mixed and limited. One trial, conducted among 107 postpartum women, showed a significant effect of a computer-delivered 20-minute intervention on illicit drug use other than cannabis, but no effect on cannabis use at 4 months.[73] Another trial, aimed at replicating these results, randomized 143 postpartum women to receive a computer-based 20-minute intervention or a 20-minute inactive control condition and showed a significant intervention effect at 3 months on 7-day point prevalence of abstinence from illicit drugs confirmed by urine screens (26.4% abstinence in intervention group, 9.9% in control group).[74]

CONCLUSION AND RECOMMENDATIONS

Alcohol

Alcohol has toxic effects on the fetus, and there is currently no safe threshold identified for its consumption during pregnancy. The current recommendation for pregnant persons, persons who might be pregnant, and persons who are trying to become pregnant is to abstain from alcohol. Given the insufficient evidence to define any threshold for low-risk drinking during pregnancy, abstinence is the prudent choice for pregnant persons or persons who might become pregnant. Physicians should inform patients of this recommendation. Healthcare professionals also have an important role in ensuring that patients who have consumed alcohol do not feel stigmatized. When alcohol consumption has happened during pregnancy, physicians should be aware of the uncertainty around the risks of low consumption during pregnancy and explain this to patients in clear but patient-centered ways.[12]

Persons of childbearing age, including pregnant persons, should be screened for alcohol use with validated tools. Brief, validated instruments (T-ACE, TWEAK, AUDIT-C) are available for screening pregnant persons and those considering pregnancy and should be used in routine practice. Beyond these tools, consideration should be given to asking directly about any substance use. In addition, patients should be advised to abstain during pregnancy given the lack of an imperative to use substances and the absence of certainty regarding safe levels of use. Persons screening positive for at-risk substance use should then receive a brief intervention. Early intervention strategies are especially recommended.[23,25,26]

Assessment of alcohol use, or pregnancy itself, may lead pregnant persons to decrease or stop drinking. In addition, brief intervention can decrease risky use in young persons (pregnant or not). Although not extensively confirmed in the literature to date, it can decrease drinking during pregnancy and associated risks, may increase abstinence, and may improve fetal outcomes. Some studies suggest that brief intervention effects are limited to those who drink the largest amounts. Even so, screening, advice to abstain from alcohol immediately before and during pregnancy, and patient education regarding potential consequences of alcohol use on the fetus should be included in routine practice, as preventing alcohol use is the only way to prevent FAS and other alcohol-related effects on infants. Depending on resources available, the screening and intervention can be repeated over a few sessions and/or include the partner, as partner involvement may have beneficial effects. Brief interventions conducted with pregnant persons should include specific feedback on consequences of drinking on the fetus and infant, as well as medical complications related to alcohol use during pregnancy, and identification of risky situations (and potential coping strategies). In 2010 consensus guidelines sponsored by the Public Health Agency of Canada and the Society of Obstetricians and Gynecologists of Canada, universal screening for alcohol consumption for all pregnant persons and subsequent brief intervention when indicated were given a level II-2B recommendation (evidence from well-designed cohort or case control studies; fair evidence to recommend the clinical preventive action).[71] Screening and brief intervention for unhealthy alcohol use in primary care, including among pregnant persons, was given a level B recommendation by the USPSTF.[23] Parents should be informed of potential legal consequences of reporting their alcohol use, if applicable (eg, risk of losing parental rights).

Other Drugs

Use of illicit drugs during pregnancy can have a negative impact on the course of pregnancy and on the fetus.[15] There is currently insufficient evidence to determine the benefits and harms of screening for illicit drug use among pregnant persons. Nevertheless, given its potential preventive benefits, it seems reasonable, if not ethically required, for physicians to give at least feedback on consequences of use as well as advice to abstain. Experts in prenatal care recommend interventions.[26] and the USPSTF recommends screening for unhealthy drug use in primary care including among pregnant persons. Routine toxicology testing is not recommended in pregnancy. Even in the absence of definitive scientific data on screening and brief intervention efficacy among pregnant persons, clinicians may consider asking about medications, illicit drug use, and alcohol and tobacco use as part of a prenatal exam. If a drug use disorder is likely after clinical examination, patients should be referred for a comprehensive assessment, in order to address substance use severity and associated psychosocial issues.[15,26] For screening, instruments have poorer performances than instruments for alcohol use. However, similar to alcohol, information on illicit drug use and tobacco use consequences on the fetus should also be provided to persons of childbearing age. It should be noted that the specific context of pregnancy and the potential legal consequences may impact the accuracy of the screening and necessary ingredients of brief intervention, and clinicians may face ethical challenges, having to balance principles of beneficence and respect for autonomy as they apply to both pregnant persons and their children.

Note: This sidebar presents recommendations for women and people with other gender identities who are pregnant or might be pregnant. Throughout the text, nongender neutral terms have been kept to reflect the context in which prior research has been conducted. More work is needed to evaluate screening and brief intervention among pregnant patients of other genders.

REFERENCES

1. Jones KL, Smith DW, Ulleland CN, Streissguth P. Pattern of malformation in offspring of chronic alcoholic mothers. *Lancet*. 1973;1(7815):1267-1271.
2. Jones KL, Smith DW. Recognition of the fetal alcohol syndrome in early infancy. *Lancet*. 1973;302(7836):999-1001.
3. Ismail S, Buckley S, Budacki R, Jabbar A, Gallicano GI. Screening, diagnosing and prevention of fetal alcohol syndrome: is this syndrome treatable? *Dev Neurosci*. 2010;32(2):91-100.
4. Flak AL, Su S, Bertrand J, Denny CH, Kesmodel US, Cogswell ME. The association of mild, moderate, and binge prenatal alcohol exposure and child neuropsychological outcomes: a meta-analysis. *Alcohol Clin Exp Res*. 2014;38(1):214-226.
5. Jacobson JL, Jacobson SW. Drinking moderately and pregnancy. Effects on child development. *Alcohol Res Health*. 1999;23(1):25-30.
6. O'Connor MJ, Kasari C. Prenatal alcohol exposure and depressive features in children. *Alcohol Clin Exp Res*. 2000;24(7):1084-1092.
7. Manning MA, Hoyme HE. Fetal alcohol spectrum disorders: a practical clinical approach to diagnosis. *Neurosci Biobehav Rev*. 2007;31(2):230-238.
8. Day NL, Jasperse D, Richardson G, et al. Prenatal exposure to alcohol: effect on infant growth and morphologic characteristics. *Pediatrics*. 1989;84(3):536-541.
9. Bradley KA, Boyd-Wickizer J, Powell SH, Burman ML. Alcohol screening questionnaires in women: a critical review. *JAMA*. 1998;280(2):166-171.
10. Feldman HS, Lyons Jones K, Lindsay S, et al. Prenatal alcohol exposure patterns and alcohol-related birth defects and growth deficiencies: a prospective study. *Alcohol Clin Exp Res*. 2012;36(4):670-676.
11. Gray R, RAS M, Rutter M. Alcohol consumption during pregnancy and its effects on neurodevelopment: what is known and what remains uncertain. *Addiction*. 2009;104(8):1270-1273.
12. Association BM. *Alcohol and Pregnancy: Preventing and Managing Fetal Alcohol Spectrum Disorders*. British Medical Association; 2016. https://www.bma.org.uk/media/2082/fetal-alcohol-spectrum-disorders-report-feb2016.pdf
13. Henderson J, Kesmodel U, Gray R. Systematic review of the fetal effects of prenatal binge-drinking. *J Epidemiol Community Health*. 2007;61(12):1069-1073.
14. Henderson J, Gray R, Brocklehurst P. Systematic review of effects of low-moderate prenatal alcohol exposure on pregnancy outcome. *BJOG*. 2007;114(3):243-252.
15. Helmbrecht GD, Thiagarajah S. Management of addiction disorders in pregnancy. *J Addict Med*. 2008;2(1):1-16.
16. Rivkin MJ, Davis PE, Lemaster JL, et al. Volumetric MRI study of brain in children with intrauterine exposure to cocaine, alcohol, tobacco, and marijuana. *Pediatrics*. 2008;121(4):741-750.
17. Patrick SW, Schumacher RE, Benneyworth BD, Krans EE, McAllister JM, Davis MM. Neonatal abstinence syndrome and associated health care expenditures: United States, 2000-2009. *JAMA*. 2012;307(18):1934-1940.
18. Huizink AC. Prenatal cannabis exposure and infant outcomes: overview of studies. *Prog Neuropsychopharmacol Biol Psychiatry*. 2014;52:45-52.
19. Gunn JK, Rosales CB, Center KE, et al. Prenatal exposure to cannabis and maternal and child health outcomes: a systematic review and meta-analysis. *BMJ Open*. 2016;6(4):e009986.
20. Patrick SW, Davis MM, Lehmann CU, Cooper WO. Increasing incidence and geographic distribution of neonatal abstinence syndrome: United States 2009 to 2012. *J Perinatol*. 2015;35(8):650-655.
21. Tolia VN, Patrick SW, Bennett MM, et al. Increasing incidence of the neonatal abstinence syndrome in U.S. neonatal ICUs. *N Engl J Med*. 2015;372(22):2118-2126.
22. Saia KA, Schiff D, Wachman EM, et al. Caring for pregnant women with opioid use disorder in the USA: expanding and improving treatment. *Curr Obstet Gynecol Rep*. 2016;5:257-263.
23. US Preventative Task Force, Curry SJ, Krist AH, Owens DK, et al. Screening and behavioral counseling interventions to reduce unhealthy alcohol use in adolescents and adults: US Preventive Services Task Force Recommendation Statement. *JAMA*. 2018;320(18):1899-1909.
24. United States Preventive Services Task Force, Krist AH, Davidson KW, Mangione CM, et al. Screening for unhealthy drug use: US Preventive Services Task Force Recommendation Statement. *JAMA*. 2020;323(22):2301-2309.
25. ACOG Committee. At-risk drinking and illicit drug use: ethical issues in obstetric and gynecologic practice. ACOG Committee Opinion No. 422. *Obstet Gynecol*. 2008;112(6):1449-1460.
26. Wright TE, Terplan M, Ondersma SJ, et al. The role of screening, brief intervention, and referral to treatment in the perinatal period. *Am J Obstet Gynecol*. 2016;215(5):539-547.
27. Ecker J, Abuhamad A, Hill W, et al. Substance use disorders in pregnancy: clinical, ethical, and research imperatives of the opioid epidemic: a report of a joint workshop of the Society for Maternal-Fetal Medicine, American College of Obstetricians and Gynecologists, and American Society of Addiction Medicine. *Am J Obstet Gynecol*. 2019;221(1):B5-B28.
28. Chang G. Maternal substance use: consequences, identification, and interventions. *Alcohol Res*. 2020;40(2):06.
29. Tough S, Tofflemire K, Clarke M, Newburn-Cook C. Do women change their drinking behaviors while trying to conceive? An opportunity for preconception counseling. *Clin Med Res*. 2006;4(2):97-105.
30. Naimi TS, Lipscomb LE, Brewer RD, Colley Gilbert B. Binge drinking in the preconception period and the risk of unintended pregnancy: implications for women and their children. *Pediatrics*. 2003;111(5 Pt 2):1136-1141.
31. Smith IE, Lancaster JS, Moss-Wells S, Coles CD, Falek A. Identifying high-risk pregnant drinkers: biological and behavioral correlates of continuous heavy drinking during pregnancy. *J Stud Alcohol*. 1987;48(4):304-309.
32. Day NL, Cottreau CM, Richardson GA. The epidemiology of alcohol, marijuana, and cocaine use among women of childbearing age and pregnant women. *Clin Obstet Gynecol*. 1993;36(2):232-245.
33. Higgins PG, Clough DH, Frank B, Wallerstedt C. Changes in health behaviors made by pregnant substance users. *Int J Addict*. 1995;30(10):1323-1333.
34. Jacobson SW, Chiodo LM, Sokol RJ, Jacobson JL. Validity of maternal report of prenatal alcohol, cocaine, and smoking in relation to neurobehavioral outcome. *Pediatrics*. 2002;109(5):815-825.
35. Skogerbø A, Kesmodel US, Wimberely T, et al. The effects of low to moderate alcohol consumption and binge drinking in early pregnancy on executive function in 5-year-old children. *BJOG*. 2012;119(10):1201-1210.
36. Mayfield D, McLeod G, Hall P. The CAGE questionnaire: validation of a new alcoholism screening instrument. *Am J Psychiatry*. 1974;131(10):1121-1123.

37. Sokol RJ, Martier SS, Ager JW. The T-ACE questions: practical prenatal detection of risk-drinking. *Am J Obstet Gynecol.* 1989;160(4):863-868. discussion 868-870.
38. Russell M, Martier SS, Sokol RJ, et al. Screening for pregnancy risk-drinking. *Alcohol Clin Exp Res.* 1994;18(5):1156-1161.
39. Chang G, Wilkins-Haug L, Berman S, Goetz MA, Hiley A. Alcohol use and pregnancy: improving identification. *Obstet Gynecol.* 1998;91(6):892-898.
40. Fabbri CE, Furtado EF, Laprega MR. Alcohol consumption in pregnancy: performance of the Brazilian version of the questionnaire T-ACE. *Rev Saude Publica.* 2007;41(6):979-984.
41. Russell M, Martier SS, Sokol RJ, Mudar P, Jacobson S, Jacobson J. Detecting risk drinking during pregnancy: a comparison of four screening questionnaires. *Am J Public Health.* 1996;86(10):1435-1439.
42. Burns E, Gray R, Smith LA. Brief screening questionnaires to identify problem drinking during pregnancy: a systematic review. *Addiction.* 2010;105(4):601-614.
43. Bush K, Kivlahan DR, McDonell MB, Fihn SD, Bradley KA. The AUDIT alcohol consumption questions (AUDIT-C): an effective brief screening test for problem drinking. Ambulatory Care Quality Improvement Project (ACQUIP). Alcohol Use Disorders Identification Test. *Arch Intern Med.* 1998;158(16):1789-1795.
44. World Health Organization. *Guidelines for Identification and Management of Substance Use and Substance Use Disorders in Pregnancy.* WHO; 2014.
45. Chasnoff IJ, Wells AM, McGourty RF, Bailey LK. Validation of the 4P's Plus screen for substance use in pregnancy validation of the 4P's Plus. *J Perinatol.* 2007;27(12):744-748.
46. Coleman-Cowger VH, Oga EA, Peters EN, Trocin KE, Koszowksi B, Mark K. Accuracy of three screening tools for prenatal substance use. *Obstet Gynecol.* 2019;133(5):952-961.
47. Yonkers KA, Gotman N, Kershaw T, Forray A, Howell HB, Rounsaville BJ. Screening for prenatal substance use: development of the Substance Use Risk Profile-Pregnancy scale. *Obstet Gynecol.* 2010;116(4):827-833.
48. Ondersma SJ, Svikis DS, LeBreton JM, et al. Development and preliminary validation of an indirect screener for drug use in the perinatal period. *Addiction.* 2012;107(12):2099-2106.
49. Chang G, Orav EJ, Jones JA, Buynitsky T, Gonzalez S, Wilkins-Haug L. Self-reported alcohol and drug use in pregnant young women: a pilot study of associated factors and identification. *J Addict Med.* 2011;5(3):221-226.
50. Chang G, Ondersma SJ, Blake-Lamb T, Gilstad-Hayden K, Orav EJ, Yonkers KA. Identification of substance use disorders among pregnant women: a comparison of screeners. *Drug Alcohol Depend.* 2019;205:107651.
51. Patnode CD, Perdue LA, Ruskin M, et al. Screening for unhealthy drug use: updated evidence report and systematic review for the US Preventive Services Task Force. *JAMA.* 2020;323(22):2310-2328.
52. Fleming MF, Barry KL, Manwell LB, Johnson K, London R. Brief physician advice for problem alcohol drinkers. A randomized controlled trial in community-based primary care practices. *JAMA.* 1997;277(13):1039-1045.
53. Manwell LB, Fleming MF, Mundt MP, Stauffacher EA, Barry KL. Treatment of problem alcohol use in women of childbearing age: results of a brief intervention trial. *Alcohol Clin Exp Res.* 2000;24(10):1517-1524.
54. Stade BC, Bailey C, Dzendoletas D, Sgro M, Dowswell T, Bennett D. Psychological and/or educational interventions for reducing alcohol consumption in pregnant women and women planning pregnancy. *Cochrane Database Syst Rev.* 2009;(2):CD004228.
55. Chang G, Wilkins-Haug L, Berman S, Goetz MA. Brief intervention for alcohol use in pregnancy: a randomized trial. *Addiction.* 1999;94(10):1499-1508.
56. Handmaker NS, Miller WR, Manicke M. Findings of a pilot study of motivational interviewing with pregnant drinkers. *J Stud Alcohol.* 1999;60(2):285-287.
57. O'Connor MJ, Whaley SE. Brief intervention for alcohol use by pregnant women. *Am J Public Health.* 2007;97(2):252-258.
58. Reynolds KD, Coombs DW, Lowe JB, Peterson PL, Gayoso E. Evaluation of a self-help program to reduce alcohol consumption among pregnant women. *Int J Addict.* 1995;30(4):427-443.
59. Gilinsky A, Swanson V, Power K. Interventions delivered during antenatal care to reduce alcohol consumption during pregnancy: a systematic review. *Addict Res Theory.* 2011;19(3):235-250.
60. Chang G, McNamara TK, Orav EJ, et al. Brief intervention for prenatal alcohol use: a randomized trial. *Obstet Gynecol.* 2005;105(5 Pt 1): 991-998.
61. Reading AE, Campbell S, Cox DN, Sledmere CM. Health beliefs and health care behaviour in pregnancy. *Psychol Med.* 1982;12(2):379-383.
62. Hankin JR. Fetal alcohol syndrome prevention research. *Alcohol Res Health.* 2002;26(1):58-65.
63. Pollick SA, Beatty JR, Sokol RJ, et al. Acceptability of a computerized brief intervention for alcohol among abstinent but at-risk pregnant women. *Subst Abus.* 2015;36(1):13-20.
64. Wouldes TA, Crawford A, Stevens S, Stasiak K. Evidence for the effectiveness and acceptability of e-SBI or e-SBIRT in the management of alcohol and illicit substance use in pregnant and post-partum women. *Front Psychiatry.* 2021;12:634805.
65. Ondersma SJ, Beatty JR, Svikis DS, et al. Computer-delivered screening and brief intervention for alcohol use in pregnancy: a pilot randomized trial. *Alcohol Clin Exp Res.* 2015;39(7):1219-1226.
66. Ondersma SJ, Svikis DS, Thacker LR, Beatty JR, Lockhart N. A randomised trial of a computer-delivered screening and brief intervention for postpartum alcohol use. *Drug Alcohol Rev.* 2016;35(6):710-718.
67. Floyd RL, Sobell M, Velasquez MM, et al. Preventing alcohol-exposed pregnancies: a randomized controlled trial. *Am J Prev Med.* 2007;32(1): 1-10.
68. Ingersoll K, Floyd L, Sobell M, et al. Reducing the risk of alcohol-exposed pregnancies: a study of a motivational intervention in community settings. *Pediatrics.* 2003;111:1131-1135.
69. Ingersoll KS, Ceperich SD, Nettleman MD, Karanda K, Brocksen S. Reducing alcohol-exposed pregnancy risk in college women: initial outcomes of a clinical trial of a motivational intervention. *J Subst Abuse Treat.* 2005;29(3):173-180.
70. Finer LB, Zolna MR. Unintended pregnancy in the United States: incidence and disparities, 2006. *Contraception.* 2011;84(5):478-485.
71. Carson G, Cox LV, Crane J, et al. Alcohol use and pregnancy consensus clinical guidelines. *J Obstet Gynaecol Can.* 2010;32(8 Suppl 3):S1-S31.
72. Saitz R. Screening for unhealthy drug use: neither an unreasonable idea nor an evidence-based practice. *JAMA.* 2020;323(22):2263-2265.
73. Ondersma SJ, Svikis DS, Schuster CR. Computer-based brief intervention a randomized trial with postpartum women. *Am J Prev Med.* 2007;32(3):231-238.
74. Ondersma SJ, Svikis DS, Thacker LR, Beatty JR, Lockhart N. Computer-delivered screening and brief intervention (e-SBI) for postpartum drug use: a randomized trial. *J Subst Abuse Treat.* 2014;46(1):52-59.

Sidebar 2

Screening and Brief Intervention in Trauma Centers, Hospitals, and Emergency Departments

Arthur F. Weissman and Richard D. Blondell

Individuals with unhealthy substance use are overrepresented among patients hospitalized for traumatic injuries[1] or acute medical conditions,[2] and among those who present to emergency departments.[3] Alcohol is a major risk factor for virtually all categories of fatal and nonfatal injury, including traffic accidents, burns, drowning, air traffic injuries, occupational injuries, homicides, suicides, domestic violence, and child abuse.[4,5] Patients with co-occurring substance use conditions have worse clinical outcomes, more complications, longer hospitalizations, and generate increased costs, suggesting an important target for screening and management.[6,7]

THE UTILITY OF SCREENING

Several randomized controlled trials of screening and brief interventions (BIs) versus "standard care" for unhealthy alcohol use in emergency departments (EDs) and trauma units have demonstrated positive effects including reduced alcohol consumption,[8,9] decreases in subsequent alcohol-related injuries,[10,11] and decreases in subsequent alcohol-related ED visits and hospitalizations.[8,12] Based on these studies, over 95% of Level I and II trauma centers in the United States routinely employ screening and BI for unhealthy alcohol use.[13] Most of these studies show either a reduction in alcohol consumption or negative consequences after alcohol BIs, but not both, and some reductions in consumption or consequences in the control "treatment as usual" groups.[14]

Although there is some research suggesting improved outcomes after screening and BI for illicit drug use in the ED, such as reductions in self-reported drug use,[15,16] at present there is a lack of randomized, controlled clinical trial data to support screening for illicit drug use in clinical settings overall.[17]

Universal toxicology screening for unhealthy substance use or substance use disorders (SUD) is generally not recommended. "Discretionary" (ie, nonuniversal) toxicology screening is done in some trauma center patients, however, without clear selection criteria.[18] One burn unit found selection bias for toxicology testing related to gender and co-occurring psychiatric disorders.[19]

There are concerns about whether positive substance screening has a meaningful impact on the acute management of the trauma patient[20,21] and about potential denial of insurance payment for hospital and surgical services if illicit drugs are detected in trauma patients.[22] Documenting illegal drug use in the medical record also has potential harms, particularly for pregnant or parenting people and those under correctional supervision.[17]

SCREENING TOOLS

Despite these limitations, knowing what substances a patient is using is still important[17] and may afford an opportunity for enhancing motivation to change. Screening tests developed for outpatient or pain management settings do not necessarily translate into reliable tests when used in emergency, trauma, or inpatient settings.[23] The Drug Abuse Screening Test (DAST) and the Alcohol, Smoking, and Substance Involvement Screening Test (ASSIST) have been validated in emergency settings.[24,25] An abbreviated version of the Alcohol Use Disorder Identification Test (AUDIT), the Screening Test for At-risk Drinking (STAD), has been validated for ED use.[26] An Australian study showed the AUDIT identified unhealthy alcohol use and was acceptable to hospitalized patients.[27] The Screener and Opioid Assessment for Patients with Pain-Revised (SOAPP-R) has been validated in a cohort of ED patients with cancer pain[28] and can be administered in a computerized tablet format in the ED.[29]

Computerized screening can integrate with existing electronic medical record systems.[30] Patients may be more at ease with computer-based screening,[31] and self-administration at a kiosk or tablet can be more effective than a face-to-face session with a staff member.[32,33] Patients report high levels of acceptance and ease-of-use with electronic screening but also have confidentiality concerns.[34]

Aside from efforts in the trauma room and ER, implementation of screening for unhealthy substance use has been uncommon.[35] Assessment tools developed for ambulatory settings, or for treatment-seeking patients, do not necessarily translate effectively to inpatients hospitalized for other reasons.[36] The prevalence of unhealthy substance use in hospitalized patients is unknown. One study, using the AUDIT-C for alcohol consumption and a single-item screening question for other drug use, identified unhealthy substance use in 16% of general medical hospitalized patients, with testing administered by nursing staff.[37]

BRIEF INTERVENTION

Once unhealthy substance use has been identified, there are several possible evidence-based brief interventions. Motivational Interviewing (MI) is a technique involving active listening, respect for autonomy, and guiding patients toward making healthier behavior changes.[38] MI can be effective in reducing alcohol intake in ED patients[39] and can reduce health care utilization and costs.[40] One ED pilot study found reductions in self-reported cannabis use, alcohol use, and substance use consequences in young adults with a combination of motivational interviewing and daily "booster" messages delivered via a mobile phone app.[41] In a multisite trauma center study, MI plus telephone "boosters" after discharge were more effective at reducing unhealthy alcohol use than brief advice to decrease alcohol consumption or MI alone.[42]

The evidence for BI is primarily for unhealthy alcohol use, with limited support for its role in unhealthy drug use, and no evidence that it is effective once someone has developed a SUD. For opioid use disorder, the gold standard treatment is opioid agonist therapy initiated in the ED; other interventions, such as a brief MI session followed by a naloxone kit or referral to treatment, are inferior. Initiating buprenorphine in the ED is associated with decreased illicit opioid use and improved treatment engagement compared to referral only,[43,44] but there can be barriers in terms of ED providers feeling ill-prepared to prescribe buprenorphine and having appropriate administrative support and patient follow-up.[45]

GAPS IN CARE

Despite evidence for the effectiveness of screening and BI, these tools remain underutilized.[46] Education on effective treatment for unhealthy alcohol and other substance use in ED and trauma settings, and skills training of staff and residents, can improve attitudes toward providing patient care and increase the frequency of screening and brief intervention.[47,48] The acute event which brings the patient with a substance problem into the hospital or ED can be an opportunity. In these high prevalence settings (ED, hospital, and trauma centers), patients should be screened for unhealthy substance use and should be counseled using a motivational approach to cut down or quit. Physicians can demonstrate an important leadership role within their own practice settings by advocating for universal screening for unhealthy substance use, by integrating screening into electronic medical record systems, and by incorporating screening and brief intervention training into resident physician education.[49]

REFERENCES

1. Guina J, Nahhas RW, Goldberg AJ, Farnsworth S. PTSD symptom severities, interpersonal traumas, and benzodiazepines are associated with substance-related problems in trauma patients. *J Clin Med.* 2016;5(8):70.
2. Isidro ML, Jorge S. Recreational drug abuse in patients hospitalized for diabetic ketosis or diabetic ketoacidosis. *Acta Diabetol.* 2013;50(2):183-187.
3. Hankin A, Daugherty M, Bethea A, Haley L. The emergency department as a prevention site: a demographic analysis of substance use among ED patients. *Drug Alcohol Depend.* 2013;130(1-3):230-233.
4. Lunetta P, Gordon S. The role of alcohol in injury deaths. In: Preedy V, Watson RR, eds. *Comprehensive Handbook of Alcohol Related Pathology.* Vol. 1. Elsevier; 2005:147-164.
5. Teeuw AH, Derkx BH, Koster WA, van Rijn RR. Educational paper: detection of child abuse and neglect at the emergency room. *Eur J Pediatr.* 2012;171(6):877-885.
6. Mahendraraj K, Durgan DM, Chamberlain RS. Acute mental disorders and short and long term morbidity in patients with third degree flame burn: a population-based outcome study of 96,451 patients from the Nationwide Inpatient Sample (NIS) Database (2001-2011). *Burns.* 2016;42(8):1766-1773.
7. Shei A, Rice JB, Kirson NY, et al. Characteristics of high-cost patients diagnosed with opioid abuse. *J Manag Care Spec Pharm.* 2015;21(10):902-912.
8. Gentilello LM, Rivara FP, Donovan DM, et al. Alcohol interventions in a trauma center as a means of reducing the risk of injury recurrence. *Ann Surg.* 1999;230(4):473-480; discussion 480-483.
9. Spirito A, Monti PM, Barnett NP, et al. A randomized clinical trial of a brief motivational intervention for alcohol-positive adolescents treated in an emergency department. *J Pediatr.* 2004;145(3):396-402.
10. Longabaugh R, Woolard RE, Nirenberg TD, et al. Evaluating the effects of a brief motivational intervention for injured drinkers in the emergency department. *J Stud Alcohol.* 2001;62(6):806-816.
11. Monti PM, Colby SM, Barnett NP, et al. Brief intervention for harm reduction with alcohol-positive older adolescents in a hospital emergency department. *J Consult Clin Psychol.* 1999;67(6):989-994.
12. Kodadek LM, Freeman JJ, Tiwary D. Alcohol-related trauma reinjury prevention with hospital-based screening in adult populations: an Eastern Association for the Surgery of Trauma evidence-based systematic review. *J Trauma Acute Care Surg.* 2020;88(1):106-112.
13. Bulger EM, Johnson P, Parker L, et al. Nationwide survey of trauma center screening and intervention practices for posttraumatic stress disorder, firearm violence, mental health, and substance use disorders. *J Am Coll Surg.* 2022;234(3):274-287.
14. Nilsen P, Baird J, Mello MJ, et al. A systematic review of emergency care brief alcohol interventions for injury patients. *J Subst Abuse Treat.* 2008;35(2):184-201.
15. Woodruff SI, Eisenberg K, McCabe CT, Clapp JD, Hohman M. Evaluation of California's alcohol and drug screening and brief intervention project for emergency department patients. *West J Emerg Med.* 2013;14(3):263-270.
16. Blow FC, Walton MA, Bohnert ASB, et al. A randomized controlled trial of brief interventions to reduce drug use among adults in a low-income urban emergency department: the HealthiER You study. *Addiction.* 2017;112(8):1395-1405.
17. Saitz R. Screening for unhealthy drug use. *JAMA.* 2020;323(22):2263.
18. Dunham CM, Chirichella TJ. Trauma activation patients: evidence for routine alcohol and illicit drug screening. *PLoS One.* 2012;7(10):e47999.
19. Williams FN, Chrisco L, Strassle PD, et al. Bias in alcohol and drug screening in adult burn patients. *Int J Burns Trauma.* 2020;10(4):146-155.
20. Bast RP, Helmer SD, Henson SR, Rogers MA, Shapiro WM, Smith RS. Limited utility of routine drug screening in trauma patients. *South Med J.* 2000;93(4):397-399.
21. Bahji A, Hargreaves T, Fitch S. Assessing the utility of drug screening in the emergency: a short report. *BMJ Open Qual.* 2018;7(4):e000414.
22. Azagba S, Shan L, Hall M, Wolfson M, Chaloupka F. Repeal of state laws permitting denial of health claims resulting from alcohol impairment: impact on treatment utilization. *Int J Drug Policy.* 2022;100:103530.
23. Sahota PK, Shastry S, Mukamel DB, et al. Screening emergency department patients for opioid drug use: a qualitative systematic review. *Addict Behav.* 2018;85:139-146.
24. Giguère CE, Potvin S; Signature Consortium. The Drug Abuse Screening Test preserves its excellent psychometric properties in psychiatric patients evaluated in an emergency setting. *Addict Behav.* 2017;64:165-170.

25. van der Westhuizen C, Wyatt G, Williams JK, Stein DJ, Sorsdahl K. Validation of the Alcohol, Smoking and Substance Involvement Screening Test in a low- and middle-income country cross-sectional emergency centre study. *Drug Alcohol Rev*. 2016;35(6):702-709.
26. Bae SJ, Kim E, Lee J. Validation of the screening test for at-risk drinking in an emergency department using a tablet computer. *Drug Alcohol Depend*. 2022;230:109181.
27. O'Brien H, di Rico R, Dean E, et al. Screening for risky drinkers among hospitalised inpatients using the AUDIT: a feasibility, point prevalence and data linkage study. *Drug Alcohol Rev*. 2022;41(1):293-302.
28. Reyes-Gibby CC, Anderson KO, Todd KH. Risk for opioid misuse among emergency department cancer patients. *Acad Emerg Med*. 2016;23(2):151-158.
29. Weiner S, Horton L, Green T, Butler SF. Feasibility of tablet computer screening for opioid abuse in the emergency department. *West J Emerg Med*. 2015;16(1):18-23.
30. Johnson JA, Woychek A, Vaughan D, Seale JP. Screening for at-risk alcohol use and drug use in an emergency department: integration of screening questions into electronic triage forms achieves high screening rates. *Ann Emerg Med*. 2013;62(3):262-266.
31. Choo E, Ranney M, Wetle T, et al. Attitudes toward computer interventions for partner abuse and drug use among women in the emergency department. *Addict Disord Their Treat*. 2015;14(2):95-104.
32. McNeely J, Marcy F, Smith JA, et al. Computer self-administered screening for substance use in a university health center: a feasibility pilot. *Addict Sci Clin Pract*. 2015;10(S2):O23.
33. Hankin A, Haley L, Baugher A, Colbert K, Houry D. Kiosk versus in-person screening for alcohol and drug use in the emergency department: patient preferences and disclosure. *West J Emerg Med*. 2015;16(2):220-228.
34. Choo EK, Ranney ML, Wong Z, Mello MJ. Attitudes toward technology-based health information among adult emergency department patients with drug or alcohol misuse. *J Subst Abuse Treat*. 2012;43(4):397-401.
35. Broyles LM, Gordon AJ. SBIRT implementation: moving beyond the interdisciplinary rhetoric. *Subst Abus*. 2010;31(4):221-223.
36. Saitz R. Candidate performance measures for screening for, assessing, and treating unhealthy substance use in hospitals: advocacy or evidence-based practice? *Ann Intern Med*. 2010;153(1):40-43.
37. Wakeman SE, Herman G, Wilens TE, Regan S. The prevalence of unhealthy alcohol and drug use among inpatients in a general hospital. *Subst Abus*. 2020;41(3):331-339.
38. Siegel R, Sullivan N, Monte AA, et al. Motivational interviewing to treat substance use disorders in the emergency department: a scoping review. *Am J Emerg Med*. 2022;51:414-417.
39. Kohler S, Hofmann A. Can motivational interviewing in emergency care reduce alcohol consumption in young people? A systematic review and meta-analysis. *Alcohol Alcohol*. 2015;50(2):107-117.
40. Barbosa C, McKnight-Eily LR, Grosse SD, Bray J. Alcohol screening and brief intervention in emergency departments: review of the impact on healthcare costs and utilization. *J Subst Abuse Treat*. 2020;117:108096.
41. Bonar EE, Cunningham RM, Sweezea EC, Blow FC, Drislane LE, Walton MA. Piloting a brief intervention plus mobile boosters for drug use among emerging adults receiving emergency department care. *Drug Alcohol Depend*. 2021;221:108625.
42. Field C, Walters S, Marti CN, Jun J, Foreman M, Brown C. A multisite randomized controlled trial of brief intervention to reduce drinking in the trauma care setting: how brief is brief? *Ann Surg*. 2014;259(5):873-880.
43. Kaczorowski J, Bilodeau J, Orkin A, Dong K, Daoust R, Kestler A. Emergency department–initiated interventions for patients with opioid use disorder: a systematic review. *Acad Emerg Med*. 2020;27(11):1173-1182.
44. D'Onofrio G, O'Connor PG, Pantalon MV, et al. Emergency department–initiated buprenorphine/naloxone treatment for opioid dependence. *JAMA*. 2015;313(16):1636-1644.
45. Im DD, Chary A, Condella AL, et al. Emergency department clinicians' attitudes toward opioid use disorder and emergency department-initiated buprenorphine treatment: a mixed-methods study. *West J Emerg Med*. 2020;21(2):261-271.
46. Broderick KB, Kaplan B, Martini D, Caruso E. Emergency physician utilization of alcohol/substance screening, brief advice and discharge: a 10-year comparison. *J Emerg Med*. 2015;49(4):400-407.
47. Seale JP, Clark DC, Dhabliwala J, et al. Impact of motivational interviewing-based training in screening, brief intervention, and referral to treatment on residents' self-reported attitudes and behaviors. *Addict Sci Clin Pract*. 2013;8(S1):A71.
48. Lukowitsky MR, Balkoski VI, Bromley N, Gallagher PA. The effects of screening brief intervention referral to treatment (SBIRT) training on health professional trainees' regard, attitudes, and beliefs toward patients who use substances. *Subst Abus*. 2022;43(1):397-407.
49. Seale JP, Shellenberger S, Clark DC. Providing competency-based family medicine residency training in substance abuse in the new millennium: a model curriculum. *BMC Med Educ*. 2010;10:33.

Sidebar 3

Implementation of Screening and Brief Intervention in Clinical Settings Using Quality Improvement Principles

Emily C. Williams and Katharine A. Bradley

Despite evidence-based recommendations that alcohol screening and brief intervention (SBI) and screening for unhealthy drug use be routinely implemented in primary care settings,[1-4] efforts to implement SBI have thus far been met with barriers at multiple levels. For instance, stigma and the related historic view of substance use as outside the purview of medicine have resulted in: the relative neglect of discussions about alcohol and other drug use in medical settings; health systems that failed to develop electronic health records with prompts and support for documentation of SBI; and inadequate training regarding alcohol and other substance use for clinicians that do not specialize in addictions.[5,6]

Implementation science frameworks and quality improvement principles and practices can serve as helpful guides for addressing these barriers. For instance, Greenhalgh's comprehensive conceptual model of dissemination of innovations in health care settings (**Fig. 31-1**)[7] outlines the importance of the nature of an *innovation* (eg, SBI), as well as the characteristics of both the *user system* (ie, clinics, clinic administrators, primary care providers, and nursing and other staff) and *innovators* (eg, researchers) and the *linkage* between the two.[7] *Innovations* are more likely to be successfully implemented if they are simple, relevant to the user, and easily transferable to the clinic setting. The setting in which implementation occurs—the *user system*—is also central to the success of innovations. Important components of *user systems* that help determine the success of innovations include system antecedents (eg, quality improvement processes, such as performance feedback and "Plan Do Study Act" [PDSA] cycles), system readiness (eg, institutional pressures for change), characteristics of adopters (eg, motivation, values, understanding of the innovation), the implementation process (eg, support from leadership, practice facilitation), and evaluation and feedback that allows the system to address consequences of implementation—both successes and failures—and iterative adaptation to improve implementation. *Innovators* typically consist of formal or informal "teams" of experts ("knowledge purveyors") and leaders able to actualize change with access to resources required to implement an innovation ("change agents"). Efforts to implement innovations are also most successful when there is strong *linkage* between the innovators and the user system, both during the development of an innovation and throughout the implementation process.

REAL WORLD APPLICATION

Some integrated health care systems (eg, the Veterans Health Administration [VA] and Kaiser Permanente [KP]), as well as some clinics engaged in pragmatic trials,[8-11] have made substantial progress toward implementation of SBI for unhealthy alcohol use and screening for drug use. For the purposes of real-world application of these quality improvement principles, we provide a retrospective analysis of the VA's implementation of alcohol SBI based on Greenhalgh's model (see **Fig. 31-1**), and briefly review efforts to implement SBI and additional follow-up care for both alcohol and drug use in other systems and clinics.

Prior to alcohol SBI implementation, the VA had undergone several quality improvement initiatives, which served as system antecedents providing an essential foundation for alcohol SBI implementation.[12] These included a nationwide electronic medical record (EMR) with embedded electronic clinical reminders, data systems (medical record reviews and patient satisfaction surveys) to monitor performance, and a system of nationwide performance feedback that incentivized recommended care with links to financial incentives for network directors. At the time, the VA also had condition-specific Quality Enhancement Research Initiative centers,[13] including one focused on substance use disorders (the SUD QUERI). These centers developed research programs to identify important gaps in the quality of VA clinical care, build strong partnerships with clinical leaders, and develop and iteratively evaluate and improve interventions to address identified gaps.

Findings from the VA's Large Health Study of Veterans—indicating VA patients who drank four or more drinks daily were not getting the help they wanted for their drinking—created pressure for VA leadership to do more to recognize and treat unhealthy alcohol use, and served as the impetus for *linkage* between VA clinical operations and quality improvement managers and SUD QUERI researchers. Via this linkage, the VA built upon its existing quality improvement structures to implement national performance measures for and electronic clinical reminders to prompt and document both screening and brief intervention (initially developed and piloted with research funding).[14-17] The QUERI infrastructure provided ongoing core funding for implementation research. However, local implementation and clinician education regarding SBI was delegated to local quality and clinical leaders without active front line clinician support. Initially, the QUERI infrastructure—with a rapid grant-funding mechanism coupled with core funding—enabled formative evaluations that identified gaps in SBI quality.[18,19] Formative evaluations highlighted the importance of ongoing attention to the educational needs of clinicians ("adopters") and feedback to clinicians regarding performance, as well as several gaps in equity (ie, disparities) in care offered and received.

Unfortunately, changes in the QUERI infrastructure, including discontinuing condition-specific funding for implementation research (and thus closing the substance use disorders QUERI center), decreased ease of ongoing SUD-focused quality improvement research. Fortunately, recent new linkages between operational leaders and clinicians are facilitating renewed focus on quality improvement (eg, a SUD Disparities Workgroup). Additionally, the VA, the Agency for Healthcare Research and Quality (AHRQ), and the National Institutes of Health (NIH) have supported ongoing research, which continues to address best practices, quality improvement, and performance measures that incentivize high-quality SBI, collaborative care, and equity.[20,21] In addition, ongoing innovation in SBI implementation and its evaluation has been supported by the Affordable Care Act, national performance measures developed by the National Committee for Quality Assurance (NCQA),[22,23] large scale demonstration projects and learning collaboratives funded by the AHRQ, the Centers for Disease Control and Prevention (CDC), and the Substance Abuse Mental Health Services Administration. Recently, increasing legalization and access to cannabis, the overdose epidemic, and the racial reckoning in response to the murders of George Floyd, Breonna, Taylor, Ahmaud Arbery, and others, have spurred further substance use related quality improvement work, importantly with increased focus on equity.[24,25]

Quality improvement processes used in the VA were subsequently used and improved in other health care systems—such as

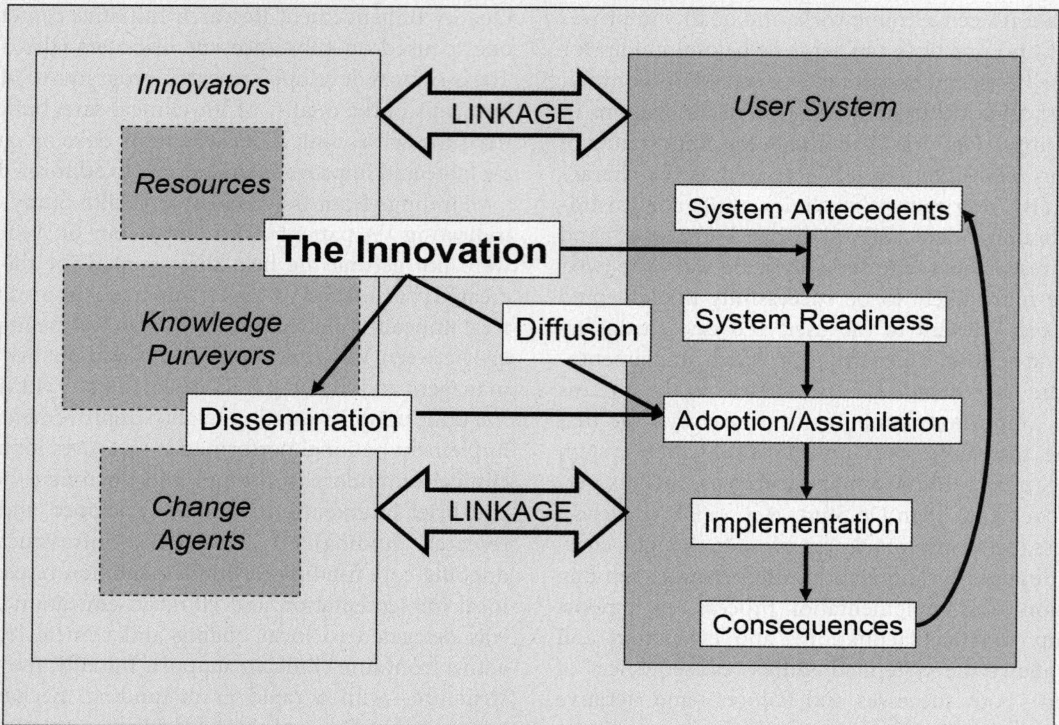

Figure 31-1. Factors that influence the success of implementation. (Adaptation of Greenhalgh Model of Diffusion of Innovations in Service Organisations. *Milbank Q.* 2004;82:581-692.)

KP. KP Northern California implemented screening for alcohol use as a "vital sign" to increase alcohol SBI in the ADVISE trial. This was supported by robust training of primary care providers, and demonstrated that primary care *screening* was best conducted by staff who room patients (eg, nurses or health techs), whereas *BI* is optimally provided by primary care providers.[26] Subsequent efforts in KP Washington used similar processes as the VA, with the addition of clinical tools targeting stigma and practice facilitation, a proven approach to primary care quality improvement.[27,28] KP Washington also implemented alcohol SBI, along with screening for depression, cannabis, and other drugs (another partnership between AHRQ-funded researchers and clinical operations leaders),[20] and used a practical, and now validated DSM-5 alcohol symptom checklist to engage patients in patient-centered discussions of alcohol use disorder symptoms, with linkage to integrated mental health clinicians or treatment, as desired.[29,30] KP Washington used patient report on paper or via an online portal for screening and assessment,[20] consistent with results from the VA,[19] KP Washington,[31,32] and another study from the NIDA Clinical Trials Network,[33] which support self-screening for patients (on paper or tablets) due to quality issues that arise when asking substance use screening questions verbally in primary care. Finally, multiple new and ongoing SUD implementation efforts in emergency departments,[34,35] hospitals,[36,37] and new primary care settings, such as Federally Qualified Health Centers,[8,9,38-41] are addressing the opioid overdose epidemics, and increasingly focused on evaluating and improving equity in SUD care.

In summary, stigma and related historic views and structures serve as ongoing barriers to implementing recommended best practices for alcohol screening and brief intervention and drug use screening, and these "structural barriers" trickle down into health care systems, clinicians, and users. However, implementation science frameworks and strategies and quality improvement principles can help health care systems and clinics design structural solutions that address barriers and facilitate implementation of high-quality care for individuals with unhealthy substance use.

REFERENCES

1. Jonas DE, Garbutt JC, Amick HR, et al. Behavioral counseling after screening for alcohol misuse in primary care: a systematic review and meta-analysis for the U.S. Preventive Services Task Force. *Ann Intern Med.* 2012;157(9):645-654.
2. National Institute for Health and Care Excellence. *Alcohol Use Disorders: Diagnosis, Assessment and Management of Harmful Drinking and Alcohol Dependence.* National Institute for Health and Care Excellence; 2015.
3. Curry SJ, Krist AH, Owens DK, et al. Screening and behavioral counseling interventions to reduce unhealthy alcohol use in adolescents and adults: US Preventive Services Task Force Recommendation Statement. *JAMA.* 2018;320(18):1899-1909.
4. Krist AH, Davidson KW, Mangione CM, et al. Screening for Unhealthy Drug Use: US Preventive Services Task Force Recommendation Statement. *JAMA.* 2020;323(22):2301-2309.
5. Williams EC, Johnson ML, Lapham GT, et al. Strategies to implement alcohol screening and brief intervention in primary care settings: a structured literature review. *Psychol Addict Behav.* 2011;25(2):206-214.

6. Chan PS, Fang Y, Wong MC, Huang J, Wang Z, Yeoh EK. Using Consolidated Framework for Implementation Research to investigate facilitators and barriers of implementing alcohol screening and brief intervention among primary care health professionals: a systematic review. *Implement Sci.* 2021;16(1):99.
7. Greenhalgh T, Robert G, Macfarlane F, Bate P, Kyriakidou O. Diffusion of innovations in service organizations: systematic review and recommendations. *Milbank Q.* 2004;82(4):581-629.
8. Austin EJ, Briggs ES, Ferro L, et al. Integrating routine screening for opioid use disorder into primary care settings: experiences from a national cohort of clinics. *J Gen Intern Med.* 2022;1-9.
9. Campbell CI, Saxon AJ, Boudreau DM, et al. PRimary Care Opioid Use Disorders treatment (PROUD) trial protocol: a pragmatic, cluster-randomized implementation trial in primary care for opioid use disorder treatment. *Addict Sci Clin Pract.* 2021;16(1):9.
10. McNeely J, Adam A, Rotrosen J, et al. Comparison of methods for alcohol and drug screening in primary care clinics. *JAMA Netw Open.* 2021;4(5):e2110721.
11. McNeely J, Troxel AB, Kunins HV, et al. Study protocol for a pragmatic trial of the Consult for Addiction Treatment and Care in Hospitals (CATCH) model for engaging patients in opioid use disorder treatment. *Addict Sci Clin Pract.* 2019;14(1):5.
12. Young GJ, Charns MP, Barbour GL. Quality improvement in the US Veterans Health Administration. *Int J Qual Health Care.* 1997;9(3):183-188.
13. Stetler CB, Mittman BS, Francis J. Overview of the VA Quality Enhancement Research Initiative (QUERI) and QUERI theme articles: QUERI Series. *Implement Sci.* 2008;3:8.
14. Bradley KA, Williams EC, Achtmeyer CE, Volpp B, Collins BJ, Kivlahan DR. Implementation of evidence-based alcohol screening in the Veterans Health Administration. *Am J Manag Care.* 2006;12(10):597-606.
15. Williams EC, Lapham G, Achtmeyer CE, Volpp B, Kivlahan DR, Bradley KA. Use of an electronic clinical reminder for brief alcohol counseling is associated with resolution of unhealthy alcohol use at follow-up screening. *J Gen Intern Med.* 2010;25(Suppl 1):11-17.
16. Williams EC, Achtmeyer CE, Kivlahan DR, et al. Evaluation of an electronic clinical reminder to facilitate brief alcohol-counseling interventions in primary care. *J Stud Alcohol Drugs.* 2010;71(5):720-725.
17. Lapham GT, Achtmeyer CE, Williams EC, Hawkins EJ, Kivlahan DR, Bradley KA. Increased documented brief alcohol interventions with a performance measure and electronic decision support. *Med Care.* 2012;50(2):179-187.
18. Williams EC, Achtmeyer CE, Young JP, et al. Local implementation of alcohol screening and brief intervention at five Veterans Health Administration primary care clinics: perspectives of clinical and administrative staff. *J Subst Abuse Treat.* 2016;60:27-35.
19. Williams EC, Achtmeyer CE, Thomas RM, et al. Factors underlying quality problems with alcohol screening prompted by a clinical reminder in primary care: a multi-site qualitative study. *J Gen Intern Med.* 2015;30(8):1125-1132.
20. Glass JE, Bobb JF, Lee AK, et al. Study protocol: a cluster-randomized trial implementing Sustained Patient-centered Alcohol-related Care (SPARC trial). *Implement Sci.* 2018;13(1):108.
21. Sterling S, Kline-Simon AH, Satre DD, et al. Implementation of screening, brief intervention, and referral to treatment for adolescents in pediatric primary care: a cluster randomized trial. *JAMA pediatrics.* 2015;169(11):e153145.
22. Hepner KA, Watkins KE, Farmer CM, Rubenstein L, Pedersen ER, Pincus HA. Quality of care measures for the management of unhealthy alcohol use. *J Subst Abuse Treat.* 2017;76:11-17.
23. National Committee for Quality Assurance. *HEDIS Measure: Unhealthy Alcohol Use Screening and Follow-Up.* Accessed October 17, 2022. https://www.ncqa.org/hedis/reports-and-research/hedis-measure-unhealthy-alcohol-use-screening-and-follow-up/
24. Blanco C, Kato EU, Aklin WM, et al. Research to move policy - using evidence to advance health equity for substance use disorders. *N Engl J Med.* 2022;386(24):2253-2255.
25. Burlew K, McCuistian C, Szapocznik J. Racial/ethnic equity in substance use treatment research: the way forward. *Addict Sci Clin Pract.* 2021;16(1):50.
26. Mertens JR, Chi FW, Weisner CM, et al. Physician versus non-physician delivery of alcohol screening, brief intervention and referral to treatment in adult primary care: the ADVISe cluster randomized controlled implementation trial. *Addict Sci Clin Pract.* 2015;10(1):26.
27. Baskerville NB, Liddy C, Hogg W. Systematic review and meta-analysis of practice facilitation within primary care settings. *Ann Fam Med.* 2012;10(1):63-74.
28. Ritchie MJ, Dollar KM, Miller CJ, et al. *Using Implementation Facilitation to Improve Care in the Veterans Health Administration (Version 2).* Veterans Health Administration, Quality Enhancement Research Initiative (QUERI) for Team-Based Behavioral Health Accessed February 20, 2020. https://www.queri.research.va.gov/tools/Facilitation-Manual.pdf
29. Hallgren KA, Matson TE, Oliver M, et al. Practical assessment of alcohol use disorder in routine primary care: performance of an alcohol symptom checklist. *J Gen Intern Med.* 2022;37:1885-1893.
30. Hallgren KA, Matson TE, Oliver M, Caldeiro RM, Kivlahan DR, Bradley KA. Practical assessment of DSM-5 alcohol use disorder criteria in routine care: high test-retest reliability of an Alcohol Symptom Checklist. *Alcohol Clin Exp Res.* 2022;46(3):458-467.
31. Bobb JF, Lee AK, Lapham GT, et al. Evaluation of a pilot implementation to integrate alcohol-related care within primary care. *Int J Environ Res Public Health.* 2017;14(9):1030.
32. Richards JE, Bobb JF, Lee AK, et al. Integration of screening, assessment, and treatment for cannabis and other drug use disorders in primary care: an evaluation in three pilot sites. *Drug Alcohol Depend.* 2019;201:134-141.
33. McNeely J, Kumar PC, Rieckmann T, et al. Barriers and facilitators affecting the implementation of substance use screening in primary care clinics: a qualitative study of patients, providers, and staff. *Addict Sci Clin Pract.* 2018;13(1):8.
34. D'Onofrio G, Edelman EJ, Hawk KF, et al. Implementation facilitation to promote emergency department-initiated buprenorphine for opioid use disorder: protocol for a hybrid type III effectiveness-implementation study (Project ED HEALTH). *Implement Sci.* 2019;14(1):48.
35. D'Onofrio G, Pantalon MV, Degutis LC, Fiellin DA, O'Connor PG. Development and implementation of an emergency practitioner-performed brief intervention for hazardous and harmful drinkers in the emergency department. *Acad Emerg Med.* 2005;12(3):249-256.
36. Weinstein ZM, Wakeman SE, Nolan S. Inpatient addiction consult service: expertise for hospitalized patients with complex addiction problems. *Medical Clinics.* 2018;102(4):587-601.
37. Wakeman SE, Metlay JP, Chang Y, Herman GE, Rigotti NA. Inpatient addiction consultation for hospitalized patients increases post-discharge abstinence and reduces addiction severity. *J Gen Intern Med.* 2017;32(8):909-916.
38. Fortney J. *Collaborating to Heal Addiction and Mental Health in Primary Care (CHAMP).* 1UF1MH121942-01. National Institute of Mental Health (NIMH); 2020.
39. Bart GB, Saxon A, Fiellin DA, et al. Developing a clinical decision support for opioid use disorders: a NIDA center for the clinical trials network working group report. Accessed August 7, 2023. https://ascpjournal.biomedcentral.com/counter/pdf/10.1186/s13722-020-0180-2.pdf
40. Rossom RC, Sperl-Hillen JM, O'Connor PJ, et al. A pilot study of the functionality and clinician acceptance of a clinical decision support tool to improve primary care of opioid use disorder. *Addict Sci Clin Pract.* 2021;16(1):1-11.
41. Hawkins EJ, Williams EC. *The SUpporting Primary care Providers in Opioid Risk reduction and Treatment (SUPPORT) Center.* Patient Safety Center of Inquiry, VHA National Center for Patient Safety; 2018.

Sidebar 4

Screening for Unhealthy Alcohol and Drug Use in Older Adults

Jennifer McNeely and Benjamin Han

EPIDEMIOLOGY

The number of older adults is estimated to continue to increase in the United States (U.S.) and by 2030, one of every five Americans is projected to be 65 years of age or older. While older adults have lower prevalence of psychoactive substance use compared to younger adults, with the aging of the Baby Boomer cohort, this prevalence has increased sharply over the past two decades. The combination of the aging of the population and increasing use of substances has created a growing public health problem: increasing numbers of older adults at risk for and experiencing unhealthy substance use, including substance use disorders (SUDs).

Table 31-5 shows recent national prevalence estimates of substance use from the National Survey on Drug Use and Health (NSDUH) among adults age 65 and over in 2019. Alcohol continues to be the most commonly used substance among older adults in the United States, and rates of high-risk drinking and alcohol use disorders have been increasing in recent years.[1,2] Tobacco is the second most used substance in this population.[2] While over the last decade cigarette smoking rates have gone down in the general adult population, they have remained relatively stable in older adults.[3] Finally, cannabis use has increased substantially among older adults; the prevalence of past-year cannabis use among adults age 65 and over was estimated to be 0.4% in 2006 and rose to 5.0% by 2019.[4] While NSDUH estimates nonalcohol or tobacco SUDs among older adults to be low, at less than 0.5%, there have been dramatic increases in harms related to substance use among older adults. The number of drug-related deaths (not including alcohol as the sole cause) in the United States among adults aged 65 and over increased from 528 in 1999 to 4,132 in 2020.[5] The United States has also experienced increases in opioid-related inpatient hospitalizations and emergency department visits and first-time SUD treatment admissions among older adults.[6,7]

TABLE 31-5 Prevalence Estimates of Psychoactive Substance Use Among Adults Age 65 and Older, United States, 2019

Substance	Prevalence in past year
Alcohol	
Any use	55.9%
Binge drinking	11.1%
Alcohol use disorder	2.0%
Tobacco use	12.5%
Cannabis use	5.0%
Psychoactive prescription drug use (nonmedical)	2.1%
Illicit drug use other than cannabis	2.6%

Source: Substance Abuse and Mental Health Services Administration. *Key substance use and mental health indicators in the United States: Results from the 2019 National Survey on Drug Use and Health (HHS Publication No. PEP20-07-01-001, NSDUH Series H-55).* Center for Behavioral Health Statistics and Quality, SAMHSA; 2019. Accessed May 15, 2022. https://www.samhsa.gov/data.

UNIQUE VULNERABILITIES TO THE HARMS OF ALCOHOL AND DRUG USE IN OLDER ADULTS

Aging affects drug and alcohol metabolism and distribution in the body. The liver and kidneys' ability to metabolize alcohol, psychoactive drugs, and medications decreases. Changes in brain structure and function (eg, diminished white matter and increased permeability of the blood-brain barrier) can increase sensitivity to the psychoactive effects of substances. Body composition also changes, with decreases in lean body mass and total body water while total body fat increases. Because alcohol is water-soluble, older adults who drink a given amount of alcohol have a higher blood alcohol level compared to younger adults who drink the same amount. Drugs that are fat-soluble, such as benzodiazepines, have a longer duration of action in older adults compared to younger adults. Therefore, substances with long half-lives, such as diazepam, can be excessively sedating. All of these factors result in older adults who consume a variety of substances having more significant risk of impairment, lower tolerance, and less awareness of their impairment than younger adults. This contributes to an increased risk of harm including confusion, falls, intoxicated driving, injuries, impaired functioning, and an increased risk for substance use-related emergency visits, hospitalizations, and nursing home admissions.[8]

Older adults are also vulnerable to the harms of substance use, as even low levels or one-time use of substances has the potential to exacerbate existing comorbidities and contribute to new conditions. Substances can worsen symptoms of insomnia (eg, alcohol, stimulants) and memory impairment (eg, benzodiazepines). They can also interact with many medications, increase medication side effects, or lessen their efficacy. These interactions are magnified when multiple substances are used. Other factors that increase risks for harm among older adults are the relatively common practice of seeing multiple medical providers, each of whom may prescribe medications without full knowledge of other medications that are being prescribed, which may be in addition to over the counter and nonmedication substances being used by the older adult. Screening for alcohol and drug use when older adults present for medical care could thus reduce the risk of medication interactions and identify patients who might benefit from substance use interventions.

APPROACH TO SCREENING, ASSESSMENT, AND DIAGNOSIS OF ALCOHOL AND DRUG USE IN OLDER ADULTS

Older adults are included in the United States Preventive Services Task Force (USPSTF) recommendations to screen adult primary care patients for both alcohol and drug use.[9,10] Yet despite the longstanding USPSTF endorsement of alcohol screening, rates of screening and counseling for alcohol remain suboptimal for older adults. One quarter of older adults who had a health care encounter in the past year were never screened or had a discussion with a medical provider about alcohol use.[11] While this represents a substantial improvement from prior decades,[12] improving screening and interventions for older adults remains important given the elevated risks of unhealthy alcohol and drug use in this population.

Screening Tools

For the purpose of this overview, screening refers to the use of standardized questionnaires to ask patients about their substance use. Because screening depends on collecting precise self-reported information from patients, validated screening questionnaires should be used, and the questions need to be delivered exactly as they were validated. Although lab tests may detect the presence of substances used very recently, (typically hours or a few days after the last use), these tests do not provide the information about quantity, frequency, or problems related to use that is needed to inform care. One exception is for patients who are prescribed medications such as benzodiazepines or opioids that pose a risk for drug-related harms or nonmedical use. In this circumstance, toxicology testing may be a useful tool for monitoring adherence and assessing for use of nonprescribed drugs.

A number of brief questionnaires have been validated and can be recommended for alcohol and drug screening in medical settings. Older adults have been included in validation studies of screening tools, though most studies have not reported results specifically for this subgroup. One of the few screening tools developed specifically for older adults is the Comorbidity Alcohol Risk Evaluation Tool (CARET), which includes items about common medications and medical conditions that could interact with alcohol, to further characterize the risky nature of alcohol use in this population. However, the performance of the CARET for identifying unhealthy alcohol use or alcohol use disorder has not been examined.[13] There is reason for concern as some studies that analyzed screening tool performance in adults age 50 and older have found lower sensitivity in this age group than in younger participants.[14,15]

While better evidence is needed to guide the selection of screening tools for older adults, in the meantime a practical approach is to rely on the same screening instruments that are used for other adult patients. It is generally recommended that screening questions that involve asking about alcohol consumption above the recommended limits (eg, single-item screening question for alcohol) should use the lower cutoff (4+ drinks daily, 7+ drinks weekly) for all adults 65 or older, regardless of sex.[10]

Approach to Administering Screening

In most populations, self-administered screening approaches (paper-based or electronic) are generally recommended over staff-administered screening. Self-administered screening can increase patient comfort and facilitate more accurate reporting,[16-18] while ensuring fidelity,[19-21] and reducing the burden on clinical staff. However, older adults may need more time and assistance with completing a self-administered screener when it is delivered electronically.[22]

Diagnosis

For patients who screen positive with a screening score or clinical presentation suggesting high-risk or daily use, further assessment is needed to determine the severity of unhealthy use and presence of a SUD. It can be challenging for geriatric or generalist practitioners to conduct a diagnostic interview during a routine visit, due to limited time or training. Symptom checklists (utilizing *Diagnostic and Statistical Manual of Mental Disorders* [DSM] criteria) have been developed that can reduce barriers and are increasingly being used in clinical care, including for older adults, though their performance and feasibility has primarily been studied in younger populations.[21,23-25]

Whether assessment is done by checklist or diagnostic interview, it is important to recognize that specific social and biological factors unique to older adults may pose challenges in the accurate diagnosis of SUDs. Symptoms of alcohol or drug use disorders in older adults may be attributed to aging or to diseases common in geriatric patients rather than substance use. Frequently, the SUD may present as a new medical diagnosis or an exacerbation of a chronic medical condition. Neurocognitive impairment, already common in this population, is worsened by excessive drinking. It is estimated that as many as 10% of patients with diagnosed Alzheimer disease may have alcohol-associated dementia, or a dementia presentation worsened by alcohol consumption.[26] **Table 31-6** reviews diseases common among older adults in which alcohol is a

TABLE 31-6 Conditions That Can Be Caused by Substance Use, and May Be Attributed to Common Coexisting Diseases in Older Adults

Depression
Delirium
Chronic fatigue
Seizures
Repeated infections
Hypertension
Malnutrition
Peripheral neuropathy
Sexual dysfunction
Cardiomyopathy

possible etiological factor or a significant contributor to worsening disease.

Diagnosis may be further challenged by DSM criteria that include consequences that are less likely to occur in older adults, including failure to meet obligations at home, school, or work, and problems with significant others. Due to the physiological and biological changes of aging that may increase the effects of substances, older adults generally experience a reduction of tolerance as they age—eliminating one of the hallmarks of DSM-5 criteria for SUDs. Given the diagnostic challenges, many older adults are "diagnostic orphans"; individuals who qualify for only one diagnostic criterion for SUD and are therefore subthreshold.[27]

In summary, when considering strategies for identifying unhealthy alcohol and drug use in older adults, clinicians should adopt an age-sensitive approach, including (1) distinguishing symptoms of alcohol or drug use disorder from other age-related conditions; (2) understanding that stigma and social isolation may delay or obscure the recognition of unhealthy substance use, and (3) adapting screening to meet the needs of this population, including by using the recommended lower cutoffs for alcohol consumption, and being prepared to offer assistance with self-administered screening tools.

INTERVENTIONS TO REDUCE UNHEALTHY ALCOHOL AND DRUG USE IN OLDER ADULTS

Brief Interventions

The USPSTF recommends alcohol screening followed by brief counseling in primary care, based on a large evidence base supporting brief interventions for unhealthy alcohol use in general adult primary care populations.[28] While there is limited evidence on brief interventions in older adults, alcohol brief intervention does appear to be effective in reducing alcohol consumption (number of drinks per week).[28] Project GOAL, conducted in parallel to Project TrEAT and based on similar methodology, showed that brief intervention can decrease self-reported alcohol use, including drinks per week and heavy drinking episodes, among older primary care patients with unhealthy alcohol use.[29] Two subsequent large trials of primary care provider-delivered alcohol brief intervention in older adults also showed reductions in alcohol consumption,[30,31] and one additionally found reductions in emergency department visits.[30]

With respect to drugs other than alcohol, no trial has been designed to assess effectiveness of interventions for substance use specifically in older adults.[32] Because the effectiveness of brief interventions for reducing substance use has not been established for adults of any age, the drug screening recommendation includes the qualifier that "screening should be implemented when services for accurate diagnosis, effective treatment, and appropriate care can be offered or referred."[9,33] Most primary care practices should have the capacity to offer this care, as they do for other complex conditions.[34] Namely, before screening the primary practice should be prepared to assess the severity of use (which can be done with standardized questionnaires), and offer treatment or refer to specialty care for patients who are found to have a SUD or to be at high risk.

Treatment of Substance Use Disorders

All older adults who meet the criteria for SUD should be offered evidence-based treatment and harm reduction interventions. As detailed elsewhere in this textbook, medications can be used in conjunction with or without psychosocial interventions to treat SUD, and have a strong evidence base for opioid use disorder, alcohol use disorder, and tobacco use disorder. Despite a robust evidence base for the benefit of several pharmacological treatments for SUDs, such treatments are severely underutilized, especially among older adults.[35] Although overall the benefits of SUD treatment seem to extend to older adults, because they are underrepresented in clinical trials, we must often extrapolate data from research on younger adult populations. However, due to higher risks for complications and adverse effects, older adults should be carefully monitored when initiating pharmacologic treatments for SUD. As such, older adults often require inpatient or closely monitored specialty care for alcohol or benzodiazepine withdrawal management. Harm reduction interventions, including overdose education and naloxone distribution, should also be offered to older adults.

SUMMARY

The use of psychoactive substances continues to increase among older adults and may present challenges for clinicians managing patients with multiple chronic diseases or serious illnesses. Screening for substance use in older adults can be challenging, and providers must consider unique aspects of aging to detect unhealthy use including physiological changes, social roles, and functional status. Most research on substance use among older adults focuses solely on alcohol and nicotine, as historically other psychoactive drug use was infrequent. Yet with the increase in substance use (including cannabis and nonmedical use of prescription medications), as well as related harms from unhealthy alcohol and drug use, more representation of older adults in substance use screening and intervention research is needed. Older adults with unhealthy substance use and SUD should be offered evidence-based treatment and harm reduction services, which may require adaptations and additional supports to optimally support this population.

ACKNOWLEDGMENTS

The authors acknowledge the contribution of James W. Campbell to the earlier version of the textbook.

REFERENCES

1. Grant BF, Chou SP, Saha TD, et al. Prevalence of 12-month alcohol use, high-risk drinking, and DSM-IV alcohol use disorder in the united states, 2001-2002 to 2012-2013: results from the national epidemiologic survey on alcohol and related conditions. *JAMA Psychiatry.* 2017;74(9):911-923.
2. Substance Abuse and Mental Health Services Administration. *Key substance use and mental health indicators in the United States: Results from the 2019 National Survey on Drug Use and Health (HHS Publication No. PEP20-07-01-001, NSDUH Series H-55).* SAMHSA; 2019.
3. Kleykamp BA, Heishman SJ. The older smoker. *JAMA.* 2011;306(8):876-877.
4. Han BH, Palamar JJ. Trends in cannabis use among older adults in the United States, 2015-2018. *JAMA Intern Med.* 2020;180(4):609-611.
5. National Center for Health Statistics. Multiple cause of death 1999-2019. *CDC WONDER Online Database.* Center for Disease Control and Prevention; 2022.
6. Weiss AJ, Heslin KC, Barrett ML, Izar R, Bierman AS. Opioid-related inpatient stays and emergency department visits among patients aged 65 years and older, 2010 and 2015: statistical brief #244. *Healthcare Cost and Utilization Project (HCUP) Statistical Briefs.* Agency for Healthcare Research and Quality; 2006.
7. Huhn AS, Strain EC, Tompkins DA, Dunn KE. A hidden aspect of the U.S. opioid crisis: rise in first-time treatment admissions for older adults with opioid use disorder. *Drug Alcohol Depend.* 2018;193:142-147.
8. Kuerbis A. Substance use among older adults: an update on prevalence, etiology, assessment, and intervention. *Gerontology.* 2020;66(3):249-258.
9. US Preventive Services Task Force. Screening for unhealthy drug use: US Preventive Services Task Force Recommendation Statement. *JAMA.* 2020;323(22):2301-2309.
10. US Preventive Services Task Force. Screening and behavioral counseling interventions to reduce unhealthy alcohol use in adolescents and adults: US Preventive Services Task Force Recommendation Statement. *JAMA.* 2018;320(18):1899-1909.
11. Mauro PM, Askari MS, Han BH. Gender differences in any alcohol screening and discussions with providers among older adults in the United States, 2015 to 2019. *Alcohol Clin Exp Res.* 2021;45(9):1812-1820.
12. Curtis JR, Geller G, Stokes EJ, Levine DM, Moore RD. Characteristics, diagnosis, and treatment of alcoholism in elderly patients. *J Am Geriatr Soc.* 1989;37(4):310-316.
13. Patnode CD, Perdue LA, Rushkin M, O'Connor EA. *Screening for Unhealthy Drug Use in Primary Care in Adolescents and Adults, Including Pregnant Persons: Updated Systematic Review for the U.S. Preventive Services Task Force.* Evidence Synthesis No. 186. Agency for Healthcare Research and Quality; 2020.
14. Beaudoin FL, Merchant RC, Clark MA. Prevalence and detection of prescription opioid misuse and prescription opioid use disorder among emergency department patients 50 years of age and older: performance of the Prescription Drug Use Questionnaire. *Patient Version. Am J Geriatr Psychiatry.* 2016;24(8):627-636.
15. McNeely J, Cleland CM, Strauss SM, Palamar JJ, Rotrosen J, Saitz R. Validation of self-administered Single-Item Screening Questions (SISQs) for unhealthy alcohol and drug use in primary care patients. *J Gen Intern Med.* 2015;30(12):1757-1764.
16. Tourangeau R, Smith TW. Asking sensitive questions: the impact of data collection mode, question format, and question context. *Public Opin Q.* 1996;60(2):275-304.
17. Spear SE, Shedlin M, Gilberti B, Fiellin M, McNeely J. Feasibility and acceptability of an audio computer-assisted self-interview version of the Alcohol, Smoking and Substance Involvement Screening Test (ASSIST) in primary care patients. *Subst Abus.* 2016;37(2):299-305.
18. McNeely J, Kumar PC, Rieckmann T, et al. Barriers and facilitators affecting the implementation of substance use screening in primary care clinics: a qualitative study of patients, providers, and staff. *Addict Sci Clin Pract.* 2018;13(1):8.
19. Bradley KA, Lapham GT, Hawkins EJ, et al. Quality concerns with routine alcohol screening in VA clinical settings. *J Gen Intern Med.* 2011;26(3):299-306.
20. Williams EC, Achtmeyer CE, Thomas RM, et al. Factors underlying quality problems with alcohol screening prompted by a clinical reminder in primary care: a multi-site qualitative study. *J Gen Intern Med.* 2015;30(8):1125-1132.
21. Bradley KA, Lapham GT, Lee AK. Screening for drug use in primary care: practical implications of the new USPSTF recommendation. *JAMA Internal Medicine.* 2020;180(8):1050-1051.
22. Adam A, Schwartz RP, Wu LT, et al. Electronic self-administered screening for substance use in adult primary care patients: feasibility and acceptability of the tobacco, alcohol, prescription medication, and other substance use (myTAPS) screening tool. *Addict Sci Clin Pract.* 2019;14(1):39.
23. Hallgren KA, Matson TE, Oliver M, Caldeiro RM, Kivlahan DR, Bradley KA. Practical assessment of DSM-5 alcohol use disorder criteria in routine care: high test-retest reliability of an Alcohol Symptom Checklist. *Alcohol Clin Exp Res.* 2022;46(3):458-467.
24. Hallgren KA, Matson TE, Oliver M, et al. Practical assessment of alcohol use disorder in routine primary care: performance of an alcohol symptom checklist. *J Gen Intern Med.* 2022;37(8):1885-1893.
25. Sayre M, Lapham GT, Lee AK, et al. Routine assessment of symptoms of substance use disorders in primary care: prevalence and severity of reported symptoms. *J Gen Intern Med.* 2020;35(4):1111-1119.
26. Meldon S, Ma J, Woolard R. *Geriatric Emergency Medicine.* New York: McGraw-Hill Medical Publications Division; 2004.
27. Kuerbis AN, Hagman BT, Sacco P. Functioning of alcohol use disorders criteria among middle-aged and older adults: implications for DSM-5. *Subst Use Misuse.* 2013;48(4):309-322.
28. O'Connor EA, Perdue LA, Senger CA, et al. Screening and behavioral counseling interventions to reduce unhealthy alcohol use in adolescents and adults: updated evidence report and systematic review for the US Preventive Services Task Force. *JAMA.* 2018;320(18):1910-1928.
29. Fleming MF, Manwell LB, Barry KL, Adams W, Stauffacher EA. Brief physician advice for alcohol problems in older adults: a randomized community-based trial. *J Fam Pract.* 1999;48(5):378-384.
30. Ettner SL, Xu H, Duru OK, et al. The effect of an educational intervention on alcohol consumption, at-risk drinking, and health care utilization in older adults: the Project SHARE study. *J Stud Alcohol Drugs.* 2014;75(3):447-457.
31. Moore AA, Blow FC, Hoffing M, et al. Primary care-based intervention to reduce at-risk drinking in older adults: a randomized controlled trial. *Addiction.* 2011;106(1):111-120.

32. Chou RD, Dana T, Blazina I, Grusing S, Fu R, Bougatsos C. *Interventions for Drug Use - Supplemental Report: A Systematic Review for the U.S. Preventive Services Task Force.* U.S. Preventive Services Task Force; 2019.
33. Saitz R. Screening for unhealthy drug use: neither an unreasonable idea nor an evidence-based practice. *JAMA*. 2020;323(22):2263-2265.
34. McLellan AT, Starrels JL, Tai B, et al. Can substance use disorders be managed using the chronic care model? review and recommendations from a NIDA Consensus Group. *Public Health Rev.* 2014;35(2).
35. Substance Abuse and Mental Health Services Administration. *Treating Substance Use Disorder in Older Adults: UPDATED 2020.* SAMHSA; 2020.

CHAPTER 32

Laboratory Assessment

Sacha N. Uljon, Eugene Lambert, and Eric Lott

CHAPTER OUTLINE

- Concepts in laboratory medicine
- Specimen types
- Methods
- Regulation of laboratory testing
- Substance-specific tests

CONCEPTS IN LABORATORY MEDICINE

Laboratory testing provides valuable evidence in assessment of substance use. A wide variety of methods are available, and many analytes can be measured; however, understanding the meaning of the result in the context of patient care is not always straightforward. Fortunately, understanding just a few laboratory terms and knowing where to find assay-specific information can help a provider to avoid most pitfalls in interpretation. This section aims to provide the tools necessary to answer the most frequent questions posed to the laboratory about drug testing.

Laboratory Terms: Understanding the Language of the Lab

Laboratory assays are described in terms of *analytical sensitivity* and *analytical specificity*. In terms of substance use testing, analytical sensitivity refers to the lowest amount of the drug or drug metabolite that can be reliably measured. Analytical specificity refers to the ability of the test to measure that drug or metabolite only (as opposed to other substances). Analytical sensitivity and clinical or diagnostic sensitivity are not always the same and the distinction is important.[1] For example, a high-sensitivity troponin assay may be able to detect 6 ng/L of troponin more than 99% of the time, but that is not the same as determining whether a patient clinically is having a heart attack.

Sensitivity is determined in part by the choice of a *cutoff value*. For a given assay, specimens that yield results above the cutoff value are considered positive. The cutoff value may be the same as or above the analytical sensitivity of the assay. This concept is especially important when tests designed for medical management of intoxication are used to assess compliance. A negative result does not mean there is no trace of a substance in a specimen. Rather, it means that the amount is less than the cutoff value.

Another frequently used term is *cross-reactivity*. Cross-reactivity describes the ability of an antibody directed against one antigen to bind to another antigen. When invoked to describe an immunoassay result, it implies that the antibody designed by the manufacturer to bind the drug or metabolite has bound another antigen. This is a typical mechanism for an analytical false positive in an immunoassay. Cross-reactivity does not occur in methods that do not use antibodies for substance recognition, such as mass spectrometry. Rather, interference can occur in mass spectrometry.

It is also important to understand the difference between *screening* tests and *confirmation* tests. The sensitivity and specificity of screening tests is highly variable and reagent dependent, but they are less sensitive and specific in general when compared with reference methods. Some rarely have cross-reactivity (eg, cocaine urine immunoassays) while some are notoriously nonspecific (eg, amphetamine immunoassays). Screening tests are typically qualitative (positive/negative). The cutoff value may vary between screening tests, even between laboratories using the same test. Screening tests in one laboratory are therefore not necessarily comparable to those in another laboratory. For example, a specimen containing 600 ng/mL of amphetamine could be positive for amphetamines in one laboratory that uses a cutoff of 500 ng/mL but negative in another laboratory whose cutoff is 1,000 ng/mL and neither result would be incorrect.

In contrast, a *confirmatory* method is highly specific to a particular substance. Typically, these tests are quantitative. Confirmatory tests are the *reference method*. Typical methods include LC-MS/MS (liquid chromatography coupled to tandem mass spectrometry) or GC/MS (gas chromatography coupled to mass spectrometry). The sensitivity and specificity of a screening test is determined by comparison to the reference method. Confirmatory tests are more sensitive as well as more specific. Depending on the quality of the screening test and the clinical suspicion, confirmation testing may or may not be necessary.

SPECIMEN TYPES

The most common sources for clinical testing are urine and blood. Other sources are oral fluid, sweat, hair, breath, meconium, umbilical cord tissue, and nails.

Urine

Urine is the most widely used fluid for drug testing. It can be collected noninvasively and in sufficient volume from most

TABLE 32-1 Urine Detection Times

Drug class	Cutoff	Detection time (days)
Amphetamines	1,000 ng/mL	1-3
Benzodiazepines Short acting Long acting	100 ng/mL	 1-2 10-20
Buprenorphine	5 ng/mL	2-3
Cocaine	150 ng/mL	2-5
Fentanyl	5 ng/mL	1-3
Opiates	300 ng/mL	2-4
Oxycodone	100 ng/mL	2-3
Methadone	300 ng/mL	5-10
THC	20 ng/mL	2-30
6-MAM	10 ng/mL	1

A note about detection times: The detection times in Table 32-1 are a good faith estimate based on institutional experience with our immunoassays and LC-MS/MS at our cutoff concentrations. They are in rough agreement with other publications.[2,3] Detection times for certain drugs, including fentanyl, cocaine, and THC, may be longer in people who use more heavily. Lower cutoff concentrations would be expected to result in longer detection times. Variations in sample creatinine concentration, route of administration, amount and chronicity of use, individual metabolism, and cumulative metabolite cross-reactivity in specific assays can all alter detection times. Most importantly, there is no way to determine the last time of use from the amount of a substance in urine or OF or to back-calculate a blood concentration.

subjects. Drugs and/or drug metabolites are generally present in high concentrations in urine long after their blood detection window has closed. Therefore, most drug screening immunoassays are for urine. Typical detection times for substances in urine are listed in **Table 32-1**.

The most significant drawback is that urine is easily adulterated (chemically altered by adding a substance to it, typically with the intent to create a false negative testing result) or substituted (the replacement of a urine specimen with a drug-free sample of urine [such as from another person], a nonurine liquid [such as tap water, colored drinks, etc.], or synthetic urine). SAMSHA requires determination of specimen validity using pH, specific gravity, and creatinine tests. Temperature at collection and appearance can also be used to determine specimen validity. However, most medical toxicology laboratories do not perform these tests unless requested by the provider, do not receive urine while it is warm, and do not have mechanisms of rejecting suspicious samples. For example, our laboratory reports creatinine with urine toxicology but not pH or specific gravity. It is left to the provider to notice if the creatinine is suspiciously low at levels of <20 mg/dL. Therefore, a patient can substitute urine for months and go unnoticed.[4]

Oral Fluid

Adulteration of urine specimens drives the need for alternative matrices, and oral fluid (OF) is now accepted by SAMSHA for workplace drug testing.[5] Although more difficult to adulterate than urine, OF is also subject to tampering. Contamination from recently ingested or smoked substances occurs if proper rinsing technique is not used by the patient before the collection.

An ultrafiltrate of plasma, OF contains a different mix of metabolites when compared to urine. The distribution of drug in OF depends on many variables, including lipid solubility and charge, and can't be predicted by either urine or whole blood values. Accordingly, analyte-specific comparisons are necessary when judging the relative value of OF and urine. Of course, which is more sensitive is dependent not only on preanalytical values but also on the cutoffs chosen and methods used for both assays. The section on specific analytes will address these concerns for specific drugs.

Blood

Blood (whole blood, serum, plasma) gives a direct measurement of drug or metabolite present in circulation. It is therefore of value in cases of acute toxicity and in pharmacokinetic studies. OF and urine cannot be used to estimate blood concentrations. Blood is also difficult to adulterate since a phlebotomist draws and labels the specimen in the presence of the patient. Unfortunately, since detection times in blood are typically much shorter than in OF or urine, blood testing is not commonly used to screen for drug use. Exceptions include indirect markers of use, such as phosphatidylethanol (PEth) for alcohol use.

Meconium and Umbilical Cord Tissue

Meconium (the first stool) is a sensitive and specific method for detecting any fetal drug exposure. Because meconium begins to form during the 12th to 16th week of gestation, it can theoretically store a long history of fetal drug exposure. However, because much more meconium is produced later in gestation, the deposition is not linear. Meconium can be captured in a diaper and multiple specimens can be pooled, if necessary, to achieve sufficient volume. It is relatively stable when frozen. Both immunoassay and LC-MS/MS methods can be used to measure drugs and metabolites in meconium. Because only a handful of specialized laboratories are equipped to process meconium, the turn-around time is rarely fast enough to inform immediate care of the newborn.

Umbilical cord tissue is not as well studied as meconium. However, it also has the advantage of being able to provide a long detection window. In addition, since it can be collected at birth immediately and noninvasively, the results are not confounded by medications administered to the newborn before the first stool. Concentrations of drugs and metabolites that have been studied in umbilical cord tissue tend to be lower than in meconium and it may be less sensitive.[6] Other studies have demonstrated reasonable agreement between the two matrices for some classes of drugs, including opiates, amphetamines, and cocaine albeit with some discrepant results in specimens obtained from the same individual.[6,7]

Sweat

As many substances are secreted into sweat, patches can be applied to the skin to absorb sweat and measure secretion. However, sweat can be collected in only relatively small amounts, and quantification of substance levels in sweat is limited by the inability to quantify the total amount of sweat secreted and lack of standard sampling procedures.[8]

Hair

Hair testing may be more applicable to forensic or research study testing than to clinical or workplace testing. Hair can be collected easily and noninvasively, and adulteration and substitution are less likely than with urine. Substances are deposited from the blood into the hair during keratinization and diffused into the hair shaft from the surrounding skin tissues and remain in the hair shaft in a fixed position indefinitely.[9] Thus, hair analysis can provide a history of the pattern of substance use over a long time span. Hair testing is not helpful in assessing acute intoxication, because significant deposition requires 1 to 2 weeks. Additionally, substance concentration in hair varies by pigmentation, cosmetic treatments, and environmental contamination.

METHODS

Immunoassays

If you work in health care, you have done an immunoassay on your own specimen. Rapid antigen tests for SARS-CoV-2 are lateral flow immunoassays, as are home pregnancy tests. In these lateral flow immunoassays, the specimen is dropped into a well and flows past conjugated antibodies that bind the antigen (spike protein, hCG, etc.), then past a second row of antibodies that binds those complexes (test line) and finally past a row of nonspecific antibodies (control line).

The initial procedure for substance use testing is usually a screening urine immunoassay. Typically, laboratories offer panels that include multiple tests for commonly used substances. Immunoassays are inexpensive, are easily automated, and yield rapid results. To increase sensitivity and enable a machine to read at a particular wavelength, most immunoassays use enzymes to multiply the signal when antibody binding occurs. This is known as an enzyme-linked immunoassay (EIA). Examples of EIAs include conventional solid phase ELISA, enzyme multiplied immunoassay technique (EMIT), cloned enzyme donor immunoassay (CEDIA), and homogeneous enzyme immunoassay (HEIA). Another type of immunoassay is kinetic interaction of microparticles in solution (KIMS), which uses particle aggregation as a readout. What they have in common is that they all rely on the ability of drug in a patient specimen to bind to an antibody. Therefore, anything that interferes with that binding can result in inaccurate results (**Table 32-2**).

Immunoassays are calibrated to a known standard, for example, amphetamine at 1,000 ng/mL. Raw signal above that is resulted as positive and signal below is resulted as negative. Unless the laboratory has specifically validated a linear range, the raw absorbance number is not meaningful in estimating the amount of drug in the specimen. In other words, the tests are qualitative not quantitative. When used to screen for a class

TABLE 32-2 Cross-reactivity

Immunoassay	Cross-reactivity
Amphetamines	Bupropion[10,11]
	Dimethylamylamine[12]
	Kavain[13]
	Labetalol[14]
	Metoprolol[15]
	Mexiletine[16]
	Promethazine[17]
	Ranitidine[18]
	Tetracaine[19]
	Trazadone[20,21]
Benzodiazepines	Efavirenz[22]
	Sertraline[23]
Buprenorphine	Codeine, morphine[22]
	Tramadol[24]
Fentanyl	Labetalol[25]
	Methamphetamine[26]
	Risperidone[27]
Methadone	Clomipramine, thioridazine, cyamemazine, alimemazine, levomepromazine, chlorpromazine, clomipramine, thioridazine[28]
	Diphenhydramine[29]
	Quetiapine[30-33]
	Verapamil[34]
	Vortioxetine[35]
Opiates	Naloxone[36]
	Ofloxacin[37,38]
	Quinolones[39]
	Rifampicin[40]
	Tapentadol[41]
THC	Efavirenz[42,43]
	Lumacaftor/ivacaftor[44]
	Pantoprazole[45]

A note about cross-reactivity: Cross-reactivity is a property of antibodies in immunoassays. Since each manufacturer uses different antibodies, cross-reactivity is assay-specific, not analyte specific. A report of cross-reactivity in one assay cannot be extrapolated to other platforms. This chart does not include drugs or substances that metabolize to the analytes of interest because they are not cross-reactivity and are not false positives (example, poppy for opiates or Adderall for amphetamines). The chart has also been purged of cross-reactivities that existed in assays that are no longer marketed. For an excellent review, please see Saitman and colleagues.[30]

of drug, the amount of sensitivity may vary by specific drug. If more than one cross-reactive drug or metabolite is present, the absorbance does not represent one substance. For example, our benzodiazepine assay was calibrated using 100 ng/mL of nordiazepam. However, it takes 163 ng/mL of lorazepam to produce a positive result, and the assay is almost completely nonreactive with the primary metabolite of lorazepam, lorazepam glucuronide. Each immunoassay has unique properties and results can't be interpreted without knowing what test was used.

Mass Spectrometry

In contrast to the ubiquity of immunoassays, most medical practitioners do not perform or interpret mass spectrometry. Because of the cost of the equipment and the specialized skill required to operate many instruments, mass spectrometry is not common in small laboratories or community hospitals. As instruments become more user-friendly and operation more automated, that may change.

Mass spectrometry is a technique in which chemicals are ionized and separated based on their mass/charge ratio (m/z). The instrument is comprised of an ion source, a separation chamber, and a detector. The analyte of interest is ionized by an ion source, separated inside a vacuum chamber by m/z, then measured on a detector. High resolution instruments can separate chemicals that differ by a single atomic mass unit (one hydrogen atom).[46] The chances that a contaminant has an identical mass/charge ratio to a compound of interest is small. This makes mass spectrometry inherently specific but also dependent on instrument resolution. Tandem mass spectrometry (or MS/MS) is a technique that adds more specificity by measuring both the ionized analyte (parent ion) and fragments of the analyte (daughter ions). Current CLSI guidelines (C62-A) suggest using the ratio of these fragments (ion ratio) to add specificity.

Letters that appear before "MS" are acronyms for separation methods to ensure that the molecule of interest is as pure as possible when it enters the ion source. This can increase sensitivity and specificity as well as protect the mass spectrometer from contamination. LC is liquid chromatography, typically HPLC. GC is gas chromatography. Prior to chromatography, an internal standard (IS), typically the analyte of interest with a heavy atom substitution, is added to the patient specimen. The IS is used for quantitation and to compensate for matrix effects, run-to-run retention time variation, and pre-analytical processing variations. Quantitation is done using a standard curve that must be re-run each time a new round of patient samples is analyzed.

Therefore, to be identified as positive by LC-MS/MS, a patient sample must contain a molecule that co-elutes through the chromatography column with the internal standard, be isobaric with the analyte, and fragment into pieces of the same size. False positives are rare by mass spectrometry and that is why it is a reference (definitive) method.

It is a common misconception that urine immunoassay materials are less expensive than mass spectrometry. Reagents (consumables) required to perform urine immunoassays are typically $3 to $8/test. By contrast, the organic solvents required to perform mass spectrometry testing are less expensive (estimated at $2/analyte for our laboratory). But, because of the skilled labor required and the initial cost of the machines, a laboratory must perform high volumes of MS testing to realize these savings. Large reference laboratories are therefore more likely to do MS and the charge to payers and/or patients is generally higher than urine immunoassays.

REGULATION OF LABORATORY TESTING

Laboratory testing in the United States is regulated by the federal government through the center for Medicare and Medicaid (CMS). The Clinical Laboratory Improvement Amendments (CLIA'67 and CLIA'88) outlined the minimum safety and quality standards that must be met by all clinical laboratories that report patient results. CMS deputizes other organizations, such as the College of American Pathologists (CAP) and the Joint Commission (JC) to accredit laboratories, ensuring that they meet or exceed the minimum standards set by CLIA. Enforcement is through periodic on-site inspections and proficiency testing programs, where unknown specimens are sent to many laboratories and the results are compared against each other for accuracy. A directory of CLIA certified laboratories is available here at https://www.cdc.gov/clia/LabSearch.html.

The only clinical laboratories that are not subject to CLIA regulations are forensic laboratories that do not report results to patients, and laboratories that do only urine toxicology under the Substance Abuse and Mental Health Services Administration (SAMHSA), which oversees drug testing of federal workers (https://www.federalregister.gov/documents/2010/04/30/2010-10118/mandatory-guidelines-for-federal-workplace-drug-testing-programs). The U.S. Department of Transportation (DOT) requires drug and alcohol testing of safety-sensitive transportation employees in aviation, trucking, mass transit, railroad, pipelines, and other transportation industries (https://www.ecfr.gov/current/title-49/subtitle-A/part-40). Both agencies have developed extensive guidelines for specimen collection, chain-of-custody procedures, specimen validation, and testing procedures. DOT and federal workplace testing must be done in laboratories certified by the National Laboratory Certification Program. A list of SAMSA-certified laboratories is available at https://www.samhsa.gov/workplace/drug-testing-resources/certified-lab-list.

Most drug immunoassays are manufactured by a few large companies. Individual laboratories need only verify that the assay meets manufacturer specifications in their hands. This includes accuracy, precision, linearity, and reference range. A list of FDA-cleared assays is available at https://www.fda.gov/medical-devices/ivd-regulatory-assistance/public-databases. Non-FDA approved tests are known as lab developed tests (LDT). These include most mass spectrometry methods.

Laboratories that report patient results using LDT must validate the tests for accuracy, precision, linearity, and reference range, but also for analytical sensitivity and specificity, specimen stability, interfering substances, and potentially more categories depending on the test. However, FDA approval is not a requirement if the assay is used exclusively by the lab that developed it.

Recently, in response to weaknesses exposed by the COVID-19 epidemic, a new regulatory framework for laboratory tests has been introduced. The Verifying Accurate Leading-edge In Vitro Clinical Tests (VALID) Act would provide FDA with greater authority to regulate diagnostic tests and change many of the current regulations. As of this writing, it has not been enacted and no consensus exists between laboratory groups or industry leaders for or against the proposed reforms.

SUBSTANCE-SPECIFIC TESTS

Ethanol

The approach to testing for ethanol or ethanol exposure depends on the clinical purpose. Testing for acute exposure in order to medically manage intoxication is relatively straightforward. Blood alcohol concentration detects alcohol use within the preceding few hours. The enzymatic analysis measures the amount of nicotinamide adenine dinucleotide formed during oxidation of ethanol; this may produce falsely elevated readings in the presence of isopropanol, methanol, and ethylene glycol. High levels of acetone, such as found in diabetic ketoacidosis or starvation, can be metabolized to isopropanol, giving falsely elevated ethanol levels by the enzymatic analysis.[47] One can also determine the amount of alcohol by analyzing the gas in a blood tube (headspace analysis) using gas chromatography and mass spectrometry (GC/MS). This method isn't practical for clinical laboratories.

Urine testing for alcohol provides a qualitative marker of recent alcohol ingestion, although it does not measure intoxication. The presence of alcohol in the urine suggests alcohol intake within the preceding 8 hours but does not provide quantitation and it is not possible to "back calculate" a blood alcohol level from a urine result. Thus, urine is not a desirable specimen for direct measurement of ethanol.

When testing is required to monitor abstinence or to rule out heavy drinking or to document abstinence, the choice of what to measure and how to interpret the results becomes complicated. Sensitivity and specificity can vary, there is no one standardized cutoff, and the consequences of false positives and false negatives can be grave.

Here, we briefly describe alcohol biomarkers currently in use, evidence regarding detection times, and common pitfalls in interpretation. For a more comprehensive discussion, the reader is referred to this excellent recent review.[48] Specialized markers of alcohol use are not recommended for screening in the general population. However, they can be used to monitor the effectiveness of intervention in individuals with known alcohol use disorder (AUD) and in special cases where abstinence is required, such as in liver transplantation candidacy.

Liver Enzymes: GGT, AST, and ALT

Because alcohol metabolism occurs mainly in the liver, heavy alcohol use (defined by SAMSHA as 3-4 drinks a day or 7-14 drinks per week depending on gender) can result in liver enzyme elevation. Specifically, a ratio of AST/ALT of more than 2 is associated with heavy alcohol use.[49] However, these are historical and nonspecific markers of alcohol use. With the availability of more sensitive and specific markers (see below), it is no longer necessary to rely on these laboratory values for clinical decision making.

Urine Ethyl Glucuronide (EtG) and Ethyl Sulfate (EtS)

EtG and EtS are not direct metabolites of ethanol. Rather, they are products of enzymatic reactions that conjugate ethanol to endogenous molecules, creating a "signature" of ethanol exposure. Urine is the matrix of choice because the concentrations of EtG and EtS are higher in urine than in other body fluids. LC-MS is the reference method for measuring EtG and EtS but immunoassays exist for both.

At relatively low cutoffs (100), urine EtG and EtS are at least 80% sensitive and 90%-100% specific for alcohol use in a 24- to 48-hour window.[50,51] Higher cutoffs (>1,000 ng/mL) increase specificity but compromise sensitivity.[50] Although the detection window may be longer (up to 3 days), the best controlled studies did not draw specimens further than 48 hours. Unfortunately, even at cutoffs of 100 and 500 ng/mL, there is no way to distinguish between recent light drinking and more remote heavy drinking.

Several publications have reported sources of false positive EtG or EtS results. EtG initially in urine can be metabolized by bacteria, and also can be produced by bacteria in contaminated urine specimens.[52,53] EtS seems to be less vulnerable to false positives caused by bacterial contamination and metabolism.[52] EtG and EtS can be present in the urine of individuals who use alcohol-based hand sanitizers although not beyond 24 hours.[54,55] Consumption of Kombucha (a fermented tea drink), predictably, can also result in positive EtS and EtG results.[56] Measuring both EtS and EtG on the same specimen can increase specificity if they are concordantly positive.

Phosphatidylethanol (PEth)

PEth is formed is formed when ethanol reacts with phosphatidylcholines, the phospholipid components of cell membranes. Thus, PEth is measured in whole blood, not urine. PEth is not a single molecule but a family of phospholipid homologues. Measurement is by LC-MS.

Because of their longer half-lives, phosphatidylethanols can reflect ethanol exposure for weeks rather than days.[57-59] Although there is no standard established cutoff concentration, high sensitivity and specificity have been reported at different cutoffs.[57-61] PEth is purported to be a reliable biomarker with the best correlation to self-reported alcohol consumption.[62,63]

PEth seemed to be less vulnerable to false positives when compared to EtS and EtG.[64] However, clinical false positives from hand sanitizer and mouthwash have been reported recently.[65,66]

To summarize, these measures are sensitive and specific for ethanol exposure, but cannot tell the difference between lighter drinking in the past 24 hours and more remote heavy drinking. There is no way to conclusively rule out a "false positive" from unintentional exposure.

Amphetamines

Amphetamines are a group of stimulants that include amphetamine; methamphetamine; "Ecstasy" or "Molly," which is MDMA (3,4-methylenedioxymethamphetamine) or MDA (3,4-methylenedioxyamphetamine); and "Eve," which is MDEA (3,4-methylenedioxy-*N*-ethylamphetamine). Amphetamine is a metabolite of methamphetamine. Both amphetamine and methamphetamine have D- and L-isomers. As the D-isomers of amphetamine and methamphetamine have stronger central nervous system effects, they are used more often than the L-isomers. In addition to nonmedical use, amphetamines are used for medical purposes such as treatment of ADHD (Adderall, Vyvanse).

Amphetamines are commonly measured in urine or OF, where they have a detection window of approximately 1 to 3 days (**Table 32-1**). Amphetamines can also be measured in meconium and cord tissue. Blood is not useful for detecting use after about 48 hours. Amphetamines can be measured as a class by immunoassays and can be individually quantitated by LC-MS.

Urine immunoassays for amphetamines are notoriously nonspecific. They are usually targeted to methamphetamine and can have variable cross-reactivity with prescribed and illicit amphetamines. Because of the wide variation between manufacturers, the reader is referred to individual package inserts. The lack of specificity is by design. Emergency departments are major consumers of amphetamine immunoassays, and the National Academy of Clinical Biochemistry laboratory guidelines suggest amphetamine assays directed against "a broad spectrum of amines as a class" for emergency department use.[67] Indeed, in the context of medical management of acute toxicity, cross-reactivity is desirable.

The list of substances that can cause analytical false positives for amphetamine immunoassays is long, and some cross-reactivities are assay specific.[68] For amphetamines, they include ranitidine, trazadone, bupropion, and labetalol.[69] See also **Table 32-2**. Finally, prescription medications, such as selegiline or benzphetamine, are metabolized to either amphetamine or methamphetamine and can also cause (clinically but not analytical) positive results.

ADHD and SUD are common co-occurring disorders, which complicates interpretation of amphetamine results in these patients.[70] First, there is no way to differentiate prescription amphetamines from nonprescribed amphetamines using common immunoassays. Second, the cutoff concentrations of immunoassays may be too high to detect prescription Adderall use, and therefore is not reliable for measuring compliance. Finally, nonprescription Adderall pills may contain methamphetamine (https://www.dea.gov/alert/sharp-increase-fake-prescription-pills-containing-fentanyl-and-meth). Laboratory professionals should be available to assist in interpretation in these complicated cases. Confirmatory testing by mass spectrometry can identify specific stimulants. Of note, Ritalin (methylphenidate) is not metabolized to amphetamine or methamphetamine and is not detected on confirmatory testing for amphetamine or methamphetamine.

Benzodiazepines

The interpretation of urine immunoassays for benzodiazepines is complicated by the multiple substances available, their variable potencies, differing half-lives, and their diverse metabolites. Urine specimens usually contain little of the parent benzodiazepine. Therefore, many metabolites have poor-cross reactivity with immunoassays directed against parent compounds. This is another situation where review of the package insert is very helpful in interpretation, but even that must be read carefully. For example, the KIMS urine benzodiazepines immunoassay detects signal equivalent to 100 ng/mL nordiazepam. It is 62% cross-reactive with lorazepam. One might logically assume that lorazepam use would be reliably detected. However, the assay is only 0.5% cross-reactive with the primary metabolite of lorazepam, lorazepam glucuronide. Therefore, although a good choice for detecting benzodiazepine overdose in an acute setting, this urine immunoassay shouldn't be used to monitor lorazepam use or to rule out diversion.

The cutoff for benzodiazepine immunoassays usually is either 200 or 300 ng/mL, which can detect high doses but may not detect therapeutic doses of all benzodiazepines. Detection windows in urine are 1 to 2 days for the short-acting benzodiazepines and 7 to 10 days for the long-acting benzodiazepines. Notably, urine immunoassay false positives can be caused by sertraline.

Benzodiazepines and their metabolites can be measured by LC-MS/MS in both urine and OF. When both are measured by LC-MS/MS, urine is more sensitive.[71]

Cocaine

Cocaine (methyl benzoylecgonine) is a stimulant made using coca leaves. Cocaine hydrochloride is the powdered form of cocaine. It is water soluble and can be inhaled nasally or mixed with water and injected. The alkaloid form of cocaine "crack" is not water soluble but vaporizes when heated and can be smoked. It can also be dissolved in acidic solution and injected.

The detection of cocaine in the urine is variable and depends on the amount of substance ingested. The usual detection time after cocaine use is 2 to 3 days but it can be longer in people with heavier use.[72] Urine immunoassays are typically directed at benzoylecgonine, the most abundant metabolite and have good specificity. Typical cutoff concentration is 150 ng/mL, in compliance with SAMSHA guidelines. Both cocaine and benzoylecgonine can be measured in oral fluid. Whether OF or urine is superior by LC-MS/MS in simultaneously collected specimens depends on cutoff concentrations chosen but both are more sensitive than the urine immunoassay.[73]

In meconium, where detection can go back for 5 months, cocaine and benzoylecgonine can both be measured by immunoassay or mass spectrometry. In addition, coca ethylene (a metabolite of cocaine that gets combined chemically when ethanol is also present) and m-hydroxy benzoylecgonine are measured using mass spectrometry. This can be confusing to review in the medical record, depending on how results are displayed. The result for cocaine itself can be negative but metabolite positive, which is a positive confirmation for cocaine exposure in utero. It is important to check for other metabolites even if the parent drug confirmation is "negative."

Fentanyl

Fentanyl is less expensive to manufacture and more potent than heroin and is now ubiquitous. Fentanyl deaths continue to increase, and a notable trend is the co-administration of fentanyl and stimulants.[74]

Blood

Because of fentanyl's very short half-life, blood is a poor matrix of choice for screening, but may be useful in cases of acute overdose.

Urine

Fentanyl and other synthetic opioids are not detected on urine opiate immunoassays and require their own immunoassays. There are currently 6 automated urine immunoassays approved by the FDA for urine fentanyl screening. The metabolite norfentanyl is present for longer and in higher concentrations in urine when compared to fentanyl. However, most urine immunoassays are targeted toward fentanyl. The ARK immunoassay does show cross-reactivity with norfentanyl, but only about 3%.[75] A newly approved immunoassay targeted against norfentanyl rather than fentanyl and may offer increased sensitivity for that reason. Manufacturer claims for sensitivity are usually very good, most <5 ng/mL. In practice, because these immunoassays cross-react with metabolites and analogues to varying extents, we sometimes see positive screens even below the official cutoffs. Note that naloxone does not cross-react with fentanyl immunoassays.

LC-MS/MS is a confirmatory method for fentanyl in urine. Methods typically quantitate both norfentanyl and fentanyl. However, many targeted methods will not detect, they will not detect most analogues that may be picked up to varying degrees by some immunoassays.[76] Specimens with positive immunoassays that do not confirm on LC-MS/MS may be false positives but may also be specimens with fentanyl analogues. Consult a laboratory professional on the specific confirmatory method used to determine exactly what drugs and metabolites are detected. This is a rare case where specificity of the LC-MS/MS method is not advantageous for clinical interpretation.

Oral Fluid

A study comparing LC-MS/MS in OF to LC-MS/MS urine in paired specimens found urine to be slightly more sensitive than OF because of the norfentanyl signal. Norfentanyl is not readily detectable in OF and so only fentanyl was measured.[77] However, when the OF cutoff was lowered slightly or the urine cutoff was raised, the sensitivity was better in OF. The take-home message is that both are quite sensitive.

The Mystery of Low but Persistent Fentanyl Positives

Are the methods *too* sensitive? Our laboratory is frequently questioned regarding "false-positive" results on urine and OF LC-MS/MS. Most of these are <5 ng/mL for both fentanyl or norfentanyl or are negative for one and positive for the other. When the run is reviewed, there is no evidence of analytical false positive. A second or third specimen will be sent to rule out an issue with patient identification. The repeat will also be positive. What is the explanation? One hypothesis is the fentanyl "leak." There is one report in the literature of a norfentanyl-only positive that persisted for nearly a month.[78] Pharmacokinetic studies of therapeutic doses in healthy individuals suggest much shorter detection times. However, ethics prohibit a controlled study of how long a positive norfentanyl remains after repeated high dose fentanyl use.

Another explanation is contamination with other substances. We know that cocaine and heroin but also oxycodone, Adderall, and other medications that are not purchased in a pharmacy are frequently contaminated with fentanyl. An ongoing but low exposure is also a reasonable explanation for the persistent positive, especially in specimens that are also positive for other substances.

Whatever the explanation, these results do not constitute "false positives" from the point of view of the laboratorian. There is indisputably fentanyl or norfentanyl in these specimens. Unfortunately, a lab result cannot measure whether the exposure was intentional or when the exposure occurred.

Opiates and Opioids

The terms opiate and opioid refer to different but overlapping constructs. Opiate is a more narrow term referring to substances derived from opium (the extract of the weeks of the opium poppy), including only morphine, codeine, and heroin. These substances can be detected from an opiate assay. The term opioid is more comprehensive and includes all agonists and antagonists with morphine like activity, including natural opiates, semisynthetic substances (eg, hydrocodone, hydromorphone, oxycodone, and oxymorphone), and synthetic

TABLE 32-3 Opioids

Drug	Classification	Metabolites	Detected opiate on IA?	Notes
Buprenorphine	Opioid agonist	Norbuprenorphine	Unlikely	IA available
Codeine	Opiate	Morphine	Yes	
Fentanyl	Synthetic opioid	Norfentanyl	Unlikely	IA available
Heroin	Opiate	6-MAM, morphine	Yes	6-MAM IA available
Hydrocodone	Opiate	Hydromorphone	Yes	May be present at low levels in oxycodone
Hydromorphone	Opiate		Yes	May be present at low levels in oxycodone
Methadone	Opioid agonist		Unlikely	
Morphine	Opiate	Hydromorphone	Yes	
Naloxone	Opiate antagonist	Noroxymorphone	Unlikely	
Oxycodone	Semi-synthetic opioid	Oxymorphone, noroxymorphone	Unlikely	IA available
Oxymorphone	Semi-synthetic opioid	Oxymorphone, Noroxymorphone	Unlikely	
Tapentadol	Synthetic opioid	Glucuronide, sulfonate	Unlikely	
Tramadol	Synthetic opioid	*O*-desmethyltramadol, others	Unlikely	

substances (eg, methadone, buprenorphine, meperidine, fentanyl, and tramadol).

Urine immunoassays for opiates are typically calibrated with morphine at 100, 300, or 1,000 ng/mL. Cross-reactivity is good for things that metabolize to morphine, hydromorphone, or codeine, but poor for compounds whose metabolites do not resemble opiates. Opiate immunoassays are unlikely to pick up oxycodone, buprenorphine, naloxone, fentanyl, or tramadol use (**Table 32-3**). Fortunately, oxycodone-, fentanyl-, and buprenorphine-specific immunoassays are available.

LC-MS/MS confirmatory testing of urine and OF specimens is available. This can be useful for confirming the presence of opiates, but it may be impossible to determine the drug ingested if the metabolites are shared by other drugs. Clinicians should take care to check exactly which opiates, opioids, or metabolites are in a specific LC-MS/MS confirmatory panel. This information can be found on the website of the reference laboratory where the specimen is to be analyzed.

Heroin metabolizes to morphine through a short-lived intermediate, 6-monoacetylmorphine (6-MAM), which then is hydrolyzed to morphine. Immunoassays that detect 6-MAM are also available and can be used to differentiate heroin use from the use of another natural opioid. 6-MAM is usually detected in the urine for up to 8 hours after heroin use, so morphine remains detectable in urine for longer.

The popular perception that poppy seed bagels and muffins can cause a positive urine opiate immunoassay is also known as the "Seinfeld Defense" after a famous episode of the series in which a character tests positive on a workplace drug screen after eating a poppy seed bagel.[79] It is true that urine immunoassays can detect poppy seed.[80-83] The SAMSHA cutoff is 2,000 ng/mL, which is difficult to reach by eating baked goods but is possible to attain by eating raw poppy seeds.[82] Thus, though unlikely, the poppy seed defense is difficult to disprove.

Oxycodone is metabolized mainly to oxymorphone and noroxymorphone and to a lesser extent noroxycodone. Oxycodone immunoassays calibrated with oxycodone or oxymorphone may have variable reactivity with other oxycodone metabolites. Because of the common metabolite, it may be oxycodone and oxymorphone use. Occasionally, with patients on very high doses of oxycodone, hydrocodone may be observed, which may cause a positive opiates immunoassay; this is thought to be a pharmaceutical impurity.[84] LC-MS/MS confirmation would be expected to yield a much smaller amount of hydrocodone as compared to oxycodone in this case.

Buprenorphine is metabolized to norbuprenorphine. Both norbuprenorphine and buprenorphine are glucuronidated. Urine immunoassays designed to detect buprenorphine use may be directed against buprenorphine or norbuprenorphine and may or may not cross-react with glucuronides. If urine adulteration is suspected, confirmatory testing can be sent to determine whether metabolites are present. Urine that is positive only because of specimen adulteration would be expected to have only the parent drug.[85] Likewise, for methadone, the presence of metabolites such as 2-ethylidene-1,5-dimethyl-3,3 diphenylpyrrolidine from methadone metabolism can indicate compliance (versus adulteration).[86] Oral fluid can also be used to detect buprenorphine and norbuprenorphine, although one study showed superior sensitivity for urine when comparing LC-MS/MS in urine to LC-MS/MS in OF.[87]

Tetrahydrocannabinol

The primary psychoactive component of the cannabis plant is tetrahydrocannabinol (THC). When smoked, THC is absorbed quickly into the circulation, with an elimination half-life estimated to be between 20 and 30 hours. THC has a highly lipophilic nature and is stored in fat tissues, where it is slowly released back into the circulation. Most commercial immunoassays measure the inactive metabolite 11-nor-Δ9-THC-9-carboxylic acid (abbreviated THC-COOH or THCA). In the past, immunoassays gave false-positive results with nonsteroidal anti-inflammatory drugs such as ibuprofen and naproxen sodium. Current immunoassays have been modified to eliminate this cross-reactivity.

Increasing specificity in THC immunoassays has eliminated many of the cross-reactivity issues seen in first generation urine immunoassays. CBD Δ9-tetrahydrocannabinol (Δ9-THC) and synthetic cannabinoids (K2, spice) are not detected on urine immunoassays unless they contain high amounts of THC.

THC testing based on SAMSHA guidelines, recommends screening cutoffs at 50 ng/mL in urine 4 ng/mL in OF (as of 2015). The mean detection time of a single cannabis cigarette sold in the 1990s is less than 2 days using a 50 ng/mL cutoff immunoassay and is 3 to 4 days using a 15 ng/mL cutoff on GC/MS.[88] This is likely an underestimate since the potency of cannabis has increased since then.[89] In people who use frequently, urine specimens were found positive for THC-COOH up to 27 days after last use using an immunoassay with a cutoff of 20 ng/mL.[90]

THC immunoassays are included on many standard urine toxicology panels. A positive urine THC-COOH test is helpful in identifying past cannabis use, but it does not correlate with level of impairment. Boston area emergency departments have been averaging more than 20% positive THC since legalization.[91] Since a positive THC screen is a qualitative result, does not imply impairment, and is extremely common, the utility of including it on a standard urine toxicology panel is unclear. Interestingly, stat testing for THC in ED patients presenting with acute symptoms is not recommended.[67]

REFERENCES

1. Saah AJ, Hoover DR. "Sensitivity" and "specificity" reconsidered: the meaning of these terms in analytical and diagnostic settings. *Ann Intern Med.* 1997;126:91-94.
2. Magnani B, Kwong TC, McMillin GA, Wu AHB. *Clinical Toxicology Testing: A Guide for Laboratory Professionals.* College of American Pathologists; 2020.
3. Verstraete AG. Detection times of drugs of abuse in blood, urine, and oral fluid. *Ther Drug Monit.* 2004;26:200-205.
4. Uljon S. An adulterated urine buprenorphine specimen. *Prim Care Companion CNS Disord.* 2022;24.
5. Flood KJ, Khaliq T, Bishop KA, Griggs DA. The new substance abuse and mental health services administration oral fluid cutoffs for cocaine and heroin-related analytes applied to an addiction medicine setting: important unanticipated findings with LC-MS/MS. *Clin Chem.* 2016;62:773-780.
6. Colby JM. Comparison of umbilical cord tissue and meconium for the confirmation of in utero drug exposure. *Clin Biochem.* 2017;50:784-790.
7. Palmer KL, Wood KE, Krasowski MD. Evaluating a switch from meconium to umbilical cord tissue for newborn drug testing: a retrospective study at an academic medical center. *Clin Biochem.* 2017;50:255-261.
8. Dolan K, Rouen D, Kimber J. An overview of the use of urine, hair, sweat and saliva to detect drug use. *Drug Alcohol Rev.* 2004;23:213-217.
9. Pragst F, Balikova MA. State of the art in hair analysis for detection of drug and alcohol abuse. *Clin Chim Acta.* 2006;370:17-49.
10. Reidy L, Walls HC, Steele BW. Crossreactivity of bupropion metabolite with enzyme-linked immunosorbent assays designed to detect amphetamine in urine. *Ther Drug Monit.* 2011;33:366-368.
11. Casey ER, Scott MG, Tang S, Mullins ME. Frequency of false positive amphetamine screens due to bupropion using the Syva EMIT II immunoassay. *J Med Toxicol.* 2011;7:105-108.
12. Vorce SP, Holler JM, Cawrse BM, Magluilo J Jr. Dimethylamylamine: a drug causing positive immunoassay results for amphetamines. *J Anal Toxicol.* 2011;35:183-187.
13. Madhavaram H, Patel T, Kyle C, Madhavaram H, Patel T, Kyle C. Kavain interference with amphetamine immunoassay. *J Anal Toxicol.* 2020;bkaa178.
14. Duenas-Garcia OF. False-positive amphetamine toxicology screen results in three pregnant women using labetalol. *Obstet Gynecol.* 2011;118:360-361.
15. LeClercq M, Soichot M, Delhotal-Landes B, et al. False positive amphetamines and 3,4-methylenedioxymethamphetamine immunoassays in the presence of metoprolol—two cases reported in clinical toxicology. *J Anal Toxicol.* 2020;44:200-205.
16. Snozek CLH, Kaleta EJ, Jannetto PJ, et al. False-positive amphetamine results on several drug screening platforms due to mexiletine. *Clin Biochem.* 2018;58:125-127.
17. Melanson SE, Lee-Lewandroski E, Griggs DA, Long WH, Flood JG. Reduced interference by phenothiazines in amphetamine drug of abuse immunoassays. *Arch Pathol Lab Med.* 2006;130:1834-1838.
18. Liu L, Wheeler SE, Rymer JA, et al. Ranitidine interference with standard amphetamine immunoassay. *Clin Chim Acta.* 2015;438:307-308.
19. Wijngaard R, Parra-Robert M, Mares L, et al. Tetracaine from urethral ointment causes false positive amphetamine results by immunoassay. *Clin Toxicol (Phila).* 2021;59:500-505.
20. Baron JM, Griggs DA, Nixon AL, Long WH, Flood JG. The trazodone metabolite meta-chlorophenylpiperazine can cause false-positive urine amphetamine immunoassay results. *J Anal Toxicol.* 2011;35: 364-368.
21. Logan BK, Costantino AG, Rieders EF, Sanders D. Trazodone, meta-chlorophenylpiperazine (an hallucinogenic drug and trazodone metabolite), and the hallucinogen trifluoromethylphenylpiperazine cross-react with the EMIT(R)II ecstasy immunoassay in urine. *J Anal Toxicol.* 2010;34:587-589.
22. Blanks A, Hellstern V, Schuster D, et al. Efavirenz treatment and false-positive results in benzodiazepine screening tests. *Clin Infect Dis.* 2009;48:1787-1789.
23. Nasky KM, Cowan GL, Knittel DR. False-positive urine screening for benzodiazepines: an association with sertraline? A two-year retrospective chart analysis. *Psychiatry (Edgmont).* 2009;6:36-39.
24. Shaikh, Hull MJ, Bishop KA, et al. Effect of tramadol use on three point-of-care and one instrument-based immunoassays for urine buprenorphine. *J Anal Toxicol.* 2008;32:339-343.
25. Wanar A, Isley BC, Saia K, Field TA. False-positive fentanyl urine detection after initiation of labetalol treatment for hypertension in pregnancy: a case report. *J Addict Med.* 2022;16(6):e417-e419.
26. Abbott DL, Limoges JF, Virkler KJ, Tracey SJ, Sarris GG. ELISA screens for fentanyl in urine are susceptible to false-positives in high concentration methamphetamine samples. *J Anal Toxicol.* 2022;46:457-459.
27. Wang BT, Colby JM, Wu AH, Lynch KL. Cross-reactivity of acetylfentanyl and risperidone with a fentanyl immunoassay. *J Anal Toxicol.* 2014;38:672-675.

28. Lancelin F, Kraoul L, Flatischler N, Brovedani-Rousset S, Piketty ML. False-positive results in the detection of methadone in urines of patients treated with psychotropic substances. *Clin Chem.* 2005;51:2176-2177.
29. Rogers SC, Pruitt CW, Crouch DJ, et al. Rapid urine drug screens: diphenhydramine and methadone cross-reactivity. *Pediatr Emerg Care.* 2010;26:665-666.
30. Cherwinski K, Petti TA, Jekelis A. False methadone-positive urine drug screens in patients treated with quetiapine. *J Am Acad Child Adolesc Psychiatry.* 2007;46:435-436.
31. Fischer M, Reif A, Polak T, Pfuhlmann B, Fallgatter AJ. False-positive methadone drug screens during quetiapine treatment. *J Clin Psychiatry.* 2010;71:1696.
32. Lasic D, Uglesic B, Zuljan-Cvitanovic M, Supe-Domic D, Uglesic L. False-positive methadone urine drug screen in a patient treated with quetiapine. *Acta Clin Croat.* 2012;51:269-272.
33. Widschwendter CG, Zernig G, Hofer A. Quetiapine cross reactivity with urine methadone immunoassays. *Am J Psychiatry.* 2007;164:172.
34. Lichtenwalner MR, Mencken T, Tully R, Petosa M. False-positive immunochemical screen for methadone attributable to metabolites of verapamil. *Clin Chem.* 1998;44:1039-1041.
35. Uljon S, Kataria Y, Flood JG. Vortioxetine use may cause false positive immunoassay results for urine methadone. *Clin Chim Acta.* 2019;499:1-3.
36. Straseski JA, Stolbach A, Clarke W. Opiate-positive immunoassay screen in a pediatric patient. *Clin Chem.* 2010;56:1220-1223.
37. Backmund M, Meter K, Zielonka M, Eichenlaub D. Ofloxacin causes false-positive immunoassay results for urine opiates. *Addict Biol.* 2000;5:319-320.
38. Meatherall R, Dai J. False-positive EMIT II opiates from ofloxacin. *Ther Drug Monit.* 1997;19:98-99.
39. Baden LR, Horowitz G, Jacoby H, Eliopoulos GM. Quinolones and false-positive urine screening for opiates by immunoassay technology. *JAMA.* 2001;286:3115-3119.
40. DePaula M, Saiz LC, Gonzalez-Revalderia J, Pascual T, Alberola C, Miravalles E. Rifampicin causes false-positive immunoassay results for urine opiates. *Clin Chem Lab Med.* 1998;36:241-243.
41. Collins AA, Merritt AP, Bourland JA. Cross-reactivity of tapentadol specimens with DRI methadone enzyme immunoassay. *J Anal Toxicol.* 2012;36:582-587.
42. Ossthuizen NM, Laurens JB. Efavirenz interference in urine screening immunoassays for tetrahydrocannabinol. *Ann Clin Biochem.* 2012;49:194-196.
43. Rossi S, Yaksh T, Bentley H, Van Den Brande G, Grant I, Ellis R. Characterization of interference with 6 commercial delta9-tetrahydrocannabinol immunoassays by efavirenz (glucuronide) in urine. *Clin Chem.* 2006;52:896-897.
44. Kissner D, LeFlore Y, Narayan SB, Marigowda G, Simard C, Le Camus C. False-positive cannabinoid screens in adult cystic fibrosis patients treated with lumacaftor/ivacaftor. *J Cyst Fibros.* 2018;17:e51-e53.
45. Gomila I, Barcelo B, Rosell A, Avella S, Sahuquillo L, Dastis M. Cross-reactivity of pantoprazole with three commercial cannabinoids immunoassays in urine. *J Anal Toxicol.* 2017;41:760-764.
46. Snozek CLH, Langman LJ, Cotton SW. An introduction to drug testing: the expanding role of mass spectrometry. *Methods Mol Biol.* 2019;1872:1-10.
47. Jones AW. Measuring alcohol in blood and breath for forensic purposes—a historical review. *Forensic Sci Rev.* 1996;8:13-44.
48. Tawiah KD, Riley SB, Budelier MM. Biomarkers and clinical laboratory detection of acute and chronic ethanol use. *Clin Chem.* 2022;68:635-645.
49. Botros M, Sikaris KA. The de ritis ratio: the test of time. *Clin Biochem Rev.* 2013;34:117-130.
50. Jatlow PI, Agro A, Wu R, et al. Ethyl glucuronide and ethyl sulfate assays in clinical trials, interpretation, and limitations: results of a dose ranging alcohol challenge study and 2 clinical trials. *Alcohol Clin Exp Res.* 2014;38:2056-2065.
51. Wurst FM, Wiesbeck GA, Metzger JW, Weinmann W. On sensitivity, specificity, and the influence of various parameters on ethyl glucuronide levels in urine—results from the WHO/ISBRA study. *Alcohol Clin Exp Res.* 2004;28:1220-1228.
52. Helander A, Dahl H. Urinary tract infection: a risk factor for false-negative urinary ethyl glucuronide but not ethyl sulfate in the detection of recent alcohol consumption. *Clin Chem.* 2005;51:1728-1730.
53. Helander A, Olsson I, Dahl H. Postcollection synthesis of ethyl glucuronide by bacteria in urine may cause false identification of alcohol consumption. *Clin Chem.* 2007;53:1855-1857.
54. Arndt T, Gruner J, Schrofel S, Stemmerich K. False-positive ethyl glucuronide immunoassay screening caused by a propyl alcohol-based hand sanitizer. *Forensic Sci Int.* 2012;223:359-363.
55. Arndt T, Schrofel S, Gussregen B, Stemmerich K. Inhalation but not transdermal resorption of hand sanitizer ethanol causes positive ethyl glucuronide findings in urine. *Forensic Sci Int.* 2014;237:126-130.
56. Li SY, Smith CR, Bartock SH, Leland McClure F, Edinboro LE, Swortwood MJ. Evaluation of alcohol markers in urine and oral fluid after regular and hard kombucha consumption. *J Anal Toxicol.* 2022;46(8):918-924.
57. Aradottir S, Asanovska G, Gjerss S, Hansson P, Alling C. Phosphatidylethanol (PEth) concentrations in blood are correlated to reported alcohol intake in alcohol-dependent patients. *Alcohol Alcohol.* 2006;41:431-437.
58. Ulwelling W, Smith K. The PEth blood test in the security environment: what it is; why it is important; and interpretative guidelines. *J Forensic Sci.* 2018;63:1634-1640.
59. Varga A, Hansson P, Lundqvist C, Alling C. Phosphatidylethanol in blood as a marker of ethanol consumption in healthy volunteers: comparison with other markers. *Alcohol Clin Exp Res.* 1998;22:1832-1837.
60. Isaksson A, Walther L, Hansson T, Anderson A, Alling C. Phosphatidylethanol in blood (B-PEth): a marker for alcohol use and abuse. *Drug Test Anal.* 2011;3:195-200.
61. Stewart SH, Reuben A, Brzezinski W, et al. Preliminary evaluation of phosphatidylethanol and alcohol consumption in patients with liver disease and hypertension. *Alcohol Alcohol.* 2009;44:464-467.
62. Rohricht M, Paschke K, Sack PM, Weinmann W, Thomasius R, Wurst FM. Phosphatidylethanol reliably and objectively quantifies alcohol consumption in adolescents and young adults. *Alcohol Clin Exp Res.* 2020;44:2177-2186.
63. Walther L, De Bejczy A, Lof E, et al. Phosphatidylethanol is superior to carbohydrate-deficient transferrin and gamma-glutamyltransferase as an alcohol marker and is a reliable estimate of alcohol consumption level. *Alcohol Clin Exp Res.* 2015;39:2200-2208.
64. Allen JP, Wurst FM, Thon N, Litten RZ. Assessing the drinking status of liver transplant patients with alcoholic liver disease. *Liver Transpl.* 2013;19:369-376.
65. Reisfield GM, Teitelbaum SA, Jones JT, Mason D, Bleiweis M, Lewis B. Blood phosphatidylethanol (PEth) concentrations following intensive use of an alcohol-based hand sanitizer. *J Anal Toxicol.* 2023;46(9):979-990.
66. Reisfield GM, Teitelbaum SA, Jones JT, Mason D, Bleiweis M, Lewis B. Blood phosphatidylethanol concentrations following regular exposure to an alcohol-based mouthwash. *J Anal Toxicol.* 2021;45:950-956.
67. Wu AH, McCkay C, Broussard LA, et al. National academy of clinical biochemistry laboratory medicine practice guidelines: recommendations for the use of laboratory tests to support poisoned patients who present to the emergency department. *Clin Chem.* 2003;49:357-379.
68. Saitman A, Park HD, Fitzgerald RL. False-positive interferences of common urine drug screen immunoassays: a review. *J Anal Toxicol.* 2014;38:387-396.
69. Marin SJ, Doyle K, Chang A, Concheiro-Guisan M, Huestis MA, Johnson-Davis KL. One hundred false-positive amphetamine specimens characterized by liquid chromatography time-of-flight mass spectrometry. *J Anal Toxicol.* 2016;40:37-42.
70. Katzman MA, Bilkey TS, Chokka PR, Fallu A, Klassen LJ. Adult ADHD and comorbid disorders: clinical implications of a dimensional approach. *BMC Psychiatry.* 2017;17:302.

71. Petrides AK, Melanson SEF, Kantartjis M, Le RD, Demetriou CA, Flood JG. Monitoring opioid and benzodiazepine use and abuse: is oral fluid or urine the preferred specimen type? *Clin Chim Acta.* 2018;481:75-82.
72. Jufer RA, Wstadik A, Walsh SL, Levine BS, Cone EJ. Elimination of cocaine and metabolites in plasma, saliva, and urine following repeated oral administration to human volunteers. *J Anal Toxicol.* 2000;24:467-477.
73. Melanson SEF, Petrides AK, Khaliq T, Griggs DA, Flood JG. Comparison of oral fluid and urine for detection of cocaine abuse using liquid chromatography with tandem mass spectrometry. *J Appl Lab Med.* 2020;5:935-942.
74. Palamar JJ, Cottler LB, Goldberger BA, et al. Trends in characteristics of fentanyl-related poisonings in the United States, 2015-2021. *Am J Drug Alcohol Abuse.* 2022;48(4):471-480.
75. Budelier MM, Franks CE, Logsdon N, et al. Comparison of two commercially available fentanyl screening immunoassays for clinical use. *J Appl Lab Med.* 2020;5:1277-1286.
76. Wharton RE, Casbohm J, Hoffmaster R, Brewer BN, Finn MG, Johnson RC. Detection of 30 fentanyl analogs by commercial immunoassay kits. *J Anal Toxicol.* 2021;45:111-116.
77. Mahowald GK, Khaliq TP, Griggs D, O M, Flood JG, Uljon S. Comparison of oral fluid and urine for detection of fentanyl use using liquid chromatography with tandem mass spectrometry. *J Appl Lab Med.* 2021;6:1533-1540.
78. Wanar A, Saia K, Field TA. Delayed norfentanyl clearance during pregnancy. *Obstet Gynecol.* 2020;136:905-907.
79. Seinfeld. In: Ackerman A. ed. *The Shower Head (TV show).*
80. Hayes LW, Krasselt WG, Mueggler PA. Concentrations of morphine and codeine in serum and urine after ingestion of poppy seeds. *Clin Chem.* 1987;33:806-808.
81. Samano KL, Clouette RE, Rowland BJ, Sample RH. Concentrations of morphine and codeine in paired oral fluid and urine specimens following ingestion of a poppy seed roll and raw poppy seeds. *J Anal Toxicol.* 2015;39:655-661.
82. Smith ML, Nichols DC, Underwood P, et al. Morphine and codeine concentrations in human urine following controlled poppy seeds administration of known opiate content. *Forensic Sci Int.* 2014;241:87-90.
83. Thevis M, Opfermann G, Schanzer W. Urinary concentrations of morphine and codeine after consumption of poppy seeds. *J Anal Toxicol.* 2003;27:53-56.
84. West R, West C, Crews B, et al. Anomalous observations of hydrocodone in patients on oxycodone. *Clin Chim Acta.* 2011;412:29-32.
85. Donroe JH, Holt SR, O'Connor PJ, Sukumar N, Tetrault JM. Interpreting quantitative urine buprenorphine and norbuprenorphine levels in office-based clinical practice. *Drug Alcohol Depend.* 2017;180:46-51.
86. George S, Parmar S, Meadway C, Braithwaite RA. Application and validation of a urinary methadone metabolite (EDDP) immunoassay to monitor methadone compliance. *Ann Clin Biochem.* 2000;37(Pt 3): 350-354.
87. Ransohoff JR, Petrides AK, Piscitello GJ, Flood JG, Melanson SEF. Urine is superior to oral fluid for detecting buprenorphine compliance in patients undergoing treatment for opioid addiction. *Drug Alcohol Depend.* 2019;203:8-12.
88. Huestis MA, Mitchell JM, Cone EJ. Urinary excretion profiles of 11-nor-9-carboxy-delta 9-tetrahydrocannabinol in humans after single smoked doses of marijuana. *J Anal Toxicol.* 1996;20:441-452.
89. ElSohly MA, Mehmedic Z, Foster S, Gon C, Chandra S, Church JC. Changes in cannabis potency over the last 2 decades (1995-2014): analysis of current data in the United States. *Biol Psychiatry.* 2016;79:613-619.
90. Smith-Kielland A, Skuterud B, Moreland J. Urinary excretion of 11-nor-9-carboxy-delta9-tetrahydrocannabinol and cannabinoids in frequent and infrequent drug users. *J Anal Toxicol.* 1999;23:323-332.
91. Tolan NV, Terebo T, Chai PR, et al. Impact of marijuana legalization on cannabis-related visits to the emergency department. *Clin Toxicol (Phila).* 2022;60:585-595.

CHAPTER

33 Assessment

Deirdre O'Sullivan and Abenaa Jones

CHAPTER OUTLINE

- Assessment of patients with substance use disorders
- Trauma-informed assessment
- Continuum of care
- Tasks of the assessment process
- Assessment needs for different providers
- Sources of assessment information
- Assessment tools
- Integrating assessment into practice
- Summary

ASSESSMENT OF PATIENTS WITH SUBSTANCE USE DISORDERS

Individualized patient assessment is an essential clinical skill and is foundational to quality patient care. Patient assessment is introduced at the earliest levels and critically evaluated in health professional training. However, these assessments can be complex and involve multidisciplinary teams and multiple forms of patient evaluations, including informal and formal methods, particularly when treating individuals with substance use disorders (SUDs). Yet, patient assessment is vital in initial treatment planning and the evolution of these plans, patient safety, and optimal treatment outcomes for people with SUD. Specifically, quality assessment bridges the gap between SUD diagnosis and the initiation of treatment, ensuring the accuracy of the initial diagnosis and identifying the most effective and efficient care. Assessment procedures should be done during the initial phase of treatment planning and ongoing to assess patient progress or changes and to revise the treatment plan accordingly. Given that addiction is among the most stigmatized illnesses, and the high rates of prior traumas among people with SUD,[1] *how* providers obtain patient information is critical. We recommend a trauma-sensitive approach to assessment for this population. We caution readers that most research conducted on assessment tools and procedures were validated using samples that may not be representative of patients from racial, socio-economic, and other marginalized backgrounds. For this reason, it is critical that providers use caution administering and interpreting assessment results with many patients. Evidence-based practice recommends that providers use validated assessments and procedures in a way that aligns with the person or community of people being served. Procedures and tools that are known to be effective and appropriate for some populations, may need to be altered or tweaked to better align with the needs of other patients.

SUD may impact the intrapersonal sense of self (self-image, self-respect, self-concept, sense of self-efficacy), interpersonal relationships (family and close friends and then social relationships suffer), avocations and hobbies, financial status, housing, criminal-legal involvement (particularly for minoritized individuals because of racism inherent in the War on Drugs), employment or school performance, and physical and mental health. Indeed, SUDs typically affect all life domains, including licensure status, insurance eligibility, prior traumas, and family relationships (CSAT TIP #27).[1] Consequently, data gathering techniques can be re-traumatizing and can inadvertently contribute to perceived provider stigma, which is often internalized and becomes a barrier to care. As such, the assessment process is a critical aspect of the approach to treating SUDs.[2] Thus, rapport building with patients and using a trauma-informed lens to obtain information is vital.

TRAUMA-INFORMED ASSESSMENT

Trauma is defined as an emotional reaction to highly distressing or threatening events. Trauma can encompass a single event (eg, a sexual assault, house fire, or natural disaster), or can be chronic and persistent, such as living with a domestically violent partner, abusive parent or caregiver, experiencing lifelong racism or other forms of oppression, or living in a combat zone. Patients receiving addiction treatment are likely to have survived multiple traumas, with childhood trauma being among the most prevalent and pernicious. Trauma is both a risk factor for SUDs and complicates addiction recovery if it is unresolved. For this reason, assessment for traumas should be included as part of the addiction assessment process, and all assessment procedures should be done using a trauma-sensitive perspective. Trauma-sensitive providers should proceed with assessments for life events, including prior traumas. Accurate and complete information is not the primary goal, but rather sensitive, open communication about trauma and its impact on survivors, aiming to promote treatment as the primary goal. This type of communication builds rapport and trust, which helps the provider gather accurate and complete information when the patient is comfortable sharing.[3] Open communication disrupts the typical provider–patient dynamic in which the provider is perceived as having all the knowledge and power, while the patient is expected to "follow orders." Dismantling this hierarchy is one way to avoid re-traumatizing patients with trauma histories.

Upwards of 90% of people in treatment for addiction report prior trauma and 35% of those report posttraumatic stress disorder,[4] necessitating trauma-informed practices. Trauma-informed practice shifts the perspective away from the problem (in this case, addiction) and toward an understanding of the underlying causes that fuel problematic use of drugs and alcohol. Primary tenets of trauma-informed care include knowledge of types of traumas and their lasting impact on the body and mind, actively avoiding re-traumatizing patients, communicating in an open, collaborative, and transparent manner with patients, and focusing on resiliency and individual strengths rather than the problems.[3] Trauma-informed communication enhances patient trust, leading to better treatment adherence and outcomes. Trauma-informed assessments then require sensitivity from providers. Specifically, they must balance the need to gather patient history to inform treatment with the recognition that asking too many invasive questions can be re-traumatizing to the patient.

CONTINUUM OF CARE

Depending on the severity of a SUD, varying levels of care are needed. In 2018 The American Society of Addiction Medicine developed a set of guidelines that provide a framework to manage the continuum of care for individuals with substance use disorders (**Table 33-1**; see Chapter 47 for more detail). Assessment of individual needs in each of these dimensions and patient preference should inform the recommendation concerning the level of care. It is important that for some patients, SUD can follow a chronic course and thus treatment should ideally be longitudinal. Specifically, recovery from SUD does not entail a singular event but rather a complex process that involves multiple life domains, each of which requires varying support levels. For those from marginalized backgrounds, additional supports may be necessary in order to maximize the likelihood of successful outcomes. For example, involving medical case management might be warranted when safe housing and/or violent environments are life factors.

TASKS OF THE ASSESSMENT PROCESS

Assessment of SUDs, contextualized within patients' life circumstances, should occur in every patient evaluation. Yet, the nature of the assessment process is influenced by patient factors, as well as clinician and organizational factors. Therefore, the tools used in an assessment may change depending upon the clinical context (ie, primary care, emergency department, hospital setting, mental health treatment center, SUD treatment center), the competency of and resources available to the clinician, and the specific characteristics of the patient presentation. However, the essential areas to be assessed remain constant.

TABLE 33-1 American Society of Addiction Medicine's Criteria: Elements of Multidimensional Assessment

	Dimension	Focus
Dimension 1	*Acute intoxication and/or withdrawal potential*	Individual's present substance use and substance use history, instances of withdrawal
Dimension 2	*Biomedical conditions and complications*	Individual's present physical condition, comprehensive health history
Dimension 3	*Emotional, behavioral, or cognitive conditions and complications*	Mental health concerns, exploration of thoughts and emotions, trauma
Dimension 4	*Readiness to change*	Individual's motivation to change
Dimension 5	*Return to use, continued use, or continued problem potential*	Consideration of recurrence of use potential and issues with sustained use of substances
Dimension 6	*Recovery and living environment*	Social and environmental aspects of the individual's recovery process

Adapted from American Society of Addiction Medicine. (n.d.). *At a Glance: The Six Dimensions of Multidimensional Assessment.* Accessed May 25, 2023. https://www.asam.org/asam-criteria/about-the-asam-criteria

As a general rule, results from one assessment tool are not very informative. Regardless of the intended purpose of the assessment task, results must be considered in the context of the patient's broader life factors and other assessment or screening results. All information gathered should be done in partnership with the patient, and verification of the provider's interpretation of assessment results is recommended for trauma-informed practice, as this further promotes collaborative patient care. Generally speaking, assessment of SUD is utilized for one or more of the following tasks: diagnostic verification, assessing for physiological dependence and the potential need for stabilization and medical withdrawal management, assessing for pharmacotherapy initiation, staging disease severity, identifying the domains of life affected by the disease, evaluating for additional medical or psychiatric diagnosis, quantifying the disease-associated morbidity, identifying characteristics of the disease that are important from a prognostic or treatment-matching perspective, quantifying the impact of treatment on disease-associated morbidity, or attempting to determine subtypes of addiction. Assessments should be repeated over time to identify treatment responses and/or the need for changes in strategy. Because of this, assessments that both provide helpful information and might be responsive to change over time and across treatment are beneficial (eg, number of heavy drinking days).

ASSESSMENT NEEDS FOR DIFFERENT PROVIDERS

Clinicians vary in their clinical decision-making strategies, particularly regarding the initial assessment of SUDs. Those who care for patients with SUDs can be generally divided into three groups: primary care clinicians, addiction medicine or psychiatry specialists, and SUD treatment providers (including social workers and counselors). Across these settings, assessment is a necessary part of evaluating patients with addiction and is a critical bridge between screening, diagnosis, and treatment planning. The application of different assessment levels reflects patient-centered care, as it provides the patient with the right degree of assessment necessary for shared decision-making between clinician and patient. It also provides more highly individualized clinical decision-making wherever the patient may access help (enhancing the use of the "no wrong door" approach). There are many tools available to assist in the assessment process. Choosing the right tool, which matches both the clinical needs of the patient and the capability of the clinician or treatment program, can be difficult. Staff training and competencies, along with the availability of time and access to assessment resources (eg, computerized database access, funding for the assessment instrument) can all impact the selection of assessment tools.

Primary Care Assessment Needs and Tools

The primary care provider (PCP) typically performs a brief patient assessment to verify the SUD diagnosis. Next, the PCP needs to gauge the severity of the disease from the perspective of assessing for psychosocial morbidity, substance-related medical conditions, risk for withdrawal, and appropriateness for medication initiation. Assessment of the patients' readiness for behavior change and screening for urgent medical or psychiatric comorbidities, including suicide risk and trauma histories, follows. These evaluations may be completed over the course of one or more office visits through a patient interview, physical examination, use of one or more validated questionnaires or assessment tools, laboratory testing including toxicology, a query of the Prescription Drug Monitoring Program (PDMP) database, and, if possible, corroboration in person or by phone from collateral sources (family, friends, other healthcare providers) after informed consent and release of information are obtained for matters related to SUD. As is the case for other medical illnesses, PCPs may differ in their expertise and involvement in assessing and managing SUDs. For example, some PCPs may choose more minimal participation, limiting their involvement to identifying the SUD(s) and drug(s) of choice, the severity of the SUD(s), impact on functional abilities, and readiness to change. Others may want to be more closely involved with the SUD management or even deliver treatment (eg, buprenorphine) and coordinate specialty counseling referrals. Specialty counseling referrals address various life domains impacted by addiction, such as treatment for co-occurring illnesses, housing, employment, legal services, and intervention for trauma. More detailed and specific assessments would be necessary to identify the life domains impacted.

The assessment resources available to the PCP are limited but quite adequate to perform an addiction assessment. As much as possible, the PCP should utilize a structured approach infused with trauma sensitivity to try to ensure an appropriately careful and thorough evaluation. A trauma-sensitive PCP introduces and explains the purpose of screening questions and reassures the patient that treatment decisions based on screening questions will be made in collaboration with the patient. Assessments with cutoff scores help determine severity levels, which may guide treatment decisions. Providers can also use follow-up questions about individual scale items to gather more information.

Many patients presenting to a PCP may not meet the criteria for a SUD. Still, they may be using alcohol or other substances at a harmful level that is hazardous to their health and well-being. The AUDIT and AUDIT-C, and other screening tools (see **Table 33-2**), can be utilized to identify these risks. Using a lower cutoff score is more sensitive to identify unhealthy use, which may need to be balanced with ideal specificity to minimize false positives in busy clinical settings. Questioning should also focus on binge drinking and risky behaviors such as driving while under the influence. Hazardous alcohol and drug use is often a precursor to addiction; and an easily recognizable symptom in a more complex array of problems (eg, suicidality, anger control, domestic violence, trauma, PTSD).

The development and deployment of evidence-based approaches for technology-assisted care of patients with SUDs are growing, increasing opportunities for enhancing assessment, referral, and treatment. They offer specific advantages to PCPs, who must maximize the efficiency of the assessment and referral process. Standardized assessment tools can be self-administered on various platforms, including websites, apps for smartphones, and computer tablets provided in waiting rooms. Ideally, these applications can be linked to the electronic health record (EHR), making the evaluation results immediately available to the provider and permitting the trending of scores over time. Increasingly, it is possible to have the patient self-administer assessments at home utilizing the EHR's patient portal. This can be done before an appointment or regularly between appointments. Clinical settings with high levels of EHR integration have successfully implemented such programs.

Technology also offers options that the PCP can use to provide brief interventions in the office or recommend that appropriate patients access directly.[3] Examples would include a decision support algorithm linked to the EHR in the Veterans Health System that guides the PCP in providing very brief feedback and assistance, as well as apps and web programs such as the Drinker's Check-up.[4] This check-up begins with a short assessment (AUDIT) and then a motivational interviewing-based presentation of feedback and options for change tailored to the patient's assessed level of need. Emerging research indicates that web- or app-based interventions are well accepted and often a practical option for some patients, particularly those at the hazardous use stage.

TABLE 33-2 Overview of Brief Screening Assessment Tools

Instrument	Purpose	Population	Strengths	Weaknesses
ACE	Screens for childhood adversity and abuse	Adults	Brief (10 items); comprehensive for abuse and adversity; widely used; free	Does not assess for other forms of adversity, such as poverty, racism, and other forms of chronic stress
ACE-ASF	Screens for emotional, sexual, and physical abuse	Adults	Brief (8 items); free; strong concurrent validity; comprehensive for childhood abuse	Typically used in higher-income countries; moderate reliability; further research needed on more diverse populations; dichotomous responses
AUDIT	Screens for unhealthy alcohol use and risk for alcohol use disorder	Recommended for 16+	Brief; free; easy to administer; offered in 28 languages; only screening available for international use; valid; reliable	Follow-up assessments and differential diagnoses are required to determine hazardous and SUD-related use; future use indicators are poor
CAGE	Screens for possible alcohol use disorder	All ages	Brief; free; easy to administer	Low reliability; insensitive, does not detect unhealthy use; lower specificity; due to brevity, follow-up assessments are recommended
CAPS CAPS-CA	Screening for PTSD symptoms can supplement the diagnosis	Adolescents and Adults (CAPS) Children and Adolescents (CAPS-CA);	Flexibility; can be used for screening and diagnosis; available in Italian; established validity and reliability	Long, structured format; cost to use; requires a level 3 qualification for administration
DAST-2	Screens for unhealthy drug use	Two item version validated in Veterans Affairs clinics and recommended for PC outpatient settings	Very brief, 2 items continuous scoring; found to have high levels of sensitivity and specificity; continuous scores prevent desirable responses, resulting in higher accuracy	Two item screener may not be sufficient for all patients; only screens for unhealthy drug use, no other symptoms or medical problems
InDUC	Screens for adverse consequences of alcohol/drugs on life domains	Recommended for sub-clinical populations	Assesses for consequences of drugs and alcohol in personal, social, physical and impulse control; strong reliability and validity	Lengthy (37 items); focus is on consequences of use, not actual use or severity
FAST	Quick screening for possible SUD	Recommended for 16+	Brief; free; beneficial to time-sensitive settings; identifies hazardous use	Variable item test-retest reliability; clarification for drink sizing needed depending on culture/ language
PHQ-9	Assesses for depression	Nonclinical adults	Includes item asking about suicidality; brief	Low sensitivity detected; wording pertaining to "several days" and "more than half the days" was reported as confusing by study participants
SASSI	Screen for SUD severity levels	Adult and Adolescent versions available	Has audio version for those who cannot read; Spanish language version available	Long format; providers will need additional assessments for comorbid conditions

Addiction Specialist Assessment Needs and Tools

The addiction medicine or psychiatry specialist will approach the assessment differently. Certainly, assessing for addiction and stage of readiness for behavior change and expert evaluation for medical withdrawal or withdrawal management needs must be accomplished. Further evaluation for co-occurring psychiatric disorders, a more thorough family assessment, impact on functional status, careful evaluation of all prior evaluations and attempts at treatment, patterns of substantial remissions and recurrences, and the potential role for pharmacotherapy should all be part of this specialist assessment.

The addiction medicine or psychiatry physician's needs require more in-depth evaluation when approaching the assessment process. They typically necessitate more formal tools for *staging* the disease and quantifying disease severity. Both the aforementioned screening and brief assessment tools and a more extensive diagnostic interview are required.

In addition, formal depression and anxiety screening with tools such as the Beck Depression Inventory or the Hamilton Anxiety Scale is often performed. Assessing for prior traumas, particularly childhood traumas, is recommended. For patients who are parents and survived childhood trauma, an assessment for harmful parenting practices may be needed to determine the welfare of the children under the patient's care. In addition, an examination for a new emergence of or change in symptoms of other psychiatric disorders should be performed. A thorough review of prior treatments, length and characteristics of remissions, patterns and triggers for recurrence, current supports, and resources available for treatment is essential. Assessment of the readiness for behavior change, commitment to a recovery program, and the possibilities for pharmacotherapy is necessary, as is careful evaluation for acute, subacute, and postacute withdrawal issues. Interviewing significant others about the patient to corroborate the history is even more essential, but still requires informed consent and a release of information to discuss addiction-related information.

Substance Use Disorder Treatment Provider Needs and Tools

Treatment programs for SUDs generally have the time and resources to emphasize assessment of prior treatment experiences, identification and management of co-occurring medical and psychiatric conditions, trauma history, family issues and the therapeutic milieu of the living environment, and past recurrence patterns (see Chapter 47). The purpose of assessment in this setting extends to details relevant to designing individualized treatment approaches.

The addiction treatment program must use a formalized addiction assessment process for quality control and accreditation reasons. A complete medical history and physical exam are mandatory, focusing on the areas mentioned earlier. Still, a structured interview such as the Addiction Severity Index (ASI) or even the Substance-Related and Addictive Disorders module of the Structured Clinical Interview for DSM-5 (SCID-5), the Mini-International Neuropsychiatric Interview (MINI),[5] or the Composite International Diagnostic Interview Substance Abuse Module (CIDI-SAM) should also be used. The SCID and the MINI have been updated to DSM-5. Programs that care for patients with a high prevalence of co-occurring psychiatric disorders will utilize the more extensive SCID or at least will need to use specific anxiety and depression screens. Assessing treatment readiness, resistance and recurrence of use patterns, and coping skills is typically part of the program assessment process.

SOURCES OF ASSESSMENT INFORMATION

As previously mentioned, SUDs affect multiple facets of an individual's life and health. It becomes incumbent on the assessment process to gather information from both conventional and atypical sources. Atypical sources are in contrast to the assessment of most medical or surgical conditions, wherein the usual and adequate references for evaluation and management are provided by the initial history and physical, followed by laboratory and diagnostic study review.

Additional sources that commonly are utilized in assessing the disease of addiction include toxicology testing, family interview, reported use of pharmacology (licit and illicit) with particular emphasis on the controlled drug use history, trauma-informed exploration of involvement with the criminal legal system, PDMP data, and educational and occupational interview, and readiness for behavior change evaluation. These areas of investigation and examination are even more critical than during routine medical care. As SUDs are highly stigmatized disorders, patient self-report reliability issues may be more problematic than with other health problems. It is vital to interview patients in ways that minimize shaming, which might well result in a defensive response style, thus limiting reliable data gathering. We urge clinicians to be particularly mindful when working with patients who have marginalized identities. Barriers such as language, education level, and health literacy can all hinder the assessment process, including obtaining informed consent in an ethical manner. We recommend taking extra time to communicate to patients that healthcare providers seek accurate health information so that the best care can be provided. Like screening and brief intervention, patient self-report reliability can be improved by using a consistent series of questions that progress from general and open-ended to specific information sought in a more closed-ended question form and utilizing the family or significant other interviews whenever possible. Additionally, there is some evidence to suggest patients may be more forthcoming with a self-report tool, including one administered by electronic means, rather than a face-to-face interview.

Owing to high rates of psychiatric symptomatology, a psychiatric screening interview, including a suicide risk assessment, is required. The cultural background, spiritual inclination, and belief system that the patient holds regarding substance use disorders are critical assessment areas. This thoughtful and comprehensive assessment process is typically extended in time and is multidisciplinary.

ASSESSMENT TOOLS

As indicated above, the natural history of addiction typically involves progressive dysfunction and disability in the significant life domains in a cascade pattern, often starting with the intrapersonal, advancing to the interpersonal, and eventually progressing to the physical in the later stages. Because of this, assessment strategies must be sensitive to the natural history of the disease of addiction. A thorough assessment should evaluate each area or domain of patient function that is necessary for the clinician performing or requesting the evaluation. In addition, the assessment tool used should be reliable, reproducible, and verifiable. Diagnostic and assessment strategies are often evaluated based upon their convergent validity (consistency with an established best practice or "gold standard") and ability to predict different outcomes (predictive validity). A high-quality assessment tool should also have face validity (seems straightforward and logical and makes sense), and retest and interrater reliability (reoffering the assessment to the same patient by the same or a different staff member should produce a consistent result).

This section suggests tools to assist the clinician in critical assessments. The clinician often begins by assessing the patient's substance use severity. Several options vary in the effort required and the range of use. The instruments highlighted are reliable and valid for the purposes suggested. Some tools (like the single screening questions, AUDIT-C, AUDIT, and DAST) are *screening instruments*. Still, the assessment process is a clear and direct extension of the screening and diagnosis process.

Consequently, extending the use of a screening tool by asking straightforward follow-up questions for each positive screening response can result in a substantial assessment without needing to use additional clinical tools. **Table 33-3** demonstrates this process of extending a screening tool (ie, CAGE questionnaire) for use in evaluation. Further information on many of these tools, and other assessment options, can be found online at niaaa.nih.gov/publications, drugabuse.gov, or samhsa.gov.

Screening Tool Results Can Provide Assessment Information

Screening tool results can be used as a bridge to the assessment process. The primary way this happens is to use positive responses for follow-up questions. The clarifying method establishes whether a positive response is a "true positive" and explores the data behind the positive response. This process of establishing "true positives" and following up on valuable data that underlies the positive response facilitates the transition from screening to assessment. For example, asking follow-up questions to the AUDIT-C positive responses can give helpful information about the quantity and frequency of use, use patterns, efforts to control usage, and adverse consequences.

Screening test results can also help start the assessment process by using the screening test "score" to identify the risk of meeting criteria for a SUD. For example, the AUDIT-C can indicate low-risk use, moderate risk use, or high risk use depending on the score.[2,6-9] For example, an AUDIT of 15 or greater and an AUDIT-C of greater than 7 have high specificity for identifying a DSM-5–defined alcohol use disorder. Similarly, a score of 27 or greater on the ASSIST or 6 and higher on the DAST-10 indicates a higher risk for drug use disorder and severity of drug-associated problems.[10-15]

Some tools formerly used for screening are probably better suited for disease staging or the assessment process. One of these is the CAGE questionnaire, where a score of two or more suggests a lifetime diagnosis of substance use disorder.[16] The F-CAGE is also a helpful tool for obtaining assessment data from friends or family members of people with substance use disorders.[17] Additional tools used in this way are the Short Michigan Alcoholism Screening Test[18] and the CAGE-AID; the CAGE questionnaire can also be adapted to assess for other drug use.[19] Realize, however, that while screening tools may be adapted for use as an aid in assessment and diagnosis, they are not endorsed by the DSM-5 as a substitute for the gold standard—a diagnostic interview and examination performed by a clinician trained in addiction-related disorders.

TABLE 33-3 Moving From Screening to Assessing

The following are simple follow-up questions that can be asked after encountering a positive response to the screening questions. The follow up interview should be conducted using a trauma-informed approach, which prioritizes transparency, patient strengths over problems, and a collaborative approach. The purpose of the follow up interview is to build trust with the patient and gather additional information, but know when to stop if the patient experiences the questions as intrusive. Patients who survived trauma are more likely to experience questions as judgmental and re-traumatizing, which will likely damage the patient-provider relationship.[3] Establishing a strong rapport by demonstrating sensitivity is a better initial outcome than gathering the most accurate and complete patient history. We suggest prefacing a follow up conversation with an explanation that you are going to ask some more questions about their drinking or drug use so that you can provide the best possible treatment in collaboration with them. A gentle reminder that you are here to help, not judge, can help set the tone. We also recommend that providers carefully watch for signs of discomfort and provide reassurance about your intent to collaboratively help them when you sense discomfort.

1. Cut down
   a. Can you tell me about a time you cut down your use? How long were you able to do this?
   b. On a scale from 1 to 10, with the 10 being the most difficult, how hard was it for you?
   c. When you cut down, was there something or someone motivating you?
2. Annoyed by comments
   a. Can you tell me about the person/people who made the annoying comments? How would you describe your relationship with them?
   b. Can you give me an example of a comment?
   c. Did this comment feel triggering to you? Or particularly hurtful because of who said it, or how it was said?
3. Embarrassed, bashful, or guilty
   a. We all feel embarrassed at times. Are you comfortable telling me about a time you felt embarrassed related to your drinking or drug use?
   b. Are you comfortable telling me about a time you felt guilt regarding your drinking or drug use?
   c. We all have regrets in life. Have there been times you wish you could forget?
4. Eye-openers
   a. Do you experience either physical or mental pain the morning after drinking or using?
   b. Is the pain so severe that you need a drink (or pill, or other) to get going?

Diagnostic Assessment Tools

Semi-structured clinical interviews designed for administration by trained evaluators are considered the "gold standard" for establishing reliable diagnoses of substance use disorders. The Substance-Related and Addictive Disorders module of the SCID-5[20,21] utilizes questions paralleling the DSM-5 diagnostic criteria and establishes lifetime and current disorder diagnoses for alcohol and each psychoactive substance included in DSM-5. Age of onset and an estimate of current severity are also obtained. Alternatively, the diagnostic portion of the Substance Abuse Outcomes Module has been shown to correlate well with the CIDI-SAM, has the advantage of being considerably shorter to administer than the CIDI-SAM, can be self-administered, and is designed to be implemented in routine clinical practice. Alternatively, the MINI can be used. It has been validated in both the United States and Europe as an alternative to the SCID and the CIDI that is shorter in administration.

Intoxication and Withdrawal Assessment

Intoxication

Both the patient history and the results of toxicology testing can be useful in assessing intoxication and withdrawal. Toxicology testing can verify recent use, involvement of more than one substance, and for some substances can provide information related to assessing current intoxication. High levels found on toxicology testing, with a relative absence of obvious physical impairment, are a strong indicator of high tolerance levels and physical dependence.

The first step in conducting an addiction assessment is establishing the degree of risk associated with withdrawal. Once the withdrawal diagnosis is made, its risk or severity should be assessed. The Clinical Institute Withdrawal Assessment for Alcohol, revised (CIWA-Ar),[22] is a brief 10-item scale that can be administered in less than 3 minutes. It quantifies the severity of the alcohol withdrawal syndrome by rating 10 common alcohol withdrawal symptoms and can be clinically valuable for monitoring progress over time. The CIWA has been adjusted to assess benzodiazepine withdrawal. The Clinical Institute Narcotic Assessment (CINA) Scale and Clinical Opiate Withdrawal Scale (COWS) have been developed to quantify opioid withdrawal symptoms. CIWA and CINA scores below 8 indicate mild withdrawal, and scores above 20 indicate severe withdrawal. COWS scores below 12 are considered a mild opioid withdrawal, and above 36 are severe withdrawal.

Assessment Tools for Co-occurring Conditions and Functioning

Patients with SUDs often present with co-occurring psychiatric disorders that require simultaneous or sequential treatment.[23] The full SCID has modules for each of the other major syndrome groups, anxiety disorders, affective disorders, and psychotic disorders, as well as other co-occurring disorders that are common in people with SUD, most notably the other disorders of impulse control, such as eating disorders and pathological gambling, and the personality disorders. Each module may stand alone for the assessment of a particular diagnostic syndrome. Administration of the full SCID can take 2 hours or more, depending on the complexity of the patient's presenting problems. The CIDI or the MINI can be shorter alternatives.

Short self-report instruments are available to measure some of the most common comorbidities. The 18-item Brief Symptom Inventory (BSI)[24] assesses psychological distress severity and includes somatization, depression, and anxiety scales. It is a powerful predictor of poor treatment outcomes among people with substance use disorders.[25]

The PHQ-9[26] assesses symptoms of depression and is highly correlated with more comprehensive assessments of current major depressive disorder. Importantly, it includes one question assessing *suicidal ideation*: "Have you thought that you would be better off dead or that you wanted to hurt yourself in some way?" The Beck Depression Inventory[27] and the Beck Anxiety Inventory are relatively short (21-item) instruments that take about 10 minutes to administer and can be re-administered over time to monitor progress. Customized versions for children (ages 7 to 14) are also available.

As noted, SUDs have broad impacts on the physical and psychosocial functioning of the patient. The Addiction Severity Index (ASI) provides a reliable measure of lifetime use and use within the past 30 days for a full range of commonly used substances.[28] It also assesses additional key dimensions of functioning: medical status, vocational, legal, family, including family history and social issues, and psychiatric status. The ASI yields composite scores for each dimension, calculated based on selected quantifiable items and a rater-generated severity score. The scores are based on structured interviews, which take approximately 1 hour to administer. The ASI sections can be re-administered to assess progress over time. More recently, modifications of the ASI have been introduced and tailored to the needs of women[29] and teenagers.[30]

Self-report instruments also provide a *broadened assessment of the consequences of use*. The Drinker Inventory of Consequences (DrInc)[31] measures the adverse effects of alcohol use in five domains: physical, social, impulsive, interpersonal, and intrapersonal. The DrInc has been used widely in clinical trials, including repeated measures design. The 50-item test takes about 10 minutes, yielding lifetime and last 3-month scores for each domain and an overall score. A companion instrument, the Inventory of Drug Use Consequences (InDUC),[32] provides similar information for a broader population of patients using drugs or drugs and alcohol. Finally, the SIP-AD (Short Inventory of Problems-Alcohol and Drugs) is a brief 15-item self-report test that measures physical, social, intrapersonal, impulsive, and interpersonal consequences of alcohol and drug consumption. Versions of the SIP exist for alcohol only, drug only, or both.

It is essential to assess the *motivational level* of the patient for engaging in treatment. Self-report instruments are available, including the Stages of Change Readiness and Treatment

Eagerness Scale (SOCRATES).[33] The 19-item short form of the self-report instrument assesses motivation to change drinking behavior. A personal drug use version is also available. The transtheoretical model of change assesses the patient's level of recognition of a problem, ambivalence, or uncertainty about changing and whether the patient is taking steps to change. It has been employed to monitor motivational levels and predicts treatment adherence and outcome. A similar instrument, the University of Rhode Island Change Assessment (URICA),[34] is slightly longer (32 items) and can readily be modified to assess motivation for change across a range of behaviors, including alcohol and other drug use, or concomitant unhealthy behaviors. Both instruments are easy to administer and have been used successfully with many patients, including patients with severe, co-occurring psychiatric disorders.[35]

When a more comprehensive assessment of *resistance to treatment* is needed, most often in the context of a specialized treatment program, the Recovery Attitude and Treatment Evaluator (RAATE)[36] provides both a 35-item semi-structured clinical interview option (RAATE-CE)[37] and a 94-item self-report version (RAATE-QI).[37] They measure five constructs: resistance to initial treatment, resistance to continuing care, the severity of biomedical problems, psychiatric/psychological problems, and social/environmental support for recovery. The RAATE-CE is designed for administration by someone with adequate SUD expertise to make the ratings required. The QI version provides a more direct patient perspective on the constructs. Both take about 30 minutes to complete.

The patient's knowledge of the situations that trigger the use of substances is an essential element in any return to use prevention plan. Assessment instruments can be valuable aids in constructing a return to use prevention plan. The Inventory of Drinking Situations[38] is a 100-item self-report instrument that allows patients to assess their tendency to drink in various situations. The measure can be categorized as urges and temptations, personal control, unpleasant emotions, pleasant emotions, conflict, social pressure, physical discomfort, and enjoyable times with others.

In helping the patient prepare a return to use prevention plan, it is also helpful to understand the *coping skills* that the patient possesses. Several instruments are available to assess coping repertoire. The Coping Response Inventory (CRI)[39] is a relatively short (48-item) self-report instrument that evaluates four types of avoidant coping (emotional discharge, cognitive avoidance, seeking alternative rewards, resigned acceptance) and four types of approach coping (logical analysis, problem-solving, seeking guidance and support, positive reappraisal). A youth version is also available. The Brief Assessment of Recovery Capital (BARC) is a 10-item instrument that measures the specific resources in a person's life that can facilitate recovery from addiction. This tool helps identify sources of support to leverage as the person engages in recovery-focused activities.

Although there is ample evidence that treatment can work, *adherence to treatment* remains a significant impediment to recovery. Self-efficacy and expectations about the effect of alcohol and drugs have been demonstrated to be related to treatment adherence across a broad range of disorders. Self-efficacy for alcohol-related situations can be measured using the Situational Confidence Questionnaire (SCQ).[40] This 39-item self-report instrument asks patients to imagine themselves in various situations and rate their confidence that they can resist the urge to drink in these situations. It takes about 15 minutes to complete. The Drug Taking Confidence Questionnaire,[41] a companion tool, assesses self-efficacy for drug-related problems. Expectations about the effect of alcohol or drugs can also influence adherence. Specific tools exist to measure expectations (eg, the Adult Alcohol Expectancy Questionnaire.[42] A shorter, 8-item version of the brief SCQ is also available and is comparable to the original version.[43]

In summary, the choice of assessment tool will depend mainly upon time constraints, the setting in which the assessment takes place, the credentials and experience of the assessor, and the intended goal of the evaluation. Additionally, state guidelines for agency certification and national accreditation standards may further dictate the exact elements that need to appear in an assessment. Agencies and treatment programs will need to incorporate these elements to meet the standards. Assessment instruments help screen for disorders, determine diagnosis and severity, and develop treatment plans—they can be used to add depth and externally validated data to the assessment process to individualize high-quality care. Notably, the assessment process should never delay or be a barrier to starting treatment.

INTEGRATING ASSESSMENT INTO PRACTICE

Given the inevitable constraints of time facing a clinician, particularly in a primary care venue, it is often necessary to prioritize the domains assessed and assessment instruments utilized. Unless the information is already known and documented, evaluating the severity and frequency of use of multiple substances is a high priority. Often, the client's level of motivation for change is also a high priority since this assessment can determine the next logical step in the treatment or referral process. Thus, if a patient seen in a primary care setting is using at levels that are at least hazardous but indicates no interest in changing use levels, the clinician may choose to work on increasing motivation. The clinician may conduct other assessments that focus on the negative impacts of use on health, vocational life, or social adjustment. These data can then impact the patient's decisional balance regarding the pros and cons of continued substance use.

Conversely, for a highly motivated patient, instruments designed to assess situations that lead to use and coping skills that will help reduce use may be an immediate high priority. Co-occurring mental health conditions are also a high priority since they should influence the type of therapies offered and the level of care that will be coordinated. As with many assessment domains highlighted above, comorbidities can first be screened for with relatively brief self-report instruments. Those who screen positive can be further assessed with more comprehensive instruments.

An assessment is just the beginning step of the treatment process and is used to inform effective treatment strategies for managing SUDs. The assessment process also promotes early engagement and longer-term retention in treatment. As a general rule, a thorough assessment can usually be completed in 1 to 2 hours. Ironically, despite the best efforts at evaluation and the appropriate recommendation for a particular level of care, many individuals cannot access all levels of care. Many communities lack the resources to fund and sustain all levels of care. For example, if the assessment reveals a severe opioid use disorder diagnosis and the recommended level of care includes pharmacotherapy with opioid agonist or partial-agonist medication, but the local community lacks qualified treatment providers, there is no alignment between the assessment results and the available resources in the community. This is the "art" of creating a workable treatment plan and an ongoing call to action to advocate for adequate treatment funding and "treatment on demand."

SUMMARY

The assessment process guides healthcare providers treating patients with SUDs along evidence-based care management pathways, ensuring the accuracy of the initial diagnosis and identifying effective and efficient patient treatment needs. Quality assessment permits the development of a comprehensive problem list and a thorough treatment plan. Evaluation of all domains of life affected by SUDs and co-occurring medical and psychiatric disorders, withdrawal management needs, prior treatment, recurrence patterns, readiness for change, and treatment resistance are critical focus areas. Similarly, specific assessment tools and rapport between patients and providers are vital to the assessment process. We advocate using a trauma-sensitive approach, which has been shown to increase provider–patient rapport and improve treatment outcomes.[44] Finally, some assessment tools can quantify the impact of addiction on the lives of patients and measure morbidity and the residual level of functioning. Repeating the use of these quantitative tools can measure improved functioning and decreased morbidity, as well as help to continue to inform the ongoing process of treatment planning.[28,32,45-48]

ACKNOWLEDGEMENT

This chapter represents an update and revision of previous chapters in this series, most recently by Theodore V. Parran, Jr., Mark Bondeson, Richard A. McCormick, and Christina M. Delos Reyes from the last edition. We are indebted to them for their work and retain much of their prose in this current edition.

REFERENCES

1. Dube SR, Felitti VJ, Dong M, Chapman DP, Giles WH, Anda RF. Childhood abuse, neglect, and household dysfunction and the risk of illicit drug use: the adverse childhood experiences study. *Pediatrics*. 2003;111(3):564-572.
2. Cook P, Dogoloff ML, Harteker L, Nelson AE, et al. *Comprehensive Case Management for Substance Abuse Treatment*. Treatment Improvement Protocol (TIP) Series 27.
3. Brown VB, Harris M, Fallot R. Moving toward trauma-informed practice in addiction treatment: a collaborative model of agency assessment. *J Psychoactive Drugs*. 2013;45(5):386-393.
4. Babor TF, Higgins-Biddle JC, Saunders JB, et al. *AUDIT: The Alcohol Use Disorders Identification Test. Guidelines for Use in Primary Care*. World Health Organization; 2001.
5. Driessen M, Schulte S, Luedecke C, et al. Trauma and PTSD in patients with alcohol, drug, or dual dependence: a multi-center study. *Alcohol Clin Exp Res*. 2008;32(3):481-488.
6. Sheehan D, Janavs J, Baker R, et al. *Mini International Neuropsychiatric Interview (MINI): English Version 5.0.0 DSM-IV*. University of South Florida; 2005.
7. Schuckit MA. Broadening the base of treatment for alcohol problems: report of a study by a committee of the institute of medicine division of mental health and behavioral medicine. *Am J Psychiatry*. 1991;148(11):1589.
8. The Joint Commission. *A Practical Guide to Documentation in Behavioral Health*. The Joint Commission; 2008.
9. Bohn MJ, Babor TF, Kranzler HR. The Alcohol Use Disorders Identification Test (AUDIT): validation of a screening instrument for use in medical settings. *J Stud Alcohol*. 1995;56(4):423-432.
10. Donovan DM, Kivlahan DR, Doyle SR, Longabaugh R, Greenfield SF. Concurrent validity of the Alcohol Use Disorders Identification Test (AUDIT) and AUDIT zones in defining levels of severity among outpatients with alcohol dependence in the COMBINE study. *Addiction*. 2006;101(12):1696-1704.
11. Cassidy CM, Schmitz N, Malla A. Validation of the alcohol use disorders identification test and the drug abuse screening test in first episode psychosis. *Can J Psychiatry*. 2008;53(1):26-33.
12. Rodriguez-Martos A, Santamariña E. Does the short form of the Alcohol Use Disorders Identification Test (AUDIT-C) work at a trauma emergency department? *Subst Use Misuse*. 2007;42(6):923-932.
13. Skinner HA. The drug abuse screening test. *Addict Behavs*. 1982;7(4):363-371.
14. Cocco KM, Carey KB. Psychometric properties of the Drug Abuse Screening Test in psychiatric outpatients. *Psychol Assess*. 1998;10(4):408.
15. Yudko E, Lozhkina O, Fouts A. A comprehensive review of the psychometric properties of the Drug Abuse Screening Test. *J Subst Abuse Treat*. 2007;32(2):189-198.
16. WHO ASSIST Working Group. The alcohol, smoking and substance involvement screening test (ASSIST): development, reliability and feasibility. *Addiction*. 2002;97(9):1183-1194.
17. Humeniuk R, Ali R, Babor TF, Farrell M, et al. Validation of the alcohol, smoking and substance involvement screening test (ASSIST). *Addiction*. 2008;103(6):1039-1047.
18. Saitz R, Cheng DM, Allensworth-Davies D, Winter MR, Smith PC. The ability of single screening questions for unhealthy alcohol and other drug use to identify substance dependence in primary care. *J Stud Alcohol Drugs*. 2014;75(1):153-157.
19. Ewing JA. Detecting alcoholism: the CAGE questionnaire. *JAMA*. 1984;252(14):1905-1907.
20. Frank SH, Graham AV, Zyzanski SJ, White S. Use of the family CAGE in screening for alcohol problems in primary care. *Arch Fam Med*. 1992;1(2):209.
21. Selzer ML, Vinokur A, van Rooijen L. A self-administered short Michigan alcoholism screening test (SMAST). *J Stud Alcohol*. 1975;36(1):117-126.
22. Spitzer RL, Williams JB, Gibbon M, First MB. The structured clinical interview for DSM-III-R (SCID) I: history, rationale, and description. *Arch Gen Psychiatry*. 1992;49(8):624-629.
23. Brown RL, Rounds LA. Conjoint screening questionnaires for alcohol and other drug abuse: criterion validity in a primary care practice. *WMJ*. 1995;94(3):135-140.

24. First MB, Spitzer RL, Gibbon M, Williams JB. *Structured Clinical Interview for DSM-IV-TR Axis I Disorders, Research Version*. patient ed. SCID-I/P; 2002.
25. Cottler LB, Robins LN, Helzer JE. The reliability of the CIDI-SAM: a comprehensive substance abuse interview. *Br J Addict*. 1989;84(7):801-814.
26. Sullivan JT, Sykora K, Schneiderman J, Naranjo CA, Sellers EM. Assessment of alcohol withdrawal: the revised clinical institute withdrawal assessment for alcohol scale (CIWA-Ar). *Br J Addict*. 1989;84(11):1353-1357.
27. Derogatis LR, Fitzpatrick M, Maruish ME, eds. *The SCL-90-R, the Brief Symptom Inventory (BSI), and the BSI-18. The Use of Psychological Testing for Treatment Planning and Outcomes Assessment: Volume 3: Instruments for Adults*. 3rd ed. Lawrence Erlbaum Associates Publishers; 2004.
28. Kroenke K, Spitzer RL, Williams JB. The PHQ-9: validity of a brief depression severity measure. *J Gen Intern Med*. 2001;16(9):606-613.
29. Beck AT, Ward CH, Mendelson M, Mock J, Erbaugh J. An inventory for measuring depression. *Arch Gen Psychiatry*. 1961;4(6):561-571.
30. Lesieur HR, Blume SB. The South Oaks Gambling Screen (SOGS): a new instrument for the identification of pathological gamblers. *Am J Psychiatry*. 1987;144:1184-1188.
31. McLellan AT, Kushner H, Metzger D. The fifth edition of the Addiction Severity Index. *J Subst Abuse Treat*. 1992;9(3):199-213.
32. Brown E, Frank D, Friedman A. *Supplementary Administration Manual for the Expanded Female Version of the Addiction Severity Index (ASI) Instrument, the ASI-F*. DHHS Publication no. (SMA); 1997.
33. Kaminer Y, Wagner E, Plummer B, Seifer R. Validation of the teen addiction severity index (T-ASI): preliminary findings. *Am J Addict*. 1993;2(3):250-254.
34. Miller WR, Tonigan JS, Longabaugh R. *The Drinker Inventory of Consequences (DrInC): An Instrument for Assessing Adverse Consequences of Alcohol Abuse*. Vol. 4. National Institute on Alcohol Abuse and Alcoholism; 1995.
35. Tonigan JS, Miller WR. The inventory of drug use consequences (InDUC): test-retest stability and sensitivity to detect change. *Psychol Addict Behav*. 2002;16(2):165.
36. Miller W, Tonigan JS. Assessing drinker's motivations for change: the Stages of Change Readiness and Treatment Eagerness Scale (SOCRATES). *Psychol Addict Behav*. 1996;10(2):81-89.
37. DiClemente CC, Hughes SO. Stages of change profiles in outpatient alcoholism treatment. *J Subst Abuse*. 1990;2(2):217-235.
38. Zhang AY, Harmon JA, Werkner J, McCormick RA. Impacts of motivation for change on the severity of alcohol use by patients with severe and persistent mental illness. *J Stud Alcohol*. 2004;65(3):392-397.
39. Mee-Lee D. An instrument for treatment progress and matching: the Recovery Attitude and Treatment Evaluator (RAATE). *J Subst Abuse Treat*. 1988;5(3):183-186.
40. Smith MB, Hoffmann NG, Nederhoed R. The development and reliability of the RAATE-CE. *J Subst Abuse*. 1992;4(4):355-363.
41. Annis HM, Graham JM, Davis CS. *Inventory of Drinking Situations (IDS): User's Guide*. Addiction Research Foundation; 1987.
42. Moos R. *Coping Response Inventory Manual*. Center for Health Care Evaluation, Department of Veterans Affairs and Stanford University Medical Center; 1992.
43. Annis HM, Graham JM. *Situational Confidence Questionnaire (SCQ-39): User's Guide*. Addiction Research Foundation; 1988.
44. Smith MB, Hoffmann NG, Nederhoed R. The development and reliability of the Recovery Attitude and Treatment Evaluator-Questionnaire I (RAATE-QI). *Int J Addict*. 1995;30(2):147-160.
45. Annis HM, Skylar Turner NE. *The Drug Taking Confidence Questionnaire: User's Guide*. Addiction Research Foundation; 1997.
46. Brown SA, Christiansen BA, Goldman MS. The Alcohol Expectancy Questionnaire: an instrument for the assessment of adolescent and adult alcohol expectancies. *J Stud Alcohol*. 1987;48(5):483-491.
47. Substance Abuse and Mental Health Services Administration. *Using Technology-Based Therapeutic Tools in Behavioral Health Services*. Treatment Improvement Protocol (TIP) Series 60. No. (SMA) 15-4924. HHS Publication, Substance Abuse and Mental Health Services Administration; 2015.
48. Hester RK, Squires DD, Delaney HD. The Drinker's check-up: 12-month outcomes of a controlled clinical trial of a stand-alone software program for problem drinkers. *J Subst Abuse Treat*. 2005;28(2):159-169.

Sidebar 1

Hospital-Based Addiction Care

Honora Englander, Jennifer McNeely, and Zoe M. Weinstein

HOSPITALIZATION AS A HIGH-RISK TOUCHPOINT

Substance use disorder (SUD)-related hospitalizations are common and costly.[1,2] At least one in nine hospitalized adults has a SUD,[3] and U.S. SUD-related hospital costs in 2017 exceeded $13 billion.[1] SUD-related hospitalizations are rising, with recent increases in hospitalizations due to opioids,[4] methamphetamines[5] and alcohol-related liver diseases.[6] Integrating addiction care as part of general hospital care is a critical part of the care continuum for people with SUDs. Hospital-based SUD care can improve physical and behavioral health, reduce harms of substance use, engage people in SUD treatment during and after hospitalization, and help to educate an interdisciplinary workforce about SUD.

People with SUD are at high risk for hospital readmission, repeat emergency department visits, and death.[7-9] Hospitalization serves as a marker that identifies people who are high risk for overdose and death, and represents an important opportunity to engage people in life-saving treatment. In a statewide study in Massachusetts, people with opioid use disorder (OUD) hospitalized for an injection-related infection had a standardized mortality ratio of 54 for fatal opioid overdose[10] compared with people who did not have an infection-related hospitalization. And, while critically important, overdose deaths represent the tip of the iceberg. A statewide study in Oregon found that 7.8% of hospitalized adults with OUD died in the year after discharge;[9] a rate similar to 1-year mortality from acute myocardial infarction.

Of those, 13% died of overdose, and 55% died of nondrug related causes, highlighting the need to create hospital systems that can support people in addressing both their SUD and their other health conditions that may be more challenging to manage in the face of untreated SUD.

Despite their frequent, high-cost health care utilization and high risk for death, most hospitalized adults with SUD are not engaged in addiction care at the time of admission.[11,12] However, many patients want SUD care and they want it to start in the hospital. In one study of adults admitted to a general hospital, 57% of people with high risk alcohol use and 68% of people with high risk drug use reported wanting to cut back or quit.[13] Many experienced hospitalization as a "wake-up call," where fear of death was motivating for change and where hospitalization offered an opportunity to disrupt use.[14]

Evidence Base

A rapidly emerging evidence base shows that hospital-based addiction care can improve patient, provider, and health system-level outcomes, both during and following a hospitalization. Hospital-based addiction care can support patients to initiate medication for opioid and alcohol use disorder,[11,15] increase patient's trust in hospital clinicians,[16,17] increase posthospital SUD treatment engagement,[18-21] reduce SUD severity,[19] and reduce mortality.[22,23] Furthermore, hospital-based addiction care can increase staff understanding of addiction and how to treat it and support hospitals to be more trauma-informed[17,24-26] and responsive to emerging population health needs.[27] Evidence for the effect of hospital-based addiction care on hospital readmission is varied,[28,29] and suggests opportunities to reduce readmission may be most promising for patients with OUD[28] or when hospital-based addiction care is combined with intensive transitional care support such as patient navigation.[30]

An array of approaches to delivering hospital-based addiction care exist. A recent scoping review and taxonomy of U.S. models described six distinct model types.[31] The first three are consult models, which include: (1) interprofessional addiction consult services (ACS), (2) psychiatry consult liaison services, and (3) individual consultants. Of these, ACS are best described in the literature and are the most comprehensive. ACS include expert addiction clinicians, a coordinator, and staff with an explicit focus on patient engagement (eg, peers with lived experience[17,32]), and support direct pathways to continue SUD care after hospitalization. Psychiatry consult liaison services are also increasingly incorporating SUD into their scope of practice, for example, by delivering medication for OUD and alcohol use disorder and developing posthospital SUD treatment pathways. In the individual consultant model, a single board-certified addiction physician offers consultation to address acute medical needs such as withdrawal and pharmacotherapy, and typically partners with general hospital staff to support posthospital treatment referrals.[31] The next two models are practice-based models, wherein general hospital staff integrate addiction care into usual practice. This approach is increasing across U.S. hospitals and includes both (4) hospital-based opioid treatment (HBOT) and (5) hospital-based alcohol treatment (HBAT). HBOT and HBAT are often implemented by hospitalists (ie, hospital-based general medicine providers), but there are also examples of infectious-disease clinicians integrating HBOT and hepatologists integrating HBAT. The final model is (6) community based in-reach, wherein community providers deliver SUD care to individuals who are currently in the hospital.[31]

Clinical Best Practices

Best practices for hospital-based addiction care include eliciting a complete SUD history and physical examination, managing acute withdrawal, initiating medication and other evidence-based treatment, and providing referral and linkage to long-term SUD supports (**Box 33-1**).[33] Hospital clinicians should offer relevant Food and Drug Administration (FDA) approved medications for SUD to hospitalized patients, including medication for opioid, alcohol,[34] and tobacco use disorders, as appropriate.[35-37] Hospital-based addiction providers can promote interdisciplinary, patient-centered care plans related to sequalae of substance use, such as long-term intravenous antibiotics,[38,39] cardiac valve surgery,[40,41] or liver transplantation.

The Imperative to Improve Hospital-Based Addictions Care

At time of writing this chapter, most U.S. hospitals do not offer evidence-based SUD treatment. Many hospitals do not have methadone or buprenorphine for OUD on formulary. In one statewide study of New Mexico hospitals, 46%

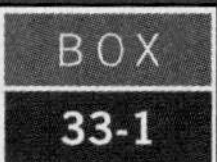

Hospital Care Standards

All hospitals should:

- Identify and treat withdrawal
- Initiate and continue evidence-based substance use disorder (SUD) medication treatments (including opioid agonist therapy, medication for alcohol use disorder, and medication for tobacco use disorder)
- Adopt trauma-informed, nondiscriminatory, evidence-based policies that facilitate patient engagement with medical care
- Develop partnerships and pathways to postacute care services for people with SUD, including having the ability for timely posthospital SUD treatment
- Support overdose prevention and harm reduction, including providing naloxone

of hospitals lacked buprenorphine-naloxone on formulary, and 10 of 26 New Mexico counties lacked any hospital with buprenorphine-naloxone available for inpatients.[42] A nationwide study in Veterans' Affairs hospitals examined rates of agonist medication for opioid use disorder (MOUD)—methadone and buprenorphine—prescribing, and found that few admissions received opioid agonist therapy during admission, and that when MOUD was provided, it was most often for withdrawal management. Among patients not on MOUD prior to admission who survived hospitalization, only 2.0% were newly initiated on methadone or buprenorphine with linkage to care after hospital discharge.[12]

Addiction medicine workforce shortages and widespread training gaps among hospital clinicians further hamper efforts to address SUD in hospitals.[43,44] SUD training gaps persist across disciplines, including medicine, nursing, pharmacy, and social work; and most hospital staff are underprepared to diagnose SUD, discuss community treatment options, and discuss overdose prevention and harm reduction.[45]

Stigma is both caused by and a consequence of unprepared hospital systems. SUDs are among the most severely stigmatized health conditions,[46] and stigma towards people who use drugs in hospitals is common and harmful.[47] People with SUD commonly avoid or delay seeking hospital care for fear of stigma and discrimination by hospital staff.[48] When hospitalized, patients with SUD often experience untreated pain and withdrawal, stigma and discrimination about substance use, and hospital restrictions including restrictions limiting visitors or time off the hospital unit.[14,49,50] This can lead to mutual mistrust between patients and staff,[51] and commonly leads to patients leaving the hospital before completing recommended treatment (also called "against medical advice").[14,49,51] These negative experiences and outcomes are not inevitable—by providing patient-centered, trauma-informed care, hospital teams can increase trust[16,17] and achieve better outcomes.

In the United States, there are wide disparities in access to SUD treatment for Black, Indigenous, Hispanic/Latinx, and other people of color,[52] which also extend to hospital-based addiction care.[53] Data from the 2018 National Survey demonstrated that, among Americans with SUD, 88% of Black people and 90% of Latinx people received no SUD treatment.[54] Another nationally representative survey demonstrated that, from 2004 to 2015, Black people with OUD were 80% less likely to be prescribed buprenorphine than White people.[55] Other studies in ambulatory settings show that Black people are more likely to be offered methadone, a treatment that is highly stigmatized and far more burdensome than buprenorphine.[52,56] Racial differences in MOUD access persist in hospitals,[53] and may reflect differences in hospital care, community treatment access, or both. Approaches to expand access to SUD treatment among communities of color must address individual clinician-, hospital-, and community-level barriers.[56-58]

These challenges are a call to action[59] for addiction specialists, general hospital clinicians, and community clinicians[31] to improve hospital-based addiction care by addressing widespread clinical gaps and structural barriers.[60]

TREATING OPIOID USE DISORDER IN HOSPITAL CARE

Offering opioid agonist medication (ie, methadone or buprenorphine) to treat hospitalized patients with OUD, whether for initiation or continuation of treatment, is best practice.[61] Though sometimes misunderstood, restrictions related to opioid prescribing in ambulatory settings—which restrict methadone administration to federally licensed opioid treatment programs (OTPs) do not apply in hospital.[62] Federal statute specifies an exception that allows for methadone dispensation as part of general hospital care. Per 1306.07 Code of Federal Regulations, hospitalized patients can be "administered or dispensed opioids for maintenance or withdrawal management as an adjunct to a condition other than addiction."[63] This means that patients must be hospitalized for an acute indication (eg, acute medical, surgical, obstetrical need). However, in hospitalized patients there are no restrictions on methadone dose, duration, or indication (eg, acute withdrawal or methadone maintenance). Patients can newly initiate methadone, have methadone dose adjusted, or have methadone continued at stable doses. Furthermore, while clinicians cannot prescribe methadone for use in the outpatient setting outside of an OTP, in March 2022 the U.S. Drug Enforcement Agency (DEA) changed existing rules to allow hospital clinicians to *dispense* up to 72 hours at a time of methadone for withdrawal management while arranging referral for ongoing treatment (called the "72-hour rule").[64] This change expanded the previous "72-hour rule," which required that practitioners administer medication *one day at a time*, now permitting practitioners to *dispense 3 days* of medication at a time.[65] As with the original "72-hour rule," this regulation applies to methadone, buprenorphine, and other opioids;[66] however, implications may be greatest for methadone, given current U.S. laws restricting methadone in general health care settings. Finally, while currently implemented in some hospitals, many hospitals are struggling to implement this rule change given challenges with medication dispensation and confusion around rule interpretation.[63]

Until December 2022, U.S. policy restricted the ability to prescribe buprenorphine to those who obtained a federal "X waiver." However, now any clinician with an active DEA license may prescribe buprenorphine for patients both in hospital and at the time of discharge (https://www.federalregister.gov/documents/2023/08/08/2023-16892/dispensing-of-narcotic-drugs-to-relieve-acute-withdrawal-symptoms-of-opioid-use-disorder). Finally, hospital clinicians can administer short acting full agonist opioids (eg, hydromorphone) as an adjunct to medications like methadone or buprenorphine—or alone—to treat pain, cravings, or withdrawal.[67,68]

Though legal and best practice, many hospital clinicians lack knowledge and confidence to offer methadone and buprenorphine. They are unfamiliar with how to discuss medication options with patients, how to initiate medications, and the nuances of coordinating post-hospital treatment linkage. Individual clinician and system-level gaps are important improvement opportunities.

Medication for opioid use disorder (MOUD) initiation is the best treatment for reducing morbidity and mortality and is superior to medically-supervised withdrawal ("detoxification"). Approaches to initiating methadone and buprenorphine during hospitalization may differ from the outpatient setting, both because rules are less restrictive and because patients have closer monitoring during hospitalization. More aggressive hospital (versus ambulatory) inductions are common in instances where patients have known tolerance (eg, fentanyl use) and can be monitored closely for signs and symptoms of over-sedation or respiratory depression.[69] For example, hospital clinicians may be more liberal in dosing methadone in the hospital, where clinicians may bring methadone naive patients to doses of 60 mg over 2 to 3 days with subsequent 10 mg increases every 3 days (versus taking weeks in the outpatient setting where increases are typically 5 mg every 5-7 days). Similarly, innovative buprenorphine induction approaches in hospitals may be necessary and possible. Traditional buprenorphine inductions—which require patients to experience acute withdrawal—may be challenging due to acute pain, anxiety, or co-occurring illness.[70] In these instances, low or very low-dose buprenorphine inductions (sometimes referred to as "microdosing" [a term no longer preferred due to risk for conflation with hallucinogen use] or the Bernese method) may be better alternatives. With low-dose inductions, patients can stay on or start full agonist opioids such as methadone, while gradually starting low doses of buprenorphine and slowly up-titrating over several days. Protocols vary, and can occur over 3 to 10 days.[70-72] Low-dose inductions also seem to have preferable risk profile in hospitalized patients who use synthetic opioids (eg, illicitly-manufactured fentanyl) and are at high risk for precipitated withdrawal, even after 24 to 48 hours of fentanyl abstinence.[73] Long-acting injectable naltrexone, an opioid antagonist that is FDA-approved for the prevention of OUD recurrence amongst individuals who have completed withdrawal management, is generally less useful in hospitalized patients, many of whom have acute pain.

Hospitalized patients commonly experience pain, and SUD is not a contraindication to using full agonist opioids (eg, hydromorphone) for acute pain. Patients with OUD may have higher opioid tolerance and hence require higher doses and more frequent dosing[74,75] to achieve analgesia. Patients who require more opioid medications can be incorrectly labeled as "drug seeking," when in reality their symptoms may reflect unmet pain needs in the setting of opioid tolerance or acute withdrawal. In addition to methadone and buprenorphine, short term full agonist opioids can also support acute withdrawal management either while MOUD is being titrated, when patients refuse MOUD, or when MOUD is contraindicated. Questions about perioperative pain management and buprenorphine are common. Generally, best practice is to continue buprenorphine and deploy additional full agonist opioids, regional anesthesia, and nonopioid pain management strategies.[76]

HARM REDUCTION

Hospitalization is a prime opportunity to support harm reduction and overdose prevention, including naloxone distribution, safer use education, sexually transmitted infection evaluation and treatment, and distribution of harm reduction supplies.[77-83] Though not yet available in the United States, some Canadian hospitals have implemented supervised consumption spaces for hospitalized patients[84,85] who continue drug use. That said, hospital systems—and more generally the biomedical model—may clash with harm reduction models.[86] Specifically, hospitals embrace a hierarchical chain of command, whereas harm reduction embraces a structural philosophy that is inclusive and community-driven. Further, hospital care centers on expert knowledge by highly trained professionals whereas harm reduction centers control and expertise with people who use drugs who are expert in their own experience. Nonetheless, these approaches should be seen as complementary, and when offered together they support patients with evidence-based care. Understanding these tensions can help support improvement, and may be important for champions of hospital-based addiction care, who may encounter resistance to harm reduction at individual and structural levels. The importance and challenges of delivering harm reduction also supports the potential role for integrating peers with lived experience as part of hospital care.[17,32]

HOSPITAL POLICIES

Hospitals are complex environments and organizational policies inform care quality and access, as well as patient and staff experience. They are critical to creating a therapeutic hospital environment. Hospital SUD policies should be grounded in evidence and principles of trauma-informed care, recognizing that addiction is a treatable chronic medical condition and not a crime or a moral failing.

Punitive hospital policies are common and often harmful; they may create a perception of control by hospital staff but may discriminate against people with SUD and likely do little to increase patient or staff safety. For example, policies that require deploying security or performing physical searches of patients or visitors in an attempt to confiscate substances may violate patient's physical and emotional safety.[87,88] They risk traumatizing patients, many of whom may have history of incarceration or trauma, they erode trust between patients and staff, and they are unlikely to recover substances. Other behavior policies such as forbidding patients with SUD from leaving the unit may make hospitalization intolerable and increase risk that patients leave the hospital before completing recommended medical therapy.[89] Further, policies around urine drug testing in pregnant patients should require patient consent.[90]

Hospital leaders can assure high quality SUD care by performing an environmental scan of local policies to ensure that policies are nondiscriminatory,[91] align with federal rules, are concordant with national recommendations, and do not introduce additional barriers to delivering evidence-based treatments such as MOUD.[92]

POSTHOSPITAL TRANSITIONS AND CARE LINKAGES

As with other chronic conditions, coordinating SUD care with outpatient providers is an important aspect of hospital-based care. Patients who start evidence-based SUD treatments in the hospital should be offered treatment linkages to continue treatment, including with medications, after discharge. To accomplish this, all hospitals should develop and sustain relationships with community SUD treatment resources and harm reduction services, and support patients to engage in timely and appropriate care after discharge. This includes identifying clinicians willing and able to prescribe buprenorphine, and developing timely treatment pathways from hospital to OTPs for methadone. As of December 2022, any clinician with an active DEA license can prescribe buprenorphine at hospital discharge. Hospital clinicians cannot prescribe methadone for OUD; however, rules allow up to 3 days of methadone dispensation while linking patients to an OTP (https://www.federalregister.gov/documents/2023/08/08/2023-16892/dispensing-of-narcotic-drugs-to-relieve-acute-withdrawal-symptoms-of-opioid-use-disorder).

Opioid treatment programs often have limited weekend hours of operation and restricted times for new patient appointments. Hospital clinicians—including physicians, social workers, and case managers—should consider the nuances of community treatment systems when developing care plans (eg, avoiding Friday or Saturday discharge to avoid missed methadone doses), and may need to advocate to assure that systems support the patient's physical health and SUD care needs. Furthermore, community treatment providers could establish care pathways that ease treatment entry for hospitalized patients, such as expediting treatment intakes, allowing patients to come directly to the treatment program from the hospital upon discharge, or assigning peer navigators to work with patients even while they are still in the hospital.[93]

Referrals of hospitalized patients with SUD to postacute medical care facilities (eg, skilled nursing facilities [SNF]) are commonly rejected due to discriminatory practices, misunderstanding of rules surrounding MOUD, and coordination challenges between SNF and OTPs for patients on methadone.[94-96] SNF rejection or delays can prolong hospital length of stay and prevent patients from accessing necessary post-acute physical and behavioral health care. This is an important area for hospital leadership, advocacy, and partnership to assure equitable and quality care.[60]

WORKFORCE EDUCATION

In addition to providing effective evidence-based care and improving health outcomes for patients with SUD, providing SUD care in hospitals can help educate multidisciplinary health care professionals working in the hospital system. The average medical school curriculum dedicates only a few hours to addiction, and barely half of the approximately 10,000 medical residency programs nationwide require curricular content on addiction prevention and treatment, leaving practicing physicians with very limited knowledge of SUD treatment.[97] However, the bulk of skill acquisition for any medical provider occurs under an apprenticeship model, and hospitals are the primary training grounds for physicians, nurses, pharmacists, social workers, and a host of other disciplines who have a role to play in addiction care. Trainees who are exposed to successful treatment for SUD can gain the required clinical knowledge and confidence to integrate this into their practices going forward, even without becoming specialized addiction providers.

CONCLUSION

There is pressing need to improve care delivery and health systems for hospitalized people with SUD, and hospitals are a long-overlooked and critical part of the care continuum for people with SUD. The opioid crisis has stimulated a proliferation of model programs and approaches.[31] However, critical research, practice, and policy gaps exist, including understanding and addressing racial and ethnic disparities for people with SUD in hospital settings. Widespread adoption of best practices and development of further improvements will require a concerted effort across addiction specialists, general hospital clinicians, hospitals and health systems, educational institutions, and policy-makers.

REFERENCES

1. Peterson C, Li M, Xu L, Mikosz CA, Luo F. Assessment of annual cost of substance use disorder in U.S. hospitals. *JAMA Netw Open*. 2021;4(3):e210242. doi:10.1001/jamanetworkopen.2021.0242
2. Ronan MV, Herzig SJ. Hospitalizations related to opioid abuse/dependence and associated serious infections increased sharply, 2002-12. *Health Aff (Millwood)*. 2016;35(5):832-837. doi:10.1377/hlthaff.2015.1424
3. Suen LW, Makam AN, Snyder HR, et al. National prevalence of alcohol and other substance use disorders among emergency department visits and hospitalizations: NHAMCS 2014-2018. *J Gen Intern Med*. 2022;37(10):2420-2428. doi:10.1007/s11606-021-07069-w
4. Singh JA, Cleveland JD. National U.S. time-trends in opioid use disorder hospitalizations and associated healthcare utilization and mortality. *PLoS One*. 2020;15(2):e0229174. doi:10.1371/journal.pone.0229174
5. Winkelman TNA, Admon LK, Jennings L, Shippee ND, Richardson CR, Bart G. Evaluation of amphetamine-related hospitalizations and associated clinical outcomes and costs in the United States. *JAMA Netw Open*. 2018;1(6):e183758. doi:10.1001/jamanetworkopen.2018.3758
6. Hirode G, Saab S, Wong RJ. Trends in the burden of chronic liver disease among hospitalized U.S. adults. *JAMA Netw Open*. 2020;3(4):e201997. doi:10.1001/jamanetworkopen.2020.1997

7. Walley AY, Paasche-Orlow M, Lee EC, et al. Acute care hospital utilization among medical inpatients discharged with a substance use disorder diagnosis. *J Addict Med*. 2012;6(1):50-56. doi:10.1097/ADM.0b013e318231de51
8. Lewer D, Freer J, King E, et al. Frequency of health-care utilization by adults who use illicit drugs: a systematic review and meta-analysis. *Addiction*. 2020;115(6):1011-1023. doi:10.1111/add.14892
9. King C, Cook R, Korthuis PT, Morris CD, Englander H. Causes of death in the 12 months after hospital discharge among patients with opioid use disorder. *J Addict Med*. 2022;16(4):466-469. doi:10.1097/ADM.0000000000000915
10. Larochelle MR, Bernstein R, Bernson D, et al. Touchpoints—opportunities to predict and prevent opioid overdose: a cohort study. *Drug Alcohol Depend*. 2019;204:107537. doi:10.1016/j.drugalcdep.2019.06.039
11. Englander H, King C, Nicolaidis C, et al. Predictors of opioid and alcohol pharmacotherapy initiation at hospital discharge among patients seen by an inpatient addiction consult service. *J Addict Med*. 2020;14(5):415-422. doi:10.1097/adm.0000000000000611
12. Priest KC, Lovejoy TI, Englander H, Shull S, McCarty D. Opioid agonist therapy during hospitalization within the veterans health administration: a pragmatic retrospective cohort analysis. *J Gen Intern Med*. 2020;35(8):2365-2374. doi:10.1007/s11606-020-05815-0
13. Englander H, Weimer M, Solotaroff R, et al. Planning and designing the improving addiction care team (IMPACT) for hospitalized adults with substance use disorder. *J Hosp Med*. 2017;12(5):339-342. doi:10.12788/jhm.2736
14. Velez CM, Nicolaidis C, Korthuis PT, Englander H. "It's been an experience, a life learning experience": a qualitative study of hospitalized patients with substance use disorders. *J Gen Intern Med*. 2017;32(3):296-303. doi:10.1007/s11606-016-3919-4
15. Nordeck CD, Welsh C, Schwartz RP, Mitchell SG, O'Grady KE, Gryczynski J. Opioid agonist treatment initiation and linkage for hospitalized patients seen by a substance use disorder consultation service. *Drug Alcohol Depend*. 2022;2:100031. doi:10.1016/j.dadr.2022.100031
16. King C, Collins D, Patten A, Nicolaidis C, Englander H. Trust in hospital physicians among patients with substance use disorder referred to an addiction consult service: a mixed-methods study. *J Addict Med*. 2021;16(1):41-48. doi:10.1097/adm.0000000000000819
17. Collins D, Alla J, Nicolaidis C, et al. "If it wasn't for him, I wouldn't have talked to them": qualitative study of addiction peer mentorship in the hospital. *J Gen Intern Med*. 2019;12:12. doi:10.1007/s11606-019-05311-0
18. Trowbridge P, Weinstein ZM, Kerensky T, et al. Addiction consultation services—linking hospitalized patients to outpatient addiction treatment. *J Subst Abuse Treat*. 2017;79:1-5. doi:10.1016/j.jsat.2017.05.007
19. Wakeman SE, Metlay JP, Chang Y, Herman GE, Rigotti NA. Inpatient addiction consultation for hospitalized patients increases post-discharge abstinence and reduces addiction severity. *J Gen Intern Med*. 2017;32(8):909-916. doi:10.1007/s11606-017-4077-z
20. Englander H, Dobbertin K, Lind BK, et al. Inpatient addiction medicine consultation and post-hospital substance use disorder treatment engagement: a propensity-matched analysis. *J Gen Intern Med*. 2019;34(12):2796-2803. doi:10.1007/s11606-019-05251-9
21. Liebschutz JM, Crooks D, Herman D, et al. Buprenorphine treatment for hospitalized, opioid-dependent patients: a randomized clinical trial. *JAMA Intern Med*. 2014;174(8):1369-1376. doi:10.1001/jamainternmed.2014.2556
22. King CA, Cook R, Wheelock H, et al. Simulating the impact of Addiction Consult Services in the context of drug supply contamination, hospitalizations, and drug-related mortality. *Int J Drug Policy*. 2022;100:103525. doi:10.1016/j.drugpo.2021.103525
23. Wilson JD, Altieri Dunn SC, Roy P, Joseph E, Klipp S, Liebschutz J. Inpatient addiction medicine consultation service impact on post-discharge patient mortality: a propensity-matched analysis. *J Gen Intern Med*. 2022;37(10):2521-2525. doi:101007/s11606-021-07362-8
24. Englander H, Collins D, Perry SP, Rabinowitz M, Phoutrides E, Nicolaidis C. "We've learned it's a medical illness, not a moral choice": qualitative study of the effects of a multicomponent addiction intervention on hospital providers' attitudes and experiences. *J Hosp Med*. 2018;13(11):752-758. doi:10.12788/jhm.2993
25. Callister C, Lockhart S, Holtrop JS, Hoover K, Calcaterra SL. Experiences with an addiction consultation service on care provided to hospitalized patients with opioid use disorder: a qualitative study of hospitalists, nurses, pharmacists, and social workers. *Subst Abus*. 2022;43(1):615-622. doi:10.1080/08897077.2021.1975873
26. Hoover K, Lockhart S, Callister C, Holtrop JS, Calcaterra SL. Experiences of stigma in hospitals with addiction consultation services: a qualitative analysis of patients' and hospital-based providers' perspectives. *J Subst Abuse Treat*. 2022;138:108708. doi:10.1016/j.jsat.2021.108708
27. Harris MTH, Peterkin A, Bach P, et al. Adapting inpatient addiction medicine consult services during the COVID-19 pandemic. *Addict Sci Clin Pract*. 2021;16(1):13. doi:10.1186/s13722-021-00221-1
28. Weinstein ZM, Cheng DM, D'Amico MJ, et al. Inpatient addiction consultation and post-discharge 30-day acute care utilization. *Drug Alcohol Depend*. 2020;213:108081. doi:10.1016/j.drugalcdep.2020.108081
29. Barocas JA, Gai MJ, Amuchi B, Jawa R, Linas BP. Impact of medications for opioid use disorder among persons hospitalized for drug use-associated skin and soft tissue infections. *Drug Alcohol Depend*. 2020;215:108207. doi:10.1016/j.drugalcdep.2020.108207
30. Gryczynski J, Nordeck CD, Welsh C, Mitchell SG, O'Grady KE, Schwartz RP. Preventing hospital readmission for patients with comorbid substance use disorder: a randomized trial. *Ann Intern Med*. 2021;174(7):899-909. doi:10.7326/m20-5475
31. Englander H, Jones A, Krawczyk N, et al. A taxonomy of hospital-based addiction care models: a scoping review and key informant interviews. *J Gen Intern Med*. 2022;37(11):2821-2833. doi:10.1007/s11606-022-07618-x
32. Englander H, Gregg J, Gullickson J, et al. Recommendations for integrating peer mentors in hospital-based addiction care. *Subst Abus*. 2020;41(4):419-424. doi:10.1080/08897077.2019.1635968
33. Weinstein ZM, Wakeman SE, Nolan S. Inpatient addiction consult service: expertise for hospitalized patients with complex addiction problems. *Med Clin North Am*. 2018;102(4):587-601. doi:10.1016/j.mcna.2018.03.001
34. Jonas DE, Amick HR, Feltner C, et al. Pharmacotherapy for adults with alcohol use disorders in outpatient settings: a systematic review and meta-analysis. *JAMA*. 2014;311(18):1889-1900. doi:10.1001/jama.2014.3628
35. Rigotti NA, Clair C, Munafò MR, Stead LF. Interventions for smoking cessation in hospitalised patients. *Cochrane Database Syst Rev*. 2012;5(5):CD001837. doi:10.1002/14651858.CD001837.pub3
36. Rigotti NA, Stoney CM. CHARTing the future course of tobacco-cessation interventions for hospitalized smokers. *Am J Prev Med*. 2016;51(4):549-550. doi:10.1016/j.amepre.2016.07.012
37. Palmer AM, Rojewski AM, Chen LS, et al. Tobacco treatment program models in U.S. hospitals and outpatient centers on behalf of the SRNT treatment network. *Chest*. 2021;159(4):1652-1663. doi:10.1016/j.chest.2020.11.025
38. Sikka MK, Gore S, Vega T, Strnad L, Gregg J, Englander H. "OPTIONS-DC", a feasible discharge planning conference to expand infection treatment options for people with substance use disorder. *BMC Infect Dis*. 2021;21(1):772. doi:10.1186/s12879-021-06514-9
39. Appa A, Barocas JA. Can I safely discharge a patient with a substance use disorder home with a peripherally inserted central catheter? *NEJM Evidence*. 2022;1(2):EVIDccon2100012. doi:10.1056/EVIDccon2100012
40. Yucel E, Bearnot B, Paras ML, et al. Diagnosis and management of infective endocarditis in people who inject drugs. *J Am Coll Cardiol*. 2022;79(20):2037-2057. doi:10.1016/j.jacc.2022.03.349
41. Weimer MB, Falker CG, Seval N, et al. The need for multidisciplinary hospital teams for injection drug use-related infective endocarditis. *J Addict Med*. 2022;16(4):375-378. doi:10.1097/ADM.0000000000000916

42. Cartmell KB, Dooley M, Mueller M, et al. Effect of an evidence-based inpatient tobacco dependence treatment service on 30-, 90-, and 180-day hospital readmission rates. *Med Care*. 2018;56(4):358-363.
43. Wakeman SE, Pham-Kanter G, Donelan K. Attitudes, practices, and preparedness to care for patients with substance use disorder: results from a survey of general internists. *Subst Abus*. 2016;37(4):635-641. doi:10.1080/08897077.2016.1187240
44. McNeely J, Schatz D, Olfson M, Appleton N, Williams AR. How physician workforce shortages are hampering the response to the opioid crisis. *Psychiatr Serv*. 2022;73(5):547-554. doi:10.1176/appi.ps.202000565
45. Englander H, Patten A, Lockard R, Muller M, Gregg J. Spreading addictions care across oregon's rural and community hospitals: mixed-methods evaluation of an interprofessional telementoring ECHO Program. *J Gen Intern Med*. 2021;36(1):100-107. doi:10.1007/s11606-020-06175-5
46. Schomerus G, Lucht M, Holzinger A, Matschinger H, Carta MG, Angermeyer MC. The stigma of alcohol dependence compared with other mental disorders: a review of population studies. *Alcohol Alcohol*. 2011;46(2):105-112. doi:10.1093/alcalc/agq089
47. van Boekel LC, Brouwers EP, van Weeghel J, Garretsen HF. Stigma among health professionals towards patients with substance use disorders and its consequences for healthcare delivery: systematic review. *Drug Alcohol Depend*. 2013;131(1-2):23-35. doi:10.1016/j.drugalcdep.2013.02.018
48. Biancarelli DL, Biello KB, Childs E, et al. Strategies used by people who inject drugs to avoid stigma in healthcare settings. *Drug Alcohol Depend*. 2019;198:80-86. doi:10.1016/j.drugalcdep.2019.01.037
49. McNeil R, Small W, Wood E, Kerr T. Hospitals as a 'risk environment': an ethno-epidemiological study of voluntary and involuntary discharge from hospital against medical advice among people who inject drugs. *Soc Sci Med*. 2014;105:59-66. doi:10.1016/j.socscimed.2014.01.010
50. Simon R, Snow R, Wakeman S. Understanding why patients with substance use disorders leave the hospital against medical advice: a qualitative study. *Subst Abus*. 2020;41(4):519-525. doi:10.1080/08897077.2019.1671942
51. Merrill JO, Rhodes LA, Deyo RA, Marlatt GA, Bradley KA. Mutual mistrust in the medical care of drug users: the keys to the "narc" cabinet. *J Gen Intern Med*. 2002;17(5):327-333. doi:10.1046/j.1525-1497.2002.10625.x
52. Andraka-Christou B. Addressing racial and ethnic disparities in the use of medications for opioid use disorder. *Health Aff (Millwood)*. 2021;40(6):920-927. doi:10.1377/hlthaff.2020.02261
53. Priest KC, King CA, Englander H, Lovejoy TI, McCarty D. Differences in the delivery of medications for opioid use disorder during hospitalization by racial categories: a retrospective cohort analysis. *Subst Abus*. 2022;43(1):1251-1259. doi:10.1080/08897077.2022.2074601
54. SAMHSA. Double Jeopardy: COVID-19 and Behavioral Health Disparities for Black and Latino Communities in the U.S. 2020. Accessed August 2, 2022. https://www.samhsa.gov/sites/default/files/covid19-behavioral-health-disparities-black-latino-communities.pdf
55. Lagisetty PA, Ross R, Bohnert A, Clay M, Maust DT. Buprenorphine treatment divide by race/ethnicity and payment. *JAMA Psychiatry*. 2019;76(9):979-981. doi:10.1001/jamapsychiatry.2019.0876
56. Peterkin A, Davis CS, Weinstein Z. Permanent methadone treatment reform needed to combat the opioid crisis and structural racism. *J Addict Med*. 2022;16(2):127-129. doi:10.1097/adm.0000000000000841
57. Jackson DS, Nguemeni Tiako MJ, Jordan A. Disparities in addiction treatment: learning from the past to forge an equitable future. *Med Clin North Am*. 2022;106(1):29-41. doi:10.1016/j.mcna.2021.08.008
58. Hagle HN, Martin M, Winograd R, et al. Dismantling racism against Black, Indigenous, and people of color across the substance use continuum: a position statement of the association for multidisciplinary education and research in substance use and addiction. *Subst Abus*. 2021;42(1):5-12. doi:10.1080/08897077.2020.1867288
59. Englander H, Priest KC, Snyder H, Martin M, Calcaterra S, Gregg J. A call to action: hospitalists' role in addressing substance use disorder. *J Hosp Med*. 2019;14(3):E1-E4. doi:10.12788/jhm.3311
60. Englander H, Davis CS. Hospital standards of care for people with substance use disorder. *N Engl J Med*. 2022;387(8):672-675. doi:10.1056/NEJMp2204687
61. Calcaterra SL, Bottner R, Martin M, et al. Management of opioid use disorder, opioid withdrawal, and opioid overdose prevention in hospitalized adults: a systematic review of existing guidelines. *J Hosp Med*. 2022;17(9):679-692. doi:10.1002/jhm.12908
62. U.S. Food & Drug Administration. *Administering or Dispensing of Narcotic Drugs*. 21 CFR Sect 130607. 2020.
63. Code of Federal Regulations. § 1306.07 Administering or Dispensing of Narcotic Drugs. Accessed May 25, 2023. https://www.ecfr.gov/current/title-21/chapter-II/part-1306/subject-group-ECFR1eb5bb3a23fddd0/section-1306.07
64. U.S. Department of Justice. Drug Enforcement Administration. Accessed May 25, 2023. https://www.deadiversion.usdoj.gov/drugreg/Instructions-to-request-exception-to-21-CFR%201306.07(b)-3-day-rule-(EO-DEA248R1).pdf
65. American College of Emergency Physicians. *Important Update on the "Three-Day" Rule for Administering Medications to Treat Opioid Use Disorder*. Accessed May 25, 2023. https://www.acep.org/federal-advocacy/federal-advocacy-overview/regs--eggs/regs--eggs-articles/regs--eggs---april-7-2022/
66. Laks J, Kehoe J, Farrell NM, et al. Methadone initiation in a bridge clinic for opioid withdrawal and opioid treatment program linkage: a case report applying the 72-hour rule. *Addict Sci Clin Pract*. 2021;16(1):73. doi:10.1186/s13722-021-00279-x
67. Thakrar AP. Short-acting opioids for hospitalized patients with opioid use disorder. *JAMA Intern Med*. 2022;182(3):247-248. doi:10.1001/jamainternmed.2021.8111
68. Kleinman RA, Wakeman SE. Treating opioid withdrawal in the hospital: a role for short-acting opioids. *Ann Intern Med*. 2022;175(2):283-284. doi:10.7326/m21-3968
69. Buresh M, Nahvi S, Steiger S, Weinstein ZM. Adapting methadone inductions to the fentanyl era. *J Subst Abuse Treat*. 2022;141:108832. doi:10.1016/j.jsat.2022.108832
70. Button D, Hartley J, Robbins J, Levander XA, Smith NJ, Englander H. Low-dose buprenorphine initiation in hospitalized adults with opioid use disorder: a retrospective cohort analysis. *J Addict Med*. 2021;16(2):e105-e111. doi:10.1097/ADM.0000000000000864
71. Wong JSH, Nikoo M, Westenberg JN, et al. Comparing rapid micro-induction and standard induction of buprenorphine/naloxone for treatment of opioid use disorder: protocol for an open-label, parallel-group, superiority, randomized controlled trial. *Addict Sci Clin Pract*. 2021;16(1):11. doi:10.1186/s13722-021-00220-2
72. Sokolski E, Skogrand E, Goff A, Englander H. Rapid low-dose buprenorphine initiation for hospitalized patients with opioid use disorder. *J Addict Med*. 2023;17(4):e278-e280. doi:10.1097/ADM.0000000000001133
73. Varshneya NB, Thakrar AP, Hobelmann JG, Dunn KE, Huhn AS. Evidence of buprenorphine-precipitated withdrawal in persons who use fentanyl. *J Addict Med*. 2022;16(4):e265-e268. doi:10.1097/ADM.0000000000000922
74. Collett BJ. Opioid tolerance: the clinical perspective. *Br J Anaesth*. 1998;81(1):58-68. doi:10.1093/bja/81.1.58
75. Martyn JAJ, Mao J, Bittner EA. Opioid tolerance in critical illness. *N Engl J Med*. 2019;380(4):365-378. doi:10.1056/NEJMra1800222
76. Lembke A, Ottestad E, Schmiesing C. Patients maintained on buprenorphine for opioid use disorder should continue buprenorphine through the perioperative period. *Pain Med*. 2019;20(3):425-428. doi:10.1093/pm/pny019
77. McNeil R, Kerr T, Pauly B, Wood E, Small W. Advancing patient-centered care for structurally vulnerable drug-using populations: a qualitative study of the perspectives of people who use drugs regarding the potential integration of harm reduction interventions into hospitals. *Addiction*. 2016;111(4):685-694. doi:10.1111/add.13214
78. Hyshka E, Morris H, Anderson-Baron J, Nixon L, Dong K, Salvalaggio G. Patient perspectives on a harm reduction-oriented addiction

medicine consultation team implemented in a large acute care hospital. *Drug Alcohol Depend.* 2019;204:107523. doi:10.1016/j.drugalcdep.2019.06.025

79. Perera R, Stephan L, Appa A, et al. Meeting people where they are: implementing hospital-based substance use harm reduction. *Harm Reduct J.* 2022;19(1):14. doi:10.1186/s12954-022-00594-9
80. Brooks HL, O'Brien DC, Salvalaggio G, Dong K, Hyshka E. Uptake into a bedside needle and syringe program for acute care inpatients who inject drugs. *Drug Alcohol Rev.* 2019;38(4):423-427. doi:10.1111/dar.12930
81. Thakarar K, Weinstein ZM, Walley AY. Optimising health and safety of people who inject drugs during transition from acute to outpatient care: narrative review with clinical checklist. *Postgrad Med J.* 2016;92(1088):356-363. doi:10.1136/postgradmedj-2015-133720
82. Sharma M, Lamba W, Cauderella A, Guimond TH, Bayoumi AM. Harm reduction in hospitals. *Harm Reduct J.* 2017;14(1):32. doi:10.1186/s12954-017-0163-0
83. Khan GK, Harvey L, Johnson S, et al. Integration of a community-based harm reduction program into a safety net hospital: a qualitative study. *Harm Reduct J.* 2022;19(1):35. doi:10.1186/s12954-022-00622-8
84. Dong KA, Brouwer J, Johnston C, Hyshka E. Supervised consumption services for acute care hospital patients. *Can Med Assoc J.* 2020;192(18):E476-e479. doi:10.1503/cmaj.191365
85. Kosteniuk B, Salvalaggio G, McNeil R, et al. "You don't have to squirrel away in a staircase": patient motivations for attending a novel supervised drug consumption service in acute care. *Int J Drug Policy.* 2021;96:103275. doi:10.1016/j.drugpo.2021.103275
86. Heller D, McCoy K, Cunningham C. An invisible barrier to integrating HIV primary care with harm reduction services: philosophical clashes between the harm reduction and medical models. *Public Health Rep.* 2004;119(1):32-39. doi:10.1177/003335490411900109
87. Koenigs KJ, Chou JH, Cohen S, et al. Informed consent is poorly documented when obtaining toxicology testing at delivery in a Massachusetts cohort. *Am J Obstet Gynecol MFM.* 2022;4(4):100621. doi:10.1016/j.ajogmf.2022.100621
88. Martin M, Snyder HR, Otway G, Holpit L, Day LW, Seidman D. In-hospital substance use policies: an opportunity to advance equity, reduce stigma, and offer evidence-based addiction care. *J Addict Med.* 2022;17(1):10-12. doi:10.1097/ADM.0000000000001046
89. Alfandre D, Stream S, Geppert C. "Doc, I'm going for a walk": liberalizing or restricting the movement of hospitalized patients-ethical, legal, and clinical considerations. *HEC Forum.* 2020;32(3):253-267. doi:10.1007/s10730-020-09398-5
90. American College of Obstetricians and Gynecologists. Opioid use and opioid use disorder in pregnancy. Committee Opinion No. 711. *Obstet Gynecol.* 2017;130:e81-e94.
91. United States Commission on Civil Rights. *Substance Abuse Under the ADA.* Accessed March 14, 2022. http://www.usccr.gov/pubs/ada/ch4.htm
92. Priest KC, Englander H, McCarty D. Hospital policies for opioid use disorder treatment: a policy content analysis and environmental scan checklist. *Gen Hosp Psychiatry.* 2021;70:18-24. doi:10.1016/j.genhosppsych.2021.02.007
93. Englander H, Gregg J, Levander XA. Envisioning minimally disruptive opioid use disorder care. *J Gen Intern Med.* 2023;38(3):799-803. doi:10.1007/s11606-022-07939-x
94. Kimmel SD, Walley AY, Li Y, et al. Association of treatment with medications for opioid use disorder with mortality after hospitalization for injection drug use-associated infective endocarditis. *JAMA Netw Open.* 2020;3(10):e2016228. doi:10.1001/jamanetworkopen.2020.16228
95. Kimmel SD, Rosenmoss S, Bearnot B, et al. Northeast postacute medical facilities disproportionately reject referrals for patients with opioid use disorder. *Health Aff (Millwood).* 2022;41(3):434-444. doi:10.1377/hlthaff.2021.01242
96. Wakeman SE, Rich JD. Barriers to post-acute care for patients on opioid agonist therapy; an example of systematic stigmatization of addiction. *J Gen Intern Med.* 2017;32(1):17-19. doi:10.1007/s11606-016-3799-7
97. Isaacson JH, Fleming M, Kraus M, Kahn R, Mundt M. A national survey of training in substance use disorders in residency programs. *J Stud Alcohol.* 2000;61(6):912-915. doi:10.15288/jsa.2000.61.912

Sidebar 2

Prevention and Early Treatment in the Workplace Setting

Marianne Cloeren, Jodi J. Frey, and Indira G. Jetton

WHAT ABOUT WORK?

Work is an important social determinant of health. We know that those with untreated substance use disorders (SUDs) are less likely to be working than those without such conditions, but research has also shown that those in stable treatment for SUD are more likely to be unemployed.[1] Studies have shown that work participation is important to maintaining health, as well as treatment adherence for those treated for SUD.[2] For optimal outcomes, physicians caring for individuals with SUDs must pay attention to planning for continuing or returning to work.

Most physicians understand the importance of effective history taking when providing patient-centered medical care. A comprehensive history universally includes past medical history, surgical history, and social history. Social history also includes a patient's occupational history, but the occupational history remains neglected in most medical notes, often limited to a single word about the patient's usual occupation. Information related to occupational history and any applicable employment medical services can be a vital part of providing precision medicine and individualized care. When working with a patient around substance use issues, it is important to explore and understand the job and sometimes the regulatory context. Understanding more about the patient's job can also shed light on treatment and recovery support resources that may be available. Finally, understanding one's job and plan for continued work or return to work may also impact how a physician will consider different treatment options, as some barriers still exist for certain types of employment, particularly around treatment with medications.

WHAT IS YOUR PATIENT'S JOB?

Sometimes, knowing your patient's usual occupation can be enough to help you understand some of the regulatory context and benefits available to that patient. For example, if your patient is a police officer, this tells you that he or she works in a safety-sensitive position, is subject to drug testing and specific physical and mental health requirements, is probably represented by a union, and likely has access to a full range of treatment benefits. You can usually assume that there are well-delineated protocols to follow before this patient will be able to return to the job following a substance-related medical issue.

What if your patient is a medical assistant in a long-term care facility? Here, the situation is not so clear. Some in this position are independent contractors, without access to employee health benefits, even if working full time. If the employer is a federal or state agency, it is more likely that your patient is an employee with benefits and may even be represented by a union. You may need to inquire specifically about these issues to better understand details that can help you support your patient. Additionally, your patient might not be covered by safety sensitive laws per se, but he or she is still involved in a job that impacts public safety.

What if your patient reports working as a laborer at a construction site? What does this mean? What does a construction laborer do? Who employs them? Are they represented by a union? The decreasing representation by unions in construction work has been tied to increased reliance on government safety net programs such as Medical Assistance.[3] This has important implications for access to treatment and other recovery services.

Is your patient self-employed in the gig economy? Most app-based gig economy jobs (think of ride share, deliveries) consider the worker an independent contractor, and do not provide benefits, although there are some proposals afoot that would provide gig workers with portable benefits, including health insurance. When patients working in the gig economy are not able to work, they are not able to make money and probably do not have health insurance to help cover costs of what is often expensive treatment.

Are there licensure considerations related to the substance use issue of your patient? For example, commercial drivers and licensed healthcare providers are subject to specific requirements for monitoring adherence to recovery plans; these requirements may also limit the choices of medication used to treat opioid use disorder. Therefore, it is important to review current laws and regulations applying to your patient's situation, as these laws and regulations are ever evolving.

What is the work environment of your patient? Those who work in the restaurant industry are usually working around alcohol and may be in a job that requires handling alcoholic beverages. Past national surveys on drug and alcohol use have shown that workers in the food services industry are people who very often use alcohol and illegal drugs.[4] How can you help your patients with SUD maintain their recovery while exposed to substances or those who use them at work? In some cases, a change in job setting or even career may need to be considered.

These are just a few examples of how your patient's work can impact treatment for SUD and recovery. Given the importance of work to health and sustained recovery, work plans need to be included in a patient-centered treatment plan. This section will provide some basic information about important occupational considerations for providers to understand to increase the chances of helping patients with SUD stay employed.

WHAT IS THE DIFFERENCE BETWEEN AN EMPLOYEE AND A CONTRACTOR?

Determining whether your patient is an employee (tax information comes on W-2) or contractor (tax information on W-9) can tell you a lot. A W-2 employee is a hired employee, who may be paid hourly or be salaried. These patients have significantly less autonomy in determining their work lifestyle, including their training and schedule. However, unlike W-9 employees, most W-2 employees receive work benefits including minimum wage, overtime protection (unless exempt, which includes most salaried positions), paid time off, and health benefits. There may also be short- or long-term disability benefits, which can help your patients make ends meet if they need to be off work for a prolonged period for treatment.

Alternatively, W-9 workers often do not have a single employer and commonly are included under the following categories: freelancers, consultants, gig workers, independent contractors, etc. These patients do not file payroll taxes, because they are on their own payroll, and they do not receive payroll benefits including health insurance.[5] It is usually safe to assume that contractors do not have employer-sponsored health insurance. They are required to pay income taxes, and typically there are no withdrawals made from their pay for this purpose—they need to set aside enough funds for income tax and may not have savings necessary to pay for healthcare and long-term recovery supports.

Another category is someone who works but who is paid "under the table." There are no protections or health benefits for such workers unless they purchase it themselves. Lack of paid time off or health benefits are important reasons that working individuals may put off entering needed treatment for SUDs.

WHAT KIND OF BENEFITS DOES YOUR PATIENT HAVE?

The Kaiser Family Foundation provides a comprehensive annual report regarding employer-sponsored health coverage. The 2020 Kaiser report collected data from mid-January through July, before the full impact of the Coronavirus pandemic (COVID-19) affected employers.[6] They found that the average annual premium for single patient coverage rose 4% to $7,470 and the average annual premium for family coverage also rose 4% to $21,342.[7] As health care providers, it is important for physicians to have conversations with their patients regarding insurance coverage and to advocate on patients' behalf by promoting an open discussion space. Encouraging patients to be knowledgeable about their insurance plans and coverage can mean prompting them to ask their employers about coverage. Patients with SUDs, who may anticipate the need for future coverage, should carefully consider options upon employment and during open enrollment season. Considerations include access to inpatient treatment as well as outpatient treatment. If the employer offers an Employee Assistance Program (EAP), this would be a confidential counseling program that is paid for by the employer (see Employer Resources section below) to discuss treatment options with the employee and/or refer to other departments such as Human Resources and Benefits, as appropriate. If the workplace is unionized, the union would also be a potential place to refer an employee to learn about benefits.

WHAT ARE YOUR PATIENT'S EMPLOYER'S POLICIES RELATED TO SUBSTANCE USE TREATMENT AND JOB PROTECTION FOR NEEDED ABSENCES?

In 1988, the U.S. Drug-Free Workplace Act set the requirement for any organizations receiving federal contracts or grants to certify that they would provide a drug-free workplace. This resulted in widespread adoption of workplace training on SUDs, as well as a dramatic increase in employee drug testing. Many companies adopted "zero-tolerance" policies, resulting in automatic termination of any employee discovered to be using illegal drugs. In recent years, there has been a movement away from universal drug testing of employees where this is not required by regulations. Reasons for this include economic pressures and difficulty finding enough qualified workers to hire/retain at the workplace, as well as the increasing prevalence of states permitting use of recreational cannabis, or cannabis used as treatment.[8] There has also been a movement toward recovery friendly workplaces (see **Box 33-2**), with policies designed to support employees in recovery.[9]

Many employers have no written policies regarding substance use, SUD, or supporting employees in recovery. Smaller employers may not have human resources departments to assist with such decision making or evaluating healthcare coverage options that would provide adequate and quality care for employees in need of treatment and/or recovery supports.

BOX 33-2 Recovery Friendly Workplaces

There is a movement away from a zero-tolerance drug-free workplace approach, to one that been called a "recovery friendly workplace."

Recovery friendly workplaces recognize that individuals in recovery can be valuable employees and that a culture that supports them is good for the whole community.

Recovery friendly workplace approaches include:

- Fostering a safe and recovery-friendly culture in the workplace.
- Retaining healthy and productive employees.
- Hiring those in recovery.
- Engaging employees in education about addiction and behavioral health.
- Promoting prevention and recovery in their local communities.

Approaches often include early identification of employees with problems and providing peer support services at work.

Physicians treating patients or evaluating employees can be very influential in helping employers consider how to support employees in recovery. With the patient's permission, the treating provider can contact the employer, often through the Employee Assistance Program (EAP) (see below) if available, to help plan for a supervised return to work.

LEGAL ASPECTS

ADA Implications

The Americans with Disabilities Act (ADA) was initially signed into law in 1990 and was modified in 2008, becoming one of the most important legislative acts protecting individuals with physical and mental disabilities as employees, customers, and public services recipients. However, the Act provides limited protection regarding active SUDs despite persons with these disorders facing persisting discrimination and differential treatment. Additionally, it is important to note that, under the current version of the ADA, there is variable treatment of individuals depending on the type of substance involved. Individuals "currently engaging in the illegal use of drugs" do not fall under the definition of disability and are therefore excluded from ADA protections. On the other hand, someone in recovery, for example, receiving opioid agonist therapy as treatment for opioid use disorder, would be covered by the ADA. This means that requests for accommodations related to such treatment (eg, attending treatment appointments) should be considered under ADA provisions. Physicians can assist such patients by providing documentation that supports reasonable accommodations requests. Unfortunately, the ADA does not provide protections in workplaces with less than 15 employees, so many of the most vulnerable working adults who are working in unstable jobs and often without health insurance, are further excluded from protections that would be offered in large workplaces through the ADA (www.ada.gov/opioid_guidance.pdf).

FMLA Protections

The Family and Medical Leave Act (FMLA) was passed in 1993 and guarantees full time employees, who have worked an approved number of hours, unpaid leave for family or medical reasons. Employees can use FMLA coverage for their own healthcare or to care for a family member with an SUD if they are seeking treatment by a health care provider or on referral from a health care provider. Employees are eligible for FMLA coverage if they have worked for the company for at least a year, worked at least 1,250 hours during the previous year, and work at a location with at least 50 employees within a 75-mile radius. As with the ADA, FMLA is not helpful to all employees. Companies with fewer than 50 employees are not required to offer FMLA and, due to the lack of requirement for paid leave, many low and even moderate-income working adults are not able to afford to take unpaid leave, even when available.

SAFETY SENSITIVE JOBS

Work classified as "safety-sensitive" means that the position requires an employee's full and unimpaired judgment and skills, and that there is the risk of danger to others if the employee is impaired in some way. Such jobs often have requirements for evaluation and testing, which are sometimes codified in federal regulations, but may also vary by state. This section will address a few common examples.

Commercial Drivers

Per regulations outlined by the Federal Motor Carrier and Safety Administration (FMCSA), all drivers who operate commercial vehicles under commercial driving licenses are subject to U.S. Department of Transportation substance and alcohol testing regulations. DOT testing includes pre-employment, postaccident, random, reasonable suspicion and return-to-work screening for a variety of substances. If an employee fails drug screening protocols, they are immediately removed from driving commercial vehicles until completion of return-to-work processes with a qualified FMCSA approved Substance Use Disorder Professional[10] Taking prescribed medication for opioid use disorder, for example, methadone or suboxone, is disqualifying, however the certified Medical Examiner is authorized to make an exception and qualify the driver. The examining physician will often seek written opinion of the treating provider about the impact of the prescribed medication on driving safety before deciding. Note that cannabis use, even under the direction of a physician, is disqualifying in all states.

Pilots

The aviation industry is governed by both the Department of Transportation procedural regulation for all transportation modes and the Federal Aviation Administration (FAA)'s drug and alcohol testing regulation specific to the aviation industry. Unlike most commercial ground drivers, where union membership is unusual, most commercial air pilots belong to a large national labor union, which provides strong support for members who are dealing with work problems related to substance use or SUD. The Human Intervention Motivational Study (HIMS) program is managed by the pilots' union, with cooperation from airline representatives, pilot peer volunteers, healthcare professionals and FAA's medical team. This program provides treatment and monitoring services to help pilots with SUDs get back to flying under FAA special rules.

Licensed Health care Workers

Most states have specific requirements for monitoring the recovery of licensed healthcare providers who need treatment for SUDs. Physician health programs or other professional health monitoring programs (PHPs) offer services for physicians, and sometimes other licensed health professionals, in almost every state (see Chapter 34). In other cases, the state professional organization representing the given type of professional offers such oversight. While not covered under DOT regulations, many healthcare facilities look to DOT regulations for guidance regarding company policy for treatment, monitoring, and return-to-work. Additionally, it is important to understand how the state licensure boards for various disciplines may become involved when a problem is identified by self-report or through a drug test or other means. These entities often coordinate with the PHP that provides monitoring and return-to-work oversight services to ensure patient safety by preventing healthcare professionals from working while impaired.

WORKERS' COMPENSATION CONSIDERATIONS

It is common for workers injured at work to be prescribed opioids. Although opioid prescribing for work-related injuries is decreasing (as is opioid prescribing overall in the U.S.), there is still a high prevalence of opioid prescribing in workers' compensation injuries.[11,12] The Workers' Compensation Research Institute found in its most recent review of opioid prescribing trends that between 32% and 70% of workers' compensation claims receiving prescriptions included opioids, varying across the 27 states included in the report. Of note, these data do not include the opioids prescribed via personal health insurance for workers' compensation injuries, an important additional source of prescriptions for patients following a work injury.[13] Indeed, work-related injury care is one of the drivers of opioid use disorder.[14] If a patient's SUD can be attributed to iatrogenic addiction following a work-related injury, the workers' compensation system should be responsible for providing treatment and covering work absence needed for treatment. There is often the need for physician advocacy for this outcome, which may require a detailed narrative account of the connections between the SUD and the work injury. Workers in this situation will often have an attorney who may be able to help orchestrate access to treatment.

On the other hand, if a worker's substance use contributed to his or her work injury, a claim for workers' compensation will usually be denied.

EMPLOYMENT DRUG TESTING

While many safety-sensitive jobs have very specific criteria for drug testing, most employment drug testing is not governed by specific regulations. Employers may choose not to conduct drug tests, or to test only new employees, or to conduct random drug testing on current employees. Many employers will conduct "reasonable suspicion" drug testing for appearance of impairment or following accidents, although the Occupational Safety and Health Administration has regulations preventing employers from having blanket policies requiring drug testing after any accident at work.

Options for drug testing include different panels of drugs to test for, and different ways to test (eg, using hair, oral fluids or urine.) Many employers default to the "DOT panel," which is a urine specimen that includes screening for cannabis, cocaine, opiates (including opium and codeine derivatives), amphetamines, methamphetamines and phencyclidine. There are different rules and protocols for collecting specimens depending on whether the collection is required under DOT regulations or not.

Each state has specific rules governing employee drug testing, and physicians supporting employee health programs should be aware of these rules. For example, in Maryland, employment drug testing for job candidates requires review of a positive drug test result by a Medical Review Officer, while testing of current employees does not have this requirement.[3]

REPORTING REQUIREMENTS

Physicians providing care for patients seen under their own volition, using their own insurance, have a different set of fiduciary responsibilities than those seeing patients referred by the employer. When there is a doctor/patient relationship, there is also the expectation of confidentiality. However, this is not necessarily the case when the evaluation or treatment occurs at the behest of the employer. Occupational health providers may see patients, for example, related to evaluation of positive employment drug tests, questions about on-the-job intoxication/impairment, or consideration of reasonable accommodations related to prescribed medications that affect cognition. Physicians providing care in this setting *may* have an obligation under the law to report substance use and/or SUD. Therefore, it is imperative to understand the rules that apply to your practice setting, and to communicate openly and honestly with patients so that they understand the limits of confidentiality and can provide informed consent to participate in their clinical care.

EMPLOYER RESOURCES

A variety of resources may be available in the workplace to assist individuals with substance-related concerns. Access to the following resources is often contingent on the type and size of their employer (**Box 33-3**).

What is an Employee Assistance Program?

An employee assistance program (EAP) is a voluntary workplace-based program offered by employers to provide free and confidential services for personal and work-related problems that are affecting employees, and often their family members. EAPs usually provide assessment, short-term problem resolution or counseling, and referral support to additional longer-term treatment. They can also provide health and wellness assessment or consultation, and higher quality EAPs often provide organizational services, including training, employee education, management consultation and crisis response services. With regard to substance use assessment and treatment in the workplace, EAPs expanded in the United States after the passage of the Drug-Free Workplace Act (DFWP), which requires all federal workplaces and federal contractors to offer an EAP. Part of the role of the EAP regarding DFWP programming was to help employers provide employee education about substance use prevention, early intervention, and treatment. The proliferation of EAPs in the workplace following passage of the DFWP Act expanded to nonfederal employers as well, and EAPs became a critical component of many employers' response to alcohol and other drugs in the workplace. EAP professionals work with employees to support and resolve a variety of issues affecting physical, mental, emotional, and social wellbeing. For

BOX 33-3 Terms Used in Workplace Substance Monitoring

EAP—Employee Assistance Program—offered by many employers to provide access to resources such as substance use disorder support groups and therapy.

MAP—Member Assistance Program—like an EAP, sponsored by a labor union.

MRO—Medical Review Officer—a licensed physician trained and certified to review laboratory results from an employment drug screening program.

SAP—Substance Abuse Professional—evaluates violations and provides recommendations including education, treatment, subsequent testing and appropriate aftercare.

substance use, employees might be referred to their EAP by their manager, HR professional, union or simply suggested to attend by a concerned co-worker. The majority of referrals to the EAP are self-referrals, but serious substance use problems, or problems related to positive drug testing at work, often result in a formal or management referral to the EAP.

Regardless of the referral source, all employees are offered a comprehensive and confidential substance use assessment. This is usually followed with recommendations for treatment, which might include short-term counseling that can be offered through the EAP, or more often, referral for longer-term treatment. In particular, EAPs work with employees to identify the appropriate level of care needed and available referral options for community-based or in-patient treatment. While the EAP services are offered at no cost to the employees (as they are paid for by the employer), any referrals to services outside of the EAP are the responsibility of the employee. EAPs often work closely with employees to find referrals that accept insurance or other community-based sliding scale payment for treatment. Once referred to treatment, the EAP can provide a liaison role between the employee and the workplace if the employee signs a release-of-information. This allows the EAP to communicate with the treatment provider and for the EAP to provide limited information to the employer, on a need-to-know only basis, about how treatment is going, additional supports needed from the workplace (eg, time off), and plan for return to work.

Employers can stipulate that they also want their EAP to provide services for family members. For SUD, this could include assessment, referral and family support for a spouse or covered dependent of an employee. Over time, employers have recognized that caring for employees' family members helps reduce stress and lost productivity from their employee. Additionally, the EAP can provide support services to family members who are concerned about an employee's substance use and/or provide support to the family while the employee is seeking or getting treatment. Support to the caregiver for substance use and other personal and health-related problems is a growing area for EAPs.[15]

EAPs are only a small part of the solution for workplace substance use. Due to lack of awareness (health literacy), stigma, and other barriers, EAPs often have lower than desired utilization[16-18]; however, when promoted throughout the company and encouraged by both leadership and through programs such as peer support, trust of such programs among employees increases. This can positively impact utilization of services and boost morale by demonstrating that the company cares about their employees and improved safety and productivity.[19-22] However, EAPs alone cannot provide all the prevention, early intervention and treatment needed; therefore, they should be offered and incorporated into a more comprehensive workplace behavioral health plan. Physicians and other healthcare providers working in the community should always ask if their patient has access to an EAP, either through their own workplace or a family member. Asking this question might open doors to return-to-work support, additional leave for treatment, requests for FMLA for flexible work schedules to support treatment needs, and more.

Peer Support

Peer support groups in the workplace grew out of a need to provide additional services in the workplace for SUD (and more recently for broader behavioral health) while working to reduce stigma about help-seeking, and to provide support for return-to-work and stay-at-work initiatives. Employers offer peer support services that allow employees who have overcome psychiatric, alcohol, and drug related problems to help co-workers currently facing similar issues. Through empowerment, support, and empathy, peer support employees foster an environment of connectedness and positive community. Services extend the reach of addiction treatment resources beyond the clinical setting and can fit comfortably into the workplace. In doing so, employee patients receive additional support, which may increase the likelihood of maintaining successful recovery processes.

Although historically peer support programs in the workplace grew out of labor union supported initiatives in the United States, including self-help groups, they expanded into crisis response services for first responder and other emergency services industries. The growth and potential future growth of peer support is critically important for today's workplace. Labor unions have been supportive of recovery efforts, starting with 12-step-based programs for abstinence since Alcoholics Anonymous was first introduced to the United States in the 1940s. The predecessor for today's EAPs were Occupational Alcohol Programs (OAPs) that were traditionally provided by peers in recovery and often financially supported and promoted by labor unions. As programs grew in number, the notion of just treating the SUD became obsolete and OAPs expanded their services to cover mental health and relationship problems that often accompanied SUDs in the workplace. These programs became known as broad-brush EAPs in the 1980s, but many peer-led EAPs and related peer support programs have continued to flourish. Connecting with peers at the workplace can help to normalize experiences that one is going through, while providing crisis (and potentially ongoing) support based on a combination of "equality of status, and shared meaningful experience, including work experience."[23]

Peer support programming can develop and grow in several ways. Given their history in unions, some workplaces' peer programs originate and live in union spaces, where employees often feel more supported because unions are not directly connected to management. Other workplaces have started to create programs through employee resource groups, which are formed to support employees with similarities or similar situations (eg, gender, sexual orientation, race, family/caregiver status, military experience) and are growing to provide additional peer support and/or mentoring programs. Employers often allow groups to meet during work times, using workplace resources, and many programs are allocated a budget to help ensure that the employees' needs are met through the peer services.

With the current strain on treatment resources, and increased stigma regarding SUD, peer support programs are experiencing a bit of a renaissance in the workplace. More and more employers are recognizing their role in supporting employees' entire health, including behavioral health, and are interested in ways to encourage early identification of problems, easy access to treatment, and continued support posttreatment to support employee retention in addition to productivity and safety. Additionally, peers are able to conduct some of the upfront triage work while employees await community-based treatment, which can have long waiting lists.

Labor Union Resources

Many employer-sponsored programs, like EAPs or benefits counseling, are underutilized by employees due to confidentiality concerns, even when confidentiality is promised and ensured (as is the case with EAPs). Therefore, employees need options to turn to for help when needed, with choices for programs that they can trust. One trusted resource is a union-sponsored program, such as a member assistance program or MAP. Like EAPs, MAPs are often designed to provide assessment, referral, and sometimes short-term counseling. They are provided at no cost to employees through the union and they offer another option for employees to seek support when seeking help through the EAP or human resources department is not viewed as a safe option. One example of a successful program that provides services through the union (that one of the authors works with) is the Flight Attendant Drug and Alcohol Program, or FADAP (www.fadap.org). FADAP provides EAP and peer based services to flight attendants—many of whom choose to access services through FADAP even when they have an employer-sponsored EAP option.[24] Unions are often designed to provide direct services. They can advocate for employees with their employer, and help support additional needs the employee might have when seeking and completing treatment (eg, financial needs, childcare, and other personal concerns).[25,26] As community medical professionals, it is important to ask questions about diverse resources that may be offered to employees through not only their workplace, but also their unions.

Screening and Brief Intervention at Work

As outlined in Chapter 31, Screening and Brief Intervention (SBI) is a comprehensive, integrated, public health approach to the delivery of screening and early intervention for persons with unhealthy substance use. SBI has been promoted as an important tool in primary care, to identify patients with potential substance use problems, provide a brief counseling message, and refer them to treatment if indicated. SBI and SBI with referral to treatment (SBIRT) have also been implemented in the workplace, primarily via EAP programs. The Brief Intervention Group (BIG) Initiative has resources to promote the universal practice of SBIRT by EAP programs.[27]

ADVOCATING FOR YOUR PATIENTS WHO WORK

Anticipating and Preventing Job Loss

Many employers differentiate between employees who seek help for their SUD, and those who are "caught," which would include those whose drug use is discovered via an employment drug test or following an employer-required evaluation for impairment on the job (sometimes called a "fitness for duty" evaluation). It is common for employers to offer assistance and support, including returning to the job after treatment, when workers come forward asking for help, but to terminate employees whose SUD was discovered by the employer. Anticipating this, providers should discuss with patients the pros and cons of approaching their employer for assistance rather than risk discovery and termination.

Plans for Returning to Work

In each encounter involving a working age patient who is not currently working, there should be consideration and discussion about a plan to return to work. Often, employees have limited communication with their workplace while in treatment and then the employee and the workplace may not be ready for a smooth transition back to work. Knowing how important work is to one's identity and how positive working is to recovery, a plan to return to the workplace (or a different workplace if necessary or desired) should be embedded in the recovery treatment plan. For employees who can return to the same workplace and have access to an EAP, treatment providers can discuss the pros and cons of having the employee sign a release of information to share limited information about medical needs and to engage the workplace in having a more active role in helping the employee return to (or stay at) work. Sometimes, employees might need accommodations under ADA or support through FMLA to continue treatment when at work or to have an opportunity to do their job with different job-offered accommodations or supports. This might be especially important for employees who take medications, such as methadone or buprenorphine, to help with their ongoing recovery. EAPs, workplace peer support persons, or other identified workplace contacts can be supportive to employees who are seeking recovery and might be out of work. The disability management field has researched the positive impact of regular communications by the employer to the employee when employees are out on short-term disability, with evidence of positive impact on morale, treatment and quicker return to work. Even helping employees return to work in a part-time or limited capacity while completing treatment has both positive psychological and overall workplace benefits.[28,29]

Plans for Monitoring Employees Returning to Work

Depending on the employee's workplace and occupation, the treatment provider or SAP under DOT might be required to provide a formal follow-up plan as part of the employee's return to work procedures and process. This could include attendance at treatment or 12-step meetings, random or scheduled drug testing, participation in an employer-sponsored monitoring program, meetings with an EAP counselor or peer or other common aspects of a treatment program. Even if not required for the employee's job, a detailed plan for ongoing recovery and support following treatment is a crucial part of any successful long-term recovery plan.[30] Identifying triggers for recurrence of use that might connect to workplace experiences and/or stressors should be folded into the plan so that the employee can predict when additional support for sustained recovery might be necessary.

Helping Employed Patients Without Treatment Health Benefits

Employed patients without health benefits who need treatment for SUD present a particular challenge. Options to explore include veteran status and union membership. Most states now have a crisis response line (in many states it is 211), which is designed to connect those with urgent health needs to available resources. Their services include navigation services to help patients enroll in health plans, as well as connecting them with free services.

SUMMARY

Work is an important social determinant of health that has known associations with substance use. In addition to providing the means to live, for most people, work can provide meaning and be an important part of a patient's identity. Loss of a job should be considered a serious adverse outcome, one that is often preventable by paying attention to work circumstances, resources, and plans when treating patients who work. Patient-centered management plans need to take into account not only the medical treatment, but the patient's social context and supports, including work.

REFERENCES

1. U.S. Department of Health and Human Services. *Integrating Substance Abuse Treatment and Vocational Services*. Substance Abuse and Mental Health Services Administration. Center for Substance Abuse Treatment; 2014.
2. Augutis M, Rosenberg D, Hillborg H. The meaning of work: perceptions of employed persons attending maintenance treatment for opiate addiction. *J Soc Work Pract Addict*. 2016;16:385-402.
3. Maryland Health—General Section 17-214. *Justia Law*. Accessed May 25, 2023. https://law.justia.com/codes/maryland/2005/ghg/17-214.html
4. Bush DM, Lipari RN. *Substance Use and Substance Use Disorder by Industry*. Accessed May 25, 2023. https://www.samhsa.gov/data/sites/default/files/report_1959/ShortReport-1959.html
5. Ames GM, Bennett JB. Prevention interventions of alcohol problems in the workplace. *Alcohol Res Health*. 2011;34:175-187.
6. KFF. *2021 Employer Health Benefits Survey*. Accessed May 25, 2023. https://www.kff.org/health-costs/report/2021-employer-health-benefits-survey/
7. Claxton G, Damico A, Rae M, Young G, McDermott D, Whitmore H. Health benefits in 2020: premiums in employer-sponsored plans grow 4 percent; Employers Consider Responses To Pandemic. *Health Aff (Millwood)*. 2020;39:2018-2028.
8. Maurer R. *Know Before You Hire: Employment-Screening Trends in 2022*. SHRM. Accessed May 25, 2023. https://www.shrm.org/resourcesandtools/hr-topics/talent-acquisition/pages/employment-screening-trends-2022-marijuana-background-checks.aspx
9. Imboden R, Frey JJ, Bazell AT, et al. Workplace support for employees in recovery from opioid use: stakeholder perspectives. *New Solut*. 2021;31(3):340-349.
10. Federal Motor Carrier safety Administration. *Substance Abuse Professionals*. Accessed May 25, 2023. https://www.fmcsa.dot.gov/regulations/drug-alcohol-testing/substance-abuse-professionals
11. Workers Compensation Research Institute. *Interstate Variations in Dispensing of Opioids*. 5th ed. Accessed May 25, 2023. https://www.wcrinet.org/reports/interstate-variations-in-dispensing-of-opioids-5th-edition
12. Centers for Disease Control and Prevention. *U.S. Opioid Dispensing Rate Maps*. Accessed May 25, 2023. https://www.cdc.gov/drugoverdose/rxrate-maps/index.html
13. Asfaw A, Quay B, Chang C-C. Do injured workers receive opioid prescriptions outside the workers' compensation system?: the case of private group health insurances. *J Occup Environ Med*. 2020;62:e515-e522.
14. Asfaw A, Boden LI. Impact of workplace injury on opioid dependence, abuse, illicit use and overdose: a 36-month retrospective study of insurance claims. *Occup Environ Med*. 2020;77:648-653.
15. Lerner DJ. *Invisible Overtime: What Employers Need to Know About Caregivers*. Accessed May 25, 2023. https://archive.hshsl.umaryland.edu/handle/10713/18402
16. Attridge M, Amaral TM, Bjornson T, et al. *Utilization of EAP Services*. Accessed May 25, 2023. https://archive.hshsl.umaryland.edu/handle/10713/5137
17. Masi DA. *EAP Utilization: EAP Field Doesn't Do Itself Justice*. Accessed May 25, 2023. https://eapmasi.com/art_masi/Inside/PDFs/EAP_Utilization_Article.pdf
18. Masi DA, Frey JJ, Harting J, Spearing M. *Data Game Changer: Current Utilization Figures Inaccurate*. Accessed May 25, 2023. https://archive.hshsl.umaryland.edu/handle/10713/17720
19. Attridge MA. Global perspective on promoting workplace mental health and the role of employee assistance programs. *Am J Health Promot*. 2019;33:622-629.
20. Attridge M, Amaral TM, Bjornson T, et al. *Implementation of EAPs*. Accessed May 25, 2023. https://archive.hshsl.umaryland.edu/handle/10713/5123
21. Frey J, Pompe J, Sharar D, Imboden R, Bloom L. Experiences of internal and hybrid employee assistance program managers: factors associated with successful, at-risk, and eliminated programs. *J Workplace Behav. Health*. 2018;33:1-23.
22. Nunes AP, Richmond MK, Pampel FC, Wood RC. The effect of employee assistance services on reductions in employee absenteeism. *J Bus Psychol*. 2018;33:699-709.
23. Spencer-Thomas S, Gaer S, Macy R, Vega E, Fox-Kemper J, Channell J. Helping the People who Help People—Mental Health Providers Working in Crisis, Disaster and Trauma Response Environments: A Peer Support Manual. MassSupport Network: Massachusetts. 2021. Accessed online August 29, 2023. https://workplacesuicideprevention.com/wp-content/uploads/2022/04/FINAL-MassSupport_Peer-Support-Manual.pdf
24. Frey JJ, Liccardo R, Healy H, Bloom L. Workplace experiences and outcomes related to participation in the flight attendant drug and alcohol program: an exploratory study. *EASNA Research Notes*. 2015;5(2):1-7.

25. Kurzman PA. Labor–social work collaboration: current and historical perspectives. *J Workplace Behav Health*. 2009;24:6-20.
26. Masi DA. The history of employee assistance programs in the United States. The Employee Assistance Research Foundation. 2020. Accessed online August 29, 2023. https://archive.hshsl.umaryland.edu/bitstream/handle/10713/12002/The_History_of_EAPs_in_the_US_022520.pdf?sequence=5&isAllowed=y
27. BIG Initiative SBIRT Education. *The BIG Initiative*. Accessed May 25, 2023. https://bigsbirteducation.webs.com/
28. Boseman J. Disability management: application of a nurse based model in a large corporation. *AAOHN J*. 2001;49:176-186.
29. Office of Disability Employment Policy. *Stay at Work/Return to Work*. U.S. Department of Labor. Accessed May 25, 2023. https://www.dol.gov/agencies/odep/initiatives/saw-rtw
30. SAMHSA. *Recovery and Recovery Support*. Accessed May 25, 2023. https://www.samhsa.gov/find-help/recovery

CHAPTER 34

Addiction Among Physicians and Physician Health Programs

Paul H. Earley and Chris Bundy

CHAPTER OUTLINE

- Introduction
- Prevalence
- Characteristics of physicians with addiction
- Risks and correlates of addiction among physicians
- Drugs used
- Co-occurring conditions
- Identification, intervention, and assessment
- Treatment
- Physician health programs
- Challenges and opportunities for further research
- Conclusion

INTRODUCTION

The available research about addiction among physicians and physician health programs (PHPs) is extensive and has been well documented in several excellent overviews[1-10] and position papers.[11-14] Bissell and Haberman,[15] Angres et al.,[16] Nace,[17] and Coombs[18] have written complete texts about addiction in physicians and other health professionals. Physicians are a convenient population to study; they are accessible both prior to and after treatment and are articulate about their disease. Research on physician addiction elucidates the natural course of addiction in a highly regulated and monitored population. At the same time, physicians differ from the general population in terms of education, income, and regulatory oversight; therefore, conclusions about the efficacy of addiction treatment among physician-patients cannot simply be generalized to the population at large. However, the highly structured and consistent treatment model developed for the care of this population does provide clues for treatment improvement with all populations. Less research is available about other health professionals; however, many of the issues and concepts described here may prove helpful for all healthcare workers as well as safety-sensitive workers in general.

PREVALENCE

We have over 30 years of debate about the actual and changing prevalence of addiction among physicians.[7] Kessler et al.[19] reported that 3.8% of the general population at any given time has any substance use disorder and 1.3% meets criteria for pre-DSM-5 defined alcohol dependence and 0.4% for drug dependence. Lifetime prevalence for alcohol use disorders has been estimated at between 8% and 13% in the general population. Prevalence studies among physicians report widely varying rates dependent upon research methodology.[7,20-25] Hughes et al.[23] reported a lifetime prevalence of alcohol use disorder or drug use disorder in physicians at 7.9%, somewhat less than the percentage reported in the general population by Kessler et al.[19] A recent and large meta-analysis reported that problematic alcohol use has increased over time from 16.3% in the time frame between 2006 to 2010 to 26.8% in the time frame of 2017 to 2020.[25]

Vaillant,[26] in his commentary on the Hughes study, rang an alarm bell by stating, "physicians are five times as likely [as the general population] to take sedatives and minor tranquilizers without medical supervision." This trend may begin before or in medical school. Merlo et al. reported that greater than 70% of medical students acknowledged binge drinking, with men reporting higher frequency than women.[27] Jackson et al. reported that over 30% of medical students developed new onset alcohol problems during medical school.[28] Early onset SUD also extends to other substances. In an earlier study, Baldwin et al. found that 90% of senior medical students who used alcohol, tobacco, cannabis, or amphetamines had initiated use prior to medical school but that tranquilizer use typically began during medical school. These findings were consistent with prior studies suggesting that patterns of substance use and unhealthy use may be established prior to entry into medical school.[29]

Another view of physician unhealthy use of alcohol and drugs can be derived from complaints reviewed by state medical boards. Morrison and Wickersham[30] noted that 14% of board disciplinary actions were alcohol or drug related and another 11% were due to inappropriate prescribing practices—many of which were? also addiction related. In 2003, Clay and Conatser[31] reported similar disciplinary rates, with 21% due to alcohol and drug issues and 10% due to inappropriate prescribing or drug possession.

In summary, the prevalence of addiction to all substances appears to be about the same among physicians as in the general population, with some data suggesting that physicians may have more alcohol-related problems and may be more likely to misuse prescription opioids and sedative–hypnotics.[32] Methodologic issues likely account for observed differences among existing prevalence data and there are no large systematic studies of SUD in physicians. Despite these limitations, the prevalence data suggest that being a physician confers no special protection against the development of addiction.

CHARACTERISTICS OF PHYSICIANS WITH ADDICTION

Age and Gender

In a 2008 analysis of more than 1,400 medical students, residents, and physicians at the same southeastern treatment program, Earley and Weaver (unpublished) noted an age range from 25.3 to 83.7 years, with a median age of 45.8, the ages distributed in a bell curve. This was a convenience sample of physician-patients who entered one treatment system and is not representative of all physicians. Physicians with SUD have similar substance use onset and history to the general public, which argues that SUD among medical professionals is not related to drug access and that treatment success in this population is not a result of later substance access.[33]

Men account for the majority of physicians entering addiction treatment, with reported ratios approximately 7 to 1.[34] This contrasts with the current 3-to-1 male-to-female ratio in the physician population at large.[35] Although fewer female than male physicians have drinking problems, data from Oreskovitch et al., show that female physicians are more likely to exhibit alcohol use disorder than women who are not physicians.[36] Concerning alcohol misuse, this apparent difference appears to be converging, according to more recent data.[25] A study from the United Kingdom reported that incoming female students were nearly twice as likely as the age-matched general public to be drinking at a moderate or greater risk level, while male students drank at levels similar to nonmedical student controls.[37]

At intake into one of four PHPs, female physicians were more likely to be younger and to have medical and psychiatric comorbidity.[38] Female physicians were more likely to have past or current suicidal ideation and were more likely to have attempted suicide regardless of whether they were under the influence or not. Wunsch et al. report that female physicians are more likely to use sedative–hypnotics than men.[38]

Sex and gender minorities have elevated rates of SUD compared to the general population, but little is known, and more research is needed, to determine the prevalence and sociodemographic correlates of SUD in physicians with marginalized sex and gender identities.

Race and Ethnicity

Race and ethnic determinants of substance use in the general population are described in the National Epidemiologic Survey on Alcohol and Related Conditions (NESARC): White people, Indigenous American people, and Hispanic/Latinx people have a higher prevalence of SUD than Asian people, but no published data about physician addiction have been reported using race or ethnicity as an independent variable.

Specialty

Bissell and Jones,[39] writing in 1976 about 98 physicians, were first to systematically parse and report this cohort by specialty. Using a follow-up questionnaire of physicians in Alcoholics Anonymous, she noted that psychiatrists and emergency medicine physicians were overrepresented in Alcoholics Anonymous (overrepresentation defined as a percentage of a cohort that is higher than predicted by the percentage of that cohort in the population of physicians at large). Hughes et al.[22] later surveyed 5,426 physicians regarding substance use; they found the self-report of SUD was highest in psychiatrists and emergency medicine physicians and lowest in surgeons and pediatricians. This questionnaire did not break down the substance used.

A synopsis of the literature on addiction rates by specialty appears in **Table 34-1**, which covers multiple authors and modes of analysis. The combined literature looks at the breakdown by specialty from multiple angles (treatment presentation, self-report, and medical board and PHP data); the data consistently report that anesthesiology, psychiatry, and emergency medicine physicians have higher rates of unhealthy substance use. **Table 34-1** also suggests that family practice physicians might be overrepresented, and pediatricians and pathologists appear to have a lower prevalence of addiction.

The problem of addiction among anesthesiologists continues to attract research and debate. Lutsky et al.[21] noted that anesthesiologists were more likely to use cannabis and psychedelics when compared with medicine and surgery physicians, but suggested caution in the interpretation of these data owing to age differences between the medicine and surgery cohort and the anesthesiology cohort. Gallegos et al.[40] noted that anesthesiologists account for 5% of all physicians, yet they account for 13% of all physician-patients in a residential treatment program. Self-report studies by Hughes et al. noted a low overall rate of substance use in anesthesiology, both in residency[23] and after completing training.[22] In an early study, Lutsky et al.[21] found that the use of fentanyl (and its congeners) occurred only in anesthesiologists. In more recent years, fentanyl (and its congeners) have found expanded medicinal use, resulting in exposure and misuse generalizing to medical specialties beyond anesthesiology.

The increasing availability of fentanyl in illegal drug supply chains, producing the most lethal addiction crisis in history, may also worsen outcomes for physicians. Historically, diversion has been the key route for fentanyl access among physicians with opioid use disorder (OUD)[45]; diversion data are commonly used to detect misuse of opioids among health professionals and drive effective intervention and treatment. With fentanyl readily available in the illegal drug supply,[46] there is less incentive for physicians to divert high-potency opioids from medicinal supplies. Future research will determine if the combination of improved anti-diversion techniques and an increased availability of illegal fentanyl will shift physician misuse to illegal opioids. Such a shift would delay SUD detection and potentially lead to devastating consequences in this population.

Anesthesiologists are strikingly overrepresented in treatment settings. Access to large quantities of these high-potency opioids (and other drugs) in the day-to-day practice of anesthesia is the most likely culprit for the prevalence of anesthesia personnel in treatment settings. Please refer to the section below on anesthesiologist reentry for additional information.

TABLE 34-1 Summary of Studies of Physicians with SUD by Specialty

Research	Year	Research type	No.	Specialties overrepresented	Specialties underrepresented
Bissell[39]	1976	Closed survey	98	Psychiatry, emergency medicine	Surgery
Gallegos et al. [40]	1987	Treatment records	1,000	Anesthesiology, family medicine/ general practice	
Shore[41]	1987	PHP/MB	34	Psychiatry	—
Pelton and Ikeda[42]	1991	PHP/MB	247	Anesthesiology, emergency medicine, family practice	—
McAullife et al.[20]	1986	Survey	489	Psychiatry, anesthesiology	
Myers and Weiss[43]	1987	Resident survey	1,805	Psychiatry, anesthesiology	Community health, emergency medicine, surgery, pediatrics
Hughes[23]	1999	Survey	1,785	Psychiatry, emergency medicine	Pediatrics, pathology, surgery
Morrison and Wickersham[30]	1998	PHP/MB	375	Anesthesiology, psychiatry	Internal medicine, pediatrics
Knight[44]	2007	PHP/MB	120	Anesthesiology, emergency medicine	Pediatrics

Note: PHP/MB = physician health program or medical board record study.

RISKS AND CORRELATES OF ADDICTION AMONG PHYSICIANS

The risk for addiction in physicians is an area rich in theory and speculation but lacking in conclusive research. While more study is needed in this area, the following sections weave together findings from physician-specific research, inferences from studies of addiction in the general population, and the authors' clinical experience, in an effort to characterize the risks and correlates of addiction among physicians.

Family History and Genetics

The strongest predictor of alcohol or drug problems in physicians is the same as in the general population; a family history of substance use disorder.[3] Genetic research literature now supports inherited genetic vulnerabilities for all major classes of addictive drugs.[47] McAuliffe et al.[48] reported that 27% of medical students and 22% of physicians had family histories of alcohol use disorder. Domino et al.[49] reported that 72% of physician and other health professionals admitted for SUD treatment had a relative with SUD, and 61% had first degree relative with SUD. Moore[50] observed several genetic and substance use factors in medical students that later correlated with unhealthy alcohol use including cigarette use of one pack or more per day (RO = 2.6), and regular use of alcohol (RO = 3.6).

Personality

All physician specialties are burdened with some common stereotypes, and it has long been tempting to speculate about causal personality factors in the development of addiction disorders among physicians. In contradistinction, decades of addiction research have never found evidence to support an "addictive personality." Observed physician personality dynamics may be a consequence of, or an epiphenomenon to the true etiology of the addictive process. With the preceding caveats, it is still interesting to review published speculations about physician personality types and addiction. Although personality issues may or may not be causative in addiction, they often play an important role in the progression, presentation, and treatment of addiction disorders and are therefore covered below.

Vaillant et al.[51] suggested that physicians commonly experience an emotionally barren childhood. Johnson and Connelly[52] identified 72% of a 50-physician sample hospitalized for SUD as experiencing parental deprivation in their childhood, echoing this postulate. Khantzian[53] eloquently depicted the physician's efforts at caring for others as a partially successful sublimation; caregiving of others becomes a partial repair of deficits in parental nurturance. Tillett[54] described this dynamic in helping professionals as a drive to "compulsively give to others what they would like to have for themself." When this transformation fails, the addiction-prone physician, lacking other methods of self-care, becomes vulnerable to substance misuse.

Clark et al.[55] reported that excessive alcohol consumption in medical students was positively associated with better grades in the first year and a strong tendency toward better scores on Part I of the National Board of Medical Examiners test. Unhealthy alcohol use was found to have no discernible impact on clinical rotations in years 3 and 4 of medical school in this study. This led Clark to speculate that heavy-drinking students may be prone to discount warnings and feel invulnerable to the effects of alcohol; their own internal experience does not match cautionary information provided to them during their medical education. This may exacerbate an emerging "us" (doctors) and "them" (patients) view of the world. These findings mirror extensive research by Schuckit, who consistently demonstrated that less intense, early-life, and adolescent reactivity to alcohol increases the risk for the later development of alcoholism.[56,57]

McAuliffe et al.[7] noted "sensation seeking" as a personality factor that is correlated with drug use among physicians in training. These authors speculate that such individuals gravitate to specialties such as emergency medicine. Emergency medicine physicians may self-select high-risk or illicit drugs owing to the same personality characteristics that draw them to their specialty. Hughes et al.[22] reported emergency medicine physicians were twice as likely to use cannabis as other specialties. Their data also suggested cocaine use was higher in this cohort. However, this hypothesis is not supported by data from other specialties also thought to attract sensation-seeking individuals, such as surgery, which is not overrepresented in treatment settings.

Bissell and Jones[39] suggest perfectionist behavior and a high class ranking are risk factors for addiction. This is supported by the work of Roche et al.,[58] who noted that anesthesiologists with addiction are often in the top 10% to 20% of their class. Udel[59] notes that obsessive compulsive personality disorder (or traits) is the most common personality diagnosis of physicians presenting for treatment. No data differentiating the occurrence of compulsive traits in physicians with or without addiction are available. However, compulsive traits may also be an asset in physician training and practice when limited in extent.

Physicians are taught in medical school and residency (and often in their childhood) to appear self-sufficient and in control. In addition, physicians in the act of saving human lives develop a varying degree of omnipotence.[17] This omnipotence, when combined with knowledge of the drugs they prescribe, may produce feelings of invulnerability regarding drug or alcohol use. Vaillant[26] has speculated that self-prescribing (related to physician self-sufficiency and false omnipotence) plays a permissive role in the development of SUD in physicians. Physicians' illusion of mastery over pharmaceuticals keeps them from appreciating their lack of control over substance use, opening the door to experimentation and, if continued, a progressive deterioration in their misuse of substances.

In addition, the drive to maintain one's sense of competency and self-mastery impacts the physician's willingness to acknowledge problematic substance use. This limits their ability to seek support (a positive coping strategy), and often results in reliance on negative and/or immature coping strategies, including more substance use, to manage the stress of hiding their addiction.

The physician's behavior deteriorates first at home, then with friends, before problems finally surface within the workplace. By the time a physician exhibits problems at work, significant familial discord (marital strife, divorce, difficulties with acting out in children) commonly exists. Despite this, it is rare for family members to share concerns about a spouse or other family member with presumptive addiction.[60] Often, a colleague or other hospital staff is the first to voice concern. The physician is then confronted at work when an undeniable incident occurs or a series of smaller incidents push colleagues and the hospital medical staff to confront the doctor.[1] Early involvement with a physician health program (PHP), especially one that is supportive and confidential, can be very beneficial in reducing the threshold for reporting to punitive agencies and, thus, can promote early detection. Physicians generally arrive at treatment following a wide range of substance-related consequences, but many continue to struggle with accepting their SUD diagnosis and identity as a patient. They often minimize concerns and may have difficulty relating to others in the treatment community. As a result, it is beneficial for physicians to seek treatment within a program with a specialized track for healthcare professionals. When entering treatment, the physician-patient has a unique blend of assets and liabilities they bring to their care.[61]

Stress and Burnout

Stress and burnout are often cited by the physician-patient as the primary agent that fuels the development of substance misuse and ultimately addiction. Burnout has been endemic among physicians for well over a decade.[62-64] The correlation between burnout and problem alcohol use appears to begin early. Thirty percent of medical students report new onset alcohol problems emerging during medical school; those with burnout being 20% more likely to report alcohol problems.[28] Oreskovich found that surgeons who screened positive for alcohol use disorder (AUD) were 25% more likely to report burnout.[65] Physicians in treatment for SUD report that the stress of medical training, when combined with social isolation, provides fertile soil for the growth of substance use.[4] Jex et al.[66] suggested that the physician's unhealthy *response* to stress is a more important determinant of addiction than the ubiquitous *presence* of stress itself. Unhealthy stress response, combined with difficulties asking for help,[15] can spiral into a vicious and self-reinforcing cycle of alcohol use, drug use,[67] and worsening stress and burnout.

Drug Access

O'Connor and Spickard[1] described a subset of physicians who began using benzodiazepines and opioids only after receiving prescribing privileges. Drug access may also account for changing addictive drugs within the opioid class over time. Green et al.[68] in 1976 and Gallegos et al.[40] in 1987 reported that the predominant opioid used by physicians at the time was meperidine. A later (2005) review of the Michigan and Alabama Physician Health Programs reported hydrocodone as the number one opioid used (40% of all opioid cases), with meperidine dropping to 10% of cases.[69] The most likely hypothesis for shifts in the drug of choice by physicians over time is the changing prescribing patterns and availability of these drugs in the marketplace.

Drug diversion is a common method of obtaining drugs for misuse among physicians. Cummings et al. described four methods of drug diversion: diverting office/hospital inventories, writing illegal prescriptions, using medication samples, and misusing valid prescriptions.[70] Multiple measures have been used to combat diversion. For example, some anesthesia training programs and hospitals have addressed diversion concerns by implementing random screening of all anesthesia personnel.[71] Auditing of hospital and office documentation, although time consuming, may help decrease institution-based access; identity check of those picking up controlled substances may decrease pharmacy prescription diversion.[70] In every case, measures to decrease misuse of prescribed drugs will have to be balanced against exploding workload and paperwork in the medical workplace. Diversion control begs the question as to whether supply side measures will be effective at decreasing physician substance use or simply shift the substances consumed and their procurement to other sources and vendors, as has been seen in the general public amidst the worsening opioid-related overdose crisis.[72]

Biologic Effect of the Drug of Choice

The neurobiological effects of drugs used by those with an addiction color the characteristics of SUD itself. Drug-of-choice characteristics also skew the characteristics of the physician-patients arriving in treatment programs. For example, all opioids produce intense tolerance, resulting in histories of ever-increasing doses. Craving and withdrawal drive the progressively tolerant physician to self-prescribe or divert increasing quantities of opioids from work and, in doing so, increases the probability of detection. This partially explains why treatment-seeking or treatment-mandated physicians tend to present disproportionately with histories of opioid use.

High-potency opioids (such as fentanyl) when consumed parenterally produce a rapid downhill course owing to the development of remarkable levels of tolerance. The accelerated course of addiction from the most potent opioids can be postulated as contributing to deaths and the high percentage of anesthesiologists seen in physician treatment programs in the past and in the lethality of fentanyl in the public at large today.[73] Collins[4] has suggested that rapid onset and the resolution of tolerance with brief periods of abstinence and/or low therapeutic ratio may account for the high mortality rate in propofol-, fentanyl-, sufentanil-, alfentanil-, and remifentanil-using anesthesiologists. Increased awareness along with checks and balances to account for the remaindered volumes of fentanyl used in hospitals may detect diversion more rapidly and save lives of anesthesia personnel.[74-76]

DRUGS USED

Alcohol

Two types of studies are used to assess the types of drugs used by physicians: anonymous questionnaires[20-23,48] and self-reports of drugs of choice of physicians as they appear in treatment or monitoring programs.[40] Both types of research underscore that alcohol is, as expected, the most frequent primary substance used by physicians, just as it is in the general population.

Tobacco and Nicotine

Tobacco use disorder has been suggested as a risk factor for alcohol and other drug use disorder in physicians[50] as in the general population.[77] In an earlier era, physicians took part in magazine advertising extolling the "soothing" and "less harsh" properties of certain cigarettes on the airway.[78] Tobacco use among physicians has decreased over time; Vaillant et al.[79] reported that 39% of physicians acknowledged smoking 10 or more cigarettes per day in 1953; this decreased to 25% in 1968.[80] Nelson et al. reported that smoking among physicians declined from 18.8% in 1976 to 3.3% in 1991.[81] In a 1996 study, Mangus reported 2% of medical school graduates were currently smoking.[82] From additional early data, emergency medicine and surgery physicians are twice as likely to smoke as are other physicians.[22] The rise in popularity and use of electronic drug delivery devices (EDDDs) such as e-cigarettes and "vaping," may reverse prior trends of declining nicotine use among medical students, residents, and physicians where some may view EDDDs as a safer alternative to tobacco products[83]; however, EDDDs are not safe either. The evidence on this topic is reviewed in chapter 22 "Electronic Drug Delivery Devices" in this textbook. Although data are lacking, this could lead to increasing nicotine use despite declining use of tobacco products. Preliminary data (with a small sample size) from Stuyt et al.[84] strongly correlate the continued use of tobacco with subsequent recurrence other drug or alcohol use, underscoring the importance of identifying and treating tobacco or nicotine use disorder in physicians recovering from other SUDs.

Opioids

Opioids are the second most frequently used substance by physicians presenting for treatment.[85] This finding has been remarkably stable over time, but the type of opioids used continues to change. Hughes et al.[23] differentiated opioid use into the "major" opioids (morphine, meperidine, fentanyl, and other injectable narcotics) and the "minor" opioids (hydrocodone, lower-dose forms of oxycodone, codeine, and other oral drugs).

Discriminating in this manner, they reported that family practice and obstetrics and gynecology specialists have a higher probability of using minor opioids. When compared with all physicians, the study reports that anesthesiologists were less likely to use minor opioids, with a trend toward an increased use of major opioids. If one assumes that use of major opioids results in a more aggressive manifestation and progression of addiction, this will partly account for the overrepresentation of anesthesiologists over other specialties in physician treatment programs.[40] Several authors[22,23,86] posit that exposure to drugs in the workplace leads to higher use of those workplace drugs. In a similar manner, family medicine and obstetrics and gynecology physicians are frequent prescribers and use more minor opioids than other specialties.[22]

Cocaine

Older literature noted that specialties that employed cocaine in the course of their work (ophthalmology, head and neck surgery, plastic surgery, and otolaryngology) showed a marginal trend for higher cocaine use.[22] Cocaine use among physicians has shifted to illegal/non-medicinal sources more recently, presumably due to decreased medical use and increased hospital pharmacy controls. Cocaine use is more common in emergency medicine physicians, presumably from street sources. Several authors[86,87] have speculated that the personality styles associated with various specialties may attract those physicians to certain drugs.

Amphetamine

Physicians primarily use amphetamines from two sources. A subset of physicians who are prescribed amphetamine and other stimulants for attentional disorders go on to develop a substance use disorder, as in the general population.[88] The pressures of premedical and medical school education and prolonged duty hours during residency may promote trial use of stimulants in another subset of physicians. Methamphetamine use is 5 to 10 times higher[89] in urban men who have sex with men. This is mirrored among physicians; most PHPs report that a large majority of physicians who use methamphetamine are men who have sex with men.

Benzodiazepines

Older, survey-based studies reported that psychiatrists have a greater misuse of benzodiazepines; 26.3% reported using unsupervised benzodiazepines in the past year, in comparison with 11.4% in other physician groups.[22] Although unsupervised use does not impute a substance use disorder, the high rate of benzodiazepine use is reflected in the overrepresentation of psychiatrists in treatment.

Propofol

Eighteen percent of anesthesia training programs report cases of propofol use among trainees[90] and its prevalence has increased fivefold in the past decade.[90] Wischmeyer et al. identified 25 anesthesia personnel with propofol use; 7 died as a direct result. This study described a positive correlation between hospitals with easy availability and subsequent propofol use. High availability was defined as little or no control over drug access within the training hospital. Although propofol use often shows up in training, use can occur later in medical practice. In contrast, propofol use in nonmedical personnel is extremely rare; until recently, only one such case had been reported in medical literature.[91]

Propofol use gained national attention after the death of pop star Michael Jackson in 2009. Increasing reports of propofol use[92] and research about its addicting qualities have resulted in the Drug Enforcement Administration (DEA) placing fospropofol[93] under Schedule IV and a proposed Schedule IV for propofol as well.[94]

Even among healthcare professionals, DSM-IV defined propofol dependence appears to occur in a relatively small proportion of physicians with SUDs, that is 1.6%, or 22 of 1,375 treated physicians, usually anesthesiologists.[95] Its incidence appears to be increasing over one 20-year study.[95] Other characteristics of this cohort of 22 physicians in SUD treatment who had used propofol was a tendency toward the female gender, higher incidence of early-life trauma, concomitant mood disorder, and physical trauma resulting from substance use.[95]

Cannabis

Lifetime and past month cannabis use is common among medical residents, second only to alcohol.[24] A 2017 US study reported cannabis use at 22.7% among medical students, with higher rates among men (27.0%) than women (18.9%).[27] Emergency medicine, orthopedics, plastic surgery, anesthesiology, and psychiatry specialty physicians display elevated odds of cannabis use over physicians as a whole.[22,96,97] Cannabis legalization for recreational use and cannabis used as treatment have raised interesting controversies about physician cannabis use that are addressed in the section "Challenges and Opportunities for Research" below.

Other Drugs

Physicians may also use drugs that are not generally available or not commonly used for non-medical purposes. Skipper[69] reported that tramadol was the third most frequent opioid mentioned by physicians presenting with SUD, "although it was rarely the primary drug of choice" in a study of 595 physicians from two state PHPs over an 8-year period. Ketamine is increasingly used in the treatment of depression despite its misuse in the population at large.[98,99] Moore and Bostwick[100] described two cases of ketamine use in anesthesiologists. Professional treatment programs and PHPs have limited experience in evaluating and treating physicians with ketamine use disorder.

CO-OCCURRING CONDITIONS

Thought and Mood Disorders

Physicians suffer from a spectrum of emotional and psychiatric problems similar to the general population. It is unclear whether physicians have higher or lower rates of unipolar depression; however, substance use disorder, self-criticism, and dependent personality characteristics are associated with depression in physicians.[101] Bipolar disorder (types I and II) may contribute to the intensity of SUD in physicians, particularly for alcohol use during manic intervals.[102] Bipolar disorder is often detected when a physician's hypomanic prodrome deteriorates into frank mania. However, physicians with addiction rarely have comorbid primary schizophrenia or related thought disorders.

Substance use disorder is strongly correlated to suicide risk.[103] As a group, physicians are more likely to die from suicide than non-physicians. These factors combine, placing physicians with SUD at a particularly elevated risk for suicide. In addition, physicians are less likely to seek care for mental health problems and more likely to deny the presence of mental health problems or see them as merely part of a stressful career choice.[104] Physicians who die from suicide are more likely to have a drug use problem in their lives, self-prescribed psychoactive substances, and/or have a recent alcohol-related problem, a history of emotional problems prior to 18 years of age, and/or a family history of unhealthy alcohol use and/or mental illness.[105] Gold et al. queried the National Violent Death Reporting System to examine drivers of physician suicide and found that a recent job-related problem was more strongly correlated with suicide in physicians compared to non-physicians. In addition, the study found that physicians who died from suicide were a staggering 20-40 times more likely than non-physicians to have antipsychotic, benzodiazepine, or barbiturate medication in their system at the time of death but *less* likely to have received any mental health treatment.[106] These data suggest that modifiable risk factors for suicide among physicians include increasing access and decreasing stigma related to mental health and substance use treatment, as well as recognizing and supporting physicians who are experiencing job-related problems or professional identity threats such as medical board complaints, "malpractice" actions, or other performance-related concerns. As will be explored later in this chapter, physician health programs (PHPs) can be a key resource to support physicians with this constellation of risk factors.

Pain

Physicians with chronic pain who use analgesic opioids are at an increased risk of physiological dependence. In turn, an unknown percentage of those go on to develop the disease of addiction. Eventual addiction is thought to be more common in patients with pain disorders,[107] and, when combined with easier access to opioids (through ready access to prescribers, prescriptions written to family and friends, and diversion) a perfect storm of high-risk factors emerges. Physicians who have significant pain and addiction disorders pose diagnostic, treatment, and management difficulties for assessors, treatment providers, and the PHPs. Regulatory issues cloud the treatment of physicians with co-occurring pain and substance use disorders. For example, should a physician in recovery who is prescribed opioid medications be allowed to practice? Is it logical for state boards to limit or prohibit ongoing methadone or buprenorphine treatment but permit potent opioids for pain management? These complex questions often result in ideological or political conclusions rather than evidence-based answers. Scientific data on the safety of physicians practicing while taking opioids for pain or SUD treatment are sorely lacking, but appropriate concern remains.[108,109]

Opioids may be necessary to maintain the quality of life when a physician is suffering with chronic non-malignant pain. However, when that same individual has a history of unhealthy opioid use or opioid diversion, their management becomes quite complex. In such cases, the PHP and treatment providers are balancing the physician's need for pain control with the safety of the public and, importantly, the fear of reprisal by an uninformed public. The decision about a physician's ability to practice in such situations should be approached with caution and thorough knowledge of the research and clinical expertise in this area. Although the use of chronic opioids may be necessary in such cases, loss of control from prescribed doses can occur. The resolution of this conundrum should rest upon the effect the medication has on the brain and behavior of the physician-patient, not upon the illness for which it is prescribed.

Childhood Trauma and Posttraumatic Stress Disorder

Posttraumatic stress disorder (PTSD) and alcohol use disorder are closely intertwined,[110] and PTSD increases the probability of return to use in stressful contexts.[111] However, no studies about the prevalence of PTSD in physicians have been published. Physicians, like anyone else, are not immune from prior trauma histories or the normalized trauma that is a common occupational hazard in medicine. Unanticipated operative mortality, suicide, lethal overdose, traumatic injury and death in children and adolescents, violent patient behaviors toward medical providers and mass casualty events are just some of the traumatic events that can have long-term psychological sequalae for physicians. Although combat exposure is known to increase the likelihood of substance use disorders in veterans, no data exist to indicate whether such trauma increases the likelihood of substance use disorders in military physicians. Importantly, treating trauma can itself be traumatizing to the caregiver.

IDENTIFICATION, INTERVENTION, AND ASSESSMENT

Identification

Physician Health Programs (PHPs) are confidential peer assistance programs for physicians (and often other health professionals) that identify, refer for evaluation and treatment, and monitor remission in physicians who have SUDs or other health conditions that could impair safe practice (see the PHP section below). One of the central activities of PHPs is to identify physicians early in the illness process, before patients are placed at risk. This is especially important because physicians present with a broad spectrum of symptom severity, ranging from a physician self-identifying alcohol use disorder during couples' therapy to a physician experiencing an opioid overdose at work. In the past, denial, shame, and fear of reprisal tended to prevent physicians from seeking proper help until significant external consequences coalesced.[2] In more recent years, the emergence of clinically-oriented, supportive, and confidential PHPs has stimulated earlier reporting, by either self- or colleague referral. Physician-patients with substance problems have often experienced years of familial and social discord while struggling to maintain acceptable work performance, until the last refuge—work—collapses. Thus, disturbances of social or familial functioning may be more sensitive indicators of early substance use disorder in the physician. Unfortunately, the family often obscures such indicators if the physician is the chief financial contributor to household income.

A variety of work-related behaviors can be clues to substance use. O'Connor and Spickard[1] describe conditions and warning signs that can help detect addiction among physicians (**Table 34-2**). Talbott and Wright[60,112] and Talbott and Benson[113] independently reported a similar list.

If problems are not addressed early, the doctor's work quality and attendance often suffer.[114] In contrast, if a physician obtains drugs at work (eg, samples from a drug closet or drugs diverted from the OR or ICU), they often display the opposite behavior—volunteering for additional shifts, arriving early for work, and signing up for more complex (ie, easier drug access) cases.

Modes of Intervention

Several comprehensive guides to physician intervention have been published.[2,5,10,115] In recent years, PHPs have become very skilled at directing the physician-patient to preliminary evaluation without overly aggressive confrontation and ultimatums. Some PHPs provide this evaluation as a service, others send the physician to a third party evaluator with experience in the complexities of such cases.[116] The physician in question is told about existing concerns (often without divulging the source of information) and the importance of resolving said concerns. Ultimately, the goal is early detection of whatever problem is causing concerns and initiation of effective treatment when indicated.[117]

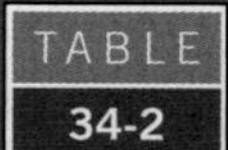

TABLE 34-2 Warning Signs of Unhealthy Substance Use in Physicians

- Positive genetic history
- Domestic problems
- Appearance of being intoxicated at social functions
- Intoxication or the odor of alcohol on the breath at work
- Highly irregular hours for rounds
- Self-prescribing
- Neglect of responsibilities
- Anger outbursts
- Frequent medical complaints without a reasonable diagnosis
- Staff concerns about physician behavior
- Depression or weight change
- Citations for driving while under the influence (DUI/DWI/OMVI)

Adapted from O'Connor PG, Spickard A. Physician impairment by substance abuse. *Med Clin North Am.* 1997;81(4):1037-1052, with permission from Elsevier.

Most physicians appreciate their duty to public safety. Once a well-being committee at a hospital or the PHP points out the need to determine if a health problem is present, this sense of duty, combined with some level of self-concern, can motivate a physician to obtain a proper evaluation. A minority of physicians, especially those who have in the past felt mistreated by a legal or employment process or have undergone previous interventions, require additional orchestration with partners or employers who then help get the physician to an evaluation and/or treatment. Regardless of the path to the door, physicians commonly arrive with a story depicting their entry into evaluation or treatment as self-motivated.

Most states have reporting laws that require hospitals and colleagues to report a physician to the state PHP or state medical board if there is reasonable concern for impairment from alcohol or drugs. Treating physicians must have knowledge of the laws in their state before beginning treatment of physicians with SUD concerns. In 2001, The Joint Commission required hospital organizations to address the wellness of their medical staff through standard MS2.6.[118] The Joint Commission standard has helped to formalize a physician health process, as well as a support network in most hospitals. Many PHPs are able to assist the hospitals in meeting this standard. Hospital wellness committees can be effective in early identification and referral of physicians if the process maintains a balance of compassion with a firm directive hand.[119]

In contrast, the primary agenda of hospital credentialing and executive committees is maintaining quality of care and minimizing risk. When concerns are raised, including concerns limited to the potential for impairment, they utilize letters of concern, sanctions, and de-credentialing to protect the hospital and the public. Wellness committees, on the other hand, focus on the health of providers within the organization. If a wellness committee attempts to get a provider help, such help would be scuttled (and appear quite disingenuous) should it become known to the organization credentialing body with the potential for resultant action. Therefore, a firewall should be maintained between the wellness and credentialing/executive committees.

If a substance use disorder is not caught in its early stages, the possibility of impairment arises. Thus, the primary public health goal of PHPs is to facilitate diagnosis and treatment of physicians early in the course of their illness, before patients are put at risk. In a study of impairment of all types (not focused solely on substance-induced impairment), Igartua reported that 7% of residents in her survey reported working with an impaired physician supervisor.[120] Reuben and Noble reported that 72% of house officers would report an impaired attending physician.[121]

Assessment

Physician responses to a request that they undergo SUD evaluation vary widely. Some physicians are quickly identified and agree to cooperate with their treatment needs or at least with an evaluation. Physicians who have more severe SUD, who have more complex presentations, or who are unable to acknowledge legitimate health concerns need a more comprehensive assessment and methodical, non-shaming discussion of their illness. In all cases, use of the ASAM Criteria can be helpful toward determination of level of care decisions.[122] Timely and proper diagnosis is best made by an interdisciplinary evaluation based upon guidelines established by the Federation of State Physician Health Programs (FSPHP).[123] Assessment can be completed at the least intensive level of care that results in a comprehensive view of the patient and his or her family and social systems. The examination process must assess for ongoing drug use and withdrawal, as well as addiction-related interpersonal challenges. Such evaluations always include a thorough examination of psychiatric concerns and diagnoses. Because of the complexity and comprehensive nature of these evaluations, in some—but not all—cases, it is helpful to conduct them in a higher level of care (such as a partial hospitalization setting) where the evaluation staff are in continuous conversation about a case, able to adjust the process rapidly, and obtain the broadest understanding of the individual. When the physician is removed from his or her work role, the evaluation team is able to observe the physician outside of the provider role; this affords a broader understanding of the individual when the protective physician cloak is removed.[123] Allowing physicians to self-select an evaluator commonly results in their choosing a friend or colleague, or someone who lacks the necessary expertise in the nuances of a physician addiction evaluation. This results in an inadequate or limited evaluation and thus a missed chance at early diagnosis. Therefore, most PHPs have established criteria and maintain a list of competent evaluators. PHPs often direct physicians to an outpatient, an intensive outpatient, or a residential evaluation based upon the complexity of the case at hand.[123]

The evaluation should include information from, but should not be carried out by, a current or past therapist, psychiatrist, or other healthcare provider. Many PHPs direct the evaluation to a multidisciplinary team composed of an addiction medicine physician and/or an addiction psychiatrist and include psychological and neuropsychological testing, family assessment, review of previous medical records, and the collection of collateral information from coworkers, hospital employees, friends, and PHPs themselves. A broad array of information from all available resources is critical to an accurate assessment.

If an evaluation is performed by a team, it is best if that team meets repeatedly during the evaluation and again when all data have been collected. Final diagnoses and recommendations are best produced by discussion among members of the evaluation team. The patient then meets with one or all members of the evaluation team to review the diagnosis and care recommendations. The patient may also elect to involve a family member. The evaluation team is best served by including the PHP in the summation session; this action decreases confusion and splitting regarding the outcome. A comprehensive, integrated report is commonly sent to both the physician-patient and other relevant parties with appropriate Release of Information authorizations.

TREATMENT

Approximately twenty substance use disorder treatment programs in the United States have experience and specialized expertise in the treatment of physicians and other health professionals; some programs have more than 40 years of experience and have treated thousands of physicians with SUD.

Clinical Considerations in Treating Addicted Physician-Patients

It has been alleged that physicians "make the worst patients."[124] Physicians may deny symptoms of illness, seek substandard care, and put off appropriate care for serious symptoms.[125] As in any other medical situation, the physician-patient who enters addiction treatment has difficulty giving up the provider role and assuming the obligations of a patient.[126,127] In treatment settings with an admixture of physician-patients and nonphysician-patients, the treatment program must set firm limits, prohibiting the physician from slipping into the provider role by offering medical advice or care to other patients. If a patient is the only physician in a given treatment setting, they will likely remain or lapse into the physician role the first moment another patient asks for medical advice or for stories from their career. This shifts focus off of the physician-patient, decreasing the efficacy of their treatment. By contrast, when a physician falls into self-diagnosis, a skilled therapist uses this as grist for the therapeutic mill.

Physicians will also attempt to fit the treatment into what they know: schooling and testing. Thus, they have little trouble learning the didactic parts of treatment. Physicians early in treatment may arrive at a group therapy session with pen and paper in hand, hoping to glean one piece of information that will rocket them into recovery or, at the very least, accelerate their discharge. They can be adept at parroting the prevailing recovery orthodoxies to the staff without meaningful integration of recovery principles. The transformation required of all patients in addiction treatment is an emotional, interpersonal, and, for some, a spiritual shift. Many physicians have little experience in this area. They often become stuck trying to obtain an "A" in treatment and, in this way, miss the necessary emotional changes needed. When staff attempt to correct the physician's approach to treatment, they risk becoming ensnared in the physician's tendency toward excess perfectionism. The resultant hostile projection produces negative transference and a thinly veiled contempt for "less educated" therapists and staff.[127]

Physicians work and interact in an environment filled with physical and emotional pain. To succeed, they must at times distance themselves from the strife around them. When combined with an achievement-oriented childhood,[51] the physician-patient defaults to intellectualization of their emotional experience or, on occasion, frank alexithymia (without words for feelings).[128,129] Treatment will necessarily reacquaint the physician with the subtle nuances of feeling states, often confused or conflated with craving or "stress."

One particularly difficult emotional state is shame. Because of pervasive stigma and discrimination towards people with SUD, patients may view their substance use and their lives through a lens of shame—and physician-patients seem to have a surfeit of shame. Fayne and Silvan[127] note that a key task in recovery is an honest appraisal of how the physician's addiction has interfered with their ability to function as a physician. This requires a vigilant therapeutic group that models self-disclosure and self-examination. The physician, owing to childhood and training-induced drives for accomplishment and perfection, risks turning the task of self-examination into self-loathing. Successful treatment of such individuals requires that the treatment staff and community encourage fearless self-examination without inadvertently pulling the hair trigger of the physician's self-loathing. When in the state of shame, an additional defense of the physician-patient is to psychologically freeze. The precarious management of shame is further complicated by the patient's transference and the therapist's countertransference that arise when a bright physician-patient seems incapable (or willfully resistant) to the self-examination necessary for recovery.

Working with addicted physicians requires understanding of the dynamics of addiction and the distinct but highly interactive elements between addiction and personality. Inexperienced or overly biased treatment providers tend to label the psychological effects of addiction as personality issues, or, conversely, they view long-standing personality dynamics in the physician-patient as addictive thoughts and actions. A balanced understanding and therapeutic approach require a healthy respect for both schools of thought. Often, specific personality dynamics of the physician-patient intensify maladaptive forces that perpetuate substance use behaviors. Conversely, the addictive process can mimic or exacerbate pathological personality traits.

Clinicians and patients are often tempted to infer a one-way, cause-and-effect relationship between non-substance-related psychiatric conditions and addiction. This narrative considers addiction to be secondary or reactive to the non-substance-related psychiatric condition. An example of this narrative is viewing addiction to alcohol as simply a means to self-medicate depression or anxiety, rather than its own unique problem. This prevents effective management because the treatment of depression or anxiety alone is unlikely to solve the addiction problem. A more powerful viewpoint is to envision a patient's SUD and other mood and personality issues as distinct disorders that are mutually reinforcing and require independent, yet coordinated, treatment.

Social and legal issues only further confound the type and course of treatment. Because of all the aforementioned issues, treatment is by its nature different in physicians. Medical boards, the general public, PHPs, and physicians themselves have low tolerance for the potential public harm that can occur when a physician develops SUD; they are exquisitely intolerant of multiple episodes of return to use. This flies in the face of the nature of addiction: a disease characterized by remission and return to use. The societal pressure to "have a perfect recovery" creates a maladaptive alliance with the physician-patient's own perfectionism.[130]

Characteristics of the Treatment Setting

The treatment of physicians involves a prolonged continuum of care, with long-term disease management extending over years in most cases. When a physician leaves his or her initial treatment setting and returns to work, this is described by the unfortunate and inaccurate vernacular of having "completed treatment." In fact, what physicians are asked to do in the second phase of treatment is, in many ways, more comprehensive care than what most patients receive during their *primary* treatment.[131] This "posttreatment" monitoring is a central function of a PHP and typically involves weekly professionally facilitated PHP group monitoring sessions, peer support groups, aftercare groups, individual and family therapy, mutual-help group attendance, random drug testing, and worksite monitor reports for 5 years or more.

The confluence of known difficulties engaging physicians in treatment, the public demand for safety, and liability issues involved in allowing a physician to work while in outpatient addiction treatment have promoted the development of physician-specific, long-term residential and partial hospital addiction treatment programs.[126] A paucity of literature exists about the efficacy of less intensive treatment, but fair results have been reported by Dilts et al.[132] and Reading.[133] Smith and Smith[134] reported a small cohort of physicians treated in low- and high-intensity care, with substantively better results when longer-term residential care was employed. DuPont et al.,[135] reviewing 16 state PHPs over 5 years, noted that 78% of physicians who required treatment went to residential treatment for 30 to 90 days, followed by less intensive outpatient treatment. The remaining 22% of treated physicians went directly to outpatient treatment. Hospitals, professional liability insurance carriers, regulatory boards, health insurance companies, and family and friends have expectations of continuous abstinence. Most medical boards and, increasingly, professional liability insurance companies (who in many states have become a more powerful threat) penalize a physician if they return to use, even a single time. Owing to concerns about the risks of return to use, and the punitive consequences that can ensue for the affected physician, higher levels of care and longer duration of treatment are typically recommended for this special population.[122] Fail-first models of care (where higher levels of care are only utilized after failing a lower level of care) that are a standard approach in the general population may confer unacceptable risks to physicians with SUD and their patients.

Skipper outlined the treatment of the impaired health professional.[136] The Federation of State Physician Health Programs revised their guidelines on the treatment of physicians in 2019.[123] Both report that most physician-specialized treatment programs use a 12-step philosophy as part of multidisciplinary, multifocal treatment. Such programs have proven effectiveness with physicians.[131,135,137,138] Studies have demonstrated that consistent involvement with mutual support meetings is the best predictor of sustained abstinence[139-144] and a recent study of physicians who successfully completed PHP monitoring reported that participation in a 12-step program was rated as the most valuable component of their recovery program.[145] All physician treatment programs reviewed by DuPont et al.[135] utilize family therapy, and most offer a brief psychoeducational family program sometime during the physician's treatment.[1] Family participation also leads to better outcomes.[146] Family members move through their own difficulties accepting the addiction diagnosis, anger at the physician-patient, and fear of loss of prestige and financial security. The initial goal of family treatment is to redirect the hostility away from the patient (as well as the treatment providers and PHP) toward the SUD itself, using this energy to build healthy and constructive family dynamics that are focused on supporting recovery.

Physician-specific groups allow self-disclosure of alcohol- and drug-related behaviors that risked or, in rare cases, caused patient harm. Such violations of the Hippocratic Oath often generate shame. Once articulated, such lapses in physician responsibility are best linked to the SUD and away from the core self. Disclosures of the deepest violations of core values in profession-specific groups can, if properly managed, provide relief and help the physician differentiate his or her SUD-related behaviors and self-concept. Physician-specific therapeutic/support groups serve a different, more pragmatic, but equally important, purpose. Most physicians have work-related triggers (eg, drug access at work, prescription pads, and locations in the office or hospital where use occurred). In these groups, participants explore work triggers and develop profession-specific plans to prevent return to use. On this practical level, physician-specific groups also address myriad issues that physicians face when returning to practice, such as the difficulties of seeing their patients in mutual help meetings, how to respond to questions from peers and other staff about their illness, Drug Enforcement Administration prescribing restrictions, and continued management of drugs and prescriptions in the office or hospital. These needs require healthcare practitioner-specific support, preferably in a group setting to increase acceptance, decrease the unique aspects of shame, and teach skills of healthy interdependence.[126]

Physician treatment programs were among the earliest adopters of the use of medications to treat addiction. Treatment providers in this space need and employ addiction medicine specialists and addiction psychiatrists,[123] which has contributed to increased utilization of needed addiction medications. Medications are especially critical in the treatment of physicians with opioid use disorder (OUD)[147-149]; and, thanks to long-term disease monitoring, physicians have a very high rate of medication compliance. Importantly, co-occurring psychiatric diseases should be detected early and managed simultaneously with SUD care. The role of medications for opioid use disorder (MOUD) is covered in the "Challenges and Opportunities" section below.

Ultimately, long-term disease monitoring may be the component of care that most contributes to the successful outcomes of physicians recovering from SUDs. The disease monitoring process will be discussed in the next section.

PHYSICIAN HEALTH PROGRAMS

History

The importance of physician health programs (PHPs) in supporting and promoting early detection and proper evaluation and treatment of physicians cannot be overstated. The heart of the physician's health movement can be traced back to the founding of the International Doctors in Alcoholics Anonymous (IDAA) by Clarence Pearson, in 1949.[150] IDAA has grown from 24 physicians, meeting in Pearson's garage in Cape Vincent, New York, to an international organization attracting thousands of physicians and other doctorate-level individuals in recovery from addiction. Equally important, and on the regulatory side, the Federation of State Medical Boards called for a model probation and rehabilitation process for "addicted physicians" in 1958. However, no meaningful change occurred until 1973, with the publication of the watershed *JAMA* article: "The sick physician. Impairment by psychiatric disorders, including alcoholism and drug dependence."[12] The American Medical Association (AMA) held its first conference on physician impairment two years later. These events led to state medical societies organizing committees on physician impairment. The American and Canadian Medical Associations have jointly sponsored conferences on physician impairment every other year since 1975. Concern from medical organizations, governing bodies, and hospital regulatory boards resulted in the state-by-state emergence of PHPs over a period of 25 years.

David Canavan, MD, started the first PHP (New Jersey) in 1982. Since that time, "all but three of the 54 US medical societies of all states and jurisdictions had authorized or implemented impaired physician programs."[151] Delaware, Nebraska, and Wisconsin remained without a PHP.[151] California moved against this trend when it decided to "sunset" the Physician Diversion Program in 2009, leaving California physicians with SUDs and other mental conditions without support and the public without a system of safety. Multiple grass roots support systems have emerged quietly to fill the void, but strong political voices continue to suggest that physicians with SUD in California deserve no "strikes" and that they are, in essence, disposable in a competitive medical economy.

All Physician Health Programs in the US and some Canadian Provinces belong to the umbrella organization called the Federation of State Physician Health Programs (FSPHP).[152] This organization promotes collaboration, research, and education among its members. In addition, the FSPHP publishes guidelines for state PHPs to drive best practices for PHPs and providers who treat physicians with SUDs.[123] Over time, PHPs have become more professional, with credibility provided by their expertise and affiliation with the FSPHP and other medical organizations, such as the American Medical Association, American Psychiatric Association, and the Federation of State Medical Boards.[153]

As professionalism has increased, so has the finesse and ability for PHPs to carry out educational programs, expanding to a broader range of topics (eg, stress, burnout, compassion fatigue, sexual misconduct, appropriate prescribing, etc.). The core concept of PHPs has become clear, to detect problems that have the potential to lead to impairment, and to intervene and encourage physicians to obtain assistance prior to damaging their careers or harming patients. Sophistication in dealing with physicians with SUDs has increased, in partnership with expert evaluators and treatment providers. Recovery monitoring has become much more sophisticated with additional technology and tools (eg, hair testing, flexible variations in drug testing, new tests for alcohol exposure, devices that detect alcohol consumption, video monitored collection systems, and so on). New software options are facilitating the aggregation and analysis of physician monitoring records, obtaining reports that aggregate data, and real-time oversight. PHP participant abstinence outcomes are among the best reported in addiction medicine,[49,85,154,155] and satisfaction with the PHP process, irrespective of whether the participant entered voluntarily or through mandate, is quite good.[156] Physician Health Programs also impact malpractice claims and, by inference, improve patient safety. This safety was confirmed by Brooks et al. who reported that after the completion of a monitoring period, those enrolled in the Colorado PHP had a 20% lower malpractice risk than a matched, disease-free cohort. In addition, physicians' annual rate of claims was significantly lower after their monitoring period.[157]

Structure

PHPs have widely different organizational structures and lines of authority, having evolved from two distinct sources. Some PHPs descended from committees of their states' medical board and have subsequently evolved, with varying degrees of autonomy from their licensing body. Other PHPs emerged from a state medical society or other concerned physician groups. Many state medical boards continue to actively monitor a limited number of physicians, referring others to their state PHP. Importantly, one comparison study of a state (Oregon) with both programs noted that access to a "voluntary diversion program for appropriately selected physicians may enhance earlier referral and intervention."[41,158] More than half (54%) of PHPs are independent nonprofit organizations. Others are part of their respective state medical association (35%) or the licensing board itself (13%).[135] All PHPs have written agreements that guide their interaction with their state licensing boards. Most (59%) PHPs evaluated in the DuPont et al. study from 2009[131] have specific laws that sanction their actions and guide their operation. Although it is common for health professionals to confuse PHPs with state medical boards, as noted above, the vast majority of PHPs are fully independent from the state medical board. That said, PHPs endeavor to have collaborative working relationships with their respective state medical boards. PHPs also have widely varying budgets, ranging from one employee with a $20,000 budget to a 1.5 million dollar budget and 19 full-time employees.[9,135] By 2007, PHP programs were monitoring more than 9,000 physicians across the United States.[135]

Function

PHPs function according to a simple yet highly effective model that provides a confidential, therapeutic alternative to discipline for physicians and other safety-sensitive health workers who have conditions that have the potential to impair their ability to practice medicine with reasonable skill and safety. Participation in a PHP interconnects healing and accountability, improving health outcomes for the participant while also providing reassurance that the professional is safe to practice. The model is predicated on a PHP's mandatory reporting obligation to their medical board when non-compliance with program requirements poses a risk to patient safety. While funding, structure, enabling legislation, and regulatory environments may differ among PHPs from one state to another, all PHPs must adhere to this basic model to qualify for state membership in the Federation of State Physician Health Programs.

Physicians should not be discouraged from seeking help outside of PHPs for emotional distress or other behavioral health problems including addiction. Indeed, PHPs were never intended nor resourced to be involved with all physicians who are ill. The expanding universe of wellness resources available to health professionals, along with decreasing stigma associated with utilizing such resources, may prevent the progression of illness and the need for PHP involvement. That said, PHPs have a unique function within the healthcare ecosystem for which there is no comparable alternative.

The impact of the COVID-19 pandemic on clinician well-being, superimposed on already high rates of clinician burnout, has galvanized increased awareness of and resources to support and sustain the well-being of the healthcare workforce. Institutional well-being committees, Physician Wellness Programs operating through state and county medical associations, and a multitude of clinical and non-clinical services have emerged over the last several years to help meet the wellness needs of the healthcare workforce. While such efforts are laudable, the increasing array of services now available can make it difficult for health professionals in distress (and concerned others) to determine which services are most appropriate.[159] Confusion and delay in accessing appropriate services can place patient safety at risk and result in devastating personal and professional consequences for the health professional. It is imperative that those involved in the health and well-being of physicians understand that which differentiates PHPs from non-PHP resources (**Table 34-3**).

TABLE 34-3 Characteristics that Differentiate PHP from Non-PHP Resources for Safety-sensitive Health Professionals

Legal Authority	PHPs typically have statutory authority to receive reports of potential impairment in lieu of a report to the state medical board. Non-PHP resources do not have such authority.
Special Accountability	PHPs have mandatory reporting obligations, set forth in contract or statute that create a higher degree of accountability for PHPs to protect public safety.
Trusted Verification	PHPs are trusted to provide ongoing verification that a health professional is safe to practice which may be a condition of licensing, credentialing, or employment. Non-PHP providers may be unwilling or unable to verify fitness for duty and those requiring such verification (such as employers or credentialing entities) may be reluctant to act in reliance upon information from a non-PHP provider.
No Treatment Relationship	PHPs do not provide treatment and therefore do not have a treatment relationship with program participants. As such, PHPs can balance the dual obligation of helping the professional and protecting the public without the added ethical and legal obligations inherent to a therapeutic relationship.
Care Management	PHPs provide oversight, communication, and coordination of health care to promote effective treatment and sustained remission of illness. Functional information from employers and key supports, toxicology testing data, and the observations of PHP clinical staff are often additional sources of data that can better inform treatment. Outside of PHPs, this level of chronic illness management is rarely available or utilized by health professionals.

Those who aim to assist physicians upstream of impairment will, sooner or later, encounter a concern for impairment and need to respond accordingly. As such, clinicians and wellness professionals who serve physicians and other health professionals outside of the purview of a PHP should:

1. Thoughtfully appraise their ability to assure safety to practice for professionals in their care and understand the legal and ethical requirements for protecting public safety within the context of the therapeutic relationship.
2. Understand the circumstances in which involvement with a PHP might offer a benefit such as the need for advocacy in employment, credentialing, or licensing matters.
3. Utilize the added layer of confidentiality protection that PHPs offer when a reportable concern for impairment arises.
4. Familiarize themselves with their state PHP and consult (anonymously if needed) if concerns of impairment arise. Proactive collaboration and relationship building with the PHP can help facilitate an excellent outcome when one is faced with a health professional in distress.

Addiction continues to be one of the most commonly identified problems addressed by PHPs.[135] In addition, PHPs often address other health conditions and circumstances that may impact safe practice including psychiatric disorders, non-psychiatric medical conditions, problematic workplace behaviors, and compassion fatigue and burnout. Some PHPs assist state medical boards with referrals related to professional sexual misconduct, but such services are combined with medical board disciplinary processes and are not part of the PHPs alternative to discipline track.[123] All PHPs offer consultation about substance use cases, coordinate intake into the PHP, make referrals for evaluation and treatment, and provide post-treatment monitoring. Some PHPs offer initial assessment, triage, and ongoing professionally facilitated monitoring groups for the physicians in their state.

Pre-Monitoring Activities

Referrals to PHPs come from a variety of sources including employers, hospital credentialing entities, physician well-being committees, families and friends, attorneys, medical schools and residency programs, and self-referrals. PHPs vary in their intake procedures, but all PHPs utilize case management systems to enter the individual into the program, track their progress, and coordinate care and communication. PHPs work with newly referred participants and their workplaces to support immediate medical leave when recommended for the well-being of the physician and their patients. PHPs then coordinate referral for additional evaluation, often utilizing multidisciplinary evaluation centers with special expertise in the assessment of substance use disorders in safety-sensitive workers. Such evaluations are useful both for ruling out a SUD diagnosis and putting concerns to rest. Alternatively, such evaluations may detect a SUD that would require additional treatment and post-treatment monitoring as a prerequisite for return to practice. When treatment is recommended, PHPs follow the physician's course in treatment, coordinate with their treatment providers to integrate treatment and post-treatment monitoring plans, and assist in identification and referral to additional treatment resources needed to support continuing care in a chronic illness management model. Treatment centers specializing in the care of physicians also provide formal practice assessment, fitness for duty evaluation, and return to work recommendations, including recommendations for accommodations. PHPs rely upon these specialized assessments and recommendations regarding the management of the physician's re-entry to clinical practice.

Recovery Monitoring

All PHPs use drug testing to track the status of physicians with SUDs in their monitoring programs. This is accomplished through the use of random body fluid analysis. The most frequent matrix is urine, but hair, nail, and blood analysis may be added for a more robust assessment. Screens commonly taper in frequency over the course of monitoring, which can be for a period of 5 or more years.[85,123] Participation in PHP monitoring is contingent upon the physician "calling in," using a smart phone app or by logging into a confidential website each day to see whether he or she has been selected for testing. Drug testing of multiple matrices and using many analysis techniques requires considerable expertise and accuracy, since physicians with addiction can use their knowledge to evade detection.[160] Most physician drug panels test for 20 to 25 drugs, including a wide variety of opioids. Specialty screens for fentanyl, alfentanil, and sufentanil are necessary in physicians who have used these drugs in the past and/or who have access to such compounds. Urine testing for fentanyl and norfentanyl may remain positive for days or even weeks among individuals with a chronic or recurrent recent use pattern. Hair testing can also be important in this regard as it provides an extended look-back for many compounds including fentanyl and its congeners. Physicians also occasionally use more unusual drugs (ketamine, propofol, tramadol, and dextromethorphan); these physicians need assessment panels specifically designed to identify recurrence of use. Toxicology testing is also broad as to the types of drugs assayed. This breadth prevents switching from one substance to another, as commonly occurs during the natural course of an addiction illness.

PHPs use multiple analytes for alcohol use by assaying for ethyl glucuronide (EtG)[161,162] and ethyl sulfate (EtS),[163] liver and lung tissue metabolites of ethyl alcohol. Newer testing for blood phosphatidyl ethanol (PEth) has provided a longer detection window for ethanol consumption. False-positive test results for EtG, EtS, and PEth have been reported owing to a combination of environmental exposure and the sensitivity of the tests (EtG, EtS, PEth) and the low-level production of EtG by urine bacteria (EtG).[164] The two most common culprits in false positives are incidental ingestion of ethanol-containing substances (eg, mouthwash) and topical application of ethanol-based hand sanitizers (especially if inhaled). The ability to differentiate incidental exposure became especially important during the COVID-19 pandemic.[165] Physicians under monitoring are counseled as to proper use of ethanol-based hand sanitizer to avoid false positives. Using an alternative to ethyl alcohol-based hand sanitizer, such as isopropyl alcohol-based sanitizers, should also be considered.

The length of time a physician should remain in monitoring is unclear. The best outcome data follow physicians for 5 years or more.[49,85,137,138,166] Looking at recurrences, Domino et al. reported 58% occurred in the first 2 years and 28% in years 3 to 5 and 14% of recurrences after year five. This suggests a cutoff of 5 years or more may be prudent. Using a 60-year prospective study of men with an alcohol use disorder (not physicians, per se), Vaillant suggested "...analogous to cancer patients, a follow-up of 5 years rather than of 1 or 2 years would appear necessary to determine stable recovery."[167] The Federation of State Physician Health Programs 2019 Guidelines recommend that monitoring duration be individualized based on severity of illness with mild illness monitored for 2 years or less and moderate to severe illness monitored for a minimum of 5 years.[123] Lastly, a 1995 policy of the Federation of State Medical Boards stated physicians involved in PHP should be supervised for a minimum of 5 years; this policy was reiterated in 2011.[168,169] Studies have shown that states do vary internally and externally as to their length of monitoring.[170] Thus, limited data, combined with a near mandate of regulatory agencies, have set a time frame of 5 years for PHP monitoring. Additional research would assist in developing more granularity in monitoring and help determine which individuals with which conditions and co-occurring disorders need what intensity of monitoring for what length of time. Some participants choose to be on extended or even career-long monitoring (often tapering its intensity), especially if their substance use has led to workplace involvement or has caused significant life consequences.

Recovery Support

In addition to toxicology monitoring, most state PHPs provide some type of group experience and behavioral monitoring (eg, attendance records at support groups and therapy). The most common of these are caduceus groups, a vague moniker that varies in its implementation from peer-led groups like 12-step meetings to large therapist-led groups whose focus varies from discussing a member's pragmatic concern to emotional process work in a large group setting. Unlike in Alcoholics Anonymous meetings, direct feedback and discussion is encouraged in most caduceus groups. Newcomers may obtain recovery sponsors or guidance from physicians that are more senior in the network of PHP support groups.

Most long-term studies of physicians underscore the importance of 12-step meetings (primarily AA and NA) as a central part of recovery support for many physicians.[85,142,143] In a study of 100 physicians with an average of 33.4 months after treatment admission, Galanter et al.[142] noted, "A.A. was apparently perceived by respondents as the most potent element of their recovery." Merlo and colleagues,[171] using an anonymous survey of PHP participants after completion of at least 5 years of monitoring, reported that 88% continued to attend 12-step meetings and that 12-step attendance was one of the top 3 rated components of the PHP process. Outcome studies that follow physicians who attend such programs show impressive abstinence rates, with one study reporting abstinence rates at 73% over an average interval of 17.3 years.[141]

Return to Use

Significant consequences to the physician and the public can result from clinically significant episodes of return to use. The PHP literature has suggested several models of staging return to use severity. DuPont et al. describe a three-category system derived from the earlier work of one of the authors (Skipper).[135] The 2019 FSPHP Guidelines modified this scale somewhat, defining these return to use levels in a manner that simultaneously highlight the most frequent indicators for professionals in a monitoring system and their effect on public safety.[123]

- Level 1—Behavior(s) without substance use that suggest pending return to use.
- Level 2—Substance use that is not in the context of active medical practice.
- Level 3—Substance use that occurs within the context of medical practice.

Among the minority of physicians who return to use while under monitoring, a "slip" or brief return to use episode seems to be the predominant pattern. If the slip is short-lived, the physician is often best placed in brief counseling or a short-term recurrence of use prevention training or other recovery support process. Here, the antecedents of substance misuse are explored and skills to support remission are strengthened. It is not uncommon for deeper or earlier life issues to emerge during this time as well. Slips (and the resultant treatment), if managed quickly with appropriate psychotherapy, can deepen the physicians' acceptance of their SUD and solidify subsequent recovery. If managed properly, singular slips are most often helpful in the long run and are not indicators of failed treatment.[172] Should a physician have more extensive return to use, they should have a more comprehensive disease management response including one or more of the following:

- Evaluation of the physician's safety to practice until they are more stable in recovery.
- Longer and tighter monitoring contract that includes behavioral monitoring, support group attendance, and more extensive toxicology testing.
- Reexamination of the patient's psychiatric status, to reassess for undiagnosed co-occurring illness, other addictive process, or past unaddressed trauma.
- Reassessment of the patient's family dynamics and support system.
- Determination of the need to modify treatment or potentially return to a higher level of care (ASAM Level 2.1, 2.5, 3.1, or 3.5).
- Reevaluation of the need for medication treatment of SUD.

While long-term abstinence is an achievable goal, especially among physicians, return to use should be evaluated non-judgmentally as part of the SUD process. Because of real or reasonable concerns about patient safety, physicians who have difficulty maintaining abstinence may be removed from the workforce until evaluators skilled in physician addiction determine that the physician is safe to return. The point in time when a physician is safe to practice is best established by a joint decision of the physician's treatment provider and the monitoring PHP. All stakeholders must be prudent and err on the side of caution when considering readiness to return to work in safety-sensitive occupations. The stability and viability of each state PHP rests on the trust it maintains with the employers, credentialing entities, and state licensing boards. These stakeholders act in reliance upon the PHP's verification of health and safety to practice. In the absence of such trust, PHPs would not be able to provide effective advocacy for participants to continue or return to clinical practice.

Return to Work

Most PHPs insist on an initial removal from the workplace during the first phases of treatment and after a complicated recurrence of use. The point in time when a physician is safe to practice is best established by a joint decision of the physician's treatment provider and the monitoring PHP. SUD disease status, co-occurring conditions, and neurocognitive concerns are taken under consideration. Stakeholders must be prudent about when to return physicians to their safety-sensitive occupations. Parameters to consider when returning a physician to his safety-sensitive occupation are reviewed in **Table 34-4**. In many cases, it is crucial to address conditioned cues in the work environment.[76,108]

PHPs and treatment providers have a wide variety of thoughts on how to structure the physician's work and home life once a return-to-work date has been determined. Issues to be considered include workplace conditions, physician's initial workload and whether shift work with rotating time frames should be allowed, his or her safety to practice in proximity to substances that were or could be misused, whether solo or group practice should be considered, any restrictions on prescribing DEA scheduled drugs, and the need for remedial training. In an effort to increase consensus on this topic, an instrument called the *Medical Professional Addiction Recovery Inventory* has been developed to balance recovery status and the workplace environment.[173]

PHP Outcome Data

Physicians have been the subject of multiple outcome studies focused on the efficacy of extended, multimodal addiction treatment and monitoring. Most addiction treatment outcome

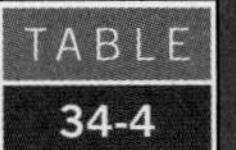

Factors to Review When Considering Returning a Physician with a Substance Use Disorder to Work

- Length of time with verified abstinence
- History of recurrences of substance use or recurrences of substance use disorder symptoms
- Tobacco or nicotine use
- Compliance with prescribed medications
- Attitude toward treatment and recovery
- Ability for honest self-appraisal of past substance use disorders and current risk for return to substance use
- Status of contributory psychiatric and medical illnesses
- Stability of family and home life
- Avocational interests
- Ability of the physician to access proper therapy, drug screening, and support groups
- Drug access in the workplace, especially for physicians who continuously handle controlled substances
- Quality of support in the workplace

studies are plagued by subjects being lost to follow-up. However, owing to the tight and long-term monitoring by PHPs, physician-based studies have excellent follow-up rates, approximating 90% in some studies.[137] Physicians appear to have responded very well to their unique treatment and monitoring processes. More sophisticated outcome analyses[44,49,85,137,138] attempt to define why physician treatment is so successful. The natural progression of this line of thought is to identify which components of the physician treatment process can be generalized to the public at large, recognizing that physicians are generally a privileged group with fewer social determinants of health and thus findings may not directly extend to other populations.[166]

Gallegos et al.[40] reported a 77% sustained abstinence rate in physicians followed for 5 years. In the North Carolina PHP, Ganley et al.[174] noted 65% of physicians had a good outcome (as defined by completing an aftercare contract), and another 26% had a good outcome with complications (eg, recurrence of use but eventually completed a monitoring contract) in a 6-year study from 1995 to 2000, resulting in a 91% good outcome. In 2002, Lloyd[141] reported an impressive follow-up of physicians with alcohol use disorder in the United Kingdom over 21 years, noting a mean sustained duration of abstinence of 17.6 years in 68 of 80 physicians reporting. He conservatively scored the 20% lost to follow-up as negative outcomes and, even with this, he noted that 73% of the physicians in his study of 80 physicians were in recovery after 21 years. Similarly, Domino et al.[49] noted that 25% of physicians in the Washington State PHP (1991-2001) had at least one episode of recurrence over the 10-year period. Family history, comorbid psychiatric disorder, and a previous recurrences increased the probability of return to use. The use of major opioids increased the probability of recurrence, but only in the presence of a comorbid psychiatric disorder. McLellan et al.[85] evaluated the outcomes among 904 physicians with SUD treated in 16 PHPs and found 78% were continuously abstinent throughout the 5- to 7-year period of evaluation; more than 90% of those physicians were still practicing medicine. Among those physicians who did have a recurrence, 74% had only one episode of substance use. A recent meta-analysis by Geuijen et al.[155] looked at 29 studies of monitoring program outcomes worldwide and found 72% abstinence and 77% work retention in pooled analysis. Despite this exhaustive analysis, the authors cited concerns about study heterogeneity and publication bias that limited their ability to draw firm conclusions about the effectiveness of monitoring programs.

Education and Outreach

Most PHPs provide education about all types of physician illness (including substance use disorders) and train local hospitals and physician organizations on techniques to help identify and report suspected impairment. Even more importantly, these educational programs afford the PHP staff the chance to personally meet and network with medical leadership throughout their state. These public relations and training efforts carried out by PHPs are important; they help individuals understand and trust the supportive goal of the PHP, which in turn promotes early referral and decreases stigma. Healthcare organizations have shown increased interest in these issues, thanks to the recent Joint Commission standard (currently MS 4.80), which mandates that "the medical staff implements a process to identify and manage matters of individual health for licensed independent practitioners. This identification process is separate from actions taken for disciplinary purposes."[118]

PHPs often provide expert consultation to state medical associations, healthcare organizations, regulators, health departments, legislators, and institutions of higher learning. They curate and convene stakeholders in coordinating initiatives to support workforce sustainability and lead initiatives to reduce barriers to help-seeking such as medical licensure question reform efforts within their states. Many PHP medical directors are clinical faculty within medical schools and residency training programs and provide educational content and training opportunities in academic settings. PHPs also contribute to written publications and media stories to advance physician health. Finally, PHPs, through membership in the Federation of State Physician Health Programs, work in collaboration with healthcare leaders at the national level to conduct physician health research and develop and disseminate education and policy relating to physician health and well-being.

CHALLENGES AND OPPORTUNITIES FOR FURTHER RESEARCH

Like all areas of medicine, physician health and addiction are fraught with challenges that reveal nuance and complexity and illuminate opportunities for further inquiry and improvement.

Tension Between Privacy and Public Safety

Physician treatment, with its mandated monitoring, illustrates the conflict between the physician-patient's need for privacy and the public's need for safety. Combined with the stigmatized view of addiction; the result is that the physician with a SUD has become (for many) synonymous with physician impairment. Many other problems among physicians can and do lead to mistakes and patient harm (eg, sleep deprivation, overwork, poor communication with hospital staff, intemperate affairs, stress, and burnout), but they are not as directly addressed and do not receive a fraction of the public or regulatory board outcry or concern. Ironically, confidentiality for treatment of physician mental illness, including substance use disorders, actually increases patient safety by encouraging early referral and safe passage into treatment.[41,158]

Conversely, many states have laws that mandate caregivers to report suspected physician impairment—a term that is not synonymous with substance use disorder, but these terms are frequently conflated. More accurately stated, impairment is a consequence of addiction if it is left untreated. Some states mandate that treatment providers report physicians to the medical board, regardless of whether impairment has been proven. In many cases, a default board action ensues. Although this may appear on superficial examination to protect patients, an excessively broad mandate for reporting actually decreases the probability that a physician will seek or accept a referral for assessment and treatment. If the perceived consequences of referral are sufficiently prejudicial, referral is delayed and ultimately only occurs when a major incident signals the transition from illness to impairment. In states with PHPs, regulatory boards allow PHP intercession, holding off disciplinary proceedings if the physician effectively addresses his or her SUD in an appropriate, structured, and accountable manner. As soon as regulatory boards tilt toward disciplinary enforcement and away from treatment, physicians who develop addiction, their colleagues, and care providers become reluctant to report. The physician with addiction and his or her family delay or avoid treatment. Their healthcare provider(s) may hesitate to report as well, believing they can handle the problem outside the purview of the PHP, or otherwise be reluctant to involve the PHP. In doing so, they lose the benefit of structured care management, monitoring, and peer support that appear to drive the excellent outcomes achieved by PHPs.

The structure of PHPs, on the other hand, facilitates a proper balance between the privacy that is critical for treatment and the public's need for safety. They hold the awkward middle ground between their medical board and treatment providers. PHPs provide confidentiality if the physician's illness does not pose a threat to public safety but report to the medical board should a physician participant become a risk to the public at large. The promise of protected and effective treatment encourages all parties to refer to the PHP before the physician who uses substances deteriorates to the point of a potential safety risk. The experience of PHPs in holding the tension between confidentiality and safety has made them effective advocates and partners in bringing about medical licensure question reform in their respective states. Such reforms, which ensure that licensure application questions only inquire about current impairment (and not past diagnoses or treatment), remove barriers to help-seeking for physicians in need and promote early intervention and treatment without increasing risk to patient safety.

Concerns About Coercion and Control

As with other areas in medicine, concerns have been expressed by the public, the media, and others that conflicts of interest could compromise decision-making and undermine the availability, utilization, and reputation of PHPs. Boyd and Knight[175] argued that impressive results do not obviate the need for scrutiny. Boyd followed this with several commentaries.[176,177] Candilis challenged this conceptualization, arguing that coercion, as an ethical construct, does not apply to the voluntary services provided by PHPs and that PHPs serve an important function in the social contract between the public and the medical profession.[178] Most PHPs address concerns of conflict of interest and bias through external reviews, oversight by their respective medical boards, and a Board of Directors with expertise in balancing effective treatment with ethical care. Additional commentary describes other trepidations such as a higher dose of initial treatment than the general public. Some of these issues appear valid on the surface but fail to account for the dual roles of PHPs in protecting the public and the unrealistic expectations many oversight bodies place on physicians (ie, where a minor return to use can result in loss of a job, hospital privileges, a medical license, or an entire career). Research, albeit limited, as opposed to opinion, points to good outcomes and a high degree of participant satisfaction among PHP participants.[11,156,179] However, there is no available research comparing PHP care versus non-PHP care, or less restrictive or expensive care in matched physician populations. In 2005 the Federation of State Physician Health Programs (FSPHP) developed[180] and in 2019 expanded[123] guidelines for state PHP members that address potential conflicts of interest and national standards of care. The FSPHP is working to standardize best practices among its members (who have varying staffing, funding, and experience) through scientific exchange, research, and ongoing revision of best practices.

Is Monitored Recovery the Same as Self-Guided Recovery?

Physicians often enter treatment claiming they are there only to protect their medical license(s). A central goal in such cases is to shift the physician from this external driver to an internalized state of recovery as a lifelong journey. During treatment and subsequent monitoring, a number of physicians do not make this shift. Once the initial consequences of active addiction remit, such individuals are held in a drug-free state by the oversight of drug screens and behavioral monitoring. In such cases, the internalization of recovery (an ongoing process of changing behaviors, attitudes, and beliefs) slows or stops; and unfortunately, the emergence of a self-motivated journey of recovery to replace the "holding cell" provided by monitoring does not occur. Such physicians have a high probability of returning to substance use when and if monitoring is discontinued. In such cases, the individual has made a commitment to abstinence only as a temporary means to an end. Such physicians may be quite compliant, assuming a false persona of acceptance to treatment providers, monitors, and PHP personnel.

Unfortunately, this state is to some degree a by-product of external pressure and the intense treatment and monitoring physicians undergo. Treatment providers should avoid pressuring patients to conform because physicians are, after all, good students who know how to give "correct answers." Instead, providers should encourage patients to verbalize their resistance and dissatisfaction with treatment and to praise honest self-disclosure, especially when the participant is describing how they feel stuck in the process of change. Physician-patients should be encouraged to discuss their ambivalence about remission, including the fallacy that they may return to drinking or using drugs in a controlled and sociable manner once they are "strong enough" or have "learned enough about myself."[181] Open discussion regarding recovery ambivalence should be a recurrent theme in group therapy as well.

Psychotherapy may help such individuals integrate how past survival techniques of false compliance to authority figures are at play in their relationship with the current authority figures, including their therapists, treatment centers, and PHPs.[54,182] In the meantime, *monitoring holds the physician behaviorally accountable* and, if properly framed as appropriate supportive care, is not only justifiable but also good medicine.

Merlo and DuPont have completed a preliminary study that attempts to differentiate between monitored abstinence and self-guided recovery, to wit: What happens after PHP monitoring is discontinued? Working with several PHPs, they contacted individuals at 5 or more years *after* they completed PHP monitoring. Of 139 anonymous respondents, 95% (n = 121) self-reported no illegal or nonmedical use of drugs since PHP completion. These findings may be impacted by response bias.[171] Once validated by additional research, these data confirm that the extended treatment and disease monitoring process in this cohort create lasting change and not just temporary interruption of the addiction illness.

How Should Physicians with Opioid Use Disorder be Treated and Managed?

Medications for opioid use disorder (MOUD) were adopted very early on by addiction treatment programs in the United States that specialize in treating physicians. Probably the most widely used medication for OUD among physicians is long-acting injectable extended-release naltrexone (XR-NTX); the reasons for this choice are multiple and complex. Studies have demonstrated that continuous naltrexone administration is associated with significantly higher rates of opioid abstinence compared to no medication.[147,183] Use of the injectable form is safe, efficient, and alleviates concerns related to temptation or forgetfulness.[184-186] Alternatives such as observed administration of oral doses of buprenorphine or oral naltrexone have been studied[147]; however, PHP experience has shown that such observation quickly becomes perfunctory or disappears completely, replacing surveillance with false security.

Most, but not all, state PHPs also consider the use of opioid agonist and partial agonist medications carefully, using them less often than is typical for other patients with OUD. This stands in contrast to the standard of care in the general population. Three issues come into play with this decision.

First, concerns about the impact of opioid agonist and partial-agonist medications on cognition have limited the acceptance of these medications among PHPs. Like any CNS-active medication, buprenorphine and methadone have the potential to affect cognition, causing subtle delays in recall and attention, particularly in older adults.[187] With methadone, deficits may persist even after maintenance has been established.[188] However, upon review of the current literature, Polles et al.[109] and Hamza and Bryson[189] concluded that concern about cognitive changes should be considered in the context of a holistic analysis including other factors, like co-prescription of other psychoactive medications, which may act synergistically to impair cognitive performance. As a result, potential side effects should be considered in light of the physician's specialty practice and duties, and balanced against concerns about the risks of ongoing opioid use. When approving use of opioid agonist or partial agonist medications for physicians in recovery, an approach sometimes utilized by PHPs to allay concerns about cognition is incorporating the use of cognitive screening or neurocognitive testing into return-to-work considerations and ongoing monitoring agreements.

Second, public perception of safety is central to an efficient medical system. Restrictions are similar to those in other safety-sensitive industries. For example, pilots cannot fly airplanes (commercial or private) if they are taking methadone or buprenorphine[190]; and, although consensus is shifting, commercial driver's licenses may be denied to individuals on opioid agonist therapy. Addiction still has a negative connotation in society, and intense stigma towards opioid agonist therapy (more so with methadone than buprenorphine) may draw unintended and counterproductive scrutiny. Further, there are professional liability concerns. Opioid agonist therapy could be perceived as opening the door to medical–legal issues and negative public attention related to "malpractice" claims.[191] As a result, management of addiction among physicians is modified by public opinion and stigma. While education is needed to address stigma and encourage the public to become more open-minded about opioid agonist therapy among physicians, education alone may not remove the public's injudicious scrutiny. An important additional lever for change is policy, with one area of increasing exploration being the protection offered under the American with Disabilities Act for people with OUD. In some cases, those treated with medication may be in a protected class under the ADA.[192] However, such protections are far from clear or absolute in safety-sensitive health care workers, where patient safety is of critical importance. Indeed, courts generally defer to carefully considered decisions by professional programs, employers, and licensing in agencies when ADA concerns arise.[193] Clarification of the law is needed to appropriately balance the protection of individuals with OUD and public safety concerns.

Third, research has consistently demonstrated that physicians with OUD who participate in PHP-coordinated care achieve high remission rates (equivalent to those with other SUDs) without use of agonist or partial agonist medications.[49,85,137,138,194,195] An earlier study of 904 physicians conducted prior to the availability of injectable naltrexone reported that only 1 physician was reported to be receiving opioid agonist treatment.[85] These results stand in sharp contrast to OUD treatment outcome studies in the population at large. Thus, from an efficacy perspective, the use of buprenorphine or methadone may be a secondary, rather than primary, treatment for this population. However, given the documented efficacy of opioid agonist therapy in other groups, such treatment does occur with physicians. Anecdotal reports and recent informal surveys of PHP directors suggest that PHPs today have adopted more permissive policies with respect to agonist/partial agonist medications and return to work, but more research is required to evaluate current practices and needs and to understand which physician-patients may benefit most from opioid agonist therapy. The FSPHP has published an expert opinion position statement, *Safety Considerations for Medication Treatment of Opioid Use Disorders in Monitored Health Professionals*, to assist PHPs and the public in navigating this important topic.[196]

Re-Entry of Physicians Diagnosed with Opioid Use Disorders

Earlier literature contained conflicting publications debating the advisability of anesthesiologists and other physicians who both misused and had high opioid access returning to the operating room or other arena of high opioid access. Menk et al.[197] reported a successful re-entry rate of only 34% for anesthesiologists using parenteral opioids versus 70% for those not using opioids. This oft-quoted 1990 study promulgated a pessimistic view of anesthesiologists returning to work but has been criticized because it was essentially a retrospective survey of anesthesia training directors, subject to recall bias. Of the 159 anesthesia training programs surveyed, 113 responded, providing 180 case reports, with most programs providing only a single case report of a resident having suffered from an opioid use disorder. Critics contend that if most programs reported only a single case, it is likely that such reports were skewed toward disasters. Collins et al.[198] also surveyed anesthesiology residencies in 2005, noting that 50% of treated anesthesiologists remained in anesthesiology after treatment, with 91% completing training and 9% dying of recurrence-related incidents.

Paris and Canavan[199] compared 32 anesthesiologists with 36 physician controls for an average of 7.5 years; they showed no difference in the recurrence rates between these two groups. When stratified by residents versus attending physicians, no significant difference was found. Domino et al.[49] examined the risk of recurrence over 11 years and 256 participants in the Washington State PHP, including 32 anesthesiologists. The recurrence rate for anesthesiologists was not statistically significantly different from other physicians. Additionally, there was not a single episode of patient harm or death from overdose by any anesthesiologist in this study. A similar report from Pelton and Ikeda[42] involving 255 physicians who had participated in the California Diversion Program over 10 years showed no difference in recurrence rates for anesthesiologists.

Domino et al.,[49] evaluating physicians in the Washington State PHP, noted that physicians who had used fentanyl had a slightly lower incidence of recurrence than those who had used other major opioids. Individuals who used potent opioids (excluding fentanyl) had a higher risk of recurrence, as did physicians with an existing comorbid psychiatric disorder or a family history of addiction. They concluded that anesthesiologists who used potent opioids and do not have other risk factors (family history, comorbid psychiatric disorder, and history of recurrence) are good candidates to return to the practice of anesthesiology. Finally, Skipper[138] reviewed data from PHPs in 16 states, culling information about anesthesia providers. They noted that anesthesiologists had outcomes similar to other physicians, with no higher mortality, recurrence rate, or disciplinary rate, and no evidence in their records of patient harm. These authors postulated that the type of treatment and monitoring that these physicians received from the 16 state PHPs accounted for the differences from earlier reports.

Oreskovich and Caldeiro,[200] in an editorial response to a call for a "one strike and you are out" response to anesthesiologists who develop OUD,[14] concluded that the research in OUD among anesthesia providers indicates success when aggressive treatment and long-term oversight is matched with sophisticated hair and nail testing for fentanyl and placement on extended release naltrexone. Indeed, studies that followed anesthesiologists under close monitoring in PHPs or by regulatory boards (Domino[49], Washington State; Paris and Canavan,[199] New Jersey; Pelton and Ikeda,[42] California; Skipper,[138] from 16 different states with active PHPs) describe outcomes for anesthesiologists that are similar to other physicians; whereas, earlier studies that were based upon a survey of the memories of anesthesiology program directors (where patients had uncertain or limited treatment and monitoring) describe poor, and at times, life-terminating outcomes. Oreskovich and Caldeiro assert that the PHP model "should be celebrated, replicated, and required for (anesthesia care providers with addiction) who seek to return to healthcare employment." The controversy about returning anesthesiologists to practice underscores the importance of sophisticated PHPs in supporting participant recovery and ensuring public safety.

Additional studies point to the importance of opioid antagonists in the long-term management of the anesthesiologist with opioid use disorder. Merlo et al.[186] in a naturalistic crossover study in one PHP showed the risk of recurrence of opioid use was significantly decreased when physicians who used parenteral opioids were treated with naltrexone (either oral naltrexone, with testing confirmed medication adherence, or injectable naltrexone) upon initial return to a high-risk practice environment. Exposure to conditioned environmental cues while protected by naltrexone may diminish conditioned cue craving.[76] Further research is needed to compare opioid agonist to antagonist therapy in physician-patient populations.

Physicians and Cannabis Use

Laws and attitudes toward cannabis in the United States are becoming more permissive, and cannabis use and cannabis use disorders in the general population have been increasing over time.[201] The trend toward legalization of cannabis in many states has raised a conundrum: Should those in oversight positions send physicians who test positive for cannabis for clinical evaluations?[97] What if the physician has a "cannabis use as treatment" authorization from their healthcare provider?

Cannabis use among people who currently use results in carryover cognitive deficits in learning, attention, concentration, processing speed and memory that extend beyond the acute effects of intoxication.[202-204] Regular use of cannabis, whether for recreational or medical purposes, may therefore result in deficits in practice performance. The Federation of State Medical Boards advises physicians to abstain from cannabis use for treatment or recreational purposes.[205] Cannabis also remains a Schedule I controlled substance with the Drug Enforcement Administration (at the time of this publication this is under scrutiny). This has resulted in institutions (including hospitals) that receive federal funding implementing zero tolerance policies regarding cannabis as a schedule I drug, thus preventing its use among employed and credentialed physicians.[206,207] In *Coats v Dish Network,* the Colorado courts set legal precedent for employers to terminate employees who use cannabis outside of work hours, even cannabis used as treatment, regardless of the legal status of cannabis at the state level.[208]

PHPs evaluate use of cannabis no differently than any other substance with psychoactive effects and addiction liability. As states liberalize cannabis laws, the question shifts from one of legality to whether the pattern of use places the physician at risk for impairment. Like other drugs of misuse, toxicology alone cannot determine problematic use. As a result, urine toxicology testing positive for cannabis metabolites may result in referral to a PHP for further evaluation. Physicians and other health professionals who use cannabis should be aware that there can be significant professional consequences of cannabis use regardless of state legal status or medical authorization.

CONCLUSION

Physicians were the first professional group to systematically address addiction within their profession; our leadership in this area continues today. Addiction among physicians follows a similar course as in the public at large, with several notable exceptions. The easy access to potent drugs is one of the most important of these exceptions. The identification, evaluation, initial treatment, and subsequent addiction monitoring in this population may afford useful elements of disease management that can be adapted to the treatment of addiction in the public at large.[172]

The treatment of physicians is different (especially in the United States), partly driven by public concern for complete and sustained remission in a disease that is chronic and recurring by nature. PHPs remain integral elements in the comprehensive disease management of physician addiction. Complexities in the management of addiction among physicians abound and call for further research in this interesting population. The long-term management systems utilized with physicians provide deep insight into the treatment of addiction in all populations. Elements of the chronic disease management of physicians should be considered for every individual suffering from this disease.

REFERENCES

1. O'Connor PG, Spickard A Jr. Physician impairment by substance abuse. *Med Clin North Am.* 1997;81(4):1037-1052.
2. Centrella M. Physician addiction and impairment—current thinking: a review. *J Addict Dis.* 1994;13(1):91-105.
3. Flaherty JA, Richman JA. Substance use and addiction among medical students, residents, and physicians. *Psychiatr Clin North Am.* 1993;16(1):189-197.
4. Collins G. Drug and alcohol use among physicians. In: Miller NS, ed. *Comprehensive Handbook of Drug and Alcohol Addiction.* Dekker; 1991:947-966.
5. Bissell L, Hankes L. Health professionals. In: Lowinson JH, Ruiz P, Millman R, eds. *Substance Abuse: A Comprehensive Textbook.* 3rd ed. Williams & Wilkins; 1997:897-908.
6. Benzer D. Healing the healer: a primer on physician impairment. *Wis Med J.* 1991;90(2): 70, 73-74, 76, 78-79.
7. McAuliffe WE, Rohman M, Breer P, Wyshak G, Santangelo S, Magnuson E. Alcohol use and abuse in random samples of physicians and medical students. *Am J Public Health.* 1991;81(2):177-182.
8. Niven R, Hurt RD, Morse RM, Swenson WM. *Alcoholism in Physicians.* Elsevier; 1984:12-16.
9. Carr GD, Bradley Hall P, Reid Finlayson AJ, DuPont RL. Physician health programs: the US model. *Physician Mental Health and Well-Being;* 2017:265-294.
10. Berge KH, Seppala MD, Schipper AM. Chemical dependency and the physician. *Mayo Clin Proc.* 2009;84(7):625-631.
11. Candilis PJ, Kim DT, Sulmasy LS; the ACP Ethics, Professionalism and Human Rights Committee. Physician impairment and rehabilitation: reintegration into medical practice while ensuring patient safety: a position paper from the American College of Physicians. *Ann Intern Med.* 2019;170(12):871-879. doi:10.7326/M18-3605
12. The Sick Physician. Impairment by psychiatric disorders, including alcoholism and drug dependence. *JAMA.* 1973;223(6):684-687.
13. American Society of Addiction Medicine. Public Policy Statement on Physicians and other Healthcare Professionals with Addiction. Accessed May 9, 2022. https://www.asam.org/docs/default-source/public-policy-statements/2020-public-policy-statement-on-physicians-and-other-healthcare-professionals-with-addiction_final.pdf?sfvrsn=5ed51c2_0
14. Berge KH, Seppala MD, Lanier WL. The anesthesiology community's approach to opioid- and anesthetic-abusing personneltime to change course. *Anesthesiology.* 2008;109(5):762-764.
15. Bissell L, Haberman PW. *Alcoholism in the Professions.* Oxford University Press; 1984.
16. Angres DH, Bettinardi-Angres K. *Healing the Healer: The Addicted Physician.* Psychosocial Press; 1998
17. Nace E. *Achievement and Addiction: A Guide to the Treatment of Professionals.* Brunner/Mazel; 1995
18. Coombs RH. *Drug-Impaired Professionals.* Harvard University Press; 1997.
19. Kessler RC, Berglund P, Demler O, Jin R, Merikangas KR, Walters EE. Lifetime prevalence and age-of-onset distributions of DSM-IV disorders in the National Comorbidity Survey Replication. *Arch Gen Psychiatry.* 2005;62(6):593-602.
20. McAuliffe WE, Rohman M, Santangelo S, et al. Psychoactive drug use among practicing physicians and medical students. *N Engl J Med.* 1986;315(13):805-810. doi:10.1056/nejm198609253151305
21. Lutsky I, Hopwood M, Abram SE, Cerletty JM, Hoffman RG, Kampine JP. Use of psychoactive substances in three medical specialties: anaesthesia, medicine and surgery. *Can J Anaesth.* 1994;41(7):561-567.
22. Hughes PH, Storr CL, Brandenburg NA, Baldwin DC Jr, Anthony JC, Sheehan DV. Physician substance use by medical specialty. *J Addict Dis.* 1999;18(2):23-37. doi:10.1300/J069v18n02_03
23. Hughes PH, Baldwin DC Jr, Sheehan DV, Conard S, Storr CL. Resident physician substance use, by specialty. *Am J Psychiatry.* 1992;149(10):1348-1354. doi:10.1176/ajp.149.10.1348

24. Hughes PH, Conard SE, Baldwin DC Jr, Storr CL, Sheehan DV. Resident physician substance use in the United States. *JAMA.* 1991;265(16):2069-2073.
25. Wilson J, Tanuseputro P, Myran DT, et al. Characterization of problematic alcohol use among physicians: a systematic review. *JAMA Netw Open.* 2022;5(12):e2244679-e2244679. doi:10.1001/jamanetworkopen.2022.44679
26. Vaillant GE. Physician, cherish thyself: the hazards of self-prescribing. *JAMA.* 1992;267(17):2373-2374. doi:10.1001/jama.1992.03480170099038
27. Merlo LJ, Curran JS, Watson R. Gender differences in substance use and psychiatric distress among medical students: a comprehensive statewide evaluation. *Subst Abus.* 2017;38(4):401-406. doi:10.1080/08897077.2017.1355871
28. Jackson ER, Shanafelt TD, Hasan O, Satele DV, Dyrbye LN. Burnout and alcohol abuse/dependence among U.S. Medical students. *Acad Med.* 2016;91(9):1251-1256. doi:10.1097/ACM.0000000000001138
29. Baldwin DC Jr, Hughes PH, Conard SE, Storr CL, Sheehan DV. Substance use among senior medical students. A survey of 23 medical schools. *JAMA.* 1991;265(16):2074-2078.
30. Morrison J, Wickersham P. Physicians disciplined by a state medical board. *JAMA.* 1998;279(23):1889-1893.
31. Clay SW, Conatser RR. Characteristics of physicians disciplined by the State Medical Board of Ohio. *J Am Osteopath Assoc.* 2003;103(2):81-88.
32. Baldisseri MR. Impaired healthcare professional. *Crit Care Med.* 2007;35(2 Suppl):S106-S116. doi:10.1097/01.Ccm.0000252918.87746.96
33. Merlo LJ, Trejo-Lopez J, Conwell T, Rivenbark J. Patterns of substance use initiation among healthcare professionals in recovery. *Am J Addict.* 2013;22(6):605-612. doi:10.1111/j.1521-0391.2013.12017.x
34. McGovern MP, Angres DH, Uziel-Miller ND, Leon S. Female physicians and substance abuse: comparisons with male physicians presenting for assessment. *J Subst Abuse Treat.* 1998;15(6):525-533.
35. Smart DR. *Physician Characteristics and Distribution in the US 2010.* American Medical Association; 2009.
36. Oreskovich MR, Shanafelt T, Dyrbye LN, et al. The prevalence of substance use disorders in American physicians. *Am J Addict.* 2015;24(1):30-38. doi:10.1111/ajad.12173
37. Newbury-Birch D, White M, Kamali F. Factors influencing alcohol and illicit drug use amongst medical students. *Drug Alcohol Depend.* 2000;59(2):125-130. doi:10.1016/s0376-8716(99)00108-8
38. Wunsch MJ, Knisely JS, Cropsey KL, Campbell ED, Schnoll SH. Women physicians and addiction. *J Addict Dis.* 2007;26(2):35-43. doi:10.1300/J069v26n02_05
39. Bissell L, Jones RW. The alcoholic physician: a survey. *Am J Psychiatry.* 1976;133(10):1142-1146.
40. Gallegos KV, Talbott GD, Wilson PO, Porter TL. The Medical Association of Georgia Impaired Physicians Program: review of the first 1000 physicians: analysis of specialty. *JAMA.* 1987;257(21):2927-2930.
41. Shore JH. The Oregon experience with impaired physicians on probation: an eight-year follow-up. *JAMA.* 1987;257(21):2931-2934.
42. Pelton C, Ikeda RM. The California Physicians Diversion Program's experience with recovering anesthesiologists. *J Psychoactive Drugs.* 1991;23(4):427-431.
43. Myers T, Weiss E. Substance use by internes and residents: an analysis of personal, social and professional differences. *Addiction.* 1987;82(10):1091-1099.
44. Knight JR, Sanchez LT, Sherritt L, Bresnahan LR, Fromson JA. Outcomes of a monitoring program for physicians with mental and behavioral health problems. *J Psychiatr Pract.* 2007;13(1):25-32. doi:10.1097/00131746-200701000-00004
45. Cummings SM, Merlo L, Cottler L. Mechanisms of prescription drug diversion among impaired physicians. *J Addict Dis.* 2011;30(3):195-202.
46. Palamar JJ, Ciccarone D, Rutherford C, Keyes KM, Carr TH, Cottler LB. Trends in seizures of powders and pills containing illicit fentanyl in the United States, 2018 through 2021. *Drug Alcohol Depend.* 2022;234:109398.
47. Tyrfingsson T, Thorgeirsson TE, Geller F, et al. Addictions and their familiality in Iceland. *Ann N Y Acad Sci.* 2010;1187:208-217. doi:10.1111/j.1749-6632.2009.05151.x
48. McAuliffe WE, Santangelo S, Magnuson BE, Sobol BA, Rohman MM, Weissman J. Risk factors of drug impairment in random samples of physicians and medical students. *Int J Addict.* 1987;22(9):825-841.
49. Domino KB, Hornbein TF, Polissar NL, et al. Risk factors for relapse in health care professionals with substance use disorders. *JAMA.* 2005;293(12):1453-1460. doi:10.1001/jama.293.12.1453
50. Moore RD, Mead L, Pearson TA. Youthful precursors of alcohol abuse in physicians. *Am J Med.* 1990;88(4):332-336.
51. Vaillant GE, Sobowale NC, McArthur C. Some psychologic vulnerabilities of physicians. *N Engl J Med.* 1972;287(8):372-375. doi:10.1056/NEJM197208242870802
52. Johnson RP, Connelly JC. Addicted physicians: a closer look. *JAMA.* 1981;245(3):253-257.
53. Khantzian EJ. The injured self, addiction, and our call to medicine: understanding and managing addicted physicians. *JAMA.* 1985;254(2):249-252.
54. Tillett R. The patient within—psychopathology in the helping professions. *Adv Psychiatr Treat.* 2003;9(4):272-279.
55. Clark DC, Eckenfels EJ, Daugherty SR, Fawcett J. Alcohol-use patterns through medical school: a longitudinal study of one class. *JAMA.* 1987;257(21):2921-2926.
56. Schuckit MA, Gold EO. A simultaneous evaluation of multiple markers of ethanol/placebo challenges in sons of alcoholics and controls. *Arch Gen Psychiatry.* 1988;45(3):211-216.
57. Schuckit MA. A longitudinal study of children of alcoholics. *Recent Dev Alcohol.* 1990;9:5-19.
58. Roche BTH. Substance abuse policies for anesthesia: time to re-evaluate your policies and curriculum. *All Anesthesia.* 2007.
59. Udel M. Chemical abuse/dependence: physicians' occupational hazard. *J Med Assoc Ga.* 1984;73(11):775-778.
60. Talbott G, Wright C. Chemical dependency in health care professionals. *Occup Med.* 1987;2(3):581-591.
61. Castro-Frenzel K. Physician-as-patient—vulnerabilities and strengths. *JAMA.* 2022;328(23):2303-2304. doi:10.1001/jama.2022.21859
62. Shanafelt TD, Boone S, Tan L, et al. Burnout and satisfaction with work-life balance among US physicians relative to the general US population. *Arch Intern Med.* 2012;172(18):1377-1385. doi:10.1001/archinternmed.2012.3199
63. Shanafelt TD, Hasan O, Dyrbye LN, et al. Changes in Burnout and satisfaction with work-life balance in physicians and the general US working population between 2011 and 2014. *Mayo Clin Proc.* 2015;90(12):1600-1613. doi:10.1016/j.mayocp.2015.08.023
64. Shanafelt TD, West CP, Sinsky C, et al. *Changes in Burnout and Satisfaction with Work-Life Integration in Physicians and the General US Working Population Between 2011 and 2017.* Elsevier; 2019.
65. Oreskovich MR, Kaups KL, Balch CM, et al. Prevalence of alcohol use disorders among American surgeons. *Arch Surg.* 2012;147(2):168-174. doi:10.1001/archsurg.2011.1481
66. Jex SM, Hughes P, Storr C, Conard S, Baldwin DC, Sheehan DV. Relations among stressors, strains, and substance use among resident physicians. *Int J Addict.* 1992;27(8):979-994.
67. Christie JD, Rosen IM, Bellini LM, et al. Prescription drug use and self-prescription among resident physicians. *JAMA.* 1998;280(14):1253-1255.
68. Green RC, Carroll GJ, Buxton WD. Drug addiction among physicians. The Virginia experience. *JAMA.* 1976;236(12):1372-1375.
69. Skipper G, Fletcher C, Rocha-Judd R. Tramadol abuse and dependence among physicians. *JAMA.* 2005;293(16):1974-1978. doi:10.1001/jama.293.16.1977-a
70. Cummings SM, Merlo L, Cottler L. Mechanisms of prescription drug diversion among impaired physicians. *J Addict Dis.* 2011;30(3):195-202. doi:10.1080/10550887.2011.581962
71. Fitzsimons MG, Baker K, Malhotra R, Gottlieb A, Lowenstein E, Zapol WM. Reducing the incidence of substance use disorders in

anesthesiology residents: 13 years of comprehensive urine drug screening. *Anesthesiology.* 2018. doi:10.1097/aln.0000000000002348
72. Cloud AM III. Cocaine, demand, and addiction: a study of the possible convergence of rational theory and national policy. *Vanderbilt Law Rev.* 1989;42(3):88.
73. Gill H, Kelly E, Henderson G. How the complex pharmacology of the fentanyls contributes to their lethality. *Addiction.* 2019;114(9):1524-1525. doi:10.1111/add.14614
74. Bryson EO, Levine A. One approach to the return to residency for anesthesia residents recovering from opioid addiction. *J Clini Anesth.* 2008;20(5):397-400.
75. Seppala MD, Oreskovich MR. Opioid-abusing health care professionals: options for treatment and returning to work after treatment. *Mayo Clin Proc.* 2012;87(3):213-215. doi:10.1016/j.mayocp.2012.02.002
76. Wilson H. Environmental cues and relapse: an old idea that is new for reentry of recovering anesthesia care professionals. *Mayo Clin Proc.* 2009;84(11):1040-1041.
77. True WR, Xian H, Scherrer JF, et al. Common genetic vulnerability for nicotine and alcohol dependence in men. *Arch Gen Psychiatry.* 1999;56(7):655-661.
78. Gardner M, Brandt A. "The doctors' choice is America's choice": the physician in US cigarette advertisements, 1930–1953. *Am J Public Health.* 2006;96(2):222-232. doi:10.2105/AJPH.2005.066654
79. Vaillant GE, Brighton JR, McArthur C. Physicians' use of mood-altering drugs. *N Engl J Med.* 1970;282(7):365-370. doi:10.1056/NEJM197002122820705
80. Vaillant GE, Brighton JR, McArthur C. Physicians' use of mood-altering drugs: a 20-year follow-up report. *N Engl J Med.* 1970;282(7):365-370.
81. Nelson D, Giovino GA, Emont SL, et al. Trends in cigarette smoking among us physicians and nurses. *JAMA.* 1994;271(16):1273-1275. doi:10.1001/jama.1994.03510400059032
82. Mangus RS, Hawkins CE, Miller MJ. Tobacco and alcohol use among 1996 medical school graduates. *JAMA.* 1998;280(13):1192-1195.
83. Kandra KL, Ranney LM, Lee JGL, Goldstein AO. Physicians' attitudes and use of e-cigarettes as cessation devices, North Carolina, 2013. *PLoS One.* 2014;9(7):e103462. doi:10.1371/journal.pone.0103462
84. Stuyt E, Gundersen D, Shore J, Brooks E, Gendel M. Tobacco use by physicians in a physician health program, implications for treatment and monitoring. *Am J Addict.* 2009;18(2):103-108.
85. McLellan AT, Skipper GS, Campbell M, DuPont RL. Five year outcomes in a cohort study of physicians treated for substance use disorders in the United States. *BMJ.* 2008;337:a2038. doi:10.1136/bmj.a2038
86. Zeldow PB, Daugherty SR. Personality profiles and specialty choices of students from two medical school classes. *Acad Med.* 1991;66(5):283-287.
87. Yufit RI, Pollock GH, Wasserman E. Medical specialty choice and personality: I. Initial results and predictions. *Arch Gen Psychiatry.* 1969;20(1):89-99.
88. Huang B, Dawson DA, Stinson FS, et al. Prevalence, correlates, and comorbidity of nonmedical prescription drug use and drug use disorders in the United States: results of the national epidemiologic survey on alcohol and related conditions. *J Clin Psychiatry.* 2006;67(7):1062-1073.
89. Shoptaw S. Methamphetamine use in urban gay and bisexual populations. *Top HIV Med.* 2006;14(2):84-87.
90. Wischmeyer PE, Johnson BR, Wilson JE, et al. A survey of propofol abuse in academic anesthesia programs. *Anesth Analg.* 2007;105(4):1066-1071, table of contents. doi:10.1213/01.ane.0000270215.86253.30
91. Fritz GA, Niemczyk WE. Propofol dependency in a lay person. *Anesthesiology.* 2002;96(2):505-506.
92. Bryson EO, Frost EA. Propofol abuse. *Int Anesthesiol Clin.* 2011;49(1):173-180. doi:10.1097/AIA.0b013e3181f2bcb0
93. Drug Enforcement Administration Department of Justice. Schedule of controlled substances; placement of fospropofol into schedule IV. Final rule. *Fed Regist.* 2009;74(192):51234-51236.
94. Drug Enforcement Administration Department of Justice. Placement of propofol into schedule IV. Proposed rule. *Fed Regist.* 2010;75:66196-66199.
95. Earley PH, Finver T. Addiction to propofol: a study of 22 treatment cases. *J Addict Med.* 2013;7(3):169-176. doi:10.1097/ADM.0b013e3182872901
96. Peckham C. *Physician Lifestyle Report 2015.* Medscape; 2015.
97. Hall W, Pacula RL. *Cannabis Use and Dependence: Public Health and Public Policy.* Cambridge University Press; 2003.
98. Swainson J, Klassen LJ, Brennan S, et al. Non-parenteral ketamine for depression: a practical discussion on addiction potential and recommendations for judicious prescribing. *CNS Drugs.* 2022;36(3):239-251. doi:10.1007/s40263-022-00897-2
99. Sassano-Higgins S, Baron D, Juarez G, Esmaili N, Gold M. A Review of Ketamine Ause and Diversion. *Depress Anxiety.* 2016;33(8):718-727. doi:10.1002/da.22536
100. Moore NN, Bostwick JM. Ketamine dependence in anesthesia providers. *Psychosomatics.* 1999;40(4):356-359.
101. Brewin CB, Firth-Cozens J. Dependency and self-criticism as predictors of depression in young doctors. *J Occup Health Psychol.* 1997;2(3):242.
102. Angres DH, McGovern MP, Shaw MF, Rawal P. Psychiatric comorbidity and physicians with substance use disorders: a comparison between the 1980s and 1990s. *J Addict Dis.* 2003;22(3):79-87.
103. Schneider B. Substance use disorders and risk for completed suicide. *Arch Suicide Res.* 2009;13(4):303-316. doi:10.1080/13811110903263191
104. Moutier C. Physician mental health: an evidence-based approach to change. *J Med Reg.* 2018;104(2):7-13. doi:10.30770/2572-1852-104.2.7
105. American Medical Association. Result and implications of the AMA-APA Physician Mortality Project Stage II. *J Am Med Assoc.* 1987;21:2949-2953.
106. Gold KJ, Sen A, Schwenk TL. Details on suicide among US physicians: data from the National Violent Death Reporting System. *Gen Hosp Psychiatry.* 2013;35(1):45-49.
107. Savage S. Addiction and pain: assessment and treatment issues. *Clin J Pain.* 2002;18(4 suppl):S28-S38.
108. Hamza H, Bryson EO. Exposure of anesthesia providers in recovery from substance abuse to potential triggering agents. *J Clin Anesth.* 2011;23(7):552-557. doi:10.1016/j.jclinane.2011.03.002
109. Polles AG, Williams MK, Phalin BR, Teitelbaum S, Merlo LJ. Neuropsychological impairment associated with substance use by physicians. *J Neurol Sci.* 2020;411:116714.
110. Volpicelli J, Balaraman G, Hahn J, Wallace H, Bux D. The role of uncontrollable trauma in the development of PTSD and alcohol addiction. *Alcohol Res Health.* 1999;23(4):256-262.
111. Norman SB, Tate SR, Anderson KG, Brown SA. Do trauma history and PTSD symptoms influence addiction relapse context? *Drug Alcohol Depend.* 2007;90(1):89-96. doi:10.1016/j.drugalcdep.2007.03.002
112. Norcini JJLR, Benson JA, Webster GD. An analysis of the knowledge base of practicing internists as measured by the 1980 recertification examination. *Ann Intern Med.* 1985;102(3):385-389.
113. Talbott GD, Benson EB. Impaired physicians: the dilemma of identification. *Postgrad Med.* 1980;68(6):56-64.
114. Pham JC, Pronovost PJ, Skipper GE. Identification of physician impairment. *JAMA.* 2013;309(20):2101-2102. doi:10.1001/jama.2013.4635
115. Fleming M. Physician impairment: options for intervention. *Am Fam Physician.* 1994;50(1):41.
116. Finlayson AJ, Dietrich MS, Neufeld R, Roback H, Martin PR. Restoring professionalism: the physician fitness-for-duty evaluation. *Gen Hosp Psychiatry.* 2013;35(6):659-663. doi:10.1016/j.genhosppsych.2013.06.009
117. Anfang SA, Faulkner LR, Fromson JA, Gendel MH. The American Psychiatric Association's resource document on guidelines for psychiatric fitness-for-duty evaluations of physicians. *J Am Acad Psychiatry Law.* 2005;33(1):85-88.
118. Joint Commission on Accreditation of Hospitals. *Accreditation Manual For Hospitals.* Joint Commission on Accreditation of Hospitals; 2020.
119. Nakagawa K, Yellowlees PM. The physician's physician: the role of the psychiatrist in helping other physicians and promoting wellness. *Psychiatr Clin North Am.* 2019;42(3):473-482. doi:10.1016/j.psc.2019.05.012
120. Igartua KJ. The impact of impaired supervisors on residents. *Acad Psychiatry.* 2000;24(4):188-194.

121. Reuben DB, Noble S. House officer responses to impaired physicians. *JAMA*. 1990;263(7):958-960.
122. Mee-Lee D, Shulman GD, Fishman M, et al. *The ASAM Criteria: Treatment for Addictive, Substance-Related, and Co-Occurring Conditions*. American Society of Addiction Medicine; 2013.
123. Federation of State Physician Health Programs. *2019 FSPHP Physician Health Program Guidelines*. Accessed May 11, 2022. https://www.fsphp.org/guidelines
124. Schneck SA. "Doctoring" doctors and their families. *JAMA*. 1998;280(23):2039-2042. doi:10.1001/jama.280.23.2039
125. Stoudemire A, Rhoads JM. When the doctor needs a doctor: special considerations for the physician-patient. *Ann Intern Med*. 1983;98(5 Pt 1):654-659.
126. Mee-Lee D; American Society of Addiction Medicine. *Persons in Safety-Sensitive occupations, Section in The ASAM Criteria: Treatment for Addictive, Substance-Related, and Co-occurring Conditions*. 3rd ed. The Change Companies; 2013.
127. Fayne M, Silvan M. Treatment issues in the group psychotherapy of addicted physicians. *Psychiatr Q*. 1999;70(2):123-135.
128. Taylor GJ, Bagby K, Parker JD. Alexithymia–state and trait. *Psychother Psychosom*. 1993;60(3-4):211-212.
129. Sifneos PE, Apfel-Savitz R, Frankel FH. The phenomenon of 'alexithymia'. *Psychother Psychosom*. 1977;28(1-4):47-57.
130. Gabbard GO. The role of compulsiveness in the normal physician. *JAMA*. 1985;254(20):2926-2929.
131. DuPont RL, McLellan AT, White WL, Merlo LJ, Gold MS. Setting the standard for recovery: physicians' Health Programs. *J Subst Abuse Treat*. 2009;36(2):159-171. doi:10.1016/j.jsat.2008.01.004
132. Dilts SL, Gendel M, Lepoff R, Clark C, Radcliff S. The colorado physician health program. Observations at 7 years. *Am J Addict*. 1994;3(4):337-345.
133. Reading E. Nine years experience with chemically dependent physicians: the New Jersey experience. *Md Med J*. 1992;41(4):325-329.
134. Smith P, Smith J. Treatment outcomes of impaired physicians in Oklahoma. *J Okla State Med Assoc*. 1991;84(12):599.
135. DuPont RL, McLellan AT, Carr G, Gendel M, Skipper GE. How are addicted physicians treated? A national survey of Physician Health Programs. *J Subst Abuse Treat*. 2009;37(1):1-7. doi:10.1016/j.jsat.2009.03.010
136. Skipper GE. Treating the chemically dependent health professional. *J Addict Dis*. 1997;16(3):67-73.
137. Buhl A, Oreskovich MR, Meredith CW, Campbell MD, Dupont RL. Prognosis for the recovery of surgeons from chemical dependency: a 5-year outcome study. *Arch Surg*. 2011;146(11):1286-1291. doi:10.1001/archsurg.2011.271
138. Skipper GE, Campbell MD, DuPont RL. Anesthesiologists with substance use disorders: a 5-year outcome study from 16 state physician health programs. *Anesth Analg*. 2009;109(3):891-896.
139. Kelly JF, Humphreys K, Ferri M. Alcoholics Anonymous and other 12-step programs for alcohol use disorder. *Cochrane Database Syst Rev*. 2020;3:CD012880. doi:10.1002/14651858.CD012880.pub2
140. Fiorentine R, Hillhouse MP. Drug treatment and 12-step program participation: the additive effects of integrated recovery activities. *J Subst Abuse Treat*. 2000;18(1):65-74. doi:10.1016/s0740-5472(99)00020-3
141. Lloyd G. One hundred alcoholic doctors: a 21-year follow-up. *Alcohol Alcohol*. 2002;37(4):370-374.
142. Galanter M, Talbott D, Gallegos K, Rubenstone E. Combined alcoholics anonymous and professional care for addicted physicians. *Am J Psychiatry*. 1990;147(1):64-68.
143. Galanter M, Dermatis H, Mansky P, McIntyre J, Perez-Fuentes G. Substance-abusing physicians: monitoring and twelve-step-based treatment. *Am J Addict*. 2007;16(2):117-123.
144. Galanter M, Dermatis H, Stanievich J, Santucci C. Physicians in long-term recovery who are members of alcoholics anonymous. *Am J Addict*. 2013;22(4):323-328. doi:10.1111/j.1521-0391.2013.12051.x
145. Merlo LJ, Campbell MD, Shea C, et al. Essential components of physician health program monitoring for substance use disorder: a survey of participants 5 years post successful program completion. *Am J Addict*. 2022;31(2):115-122.
146. Enders LE, Mercier JM. Treating chemical dependency: the need for including the family. *Int J Addict*. 1993;28(6):507-519.
147. Merlo LJ, Greene WM, Pomm R. Mandatory Naltrexone treatment prevents relapse among opiate-dependent anesthesiologists returning to practice. *J Addict Med*. 2011;5(4):279-283. doi:10.1097/ADM.0b013e31821852a0
148. FSPHP. *FSPHP Physician Health Program Guidelines*. FSPHP; 2019 Accessed May 26, 2023. https://www.fsphp.org/guidelines.
149. Kan D, Zweben J, Stine S. Pharmacological and psychosocial treatment for opioid use disorder. *The ASAM Principles of Addiction Medicine*. Lippincott Williams and Wilkins; 2018.
150. International Doctors in Alcoholics Anonymous. *IDAA History and Objectives*. IDAA. Accessed May 26, 2023. http://www.idaa.org/
151. Federation of State Physician Health Programs. List of State Programs. Accessed November 18, 2018. http://www.fsphp.org/state-programs
152. Federation of State Physician Health Programs. About the FSPHP. Accessed November 12, 2016. http://www.fsphp.org/about
153. Federation of State Physician Health Programs. Other Organizations' Statements Supporting Physician Health. Accessed May 9, 2022. https://www.fsphp.org/other-organizations--statements---revised-dec-2020
154. Knight JR, Sanchez LT, Sherritt L, Bresnahan LR, Fromson JA. Outcomes of a monitoring program for physicians with mental and behavioral health problems. *J Psychiatr Pract*. 2007;13(1):25-32.
155. Geuijen PM, van den Broek SJ, Dijkstra BA, et al. Success rates of monitoring for healthcare professionals with a substance use disorder: a meta-analysis. *J Clin Med*. 2021;10(2):264.
156. Knight JR, Sanchez LT, Sherritt L, Bresnahan LR, Silveria JM, Fromson JA. Monitoring physician drug problems: attitudes of participants. *J Addict Dis*. 2002;21(4):27-36. doi:10.1300/J069v21n04_03
157. Brooks E, Gendel MH, Gundersen DC, et al. Physician health programmes and malpractice claims: reducing risk through monitoring. *Occup Med (London)*. 2013;63(4):274-280. doi:10.1093/occmed/kqt036
158. Nelson HD, Matthews AM, Girard DE, Bloom JD. Substance-impaired physicians-Probationary and voluntary treatment programs compared. *West J Med*. 1996;165(1):31-36.
159. Polles A, Bundy C, Jacobs W, Merlo LJ. Adaptations to substance use disorder monitoring by physician health programs in response to COVID-19. *J Subst Abuse Treat*. 2021;125:108281.
160. Jaffee WB, Trucco E, Levy S, Weiss RD. Is this urine really negative? A systematic review of tampering methods in urine drug screening and testing. *J Subst Abuse Treat*. 2007;33(1):33-42. doi:10.1016/j.jsat.2006.11.008
161. Skipper GE, Weinmann W, Thierauf A, et al. Ethyl glucuronide: a biomarker to identify alcohol use by health professionals recovering from substance use disorders. *Alcohol Alcohol*. 2004;39(5):445-449.
162. Wurst FM, Skipper GE, Weinmann W. Ethyl glucuronide—the direct ethanol metabolite on the threshold from science to routine use. *Addiction*. 2003;98(s2):51-61.
163. Wurst F, Dresen S, Allen J, Wiesbeck G, Graf M, Weinmann W. Ethyl sulphate: a direct ethanol metabolite reflecting recent alcohol consumption. *Addiction*. 2005;101:204-211. doi:10.1111/j.1360-0443.2005.01245.x
164. Helander A, Dahl H. Urinary tract infection: a risk factor for false-negative urinary ethyl glucuronide but not ethyl sulfate in the detection of recent alcohol consumption. *Clin Chem*. 2005;51(9):1728-1730.
165. Reisfield GM, Goldberger BA, Crews BO, et al. Ethyl glucuronide, ethyl sulfate, and ethanol in urine after sustained exposure to an ethanol-based hand sanitizer. *J Anal Toxicol*. 2011;35(2):85-91. doi:10.1093/anatox/35.2.85
166. DuPont RL, Compton WM, McLellan AT. Five-year recovery: a new standard for assessing effectiveness of substance use disorder treatment. *J Substance Abuse Treat*. 2015;58:1-5.
167. Vaillant GE. A 60-year follow-up of alcoholic men. *Addiction*. 2003;98(8):1043-1051. doi:10.1046/j.1360-0443.2003.00422.x

168. Federation of State Medical Boards. Policy on Physician Impairment—1995. Accessed November 21, 2016. https://www.fsmb.org/Media/Default/PDF/FSMB/Advocacy/1995_grpol_Physician_Impairment.pdf
169. Federation of State Medical Boards. Policy on Physician Impairment—2011. Accessed November 21, 2016. https://www.fsmb.org/Media/Default/PDF/FSMB/Advocacy/grpol_policy-on-physician-impairment.pdf
170. Brooks E, Early SR, Gundersen DC, Shore JH, Gendel MH. Comparing substance use monitoring and treatment variations among physician health programs. *Am J Addict.* 2012;21(4):327-334. doi:10.1111/j.1521-0391.2012.00239.x
171. Merlo LJ, Campbell MD, Shea C, et al. Essential components of physician health program monitoring for substance use disorder: a survey of participants 5 years post successful program completion. *Am J Addict.* 2022;31(2):115-122. doi:10.1111/ajad.13257
172. DuPont RL, Skipper GE. Six lessons from state physician health programs to promote long-term recovery. *J Psychoactive Drugs.* 2012;44(1):72-78. doi:10.1080/02791072.2012.660106
173. Earley P. MPARI History, Part One. Accessed June 10, 2012. http://www.earleyconsultancy.com/portal/mpari/mpari-history-part-one
174. Ganley OH, Pendergast WJ, Wilkerson MW, Mattingly DE. Outcome study of substance impaired physicians and physician assistants under contract with North Carolina Physicians Health Program for the period 1995–2000. *J Addict Dis.* 2005;24(1):1-12. doi:10.1300/J069v24n01_01
175. Boyd JW, Knight JR. Ethical and managerial considerations regarding state physician health programs. *J Addict Med.* 2012;6(4):243-246. doi:10.1097/ADM.0b013e318262ab09
176. Boyd JW. A call for national standards and oversight of state physician health programs. *J Addict Med.* 2015;9(6):431-432.
177. State BJ. Physician health programs require national standards and external oversight. *J Psychiatry.* 2016;19(346):2.
178. Candilis PJ. Physician health programs and the social contract. *AMA J Ethics.* 2016;18(1):77.
179. Merlo LJ, Greene WM. Physician views regarding substance use-related participation in a state physician health program. *Am J Addict.* 2010;19(6):529-533. doi:10.1111/j.1521-0391.2010.00088.x
180. Programs FoSPH. *FSPHP Physician Health Program Guidelines.* FSPHP; 2016. https://www.fsphp.org/assets/docs/2005_fsphp_guidelines-master_0.pdf
181. Martino F, Caselli G, Fiabane E, et al. Desire thinking as a predictor of drinking status following treatment for alcohol use disorder: a prospective study. *Addict Behav.* 2019;95:70-76. doi:10.1016/j.addbeh.2019.03.004
182. Malan D. *Individual Psychotherapy and the Science of Psychodynamics.* Hodder Education; 1995.
183. Earley PH, Zummo J, Memisoglu A, Silverman BL, Gastfriend DR. Open-label study of injectable extended-release naltrexone (XR-NTX) in healthcare professionals with opioid dependence. *J Addict Med.* 2017;11(3):224-230.
184. Merlo LJ, Gold MS. Prescription opioid abuse and dependence among physicians: hypotheses and treatment. *Harv Rev Psychiatry.* 2008;16(3):181-194. doi:10.1080/10673220802160316
185. Earley PH, Zummo J, Memisoglu A, Silverman BL, Gastfriend DR. Open-label study of injectable extended-release naltrexone (XR-NTX) in healthcare professionals with opioid dependence. *J Addict Med.* 2017;11(3):224-230. doi:10.1097/ADM.0000000000000302
186. Merlo LJ, Greene WM, Pomm R. Mandatory naltrexone treatment prevents relapse among opiate-dependent anesthesiologists returning to practice. *J Addict Med.* 2011;5(4):279-283. doi:10.1097/ADM.0b013e31821852a0
187. Cherrier MM, Amory JK, Ersek M, Risler L, Shen DD. Comparative cognitive and subjective side effects of immediate-release oxycodone in healthy middle-aged and older adults. *J Pain.* 2009;10(10):1038-1050.
188. Schindler SD, Ortner R, Peternell A, Eder H, Opgenoorth E, Fischer G. Maintenance therapy with synthetic opioids and driving aptitude. *Eur Addict Res.* 2004;10(2):80-87. doi:10.1159/000076118
189. Hamza H, Bryson EO. Buprenorphine maintenance therapy in opioid-addicted health care professionals returning to clinical practice: a hidden controversy. *Mayo Clinic Proc.* 2012;87(3):260-267. doi:10.1016/j.mayocp.2011.09.007
190. Federal Aviation Regulations – FAR 61.53 (2022). Accessed May 26, 2023. https://www.ecfr.gov/current/title-14/chapter-I/subchapter-D/part-61/subpart-A/section-61.53
191. Haston S. Impaired physicians and the scope of informed consent: balancing patient safety with physician privacy. *Fla St UL Rev.* 2013;41:1125.
192. U.S. Department of Justice. Justice Department Issues Guidance on Protections for People with Opioid Use Disorder under the Americans with Disabilities Act. 2022. Accessed 26 May, 2023. https://www.justice.gov/opa/pr/justice-department-issues-guidance-protections-people-opioid-use-disorder-under-americans
193. Rothstein L. Impaired physicians and the ADA. *JAMA.* 2015;313(22):2219-2220. doi:10.1001/jama.2015.4602
194. Merlo LJ, Campbell MD, Skipper GE, Shea CL, DuPont RL. Outcomes for physicians with opioid dependence treated without agonist pharmacotherapy in physician health programs. *J Subst Abuse Treat.* 2016;64:47-54. doi:10.1016/j.jsat.2016.02.004
195. Kauffman M, Brewster J. Physician health: characteristics and outcomes of a canadian monitoring program for substance dependent doctors. *Can J Addict.* 2009;1(1):42-43.
196. Federation of State Physician Health Programs. Safety Considerations for Medication Treatment of Opioid Use Disorders in Monitored Health Professionals. Accessed May 26, 2023. https://fsphp.memberclicks.net/assets/MEMBERPORTAL/FSPHP%20Safety%20Considerations%20and%20Medication-Assisted%20Treatment%20for%20SUD%20among%20Physicians%20Monitored%20by%20PHPs%20August%202022.pdf
197. Menk EJ, Baumgarten R, Kingsley CP, Culling RD, Middaugh R. Success of reentry into anesthesiology training programs by residents with a history of substance abuse. *JAMA.* 1990;263(22):3060-3062.
198. Collins GB, McAllister MS, Jensen M, Gooden TA. Chemical dependency treatment outcomes of residents in anesthesiology: results of a survey. *Anesth Analg.* 2005;101(5):1457-1462. doi:10.1213/01.ANE.0000180837.78169.04
199. Paris RT, Canavan DI. Physician substance abuse impairment: anesthesiologists vs. other specialties. *J Addict Dis.* 1999;18(1):1-7.
200. Oreskovich MR, Caldeiro RM. Anesthesiologists recovering from chemical dependency: can they safely return to the operating room? *Mayo Clin Proc.* 2009;84(7):576-580.
201. Hasin DS, Sarvet AL, Cerda M, et al. US adult Illicit Cannabis use, Cannabis use disorder, and medical Marijuana laws: 1991–1992 to 2012–2013. *JAMA Psychiatry.* 2017;74(6):579-588. doi:10.1001/jamapsychiatry.2017.0724
202. National Academies of Sciences, Engineering, and Medicine. *The Health Effects of Cannabis and Cannabinoids: The Current State of Evidence and Recommendations for Research.* The National Academies Press; 2017.
203. Petker T, Owens MM, Amlung MT, Oshri A, Sweet LH, MacKillop J. Cannabis involvement and neuropsychological performance: findings from the Human Connectome Project. *J Psychiatry Neurosci.* 2019;44(6):414-422. doi:10.1503/jpn.180115
204. Yesavage JA, Leirer VO, Denari M, Hollister LE. Carry-over effects of marijuana intoxication on aircraft pilot performance: a preliminary report. *Am J Psychiatry.* 1985;142(11):1325-1329. doi:10.1176/ajp.142.11.1325
205. Federation of State Medical Boards. Physicians' Use of Marijuana. Accessed May 9, 2022. https://www.fsmb.org/siteassets/advocacy/policies/physicians-use-of-marijuana.pdf
206. Executive Order of the President if the United States. *Drug Free Workplace*; 1986:12564. Accessed May 26, 2023. https://www.archives.gov/federal-register/codification/executive-order/12564.html
207. Drug-Free Workplace Act of 1988. Accessed May 26, 2023. https://www.govinfo.gov/content/pkg/USCODE-2009-title41/pdf/USCODE-2009-title41-chap10.pdf
208. Lexis-Nexis. *Brandon Coats v. Dish Network*, LLC - 2015 CO 44, 350 P.3d 849. Accessed May 11, 2022. https://www.lexisnexis.com/community/casebrief/p/casebrief-brandon-coats-v-dish-network-llc

Sidebar

Health care Professional Wellness After Patient Overdose Death

Amy M. Yule and Frances Rudnick Levin

INTRODUCTION

Health care professionals who work with individuals with substance use disorders (SUD) are dedicated to decreasing acute risks associated with substance use, such as drug overdose. Drug overdoses commonly involve opioids,[1] and medication treatment for opioid use disorders can decrease opioid overdose risk.[2] However, individuals with an opioid use disorder may still be at high risk for overdose due to difficulty stabilizing on medication[3] or difficulty consistently accessing medication.[3,4] Given the high and increasing number of drug overdose deaths in the United States,[5] the dynamic nature of the key substances involved in drug overdose deaths,[6] and barriers to accessing multimodal treatment for opioid use disorders and other SUDs,[4] health care professionals need to be prepared for a patient overdose death in their practice. Furthermore, substance use treatment program leaders, frequently physicians, need to be prepared to support clinical teams after a patient drug overdose death.

THE IMPACT OF A PATIENT DRUG OVERDOSE DEATH ON HEALTH CARE PROFESSIONALS

Although SUDs are associated with substantial morbidity, drug overdose deaths are still unexpected, sudden, and stigmatized.[7] It is important that health care professionals be prepared for a patient overdose death since there is increasing evidence that the experience is stressful for the clinician. For example, a qualitative study of Irish physicians, counselors, and case managers who worked with individuals with SUDs who were experiencing being unhoused, found they experienced anxiety and self-blame after a patient overdose death.[8] Likewise, a survey of health care professionals in Scotland who worked with individuals with SUDs found 88% experienced a grief-related reaction after a patient overdose death.[9] Feelings of sadness, guilt, anger, and helplessness, as well as thoughts regarding their own morbidity, were commonly endorsed.[9] Furthermore, clinicians with past lived experience of a SUD, whether themselves or with a family member and/or close friend who has a SUD, may be more vulnerable to experience high stress or a more complicated grief-related reaction after a patient overdose death.

Importantly, stress associated with a patient overdose death may impact the clinical care a health care professional provides to other individuals in their practice. For instance, half of health care professionals in a substance use treatment program reported the emotions they experienced after a patient overdose death affected their relationships with other patients "somewhat or a lot."[9] Another survey of health care professionals working with individuals with a SUD in the United States observed differences in clinical practice related to stress after a patient overdose death.[10] Clinicians with high stress after a patient overdose death, when compared to those with low stress, were more likely to focus on overdose and suicide risk factors during clinical encounters, and more likely to refer patients to a higher level of care.[10] Although increased focus on risk factors for adverse events may be a positive consequence, increased frequency of recommending a higher level of care could be less patient-centered than intended, as there is increasing recognition that recommending a higher level of care when a patient is not interested or ready for more intensive treatment may result in them leaving treatment.

To our knowledge, no current research has examined risk factors associated with increased stress after a patient overdose death among health care professionals. However, research on stress associated with a patient death by suicide is informative since suicide deaths are also unexpected, sudden, and stigmatized.[7] A study of stress associated with a patient death by suicide among mental health professionals working in an outpatient or hospital setting found an association between stress severity and the professional's relationship to the patient, exposure and support after the suicide, and level of training.[11] Mental health professionals who were highly impacted by patient death by suicide were more commonly emotionally close with the patient, had experienced a greater number of patient deaths by suicide, lacked support after the suicide death, and had less education and clinical training. This research suggests support and education about risk and adverse outcomes, particularly for those earlier in their career, may be important strategies to mitigate the stress associated with a patient drug overdose death.

Even if a health care professional does not experience high levels of acute stress after a patient overdose death, research on the experiences of community health workers and emergency services first responders suggests frequent exposure to nonfatal and fatal overdoses is associated with secondary traumatic stress.[12,13] This is noteworthy because secondary traumatic stress impacts health care professional wellbeing, and can contribute to burnout and compassion fatigue if not addressed.[14] Burnout and compassion fatigue are concerning, in part because they are associated with lower quality of care and health care professional turnover.[14] Considering the existing shortage of health care professionals prepared to care for individuals with SUD,[15] it is important that the addiction field provide health care professionals with support to cope with stressful events/experiences associated with this work.

SUGGESTED SUPPORT FOR HEALTH CARE PROFESSIONALS AFTER A PATIENT DRUG OVERDOSE DEATH

Unfortunately, despite the rising number of drug overdose deaths in the United States, there has been relatively little attention focused on developing standard procedures for health care professionals following a patient overdose death. When procedures are developed and agreed upon before an adverse event, they can help decrease additional stress by ensuring a standardized, predictable, and consistent response. Guidance on procedures after a patient overdose death can be drawn from the literature on procedures after a patient suicide, referred to as postvention, and procedures after medical error. Medical errors in the acute hospital setting, whether fatal or nonfatal, also have similar features to deaths due to suicide and drug overdose—they are unexpected, sudden, and stigmatized.[16] Postvention following patient suicide and procedures after medical error both focus on the importance of *structured notification, case review, and support*.[17-20]

Within the health care setting, structured notification after a patient overdose death includes prompt notification of individuals who frequently interacted with the patient.[20] Addiction care is often multidisciplinary, and a patient may have interacted with multiple members within a clinical system including a physician, an individual therapist, nurse(s), medical assistant(s), and front desk administrative staff. The health care team should be notified in a timely manner, and if possible, in person to allow for observations of body language and other nonverbal responses to the news to guide initial offers of support. With increased use of telehealth modalities, many health care teams now have fewer opportunities to communicate in person. Consequently, health care teams may benefit from identifying ways to increase virtual or in person interactions to allow staff time and space to support one another and express their emotions after a stressful clinical event.

Formal notifications within the health care setting after a patient overdose death are important since an overdose death is an adverse event. Formal notifications may include contacting clinic or department leadership to make them aware of the death, filing an incident report, and notifying state agencies that oversee substance use treatment if required, such as the Department of Public Health.[20] An incident report may lead to a formal department quality improvement/quality assurance case review. Formal notifications also present an opportunity for feedback through case review from individuals outside of the clinical team. Additionally, they can help increase awareness within the health care system of the clinical acuity and risks associated with treating individuals with SUDs. Notification and/or consultation with a health care professional liability insurance carrier can also be considered, particularly for health care professionals who work alone or in a small practice setting with less infrastructure support to review adverse events.

In addition to a larger department quality improvement/assurance review, once ample time has passed for the health care team to initially process their emotions, it can be important for the team to review the clinical case to identify if there are changes to consider regarding clinic policies/procedures and education. However, descriptions of postvention interventions emphasize the importance of staff not blaming one another and respecting each individual's adaptive style when responding to stress.[21,22] One challenge for health care professionals as they process their initial emotions and prepare to review the case is that there may be little known about the overdose death. For example, in our experience, it is not uncommon for opioid treatment programs to find out that a patient has died only after reading an obituary announcement. When information about the death is limited, and/or there were not things that the health care team could have clearly done to decrease a patient's risk for overdose, it can be difficult for health care professionals to have closure with this type of ambiguous loss.

In the setting of ambiguous loss and grief generally, it can be helpful to try to find meaning and acknowledge the patient's death in a formal way.[23] Health care professionals may choose to attend formal memorial events organized by the patient's friends and/or family that are open to the public. A limited literature on health care professional experiences after a patient death by suicide suggests funeral attendance can help clinicians process their grief.[22,24] Substance use treatment teams may also choose to have an annual memorial event or create a memorial space within a staff room or other clinical area. Examples of memorials include attaching ribbons that represent the patient who died to a tree or collecting obituaries that are kept in a binder and stored in a secure space to maintain patient confidentiality.

Peer support from colleagues is also important after a patient overdose death. Research on peer support after a patient suicide death has found that it is helpful when colleagues share their own experience with the suicide of a patient.[25] However, other studies have found it is not helpful when colleagues provide premature reassurance that a clinician did nothing wrong.[26,27]

Formal models of support after a patient death from suicide or a medical error include formalizing discussions about loss as part of regular clinical supervision, and using peer supporters.[18] After a medical error, peer supporters are trained to provide psychological first aid to reduce acute distress and strengthen an individual's coping strategies.[18] Psychological first aid was initially developed for individuals in disaster settings and has since been adapted for humanitarian workers and health care professionals experiencing distress.[28,29] The model emphasizes reflective listening, normalization of an individual's reaction, as well as linkage to more formal mental health support if indicated.

Finally, it is beneficial for health care professionals who work with individuals with SUDs to consistently engage in self-care given the overall stress associated with repeated exposure to nonfatal and fatal overdoses. For other health care professionals who have repeated exposure to trauma and death, for example, mental health clinicians, oncologists, and palliative care physicians, the importance of education on strategies to support self-care has been emphasized.[30,31] Self-care includes good health habits such as adequate sleep and regular exercise, as well as engaging in activities that bring joy and connection.[32] Within substance use treatment programs it is important to discuss what programs can do to support self-care,[32] and consider how health care professionals are incorporating self-care into their life.

CONCLUSION

Experiencing a patient death by overdose is associated with acute stress and can contribute to secondary traumatic stress over time. Therefore, health care professionals and substance use treatment programs should prepare by developing standard procedures to follow after a patient overdose death that include *structured notification, case review, and support* to ensure that they and their colleagues are well supported. Due to limited research on the experience of health care professionals after a patient overdose death, it will be important to evaluate the effectiveness of new procedures and processes to promote continuous quality improvement.

REFERENCES

1. Mattson CL. Trends and geographic patterns in drug and synthetic opioid overdose deaths—United States, 2013-2019. *MMWR Morb Mortal Wkly Rep.* 2021;70(6):202-207. doi:10.15585/mmwr.mm7006a4
2. Sordo L, Barrio G, Bravo MJ, et al. Mortality risk during and after opioid substitution treatment: systematic review and meta-analysis of cohort studies. *BMJ.* 2017;357:j1550. doi:10.1136/bmj.j1550
3. Strang J, Volkow ND, Degenhardt L, et al. Opioid use disorder. *Nat Rev Dis Primers.* 2020;6(1):1-28. doi:10.1038/s41572-019-0137-5
4. Mackey K, Veazie S, Anderson J, Bourne D, Peterson K. Barriers and facilitators to the use of medications for opioid use disorder: a rapid review. *J Gen Intern Med.* 2020;35(Suppl 3):954-963. doi:10.1007/s11606-020-06257-4
5. Ahmad FB, Rossen LM, Sutton P. *Provisional Drug Overdose Death Counts*; 2022. Accessed May 13, 2022. https://www.cdc.gov/nchs/nvss/vsrr/drug-overdose-data.htm
6. Hedegaard H, Miniño AM, Warner M. Co-involvement of opioids in drug overdose deaths involving cocaine and psychostimulants. *NCHS Data Brief.* 2021;406:1-8.
7. Kheibari A, Cerel J, Victor G. Comparing attitudes toward stigmatized deaths: suicide and opioid overdose deaths. *Int J Ment Health Addict.* 2022;20(4):2291-2305. doi:10.1007/s11469-021-00514-1
8. O'Callaghan D, Lambert S. The impact of COVID-19 on health care professionals who are exposed to drug-related deaths while supporting clients experiencing addiction. *J Subst Abuse Treat.* 2022;138:108720. doi:10.1016/j.jsat.2022.108720
9. Mcauley A, Forsyth AJ. The impact of drug-related death on staff who have experienced it as part of their caseload: an exploratory study. *J Subst Use.* 2011;16(1):68-78. doi:10.3109/14659891.2010.487555
10. Yule AM, Basaraba C, Mail V, Bereznicka A, Cates-Wessel K, Levin FR. A cross sectional survey of provider experiences with patient drug overdose death. *J Subst Addict Treat.* doi:10.1016/j.josat.2023.209008
11. Castelli Dransart DA, Heeb JL, Gulfi A, Gutjahr EM. Stress reactions after a patient suicide and their relations to the profile of mental health professionals. *BMC Psychiatry.* 2015;15:265. doi:10.1186/s12888-015-0655-y
12. Kolla G, Strike C. It's too much, I'm getting really tired of it: overdose response and structural vulnerabilities among harm reduction workers in community settings. *Int J Drug Policy.* 2019;74:127-135. doi:10.1016/j.drugpo.2019.09.012
13. Pike E, Tillson M, Webster JM, Staton M. A mixed-methods assessment of the impact of the opioid epidemic on first responder burnout. *Drug Alcohol Depend.* 2019;205:107620. doi:10.1016/j.drugalcdep.2019.107620
14. Winstanley EL. The bell tolls for thee & thine: compassion fatigue & the overdose epidemic. *Int J Drug Policy.* 2020;85:102796. doi:10.1016/j.drugpo.2020.102796
15. Volkow ND, McLellan T, Blanco C. How academic medicine can help confront the opioid crisis. *Acad Med.* 2022;97(2):171-174. doi:10.1097/ACM.0000000000004289
16. Wu AW. Medical error: the second victim. The doctor who makes the mistake needs help too. *BMJ.* 2000;320(7237):726-727. doi:10.1136/bmj.320.7237.726
17. Cazares PT, Santiago P, Moulton D, Moran S, Tsai A. Suicide response guidelines for residency trainees: a novel postvention response for the care and teaching of psychiatry residents who encounter suicide in their patients. *Acad Psychiatry.* 2015;39(4):393-397. doi:10.1007/s40596-015-0352-7
18. Busch IM, Moretti F, Campagna I, et al. Promoting the psychological well-being of healthcare providers facing the burden of adverse events: a systematic review of second victim support resources. *Int J Environ Res Public Health.* 2021;18(10):5080. doi:10.3390/ijerph18105080
19. Seys D, Wu AW, Van Gerven E, et al. Health care professionals as second victims after adverse events: a systematic review. *Eval Health Prof.* 2013;36(2):135-162. doi:10.1177/0163278712458918
20. Yule AM, Levin FR. Supporting providers after drug overdose death. *Am J Psychiatry.* 2019;176(3):173-178. doi:10.1176/appi.ajp.2018.18070794
21. Coverdale JH, Roberts LW, Louie AK. Encountering patient suicide: emotional responses, ethics, and implications for training programs. *Acad Psychiatry.* 2007;31(5):329-332. doi:10.1176/appi.ap.31.5.329
22. Kaye NS, Soreff SM. The psychiatrist's role, responses, and responsibilities when a patient commits suicide. *Am J Psychiatry.* 1991;148(6):739-743. doi:10.1176/ajp.148.6.739
23. Boss P, Carnes D. The myth of closure. *Fam Process.* 2012;51(4):456-469. doi:10.1111/famp.12005
24. Markowitz JC. Attending the funeral of a patient who commits suicide. *Am J Psychiatry.* 1990;147(1):122-123. doi:10.1176/ajp.147.1.122b
25. Biermann B. When depression becomes terminal: the impact of patient suicide during residency. *J Am Acad Psychoanal Dyn Psychiatry.* 2003;31(3):443-457. doi:10.1521/jaap.31.3.443.22130
26. Hendin H, Lipschitz A, Maltsberger JT, Haas AP, Wynecoop S. Therapists' reactions to patients' suicides. *Am J Psychiatry.* 2000;157(12):2022-2027. doi:10.1176/appi.ajp.157.12.2022
27. Tillman JG. When a patient commits suicide: an empirical study of psychoanalytic clinicians. *Int J Psychoanal.* 2006;87(Pt 1):159-177. doi:10.1516/6ubb-e9de-8ucw-uv3l
28. Malik M, Peirce J, Wert MV, Wood C, Burhanullah H, Swartz K. Psychological first aid well-being support rounds for frontline healthcare workers during COVID-19. *Front Psychiatry.* 2021;12:669009. doi:10.3389/fpsyt.2021.669009

29. Corey J, Vallières F, Frawley T, De Brún A, Davidson S, Gilmore B. A rapid realist review of group psychological first aid for humanitarian workers and volunteers. *Int J Environ Res Public Health.* 2021;18(4):1452. doi:10.3390/ijerph18041452
30. Posluns K, Gall TL. Dear mental health practitioners, take care of yourselves: a literature review on self-care. *Int J Adv Couns.* 2020;42(1): 1-20. doi:10.1007/s10447-019-09382-w
31. Sanchez-Reilly S, Morrison LJ, Carey E, et al. Caring for oneself to care for others: physicians and their self-care. *J Support Oncol.* 2013;11(2):75-81. doi:10.12788/j.suponc.0003
32. U.S. Department of Health and Human Services. 2022 *Addressing Health Worker Burnout*. Accessed November 8, 2022. https://www.hhs.gov/surgeongeneral/priorities/health-worker-burnout

SECTION

5

Overview of Addiction Treatment

Associate Editor: Jeanette M. Tetrault

Lead Section Editor: Deborah S. Finnell

Section Editors: Wilson M. Compton and Karran A. Phillips

CHAPTER

35 Addiction Medicine in America: Its Birth, Early History, and Current Status (1750-2022)

Kevin Kunz, Hoover Adger, William L. White, Timothy K. Brennan, Annie Lévesque, and Jacqueline Deanna Wilson

CHAPTER OUTLINE

- Chapter overview
- Introduction
- The birth of addiction medicine
- Early professionalism and medical advancements (1830-1900)
- Demedicalization and the collapse of addiction treatment (1900-1935)
- The rebirth of addiction treatment (1935-1970)
- Addiction medicine comes of age (1970-2023)
- Organized addiction medicine today
- Historic racism, discriminatory laws and policies and the importance of anti-racism, diversity, equity, and inclusion
- Future status of organized addiction medicine in America

CHAPTER OVERVIEW

The birthing and organization of addiction medicine have evolved in concert with advances in neuroscience, public health policy—or lack of such—physician and other health care professional interest, serial epidemics, endemic substance use, and societal understanding.

1. Scientific research from the bench to bedside to the community has informed a modern understanding of addiction as a brain disease for which prevention and treatment are possible and effective. Terminology, attitudes, and practices have evolved with increased knowledge allowing the condition and persons affected by it to benefit from the spectrum of attention and care given to other conditions with less morbidity and mortality.
2. As is true for many medical fields, the 18th and 19th centuries were relatively "dark ages" preceding the maturation of science and medical practice in the 20th century and a new era in practice and organization that occurred as the century closed and the 21st century opened.
3. Organized medicine increasingly addressed unhealthy substance use and addiction beginning in the 1950s, when physicians organized the forerunners of today's addiction-related medical organizations. Governmental and health care systems followed the lead of physicians.

INTRODUCTION

The recent recognition of addiction medicine by the American Board of Medical Specialties and the Accreditation Council for Graduate Medical Education presents a timely backdrop to this review of American physicians' involvement in the prevention and treatment of alcohol and other drug-related problems over the last two centuries. This chapter describes the birth of addiction medicine in the late 18th century, the professionalization of addiction medicine in the second half of the 19th century, its virtual collapse in the opening decades of the 20th century, and its reemergence as a fully legitimized medical subspecialty at the opening of the 21st century. "What is past is prologue" is a saying of prescient value in medicine and public health. (This quotation by William Shakespeare, which in present-day use emphasizes that history sets the context for the present, is engraved on the National Archives Building in Washington, DC). This chapter represents history still evolving and in which the reader is a participant. Indeed, William Faulkner was correct: "the past is never dead – it is never even past" (William Faulkner, *Requiem for a Nun.* London: Chatto & Windus; 1919). 1A. The modern field of addiction medicine can trace its lineage from the scholars of ancient civilizations, through Indigenous Americans on to Drs Benjamin Rush, Ruth Fox, Robert Smith, and American Surgeon Generals, It includes today some 5,000 practicing addiction physician specialists and thousands of other health professionals across disciplines who have brought the field to its new standing in mainstream medicine and health care.

This review includes early pioneers of addiction medicine, conceptual and clinical breakthroughs, the evolving settings in which addiction medicine was practiced, the larger currents in American medicine, and the evolving social policies that influenced the early practice of addiction medicine. That this brief history ends with an update of the field's progress within the American "House of Medicine" is especially poignant, as time has amply demonstrated the multisystem biological, behavioral, and societal impact of unhealthy substance use and addiction within the purview of every health professional.

THE BIRTH OF ADDICTION MEDICINE

The roots of addiction medicine began not in a young America but in the ancient civilizations of Africa and Europe. Special methods to care for persons addicted to alcohol were developed in ancient Egypt, and references to chronic intoxication as a sickness that enslaved the body and soul date to Herodotus (5th century BCE), Aristotle (384-322 BCE), and Seneca (4 BCE-65 CE). St John Chrysostom (1st century CE) provided one of the earliest comparisons of chronic alcohol inebriety to other diseases.[1] These earliest intimations of the concept of addiction and its treatment reflect the fleeting observations of individuals rather than an organized cultural response to alcohol and other drug problems. To preserve the historic perspective of this chapter, terms such as inebriety and intemperance have been maintained despite their current obsolescence. However, terms such as chronic drunkenness, drunkards, alcoholic, addict, and others have been updated in an effort to reflect modern terminology and current understanding of the disease of addiction and the persons afflicted by it (see Chapter 2 "Recommended Use of Terminology in Addiction Medicine").

The earliest American medical responses to alcoholism emerged within the systems of medicine practiced by Indigenous American tribes. Alcohol-related problems rose dramatically in early America as alcohol became increasingly used as a tool of economic, political, and sexual exploitation in the 18th and early 19th centuries.[2,3] Indigenous tribes actively resisted these problems through political and legal advocacy, organizing abstinence-based cultural revitalization movements, and through the medical treatment of those affected. Indigenous American healers used botanical agents to suppress cravings for alcohol (hop tea), to induce an aversion to alcohol (the root of the trumpet vine), and to facilitate personal transformation within abstinence-based cultural and religious revitalization movements.[4]

By the time the American Declaration of Independence was penned in 1776, there were merging parallel social trajectories and disruptions as alcohol was used to purchase enslaved Africans to work in the fields producing the new nation's major exported commodity, tobacco.

In colonial America, there was pervasive consumption of alcoholic beverages but no recognition of excessive drinking as a distinct medical problem.[5] This changed in response to increased alcohol consumption (a near tripling of annual per capita alcohol consumption between 1780 and 1830), a shift in preference from fermented to more potent forms of distilled alcohol, and the emergence of a pattern of socially disruptive "frontier drinking."[6,7] It was in this changing context that several prominent Americans "discovered" the phenomenon of addiction.[8]

In 1774, the philanthropist and social reformer Anthony Benezet published a treatise, *Mighty Destroyer Displayed*, that recasts alcohol from its status as a gift from God to that of a "bewitching poison." He noted the presence of "unhappy dram-drinkers bound in slavery" and observed that intoxication had a tendency to self-accelerate: "Drops beget drams, and drams beget more drams, till they become to be without weight or measure."[9]

Benezet's warning was followed by a series of publications by Dr Benjamin Rush. Rush's work is particularly important given his prominence in colonial society and his role in the history of American medicine and psychiatry. Rush's 1784 pamphlet, *Inquiry into the Effects of Ardent Spirits on the Human Mind and Body*, was the first American treatise on alcoholism, and it almost single-handedly launched the American temperance movement. In this pamphlet, Rush catalogued the symptoms of acute and chronic intoxication, described the progressiveness of these symptoms, and suggested that chronic intoxication was a "disease induced by a vice."[10] Rush was the first prominent physician to claim that many persons with alcohol addiction could be restored to full health and responsible citizenship through proper medical treatment and to call for the creation of a special facility (a "Sober House") to care for these persons.[11]

Rush's writings were mirrored in the work of physicians in other countries, most notably the Edinburgh physician Dr Thomas Trotter, whose 1788 publication, *An Essay, Medical, Philosophical, and Chemical, on Drunkenness and Its Effects on the Human Body*, shared many of Rush's ideas.[12] Another contribution that influenced the subsequent development of addiction medicine in America was the work of Christopher Wilhelm Hufeland, who in 1819 described a clinical condition characterized by uncontrollable cravings for alcoholic spirits that triggered periodic "drink storms." Hufeland labeled this condition *dipsomania*. During the same decade, Lettsom, Armstrong, and Pearson described the condition that Thomas Sutton subsequently christened *delirium tremens*.[13]

By the late 1820s, the subject of chronic intoxication was taken up in a number of medical dissertations. Most notable among these were the works of Drs Daniel Drake and William Sweetser. Drake speculated on the causes of "habitual drinking" and hinted at what would later become the concepts of *inability to abstain* and *loss of control* ("the habit being once established, he will not, I almost say cannot, refrain").[14] In 1828, Sweetser provided a detailed account of the pathophysiology of chronic alcohol intoxication, including depictions of the addictiveness of alcohol and the potential role of heredity. He concluded that intemperance created a "morbid alteration" in nearly all the major structures and functions of the human body. Cycles of compulsive drinking were viewed by Sweetser as the product of a devastating paradox: the poison (alcohol) was itself its only antidote.[15]

The 1827 publication of the Reverend Lyman Beecher's *Six Sermons on the Nature, Occasion, Signs, and Remedy of Intemperance* exerted their own influence on the emerging concept of addiction. Bridging the gap between moral and medical models, Beecher described the intemperate as being "addicted to the sin" and suffering from an "insatiable desire for drink." Beecher also described the early warning signs of addiction, linking these to the later signs that Rush, Drake, Sweetser, and others had catalogued. Second, he challenged these very physicians who, as in the case of Rush, had tried to get their patients to moderate their drinking by switching from distilled alcohol to fermented drinks such as wine or beer. Beecher's declaration, "There is no remedy for intemperance but the cessation of it," marked the call for complete abstinence as a personal and social strategy for the resolution of alcohol problems.[16]

Between 1774 and 1829, America "discovered" addiction through the collective observations of her physicians, clergy, and social activists. There was an emerging view that chronic intoxication was a problem with biological roots and consequences and thus the province of the physician. These earliest pioneers declared that chronic intoxication was a diseased state, and they articulated the major elements of an addiction disease concept: biological predisposition, drug toxicity, physical tolerance, disease progression, morbid appetite (craving), loss of volitional control of intake, and the pathophysiological consequences of sustained alcohol and opiate ingestion. Though their treatments could involve such "heroic" methods as purging, blistering, bleeding, and the use of toxic medicines, they also used surprisingly modern strategies (eg, aversive conditioning) and recognized many pathways to the initiation of abstinence (eg, from religious conversion to witnessing an alcohol-related death). The writings of this period portray addiction recovery not as an enduring process but as a climactic decision. This view focused the attention of the emerging temperance movement on the pledge of lifetime abstinence (from distilled alcohol) as a central strategy in early attempts at disease recovery.

Addiction medicine emerged in the shift, which continues today, from treating medical consequences to also treating the alcohol addiction itself. The earliest practice of addiction medicine predated institutional treatment and was practiced out of the private offices of individual physicians. Alcohol was not the only drug of concern to these physicians. During the 16th and 17th centuries, physicians in Germany, Holland, Portugal, and England had begun to conceptualize opium as "a kind of poison" requiring regular and increasing use that, when stopped, created a unique sickness that drove people to return to the drug.[17] In 1701, the English physician John Jones provided a detailed account of opiate withdrawal in his book, *The Mysteries of the Opium Reveal'd*.[18] Three events between the early- and mid-19th century profoundly altered the future of narcotic addiction in America: the isolation of morphine from opium, the introduction of the hypodermic syringe, and the emergence of a patent drug industry. These events produced drugs of greater potency, created a more efficient and euphorigenic method of drug ingestion, and increased the availability and promotion of psychoactive drugs.[19,20] "Narcotic" in current medical terminology refers to opioids. It has been used to legally categorize other substances, including other drugs causing altered mental states, such as stupor.

EARLY PROFESSIONALISM AND MEDICAL ADVANCEMENTS (1830-1900)

In 1828, Dr Eli Todd, superintendent of the Hartford Retreat for the Insane, called for the creation of physician-directed asylums for persons with severe alcohol addiction. Under his influence, the Connecticut State Medical Society gave support to this idea in 1830.[21] A year later, Dr Samuel Woodward, superintendent at the Hospital for the Insane at Worcester, Massachusetts, wrote a series of influential essays echoing the Connecticut recommendations. He declared:

> "A large proportion of the intemperate in a well-conducted institution would be radically cured, and would again go into society with health reestablished, diseased appetites removed, with principles of temperance well-grounded and thoroughly understood, so that they would be afterwards safe and sober men."[22]

Woodward argued that intemperance was a physical disease requiring medical remedies and, siding with Beecher, declared that "the grand secret of the cure for intemperance is total abstinence from alcohol in all its forms."[22] This total abstinence position gained influence in light of the failed efforts to cure alcoholism through the use of public pledges to refrain only from distilled alcohol. Indeed, the continuing variant social behaviors resulting from fermented alcoholic drinks contributed to the temperance movement's shift from the partial pledge to the T-total pledge (teetotalism).[23]

In the 1830s and 1840s, a series of clinical contributions to the understanding of chronic intoxication exerted considerable influence on the emerging field of addiction medicine.[24] First, there were new experiments and clinical observations on the pathophysiology of alcohol, such as those of Prout, Beaumont, and Percy on the effects of alcohol on the stomach and the blood.[25] Dr Robert Macnish's *Anatomy of Drunkenness* (1835)[26] offered one of the earliest typologies of alcohol addiction, noting seven clinical subtypes.

In 1838, France's leading expert on alcoholism, Dr Jean-Étienne Dominique Esquirol, argued that the disease of intemperance was a "monomania"—a "mental illness whose principal character is an irresistible tendency toward fermented beverages."[27] This was followed in 1840 by Dr R.B. Grindrod's text, *Bacchus*, in which he declared "I am more than ever convinced that drunkenness is a disease, physical as well as moral, and consequently requires physical as well as moral remedies."[28,29]

One of the most significant milestones in the history of addiction medicine was the 1849 publication of Magnus Huss' text, *Chronic Alcoholism*. After an extensive review of the chronic effects of intoxication, Huss declared:

> "These symptoms are formed in such a particular way that they form a disease group in themselves and thus merit being designated and described as a definite disease … It is this group of symptoms which I wish to designate by the name Alcoholismus chronicus."[30,31]

Huss's text stands as the landmark addiction medicine text of the mid-19th century. It contributed a clinical term—*alcoholism*—that came into increasing medical and public popularity in the transition between the 19th and 20th centuries.

The Washingtonian Revival of the 1840s and the fraternal temperance societies and reform clubs that followed brought the issue of recovery from alcoholism onto center cultural stage. Local Washingtonian groups encountering "hard cases" needing more than an occasional abstinence support meeting began organizing lodging houses that evolved into America's first addiction treatment institutions. A multi-branched treatment field emerged in the mid-19th century. Homes for the chronically inebriated emerged out of mutual aid societies that viewed addiction recovery as a process of moral reformation.[32] There were medically directed "inebriate asylums," the first of which was the New York State Inebriate Asylum, chartered in 1857 and opened in 1864.[33,34] There were also privately franchised, for-profit addiction cure institutions such as the Keeley, Neal, Gatlin, and Oppenheimer Institutes. These institutions generated considerable controversy over their claim to have medicinal specifics that could cure addiction and their practice of hiring physicians who were in recovery from addiction.[35,36] Homes established by mutual aid societies, asylums, and the private addiction cure institutes competed with bottled patent medicine addiction cures (most containing alcohol, opium, morphine, or cocaine), some of which were promulgated by physicians, and religiously sponsored recovery colonies and rescue missions.[21] By the late 1870s, large urban hospitals, such as Bellevue Hospital in New York City, had also started opening wards designed to treat chronic addiction.[37] Annual admissions of persons with alcoholism at Bellevue rose to 4190 by 1895—a number that continued to climb to more than 11,300 per year in the opening decade of the 20th century.[21]

In 1870, Dr Joseph Parrish led the creation of the American Association for the Cure of Inebriety (AACI), which brought together the heads of America's most prominent inebriate homes and asylums. The AACI bylaws posited that:

a. Intemperance is a disease.
b. It is curable in the same sense that other diseases are.
c. Its primary cause is a constitutional susceptibility to the alcoholic impression.
d. This constitutional tendency may be either inherited or acquired.[38]

The AACI published the first specialized medical journal on addiction—the *Journal of Inebriety*. The journal, edited by Dr T.D. Crothers during its entire publication life (1876-1914), was filled with essays by addiction medicine specialists and with advertisements promoting various treatment institutions.[39,40] A similar inebriety treatment movement was under way in Europe, and the first international meetings of addiction medicine specialists were held during this period.[41]

American physicians specializing in addiction began releasing texts on addiction and treatment methods in the 1860s: Dr Albert Day's *Methomania: A Treatise on Alcoholic Poisoning* and Dr W. Marcet's *On Chronic Alcoholic Intoxication.* The production of such literature virtually exploded in the 1880s and 1890s. Among the most prominent texts either written in America or that exerted a significant influence on the practice of addiction medicine in America during this period were Dr H.H. Kane's *Drugs That Enslave: The Opium, Morphine, Chloral and Hashish Habits*; Dr Fred Hubbard's *The Opium Habit and Alcoholism*; Dr Asa Meyerlet's *Notes on the Opium Habit*; Dr T.L. Wright's *Inebriism*; Franklin Clum's *Inebriety: Its Causes, Its Results, Its Remedy*; Dr T.D. Crothers' *The Disease of Inebriety from Alcohol, Opium and Other Narcotic Drugs*; Dr Norman Kerr's *Inebriety or Narcomania: Its Etiology, Pathology, Treatment, and Jurisprudence*; and Dr Charles Palmer's *Inebriety: Its Source, Prevention, and Cure.*[21]

The central organizing concept of 19th-century addiction medicine specialists was that of *inebriety*. Inebriety was viewed as a disease that manifested itself in numerous varieties. These varieties were meticulously detailed by clinical subpopulation and drug choice. Addiction medicine texts were often organized under such headings as *alcoholic inebriety*, *opium inebriety*, *cocaine inebriety*, and *ether inebriety*. Inebriety was viewed as a disease that sprang from multiple etiological pathways, unfolded in many diverse patterns, and had a variable course and outcome. Inebriety specialists talked eloquently about the need to individualize treatment and, by the 1880s, had begun to recognize and study the problem of posttreatment recurrence of use.[42]

The treatment methods of the two physician-directed branches of the inebriety movement (the inebriate asylums and the private addiction cure institutes) were quite different, and the conflicts between these branches reflected allopathic and homeopathic approaches to medicine in this period. The inebriate asylum physicians advocated a sustained (1-3 years), legally enforced course of treatment that consisted of withdrawal management, collateral medical treatments, and a period of institutional convalescence. The addiction cure institute physicians boasted medicinal specifics (hypodermic injections and liquid tonics) that could "unpoison" the cells and destroy the craving and compulsion to use alcohol, opiates, and cocaine—all in 4 short weeks, cash in advance. Drug treatments within both branches included such substances as cannabis, cocaine, chloral hydrate, paraldehyde, strychnine, atropine, and apomorphine. Although some addiction medicine specialists used cocaine as a tonic during withdrawal management, most warned of the addictive properties of the drug.[21]

Most inebriate asylums and addiction cure institutes treated all drug addiction, whereas others, such as Dr Jansen Mattison's Brooklyn Home for Habitues (opened in 1891), specialized in the treatment of opiate and cocaine addiction.[43] The inebriety literature of this period is filled with debates over whether medically supervised opiate withdrawal should be abrupt, rapid (over days), or sustained (over weeks and months). One also finds discussions of such contemporary issues as the problems of drug substitution and the management of the people who have a recurrence of use.[41]

Understanding of the potential physiological foundations and consequences of addiction increased during the last two decades of the 19th century. Carl Wernicke's 1881 discovery of a psychosis with polyneuritis that resulted from chronic alcoholism and Sergei Korsakoff's 1887 description of an alcoholism-induced psychosis characterized by confusion, memory impairment, confabulation, hallucinations, and stereotyped and superficial speech both underscored the potential organic basis of behavior in persons with chronic alcoholism. There was considerable discussion about the potential hereditary transmission of inebriety.[44]

The American Medical Temperance Association (AMTA) was founded in Washington, DC, in 1891 at the annual meeting of the American Medical Association (AMA). Dr N.S. Davis of Chicago was its founder and first president. The AMTA published the *Bulletin of the American Medical Temperance Association* under the editorship of Dr J.H. Kellogg, director of the Battle Creek Sanitarium.[45]

In summary, the field of addiction medicine experienced professionalization and specialization between 1830 and 1900. There were many addiction medicine pioneers who founded medically directed treatment institutions, men such as Turner, Parrish, Crothers, and Day and, later, Dr Agnes Sparks, one of the first female physicians specializing in addiction medicine. The practice of addiction medicine shifted from the private physician's practice to the institutional setting. Within this institutional practice, there was a growing understanding of the physiological consequences of chronic alcoholism and an extension of the concept of inebriety to embrace dependence upon opium, morphine, cocaine, chloral hydrate, chloroform, and ether. There was a well-articulated addiction disease concept with elaborate protocols for withdrawal management and rehabilitation, though there was considerable conflict between allopathic and homeopathic approaches to addiction treatment.

The growing field of addiction medicine was infused with optimism in the early 1890s. Dr T.D. Crothers proclaimed, "The future looks promising, and it is believed that the public will support inebriate asylums with increasing generosity."[46] There were reasons for Crothers' optimism. There was a new and feasible disease concept of inebriety and two addiction-related medical organizations that embraced a field that had grown from a handful of specialized treatment institutions in 1870 to several hundred by the turn of the century. But forces outside the medical profession that were stirring would drive a wedge between the physician and those addicted to alcohol and other drugs.

DEMEDICALIZATION AND THE COLLAPSE OF ADDICTION TREATMENT (1900-1935)

There was a further profusion of addiction medicine texts in the first decade of the 20th century: J.B. Mattison's *The Mattison Method in Morphinism: A Modern and Humane Treatment of the Morphine Disease*; T.D. Crothers' *The Drug Habits and Their Treatment*; T.D. Crothers' *Morphinism*; and George Cutten's *The Psychology of Alcoholism*. The proliferation of addiction literature could not hide the fact that America's response to alcohol and other drug problems was shifting. Between 1900 and 1920, addiction treatment institutions closed in great numbers in the wake of a weakened infrastructure of the field, rising therapeutic pessimism, economic austerity triggered by unexpected depressions, and a major shift in national policy. The country turned its gaze to state and national prohibition laws as the solution to alcohol and other drug-related problems.

As inebriate homes, asylums, and the private addiction cure institutes closed in tandem with the spread of local and state prohibition laws, persons with alcoholism were relegated to other institutions. These included the "foul wards" of large city hospitals, the back ward of aging state psychiatric asylums, and the local psychopathic hospital, all of which did everything possible to discourage admission for the treatment of alcoholism. Wealthy persons with alcoholism or other addiction sought discrete withdrawal management in a new genre of private hospitals or sanitariums. These latter institutions were known as "dip shops" (from *dipsomania*), "jitter joints," or "jag farms."[21] There were also efforts to integrate medicine, religion, and psychology in the treatment of alcoholism, most notably within the Emmanuel Clinics in New England.[47] For all but the most affluent, the management of alcoholism shifted from a strategy of treatment to a strategy of control and punishment via inebriate penal colonies. The large public hospitals also bore much of the responsibility for the medical care of chronic alcoholism.[48]

The shift from viewing the alcohol addicted person as a person with a disease in need of help to a person of weak character was reflected in the medical literature of the early 20th century. Kurtz and Kraepelin coined the term *alcohol addiction* to depict those whose will was "not strong enough to abandon the use of alcohol even if drinking causes them serious economic, social and somatic changes."[31] Addiction medicine organizations struggled in this shifting cultural climate. The AMTA and the American Association for the Study and Cure of Inebriety merged in 1904 to create the American Medical Society for the Study of Alcohol and Other Narcotics. In 1907, the *Journal of Inebriety* merged with *The Archives of Physiological Therapy*. This marked the progressive demise of both the *Journal of Inebriety* and its parent organization. The last issue of the *Journal of Inebriety* was published in 1914, and the American Association for the Study and Cure of Inebriety collapsed in the early 1920s after a subsequent sharp decline in demand for treatment after passage of The National Prohibition Act, also known as the Volstead Act, which promulgated prohibition in keeping with the 18th Amendment of the U.S. Constitution. Alcohol-related problems decreased dramatically in the early 1920s but rose to preprohibition levels by the late 1920s.[21] The 18th Amendment transferred cultural ownership of alcohol problems from physicians to law enforcement authorities. A similar process was underway with drugs other than alcohol, but it took two decades for this shift in approach to fully emerge.

Early 20th-century addiction texts by physicians such as George Pettey and Ernest Bishop boldly proclaimed that narcotic addiction was a disease, and Dr Foster Kennedy in 1914 declared that morphinism was "a disease, in the majority of cases, initiated, sustained and left uncured by members of the medical profession."[49-51] An early cohort of physicians had already begun operationalizing this addiction disease concept by advocating and offering clinic-directed withdrawal management and maintenance for persons with "incurable" narcotic addiction.[52-55] The medical treatment of persons addicted to narcotics was dramatically altered by passage of the Harrison Anti-Narcotic Act of 1914. This federal act designated physicians and pharmacists as the gatekeepers for the distribution of opioids and cocaine. Although this law was not presented as a prohibition law, a series of Supreme Court interpretations of the Harrison Act (particularly the 1919 *Webb v the United States* case) declared that for a physician to maintain a person with addiction on his or her customary dose is not "good faith" medical practice under the Harrison Act and therefore an indictable offense.[19]

Despite the federal mandate against prescribing narcotics to addicted persons, physicians in 44 communities operated morphine maintenance clinics between 1919 and 1924. These clinics, which were sponsored by local health departments and even local police departments, all eventually closed under the threat of federal indictment.[19-21] The Harrison Act, in effect if not intent, transferred responsibility for the care of addicted persons from physicians to criminal syndicates and the criminal justice system by threatening physicians with both loss of license and incarceration if they provided maintenance rather than rapid withdrawal management of addicted persons.[56]

Physician culpability in the problem of addiction to opioids made it difficult for the AMA to oppose this government infringement in medical practice. In 1919, the AMA passed a resolution opposing ambulatory treatment, in effect opposing narcotic maintenance as treatment. There were, however, many physicians who became harsh critics of the Harrison Act and this new era of criminalization. Such criticism was reflected in the new addiction medicine texts that emerged in the 1920s, such as Dr Ernest Bishop's *The Narcotic Drug Problem* and Dr E.H. Williams' *Opiate Addiction: Its Handling and Treatment*.[57-59]

The influence of psychiatry on the characterization and treatment of addiction increased in tandem with the decline of a specialized field of addiction medicine. Karl Abraham's 1908 essay, *The Psychological Relations between Sexuality and Alcoholism*, marked the shift from seeing alcoholism as a primary medical disorder to seeing the condition as a symptom of underlying psychiatric disturbance.[60] Abraham's essay marked a long series of psychoanalytic writings that viewed alcoholism as a manifestation of latent homosexuality. In the mid-1920s, a Public Health Service psychiatrist, Dr Lawrence Kolb, published a series of articles challenging earlier physiological explanations of narcotic addiction. Kolb portrayed addiction as a product of defects in personality—a characterization that reflected the growing portrayal of addicted persons as psychopathic and constitutionally inferior.[61] The first American Standard Classified Nomenclature of Disease (1933) included the diagnoses of "alcohol addiction," "alcoholism without psychosis," and "drug addiction" and classified these conditions as personality disorders.[62]

Few institutional resources existed for the treatment of alcoholism and narcotic addiction during the 1920s and early 1930s, but the growing visibility of these problems began to generate new proposals for their management. The opening of the California Narcotics Hospital at Spadra in 1928 marked the beginning of state support for addiction treatment.[63] Physicians working within the federal prison system were writing about the problems posed by a growing population of incarcerated persons with addiction and advocating more specialized treatment of these individuals.[64]

There were important addiction-related research studies in the 1920s. Drs Arthur B. Light and Edward G. Torrance conducted research on opioid addiction at the Philadelphia General Hospital under the auspices of the Philadelphia Committee for the Clinical Study of Opium Addiction Research. They demonstrated that withdrawal from opiates is not life-threatening and usually not dangerous—a finding that was misused by policy makers to withhold medical care for persons addicted to opioids.[65] In 1928, the Bureau of Social Hygiene published Charles Terry and Mildred Pellens' work, *The Opium Problem*.[66] In this important report, Terry and Pellens made a strong argument in favor of opioid maintenance therapy as the most appropriate treatment for persons not able to sustain abstinence. Their views were viciously attacked, and it would only be years later that *The Opium Problem* would be recognized as one of the best treatises on opiate addiction ever written.[54]

Medical treatments for addiction to narcotics in the first three decades of the 20th century continued to focus on managing the mechanics of narcotic withdrawal. Heroin was briefly used for withdrawal management from morphine, and its subsequent emergence as the drug of preference among opioid addicted persons bred caution in the choice of any narcotic as a withdrawal agent. This fear of exposing patients to other addicting agents led to the experimentation with a wide variety of nonnarcotic withdrawal procedures. These procedures included various belladonna treatments (scopolamine and hyoscine) that were known to induce hallucinations, peptization treatments (sodium thiocyanate) that could induce long-lasting psychosis, sleep treatments (sodium bromide) that had a 20% mortality rate, injected Narcosan, a lipoid treatment thought to eliminate toxins and stimulate new blood formation but which actually worsened withdrawal, insulin treatments that had no effect on the withdrawal process, and serum and blood therapies in which either previously drawn blood or serum (the latter drawn from induced blisters) was reinjected as a purported aid to withdrawal management.[67-69]

The first decades of the 20th century were marked by a profound therapeutic pessimism regarding treatment of alcoholism and narcotic addiction. Biological views of addiction fell out of favor and were replaced by psychiatric and criminal models that placed the source of addiction within the addicted persons' character and argued for control and sequestration of this group.

THE REBIRTH OF ADDICTION TREATMENT (1935-1970)

After the early 20th-century collapse of systems of care for those addicted to alcohol and other drugs, addiction medicine was revived within the larger context of two movements.

The "modern alcoholism movement" was ignited by the founding of Alcoholics Anonymous (1935), a new scientific approach to alcohol problems in postrepeal America led by the Research Council on Problems of Alcohol (1937) and the Yale Center of Alcohol Studies (1943) and by a national recovery advocacy effort led by the National Committee for Education on Alcoholism (1944). Two goals of this movement were to encourage local hospitals to manage the withdrawal from use of alcohol-dependent patients and to encourage local communities to establish post hospitalization alcoholism rehabilitation centers.[70] The establishment of a successful community-based noninstitutional mutual support organization for alcohol use disorders, Alcoholic Anonymous, was cofounded by Dr Robert Smith, a physician in recovery from severe alcohol dependence. This "12-step" prototype and burgeoning movement of broader institutional and community attention to alcoholism spawned new resources for treatment from the mid-1940s through the 1960s, including "AA wards" in local hospitals, model outpatient clinics for alcoholism developed in Connecticut and Georgia, and a community-based residential model pioneered by three alcoholism programs in Minnesota: Pioneer House (1948), Hazelden (1949), and Willmar State Hospital (1950). Dr Nelson Bradley, who led the developments at Willmar, later adapted the Minnesota Model for delivery within a community hospital. That adapted model was franchised throughout the United States in the 1980s via Parkside Medical Services[71] and was replicated by innumerable hospital-based treatment programs.

The spread of these models nationally was aided by efforts to legitimize the work of physicians in the treatment of alcoholism. Early milestones in this movement included landmark resolutions on alcoholism passed by the AMA (1952, 1956, 1967) and the American Hospital Association (1944, 1951, 1957) that paved the way for hospital-based treatment of alcoholism. The former were championed by Dr Marvin Block, chairman of the AMA's first Committee on Alcoholism. Midcentury alcoholism treatments included nutritional therapies, brief experiments with chemical and electroconvulsive therapies, psychosurgery, and new drug therapies, including the use of disulfiram, stimulants, sedatives, tranquilizers, and lysergic acid diethylamide (LSD).[21]

A mid–20th-century reform movement advocating medical rather than penal treatment of the person opioid-addiction also helped spawn the rebirth of addiction medicine. This began with the founding of state-sponsored addiction treatment hospitals and led to the creation of two U.S. Public Health Hospitals within the Bureau of Prisons—one in Lexington, Kentucky (1935), and the other in Fort Worth, Texas (1938). Many of the pioneers of modern addiction medicine and addiction research—Drs Marie Nyswander, Jerry Jaffe, George Vaillant, and Patrick Hughes—received their initial training at these facilities. The documentation of substance recurrence rates after community reentry from Lexington and Fort Worth confirmed the need for community-based treatment. Three replicable models of treatment emerged: therapeutic communities directed by persons in sustained recovery, methadone maintenance pioneered by Drs Vincent Dole and Marie Nyswander, and outpatient drug-free counseling.[21]

State and federal funding for alcoholism and addiction treatment slowly increased from the late 1940s through the 1960s and was followed by landmark legislation in the early 1970s that created the National Institute on Alcohol Abuse and Alcoholism (NIAAA) and the National Institute on Drug Abuse (NIDA)—the beginning of the federal, state, and local community partnership that has been the foundation of modern addiction treatment. Parallel efforts were under way to provide insurance coverage for the treatment of alcoholism and other drug dependencies. The expansion of such insurance coverage in the 1960s and 1970s and the establishment of accreditation standards for addiction treatment programs by the Joint Commission on Accreditation of Hospitals set the stage for the dramatic growth of hospital-based and freestanding, private addiction treatment programs in the 1980s. NIAAA and NIDA also made heavy investments in research that led to dramatic breakthroughs in understanding the neurobiology of addiction that encouraged more medicalized approaches to severe alcohol and other drug problems.[72]

The growing sophistication of addiction science was aided by other key organizations. The College on Problems of Drug Dependence, which dates from the Committee on Problems of Drug Dependence established in 1929, hosts an annual scientific meeting and publishes the journal *Drug and Alcohol Dependence*. The Research Society on Alcoholism, founded in 1976, also holds an annual scientific conference and publishes the journal *Alcoholism: Clinical and Experimental Research*.

ADDICTION MEDICINE COMES OF AGE (1970-2023)

Many factors were involved with the modernization of organized addiction medicine practice. Insights from basic, clinical, and epidemiological science and the availability of evidence-based prevention and treatment interventions provided new understanding and tools. The pioneering brain imaging studies of Volkow and others[73] demonstrated even to the casual observer that addiction was more than a moral failing, behavioral, or criminal problem. Elucidating the addicted brain neurocircuitry also suggested prevention and intervention strategies. These imaging studies added to the emerging consensus that substance use disorder is a unified etiological and diagnostic disease state and that sub classifications based on the particular substances used, although useful, are insufficient. A further insight from neuroimaging is that so-called behavioral addiction, such as gambling and some eating disorders, appears to involve the same brain neurocircuitry as addictive substances. Thus, these disorders, which represent significant medical and public health problems, are being increasingly addressed by physician addiction specialists. Another example of cross-substance commonality is the early work of Dr Heather Ashton[74] who through close clinical attention described in detail a protracted withdrawal syndrome from benzodiazepines. This was followed by reports of an often-similar protracted withdrawal syndrome from other substance classes. Perhaps the cap to the unified theory of addiction came from the Nobel Laureate Dr Paul Greengard, who was able to demonstrate the role of the protein DARPP-32 in the actions of multiple dependence producing drugs.[75] Finally, the unified view of substance use disorders is exemplified in the 2016 Surgeon General's Report on Alcohol, Drugs, and Health: Facing Addiction in America.[76] Previous U.S. Surgeon General Reports had focused only on tobacco/nicotine, and most reports from the National Institutes of Health were also substance specific. In the 2016 report, Surgeon General Vivek Murthy addressed *all* nontobacco/nicotine substances (there were two recent tobacco/nicotine and health reports, in 2014 and 2016).

Also occurring and adding to a shift in appreciation for drugs in American culture has been a series of highly visible American drug use crises and controversies with which society and medicine have had serial struggles: heroin use by U.S. soldiers in Vietnam, the powder and crack cocaine epidemics, the national methamphetamine epidemic, and scientific and public consideration of tobacco and cannabis use. Perhaps no substance use disorder better represents the potential for the critical role of medicine and physicians in attenuating substance use harm as that of tobacco use over the last 60 years. The direct medical consequences of tobacco use are still responsible for more than 480,000 annual deaths in America. Yet, beginning with the first Surgeon General's Report on Tobacco in 1964 and carrying through this last decade, both the prevalence of tobacco use and the public's acceptance of it has plummeted. Contrasting with this is the changing status of cannabis from an illegal to a legal substance in some states and even as cannabis used as treatment made legal legislatively. As we bring this history to the present, it must unfortunately be noted that beginning in the 1990s, another devastating prescription opioid epidemic began its sweep across America. Illicitly manufactured, powder fentanyl then emerged as other opioids became difficult to acquire. Illicit fentanyl, and other high potency synthetic opioids, are cut into illicit substances and pressed into fake pills to engage the individuals who use substances and who are accustomed to buying diverted prescription medications. For this century's opioid epidemic, still raging at the time this chapter was written, the words of Dr Foster Kennedy 100 years ago are worth repeating. Opioid addiction is, he said, "a disease, in the majority of cases, initiated, sustained and left uncured by members of the medical profession." Whereas physician complicity in the previous opioid epidemic made it difficult for organized medicine to oppose a criminal justice solution in the early 1900s, in 2016-2017, modern organized medicine responded by addressing the role of physicians in the modern opioid epidemic by advancing physician credentialing and training in addiction medicine. Thus, the current response of medicine brought physicians into the solution, rather than defaulting to a historically flawed and ineffective criminal justice approach. This response helped usher addiction medicine into new relevance and importance in medicine and public health.

ORGANIZED ADDICTION MEDICINE TODAY

Addiction medicine as an organized subspecialty of medical practice has been significantly advanced by five entities: the American Society of Addiction Medicine (ASAM), The American Academy of Addiction Psychiatry, the American Board of Addiction Medicine (ABAM), The American College of Academic Addiction Medicine (ACAAM, formerly the Addiction Medicine Foundation [TAMF]), and The American Board of Preventive Medicine (ABPM).

The American Society of Addiction Medicine

The American Society of Addiction Medicine can trace its roots to the establishment of the New York City Medical Committee on Alcoholism in 1951 and the 1954 founding of the New York State Medical Society on Alcoholism under the leadership of Dr Ruth Fox, which in 1967 established itself as a national organization—the American Medical Society on Alcoholism (AMSA). AMSA evolved into the AMSA and Other Drug Dependencies and then into ASAM.

ASAM's achievements include:

- Offering the first national certification and recertification process for addiction medicine.
- Hosting its Annual Medical–Scientific Conference, State of the Art Course, Review Course, and a variety of other continuing education courses.
- Publishing *The Principles of Addiction Medicine*, now in its seventh edition; *The Essentials of Addiction Medicine*, now in its third edition; Publishing first the *Journal of Addictive Diseases* and presently the *Journal of Addiction Medicine*.
- Effectively advocating for national policies to broaden access to care.
- Creation of *The ASAM Standards of Care for the Addiction Specialist Physician*.

The American Academy of Addiction Psychiatrists

The AAAP (formerly the American Academy of Psychiatrists in Alcoholism and the Addictions) was established in 1985 with the goal of elevating the quality of clinical practice in addiction psychiatry. The AAAP's contributions include successfully advocating that the American Board of Psychiatry and Neurology grant addiction psychiatry (ADP) subspecialty status (1991) to psychiatrists who meet the eligibility criteria and administering an ADP certification and maintenance of certification (MOC) process. As of 2021, there were 1,393 ABPN diplomates holding active subspecialty certification in ADP, with an annual average of 35 new certificants from 2011 through 2021.

The American Board of Addiction Medicine

By 2006, ASAM had held as an organizational priority for nearly three decades the acceptance of addiction medicine within the "House of Medicine"—recognition of the field by the American Board of Medical Specialties (ABMS). On three occasions since the 1980s, ASAM explored pathways for bringing addiction medicine forward through formal recognition as a specialized field of practice by the ABMS. Recognition by ABMS of a subspecialty indicates special expertise is necessary to practice in the field. Certification of a physician by an ABMS member board signifies that the physician has achieved the highest measurable American standard for competency in a field. The ASAM Directors believed that ABMS recognition was critical in bringing the field to its greatest benefit in advancing patient care and the public health. The ASAM leadership understood that if patients were to have access to qualified addiction medicine physicians and that if health systems and insurers were to offer and compensate addiction medicine services, then training and credentialing standards would need to be established as they are for other medical fields. Addiction medicine would thus have to become an ABMS and Accreditation Council for Graduate Medical Education (ACGME) recognized field for physician certification and training.

ASAM was aware that the newly incorporated American Board of Addiction Medicine (ABAM) would work to gain recognition by ABMS and thus launch the field into full membership and participation in American medicine and health care, setting the stage for the availability of prevention and treatment services by identifiable, qualified physicians. ABMS recognition would bring four critical avenues of parity to the prevention and treatment of unhealthy substance use and addiction: availability of addiction prevention and care services equivalent to those of other disease states, availability of physicians who can attend to these medical conditions, patient payment coverage for addiction medicine services through third parties on par with other conditions, and reimbursement to physicians, systems, and others who provide specialized addiction medicine services. Without parity in these dimensions, patients with unhealthy substance use and addiction would not benefit from the many available evidence-based prevention and treatment modalities catalogued in other chapters of this text.

The American Board of Addiction Medicine—a freestanding and independent organization—was incorporated in 2007 as a nonprofit entity for the purposes of promoting the public welfare by contributing to the improvement of the quality of care in the medical specialty of addiction medicine, establishing and maintaining standards of excellence in the field, establishing and maintaining standards and procedures for certification and MOC, granting to qualified physicians documents certifying that they are Diplomates of the Board, granting and issuing other documentation of recognition of special knowledge and skills in addiction medicine, suspending or revoking diplomate certificates, serve the public, physicians, hospitals, and other health care organizations by furnishing lists of the Diplomates of the Board, and communicating to and with health professional and relevant organizations the importance of the standards, certification, and practice in addiction medicine as a means to confirm and advance the quality of care received by patients with substance use disorders.

In 2009, ASAM transferred its addiction medicine certification examination to ABAM. The ABAM Credentials Committee set the exam eligibility criteria to be consistent with the other national licensure, training, and experience requirements. The ABAM certification examination was continuously updated by collaboration between the National Board of Medical Examiners (NBME) and the ABAM Examination Committee. Clinical relevance was added to the evaluation process for all questions, and the committee was enlarged to assure that the content of the examination reflected the range of issues faced by addiction medicine physicians, including medical and psychiatric complications, observed across all medical specialties. Committee members included physicians from the specialties most usually encountering substance use disorders and their complications and basic and clinical scientists. Applicants for the examination were accepted from all medical specialties, with significant representation from family medicine, internal medicine and psychiatry. ABAM certified just over 4,000 physicians between 2009 and 2016.

As noted above, certification of physicians by an ABMS member board and The Accreditation Council for Graduate Medical Education (ACGME) accreditation of postgraduate physician training (residencies and fellowships) are the highest standards of measurement for physician competencies and training in a field. Acquisition of these recognitions is an acknowledgment that the field is meeting the highest available training and practice certification standards, thus expanding the pool of physicians who can provide high quality specialty care to patients with substance use disorders. Thus, the goals of gaining ABMS level certification of physicians who practice addiction medicine and accreditation of addiction medicine fellowships by the ACGME were critical to advancing the field. ABMS board certification in addiction medicine could become available to physicians of all specialties, adding substantially to the available number of certified psychiatrists in addiction psychiatry

The ABAM certification and Maintenance of Certification processes were developed and executed in the format of and with the standards promulgated by ABMS, thus setting up the recognition of the field within this room of the "House of Medicine."

With the formal ABMS recognition of addiction medicine in 2016, ABAM discontinued its certification exam, to be administered in the future by the ABMS member board, the ABPM.

The American College of Academic Addiction Medicine

The American College of Academic Addiction Medicine (ACAAM, formerly the ABAM Foundation and The Addiction Medicine Foundation or TAMF) was incorporated in 2007 as a nonprofit entity to support the advance of addiction medicine through (1) defining the field of addiction medicine and developing and accrediting addiction medicine fellowships, (2) advancing eventual ABMS and ACGME recognition of addiction medicine, (3) promoting prevention as a core principle for the field, and (4) aligning key stakeholders in medicine, government, philanthropy, and public health in collaborative activities to more successfully address substance use disorders and their sequelae, and to serve as an academic association for fellowships and board-certified practitioners of addiction medicine.

Defining the Field

In July 2010, ACAAM held a retreat attended by representatives of government, academic medical education, prevention, treatment, and research organizations in the field, directors of fellowship programs in addiction medicine, addiction psychiatry, internal medicine, family medicine, and pediatrics, clinicians and trainees (residents), and clinicians in these and other specialties, including pain medicine. The purpose of the meeting was to construct the documents that define addiction medicine and its training programs. Core documents of a new field include the core competencies, educational objectives, core content, scope of practice, training program requirements, and training program accreditation policies and procedures.

The documents produced include the Addiction Medicine Scope of Practice, Addiction Medicine Core Content, and the Core Competencies for Addiction Medicine: Compendium of Educational Objectives for Addiction Medicine Fellowship Training Program Requirements for Graduate Medical Education in Addiction Medicine, and the Program Accreditation Application Form.

Accredited Addiction Medicine Fellowships

The American College of Academic Addiction Medicine fostered the development of the nation's first addiction medicine fellowship programs, and their eventual accreditation by The Accreditation Council of Graduate Medical Education (ACGME). As of July, 2022, ACGME has accredited 93 addiction medicine fellowships. Graduated fellows are majority family medicine physicians and internists yet include pediatricians, psychiatrists, obstetrician-gynecologists, preventive medicine physicians, anesthesiologists, and others. The program directors are primarily family medicine physicians, internists, and psychiatrists.

As of 2022 approximately two dozen of the 93 ACGME fellowship programs had a parallel addiction psychiatry fellowship at their institution. A preliminary survey of graduated fellows indicated that (1) the majority are internists and family medicine physicians, (2) fellows were generally young career physicians, usually entering the fellowship within 10 years of completing a primary residency, (3) fellows had a high likelihood of remaining at the institution they trained in and in the state where they trained, and (4) the numbers of female and male fellows were almost equal, a contrast to the existing pool of ABAM diplomates who are mostly male. (Private communication with Mr Andrew Danzo, Fellowship Specialist, ACAAM, 2022).

A problem not unique to fellowships in a new field was encountered: securing funding for the start-up and expansion of accredited fellowship positions. At the state and local level this was spearheaded by fellowship directors who sought institutional, state and federal funding. At the national level, after a number of milestone grants were awarded from NIAAA, NIDA and philanthropies, a 10-year effort seeking federal legislative and agency support resulted in a $1,000,000 grant award from HRSA in 2020.

ACAAM has estimated that 125 addiction medicine fellowships will be needed to train an adequate workforce of addiction medicine subspecialists.

ACAAM continues to serve as the home of academic addiction medicine. Its mission is to promote academic excellence and inspire leadership in addiction medicine with a vision of providing high-quality equitable prevention and care for all. The organization values are: excellence, leadership, social justice, integrity and equity. ACAAM provides support to ACGME fellowships and credentialed faculty, promotes high standards and evidence-informed science free of outside influence or bias, promotes integration and teaching of an addiction medicine curriculum in all medical schools and residencies, represents the interests of academic addiction medicine to stakeholders, including the public, and advances a formal presence of addiction medicine across medicine and health care.

After the transfer of physician credentialing to ABMS and fellowship accreditation to ACGME, ACAAM has continued to serve as the central organization for academic addiction medicine. Its most popular activities include providing weekly evidence-based didactic fellowship and specialists sessions, bringing fellowships together for issues of mutual interest (ie, serving as the sponsor for the first National Residency Matching Program addiction medicine match for the 2023-2024 academic year), and convening regional and national gatherings of fellows, faculty fellowship staff, and board-certified addiction medicine physicians.

The American Board of Preventive Medicine: Home to Addiction Medicine

The early successes of the newly revitalized field of addiction medicine led to optimism that an enduring new medical field of medical practice could be firmly established.[77]

In 2014 at the request of ACAAM, the ABPM, an ABMS member board, agreed to review the readiness of the field to acquire ABMS recognition, possibly through the sponsorship of the ABPM. For acceptance as an ABMS field, addiction medicine would have to demonstrate a sufficient group of credentialed physicians practicing in the field, a complete set of addiction medicine competencies and educational content, detailed program requirements for fellowship accreditation, a sufficient number of established fellowships, and the support of multiple medical and public health organizations, associations, and academic medical institutions. With these prerequisites met, ABPM began the process of seeking ABMS recognition of the field. In May 2015, ABPM's President, Dr Denece Kesler, submitted to ABMS an application for the new field, and in March 2016, ABMS announced recognition of addiction medicine as a multispecialty subspecialty.

The first annual ABPM addiction medicine certifying exam, open to current ABMS diplomates from any field, was administered in October 2017. Thirteen hundred (1,300) physicians passed the exam and became the first ABMS level diplomates in the new field: by 2023 there were 4,420 diplomates.[78] During the initial years of the ABPM certification exam being administered, "time in practice" in the field of addiction medicine is an alternative to fellowship training (through 2025). Known as the ABPM Practice Pathway, applicants without a fellowship who could demonstrate sufficient practice time in addiction medicine—at least 1920 hours over the previous 5 years—as well as meeting other eligibility criteria can take the certification exam without completing an addiction medicine fellowship.

With the transition of certification in addiction medicine passing from ABAM to ABPM, ABAM no longer offered a certification exam. The American Osteopathic Association (AOA) also now offers addiction medicine certification by examination and through a similar "practice pathway."

Transition to Accreditation of Addiction Medicine Fellowships by the Accreditation Council for Graduate Medical Education

In December 2015, ABPM submitted an application to the Accreditation Council for Graduate Medical Education (ACGME) for recognition of addiction medicine as a field for which fellowship training could be accredited by ACGME. ACGME "is an independent, not-for-profit, physician-led organization that sets and monitors the professional educational standards essential in preparing physicians to deliver safe, high-quality medical care to all Americans."[79] ACGME is the "gold standard" accreditation of all postmedical school physician training in the United States. As noted above, there are now 93 addiction medicine fellowships, which are ACGME accredited and there are an additional 9 that are ACAAM accredited, pending transition to ACGME accreditation.

In June 2016, ACGME initiated the process to offer accreditation to addiction medicine fellowship training programs. The first programs applied for accreditation in early 2018. Concurrent with ACGME-accreditation becoming available, TAMF stopped accrediting new programs and instead encourages and assists interested institutions to obtain ACGME accreditation. As of 2023, there are currently 93 ACGME accredited addiction medicine fellowships across the United States, from as far east as Bayamón, Puerto Rico, and as far west as Honolulu, Hawaii.

Federal Collaboration and AMERSA

Finally, several other historical initiatives should be mentioned that have advanced addiction-related medical education.

ACAAM, immediately after it's incorporation, initiated a relationship with the Office of National Drug Control Policy (ONDCP) and this has continued through the most recent 4 administrations, providing education on the field of addiction medicine and the positive impact it can have on the health of the nation. Through ONDCP, the leadership of the field was able to collaborate with other agencies, such as HRSA and SAMSHA, to advance the care of patients with substance use disorders and the training of physicians in addiction medicine.

The NIAAA and the NIDA have been a continuous force in the field since their establishment, bringing state and federal government and academic and community physicians into effective collaborative partnerships. In 1971, these institutes created the Career Teacher Program (1971-1981) that developed addiction-related curricula for the training of physicians in 59 US medical schools.

In 1976, career teachers and others involved in addiction-related medical education and research established the Association for Multidisciplinary Education and Research in Substance use and Addictions (AMERSA). AMERSA has expanded from the small group of founding physicians to membership that represents the various disciplines that make up interdisciplinary teams in the prevention, intervention, treatment, and recovery support for persons across the continuum of substance use. AMERSA's mission is to improve health and well-being through leadership and advocacy in substance use education, research, clinical care and policy. AMERSA hosts an annual conference and publishes the journal, *Substance Abuse*.

HISTORIC RACISM, DISCRIMINATORY LAWS AND POLICIES AND THE IMPORTANCE OF ANTI-RACISM, DIVERSITY, EQUITY, AND INCLUSION

As with so much of society, and virtually all fields in medicine and health care, addiction medicine has an unfortunate and sad history of neglect for "invisible" patient populations and systemically marginalized persons. It is of course impossible in the United Sates today to be unaware of the extraordinary moral and social costs of these omissions.

Racism is a normative experience for minoritized populations in the United States. While minoritized and marginalized populations use substances at rates similar to White individuals, minoritized populations have been and are more likely to experience more severe consequences due to their substance use. Compared to their White counterparts, Black, Latinx, and Indigenous American/Alaska Native populations experience greater mortality rates from substance use, greater severity of substance use disorders, and increased vulnerability to criminal justice system involvement. Black and Latinx populations, in particular, have more significant barriers accessing and completing substance use treatment and fewer minoritized individuals report satisfactory experiences within substance use treatment than Whites. These disparities are driven by long-existing intersectional racism and drug-related stigma. Structural racism is manifested in unequal enforcement of drug laws, lower access to evidence-based treatments, and greater odds of experiencing adverse substance-related health outcomes among minoritized and marginalized populations. Structural violence is expressed through stigma enacted against people with substance use disorders and through policies that disqualify people with substance use histories from access to public services, employment, education, and housing. These policies contribute to the poor outcomes and health disparities seen among minoritized populations with substance use disorders.

Minoritized populations experience discrimination at every stage of the judicial system and are more likely to be stopped, searched, arrested, convicted, harshly sentenced and/or burdened with a lifelong criminal record. This is particularly the case for drug law violations.[80,81] Although Black people comprise 13% of the U.S. population[82,83] and use drugs at similar rates to people of other races,[84,85] Black people comprise 29% of those arrested for drug law violations,[86] and nearly 40% of those incarcerated in state or federal prison for drug law violations.[87] With less than 5% of the world's population, but over 20% of its incarcerated population, the United States imprisons more people than any other nation in the world.[87] Racialized drug policies with harsh and disparate sentencing requirements have led to profoundly unequal criminal justice outcomes for minoritized populations with substance use disorders. Although rates of drug use and sales are similar across racial and ethnic lines, Black and Latinx individuals are far more likely to have criminal justice involvement and experience stricter consequences compared to White individuals.[80-81, 84-85, 87-90]

American history has a legacy of discriminatory laws and policies driven by unjust practices and institutional racism, which contribute to disparities for minoritized populations with substance use and substance use disorders. One of many examples, was the motivation to pass a tax on cannabis through the Marijuana Tax Act-1937. This was not solely a public health effort to decrease drug use but was instead motivated by widespread racial discrimination against Mexican-Americans and Black populations and a way to penalize these populations.[91]

The U.S. "war on drugs" began in 1971. This ineffective, counterproductive effort had its origin in social and political racism. America has criminalized specific drug classes since the 1875 anti-opium law in San Francisco. In that instance, the law was aimed at immigrant Chinese neighborhoods.

In 1994 a Nixon deputy, John Erlichman, stated: "The Nixon campaign in 1968, and the Nixon White House after that, had two enemies: the antiwar left and Black people. We knew we couldn't make it illegal to be either against the war or Black, but by getting the public to associate the hippies with cannabis and Blacks with heroin, and then criminalizing both heavily, we could disrupt those communities. We could arrest their leaders, raid their homes, break up their meetings, and vilify them night after night on the evening news. Did we know we were lying about the drugs? Of course we did."[92]

One of most widely cited examples of structural racism in federal policy around drugs are the mandatory minimum sentencing laws widely adopted in the 1980s and 1990s. The disparate sentencing requirements written into these laws codified structural racism into judicial policy and contributed greatly to escalating incarceration rates for minoritized individuals.[93] Prompted by the death of Len Bias, a basketball star who died from what was believed to be a crack cocaine overdose days after being drafted into the NBA, Congress passed and President Reagan signed into law the Anti-Drug Abuse Act. Federal laws required the same mandatory prison sentence for five grams of crack cocaine as 500 g of powder cocaine. The 100-to-1 sentencing disparity between crack and power cocaine were not informed by any public safety or public health benefits. Over the years, this sentencing disparity served to propagate racial disparities in the criminal justice system and increased mass incarceration rates, particularly among Black communities.

The ongoing consequences from these policies drive not only mass incarceration, but also perpetuate differential racial access to employment, business loans, licensing, student aid, public housing and other public assistance often denied to individuals with incarceration histories. Drug convictions, separate from jail or prison time, often leads to a lifelong ban on accessing many social, economic and political benefits, such as voting.[94]

Organized addiction medicine now has taken several key steps in outlining a path to the future that recognizes the importance of a workforce that not only understands the unique needs and lived experiences of the multiple populations we serve, but that also mirrors the patient populations for whom we provide care. There is now a push to transform the substance use prevention and treatment system to meet the needs of affected individuals in the spaces and communities where they reside. With a new historic and real-time perspective there is momentum to address the lack of racial, ethnic, language and cultural diversity within our institutions and training programs and to develop a robust workforce able to effectively care for minoritized and marginalized populations.[95] Moreover, we are moving from the past default acceptance to tailor the provision of addiction-related care to address the differential access among minoritized populations to social determinants of health that constrain access to substance use treatment and early intervention services. The historic failure to support efforts to decriminalize substance use disorders as a means to better support and engage individuals in treatment is currently a new and broadly accepted goal of addiction medicine. In order to reduce health disparities and overcome past deficits, we must identify and promote the delivery of innovative services that acknowledge a patient's needs and preferences, and also understand and address the social context and social needs of their substance use.[96] The American College of Academic Addiction Medicine (ACAAM), the American Society of Addition Medicine (ASAM) and AMERSA have developed policies and position statements that serve as models for addressing these gaps and ensuring that there is accountability and standards to ensure our own field takes action steps to address the important and emerging transformation in the field that is occurring.[97]

This textbook contains chapters that directly address racism and social disparities of heath–Chapters 38 and 49.

FUTURE STATUS OF ORGANIZED ADDICTION MEDICINE IN AMERICA

As this history has reviewed, addiction medicine rose in the United States in the mid-19th century, collapsed in the opening decades of the 20th century, yet reemerged and became increasingly professionalized in the late 20th century. Now, 23 years in to the 21st century, addiction medicine has been formally recognized and accepted within the "House of Medicine." The field is now positioned to integrate prevention, treatment and recovery support for unhealthy substance use and addiction into health care and public health systems nationally. Concurrent with this recognition of addiction medicine into the fabric of American health care has been the tragic rise of the "Opioid Crisis" reflected in the escalating overdose mortality across some 40+ years.[98] Fentanyl and fentanyl-analogues are increasingly implicated in the majority of opioid overdose deaths, vaping use among adolescents is at historic highs, and tobacco remains a major cause of premature mortality. It is a certainty that other reformulated or novel addictive substances will continue to appear. As this edition is being published, one example stands out: the addition of the veterinary tranquilizer xylazine to illicit opioids. Fortunately modern addiction medicine has organized itself and stands ready to address these issues in real time.

REFERENCES

1. Crothers TD. *The Disease of Inebriety From Alcohol, Opium and Other Narcotic Drugs: Its Etiology, Pathology, Treatment and Medico-legal Relations*. E.B. Treat Publisher; 1893.
2. Mancall P. *Deadly Medicine: Indians and Alcohol in Early America*. Cornell University Press; 1995.
3. Unrau W. *White Man's Wicked Water: The Alcohol Trade and Prohibition in Indian Country, 1802–1892*. University Press of Kansas; 1996.
4. Coyhis D, White W. *Alcohol Problems in Native America: The Untold Story of Resistance and Recovery*. White Bison; 2006.
5. Lender M, Martin J. *Drinking in America*. The Free Press; 1982.
6. Rorabaugh W. *The Alcoholic Republic: An American Tradition*. Oxford University Press; 1979.
7. Winkler AM. Drinking on the American frontier. *Q J Stud Alcohol*. 1968;29:413-445.
8. Levine H. The discovery of addiction: changing conceptions of habitual drunkenness in America. *J Stud Alcohol*. 1978;39(2):143-174.
9. Benezet A. *A Lover of Mankind. Mighty Destroyer Displayed in Some Account, of the Dreadful Havock Made by the Mistaken Use as Well as Abuse of Distilled Spirituous Liquors*. Joseph Crukshank; 1774.
10. Rush B. *An Inquiry Into the Effect of Ardent Spirits Upon the Human Body and Mind, With an Account of the Means of Preventing and of the Remedies for Curing Them*. 8th rev. ed. E. Merriam & Co; 1814.
11. Rush B. Plan for an asylum for drunkards to be called the Sober House. In: Corner G, ed. *The Autobiography of Benjamin Rush*. Princeton University Press; 1948.
12. Trotter T. *An Essay, Medical, Philosophical, and Chemical, on Drunkenness and its Effects on the Human Body*. University of Edinburgh; 1788.
13. Romano J. Early contributions to the study of delirium tremens. *Ann Med Hist*. 1941;3:128-139.
14. Drake D. A discourse on intemperance. In: Grob G, ed. *Nineteenth Century Medical Attitudes Toward Alcohol Addiction*. Arno Press; 1981:54.
15. Sweetser W. A dissertation on intemperance. In: Grob G, ed. *Nineteenth Century Medical Attitudes Toward Alcohol Addiction*. Arno Press; 1981.
16. Beecher L. *Six Sermons on the Nature, Occasions, Signs, Evils and Remedy of Intemperance*. 3rd ed. T.R. Martin; 1828.
17. Sonnedecker G. Emergence of the concept of opiate addiction. *J Mondial Pharm*. 1962;3:275-290.
18. Jones J. *The Mysteries of the Opium Reveal'd*. Printed for Richard Smith; 1701.
19. Musto D. *The American Disease: Origins of Narcotic Controls*. Yale University Press; 1973.
20. Howard-Jones N. A critical study of the origins and early development of hypodermic medication. *J Hist Med*. 1947;2(2):201-249.
21. White W. *Slaying the Dragon: The History of Addiction Treatment and Recovery in America*. Chestnut Health Systems; 1998.
22. Woodward SB. Essays on asylums for inebriates (1836). In: Grog G, ed. *Nineteenth-century Medical Attitudes Toward Alcohol Addiction*. Arno Press; 1981.
23. Blair H. *The Temperance Movement*. William E. Smythe Company; 1888.
24. Bynum W. Chronic alcoholism in the first half of the 19th century. *Bull Hist Med*. 1968;42:160-185.
25. Wilkerson A. *A History of the Concept of Alcoholism as a Disease* [DSW dissertation]. University of Pennsylvania; 1966.
26. MacNish R. *Anatomy of Drunkenness*. William Pearson & Co; 1835.
27. Paredes A. The history of the concept of alcoholism. In: Tarter R, Sugerman A, eds. *Alcoholism: Interdisciplinary Approaches to an Enduring Problem*. 3rd ed. Addison-Wesley; 1976:9-52.
28. Grindrod R. *Bacchus: An Essay on the Nature, Causes, Effects and Cure of Intemperance*. J & H Langley; 1840.
29. Hargreaves W. *Alcohol and Science*. National Temperance Society and Publication House; 1884.
30. Huss M. *Alcoholismus Chronicus: Chronisk Alcoholisjudkom: Ett Bidrag Till Dyskrasiarnas Känndom*. Bonner/Norstedt; 1849.
31. Marconi J. The concept of alcoholism. *Q J Stud Alcohol*. 1959;20(2):216-235.
32. Baumohl J, Room R. Inebriety, doctors, and the state: alcoholism treatment institutions before 1940. In: Galanter M, ed. *Recent Developments in Alcoholism*. Vol. 5. Plenum Publishing; 1987:135-174.
33. Turner J. *History of the First Inebriate Asylum in the World*. Privately printed; 1888.
34. Crowley J, White W. *Drunkard's Refuge: The Lessons of the New York Inebriate Asylum*. University of Massachusetts Press; 2004.
35. Crothers TD. Reformed men as asylum managers. *J Inebriety*. 1897;19(79):897.
36. White WL. The role of recovering physicians in 19th century addiction medicine: an organizational case study. *J Addict Dis*. 1999;19(2):1-10.
37. Dana C. A study of alcoholism as it occurs in the Belleville Hospital Cells. *N Y Med J*. 1890;51:564-647.
38. American Association for the Cure of Inebriates. *Proceedings 1870–1875*. Reprinted Arno Press; 1981.
39. Crothers TD. A review of the history and literature of inebriety, the first journal and its work to present. *J Inebriety*. 1912;33:139-151.

40. Weiner B, White W. The journal of inebriety (1876–1914): history, topical analysis and photographic images. *Addiction*. 2007;102:15-23.
41. Crothers TD. Inebriate asylums. In: Stearns JN, ed. *Temperance in all Nations*. National Temperance Society and Publication House; 1893.
42. Parrish J. *Alcoholic Inebriety: From a Medical Standpoint with Cases from Clinical Records*. P. Blakiston, Son & Co; 1883.
43. Brooklyn home for habitues. *Q J Inebriety*. 1891;3:271-272.
44. Jellinek EM, ed. *Alcohol Addiction and Chronic Alcoholism*. Yale University Press; 1942.
45. Weiner B, White W. The history of addiction/recovery-related periodicals in America: literature as cultural/professional artifact. *Contemp Drug Probl*. 2002;28:531-557.
46. Crothers TD. Inebriate asylums. In: Spooner WW, ed. *Cyclopaedia of Temperance and Prohibition*. Funk and Wagnall's; 1891:247-248.
47. Worcester E, McComb S, Coriat I. *Religion and Medicine*. Funk & Wagnall's; 1908.
48. Moore M, Gray M. The problem of alcoholism at the Boston City Hospital. *N Engl J Med*. 1937;217:381-388.
49. Pettey G. *Narcotic Drug Diseases and Allied Ailments*. F.A. Davis Co; 1913.
50. Bishop E. *The Narcotic Drug Problem*. The Macmillan Company; 1920.
51. Kennedy F. The effects of narcotic drug addiction. *N Y Med J*. 1914;22:20-22.
52. Terry C. Some recent experiments in narcotic control. *Am J Public Health*. 1921;11:35.
53. Butler W. How one American city is meeting the public health problems of narcotic addiction. *Am Med*. 1922;28:154-162.
54. Courtwright D. Charles Terry: the opium problem and American narcotic policy. *J Drug Issues*. 1986;16:422-425.
55. Courtwright D. Willis Butler and the Shreveport narcotic clinic. *Soc Pharmacol*. 1987;1:13-24.
56. King R. *The Narcotics Bureau and the Harrison Act: jailing the healers and the sick. Yale Law Rev*. 1953;62:736-749.
57. Bishop E. Morphinism and its treatment. *JAMA*. 1912;58:1499-1504.
58. Williams EH. *Opiate Addiction*. Arno Press; 1922.
59. Williams H. *Drug Addicts are Human Beings*. Shaw Publishing Company; 1938.
60. Abraham K. The psychological relations between sexuality and alcoholism. *Int J Psychoanal*. 1926;7:2-10.
61. Kolb L. Clinical contributions to drug addiction: the struggle for care and the conscious reasons for relapse. *J Nerv Ment Dis*. 1927;66:22-43.
62. Schuckit M, Nathan PE, Helzer JE, et al. Evolution of the DSM diagnostic criteria for alcoholism. *Alcohol Health Res World*. 1991;15:278-283.
63. Joyce T. California State Narcotic Hospital. *Calif West Med*. 1929;31:190-192.
64. Bennett C. Hospitalization of narcotic addicts, U.S. Penitentiary, Leavenworth, KS. *J Kans Med Soc*. 1929;30:341-345.
65. Acker C. *Creating the American Junkie: Addiction Research in the Classical Era of Narcotic Control*. The Johns Hopkins University Press; 2002.
66. Terry C, Pellens M. *The Opium Problem*. Patterson Smith; 1928.
67. Reddish W. The treatment of morphine addiction by blister fluid injection. *Ky Med J*. 1931;29:504.
68. Kolb L, Himmelsbach C. Clinical studies of drug addiction: a critical review of the withdrawal treatment with method of evaluating abstinence syndromes. *Am J Psychiatry*. 1938;94:759-797.
69. Kleber H, Riordan C. The treatment of narcotic withdrawal: a historical review. *J Clin Psychiatry*. 1982;43(6):30-34.
70. Mann M. Formation of a National Committee for education on alcoholism. *Q J Stud Alcohol*. 1944;5(2):354.
71. White W. Listening to history: lessons for the EAP/managed care field. *EAP Digest*. 2000;20(1):16-26.
72. Chou I-H, Narasimha K. Neurobiology of addiction. *Nat Neurosci*. 2005;8(11):1427.
73. Volkow ND, Fowler JS, Wang GJ. The addicted human brain viewed in the light of imaging studies: brain circuits and treatment strategies. *Neuropharmacology*. 2004;47(Suppl 1):3-13.
74. Ashton H. Protracted withdrawal from benzodiazepines: the post-withdrawal syndrome. *Psychiatr Ann*. 1995;25(3):174-179.
75. Nairn AC, Svenningsson P, Nishi A, Fisone G, Girault JA, Greengard P. The role of DARPP-32 in the actions of drugs of abuse. *Neuropharmacology*. 2004;47(Suppl 1):14-23.
76. US Department of Health and Human Services. Office of the Surgeon General. *Facing Addiction in America: The Surgeon General's Report on Alcohol, Drugs and Health*. HHS; 2016.
77. Galanter M, Frances R. Addiction psychiatry: challenges for a new psychiatric subspecialty. *Hosp Commun Psychiatry*. 1992;43(11):1067-1070.
78. *ABMS Certification Report 2022-2023*. American Board of Medical Specialties; 2023. https://www.abms.org/abms-board-certification-report/
79. O'Connor PG, Sokol RJ, D'Onofrio G. Addiction medicine: the birth of a new discipline. *JAMA Intern Med*. 2014;174(11):1717-1718.
80. Jamie Fellner, *Decades of disparity: drug arrests and race in the United States*. Human Rights Watch; 2009.
81. Meghana Kakade et al, *Adolescent Substance Use and Other Illegal Behaviors and Racial Disparities in Criminal Justice System Involvement: Findings From a U.S. National Survey, Am J Pub Health*. 2012;102(7):1307-1310.
82. Roy Walmsley, *World Population List*. 10th ed. International Centre for Prison Studies; 2013.
83. United States Census. Quick Facts. https://www.census.gov/quickfacts/fact/table/US/PST045222
84. Substance Abuse and Mental Health Services Administration. *Results from the 2015 National Survey on Drug Use and Health*. Substance Abuse and Mental Health Services Administration; 2015 Table 1.31B.
85. Substance Abuse and Mental Health Services Administration. *Results From the 2014 National Survey on Drug Use and Health: Detailed Tables*. Substance Abuse and Mental Health Services Administration; 2015. Table 1.19B.
86. Federal Bureau of Investigation. Uniform Crime Reports; Bureau of Justice Statistics, Arrest Data Analysis Tool; Federal Bureau of Investigation. *Crime in the United States, 2016 U.S. Census*.
87. National Research Council, *The Growth of Incarceration in the United States: Exploring Causes and Consequences* The National Academies Press; 2014.
88. Federal Bureau of Investigation. *Crime in the United States, 2015*: Table 49A. Accessed May 26, 2023. https://ucr.fbi.gov/crime-in-the-u.s/2015/crime-in-the-u.s.-2015/tables/table-49
89. Bureau of Justice Statistics, Federal Justice Statistics Program; Carson EA *Prisoners in 2014*.
90. Taxy S, Samuels J, Adams WP *Drug Offenders in Federal Prison: Estimates of Characteristics Based on Linked Data*. US Department of Justice, Bureau of Justice Statistics, 2015. Accessed May 26, 2023. http://www.bjs.gov/fjsrc/
91. Musto D. The Marijuana Tax Act of 1937. *Arch Gen Psychiatry*. 1972;26(2):101-108.
92. Baum D. Legalize it now: how to win the war on drugs. *Harpers Magazine*. April, 2016.
93. Mauer M. The impact of mandatory minimum penalties in federal sentencing. *Judicature*. 2010;94(1):6.
94. Chesney-Lind M, Mauer M. *Invisible Punishment: The Collateral Consequences of Mass Imprisonment*. The New Press; 2011.
95. Alegria M. Transforming mental health and addiction services. *Health Aff (Millwood)*. 2021;40(2):226-234.
96. Hagle HN, Martin M, Winograd R, et al. Dismantling racism against black, indigenous, and people of color across the substance use continuum: a position statement of the association for multidisciplinary education and research in substance use and addiction. *Subst Abus*. 2021;42(1):5-12.
97. Alegria M. Removing obstacles to eliminating racial and ethnic disparities in behavioral health. *Health Aff (Millwood)*. 2016;35(6):991-999.
98. Compton WM, Einstein EB, Jones CM. Exponential increases in drug overdose: implications for epidemiology and research. *Int J Drug Policy*. 2022;104:103676.

CHAPTER

36 The Treatment of Substance Use Disorders: An Overview

Lawrence S. Brown Jr, Andrea G. Barthwell, and Ana Ventuneac

CHAPTER OUTLINE

- Introduction
- Goals of substance use disorder treatment
- Treatment settings
- Residential programs, including the therapeutic community
- Treatment services
- Pharmacological therapies
- Conclusion

INTRODUCTION

Substance use disorders (SUDs) are complex illnesses. Compulsive (at times uncontrollable) drug seeking and use, which persist even in the face of negative consequences, characterize the disorder. For many patients, SUD is a chronic disease, with recurrences possible even after long periods of abstinence. Patients with SUDs are heterogeneous in a number of clinically important features and domains. Because SUDs have many dimensions and disrupt many aspects of an individual's life, treatment may not be simple; generally, a multimodal approach to treatment is indicated. Treatment helps the individual stop using drugs and maintain a drug-free lifestyle while achieving productive functioning in the family, work, and societal settings. Like with other chronic diseases, after repeated attempts with appropriately matched treatment, some individuals remain unable to achieve treatment goals. In this instance, it is appropriate to work to achieve outcomes that include a reduction in the use and harm related to use, reduction in frequency and severity of recurrences of substance use, and improvement in psychological and social functioning, and quality of life.

Effective treatment programs incorporate many components, each directed to an aspect of the illness and its consequences. In practice, specific pharmacological and psychosocial treatments are often combined because combined treatments lead to better treatment retention and outcomes.[1-3] Eight decades of research and clinical practice have yielded a variety of approaches to SUD treatment; patient-centered approaches match the patient's assessed needs to evidence-based services that have the greatest potential for success. Evidence suggests that individuals with SUD who achieve sustained abstinence have the best long-term outcomes.[4-8] Extensive data[9] show that SUD treatment is as effective as treatment for most other chronic medical conditions.[10] Of course, not all SUD treatment is equally effective or applied in a standardized way. In 1999, the National Institute on Drug Abuse (NIDA) published a set of overarching principles that characterized the most effective SUD treatments and their implementation. The principles have been updated but remain engrained in SUD treatment policy and practice today (**Table 36-1**).

GOALS OF SUBSTANCE USE DISORDER TREATMENT

SUDs are complex disorders that can impact virtually every aspect of an individual's functioning. Because of the complexity and pervasive consequences of SUD, treatment typically may involve many components. Some components focus directly on the individual's alcohol or other substance use, whereas others, such as employment training, focus on restoring the patient to health, well-being, and productivity (**Fig. 36-1**). Treatment of SUD is delivered in different settings, using a variety of behavioral and pharmacological approaches. In the United States, specialized drug treatment facilities provide rehabilitation, counseling, behavioral therapy, medication management, case management, and other types of services to persons with substance use and gambling disorders.[11] Among the 41.1 million people aged 12 or older in 2020 who needed substance use treatment in the past year, 6.5% (or 2.7 million people) received substance use treatment at a specialty facility in the past year.[11]

Care of individuals with SUD includes assessing needs, providing treatment for intoxication and withdrawal, and developing, with appropriate support, the treatment plan that may consist of referrals to psychosocial care or for co-occurring medical conditions or complications. The treatment plan should address how the patient can work toward abstinence without medical compromise, achieve and maintain abstinence after withdrawal (if indicated), and gain improvement in functioning in, for instance, the medical, social, and psychological domains.

TREATMENT SETTINGS

Historically, the SUD treatment delivery system was primarily a specialty care delivery system, often separate from the medical-surgical delivery system. Funding for care in the system was usually separate, and the professionals in the system

TABLE 36-1 Principles of Effective Treatment

1.	Addiction is a complex but treatable disease that affects brain function and behavior.	Addictive substances alter the brain's structure and function, resulting in changes that persist long after substance use has ceased. This may explain why people who use substances are at risk for recurrence even after long periods of abstinence and despite the potentially devastating consequences.
2.	No single treatment is appropriate for everyone.	Treatment varies depending on the type of substance and the characteristics of the patients. Matching treatment settings, interventions, and services to an individual's particular problems and needs is critical to their ultimate success in returning to productive functioning in the family, workplace, and society.
3.	Treatment needs to be readily available.	Because people with addiction disorders may be uncertain about entering treatment, taking advantage of available services the moment people are ready for treatment is critical. Potential patients can be lost if treatment is not immediately available or readily accessible. As with other chronic diseases, the earlier the treatment is offered in the disease process, the greater the likelihood of positive outcomes.
4.	Effective treatment attends to multiple needs of the individual, not just their addiction.	To be effective, treatment must address the individual's substance use or gambling and any associated medical, psychological, social, vocational, and legal problems. It is also important that treatment be appropriate to the individual's age, gender, ethnicity, and culture.
5.	Remaining in treatment for an adequate period of time is critical.	The appropriate treatment duration for an individual depends on the type and degree of the patient's problems and needs. Research indicates that most individuals with SUD need at least 3 months in treatment to significantly reduce or stop their substance use or gambling and that the best outcomes occur with longer durations of treatment. Recovery from SUD is a long-term process and frequently requires multiple episodes of treatment. As with other chronic illnesses, recurrence can occur and should signal a need for treatment to be reinstated or adjusted. Because individuals often leave treatment prematurely, programs should include strategies to engage and keep patients in treatment.
6.	Behavioral therapies including individual, family, or group counseling are the most commonly used forms of treatment.	Behavioral therapies vary in their focus and may involve addressing a patient's motivation to change, providing incentives for abstinence, building skills to resist recurrence, replacing addiction-related activities with constructive and rewarding activities, improving problem-solving skills, and facilitating better interpersonal relationships. Also, participation in group therapy and other peer support programs during and following treatment can help maintain abstinence.
7.	Medications are an important element of treatment for many patients, especially when combined with counseling and psychotherapies.	There is evidence that medications significantly improve remission rates for both gambling disorder and many substance use disorders. Often the best approaches include combining both pharmacotherapy and various psychotherapies and other psychosocial approaches.
8.	An individual's treatment plan must be assessed continually and modified as necessary to ensure that it meets his or her changing needs.	A patient may require varying combinations of services and treatment components during the course of treatment and recovery. In addition to counseling or psychotherapy, a patient may require medication, medical services, family therapy, parenting instruction, vocational rehabilitation, and legal services. For many patients, a continuing care approach provides the best results, with the treatment intensity varying according to a person's changing needs.
9.	Many people with addiction disorders also have other mental disorders.	Because substance use disorder and gambling disorder—both of which are mental disorders—often co-occur with other mental disorders, patients presenting with one condition should be assessed for use of medications as appropriate.
10.	Medical withdrawal management is only the first stage of addiction treatment and by itself does little to change long-term drug use.	Although medical withdrawal management can safely manage the acute physical symptoms of withdrawal and can, for some, pave the way for effective long-term addiction treatment, withdrawal management alone is rarely sufficient to help achieve long-term abstinence. Thus, patients should be encouraged to continue treatment following withdrawal management. Motivational enhancement and incentive strategies, begun at initial patient intake, can improve treatment engagement.
11.	Treatment does not need to be voluntary to be effective.	Sanctions or enticements from family, employment settings, or the criminal legal system can significantly increase treatment entry, retention rates, and the ultimate success of treatment interventions.

(Continued)

TABLE 36-1 Principles of Effective Treatment (Continued)

12.	Drug use during treatment must be monitored continuously, as lapses during treatment do occur.	Because addiction is a disease, remission is expected, and good medical care includes monitoring for both. Knowing their drug use is being monitored can be a powerful incentive for patients and can help them withstand urges to use drugs. Monitoring also provides an early indication of a return to drug use, signaling a possible need to adjust an individual's treatment plan to better meet his or her needs.
13.	Treatment should include testing patients for the presence of HIV/AIDS, hepatitis B and C, tuberculosis, and other infectious diseases as well as provide targeted risk reduction counseling, linking patients to treatment for other conditions if necessary.	Typically, treatment addresses some of the drug-related behaviors that put people at risk of infectious diseases. Targeted counseling focused on reducing infectious disease risk can help patients further reduce or avoid substance-related and other high-risk behaviors. Counseling can also help those who are already infected to manage their illness. Moreover, engaging in substance use disorder treatment can facilitate adherence to other medical treatments. Treatment providers should provide on-site, rapid HIV testing rather than referrals to off-site testing—research shows that doing so increases the likelihood that patients will be tested and receive their test results. Treatment providers should also inform patients that highly active antiretroviral therapy (HAART) has proven effective in treating HIV, including among drug-using populations, and help link them to HIV treatment if they test positive.

Adapted from *Principles of Drug Addiction Treatment A Research-based Guide.* 3rd ed. National Institute on Drug Abuse, National Institutes of Health, U.S. Department of Health and Human Services, NIH Publication No 12-4180. 2012:8.

were often not healthcare professionals. Today treatment settings vary with regard to available services and medical support. For clinicians, patient assessment, treatment matching, and knowledge of referral opportunities in the community are important, as every community is different.

While this chapter addresses treatment for all substances, it is important to recognize that the utilization and capacity of treatment vary by setting and other factors such as race, ethnicity, and socioeconomic status (SES). For instance, buprenorphine prescribed in an Office-Based Opioid Treatment (OBOT) setting and methadone provided in an Opioid Treatment Program (OTP) setting both treat Opioid Use Disorder (OUD), but they vary greatly in the population served. The variance represents the background and resources of the individual patients more than the clinical needs of the populations served. Both services combined still fall short of the capacity needed to treat the number of individuals with OUD in this country.[12,13]

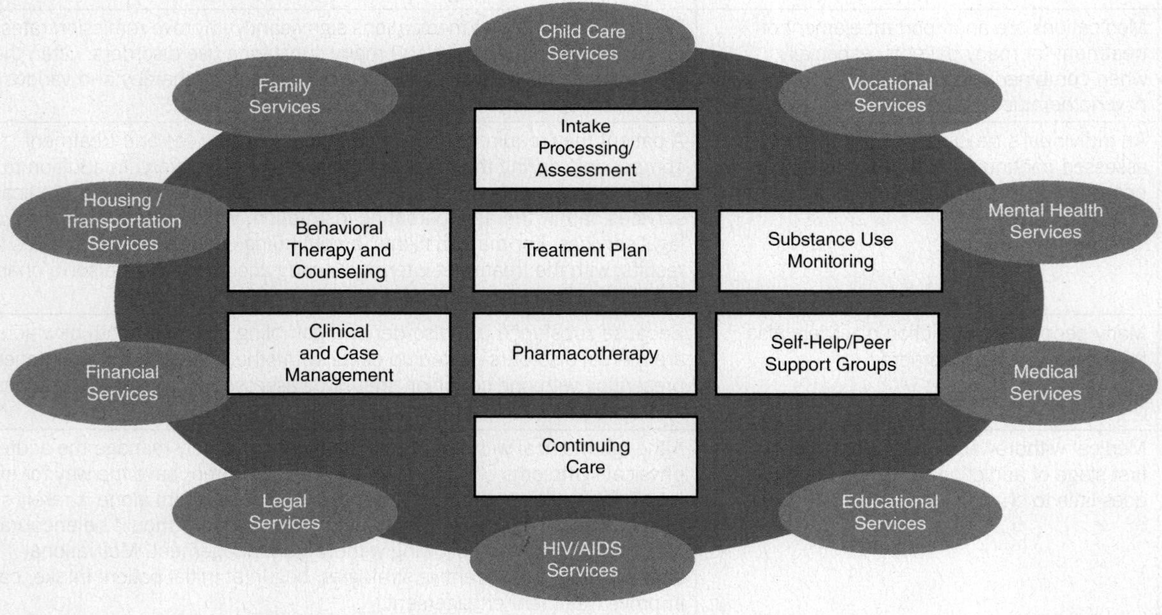

Figure 36-1. Components of addiction treatment. (From National Institute on Drug Abuse. *Principles of Drug Addiction Treatment—A Research-based Guide*. 3rd ed. NIH Publication No. 12-4180. NIDA; 2012.)

Decisions regarding the site of care should be based on the patient's ability to adhere with and benefit from the treatment offered, to refrain from use of substances, and to avoid high-risk behaviors, as well as the patient's need for structure and support or treatment preference. Patients can move from one level of care to another based on these factors and an assessment of their ability to benefit from a different level of care. Delivery system discontinuities occur when coverage is available for a limited number of levels of care, but not the one indicated based on the assessment carried out using a standardized system such as the American Society of Addiction Medicine (ASAM) Criteria. The ASAM Criteria (Chapter 47) describes four levels of care: (1) outpatient services, (2) intensive outpatient/partial hospitalization services, (3) residential/inpatient services, and (4) medically managed intensive inpatient services. An addiction medicine consultant or a member of the medical staff who is knowledgeable in the diagnosis and treatment of SUD make criterion-based placement decisions.

Hospital-based clinicians may find management of SUD limited to withdrawal management and referral. It may be challenging to refer outside of the hospital, because either the payer requires referral to a contracted provider, or the patient lacks coverage and needs referral to the public system of care. Hospital-based clinicians can create an inpatient Addiction Medicine Consultation Service with specialty-trained clinicians who assess severity and withdrawal potential, manage withdrawal, and refer to posthospital SUD care when the patient no longer requires care in the hospital setting.

Withdrawal Management

According to the ASAM Criteria, withdrawal management refers not only to the attenuation of the physiological and psychological features of withdrawal syndromes but also to the process of interrupting the momentum of compulsive use in people diagnosed with substance use disorder.[14] Because withdrawal management is not an adequate approach to addressing a substance use disorder as a stand-alone level of care, it must be conceived as an entry point into treatment, not a separate level of care. This phase frequently requires a great intensity of services to establish treatment engagement. It may be delivered in ambulatory settings with extended on-site monitoring. In residential or inpatient settings, is delivered under clinically managed, medically monitored, or medically managed conditions. There is increasing intensity of services and involvement of nursing and medical personnel across the latter continuum.

Hospital Settings

Hospitalization is appropriate for patients whose assessed need cannot be treated safely in an outpatient or emergency department setting because of (1) acute intoxication, (2) severe or medically complicated withdrawal potential, (3) co-occurring medical or psychiatric conditions that complicate withdrawal management or impair treatment engagement and response, (4) failure of engagement in treatment at a lower level of care, (5) life- or limb-threatening medical conditions that would require hospitalization, (6) psychiatric disorders that make the patient an imminent threat to self or others, and (7) failure to respond to care at any level such that the patient endangers others or poses a self-threat. Aside from withdrawal management and management of overdose or intoxication, most hospitalized patients receive services incident to a medical-surgical need or a psychiatric need. The clinician must evaluate the timing and intensity of addiction medicine services in the context of other pressing medical and psychiatric concerns.

Outpatient Settings

Outpatient treatment varies in the type and intensity of services offered, ranging from specialty programs to individual clinician offices and other general medical settings. Outpatient services typically costs less than residential or inpatient treatment and often is more suitable for individuals who show insight into their disease, a high degree of predicted compliance, low symptomatology, high resource availability and use, and a supportive structure in home environment. Low-intensity programs may offer little more than education and encouragement and support; however, as in the other treatment settings, a comprehensive approach is optimal, using—where indicated—a variety of psychotherapeutic and pharmacological interventions along with behavioral and laboratory monitoring. High rates of attrition can be problematic, particularly in the early phase. Because outcomes are highly correlated with time in treatment, retention should be one focus of treatment,[15] along with self-efficacy regarding adherence to the treatment plan. Participation in mutual groups is an evidence-based element of treatment.[16]

Other outpatient models, such as intensive day treatment, can be comparable to residential programs (see below "Residential Programs, Including the Therapeutic Community") in services and effectiveness, depending on the individual patient characteristics and needs. In many outpatient programs, as in treatment in general, group counseling is emphasized. Some outpatient programs are designed to treat patients who have medical or mental health problems in addition to their substance use or gambling disorder.[17]

Most alcohol use disorders are treated outside of the hospital after medical complications associated with withdrawal management are addressed.[18,19] Similarly, cocaine,[20] nicotine,[21] and cannabis use disorders are often treated on an outpatient basis as long as the focus on reduced substance use can be maintained and there are no other reasons for hospitalization.[22,23]

Partial Hospital Programs and Intensive Outpatient Settings

Partial hospitalization programs (PHPs) are considered for patients who require intensive treatment but have a reasonable chance of making progress on treatment goals in the between visit, or intertreatment, interval. PHPs are often provided to individuals whose treatment was hospital- or residential-initiated and who, after discharge, still require frequent and concentrated contact with treatment professionals for support, monitoring, and risk management. These patients often have a history of recurrences of substance use after completion of treatment or are returning to a high-risk environment and need to develop support for their recovery-focused efforts beyond the residential treatment system. Waning motivation to build on the gains made in treatment, allowing the treatment effect to erode, is often a cause to continue the patient in this highly intensive and structured setting. The difference between partial hospital programs and intensive outpatient programs is in intensity, number of hours per day, setting of the program, and structure of the program. Intensive outpatient programs have been proven effective when working with special subgroups of patients, such as those who are economically disadvantaged, have psychiatric comorbidities, are pregnant, or have been mandated into treatment by the criminal legal system or outside parties.[24,25] Patients who are not successful in intensive outpatient care may have clinical contact increased by transfer to partial hospital programs.

RESIDENTIAL PROGRAMS, INCLUDING THE THERAPEUTIC COMMUNITY

Residential programs provide care 24 hours a day, generally in nonhospital settings. Residential care is provided to patients who do not meet the clinical criteria for acute hospitalization but whose lives are also transformed by and focused on substance use. ASAM Criteria are used to determine the appropriate level of residential treatment with higher levels of care corresponding with greater medical need. Individuals for whom a residential level of care is necessary are typically unlikely to maintain abstinence in the absence of continued application of a variety of therapeutic techniques in a highly structured and supportive environment. Short-term programs provide intensive but relatively brief residential treatment based on a modified mutual aid approach and may or may not include elements of therapeutic communities (TCs). The duration of residential treatment should be determined by the clinical response to therapy and the length of time necessary for the patient to meet specific criteria predictive of success in a lower level of care according to the ASAM Criteria. The relationship between length of treatment and clinical outcomes is mixed, largely due to differences in study designs.[26-28] Residential programs originally were designed to treat alcohol use disorder, but at the start of the cocaine epidemic of the mid-1980s, many began to treat other substance use disorders. The original residential treatment model consisted of a 3- to 6-week hospital-based inpatient treatment phase, followed by extended outpatient therapy and participation in a mutual aid group such as Alcoholics Anonymous. Health insurers' restrictions on coverage of residential SUD treatment have resulted in a diminished number of these programs, and the average length of stay under managed care review is much shorter than in early programs.

One residential treatment model is the therapeutic community (TC),[29] but residential treatment programs also employ other approaches, such as cognitive-behavioral therapy. Note that TCs are different from "sober houses," which may not be accredited or provide evidence-based treatment. TCs are residential programs with planned lengths of stay from 6 to 12 months. TCs focus on the "resocialization" of the individual and use the program's entire "community"—including other residents, staff, and the social context—as active components of treatment. SUD is viewed in the context of an individual's social and psychological needs, so treatment focuses on developing personal accountability, responsibility, and socially productive lives. Treatment is highly structured and can at times be confrontational, with activities designed to help residents examine damaging beliefs, self-concepts, and patterns of behavior and to adopt new, more harmonious and constructive ways to interact. Many TCs are quite comprehensive and include employment training and other support services onsite or through formal linkage agreements. Research shows that TCs can be modified to treat individuals with special needs, including adolescents, women,[30,31] those with severe mental health disorders,[32] and individuals in the criminal legal system.[33,34] Elements of TCs have been incorporated into shorter-term residential programs and institutional criminal legal settings.

Opioid use disorder related to heroin has been effectively reduced in the TC; however, return to use after TC treatment is higher than 80% in most long-term follow-up studies, indicating a need for selectivity in application of this modality over clinical settings that provide medication.[35] Data regarding the effectiveness of traditional long-term TC are limited by the low completion rates of 15% to 25%, with most attrition occurring during the first 3 months. Retention lengths predict outcomes on abstinence with abstinence success rates of 90% for graduates of 2-year programs and 25% for participants who complete less than 1 year in the same program.[36] Retention rates differ by program site.[37,38]

Community Residential Rehabilitation

Community residential rehabilitation facilities provide supportive environments to people in the early stages of recovery but do not provide treatment per se. These facilities are also called "recovery residences," "sober living facilities," or "halfway houses." Individuals referred to these settings are generally deemed to be at risk for recurrence without such support. Often, this setting is offered to the individual whose environmental risk is great or those needing a number of services after primary treatment to address vocational, employment, and social support needs. These services have been shown to significantly improve substance use outcomes for both sexes but are variable in their impact on young people.[39-42] There is wide variability in the quality of these programs, as some facilities lack licensure or accreditation.

Case Management

Case management is a collaborative process that assesses, plans, implements, coordinates, monitors, and evaluates the options and services to meet an individual's health needs.[43-45] It uses communication and available resources to promote quality, cost-effective outcomes.

Case management, although difficult to assess for effectiveness in a rigorous fashion, has been shown to be an effective adjunctive treatment for some patients with alcohol use disorders, patients with substance use disorders co-occurring with psychiatric disorders,[46] and adolescents.[47] Several meta-analyses reveal variable results. In one meta-analysis, using data from 15 studies that included information on illicit drug use among 2,391 patients, case management was found to be superior to psychoeducation and drug counseling alone, although a direct causal link was not clearly established.[48] In another meta-analysis, limited by highly variable data collection techniques, treatment adherence was most highly correlated with receipt of case management.[49] Finally, case management was found to be more effective than treatment as usual relative to treatment-related tasks over personal functioning.[50] These results support case management as a useful service in SUD treatment but fail to provide clear evidence-based guidance on the nature and extent of the service. In most instances, case management is provided to individuals whose social situation and complex needs impair their ability to adhere to a prescribed treatment plan and follow-up care. Basic needs are often met as part of the service array, which includes psychoeducation and assistance in comprehension of the extent and nature of the disease for which treatment is provided.

Aftercare Programs

Aftercare generally follows an episode of care and is focused on maintenance of gains made in treatment over a prescribed period with less frequent contact than the primary episode of care (eg, once-weekly monitoring and group therapy after a 6-week intensive outpatient program in which the patient is seen nightly for 3 hours). The patient's engagement with a mutual aid is encouraged, and the transition to self-efficacy is monitored. Many professionals view the term "aftercare" as outdated, in that it suggests that care has somehow ended. Other terms for such programs are "continuing care" and "recovery support," reflecting that recovery is a process of change through which individuals improve their health and wellness, live self-directed lives, and strive to reach their full potential.[51]

Peer Recovery Specialists, Recovery Coaches, and Other Support Services

Peer recovery specialists, recovery coaches, and other such aides provide nonmedical guidance to individuals considering treatment or going through the treatment or recovery process. The aides' role may include offering to provide persons with active SUD "warm handoffs" to treatment, connecting people who are not yet ready for SUD treatment with care and services, supporting patients in accessing and participating in treatment, and encouraging healthy structure and habits within a recovery-oriented framework. Peer recovery specialists and similar aides are best deployed as part of comprehensive, multidisciplinary treatment and support plans that address the multifaceted needs of individuals in the pretreatment, active treatment, or recovery phases of SUD management.

For example, Tennessee Recovery Navigators are people in long-term recovery who meet in hospitals with patients who have recently experienced drug poisoning.[52] Navigators connect patients with medical, social, and other services they may need.[53] Navigators can also provide direct support services, such as helping a person develop recovery goals, introducing a person to a local mutual aid group, and assisting a person in navigating the behavioral health care system to access individually appropriate treatment.[54] Navigators maintain a Certified Peer Recovery Specialist certification from the Tennessee Department of Mental Health and Substance Abuse Services.[52]

Peer recovery specialists and similar aides fulfill needs otherwise unmet by health care professionals, social workers, or other service providers. Peer recovery services are evidence based and shown to be effective, and may be covered by health insurance, including state Medicaid plans.[55] The development and activation of a peer-to-peer workforce in behavioral health may serve as a model that can be replicated within other medical specialties to address the needs of patients with other health conditions.

Treatment in the Outpatient Office, Including Screening and Brief Intervention

Federal, state, and local laws have long impeded the treatment of individuals with SUD within conventional medical settings and using opioid medications in the treatment of OUD. For example, the Harrison Narcotics Tax Act of 1914 was a U.S. federal law that regulated and taxed the production, importation, and distribution of opioids. The courts interpreted the law to mean that clinicians could prescribe opioids to patients in the course of medical treatment but not for the treatment of OUD.[56] Despite long-standing barriers, clinicians have recognized a need to provide treatment to individuals with SUD, including with medications when appropriate and available. Methadone, buprenorphine, and naltrexone are FDA-approved medications for the treatment of OUD. Methadone and buprenorphine are opioids. Under federal law, methadone can only be dispensed in certified OTPs. Medications are also available for office-based treatment of other substance use and gambling disorders.[9,57-59]

Brief interventions for at-risk drinking were studied before being adopted and expanded for other substance use disorders.[60] These first interventions were intended to help reduce at-risk drinking by addressing the behavior in settings other than those where SUD treatment typically took place (eg, mental health clinics, outpatient medical offices).[61,62] Today, brief interventions include assessment, feedback, responsibility for change, advice, and a menu of options provided using empathic listening and encouraging self-efficacy.[63] A more extensive review of this area is offered elsewhere in this textbook.

Legally Mandated Treatment

Research has shown that combining criminal legal sanctions with drug treatment can be effective in decreasing drug use and related crime. Individuals under legal mandates tend to stay in treatment for a longer period and do as well as or better than others not under legal pressure.[33,34,64] Often, people with SUDs encounter the criminal legal system earlier than other health or social systems, and intervention by the criminal legal system to engage the individual in treatment may help to interrupt and shorten the duration of drug use.[65,66] SUD treatment may be delivered before, during, after, or in lieu of incarceration.

Treatment in Carceral Settings

Incarcerated individuals with SUDs may encounter a number of treatment options, including medications for opioid use disorder (MOUD),[67] while incarcerated, as well as didactic drug education classes, mutual aid programs, and treatment based on TC or residential milieu therapy models. The TC model has been studied extensively and found to be quite effective in reducing drug use and recidivism to criminal behavior.[68] Those in treatment are generally segregated from the general prison population, so that the "prison culture" does not overwhelm progress toward recovery. As might be expected, treatment gains can be lost if participants are returned to the general prison population after treatment. Research shows that recurrence of substance use and return to crime are significantly lower if the incarcerated individual with a substance use disorder continues treatment after returning to the community.[69,70]

Community-Based Treatment for Criminal Legal Populations, Including Drug Courts

Several criminal legal alternatives to incarceration have been tried with individuals who have SUDs, including limited diversion programs, pretrial release conditional on entry into treatment, and conditional probation with sanctions. The drug court is a specific community-based approach. Drug courts mandate and arrange for SUD treatment, actively monitor progress in treatment, and arrange other services for drug-involved individuals. Federal support for planning, implementation, and enhancement of drug courts is provided under the U.S. Department of Justice's Drug Courts Program Office. As a well-studied example, the Treatment Accountability for Safer Communities program provides an alternative to incarceration by addressing the multiple needs of individuals with SUD in a community-based setting.[71] Treatment Accountability for Safer Communities programs typically include counseling, medical care, parenting instruction, family counseling, school and job training, and legal and employment services. The key features of Treatment Accountability for Safer Communities include coordination between the law enforcement and drug treatment communities; early identification, assessment, and referral of drug-involved individuals; monitoring through drug testing; and use of legal sanctions as inducements to remain in treatment.

TREATMENT SERVICES

This section presents several examples of evidence-based treatment approaches and components that have been developed and tested through research supported by the National Institute on Drug Abuse. Each approach is designed to address certain aspects of SUD and the consequences for the individual, family, and society. This section is not a complete list of empirically supported treatment approaches, but rather provides an overview of some types of treatment services.

Clinical Monitoring

As with the treatment of other medical disorders and irrespective of the therapeutic approach chosen, clinical monitoring is extremely important in achieving successful and safe clinical outcomes. Although many studies have underscored the limitations of relying solely on a patient's self-report,[72] self-reports can be useful in the context of a nonconfrontational, nonjudgmental, patient-provider relationship based on openness, understanding, and empathy. It should also be explicitly recognized that patients receiving care for other chronic disorders also underreport unhealthy behaviors to their caregivers, and because substance use is stigmatized and often illegal, underreporting is understandable.

Because of the limitations of self-report in the initial assessment and during clinical monitoring, clinical drug testing represents an important tool for addiction medicine specialists[73,74] but is underused and often misunderstood by primary care providers.[75,76] When used by an experienced practitioner in concert with a good history, physical examination, and biomarkers, clinical drug testing facilitates screening, assessment, diagnosis, and clinical monitoring of a substance use disorder. Drug testing provides useful information about a patient's potential for achieving desirable clinical outcomes with co-occurring medical or psychiatric disorders. Drug testing is also an important safety tool allowing detection of potentially harmful substances to which a patient may have unknowingly been exposed.

Managing Intoxication and Withdrawal

Similar to the treatment of other clinical disorders, patients with SUDs exhibit varied clinical presentations, from acute and subacute to chronic manifestations. Some manifestations, such as intoxication and withdrawal, can be life-threatening without appropriate, if not emergent, intervention. The therapeutic response is contingent on the substance used, the presence or absence of evidence of a compromised cardiopulmonary system, and the underlying health status of the patient. Pharmacotherapy is the cornerstone for patients with either intoxication or withdrawal. Effective treatment for intoxication typically requires a hospital setting, whereas withdrawal can be treated in either an inpatient or outpatient setting.

Withdrawal management is a commonly used approach in responding to patients with clinical signs of intoxication or withdrawal. It is a process in which, under the care of a clinician, individuals are systematically withdrawn from addictive drugs in an inpatient or outpatient setting. Withdrawal management is intended to reduce or eliminate the medical consequences of withdrawal, the pain of withdrawal, and the acute increase in craving experienced by the patient while establishing a therapeutic alliance with the patient and enabling the patient's own motivation toward rehabilitation therapies that follow. Medications are available for withdrawal management or tapering from opioids, nicotine, benzodiazepines, alcohol, barbiturates, and other sedatives. Withdrawal management alone does not address the associated psychological, social, and behavioral problems; therefore, this clinical approach does not typically produce the type of lasting behavioral changes necessary for recovery. Withdrawal management is most useful when it incorporates formal processes of assessment and referral to subsequent SUD treatment[77] as recurrence rates are high following withdrawal management alone. It may be better conceived as early treatment engagement, preceding a full continuum of services.

Behavioral Therapy

Numerous studies have demonstrated that therapy or counseling can be an effective treatment for some substance use disorders. Therapy and counseling attempt to arrest compulsive substance use through modification of behaviors, feelings, social functioning, and thoughts. They address a set of common tasks and attempt to increase motivation, expand the coping repertoire, change reinforcement contingencies to increase the frequency of positive behaviors, improve mood, and enhance interpersonal connection and the number of social supports. Lack of knowledge regarding how to match patients to the various techniques should not be an excuse to avoid referral for consideration of SUD-specific psychotherapies.

Cognitive-Behavioral Therapy

Cognitive-behavioral therapy is based on the theory that learning processes play a critical role in the development of maladaptive patterns of behavior. Cognitive-behavioral therapy targets two processes: dysfunctional thoughts and maladaptive behaviors. Thought-based interventions focus on increasing the patient's resolve not to use substances—based on negative and positive consequences of use—and confronting thoughts about use. Relapse prevention (RP) is a term used in the literature to describe a specific cognitive-behavioral therapy. Variations of this approach aim to reduce the risk of a patient returning to substance use (or gambling or other behaviors) after a period of change.

When not referring to the specific RP intervention more appropriate terminology includes "recurrence of symptoms" and "return to use." RP was developed for the treatment of unhealthy alcohol use and later adapted to other substance use disorders. RP encompasses several cognitive-behavioral strategies that facilitate abstinence as well as provide help for persons who experience recurrence of substance use. The goal of RP is to help addicted individuals learn to identify and correct problematic behaviors. For example, the RP approach to the treatment of cocaine use disorders consists of a collection of strategies intended to enhance self-control.[78] Specific techniques include exploring the positive and negative consequences of continued use, self-monitoring to recognize drug cravings early on and to identify situations that pose high risk of use and developing strategies for coping with and avoiding high-risk situations and the desire to use. A central element of this treatment is anticipating the problems patients are likely to confront and helping them develop effective coping strategies. Research indicates that the skills individuals learn through RP therapy remain after the completion of treatment.[79] In one study, most persons receiving a cognitive-behavioral approach maintained the gains they made in the treatment throughout the year after discharge.[80]

Motivational Enhancement Therapy

Motivational enhancement therapy is a patient-centered counseling approach that attempts to initiate behavior change by helping patients resolve their ambivalence about engaging in treatment and stopping drug use. This approach employs strategies to evoke rapid and internally motivated change in the patient, rather than guiding the patient stepwise through the recovery process. These strategies include exploration of the extent and nature of one's problems and the source of the same, creating lists of reasons to change, defining activities that will bring about change, and monitoring success at keeping to one's goals. The therapy provides feedback generated from an initial assessment to stimulate discussion regarding personal substance use and to elicit self-motivational statements. Motivational interviewing principles are used to strengthen motivation and build a plan for change. Coping strategies for high-risk situations are suggested and discussed with the client. Over time, the therapist monitors change, reviews abstinence strategies being used, and continues to encourage commitment to change or to sustained abstinence. Patients sometimes are encouraged to bring a spouse, partner, or family member to sessions. This approach was developed for tobacco use disorder and has been used successfully with individuals with alcohol and cannabis use disorders.[81]

Community Reinforcement Approach Plus Voucher-Based Reinforcement Therapy (Chapter 73)

The community reinforcement approach (CRA) is an outpatient therapy for the treatment of cocaine,[82] alcohol,[83] opiate,[84] and cannabis use disorder.[85,86] The treatment has dual goals: to achieve abstinence long enough for patients to learn new life skills that will help sustain abstinence and to reduce consumption. Patients attend one or two individual counseling sessions per week, where they focus on improving family relations, learning a variety of skills to minimize drug use, receiving vocational counseling, and developing new recreational activities and social relationships. Those with unhealthy alcohol use receive clinic-monitored disulfiram therapy. Patients submit urine samples two or three times per week and receive vouchers for negative samples. The value of the vouchers increases with consecutive negative samples. Patients may exchange their vouchers for retail goods that are consistent with a substance-free lifestyle. This approach facilitates patients' engagement in treatment and systematically aids them in gaining substantial periods of abstinence.[87] The approach has been tested in urban and rural areas and used successfully in outpatient withdrawal management of adults with OUD and with urban patients receiving methadone who have high rates of intravenous cocaine use.[88]

A computer-based version of CRA plus vouchers called the therapeutic education system was found to be nearly as effective as treatment administered by a therapist in promoting abstinence from opioids and cocaine among individuals with OUD in outpatient treatment.[89] A version of CRA for adolescents addresses problem solving, coping, and communication skills and encourages active participation in positive social and recreational activities.[90]

Voucher-Based Reinforcement Therapy

Voucher-based reinforcement therapy helps patients achieve and maintain abstinence from substances by providing them with a voucher each time they provide a drug-free urine sample. The voucher has monetary value and can be exchanged for goods and services consistent with the goals of treatment. Initially, the voucher values are low, but their value increases with the number of consecutive drug-free urine specimens the individual provides. Cocaine- or heroin-positive urine specimens reset the value of the vouchers to the initial low value. The contingency of escalating incentives is designed specifically to reinforce periods of sustained abstinence. Studies show that patients receiving vouchers for drug-free urine samples achieved significantly more weeks of abstinence and significantly more weeks of sustained abstinence than patients who were given vouchers independent of urine toxicology results. In another study, urine toxicology positive for heroin decreased significantly when the voucher program was started and increased significantly when the program was stopped.[91]

Day Treatment With Abstinence Contingencies and Voucher-Based Reinforcement Therapy

This approach was developed to treat crack cocaine use disorder among unhoused persons.[92] For the first 2 months, participants were required to spend 5.5 hours daily in the program, which provided lunch and transportation to and from shelters. Interventions included individual assessment and goal setting, individual and group counseling, multiple psychoeducational groups and patient-governed community meetings, in which patients reviewed contract goals and provided support and encouragement to each other. Individual counseling occurred once per week, and group therapy sessions were held three times per week. After 2 months of day treatment and at least 2 weeks of abstinence, participants graduated to a 4-month work component that paid wages, which could be used to rent inexpensive, drug-free housing. A voucher system also rewarded drug-free social and recreational activities. This innovative day treatment was compared with treatment consisting of twice-weekly individual counseling and mutual aid groups, medical examinations and group and individual counseling, and referral to community resources for housing and vocational services. Innovative day treatment followed by work and housing (dependent on drug abstinence) had a more positive effect on alcohol use, cocaine use, and days of being unhoused.[93]

Individual Psychotherapies

Individualized counseling focuses directly on reducing or stopping the patient's substance use. It also addresses related areas of impaired functioning—such as employment status, illegal activity, and family and social relations—as well as the content and structure of the patient's recovery program. Through its emphasis on short-term behavioral goals, individualized drug counseling helps the patient develop coping strategies and tools for abstaining from drug use and then maintaining abstinence. This can be achieved with and without formal psychotherapy. The licensed provider trained in such therapy encourages mutual aid program participation and makes referrals for needed supplemental medical, psychiatric, employment, and other services. Individuals are encouraged to attend sessions one or two times per week. In a study comparing patients with DSM-IV–defined opioid dependence receiving methadone alone with those receiving methadone coupled with counseling, individuals who received methadone alone showed minimal improvement in reducing opioid use.[94] The addition of counseling produced significantly more improvement. The addition of on-site medical, psychiatric, employment, and family services further improved outcomes. In another study with patients with DSM-IV–defined cocaine dependence, individualized drug counseling, together with group counseling, was quite effective in reducing cocaine use.[95] Thus, it appears that this approach has great utility in outpatient treatment for both heroin and cocaine use disorders.

Supportive expressive psychotherapy is a time-limited, focused psychotherapy that has been adapted for individuals with heroin and cocaine use disorders.[96] The therapy has two main components: supportive techniques to help patients feel comfortable in discussing their personal experiences and expressive techniques to help patients identify and work through interpersonal relationship issues. Special attention is paid to the role of drugs in relation to problem feelings and behaviors and how problems may be solved without recourse to drugs. The efficacy of individual supportive-expressive psychotherapy has been tested with patients receiving methadone treatment who had co-occurring psychiatric disorders.[97] In a comparison with patients receiving drug counseling only (with no psychotherapy versus those with drug counseling and psychotherapy), both groups fared similarly with regard to opioid use, but the supportive-expressive psychotherapy group had lower cocaine use and required lower doses of methadone. In addition, the patients who received supportive-expressive psychotherapy maintained many of the gains they had made after the end of the trial. In an earlier study, supportive-expressive psychotherapy, when added to drug counseling, improved outcomes for opioid-dependent patients in methadone treatment with moderately severe psychiatric problems.[98]

Treatment of the Adolescent With Multidimensional Family Therapy

Multidimensional family therapy is an outpatient, family-based drug treatment approach for adolescents. It approaches adolescent drug use in terms of a network of influences (individual, family, peer, and community) and suggests that reducing unwanted behavior and increasing desirable behavior occur in multiple ways in different settings. Treatment includes individual and family sessions held in the clinic, in the home, or with family members at the family court, school, or other community locations. During individual sessions, the therapist and adolescent work on important developmental tasks, such as decision-making, negotiation, and problem-solving skills. Teens acquire skills in communicating their thoughts and feelings to deal better with life stressors and vocational skills. Parallel sessions are held with family members. Parents examine their particular parenting styles, learn to distinguish influence from control, and learn how to have a positive and developmentally appropriate influence on their child.[99]

Treatment of the Adolescent With Multisystemic Therapy

Multisystemic therapy addresses the factors associated with serious antisocial behavior in children and adolescents who use drugs. These factors include characteristics of the adolescent (eg, favorable attitudes toward drug use), the family (poor discipline, family conflict, or parental drug use), peers (positive attitudes toward drug use), school (dropout, poor performance), and neighborhood (criminal subculture).[90] By participating in intense treatment in natural environments (homes, schools, and neighborhood settings), most youth and families complete a full course of treatment. Multisystemic therapy significantly reduces adolescent drug use during treatment and for at least six months after treatment. Reduced numbers of incarcerations and out-of-home placements of juveniles[100] offset the cost of providing this intensive service and maintaining the clinicians' low caseloads.[101] For more information on treatment of adolescents, see Section 14 of this textbook.

Computer-Assisted Therapy

There is a growing body of literature that supports the use of technology in the treatment of SUD, using computer-assisted therapies (CAT) through online counseling and mutual aid resources, as well as mobile therapies through smartphone applications and text messaging. A number of randomized controlled trials (RCTs) have been conducted in recent years examining the efficacy of CAT for SUD related to a number of substances, with some of these demonstrating that this intervention approach may significantly reduce substance use. Formal CAT programs are usually clinician-facilitated, although some are developed to be used independently by the individual with SUD. A number of online CAT programs were developed and evaluated in RCTs, including a smoking abstinence and other substance use program, CHESS,[102] and a computerized version of cognitive-behavioral therapy (CBT4CBT). When compared with participants receiving standard treatment, participants receiving the CBT4CBT or the CHESS program provided a significantly higher number of negative urine samples and achieved longer periods of abstinence.[103] Other CAT programs are used throughout the SUD treatment field, although many of them are proprietary and there is a paucity of RCT data to support their use. For example, the MAP Program at the Origins Recovery Centers and Hazelden MORE (My Ongoing Recovery Experience) program are CAT programs used within these treatment centers that are not available to individuals who are not receiving such "in-house" treatment.

In addition to formal CAT, online counseling and information programs have also been evaluated. In an RCT with 206 young people with cannabis use problems, the "quit the shit" program[104] was evaluated. This program incorporates mutual aid, counseling, keeping a diary of cannabis consumption, and monitoring of a range of mental health outcomes such as anxiety and depression. Compared to wait-list controls, participants randomized to the "quit the shit" program were demonstrated to have significantly reduced self-reported cannabis use, and there were some small improvements in mental health outcomes.

Removing the need for direct therapist involvement, online self-help resources for SUD have also been evaluated in a number of studies. For example, an RCT of an online, multicomponent, self-help program for problem alcohol consumption[105] with 261 problem drinkers provided some support for the efficacy of this kind of intervention. When compared with control participants exposed to an online brochure regarding the effects of unhealthy alcohol consumption, participants exposed to the self-help program reduced their self-reported alcohol consumption significantly more than the control group.

The internet may also provide a useful format for screening for substance problems and for providing brief interventions. An RCT of a web-based alcohol screening and brief intervention program[106] with 576 problem drinking university students found that compared to no-treatment controls, those using the program experienced a reduction in problem drinking. This reduction in drinking was accompanied by a reduction in associated psychosocial problems, with both of these outcomes being maintained at 6- and 12-month follow-up.

Moving beyond online programs, the use of technology to treat SUD has extended into the use of cell phones and text messaging interventions. For example, the "txt2stop" tobacco treatment program was evaluated using an RCT methodology with 5,524 smokers. Compared to controls, significantly more participants using the "txt2stop" program achieved abstinence from smoking at 6-month follow-up, with this abstinence being biochemically verified. These findings appear to be partially verified by a Cochrane review,[107] in which five studies were included in a meta-analysis, resulting in an outcome indicating an overall benefit at 6-month follow-up in terms of abstinence. However, the authors of the review report that this finding should be interpreted with caution due to some heterogeneity across the five studies included. There is some research looking at the efficacy of using cell phone technology in treating unhealthy alcohol[108] and cannabis use,[100] although more is needed before any firm conclusions can be drawn regarding the efficacy of such a treatment approach for the SUD.

PHARMACOLOGICAL THERAPIES

Medications for Opioid Use Disorder

Treatment with Medications for Opioid Use Disorder (MOUD) is usually conducted in outpatient treatment settings, such as federally-regulated opioid treatment programs (OTPs, also known as methadone clinics, which may also provide buprenorphine or naltrexone) or a clinician's office (which may provide buprenorphine or naltrexone). These services are discussed in more detail elsewhere in the textbook, including Section 7. OTPs most often provide methadone[109] or buprenorphine[110-113] for a sustained period of months to years and at a dose sufficient to prevent opioid withdrawal while also blocking the effects of nonprescribed opioid use to reduce reinforcement of continued use. Also, these medications decrease opioid craving. Buprenorphine is currently available in formulations that are taken sublingually and buccally or in depot formulations. Sublingual and buccal formulations most commonly combine buprenorphine with the drug naloxone, an opioid receptor antagonist. Naloxone has no effect when the combination medications are taken as prescribed, but if an individual with opioids in their system attempts to inject the buprenorphine/naloxone combination, the naloxone will produce severe withdrawal symptoms. This formulation lessens the likelihood that the drug will be used for self-reward or be diverted to others for misuse. Office-based treatment for OUD is a cost-effective approach that is generally more available in many communities than methadone.[114]

Previously, U.S. federal law required health care practitioners to obtain a waiver for office-based prescribing of buprenorphine for OUD. Practitioners were required to complete an approved training and submit an application to the Substance Abuse and Mental Health Services Administration. Once approved, the Drug Enforcement Administration (DEA) issued a registration number beginning with X (often referred to as an "X-waiver") for office-based prescribing of buprenorphine for OUD. Prescribers of buprenorphine for OUD were subject to additional federal requirements, such as discipline restrictions, numeric patient limits, and certification related to the provision of counseling.

In December 2022, Congress passed Section 1262 of the Consolidated Appropriations Act of 2023, which eliminated the federal requirement for practitioners to obtain an X-waiver prior to prescribing buprenorphine for OUD.[115] Prescribers who have a current DEA registration that includes Schedule III authority may prescribe buprenorphine for OUD if permitted by applicable state law.[115] Separately, section 1263 of the Consolidated Appropriations Act of 2023 requires practitioners seeking a new or renewal DEA registration to prescribe controlled substances (of any type, not just for the treatment of OUD) to have at least 8 hours of training on opioid or other substance use disorders, or board certification in addiction medication or addiction psychiatry.[116]

Patients stabilized on adequate, sustained doses of methadone or buprenorphine can function at previous levels. Data shows that patients in MOUD treatment can hold jobs, avoid crime and the drug culture, and reduce their exposure to HIV and hepatitis C by stopping or decreasing injection drug use and drug-related high-risk sexual behaviors.[117-123] Indeed, the infection-reducing benefit of substance use treatment programs is most robust in those programs providing MOUD.[103-106] Patients stabilized on MOUD can engage more readily in counseling and other behavioral interventions that are essential to recovery and rehabilitation. The most effective OTPs include individual or group counseling and provision of, or referral to, other needed medical, psychological, and social services. Criteria for management in the physician's office have been described, and is being considered under the Modernization of Methadone (as of this writing in 2023). Clinicians are advised to engage with local providers of substance use disorder care to provide services that may be beyond the scope or ability of the office-based practice.

Antagonist Treatment Using Naltrexone

Antagonist therapies are used to block or counteract the physiological or subjective reinforcing effects of substances. Treatment of patients with OUD with naltrexone usually is conducted in outpatient settings, although initiation of the medication often begins after medical withdrawal management or in a residential setting. Naltrexone is a long-acting synthetic opioid antagonist with few side effects that is taken orally, either daily or three times per week, for a sustained period. An extended-release injectable, formulation of naltrexone is also available and has shown some efficacy in select populations.[124] Candidates for therapy with naltrexone must be opioid-free for several days before the drug can be given, to avoid precipitating opioid withdrawal. Naltrexone blocks the effects of self-administered opioids, including euphoria. The theory behind this treatment is that the repeated lack of the desired opioid effects, as well as the perceived futility of using the opioid, will gradually extinguish the desire to use opioids. Naltrexone itself has no subjective effects or potential for misuse and is not addictive. Patient noncompliance is a common problem; therefore, a favorable treatment outcome requires that there also be a positive therapeutic relationship, effective counseling or therapy, and careful monitoring of medication compliance.[125] Many experienced clinicians have found naltrexone most useful for highly motivated, recently detoxified patients who desire total abstinence because of external circumstances, including impaired professionals, parolees,[126] probationers, and prisoners in work release status. Patients stabilized on naltrexone can function normally. They can hold jobs, avoid crime and violence, and reduce their exposure to HIV by stopping injection drug use and drug-related high-risk sexual behaviors.

A NIDA study comparing the effectiveness of a buprenorphine/naloxone combination with extended-release naltrexone for OUD found that both medications were comparably effective in treating OUD once treatment was initiated. Because naltrexone requires waiting at least seven days after last use of short-acting opioids and 10 to 14 days after long-acting opioids, initiating treatment among individuals actively using opioids was more difficult with this medication; however, once withdrawal management was complete, the naltrexone formulation had a similar effectiveness as the combo product.[127,128]

CONCLUSION

There is a wide scope of other SUD-specific therapies discussed elsewhere in this textbook (see Section 9). Although this chapter has not been exhaustive in its coverage of all the behavioral or pharmacological treatments currently available, many of them are covered in more detail elsewhere in this book, and new pharmacotherapies and psychotherapies are in various stages of development. Dissemination and implementation of evidence-based treatment to ensure access to all populations remains a challenge that requires the highest priority if patients with substance use disorders in various clinical settings are to benefit from the advances made since the 1960s and those in the future.

REFERENCES

1. Siqueland L, Crits-Christoph P. Current developments in psychosocial treatments of alcohol and substance abuse. *Curr Psychiatry Rep.* 1999;1:179-184.
2. Carroll KM, Onken LS. Behavioral therapies for drug abuse. *Am J Psychiatry.* 2005;162(8):1452-1460.
3. Volkow ND. Personalizing the treatment of substance use disorders. *Am J Psychiatry.* 2020;177(2):113-116.
4. Vaillant GE. A long-term follow-up of male alcohol abuse. *Arch Gen Psychiatry.* 1996;53:243-249.
5. Vaillant GE. A 60-year follow-up of alcoholic men. *Addiction.* 2003;98:1043-1051.
6. Laudet AB, White W. What are your priorities right now? Identifying service needs across recovery stages to inform service development. *J Subst Abuse Treat.* 2010;38(1):51-59.
7. McKay JR. Is there a case for extended interventions for alcohol and drug use disorders? *Addiction.* 2005;100(11):1594-1610.
8. Dennis ML, Foss MA, Scott CK. An eight-year perspective on the relationship between the duration of abstinence and other aspects of recovery. *Eval Rev.* 2007;31(6):585-612.
9. Sigmon SC. The untapped potential of office-based buprenorphine treatment. *JAMA Psychiatry.* 2015;72(4):395-396.
10. McLellan AT, Lewis DC, O'Brien CP, Kleber HD. Drug addiction as a chronic medical illness: implications for treatment, insurance, and evaluation. *JAMA.* 2000;284:1689-1695.
11. Substance Abuse and Mental Health Services Administration. *Key substance use and mental health indicators in the United States: Results from the 2020 National Survey on Drug Use and Health.* HHS Publication No. PEP21-07-01-003, NSDUH Series H-56. Center for Behavioral Health Statistics and Quality, SAMHSA. Accessed September 6, 2023. https://www.samhsa.gov/data/sites/default/files/reports/rpt35325/NSDUHFFRPDFWHTMLFiles2020/2020NSDUHFFR1PDFW102121.pdf
12. Jones CM, Campopiano M, Baldwin G, McCance-Katz E. National and state treatment need and capacity for opioid agonist medication-assisted treatment. *Am J Public Health.* 2015;105:e55-e63.
13. Wakeman SE, Larochelle MR, Ameli O, et al. Comparative effectiveness of different treatment pathways for opioid use disorder. *JAMA Netw Open.* 2020;3(2):e1920622.
14. Gastfriend DR, Mee-Lee D. Patient placement criteria. In: Galanter G, Kleber HD, eds. *Psychotherapy for the Treatment of Substance Abuse Treatment.* 4th ed. American Psychiatric Publishing, Inc; 2010:99-113.
15. Kritz S, Chu M, John-Hull C, Madray C, Louie B, Brown LS. Opioid dependence as a chronic disease: the interrelationships between length of stay, methadone dose and age on treatment outcome at an urban opioid treatment program. *J Addict Dis.* 2009;28(1):53-56.
16. Klamen DL. Education and training in addictive diseases. *Psychiatr Clin North Am.* 1999;22(2):471-480.
17. Kleber H, Slobetz F. Outpatient drug-free treatment. In: DuPont RL, Goldstein A, O'Donnell J, eds. *Handbook on Drug Abuse.* National Institute on Drug Abuse; 1979:31-38.
18. Institute of Medicine. *Treating Drug Problems.* National Academy Press; 1990.
19. McLellan AT, Grissom GR, Brill P, Durell J, Metzger DS, O'Brien CP. Private substance abuse treatments: are some programs more effective than others? *J Subst Abuse Treat.* 1993;10:243-254.
20. Higgins ST, Budney AJ, Bickel WK, Foerg FE, Donham R, Badger GJ. Incentives improve outcome in outpatient behavioral treatment of cocaine dependence. *Arch Gen Psychiatry.* 1994;51:568-576.
21. Fiore MC, Smith SS, Jorenby DE, Baker TB. The effectiveness of the nicotine patch for smoking cessation: a meta-analysis. *JAMA.* 1994;271:1940-1947.
22. Miller WR, Wilbourne PL, Hettema JE. What works? A summary of alcohol treatment outcome research. In: Hester RK, Miller WR, eds. *Handbook of Alcoholism Treatment Approaches: Effective Alternatives.* 3rd ed. Allyn & Bacon; 2003:13-63.
23. Center for Substance Abuse Treatment. *Substance Abuse: Clinical Issues in Intensive Outpatient Treatment.* Substance Abuse and Mental Health Services Administration (US). Accessed September 6, 2023. http://www.ncbi.nlm.nih.gov/books/NBK64093
24. Washton AM. Evolution of intensive outpatient treatment (IOP) as a "legitimate" treatment modality. *J Addict Dis.* 1997;16(2):xxi-xxvii. doi:10.1300/J069v16n02_b

25. McLellan AT, Hagan TA, Meyers K, Randall M, Durell J. "Intensive" outpatient substance abuse treatment. *J Addict Dis.* 1997;16(2):57-84. doi:10.1300/J069v16n02_05
26. Lewis BF, McCusker J, Hindin R, et al. Four residential drug treatment programs: project IMPACT. In: Inciardi JA, Tims FM, Fletcher BM, eds. *Innovative Approaches in the Treatment of Drug Abuse.* Greenwood Press; 1993:45-60.
27. Lukefeld C, Pickens R, Schuster CR. Improving drug abuse treatment: recommendations for research and practice. In: Pickens RW, Lukefeld CG, Schuster CR, eds. *Improving Drug Abuse Treatment.* NIDA Research Monograph Series. National Institute on Drug Abuse; 1991.
28. Harris AHS, Kivlahan D, Barnett PG, Finney JW. Longer length of stay is not associated with better outcomes in VHA's substance abuse residential rehabilitation treatment programs. *J Behav Health Serv Res.* 2012;39:68-79.
29. De Leon G. Therapeutic communities. In: Galanter M, Kleber HD, Brady KT, eds. *The American Psychiatric Publishing Textbook of Substance Abuse Treatment.* American Psychiatric Publishing, Inc; 2015.
30. Stevens S, Arbiter N, Glider P. Women residents: expanding their role to increase treatment effectiveness in substance abuse programs. *Int J Addict.* 1989;24(5):425-434.
31. Stevens SJ, Glider PJ. Therapeutic communities: substance abuse treatment for women. In: Tims FM, De Leon G, Jainchill N, eds. *Therapeutic Community: Advances in Research and Application.* NIDA Research Monograph 144. National Institute on Drug Abuse; 1994; 162-180.
32. Sacks S, Sacks J, De Leon G, Bernhardt AI, Staines GL. Modified therapeutic community for mentally ill chemical abusers: background; influences; program description; preliminary findings. *Subst Use Misuse.* 1998;32(9):1217-1259.
33. Welsh WN. A multisite evaluation of prison-based therapeutic community drug treatment. *Crim Justice Behav.* 2007;34(11):1481-1498.
34. Inciardi JA, Martin SS, Butzin CA. Five-year outcomes of therapeutic community treatment of drug-involved offenders after release from prison. *Crime Delinq.* 2004;50(1):88-107.
35. Simpson DD, Sells S. *Opioid Addiction and Treatment: A 12-year Follow-up.* Robert E. Krieger; 1990.
36. De Leon G, Schwartz S. Therapeutic communities: what are the retention rates? *Am J Drug Alcohol Abuse.* 1984;10:267-284.
37. De Leon G. *The Therapeutic Community: Study of Effectiveness.* National Institute on Drug Abuse; 1984.
38. Friedmann PD, Hendrickson JC, Gerstein DR, Zhang Z. The effect of matching comprehensive services to patients' needs on drug use improvement in addiction treatment. *Addiction.* 2004;99:962-972.
39. Lemke S, Moos RH. Treatment and outcomes of older patients with alcohol use disorders in community residential programs. *J Stud Alcohol.* 2003;64:219-226.
40. Lewis BF, McCusker J, Hindin R, Frost R, Garfield F. Four residential drug treatment programs: project IMPACT. In: Inciardi JA, Tims FM, Fletcher BW, eds. *Innovative Approaches in the Treatment of Drug Abuse.* Greenwood Press; 1993:45-60.
41. Moos RH, King MJ. Participation in community residential treatment and substance abuse patients' outcomes at discharge. *J Substance Abuse Treat.* 1997;14(1):71-80.
42. Jason LA, Davis MI, Ferrari JR, Bishop PD. Oxford house: a review of research and implications for substance abuse recovery and community research. *J Drug Educ.* 2001;31:1-27.
43. National Case Management Task Forces. *CCM Certification Guide.* CIRSC/Certified Case Manager; 1993.
44. Graham K, Timney CB. Case management in addictions treatment. *J Subst Abuse Treat.* 1990;7:181-188.
45. McNeese-Smith DK. Case management within substance abuse treatment programs in Los Angeles County. *Care Manag J.* 1999;1:10-18.
46. Drake RE, Mercer-McFadden C, Mueser KT, McHugo GJ, Bond GR. Review of integrated mental health and substance abuse treatment for patients with dual disorders. *Schizophr Bull.* 1998;24:589-608.
47. Weiner DA, Abraham ME, Lyons J. Clinical characteristics of youths with substance use problems and implications for residential treatment. *Psychiatr Serv.* 2001;52:793-799.
48. Hesse M, Vanderplasschen W, Rapp RC, Broekaert E, Fridell M. Case management for persons with substance use disorders. *Cochrane Database Syst Rev.* 2007;4:CD006265.
49. Penzenstadler L, Machado A, Thorens G, Zullino D, Khazaal Y. Effect of case management interventions for patients with substance use disorders: a systematic review. *Front Psychiatry.* 2017;8:51.
50. Vanderplasschen W, Rapp RC, De Maeyer J, Van Den Noortgate W. A meta-analysis of the efficacy of case management for substance use disorders: a recovery perspective. *Front Psychiatry.* 2019;10:186.
51. Substance Abuse and Mental Health Services Administration. *Recovery and Recovery Support.* Accessed May 22, 2023. https://www.samhsa.gov/find-help/recovery
52. Department of Mental Health and Substance Abuse Services. *Tennessee recovery navigators.* Accessed May 11, 2023. https://www.tn.gov/behavioral-health/substance-abuse-services/treatment---recovery/treatment---recovery/tennessee-recovery-navigators.html
53. Department of Mental Health and Substance Abuse Services. *HIV/AIDS Early Intervention Services.* Accessed May 11, 2023. https://www.tn.gov/behavioral-health/substance-abuse-services/prevention/hiv-aids.html
54. Department of Mental Health and Substance Abuse Services. *What is a Certified Peer Recovery Specialist?* Accessed May 11, 2023. https://www.tn.gov/content/tn/behavioral-health/cprs/what-is-a-cprs.html
55. Washington State Health Care Authority. *Peer support.* Accessed May 11, 2023. https://www.hca.wa.gov/billers-providers-partners/program-information-providers/peer-support#:~:text=As%20of%20July%201%2C%202019%2C%20peer%20support%20services,disorders%20and%20bill%20them%20as%20Medicaid%20reimbursable%20encounters
56. Reif S, Braude L, Lyman DR, et al. Peer recovery support for individuals with substance use disorders: Assessing the evidence. *Psychiatr Serv.* 2014;65(7):853-861.
57. Wesson DR, Smith DE. Buprenorphine in the treatment of opiate dependence. *J Psychoactive Drugs.* 2010;42(2):161-175.
58. Turner L, Kruszewski SP, Alexander GC. Trends in the use of buprenorphine by office-based physicians in the United States, 2003–2013. *Am J Addict.* 2015;24(1):24-29.
59. Fiellin DA, Kleber H, Trumble-Hejduk JG, McLellan AT, Kosten TR. Consensus statement on office-based treatment of opioid dependence using buprenorphine. *J Subst Abuse Treat.* 2004;27(2):153-159.
60. Jonas DE, Garbutt JC, Amick HR, et al. Behavioral counseling after screening for alcohol misuse in primary care: a systematic review and meta-analysis for the U.S. Preventive Services Task Force. *Ann Intern Med.* 2012;157(9):645-654.
61. Miller WR, Rollnick S. *Motivational Interviewing: Preparing People for Change.* 2nd ed. Guilford Press; 2002.
62. Edwards G, Orford J, Egert S, et al. Alcoholism: a controlled trial of "treatment" and "advice". *J Stud Alcohol.* 1977;38:1004-1031.
63. Bien TH, Miller WR, Tonigan JS. Brief interventions for alcohol problems: a review. *Addiction.* 1993;88:315-335.
64. National Institute on Drug Abuse. *Principles of Drug Addiction Treatment: A Research-Based Guide.* Accessed September 6, 2023. https://nida.nih.gov/sites/default/files/675-principles-of-drug-addiction-treatment-a-research-based-guide-third-edition.pdf
65. Anglin MD, Hser Y. Treatment of drug abuse. In: Tonry M, Wilson JQ, eds. *Drugs and Crime.* University of Chicago Press; 1990:393-460.
66. Simpson DD, Joe GW, Brown BS. Treatment retention and follow-up outcomes in the Drug Abuse Treatment Outcome Study. *Psychol Addict Behav.* 1997;11:294-307.
67. Rich JD, McKenzie M, Larney S, et al. Methadone continuation versus forced withdrawal on incarceration in a combined U.S. prison and jail: a randomized, open-label trial. *Lancet.* 2015;386:350-359.
68. Inciardi JA, Martin SS, Butzin CA, Hooper RM, Harrison LD. An effective model of prison-based treatment for drug-involved offenders. *J Drug Issues.* 1997;27(2):261-278.

69. Wexler HK. Therapeutic communities in American prisons. In: Cullen E, Jones L, Woodward R, eds. *Therapeutic Communities in American Prisons.* John Wiley & Sons; 1997.
70. Hiller ML, Knight K, Broome KM, Simpson DD. Compulsory community-based substance abuse treatment and the mentally ill criminal offender. *Prison J.* 1996;76(2):180-191.
71. Center for Substance Abuse Treatment. *Substance Abuse Treatment for Adults in the Criminal Justice System.* Substance Abuse and Mental Health Services Administration (US). Treatment Improvement Protocol (TIP) Series, No. 44.
72. Chen JT, Fang CC, Shyu RS, Lin KC. Underreporting of illicit drug use by patients at emergency departments as revealed by two-tiered urinalysis. *Addict Behav.* 2006;31:2304-2308.
73. Brown RL. Identification and office management of alcohol and drug disorders. In: Fleming MF, Barry KL, eds. *Addictive Disorders.* Mosby Yearbook; 1992.
74. Warner EA, Friedmann PD. Laboratory testing for drug abuse. *Arch Pediatr Adolesc Med.* 2006;160:854-864.
75. Cone EJ. New developments in biological measures of drug prevalence. In: Harrison L, Hughes A, eds. *The Validity of Self-reported Drug Use: Improving Accuracy of Survey Estimates.* NIDA Research Monograph 167. National Institute on Drug Abuse; 1997.
76. Reisfield GM, Bertholf R, Barkin RL, Webb F, Wilson G. Urine drug test interpretation: what do physicians know? *J Opioid Manag.* 2007;3:80-86.
77. Kleber HD. Outpatient detoxification from opiates. *Prim Psychiatry.* 1996;1:42-52.
78. Carroll K, Rounsaville B, Keller D. Relapse prevention strategies for the treatment of cocaine abuse. *Am J Drug Alcohol Abuse.* 1991;17(3):249-265.
79. Marlatt G, Gordon JR, eds. *Relapse Prevention: Maintenance Strategies in the Treatment of Addictive Behaviors.* Guilford Press; 1985.
80. Carroll K, Rounsaville B, Nich C, Gordon LT, Wirtz PW, Gawin F. One-year follow-up of psycho-therapy and pharmacotherapy for cocaine dependence: delayed emergence of psychotherapy effects. *Arch Gen Psychiatry.* 1994;51:989-997.
81. Miller WR. Motivational interviewing: research, practice and puzzles. *Addict Behav.* 1996;61(6):835-842.
82. Higgins ST, Budney AJ, Bickel WK, Badger GJ, Foerg FE, Ogden D. Outpatient behavioral treatment for cocaine dependence: one-year outcome. *Exp Clin Psychopharmacol.* 1995;3(2):205-212.
83. Meyers RJ, Roozen HG, Smith JE. The community reinforcement approach: an update of the evidence. *Alcohol Res Health.* 2011;33:380-388.
84. Abbott PJ. A review of the community reinforcement approach in the treatment of opioid dependence. *J Psychoactive Drugs.* 2009;41:379-385.
85. Budney AJ, Kandel DB, Cherek DR, Martin BR, Stephens RS, Roffman R. College on problems of drug dependence meeting, Puerto Rico (June 1996). Marijuana use and dependence. *Drug Alcohol Depend.* 1997;45:1-11.
86. Stephens RS, Roffman RA, Simpson EE. Treating adult marijuana dependence: a test of the relapse prevention model. *J Consult Clin Psychol.* 1994;62(1):92-99.
87. Fuller RK, Branchey L, Brightwell DR, et al. Disulfiram treatment of alcoholism: a Veteran's Administration cooperative study. *JAMA.* 1986;256:1449-1455.
88. Silverman K, Higgins ST, Brooner RK, et al. Sustained cocaine abstinence in methadone maintenance patients through voucher-based reinforcement therapy. *Arch Gen Psychiatry.* 1996;53:409-415.
89. Marsch LA, Guarino H, Acosta M, et al. Web-based behavioral treatment for substance use disorders as a partial replacement of standard methadone maintenance treatment. *J Subst Abuse Treat.* 2014;46:43-51.
90. Godley SH, Smith JE, Meyers RJ, Godley MD. Adolescent community reinforcement approach. In: Springer DW, Rubin A, eds. *Substance Abuse Treatment for Youth and Adults: Clinician's Guide to Evidence-Based Practice.* John Wiley & Sons, Inc; 2009:109-201.
91. Silverman K, Wong C, Higgins S, et al. Increasing opiate abstinence through voucher-based reinforcement therapy. *Drug Alcohol Depend.* 1996;41:156-165.
92. Milby JB, Schumacher JE, McNamara C, et al. *Abstinence Contingent Housing Enhances Day Treatment for Homeless Cocaine Abusers.* NIDA Research Monograph Series 174. National Institute on Drug Abuse; 1996.
93. Milby JB, Schumacher JE, Raczynski JM, et al. Sufficient conditions for effective treatment of substance abusing homeless. *Drug Alcohol Depend.* 1996;43:39-47.
94. Woody GE, Luborsky L, McLellan AT, et al. Psychotherapy for opiate addicts: does it help? *Arch Gen Psychiatry.* 1983;40:639-645.
95. McLellan AT, Arndt I, Metzger DS, Woody GE, O'Brien CP. The effects of psychosocial services in substance abuse treatment. *JAMA.* 1993;269(15):1953-1959.
96. Luborsky L. *Principles of Psychoanalytic Psychotherapy: A Manual for Supportive-Expressive (SE) Treatment.* Basic Books; 1984.
97. Woody GE, McLellan AT, Luborsky L, O'Brien CP. Twelve-month follow-up of psychotherapy for opiate dependence. *Am J Psychiatry.* 1987;144:590-596.
98. Woody GE, McLellan AT, Luborsky L, O'Brien CP. Psychotherapy in community methadone programs: a validation study. *Am J Psychiatry.* 1995;152(9):1302-1308.
99. Diamond GS, Liddle HA. Resolving a therapeutic impasse between parents and adolescents in multidimensional family therapy. *J Consult Clin Psychol.* 1996;64(3):481-488.
100. Schmidt SE, Liddle HA, Dakof GA. Effects of multidimensional family therapy: relationship of changes in parenting practices to symptom reduction in adolescent substance abuse. *J Fam Psychol.* 1996;10(1):1-16.
101. McLellan AT, Woody GE, Luborsky L, Goehl L. Is the counselor an "active ingredient" in substance abuse treatment? *J Nerv Ment Dis.* 1988;176:423-430.
102. Japuntich SJ, Zehner ME, Smith SS, et al. Smoking cessation via the internet: a randomized clinical trial of an internet intervention as adjuvant treatment in a smoking cessation intervention. *Nicotine Tob Res.* 2006;8:S59-S67.
103. Carroll K, Ball S, Martino S, et al. Computer-assisted delivery of cognitive-behavioral therapy for addiction: a randomized trial of CBT4CBT. *Am J Psychiatry.* 2008;165(7):881-888.
104. Tossmann HP, Jonas B, Tensil MD, Lang P, Strüber E. A controlled trial of an internet-based intervention program for cannabis users. *Cyberpsychol Behav Soc Netw.* 2011;14(11):673-679.
105. Riper H, Kramer J, Smit F, Conijn B, Schippers G, Cuijpers P. Web-based self-help for problem drinkers: a pragmatic randomized trial. *Addiction.* 2008;103(2):218-227.
106. Kypri K, Langley JD, Saunders JB, Cashell-Smith ML, Herbison P. Randomized controlled trial of web-based alcohol screening and brief intervention in primary care. *Arch Intern Med.* 2008;168(5):530-536.
107. Whittaker R, Borland R, Bullen C, Rodgers A, Gu Y. Mobile phone-based interventions for smoking cessation. *Cochrane Database Syst Rev.* 2009;4:CD006611.
108. McTavish FM, Chih MY, Shah D, Gustafson DH. How patients recovering from alcoholism use a smartphone intervention. *J Dual Diagn.* 2012;8(4):294-304.
109. The Rockefeller University. *The first pharmacological treatment for narcotic addiction: Methadone maintenance.* The Rockefeller University Hospital Centennial; 2010 Accessed September 6, 2023. https://centennial.rucares.org/index.php?page=Methadone_Maintenance
110. Fiellin DA, Pantalon MV, Chawarski MC, et al. Counseling plus buprenorphine–naloxone maintenance therapy for opioid dependence. *N Engl J Med.* 2006;355(4):365-374.
111. Fudala P, Bridge TP, Herbert S, et al. Buprenorphine/Naloxone Collaborative Study Group: office-based treatment of opiate addiction with a sublingual-tablet formulation of buprenorphine and naloxone. *N Engl J Med.* 2003;349(10):949-958.
112. Kosten TR, Fiellin DA. Buprenorphine for office-based practice: consensus conference overview. *Am J Addict.* 2004;13(S1):S1-S7.
113. McCance-Katz EF. Office-based buprenorphine treatment for opioid-dependent patients. *Harvard Rev Psychiatry.* 2004;12(6):321-338.

114. Fiellin DA, Barthwell AG. Guideline development for office-based pharmacotherapies for opioid dependence. *J Addict Dis.* 2003;22(4):109-120. doi:10.1300/J069v22n04_09
115. Substance Abuse and Mental Health Services Administration. Removal of DATA waiver (X-waiver) requirement. Accessed May 19, 2023. https://www.samhsa.gov/medications-substance-use-disorders/removal-data-waiver-requirement
116. Congress.gov. H.R.2617 – Consolidated Appropriations Act, 2023. 117th Congress (2021-2022). Accessed May 19, 2023. https://www.congress.gov/bill/117th-congress/house-bill/2617/text
117. Dole VP, Nyswander M, Kreek MJ. Narcotic blockade. *Arch Intern Med.* 1996;118:304-309.
118. Lowinson JH, Payte JT, Joseph H, et al. Methadone maintenance. In: Lowinson JH, Ruiz P, Millman RB, Langrod JG, eds. *Substance Abuse: A Comprehensive Textbook*. Lippincott Williams & Wilkins; 1996:405-414.
119. Simpson DD. Treatment for drug abuse: follow-up outcomes and length of time spent. *Arch Gen Psychiatry.* 1981;38(8):875-880.
120. Simpson DD, Joe GW, Bracy SA. Six-year follow-up of opioid addicts after admission to treatment. *Arch Gen Psychiatry.* 1982;39(11):1318-1323.
121. Novick DM, Joseph J, Croxson TS, et al. Absence of antibody to human immunodeficiency virus in long-term, socially rehabilitated methadone maintenance patients. *Arch Intern Med.* 1990;150(1):97-99.
122. Brown LS, Kritz SA, Goldsmith RJ, et al. Health services for HIV/AIDS, hepatitis C virus, and sexually transmitted infections in substance abuse treatment programs. *Public Health Rep.* 2007;122:441-451.
123. Brown LS, Kritz SA, Goldsmith JR, et al. Characteristics of substance abuse treatment programs providing services for HIV/AIDS, hepatitis C virus infection, and sexually transmitted infections: the National Clinical Trials Network. *J Subst Abuse Treat.* 2006;30:315-321.
124. Lee JD, Friedmann PD, Kinlock TW, et al. Extended-release naltrexone to prevent opioid relapse in criminal justice offenders. *N Engl J Med.* 2016;374:1232-1242.
125. Greenstein RA, Arndy IC, McLellan AT, O'Brien CP, Evans B. Naltrexone: a clinical perspective. *J Clin Psychiatry.* 1984;45(9 Pt 2):25-28.
126. Cornish JW, Metzger D, Woody GE, et al. Naltrexone pharmacotherapy for opioid dependent federal probationers. *J Subst Abuse Treat.* 1997;14(6):529-534.
127. Nunes EV, Lee JD, Sisti D, et al. Ethical and clinical safety considerations in the design of an effectiveness trial: a comparison of buprenorphine versus naltrexone treatment for opioid dependence. *Contemp Clin Trials.* 2016;51:34-43.
128. Lee JD, Nunes EV, Novo P, et al. Comparative effectiveness of extended-release naltrexone versus buprenorphine-naloxone for opioid relapse prevention (X: BOT): a multicentre, open-label, randomised controlled trial. *Lancet.* 2018;391(10118):309-318.

CHAPTER 37

Identification and Treatment of High-Risk Alcohol Use and Alcohol Use Disorder: An Overview

Mark Willenbring

CHAPTER OUTLINE

- Introduction
- The spectrum of severity in unhealthy alcohol use
- Modern approaches to treatment
- Defining the problem: What are treatment outcomes?
- Measuring drinking outcomes
- Tailoring treatment to the continuum of severity
- Treatment and behavior change
- Systems of care
- Integrating the evidence and personalizing practice

INTRODUCTION

For millennia, alcohol has been one of the most popular and dangerous substances ingested by humans. Inevitably, some individuals drink too much, causing individual and social harm. In response to mental illness and chronic intoxication, societies have vacillated between rehabilitation and punitive approaches over the years. In the middle of the 1800s, there was a period of "moral therapy" with a rehabilitation focus, followed by a period of more custodial and punitive approaches. During this time, the funding applied to rehabilitative efforts diminished, and affected individuals were more likely to be incarcerated.

In the middle of the last century, the United States went through a period whereby persons with chronically excessive alcohol use and functional impairment were seen as "ill." Alcoholics Anonymous (AA) was founded in 1935, followed by the organization of "treatment centers" using an AA-based model for "treatment." In the 1950s and 1960s, modern research revealed knowledge of the nature, course, and treatment of excessive alcohol use and Alcohol Use Disorder (AUD). Indeed, considerable progress toward more humane and effective treatment has been made in a relatively short time. Nevertheless, the history of treatment for AUD presents some unique obstacles that have proved resistant to reform. Although 12-Step based treatment programs offer a form of "treatment," most of their clients are "referred" by the criminal justice system.[1,2]

A large majority of community programs only offer the Minnesota Model for the treatment of AUD in a form little different from that in 1955.[3-5] In many cases, physician involvement is limited to treating alcohol withdrawal. Furthermore, regardless of theoretical orientation, treatment programs offer a time-limited treatment focused on inducing and maintaining early remission and offer little except repetition for patients who do not respond. Treatment failure is often attributed to a patient's lack of "motivation" or "insight," rather than to shortcomings in the therapeutic approach. For example, why would 30 days of didactic lectures, limited counseling, and an introduction to Alcoholics Anonymous (AA) be expected to change the course of a chronic illness? While often reported as evidence-based, the quality of counseling in community programs is often poor, consisting of casual talk unrelated to therapy and supervision of counseling staff is minimal.[6] Integration with healthcare systems is rare, so identification and management of coexisting mental and physical disorders are uncommon and highly fragmented, despite the high prevalence and societal cost of such conditions in treatment-seeking populations. Few community treatment programs offer pharmacotherapy for AUD, and most fail to educate their patients about it.[7] Because of these and other shortfalls, lifetime exposure to professional treatment for AUD is around 10%, a figure that has not changed in 70 years. In sum, although progress has been made, more remains to be done. Without a major change in how, where, and by whom treatment is delivered, research findings will remain unimplemented and unavailable to the patients and families who need them. Some hope can be found in the recent implementation of pharmacotherapy for opioid use disorders (most of which is prescribed by clinicians who are not addiction specialists) and in internet-based start-ups that integrate mental health and substance use treatment.

This chapter provides an overview of current research on treatment for unhealthy alcohol use. The various behavioral and pharmacological treatments are addressed in detail in other chapters of this textbook. The goal of this overview is to provide a context to help guide the interpretation of the research and guidelines provided in other chapters. First, an overview of the spectrum of alcohol use is presented. Then, a brief review of the history of therapy for AUD and ways of measuring alcohol use to contextualize potential treatment goals is provided. Next, a continuum of care is presented that corresponds to the spectrum of alcohol use with comment on how it may relate to mechanisms of behavior change. This is followed by how changes in healthcare policy are affecting the treatment infrastructure for changing drinking behavior. The chapter concludes by exploring how research findings may be applied to individual patients, that is, the art of evidence-based medicine.

THE SPECTRUM OF SEVERITY IN UNHEALTHY ALCOHOL USE

Recent research has provided a new and more complete view of the range of drinking, AUD, and alcohol-related harms in the community. However, some definitions are needed to understand drinking behavior and relate it to adverse events. In the United States, a "standard drink" is defined as the amount of ethanol in 1.5 oz (45 mL) of 80-proof spirits, 12 oz of beer, or 5 oz of table wine, each containing about 14.5 g of absolute ethanol (see **Table 37-1**).

Since actual alcohol levels in beer and wine vary, these amounts are meant to be approximate. A "standard drink" varies widely across the world, and there is no universal definition. For example, in the United Kingdom and Australia, a drinking "unit" is defined as 30 mL (1 oz) of 80-proof spirits, equal to about 10 g of absolute ethanol. Thus, for cross-national comparisons, it is best to focus on grams of absolute ethanol (per day, per drink, etc.). The National Institute of Alcohol Abuse and Alcoholism (NIAAA) recommends that men drink no more than 4 drinks per day and 14 drinks per week and that women (and men 65 and older) drink no more than 3 drinks per day and 7 drinks per week (see **Table 37-1**). Differences between men, women, and others are based entirely on epidemiology. The reasons for this are complex and not fully understood. How to apply them to transgender and nonbinary people is unknown, although using 50 g/day of absolute ethanol as an upper limit is likely a good idea. The daily limit amounts to approximately 50 g of absolute ethanol per day. Drinking within these limits is considered "lower-risk" drinking. Lower limits or abstinence may be indicated in the presence of coexisting medical or psychiatric disorders, in older people, or when medication interactions are a concern. Women who are pregnant or at risk of becoming pregnant are advised to abstain. In this chapter, a day on which the limit is exceeded is considered a "heavy drinking day," and "heavy drinking" is defined as drinking more than the maximum limits on a regular basis, such as exceeding the daily limits weekly or more often. Drinking more than advised itself is not considered a disorder. Instead, DSM-5-TR[8] recommends that drinking causes "clinically significant impairment or distress" and that an individual endorse at least 2 out of 11 diagnostic criteria for AUD to make a diagnosis. Drinking more than the recommended limits in the absence of a disorder is considered "high-risk or hazardous" alcohol use.

TABLE 37-1 Volume of Common Beverages Containing About 14.5 g of Absolute Ethanol (a U.S. "Standard Drink") and the Maximum Recommended Drinking Limits From The National Institute on Alcohol Abuse and Alcoholism

	Beverage size	Maximum limits	
U.S. lager beer	12 oz	Women[a]	Daily ≤3 drinks Weekly ≤7 drinks
Table wine (eg, Chardonnay)	5 oz (5 drinks per 750 mL)	Men	Daily ≤4 drinks Weekly ≤14 drinks
80 Proof spirits (eg, vodka)	1.5 oz (17 drinks per 750 mL)		

[a]And those 65 or older.

Data from The National Institute on Alcohol Abuse and Alcoholism. https://www.niaaa.nih.gov/alcohols-effects-health/alcohol-topics-a-to-z

Interpretation of most previous studies of the epidemiology of heavy drinking and AUD are complicated by the 2013 changes in the DSM (in DSM-5, dissolving Alcohol Abuse and Alcohol Dependence as one single diagnostic entity, newly named Alcohol Use Disorder/AUD, with levels of severity identified by number of diagnostic criteria met). Consequently, a DSM-IV-TR[9] diagnosis of alcohol dependence is difficult to relate to a DSM-5 diagnosis of AUD. Nevertheless, the number of positive DSM-5 criteria is a good reflection of the severity and disability related to drinking.[10] Given the marked changes in epidemiology that resulted from a new sample of the National Epidemiological Study of Alcohol and Related Conditions (NESARC) in 2011-2012, it is perhaps best to use the National Study on Drug Use and Health (NSDUH) data for reliable estimates of the prevalence of AUD.[11] According to the 2020 version of NSDUH, 28.3 million people 12 and older met DSM-5 criteria for AUD. In other words, about 70% of all SUDs were in individuals who use alcohol. Most of the others (about 14 million people) met the diagnostic criteria for cannabis use disorder, while other SUDs (about 4 million) were distributed among other drugs. Binge drinking (1 or more days in the past month with more than the recommended limits by NIAAA) is more common than AUD. In 2020, nearly half of individuals who use alcohol (61.6 million, or 22%) exhibited binge drinking, a number that has not changed in the past 5 years. Binge drinking, while not a diagnosis, is responsible for more acute problems stemming from drinking alcohol than AUD.[12] Hazardous alcohol use and AUD result in a burden of disease estimated at 4.9% of all deaths and 6.8% of all Disability-Adjusted Years of Life lost.[13]

MODERN APPROACHES TO TREATMENT

Professional treatment for AUD that is supported by a base of basic and clinical research is a relatively new field compared to other areas of medicine. It is helpful to understand the historical context of our current treatment and outcome paradigms to understand opportunities and controversies within the field.

For most of history, only custodial treatment for AUD was available. Modern behavioral treatment approaches grew out of AA on one hand and the growth of academic psychiatry and psychology after World War II on the other. AA rapidly spread from its roots in an evangelical Christian movement in 1935, publishing its *The Big Book* in 1939. The 12 Steps of AA, counseling, and education were combined to create the "Minnesota Model" of treatment in the 1950s in a collaboration between providers at Willmar State Hospital, the Pioneer House, and Hazelden—the latter two early AA recovery centers. In 1961, Dan Anderson, a cocreator of the model, became the CEO of the Hazelden Foundation, an organization that has been influential in its spread. The Johnson Institute, another Minnesota organization, was established in 1966 to help spread the Minnesota Model; it also developed the procedure known as an "intervention," where people close to someone with an AUD come together to share their concerns (and usually shuttle the soon-to-be patient off to a program). Subsequently, the Minnesota Model has been adopted internationally, and it is the most prevalent form of treatment available in the United States. For many U.S. residents, programs based on the Minnesota Model may be the only available approach to treatment.[14]

Key features of the Minnesota Model are the use of both professional staff and individuals with a personal history of AUD to provide group counseling as well as patient and family education. Model programs also include a strong linkage to AA, a requirement of abstinence from all psychoactive substances other than tobacco and caffeine, and belief that alcoholism is a "primary, progressive disease that cannot be cured, although it can be arrested through abstinence and AA." This approach was initially provided only in 28-day programs in hospitals or residential facilities but is now provided in a wider range of durations and settings. These programs are often referred to as rehabilitation ("rehab") programs. Twelve-Step Facilitation is a manualized version of the Minnesota Model that has been adapted for research using an individual outpatient approach.[15] Note that 12-step facilitation resembles community 12-step programs in its focus on AA and abstinence. It is different in many other ways, including using individual counseling by highly trained and supervised therapists with advanced clinical training. In contrast, community programs are almost completely group-based, and the counselors have minimal training and no meaningful supervision. Thus, it is difficult to generalize from studies of 12-step facilitation to community-based 12-step rehabilitation programs.

The fields of psychology and psychiatry have undergone substantial development and expansion as well, primarily because the Veterans Administration (VA) rapidly expanded mental health services following World War II. Pavlov discovered classical conditioning in the 1920s,[16] and B.F. Skinner first published on operant conditioning in 1935.[16] The concepts of group therapy and therapeutic community were first proposed in the mid-1940s, with subsequent development and spread in the 1950s and 1960s.[17] Albert Ellis developed the first type of cognitive-behavior therapy, Rational-Emotive Therapy, in the mid-1950s,[18] and Aaron Beck developed cognitive therapy for depression in the 1960s.[19] Specific therapies for AUD based on these earlier psychological theories include therapeutic communities, aversion therapy, cognitive-behavior therapy, skills training, community reinforcement, and contingency management. More recently, William Miller and colleagues developed an approach, motivational enhancement therapy, based on stages of change and encouraging motivation to change.[20] There are several others that have some evidence of effectiveness, although most studies are small and have a high potential for bias (such as the originator of the therapy serving as principal investigator). Manualization and sophisticated monitoring of the application of behavioral techniques have allowed true comparisons of efficacy with a high degree of confidence in the validity of the trials. The main conclusion from this work is that a variety of validated therapy approaches and techniques all produce similar outcomes.[21,22] Thus, the best therapy approach is to use the most relevant aspects of all available therapies, rather than focusing on one type over others. This approach allows greater individualization based on patient preferences.

Pharmacotherapy for AUD has experienced halting advancement. Many older psychiatric medications have been tested including lithium carbonate, anxiolytics, tricyclic antidepressants, antipsychotics, and phenytoin. Although initial open-label studies for many reported efficacy, subsequent research for all except disulfiram failed to substantiate early claims. Disulfiram was approved for use in the United States as a deterrent agent in 1949. It took until 1995 for the next medication, naltrexone, to be approved by the U.S. Food and Drug Administration (FDA) for treatment of AUD. Since then, acamprosate and an injectable depot formulation of naltrexone have been FDA approved, and other primary or adjuvant agents including topiramate, varenicline, baclofen, and gabapentin have demonstrated variable degrees of efficacy in randomized controlled trials.[23] Available antirecurrence medications have a degree of efficacy in reducing risk of recurrences like antidepressants for major depression, statins for prevention of coronary events, and nonsteroidal anti-inflammatory drugs for arthritis pain. But because of deficiencies of the current system, they very seldom are prescribed.[24] In addition, pharmacotherapy has been stuck at the current level for the past 15 years, with no new drugs approved. Heilig et al. have commented on this lag in treatment development.[25]

Research on the nature, causes, consequences, and course of AUD has slowly grown. Major advances have been made in identifying genetic, developmental, and environmental risk factors for AUD and describing its natural history and treatment response, as well as biopsychosocial consequences of heavy drinking and AUD. Excellent animal models continue to underpin research on the biological mechanisms underlying behavior. The clinical criteria defining AUD and its relationship to the timing, frequency, and quantity of heavy drinking have evolved. However, we still do not understand the underlying processes of behavior change in drinking or other behaviors.

DEFINING THE PROBLEM: WHAT ARE TREATMENT OUTCOMES?

The primary goal of treatment for AUD is reduction of alcohol use. However, given the cultural heritage of treatment in the United States, as well as the range of beliefs around the origins of addiction, achieving consensus on specific treatment goals and more comprehensive outcome definitions has been difficult. Topics in these debates include the nature of addictive behavior, the role of spirituality in recovery, and the relationship of specific drinking behaviors to functional outcomes. Commonly considered outcomes are drinking behavior, the number of positive diagnostic criteria of AUD, functional consequences of drinking, and "recovery" versus abstinence or remission (the absence of a disease once present).

Drinking behavior is the most common outcome of interest. The oldest conceptual definition of treatment success is continuous, lifelong abstinence. The origins of this belief are complex, but it emerged in part from the belief among puritanical American Protestants that only through lifelong abstinence could a "habitual drunkard" attain moral redemption and salvation. Indeed, it was to his experience with the evangelical Christian Oxford Group that Bill Wilson attributed his "hot flash" of spiritual awakening, his subsequent abstinence from alcohol, and later many aspects of AA's 12 steps.[26,27] The AA community still considers any return to drinking to be an absolute failure, requiring the individual to restart their recovery process.

Abstinence is not always mandatory, though, and nonabstinent remission (NAR) is a frequent outcome.[28-31] In a retrospective study, Dawson and colleagues[28] found NAR to be the most frequent outcome, while abstinent remission (AR) was a close second. More recently, Wietkewicz[32] and colleagues used samples from the MATCH trial and determined that three years after initiating of a research treatment, four patterns were discernable: low-functioning people who frequently use alcohol (13.9%), low-functioning people who infrequently use alcohol (15.8%), high-functioning people who frequently use alcohol (19.4%), and high-functioning people who infrequently use alcohol (51.8%). It should be noted that the sample was older (mean age = 45 + 11 years), and NAR is more frequent among this group. A recent study of AUD outcomes with a DSM-5 sample found rates of persistent AUD (34%) that were comparable to prior studies. Also, the rate of NAR was similarly high, about half of those in recovery, and about one quarter of those in recovery did not seek any help at all. Duration of recovery was associated with a gradual reduction in the prevalence of persistent AUD. The severity of AUD predicted both seeking help and abstinent outcomes.[33] These findings add weight to the notion that NAR is a reasonable outcome, especially among those with a less severe course. More work is clearly needed to determine the characteristics and methods for helping those people achieve NAR.

In the past few years, numerous interventions have been tested in RCTs. There is research support for combining treatment for social anxiety disorders and AUD,[34] more frequent and comprehensive follow up research interviews, a harm-reduction approach, and psychodynamic treatment for AUD. Some interventions with promise include ketamine treatment and the gabapentinoids[35,36] The following were determined to be ineffective: prazosin, exercise, mecamylamine, combined treatment for PTSD and AUD, transcranial magnetic stimulation, pioglitazone, eye-movement desensitization and reprocessing therapy, and attentional bias training.

The impact of alcohol use on medical and psychiatric outcomes, including all-cause mortality, seems closely tied to the frequency and quantity consumed.[37] A recent study on the global burden of disease found that alcohol was the sixth leading cause of disability globally, including a 41% increase in attributable mortality and a 31% increase in disability-adjusted life years since 1990.[38,39] More premature deaths are due to acute events related to alcohol intoxication (53%) with the remainder due to sequelae of chronic heavy alcohol use.[40] From a medical perspective, it follows that a reasonable treatment goal would be to reduce the frequency and/or volume of alcohol consumed, regardless of whether abstinence is an explicit goal of the patient, like the exposure reduction goals of treatment for diabetes and hypertension. Indeed, even among people with moderate to severe AUD, all-cause mortality is reduced with decreases in alcohol consumption.[41] These studies do not support a dualistic view of outcomes. They suggest that working with patients to achieve any reduction in drinking is better than doing nothing.

Complicating matters, alcohol consumption may provide benefits at lower-risk levels. Lower-risk alcohol consumption in middle-aged adults is associated with decreased incidence of ischemic cardiovascular disease and death, diabetes, Alzheimer disease, and stroke, although heavy drinking increases risk for these disorders.[39,42-44] Thus, one must subtract potential beneficial effects of drinking from potential risk for adverse events when developing risk estimates.

Compared to measures of consumption, the presence or absence of DSM-5 diagnostic criteria for AUD are less frequently discussed as a measure of treatment success. Using the DSM criteria, full sustained remission is defined as no longer meeting any of the 11 criteria of AUD for a period of 12 months or more other than cravings/strong desire or urge for alcohol, and someone in partial remission displays the same history as above, except that the time course is at least 3 months but still less than 12 months. Note that the quantity and frequency of alcohol use are not DSM-5 criteria. Indeed, as previously discussed NAR is the most frequent longer-term outcome among individuals with AUD. Most direct estimates of mortality among people with AUD have been obtained with samples of people seeking treatment. In this group, annual mortality is 1.4 to 4.7 times that of matched controls.[39,45] Since individuals who seek help have more severe AUD, a higher prevalence of co-occurring conditions, and less social capital than do those who do not seek help, information obtained by studying treatment populations applies only to the small proportion of people with severe, recurring AUD. Consequently, there is a need for additional research into multilevel outcomes that include drinking behaviors, symptoms of AUD, and function among community dwellers who have not sought treatment.

Social consequences are mediated by co-occurring mental disorders, especially antisocial personality disorder, and social context. Societies vary markedly in their tolerance for various forms of behavior associated with intoxication or AUD.

For example, whether an individual is arrested for driving while intoxicated depends on local laws and how they are enforced. However, social problems associated with alcohol use are strongly related to mortality, the health of the family and friends of an individual who drinks alcohol, as well as their quality of life. In a large community sample, as the number of diagnostic criteria met increased, disability increased, and functional impairment for DSM-IV Alcohol Dependence (with the highest end of criteria met—6-7 dependence criteria) was similar to that for anxiety disorders and depression.[46]

MEASURING DRINKING OUTCOMES

Methods for measuring drinking behavior and how it affects other outcomes have remained stable, with structured retrospective self-report being the most common tool. This approach is used in most treatment trials, and research supports its validity and reliability.[47] The most common instrument used is the Timeline Follow-Back.[48] Using methods that collect data in real time using interactive voice response, personal digital assistants (eg, smartphones), and ecological momentary assessment reduced memory errors by minimizing the time and distractions between drinking episodes and reporting.[49] Recent research demonstrated that ecological momentary assessment was more accurate than retrospective self-report.[50,51] An RCT reported that following a time-limited rehabilitation program, smartphone, smartphone plus telephone and telephone only follow up were all superior to treatment as usual for drinking behavior.[52] Although smartphone app development continues, currently there is not an evidence base for using or selecting them.

Laboratory tests, despite ongoing research, have not yet delivered significant advances. Serum or exhaled alcohol concentrations continue to be useful markers of alcohol consumption in the hours before the test is performed. The refinement of biosensors that measure BAC transcutaneously may improve accuracy in the assessment of drinking behavior[53,54] but may also cause decreases in drinking. Other traditional lab tests and calculations such as gamma-glutaryl transferase (GGT), mean corpuscular volume (MCV), and the ratio of aspartate aminotransferase (AST) to alanine aminotransferase (ALT) all have poor test characteristics and may be elevated or altered by other common liver conditions.[55] Those tests should not be relied upon in clinical practice to detect or monitor unhealthy alcohol use. Some promising clinical measures include ethyl glucuronide (EtG), ethyl succinate (EtS), percent carbohydrate-deficient transferrin (%CDT), and phosphatidylethanol (PEth). Caution must be observed in using any of these tests, however, particularly EtG/EtS and PEth. None of the biomarkers have adequate sensitivity and specificity to detect low to moderate drinking levels. Even at high levels, systematic self-report is more accurate.[56] High-quality studies of sensitivity and specificity by multiple investigators at different sites are needed. Until more research is done, a "positive" should be taken as suggestive and requires clinical confirmation. In particular, they should not be used in administrative or clinical decisions as the sole reason for adverse actions.

In early treatment studies of AUD, drinking behavior was grouped into dichotomous categories of abstinence or drinking. Over time, these simple categories were supplanted by more complex variable-based approaches, where average values of a continuous drinking variable were compared among groups using increasingly sophisticated statistical techniques. Percent days abstinent and percent days heavy drinking are common examples. This variable-centered approach has advantages, such as using more data and allowing use of parametric statistics, thus increasing statistical power. This approach also allows for a wider range of outcomes to be considered, as discussed above.

However, variable-based approaches will not capture individual heterogeneity within the study population if only mean values are considered. In many treatment trials, a portion of the study population will demonstrate a response, but the majority may not respond at all. A robust response in a minority of individuals may only move the average outcome a small distance, suggesting that the treatment is only minimally effective overall (which is true for the study population overall). Variable-centered analyses using either a dichotomous measure or means of a continuous drinking measure are not designed to capture such an effect.

Trajectory analyses characterize samples into groups with different courses. This approach has become increasingly popular in recent years, and has been used to compare different alcohol use over time in UK armed forces,[57] different courses of problematic alcohol use after a natural disaster,[58] COVID-19,[59] disparities in functioning from alcohol and cannabis use in a racially diverse sample,[60] the course of employment following treatment for AUD,[61] intervention impact on alcohol use and harms,[62] and the impact of parental behavior on teen alcohol outcomes.[63] One advantage of trajectory analyses is that they lend themselves to figures that show the response of different groups over time. Another advantage is that they are much easier to understand. Most important, trajectory analysis can help break down the variability within a sample in a way that variable-centered analyses do not.

Another new method that has exploded in recent use is machine learning and deep neural networks. Machine learning has been used to identify noninvasive proteomic biomarkers for alcohol-related liver disease,[64] detecting intoxication with passive smartphone and wristband activity devices[65] predicting imminent driving (and drinking),[66] predicting drop-out of outpatient alcohol care,[67] predicting remission of AUD,[68] and to predict bleeding of esophageal varices in cirrhosis,[69] among many others. Although most of these studies are still preliminary, over time they will become more refined and will be used in research and treatment of AUD.

Interpretation of randomized controlled treatment studies requires consideration of the mechanism of behavior change and the nature of the control group. As discussed, there are numerous ways to measure different types of outcomes during and after intervention. However, what happens before treatment should not be ignored. Arguably, what happened before a trial starts may best predict how well a treatment works. In several trials, subjects' drinking trajectories prior to treatment entry significantly predicted outcome independent of treatment condition.[70-74] Another large study in the VA Healthcare System found that brief intervention (the primary independent variable) likely played no role in the 48% reduction in prevalence of heavy drinking among patients.[75] Keeping this in mind may affect how policymakers and clinicians apply research results to patients either seeking help or being mandated to treatment.

TAILORING TREATMENT TO THE CONTINUUM OF SEVERITY

Multiple treatment modalities are used in the treatment of AUD. However, the best way to match the type and intensity of treatment to the individual needs of a patient with AUD remains unclear. For example, no systematic outcome advantage has been demonstrated for residential or intensive day program treatment compared to once or twice weekly outpatient treatment. No behavioral treatment has been shown to be better than others that are conceptually distinct and use different behavioral techniques. Attempts to match specific behavioral therapies with clinical characteristics of patients have yielded little. Several medications are efficacious in reducing recurrence of alcohol use or heavy drinking during early recovery, but none are clearly better than others, and there is not yet a way to predict how likely a patient is to respond to one rather than another. Finally, approximately 10% of people with AUD have a severe chronic form of the disorder, yet most treatment programs offer a few weeks or months of treatment, and information on management of AUD as a chronic illness is limited with mixed results. In sum, current recommendations and practice regarding the selection and sequencing of treatments are based upon clinical experience and expert consensus and not randomized controlled trials.[76] In practical terms, the addiction treatment offered or available likely depends on patient preference, availability, access, coercion, urgent needs such as imminent withdrawal or suicide risk, and clinician orientation rather than on scientific evidence. One of the key research challenges ahead is to develop methods to compare the effectiveness of different stepwise or adaptive strategies for deploying treatment modalities with demonstrated efficacy.

In current models, the goal and approach of treatment depends upon the nature, extent, and severity of the disorder. The continuum of severity as presented in **Figure 37-1** serves as a template upon which to project a continuum of care.

Persons Who Abstain, Engage in Lower-Risk Use, or in At-Risk/Hazardous Alcohol Use

Persons who abstain, or engage in lower-risk use, or at-risk/hazardous alcohol use require health promotion, such as

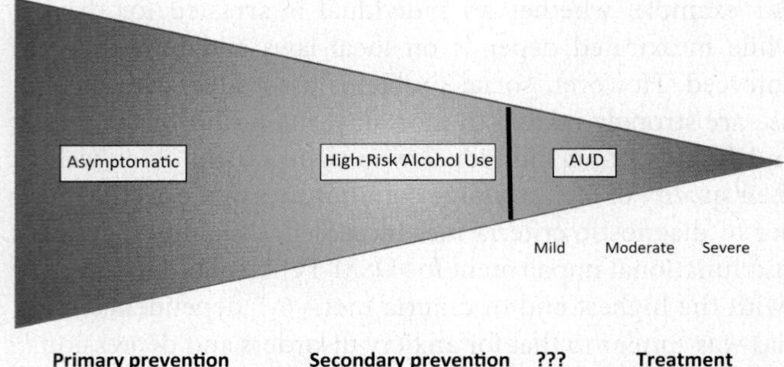

Figure 37-1. A diagram of the spectrum of alcohol use. Most people are asymptomatic, and those who use alcohol in a high-risk manner and those with an AUD are about equal. However, only about 10% of people with an AUD end up making use of current "rehabilitation" centers. The text below the figure is the appropriate intervention to use. Treatment here means interventions by physicians and other prescribers, not necessarily current "rehabilitation" centers. For the mildest form of AUD, it is not clear what intervention to use, although secondary prevention approaches have been somewhat helpful among college students.

education about the recommended maximum limits adjusted for that person's individual situation. Health promotion is especially important for adolescents and women who are pregnant or at risk of becoming pregnant. The goal for those engaging in at-risk/hazardous alcohol use is to reduce consumption, preferably below recommended maximum limits, to reduce risk of future harm. Individuals in this at-risk group may respond well to facilitated self-change and brief counseling by their health care provider but primarily among those who are young and do not meet criteria for AUD. Brief counseling in emergency departments or with hospital inpatients has unclear efficacy. Studies vary in their findings. Most find significant reductions in alcohol use in both brief counseling and comparison groups. Some studies find between-group differences and some do not.[77,78] The efficacy of internet-based interventions is also unclear. More research in these areas is needed.

People With Alcohol Use Disorder

Treatment of DSM-5 mild AUD is not well studied. Most studies of treatment of DSM-IV alcohol dependence have been conducted with middle-aged, treatment-seeking adults, especially White males and veterans who have a more severe disorder. Thus, findings from most treatment studies cannot be generalized to most adults with AUD. A pressing need is to develop and test treatment approaches for people with mild to moderate AUD and relatively few comorbidities.

About two-thirds of individuals who develop DSM-5 AUD do so in adolescence or young adulthood. However, only about one-half of them go on to a chronic course.[46] Those who do progress are more likely to have a family history of AUD and antisocial personality traits and to have started drinking in early adolescence.[44] More research on intervening earlier in the course of illness for those at high risk for chronicity is another priority. About 40% of those meeting criteria for AUD have midlife onset of mild to moderate AUD, and those who do are more likely to have coexisting psychopathology and/or a family history of AUD. This suggests that primary care and general psychiatry may be ideal settings in which to evaluate strategies to identify and treat this group.

For those who do not respond to self-change efforts and less intensive treatment, referral to specialty addiction treatment is needed. This type of stepped-care approach is implied in the American Society of Addiction Medicine's (ASAM) Criteria[76] (further information on The ASAM Criteria are covered in Chapter 47 "The ASAM Criteria and Matching Patients to Treatment"). However, although the stepped-care approach makes sense intuitively, it has not been adequately examined for its effectiveness. (The ASAM Criteria are currently being updated.) However, mental health care, substance use care, and general medical care remain poorly integrated into time-limited rehabilitation programs. Attempts to improve outcomes by matching patient characteristics to treatment type have not yet yielded information of much use to clinicians, but such a body of knowledge may develop over time.

For those who do not respond to self-change efforts and nonintensive treatment, the appropriate next steps are specified by the VA/DOD Clinical Practice Guideline.[79]

Since 12-step rehabilitation is the only other available treatment option in most places, clinical practice is to refer to one. The ASAM Criteria describe how patients can be triaged to various intensities of rehabilitation programs and medical care. Although this has helped rehabilitation programs and payers to agree on placement, the criteria merely reflect current practice and have no scientific basis. For example, the first study was published in 1977, and it found that intensive outpatient and/or residential treatment offers no outcome advantage for AUD over less intensive outpatient care.[80] In general, length of engagement in treatment is a better predictor of outcome than intensity. There is no empirical basis for residential rehabilitation, which consists of an intensive outpatient rehabilitation program in a house. Although some individuals undoubtedly require structured sober housing to stabilize, it makes more sense to determine type and intensity of treatment independent of housing needs. That way, they can both be varied to fit the needs of the patient.

At the most severe end of the spectrum are individuals with severe and persistent or recurrent AUD. In this group, coexisting substance, mental and physical disorders, and social disabilities are common (including antisocial personality), as is a family history of AUD and very early onset AUD. Not surprisingly, this group are the most likely to seek and receive treatment, often due to overt coercion. Even though most of this group has a chronic or recurrent course, addiction treatment programs typically offer treatment for only a few weeks or months. Furthermore, few programs are staffed to address the serious comorbidities present, so they are often ignored or dealt with through referral. The effectiveness of treatment programs for this group is difficult to evaluate because there are many factors present that may be driving change. For example, serious physical illness, legal mandates, lack of housing, unemployment, poverty, and family pressure frequently cause or contribute to a decision to seek treatment. Many of these factors are quite powerful and could account for much of whatever change occurs. More research is needed on the mechanisms of behavior change among individuals with heavy alcohol use across the spectrum of AUD severity.

Research on long-term care management strategies, like those used for other chronic disorders, is promising, especially for people with severe AUD and serious mental or physical disorders. For example, studies of individuals with heavy alcohol use with severe medical complications such as liver cirrhosis suggest that addressing drinking using a care management approach in the context of general medical care is effective at reducing drinking and inducing abstinence. In two studies of this approach, 2-year mortality was about two-thirds of that in comparison groups receiving usual medical care.[81,82] Integrating substance use interventions into community support programs for severely mentally ill people also has some support. These studies suggest that for individuals with heavy alcohol use and serious medical or psychiatric illnesses, addressing drinking directly in the context of medical or psychiatric treatment is preferable to referral to a standard addiction treatment program, which are not often staffed to be able to address serious medical or psychiatric illnesses. There are no treatment approaches shown to be effective with severe and persistent AUD in the absence of comorbidities that cause serious dysfunction.[83] Since people with severe AUD frequently consume a great deal of healthcare, social, and criminal justice services, development of more effective treatments is a priority. It may be that external motivating factors, such as skillful application of legal requirements (whether civil commitment or, with consent, the criminal legal system), contingency management may be effective with this group, especially when combined with "wrap-around" services that integrate addiction, psychiatric and medical care as well as social services and sober housing. At this time, it is clear that treatment for these individuals needs to be structured with the goal of providing services intermittently or continuously for years to decades rather than weeks or months.

To summarize, recent research has shown that drinking and associated symptoms and problems occur along a continuum ranging from none to mild, moderate, and severe. A large majority of U.S. adults abstains or uses alcohol at lower-risk levels. Many with hazardous alcohol use are without current symptoms or problems but are at increased risk for physical, mental, and substance use disorders developing over time. In contrast to popular belief, most people who meet AUD criteria do not have a chronic course and most recover without professional treatment or even attendance at mutual help groups.[46] It appears that most people, upon recognizing a problem, attempt to change alone or with informal help, and the majority are eventually successful, albeit after several years of active disorder. Seeking help from mutual help groups or nonaddiction professionals (about 25%) and/or professional treatment programs (10%) occurs when informal attempts to change fail or an external contingency is applied, such as a charge for driving while intoxicated, or family demands. A significant proportion of individuals who seek treatment responds with improvement or remission, although this often takes years, with multiple quit attempts and recurrences prior to achieve stable remission. There is a small but important group with severe and persistent AUD. This continuum of drinking and associated symptoms and problems suggests a corresponding continuum of care.

Unfortunately, most of this continuum of care is not yet implemented or available. The quality of care for persons with at-risk alcohol use and AUD in primary care is the lowest among thirty chronic conditions,[84] and attempts to increase screening and brief intervention for at-risk drinking have met with little success, in part due to lack of efficacy. Among people with severe AUD, the proportion of people receiving treatment of any type increased from 24% to 34% between 2001-2002 and 2012-2013,[85] but the prevalence or public health burden of at-risk drinking or AUD also increased.[86] Thus, much remains to be done and many challenges lie ahead. Nevertheless, this fuller understanding of the spectrum of drinking, disorders, and treatment approaches provides one possible conceptual framework for advancing investment and development of the continuum of care.

A major public health challenge is to provide earlier identification and appropriate treatment to a much broader spectrum of individuals with unhealthy alcohol use than is currently the case. There is a pressing need to identify early intervention strategies for youth who begin drinking in early adolescence and who are at high risk for later development of severe chronic AUD. Early identification and treatment of high risk alcohol use and AUD in primary care and general mental health care would provide access for millions of people who otherwise will not receive treatment. Needed also is a better understanding of the factors driving change in persons with heavy alcohol use and how to facilitate that change both in addiction treatment and in other settings. Finally, effective, and cost-effective care management strategies for managing chronic severe AUD need to be implemented. To provide this type of comprehensive care, the specialty addiction treatment sector will require substantial development so that addiction, psychiatric, medical, and social services can be provided in an integrated way over longer periods of time.

TREATMENT AND BEHAVIOR CHANGE

The outcome of treatment varies based on the diagnostic severity of illness. In a typical treatment study, about one-third of subjects will be in full abstinent or nonabstinent remission for the following year, 30%-40% will show substantial improvement but will have at least some episodes of heavy drinking, and 20%-30% will not show an effect.[53,54] However, over the course of the ensuing 5-10 years, most will suffer at least some recurrences.[87] Detailed information about each different behavioral (especially sections 9 and 10 of this textbook) and pharmacological modality (especially sections 7 and 8 in this textbook) is provided in the appropriate chapters of this textbook. However, no one technique has proved to be overall more effective than others, thus raising the question of what the mechanisms of change really are. In fact, many people start reducing their drinking prior to treatment entry, and both study protocols and treatment programs require that someone be abstinent at treatment entry. For that matter, there are no clear criteria for distinguishing "still drinking" from "abstinent," since treatment cannot take place if an individual is intoxicated. In other words, it is arbitrary how long abstinence is required to qualify as "abstinent." Even most individuals with daily or near daily alcohol use will have a negative blood alcohol level at some point each day. One could thus conceptualize the start of drinking each day as a "recurrence of drinking" (using drinking as the outcome indicator). In yet another randomized controlled trial of two behavioral treatments for AUD that showed no difference between brief motivational counseling versus a more extensive multimodal program of care, Orford and colleagues qualitatively examined the process leading to help seeking in study subjects.[88] They identified a "catalyst system" consisting of increasing problems and distress related to drinking, pressure from others, and a trigger event, which in turn led to the realization "I cannot do this on my own." Factors outside the treatment context continued to be important throughout the recovery process, especially after the discontinuation of treatment services. In another study of 15 community treatment programs, 5-year outcomes of patients who dropped out of treatment early did not differ from those who completed the program.[89] These findings suggest that the process of deciding to seek help is itself part of the change process and is arguably the most important factor determining the future course, although it is not well understood.

Treatment seeking is strongly associated with increased odds of achieving and maintaining abstinence. Those who seek help on average are older and have more severe AUD and more coexisting mental and physical disorders as well as less social support.[90,91] In this group, both professional treatment and 12-step support group participation are associated with increased likelihood of abstinent remission. For individuals older than 35 years, abstinence is a much more stable outcome than even light drinking without problems, while in younger persons, lower-risk drinking without problems (nonabstinent remission) is similar to abstinence in predicting continued remission 3 years later.[92] Thus, remission, whether abstinent or nonabstinent, should be the goal of treatment for AUD, tempered with the recognition that full remission cannot always be achieved or sustained.

Unfortunately, such studies are not able to establish causality. Although help seeking and participation in treatment and Twelve Step community support groups are associated with improved outcomes, including decreased mortality, it is just as likely that people who have decided to change will seek treatment, while those who do not want to change do not, or that people who respond to treatment early develop more hope and motivation to continue. That is, treatment participation or continuation may be more a result of change rather than the converse. There may be other unmeasured differences between the groups, as well. Regardless, people who achieve full remission of AUD have much better overall functional and medical outcomes than those with partial or no response. Furthermore, it appears that treatment followed by Twelve Step support group participation is a frequent and effective (but not the only) path to recovery for many people.[93] Rudolf Moos has emphasized the importance of personal and social resources to the achievement of remission.[91] Specific theories and treatment components he identifies include social control theory (support, goal direction, and structure), behavioral economics and behavioral choice theory (an emphasis on rewards that compete with substance use), social learning theory (focus on abstinence-oriented norms and models), and stress and coping theory (attempts to develop self-efficacy and coping skills). Conceptualizations such as this provide guidance for both research and clinical practice and are particularly helpful to approach the relationship of factors at different levels of analysis (neurobiological, personal, and social). This type of integrative thinking and research will become increasingly important as determinants of change are further explored. As an indication of this trend, the National Institutes of Health has undertaken a major research initiative to promote interdisciplinary research into mechanisms of behavior change related to initiation of positive change among people with unhealthy behaviors.

SYSTEMS OF CARE

An ongoing opportunity within the field of addiction medicine is how and where tailored treatments should be provided to catalyze behavior change. Historically, rehabilitation programs independent of the healthcare system have been the cornerstone of care for people with alcohol or other substance use disorders.[94] About two-thirds of these programs are publicly funded, relying primarily on government block grants and state contracts to provide services. The remaining privately funded programs largely depend on revenues from private insurance and self-paying patients. Most people with AUD are treated in the publicly funded treatment sector.

Federal legislative changes have had substantial impacts on the funding and structure of both publicly and privately funded treatment programs. In 2008, the Paul Wellstone and Pete Domenici Mental Health Parity and Addiction Equity Act (MHPAEA) required Medicaid managed care organizations to provide coverage benefits for mental health and substance use comparable to those offered for physical medical services if they were offered at all. The passage of the Affordable Care Act (ACA) in 2010 extended these coverage requirements to commercial health plans and Medicaid's Alternative Benefit Plans (ABPs). Coverage of substance use disorder treatment for people enrolled in traditional Medicaid fee-for-service plans remains at each state's discretion. It is important to note that future coverage requirements are uncertain given current Congressional debates regarding the future of the ACA and other potential changes in the structure of healthcare law. Unfortunately, people with AUD are unusually vulnerable to changes in health law and policy.

State authorities significantly influence the organization and structure of community treatment programs. Each state, and the District of Columbia, has a single state authority (SSA) funded by both federal and state monies that is charged with overseeing substance use treatment programs. SSAs contract with or license almost all programs—either directly or indirectly through counties and other organizations—to ensure service delivery. In their regulatory and funding roles, SSAs play a major role determining how evidence-based practices and patient values are integrated into treatment programs. Although most SSAs provide technical assistance to foster collaborations between publicly funded addiction treatment programs, mental health programs, and the criminal justice system, about 40% of the agencies do not provide support to facilitate collaborations with medical programs or federally qualified health centers.

Most care for AUD occurs in programs where it is uncertain whether a medical professional would be involved in their care, despite legislative and reimbursement efforts to promote a medical model of care. However, uptake of medication treatment remains very low, either in a treatment program or primary care. Providers do not feel competent to decide who might benefit, and a surprising number believe that medications either do not work or that a treatment program is a better alternative.[95] This limitation is accentuated by the time-limited care standard in most treatment programs, whereby patients are often discharged to follow-up with AA only, or with providers unfamiliar with how to support recovery. Similarly, implementation of Screening, Brief Intervention, and Referral to Treatment (SBIRT) has been stalled. In most cases, even when it is done, such as in VA care or in large private HCOs with Medicaid populations,[96] it seldom results in a successful referral.[97] SBIRT appears to be most effective with young people who do not have an AUD.[98] The changes initiated by the Affordable Care Act (ACA) and other legislation were supposed to make innovations such as SBIRT more appealing, but intervening events such as the Trump presidency eroded the effects of the legislation. Consequently, realizing the potential value of screening, brief intervention, and referral to treatment (SBIRT) has been difficult to achieve in practice.[99]

INTEGRATING THE EVIDENCE AND PERSONALIZING PRACTICE

Given the proliferation of new research, it is a challenge to understand and incorporate new findings into practice. Unfortunately, although studies of the efficacy of various treatments may help determine how one treatment compares to another treatment or to no treatment, there are few studies that directly address questions of central importance to clinicians. For example, should one recommend a few sessions of motivational enhancement therapy or an intensive day program for the treatment of AUD? If a person with at-risk drinking does not respond to brief motivational counseling, what is the appropriate next step? Is the stepped care strategy, where the least restrictive and expensive option for a situation is offered first, the best approach? How much evidence is required before recommending a new treatment? How much evidence is required before failure to offer or recommend a treatment based on personal taste or ideology is ethically indefensible?

Although it is not yet possible to provide definitive answers to these questions, certain conclusions emerge from available evidence. Although there is no systematic advantage of one type of behavioral therapy to another, the quality of the behavioral treatment provided is important. Specifically, empathic, skillful therapy is more effective than confrontation and education. Furthermore, it is more important to engage someone with AUD in treatment than which treatment is used. Therefore, it makes sense to offer a variety of treatment options, since patients are likely to vary in their preferences. The same holds true for the setting of treatment. Unless someone is unable to abstain from alcohol while living in the community, there is no advantage of residential versus outpatient treatment, or of intensive versus less intensive outpatient treatment. Second, medications offer clinically important benefits in early recovery and therefore patients should routinely be made aware of them and offered the opportunity to use them. Current evidence provides no guidance, however, on choosing one medication over another, or what the sequence of subsequent medications should be. For appropriate patients (mild to moderate levels of AUD, little or no coexisting psychopathology, socially stable, and motivated to change drinking), medication with medical care management and encouragement to abstain, adhere to treatment, and attend community support groups is as effective as "specialized" alcohol counseling. Third, a social network supportive of abstinence is at least as important as whatever treatment occurs in determining outcome.[100] Except for referral to community support groups, this aspect of treatment tends to be neglected, to the detriment of our patients. Finally, for any given diagnosis (eg, high-risk drinking versus AUD), there is not yet a way to identify patient characteristics that reliably predict differential response to different treatments.

REFERENCES

1. Evans E, Anglin MD, Urada D, Yang J. Promising practices for delivery of court-supervised substance abuse treatment: perspectives from six high-performing California counties operating proposition 36. *Eval Program Plan.* 2011;34(2):124-134.
2. Ferri M, Amato L, Davoli M. Alcoholics anonymous and other 12-step programmes for alcohol dependence. *Cochrane Database Syst Rev.* 2006;3:CD005032.
3. McLellan AT, Meyers K. Contemporary addiction treatment: a review of systems problems for adults and adolescents. *Biol Psychiatry.* 2004;56(10):764-770.
4. CASA. *Addiction Medicine: Closing the Gap Between Science and Practice.* The National Center for Addiction and Substance Abuse at Columbia University; 2012.
5. Facing Addiction in America. *The Surgeon General's Report on Alcohol, Drugs, and Health.* U.S. Department of Health and Human Services; 2016.
6. Santa Ana EJ, Martino S, Ball SA, Nich C, Frankforter TL, Carroll KM. What is usual about "treatment-as-usual"? Data from two multisite effectiveness trials. *J Subst Abuse Treat.* 2008;35(4):369-379.
7. Abraham AJ, Andrews CM, Harris SJ, Friedmann PD. Availability of medications for the treatment of alcohol and opioid use disorder in the USA. *Neurotherapeutics.* 2020;17(1):55-69.
8. American Psychiatric Association. *Diagnostic and Statistical Manual of Mental Disorders: DSM-5-TR.* 5th ed. American Psychiatric Association Publishing; 2022.
9. American Psychiatric Association. *Diagnostic and Statistical Manual of Psychiatric Disorders.* 4th ed., *Text Revision.* American Psychiatric Publishing; 2000.
10. Saha TD, Harford T, Goldstein RB, Kerridge BT, Hasin D. Relationship of substance abuse to dependence in the U.S. general population. *J Stud Alcohol Drugs.* 2012;73(3):368-378.
11. SAMHSA Key substance use and mental health indicators in the United States: Results from the 2019 National Survey on Drug Use and Health. 2020. Accessed May 26, 2023. https://www.samhsa.gov/data/sites/default/files/reports/rpt29393/2019NSDUHFFRPDFWHTML/2019NSDUHFFR090120.htm
12. Sacks JJ, Gonzales KR, Bouchery EE, Tomedi LE, Brewer RD. 2010 national and state costs of excessive alcohol consumption. *Am J Prev Med.* 2015;49(5):e73-e79.
13. Chrystoja BR, Monteiro M, Rehm J, Shield K. Alcohol-attributable burden of disease in the Americas in 2000 and 2016. *J Stud Alcohol Drugs.* 2022;83(1):45-54.
14. Fletcher AM. *Inside Rehab: The Surprising Truth About Addiction Treatment—And How to Get Help That Works.* The Penguin Group; 2013.
15. Nowinski J, Baker S, Carroll K. *Twelve Step Facilitation Therapy Manual.* U.S. Department of Health and Human Services; 1999.
16. Pavlov IP. *Conditioned Reflexes: An Investigation of the Physiological Activity of the Cerebral Cortex.* Oxford University Press: Humphrey Milford; 1927.
17. Pines M. *Forgotten pioneers: The unwritten history of the therapeutic community movement. Ther Commun.* 1999;20:23-42.
18. Ellis A. *Reason and Emotion in Psychotherapy.* Citadel; 1962.
19. Beck AT. *Cognitive Therapy and the Emotional Disorders.* International Universities Press; 1976.
20. Miller WR, Rollnick S. *Motivational Interviewing: Preparing People to Change Addictive Behavior*; 1991.
21. Wampold BE. *The Great Psychotherapy Debate: Models, Methods, and Findings.* Lawrence Erlbaum Associates; 2001.
22. Anton RF, O'Malley SS, Ciraulo DA, et al. Combined pharmacotherapies and behavioral interventions for alcohol dependence: the COMBINE study: a randomized controlled trial. *JAMA.* 2006;295(17):2003-2017.
23. Burnette EM, Nieto SJ, Grodin EN, et al. Novel agents for the pharmacological treatment of alcohol use disorder. *Drugs.* 2022;82(3):251-274.
24. Abraham AJ, Yarbrough CR. Availability of medications for the treatment of alcohol use disorder in U.S. counties, 2016-2019. *J Stud Alcohol Drugs.* 2021;82(6):689-699.
25. Heilig M, Augier E, Pfarr S, Sommer WH. Developing neuroscience-based treatments for alcohol addiction: a matter of choice? *Transl Psychiatry.* 2019;9(1):255.
26. Pittman B. *AA: The Way It Began.* Glen Abbey Books; 1988.
27. Alcoholics Anonymous. *The Big Book.* 3rd ed. Alcoholics Anonymous World Services; 1976.
28. Dawson DA, Grant BF, Stinson FS, Chou PS, Huang B, Ruan WJ. Recovery from DSM-IV alcohol dependence: United States, 2001-2002. *Addiction.* 2005;100(3):281-292.
29. Witkiewitz K, Pearson MR, Wilson AD, et al. Can alcohol use disorder recovery include some heavy drinking? A replication and extension up to 9 years following treatment. *Alcohol Clin Exp Res.* 2020;44(9):1862-1874.

30. Tucker JA, Cheong JW, James TG, Jung S, Chandler SD. Preresolution drinking problem severity profiles associated with stable moderation outcomes of natural recovery attempts. *Alcohol Clin Exp Res.* 2020;44(3):738-745.
31. Tucker JA, Cheong JW, Chandler SD, et al. Prospective analysis of behavioral economic predictors of stable moderation drinking among problem drinkers attempting natural recovery. *Alcohol Clin Exp Res.* 2016;40(12):2676-2684.
32. Witkiewitz K, Wilson AD, Pearson MR, et al. Profiles of recovery from alcohol use disorder at three years following treatment: can the definition of recovery be extended to include high functioning heavy drinkers? *Addiction.* 2019;114(1):69-80.
33. Fan AZ, Chou SP, Zhang H, Jung J, Grant BF. Prevalence and correlates of past-year recovery from DSM-5 alcohol use disorder: results from national epidemiologic survey on alcohol and related conditions-III. *Alcohol Clin Exp Res.* 2019;43(11):2406-2420.
34. Stapinski LA, Sannibale C, Subotic M, et al. Randomised controlled trial of integrated cognitive behavioural treatment and motivational enhancement for comorbid social anxiety and alcohol use disorders. *Aust N Z J Psychiatry.* 2021;55(2):207-220.
35. Grabski M, McAndrew A, Lawn W, et al. Adjunctive ketamine with relapse prevention-based psychological therapy in the treatment of alcohol use disorder. *Am J Psychiatry.* 2022;179(2):152-162.
36. Cheng YC, Huang YC, Huang WL. Gabapentinoids for treatment of alcohol use disorder: a systematic review and meta-analysis. *Hum Psychopharmacol.* 2020;35(6):1-11.
37. Sohi I, Franklin A, Chrystoja B, Wettlaufer A, Rehm J, Shield K. The global impact of alcohol consumption on premature mortality and health in 2016. *Nutrients.* 2021;13(9):3145.
38. Rehm J, Imtiaz S. A narrative review of alcohol consumption as a risk factor for global burden of disease. *Subst Abuse Treat Prev Policy.* 2016;11(1):37.
39. Timko C, Debenedetti A, Moos BS, Moos RH. Predictors of 16-year mortality among individuals initiating help-seeking for an alcoholic use disorder. *Alcohol Clin Exp Res.* 2006;30(10):1711-1720.
40. Rivara FP, Garrison MM, Ebel B, McCarty CA, Christakis DA. Mortality attributable to harmful drinking in the United States, 2000. *J Stud Alcohol.* 2004;65(4):530-536.
41. Stewart SH, Latham PK, Miller PM, Randall P, Anton RF. Blood pressure reduction during treatment for alcohol dependence: results from the Combining Medications and Behavioral Interventions for Alcoholism (COMBINE) study. *Addiction.* 2008;103(10):1622-1628.
42. Rehm J, Shield KD, Roerecke M, Gmel G. Modelling the impact of alcohol consumption on cardiovascular disease mortality for comparative risk assessments: an overview. *BMC Public Health.* 2016;16(1):363.
43. Dawson DA. Alcohol consumption, alcohol dependence, and all-cause mortality. *Alcohol Clin Exp Res.* 2000;24(1):72-81.
44. Rogers RG, Boardman JD, Pendergast PM, Lawrence EM. Drinking problems and mortality risk in the United States. *Drug Alcohol Depend.* 2015;151:38-46.
45. Saitz R, Gaeta J, Cheng DM, Richardson JM, Larson MJ, Samet JH. Risk of mortality during four years after substance detoxification in urban adults. *J Urban Health.* 2007;84(2):272-282.
46. Hasin DS, Stinson FS, Ogburn E, Grant BF. Prevalence, correlates, disability, and comorbidity of DSM-IV alcohol abuse and dependence in the United States: results from the national epidemiologic survey on alcohol and related conditions. *Arch Gen Psychiatry.* 2007;64(7):830-842.
47. Sobell MB, Sobell LC, Klajner F, Pavan D, Basian E. The reliability of the timeline method of assessing normal drinker college students recent drinking history: utility for alcohol research. *Addict Behav.* 1986;21:149-161.
48. Perrine MW, Mundt JC, Searles JS, Lester LS. Validation of daily self-reported alcohol consumption using interactive voice response (IVR) technology. *J Stud Alcohol.* 1995;56(5):487-490.
49. Searles JS, Helzer JE, Rose GL, Badger GJ. Concurrent and retrospective reports of alcohol consumption across 30, 90 and 366 days: interactive voice response compared with the timeline follow back. *J Stud Alcohol.* 2002;63(3):352-362.
50. Serre F, Fatseas M, Debrabant R, Alexandre J-M, Auriacombe M, Swendsen J. Ecological momentary assessment in alcohol, tobacco, cannabis and opiate dependence: a comparison of feasibility and validity. *Drug Alcohol Depend.* 2012;126(1-2):118-123.
51. McKay JR. Continuing care research: what we have learned and where we are going. *J Subst Abuse Treat.* 2009;36(2):131-145.
52. McKay JR, Gustafson DH, Ivey M, et al. Efficacy and comparative effectiveness of telephone and smartphone remote continuing care interventions for alcohol use disorder: a randomized controlled trial. *Addiction.* 2022;117(5):1326-1337.
53. Cisler RA, Kowalchuk RK, Saunders SM, Zweben A, Trinh HQ. Applying clinical significance methodology to alcoholism treatment trials: determining recovery outcome status with individual- and population-based measures. *Alcohol Clin Exp Res.* 2005;29(11):1991-2000.
54. Group PMR. Matching alcoholism treatments to client heterogeneity: treatment main effects and matching effects on drinking during treatment. *J Stud Alcohol.* 1998;59(6):631-639.
55. Gough G, Heathers L, Puckett D, et al. The utility of commonly used laboratory tests to screen for excessive alcohol use in clinical practice. *Alcohol Clin Exp Res.* 2015;39(8):1493-1500.
56. Mastrovito R, Strathmann FG. Distributions of alcohol use biomarkers including ethanol, phosphatidylethanol, ethyl glucuronide and ethyl sulfate in clinical and forensic testing. *Clin Biochem.* 2020;82:85-89.
57. Palmer L, Norton S, Jones M, Rona RJ, Goodwin L, Fear NT. Trajectories of alcohol misuse among the UK Armed Forces over a 12-year period. *Addiction.* 2022;117(1):57-67.
58. Morishima R, Usami S, Ando S, et al. Trajectory and course of problematic alcohol use after the Great East Japan Earthquake: Eight-year follow-up of the Higashi-Matsushima cohort study. *Alcohol Clin Exp Res.* 2022;46(4):570-580.
59. Leventhal AM, Cho J, Ray LA, et al. Alcohol use trajectories among U.S. adults during the first 42 weeks of the COVID-19 pandemic. *Alcohol Clin Exp Res.* 2022;46(6):1062-1072.
60. D'Amico EJ, Rodriguez A, Tucker JS, Dunbar MS, Pedersen ER, Seelam R. Disparities in functioning from alcohol and cannabis use among a racially/ethnically diverse sample of emerging adults. *Drug Alcohol Depend.* 2022;234:109426.
61. Christiansen SG, Moan IS. Employment trajectories among those treated for alcohol use disorder: a register-based cohort study. *Addiction.* 2022;117(4):913-924.
62. Padgett RN, Andretta JR, Cole JC, Percy A, Sumnall HR, MT MK. Intervention impact on alcohol use, alcohol harms, and a combination of both: a latent class, secondary analysis of results from a randomized controlled trial. *Drug Alcohol Depend.* 2021;227:108944.
63. Lemoine M, Gmel G, Foster S, Marmet S, Studer J. Multiple trajectories of alcohol use and the development of alcohol use disorder: do Swiss men mature-out of problematic alcohol use during emerging adulthood? *PLoS One.* 2020;15(1):e0220232.
64. Niu L, Thiele M, Geyer PE. Noninvasive proteomic biomarkers for alcohol-related liver disease. *Nat Med.* 2022;28(6):1277-1287.
65. Lin Y, Sharma B, Thompson HM, et al. External validation of a machine learning classifier to identify unhealthy alcohol use in hospitalized patients. *Addiction.* 2022;117(4):925-933.
66. Walters ST, Businelle MS, Suchting R, Li X, Hébert TH, Mun E-Y. Using machine learning to identify predictors of imminent drinking and create tailored messages for at-risk drinkers experiencing homelessness. *J Subst Abuse Treat.* 2021;127:108417.
67. Park SJ, Lee SJ, Kim H, et al. Machine learning prediction of dropping out of outpatients with alcohol use disorders. *PLoS One.* 2021;16(8):e0255626.
68. Kinreich S, McCutcheon VV, Aliev F, et al. Predicting alcohol use disorder remission: a longitudinal multimodal multi-featured machine learning approach. *Transl Psychiatry.* 2021;11(1):166.
69. Agarwal S, Sharma S, Kumar M, et al. Development of a machine learning model to predict bleed in esophageal varices in compensated advanced chronic liver disease: a proof of concept. *J Gastroenterol Hepatol.* 2021;36(10):2935-2942.

70. Schlauch RC, Crane CA, Connors GJ, Dearing RL, Maisto SA. The role of craving in the treatment of alcohol use disorders: the importance of competing desires and pretreatment changes in drinking. *Drug Alcohol Depend.* 2019;199:144-150.
71. Stasiewicz PR, Schlauch RC, Bradizza CM, Bole CW, Coffey SF. Pretreatment changes in drinking: relationship to treatment outcomes. *Psychol Addict Behav.* 2013;27(4):1159-1166.
72. Berger L, Brondino M, Fisher M, Gwyther R, Garbutt JC. Alcohol use disorder treatment: the association of pretreatment use and the role of drinking goal. *J Am Board Fam Med.* 2016;29(1):37-49.
73. Dunn KE, Strain EC. Pretreatment alcohol drinking goals are associated with treatment outcomes. *Alcohol Clin Exp Res.* 2013;37(10):1745-1752.
74. Worden BL, Epstein EE, McCrady BS. Pretreatment assessment-related reductions in drinking among women with alcohol use disorders. *Subst Use Misuse.* 2015;50(2):215-225.
75. Sobell MB, Sobell LC. Guided self-change model of treatment for substance use disorders. *J Cogn Psychother.* 2005;19(3):199-210.
76. Mee-Lee D. *The ASAM Criteria.* 3rd ed. The American Society for Addiction Medicine; 2003.
77. Elzerbi C, Donoghue K, Boniface S, Drummond C. Variance in the Efficacy of brief interventions to reduce hazardous and harmful alcohol consumption between injury and noninjury patients in emergency departments: a systematic review and meta-analysis of randomized controlled trials. *Ann Emerg Med.* 2017;70(5):714-723. e13.
78. Heather N. The efficacy-effectiveness distinction in trials of alcohol brief intervention. *Addict Sci Clin Pract.* 2014;9:13.
79. US Department of Veterans Affairs. *VA/DoD Clinical Practice Guideline for the Management of Post-Traumatic Stress.* Department of Veterans Affairs; 2010.
80. Edwards G, Orford J, Guthrie S, et al. Alcoholism: a controlled trial of "treatment" and "advice". *J Stud Alcohol.* 1977;38(5):1004-1031.
81. Willenbring ML, Olson DH. A randomized trial of integrated outpatient treatment for medically ill alcoholic men. *Arch Intern Med.* 1999;159(16):1946-1952.
82. Willenbring ML, Olson DH, Bielinski J. Integrated outpatient treatment for medically ill alcoholic men: results from a quasi-experimental study. *J Stud Alcohol.* 1995;56(3):337-343.
83. Saitz R, Cheng DM, Winter M, et al. Chronic care management for dependence on alcohol and other drugs: the AHEAD randomized trial. *JAMA.* 2013;310(11):1156-1167.
84. McGlynn EA, Asch SM, Adams J, et al. The quality of health care delivered to adults in the United States. *N Engl J Med.* 2003;348(26):2635-2645.
85. Dawson DA, Goldstein RB, Saha TD, Grant BF. Changes in alcohol consumption: United States, 2001–2002 to 2012–2013. *Drug Alcohol Depend.* 2015;148:56-61.
86. Rehm J, Dawson D, Frick U, et al. Burden of disease associated with alcohol use disorders in the United States. *Alcohol Clin Exp Res.* 2014;38(4):1068-1077.
87. Vaillant GE. A 60-year follow-up of alcoholic men. *Addiction.* 2003;98(8):1043.
88. Orford J, Hodgson R, Copello A, et al. The clients' perspective on change during treatment for an alcohol problem: qualitative analysis of follow-up interviews in the UK Alcohol Treatment Trial. *Addiction.* 2006;101(1):60-68.
89. McKellar JD, Harris AH, Moos RH. Predictors of outcome for patients with substance-use disorders five years after treatment dropout. *J Stud Alcohol.* 200667(5):685-693.
90. Fein G, Landman B. Treated and treatment-naive alcoholics come from different populations. *Alcohol.* 2005;35(1):19-26.
91. Moos RH. Theory-based active ingredients of effective treatments for substance use disorders. *Drug Alcohol Depend.* 2007;88(2-3):109-121.
92. Dawson DA, Stinson FS, Chou SP, Grant BF. Three-year changes in adult risk drinking behavior in relation to the course of alcohol-use disorders. *J Stud Alcohol Drugs.* 2008;69(6):866-877.
93. Moos RH. Theory-based processes that promote the remission of substance use disorders. *Clin Psychol Rev.* 2007;27(5):537-551.
94. White WL. *Slaying the Dragon: The History of Addiction Treatment and Recovery in America.* 2nd ed. Chestnut Health Systems/Lighthouse Institute; 2014.
95. Williams EC, Achtmeyer CE, Young JP, et al. Barriers to and facilitators of alcohol use disorder pharmacotherapy in primary care: a qualitative study in five VA clinics. *J Gen Intern Med.* 2018;33(3):258-267.
96. Moberg DP, Paltzer J. Clinical recognition of substance use disorders in Medicaid primary care associated with universal screening, brief intervention and referral to treatment (SBIRT). *J Stud Alcohol Drugs.* 2021;82(6):700-709.
97. Frost MC, Glass JE, Bradley KA, Williams EC. Documented brief intervention associated with reduced linkage to specialty addictions treatment in a national sample of VA patients with unhealthy alcohol use with and without alcohol use disorders. *Addiction.* 2020;115(4):668-678.
98. Chi FW, Parthasarathy S, Palzes VA, et al. Alcohol brief intervention, specialty treatment and drinking outcomes at 12 months: results from a systematic alcohol screening and brief intervention initiative in adult primary care. *Drug Alcohol Depend.* 2022;235:109458.
99. Tanner-Smith EE, Parr NJ, Schweer-Collins M, Saitz R. Effects of brief substance use interventions delivered in general medical settings: a systematic review and meta-analysis. *Addiction.* 2022;117(4):877-889.
100. Zywiak WH, Longabaugh R, Wirtz PW. Decomposing the relationships between pretreatment social network characteristics and alcohol treatment outcome. *J Stud Alcohol.* 2002;63(1):114-121.

CHAPTER

38

Race, Ethnicity, Gender, and Social Determinants of Health, Disparities, and Access to Care

Oluwole O. Jegede, Myra L. Mathis, Richard Youins, Kimberly Guy, Skylar Gross, and Ayana Jordan

CHAPTER OUTLINE

- Introduction
- Racism as a social determinant of health
- Definitions and concepts: race and ethnicity, and levels of racism
- Systemic racism in addiction
- Gender biases in addiction
- Cultural integration and structural competency in addiction treatment and research
- We *walk the walk*—firsthand accounts from racial, gender, and sexually minoritized people in recovery
- Summary

INTRODUCTION

Discussions around inequality in health outcomes gained prominence as a public health concern in the 1990s and were spurred into a larger, global discussion—specifically within addiction, after the killing of George Floyd.[1] Health inequality refers to specific differences resulting in poor health among socially disadvantaged groups of people.[2] Although inequality and inequities are often used interchangeably, they represent different constructs. Health inequities are inequalities that result from avoidable systemic, and unjust policies and practices.[3] The subtle difference between these terms highlights an important shift in health disparities literature over the last few years and have important consequences in policy, distribution of resources, clinical care, and research.

Overwhelming evidence shows that structural and institutional factors are the biggest drivers of inequities among minoritized populations. In fact the risk of negative health outcomes, has been shown to persist as individuals and minoritized groups interface with socioeconomic, political, and cultural/normative hierarchies.[4] In the field of addiction, social factors continue to drive access to treatment and treatment outcomes. Since 2015, Black, Latinx, Indigenous American, and Alaskan Native communities have seen the fastest rate of drug overdose mortality,[5] are more likely to be involved in the carceral system/law enforcement and incarcerated for minor drug offenses,[6] far less likely to be treated with evidence-based medication for any substance use disorder SUD) including medications for opioid use disorder (MOUD),[7] less likely to engage in addiction treatment and must invariably navigate a "trifecta of stigmas" while they do so.[8]

In this chapter, we discuss the impact of racism, and the intersection of gender, racism, culture, and related concepts in addiction, while presenting case scenarios of lived experiences of people with addiction who have navigated these intersections.

RACISM AS A SOCIAL DETERMINANT OF HEALTH

Race and ethnicity were introduced as independent social determinants of health outcomes in scientific literature in 1985 in the Heckler report, thus providing validation for an age-long observation recognized years earlier.[9] The 2003 landmark publication of the Institutes of Medicine (IOM), *Unequal Treatments*,[10] outlined the causes of disparities in health outcomes among underrepresented and minoritized populations. This IOM report showed that racial and ethnic minoritized people received far less optimal medical care and had worse overall health indices compared to nonminoritized people even when access to care was controlled.[10] Racism, a system that preferentially benefits one group of people (usually White people), while simultaneously disadvantaging another group (racial and ethnic minoritized people), runs quite deep in health care. Its legacy in health care has persisted to this day, beginning with the despicable institution of slavery, allowable medical experimentations on Black bodies and the mass incarceration and murder of Black people for minor drug-related infractions.[11,12] Over the last decade, the attention of social commentators, academic researchers, and the country has been drawn to the impact of systemic racism as a significant social determinant of health. In the field of cardiovascular medicine, people of African ancestry are less likely to get lifesaving procedures such as coronary artery bypass graft (CABG) and angioplasty[13]; in obstetrics, Black women are three times more likely to die due to childbirth than White women[14]; in nephrology and urology, race-based calculations of estimated glomerular filtration rates (eGRF) have limited the access of Black people to renal transplantations[15]; in psychiatry, Black people are more likely to be diagnosed with psychotic spectrum disorders,[16,17] and restrained for "disorganized and disruptive behaviors."[18,19] Similar to these discriminatory practices in other medical specialties, the addiction field is not unique, White men are more likely to receive and to be offered MOUD compared with other racial and ethnic minoritized groups.[7]

DEFINITIONS AND CONCEPTS: RACE AND ETHNICITY, AND LEVELS OF RACISM

To adequately address and deconstruct endemic racism within health care, and more specifically, addiction, it is critical to clearly define concepts of race, and describe the levels of racism. By doing so, we make a very important distinction between race—a social construct and systemic racism in health care, as the foundation and root cause of health disparities.[20,21] The classification of humanity based on race has been fraught with problematic innuendoes and outright falsehoods that claim "fixed biological" characteristics as the basis of such classification, while using the same as a justification for racism.[3,22] Currently, five categories of race are described: Indigenous American and Alaskan Native, Asian, Black or African American, Native Hawaiian, and Other Pacific Islander and White. However, a "multirace" category was included in the 2000 census and two categories identified for ethnicity: Hispanic/Latino and Not Hispanic/Latino.

Phelan and Link discussed racism as the fundamental cause of inequalities in health, predicated upon the effects on socioeconomic status.[21] In a recent systematic review and meta-analysis, racism was reported to be associated with poorer mental and physical health with ethnicity moderating these effects mainly among Black/African Americans and Latinx individuals.[23] In other words, health inequities persist *only* because of racism. Structural racism not only results in differential poor health outcomes in minoritized patients but also exists and propagates inequalities in health via complex interrelated pathways.

Dr Camara Jones presents a useful theoretical framework for understanding racism and race-based differences on three levels: internalized, personally mediated, and institutionalized.[24] Internalized racism is defined as self-directed racism of a minoritized individual or toward persons of their own race based on accepting an overwhelming negative imagery of that minoritized population; personally mediated racism is defined as prejudice (assumptions about the abilities, motives, and intentions of people based on their races); and institutionalized racism is based on structures that perpetuate differential health outcomes among minoritized populations such as differing socioeconomic status, housing segregation, and mass incarceration.

SYSTEMIC RACISM IN ADDICTION

The pathways from structural racism to addiction include biological system (stress-related) pathways, trauma, and micro-trauma (biopsychosocial), economic/social status and intergenerational transfer of disadvantage.[25,26] Structural racism may result in the development and perpetuation of a substance use disorders (SUD) as well as poorer health and health outcomes among individuals with SUDs; these causal pathways are complex, variable, and interrelated. The impact of stress on addiction (initiation of substance use and return to substance use after a period of stability) has been demonstrated in many preclinical and clinical studies.[27,28] One impact of structural racism (among others) is racial segregation through red-lining—a government sanctioned systematic, discriminatory and racist practice that mapped and allocated risk values to neighborhoods based on race thus resulting in inability to obtain loans and Black and Latinx people living in impoverished neighborhoods with low-resourced schools leading to lower educational attainment.[26] Segregated neighborhoods have also been directly linked to the prevalence of injection drug use in Black communities.[29] Beyond structural racism among people with SUD, personally mediated racism is quite present, leading to differential outcomes for White people compared to other racial and ethnic minoritized groups. For example, buprenorphine is more likely to be prescribed in White, middle class communities while methadone is more likely in poorer Black and Latinx neighborhoods.[30,31] In addition, recent data suggest that Black individuals were far less likely to receive buprenorphine, and although uptake of buprenorphine as MOUD continues to rise, it has risen far less in areas where Black and Latinx people live.[7,31] Some of the reasons for this disparity include provider bias that assumes that buprenorphine is more appropriate for individuals deemed to have social stability (employed, stable housing) and less likely to divert the medication[32]; unavailability of buprenorphine providers in Black and Latinx communities; strategic pattern of pharmaceutical marketing of buprenorphine to White individuals and the consistent negative media depictions and criminalization of urban Black and Latinx people as people who use heroin of heroin in contrast with the thoughtful, attentive and considerate depictions of suburban White people as people who use nonprescribed prescription opioids.[33]

GENDER BIASES IN ADDICTION

In addition to the concepts of race and racism, compounding minoritized identities (gender identity, sexual status) further potentiate discrimination and further exacerbate poor health outcomes.[34] Intersectionality, originally articulated by Kimberlé Crenshaw, refers to the ways in which gender, race, class, ethnicity, nationality, sexual orientation, ability, and other markers of identity intersect to shape lived experiences.[35] Many believe this concept offers a way forward to first identifying, then understanding how multiple intersecting identities can impact health and behavior, for improved health outcomes.[36] As defined by the World Health Organization, gender refers to the socially constructed characteristics of women, men, girls, and boys, which include social norms, behaviors and roles that vary from society to society and change over time.[37] While gender interacts with sex, they are different from one another as sex refers to biological and physiological characteristics such as chromosomes, hormones, and reproductive organs.[37] Gender classifications and their relationships to one another are hierarchical, intersecting with other societal structures that produce inequities. For example, a Black woman's experience of sexism is distinct from that of a White woman. Similarly, a Black woman's experience of racism is different from that of a Black man. These points become salient as it impacts how one's identity impacts treatment initiation and subsequent engagement.[34] The intersection of race and gender informs how one experiences these separate yet connected systems of oppression. When discussing the impact of gender in addiction and the varied social considerations that affect access to and engagement in addiction treatment, the intersectional frame must be employed.[34]

Forty percent of people who use substances identify as women, with substance use among women increasing at faster rates than any other demographic.[38] In 2019, 7.8 million U.S. women above age 12 (~5.6%) met criteria for a SUD. During that year only 10.8% of women with a SUD received any treatment.[39] Compared to men, women seeking SUD treatment spend longer times on waitlists, and while they often enter treatment with shorter use histories, their disorders tend to be more severe, with greater psychological, social and relational consequences of their use. Additional barriers exist for pregnant and parenting people in need of addiction treatment as doing so may lead to the involvement of child welfare systems.[40] This risk is greatest for non-White women, with one in ten Black children being separated from their parents through these systems.[41] For those who do access and engage in treatment, special consideration must be given to co-occurring mental health conditions including depression, anxiety, and trauma-related disorders.[42] Gender-responsive addiction treatment must also attend to coexisting substance use and intimate partner violence (IPV) as lifetime rates of IPV among women receiving treatment range from 47% to 90%.[43] Addiction treatment was historically designed to meet the needs of White men,[44] however, attending to the needs of intersecting identities can be immensely impactful in improving overall health outcomes such as increased engagement of people in treatment, favorable treatment outcomes, and reduction of substance use treatment attrition rates. For instance, women in treatment are less likely to have episodes of use compared to men, demonstrating similar or greater treatment success rates.[45] Additionally, women who complete treatment have a nine times higher rate of not using substances, compared with men who complete treatment who are three times more likely to remain abstinent.[45]

CULTURAL INTEGRATION AND STRUCTURAL COMPETENCY IN ADDICTION TREATMENT AND RESEARCH

While understanding the impact of racism as a foundational contributor to inequities in addiction treatment remains paramount, familiarizing oneself with the concept of intersectionality offers a tangible tool to integrate race, class, gender, and other statuses to eliminate these existing disparities. Another tangible tool in achieving this goal is structural competency,[46] forming partnerships with organizations outside of health care that can address the social determinants of health, to create systemic solutions to inequities that arise due to race, class, gender, and other factors. Partnering with community agencies, people with lived experience and not-for-profit and/or advocacy organizations can be invaluable in offering support to people from multiple intersecting identities, who don't always benefit from care provided in traditional systems that preferentially favor the dominant group. Structural competency also bridges research on the social determinants of health to tangible clinical interventions, and prepares all health care professionals, including addiction specialists, to act systemically to address the fundamental cause of health inequalities.[46] While a critical mass of health care professionals, such as social workers and public health scholars and clinicians, have been practicing structural competency (focusing on structural drivers of health) for some time, much of the training in addiction and in medicine at large continues to focus on individual factors, thereby limiting the scope of practice and resultant impact on eliminating disparities in addiction. Structural competency offers a tangible frame to develop a shared mental model and set of interventions to reduce health inequalities at the level above the patient, taking into account neighborhoods, institutions, and policies.[47]

As we build on cultural competency (awareness and understanding of how a patient's cultural background and worldview impacts health and behavior)[48] and incorporate a more structural understanding of how system level factors influence health, access to a working diagram can be useful (see **Fig. 38-1**). Coined initially by Hansen and Metzl in 2014,[46] structural competency builds on five main principles:

1. Recognizing the structures that shape clinical interactions
2. Developing an extra-clinical language of structure
3. Rearticulating "cultural" formulations in structural terms
4. Observing and imagining structural interventions
5. Developing structural humility which is to be differentiated from the traditional concept of *structural/cultural competence* describing the capacity for health care professionals to engage with structures and individuals across varying contexts and cultures; *structural/cultural humility* indicates a lifelong, ongoing commitment to patient care through self-reflection and developing partnerships with communities[49]

Assessing racial and ethnic minoritized people with SUDs for inequities in the social determinants of health using the social vulnerability tool[4] is the first step. Then developing language to reconsider cultural formulations, allows for the forming of relationships with community organizations to address these structural factors and intervene at the systematic level. By developing a treatment plan to track and assess change in health outcomes over time, structural competency provides a tangible tool to eliminate disparities in addiction. Not only is

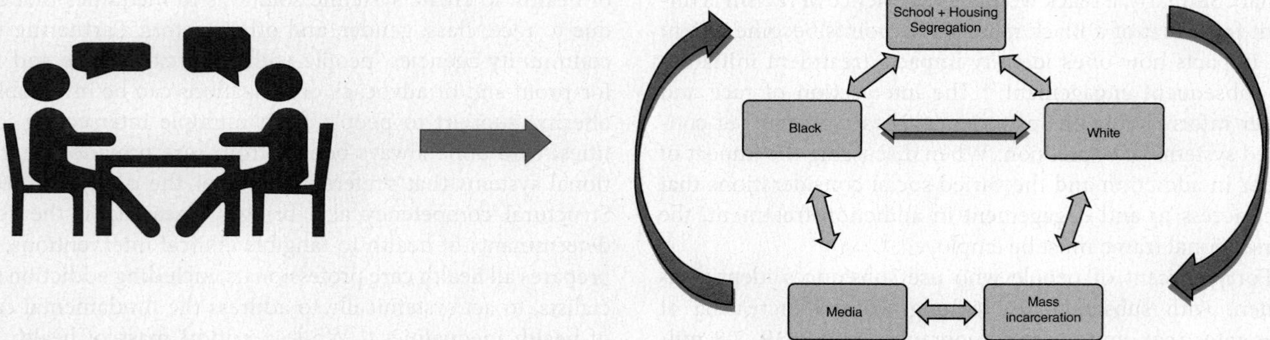

Figure 38-1. Transitioning From Cultural Competency to Structural Competency. (Adapted from Structural Competency lecture with permission from Dr. Helena Hansen)

structural competency a viable goal for the health care system, it also helps minimize physician and provider burnout while optimizing the health and well-being of both providers and patients alike.[46]

Many outside factors influence how patients receive addiction treatment. Examples include neighborhood resources (where people attend school, which medical facilities are available) and housing stability. Other examples include media and the influence therein on the understanding of drug epidemics (eg, how the opioid crisis was covered compared to the cocaine crisis). Mass incarceration and the impact of drug policy laws on Black and other racial and ethnically minoritized people being jailed instead of receiving treatment contribute greatly to current addiction disparities and health outcomes. Other salient factors include socioeconomic status, racism, legal status, education, food access, and housing stability. Evolution from Cultural Competence to Structural Competence (considering SDOH) provides a tangible tool to improve outcomes for both patients and providers alike.

WE *WALK THE WALK*—FIRSTHAND ACCOUNTS FROM RACIAL, GENDER, AND SEXUALLY MINORITIZED PEOPLE IN RECOVERY

In the final section of our chapter, we include first-hand accounts (as told to one of the coauthors and summarized herein) of two people from multiple intersecting backgrounds (of race, gender, and sexually minoritized individuals) who have interacted over the past 30 years with the U.S. addiction treatment system and provide key insights into their experiences and barriers faced and offer ways foreword. We are grateful for their contribution to the work and include first-hand accounts of their personal narratives, with pseudonyms to preserve their anonymity while promoting the authenticity of their experience.

According to Richard (Black, queer man), the interaction between addiction treatment and community has evolved over time. Although treatment is more accessible now than ever before, barriers to treatment are plentiful. When discussing access to treatment in his community, Richard expressed that he must travel on many buses to receive his treatment because the location is not near his community. He then revealed how the bus would often run behind schedule, and the service provider would not only cancel his appointment, but also blame and scold him, instead of attempting to understand the external circumstances. He described this lack of cultural and structural humility and compassion from service providers as a barrier to treatment.

When discussing service providers, Richard stated they "are racist and fear people like me, they only see me as someone who is Black and uses drugs, not as a person." Stigma, bias, and racism from service providers is a barrier for individuals who use drugs to seek and continue mental health and addiction treatment. By not going into the community, service providers neglect opportunities to educate themselves (about individual and structural barriers to treatment) and the community about services and treatments available. Richard believes that understanding the community is important to successful treatment because "how can you serve something you don't know?" By service providers understanding and becoming better acquainted with the community, mental health and addiction treatment could be more effective, and education could be more wide-reaching.

Although there are numerous barriers to treatment, a new initiative surrounding spirituality and culture was founded in a church near Richard's community.[50] Due to the trauma Richard's community has experienced, he believes "vulnerability is important to treatment, and that vulnerability is founded in religion, spirituality, and culture." Furthermore, Richard believes that impactful treatment is rooted in spirituality and culture, and those leading the initiative are essential to its success. Richard believes an initiative guided by community leaders is important because they understand the community they are serving and embrace cultural humility and compassion. Based on Richard's experience, for treatment to be effective, it needs to be spiritually and culturally based, and service providers need to be rooted in the community.

When discussing family life with Kim (Black cis-gender woman), she portrayed how addiction and trauma "is generational." Her mother was "addicted" to heroin, and unfortunately died from her addiction. Not even 2 days later, her father died. The trauma she endured from losing both parents days apart ended up being a contributing factor to her own substance use disorder. In her 20s, she became addicted to crack cocaine. Kim conferred that she "didn't know anything about posttraumatic stress disorder (PTSD), but that was what I was experiencing." After 7 years, she was able to overcome her addiction. She had been in and out of rehab, but the final rehab she went to made her realize she did not want to continue with drug use. Although she described herself as a "functional addict" and was able to maintain her addiction, she described how none of that could take away her pain. Kim also started to realize how her addiction played roles in her children's lives—her daughter had also started to struggle with an addiction as well and sadly, at the age of 27 years old, died from a fentanyl overdose.

According to Kim, there were many areas in the system that failed her and her family. While she navigated the system, no one asked about her trauma, other mental health diagnoses, structural drivers of poor health, racism, or gender identity. When her mother was growing up, people "didn't talk about mental health, " Kim says. "Our neighborhood was infested with drugs, but back then, helping Black people and other people who were not White was not the focus of treatment." Similarly, Kim's daughter was in and out of the Department of Children Youth Services (DCYS) system for more than half of her life as she tried to seek help. They would place her daughter in inpatient care, but after 3 days, she would be released.

As explained by Kim, "there was no stable place for my daughter's recovery". However, Kim was able to discover a program that she wishes was around for both her mother and daughter. The program focuses on the eight dimensions of wellness and gives an opportunity for participants with lived experience in mental health conditions including addiction to facilitate individual and group coaching sessions.[51] Kim believes "if more programs were geared toward wellness, they would be much more successful." In conclusion, Kim depicted how important it is to share her story, not only is it powerful, but also it helps people become more culturally aware. One lasting quote Kim shared is "if you want to know about the book, go to the author."

The experiences above are representative of two people with lived experience in addiction from multiple minoritized identities, and the similarities between the two accounts, overwhelmingly reflect the need to focus on community as a source of strength while also addressing the structural barriers that impede access to positive health outcomes.

SUMMARY

When considering addiction treatment, especially when taking care of people from racial and ethnic minoritized backgrounds, having an appreciation of how racism, NOT race, contributes to the existence and propagation of inequities in health is paramount.[3] Various levels of racism exist, internalized, personally mediated, and institutionalized, that preferentially advantage health outcomes for White people with addiction, over racial and ethnic minoritized people with SUDs. As such, racism contributes to health inequities and resultant inequalities that result from systemic, avoidable, and unjust policies and practices. Having a deep appreciation for the concept of intersectionality, as a lens toward examining power and how varying aspects of someone's identity (race, gender, sexual status) affects addiction care, provides one way to eliminate these disparities. Structural competency (articulating the systemic factors that cause poor health outcomes) provides yet another way to re-envision addiction treatment and provide informed care to racial and ethnic minoritized people.

REFERENCES

1. Weine S, Kohrt BA, Collins PY, et al. Justice for George Floyd and a reckoning for global mental health. *Global Mental Health.* 2020;7:e22.
2. Braveman P. What are health disparities and health equity? We need to be clear. *Public Health Rep*. 2014;129(Suppl 2):5-8.
3. Shim RS. Dismantling structural racism in psychiatry: a path to mental health equity. *Am J Psychiatry.* 2021;178(7):592-598.
4. Bourgois P, Holmes SM, Sue K, Quesada J. Structural vulnerability: operationalizing the concept to address health disparities in clinical care. *Acad Med.* 2017;92(3):299-307.
5. Friedman JR, Hansen H. Evaluation of increases in drug overdose mortality rates in the us by race and ethnicity before and during the COVID-19 pandemic. *JAMA Psychiatry.* 2022;79(4):379-381.
6. James K, Jordan A. The opioid crisis in black communities. *J Law Med Ethics.* 2018;46(2):404-421.
7. Lagisetty PA, Ross R, Bohnert A, Clay M, Maust DT. Buprenorphine treatment divide by race/ethnicity and payment. *JAMA Psychiatry.* 2019;76(9):979-981.
8. Andraka-Christou B. Addressing racial and ethnic disparities in the use of medications for opioid use disorder: study examines racial and ethnic disparities in the use of medications for opioid use disorder. *Health Affairs.* 2021;40(6):920-927.
9. Dankwa-Mullan I, Perez-Stable EJ, Gardner KL, Zhang X, Rosario AM. *The Science of Health Disparities Research*. Wiley; 2021.
10. Smedley BD, Stith AY, Nelson AR, eds. *Unequal Treatment: Confronting Racial and Ethnic Disparities in Health Care.* Institute of Medicine of the National Academies. National Academies Press; 2003.
11. Washington HA. *Medical Apartheid: The Dark History of Medical Experimentation on Black Americans From Colonial Times to the Present.* Doubleday Books; 2006.
12. Alexander M. The new Jim Crow. *Ohio St J Crim L.* 2011;9:7.
13. Peterson ED, Shaw LK, DeLong ER, Pryor DB, Califf RM, Mark DB. Racial variation in the use of coronary-revascularization procedures. Are the differences real? Do they matter? *N Engl J Med.* 1997;336(7):480-486.
14. MacDorman MF, Thoma M, Declcerq E, Howell EA. Racial and ethnic disparities in maternal mortality in the united states using enhanced vital records, 2016-2017. *Am J Pub Health.* 2021;111(9):1673-1681.
15. Tsai JW, Cerdeña JP, Goedel WC, et al. Evaluating the impact and rationale of race-specific estimations of kidney function: estimations from US NHANES, 2015-2018. *EClinicalMedicine.* 2021;42:101197.

16. Schwartz RC, Blankenship DM. Racial disparities in psychotic disorder diagnosis: a review of empirical literature. *World J Psychiatry.* 2014;4(4):133.
17. Heun-Johnson H, Menchine M, Axeen S, et al. Association between race/ethnicity and disparities in health care use before first-episode psychosis among privately insured young patients. *JAMA Psychiatry.* 2021;78(3):311-319.
18. Nash KA, Tolliver DG, Taylor RA, et al. Racial and ethnic disparities in physical restraint use for pediatric patients in the emergency department. *JAMA Pediatrics.* 2021;175(12):1283-1285.
19. Schnitzer K, Merideth F, Macias-Konstantopoulos W, Hayden D, Shtasel D, Bird S. Disparities in care: the role of race on the utilization of physical restraints in the emergency setting. *Acad Emerg Med.* 2020;27(10):943-950.
20. Williams DR, Rucker TD. Understanding and addressing racial disparities in health care. *Health Care Financ Rev.* 2000;21(4):75-90.
21. Phelan JC, Link BG. Is racism a fundamental cause of inequalities in health? *Annu Rev Sociol.* 2015;41:311-330.
22. Morning A. *The Nature of Race: How Scientists Think and Teach About Human Difference.* University of California Press; 2011.
23. Paradies Y, Ben J, Denson N, et al. Racism as a determinant of health: a systematic review and meta-analysis. *PLoS One.* 2015;10(9):e0138511.
24. Jones CP. Levels of racism: a theoretic framework and a gardener's tale. *Am J Public Health.* 2000;90(8):1212-1215.
25. Coley RL, Sims J, Thomson D, Votruba-Drzal E. The intergenerational transmission of socioeconomic inequality through school and neighborhood processes. *J Child Poverty.* 2019;25(2):79-100. up to here.
26. Braveman P, Egerter S, Williams DR. The social determinants of health: coming of age. *Annu Rev Public Health.* 2011;32(1):381-398.
27. Sinha R. How does stress increase risk of drug abuse and relapse? *Psychopharmacology (Berl).* 2001;158(4):343-359.
28. Sinha R, Garcia M, Paliwal P, Kreek MJ, Rounsaville BJ. Stress-induced cocaine craving and hypothalamic-pituitary-adrenal responses are predictive of cocaine relapse outcomes. *Arch Gen Psychiatry.* 2006;63(3):324-331.
29. Cooper HL, Friedman SR, Tempalski B, Friedman R. Residential segregation and injection drug use prevalence among Black adults in U.S. metropolitan areas. *Am J Public Health.* 2007;97(2):344-352.
30. Hansen HB, Siegel CE, Case BG, Bertollo DN, DiRocco D, Galanter M. Variation in use of buprenorphine and methadone treatment by racial, ethnic, and income characteristics of residential social areas in New York City. *J Behav Health Serv Res.* 2013;40(3):367-377.
31. Hansen H, Siegel C, Wanderling J, DiRocco D. Buprenorphine and methadone treatment for opioid dependence by income, ethnicity and race of neighborhoods in New York City. *Drug Alcohol Depend.* 2016;164:14-21.
32. Doernberg M, Krawczyk N, Agus D, Fingerhood M. Demystifying buprenorphine misuse: has fear of diversion gotten in the way of addressing the opioid crisis? *Subst Abus.* 2019;40(2):148-153.
33. Netherland J, Hansen HB. The war on drugs that wasn't: wasted whiteness, "dirty doctors," and race in media coverage of prescription opioid misuse. *Cult Med Psychiatry.* 2016;40(4):664-686.
34. López N, Gadsden VL. *Health inequities, social determinants, and intersectionality.* Discussion Paper. National Academy of Medicine Accessed August 11, 2023. https://nam.edu/wp-content/uploads/2016/12/Health-Inequities-Social-Determinants-and-Intersectionality.pdf
35. Crenshaw KW. Mapping the margins: intersectionality, identity politics, and violence against women of color. In: Fineman MA, ed. *The Public Nature of Private Violence.* Routledge; 2013:93-118.
36. Kelly UA. Integrating intersectionality and biomedicine in health disparities research. *Adv Nurs Sci.* 2009;32(2):E42-E56.
37. World Health Organization. *Gender and Health.* Accessed January 13, 2023. https://www.who.int/health-topics/gender#tab=tab_1
38. Ait-Daoud N, Blevins D, Khanna S, Sharma S, Holstege CP, Amin P. Women and addiction: an update. *Med Clin North Am.* 2019;103(4):699-711.
39. Substance Abuse and Mental Health Services Administration. *Key substance use and mental health indicators in the United States: results from the 2019 National Survey on Drug Use and Health.* SAMHSA; 2020.
40. Baskin C, Strike C, McPherson B. Long time overdue: an examination of the destructive impacts of policy and legislation on pregnant and parenting aboriginal women and their children. *Int Indig Policy J.* 2015;6(1):1-19.
41. Roberts D. *Torn Apart: How the Child Welfare System Destroys Black Families--and How Abolition Can Build a Safer World.* Basic Books; 2022.
42. Covington S. Helping women recover: creating gender-responsive treatment. In: Straussner SLA, Brown S, eds. *The Handbook of Addiction Treatment for Women: Theory and Practice.* Wiley; 2002:52-72.
43. Rivera E, Phillips H, Warshaw C, Lyon E, Bland P, Kaewken O. *An applied research paper on the relationship between intimate partner violence and substance use.* National Center on Domestic Violence, Trauma & Mental Health; 2015.
44. Netherland J, Hansen H. White opioids: pharmaceutical race and the war on drugs that wasn't. *BioSocieties.* 2017;12(2):217-238.
45. Green CA. Gender and use of substance abuse treatment services. *Alcohol Res Health.* 2006;29(1):55.
46. Metzl JM, Hansen H. Structural competency: theorizing a new medical engagement with stigma and inequality. *Soc Sci Med.* 2014;103:126-133.
47. structuralcompetency.org. *Structural Competency: Related Organizations.* Accessed October 21, 2022. https://structuralcompetency.org/resources-2/
48. Gainsbury SM. Cultural competence in the treatment of addictions: theory, practice and evidence. *Clin Psychol Psychother.* 2017;24(4):987-1001.
49. Lekas HM, Pahl K, Fuller LC. Rethinking cultural competence: shifting to cultural humility. *Health Serv Insights.* 2020;13:1178632920970580.
50. Jordan A, Babuscio T, Nich C, Carroll KM. A feasibility study providing substance use treatment in the Black church. *J Subst Abuse Treat.* 2021;124:108218.
51. Bellamy CD, Costa M, Wyatt J, et al. A collaborative culturally-centered and community-driven faith-based opioid recovery initiative: the Imani Breakthrough project. *Soc Work Ment Health.* 2021;19(6):558-567.

CHAPTER

39 Cultural Issues in Addiction Medicine

Andrea G. Barthwell

CHAPTER OUTLINE

- Introduction
- Background and significance
- Culture and patterns of substance use
- Cultural aspects of clinical assessment
- Culture, treatment, and recovery
- Conclusions

INTRODUCTION

This chapter is a revision of Chapter 42 authored by Joseph Westermeyer and Patricia Jean Dickmann in *The ASAM Principles of Addiction Medicine*, 6th edition. Westermeyer's research has grounded and advanced our understanding of the cultural and social factors contributing to substance use disorder (SUD). This revision attempts to retain the rich understanding of culture as contributor to in the acquisition and expression of substance use patterns while acknowledging the unique American experience of structural racism and its effects on the environment and life experiences of Black, Hispanic/Latinx, Asian, Pacific Islander, Indigenous American and other racially oppressed and disenfranchised people (hereinafter referred to as Black, Indigenous, People of Color [BIPOC]), their access to evidence-based addiction treatment services. The full definition of "structural racism" is:

> A system in which public policies, institutional practices, cultural representations, and other norms work in various, often reinforcing ways to perpetuate racial group inequity. It identifies dimensions of our history and culture that have allowed privileges associated with "whiteness" and disadvantages associated with "color" to endure and adapt over time. Structural racism is not something that a few people or institutions choose to practice. Instead, it has been a feature of the social, economic, and political systems in which we all exist.[1]

The term BIPOC acknowledges that all ethnic groups have the potential to be different and that those differences should be valued. These differences, historically, have been responses to diverse environmental contexts of the lives of people over many years. Each group has developed a culture that is appropriate to its time, external stressors, internal questions, world view, uncertainty, and environment. These cultures have come together in the United States for vastly varied reasons (eg, to escape tyranny, to be enslaved against their will, to escape poverty and oppression, to labor, etc.). In the United States, these groups have not had equal access to resources; nor do they share power equally compared to the majority population with common European ancestry. BIPOC have a greater probability of being from a lower-status social class.[2]

This chapter endeavors to help clinicians incorporate cultural factors when treating substance use disorders. Cultural factors may predict the substances one is exposed to and experiments with, and how a person's environment, tradition, and ritual influence use within the community. Clinicians should know how cultural factors can potentially serve as pathogenic agents or therapeutic resources. Acquiring the necessary clinical knowledge, attitudes, and skills depends on learning several sociocultural concepts relevant to substance use. Clinicians who know and can apply these concepts possess "clinical cultural competence," which empowers clinicians in engaging, retaining, and fostering optimal clinical outcomes among culturally diverse patients. The clinical goal is to enable the patient to return to health, psychological competence, and full sociocultural function.

SUD can vary widely across nations and cultures. For example, high rates of alcohol use disorders occur in several countries of Eastern Europe, especially Hungary, Poland, and Romania[3]; the Aboriginal Australians[4]; and the Northern Plains tribes of North America[5]. Likewise, ethnic groups in Southeast Asia that traditionally raised poppies as a cash crop (eg, Hmong and Iu Mien) may have high rates of opioid use disorder.[6] At times, subgroups within a culture can manifest high rates. For example, full-time college students tend to drink more than others in their age group. In 2019, 53% of full-time college students drank alcohol in the past month. Among individuals ages 18 to 22 not enrolled fulltime in college, the percentage was 44%.[7]

Many national governments are devoting more attention to culture and health services, including SUD treatment. In the United States, for example, the National Standards for Culturally and Linguistically Appropriate Services (National CLAS Standards) are a set of 15 action steps intended to advance health equity, improve quality, and help eliminate health care disparities by providing a blueprint for individuals and health care organizations to implement culturally and linguistically appropriate services.[8] The pillars of CLAS are to respect the individual and respond to the individual's health needs and preferences.[8]

This chapter highlights cultural factors influencing the prevalence of SUD across nations and cultures, plus the importance of providing culturally competent care to reduce health disparities and achieve health equity. It recognizes and accepts the concept that, while addiction involves complex interactions among an individual's brain circuits, genetics, the environment, and their life experiences, racism influences the environment and life experiences of BIPOC, and that "structural competency" can mitigate these effects (see Chapter 53). Our objectives include to:

- Describe linkages between culture and addiction.
- Explain clinical skills needed to take a substance use history and inquire about each patient's unique cultural characteristics.
- Articulate therapeutic attitudes and approaches that can engage people across cultures.[9]
- Enhance clinician awareness of cross-cultural interactions, which may promote improved communication, reduce bias, and reinforce healing relationships.
- Increase structural competency, defined as the capacity to recognize and respond to health and illness as downstream effects of social, political, and economic structures.[10,11]

BACKGROUND AND SIGNIFICANCE

The cultural background of a patient may profoundly influence the availability of alcohol or substances; patterns of use; and health consequences and complications of use, which may be intensified due to pre-existing conditions or socioeconomic contributors to health. The degree to which cultural background influences use patterns, independent of socioeconomic factors, such as employment and poverty, is not well understood.

Clinicians are taught to recognize patterns (ie, clusters of signs and symptoms) as a basis of diagnosis and treatment. Variances in patterns observed across cultures may adversely influence a clinician's ability to formulate an individually appropriate clinical approach. To overcome this possibility, it is helpful first to acknowledge that these cultural variances exist.

Several tenets underlie the understanding of cultural variances. First, all patients are not equal clinically, pathologically, socio-culturally, environmentally, or biogenetically. Second, in order to identify SUD in diverse individuals who may vary culturally from the clinician, one must respect cultural differences and combine that respect with effective screening and assessment tools modified as necessary to foster effective communication across culture and experiences. Third, across individuals and cultural groups, substance use along a continuum (ie, incidental use, experimental use, regular use, and use disorders) can vary significantly. Fourth, clinicians may have to adapt their usual therapeutic approaches or methods to account for the beliefs and experiences of the patient, and to allow the patient to see themselves in the discussion. Fifth and finally, SUD may present at any point in life, its onset and progression are influenced by culture and yield varying consequences, and SUD management strategies must account for the stage and severity of substance misuse.[12]

Cultural Definitions Related to Substance Use

Several concepts can aid clinicians in perceiving how culture may contribute to or alleviate SUD (see **Table 39-1** for a list of these concepts and their definitions). *Cultures* typically have rules and traditions regarding substance production,

TABLE 39-1 Definition of Culture-Related Terms With Utility in Understanding, Assessing, and Treating Substance Use Disorder and Gambling Disorder

Term	Definition
Culture	The sum total of a people's way of life, including their geography, topography, climate, work and recreation, technology and economic production, formal and informal political organization, law and law enforcement, family organization and function, child raising and education, life cycle patterns and age–sex roles, language and communication, clothing, beliefs and norms, customs and ceremonies, recreation and "time-out" from social roles, diet, and health care. In sum, it is the advanced structure of language, behavior, customs, knowledge, symbols, ideas, values, matter, and mind that provide a group of people with a general design for living and with patterns for interpreting their reality. Cultures differ in world views, in perspectives on the rhythms and patterns of life, and in concepts of the essential nature of the human condition. These customs, beliefs, values, knowledge, and skills guide a people's behavior along shared paths.
Ethnicity	Ethnicity refers to the social characteristics that people may have in common, such as language, religion, regional background, culture, foods, etc. Ethnicity is revealed by the traditions one follows, a person's native language, and so on. Race, on the other hand, describes categories assigned to demographic groups based mostly on observable physical characteristics, like skin color, hair texture, and eye shape.[1] Ethnic groups are socially distinguishable or set apart by others or itself primarily on the basis of cultural characteristics or nationality. Ethnicity, in contrast to race, is therefore, intricately connected to groups within a culture who share their own unique cultural characteristics, including national origin, language, shared ancestors, religion, traditions, clothing, and/or beliefs or norms. A racial group is not naturally generated as a part of the self-evident order of the universe but is a social group in which persons inside or outside have decided that it is important to single themselves out as inferior or superior, typically on the basis of real or alleged physical characteristics that are objectively selected. Ethnic and racial groups are bound together by the intangible nonmaterial elements of culture.

(Continued)

TABLE 39-1 Definition of Culture-Related Terms With Utility in Understanding, Assessing and Treating Substance Use Disorder and Gambling Disorder *(Continued)*

Term	Definition
Subculture	Groups within a culture that share major sociocultural characteristics, such as occupation, identity, or values. Examples include professional groups, guilds or unions, political parties, recovery organizations, commercial groups, age cohorts, school cliques, or recreational associations. Subcultures depend on the majority culture for their existence; they are not freestanding and cannot sustain themselves.
Norms	Values, beliefs, and behaviors within a culture that possess positive or negative valance; norms exist with behaviors that are viewed in a judgmental way or have moral overtones. These shared rules specify appropriate and inappropriate behavior. Social mores are norms that people consider *vital* to their well-being and to their most cherished values (eg, a woman as a model of virtue and sobriety). Sanctions are used within cultures to *compel* people to comply with norms. Sanctions applied to subgroups can act as *protective factors* against the development of, for example, alcoholism.
Ideal norms	These norms describe the manner in which a person should behave.
Behavioral norms	These norms describe the manner in which the people in a group actually do behave, regardless of expressed ideal norms.
Identity	An individual's view of themselves based on group affiliations
Enculturation	Training of children to become culturally competent
Acculturation	A process by which two adjacent cultural groups adapt certain aspects of one another's culture; also applied to migrants into a new culture, who must acquire attitudes, knowledge, and skill of the new culture to function as an adult
Minority	Minority is avoided in this article because it connotes inferiority and has been linked to groups most impacted by racism and poverty with misattribution of the effects of racism and poverty. Minority status is also a view of ethnicity from a dominant group and position of power. We avoid reinforcing the notions of superiority and inferiority, better and worse, good and bad, desirable and undesirable characteristics by referring to *ethnic groups of color* as *BIPOC* who are collectively the *majority of people worldwide*.
Racism	The belief that all members of a purported race possess characteristics, abilities, or qualities specific to a race, a particular form of prejudice directed toward a person or group of people based upon their membership in a particular racial or ethnic group.
Antiracism	Strategies, theories, actions, and practices that challenge or counter racism, inequalities, prejudices, and discrimination based on race
Structural racism	Public policies, institutional practices, cultural repression, and other societal norms that contribute to and perpetuate group inequality
Socioeconomic contributors to health	Social determinants of health (SDOH) are the conditions in the environments where people are born, live, learn, work, play, worship, and age that affect a wide range of health, functioning, and quality-of-life outcomes and risks. SDOH also contribute to wide health disparities and inequities. There are five domains: economic stability, education access and quality, heath care access and quality, neighborhood and built environment, and social and community context.[13]
Structural competency	A paradigm for medical education in which inequalities in health care are conceptualized in relation to the institutions and social conditions that determine health-related resources (see Chapter 53).[10,11]
Cultural representation	Popular stereotypes, images, frames, and narratives that are socialized and reinforced by media, language, and other forms of mass communication are cultural representations. They can be positive or negative, but too often cultural representations depict people of color in ways that are dehumanizing, perpetuate inaccurate stereotypes, and have the overall effect of allowing unfair treatment within the society as a whole to seem fair, or "natural."[1]

distribution, and consumption. Most nations encompass numerous cultures, or *ethnicities*. The role of alcohol and psychoactive substances, for example, differs within cultures and ethnicities particularly when it comes to rituals and traditions. A *subculture*'s traditions, rituals, attitudes, values, and practices toward substances may resemble or differ from those of its culture at large.[14]

Groups of people with SUD can comprise *subcultures* with their own values, loyalties, beliefs, and traditions. Examples include neighborhood bars, places where people gather to use substances, or college party houses.[15] These subcultures may demonstrate preferential availability and use of certain substances based on the norms and habits of the group.

One factor in drug use initiation is drug availability, and communities vary in the substances presenting in ample supply that people can access. For example, in some communities during the 1990s, "crack" cocaine was an economic commodity in ample supply. Often the low cost of a "dose" of crack packaged in a $10 unit made the "cost of admission" low enough to enable use, and potentially encourage use, by impoverished individuals and young people. According to a personal communication from W. Clark in October 2022, in poorer communities, cocaine use could be as prevalent as youth use of alcohol from a parent's home. Just as subcultures can furnish environments for the spread of substance use, recovery subcultures can impart opportunities to abstain from use. Affiliating with mutual aid groups, such as Alcoholics Anonymous, Narcotics Anonymous, and SMART Recovery can reinforce healthy norms and reduce return to use.

An *ideal norm* might support and promote use of a substance under certain circumstances, such as drinking wine during Jewish Passover or consuming peyote in the Indigenous American Church. Another ideal norm may demand abstinence, such as abstention from alcohol by many Muslim sects, or from tobacco by Seventh Day Adventists. *Behavioral norms* are those things that people actually do.[16] A *norm gap* or *conflict* occurs if the ideal norm and behavioral norm diverge. In cultures with norm conflicts regarding substance use, SUD predictably ensues.[17] Bringing norm dissonance to patients' awareness can aid the journey to a culturally appropriate recovery.

Exploring an individual's *cultural identity* during motivational interviewing can lead to valuable insights that can guide interventions. For example, if a physician asks a patient about their identity, the patient could reply, "I'm a heavy drinker, but I'm not an alcoholic." This response may support a useful conversation regarding the patient's criteria for these categories and why they were willing to accept one identity while rejecting the other. Entrenched stigmatizing language and cultural identities (eg, "drunk" and "addict") can negatively influence one's self-esteem, sense of hope, and ongoing patterns of substance use.[18]

CULTURE AND PATTERNS OF SUBSTANCE USE

When ideal and behavioral norms regarding substance use are congruent, SUD is less common. On the other hand, groups that prohibit use of a substance in theory, yet foster its use in practice, invite individuals to decide on their own use patterns, which may subject the individuals to the reinforcing nature of using the substance. Examples of norm conflict fostering increased substance use in the United States include cannabis legalization and socially promoted patterns of use,[19] excessive prescribing of opioid pain relievers,[20] and college binge drinking.[7] **Table 39-2** shows the characteristics of substance use in relation to ideal norms.[21]

Despite similarities and differences among cultural groups, clinicians must assess each patient as a unique individual who may differ from others in the group.[22] Stereotyping patients is never warranted, as relying on general trends or expectations can be clinically misleading:

- Within any large population, considerable differences can exist among subgroups. For example, Korean Americans tend to have higher rates of SUD than other Asian American groups.[23]
- Rates of SUD may change with the generations since immigration. For example, Mexican American women have extremely low rates of SUD in the first generation after immigration, but rates comparable to other American women in the second and subsequent generations.[24]
- Sociocultural changes within ethnic groups can affect the pattern of substance use and SUD over time. For example, some Hispanic Americans have abandoned Roman Catholicism for abstinence-oriented Protestantism in an effort to resolve alcohol use disorder.[25] The Hmong, an Asian American immigrant group, formerly had no norm gap with regard to alcohol use and virtually no alcohol use disorder. However, widespread conversion to abstinence-oriented Protestantism resulted in a norm conflict regarding drinking and the appearance of alcohol use disorder.[26]

Clinicians must conduct individual assessments for each patient while avoiding stereotyping. Failure to do so can result in missed diagnosis (eg, in patients from groups with low rates of SUD) and erroneous diagnosis (eg, in patients from groups with high rates of SUD). Person- and family-centered care enable clinicians to individualize assessments, diagnoses, treatment, and supportive services in culturally appropriate ways.

Person-centered care enables health care consumers to make decisions about their treatment and overall care, such as choice of provider and amount, scope, and duration of services. Person-centered care is respectful and responsive to the cultural, linguistic, and other social and environmental needs of the individual. Person-centered care may account for a patient's ethnicity, race, age, sexual orientation, and gender identity, and it may include family and peer involvement.[27]

TABLE 39-2 Characteristics of Substance Use Depending on Presence Versus Absence of Norm Conflict

Characteristic	Source of norm gap	Ideal norm
Enculturation	Peers teach substance use	Family teaches substance use
Context of use	Surreptitious, hidden	Open, acknowledged
Ritual focus	Secular; substance use is the primary activity	Religious or communal eating or celebration
Locus of control	The individual controls frequency and amount of use	Family or community expectations influence use
Psychological correlates	Shame, guilt, denial, negative or "outlaw" identity	Satisfaction, group cohesion, positive identity
Health risk	Risk is high	Risk is low

Similarly, family-centered care recognizes the important role of family members and caregivers, and upon the direction of the patient, includes them in the development of treatment goals and selection of services to be provided. Person- and family-centered care are respectful and responsive to the needs of the individual, yet occur within the professional responsibilities of treatment providers and care teams.[27]

CULTURAL ASPECTS OF CLINICAL ASSESSMENT

Taking a Cultural History

Many researchers now acknowledge that heterogeneity among and within European immigrant and BIPOC populations exists, and this acknowledgment is represented in descriptions of study samples and incorporated in research designs. The heterogeneity within ethnic groups may derive from socioeconomic status, education, acculturation, country of origin, years since arrival in the United States, and racial makeup. These variables may interact to complicate treatment of individuals within discrete groups. If diversity within groups is acknowledged, it can temper an inclination to generalize characteristics and expectations while also serving to negate stereotypes. For example, African Americans have encountered a variety of experiences that have contributed to the creation of cultural hybrids. The immigration status, migratory patterns, and personal struggles of African Americans give them an authentic (natural) African cultural base, adopted (survivalist) European American cultural subtype, and adapted (developmentally) African American culture. Cultural hybrids, deriving from ethnicity and racial or biogenetic mixing, are common and must be accounted for in assessing, diagnosing, and treating individual patients.[28]

Cultural factors can be protective against loss of control over one's use. Culture, tradition, and rituals set the patterns of use that are normative for a collective group and provide control to protect the individual from ill effects of the substance. They serve to protect others from an individual who is affected by the mood- or mind-altering chemical. When that control is lifted, individual control over use patterns may be difficult, if not impossible, for some members of the group. Understanding the importance of culture supports assessments of potential and actual substance use.

The first step in conducting a cultural history consists of asking the patient about the ethnic origins of their parents and grandparents, or their surrogates. Relevant information includes place of birth, national origin, language spoken at home, migrations, roles and affiliations in the ethnic community, and roles and affiliations in the community at large. Educational experiences or relationship history (eg, marital status) may also be relevant. The second step consists of assessing the family's overall enculturation and that of the patient into their ethnic groups of origin.[29]

Many studies conducted by individuals who are not part of the racial and ethnic groups being studied do not attach significance to the degree to which individuals within that group are acculturated.[30-34] Acculturation is a complex process that occurs when an individual makes a deliberate decision to move away from one's cultural norm. One example is moving to a subculture within that culture and immersing oneself in either a negative or positive iteration of the original culture. Another is an individual who moves away from the culture toward a more predominant culture. The movement can occur through assimilation due to attraction to the new culture or away from the original culture out of dissatisfaction. The endpoints may be the same, but the motivational base can be vastly different.[35] The acculturation itself may be a source of information relevant to the assessment, diagnosis, or treatment of SUD. Acculturation can involve stressors that may precipitate unhealthy substance use.[36] During late adolescence and early adulthood, relocation to college, military service, or cross-ethnic marriage can alter previously learned substance use norms and behaviors.[37] Likewise, a BIPOC person who was adopted into a family that believes that race and ethnicity are not important contributors to social or economic opportunities or outcomes may be frustrated by experiences outside of the household that prove otherwise. This frustration may predispose the person to self-medication through drug use.

The rationale for a person's acculturation may also provide clinically significant information. For example, parental SUD may provide a basis for acculturation. Parental SUD can disrupt a healthy identity formation and undermine cultural competence.[38] It can result in lower ability to develop meaningful relationships, which can increase the risk of SUD.[39] In an effort to reduce their own risk of developing SUD, a person whose parent had SUD may spurn the parent's culture in favor of one in which ideal norms are more commonly reinforced and followed. A clinician who asks such a patient about their culture of origin, current culture, and the rationale for acculturation can elicit information about the patient's biology, adverse childhood experiences, corresponding predisposition to SUD, and commitment to healthful living. All of these data points are germane to SUD assessment, diagnosis, and treatment.

CULTURE, TREATMENT, AND RECOVERY

Addiction, Recovery, and the Intimate Social Network

Research conducted in the 1970s and 1980s (before widespread use of the Internet) determined that the normal "intimate social network" (ISN) of one person (or "proband") consists of 20 to 30 people organized into four or five groups[40] (see **Table 39-3**). Typical subgroups include the people with whom the proband interacts face-to-face, namely relatives, friends, coworkers, and another group or two (eg, neighbors, church members, or a recreational group). The chance that any one person knows another in the proband's ISN (termed "connectedness") is about 80%. Such groups tend to be stable over time.

TABLE 39-3 Characteristics of the Intimate Social Network in Relation to Clinical Characteristics

Category	Number of people	Number of groups	Reciprocity	Connectedness[a]	Other
Normal	20-30	4-5	Symmetric	80%	Stable, long lasting
Dysfunctional (in outpatient, self-help group)	10-19	2-3	Symmetric	60%	Unstable, may include pets, caregivers, and deceased
Disabled (in residential or day program)	1-9	1	Asymmetric	100%	Easily destabilizes
Isolated (in hospital, jail, homeless, ER)	0	0	Absent	0	Presents in crisis, suicidal

[a]Likelihood that any one person in the intimate social network (ISN) knows anyone else in the ISN.

Middle-class, middle-aged, married, employed men with alcohol use disorder were noted to have normal ISN size upon entering SUD treatment.[41] However, they lost about half of their ISN members (mostly other people who drink heavily) during early recovery, precipitating feelings of loss, loneliness, and lack of support.

Progressive SUD and growing dysfunction often reduce the ISN to fewer than 20 people, with two or three groups (eg, family and relatives) plus some one-to-one relationships. Although the element of reciprocity persists, the proband may become more of a client vis-a-vis other people in the ISN. The latter may consist of drug dealers, bartenders, hair stylists, clergy, social workers, and health professionals. These patients sometimes report ISN members not ordinarily reported, such as deceased persons, pets, or people who were close friends years ago.[42]

With disability, the ISN often declines further to ten or fewer people. Their common link involves nonreciprocal relationships with the proband, who receives but seldom returns their courtesies. For example, a parent, social worker, homeless shelter manager, and police officer may all know one another through their respective efforts to help the proband. Eventually, the alienated proband may become isolated to the point of not having anyone to call upon—a grave prognostic sign.[43]

ISN reconstruction offers a potent means for intervening in the SUD progression and supporting recovery.[44] A key element involves eliminating companions who use drugs from the ISN, with retention of those committed to the patient's ultimate recovery.[45] This approach has proven useful even in cases with limited family or economic resources.[46] Recovery communities, including recovery residences, depend on this powerful strategy.

With sobriety, support from family and peers, and sufficient time, persons with SUD can rebuild a functional, supportive ISN, as in the following case.

A surgeon referred a veteran to SUD treatment who reported that the preoperative sedative provided him with the first full night of sleep that he had experienced in years. The patient, in for surgical repairs related to shrapnel injuries, had been seriously wounded in combat, with polytrauma and blast injury. After his return to civilian life, he completed postcollege professional training. Despite his many successes, he went to his basement once or twice a month to drink a quart of whiskey alone and think about his experiences and deceased comrades-in-arms.

Aside from his spouse and two children, he had minimal social contacts or commitments outside of his professional work. Evaluation revealed chronic posttraumatic stress disorder and alcohol use disorder. After a 3-month period of sobriety and relief from his posttraumatic stress disorder and insomnia, he began reconstructing his ISN. He chose first to expand his affiliations with his former combat unit. This choice provided opportunities to obtain support from those with similar experiences and, eventually, to provide support to others (similar to the role of sponsors in Alcoholics Anonymous). A few years later, he became active with the alumni group where he received his professional training, providing him with opportunities to "pay back" that institution. This gradual process required over a decade.

This case demonstrates principles of ISN reconstruction. First, the patient had a period of sobriety and psychological recovery from his alcohol use disorder and posttraumatic stress disorder before initiating a process that could be stressful and result in rejection or failure. Second, he chose to join identity groups (veterans first and alumni second). He believed (and rightly, as it turned out) that his veteran group would accept him whatever his circumstances, given their shared combat experience and injuries. The alumni group posed a greater risk of social rejection; therefore, he pursued re-entry into that group after he was more stable in recovery and better prepared to manage a negative outcome.

Cultural Recovery in Substance Use Disorders

Reconstruction of the ISN can pose a serious challenge. Most adults have a full complement of people with whom they have stable relationships. Thus, they do not readily take on another person outside of their current ISN. Nonetheless, a number of strategies have proven useful to ISN reconstruction during recovery:

- Joining a recovery group whose members are looking for new associates (eg, Alcoholics Anonymous, Narcotics Anonymous, and SMART Recovery)

- Participating in a sports or exercise club, or occupational association
- Supporting a charitable organization or social group with a charitable purpose
- Volunteering at a school, clinic, hospital, or nursing home
- Returning to an ethnic association or church group
- Taking a job (part time or full time) that leads to new contacts

These strategies replace the groups associated with psychoactive substance use in the person's previous life.[47] They lead to affiliations with new people and groups, affording the recovering person new opportunities for success.

A more challenging task can occur in rebuilding bridges with relatives and family members. Previous SUD-related affronts may have alienated them. Relatives and family members need evidence that the recovering person can follow through on commitments, engage in reciprocal acts of mutual support, and adopt a predictable lifestyle. Accordingly, it may be wise to delay rebuilding certain relationships until stability (ie, 6-24 months) has been established. If the recovering person resumes substance use—common in the early months of recovery—the occurrence may demoralize previously optimistic family and friends. For those involved in 12-step recovery, several early steps prepare the recovering person for making amends to disheartened family and estranged friends.

Digital social networks comprise an increasingly popular means for recovering people to join with like-minded people, chat on social media, play competitive games, acquire information, begin new relationships, and attend mutual aid groups. However, overuse, risky use, or too trusting use of the Internet may lead to problems that precipitate a return to substance use.[48] A lonely person might buy into the illusion of real relationships, which turn out to be Internet fictions. Having 1000+ "friends" on Facebook typically does not replicate the commitment, continuity, and reciprocity existing within one's real-life ISN.

Evolution of Sociocultural Interventions

Sociocultural therapies outside of traditional clinics and hospitals have evolved. Mutual aid groups (from 19th century England), day hospitals (from WWII Moscow), and workplace programs (from former Yugoslavia) remain common today. Newer approaches to treatment and recovery are now supported by an evidence base.

As a current example in North America, the "Housing First" model has gained an evidence base, increased in popularity, and serves hundreds of thousands of individuals with SUD. This model involves first providing "permanent independent housing" to homeless people with SUD, then following up with optional treatment services.

Culture-Specific Treatment

Therapies specific to particular cultures can contribute to recovery from SUD. Participation aids the recovering person in several ways: providing a recovery-supportive environment, engaging in meaningful activity, receiving emotional support from others with whom the person may identify, and building a new identity as a recovering person. Referral to treatment that undermines positive cultural or ethnic values or that introduces unacceptable risks can be counterproductive. For example, some people may dislike the "higher power" emphasis in Alcoholics Anonymous but accept the biosocial paradigms in SMART Recovery.

CONCLUSIONS

Across history, cultural groups have fostered specific norms with regard to substance use.

Clinicians can increase their effectiveness by inquiring about the cultural elements that accompany the patient into the consultation room. This task begins with understanding patients' enculturation experiences from childhood to present day. Patients' past and current cultural affiliations can help clinicians in conducting assessments, making diagnoses, and devising successful treatment and recovery plans. As part of this process, assessing the patient's ISN can inform clinicians as to the severity of SUD, therapeutic resources readily at hand, and formulation of realistic treatment goals and recovery. As cultural factors have contributed to the onset of substance misuse or SUD, likewise communities and cultural resources can aid clinicians and patients in the challenging processes of treatment and recovery.

REFERENCES

1. Aspen Institute. *Glossary for Understanding the Dismantling Structural Racism/Promoting Racial Equity Analysis*. Accessed October 17, 2022. https://www.aspeninstitute.org/wp-content/uploads/files/content/docs/rcc/RCC-Structural-Racism-Glossary.pdf
2. Hirschl TA, Rank MR. The life course dynamics of affluence. *PLoS One*. 2015;10(1):e0116370. doi:10.1371/journal.pone.0116370
3. Popova S, Rehm J, Patra J, Zatonski W. Comparing alcohol consumption in central and eastern Europe to other European countries. *Alcohol Alcohol*. 2007;42:465-473.
4. Kahn MW, Hunter E, Heather N, Tebbutt J. Australian Aborigines, and alcohol: a review. *Drug Alcohol Rev*. 1991;10:351-366.
5. Landen M, Roeber J, Naimi T, Nielsen L, Sewell M. Alcohol-attributable mortality among American Indians and Alaska Natives in the United States, 1999-2009. *Am J Public Health*. 2014;104:343-349.
6. Westermeyer J, Lyfoung T, Westermeyer M, Neider J. Opium addiction among Indochinese refugees in the U.S.: characteristics of addicts and their opium use. *Am J Drug Alcohol Abuse*. 1991;17:267-277.
7. SAMHSA. *FACTS on college student drinking*. Accessed August 11, 2023. https://store.samhsa.gov/sites/default/files/pep21-03-10-006.pdf
8. U.S. Department of Health and Human Services. Think Cultural Health. *National CLAS Standards*. Accessed August 11, 2023. https://thinkculturalhealth.hhs.gov/clas
9. Westermeyer J. The role of cultural and social factors in the cause of addictive disorders. *Psychiatr Clin North Am*. 1999;22:253-273.
10. Neff J, Holmes SM, Knight KR, et al. Structural competency: curriculum for medical students, residents, and interprofessional teams on the structural factors that produce health disparities. *MedEdPORTAL*. 2020;16:10888. doi:10.15766/mep_2374-8265.10888

11. Metzl JM, Hansen H. Structural competency: theorizing a new medical engagement with stigma and inequality. *Soc Sci Med.* 2014;103:126-133. doi:10.1016/j.socscimed.2013.06.032
12. Barthwell AG, Hewitt W, Jilson I. An introduction to ethnic and cultural diversity. *Pediatr Clin North Am.* 1995;42(2):431-451.
13. U.S. DHHS, Office of Disease Prevention and Health Promotion: Healthy People 2030. Accessed 11 August, 2023. https://health.gov/healthypeople/priority-areas/social-determinants-health
14. Caetano R, Clark CL. Trends in alcohol consumption patterns among whites, blacks, and Hispanics: 1984 and 1995. *J Stud Alcohol.* 1998;59:659-668.
15. Dumont M. Tavern culture: the sustenance of homeless men. *Am J Orthopsychiatry.* 1967;37:938-945.
16. Kulis S, Napoli M, Marsiglia EF. Ethnic pride, biculturalism, and drug use norms in urban American Indian adolescents. *Soc Work Res.* 2002;26:101-112.
17. Gonzales NA, German M, Kim SY, et al. Mexican American adolescents' cultural orientation, externalizing behavior and academic engagement: the role of traditional cultural values. *Am J Community Psychol.* 2008;41:151-164.
18. Larimer ME, Cronce JM. Identification, prevention, and treatment: a review of individual-focused strategies to reduce problematic alcohol consumption by college students. *J Stud Alcohol Suppl.* 2002;14:148-163.
19. Kleber HD, DuPont RL. Physicians and medical marijuana. *Am J Psychiatry.* 2012;169:564-568.
20. Nuckols TK, Anderson L, Popescu I, et al. Opioid prescribing: a systemic review and critical appraisal of guidelines for chronic pain. *Ann Intern Med.* 2014;160:38-47.
21. Arif A, Westermeyer J. *A Manual for Drug and Alcohol Abuse: Guidelines for Teaching.* Plenum; 1988.
22. Gaw A. *Culture and Ethnicity.* Praeger Press; 1993.
23. Chi I, Lubben J, Kitano H. Differences in drinking behavior among three Asian-American groups. *J Stud Alcohol.* 1989;50:15-23.
24. Markides KS. Acculturation and alcohol consumption among Mexican Americans: a three-generation study. *Am J Public Health.* 1988;78:1178-1181.
25. Kearny M. Drunkenness and religious conversion in a Mexican village. *Q J Stud Alcohol.* 1970;31:248-249.
26. Bennett LA, Ames GM, eds. *The American Experience with Alcohol: Contrasting Cultural Perspectives.* Plenum; 1985.
27. Substance Abuse and Mental Health Services Administration. *Person-and Family-Centered Care and Peer Support.* Accessed May 22, 2023. https://www.samhsa.gov/certified-community-behavioral-health-clinics/section-223/care-coordination/person-family-centered
28. Barthwell AG. Alcoholism in the family: a multicultural exploration. In: Galanter M, Begleiter H, Dietrich R, et al., eds. *Recent Developments in Alcoholism.* Vol. 12 Springer; 1995:387-407.
29. Westermeyer J. Cultural aspects of substance abuse and alcoholism: assessment and management. *Psychiatr Clin North Am.* 1995;18:589-605.
30. Parrish KM, Jiguchi S, Stinson FS, et al. The association of drinking levels and drinking attitudes among Japanese in Japan and Japanese Americans in Hawaii in California. *J Subst Abuse.* 1992;4:165-177.
31. Atkinson DR, Whitley S, Gin RH. Asian-American acculturation and preferences for health providers. *J Coll Stud Dev.* 1990;31:155-161.
32. Sasaki T. Intercultural research of drinking between Japanese American and mainland Japanese: 1 Drinking patterns in problem drinking. *Jpn J Alcohol Drug Depend.* 1985;20(1):28-39.
33. Attneave C. American Indians and Alaska Native families: immigrants in their own homeland. In: McGoldrick M, Pierce J, Giordano J, eds. *Ethnicity and Family Therapy.* Guilford Press; 1982:55-83.
34. Szapocznik J, Kurtines W. Acculturation, biculturalism, and adjustment among Cuban Americans. In: Padilla AM, ed. *Acculturation, Theory, Models and Some New Findings.* Westview Press; 1980:139-160.
35. Rogler LH, Malgady RG, Constantino G, Blumentah R. What do culturally sensitive mental health services mean? The case of Hispanics. *Am Psychol.* 1987;42:565-570.
36. Berry JW, Kim V, Minde T, Mok D. Comparative studies of acculturative stress. *Int Migr Rev.* 1987;21:491-511.
37. Silverman I, Lief VF, Shah RK. Migration and alcohol use: a careers analysis. *Int J Addict.* 1971;6:195-213.
38. Ornoy A, Daka L, Goldzweig G, Greenbaum CW. Neurodevelopmental and psychological assessment of adolescents born to drug-addicted parents: effects of SES and adoption. *Child Abuse Neglect.* 2010;34:354-368.
39. Caetano R. Acculturation and drinking patterns among U.S. Hispanics. *Br J Addict.* 1987;82:789-799.
40. Speck RV, Attneave CL. *Family Networks.* Pantheon; 1973.
41. Favazza A, Thompson JJ. Social networks of alcoholics: some early findings. *Alcohol Clin Exp Res.* 1984;8:9-15.
42. Westermeyer J, Pattison EM. Social networks and mental illness in a peasant society. *Schizophr Bull.* 1981;7:125-134.
43. Kroll J, Carey K, Hagedorn D, Dog PF, Benavides E. A survey of homeless adults in urban emergency shelters. *Hosp Community Psychiatry.* 1986;37:283-286.
44. Pattison EM. Clinical social systems interventions. *Psychiatry Dig.* 1977;38:25-33.
45. Galanter M. *Network Therapy for Alcohol and Drug Abuse.* Basic Books; 1993.
46. Red HY. A cultural network model: perspectives for adolescent services and para-professional training. In: Manson S, ed. *New Directions in Prevention among American Indian and Alaska Native Communities.* University of Oregon; 1982:173-185.
47. Pattison EM. Social system psychotherapy. *Am J Psychother.* 1973;27:396-409.
48. Black DW, Belsare G, Schlosser S. Clinical features, psychiatric comorbidity, and health related quality of life in persons reporting compulsive computer use behavior. *J Clin Psychiatry.* 1999;60:839-843.

CHAPTER

40 Substance Use and Co-occurring Conditions in Women

Joan E. Zweben

CHAPTER OUTLINE

- Introduction
- Epidemiology
- Special populations
- Substance use-related consequences
- Common mental disorders
- HIV and sexually-transmitted infections
- Interpersonal violence
- Treatment
- Conclusions

INTRODUCTION

From a clinical and epidemiological perspective, substance use among women is a distinct phenomenon with its own unique causes and consequences.[1] Specialized services for women with substance use and co-occurring conditions have been evolving for many decades. Gender disparities were largely ignored until the 1970s, when interest grew in the biomedical and psychosocial aspects of women's use of alcohol and other drugs. Pressed by the women's movement, the federal government launched efforts to focus scientific and public attention on women's issues.[2,3] This emphasis generated new research and services specifically focused on women's needs to inform clinical care, new materials for clinicians in the field, and reconsideration of public policy. Much of the basic work on women's issues was done during that time.

Although a growing number of programs are providing gender-related services, there still are unmet needs for women in alcohol and drug treatment. According to 2022 data from Substance Abuse and Mental Health Services Administration's (SAMHSA) Facility Locator, a little over half (55%) of the 12,177 substance use treatment programs listed offered specific services for women, up from 44% in 2016.[4] Women with OUD are at high risk of getting no treatment at all if they have commercial insurance.[5] There is a clear need for programs for women that assess and manage trauma, medical and psychiatric comorbidities, financial independence, and pregnancy and child care.[6]

This chapter examines the scope of the problem based on epidemiological data for women including marginalized populations, the gender-specific consequences of alcohol and other drug use, comorbid mental disorders, and other social and general health consequences. The chapter concludes with a review of treatments for this population.

EPIDEMIOLOGY

Women account for nearly half of the total population in the United States (statista.com). As federal agencies have pushed for women to be included in research, more reliable data are available to estimate the prevalence of alcohol and other drug use related to sex (ie, biologically based factors) and gender (ie, factors that affect how women, girls, and gender-diverse people experience roles, relations, opportunities, customs, and expectations).[7] In the U.S. women are a rapidly growing population of individuals who use substances and need tailored programs that assess and manage trauma, medical and psychiatric comorbidities, pregnancy, childcare and financial independence.

According to SAMHSA, in 2019, 34.3 million adult women had a substance use disorder (SUD) and/or a mental health disorder, an increase of 6.8% over 2018. For the years spanning 2016 through 2019, for individuals 12 years of age and older, alcohol use was highest in women ages 18 to 25 years. In 2019, more than nine million women reported alcohol use in the past month, a decline from 9.7 million in 2016. Reports of past-year alcohol use disorders have also been highest among that same age group with 1.4 million women in 2019.[8] In terms of substance use, 21 million women reported cannabis use in the past year, an increase of 13.4% from 2018 (NSDUH). Across ages 12 years and older, women ages 18 to 25 years represented the highest past-month cannabis use: 3.6 million in 2019.

Using data from the National Survey on Drug Use and Health (NSDUH) for 2015 to 2018, Martin et al. reported that although a greater percentage of women than men needed treatment for opioid use disorder (11.9% versus 9.9%), receipt of SUD treatment was lowest among women with alcohol use disorder followed by men with alcohol use disorder (7.5% versus 8.9%). Black women had significantly lower odds of receiving SUD treatment than non-Latinx White women.[9]

SPECIAL POPULATIONS

Lesbian, Gay, Bisexual, Transexual, Questioning, Queer, Intersex, Asexual, Pansexual, and Allies (LGBTIA+)

Several studies report that bisexual women report elevated alcohol and other drug use compared to other sexual minority women.[10-12] They may experience unique sexual discrimination, described as "bi-negativity," contributing to stress and victimization. Microaggressions are associated with greater same day alcohol use and negative consequences. Adverse outcomes for these women include poor mental health and adverse alcohol related outcomes.[11,13]

LGBTQIA+ women are at particular risk because extensive use of alcohol and drugs is often part of the culture.[14] Socializing patterns built around bars and drug sharing increase the risk of addiction but do not necessarily lead to recognition of the attendant problems. These women generally are more dependent on LGBTQIA+ friendship networks than on families or marital bonds, and it is important not to pathologize their adaptive system of mutual reliance as "codependence." Historically, LGBTQIA+ bars were seen as gathering places and safe arenas for self-expression and, in many areas, they still are the only place where such behavior can occur. A study of college undergraduates confirms increased use of alcohol, tobacco, and other drugs among sexual minority women, with bisexual women having the highest use.[15] A community sample also indicated that sexual minority women are at elevated risk for higher rates of heavy episodic drinking. Adverse outcomes include poor mental health and adverse alcohol-related outcomes.[11,13]

Even when problems are recognized, women may avoid treatment agencies if they fear discrimination or lack of understanding about their specific needs.[16] However, data suggest that lesbian and bisexual women, with and without psychiatric disorders, are quite successful in accessing treatment.[17]

According to 2017 estimates, there are approximately one million transgender persons in the United States, and they are considered a highly vulnerable population.[18] Many of the studies focus on the high rates of HIV in this population, but rates of substance use are also elevated.[19,20] Among the contributing factors are family rejection, lack of social support, stigma, and minority stress.[21] A lack of NIH-funded research on illicit drug use in the LGBTQIA+ populations[22] contributes to gaps in knowledge, particularly in the area of effective treatment interventions. There is a scarcity of well-designed, culturally sensitive research on treatment interventions for transgender women. The Minority Stress Model suggests that clinicians should focus on promoting a positive identification of the transgender community while addressing issues such as transphobia, discrimination, and lack of social support that elevates health risks for this group.[23]

Transgender women experience trauma at disproportionate rates. Social support, defined as the judgment that social network members will be helpful when needed, appears to reduce the association between trauma symptoms and alcohol use.[24]

Connolly et al. did a systematic review, examining the prevalence and correlates of substance use among transgender adults.[18,25] Prevalence of substance use was high compared with cisgender people, with correlates that support the utility of the Minority Stress model. Challenges include stigma, transphobic discrimination or violence, family rejection and lack of other social support, gender dysphoria, unemployment and sex work, and high visual gender nonconformity, and intersectional sexual minority status.[25] A lack of NIH-funded research on drug use in the LGBTQIA+ populations[22] contributes to gaps in knowledge, particularly in the area of effective treatment interventions.

Immigrants

Gender roles vary greatly, especially among immigrant groups, in which the degree of acculturation determines many of the constraints on the woman's role. Use of alcohol and other drugs may be taboo for women, so recognition of their use, or seeking treatment for problems related to use, may be challenging. Those from patriarchal cultures can face strong taboos about disclosing family secrets, especially around interpersonal violence. Women can fear abandonment and violence if they violate cultural norms. Those disclosing sexual violations can risk severe devaluation within, or expulsion from, their community, and they can lack the hope for improvement that could propel them past this barrier. Many fear institutions such as the police, social services, and mental health agencies that might provide alternative resources.[26-28] Culturally sensitive and specific education and prevention messages have begun to be developed for women in some subgroups, but much more work in this area remains to be done.

SUBSTANCE USE-RELATED CONSEQUENCES

A steadily growing body of evidence indicates women are at higher risk for developing health problems in multiple organ systems from a variety of substances. In addition, women may be more vulnerable to the side effects of medications used to treat SUDs, and doses need to be adjusted accordingly.[29]

Alcohol

The National Institute on Alcoholism and Alcohol Abuse (NIAAA) had conducted research on alcohol since its founding in December 1970. Their recent recommendations are for men to limit their drinks to two drinks per day and women to limit themselves to one drink per day. The Rethinking Drinking website offers a calculator to check out the drink size and alcohol content.[30] Differences between men and women are due to how alcohol is metabolized. No amount of alcohol is safe for women who are pregnant or may become pregnant. As of this writing, research is lacking to offer clinical recommendations for use with transgender populations.[31]

The influence of alcohol on women's health has been more extensively studied than other substance use. Women with heavy alcohol use are more vulnerable to alcohol-related liver damage, cardiovascular disease, and neurological problems. Alcohol increases women's susceptibility to myopathy and cardiomyopathy, and studies suggest that females with alcohol use disorder suffer from a generalized skeletal fragility that increases their risks of fracture from falls.[32]

A large prospective study that followed 13,000 adults in Copenhagen for 12 years found that women developed alcohol-related liver disease (ALD) at approximately half the consumption levels of men. For women, the risk of alcohol-induced liver disease and alcohol-related cirrhosis (AC) rose once consumption levels exceeded 7 to 13 standard drinks (84-156 g of alcohol) per week.[33] ALD the leading indication for liver transplantation in the U.S., increased more rapidly among women, with alcohol-related hepatitis (AH) rising the most. Changes in AC and AH were greater in women in nearly all age groups. Similar increases were present, notably for Indigenous American and Asian women. AH mortality increased in women in almost all age groups. The authors recommend intensive public health interventions for these groups.[34]

Negative consequences occur at lower levels of consumption and after much shorter periods of drinking among women. This is referred to as the "telescoped course" in women. For a long time, there has been evidence that women develop many of the pathological effects of alcohol more rapidly than men, including fatty liver, hypertension, anemia, malnutrition, gastrointestinal hemorrhage, and peptic ulcers requiring surgery.[6,35] Some of the proposed mechanisms include a lower body mass index, a smaller volume of total body water (more fat and smaller water compartment for distribution), and lower rates of gastric alcohol dehydrogenase,[36] such that after an equivalent dose of alcohol, women have a higher blood alcohol level than men.

One review of studies of alcohol absorption, distribution, elimination, and impairment explored the mechanisms by which women achieve higher blood alcohol concentrations than men after drinking equivalent amounts of alcohol, even when doses are adjusted for body weight.[37] Women tend to have lower levels of gastric alcohol dehydrogenase and lower volumes of water compartment distribution leading to an increased effect of alcohol from an equivalent exposure in a man. These authors noted women demonstrate a relatively greater susceptibility to alcohol's effects on cognitive function, such as impaired memory. They concluded that the menstrual cycle is not likely to affect alcohol pharmacokinetics and is not a significant influence on alcohol's effects on performance.

Alcohol consumption raises breast cancer risk even after adjustment for age, family history, and other known dietary and reproductive risk factors.[32,38,39] The increased risk appears to be modest and dose-related, and the form of alcohol appears to be irrelevant. Increases in alcohol consumption later in life among postmenopausal women appears to be associated with greater risk.

The NIAAA conducted an extensive review of drinking patterns in minority women.[40] Prevalence studies suggest that Indigenous American women from certain tribes drink the most, African American and Latinx women are in the middle, and Asian American women drink the least.

A complex interplay of variables determines minority women's drinking behavior. A different factor influences behavior for each of these groups. For African American women, participation in religious activities appears to serve a protective function, buffering them from higher rates of alcohol use. For Asian American women, the facial flushing response emerges as an important protective factor. For Latinas, the level of acculturation to U.S. society is of major importance. For Indigenous American women, a variety of historical, social, and policy influences affect their drinking behavior. These include tribal affiliation, and residence on or off the reservation. More recent studies focus on sexual minority women. These will be discussed below.

It is important that clinicians make use of opportunities to educate women about their greater risks, even for those who are highly educated and articulate.[41] There is still widespread public naivete about what constitutes moderate- or low-risk drinking. Women surveyed interpreted their increased tolerance or the absence of short-term negative consequences to mean they are drinking moderately. None of the 150 respondents discussed gender differences in their in-depth interview,[41] indicating a surprising lack of awareness given how long the public information on differential impact has been available.

Prenatal Alcohol Exposure

There is no demonstrated safe level of alcohol consumption at any time during pregnancy. Drinking during pregnancy remains a serious concern, with health care professionals in a key position to reinforce social norms that encourage the elimination of drinking during this time.

Fetal alcohol spectrum disorder (FASD) refers to a group of conditions that include both physical and behavioral problems. The most serious of the FASDs, fetal alcohol syndrome (FAS), is a set of birth defects considered the single leading nonhereditary cause of mental delay. The growth deficiency and characteristic set of facial traits tend to appear more normal over time, but the alcohol-induced damage to the developing brain is enduring. Other fetal alcohol impairments are dose related and include some physical abnormalities as well as difficulties in learning and remembering, understanding and following directions, controlling emotions, and communicating a socializing, daily life skill, such as feeding and bathing.[42]

The caregiving challenges for the child with FASD will be even greater if one or both of the child's parents are drinking heavily. Thus, interventions will need to be directed toward the parent(s) while ensuring a safe and nurturing environment for the child. The risks to the child include inconsistent nurturance; poor parental support, inconsistent monitoring, and communication; high levels of family conflict; and higher rates of physical and sexual abuse.[43] Comprehensive treatment of the woman with active substance use needs to address these contextual needs and to assess for antecedent traumas, as described later in this chapter.

Drugs

SAMHSA reports show a significant increase in cocaine, methamphetamine, prescription stimulant use and LSD in women 18 to 25 between 2016 and 2019.[8] There are no trend tables comparing estimates to years after 2019 because changes in survey methodology mean the indicators are not comparable to past NSDUH estimates. Although evidence for gender differences in the effects of drug use is not as extensive as alcohol, there are indications that gender may be a factor. Greenfield and colleagues[44] summarize sex differences related to responsivity to substance use and to return to use, citing differences in hormonal activity, stress reactivity, and neurobiological correlates documented in neuroimaging studies. Compared to men, women also show a telescoped course, an accelerated progress from the initiation to the onset of SUD and first admission to treatment.[44]

Health consequences associated with specific drugs are described in the following sections.

Stimulants

Women may be more at risk for using stimulants due to a combination of their pleasurable reinforcing effects and the weakening influence of social protective factors. A study of treatment-seeking women who use cocaine concluded that some women may have greater vulnerability to the effects of cocaine compared to men, resulting in more rapid progression of pathology.[45,46]

A study of long term cardiovascular risks of cocaine use in women found that women with cocaine use disorders have a high risk of cardiovascular hospitalization up to three decades later.[47]

A large-scale study of individuals with methamphetamine use (N = 1016) participating in a multisite treatment study reported high levels of psychiatric symptoms. Depression, including attempted suicide, was common, as well as anxiety and psychotic symptoms. Participants reported high levels of problems controlling anger and violent behavior, with a correspondingly high frequency of assault and weapons charges. Findings continue to support the value of integrated treatment for co-occurring conditions, especially the importance of training counseling staff to handle psychotic symptoms when needed.[48] A more recent study of pregnant women confirmed the importance of integrated care, making resources for psychiatric, obstetric and pediatric care and assistance from community and government agencies easily available. The authors reported that after an average of seven months in treatment with readily available resources, nearly half of the participants reported stable abstinence and functional recovery.[49]

Opioids

With rates of opioid use disorder (OUD) at a national high, communities are struggling with significant morbidity and mortality. In women, rates of opioid use have been steadily increasing to be at par with OUD rates in men. Women tend to have a shorter duration between onset of opioid use and development of OUD, as well as shorter duration to adverse outcomes. As with other alcohol and other drug use, treatment of women has the best outcomes when it is gender-specific, trauma-informed, connected with access to psychiatric services, and integrated into the medical home.[50]

Women report more acute and chronic pain and are more likely than men to be prescribed opioids for pain. The use of these medications has become a concerning pathway for development of OUD women. In an effort to stem the opioid overdose crisis, availability of these medications was reduced. Treatment opportunities for chronic pain became limited, and many women turned to heroin and fentanyl.[51] Women seeking treatment began to constitute a significant segment of the population using heroin, leading to an increase by a factor of three for the number of women dying from heroin overdose between 2010 and 2013.[6,52]

Grella[53] documented that women who use heroin report significantly more chronic health problems and psychological distress, and overall poorer health status and mental health problems. They frequently report using substances to cope with emotional abuse and interpersonal violence, thus increasing their risk of recurrence of use and difficulties engaging in treatment. Their greater impairment in functioning reduces their capacity to maintain housing and employment, as well supportive social connections.[51]

It is well known that a woman's substance use is heavily influenced by her male partner,[54-57] and she can underestimate her level of harm if her main reference point is comparing her own use to her partner's behavior.

Unhealthy prescription medication use and opioid treatment has been covered in detail elsewhere in this textbook.

Cannabis

Little attention has been given to cannabis use among women, especially during pregnancy. It appears that women in treatment for OUD, and those who consume alcohol, are quite likely to use cannabis as well.[58] Adolescents and young adults under age 25 were more likely to use cannabis during pregnancy, as were those who smoke cigarettes.[59]

Damage to the respiratory system is the major adverse health problem associated with smoking cannabis. Respiratory illness increased with the number of days and with the number of days per month of smoking. Although no links have been shown between cannabis and chronic obstructive pulmonary disease (COPD) or cancer, airway inflammation, decreased airway conductance, and airway edema have been reported. Cannabis increases heart rate and leads to orthostatic hypotension, making the drug less safe in patients with cardiac conditions, particularly if they are older. Patients with liver disease who smoke cannabis daily can have fibrosis progression, which can slow the metabolism of some drugs.[60]

COMMON MENTAL DISORDERS

The need for treatment interventions that are sensitive to gender differences has brought increased attention to co-occurring disorders in women. Although, in the last several decades, the addiction treatment field has made great progress in addressing co-occurring disorders, advances in understanding and practice vary greatly in their degree of dissemination. It is still common for public sector addiction and psychiatric treatment to remain in separate silos, with psychiatric resources focused on those with severe and persistent mental illness. Many with SUD and other mental disorders fall into the addiction treatment system, where access to psychiatry services can be limited. Clinicians can expect wide variation in sophistication and responsiveness among community providers and should attempt to refer or place the patient where she is likely to get the specific services indicated by her specific conditions and behaviors. These are described in the most recent revision of ASAM Criteria[61] (see also Chapter 47, "The ASAM Criteria and Matching Patients to Treatment").

The most common psychiatric disorders found in women with unhealthy substance use are anxiety disorders (especially PTSD), mood disorders, eating disorders, and borderline personality disorder.

Anxiety Disorders

As a group, these disorders constitute the most common psychiatric disorders among women, with a total lifetime prevalence of 30.5% and a 12-month prevalence of 22.6%.[62] A meta-analysis of community-based studies examining the prevalence of anxiety in the COVID-19 pandemic showed that most studies reported significantly higher anxiety levels in women compared with men. Those findings were consistent with previous epidemiological data.[63] The experience of anxiety is characterized by sensations of nervousness, tension, apprehension, and fear that arise from the anticipation of internal or external danger. These feelings constitute important survival signals (fight/flight responses), so the task is to distinguish what is normal and appropriate from states that require intervention. Certainly, women in early recovery will experience heightened distress as they try to cope with situations in which they previously relied on alcohol and other substances and also as they more clearly see the impact of their self-destructive behaviors. However, overwhelming anxiety is debilitating, interferes with new learning, and contributes to recurrence of use. Severe anxiety is associated with premature departure from residential treatment.[64]

Psychosocial strategies are beneficial for the management of anxiety regardless of whether it is normal or excessive. The task for the woman and the treating clinician is to determine when the level is high enough to impair daily function and to justify medication. Fortunately, the first-line medications for anxiety and panic disorders are no longer benzodiazepines, rather the selective serotonin reuptake inhibitors (SSRIs) and serotonin norepinephrine reuptake inhibitors (SNRIs) are now first-line.

Both depression and anxiety can occur in the context of a wide variety of other disorders, and it may be difficult to disentangle the interacting elements and identify the predominant disorders. When anxiety symptoms do not resolve with abstinence or a reduction in substance use, a variety of psychosocial interventions can be used, selected to address the tasks specific to the woman's stage of recovery. Calming reassurance, reality-oriented support, exercise, meditation, breathing management and other relaxation techniques can be helpful when added to group activities designed to encourage exchange of experiences and transmission of skills such as provided in cognitive–behavior therapy.

With more severe disease, a variety of supportive, cognitive, and psychodynamic therapies can be used, but anxiety-arousing explorations should be avoided in early recovery. Insight-oriented therapy should be used in the context of a firm recovery support system (including regular mutual-help group attendance) by a therapist familiar with recovery issues. Familiarity with hazards that may lead to a return to use, warning signs, and prevention strategies are important. Severe or chronic anxiety can be a significant risk for recurrence of use, so it is important to develop a medication stance that does not make a virtue out of excessive suffering. It is important for the patient to develop new ways of coping with everyday distress, and it is not desirable to seek to eliminate most of the unpleasant feeling states that are inevitable in recovery.

SSRIs, especially sertraline, are the first line medications recommended by the National Collaborating Centre for Mental Health.[65] These authors note that sertraline is preferred, followed by an alternative SSRI or SNRI. They recommend pregabalin for anxiety if these medications are not well tolerated. They caution against the use of benzodiazepines for anything other than short term management of crises.

Benzodiazepines, once commonly prescribed for anxiety disorders, are no longer first-line drugs for the treatment of anxiety, and they can be particularly problematic for those with a personal or family history of SUD. Benzodiazepines should be judiciously considered after screening of relevant risk factors for negative outcomes, including history of SUD, current use of opioids and alcohol or other central nervous system depressants, older age (65 years or older), risk of falls, and cognitive impairment,[66] and sleep apnea.

Posttraumatic Stress Disorder

Of all the anxiety disorders, posttraumatic stress disorder (PTSD) is arguably the most difficult and complex to manage. In the original National Comorbidity Study, the estimated lifetime prevalence of PTSD was 7.8%, with a striking gender difference—a prevalence of 10.4% in women as compared with 5.0% in men.[67] An exception to this, in this era of sustained international wars, may be found in male combat veterans who have higher rates of deployment-related PTSD and women veterans who report high rates of military sexual trauma (MST). This finding is consistent with several studies by Breslau and colleagues.[68-70] Wasserman and colleagues[71] concluded that the association between female gender and PTSD is robust across patient populations. Rape and sexual molestation were the most frequently reported "most upsetting event(s)," with childhood parental neglect and childhood physical abuse reported more frequently by women. Female victims were more than twice as likely as male victims to develop PTSD (20% compared with 8.2%). A lifetime history of at least one other disorder was present in 79% of women with PTSD, and more than a third of the women with PTSD failed to recover from their PTSD, even after many years and even if they received professional treatment.

Participants in addiction treatment have long been known to have much higher rates of traumatic experiences and PTSD than the general population. Studies of both residential and outpatient treatment programs that serve both middle-class insured and indigent populations show high levels of childhood abuse and adult trauma.[71-77] These findings require treatment providers to equip themselves to meet complex needs. As Brown and colleagues[78] demonstrated, such a high "level of burden" promotes early dropout, increases the difficulty of treatment in a variety of ways, and makes it more difficult to obtain a positive outcome.

Childhood traumatic experiences set the stage for later manifestation of a wide range of disorders and enhance the likelihood of dysfunctional coping responses in adulthood.[79,80] Studies differ in terms of the types of trauma they consider and how they measure it, making it difficult to compare across studies. Russell and Wilsnack[81] discuss the methodological problems in comparing the studies that started to emerge in the 1990s. They examined available studies using a conservative definition of Childhood Sexual Abuse (CSA) that included both intrafamilial and extrafamilial sexual abuse, but excluded noncontact experiences, before the age of 18. By these criteria, in community samples, more than one-third of female children experienced sexual abuse by the age of 18 years. This included incest, defined as sexual abuse by a relative before the age of 18.

Subsequent studies and reviews support these findings. In a population-based study of female twins, Kendler and his colleagues[82] found that 30.4% reported CSA of a variety of kinds (sexual invitation, sexual kissing, fondling, exposing, sexual touching), and 8.4% reported intercourse. They analyzed their data to examine the relationship of CSA and common psychiatric disorders and SUDs, controlling for background familial factors. They concluded that women with CSA are at high risk for developing a wide range of psychopathology. In their 1995 National Comorbidity Study, Kessler and colleagues[67] came to similar conclusions regarding the relationship between sexual trauma, PTSD, and other psychiatric disorders in women. It is also worth noting that the ACE (Adverse Childhood Experiences) Study documented that persons exposed to one category of adverse experiences (abuse or family dysfunction) were likely to have been exposed to others, and this was associated with greater health risk factors for leading causes of death in adults, including heart disease, cancer, skeletal fractures, and liver disease.[83] Thus, the impact of abuse extends far beyond psychological injury.

Women in SUD treatment show higher rates of CSA than the general population.[84,85] SUD is only one of many sequelae. Others include low self-esteem, depression, suicidal thoughts and attempts, anxiety, difficulties in interpersonal relationships, sexual dysfunction, and a tendency toward revictimization.[71] These females are at nearly a fourfold increased risk of any psychiatric disorder and a threefold risk of a SUD.[86]

It appears that among adult stressors, rape is the most consistently severe in its effect[68,87] and is associated with a range of psychiatric symptoms.[88] Koss and Burkart[89] noted that almost half of the victims of rape seek some type of professional psychotherapy, often years after the assault. Women with histories of sexual assault in both childhood and adulthood reported significantly greater odds of lifetime suicide attempts.[90] Intimate partner violence is especially associated with suicidal ideation and other psychiatric symptoms.[91]

Mood Disorders

Major depressive episodes increased for women under 50, with severe impairment reported for those at the younger end of the range.[8] Women with depression were much more likely to receive treatment in the mental health system than in the SUD treatment system. However, young women from minoritized backgrounds were less likely to receive treatment for either condition.[92]

In assessing depressive symptoms, it is important to rule out the direct effects of alcohol, nonprescribed drugs, or medications, as well as general medical conditions, such as hypothyroidism and low vitamin D.[93] Providers should have protocols for assessing risk factors and protective factors for suicide. Risk factors are not predictors per se; they are reminders for more complete evaluation. These risks are often, but not exclusively, linked to mood disorders. One may consider suicide out of shame or failure as well as depression.

Pregnant patients with mood disorders fared worse on drug use outcomes than those with an anxiety disorder or no co-occurring disorder,[94] highlighting the importance of rapid identification and intervention during pregnancy. When antidepressant management is required during pregnancy, there is a substantial literature on known pregnancy risks of common antidepressants.[95-97]

For diagnostic purposes, negative mood states that are the direct effect of alcohol or drugs generally clear within 2 to 3 weeks from the last use, with symptoms of longer duration suggesting an independent mood disorder.[98] Distress or dysphoria or guilt, which is not the same as major depression, can persist for a long time. It is important to inquire carefully, because women in recovery often use the term "depressed" to describe brooding anxiety, misery, obsessive guilt, apprehension, and other forms of wretchedness that are not synonymous with major depression.

It also is important to remember that a sad or depressed mood is only one of many signs and symptoms of a clinically significant depression and may not be the most prominent feature. Other indications include disturbances in emotional, cognitive, behavioral, or somatic regulation. The mood disturbance itself can include apathy, anxiety, or irritability along with, or instead of, sadness. Not all clinically depressed patients feel sad, and many who feel sad are not clinically depressed. Clinicians need to have good skills for drawing patients out and helping them describe their feelings. Women in subcultures that place a high value on functioning can mask depressive symptoms. Those in leadership or caregiver roles can initially manifest depression in more disguised forms, especially if they have a high investment in performance or in continuing to function despite distress. Some women who are depressed do not describe a low mood, but their interest in or capacity for pleasure or enjoyment may be markedly reduced, making it difficult for them to experience rewards in recovery or to invest in new social relationships with others who do not drink alcohol or use drugs.

Eating Disorders

Despite the recognition that eating disorders are relatively common in women with SUDs, careful assessment is not routine and integrated treatment is unusual. Eating disorders are more prevalent among women who use substances than in the general population, and women with SUDs report more disordered eating behavior than women in the general population. Stimulants and over-the-counter diet preparations are particularly appealing to women seeking to lose or control weight. In many cases, the early appeal of stimulant use is the associated loss of appetite. In another era, cigarette manufacturers touted the anorectic benefits of smoking.

An early review of the comorbidity of eating disorders and SUDs[99] indicated that bulimia is more common than anorexia. Women with bulimia and alcohol use disorder are more likely to have major depression, tobacco and other drug use, and obsessive compulsive disorder than women with either disorder alone.[100,101] Krahn and colleagues[101,102] studied eating abnormalities and substance use (including alcohol use disorder) and suggested that levels of symptoms below the threshold required to meet criteria for eating disorders are important for the clinician to address. They caution that dieting-related attitudes and behaviors in young women may be related to increased susceptibility to alcohol and other drug use.

Among women who use alcohol and other drugs, there are many possible relationships between substance use and eating disorders. The eating disorder may present before the onset of alcohol or drug problems. Eating disorders can coexist with substance use in a variety of ways. Some patients report that opioids are appealing because they facilitate vomiting. Drinking alcohol can provide the feeling of release also gained from vomiting. Stimulants are attractive because they make women feel capable and energetic and suppress the appetite. Alcohol can be used to suppress the panic associated with bingeing and vomiting or to quash the shame that follows an episode. Eating disorders also can be part of a pattern of symptom substitution in abstinent substance users. For example, women concerned about weight gain once abstinent from stimulants may begin to vomit or purge to cope with their anxiety about body image.

It is important for clinicians caring for women to develop proficiency in addressing eating disorders and obesity, especially given the difficulty of finding specialized eating disorder programs in many communities. Because secrecy is a feature of both disorders, careful inquiry is important during the initial assessment, and observation by staff members is necessary throughout treatment. A woman in treatment may gain or lose 20 lb without a disorder being assessed and addressed by her individual clinician, counselor, or in her groups. Eating disorder specialists agree that treatment of these conditions requires specialized training. A thorough medical evaluation should assess possible problems, including metabolic abnormalities and menstrual history, and be part of a plan for nutritional stabilization, including strategies to stop aberrant eating behaviors, as well as medication planning and discharge planning that actively addresses both disorders.[103,104]

Addiction specialists should avoid application of the Twelve Step model as the sole treatment for eating disorders and should be selective about which elements are applied. Cognitive-behavioral approaches to eating disorders, which are well supported by empirical evidence,[105] are designed to reduce dietary restraint (in contrast with promoting abstinence from particular foods), address abnormal attitudes about body weight and shape, and alter thinking about eating and personal control. Claudat et al. provide a rationale for the usefulness of DBT to target eating disorders and SUD concurrently. They note that these patients had a higher number of co-occurring psychiatric conditions and more difficulty with emotion regulation. This included more difficulty engaging in goal-directed activity, higher impulsivity, and more limited access to strategies for emotion regulation. They recommend integrated treatment for both disorders.[106] An earlier study described a viable adaptation of CBT for individuals with bulimia and SUD, with modules to address common features such as motivation, relationship difficulties, reward sensitivity and impulsivity.[107]

Psychotherapy to address related personal issues is encouraged much earlier in the recovery process than is the case with SUD, and a strong therapeutic alliance increases the likelihood of remission.[108,109]

Borderline Personality Disorder

When receiving a patient with a diagnosis of borderline personality disorder, it is important to review the diagnosis for accuracy. Unfortunately, misdiagnosis of borderline personality disorder has been quite common, because of conflation of borderline characteristics with the demanding and manipulative behaviors exhibited during active alcohol and drug use and early recovery. It was not until 1994, in the DSM-IV, that clear criteria for differential diagnosis were introduced. These were retained in the subsequent edition, DSM-5-TR.[110] Diagnoses prior to that time, or from settings in which diagnostic rigor is not the norm, may be improperly classified. It is often a residual term of art applied to the most difficult of behavioral presentations. Thus, it may be advisable to reconsider the diagnosis. This reconsideration is especially important because these patients are viewed in many settings as unrewarding to treat. Clinicians treating SUD are accustomed to seeing women present with behaviors consistent with borderline personality disorder, who settle down markedly and look far less pathological with a year or so of sobriety and a good recovery program.

Enduring characteristics of borderline personality disorder include unstable mood and self-image; unstable, intense, interpersonal relationships; extremes of over-idealization and devaluation; and marked shifts from baseline to impulsive outbursts, anxiety states, or other extreme moods. Prevalence of borderline personality disorder is estimated to be about 2% of the general population, 10% of those seen in outpatient mental health clinics, and 20% of psychiatric inpatients. Although it was previously reported that women constitute about 75% of those with the diagnosis,[110] subsequent studies indicate no differences by gender.[111] An estimated 57.4% of persons with borderline personality disorder meet criteria for an SUD, and multiple studies confirm that significant percentage are women.[112]

Initial formulations and discussion of borderline personality disorder emerged from the psychoanalytic tradition and downplayed the possibility that abuse experiences were real, in favor of the view that fantasy distortion, strong impulses in a weak ego structure, maternal conflicts, and separation and loss experiences were decisive. The possibility that fearfulness, anger, and suspicion of the borderline patient might have its roots in real childhood trauma was minimized.[113] Cultural denial of childhood abuse was pervasive until the attention to PTSD created a knowledge base that revised earlier notions about abuse as mere fantasy. Herman, van der Kolk, and others have explored the possibility that actual traumatic experiences play a key role in the etiology of borderline pathology. Subsequently, a literature has emerged that described a relationship between borderline personality disorder and childhood physical and sexual abuse. Although childhood trauma is not a necessary cause for borderline personality disorder, it can be a sufficient contributing factor.[114-119] A history of CSA and a family history of SUD are associated with longer time to clinical improvement of borderline personality disorder.[120]

In summary, the prevalence of co-occurring disorders in women underlines the importance of offering psychiatric services well integrated into outpatient, inpatient, and residential (nonmedical) treatment services. Many barriers persist and resources for this population are often inadequate. In addition to education about addiction, providers should include material on co-occurring mental disorders and how they can influence relapse and recovery. This education should have many of the same components as substance use topics: (1) nature of the disorders commonly found in women; their usual course and prognosis; (2) important factors such as genetics, environmental stressors, and traumatic experiences; (3) misunderstandings about medication; (4) relapse warning signs; and (5) how to maximize recovery potential. Patients benefit from clarification of what constitutes effective teamwork with the physician (log of symptoms, notes about MD recommendations, when to call and when to wait, etc.)

HIV AND SEXUALLY-TRANSMITTED INFECTIONS

According to the Centers for Disease Control (2022), women accounted for 18% (6,400) of estimated new HIV infections in the U.S. The annual number of new infections has been slowly decreasing in women (from 6,800 in 2015 to 6,400 in 2019). HIV prevention and treatment are still not reaching all women who could benefit; major racial disparities still exist. Black and African American women made up more than half (53%; 3,400) of estimated new HIV infections among all women in 2019. HIV disproportionally affects with transgender women. Among transgender women interviewed in seven U.S. cities in 2019 to 2020, 42% reported having HIV. Among Black and African American transgender women, 62% reported having HIV, and among Hispanic/Latina transgender women, 35% reported having HIV.[121]

Among women of color, alcohol intoxication is a risk factor evidenced by those women reporting high risk intentions, such as inconsistent condom use. The sense of belonging to one's ethnicity can be a risk or protective factor, depending on the behavioral norms within the group. The perception of high risk for sexually transmitted infections has been reported to be negatively associated with sexual risk intentions, leading to the recommendation for prevention initiatives to address sexually transmitted infection-risk perception, condom assertion behaviors, and alcohol use, to reduce women's sexual risk behaviors.[122]

Socially sanctioned imbalance of power plays a major role in inhibiting risk reduction actions in women. Because condoms remain the major method to reduce sexual transmission of HIV, women remain at a disadvantage. Women either must gain the cooperation of their male partners in using a condom or must either decide *not* to have sexual relations if the man refuses or use other forms of barrier methods that may provide less protection.[123,124] Many women may lack the self-esteem and communication skills to negotiate condom use. Young women, in particular, often lack the fortitude to insist if their partners balk. Women with SUD are at an additional disadvantage in attempting to practice safer sex. Many women fear emotional or physical abuse if they do so. The future development of an effective protective method that is under the woman's control and can be used without the knowledge of her sexual partner is a key goal for reducing women's risk.

For HIV-infected women, managing caretaking responsibilities often is an issue added to the physical and psychiatric burdens of the disease. They worry about transmission of the virus to family members and must be both well informed and reassured. They struggle with how to address their health issues and their possible death with their children. Women who have given birth to HIV-infected children have an added layer of anxiety and guilt. After delivery, women in these circumstances are often socially isolated and welcome the opportunity to share with other women in a support group, which can help to reduce their shame and express their feelings more openly, with less fear of rejection.[125]

INTERPERSONAL VIOLENCE

There is now very strong evidence that substance use plays an important role in interpersonal violence, though it may be only one of many contributing factors. If a comprehensive assessment indicates it is a major factor, integrated substance use treatment is likely to yield the best results, though this may be relatively rare in community programs.[126]

Domestic violence accounts for 21% of all violent crime, and the majority (76%) is committed against women.[127] Many of these women endure abuse for many years, because they have difficulty effecting separations and utilizing shelters to get away from their abusers. Women who have been abused report that their general health is fair or poor, that they have had sexually transmitted diseases and other gynecological problems, and that they have needed medical care that they have not received. Chronic headaches, as well as hearing, vision, and concentration problems, are common sequelae. A variety of stress-related symptoms, such as irritable bowel syndrome, anxiety, and depression can also manifest. For these reasons, psychosocial treatment must be integrated with good medical care.

Women with a history of childhood trauma report a variety of betrayals in their accounts. These include direct victimization by the perpetrator; complicity or denial of another adult; failure of responsibility on the part of others in a position to help in community settings. The adolescent may remain silent and turn to alcohol and drugs for solace. The authors stress the importance of early interventions for childhood and adolescent trauma to prevent lifelong consequences.[128]

Violence in the family of origin, antisocial and/or aggressive behavior as a teen, anger, substance use, relationship dissatisfaction, psychological aggression, and power/control tactics have been shown to predict partner violence.[129] Careful assessment is needed because of patterns of secrecy and because differing levels of partner violence will require different types of interventions. The Conflict Tactics Scale (CTS) is well validated and widely used for identifying partner violence.[130] Clinicians need to know how to develop a safety plan with the patients, when and how to treat the substance use, when to utilize marital therapy, and how to avoid common mistakes such as confronting the partner directly or allowing the partner to join the medical or psychiatric interview. A special technical problem often confronted by clinicians is a revelation of previously secret violence but linked to a plea not to reveal any of that to the partner. Often, such "binds" can be discussed in team staff meetings, so that a clinical consensus may be established and documented. Clinicians need to know contact information for local shelters and other community resources, and they need to be familiar with state reporting requirements for domestic violence.

TREATMENT

The 1970s brought a focus on women's issues and funding, likely related to the entry of more women into Congress. In a review of 280 articles published between 1975 and 2005, and in a review chapter, Greenfield and her colleagues examined substance use treatment entry, retention, and outcomes in women.[44,131] Most studies reported a higher ratio of men to women entering treatment, on average, 3:1. Population studies reported a smaller gender gap, but this may be in part because of women's tendency to seek help in medical or mental health settings.[132] Barriers varied but include lack of pregnancy services, lack of childcare, fears of loss of custody or of prosecution, and inadequate services for women with co-occurring disorders. Therefore, specialized approaches are important for women who seek treatment for a variety of social, family and health problems. These situations include the death of a loved one, violence from partners, cognitive and medical problems. Emotional and material losses during the period of addiction have been identified as influential motivators.[133] Although most research focuses on clinical samples, a study of a community sample reported similar findings. While men tended to respond more to financial consequences, women responded to intrapersonal consequences.[134]

Yet, with respect to treatment retention, Greenfield and colleagues conclude that larger studies suggest gender is not a significant predictor of outcomes overall, but specific treatment elements improve outcomes for various subgroups. For example, inclusion of children enhances engagement and retention for women seeking residential treatment or intensive day treatment. Some of these key issues are explored further below.

Management and Retention Issues

The finding that women have high rates of three or more disorders has consequences for treatment. Work on readiness to change shows promise for improving women's treatment. Brown et al.[135] noted that candidates for addiction treatment can vary in their commitment to make changes in a variety of areas that will affect their prospects. They have developed a *Steps of Change Model* that covers four areas in which changes may be relevant: (1) domestic violence, (2) risky sexual behaviors, (3) addictive disorder behaviors, and (4) emotional problems. Their work supports the hypothesis that the most immediate or threatening problems will be what a woman focuses on first, and she selects her treatment modality accordingly. Women with SUD who are in domestic violence situations may be relatively resistant to extricating themselves and also to addressing their alcohol and drug use. Once they make the decision to move, they are preoccupied with achieving greater safety and keeping or maintaining access to their children and see their alcohol and other drug problems as secondary. By contrast, women with other mental health problems are more receptive to treatment for their SUD. Treatment providers need to be willing to start by addressing those problems the woman is most ready to change while cultivating readiness in other areas identified by the clinician as important for long-term success.

The number and severity of problems experienced by women can be translated into a measure of level of burden. In studies of patients with a high burden, such women tend to be at greatest risk of early termination and poor outcomes even when they do remain in treatment for longer periods of time.[78] Integrated treatment for multiple disorders thus is especially important in designing or selecting a treatment program to meet women's needs. It generally is agreed by providers that women-only programs or activities are an important aspect of effective treatment. Research on this question does not yield definitive findings and many important questions remain to be carefully explored. An examination of the services offered in women-only programs compared with mixed-gender programs in southern California found that the most consistent difference was the provision of services specific to women's needs, particularly those associated with pregnancy and parenting.[136] These services included parenting classes, children's activities, and pediatric, prenatal, and postpartum services. Women-only programs also were more likely to assist with housing, transportation, job training, and practical skills training. Thus, even though programs can present themselves as doing individualized treatment planning, women-only programs appeared to be better equipped to meet women's needs. These programs also were more likely to be funded through the Medicaid system instead of fees or private insurance, reflecting the lower socioeconomic status of their client population. Indeed, Greenfield and colleagues report that women in general are more dependent on public insurance for treatment.[44]

Interprofessional Coordination

It is especially important that residential and outpatient programs without care targeted toward women on site develop methods or liaisons for effective case management. Addiction medicine specialists can help such programs develop protocols and procedures to ensure that the counseling staff members review a woman's medical status and are clear in their role as facilitators of integrated services. Larger programs have found that a medical coordinator who functions as a medical case manager can provide more systematic attention for medical concerns.

Child Reunification

Retention in treatment and provision of specific services appear to be predictors of child reunification. A large-scale study of 1,115 mothers and their children documented that mothers who were treated in programs with a high level of family-related, education, or employment services were approximately twice as likely to be reunified with their children. A high-risk group of mothers with employment and psychiatric problems were less likely to be reunified with their children; however, completion of 90 or more days in treatment approximately doubled their rates of reunification.[137] It is important for funders to have good data on the impact of their decisions when they consider shortening length of stay.

Treatment Interventions

Do women-only programs produce better results than mixed-gender programs? This question has evolved into consideration of whether specific program elements yield better results. For example, inclusion of children enhances engagement and retention for women seeking residential treatment or intensive day treatment. Practical assistance with transportation and childcare makes it possible for women to participate more consistently. These elements can be added to both residential and outpatient programs. In addition, several carefully developed treatment manuals have become available and are often enthusiastically welcomed by treatment staff and program participants. They facilitate staff training and give participants practical tools to advance their recovery.

Problem severity is often assumed to lead to worse outcomes, but this is not necessarily the case. One of the first prospective longitudinal studies examining service needs, utilization, and outcomes in women-only and mixed-gender programs found that those in women-only programs had greater problem severity but better outcomes in the areas of drug use and legal problems.[137,138] This study had a large, ethnically diverse sample of women in community-based treatment in eight different programs in California. The 189 women in women-only programs tended to be in residential treatment, while the 871 women in mixed-gender programs were in outpatient treatment. Those in women-only programs had greater addiction severity index severity scores in the areas of alcohol, drug, family, medical, and psychiatric domains, but nonetheless had good outcomes.

A study that recruited and followed 259 women continues the mixed picture about effectiveness of single-gender treatment. Those in women-only treatment reported significantly less substance use and criminal activity, but there were no differences in arrest or employment status at follow-up.[139]

Treatment manuals allow for more consistency in clinical practice, even if implementation is imperfect. In a series of trials, Greenfield and colleagues[140,141] compared a manual-based 12-session Women's Recovery Group (WRG) and a mixed-gender Group Drug Counseling (GDC). Both groups reduced drug use while in treatment, but the WRG demonstrated significant improvement in reducing alcohol and other drug use during the 6-month and posttreatment phase. Although both groups were satisfied with their treatment, women were significantly more satisfied with WRG. The WRG demonstrated comparable effectiveness to standard mixed-gender treatment (ie, GDC) and is feasibly delivered in an open-group format typical of community treatment. Based on her research, Dr Greenfield has provided a comprehensive manual for clinicians conducting WRGs.[142] It covers a range of topics, including management of triggers and high-risk situations, relationships with partners, coping with stress, violence and abuse and other important topics. This is a significant contribution to women's treatment.

A preliminary assessment of another manualized treatment, The Art of Addiction Recovery Program, indicated that it was effective in conveying knowledge about substance use and recovery for pregnant and parenting women. Sessions focused on 14 different topics, such as health, social relationships, the recovery process, well-being and introspection. Participants agreed that the program was useful.[143]

Seeking Safety, another widely used manualized treatment manual with demonstrable benefits, will be discussed below in the section entitled, "Trauma-Informed Systems and Interventions."

It appears that gender-specific treatment is also associated with higher rates of continuing care. In a quasi-experimental retrospective study of women and children in residential treatment, those in specialized, women-only programs who completed the residential phase were more likely to continue appropriate care than those in mixed-gender programs.[144]

Aside from the different needs and characteristics of male and female individuals with substance use, there is reason to think that women-only groups tend to foster greater interaction, emotional and behavioral expression, and more variability in style than mixed-gender groups. Women in mixed groups tend to engage in a more restricted type of behavior, whereas the behavior of the men shows a wider variability.[145]

It is currently not known whether these differences are most influenced by the overall characteristics of the women-only treatment setting or by specific services provided by these programs. As McLellan and colleagues have shown, the tightness of fit between the individual's problem profile and the actual services received is more relevant than the specific treatment setting.[146,147] It is also possible that women-only programs create a distinctive type of synergy that makes it difficult to disentangle the active ingredients. Veterans and members of sexual or ethnic minorities are often enthusiastic about homogenous groups, though research has not determined whether there is consistently greater effectiveness.

Web-based interventions are receiving attention an offer promising increases in access to treatment. A study of college women with sexual assault histories explored the usefulness of a Web-based alcohol intervention that included strategies to reduce drinking and improve regulatory skills. The intervention group received a brief skill module each day. This resulted in short term reductions in drinking and PTSD symptoms as well as improvements in regulatory abilities.[148]

Physical and Sexual Abuse and Domestic Violence

Although more than a third of women with PTSD fail to recover after many years, even with professional treatment, the average duration of symptoms was shorter among women in treatment[67] even in the early stages of treatment development. This suggests that the treatments that existed then did confer some benefit. Co-occurring psychopathology typically is associated with less-favorable addiction treatment outcomes. However, in a study of clients with history of abuse, they were more likely than their counterparts who were not abused to participate in counseling and just as likely to complete treatment and remain drug-free during and up to six months after treatment.[74]

Preschool children are more vulnerable to the effects of domestic violence[149] than older children. It has been noted that children with mothers with a history of abuse experience posttraumatic stress reactions themselves. These children often are subjected to ongoing marital conflict, family dysfunction, dislocations and relocations of home, lack of parental care, economic and social disadvantage, and interactions with the police and court.

The extensive variety and complexity of children's reactions to domestic violence argue for routine assessment and case management for these families. Partnerships between substance use treatment programs and organizations focused on children can be excellent ways of bringing specialized services to augment what can be provided in-house. Children can develop a variety of other problems in response to traumatic events, including thought suppression, sleep problems, exaggerated startle responses, developmental regressions, deliberate avoidances, panic, irritability, psychophysiological disturbances, hypervigilance, and fear of recurrence. Children can engage in repetitive play in which the trauma is re-enacted, cope by psychic numbing and withdrawal, show uncharacteristic behavior patterns, and/or become fearful of mundane things. Cognitive and emotional problems include a preoccupation with physical aggression, withdrawal and suicidal ideation, anxiety, depression, and social withdrawal. Behavioral problems include conduct problems, hyperactivity, diminished social competence, school problems, bullying, truancy, clinging behaviors, and speech disorders. Physical symptoms include bed-wetting, sleep disturbances, headaches, gastrointestinal problems, and failure to thrive.[149] Women's programs are encouraged to utilize public funding available to address the needs of at-risk children and integrate their services into adult treatment programs.

Parenting and Attachment

Trauma-related difficulties can impair parenting in a variety of ways.[80] Women with histories of childhood trauma can have attachment problems that impact their own parenting, particularly their ability to nurture. They often lack appropriate role models, which can lead to reliance on physical punishment, difficulties setting appropriate boundaries, and neglect. They may be unable to integrate protective discipline and affection. Women with sexual abuse histories may be deeply mistrustful of men but at the same time miss danger signs that their children are at risk. Obviously, current alcohol and other drug use will exacerbate these vulnerabilities. It is important to keep in mind that not all women with histories of abuse will abuse their children. Clinicians should be observant but avoid conveying a pessimistic attitude toward a woman's prospects for being a good parent.

Trauma-Informed Systems and Interventions

Many efforts have been underway to modify service systems to meet the needs of clients with histories of abuse and violence. At minimum, these systems need to be *trauma-informed* or knowledgeable about and sensitive to trauma-related issues present in survivors. Most importantly, these services will be delivered in a way that avoids re-traumatization and encourages patient participation in treatment. *Trauma-specific services* include appropriate assessment methods and specific interventions to address trauma issues.[150] Parenting classes offered to women should be trauma informed.

Seeking Safety[151-153] is a well-accepted and widely disseminated trauma-specific treatment intervention for those with substance use and a trauma history. It is an early-stage intervention designed to stabilize the patient (create safety) with respect to both substance use and PTSD, integrated within a manualized but flexible treatment approach. It has been well accepted by clinical staff and clients alike. Najavits has developed a manual and other materials for the second stage, *Creating Change*, which focuses on processing trauma issues and forming a new identity (see https://www.treatment-innovations.org/creating-change.html).

The harmful aspects of trauma have been well documented, but more recently, some researchers have focused on positive outcomes, described as posttraumatic growth (PTG). One study focused on women with histories of addiction and victimization living in trauma-informed sober living homes. Most participants reported less depression, PTSD symptoms, financial worries, and greater active coping and a sense of community.[154] Women often lack social supports, so participation in a positive community, whether in a residential facility, mutual help group, or other vehicle can have important consequences.

Preschool children are more vulnerable to the effects of domestic violence[149] than older children. It has been noted that children with abused mothers experience posttraumatic stress reactions themselves. These children often are subjected to ongoing marital conflict, family dysfunction, dislocations and relocations of home, lack of parental care, economic and social disadvantage, and interactions with the police and court.

The extensive variety and complexity of children's reactions to domestic violence argue for routine assessment and case management for these families. Partnerships between substance use treatment programs and organizations focused on children can be excellent ways of bringing specialized services to augment what can be provided in-house. Children can develop a variety of other problems in response to traumatic events, including thought suppression, sleep problems, exaggerated startle responses, developmental regressions, deliberate avoidances, panic, irritability, psychophysiological disturbances, hypervigilance, and fear of recurrence. Children can engage in repetitive play in which the trauma is re-enacted, cope by psychic numbing and withdrawal, show uncharacteristic behavior patterns, and/or become fearful of mundane things. Cognitive and emotional problems include a preoccupation with physical aggression, withdrawal and suicidal ideation, anxiety, depression, and social withdrawal. Behavioral problems include conduct problems, hyperactivity, diminished social competence, school problems, bullying, truancy, clinging behaviors, and speech disorders. Physical symptoms include bed-wetting, sleep disturbances, headaches, gastrointestinal problems, and failure to thrive.[149] Women's programs are encouraged to utilize public funding available to address the needs of at-risk children and integrate their services into adult treatment programs.

Treatment Culture

Women and treatment providers have noted that the male-dominated treatment culture characteristic of some programs (particularly some therapeutic communities and veterans' programs) is not conducive to meeting women's needs.[155] They stress the importance of a more supportive and gentle approach to feedback in treatment. In addition to the gender imbalance in the client population, reliance on aggressive confrontation contributed to premature dropout and a treatment environment that can be experienced as disrespectful at best and abusive at worst. An emphasis on harsh confrontation is particularly problematic for populations with a high frequency of traumatic experiences. Treatment methods that exacerbate a woman's sense of powerlessness discourage her from revealing and exploring key issues. In addition, women with severe psychiatric disorders can decompensate and leave treatment if confrontation is too intense. Reducing the emphasis on confrontation and broadening the skill base of clinicians can be a difficult task in some treatment modalities, particularly those that rely primarily on staff members without advanced professional training. Although these practitioners may have extensive training and many have acquired addiction credentials, the style of intervention they learned first can be difficult to change, particularly if it involves charismatic or dogmatic personal role models of recovery.

Both the National Institute on Drug Abuse (NIDA) and the Center for Substance Abuse Treatment (CSAT) have funded specialized research and treatment demonstration programs focused on women, and these programs have enhanced the development of provider groups committed to improving women's treatment. Additional resources made available through CSAT's Addiction Technology Transfer Centers (ATTCs) made it easier to broaden the skill base of frontline practitioners working with an indigent population. There appears to be less coordinated activity focused on women in treatment facilities that serve the insured population. Provider groups serving women also emphasize the importance of female leadership at all levels of the organization to serve as role models and to avoid perpetuating the view that major decision-making influence is reserved for men. Some programs hire only female staff members to facilitate the task of dealing with sensitive issues such as incest, rape, and battering. This eliminates the potential benefits of positive male interactions for the women and their children when included in the treatment. Male staff members in a residential program are in a difficult position and must have clear boundaries and a supervision structure that protects them and the patients from potential boundary violations. This situation also is an issue for female staff members, particularly in areas with a large lesbian population, since boundary violations among women can be more taboo to reveal.

Pregnant Women With Opioid Use Disorder

It is especially important to reduce early treatment departure in pregnant women because participation in treatment is associated with better maternal and neonatal outcomes. Drug craving and withdrawal were important precipitants of early treatment departure and return to substance use, especially for individuals using heroin who did not receive pharmacotherapy.[156] Medical management of withdrawal can be an important tool to reduce early treatment departure.

Methadone and Buprenorphine

The American Society of Addiction Medicine (ASAM) recommends methadone or buprenorphine as the standard of care for pregnant women with active OUD. Those with a history of OUD are also candidates if they are at-risk of return to opioid use. Women who chose psychosocial interventions without medication should be closely monitored.[157]

It is important that the dose is adequate in the context of metabolic alterations in pregnancy. Contrary to common expectations, higher doses of methadone are not associated with increased risks of neonatal opioid withdrawal syndrome (NOWS). Although single daily dosing is the most common, a protocol that increased methadone dose and dose frequency in response to maternal reports of withdrawal is associated with lower severity of NOWS.[158] Despite the fact that some of the women were on relatively high doses of methadone (up to 180 mg/d), levels in breast milk were small and no adverse events were detected.[159] Women should not be discouraged from breastfeeding if they are not using substances and do not have specific contraindications. Stereotypes about methadone being replacing one opioid with another ca n have prejudicial influence on medical decisions. The American College of Obstetricians and Gynecologists also considers opioid agonist therapy the standard of care.[160]

A large-scale, multisite study (the MOTHER study) to evaluate safety and efficacy of buprenorphine in pregnancy found that compared to methadone, outcomes were largely similar but the newborns of buprenorphine patients had lower severity of neonatal abstinence symptoms, thus requiring less medication and less time in the hospital.[161] However, the retention rates of the mothers treated with methadone were significantly better than for those mothers in the buprenorphine group (33% versus 18%) and the careful, hospital-based induction required by the research study may make it difficult to implement in the community.

Inasmuch as women taking buprenorphine may become pregnant or may prefer buprenorphine to methadone, the MOTHER project sought to develop guidelines based on risk–benefit ratios. The authors recommended using buprenorphine alone rather than the buprenorphine/naloxone combination to avoid any risk of prenatal exposure to naloxone. Subsequently, ASAM noted that although there is limited evidence about naloxone in pregnancy, it is minimally absorbed and hence the combination product can be used.

Transferring a patient receiving methadone to buprenorphine is challenging because of the need for the mother to remain off methadone for a protracted period prior to buprenorphine induction and due to the risk of a precipitated withdrawal. Although there are case reports in the literature looking at methadone to buprenorphine transitions, none are without risk for pregnant women, and the associated risks of fetal distress, miscarriage, and stillbirth. In research studies, this transition has been accomplished using intravenous morphine in a hospital,[162] but this is not a practical option for community treatment providers. Buprenorphine and methadone in pregnancy are covered in more detail in Section 8 of this textbook.

In summary, opioid agonist treatment, with either methadone or buprenorphine, is the treatment of choice for pregnant women with OUD. The use of buprenorphine is an option with potential to expand treatment access in rural areas and in other circumstances where methadone is not available. For women in the transition between pregnancy and postpartum, psychosocial services are very important. These include resources to address anxiety and depression causing mood changes, stigma and mistrust among health care providers, problems with child welfare. A robust support system is needed for a positive outcome.[163]

Women and the Criminal Legal System

Research attention turned to women in the criminal legal system in the 1990s and documented that women constituted the fastest-growing segment nationally. At that time, there were few appropriate social services available to them.[164,165] For some time, women were more likely than men to serve time in jail or prison for drug-related offenses.[166] Between 1982 and 1991, the number of women arrested for drug offenses increased 89%.[164] Since 1991, increasing numbers of women have been incarcerated for crimes committed in the service of drug use. Half the women reported committing their crimes while under the influence of drugs or alcohol, and about 40% reported using drugs daily before arrest. Fifty-three percent of the women in federal prison were unemployed at the time of arrest.[166]

More recently, the number of persons held in federal or state prisons declined, and by 2020, the imprisonment rate was the lowest since 1992. The COVID-19 pandemic was largely responsible, due to significant changes in the operation of the courts. Delays in trials and/or sentencing and COVID-19 mitigation measures contributed to a decline in the U.S. prison population. The number of women in prison at the end of 2020 decreased in all states and the federal Bureau of Prisons, and the percentage of decrease for women exceeded that of men.[167]

Early research described the characteristics of incarcerated women. Typically, they report that they started using drugs at an early age. These women commonly were confronted with obstacles such as absent parents, educational setbacks, parenthood, poverty, drug accessibility, and minimal social resources. Most came from communities in which crime was rampant. Additionally, most were victims of childhood sexual and/or physical abuse, as well as traumatic experiences as adults. Consequently, they had high rates of depressive and other psychiatric disorders.[168] They often suffered from low self-esteem, depression, addiction, and shame.

Insufficient job skills, resulting from poor education, undermine self-esteem in incarcerated women. Low income or poverty results in desperation, thus making illegal activities more acceptable, especially in the service of drug use. Major child-rearing responsibilities with inadequate social support systems contribute to the development of psychiatric disorders in mothers and behavior problems in children.[168] Is there sexual assault in women's prisons? A bipartisan Senate investigation has found widespread sexual abuse of women in prison by the wardens, officers and volunteers tasked to protect them, uncovering incidents inside at least two-thirds of the federal facilities that housed women over the past decade.

Women's social status and gender roles affect sexual risk behaviors and the ability to take steps to reduce the risk of HIV infection,[123] contributing to the high incidence of HIV in drug-using and incarcerated women. A subsequent study of 3,315 subjects found rates of 7.5% in incarcerated women, several times higher than found in community samples.[169]

Intergenerational and familial transmission of drug use and associated criminality makes the obstacles confronting these women more debilitating. National data on women in prison show that 40% of the women reported that an immediate family member also was in jail.[166]

In California, 59% of inmate women reported that family members were currently incarcerated.[170] One-third of the inmates reported that a parent or guardian had problems related to drugs or alcohol. For these and other complex and interwoven factors, it is necessary to intervene decisively in prison prerelease programs to break the cycle of drug use and criminality and to include family members in the treatment experience whenever possible. Various states have invested in treatment in custody and postrelease, but many challenges remain to be surmounted (such as a trained workforce of adequate size), and the data currently support only modest benefits. However, a recent quasi-experimental study of 2,726 women indicated that they did better for psychiatric, trauma, and substance use outcomes with integrated treatment and mandated treatment.[171]

Prison-based treatment is growing rapidly, and specialized programs for women are included in this development.[172] A 2016 meta-analysis of gender-neutral compared to gender-informed approaches indicated that women and girls, especially those with trauma histories, are more likely to respond well to gender-informed treatment.[173]

Both research and clinical experience indicate that community-based services after treatment in prison significantly increase the percentage of offenders who remain drug-free 18 months after release. Thus, programs in large states such as California emphasize the importance of a seamless transition to services in the community and provide substantial funding to accomplish these goals.[174] Although the implementation remains imperfect, segments of the criminal justice system are increasing their understanding of what it takes to achieve and maintain positive outcomes. Drug courts and diversion initiatives such as California's Proposition 36 (treatment rather than incarceration) have also shown success in reducing recidivism, likely in proportion to their access to psychiatric and social services.

CONCLUSIONS

Although gender differences have been well studied in specific areas, there are many gaps in our understanding. Biomedical effects are far better understood for alcohol than for other drugs. Research and treatment funding incentives over the past 25 years have provided a much better understanding of women's treatment needs and preferences, but much work on implementation needs to be done. Removing obvious treatment barriers, such as transportation and childcare, increases women's participation in treatment. Treatment for women should be comprehensive, including their spouses, partners, and children. Research on children is needed to determine how to reduce the negative effects of their parents' SUD. Programs need to be capable of addressing co-occurring mood and anxiety disorders, particularly PTSD and eating disorders. When queried, women report that women-only groups and other activities and role models at all levels of decision-making in the organization are important to them. Advocacy is still needed for research to clarify which gender-specific treatment components are most influential in improving outcomes.

REFERENCES

1. Martin FS, Aston S. A "special population" with "unique treatment needs": dominant representations of "women's substance abuse" and their effects. *Contemp Drug Probl.* 2014;41(3):335-360.

2. Blume S. Alcohol and other drug problems in women. In: Lowinson JH, Ruiz P, Millman RB, Langrod JG, eds. *Substance Abuse: A Comprehensive Textbook*. Williams and Wilkins; 1992:794-807.
3. Blume SB. Understanding addictive disorders in women. In: Graham AW, Schultz TK, eds. *Principles of Addiction Medicine*. 2nd ed. American Society of Addiction Medicine; 1998.
4. Substance Abuse and Mental Health Services Administration. Facility Locator. Accessed August 14, 2023. https://www.samhsa.gov/resource/dbhis/behavioral-health-treatment-services-locator
5. Busch AB, Greenfield SF, Reif S, Normand ST, Huskamp HA. Outpatient care for opioid use disorder among the commercially insured: use of medication and psychosocial treatment. *J Subst Abuse Treat.* 2020;115:108040.
6. Ait-Daoud N, Blevins D, Khanna S, Sharma S, Holstege CP, Amin P. Women and addiction: an update. *Med Clin North Am.* 2019;103(4):699-711.
7. Greaves L. Missing in action: sex and gender in substance use research. *Int J Environ Res Public Health.* 2020;17(7):2352.
8. Substance Abuse and Mental Health Services Administration. *2019 National Survey on Drug Use and Health: Women*. U.S. Department of Health & Human Services; 2020.
9. Martin CE, Parlier-Ahmad AB, Beck L, Scialli A, Terplan M. Need for and receipt of substance use disorder treatment among adults, by gender, in the United States. *Public Health Rep.* 2021;137(5):955-963.
10. Ehlke SJ, Kelley ML, Lewis RJ, Braitman AL. The role of alcohol demand on daily microaggressions and alcohol use among emerging adult bisexual+ women. *Psychol Addict Behav.* 2022;36(2):209-219.
11. Schulz CT, Glatt EM, Stamates AL. Risk factors associated with alcohol and drug use among bisexual women: a literature review. *Exp Clin Psychopharmacol.* 2022;30(5):740-749.
12. Schuler MS, Stein BD, Collins RL. Differences in substance use disparities across age groups in a national cross-sectional survey of lesbian, gay, and bisexual adults. *LGBT Health.* 2019;6(2):68-76.
13. Scheer JR, Batchelder AW, Bochicchio LA, Kidd JD, Hughes TL. Alcohol use, behavioral and mental health help-seeking, and treatment satisfaction among sexual minority women. *Alcohol Clin Exp Res.* 2022;46(4):641-656.
14. Wilsnack SC, Hughes TL, Johnson TP, et al. Drinking and drinking-related problems among heterosexual and sexual minority women. *J Stud Alcohol Drugs.* 2008;69(1):129-139.
15. Kerr D, Ding K, Burke A, Ott-Walter K. An alcohol, tobacco, and other drug use comparison of lesbian, bisexual, and heterosexual undergraduate women. *Subst Use Misuse.* 2015;50(3):340-349.
16. Hall JM. Lesbians and alcohol: patterns and paradoxes in medical notions and lesbians' beliefs. *J Psychoactive Drugs.* 1993;25(2):109-119.
17. Grella CE, Greenwell L, Mays VM, Cochran SD. Influence of gender, sexual orientation, and need on treatment utilization for substance use and mental disorders: findings from the California Quality of Life Survey. *BMC Psychiatry.* 2009;9:52.
18. Meerwijk EL, Sevelius JM. Transgender population size in the United States: a meta-regression of population-based probability samples. *Am J Public Health.* 2017;107(2):216.
19. Institute of Medicine Committee on Lesbian, Gay, Bisexual, and Transgender, Health Issues and Research Gaps and Opportunities. *The Health of Lesbian, Gay, Bisexual and Transgender People: Building a Foundation for Better Understanding.* The National Academies Press; 2014.
20. Hoffman BR. The interaction of drug use, sex work, and HIV among transgender women. *Subst Use Misuse.* 2014;49(8):1049-1053.
21. Stevens S. Meeting the substance abuse treatment needs of lesbian, bisexual and transgender women: implications from research to practice. *Subst Abuse Rehabil.* 2012;3(Suppl 1):27-36.
22. Coulter RW, Kenst KS, Bowen DJ, Scout. Research funded by the National Institutes of Health on the health of lesbian, gay, bisexual, and transgender populations. *Am J Public Health.* 2014;104(2):e105-e112.
23. Hendricks ML, Testa RJ. A conceptual framework for clinical work with transgender and gender nonconforming clients: an adaptation of the Minority Stress Model. *Prof Psychol Res Pr.* 2012;43(5):460-467.
24. Johnson EEH, Wilder SMJ, Andersen CVS, et al. Trauma and alcohol use among transgender and gender diverse women: an examination of the stress-buffering hypothesis of social support. *J Prim Prev.* 2021;42(6):567-581.
25. Connolly D. Prevalence and correlates of substance abuse among transgender adults: a systematic review. *Addict Behav.* 2020;111:1-11.
26. Held ML, Nulu S, Faulkner M, Gerlach B. Climate of fear: provider perceptions of Latinx immigrant service utilization. *J Racial Ethn Health Disparities.* 2020;7(5):901-912.
27. Comas-Dias L, Greene B, eds. *Women of Color: Integrating Ethnic and Gender Identities in Psychotherapy*. Guilford Press; 1994.
28. Khullar D, Chokshi DA. Challenges for immigrant health in the USA-the road to crisis. *Lancet.* 2019;393(10186):2168-2174.
29. Agabio R, Campesi I, Pisanu C, Gessa GL, Franconi F. Sex differences in substance use disorders: focus on side effects. *Addict Biol.* 2016;21(5):1030-1042.
30. NIAAA. Rethinking Drinking. Accessed August 14, 2023. https://www.rethinkingdrinking.niaaa.nih.gov/
31. Arellano-Anderson J, Keuroghlian AS. Screening, counseling, and shared decision making for alcohol use with transgender and gender-diverse populations. *LGBT Health.* 2020;7(8):402-406. doi:10.1089/lgbt.2020.0179
32. National Institute on Alcohol and Alcohol Abuse. *10th Special Report to the U.S. Congress on Alcohol and Health.* U.S. Department of Health and Human Services; 2000.
33. Becker U, Deis A, Sorensen TI, et al. Prediction of risk of liver disease by alcohol intake, sex and age: a prospective population study. *Hepatology.* 1996;23(5):1025-1029.
34. Bertha M, Shedden K, Mellinger J. Trends in the inpatient burden of alcohol related liver disease among women hospitalized in the United States. *Liver Int.* 2022;42(7):1557-1561.
35. Blume SB, Zilberman ML. Alcohol and women. In: Lowinson JH, Ruiz P, Millman RB, Langrod JG, eds. *Substance Abuse: A Comprehensive Textbook.* 4th ed. Lippincott Williams & Wilkins; 2005:1049-1064.
36. Frezza M, di Padova C, Pozzato G, Terpin M, Baraona E, Lieber CS. High blood alcohol levels in women. The role of decreased gastric alcohol dehydrogenase activity and first-pass metabolism. *N Engl J Med.* 1990;322(2):95-99.
37. Mumenthaler MS, Taylor JL, O'Hara R, Yesavage JA. Gender differences in moderate drinking effects. *Alcohol Res Health.* 1999;23(1):55-64.
38. Donat-Vargas C, Guerrero-Zotano A, Casas A, et al. Trajectories of alcohol consumption during life and the risk of developing breast cancer. *Br J Cancer.* 2021;125(8):1168-1176.
39. Terry K, Mayer DK, Wehner K. Alcohol consumption: discussing potential risks for informed decisions in breast cancer survivors. *Clin J Oncol Nurs.* 2021;25(6):672-679.
40. National Institute on Alcohol Abuse and Alcoholism. *Minority Women and Alcohol Use.* NIAAA; 2003.
41. Green CA, Polen MR, Janoff SL, Castleton DK, Perrin NA. "Not getting tanked": definitions of moderate drinking and their health implications. *Drug Alcohol Depend.* 2007;86:265-273.
42. Centers for Disease Control and Prevention. *Fetal Alcohol Spectrum Disorders.* U.S. National Library of Medicine; 2017.
43. Young NK. Effects of alcohol and other drugs on children. *J Psychoactive Drugs.* 1997;29(1):23-42.
44. Greenfield S, Back SE, Lawson K, Brady KT. Women and addiction. In: Ruiz P, Strain E, eds. *Substance Abuse: A Comprehensive Textbook.* 5th ed. Lippincott Williams & Wilkins; 2011.
45. McCance-Katz EF, Carroll KM, Rounsaville BJ. Gender differences in treatment-seeking cocaine abusers--implications for treatment and prognosis. *Am J Addict.* 1999;8(4):300-311.
46. Lynch WJ, Potenza MN, Cosgrove KP, Mazure CM. Sex differences in vulnerability to stimulant abuse: a translational perspective. In: Brady KT, Back SE, Greenfield SF, eds. *Women and Addiction.* Guilford Press; 2009:407-418.
47. Ukah UV, Potter BJ, Paradis G, Low N, Ayoub A, Auger N. Cocaine and the long-term risk of cardiovascular disease in women. *Am J Med.* 2022;135(8):993-1000.

48. Zweben JE, Cohen JB, Christian D, et al. Psychiatric symptomatology in methamphetamine users. *Am J Addict.* 2004;13:181-190.
49. Petzold J, Spreer M, Kruger M, et al. Integrated care for pregnant women and parents with methamphetamine-related mental disorders. *Front Psychiatry.* 2021;12:762041.
50. Jacobs AA, Cangiano M. Medication-assisted treatment considerations for women with opiate addiction disorders. *Prim Care.* 2018;45(4):731-742.
51. Goetz TG, Becker JB, Mazure CM. Women, opioid use and addiction. *FASEB J.* 2021;35(2):e21303.
52. Cicero TJ, Ellis MS, Surratt HL, Kurtz SP. The changing face of heroin use in the United States: a retrospective analysis of the past 50 years. *JAMA Psychiatry.* 2014;71(7):821-826.
53. Grella CE, Lovinger K. Gender differences in physical and mental health outcomes among an aging cohort of individuals with a history of heroin dependence. *Addict Behav.* 2012;37(3):306-312.
54. Anglin MD, Hser YI, Booth MW. Sex differences in addict careers. 4. Treatment. *Am J Drug Alcohol Abuse.* 1987;13(3):253-280.
55. Anglin MD, Hser YI, McGlothlin WH. Sex differences in addict careers. 2. Becoming addicted. *Am J Drug Alcohol Abuse.* 1987;13(1-2):59-71.
56. Hser YI, Anglin MD, Booth MW. Sex differences in addict careers. 3. Addiction. *Am J Drug Alcohol Abuse.* 1987;13(3):231-251.
57. Hser YI, Anglin MD, McGlothlin W. Sex differences in addict careers. 1. Initiation of use. *Am J Drug Alcohol Abuse.* 1987;13(1-2):33-57.
58. Page K, Murray-Krezan C, Leeman L, Carmody M, Stephen JM, Bakhireva LN. Prevalence of marijuana use in pregnant women with concurrent opioid use disorder or alcohol use in pregnancy. *Addict Sci Clin Pract.* 2022;17(1):3.
59. Gupta PS, Upadhya K, Matson P, Magee S, Adger H Jr, Trent M. Higher marijuana use among young adults persists even during pregnancy. *J Gynaecol Obstet Adv.* 2021;1(1):23-29.
60. Welch SP, Tricia HS, Malcolm R, Lichtman A. The pharmacology of cannabinoids. In: Miller S, Fiellin DA, Rosenthal RN, Saitz R, eds. *The ASAM Principles of Addiction Medicine.* 6th ed. Wolters Kluwer; 2019.
61. Mee-Lee D, Shulman G, Fishman M, Gastfriend DR, Miller M. *The ASAM Criteria: Treatment Criteria for Addictive, Substance-Related, and Co-Occurring Conditions.* 3rd ed. The Change Companies; 2013.
62. Kessler RC, McGonagle KA, Zhao S, et al. Lifetime and 12 month prevalence of DSM-III-R psychiatric disorders in the United States. *Arch Gen Psychiatry.* 1994;51:8-19.
63. Santabárbara J, Lasheras I, Lipnicki D, et al. Prevalence of anxiety in the COVID-19 pandemic: an updated meta-analysis of community-based studies. *Prog Neuro-Psychopharmacol Biol Psychiatry.* 2021;109:110207.
64. Elmquist J, Shorey RC, Anderson SE, Stuart GL. The relationship between generalized anxiety symptoms and treatment dropout among women in residential treatment for substance use disorders. *Subst Use Misuse.* 2016;51(7):835-839.
65. Hartwell KJ, Orwat DE, Brady KT. Co-occurring substance use and anxiety disorders. In: Miller S, Fiellin D, Rosenthal RK, Saitz R, eds. *Principles of Addiction Medicine.* 6th ed. American Society of Addiction Medicine; 2019:1389.
66. Balon R, Starcevic V. Role of benzodiazepines in anxiety disorders. *Adv Exp Med Biol.* 2020;1191:367-388.
67. Kessler RC, Sonnega A, Bromet E, Hughes M, Nelson CB. Posttraumatic stress disorder in the National Comorbidity Survey. *Arch Gen Psychiatry.* 1995;52(12):1048-1060.
68. Breslau N, Davis GC, Andreski P, Peterson E. Traumatic events and posttraumatic stress disorder in an urban population of young adults. *Arch Gen Psychiatry.* 1991;48:216-222.
69. Breslau N, Davis GC, Andreski P, Peterson EL, Schultz LR. Sex differences in posttraumatic stress disorder. *Arch Gen Psychiatry.* 1997;54(11):1044-1048.
70. Breslau N, Davis GC, Peterson EL, Schultz L. Psychiatric sequelae of posttraumatic stress disorder in women. *Arch Gen Psychiatry.* 1997;54(1):81-87.
71. Wasserman DA, Havassy BE, Boles SM. Traumatic events and post-traumatic stress disorder in cocaine users entering private treatment. *Drug Alcohol Depend.* 1997;46(1-2):1-8.
72. Boyd CJ, Blow F, Orgain LS. Gender differences among African-Americans. *J Psychoactive Drugs.* 1993;25(4):301-305.
73. Dansky BS, Brady KT, Saladin ME, Killeen T, Becker S, Roitzsch J. Victimization and PTSD in individuals with substance use disorders: gender and racial differences. *Am J Drug Alcohol Abuse.* 1996;22(1):75-93.
74. Gil-Rivas V, Fiorentine R, Anglin MD, Taylor E. Sexual and physical abuse: do they compromise drug treatment outcomes? *J Subst Abuse Treat.* 1997;14(4):351-358.
75. Janikowski TP, Glover NM. Incest and substance abuse: implications for treatment professionals. *J Subst Abuse Treat.* 1994;11(3):177-183.
76. Teets JM. The incidence and experience of rape among chemically dependent women. *J Psychoactive Drugs.* 1997;29(4):331-336.
77. Yandow V. Alcoholism in women. *Psychiatr Ann.* 1989;19:243-247.
78. Brown VB, Huba GJ, Melchior LA. Level of burden: women with more than one co-occurring disorder. *J Psychoactive Drugs.* 1995;27(4):321-325.
79. Zweben JE, Clark HW, Smith DE. Traumatic experiences and substance abuse: mapping the territory. *J Psychoactive Drugs.* 1994;26(4):327-345.
80. Hien D, Litt LC, Cohen LR, Miele G, Campbell A. *Trauma services for women in substance abuse programs: an integrated approach.* APA Books; 2009.
81. Russell SA, Wilsnack S. Adult survivors of childhood sexual abuse: substance abuse and other consequences. In: Roth P, ed. *Alcohol and Drugs are Women's Issues: Volume I.* Women's Action Alliance and the Scarecrow Press; 1991.
82. Kendler KS, Bulik CM, Silberg J, Hettema JM, Myers J, Prescott CA. Childhood sexual abuse and adult psychiatric and substance use disorders in women. *Arch Gen Psychiatry.* 2000;57:953-959.
83. Felitti VJ, Anda RF, Nordenberg D, et al. Relationship of childhood abuse and household dysfunction to many of the leading causes of death in adults. The Adverse Childhood Experiences (ACE) Study. *Am J Prev Med.* 1998;14(4):245-258.
84. Najavits LM, Weiss RD, Shaw SR. The link between substance abuse and posttraumatic stress disorder in women. A research review. *Am J Addict.* 1997;6(4):273-283.
85. Wilsnack SC, Wonderlich SA, Kristjanson AF, Vogeltanz-Holm ND, Wilsnack RW. Self-reports of forgetting and remembering childhood sexual abuse in a nationally representative sample of US women. *Child Abuse Negl.* 2002;26(2):139-147.
86. Finkelhor D, Dziuba-Leatherman D. Victimization of children. *Am Psychol.* 1994;49(3):173-183.
87. Chaudhury S, Bakhla A, Murthy P, Jagtap B. Psychological aspects of rape and its consequences. *Psychol Behav Sci Int J.* 2017;2(3):555586.
88. Faravelli C, Giugni A, Salvatori S, Ricca V. Psychopathology after rape. *Am J Psychiatry.* 2004;161(8):1483-1485.
89. Koss MP, Burkhart BR. A conceptual analysis of rape victimization. *Psychol Women Q.* 1989;13:27-40.
90. Ullman SE, Brecklin LR. Sexual assault history and suicidal behavior in a national sample of women. *Suicide Life Threat Behav.* 2002;32(2):117-130.
91. Weaver TL, Allen JA, Hopper E, et al. Mediators of suicidal ideation within a sheltered sample of raped and battered women. *Health Care Women Int.* 2007;28(5):478-489.
92. Martin CE, Scialli A, Terplan M. Addiction and depression: unmet treatment needs among reproductive age women. *Matern Child Health J.* 2020;24(5):660-667.
93. Srifuengfung M, Srifuengfung S, Pummangura C, Pattanaseri K, Oon-arom A, Srisurapanont M. Efficacy and acceptability of vitamin D supplements for depressed patients: a systematic review and meta-analysis of randomized controlled trials. *Nutrition.* 2023;108:111968. doi:10.1016/j.nut.2022.111968
94. Fitzsimons HE, Tuten M, Vaidya V, Jones HE. Mood disorders affect drug treatment success of drug-dependent pregnant women. *J Subst Abuse Treat.* 2007;32(1):19-25.
95. ACOG Committee on Practice Bulletins—Obstetrics. ACOG Practice Bulletin: clinical management guidelines for obstetrician-gynecologists number 92, April 2008 (replaces practice bulletin number 87, November 2007). Use of psychiatric medications during pregnancy and lactation. *Obstet Gynecol.* 2008;111(4):1001-1020.

96. Misri S, Kendrick K. Treatment of perinatal mood and anxiety disorders: a review. *Can J Psychiatry.* 2007;52(8):489-498.
97. American College of Obstetricians and Gynecologists. *The Management of Depression During Pregnancy.* ACOG; 2014.
98. Brown SS, Inaba RK, Gillin JC, Schuckit MA, Stewart MA, Irwin MR. Alcoholism and affective disorder; clinical course of depressive symptoms. *Am J Psychiatry.* 1995;152(1):45-51.
99. Holderness CC, Brooks-Gunn J, Warren MP. Co-morbidity of eating disorders and substance abuse review of the literature. *Int J Eat Disord.* 1994;16(1):1-34.
100. Duncan AE, Neuman RJ, Kramer JR, Kuperman S, Hesselbrock VM, Bucholz KK. Lifetime psychiatric comorbidity of alcohol dependence and bulimia nervosa in women. *Drug Alcohol Depend.* 2006;84(1):122-132.
101. Krahn D, Kurth C, Demitrack M, Drewnowski A. The relationship of dieting severity and bulimic behaviors to alcohol and other drug use in young women. *J Subst Abuse.* 1992;4(4):341-353.
102. Krahn DD. The relationship of eating disorders and substance abuse. *J Subst Abuse.* 1991;3(2):239-253.
103. Marcus RN, Katz JL. Inpatient care of the substance-abusing patient with a concomitant eating disorder. *Hosp Community Psychiatry.* 1990;41(1):59-63.
104. Gregorowski C, Seedat S, Jordaan GP. A clinical approach to the assessment and management of co-morbid eating disorders and substance use disorders. *BMC Psychiatry.* 2013;13:289.
105. Atwood ME, Friedman A. A systematic review of enhanced cognitive behavioral therapy (CBT-E) for eating disorders. *Int J Eat Disord.* 2020;53(3):311-330.
106. Claudat K, Brown TA, Anderson L, et al. Correlates of eating disorders and substance use disorders: a case for dialectical behavior therapy. *Eat Disord.* 2020;28(2):142-156.
107. Sysko R, Hildebrandt T. Cognitive-behavioural therapy for individuals with bulimia nervosa and a co-occurring substance use disorder. *Eur Eat Disord Rev.* 200917(2):89-100. doi:10.1002/erv.906
108. Wilson GT, Loeb KL, Walsh BT, et al. Psychological versus pharmacological treatments of bulimia nervosa: predictors and processes of change. *J Consult Clin Psychol.* 1999;67(4):451-459.
109. Wilson GT. Eating disorders and addictive disorders. In: Brownell KD, Fairburn CG, eds. *Eating Disorders and Obesity: A Comprehensive Handbook.* Guilford Press; 1997.
110. American Psychiatric Association. *Diagnostic and Statistical Manual of Mental Disorders (DSM 5 TR).* American Psychiatric Association Publishing; 2022.
111. Sansone RA, Sansone LA. Gender patterns in borderline personality disorder. *Innovations in clinical neuroscience.* 2011;8(5):16-20.
112. Trull TJ, Sher KJ, Minks-Brown C, Durbin J, Burr R. Borderline personality disorder and substance use disorders: a review and integration. *Clin Psychol Rev.* 2000;20(2):235-253.
113. Van der Kolk BA. The body keeps score: memory and the evolving psychobiology of posttraumatic stress. *Harv Rev Psychiatry.* 1994;1(5):253-265.
114. Herman J. *Trauma and Recovery.* Basic Books; 1992.
115. Herman J. Complex PTSD: a syndrome in survivors of prolonged and repeated trauma. *J Traumatic Stress.* 1992;5:377-391.
116. Bandelow B, Krause J, Wedekind D, Broocks A, Hajak G, Ruther E. Early traumatic life events, parental attitudes, family history, and birth risk factors in patients with borderline personality disorder and healthy controls. *Psychiatry Res.* 2005;134(2):169-179.
117. Bradley R, Jenei J, Westen D. Etiology of borderline personality disorder: disentangling the contributions of intercorrelated antecedents. *J Nerv Ment Dis.* 2005;193(1):24-31.
118. Grover KE, Carpenter LL, Price LH, et al. The relationship between childhood abuse and adult personality disorder symptoms. *J Personal Disord.* 2007;21(4):442-447.
119. Golier JA, Yehuda R, Bierer LM, et al. The relationship of borderline personality disorder to posttraumatic stress disorder and traumatic events. *Am J Psychiatry.* 2003;160(11):2018-2024.
120. Zanarini MC, Frankenburg FR, Hennen J, Reich DB, Silk KR. Prediction of the 10-year course of borderline personality disorder. *Am J Psychiatry.* 2006;163(5):827-832.
121. Centers for Disease Control and Prevention. *Women and HIV.* Accessed August 14, 2023. https://www.cdc.gov/hiv/group/gender/women/index.html
122. Eakins DR, Neilson EC, Stappenbeck CA, Nguyen HV, Cue Davis K, George WH. Alcohol intoxication and sexual risk intentions: Exploring cultural factors among heavy drinking women. *Addict Behav.* 2022;131:107314.
123. Amaro H. Love, sex and power. Considering women's realities in HIV prevention. *Am Psychol.* 1995;50(6):437-447.
124. Amaro H, Hardy-Fanta C. Gender relations in addiction and recovery. *J Psychoactive Drugs.* 1995;27(4):325-356.
125. Chung JY, Magraw MM. A group approach to psychosocial issues faced by HIV-positive women. *Hosp Community Psychiatry.* 1992;43(9):981-894.
126. Fals-Stewart W, Klostermann K, Sherrod MC. Substance abuse and intimate partner violence. In: O'Leary KD, Woodin EM, eds. *Psychological and Physical Aggression in Couples.* American Psychological Association; 2009.
127. Truman JL, Morgan RE. *Nonfatal Domestic Violence, 2003-2012.* Report No: NCJ 244697. US Department of Justice; Office of Justice Programs; Bureau of Justice Statistics; 2014.
128. Grabbe L, Ball J, Hall JM. Girlhood betrayals of women childhood trauma survivors in treatment for addiction. *J Nurs Scholarsh.* 2016; 48(3):232-243.
129. O'Leary KD, Kar HL. Partner abuse. In: O'Leary KD, Kar HL, eds. *Partner Abuse: Assessment and Treatment.* American Psychological Association; 2010:1039-1061.
130. Straus MA, Hamby SL, Boney-McCoy S, Sugarman BB. The revised conflict tactics scales (CTS2): development and preliminary psychometric data. *J Fam Issues.* 1996;17(3):283.
131. Greenfield SF, Brooks AJ, Gordon SM, et al. Substance abuse treatment entry, retention, and outcome in women: a review of the literature. *Drug Alcohol Depend.* 2007;86(1):1-21.
132. Weisner C. Toward an alcohol treatment entry model: a comparison of problem drinkers in the general population and in treatment. *Alcohol Clin Exp Res.* 1993;17(4):746-752.
133. Moll MF, Santos VO, Duarte CF, Silva PS, Ventura CAA. Situations that lead women to seek treatment for drug addiction. *J Addict Nurs.* 2021;32(2):126-131.
134. Conner KR, Abar B, Aldalur A, et al. Alcohol-related consequences and the intention to seek care in treatment naive women and men with severe alcohol use disorder. *Addict Behav.* 2022;131:107337.
135. Brown VB, Melchior LA, Panter AT, Slaughter R, Huba GJ. Women's steps of change and entry into drug abuse treatment. A multidimensional stages of change model. *J Subst Abuse Treat.* 2000;18(3):231-240.
136. Grella CE, Polinsky ML, Hser YI, Perry SM. Characteristics of women-only and mixed-gender drug abuse treatment programs. *J Subst Abuse Treat.* 1999;17(1-2):37-44.
137. Grella CE, Needell B, Shi Y, Hser YI. Do drug treatment services predict reunification outcomes of mothers and their children in child welfare? *J Subst Abuse Treat.* 2009;36(3):278-293.
138. Niv N, Hser YI. Women-only and mixed-gender drug abuse treatment programs: service needs, utilization and outcomes. *Drug Alcohol Depend.* 2007;87(2-3):194-201.
139. Prendergast ML, Messina NP, Hall EA, Warda US. The relative effectiveness of women-only and mixed-gender treatment for substance-abusing women. *J Subst Abuse Treat.* 2011;40(4):336-348.
140. Greenfield SF, Trucco EM, McHugh K, Lincoln M, Gallup RJ. The Women's Recovery Group Study: a Stage I trial of women-focused group therapy for substance use disorders versus mixed-gender group drug counseling. *Drug Alcohol Depend.* 2007;90:39-47.
141. Greenfield SF, Sugarman DE, Freid CM, et al. Group therapy for women with substance use disorders: results from the Women's Recovery Group Study. *Drug Alcohol Depend.* 2014;142:245-253.
142. Greenfield S. *Treating Women with Substance Use Disorders: The Women's Recovery Group Manual.* Guilford Press; 2016.

143. Jones HE, Apsley HB, Cocowitch A, et al. Increasing knowledge about recovery-related life domains among pregnant and parenting women in comprehensive substance use disorder treatment: the Art of Addiction Recovery Program. *Drug Alcohol Depend.* 2021;232:109252.
144. Claus RE, Orwin RG, Kissin W, Krupski A, Campbell K, Stark K. Does gender-specific substance abuse treatment for women promote continuity of care? *J Subst Abuse Treat.* 2007;32(1):27-39.
145. Hodgins DC, el-Guebaly N, Addington J. Treatment of substance abusers: single or mixed gender programs? *Addiction.* 1997;92(7):805-812.
146. McLellan AT, Grisson GR, Zanis D, Randall M, Brill P, O'Brien CP. Problem-service matching in addiction treatment. *Arch Gen Psychiatry.* 1997;54:730-735.
147. McLellan AT, Hagan TA, Levine M, et al. Supplemental social services improve outcomes in public addiction treatment. *Addiction.* 1998;93(10):1489-1499.
148. Stappenbeck CA, Gulati NK, Jaffe AE, Blayney JA, Kaysen D. Initial efficacy of a web-based alcohol and emotion regulation intervention for college women with sexual assault histories. *Psychol Addict Behav.* 2021;35(7):852-865.
149. Campbell JC, Lewandowski LA. Mental and physical health effects of intimate partner violence on women and children. *Psychiatr Clin North Am.* 1997;20(2):353-374.
150. Jennings A. *Models for Developing Trauma-Informed Behavioral Health Systems and Trauma Specific Services.* U.S. Department of Health and Human Services; 2004.
151. Najavits LM, Weiss RD, Shaw SR, Muenz LR. "Seeking safety": outcome of a new cognitive-behavioral psychotherapy for women with posttraumatic stress disorder and substance dependence. *J Trauma Stress.* 1998;11(3):437-456.
152. Najavits LM. *A Woman's Addiction Workbook: Your Guide to In-Depth Healing.* New Harbinger Publications; 2002.
153. Najavits LM. *Seeking Safety: A Treatment Manual for PTSD and Substance Abuse.* Guilford Press; 2002.
154. Edwards KM, Siller L, Murphy SB. Reactions to participating in trauma and addiction research among women in a sober living home: a brief report. *J Interpers Violence.* 2021;36(23-24):11781-11791.
155. Brown V, Sanchez S, Zweben JE, Aly T. Challenges in moving from a traditional therapeutic community to a women and children's TC model. *J Psychoactive Drugs.* 1996;28(1):39-46.
156. Kissin WB, Svikis DS, Moylan P, Haug NA, Stitzer ML. Identifying pregnant women at risk for early attrition from substance abuse treatment. *J Subst Abuse Treat.* 2004;27(1):31-38.
157. American Society of Addiction Medicine. *National Practice Guideline for the Treatment of Opioid Use Disorder: 2020 Focused Update.* ASAM; 2020.
158. McCarthy JJ, Leamon MH, Willits NH, Salo R. The effect of methadone dose regimen on neonatal abstinence syndrome. *J Addict Med.* 2015; 9(2):105-110.
159. McCarthy JJP, Posey BL. Methadone levels in human milk. *J Hum Lact.* 2000;16(2):115-120.
160. American College of Obstetricians and Gynecologists. *Opioid Use and Opioid Use Disorder in Pregnancy: Committe Opinion #17.* ACOG; 2017.
161. Jones HE, Kaltenbach K, Heil SH, et al. Neonatal abstinence syndrome after methadone or buprenorphine exposure. *N Engl J Med.* 2010;363(24):2320-2331.
162. Jones HE, Suess P, Jasinski DR, Johnson RE. Transferring methadone-stabilized pregnant patients to buprenorphine using an immediate release morphine transition: an open-label exploratory study. *Am J Addict.* 2006;15(1):61-70.
163. Martin CE, Almeida T, Thakkar B, Kimbrough T. Postpartum and addiction recovery of women in opioid use disorder treatment: a qualitative study. *Subst Abus.* 2022;43(1):389-396.
164. Wellisch J, Anglin MD, Prendergast ML. Numbers and characteristics of drug-using women in the criminal justice system: implications for treatment. *J Drug Issues.* 1993;23:7-30.
165. Swavola E, Riley K, Subramanian R. *Overlooked: Women and Jails in an Era of Reform.* Vera Institute of Justice; 2016.
166. Bureau of Justice Statistics. *Women in Prison.* U.S. Department of Justice; 1994.
167. Bureau of Justice Statistics. *Prisoners in 2020 - Statistical Tables.* U.S. Department of Justice; 2020.
168. Jordan K, Schlenger WE, Fairbank JA, Caddell JM. Prevalence of psychiatric disorders in incarcerated women. II. Convicted felons entering prison. *Arch Gen Psychiatry.* 1996;53:513-519.
169. Altice FL, Marinovich A, Khoshnood K, Blankenship KM, Springer SA, Selwyn PA. Correlates of HIV infection among incarcerated women: implications for improving detection of HIV infection. *J Urban Health.* 2005;82(2):312-326.
170. Arnaudy M, Lee S, Relojo E. *Report on the health care status of incarcerated women.* San Francisco Department of Public Health; 1996.
171. Clark C, Young MS. Outcomes of mandated treatment for women with histories of abuse and co-occurring disorders. *J Subst Abuse Treat.* 2009;37(4):346-352.
172. Zweben JE. Women's treatment in criminal justice settings. In: Leukefeld C, Gullotta TP, Gregrich JS, eds. *Handbook on Evidence Based Substance Abuse Treatment Practice in Criminal Justice Settings.* Springer; 2011: 229-244.
173. Gobeil R, Blanchette K, Stewart L. A meta-analytic review of correctional interventions for women offenders. *Crim Justice Behav.* 2016;43(3):301-322.
174. Saxena P, Grella CE, Messina NP. Continuing care and trauma in women offenders' substance use, psychiatric status, and self-efficacy outcomes. *Women Crim Justice.* 2016;26(2):99-121.

CHAPTER

41 Treatment of Substance Use Disorders in Older Adults

Frederic C. Blow, Kristen J. Barry, and Angela M. Tiberia

CHAPTER OUTLINE

- Introduction
- Scope of the problem
- Issues unique to older adults
- Identification
- Brief intervention
- Treatment
- Pharmacotherapy
- Recovery support
- Prevention of return to use for older adults
- Conclusion

INTRODUCTION

When it comes to unhealthy substance use (see **Table 41-1** for key definitions), older adults (ages 65+) are a unique, unrecognized, and undertreated population. In 2020, nearly 3.5 million older adults were living with a substance use disorder (SUD)—yet only 245,000 reported receiving any type of SUD treatment,[1] signifying a major gap in care and a growing problem from both a public health and clinical perspective. Ageist beliefs, stigma (including self-stigma), and lack of treatment resources often prevent older adults from experiencing lifesaving treatment. Societal views of older adults are often stereotypical and inaccurate despite the fact older adults, like other age groups, are diverse in terms of health, lifestyle, ethnicity, and socioeconomic status. Although older adults do have unique health concerns and treatment needs, they are just as, if not more likely than their younger counterparts, to experience stable recovery.

SCOPE OF THE PROBLEM

Aging is not a protective factor against the development of SUDs.[2] Individuals can develop problems at an age or stage. Although overall rates of substance use are lower in older adults versus younger cohorts, the natural aging process involves physiological, psychological, and psychosocial changes that make the use of alcohol and/or other drugs particularly risky for older adults. Research indicates that the baby boom cohort (persons born between 1946 and 1964), have higher rates of drug and alcohol use than prior generations.[3] These higher rates may be partially due to changes in attitudes and behaviors toward the use of alcohol and other drugs during this "coming of age" period, as well as increases in life expectancy.[4,5] A further complication is that many of the comorbid medical and mental health problems that are common in older adults (ie, cognitive changes, sleep problems, injury, and depression) are greatly influenced by the use of alcohol, prescription medications, and other drugs.

Alcohol

Alcohol is the most used psychoactive substance among older adults. In 2020, nearly 58% of older adults in the United States used alcohol in the past year, 45% used alcohol in the past month. Nearly 10% reported binge alcohol use (5 or more drinks for men, 4 or more for women in one occasion) and 3.4% reported heavy alcohol use (binge drinking 5 or more days in the past month).[1] Although unhealthy alcohol use (ie, binge, heavy use, at-risk use) increases the potential for developing problems and complications at any age, there is growing evidence that no amount of alcohol is safe for older adults. That is, the metabolic changes that are part of the natural aging process impact the ability of the older adult to tolerate the effects of alcohol on the body and brain. Additionally, life events such as bereavement and serious illnesses can put the most stress on individuals, but any changes (ie, retirement, change in income, etc.) can affect alcohol use patterns.

The National Institute on Alcohol Abuse and Alcoholism (NIAAA) and the Substance Abuse and Mental Health Services Administration (SAMHSA) Center for Substance Abuse Treatment (CSAT) on older adults recommends that persons on any given day, regardless of gender, age 65 and older consume no more than one standard drink per day. However, recommendations include no alcohol intake for those who are in recovery from any SUD, as well as those take who take alcohol-interactive prescriptions (ie, opioids, benzodiazepines, etc.), for those who have medical conditions that are worsened by alcohol (diabetes, cognitive problems, etc.), and for those who participate in any activity that requires alertness/coordination/skill.[6] Signs and symptoms of issues that could be related to alcohol and other substance use in older adults are shown in **Table 41-2**.

Prescription Drugs

Data from 2015 to 2016 showed that 87.5% of older adults took at least 1 prescription drug in the past 30 days. A little less than half (47.7%) took 1 to 4 and nearly 40% reported taking 5 or more prescription drugs.[7] The nonmedical use of

TABLE 41-1 Key Definitions: Cons

Term	Definition
Drug misuse	Improper, unhealthy, and/or nonmedical use of prescription medication or any use of illegal drugs (ie, heroin, cocaine, etc.).
Alcohol misuse	Any pattern of drinking those results in harm to one's health, interpersonal relationships or ability to work, including binge drinking and heavy alcohol use. For women, more than 1 drink per day on average. For men, more than 2 drinks per day on average.
Substance use disorder	A medical illness characterized by a cluster of cognitive, behavioral, and physiological symptoms indicating that the individual continues using the substance despite significant substance-related problems.

prescription drugs among older adults, whether obtained by prescription or otherwise, is very concerning. Unhealthy use can include the spectrum from risky/at-risk/hazardous use through disorder.[8] Although older adults are more likely to be prescribed medications, they are less likely than younger groups to exhibit unhealthy use of prescription medications. Nonetheless, older adults can still be at risk for having unhealthy use of prescriptions drugs including opioids, sedatives, tranquilizers, or amphetamines. Many older adults unintentionally use prescription drugs in a manner other than intended due to pain, insomnia, sleep problems, or anxiety.[9] Older adults with co-occurring unhealthy prescription drug use and chronic pain often find it hard to accept that they have/are developing a SUD. For example, rather than finding treatment for opioid use disorder (OUD), they may seek alternative ways to obtain opioids, furthering progression to OUD. The medications that carry the most risk for older adults are prescription medications that affect brain function, resulting in changes in perception, pain, mood, consciousness, cognition, and behavior. Of greatest concern are the opioid analgesics, used to treat acute and chronic pain, and benzodiazepines (BZDs) used to treat anxiety and insomnia. These two classes of medications are important foci because they are frequently prescribed to older adults, have a high addiction potential, and interact with alcohol, increasing the risk of negative outcomes.[10] Although rates of opioid use and unhealthy use of prescription opioids are lower in older adults when compared to younger adults, according to Medicare data the prevalence of OUD among older adults tripled from 4.6% to 15.7% from 2013 to 2018.[11] Rates of opioid overdose deaths among older adults ages 55+ are consistently higher for men, with disproportionate increases among non-Hispanic black men since 2013.[12] Benzodiazepines have a very high addiction potential, and are linked to a number of adverse effects in older adults such as cognitive problems, falls, driving issues, and overdose.[6] According to the 2020 NSDUH data, 10.7% of older adults reported past year benzodiazepine use, 0.3% reported misuse, 18.9% reported prescription tranquilizer use or prescription sedative use, and 0.8% reported misuse in the past year.[1]

TABLE 41-2 Signs and Symptoms of Potential Alcohol and Substance Use Problems in Older Adults: Time to Ask Questions

Mental/cognitive/ relationship changes	Physical health	Alcohol and medication
Anxiety	Poor hygiene	Increased alcohol tolerance
Depression	Falls, bruises	Unusual medication response
Social isolation	Poor nutrition	
Excessive mood swings	Incontinence	
Disorientation	Sleep problems	
Memory loss	Increased heart rate	
New decision-making problems	Elevated blood pressure	
Idiopathic seizures	Falls/injuries	

Adapted from Barry KL, Oslin D, Blow FC. *Alcohol Problems in Older Adults: Prevention and Management.* Springer Publishing; 2001.

Cannabis

With the increased statewide legalization and widespread availability of cannabis, for both use as treatment and recreational purposes, many older adults use it to treat pain and promote relaxation. As a result, past year use among older adults increased dramatically from 0.4% in 2006 and 2007 to 6% in 2020.[1,13] Ahamed et al. performed a secondary analysis NSDUH data from 2015-2018 and found a 75% relative increase in past-year cannabis use in older adults, with marked increases among racial/ethnic minorities, those with mental health problems, women, individuals with diabetes, higher family incomes, and those who use alcohol.[13] As the baby boom population ages, it is estimated that rates of cannabis use among older adults will continue to increase. Cannabis has been shown to affect both the central nervous system and peripheral processes, cognition, learning, and motor coordination. Its use is associated with anxiety, depression, increased injury and short-term memory deficits.[14 15] Although it is not well known if cannabis interacts with specific prescription drugs, it can intensify the effects of alcohol. A recent study by Croker et al. on adults aged 60+ who use cannabis as treatment and found that they reported a range of positive and negative self-reported outcomes simultaneously or independently.[16] Preexisting positive opinions or expectations about cannabis use as a potential therapeutic could lead to social desirability bias and is an area of further study.[16]

Other Drugs

Most research conducted on substance use in older adults has focused on alcohol. Rates of substance use disorder, other than cannabis and opioids in older adults are poorly documented and thought to be very low. However, Chhatre and colleagues reported decreased alcohol admissions (77% to 64%) among older adults (age 55 years or older) from 2000 to 2012, and increased admissions for cannabis/hashish (150% increase), cocaine/crack (63% increase), heroin (26% increase), non-prescription methadone (200% increase), other opioids and synthetics (221% increase), and benzodiazepines (67% increase).[17] However, economic and social changes resulting from the COVID-19 pandemic resulted in multiple levels of barriers to treatment for people with SUDs. Lock down policies, social isolation and social distancing disrupted access and continuity of care and support disrupted the treatment landscape. The shift to telehealth helped to alleviate treatment gaps, but only for those who are technologically literate.[18,19]

Nicotine

Nicotine/tobacco use disorder remains prevalent across age groups. Most people who use tobacco daily have nicotine/tobacco use disorder. In an analysis of the 2020 National Health Interview Survey, the Centers for Disease Control and Prevention (CDC) estimated that nearly 12% of adults ages 65 and older reported tobacco product use "every day" or "some days" and 9.0% smoke cigarettes.[20] Older adults who smoke tobacco face health consequences such as increased risks of lung cancer and chronic obstructive pulmonary disease and decreased cognitive functioning.[21] Although nicotine replacement therapies and other medications such as bupropion or varenicline have advanced rapidly, there remains little information specific to older adults on ideal dosing, adherence, and adverse events. Evidence on the use of electronic drug delivery devices (e-cigarettes) or nicotine vaping products as potential aids to stop smoking have been mixed, which may be due to a lack of well-designed randomized controlled trials and longitudinal studies.[22] Further, the American Lung Association advises against the use of these products due the health risks that can lead to irreversible lung damage and lung disease.[23] Behavioral interventions for stopping smoking such as contingency management and cognitive behavioral therapy can provide tremendous health benefits.[24-27] Research shows that older adults who are persistent smokers have significantly higher levels of psychological distress when compared to quitters, which should be kept in mind when implementing a treatment intervention.[28]

Early- Versus Late-Onset Substance Use

It is important for diagnosis and treatment planning to distinguish older adults who have a history of unhealthy substance use (ie, binge, heavy use, at-risk use; early onset) compared to those that do not develop problems until later in life (late-onset). It is estimated that two-thirds of older adults with an alcohol use disorder (AUD) have early onset.[29] Individuals with early onset had unhealthy substance use patterns prior to the age of 50, while those with late onset did not misuse substances until later in life, often due to the stressors that develop with aging (eg, retirement, loss of income, loss of partner, etc).[3] Treatment for people who experience early onset may be complicated by long-term denial, medical and psychiatric comorbidities, limited social support, poor emotional skills, and cognitive impairment. Older adults with late-onset unhealthy substance use may have had problems with alcohol and/or drugs at various periods earlier in life but have had stable periods of abstinence or low-level drinking for extended periods of time.[30,31]

Clinicians should obtain information from older adults about lifetime substance use patterns, because problems can arise or reappear with stressors in older adulthood. Substance use among older adults with late-onset, for example, can be overlooked when the individual appears healthy. Thus, universal screening, which is asking all older adults about their alcohol and other drug use is an important standard of care. Because patients with a previous history of unhealthy substance use are at risk for an exacerbation of these problems with additional stressors, establishing a history of use can provide important clues for future substance use concerns and can provide the opportunity to provide prevention messages and encouragement to individuals who are maintaining abstinence or very low use.[30]

ISSUES UNIQUE TO OLDER ADULTS

Metabolic Changes

The aging process causes changes in the body that increase older adults' sensitivity to alcohol and other drugs, and prescription medications. Compared to younger individuals, older adults have lower body water volume. Thus, when consuming the same amount of alcohol as a younger person, older adults will have a higher blood alcohol concentration. As such, older adults will be more sensitive to the effects of alcohol than when they were younger. Since older adults often take over the counter and prescription medications, interactions with alcohol are concerning. Older adults are at risk for adverse drug reactions involving alcohol due to age-related changes in alcohol and medication absorption and metabolism, and the exacerbation of or interference with the effects of medication when combined with alcohol.[32] The results of a systematic review suggest that between one-in-five and one-in-three older adults may be susceptible to alcohol-medication interactions. There are little data regarding the interactions between common nonmedical drugs and prescription medications. However, a review of clinical literature suggests that such interactions can lead to toxic effects or a reduction in the prescription medication's therapeutic activity.[33] Again, the substance-prescription medication interaction risks points to the importance of asking older adults about any alcohol and drug use.

Co-occurring Disorders

Life events such as illness, bereavement, job loss, and retirement can all worsen depressive symptoms. However, mental health disorders such as depression and anxiety are not a normal part of aging and have been recognized as major public health concerns. There are significant associations between mental health disorders and SUDS both in the general population[34-37] and in older adults.[38,39] Further, having a current SUD has been associated with the development of a new-onset psychiatric disorder.[39] Co-occurring substance use disorders and mental health disorders among older adults are associated with poor health outcomes, higher health care utilization, increased complexity, poorer prognosis of mental illness, heightened mortality, higher rates of active suicidal ideation, and social dysfunction compared to individuals with either disorder alone.[40,41] Co-occurring disorders often complicate interventions, treatments, and relapse prevention, as well.[37]

There is a strong association between depression and an AUD across age cohorts that continues into later life.[42,43] Even when drinking within NIAAA guidelines, alcohol use can aggravate affective disorders, such as depression, among some older adults. One study looked at rates of depressive episodes over 10 years among adults ages 50 years and older from 19 countries and found that rates of depressive episodes were the highest among high and low alcohol consumers, especially among women and people who smoke, underscoring the importance of systematic screening for alcohol issues and comorbid psychiatric conditions.[44]

Comorbidity and Suicidality

The risk of dying by suicide increases with age, with the highest rates among older adults. Despite the fact that overall rates of suicide in the United States declined since their peak in 2018 from 14.2 to 13.5 per 100,000 population in 2020, suicide rates in adults aged 75 and older increased.[45] Factors such as loss and grieving, depression, injury, trauma, and dementia[46,47] contribute to high suicide rates among older adults. The COVID-19 pandemic worsened the already vulnerable physical and emotional well-being of older adults, leading to an increased risk of suicidal behaviors, particularly among individuals with SUDs.[42,48-51] However, detecting suicidal ideation among people who have unhealthy alcohol use is often complicated due to comorbid physical, mental, or cognitive problems, as well as the tendency to hide or underreport.[48,52]

Cognitive Impairment

Due to age-related sensitivities to drugs and alcohol, older adults who use substances or with nonmedical prescription use are at an increased risk of serious cognitive impairment, beyond the type of changes that occur as a normal part of aging.[3] The risk is further complicated when a mental health disorder such as posttraumatic stress disorder (PTSD), anxiety, or depression, all of which can cause cognitive problems, co-occur with SUDs.

Chronic Pain

Chronic pain is an issue that is extremely prevalent and problematic in older adults. The prevalence of chronic pain among older adults vary widely, from 5% to 52%, depending on the type of condition and how it was assessed.[53,54] As individuals age, they are at an increased risk of physical pain resulting from degenerative problems, increasing their likelihood of being prescribed opioid analgesics, and/or increasing their use of substances such as the use of alcohol or cannabis to help alleviate pain-related issues.

Sleep Problems

Although physiological changes in sleep-wake patterns can occur as part of the normal aging process, sleep problems that lead to impairments in daytime functioning, mood, and fatigue are not. Some older adults develop a SUD from nonmedical use of prescription medication that have been prescribed to address their sleep problems. Conversely, any alcohol use, smoking, cocaine use, and chronic opioid use have all be closely linked to sleep problems.[6] Although psychological interventions such as cognitive behavioral therapy have been shown to improve perceived sleep in older adults, medications that treat insomnia include melatonin, herbs, nonbenzodiazepines, and sedating antidepressants. Among them, sedative–hypnotic medications, such as barbiturates or benzodiazepines (BZDs), are the most prescribed treatment approaches for insomnia among older adults. The use of benzodiazepines in older adults have side effects such as balance issues/falls and cognitive decline, worsening sleep quality with long-term use, and significant addiction potential.[55] The American Geriatric Society issued warnings to avoid BDZ use in older adults, yet this medication continues to be prescribed to older adults, especially older women.[46-56]

Alcohol and Prescription Medications

Older adults who drink alcohol have an increased likelihood of being prescribed alcohol-interactive (AI) medications.[57] Most older adults who are experiencing problems related to their alcohol consumption may not technically meet criteria for an AUD. Even small amounts of alcohol can increase risks for problems due to medication interactions. Some medications and dietary supplements interact directly with alcohol and can intensify side effects causing dizziness or vomiting, others may not cause any noticeable side effects but are silently causing liver damage.[58] One study using the National Health and Nutrition Examination Survey (NHANES) data showed a striking 77.8% of older adults who drink used AI medications.[59] AI medications can include benzodiazepines, antidepressants, diuretics and narcotics. Individuals can experience adverse reactions including falls, heart problems, and liver damage. Taking alcohol interactive medications on a regular basis and taking multiple alcohol interactive medications further increase the risk of adverse reactions, especially among people who drink frequently. One study found that only 9.3% of adults aged 65 years and older had ever discussed alcohol use with a health professional.[60] These data emphasize the need for the broad range of healthcare providers, not just physicians, to discuss the potential risks of combining alcohol with prescription medications that interact with alcohol for their patients, especially if the patient has a past or current history of alcohol use.

Alcohol in Social Settings

Alcohol in moderate amounts (ie, no more than one standard drink per day for women and two standard drinks for men) may improve self-esteem or provide relaxation. As such, it is common for retirement communities, assisted living facilities, and nursing homes offer a "happy hour" to encourage socialization among residents. Such programs aimed at increasing sociability among residents may unwittingly give rise to alcohol problems in some older adults. Some individuals might feel pressured to drink to feel like they belong to the group, especially when nonalcoholic beverages are not offered. There has been little research on alcohol policies in residential living facilities. Empirical studies have found that some facilities require nursing staff to retain and manage residents' personal supplies of alcohol (similar to medication dispensing), while staff at other facilities provide very little oversight of residents' alcohol possession and consumption.[61] More studies that examine alcohol-related policies and patterns within retirement communities, assisted living, and nursing homes are needed. Training staff on best practices for the identification and referral to treatment of alcohol-related issues is essential in this fast-growing aging adult population.

With the mixed opinions regarding the detrimental effects and potential benefits of alcohol use, clinicians may feel confused regarding whether they should recommend no change in consumption or a reduction in consumption for older adults who do not meet criteria for a SUD.

IDENTIFICATION

The process known as SBIRT—Screening, Brief Interventions, and Referral to Treatment. is a comprehensive, integrated public health approach to the delivery of early intervention for persons whose substance use puts them at-risk.[62] Screening measures are used to identify the level of risk based on the results, determining the need for diagnostic evaluation, treatment, evidence-based medications, recovery support, and return to use prevention.

Screening

In order to identify current or potential problems, screening should be done as part of routine mental and physical health care and updated annually, before beginning any new medications, or in response to problems that may be alcohol- or substance use-related. The SAMHSA CSAT *TIP #26* expert panel on Substance Abuse Among Older Adults[6] recommends screening all adults over age 60 on a yearly basis and when there are changes that warrant additional screening such as major life events (ie, retirement, loss of partner/spouse, etc.), changes in health (ie, injury or accidents, onset of mental health problems, etc.) and before starting a new medication. Brief screening measures such as single-item screening tests for alcohol or drugs are a useful way to identify unhealthy use in busy settings.[63,64] Alcohol screening measures that can help detect problems in older adults include the Alcohol Use Disorders Identification Tests (AUDIT and AUDIT-C), The NIAAA Single Alcohol Screening Question (SASQ), and the Short Michigan Alcoholism Screening Test-Geriatric Version (SMAST-G).[65-68] To screen for multiple substances, providers can use screeners such as the Alcohol, Smoking, and Substance Involvement (ASSIST),[69] Brief Addiction Monitor (BAM),[70] and the self-administered Substance Use Brief Screen (SUBS).[71]

Screening questions can be asked by verbal interview, paper-and-pencil questionnaire, or computerized questionnaire. All three methods are reliable and valid,[72] as long as the provider is mindful of the clients level of comfort when using computers/tablet technology. Before asking any screening questions, the following conditions are helpful: the interviewer needs to be empathetic and nonthreatening, the purpose of the questions should be clearly related to health status, the information must be confidential, and the questions need to be easy to understand. In some settings (such as waiting rooms), screening instruments are administered as self-report questionnaires with instructions for patients to discuss the meaning of the results with their healthcare providers. However, screening instruments need larger typefaces to accommodate patients with visual problems.

Clinicians should assess the quantity, frequency, and pattern for each substance used (including medications that are prescribed or not). More accurate histories can be obtained by asking questions about the recent past. Questions related to substance use can be asked in the context of other health behaviors (ie, exercise, weight, smoking, alcohol use), and asking straightforward questions in a nonjudgmental manner. Additionally, a "brown bag approach," where the clinician asks the patient to bring in all medications, over-the-counter (OTC) preparations, and herbs in a bag to the next clinical visit, is one potential means of getting reliable information about all medication use—medical or nonmedical use. Real-time information on controlled substance prescriptions can be obtain from the prescription drug monitoring program, a database that can reveal multiple prescribers for controlled substances, such as opioid analgesics or sedative-hypnotics. Today, one must also ask about any cannabis as medicine recommendations, prescriptions, or use. Used together, these strategies allow the provider to determine what the patient is taking and what, if any, interaction effect these medications, OTCs, and herbs may have with each other and with alcohol. OTC preparation use often remains unevaluated in clinical settings, and the use of some OTC preparations (particularly anticholinergic agents) can be problematic in combinations with alcohol or prescriptions.

All members of the healthcare team are essential for identifying older adults with unhealthy substance use as well as those in need of treatment, yet most older adults experiencing issues related to substance use are unidentified by their health care personnel. To successfully incorporate alcohol, prescription medication, and other drug screening into clinical practice with older adults, simple and consistent routines can be used along with other screening procedures already in place.[73] The addition of chronic medical conditions may make it more difficult for clinicians to recognize the role of alcohol and/or other drugs in decreased functioning and quality of life. These issues present identification barriers for both clinicians and older adults in identifying the need for change. The American Psychiatric Association's *Diagnostic and Statistical Manual of Mental Disorders*, Fifth Edition-Revised Text Revision (DSM-5-TR) is the gold standard for diagnosing substance use-related disorders. However, classifying older adults remains a concern.[74,75] For example, the criteria for SUD may not apply to older adults with substance use problems because older adults may not experience a use of substances that results in a failure to fulfill major role obligations at work, school, or at home. Individuals who are retired may have fewer familial and work obligations.[76] See Table 38.1 for a list of signs and symptoms of SUDs in older adults.

BRIEF INTERVENTION

A brief intervention is an efficient, cost-effective and are an overall accepted approach in most outpatient general settings and suitable for older adults.[6] Brief interventions can range from a few brief comments from a health care provider about the older adult's alcohol or other drug use to several brief counseling sessions and follow-up. There is a large body of research testing brief motivational interventions in a variety of healthcare and social service settings. Studies have shown that older adults can be engaged in brief intervention protocols; such protocols are acceptable in this population and include reductions in alcohol consumption among persons with unhealthy substance use compared with a control group.[77-79] Brief interventions have had the most success across age groups and over time in primary care settings.[80-82] In general, brief interventions with older adults have seen statistically significant changes in alcohol use, but the actual number differences are small. Individuals with AUD generally require continuity of care and a higher level of support to maintain changes. However, brief interventions can serve as a bridge into more intensive treatment.[83] One example is the brief negotiated interview (BNI), which is designed to help providers discuss unhealthy alcohol and/or other drug use in a way that motivates the individual to identify their own reasons to cut back or stop using, along with individualized action steps.[84]

TREATMENT

It is a common stereotype that older adults are not open to accepting SUD treatment, yet research has shown that when treatment programs are age-sensitive and delivered by providers who are knowledgeable about age-related issues, older adults can and do achieve their recovery goals.[83,85,86] In fact, older adults are just as—if not more—likely than their younger counterparts to have positive outcomes from SUD treatment.[87,88] The SAMHSA Treatment Improvement Protocol (TIP) #26 consensus panel recommends that treatment providers provide age-sensitive options for older adults.[6] As the demand for treatment increases, age-sensitive SUD treatments that can address the complexities treating older adults with medical comorbidities and other age-related concerns are needed. Models of care are needed for older adults that take a multidisciplinary approach informed by geriatric medicine (including geriatric psychiatry), addiction medicine, and primary care.[89]

There are several potential barriers that can prevent or delay lifesaving SUD treatment for older adults. Many of these barriers are common across all age groups—and must be addressed. For older adults, ageism is a form of stigma that many experience. It is common for caretakers, family members, and/or providers to hold ageist beliefs that older adults "cannot change" or that it's "not worth the effort to try." Other barriers such as inability to pay/insurance limitations, geographic isolation/transportation issues, lack of treatment options tailored to the needs of older adults, and providers who are not equipped to manage older adults with complex medical and psychosocial issues.[6]

Treatment Within Primary Care Settings

Primary care clinicians can play a critical role in the identification and treatment of SUDs in older adults. Such actions include conducting brief interventions, offering referrals to mental health care and treatment programs, performing laboratory tests to detect alcohol-related health problems, prescribing evidence-based medications, educating clients on the risks of substance use including providing educational resources, and linking clients to community supports. However, there can be several unique challenges when treating older adults for SUDs. Some older adults find it particularly difficult to recognize and/or acknowledge that they might have a problem. When working with resistant patients who do not recognize a problematic level of alcohol or drug use, clinicians can begin by teaching about changes in metabolism with aging, the interactions between alcohol and specific medications (especially sedatives), the potential for falls, and the relationship between alcohol and some medical problems (ie, hypertension, liver issues, cognitive decline, etc). Providing the results of laboratory tests that detect problematic levels of alcohol use can be used to motivate clients to consider treatment but should not be the sole screening method or domain used to enhance motivation. The use of nonjudgmental, motivational approaches is key to successfully engaging older adults patients in care, along with periodic follow up, especially in the early stages of recovery.[90]

Older adults whose alcohol use is above recommended guidelines can pose challenges for clinicians on how to approach the topic. Yet, this level of alcohol use provides the opportunity for clinicians to intervene to prevent the escalation of use to more consequential use or a diagnosable disorder. For example, Conigliaro and colleagues surveyed patients with a positive AUDIT score one-month after being seen by a primary care physician. The majority (78%) of the patients remembered having a discussion with their physician about their alcohol use, but a little over half (58%) remembered being advised to reduce consumption.[91] For older adults who are more susceptible to both the physiological and the psychosocial effects of substance use, erring on the side of caution with nonconfrontational messages about alcohol consumption guidelines and following up if there are concerns is generally the most practical and effective approach.

Person-Centered Treatment Planning

When planning the course of treatment, it is best to take a systematic approach that considers the preferences and unique needs of the older adult. A stepped-care approach is one that starts with the least intensive option that best fits the individual needs, then increasing the level of intensity if needed.[6] Individualized treatment planning should be can be done using tools such as the American Society of Addiction Medicine (ASAM) Continuum of Care for adults, or the LOCUS 20, which allows the provider to systematically plan for treatment, keeping in mind that specific recommendations may need to be adjusted for older adults (ie, handicap accessible treatment settings, therapy tailored to individuals who are Deaf or Hard of Hearing, etc.[6,92,93] The ASAM Continuum of Care is structured around ASAM Criteria, which is comprised of the following six dimensions:

1. Acute intoxication and/or withdrawal potential
2. Biomedical conditions and complications
3. Emotional, behavioral, or cognitive conditions and complications
4. Readiness to change
5. Recurrence of substance use, continued use or continued problem potential
6. Recovery/living environment

For treatment planning to be successful, providers should take specific steps to identify and develop linkages to the resources within their communities that provide age-appropriate care. If age-specific treatment programs are not available, providers can create a plan within the resources that are available. Although the clinical recommendation might be for the individual to completely abstain from all substances, the goals of treatment should depend on the individual. One person might need withdrawal management to abstain from opioids but will not be ready or willing to give up alcohol, at least at first. Others will need to completely abstain from all substances. Having a dedicated individual within one's own organization who can help with care coordination and guide their clients through an often overwhelming and confusing process will help the process. See **Table 41-3** for more information on referral management and care coordination.

Specialized Addiction Treatment in Older Adulthood

Older adults with SUDs are at an elevated risk for more severe or complicated withdrawal due to their age.[94] Their vulnerability increases by the presence of additional risk factors such as having a comorbid medical or psychiatric disorder, prescription medication interactions, and concomitant use of substances (ie, alcohol, benzodiazepines, opioids), long duration of heavy and regular alcohol consumption, and/or a history of numerous prior withdrawal episodes in their lifetime. Management of alcohol withdrawal should only be done under close medical supervision. Older adults with AUD are at a higher risk for severe alcohol withdrawal syndrome (AWS), which includes complications such as seizures and delirium. Providers are encouraged to use the Prediction of Alcohol Withdrawal Severity Scale (PAWSS) to determine of the individual is at risk for severe AWS and in need of medically assisted withdrawal (MAW).[95,96]

Because traditional residential SUD treatment programs generally provide services to few older adults, there have been few studies with sufficient sample sizes to determine the effectiveness of residential programming in this age group. Older adults also seem to do best in programs that offer age-appropriate care with providers who are knowledgeable about aging issues.[97,98] A number of the studies of midlife to older adult treatments have been conducted in the VA setting. For example, one of the few randomized controlled trials of treatment outcomes for older adults is a study of 137 male veterans (age 45–59 years, $n = 64$; age 60–69 years, $n = 62$; age 70 years and older, $n = 11$) with DSM-IV–defined alcohol dependence who were randomly assigned after withdrawal management to age-specific treatment or standard mixed-age treatment.[99] Outcome data showed that those in the age-specific treatment programs were 2.1 times more likely at 1 year to report abstinence compared with patients in mixed-age groups.

D'Agostino and colleagues[100] created a model community-based intervention program, the Geriatric Addictions Program (GAP), designed to assist older adults who have SUDs and co-occurring mental health problems in accessing services and changing health behaviors. In their study, 120 older adults were randomly assigned into a traditional referral approach with an assessment and linkage model or a multidimensional approach incorporating geriatric care management assessment, motivational counseling, and the combination of aging service and addiction treatment linkages. Outcome data showed that those in the second group, with the multidimensional approach, had greater rates of linkage to both outpatient and inpatient treatments.

Most of the treatment outcome research on older adults with SUDs has focused on compliance with treatment program

TABLE 41-3 Referral Management and Care Coordination for Older Adult With Unhealthy Substance Use

Organizational level	
Identify care manager	Assign a clinician who is sensitive to the unique needs of older adults to manage the referrals and care coordination for older adult clients. This approach includes following up with clients to ensure referral success, guiding them through the process, and making new referrals as needed. If you are not a part of an integrated care team, be prepared to take on the responsibility.
Identify and develop linkages to local programs and services	Identify the services available within your local community that have age-sensitive treatment, mental health services, and recovery support. Reach out and develop ongoing relationships and linkages. Gather information from each program (ie, insurance eligibility criteria, type(s) of treatment/services offered, length of treatment, etc.). If age-specific resources do not exist, work with local social service and recovery programs to expand their offerings.
Keep an updated referral list	Keep a list of services offered, including important details such as their cost, eligibility, schedule, location, and contacts. Periodically check the list for updates, additions, etc.
Patient level	
Match client to services	In the context of available resources, treatment needs identify the appropriate level of treatment and services that best fit the older client's unique situation.
Include client and caregivers in treatment plan	Provide clients with a thorough overview of treatment plan. With their permission, include their family and/or caregivers. Ask them questions, provide opportunities for questions, and use reflective listening techniques to help alleviate concerns.
Provide a "warm handoff"	Introduce client to the care manager and service providers whenever possible.
Track clients treatment progress	Make linkages with treatment providers to keep track of client's progress. Follow up with clients, especially in the beginning, and offer additional care as needed.

Adapted from SAMHSA. *TIP 26 Treating Substance Use Disorder in Older Adults.* Chapter 4. Referral and care coordination. 2020:104-105.

expectations, in particular the patient's fulfillment of prescribed treatment activities and goals, including drinking behavior. Results from compliance studies have shown that age-specific programming improved treatment completion and resulted in higher rates of attendance at group meetings compared to mixed-age treatment.[101] In addition, older adults with SUDs were significantly more likely to complete treatment than younger patients. Atkinson et al.[102] also found that the proportion of older male with DSM-IV–defined alcohol dependence completing treatment was twice that of younger men.

Limitations of Treatment Outcome Research

There are few recent studies that have examined the factors related to treatment compliance in older adults. Major limitations remain in the treatment compliance literature, including a lack of alcohol consumption outcome data, failure to report on treatment dropouts, and variations in definitions of treatment completion. More controlled studies that include sufficiently large numbers of older subjects are needed to identify the characteristics of those who remain in treatment, as well as studies that examine the underlying mechanisms for low treatment engagement and recurrence of use.[90,103,104]

Many existing studies have an inherent selectivity bias and provide no information on treatment dropouts or on short- or long-term treatment outcomes. Other issues with sampling may also limit the generalizability of previous studies. For example, most reports on alcoholism treatment outcome for older adults have included only male subjects. Furthermore, age cutoffs for inclusion in studies have varied widely and have included individuals at midlife in the "older" category. In addition to these issues, many studies have used relatively unstructured techniques for assessing alcohol-related symptoms and the consequences of drinking behavior. Finally, the way outcomes have been assessed has been narrow in focus. Most studies have dichotomized treatment outcome (abstention versus recurrence) based solely on drinking behavior. Several studies have taken place in VA treatment facilities limiting generalizability to the general population and to women.

Given evidence that unhealthy alcohol use is more strongly related to alcohol consequences than is average alcohol consumption, it is possible that there are important differences in outcomes for individuals who are not abstinent, depending on whether their return to alcohol consumption after treatment involves return to unhealthy alcohol use. Furthermore, most studies have not addressed other relevant domains that may be positively affected by treatment, such as physical and mental health status, and psychological distress.

PHARMACOTHERAPY

Pharmacological agents can be prescribed to younger and middle aged adults to help them better manage the effects of SUD withdrawal and/or can be used as part of their recovery maintenance program.[105] Yet there have been very few systematic studies on the safety and efficacy of medication treatments for older adults with SUDs.[103] As the demand for

SUD treatment among older adults grows, further research is needed on the safety and efficacy of pharmacotherapy options for older adults. The following section presents some of the medications used in treating SUDs.

Alcohol Use Disorder Pharmacotherapy

Disulfiram, acamprosate and naltrexone are all approved by the Food and Drug Administration (FDA) for the treatment of AUDs. Naltrexone and acamprosate were originally approved for treatment of alcohol dependence (as defined by DSM-IV criteria) and have been shown to improve alcohol consumption outcomes over time. However, these treatments are underutilized in the treatment of older adults with AUD due to the lack of randomized controlled trials (RCTs) on the safety and effectiveness.[6,106]

Disulfiram causes acute sensitivity to alcohol, but its effects can be harmful to older adults. When alcohol is ingested, disulfiram will cause the patient to feel effects similar to a hangover, which deters the individual from drinking. Such effects can put stress on the cardiovascular system and can cause hypotension and arrhythmia, which makes it risky for older adults.[107] Disulfiram is also a medication that needs to be closely monitored and taken according to a strict protocol, which makes it less ideal for older adults with cognitive impairment.[6]

Naltrexone is an opioid antagonist that reduces craving for alcohol and decreases the rate of return to use. It has been well studied in the general adult population, but very few studies to date have tested its safety, tolerability and effectiveness in older adults.[108] One of the few studies testing naltrexone (50 mg/d) in older adults was conducted by Oslin et al. who enrolled 44 veterans older than age 50 in a 12-week double-blind placebo-control efficacy trial. The study found that naltrexone was well-tolerated by older adults and had efficacy in preventing recurrence.[109] A small study (N =18) of older adults (mean age = 73) treated with naltrexone for severe pruritus for two months. Five patients reported mild side effects that either resolved within the first two weeks or were well managed.[110] Another study (N = 74) of older adults (ages 55+) who met the criteria for major depressive disorder (primary major depression or substance-induced) and DSM-IV alcohol dependence were given sertraline combined with naltrexone. No subjects experienced recurrence of alcohol use during the 12 weeks of treatment.[111] It's important to note that naltrexone it is metabolized through the liver and thus must be used with caution with individuals who impaired liver function. Naltrexone is also an opioid blocker; therefore, it cannot be used in patients taking opioid analgesics because concomitant use may provoke significant opioid withdrawal symptoms.[112]

Acamprosate is used in the general adult population for reduction of recurrence of alcohol use, by reducing cravings for alcohol. To date, there are no randomized controlled trials on the efficacy or safety of acamprosate with older patients. Research may be lacking because acamprosate is contraindicated in patients with renal impairment, and renal function is diminished in older adults.[6,113]

Opioid Use Disorder Pharmacotherapy

Medication for older adults with OUD can reduce the risk of recurrence of use and prevent an opioid overdose.[114] Three FDA-approved medications are methadone, buprenorphine, and naloxone. Used to reverse an opioid overdose, naloxone has been found to be safe and effective for older adults and is considered essential for the reversal of opioid overdose.[115] Although RCTs on the safety and effectiveness methadone and buprenorphine in older adults are limited, an adequate amount of observational data exists that have given way to treatment guidelines that recommend the use of opioid agonist therapy (OAT) for both acute withdrawal management and maintenance therapy in older adults.[114]

Buprenorphine is also an opioid agonist, and can be used to treat withdrawal, for long-term maintenance of OUD, as well as chronic pain in older adults. Compared to methadone, buprenorphine may be safer and more in older adults and is thus recommended as the first line medication management.[114] Due to the various formulations offered (long lasting and self-administered options), buprenorphine can be more accessible to older adults. Although buprenorphine has been studied in adults ages 50+ and found to be safe, studies on the safety and benefits of its use in adults ages 65+ are needed.

Methadone is an opioid agonist and is used to treat OUD withdrawal, reduce cravings, and treat chronic pain, but is not widely used in older adults. Federal regulations for methadone treatment programs, such as same-day screening and mandated counseling, can be a barrier for older adults. Other barriers to methadone treatment for OUD include lack of insurance coverage, and several medication interactions, risk of overdose with first-time use, and the risk of falls.[114,116] Although there are a number of observational studies on methadone use for older adults with OUD that showed reductions in substance use, there are currently no RCTs to examine the safety and effectiveness of medication management for OUD in older adults.[117] It is highly recommended that older adults who are provided methadone treatment should be closely monitored for toxicities and adverse events on a routine basis.[118]

Treatment for Benzodiazepines

As discussed previously, BDZs should be avoided in the older adult population. Reduction or discontinuation of BDZs can precipitate a withdrawal and can include serious adverse events such as seizures.[119] Older adults who choose reduce or discontinue their use of benzodiazepines such as clonazepam, lorazepam, and alprazolam, should undergo a medically supervised withdrawal, which should include client education about BZDs and withdrawal, a stepped or tapered withdrawal schedule, and counseling.[55] In order to reduce the risk of serious complications, providers should have a thorough understanding of the clients' co-occurring conditions, substance use history, risk of falls, etc. A tapered approach should be gradual, lasting a minimum of 4 weeks and can last up to 22 weeks. The length of time for that taper will depend on individual considerations such as the BZD dosage and the length of time that the BZD has been used. Importantly, the discontinuation of even low doses of BZDs or BZDs used for a brief duration can cause still withdrawal symptoms in some older adults.

RECOVERY SUPPORT

Mutual help groups, including 12-Step recovery support groups, can help with a sense of community and help older adults obtain and maintain stable recovery with a network of their peers. The generational or age-related differences between older and younger adults can make mixed-age group therapy settings uncomfortable for older adults. Most older adults grew up in an environment were talking about mental health and substance use issues are highly stigmatized and hidden from society, while younger generations may be very open about their issues and experiences and might tend to use language that older adults find offensive. Providers are encouraged to identify the older-adult focused mutual help groups in their own communities and have this information on hand for their older adult clients.

Alcoholics Anonymous (AA) and Narcotics Anonymous (NA) are the most common and widely used 12-Step, community-based support groups in the recovery community. A Cochrane review including 27 AA and twelve-step facilitation interventions (TSF) reported that AA/TSF would often produce greater periods of continuous abstinence, fewer alcohol-related consequences, lower addiction severity, and some reductions in drinking intensity than other established psychosocial interventions. These findings were consistent whether the study participants were young, elderly, male, female, veterans, or civilians and held up across five different countries.[95] Other programs such as Seniors in Sobriety, an extension of AA, provide online meeting lists and resources for older adults. Some groups meet online or via phone. Some individuals do not prefer the spiritual foundation embedded in 12-Step programs such as AA and NA. SMART Recovery is a secular recovery program that can be a good alternative. SMART stands for Self-Management and Recovery Training. It is a 4-Point program that uses a combination of cognitive behavioral therapy (CBT) and motivational methods.

Peer support specialists (PSS) or peer recovery coaches (PRC) are individuals in recovery, who use their lived experience to support another on their recovery journey. The literature supports their use for both mental health and substance use support, as part of a collaborative effort with clinical and social support services.[120]

PREVENTION OF RETURN TO USE FOR OLDER ADULTS

For older adults with a history of SUDs, recovery is an ongoing process. Due to their age-related risks for return to substance use, recovery management and social support is particularly important for older adults. Life stressors, common in older age, such as social isolation, loneliness, loss/grief, and depression, can be antecedents to substance use as a way of self-medicating to alleviate negative emotional states. Comorbid medical conditions such as pain also put older adults at higher risk for return to use.[121] A continuing care approach, similar to other chronic disease management, can help older adults maintain stable recovery. Self-help groups and family therapies that focus on social support can greatly benefit older adults.[112]

Clinicians can help prevent or reduce the risk for return to use in older adults by helping to expand and strengthen their social networks. Older adults are already at risk of decreased psychosocial supports through common life events such as retirement, loss of a spouse, and/or friends and loved ones. Positive social support and social networks can help individuals in recovery increase social functioning, reduce social isolation, and promote positive behavior change.[122] Expanding and solidifying their networks can be done by connecting older adults to community supports (local programs, area agencies for aging, recovery-specific mutual aid groups, etc) and including families and caretakers (with permission) in their treatment plan and recovery-related activities. Online social networks, geared toward older adults, can also help individuals grow their social supports from any location.

Other areas of health and wellbeing that can help support recovery can include nutrition and exercise (physical health), spirituality, finances, complementary therapies (massage, animal-assisted therapy, meditation, etc.), work (including volunteer work), continuing education (community education, college courses, adult education, etc.) and emotional health. There are many paths to recovery. Providers are encouraged to take time to brainstorm with older adult clients and make suggestions based on their unique needs (ie, physical, cognitive, financial, etc.) and interests.

CONCLUSION

As the baby boom cohort ages, as well as the increasing need for care due to COVID-19, the number of older adults in need of SUD treatment is increasing and is an area of major public health concern.[123] Although significant advances have been made in understanding the aging process, there is a growing need for new models of care that intersect the fields of gerontology/geriatrics, addiction medicine, primary care and other disciplines (eg, psychiatry, pharmacy, social work), ideally in interprofessional teams. More research on best practices to treat older adults with previous trauma and SUDs, within the broader context of aging are also needed. There also remains a need for research on medication treatment older adults with SUDs, especially those with comorbid health conditions.[124,125] Fortunately, there are several venues in which to detect and address substance-related problems in older adults, including primary care clinics, specialty care settings, home health care, elder housing, and senior center programs. The challenge remains that providers are expected to deliver quality health care for a wide variety of problems within greater time constraints. Therefore, the application of consistent, short, effective techniques to prevent, identify and address SUDs in this growing population continues to be an important focus for all providers interacting with older adults. When successfully implemented, evidence-based screening, brief interventions, and brief treatments are key steps in the process of assuring that current and future generations have the opportunity for improved physical and emotional health. The challenge to the system will be moving from the development of these evidence-based programs to implementing them in the real world—the "bench to bedside" dilemma.

REFERENCES

1. *Results from the 2020 National. Survey on Drug Use and Health: Detailed Tables*. SAMHSA; 2021.
2. Wu L-T, Blazer DG. Illicit and nonmedical drug use among older adults: a review. *J Aging Health.* 2011;23(3):481-504.
3. Barry KL, Blow FC. Drinking over the lifespan: focus on older adults. *Alcohol Res.* 2016;38(1):115-120.
4. Gee EM. Misconceptions and misapprehensions about population ageing. *Int J Epidemiol.* 2002;31(4):750-753.
5. Slagsvold B, Hansen T. The Baby-boomer generation: another breed of elderly people? In: Falch-Eriksen A, Takle M, Slagsvold B, eds. *Generational Tensions and Solidarity Within Advanced Welfare States.* Routledge; 2021:153-172.
6. SAMHSA. *Treating Substance Use Disorder in Older Adults. Treatment Improvement Protocol (TIP) Series*, vol. 26; 2020.
7. National Center for Health Statistics (US). Health, United States, 2018, [Internet]. 2019.
8. Saitz R, Miller SC, Fiellin DA, Rosenthal RN. Recommended use of terminology in addiction medicine. *J Addict Med.* 2021;15(1):3-7.
9. Levi-Minzi MA, Surratt HL, Kurtz SP, Buttram ME. Under treatment of pain: a prescription for opioid misuse among the elderly? *Pain Med.* 2013;14(11):1719-1729. doi:10.1111/pme.12189
10. Maree RD, Marcum ZA, Saghafi E, Weiner DK, Karp JF. A systematic review of opioid and benzodiazepine misuse in older adults. *Am J Geriatr Psychiatry.* 2016;24(11):949-963.
11. Shoff C, Yang T-C, Shaw BA. Trends in opioid use disorder among older adults: analyzing Medicare data, 2013–2018. *Am J Preve Med.* 2021;60(6):850-855.
12. Mason M, Soliman R, Kim HS, Post LA. Disparities by sex and race and ethnicity in death rates due to opioid overdose among adults 55 years or older, 1999 to 2019. *JAMA Netw Open.* 2022;5(1):e2142982-e2142982.
13. Han BH, Palamar JJ. Trends in cannabis use among older adults in the United States, 2015–2018. *JAMA Intern Med.* 2020;180(4):609-611.
14. Choi NG, Marti CN, DiNitto DM, Choi BY. Older adults' marijuana use, injuries, and emergency department visits. *Am J Drug Alcohol Abuse.* 2018;44(2):215-223.
15. Minerbi A, Häuser W, Fitzcharles M-A. Medical cannabis for older patients. *Drugs Aging.* 2019;36(1):39-51.
16. Croker JA, Bobitt JL, Arora K, Kaskie B. Assessing health-related outcomes of medical Cannabis use among older persons: findings from Colorado and Illinois. *Clin Gerontol.* 2021;44(1):66-79. doi:10.1080/07317115.2020.1797971
17. Chhatre S, Cook R, Mallik E, Jayadevappa R. Trends in substance use admissions among older adults. *BMC Health Serv Res.* 2017;17(1):584. doi:10.1186/s12913-017-2538-z
18. Rosen D. Addressing the crises in treating substance use disorders in later-life: Tele-medication Assisted Treatment (TELE-MAT) for an older adult population. *Am J Geriatr Psychiatry.* 2022;30(10):1064-1066.
19. Lau-Ng R, Day H, Alford DP. Barriers facing older adults with substance use disorders in post–acute care settings. *Generations.* 2021;44(4):1-10.
20. Cornelius ME, Loretan CG, Wang TW, Jamal A, Homa DM. Tobacco product use among adults—United States, 2020. *MMWR Morb Mortal Wkly Rep.* 2022;71(11):397-405. doi:10.15585/mmwr.mm7111a1
21. Burns DM. Cigarette smoking among the elderly: disease consequences and the benefits of cessation. *Am J Health Promot.* 2000;14(6):357-361. doi:10.4278/0890-1171-14.6.357
22. Chan GCK, Stjepanović D, Lim C, et al. A systematic review of randomized controlled trials and network meta-analysis of e-cigarettes for smoking cessation. *Addict Behav.* 2021;119:106912. doi:10.1016/j.addbeh.2021.106912
23. American Lung Association. Do Not Use E-Cigarettes. 2019.
24. Cawkwell PB, Blaum C, Sherman SE. Pharmacological smoking cessation therapies in older adults: a review of the evidence. *Drugs Aging.* 2015;32(6):443-451.
25. Zhong G, Wang Y, Zhang Y, Guo JJ, Zhao Y. Smoking is associated with an increased risk of dementia: a meta-analysis of prospective cohort studies with investigation of potential effect modifiers. *PloS One.* 2015;10(3):e0118333.
26. Aonso-Diego G, González-Roz A, Krotter A, García-Pérez A, Secades-Villa R. Contingency management for smoking cessation among individuals with substance use disorders: in-treatment and post-treatment effects. *Addict Behav.* 2021;119:106920. doi:10.1016/j.addbeh.2021.106920
27. García-Fernández G, Krotter A, García-Pérez Á, Aonso-Diego G, Secades-Villa R. Pilot randomized trial of cognitive-behavioral treatment plus contingency management for quitting smoking and weight gain prevention among smokers with overweight or obesity. *Drug Alcohol Depend.* 2022;236:109477.
28. Sachs-Ericsson N, Schmidt NB, Zvolensky MJ, Mitchell M, Collins N, Blazer DG. Smoking cessation behavior in older adults by race and gender: the role of health problems and psychological distress. *Nicotine Tob Res.* 2009;11(4):433-443.
29. Kinney J, Leaton G. *Loosening the Grip: A Handbook of Alcohol Information.* 10th ed. McGraw Hill Education; 2011.
30. Babatunde OT, Outlaw KR, Forbes B, Gay T. Revisiting baby boomers and alcohol use: emerging treatment trends. *J Hum Behav Soc Environ.* 2014;24(5):597-611.
31. Wang Y-P, Andrade LH. Epidemiology of alcohol and drug use in the elderly. *Curr Opin Psychiatry.* 2013;26(4):343-348.
32. Moore AA, Whiteman EJ, Ward KT. Risks of combined alcohol/medication use in older adults. *Am J Geriatr Pharmacother.* 2007;5(1):64-74.
33. Lindsey WT, Stewart D, Childress D. Drug interactions between common illicit drugs and prescription therapies. *Am J Drug Alcohol Abuse.* 2012;38(4):334-343.
34. Dierker L, Selya A, Lanza S, Li R, Rose J. Depression and marijuana use disorder symptoms among current marijuana users. *Addict Behav.* 2018;76:161-168.
35. Feingold D, Weinstein A. Cannabis and depression. *Adv Exp Med Biol.* 2021;1264:67-80.
36. Guertler D, Moehring A, Krause K, et al. Latent alcohol use patterns and their link to depressive symptomatology in medical care patients. *Addiction.* 2021;116(5):1063-1073.
37. Choi NG, DiNitto DM, Marti CN, Choi BY. Relationship between marijuana and other illicit drug use and depression/suicidal thoughts among late middle-aged and older adults. *Int Psychogeriatr.* 2016;28(4):577-589.
38. Blazer DG, Wu L-T. The epidemiology of substance use and disorders among middle aged and elderly community adults: national survey on drug use and health. *Am J Geriatr Psychiatry.* 2009;17(3):237-245.
39. Chou K-L, Mackenzie CS, Liang K, Sareen J. Three-year incidence and predictors of first-onset of DSM-IV mood, anxiety, and substance use disorders in older adults: results from Wave 2 of the National Epidemiologic Survey on Alcohol and Related Conditions. *J Clin Psychiatry.* 2011;72(2):20965.
40. Pompili M, Serafini G, Innamorati M, et al. Suicidal behavior and alcohol abuse. *Int J Environ Res Public Health.* 2010;7(4):1392-1431.

41. Esang M, Ahmed S. A closer look at substance use and suicide. *Am J Psychiatry Resid J.* 2018. doi:10.1176/appi.ajp-rj.2018.130603
42. Wu L-T, Blazer DG. Substance use disorders and psychiatric comorbidity in mid and later life: a review. *Int J Epidemiol.* 2014;43(2):304-317.
43. Caputo F, Vignoli T, Leggio L, Addolorato G, Zoli G, Bernardi M. Alcohol use disorders in the elderly: a brief overview from epidemiology to treatment options. *Exp Gerontol.* 2012;47(6):411-416. doi:10.1016/j.exger.2012.03.019
44. Keyes KM, Allel K, Staudinger UM, Ornstein KA, Calvo E. Alcohol consumption predicts incidence of depressive episodes across 10 years among older adults in 19 countries. *Int Rev Neurobiol.* 2019;148:1-38.
45. Ehlman DC. Changes in suicide rates—United States, 2019 and 2020. *MMWR Morb Mortal Wkly Rep.* 2022;71(8):306-312.
46. Schmutte T, Olfson M, Maust DT, Xie M, Marcus SC. Suicide risk in first year after dementia diagnosis in older adults. *Alzheimers Dement.* 2022;18(2):262-271. doi:10.1002/alz.12390
47. Bickford D, Morin RT, Nelson JC, Mackin RS. Determinants of suicide-related ideation in late life depression: associations with perceived stress. *Clin Gerontol.* 2020;43(1):37-45. doi:10.1080/07317115.2019.1666442
48. Rahoof FV, Cherian AV, Kandasamy A, Ezhumalai S, Dhanasekara RP. Suicidal ideation among persons with alcohol use disorder: a cross-sectional study. *J Psychosoc Well Being.* 2021;2(2):30-41. doi:10.55242/jpsw.2021.2206
49. Sorrell JM. Losing a generation: the impact of COVID-19 on older Americans. *J Psychosoc Nurs Ment Health Serv.* 2021;59(4):9-12.
50. Troutman-Jordan M, Kazemi DM. COVID-19's impact on the mental health of older adults: increase in isolation, depression, and suicide risk. An urgent call for action. *Public Health Nurs.* 2020;37(5):637-638.
51. Kim M-J, Paek S-H, Kwon J-H, Park S-H, Chung H-J, Byun Y-H. Changes in suicide rate and characteristics according to age of suicide attempters before and after CoViD-19. *Children.* 2022;9(2):151.
52. Woo SH, Lee WJ, Jeong WJ, Kyong YY, Choi SM. Blood alcohol concentration and self-reported alcohol ingestion in acute poisoned patients who visited an emergency department. *Scand J Trauma Resusc Emerg Med.* 2013;21(1):1-6.
53. Domenichiello AF, Ramsden CE. The silent epidemic of chronic pain in older adults. *Prog Neuropsychopharmacol Biol Psychiatry.* 2019;93:284-290.
54. Shmagel A, Krebs E, Ensrud K, Foley R. Illicit substance use in US adults with chronic low back pain. *Spine.* 2016;41(17):1372.
55. Gerlach LB, Wiechers IR, Maust DT. Prescription benzodiazepine use among older adults: a critical review. *Harv Rev Psychiatry.* 2018;26(5):264.
56. American Geriatrics Society 2012 Beers Criteria Update Expert Panel. American Geriatrics Society updated beers criteria for potentially inappropriate medication use in older adults. *J Am Geriatr Soc.* 2012;60(4):616-631.
57. Slattum PW, Hassan OE. Medications, alcohol, and aging. In: *Alcohol and Aging.* Springer; 2016:117-129.
58. Meier P, Seitz HK. Age, alcohol metabolism and liver disease. *Curr Opin Clin Nutr Metab Care.* 2008;11(1):21-26.
59. Breslow RA, Dong C, White A. Prevalence of alcohol-interactive prescription medication use among current drinkers: United States, 1999 to 2010. *Alcohol Clin Exp Res.* 2015;39(2):371-379.
60. McKnight-Eily LR, Liu Y, Brewer RD, et al. Vital signs: communication between health professionals and their patients about alcohol use—44 states and the District of Columbia, 2011. *MMWR Morbid Mortal Wkly Rep.* 2014;63(1):16.
61. Klein WC, Jess C. One last pleasure? Alcohol use among elderly people in nursing homes. *Health Soc Work.* 2002;27(3):193-203.
62. SAMHSA. *Screening, Brief Intervention and Referral to Treatment (SBIRT) in Behavioral Healthcare.* 2011 White paper. Accessed May 29, 2023. https://www.samhsa.gov/sites/default/files/sbirtwhitepaper_0.pdf
63. Smith PC, Schmidt SM, Allensworth-Davies D, Saitz R. A single-question screening test for drug use in primary care. *Arch Intern Med.* 2010;170(13):1155-1160.
64. Smith PC, Schmidt SM, Allensworth-Davies D, Saitz R. Primary care validation of a single-question alcohol screening test. *J Gen Intern Med.* 2009;24(7):783-788.
65. Aalto M, Alho H, Halme JT, Seppä K. The alcohol use disorders identification test (AUDIT) and its derivatives in screening for heavy drinking among the elderly. *Int J Geriatr Psychiatry.* 2011;26(9):881-885.
66. Van Gils Y, Franck E, Dierckx E, Van Alphen SP, Saunders JB, Dom G. Validation of the AUDIT and AUDIT-C for hazardous drinking in community-dwelling older adults. *Int J Environ Res Public Health.* 2021;18(17):9266.
67. Blow F, Gillespie B, Barry K, Mudd S, Hill E. Brief screening for alcohol problems in elderly populations using the Short Michigan Alcoholism Screening Test-Geriatric Version (SMAST-G). *Alcohol Clin Exp Res.* 1998;22(suppl 3):131A.
68. National Institute on Alcohol Abuse and Alcoholism. *Helping Patients Who Drink Too Much, A Clinician's Guide.* 2007.
69. Humeniuk R, Ali R, Babor TF, et al. Validation of the alcohol, smoking and substance involvement screening test (ASSIST). *Addiction.* 2008;103(6):1039-1047. doi:10.1111/j.1360-0443.2007.02114.x
70. Cacciola JS, Alterman AI, DePhilippis D, et al. Development and initial evaluation of the Brief Addiction Monitor (BAM). *J Subst Abuse Treat.* 2013;44(3):256-263.
71. McNeely J, Strauss SM, Saitz R, et al. A brief patient self-administered substance use screening tool for primary care: two-site validation study of the Substance Use Brief Screen (SUBS). *Am J Med.* 2015;128(7):784. e9-e19.
72. Barry K, Fleming M. Computerized administration of alcoholism screening tests in a primary care setting. *J Am Board Fam Pract.* 1990;3(2):93-98.
73. Barry K, Blow F. Screening and assessment of alcohol problems in older adults. In: Lichtenberg PA, ed. *Handbook of Assessment in Clinical Gerontology*; 1999:243-269.
74. Grant BF, Saha TD, Ruan WJ, et al. Epidemiology of DSM-5 drug use disorder: results from the National Epidemiologic Survey on Alcohol and Related Conditions–III. *JAMA Psychiatry.* 2016;73(1):39-47.
75. Hasin DS, O'Brien CP, Auriacombe M, et al. DSM-5 criteria for substance use disorders: recommendations and rationale. *Am J Psychiatry.* 2013;170(8):834-851.
76. Kuerbis AN, Hagman BT, Sacco P. Functioning of alcohol use disorders criteria among middle-aged and older adults: implications for DSM-5. *Subst Use Misuse.* 2013;48(4):309-322.
77. Schonfeld L, Hazlett RW, Hedgecock DK, Duchene DM, Burns LV, Gum AM. Screening, brief intervention, and referral to treatment for older adults with substance misuse. *Am J Public Health.* 2015;105(1):205-211. doi:10.2105/ajph.2013.301859
78. Kuerbis AN, Yuan SE, Borok J, et al. Testing the initial efficacy of a mailed screening and brief feedback intervention to reduce at-risk drinking in middle-aged and older adults: the Comorbidity Alcohol Risk Evaluation Study. *J Am Geriatr Soc.* 2015;63(2):321-326.
79. Ettner SL, Xu H, Duru OK, et al. The effect of an educational intervention on alcohol consumption, at-risk drinking, and health care utilization in older adults: the Project SHARE study. *J Stud Alcohol Drugs.* 2014;75(3):447-457.
80. Jonas DE, Garbutt JC, Amick HR, et al. Behavioral counseling after screening for alcohol misuse in primary care: a systematic review and meta-analysis for the US Preventive Services Task Force. *Ann Intern Med.* 2012;157(9):645-654.
81. Whitlock EP, Polen MR, Green CA, Orleans T, Klein J. Behavioral counseling interventions in primary care to reduce risky/harmful alcohol use by adults: a summary of the evidence for the US Preventive Services Task Force. *Ann Intern Med.* 2004;140(7):557-568.
82. Kaner EF, Beyer FR, Muirhead C, et al. Effectiveness of brief alcohol interventions in primary care populations. *Cochrane Database Syst Rev.* 2018;2:CD004148.
83. Schutte K, Lemke S, Moos RH, Brennan PL. Age-sensitive psychosocial treatment for older adults with substance abuse. In: Crome I, Wu L-T, Rao R, Crome P, eds. *Substance Use and Older People.* Wiley-Blackwell; 2015:314-339.
84. Finnell DS. Something to talk about: reducing risk in alcohol consumption using education and conversation. *Generations.* 2021;44(4):1-8.
85. Oslin DW, Zanjani F. Treatment of unhealthy alcohol use in older adults. *Alcohol Aging.* 2016;181-199.

86. Kuerbis A, Sacco P. A review of existing treatments for substance abuse among the elderly and recommendations for future directions. *Subst Abuse*. 2013;7:SART.S7865.
87. Weiss L, Petry NM. Older methadone patients achieve greater durations of cocaine abstinence with contingency management than younger patients. *Am J Addict*. 2013;22(2):119-126.
88. Kuerbis A, Sacco P, Blazer DG, Moore AA. Substance abuse among older adults. *Clin Geriatr Med*. 2014;30(3):629-654.
89. De Jong CA, Goodair C, Crome I, et al. Focus: the aging brain: substance misuse education for physicians: why older people are important. *Yale J Biol Med*. 2016;89(1):97.
90. Moore AA, Blow FC, Hoffing M, et al. Primary care-based intervention to reduce at-risk drinking in older adults: a randomized controlled trial. *Addiction*. 2011;106(1):111-120.
91. Conigliaro J, Lofgren RP, Hanusa BH. Screening for problem drinking: impact on physician behavior and patient drinking habits. *J Gen Intern Med*. 1998;13(4):251-256.
92. Mee-Lee D. *The ASAM Criteria: Treatment Criteria for Addictive, Substance-Related, and Co-Occurring Conditions*. 3rd ed. The Change Companies; 2013.
93. Sowers W, George C, Thompson K. Level of care utilization system for psychiatric and addiction services (LOCUS): a preliminary assessment of reliability and validity. *Commun Ment Health J*. 1999;35(6): 545-563.
94. Alvanzo A, Kleinschmidt K, Kmiec J. The ASAM Clinical Practice Guideline on Alcohol Withdrawal Management. 2020 Accessed May 29, 2023. https://www.asam.org/docs/default-source/quality-science/the_asam_clinical_practice_guideline_on_alcohol-1.pdf
95. Kelly JF, Humphreys K, Ferri M. Alcoholics Anonymous and other 12-step programs for alcohol use disorder. *Cochrane Database Syst Rev*. 2020;3(3):CD012880.
96. Butt PR, White-Campbell M, Canham S, et al. Canadian guidelines on alcohol use disorder among older adults. *Can Geriatr J*. 2020; 23(1):143.
97. Lemke S, Moos RH. Treatment and outcomes of older patients with alcohol use disorders in community residential programs. *J Stud Alcohol*. 2003;64(2):219-226.
98. MacFarland NS. *Outpatient Treatment Approaches, Services and Outcomes for Older Addicted Adults*. State University of New York at Albany; 2014
99. Kashner TM, Rodell DE, Ogden SR, Guggenheim FG, Karson CN. Outcomes and costs of two VA inpatient treatment programs for older alcoholic patients. *Hosp Commun Psychiatry*. 1992;43(10):985-989.
100. D'Agostino CS, Barry KL, Blow FC, Podgorski C. Community interventions for older adults with comorbid substance abuse: the Geriatric Addictions Program (GAP). *J Dual Diagn*. 2006;2(3):31-45.
101. Wiens AN, Menustik CE, Miller SI, Schmitz RE. Medical-behavioral treatment of the older alcoholic patient. *Am J Drug Alcohol Abuse*. 1982;9(4):461-475.
102. Atkinson RM, Tolson RL, Turner JA. Factors affecting outpatient treatment compliance of older male problem drinkers. *J Stud Alcohol*. 1993;54(1):102-106.
103. Tampi RR, Chhatlani A, Ahmad H, et al. Substance use disorders among older adults: a review of randomized controlled pharmacotherapy trials. *World J Psychiatry*. 2019;9(5):78.
104. Arndt S. *Minority Clients Entering Substance Abuse Treatment for the First Time: 10 Year Trends*. Iowa Consortium for Substance Abuse Research and Evaluation; 2010.
105. Jonas DE, Amick HR, Feltner C, et al. Pharmacotherapy for adults with alcohol use disorders in outpatient settings: a systematic review and meta-analysis. *JAMA*. 2014;311(18):1889-1900.
106. Crome I. Substance misuse in the older person: setting higher standards. *Clin Med*. 2013;13(Suppl 6):s46-s49.
107. Skinner MD, Lahmek P, Pham H, Aubin H-J. Disulfiram efficacy in the treatment of alcohol dependence: a meta-analysis. *PloS One*. 2014;9(2):e87366.
108. Mitra P. Naltrexone as an adjunctive treatment for older patients with alcohol dependence. In: Tampi RR, Tampi DJ, Young JJ, Balasubramaniam M, Joshi P, eds. *Essential Reviews in Geriatric Psychiatry*. Springer; 2022:413-416.
109. Oslin D, Liberto JG, O'Brien J, Krois S, Norbeck J. Naltrexone as an adjunctive treatment for older patients with alcohol dependence. *Am J Geriatr Psychiatry*. 1997;5(4):324-332.
110. Lee J, Shin JU, Noh S, Park CO, Lee KH. Clinical efficacy and safety of naltrexone combination therapy in older patients with severe pruritus. *Ann Dermatol*. 2016;28(2):159-163.
111. Oslin DW. Treatment of late-life depression complicated by alcohol dependence. *Am J Geriatr Psychiatry*. 2005;13(6):491-500.
112. Barrick C, Connors GJ. Relapse prevention and maintaining abstinence in older adults with alcohol-use disorders. *Drugs Aging*. 2002;19(8):583-594. doi:10.2165/00002512-200219080-00004
113. Rösner S, Hackl-Herrwerth A, Leucht S, Lehert P, Vecchi S, Soyka M. Acamprosate for alcohol dependence. *Cochrane Database of Syst Rev*. 2010;9:CD004332.
114. Rieb LM, Samaan Z, Furlan AD, et al. Canadian guidelines on opioid use disorder among older adults. *Can Geriatr J*. 2020;23(1):123.
115. World Health Organization. *World Health Organization Model List of Essential Meedicines for Children: 7th List 2019*. 2019. Accessed May 29, 2023. https://apps.who.int/iris/bitstream/handle/10665/325772/WHO-MVP-EMP-IAU-2019.07-eng.pdf
116. Joshi P, Shah NK, Kirane HD. Medication-assisted treatment for opioid use disorder in older adults: an emerging role for the geriatric psychiatrist. *Am J Geriatr Psychiatry*. 2019;27(4):455-457.
117. Carew AM, Comiskey C. Treatment for opioid use and outcomes in older adults: a systematic literature review. *Drug Alcohol Depend*. 2018;182:48-57.
118. Chou R, Cruciani RA, Fiellin DA, et al. Methadone safety: a clinical practice guideline from the American Pain Society and College on problems of drug dependence, in collaboration with the Heart Rhythm Society. *J Pain*. 2014;15(4):321-337. doi:10.1016/j.jpain.2014.01.494
119. Jobert A, Laforgue E-J, Grall-Bronnec M, et al. Benzodiazepine withdrawal in older people: what is the prevalence, what are the signs, and which patients? *Eur J Clin Pharmacology*. 2021;77(2): 171-177.
120. Shalaby RAH, Agyapong VI. Peer support in mental health: literature review. *JMIR Ment Health*. 2020;7(6):e15572.
121. Brennan PL, Schutte KK, Moos RH. Pain and use of alcohol to manage pain: prevalence and 3-year outcomes among older problem and non-problem drinkers. *Addiction*. 2005;100(6):777-786.
122. Jarnecke AM, Brown DG, Melkonian AJ. Family and social processes in recovery from alcohol use disorder. In: Jarnecke AM, Brown DG, Melkonian AJ, eds. *Dynamic Pathways to Recovery from Alcohol Use Disorder: Meaning and Methods*. 2021:200.
123. Blow FC, Barry KL. Alcohol and substance misuse in older adults. *Curr Psychiatry Rep*. 2012;14(4):310-319.
124. Huhn AS, Ellis JD. Commentary on Zolopa et al.: trauma as an impediment to successful aging and a precipitant of opioid and stimulant use among older adults. *Addiction*. 2022;117(8):2189-2190. doi:10.1111/add.15877
125. Zolopa C, Høj SB, Minoyan N, Bruneau J, Makarenko I, Larney S. Ageing and older people who use illicit opioids, cocaine or methamphetamine: a scoping review and literature map. *Addiction*. 2022;117(8):2168-2188. doi:10.1111/add.15813

CHAPTER 42

Treatment Considerations for LGBTQ Patients

Timothy M. Hall, Maliha Khan, and Steven Shoptaw

CHAPTER OUTLINE

- Introduction
- Notes on language
- History and context of substance use among LGBTQ communities
- Epidemiology of substance use and substance use disorders
- What to do? Evidence-supported recommendations for clinicians
- Mitigating risk of HIV and STIs: PrEP, TasP, and emerging technologies
- Conclusions
- Select LGBTQ documentaries for further viewing

INTRODUCTION

Alcohol, nicotine, and a variety of other psychoactive substances have long and complex social histories in lesbian, gay, bisexual, transgender, and queer communities, henceforth, LGBTQ (see below for "Notes on Language"). Some of these communities also have cultural practices of diverting prescription medications such as anabolic steroids or estrogens to modify bodily appearance to be more congruent with their self-image or experienced gender. Some substances, such as alkyl nitrite "poppers," are mainly used by some LGBTQ groups. Substances such as crystal methamphetamine have an outsized impact on cisgender men who have sex with men (MSM) and transgender persons with male partners. Clinicians need to understand the social context of substance use and substance use disorders (SUD) in LGBTQ communities in order to appropriately screen for SUD and associated behaviors, and to understand individual and structural challenges to care and recovery.

Many sexual and gender minority individuals, as well as LGBTQ communities, have complicated or even frankly traumatic individual and collective experiences of social discrimination and legal persecution, as well as mistreatment by medical authorities. Same-sex sexual orientation was categorized as a mental illness under the DSM prior to 1973.[1] Mental health and medical professionals have been even slower to fully recognize transgender experiences as part of normal human variation, with continuing debates over the categorization of gender dysphoria and medical gatekeeping of gender-affirming care. Health care institutions and government agencies have neglected LGBTQ health concerns, most notably during the HIV/AIDS epidemic in the 1980s and 1990s.[2] LGBTQ individuals may thus have quite understandable mistrust of health care professionals,[3] as well as a habit of weighing medical advice against community norms that include higher tolerance for social drinking and casual drug use. LGBTQ individuals may feel unsafe disclosing their sexual behavior or their gender identity to clinicians in mainstream health settings based on prior adverse experiences,[4] or they may be in early phases of their coming out process and not ready to disclose these to anyone, even though these may be significant for their health care.

Despite this history of significant discrimination and health disparities, LGBTQ communities have also been sources of resilience and innovation, and the process of coming out as LGBTQ can foster personal growth. There is enormous heterogeneity of experience, self-understanding, and behaviors within LGBTQ populations. This diversity increases when we consider intersections of sexual behavior, sexual orientation, and gender experience with statuses such as generational cohort,[5] social class,[6,7] cultural or religious background,[8] urban/suburban/rural residence,[9] involvement with the carceral system,[10] and disability status, among others.[11]

In this chapter, we discuss common considerations when working with LGBTQ persons, the roles that particular substances play in certain LGBTQ subcultures, and ways clinicians can build LGBTQ cultural competence. We remind readers that any specific LGBTQ individual may have very different experiences than those described here. We review: (1) the history and social contexts of substance use in LGBTQ individuals and in LGBTQ communities; (2) epidemiology of substance use and addiction for LGBTQ individuals; (3) links between substance use or addiction and sexual behaviors that may involve increased risk for HIV and other sexually transmitted infections (STIs), as well as mitigation strategies (including preexposure prophylaxis for HIV, or PrEP); and (4) evidence-based treatments for LGBTQ patients and the value of cultural competence when delivering those treatments. At the end of this chapter, we provide a list of accessible LGBTQ documentaries for clinicians who wish to increase their cultural competency with these communities.

Throughout, we take a pragmatic, principles-oriented approach rather than focusing on detailed estimates of prevalence or an exhaustive enumeration of risks—all of which are limited by challenges with sampling.[12] The social and cultural milieux of LGBTQ persons is constantly evolving, as is our medical knowledge. For example, at the time of this writing, human monkeypox virus (hMPXV) is an emerging infectious disease disproportionately affecting MSM and transgender persons with male partners, and raising the specter of renewed stigmatization of an infectious disease associated with LGBTQ communities.[13] Conversely, PrEP and treatment as prevention (TasP) have profoundly changed both the medical risks and social construction of HIV disease and normalized the experiences of many gay and bisexual men.[11] Civil rights of transgender persons, and debates over the best way to support transgender and gender dysphoric children and adolescents,[14,15] have featured prominently in national political discourse. These are not static facts to be learned by rote. We encourage clinicians to learn more about LGBTQ cultures and history, to stay current with relevant social and medical developments, and to engage respectfully with their patients as individuals—who may have some of the experiences that we describe herein.

NOTES ON LANGUAGE

Recent scholarship in public health has tended to use behaviorally based terms, such as MSM, which recognize that sexual behavior is not fully determined by one's sexual orientation, nor is sexual identity necessarily determined by one's behavior.[16] For instance, some individuals may have transactional sex with nonpreferred partners in exchange for drugs or money; there is also a phenomenon of otherwise heterosexually identified men who engage in sex with male partners only when using methamphetamine or other stimulants.[17] These men would be included behaviorally in "MSM," but likely do not see themselves as belonging to a gay or LGBTQ community.[11] Other individuals may feel a "gay" or "lesbian" identity does not fit their self-understanding or cultural background, or carries unwelcome political or cultural associations. Bisexual individuals are less likely than gay or lesbian persons to openly disclose their sexuality, may have particularly increased rates of substance use (compared to non-LGBTQ and other LGBTQ groups), and are less likely to be engaged in LGBTQ social networks; despite being the largest block of LGBTQ individuals, bisexual persons have often been left out of health research and community interventions ostensibly focused on LGBTQ populations.[18,19] Research and clinical work need to engage with this diversity.[20] Additionally, behavior and identity carry different relevance for health: sexual behavior may be most relevant for potential transmission of STIs, for instance, but identity shapes social–sexual networks as well as affecting an individual's receptivity to messaging around health or comfort with engaging particular services. Sexual identity, sexual orientation, sexual behavior, and gender identity are not interchangeable. Competent clinicians know these distinctions.

Transgender individuals may understand and express their gender identities in multiple ways, and their gender identity may coexist with any kind of sexual orientation. Some transgender persons identify as heterosexual and do not participate in communities of bisexual, lesbian, or gay persons. Other transgender persons may identify as bisexual, gay, lesbian, pansexual, etc. and participate in those communities. Transgender persons of any sexual orientation may have a significant community of transgender friends and peers or may not. Nonbinary or "NB" (or "enby") identities have become more visible in recent years; there is limited data on how nonbinary identities may interact with risk for SUD, but recent studies have found worse overall mental health and greater risk for SUD.[21] A great deal of transgender organizing and community building has taken place online, facilitated by social media. The risky or protective impact of social media on SUD or other mental health conditions among transgender persons needs more research.

Terminology and recommended best practices around transgender experiences and identities are evolving rapidly.[22] Identifying one's preferred pronouns (most commonly she/her/hers, he/him/his, or they/them/theirs) in verbal introductions, email signatures, or videoconference names, has become standard in some settings; this normalizes the practice of not assuming someone's gender identity from appearance (and can also clarify gender identity for an unseen person or someone with a gender-ambiguous name). We recommend listening to your patients and addressing them by the names, terms, and pronouns that they prefer[22]—which may evolve over time. This practice accords best with respect for persons and autonomy and is the best way to earn trust and maintain rapport with patients who have often had negative experiences around nonacceptance of their gender identity.

It can be helpful to shift your clinic templates toward gender neutrality. Review office forms and electronic templates for gendered language such as "patient is an X-year-old woman," or requiring a binary choice of "male or female" as gender. Changing these to "adult" or "patient," and changing pronouns in templates to generic "they" or "the patient" instead of "he/she," reduce the risk of inadvertently misgendering patients. Consider limiting gender-specific labels to situations in which they clearly guide clinical management.

Throughout this chapter, we use LGBTQ as a broad term that is more succinct and less clinically distancing than "sexual orientation and gender identity" (SOGI) minorities. We recognize that LGBTQ emphasizes identity over behavior, whereas behavior is sometimes the most salient factor. When citing particular studies focusing on behavior, or when referring specifically to a subset of LGBTQ persons, we use MSM or other specific language such as lesbian women.[16] We do not use some longer forms such as LGBTQIA2+, which aim to include groups such as individuals with intersex conditions (or difference of sexual development), asexual persons, and individuals who identify as Two-Spirit. Doing so would falsely imply that we have an adequate empirical knowledge base to talk about SUD in these populations. It also falls into what anthropologist Tom Boellstorff calls the "fallacy of enumeration," implying that we can capture an ever-evolving social phenomenon if we just add enough letters to the acronym, rather than attending to the particular real persons in front of us.[23]

HISTORY AND CONTEXT OF SUBSTANCE USE AMONG LGBTQ COMMUNITIES

From alcohol and cigarettes to alkyl nitrite poppers and amphetamine-type stimulants, psychotropic substances can play many roles in the lives of LGBTQ individuals. These relate to three foundational principles. First, LGBTQ communities historically often began organizing around bars and later nightclubs, with evidence going back to the 1700s in Europe[24] and the 1800s in the United States.[25] Alcohol consumption was normative in these settings. As these venues were often illegal or at least tolerated criminalized behavior, they often also tacitly tolerated illegal drug use.[26,27] Such bars and nightclubs were the easiest entry point to LGBTQ social networks and communities for individuals in their processes of coming out, though online dating sites and apps have been slowly replacing these venues since the 2000s.[28] Alcohol and cigarettes can be used as icebreakers to facilitate interactions. Until very recently, many LGBTQ persons were acculturated into LGBTQ communities partly structured around bars that normalized alcohol consumption and often tolerated some degree of drug use. Second, growing up in societies that strongly stigmatized or even criminalized same-sex sexuality and diverse gender expressions, many LGBTQ persons used alcohol and other substances to cope with psychological distress, to mitigate internalized homophobia or transphobia,[27,29] or to decrease anxiety in social and sexual situations.[6,24,30] Third, certain drugs, including alkyl nitrite poppers, amphetamine-type stimulants, and club drugs, are used particularly by some MSM and transgender persons to reduce sexual inhibitions and enhance sexual experiences.[27,31] MSM and transgender women have a cultural history of using cannabis to mitigate effects of HIV disease and of some HIV medications (such as neuropathy, nausea, and poor appetite). LGBTQ communities in general had a higher tolerance for casual cannabis use, prior to the process of gradual legalization and social acceptance in many jurisdictions since the 1990s.

The generally greater acceptance of the use of drugs and of heavy or hazardous alcohol drinking among LGBTQ communities[32] increases risks for exposure to substances through social and sexual networks. In turn, this greater cultural acceptance of substance use presents unique challenges to LGBTQ persons seeking recovery. Triggers to drug use and access to substances occur in multiple settings—for instance, coded messages in dating app profiles. Following initiation of abstinence, building and maintaining a social network comprised of sober LGBTQ peers takes time and consistent effort, which increases feelings of isolation. Substance-free social events may be perceived as less interesting and more restricted in frequency and availability compared to LGBTQ events that incorporate substance use. Still more challenging, patients and their current or former sexual or romantic partners may not be ready to give up sexual experiences enhanced by substance use, forcing LGBTQ persons in recovery to choose between important interpersonal connections and their sobriety. While being aware of cultural factors, it is important not to assume a patient's substance use is founded in their minority sexual behavior or gender identities; LGBTQ persons also use drugs for same reasons as their cisgender, heterosexual peers.[22]

Syndemic was coined by anthropologist Merrill Singer in the 1990s to describe the synergistic interaction of two or more epidemics that cooccur and exacerbate or complicate one another. The term has subsequently been broadened to include epidemics that interact synergistically with behavioral disorders such as SUD, or with social phenomena such as poverty, structural violence, and systemic lack of access to health care (or a history of medical mistrust).[33] A frequent example is the syndemic interaction of HIV and crystal methamphetamine use in communities minoritized on the basis of race and/or sexual orientation. Each component of a syndemic complicates efforts to address other components. According to syndemic theory, negative health consequences linked with substance use, HIV and other STIs, depression, and adverse childhood experiences (ACES),[34] sustain poor health outcomes among MSM.[35]

For clinicians, this implies that focusing intervention on one or two aspects of the syndemic is likely to be insufficient. An LGBTQ patient may abstain from substance use, yet continue to face health risks due to other syndemic conditions (eg, discrimination, intimate partner violence, or internalized homophobia).[36] Syndemic effects may be greatest among LGBTQ individuals who are also persons of color,[36] or who have other intersecting minoritized or stigmatized statuses.[37] Local LGBTQ-oriented services may be predominantly oriented toward white clientele (implying discrimination by race), while medical and other services in predominantly non-white neighborhoods may not be welcoming toward LGBTQ clients (implying discrimination by homophobia). Few health care venues are available that specifically serve LGBTQ clients of color. While explicit biases against lesbian women and gay men in health care are less common than implicit biases,[38] it remains that primary health care settings present barriers to LGBTQ patients that are even greater when seeking services, delivered with cultural competence, for problems with substance use.

Personal Resilience

Despite the potential challenges of addiction and related syndemic conditions, many LGBTQ individuals have learned to manage some or all of these with resiliency. Much of the literature on SUD and mental health issues in LGBTQ populations prior to the 1980s pathologized same-sex sexuality per se, while research since then has often focused on same-sex sexuality as mediators of risk for HIV and STIs.[39] Nonetheless, most LGBTQ persons do not have SUDs or HIV despite greater potential exposures to both. LGBTQ communities have shown strength in mobilizing against social discrimination and stigma over addiction and HIV/AIDS. LGBTQ cultures can buffer against sexual minority stress.[40] The process of coming out often helps develop skills in self-awareness and in communication, with corresponding benefits that include a secure sense of self and access to networks of social support.[41]

Cultural Resilience

It is also important to attend to changes in patterns of substance use over the lifespan and cultural changes experienced by successive generations of LGBTQ individuals.[42] Ritch Savin-Williams and others have documented the resilience of contemporary LGBTQ youth, and have critiqued the existing literature for focusing on subgroups that are most likely to be experiencing problems, such as youth seeking support services, rather than more representative community samples.[43] Qualitative and mixed-methods studies suggest that the social context and developmental experiences of LGBTQ persons in Western countries since the 1960s have been changing with each cohort, such that LGBTQ persons born in different decades or coming out at different ages face very different sets of challenges and resources.[44,45] Clinicians should be aware that LGBTQ communities can provide substantial support to their members.

Cultural Competence

Persons who are not themselves LGBTQ can still provide culturally competent addiction treatment to LGBTQ individuals. This requires, however, more than a passing familiarity regarding some important issues experienced by LGBTQ persons with SUD. For many LGBTQ persons, current and former sexual partners make up key parts of their social-sexual networks—sometimes a majority of those networks.[41,46] Consequently, it is important for clinicians to be able to discuss sexual behaviors in the context of an LGBTQ person's overall social life in a nonjudgmental way, and specifically in relation to their substance use. However, many non–evidence-based strategies (such as some 12-step approaches) avoid talking about sex or even proscribe sex for some period—up to a year or more—after starting treatment. This can present conflicts in personal identity while striving to reduce or stop using substances. Conversely, discussion of chemsex (sex in the context of drug use) may be triggering to such an extent that LGBTQ clients may prefer non-LGBTQ support groups. These cultural factors present real challenges to clinicians in establishing a behavioral treatment framework that affirms the patient while meeting goals to stop or reduce substance use.

EPIDEMIOLOGY OF SUBSTANCE USE AND SUBSTANCE USE DISORDERS

Perceptions of a unique vulnerability among LGBTQ individuals to addiction stem from early views in psychiatry that homosexuality itself was a marker or result of mental illness.[47] Early studies overestimated prevalence of SUD by conducting epidemiological surveys in gay bars.[48] Better definitions of SUD, better sampling frames, and inclusion of questions regarding same-sex sexual behaviors in probability framed surveys have yielded estimates of prevalence among LGBTQ persons closer to those in the general population,[49] although the prevalence is still documented to be significantly higher for many categories of substance use among LGBTQ persons compare to non-LGBTQ.[17,50] These may also contribute to greater risk for exposure to HIV, viral hepatitis, and other STIs.

Since the 1980s, stimulants and the so-called club drugs have been a significant aspect of the "circuit party" scene.[27] The terms "to party," "party & play," or "PnP" have come to signify sexual encounters under the influence of drugs—particularly stimulants, GHB, dissociatives such as ketamine, nitrite poppers, and empathogens like MDMA, which all reduce inhibitions and enhance sexual experience.[27] More recently, the British term "chemsex" has been gaining currency both in LGBTQ slang and in public health discourses.[51] (See further discussion of this in Chapter 53 "Compulsive Sexual Behaviors".) This practice is doubly problematic. First, the decreased inhibitions and increased stamina (with stimulants) may predispose to sexual behaviors with high risks for HIV and other STIs.[52] Second, the incorporation of drug-altered consciousness with intense sexual experiences can be powerful and mutually reinforcing. Powerful emotional linkages among drug use, sex, and experience of community can complicate efforts to become substance abstinent. Sexual or emotional intimacy may trigger drug use, and there may be no opportunities for drug-free experiences of similarly intense emotional connections. There is a robust association between sexualized use of methamphetamine, amphetamine, ecstasy, cocaine and/or poppers, and increased HIV incidence.[53,54] Subjectively, many users of stimulants, club drugs, and poppers report increased libido, decreased anxiety, and increased sexual pleasure (including access to extreme sexual behaviors) that are only possible when using these drugs. Some users report increased anxiety, while chronic use can cause erectile dysfunction.[55]

In the following, we list substances alphabetically (see also **Table 42-1**). We devote more space to several substances that are more commonly used among LGBTQ persons (alkyl nitrites, pro-erectile drugs, and sex hormones), and refer readers to the specific chapters in this volume for general information on presentation and management of other intoxicating substances.

Specifics about pharmacology of these various drug classes can be found in section 2 of this textbook.

Alcohol

Alcohol is embedded in many social interactions, and it has particular significance in some LGBTQ subcultures. It remains to be seen how the decline of brick-and-mortar LGBTQ bars and nightclubs, and their partial replacement by dating apps, will affect socialization of LGBTQ persons around alcohol consumption for cohorts born since the 1990s. LGBTQ individuals consume alcohol and engage in heavy drinking at higher rates,[56] although more recent data suggest that rates of heavy drinking may be similar for some LGBTQ groups as non-LGBTQ persons.[17] While alcohol use has decreased among U.S. teens and young adults since the 2000s, LGBTQ teens continue to consume more than their non-LGBTQ peers.[57]

TABLE 42-1 Substance Use by Specific LGBTQ Populations

Substance	LGBTQ population	Notes
Alcohol	All LGBTQ groups	As a group, higher alcohol consumption; lesbian and bisexual women at higher risk for alcohol use disorder; transgender men and women, and nonbinary persons, likely also at higher risk
Alkyl nitrite "poppers"	MSM, transgender persons with male partners	Much more likely to use poppers than any other population. Used to enhance sexual experiences
Amphetamine-type stimulants: methamphetamine	MSM, transgender women	Used at circuit parties and to enhance sexual experiences. May also be used as part of survival sex work. Links with HIV, STIs among MSM and transgender persons with male partners
Cocaine	MSM	Links with HIV, STIs among MSM and transgender persons with male partners
Dissociatives: ketamine	MSM	Used at circuit parties and to enhance sexual experiences
Nicotine: cigarettes, vaping	All groups	LGBTQ groups slightly more likely to use than general population, particularly notable for LGBTQ youth
Pro-erectile drugs	MSM	Used to enhance sexual experiences and mitigate impact of other drugs on erectile function. May interact with other drugs to cause hypotension
Sex hormones	Transgender persons, MSM (bodybuilders)	Transgender persons may obtain these from illicit sources or use at supraphysiologic doses MSM may do the same to facilitate bodybuilding

Many surveys find that lesbian and bisexual (LB) women report greater consumption of alcohol and more binge drinking.[56] Data from the 2015 to 2019 National Survey on Drug Use and Health, found an intersectional effect: Black and Hispanic women who identified as lesbian or bisexual reported the highest prevalence of binge drinking (45.4% and 43.4%, respectively)—more than white LB women (35.7%) and much more than white heterosexual women (23%).[58] While the long-term effects of social stresses during the COVID-19 pandemic remain to be seen, early studies indicate that LGBTQ communities were more heavily impacted by psychosocial stressors; among other effects, greater increased alcohol consumption has been noted in LGBTQ persons during the pandemic.[59]

All studies of transgender persons are subject to significant methodological challenges; nonetheless, several good probability-sampling studies including the 2018 Global Drug Survey have found that transgender men, transgender women, and nonbinary persons were more likely than cisgender respondents to report heavy drinking or likely alcohol use disorder.[60] Experience of transphobic discrimination has been associated with increased binge-drinking.[61]

Alkyl Nitrites (Poppers)

Amyl nitrite is used medically to alleviate angina and to treat acute cyanide poisoning. It causes production of nitrous oxide (NO) in endothelial cells of blood vessels, acting as a local vasodilator. Initially produced in glass ampules that were broken or "popped" and the vapors inhaled, it became popular as a club drug among both heterosexual and LGBTQ club-goers during the 1970s. Since the end of the Disco era, poppers have been used predominantly by gay/bisexual men, with some studies finding up to a quarter of gay/bisexual men using poppers on a regular basis, compared to about 3% of the general population.[62]

Amyl nitrite has been illegal to sell without a prescription in the U.S. since 1988, but congeners including cyclohexyl nitrite, butyl nitrite, isobutyl nitrite, and isopropyl nitrite are sold over the counter in sex shops under a number of brand names as "room odorizer" or other euphemisms. Poppers are typically sold in small bottles of dark glass to slow the breakdown of the nitrites from exposure to light and are administered by inhaling or "sniffing" from the bottle. Subjective effects lasting a few minutes per inhalation include warmth, mild to substantial behavioral disinhibition, and relaxation of muscles including anal sphincter muscles, which explains their use as an adjunct to anal sex.[63] Use of poppers was once implicated as a specific risk factor for HIV/AIDS, but consensus now sees them primarily as a marker for other risk behaviors.[63]

Poppers can cause chemical burns if spilled or inhaled. Poppers can also trigger migraines and can temporarily impair erectile function. Poppers can cause clinically significant hemolysis or rupture of red blood cells in persons with a genetic condition called G6PD deficiency, more common in those with ancestry in the Mediterranean and sub-Saharan Africa, including about 10% of African Americans.[64] Although rare, visual changes ranging from temporary bright spots in the visual field (phosphenes) to permanent retinal damage have been reported with chronic use. A systematic review of 64 published cases found that one third of poppers-associated maculopathy appeared to be an acute reaction to one-time use, while most appeared related to chronic use.[65] Most of the reports were from Europe, and most affected individuals were middle-aged men (median age 38.7, SD = 10.5 years). Some of the cases appeared reversible with abstinence from poppers use. Rare case reports of oral ingestion or intravenous injection of poppers carry much more deleterious effects including methemoglobinemia.[66]

Amphetamine-Type Stimulants

Amphetamine, methamphetamine, and related drugs collectively called *amphetamine-type stimulants* (ATS) are synthetic substances that inhibit reuptake of dopamine and transport of dopamine into vesicles. These produce potent stimulant effects similar to cocaine, but typically with a longer duration. ATS can be snorted as a powder, smoked, inhaled in a freebase form (crystal methamphetamine), inserted anally ("booty bump"), or injected. Methamphetamine in particular has been associated with risky sexual behaviors.[67] It has displaced cocaine in many populations, including white and Latino gay/bisexual men, because its longer half-life (more than 9-12 hours) provides a much longer subjective effect from a single dose than for a similarly priced amount of cocaine.

Benzodiazepines and Other CNS Depressants

Benzodiazepines are used medically as sedatives, anxiolytics, and anticonvulsants. Benzodiazepines have amnestic effects, acutely preventing encoding of memory (contributing to "blackout" states).[68] Benzodiazepines have been used for their amnestic, sedating, and disinhibiting effects as date-rape drugs, surreptitiously slipped into a drink or given under false pretenses to make someone more likely to acquiesce to sexual intercourse or to forget it afterward. This is also known colloquially as "roofies" and in the public health literature as drug-facilitated sexual assault. Rates are unknown, as many cases likely go unreported.[69]

Cocaine

Cocaine is associated with significantly elevated rates of unprotected anal sex and heightened risks for HIV transmission among MSM.[70,71] Transgender women and MSM with DSM-IV–defined stimulant dependence may be motivated to exchange sex for drugs. In this situation, they may feel less able to insist on safer sex practices, particularly if they receive higher compensation for unprotected intercourse or are disinhibited while using or in withdrawal. Adherence to antiretroviral medications (ARV) for persons living with HIV is eroded, particularly for those who have multiple syndemic conditions.

Club Drugs/Empathogens

MDMA and relatives. MDMA, or 3,4 methylenedioxy-N-methamphetamine, is chemically related to amphetamine, has a short half-life (1-2 hours) and has distinct subjective effects, particularly empathogenic properties that facilitate subjective feelings of closeness to others, accounting for its popularity at circuit parties. Individuals taking MDMA in the context of a circuit party may experience dehydration (related to continued dancing or moving about without rehydrating), hyponatremia (from excessive water intake because of fear of dehydration, without repleting electrolytes), bruxism (grinding teeth), and sexual disinhibition (with corresponding incident HIV/STIs). In practice, what is sold as "Ecstasy," "E", or "Molly," may contain anything from caffeine to methamphetamine or fentanyl.[72]

Dissociatives

Ketamine ("K," "Special K") is a synthetic chemical that is used medically (and in veterinary medicine) as a dissociative anesthetic and recently has been investigated for use in treatment-resistant depression.[73] Ketamine is commonly used in the circuit party and rave scenes. Subjective effects last about an hour and may include derealization or hallucinations at higher doses, sometimes called a "K-hole." Other potential side effects include abdominal cramps ("K-cramps"). Heavy chronic use is associated with a potentially irreversible inflammation of the bladder and urinary tract (ketamine cystitis).[74] Ketamine can be insufflated or injected intravenously. Ketamine popularity shifts over time and has been particularly associated with MSM as a club drug.

GHB

Commonly included among club drugs, γ-hydroxy-butyrate or GHB ("G", "liquid Ecstasy") occurs naturally in the body as a neurotransmitter. It acts on specific GHB receptors and has indirect effects at $GABA_B$ receptors.[75] GHB has an unusual legal status in the United States: it is classified as Schedule I—unless it is prescribed to treat narcolepsy, in which case it is Schedule III. Metabolic precursors of GHB such as γ-butyrolactone (GBL) and 1,4-butanediol may be purchased over the internet as nutritional supplements. Bodybuilders and gay/bisexual men involved in the gym culture sometimes take GHB or its precursors in hopes of enhancing muscle mass, as it increases endogenous release of human growth hormone. GHB has also been used by gay/bisexual men at circuit parties and to enhance sexual experiences, reportedly by decreasing inhibitions. Physical tolerance and dependence can develop rapidly, with potential for seizures during withdrawal; it is easy to overdose on GHB as concentrations in illicit supplies are hard to estimate, and it acts synergistically with other CNS depressants.[76] GHB has also been implicated in drug-facilitated sexual assault due to its CNS depressant effects, erosion of retrograde memory, and very brief window of detection in urine. Intoxication with GHB or its prodrugs has a non-specific presentation similar to intoxication with alcohol or central nervous system depressants. GHB is also commonly used along with other intoxicants, which complicates diagnosis. We recommend the following review[77] and the relevant chapters in this volume for specifics of diagnosis and management.

Nicotine and Tobacco Products

LGBTQ individuals are more likely to use tobacco and nicotine products.[78] LGBTQ communities have been specifically targeted in tobacco advertising, contributing to these higher rates.[79] National survey data from 2016 to 2019 found that 13% of LGBTQ respondents reported using e-cigarettes, roughly double the rate of non-LGBTQ adults.[80] LGBTQ youth are more likely than non-LGBTQ peers to smoke cigarettes or use nicotine products; LB women appear to do so at the highest rates.[81]

Pro-Erectile Drugs

Sildenafil, tadalafil, and vardenafil act by inhibiting phosphodiesterase-type 5 (PDE5) and thereby increasing blood flow, which can enhance erectile function in males. Among gay/bisexual men in particular, PDE5 inhibitors have been used to overcome the adverse effects of stimulants or other drug use on male erections. They are frequently integrated with stimulant use among MSM in order to ensure erectile function during long sex sessions. One study found that 49% of MSM surveyed in nightclubs in London had used PDE5 inhibitors during the previous year.[82] This practice has been implicated in risk behavior for HIV and other STIs, by promoting continuing sexual activity while in a disinhibited state.[83]

PDE5 inhibitors were initially developed to lower blood pressure. They can have life-threatening interactions if combined with some other antihypertensives, particularly nitroglycerin and related medications. Based on this, there have been warnings about the potential risk of combining PDE5 inhibitors with nitrite poppers; however, there are no published case reports of deaths due to this combination. The actual risk of combining nitrite poppers with PDE5 inhibitors is unclear.

Other substances may also be used to promote erectile function, including a number of traditional herbal remedies: yohimbine (*Pausinystalia johimbe*), horny goat weed (*Epimedium* species), and maca (*Lepidium meyenii*).[84] Several, including horny goat weed, have PDE5 inhibitor activity in vitro, though less potent than prescription PDE5 inhibitors and of unclear efficacy. Accuracy of labeling and purity of herbal remedies is questionable: some do not contain the plants they claim to contain, and one study found up to 61% of herbal sexual enhancing remedies contained illicit prescription-controlled medications, including PDE5 inhibitors.[85] It is consequently difficult to predict potential drug-drug interactions. These substances are not unique to LGBTQ consumers, but they may be used by LGBTQ patients, particularly in the context of other sexualized drug use.

Sex Hormones

Sex hormones are natural or synthetic androgens (testosterone and other male hormones), estrogens, and progesterones, taken to enhance or alter secondary sexual physiognomy and sexual function. All sex hormones are steroids. Estrogens and progesterone are readily available in pill forms, often as oral contraceptives. Testosterone can be administered in a topical gel or as either depot or immediate-release injections.[86] Use of injected sex hormones carries the same risks of other injection drugs if needles are shared or reused: transmission of blood-borne pathogens like HIV and viral hepatitis, or local infections with skin flora such as MRSA.[87]

Exogenously administered sex hormones have four main uses in an LGBTQ context: androgen supplementation for treatment of HIV-related hypogonadism and wasting in men; attempts by gay/bisexual men to gain a more muscular physique from bodybuilding with anabolic steroids; use by transgender women or nonbinary persons to achieve or maintain female secondary sexual characteristics; and use by transgender men or nonbinary persons to achieve or maintain male secondary sexual characteristics.

Androgen Supplementation: Hypogonadism and Bodybuilding

Deleterious effects of exogenous androgens include acne, cholestatic jaundice, dyslipidemia (particularly increased LDL), gynecomastia, testicular atrophy, mood instability,[88] increased hemoglobin levels with potential increase in risk of blood clots, and other cardiovascular problems.[89] Prevalence rates of these deleterious effects of 5.2% to 15.2% have been cited,[90] with one study finding a lifetime prevalence rate of 21% among gay/bisexual adolescents.[91] A large cross-sectional survey examining anabolic androgen supplementation use in gay/bisexual men in Australia and New Zealand found that the highest predictor of use related to those individuals experiencing eating disorder symptoms.[92]

Hormone Supplementation in Transgender Persons

Transgender women may take estrogen, sometimes with progesterone and/or antiandrogens as part of the process of feminizing their physical characteristics to better match their gender identity. For reasons of cost or difficulty in accessing medical care, some purchase these over the internet or other illicit sources, often in the form of oral contraceptives. In the presence of functioning testes, transgender women may take estrogens up to several times normal physiologic doses. Estrogens promote blood clotting and may raise the risk of stroke, myocardial infarction, and pulmonary embolism. This is greatly exacerbated in people who smoke tobacco.[93]

Transgender men and nonbinary persons may take testosterone ("T") as part of the process of masculinizing their bodies to match their gender identity. In addition to the virilizing effects (lowering voice, growing body and facial hair in a male pattern, amenorrhea, and increasing muscle mass), exogenous androgens can cause the effects noted above, including male pattern baldness, acne, and mood swings.[93] Transgender persons who no longer have functioning ovaries or testes—whether due to surgical removal or the effects of exogenous hormones—need to take lifelong sex hormone supplementation. This is not only to maintain their appearance in matching their gender identity but also to protect against loss of muscle mass, cardiac problems, and osteoporosis. It is important that their care be managed by competent clinicians because of the sometimes complex and unique health issues faced by transgender persons.[93]

The nonprescription use of hormones in transgender individuals is poorly characterized. Transfeminine individuals appear more likely than transmasculine individuals to obtain nonprescribed hormones for the purposes of gender affirming effects.[94,95] Factors that have been linked to nonprescribed hormone use include younger age,[96,97] lower education,[98] homelessness,[98] Black/African American individuals,[96] and persons with sex work as a main source of income.[96,97] Nonprescription use of hormones may be more common in individuals living with HIV.[94] Some of the reasons for obtaining nonprescribed sex hormones cited include lack of access to health care, long wait times to get established into care, and discrimination.[99] Sources of these hormones primarily include the internet, friends, and other community members. Risks involved with unsupervised usage of nonprescribed hormones include receiving unsafe or counterfeit products, improper injection administration, and lack of knowledge regarding side effects.[95,99] Further research is needed.

WHAT TO DO? EVIDENCE-SUPPORTED RECOMMENDATIONS FOR CLINICIANS

Other chapters of this volume address evidence-based best practices for treatment of particular substances, as well as ASAM consensus criteria to match patient needs with appropriate levels of care for SUD treatment. In this section, we review some evidence-based treatments and treatment considerations specifically tailored for LGBTQ patients.

Screening, Brief Intervention, Referral to Treatment (SBIRT)

The most important step in addressing substance use in patients in general care settings is simply to ask about it. An emerging consensus advises primary care and mental health providers to incorporate assessment of substance use behaviors into their practice at regular intervals. Normalizing inquiries about substance use as part of ongoing basic health assessment reduces potential defensiveness on the part of the patient and recognizes that substance use is common. Periodic reassessment is useful, and it is helpful to be mindful of higher prevalence of substance among LGBTQ individuals when interpreting self-reports in SBIRT assessments. Recognizing this with patients may lead to more comfortable discussions regarding substance use, as they develop a relationship with a provider. Patterns of substance use also change over time.

Treatment

Referring LGBTQ individuals to treatment raises challenges, as most patients prefer culturally competent clinicians and agencies that not only deliver evidence-based treatments but also recognize LGBTQ-specific concerns. Mainstream health care clinicians rarely discuss issues related to sexual identity with their LGBTQ clients, nor do they discuss concerns related to legal and family issues that can impact treatment, including same-sex marriage (and divorce), power of attorney, or relationships with family of origin. In both U.S.-based and international studies, many LGBTQ individuals report experience of discriminatory attitudes in health care settings generally[100] and report avoiding or delaying seeking health care services out of concern for this.[3,101] Finally, few agencies outside major cities provide specialized addiction treatment services for LGBTQ clients.

Pharmacotherapies

Choice of pharmaceutical interventions and dosing are not generally affected by sexual orientation and sexual identity; however, anatomy and hormonal status may need to be considered when selecting regimens for transgender persons, and medication interactions need to be considered when prescribing for persons taking medication for treatment or prevention of HIV. Some medications have different dosing recommendations for cisgender women compared to cisgender men, and differences have been noted in volume of distribution, rates of oral absorption and of both renal and hepatic drug clearance, and expression of some receptors.[102] Most medications have not been adequately studied specifically in transgender persons, and information is particularly lacking to guide care for persons in early stages of hormonal therapy, or taking intermediate hormonal regimens, such as a nonbinary person taking a low dose of testosterone. One review of pharmacologic studies finds that after 6 months of gender-affirming hormone therapy (GAHT), dosing should be based on creatinine clearance (CLcr) and ideal body weight (IBW) as calculated for their gender identity; with less than 6 months of GAHT, consider making calculations based on sex as assigned at birth.[102]

For patients taking ARVs to treat or prevent HIV, remember that many ARV regimens include one or more medications that affect hepatic metabolism, in order to slow the clearance of the ARVs and allow for once-daily dosing. This effect may raise or lower levels of other medications. Older persons living with HIV are more likely to have lower baseline renal function, more polypharmacy, and more health comorbidities, and may be even more vulnerable; also, women living with HIV experience more problems from inappropriate prescribing, possibly due to higher rates of anxiety, depression, renal impairment, and lower bone density.[103]

Methadone metabolism is complex, with a very long half-life and risk of respiratory depression, QT prolongation, and seizures at higher doses or interacting with other drugs.[104] Methadone has many interactions with other drugs, too numerous to list here. This is one reason it should only be managed by a methadone specialist. Prescribers should check potential interactions for any patients taking methadone. Ritonavir/atazanavir and delavirdine may increase levels of buprenorphine but may not lead to withdrawal symptoms.[104] Conversely efavirenz and etravirine may decrease buprenorphine levels.[105] Lenacapavir, a capsid inhibitor, is a relatively new medication used as a long-acting injectable treatment for HIV and is currently under investigation for use as long-acting PrEP. It is a moderate CYP3A4 inhibitor and may increase levels of buprenorphine, methadone, or other opioids.[106]

We note as well that ritonavir, which is included in many ARV regimens due to its inhibition of CYP2D6 metabolism, has potential interactions with many medications and some illegal drugs. In particular, unexpected overdoses have been documented in individuals taking GHB or MDMA while on ritonavir; it also increases levels of alprazolam.[104] Conversely, naltrexone, commonly used for both alcohol use disorder and opioid use disorder, does not appear to have clinically significant drug interactions with antiretrovirals; naltrexone does have a boxed warning for possible hepatoxicity and should not be in used in patients with severe hepatic dysfunction.[107] Bupropion, prescribed for nicotine use disorder and used off-label for stimulant use disorders, may be decreased with ritonavir, nelfinavir, and efavirenz due to CYP2B6 interactions.[108] ARVs including ritonavir, nelfinavir, and efavirenz can increase bupropion levels by inhibiting CYP2B6, with theoretical risk of seizures.[109] We recommend as best practice always checking drug-drug interactions when prescribing for persons on ARVs.

Pharmacotherapies are approved by the FDA for treatment of alcohol, nicotine, and opioid use disorders, as noted in the relevant chapters in this volume. There are no FDA-approved pharmacologic treatments for stimulant, cannabis, or hallucinogen use disorders. Most pharmacotherapies have not been studied specifically in LGBTQ populations. We review some of the exceptions here.

There has been progress in pharmacotherapies for stimulant use disorders, which merits special mention given the strong link between stimulant use, stimulant use disorder, chemsex and corresponding infectious diseases among MSM and transgender individuals. Two RCTs showed reduction in methamphetamine use and in concomitant high-risk sexual behaviors compared to placebo for gay/bisexual men and transgender women in San Francisco treated with mirtazapine 30 mgs daily,[110,111] with number needed to treat (NNT) = 8 at 12 weeks.[111] For MSM and heterosexual individuals with methamphetamine use disorder, a large (N = 403) 12-week randomized controlled trial showed combination of long-acting injectable naltrexone every 3 weeks plus daily bupropion 450 mg/day significantly reduced methamphetamine use over placebo; the NNT was nine.[112] A similar signal was seen for cocaine use disorder in two 12-week RCTs evaluating combined extended-release mixed amphetamine salts (ER-MAS) 60 mg/day plus topiramate 200 mg/day.[113,114] A dose-response finding for ER-MAS (0 mg, 60 mg, 80 mg) as measured by positive urine test results over 12 weeks was shown for persons with cocaine use disorder and cooccurring Adult Attention Deficit Hyperactivity Disorder (ADHD).[115] While these studies have not yet resulted in FDA approval for treatment indications for stimulant use disorders, they are encouraging developments in what otherwise has been a long series of negative results.

Behavioral Therapies

Evidence-based behavioral therapies for treating SUD are from three broad areas: cognitive-behavioral therapy (CBT), contingency management (CM), and motivational interviewing (MI); these are not specific to LGBTQ populations. Other behavioral approaches such as mindfulness have also shown some benefit.[116] Integrating behavioral interventions with efficacious pharmacotherapies bring potential for maximizing both treatment efficacy. Behavioral interventions with efficacy comprise individual and group psychotherapies as well as support groups and are effective alone or can enhance efficacy of pharmacologic interventions.

Cognitive-Behavioral Therapy

CBT approaches are didactic, teaching skills and information necessary to initiate abstinence and prevent relapse. Techniques are closely related to CBT used for major depressive disorder. Meta-analyses show CBT has small but significant effects in reducing substance use compared to standard of care.[117] CBT shows few effects when compared to low-intensity interventions for amphetamine-dependent individuals, but substantial benefit when compared to high-intensity interventions among gay/bisexual men.[118] CBT requires trained therapists when delivering the intervention. The model is easily adapted to incorporate cultural or behavioral specifics that can enhance acceptability. One example of this is "Getting Off," a behavioral intervention for gay/bisexual men who use methamphetamine.[119] The adaptation of this model began with a mainstream CBT approach to DSM-IV defined stimulant dependence, the Matrix Model. Using a consultative approach, it was tailored it to arrive at a manual that retained key CBT elements while integrating cultural and behavioral referents to enhance its acceptability. This treatment approach addresses links among methamphetamine use, concomitant sexual risk behaviors, and HIV. Effects show a roughly 50% reduction in the number of days of methamphetamine use up to one year, along with comparable reductions in use of alcohol and cannabis, and reduction in sexual risk behaviors.[120]

Motivational Interviewing

MI is a client-centered, directive approach to treatment that helps clinicians identify the factors that work for ("pros") and against ("cons") continued substance use.[121] Techniques to deliver MI include OARS-E: open-ended questions, affirmations, reflective listening, summarizing, and eliciting "change talk" (client statements that recognize the need for change). In meta-analyses, MI produced 29% reduction in substance use compared to standard care.[122] Meta-analyses of applications of MI to substance use problems among gay/bisexual men, however, showed no consistent findings.[123]

Contingency Management

CM is based on operant conditioning. Clients earn increasingly valuable reinforcements with consecutive biological samples (such as urine drug screens) that document abstinence. It remains one of the most effective forms of treatment for cocaine and amphetamine use disorders; meta-analyses show that contingency management has an effect size of about 0.6 (ie, is 60% better) compared to usual treatments.[124] CM can be easily incorporated with other standard substance use therapies, including CBT and most recently with efficacious stimulant medications.

Contingency management has been used with gay/bisexual males with DSM-IV defined methamphetamine dependence, alone and in combination with CBT, to significantly reduce drug use at one-year follow-up evaluations.[119] Lower cost CM treatments also are effective for treating methamphetamine dependence among gay/bisexual men.[125] There also appear to be limits for contingency management solely as a treatment for SUD, as it shows no significant effects when implemented in public health settings in nontreatment-seeking, stimulant-using gay/bisexual men.[126]

MITIGATING RISK OF HIV AND STIs: PrEP, TasP, AND EMERGING TECHNOLOGIES

SUDs can increase risks for contracting HIV or other STIs through a variety of means. Substance use can increase impulsivity, lower inhibitions, and increase the likelihood of engaging in sexual intercourse without barrier methods of protection (such as condoms). Persons with SUD may engage in survival sex work or exchange sex for drugs, during which they may be less able to protect themselves from HIV and STIs. For persons living with HIV, SUD can also interfere with adherence to their antiviral medications and with consistent attendance at medical appointments, potentially compromising their ability to maintain viral suppression. Injection drug use can also transmit HIV, viral hepatitis, and other infections. These risks are all increased for LGBTQ persons, particularly for sexual transmission for MSM and for transgender persons with male partners. Assessing these risks and attempting to mitigate them appropriately fall within the scope of addiction medicine practice.

Fortunately, medical interventions to reduce risk of HIV transmission have advanced substantially since the 2000s. Several medications have now been approved by the U.S. FDA and in multiple other countries for use as PrEP. A combination pill containing tenofovir disoproxil fumarate (TDF) and emtricitabine (FTC) and a related medication containing FTC and tenofovir alafenamide (TAF) are both used as a daily preventive medication. TDF/FTC has also shown benefit when taken "on demand," or "event-based dosing," operationalized as two pills on the day of potential exposure through sexual intercourse, and one pill daily up to 72 hours after the last potential exposure.[127] Oral preexposure prophylaxis for HIV (PrEP) has demonstrated efficacy in greatly reducing the risk of contracting HIV for MSM and for persons sharing needles used to inject drugs.[128] More recently, long-acting injectable (LAI) cabotegravir has also demonstrated efficacy as PrEP in both MSM and transgender women.[129] Note that long-acting cabotegravir is also used for HIV treatment, but with a different dose and schedule. Cabotegravir is injected every 2 months at a dose of 600 mg for prevention,[130] and every month at a dose of 600 mg (plus injection of 900 mg rilpivirine) as treatment for persons living with HIV.[130] Other longer-acting formulations of PrEP are actively under investigation. Long-acting formulations for PrEP (and for treatment) may be particularly helpful for persons with SUD, unstable housing, or who live in situations where they may be at risk if others find out they are taking a medication used to treat or prevent a stigmatized condition like HIV.

Clinical trials of PrEP in cisgender women with male partners have been less successful, for several reasons, a point of most relevance to bisexual women. Adherence, as measured by blood levels of medication, has been much lower in trials with cisgender women. Anatomy plays a role: FTC/TDF reaches peak levels in rectal tissue within seven days, while it takes 21 days of consistent dosing to reach peak levels in vaginal tissue.[131] Transgender women were included in some of the early trials that focused on PrEP in MSM, and have been explicitly recruited for participation in more recent trials, some of which also actively include transgender men. Studies of PrEP in transgender persons have found that estrogens have minor drug-drug interactions, slightly lowering levels of tenofovir/emtricitibine, though these remained at levels expected to be effective; no drug-drug interactions were found in transgender men taking testosterone.[132]

Complementary to PrEP is postexposure prophylaxis (PEP), which is the practice of taking certain ARVs within 72 hours after a potential exposure to HIV and for 30 days after. Specific guidelines vary by country, based on patterns of viral resistance prevalence and estimates of cost-effectiveness. The United States Centers for Disease Control and Prevention (CDC) maintains a website (https://www.cdc.gov/hiv/risk/pep/index.html) and hotline (+1-888-448-4911) for clinicians to guide PEP prescribing. Treatment as prevention (TasP), is the practice of connecting individuals to HIV care and initiating treatment with ARVs as soon as possible after diagnosis with HIV; this has been found to greatly reduce potential transmission of HIV, with a slogan "Undetectable = Untransmittable" (U = U).[133,134]

CONCLUSIONS

LGBTQ people with at-risk substance use or with frank SUD face multiple challenges to finding culturally competent, high-quality treatment services to meet their substance use goals. At the level of the patient, experiences with both implicit and explicit discrimination, homophobia, and transphobia interfere with seeking formal treatment services. At the level of the clinic, there are few clinicians who are culturally competent in understanding the unique space that substance use occupies in the communities of LGBTQ persons.

At the same time, the emergence of pharmacotherapies for psychostimulant use disorders offers exciting new potential for integrating treatments with effective behavioral treatments to help LGBTQ patients to meet their substance use goals. PrEP, PEP, and TasP provide powerful tools to reduce risk of HIV transmission. Treatment materials specifically designed to address key cultural issues faced by gay and bisexual men when reducing or stopping their substance use are available and have demonstrated efficacy. The availability of clinicians with LGBTQ expertise, the interests of LGBTQ clinicians, and the recognition of multiple identities (ie, sexual orientation, gender, racial/ethnic) are encouraging factors that emerged over the past 10 years and offer real opportunities for those seeking care. What remains to be done is to scale-up use of efficacious and culturally adapted treatments for LGBTQ patients and lower barriers to accessing these treatments in traditional health care settings.

SELECT LGBTQ DOCUMENTARIES FOR FURTHER VIEWING

- *A Place to Live: The Story of Triangle Square*. Directed by Carolyn Coal. Elder Housing Project; 2008. Available via streaming on Tubitv.com: https://tubitv.com/movies/500808/a-place-to-live-the-story-of-triangle-square. Documentary about several LGBTQ seniors trying to get into supported housing in Los Angeles, with reflections on their diverse life experiences during the 20th century.
- *Gen Silent*. Directed by Stu Maddox. Performance by Lois Johnson. Interrobang Productions; 2011. https://pluto.tv/en/on-demand/movies/gensilent-2011-1-1. Documentary about LGBTQ older adults in Boston facing challenges in accessing medical and housing services.
- *How to Survive a Plague*. Directed by David France. Performances by Larry Kramer, Peter Staley, Iris Long, Bill Bahlman, David Barr. IFC Independent Film; 2012. Academy Award®-nominated documentary about LGBTQ activism in the response to the HIV/AIDS epidemic. Available from multiple streaming sites.
- *Paris Is Burning*. Directed by Jennie Livingston. Distributed by Miramax; 1991. https://www.amazon.com/Paris-Burning-Jennie-Livingston/dp/B007L739EE/. Documentary about African American and Latinx drag queens and transgender women in the "house and ball" scene in late 1980s New York City.
- *Pray Away*. Directed by Kristine Stolakis. Multitude Films; 2021. Streaming on Netflix. Documentary about the ex-gay movement and the harms of sexual orientation and gender identity conversion therapy.

REFERENCES

1. Spitzer RL. The diagnostic status of homosexuality in DSM-III: a reformulation of the issues. *Am J Psychiatry*. 1981;138(2):210-214.
2. Shilts R. *And the Band Played On: Politics, People, and the AIDS Epidemic*. St. Martin's Press; 1987.
3. Mirza SA, Rooney C. *Discrimination Prevents LGBTQ People from Accessing Health Care*. Center for American Progress; 2018.
4. Casey LS, Reisner SL, Findling MG, et al. Discrimination in the United States: Experiences of lesbian, gay, bisexual, transgender, and queer Americans. *Health Serv Res*. 2019;54(Suppl 2):1454-1466.
5. Hammack PL, Toolis EE, Wilson BDM, Clark RC, Frost DM. Making meaning of the impact of pre-exposure prophylaxis (prep) on public health and sexual culture: narratives of three generations of gay and bisexual men. *Arch Sex Behav*. 2019;48(4):1041-1058.
6. Kennedy EL, Davis MD. *Boots of Leather, Slippers of Gold: The History of a Lesbian Community*. Routledge; 1993.
7. Malebranche DJ. Bisexually active Black men in the United States and HIV: acknowledging more than the "Down Low". *Arch Sex Behav*. 2008;37(5):810-816.
8. Dolezal C, Carballo-Dieguez A, Nieves-Rosa L, Diaz F. Substance use and sexual risk behavior: understanding their association among four ethnic groups of Latino men who have sex with men. *J Subst Abuse*. 2000;11(4):323-336.
9. Gray M. *Out in the Country: Youth, Media, and Queer Visibility in Rural America*. New York University Press; 2009.
10. Gideonse TK. Survival tactics and strategies of methamphetamine-using hiv-positive men who have sex with men in San Diego. *PloS One*. 2015;10(9):e0139239.
11. Schnarrs PW, Jones SS, Parsons JT, et al. Sexual subcultures and hiv prevention methods: an assessment of condom use, PrEP, and TasP among gay, bisexual, and other men who have sex with men using a social and sexual networking smartphone application. *Arch Sex Behav*. 2021;50(4):1781-1792.
12. National Academies of Sciences, Engineering and Medicine. *Measuring Sex, Gender Identity, and Sexual Orientation*. National Academies Press; 2022.
13. Chang CT, Thum CC, Lim XJ, Chew CC, Rajan P. Monkeypox outbreak: preventing another episode of stigmatisation. *Trop Med Int Health*. 2022;27(9):754-757.
14. Yarbrough E. *Transgender Mental Health*. American Psychiatric Association Publishing; 2018.
15. Lemma A. *Transgender Identities: A Contemporary Introduction*. Routledge; 2022.
16. Young R, Meyer I. The trouble with "MSM" and "WSW": erasure of the sexual-minority person in public health discourse. *Am J Public Health*. 2005;95(7):1144-1149.
17. Compton WM, Jones CM. Substance use among men who have sex with men. *N Engl J Med*. 2021;385(4):352-356.
18. Bostwick WB, Dodge B. Introduction to the special section on bisexual health: can you see us now? *Arch Sex Behav*. 2019;48(1):79-87.
19. Boyd CJ, Veliz PT, Stephenson R, Hughes TL, McCabe SE. Severity of alcohol, tobacco, and drug use disorders among sexual minority individuals and their "not sure" counterparts. *LGBT Health*. 2019;6(1):15-22.
20. Hammack PL, Frost DM, Hughes SD. Queer intimacies: a new paradigm for the study of relationship diversity. *J Sex Res*. 2019;56(4-5):556-592.
21. Newcomb ME, Hill R, Buehler K, Ryan DT, Whitton SW, Mustanski B. High burden of mental health problems, substance use, violence, and related psychosocial factors in transgender, non-binary, and gender diverse youth and young adults. *Arch Sex Behav*. 2020;49(2):645-659.
22. American Psychological Association. Guidelines for psychological practice with transgender and gender nonconforming people. *Am Psychol*. 2015;70(9):832-864.
23. Boellstorff T. But do not identify as gay: a proleptic genealogy of the MSM category. *Curr Anthropol*. 2011;26(2):287-312.
24. Norton R. *Mother Clap's Molly House: The Gay Subculture in England, 1700-1830*. GMP; 1992.
25. Chauncey G. *Gay New York: Gender, Urban Culture, and the Making of the Gay Male World, 1890-1940*. Basic Books; 1994.

26. Read K. *Other Voices: The Style of a Male Homosexual Tavern.* Chandler & Sharp; 1980.
27. Race K. *Pleasure Consuming Medicine: The Queer Politics of Drugs.* Duke University Press; 2009.
28. Durbin A. At the Gay Bar. *London Review of Books.* 2022;44(1).
29. Gideonse TK. Pride, shame, and the trouble with trying to be normal. *Ethos.* 2015;43(4):332-352.
30. Newton E. *Cherry Grove, Fire Island: Sixty Years in America's First Gay and Lesbian Town.* Beacon Press; 1993.
31. Hall TM, Shoptaw S, Reback CJ. Sometimes poppers are not poppers: huffing as an emergent health concern among MSM substance users. *J Gay Lesbian Ment Health.* 2014;19(1):118-121.
32. Cochran S, Grella C, Mays V. Do substance use norms and perceived drug availability mediate sexual orientation differences in patterns of substance use? Results from the California Quality of Life Survey II. *J Stud Alcohol Drugs.* 2012;73(4):675-685.
33. Singer M. *Introducing Syndemics: A Critical Systems Approach to Public and Community Health.* Wiley; 2009.
34. Tran NM, Henkhaus LE, Gonzales G. Adverse childhood experiences and mental distress among US adults by sexual orientation. *JAMA Psychiatry.* 2022;79(4):377-379.
35. Stall R, Friedman M, Catania JA. Intersecting epidemics and gay men's health: a theory of syndemic production among urban gay men. In: Richard J, Wolitski RS, Valdeserri RO, eds. *Unequal Opportunity: Health Disparities Affecting Gay and Bisexual Men in the United States.* Oxford University Press; 2008:251-274.
36. Dyer TP, Shoptaw S, Guadamuz TE, et al. Application of syndemic theory to black men who have sex with men in the Multicenter AIDS Cohort Study. *J Urban Health.* 2012;89(4):697-708.
37. Mericle AA, Carrico AW, Hemberg J, de Guzman R, Stall R. Several common bonds: addressing the needs of gay and bisexual men in LGBT-specific recovery housing. *J Homosex.* 2020;67(6):793-815.
38. Sabin JA, Riskind RG, Nosek BA. Health care providers' implicit and explicit attitudes toward lesbian women and gay men. *Am J Public Health.* 2015;105(9):1831-1841.
39. Herrick AL, Lim SH, Wei C, et al. Resilience as an untapped resource in behavioral intervention design for gay men. *AIDS Behav.* 2011;15(Suppl 1):S25-S29.
40. D'Augelli AR. *Identity Development And Sexual Orientation: Toward a Model Of Lesbian, Gay, and Bisexual Development.* Jossey-Bass; 1994.
41. Nardi PM. *Gay Men's Friendships: Invincible Communities.* University of Chicago Press; 1999.
42. Cohler BJ, Galatzer-Levy RM. *The Course of Gay and Lesbian Lives: Social and Psychoanalytic Perspectives.* University of Chicago Press; 2000.
43. Savin-Williams RC. A critique of research on sexual-minority youths. *J Adolesc.* 2001;24(1):5-13.
44. Grierson J, Smith AMA. In from the outer: generational differences in coming out and gay identity formation. *J Homosex.* 2005;50(1):53-70.
45. Hall TM. Stories from the Second World: narratives of sexual identity across three generations of Czech men who have sex with men. In: Cohler BJ, Hammack PL, eds. *The Story Of Sexual Identity: Narrative Perspectives on the Gay and Lesbian Life Course.* Oxford University Press; 2009:77-130.
46. Weston K. *Families We Choose: Lesbians, Gays, Kinship.* Columbia University Press; 1991.
47. Lewes K. *Psychoanalysis and Male Homosexuality.* 20th anniversary ed. J. Aronson; 2009.
48. Bux DA. The epidemiology of problem drinking in gay men and lesbians: a critical review. *Clin Psychol Rev.* 1996;16(4):277-298.
49. Green KE, Feinstein BA. Substance use in lesbian, gay and bisexual populations: an update on empirical research and implications for treatment. *Psychol Addict Behav.* 2012;26(2):265-278.
50. National Academies of Sciences, Engineering, and Medicine. *Understanding the Well-Being of LGBTQI+ Populations.* National Academies Press; 2020.
51. Edmundson C, Heinsbroek E, Glass R, et al. Sexualised drug use in the United Kingdom (UK): a review of the literature. *Int J Drug Policy.* 2018;55:131-148.
52. Frosch D, Shoptaw S, Huber A, Rawson RA, Ling W. Sexual HIV risk among gay and bisexual male methamphetamine abusers. *J Subst Abuse Treat.* 1996;13(6):483-486.
53. Plankey MW, Ostrow DG, Stall R, et al. The relationship between methamphetamine and popper use and risk of HIV seroconversion in the multicenter AIDS cohort study. *J Acquir Immune Defic Syndr.* 2007;45(1):85-92.
54. Koblin BA, Husnik MJ, Colfax G, et al. Risk factors for HIV infection among men who have sex with men. *AIDS.* 2006;20:731-739.
55. Reback CJ. *The Social Construction of a Gay Drug: Methamphetamine Use Among Gay & Bisexual Males in Los Angeles.* Report for the City of Los Angeles; 1997.
56. Drabble LA, Mericle AA, Karriker-Jaffe KJ, Trocki KF. Harmful drinking, tobacco, and marijuana use in the 2000-2015 National Alcohol Surveys: Examining differential trends by sexual identity. *Subst Abus.* 2021;42(3):317-328.
57. Phillips Ii G, Turner B, Felt D, Han Y, Marro R, Beach LB. Trends in alcohol use behaviors by sexual identity and behavior among high school students, 2007-2017. *J Adolesc Health.* 2019;65(6):760-768.
58. Greene N, Jackson JW, Dean LT. Examining disparities in excessive alcohol use among black and hispanic lesbian and bisexual women in the United States: an intersectional analysis. *J Stud Alcohol Drugs.* 2020;81(4):462-470.
59. Akré ER, Anderson A, Stojanovski K, Chung KW, VanKim NA, Chae DH. Depression, anxiety, and alcohol use among LGBTQ+ people during the COVID-19 pandemic. *Am J Public Health.* 2021;111(9):1610-1619.
60. Connolly DJ, Davies E, Lynskey M, et al. Differences in alcohol and other drug use and dependence between transgender and cisgender participants from the 2018 Global Drug Survey. *LGBT Health.* 2022;9(8):534-542.
61. Kcomt L, Evans-Polce RJ, Boyd CJ, McCabe SE. Association of transphobic discrimination and alcohol misuse among transgender adults: results from the U.S. Transgender Survey. *Drug Alcohol Depend.* 2020;215:108223.
62. Le A, Yockey A, Palamar JJ. Use of "Poppers" among adults in the United States, 2015-2017. *J Psychoactive Drugs.* 2020;52(5):433-439.
63. Romanelli F, Smith KM, Thornton AC, Pomeroy C. Poppers: epidemiology and clinical management of inhaled nitrite abuse. *Pharmacotherapy.* 2004;24(1):69-78.
64. Nkhoma ET, Poole C, Vannappagari V, Hall SA, Beutler E. The global prevalence of glucose-6-phosphate dehydrogenase deficiency: a systematic review and meta-analysis. *Blood Cells, Mol Dis.* 2009;42(3):267-278.
65. Gonzalez-Martin-Moro J, Almagro EG, Abreu NV, Serrano FN. Poppers maculopathy: a quantitative review of previous literature. *Semin Ophthalmol.* 2022;37(3):391-398.
66. Reisinger A, Vogt S, Essl A, et al. Lessons of the month 3: intravenous poppers abuse: case report, management and possible complications. *Clin Med (Lond).* 2020;20(2):221-223.
67. Quinn B, Gorbach PM, Okafor CN, Heinzerling KG, Shoptaw S. Investigating possible syndemic relationships between structural and drug use factors, sexual HIV transmission and viral load among men of colour who have sex with men in Los Angeles County. *Drug Alcohol Rev.* 2020;39(2):116-127.
68. Fisher J, Hirshman E, Henthorn T, Arndt J, Passannante A. Midazolam amnesia and short-term/working memory processes. *Conscious Cogn.* 2006;15(1):54-63.
69. Busardò FP, Varì MR, di Trana A, Malaca S, Carlier J, di Luca NM. Drug-facilitated sexual assaults (DFSA): a serious underestimated issue. *Eur Rev Med Pharmacol Sci.* 2019;23(24):10577-10587.
70. Berry MS, Johnson MW. Does being drunk or high cause HIV sexual risk behavior? A systematic review of drug administration studies. *Pharmacol Biochem Behav.* 2018;164:125-138.
71. Tobin KE, German D, Spikes P, Patterson J, Latkin C. A comparison of the social and sexual networks of crack-using and non-crack using African American men who have sex with men. *J Urban Health.* 2011;88(6):1052-1062.

72. Saleemi S, Pennybaker SJ, Wooldridge M, Johnson MW. Who is 'Molly'? MDMA adulterants by product name and the impact of harm-reduction services at raves. *J Psychopharmacol.* 2017;31(8):1056-1060.
73. McIntyre RS, Rosenblat JD, Nemeroff CB, et al. Synthesizing the evidence for ketamine and esketamine in treatment-resistant depression: an international expert opinion on the available evidence and implementation. *Am J Psychiatry.* 2021;178(5):383-399.
74. Morgan CJA, Curran HV. Independent scientific committee on drugs. Ketamine use: a review. *Addiction.* 2012;107(1):27-38.
75. Schep LJ, Knudsen K, Slaughter RJ, Vale JA, Megarbane B. The clinical toxicology of gamma-hydroxybutyrate, gamma-butyrolactone and 1,4-butanediol. *Clin Toxicol.* 2012;50(6):458-470.
76. Busardò FP, Jones AW. GHB pharmacology and toxicology: acute intoxication, concentrations in blood and urine in forensic cases and treatment of the withdrawal syndrome. *Curr Neuropharmacol.* 2015;13(1):47-70.
77. Marinelli E, Beck R, Malvasi A, Lo Faro AF, Zaami S. Gamma-hydroxybutyrate abuse: pharmacology and poisoning and withdrawal management. *Arh Hig Rada Toksikol.* 2020;71(1):19-26.
78. McCabe SE, Hughes TL, Matthews AK, et al. Sexual orientation discrimination and tobacco use disparities in the United States. *Nicotine Tob Res.* 2019;21(4):523-531.
79. Emory K, Buchting FO, Trinidad DR, Vera L, Emery SL. Lesbian, Gay, Bisexual, and Transgender (LGBT) view it differently than non-LGBT: exposure to tobacco-related couponing, e-cigarette advertisements, and anti-tobacco messages on social and traditional media. *Nicotine Tob Res.* 2019;21(4):513-522.
80. Al Rifai M, Mirbolouk M, Jia X, et al. E-cigarette use and risk behaviors among Lesbian, Gay, Bisexual, and Transgender adults: the Behavioral Risk Factor Surveillance System (BRFSS) Survey. *Kans J Med.* 2020;13:318-321.
81. Delahanty J, Ganz O, Hoffman L, Guillory J, Crankshaw E, Farrelly M. Tobacco use among lesbian, gay, bisexual and transgender young adults varies by sexual and gender identity. *Drug Alcohol Depend.* 2019;201:161-170.
82. Chan WL, Wood DM, Dargan PI. Significant misuse of sildenafil in London nightclubs. *Subst Use Misuse.* 2015;50(11):1390-1394.
83. Rosen RC, Catania JA, Ehrhardt AA, et al. The Bolger conference on PDE-5 inhibition and HIV risk: implications for health policy and prevention. *J Sex Med.* 2006;3(6):960-975. discussion 973-965.
84. Kuchakulla M, Narasimman M, Soni Y, Leong JY, Patel P, Ramasamy R. A systematic review and evidence-based analysis of ingredients in popular male testosterone and erectile dysfunction supplements. *Int J Impot Res.* 2021;33(3):311-317.
85. Gilard V, Balayssac S, Tinaugus A, Martins N, Martino R, Malet-Martino M. Detection, identification and quantification by 1H NMR of adulterants in 150 herbal dietary supplements marketed for improving sexual performance. *J Pharm Biomed Anal.* 2015;102:476-493.
86. Tijerina AN, Srivastava AV, Patel VR, Osterberg EC. Current use of testosterone therapy in LGBTQ populations. *Int J Impot Res.* 2021.
87. Ip EJ, Yadao MA, Shah BM, Lau B. Infectious disease, injection practices, and risky sexual behavior among anabolic steroid users. *AIDS Care.* 2016;28(3):294-299.
88. Lumia AR, McGinnis MY. Impact of anabolic androgenic steroids on adolescent males. *Physiol Behav.* 2010;100(3):199-204.
89. Angell P, Chester N, Green D, Somauroo J, Whyte G, George K. Anabolic steroids and cardiovascular risk. *Sports Med.* 2012;42(2):119-134.
90. Ip EJ, Yadao MA, Shah BM, et al. Polypharmacy, infectious diseases, sexual behavior, and psychophysical health among anabolic steroid-using homosexual and heterosexual gym patrons in San Francisco's Castro district. *Subst Use Misuse.* 2017;52(7):959-968.
91. Blashill AJ, Safren SA. Sexual orientation and anabolic-androgenic steroids in U.S. adolescent boys. *Pediatrics.* 2014;133(3):469-475.
92. Griffiths S, Murray SB, Dunn M, Blashill AJ. Anabolic steroid use among gay and bisexual men living in Australia and New Zealand: associations with demographics, body dissatisfaction, eating disorder psychopathology, and quality of life. *Drug Alcohol Depend.* 2017;181:170-176.
93. Hembree WC, Cohen-Kettenis PT, Gooren L, et al. Endocrine treatment of gender-dysphoric/gender-incongruent persons: an Endocrine Society clinical practice guideline. *J Clin Endocrinol Metab.* 2017;102(11):3869-3903.
94. Benotsch EG, Zimmerman R, Cathers L, et al. Non-medical use of prescription drugs, polysubstance use, and mental health in transgender adults. *Drug Alcohol Depend.* 2013;132(1-2):391-394.
95. Mepham N, Bouman WP, Arcelus J, Hayter M, Wylie KR. People with gender dysphoria who self-prescribe cross-sex hormones: prevalence, sources, and side effects knowledge. *J Sex Med.* 2014;11(12):2995-3001.
96. Clark K, Fletcher JB, Holloway IW, Reback CJ. Structural inequities and social networks impact hormone use and misuse among transgender women in Los Angeles County. *Arch Sex Behav.* 2018;47(4):953-962.
97. Silva RAD, Silva L, Soares F, Dourado I. Use of unprescribed hormones in the body modification of travestis and transsexual women in Salvador/Bahia, Brazil. *Cien Saude Colet.* 2022;27(2):503-514.
98. Costa MCB, McFarland W, Wilson EC, et al. Prevalence and correlates of nonprescription hormone use among trans women in São Paulo, Brazil. *LGBT Health.* 2021;8(2):162-166.
99. Metastasio A, Negri A, Martinotti G, Corazza O. Transitioning bodies. The case of self-prescribing sexual hormones in gender affirmation in individuals attending psychiatric services. *Brain Sci.* 2018;8(5):88.
100. Ayhan CHB, Bilgin H, Uluman OT, Sukut O, Yilmaz S, Buzlu S. A systematic review of the discrimination against sexual and gender minority in health care settings. *Int J Health Serv.* 2020;50(1):44-61.
101. Streed CG Jr, McCarthy EP, Haas JS. Association between gender minority status and self-reported physical and mental health in the United States. *JAMA Intern Med.* 2017;177(8):1210-1212.
102. Webb AJ, McManus D, Rouse GE, Vonderheyde R, Topal JE. Implications for medication dosing for transgender patients: a review of the literature and recommendations for pharmacists. *Am J Health Syst Pharm.* 2020;77(6):427-433.
103. Livio F, Deutschmann E, Moffa G, et al. Analysis of inappropriate prescribing in elderly patients of the Swiss HIV Cohort Study reveals gender inequity. *J Antimicrob Chemother.* 2021;76(3):758-764.
104. Gruber VA, McCance-Katz EF. Methadone, buprenorphine, and street drug interactions with antiretroviral medications. *Current HIV/AIDS reports.* 2010;7(3):152-160.
105. Bositis CM, St Louis J. HIV and substance use disorder: role of the HIV physician. *Infect Dis Clin North Am.* 2019;33(3):835-855.
106. Dvory-Sobol H, Shaik N, Callebaut C, Rhee MS. Lenacapavir: a first-in-class HIV-1 capsid inhibitor. *Curr Opin HIV AIDS.* 2022;17(1):15-21.
107. Tetrault JM, Tate JP, McGinnis KA, et al. Hepatic safety and antiretroviral effectiveness in HIV-infected patients receiving naltrexone. *Alcohol Clin Exp Res.* 2012;36(2):318-324.
108. Hill L, Lee KC. Pharmacotherapy considerations in patients with HIV and psychiatric disorders: focus on antidepressants and antipsychotics. *Ann Pharmacother.* 2013;47(1):75-89.
109. Hesse LM, von Moltke LL, Shader RI, Greenblatt DJ. Ritonavir, efavirenz, and nelfinavir inhibit CYP2B6 activity in vitro: potential drug interactions with bupropion. *Drug Metab Dispos.* 2001;29(2):100-102.
110. Colfax GN, Santos GM, Das M, et al. Mirtazapine to reduce methamphetamine use: a randomized controlled trial. *Arch Gen Psychiatry.* 2011;68(11):1168-1175.
111. Coffin PO, Santos GM, Hern J, et al. Effects of mirtazapine for methamphetamine use disorder among cisgender men and transgender women who have sex with men: a placebo-controlled randomized clinical trial. *JAMA Psychiatry.* 2020;77(3):246-255.
112. Trivedi MH, Walker R, Ling W, et al. Bupropion and naltrexone in methamphetamine use disorder. *N Engl J Med.* 2021;384(2):140-153.
113. Levin FR, Mariani JJ, Pavlicova M, et al. Extended release mixed amphetamine salts and topiramate for cocaine dependence: a randomized clinical replication trial with frequent users. *Drug Alcohol Depend.* 2020;206:107700.
114. Mariani JJ, Pavlicova M, Bisaga A, Nunes EV, Brooks DJ, Levin FR. Extended-release mixed amphetamine salts and topiramate for

cocaine dependence: a randomized controlled trial. *Biol Psychiatry.* 2012;72(11):950-956.

115. Levin FR, Mariani JJ, Specker S, et al. Extended-release mixed amphetamine salts vs placebo for comorbid adult attention-deficit/hyperactivity disorder and cocaine use disorder: a randomized clinical trial. *JAMA Psychiatry.* 2015;72(6):593-602.
116. Mutumba M, Moskowitz JT, Neilands TB, Lee JY, Dilworth SE, Carrico AW. A mindfulness-based, stress and coping model of craving in methamphetamine users. *PloS One.* 2021;16(5):e0249489.
117. McGill M, Ray LA. Cognitive-behavioral treatment with adult alcohol and illicit drug users: a meta-analysis of randomized controlled trials. *J Stud Alcohol Drugs.* 2009;70(4):516-527.
118. Colfax G, Santos G-M, Chu P, et al. Amphetamine-group substances and HIV. *Lancet.* 2010;376(9739):458-474.
119. Shoptaw S, Reback CJ, Peck JA, et al. Behavioral treatment approaches for methamphetamine dependence and HIV-related sexual risk behaviors among urban gay and bisexual men. *Drug Alcohol Depend.* 2005;78(2):125-134.
120. Shoptaw S, Reback CJ, Larkins S, et al. Outcomes using two tailored behavioral treatments for substance abuse in urban gay and bisexual men. *J Subst Abuse Treat.* 2008;35(3):285-293.
121. Miller W, Rollnick S. *Motivational Interviewing: Preparing People to Change Addictive Behavior.* Guilford Press; 1991.
122. Smedslund G, Berg RC, Hammerstrøm KT, et al. Motivational interviewing for substance abuse. *Cochrane Database Syst Rev.* 2011;11(5):CD008063.
123. Berg RC, Ross MW, Tikkanen R. The effectiveness of MI4MSM: how useful is motivational interviewing as an HIV risk prevention program for men who have sex with men? A systematic review. *AIDS Educ Prev.* 2011;23(6):533-549.
124. Dutra L, Stathopoulou G, Basden SL, Leyro TM, Powers MB, Otto MW. A meta-analytic review of psychosocial interventions for substance use disorders. *Am J Psychiatry.* 2008;165(2):179-187.
125. Reback CJ, Shoptaw S. Development of an evidence-based, gay-specific cognitive behavioral therapy intervention for methamphetamine-abusing gay and bisexual men. *Addict Behav.* 2014;39(8):1286-1291.
126. Menza TW, Jameson DR, Hughes JP, Colfax GN, Shoptaw S, Golden MR. Contingency management to reduce methamphetamine use and sexual risk among men who have sex with men: a randomized controlled trial. *BMC Public Health.* 2010;10:774.
127. Molina JM, Capitant C, Spire B, et al. On-demand preexposure prophylaxis in men at high risk for HIV-1 infection. *N Engl J Med.* 2015;373(23):2237-2246.
128. Murchu EO, Marshall L, Teljeur C, et al. Oral pre-exposure prophylaxis (PrEP) to prevent HIV: a systematic review and meta-analysis of clinical effectiveness, safety, adherence and risk compensation in all populations. *BMJ open.* 2022;12(5):e048478.
129. Landovitz RJ, Donnell D, Clement ME, et al. Cabotegravir for HIV prevention in cisgender men and transgender women. *N Engl J Med.* 2021;385(7):595-608.
130. Swindells S, Andrade-Villanueva JF, Richmond GJ, et al. Long-acting cabotegravir and rilpivirine for maintenance of HIV-1 suppression. *N Engl J Med.* 2020;382(12):1112-1123.
131. Buchbinder SP. Maximizing the benefits of HIV preexposure prophylaxis. *Top Antivir Med.* 2018;25(4):138-142.
132. Yager JL, Anderson PL. Pharmacology and drug interactions with HIV PrEP in transgender persons receiving gender affirming hormone therapy. *Expert Opin Drug Metab Toxicol.* 2020;16(6):463-474.
133. Cohen MS, Gamble T, McCauley M. Prevention of HIV transmission and the HPTN 052 study. *Annu Rev Med.* 2020;71:347-360.
134. Bor J, Fischer C, Modi M, et al. Changing knowledge and attitudes towards HIV treatment-as-prevention and "undetectable = untransmittable": a systematic review. *AIDS Behav.* 2021;25(12):4209-4224.

CHAPTER

43

Military Sexual Trauma

Joan E. Zweben

CHAPTER OUTLINE

- Introduction
- Barriers to reporting sexual assault and MST
- Military culture
- Clinical issues
- Getting help at the VA
- Conclusions

INTRODUCTION

With over 17.42 million veterans in the United States as of 2022,[1] the high demand for health care services among this population is met by the U.S. Department of Veterans Affairs (VA) and community clinicians. Although the VA can offer excellent comprehensive care in many communities, including VA clinicians who are specially trained and credentialed in military sexual trauma (MST), those who have experienced sexual trauma in the military may refuse to seek help at the VA because of their complex feelings about such trauma.[2] When these individuals present to community health care systems or private practitioners, it is essential that they are met by professionals who understand their culture and the trauma they have experienced and how that trauma may be related to substance use or other addictive behaviors.

This chapter will focus on the scope of MST and the importance of a community clinicians' role in recognizing and addressing health concerns, including substance use, when veterans seek help for MST or any other reason. It will describe the unique aspects of military culture and the barriers to reporting sexual assault while still serving. It will review common medical and psychological issues and how they can be addressed, and give examples of evidence-based treatments. It will then describe the VA model as an example of how to facilitate access and provide trauma-informed treatment. Information on how to get help within the VA is included and well as other resources and supports.

Military sexual trauma, or MST, is the term used by VA to refer to "experiences of sexual assault or sexual harassment experienced during military service." More concretely, MST includes any unwilling sexual activity including the following:

- Being pressured into sexual activities (such as with threats of negative treatment if you refuse to cooperate or promises of better treatment in exchange for sex).
- Sexual contact or activities without your consent, including when you were asleep or intoxicated.
- Being overpowered or physically forced to have sex.
- Being touched or grabbed in a sexual way that made you uncomfortable, including during hazing experiences.
- Comments about your body or sexual activities that you found threatening.
- Unwanted sexual advances that you found threatening.

The identity or characteristics of the perpetrator, whether you were on or off duty at the time, and whether you were on or off base at the time do not matter." (https://www.mentalhealth.va.gov/docs/mst_general_factsheet.pdf). For fiscal year (FY) 2020, the Department of Defense (DoD) reported 6,290 sexual assaults involving members of the U.S. Armed Services, an increase of 59 from FY2020.[3,4] Across the years reported, from FY2012 to FY2020, reports of sexual assaults were higher among women compared to men (eg, 6.2% versus 0.7% in FY2019).[4] A meta-analysis identified that women evidenced significantly larger prevalence rates of MST compared to men. That meta-analysis indicated that 38.4% of women and 3.9% of men reported MST when the measure includes both harassment and assault. When the measures focused only on assault, 23.6% of women and 1.9% of men reported victimization.[4]

The risk of sexual assault is highest among those aged 17-24 years. A significantly higher percentage of women are assaulted while serving compared to men. But men outnumber women in the military; and although the percentages of men reporting assault are lower than women, the actual numbers are almost equal.[3,5] Outside of the VA, men may be less likely to be screened for sexual trauma than women.

There is a significant impact on physical and mental health among veterans with MST.[6]

Since 2012, the Department of Defense (DoD) has devoted a great deal of attention to preventing and appropriately addressing sexual harassment and assault and has demonstrated steady improvement. The estimated number of service member victims was 26,000 in FY 2012, and 6,290 in FY 2020.[3] The DOD began implementing strategies to reduce barriers to reporting, and since 2012, there was a significant decrease in victim reports of sexual assault. Service members have several pathways open to them. A restricted report allows victims to confidentially access medical care and advocacy services without triggering an investigation. An unrestricted report is provided to command and/or law enforcement for investigation. Service members may reclassify their report as unrestricted at any time and participate in the military justice process. Over time, the rate of unrestricted reports has risen, and restricted reports have converted more quickly.

BARRIERS TO REPORTING SEXUAL ASSAULT AND MST

Despite the strong commitment of the U.S. DoD to address sexual assault, both men and women continue to report devastating experiences of sexual assault. DoD is making comprehensive prevention and intervention efforts[3] to address barriers to reporting, failure to hold perpetrators accountable, and retaliation against victims but the legacy will remain for some time.

While many of the barriers to reporting are common to other victims of sexual assault, some are more characteristic of military members. Service members may minimize the seriousness of the experience or be too embarrassed to report it. Additional barriers include fear not being believed, of being blamed, or of having their reputation suffer. As active duty military service members may have a well-founded fear of harm or retribution if they report it, evident by the numerous examples often shared by military members among themselves and discussed in the media.[7,8] Ultimately, these service members may fear for their career. Additionally, service members may be concerned that their own behavior, such as alcohol and other drug use and fraternization offenses, may undermine their efforts to hold perpetrators accountable. For all these reasons, they may seek help in community settings either during their period of service or once they leave active duty.

MILITARY CULTURE

Clinicians can identify U.S. military members and veterans by asking every adult patient, "Have you ever served in the military?"[9] and follow with additional questions related to that experience.[10] Clinicians are beginning to acknowledge that the military has a distinctive culture as complex as others routinely discussed under the theme of cultural competence. It is important to engage in continuing education and learn from the patient's experience. Because of the nature of the war veterans can have combat-related experiences, even if they did not engage directly in combat. Clinicians should explore specific experiences for veterans of Iraq (Operational Iraqi Freedom; OIF), Afghanistan (Operation Enduring Freedom; OEF), and Operation New Dawn. Many MST events occur during training (while in a very subordinate role) or during peacetime experiences.

Cultural values in the military include a strong emphasis on honor, respect, and obeying the chain of command. These values can be positive forces in treatment. Community programs working with unhoused veterans have noted a heartening level of follow-through once treatment plans have been collaboratively developed. The value placed on "leave no one behind" can be a positive factor in recognizing the value of cohesion in treatment groups and working to promote it. However, military values can also be impediments to seek and utilize help. The value placed on self-protection may add to the shame the patient feels about the sexual assault and make it more difficult for them to report it. They may feel like they "should have been able to fight my perpetrator off." This is particularly true for men, who are even more likely to feel they should have been able to overpower the assailant and prevent the assault.[11] Respect for authority turns to a profound sense of betrayal when commanding officers actively discourage reports, avoid investigating, or if they or the military courts fail to impose serious consequences on allegations of MST.

CLINICAL ISSUES

Screening

It is important to screen for MST when patients seek care for physical or psychiatric conditions. This standard practice in the VA should also be a community health care standard. This process requires creating a comfortable climate for disclosure, unhurried, with adequate privacy. Interruptions should be minimized as much as possible. In general, patients are willing to answer specific questions if the clinician is perceived as nonjudgmental and potentially helpful. Questions can be asked as part of the social history, explaining to the patient that these experiences are sufficiently common in the military and that the questions are routine. At Veterans Affairs Medical Centers, two standardized questions are asked to screen for MST.[12]

These are as follows:

- Did you receive uninvited and unwanted sexual attention, such as touching or cornering, pressure for sexual favors, or verbal remarks?
- Did someone ever use force or the threat of force to have sexual contact with you against your will?

It is important to manage and limit the initial disclosure process, to assess current status and safety, and to be prepared to offer mental health services or make an appropriate referral.

Assessment

Substance Use

There is a strong association between MST and substance use in both men and women.[13] But the health risk disparity was greater for women, especially for alcohol use disorder.[14] A systematic review assessed MST in relation to substance use (alcohol, other drugs, including tobacco smoking). Most of the included studies found significantly increased associations between MST and use of alcohol, drugs, tobacco smoking, and substance use disorders.[15]

Posttraumatic Stress Disorder

Posttraumatic stress disorder (PTSD) is associated with MST.[13] There are high rates of childhood trauma among veterans in general, particularly those who experience MST.[16] Multiple traumatic experiences in childhood and adulthood complicate the presentation and treatment of the PTSD and often increase the severity of concomitant substance use.

In the military, as in other situations, a victim may be continually seeing and working with the perpetrator during workplace or other military settings, adding to the trauma. Male service members more likely than females to report symptoms of PTSD and depression.[17]

Suicide risk is high among both men and women who have experienced MST, regardless of mental health diagnosis or treatment.[18] Co-occurring PTSD and depression elevate the risk of intentional self-injury.[19] Beliefs of unlovability, unbearability and unsolvability strongly predict suicidal ideation and future suicidal behavior.[20] Given the potential for severe PTSD symptoms and the high suicide rates of military members compared to nonmilitary populations, clinicians must address the issue of lethal weapons. It is important to ask about readily accessible weapons. Whether male or female, military members are more likely than nonmilitary to have at least one gun in their home; and it may serve as an important part of their identity. Ask specific questions about how the weapon and the bullets are stored, and how safety is maintained. If lethality is an issue, the clinician should negotiate storing ammunition with a friend or obtaining a trigger lock. The VA provides free gun locks to all veterans to enhance gun safety. Weapons may be turned into the VA police, but they will not be stored and returned. Check with local police to learn their policy. It is advisable to ask how guns will be stored and locked, and what additional safety measures the patient is willing to implement into a "safety plan" documented in the record. Such a safety plan documents risk and protective factors relating to suicide or violence risk, and is structured to increase protective factors and to construct safety measures in advance, before any crisis, in a way that the patient is comfortable following should their condition deteriorate.

Medical Problems

A study of both men and women reports that MST may intensify the overall burden of chronic pain, with younger veterans particularly affected. Participants in this study reported challenges in performing daily, social or work-related tasks. The group of younger veterans seems somewhat less likely to benefit from pain rehabilitation.[21] Gastrointestinal symptoms include diarrhea, indigestion, nausea, and difficulty swallowing. Other complaints can include chronic fatigue, sudden weight changes, and heart palpitations.[22] These complaints may be the vehicle through which the victim seeks help and provides the opportunity for the health care team member to address MST.

Men who reported either sexual harassment or assault were more likely to have poor baseline physical health, reported stronger symptoms at the beginning of treatment, and perceive their general health as more damaged.[11] They may be more likely to report symptoms of PTSD and depression.[17]

Sexual Health/Behaviors

Both males and female MST survivors report lower sexual satisfaction, with depression identified as a key confounding factor to address.[23] Males with MST are more likely to have sexually transmitted diseases, such as HIV/AIDS, syphilis, and herpes, as well as disorders of sexual desire and arousal.[11] Females can have a variety of gynecological problems: sexual dysfunctions, menstrual abnormalities, menopausal symptoms, or reproductive symptoms.[22]

Compulsive sexual behavior is also an issue in men, and is associated with low relationship satisfaction.[24]

Physical Examination Procedures

Conducting a physical examination or doing medical procedures can also present challenges. It is important to make the medical encounter as safe as possible by providing a private, calm setting and explaining what to expect. If the patient becomes upset, or begins to dissociate, it is important to stop touching the patient or discontinue the procedure and then reorient and verbally soothe the patient. A well-established pathway for mental health referrals and a "warm handoff" is part of good care, as these patients may be reluctant to seek this kind of help and give up easily if the referral is not guided at each point that obstacles might occur.

Psychosocial Treatment

Studies of treatment have increased in recent years. Some highlights:

- Both Cognitive Processing Therapy and Prolonged Exposure have been shown to be effective.[25,26]
- Matching patient gender preferences with the assigned clinician increases a sense of comfort and confidence in clinicians competency.[27] However, very often the gender of the clinician is not an impasse that cannot be worked through in the therapy.
- Trauma-sensitive Yoga for PTSD is an innovative approach that appears to be an effective treatment for women with MST related trauma. It yielded improvement more quickly than CPT, had higher retention, and had a sustained effect.[28]
- Seeking safety—early stage stabilization for patients with PTSD and unhealthy substance use.[29]

Treatment of patients with MST must be prepared to manage affective lability and other expected emotions. Patients with MST may experience anxiety and irritability and may be prone to angry outbursts. It can be challenging to establish a therapeutic alliance of trust, particularly if the therapist is of the same gender as the perpetrator. Working with a treatment team is helpful, as multiple treatment contacts with different individuals may be necessary to address the complex physical and mental health needs. A multidisciplinary team can also assist a solo practitioner in the community in identifying and securing referrals to specialty treatment. Patients with MST can be highly crisis prone, and a treatment team can help in the assessment of their needs and collaborate on a patient-centered plan of care. A treatment team can also help the clinician to avoid becoming too self-critical and discouraged, while providing a forum to explore the strong feelings these patients can engender.

GETTING HELP AT THE VA

There is a subset of veterans who are concerned about seeking MST treatment because of stigma and shame. Some veterans have reservations about using VA care, based on negative perceptions of the VA health care system. Participants of a qualitative study expressed concerns regarding distrust, clinician compassion, privacy, stigma, shame, and continuity of care. Women who experienced MST may describe feeling anxious or out of place, preferring separate facilities.[8]

Although some women veterans will emphatically refuse to go to the VA, health care clinicians are in key positions to convey what the VA provides and their outcomes of care. It is important for them to know what it has to offer, particularly if other resources in the community are scarce. A pioneer in the use of electronic records in the 1980s, and clinical practice guidelines, the VA has used them to identify the factors involved in good outcomes and then formulate and disseminate protocols to improve care across the system. The result is that VA care produces better outcomes for chronic conditions such as diabetes and hypertension than Medicaid and the private sector.[30,31] All veterans seen in VA health care are asked if they experienced MST, which then prompts a referral to specialized and empathic MST care. All treatment for physical or mental health conditions related to MST is free. Every VA health care facility has a designated MST coordinator who serves as the contact person for MST-related issues. Veterans who may be unsure of their eligibility for VA services and other benefits should be informed of the resources shown in **Table 43-1**, in case they lose their current insurance or later need care they cannot access in the community.

CONCLUSIONS

Clinicians can expect to see veterans who experienced MST and should be prepared to address their complex needs. Many patients will have highly conflicted feelings about their military experience and may not even share they are a veteran unless specifically asked "have you served in the military?" Although the VA provides excellent services to these patients, many will not consider seeking help in that setting. Community clinicians who are knowledgeable about the culture of the military will be better able to engage this population in their community setting or encourage them to engage with the VA. Their traumatic experiences will influence their efforts to address their physical and emotional problems, as it affects everything from their ability to tolerate a physical exam to their emotional stability and participation in a recovery process. Expertise in assessing and addressing co-occurring issues, including substance use, are critical in treating this vulnerable population.

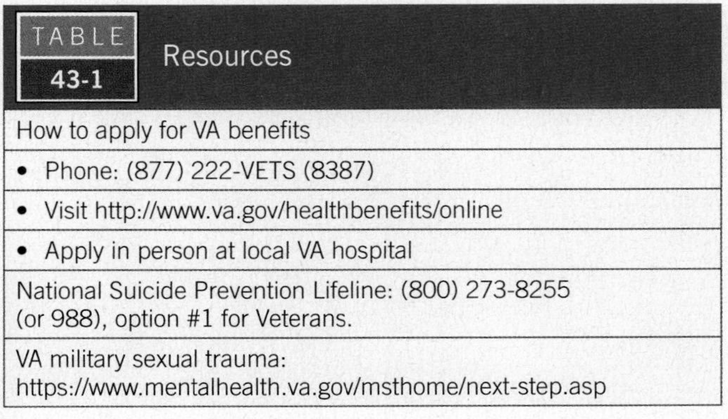

TABLE 43-1 Resources
How to apply for VA benefits
• Phone: (877) 222-VETS (8387)
• Visit http://www.va.gov/healthbenefits/online
• Apply in person at local VA hospital
National Suicide Prevention Lifeline: (800) 273-8255 (or 988), option #1 for Veterans.
VA military sexual trauma: https://www.mentalhealth.va.gov/msthome/next-step.asp

ACKNOWLEDGMENTS

The author thanks John Straznickas, MD, Associate Clinical Professor, University of California, San Francisco and Team Leader, Substance Use Posttraumatic Stress Disorder Team, San Francisco Veteran's Affairs Medical Center.

REFERENCES

1. Statista Research Department. Veterans in the United States—Statistics & Facts. 2022. Accessed March 14, 2022. https://www.statista.com/topics/3450/veterans-in-the-united-states/#dossierKeyfigures
2. Monteith LL, Holliday R, Schneider AL, Miller CN, Bahraini NH, Forster JE. Institutional betrayal and help-seeking among women survivors of military sexual trauma. *Psychol Trauma*. 2021;13(7):814-823.
3. Department of Defense. *Annual Report on Sexual Assault in the Military: Fiscal Year 2020*. Department of Defense; 2021.
4. Wilson LC. The prevalence of military sexual trauma: a meta-analysis. *Trauma Violence Abuse*. 2018;19(5):584-597.
5. Department of Defense. *Department of Defense Annual Report on Sexual Assault in the Military*. Department of Defense; 2017.
6. Nichter B, Holliday R, Monteith LL, et al. Military sexual trauma in the United States: results from a population-based study. *J Affect Disord*. 2022;306:19-27.
7. O'Toole M. *Military Sexual Assault Epidemic Continues to Claim Victims as Defense Department Fails Females*. Huffington Post; 2012.
8. Monteith LL, Bahraini NH, Gerber HR, et al. Military sexual trauma survivors' perceptions of veterans health administration care: a qualitative examination. *Psychol Serv*. 2020;17(2):178-186.
9. Collins E, Wilmoth M, Scwartz L. "Have you ever served in the military?" Campaign in partnership with the Joining Forces initiative. *Nurs Outlook*. 2013;61(5):375-376.
10. Sheehy, Schwartz LS. Ask the question: 'have you ever served?' Caring for military members and veterans in civilian healthcare. *Nursing*. 2021;51(11):28-35.
11. Morris EE, Smith JC, Farooqui SY, Suris AM. Unseen battles: the recognition, assessment, and treatment issues of men with military sexual trauma (MST). *Trauma Violence Abuse*. 2014;15(2):94-101.
12. McIntyre LM, Butterfield MI, Nanda K, et al. Validation of a Trauma Questionnaire in veteran women. *J Gen Intern Med*. 1999;14(3):186-189. doi:10.1046/j.1525-1497.1999.00311.x
13. Banducci AN, McCaughey V, Gradus JL, Street AE. The associations between deployment experiences, PTSD, and alcohol use among male and female veterans. *Addict Behav*. 2019;98:106032.
14. Goldberg SB, Livingston WS, Blais RK, et al. A positive screen for military sexual trauma is associated with greater risk for substance use disorders in women veterans. *Psychol Addict Behav*. 2019;33(5):477-483.
15. Forkus SR, Weiss NH, Goncharenko S, Mammay J, Church M, Contractor AA. Military sexual trauma and risky behaviors: a systematic review. *Trauma Violence Abuse*. 2021;22(4):976-993.
16. Sadler AG, Booth BM, Cook BL, Doebbeling BN. Factors associated with women's risk of rape in the military environment. *Am J Ind Med*. 2003;43(3):262-273.

17. Millegan J, Wang L, LeardMann CA, Miletich D, Street AE. Sexual trauma and adverse health and occupational outcomes among men serving in the U.S. Military. *J Trauma Stress.* 2016;29(2):132-140.
18. Decker SE, Ramsey CM, Ronzitti S, et al. Military sexual trauma and suicidal ideation in VHA-care-seeking OEF/OIF/OND veterans without mental health diagnosis or treatment. *Psychiatry Res.* 2021;303:114089.
19. Livingston WS, Fargo JD, Gundlapalli AV, Brignone E, Blais RK. Comorbid PTSD and depression diagnoses mediate the Association of Military Sexual Trauma and Suicide and Intentional Self-Inflicted Injury in VHA-enrolled Iraq/Afghanistan Veterans, 2004-2014. *J Affect Disord.* 2020;274:1184-1190.
20. Holliday R, Holder N, Monteith LL, Suris A. Decreases in suicide cognitions after cognitive processing therapy among veterans with posttraumatic stress disorder due to military sexual trauma: a preliminary examination. *J Nerv Ment Dis.* 2018;206(7):575-578.
21. Turner AP, Harding KA, Brier MJ, Anderson DR, Williams RM. Military sexual trauma and chronic pain in veterans. *Am J Phys Med Rehabil.* 2020;99(11):1020-1025.
22. Lofgreen AM, Carroll KK, Dugan SA, Karnik NS. An overview of sexual trauma in the U.S. Military. *Focus.* 2017;15(4):411-419.
23. Blais RK, Zalta AK, Livingston WS. Interpersonal trauma and sexual function and satisfaction: the mediating role of negative affect among survivors of military sexual trauma. *J Interpers Violence.* 2022;37(7-8):NP5517-NP5537.
24. Blais RK, Livingston WS. The association of assault military sexual trauma and sexual function among partnered female service members and veterans: the mediating roles of depression and sexual self-schemas. *Eur J Psychotraumatol.* 2021;12(1):1872964.
25. Khan AJ, Holder N, Li Y, et al. How do gender and military sexual trauma impact PTSD symptoms in cognitive processing therapy and prolonged exposure? *J Psychiatr Res.* 2020;130:89-96.
26. Boehler J. The efficacy of cognitive processing therapy for ptsd related to military sexual trauma in veterans: a review. *J Evid Based Soc Work.* 2019;16(6):595-614.
27. McBain SA, Garneau-Fournier J, Turchik JA. The relationship between provider gender preferences and perceptions of providers among veterans who experienced military sexual trauma. *J Interpers Violence.* 2022;37(5–6):NP2868-NP2890.
28. Kelly U, Haywood T, Segell E, Higgins M. Trauma-sensitive yoga for post-traumatic stress disorder in women veterans who experienced military sexual trauma: interim results from a randomized controlled trial. *J Altern Complement Med.* 2021;27(S1):S45-S59.
29. Najavits LM. *Seeking Safety: A Treatment Manual for PTSD and Substance Abuse.* New Guilford Press; 2002.
30. Longman P. *Best Care Anywhere: Why VA Health Care Would Work Better for Everyone.* 3rd ed. Berrett-Koehler Publishers, Inc; 2012.
31. Association of VA Psychologist Leaders. *Comparison of VA to Community Healthcare: Summary of Research, 2000-2016*; 2016.

CHAPTER

44 Traumatic Brain Injury and Substance Use Disorders

David L. Pennington, Amy A. Herrold, and Angela M. Mueller

CHAPTER OUTLINE

- Introduction
- Definition of traumatic brain injury
- Epidemiology of TBI
- Prevalence of SUD and TBI
- Risk factors influencing co-occurrence
- Harms associated with co-occurrence of SUD and TBI
- Assessment of co-occurring TBI and SUD
- Treatment approaches for TBI and SUD
- Conclusions

INTRODUCTION

Traumatic brain injury (TBI) is a major cause of death and disability in the United States. In 2010, the Centers for Disease Control and Prevention (CDC) estimated that TBIs accounted for approximately 2.5 million hospital emergency department (ED) visits in the United States. Among TBIs that occurred in community settings in the United States, falls accounted for 41% of TBIs (disproportionately affecting the youngest and oldest age groups), followed by blunt trauma (16%) and motor vehicle accidents (14%). Direct costs for TBI hospital care, extended care, and other medical care and services, coupled with indirect costs such as lost productivity, were estimated by the CDC to be $76.5 billion annually.[1,2] These numbers likely underestimate the occurrence and associated cost of TBIs since they do not account for those who did not receive medical care in ED, those who had only outpatient medical care or those who received care at a federal facility, such as a U.S. military hospital or a Veterans Affairs hospital.[3]

Those who serve in the military are at significant risk for TBI. Between 2000 and 2022, the U.S. Department of Defense (DOD) data indicate that 458,894 service members were diagnosed with a TBI. Internationally, continuing conflicts have increased the likelihood of exposure to high-energy blasts and explosions. As a result of this increasingly common mechanism of injury, more service members wounded in war are returning with multiple complex injuries including TBI, spinal cord injuries, eye injuries, musculoskeletal injuries, and mental health problems. The term "polytrauma" has been introduced to encompass injuries to more than one physical region or organ system that result in physical, cognitive, psychological, or psychosocial impairments and functional disability. Mental health comorbidities are common in this patient population including posttraumatic stress disorder (PTSD), depression, anxiety, and substance use disorders (SUDs).

There is a growing body of literature indicating that as many as 60% of persons with TBI have significant problems with alcohol and/or other substances.[4-7] The relationship between TBI and SUDs is bidirectional, with evidence for higher rates of TBI in individuals with preexisting SUD and also higher rates of SUD in individuals following a TBI. Although it is well demonstrated that TBI is a common co-occurrence with alcohol and SUD,[8] little is known, and even less is disseminated, regarding prevalence, associated harms, or treatment strategies for patients with both TBI and unhealthy substance use. Knowing about TBI and the clinical strategies required to address it appropriately is a needed skill set for addiction medicine professionals.

This chapter defines and classifies TBI, discusses the prevalence and neurobehavioral harms related to TBI and alcohol and other substance use, and provides an overview of assessment aimed at identifying symptoms during acute-stage injury. We also discuss potential cognitive and pharmacotherapy treatment approaches for patients with TBI and unhealthy alcohol use. Recommendations for early screening and assessment of TBI and substance use are highlighted.

DEFINITION OF TRAUMATIC BRAIN INJURY

A TBI is an injury that disrupts the normal function of the brain. It can be caused by a hit, explosive blast, jolt to the head, or a penetrating injury.[9] The DOD and Department of Veterans Affairs (VA)[10] have defined TBI as any traumatically induced injury and/or physiological disruption of brain function that involves new onset or worsening of at least one of the following clinical signs, immediately following the event:

1. Any period of loss of or a decreased level of consciousness.
2. Any loss of memory for events immediately before or after the injury.
3. Any alteration in mental state at the time of the injury (eg, confusion, disorientation, slowed thinking).
4. Neurological deficits (eg, balance disturbance, change in vision, other sensory alterations, aphasia) that may or may not be transient.
5. Intracranial lesion secondary to head trauma (excluding other acquired conditions, eg, stroke, tumor).

Classification

TBIs are heterogeneous, and there are several ways to categorize patients in terms of clinical severity, mechanism of injury, and pathophysiology. Mild TBIs (synonymous with concussions) are the most frequent TBIs, accounting for 70% to 90% of all brain injuries treated in hospitals worldwide with incidence likely more than 600/100,000/year.[11] Regardless of injury mechanism, TBI severity grade at the time of the injury (mild, moderate, or severe) is determined by using four indices:

- **Glasgow Coma Scale (GCS)**—The GCS is a 15-point scale based upon ratings of the patient's best motor, eye opening, and verbal responses following an injury.
- **Length of coma (LOC)** (duration of unconsciousness)—Coma or unconsciousness is the time a patient is nonresponsive after injury.
- **Length of period of altered consciousness or mental status**—Following a TBI, an individual may be conscious but may nonetheless be confused, disoriented, feel dazed, have difficulty tracking events, and may respond in a confused manner to questions.
- **Length of posttraumatic amnesia (PTA)**—PTA is the time interval from when the person regains consciousness until he or she is able to consistently form memories for ongoing events.[12] Of note, PTA can be influenced by medications that are given in routine trauma care (ie, pain medication).

The classification provided in the following table has been accepted by DOD/VA and the American College of Rehabilitation Medicine (ACRM)[13] (**Table 44-1**).

TABLE 44-1 Classification of TBI

Severity index	Mild TBI/ concussion	Moderate TBI	Severe TBI
Neuroimaging findings	Normal structural imaging	Normal *or* abnormal structural imaging	Normal *or* abnormal structural imaging
Initial Glasgow Coma Scale	13-15	9-12	<9
Loss of consciousness (LOC)	0-30 min	>30 min and <24 h	>24 h
Length of alteration of consciousness (AOC)	A moment up to 24 h	AOC > 24 h (use other criteria)	
Length of posttraumatic amnesia (PTA)	0–1 d	>1 and <7 d	>7 d

DoD/DVA/ACRM consensus-based classification of TBI severity.

Diagnosis of TBI

In cases of moderate or severe TBI, the diagnosis is readily assessed through history and examination in the emergency medical setting. TBI diagnosis may be complicated in cases of closed head injury accompanied by other life-threatening injury, particularly in the case of mild TBI (mTBI). In such cases, mTBI might not be diagnosed until days to weeks following the injury, when neurobehavioral problems are noticed, and sometimes only after other emergent medical problems are resolved. Such patients may require detailed neurological exam, brain imaging, and/or formal neurocognitive evaluation by a neuropsychologist to establish the presence and associated symptoms of a TBI.

Acute-stage injury parameters of LOC, PTA, and GCS are strongly predictive of long-term recovery and form the basis for establishing a diagnosis of TBI.[14] Other TBI symptoms may be physical (eg, fatigue, headache, vertigo, dizziness, or disordered sleep), cognitive (eg, deficits in attention or memory), or emotional (depression, anxiety, affective lability, apathy, or other changes in personality), commonly referred to as postconcussional disorder[15] or "postconcussion syndrome" (PCS).[16] Although these symptoms can be used to support a mTBI diagnosis, this should only be done to the extent that these symptoms cannot be accounted for by causes other than mTBI itself such as psychological reaction to physical or emotional stress.[14] The frequent psychological trauma that can accompany head injuries may also make it difficult to accurately determine the degree of altered mental status and complicates assessment of causality for symptoms. In sum, behavioral, cognitive, and emotional symptoms can be nonspecific and therefore must not be used in isolation to establish a TBI diagnosis.

Military Populations

Diagnosis of mTBI in military populations is even more complex due to reluctance to report brain injuries for fear of removal from duty, delays between time of TBI and discharge from military service, and because of the unique mechanisms of injury, often including repeated exposure to blasts. It is estimated that 50% to 80% of battlefield injuries in U.S. veterans are now due to blast exposure.[17,18] Worldwide, blast-induced traumatic brain injury (bTBI) is considered the "signature wound" of modern warfare.[19] Primary blast injury refers to injury that is caused by exposure to a blast wave, a sudden change in atmospheric pressure.[14] This blast wave is thought to account for unique injury to the brain resulting in behavioral traits similar to PTSD in humans and biochemical, pathological, and physiological effects on the nervous system in animal models.[20] Primary blast injury is often accompanied by blunt or penetrating trauma from material propelled by the blast wave (secondary blast injury), by the body being thrown to the ground or against an object from the wave (tertiary blast injury), or from other injury mechanisms attributable to the blast such as burns, wounds, broken bones, or breathing toxic fumes (quaternary blast injury). All of these injuries may contribute to symptom development following bTBI and add to the complexity of diagnoses. There are currently no specific bTBI treatment strategies, but research aimed at understanding the mechanisms underlying bTBI is steadily growing and will aid in the development of specific treatment strategies for this type of injury. See Courtney and Courtney[20] for a review of the potential underlying mechanisms of primary bTBI.

High-Impact Sports

Repeated exposure to TBIs (including mild) have been associated with the development of a progressive, neurodegenerative disease called chronic traumatic encephalopathy (CTE). The majority of confirmed CTE cases have been among athletes competing in high-impact sports, such as football, boxing, soccer, ice hockey, wrestling, and rugby.[21] Symptoms associated with CTE include disruptions in mood, behavior, cognition, and motor function. It typically takes 8-10 years after repeated exposures to present; severity can range from mild symptoms to those that produce a parkinsonian-like syndrome.[22] Currently, CTE can be diagnosed only via postmortem examination and can be challenging to diagnose due to its overlap with other neurodegenerative diseases such as Alzheimer dementia.[22] See Murray et al.,[23] Blennow et al.,[24] and Safinia et al.[22] for a review of CTE pathology. Although there are no established clinical criteria or biomarkers that support the diagnosis of CTE,[24] increased attention in the media and medical research has resulted in more studies that may soon provide a pathway for diagnosing CTE in living patients, including the use of PET imaging to identify tau-specific ligands indicative of CTE.[22,25] Ultimately, prevention may prove to be the most beneficial approach to reducing CTE. Prevention methods include the use of optimal helmets with adequate shock absorption, modifications to rules in high-impact sports, and the use of more sensitive neurobehavioral assessment tools and routine cognitive testing.[22]

Assessment

Civilian-related mTBI can be assessed using the *Ohio State University TBI Identification Method*,[26,27] a structured interview, which allows for breadth of assessment (number and severity of TBIs, age of onset, and duration of symptoms). The *Boston Assessment of Traumatic Brain Injury-Lifetime* (BAT-L)[28] is also a retrospective tool used to characterize and diagnose lifetime TBI. The BAT-L is unique in that it guides the examiner to distinguish between physiological disruption of consciousness and the psychological response to co-occurring traumatic events. The BAT-L also includes assessment of blast injury common to veterans.

To date, the diagnosis of mTBI in veterans returning to the United States relies on data acquired from self-report through the use of a limited set of validated semistructured interviews. The *VA TBI Identification Clinical Interview*,[29] the *Warrior-Administered Retrospective Casualty Assessment Tool* (WAR-CAT),[30] and the *Structured Interview for TBI Diagnosis*[31] are structured clinical interviews, which focus on military-related head injury and can be administered post-deployment.

The most widely researched and used tool for assessment of concussion (mTBI) in athletes is the *Sports Concussion Assessment Tool-V3* (SCAT-3).[32] The SCAT-3 combines the GCS, Maddocks score (a set of orientation questions, eg, at what venue are we today, which half is it now, who scored last in the match, did your team win the last game), symptom checklist, a standardized assessment of concussion,[33] and the balance error scoring system.[34] Although this is a well-validated assessment for sports injury–related concussion, it has been developed to assess a younger, healthier, and more homogenous cohort, not the general civilian or military population.[35]

All of the abovementioned tools assess for GCS, LOC, and AOS in relation to a type of trauma (eg, blunt, fall, motor vehicle accident). Some include the acquisition of information related to blast injury, and the SCAT-3 is specific to sports-related injury. Although all these instruments possess some degree of validity in assessing mTBI, there is a need for cross-validation of their accuracy to assess mTBI in patients with SUD and across the lifetime.

EPIDEMIOLOGY OF TBI

Approximately 80% of patients who sustain TBIs have had a mild case.[3] Individuals with uncomplicated mTBI/concussion typically recover fully within the first 3 months.[36] However, about 10% to 15% continue to report symptoms for months[37,38] or years postinjury.[39,40] Individuals with repeated mTBI have an increased risk for persistent symptoms.

Persisting functional limitations are also common in patients with moderate to severe TBI. Among patients with TBI-related postconcussive symptoms requiring acute care hospitalization, functional limitations were found in up to 47% of patients discharged at 1-year follow-up.[41] In another sample of persons hospitalized with moderate or severe TBI,[42] 24% had failed to return to work at 1-year follow-up. Similarly, in a 15-year follow-up study of a cohort of U.S. veterans from the war in Vietnam, only 56% of those with TBI were employed compared with 82% of the uninjured controls.[43]

PREVALENCE OF SUD AND TBI

Literature addressing illicit substance use at the time of head injury is limited. Currently, there remains no standard for assessment or reporting of substance use for patients presenting with TBI. Thus, rates of illicit substance use at time of injury remain largely unknown; however, it *is* known that alcohol intoxication at the time of a TBI is common.[8] Studies indicating alcohol use at the time of injury range from as low as 37% to as high as 50% of all cases.[44-49] Rates of preinjury nonalcohol SUDs range from 21% to 40% and preinjury alcohol use disorders (AUDs) range from 44% to 79%.[50-54] Likewise, studies examining preinjury AUD and SUD suffer from a lack of uniformity in assessment methods and diagnostic criteria limiting their interpretability. Overall, current rates of SUD in patients with TBI are estimated to range up to 50%[8] but should be considered with caution given the methodological limitations.

Regarding military populations, U.S. military service members with a hospital diagnosis of TBI are 2.6 to 5.4 times more likely to be discharged from the military for alcohol or drug use when compared to the total discharged population.[55] The prevalence of SUD and unhealthy alcohol use is approximately twice greater in veterans with TBI than in those without. There is a 26% rate of substance-related disorders in U.S. veterans with a positive TBI screen compared to 9.7% in those with a negative screen (risk ratio of 2.27).[6] In a study of over 300,000 *Operation Enduring Freedom* and *Operation Iraqi Freedom* veterans, the rate of SUD diagnoses in veterans with TBI was more than twice that of veterans without TBI (22% versus 8%).[7] A TBI also increases service members' risk of being diagnosed with AUD in the 12 months following head injury by 50%.[56]

Rates of head injury in populations with SUD range from 31% to as high as 68%.[57-60] Studies examining TBI in population with SUD have similar methodological problems to studies examining rates of SUD in populations with TBI. Most reports of head injury in populations with SUD are retrospective, lack specificity regarding the severity of head injury, and rely on self-report methods for the documentation of a head injury. These reports often loosely define TBI as any head injury with loss of consciousness, and samples consist primarily of those seeking treatment for SUD. Although the research in prevalence rates of TBI and SUD have methodological limitations, studies consistently find high correlations between these diagnoses.

RISK FACTORS INFLUENCING CO-OCCURRENCE

Those with unhealthy substance use are more likely to engage in high-risk behaviors that result in TBI, that is, motor vehicle accidents, falls, and blunt trauma from violent acts.[5] There is substantial literature demonstrating that substance use often declines immediately following brain injury but later increases commensurate with improvement in functional status.[5,61] However, not all subpopulations of patients with TBI and SUD exhibit this immediate drop in substance use; there is emerging evidence showing that TBI increases the risk of heavy drinking immediately following TBI in young men with a previous history of SUD problems and diagnosis of depression.[61]

TBI Increases Risk of Developing an SUD

There is a growing body of literature showing that TBI alone can result in increased risk for substance-related problems postinjury.[62] Hibbard et al.[52] reported that patients without a history of DSM-IV Axis I disorder (including SUD) had increased rates of postinjury SUD relative to community controls. After controlling for alcohol use prior to injury, Silver et al.[63] also found that TBI was associated with increased rates of SUD compared with community controls, evident up to 36 months postinjury.[64] Patients with TBI are also more likely than individuals without TBI to be treated with potentially addictive medication such as opioids, as has been shown in a study of U.S. veterans of the Iraq and Afghanistan conflicts.[65]

Risk for SUD following TBI may be greater in those with mild to moderate TBI.[66] The increase in alcohol- and drug-related discharges among service members is specific to those with a history of mild or moderate TBI. Subjects with severe TBI have *not been shown* to have increased incidence of substance-related discharge.[55] In fact, less severe functional disability following TBI is related to worse SUD-related behaviors. Increased rates of substance- and alcohol-related problems in those with mild to moderate TBI can be partially attributed to psychiatric comorbid disorders such as depression and PTSD and physical discomfort of postinjury chronic pain.[67] There is also early evidence showing that this increased SUD risk is related to the neurobiological and related neurocognitive mechanisms underlying TBI.[68-70] The *decreased* risk of SUD among those with a *severe* TBI is likely due to the inability to seek or access drugs and alcohol because of the debilitating nature of the head injury.

Neurocircuitry of TBI

Many of the neurological deficits associated with severe TBI are a result of direct anatomical damage. However, changes in neurotransmitter systems, particularly in the long axonal projections of the dopamine pathways (easily injured by acceleration and deceleration shearing force), appear to be vulnerable to mild/moderate TBI.[68] Additionally, the secondary damage induced by TBI includes excitotoxicity resulting from release of excitatory neurotransmitters (primarily glutamate[69]), which can last for a week or longer.[70] Increased glutamate and subsequent binding to *N*-methyl-D-aspartate (NMDA) receptors leads to an influx in calcium ions, which can ultimately lead to cell death.[71] This period of excitotoxicity can be followed by a depression in glutamatergic transmission.[70] Many other transmitter systems are disrupted including dopamine.[72,73] GABA, acetylcholine, norepinephrine, and serotonin (for review, see[70,71]). Disruption across transmitter systems, which can evolve over time, leads to a host of symptoms including cognitive and emotional deficits.[70]

Emerging Evidence for Dopaminergic Agonist Treatment for TBI

Preclinical and clinical trials have begun to look at dopamine pathway drugs to target pathophysiological and functional outcomes of TBI.[74] Dopamine is the most common catecholamine found in the central nervous system and has been the most studied neurotransmitter target for TBI treatment to date, but it should be noted that other catecholamines such as epinephrine, norepinephrine, and monoamine agonists are also being evaluated for TBI intervention.[75]

Evidence showing that dopamine agonists improve cellular and functional deficits associated with TBI is growing. Dopamine agonists studied for post TBI treatment include bromocriptine, amantadine, dopamine agonists used in Parkinson disease such as ropinirole and pramipexole, stimulants such as methylphenidate and amphetamine, and dopamine reuptake inhibitors.[75] Preclinical and clinical trials of these medications have been examined to target a wide range of TBI-related symptoms including impaired cognitive function (eg, spatial memory, working memory, attention, executive function), impaired motor deficits, agitation, sleep disorders, depression, and neuroinflammation and to promote neurogenesis, postinjury plasticity, and synaptogenesis.[75] Evidence is primarily from case reports, case series or open label trials.[74] There are also a few early investigations into the role of genetic factors in response to trauma given that functional outcomes can vary between patients with similar degrees of TBI, and that individual response to medications can also vary widely.[74]

Neuroprotective and therapeutic dopaminergic targeting strategies have been beneficial for memory and attention recovery.[68] However, the clinical trials conducted in this line of work have limitations including replication failure, lack of specificity, lack of examination into moderating characteristics such as genetic factors, and difficulty translating therapies into clinical practice.[75] At this time, there is a lack of rigorous evaluation of dopaminergic therapy in large double-blind randomized clinical trials for improving outcomes in TBI, and thus insufficient evidence to support specific medication intervention recommendation. If future dopaminergic medications prove to be efficacious for TBI, then they are worth investigating in the treatment of both SUD and TBI, given the overlap of both conditions in relation to cognitive dysfunction (learning, memory, and executive dysfunction) and propensity for neuroplastic recovery.[74]

Evidence for Increased Risk of SUD Among Patients With a History of Adolescent TBI

In the United States, adolescents are at the highest risk for developing a SUD. The prevalence of SUD in the United States peaks during the period from adolescence to young adulthood (15-30 years of age) and then decreases steadily by age.[76] Likewise, young children (0-4 years) and adolescents (15-24) belong to the three age groups with the highest risk to sustain a TBI.[77] As data from 2013 show, the incidence rate in children and adolescents (1,591 and 1,080 per 100,000 population per year) were only surpassed by persons aged 75 of years and older (2,232). As these rates show, adolescents have a higher risk than all other age-groups for experiencing both TBI and SUD, and this is a stage of their life when the brain is particularly vulnerable to environmental effects.

Adolescence is a phase of heightened sensation seeking, impulsivity and boundary testing, which is associated in the brain with intensive maturation processes characterized by intensive structural and functional reorganization, particularly in the prefrontal cortex, which is involved in cognition and in control of motivation and emotions. Two processes, myelination and pruning, underlie the reorganization of brain during adolescence, and both are highly vulnerable to the immediate and long-term effects of TBI and substance use.[78-82]

Myelination, the acquisition of the myelin membrane around the axons, starts in the visual and motor cortex and is the last to occur in the prefrontal cortex beginning at adolescence and continuing into early adulthood. Of particular importance in the context of adolescent SUD and TBI is that the dopamine innervation to the prefrontal cortex is still ongoing in that stage of life, which is unique as all other neuromodulators have already reached their maximum innervation level at the end of childhood.[83] The dopaminergic innervation of the prefrontal cortex during adolescence is orchestrated by a complex interplay of the guidance clue protein Netrin-1 in the frontal cortex and the receptor DCC in the axons[84,85] that grow from the nucleus accumbens to the medial prefrontal cortex. If this orchestrated interplay is disturbed by external events, then maladaptive or even ectopic interconnections can occur with more or less subtle effects on cognition and behavior.[86]

Adolescence is also the phase during which the highest rate of synaptic pruning occurs.[87] Microglia, the brain resident immune cells, play a major role in the pruning process.[88] Insufficient or disturbed pruning during this period is associated with impairment of synaptic spine density in the prefrontal cortex[89] and nucleus accumbens[90] with consequences cognitive functioning later in adulthood.[91] Neuroinflammation, a process characterized by heightened microglial activity is a common sequelae of both, TBI[80,82,92] and substance use,[78] and can persist for months after a TBI.[93] As such, neuroinflammation has the potential to disrupt or maladaptively interact with the ongoing pruning process in the adolescent brain.

Adolescence is a highly vulnerable developmental stage due to the fact of the ongoing maturation of the prefrontal cortex. There is mounting evidence that TBI and problematic substance consumption during this developmental stage leads to long-standing alterations in brain morphology and function. Evidence suggests that patients with a history of adolescent TBI and substance use disorder neurobiologically differ from SUD patients who started using substances or acquired a TBI after brain maturation was completed.

TBI-Related Neurobehavioral Risks of Developing Addiction

The orbitofrontal cortex (OFC) is a component structure of the prefrontal cortex, which underlies the reflective control system implicated in addiction. The OFC is also especially vulnerable to direct blunt trauma to the head and to shearing along the sharp edges of the orbital surface of the skull that can occur following percussive shock waves to the brain.[62] TBI structural damage to the OFC can result in organic personality changes including impaired empathy, increased problems with interpersonal functioning, antisocial behavior, poor distress tolerance, apathy, increased mood lability, and hostility.[50,62,94-102]

OFC damage is also associated with impulsive responding.[103-105] Patients with TBI have been shown to prefer small immediate rewards over larger delayed rewards, have prolonged decision-making, make poor quality of decisions, and display impulsive-responding compared to controls.[106-109] Patients with TBI in comparison to healthy controls have also been shown to have difficultly discriminating between contingencies and altering behavior based on past experience, thus not being able to maximize future reward.[110] These complex deficits in decision-making may contribute to difficulties with poor judgment and inhibition in patients with TBI. Thus, patients with TBI with frontal damage may demonstrate impaired ability to delay gratification and seek immediate reward related to drug and alcohol use. This is similar to behavior typically associated with abnormalities of the dopamine system found in patients with OFC lesions.[106,111,112] In the OFC, dopamine enables shifting from immediate versus delayed reward through the processing of salience attribution and in the insula through interceptive information processing.

In sum, decision-making and risk-aversion are dependent on dopamine signaling in the OFC. Dopamine neurocircuitry in the OFC is disrupted by TBI in at least a subset of patients; disruption of dopaminergic signaling in the frontolimbic reward system is thought to bring about addictive behavior.[113] There may be a subset of patients with TBI that have disrupted executive function, leaving them at risk for development of psychological disorders including unhealthy substance use following injury. Identifying these patients and providing treatment aimed at improving executive function may aid in reducing risk for development or re-emergence of SUDs.

HARMS ASSOCIATED WITH CO-OCCURRENCE OF SUD AND TBI

Substance use in those with TBI presents an even greater challenge and is associated with increased risks of adverse medical, neurobehavioral, vocational, and life satisfaction outcomes.

Mortality

In studies examining predictors of mortality in patients with TBI, excessive alcohol use is independently predictive of mortality.[114,115] Younger age and a previous history of substance use have also been associated with increased mortality rates in TBI.[50,116,117] For instance, patients with TBI who demonstrate unhealthy alcohol use had 41% mortality rate compared to 13% to 23% for those with no, occasional, or regular alcohol use at 700 days postinjury.[118] Additionally, in comparison to the general population, the risk of death by suicide has been reported as being four times higher for patients with TBI with substance use at the time of hospital admission.[119]

Violence

There is an increased risk of violent behavior following head injury mediated by substance and/or AUDs in individuals with TBI compared to the general population.[120] In a large study conducted by Kreutzer et al.,[121] moderate to heavy drinking both pre- and postinjury increased the rates of aggressive behavior and arrest postinjury, a threefold increase compared to the general population.[121] Individuals who report drug use or drug use in combination with alcohol are also more likely to have sustained violent injuries than those who report alcohol use alone or deny any substance use.[53] Additionally, the incidence of fatal brain injuries due to violent acts is increasing.[51] Almost 80% of persons with TBIs from violence-related causes had a history of substance use.[51] Alcohol use alone is also associated with violent acts causing TBI. In a large study of persons who were hospitalized or died due to TBI, 60% of those with assault-related TBI had positive blood alcohol concentration upon postinjury testing.[46] Positive blood alcohol upon hospital entry is also associated with longer hospital stays, acute complications (eg, intubation, pneumonia, respiratory distress, intracranial pressure), and greater incidence of neurological impairments at discharge.[5]

An additional important issue to highlight is the high rates of TBI among victims of intimate partner violence (IPV). TBI among the IPV population is under reported. Prevalence estimates are inconsistent and range between 32% and 92%.[122] Additionally, women experiencing a TBI are at increased risk for IPV.[123] Substance use is also associated with risk of TBI and co-occurs among the IPV population.[122]

Neurocognitive Performance

Preexisting alcohol and other SUDs are associated with lower scores on the GCS, increased brain tissue atrophy, and poorer performance on a variety of neurocognitive assessments among persons with TBI.[8] In 129 people who injected drugs, those with histories of multiple head traumas involving LOC performed worse than both a control group and a reference group with only a single episode of loss of consciousness on multiple cognitive domains including working memory (digit span), fine motor speed (Grooved Pegboard), processing speed (Trail-Making Test A), and visuospatial ability and memory (Rey Complex Figure Recall).[124] Group differences were apparent up to 11 years postinjury.[124] Higher blood alcohol levels at time of injury have also been associated with worse performance on orientation and naming (Neurobehavioral Cognitive Status Examination, NCSE), auditory-verbal learning (Rey auditory verbal learning test), and processing speed (Trail-Making Test A)[125] at 30 days postinjury. Similar relationships were observed in patients tested 31-60 days postinjury on the verbal memory and similarities subtest of the NCSE.[125] Additionally, patients with a positive urine screen for illicit drug use upon TBI hospital admission performed significantly worse on WAIS-R Full-Scale IQ and Verbal IQ Indices than patients with a negative drug and alcohol screen.

Finally, in a retrospective analysis, TBI inpatients with a blood alcohol level at or below the legal limit and a positive cocaine screen upon hospital admission performed significantly worse on auditory-verbal learning (Rey auditory verbal learning test) than those with similar blood alcohol level but negative for cocaine.[125] In sum, both TBI and SUD have discrete and overlapping impact on cognitive performance; the combination appears particularly deleterious.

Life Satisfaction and Vocation

Only 40% of patients with TBI and unhealthy alcohol use have been shown to return to work postinjury compared to 73% of patients with TBI without unhealthy alcohol use.[5] Similar effects are seen regarding drug use. Patients with preinjury substance use are eight times less likely to be employed at follow-up than patients without preinjury substance use.[5] Further, patients with preinjury substance use report lower productivity and life satisfaction 2 years postinjury.[5]

Mood/Affect Impairment

Mood disorders are common consequences of TBI and are related to preinjury vulnerability, type and extent of brain damage, and levels of family and social support following head injury.[126] Depressive disorders are the most common mood disorder among patients with TBI and range from 25% to 50% in the first year postinjury and 26% to 64% over the lifetime.[126] Major depression is also frequently associated with anxiety, aggression, and a history of substance-related problems.[126] In a significant number of cases, mood disorders following TBI become chronic and resistant to treatment, with a negative impact on community reintegration and quality of life.[126]

Chronic Pain

Chronic pain is associated with both TBI and SUD in civilian and military populations.[127] It is often comorbid with a range of chronic mental health disorders including depression, PTSD, and SUD.[127] As of mid-2017, published studies examining the co-occurrence of pain and mental health conditions have typically examined one or two conditions (chronic pain and TBI or chronic pain and SUD) rather than the co-occurrence of all three. Similarly, there have been no studies that have prospectively examined the risk and relationship between unhealthy substance use and pain following TBI.[67] Research involving nonopioid treatment for TBI-related chronic pain is also limited. However, there is evidence that the acceptance of chronic pain can be beneficial for reducing disability and improving quality of life in veteran patients with unhealthy alcohol use and mTBI.[128]

Summary of TBI and SUD Harms

The co-occurrence of SUD and TBI is common and is associated with worse psychosocial and medical outcomes, recurrence of substance use, and higher rates of hospitalization.[129] A history of preinjury problems with alcohol and/or substance use is related to greater mortality rates, postinjury emotional and cognitive problems, chronic pain, less work productivity, greater associations with crime, and less life satisfaction following TBI. Collaboration among specialists in pain management, SUD treatment, and neurology is recommended.[130]

ASSESSMENT OF CO-OCCURRING TBI AND SUD

Within the alcohol literature, there is robust evidence that screening, brief intervention, and referral for treatment (SBIRT) for at-risk alcohol use, particularly in primary care settings, is highly efficacious and results in clinically meaningful reductions in alcohol use, increased health care utilization, fewer motor vehicle accidents, and large economic savings.[131-133] The Substance Abuse and Mental Health Services Administration (SAMHSA) recommends SBIRT for medical settings (inpatient, emergency departments, ambulatory, primary and specialty health care settings, and community health clinics).[134] In 1999, the National Institutes of Health (NIH) made a recommendation for the inclusion of SUD evaluation and treatment in rehabilitation programs for TBI.[135] Beginning in 2006, the American College of Surgeons required level I and level II trauma centers to attempt to identify patients with unhealthy alcohol use and level I centers to provide an intervention for patients with unhealthy alcohol use. Screening patients with TBI acutely after injury for both the presence of preinjury substance use and development of new-onset substance use may promote early detection and facilitate adequate follow-up health care.[136] In regard to screening, few studies have examined and identified appropriate and standardized screening instruments that adequately assess for substance use in patients with TBI despite the fact that both diagnoses can share similar impacts on cognitive function, mood, and disinhibition.[8]

Future research will need to develop uniformity in assessment, reporting, and development of alcohol and substance use screening tools specific for TBI populations.[8] Until such tools are developed, we recommend that clinicians continue to use standard tools used in general medical and surgical settings.

Investigators who study SUD have made similar omissions in not adequately assessing the specific symptoms and severity needed to establish TBI.[8] Such mistakes include the reliance on a singular self-report question (typically "loss of consciousness") to identify brain injury and failure to classify the degree and extent of injury.[8] There are only three prospective studies examining the prevalence of brain injury among patients entering substance use treatment programs. The first, part of a large-scale NIDA-funded health services study, examined rates of TBI among patients with SUD was conducted in 652 inmates who used drugs.[137] In this cohort, 446/652 (68%) reported at least one head injury, and 201/653 (31%) reported two or more injuries.[137] Patients with TBI reported significantly higher levels of alcohol, cannabis, and sedative use in the 12 months preceding incarceration, along with other lifetime health-related problems including respiratory, musculoskeletal, circulatory, gastrointestinal, neurological, and skin disorders.[137] Those with two or more injuries had significantly more lifetime health problems than those with one or no injuries.[137]

A second study examined TBI rates among 7,784 adults entering SUD treatment in a state-funded community substance use treatment center.[60] Out of 7,784 patients, 31.7% reported one or more TBI with loss of consciousness.[60] Patients reporting two or more TBIs with loss of consciousness were more likely to have depression, anxiety, suicidal thoughts and attempts, violent behavior, trouble concentrating, and more substance use compared to those with none or one TBI.[60] In a third study, rates of TBI were higher (30%) in 95 patients with a cocaine use disorder than in 75 healthy control subjects (8%), and TBI often preceded initiation of cocaine use.[138]

These findings suggest that TBI screening should be considered as part of a routine intake process to facilitate early detection of head injury. As previously mentioned, screening instruments range in length and comprehension, but they all inquire about history of head injury, and associated loss of consciousness, change in behavior, and difficulty in concentration, thinking, or remembering. At the least, early detection could identify patients with TBI treatment needs, allowing clinicians to consult with specialty care providers and/or to provide education regarding symptoms of both conditions and coping strategies to minimize symptom impact.[139]

In practice, SUD clinical staff are typically not adequately trained in the assessment of TBI and are not familiar with acceptable screening/assessment tools and diagnostic criteria. Both SUD and TBI can present with overlapping and complicated neurocognitive and behavioral problems, which are difficult to discriminate. Both diagnoses also commonly present with other comorbidities such as anxiety, depression, and PTSD, further complicating the TBI diagnostic assessment. Therefore, properly trained clinicians are advised to use one of the following standard measures of TBI assessment: The *VA TBI Identification Clinical Interview*,[29] WARCAT,[30] *Structured Interview for TBI Diagnosis*,[31] *Ohio State University TBI Identification Method*,[26,27] or BAT-L.[28] Additional neurocognitive testing and/or neuroimaging may be used to establish the presence of and track change in the associated symptoms of a TBI but can be used only to support a TBI diagnosis to the extent that these symptoms cannot be accounted for by causes other than TBI itself. In sum, each clinician will use TBI assessment tools differently depending upon their role and degree of training. One potential goal is to identify clinical characteristics that may require special treatment accommodations or varying treatment approaches.[60] Clinical staff are advised to consult with neurology and neuropsychology specialty providers in the management of uncovered TBI symptomology accordingly.

Uncovering of a self-reported head injury may provide an indicator that other mental health and cognitive problems are present and may need proper evaluation and management.[137] Upon identification of TBI, SUD clinicians can offer treatments that emphasize the prevention of risk-taking behaviors that may lead to reinjury, the resumption of work, social and other interpersonal obligations, and accommodation strategies for limitations related to poor cognitive function.

TREATMENT APPROACHES FOR TBI AND SUD

Although NIH and the American College of Surgeons call for the inclusion of SUD treatment in patients with brain injury, little work has been done to determine if traditional SUD interventions are effective for patients with TBI.[135,136,140] In fact, some results have shown that traditional SUD treatment may be relatively ineffective for patients with TBI due to cognitive, behavioral, physical, and emotional deficits that occur after brain injury.[140] More effective care may be provided by accommodating or matching patients with treatment approaches that address specific deficits. However, the literature pertaining to treatment matching is nonexistent and much work needs to be done prior to making evidence-based recommendations. In this section, we will provide an overview of special cognitive, rehabilitative, and pharmacotherapy approaches for TBI and SUD and cotreatment of both TBI and SUD where evidence is available.

Cognitive Rehabilitation for TBI

In reviewing 370 published studies on cognitive rehabilitation in 1246 participants with TBI and stroke, Cicerone et al.[141] concluded that cognitive rehabilitation is clearly the best available form of treatment for people who exhibit neurocognitive impairment and functional limitations following TBI. It is further noted that there is substantial evidence to support interventions for attention, memory, executive function, social communication skills, and comprehensive-holistic rehabilitation after TBI. We present a brief overview of cognitive rehabilitation techniques for TBI that overlap with three common cognitive deficits also occurring in SUD: attention, memory, and executive function.

Attention Training

Although attention training has its limitations,[141,142] ACRM Cognitive Rehabilitation Task Force recommends remediation of attention as a standard practice during postacute rehabilitation from TBI.[141,142] ACRM further recommended that remediation of attention deficits should include both direct attention training and cognitive training as an adjunct to clinician-guided treatment to promote development of compensatory strategies and foster generalization to real-world tasks.[141]

Memory Exercises

Memory training has a controversial past. Therapies based on repetitive drills have shown little evidence of efficacy. However, other approaches to memory training, including mnemonic techniques and other memory-enhancing strategies fostering development of techniques to enhance registration and encoding of information and development of memory search methods, have shown efficacy. Memory strategy training appears to be most effective for persons with mTBI and/or mild memory impairment, with decreasing effectiveness as injury severity and memory impairment increase.[141,143]

External aids have been used to address memory impairments.[144] The majority of more recent memory training studies have focused upon the use of memory notebook and electronic equivalents, essentially serving as "memory prosthetics."

Executive Functions

Executive functions refer to those cognitive abilities required for formulating goals, planning how to achieve them, and carrying out the plans effectively. These functions are critically important in social and vocational situations and are a specific target of cognitive remediation. There is increasing support for the proposition that training-based therapies targeting problem solving may improve functioning in individuals with traumatic brain injury. Programs that allow individuals to practice planning, analyzing, and applying personally and functionally relevant tasks and goals, monitor task performance, and evaluate outcomes have been associated with improved functional skills.

Several interventions have been developed and successfully implemented with such an approach. For example, *Goal Management Training* (GMT) emphasizes the cessation of ongoing activity, and a cognitive strategy for breaking down goals into manageable substeps; learning of these strategies improves goal management on tasks.[145] A second intervention combines attention and problem solving (APS) as targets of therapy in a group-based training protocol. Initial group sessions address attentional difficulties, and later sessions introduce and practice the use of problem-solving strategies. During group sessions, participants are encouraged to adopt a systematic approach to solving problems and to manage and monitor goal achievement through periodic mental checking.[146]

Goal-oriented attentional self-regulation (GOALS) is another manualized group intervention that targets attention regulation skills during the first phase of training, and application of trained attention regulation and goal management strategies to individually defined real-life goals during the second part of training. GOALS participants with chronic brain injury show improvements in cognitive domains such as attention and executive function, performance on complex "real-life" functional tasks, and self-reported use of trained strategies in daily lives, including ability to stop, relax, and refocus (SRR) during stressful times.[147]

Cognitive Rehabilitation for SUD

Cognitive training strategies that target cognitive dysfunctions have shown promise to restore cognitive alterations and help maintain abstinence in SUD[148] by enhancing neuroplasticity and supporting more adaptive decision-making ability.[148,149] Working-memory training (WMT) has been the most studied executive function-based cognitive training tool[148] and has demonstrated promise for near-transfer effects, including improved performance on related tasks of working memory[150] and some far-transfer effects related to reduced alcohol consumption among individuals with heavy drinking following one month of training.[149] WMT often involves a series of computerized tasks that requires participants to repeatedly manipulate and recall stimuli (eg, shapes, numbers) with increasing challenge. Despite having some evidence of far-transfer effects (eg, robust change in alcohol use behavior), findings indicate that WMT is associated with design and compliance issues, as the tasks are often repetitive and require significant time to achieve the desired effects.[151] Thus, study retention is often poor, which raises concerns about WMT generalizability and its transferability toward other behaviors, including increased self-control over substance use.[151] Other cognitive trainings have been shown to improve cognitive performance but have failed to show transferability to real-world tasks.[152]

Cognitive bias modification (CBM) studies have targeted attentional bias training for substance-related cues. Studies training alcohol attentional bias have shown delay in time to return to use (but not in rates of return to alcohol use)[153] and reduced rates of return to alcohol use at a 1-year follow-up relative to a sham training condition in a sample of individuals with AUD seeking treatment.[154] Approach bias (the automatic action tendency to approach alcohol-related cues) is also a target for CBM as alcohol-related cues can trigger automatic tendencies to approach and ultimately consume alcohol.[155] Approach bias training (4-12 CBM sessions lasting 15 minutes) can reduce return to alcohol use rates by 8% to 17% at 1-year follow-up.[154,156,157] Approach bias training is currently being tested among other SUDs, including for methamphetamine.[158]

These promising results for CBM and research gaps in executive function training illuminate the need for more treatment studies on cognitive training overall, as well as the development of innovations to enhance cognitive training acceptability and potential long-term effectiveness.

Cognitive Rehabilitation for SUD and TBI

There has only been one pilot study that has examined the effects of a virtual reality cognitive training and exercise intervention on improving executive function and reducing alcohol use and postconcussive symptoms in veterans with TBI and AUD.[159] It was found that delivering an exercise and virtual reality executive function intervention to U.S. veterans with co-occurring AUD and TBI was feasible with moderate usability and high acceptability ratings. There was also preliminary indication that the training was associated with cognitive improvement in domains related to the specific cognitive challenges of the task, that is, visual scanning and cognitive inhibition-switching. The study was preliminary, and changes may have been partially driven by natural recovery, practice effects, and nonspecific effects, such as participant expectancy, interaction with study staff, and close monitoring. However, these findings lend support for further investigation into the beneficial effects of cognitive training among U.S. veterans with AUD and TBI.[159]

Cognitive Rehabilitation Summary and New Directions

The rehabilitation of cognitive deficits following brain injury has shown significant growth over the last three decades, despite the complexity of the problems being treated and the difficulty in designing valid scientific studies to guide therapy. Cognitive rehabilitation training has been repeatedly shown to improve processes such as attention, memory, and executive functions after brain injury. Compensatory interventions, such as electronic or prosthetic memory book devices and electronic alerting systems, also help improve functional skills. Furthermore, cognitive rehabilitation therapy techniques have been successfully applied to the problems of social integration and vocational training. Experience suggests that the most effective therapy occurs when cognitive training is conducted in real-life situations and has high interest to the individual. Despite the promise, there has been only one pilot cognitive training study for co-occurring SUD and TBI. Preliminary results are promising and there is value to examining strategies which target impairments characteristic to both SUD and TBI patient populations.

Neuromodulation Treatments for SUD and Potential for TBI

Transcranial magnetic stimulation (TMS) is a noninvasive neuromodulation technique that was cleared by the FDA for treatment-resistant depression in 2008. TMS uses the principles of electromagnetic induction of a magnetic pulse delivered through a coil on the scalp to induce an electric current in underlying brain tissue.[160] In August of 2020, the FDA cleared[161] the Brainsway H4 TMS coil for treating tobacco use disorder based on positive findings from an industry sponsored multisite clinical trial (ClinicalTrials.gov, #NCT02126124).[162,163] The Brainsway H4 coil was applied to the bilateral lateral prefrontal and insular cortices[162] and showed significant ($P < 0.001$) improvement between active versus sham conditions in the continuous quit rate for individuals completing treatment on two follow-up assessment points at 6 and 18 weeks.[162] A recent (2022) systematic review and meta-analysis found that tobacco-using participants receiving noninvasive brain stimulation (including both TMS and transcranial direct current stimulation) are 139% more likely to be abstinent with active stimulation relative to placebo stimulation 3-6 months after stopping smoking.[164]

Given the ability of TMS to modulate the neurocircuitry involved with SUD,[165-167] TMS has also been studied as a potential treatment for a variety of other SUDs including alcohol, cocaine, methamphetamine, and heroin/opioids.[168] The co-occurrence of TBI with SUDs adds additional heterogeneity to the pathophysiology of diseases as well as clinical course and outcomes.[167] To that extent, neuromodulatory techniques like TMS and other forms of noninvasive brain stimulation, may be ideal because of the ability to customize treatment paradigms even at the individual level.[169,170] TMS adverse events (5.7%-66.7% rate) are often transient in nature and include headache, tinnitus, physical discomfort, nausea, increased use of analgesics, increased compulsion to over-eat, anxiety/agitation, mood disturbance, blurry vision, and muscle-twitching.[164] It is important to point out that seizure is a known risk for TMS. While this risk is very low when following published safety guidelines, TBI, substance intoxication and withdrawal and indirect effects on sleep loss can garner additional seizure risks.[171,172] Therefore, TMS studies for SUDs and TBI should carefully consider and add additional measures to mitigate seizure risk. Therefore, while promising, additional, larger studies on TMS and other forms of noninvasive brain stimulation for tobacco use disorder smoking and other SUDs with and without co-occurring TBI are needed.[168]

Pharmacological Interventions for SUD and TBI

Very little is known about the pharmacological treatment of SUDs in individuals with TBI and there is limited evidence to inform clinical care.

Possible medications for treating SUD in individuals with TBI can be broadly lumped into two categories: (1) *SUD pharmacotherapies*—medications that are known to be effective for SUD and that are used in patients without TBI and (2) *TBI pharmacotherapies*—medications that have been shown to have some utility for TBI treatment in patients without SUDs.

Pharmacotherapy of Alcohol Use Disorder in Individuals With TBI

The following discussion focuses on the available published data on the treatment of individuals with TBI and SUDs with medications that are either known SUD pharmacotherapies or TBI pharmacotherapies.

Although there are four FDA-approved medications for the treatment of AUD, including disulfiram, acamprosate, and both oral and extended-release injectable naltrexone, there are not any published reports of the use of any of the four FDA-approved AUD treatments in patients with AUD and history of TBI.[173]

One study sought to examine the efficacy of valproate (an anticonvulsant medication with a role in the treatment of addiction disorders, likely through glutamatergic and GABAergic neurotransmission) compared to naltrexone to reduce heavy drinking among U.S. veterans with AUD and common co-occurring conditions including TBI and PTSD.[173] Of the 62 patients randomized, 60% had a history of TBI and were more likely to return to heavy drinking compared with those with no TBI.[173] Although the results did not reach significance, the authors noted that valproate appears to be less effective than naltrexone to prevent return to heavy drinking.[173] Valproic acid, has also been tested in one other small open-label pilot trial focusing on alcohol use in individuals with TBI and found pre/postreductions in alcohol use and in symptoms of mood lability.[174]

A fifth medication, topiramate, although not FDA-approved for AUD treatment, is also known to be efficacious[175] in reducing alcohol use. Topiramate is thus an off-label AUD pharmacotherapy. It is also a form of "TBI pharmacotherapy" when it is used to treat TBI-related headache.[176] To date, topiramate is the only medication that has been tested in a prospective controlled trial to treat AUD in patients with mTBI (AUD/TBI). In a double-blind, randomized controlled study of 32 veterans with AUD and mTBI, topiramate in doses up to 300 mg/d significantly reduced alcohol use (drinks per week) compared to placebo.[177] However, topiramate treatment was also associated with negative effects on cognition, with dysfunction observed in verbal learning and memory but appeared to resolve with tapering off medication. In conclusion, while topiramate may help reduce alcohol use, it may aggravate cognitive dysfunction in individuals with mTBI. Difficulties with cognition should be regularly monitored when using topiramate to treat AUD in patients with a history of TBI, and treatment modified if significant functional impairment is observed.

Pharmacotherapy of Nonalcohol SUDs in TBI

To date, there are no published reports of clinical trials employing pharmacotherapy to treat SUDs other than AUD. Specifically, there are no reports of pharmacological treatment of opioid, stimulant, sedative-hypnotic, cannabis, or other nonalcohol SUDs in patients with TBI.

SUD Pharmacotherapies Used to Treat Non-SUD Symptoms in TBI

Regarding the use of SUD pharmacotherapies for non-SUD indications in patients with TBI, there are two published reports of naltrexone treatment, describing a total of three cases.[178,179] These case reports describe the use of naltrexone, an opioid antagonist, to improve TBI symptoms, not SUD. The experimental use of naltrexone was based on animal studies that suggest that opioid antagonists such as naloxone may be helpful in reducing the effects of acute brain injury.[178,180] Tennant[179] described placebo-controlled within-case studies involving two patients whose postconcussion symptoms (including headache, amnesia, disorientation, depression, and problems with speech) were improved by naltrexone treatment. Another case report[178] described the open-label use of oral naltrexone for a non-SUD indication in a patient after severe brain injury, to enhance motor, speech, and overall functional recovery, not as a treatment for SUD. The patient in this case was described as showing accelerated improvement in functional status following naltrexone treatment. There are no reports on the use of partial or full opioid agonist pharmacotherapies such as buprenorphine or methadone treatment in patients with TBI. Nor are reports available for tobacco use disorder pharmacotherapies in patients with TBI.

Pharmacotherapy for SUD and TBI: Future Directions

The use of catecholaminergic (particularly dopaminergic medications) remains a research approach to pharmacotherapy of both TBI-related cognitive impairments[75] as well as SUDs. These medications include stimulants and other dopaminergic agents such as antiparkinsonian medications, some of which have been shown to have modest efficacy in trials in stimulant use disorders. Examples are D-amphetamine and bupropion-dopaminergic medications that have been found to have modest efficacy in cocaine use disorder.[181] Stimulants and bupropion have also been judged to have modest efficacy in methamphetamine use disorder.[182]

Clinical research on the feasibility and effectiveness of both known and experimental SUD pharmacotherapies is needed in order to guide practitioners in the use of medications for these co-occurring disorders. No clear evidence exists that would prevent the use of currently approved pharmacotherapies for nicotine, opioid, or AUDs in patients with TBI, but nor is there evidence regarding their effectiveness in this population.

CONCLUSIONS

The co-occurrence of SUD and TBI is common and carries great neurocognitive, neurobiological, affective, and functional harms along with higher rates of mortality than either diagnosis alone. Numerous studies document a high incidence of preinjury drug and alcohol use in patients with TBI, with high rates of intoxication upon hospital admission. Both SUD and TBI are highly comorbid with other medical and mental health problems including chronic pain, depression, PTSD, and anxiety. Although the prevalence and associated harms of these co-occurring disorders are beginning to be examined, much work is needed to identify factors that may enhance current treatment interventions.

Patients with preinjury histories of substance use are at higher risk for return to substance use following TBI. More research is needed on the prevalence of SUD following TBI and to determine if the development of SUD postinjury is an attempt to assuage TBI-related symptoms.[183] If this is true, treatments aimed at recovery of dysfunction and on improving emotional and pain distress tolerance, coping, and accommodation are likely treatment targets. Barriers to accessing these routine clinical treatments for SUD and TBI need to be identified and reduced.

It's imperative that current SUD and TBI screening and treatment interventions (eg, pharmacotherapy and cognitive rehabilitation) are tested for accuracy and efficacy in patients with these dual diagnoses. If current tools are ineffective, it will be necessary to adapt or develop new interventions for this unique patient population. Until these tools are available, SUD treatment providers should, at a minimum, screen for TBI in patients seeking SUD treatment. Upon discovery of TBI, clinicians should offer treatment emphasizing reduction of risk-taking behavior and accommodate for any limitations that prevent full benefit from known drug and alcohol treatments. Providers are also encouraged to seek consultation from specialty services such as neurology, neuropsychology, and rehabilitation medicine and modify current treatment approaches to accommodate the neurocognitive deficits common in these dually diagnosed patients.

In sum, the problems associated with co-occurring TBI and SUD are bidirectional and complex. Our understanding of the underlying neural mechanisms and associated dual treatment options for these comorbidities is in its infancy. Recent academic and media attention have resulted in a growing literature examining these conditions with the aim of developing new innovative treatment strategies, ultimately reducing the harm and burden associated with these co-occurring conditions.

REFERENCES

1. Finkelstein E, Corso PS, Miller TR. *The Incidence and Economic Burden of Injuries in the United States.* Oxford University Press; 2006.
2. Coronado VG, McGuire LC, Faul M, Sugerman DE, Pearson WS. Traumatic brain injury epidemiology and public health issues. In: *Brain Injury Medicine: Principles and Practice.* Demos Medical Publishing; 2012.
3. Faul M, Xu L, Wald MM, Coronado VG. *Traumatic Brain Injury in the United States: Emergency Department Visits, Hospitalizations and Deaths 2002–2006.* Centers for Disease Control and Prevention, National Center for Injury Prevention and Control; 2010.
4. Kolakowsky-Hayner SA, Gourley EV III, Kreutzer JS, Marwitz JH, Meade MA, Cifu DX. Post-injury substance abuse among persons with brain injury and persons with spinal cord injury. *Brain Inj.* 2002;16(7):583-592.
5. Taylor LA, Kreutzer JS, Demm SR, Meade MA. Traumatic brain injury and substance abuse: a review and analysis of the literature. *Neuropsychol Rehabil.* 13(1-2):165-188. doi:10.1080/09602010244000336
6. Carlson K, Nelson D, Orazem RJ, Nugent S, Cifu DX, Sayer NA. Psychiatric diagnoses among Iraq and Afghanistan war veterans screened for deployment-related traumatic brain injury. *J Trauma Stress.* 2010;23(1):17-24.
7. Taylor BC, Hagel EM, Carlson KF. Prevalence and costs of co-occurring traumatic brain injury with and without psychiatric disturbance and pain among Afghanistan and Iraq War Veteran V.A. users. *Med Care.* 2012;50(4):342-346. doi:10.1097/MLR.0b013e318245a558
8. West SL. Substance use among persons with traumatic brain injury: a review. *NeuroRehabilitation.* 2011;29(1):1-8. doi:10.3233/nre-2011-0671
9. Marr A, Coronado VG, eds. *Central Nervous System Injury Surveillance Data Submission Standards-2002.* Vol. Vol 62 Centers for Disease Control and Prevention, National Center for Injury Prevention and Control; 2004:549-552.
10. Defense Centers of Excellence for Psychological Health and Traumatic Brain Injury. *Mild Traumatic Brain Injury Pocket Guide (CONUS).* Defense Technical Information Center; 2010.
11. Cassidy JD, Carroll LJ, Peloso PM, et al. Incidence, risk factors and prevention of mild traumatic brain injury: results of the WHO Collaborating Centre Task Force on Mild Traumatic Brain Injury. *J Rehabil Med.* 2004;(43 Suppl):28-60.
12. Zuccarelli LA. Altered cellular anatomy and physiology of acute brain injury and spinal cord injury. *Crit Care Nurs Clin North Am.* 2000;12(4):403-411.
13. Stocco A, Fum D, Napoli A. Dissociable processes underlying decisions in the Iowa Gambling Task: a new integrative framework. *Behav Brain Funct.* 2009;5:1. doi:10.1186/1744-9081-5-1
14. Nelson NW, Davenport ND, Sponheim SR, Anderson CR. Blast-related mild traumatic brain injury: neuropsychological evaluation and findings. In: Kobeissy FH, ed. *Brain Neurotrauma Molecular, Neuropsychological, and Rehabilitation Aspects.* Taylor & Francis; 2015.
15. American Pyschiatric Association. *Diagnostic and Statistical Manual of Mental Disorders IV.* American Psychiatric Publishing; 2000.
16. Mittenberg W, Strauman S. Diagnosis of mild head injury and the postconcussion syndrome. *J Head Trauma Rehabil.* 2000;15(2):783-791.
17. Murray CK, Reynolds JC, Schroeder JM, Harrison MB, Evans OM, Hopenthal DR. Spectrum of care provided at an echelon II Medical Unit during Operation Iraqi Freedom. *Mil Med.* 2005;170(6):516-520.
18. Galarneau MR, Woodruff SI, Dye JL, Mohrle CR, Wade AL. Traumatic brain injury during Operation Iraqi Freedom: findings from the United States Navy-Marine Corps Combat Trauma Registry. *J Neurosurg.* 2008;108(5):950-957. doi:10.3171/jns/2008/108/5/0950
19. Zhao Y, Wang ZG. Blast-induced traumatic brain injury: a new trend of blast injury research. *Chin J Traumatol.* 2015;18(4):201-203.
20. Courtney A, Courtney M. The complexity of biomechanics causing primary blast-induced traumatic brain injury: a review of potential mechanisms. *Front Neurol.* 2015;6:221. doi:10.3389/fneur.2015.00221
21. Maroon JC, Winkelman R, Bost J, Amos A, Mathyssek C, Miele V. Chronic traumatic encephalopathy in contact sports: a systematic review of all reported pathological cases. *PLoS One.* 2015;10(2):e0117338.
22. Safinia C, Berhsad EM, Clark HB, et al. Chronic traumatic encephalopathy in athletes involved with high-impact sports. *J Vasc Interv Neurol.* 2016;9(2):34-48.
23. Murray HC, Osterman C, Bell P, Vinnell L, Curtis MA. Neuropathology in chronic traumatic encephalopathy: a systematic review of comparative post-mortem histology literature. *Acta Neuropathol Commun.* 2022;10(1):108. doi:10.1186/s40478-022-01413-9
24. Blennow K, Brody DL, Kochanek PM, et al. Traumatic brain injuries. *Nat Rev Dis Primers.* 2016;2:16084. doi:10.1038/nrdp.2016.84
25. Sparks P, Lawrence T, Hinze S. Neuroimaging in the diagnosis of chronic traumatic encephalopathy: a systematic review. *Clin J Sport Med.* 2020;30(Suppl 1):S1-s10. doi:10.1097/jsm.0000000000000541
26. Corrigan JD, Bogner J. Initial reliability and validity of the Ohio State University TBI identification method. *J Head Trauma Rehabil.* 2007;22(6):318-329.
27. Corrigan JD, Selassie AW, Lineberry LE, et al. Comparison of the traumatic brain injury (TBI) model systems national dataset to a population-based cohort of TBI hospitalizations. *Arch Phys Med Rehabil.* 2007;88(4):418-426. doi:10.1016/j.apmr.2007.01.010
28. Fortier CB, Amick MM, Grande L, et al. The Boston assessment of traumatic brain injury-lifetime (BAT-L) semistructured interview: evidence of research utility and validity. *J Head Trauma Rehabil.* 2014;29(1):89-98. doi:10.1097/HTR.0b013e3182865859
29. Vanderploeg RD, Groer S, Belanger HG. Initial developmental process of a VA semistructured clinical interview for TBI identification. *J Rehabil Res Dev.* 2012;49(4):545-556.
30. Terrio H, Brenner LA, Ivins BJ, et al. Traumatic brain injury screening: preliminary findings in a US Army Brigade Combat Team. *J Head Trauma Rehabil.* 2009;24(1):14-23. doi:10.1097/HTR.0b013e31819581d8
31. Donnelly KT, Donnelly JP, Dunnam M, et al. Reliability, sensitivity, and specificity of the VA traumatic brain injury screening tool. *J Head Trauma Rehabil.* 2011;26(6):439-453. doi:10.1097/HTR.0b013e3182005de3
32. SCAT3. *Br J Sports Med.* 2013;47(5):259.
33. McCrea M, Kelly JP, Randolph C, et al. Standardized assessment of concussion (SAC): on-site mental status evaluation of the athlete. *J Head Trauma Rehabil.* 1998;13(2):27-35.
34. Hunt TN, Ferrara MS, Bornstein RA, Baumgartner TA. The reliability of the modified balance error scoring system. *Clin J Sport Med.* 2009;19(6):471-475. doi:10.1097/JSM.0b013e3181c12c7b

35. Bin Zahid A, Hubbard ME, Dammavalam VM, et al. Assessment of acute head injury in an emergency department population using sport concussion assessment tool. 3rd ed. *Appl Neuropsychol Adult.* 2016;25(2):110-119. doi:10.1080/23279095.2016.1248765
36. Belanger HG, Curtiss G, Demery JA, Lebowitz BK, Vanderploeg RD. Factors moderating neuropsychological outcomes following mild traumatic brain injury: a meta-analysis. *J Int Neuropsychol Soc.* 2005;11(3):215-227. doi:10.1017/s1355617705050277
37. Dikmen S, McLean A, Temkin N. Neuropsychological and psychosocial consequences of minor head injury. *J Neurol Neurosurg Psychiatry.* 1986;49(11):1227-1232.
38. Powell JH, al-Adawi S, Morgan J, Greenwood RJ. Motivational deficits after brain injury: effects of bromocriptine in 11 patients. *J Neurol Neurosurg Psychiatry.* 1996;60(4):416-421.
39. Vanderploeg RD, Curtiss G, Luis CA, Salazar AM. Long-term morbidities following self-reported mild traumatic brain injury. *J Clin Exp Neuropsychol.* 2007;29(6):585-598. doi:10.1080/13803390600826587
40. Hartlage LC, Durant-Wilson D, Patch PC. Persistent neurobehavioral problems following mild traumatic brain injury. *Arch Clin Neuropsychol.* 2001;16(6):561-570.
41. Pickelsimer EE, Selassie AW, Gu JK, Langlois JA. A population-based outcomes study of persons hospitalized with traumatic brain injury: operations of the South Carolina Traumatic Brain Injury Follow-up Registry. *J Head Trauma Rehabil.* 2006;21(6):491-504.
42. Whiteneck G, Brooks CA, Mellick D, Harrison-Felix C, Terrill MS, Noble K. Population-based estimates of outcomes after hospitalization for traumatic brain injury in Colorado. *Arch Phys Med Rehabil.* 2004;85(4 Suppl 2):S73-S81.
43. Schwab K, Grafman J, Salazar AM, Kraft J. Residual impairments and work status 15 years after penetrating head injury: report from the Vietnam Head Injury Study. *Neurology.* 1993;43(1):95-103.
44. Gurney JG, Rivara FP, Mueller BA, Newell DW, Copass MK, Jurkovitch GJ. The effects of alcohol intoxication on the initial treatment and hospital course of patients with acute brain injury. *J Trauma.* 1992;33(5):709-713.
45. Kaplan CP, Corrigan JD. Effect of blood alcohol level on recovery from severe closed head injury. *Brain Injury.* 1992;6(4):337-349.
46. Kraus JF, Morgenstern H, Fife D, Conroy C, Nourjah P. Blood alcohol tests, prevalence of involvement, and outcomes following brain injury. *Am J Public Health.* 1989;79(3):294-299.
47. Sparadeo FR, Gill D. Effects of prior alcohol use on head injury recovery. *J Head Trauma Rehabil.* 1989;4:75-81.
48. Rimel RW, Giordani B, Barth JT, Jane JA. Moderate head injury: completing the clinical spectrum of brain trauma. *Neurosurgery.* 1982;11(3):344-351.
49. Gordon WA, Mann N, Willer B. Demographic and social characteristics of the traumatic brain injury model system database. *J Head Trauma Rehabil.* 1993;8:26-33.
50. Corrigan JD. Substance abuse as a mediating factor in outcome from traumatic brain injury. *Arch Phys Med Rehabil.* 1995;76(4):302-309.
51. Bogner JA, Corrigan JD, Mysiw WJ, Clinchot D, Fugate L. A comparison of substance abuse and violence in the prediction of long-term rehabilitation outcomes after traumatic brain injury. *Arch Phys Med Rehabil.* 2001;82(5):571-577. doi:10.1053/apmr.2001.22340
52. Hibbard MR, Uysal S, Kepler K, Bogdany J, Silver J. Axis I psychopathology in individuals with traumatic brain injury. *J Head Trauma Rehabil.* 1998;13(4):24-39.
53. Drubach DA, Kelly MP, Winslow MM, Flynn JP. Substance abuse as a factor in the causality, severity, and recurrence rate of traumatic brain injury. *Md Med J.* 1985;42(10):989-993.
54. Kreutzer JS, Witol AD, Marwitz JH. Alcohol and drug use among young persons with traumatic brain injury. *J Learn Disabil.* 1996;29(6):643-651.
55. Ommaya AK, Salazar AM, Dannenberg AL, Ommaya AK, Chervinsky AB, Schwab K. Outcome after traumatic brain injury in the U.S. military medical system. *J Trauma.* 1996;41(6):972-975.
56. Johnson LA, Eick-Cost A, Jeffries V, Russell K, Otto JL. Risk of alcohol use disorder or other drug use disorder among U.S. Service members following traumatic brain injury, 2008-2011. *Mil Med.* 2015;180(2):208-215. doi:10.7205/milmed-d-14-00268
57. Alterman AI, Tarter RE. Relationship between familial alcoholism and head injury. *J Stud Alcohol.* 1985;46(3):256-258.
58. Walker R, Staton M, Leukefeld CG. History of head injury among substance users: preliminary findings. *Subst Use Misuse.* 2001;36(6-7):757-770.
59. Hillbom M, Holm L. Contribution of traumatic head injury to neuropsychological deficits in alcoholics. *J Neurol Neurosurg Psychiatry.* 1986;49(12):1348-1353.
60. Walker R, Cole JE, Logan TK, Corrigan JD. Screening substance abuse treatment clients for traumatic brain injury: prevalence and characteristics. *J Head Trauma Rehabil.* 2007;22(6):360-367. doi:10.1097/01.htr.0000300231.90619.50
61. Horner MD, Ferguson PL, Selassie AW, Labbate LA, Kniele K, Corrigan JD. Patterns of alcohol use 1 year after traumatic brain injury: a population-based, epidemiological study. *J Int Neuropsychol Soc.* 2005;11(3):322-330. doi:10.1017/s135561770505037x
62. Bjork JM, Grant SJ. Does traumatic brain injury increase risk for substance abuse? *J Neurotrauma.* 2009;26(7):1077-1082. doi:10.1089/neu.2008-0849 10.1089/neu.2008.0849
63. Silver JM, Kramer R, Greenwald S, Weissman M. The association between head injuries and psychiatric disorders: findings from the New Haven NIMH Epidemiologic Catchment Area Study. *Brain Inj.* 2001;15(11):935-945. doi:10.1080/02699050110065295
64. Fann JR, Burington B, Leonetti A, Jaffe K, Katon WJ, Thompson RS. Psychiatric illness following traumatic brain injury in an adult health maintenance organization population. *Arch Gen Psychiatry.* 2004;61(1):53-61. doi:10.1001/archpsyc.61.1.53
65. Seal KH, Bertenthal D, Samuelson K, Maguen S, Kumar S, Vasterling JJ. Association between mild traumatic brain injury and mental health problems and self-reported cognitive dysfunction in Iraq and Afghanistan Veterans. *J Rehabil Res Dev.* 2016;53(2):185-198. doi:10.1682/jrrd.2014.12.0301
66. Miller SC, Baktash SH, Webb TS, et al. Risk for addiction-related disorders following mild traumatic brain injury in a large cohort of active-duty U.S. airmen. *Am J Psychiatry.* 2013;170(4):383-390. doi:10.1176/appi.ajp.2012.12010126
67. Nampiaparampil DE. Prevalence of chronic pain after traumatic brain injury: a systematic review. *JAMA.* 2008;300(6):711-719. doi:10.1001/jama.300.6.711
68. Chen Y-H, Huang EY-K, Kuo T-T, Miller J, Chiang Y-H, Hoffer BJ. Impact of traumatic brain injury on dopaminergic transmission. *Cell Transplant.* 2017;26(7):1156-1168.
69. Blennow K, Hardy J, Zetterberg H. The neuropathology and neurobiology of traumatic brain injury. *Neuron.* 2016;76(12):886-899. doi:10.1016/j.neuron.2012.11.021
70. McGuire JL, Ngwenya LB, McCullumsmith RE. Neurotransmitter changes after traumatic brain injury: an update for new treatment strategies. *Mol Psychiatry.* 2019;24(7):995-1012. doi:10.1038/s41380-018-0239-6
71. Bagri K, Kumar P, Deshmukh R. Neurobiology of traumatic brain injury. *Brain Inj.* 2021;35(10):1113-1120. doi:10.1080/02699052.2021.1972152
72. Wagner AK, Sokoloski JE, Ren D, et al. Controlled cortical impact injury affects dopaminergic transmission in the rat striatum. *J Neurochem.* 2005;95(2):457-465. doi:10.1111/j.1471-4159.2005.03382.x
73. Jenkins PO, Mehta MA, Sharp DJ. Catecholamines and cognition after traumatic brain injury. *Brain.* 2016;139(Pt 9):2345-2371. doi:10.1093/brain/aww128
74. Lan YL, Li S, Lou JC, Ma XC, Zhang B. The potential roles of dopamine in traumatic brain injury: a preclinical and clinical update. *Am J Transl Res.* 2019;11(5):2616-2631.
75. Osier ND, Dixon CE. Catecholaminergic based therapies for functional recovery after TBI. *Brain Res.* 2016;1640(Pt A):15-35. doi:10.1016/j.brainres.2015.12.026
76. Vasilenko SA, Evans-Polce RJ, Lanza ST. Age trends in rates of substance use disorders across ages 18-90: differences by gender and race/ethnicity. *Drug Alcohol Depend.* 2016;180:260-264. doi:10.1016/j.drugalcdep.2017.08.027

77. Taylor CA, Bell JM, Breiding MJ, Xu L. Traumatic brain injury-related emergency department visits, hospitalizations, and deaths—United States, 2007 and 2013. *MMWR Surveill Summ.* 2017;66(9):1-16. doi:10.15585/mmwr.ss6609a1
78. Merkel SF, Razmpour R, Lutton EM, et al. Adolescent traumatic brain injury induces chronic mesolimbic neuroinflammation with concurrent enhancement in the rewarding effects of cocaine in mice during adulthood. *J Neurotrauma.* 2017;34(1):165-181. doi:10.1089/neu.2015.4275
79. Merkel SF, Cannella LA, Razmpour R, et al. Factors affecting increased risk for substance use disorders following traumatic brain injury: what we can learn from animal models. *Neurosci Biobehav Rev.* 2017;77:209-218. doi:10.1016/j.neubiorev.2017.03.015
80. Cannella LA, McGary H, Ramirez SH. Brain interrupted: Early life traumatic brain injury and addiction vulnerability. *Exp Neurol.* 2019;317:191-201. doi:10.1016/j.expneurol.2019.03.003
81. Cannella LA, Andrews AM, Tran F, et al. Experimental traumatic brain injury during adolescence enhances cocaine rewarding efficacy and dysregulates dopamine and neuroimmune systems in brain reward substrates. *J Neurotrauma.* 2020;37(1):27-42. doi:10.1089/neu.2019.6472
82. Weil ZM, Karelina K, Corrigan JD. Does pediatric traumatic brain injury cause adult alcohol misuse: combining preclinical and epidemiological approaches. *Exp Neurol.* 2019;317:284-290. doi:10.1016/j.expneurol.2019.03.012
83. Hoops D, Flores C. Making dopamine connections in adolescence. *Trends Neurosci.* 2017;40(12):709-719. doi:10.1016/j.tins.2017.09.004
84. Reynolds LM, Flores C. Mesocorticolimbic dopamine pathways across adolescence: diversity in development. *Front Neural Circuits.* 2021;15:735625. doi:10.3389/fncir.2021.735625
85. Vosberg DE, Leyton M, Flores C. The Netrin-1/DCC guidance system: dopamine pathway maturation and psychiatric disorders emerging in adolescence. *Mol Psychiatry.* 2020;25(2):297-307. doi:10.1038/s41380-019-0561-7
86. Kaukas L, Holmes JL, Rahimi F, Collins-Praino L, Corrigan F. Injury during adolescence leads to sex-specific executive function deficits in adulthood in a pre-clinical model of mild traumatic brain injury. *Behav Brain Res.* 2021;402:113067. doi:10.1016/j.bbr.2020.113067
87. Penzes P, Cahill ME, Jones KA, VanLeeuwen JE, Woolfrey KM. Dendritic spine pathology in neuropsychiatric disorders. *Nat Neurosci.* 2011;14(3):285-293. doi:10.1038/nn.2741
88. Paolicelli RC, Bolasco G, Pagani F, et al. Synaptic pruning by microglia is necessary for normal brain development. *Science.* 2011;333(6048):1456-1458. doi:10.1126/science.1202529
89. Mallya AP, Wang HD, Lee HNR, Deutch AY. Microglial pruning of synapses in the prefrontal cortex during adolescence. *Cereb Cortex.* 2019;29(4):1634-1643. doi:10.1093/cercor/bhy061
90. Kopec AM, Smith CJ, Ayre NR, Sweat SC, Bilbo SD. Microglial dopamine receptor elimination defines sex-specific nucleus accumbens development and social behavior in adolescent rats. *Nat Commun.* 2018;9(1):3769. doi:10.1038/s41467-018-06118-z
91. Schalbetter SM, von Arx AS, Cruz-Ochoa N, et al. Adolescence is a sensitive period for prefrontal microglia to act on cognitive development. *Sci Adv.* 2022;8(9):eabi6672. doi:10.1126/sciadv.abi6672
92. Vonder Haar C, Ferland J-MN, Kaur S, Riparip L-K, Rosi S, Winstanley CA. Cocaine self-administration is increased after frontal traumatic brain injury and associated with neuroinflammation. *Eur J Neurosci.* 2019;50(3):2134-2145. doi:10.1111/ejn.14123
93. Ware AL, Yeates KO, Tang K, et al. Longitudinal white matter microstructural changes in pediatric mild traumatic brain injury: an A-CAP study. *Hum Brain Mapp.* 2022;43(12):3809-3823. doi:10.1002/hbm.25885
94. Franulic A, Horta E, Maturana R, Scherpenisse J, Carbonell C. Organic personality disorder after traumatic brain injury: cognitive, anatomic and psychosocial factors. A 6 month follow-up. *Brain Inj.* 2000;14(5):431-439.
95. Neumann D, Zupan B, Babbage DR, et al. Affect recognition, empathy, and dysosmia after traumatic brain injury. *Arch Phys Med Rehabil.* 2012;93(8):1414-1420. doi:10.1016/j.apmr.2012.03.009
96. Wood RL, Williams C. Inability to empathize following traumatic brain injury. *J Int Neuropsychol Soc.* 2008;14(2):289-296. doi:10.1017/s1355617708080326
97. Milders M, Fuchs S, Crawford JR. Neuropsychological impairments and changes in emotional and social behaviour following severe traumatic brain injury. *J Clin Exp Neuropsychol.* 2003;25(2):157-172. doi:10.1076/jcen.25.2.157.13642
98. Henry JD, Phillips LH, Crawford JR, Theodorou G, Summers F. Cognitive and psychosocial correlates of alexithymia following traumatic brain injury. *Neuropsychologia.* 2006;44(1):62-72. doi:10.1016/j.neuropsychologia.2005.04.011
99. Lippert-Gruner M, Kuchta J, Hellmich M, Klug N. Neurobehavioural deficits after severe traumatic brain injury (TBI). *Brain Inj.* 2006;20(6):569-574. doi:10.1080/02699050600664467
100. Geva S, Cooper JM, Gadian DG, Mishkin M, Vargha-Khadem F. Impairment on a self-ordered working memory task in patients with early-acquired hippocampal atrophy. *Dev Cogn Neurosci.* 2016;20:12-22. doi:10.1016/j.dcn.2016.06.001
101. Hornak J, Bramham J, Rolls ET, et al. Changes in emotion after circumscribed surgical lesions of the orbitofrontal and cingulate cortices. *Brain.* 2003;126(Pt 7):1691-1712. doi:10.1093/brain/awg168
102. Anderson SW, Barrash J, Bechara A, Tranel D. Impairments of emotion and real-world complex behavior following childhood- or adult-onset damage to ventromedial prefrontal cortex. *J Int Neuropsychol Soc.* 2006;12(2):224-235. doi:10.1017/s1355617706060346
103. Crowe SF, Crowe LM. Does the presence of posttraumatic anosmia mean that you will be disinhibited? *J Clin Exp Neuropsychol.* 2013;35(3):298-308. doi:10.1080/13803395.2013.771616
104. Varney NR. Prognostic significance of anosmia in patients with closed-head trauma. *J Clin Exp Neuropsychol.* 1998;10(2):250-254. doi:10.1080/01688638808408239
105. Rolls ET. The functions of the orbitofrontal cortex. *Brain Cogn.* 2004;55(1):11-29. doi:10.1016/s0278-2626(03)00277-x
106. Rogers RD, Everitt BJ, Baldacchino A, et al. Dissociable deficits in the decision-making cognition of chronic amphetamine abusers, opiate abusers, patients with focal damage to prefrontal cortex, and tryptophan-depleted normal volunteers: evidence for monoaminergic mechanisms. *Neuropsychopharmacology.* 1999;20(4):322-339. doi:10.1016/s0893-133x(98)00091-8
107. Salmond CH, Menon DK, Chatfield DA, Pickard JD, Sahakian BJ. Deficits in decision-making in head injury survivors. *J Neurotrauma.* 2005;22(6):613-622. doi:10.1089/neu.2005.22.613
108. McHugh L, Wood RL. Using a temporal discounting paradigm to measure decision-making and impulsivity following traumatic brain injury: a pilot study. *Brain Inj.* 2008;22(9):715-721. doi:10.1080/02699050802263027
109. Dixon MR, Jacobs EA, Sanders S, et al. Impulsivity, self-control, and delay discounting in persons with acquired brain injury. *Behav Intervent.* 2005;20(1):101-120. doi:10.1002/bin.173
110. Schlund MW. Effects of acquired brain injury on adaptive choice and the role of reduced sensitivity to contingencies. *Brain Inj.* 2002;16(6):527-535. doi:10.1080/02699050110113679
111. Manes F, Sahakian B, Clark L, et al. Decision-making processes following damage to the prefrontal cortex. *Brain.* 2002;125(Pt 3):624-639.
112. McDowell S, Whyte J, D'Esposito M. Differential effect of a dopaminergic agonist on prefrontal function in traumatic brain injury patients. *Brain.* 1998;121(Pt 6):1155-1164.
113. Volkow ND, Baler RD. NOW vs LATER brain circuits: implications for obesity and addiction. *Trends Neurosci.* 2015;38(6):345-352. doi:10.1016/j.tins.2015.04.002
114. McMillan TM, Teasdale GM. Death rate is increased for at least 7 years after head injury: a prospective study. *Brain.* 2007;130(Pt 10):2520-2527. doi:10.1093/brain/awm185

115. McMillan TM, Weir CJ, Wainman-Lefley J. Mortality and morbidity 15 years after hospital admission with mild head injury: a prospective case-controlled population study. *J Neurol Neurosurg Psychiatry*. 2014;85(11):1214-1220. doi:10.1136/jnnp-2013-307279
116. Spitz G, Downing MG, McKenzie D, Ponsford JL. Mortality following traumatic brain injury inpatient rehabilitation. *J Neurotrauma*. 2015;32(16):1272-1280. doi:10.1089/neu.2014.3814
117. Kraus J, McArthur D. Incidence and prevalence of, and costs associated with, traumatic brain injury. In: Rosenthal M, Griffith ER, Kreutzer JS, Pentland B, eds. *Rehabilitation of the Adult and Child With Traumatic Brain Injury*. 3rd ed. 1999:3-18.
118. Ruff RM, Marshall LF, Klauber MR, et al. Alcohol abuse and neurological outcome of the severely head injured. *J Head Trauma Rehabil*. 1990;5(3):21-31.
119. Teasdale TW, Engberg AW. Suicide after traumatic brain injury: a population study. *J Neurol Neurosurg Psychiatry*. 2001;71(4):436-440.
120. Fazel S, Lichtenstein P, Grann M, Langstrom N. Risk of violent crime in individuals with epilepsy and traumatic brain injury: a 35-year Swedish population study. *PLoS Med*. 2011;8(12):e1001150. doi:10.1371/journal.pmed.1001150
121. Kreutzer JS, Marwitz JH, Witol AD. Interrelationships between crime, substance abuse, and aggressive behaviours among persons with traumatic brain injury. *Brain Inj*. 1995;9(8):757-768.
122. St Ivany A, Schminkey D. Intimate partner violence and traumatic brain injury: state of the science and next steps. *Fam Community Health*. 2016;39(2):129-137. doi:10.1097/fch.0000000000000094
123. Toccalino D, Haag HL, Estrella MJ, et al. The intersection of intimate partner violence and traumatic brain injury: findings from an emergency summit addressing system-level changes to better support women survivors. *J Head Trauma Rehabil*. 2022;37(1):E20-E29. doi:10.1097/htr.0000000000000743
124. Hestad K, Updike M, Selnes OA, Royal W 3rd. Cognitive sequelae of repeated head injury in a population of intravenous drug users. *Scand J Psychol*. 1995;36(3):246-255.
125. Parry-Jones BL, Vaughan FL, Miles CW. Traumatic brain injury and substance misuse: a systematic review of prevalence and outcomes research (1994-2004). *Neuropsychol Rehabil*. 2006;16(5):537-560. doi:10.1080/09602010500231875
126. Jorge RE, Arciniegas DB. Mood disorders after TBI. *Psychiatr Clin North Am*. 2014;37(1):13-29. doi:10.1016/j.psc.2013.11.005
127. Higgins DM, Kerns RD, Brandt CA, et al. Persistent pain and comorbidity among operation enduring freedom/operation Iraqi freedom/operation new dawn veterans. *Pain Med*. 2014;15(5):782-790. doi:10.1111/pme.12388
128. Cook AJ, Meyer EC, Evans LD, et al. Chronic pain acceptance incrementally predicts disability in polytrauma-exposed veterans at baseline and 1-year follow-up. *Behav Res Ther*. 2015;73:25-32. doi:10.1016/j.brat.2015.07.003
129. Tanielian T, Jaycox LH, Schell TL, et al. Invisible wounds of war: summary and recommendations for addressing psychological and cognitive injuries. *Rand Corp*. 2008.
130. Galloway K, Buckenmaier C III, Gallagher R. War on Pain: pain management across the military continuum. *Am Nurse Today*. 2011; 6:8-12.
131. Fleming MF, Mundt MP, French MT, Manwell LB, Stauffacher EA, Barry KL. Brief physician advice for problem drinkers: long-term efficacy and benefit-cost analysis. *Alcohol Clin Exp Res*. 2002;26(1):36-43.
132. Gentilello LM, Ebel BE, Wickizer TM, Salkever DS, Rivara FP. Alcohol interventions for trauma patients treated in emergency departments and hospitals: a cost benefit analysis. *Ann Surg*. 2005;241(4):541-550.
133. Corrigan JD, Bogner J, Hungerford DW, Schomer K. Screening and brief intervention for substance misuse among patients with traumatic brain injury. *J Trauma*. 2010;69(3):722-726. doi:10.1097/TA.0b013e3181e904cc
134. Madras BK, Compton WM, Avula D, Stegbauer T, Stein JB, Clark HW. Screening, brief interventions, referral to treatment (SBIRT) for illicit drug and alcohol use at multiple healthcare sites: comparison at intake and 6 months later. *Drug Alcohol Depend*. 2009;99(1-3):280-295. doi:10.1016/j.drugalcdep.2008.08.003
135. Consensus conference. Rehabilitation of persons with traumatic brain injury. NIH Consensus Development Panel on Rehabilitation of Persons With Traumatic Brain Injury. *JAMA*. 1999;282:974-983.
136. King PR, Wray LO. Managing behavioral health needs of veterans with traumatic brain injury (TBI) in primary care. *J Clin Psychol Med Settings*. 2012;19(4):376-392. doi:10.1007/s10880-012-9345-9
137. Walker R, Hiller M, Staton M, Leukefeld CG. Head injury among drug abusers: an indicator of co-occurring problems. *J Psychoactive Drugs*. 2003;35(3):343-353. doi:10.1080/02791072.2003.10400017
138. Ramesh D, Keyser-Marcus LA, Ma L, et al. Prevalence of traumatic brain injury in cocaine-dependent research volunteers. *Am J Addict*. 2015;24(4):341-347. doi:10.1111/ajad.12192
139. Olson-Madden JH, Brenner LA, Corrigan JD, Emrick CD, Britton PC. Substance use and mild traumatic brain injury risk reduction and prevention: a novel model for treatment. *Rehabil Res Pract*. 2012;2012:174579. doi:10.1155/2012/174579
140. Graham DP, Cardon AL. An update on substance use and treatment following traumatic brain injury. *Ann N Y Acad Sci*. 2008;1141:148-162. doi:NYAS1141029 10.1196/annals.1441.029
141. Cicerone KD, Langenbahn DM, Braden C, et al. Evidence-based cognitive rehabilitation: updated review of the literature from 2003 through 2008. *Arch Phys Med Rehabil*. 2011;92(4):519-530. doi:10.1016/j.apmr.2010.11.015
142. Haskins EC. *Cognitive Rehabilitation Manual; Translating Evidence-Based Recommendations into Practice*. ACRM Publishing; 2012.
143. Ehlhardt LA, Sohlberg MM, Kennedy M, et al. Evidence-based practice guidelines for instructing individuals with neurogenic memory impairments: what have we learned in the past 20 years? *Neuropsychol Rehabil*. 2008;18(3):300-342. doi:10.1080/09602010701733190
144. Thickpenny-Davis KL, Barker-Collo SL. Evaluation of a structured group format memory rehabilitation program for adults following brain injury. *J Head Trauma Rehabil*. 2007;22(5):303-313. doi:10.1097/01.htr.0000290975.09496.93
145. Levine B, Robertson IH, Clare L, et al. Rehabilitation of executive functioning: an experimental-clinical validation of goal management training. *J Int Neuropsychol Soc*. 2000;6(3):299-312.
146. Miotto EC, Evans JJ, de Lucia MC, Scaff M. Rehabilitation of executive dysfunction: a controlled trial of an attention and problem solving treatment group. *Neuropsychol Rehabil*. 2009;19(4):517-540. doi:10.1080/09602010802332108
147. Novakovic-Agopian T, Chen AJ-W, Rome S, et al. Rehabilitation of executive functioning with training in attention regulation applied to individually defined goals: a pilot study bridging theory, assessment, and treatment. *J Head Trauma Rehabil*. 2011;26(5):325-338. doi:10.1097/HTR.0b013e3181f1ead2
148. Verdejo-Garcia A, Lorenzetti V, Manning V, et al. A roadmap for integrating neuroscience into addiction treatment: a consensus of the neuroscience interest group of the international society of addiction medicine. *Front Psychiatry*. 2019;10:877. doi:10.3389/fpsyt.2019.00877
149. Houben K, Nederkoorn C, Wiers RW, Jansen A. Resisting temptation: decreasing alcohol-related affect and drinking behavior by training response inhibition. *Drug Alcohol Depend*. 2011;116(1-3):132-136. doi:10.1016/j.drugalcdep.2010.12.011
150. Lechner WV, Sidhu NK, Kittaneh AA, Anand A. Interventions with potential to target executive function deficits in addiction: current state of the literature. *Curr Opin Psychol*. 2019;30:24-28. doi:10.1016/j.copsyc.2019.01.017
151. Wanmaker S, Leijdesdorff SMJ, Geraerts E, van de Wetering BJM, Renkema PJ, Franken IHA. The efficacy of a working memory training in substance use patients: a randomized double-blind placebo-controlled clinical trial. *J Clin Exp Neuropsychol*. 2018;40(5):473-486. doi:10.1080/13803395.2017.1372367
152. Ball K, Berch DB, Helmers KF, et al. Effects of cognitive training interventions with older adults: a randomized controlled trial. *JAMA*. 2002;288(18):2271-2281. doi:10.1001/jama.288.18.2271

153. Schoenmakers TM, de Bruin M, Lux IFM, Goertz AG, Van Kerkhof DHAT, Wiers RW. Clinical effectiveness of attentional bias modification training in abstinent alcoholic patients. *Drug Alcohol Depend.* 2010;109(1-3):30-36. doi:10.1016/j.drugalcdep.2009.11.022
154. Rinck M, Wiers RW, Becker ES, Lindenmeyer J. Relapse prevention in abstinent alcoholics by cognitive bias modification: clinical effects of combining approach bias modification and attention bias modification. *J Consult Clin Psychol.* 2018;86(12):1005-1016. doi:10.1037/ccp0000321
155. Wiers RW, Gladwin TE, Hofmann W, Salemink E, Ridderinkhof KR. Cognitive bias modification and cognitive control training in addiction and related psychopathology: mechanisms, clinical perspectives, and ways forward. *Clin Psychol Sci.* 2013;1(2):192-212.
156. Eberl C, Wiers RW, Pawelczack S, Rinck M, Becker ES, Lindenmeyer J. Approach bias modification in alcohol dependence: do clinical effects replicate and for whom does it work best? *Dev Cogn Neurosci.* 2013;4:38-51. doi:10.1016/j.dcn.2012.11.002
157. Wiers RW, Eberl C, Rinck M, Becker ES, Lindenmeyer J. Retraining automatic action tendencies changes alcoholic patients' approach bias for alcohol and improves treatment outcome. *Psychol Sci.* 2011;22(4):490-497. doi:10.1177/0956797611400615
158. Manning V, Garfield JBB, Mroz K, et al. Feasibility and acceptability of approach bias modification during methamphetamine withdrawal and related methamphetamine use outcomes. *J Subst Abuse Treat.* 2019;106:12-18. doi:10.1016/j.jsat.2019.07.008
159. Pennington DL, Reavis JV, Cano MT, Walker E, Batki SL. The impact of exercise and virtual reality executive function training on cognition among heavy drinking veterans with traumatic brain injury: a pilot feasibility study. *Front Behav Neurosci.* 2022;16:802711. doi:10.3389/fnbeh.2022.802711
160. Hallett M. Transcranial magnetic stimulation: a primer. *Neuron.* 2007;55(2):187-199. doi:10.1016/j.neuron.2007.06.026
161. United States Food & Drug Administration. 2023 FDA approval letter, https://www.accessdata.fda.gov/scripts/cdrh/cfdocs/cfpmn/pmn.cfm?ID=K200957
162. Zangen A, Moshe H, Martinez D, et al. Repetitive transcranial magnetic stimulation for smoking cessation: a pivotal multicenter double-blind randomized controlled trial. *World Psychiatry.* 2021;20(3):397-404. doi:10.1002/wps.20905
163. Office on Smoking and Health, Centers for Disease Control and Prevention (CDC). 2023 *Smoking Cessation: Fast Facts.* Accessed May 30, 2023. https://www.cdc.gov/tobacco/data_statistics/fact_sheets/cessation/smoking-cessation-fast-facts
164. Petit B, Dornier A, Meille V, Demina A, Trojak B. Non-invasive brain stimulation for smoking cessation: a systematic review and meta-analysis. *Addiction.* 2022;117(11):2768-2779. doi:10.1111/add.15889
165. Diana M, Raij T, Melis M, Nummenmaa A, Leggio L, Bonci A. Rehabilitating the addicted brain with transcranial magnetic stimulation. *Nat Rev Neurosci.* 2017;18(11):685-693. doi:10.1038/nrn.2017.113
166. Hanlon CA, Dowdle LT, Henderson JS. Modulating neural circuits with transcranial magnetic stimulation: implications for addiction treatment development. *Pharmacol Rev.* 2018;70(3):661-683. doi:10.1124/pr.116.013649
167. Herrold AA, Kletzel SL, Harton BC, Chambers RA, Jordan N, Bender Pape TL. Transcranial magnetic stimulation: potential treatment for co-occurring alcohol, traumatic brain injury and posttraumatic stress disorders. *Neural Regen Res.* 2014;9(19):1712-1730. doi:10.4103/1673-5374.143408
168. Ekhtiari H, Tavakoli H, Addolorato G, et al. Transcranial electrical and magnetic stimulation (tES and TMS) for addiction medicine: a consensus paper on the present state of the science and the road ahead. *Neurosci Biobehav Rev.* 2019;104:118-140. doi:10.1016/j.neubiorev.2019.06.007
169. Herrold AA, Siddiqi SH, Livengood SL, et al. Customizing TMS applications in traumatic brain injury using neuroimaging. *J Head Trauma Rehabil.* 2020;35(6):401-411. doi:10.1097/HTR.0000000000000627
170. Bender Pape TL, Herrold AA, Guernon A, Aaronson A, Rosenow JM. Neuromodulatory interventions for traumatic brain injury. *J Head Trauma Rehabil.* 2020;35(6):365-370. doi:10.1097/HTR.0000000000000643
171. Rossi S, Antal A, Bestmann S, et al. Safety and recommendations for TMS use in healthy subjects and patient populations, with updates on training, ethical and regulatory issues: expert guidelines. *Clin Neurophysiol.* 2021;132(1):269-306. doi:10.1016/j.clinph.2020.10.003
172. Rossi S, Hallett M, Rossini PM, Pascual-Leone A. Safety, ethical considerations, and application guidelines for the use of transcranial magnetic stimulation in clinical practice and research. *Clin Neurophysiol.* 2009;120(12):2008-2039. doi:10.1016/j.clinph.2009.08.016
173. Jorge RE, Li R, Liu X, et al. Treating alcohol use disorder in U.S. veterans: the role of traumatic brain injury. *J Neuropsychiatry Clin Neurosci.* 2019;31(4):319-327. doi:10.1176/appi.neuropsych.18110250
174. Beresford TP, Arciniegas D, Clapp L, Martin B, Alfers J. Reduction of affective lability and alcohol use following traumatic brain injury: a clinical pilot study of anti-convulsant medications. *Brain Inj.* 2005;19(4):309-313.
175. Blodgett JC, Del Re AC, Maisel NC, Finney JW. A meta-analysis of topiramate's effects for individuals with alcohol use disorders. *Alcohol Clin Exp Res.* 2014;38(6):1481-1488. doi:10.1111/acer.12411
176. Minen MT, Boubour A, Walia H, Barr W. Post-concussive syndrome: a focus on post-traumatic headache and related cognitive, psychiatric, and sleep issues. *Curr Neurol Neurosci Rep.* 2016;16(11):100. doi:10.1007/s11910-016-0697-7
177. Pennington DL, Bielenberg J, Lasher B, et al. A randomized pilot trial of topiramate for alcohol use disorder in veterans with traumatic brain injury: effects on alcohol use, cognition, and post-concussive symptoms. *Drug Alcohol Depend.* 2020;214:108149. doi:10.1016/j.drugalcdep.2020.108149
178. Calvanio R, Burke DT, Kim HJ, et al. Naltrexone: effects on motor function, speech, and activities of daily living in a patient with traumatic brain injury. *Brain Inj.* 2000;14(10):933-942.
179. Tennant FS Jr, Wild J. Naltrexone treatment for postconcussional syndrome. *Am J Psychiatry.* 1987;144(6):813-814. doi:10.1176/ajp.144.6.813
180. Zhang H, Wang X, Li Y, et al. Naloxone for severe traumatic brain injury: a meta-analysis. *PLoS One.* 2014;9(12):e113093. doi:10.1371/journal.pone.0113093
181. Castells X, Cunill R, Pérez-Mana C, Vidal X, Capellà D. Psychostimulant drugs for cocaine dependence. *Cochrane Database Syst Rev.* 2016;9(9):CD007380. doi:10.1002/14651858.CD007380.pub4
182. Courtney KE, Ray LA. Methamphetamine: an update on epidemiology, pharmacology, clinical phenomenology, and treatment literature. *Drug Alcohol Depend.* 2014;143:11-21. doi:10.1016/j.drugalcdep.2014.08.003
183. Olsen CM, Corrigan JD. Does traumatic brain injury cause risky substance use or substance use disorder? *Biol Psychiatry.* 2022;91(5):421-437. doi:10.1016/j.biopsych.2021.07.013

CHAPTER

45 Integrated Care for Substance Use Disorder

Emma E. McGinty, Rachel H. Alinsky, and Mark McGovern

CHAPTER OUTLINE

- Introduction
- A brief history of 20th century addiction treatment in the United States
- Toward integrated care for the population of people with SUDs
- Conclusion

INTRODUCTION

Substance use disorder (SUD) involving alcohol or other drugs is common, affecting 15% of the U.S. population aged 12 years or older 2020.[1] The large majority of people with SUD—93% in 2020—do not receive treatment.[1] The historic separation of SUD treatment from the general medical system is one key barrier to treatment. While important progress toward integrating SUD care into primary care and other general medical settings, such as emergency departments, has been made in recent years, much work remains.

The bulk of the U.S. health care system revolves around chronic health conditions. Primary care clinicians screen for conditions and treat identified cases to the limits of their knowledge and ability. In working to manage such conditions in collaboration with patients, primary care clinicians are backed up by specialists with whom they share information and with whom they collaborate when cases are more severe or complex. This guideline- and protocol-driven approach to managing chronic health conditions is the norm across most of health care.

But in most of the health care system, this model has not been optimally applied to SUDs. This chapter describes the evolution of the SUD treatment system in the United States, including recent progress toward integration, a scalable model for the continuum of integrated SUD care, and strategies for expanding integration moving forward.

A BRIEF HISTORY OF 20TH CENTURY ADDICTION TREATMENT IN THE UNITED STATES

In describing how addiction treatment evolved in the health care system, one has to begin by observing the long-term cultural ambivalence about situating it in health care at all. Following from the view that people with SUDs have "bad character" for which they should be punished, criminal justice has often been the lead public entity tasked with responding to people with SUDs. This punitive approach has been exacerbated by the systemic racism underlying the "drug war" approach to substance use in the United States, which has produced policies and systems that disproportionately punish racially and ethnically minoritized groups in the United States. One well-known example is tougher federal criminal penalties for the form of cocaine more commonly used by minoritized people—"crack" cocaine, created by dissolving powder cocaine and baking soda in boiling water and drying the resulting paste—relative to the powdered form of cocaine more frequently used by White people. Concentration of drug possession arrests, and resulting incarceration, among Black, Latinx and Hispanic, and Indigenous American/Alaska Native people relative to White people is another example of how the punitive consequences of substance use have disproportionately fallen among racially and ethnically minoritized individuals and communities, who are also less likely to receive evidence-based SUD treatment than White people.[2,3]

SUD treatment has also sometimes been considered part of social welfare, for example, outreach and counseling done in shelters for those who are unhoused and Salvation Army soup kitchens. This framework is gentler than punitive interventions and has often been applied by dedicated people in some of the most resource-poor parts of the country. Without demeaning the commitment of such programs to helping people in need, it is descriptively correct to say they are not part of the health care system. They generally employ no medically trained individuals, provide no medical interventions, and do not typically think of themselves as treating a health condition.

Even psychiatric medicine did not make SUD a genuine part of health care for much of the 20th century. From the time of Freud, psychiatrists generally conceptualized substance use as a symptom, perhaps a maladaptive attempt at "self-medication" of an underlying condition. The (empirically unsupported) premise was that when the "real problem" is resolved, SUD will be cured in tow.

SUD treatment did not gain a significant foothold as a specialized form of health care until around 1970.[4,5] The main drivers of the change were the emergence of a drug culture among college-aged baby boomers, the return of U.S. Veterans with opioid use disorder from Vietnam, a flood of federal government money for SUD treatment and research (the National Institutes focusing on alcohol and other drugs were founded in the early 1970s), and the dissemination of an effective, scalable medical intervention for opioid use disorder: methadone treatment.

With the exception of the Veterans Health Administration and the Department of Defense, the mainstream health care systems of the 1970s were neither equipped for nor particularly eager to accept patients with SUD. Thus, at the time, the new system was designed and financed separately. Originally, state systems were well-funded and organizationally placed at the highest levels of government bureaucracy, reflecting the political importance of the issue. The treatments that emerged were largely based upon the prevailing schools of thought from a very wide range of care clinicians (eg, psychiatrists and other physicians, psychologists, nurses, correctional counselors) and perhaps even more based upon the individual experiences with personal recovery from SUDs.[5]

SUD treatment advocates had their own reasons to want a segregated system. Because there were concerns among federal and state policy makers that funds for SUD treatment would be quickly appropriated by politically stronger mental health, more highly trained, and mainstream medical practitioners, special efforts were made to create targeted funding streams. In parallel, legitimate concerns that sharing health information about SUDs could lead to harm to patients (eg, police staking out opioid treatment programs and arresting patients suspected of possessing illegal substances), health information that would normally be in a patient's record was walled off such that SUD treatment professionals only communicated among themselves (ie, under Section 42 of the Code of Federal Regulations). Unique regulations for SUD treatment went beyond health information to cover many other matters regarding the delivery, staffing, and outcomes of health care. Channels that connected other specialties to the health care system—funding streams, shared information, professional collaboration, and common regulations—were thus cut off for SUD treatment.

Being isolated had downsides. The much-heralded treatments of the period failed to "cure" SUDs in the fashion expected of treatments for acute illnesses, and the field did not have the alliances needed to continue to make the case for resources. Health care spending became an increasingly important issue within the private sector. Employers became disenchanted with Employee Assistance Program efforts to control workplace substance use and began to reduce employee health care benefits for SUD treatment through managed care organizations.[6] Meanwhile, in the public sector, the political positions of most state alcohol and drug prevention and treatment authorities became reduced in status, visibility, budget, and organizational power.[7] By the first decade of the new century, there were only two states whose substance use treatment agencies remained in the cabinet.[8] Addiction treatment programs and professionals became stigmatized and marginalized in much the same way as were the patients for whom they cared.

In the rest of the health care system, the expansion of pharmacotherapy benefits in private insurance packages fostered the development of new medications with the potential for significant cost savings from reduced hospital stays and fewer retreatments. However, in the SUD field, care was already very inexpensive; there were few addiction specialists and enduring ideological conflicts among those specialists regarding the appropriateness of medications for SUDs. These belief-based disputes fractionated an already small market. Thus, there was little political pressure within the field for insurers (public or private) to include medication benefits—thus, no incentive for pharmaceutical firms to invest in SUD pharmacotherapies. Consequently, until the late 1990s, there were very few existing medications available to treat SUDs and little active research to develop new ones.[9,10]

Another critical consequence of SUD treatment's historical isolation is that it tended to care only for high-severity cases. For decades after the specialty system emerged to care for severe cases within its own silo, no empirically grounded technologies were developed for primary care clinicians to screen for and intervene with people at risk of or experiencing mild to moderately severe SUDs. Furthermore, there were no clear clinical pathways or protocols as to how patients with severe SUD identified in primary care could be connected to specialty treatment. Individuals with SUDs thus tended to receive little help until they were in an acute situation, for example, if they required an inpatient withdrawal management or were arrested on a substance-related charge. As with most other disorders, providing care only when patients are at their worst and their condition at the most advanced stage results in poor outcomes. This fosters health care clinician perceptions that SUD treatment is ineffective and that people with SUDs are "hopeless cases."

The lack of a connection of SUD treatment to the rest of the health care system also had negative implications even when initial outcomes were positive. SUD treatment programs usually had nowhere to send successfully treated patients in early recovery for ongoing management within the health care system. Many people went to and benefitted from peer recovery support groups, but those are outside the formal health system. In stark contrast to other chronic conditions like hypertension or diabetes, if a primary care clinician was caring for a patient who had just spent 28 days in an alcohol rehabilitation unit or was concurrently receiving methadone from an opioid agonist treatment program, the clinician would usually not know it unless the patient volunteered the information. Practically, this meant that the usual follow-up procedures that would help after other specialty care did not happen for SUD, which likely reduced the number of individuals who translated their specialty treatment gains into sustained recovery. It probably also sometimes unwittingly resulted in iatrogenic harms such as primary care clinicians prescribing medications that undermined the potential benefit of SUD pharmacotherapies or themselves could lead to substance use disorder (eg, narcotics for pain).

TOWARD INTEGRATED CARE FOR THE POPULATION OF PEOPLE WITH SUDS

In recent decades, opportunities to better integrate SUD treatment with the rest of health care system have increased, for five main reasons. First, there have been improvements in insurance coverage for SUD through several laws and other policy changes, including the Wellstone-Domenici Mental Health Parity and Addiction Equity Act of 2008, the 2010 Affordable Care Act, the Substance Use Disorder Prevention that Promotes Opioid Recovery and Treatment for Patients and Communities (SUPPORT) Act of 2018, and Medicaid section 1115 demonstrations.

Second, there have been new developments in SUD tools, technologies, and treatments such as improved screening instruments, brief interventions for early-stage or less severe problems, medical management strategies for SUD that are usable in primary care, promising but as yet poorly scaled digital health tools, including FDA-approved digital therapeutics for substance use disorder, and evidence-based pharmaco- and psychotherapies that can be deployed in a range of settings. Third, U.S. society has begun to shift away from the primarily punitive "War on Drugs" approach to substance use to a more public health-based approach, a change due at least in part to the large swaths of White, middle and upper-class people affected by the ongoing opioid crisis.[11]

Fourth, team-based care, a central component of integrated SUD care, is increasingly becoming the norm across the health care system, a change accelerated by changes in privacy regulation and information technology that facilitate information sharing across providers, as well as by rapid health care market consolidation that is greatly decreasing solo-practitioner models. Fifth, primary care has undergone a paradigm shift around treatment of mental health, leading to increased recognition of co-occurring substance use; in combination with the opioid crisis, this shift has increased momentum for primary care-based substance use treatment in general and adoption of medication for opioid use disorder, specifically, in primary care and other general medical settings. Policy changes facilitating office-based prescribing of buprenorphine and professional societies' widespread endorsement of integrating opioid use disorder care have further supported implementation of integrated SUD care.

Despite these opportunities, barriers to integrated SUD remain in place. Insurance barriers persist, including inadequate coverage of SUD treatment and administrative processes that can impede access to care like prior authorization requirements for buprenorphine and dispensing and dosing limits not based on clinical evidence. Many SUD "treatment" providers offer services that are not evidence-based, such as withdrawal management without subsequent treatment or abstinence-only approaches for treatment of opioid use disorder.[12] Stigma toward SUD is a key barrier to treatment in general and integrated care specifically; primary care clinicians report high levels of stigma toward people with SUD.[13-15]

A well-known model for managing chronic conditions that has been shown to be effective for a range of conditions including SUD is the chronic care management model (CCM).[16] The CCM model is a long-term, proactive strategy involving multidisciplinary teams. Methods include patient registries, standardized protocols and metrics, measurement-based care, and an expectation of a long-term relationship.[16,17] The ultimate goal of the CCM model is engaging patients and their families and providing them with the necessary information, options, strategies, and supports necessary for continued self-management of their chronic condition. Rather than providing reactive, acute care episodes of expensive hospital care following a serious worsening of the condition, the CCM is decidedly proactive, using a range of mechanisms to stay in contact with patients and to provide anticipatory clinical care options to maximize disease control and to prevent recurrence of use that can lead to emergency department visits, hospitalizations, and poor health outcomes.[18] The CCM model has been shown to support integrated delivery of SUD care and to improve patient outcomes in research studies,[19,20] but these models are not yet widely implemented. In the remainder of this chapter, we describe the stages of SUD care and how patients might be managed, throughout all stages, using a CCM model. In this regard, four linked clinical stages are suggested (see **Table 45-1**), each with a specific clinical purpose that is related to the overall goal: patient empowerment through self-management to maximize functioning and reduce risk of recurrence of substance

TABLE 45-1 Four Stages of CCM for Substance Use Disorders

Stage	Goals	Clinical methods
Early identification/ intervention	Identify "unhealthy" substance use through screening Educate and motivate the patient to reduce substance use Engage the patient in healthy alternative behaviors and continuing self-management	Screening instruments—verbal or electronic Brief motivational interviewing Office-based and off-site (through electronic media) monitoring with consequences
Stabilization	Reduce substance use Safe reduction of withdrawal symptoms; improve patient health Educate/manage patient to accept problem	Medications to manage withdrawal, craving Initiate medication maintenance if needed Brief motivational interviewing Individual therapy Address acute social determinants of health needs
Clinical management/ monitoring	Maintain reductions in use and related medical consequences Educate the patient and family to maintain no/low-level use Engage the patient in health behaviors and continued self-management	Medications—maintenance medications Brief motivational interviewing Family and couple therapy Individual therapy Monitoring (on-site and off-site) with consequences
Recovery and personal management	Maintain reductions in use and related consequences Prevent emotional or social threats that reinitiate use	Medications—maintenance medications Self-help groups and activities Individual, family, and couple therapy as needed

use. The stages are Early Identification/ Intervention, Stabilization, Clinical Monitoring/Management, and Patient Self-Management.

Five introductory points are important prior to discussion of the stages of care. First, primary care clinicians will notice that these stages of care, and many of the clinical activities that occur within each, are nearly identical to those associated with the management of other chronic illnesses. Of course, there are special clinical issues associated with SUDs—as there are special issues associated with chronic noncancer pain, sleep disorders, diabetes, and asthma. But the overall goals for the CCM model are similar across virtually all chronic illnesses.

Second, the CCM model and the suggested stages are not just for the management of "addiction" but rather for that of the full spectrum of unhealthy substance use and SUDs. This can be a difficult issue for both general and specialist practitioners. Many general practitioners have learned only about SUD of the higher-severity levels and fail to recognize the more highly prevalent, lower-severity SUDs in their practices. Experienced SUD professionals sometimes dichotomize any inappropriate substance use as definitive evidence for "addiction." This too can limit the possible benefits of care. Through a shared decision-making process, a customized, patient-centered variety of clinical goals can be attractive to and appropriate for individuals with lower-severity hazardous substance use (eg, lower-risk use) even though they are generally not appropriate for those who meet criteria for serious SUDs. Treatment of nicotine/tobacco use (including electronic drug/nicotine delivery devices/EDDDs) and disorder is unique in that management of the full spectrum of unhealthy tobacco use to severe addiction has already been fully incorporated into and embraced by primary care. This process began over 40 years ago with numerous large studies in the 1980s demonstrating the effectiveness of treating tobacco use in primary care settings toward improving population health, and has continued to evolve.[21] There is extensive evidence compiled by the United States Preventive Services Task Force to support their recommendation for primary care screening and management of tobacco use,[22] which has led to the general acceptance of this work as the standard of care, whereas integrated care for other types of substance use has lagged behind.

Third, because these stages and their clinical goals are conceptually linked, many treatment practices will have a role in more than one stage—but to address different problems. For example, one medication may be prescribed within the stabilization stage to reduce withdrawal symptoms, whereas a different medication may be appropriate in the clinical management stage to ameliorate the intensity of craving episodes. Outcome expectations and evaluation methods are most useful when tied directly to a specific stage of care. For example, under the CCM model, it is not informative to ask "Is naltrexone effective in the treatment of alcohol use disorder?" A much more informative question would be "Is naltrexone effective in reducing alcohol craving among well-stabilized patients receiving clinical monitoring and management?"

Fourth, there are as yet very few clear biological or behavioral markers to guide clinical decision-making in questions of transition among these stages. For example, an HgA1c reading below 6% and a blood pressure of 130/80 are good markers of control in other medical disorders. Biological measures for substance use (eg, breath, blood, urine, and/or hair samples) and physical consequences (eg, liver function tests) are available, but they have not been integrated with care monitoring protocols as well. This is in part because SUDs have only recently been studied as chronic illnesses, and standards for "optimal control" of SUDs have not been established. Even if there were established measures for SUD management, as is true with many other chronic illnesses, an individual's co-occurring conditions, genetic factors, and social determinants of clinical progress add complexity to clinical management.

The final point—a new one for experienced "addiction" treatment providers—is that the clinical stages are not isomorphic with specific settings or modalities of care. Changes in insurance coverage, advances in medication and intervention development, and new forms of care delivery and electronic communication and information exchange offer new opportunities to achieve the goals of every stage of care in different settings (eg, primary care office) or with previously unavailable modalities of care (eg, telemedicine, nursing home visits, new medications, a next generation of peer recovery support groups, including via connections through social media).

The Early Identification/Intervention Stage of Care

Clinical Goals in the Early Identification/ Intervention Stage

The main goals of this stage of the care continuum are to identify individuals (adolescents or adults) whose substance use is frequent and/or intense enough to risk their health and well-being and to motivate change among these individuals. This may be particularly important for those with other diagnosed medical or psychiatric conditions whose conditions may be worsened due to their substance use. Also, primary care practitioners can often improve the outcomes and reduce the costs of treating other illnesses simply by identifying and managing co-occurring substance use problems.[23,24]

This early identification stage is an adaptation of the SBIRT model,[25] or substance use screening, brief intervention, and referral to treatment, with the goal of this chronic care model being that most identified substance use can actually be managed within the medical home rather than necessitating a referral to outside addiction treatment. This first component of the SBIRT approach parallels the "ask" component of the "5 A's" approach to abstinence from tobacco.[21,26] Once unhealthy substance use has been identified, the first goal of this stage of treatment is to capitalize on the power of the health teaching moment as well as clinical techniques such as empathic listening and motivational interviewing to help patients consider that their substance use could be a problem and recognize that they can reduce their use. For tobacco use, the next "A" would be to "advise" to quit through clear personalized messages, and "assess" willingness to change.[21,26] Whether for tobacco use or other substances, this approach is often based on patient education, connecting the dots between a patient's substance use and other life problems. Initial screening and brief motivational interventions should conclude with an agreed-upon target for use frequency and amount, and an identified plan by which the patient will reduce their use with the support of the medical home. It is critical that the patient is frequently monitored for substance use frequency, risk, and consequences, in the early stages of change. The monitoring can occur through telephone, telemedicine, or other electronic contact methods to check the effectiveness of the patient's efforts and to offer support and encouragement for those efforts.

Screening

Unhealthy alcohol and other substance use can now be reliably and accurately identified through standard screening instruments available in computerized, paper and pencil, or individual interview formats. Numerous validated tools have been integrated with health care system electronic health records (EHR) to facilitate integration with clinical care delivery.[25] Implementation guides have been developed for nearly every type of health care setting including primary care of both adult and pediatric populations.[25] These guides can assist practices in every phase of implementation, starting with initial adoption of screening and the determination of which tool or tools to use, how to integrate screening into clinical care, and how to train providers. Facilitators to implementation as well as sustainment of this process include adequate training and education of providers, development of multidisciplinary teams, and use of clinical decision support within the EHR. To best support a particular clinical setting, provider education and training materials can be adapted, as can the EHR integration of the screening tools and decision support regarding management of identified unhealthy substance use.

Brief Motivational Intervention(s)

After identification of potentially problematic substance use, brief intervention follows. There has now been broad development and testing of several brief therapies typically consisting of two to six sessions. One-session interventions such as motivational interviewing are considered advice and are typically administered within medical contexts.[23] Brief therapies such as motivational enhancement therapy[27] are designed to promote problem recognition among reluctant or unaware patients with SUDs, to foster a sense of willingness and ability to address the problem, and, often, to promote engagement in treatment.

Brief interventions have been tested extensively in over one hundred trials with people with alcohol and other substance use disorders, usually as a strategy for encouraging non–treatment-seeking individuals to enter into formal treatment but also as a treatment intervention.[28-30] Because of their brevity and low reliance on treatment compliance, they have been particularly attractive to physicians caring for patients with alcohol use disorder in emergency medical settings, but they have also been used successfully in primary care settings.[31] The effect of brief intervention (ie, educational and motivational interventions lasting less than 10 minutes) and brief treatment (similar interventions of two to five sessions) studies within these populations have shown mixed results, with some studies showing significant reductions in substance use, particularly alcohol and tobacco, with less favorable results for other drugs and polysubstance use.[32] While the evidence at this time remains mixed, SBIRT including brief interventions remain a useful process or pathway for structuring the identification and management of SUDs in health care settings.

Clinical Practices Associated With the Identification and Early Intervention Stage

Screening and brief interventions are targeted at patients with unhealthy substance use (particularly at-risk alcohol use) and no study shows they are effective with people who have high-severity SUDs. Thus, post-screening monitoring of substance use is an essential part of clinical decision-making in these cases. If monitoring reveals that a patient cannot even with great effort reduce substance use to levels that no longer pose risk to health and well-being, this is an indication of a more serious problem. In fact, this loss of personal control, and continued use despite consequences, is suggestive of a SUD. Much as antibiotic-resistant infections are diagnosed in part by the failure of first-line antibiotics, failure of brief intervention is an indicator that a SUD is likely more than mild in severity. In these cases, an important secondary goal from this stage of care is to have those patients be open to recognize and self-observe that they may have a more serious SUD and come to appreciate that more intensive treatment is necessary. Therefore, in practice, achieving this level of patient acceptance generally involves collaboration, repeated motivational interviewing sessions, engaging supportive significant others, and offering practical suggestions for coping with urges and cravings as well as high-risk situations—always accompanied by reviewing the patient's personally accumulating evidence. Clinical practices that have been effective in this stage of care are screening for substance use and brief motivational interventions to increase awareness and promote reductions in use.

At this stage, it is crucial for the health care provider to empathize with the patient including any shame and guilt about the struggle to control their substance use. Historical remnants of the "addiction as character flaw" remain pervasive, and much work remains to be done to reduce the stigma of addiction. In addition, at a cognitive neurobiological level, brain impingement accrues and causes deficits in insight, judgment, memory, and, most significantly, the self-control regarding the substance to which the person is addicted.

Indications for Transition to a Different Stage of Care

In cases in which monitoring after a brief intervention reveals significant reductions in the quantity and frequency of substance use below the levels that may be medically or socially harmful, this will signal a transition to the patient management stage of care. In that stage, formal clinical interventions are typically not needed. The patient is educated and motivated to keep substance use at low levels, has a number of techniques to achieve these reductions, and, ideally, is well supported by family and social relationships to control their use.

Conversely, failure of lower-level brief intervention indicates that there may be a more serious SUD. Among the first follow-up activities suggested in such circumstances is a full, standardized assessment to determine their needs as they transition into the stabilization stage of care.

The Stabilization Stage of Care

Finding the Appropriate Treatment Setting Within the Continuum of Care

The gold standard guideline for determining the appropriate treatment setting for an individual with a substance use disorder is The ASAM (American Society of Addiction Medicine) Criteria.[33] This set of guidelines describes the aspects of a full substance use assessment including an individual's substance use history and their use-related medical, personal, and social problems, as well as resources for recovery. This includes consideration of their potential for withdrawal, comorbid conditions, and complicating factors. The result of this assessment then determines where within the ASAM continuum of care an individual should receive treatment: early intervention, outpatient, intensive outpatient/partial hospitalization, residential/inpatient, and intensive inpatient. The ASAM Criteria offer rationale as to placement of patients by level of care; however, there are few empirically derived guidelines on which of these options is better or for which types of patients and problems. Regardless of setting, the goal is to help the patient develop the capability, with professional help, to manage their substance use. After an individual has been identified as needing treatment for their substance use disorder, and they have committed to change, providers can use the ASAM Criteria to help determine the optimal placement for initial treatment to begin. For many patients, outpatient primary care through the CCM model will be appropriate. For others at high risk of dangerous withdrawal from alcohol or benzodiazepines, or with significant co-occurring physical or mental health conditions, a higher level of care such as inpatient treatment may be the first step, followed by return to the medical home for chronic care management after initial acute stabilization.

Clinical Goals in the Stabilization Stage

Alcohol and other substances with addictive potential often cause significant physical and emotional problems directly due to the development of tolerance and/or indirectly due to long periods of sleep disturbances, poor nutrition, and general lack of personal care. The purpose of the stabilization stage of treatment is not to produce cure or lasting abstinence, but rather to prepare a patient with clinical instability to do well in a subsequent clinical monitoring/management stage of care. Significant physiological withdrawal is not present in all cases—even in those with more serious forms of SUD. However, prolonged, heavy alcohol, opioid, or sedative/tranquilizer use may produce a characteristic physiological withdrawal syndrome of several hours to several days or even weeks following the last use of the substance (depending upon the type, dose, and duration/frequency of use). Individuals who use nicotine, amphetamine, cocaine, and cannabis may also experience substantial emotional and physiological symptoms requiring a period of stabilizing care.

Sustaining motivation and ultimately engaging the stabilized patient into some form of continuing care involving monitoring and management (in a residential or outpatient specialty care setting or in a primary care setting) are important clinical goals of this stage of treatment because stabilization alone is rarely effective in helping patients achieve lasting recovery—particularly patients with more severe and/or chronic SUD. Thus, this stage of treatment is the best considered preparation for continued rehabilitation.

The ultimate goal of recovery is patient-specific. It may be possible for early stage, less chronically or severely affected patients to achieve "control" through careful moderation of their use.[34] Most patients will seek "normal" use as a goal, but after a series of behavioral experiments or repeated unsuccessful attempts, this may prove unattainable. For patients with more protracted and/or severe use problems, abstinence may be the only way to reduce risk and lead a functional life. It will be important to negotiate frankly with the patient and their family about their options for attaining and maintaining some relief and stability. The response to treatment will shape subsequent and ongoing treatment decision-making.

Clinical Practices Associated With the Stabilization Stage

The major components of this stage of care include medications to relieve physical and emotional distress symptoms and to reduce craving. These medications are typically accompanied by rest, patient education, and motivational forms of therapy. Stabilization may occur in the context of a residential or hospital setting, or it may be appropriately managed in the primary care setting for patients at lower risk of complications. There have been significant advances in the use of medications to reduce the medical dangers of withdrawal and also to alleviate the associated discomfort. This area of addiction medicine is quite specialized and has been reviewed elsewhere,[9,10] including in Section 7 of this textbook.

Medical practices may implement protocols and tools to aid in the seamless provision of stabilization services including medications.[19] For example, numerous protocols for in-office or at-home buprenorphine inductions have been developed that offer standard practices for dosing and monitoring. Practices should also consider behavioral contracts that outline expectations for both patients and providers, as well as standards for how the practices will handle after-hour calls (particularly during home-inductions), reports of stolen medications, missed appointments, unexpected toxicology findings, and other potentially difficult situations that may arise.

Because stabilization is typically short (3-7 days) and patients' attention and concentration may be compromised for much of this period, extended behavioral/psychosocial therapies within this context are not typically possible. However, the same brief interventions and brief therapies described in the early identification/intervention stage of care are also practical in this context. In this stage, the goal of psychosocial therapy should generally be to help the patient understand and accept that they have a SUD and that they have the ability to manage the problem through continued participation in some form of continuing care involving monitoring and management. Additional psychosocial supports may be necessary for patients with co-occurring mental illness.

Similar to the provision of directed behavioral supports during the stabilization phase, it is crucial to address the most pressing social determinants of health that could interfere with a patient's ability to engage in care. A multidisciplinary team may be able to help patients with acute concerns such as housing or food insecurity.[35]

Transitioning to and From the Stabilization Stage of Care

What are the indications for transition to the next stage of care? There are typically clear and standard biological and behavioral indicators of both physiological and emotional stabilization (vital signs, sleep pattern, appetite, mood). There is great variability in the time required to achieve physical and emotional stabilization depending upon the nature, duration, and intensity of the substance(s) used and the general physical and emotional health of the affected patient. However, most patients make rapid improvements in the standard indicators within 3-7 days of medical care. It is also possible that patients may be lost to follow-up within the stabilization stage before the transition to the monitoring stage can occur, or even when they are in later stages. Proactive outreach from members of the multidisciplinary team, such as peer recovery coaches,[36] may help to decrease this attrition. However, given that return to substance use is common and even expected in the recovery process, clinicians should consider having a flexible model that will easily facilitate a patient's re-engagement in care when they are ready.[37] These patients should be integrated back into the stabilization stage of care with added recovery supports.

Any patient who has required physiological and emotional stabilization will need some form of clinical monitoring/management, as it is unlikely for the patient to do well with a less intensive stage of care. The clinical monitoring/management stage of care may occur within the primary care setting or within a specialty addiction treatment program.

The Clinical Monitoring/Management Stage of Care

Clinical Goals in the Monitoring/Management Stage

Clinical monitoring and management are the most variable—in time, procedure, and patient eligibility—of all the stages of care. It is appropriate for patients who are physically and emotionally stabilized and who have gained some capacity for self-regulation of their urges to use substances—through clinical care provided in the early identification/intervention or stabilization stages. Clinical goals for this stage of care are to maintain the reductions in (or elimination of) substance use, by providing care for the medical and psychiatric as well as social and environmental problems that were identified in the assessment as contributors to the substance use problems, and to continue monitoring for recurrence of use threats. In practice, this stage of care may last many months and can involve varying numbers and frequencies of medications, psychosocial therapies, and adjunctive social services.

An additional and important goal from this stage of care is to educate and engage the patient's family and social relationships to assist in the monitoring and support of the patient's recovery. Several long-term studies have identified ongoing support from family and social networks as key factors in recovery, as well as the development of prosocial, healthy activities and behaviors that are inconsistent with substance use.[38-40] The continued maintenance of abstinence or markedly reduced substance use, good health—including mental health—and good social function in the clinical management/monitoring stage of care has the following four goals:

1. Maintain physical and emotional stability initiated during stabilization.
2. Enhance and sustain reductions in alcohol and drug use (more severe and chronic patients will require complete abstinence).
3. Teach, model, and support behaviors that lead to improved personal physical and mental health, family, and social function and reduced threats to public health and public safety.
4. Motivate behavioral and lifestyle changes that are incompatible with substance use.

Clinical Practices Associated With the Clinical Management/Monitoring Stage

Regardless of the care setting, patients entering (or reentering) the clinical monitoring/management stage of care will likely require a rather intensive combination of individual, group, or family therapies, contingency contracting, stabilization of physical and psychiatric comorbidities, and/or one or more medications. FDA has approved a moderate number of medications for treating SUDs, largely for tobacco, alcohol, and opioid use disorders. These medications have been demonstrated to be safe and effective, and their provision can be integrated into primary care.[19,24,41] The duration of treatment may vary; however, medication for opioid use disorder enhances retention in care and may be safely continued for years.[41] We will not review these medications extensively here, but they are the subject of much greater review in other sections of this textbook, including section 8.

Individuals with SUDs and concurrent psychiatric problems are more likely to prematurely disengage from standard SUD treatments, less likely to benefit from those treatments, and more likely to experience recurrence of use early following those treatments. There is increasing evidence that the prescription of appropriate psychotropic medications can alter that prognosis.[24,25] Integrated psychosocial therapies, which address both the mental health and substance use issues within the same approach, may also be effective.

Clinical management and monitoring will often involve the provision of behavioral/psychological therapies. Significant clinical research over the past two decades has led to the development, testing, and wide availability of psychosocial therapies to help patients control their urges to use substances and improve skills to manage emotional and relationship problems that so often accompany SUDs. Effective models (described in section 9 of this textbook) include contingency management approaches, cognitive–behavioral therapy, 12-step facilitation counseling, and behavioral marital therapy. Most of these therapies have been studied in outpatient specialty care settings—and it remains for additional research to investigate their role in other settings within the clinical management/monitoring stage of care.

It is extremely common for the SUD-focused psychological therapy and pharmacotherapy providers to be different individuals (eg, a physician and a clinical social worker). This multidisciplinary collaborative team-based approach[24] creates advantages in terms of cost and efficiency but also requires more coordination, which can be challenging depending on how the care system handles information-sharing regulations, whether the various disciplines have a compatible approach to care, and whether a positive and respectful interdisciplinary atmosphere prevails on the care team. As problems on any of these fronts can result in worse care for the patients, the care team must prioritize the smooth working of their own relationship (see the Chapter 45 for more information on this subject). Mutual respect for one another's professional voice and expertise, good communication skills, and a sense of a common purpose are key ingredients to team-based care. System managers should also monitor the formal procedures and informal norms governing such care arrangements, as they are likely to influence not only patient outcomes, but those for staff (eg, morale, burnout, productivity). Lack of treatment collaboration can even place the provider at increased risk for malpractice claims.

The monitoring and management stage is also well-suited to address patients' social determinants of health more comprehensively than possible during the acute stabilization phase. An important resource within this stage of care is the availability of a living environment that is free from active use, as this is a risk factor for recurrence of substance use. This type of living arrangement may be available within the family home, in drug-free housing, or in a residential specialty SUD treatment setting.

Indications for Transition to a Different Stage of Care

Patients with more severe, complex, and chronic SUDs will likely require a greater number and frequency of clinical visits to achieve and sustain clinical goals and will likely require a longer period of successful maintenance of these goals prior to transfer to a less intensive stage of care. However, even these intuitive assumptions have received very little research attention. There are important opportunities to study the specific behavioral indicators of high likelihood for successful transition to the patient management stage of care and the particular sets of clinical interventions that are most likely to produce patient changes that reach the designated performance threshold for transition.

Though important in all earlier stages of care, monitoring of substance use through biological tests and patient self-report is critical in the clinical monitoring/management stage for important clinical determinations such as whether to increase or decrease the intensity or change the composition of clinical practices provided to a patient and particularly whether to transition a patient to a more intensive or less intensive stage of care. Again, there has been little research regarding the appropriate behavioral and biological criteria for these transitions. There are thus important opportunities for practical research in this area.

In general, self-disclosed or positive biological tests for substances with addictive potential or liability are an indication that there is a need for more frequent monitoring and likely more intensive clinical interventions. As indicated above, recurrence of substance use is common within the recovery process, and there are already many types of medications, psychosocial therapies, and clinical services that may be recommended to further support the patient's goal of reducing substance use and related problems. The question of how long to continue any level of clinical management/monitoring in the face of continued positive biological test results will always be an individual clinical determination. However, in general, it is wise to negotiate in advance of care initiation regarding the specific behavioral goals and to get patient acceptance for more intensive clinical options if there is not progress toward the agreed-upon goals (perhaps referral to specialty SUD care if the patient is being managed in a primary care office or to a residential treatment program if the patient is being managed in an outpatient treatment program).

A more welcome but no more informed question is when to refer a patient with high degree of functioning and with few to no indications of substance use to the personal management stage of care. It is currently not known how long a period of sustained abstinence or significantly reduced use should be achieved before a stable, well-motivated patient can be expected to continue good function with little or no clinical management. Even when clinically managed and monitored patients are able to achieve stable periods of abstinence, the transition to personal management can be difficult and unsettling. Among the most reliable and robust findings from clinical studies of patients with SUDs is that continued, active participation in mutual support groups is an excellent predictor of sustained abstinence and positive psychosocial outcomes.[42-45] The peer support and life skills are valuable for initiating and maintaining positive lifestyle changes and functioning.[46]

The Recovery or Patient Self-Management Stage

This final phase may look very different for different patients depending on their individual needs and goals. Prior concepts of recovery were very much focused on abstinence and being able to manage oneself without medical support. The term "patient self-management" historically indicated the transition from some/any form of clinically directed care and monitoring, toward self-management by the patient of substance use and related problems, likely with the informed assistance of family, friends, and other community resources (eg, mutual help groups and recovery support services). This focus on being free of medication and medical care unfortunately leads to a false dichotomy and debate over what constitutes "real recovery." In truth, recovery is a much broader concept that involves remission from previous problematic behaviors and overall improved biopsychosocial functioning.[42] The support that will be needed to maintain this recovery will vary between individuals, and even within one individual over time. Self-management does not have to mean departure from the medical home, but rather ownership of the tasks involved in managing a chronic illness, including the medical, behavioral, and emotional components.[47] For some patients, this may involve routine medical visits and continued pharmacotherapy; for them, self-management may mean that are able to independently problem-solve and seek out resources for their SUD when challenges arise. For others, recovery and self-management may not include the medical home and will rely upon the support of peer recovery groups. Key to the concept of recovery within the chronic care model is the understanding that like any other chronic illness, SUD recovery may involve cycles through these stages of care rather than a linear trajectory.

Goals of the Recovery or Personal Self-Management Stage

The recovery and self-management stage of care shares many of the goals of the clinical management stage of care—the essential difference is that in the latter stage, responsibility and capability for management rest on the patient and his or her family and social circle. In turn, it follows that one of the goals of the later phases of the clinical management/monitoring stage is to inform, train, engage, and practice the family and other social supports to take on these responsibilities in a practical and effective manner. Personal management has the following four goals:

1. Maintain physiological and emotional improvements initiated during earlier stages.
2. Self-monitor threats toward recurrence of substance use and make corrections where appropriate.
3. Learn and practice more effective coping behaviors and self-care.
4. Maintain healthy relationships and social behaviors incompatible with substance use.

Clinical Practices Associated With the Personal Self-Management Stage

All FDA-approved medications mentioned in the prior section may also be useful in supporting patients in this recovery and self-management phase. As stated above, the fact that a patient remains on medication for a SUD does not negate their ability to engage in other aspects of self-management. In addition, co-occurring mood disorders are prevalent and may reoccur, particularly at times of significant life stress. Psychotropic medications can be important in such instances, which, if handled well, will reduce likelihood of substance use reinstatement. The assistance of these medications may provide pharmacological support for the benefits of psychosocial interventions and peer recovery support groups such as 12-step recovery fellowships.

Psychosocial therapies designed to engage family supports and to forge new, healthy peer relationships may be particularly valuable as recovering patients attempt to integrate a new recovering lifestyle into their historical environment and relationships. However, as is true of so much of the clinical practice in this developing field, there has been little systematic research to guide patients or their clinicians in suggesting or selecting continuing care interventions or practices (other than mutual help group attendance) that a patient and his or her family can manage independently.

Peer recovery support group participation is important for many individuals. Among 12-step programs, AA remains the most prevalent form of continuing care for individuals who are dealing with alcohol and/or other substance use problems, and these and other mutual support organization meetings can be very helpful to a wide range of individuals including those considering reducing their substance use, those actively participating in earlier stages of the care continuum, those on psychotropic and/or addiction medicines, and particularly those in the personal self-management stage. Mutual support groups can be found in most towns and cities and are now even offered through virtual platforms. Some groups may cater to particular groups (ie, LGBTQIA+ individuals, people who do not smoke, atheists, individuals with co-occurring substance use and mental health problems, etc.). Within any single group, it is common that some meetings will be "open" to all individuals regardless of whether they have a SUD; some will feature speakers who will share their stories and topic meetings where the group discusses views on a particular aspect of recovery from substance use. Patients should consider attending several groups in several locations before deciding whether to become an active participant and which group to use as their home group. In general, peer recovery support groups, including AA, provide support for not only abstinence, but also positive behavioral, interpersonal and attitude changes. Furthermore, a core value in 12-step programs is citizenship and service to others.

CONCLUSION

To widely integrate and scale up SUD care using the CCM model, policy and implementation supports are needed. Financing barriers to core CCM model components not traditionally reimbursed by insurance, like care coordination and management, impede widespread adoption. Recent innovations like the CMS behavioral health integration billing codes and the Affordable Care Act Medicaid Health Home waiver represent progress on this front. However, these mechanisms, which provide modest monthly payments for integrated care activities, are often insufficient to cover the costs of the structural elements of the CCM model, like patient registries and shared electronic health records. Innovative bundled payment mechanisms could overcome this issue; the American College of Physicians has recommended separate prospective bundled payments for the structural and process-of-care elements of the CCM.

In our current system, neither general medical nor specialty behavioral health providers are held accountable for health outcomes among people with SUD. Moving forward, we need to study the potential for value-based financing arrangements structured so that both groups of providers are subject to the same incentives. For example, including SUD treatment providers in accountable care organization networks alongside general medical providers and aligning payment with SUD performance measures could incentivize integration.

Implementation supports are also needed. Strategies such as facilitation, coaching, training, and performance feedback have been shown to support scale-up of evidence-based SUD care in other contexts, for example contingency management adoption among opioid treatment providers[48] and integrated mental health and SUD treatment in addiction treatment organizations.[49]

Electronic decision support tools within the context of a health system or primary care network EHR would also contribute to standardized care and incorporation of CCM SUD care into regular workflow. To the extent, the components of CCM are constructed in parallel to the EHR, such as with patient registries, they are not sustainable.

To build integrated care workforce capacity, general medical training needs to include increased emphasis on SUD treatment and on team-based and integrated care competencies. Digital health innovations, including SUD treatment via telehealth technology, self-management applications, and digital therapeutics, have the potential to play important roles in the implementation of integrated care by increasing flexibility for provider-patient interactions and by augmenting care delivered in clinical settings, for example, through symptom tracking or cognitive behavioral therapy practice activities (sometimes called "homework") completed via a digital application. But thus far, digital therapeutics have been challenging to implement in routine care, in part due to payment barriers, and have yet to fulfill their promise.

Equity must be front and center within integrated SUD care, from delivery of culturally appropriate treatment, to financing policies explicitly designed to support equity, to implementation focused on correcting historic inequities in access to treatment. Brownson and colleagues propose a set of highly applicable recommendations to advance health equity within implementation of health care services, including but not limited to the importance of using equity-relevant metrics to gauge implementation success and connecting with systems and sectors outside of health to address social determinants of health.[50] This last point is critical in the context of SUD care: many people with SUD need a range of supports in tandem with treatment, such as housing and childcare.

A pragmatic and implementable approach with the CCM model may be one that considers the most common SUDs and/or mental health conditions encountered by general medical practices. Epidemiological studies confirm these conditions frequently co-occur with one another and with general medical conditions, yet clinical research is largely based on singular disorders and specific treatments.[51] Unfortunately, this does not match the clinical reality of at least comorbidity, if not multimorbidity, among the more typical complex patients in routine practice settings. A unified CCM model that builds upon and braids the evidence-based approaches for a variety of common conditions is needed to guide providers and patients across the stages outlined here. Especially if we consider general medical settings such as primary care, a unified model would likely be more implementable by considering aspects of workflow and workforce, unlike the more single disorder, specific targeted approaches that presently exist. Such a unified model would build across well-defined disorder-specific approaches but more realistically address the typical patient, the typical provider, and the typical setting within which health care takes place.[52]

In conclusion, progress has been made toward integration of SUD into general health care, particularly in the context of the ongoing opioid epidemic. But much work remains to be done, with a blueprint focused on creating adequate financing models to support CCM-based integrated care, building the integrated care workforce, centering equity, and reducing stigma.

ACKNOWLEDGMENTS

The authors acknowledge the authors of the prior edition's chapter of the same title, Keith Humphreys, Mark McGovern, and A. Thomas McLellan. This version builds on their excellent work, primarily by updating content focused on developments in integrated SUD care since the prior publication.

REFERENCES

1. Substance Abuse and Mental Health Services Administration. Key Substance Use and Mental Health Indicators in the United States: Results From the 2020 National Survey on Drug Use and Health. HHS Publication No PEP21-07-01-003, NSDUH Series H-56. Center for Behavioral Health Statistics and Quality, Substance Abuse and Mental Health Services Administration; 2023. Accessed May 29, 2023. https://www.samhsa.gov/data/
2. Camplain R, Camplain C, Trotter RT II, et al. Racial/ethnic differences in drug- and alcohol-related arrest outcomes in a southwest county from 2009 to 2018. *Am J Public Health*. 2020;110(S1):S85-S92.
3. Saini J, Johnson B, Qato DM. Self-reported treatment need and barriers to care for adults with opioid use disorder: the US National Survey on Drug Use and Health, 2015 to 2019. *Am J Public Health*. 2022;112(2):284-295.
4. Musto DF. *The American Disease: Origins of Narcotic Control*. Oxford University Press; 1999.
5. White WL. *Slaying the Dragon: The History of Addiction Treatment and Recovery in America*. Chestnut Health Systems/Lighthouse Institute; 1998.
6. Weisner C, Hinman A, Lu Y, Chi FW, Mertens J. Addiction treatment ultimatums and US health reform: a case study. *Nordisk Alkohol Nark*. 2010;27(6):685-698.
7. McGlynn EA, Asch SM, Adams J, et al. The quality of health care delivered to adults in the United States. *N Engl J Med*. 2003;348(26):2635-2645.
8. Kerwin ME, Walker-Smith K, Kirby KC. Comparative analysis of state requirements for the training of substance abuse and mental health counselors. *J Subst Abuse Treat*. 2006;30(3):173-181.
9. Willenbring ML. Medications to treat alcohol dependence: adding to the continuum of care. *JAMA*. 2007;298(14):1691-1692.
10. O'Brien CP, McKay J. Psychopharmacological treatments for substance use disorders. In: Nathan PE, Gorman JM, eds. *A Guide to Treatments That Work*. Oxford University Press; 2007.
11. Beckett K, Brydolf-Horwitz M. A kinder, gentler drug war? Race, drugs, and punishment in 21st century America. *Punish Soc*. 2020;22(4): 509-533.
12. Mojtabai R, Mauro C, Wall MM, Barry CL, Olfson M. Medication treatment for opioid use disorders in substance use treatment facilities. *Health Affairs*. 2019;38(1):14-23.
13. Kennedy-Hendricks A, Busch SH, McGinty EE, et al. Primary care physicians' perspectives on the prescription opioid epidemic. *Drug Alcohol Depend*. 2016;165:61-70.
14. McGinty EE, Stone EM, Kennedy-Hendricks A, Bachhuber MA, Barry CL. Medication for opioid use disorder: a national survey of primary care physicians. *Ann Intern Med*. 2020;173(2):160-162.
15. Stone EM, Kennedy-Hendricks A, Barry CL, Bachhuber MA, McGinty EE. The role of stigma in US primary care physicians' treatment of opioid use disorder. *Drug Alcohol Depend*. 2021;221:108627.
16. Davy C, Bleasel J, Liu H, Tchan M, Ponniah S, Brown A. Effectiveness of chronic care models: opportunities for improving healthcare practice and health outcomes: a systematic review. *BMC Health Serv Res*. 2015;15(1):1-11.
17. Wagner EH, Austin BT, Von Korff M. Organizing care for patients with chronic illness. *Milbank Q*. 1996;74(4):511-544.
18. Dobscha SK, Corson K, Perrin NA, et al. Collaborative care for chronic pain in primary care: a cluster randomized trial. *JAMA*. 2009;301(12):1242-1252.
19. Alford DP, LaBelle CT, Kretsch N, et al. Collaborative care of opioid-addicted patients in primary care using buprenorphine: five-year experience. *Arch Intern Med*. 2011;171(5):425-431.
20. Watkins KE, Ober AJ, Lamp K, et al. Collaborative care for opioid and alcohol use disorders in primary care: the SUMMIT randomized clinical trial. *JAMA Intern Med*. 2017;177(10):1480-1488.
21. Office USPHS. *Smoking Cessation: A Report of the Surgeon General [Internet]*. 2020.
22. Patnode CD, Henderson JT, Coppola EL, Melnikow J, Durbin S, Thomas RG. Interventions for tobacco cessation in adults, including pregnant persons: updated evidence report and systematic review for the US preventive services task force. *JAMA*. 2021;325(3):280-298.
23. Fleming MF, Barry KL, Manwell LB, Johnson K, London R. Brief physician advice for problem alcohol drinkers: a randomized controlled trial in community-based primary care practices. *JAMA*. 1997;277(13):1039-1045.
24. Watkins KE, Ober AJ, Lamp K, et al. Implementing the chronic care model for opioid and alcohol use disorders in primary care. *Prog Community Health Partnersh*. 2017;11(4):397-407.
25. Thoele K, Moffat L, Konicek S, et al. Strategies to promote the implementation of screening, brief intervention, and referral to treatment (SBIRT) in healthcare settings: a scoping review. *Subst Abuse Treat Prev Policy*. 2021;16(1):42.
26. US Preventative Services Task Force. *Tobacco Smoking Cessation in Adults, Including Pregnant Persons: Interventions*. 2023. Accessed May 29, 2023. https://www.uspreventiveservicestaskforce.org/uspstf/recommendation/tobacco-use-in-adults-and-pregnant-women-counseling-and-interventions
27. Bertholet N, Daeppen J-B, Wietlisbach V, Fleming M, Burnand B. Reduction of alcohol consumption by brief alcohol intervention in primary care: systematic review and meta-analysis. *Arch Intern Med*. 2005;165(9):986-995.
28. Bien TH, Miller WR, Tonigan JS. Brief interventions for alcohol problems: a review. *Addiction*. 1993;88(3):315-336.
29. Moyer A, Finney JW, Swearingen CE, Vergun P. Brief interventions for alcohol problems: a meta-analytic review of controlled investigations in treatment-seeking and non-treatment-seeking populations. *Addiction*. 2002;97(3):279-292.
30. Shorter GW, Bray JW, Giles EL, et al. The variability of outcomes used in efficacy and effectiveness trials of alcohol brief interventions: a systematic review. *J Stud Alcohol Drugs*. 2019;80(3):286-298.
31. Saitz R, Horton NJ, Larson MJ, Winter M, Samet JH. Primary medical care and reductions in addiction severity: a prospective cohort study. *Addiction*. 2005;100(1):70-78.
32. Tanner-Smith EE, Parr NJ, Schweer-Collins M, Saitz R. Effects of brief substance use interventions delivered in general medical settings: a systematic review and meta-analysis. *Addiction*. 2022;117(4):877-889.
33. American Society of Addiction Medicine. *2022 ASAM Criteria*. Accessed September 11, 2022. https://www.asam.org/asam-criteria/about-the-asam-criteria
34. Humphreys K, Lingford-Hughes A. *Edwards' Treatment of Drinking Problems: A Guide for the Helping Professions*. Cambridge University Press; 2016.
35. Tofighi B, Williams AR, Chemi C, Suhail-Sindhu S, Dickson V, Lee JD. Patient barriers and facilitators to medications for opioid use disorder in primary care. *Subst Use Misuse*. 2019;54(14):2409-2419.
36. Stanojlović M, Davidson L. Targeting the barriers in the substance use disorder continuum of care with peer recovery support. *Subst Abuse*. 2021;15:1178221820976988.
37. Bagley SM, Hadland SE, Schoenberger SF, et al. Integrating substance use care into primary care for adolescents and young adults: lessons learned. *J Subst Abuse Treat*. 2021;129:108376.
38. Anglin MD, Hser Y-I, Grella CE. Drug addiction and treatment careers among clients in the Drug Abuse Treatment Outcome Study (DATOS). *Psychol Addict Behav*. 1997;11(4):308.
39. McLellan AT, Lewis DC, O'Brien CP, Kleber HD. Drug dependence, a chronic medical illness: implications for treatment, insurance, and outcomes evaluation. *JAMA*. 2000;284(13):1689-1695.
40. Moos RH, Moos BS. Participation in treatment and alcoholics anonymous: a 16-year follow-up of initially untreated individuals. *J Clin Psychol*. 2006;62(6):735-750.
41. Mirer AG, Tiemstra JD, Hammes NE, Cloum HM, LaFavor KJ. Integrating buprenorphine treatment for opioid use with primary care is associated with greater retention in treatment. *J Am Board Fam Med*. 2022;35(1):206-208.

42. US Public Health Services. Vision for the future. *Facing Addiction in America: The Surgeon General's Report on Alcohol, Drugs, and Health.* 2023. Accessed May 30, 2023. https://addiction.surgeongeneral.gov/vision-future
43. Kelly JF, White WL. Recovery management and the future of addiction treatment and recovery in the USA. In: Kelly JF, White WL, eds. *Addiction Recovery Management*. Springer; 2010:303-316.
44. Timko C, Moos RH, Finney JW, Moos BS. Outcome of treatment for alcohol abuse and involvement in alcoholics anonymous among previously untreated problem drinkers. *J Ment Health Adm.* 1994;21(2):145-160.
45. Tonigan JS, Toscova R, Miller WR. Meta-analysis of the literature on alcoholics anonymous: sample and study characteristics moderate findings. *J Stud Alcohol.* 1996;57(1):65-72.
46. Humphreys K. *Circles of recovery: self-help organizations for addictions.* Cambridge University Press; 2003.
47. Anekwe TD, Rahkovsky I. Self-management: a comprehensive approach to management of chronic conditions. *Am J Public Health.* 2018;108(Suppl 6):S430-S436.
48. Becker SJ, Kelly LM, Kang AW, Escobar KI, Squires DD. Factors associated with contingency management adoption among opioid treatment providers receiving a comprehensive implementation strategy. *Subst Abuse.* 2019;40(1):56-60.
49. Assefa MT, Ford JH, Osborne E, et al. Implementing integrated services in routine behavioral health care: primary outcomes from a cluster randomized controlled trial. *BMC Health Serv Res.* 2019;19(1):1-13.
50. Brownson RC, Kumanyika SK, Kreuter MW, Haire-Joshu D. Implementation science should give higher priority to health equity. *Implement Sci.* 2021;16(1):1-16.
51. Moberg CA, Humphreys K. Exclusion criteria in treatment research on alcohol, tobacco and illicit drug use disorders: a review and critical analysis. *Drug Alcohol Rev.* 2017;36(3):378-388.
52. McGovern M, Dent K, Kessler R. A unified model of behavioral health integration in primary care. *Acad Psychiatry.* 2018;42(2):265-268.

CHAPTER

46 Substance Use–Related Care—Interprofessional Collaborative Practice

Deborah S. Finnell, Jeffrey Bratberg, and Lisa K. Berger

CHAPTER OUTLINE

- Introduction
- Competencies for health care clinicians
- Interprofessional substance use–related education
- Interprofessional practice models
- Interprofessional collaborative practice research
- Recommendations
- Summary

INTRODUCTION

The high prevalence of alcohol and other drug use in the United States puts health care clinicians from different disciplines and across diverse settings in key positions to identify persons who may be at risk because of substance use and intervene accordingly. Various health care clinicians engage in prevention, intervention, treatment, harm-reduction, and recovery support for persons across the continuum of substance use. Interprofessional collaborative practice occurs when clinicians from different professional backgrounds deliver comprehensive coordinated services working with patients, families, and communities to provide the highest quality of care across settings.[1] Johnson et al. identified common characteristics of interprofessional collaboration including trust and respect, communication, and shared vision.[2] They posit that trust develops over time through role clarity and reliance on each member's competence in fulfilling those roles. In turn, that trust reflects respect for each team member's expertise and the decisions they make in enacting their role. Respectful and constant communication among team members was identified across all studies included in the review by Johnson et al. as essential in coordinating care and enhancing collaboration. Team members with clearly articulated shared vision and common goals are able to set a clear direction and be action-oriented.[2]

This chapter provides an overview of the knowledge, skills, and attitudes that are essential for various health care clinicians working with persons who are at risk because of substance use, including those with a substance use disorders. Examples of curricular innovations and continuing education to prepare the current and future health care workforce are provided. Pragmatic strategies and models of care are discussed, which promote feasible and effective approaches for persons who are at any point along the continuum of substance use. With an overall goal to improve the quality of care and outcomes for these populations, the chapter concludes with recommendations for education, practice, research, and policy.

COMPETENCIES FOR HEALTH CARE CLINICIANS

Competencies help define how a person should effectively perform their role. The first competencies for health care clinicians working with individuals with substance use disorders were published in 2002.[3] Two decades later, the Association for Multidisciplinary Education and Research in Substance use and Addictions (AMERSA) led efforts to document the knowledge, skills, and attitudes (KSA) recommended for newly licensed entry-level and advance practice nurses,[4] pharmacists,[5] physicians,[6] physician assistants,[7] and social workers.[8] The AMERSA competencies for the pharmacists, physicians, physician assistants, and social workers were organized in accord with the KSA framework. The AMERSA nursing competencies were organized in accord with the American Nurses Association's standards of practice[9] and delineated the KSAs required to meet the standards of practice and standards of performance.

Unlike multidisciplinary teams in which clinicians have an awareness of other disciplines, but do not share care planning and coordination,[10] interprofessional teams cooperate, collaborate, communicate and integrate care.[11] This interprofessional approach is particularly suited for populations with multiple and complex health problems including substance use. Rutkowski identified substance use–related core competencies shared by two or more disciplines despite differences in their scope of practice.[12] The commonality of competencies underscores the importance of clinicians from various disciplines working collaboratively (ie, interprofessional) rather than independently (ie, multidisciplinary). Thus, the provision of integrated, evidence-based, and patient-centered care is optimally provided by interdisciplinary teams that cooperate, collaborate and communicate effectively.

More recently acknowledged members of the interprofessional team are individuals in peer support positions with core competencies for persons in this role documented by the Substance Abuse and Mental Health Services Administration (SAMHSA).[13] Peer-based recovery support services have gained prominence in the United States since 1998.[14] The Institute of Medicine has since recommended that mental health/substance use treatment services include peer support.[15] Various titles are used to refer to the person in this role, herein referred to as peer support specialists. Their success in their own recovery process, or their lived experience, is fundamental for their role in helping others experiencing similar situations. The role of the peer support specialist is to intervene early with persons with substance use, to support sustained stability, and to improve the health and wellness of individuals and families.[16] A systematic review by Eddie et al. conveyed the positive findings of research associated with peer support services including reduced substance use and substance use disorder recurrence rates, improved relationships with treatment providers and social supports, increased treatment retention, and treatment satisfaction.[17] Jack et al. sought to understand the activities of persons in the peer support role (ie, peer recovery coaches) through patient and coach interviews.[18] Core activities identified included system navigation, supporting behavior change, harm reduction, and relationship building.[18] Slater et al. summarized the activities carried out by the peer support specialist engaged as members of the team caring for persons with opioid use.[19] Importantly, many of those peer support specialists' responsibilities, including screening, delivery of brief intervention, and referral to treatment overlapped with the common AMERSA substance-related competencies across the five disciplines.[12]

Interprofessional collaboration among clinicians working with persons with alcohol and other substance use is influenced by the complexity of the patient's needs and the context in which the patient presents. For example, a brief motivational conversation may be appropriate for a patient in primary care who is identified to be at low risk because of alcohol use. That brief intervention can be delivered by one of several health care clinicians competent to do so. A more complex situation requiring greater interprofessional collaboration may be the person seen by a peer support specialist after their opioid overdose has been reversed in the community who is then assessed by a registered nurse to be in opioid withdrawal after admission to the emergency department, initiated on buprenorphine, assisted by the social worker in referral to ongoing treatment in the community, and then accompanied by the peer support specialist to treatment to ensure follow-up.

INTERPROFESSIONAL SUBSTANCE USE–RELATED EDUCATION

Higher Education

Higher education is beginning to support the interprofessional training of future health care workers. The transformation has been crystalized, in part, due to the Quality Chasm series by the US Institute of Medicine.[20] The series, which includes *Improving the Quality of Health Care for Mental and Substance-Use Conditions*[15] recommends patient-centered, team-based care as a mechanism for improving health care quality.[20] Interprofessional education (IPE) is defined as students from different professions learning together and from each other to collaborate and improve health outcomes[21] and IPE is regarded as effective.[22] Colleagues in Canada have been leading the way for decades in IPE.[20] For example, the University of Toronto (UT) Interprofessional Education Curriculum includes almost a dozen professions, is competency based, and developmental.[23]

Table 46-1 provides examples of U.S. universities that have implemented and evaluated substance use–related IPE that is taught by faculty with this expertise and persons with lived experience.[24-29] The form of the education ranges from a standalone IPE course to content in profession-specific courses. The targeted groups of professions for the IPE point to the importance of understanding the unique roles and functions of team members as well as commonalities of competencies. Such understanding is critically important in delivering coordinated patient-centered care. In the examples provided, educational content is directed at advancing the knowledge and skills future health care clinicians who will care for persons at risk across the continuum of care. Learning activities center on teamwork, effective communication, and case-based examples including the use of standardized patients and simulation. Real-life experiences provide an opportunity for students to learn and practice essential collaboration skills for interprofessional teams. The types of learning outcomes for IPE (eg, often based on self-report versus observed practice behaviors) reflect that IPE is in early stages in higher education.[25,30,31] Efforts are needed to motivate future health care clinicians to care for those at risk because of substance use and ensure that future clinicians are equipped with the knowledge and skills to do so within the context of interprofessional teams. As IPE related to the substance use continuum grows, training the existing workforce through higher education programs or continuing education programs is necessary.

Continuing Education

At present, there are many continuing education (CE) programs focused on substance use education available for health care clinicians. Some CEs are interprofessional with clinicians from different professions learning together as colocated training participants. Fewer focus on substance use–related IPE, which includes substance use care and communication in interprofessional teams. **Table 46-2** provides two examples of such IPE, both of which utilized distance learning and distributed content over a series of weeks to accommodate busy health care clinicians.[32,33] Unlike the IPE examples in higher education, the Extension for Community Healthcare outcomes in **Table 46-2** included hospital leadership and quality improvement staff, thus encouraging substance use interprofessional practice at the systems level.[32,34] Training content across the two examples was tailored to health care settings. For example, one training focused on medications for opioid use disorder (MOUD) in hospital settings,[32] and another on Screening, Brief Intervention, and Referral to Treatment for clinicians in various health settings, including community health centers.[33] Evaluation outcomes suggest a need for increased knowledge and skill on substance use and patient-centered communication,[32,33] plus perceived need for and importance of interprofessional practice.[34] Given the few substance use–related IPE opportunities available for CE, this is an area for continued growth.[35,36]

TABLE 46-1 Examples of Interprofessional Substance Use–Related Education

Authors	Training type/educators	Professions included	Training content	Evaluation outcome
Monteiro K, Dumenco L, Collins S, et al.[24]	4-hour workshop/faculty from several institutions and professions	Preclinical medical students, nursing, pharmacy, physical therapy, and social work	Patient panel; naloxone training; standardized patient case and case study; Interprofessional Collaborative Practice four compentencies[60]	Medical students increased their knowledge on opioid overdose; high degree of training satisfaction; medical students favored the standardized patient case
Muzyk A, Mullan P, Andossek KM, et al.[25]	4 classes (6 hours total) as part of a 1-month psychiatry clerkship, attendance at a 12-step meeting, plus an optional patient counseling opportunity/interprofessional faculty	Accelerated bachelor of science in nursing, medicine, pharmacy, physician assistant, and social work	Recognizing at-risk substance use, SUD treatment; behavior change counseling; role-playing and case examples; empathy and recognizing bias	Improved attitudes on the following: Patients • Nonmoralizing • Treatment optimism • Treatment intervention • Nonstereotyping Interprofessional Collaboration • Teamwork • Roles/responsibilities • Patient outcomes
Muzyk AJ, Tew C, Thomas-Fannin A, et al.[26]	6 1-hour classes as part of a 1-month psychiatry clerkship, plus attendance at a 12-step meeting/interdisciplinary faculty, including licensed addiction specialists	Medicine, physician assistant, pharmacy, and social work	Recognizing at-risk substance use, social determinants of health/neurobiology, and treatment; observed practice of motivational interviewing; screening; empathy and recognizing bias through standardized clinical cases and guided reflection	Improved attitudes on the following: Patients • Nonmoralizing, • Treatment optimism • Treatment intervention Interprofessional Collaboration • Teamwork • Roles • Responsibilities
Sherwood DA, Kramlich D, Rodriquez K, Graybeal C[27]	Educational modules integrated into curriculum/faculty champions from each professional program	Dental hygiene, dental medicine, health, wellness and occupational studies, nursing, occupational therapy, osteopathic medicine, pharmacy, physical therapy, physician assistant, and social work	Substance use–related SBIRT; motivational interviewing; simulated interprofessional team immersion with standardized patients; leadership development	Formative to improve the training; one-day interprofessional simulation experience dispersed over 2-hour sessions; addition of MI practice sessions
Stoddard-Dare P, DeBoth KK, Wendland M, et al.[28]	2 ½ hour workshop/clinical experts, persons with lived experience	Medicine, nursing, occupational therapy, pharmacy, physical therapy, social work, and speech-language pathology	Professional role in the opioid epidemic; evidence-based treatments, harm reduction; case example; understanding personal values and beliefs relative to at-risk substance use and reflection	Increased confidence on four outcomes: • Values and beliefs • Appropriate response to persons with SUD • Finding harm reduction resources • Finding SUD treatment resources
Weller BE, Carver JN, Harrison, J, Chapleau A[29]	Programs (2 to 6 hours) that train students to serve individuals with SUD/faculty from target disciplines	Occupational therapy, social work plus community providers and peer support	Knowledge on opioid use disorder; motivational interviewing; relevant field placement; culturally competence practice	Self-evaluation of learning using Goal Attainment Scaling

TABLE 46-2 Example of Interprofessional Continuing Education on Substance Use

Authors	Training type/educators	Professions included	Training content	Evaluation outcome
Englander H, Patten A, Lockard R, et al.[32]	10 to 12 weekly 1-hour long sessions delivered through ECHO/nurse, pharmacist, physicians, social worker, and peer mentor	Hospital leadership, nurses, nurse practitioners, peer/outreach coordinators, pharmacists, physical therapists, physicians, physician assistants, quality improvement staff, and social workers/counselors	Brief didactics on opioid withdrawal, opioid overdose, acute pain, harm reduction; plus OUD medications, treatment settings, care delivery systems; case presentations; trauma-informed care	ECHO was feasible and acceptable; 2 additional sessions added Increased knowledge of treatment (quantitative); and knowledge and skills on use of OUD medications, patient-centered communication, and harm reduction (qualitative)
Puskar K, Mitchell AM, Albrecht SA, et al.[33]	Online program (spread over 6 hours) with educational modules, case scenarios, facilitated dialogues/Developed by faculty with expertise in addictions	Behavioral health counselors, nurses, public health professionals	SBIRT and Interprofessional Collaborative Practice four competencies[60]; online technologies; case scenarios; interprofessional interaction	Increased competence, perceived need for and actual cooperation, and understanding of value of other professions

INTERPROFESSIONAL PRACTICE MODELS

This section presents models of interprofessional care for persons with substance use, with the acknowledgement that randomized clinical trials (RCT) comparing interprofessional practice models are lacking. Three models are discussed including (1) screening, brief intervention, treatment and referral to treatment, (2) the Chronic Care Model, and (3) The Massachusetts Collaborative Care Model.

Screening, Brief Intervention, Treatment and Referral to Treatment

Efforts have been made to shift from an exclusive focus on the most severe end of the substance use continuum to a public health prevention approach to identify persons who are at risk due to the consequences of alcohol and other drug use and intervene accordingly. These prevention efforts are increasingly possible with the promotion of brief, validated screening measures for alcohol and drug use[37] and evidence for the efficacy of brief alcohol interventions,[38] and pharmacotherapy for alcohol use disorder,[39] opioid use disorder,[40] and tobacco use disorder.[41] However, implementing strategies from screening to brief intervention to referral to treatment (SBIRT) for those needing more extensive treatment, has presented a challenge to health care systems. Hargraves et al. analyzed the SBIRT process flow in 10 primary care practices and reported on best practices.[42] A key finding was the utilization of an interprofessional team. They state, "coordination and communication across disciplines and between diverse skillsets is necessary for seamless and complete delivery of all SBIRT states."[42] An additional best practice was to define and communicate details of each step within the team.[42]

Aligning SBIRT within the flow of the clinical practice is another best practice identified by Hargraves et al.[42] and can be done by defining ownership of various SBIRT components. Del Boca et al. proposed a conceptual framework to guide SBIRT translational research in which they point out that with the expansion of SBI to include referral to treatment and brief treatment; different types of clinicians often delivered different components within the same program.[43] Similarly, in describing SBIRT processes across 14 acute care facilities, Keen, Theole, and Newhouse reported differences in the interprofessional clinician responsible for executing each step of the intervention.[44] In all 14 facilities the registered nurse admitting the patient completed the initial screening for alcohol, drug, and tobacco use, while the brief intervention was completed by a registered nurse or social worker after a positive screen, and referral to treatment led by a social worker, a registered nurse, or a case manager.[44]

In their lessons learned from 10 years of implementing SBIRT in Colorado, Nunes et al. recommended engaging staff at multiple levels for the practice to be sustained.[45] The authors pointed out that following up on positive screens including providing brief intervention can be conducted effectively by a wide variety of staff regardless of their discipline as well as paraprofessionals.[45] Screening, intervention, treatment, and linkages to specialty treatment were identified as common competencies and as such the full set of these clinical strategies can be delivered by an interprofessional team.

Chronic Care Model

The Chronic Care Model (CCM) was based on the premise that high quality chronic illness care is characterized by productive interactions between practice team members who organize and coordinate care, and patients.[46] In 2008, Saitz et al. proposed a model of care based on the CCM in guiding comprehensive and coordinated care to address the complex needs of persons with substance use disorders (SUD) wherein informed, motivated patients and a prepared, practice team and delivery system would lead to optimal outcomes.[47] In 2014, a consensus group from the National Institute on Drug Abuse examined whether and how the core elements of the CCM could be applied to the treatment of persons with SUD in primary care, underscoring that the CCM involves teams of health care clinicians from various disciplines to anticipate and prevent recurrence of serious and expensive returns to use.[48] Importantly, the consensus group acknowledged the continuum of substance use and emphasized that SBIRT is consonant with both the CCM and good clinical practice. Tai and Volkow similarly stated that a comprehensive CCM for persons with SUD should start from routine SBI to detect early risk, and care for persons with SUD should follow with effective coordination and collaboration between the primary care team and specialty services to ensure continuity of care.[49]

Two studies have tested the impact of chronic care management delivered to patients with substance use disorders with comorbid depressive disorder or post-traumatic stress disorder [50] and women with hazardous alcohol use (ie, AUDIT-C score of three or above) engaged in a health care for the unhoused program.[51] While neither found that the chronic care management intervention impacted outcomes, neither trial implemented the chronic care model as originally conceptualized. For example, a key component of the CCM is delivery system design. That is, the roles of team members need to be clearly defined and tasks distributed accordingly. Busetto et al. undertook a study to identify what should be implemented as part of integrated chronic care interventions, interventions that targeted components of the CCM.[52] Based on their literature review, questionnaires from experts, and case reports, the authors identified seven workforce changes: (1) involvement of a nurse in the delivery of care, (2) multidisciplinary staff including health care clinicians from different disciplines, (3) multidisciplinary protocols/pathways involving tasks for health care clinicians from different disciplines, (4) provider training such as on-the-job training, educational seminars or materials for health professionals, (5) involvement of a case manager/care coordinator in the delivery of care, (6) regular team meetings to discuss patient treatment; and (7) the creation of a new position, role or function specifically to deliver integrated chronic care.[52] Though the term "multidisciplinary" was used to describe staff and protocols in the recommendations, the inclusion of regular team meetings is consistent with interprofessional collaborative practice. That is, interprofessional collaborative practice is when clinicians from different professional backgrounds deliver comprehensive coordinated services working with patients, families, and communities to deliver the highest quality of care across settings.[1] These publications focusing on chronic care management highlight the imperative to evaluate delivery system design to effectively manage the complex interventions needed for patients with chronic health conditions at any point along the continuum of substance use.

Massachusetts Collaborative Care Model

The prescribing of buprenorphine for office-based treatment of persons with opioid use disorder (OUD) was initially restricted to qualified physician prescribers.[53] The Massachusetts Collaborative Care Model (MCCM) was developed in recognition of the need for an interprofessional team to address the complex needs of and provide comprehensive collaborative care to patients with OUD.[54] Implemented in 2003, the program staff included a full-time nurse program director, nurse care managers, program coordinator, physicians, and collaboration with pharmacists, each staff carrying out tasks based on protocols and specific to their role and scope of practice.[55] Their 5-year experience with 382 patients receiving treatment guided by the MCCM demonstrated successful retention in treatment (51.3%) and some (2.4%) patients successfully tapered off medication after 6 months abstinence from drug use. Importantly, the MCCM ensured compliance with the federal law in existence at that time limiting the number of patients treated per prescribing physician yet allowed the clinic to treat many patients with complex needs. The success of the MCCM led to expansion of the model to 14 community health centers successfully initiating office-based treatment, and over a 5-year period (2007-2013), serving more than 10,000 patients[55] and establishing a sustainable reimbursement model.[56] While abstinence and treatment retention outcomes are important, future studies evaluating the MCCM and other substance use interventions should include patient-centered outcomes such as decreased substance use, attainment of stable housing, employment, relationships, and quality of life.

Bailey et al. evaluated an interdisciplinary model of OUD treatment, an adaptation of the MCCM.[57] Prior to implementing their model, treatment primarily consisted of buprenorphine prescribed by a primary care provider with behavioral health services provided on an ad-hoc basis. Their adapted program included primary care providers who prescribed medications for OUD. These providers included physicians, and with changed legislation allowing expanded prescribing to include nurse practitioners and physician's assistants in 2016[58] and all advanced practice nurses through the SUPPORT Act in 2018.[59] Each primary care team also included behavioral health clinicians (eg, psychologists, social workers) who focused on improving coping skills, recurrence of use prevention, and resilience strategies to facilitate recovery, and a registered nurse who focused on care management.[57] A retrospective observational study using data from 494 patients with OUD and at least one buprenorphine prescription order revealed that 53.2% were retained for at least 6 months.[57] The study findings also highlighted the applicability of the MCCM for guiding the care of patients with complex needs. The majority (68.7%) of the sample had one or more psychiatric comorbidity and in that subsample, 43.5% were retained for 6 months or more[57] consistent with findings from Weinstein et al. of an increased odds of 1 year or more treatment retention for patients with a psychiatric diagnosis in their MCCM-based program.[60]

INTERPROFESSIONAL COLLABORATIVE PRACTICE RESEARCH

Although the goal of IPE studies is to enable professionals to achieve competency to successfully practice collaboratively, and care models have successfully shown positive clinical patient and system benefits, the literature on evaluation and/or outcomes of the people involved in interprofessional collaborative practice (IPCP) remains sparse, especially in patients with SUD. However, existing models of SUD interprofessional care coordination may serve as platforms for future and ongoing IPCP scholarship.

IPCP often goes beyond care coordination. Care coordination works best when health care clinicians work together as a team with patients and their caregivers to achieve positive outcomes for all involved. The most severe outcomes that are studied are those with the most likelihood of cost containment for health systems, such as urgent medical appointments, emergency department visits, hospitalization, and readmissions.[61] Despite its moniker, care coordination may only integrate care provision for chronic diseases and comorbidities by different disciplines, through enhanced communication and referrals and/or colocation instead of "laboring together for a common goal," or true IPCP.[62]

As robust IPE programs become implemented, and health care clinicians addressing SUD integrate their knowledge, skills and roles beyond care coordination to improve patient outcomes, researchers should focus on systematic documentation and evaluation of these outcomes. Benefits to patients, interprofessional care team members, and health care system should be documented and evaluated to enable replication and sustainability in resource-limited environments characterized by increasing burnout across professions.[63] This, in turn, not only helps justify and expand IPE so that IPCP models function smoothly with clinicians already familiar with each discipline's roles, but also fosters an environment for establishment of best practices and reimbursement models.

Examples and summaries of reviews and other studies of SUD and/or SUD-related IPCP are listed in **Table 46-3**. Examples were chosen to reflect different research types, disciplines, and patient types. The significant overlap between people living with chronic pain and people diagnosed with OUD parallels the overlap between successful models of IPCP for chronic pain and OUD.[64] Becker et al. evaluated the holistic success of an outpatient referral clinic for people with chronic pain, that employed a team of pain and addiction specialists from different disciplines. Even though this model may not be replicable outside the setting described, it shows how IPCP is facilitated and sustained by evaluation and, at minimum, colocation.[65]

Englander et al. led a team of researchers to characterize and catalog the typologies of inpatient SUD care team models in a published scoping review supported by key informant interviews.[66] Interprofessional addiction consult services (ACS) utilized a wide variety and breadth of disciplines to initiate care for admitted patients with SUD and included roles unique to SUD IPCP: peer mentors and community partners. Patients on one ACS were interviewed by Collins, et al. on their views of peer mentors and described their role as essential for "translating" care decisions between providers and patients. The peer mentors were also interviewed and reported professional isolation from the team as nonclinicians, despite their connections to the patients.[67]

Measuring IPCP outcomes should include changes in and maintenance of improved team dynamics and patient viewpoints using qualitative research methods such as interviews and focus groups. SUD patient outcomes can be quantitatively compared before and after implementation of IPCP and include both clinical and financial variables. Randomization of patients to a usual care model (either care coordination/multidisciplinary care or fragmented/single-discipline care) and to a IPCP model is possible. The IPCP model could take the form of one or more additional disciplines to form and/or expand the team, or alternatively, add professionals or people particularly unique to IPCP SUD care, such as peer mentors and/or (other) people with lived experience.

In a report from Caron et al., clinical pharmacists integrated into office-based opioid treatment (OBOT) in four different practice settings (academic family medicine, private family medicine practice, a federally qualified health center (FQHC), and an academic obstetrics-gynecology residency) were surveyed to collect and compare their roles.[68] Although there were patterns of patient care activities consistent with IPCP, it is difficult to characterize these activities as IPCP in any of the practice settings. For comparison, Tran and colleagues clearly pointed out that their interprofessional team was comprised of physicians, nurse practitioners, clinical pharmacist, social workers, and a nurse.[69] More research is needed to establish the value of IPCP in ambulatory care settings, and specify the composition of the team. Goodman described an innovative and feasible integration of addiction professionals and reproductive health clinicians to make care easier for patients.[70] To assess IPCP effectiveness, all IPCP participants, in particular patients, should have their experiences documented and analyzed. For example, Wenaas, et al. found in their study of patients participating in interprofessional team meetings, that patients had far different experiences, knowledge, and expectations of the meetings than expected, demonstrating the need for continuous quality improvement and evaluation when implementing IPCP models.[71]

TABLE 46-3 Example of Studies of Interprofessional Collaborative Practices (IPCP)

Authors	Study design Practice setting sample size	Study objective	Professions included	Results outcomes limitations
Becker W, Edmond S, Cervone D, et al.[65]	Brief Research Report Veterans' Administration outpatient clinic $N = 87$ referred patients from 2012-2014	Evaluate a novel multidisciplinary, patient-centered, opioid reassessment clinic (ORC) at patient, provider, clinic, and health-system levels	• Internist (MD) with addiction and pain training • Addiction psychiatrist • Behavioral health advanced practice nurse/addiction training • Clinical health psychologist • Nurse care manager	• 84% ($N = 73$) had SUD history • 70% ($N = 61$) of patients currently misuse opioids prescribed for pain • All patients with current SUD diagnosis engaged in addiction treatment • Mean patient treatment satisfaction 3.8 (1-5 scale) • Mean change in milligram MEDD* 33.4 • 48% of PCP referred patients to ORC • Hired nurse care manager Design limitations: Health care utilization, clinical and cost outcomes were not measured. No control group Outcome limitations: Intensive resources required may limit implementation of model

Englander H, Jones A, Krawczyk N, et al.[66]	Scoping literature review and key informant interviews to generate a taxonomy of hospital-based, inpatient addiction care models	Construct a taxonomy of hospital-based addiction care models	Interprofessional Addiction Consult Service (ACS) only:
			
			• Addiction medicine expert (MD, NP)
			• Coordinator with addiction expertise: (licensed clinical social worker [LCSW]), navigator, peer mentor, and/or pharmacist
			• Patient engagement peer
			• Community partner
			• Trainees
				• 87 papers identified
				• 6 models described
				  • Interprofessional addiction consult service
				  • Psychiatry consult liaison service
				  • Individual consultant
				  • Hospital-based opioid treatment
				  • Hospital-based alcohol treatment
				  • Community-based in-reach
				• 15 key informants interviewed
				
				Design limitations: Models can coexist. Key informants may not be representative of all models; some models may not be described. Comparative model effectiveness unknown.
				Outcome limitations: In all of the models, patients must access postdischarge care to sustain treatment, which may be limited by provider type and access, insurance barriers, geography, stigma and/or discrimination.

(Continued)

TABLE 46-3 Example of Studies of Interprofessional Collaborative Practices (IPCP) *(Continued)*

Authors	Study design Practice setting sample size	Study objective	Professions included	Results outcomes limitations

Collins D, Alla J, Nicolaidis C, et al.[67]	Qualitative thematic analysis of 46 pre- and posthospitalization patients' views of peer mentors (PM) who were part of the Improving Addiction Care Team (IMPACT) using focus groups, interviews, and patient observation	Evaluate how peer mentorship affects care for hospitalized patients with SUD
		• How does working in a hospital affect PMs' sense of professional identity?
			IMPACT team (ref *J Hosp Med*)
			• LCSW
			• Addiction physician
			• Peer mentors
				• PMs bonded with SUD inpatients and earned trust through shared lived experiences, often contrary to typical provider-patient interactions
				• Trust facilitates provider-patient communication where the PM "translates" shared goals of care to result in:
				  • Reduced patient-directed discharges
				  • Increased patient follow-through and follow-ups
				  • Reduced clinician stigma
				  • Role on the team was professionally and personally satisfying, "meeting patients where they are at," yet
				  • Compassion fatigue led to burnout and emotional strain
				  • Inpatient hierarchy isolated nonclinical PM
				  • Peer supervision was key to enhancing "translator" role and mitigating professional isolation
				Design Limitations: inpatient only; single site academic medical center in urban area. Patient data collected as part of larger study. Limited racial and ethnic makeup of sample.
				Outcome Limitations: Peer mentor models, background, training, and inpatient integration and access vary across jurisdictions.

Caron O, Fay A, Pressley H, et al.[68]	A survey of 4 pharmacists who implemented office-based opioid treatment (OBOT) in four outpatient practice types
	• Family medicine (FM) residency
	• Obstetrics-gynecology residency
	• Physician-owned FM practice
	• Federally qualified health center (FQHC)
		Identify common roles, clinical background, and barriers of pharmacists integrated into four different OBOT services	• Pharmacists
			• Physicians
			• Resident physicians
			• Nurse practitioners
			• LCSW
			• Certified nurse midwives
			• Physician assistants
				• None of the pharmacists is directly funded for their role
				• 5-20 h/week spent performing OBOT
				• 30 to more than 100 patients in treatment
				• Wide range of direct patient care activities, four were universal
				  • Monitoring Adverse drug interactions/experiences
				  • Developing/adjusting treatment care Plan
				  • Patient counseling and education
				  • Urine toxicology interpretation
				Design Limitations: Pharmacists recruited were located in a small geographic area and intentionally recruited, and thus may not represent all models of pharmacist OBAT clinic integration.
				Outcome Limitations: Pharmacists are prohibited by law from obtaining an X-waiver to prescribe buprenorphine, thus limiting their integration.

Goodman D[70]	Review of outpatient Perinatal Addiction Treatment Program at one academic medical center	Describe the structure, function and outcomes of a multidisciplinary perinatal addiction treatment program	• Certified nurse-midwife (CNM) • Maternal-fetal medicine physician -LCSW • Addiction psychiatrist • Pediatric hospitalist • Licensed drug and alcohol counselor • Behavioral health specialist	• Improved coordination of care • Increased satisfaction among both pregnant women and providers • Higher proportion of recommended prenatal visits attended • Improved patient satisfaction for colocation of prenatal care and addiction treatment Design Limitations: unpublished data on outcomes, no methods nor quantitative data reported; single-center description. Outcome Limitations: Overall perinatal care, much less substance use disorder care in the perinatal period is limited, especially for historically marginalized groups. Multidisciplinary perinatal care, while innovative, requires further study, perhaps using different access models such as telemedicine.

Wenaas M, Andersson HW, Kiik R, et al.[71]	In 2016 in central Norway, 16 people with comorbid SUD and psychiatric disorders admitted to the hospital were interviewed about their participation in interprofessional SUD team meetings; data from first 5 people recruited are reported Meetings were also observed by videoconference	Using an ethnographic approach, evaluated the experience of and identified barriers to SUD service users' participation and/or collaboration with members of the inter-professional team in team meeting	• Inpatient and outpatient SUD service users
			Teams
			• Specialty health care professionals (MD)
			• Social services (LCSW)
			• Primary health care staff
				• Meeting purpose was perceived differently by attendees
				• Several barriers to involvement found
				  • Unclear roles and expectations
				  • Unclear, non-patient-centered routines and rules
				  • Lack of user knowledge and skills
				  • Provider paternalism
				  • Use of professional jargon
				• Meetings were not useful nor productive
				• Providers should involve people in their care meeting with clearly established expectations, roles, baseline knowledge, and effective communication
				Design Limitations: Small convenience sample in single site
				Outcome Limitations: Additional research is needed to replicate the results

*MEDD, morphine equivalent daily dose.

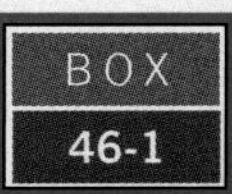

BOX 46-1 Recommendations for Promoting an Interprofessional Workforce to Address the Substance Use Continuum

Education

Include peers or peer support specialists in developing and delivering education
Incorporate reflection on content and its influence on one's future practice to minimize personal bias/stigma
Emphasize existing treatment resources in the local community
Employ rapid cycle quality improvement
Utilize substance use–related interprofessional competencies as a framework for curricular enhancements and continuing education programs
Expand evaluation to include practice behaviors

Practice in the Field

Identify and document core competencies for interprofessional collaborative practice across the continuum of substance use practice
Disseminate and evaluate evidence-based practice models

Research

Examine methods for improving the efficiency of interprofessional care and how care responsibilities are distributed across team members.
Identify outcomes to allow greater ability to compare practice models, such as engagement, retention, treatment acceptance, substance use, and quality of life

Policy

Promote the recognition of interprofessional substance use–related competencies by accrediting bodies

RECOMMENDATIONS

Ongoing efforts are needed to ensure an interprofessional workforce that has the requisite competencies to address the needs of persons across the continuum of substance use. The recommendations in Box 46-1 are offered to help realize that goal and to build upon the growing evidence in support of interprofessional practice models.

SUMMARY

Interprofessional collaborative practice entails multiple health care clinicians from different professional backgrounds working together with patients, families and communities to deliver the highest quality of care. The needs of persons who are at-risk because of substance use, persons with a substance use disorder, and persons in recovery are best addressed through cooperative, coordinated, and collaborative relationships between clinicians of various professions and peer specialists in delivering patient-centered care. Education and practice models, driven by interprofessional competencies that specify substance use–related knowledge, skills, and attitudes will help shape a more efficient and effective care delivery system for this population.

REFERENCES

1. World Health Organization. *Framework for Action on Interprofessional Education and Collaborative Practice.* 2010.
2. Johnson JM, Hermosura BJ, Price SL, Gougeon L. Factors influencing interprofessional team collaboration when delivering care to community-dwelling seniors: a metasynthesis of Canadian interventions. *J Interprof Care.* 2021;35(3):376-382.
3. Haack MR, Adger H, eds. *Strategic Plan for Interdisciplinary Faculty Development: Arming the Nation's Health Professional Workforce for a New Approach to Substance Use Disorders.* Association for Medical Education and Research in Substance Abuse; 2002.
4. Finnell DS, Tierney M, Mitchell AM. Nursing: addressing substance use in the 21st century. *Subst Abuse.* 2019;40(4):412-420.
5. Bratberg J. Pharmacy: addressing substance use in the 21st century. *Subst Abuse.* 2019;40(4):421-434.
6. Levy S, Seale JP, Alford DP. Medicine, with a focus on physicians: addressing substance use in the 21st century. *Subst Abuse.* 2019;40(4):396-404.
7. Mattingly JR. Medicine, with a focus on physician assistants: addressing substance use in the 21st century. *Subst Abuse.* 2019;40(4):405-411.
8. Osborne-Leute V, Pugatch M, Hruschak V. Social work: addressing substance use in the 21st century. *Subst Abuse.* 2019;40(4):435-440.
9. American Nurses Association. *Nursing: Scope and Standards of Practice.* 3rd ed. American Nurses Association; 2015.
10. Ray MD. Shared borders: achieving the goals of interdisciplinary patient care. *Am J Health Syst Pharm.* 1998;55(13):1369-1374.
11. Committee on the Health Professions Education Summit. *Health Professions Education: A Bridge to Quality.* National Academies Press; 2003.
12. Rutkowski BA. Specific disciplines addressing substance use: AMERSA in the 21st century. *Subst Abuse.* 2019;40(4):392-395.
13. Substance Abuse and Mental Health Services Administration. *Core Competencies for Peer Health Workers.* SAMHSA; 2015.
14. White WL, Evans AC. The recovery agenda: The shared role of peers and professionals. *Public Health Rev.* 2013;35(2):4.
15. Institute of Medicine. *Improving the Quality of Health Care for Mental and Substance-Use Conditions.* National Academies Press; 2006.
16. Laudet A, Best D. Addiction recovery in services and policy: an international overview. In: el-Guebaly N, Carrà G, Galanter M, Baldacchino AM, eds. *Textbook of Addiction Treatment: International Perspectives.* Springer; 2015:1065-1083.
17. Eddie D, Hoffman L, Vilsaint C, et al. Lived experience in new models of care for substance use disorder: a systematic review of peer recovery support services and recovery coaching. *Front Psychol.* 2019;10:1052.
18. Jack HE, Oller D, Kelly J, Magidson JF, Wakeman SE. Addressing substance use disorder in primary care: the role, integration, and impact of recovery coaches. *Subst Abuse.* 2018;39(3):307-314.
19. Slater T, Rodney T, Kozachik SL, Finnell DS. Recommendations for emergency departments caring for persons with opioid use and opioid use disorders: an integrative review. *J Emerg Nurs.* 2022;48:129-144.
20. Schmitt MH, Gilbert JH, Brandt BF, Weinstein RS. The coming of age for interprofessional education and practice. *Am J Med.* 2013;126(4):284-288.
21. Health Professions Networks Nursing & Midwifery Human Resources for Health. *Framework for Action on Interprofessional Education & Collaborative Practice.* World Health Organization; 2010.
22. Remington TL, Foulk MA, Williams BC. Evaluation of evidence for interprofessional education. *Am J Pharm Educ.* 2006;70(3):66.
23. Adamson K, Ashcroft R, Langlois S, Lising D. Integrating social work into interprofessional education: a review of one university's curriculum to prepare students for collaborative practice in healthcare. *Adv Soc Work.* 2020;20(2):454-472.
24. Monteiro K, Dumenco L, Collins S, et al. Substance use disorder training workshop for future interprofessional health care providers. *MedEdPORTAL.* 2017;13:10576.
25. Muzyk A, Mullan P, Andolsek KM, et al. An interprofessional substance use disorder course to improve students' educational outcomes and patients' treatment decisions. *Acad Med.* 2019;94(11):1792-1799.

26. Muzyk AJ, Tew C, Thomas-Fannin A, et al. An interprofessional course on substance use disorders for health professions students. *Acad Med.* 2017;92(12):1704-1708.
27. Sherwood DA, Kramlich D, Rodriguez K, Graybeal C. Developing a Screening, Brief Intervention, and Referral to Treatment (SBIRT) program with multiple health professions programs. *J Interprof Care.* 2019;33(6):828-831.
28. Stoddard-Dare P, Niederriter J, DeBoth KK, et al. An interprofessional learning opportunity regarding pain and the opioid epidemic. *Adv Soc Work.* 2020;20(2):215-234.
29. Weller BE, Carver JN, Harrison J, Chapleau A. Addressing opioid misuse and mental health conditions through interdisciplinary workforce development programs. *Soc Work Ment Health.* 2021;19(3):220-229.
30. Broyles LM, Conley JW, Harding JD Jr, Gordon AJ. A scoping review of interdisciplinary collaboration in addictions education and training. *J Addict Nurs.* 2013;24(1):29-36.
31. Muzyk A, Smothers ZPW, Andolsek KM, et al. Interprofessional substance use disorder education in health professions education programs: a scoping review. *Acad Med.* 2020;95(3):470-480.
32. Englander H, Patten A, Lockard R, Muller M, Gregg J. Spreading addictions care across Oregon's rural and community hospitals: mixed-methods evaluation of an interprofessional telementoring ECHO program. *J Gen Intern Med.* 2021;36(1):100-107.
33. Puskar K, Mitchell AM, Albrecht SA, et al. Interprofessional collaborative practice incorporating training for alcohol and drug use screening for healthcare providers in rural areas. *J Interprof Care.* 2016;30(4):542-544.
34. Lindsey AC, Janich N, Macchi CR, et al. Testing a Screening, Brief Intervention, and Referral to Treatment (SBIRT) interdisciplinary training program model for higher education systems. *Fam Syst Health.* 2021;39(2):212-223.
35. Regnier K, Chappell K, Travlos DV. The role and rise of interprofessional continuing education. *J Med Regul.* 2019;105(3):6-13.
36. Safabakhsh L, Irajpour A, Yamani N. Designing and developing a continuing interprofessional education model. *Adv Med Educ Pract.* 2018;9:459-467.
37. McNeely J, Hamilton L. Screening for unhealthy alcohol and drug use in general medicine settings. *Med Clin.* 2022;106(1):13-28.
38. Bertholet N, Daeppen J, Wietlisbach V, Fleming M, Burnand B. Reduction of alcohol consumption by brief alcohol intervention in primary care: systematic review and meta-analysis. *Arch Intern Med.* 2005;165(9):986-995.
39. Maisel NC, Blodgett JC, Wilbourne PL, Humphreys K, Finney JW. Meta-analysis of naltrexone and acamprosate for treating alcohol use disorders: when are these medications most helpful? *Addiction.* 2013;108(2):275-293. doi:10.1111/j.1360-0443.2012.04054.x
40. Mattick RP, Breen C, Kimber J, Davoli M. Buprenorphine maintenance versus placebo or methadone maintenance for opioid dependence. *Cochrane Database Syst Rev.* 2014;3:CD002207.
41. Stead LF, Perera R, Bullen C, et al. Nicotine replacement therapy for smoking cessation. *Cochrane Database Syst Rev.* 2012;11:CD000146.
42. Hargraves D, White C, Frederick R, et al. Implementing SBIRT (Screening, Brief Intervention and Referral to Treatment) in primary care: lessons learned from a multi-practice evaluation portfolio. *Public Health Rev.* 2017;38(1):1-11.
43. Del Boca FK, McRee B, Vendetti J, Damon D. The SBIRT program matrix: a conceptual framework for program implementation and evaluation. *Addiction.* 2017;112:12-22.
44. Keen A, Thoele K, Newhouse R. Variation in SBIRT delivery among acute care facilities. *Nurs Outlook.* 2020;68(2):162-168.
45. Nunes AP, Richmond MK, Marzano K, Swenson CJ, Lockhart J. Ten years of implementing screening, brief intervention, and referral to treatment (SBIRT): lessons learned. *Subst Abus.* 2017;38(4):508-512.
46. Wagner EH, Austin BT, Davis C, Hindmarsh M, Schaefer J, Bonomi A. Improving chronic illness care: translating evidence into action. *Health Aff.* 2001;20(6):64-78.
47. Saitz R, Larson MJ, Labelle C, Richardson J, Samet JH. The case for chronic disease management for addiction. *J Addict Med.* 2008;2(2):55-65.
48. McLellan AT, Starrels JL, Tai B, et al. Can substance use disorders be managed using the chronic care model? review and recommendations from a NIDA consensus group. *Public Health Rev.* 2014;35:8.
49. Tai B, Volkow ND. Treatment for substance use disorder: opportunities and challenges under the affordable care act. *Soc Work Public Health.* 2013;28(3–4):165-174.
50. Park TW, Cheng DM, Samet JH, Winter MR, Saitz R. Chronic care management for substance dependence in primary care among patients with co-occurring disorders. *Psychiatr Serv.* 2015;66(1):72-79.
51. Upshur C, Weinreb L, Bharel M, Reed G, Frisard C. A randomized control trial of a chronic care intervention for homeless women with alcohol use problems. *J Subst Abuse Treat.* 2015;51:19-29.
52. Busetto L, Luijkx K, Calciolari S, Ortiz LGG, Vrijhoef HJM. Exploration of workforce changes in integrated chronic care: findings from an interactive and emergent research design. *PloS One.* 2017;12(12):e0187468.
53. 106th Congress. Drug Addiction Treatment Act of 2000. Public Law H.R.2634; July 19, 2019.
54. LaBelle CT, Han SC, Bergeron A, Samet JH. Office-based opioid treatment with buprenorphine (OBOT-B): statewide implementation of the Massachusetts collaborative care model in community health centers. *J Subst Abuse Treat.* 2016;60:6-13.
55. Alford DP, LaBelle CT, Kretsch N, et al. Collaborative care of opioid-addicted patients in primary care using buprenorphine: five-year experience. *Arch Intern Med.* 2011;171(5):425-431.
56. Substance Abuse and Mental Health Services Administration. *Medicaid Coverage and Financing of Medications to Treat Alcohol and Opioid Use Disorders.* HHS Publication No. SMA-14-4854; 2014.
57. Bailey SR, Lucas JA, Angier H, et al. Associations of retention on buprenorphine for opioid use disorder with patient characteristics and models of care in the primary care setting. *J Subst Abuse Treat.* 2021;131:108548.
58. 114th Congress. Comprehensive Addiction and Recovery Act. 2016 July 22, 2016; H.R. 6311.
59. 115th Congress. Substance Use Disorder Prevention that Promotes Opioid Recovery and Treatment for Patients and Communities Act (SUPPORT). October 24, 2018; H.R. 6.
60. Weinstein ZM, Kim HW, Cheng DM, et al. Long-term retention in office based opioid treatment with buprenorphine. *J Subst Abuse Treat.* 2017;74:65-70.
61. The Pew Charitable Trusts. Care coordination strategies for patients can improve substance use disorder outcomes. Accessed May 30, 3023. https://www.pewtrusts.org/en/research-and-analysis/issue-briefs/2020/04/care-coordination-strategies-for-patients-can-improve-substance-use-disorder-outcomes
62. Agency for Healthcare Research and Quality. (AHRQ). *Integration of Mental Health/Substance Abuse and Primary Care: Evidence Report/Technology 173.* AHRQ; 2008.
63. Sullivan EE, Phillips RS. Sustaining primary care teams in the midst of a pandemic. *Isr J Health Policy Res.* 2020;9(1):77.
64. Rehman S, Dhanjal-Reddy A, Okvat HA, et al. Flipping the pain care model: a sociopsychobiological approach to high-value chronic pain care. *Pain Med.* 2020;21(6):1168-1180.
65. Becker WC, Edmond SN, Cervone DJ, et al. Evaluation of an integrated, multidisciplinary program to address unsafe use of opioids prescribed for pain. *Pain Med.* 2018;19(7):1419-1424.
66. Englander H, Jones A, Krawczyk N, et al. A taxonomy of hospital-based addiction care models: a scoping review and key informant interviews. *J Gen Intern Med.* 2022;37(11):2821-2833.
67. Collins D, Alla J, Nicolaidis C, et al. "If It Wasn't for Him, I Wouldn't Have Talked to Them": qualitative study of addiction peer mentorship in the hospital. *J Gen Intern Med.* 2019; doi:10.1007/s11606-019-05311-0
68. Caron O, Fay AE, Pressley H, Seamon G, Taylor SR, Wilson CG. Four models of pharmacist-integrated office-based opioid treatment. *J Am Coll Clin Pharm.* 2022;5(4):413-421. doi:10.1002/jac5.1607

69. Tran TH, Swoboda H, Perticone K, et al. The substance use intervention team: a hospital-based intervention and outpatient clinic to improve care for patients with substance use disorders. *Am J Health Syst Pharm.* 2021;78(4):345-353.
70. Goodman D. Improving access to maternity care for women with opioid use disorders: colocation of midwifery services at an addiction treatment program. *J Midwifery Womens Health.* 2015;60(6):706-712.
71. Wenaas M, Andersson HW, Kiik R, Juberg A. User involvement in interprofessional team meetings within services for substance use disorders. *Nordisk Alkohol Nark.* 2021;38(2):190-203.

CHAPTER 47

The ASAM Criteria and Matching Patients to Treatment

David R. Gastfriend and R. Corey Waller

CHAPTER OUTLINE

- Introduction
- Selecting appropriate services
- Understanding *The ASAM Criteria*
- Assessment dimensions
- Levels of care
- Research on *The ASAM Criteria*
- *The ASAM Criteria* standard implementation, ASAM CONTINUUM
- Social impact
- Evolution of standardized toolkit
- Conclusions
- Brief summary

INTRODUCTION

Today, *The ASAM Criteria* for the treatment of addiction-related and co-occurring conditions consists of an extensive toolkit of books, trainings, decision rules, assessment software, and certification processes.[1] But the roots of this system began growing in the mid-1980s, when developers of two sets of placement criteria joined with the American Society of Addiction Medicine (ASAM) to develop a single national set of criteria that would unify the addiction treatment field.[2,3]

In 1991, the ASAM published the *Patient Placement Criteria for the Treatment of Psychoactive Substance Use Disorders.*[4] ASAM formed multidisciplinary groups of addiction treatment specialists to develop consensus criteria to promote a common language and guidelines for assigning a given patient to specific levels and types of treatment services for all persons with substance use disorders (SUDs). *The ASAM Criteria* were designed to help clinicians, payers, and regulators shift from:

1. One-dimensional to six-dimensional assessment—from treatment based solely on diagnosis to treatment that addresses multiple needs
2. A Program-driven approach to clinical and outcome-driven treatment—from programs with fixed lengths of stay to variable length of stay (LOS), person-centered, individualized treatment responsive to specific needs and progress and outcome in treatment
3. A limited number of discrete levels of care (LOCs) to a broad and flexible continuum of care

A second edition was developed in 1996, the *ASAM PPC-2,*[5] and a revision of that, the *ASAM PPC-2R*, was released in 2001.[6] The 2013 third edition[7] expanded the criteria to address special populations of older adults, parents receiving treatment concurrently with their children, people in safety-sensitive occupations, and criminal justice populations. There were also sections on tobacco use disorder and gambling disorder to promote a necessary continuum of services that are still not funded and reimbursed like other substance-related and addiction disorders. An updated Opioid Treatment Services section included opioid treatment programs (methadone), office-based opioid treatment (buprenorphine), and antagonist medication (naltrexone). The ongoing goal was to promote individualized, person-centered, and outcome-driven care.[7]

Adoption of *The ASAM Criteria* in some form proceeded throughout the late 1990s and 2000s, with managed care pressure and accreditation being leading reasons for program adoption.[8] In 2006, a survey of all 50 U.S. state authorities was conducted for the National Association of State Alcohol and Drug Abuse Directors (NASADAD). By then, 43 states (84%) required the use of standard patient placement criteria.[9] Among the states that require patient placement criteria, approximately two-thirds required providers to use *The ASAM Criteria*, and this percentage has grown since the time of the survey. Some developed their own criteria or used criteria based on the Addiction Severity Index (ASI), the Global Assessment of Individual Needs, and the Treatment Demand Indicator.[9] Since the 2006 NASADAD study, some states that had their own criteria have since switched to using *The ASAM Criteria*. The U.S. Department of Defense endorsed *The ASAM Criteria*, and a national survey of the U.S. Veterans Health Administration (VA) addiction program leaders reported that 48% were very familiar with *The ASAM Criteria.*[10]

In 2015 and again in 2017, the Centers for Medicare and Medicaid Services (CMS) recommended that states use *The ASAM Criteria* in the CMS 1115 Waiver program.[11] This led nearly 30 states to design alternative Medicaid payment models using *The ASAM Criteria.*[12] At this point, the Substance Abuse and Mental Health Services Administration (SAMHSA) considers *The ASAM Criteria* to be "the most widely used and comprehensive set of guidelines for placement, continued stay, and transfer/discharge of patients with addiction and co-occurring conditions" as listed in SAMHSA's Evidence-Based Practices Resource Center.[13]

In 2020, ASAM began the process of updating the ASAM Criteria to the fourth edition. The development process for this new edition included 17 writing groups, structured literature reviews, a modified Delphi methodological process, an open public comment period, and the involvement of those with lived experience, all national addiction-related societies, regulatory bodies (both state and federal), and payer viewpoints.

It was determined that the effective treatment of adolescents, those in jails and prisons, and those with behavioral addictions was different enough that the next edition of the fourth edition will be divided into four volumes:

1. The ASAM Criteria for Adults and Special Populations
2. The ASAM Criteria for Jails and Prisons
3. The ASAM Criteria for Adolescents
4. The ASAM Criteria for Behavioral Addictions

This division will allow evidence-based, population-specific criteria to be developed, allowing for a more patient-centered and higher fidelity approach to care for these unique populations.

SELECTING APPROPRIATE SERVICES

All patients with addiction require access to four major components of care. These include medical, psychotherapy, psychoeducation, and recovery support services. Depending on the addiction and that person's needs, the amount and specifics of each component can be modified to fit an individual's unique circumstances. Luckily, the patterns of dysfunction associated with SUDs and behavioral addictions are relatively consistent. Given this consistency, care can be grouped into the most common patterns found in our populations. The correct types, intensities, and locations of services can be identified by completing a dimensional analysis. In the fourth edition, the dimensions have been arranged in a descending order that best aligns with rapidly identifying initial placement and decreasing the risk of mortality to the patient. Described below are the six dimensions and their related "subdimensions." A deeper description of the dimensions and the associated subdimensions is found in the section entitled "Assessment Dimensions."

Dimensions

Dimension 1—Acute intoxication and withdrawal potential

- Intoxication and associated risks (including overdose)
- Withdrawal risks
  - Alcohol withdrawal risks
  - Sedative/hypnotic withdrawal risks
  - Opioid withdrawal risk, including need for MOUD initiation
  - Stimulant withdrawal risks
  - Other withdrawal risks

Dimension 2—Biomedical conditions

- Acute physical health concerns
- Acute or uncontrolled pain
- Pregnancy-related concerns
- Chronic physical health concerns
- Sleep problems

Dimension 3—Psychiatric and cognitive conditions

- Acute mental health concerns
- Chronic mental health concerns
- Cognitive functioning
- Trauma-related needs
- Psychiatric history

Dimension 4—Substance use–related risks

- Risky behaviors (including recent patterns of use and other behaviors that pose risks to self or others)
- Ability to cope with stressors, cues, and cravings
- Social and interpersonal skills
- Skills of daily living
- Patient perceptions of drug use and addiction

Dimension 5—Recovery environment

- Social support system and related risks
- Daily structure (work, school, etc.)
- Safety in current environment (interpersonal violence risk)
- Current/likely exposure to cues/triggers/stressors in daily environment
- Access to substances
- Cultural perceptions of drug use and addiction

Dimension 6—Readiness and resources

- Internal motivation to address substance use concerns
- Internal motivation to address mental health concerns
- Internal motivation to address physical health concerns
- Internal motivation to address life concerns
- Barriers to accessing care including:
  - Responsibilities for care of others (children, elders, etc.)
  - Employment or educational responsibilities
  - Transportation
  - Criminal justice–related restrictions
- Underlying social and structural determinants of health that impact recovery
  - Housing stability
  - Food insecurity
  - Poverty
- External motivators for treatment participation
  - Social encouragement
  - Drug court participation and other criminal-legal–related motivators
  - Involvement in community-based services (eg, child protective services)
  - Other incentives
- "Hope" or "belief" that treatment can make a difference
- "Hope" or "belief" that they deserve to be healthy

UNDERSTANDING *THE ASAM CRITERIA*

Principles Guiding the Criteria

Individualized Treatment Plan

The ASAM Criteria promote patient-centered care[14] in which each patient's treatment plan prioritizes their problems according to:

- Severity (such as obstacles to recovery, knowledge or skill deficits, dysfunction, or loss)
- Strengths (such as peer refusal skills, social supports, and a source of spiritual support)
- Individualized needs (including gender, age, race, ethnicity, culture, marital status, reproductive history, and level of understanding)
- Goals (realistic, achievable, short-term resolution of problems or attainment of positive outcomes)
- Objectives, methods or strategies (what the patient will do, the treatment services to be provided, the site of those services, the staff responsible for delivering treatment)
- A timetable for follow-through with the treatment plan that promotes accountability[7]

Choice of Treatment Levels

For both clinical and financial reasons, the preferred LOC is *the least intensive level that meets treatment objectives while providing safety and security* for the patient. Moreover, while the LOCs are presented as discrete levels, in reality, they represent benchmarks or points along a continuum of treatment services that could be used in a variety of ways, depending on a patient's needs and response. Particular consideration is given to special populations, including older adults, individuals receiving treatment concurrently with their children, persons in safety-sensitive occupations, and persons in criminal justice settings.

Patients could begin at a more intensive level and move to a more or less intensive LOC, depending on their individual needs and progress. For patients with a history of recurrence, the current LOC and LOS should be chosen based on an assessment of the patient's history and current functioning, rather than automatic placement in a more intensive LOC and fixed LOS. Such "placement-by-policy" assumes that recurrence of use after treatment indicates that the previous LOC was of insufficient intensity. In fact, poorly matched services may have been the problem, for example, recovery and recurrence prevention services for a patient at an early stage of change who does not acknowledge that substance use is a problem.[7,15]

Continuum of Care

A continuum of care provides the most clinically appropriate and cost-effective treatment system, whether via a single provider or multiple providers. Clinical offerings need to reflect the diversity of patients with needs in multiple clinical and functional dimensions. An effective continuum is distinguished by three characteristics: (a) seamless transfer between LOCs, (b) philosophical congruence among the various providers of care, and (c) timely arrival of the patient's clinical record at the next provider. In the best systems, providers envision admitting the patient into the continuum through their program versus admitting the patient *to* their program.

Many providers offer only one LOC. This necessitates referring the patient out of the provider's own network of care. This may be impossible, unfortunately, due to lack of reimbursement for or lack of availability of other LOCs. For states and counties, an effective continuum of care necessitates that licensing, contracting, and reimbursement for services establish equity in supporting the diversity of communities—based on public health needs. This necessitates good access to care—both in geographic proximity and payer network adequacy. This includes correcting access disparities based on stigma, inadequate funding, racism, criminalization, and other inequities.[16]

Progress Through the Levels of Care

Each program, at a given LOC, needs to continually assess patients in all six dimensions. Residual issues or new problems may require services that can be effectively provided at the same LOC or that require a more or less intensive LOC. This avoids a fixed LOS, which is not individualized and may be less effective for patients.[17]

When patients fail to improve or worsen, changes in the LOC or program should be based on a multidimensional reassessment of the treatment plan, including consideration of transfer to another LOC or different treatment.[7]

Should a patient use alcohol or other drugs during treatment, automatically changing the LOC or administrative discharge represents program-driven treatment—not assessment-driven or outcome-driven treatment. Some benefit managers require that a patient be "motivated for sobriety" as a requirement for admission to a program. A *sine qua non* of SUD, however, is ambivalence. Given the disease's direct impairment of self-awareness and healthy volition, the rational requirement should be the lower threshold willingness to enter treatment—not the more restrictive motivation for sobriety. It is the role of treatment to facilitate the patient's progress along the stages of change via motivational enhancement strategies.

Clinical Versus Reimbursement Considerations

The ASAM Criteria describe a wide range of levels and types of care. To achieve this, payers and treatment systems must address the challenges posed by social determinants of health (SDOH), including both staffing and patient population issues of diversity, equity, and inclusion. If the criteria only covered the LOCs commonly reimbursable by private insurance carriers, they would tacitly endorse inappropriate care by limiting recommendations for the complete continuum of care. Systems including Los Angeles County[18] and Arizona[19] have found it necessary to issue crosswalk guides that indicate, for a given

ASAM Criteria LOC, what type of service in their particular locality corresponds most closely—while working toward implementation of the full ASAM CONTINUUM over time.

"Treatment Failure"

Two incorrect assumptions are associated with the concept of "treatment failure." The first is that the disorder is acute rather than chronic, so that the only criterion for success is total and complete cure and elimination of the problem. Such expectations are recognized as inappropriate in the treatment of other chronic disorders, such as diabetes, asthma, or hypertension. By applying the same understanding of chronicity to the treatment of addiction, progress is manifested when recurrences are less intensive, severe, frequent, and shorter in duration.

The second assumption is that responsibility for treatment "failure" always rests with the patient (as in, "the patient was not ready"). Poor treatment outcomes also may be related to a provider's failure to provide evidence-based services tailored to the patient's needs.

Finally, some benefit managers require that a patient "fail-first" at one LOC as a prerequisite for approving admission to a more intensive LOC (eg, "failure" in outpatient treatment as a prerequisite for admission to inpatient treatment). Such a strategy threatens patient safety. It delays care at a more appropriate level of treatment and potentially increases health care costs, given the natural tendency of the disease of addiction to progress.

ASSESSMENT DIMENSIONS

The ASAM Criteria identify six assessment areas (dimensions) as the most important in formulating an individualized treatment plan and in making subsequent patient placement decisions. **Table 47-1** outlines the six dimensions and the assessment and treatment planning focus of each dimension.

With increased focus on recovery and strength-based, person-centered assessments and services, a multidimensional assessment should address not only a patient's needs, obstacles, and liabilities but also their strengths, skills, resources, and supports to promote recovery. For example, in assessing a patient's substance use–related risks (Dimension 4), the focus should not restrict the inquiry to cravings, peer refusal skill problems, recurrence triggers, or other impulses but also to the identification of any periods of sobriety or mental health wellness and what skills and resources produced a good outcome. Even if these were for relatively short periods of time, assessment of how the patient changed attitudes, knowledge, skills, or behavior to achieve success identifies strategies that can be included in the individualized service plan.

Similarly, if a person has been suicidal before but has never needed hospitalization or medical care for serious cutting or overdose behavior, this may suggest a level of impulse control that can be harnessed in the psychiatric and cognitive conditions (Dimension 3) part of the treatment plan. Or if a patient is homeless but has one family member who is still invested in the patient's well-being, that family member is a recovery support (Dimension 5) who should be involved in the patient's treatment.

The dimensional assessment should also help to "drive" the determination of the LOC. With the updates to the LOCs in the fourth edition, we can quickly identify the primary focus of care (medical, psychotherapy, psychoedication, or recovery supports) needed to help stabilize a person in acute distress. Identifying these dimensional drivers can also help to narrow the focus of treatment to those behaviors or situations most relevant to the patient's needs.

TABLE 47-1 The ASAM Criteria Assessment Dimensions

Assessment dimensions	Treatment planning focus
1. Acute intoxication and/or withdrawal potential, need for medication initiation	Withdrawal management in a variety of Levels of Care and preparation for continued addiction services Initiation of medications for persons with substance use disorders with FDA-approved medications
2. Biomedical conditions and complications	Treatment provided within the level of care or through coordination with physical health services
3. Psychiatric and cognitive conditions	Treatment provided within the level of care or through coordination of mental health services for subdiagnostic, diagnosed, or unstable conditions or complications
4. Substance use–related risks	Identify previous periods of sobriety or wellness and what worked to achieve this. If still at early stages of change, focus on raising consciousness of consequences of continued use or continued problems as part of motivational enhancement strategies
5. Recovery environment	Assess the need for specific individualized family or significant other, housing, financial, vocational, educational, legal, transportation, and childcare services. Identify any supports and assets in any or all of the areas
6. Patient-centered considerations	Evaluates patient's social determinants of health (SDOH) needs and barriers to care as well as where they sit on the trans-theoretical model of change. If not ready and able to commit to full recovery, engage in treatment using motivational enhancement strategies. If ready for recovery, consolidate and expand action for change.

A simple example of this would be a person who needs treatment for acute alcohol withdrawal (Dimension 1) and has diabetes (Dimension 2). This person would need medically managed care to meet their needs. As we will see in the following section, this need corresponds to specific LOCs and staffing models that best fit the patient's treatment needs.

Interactions Across Dimensions in Assessing for Level of Care

While *The ASAM Criteria* recommends assessing individuals in each dimension independently, a fundamental strength of the system is how it takes into account interactions across dimensions. Such interaction is explained in "Determining Dimensional Interaction and Priorities".[7]

For example, a patient's significant problems with readiness and resources (Dimension 6), moderate problems with substance use–related risks (Dimension 4), and poor recovery environment (Dimension 5) may interact to pose a considerable risk of an acute exacerbation of addiction.

Another common interaction involves problems in Dimension 2 (such as chronic pain that drives opioid craving or rationalization of use) coupled with problems in Dimension 1, 4, 5, or 6.

The converse also is true. For example, problems with potential substance use–related risks (Dimension 4) may be offset by low barriers to care (Dimension 6) or a very supportive recovery environment (Dimension 5). The interaction of these factors may result in a lower level of severity than in any dimension alone.[7]

The lesson here is that assessments are most accurate when they consider all of the factors (Dimensions) that affect each individual's receptivity and ability to engage in treatment at each particular time point in the trajectory of illness and recovery.

Continued Service and Transfer/Discharge Criteria

The ASAM Criteria, since the first edition in 1991, have consistently indicated that the duration of treatment must vary with the severity of illness and the individual's response to treatment. Thus, fixed LOS programs are inconsistent with individualized, person-centered, and outcome-driven treatment. Patients, especially individuals, mandated to treatment, in fixed LOS programs often focus more on "doing time" rather than "doing treatment." The ASAM Criteria does not support this approach to care.

The assessment process for continued service or transfer/discharge is the same as for admission, with the reassessment of multidimensional severity determining the treatment priorities, the intensity of needed services, and the decision about the ongoing LOC. Decisions concerning continued service, transfer, or discharge involve a review of the treatment plan and assessing the patient's progress. That is, they require the same multidimensional assessment process that led to admission to the current LOC. Using the concept of the dimensional driver will make this reassessment more efficient and easier to translate to payers and state agencies.

The ASAM Criteria and State Licensure or Certification

The ASAM Criteria specify the characteristics of treatment programs at each LOC. These specifications include (1) the setting, (2) staffing, (3) support systems, (4) therapies, (5) assessments, and the (6) documentation and treatment plan reviews typically found at that level. This information should be useful to referrers, providers, and payers. The descriptions are not intended to replace or supersede the relevant statutes or licensure requirements of any state. They are, however, increasingly becoming standards for certification under a collaborative program between ASAM and the Commission on Accreditation of Rehabilitation Facilities (CARF).[20-22]

LEVELS OF CARE

The ASAM Criteria fourth edition conceptualizes treatment as a continuum marked by five basic LOCs, which are numbered from levels 0.5 through level 4, as listed in **Table 47-2**. This provides the addiction field with a standard nomenclature for describing the continuum of addiction services. Within each level, *The ASAM Criteria* employs decimal numbers comprised of 0.1, 0.5, and 0.7 to express the focus of care (medical, psychotherapy, psychoeducation, and recovery supports) within the LOCs. This structure allows improved precision of, description about, and better interrater reliability. For example, a 2.1 LOC provides a benchmark for intensive care (the 2.) that is focused on psychoeducation (the .1). For the fourth edition, we have "rolled" withdrawal management and biomedically enhanced treatment services (BIO) into the .7s (1.7, 2.7, 3.7), which will improve the consistency and predictability of the addiction treatment system. Only level 3.7 has the addition of "BIO" to distinguish programs that have the ability to provide IV medications.

Objectivity

The ASAM Criteria have increasingly sought to be as objective, measurable, and quantifiable as possible. Certain aspects of the criteria require subjective interpretation. In this regard, the assessment and treatment of substance-related and addiction disorders are no different from biomedical or psychiatric conditions in which diagnosis or assessment and treatment are a mix of objectively measured criteria and experientially based professional judgments.

Co-occurring Disorders

Clinical reality, such as seen with the opioid epidemic, suggests that programs and practitioners must be able to meet the needs

TABLE 47-2 The ASAM Criteria Levels of Care

ASAM criteria levels of care	Level	Same levels of care for adolescents except level 3.3
Early intervention	NA	Assessment and education for at-risk individuals who do not meet diagnostic criteria for substance-related disorder
Long-term recovery support	1	<9 hours of service/week (adults); <6 hours/week (adolescents) for recovery or motivational enhancement therapies/strategies
Low-intensity clinically managed care	1.5	Low-intensity delivery of psychotherapy and psychoeducation as needed for generally stable patients with mild- to low-moderate disease
Low intensity medically managed care	1.7	Low-intensity delivery of medical care with on-site or formally coordinated psychotherapy and psychoeducation as needed for generally stable patients with mild- to low-moderate disease. This level includes low-intensity withdrawal management
Intensive outpatient	2.1	9 or more hours of service per week (adults); 6 or more hours per week (adolescents) in a structured program to treat multidimensional instability with a focus on psychoeducation
High-intensity outpatient	2.5	20 or more hours of service per week in a structured program for multidimensional instability not requiring 24-hour care, with a focus on psychotherapy
Medically managed intensive outpatient	2.7	High-intensity delivery of medical care with on-site psychotherapy and psychoeducation as needed for patients with moderate to severe disease. This level also incorporates withdrawal management. This level would include opioid treatment programs (OTP)
Clinically managed low-intensity residential	3.1	24-hour structure with available trained personnel with emphasis on re-entry to the community; at least 9 hours of clinical service per week with a focus on psychoeducation
Clinically managed high-intensity residential	3.5	24-hour care with trained therapists and counselors to stabilize multidimensional imminent risks of relapse or danger and prepare for outpatient treatment. Able to tolerate and use a full active milieu or therapeutic community. This level has a focus on psychotherapy
Medically managed residential	3.7 and 3.7 BIO	24-hour nursing care with physician availability for significant problems in Dimensions 1, 2, or 3. This includes nursing care, continued care of stable medical issues (IV medications and wound vac management are 3.7 BIO)
Medically managed intensive inpatient	4	This is a hospital level of care with 24-hour nursing care and daily physician care for severe, unstable problems in Dimensions 1, 2, or 3. Counseling available to engage the patient in treatment

ASAM, American Society of Addiction Medicine Criteria.

of people with co-occurring and complex disorders, such as pain, either directly or through referral or consultation. Other population health realities include the expansion of SUD and substance-induced disorders in younger populations; greater sensitivity to substance use and addiction problems in the mental health, welfare, and criminal justice systems; greater awareness of the role of trauma in addiction; and increased commitment to earlier intervention in addiction in preference to fragmented services and incarceration. A greater understanding of the uses and effects of psychosocial and cognitive-behavioral strategies also have heightened awareness of a broadened range of modalities to meet individual needs.

The ASAM Criteria fourth edition, therefore, also addresses the needs of populations that present for treatment with co-occurring SUDs and co-occurring mental disorders. As compared to the third edition, the fourth edition integrates co-occurring capable care into all levels, while defining parallel levels of co-occurring enhanced (COE) care. **Table 47-3** summarizes what kinds of patients with co-occurring mental and substance-related disorders are best treated in COE services. Two cases that represent the approach to a basic ASAM Criteria evaluation and LOC placement are provided in **Table 47-4**.

Assessment of Imminent Danger

In *The ASAM Criteria*, residential treatment is reserved for the stabilization of patients who have a strong probability, in the very near future, that certain behaviors, such as continued use will occur, and for whom such behaviors will present a significant risk of adverse consequences to the individual and/or others.[7] Risks of adverse consequences may include imminent physical or medical dangers but are not limited to these. Alternatively, they may include dangers such as emotional or sexual abuse, neglect, or likely criminal activity and rearrest; inability to care for or loss of custody of dependents; psychiatric deterioration; or simply a high likelihood of current- or near-term (ie, within hours or the next days) relapse with

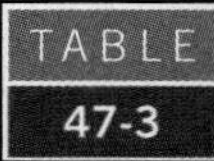

TABLE 47-3 Matching Patients With Co-occurring Disorders to Services

Characteristics of co-occurring disorders	
Patients	**Services**
Patients with Co-occurring mental health problems of *mild to moderate* severity: Individuals who exhibit (a) *subthreshold* diagnostic (ie, traits, symptoms) mental disorders (b) diagnosable but *stable* mental disorders (ie, bipolar disorder but adherent with and stable on lithium)	**Co-occurring Capable (COC) Services that are *now incorporated into all levels of care*:** Primary focus on substance use disorder (SUD) but capable of treating patients with subthreshold or diagnosable but stable mental disorders. Psychiatric services are available on-site or by consultation; at least some staff are competent to understand and identify signs and symptoms of acute psychiatric conditions.
Patients with co-occurring mental health problems of *moderate to high* severity: Individuals who exhibit moderate to severe diagnosable mental disorders, who are *not stable* and require mental health as well as addiction treatment	**Co-occurring Enhanced (COE) Services**: Psychiatric services available on-site or closely coordinated; all staff are cross-trained in SUD and mental health and are competent to understand and identify signs and symptoms of acute psychiatric conditions and treat mental health problems along with the SUDs. Treatment for both mental health and SUD is integrated.

TABLE 47-4 Application of *The ASAM Criteria* to Clinical Presentations

Use of *The ASAM Criteria* involves (1) six-dimensional assessment, (2) determining needs and strengths, (3) with integration of the interactions between the Dimensions, (4) determining needed services, (5) using *The ASAM Criteria* Decision Rules to select the recommended Level(s) of Care, (6) using these data to construct the treatment plan, and (7) ongoing reassessment. The following vignettes illustrate some key issues in this process.

Case 1: Mr. A

Mr. A is a 58-year-old male who meets diagnostic criteria for "Alcohol Use Disorder, Moderate." In Dimension 1, he is currently in mild withdrawal from alcohol (Clinical Institute Withdrawal Assessment for Alcohol, Revised, CIWA-Ar score of 7) with a history of no more than moderate-severity withdrawal. However, he stopped drinking only 2 hours ago. Mr. A is hypertensive by history and not well controlled with medication even when sober, and his current blood pressure is 140/100. Severity in Dimensions 3 through 6 is low.

Initial Response: Based on only mild withdrawal severity in Dimension 1, Mr. A might be referred for Level 1.7, low-intensity medically managed care. For his Dimension 2 problem, he might be referred back to his primary care provider for a review of his hypertension or evaluated by the program provider.

Discussion: Given that Mr. A is withdrawing from alcohol, a sedative drug, the resultant autonomic arousal will create an increase in blood pressure. His current blood pressure reading is only 2 hours since his last drink, and insufficient time has elapsed for the full withdrawal syndrome to develop. It can be assumed, therefore, that the autonomic arousal could markedly increase his blood pressure, and because his baseline blood pressure is already elevated, the interaction between Dimensions 1 and 2 increases his overall severity.

Recommendation, Based on the ASAM Criteria Decision Rules:
Dimension 1 and Dimension 2 interact to pose a high severity for Mr. A.
Best Recommendation: L3.7—Medically Managed Residential Service.
Also Consider: L2.7 Ambulatory Withdrawal Management with Extended On-Site Monitoring—if Mr. A enters treatment early in the week and could be observed for a number of days OR if the 2.7 service operates 7 days a week.

Case 2: Ms. P

An 18-year-old girl is brought to the emergency department (ED) after an argument with her parents and throwing a chair. Her parents suspect drug intoxication is the cause. They report that she has been staying out unusually late at night and mixing with "the wrong crowd." They describe much family discord, anger, and frustration, particularly directed by the young woman toward her father. Ms. P has no history of psychiatric or addiction treatment.

Ms. P was brought in by the police after her mother called for help. An ED physician and a nurse from the psychiatric unit agree that Ms. P needs to be hospitalized in view of the animosity at home, her violent behavior, and the possibility that she is using an unknown drug.

Following the ASAM assessment dimensions, they organize the clinical information as follows:

Dimension 1: Acute Intoxication and/or Withdrawal Potential: Although she was intoxicated when she threw the chair, Ms. P no longer is intoxicated and has not been using alcohol or other drugs in sufficient quantities or duration to suggest the possibility of a withdrawal syndrome.

Dimension 2: Biomedical Conditions and Complications: Ms. P is not taking any medications, is physically healthy, and has no current complaints.

(Continued)

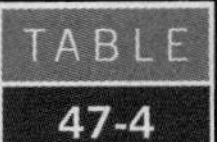

TABLE 47-4 Application of *The ASAM Criteria* to Clinical Presentations (*Continued*)

Dimension 3: Emotional, Behavioral, or Cognitive Conditions and Complications: Ms. P has complex problems with anger management, as evidenced by the chair-throwing incident, but is not impulsive at present if separated from her parents, especially her father.

Dimension 4: Relapse, Continued Use, or Continued Problem Potential: The team perceives an imminent risk of return to drug use if released. They believe that, if she returns home immediately, fighting and possibly violence may reoccur.

Dimension 5: Recovery Environment: Ms. P's parents are frustrated, angry, mistrustful of their daughter, and want her hospitalized.

Dimension 6: Readiness and Resources: Ms. P is willing to talk to a therapist, blames her parents for being overbearing and not trusting her, and agrees to come into treatment but does not want to be at home with her father. No barriers otherwise.

Initial Response: Based on Ms. P's recent history of violent acting out, the ED physician and the psychiatric nurse recommend admission to the L4 inpatient psychiatric unit, at least for the night.

Discussion: Ms. P's acting out occurred when she was intoxicated, which she no longer is. The major conflict appears to be a family issue, particularly between Ms. P and her father. Nothing indicates that Ms. P suffers from a diagnosable substance use disorder. Her conflict with her parents may reflect normal adolescent struggles rather than psychopathology.

To adwwdress this, outpatient family counseling should be considered. In crisis or mandated treatment situations, clinicians often come under pressure from family or referral agencies to provide a certain level of care. But when the essential information is organized according to the ASAM dimensions, the patient's real severity and needs are more easily identified. This leads to a more appropriate clinical plan and avoids wasteful use of resources by focusing on the services needed to meet the patient's individual needs.

Recommendation, Based on the ASAM Criteria Decision Rules:

Dimension 1, Dimension 2, or Dimension 3: There are no signs of severe withdrawal, biomedical, or emotional problems, respectively, that call for L4 Medically Managed Intensive Inpatient Services.

Dimension 5, Dimension 6: There is no evidence of a moderate or severe SUD and anticipated imminent risk of consequential substance use or problem that requires the resources of L3 Clinically Managed Residential Services (or L2.1 Intensive Outpatient Treatment or L2.5 Partial Hospitalization).

Recommendation: L1.5 Clinically Managed Outpatient Care, with separation of Ms. P from her father, eg, by arranging for Ms. P to stay with a relative or family friend overnight or by having Ms. P and her mother stay at a motel for the night or her father to do so.

resulting implausibility of maintaining recovery effort. Any of these examples constitute a basis for imminent danger and need for residential care per *The ASAM Criteria*. Risk assessment for imminent danger has been incorporated into the "rules" that govern the LOC recommendation, thus eliminating the need for separate evaluations.

Mandated Level of Care or Length of Service

A fixed LOS in a treatment center, even if mandated or court-ordered, is not based on clinical considerations and thus is inconsistent with *The ASAM Criteria*. In such a case, the provider should attempt to have the order amended to reflect the assessed clinical level or length of service.

Suppose the court order or other mandate cannot be amended. In that case, staff should note in the record the patient's readiness for discharge or transfer and the staff's attempts to implement a clinically appropriate placement, and the treatment plan should be updated.

Logistical Impediments

Dimension 6 was specifically designed to evaluate not only readiness to change but most of the SDOH factors that impact persons with SUDs and addictions. When logistical considerations impede the indicated services (eg, lack of transportation), an outpatient service combined with unsupervised/minimally supervised housing may be a necessary compromise. In cities or towns, such a domiciliary option might be found in a group living situation (such as a Salvation Army program, motel accommodations, YMCA/YWCA, or mission). In rural and other underserved areas, options could include (a) the creation of a supervised housing situation by using unused treatment beds, (b) assertive community treatment models in which the treatment is brought to rural areas (such as Native American settlements) and provided in weekend intensive models at sites such as community centers and churches, (c) van or approved ride-share transport, and (d) using van- or motor home-based traveling offices.

The Need for a Safe Recovery Environment

When a patient lives in an environment that is so toxic as to preclude recovery efforts (as through victimization or exposure to a person with active substance use), and a Level 1 or 2 outpatient service is indicated, the patient may need placement in a recovery residency LOC or need a referral to a safe place to live while in treatment, as well as to treatment itself (eg, combining a women's shelter with a Level 2.1 or 2.5 treatment program).

Gathering Data to Improve Systems of Care

There are no ideal systems of care that have seamless LOCs and where all policy, licensure, and funding obstacles have

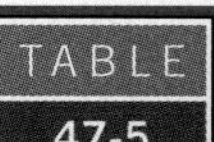

TABLE 47-5 Data Gathering on Discrepancy Between Needed and Available Services: Placement Summary

Data Gathering on Discrepancy Between Needed and Available Services: Placement Summary
Level of Care/Service Indicated: Insert the ASAM Level number that offers the most appropriate level of care/service that can provide the service intensity needed to address the client's current functioning/severity and/or the service needed (eg, shelter, housing, vocational training, transportation, language interpreter).
Level of Care/Service Received: ASAM Level number—If the most appropriate level or service is not utilized, insert the most appropriate placement or service available and circle the reason for difference between indicated and received level or service and the anticipated outcome if service cannot be provided.
Reason for Difference: Circle only one number—1. Service not available. 2. Provider judgment. 3. Client preference. 4. Client is on waiting list for appropriate level. 5. Service available, but no payment source. 6. Geographic accessibility. 7. Family responsibility. 8. Language. 9. Not applicable. 10. Not listed (specify).
Anticipated Outcome If Service Cannot Be Provided: Circle only one number—1. Admitted to acute care setting. 2. Discharged to street. 3. Continued stay in acute care facility. 4. Incarcerated. 5. Client will dropout until next crisis. 6. Not listed (specify).

From Mee-Lee D, Shulman GD, Fishman MJ, et al., eds. *The ASAM Criteria: Treatment Criteria for Addictive, Substance-Related, and Co-Occurring Conditions*. 3rd ed. The Change Companies; 2013:126.

been removed. If an appropriately matched LOC is unavailable, it is imperative for programs to drive systems change. This can be done by noting the date and patient's name and case number, the clinically indicated LOC or service and the LOC or service actually received, and the reason(s) for the discrepancy and any consequences of the mismatch. These data can identify the greatest gaps in services and prioritize where resources need to be concentrated to improve the system of care (Table 47-5).

RESEARCH ON *THE ASAM CRITERIA*

The ASAM Criteria are the most intensively studied set of addiction placement criteria. Scientists began the crucial process of testing *The ASAM Criteria* in the early 1990s through an international collaboration of data gathering, quantitative analysis, and empirical feedback.[23]

In the intervening three decades, dozens of reports published in the peer-reviewed literature have been supported by over $10 million of U.S. government funding. Project funding came from the National Institute on Drug Abuse and the National Institute on Alcohol Abuse and Alcoholism and SAMHSA's Center for Substance Abuse Treatment.[23] Consultation or training projects were funded by Aetna Behavioral Health, Harvard Business School,[24] the Oklahoma Department of Mental Health and Substance Abuse Services, and the U.S. Veterans Administration. Additional studies were subsequently supported by the federal governments of Belgium[25] and Norway[26-28] and the criteria have influenced placement criteria as far away as Korea.[29] Research training fellowships have been funded by the World Health Organization and Israel, and scientific review conferences have been conducted in Iceland and Switzerland.

Research confirms that patients who undergo ASAM-based assessments are more likely to be evaluated for their withdrawal symptoms, substance use, psychiatric history, and recurrence of use and recovery environment.[30] Patient centeredness is also supported by the approach, which presents patient with treatment options and their rationale. As a result, patients have reported feeling that the interviewer "wanted to learn about my situation," "asked good questions to understand my needs," "showed respect for what I had to say," and "discussed what they learned about my addiction."[30]

A considerable body of outcome research exists to date on *The ASAM Criteria*. By 2011, there were at least 10 evaluations involving a total of 3,672 adult subjects.[24] The smallest of these, a matched-sample pilot ($N = 16$) found that, in veterans experiencing homelessness, patients who received services according to *The ASAM Criteria* recommendations "improved considerably," whereas those receiving a housing-first intervention "deteriorated rapidly" with events including "readdiction, lost housing, new substance-related medical diagnoses, loss of intimate partners, hospitalization, detoxification, felony offenses and/or incarceration in prison, leaving the state, suicide attempt, and death" occurring only in the former group.[31] Larger studies included patients with a variety of SUDs and have examined a variety of time periods, including immediate dropout, 1 month, 3 months, and 1 year. A large naturalistic study ($N = 14,676$) in Milwaukee County found that *The ASAM Criteria* showed good ability to distinguish between patients with versus without psychiatric disorders and between degrees of psychiatric severity, yielding a sensitivity of .89 and specificity of .44 (AUC = .73). The authors concluded that *The ASAM Criteria* had "the clinical dexterity to assist in identifying and placing individuals with co-occurring SUDs to the appropriate level of dual diagnosis care."[32] Controlled studies have found that when treatment was matched according to *The ASAM Criteria* versus ASI-based and clinician-based placement approaches, patients have experienced a variety of superior outcomes, including better initial engagement, better retention, reduced substance use, less morbidity, better client functioning, and more efficient service utilization than mismatched treatment.[12,23,25,28,33-38] Furthermore, *The ASAM Criteria* have proven to be patient-centered; California Medicaid beneficiaries (N = 851) across 10 counties reported greater satisfaction with their treatment when *The ASAM Criteria* were used.[30]

Attention is also being directed toward the use of the criteria with adolescents,[39] which appear to be the most widely used treatment planning approach for highly rated adolescent treatment programs.[40] Adolescents were studied in a pilot comparing two matched adolescent residential (Level 3) programs; better clinical outcomes were found in the program that used regular patient assessment and treatment plan adjustment according to the ASAM dimensions.[37]

A large evaluation naturalistically compared two different automated ASAM-related software approaches, based on an enhanced ASI.[34] Patients first completed an intake ASI (N = 2,429) in 78 addiction treatment programs in Arkansas, New Hampshire, Rhode Island, and Utah. Then, they were naturalistically assigned to a LOC based on availability and clinical considerations. Two placement recommendations were independently calculated: using either ASI summary scores or an algorithm approximating *The ASAM Criteria*. Both structured approaches showed evidence of predictive validity. Patients who were undertreated, meaning that they were actually placed in a LOC less intense than recommended according to the matching calculations, had consistently worse treatment completion and self-reported abstinence.

The largest evaluation (N = 407,792 treatment episodes) examined California Medicaid beneficiaries in SUD treatment, using a comparative interrupted time series analysis. This naturalistic study compared counties that were using (nonsoftware) ASAM-based assessments versus counties that used non-ASAM approaches. In residential placements, ASAM approaches showed a 9% increase in 30-day retention. Outpatient placements showed similar magnitudes of outcome coefficients, although not reaching significance. The authors concluded that the results "may be encouraging to the many state Medicaid programs that are adopting ASAM-based criteria."[12]

These studies indicate that *The ASAM Criteria* achieve good feasibility and reliability through standardized computerized structured interviewing and good concurrent validity with other validated assessments.[41] Undertreatment has been found to be clinically adverse in multiple studies.[27,35,36,42] Overtreatment causes unnecessary and expensive treatment[27,38,43] which can be dramatic (eg, a day in Level 4 may equal a week or weeks in Levels 2.7 or 1.7). In one study of 281 patients, the majority (59%) was overtreated (placed in a LOC more intensive than indicated by ASAM Criteria), and the reason for 93% of these was because Medicaid covered residential care.[43]

Two controlled studies found that overtreatment is not simply a financial waste—it can also be associated with adverse clinical outcomes.[27,38] Overall, it is important for systems to detect, report, and overcome the reasons for such mismatches, which can include issues of patient choice, payer rejection, and limited access. When clinicians use the standardized software application of *The ASAM Criteria*, CONTINUUM, the software systematically gathers the incidence of and various causes of discrepant treatment, permitting research, evaluation, and data-driven system improvement.

THE ASAM CRITERIA STANDARD IMPLEMENTATION, ASAM CONTINUUM

With widespread training, *The ASAM Criteria* raised providers' consciousness of the need for multidimensional assessment but did not necessarily achieve widespread practice.[7] There were many challenges to adoption, for example, diverse training levels, service fragmentation, and high rates of staff turnover. These challenges led to the search for technology that could advance *The ASAM Criteria* empirically. States and counties were developing ASAM-based assessment tools, but these either failed to properly implement *The ASAM Criteria* or lacked reliability and/or validity.[44]

Evaluators also found that, despite trainings, providers and managed care organizations tended to showed poor fidelity in using *The ASAM Criteria*. Even the textbook's Risk Assessment Matrix Format is misunderstood and misused, undermining fidelity. Provided only as a simplified instructional tool, the Risk Ratings are conceptual and lack any reliability or validity. Proper use of *The ASAM Criteria* requires users to read and apply the decision rules, which use precise definitions, operationalize functional patient characteristics, and concretely specify how to combine the patient's needs and strengths across the dimensions (**Table 47-4**).

States found that providers were used to really almost no criteria, so rather than attempting to secure fidelity, stakeholders compromised adoption goals to merely developing a "cultural understanding about substance use disorder as a chronic illness…"[45] As a result, despite the face validity of *The ASAM Criteria*, research using partial or abbreviated attempts to implement its dimensions or decision rules were met with only mixed success in formal validity testing.[34,46,47] Clearly, the field needed a more comprehensive, reliable standard solution.

By the late 1990s, a comprehensive computerized research tool emerged, with funding from NIH-NIDA. The structured interview and decision analysis algorithm operationalized all 266 discrete decision rules in the adult admission criteria of PPC-1. Constructed by Gastfriend et al. at Massachusetts General Hospital, it demonstrated feasibility for comprehensively standardizing *The ASAM Criteria*[48] with good inter-rater reliability (ie, intraclass correlation coefficient = 0.77; $P < 0.01$).[49] This compared favorably with DSM diagnosis and severity ratings, despite measuring a more complex construct.[50] This tool proved to be an important contributor to validity, as subsequently noted in a series of reports.[25,27,36,38,42,43,48,49,51,52]

Based on the success of the research tool, ASAM authorized the creation of a new, end-user software product to serve as the authorized, standard implementation of *The ASAM Criteria*. After translation into Norwegian and use in 10 treatment programs across Norway over 3 years, this software showed good convergent and predictive validity and also received high satisfaction ratings from both patients and counselors.[26-28] In Uzbekistan, translated into both Uzbek and Russian, use of the PPC-2R software reportedly increased individualization of placements compared with the mandated treatment that was not based on an individualized assessment.[53] Using Dutch and French translations, 201 Belgian patients who received matched or a more intensive LOC had significantly better 30-day global outcomes than patients who were undermatched.[25]

This software, which became known as ASAM CONTINUUM, incorporated the changes of The ASAM Criteria third edition.[7] The structured interview incorporated the ASI, which supports the predictive validity of the system,[34] the Clinical Institute Withdrawal Assessment[54] and the Clinical Institute Narcotic Assessment[55] instruments. The tool used an intricate, asymmetric, branched-tree algebraic algorithm to generate a formal DSM-5 SUD diagnosis,[56] withdrawal scores, a summary report suitable for submission to managed care review, a comprehensive biopsychosocial evaluation report, recommended LOC determination(s), and a formal problem list.

SAMHSA and ASAM's technology partners supported the updating of the software with nearly a million dollars of investment to prepare the software for integration into electronic health records for the Health Information Technology Act, the federal Parity Act, healthcare reform, and new rules allowing states flexible waivers to create new payment models for Medicaid.

This new software, for the first time, allowed both SUD clinicians and researchers to speak the same language and arrive at the same LOC determinations. The software included confidential data uploads to an ASAM-authorized database, which facilitated aggregate analyses of patient placements, service utilization, and clinical outcomes. This database has two simultaneous benefits for the field. It will permit treatment programs to understand their utilization patterns and needs. At the same time, the data are beginning to offer researchers a precise, objective look at the validity of *The ASAM Criteria* and empirical guidance on how to improve it.

In 2014, 20 addiction treatment systems across the United States used CONTINUUM in a 6-month National Demonstration Project.[57] The largest pilot was conducted by Los Angeles County, with independent evaluation by UCLA researchers. They highlighted the importance of training and reported that the learning curve for efficient interviewing with CONTINUUM was 18 interviews, at which point the average duration of assessment was 60 minutes.[58] This project reported good adoption by participating programs, acceptance by intake clinicians, and satisfaction among patients. Provider response indicated that the software provided "direction beyond what might be just our gut instinct ... the tool has been easy to use. Intake is a bit longer on the front end ... But it saves time ... during assessment and continuous assessment."[59]

CONTINUUM subsequently underwent commercial release throughout the United States, with large initial pilots by county and state systems, informed by the Coalition for National Clinical Criteria, which includes major provider, professional, and government agencies and organizations.

CONTINUUM's growth in adoption led to the commissioning of two derivative tools. Los Angeles County called for a 10-minute telephone or inperson brief provisional assessment, CO-Triage. California's Department of Corrections and Rehabilitation requested the RISE (Re-entry Interview Script Enhancement) for its 30 state prisons, to assess patients in controlled environments just prior to or upon re-entry. In California's prisons, residents (N = 38,638) underwent initial assessments and/or re-entry evaluations, with the findings used to determine eligibility for medication for opioid use disorder (MOUD), housing, and other services. The state reported that overdose deaths dropped 58% over the 2 years after the program began and hospitalizations were 48% lower, among residents receiving MOUD (vs wait-list residents), results that occurred even in the challenging context of the COVID-19 pandemic.[60]

By mid-2022, ASAM reported that these tools had been adopted county-wide or state-wide for routine assessment in publicly funded treatment and correctional systems in 8 states (AK, AZ, CA, DC, FL, MI, NH, and WV). Other private and public systems had also adopted these tools in 12 other states (CO, KY, MD, ME, MT, NC, OH, PA, TN, UT, VA, and WA). The CONTINUUM system was generating over 10,000 new patient assessments per month. Across all three software tools, with over 6,000 software subscriptions, interviewers had entered over 212,000 patient assessments in its database.

Empirical analysis indicated that the software yields recommendations that are consistent with ASAM's Practice Guidelines.[61,62] ASAM's Science Team of internal researchers, seeking to help guide the ASAM Criteria fourth edition, performed a multistate analysis of a single month's data (July 2021; N = 5,154 unique individuals' assessments). Of these patients, 48% had active DSM-5 opioid use disorder (OUD), almost 100% were computer-recommended to receive MOUD, and 70% were also recommended for other clinical treatment services, for example, 26% for Level 3 residential or Level 4 hospital-type care. A third of patients were recommended for additional co-occurring behavioral health services. These data indicated that patients with OUD frequently needed services beyond pharmacotherapy. The data also highlight the importance of "unbundling," that is, combining services from different specialists or sources, rather than through fixed but incomplete resources.[63]

These empirical mechanisms are facilitating continuous quality improvement of *The ASAM Criteria*. The result is that patients are benefitting not only from the art of addiction medicine, for example, ASAM's expert consensus, but by ASAM's own contributions to science as well.

SOCIAL IMPACT

Over 30 years, *The ASAM Criteria* has progressed from a theoretical construct[41] to generating wide-spread educational efforts.[64] It has broadened the differentiation of services to address diverse patient needs[65] and introduced standardization of patient assessment in both clinical[58,66,67] and justice[60] settings. It has driven accreditation,[68] reimbursement reform,[69] and behavioral health care standardization beyond SUD (via the LOCUS Level of Care Utilization System[70]). The largest federal court class action lawsuit, on behalf of 67,000 mental health and SUD plaintiffs, challenged the nation's largest payer for obstructing access to the full continuum of *The ASAM Criteria*[71] While the outcome of that case is subject to appeal, nevertheless, *The ASAM Criteria* now has the potential to drive measurement-based care, outcomes-based treatment, and value-based contracting in addiction treatment.[72] Its influence has steadily grown, impacting patients, providers, payers, states, U.S. federal agencies and other countries.

EVOLUTION OF STANDARDIZED TOOLKIT

With growing demand from the field for a unified language and standards to facilitate adoption of *The ASAM Criteria*, ASAM has supported the *ASAM Criteria* textbook with a coordinated set of live and online trainings,[64] a direct online patient self-assessment (ATNA—the Addiction Treatment Needs Assessment),[73] a managed care guide (The ASAM Criteria—Powered by InterQual),[74] and the ASAM–CARF Level of Care Certification Program.[20-22] Fidelity problems created by many jurisdictions' "home grown" attempts at simplified assessments[45] led to the creation of a paper-based ASAM Criteria Assessment Interview Guide.[75] These are all described, along with models and strategies for adoption, in *Speaking the Same Language: A Toolkit for Strengthening Patient-Centered Addiction Care in the United States.*[1]

The next advance for *The ASAM Criteria* will be a fourth edition.[76] This will incorporate rigorous empirical data from the literature and CONTINUUM's dataset and a formal modified Delphi process for developing expert consensus. It will build training salience using case-based learning, draw on empirically driven quality improvement, and increase the objectivity of managed care, prior approval and utilization management processes. Goals include improving coherence and reducing the complexity of the decision rules, and streamlining the CONTINUUM interview process. Improvements are contemplated regarding adolescents, nicotine and cannabis use, justice-involved populations, and recovery support services. Finally, it will connect assessment with treatment planning and outcome measurement. The goal for this next stage in the evolution of *The ASAM Criteria* is to become the standard vehicle for real-time, patient- and population-based outcome measurement, in order to drive comprehensive care.

CONCLUSIONS

Four important missions underlie *The ASAM Criteria*: (a) to enable patients to receive the most appropriate and highest quality treatment services, (b) to encourage the development of a broad continuum of care, (c) to promote the effective and efficient use of care resources, and (d) to help protect appropriate access to and funding for care. Further goals include patient centeredness and addressing SDOH. Evidence supports the benefit of standardized implementation for these objectives.

Effective implementation of *The ASAM Criteria* will require continued adoption of assessment and decision-assistance technology, as has already been undertaken elsewhere in health care, and a shift in thinking toward outcome-driven case management. A variety of entities will need to make this shift, including regulatory agencies, clinical and medical staff, and referral sources, such as courts, probation officers, child protective services, employers, and employee assistance professionals.[67] *The ASAM Criteria* and its software implementation offer a system for improving patient-centered, collaborative care. With improved outcome analysis driving treatment decisions, the problem of access to care and funding of treatment can be championed more effectively.

BRIEF SUMMARY

For individuals suffering from SUDs, *The ASAM Criteria* is the most widely used approach for assessment, determining needs, recommending treatment, and securing reimbursement coverage. Its foundational principle is that patients should be treated with the least intensive set of services that will safely and effectively meet their needs. This principle is implemented via a six-dimensional assessment model and a formally specified continuum of care. This care continuum ranges from brief intervention to hospital-based services. Over 30 years, *The ASAM Criteria* has impacted society by fostering patient-centered care, differentiation of services to address diverse patient needs, standardization of patient assessment, accreditation and certification, and payment reform. The result is empirically demonstrated improvement in patient outcomes in clinical and justice settings. *The ASAM Criteria* now has the potential to drive treatment planning, measurement-based care, outcomes-based treatment, and value-based contracting in the United States and internationally.

ACKNOWLEDGMENTS

The authors would like to recognize the work on the prior edition version of this chapter, authored by David Mee-Lee, M.D., DFASAM, and Gerald D. Shulman, M.A., M.A.D., FACATA. In this new edition, this chapter describes the considerable progress that has been made with the development of new tools, the growing adoption of the standard implementation of The ASAM Criteria, the empirical evidence of validity and expanding social impact on clinical care and outcomes, and the development of The ASAM Criteria fourth edition.

REFERENCES

1. Guyer J, Traube A, Deshchenko. *Speaking the Same Language: A Toolkit for Strengthening Patient-Centered Addiction Care in the United States.* American Society of Addiction Medicine; 2021.

Accessed November 9, 2021. https://www.asam.org/docs/default-source/quality-science/final---asam-toolkit-speaking-same-language.pdf?sfvrsn=728c5fc2_2#page=13

2. Hoffmann NG. *The Cleveland Admission, Discharge & Transfer Criteria: Model for Chemical Dependency Treatment Programs.* Greater Cleveland Hospital Assn.; 1987.
3. Weedman R. *Admission, Continued Stay and Discharge Criteria for Adult Alcoholism and Drug Dependence Treatment Services.* National Association of Addiction Treatment Providers; 1987.
4. Hoffman NG, Halikas JA, Mee-Lee D. *ASAM Patient Placement Criteria for the Treatment of Psychoactive Substance Use Disorders.* American Society of Addiction Medicine; 1991.
5. Mee-Lee D. *ASAM (American Society of Addiction Medicine) Patient Placement Criteria for the Treatment of Substance-Related Disorders.* American Society of Addiction Medicine; 1996.
6. Mee-Lee D. *ASAM Patient Placement Criteria for the Treatment of Substance-Related Disorders.* 2nd ed.-Revised. American Society of Addiction Medicine; 2001.
7. Mee-Lee D, Shulman GD, Fishman M, Gastfriend DR, Miller MM. *The ASAM Criteria: Treatment for Addictive, Substance-Related, and Co-Occurring Conditions.* 3rd ed. The Change Companies; 2013.
8. Chuang E, Wells R, Alexander JA, Friedmann PD, Lee IH. Factors associated with use of ASAM criteria and service provision in a national sample of outpatient substance abuse treatment units. *J Addict Med.* 2009;3(3):139-150. doi:10.1097/ADM.0b013e31818ebb6f
9. Kolsky GD. *Current State AOD Agency Practices Regarding the Use of Patient Placement Criteria (PPC).* NASADAD—The National Association of State Alcohol and Drug Abuse Directors; 2006:17. Accessed January 25, 2022. https://nasadad.org/pageviewer/?target=resources/PPC_Report.pdf
10. Willenbring ML, Kivlahan D, Kenny M, Grillo M, Hagedorn H, Postier A. Beliefs about evidence-based practices in addiction treatment: a survey of Veterans Administration program leaders. *J Subst Abuse Treat.* 2004;26(2):79-85. doi:10.1016/S0740-5472(03)00161-2
11. Wachino V. *New Service Delivery Opportunities for Individuals with a Substance Use Disorder.* Published online July 27, 2015. Accessed November 30, 2016. https://www.medicaid.gov/federal-policy-guidance/downloads/smd15003.pdf
12. Mark TL, Hinde JM, Barnosky A, Joshi V, Padwa H, Treiman K. Is implementation of ASAM-based addiction treatment assessments associated with improved 30-day retention and substance use? *Drug Alcohol Depend.* 2021;226:108868. doi:10.1016/j.drugalcdep.2021.108868
13. *ASAM Criteria.* SAMHSA's Evidence-Based Practices Resource Center. Accessed May 13, 2022. https://www.samhsa.gov/resource/ebp/asam-criteria
14. NIDA-The National Institute on Drug Abuse. *Principles of Drug Addiction Treatment: A Research-Based Guide.* 3rd ed. National Institute on Drug Abuse; 2018:60. Accessed January 25, 2022. https://www.drugabuse.gov/publications/principles-drug-addiction-treatment-research-based-guide-third-edition/preface
15. Miller WR. Sacred cows and greener pastures: reflections from 40 years in addiction research. *Alcohol Treat Q.* 2016;34(1):92-115. doi:10.1080/07347324.2015.1077637
16. *ASAM Public Policy Statement on Advancing Racial Justice in Addiction Medicine.* American Society of Addiction Medicine; 2021:6. Accessed May 23, 2022. https://www.asam.org/docs/default-source/public-policy-statements/asam-policy-statement-on-racial-justiced7a33a9472bc604ca5b7ff000030b21a.pdf?sfvrsn=5a1f5ac2_2
17. Boswell JF, Kraus DR, Miller SD, Lambert MJ. Implementing routine outcome monitoring in clinical practice: benefits, challenges, and solutions. *Psychother Res.* 2015;25(1):6-19. doi:10.1080/10503307.2013.817696
18. *ASAM CONTINUUM™ to SAPC Level of Care Crosswalk.* Published online August 28, 2018. Accessed May 16, 2022. http://publichealth.lacounty.gov/sapc/NetworkProviders/ClinicalForms/TS/ASAMCONTINUUMSAPCLOCCrosswalk.pdf
19. *Overview of Substance Use Disorder (SUD) Care Clinical Guidelines: A Resource for States Developing SUD Delivery System Reforms*; 2017:26. Accessed May 16, 2022. https://www.medicaid.gov/state-resource-center/innovation-accelerator-program/iap-downloads/reducing-substance-use-disorders/asam-resource-guide.pdf
20. Merrifield C. *ASAM and CARF Launch Transformative Residential Addiction Treatment Certification Nationwide*; 2020. Accessed January 28, 2022. http://carf.org/LOC-certification-launch/
21. Knopf A. CARF adds OBOT accreditation and ASAM certification. *Alcoholism & Drug Abuse Weekly.* 2019;31(5):3-4. doi:10.1002/adaw.32246
22. *ASAM LOC Certification.* Accessed January 28, 2022. http://www.carf.org/LOCcertification/
23. Gastfriend DR, Mee-Lee D. The ASAM patient placement criteria: context, concepts and continuing development. *J Addict Dis.* 2003;22(Suppl 1):1-8.
24. Hoopfer S, Ryan M, Lucena A, Gastfriend EE. *ASAM PPC Assessment Software Business Plan.* Harvard Business School Volunteer Consulting Organization; 2011:30.
25. Reggers J, Ansseau M, Gustin F. Adaptation and validation of the ASAM PPC-2R Criteria in French and Dutch speaking Belgian drug addicts. Presented at: The 65th Annual Meeting of the College on Problems of Drug Dependence; June 14, 2003; Bal Harbor, FL.
26. Stallvik M, Nordahl HM. Convergent validity of the ASAM criteria in co-occurring disorders. *J Dual Diagn.* 2014;10(2):68-78. doi:10.1080/15504263.2014.906812
27. Stallvik M, Gastfriend DR, Nordahl HM. Matching patients with substance use disorder to optimal level of care with the ASAM Criteria software. *J Subst Use.* 2015;20(6):389-398. doi:10.3109/14659891.2014.934305
28. Stallvik M, Gastfriend DR. Predictive and convergent validity of the ASAM criteria software in Norway. *Addict Res Theory.* 2014;22(6):515-523. doi:10.3109/16066359.2014.910512
29. Park SW, Na E, Roh S, et al. Development of Korean patient placement criteria for the treatment of alcohol use disorder. *Korean Acad Addict Psychiatry.* 2021;25(1):18-27. doi:10.37122/kaap.2021.25.1.18
30. Mark TL, Hinde J, Henretty K, Padwa H, Treiman K. How patient centered are addiction treatment intake processes? *J Addict Med.* 2021;15(2):134-142. doi:10.1097/ADM.0000000000000714
31. Westermeyer J, Lee K. Residential placement for veterans with addiction: American Society of Addiction Medicine Criteria vs. a veterans homeless program. *J Nerv Ment Dis.* 2013;201(7):567-571. doi:10.1097/NMD.0b013e3182982d1a
32. Drymalski WM, Nunley MR. Sensitivity of the ASAM criteria to psychiatric need. *Int J Ment Health Addict.* 2018;16(3):617-629. doi:10.1007/s11469-017-9801-8
33. Gastfriend DR, ed. *Addiction Treatment Matching: Research Foundations of the American Society of Addiction Medicine (ASAM) Criteria.* 1st ed. Haworth Pr Inc; 2004.
34. Camilleri AC, Cacciola JS, Jenson MR. Comparison of two ASI-based standardized patient placement approaches. *J Addict Dis.* 2012;31(2):118-129. doi:10.1080/10550887.2012.665727
35. Magura S, Staines G, Kosanke N, et al. Predictive validity of the ASAM patient placement criteria for naturalistically matched vs. mismatched alcoholism patients. *The American Journal on Addictions.* 2003;12(5):386-397. doi:10.1111/j.1521-0391.2003.tb00482.x
36. Sharon E, Krebs C, Turner W, et al. Predictive validity of the ASAM Patient Placement Criteria for hospital utilization. *J Addict Dis.* 2003;22(Suppl 1):79-93. doi:10.1300/j069v22s01_06
37. Coll KC, Freeman BJ, Juhnke GA, Sass M, Thobro P, Hauser N. *Evaluating American Society of Addiction Medicine (ASAM) Dimension Assessment as an Outcome Measure: A Pilot Study with Substance Abusing Adolescents in Two Matched Residential Treatment Centers.* Published 2015. Accessed January 26, 2022. https://www.counseling.org/knowledge-center/vistas/by-subject2/vistas-substance-abuse/docs/default-source/vistas/article_679b5a22f16116603abcacff0000bee5e7
38. Angarita GA, Reif S, Pirard S, Lee S, Sharon E, Gastfriend DR. No-show for treatment in substance abuse patients with comorbid

symptomatology: validity results from a controlled trial of the ASAM patient placement criteria. *J Addict Med.* 2007;1(2):79-87. doi:10.1097/ADM.0b013e3180634c1d

39. Garner BR, Godley MD, Funk RR, Lee MT, Garnick DW. The Washington Circle continuity of care performance measure: predictive validity with adolescents discharged from residential treatment. *J Subst Abuse Treat.* 2010;38(1):3-11. doi:10.1016/j.jsat.2009.05.008
40. Gans J, Falco M, Shackman BR, Winters KC. An in-depth survey of the screening and assessment practices of highly regarded adolescent substance abuse treatment programs. *J Child Adolesc Subst Abuse.* 2010;19(1):33-47. doi:10.1080/10678280903400578
41. Gastfriend DR, McLellan AT. Treatment matching. Theoretic basis and practical implications. *Med Clin North Am.* 1997;81(4):945-966. doi:10.1016/s0025-7125(05)70557-5
42. Staines G, Kosanke N, Magura S, Bali P, Foote J, Deluca A. Convergent validity of the ASAM Patient Placement Criteria using a standardized computer algorithm. *J Addict Dis.* 2003;22(Suppl 1):61-77. doi:10.1300/j069v22s01_05
43. Kosanke N, Magura S, Staines G, Foote J, DeLuca A. Feasibility of matching alcohol patients to ASAM levels of care. *Am J Addict.* 2002;11(2):124-134. doi:10.1080/10550490290087893
44. Padwa H, Treiman K, Mark TL, Tzeng J, Gilbert M. Assessing assessments: substance use disorder treatment providers' perceptions of intake assessments. *Substance Abuse.* 2022;43(1):451-457. doi:10.1080/08897077.2021.1946891
45. Crable EL, Benintendi A, Jones DK, Walley AY, Hicks JM, Drainoni ML. Translating Medicaid policy into practice: policy implementation strategies from three US states' experiences enhancing substance use disorder treatment. *Implement Sci.* 2022;17(1):3. doi:10.1186/s13012-021-01182-4
46. McKay JR, Cacciola JS, McLellan AT, Alterman AI, Wirtz PW. An initial evaluation of the psychosocial dimensions of the American Society of Addiction Medicine criteria for inpatient versus intensive outpatient substance abuse rehabilitation. *J Stud Alcohol.* 1997;58(3):239-252. doi:10.15288/jsa.1997.58.239
47. May WW. A field application of the ASAM placement criteria in a 12-step model of treatment for chemical dependency. *J Addict Dis.* 1998;17(2):77-91. doi:10.1300/J069v17n02_06
48. Turner WM, Turner KH, Reif S, Gutowski WE, Gastfriend DR. Feasibility of multidimensional substance abuse treatment matching: automating the ASAM Patient Placement Criteria. *Drug Alcohol Depend.* 1999;55(1):35-43. doi:10.1016/S0376-8716(98)00178-1
49. Baker SL, Gastfriend DR. Reliability of multidimensional substance abuse treatment matching. *J Addict Dis.* 2004;22(suppl 1):45-60. doi:10.1300/J069v22S01_04
50. Corty E, Lehman AF, Myers CP. Influence of psychoactive substance use on the reliability of psychiatric diagnosis. *J Consult Clin Psychol.* 1993;61(1):165-170. doi:10.1037//0022-006x.61.1.165
51. Mee-Lee D. Development and implementation of patient placement criteria in new developments in addiction treatment. *J Clin Psychiatry.* 2006;67(11):4357.
52. Gastfriend DR, Lu S, Sharon E. Placement matching: challenges and technical progress. *Substance Use Misuse.* 2000;35(12-14):2191-2213. doi:10.3109/10826080009148254
53. Boltaev A, Bakhtiyor S, Gromov I, Lefebvre R, Gastfriend DR. Comparative analyses of ASAM PPC-2r Software Derived Level of Care with Actual of Clients on Mandatory Substance Addiction Treatment in Bukhara. Presented at: Proceedings of the 6th Annual Scientific Meeting of the International Society of Addiction Medicine; June 2, 2004; Helsinki, Finland.
54. Sullivan JT, Sykora K, Schneiderman J, Naranjo CA, Sellers EM. Assessment of alcohol withdrawal: the revised clinical institute withdrawal assessment for alcohol scale (CIWA-Ar). *Addiction.* 1989;84(11):1353-1357. doi:10.1111/j.1360-0443.1989.tb00737.x
55. Peachey JE, Lei H. Assessment of opioid dependence with naloxone. *Br J Addict.* 1988;83(2):193-201. doi:10.1111/j.1360-0443.1988.tb03981.x
56. *Diagnostic and Statistical Manual of Mental Disorders: DSM-5™*. 5th ed. American Psychiatric Publishing, Inc.; 2013:xliv, 947. doi:10.1176/appi.books.9780890425596
57. American Society of Addiction Medicine. *The ASAM Criteria Software National Demonstration Launch. Default.* Published August 9, 2021. Accessed May 18, 2022. https://www.asam.org/blog-details/article/2021/08/09/the-asam-criteria-software-national-demonstration-launch
58. Tsai G, Kim T, DA C-MP. Electronic ASAM Assessments for Substance Use Disorders: Innovative Pilots. Slide Deck Presentation presented at: Los Angeles, CA. Accessed May 18, 2022. https://www.uclaisap.org/slides/psattc/cod/2017/Workshop_I.pdf
59. Miller J. ASAM criteria becomes electronic tool: hosted by EHR vendors, the interactive program leads counselors to level of care recommendations. *Behav Healthc.* 2015;35(1):25-26.
60. Kanan R, Lambert A, Kalauokalani D, Allen D. *Impacts of the Integrated Substance Use Disorder Treatment Program 2019-2021.* CDCR-California Department of Corrections and Rehabilitation and California Correctional Health Care Services; 2022:24. Accessed May 15, 2022. https://cchcs.ca.gov/wp-content/uploads/sites/60/ISUDT/Impacts-ISUDT-Program2019-22.pdf
61. Kampman K, Jarvis M. American Society of Addiction Medicine (ASAM) national practice guideline for the use of medications in the treatment of addiction involving opioid use. *J Addict Med.* 2015;9(5):358-367. doi:10.1097/ADM.0000000000000166
62. *The ASAM National Practice Guideline for the Treatment of Opioid Use Disorder: 2020 Focused Update.* American Society of Addiction Medicine; 2020:91.
63. Denny R, Timko R, Pagano A, Niculescu M, Sagar R, Gastfriend DR. Individual and population opioid use disorder needs: a multi-state ASAM Criteria database. In: *Innovations in Addiction Medicine and Science.* Vol. (Poster). American Society of Addiction Medicine; 2022:1. Accessed May 19, 2022. https://annualconference.asam.org/2022/ASAM/fsPopup.asp?efp=Q0NUS01HUUYxMDIwNA&PosterID=459502&rnd=2.4122E-04&mode=posterinfo
64. *ASAM eLearning: ASAM Criteria.* Accessed May 22, 2022. https://elearning.asam.org/asam-criteria
65. Deck D, Gabriel R, Knudsen J, Grams G. Impact of patient placement criteria on substance abuse treatment under the Oregon Health Plan. *J Addict Dis.* 2004;22(Suppl 1):27-44. doi:10.1300/J069v22S01_03
66. Urada D, Antonini VP, Teruya C, et al. *Drug Medi-Cal Organized Delivery System 2019 Evaluation Report.* UCLA Integrated Substance Abuse Programs. http://www.uclaisap.org/dmc-ods-eval/html/reports-presentations.html
67. Heatherton B. Implementing the ASAM Criteria in community treatment centers in Illinois: opportunities and challenges. American Society of Addiction Medicine. *J Addict Dis.* 2000;19(2):109-116. doi:10.1300/j069v19n02_09
68. The Joint Commission. *Enhanced Substance Use Disorders Standards for Behavioral Health Organizations.* The Joint Commission; 2019:7. Accessed January 31, 2022. https://www.google.com/search?q=SAMHSA+ASAM+Criteria+software&oq=SAMHSA+ASAM+Criteria+software&aqs=chrome..69i57j33i160.10264j0j7&sourceid=chrome&ie=UTF-8
69. Cohen C, Hernández-Delgado H, Robles-Fradet A. *Medicaid Section 1115 Waivers for Substance Use Disorders: A Review.* National Health Law Program; 2021:42.
70. American Association of Community Psychiatrists. *LOCUS-Level of Care Utilization System for Psychiatric and Addiction Services.* Vol. Adult Version, 2010. American Association of Community Psychiatrists; 2009.
71. Enos G. Ruling against UBH in class action resonates within treatment community. *Alcoholism & Drug Abuse Weekly.* Published August 5, 2019. Accessed September 4, 2020. https://onlinelibrary.wiley.com/doi/abs/10.1002/adaw.32445
72. Gastfriend DR, Mee-Lee D. Thirty years of the ASAM criteria: a report card. *Psychiatr Clin North Am.* 2022;45(3):593-609.

73. *About the Addiction Treatment Needs Assessment*. Accessed January 31, 2022. https://www.shatterproof.org/need-help/about-addiction-treatment-needs-assessment
74. *Change Healthcare Partners with the American Society of Addiction Medicine to Transform Utilization Management for SUD*. Recent News & Press Releases. Accessed January 31, 2022. https://newsroom.changehealthcare.com/press-releases/change-healthcare-partners-with-the-american-society-of-addictio
75. *ASAM Releases New Free Paper-Based ASAM Criteria Assessment Interview Guide*. Default. Published February 6, 2022. Accessed May 21, 2022. https://www.asam.org/news/detail/2022/02/16/asam-releases-new-free-paper-based-asam-criteria-assessment-interview-guide
76. *ASAM Criteria 4th Edition Development*. Default. Accessed May 21, 2022. https://www.asam.org/asam-criteria/4th-edition-development

CHAPTER

48

Linking Addiction Treatment With Other Medical and Psychiatric Treatment Systems

Alyssa F. Peterkin, Karran A. Phillips, Peter D. Friedmann, and Jeffrey H. Samet

CHAPTER OUTLINE

- Introduction
- Potential benefits of linked services
- Barriers to optimal linkage
- Models of linked services
- Prospects for improved linkage

INTRODUCTION

Persons with substance use disorders (SUDs) are at substantial risk for coexisting medical and mental health conditions and often present to both medical and mental health care settings. Similarly, patients in addiction treatment commonly experience medical and psychiatric problems, which can increase risk of return to use.[1-3] In both medical and addiction treatment settings, the provision of comprehensive care for individuals with SUDs presents challenges to clinicians who traditionally have focused primarily on issues reflecting their own training and perspectives. For example, medical practitioners typically address the harmful effects of a particular substance, such as seizures from benzodiazepine withdrawal or cirrhosis from alcohol use, or the medical consequences of high-risk behaviors, such as viral hepatitis or HIV. Mental health professionals emphasize the psychological and psychiatric issues that are prevalent among patients with SUDs. Meanwhile, addiction specialists may focus on the individual's destructive preoccupation with obtaining and consuming a substance and the negative consequences of such actions. For the patient, these issues are inseparable and often interrelated, yet many clinicians operate in distinct systems of care, each with its own—at times exclusive—focus. For example, the medical literature describes medical practitioners not attending to their patients' addiction by failing to consider the diagnosis, intervene with medication, or refer for further treatment.[4-6] Similarly, patients in addiction treatment programs report unmet psychological and medical needs.[7,8] Patients with SUDs and medical or psychiatric conditions are sometimes bounced between systems and given contradictory and unhelpful recommendations—told that they must be abstinent before they can receive treatment for their psychiatric and medical problems, that they cannot receive treatment if they are taking particular medications, or that they are too sick (medically or psychiatrically) to get into an addiction treatment program—resulting in a clinical "Catch-22."

Patients who present with complex, interrelated, comorbid problems highlight the disconnections between these often-separate systems of care. Health care reform such as the Patient Protection and Affordable Care Act[9] includes addiction as an "essential health benefit" and increased the number of individuals with addiction presenting to primary care and other health care settings.[10,11] The resulting increased demand for addiction, medical and psychiatric services is being met, in part, by the arrival of addiction medicine as a board-certified subspecialty joining the ranks of addiction psychiatry. However, given that many systems lack access to certified addiction physicians,[12] further addiction training for generalists is key. Generalist physicians and their health care colleagues' willingness to provide addiction care, and create linkages across the systems of medical, mental health, and addiction are essential to improve quality of care for patients with addiction.[13] This chapter reviews the potential benefits of linkages between primary medical care, mental health, and addiction services; the potential barriers to such linkages; and published linkage models.

POTENTIAL BENEFITS OF LINKED SERVICES

Effective linkage may benefit individuals using substances in the following common scenarios: when issues related to substance use are not addressed in primary care, hospitals, emergency departments and mental health settings; when medical and mental health issues are not addressed in addiction treatment; and when patient care occurs in two or more of these settings without effective communication between settings.

From a patient's perspective, the potential for improved care is motivation for linkage of systems (**Table 48-1**). For example, other medications can impact methadone metabolism (eg, rifampin can decrease serum methadone levels), and without coordination of care, the patient might experience opioid withdrawal. Chronic pain and pain-related dysfunction are common in primary care with nearly one-third of primary care patients who screened positive for drug use reporting severe pain and pain-related dysfunction.[14] Improved pain control and decreased substance use in a patient receiving substance use treatment services is another possible benefit of linked care. Proper attribution of symptoms to causes

TABLE 48-1 Potential Benefits of Linking Addiction Treatment With Other Medical and Psychiatric Services

From the patient's perspective • Promotes structured format • Improves overall quality of care • Facilitates access to addiction treatment for patients in medical care settings • Enhances access to primary medical care for patients receiving addiction treatment • Improves patient well-being in terms of addiction severity and medical problems • Provides care that may be easier to access • Increases the patient's satisfaction with his or her health care
From the primary care provider's perspective • Promotes screening of all patients for alcohol-related problems • Facilitates inclusion of substance related causes when considering a differential diagnosis • Allows more achievable access to the addiction treatment system • Supports the prevention of return to alcohol and substance use • Encourages other mental health services for primary care patients • Enhances adherence with appointments and medical regimens • Provides addiction training opportunities for personnel
From the addiction treatment provider's perspective • Improves addiction treatment outcomes • Reduces stigma about addiction among medical providers • Provides training opportunities about addiction-related medical problems • Promotes healthier behaviors • Enhances medical providers' appreciation of the value of addiction treatment • Creates support for reimbursement parity for addiction services • Develops ongoing quality improvement efforts within addiction programs
From a societal perspective • Reduces costs of health care and loss of productivity • Reduces duplication of services and administrative costs • Improves health outcomes of specific populations

(eg, cocaine causing uncontrolled hypertension), and better access to medically managed withdrawal and treatment for patients in the medical system are other benefits from such linkages. Uncoordinated care creates potential risk for medical errors such as serious medication interactions by clinicians who are unaware of each other. Linked systems hold the potential for achieving improved well-being of patients regarding addiction severity, medical and psychiatric condition severity, and overall quality of life.[15,16] Additional benefits include the provision of convenient, comprehensive, and coordinated care to patients and the entry of new patients into treatment.[17] Finally, linking services may decrease stigma, as all clinicians would recognize and support the patient's addiction, medical and psychiatric treatment goals in all treatment locations.

From the perspectives of primary care and mental health clinicians, possible benefits of linkage include early identification of SUDs and prevention of return to use,[18] increased consideration of substance use related conditions in differential diagnoses, better access to addiction treatment services, enhanced patient adherence to appointments and medications, and improved addiction knowledge for clinical personnel. From an addiction treatment clinician's perspective, stronger linkages could yield improved addiction treatment outcomes, as seen with the addition of needed psychosocial services.[19,20] Ready availability of needed medical and mental health services also would allow addiction professionals to focus on core substance use issues. Exposure to successful recovery could reduce stigma from health care professionals and enhance their appreciation of the value of addiction treatment. Bringing addiction treatment into mainstream medical care would make explicit its similarities to the care of other chronic illnesses.[21] Finally, linkage of services could enhance quality improvement efforts within addiction treatment systems—as articulated in an accreditation requirement from the Joint Commission (that accredits health care organizations)[22] and by the focus of an Institute of Medicine (IOM) report[23]—by taking lessons from medical care systems that have grappled with these issues.

From a societal perspective, stronger linkages might lower long-term costs, including savings from reduced HIV and hepatitis incidence and other health-related sequelae of averted substance use, reduced incarceration and other criminal legal expenditures, and increased productivity.[24,25] Another possible benefit is reduced duplication of services across systems. Finally, a potential public health achievement would be improved health outcomes for populations with substantial morbidity associated with SUDs.

BARRIERS TO OPTIMAL LINKAGE

Medical Training

Many barriers impede optimal linkage of services. One well-documented challenge has been the perspective of many medical clinicians that substance use is a social issue rather than a medical condition and thus outside of their purview.[26,27] This viewpoint has declined over the past 20 years. Efforts to increase medical education about addiction have been under way, most notably in the past two decades, with development of core competencies, curricula for the prevention and management of drug use,[28-30] and increasing the number of addiction educators across disciplines. Recently, the Accreditation Council for Graduate Medical Education (ACGME) has required all training programs to develop effective educational interventions about recognizing and treating SUDs.[31] The American Board of Medical Specialties (ABMS) officially recognized Addiction Medicine as a subspecialty in 2015, which allows physicians from any of the 24 Member Boards to become board certified in addiction medicine. It also allows for accreditation by the ACGME for addiction medicine fellowship programs, which will result in an increased addiction physician workforce and improved access to care. The emergence of the American College of Academic Addiction Medicine has energized these efforts to enable addiction medicine physicians to work alongside addiction psychiatrists to treat this population and model excellent care to medical trainees.

Compared to mental health services, substance use services tend to be less integrated with primary care and rated as significantly less effective; the perceived difference in effectiveness appeared to be related to clinician training.[32] Physicians report having received minimal training in SUDs, resulting in inadequate screening for preclinical cases.[33-35] Many physicians have had minimal experience with few successful patients with SUDs because they do not identify patients with less severe addiction or follow up those who have had success in treatment. This limited exposure biases the spectrum of medical clinicians' clinical experience and further discourages physician involvement. As a result, only patients with poor treatment response who develop severe medical and psychosocial consequences are "visible."[36] In such an environment, it is difficult to convince even well-meaning physicians that the diagnosis and management of these disorders are within their scope of practice. Training can help overcome these barriers.[37-43] Further, the highly visible overdose crisis, and complex issues surrounding pain and opioid prescribing, have served as opportunities to expand addiction training[44-47] including training related to prescribing required in some states for licensure. In 2015, the Massachusetts Medical Society developed Opioid Therapy and Physician Communication Guidelines to assist physicians in developing and practicing safe opioid prescribing, which are now incorporated into the Massachusetts Board of Registration in Medicine's comprehensive advisory to physicians on prescribing best practices.[48]

Diversity in the Work Force and Facilitating Linkage to Addiction Treatment

Currently, the United States addiction workforce does not reflect the demographics of the affected population. Approximately 33% of the U.S. population identifies as Black/African American, Latinx or Indigenous; yet, only 12% of addiction trained physicians represent those groups. Asian, Black and Indigenous physicians are less likely to obtain addiction board certifications.[49] Building diversity within the field of addiction requires deliberate efforts such as increasing funding for medical schools in under-resourced areas, mentorship and pipeline programs. Exposing students to the field of addiction, evaluating workplace diversity[49] in addition to developing direct training programs focused on supporting underrepresented individuals in medicine with a specific interest in addiction will also promote diversity within the field. One such Substance Abuse and Mental Health Services Administration (SAMHSA) funded program, Recognizing and Eliminating disparities in Addiction through Culturally informed Healthcare (REACH) (https://reachgrant.org) aims to increase the number of addiction specialists, including advanced practice practitioners, adequately trained to work with patients from underrepresented groups and increase the overall number of underrepresented minority addiction specialists in the workforce.[50]

Black/African Americans and Latinx people are less likely to complete SUD treatment when compared to White people.[51] In a retrospective, observational cohort study ($N = 785$) White patients ($N = 617$) were more likely to be engaged in addiction treatment by Peer Support Specialists compared to Black patients ($N = 168$) in the emergency department (adjusted odds ratio: [95% confidence interval] = 1.61 [1.11-2.34] $p = 0.12$).[52] Additionally, despite efforts to increase access to the less restrictive yet effective medication, buprenorphine treatment has been disproportionately higher in geographic areas with a larger percentage of White people.[53,54] Lagisetty et al. found that White patients (between 2012 and 2015) had 35-fold more buprenorphine-related office visits compared to patients of other races and ethnicities revealing a treatment divide.[55] In contrast, methadone treatment which is largely concentrated in areas with larger African American and Latinx populations is subject to inconsistent regulations that vary by state.[53,54] As the disparities of opioid overdose fatalities continue to widen with 2020 rates of overdose mortality among Black individuals exceeding those among White individuals for the first time since 1999,[56] there is a critical need for more equitable treatment opportunities and well-equipped addiction specialists to care for these under-resourced populations.

Stigma and Concerns About Confidentiality

Stigma remains a fundamental barrier in the treatment of any patient, particularly those using substances. Stigma comes in many forms (eg, public, self-perceived, anticipated, by association, structural, and health care provider) and individuals with SUD can face them all.[57,58] Individuals with SUD also face another type of stigma, intervention stigma, where the treatment for the disorder is the focus of the stigma. Medications for opioid use disorder (MOUD) are often the focus of intervention stigma. Examples include opioid use disorder (OUD) treatment with methadone automatically disqualifying an individual for a Commercial Driver's License and people taking methadone for OUD being denied the following: custody rights of their children, access to housing and shelter, admission to residential SUD treatment facilities, and acceptance by subacute skilled nursing facilities.[59-62] In addition to effects on patient behavior, such as limiting recognition of needs and readiness to accept services, stigma might result in medical clinicians' disinclination toward spending time addressing drug and alcohol concerns. Both outgrowths of stigma impede overall progress.

Medical and mental health clinicians may not fully appreciate the efficacy of addiction treatment despite an overwhelming supportive body of research. For example, the therapeutic value of treatment for SUDs is comparable to treatment for other chronic disorders, such as diabetes mellitus.[21,63-65] Interventions to address stigma have been effective in achieving wider understanding of the comparable effectiveness of SUD treatment. Friedmann et al. found that knowledge, perceptions, and information training plus interorganizational strategic planning interventions were effective in changing attitudes and the intent to refer patients for medication treatment for addiction in community corrections settings, especially among corrections staff.[40] Additionally, mentorship programs for health professions students (including medical, nursing and physician assistant) and substance use related curriculum have helped transform negative attitudes and promote empathy for patients with SUD.[66-68]

Well-meaning concerns about patient confidentiality can be barriers to effectively linked medical, mental health, and addiction care. Practical difficulties interfere with obtaining timely two-way written releases of information. Title 42 of the Code of Federal Regulations (CFR) part 2 (42 CFR part 2), the Confidentiality of Alcohol and Drug Abuse Patient Records, was promulgated in 1975 (40 FR 27802) and revised in 1987 (52 FR 21796) to protect the privacy rights of patients who receive treatment for a SUD. On February 17, 2017, the 1987 version was replaced with a revised CFR part 2 renamed the Confidentiality of Substance Use Disorder Patient Records (82 FR 6052).[69] Although the protection of patient confidentiality is noble, it can impede integrated care. Special protection for addiction information may inadvertently reinforce stigma against patients by supporting the misconception that SUDs are different from other health conditions, and further inhibit the delivery of comprehensive integrated care.[70,71]

The dissemination of electronic health records (EHRs) has resulted in a major evolution in information sharing across systems. The Cures Act of 2016, mandates sharing of health care information across health care systems and patient access to clinical notes, labs and imaging through electronic portals by December 2022.[72] While privacy regulations under 42 CFR Part 2 have limited the dissemination of these innovations in specialty addiction treatment settings, the Cures Act has increased access to documentation in nonaddiction specialty care settings by generalists (eg, primary care office-based addiction treatment). The increased transparency with OpenNotes, that is online portals to clinical records, may encourage less stigmatizing, more objective, patient-centered documentation of substance use patterns in the medical record.[73] The integration of addiction information into electronic medical records will continue to be a challenging but worthwhile effort. Regulators and clinicians will continue to struggle to balance protections against discrimination with the need for information sharing.

In summary, the barriers to an integrated system of care for patients with SUDs are manifold. Barriers include clarity about professional responsibility, education for clinicians, lack of clinician diversity, concerns about confidentiality, and stigma, among others. Though extensive, the barriers are not insurmountable. Educational barriers might be addressed through active learning educational programs,[43] e-learning technology, the development of clear guidelines, the development of supportive materials,[64,74] role models,[66] the growth of addiction specialists and greater integration of biopsychosocial model into health care education. Deliberate efforts to build diversity within the field of addiction and community partnerships addressing inequities can improve addiction treatment outcomes.[75] At the "macro" level, addressing systems linkages would go a long way toward improving integrated care. Examples of system approaches include implementation of the following: linkage models of care, payment systems that encourage linkage, and quality measures valuing coordinated care.

Confidentiality issues can be addressed at the system level by having all care occur under one health system umbrella, with informatics and office procedures that prompt clinicians and staff to obtain releases to allow health care providers to share information. Published and future studies demonstrating the feasibility and effectiveness of these models should help convince payers and practitioners to move in this direction.

The growth of office-based addiction treatment has enhanced communication between some primary medical care clinicians and opioid treatment staff members highlighting the opportunity for integrating addiction treatment into medical care. Active learning education programs can change health care provider attitudes, skills, and practices.[37,38] Convincing theoretical and empirically proven benefits of linked services also will lead clinicians to favor better-integrated care.[76,77]

MODELS OF LINKED SERVICES

Persons with SUD at times utilize services in "inefficient" ways (eg, emergency department [ED] presentations rather than outpatient clinic visits), and have challenges engaging in continuous, longitudinal, and comprehensive care.[78-81] Two models have been proposed to bring the system of care for patients with SUDs closer to a primary care or chronic disease management (CDM) model (**Table 48-2**). One model uses a

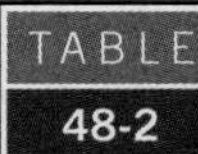

TABLE 48-2 Features of Centralized and Distributive Integrated Service Models

Centralized models

- Addiction treatment and pharmacotherapy in primary medical care and mental health services sites
- Addiction providers located in group health maintenance organizations (HMOs), private practices, or clinics
- Behavioral medicine and primary medical provider offices co-located in shared space
- Addiction treatment delivered at public health clinics (eg, sexually transmitted infections, HIV, or tuberculosis care)
- Addiction treatment delivered in a general hospital with proximate medical and mental health clinics
- Addiction treatment and primary care services co-located in a community mental health setting
- Addiction-trained advanced practice practitioner or physician available in a primary care practice to prescribe and monitor naltrexone, to prescribe and monitor buprenorphine, and to initiate and manage withdrawal management
- Addiction and mental health specialty teams present in medical care sites (eg, consult teams in EDs or hospitals)
- Nicotine/tobacco use counseling and pharmacotherapy delivered as part of primary care
- Brief interventions and advice for unhealthy substance use in doctor's offices, EDs, and hospitals
- Primary medical care and mental health services delivered at addiction treatment sites
- Medical and mental health providers or clinic located at a methadone treatment program
- Collocated primary care and addiction care
- An integrated alcohol and medical clinic
- An addiction medicine physician with psychiatric skills
- A multiservice community agency with a central location

Distributive

- HMOs or preferred provider organizations with defined, yet decentralized, referral networks
- Addiction triage and referral or central intake and assessment centers that perform medical and mental health assessments and referral for multiple addiction treatment programs
- Community-based case management
- Evaluation at addiction treatment sites with external referral for ongoing medical and mental health care
- Defined networks of providers with facilitated communication and financial/contractual links and systems
- Informal links between clinicians or agencies facilitated by releases of information, transportation, and case management
- A multiservice community agency with a single owner but several locations
- Low threshold substance use disorder clinics
- Harm reduction services

centralized approach in which addiction treatment, primary medical care, and mental health services are located within a single site. A second model uses a distributive approach to facilitate effective patient referrals to services at different sites. This section describes these models of linked primary medical, mental health, and addiction services and reviews evidence of their success in facilitating the multidisciplinary care of patients with SUD.[23,82]

Centralized Models

Centralized or on-site models bring primary care, mental health, and/or addiction services together at a single site. This integrated, "one-stop-shopping" model has been best described in primary care clinics and addiction treatment programs. In addition to overcoming the substantial political, bureaucratic, attitudinal, and financial barriers that separate persons with SUD from needed services, centralized delivery mitigates the problems of geographic separation and patient challenges of keeping outside appointments.[83-86] Korthuis et al. reviewed 12 models of integration of medication for addiction treatment into primary care and found that all included pharmacotherapy, psychosocial services, integration of care, education, and outreach. The ideal model of care for a particular setting depended on local factors including available expertise, the population, proximity to an addiction center of excellence, reimbursement policies, and geography.[87]

Willenbring and Olson[88] reported favorable results for a model of integrated medical and alcohol treatment in a specialty clinic. Their model included at least monthly visits, outreach to patients who missed appointments, clinic notes that cued the primary care provider (PCP) to monitor alcohol consumption at each visit, provider-delivered brief advice that emphasized reducing the harm from alcohol use and cutting down rather than strict abstinence, verbal and graphic feedback of change in biological markers such as gamma-glutamyl transferase (GGT),[89] and on-site mental health services as needed.[90] In a randomized design, medically ill patients with alcohol use disorder in the integrated clinic were compared with similar patients referred to traditional alcohol use disorder treatment and ambulatory medical care. Patients in the integrated clinic had improved alcohol treatment outcomes (including greater abstinence), improved outpatient visit adherence, and lower mortality.[91] This model serves as a starting point for a disease management system for SUDs, perhaps a specialty disease management clinic like those established for asthma, diabetes mellitus, and congestive heart failure. Clinical trials of similar approaches have yielded mixed results but merit further and longer testing to understand the cost-effectiveness of such an approach for patients with severe SUD.[92,93]

Less resource-intensive intervention models for individuals in primary care who exhibit unhealthy alcohol use have proved feasible. The cost analysis of Project TrEAT, Trial for Early Alcohol Treatment, a randomized study of physician-delivered brief interventions, showed modest improvements in self-reported drinking and estimated substantial savings for society and health systems.[94] A primary care study reported that 2.5 hours of primary care clinician training in patient-centered alcohol brief intervention was feasible[37] and reduced self-reported alcohol consumption among individuals who exhibit problem drinking.[95] Saitz et al.[96] demonstrated that a systems intervention (physician prompting with suggested courses of action) can improve counseling about alcohol and reduce drinking. Generalizing these efforts to primary care settings would require substantial training of clinicians as they often estimate their competence in promoting alcohol-related behavior change lower than in other health-related behavior change such as abstinence from tobacco, stress, exercise, and weight management.[97]

Other studies have demonstrated the effectiveness of pharmacological treatment for alcohol use disorder in the primary care setting. Lee et al.[98] found that 62% of participants completed a 12-week observational study of long-term extended-release naltrexone plus medical management in adults with alcohol use disorder in two public primary care clinics. During an additional 48-week active extension phase, 29% continued treatment for a median of 38 weeks total (range, 16-72 weeks). In the active extension phase participants, self-reported drinking days were low compared to 30-day pretreatment baseline (median 0.2 versus 6.0 drinks per day; 82% versus 38% days abstinent; 11% versus 61% heavy drinking days) demonstrating that long-term extended-release naltrexone in a primary care medical management model was feasible and may promote reductions in drinking and increased abstinence from alcohol.[98] In a randomized trial, engagement was higher and heavy drinking lower in those treated by a behavioral health specialist working with a primary care physician compared with specialty clinic referral.[99]

Prior to the Drug Addiction Treatment Act of 2000, few U.S. practices had integrated treatment of OUD into primary care. Though generalists have frequently participated in the management of OUD elsewhere in the world, it only occurred in the United States after the enactment of legislation permitting office-based treatment with Schedule III, IV, or V pharmacotherapy approved for the treatment of DSM-IV–defined opioid dependence by the U.S. Food and Drug Administration. Buprenorphine alone and a combination of buprenorphine and naloxone have been available for this purpose in the United States since 2003. Several studies have found that buprenorphine works as well as methadone for patients with mild to moderate OUD. In a 12-week randomized trial of 46 patients treated with buprenorphine, retention was higher in the primary care setting compared to a drug treatment program (78% versus 52%; $p = 0.06$) and rates of opioid use based on urine toxicology were lower (63% versus 85%; $p < 0.01$).[88] Furthermore, treatment with buprenorphine appears to be the effective element, as specialized counseling has shown no benefit over-and-above medication management alone.[100] Barry surveyed 142 patients receiving primary care–based buprenorphine/naloxone for OUD and found the mean overall satisfaction with treatment was 4.4 (out of 5).[101] Patients were most satisfied with the medication and ancillary services; and they indicated a strong willingness to refer a friend for the same treatment.[101]

Methadone is an effective treatment for OUD; however, its use is heavily regulated in the United States. A study by Merrill et al.[102] received regulatory exemptions to establish a methadone treatment program in primary care. The study enrolled 30 stable patients treated with methadone who transferred to a medical office for care. Twenty-eight of the patients remained connected to the health care center after 1 year and only two patients had nonprescribed opioid-positive urine tests. Unmet medical needs were attended to demonstrated by an improvement in the medical composite score of the Addiction Severity Index ($p = 0.02$), and patient and physician satisfaction was high with an improved attitude of physicians toward methadone maintenance ($p = 0.007$). Despite these promising findings, and calls for changes in extensive regulations, regulatory restrictions have prevented further experience with methadone as a treatment for OUD in U.S. outpatient medical practices.[103] In 2020, in response to the COVID-19 public health emergency, SAMHSA relaxed methadone regulations by allowing up to 28 days of take-home doses for stable patients and 14 take-home doses for less stable patients.[104] The methadone take-home dose expansion has not been associated with negative outcomes including fatal overdoses,[105,106] which has prompted addiction specialists to advocate for permanent regulatory changes.

Centralizing primary medical care, SUD treatment, and psychiatric services has proven an effective way to manage concomitant medical conditions such as hepatitis C virus (HCV), tuberculosis, and HIV. A 2012 Centers for Disease Control and Prevention report argued that integration of prevention services for HIV, viral hepatitis, sexually transmitted infections, and tuberculosis in persons who use drugs could improve quality, reduce duplication, increase access, and improve timeliness of service delivery. It could also increase the effectiveness of efforts to prevent infectious diseases that share common risk factors, behaviors, and social determinants.[107] Addiction treatment physicians often perform initial hepatitis C management including screening for HCV antibodies and integrate treatment in addition to recommending hepatitis A and B vaccines.[108-110]

Given the safety, tolerability, and effectiveness of direct-acting agents (DAAs), patients with HCV can be treated in general medicine settings.[111,112] Patients can achieve greater than 90% sustained virologic response with DAAs without toxicity related to concomitant alcohol use. Studies have also shown that current and former people who inject drugs (PWID) can engage successfully in evaluation and treatment of HCV infection in a number of treatment settings including co-located with methadone treatment.[113-117] Less is known about tuberculosis management within a centralized medical care and SUD setting. However, O'Connor et al.[118] demonstrated that by utilizing an admixture of isoniazid and methadone, 72% of patients receiving methadone who were eligible for tuberculosis chemoprophylaxis completed therapy.

Centralized models of primary medical and mental health care in addiction treatment settings improve patients with SUD access to these services.[119] Umbricht-Schneiter et al.[84] found that 92% of patients randomly assigned to a centralized model in a methadone treatment program received medical services, compared with only 35% of patients referred to a local clinic. A trial of veterans found that primary care on-site in an addiction treatment program increased attendance at primary care (adjusted odds ratio [OR] = 2.20; 95% confidence interval [CI] = 1.53-3.15) and engagement in addiction treatment at 3 months (adjusted OR = 1.36; 1.00-1.84) but showed no effect on overall health status or costs.[120] Among patients with substance use–related medical conditions, integrated care models compared to independent care models have shown significant decreases in hospitalization rates ($p = 0.04$), inpatient days ($p = 0.05$), and emergency room use ($p = 0.02$).[121] Other work suggests that integration of addiction treatment and community mental health services reduces return to use and improves stability for patients with co-occurring mental illness.[20,122-124] A study comparing on-site, integrated psychiatric and substance use services in a methadone treatment setting versus off-site, nonintegrated care demonstrated that on-site participants were more likely to initiate psychiatric care (96.9% versus 79.5%; $p < 0.001$), remain longer in treatment (195.9 versus 101.9 days; $p < 0.001$), attend more psychiatrist appointments (12.9 versus 2.7; $p < 0.001$), and have greater reductions in Global Severity Index (GSI) scores (4.2 versus 1.7; $p = 0.003$) than were off-site participants.[125]

Integrated models also promote delivery of HIV-related care, medication adherence, and outpatient medical services.[126,127] Lucas et al. compared HIV clinic-based buprenorphine treatment with referral to an opioid treatment program and found that the HIV clinic-based group receiving on-site buprenorphine had increased access to opioid agonist treatment (buprenorphine) and improved addiction treatment outcomes.[128] An analysis of New York State Medicaid claims data found that regular substance use treatment and medical care reduced hospitalizations by about 25% among HIV-positive and HIV-negative patients with drug use diagnoses.[129] In a study investigating patient satisfaction and experience with buprenorphine/naloxone treatment and integrated care, patients described being more engaged with both their substance use treatment and HIV care, including greater ability to manage their own treatment, keep up with appointments, and adhere to antiretroviral medication regimes.[130]

In general, nicotine use, at-risk drinking, and low-severity substance use can be managed in primary care settings without subspecialty addiction medicine training or consultation. Conversely, patients with severe SUDs generally should be cared for in collaboration with addiction specialists and/or treatment counselors (whether integrated in a primary care office or located elsewhere). However, it is uncertain when such specialty care is necessary, except in severe cases and cases with poor treatment response. Recent advances support and encourage a major role for primary care and mental health clinicians (including medical doctors, advanced practice registered nurses, and physician assistants) in the pharmacological management of patients with opioid or alcohol use disorder in collaboration and coordination with addiction treatment providers. For example, with the availability of office-based buprenorphine/naloxone, the primary care physician or general psychiatrist can prescribe MOUD while counseling is delivered by the physician, a health behavior expert in the practice, or referral. Similarly, medications for alcohol use disorder are effective when given along with low-intensity medication management counseling that addresses adherence, side effects, and alcohol use[96] in medical settings, similar to medication adherence counseling for other chronic conditions (eg, hypertension).

All patients should have primary and preventive health care—again, where this care is delivered will depend on the system of care. An ideal centralized model of care can provide addiction, mental health, and medical care at a single site. Whether specialty addiction medicine or addiction psychiatry services are delivered at an addiction specialty treatment site or within the primary care setting, the key is that systems are integrated to deliver the most appropriate and efficient care.

Chronic Disease Management Model

Chronic Disease Management (CDM), also referred to as chronic care management (CCM), is a care delivery approach that links, integrates, and coordinates primary and specialty care.[131,132] It is also sometimes described as a collaborative care model. The key components are an informed patient, a proactive team, and an established delivery system resulting in maximized CDM and outcomes. Such an approach has been successfully applied to many chronic diseases including SUDs. In the AHEAD (Alcohol Health Evaluation and Disease management) study, Saitz et al.[92,93] proposed that CDM focused on SUDs should include attention to (1) systems of care; (2) addressing medical, psychiatric, and social problems; and (3) addiction-specific treatments. The systems component addresses the fragmentation of care through on-site longitudinal service delivery, referral agreements, multidisciplinary teams, coordination of an explicit care plan, patient reminders, electronic medical records, and collaboration of addiction, medical, and psychiatric physicians. Medical, psychiatric, and social components include assessment, management, and coordination of care with specialty referral. Addiction-specific components include all known effective treatments such as medications for opioid and alcohol use disorders, motivational interviewing, recurrence of use prevention counseling, ambulatory withdrawal management, and appropriate referral. In the AHEAD randomized trial of CCM for SUDs, investigators found few benefits for the group that received care management versus a control group receiving usual care.[92] However, a secondary data analysis,[133] demonstrated that high-quality CDM for SUDs may improve addiction outcomes and that chronic care model quality measures may better reflect effective CDM than measures such as visit frequency. The Substance Use Motivation and Medication Integrated Treatment (SUMMIT) study is a randomized clinical trial comparing the effect of collaborative care versus usual care on primary care-based opioid and alcohol use disorder treatment utilization and self-reported abstinence. At 6 months, 39.0% (73/187) in the collaborative care arm versus 16.8% (32/190) in the usual care arm received any treatment for alcohol or OUD and a higher proportion of participants in the collaborative care arm reported abstinence (32.8% versus 22.3%).[93] These findings suggest that CDM may be effective for SUDs when delivered with high quality and fidelity. A functional addiction CDM approach may also require the health system at large to improve facilitation of care for patients with complex chronic conditions.

Additional guidance may be found in implementation science, which studies the best methods to promote the systematic uptake of clinical research findings and other evidence-based practices into routine care.[134] LaBelle et al. studied the Massachusetts Collaborative Care Model in which nurses working with physicians and advanced practice providers play a central role in the evaluation and monitoring of individuals with OUD treated with buprenorphine and found that program expansion into 14 community health centers increased the number of physicians who were waivered to prescribe buprenorphine by 375% within 3 years.[135] Additionally, the addiction trained nurse care manager model expands access to treatment and supports retention in treatment. In an office-based opioid treatment program using the nurse care manager model, nearly half of patients (187/382) enrolled remained engaged in treatment and 91.1% (154/169) were abstinent based on urine drug test results at 12 months.[77] In a clinician-randomized trial of the chronic care model for disease management for alcohol related problems among women in a "Health Care for the Homeless" clinic, women with risky alcohol use received usual care or an intervention consisting of a PCP brief intervention based on National Institute on Alcohol Abuse and Alcoholism's guidelines, referral to addiction services, and ongoing support from a care manager for 6 months. While baseline differences and small sample size limit generalizability, both groups significantly reduced their alcohol consumption, with a small effect size favoring the intervention at 3 months; intervention women also had significantly more participation in substance use treatment services.[136] Studies using implementation indices (eg, the Behavioral Health Integration in Medical Care [BHIMC] index) to measure integration capability at baseline and follow-up may help to target technical assistance and resources.[137] In 2014, a National Institute on Drug Abuse (NIDA) consensus group[138] supported CDM as a framework for primary care management of SUD and recommended: (1) implementing screening and brief intervention, (2) expanding and restructuring the health care team and (3) collaborating with local addiction specialists. To further demonstrate benefits of CDM on SUD outcomes, the care system would benefit from focused approaches based on specific diagnoses, patient needs and severity, and implementation details.

Distributive Models

Most settings lack resources to provide comprehensive, centralized services for patients with SUD. Therefore, the development and dissemination of effective decentralized or distributive models is key to quality service delivery in the current health care environment. Successful referral is the central task of the distributive model. Anecdote and limited data suggest that simple referral alone cannot integrate the care of patients with addiction in primary care settings. Historically, the treatment systems for medical and addiction care did not communicate effectively. Substance use disorder is underrecognized in medical settings. Studies have demonstrated that nearly 50% of the patients report that their primary care physician was unaware of their addiction.[139,140] This finding suggests that the substantial interorganizational distance between addiction treatment programs and mainstream health care presents great barriers to successful referral. Community-based case management can effectively overcome these barriers and link patients to needed services.[141,142]

Low Threshold Treatment Models

In recent years, low threshold treatment models have emerged to improve just-in-time engagement of individuals with SUD. These innovative care models promote rapid, same day entry into treatment, without waiting lists or abstinence requirements.[143] Low threshold programs utilize a flexible and patient-centered approach by providing medications for SUD and harm reduction services at initial presentation. Low threshold treatment settings often also offer screening for HIV, HCV and other sexually transmitted infections as well as case management to patients who might be reluctant to access care in a traditional treatment setting.[144] Patients engaging in care at a low threshold program are often Medicaid-insured and experiencing lack of housing.[145] In a retrospective observational study of low barrier access addiction clinics in an academic medical center, 82% of patients arrived at their appointment when they were given an appointment with same day access.[146]

Bridge clinics are one example of low barrier access programs that rapidly link people with SUD to treatment. Referrals to bridge clinics occur from jails or prisons, emergency departments, withdrawal management centers, social service agencies, medical and mental health providers, inpatient settings, word of mouth and self-referral.[146,147] In addition to medications, these low threshold programs may offer peer support and social support services such as connecting to health insurance, access to food, transportation vouchers and hygiene products to encourage care engagement.[143] Counseling and attending mutual help groups may be encouraged but are not typically required.[148] Patients often remain engaged in care at bridge clinics for several weeks to months. Snow and colleagues found that a majority of patients transitioned to a longer-term or more permanent treatment setting after a median of 73 days; however, 25% of patients remained in care at the bridge clinic for over one year.[148] A study evaluating low threshold buprenorphine (ie, unobserved inductions, weekly then less frequent follow-up, no requirement for additional psychosocial treatment) found that over half of patients were retained in treatment at 24 weeks and 20% retained for greater than 3 years.[145]

Referral to bridge clinics reduces utilization of higher acuity settings. Sullivan et al. found a 42% reduction in emergency department visits for patients referred to a bridge clinic.[147] In a qualitative study describing the patient experience in a bridge clinic, patients appreciated the accessibility, flexibility and harm reduction focus of a transitional clinic care setting.[148] Immediate access to MOUD and continued treatment despite ongoing challenges with recovery were rated highly by patients.[148]

Recently, a bridge clinic in Massachusetts has promoted increased utilization of the 72-hour rule (21 CFR 1306.07), which permits nonopioid treatment program prescribers to administer methadone for opioid withdrawal symptoms for up to 72 hours while arranging opioid treatment program referral.[149,150] This innovative treatment pathway has achieved high rates of linkage (93.1% patients [94/101] presented within 48 hours of scheduled appointment time and received methadone at opioid treatment program) and good retention in care (57.9% [70/121] of total referrals remained in care at opioid treatment program at one month).[149]

Harm Reduction Services and Overdose Prevention Centers

Harm reduction services aim to reduce the adverse consequences and risks associated with substance use through a range of services.[151] Syringe service programs (also called needle exchanges) prevent disease transmission, reduce risky behaviors, engage out-of-treatment persons who use drugs, and promote linkage to treatment services. A meta-analysis of 12 studies found that syringe service programs were associated with a reduction in HIV transmission with a pooled effect size 0.66 (95% confidence interval 0.43, 1.01).[152] In a cohort study of persons who inject drugs in Seattle, new exchangers were 5 times more likely to enter a methadone treatment program (absolute risk reduction = 5.05, 95% confidence limit = 1.44-17.7) during the next 12 months than were never-exchangers.[153]

In 2021, the first U.S. government-sanctioned overdose prevention center opened in New York City.[154,155] Within the first two months of operation, 613 individuals accessed services 5,975 times across the two sites; 52.5% of individuals received support including hepatitis C testing, counseling, and holistic services such as acupuncture.[155] Overdose prevention centers (also called safe consumption sites or supervised injection facilities) have been present in various countries including Canada and are effective in reducing overdose mortality (35% reduction in the vicinity closest to the site).[156]

Addiction Consult Services

Hospitalizations are opportunities to engage persons with SUD in treatment and create opportunities to establish linkages between traditional medical care and addiction treatment.[157-159] The expanding addiction treatment provider workforce in the setting of increasing substance use related hospitalizations has spurred the growth of inpatient Addiction Consult Services. Addiction Consult Services provide evidence-based addiction treatment to reduce substance use-associated morbidity and mortality and link affected patients to posthospitalization care.[160,161] Addiction Consult Services are comprised of interprofessional teams including addiction physicians and/or advance practice providers, medical trainees (fellows, residents and medical students), social workers and peer navigators who assist with biopsychosocial interventions and transitions to care in the community. Common interventions by Addiction Consult Services include inpatient withdrawal management, medication induction and counseling, bridge prescriptions (ie, a prescription for buprenorphine at the time of discharge until care in the community is established), and warm referrals to community-based services, bridge clinics and transitional programs.[162] Addiction Consult Services have been instrumental in changing hospital culture and policies, increasing the understanding of addiction, debunking misconceptions and reducing stigma among providers.[162,163]

Studies show that inpatient addiction consultation reduces patient-initiated discharge and readmission rates,[157,159,161] increases engagement in care and abstinence,[158] and promotes linkage to care and treatment retention. Management of withdrawal symptoms increases the likelihood that patients will remain hospitalized to complete medical treatment.[161,164] Liebschutz et al. found that inpatient initiation of buprenorphine treatment engaged medically hospitalized patients who are not seeking addiction treatment and reduced illicit opioid use 6 months after hospitalization.[165] Trowbridge et al. noted that 54% and 39% of patients linked to methadone and buprenorphine treatment, respectively, remained engaged in care at 30 days.[166] When Addiction Consult Services are unavailable, generalists should initiate MOUD and facilitate linkage to care in the community. In a study at an urban safety net hospital, generalists initiated MOUD for 31.8% of hospitalized patients with OUD (241/747), which was associated with presenting to an opioid treatment program within 30 (28.0% $p < 0.001$) and 90-days (30.6% $p < 0.001$).[167]

Recently, addiction specialists have collaborated with infectious disease specialists, cardiothoracic surgeons, and cardiologists to develop multidisciplinary teams to manage patients with injection-related infectious endocarditis. Multidisciplinary endocarditis teams aim to optimize the clinical decision making for hospitalized patients with injection related endocarditis, which includes cardiac surgery as a standard when indicated, antimicrobials and treatment of the underlying SUD. These teams may also include case management, nursing, social work and anesthesia.[168] Additionally, the collaboration between infectious disease and addiction specialists may provide people who inject drugs requiring long term intravenous therapy with more options including outpatient parenteral antimicrobial therapy (OPAT).[169] A pilot randomized control trial compared OPAT (N = 10) to usual care (N = 10) for people with SUD treated with buprenorphine admitted with a severe injection related infection.[170] In OPAT participants, hospital length of stay was shortened by 23.5 days and the proportion of urine samples negative for non-prescribed opioids was significantly greater; however, in both cases treatment retention was similar.[170]

Growing evidence supports that linkage between the ED and addiction treatment services is similarly beneficial. D'Onofrio et al. found that ED-initiated buprenorphine treatment significantly increased engagement in addiction treatment, reduced self-reported nonprescribed opioid use, and decreased use of inpatient addiction treatment services compared to brief intervention and referral. ED-initiated buprenorphine treatment did not significantly decrease the rates of opioid-positive urine samples or HIV risk behaviors.[171] Other studies have replicated these results with rates of follow up attendance as high as 77% for patient receiving ED-initiated buprenorphine.[172] Furthermore, the benefit of ED-initiated buprenorphine persists at 2 months with referral for continued treatment in primary care—consistent with primary care-based buprenorphine outcomes.[173] For example, in a primary care-based buprenorphine treatment study, 66% of those maintained on buprenorphine (37/56) were retained in treatment at 14 weeks.[174] Consequently in 2021, the American College of Emergency Physicians recommended that emergency physicians initiate buprenorphine for individuals with untreated OUD and provide direct linkage to treatment.[175] Although many EDs have opted to initiate buprenorphine, more intentional interventions such as an EHR Best Practice advisory, public messaging in ED, clinician feedback on patient outcomes and email reminders about buprenorphine prescription initiatives are needed to augment ED clinician buprenorphine prescribing.[176]

Addiction treatment programs commonly use distributive arrangements to link patients to medical and mental health services.[177,178] Examples of distributive arrangements range from an addiction treatment unit contracting with a local practice to provide physical examinations and routine medical care to one sending ad hoc referrals to a local community mental health center. The advantage of this model is its use of existing health care systems. For example, patients in an inpatient withdrawal management unit who received a facilitated referral to primary care in the local community from a multidisciplinary team (physician, nurse, and social worker) were more likely to link with primary medical care.[179] This model requires no rearrangement of existing health care delivery systems; however, it does require efforts (and therefore costs) to assure that linkage is completed. Case management or transportation assistance can facilitate these referrals.[180,181] A study of public addiction treatment programs found that contracted referral with case management increased medical services utilization two- to threefold over ad hoc referrals.[182]

There is also some evidence for combining centralized and distributive approaches. A primary health care facility implementing a hepatitis C treatment assessment plan serving PWID resulted in successful referrals to a tertiary liver clinic (71% of those referred attended). Staff facilitated appointment scheduling, phone and SMS appointment reminders, attendance confirmation, and referral outcome communication. Additionally, missed appointments were immediately rescheduled.[183]

Recently, innovative models connecting people remotely have emerged. ECHO (Extension for Community Healthcare Outcomes) has emerged to improve access to addiction treatment through teams of specialists at academic centers providing clinical expertise for specific cases using videoconferencing, an approach particularly useful for rural areas.[184] During the COVID-19 pandemic, U.S. Center for Medicare and Medicaid Services expanded access to telehealth to include audio-only visits and Drug Enforcement Administration relaxed regulations allowing for remote buprenorphine prescribing for new patients without an in-person examination.[185,186] These changes contributed to a 35-fold increase OUD related telehealth services which was associated with increased odds of retention in addiction treatment (adjusted odds ratio, 1.27; 95% confidence interval, 1.14-1.41).[187]

At Risk Populations

Integrated models may show the most benefit for at-risk populations, including those experiencing lack of housing, pregnant people, people who are incarcerated and young adults. People experiencing lack of housing have a high prevalence of SUDs and unique needs requiring tailored interventions.[188] Public policies that bar persons with prior felony convictions from housing assistance programs likely contribute to the strong association between substance use and being unhoused. People experiencing being unhoused often have unpredictable lifestyles, co-occurring conditions, and substance use, which make them ideally suited for integrated care. A retrospective review of 44 patients experiencing lack of housing and 41 patients with housing enrolled in office-based opioid treatment receiving buprenorphine/naloxone found that treatment failure did not differ for patients experiencing homelessness (21%) compared to patients with housing (22%) (p = 0.94).[189] Both groups had similar proportions with nonprescribed opioid use (OR, 0.9; 95% CI, 0.5-1.7 p = 0.8), utilization of counseling (homeless, 46%; housed, 49%; p = 0.95), and participation in mutual help groups (unhoused, 25%; housed, 29%; p = 0.96) at 12 months. A low barrier to entry and access to harm reduction-oriented programming are important.[190] Additionally assertive outreach (eg, mobile medical vans and shelter-based programs) have been helpful in linking people experiencing being unhoused to SUD treatment.[191,192,193] A New York City based mobile medical outreach clinic noted reductions in past 30-day substance use (4.1 versus 2.2 fewer days) and number of medical complaints (6.3 versus 4.8) at 4 months (N = 128/250).[194] Additionally, the Community Care in Reach program, a mobile health initiative targeting opioid overdose "hotspots" in Boston through harm reduction and on demand primary care and addiction treatment found that participants strongly preferred the mobile program to traditional office-based care. This preference was attributed to the perception of less wait time and more respect for people experiencing a lack of housing with addiction.[193,195]

Centralization of addiction services within existing primary care systems may also benefit people released from jail or prison by decreasing emergency room visits and hospitalizations and improving care of SUDs and other chronic conditions. SUD is common among people who are incarcerated, ranging from 10% to 60%[196]; however, one study found only 8% are connected to treatment at time of release.[197] In 2021, 28 states had policies regarding SUD treatment for people who were incarcerated, primarily in state prisons. Policies vary; some states only permit extended-release naltrexone, others only provide medications for withdrawal management and others do not offer any medications for addiction treatment.[198] Lack of agonist treatment for OUD in jails and prisons places people who are incarcerated at high risk for recurrence of use, overdose, hospitalization and death following release.[199,200] In the first 2 weeks of release, Binswanger et al. found the risk of death was 12.7 times higher among former inmates compared to the general population; drug overdose was a leading cause of death.[201] In a randomized trial of continuation of methadone versus forced withdrawal among people who are incarcerated, the former was found to increase treatment engagement after release yielding the potential to reduce risky behaviors, overdose, and death.[202] Initiating buprenorphine during incarceration increases the likelihood of treatment retention at 6 months postrelease and decreases chances of re-arrest within 30 days.[203,204] Boyd et al. showed that within the year following jail release, the presence of a SUD increased the frequency of ED use, while being retained in HIV primary care decreased the frequency of ED use.[205] Addressing high overdoses and deaths post release have been motivators for carceral systems. In 2019, Massachusetts legislation established a pilot program to provide medications for addiction treatment in county jails. Through a 3-year pilot, participating correctional facilities can offer all FDA-approved forms of medications for addiction treatment and arrange post release treatment services for participants.[206] Dedicated resources for collaborating with community-based treatment organizations to provide onsite services and smooth transitions of care into the community at the time of release may be key to increasing rates of treatment.[207]

Substance use during pregnancy is rising. Pregnant people using substances experience several barriers to care including stigma, paucity of providers with obstetrics and addiction treatment expertise and fear of child welfare consequences.[208] Dignified, trauma informed, integrated, multidisciplinary treatment care models such as the Project RESPECT (Recovery, Empowerment, Social Services, Prenatal care, Education, Community and Treatment), substance use disorder treatment in pregnancy clinic is essential for caring for pregnant people using substances.[208-210] This centralized model integrates SUD treatment and pre-natal care through a team of addiction focused obstetric providers, a psychiatrist and a social worker. Patients are scheduled for prenatal care and formal recurrence of use prevention visits every 1–3 weeks from initiation of care until delivery. In the RESPECT Clinic, the percentage of pregnant people with OUD receiving buprenorphine from 2006 to 2010 increased from 3% to 41%.[209]

The overdose epidemic has also impacted youth. Polysubstance use is common among adolescents and young adults, leading to 760% increase in overdose deaths from 1999 to 2018.[211] Treatment initiation for youth with SUD ranges from 24%-27% and retention in care is very challenging.[212,213] The American Academy of Pediatrics (AAP)'s Committee on Substance Use and Prevention has called on pediatricians to address substance use in primary health care settings.[214] Bagley et al. found that one in ten young people were retained in care at 12 months in a primary care-based model inclusive of medical, SUD treatment and behavioral health supported by a nurse care manager; of those lost to follow up 28.5% re-engaged in care.[212] To improve engagement and retention for youth, SUD treatment settings and services should be tailored to young people. Clinical care providers should be collaborative and culturally diverse, and programs should engage families.[212,215,216]

In summary, effective models exist for centralized and distributive linkage in both medical and specialty addiction treatment settings. Addiction interventions in medical settings are appropriate for patients with unhealthy alcohol use and those with mild to moderate SUDs, medically ill patients with SUD who decline formal treatment referral, and patients with SUDs who receive rehabilitative counseling elsewhere yet would benefit from addiction-related pharmacotherapy and management of their medical conditions. With adequate support, primary care physicians can have a productive role in outpatient withdrawal management.[217] Additionally, patients who are solely interested in harm reduction interventions can benefit from primary care management. For patients in formal addiction treatment, linkage to needed medical and psychological services may improve access, physical and mental health, and outcomes, including substance use. Both centralized and distributive models show promise for integrating care across these systems. While the distributive model predominates,[218] it can be less effective than the centralized model in linking patients with SUD to needed services.[83,179] However, given its low cost, flexibility, and adaptability (especially to integration of secondary and tertiary care services) the distributive model is likely to remain the predominant approach to service linkage. With increasing adoption of office-based addiction pharmacotherapy, the integrated model of care within medical settings will be of increasing interest to patients, physicians, other providers, as well as policy makers and researchers.[219]

PROSPECTS FOR IMPROVED LINKAGE

Momentum is building for a transformation in the delivery of addiction treatment and health care services. The rising prevalence of SUDs and the staggering number of co-occurring medical, mental health and social problems is well-documented, from drug overdose, HIV, hepatitis C to depression, anxiety, and discrimination.[75,220,221] The enormous economic burden that substance-related problems place on our society, through costs related to health care, incarceration, family disintegration, and loss of productivity, is increasingly recognized and forces policymakers to consider alternative approaches to the care of this population.[222,223] Furthermore, advances in the diagnosis and treatment of SUDs, including pharmacological and behavioral approaches effective in the primary care, hospital and community settings, promise to change the approach to management of these disorders. A report from the IOM, "Improving the quality of healthcare for mental and substance use conditions: The quality chasm" series noted that the current century is an opportune time to advance the linkage of substance use treatment with mental health and medical care.[23] The IOM said that only by addressing substance use and mental health problems can one achieve optimal benefit for patients engaged in medical care. Primary care and disease management systems are achievable only if adopted by physicians as part of multidisciplinary teams. Thus, the concern of overburdening physicians should not preclude the development of linkage systems, but rather influence their development so that their implementation does not solely rely on physicians' functions.[224] Increased attention to the improvement of quality in health care systems also presents opportunities to address linkage to addiction treatment as a quality issue. The treatment of addiction in less intensive settings will further promote cost-saving and cost-effectiveness. These innovations will drive the delivery of high-quality, comprehensive, and coordinated care for all patients with SUDs.

REFERENCES

1. Friedmann PD, Zhang Z, Hendrickson J, Stein MD, Gerstein DR. Effect of primary medical care on addiction and medical severity in substance abuse treatment programs. *J Gen Intern Med.* 2003;18(1):1-8. doi:10.1046/j.1525-1497.2003.10601.x
2. Bradizza CM, Stasiewicz PR. Qualitative analysis of high-risk drug and alcohol use situations among severely mentally ill substance abusers. *Addict Behav.* 2003;28(1):157-169. doi:10.1016/s0306-4603(01)00272-6
3. Saxon AJ, Wells EA, Fleming C, Jackson TR, Calsyn DA. Pre-treatment characteristics, program philosophy and level of ancillary services as predictors of methadone maintenance treatment outcome. *Addiction.* 1996;91(8):1197-1210. doi:10.1046/j.1360-0443.1996.918119711.x
4. Harris SK, Herr-Zaya K, Weinstein Z, et al. Results of a statewide survey of adolescent substance use screening rates and practices in primary care. *Subst Abuse.* 2012;33(4):321-326. doi:10.1080/08897077.2011.645950
5. Smothers BA, Yahr HT, Ruhl CE. Detection of alcohol use disorders in general hospital admissions in the United States. *Arch Intern Med.* 2004;164(7):749-756. doi:10.1001/archinte.164.7.749
6. Mendiola CK, Galetto G, Fingerhood M. An exploration of emergency physicians' attitudes toward patients with substance use disorder. *J Addict Med.* 2018;12(2):132-135. doi:10.1097/ADM.0000000000000377
7. Etheridge RM, Craddock SG, Dunteman GH, Hubbard RL. Treatment services in two national studies of community-based drug abuse treatment programs. *J Subst Abuse.* 1995;7(1):9-26. doi:10.1016/0899-3289(95)90303-8
8. Rowe TA, Jacapraro JS, Rastegar DA. Entry into primary care-based buprenorphine treatment is associated with identification and treatment of other chronic medical problems. *Addict Sci Clin Pract.* 2012;7(1):22-22. doi:10.1186/1940-0640-7-22
9. *Patient Protection and Affordable Care Act, 42 USC §18001.* 2010.
10. Ghitza UE, Tai B. Challenges and opportunities for integrating preventive substance-use-care services in primary care through the Affordable Care Act. *J Health Care Poor Underserved.* 2014;25(1 Suppl):36-45. doi:10.1353/hpu.2014.0067
11. Beronio K, Glied S, Frank R. How the Affordable Care Act and Mental Health Parity and Addiction Equity Act greatly expand coverage of behavioral health care. *J Behav Health Serv Res.* 2014;41(4):410-428. doi:10.1007/s11414-014-9412-0
12. Laine C, Newschaffer C, Zhang D, Rothman J, Hauck WW, Turner BJ. Models of care in New York State Medicaid substance abuse clinics: range of services and linkages to medical care. *J Subst Abuse.* 2000;12(3):271-285. doi:10.1016/s0899-3289(00)00054-7
13. Compton WM, Blanco C, Wargo EM. Integrating addiction services into general medicine. *JAMA.* 2015;314(22):2401. doi:10.1001/jama.2015.12741
14. Alford DP, German JS, Samet JH, Cheng DM, Lloyd-Travaglini CA, Saitz R. Primary care patients with drug use report chronic pain and self-medicate with alcohol and other drugs. *J Gen Intern Med.* 2016;31(5):486-491. doi:10.1007/s11606-016-3586-5
15. Druss BG, von Esenwein SA. Improving general medical care for persons with mental and addictive disorders: systematic review. *Gen Hosp Psychiatry.* 2006;28(2):145-153. doi:10.1016/j.genhosppsych.2005.10.006
16. Samet JH, Friedmann P, Saitz R. Benefits of linking primary medical care and substance abuse services. *Arch Intern Med.* 2001;161(1):85. doi:10.1001/archinte.161.1.85
17. Sullivan LE, Chawarski M, O'Connor PG, Schottenfeld RS, Fiellin DA. The practice of office-based buprenorphine treatment of opioid dependence: is it associated with new patients entering into treatment? *Drug Alcohol Depend.* 2005;79(1):113-116. doi:10.1016/j.drugalcdep.2004.12.008
18. Pace CA, Samet JH. In the clinic. Substance use disorders. *Ann Intern Med.* 2016;164(7):ITC49-ITC64. doi:10.7326/AITC201604050
19. Alegría M, Frank RG, Hansen HB, Sharfstein JM, Shim RS, Tierney M. Transforming mental health and addiction services. *Health Aff (Millwood).* 2021;40(2):226-234. doi:10.1377/hlthaff.2020.01472
20. Dugosh K, Abraham A, Seymour B, McLoyd K, Chalk M, Festinger D. A systematic review on the use of psychosocial interventions in conjunction with medications for the treatment of opioid addiction. *J Addict Med.* 2016;10(2):91-101. doi:10.1097/ADM.0000000000000193
21. McLellan AT, Lewis DC, O'Brien CP, Kleber HD. Drug dependence, a chronic medical illness. *JAMA.* 2000;284(13):1689. doi:10.1001/jama.284.13.1689
22. The Joint Commission. *Behavioral Health Care and Human Services.* Accessed March 17, 2023. https://www.jointcommission.org/what-we-offer/accreditation/health-care-settings/behavioral-health-care
23. Institute of Medicine (US). Committee on crossing the quality chasm: adaptation to mental health and addictive disorders. *Improving the Quality of Health Care for Mental and Substance-Use Conditions: Quality Chasm Series.* National Academies Press; 2006. Accessed July 15, 2022. http://www.ncbi.nlm.nih.gov/books/NBK19830/
24. Friedmann PD, Hendrickson JC, Gerstein DR, Zhang Z, Stein MD. Do mechanisms that link addiction treatment patients to primary care

influence subsequent utilization of emergency and hospital care? *Med Care.* 2006;44(1):8-15. doi:10.1097/01.mlr.0000188913.50489.77
25. Schermer CR, Moyers TB, Miller WR, Bloomfield LA. Trauma center brief interventions for alcohol disorders decrease subsequent driving under the influence arrests. *J Trauma Inj Infect Crit Care.* 2006;60(1):29-34. doi:10.1097/01.ta.0000199420.12322.5d
26. van Boekel LC, Brouwers EPM, van Weeghel J, Garretsen HFL. Stigma among health professionals towards patients with substance use disorders and its consequences for healthcare delivery: systematic review. *Drug Alcohol Depend.* 2013;131(1):23-35. doi:10.1016/j.drugalcdep.2013.02.018
27. McNeely J, Kumar PC, Rieckmann T, et al. Barriers and facilitators affecting the implementation of substance use screening in primary care clinics: a qualitative study of patients, providers, and staff. *Addict Sci Clin Pract.* 2018;13:8. doi:10.1186/s13722-018-0110-8
28. Governor's Medical Education Working Group on Prescription Drug Misuse. *Medical Education Core Competencies for the Prevention and Management of Prescription Drug Misuse.* Commonwealth of Massachusetts; 2015. Accessed March 17, 2023. https://www.mass.gov/files/documents/2017/01/vh/governors-medical-education-working-group-core-competencies.pdf
29. Association of American Medical Colleges. *How Academic Medicine is Addressing the Opioid Epidemic.* 2019. Accessed March 17, 2023. https://www.aamc.org/system/files/d/1/63-opioids_-_how_academic_medicine_is_addressing_the_opioid_epidemic_-_20190222.pdf
30. Wakeman SE, Pham-Kanter G, Baggett MV, Campbell EG. Medicine resident preparedness to diagnose and treat substance use disorders: impact of an enhanced curriculum. *Subst Abuse.* 2015;36(4):427-433. doi:10.1080/08897077.2014.962722
31. Accreditation Council for Graduate Medical Education. *Opioid Use Disorder.* Accessed July 3, 2022. https://www.acgme.org/meetings-and-educational-activities/opioid-use-disorder/
32. Urada D, Teruya C, Gelberg L, Rawson R. Integration of substance use disorder services with primary care: health center surveys and qualitative interviews. *Subst Abuse Treat Prev Policy.* 2014;9:15-15. doi:10.1186/1747-597X-9-15
33. Isaacson JH, Fleming M, Kraus M, Kahn R, Mundt M. A national survey of training in substance use disorders in residency programs. *J Stud Alcohol.* 2000;61(6):912-915. doi:10.15288/jsa.2000.61.912
34. Friedmann PD, McCullough D, Chin MH, Saitz R. Screening and intervention for alcohol problems. A national survey of primary care physicians and psychiatrists. *J Gen Intern Med.* 2000;15(2):84-91. doi:10.1046/j.1525-1497.2000.03379.x
35. Wakeman SE, Pham-Kanter G, Donelan K. Attitudes, practices, and preparedness to care for patients with substance use disorder: results from a survey of general internists. *Subst Abuse.* 2016;37(4):635-641. doi:10.1080/08897077.2016.1187240
36. Cohen P. The clinician's illusion. *Arch Gen Psychiatry.* 1984;41(12):1178. doi:10.1001/archpsyc.1984.01790230064010
37. Adams A, Ockene JK, Wheller EV, Hurley TG. Alcohol counseling: physicians will do it. *J Gen Intern Med.* 1998;13(10):692-698. doi:10.1046/j.1525-1497.1998.00206.x
38. Saitz R, Sullivan LM, Samet JH. Training community-based clinicians in screening and brief intervention for substance abuse problems: translating evidence into practice. *Subst Abuse.* 2000;21(1):21-31. doi:10.1080/08897070009511415
39. D'Onofrio G, Nadel ES, Degutis LC, et al. Improving emergency medicine residents' approach to patients with alcohol problems: a controlled educational trial. *Ann Emerg Med.* 2002;40(1):50-62. doi:10.1067/mem.2002.123693
40. Friedmann PD, Wilson D, Knudsen HK, et al. Effect of an organizational linkage intervention on staff perceptions of medication-assisted treatment and referral intentions in community corrections. *J Subst Abuse Treat.* 2015;50:50-58. doi:10.1016/j.jsat.2014.10.001
41. Alford DP, Carney BL, Jackson AH, et al. Promoting addiction medicine teaching through functional mentoring by co-training generalist chief residents with faculty mentors. *Subst Abuse.* 2018;39(3):377. doi:10.1080/08897077.2018.1439799
42. Roy P, Jackson AH, Baxter J, et al. Utilizing a faculty development program to promote safer opioid prescribing for chronic pain in internal medicine resident practices. *Pain Med.* 2019;20(4):707-716. doi:10.1093/pm/pny292
43. Alford DP, Bridden C, Jackson AH, et al. Promoting substance use education among generalist physicians: an evaluation of the Chief Resident Immersion Training (CRIT) Program. *J Gen Intern Med.* 2009;24(1):40-47. doi:10.1007/s11606-008-0819-2
44. Providers Clinical Support System. Accessed April 3, 2022. https://pcssnow.org/
45. Centers for Disease Control and Prevention. *CDC Guideline for Prescribing Opioids for Chronic Pain—United States, 2016.* Accessed April 3, 2022. https://www.cdc.gov/mmwr/volumes/65/rr/rr6501e1.htm
46. Chobanian & Avedisian School of Medicine. *Scope of Pain: Safer/Competent Opioid Prescribing Education.* Accessed April 3, 2022. https://www.scopeofpain.org/
47. Surgeon General.gov. *Facing Addiction in America: The Surgeon General's Spotlight on Opioids.* Accessed April 3, 2022. https://addiction.surgeongeneral.gov/
48. Massachusetts Medical Society. *New Opioid Prescribing Guidelines in Practice.* Accessed April 3, 2022. http://www.massmed.org/Continuing-Education-and-Events/Online-CME/Courses/New-Opioid-Prescribing-Guidelines/New-Opioid-Prescribing-Guidelines-in-Practice/
49. Garcia ME, Coffman J, Jordan A, Martin M. Lack of racial and ethnic diversity among addiction physicians. *J Gen Intern Med.* 2022;37(12):3214-3216. doi:10.1007/s11606-022-07405-8
50. Jordan A, Jegede O. Building outreach and diversity in the field of addictions. *Am J Addict.* 2020;29(5):413-417.
51. Center for Behavioral Health Statistics and Quality. *Racial/Ethnic Differences in Substance Use, Substance Use Disorders, and Substance Use Treatment Utilization among People Aged 12 or Older (2015-2019).* Substance Abuse and Mental Health Services Administration; 2021. https://www.samhsa.gov/data/sites/default/files/reports/rpt35326/2021NSDUHSUChartbook.pdf
52. Webb CP, Huecker M, Shreffler J, McKinley BS, Khan AM, Shaw I. Racial disparities in linkage to care among patients with substance use disorders. *J Subst Abuse Treat.* 2022;137. doi:10.1016/j.jsat.2021.108691
53. Schuler MS, Dick AW, Stein BD. Growing racial/ethnic disparities in buprenorphine distribution in the United States, 2007–2017. *Drug Alcohol Depend.* 2021;223:108710. doi:10.1016/j.drugalcdep.2021.108710
54. Jackson JR, Harle CA, Silverman RD, Simon K, Menachemi N. Characterizing variability in state-level regulations governing opioid treatment programs. *J Subst Abuse Treat.* 2020;115:108008. doi:10.1016/j.jsat.2020.108008
55. Lagisetty PA, Ross R, Bohnert A, Clay M, Maust DT. Buprenorphine treatment divide by race/ethnicity and payment. *JAMA Psychiatry.* 2019;76(9):979. doi:10.1001/jamapsychiatry.2019.0876
56. Friedman JR, Hansen H. Evaluation of increases in drug overdose mortality rates in the us by race and ethnicity before and during the COVID-19 pandemic. *JAMA Psychiatry.* 2022;79(4):379-381. doi:10.1001/jamapsychiatry.2022.0004
57. Overcoming Stigma. NAMI: National Alliance on Mental Illness. Accessed September 4, 2022. https://www.nami.org/Blogs/NAMI-Blog/October-2018/Overcoming-Stigma
58. Tsai AC, Kiang MV, Barnett ML, et al. Stigma as a fundamental hindrance to the United States opioid overdose crisis response. *PLOS Med.* 2019;16(11):e1002969. doi:10.1371/journal.pmed.1002969
59. Kimmel SD, Rosenmoss S, Bearnot B, et al. Northeast postacute medical facilities disproportionately reject referrals for patients with opioid use disorder. *Health Aff (Millwood).* 2022;41(3):434-444. doi:10.1377/hlthaff.2021.01242
60. Child Welfare Information Gateway. *Parental Substance Use as Child Abuse.* Accessed May 30, 2023. https://www.childwelfare.gov/pubPDFs/parentalsubstanceuse.pdf
61. *What Medications Disqualify a CMV Driver?* FMCSA. Accessed September 4, 2022. https://www.fmcsa.dot.gov/faq/what-medications-disqualify-cmv-driver

62. Feldman N. *Many "Recovery Houses" Won't Let Residents Use Medicine to Quit Opioids*. NPR. Accessed September 19, 2022. https://www.npr.org/sections/health-shots/2018/09/12/644685850/many-recovery-houses-wont-let-residents-use-medicine-to-quit-opioids
63. Harris AHS, Reeder RN, Ellerbe LS, Bowe TR. Validation of the treatment identification strategy of the HEDIS addiction quality measures: concordance with medical record review. *BMC Health Serv Res.* 2011;11:73-73. doi:10.1186/1472-6963-11-73
64. Abidi L, Oenema A, Nilsen P, Anderson P, van de Mheen D. Strategies to overcome barriers to implementation of alcohol screening and brief intervention in general practice: a Delphi study among healthcare professionals and addiction prevention experts. *Prev Sci.* 2016;17(6):689-699. doi:10.1007/s11121-016-0653-4
65. McLellan AT. Have we evaluated addiction treatment correctly? Implications from a chronic care perspective. *Addiction.* 2002;97(3):249-252. doi:10.1046/j.1360-0443.2002.00127.x
66. Schuler MS, Horowitz JA. Nursing students' attitudes toward and empathy for patients with substance use disorder following mentorship. *J Nurs Educ.* 2020;59(3):149-153. doi:10.3928/01484834-20200220-05
67. Finnell D, Sanchez M, Hansen B, et al. Changes in nursing students' attitudes and perceptions after receipt of enhanced substance use-related curricular content. *J Addict Nurs.* 2022;33(2):62-69. doi:10.1097/JAN.0000000000000427
68. Muzyk A, Mullan P, Andolsek KM, et al. An interprofessional substance use disorder course to improve students' educational outcomes and patients' treatment decisions. *Acad Med J Assoc Am Med Coll.* 2019;94(11):1792-1799. doi:10.1097/ACM.0000000000002854
69. Federal Register. *Confidentiality of Substance Use Disorder Patient Records.* Department of Health and Human Services; 2017. Accessed April 3, 2022. https://www.federalregister.gov/documents/2017/01/18/2017-00719/confidentiality-of-substance-use-disorder-patient-records
70. Schaper E, Padwa H, Urada D, Shoptaw S. Substance use disorder patient privacy and comprehensive care in integrated health care settings. *Psychol Serv.* 2016;13(1):105-109. doi:10.1037/a0037968
71. Wakeman SE, Friedmann P. *Outdated Privacy Law Limits Effective Substance Use Disorder Treatment: The Case Against 42 CFR Part 2.* Forefront Group; 2017. doi:10.1377/forefront.20170301.058969
72. One Hundred Fourteenth Congress of the United States of America. H. R. 34. GovInfo. 2016. Accessed April 3, 2022. https://www.govinfo.gov/content/pkg/BILLS-114hr34enr/pdf/BILLS-114hr34enr.pdf
73. Chan CA, Tetrault JM, Fiellin DA, Weimer MB. SOAPs and SUDs: patients with substance use disorders and what clinicians should know about the Cures Act. *J Addict Med.* 2022;16(2):141-142. doi:10.1097/ADM.0000000000000879
74. Wason K, Potter A, Alves J, et al. Addiction nursing competencies: a comprehensive toolkit for the addictions nurse. *J Nurs Adm.* 2021;51(9):424-429. doi:10.1097/NNA.0000000000001041
75. Jackson DS, Nguemeni Tiako MJ, Jordan A. Disparities in addiction treatment: learning from the past to forge an equitable future. *Med Clin North Am.* 2022;106(1):29-41. doi:10.1016/j.mcna.2021.08.008
76. Gourevitch MN, Chatterji P, Deb N, Schoenbaum EE, Turner BJ. On-site medical care in methadone maintenance: associations with health care use and expenditures. *J Subst Abuse Treat.* 2007;32(2):143-151. doi:10.1016/j.jsat.2006.07.008
77. Saitz R, Horton NJ, Larson MJ, Winter M, Samet JH. Primary medical care and reductions in addiction severity: a prospective cohort study. *Addiction.* 2005;100(1):70-78. doi:10.1111/j.1360-0443.2005.00916.x
78. Alford DP, LaBelle CT, Kretsch N, et al. Collaborative care of opioid-addicted patients in primary care using buprenorphine: five-year experience. *Arch Intern Med.* 2011;171(5):425-431. doi:10.1001/archinternmed.2010.541
79. Bodenheimer T. Disease management in the American market. *BMJ.* 2000;320(7234):563-566. doi:10.1136/bmj.320.7234.563
80. Saitz R, Mulvey KP, Samet JH. The substance-abusing patient and primary care: linkage via the addiction treatment system? *Subst Abuse.* 1997;18(4):187-195. doi:10.1080/08897079709511365
81. Walley AY, Paasche-Orlow M, Lee EC, et al. Acute care hospital utilization among medical inpatients discharged with a substance use disorder diagnosis. *J Addict Med.* 2012;6(1):50-56. doi:10.1097/ADM.0b013e318231de51
82. Ducharme LJ, Chandler RK, Harris AHS. Implementing effective substance abuse treatments in general medical settings: mapping the research terrain. *J Subst Abuse Treat.* 2016;60:110-118. doi:10.1016/j.jsat.2015.06.020
83. McKay JR. Continuing care research: what we have learned and where we are going. *J Subst Abuse Treat.* 2009;36(2):131-145. doi:10.1016/j.jsat.2008.10.004
84. Umbricht-Schneiter A, Ginn DH, Pabst KM, Bigelow GE. Providing medical care to methadone clinic patients: referral vs on-site care. *Am J Public Health.* 1994;84(2):207-210. doi:10.2105/ajph.84.2.207
85. Teitelbaum M, Walker A, Gabay M. *Analysis of Barriers to the Delivery of Integrated Primary Care Services and Substance Abuse Treatment: Case Studies of Nine Linkage Program Projects.* Health Resources and Services Administration and Abt Associates, Inc; 1992.
86. Substance Abuse and Mental Health Services Administration. *Federal Guidelines for Opioid Treatment Programs.* Substance Abuse and Mental Health Services Administration; 2015. Accessed September 6, 2022. https://store.samhsa.gov/sites/default/files/d7/priv/pep15-fedguideotp.pdf
87. Korthuis PT, McCarty D, Weimer M, et al. Primary care-based models for the treatment of opioid use disorder: a scoping review. *Ann Intern Med.* 2017;166(4):268-278. doi:10.7326/M16-2149
88. Willenbring ML, Olson DH. A randomized trial of integrated outpatient treatment for medically ill alcoholic men. *Arch Intern Med.* 1999;159(16):1946. doi:10.1001/archinte.159.16.1946
89. Anton RF, O'Malley SS, Ciraulo DA, et al. Combined pharmacotherapies and behavioral interventions for alcohol dependence. *JAMA.* 2006;295(17):2003. doi:10.1001/jama.295.17.2003
90. Center for Substance Abuse Treatment. *Substance Abuse Treatment for Persons with Co-Occurring Disorders.* Substance Abuse and Mental Health Services Administration (US); 2005. Accessed August 10, 2022. http://www.ncbi.nlm.nih.gov/books/NBK64197/
91. Willenbring M, Olson D, Bielinski J. Treatment of medically ill alcoholics in the primary-care setting. In: Beresford T, Gomberg E, eds. *Alcohol and Aging.* Oxford University Press; 1995:249-259.
92. Saitz R, Cheng DM, Winter M, et al. Chronic care management for dependence on alcohol and other drugs: the AHEAD randomized trial. *JAMA.* 2013;310(11):1156-1167. doi:10.1001/jama.2013.277609
93. Watkins KE, Ober AJ, Lamp K, et al. Collaborative care for opioid and alcohol use disorders in primary care: the SUMMIT randomized clinical trial. *JAMA Intern Med.* 2017;177(10):1480-1488. doi:10.1001/jamainternmed.2017.3947
94. Fleming MF, Mundt MP, French MT, Manwell LB, Stauffacher EA, Barry KL. Benefit-cost analysis of brief physician advice with problem drinkers in primary care settings. *Med Care.* 2000;38(1):7-18. doi:10.1097/00005650-200001000-00003
95. Reiff-Hekking S, Ockene JK, Hurley TG, Reed GW. Brief physician and nurse practitioner–delivered counseling for high-risk drinking. *J Gen Intern Med.* 2005;20(1):7-13. doi:10.1111/j.1525-1497.2005.21240.x
96. Saitz R, Horton NJ, Sullivan LM, Moskowitz MA, Samet JH. Addressing alcohol problems in primary care: a cluster randomized, controlled trial of a systems intervention: the screening and intervention in primary care (SIP) study. *Ann Intern Med.* 2003;138(5):372. doi:10.7326/0003-4819-138-5-200303040-00006
97. Geirsson M, Bendtsen P, Spak F. Attitudes of Swedish general practitioners and nurses to working with lifestyle change, with special reference to alcohol consumption. *Alcohol Alcohol.* 2005;40(5):388-393. doi:10.1093/alcalc/agh185
98. Lee JD, Grossman E, Huben L, et al. Extended-release naltrexone plus medical management alcohol treatment in primary care: findings at 15 months. *J Subst Abuse Treat.* 2012;43(4):458-462. doi:10.1016/j.jsat.2012.08.012
99. Oslin DW, Lynch KG, Maisto SA, et al. A randomized clinical trial of alcohol care management delivered in Department of Veterans Affairs primary care clinics versus specialty addiction treatment. *J Gen Intern Med.* 2014;29(1):162-168. doi:10.1007/s11606-013-2625-8

100. Fiellin DA, Barry DT, Sullivan LE, et al. A randomized trial of cognitive behavioral therapy in primary care-based buprenorphine. *Am J Med.* 2013;126(1):74.e11-74.e17. doi:10.1016/j.amjmed.2012.07.005
101. Barry DT, Moore BA, Pantalon MV, et al. Patient satisfaction with primary care office-based buprenorphine/naloxone treatment. *J Gen Intern Med.* 2007;22(2):242-245. doi:10.1007/s11606-006-0050-y
102. Merrill JO, Jackson TR, Schulman BA, et al. Methadone medical maintenance in primary care. An implementation evaluation. *J Gen Intern Med.* 2005;20(4):344-349. doi:10.1111/j.1525-1497.2005.04028.x
103. Samet JH, Botticelli M, Bharel M. Methadone in primary care—one small step for congress, one giant leap for addiction treatment. *N Engl J Med.* 2018;379(1):7-8. doi:10.1056/NEJMp1803982
104. Methadone Take-Home Flexibilities Extension Guidance, SAMHSA. 2023. Accessed January 20, 2023. https://www.samhsa.gov/medication-assisted-treatment/statutes-regulations-guidelines/methadone-guidance
105. Brothers S, Viera A, Heimer R. Changes in methadone program practices and fatal methadone overdose rates in Connecticut during COVID-19. *J Subst Abuse Treat.* 2021;131:108449. doi:10.1016/j.jsat.2021.108449
106. Joseph G, Torres-Lockhart K, Stein MR, Mund PA, Nahvi S. Reimagining patient-centered care in opioid treatment programs: lessons from the Bronx during COVID-19. *J Subst Abuse Treat.* 2020;122. doi:10.1016/j.jsat.2020.108219
107. Centers for Disease Control and Prevention (CDC). Integrated prevention services for HIV infection, viral hepatitis, sexually transmitted diseases, and tuberculosis for persons who use drugs illicitly: summary guidance from CDC and the U.S. Department of Health and Human Services. *MMWR Recomm Rep.* 2012;61(RR-5):1-40.
108. Butner JL, Gupta N, Fabian C, Henry S, Shi JM, Tetrault JM. Onsite treatment of HCV infection with direct acting antivirals within an opioid treatment program. *J Subst Abuse Treat.* 2017;75:49-53. doi:10.1016/j.jsat.2016.12.014
109. Haque LY, Butner JL, Shi JM, et al. Primary care associated with follow up viral load testing in patients cured of hepatitis c infection with direct acting antivirals at a multidisciplinary addiction treatment program: insights from a real-world setting. *J Addict Med.* 2022;16(3):333-339. doi:10.1097/ADM.0000000000000910
110. Jiang X, Vouri SM, Diaby V, Lo-Ciganic W, Parker R, Park H. Health care utilization and costs associated with direct-acting antivirals for patients with substance use disorders and chronic hepatitis C. *J Manag Care Spec Pharm.* 2021;27(10):1388-1402. doi:10.18553/jmcp.2021.27.10.1388
111. Lasser KE, Heinz A, Battisti L, et al. A hepatitis c treatment program based in a safety-net hospital patient-centered medical home. *Ann Fam Med.* 2017;15(3):258-261. doi:10.1370/afm.2069
112. McGinn TG, Gardenier D, McGinn LK, et al. Treating chronic hepatitis c in the primary care setting. *Semin Liver Dis.* 2005;25(01):65-71. doi:10.1055/s-2005-864782
113. Litwin AH, Kunins HV, Berg KM, et al. Hepatitis C management by addiction medicine physicians: results from a national survey. *J Subst Abuse Treat.* 2007;33(1):99-105. doi:10.1016/j.jsat.2006.12.001
114. Sylvestre DL, Clements BJ. Adherence to hepatitis C treatment in recovering heroin users maintained on methadone. *Eur J Gastroenterol Hepatol.* 2007;19(9):741-747. doi:10.1097/meg.0b013e3281bcb8d8
115. Stein MR, Soloway IJ, Jefferson KS, Roose RJ, Arnsten JH, Litwin AH. Concurrent group treatment for hepatitis C: implementation and outcomes in a methadone maintenance treatment program. *J Subst Abuse Treat.* 2012;43(4):424-432. doi:10.1016/j.jsat.2012.08.007
116. Harris KA Jr, Arnsten JH, Litwin AH. Successful integration of hepatitis C evaluation and treatment services with methadone maintenance. *J Addict Med.* 2010;4(1):20-26. doi:10.1097/ADM.0b013e3181add3de
117. Martinez AD, Dimova R, Marks KM, et al. Integrated internist-addiction medicine-hepatology model for hepatitis C management for individuals on methadone maintenance. *J Viral Hepat.* 2012;19(1):47-54. doi:10.1111/j.1365-2893.2010.01411.x
118. O'Connor PG, Shi JM, Henry S, Durante AJ, Friedman L, Selwyn PA. Tuberculosis chemoprophylaxis using a liquid isoniazid-methadone admixture for drug users in methadone maintenance. *Addiction.* 1999;94(7):1071-1075. doi:10.1046/j.1360-0443.1999.947107112.x
119. Friedmann PD, Alexander JA, Jin L, D'Aunno TA. On-site primary care and mental health services in outpatient drug abuse treatment units. *J Behav Health Serv Res.* 1999;26(1):80-94. doi:10.1007/bf02287796
120. Saxon AJ, Malte CA, Sloan KL, et al. Randomized trial of onsite versus referral primary medical care for veterans in addictions treatment. *Med Care.* 2006;44(4):334-342. doi:10.1097/01.mlr.0000204052.95507.5c
121. Parthasarathy S, Mertens J, Moore C, Weisner C. Utilization and cost impact of integrating substance abuse treatment and primary care. *Med Care.* 2003;41(3):357-367. doi:10.1097/01.mlr.0000053018.20700.56
122. Baker F. *Coordination of Alcohol, Drug Abuse, and Mental Health Services.* (Publication No. SMA 00–3360, Technical Assistance Publication Series, No. 4). CSAT, Substance Abuse and Mental Health Services Administration; 1991
123. Center for Substance Abuse Treatment. *Comprehensive Case Management for Substance Abuse Treatment Protocol (TIP) Series, No 27.* Center for Substance Abuse Treatment; 2000.
124. Harvey LM, Fan W, Cano MÁ, et al. Psychosocial intervention utilization and substance abuse treatment outcomes in a multisite sample of individuals who use opioids. *J Subst Abuse Treat.* 2020;112:68-75. doi:10.1016/j.jsat.2020.01.016
125. Brooner RK, Kidorf MS, King VL, et al. Managing psychiatric comorbidity within versus outside of methadone treatment settings: a randomized and controlled evaluation. *Addiction.* 2013;108(11):1942-1951. doi:10.1111/add.12269
126. Simeone C, Shapiro B, Lum PJ. Integrated HIV care is associated with improved engagement in treatment in an urban methadone clinic. *Addict Sci Clin Pract.* 2017;12(1):19. doi:10.1186/s13722-017-0084-y
127. Drainoni ML, Farrell C, Sorensen-Alawad A, Palmisano JN, Chaisson C, Walley AY. Patient perspectives of an integrated program of medical care and substance use treatment. *AIDS Patient Care STDs.* 2014;28(2):71-81. doi:10.1089/apc.2013.0179
128. Lucas GM. Clinic-based treatment of opioid-dependent HIV-infected patients versus referral to an opioid treatment program. *Ann Intern Med.* 2010;152(11):704. doi:10.7326/0003-4819-152-11-201006010-00003
129. Laine C. Regular outpatient medical and drug abuse care and subsequent hospitalization of persons who use illicit drugs. *JAMA.* 2001;285(18):2355. doi:10.1001/jama.285.18.2355
130. Egan JE, Netherland J, Gass J, Finkelstein R, Weiss L. Patient perspectives on buprenorphine/naloxone treatment in the context of HIV care. *J Acquir Immune Defic Syndr.* 2011;56(Supplement 1):S46-S53. doi:10.1097/qai.0b013e3182097561
131. Wagner EH. The role of patient care teams in chronic disease management. *BMJ.* 2000;320(7234):569-572. doi:10.1136/bmj.320.7234.569
132. Wagner EH, Austin BT, Korff MV. Organizing care for patients with chronic illness. *Milbank Q.* 1996;74(4):511. doi:10.2307/3350391
133. Kim TW, Saitz R, Cheng DM, Winter MR, Witas J, Samet JH. Effect of quality chronic disease management for alcohol and drug dependence on addiction outcomes. *J Subst Abuse Treat.* 2012;43(4):389-396. doi:10.1016/j.jsat.2012.06.001
134. Hunter SB, Schwartz RP, Friedmann PD. Introduction to the special issue on the studies on the implementation of integrated models of alcohol, tobacco, and/or drug use interventions and medical care. *J Subst Abuse Treat.* 2016;60:1-5. doi:10.1016/j.jsat.2015.10.001
135. LaBelle CT, Han SC, Bergeron A, Samet JH. Office-based opioid treatment with buprenorphine (Obot-b): statewide implementation of the Massachusetts collaborative care model in community health centers. *J Subst Abuse Treat.* 2016;60:6-13. doi:10.1016/j.jsat.2015.06.010
136. Upshur C, Weinreb L, Bharel M, Reed G, Frisard C. A randomized control trial of a chronic care intervention for homeless women with alcohol use problems. *J Subst Abuse Treat.* 2015;51:19-29. doi:10.1016/j.jsat.2014.11.001
137. Chaple M, Sacks S, Randell J, Kang B. A technical assistance framework to facilitate the delivery of integrated behavioral health services in federally qualified health centers (FQHCs). *J Subst Abuse Treat.* 2016;60:62-69. doi:10.1016/j.jsat.2015.08.006
138. McLellan AT, Starrels JL, Tai B, et al. Can substance use disorders be managed using the chronic care model? Review and recommendations from a NIDA consensus group. *Public Health Rev.* 2014;35(2). doi:10.1007/BF03391707

139. Saitz R, Mulvey KP, Plough A, Samet JH. Physician unawareness of serious substance abuse. *Am J Drug Alcohol Abuse.* 1997;23(3):343-354. doi:10.3109/00952999709016881
140. National Center on Addiction and Substance Abuse. *Missed Opportunity: National Survey of Primary Care Physicians and Patients on Substance Abuse.* Columbia University; 2000. Accessed January 22, 2023. https://files.eric.ed.gov/fulltext/ED452442.pdf
141. Vanderplasschen W, Rapp RC, Wolf JR, Broekaert E. The development and implementation of case management for substance use disorders in North America and Europe. *Psychiatr Serv Wash DC.* 2004;55(8):913-922. doi:10.1176/appi.ps.55.8.913
142. McLellan AT, Weinstein RL, Shen Q, Kendig C, Levine M. Improving continuity of care in a public addiction treatment system with clinical case management. *Am J Addict.* 2005;14(5):426-440. doi:10.1080/10550490500247099
143. Jakubowski A, Fox A. Defining low-threshold buprenorphine treatment. *J Addict Med.* 2020;14(2):95-98. doi:10.1097/ADM.0000000000000555
144. Harvey L, Taylor JL, Assoumou SA, et al. Sexually transmitted and blood-borne infections among patients presenting to a low-barrier substance use disorder medication clinic. *J Addict Med.* 2021;15(6):461-467. doi:10.1097/ADM.0000000000000801
145. Bhatraju EP, Grossman E, Tofighi B, et al. Public sector low threshold office-based buprenorphine treatment: outcomes at year 7. *Addict Sci Clin Pract.* 2017;12:7. doi:10.1186/s13722-017-0072-2
146. Roy PJ, Choi S, Bernstein E, Walley AY. Appointment wait-times and arrival for patients at a low-barrier access addiction clinic. *J Subst Abuse Treat.* 2020;114:108011. doi:10.1016/j.jsat.2020.108011
147. Sullivan RW, Szczesniak LM, Wojcik SM. Bridge clinic buprenorphine program decreases emergency department visits. *J Subst Abuse Treat.* 2021;130:108410. doi:10.1016/j.jsat.2021.108410
148. Snow RL, Simon RE, Jack HE, Oller D, Kehoe L, Wakeman SE. Patient experiences with a transitional, low-threshold clinic for the treatment of substance use disorder: a qualitative study of a bridge clinic. *J Subst Abuse Treat.* 2019;107:1-7. doi:10.1016/j.jsat.2019.09.003
149. Taylor JL, Laks J, Christine PJ, et al. Bridge clinic implementation of "72-hour rule" methadone for opioid withdrawal management: impact on opioid treatment program linkage and retention in care. *Drug Alcohol Depend.* 2022;236:109497. doi:10.1016/j.drugalcdep.2022.109497
150. Laks J, Kehoe J, Farrell NM, et al. Methadone initiation in a bridge clinic for opioid withdrawal and opioid treatment program linkage: a case report applying the 72-hour rule. *Addict Sci Clin Pract.* 2021;16(1):73. doi:10.1186/s13722-021-00279-x
151. *Why Would You Give Clean Needles to Someone Who Uses Drugs?* 2022. Accessed September 6, 2022. https://www.opensocietyfoundations.org/explainers/what-harm-reduction
152. Aspinall EJ, Nambiar D, Goldberg DJ, et al. Are needle and syringe programmes associated with a reduction in HIV transmission among people who inject drugs: a systematic review and meta-analysis. *Int J Epidemiol.* 2014;43(1):235-248. doi:10.1093/ije/dyt243
153. Hagan H, McGough JP, Thiede H, Hopkins S, Duchin J, Alexander ER. Reduced injection frequency and increased entry and retention in drug treatment associated with needle-exchange participation in Seattle drug injectors. *J Subst Abuse Treat.* 2000;19(3):247-252. doi:10.1016/s0740-5472(00)00104-5
154. Samuels EA, Bailer DA, Yolken A. Overdose prevention centers: an essential strategy to address the overdose crisis. *JAMA Netw Open.* 2022;5(7):e2222153. doi:10.1001/jamanetworkopen.2022.22153
155. Harocopos A, Gibson BE, Saha N, et al. First 2 months of operation at first publicly recognized overdose prevention centers in US. *JAMA Netw Open.* 2022;5(7):e2222149. doi:10.1001/jamanetworkopen.2022.22149
156. Marshall BDL, Milloy MJ, Wood E, Montaner JSG, Kerr T. Reduction in overdose mortality after the opening of North America's first medically supervised safer injecting facility: a retrospective population-based study. *Lancet.* 2011;377(9775):1429-1437. doi:10.1016/S0140-6736(10)62353-7
157. Wakeman SE, Kane M, Powell E, Howard S, Shaw C, Regan S. Impact of inpatient addiction consultation on hospital readmission. *J Gen Intern Med.* 2021;36(7):2161-2163. doi:10.1007/s11606-020-05966-0
158. Wakeman SE, Metlay JP, Chang Y, Herman GE, Rigotti NA. Inpatient addiction consultation for hospitalized patients increases post-discharge abstinence and reduces addiction severity. *J Gen Intern Med.* 2017;32(8):909-916. doi:10.1007/s11606-017-4077-z
159. Bahji A, Reshetukha T, Newman A, et al. The Substance Treatment and Recovery Team (START): measuring the effectiveness and feasibility of an inpatient addiction consult service at an academic general hospital. *Gen Hosp Psychiatry.* 2020;67:160-161. doi:10.1016/j.genhosppsych.2020.05.009
160. Weinstein ZM, Wakeman SE, Nolan S. Inpatient addiction consult service: expertise for hospitalized patients with complex addiction problems. *Med Clin North Am.* 2018;102(4):587-601. doi:10.1016/j.mcna.2018.03.001
161. Marks LR, Munigala S, Warren DK, Liang SY, Schwarz ES, Durkin MJ. Addiction medicine consultations reduce readmission rates for patients with serious infections from opioid use disorder. *Clin Infect Dis.* 2019;68(11):1935-1937. doi:10.1093/cid/ciy924
162. Priest KC, McCarty D. Role of the hospital in the 21st century opioid overdose epidemic: the addiction medicine consult service. *J Addict Med.* 2019;13(2):104-112. doi:10.1097/ADM.0000000000000496
163. Wakeman SE, Kanter GP, Donelan K. Institutional substance use disorder intervention improves general internist preparedness, attitudes, and clinical practice. *J Addict Med.* 2017;11(4):308-314. doi:10.1097/ADM.0000000000000314
164. McNeil R, Small W, Wood E, Kerr T. Hospitals as a "risk environment": an ethno-epidemiological study of voluntary and involuntary discharge from hospital against medical advice among people who inject drugs. *Soc Sci Med. 1982*;2014(105):59-66. doi:10.1016/j.socscimed.2014.01.010
165. Liebschutz JM, Crooks D, Herman D, et al. Buprenorphine treatment for hospitalized, opioid-dependent patients: a randomized clinical trial. *JAMA Intern Med.* 2014;174(8):1369-1376. doi:10.1001/jamainternmed.2014.2556
166. Trowbridge P, Weinstein ZM, Kerensky T, et al. Addiction consultation services—linking hospitalized patients to outpatient addiction treatment. *J Subst Abuse Treat.* 2017;79:1-5. doi:10.1016/j.jsat.2017.05.007
167. Tierney HR, Rowe CL, Coffa DA, Sarnaik S, Coffin PO, Snyder HR. Inpatient opioid use disorder treatment by generalists is associated with linkage to opioid treatment programs after discharge. *J Addict Med.* 2022;16(2):169-176. doi:10.1097/ADM.0000000000000851
168. Weimer MB, Falker CG, Seval N, et al. The need for multidisciplinary hospital teams for injection drug use-related infective endocarditis. *J Addict Med.* 2022;16(4):375-378. doi:10.1097/ADM.0000000000000916
169. Cortes-Penfield N, Cawcutt K, Alexander BT, Karre VMM, Balasanova AA. A proposal for addiction and infectious diseases specialist collaboration to improve care for patients with opioid use disorder and injection drug use-associated infective endocarditis. *J Addict Med.* 2022;16(4):392-395. doi:10.1097/ADM.0000000000000936
170. Fanucchi LC, Walsh SL, Thornton AC, Nuzzo PA, Lofwall MR. Outpatient parenteral antimicrobial therapy plus buprenorphine for opioid use disorder and severe injection-related infections. *Clin Infect Dis.* 2020;70(6):1226-1229. doi:10.1093/cid/ciz654
171. D'Onofrio G, O'Connor PG, Pantalon MV, et al. Emergency department-initiated buprenorphine/naloxone treatment for opioid dependence: a randomized clinical trial. *JAMA.* 2015;313(16):1636-1644. doi:10.1001/jama.2015.3474
172. Jennings LK, Lane S, McCauley J, et al. Retention in treatment after emergency department-initiated buprenorphine. *J Emerg Med.* 2021;61(3):211-221. doi:10.1016/j.jemermed.2021.04.007
173. D'Onofrio G, Chawarski MC, O'Connor PG, et al. Emergency department-initiated buprenorphine for opioid dependence with continuation in primary care: outcomes during and after intervention. *J Gen Intern Med.* 2017;32(6):660-666. doi:10.1007/s11606-017-3993-2
174. Fiellin DA, Schottenfeld RS, Cutter CJ, Moore BA, Barry DT, O'Connor PG. Primary care–based buprenorphine taper vs maintenance therapy for prescription opioid dependence: a randomized clinical trial. *JAMA Intern Med.* 2014;174(12):1947-1954. doi:10.1001/jamainternmed.2014.5302

175. Hawk K, Hoppe J, Ketcham E, et al. Consensus recommendations on the treatment of opioid use disorder in the emergency department. *Ann Emerg Med.* 2021;78(3):434-442. doi:10.1016/j.annemergmed.2021.04.023
176. Butler K, Chavez T, Wakeman S, et al. Nudging emergency department initiated addiction treatment. *J Addict Med.* 2022;16(4):e234-e239. doi:10.1097/ADM.0000000000000926
177. Samet JH, Saitz R, Larson MJ. A case for enhanced linkage of substance abusers to primary medical care. *Subst Abuse.* 1996;17(4):181-192. doi:10.1080/08897079609444748
178. Friedmann PD, Lemon SC, Stein MD, Etheridge RM, D'Aunno TA. Linkage to medical services in the drug abuse treatment outcome study. *Med Care.* 2001;39(3):284-295. doi:10.1097/00005650-200103000-00008
179. Samet JH, Larson MJ, Horton NJ, Doyle K, Winter M, Saitz R. Linking alcohol- and drug-dependent adults to primary medical care: a randomized controlled trial of a multi-disciplinary health intervention in a detoxification unit. *Addiction.* 2003;98(4):509-516. doi:10.1046/j.1360-0443.2003.00328.x
180. Brindis C, Pfeffer R, Wolfe A. A case management program for chemically dependent clients with multiple needs. *J Case Manag.* 1995;4(1):22-28.
181. Friedmann PD, D'Aunno TA, Jin L, Alexander JA. Medical and psychosocial services in drug abuse treatment: do stronger linkages promote client utilization? *Health Serv Res.* 2000;35(2):443-465.
182. Shwartz M, Baker G, Mulvey KP, Plough A. Improving publicly funded substance abuse treatment: the value of case management. *Am J Public Health.* 1997;87(10):1659-1664. doi:10.2105/ajph.87.10.1659
183. Islam MM, Topp L, Conigrave KM, et al. Linkage into specialist hepatitis C treatment services of injecting drug users attending a needle syringe program-based primary healthcare centre. *J Subst Abuse Treat.* 2012;43(4):440-445. doi:10.1016/j.jsat.2012.07.007
184. Komaromy M, Duhigg D, Metcalf A, et al. Project ECHO (Extension for Community Healthcare Outcomes): a new model for educating primary care providers about treatment of substance use disorders. *Subst Abuse.* 2016;37(1):20-24. doi:10.1080/08897077.2015.1129388
185. *Medicare Payment Policies During COVID-19.* Telehealth.HHS.gov. Accessed September 5, 2022. https://telehealth.hhs.gov/providers/billing-and-reimbursement/medicare-payment-policies-during-covid-19/
186. Drug Enforcement Administration. *Use of Telephone Evaluations to Initiate Buprenorphine Prescribing.* Accessed September 5, 2022. https://www.deadiversion.usdoj.gov/GDP/(DEA-DC-022)(DEA068)%20DEA%20SAMHSA%20buprenorphine%20telemedicine%20%20(Final)%20+Esign.pdf
187. Jones C, Shoff C, Hodges K, et al. Receipt of telehealth services, receipt and retention of medications for opioid use disorder, and medically treated overdose among Medicare beneficiaries before and during the Covid-19 pandemic. *JAMA Psychiatry.* 2022;79(10):981-992. doi:10.1001/jamapsychiatry.2022.2284
188. O'toole TP, Conde-Martel A, Gibbon JL, Hanusa BH, Freyder PJ, Fine MJ. Substance-abusing urban homeless in the late 1990s: how do they differ from non-substance-abusing homeless persons? *J Urban Health Bull N Y Acad Med.* 2004;81(4):606-617. doi:10.1093/jurban/jth144
189. Alford DP, LaBelle CT, Richardson JM, et al. Treating homeless opioid dependent patients with buprenorphine in an office-based setting. *J Gen Intern Med.* 2007;22(2):171-176. doi:10.1007/s11606-006-0023-1
190. Carver H, Ring N, Miler J, Parkes T. What constitutes effective problematic substance use treatment from the perspective of people who are homeless? A systematic review and meta-ethnography. *Harm Reduct J.* 2020;17(1):10. doi:10.1186/s12954-020-0356-9
191. Fisk D, Rakfeldt J, McCormack E. Assertive outreach: an effective strategy for engaging homeless persons with substance use disorders into treatment. *Am J Drug Alcohol Abuse.* 2006;32(3):479-486. doi:10.1080/00952990600754006
192. Miescher A, Galanter M. Shelter-based treatment of the homeless alcoholic. *J Subst Abuse Treat.* 1996;13(2):135-140. doi:10.1016/0740-5472(96)00034-7
193. Fine DR, Weinstock K, Plakas I, et al. Experience with a mobile addiction program among people experiencing homelessness. *J Health Care Poor Underserved.* 2021;32(3):1145-1154. doi:10.1353/hpu.2021.0119
194. Rosenblum A, Nuttbrock L, McQuistion H, Magura S, Joseph H. Medical outreach to homeless substance users in New York City: preliminary results. *Subst Use Misuse.* 2002;37(8-10):1269-1273. doi:10.1081/ja-120004184
195. Regis C, Gaeta JM, Mackin S, Baggett TP, Quinlan J, Taveras EM. Community care in reach: mobilizing harm reduction and addiction treatment services for vulnerable populations. *Front Public Health.* 2020;8:501. doi:10.3389/fpubh.2020.00501
196. Fazel S, Bains P, Doll H. Substance abuse and dependence in prisoners: a systematic review. *Addiction.* 2006;101(2):181-191. doi:10.1111/j.1360-0443.2006.01316.x
197. Rich JD, Boutwell AE, Shield DC, et al. Attitudes and practices regarding the use of methadone in US state and federal prisons. *J Urban Health.* 2005;82(3):411-419. doi:10.1093/jurban/jti072
198. Weizman S, Perez J, Manoff I, Baney M, El-Sabawi T. *National Snapshot: Access to Medications for Opioid Use Disorder in U.S. Jails And Prisons.* O'Neill Institute for National and Global Health Law at Georgetown Law Center; 2021:32.
199. Wang EA, Wang Y, Krumholz HM. A high risk of hospitalization following release from correctional facilities in Medicare beneficiaries: a retrospective matched cohort study, 2002 to 2010. *JAMA Intern Med.* 2013;173(17):1621-1628. doi:10.1001/jamainternmed.2013.9008
200. Chandler RK, Finger MS, Farabee D, et al. The SOMATICS collaborative: Introduction to a National Institute on Drug Abuse cooperative study of pharmacotherapy for opioid treatment in criminal justice settings. *Contemp Clin Trials.* 2016;48:166-172. doi:10.1016/j.cct.2016.05.003
201. Binswanger IA, Heagerty PJ, Koepsell TD. Release from prison—a high risk of death for former inmates. *N Engl J Med.* 2007;9.
202. Rich JD, McKenzie M, Larney S, et al. Methadone continuation versus forced withdrawal on incarceration in a combined US prison and jail: a randomised, open-label trial. *Lancet.* 2015;386(9991):350-359. doi:10.1016/S0140-6736(14)62338-2
203. Zaller N, McKenzie M, Friedmann PD, Green TC, McGowan S, Rich JD. Initiation of buprenorphine during incarceration and retention in treatment upon release. *J Subst Abuse Treat.* 2013;45(2):222-226. doi:10.1016/j.jsat.2013.02.005
204. Evans EA, Wilson D, Friedmann PD. Recidivism and mortality after in-jail buprenorphine treatment for opioid use disorder. *Drug Alcohol Depend.* 2022;231:109254. doi:10.1016/j.drugalcdep.2021.109254
205. Boyd AT, Song DL, Meyer JP, Altice FL. Emergency department use among HIV-infected released jail detainees. *J Urban Health.* 2015;92(1):108-135. doi:10.1007/s11524-014-9905-4
206. Session Law—Acts of 2018 Chapter 208. Accessed July 14, 2022. https://malegislature.gov/Laws/SessionLaws/Acts/2018/Chapter208
207. Ferguson WJ, Johnston J, Clarke JG, et al. Advancing the implementation and sustainment of medication assisted treatment for opioid use disorders in prisons and jails. *Health Justice.* 2019;7(1):19. doi:10.1186/s40352-019-0100-2
208. Saia KA, Schiff D, Wachman EM, et al. Caring for pregnant women with opioid use disorder in the USA: expanding and improving treatment. *Curr Obstet Gynecol Rep.* 2016;5:257-263. doi:10.1007/s13669-016-0168-9
209. Saia K, Bagley SM, Wachman EM, Patel PP, Nadas MD, Brogly SB. Prenatal treatment for opioid dependency: observations from a large inner-city clinic. *Addict Sci Clin Pract.* 2017;12:5. doi:10.1186/s13722-016-0070-9
210. Ramage M, Tak C, Goodman D, Johnson E, Barber C, Jones H. Improving access to care through Advanced Practice Registered Nurses: focus on perinatal patients with opioid use disorder. *J Adv Nurs.* 2021;77(1):4-10.
211. Lim JK, Earlywine JJ, Bagley SM, Marshall BDL, Hadland SE. Polysubstance involvement in opioid overdose deaths in adolescents and young adults, 1999–2018. *JAMA Pediatr.* 2021;175(2):194-196. doi:10.1001/jamapediatrics.2020.5035
212. Bagley SM, Hadland SE, Schoenberger SF, et al. Integrating substance use care into primary care for adolescents and young adults: lessons learned. *J Subst Abuse Treat.* 2021;129:108376. doi:10.1016/j.jsat.2021.108376
213. Wenren LM, Rodean J, Zima BT, Bagley SM, Nurani A, Hadland S. 33. Treatment initiation and engagement for youth with substance use disorders. *J Adolesc Health.* 2022;70(4):S18. doi:10.1016/j.jadohealth.2022.01.146

214. Levy S, Botticelli M. Moving to a medical model of substance use treatment of youth. *Pediatrics.* 2021;147(Suppl. 2):S262-S264. doi:10.1542/peds.2020-023523J
215. Hawke LD, Mehra K, Settipani C, et al. What makes mental health and substance use services youth friendly? A scoping review of literature. *BMC Health Serv Res.* 2019;19(1):257. doi:10.1186/s12913-019-4066-5
216. Ventura AS, Bagley SM. To improve substance use disorder prevention, treatment and recovery: engage the family. *J Addict Med.* 2017;11(5):339-341. doi:10.1097/ADM.0000000000000331
217. Buresh M, Stern R, Rastegar D. Treatment of opioid use disorder in primary care. *BMJ.* 2021;373:n784. doi:10.1136/bmj.n784
218. Weisner C, Schmidt LA. Expanding the frame of health services research in the drug abuse field. *Health Serv Res.* 1995;30(5):707-726.
219. Guerrero E, Aarons G, Palinkas L. Organizational capacity for service integration in community-based addiction health services. *AJPH.* 2014;104(4):e40-e47. Accessed August 8, 2022. https://ajph.aphapublications.org/doi/abs/10.2105/AJPH.2013.301842
220. Jones CM, McCance-Katz EF. Co-occurring substance use and mental disorders among adults with opioid use disorder. *Drug Alcohol Depend.* 2019;197:78-82. doi:10.1016/j.drugalcdep.2018.12.030
221. Peterkin A, Laks J, Weinstein ZM. Current best practices for acute and chronic management of patients with opioid use disorder. *Med Clin North Am.* 2022;106(1):61-80. doi:10.1016/j.mcna.2021.08.009
222. Peterson C, Li M, Xu L, Mikosz CA, Luo F. Assessment of annual cost of substance use disorder in US Hospitals. *JAMA Netw Open.* 2021;4(3):e210242. doi:10.1001/jamanetworkopen.2021.0242
223. Weisner C, Mertens J, Parthasarathy S, Moore C, Lu Y. Integrating primary medical care with addiction treatment: a randomized controlled trial. *JAMA.* 2001;286(14):1715-1723. doi:10.1001/jama.286.14.1715
224. St. Peter RF, Reed MC, Kemper P, Blumenthal D. Changes in the scope of care provided by primary care physicians. *N Engl J Med.* 1999;341(26):1980-1985. doi:10.1056/nejm199912233412606

CHAPTER 49

Reducing Inequities of Care Through Changes in Practice

Kimberly Sue, Amanda Latimore, and India Perez-Urbano

CHAPTER OUTLINE

- Background: theoretical frameworks
- Limitations to change in practice: understanding policy and regulations
- Conclusion

BACKGROUND: THEORETICAL FRAMEWORKS

People who use drugs (PWUD) face stigma from families, friends, health care professionals, institutions and the community at large. It is critical for clinicians to understand systems of care, particularly for historically stigmatized groups of individuals, and the ways in which bias and prejudice affect PWUD and their families, including patients with substance use disorders. Fortunately, there are evidence-based ways in which practitioners can reduce inequities of care through changes in personal, clinical, health system and community-level practice. In this chapter we first provide a theoretical framework for considering the factors that produce disparate health outcomes. Then we review opportunities to address inequities in care at each of those levels.

Structural determinants are the cultural, historical, and normative scaffolding that dictate the way that care can be provided at the *institutional* level through *interpersonal* interactions, which facilitate or provide barriers to social and material resources. Health inequities occur when individuals in one group differentially experience these health risks and benefits. Structural, institutional, and interpersonal factors can each directly and indirectly influence individual health through behavior, psychosocial, and physiological mechanisms. **Figure 49-1** provides examples of structural, institutional, and interpersonal factors that can influence service provision and inequities in care.

Structural Determinants of Care

Structural determinants of care include culture, laws, stigma, and norms—historical and current societal conditions—that can directly influence the delivery of services. PWUD face many barriers to their well-being because of long-standing historical attitudes and policies. Historically, prohibition of certain substances, including alcohol, cocaine, cannabis, and heroin, among others, has been promulgated for over 50 years at great economic and social cost while failing to curb drug use or improve health.[1,2] Experts have argued that punitive drug policies that focus less on supports and more on harsh penalties for possession paradoxically lead to the development of more potent/toxic drug supply, drive violence, create social and economic isolation for PWUD, and ironically deter treatment-seeking and other health-promoting behaviors.[3-5]

Stigma is a fundamental structural cause of health inequities.[6] What is defined as criminal activity by laws, regulations and practice and who is designated by law to receive harsh penalties signals to the entire society how certain groups can be marked as deviant, immoral or wrong. The definition of criminality and associated negative stereotypes has been used throughout history to justify the social and economic exclusion, disenfranchisement, and demotion in social status of those designated as criminals or wrong-doers. As such, punitive drug policies drive stigma against PWUD, have wrongly normalized jail or prison time as an appropriate response to a chronic illness condition, and as such are a root cause of ongoing inequities in addiction care.

In the United States, public support for drug policy has historically been amplified through narratives that tap into the predominant xenophobic and racist stereotypes about minoritized groups.[7,8] Drugs like opium, heroin, cannabis, and cocaine have been associated with the wholly unsubstantiated criminality of Chinese and Mexican immigrants and Black people to justify the inequitable surveillance, raids, and imprisonment of these groups.[1,2,9] Today, although drug laws are seemingly race-neutral, they are inequitably implemented at the institutional level such that Black, Indigenous and People of Color (BIPOC) make up a disproportionate amount of the population incarcerated for drug-related charges compared to White individuals although they use illegal drugs at similar rates.[10] Populations experiencing oversurveillance and high rates of incarceration have diminished opportunities for treatment, housing, social support, education, harm reduction, and ultimately wellness.[11]

Structural determinants can have an indirect impact on health through access to social and material resources and ultimately health behavior. But they can also have a direct impact on health, triggering neurologic stress responses tied to psychological wellbeing, mental illness, and substance use.[12,13]

Institutional Determinants of Care

Laws, culture, norms, and other structural determinants are translated through institutional determinants of health—the practices of organizations and groups of people in settings such as addiction treatment clinics, academic institutions,

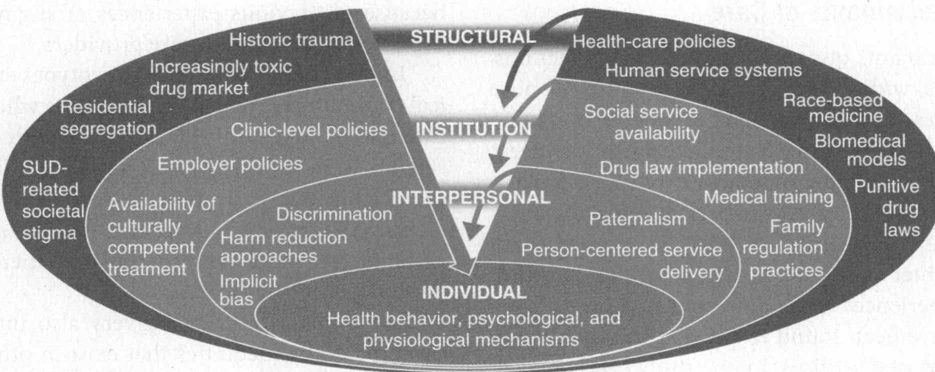

Figure 49-1. Example structural, institutional, and interpersonal determinants of inequities in care.

licensing boards, places of employment, child welfare agencies, law enforcement agencies, and housing and government benefits programs.

Unintentional injuries were the 3rd leading cause of death in 2019 with drug overdoses making the greatest contribution to the increase in unintentional injuries between 2019 and 2020.[14] Despite this, there is a clear lack of training in addiction within undergraduate medical education as well as within the workforce despite recent attempts to change this. Substance use disorder content remains relatively limited during foundational medical training[15,16] and leaves many medical professionals feeling under-prepared to address the needs of PWUD.[17] Similarly, medical professionals are often provided limited training and experience for understanding and addressing structural and social factors that underpin racial inequities in care.[18] In one survey of primary care physicians (PCPs), many clinicians held stigmatizing beliefs about people with opioid use disorder, which correlated with not providing medication for opioid use disorder such as buprenorphine.[19]

Restrictions within treatment institutions that raise barriers for those seeking services are often not driven by science and best practice, but instead have origins in society-level paternalistic medical models and prohibition-driven structural determinants. For example, addiction clinic policies such as random pill-checking and abstinence-only requirements are institutional determinants that make it difficult for people to enter or sustain treatment. Institutional factors can also facilitate care, such as the availability of social services in combination with medical care—see Case Study Drug User Health Hubs as an Institutional Determinant of Care.

Drug User Health Hubs as an Institutional Determinant of Care

New York State has long-funded a model for comprehensive health and social services for PWUD, including funding syringe service programs throughout cities and rural areas alike. This model is called the Drug User Health Hub model and funds 12 programs to provide syringe services, additional harm reduction supplies, mental health, medical care, and medication for opioid use disorder including buprenorphine, and are often available on-site. These programs are individualized, according to the community or individual needs of PWUD. According to their website, "categories of services may include buprenorphine; opioid overdose prevention; supportive services and counseling for individuals who have experienced an overdose; referrals from law enforcement, emergency departments (EDs), families and emergency services; and anti-stigma activities related to drug use and people who use drugs (PWUD)." Many of these programs, distributed across a range of New York cities and towns, have the potential to reach populations that often do not interface with traditional health care or social services, and in the pandemic, many of them expanded to provide telehealth or mail delivery. These programs also epitomize ways in which harm reduction and treatment interventions can be delivered concurrently, when viewed as a toolkit or menu of multiple options that people can use simultaneously to reduce their risk of harm. For example, a patient might access the program and obtain both buprenorphine as well as sterile syringes and other equipment during a visit; this is a model example of harm reduction and treatment services offered in a nonpunitive, compassionate and evidence-based manner.

Please read more about this work here: https://www.health.ny.gov/diseases/aids/consumers/prevention/

Interpersonal Determinants of Care

Interpersonal determinants of care consist of the interactions between an individual with service providers, families, friends, employers, colleagues, and others, that can deter or facilitate engagement with health care or public health providers. PWUD commonly report feeling stigmatized for substance use when they encounter health care providers in hospitals, ERs, or clinics; specifically, they report feeling the language and attitudes they encounter as pejorative, derogatory or demeaning.[20,21] Negative experiences while accessing harm reduction or social services have been found to prevent health-seeking behavior or uptake of vital services. In one study conducted at a syringe service program, researchers found that people with skin and soft tissue infections avoided coming for health care because of previous experiences of stigma and overall poor experiences with health care providers.[22]

Implicit biases and racial stereotypes exist within the medical community,[23] which can influence who is offered care. For example, in one study, Black people with opioid use disorder (OUD) were less likely to receive the office-based addiction medication buprenorphine than their White counterparts.[24] A recent study of 1,300 patients in Oregon found that White patients were more likely than Black patients to be initiated on buprenorphine in the hospital.[25]

Inequities in service delivery also interact with and are exacerbated by inequities that exist in other settings, such as the family regulation system (see Case Study Family Regulation System as a Structural Determinant of Care).

Family Regulation System as a Structural Determinant of Care

Societal stigma, state-level reporting requirements, structural racism, and implicit bias in the family regulation system drive inequities in care.

Parental drug use has been highly moralized and politicized. Punitive civil, and even criminal, penalties have utilized misinformation on drugs purporting fetal harm—positions that research has since invalidated.[26] False moral justifications and erroneous beliefs that any drug use is equivalent to child maltreatment have perpetuated inhumane state policies, such as the triggered automatic reporting for perinatal medications for OUD (MOUD) treatment despite strong evidence that MOUD are known to be one of the most effective treatments for maternal OUD.[27]

Substance use is associated with a majority of child welfare case worker case-loads.[28] Although Black people do not use drugs at a higher rate than White people, and Black children represent 14% of the general population of children, Black children are over-represented at 23% of the foster care system.[29] Some debate exists on whether Black-White disparities in the family regulation system exist purely due to structural social and economic inequities,[30] or whether implicit bias plays a role in the higher exposures to screening, reporting, substantiated charges, and family separation.[31] Racial biases persists in medical care[32] and research suggests that doctors may have a lower threshold for suspicion of child abuse for Black compared to White children receiving X-rays for traumatic brain injuries.[33] Therefore, it is unlikely that medical provider assessments related to the family regulations system are somehow immune to implicit bias, particularly in the context of high-stress environments where implicit racial bias is more likely to play a role in decision-making.[34] Regardless of the role of implicit bias in entering the family regulations system, Black children stay in foster care longer and are less likely to be reunified with their families compared to White children.[35]

Stigma, racism, and fear of loss of custody are significant barriers to care for parents with substance use disorder.[36,37] Custody loss has consistently been found to have a negative impact on drug use[38-40] in contrast to women with SUD who identified maintaining connection to their children as a primary source of motivation. The collateral consequences of drug charges, restrictive medication policies, lack of access to economic opportunity, lack of affordable housing and childcare, and policies that do not protect family connections can reduce the chances for reunification and amplify poor outcomes for the families.

Scholars have called for a more universal approach that emphasizes early assessment and voluntary prevention and parental assistance interventions over mandatory interventions targeted towards parents who are suspected of placing their children at risk of harm.[41] To better serve parents with SUD, and interrupt the intergenerational transmission of poverty and trauma, clinicians must be trained on structural competency and have sufficient resources at the institutional level so that child welfare reporting is not the only tool at their disposal. States have also begun to put into place infrastructure that allows providers to meet federal Child Abuse Prevention and Treatment Act (CAPTA) requirements while disentangling drug use and assumptions of harm by allowing anonymous reporting of substance exposure when no concerns exist for abuse or neglect.[27] Some hospital-based programs are attempting to try to change the criminalization of substance use during pregnancy by providing another model. For example, the Project Respect Clinic at Boston Medical Center combines clinicians providing buprenorphine, psychiatrists, nurse clinical managers, clinical social workers, and child life specialists working together in order to support patients and their families from pregnancy throughout the entire first year postpartum. More details about their work can be found at: https://www.bmc.org/obstetrics/pregnancy/addiction.

LIMITATIONS TO CHANGE IN PRACTICE: UNDERSTANDING POLICY AND REGULATIONS

The lasting impacts of the War on Drugs in the United States, compounded by institutions of systemic and racial oppression, continue to limit and complicate efforts to reduce inequities in substance use and harm reduction care. The racialized criminalization of substance use affects all institutions and has led to the disenfranchisement of countless Americans, further distancing them from drug safety resources and therapeutic modalities for addressing disordered drug use. Until there is a societal commitment to sustained systemic and ideologic transformation around protecting the health and humanity of PWUD, they and practitioners will continue to have to innovate around such policy and legal limitations.

The decriminalization of illegal drug possession in conjunction with increased substance use health services has the potential to: reduce incarceration rates (while reducing related racial/ethnic disparities), increase connection to substance use treatment, allow for the redirection of legal system funds and resources to prevent serious and violent crimes, and contribute to the destigmatization of substance use. There is no evidence that decriminalizing drug possession leads to increased drug use and, similarly, more stringent drug laws are not associated with decreased use.[42] In 2001, Portugal enacted national policy that decriminalized illegal drug possession for personal use by considering it an administrative offense. This reform was accompanied by the expansion of harm reduction services, substance use treatment, specialist training, and research funding. From 2000 to 2010, Portugal saw decreased problematic and adolescent substance use, decreased incarceration rates, increased substance use treatment utilization, decreased HIV/AIDS incidence, and a 18% decrease in total social costs related to illegal drug use.[43]

In recent years, there have been historic efforts to decriminalize illegal substance use in the United States. In 1996, California became the first state to legalize cannabis used as treatment. As of March 2023, 19 states, two territories and the District of Columbia have legalized cannabis for recreational use; yet it remains illegal on the federal level. In 2021, the first American overdose prevention centers (also known as safe consumption sites, which are locations where people can bring and consume unregulated substances under supervision of medical staff or peer health workers) began operating in New York City, although overdose prevention centers continue to be illegal on the federal level. In 2020, Oregon passed "Measure 110," which enacted policies similar to Portugal, which enforces a maximum punishment of a US$100 fine for possession of small amounts of illegal substances and invests in substance use treatment and harm reduction services.[44] Emerging outcomes of Oregon's historic legal reform could have a significant impact on national drug policy in the United States. The Oregon Criminal Justice Commission estimates a 90.7% reduction in the total number of convictions for the possession of controlled substances; the greatest reduction being among Black and Indigenous Americans (decreases of 93.7% and 94.2%, respectively), who were both overrepresented in drug possession-related convictions prior to the enactment of Measure 110.[45]

The criminalization of drug use has also resulted in the overregulation of life-saving treatment modalities, as well as the reliance on ill-equipped penal institutions (ie, prisons, jails) to provide addiction treatment or other modalities of care.[46] Racially minoritized communities are disproportionately represented in these institutions. Few jails and prisons across the United States offer at least one form of medication for OUD[47]; many of these institutions have a preference for "detoxification" or abstinence-based treatment programs over evidence-based medication programs.

In addition, drug criminalization results in discrimination and inequities in employment, education and housing—further exacerbating health disparities. The use of involuntary biologic drug testing in settings such as the workplace, prenatal care, educational institutions, and for public benefit eligibility is pervasive, inappropriate, inhumanely surveillant, and poses significant legal consequences to individuals. Services and resources that increase access to basic needs (eg, housing, food, shelter, health care) should not be contingent on substance use behavior or having a history of involvement with the legal system.

Punitive policies that equate substance use during pregnancy to child abuse—which currently exists in 19 states and the District of Columbia—result in the routine forced separation of children from their families, and even incarceration of parents, in ways that disproportionately affect racially and ethnically minoritized communities.[48] Further, the societal and media inflation of substance use in pregnancy (ie, the "crack baby epidemic") perpetuates barbaric racial imagery and disparages Black parenthood.[49,50] Fear of legal repercussions contributes to the avoidance of care and the underdiagnosis and undertreatment of substance use disorders during pregnancy, further contributing to poor maternal and neonatal outcomes.

The 2022 landmark U.S. Supreme Court decision in *Dobbs v. Jackson Women's Health Organization* to overturn *Roe v. Wade* and reverse any constitutional rights to abortion will only further exacerbate these injustices, particularly for people of color. The War on Drug's deliberate racialization, demonization, and surveillance of substance use behaviors in pregnancy paved the way for the pro-life notion of "personhood:" the assertion that a fetus holds rights that are separate from, and above, that of the pregnant person. As a result, substance use continues to pose significant legal threat to pregnant people without critical evaluation of the extent or impact of substance use nor the prioritization of comprehensive addiction treatment for those who may benefit from it. For some, fear of such legal repercussions has contributed to or motivated the decision to seek an abortion; however, in the setting of severely restricted access to legal abortion care, the dependence on illegal abortion can beget life-threatening medical consequences—ones that are only exacerbated by the *Dobbs v. Jackson Women's Health Organization* decision.[51]

Addressing inequities in care for people with substance use disorder and minoritized people with substance use disorder means understanding the root causes of inequities and appreciating the most influential lever may be upstream of individual behavior. As the medical community expands the biomedical view to recognize that psychosocial and economic context plays a role in addiction and health inequities,[52] health care providers are uniquely positioned to make a long-lasting impact on the health of communities. Service providers can consider acting at various levels of influence.

Individual and Interpersonal Strategies for Addressing Inequities in Care

Recognize Implicit Bias and Discrimination

Self-reflective practitioners who remain curious, engaged, and critical of themselves and their colleagues are a necessary part of quality improvement within health care settings. Understanding that stigma against PWUD is pervasive and that they often report feeling violence and hostility within the health care system is a critical first step. Then it is necessary to recognize and articulate that implicit bias, racism, and discrimination might be occurring within one's practice or that of colleagues or the institution. This can be achieved by integrating structured time for reflection and team debriefing into clinical workflow. For example, requiring that structural determinants of health be considered in the problem list of clinical plan/management section of medical notes (with accompanying action items); mandating all morbidity and mortality presentations include a consideration of the structural factors that may have contributed to the outcomes of the case; and including literature that relates to bias, discrimination and structural oppression during teaching rounds or journal clubs.

Continuous learning and introspection are necessary steps in commitment to a clinical culture that values health equity and ongoing education. Similar to the ways in which clinicians keep abreast of scientific developments in their respective fields, it is important to continually engage in scholarship around structural competency, health disparities, and race theory. Other forms of proactive and consistent self-education include: conducting research or quality improvement initiatives that expand our understanding and tools for this population and the pursuit of formalized training (eg, implicit bias training, buprenorphine training, addiction medicine fellowship). There is widespread stigma (ie, disregard, negative attitudes) held towards PWUD within health care system providers[53]; addiction clinicians have shown more compassionate views than general practitioners,[54] however, there is significant need for critical inquiry of oneself and others while striving to provide compassionate and evidence-based care. Using this spirit of critical self-inquiry, clinicians may be more likely to adopt nonjudgmental, evidence-based interpersonal, practice and policy stances that can advance better care and outcomes for PWUD.

Use Person-Centered Language

One essential way that providers can create safe, compassionate care for PWUD is using accurate language that respects patient's humanity and is clinically appropriate. Over the past 10 years, there has been a shift generally towards person-first language, as outlined by ASAM, NIDA and SAMHSA.[55] The Recovery Research Institute offers an "addictionary" of terms and the evidence behind using current or new terms (https://www.recoveryanswers.org/addiction-ary/).

Provide Harm Reduction-Informed Support Services

A critical philosophical foundation for reducing inequities of care is harm reduction. Harm reduction can be viewed as both a philosophy and a practice of reducing the harms of substance use and harmful social and legal policies towards PWUD.[56] Harm Reduction International defines harm reduction as "policies, programmes and practices that aim to minimise negative health, social and legal impacts associated with drug use, drug policies and drug laws."[57] Harm reduction includes a wide range of strategies, such as overdose education and community-based naloxone distribution, syringe service provision, drug checking (eg, fentanyl and other drug contaminant test strips), overdose prevention centers, housing first programs, and safer supply provision. In the clinic, providers can adopt and utilize a harm reduction philosophy that does not require or mandate abstinence, and support patients with harm reduction education and safer use strategies. Importantly, harm reduction and treatment modalities, such as medication and other therapies, are not mutually exclusive and this should be articulated.

Clinic-Based and Institutional Strategies for Addressing Inequities in Care

There are also measures that can be taken within one's medical practice or at the clinic level that can be powerful levers for change and directly address many of the inequities that patients might face.[58]

Integrate Structural Competency in Training

One useful theoretical approach for clinical practice is "structural competency," which is a framework developed by physician–anthropologists Helena Hansen and Jonathan Metzl. This framework is useful in guiding learners to focus on structures that contribute to health inequalities—such as structural racism, class, being part of a stigmatized community group—rather than individual level factors or behaviors.[59] This approach can be useful in examining the systems of care for PWUD, as conventional cultural approaches to substance use disorders can focus disproportionately on choice or willpower. One group of physician-anthropologists developed a structural competency checklist that helps front line clinicians think about how to assess domains of structural vulnerability when working with patients.[60] Such training can, and should, begin at the undergraduate (UME) and graduate (GME) medical education levels and throughout the spectrum of education for other health professional trainees including nurses and physician assistants.

Institutionalize Health Equity

Medical systems can take on structural changes that can minimize differential management of marginalized patient populations. Examples relevant to addiction include: (1) eliminating abstinence requirements and as a prerequisite for accessing life-saving or life-preserving treatment, such as a liver transplant,[61,62] (2) removing police presence from clinical settings and increasing training on de-escalation practices,[63] (3) instituting universal and evidence-based substance use disorder screening across all clinical settings, accompanied by robust referral systems, (4) instituting universal screening of other important threats such as interpersonal violence, depression, anxiety and trauma (eg, physical violence, sexual assault, interactions with the carceral system) and (5) creating centralized bias reporting systems to identify and act on instances of discrimination, maltreatment and microaggression. Some practitioners see themselves as part of "abolition medicine," or practicing medicine in a way that recognizes oppression and stigma outlined in race-based algorithms, tools, or programs that perpetuate police or carceral power.[64] An example of a race-based algorithm is the race-based estimated glomerular filtration rates (eGFR) equations, which many health systems like UCSF and Yale have recently eliminated as it treats race as a biologic entity and disadvantages Black Americans.[65]

Reassess the Use of Routine Toxicology

Screening for substance use disorders is important in order to identify patients that could be offered medical treatment or risk reduction resources. Unfortunately, screening is often conflated with performing toxicology. Many clinicians utilize urine toxicology regularly to screen or monitor substance use disorders; however, some clinicians within the addictions field have called for the reassessment of routine toxicology.[66] Many PWUD feel that toxicology is a form of policing, a tool of punishment, and a violation void of respect and dignity, especially when the urine specimen is collected while being observed.[67] PWUD are often not asked for written or verbal consent for toxicology. While urine toxicology can provide valuable information, such as the presence or absence of fentanyl or other unintended substances, it should never be performed without the patient's consent.[68] There are validated questionnaires that can effectively screen for substance use (ie, AUDIT-C and single item screener).[69,70] Some studies indicate that self-report of substance use can be correlated with urine toxicology.[71,72]

It is important for clinicians to understand that toxicology results, of patients as well as infants or others, can be applied and utilized in a variety of nonclinical realms, including employment, housing, assistance programs, probation/parole, and family regulation systems. Furthermore, toxicology can be applied differentially. For example, one study found that urine toxicology was more likely to be done on Black women and their newborns than non-Black women and their newborns,[73] which contributes to disproportionately higher rates of family regulation system involvement and forced removal of children among Black families. Understanding the conditions in which toxicology is used, obtaining patient consent and permission, and minimizing its use when not necessary, are important factors to consider. In fact, in response to the COVID-19 pandemic, one low-barrier buprenorphine program in Baltimore, MD, suspended in-person visits and accompanying oral toxicology and, under clinical guidance provided by American Society of Addiction Medicine, did not include routine toxicology in telehealth visits. This study had 63% retention in buprenorphine telehealth visits at 30-day follow-up, among a population comprised of largely Black men with OUD.[74]

Toxicology can be used in a nonpunitive, harm reduction-oriented manner, where patients are never "fired" or unable to access medications based on toxicology results, where patients are able to correlate the toxicology with their use, where patients can refuse a recommended toxicology test or request one, and the results can be used to support a person's goals, such as decreased use or abstinence (ie, contingency management).

Reduce Unnecessary Barriers to Treatment

Low-barrier approaches to medication for OUD are critical in reducing inequities of care through changes in practice. This includes tenets such as providing medication despite ongoing substance use or polysubstance use, despite intermittent or irregular engagement with the clinic, flexibility and same day access.[75,76] Creating and providing services that people need where they need them (ie, literally "meeting people where they are"), whether it be in housing encampments, soup kitchens, mobile vans, churches, and creating one-stop-shop models for service provision, can be important models for reducing inequities of care.

Recognize Intersecting Racial Inequities

Addiction care intersects with other axes of social inequity. For example, in areas of kidney and liver transplants, widespread disparities in access to these organs exist for minoritized groups and people lacking insurance as well as "social support."[77]

There are many examples of groups and approaches to innovating changes in practice to address health injustice and improve the health of PWUD. See **Table 49-1** for model examples of some leaders in the field.

Structural Strategies for Addressing Inequities in Care

Advocate for the Removal of Punitive Policies

People create policies, but policies also create people. For example, policies related to tobacco control contributed

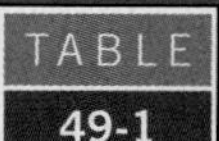

TABLE 49-1 Resources
California Bridge: A $40 million dollar program funded by California legislature to bring medication for OUD treatment, patient navigators, buprenorphine champions, harm reduction services and more into more than 155 rural and urban emergency rooms and hospitals.
Camden Coalition Core Model: A multidisciplinary model that focuses on patients with high utilization of acute hospital care and aims to prevent further hospitalizations by addressing social determinants of health, language barriers, behavioral health with home visits and increased care coordination and supports.
Cannabis Equity: Several states have passed legislation that seeks to not only decriminalize simple drug possession but restore justice in communities that have been targeted by decades of punitive drug laws and police surveillance. A growing number of states including California, New Jersey, New York, and Illinois have enacted legislation that ensures tax revenue from the regulation of cannabis is reinvested in social and economic innovation, is used to address health inequities, and benefits communities within the state that have been disproportionately affected by the criminalization of drugs.[82]
Housing First: An evidence-based approach to homelessness where permanent housing is provided to individuals experiencing homelessness without prerequisites, such as substance use or mental health treatment.
Imani Breakthrough Recovery: Imani Breakthrough is a faith-based, person-centered, culturally informed harm reduction recovery program and is a collaboration between churches in New Haven, CT and Yale University researchers. This program provides an innovative approach to engaging vulnerable groups into SUD treatment, by focusing on SAMHSA's eight dimensions of wellness (social determinants of health or SDOH), seven domains of citizenship, culturally informed education, and referral to medication for addiction treatment (MAT) or any FDA-approved pharmacotherapy for treating a SUD.
Missouri Medication First ("NoMoDeaths") program: Led by the Missouri Department of Mental Health and Opioid State Targeted Response/State Opioid Response grant partners, this program seeks to ensure low threshold access to medication for OUD as quickly as possible, "without arbitrary tapering or time limits"; across 69 treatment sites in the state.
Movement for Family Power: A community coalition and advocacy group that addresses the family regulatory system; their goal is to "end the Foster System's policing and punishment of families and to create a world where the dignity and integrity of all families is valued and supported."
Next Distro: An online, mail-based harm reduction platform that brings education, supplies, and naloxone to people who cannot access brick-and-mortar syringe service programs. The program seeks to combat the stigma that PWUDs often face accessing traditional services. They have reached approximately 63% of U.S. counties with their services and have gotten naloxone into the hands of people most at need (76% of the requestors had witnessed an overdose in the previous year).

significantly to a cultural shift that reduced smoking-related deaths without criminalizing the personal choice to smoke tobacco.[78] Similarly, decriminalization of many illegal drugs could support a cultural shift towards viewing addiction as a chronic condition and prevent the collateral consequences of drug charges. The U.S. Government Accountability Office recognizes 671 collateral consequences of a nonviolent drug conviction, including negative impacts on professional licensure, housing, transportation, and family and domestic rights.[79] The key to structural change is not only the removal of punitive polices but the restoration of justice. Many individuals are still incarcerated or have criminal records that diminish their opportunities for activities that states have since determined are legal. Advocates should insist on retroactive decriminalization policies that release individuals from incarceration and expunge records that have served as barriers to health and wellbeing.

Advocate for Primary Prevention and More Appropriate Family Regulation Policies

Universal prevention policies avert discriminatory practices and address structural racism[27,41] through broad-based screening and the delivery of services that more appropriately address the root causes. Abuse and neglect are often caused and/or complicated by pervasive contextual challenges faced by families such as severe poverty. Community-based prevention provides a more effective and less discriminatory approach and offers a five-to-one return on investment.[80] The returns on prevention for substance use disorder are even greater; there is a savings of $18 for every dollar spent on youth before problems occur.[81]

Develop Priorities Grounded in Lived Experience

Programmatic, clinical, policy, and research priorities should be grounded in the lived and living experience of PWUD. Advocating for policy, funding research and delivering services that addresses upstream social determinants of health, that meaningfully engages and works with communities actively experiencing the overdose death crisis, is critical. Working with groups of individuals who use drugs, such as the National Survivors Union, local drug users' unions and recovery groups, ensures critical participation of people at the forefront of the overdose crisis. Given the rapidly evolving and shifting toxic drug supply, to include adulterants such as xylazine and isotonitazene, it is even more important that research be flexible, nimble, and responsive to people on the ground. Identifying meaningful ways to engage and compensate people for their expertise and time without tokenizing groups of people in conducting such research is critical. How can PWUD inform the methodology, instruments, tools, data collection, and dissemination of research into clinical and policy settings? Finally, many clinicians and researchers find it meaningful and important to engage in social advocacy on behalf of, and with, impacted communities. This might involve testimony at local city council or state hearings for essential services, such as syringe service programs, or working with groups addressing upstream social determinants of health, such as groups working for Medicaid expansion or housing justice. Learning what active groups on the ground need, including local drug user unions, is critical.

CONCLUSION

This chapter has presented theoretical frameworks for understanding health and racial inequities in access to healthy environments, treatment, and harm reduction services for PWUD. It outlines and provides examples of ways in which both addiction medicine specialists and general health care practitioners can change their practice and attitudes, from internal implicit bias work to changes within the clinic to advocating for systemic and structural change. Partnering with people with lived and living experience across these spheres of research, treatment, teaching and advocacy are essential for meaningful, sustained and impactful changes in practice to address historical and ongoing health inequities.

REFERENCES

1. Courtwright DT. *Dark Paradise: A History of Opiate Addiction in America.* Enlarged edition. Harvard University Press; 2001.
2. Acker CJ. *Creating the American Junkie: Addiction Research in the Classic Era of Narcotic Control.* The Johns Hopkins University Press; 2002.
3. Cowan R. How the Narcs Created Crack. *Natl Rev Mag.* 1986;38:26-31.
4. Beletsky L, Davis CS. Today's fentanyl crisis: Prohibition's Iron Law, revisited. *Int J Drug Policy.* 2017;46:156-159. doi:10.1016/j.drugpo.2017.05.050
5. Csete J, Kamarulzaman A, Kazatchkine M, et al. Public health and international drug policy. *Lancet.* 2016;387(10026):1427-1480. doi:10.1016/S0140-6736(16)00619-X
6. Hatzenbuehler ML, Phelan JC, Link BG. Stigma as a fundamental cause of population health inequalities. *Am J Public Health.* 2013;103(5):813-821. doi:10.2105/AJPH.2012.301069
7. Nunn K. Race, crime and the pool of surplus criminality: or why the "War on Drugs" was a "War on Blacks". *UF Law Fac Publ.* 2002;381.
8. Netherland J, Hansen HB. The war on drugs that wasn't: wasted whiteness, "dirty doctors," and race in media coverage of prescription opioid misuse. *Cult Med Psychiatry.* 2016;40(4):664-686. doi:10.1007/s11013-016-9496-5
9. El-Sabawi T, Oliva JD. The influence of white exceptionalism on drug war discourse. *Temple Law Review.* 2022;649. Accessed July 7, 2022. https://papers.ssrn.com/abstract=4128076
10. Substance Abuse and Mental Health Services Administration. *Key Substance Use and Mental Health Indicators in the United States: Results from the 2019 National Survey on Drug Use and Health.* Center for Behavioral Health Statistics and Quality, SAMHSA; 2020. Accessed August 15, 2023. https://www.samhsa.gov/data/sites/default/files/reports/rpt29393/2019NSDUHFFRPDFWHTML/2019NSDUHFFR1PDFW090120.pdf
11. Jalali MS, Botticelli M, Hwang RC, Koh HK, McHugh RK. The opioid crisis: a contextual, social-ecological framework. *Health Res Policy Syst.* 2020;18(1):87. doi:10.1186/s12961-020-00596-8
12. Geller A, Fagan J, Tyler T, Link BG. Aggressive policing and the mental health of young urban men. *Am J Public Health.* 2014;104(12):2321-2327. doi:10.2105/AJPH.2014.302046
13. Hatzenbuehler ML, O'Cleirigh C, Grasso C, Mayer K, Safren S, Bradford J. Effect of same-sex marriage laws on health care use and expenditures in sexual minority men: a quasi-natural experiment. *Am J Public Health.* 2012;102(2):285-291. doi:10.2105/AJPH.2011.300382
14. Centers for Disease Control and Prevention. WISQARS Injury Data Visualization Tools. Accessed December 6, 2022. https://wisqars.cdc.gov/data/non-fatal/home
15. Lembke A, Humphreys K. The opioid epidemic as a watershed moment for physician training in addiction medicine. *Acad Psychiatry.* 2018;42(2):269-272. doi:10.1007/s40596-018-0892-8
16. Morreale MK, Balon R, Aggarwal R, et al. Substance use disorders education: are we heeding the call? *Acad Psychiatry.* 2020;44(2):119-121. doi:10.1007/s40596-020-01204-1
17. Miller NS, Sheppard LM, Colenda CC, Magen J. Why physicians are unprepared to treat patients who have alcohol- and drug-related disorders. *Acad Med.* 2001;76(5):410-418. doi:10.1097/00001888-200105000-00007
18. Hansen HB, Metzl J. *Structural Competency in Mental Health and Medicine A Case-Based Approach to Treating the Social Determinants of Health.* Springer; 2019.
19. Stone EM, Kennedy-Hendricks A, Barry CL, Bachhuber MA, McGinty EE. The role of stigma in U.S. primary care physicians' treatment of opioid use disorder. *Drug Alcohol Depend.* 2021;221:108627. doi:10.1016/j.drugalcdep.2021.108627
20. Biancarelli DL, Biello KB, Childs E, et al. Strategies used by people who inject drugs to avoid stigma in healthcare settings. *Drug Alcohol Depend.* 2019;198:80-86. doi:10.1016/j.drugalcdep.2019.01.037
21. Bergstein RS, King K, Melendez-Torres GJ, Latimore AD. Refusal to accept emergency medical transport following opioid overdose, and conditions that may promote connections to care. *Int J Drug Policy.* 2021;97:103296. doi:10.1016/j.drugpo.2021.103296
22. Figgatt MC, Salazar ZR, Vincent L, et al. Treatment experiences for skin and soft tissue infections among participants of syringe service programs in North Carolina. *Harm Reduct J.* 2021;18(1):80. doi:10.1186/s12954-021-00528-x
23. Hall WJ, Chapman MV, Lee KM, et al. Implicit racial/ethnic bias among health care professionals and its influence on health care outcomes: a systematic review. *Am J Public Health.* 2015;105(12):e60-e76. doi:10.2105/AJPH.2015.302903
24. Lagisetty PA, Ross R, Bohnert A, Clay M, Maust DT. Buprenorphine treatment divide by race/ethnicity and payment. *JAMA Psychiatry.* 2019;76(9):979-981. doi:10.1001/jamapsychiatry.2019.0876
25. Priest KC, King CA, Englander H, Lovejoy TI, McCarty D. Differences in the delivery of medications for opioid use disorder during hospitalization by racial categories: a retrospective cohort analysis. *Subst Abuse.* 2022;43(1):1251-1259. doi:10.1080/08897077.2022.2074601
26. Carroll JJ, El-Sabawi T, Ostrach B. The harms of punishing substance use during pregnancy. *Int J Drug Policy.* 2021;98:103433. doi:10.1016/j.drugpo.2021.103433
27. Wakeman SE, Bryant A, Harrison N. Redefining child protection: addressing the harms of structural racism and punitive approaches for birthing people, dyads, and families affected by substance use. *Obstet Gynecol.* 2022;140(2):167-173. doi:10.1097/AOG.0000000000004786
28. Freisthler B, Maguire-Jack K, Yoon S, Dellor E, Wolf JP. Enhancing Permanency in Children and Families (EPIC): a child welfare intervention for parental substance abuse. *BMC Public Health.* 2021;21(1):780. doi:10.1186/s12889-021-10668-1
29. Children's Defense Fund. The State of America's Children 2021. Accessed August 15, 2023. https://www.childrensdefense.org/the-state-of-americas-children/
30. Barth RP, Berrick JD, Garcia AR, et al. Research to consider while effectively re-designing child welfare services. *Res Soc Work Pract.* 2022;32(5):483-498. doi:10.1177/10497315211050000
31. Roberts DE. *Torn Apart by Dorothy Roberts.* Basic Books; 2022.

32. Hoffman KM, Trawalter S, Axt JR, Oliver MN. Racial bias in pain assessment and treatment recommendations, and false beliefs about biological differences between blacks and whites. *Proc Natl Acad Sci.* 2016;113(16):4296-4301. doi:10.1073/pnas.1516047113
33. Lane WG, Rubin DM, Monteith R, Christian CW. Racial differences in the evaluation of pediatric fractures for physical abuse. *JAMA.* 2002;288(13):1603-1609. doi:10.1001/jama.288.13.1603
34. Johnson TJ, Hickey RW, Switzer GE, et al. The impact of cognitive stressors in the emergency department on physician implicit racial bias. *Acad Emerg Med.* 2016;23(3):297-305. doi:10.1111/acem.12901
35. Wulczyn F, Parolini A, Schmits F, Magruder J, Webster D. Returning to foster care: age and other risk factors. *Child Youth Serv Rev.* 2020;116:105166. doi:10.1016/j.childyouth.2020.105166
36. Jackson A, Shannon L. Barriers to receiving substance abuse treatment among rural pregnant women in Kentucky. *Matern Child Health J.* 2012;16(9):1762-1770. doi:10.1007/s10995-011-0923-5
37. Seay KD, Iachini AL, DeHart DD, Browne T, Clone S. Substance abuse treatment engagement among mothers: perceptions of the parenting role and agency-related motivators and inhibitors. *J Fam Soc Work.* 2017;20(3):196-212. doi:10.1080/10522158.2017.1300113
38. Mackay L, Ickowicz S, Hayashi K, Abrahams R. Rooming-in and loss of child custody: key factors in maternal overdose risk. *Addiction.* 2020;115(9):1786-1787. doi:10.1111/add.15028
39. Harp KLH, Oser CB. A longitudinal analysis of the impact of child custody loss on drug use and crime among a sample of African American mothers. *Child Abuse Negl.* 2018;77:1-12. doi:10.1016/j.chiabu.2017.12.017
40. Kenny KS, Barrington C, Green SL. "I felt for a long time like everything beautiful in me had been taken out": women's suffering, remembering, and survival following the loss of child custody. *Int J Drug Policy.* 2015;26(11):1158-1166. doi:10.1016/j.drugpo.2015.05.024
41. Daro D. A shift in perspective: a universal approach to child protection. *Future Child.* 2019;29(1):17-40.
42. Larney S, Peacock A, Leung J, et al. Global, regional, and country-level coverage of interventions to prevent and manage HIV and hepatitis C among people who inject drugs: a systematic review. *Lancet Glob Health.* 2017;5(12):e1208-e1220. doi:10.1016/S2214-109X(17)30373-X
43. Gonçalves R, Lourenço A, da Silva SN. A social cost perspective in the wake of the Portuguese strategy for the fight against drugs. *Int J Drug Policy.* 2015;26(2):199-209. doi:10.1016/j.drugpo.2014.08.017
44. Netherland J, Kral AH, Ompad DC, et al. Principles and metrics for evaluating oregon's innovative drug decriminalization measure. *J Urban Health.* 2022;99(2):328-331. doi:10.1007/s11524-022-00606-w
45. Oregon Criminal Justice Commission. Racial and Ethnic Impact Statement: Supplemental Document. Accessed August 12, 2022. https://drive.google.com/file/d/1CDKzOBb-3RHTaVUT9wnFP4hxTtsu8yYd/view
46. Wakeman SE, Rich JD. Addiction treatment within U.S. correctional facilities: bridging the gap between current practice and evidence-based care. *J Addict Dis.* 2015;34(2-3):220-225. doi:10.1080/10550887.2015.1059217
47. Pew Charitable Trusts. Opioid Use Disorder Treatment in Jails and Prisons. Accessed August 12, 2022. https://pew.org/2VJkT5F
48. Welfare C. The drug war breaks up families. *Uprooting The Drug War.* Accessed July 4, 2022. https://uprootingthedrugwar.org/child-welfare/
49. Logan E. The wrong race, committing crime, doing drugs, and maladjusted for motherhood: the nation's fury over "crack babies.". *Soc Justice.* 1999;26(1):115-138.
50. Roberts DE. Punishing drug addicts who have babies: women of color, equality, and the right of privacy. *Harv Law Rev.* 1991;104(7):1419-1482.
51. Paltrow LM. The war on drugs and the war on abortion: some initial thoughts on the connections, intersections and effects. *Reprod Health Matters.* 2002;10(19):162-170.
52. American Society of Addiction Medicine. *Advancing Racial Justice and Health Equality.* Accessed March 7, 2023. https://www.asam.org/advocacy/national-advocacy/justice
53. van Boekel LC, Brouwers EPM, van Weeghel J, Garretsen HFL. Stigma among health professionals towards patients with substance use disorders and its consequences for healthcare delivery: systematic review. *Drug Alcohol Depend.* 2013;131(1-2):23-35. doi:10.1016/j.drugalcdep.2013.02.018
54. van Boekel LC, Brouwers EPM, van Weeghel J, Garretsen HFL. Healthcare professionals' regard towards working with patients with substance use disorders: comparison of primary care, general psychiatry and specialist addiction services. *Drug Alcohol Depend.* 2014;134:92-98. doi:10.1016/j.drugalcdep.2013.09.012
55. National Institute on Drug Abuse. *Words Matter - Terms to Use and Avoid When Talking About Addiction.* Accessed August 14, 2022. https://nida.nih.gov/nidamed-medical-health-professionals/health-professions-education/words-matter-terms-to-use-avoid-when-talking-about-addiction
56. Chan CA, Canver B, McNeil R, Sue KL. Harm reduction in health care settings. *Med Clin North Am.* 2022;106(1):201-217. doi:10.1016/j.mcna.2021.09.002
57. Harm Reduction International. *What is Harm Reduction?* Accessed August 12, 2022. https://www.hri.global/what-is-harm-reduction
58. Garzón-Orjuela N, Samacá-Samacá DF, Luque Angulo SC, Mendes Abdala CV, Reveiz L, Eslava-Schmalbach J. An overview of reviews on strategies to reduce health inequalities. *Int J Equity Health.* 2020;19(1):192. doi:10.1186/s12939-020-01299-w
59. Metzl JM, Hansen H. Structural competency: theorizing a new medical engagement with stigma and inequality. *Soc Sci Med 1982.* 2014;103:126-133. doi:10.1016/j.socscimed.2013.06.032
60. Bourgois P, Holmes SM, Sue K, Quesada J. Structural vulnerability: operationalizing the concept to address health disparities in clinical care. *Acad Med.* 2017;92(3):299-307. doi:10.1097/ACM.0000000000001294
61. Obed A, Stern S, Jarrad A, Lorf T. Six month abstinence rule for liver transplantation in severe alcoholic liver disease patients. *World J Gastroenterol.* 2015;21(14):4423-4426. doi:10.3748/wjg.v21.i14.4423
62. Herrick-Reynolds KM, Punchhi G, Greenberg RS, et al. Evaluation of early vs standard liver transplant for alcohol-associated liver disease. *JAMA Surg.* 2021;156(11):1026-1034. doi:10.1001/jamasurg.2021.3748
63. Song JS. *Policing the Emergency Room.* Accessed March 26, 2023. https://harvardlawreview.org/2021/06/policing-the-emergency-room/
64. Iwai Y, Khan ZH, DasGupta S. Abolition medicine. *Lancet.* 2020;396(10245):158-159. doi:10.1016/S0140-6736(20)31566-X
65. Tsai JW, Cerdeña JP, Goedel WC, et al. Evaluating the impact and rationale of race-specific estimations of kidney function: estimations from U.S. NHANES, 2015-2018. *eClinicalMedicine.* 2021;42. doi:10.1016/j.eclinm.2021.101197
66. Incze MA. Reassessing the role of routine urine drug screening in opioid use disorder treatment. *JAMA Intern Med.* 2021;181(10):1282-1283. doi:10.1001/jamainternmed.2021.4109
67. Brico E. Witnessed urine screens in drug treatment: humiliating and harmful. *Filter.* Accessed March 26, 2023. https://filtermag.org/urine-screen-drug-treatment/
68. Strike C, Rufo C. Embarrassing, degrading, or beneficial: patient and staff perspectives on urine drug testing in methadone maintenance treatment. *J Subst Use.* 2010;15(5):303-312. doi:10.3109/14659890903431603
69. Frank D, DeBenedetti AF, Volk RJ, Williams EC, Kivlahan DR, Bradley KA. Effectiveness of the AUDIT-C as a screening test for alcohol misuse in three race/ethnic groups. *J Gen Intern Med.* 2008;23(6):781-787. doi:10.1007/s11606-008-0594-0
70. Smith PC, Schmidt SM, Allensworth-Davies D, Saitz R. A single-question screening test for drug use in primary care. *Arch Intern Med.* 2010;170(13):1155-1160. doi:10.1001/archinternmed.2010.140
71. Skelton KR, Donahue E, Benjamin-Neelon SE. Validity of self-report measures of cannabis use compared to biological samples among women of reproductive age: a scoping review. *BMC Pregnancy Childbirth.* 2022;22(1):344. doi:10.1186/s12884-022-04677-0
72. McLouth CJ, Oser CB, Stevens-Watkins D. Concordance between self-reported drug use and urinalysis in a sample of Black American women.

Subst Use Misuse. 2022;57(4):495-503. doi:10.1080/10826084.2021.2019778

73. Kunins HV, Bellin E, Chazotte C, Du E, Arnsten JH. The effect of race on provider decisions to test for illicit drug use in the peripartum setting. *J Womens Health (Larchmt).* 2007;16(2):245-255. doi:10.1089/jwh.2006.0070
74. Rosecrans A, Harris R, Saxton RE, et al. Mobile low-threshold buprenorphine integrated with infectious disease services. *J Subst Abuse Treat.* 2022;133. doi:10.1016/j.jsat.2021.108553
75. Martin SA, Chiodo LM, Bosse JD, Wilson A. The next stage of buprenorphine care for opioid use disorder. *Ann Intern Med.* 2018;169(9):628-635. doi:10.7326/M18-1652
76. Jakubowski A, Fox A. Defining low-threshold buprenorphine treatment. *J Addict Med.* 2020;14(2):95-98. doi:10.1097/ADM.0000000000000555
77. Mathur AK, Sonnenday CJ, Merion RM. Race and ethnicity in access to and outcomes of liver transplantation: a critical literature review. *Am J Transplant.* 2009;9(12):2662-2668. doi:10.1111/j.1600-6143.2009.02857.x
78. Ward K. Reflections on 15 years in the global tobacco trenches. *Health Behav Res.* 2017;1(1). doi:10.4148/2572-1836.1007
79. U.S. Government Accountability Office. *Nonviolent Drug Convictions: Stakeholders' Views on Potential Actions to Address Collateral Consequences.* Accessed August 14, 2022. https://www.gao.gov/products/gao-17-691
80. Trust for America's Health. Prevention for a Healthier America: Investments in Disease Prevention Yield Significant Savings, Stronger Communities. Accessed August 14, 2022. https://www.preventioninstitute.org/sites/default/files/publications/Prevention%20for%20a%20Healthier%20America_0.pdf
81. Substance Abuse and Mental Health Services Administration. *Substance Abuse Prevention Dollars and Cents: A Cost-Benefit Analysis.* Accessed August 14, 2022. https://www.samhsa.gov/sites/default/files/cost-benefits-prevention.pdf
82. Marijuana Policy Project. *Cannabis Tax Revenue in States that Regulate Cannabis for Adult Use.* Accessed August 12, 2022. https://www.mpp.org/issues/legalization/cannabis-tax-revenue-states-regulate-cannabis-adult-use/

CHAPTER

50 Quality Improvement for Addiction Treatment

James H. Ford II, Kim A. Hoffman, Kimberly Johnson, and Javier Ponce Terashima

CHAPTER OUTLINE

- Introduction
- Framework for change
- Defining and measuring organizational quality treatment and outcomes
- Accreditation of treatment programs
- Building system capacity to deliver effective care
- Using quality improvement principles to improve patient outcomes
- Ensuring primary care clinicians can identify, treat or refer, and monitor substance use disorder
- International efforts: The International Center for Credentialing and Education of Addiction Professionals
- Conclusions

INTRODUCTION

Outcomes from addiction treatment services compare favorably with treatments for other chronic conditions such as hypertension, diabetes, and asthma.[1] Addiction traditionally has been treated under an acute care model where treatment is short-term, and post acute support occurs within self-help groups. A consequence of the discrepancies between the treatment of addiction and other chronic illnesses is a persistent expectation that patients with diagnosed substance use disorders (SUDs) remain substance free after their treatment begins and without substance use after their treatment ends. For most other chronic health conditions, the expectation is for long-term symptom management rather than symptom elimination. A contemporary understanding of addiction as a treatable, chronic health condition includes a recognition that withdrawal of treatment or related supports may promote a reemergence of symptoms; continuing care by a clinician as well as active self-management and recovery supports is essential for sustaining positive outcomes associated with treatment.[2,3] Improvement in the quality of addiction treatment, which has improved over the past 15 years, still lags behind that of general health care[4] though, as this chapter will discuss, advancements have been made in recent years.

Efforts to improve the quality of addiction treatment and enhance effectiveness generally fall into seven categories:

1. Framework for change
2. Defining and measuring organizational quality and treatment outcomes
3. Accreditation of treatment programs
4. Building system capacity to deliver effective care
5. Utilizing quality improvement principles to improve patient outcomes
6. Ensuring primary care clinicians can identify, treat or refer, and monitor substance use disorder
7. International efforts: The International Center for Credentialing and Education of Addiction Professionals

This chapter covers each of these categories. It reviews efforts to define appropriate outcomes and current trends in accrediting and licensing and efforts to increase the focus on quality improvement in addiction treatment.

FRAMEWORK FOR CHANGE

National Academy of Medicine Reports

The National Academy of Medicine (NAM, formerly known as Institute of Medicine [IOM]) within the National Academy of Sciences advises federal policy makers about health concerns and public health policy issues. In a series of reports, the IOM identified needs for better health care and outlined strategies to improve the quality of health care in America. *To Err is Human: Building a Safer Health System*[4] found that medical error was a major source of morbidity and mortality in the U.S. health care system and challenged health care systems to track and eliminate error through implementation of performance standards that emphasize patient safety. *Crossing the Quality Chasm: A New Health System for the 21st Century*[5] provided guidance on redesigning systems of health care to better address chronic care, make greater use of information and technology, coordinate care, incorporate process and outcome measures into systems of care, and continually improve the effectiveness of clinicians. Six dimensions of quality were specified: care should be safe, effective, patient centered, timely, efficient, and equitable (**Table 50-1**). A third report, *Improving the Quality of Health Care for Mental Health and Substance Use Conditions*,[6] asserts that the *Crossing the Quality Chasm*[5] framework can be extended to treatments for SUDs and other mental health disorders. The report notes that proven science-based treatments are not used routinely, services are often fragmented, and substandard care leads to greater expense and suffering. In addition to the human costs associated with this treatment gap, there are implications for employers and the workforce, for the nation's economy, as well as for the education, welfare, and justice systems. The report, sponsored by

TABLE 50-1 Summary of NAM Dimensions of Care

NAM dimensions	Addiction medicine examples
Safety: Avoid allowing the system of care to cause injury to the patient	Access to care, delays in appointment scheduling, or medication errors
Effectiveness: Provide evidence-based treatment to all patients and avoid services with limited patient benefits .	The use of addiction medications; screening and brief intervention in primary care, case management, and posttreatment aftercare; and offer psychological interventions such as structured family therapy, motivational interviewing, or contingency management
Patient centered: Provide care that is based on and guided by patient needs, preferences, and values	Establish clear two-way expectations; include family and friends in treatment process, or work with clients to create treatment plans
Timely: Reduce waits and delays for both the patients and staff alike	Establish walk-in hours; offer interim services; add additional groups
Efficient: Evaluate the process of care to create an efficient process that reduces waste and conserves resources	Eliminate excessive paperwork, reassign tasks, cross-train staff, or develop a process for a seamless transition across treatment providers
Equitable: Ensure that processes of care are consistently applied across gender and racial/ethnic groups	Address cultural differences by offering treatment groups in multiple languages or integrating cultural customs into groups

the Substance Abuse and Mental Health Services Administration (SAMHSA), explicitly recommends that SUD and mental health treatment systems emphasize the six dimensions of quality of care and that these public agencies and other payers promote the development of process and outcome measures that track quality of care.[6] Since this report, significant efforts have been taken to improve measurement and quality although much work is yet to be done.

Subsequent reports from the NAM focused on *Psychosocial Interventions for Mental and Substance Use Disorders*[7] and *Substance Use Disorders in the U.S. Armed Forces*.[8] The first report places the patient at the center of a process to identify outcomes that are important, research methods that identify key elements of interventions, and translation efforts that ensure fidelity. The U.S. Armed Forces report[8] recognized the effect of combat on substance use among veterans, encouraged the adoption of Department of Defense evidence-based clinical practice guidelines for treating SUDs, and identified some of the barriers to care that currently exist in the military. Report recommendations to address these systemic barriers to care include (1) enhancing the use of technology, (2) providing confidential care, (3) making greater use of continuing care, (4) expanding access to care, and (5) creating a 21st century workforce.[8] These recommendations align with two Surgeon General reports, *Facing Addiction: The Surgeon General's Report on Alcohol, Drugs, and Health*, which presented "a call to action to end the public health crisis of addiction"[9] and the follow-up report Spotlight on Opioids.[10]

One important common theme that carried across all NAM reports on quality is that system design, reimbursement processes, and service delivery have more impact on treatment results (patient outcomes) than variation in individual clinician knowledge or behavior. In other words, improved outcomes will come more readily from improved service delivery systems than from additional training. Though human resource development is important, better system design trumps improvement of skills as a leverage point for improving outcomes for populations.[11]

Since the release of the earlier NAM and U.S. Surgeon General reports, significant efforts have been taken to improve measurement and quality. However, the ongoing opioid overdose crisis resulted the NAM releasing a series of discussion papers,[12,13] commentaries,[14,15] and a research agenda[16] focused on addressing the issues and challenges that the treatment system faces while trying to address the opioid overdose epidemic. These publications highlight that much work is yet to be done to address this systemic public health crisis.

DEFINING AND MEASURING ORGANIZATIONAL QUALITY TREATMENT AND OUTCOMES

Public expectations, demands for accountability from payers and policy makers, and a strong desire from within the field of addictions to improve performance drive efforts to define and measure effective treatments and treatment outcomes. Measurement is a key to improvement. Measures of performance before and after the introduction of changes enable managers to verify desired impacts and to monitor, track, and maintain performance over time. The National Committee for Quality Assurance (NCQA), National Quality Forum (NQF), and payers (eg, SAMHSA and its Center for Substance Abuse Treatment [CSAT], Veterans Health Administration [VHA], state and county governments, private insurance payers) collaborate with researchers, clinicians, and professional trade groups to construct and evaluate measurement systems and to promote quality improvements.

Measuring Performance in Addiction Treatment Provider Organizations

NQF has endorsed 11 different measures for SUDs. **Table 50-2** shows the NQF measures. The initiation and engagement (IET) measures have been tracked for various health plans under HEDIS requirements for nearly 20 years, but for most plans there has been no improvement in the measures at the health plan level, and in many cases performance has gotten worse.[17] CMS requires Medicaid adult and home health plans to report on the IET measures as well as follow-up from emergency department visits and continuity of pharmacotherapy measures. All of the measures that have been endorsed by NQF and are used at the system level are process measures. There is little agreement about appropriate outcomes to measure at either the population health or individual patient level.[18,19]

Recently, there has been an effort to assess the system of care using a cascade or continuum of care model to assess patient flow through the system from problem identification through treatment outcome.[20,21] Efforts to quantify measures for the cascade of care have focused on OUD where continuity of pharmacotherapy is evidence-based and relatively easy to measure. Lack of evidence for the length of care necessary and ability to measure whether psychosocial interventions delivered are evidence based make it difficult to use this mechanism for other substance use disorders.

The cascade of care method provides a link or a pathway between process measures and expected outcomes.

The Veterans Health Administration (VHA) examined relationships between center performance on the IET measures and improvements in patient outcomes. Study results are mixed. For example, one study found no significant influence: better rates of identification, initiation, and engagement were not related to greater improvement on outcomes as measured by the Addiction Severity Index (ASI).[22] Another study compared the VHA continuity of care and the HEDIS engagement measure and found that improvement in ASI measures was associated with the HEDIS but not the VHA measure.[23,24] Conversely, the continuity of care measure was associated with a significantly lower mortality rate.[25]

Improvements in initiation and engagement in treatment often have little to do with the treating clinician's knowledge and skills in treating addiction but are instead related to organizational issues involving the intake process, eligibility requirements, waiting lists, office hours and transportation.[26-28] To address these issues, it is important to explore existing processes and implement system changes that enhance these outcomes. For example, a provider could offer "minimal treatment" or "interim maintenance" for individuals placed on opioid treatment program waiting lists, examine and improve their existing paperwork process, or offer walk-in appointments or open access models to clients which abolish waiting lists.[29] Other promising practice examples can be found on the NIATx (an acronym derived from its origins as the Network for the Improvement of Addiction Treatment) website.[30]

Certification of Office-Based Opioid Treatment Clinicians

The Drug Addiction Treatment Act,[31] passed in 2000 (DATA 2000), permitted clinicians to obtain a waiver from the separate registration requirements of the 1974 Narcotic Addict Treatment Act[32] to treat opioid use disorder with Schedule III, IV, and V medications or combinations of such medications that have been approved by the U.S. Food and Drug Administration (FDA) for that indication. Currently the only medication that meets these criteria is buprenorphine (in various formulations). To further increase access to buprenorphine, the Support for Patients and Communities Act makes permanent

TABLE 50-2 National Quality Forum Measure Definitions

Measure number	Measure title and description	Date endorsed
4	Initiation and Engagement of Alcohol and Other Drug Abuse or Dependence Treatment	6/10/2019
2152	Preventive Care and Screening: Unhealthy Alcohol Use: Screening and Brief Counseling	5/5/2021
2600	Tobacco Use Screening and Follow-up for People with Serious Mental Illness or Alcohol or Other Drug Dependence	9/21/2021
2605	Follow-Up After Emergency Department Visit for Mental Illness or Alcohol and Other Drug Abuse or Dependence	6/30/2018
3175	Continuity of Pharmacotherapy for Opioid Use Disorder	11/30/2021
3312	Continuity of Care after Medically Managed Withdrawal for Alcohol or Drugs	11/9/2020
3400	Use of Pharmacotherapy for Opioid Use Disorder	7/1/2021
3488	Follow up after Emergency Department Visit for AOD Abuse or Dependence	6/19/2020
3589	Prescription or Administration of Pharmacotherapy to Treat Opioid Use Disorder (OUD)	7/1/2021
3590	Continuity of Care After Receiving Hospital or Residential Substance Use Disorder (SUD) Treatment	7/1/2021
0028 & 0028e	Preventive Care and Screening: Tobacco Use: Screening and Cessation Intervention	5/5/2021

the authorization of nurse practitioners and physician assistants to prescribe buprenorphine and included authorization for other advanced practice nurses (ie, clinical nurse specialists, certified registered nurse anesthetists, certified nurse midwives) through October 1, 2023.[33]

Regulations allow prescribers to obtain a waiver to treat up to 30 patients without additional training. Providing care to more than 30 patients requires proof of having obtained additional training. Advocacy has focused on further reducing constraints for prescribing buprenorphine, and changes to these requirements are likely in the coming years.

ACCREDITATION OF TREATMENT PROGRAMS

Performance measures are often examined in accreditation reviews. Accreditation is recognition by peers that an organization meets standards of performance that represent safe and competent treatment. Three bodies—the Joint Commission (TJC), the Commission on Accreditation of Rehabilitation Facilities (CARF), and the Council on Accreditation for Children and Family Services (COA)—are the primary entities that provide peer-reviewed accreditation for addiction treatment programs.[34] The 2020 National Survey of Substance Abuse Treatment Services (N-SSATS) notes that 94% of facilities reported accreditation by a state substance abuse agency (77%), department of health (48%), or mental health department (39%); CARF (30%): TJC (23%); hospital licensing (5%); COA (4%); NCQA (2%); Healthcare Facilities Accreditation Program (HFAP, 1%); or another agency (5%).[35]

Accreditation Process

Accreditation requires an organization to conduct an extensive internal analysis of its performance. Accreditation standards focus on broad domains, including governance, consumer rights and privacy, human resource development, the use of treatment and/or clinical interventions, methods to continually improve quality, maintenance and use of records, business systems, and facilities. The standards are aimed at minimum to promote patient safety and optimally to improve patient outcomes. The organizational self-analysis is followed by a site visit by peers or accreditation surveyors, who independently verify the existence and performance of components noted in the self-assessment. Surveyors identify strengths and the need for improvement and then present a recommendation to the accrediting body for multiyear, limited, conditional, or denial of accreditation.

Accreditations of Opioid Treatment Programs

As a result of a transfer of authority from the FDA to SAMHSA in 2001, federal regulations (42 CFR Part 8) require that opioid treatment programs (OTPs) receive certification from a national accreditation organization or state agency documenting that the treatment program meets regulatory standards and will comply with the standards. The Division of Pharmacologic Therapies, a division of CSAT, oversees accreditation of opioid treatment programs. Published guidelines require OTPs to have a current and valid accreditation, SAMHSA certification, and Drug Enforcement Administration registration before dispensing opioid medications.[36] There are six approved accrediting bodies including CARF, TJC, and COA as well as the National Commission on Correctional Health Care, the Healthcare Facilities Accreditation Program, and two states.[37] They review OTPs to confirm that the services comply with federal standards across a wide range of topics including but not limited to continuous quality improvement, telemedicine, clinical assessment and treatment planning, and recovery oriented systems of care.[36]

BUILDING SYSTEM CAPACITY TO DELIVER EFFECTIVE CARE

Since 2001, several national-level efforts have focused on improving the quality of treatment offered, particularly among the state-implemented, SAMHSA block grant-funded programs. Contemporary quality improvement strategies begin with recognition that insufficient quality often reflects poor system and process design. As in other industries, process improvement strategies in addiction treatment strive to construct processes that minimize variability and eliminate error to improve efficiency and enhance customer satisfaction with the product or service. Shewhart[38,39] and his students Deming[40] and Juran[41] were pioneers in the application of these techniques to manufacturing. Over time, the concepts have been extended to service industries including health care.[42,43] The Institute of Healthcare Improvement (IHI) is one such organization that utilizes a science of improvement[44] approach when working with its member organizations. Their efforts focus on three key questions: What are we trying to accomplish? How will we know that a change is an improvement? What changes can we make that will result in improvement?

The NIATx Model of Process Improvement

NIATx is the primary mechanism that has been used to apply process improvement strategies to the programs that treat alcohol and other substance use disorders. Change teams within participating organizations learn to use process improvement tools and techniques to meet quality measures including reduced time to admission, decreased no-shows, enhanced retention in care, increased admissions, and increased use of evidence-based practices.[45,46] Five key process improvement principles have been identified through meta-analysis to facilitate organizational changes to enhance the quality of addiction treatment services: understanding the customer, fixing key problems, picking a powerful change leader, seeking outside ideas and encouragement, and using rapid Plan, Do, Study, Act (PDSA) cycles.[47,48] Together, these principles have the potential to influence organizational culture and reflect an orientation to continuous improvement. The use of the NIATx approach for quality improvement, an IHI-like approach for addiction treatment, is also applicable for clinicians as they seek to address the NAM six dimensions of care.[49]

Understand the Customer

Process improvement stresses the need to understand and involve customers in identifying and fixing problems. Focus groups and interviews with patients can help increase understanding of treatment experiences. Another useful tool is the walk-through; observers simulate the patient experience and participate in the processes that are required for patients, documenting their experiences. Change leaders use a walk-through to gain insight into problems in treatment processes. Walk-through protocols typically start with the admission process. A senior manager develops a patient script (description of the patient and the presenting problems), calls the treatment center for an appointment, completes the admission process, and notes positive and negative findings. Typically, the walk-through scenario includes a "family member" (eg, sibling, spouse, or parent) who shares the experience and makes additional observations. Individuals who conduct the walk-through should record notes about all stages of the experience (eg, initial assessment, first treatment session) and identify what surprised them as well as opportunities for improvement. For example, the front office staff was friendly and efficient, or the intake process involved multiple steps with redundant paperwork. As part of the walk-through process, they should ask staff about their ideas to change or improve the process. These walk-through notes create stories with impact and illuminate problematic facets of the process that can then be addressed in process improvement protocols.

A review of NIATx walk-through reports revealed a number of issues that treatment programs needed to improve, including conflicting and incorrect information provided to patients, redundant and burdensome intake forms, unanswered telephone lines, and unreturned voice mails.[50] There were also challenges addressing complex patient needs (such as co-occurring disorders) and weaknesses in agency infrastructure.[50,51] Change teams use the results of walk-through to identify process problems that can be corrected and improved.

Fix Key Problems

Agency change requires active support from the highest levels of the organization. The chief executive will often be supportive of change that addresses issues that affect revenue and costs.[51] Missed appointments, for example, reduce counselor productivity, and anticipated revenue is lost. Strategies to reduce no-show rates, therefore, can lead to increased revenues and improved counselor productivity.

Phoenix Center in Greenville, South Carolina, for example, completed a walk-through and found that they had a waiting list for withdrawal management beds at the same time as having five empty beds. To reduce the waiting list and fill the beds, the program implemented a series of change cycles. The specific changes were to eliminate scheduled withdrawal management admission appointment, reduce phone screen questions, adjust staff schedules during peak admission times, post bed availability, and ask clients "What time can you be here today?" versus "We have an appointment available on." As a result of the change, bed utilization increased almost 10% from 90% to 99%, and monthly program revenues increased by 11%. In another example, the Aegis Medical System that operates 25 OTPs across California conducted a walk-through of the admission process. The results found that the first appointment, which included paperwork and a medical assessment, lasted 4 hours and the first clinical intervention was scheduled for 1 to 3 weeks later. They also analyzed 17 months of discharge data and set as a goal to reduce the first 90-day attrition rate by 10% over a 6-month period. The staff tested a change called "Five in Five" where the client had their medical assessment on day one and then on 4 subsequent days met with the clinician to tell their story and establish a relationship. As a result of the change, the attrition rate fell by 75% from 16% to 4% in 2 months with a projected increase in the annual revenue of $388,000. The change was diffused to all Aegis OTPs.

Pick a Powerful Change Leader

The change leader (the individual who leads a team in creating and implementing organizational change) is an integral part of the successful change effort in the organization. It can also be an excellent career development opportunity. To help prepare individuals, NIATx developed a Change Leader Academy designed to teach the skills to become an effective change leader.[52] Not every counselor or employee has the skill to lead change, and many do not seek the responsibility of leading change. It is important, therefore, to choose individuals with the right mix of aptitude and ability. Change leaders should have the respect of their peers and of staff and leaders throughout the organization. They must also have access to agency management. Within the organization, the change leader is responsible for running the change team meetings, and as such, they should have effective project management skills including being organized, a good delegator, and comfortable with using data to guide improvement efforts. Over time, a well-developed organization will use the opportunity to lead change teams as a strategy for grooming future managers and leaders within the organization.

Seek Outside Ideas and Encouragement

NIATx members get ideas for service improvements from other NIATx participants (ie, inside the field) and from other industries (ie, outside the field). The vice president of quality improvement at the Ritz Carlton spoke at a NIATx conference and shared his perspectives on serving hotel guests and the hotel's expectations for customer orientation among all employees: "Ladies and Gentlemen Serving Ladies and Gentlemen." Though the Ritz typically serves a clientele different from that found in most publicly funded substance use treatment services, its emphasis on treating guests and staff as ladies and gentlemen can be applied in any business, including addiction treatment. Opportunities to learn from others are not limited to the hospitality field. For example, an organization might be able to learn from a local car dealer how to engage clients, from an air traffic control how to hand-off clients within or across organizations, or from retailers who open up new lines when the queue gets too long. Leveraging these ideas requires an ability to think outside the box, recognize that other organizations experience similar problems, and adapt those solutions to the specific situation in their organization.

Use Rapid Plan, Do, Study, Act Cycles

Plan, Do, Study, Act (PDSA) cycles are a central component of process improvement. Planning includes specification of the problem that will be fixed, collection of data to assess the extent of the problem, and development of a change that will be implemented. Process improvement is about action. Change teams test the proposed change (do). A key facet is that the test is for a limited time and limited number of patients. Initially, it is a feasibility test. Can we make the change, and does the change produce the desire effect? A few simple measures are collected and analyzed (study): did a change occur in the frequency or extent of the problem? Based on the planning, doing, and studying, the change team decides what to do next (act). The change can be abandoned if it does not work. It may be modified to enhance the effect. If the pilot was successful, it expands to include more patients and more counselors or more sites and, eventually, is institutionalized through changed policy and procedure manuals. PDSA cycles are rapid. Two weeks or less is usually sufficient to learn whether the change is viable and if additional time and resources should be invested.

An analysis from the first cohort of NIATx participants over a 15-month reporting period found a 37% decline in days to treatment and significant improvements in retention in care were also observed.[46] Further analysis with a second cohort of NIATx participants replicated these findings and showed that participants from the first cohort sustained the improvements.[53] Although gains may appear to be modest, the impact of process improvement seemed to increase over time suggesting that programs can sustain the improvements in access and retention. Additional analysis suggests that reduction in days to treatment enhances the likelihood that individuals will complete at least four treatment sessions.[54]

Research on Quality Improvement in Addiction Treatment

Since its establishment in 2003, NIATx has become an evidence-based implementation strategy to improve the quality of care in specialty addiction clinics. A randomized controlled trial funded by the National Institute on Drug Abuse examined the effectiveness of four implementation strategies (interest circles, coaching, learning sessions or a combination of interest circles, coaching and learning sessions) in 201 treatment programs.[55] Analyses assessed the influence of each study condition on change in days to treatment and retention in care. Results indicated significant improvements in wait time for each level of support except interest circle calls.[56] While none of the levels of support resulted in a significant improvement in continuation defined as the percent of clients retained from the first to fourth treatment session, clinicians in the coaching and combination levels of support significantly increased the number of new patients. A calculation of the benefit-cost ratios found that the coaching level of support was more cost-effective than the learning session or combination supports at reducing wait time or improving the number of new patients.

Building on this success, NIATx implementation strategies were evaluated along with five levers of change to guide efforts to improve access to medications in specialty addiction clinics and to provide structure for state and clinician initiatives designed to support efforts to increase access to medication.[57] Research studies found that specialty addiction clinics successfully applied NIATx implementation strategies, most often a combination of coaching, learning sessions and group coaching calls to improve client access to medications for opioid use or alcohol use disorder.[58-62]

NIATx implementation strategies have also been utilized to improve co-occurring capacity, increase access to substance use and psychotropic medications, and reduce medication wait times in specialty addiction clinics.[63-66] NIATx has been applied in research studies in HIV clinics,[67] the criminal justice setting,[68,69] medical withdrawal programs,[70] and in county mental health organizations[71] to address key problems such as no-shows, screening for alcohol and opioid use disorder, or the perceived value of HIV services. Qualitative analyses examined facilitators and barriers to using NIATx in specialty addiction clinics as well as other organizational settings.[72-78]

The evidence of NIATx as a quality improvement approach is substantial. Almost every successful application of NIATx utilizes coaching to guide the organization through the change process and relies, as needed, on learning sessions and group coaching calls to provide opportunities for organizations to learn from their peers, a critical element of getting ideas from inside and outside the field.

USING QUALITY IMPROVEMENT PRINCIPLES TO IMPROVE PATIENT OUTCOMES

Though the measurement of performance measures within addiction health care practices and organizations was recognized as important decades ago, the use of these measures in evaluating processes and outcomes of substance use treatment services has lagged behind other trends in health care. This is in part due to the struggle within the field about how to establish clinically meaningful outcomes.[19] Indicators of quality treatment may vary over time and context, for example, early treatment indicators of cravings versus later stage quality of life measures. Given that recovery may take years or a lifetime, metrics that measure personal patient progress and community integration can be considered appropriate measures of quality care.

Questions remain as to how patient outcomes should be assessed and understood in relation to other components of health care, especially given the movement toward more harm reduction strategies within the field. For example, some OTPs may have strict definitions of successful treatment such as long-term abstinence while others may have other criteria such as reductions in overdoses. Generally, programs that tend to create fewer barriers to treatment, such as not requiring drug abstinence or ensuring adequate methadone dosing, have seen improved retention and lower rates of adverse events compared to programs with greater restrictions.[79] Additionally, quality care may need more a more expansive definition than simply monitoring the services provided; patient outcome measures can include variables such as stable housing, employment and quality of life[80] such as the WHO QOL.[81] Some of these measures are currently incorporated into the Government Performance and Results Act (GPRA) Client Outcome Measures for Discretionary Programs.

Recovery capital (RC) has gained attention as a potential metric for measuring patient recovery as a result of treatment. RC is an asset-based model based focused on initiating or sustaining recovery through increasing individual resources and capacities. Though the term first emerged 20 years ago, the domains, best practices, and applications are not established.[82] The most widely used RC instrument is the 50-item Assessment of Recovery Capital (ARC), along with its 10-item abbreviated version among the six instruments in the literature. Using these instruments, clinicians can evaluate the results to incorporate strengths-based connections that further treatment engagement such as linkages to peer-based support services, housing services, psychiatric services, and other community supports.

Measurement Based Care (MBC) is the measurement of standardized patient-reported outcomes (PROs) to identify patient symptoms and function. Results can then be used by practitioners to adjust and improve care.[83] Use of MBC in treatment planning has been shown to improve the quality of care and outcomes for patients.[84,85] The Addiction Medicine Practice-based Research Network (AMNet) is a joint initiative of the American Psychiatric Association (APA), American Society of Addiction Medicine (ASAM), and Friends Research Institute seeking to further performance improvement in addiction medicine and addiction psychiatry.[86] Measures in the framework include the Brief Addiction Monitor, Tobacco, Alcohol and Prescription Medication and Other Substance Use Tool, Treatment Effectiveness Assessment, Short Opiate Withdrawal Scale, Clinical Opiate Withdrawal Scale, Visual Analogue Scale for Opioid Craving, Patient Health Questionnaire (PHQ-2), PROMIS Pain Interference, and three psychiatric measures including the DSM-5 Cross-cutting measure, PHQ-9, and the Generalized Anxiety Disorder (GAD-7).

ASAM Standard Workgroup

ASAM has released two reports: *Standards of Care for the Addiction Specialist Physician* and *Performance Measures for the Addiction Specialist Physician*. These documents outline the standards of care and how to measure performance in meeting the standards for addiction specialists. The standards cover the activities expected to be conducted for diagnosis, withdrawal management, treatment planning and management, continuing care and transitions, and care coordination.[87,88]

Impact of COVID-19 on How We Define Quality Care

The COVID-19 pandemic has raised questions about what would be considered quality measurements for patient care, as medication regulations have been eased for treatment of SUD. For example, telehealth has expanded, buprenorphine treatment initiation can occur remotely, and OTPs may dispense take-home supplies of methadone to patients that had previously been considered not eligible due to only partial adherence to treatment. Current data show that virtual behavioral health visits may deliver equivalent quality treatment to patients and lower the rate of no-shows,[89] improve retention, and decrease UDT opioid positive results[90] demonstrating how diverse modalities maintain quality treatment delivery. Moreover, patient level assessment of quality care can be related to other dimensions of well-being which may be improving because of changes in treatment modality. For example, Levander et al.[91] found that patients who received more take-home methadone doses and received telehealth services because of the SAMHSA blanket exceptions felt the changes benefited their recovery, reduced time traveling, and enabled them to have more time for family and for work responsibilities. These important patient outcomes should be measured as quality-of-care indicators.

ENSURING PRIMARY CARE CLINICIANS CAN IDENTIFY, TREAT OR REFER, AND MONITOR SUBSTANCE USE DISORDER

There is an increasing recognition that practitioners across all settings should be able to screen for and monitor and provide medication for SUDs. A multisite study found a high prevalence of alcohol (62%) and other drug use (27.9%) in primary care settings. The prevalence of any 12-month SUD was 36.0% (mild disorder 14.2%, moderate to severe disorder 21.8%).[92] Patients with SUDs have a higher prevalence of heart, liver, and gastrointestinal disorders.[93] Specialty addiction treatment centers developed because the patient's SUDs were not addressed in general health care settings. However, primary health care clinicians regularly see patients who have (or risk having) a substance use problem or health conditions that are exacerbated by substance use.

The separation of treatment for medical and behavioral illness is an area that is increasingly being addressed. For example, the White House Office of National Drug Control

Policy (ONDCP) 2015 National Drug Control Strategy asserts that SUDs are medical conditions and that treatment should be integrated into mainstream health care and suggests concrete steps toward the goal of improved access to addiction treatment services,[94] including the integration of Screening, Brief Intervention, and Referral to Treatment (SBIRT) into all health care settings. At its core, SBIRT has three goals: (1) screening to rapidly assess the severity of substance use and identify the appropriate level of treatment, (2) a brief intervention that focuses on increasing insight and awareness regarding substance use and motivation toward behavioral change, and (3) referral to specialty treatment.[95] The Health Resources and Services Administration has taken steps to promote the use of screening services, such as including codes for BI in the Uniform Data Systems to track screening activity in Federally Qualified Health Centers. States are encouraged to adopt SBIRT as a reimbursable service and train more clinicians in SBIRT. Lastly, the ONDCP strategy also stressed the importance of screening and early intervention in women's health care settings, as this has the potential to reduce the estimated 400,000 to 440,000 infants affected by prenatal alcohol or illicit drug exposure.

Although there has been some movement to offer primary care services in addiction specialty clinics, the ONDCP Strategy reflects the general trend of incorporating addiction-focused resources into primary care settings rather than the other way around. An advantage to this arrangement concerns the reduction in the stigma that may occur for individuals obtaining SUD treatment from a primary care clinician, compared to a stand-alone specialized service. Yet, many clinicians, including physicians, are not trained in how to identify or treat addiction. With new research into how substance use and addiction affect the body and the brain, more doctors are coming to an understanding of addiction as a medical problem and addressing it as a chronic health condition. Until recently, there have been no national standards for training in addiction medicine, and medical students receive little addiction training. In 2016, the American Board of Medical Specialties recognized addiction medicine as a new subspecialty under the American Board of Preventative Medicine. This replaced the American Board of Addiction Medicine (ABAM) subspecialty process for becoming certified in Addiction Medicine.

These same specialty boards require that clinicians at the time of recertification and licensing requirements implement a performance in practice project.[96,97] From 2006 to 2010, Improving Performance in Practice initiative uses quality improvement tools and techniques including PDSA cycles designed to improve processes of care.[98] The tools and techniques outlined in this chapter provide an approach that clinicians could use to achieve their maintenance of certification requirements. More recently the American Academy of Addiction Psychiatry and the Providers Clinical Support System has created a Performance-in-Practice (PIP) activity to help clinicians treat opioid use disorder in their practices, determining individual practice gaps and addressing them through a performance improvement plan designed to increase competence, performance, and patient outcomes. The PIP walks participants through three steps in a process to enhance practice of the treatment of patients with opioid use disorder. It is recommended that the PIP take 3 months or more to complete, though it may take significantly longer (as long as deemed necessary to plan, implement, and evaluate your educational plan). This PIP follows the AMA-standardized three-stage process: (1) Assess current practice against current evidence and expert consensus, (2) Develop and follow your own improvement plan, (3) Reassess your practice to measure the effects of your improvement plan. Addiction psychiatrists can also leverage the Maintenance of Certification process to improve clinical care.[99] In 2019, the Accreditation Council for Graduate Medical Education released guidelines that require all medical specialties to teach competencies related to addiction and pain. These efforts could increase clinician skills in talking to patients about these topics. Additionally, the National Association of Addiction Treatment Providers endorses value-based practices, which includes a code of ethics that discourages certain practices such as the unethical recruitment of patients.

There are a number of tools for clinicians to ensure quality in office-based addiction treatment. The CSAT offers Treatment Improvement Protocols (TIPs), three of which are for prescribers treating either alcohol or opioid addiction.[100-102] Each of these manuals comes with a Knowledge Application Program (KAP) Key that is a short version of the critical clinical information outlined in the TIP. In 2017, TIP 40 (on guidelines for prescribing buprenorphine) and TIP 43 (on medication use in opioid treatment programs) were combined into one manual and updated to include the new formulations of medications recently made available.

The Provider's Clinical Support System for Medication Assisted Treatment (PCSS-MAT) provides clinicians with training, support, and mentoring in treating patients with opioid use disorder using medication. Though the requirements for buprenorphine prescribing no longer require an 8-hour training, an application for a waiver from the Drug Enforcement Administration must still be made by clinicians intending to prescribe buprenorphine. Qualified clinicians include physicians, Nurse Practitioners, Physician Assistants, Clinical Nurse Specialists, Certified Registered Nurse Anesthetist, and Certified Nurse-Midwives. Training, waiver process, and PCSS-MAT are all part of an effort to ensure quality in the treatment of patients with opioid use disorder.[103] The PCSS training is geared toward those seeking to prescribe buprenorphine, all three currently available medications (methadone, buprenorphine, and naltrexone) are included so that practitioners are knowledgeable about the choices available to their patients and the rationale for prescribing one medication over another for specific patients.

One final tool that is being used increasingly by clinicians in primary care who wish to treat patients with SUDs is prescription drug monitoring programs (PDMPs). PDMPs provide clinicians with timely information on the scheduled drugs their patients have been prescribed by other clinicians as well as themselves. Requesting data from the PDMP on prescriptions filled by a patient with SUDs, in addition to drug testing, can serve as a risk management tool but also as a quality management tool. Treatment may need to be adjusted if patients are not filling their prescriptions or are on multiple medications prescribed by other medical professionals. Active engagement of patients into SUD treatment should also be considered when such prescription behaviors are uncovered.

The use of medications to treat SUDs needs to continue to be integrated into the treatment system at a faster pace and for more patients. The pace that changes are made will be impacted by individuals' ability to pay and payers' willingness to include these medications and services in their plans. The U.S. Preventive Services Task Force has endorsed screening for various SUD conditions. For primary care clinicians, understanding of these screening recommendations is important considering the implications for insurance coverage.

INTERNATIONAL EFFORTS: THE INTERNATIONAL CENTER FOR CREDENTIALING AND EDUCATION OF ADDICTION PROFESSIONALS

The United Nations Office on Drugs and Crime (UNODC) in conjunction with the World Health Organization (WHO) has conducted extensive efforts to improve the quality of care for people who use drugs worldwide. In 2020, they jointly published the International Standards for the Treatment of Drug Use Disorders.[104] The standards include requirements for system design that includes five levels of care: self-care, informal community care, generic health and human services, specialized drug dependence services and long stay residential services. It provides definitions and expectations for what should be available at each level. For each level it describes specific services necessary to address specific needs including pharmacotherapy and recovery supports. These standards will provide a guideline for the global effort to improve the quality of care. UNODC provides training and technical assistance to governments on how to create systems of care and provide quality assurance mechanisms based on the standards.

Established in February 2009, the Global Center for Credentialing and Certification (GCCC), formerly the International Center for Credentialing and Education of Addiction Professionals (ICCE), is a global initiative funded by the Bureau of International Narcotics and Law Enforcement Affairs (INL), U.S. Department of State. GCCC's mission is to ensure the workforce can demonstrate the knowledge, skills and attitudes necessary to provide the standard of care proposed by WHO and UNODC.

GCCC collaborates with international experts that provide training in substance use disorders. The Universal Prevention Curricula and the Universal Treatment Curricula are multimodule training programs designed to equip prevention and addiction treatment professionals with knowledge, skills, and competencies to efficiently deliver drug demand reduction services. Both the UPC and UTC were developed by a team of experts in the field and approved by three international organizations, namely, United Nations Office on Drugs and Crime (UNODC), Organization of American States (OAS), and Colombo Plan. Each curriculum is piloted, adapted, and adopted by the region or country implementing the initiative. The curriculum content of the UPC and UTC has been found to meet the national and international certification standards set by the U.S. National Certification Commission of Addiction Professionals (NCCAP).

In addition to the postemployment training offered by these international organizations, there is an effort to incorporate SUD knowledge in university curricula and to create addiction specialty education programs for the rapid improvement in competencies and skills among current and future professionals in the field of addictions. These efforts are led by the International Consortium of Universities for Drug Demand Reduction (ICUDDR). These different bodies together are working to create quality design, assessment and improvement into the systems that provide care to people who use alcohol and other drugs across the globe.

CONCLUSIONS

Quality improvement efforts are affecting the organization and delivery of treatment for SUDs. These efforts should include a focus ensuring that the care delivered is consistent with the NAM's six dimensions of quality. Strategies to define, measure, and improve the quality of addiction treatment services influence standards of care and the ways in which quality is evaluated. Quality interventions that build on the foundation of the NIATx model have been widely adopted, which is supported by a growing body of research on the effectiveness of implementation strategies that are a part of the NIATx model. Treatment programs engaged in NIATx gain encouragement and ideas from participation in learning communities and support the application of process improvement to systems of care for these disorders. Outcome studies including those at the organizational and patient levels suggest that process changes can lead to reductions in days to admission and to improvements in retention in care, access the medications, and the adoption of evidence-based practices. Organizational NIATx change initiatives have many advantages and the NIATx model provides the key resources needed to widely spread and sustain changes.

The NIATx approach also attempts to promote a spread of process improvements across a variety of organizational settings including HIV-AIDS organizations, the criminal justice system, and statewide treatment systems. The key NIATx principles of change work for individual organizations and are also applicable to multi-organizational system changes to facilitate adoption of evidence-based practices. Additional principles, however, also need to be considered when addressing statewide adaptations/changes or supporting changes in unique treatment environments or the implementation of evidence-based practices (eg, motivational interviewing or co-occurring capacity).

Continuing education is evolving to be more practice oriented in general, focusing less on information provision and more on supporting change in practice and development of skills. As clinicians are asked to demonstrate their ability to institute change and ensure quality treatment, demonstration of the use of the tools of quality management including the institutionalization of quality improvement mechanism becomes an essential component of their practice.

Additionally, technology is a growing factor in ensuring consistency in practice. There are many efforts to automate and streamline service delivery: computer-based screening and brief interventions, mobile phone applications for return to use prevention, web-based delivery of therapy sessions, development of predictive models that use real-time data from sensors or ecological momentary assessments, and the use of games to increase engagement in the recovery process. These leaps forward are dramatically changing the landscape of addiction care and shifting the criteria for defining quality as well as the way we measure it.

REFERENCES

1. McLellan AT, Lewis DC, O'Brien CP, Kleber HD. Drug dependence, a chronic medical illness: implications for treatment, insurance, and outcomes evaluation. *JAMA*. 2000;284(13):1689-1695. doi:10.1001/jama.284.13.1689
2. Strang J, Volkow ND, Degenhardt L, et al. Opioid use disorder. *Nat Rev Primer*. 2020;6(1):3. doi:10.1038/s41572-019-0137-5
3. Volkow ND, Boyle M. Neuroscience of addiction: relevance to prevention and treatment. *Am J Psychiatry*. 2018;175(8):729-740. doi:10.1176/appi.ajp.2018.17101174
4. Institute of Medicine (US) Committee on Quality of Health Care in America; Kohn LT, Corrigan JM, Donaldson MS, eds. *To Err is Human: Building a Safer Health System*. National Academies Press; 2000.
5. Institute of Medicine (US) Committee on Quality of Health Care in America. *Crossing the Quality Chasm: A New Health System for the 21st Century*. National Academies Press; 2001.
6. Institute of Medicine (US) Committee on Crossing the Quality Chasm: Adaptation to Mental Health and Addictive Disorders. *Improving the Quality of Health Care for Mental and Substance-Use Conditions: Quality Chasm Series*. National Academies Press; 2006.
7. England MJ, Butler AS, Gonzalez ML; Committee on Developing Evidence-Based Standards for Psychosocial Interventions for Mental Disorders; Board on Health Sciences Policy; Institute of Medicine, eds. *Psychosocial Interventions for Mental and Substance Use Disorders: A Framework for Establishing Evidence-Based Standards*. National Academies Press; 2015.
8. O'Brien CP, Oster M, Morden E; Committee on Prevention, Diagnosis, Treatment, and Management of Substance Use Disorders in the U.S. Armed Forces; Board on the Health of Select Populations; Institute of Medicine, eds. *Substance Use Disorders in the U.S. Armed Forces*. National Academies Press; 2013.
9. Substance Abuse and Mental Health Services Administration (US); Office of the Surgeon General (US). *Facing Addiction in America: The Surgeon General's Report on Alcohol, Drugs, and Health*. US Department of Health and Human Services; 2016.
10. Substance Abuse and Mental Health Services Administration (US); Office of the Surgeon General (US). *Facing Addiction in America: The Surgeon General's Spotlight on Opioids*. US Department of Health and Human Services; 2018.
11. Health Resources & Services Administration Health Center Program. *Clinical Quality Improvement*. Accessed September 19, 2022. https://bphc.hrsa.gov/technical-assistance/clinical-quality-improvement
12. Madras BK, Ahmad NJ, Wen J, Sharfstein JS. Improving access to evidence-based medical treatment for opioid use disorder: strategies to address key barriers within the treatment system. *NAM Perspect*. 2020. doi:10.31478/202004b
13. Blanco C, Ali MM, Beswick A, et al. The American opioid epidemic in special populations: five examples. *NAM Perspect*. 2020. doi:10.31478/202010b
14. Woodruff AE, Tomanovich M, Beletsky L, Salisbury-Afshar E, Wakeman S, Ostrovsky A. Dismantling buprenorphine policy can provide more comprehensive addiction treatment. *NAM Perspect*. 2019. doi:10.31478/201909a
15. Atkins J, Dopp AL, Temaner EB. Combatting the stigma of addiction—the need for a comprehensive health system approach. *NAM Perspect*. 2020. doi:10.31478/202011d
16. National Academy of Medicine. *National Academy of Medicine Action Collaborative on Countering the U.S. Opioid Epidemic: Research Agenda*. National Academy of Medicine. Accessed April 14, 2022. 2022 https://nam.edu/programs/action-collaborative-on-countering-the-u-s-opioid-epidemic/opioid-collaborative-agenda/
17. The National Committee for Quality Assurance (NCQA). *Initiation and Engagement of Alcohol and Other Drug Abuse or Dependence Treatment (IET)*. Accessed April 22, 2022. https://www.ncqa.org/hedis/measures/initiation-and-engagement-of-alcohol-and-other-drug-abuse-or-dependence-treatment/
18. Schmidt EM, Liu P, Combs A, Trafton J, Asch S, Harris AHS. Surveying the landscape of quality-of-care measures for mental and substance use disorders. *Psychiatr Serv*. 2022;73(8):880-888. doi:10.1176/appi.ps.202000913 3
19. Kiluk BD, Fitzmaurice GM, Strain EC, Weiss RD. What defines a clinically meaningful outcome in the treatment of substance use disorders: reductions in direct consequences of drug use or improvement in overall functioning? *Addiction*. 2019;114(1):9-15. doi:10.1111/add.14289
20. Socías ME, Volkow N, Wood E. Adopting the "cascade of care" framework: an opportunity to close the implementation gap in addiction care? *Addiction*. 2016;111(12):2079-2081. doi:10.1111/add.13479
21. Williams AR, Nunes EV, Olfson M. *To Battle The Opioid Overdose Epidemic, Deploy The 'Cascade of Care' Model*. Health Affairs Blog. Accessed April 14, 2022. https://www.healthaffairs.org/do/10.1377/forefront.20170313.059163
22. Harris AH, Humphreys K, Finney JW. Veterans affairs facility performance on Washington circle indicators and casemix-adjusted effectiveness. *J Subst Abuse Treat*. 2007;33(4):333-339. doi:10.1016/j.jsat.2006.12.015
23. Harris AH, Humphreys K, Bowe T, Tiet Q, Finney JW. Does meeting the HEDIS substance abuse treatment engagement criterion predict patient outcomes? *J Behav Health Serv Res*. 2010;37(1):25-39. doi:10.1007/s11414-008-9142-2
24. Harris AH, Humphreys K, Bowe T, Kivlahan DR, Finney JW. Measuring the quality of substance use disorder treatment: evaluating the validity of the Department of Veterans Affairs continuity of care performance measure. *J Subst Abuse Treat*. 2009;36(3):294-305. doi:10.1016/j.jsat.2008.05.011
25. Harris AH, Gupta S, Bowe T, et al. Predictive validity of two process-of-care quality measures for residential substance use disorder treatment. *Addict Sci Clin Pr*. 2015;10:22. doi:10.1186/s13722-015-0042-5
26. Chang JS, Sorensen JL, Masson CL, et al. Structural factors affecting Asians and Pacific Islanders in community-based substance use treatment: treatment provider perspectives. *J Ethn Subst Abuse*. 2017;16(4):479-494. doi:10.1080/15332640.2017.1395384
27. Masson CL, Shopshire MS, Sen S, et al. Possible barriers to enrollment in substance abuse treatment among a diverse sample of Asian Americans and Pacific Islanders: opinions of treatment clients. *J Subst Abuse Treat*. 2013;44(3):309-315. doi:10.1016/j.jsat.2012.08.005
28. Wisdom JP, Hoffman K, Rechberger E, Seim K, Owens B. Women-focused treatment agencies and process improvement: strategies to increase client engagement. *Women Ther*. 2009;32(1):69-87. doi:10.1080/02703140802384693

29. Madden LM, Farnum SO, Eggert KF, et al. An investigation of an open-access model for scaling up methadone maintenance treatment. *Addiction.* 2018;113(8):1450-1458. doi:10.1111/add.14198
30. University of Wisconsin-Madison. NIATx. https://www.niatx.net/
31. 106th Congress. *Drug Addiction Treatment Act of 2000.* Accessed April 22, 2022. https://www.congress.gov/bill/106th-congress/house-bill/2634
32. 93rd Congress. *Narcotic Addict Treatment Act.* Accessed May 31, 2023. https://www.congress.gov/bill/93rd-congress/senate-bill/1115
33. 115th Congress. SUPPORT for Patients and Communities Act. Accessed September 19, 2022. https://www.congress.gov/bill/115th-congress/house-bill/6/actions
34. Institute of Medicine (US) Committee on Quality Assurance and Accreditation Guidelines for Managed Behavioral Health Care; Edmunds M, Frank R, Hogan M, et al., eds. *Managing Managed Care: Quality Improvement in Behavioral Health.* National Academies Press; 1997.
35. Substance Abuse and Mental Health Services Administration. National Survey of Substance Abuse Treatment Services (N-SSATS): 2020. Data on Substance Abuse Treatment Facilities. Accessed May 31, 2023. https://www.samhsa.gov/data/sites/default/files/reports/rpt35313/2020_NSSATS_FINAL.pdf
36. Wechsberg WM, Kasten JJ, Berkman ND, Roussel AE. *Methadone Maintenance Treatment in the U.S.: A Practical Question and Answer Guide.* Springer; 2007.
37. SAMHSA. *Approved Accreditation Bodies.* Substance Abuse and Mental Health Services Administration. Published March 30, 2022. Accessed April 14; 2022. https://www.samhsa.gov/medication-assisted-treatment/become-accredited-opioid-treatment-program/approved-accreditation-bodies
38. Shewhart WA. *Economic Control of Quality of Manufactured Product.* Martino Publishing; 2015.
39. Shewhart WA. *Statistical Method from the Viewpoint of Quality Control.* Dover Publications; 2012.
40. Deming WE, Cahill KE, Allan KL. *Out of the Crisis Reissue.* MIT Press; 2018.
41. Juran JM, Gryna FM. *Juran's Quality Control Handbook.* McGraw Hill; 1988.
42. Barney M, McCarty T. *The New Six Sigma: A Leader's Guide to Achieving Rapid Business Improvement and Sustainable Results.* Prentice Hall PTR; 2003.
43. Berwick DM. *Escape Fire: Designs for the Future of Health Care.* Wiley; 2010.
44. Institute for Healthcare Improvement. *Science of Improvement.* Accessed April 14, 2022. http://www.ihi.org/about/Pages/ScienceofImprovement.aspx
45. Capoccia VA, Cotter F, Gustafson DH, et al. Making "stone soup": improvements in clinic access and retention in addiction treatment. *Jt Comm J Qual Patient Saf.* 2007;33(2):95-103. doi:10.1016/s1553-7250(07)33011-0
46. McCarty D, Gustafson DH, Wisdom JP, et al. The Network for the Improvement of Addiction Treatment (NIATx): enhancing access and retention. *Drug Alcohol Depend.* 2007;88(2-3):138-145. doi:10.1016/j.drugalcdep.2006.10.009
47. Gustafson DH, Johnson KA, Capoccia V, et al. *The Niatx Model: Process Improvement in Behavioral Health.* Center for Health Enhancement Systems Studies, University of Wisconsin; 2012.
48. Hoffman KA, Green CA, Ford JH, Wisdom JP, Gustafson DH, McCarty D. Improving quality of care in substance abuse treatment using five key process improvement principles. *J Behav Health Serv Res.* 2012;39(3):234-244. doi:10.1007/s11414-011-9270-y
49. McCarty D, Gustafson D, Capoccia VA, Cotter F. Improving care for the treatment of alcohol and drug disorders. *J Behav Health Serv Res.* 2009;36(1):52-60. doi:10.1007/s11414-008-9108-4
50. Ford JH, Green CA, Hoffman KA, et al. Process improvement needs in substance abuse treatment: admissions walk-through results. *J Subst Abuse Treat.* 2007;33(4):379-389. doi:10.1016/j.jsat.2007.02.003
51. Quanbeck AR, Madden L, Edmundson E, et al. A business case for quality improvement in addiction treatment: evidence from the NIATx collaborative. *J Behav Health Serv Res.* 2012;39(1):91-100. doi:10.1007/s11414-011-9259-6
52. Evans AC, Rieckmann T, Fitzgerald MM, Gustafson DH. Teaching the NIATx model of process improvement as an evidence-based process. *J Teach Addict.* 2008;6(2):21-37. doi:10.1080/15332700802127912
53. Hoffman KA, Ford JH, Choi D, Gustafson DH, McCarty D. Replication and sustainability of improved access and retention within the Network for the Improvement of Addiction Treatment. *Drug Alcohol Depend.* 2008;98(1-2):63-69. doi:10.1016/j.drugalcdep.2008.04.016
54. Hoffman KA, Ford JH, Tillotson CJ, Choi D, McCarty D. Days to treatment and early retention among patients in treatment for alcohol and drug disorders. *Addict Behav.* 2011;36(6):643-647. doi:10.1016/j.addbeh.2011.01.031
55. Quanbeck AR, Gustafson DH, Ford JH, et al. Disseminating quality improvement: study protocol for a large cluster-randomized trial. *Implement Sci.* 2011;6:44. doi:10.1186/1748-5908-6-44
56. Gustafson DH, Quanbeck AR, Robinson JM, et al. Which elements of improvement collaboratives are most effective? A cluster-randomized trial. *Addiction.* 2013;108(6):1145-1157. doi:10.1111/add.12117
57. Schmidt LA, Rieckmann T, Abraham A, et al. Advancing recovery: implementing evidence-based treatment for substance use disorders at the systems level. *J Stud Alcohol Drugs.* 2012;73(3):413-422. doi:10.15288/jsad.2012.73.413
58. Molfenter T, Kim JS, Quanbeck A, Patel-Porter T, Starr S, McCarty D. Testing use of payers to facilitate evidence-based practice adoption: protocol for a cluster-randomized trial. *Implement Sci.* 2013;8:50. doi:10.1186/1748-5908-8-50
59. Molfenter T, McCarty D, Jacobson N, Kim JS, Starr S, Zehner M. The payer's role in addressing the opioid epidemic: it's more than money. *J Subst Abuse Treat.* 2019;101:72-78. doi:10.1016/j.jsat.2019.04.001
60. Molfenter T, Sherbeck C, Zehner M, et al. Implementing buprenorphine in addiction treatment: payer and provider perspectives in Ohio. *Subst Abuse Treat Prev Policy.* 2015;10:13. doi:10.1186/s13011-015-0009-2
61. Ford JH, Abraham AJ, Lupulescu-Mann N, et al. Promoting adoption of medication for opioid and alcohol use disorders through system change. *J Stud Alcohol Drugs.* 2017;78(5):735-744. doi:10.15288/jsad.2017.78.735
62. Alanis-Hirsch K, Croff R, Ford JH, et al. Extended-release naltrexone: a qualitative analysis of barriers to routine Use. *J Subst Abuse Treat.* 2016;62:68-73. doi:10.1016/j.jsat.2015.10.003
63. Chokron Garneau H, Assefa MT, Jo B, Ford JH, Saldana L, McGovern MP. Sustainment of integrated care in addiction treatment settings: primary outcomes from a cluster-randomized controlled trial. *Psychiatr Serv.* 2022;73(3):280-286. doi:10.1176/appi.ps.202000293
64. Ford JH, Kaur A, Rao D, et al. Improving medication access within integrated treatment for individuals with co-occurring disorders in substance use treatment agencies. *Implement Res Pract.* 2021;2: doi:10.1177/26334895211033659
65. Assefa MT, Ford JH, Osborne E, et al. Implementing integrated services in routine behavioral health care: primary outcomes from a cluster randomized controlled trial. *BMC Health Serv Res.* 2019;19(1):749. doi:10.1186/s12913-019-4624-x
66. Ford JH 2nd, Rao D, Gilson A, et al. Wait no longer: reducing medication wait-times for individuals with co-occurring disorders. *J Dual Diagn.* 2022;18(2):101-110. doi:10.1080/15504263.2022.2052225
67. Garner BR, Gotham HJ, Chaple M, et al. The implementation and sustainment facilitation strategy improved implementation effectiveness and intervention effectiveness: results from a cluster-randomized, type 2 hybrid trial. *Implement Res Pract.* 2020;1: doi:10.1177/2633489520948073
68. Pearson FS, Shafer MS, Dembo R, et al. Efficacy of a process improvement intervention on delivery of HIV services to offenders: a multisite trial. *Am J Public Health.* 2014;104(12):2385-2391. doi:10.2105/ajph.2014.302035
69. Visher CA, Hiller M, Belenko S, et al. The effect of a local change team intervention on staff attitudes towards HIV service delivery in correctional settings: a randomized trial. *AIDS Educ Prev.* 2014;26(5):411-428. doi:10.1521/aeap.2014.26.5.411

70. Molfenter T, Kim JS, Zehner M. Increasing engagement in post-withdrawal management services through a practice bundle and checklist. *J Behav Health Serv Res*. 2021;48(3):400-409. doi:10.1007/s11414-020-09700-w
71. Molfenter T, Connor T, Ford JH, Hyatt J, Zimmerman D. Reducing psychiatric inpatient readmissions using an organizational change model. *WMJ*. 2016;115(3):122-128.
72. Manwell LB, Fleming MF, Johnson K, Barry KL. Tobacco, alcohol, and drug use in a primary care sample: 90-day prevalence and associated factors. *J Addict Dis*. 1998;17(1):67-81. doi:10.1300/J069v17n01_07
73. Molfenter T, Fitzgerald M, Jacobson N, McCarty D, Quanbeck A, Zehner M. Barriers to buprenorphine expansion in Ohio: a time-elapsed qualitative study. *J Psychoactive Drugs*. 2019;51(3):272-279. doi:10.1080/02791072.2019.1566583
74. Jacobson N, Horst J, Wilcox-Warren L, et al. Organizational facilitators and barriers to medication for opioid use disorder capacity expansion and use. *J Behav Health Serv Res*. 2020;47(4):439-448. doi:10.1007/s11414-020-09706-4
75. Croff R, Hoffman K, Alanis-Hirsch K, Ford J, McCarty D, Schmidt L. Overcoming barriers to adopting and implementing pharmacotherapy: the medication research partnership. *J Behav Health Serv Res*. 2019;46(2):330-339. doi:10.1007/s11414-018-9616-9
76. Fleddermann K, Molfenter T, Jacobson N, et al. Clinician perspectives on barriers and facilitators to implementing e-health technology in substance use disorder (SUD) treatment facilities. *Subst Abus*. 2021;15. doi:10.1177/11782218211053360
77. Madden L, Bojko MJ, Farnum S, et al. Using nominal group technique among clinical providers to identify barriers and prioritize solutions to scaling up opioid agonist therapies in Ukraine. *Int J Drug Policy*. 2017;49:48-53. doi:10.1016/j.drugpo.2017.07.025
78. Pankow J, Willett J, Yang Y, et al. Evaluating fidelity to a modified NIATx process improvement strategy for improving HIV services in correctional facilities. *J Behav Health Serv Res*. 2018;45(2):187-203. doi:10.1007/s11414-017-9551-1
79. Gostin LO, Hodge JG, Gulinson CL. Supervised injection facilities: legal and policy reforms. *JAMA*. 2019;321(8):745-746. doi:10.1001/jama.2019.0095
80. Bray JW, Aden B, Eggman AA, et al. Quality of life as an outcome of opioid use disorder treatment: a systematic review. *J Subst Abuse Treat*. 2017;76:88-93. doi:10.1016/j.jsat.2017.01.019
81. Tracy EM, Laudet AB, Min MO, et al. Prospective patterns and correlates of quality of life among women in substance abuse treatment. *Drug Alcohol Depend*. 2012;124(3):242-249. doi:10.1016/j.drugalcdep.2012.01.010
82. Best D, Hennessy EA. The science of recovery capital: where do we go from here? *Addiction*. 2022;117(4):1139-1145. doi:10.1111/add.15732
83. Lewis CC, Boyd M, Puspitasari A, et al. Implementing measurement-based care in behavioral health: a review. *JAMA Psychiatry*. 2019;76(3):324-335. doi:10.1001/jamapsychiatry.2018.3329
84. Marsden J, Tai B, Ali R, Hu L, Rush AJ, Volkow N. Measurement-based care using DSM-5 for opioid use disorder: can we make opioid medication treatment more effective? *Addiction*. 2019;114(8):1346-1353. doi:10.1111/add.14546
85. Scott K, Lewis CC. Using measurement-based care to enhance any treatment. *Cogn Behav Pract*. 2015;22(1):49-59. doi:10.1016/j.cbpra.2014.01.010
86. Schwartz RP, Gibson D, Pagano A, et al. Addiction Medicine Practice-Based Research Network (AMNet): building partnerships. *Psychiatr Serv*. 2021;72(7):845-847. doi:10.1176/appi.ps.202000390
87. American Society of Addiction Medicine. *The ASAM Performance Measures for the Addiction Specialist Physician*. Accessed April 22, 2022. https://www.asam.org/docs/default-source/advocacy/performance-measures-for-the-addiction-specialist-physician.pdf?sfvrsn=0
88. American Society of Addiction Medicine. *The ASAM Standards of Care for the Addiction Specialist Physician*. Accessed April 22, 2022. https://www.asam.org/docs/default-source/practice-support/quality-improvement/asam-standards-of-care.pdf?sfvrsn=10
89. Silver Z, Coger M, Barr S, Drill R. Psychotherapy at a public hospital in the time of COVID-19: telehealth and implications for practice. *Couns Psychol Q*. 2020;34:1-9. doi:10.1080/09515070.2020.1777390
90. Hoffman KA, Foot C, Levander XA, et al. Treatment retention, return to use, and recovery support following COVID-19 relaxation of methadone take-home dosing in two rural opioid treatment programs: a mixed methods analysis. *J Subst Abuse Treat*. 2022;141:108801. doi:10.1016/j.jsat.2022.108801
91. Levander XA, Hoffman KA, McIlveen JW, McCarty D, Terashima JP, Korthuis PT. Rural opioid treatment program patient perspectives on take-home methadone policy changes during COVID-19: a qualitative thematic analysis. *Addict Sci Clin Pr*. 2021;16(1):72. doi:10.1186/s13722-021-00281-3
92. Wu LT, McNeely J, Subramaniam GA, et al. DSM-5 substance use disorders among adult primary care patients: results from a multisite study. *Drug Alcohol Depend*. 2017;179:42-46. doi:10.1016/j.drugalcdep.2017.05.048
93. Gourevitch MN, Arnsten JH. Medical complications of drug use. In: Lowinson JH, Ruiz P, Langrod J, Millman R, eds. *Substance Abuse: A Comprehensive Textbook*. 4th ed. Lippincott Williams & Wilkins; 2005:840-862.
94. Office of National Drug Control Policy. *National Drug Control Strategy*; 2015. Accessed April 14, 2022. https://obamawhitehouse.archives.gov/sites/default/files/ondcp/policy-and-research/2015_national_drug_control_strategy_0.pdf
95. Babor TF, McRee BG, Kassebaum PA, Grimaldi PL, Ahmed K, Bray J. Screening, Brief Intervention, and Referral to Treatment (SBIRT): toward a public health approach to the management of substance abuse. *Subst Abus*. 2007;28(3):7-30. doi:10.1300/J465v28n03_03
96. Josephson SA, Engstrom JW. Residency training: developing a program of quality and safety to train resident neurologists for the future. *Neurology*. 2012;78(8):602-605. doi:10.1212/WNL.0b013e318247cc69
97. Duffy F, Joyce C, West M, et al. Performance in practice: physician practice assessment tool for the care of adults with schizophrenia. *Focus San Franc Calif*. 2012;10:157-171.
98. American Board of Medical Specialties. *Improving Performance in Practice (IPIP)*. American Board of Medical Specialties. Accessed April 14, 2022. 2022 https://www.abms.org/about-abms/research-and-education-foundation/foundation-initiatives/improving-performance-in-practice-ipip/
99. Ford JH, Oliver KA, Giles M, Cates-Wessel K, Krahn D, Levin FR. Maintenance of certification: how performance in practice changes improve tobacco cessation in addiction psychiatrists' practice. *Am J Addict*. 2017;26(1):34-41. doi:10.1111/ajad.12480
100. Center for Substance Abuse Treatment. *Incorporating Alcohol Pharmacotherapies Into Medical Practice*. Substance Abuse and Mental Health Services Administration; 2009.
101. Center for Substance Abuse Treatment. *Medication-Assisted Treatment for Opioid Addiction in Opioid Treatment Programs*. Substance Abuse and Mental Health Services Administration; 2005.
102. Center for Substance Abuse T. SAMHSA/CSAT treatment improvement protocols. *Clinical Guidelines for the Use of Buprenorphine in the Treatment of Opioid Addiction*. Substance Abuse and Mental Health Services Administration; 2004.
103. Executive Office of the President of the United States. *The Mental Health and Substance Use Disorder Task Force Final Report*; 2016. Accessed May 31, 2023. https://obamawhitehouse.archives.gov/the-press-office/2016/03/29/presidential-memorandum-mental-health-and-substance-use-disorder-parity
104. World Health Organization, United Nations Office on Drugs and Crime. *International Standards for the Treatment of Drug Use Disorders: Revised Edition Incorporating Results of Field-Testing*. World Health Organization; 2020. Accessed April 14, 2022. https://apps.who.int/iris/handle/10665/331635

Sidebar

Delivery of Addiction Medicine Care via Video or Phone

Christopher M. Jones and Yngvild Olsen

INTRODUCTION

The increasingly widespread availability of highly potent synthetic opioids, primarily illicitly manufactured fentanyl and fentanyl analogs (IMFs), and the resurgence of stimulants such as methamphetamine are escalating the U.S. overdose crisis.[1,2] Provisional data from the Centers for Disease Control and Prevention (CDC) estimate more than 107,000 overdose deaths in the 12 months ending December 2021.[3] Many of the people losing their lives have an underlying opioid use disorder (OUD) and other substance use disorders (SUDs). In 2020, an estimated 40.3 million people aged 12 or older met diagnostic criteria for an SUD in the past year, including 28.3 million with an alcohol use disorder (AUD) and 18.4 million with an illicit drug use disorder. Among this latter group, cannabis use disorder was the most common (14.2 million); 2.7 million met criteria for an OUD, and 1.3 to 1.5 million had a stimulant use disorder (cocaine or methamphetamine, respectively).[4]

In addition to overdose mortality, substance use contributes to substantial health, social, criminal justice, and economic costs to society each year.[5,6] Thus, expanding access to, provision of, and retention in evidence-based SUD treatment, including medications for opioid use disorder (MOUD), and recovery support services are central components of the U.S. response to the substance use and overdose crisis.[7] The need here is significant. Only a minority of individuals with a SUD in 2020 reported receipt of treatment in the past year.[4] The reasons are myriad: not feeling treatment was needed, limited acceptable treatment choices, lack of health insurance or ability to afford treatment, transportation and distance barriers, inconvenient service hours, and concerns about stigma from family, friends and neighbors.[4] Prior research has also identified structural, economic, geographic, and social barriers to receiving SUD treatment, with barriers often disproportionately affecting communities of color, individuals living in rural areas, those with disabilities, and those with greater socioeconomic disadvantage.[8-13]

TELEHEALTH AS A TOOL TO HELP ADDRESS ACCESS BARRIERS

Telehealth is a strategy that may help address some of the treatment and recovery support services access barriers. Telehealth as a mode of health care delivery to reach patients at home, in private spaces within a clinical setting, or another location in the community, became more common in general health care many years ago, even prior to the COVID-19 pandemic.[14] Telehealth is often defined as two-way, synchronous, real time interactive communication between a patient and a provider at a distant site using audio and/or video equipment.[15] Telehealth can also include asynchronous patient-provider interactions using various forms of technology (eg, store-and-forward technology).[14] Providers can use telehealth as a stand-alone service delivery modality or integrate it into traditional in-person practice. For SUD services, telehealth can facilitate low-barrier access and more convenient ability to assess treatment needs, create treatment plans, initiate care, and provide ongoing support that complement or supplement in-person interactions.[14]

Given the rapid evolution of technology, and spurred by the COVID-19 pandemic, the definition of telehealth has also broadened to involve delivery of health care through electronic means that can include telephonic video, remote monitoring, video communication, remote consultation, apps, and web-based platforms.[16]

TELEHEALTH FOR SUD-RELATED SERVICES PRIOR TO THE COVID-19 PANDEMIC

Prior to the COVID-19 pandemic, the pace of telehealth use in general medical or mental health care settings eclipsed that by specialty SUD providers. In an analysis of a large cohort of privately insured and Medicare Advantage enrollees with SUD, Huskamp et al. found that, while the number of telehealth visits for SUD increased rapidly between 2010 and 2017 (0.6 visits per 1,000 people to 3.1 visits per 1,000 people, respectively), as a proportion of all SUD visits, those conducted via telehealth accounted for only 0.1% of visits during the study period.[17] Of the SUD-related telehealth visits, family practice physicians or internists provided 45.6% of them; psychiatrists provided 29.2%; social workers provided 11.8%; and psychologists provided 1.4%.[17]

Multiple factors limited the pre-COVID pandemic adoption of SUD-related telehealth services, particularly among specialty SUD providers. These include reimbursement and coverage restrictions, licensure requirements, regulations pertaining to who can provide telehealth services and under what context, and requirements for in-person examinations prior to prescribing controlled medications.[18] In addition, providers reported concerns related to forming a therapeutic alliance with patients, suboptimal patient outcomes, and integrating costly technology into clinical workflows, as well as patient concerns related to digital privacy and access to the internet and appropriate technology to engage in telehealth.[18]

Despite these barriers, the prepandemic era saw some increase in the use of telehealth for SUD-related services. SAMHSA's 2013 National Survey of Substance Abuse Treatment Services (NSSATS) reported that approximately 4% of substance use treatment facilities reported often or always using computerized treatment in the past year.[19] By 2019, that proportion had increased to 27%, with the percentage varying across states with a low of 8.2% of treatment facilities in Connecticut and a high of 59.6% in Wyoming.[20]

TELEHEALTH FOR SUD-RELATED SERVICES DURING THE COVID-19 PANDEMIC

The emergence of the COVID-19 pandemic and the societal response to limit its spread led to rapid regulatory and policy changes that greatly affected the delivery of SUD treatment. To facilitate access and continuity of care for people with SUD as COVID-19 spread in the United States, providers, health systems, and community organizations increasingly turned to telehealth. Federal level actions shortly following the declaration of the COVID-19 Public Health Emergency (PHE) on January 27, 2020[21] largely facilitated this shift. Specifically, the Centers for Medicare & Medicaid Services (CMS) expanded payment for telehealth services and provided flexibility on accepted communication technologies for clinical care, including a waiver allowing the use of audio-only platforms[22]; the Substance Abuse and Mental Health Services Administration (SAMHSA) relaxed policies related to take-home methadone and buprenorphine doses for OUD from opioid treatment programs (OTPs) and the use of telehealth at OTPs[23]; the Office for Civil Rights (OCR) at the U.S. Department of Health and Human Services (HHS) announced a waiver of potential penalties for HIPAA violations against providers that serve patients through everyday communications technologies[24]; and the Drug Enforcement Administration (DEA) provided an exemption to the requirement for an in-person examination prior to initiating buprenorphine for OUD for clinicians with a Drug Addiction Treatment Act (DATA) waiver to prescribe the medication, enabling practitioners to remotely treat new patients evaluated via telehealth.[25] States also took regulatory action to facilitate use of telehealth.[18]

The field responded to these flexibilities and opportunities. By the end of 2020, the percentage of substance use treatment facilities providing telehealth services increased substantially, rising to 58.6% nationally. All states saw adoption, from a low of 32.3% of facilities providing telehealth services frequently in Hawaii to a high of 85.3% of facilities in Montana.[26] Similar to findings prior to COVID-19, states with large rural and remote areas had some of the highest rates of offering telehealth service in this survey, underscoring the potential value of telehealth in expanding SUD treatment access particularly in rural communities.

Emerging research indicates that adoption of telehealth increased among a range of SUD treatment settings, including traditional outpatient programs, inpatient addiction services, opioid treatment programs, among DATA-waived providers, and recovery and mutual-help organizations, and has been used to support an array of formal treatment and recovery support services.[27-39]

In a large cohort study of Medicare patients with OUD before (March 2019-February 2020) and during the COVID-19 pandemic (March 2020-February 2021), the percentage of patients receiving OUD-related telehealth services at their index visit where an OUD diagnosis was made was significantly higher in the pandemic cohort (12.07%) compared to the prepandemic cohort (0.12%). The study also found an increase in receipt of OUD-related telehealth services across the study period (19.61% of patients in the pandemic cohort versus 0.56% of patients in the prepandemic cohort).[27]

In a survey of SUD treatment facilities and recovery and mutual-help organizations, Molfenter et al. found uptake of telehealth, both telephone- and video-based, across multiple settings and services, including medication-related, peer support services and case management (**Fig. 50-1**).

Providers of OUD treatment particularly responded to the pandemic regulatory flexibilities. Jones et al. found that 33.0% of DATA-waived providers responding to a national survey in summer of 2020 had prescribed buprenorphine remotely to new patients without first conducting an in-person exam. Survey respondents also identified adopting a range of audio-visual technologies (eg, laptop/desktop with video, phone with video, tablets) and audio-only platforms, to engage new and established patients in OUD treatment (**Fig. 50-2**).[29]

In a study of OTPs across the United States conducted in June-July 2020, Cantor and Laurito found that 80.8% of responding OTPs offered telehealth services.[30] Among OTPs in Pennsylvania, Krawczyk et al. found that for patients receiving methadone, 84% of OTPs offered telehealth counseling/self-help groups, 61% offered telephone follow-up appointments, and 50% offered video follow-up appointments. For patients receiving buprenorphine in OTPs, 70% offered virtual counseling/self-help groups, 50% offered telephone follow-up appointments, 40% offered video follow-up appointments, 25% offered video appointments for buprenorphine initiation, and 10% offered telephone appointments for buprenorphine initiation.[31]

However, by January 2021, despite these significant changes in telehealth adoption among SUD programs, an estimated 49% of counties in the United States, accounting for 11% of the total U.S. population, still did not have a SUD treatment facility offering telehealth.[32]

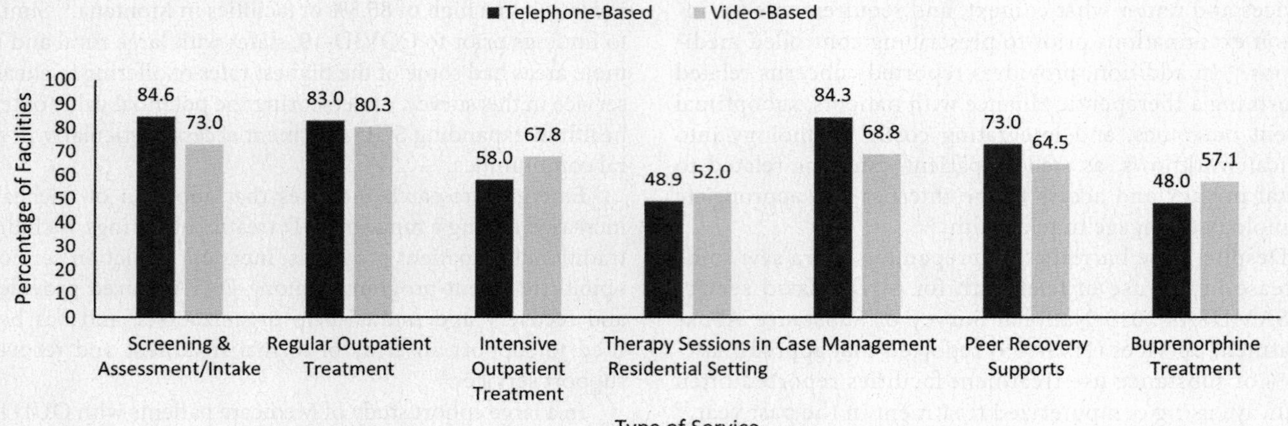

Figure 50-1. Rates of use of different telehealth services. (Adapted from Molfenter T, Roget N, Chaple M, et al. Use of telehealth in substance use disorder services during and after COVID-19: online survey study. *JMIR Mental Health.* 2021;8(2):e25835.)

RESEARCH ON THE EFFECTIVENESS AND BENEFITS OF TELEHEALTH FOR SUD

Multiple benefits of telehealth for patients and providers have been identified (Table 50-3).[14]

Although further research is needed, with the rapid adoption of telehealth during the COVID-19 pandemic, numerous studies are emerging that document patient and provider impacts of telehealth on SUD-related services and outcomes. These studies largely report on impacts in three areas: (1) patient acceptability, satisfaction, and outcomes, (2) provider receptivity and satisfaction, and (3) challenges and barriers related to telehealth implementation.

Patient Acceptability, Satisfaction, and Outcomes

Studies have found that patients are generally satisfied with telehealth-based services for SUD.[40] In a qualitative study of patients with OUD engaging in treatment and harm reduction services in Portland, OR, Lockard et al. found that when compared to in-person visits, patients perceived virtual visits as more readily available, more convenient, and more accommodating to their life circumstances. Patients described virtual visits as more comfortable and fostering self-empowerment and mutual respect between the patient and provider. For some, the acceptability of virtual visits was driven by prior experiences of stigma and discrimination when accessing OUD treatment. Some participants believed that the patient–provider relationship successfully translated into virtual environments and that virtual visits implied mutual trust. Importantly, while most patients indicated virtual care was their preferred way to engage with clinicians, others endorsed the importance of having the flexibility to choose in-person or virtual services.[41]

Among clinics affiliated with academic medical centers in New York City, Philadelphia, San Francisco, and Rhode Island,

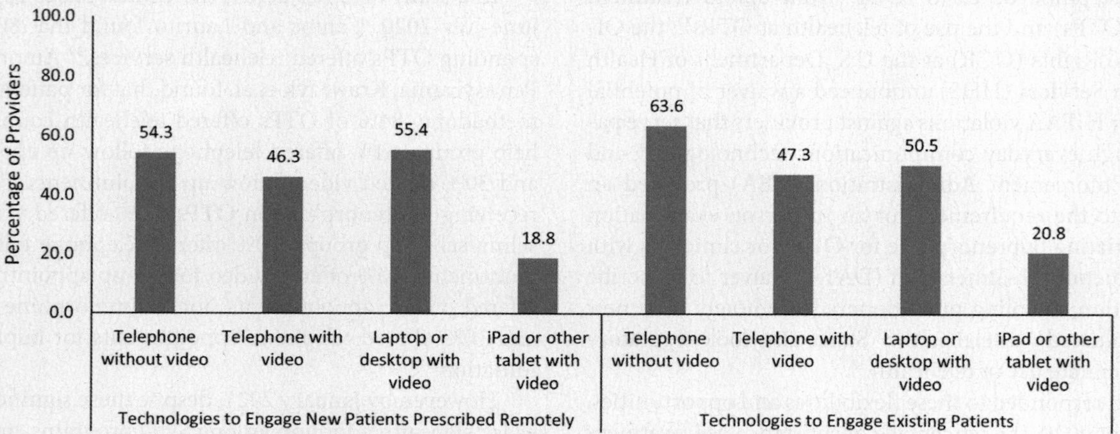

Figure 50-2. Telehealth approaches used by DATA-waived providers. (Adapted from Jones CM, Diallo MM, Vythilingam M, Schier JG, Eisenstat M, Compton WM. Characteristics and correlates of U.S. clinicians prescribing buprenorphine for opioid use disorder treatment using expanded authorities during the COVID-19 pandemic. *Drug Alcohol Depend.* 2021;225:108783.)

TABLE 50-3 Benefits of Telehealth for Patients and Providers

Patient benefits	Provider benefits
• Increased access to experienced providers and high-quality care • Improved access to care and continuity of care • Increased convenience that removes traditional barriers to care, including barriers related to geography, psychological, accessibility, employment, child, and caregiver responsibilities • Increased access to team-based services and group-based interventions • Reduction in stigma associated with conditions such as substance use disorder • Improved satisfaction with care consistent with in-person treatment	• Provision of timely patient care • Effective and efficient coordination of care • Reduction in workforce shortages • Ability to assess a patient's home environment • Ability to share information for psychoeducation and assessment • Efficient connections to crisis services • Reduction in provider burnout

Adapted from SAMHSA's Evidence-Based Resource Guide Series. *Telehealth for the Treatment of Serious Mental Illness and Substance Use Disorders*; 2022.

researchers found that use of audiovisual and audio-only telehealth allowed for rapid scaleup of services, including initiation of treatment, for vulnerable patients. Approximately 85% of patients, including patients experiencing a lack of housing, leaving incarceration, and those receiving Medicaid, who remotely started MOUD treatment with buprenorphine during the pandemic, continued to engage in care within 30 days of initiation.[42]

Multiple studies have shown either similar or improved appointment cancellation or no-show rates as a result of telehealth implementation. For example, the Substance Treatment and Recovery (STAR) clinic documented equivalent no show rates for existing patients comparing pandemic to prepandemic trends and new patient no show rates declined to zero by May 2020 after implementation of virtual service delivery.[43] Among patients with SUD treated in the New York Health + Hospital system, implementation of televisits during COVID-19 became essential to continuing care for patients with SUD. An analysis of nearly 20,000 health care visits found that televisit availability improved attendance rates for SUD treatment, with patients more likely to attend televisit appointments compared to in-person appoints during the pandemic and the prepandemic periods, regardless of age, sex, race, and insurance status.[44]

In the inpatient acute care hospital setting, an addiction consultation service shift to telehealth found that remote consultations resulted in comparable quality of care and patient acceptability compared to in-person consultative services prior to the pandemic. Specifically, the 78.1% reduction in the 30-day readmission rate among patients who received a virtual addiction compared to patients not receiving such a consultation during the pandemic was consistent with readmission rate reductions seen with in-person addiction consult services prior to COVID-19.[45]

In addition to patient acceptability and satisfaction, studies are increasingly documenting the benefits of telehealth-delivered services on patient outcomes. Among a large cohort of patients enrolled in an intensive outpatient treatment program from January 2020 to March 2021, no differences emerged in self-reported continuous abstinence, adherence with medications for opioid or alcohol use disorder, or in the quality of life or well-being across in-person only, virtual only, or hybrid treatment modalities at 3-month follow-up.[46]

Cunningham et al. compared patients referred to buprenorphine treatment clinics in NYC from March-August 2019 (in-person visits) and March 2020 to August 2020 (telehealth-based visits) and found no differences between the two cohorts in the percentage of patients who completed each step of the OUD cascade of care (initial visit scheduled, initial visit completed, treatment initiated, and treatment retention at 90 days). Further, patients initiating buprenorphine via telehealth through a referral during the pandemic were more likely to be retained in treatment at 90 days compared to those starting the medication as part of an in-person visit and referral in 2019 (68.0% versus 42.9%, $p < 0.05$).[47]

In the largest longitudinal cohort study to date examining outcomes for Medicare patients with OUD engaging in initial services during the COVID-19 pandemic compared to a cohort initiating an episode of OUD care prepandemic, Jones et al. found substantially higher rates of receiving OUD-related telehealth services, similar rates of nonfatal overdose, increased likelihood of receiving MOUD, and among those that received MOUD, no difference or higher retention on MOUD, depending on type of medication received. Importantly, patients in the pandemic cohort that received OUD-related telehealth services had lower odds of experiencing a nonfatal overdose, were more likely to receive MOUD, and among those that did receive MOUD, had better retention than those not receiving OUD-related telehealth services. This protective effect remained after controlling for baseline demographic, substance use, mental health, and physical health conditions.[27]

Provider Receptivity and Satisfaction

Studies have generally found positive receptivity and satisfaction with use of telehealth among providers.[14,45,48-50] Deng et al. documented the perceived feasibility and effectiveness of transitioning to a virtual addiction consult service for inpatient hospitalized patients, with a resulting strengthening of the interdisciplinary team approach where peer support and complex case management services enhanced inpatient and postdischarge outreach.[45] Goldsamt et al. found a majority of geographically diverse OTP program directors generally supported the regulatory changes allowing for increased use of telehealth, with only 28% reacting negatively.[50] In this survey, OTP program directors also noted that both staff and patients liked telehealth sessions and that staff were able to maintain their caseload despite the transition.[50] Among Pennsylvania OTPs, 88% of respondents agreed that virtual buprenorphine prescribing provided for less burdensome access for patients and 55% endorsed maintaining buprenorphine initiation via telehealth if video were required, with 39% supportive of maintaining starting the medication via audio-only platforms.[31]

Many respondents of a large, geographically diverse survey of SUD and mental health treatment organizations expressed a sense of relief that they were able to continue providing services to clients during COVID-19 and that lives were saved as a result. Some respondents noted positive experiences with telehealth integration into their organizational workflow; others expressed positive feedback about their organization's access to technology, allowing for easy engagement with various telehealth platforms. Several respondents indicated that telehealth and virtual services implementation opened the treatment access door for new populations, such as patients with severe anxiety, those wishing to avoid stigma associated with seeking treatment, and those with transportation or other geographic distance barriers.[51]

Challenges and Barriers Related to Telehealth Implementation

While emerging evidence supports benefits for telehealth and general receptivity and acceptance among patients and providers, concerns about exacerbating pre-existing disparities in access to care or creating new disparities in access remain, especially among communities of color, those with low digital literacy, limited economic means, disabilities, and limited access to the internet or broadband.[8,14,50] An estimated quarter of adults with incomes below $30,000 a year do not own a smartphone, and, among adults with lower incomes, 43% do not have home broadband and 41% cannot access a private laptop.[14,52]

Chang et al. found that several patient groups are more likely to rely on audio-only rather than video as their primary means of engaging in MOUD. This includes patients over age 50, those with unstable housing or unemployment/looking for work, less education, or mobility limitations.[52] Jones et al. found, in a study of Medicare beneficiaries initiating OUD care, males, people older than 44 years, non-Hispanic African American persons, and people living in the South were less likely to receive OUD-related telehealth services during the pandemic, after controlling for other demographic and clinical characteristics.[27]

Technology-related barriers may affect providers as well as patients. A survey of DATA-waivered providers in the summer of 2020 found that barriers to remote initiation of buprenorphine for new patients included inadequate remote technology for patients (10.6% of providers), inadequate broadband or internet in the practice (3.4%), and concerns about security or privacy (3.7%). Providers in this survey noted the technology-related challenges among their patients: challenges with unreliable phone, computer, or internet service (48.2% of providers); cancellation of in-person mutual support or counseling groups (39.2% of providers); and inability to find remote mutual support or counseling groups (29.0% of providers).[29]

In a large survey of treatment organizations, Kisicki et al. reported that some respondents struggled to integrate telehealth into their organization's usual operations, and shared concerns about confidentiality, security, and encryption on various platforms. Several respondents stated receiving limited support and training on telehealth technologies, lack of equipment necessary for seamless and proper use of telehealth, and difficulty managing multiple platforms.[51] OTP program directors raised concerns about telehealth in the context of group counseling, with some respondents indicating greater difficulties implementing telehealth group counseling compared to individual sessions and patient's acceptance of this modality for use with groups.[50]

Among a study of individuals providing peer recovery support services during the pandemic, Anvari et al. found that despite peer specialists noting a number of positive aspects related to the transition to telehealth and virtual service delivery, a majority noted witnessing a decrease in interpersonal connection between themselves and their clients as well as their clients and recovery networks, the lack of access to technology among some of their clients, and the resistance by some in transitioning to a virtual environment, resulting in disconnection from SUD-related services.[49]

FUTURE DIRECTIONS

Although emerging evidence supports the benefits and acceptability of telehealth delivery of SUD-related services, the full implications of the rapid adoption of telehealth during the COVID-19 pandemic remain unclear. Future research should examine the impact of telehealth on substance use, health, and social outcomes, identify which populations are more likely to benefit from remote versus in-person versus hybrid models of care, how best to implement, integrate, and scale telehealth services in different clinical and community settings, and identify disparities in access to telehealth and other virtual services. In addition, the pandemic has seen the emergence of new business models that solely provide telehealth-based OUD and SUD care. Future research should rigorously evaluate the impacts of these models of care on patient access and outcomes as compared to in-person and hybrid care delivery.

In addition, at present, uncertainty about the future scope of telehealth-based services exists, in part related to the complex federal and state regulatory requirements and decisions about regulatory flexibilities afforded during the COVID-19 pandemic that may bar health systems and providers from offering the full breadth of available telehealth services to patients. However, telehealth clearly will be part of the clinical tool kit in an increasingly growing number of SUD treatment and recovery settings. For providers, health systems, or organizations interested in implementing telehealth services, the Substance Abuse and Mental Health Services Administration has released a resource, "Telehealth for the Treatment of Serious Mental Illness and Substance Use Disorders" that includes practical suggestions and considerations for implementation in various practice settings.[14]

REFERENCES

1. O'Donnell J, Tanz LJ, Gladden RM, David NL, Bitting J. Trends in and characteristics of drug overdose deaths involving illicitly manufactured fentanyls—United States, 2019–2020. *MMWR Morb Mortal Wkly Rep.* 2021;70(50):1740-1746.
2. Jones CM, Houry D, Han B, Baldwin G, Vivolo-Kantor A, Compton WM. Methamphetamine use in the United States: epidemiological update and implications for prevention, treatment, and harm reduction. *Ann NY Acad Sci.* 2022;1508(1):3-22.
3. Centers for Disease Control and Prevention. *Vital Statistics Rapid Release*. 2022. Accessed May 31, 2023. https://www.cdc.gov/nchs/nvss/vsrr/drug-overdose-data.htm
4. Substance Abuse and Mental Health Services Administration. *National Survey on Drug Use and Health Annual National Report*. 2020. Accessed May 31, 2023. https://www.samhsa.gov/data/report/2020-nsduh-annual-national-report
5. Manthey J, Hassan SA, Carr S, Kilian C, Kuitunen-Paul S, Rehm J. Estimating the economic consequences of substance use and substance use disorders. *Expert Rev Pharmacoecon Outcomes Res.* 2021;21(5):869-876.
6. Peterson C, Luo F, Florence C. State-level economic costs of fatal injuries—United States, 2019. *MMWR Morb Mortal Wkly Rep.* 2021;70(48):1660-1663.
7. U.S. Department of Health and Human Services. *Overdose Prevention Strategy*. Accessed May 31, 2023. https://aspe.hhs.gov/sites/default/files/documents/101936da95b69acb8446a4bad9179cc0/overdose-prevention-strategy.pdf
8. Kang AW, DeBritz AA, Hoadley A, et al. Barriers and poor telephone counseling experiences among patients receiving medication for opioid use disorders. *Patient Educ Couns.* 2022;105(7):2607-2610.
9. Cernasey A, Hohmeier KC, Frederick K, Jasmin H, Gatwood J. A systematic literature review of patient perspectives of barriers and facilitators to access, adherence, stigma, and persistence to treatment for substance use disorder. *Explor Res Clin Soc Pharm.* 2021;2:100029.
10. Pilarinos A, Bromberg DJ, Karamouzian M. Access to medications for opioid use disorder and associated factors among adolescents and young adults: a systematic review. *JAMA Pediatr.* 2022;176(3):304-311.
11. Park JN, Rouhani S, Beletsky L, Vincent L, Saloner B, Sherman SG. Situating the continuum of overdose risk in the social determinants of health: a new conceptual framework. *Milbank Q.* 2020;98(3):700-746.
12. Chang JE, Franz B, Cronin CE, Lindenfeld Z, Lai AY, Pagán JA. Racial/ethnic disparities in the availability of hospital based opioid use disorder treatment. *J Subst Abuse Treat.* 2022;138:108719.
13. Soto C, West A, Unger J, et al. *Addressing the Opioid Crisis in American Indian & Alaska Native Communities in California: A Statewide Needs Assessment*. Accessed May 31, 2023. https://ipr.usc.edu/wp-content/uploads/2019/11/USC_AI_Report.pdf
14. Substance Abuse and Mental Health Services Administration. *Telehealth for the Treatment of Serious Mental Illness and Substance Use Disorders*. Accessed May 31, 2023. https://store.samhsa.gov/sites/default/files/pep21-06-02-001.pdf

Disclaimers: The findings and conclusions of this study are those of the authors and do not necessarily reflect the views of the Centers for Diseases Control and Prevention, the Substance Abuse and Mental Health Services Administration, and the U.S. Department of Health and Human Services.

15. U.S Code of Federal Regulations. 42 CFR 410.78. Accessed May 31, 2023. https://www.ecfr.gov/current/title-42/chapter-IV/subchapter-B/part-410/subpart-B/section-410.78
16. Haque SN. Telehealth beyond COVID-19. *Psychiatr Serv.* 2020;72(1):100-103.
17. Huskamp HA, Busch AB, Souza J, et al. How is telemedicine being used in opioid and other substance use disorder treatment. *Health Aff.* 2018;37(12):1940-1947.
18. Legislative Analysis and Public Policy Association. *Telehealth and Substance Use Disorder Services in the Era of COVID-19: Review and Recommendations*. Accessed May 31, 2023. https://www.samhsa.gov/resource/dbhis/telehealth-substance-use-disorder-services-era-covid-19-review-recommendations
19. Substance Abuse and Mental Health Services Administration. *National Survey of Substance Abuse Treatment Services (N-SSATS): 2013*. 2013. https://www.samhsa.gov/data/sites/default/files/2013_nssats_rpt.pdf
20. Substance Abuse and Mental Health Services Administration. *National Survey of Substance Abuse Treatment Services (N-SSATS): 2019*. 2020. Accessed May 31, 2023. https://www.samhsa.gov/data/sites/default/files/2013_nssats_rpt.pdf
21. U.S. Department of Health and Human Services. *Public Health Emergency Determination for 2019 Novel Coronavirus*. Accessed May 31, 2023. https://www.phe.gov/emergency/news/healthactions/phe/Pages/2019-nCoV.aspx
22. Centers for Medicare and Medicaid Services. Centers for Medicare & Medicaid Services (CMS) and Substance Abuse and Mental Health Services Administration (SAMHSA): leveraging existing health and disease management programs to provide mental health and substance use disorder resources during the COVID-19 Public Health Emergency (PHE). Accessed May 31, 2023. https://www.cms.gov/CCIIO/Programs-and-Initiatives/Health-Insurance-Marketplaces/Downloads/Mental-Health-Substance-Use-Disorder-Resources-COVID-19.pdf
23. Substance Abuse and Mental Health Services Administration. *Opioid Treatment Program (OTP): Guidance (March 16, 2020)*. 2020. Accessed May 31, 2023. https://www.samhsa.gov/sites/default/files/otp-guidance-20200316.pdf
24. U.S. Department of Health and Human Services, Office for Civil Rights. *FAQs on Telehealth and HIPAA During the COVID-19 Nationwide Public Health Emergency*. 2020. Accessed May 31, 2023. https://public3.pagefreezer.com/content/HHS.gov/31-12-2020T08:51/https:/www.hhs.gov/sites/default/files/telehealth-faqs-508.pdf
25. Drug Enforcement Administration. *Use of Telephone Evaluations to Initiate Buprenorphine Prescribing*. 2020. Accessed May 31, 2023. https://www.deadiversion.usdoj.gov/GDP/(DEA-DC-022)(DEA068)%20DEA%20SAMHSA%20buprenorphine%20telemedicine%20%20(Final)%20+Esign.pdf
26. Substance Abuse and Mental Health Services Administration. *National Survey of Substance Abuse Treatment Services (N-SSATS): 2020*. 2021. Accessed May 31, 2023. https://www.samhsa.gov/data/sites/default/files/reports/rpt35313/2020_NSSATS_FINAL.pdf
27. Jones CM, Shoff C, Hodges K, et al. Receipt of telehealth services, receipt and retention on medications for opioid use disorder, and medically treated overdose among Medicare beneficiaries before and during the COVID-19 pandemic. *JAMA Psychiatry.* 2022;79(10):981-992.
28. Molfenter T, Roget N, Chaple M, et al. Use of telehealth in substance use disorder services during and after COVID-19: online survey study. *JMIR Mental Health.* 2021;8(2):e25835.
29. Jones CM, Diallo MM, Vythilingam M, Schier JG, Eisenstat M, Compton WM. Characteristics and correlates of U.S. clinicians prescribing buprenorphine for opioid use disorder treatment using expanded authorities during the COVID-19 pandemic. *Drug Alcohol Depend.* 2021;225:108783.
30. Cantor J, Laurito A. The new services that opioid treatment programs have adopted in response to COVID-19. *J Subst Abuse Treat.* 2021;130:108393.
31. Krawczyk N, Maniates H, Hulsey E, et al. Shifting medication treatment practices in the COVID-19 pandemic: a statewide survey of Pennsylvania opioid treatment programs. *J Addict Med.* 2022;16(6):645-652. doi:10.1097/ADM.0000000000000981

32. Cantor J, McBain RK, Kofner A, Hanson R, Stein BD, Yu H. Telehealth adoption by mental health and substance use disorder treatment facilities in the COVID-19 pandemic. *Psychiatr Serv.* 2022;73(4):411-417.
33. Oesterle TS, Kolla B, Risma CJ, et al. Substance use disorders and telehealth in the COVID-19 pandemic era: a new outlook. *May Clin Proc.* 2020;95(12):2709-2718.
34. Melamed OC, deRuiter WK, Buckley L, Selby P. Coronavirus disease 2019 and the impact on substance use disorder treatments. *Psychiatr Clin North Am.* 2022;45(1):95-107.
35. Uscher-Pines L, Sousa J, Raja P, Mehrotra A, Barnett M, Huskamp HA. Treatment of opioid use disorder during COVID-19: experiences of clinicians transitioning to telemedicine. *J Subst Abuse Treat.* 2020;118:108124.
36. Wang L, Weiss J, Ryan EB, Waldman J, Rubin S, Griffin JL. Telemedicine increases access to buprenorphine initiation during the COVID-19 pandemic. *J Subst Abuse Treat.* 2021;124:108272.
37. Lin LA, Casteel D, Shigekawa E, Weyrich MS, Roby DH, McMenamin SB. Telemedicine-delivered treatment interventions for substance use disorders: a systematic review. *J Subst Abuse Treat.* 2019;101:38-49.
38. Uhl S, Bloschichak A, Moran A, et al. Telehealth for substance use disorders: a rapid review for the 2021 U.S. Department of Veterans Affairs and U.S. Department of Defense Guidelines for Management of Substance Use Disorders. *Ann Intern Med.* 2022;175(5):691-700.
39. Mark TL, Treiman K, Padwa H, Henretty K, Tzeng J, Gilbert M. Addiction treatment and telehealth: review of efficacy and provider insights during the COVID-19 pandemic. *Psychiatr Serv.* 2022;73(5):484-491.
40. Colegee TO, Robinson D, Kelley-Freeman A, et al. Patient satisfaction with medications for opioid use disorder treatment via telemedicine: brief literature review and development of a new assessment. *Front Public Health.* 2021;8:557275.
41. Lockard R, Priest KC, Gregg J, Buchheit BM. A qualitative study of patient experiences with telemedicine opioid use disorder treatment during COVID-19. *Subst Abus.* 2022;43(1):1150-1157.
42. Samuels EA, Khatri UG, Synder H, Wightman RS, Tofighi B, Kraawczyk N. Buprenorphine telehealth initiation and follow-up during COVID-19. *J Gen Intern Med.* 2022;37(5):1331-1333.
43. Fiacco L, Pearson BL, Jordan RJ. Telemedicine works for treating substance use disorder: the STAR clinic experience during COVID-19. *J Subst Abuse Treat.* 2021;125:108312.
44. Avalone L, King C, Popeo D, et al. Increased attendance during rapid implementation of telehealth for substance use disorders during COVID-19 at the largest public hospital system in the United States. *Subst Use Misuse.* 2022;57(8):1322-1327.
45. Deng H, Raheemullah A, Fenno LE, Lembke A. A telehealth inpatient addiction consult service is both feasible and effective in reducing readmission rates. *J Addict Dis.* 2023;41(3):225-232.
46. Gliske K, Welsh JW, Braughton JE, Waller LA, Ngo QM. Telehealth services for substance use disorders during the covid-19 pandemic: longitudinal assessment of intensive outpatient programming and data collection practices. *JMIR Ment Health.* 2022;9(3):e36263.
47. Cunningham CO, Khalid L, Deng Y, et al. A comparison of office-based buprenorphine treatment outcomes in Bronx community clinics before versus during the COVID-19 pandemic. *J Subst Abuse Treat.* 2022;135:108641.
48. Henretty K, Padwa H, Treiman K, Gilbery M, Mark TL. Impact of the Coronavirus pandemic on substance use disorder treatment: findings from a survey of specialty providers in California. *Subst Abuse.* 2021;15:117822182.
49. Anvari MS, Seitz-Brown CJ, Spencer J, et al. "How can I hug someone now [over the phone]?": impacts of COVID-19 on peer recovery specialists and clients in substance use treatment. *J Subst Abuse Treat.* 2021;131:108649.
50. Goldsamt LA, Rosenblum A, Appel P, Paris P, Nazia N. The impact of COVID-19 on opioid treatment programs in the United States. *Drug Alcohol Depend.* 2021;228:109049.
51. Kisicki A, Becker S, Chaple M, et al. Behavioral healthcare organizations' experiences related to use of telehealth as a result of the COVID-19 pandemic: an exploratory study. *BMC Health Serv Res.* 2022;22(1):775.
52. Chang JE, Lindenfeld Z, Thomas T, Waldman J, Griffin J. Patient characteristics associated with phone versus video telemedicine visits for substance use treatment during COVID-19. *J Addict Med.* 2022;16(6):659-665. doi:10.1097/ADM.0000000000000098

SECTION

6

Nonsubstance Addiction-Related Disorders

Associate Editor: Jeanette M. Tetrault
Lead Section Editor: Jon E. Grant
Section Editor: Sarah W. Yip

CHAPTER

51 Understanding Nonsubstance Addictions

Luis C. Farhat, Sarah W. Yip, and Marc N. Potenza

CHAPTER OUTLINE

- Introduction
- Gambling disorder
- Internet gaming disorder
- Problematic internet use
- Compulsive buying disorder
- Compulsive sexual behavior disorder
- Binge eating disorder
- Overall conclusion

INTRODUCTION

The term "addiction" is derived from the Latin word *addicere*, meaning "bound to" or "enslaved by."[1] In its original formulation, the word was not linked to substance use behaviors. Several hundred years ago, the word became associated first with excessive use of alcohol and then drugs.[2] By the time of the 1980s, the word was almost exclusively linked to excessive patterns of substance use, with experts involved in generating diagnostic criteria for drug dependence, as defined in editions of the Diagnostic and Statistical Manual (DSM) prior to the fifth edition (DSM-5), showing good agreement that the term applied to the condition of compulsive drug-taking.[3]

Nonetheless, addictive disorders have been proposed to have several defining components such as poor control, sustained engagement, and appetitive urges or cravings prior to the engagement in the behavior.[1] If these elements are considered the core features of addiction, then excessive patterns of gambling and engagement in other non–substance-related motivated behaviors such as gaming, internet use, sex, and shopping might be considered addictions. Thus, the term "behavioral addiction" has been used to describe patterns of engagement with these short-term rewarding behaviors characterized by core elements of addiction.[4]

Many disorders under the "behavioral addiction" umbrella terminology have been previously considered impulse control disorders (ICDs) and were previously classified in the fourth edition of the DSM as "Impulse Control Disorders Not Elsewhere Classified."[5] The ICDs within the "not elsewhere classified" section included intermittent explosive disorder, kleptomania, pathological gambling (PG), pyromania, trichotillomania, and ICD not otherwise specified. However, by the early part of the 2000s, a growing movement to consider some of these disorders as addictions emerged.[6] Aided by data from neurobiological studies, this view gained momentum, leading to the consideration of a renaming of the "Substance-Related Disorders" diagnostic category to "Substance-Related and Addictive Disorders" in the DSM-5.[7] Currently, only PG was proposed for inclusion in this category by the American Psychiatric Association (APA),[8] and gambling disorder (GD, as the entity is currently named in the DSM-5) is classified together with substance use disorders (SUDs) in the DSM-5.[9] Another nondrug behavior, internet gaming disorder (IGD), was considered for the DSM-5 and included in Section 3 of the DSM-5 (in which conditions that require further research are included).[9]

Additional ICDs/behavioral addictions that were under consideration for DSM-5 as independent mental health conditions included ones related to excessive internet use (problematic internet use, PIU), buying/shopping (compulsive buying disorder, CBD), sex (compulsive sexual behavior disorder, CSBD, or hypersexual disorder or sex addiction), and nail-biting.[10] A case for the inclusion of obesity was forwarded and debated. Nonetheless, ultimately all these candidate disorders were rejected as independent mental health conditions. Of note, in the case of obesity, binge eating disorder (BED) was included in the DSM-5 as an eating disorder. While there are strong links between BED and obesity,[11] it is important to note that obesity and addiction are not necessarily related and that for some individuals, overeating is a relatively passive event that takes the form of liberal snacking and eating large portions.[12] Likewise, some individuals with BED are not obese. BED may be a specific subtype of obesity driven by a biologically based hyperreactivity to the hedonic properties of food, coupled with an enhanced motivation to encourage appetitive behaviors that is related to neurobiological differences in reward and control circuitry.[13]

Similarly, the eleventh edition of the International Classification of Diseases (ICD-11) only classified gambling and gaming disorders as "disorders due to addictive behaviors." A separate, nonspecific category was created to represent behaviors that may be considered addictive in nature—"other specified behaviors due to addictive behaviors." However, no specific description of what behaviors would be appropriate for this code was provided.[14]

Among issues that were considered within research workgroups were whether the ICDs might be best categorized separately, with SUDs as addictions, or with obsessive-compulsive disorder (OCD) as obsessive-compulsive–related disorders (OCRDs) as well as the potential clinical relevance of these classifications.[15] Although the conceptualizations of ICDs as addictions or OCRDs are not mutually exclusive and data exist to support each formulation in line with impulsive/compulsive transdiagnostic domains,[16] these classificatory frameworks have important clinical implications with respect to prevention and treatment strategies.[4]

Despite the ongoing nosology debate, mental health professionals have noted that some individuals experience negative personal, social, academic/occupational, physical, and/or mental health consequences due to problematic engagement with candidate or established behavioral addictions. Therefore, additional recognition of behavioral addictions is important to understand these potentially impairing conditions and contribute to the advancement of the current state of knowledge of these conditions.

In the following sections, we review behavioral addictions, their main clinical features, and what is currently known regarding their biologies. Evidence from neurobiological research, epidemiological reports, and treatment (psychotherapy and psychopharmacology) studies regarding these conditions are reviewed. In reviewing the individual disorders, consideration is given to disorders for which there have been arguably the most data supporting similarities with SUDs (eg, in the areas of gambling, gaming, internet use, shopping, sex, and eating). A particular emphasis is placed on GD as it is arguably the best studied of the behavioral addictions to date and the only one formally classified as such in the DSM-5. We note that additional details for some of these behavioral addictions are provided in other chapters in this textbook. We refer interested readers to Chapter 52 "Gambling Disorder: Clinical Characteristics and Treatment," Chapter 53 "Compulsive Sexual Behaviors," and Chapter 54 "Disorders Associated With Technology and Social Media" for additional information pertaining some of the behavioral addictions outlined below.

GAMBLING DISORDER

Definition and Conceptualization

Gambling is defined as an activity that involves placing something of value at risk in the hopes of gaining something of greater value in return.[17] Gambling activities are commonly endorsed by a sizable proportion of the general population across the world.[18] In the United States, telephone surveys of adults conducted in 1999 to 2000 and 2011 to 2013 indicated that as many as 80% of surveyed adults had gambled in the past year.[19]

Notably, fewer individuals will experience a persistent, recurrent pattern of gambling that is associated with substantial distress or impairment. The DSM-5 adopted the term GD to describe such a disordered pattern of engagement in gambling. The operational criteria for GD are related to those for SUDs. According to the DSM-5,[9] a diagnosis of GD requires that the patient display four or more of the following: preoccupation with gambling, gambling with greater amounts of money to receive the same level of desired experience (tolerance), repeated, unsuccessful attempts to reduce or quit gambling, restlessness/irritability when trying to stop gambling (withdrawal), gambling to escape from a dysphoric state, gambling to regain gambling-related losses ("chasing" losses), lying in significant relationships about gambling, jeopardizing of a job or significant other due to gambling, and reliance on others to fund gambling. An exclusion criterion exists to specify that the gambling behavior is not better accounted for by manic episodes. Additionally, the severity of GD may be specified based on the number of criteria met as mild (4-5 criteria), moderate (6-7 criteria), or severe (8-9 criteria).

Of note, the term "problem gambling" has been commonly used in the literature to describe a recurrent and interfering pattern of gambling in which the presence of formal diagnostic criteria are not determined, and therefore, individuals may not necessarily meet diagnostic criteria for GD, for example, have subthreshold symptomatology.[17]

Neurobiology

Genetics

Family studies of addiction indicate that genetic and environmental factors are important in the development of drug- and alcohol use disorders. Similarly, family studies of GD suggest a significant parental influence on the development of offspring gambling behaviors.[20] Twin studies are particularly useful as they allow for the estimation of the relative influences of genetic and environmental factors. Given there are continuing changes in the gambling environment that might increase the overall access to different types of gambling (eg, internet gambling),[21] understanding the magnitude of genetic and environmental factors in the genesis of GD separately may be informative.

Data derived from the Vietnam Twin Era Registry found that between 35% and 54% of the probability of meeting the criteria for a DSM-III-R diagnosis of GD was attributable to heritable factors,[22] and a similar but slightly lower figure (34%) was found for data from the same sample regarding DSM-IV-defined drug dependence, suggesting similar degrees of heritability for GD and SUDs.[23] This finding has been replicated in independent samples since then, for example, 49% heritability for GD.[24] Evidence from twin studies also indicates that there exists a significant genetic correlation between GDs and SUDs such as those involving alcohol,[25] a finding replicated in an independent sample,[26] cannabis, tobacco, and stimulants,[27] also consistent with findings from another sample.[28] Shared genetic and environmental factors may not be limited to SUDs, with both contributing to externalizing conditions like conduct and antisocial personality disorders as well as internalizing conditions like anxiety disorders, although genetic factors may contribute more prominently to the co-occurrence of GD and some internalizing disorders.[29]

Unfortunately, there have not been significant advancements in the identification of variants associated with GD through molecular genetic research. To date, well-powered genome-wide studies, for example, genome-wide association studies (GWASs), are currently lacking which precludes the identification of high-confidence risk genes for GD. To date, there are only two GWASs of GD[30,31] and neither was able to identify genome-wide-significant single nucleotide polymorphisms, although sample sizes of ten thousand or more may be needed. As such, additional collaborative efforts across GD research centers are required to characterize the genetic architecture of GD.

Currently, available evidence for variants associated with GD involves data from candidate gene studies which are limited and have provided nonreplicable and low-confidence findings in other psychiatric conditions such as depression.[32] Consequently, these findings should be interpreted with caution. Genetic polymorphisms related to genes encoding for the dopamine-related moieties (*DRD1*Ddel, *DRD2* Taq I A, *DRD4* [exon III]) were hypothesized to contribute to GD with mixed results observed.[33,34] Variants of the serotonin transporter gene promoter region (*5HTTLPR*)[35] and MAOA enzymes (*MAO-A* [intron I], *MAO-A* [promoter], *MAO-B* [intron II])[36] have been reported in association with GD. Similarities concerning allelic distributions have been reported in GD and DSM-IV–defined drug and alcohol dependence; for example, variations in *DRD2* and *MAOA* genes have been linked to GD and alcohol-use disorders, and *DRD4* variants have been linked to GD and alcohol, cocaine, and heroin use disorders.[37]

Neurocognition

The study of neurocognitive correlates of GD is significant because it provides insight into neurobiological functioning.[38] Currently, available evidence indicates that individuals with GD demonstrate impaired functioning regarding impulsivity,[39] which may be associated with a dysregulation of the ventromedial prefrontal cortex (vmPFC) and orbitofrontal cortex (OFC) in these individuals.[40]

Impulsivity is a multifaceted construct[41] characterized by a predisposition to rapid reactions to stimuli without forethought or regard for the consequences associated with such reactions.[42] Different neurocognitive tasks can be employed to evaluate different domains of impulsivity (eg, impulsive choices and decision-making).

Impulsive choices may be evaluated through monetary tasks in which an individual is offered options to choose hypothetical dollar amounts delivered immediately or larger amounts after specified delays. The rapid temporal discounting of rewards has been termed delay discounting, as rewards are more steeply discounted as a function of delay duration.[43] Delay discounting involves aspects of reward evaluation, and multiple brain regions contribute to reward processing in humans.[44] One implicated brain region in subjective reward valuation is the nucleus accumbens (NAcc), situated in the ventral striatum.[45] The anticipation of working for or receiving monetary rewards is associated with ventral striatal activation, whereas an increase in vmPFC activation is associated with the processing of actual reward outcomes during the performance of a monetary incentive delay task.[46] An effective functional balance between these reciprocally connected neural regions may mediate appropriate and advantageous behavioral responses to varying reward contingencies. Risk-reward decision-making may be evaluated using the Iowa gambling task (IGT) in which individuals choose between four decks of cards: two with big, but unlikely, wins and larger losses and another with small, but probable, wins and smaller losses, with selections from the latter two decks associated with more money being accrued over time.

Individuals with GD often make disadvantageous decisions in real life (eg, "I'll go gambling one last time") and select small immediate rewards over larger delayed rewards (eg, preferring $20 now as compared with $40 in a month). Delay discounting among individuals with GD has been associated with decreased activations in the ventral striatum and OFC compared to matched controls.[44] Individuals with GD have also shown disadvantageous decision-making on the IGT.[47] Importantly, neurocognitive measures of disinhibition and decision-making have been positively associated with problem-gambling severity[48] and have been associated with GD recurrence.[49]

Individuals with SUDs also display greater propensities to make risky decisions.[50] A dose-dependent relationship has been found between severity of alcohol use problems and delay discounting.[51] A similar effect has been reported among people who use heroin regarding needle sharing, with people who shared needles showing steeper delay-discounting tendencies.[51] Individuals with comorbid SUDs and GD discount rewards more rapidly than do GD individuals without SUDs,[43,52] although whether co-occurring SUDs and GD promote delay discounting or delay discounting is a vulnerability factor for such co-occurrence is unclear.

Taken together, impulsivity represents a multi-faceted transdiagnostic domain spanning addictive disorders.[53] These data highlight some of the similarities between GD and SUDs and suggest similarities in underlying neurobiological features.[54] As such, neurocognitive research may be a useful tool in the identification of brain regions of interest warranting further investigation via more direct imaging-based modalities.

Neurochemistry

Serotonin (5-Hydroxytryptamine)

Serotonergic neurons project from the raphe nucleus of the brain stem to multiple brain regions including the hippocampus, amygdala, and prefrontal cortex (PFC). It has been hypothesized that dysregulated serotonergic functioning may mediate behavioral inhibition and impulsivity in GD.[55] Data from studies of cerebrospinal fluid (CSF), pharmacological challenge studies, and preclinical investigations together suggest a role for serotonin in GD.

Low CSF levels of the serotonin metabolite 5-hydroxyindoleacetic acid (5-HIAA) have been reported in individuals with GD.[56] Low CSF levels of 5-HIAA in humans have been associated with violence, suicidality, and impulsive aggression and observed in other psychiatric disorders including ICDs and alcohol use disorder.[57] Preclinical research has identified a correlation between risk-taking behaviors and lowered CSF levels of 5-HIAA in monkeys[57] and rats.[58] Low levels of platelet monoamine oxidase (MAO) activity, considered a peripheral marker of serotonin activity, have been reported among males with GD.[36,59] Consistent with findings of 5-HIAA CSF levels, lowered levels of platelet MAO have additionally been reported in both suicidal and risk-taking individuals.[35]

Serotonin receptor sensitivity has been investigated via the administration of the 5-HT1/5-HT2 receptor partial agonist meta-chlorophenylpiperazine (m-CPP). Individuals with GD, like those with SUDs, report a euphoric or "high" response to the m-CPP, whereas control subjects report an unpleasant response,[60] along with an enhanced prolactin response.[61] In GD, this differential response was associated with severity of GD symptomatology, with higher scores on the Yale-Brown Obsessive-Compulsive Scale Modified for PG, a GD severity rating scale, significantly correlating with increased prolactin responses. In response to the 5-HT1B/1D receptor agonist sumatriptan, blunted growth hormone and prolactin responses were observed among individuals with GD (versus controls), a response that suggests decreased serotonin receptor sensitivity,[62] similar to that observed among individuals with alcohol use disorder.[63] Furthermore, disturbances in serotonin function, as reflected by blunted prolactin response to m-CPP, appear associated with the severity of drug use among individuals with cocaine use disorder.[64] Taken together, these studies suggest that responses to serotonin agonist administration are similar to those reported for substance-related addictions.

Lastly, among individuals with GD, 5-HT1B receptor availability within both the ventral striatum/pallidum and the anterior cingulate cortex (ACC) have been positively correlated with problem-gambling severity (as assessed using the South Oaks Gambling Screen).[65]

Dopamine

Dopamine has been implicated in rewarding and reinforcing processes in drug addiction. There have been several ligand-based studies investigating dopamine functioning among individuals with GD versus healthy controls. Linnet et al.[66] reported in a very small sample a positive association between self-reported excitement levels during IGT performance and dopamine release within the ventral striatum among individuals with GD. Joutsa et al.[67] reported that whereas individuals with GD and healthy controls showed similar levels of dopamine release during a slot-machine task performance, dopamine release was positively correlated with problem-gambling severity among individuals with GD. Similarly, there have been two reports of no alterations in overall dopamine receptor binding within the striatum among individuals with GD,[68,69] despite significant correlations between D3 receptor binding and both problem-gambling severity and impulsivity within the dorsal striatum,[68] as well as between mood-related impulsivity and D2/D3 receptor binding within the striatum[69] among individuals with GD. Taken together, these preliminary data raise questions regarding the centrality of dopamine in GD.[70]

Psychopharmacological data suggest that the dopamine system may influence impulsive behavior, although the precise manner is not completely understood. Stimulants such as amphetamine increase dopamine release and prevent dopamine uptake within the synaptic cleft and lead to improved impulse control in individuals with ADHD.[57] However, amphetamine administration in GD has been associated with the priming of gambling motivations.[71] Whereas dopamine agonists have been associated with GD and ICDs in the treatment of Parkinson disease (PD),[72] the dopamine D2-like receptor antagonist haloperidol has been reported to enhance the rewarding and priming effects of gambling in non-PD GD,[71] though individual differences may be important.[73] Investigations of CSF dopamine levels in GD have also yielded equivocal findings. Decreased CSF levels of dopamine and increased levels of the dopamine metabolites homovanillic acid (HVA) and 3,4-dihydroxyphenylacetic acid have been reported in GD.[74] However, these findings were no longer present when correcting for CSF flow rates.[56] A subsequent investigation reported increased levels of CSF HVA among individuals with GD.[75] The authors additionally reported enhanced levels of 5-HIAA, a finding different from their earlier investigations of CSF serotonin metabolite concentration levels.[56] These data highlight the need for studies using larger carefully controlled samples while accounting for potentially confounding factors such as co-occurring pathologies and CSF flow rate.

Norepinephrine and Arousal in GD

Dysregulation of norepinephrine—a neurotransmitter implicated in arousal, attention, and sensation-seeking behaviors—has been reported in individuals with GD. Individuals with GD have elevated urinary concentrations of norepinephrine, as well as elevated CSF levels of a metabolite of norepinephrine (metabolite 4-hydroxy-3-methoxyphenyl glycol).[76] Research supports dysregulated hypothalamic-pituitary-adrenal axis regulation in GD. Meyer et al.[77] measured the neuroendocrine responses to "real-life" casino gambling in people with gambling problems and found that people with gambling problems had higher heart rates and elevated norepinephrine and dopamine levels in comparison to controls. In a separate study, individuals with GD (versus controls) showed a higher growth hormone peak response to clonidine—an adrenergic agonist used to investigate norepinephrine function—the magnitude of which was positively correlated with problem-gambling severity.[78] Together, these data suggest that there may be an elevation of norepinephrine activity in GD that may be potentiated by gambling behaviors.

Opioids

Opioid systems have also been implicated in the pathophysiology of GD as challenge studies with oral amphetamine showed a blunted opioid response in individuals with GD,[79] a transdiagnostic finding that is also observed among individuals with other addictive behaviors, for example, SUDs.[80] Clinical trials have also implicated opioids in GD pathophysiology as randomized controlled trials (RCTs) show opioid antagonists such as naltrexone and naloxone may have efficacy in comparison to placebo for GD, although findings are mixed.[81] Additional research is further warranted to clarify the role of the opioid system in GD.

Neurocircuitry and Structure

Corticostriatal and forebrain neuromodulatory systems have been implicated in delayed and probabilistic reward (ie, delay discounting).[57] Dysregulation of the mesocorticolimbic (MCL) dopamine system has been hypothesized to contribute to GD and SUDs,[82] although more recent data suggest that dopamine may not contribute a central role as previously hypothesized.[83] Given the phenomenological (eg, craving, tolerance) and neurocognitive (eg, delay discounting) similarities between GD and SUDs, it is possible that these disorders may share similar neurobiological abnormalities, and current investigations examining this hypothesis have identified both similarities and differences.[84]

There have been several fMRI studies that suggest that specific brain regions contribute to the pathophysiology of GD. For example, reduced frontal cortical, basal ganglia, and thalamic activations in response to gambling videos—during the period prior to the subjective onset of emotional or motivational response—have been reported among GD subjects (versus controls).[85] This finding differed from those observed in similar studies involving subjects with OCD in which relatively increased activation of these regions was observed in the patient group. In particular, when viewing the portion of the videotapes during which the most robust gambling stimuli (eg, video clips of a gambling public service announcement involving slot machines or an advertisement for a casino in which table gambling is shown) were presented, individuals with GD displayed relatively less activation of the vmPFC. Diminished activations of the vmPFC among individuals with GD as compared to control subjects have also been observed in other studies across a range of fMRI tasks, including the Stroop color-word interference task,[86] a monetary incentive delay task,[87] and a simulated gambling task.[82] Similarly, individuals with SUDs either with or without co-occurring GD show relatively diminished activation of the vmPFC during performance of the IGT,[88] in comparison to control subjects. Together, these data indicate an important role for the vmPFC in GD.

Multiple studies also implicate the striatum in GD. For example, Reuter et al.[82] observed significantly less vmPFC and ventral striatal activation in GD participants compared to control subjects during a simulated gambling task. Both right ventral striatal activation and vmPFC activation were inversely correlated with severity of gambling symptomatology in GD subjects, indicating that the less the activation of these brain regions, the greater the gambling pathology. Other fMRI studies during gambling-cue exposure have similarly observed diminished activation in the ventral[89] and dorsal striatum[90] in GD participants (versus controls).

In recent years, multiple studies have investigated the neurostructural correlates of psychiatric disorders using either diffusion tensor imaging (DTI) or voxel-based morphometry (VBM) to assess white and gray matter structures, respectively. Findings from DTI studies indicate similar alterations in white matter microstructures encompassing regions of callosal, association, and projection fiber tracts between GD[91] and SUDs.[92] Among individuals with GD, a history of alcohol use disorder has been associated with a greater magnitude of white matter microstructural alterations within regions of the corpus callosum, and white matter integrity within the corpus genu has been associated with increased levels of self-reported impulsivity.[91] More recently in a larger sample, similar white matter–related alterations were observed in secondary crossing fibers in individuals with GD and cocaine use disorder.[93] Together, these data provide evidence for white matter involvement in the pathophysiology of GD.

Several VBM studies have been conducted among individuals with GD.[94] In contrast to a region-of-interest study finding smaller hippocampal and amygdalar volumes in GD,[95] no significant differences were reported in gray matter volumes between individuals with and without GD in the VBM studies. In comparison to individuals with alcohol or cocaine use disorders, those with GD showed relatively greater gray matter volumes including within the PFC, with measures similar to those in healthy populations.[94] These data therefore suggest differences in gray matter macrostructures in GD as compared with SUDs and raise the possibility that some of the volumetric differences in SUDs may be specific to these disorders, perhaps via substance-related neurotoxicities.

Epidemiology

Epidemiological studies evaluating the distribution of gambling and problem gambling behaviors in adults are heterogeneous. A recent systematic review concluded that studies reported prevalence ratios from 0.12% to 5.8% for past-year problem gambling in different countries.[18] On one hand, it is possible that unequal distributions in exposure to risk factors could explain these differences, but on the other hand, methodological variations should also be considered as heterogeneous sampling procedures and diagnostic assessments could partially explain seemingly contrasting findings. In the United States, a well-estimated prevalence of lifetime PG (as defined in the DSM-IV) among adults probably comes from the National Comorbidity Survey Replication (NCS-R), a face-to-face household survey of 9,282 English-speaking respondents aged 18 years and older conducted between February 2001 and April 2003 in a nationally representative multistage clustered area probability sample of the U.S. household population. In that survey, 2.3% met at least one DSM-IV criterion for PG, while only 0.6% met criteria for PG.[96] These findings reinforce the public health importance of PG and problem gambling.

It is likely that with less restrictive DSM-5 criteria for GD (as is the case for SUDs), the prevalence of GD would be higher.

GD often begins in adolescence and young adulthood, and prevalence estimates of GD tend to decrease across the life span.[97] In particular, adolescents are considered a vulnerable group to develop gambling problems, and a similar vulnerability with SUDs is also observed, likely due to common vulnerability factors (eg, impaired impulse control) for both SUDs and GD. Early age of onset has been associated with increased risk of GD in adulthood, for example, as reported in the NCS-R. This is particularly important because it underlines the importance of adolescent gambling as a risk factor for GD. Adolescent gambling frequently goes unnoticed[98] and is usually underestimated as a youth mental health problem by parents[99] and teachers,[100] although the immediate and longer-term problems associated with adolescent recreational problem gambling have been reported.[101] Early recognition and early intervention of adolescent problem gambling are in line with public health needs and initiatives.

The NCS-R also identified important demographic characteristics associated with GD. Being young and male were identified as risk factors, and these findings have been replicated in other independent studies.[102] Nevertheless, it is important to recognize that females are also at risk of GD and may show a faster progression between initiation and problematic engagement in addictive behavior, a phenomenon called "telescoping," which is also observed in SUDs.[103]

The NCS-R also identified that individuals who self-identified as non-Hispanic Black showed elevated odds of experiencing GD. This finding is in line with other studies in the United States[104] and other countries,[105] which have reported that racial/ethnic minorities have elevated odds of experiencing gambling-related problems. Particularly, the National Epidemiologic Survey on Alcohol and Related Conditions (NESARC) showed that the prevalence estimates of GD in Black and Native/Asian American people were nearly twofold that in White individuals.[104] It is possible that the increased vulnerability of minorities (eg, language barriers, unemployment) could predispose them to gambling-related problems or other psychiatric conditions that frequently co-occur with GD, such as SUDs. Regarding sexual orientation, there is some evidence that lesbian, gay, bisexual, transgender, intersex, and queer (LGBTIQ) individuals may be at increased risk of GD,[106] although conflicting findings have been reported,[107] and GD among gay and bisexual men may show worse prognosis as individuals experience more impairment and co-occurring ICDs.[108] Additional research is warranted to clarify the impacts of race/ethnicity and sexual orientation in the occurrence and course of GD. Regardless, these findings highlight the importance of considering race/ethnicity and sexual orientation in GD.

There additionally exist frequent co-occurrence between GD and SUDs, with co-occurrence estimates as high as 39.0% in clinical populations[109] and elevated odds observed in community samples.[110] Frequent co-occurrence is also observed with mood, anxiety, impulse-control, and personality disorders. Considering the longitudinal course of GD, few prospective studies have been conducted to date,[111] and additional efforts are required to characterize the persistence of and recovery from GD and related factors across the lifespan.

Treatment

Psychotherapeutic and psychopharmacological interventions have been evaluated for the treatment of GD. Among the different types of psychotherapeutic interventions, cognitive (CT), cognitive-behavioral (CBT), and motivational interviewing (MI) strategies comprise the largest proportion of interventions tested in RCTs of psychotherapy for GD. CT attempts to correct gambling-related cognitive distortions (erroneous beliefs that one can control and predict outcomes of chance events), while CBT attempt to address both gambling-related cognitive distortions and gambling-related behavioral aspects (eg, identifying triggers, promoting gambling alternatives).[17] MI adopts a nonjudgmental/nonconfrontational position with patients to assess their readiness for change and enhance engagement through open-ended questions, affirmations, reflective listening, and brief summarizations.[17] A systematic review of psychotherapeutic interventions published in 2017 provides a comprehensive summary of available RCTs of psychotherapies for GD.[112] Regarding psychopharmacological interventions, multiple medications have been evaluated in RCTs including selective serotonin reuptake inhibitors (SSRIs) (eg, escitalopram, fluvoxamine, paroxetine, sertraline); tricyclic (eg, clomipramine) and atypical (eg, bupropion) antidepressants; opioid receptor antagonists (eg, naltrexone and nalmefene); glutamatergic agents (eg, *N*-acetyl-cysteine); mood stabilizers including lithium, valproate, and others (eg, topiramate, olanzapine). A pharmacotherapy algorithm based in part on co-occurring disorders has been proposed,[113] and a meta-analysis was published in 2019.[114]

Overall, the literature focused on the management of GD has been limited to short-term trials that have heterogeneous methodologies. Most interventions have been administered differently and therefore have been mostly examined in single studies. Also, different rating scales and assessments have been used to measure outcomes, which creates difficulties when comparing findings across trials. For psychotherapies specifically, suboptimal control conditions such as waiting lists have been used. For pharmacotherapies specifically, trials have been hampered by high placebo response rates,[115] and there are no clear first-line agents.

These limitations of existing studies highlight the need for more, and better, RCTs for GD in the future. Regardless, practitioners are currently faced with patients who require assistance and may still desire some practical guidance regarding the pharmacological treatment of GD. For psychotherapeutic interventions, Petry and colleagues[112] concluded that 6 to 8 sessions of CBT should be considered for patients with severe gambling problems, whereas minimal interventions (eg, feedback related to one's gambling) may have sufficient efficacy. For pharmacotherapy, Bullock and Potenza[113] proposed an empirically based algorithm—updated in Potenza et al. (2019)[17]—which may be used as a reference to guide prescribing practices, although no medication has a formal indication for GD. Briefly, because some pharmacotherapy trials have selected patients based on patterns of co-occurring disorders (eg, anxiety, SUDs), pharmacotherapy recommendations stemming from the presence or absence of specific disorders may be generated. This approach of employing pharmacological interventions based on co-occurring disorders is likely to resonate with prescribing physicians trained to evaluate patients systematically for the presence or absence of specific disorders and hence may be particularly useful for practitioners. We encourage readers to refer to these pieces for additional details.

Conclusion

GD defines a persistent, recurrent pattern of gambling that is associated with substantial distress or impairment. Although PG (as formerly defined in the DSM) was initially recognized as an ICD, advances in neurobiological research (eg, neurocognitive, neurochemical, neuroimaging, and genetics) have indicated similarities with SUDs and contributed to the reclassification of GD as an addictive disorder along SUDs. Nevertheless, there remains much to be clarified regarding the neurobiology, epidemiology, and treatment of GD. Considering the public health importance of GD, additional research efforts are required.

INTERNET GAMING DISORDER

Definition and Conceptualization

The DSM-5 SUD workgroup introduced internet gaming disorder (IGD) as a condition for further study in the DSM-5. According to the DSM-5,[9] the following operational criteria, which resemble those for SUDs/GD, were proposed for IGD: persistent and recurrent thoughts about previous or future gaming activities, irritability, anxiety, or sadness when gaming is ceased, the need to spend increasing amounts of time gaming, unsuccessful attempts to cut down gaming, loss of interest in previous hobbies and other entertainment as a result of gaming, continued excessive gaming despite adverse consequences, deception about the extent of gaming (eg, lied to family members), usage of gaming to escape reality, endangerment of a relationship or job/educational/career opportunity because of gaming. In these instances, gaming refers to videogames and is focused on multiplayer games, as detailed in the DSM-5.

The existence of IGD as a distinct psychiatric diagnosis and its diagnostic characteristics have been debated. This DSM-5 workgroup considered debates regarding the differences between generalized and specific forms of PIU. Some authors have contended that IGD fits in the latter.[116] This situation has been complicated in that some studies, including treatment research, for example, Wolfling et al.[117] have included participants with both PIU and IGD and it is thus sometimes difficult to separate findings which apply specifically to IGD.

Nonetheless, problematic gaming behavior including IGD has been linked to poor social competence, low academic performance, and, in the case of violent video games, aggression or violence.[118] Extreme cases of IGD have been cited as a possible contributing factor in deaths in South Korea and the United States. IGD is also frequently accompanied by co-occurring psychiatric conditions including ADHD,[119] mood disorders,[120] and SUDs.[120] These associations underscore the importance of studying further IGD.[121]

Neurobiology

Genetics

There exists limited research regarding the genetics of IGD. To date, no family or twin studies have been conducted investigating IGD. Considering molecular genetic studies, there have been some investigations evaluating specific candidate genes, which suggest that polymorphisms of the TaqIA1 allele of the *DRD2* receptor gene and Val158Met in the catecholamine-*O*-methyltransferase (*COMT*) gene could be implicated in IGD.[122,123] Interestingly, both alleles have been also implicated in other addictive behaviors including SUDs (eg, alcohol use disorder)[124] and GD.[109] However, candidate gene approaches notably do not yield high-confidence results. To date, no GWAS of IGD has been conducted. Further research concerning the genetic factors relating to IGD is needed.

Neurochemistry

Despite questions about the role of dopamine in GD,[83] the dopaminergic system has been proposed to contribute to reward processing in IGD.[125] An early study using the D2-like dopamine receptor radioligand [11C]raclopride during PET scanning reported findings consistent with increased release of dopamine, particularly in the ventral striatum, following a 50-minute video-game play in eight healthy adult males.[126] More recently, researchers used SPECT and suggested that dopamine release in the ventral striatum during a motorbike riding computer game[127] may be comparable to that induced by psychostimulant drugs such as amphetamines[128] and methylphenidate.[129] How this relates to IGD has yet to be investigated, and no study has directly compared dopamine release following computer gaming versus following amphetamine in the same individuals.

Neurocognition

There have been few studies evaluating the neurocognitive characteristics of IGD. Although part of the available evidence seems to corroborate to some extent the hypothesis that IGD is characterized by deficits in response inhibition,[130] this finding has been mixed across studies.[131] Nevertheless, a meta-analysis published in 2017 identified that individuals with IGD displayed diminished response inhibition when findings from multiple studies were pooled together.[132] Individuals with IGD have been shown to be prone to risky decision-making[133] although this finding also warrants additional replication.

Neurocircuitry and Structure

The ventral striatum has been frequently implicated in fMRI studies of IGD. In one MRI study, both structural and functional differences were observed in people with frequent (>9 hours per week) compared to infrequent (≤9 hours per week) gaming.[134] Greater left ventral striatal gray matter volume was associated with frequent as opposed to infrequent gaming, and volume of this region was negatively correlated with deliberation time during the Cambridge Gambling Task. Activation in the same region was also greater during feedback of loss compared to no loss during performance of a monetary incentive delay task among participants with frequent compared to infrequent gaming.

Other brain regions have also been implicated in IGD. Among 19 healthy male adults who played a novel video game for 60 minutes per day for 10 days, increased activations to video game versus neutral stimuli were observed in the left inferior frontal gyrus, left parahippocampal gyrus, right and left parietal lobe, right and left thalamus, and right cerebellum.[135] Greater activation of the right OFC, right NAcc, bilateral ACC, medial frontal cortex, right dorsolateral prefrontal cortex (dlPFC), and right caudate in response to video-game cues has also been reported among adult males who spent more than 30 hours per week playing World of Warcraft (a Massive Multiplayer Online Role-Playing Game), in comparison to those with nonheavy play (<2 hours per day).[136] Subsequent studies have similarly reported greater activation in these regions among individuals with current IGD[137] and among individuals in remission from online IGD[138] in response to video-game cues, in comparison to controls.

While many early studies examined participants with frequent versus infrequent gaming, limiting the generalizability of findings to IGD, more recent studies have examined individuals with IGD. These studies have suggested differences in reward processing and control that at times have been linked to cognitive processes and treatment outcome.[139] For example, a resting-state fMRI study found that individuals with IGD as compared to those without had relatively decreased functional connectivity within executive-control networks and that the strength of connectivity was inversely linked to Stroop performance, a measure of cognitive control.[140] Furthermore, a meta-analysis showed that individuals with IGD demonstrated hyperactivity in the anterior and posterior cingulate cortices, caudate and posterior inferior frontal gyrus as well as hypoactivation of the posterior insula, somatomotor and somatosensory cortices in studies measuring reward.[141] Besides, individuals with IGD also demonstrated hyperactivation of the same areas in relation to cold-executive function and hypoactivation of the anterior inferior frontal gyrus in relation to hot-executive function.[141] Also, individuals with IGD have also been shown to display gray matter volume and white matter density alterations in brain regions associated with impulse control, emotional regulation and motor function.[141] Whether these pieces of information could be harnessed to develop meaningful changes in current diagnostic methods and treatments for IGD remains to be seen. One study showed that individuals with IGD who received a craving behavioral intervention that included elements of cognitive behavioral therapy and mindfulness training demonstrated relatively increased activation of the insula to gaming cues following treatment as compared to before and as compared to the test-retest comparison group,[142] perhaps suggesting a mechanism for how a promising treatment for IGD might operate at a biological level.

Epidemiology

A range of prevalence estimates has been reported for adolescents (4.2%-20.0%), with published adult estimates (11.9%) falling in this range.[118] In a recent systematic review with meta-analysis, the pooled prevalence of IGD was estimated at 3.05%.[143] However, the authors found heterogeneity across studies, which was largely explained by differences in screening tools used to evaluate IGD. Indeed, because of the inconsistencies in the definition and conceptualization of IGD, multiple assessments tools have been developed and used to screen for IGD in the general population. Assessment tools for IGD were initially based on the DSM-IV definitions for SUDs and PG,[144] with more recent assessment instruments for DSM-5 IGD.[145] Standardization of instruments used to measure IGD will contribute to identifying the true prevalence of this condition in the general population. However, considering the available evidence, IGD is likely a prevalent condition in the general population. Currently available estimates also indicate IGD may be more prevalent in Asia than in Europe,[143] suggesting that differences in socio-cultural factors or environment might play an important role in the development and prevalence of IGD. This is a particularly important remark because there have been increasing changes in the gaming environment over the past 30 years. Studies should examine how the prevalence of IGD will change with modifications in the gaming environment in the future.

While adolescent boys are more likely to endorse IGD symptoms, no associations with negative health measures were observed among adolescent boys suggesting that video gaming may be a normative behavior among boys.[119] However, gaming may be associated with measures of aggression and violence among adolescent girls.[120] Research pertaining to gender-related differences in adults has yielded mixed results.[118] IGD and gaming behaviors in girls are under-researched and additional investigations considering gender-related differences are currently required.[146] There is a paucity of research examining race/ethnicity in the distribution of IGD. Desai, Krishnan-Sarin, Cavallo, and Potenza[120] reported that youth belonging to racial and ethnic minorities had higher rates of IGD in a high school survey from Connecticut. Individuals pertaining to different race and ethnic groups tend to display different rates of use of the internet and videogames, and minorities have been shown to use videogames and the internet with more frequency than White youth.[147] Whether these differences in exposure account for the possible higher frequency of IGD in minority groups is unknown. Regardless, these findings underscore the importance of considering race/ethnicity in IGD. Additional empirical research is required to expand our understanding on this topic and extend it to other groups (eg, individuals of diverse sexuality).

Treatment

A systematic review compiled treatment studies for PIU including IGD and reported that psychotherapy studies outnumbered pharmacotherapy studies 3:1.[148] Indeed, CBT aimed at modifying maladaptive cognitions related to gaming, fostering coping strategies to reduce withdrawal and unpleasant mood states, and developing social skills and new routines has been recommended for IGD.[149] Few RCTs have investigated pharmacological agents, and currently available findings do not enable evidence-based conclusions in favor of any medication. To date, only escitalopram and bupropion have been evaluated in controlled trials in a few small studies, and although promising findings have been reported, additional RCTs studies are needed.

Conclusion

IGD is a candidate behavioral addiction characterized by persistent and disordered engagement with internet games. Although there is considerable debate considering its nosology and classification, IGD has been associated with negative outcomes across the lifespan and psychiatric comorbidity. Preliminary evidence suggests alterations in brain structure and function among individuals with IGD and possible dopaminergic and serotonergic involvement in video-gaming behaviors similarly to other addictions. Treatment research of IGD is in early stages and additional efforts are required.

PROBLEMATIC INTERNET USE

Definition and Conceptualization

Problematic internet use (PIU) or "internet addiction" (IA) was not included in the DSM-5 as there is considerable debate as to whether IA is a misnomer as individuals would not be addicted to the internet per se but rather would use the internet to engage in specific addictive behaviors related to gambling, shopping, and sex.[150] PIU often involves excessive engagement in socially normative activities and as such, it may be hard to identify, and patients may be reticent to disclose PIU due to embarrassment, lack of awareness, or ambivalence over reducing use.

While moderate internet use may enhance one's quality of life by widening social circles and enhancing psychological well-being,[151] some individuals demonstrate excessive internet use may be problematic and impact negatively on daily function, family relationships, and emotional stability.[151] The term PIU may be used to describe such an excessive or poorly controlled urges and a maladaptive use of the internet.[152] Moreover, PIU may be positively associated with SUDs, incarceration and legal troubles, and poor physical and mental health.[152] As such, additional efforts to understand this under-researched and infrequently addressed clinical problem is warranted.

There are no uniformly agreed-upon diagnostic criteria for PIU. The term PIU has been used to describe an excessive or poorly controlled urges and a maladaptive use of the internet. Operational definitions of PIU were initially often based on DSM-IV criteria for PG.[153] Of these, Young's Internet Addiction Scale[154] was often used and has demonstrated sufficient reliability.[155] Based on the DSM-IV definitions of SUDs and PG, Young[154] proposed the following criteria for IA: withdrawal, tolerance, preoccupation with the internet, longer than intended spent on the internet, risk to significant other relationships and/or employment, lying about internet use, and repeated, unsuccessful attempts to stop internet use. However, other studies (including some that are cited below) have adopted different operational definitions of PIU from the one mentioned above.

Neurobiology

Genetics

Twin studies from China[156] and the Netherlands[157] indicate considerable heritability of PIU—between 50% and 60%. However, there has been little advance in identifying risk genes associated with PIU as available evidence is still based on candidate genes rather than hypothesis-free GWASs. In candidate gene approaches, the short allelic variant of the gene encoding the serotonin transporter (SS-5HTTLPR) has been reported to be more prevalent among 91 adolescent males with PIU compared to 75 matched controls.[158] Within the PIU group, the authors also reported that those with the SS-5HTTLPR showed higher harm avoidance and scored higher on Young's Internet Addiction Scale compared to those expressing other 5HTTLPR allelic variants. The T-variant (CC genotype) polymorphism of the nicotinic acetylcholine receptor subunit alpha-4 (*CHRNA4*) gene has also been implicated, with increased frequencies among individuals with PIU compared to controls; further analyses revealed that this finding was driven by females, suggesting sex-related genetic effects.[159] Replication of these findings is needed in future studies before definitive conclusions can be drawn. Other genes implicated in IGD have been implicated in PIU (eg, *DRD2*, *COMT*), in part because research examining IGD may also include individuals with PIU.[160]

Neurochemistry

There have been ligand-based studies of dopaminergic functioning among individuals with PIU. A small-scale single-photon emission computed tomography (SPECT) study reported reduced dopamine transporter expression within the striatum among young adult males who used the internet almost every day and spent more than 8 hours per day online, compared to matched controls.[161] Another small-scale study using [11C]raclopride during PET scanning reported that adult males with PIU had reduced dopamine D2-like receptor availability in the bilateral caudate and left putamen compared to controls and that the degree of dopamine receptor availability was inversely correlated with the severity of PIU.[162] These preliminary findings suggest that PIU may be associated with dopaminergic neural systems in a fashion similar to substance-related addiction.

Neurocognition

Studies investigating the neurocognitive profile of individuals with PIU suggest a similar impaired "top-down" cortical behavioral control in PIU similar to that observed in other addictive behaviors. In a recent systematic review and meta-analysis,[163] individuals with PIU demonstrated impaired inhibitory control and decision-making irrespective of whether gaming was the predominant type of online behavior, that is likely independently of IGD. These findings are in line with evidence for other addictive behaviors, including SUDs and GD, as reflected in current theoretical models.[164]

Neurocircuitry and Structure

While evidence remains scarce and frequently mixed with findings from IGD, studies implicate areas involved in executive control including the superior temporal gyrus and the middle frontal gyrus (as reviewed in Peng et al.[165]). For instance, in an fMRI study, increased resting-state regional homogeneity involving the right frontal region, left superior frontal gyrus, right cingulate gyrus, bilateral parahippocampus, and other regions was observed among PIU individuals (versus controls).[166]

Other studies also suggest differences in brain function during cognitive tasks. Greater activation of the anterior and posterior cingulate cortices during the Stroop color-word interference task has been observed.[167] Greater ACC activation was associated with slower incongruent reaction time and more severe scores on the Young's Internet Addiction Scale across all participants.[167] In a monetary gain and loss guessing task, increased activation of the OFC to gain trials and decreased ACC to loss trials was observed among PIU subjects compared to controls, suggesting sensitization to reward and desensitization to loss.[168]

A VBM study reported decreased gray matter density in the left ACC, left posterior cingulate cortex, left insula, and left lingual gyrus among individuals with PIU in comparison to age- and gender-matched comparison participants.[169] Similarly, an independent study reported among adolescents with IA relatively decreased gray matter volumes in the left ACC—as well as in regions of the dorsolateral and orbitofrontal PFC, supplementary motor area, and cerebellum.[170]

Fractional anisotropy (FA)—a widely used measure of white matter integrity based on DTI—was increased within a region of the left internal capsule and decreased within a region of the right parahippocampal gyrus among adolescents with IA (versus controls).[170] By contrast, Lin et al.[171] reported widespread impairments in white matter microstructures—as indexed by decreased FA and increased radial diffusivity—encompassing callosal, association, and projection fiber tracts among adolescents with IA. Together, these data suggest involvement of white matter microstructures in the pathophysiology of PIU. However, given the differences in anatomical loci reported between studies, further research into the precise relationship between scalar indices of white matter microstructural integrity (eg, FA) and PIU are warranted.

Epidemiology

The lack of a universal assessment tool may contribute to the wide range of prevalence estimates reported among adolescents (4.0%-19.1%) and adults (0.7%-18.3%) (reviewed by Yau et al.[118]). Some data suggest that internet use is higher among men than among women, with men being more likely to have PIU,[172] although this gender gap has not been observed consistently. Regardless, a recent systematic review with meta-analysis showed that men were more likely to demonstrate PIU,[173] although this finding could likely be attributed to gender-related differences in social norms. Indeed, another meta-analysis demonstrated that while males were more likely to show higher levels of IGD, females were more likely to show higher levels of social media addiction.[174] These findings reinforce the importance of considering gender-related differences in the distribution of behavioral addictions including PIU. Additionally, it is also important to recognize potential race/ethnicity-related differences in the distribution of PIU. Individuals from different racial and ethnic backgrounds may be differentially exposed to internet use,[147] which may contribute to different susceptibilities to PIU across racial and ethnic groups. More specifically, minoritized groups such as Hispanic and Latinx and Asian American individuals have been shown to use the internet more frequently and to have higher rates of PIU than White and non-Latinx individuals, respectively.[175] More research aimed at understanding the distribution of PIU across minority groups is warranted.

PIU frequently co-occurs not only with SUDs[176] but also with various psychiatric conditions including impulse-control, mood, and personality disorders.[177] There also seems to exist gender-related differences in the comorbidity distribution as higher rates of aggression were associated with increased severity of PIU only among males (while ADHD and depression were associated with PIU across genders).[178]

Treatment

To date, there are no RCTs evaluating the efficacy of pharmacological interventions for PIU. Considering that psychotherapy studies frequently administered interventions to populations of IGD and PIU together[117] CBT is also the recommended therapy for individuals with PIU,[149] although additional research is required to evaluate the benefits and functional improvements over longer periods of follow-up.

Conclusion

Although not included in the DSM-5, PIU is associated with significant psychological distress. Preliminary evidence suggests neurobiological similarities with SUDs; however, further research is needed to support this hypothesis. Standardization of definitions and criteria of PIU is warranted to enable further research aimed at identifying better treatments. To that end, researchers in the field have been working collaboratively to reach a consensus on conceptualization, description and definition of diagnostic criteria for PIU and there exist expectations that progress will be made through the establishment of shared multinational databases.[179]

COMPULSIVE BUYING DISORDER

Definition and Conceptualization

Classically referred to as "oniomania," compulsive buying disorder (CBD) has been clinically recognized for at least a century[180] (reviewed by Lejoyeux et al.[181]). CBD may be characterized by excessive shopping cognitions and buying behaviors that lead to distress and/or impairment.[182]

There is debate regarding the classification of CBD. Currently, CBD is also not formally recognized in the DSM-5, and therefore represents a candidate behavioral addiction. Although there are data supporting its classification as a behavioral addiction,[14] some others contend that an ICD classification may be more appropriate.[183] Despite nosologic debates, diagnostic criteria have been proposed,[184] which has facilitated the development of research on CBD. These criteria include preoccupations with buying or buying-related obsessions/urges; shopping for unnecessary items or more than can be afforded; shopping for longer periods than originally intended; shopping despite adverse consequences (eg, occupational, relational, or financial).

Neurobiology

Neurocircuitry

Using fMRI, Raab et al.[185] compared signal responses between individuals with CBD versus those of healthy controls during performance of a multiphase purchasing task. During an initial product presentation phase, CBD individuals showed stronger NAcc activity compared to controls. During the subsequent price presentation phrase, CBD individuals showed attenuated activation of the insula and ACC compared to controls. In contrast, individuals with CBD had increased ACC activity while making purchasing decisions, in comparison to controls. More recent studies suggest that constructs related to addiction (eg, craving, decision-making, and other executive functions) hold relevance for CBD.[186]

Epidemiology

A prevalence estimate of CBD in the United States comes from a random sample, national household survey involving 2,513 adults.[187] The authors used the proposed criteria mentioned above.[184] The study reported a point prevalence of 5.8%, suggesting more than 1 in 20 individuals in the United States had CBD. Importantly, this study was conducted about 20 years ago and it is possible that changes in shopping behaviors (eg, online shopping) over this time could influence the distribution of CBD in the general population. Nonetheless, a meta-analysis published in 2016 with 40 studies from 16 countries identified a similar prevalence ratio of 4.9%.[188]

CBD has been frequently associated with female gender in the literature, although few studies have examined empirically gender-related differences in CBD. Currently, it remains unknown whether women are at increased risk of CBD in comparison to men. For instance, in Koran et al.,[187] women did not have a substantially higher prevalence of CBD (6%) in comparison to men (5.5%). Regardless, it is possible that women and men differ in buying behaviors and motives, which could underlie different pathways *en route* to CBD. A study of Chinese college students demonstrated avoidance coping partially mediated the link between psychological distress and compulsive buying in females only.[189] Additional research is warranted to clarify the roles of gender in CBD. Similarly, more research is required to characterize the differential distribution of CBD across minoritized groups. Hispanic and Latinx individuals may be more likely to engage in problematic shopping behaviors, although there is scant empirical evidence to support this possibility.[190]

Treatment

There are no clear evidence-based treatments for CBD. In a recent review of psychotherapy and pharmacotherapy interventions for CBD,[191] few RCTs were identified. Regarding psychotherapy, group CBT was the most frequently tested intervention, and a meta-analysis reported a large effect size in favor of this treatment. However, there was evidence of publication bias which suggests that there may be an overestimation of the true effect of CBT in CBD considering the currently available literature. Regarding pharmacotherapy, RCTs have tested SSRIs and did not demonstrate between-group differences in outcomes with fluvoxamine[192] or escitalopram.[193] It is possible that a substantial placebo effect has contributed to the lack of comparative efficacy. Although these findings from controlled studies raise questions regarding the clinical utility of SSRIs in the treatment of CBD, they also highlight the need for further studies.

Conclusion

CBD is a candidate behavioral addiction that has been recognized for centuries, although there remains debate regarding its delineation as a separate mental health condition. It is estimated that about 5% of individuals in the general population experience CBD. However, little is known about its pathophysiology or treatment. Preliminary research suggests altered neurofunctional responses to shopping stimuli. There are few treatment studies, and future research should explore the efficacy of medications such as naltrexone in RCTs. The availability of assessment tools for CBD should aid in clinical and research efforts.

COMPULSIVE SEXUAL BEHAVIOR DISORDER

Definition and Conceptualization

Compulsive sexual behavior disorder (CSBD) is characterized by excessive engagement in normative sexual behaviors. Clinically relevant sexual behaviors may be divided into paraphilic and nonparaphilic behaviors. In paraphilic sexual behaviors, there is a disturbance in the object selection (eg, an animal, unwilling person, inanimate object), whereas in nonparaphilic sexual behaviors, the individual engages in socially normative sexual behaviors in an excessive, obsessive, or compulsive manner, without a disturbance of object choice.

Paraphilic disorders are a distinct category of disorders, included in the DSM-5, and are outside the scope of this chapter. Nonparaphilic impulsive or compulsive sexual disorders are not specifically listed in the DSM-5. While hypersexual disorder was considered for inclusion in DSM-5, it was omitted. However, CSBD was defined in the eleventh revision of the International Classification of Diseases (ICD-11) as an ICD characterized by a persistent pattern of failure to control intense, repetitive sexual urges and behaviors. The following operational criteria were provided in the ICD-11 as essential features of CSBD: continued engagement in sexual behaviors leading to neglect of health or personal care and other interests, activities, and responsibilities, repeated unsuccessful attempts to cut down on the behavior, continued engagement in sexual behaviors despite adverse consequences (eg, marital conflict, financial, legal or general negative health impact) and despite little or no of satisfaction from it. As with other ICDs (as discussed in the Introduction of this chapter), CSBD can be conceptualized along an impulsive-compulsive spectrum as addictive behaviors or OCRDs.[194] Regardless, these criteria are in line with those of hypersexual disorder that were proposed for DSM-5.[195]

Phenomenological similarities between CSBD and SUDs or other behavioral addictions have been described.[194] Individuals suffering from CSBD often report feeling "out of control." Estimates of co-occurrence rates for SUDs and CSBD range from 25% to 71%.[196] CSBs are aimed at reward seeking and anxiety reduction. Individuals with CSBD report feelings of regret and fear over losing loved ones or employment as a result of their behaviors.

Neurobiology

Neurochemistry

Dopamine, serotonin, norepinephrine, and the opioid system contribute to human sexual behavior, though systematic studies of their involvement in CSBD are largely lacking (for a review, refer to Chatzittofis et al.[197]). Serotonin is implicated in sexual functioning and desire, and sexual dysfunctions, such as decreased libido, anorgasmia, and delayed ejaculation, are reported as adverse effects of SSRI treatment.[198] Increased sexual desire and impulse control behaviors have been observed in patients with PD or restless leg syndrome (RLS) taking dopaminergic medications.[199] Voon and Fox[200] estimated that 2.4% of PD patients taking dopamine agonists meet the criteria for hypersexuality or pathological sexual behavior. In a study of 70 RLS patients without comorbid PD, 5% of respondents reported a high level of sexual desire and 4% reported that their desire had increased subsequent to taking dopaminergic medication (pramipexole, ropinirole, and levodopa).[199] None of the patients with high levels of sexual desire had a personal or family history of CSBD or sexual paraphilia. However, impulse control behaviors (including hypersexuality) have been associated with demographic and clinical features of PD independent of medication, supporting the notion that multiple factors contribute to the development of ICDs in PD.[201] Further research is needed to examine the potential role of dopamine in the pathophysiology of CSBD and other sexual behaviors in PD and RLS as well as in individuals without these disorders, particularly as dopamine pathology is central to PD. Oxytocin has also been implicated in sexual behavior as its release is increased during penile erection and ejaculation and it is associated with sexual satiety. In CSBD, a recent study demonstrated that individuals with hypersexual disorder exhibited significantly higher oxytocin plasma levels compared to healthy volunteers, reinforcing the possibility that this peptide is implicated in CSBD.[202] Intriguingly, relatively little research has investigated the role of hormones from the hypothalamus-pituitary-gonadal axis such as testosterone and luteinizing hormone (LH) in CSBD. One recent study compared basal morning plasma levels of these hormones and reported significantly higher LH plasma levels in CSBD, but no significant differences in testosterone. Additional research is required to clarify the role of these hormones in CSBD. Lastly, additional neurotransmitter systems warrant consideration. For example, arginine vasopressin has been associated with problematic pornography use in men with CSBD, whereas diminished empathy may link low levels of oxytocin to problematic pornography use in the same sample.[203]

Neurocircuitry and Structure

In human and preclinical populations, bilateral temporal lesions are associated with placidity, hyperorality, visual agnosia, and hypersexuality.[204] Together, this constellation of symptoms has been termed Klüver-Bucy syndrome and has also been observed in amygdala-lesioned patients.[196] Extremely rare in humans, Klüver-Bucy syndrome's associated hypersexuality, although infrequent, suggests possible involvement of temporal lobe function in CSBD and other paraphilia-related disorders.

Functional imaging studies of CSBD have been published,[205] with findings suggesting significant parallels with addictions. Attentional biases toward sexual cues have been linked to CSBD and neural regions implicated in motivational processes.[206] During exposure to sexual cues, men with CSBD, as compared to those without, activate to a greater degree brain regions previously implicated in reward and craving, with subjective responses suggesting greater wanting than liking, consistent with incentive salience models of addiction.[207] For instance, among men with problematic pornography use as compared to those without, greater ventral striatal activation to cues associated with sexual reward images was observed, but no between-group differences were associated with monetary cues or sexual or monetary reward outcomes.[208] Furthermore, the differences in ventral striatal activation to sexual versus monetary cues were associated with faster reaction times to receive sexual rewards and out-of-magnet measures relating to hypersexuality and masturbation frequency.[208] Individuals with CSBD also demonstrate poor response inhibition in go/no-go tasks related to decreased brain activation in the inferior frontal gyrus when response inhibition is required.[209] Thus, findings link CSBD to theoretical aspects of addiction and habit formations where salience may shift from rewards to cues.

There has been a DTI study of white matter microstructures in CSBD. Miner et al.[210] reported significantly higher mean diffusivity in a superior frontal region among individuals with CSBD in comparison to controls. Correlational analyses revealed a significant negative association between fractional anisotropy (FA) within an inferior frontal region and self-reported impulsivity. However, given the small sample size of this study (ie, eight patients with CSBD and eight controls), further research is needed.

Epidemiology

CSBD has not been included in large-scale, nationally representative studies, and the existence of heterogeneous assessments of CSBD has created difficulties for further advancements. For instance, older studies used to assess sexual behaviors through frequency[211] and the number of orgasms/week.[212] More recently, the Minnesota Impulsive Disorders Inventory (MIDI)[213] and clinician-designed "hypersexuality" (ie, CSBD) questionnaires[200] have been available for use in epidemiological studies. Those instruments more closely resemble the diagnostic criteria for SUDs and GD and should contribute to advance the current knowledge on the distribution of CSBD in the general population. Indeed, in a recent study on a college sample, Odlaug and Grant[214] evaluated the prevalence of ICDs using the MIDI and reported a CSBD prevalence ratio of 3.66%. The same authors later conducted another study with college students and reported a prevalence ratio of 2%.[215] More recent instruments include ones for ICD-11–defined CSBD and problematic pornography use.[216]

There seems to exist an important male preponderance in individuals affected by CSBD (80% or higher). Indeed, the prevalence of CSBD among men (3%) seems to be higher than that among women (1%). Although there are few longitudinal studies evaluating CSBD, individuals seem to report dysregulated sexual fantasies, urges, and behaviors prior to adulthood, suggesting an early onset.[217] It is also possible that CSBD behaviors are stable over time. Particularly, studies conducted during the COVID-19 pandemic did not demonstrate increased pornography use during periods of lockdown or stay-at-home orders. Instead, these studies demonstrated relatively stable levels of pornography use, including when considering engagement with behaviors prior to the pandemic.[218]

Regarding race and ethnicity, in a survey study published in 2018 involving a nationally representative sample of the United States, Hispanic and Latinx and Black individuals were found at increased risk of experiencing clinically relevant levels of distress and impairment associated with difficulty of controlling sexual feelings, urges, and behaviors.[219] Regarding sexual orientation, LGBTIQ individuals seem to be at increased risk of experiencing distress related to sexual behaviors.[220] Additional research is warranted to clarify the distribution of CSBD across different racial/ethnic and sexual orientation groups.

Treatment

Open-label prescriptions of lithium, tricyclic antidepressants, SSRIs, nefazodone, naltrexone, and atypical antipsychotics have all been explored in CSBD treatment,[221] but their efficacy in treating CSBD remains to be systematically examined. At present, most data on pharmacological treatment for CSBD are from individual case reports, and more research is needed to identify empirically validated pharmacotherapies.

There is mixed evidence to support the efficacy of SSRIs in treating CSBD. In an RCT, gay men with CSBD reported a greater reduction in sexual desire after taking citalopram, without a lessening in sexual satisfaction, than did individuals taking placebo.[222] It is presently not clear whether the efficacy of SSRI administration in reducing CSBD symptoms may be attributed to a reduction in sexual thoughts or to sexual "side effects" of the medication.[223] Positive results have been noted with nefazodone, a phenylpiperazine antidepressant that antagonizes serotonin receptors and influences serotonin and norepinephrine reuptake, in reducing sexual thoughts without the presence of substantial sexual side effects over the longer term.[224] Because sexual side effects may deter CSBD patients from continuing SSRI treatment, nefazodone may be particularly preferred in treating CSBD. However, controlled trials are needed to further determine the efficacy and tolerability of nefazodone in treating CSBD.

Pharmacological tolerance to SSRI treatment has been reported in men with CSBD, and ADHD co-occurs with CSBD. Kafka and Hennen[225] examined the effect of psychostimulant augmentation during SSRI treatment in a sample of men with paraphilic or paraphilia-related (eg, CSBD) disorders. They found a significant reduction in paraphilic or paraphilia-related behaviors in response to SSRI treatment alone and reported a significant improvement subsequent to methylphenidate SR (sustained release). These preliminary data suggest an additive effect of methylphenidate administration in CSBD populations that may help to counteract pharmacological tolerance to SSRIs, and they additionally implicate a dysregulation of dopamine, serotonin, and norepinephrine systems in CSBD. The SSRI paroxetine was explored in the treatment of three men with CSBD relating to pornography use and while reductions in pornography use were observed, non–pornography-related problematic sexual behaviors emerged.[226] Given these findings, controlled trials with careful monitoring of a range of sexual behaviors are needed to examine the efficacy and tolerability of these medications in treating CSBD.

In a randomized, double-blind crossover design, naltrexone (25 mg/d), an opioid receptor antagonist, or placebo was administered to a sample of 20 sexually active men over a 3-day time period.[227] After 14 days, participants were administered either naltrexone or placebo (ie, whichever they did not receive in the initial phase). As assessed via subject self-report, naltrexone administration was associated with increased sexual arousal, greater frequency of orgasms, and orgasm intensity in response to masturbatory behaviors, which may indicate that the opioid system could inhibit ejaculation (eg, through analgesic effects).[227] Topiramate, an anticonvulsant hypothesized to partially inhibit GABAergic input into the NAcc in a similar fashion to opioid receptor antagonists,[228] may also alleviate symptoms of CSBD, although these effects were not maintained following topiramate discontinuation.[221] Conversely, preliminary open-label studies of opioid receptor antagonists in CSBD populations suggest possible efficacy at high doses; for example, administration of naltrexone at 150 mg/d[229] and 100 to 200 mg/d[230] have been reported to reduce CSBD symptoms and decrease sexual fantasies and masturbation. Together, these potentially contradictory findings suggest the involvement of endogenous opioids in CSBD, although the precise relationship remains unclear. Other factors, including differences in patient populations and dosing durations, also warrant consideration.

Conclusion

CSBD has been clinically acknowledged for years and is recognized in the ICD-11 as an ICD, although it is not included in the DSM-5. Like other behavioral addictions, CSBD is associated with distress and may interfere with personal and professional life. Relatively little is currently known about the neurobiology of CSBD, and further research is needed to determine effective therapeutic interventions.

BINGE EATING DISORDER

Definition and Conceptualization

Data suggest that both substance use and eating behaviors may be modulated by similar motivational neurocircuitry, leading to the conceptualization of "foods as drugs"[231] and "food addiction," albeit with debate. The DSM-IV-TR category of eating disorders included anorexia nervosa (AN), bulimia nervosa (BN), and eating disorder NOS, with BED being added in the DSM-5.

The diagnostic features of BED share similarities to those of SUDs and ICDs. The DSM-5 criteria include recurrent episodes, impaired control, and marked distress in relation to binge eating. Individuals may make repeated unsuccessful attempts to stop binge eating, and they may report that their binge eating has detrimental social and occupational effects—two important criteria for SUDs. Over a quarter of clinicians report often or always using addiction-based therapies for BED,[232] further suggesting phenomenological and clinical similarities between BED and SUDs. Given that BED has an important element of episodic behavioral loss of control similar to candidate and recognized behavioral and substance addictions, this section focuses primarily on this disorder.

Neurobiology

Neurochemistry

Leptin

Leptin, an adipose-derived hormone, is a chemical modulator involved in the maintenance of energy homeostasis and feeding behaviors.[233] Leptin is also implicated in other reward-seeking behaviors[233] including SUDs.[234] Leptin acts as a peripheral metabolic cue within the central nervous system to modulate neuronal activity in brain areas involved in appetite control, including the hypothalamus. Administration of exogenous leptin increases energy expenditure and reduces hyperphagia and obesity in genetically leptin-deficient mice and humans (*ob*/*ob*).[235] However, leptin deficiency syndrome is extremely rare in humans.[236]

Whereas leptin-modulated hypothalamic activity has been well documented, research suggests that leptin acts directly on other brain regions, including the substantia nigra pars compacta (SNc) and ventral tegmental area (VTA) of the midbrain. Dopamine neurons in the VTA and SNc project to the striatum and are implicated in reward, motivation, and addiction. Preclinical data[237] have demonstrated that dopamine neurons within the VTA express mRNA encoding for both leptin and insulin receptors. Exogenous leptin administration to the VTA results in a decrease in food consumption, and intravenous exogenous leptin administration reduces the firing of VTA dopaminergic neurons.[238] The expression of mRNA encoding the long form of the leptin receptor (ObRb) has additionally been reported in regions including the hippocampus, brain stem, cortex, thalamus, cerebellum, and substantia nigra.[239] Leptin has additionally been reported to enhance synaptic plasticity in brain regions such as the hippocampus.[240] Besides, preclinical research using pharmacological and genetic knockout strategies suggests that D2 dopamine receptor blockade attenuates the acute hypophagic effect of leptin in fasted mice.[241] These data suggest that, in addition to its metabolic function, leptin may help to modulate mesolimbic reward circuits that may relate to both palatability and substance use.

Orexins

Partially modulated by adipose-derived hormones such as leptin and ghrelin, the hypothalamic neuropeptides orexin-A and orexin-B—also referred to as hypocretin 1 and hypocretin 2—are important modulators of eating behavior and help to maintain energy homeostasis. The hypothalamus is the primary site of hypocretin-containing neurons, though these neurons project to other brain regions.[242] Orexin administration has been demonstrated to increase feeding behaviors,[242] while orexin antagonists have been shown to impair operant responses to food reinforcers[243] in preclinical populations.

Preclinical research has demonstrated that administration of orexin-A reinstates cocaine-seeking behaviors in a dose-dependent manner.[244] Similar research has demonstrated that the administration of an orexin receptor antagonist abolishes reinstatement of cue-induced alcohol-seeking[245] and heroin-seeking[246] behaviors in rodents, further implicating orexin in substance-seeking behaviors. Preclinical research also indicates a significant increase in hypothalamic orexin-containing neurons after preference conditioning for food, cocaine, or morphine, suggesting important similarities between the development of food and drug preferences.[247] Direct administration of orexin-A or orexin-B produces locomotor-enhancing effects in mice that were prevented by prior administration of a dopamine receptor antagonist.[248] The same study additionally demonstrated a lack of hyperlocomotion and a significantly lessened increase in dopamine in response to morphine.[248] Increases in PFC dopamine subsequent to orexin-A administration to the VTA have also been reported.[249] Together, these data suggest that orexin may directly influence mesolimbic dopamine pathways implicated in reward and drug addiction. However, further research investigating the relationship between orexinergic and dopaminergic signaling in clinical populations is needed.

Ghrelin

Ghrelin is a gastrointestinal hormone that helps to maintain energy homeostasis and may contribute importantly to the initiation of eating. Unlike leptin and orexin, which are anorexigenic, ghrelin is orexigenic and increases food intake and body weight.[250] Reduced levels of circulating ghrelin have been reported in obese individuals, with an inverse correlation between body mass index (BMI) and ghrelin levels observed.[251] Interestingly, preclinical research suggests that whereas ghrelin administration increases the motivation to eat, it does not alter perceived food palatability.[252]

Although ghrelin is primarily synthesized in the stomach, research suggests that it may also mediate feeding behaviors via direct action on certain brain regions. Preclinical research has identified a ghrelin receptor, growth hormone secretagogue 1 receptor (GHSR), in the hypothalamus and VTA. Ghrelin has been linked to increased synapse formation and dopamine turnover in the NAcc.[253] Administration of exogenous ghrelin in the VTA prompted feeding behavior, and GHSR antagonist administration reduced feeding subsequent to food deprivation.[253] Direct administration of ghrelin into the VTA, but not into the NAcc, was reported to motivate behavior for sucrose reward in an operant conditioning paradigm in rats, suggesting that ghrelin signaling within the VTA contributes to incentive-motivated behavior for a food reward.[254] Ghrelin administration-induced increases in motivation to eat are eliminated following pretreatment with a dopamine D1 receptor antagonist, suggesting that the orexigenic effects of ghrelin are mediated by dopamine signaling.[252] Conversely, ghrelin-deficient mice display attenuated responses to chronic and acute cocaine administration, indicating that dopaminergic neurotransmission is disrupted by deletion of the ghrelin gene.[255] Overall, these findings suggest that ghrelin may help to modulate the warding properties of food via interaction with dopaminergic neurons.

Serotonin

Increases in both exogenous and endogenous serotonin are associated with reductions in food intake and weight gain and an increase in energy expenditure.[256] Medial hypothalamic serotonin has been implicated in the temporal management of eating behavior, in particular with meal termination, as opposed to initiation. Preclinical research has demonstrated that d-fenfluramine (d-FEN), an exogenous agent that increases serotonin release while also blocking reuptake, may exert its anorexigenic effects via $5HT_{2C}$ receptor activation of proopiomelanocortin (POMC) neurons in lateral hypothalamic regions.[257] Serotonin has also been implicated in food preference. For example, preclinical studies have demonstrated that the injection of either exogenous serotonin or drugs that increase serotonin availability (such as fluoxetine) into the medial hypothalamus selectively inhibits carbohydrate intake but has no significant effect on fat or protein intake.[258] Conversely, elevated levels of tryptophan (TRP), a serotonin amino acid precursor and hypothalamic serotonin, are associated with high-carbohydrate intake (reviewed in Wurtman and Wurtman[259]).

Opioids

Research suggests that opioid receptors in the NAcc region of the ventral striatum may be particularly important for the encoding of food palatability. Stimulation of NAcc opioid receptors has been found to increase food intake.[260] Administration of opioid receptor antagonists, such as naloxone or naltrexone, extinguishes previously established preferences for sweetened versus unsweetened water in rats, whereas morphine has been demonstrated to enhance palatability and preference for sweet food.[260] Importantly, such preclinical data demonstrate opioid involvement in the palatability—or reward value—encoding of food that does not appear to directly affect caloric intake. Rather, the opioid system may be involved in general reward processing, as opposed to specific appetitive control. These data nonetheless suggest shared neurobiological mechanisms in eating and substance use behaviors.

Cannabinoids

Human and animal studies also implicate the endocannabinoid system (composed of cannabinoid receptors, endocannabinoids, and associated enzymes) in eating behaviors.[12] Preclinical research suggests that CB1 receptors influenced by leptin[261] are involved in the presynaptic modulation of release for the neurotransmitters GABA, glutamate, dopamine, noradrenaline, and serotonin[262] and has identified cannabinoid receptors (CB1/2) in the limbic forebrain, striatum, and NAcc (reviewed in Mahler et al.[263]). Colocalization of opioid and CB1 receptors in the striatum has also been reported (reviewed in Mahler et al.[263]). Preclinical investigations have additionally reported increases in feeding behaviors subsequent to administration of Δ9-THC and anandamide (an endogenous cannabinoid neurotransmitter) (reviewed in Mahler et al.[263]). Cannabinoids have been associated with rewarding psychotropic effects and increases in food intake. In addition to cannabinoid-induced increases in feeding behaviors, studies have implicated endogenous cannabinoids in the experience and encoding of food-associated reward. For example, direct anandamide administration to the NAcc shell has been found to significantly enhance "hedonistic" reward and increase feeding behaviors in rats.[263] Preclinical research has suggested that the neutral CB1R antagonist NESS0327 may be as effective as rimonabant in reducing weight gain and food intake and lack potentially harmful effects on anxiety and motivation.[264]

Neurocognition

Neurocognitive research implicates frontal lobe involvement in binge eating. Similar to impulse-control–related disorders (eg, SUDs, GD), disadvantageous decision-making have been reported in BED and obesity. In a sample of 41 healthy adult women, both a tendency to overeat in response to stress and higher BMI significantly predicted poorer IGT performance.[265] In other studies, obese (versus nonobese) individuals also performed significantly worse on the IGT and showed no improvement in performance over time.[266] Similar decision-making deficits on the IGT have been reported in both AN and BN.[267] Similar performance deficits among individuals with BN were also reported in a study using the Game of Dice Task,[268] a decision-making assessment that, unlike the IGT, provides explicit information of reward-loss contingencies.[269] A systematic review suggested that choice impulsivity may relate to BED relative to other forms of impulsivity and compulsivity.[270]

Neurocircuitry and Structure

Research from neuroimaging, neurocognitive, and lesion studies implicates circuits involved in impulsivity and cognitive control in the modulation of eating behaviors. The striatum and insula have been implicated in BED as individuals with this condition have been shown to demonstrate activation in the left ventral striatum and right insula during exposure to high-caloric food images in comparison to obese individuals or individuals with BN.[13] Therefore, it has been hypothesized that those regions are implicated in reward sensitivity and impulsivity in BED. Besides, the prefrontal cortex has also been implicated in BED. Individuals with frontotemporal dementia (FTD), a degenerative disorder involving atrophy of frontal, insular, and temporal cortical regions, demonstrate behavioral changes in eating and behaviors[271] such as increases in weight, food cravings/obsessions, and gluttony.[272] Evidence derived from positron emission tomography (PET) research additionally suggests a relationship between frontal lobe activity and eating behaviors. In weight-loss studies, "successful" as compared to "nonsuccessful" weight-loss dieters/maintainers had significantly greater activation in the dlPFC, dorsal striatum, and anterior cerebellar lobe brain regions following meal consumption[273] and food visualization.[274] Conversely, unsuccessful dieters had significantly greater OFC activation following meal consumption.[273] These data suggest differential modulation of eating behaviors by prefrontal regions. Further investigation is required to fully understand interactions between PFC regions in relation to eating behaviors.

Consistent with the finding that greater dietary restraint is negatively correlated with OFC activation and positively correlated with dlPFC activation, one RCT using repetitive transcranial magnetic stimulation found reduced self-reported craving sensations in response to exposure to craving-inducing foods subsequent to left dlPFC stimulation.[275] dlPFC stimulation has also been reported to be effective in reducing cravings for nicotine, alcohol, and cocaine, suggesting potentially similar neurobiological mechanisms for food and drug craving (reviewed in Barr et al.[276]).

Epidemiology

Obesity, often associated with binge eating, has become increasingly common. Defined as "abnormal" or excessive fat accumulation that may impair health, it is estimated that up to 41.9% of the U.S. population meets the criteria for obesity.[277] Globally, estimates from 2017 suggest that 4.7 million deaths were caused by high BMI due to associated medical conditions such as cardiovascular diseases, diabetes, and kidney diseases.[278]

Frequently co-occurring psychiatric disorders include depression, anxiety, personality disorders, and lifetime SUDs.[279]

Features of GD among individuals with BED are associated with decreased self-esteem and substance use problems.[280]

Treatment

Along with the recent rise in the prevalence of obesity, there has been a concurrent rise in the number and diversity of proposed interventions. Such interventions range from preventive interventions, such as the incorporation of nutrition classes into school curricula, to pharmaceutical interventions, such as the administration of appetite-suppressing drugs and the use of surgical interventions, like gastric bypass surgery. Because some treatments for obesity are highly invasive (eg, gastric bypass, jaw wiring), it is important to examine and assess not only efficacy, but also tolerability and impact on quality of life. Indeed, psychostimulants such as d-amphetamine have a long well-documented history of use in the treatment of obesity; however, they are also associated with significant adverse events which hinder their use.[281] A positive trial of semaglutide was published and raised optimism about a potential efficacious pharmacological treatment for obesity.[282] Other FDA-approved treatments for overweight/obesity include orlistat and naltrexone-bupropion. Nonetheless, it is important to understand the pathophysiology underlying obesity, particularly if individual differences contribute to the selection of effective interventions.

Considering BED specifically, lisdexamfetamine is approved by the U.S. Food and Drug Administration (FDA) for the treatment of BED as it has been shown to reduce binge eating behaviors and weight in placebo-controlled trials.[283] Placebo-controlled trials have also demonstrated efficacy of topiramate for the treatment of BED,[284] including when used as an adjunctive treatment to cognitive-behavioral therapy.[285] However, topiramate has been associated with decreased tolerability and increased discontinuation rates in the long-term.[286] A trial published in 2022 evaluated the comparative effects of naltrexone-bupropion combination for the treatment of BED and reported promising findings,[287] but those have yet to be confirmed by large scale studies.

Conclusion

Binge eating and obesity are common phenomena with wide-ranging public health implications. Recent neurobiological findings, such as the involvement of the adipose-derived hormone leptin in the dopaminergic reward system, suggest that BED is a brain-based disorder that may share many of the same neurobiological features as SUDs. Such findings have important treatment implications, and further investigation is required to optimize treatment interventions.

OVERALL CONCLUSION

In conclusion, this chapter provides an overview of several psychiatric conditions which have been grouped under the umbrella-term "behavioral addictions." We focused on aspects concerning the neurobiology, epidemiology, and treatment of these conditions. Although most of these behavioral addictions are not formally recognized as addictive behaviors, throughout the chapter we outlined several pieces of evidence which indicate these behavioral conditions share several similarities with SUDs. Irrespective of nosological debates, behavioral addictions are associated with considerable heath burden and social impact. Although the scientific community has been increasingly interested in the topic of behavioral addictions, there remains considerable gaps to fill out, which underscores the importance of continued research on the field.

REFERENCES

1. Potenza MN. Should addictive disorders include non-substance-related conditions? *Addiction*. 2006;101(Suppl 1):142-151. doi:10.1111/j.1360-0443.2006.01591.x
2. Maddux JF, Desmond DP. Addiction or dependence? *Addiction*. 2000;95(5):661-665. doi:10.1046/j.1360-0443.2000.9556611.x
3. O'Brien CP, Volkow N, Li TK. What's in a word? Addiction versus dependence in DSM-V. *Am J Psychiatry*. 2006;163(5):764-765. doi:10.1176/ajp.2006.163.5.764
4. Grant JE, Potenza MN, Weinstein A, Gorelick DA. Introduction to behavioral addictions. *Am J Drug Alcohol Abuse*. 2010;36(5):233-241. doi:10.3109/00952990.2010.491884
5. Grant JE, Potenza MN. Overview of the impulse control disorders not elsewhere classified and limitations of knowledge. In: Grant JE, Potenza MN, eds. *The Oxford Handbook of Impulse Control Disorders*. Oxford University Press; 2012:3-10.
6. Holden C. 'Behavioral' addictions: do they exist? *Science*. 2001; 294(5544):980-982. doi:10.1126/science.294.5544.980
7. American Psychiatric Association. *Proposed Revisions—Substance Use and Addictive Disorders*. Accessed June 2, 2023. https://www.psychiatry.org/psychiatrists/practice/dsm
8. Psychiatry HC. Behavioral addictions debut in proposed DSM-V. *Science*. 2010;327(5968):935. doi:10.1126/science.327.5968.935
9. American Psychiatric Association. *Diagnostic and Statistical Manual of Mental Disorders: DSM-5*. American Psychiatric Publishing; 2013.
10. Hollander E, Kim S, Zohar J. OCSDs in the forthcoming DSM-V. *CNS Spectr*. 2007;12(5):320-323. doi:10.1017/s109285290002109x
11. Bean MK, Stewart K, Olbrisch ME. Obesity in America: implications for clinical and health psychologists. *J Clin Psychol Med Settings*. 2008;15(3):214-224. doi:10.1007/s10880-008-9124-9
12. Drewnowski A, Darmon N. The economics of obesity: dietary energy density and energy cost. *Am J Clin Nutr*. 2005;82(1 Suppl):265s-273s. doi:10.1093/ajcn/82.1.265S
13. Kessler RM, Hutson PH, Herman BK, Potenza MN. The neurobiological basis of binge-eating disorder. *Neurosci Biobehav Rev*. 2016;63:223-238. doi:10.1016/j.neubiorev.2016.01.013
14. Brand M, Rumpf HJ, Demetrovics Z, et al. Which conditions should be considered as disorders in the International Classification of Diseases (ICD-11) designation of "other specified disorders due to addictive behaviors"? *J Behav Addict*. 2020;11(2):150-159. doi:10.1556/2006.2020.00035
15. Grant JE, Atmaca M, Fineberg NA, et al. Impulse control disorders and "behavioural addictions" in the ICD-11. *World Psychiatry*. 2014;13(2):125-127. doi:10.1002/wps.20115
16. Chamberlain SR, Stochl J, Redden SA, Grant JE. Latent traits of impulsivity and compulsivity: toward dimensional psychiatry. *Psychol Med*. 2018;48(5):810-821. doi:10.1017/s0033291717002185
17. Potenza MN, Balodis IM, Derevensky J, et al. Gambling disorder. *Nat Rev Dis Primers*. 2019;5(1):51. doi:10.1038/s41572-019-0099-7

18. Calado F, Griffiths MD. Problem gambling worldwide: an update and systematic review of empirical research (2000-2015). *J Behav Addict.* 2016;5(4):592-613. doi:10.1556/2006.5.2016.073
19. Welte JW, Barnes GM, Tidwell MC, Hoffman JH, Wieczorek WF. Gambling and problem gambling in the United States: changes between 1999 and 2013. *J Gambl Stud.* 2015;31(3):695-715. doi:10.1007/s10899-014-9471-4
20. Gupta R, Derevensky J. Familial and social influences on juvenile gambling behavior. *J Gambl Stud.* 1997;13(3):179-192. doi:10.1023/a:1024915231379
21. Potenza MN, Wareham JD, Steinberg MA, et al. Correlates of at-risk/problem internet gambling in adolescents. *J Am Acad Child Adolesc Psychiatry.* 2011;50(2):150-159.e3. doi:10.1016/j.jaac.2010.11.006
22. Eisen SA, Lin N, Lyons MJ, et al. Familial influences on gambling behavior: an analysis of 3359 twin pairs. *Addiction.* 1998;93(9):1375-1384. doi:10.1046/j.1360-0443.1998.93913758.x
23. Tsuang MT, Lyons MJ, Eisen SA, et al. Genetic influences on DSM-III-R drug abuse and dependence: a study of 3,372 twin pairs. *Am J Med Genet.* 1996;67(5):473-477. doi:10.1002/(sici)1096-8628(19960920)67:5<473::Aid-ajmg6>3.0.Co;2-l
24. Slutske WS, Eisen S, Xian H, et al. A twin study of the association between pathological gambling and antisocial personality disorder. *J Abnorm Psychol.* 2001;110(2):297-308. doi:10.1037//0021-843x.110.2.297
25. Slutske WS, Eisen S, True WR, Lyons MJ, Goldberg J, Tsuang M. Common genetic vulnerability for pathological gambling and alcohol dependence in men. *Arch Gen Psychiatry.* 2000;57(7):666-673. doi:10.1001/archpsyc.57.7.666
26. Slutske WS, Ellingson JM, Richmond-Rakerd LS, Zhu G, Martin NG. Shared genetic vulnerability for disordered gambling and alcohol use disorder in men and women: evidence from a national community-based Australian Twin Study. *Twin Res Hum Genet.* 2013;16(2):525-534. doi:10.1017/thg.2013.11
27. Xian H, Giddens JL, Scherrer JF, Eisen SA, Potenza MN. Environmental factors selectively impact co-occurrence of problem/pathological gambling with specific drug-use disorders in male twins. *Addiction.* 2014;109(4):635-644. doi:10.1111/add.12407
28. Blanco C, Myers J, Kendler KS. Gambling, disordered gambling and their association with major depression and substance use: a web-based cohort and twin-sibling study. *Psychol Med.* 2012;42(3):497-508. doi:10.1017/s0033291711001401
29. Giddens JL, Xian H, Scherrer JF, Eisen SA, Potenza MN. Shared genetic contributions to anxiety disorders and pathological gambling in a male population. *J Affect Disord.* 2011;132(3):406-412. doi:10.1016/j.jad.2011.03.008
30. Lang M, Leménager T, Streit F, et al. Genome-wide association study of pathological gambling. *Eur Psychiatry.* 2016;36:38-46. doi:10.1016/j.eurpsy.2016.04.001
31. Lind PA, Zhu G, Montgomery GW, et al. Genome-wide association study of a quantitative disordered gambling trait. *Addict Biol.* 2013;18(3):511-522. doi:10.1111/j.1369-1600.2012.00463.x
32. Border R, Johnson EC, Evans LM, et al. No support for historical candidate gene or candidate gene-by-interaction hypotheses for major depression across multiple large samples. *Am J Psychiatry.* 2019;176(5):376-387. doi:10.1176/appi.ajp.2018.18070881
33. da Silva Lobo DS, Vallada HP, Knight J, et al. Dopamine genes and pathological gambling in discordant sib-pairs. *J Gambl Stud* 2007;23(4):421-433. doi:10.1007/s10899-007-9060-x
34. Lobo DS, Souza RP, Tong RP, et al. Association of functional variants in the dopamine D2-like receptors with risk for gambling behaviour in healthy Caucasian subjects. *Biol Psychol.* 2010;85(1):33-37. doi:10.1016/j.biopsycho.2010.04.008
35. Pérez de Castro I, Ibáñez A, Saiz-Ruiz J, Fernández-Piqueras J. Genetic contribution to pathological gambling: possible association between a functional DNA polymorphism at the serotonin transporter gene (5-HTT) and affected men. *Pharmacogenetics.* 1999;9(3):397-400.
36. Pérez de Castro I, Ibáñez A, Saiz-Ruiz J, Fernández-Piqueras J. Concurrent positive association between pathological gambling and functional DNA polymorphisms at the MAO-A and the 5-HT transporter genes. *Mol Psychiatry.* 2002;7(9):927-928. doi:10.1038/sj.mp.4001148
37. Kreek MJ, Nielsen DA, Butelman ER, LaForge KS. Genetic influences on impulsivity, risk taking, stress responsivity and vulnerability to drug abuse and addiction. *Nat Neurosci.* 2005;8(11):1450-1457. doi:10.1038/nn1583
38. Potenza MN. Clinical neuropsychiatric considerations regarding nonsubstance or behavioral addictions. *Dialogues Clin Neurosci.* 2017;19(3):281-291. doi:10.31887/DCNS.2017.19.3/mpotenza
39. Ioannidis K, Hook R, Wickham K, Grant JE, Chamberlain SR. Impulsivity in gambling disorder and problem gambling: a meta-analysis. *Neuropsychopharmacology.* 2019;44(8):1354-1361. doi:10.1038/s41386-019-0393-9
40. Chambers RA, Taylor JR, Potenza MN. Developmental neurocircuitry of motivation in adolescence: a critical period of addiction vulnerability. *Am J Psychiatry.* 2003;160(6):1041-1052. doi:10.1176/appi.ajp.160.6.1041
41. Fineberg NA, Chamberlain SR, Goudriaan AE, et al. New developments in human neurocognition: clinical, genetic, and brain imaging correlates of impulsivity and compulsivity. *CNS Spectr.* 2014;19(1):69-89. doi:10.1017/s1092852913000801
42. Moeller FG, Barratt ES, Dougherty DM, Schmitz JM, Swann AC. Psychiatric aspects of impulsivity. *Am J Psychiatry.* 2001;158(11):1783-1793. doi:10.1176/appi.ajp.158.11.1783
43. Andrade LF, Petry NM. Delay and probability discounting in pathological gamblers with and without a history of substance use problems. *Psychopharmacology (Berl).* 2012;219(2):491-499. doi:10.1007/s00213-011-2508-9
44. Miedl SF, Peters J, Büchel C. Altered neural reward representations in pathological gamblers revealed by delay and probability discounting. *Arch Gen Psychiatry.* 2012;69(2):177-186. doi:10.1001/archgenpsychiatry.2011.1552
45. Clark AM. Reward processing: a global brain phenomenon? *J Neurophysiol.* 2013;109(1):1-4. doi:10.1152/jn.00070.2012
46. Knutson B, Fong GW, Bennett SM, Adams CM, Hommer D. A region of mesial prefrontal cortex tracks monetarily rewarding outcomes: characterization with rapid event-related fMRI. *Neuroimage.* 2003;18(2):263-272. doi:10.1016/s1053-8119(02)00057-5
47. Goudriaan AE, Oosterlaan J, de Beurs E, van den Brink W. Decision making in pathological gambling: a comparison between pathological gamblers, alcohol dependents, persons with Tourette syndrome, and normal controls. *Brain Res Cogn Brain Res.* 2005;23(1):137-151. doi:10.1016/j.cogbrainres.2005.01.017
48. Odlaug BL, Chamberlain SR, Kim SW, Schreiber LR, Grant JE. A neurocognitive comparison of cognitive flexibility and response inhibition in gamblers with varying degrees of clinical severity. *Psychol Med.* 2011;41(10):2111-2119. doi:10.1017/s0033291711000316
49. Goudriaan AE, Oosterlaan J, De Beurs E, Van Den Brink W. The role of self-reported impulsivity and reward sensitivity versus neurocognitive measures of disinhibition and decision-making in the prediction of relapse in pathological gamblers. *Psychol Med.* 2008;38(1):41-50. doi:10.1017/s0033291707000694
50. Lawrence AJ, Luty J, Bogdan NA, Sahakian BJ, Clark L. Problem gamblers share deficits in impulsive decision-making with alcohol-dependent individuals. *Addiction.* 2009;104(6):1006-1015. doi:10.1111/j.1360-0443.2009.02533.x
51. Reynolds B. A review of delay-discounting research with humans: relations to drug use and gambling. *Behav Pharmacol.* 2006;17(8):651-667. doi:10.1097/FBP.0b013e3280115f99
52. Petry NM. Pathological gamblers, with and without substance use disorders, discount delayed rewards at high rates. *J Abnorm Psychol.* 2001;110(3):482-487. doi:10.1037//0021-843x.110.3.482
53. Yücel M, Oldenhof E, Ahmed SH, et al. A transdiagnostic dimensional approach towards a neuropsychological assessment for addiction: an international Delphi consensus study. *Addiction.* 2019;114(6):1095-1109. doi:10.1111/add.14424
54. Balodis IM, Potenza MN. Anticipatory reward processing in addicted populations: a focus on the monetary incentive delay task. *Biol Psychiatry.* 2015;77(5):434-444. doi:10.1016/j.biopsych.2014.08.020

55. Brewer JA, Potenza MN. The neurobiology and genetics of impulse control disorders: relationships to drug addictions. *Biochem Pharmacol.* 2008;75(1):63-75. doi:10.1016/j.bcp.2007.06.043
56. Nordin C, Eklundh T. Altered CSF 5-HIAA Disposition in pathologic male gamblers. *CNS Spectr.* 1999;4(12):25-33. doi:10.1017/s1092852900006799
57. Cardinal RN. Neural systems implicated in delayed and probabilistic reinforcement. *Neural Netw.* 2006;19(8):1277-1301. doi:10.1016/j.neunet.2006.03.004
58. Ettenberg A, Ofer OA, Mueller CL, Waldroup S, Cohen A, Ben-Shahar O. Inactivation of the dorsal raphé nucleus reduces the anxiogenic response of rats running an alley for intravenous cocaine. *Pharmacol Biochem Behav.* 2011;97(4):632-639. doi:10.1016/j.pbb.2010.11.008
59. Ibañez A, Perez de Castro I, Fernandez-Piqueras J, Blanco C, Saiz-Ruiz J. Pathological gambling and DNA polymorphic markers at MAO-A and MAO-B genes. *Mol Psychiatry.* 2000;5(1):105-109. doi:10.1038/sj.mp.4000654
60. DeCaria CM, Begaz T, Hollander E. Serotonergic and noradrenergic function in pathological gambling. *CNS Spectr.* 1998;3(6):38-47. doi:10.1017/S1092852900006003
61. Pallanti S, Bernardi S, Quercioli L, DeCaria C, Hollander E. Serotonin dysfunction in pathological gamblers: increased prolactin response to oral m-CPP versus placebo. *CNS Spectr.* 2006;11(12):956-964. doi:10.1017/s1092852900015145
62. Pallanti S, Bernardi S, Allen A, Hollander E. Serotonin function in pathological gambling: blunted growth hormone response to sumatriptan. *J Psychopharmacol.* 2010;24(12):1802-1809. doi:10.1177/0269881109106907
63. Moss HB, Hardie TL, Dahl JP, Berrettini W, Xu K. Diplotypes of the human serotonin 1B receptor promoter predict growth hormone responses to sumatriptan in abstinent alcohol-dependent men. *Biol Psychiatry.* 2007;61(8):974-978. doi:10.1016/j.biopsych.2006.08.029
64. Patkar AA, Mannelli P, Hill KP, Peindl K, Pae CU, Lee TH. Relationship of prolactin response to meta-chlorophenylpiperazine with severity of drug use in cocaine dependence. *Hum Psychopharmacol.* 2006;21(6):367-375. doi:10.1002/hup.780
65. Potenza MN, Walderhaug E, Henry S, et al. Serotonin 1B receptor imaging in pathological gambling. *World J Biol Psychiatry.* 2013;14(2):139-145. doi:10.3109/15622975.2011.598559
66. Linnet J, Peterson E, Doudet DJ, Gjedde A, Møller A. Dopamine release in ventral striatum of pathological gamblers losing money. *Acta Psychiatr Scand.* 2010;122(4):326-333. doi:10.1111/j.1600-0447.2010.01591.x
67. Joutsa J, Johansson J, Niemelä S, et al. Mesolimbic dopamine release is linked to symptom severity in pathological gambling. *Neuroimage.* 2012;60(4):1992-1999. doi:10.1016/j.neuroimage.2012.02.006
68. Boileau I, Payer D, Chugani B, et al. The D2/3 dopamine receptor in pathological gambling: a positron emission tomography study with [11C]-(+)-propyl-hexahydro-naphtho-oxazin and [11C]raclopride. *Addiction.* 2013;108(5):953-963. doi:10.1111/add.12066
69. Clark L, Stokes PR, Wu K, et al. Striatal dopamine D_2/D_3 receptor binding in pathological gambling is correlated with mood-related impulsivity. *Neuroimage.* 2012;63(1):40-46. doi:10.1016/j.neuroimage.2012.06.067
70. Potenza MN. How central is dopamine to pathological gambling or gambling disorder? *Front Behav Neurosci.* 2013;7:206. doi:10.3389/fnbeh.2013.00206
71. Zack M, Poulos CX. A D2 antagonist enhances the rewarding and priming effects of a gambling episode in pathological gamblers. *Neuropsychopharmacology.* 2007;32(8):1678-1686. doi:10.1038/sj.npp.1301295
72. Voon V, Gao J, Brezing C, et al. Dopamine agonists and risk: impulse control disorders in Parkinson's disease. *Brain.* 2011;134(Pt 5):1438-1446. doi:10.1093/brain/awr080
73. Tremblay AM, Desmond RC, Poulos CX, Zack M. Haloperidol modifies instrumental aspects of slot machine gambling in pathological gamblers and healthy controls. *Addict Biol.* 2011;16(3):467-484. doi:10.1111/j.1369-1600.2010.00208.x
74. Bergh C, Eklund T, Södersten P, Nordin C. Altered dopamine function in pathological gambling. *Psychol Med.* 1997;27(2):473-475. doi:10.1017/s0033291796003789
75. Nordin C, Sjödin I. CSF monoamine patterns in pathological gamblers and healthy controls. *J Psychiatr Res.* 2006;40(5):454-459. doi:10.1016/j.jpsychires.2005.06.003
76. Roy A, Pickar D, De Jong J, Karoum F, Linnoila M. Norepinephrine and its metabolites in cerebrospinal fluid, plasma, and urine. Relationship to hypothalamic-pituitary-adrenal axis function in depression. *Arch Gen Psychiatry.* 1988;45(9):849-857. doi:10.1001/archpsyc.1988.01800330081010
77. Meyer G, Schwertfeger J, Exton MS, et al. Neuroendocrine response to casino gambling in problem gamblers. *Psychoneuroendocrinology.* 2004;29(10):1272-1280. doi:10.1016/j.psyneuen.2004.03.005
78. Pallanti S, Bernardi S, Allen A, et al. Noradrenergic function in pathological gambling: blunted growth hormone response to clonidine. *J Psychopharmacol.* 2010;24(6):847-853. doi:10.1177/0269881108099419
79. Mick I, Myers J, Ramos AC, et al. Blunted endogenous opioid release following an oral amphetamine challenge in pathological gamblers. *Neuropsychopharmacology.* 2016;41(7):1742-1750. doi:10.1038/npp.2015.340
80. Gorelick DA, Kim YK, Bencherif B, et al. Imaging brain mu-opioid receptors in abstinent cocaine users: time course and relation to cocaine craving. *Biol Psychiatry.* 2005;57(12):1573-1582. doi:10.1016/j.biopsych.2005.02.026
81. Bartley CA, Bloch MH. Meta-analysis: pharmacological treatment of pathological gambling. *Expert Rev Neurother.* 2013;13(8):887-894. doi:10.1586/14737175.2013.814938
82. Reuter J, Raedler T, Rose M, Hand I, Gläscher J, Büchel C. Pathological gambling is linked to reduced activation of the mesolimbic reward system. *Nat Neurosci.* 2005;8(2):147-148. doi:10.1038/nn1378
83. Potenza MN. Searching for replicable dopamine-related findings in gambling disorder. *Biol Psychiatry.* 2018;83(12):984-986. doi:10.1016/j.biopsych.2018.04.011
84. Kober H, Lacadie CM, Wexler BE, Malison RT, Sinha R, Potenza MN. Brain activity during cocaine craving and gambling urges: an fMRI study. *Neuropsychopharmacology.* 2016;41(2):628-637. doi:10.1038/npp.2015.193
85. Potenza MN, Steinberg MA, Skudlarski P, et al. Gambling urges in pathological gambling: a functional magnetic resonance imaging study. *Arch Gen Psychiatry.* 2003;60(8):828-836. doi:10.1001/archpsyc.60.8.828
86. Potenza MN, Leung HC, Blumberg HP, et al. An FMRI Stroop task study of ventromedial prefrontal cortical function in pathological gamblers. *Am J Psychiatry.* 2003;160(11):1990-1994. doi:10.1176/appi.ajp.160.11.1990
87. Balodis IM, Kober H, Worhunsky PD, Stevens MC, Pearlson GD, Potenza MN. Diminished frontostriatal activity during processing of monetary rewards and losses in pathological gambling. *Biol Psychiatry.* 2012;71(8):749-757. doi:10.1016/j.biopsych.2012.01.006
88. Tanabe J, Thompson L, Claus E, Dalwani M, Hutchison K, Banich MT. Prefrontal cortex activity is reduced in gambling and nongambling substance users during decision-making. *Hum Brain Mapp.* 2007;28(12):1276-1286. doi:10.1002/hbm.20344
89. Potenza MN. Review. The neurobiology of pathological gambling and drug addiction: an overview and new findings. *Philos Trans R Soc Lond B Biol Sci.* 2008;363(1507):3181-3189. doi:10.1098/rstb.2008.0100
90. de Greck M, Enzi B, Prösch U, Gantman A, Tempelmann C, Northoff G. Decreased neuronal activity in reward circuitry of pathological gamblers during processing of personal relevant stimuli. *Hum Brain Mapp.* 2010;31(11):1802-1812. doi:10.1002/hbm.20981
91. Yip SW, Lacadie C, Xu J, et al. Reduced genual corpus callosal white matter integrity in pathological gambling and its relationship to alcohol abuse or dependence. *World J Biol Psychiatry.* 2013;14(2):129-138. doi:10.3109/15622975.2011.568068
92. Moeller FG, Hasan KM, Steinberg JL, et al. Diffusion tensor imaging eigenvalues: preliminary evidence for altered myelin in cocaine

dependence. *Psychiatry Res.* 2007;154(3):253-258. doi:10.1016/j.pscychresns.2006.11.004

93. Yip SW, Morie KP, Xu J, et al. Shared microstructural features of behavioral and substance addictions revealed in areas of crossing fibers. *Biol Psychiatry Cogn Neurosci Neuroimaging.* 2017;2(2):188-195. doi:10.1016/j.bpsc.2016.03.001
94. Yip SW, Worhunsky PD, Xu J, et al. Gray-matter relationships to diagnostic and transdiagnostic features of drug and behavioral addictions. *Addict Biol.* 2018;23(1):394-402. doi:10.1111/adb.12492
95. Rahman AS, Xu J, Potenza MN. Hippocampal and amygdalar volumetric differences in pathological gambling: a preliminary study of the associations with the behavioral inhibition system. *Neuropsychopharmacology.* 2014;39(3):738-745. doi:10.1038/npp.2013.260
96. Kessler RC, Hwang I, LaBrie R, et al. DSM-IV pathological gambling in the National Comorbidity Survey Replication. *Psychol Med.* 2008;38(9):1351-1360. doi:10.1017/s0033291708002900
97. Grant BF, Odlaug BL, Potenza MN. Pathological gambling: clinical characteristics and treatment. In: Ries RK, Miller SC, Fiellin DA, eds. *Principles of Addiction Medicine.* Lippincott Williams & Wilkins; 2009.
98. Derevensky JL. Youth gambling: an important social policy and public health issue. In: O'Dea J, ed. *Current Issues and Controversies in School and Community Health, Sport and Physical Education.* Nova Science Publishers; 2012:115-130.
99. Campbell C, Derevensky J, Meerkamper E, Cutajar J. Parents' perceptions of adolescent gambling: a Canadian national study. *J Gambl Issues.* 2011;25:36-53.
100. Derevensky JL, St-Pierre RA, Temcheff CE, Gupta R. Teacher awareness and attitudes regarding adolescent risky behaviours: is adolescent gambling perceived to be a problem? *J Gambl Stud.* 2014;30(2):435-451. doi:10.1007/s10899-013-9363-z
101. Lynch WJ, Maciejewski PK, Potenza MN. Psychiatric correlates of gambling in adolescents and young adults grouped by age at gambling onset. *Arch Gen Psychiatry.* 2004;61(11):1116-1122. doi:10.1001/archpsyc.61.11.1116
102. Dowling NA, Merkouris SS, Greenwood CJ, Oldenhof E, Toumbourou JW, Youssef GJ. Early risk and protective factors for problem gambling: a systematic review and meta-analysis of longitudinal studies. *Clin Psychol Rev.* 2017;51:109-124. doi:10.1016/j.cpr.2016.10.008
103. Zakiniaeiz Y, Cosgrove KP, Mazure CM, Potenza MN. Does telescoping exist in male and female gamblers? Does it matter? *Front Psychol.* 2017;8:1510. doi:10.3389/fpsyg.2017.01510
104. Alegria AA, Petry NM, Hasin DS, Liu SM, Grant BF, Blanco C. Disordered gambling among racial and ethnic groups in the US: results from the national epidemiologic survey on alcohol and related conditions. *CNS Spectr.* 2009;14(3):132-142. doi:10.1017/s1092852900020113
105. Volberg RA, Abbott MW, Rönnberg S, Munck IM. Prevalence and risks of pathological gambling in Sweden. *Acta Psychiatr Scand.* 2001;104(4):250-256. doi:10.1034/j.1600-0447.2001.00336.x
106. Richard J, Martin-Storey A, Wilkie E, Derevensky JL, Paskus T, Temcheff CE. Variations in gambling disorder symptomatology across sexual identity among college student-athletes. *J Gambl Stud.* 2019;35(4):1303-1316. doi:10.1007/s10899-019-09838-z
107. Broman N, Prever F, di Giacomo E, et al. Gambling, gaming, and internet behavior in a sexual minority perspective. A cross-sectional study in seven European countries. *Front Psychol.* 2021;12:707645. doi:10.3389/fpsyg.2021.707645
108. Grant JE, Potenza MN. Sexual orientation of men with pathological gambling: prevalence and psychiatric comorbidity in a treatment-seeking sample. *Compr Psychiatry.* 2006;47(6):515-518. doi:10.1016/j.comppsych.2006.02.005
109. Comings DE, Rosenthal RJ, Lesieur HR, et al. A study of the dopamine D2 receptor gene in pathological gambling. *Pharmacogenetics.* 1996;6(3):223-234. doi:10.1097/00008571-199606000-00004
110. Dowling NA, Cowlishaw S, Jackson AC, Merkouris SS, Francis KL, Christensen DR. Prevalence of psychiatric co-morbidity in treatment-seeking problem gamblers: a systematic review and meta-analysis. *Aust N Z J Psychiatry.* 2015;49(6):519-539. doi:10.1177/0004867415575774
111. LaPlante DA, Nelson SE, LaBrie RA, Shaffer HJ. Stability and progression of disordered gambling: lessons from longitudinal studies. *Can J Psychiatry.* 2008;53(1):52-60. doi:10.1177/070674370805300108
112. Petry NM, Ginley MK, Rash CJ. A systematic review of treatments for problem gambling. *Psychol Addict Behav.* 2017;31(8):951-961. doi:10.1037/adb0000290
113. Bullock SA, Potenza MN. Pathological gambling: neuropsychopharmacology and treatment. *Curr Psychopharmacol.* 2012;1(1): doi:10.2174/2211556011201010067
114. Goslar M, Leibetseder M, Muench HM, Hofmann SG, Laireiter AR. Pharmacological treatments for disordered gambling: a meta-analysis. *J Gambl Stud.* 2019;35(2):415-445. doi:10.1007/s10899-018-09815-y
115. Grant JE, Chamberlain SR. The placebo effect and its clinical associations in gambling disorder. *Ann Clin Psychiatry.* 2017;29(3):167-172.
116. Griffiths MD. Conceptual issues concerning internet addiction and internet gaming disorder: further critique on Ryding and Kaye (2017). *Int J Ment Health Addict.* 2018;16(1):233-239. doi:10.1007/s11469-017-9818-z
117. Wölfling K, Müller KW, Dreier M, et al. Efficacy of short-term treatment of internet and computer game addiction: a randomized clinical trial. *JAMA Psychiatry.* 2019;76(10):1018-1025. doi:10.1001/jamapsychiatry.2019.1676
118. Yau YH, Crowley MJ, Mayes LC, Potenza MN. Are internet use and video-game-playing addictive behaviors? Biological, clinical and public health implications for youths and adults. *Minerva Psichiatr.* 2012;53(3):153-170.
119. Gentile DA, Choo H, Liau A, et al. Pathological video game use among youths: a two-year longitudinal study. *Pediatrics.* 2011;127(2):e319-e329. doi:10.1542/peds.2010-1353
120. Desai RA, Krishnan-Sarin S, Cavallo D, Potenza MN. Video-gaming among high school students: health correlates, gender differences, and problematic gaming. *Pediatrics.* 2010;126(6):e1414-e1424. doi:10.1542/peds.2009-2706
121. King DL, Delfabbro PH, Potenza MN, Demetrovics Z, Billieux J, Brand M. Internet gaming disorder should qualify as a mental disorder. *Aust N Z J Psychiatry.* 2018;52(7):615-617. doi:10.1177/0004867418771189
122. Kim E, Lee D, Do K, Kim J. Interaction effects of DRD2 genetic polymorphism and interpersonal stress on problematic gaming in college students. *Genes (Basel).* 2022;13(3):449. doi:10.3390/genes13030449
123. Yen JY, Lin PC, Lin HC, Lin PY, Chou WP, Ko CH. Association of internet gaming disorder with catechol-O-methyltransferase: role of impulsivity and fun-seeking. *Kaohsiung J Med Sci.* 2022;38(1):70-76. doi:10.1002/kjm2.12454
124. Wang T, Franke P, Neidt H, et al. Association study of the low-activity allele of catechol-O-methyltransferase and alcoholism using a family-based approach. *Mol Psychiatry.* 2001;6(1):109-111. doi:10.1038/sj.mp.4000803
125. Weinstein AM. An update overview on brain imaging studies of internet gaming disorder. *Front Psych.* 2017;8:185. doi:10.3389/fpsyt.2017.00185
126. Koepp MJ, Gunn RN, Lawrence AD, et al. Evidence for striatal dopamine release during a video game. *Nature.* 1998;393(6682):266-268. doi:10.1038/30498
127. Weinstein AM. Computer and video game addiction—a comparison between game users and non-game users. *Am J Drug Alcohol Abuse.* 2010;36(5):268-276. doi:10.3109/00952990.2010.491879
128. Farde L, Nordström AL, Wiesel FA, Pauli S, Halldin C, Sedvall G. Positron emission tomographic analysis of central D1 and D2 dopamine receptor occupancy in patients treated with classical neuroleptics and clozapine. Relation to extrapyramidal side effects. *Arch Gen Psychiatry.* 1992;49(7):538-544. doi:10.1001/archpsyc.1992.01820070032005
129. Volkow ND, Wang GJ, Fowler JS, et al. Imaging endogenous dopamine competition with [11C]raclopride in the human brain. *Synapse.* 1994;16(4):255-262. doi:10.1002/syn.890160402
130. Littel M, van den Berg I, Luijten M, van Rooij AJ, Keemink L, Franken IH. Error processing and response inhibition in excessive computer game players: an event-related potential study. *Addict Biol.* 2012;17(5):934-947. doi:10.1111/j.1369-1600.2012.00467.x

131. Irvine MA, Worbe Y, Bolton S, Harrison NA, Bullmore ET, Voon V. Impaired decisional impulsivity in pathological videogamers. *PloS One*. 2013;8(10):e75914. doi:10.1371/journal.pone.0075914
132. Argyriou E, Davison CB, Lee TTC. Response inhibition and internet gaming disorder: a meta-analysis. *Addict Behav*. 2017;71:54-60. doi:10.1016/j.addbeh.2017.02.026
133. Bailey K, West R, Kuffel J. What would my avatar do? Gaming, pathology, and risky decision making. *Front Psychol*. 2013;4:609. doi:10.3389/fpsyg.2013.00609
134. Dong G, Potenza MN. A cognitive-behavioral model of internet gaming disorder: theoretical underpinnings and clinical implications. *J Psychiatr Res*. 2014;58:7-11. doi:10.1016/j.jpsychires.2014.07.005
135. Han DH, Bolo N, Daniels MA, Arenella L, Lyoo IK, Renshaw PF. Brain activity and desire for internet video game play. *Compr Psychiatry*. 2011;52(1):88-95. doi:10.1016/j.comppsych.2010.04.004
136. Ko C-H, Liu G-C, Hsiao S, et al. Brain activities associated with gaming urge of online gaming addiction. *J Psychiatr Res*. 2009;43(7):739-747. doi:10.1016/j.jpsychires.2008.09.012
137. Han DH, Kim YS, Lee YS, Min KJ, Renshaw PF. Changes in cue-induced, prefrontal cortex activity with video-game play. *Cyberpsychol Behav Soc Netw*. 2010;13(6):655-661. doi:10.1089/cyber.2009.0327
138. Ko CH, Liu GC, Yen JY, Chen CY, Yen CF, Chen CS. Brain correlates of craving for online gaming under cue exposure in subjects with Internet gaming addiction and in remitted subjects. *Addict Biol*. 2013;18(3):559-569. doi:10.1111/j.1369-1600.2011.00405.x
139. Schiebener J, Brand M. Decision-making and related processes in internet gaming disorder and other types of internet-use disorders. *Curr Addict Rep*. 2017;4(3):262-271. doi:10.1007/s40429-017-0156-9
140. Dong G, Lin X, Potenza MN. Decreased functional connectivity in an executive control network is related to impaired executive function in internet gaming disorder. *Prog Neuropsychopharmacol Biol Psychiatry*. 2015;57:76-85. doi:10.1016/j.pnpbp.2014.10.012
141. Yao YW, Liu L, Ma SS, et al. Functional and structural neural alterations in Internet gaming disorder: a systematic review and meta-analysis. *Neurosci Biobehav Rev*. 2017;83:313-324. doi:10.1016/j.neubiorev.2017.10.029
142. Zhang JT, Yao YW, Potenza MN, et al. Effects of craving behavioral intervention on neural substrates of cue-induced craving in internet gaming disorder. *Neuroimage Clin*. 2016;12:591-599. doi:10.1016/j.nicl.2016.09.004
143. Stevens MW, Dorstyn D, Delfabbro PH, King DL. Global prevalence of gaming disorder: a systematic review and meta-analysis. *Aust N Z J Psychiatry*. 2021;55(6):553-568. doi:10.1177/0004867420962851
144. Pápay O, Urbán R, Griffiths MD, et al. Psychometric properties of the problematic online gaming questionnaire short-form and prevalence of problematic online gaming in a national sample of adolescents. *Cyberpsychol Behav Soc Netw*. 2013;16(5):340-348. doi:10.1089/cyber.2012.0484
145. Király O, Sleczka P, Pontes HM, Urbán R, Griffiths MD, Demetrovics Z. Validation of the Ten-Item Internet Gaming Disorder Test (IGDT-10) and evaluation of the nine DSM-5 Internet Gaming Disorder criteria. *Addict Behav*. 2017;64:253-260. doi:10.1016/j.addbeh.2015.11.005
146. King DL, Potenza MN. Gaming disorder among female adolescents: a hidden problem? *J Adolesc Health*. 2020;66(6):650-652. doi:10.1016/j.jadohealth.2020.03.011
147. Carson N, Cook BL, Chen CN, Alegria M. Racial/ethnic differences in video game and Internet use among US adolescents with mental health and educational difficulties. *J Child Media*. 2012;6(4):450-468. doi:10.1080/17482798.2012.724592
148. King DL, Delfabbro PH, Wu AMS, et al. Treatment of internet gaming disorder: an international systematic review and CONSORT evaluation. *Clin Psychol Rev*. 2017;54:123-133. doi:10.1016/j.cpr.2017.04.002
149. King DL, Wölfling K, Potenza MN. Taking gaming disorder treatment to the next level. *JAMA Psychiatry*. 2020;77(8):869-870. doi:10.1001/jamapsychiatry.2020.1270
150. Griffiths MD. Internet use disorders: what's new and what's not? *J Behav Addict*. 2020;9(4):934-937. doi:10.1556/2006.2020.00072
151. Willoughby T. A short-term longitudinal study of Internet and computer game use by adolescent boys and girls: prevalence, frequency of use, and psychosocial predictors. *Dev Psychol*. 2008;44(1):195-204. doi:10.1037/0012-1649.44.1.195
152. Ko CH, Yen JY, Yen CF, Chen CS, Chen CC. The association between internet addiction and psychiatric disorder: a review of the literature. *Eur Psychiatry*. 2012;27(1):1-8. doi:10.1016/j.eurpsy.2010.04.011
153. Tao R, Huang X, Wang J, Zhang H, Zhang Y, Li M. Proposed diagnostic criteria for internet addiction. *Addiction*. 2010;105(3):556-564. doi:10.1111/j.1360-0443.2009.02828.x
154. Young KS. Internet addiction: the emergence of a new clinical disorder. *Cyberpsychol Behav*. 1998;1(3):237-244. doi:10.1089/cpb.1998.1.237
155. Han DH, Lee YS, Na C, et al. The effect of methylphenidate on internet video game play in children with attention-deficit/hyperactivity disorder. *Compr Psychiatry*. 2009;50(3):251-256. doi:10.1016/j.comppsych.2008.08.011
156. Li M, Chen J, Li N, Li X. A twin study of problematic internet use: its heritability and genetic association with effortful control. *Twin Res Hum Genet*. 2014;17(4):279-287. doi:10.1017/thg.2014.32
157. Vink JM, van Beijsterveldt TC, Huppertz C, Bartels M, Boomsma DI. Heritability of compulsive internet use in adolescents. *Addict Biol* 2016;21(2):460-468. doi:10.1111/adb.12218
158. Lee YS, Han DH, Yang KC, et al. Depression like characteristics of 5HTTLPR polymorphism and temperament in excessive internet users. *J Affect Disord*. 2008;109(1-2):165-169. doi:10.1016/j.jad.2007.10.020
159. Montag C, Kirsch P, Sauer C, Markett S, Reuter M. The role of the CHRNA4 gene in Internet addiction: a case-control study. *J Addict Med*. 2012;6(3):191-195. doi:10.1097/ADM.0b013e31825ba7e7
160. Han DH, Lee YS, Yang KC, Kim EY, Lyoo IK, Renshaw PF. Dopamine genes and reward dependence in adolescents with excessive internet video game play. *J Addict Med*. 2007;1(3):133-138. doi:10.1097/ADM.0b013e31811f465f
161. Hou H, Jia S, Hu S, et al. Reduced striatal dopamine transporters in people with internet addiction disorder. *J Biomed Biotechnol*. 2012;2012:854524. doi:10.1155/2012/854524
162. Kim SH, Baik SH, Park CS, Kim SJ, Choi SW, Kim SE. Reduced striatal dopamine D2 receptors in people with internet addiction. *Neuroreport*. 2011;22(8):407-411. doi:10.1097/WNR.0b013e328346e16e
163. Ioannidis K, Hook R, Goudriaan AE, et al. Cognitive deficits in problematic internet use: meta-analysis of 40 studies. *Br J Psychiatry*. 2019;215(5):639-646. doi:10.1192/bjp.2019.3
164. Brand M, Wegmann E, Stark R, et al. The Interaction of Person-Affect-Cognition-Execution (I-PACE) model for addictive behaviors: update, generalization to addictive behaviors beyond internet-use disorders, and specification of the process character of addictive behaviors. *Neurosci Biobehav Rev*. 2019;104:1-10. doi:10.1016/j.neubiorev.2019.06.032
165. Peng W, Hao Q, Gao H, et al. Functional neural alterations in pathological internet use: a meta-analysis of neuroimaging studies. *Front Neurol*. 2022;13:841514. doi:10.3389/fneur.2022.841514
166. Liu J, Gao XP, Osunde I, et al. Increased regional homogeneity in internet addiction disorder: a resting state functional magnetic resonance imaging study. *Chin Med J (Engl)*. 2010;123(14):1904-1908.
167. Dong G, Devito EE, Du X, Cui Z. Impaired inhibitory control in 'internet addiction disorder': a functional magnetic resonance imaging study. *Psychiatry Res*. 2012;203(2-3):153-158. doi:10.1016/j.pscychresns.2012.02.001
168. Dong G, Huang J, Du X. Enhanced reward sensitivity and decreased loss sensitivity in Internet addicts: an fMRI study during a guessing task. *J Psychiatr Res*. 2011;45(11):1525-1529. doi:10.1016/j.jpsychires.2011.06.017
169. Zhou Y, Lin FC, Du YS, et al. Gray matter abnormalities in Internet addiction: a voxel-based morphometry study. *Eur J Radiol*. 2011;79(1):92-95. doi:10.1016/j.ejrad.2009.10.025

170. Yuan K, Qin W, Wang G, et al. Microstructure abnormalities in adolescents with internet addiction disorder. *PloS One*. 2011;6(6):e20708. doi:10.1371/journal.pone.0020708
171. Lin F, Zhou Y, Du Y, et al. Abnormal white matter integrity in adolescents with internet addiction disorder: a tract-based spatial statistics study. *PloS One*. 2012;7(1):e30253. doi:10.1371/journal.pone.0030253
172. Bakken IJ, Wenzel HG, Götestam KG, Johansson A, Oren A. Internet addiction among Norwegian adults: a stratified probability sample study. *Scand J Psychol*. 2009;50(2):121-127. doi:10.1111/j.1467-9450.2008.00685.x
173. Su W, Han X, Jin C, Yan Y, Potenza MN. Are males more likely to be addicted to the internet than females? A meta-analysis involving 34 global jurisdictions. *Comput Hum Behav*. 2019;99:86-100. doi:10.1016/j.chb.2019.04.021
174. Su W, Han X, Yu H, Wu Y, Potenza MN. Do men become addicted to internet gaming and women to social media? A meta-analysis examining gender-related differences in specific internet addiction. *Comput Hum Behav*. 2020;113:106480. doi:10.1016/j.chb.2020.106480
175. Liu TC, Desai RA, Krishnan-Sarin S, Cavallo DA, Potenza MN. Problematic internet use and health in adolescents: data from a high school survey in Connecticut. *J Clin Psychiatry*. 2011;72(6):836-845. doi:10.4088/JCP.10m06057
176. Yen JY, Ko CH, Yen CF, Chen CS, Chen CC. The association between harmful alcohol use and internet addiction among college students: comparison of personality. *Psychiatry Clin Neurosci*. 2009;63(2):218-224. doi:10.1111/j.1440-1819.2009.01943.x
177. Dowling NA, Brown M. Commonalities in the psychological factors associated with problem gambling and internet dependence. *Cyberpsychol Behav Soc Netw*. 2010;13(4):437-441. doi:10.1089/cyber.2009.0317
178. Yen JY, Ko CH, Yen CF, Wu HY, Yang MJ. The comorbid psychiatric symptoms of Internet addiction: attention deficit and hyperactivity disorder (ADHD), depression, social phobia, and hostility. *J Adolesc Health*. 2007;41(1):93-98. doi:10.1016/j.jadohealth.2007.02.002
179. Fineberg NA, Demetrovics Z, Stein DJ, et al. Manifesto for a European research network into problematic usage of the internet. *Eur Neuropsychopharmacol*. 2018;28(11):1232-1246. doi:10.1016/j.euroneuro.2018.08.004
180. Kraepelin R. *Psychiatrie*. Barth; 1915.
181. Lejoyeux M, Adès J, Tassain V, Solomon J. Phenomenology and psychopathology of uncontrolled buying. *Am J Psychiatry*. 1996;153(12):1524-1529. doi:10.1176/ajp.153.12.1524
182. Black DW. A review of compulsive buying disorder. *World Psychiatry*. 2007;6(1):14-18.
183. Starcevic V, Aboujaoude E. Internet gaming disorder, obsessive-compulsive disorder, and addiction. *Curr Addict Rep*. 2017;4(3):317-322. doi:10.1007/s40429-017-0158-7
184. McElroy SL, Keck PE, Pope HG, Smith JMR, Strakowski SM. Compulsive buying: a report of 20 cases. *J Clin Psychiatry*. 1994;55(6):242-248.
185. Raab G, Elger CE, Neuner M, Weber B. A neurological study of compulsive buying behaviour. *J Consum Policy*. 2011;34(4):401. doi:10.1007/s10603-011-9168-3
186. Trotzke P, Brand M, Starcke K. Cue-reactivity, craving, and decision making in buying disorder: a review of the current knowledge and future directions. *Curr Addict Rep*. 2017;4(3):246-253. doi:10.1007/s40429-017-0155-x
187. Koran LM, Faber RJ, Aboujaoude E, Large MD, Serpe RT. Estimated prevalence of compulsive buying behavior in the United States. *Am J Psychiatry*. 2006;163(10):1806-1812. doi:10.1176/ajp.2006.163.10.1806
188. Maraz A, Griffiths MD, Demetrovics Z. The prevalence of compulsive buying: a meta-analysis. *Addiction*. 2016;111(3):408-419. doi:10.1111/add.13223
189. Ching TH, Tang CS, Wu A, Yan E. Gender differences in pathways to compulsive buying in Chinese college students in Hong Kong and Macau. *J Behav Addict*. 2016;5(2):342-350. doi:10.1556/2006.5.2016.025
190. Grant JE, Potenza MN, Krishnan-Sarin S, Cavallo DA, Desai RA. Shopping problems among high school students. *Compr Psychiatry*. 2011;52(3):247-252. doi:10.1016/j.comppsych.2010.06.006
191. Hague B, Hall J, Kellett S. Treatments for compulsive buying: a systematic review of the quality, effectiveness and progression of the outcome evidence. *J Behav Addict*. 2016;5(3):379-394. doi:10.1556/2006.5.2016.064
192. Black DW, Gabel J, Hansen J, Schlosser S. A double-blind comparison of fluvoxamine versus placebo in the treatment of compulsive buying disorder. *Ann Clin Psychiatry*. 2000;12(4):205-211. doi:10.1023/a:1009030425631
193. Koran LM, Aboujaoude EN, Solvason B, Gamel NN, Smith EH. Escitalopram for compulsive buying disorder: a double-blind discontinuation study. *J Clin Psychopharmacol*. 2007;27(2):225-227. doi:10.1097/01.jcp.0000264975.79367.f4
194. Kraus SW, Voon V, Potenza MN. Should compulsive sexual behavior be considered an addiction? *Addiction*. 2016;111(12):2097-2106. doi:10.1111/add.13297
195. Gola M, Lewczuk K, Potenza MN, et al. What should be included in the criteria for compulsive sexual behavior disorder? *J Behav Addict*. 2020;11(2):160-165. doi:10.1556/2006.2020.00090
196. Mick TM, Hollander E. Impulsive-compulsive sexual behavior. *CNS Spectr*. 2006;11(12):944-955. doi:10.1017/S1092852900015133
197. Chatzittofis A, Boström ADE, Savard J, Öberg KG, Arver S, Jokinen J. Neurochemical and hormonal contributors to compulsive sexual behavior disorder. *Curr Addict Rep*. 2022;9(1):23-31. doi:10.1007/s40429-021-00403-6
198. Hirschfeld RM. Long-term side effects of SSRIs: sexual dysfunction and weight gain. *J Clin Psychiatry*. 2003;64(Suppl 18):20-24.
199. Driver-Dunckley ED, Noble BN, Hentz JG, et al. Gambling and increased sexual desire with dopaminergic medications in restless legs syndrome. *Clin Neuropharmacol*. 2007;30(5):249-255. doi:10.1097/wnf.0b013e31804c780e
200. Voon V, Fox SH. Medication-related impulse control and repetitive behaviors in Parkinson disease. *Arch Neurol*. 2007;64(8):1089-1096. doi:10.1001/archneur.64.8.1089
201. Leeman RF, Potenza MN. Impulse control disorders in Parkinson's disease: clinical characteristics and implications. *Neuropsychiatry (London)*. 2011;1(2):133-147. doi:10.2217/npy.11.11
202. Flanagan J, Chatzittofis A, Boström ADE, et al. High plasma oxytocin levels in men with hypersexual disorder. *J Clin Endocrinol Metab*. 2022;107(5):e1816-e1822. doi:10.1210/clinem/dgac015
203. Kor A, Djalovski A, Potenza MN, Zagoory-Sharon O, Feldman R. Alterations in oxytocin and vasopressin in men with problematic pornography use: the role of empathy. *J Behav Addict*. 2022;11(1):116-127. doi:10.1556/2006.2021.00089
204. Chou CL, Lin YJ, Sheu YL, Lin CJ, Hseuh IH. Persistent Klüver-Bucy syndrome after bilateral temporal lobe infarction. *Acta Neurol Taiwan*. 2008;17(3):199-202.
205. Kowalewska E, Grubbs JB, Potenza MN, Gola M, Draps M, Kraus SW. Neurocognitive mechanisms in compulsive sexual behavior disorder. *Curr Sex Health Rep*. 2018;10(4):255-264. doi:10.1007/s11930-018-0176-z
206. Banca P, Morris LS, Mitchell S, Harrison NA, Potenza MN, Voon V. Novelty, conditioning and attentional bias to sexual rewards. *J Psychiatr Res*. 2016;72:91-101. doi:10.1016/j.jpsychires.2015.10.017
207. Voon V, Mole TB, Banca P, et al. Neural correlates of sexual cue reactivity in individuals with and without compulsive sexual behaviours. *PloS One*. 2014;9(7):e102419. doi:10.1371/journal.pone.0102419
208. Gola M, Wordecha M, Sescousse G, et al. Can pornography be addictive? An fMRI study of men seeking treatment for problematic pornography use. *Neuropsychopharmacology*. 2017;42(10):2021-2031. doi:10.1038/npp.2017.78
209. Seok JW, Sohn JH. Response inhibition during processing of sexual stimuli in males with problematic hypersexual behavior. *J Behav Addict*. 2020;9(1):71-82. doi:10.1556/2006.2020.00003
210. Miner MH, Raymond N, Mueller BA, Lloyd M, Lim KO. Preliminary investigation of the impulsive and neuroanatomical characteristics of compulsive sexual behavior. *Psychiatry Res*. 2009;174(2):146-151. doi:10.1016/j.pscychresns.2009.04.008
211. Kinsey AC, Pomeroy WR, Martin CE. Sexual behavior in the human male. 1948. *Am J Public Health*. 2003;93(6):894-898. doi:10.2105/ajph.93.6.894

212. Kafka MP. Hypersexual disorder: a proposed diagnosis for DSM-V. *Arch Sex Behav*. 2010;39(2):377-400. doi:10.1007/s10508-009-9574-7
213. Grant JE, Levine L, Kim D, Potenza MN. Impulse control disorders in adult psychiatric inpatients. *Am J Psychiatry*. 2005;162(11):2184-2188. doi:10.1176/appi.ajp.162.11.2184
214. Odlaug BL, Grant JE. Impulse-control disorders in a college sample: results from the self-administered Minnesota Impulse Disorders Interview (MIDI). *Prim Care Companion J Clin Psychiatry*. 2010;12(2). doi:10.4088/PCC.09m00842whi
215. Odlaug BL, Lust K, Schreiber LR, et al. Compulsive sexual behavior in young adults. *Ann Clin Psychiatry*. 2013;25(3):193-200.
216. Bőthe B, Potenza MN, Griffiths MD, et al. The development of the Compulsive Sexual Behavior Disorder Scale (CSBD-19): an ICD-11 based screening measure across three languages. *J Behav Addict*. 2020;9(2):247-258. doi:10.1556/2006.2020.00034
217. Reid RC, Carpenter BN, Hook JN, et al. Report of findings in a DSM-5 field trial for hypersexual disorder. *J Sex Med*. 2012;9(11):2868-2877. doi:10.1111/j.1743-6109.2012.02936.x
218. Grubbs JB, Perry SL, Grant Weinandy JT, Kraus SW. Porndemic? A longitudinal study of pornography use before and during the COVID-19 pandemic in a nationally representative sample of Americans. *Arch Sex Behav*. 2022;51(1):123-137. doi:10.1007/s10508-021-02077-7
219. Dickenson JA, Gleason N, Coleman E, Miner MH. Prevalence of distress associated with difficulty controlling sexual urges, feelings, and behaviors in the United States. *JAMA Netw Open*. 2018;1(7):e184468. doi:10.1001/jamanetworkopen.2018.4468
220. Bőthe B, Bartók R, Tóth-Király I, et al. Hypersexuality, gender, and sexual orientation: a large-scale psychometric survey study. *Arch Sex Behav*. 2018;47(8):2265-2276. doi:10.1007/s10508-018-1201-z
221. Fong TW, De La Garza R II, Newton TF. A case report of topiramate in the treatment of nonparaphilic sexual addiction. *J Clin Psychopharmacol*. 2005;25(5):512-514. doi:10.1097/01.jcp.0000177849.23534.bf
222. Wainberg ML, Muench F, Morgenstern J, et al. A double-blind study of citalopram versus placebo in the treatment of compulsive sexual behaviors in gay and bisexual men. *J Clin Psychiatry*. 2006;67(12):1968-1973. doi:10.4088/jcp.v67n1218
223. Serretti A, Chiesa A. Treatment-emergent sexual dysfunction related to antidepressants: a meta-analysis. *J Clin Psychopharmacol*. 2009;29(3):259-266. doi:10.1097/JCP.0b013e3181a5233f
224. Coleman E, Gratzer T, Nesvacil L, Raymond NC. Nefazodone and the treatment of nonparaphilic compulsive sexual behavior: a retrospective study. *J Clin Psychiatry*. 2000;61(4):282-284.
225. Kafka MP, Hennen J. Psychostimulant augmentation during treatment with selective serotonin reuptake inhibitors in men with paraphilias and paraphilia-related disorders: a case series. *J Clin Psychiatry*. 2000;61(9):664-670. doi:10.4088/jcp.v61n0912
226. Gola M, Potenza MN. Paroxetine treatment of problematic pornography use: a case series. *J Behav Addict*. 2016;5(3):529-532. doi:10.1556/2006.5.2016.046
227. Sathe RS, Komisaruk BR, Ladas AK, Godbole SV. Naltrexone-induced augmentation of sexual response in men. *Arch Med Res*. 2001;32(3):221-226. doi:10.1016/s0188-4409(01)00279-x
228. Dannon PN. Topiramate for the treatment of kleptomania: a case series and review of the literature. *Clin Neuropharmacol*. 2003;26(1):1-4. doi:10.1097/00002826-200301000-00001
229. Grant JE, Kim SW. A case of kleptomania and compulsive sexual behavior treated with naltrexone. *Ann Clin Psychiatry*. 2001;13(4):229-231. doi:10.1023/a:1014626102110
230. Ryback RS. Naltrexone in the treatment of adolescent sexual offenders. *J Clin Psychiatry*. 2004;65(7):982-986. doi:10.4088/jcp.v65n0715
231. Davis C, Carter JC. Compulsive overeating as an addiction disorder. A review of theory and evidence. *Appetite*. 2009;53(1):1-8. doi:10.1016/j.appet.2009.05.018
232. von Ranson KM, Robinson KE. Who is providing what type of psychotherapy to eating disorder clients? A survey. *Int J Eat Disord* 2006;39(1):27-34. doi:10.1002/eat.20201
233. Enriori PJ, Evans AE, Sinnayah P, Cowley MA. Leptin resistance and obesity. *Obesity (Silver Spring)*. 2006;14(Suppl 5):254s-258s. doi:10.1038/oby.2006.319
234. Kiefer F, Jahn H, Otte C, Demiralay C, Wolf K, Wiedemann K. Increasing leptin precedes craving and relapse during pharmacological abstinence maintenance treatment of alcoholism. *J Psychiatr Res*. 2005;39(5):545-551. doi:10.1016/j.jpsychires.2004.11.005
235. Halaas JL, Gajiwala KS, Maffei M, et al. Weight-reducing effects of the plasma protein encoded by the obese gene. *Science*. 1995;269(5223):543-546. doi:10.1126/science.7624777
236. Unger RH, Clark GO, Scherer PE, Orci L. Lipid homeostasis, lipotoxicity and the metabolic syndrome. *Biochim Biophys Acta*. 2010;1801(3):209-214. doi:10.1016/j.bbalip.2009.10.006
237. Figlewicz DP, Evans SB, Murphy J, Hoen M, Baskin DG. Expression of receptors for insulin and leptin in the ventral tegmental area/substantia nigra (VTA/SN) of the rat. *Brain Res*. 2003;964(1):107-115. doi:10.1016/s0006-8993(02)04087-8
238. Hommel JD, Trinko R, Sears RM, et al. Leptin receptor signaling in midbrain dopamine neurons regulates feeding. *Neuron*. 2006;51(6):801-810. doi:10.1016/j.neuron.2006.08.023
239. Elmquist JK, Bjørbaek C, Ahima RS, Flier JS, Saper CB. Distributions of leptin receptor mRNA isoforms in the rat brain. *J Comp Neurol*. 1998;395(4):535-547.
240. Shanley LJ, Irving AJ, Harvey J. Leptin enhances NMDA receptor function and modulates hippocampal synaptic plasticity. *J Neurosci*. 2001;21(24):Rc186. doi:10.1523/JNEUROSCI.21-24-j0001.2001
241. Billes SK, Simonds SE, Cowley MA. Leptin reduces food intake via a dopamine D2 receptor-dependent mechanism. *Mol Metab*. 2012;1(1-2):86-93. doi:10.1016/j.molmet.2012.07.003
242. Sakurai T, Amemiya A, Ishii M, et al. Orexins and orexin receptors: a family of hypothalamic neuropeptides and G protein-coupled receptors that regulate feeding behavior. *Cell*. 1998;92(4):573-585. doi:10.1016/s0092-8674(00)80949-6
243. Sharf R, Sarhan M, Brayton CE, Guarnieri DJ, Taylor JR, DiLeone RJ. Orexin signaling via the orexin 1 receptor mediates operant responding for food reinforcement. *Biol Psychiatry*. 2010;67(8):753-760. doi:10.1016/j.biopsych.2009.12.035
244. Boutrel B, Kenny PJ, Specio SE, et al. Role for hypocretin in mediating stress-induced reinstatement of cocaine-seeking behavior. *Proc Natl Acad Sci U S A*. 2005;102(52):19168-19173. doi:10.1073/pnas.0507480102
245. Lawrence AJ, Cowen MS, Yang HJ, Chen F, Oldfield B. The orexin system regulates alcohol-seeking in rats. *Br J Pharmacol*. 2006;148(6):752-759. doi:10.1038/sj.bjp.0706789
246. Smith RJ, Aston-Jones G. Orexin/hypocretin 1 receptor antagonist reduces heroin self-administration and cue-induced heroin seeking. *Eur J Neurosci*. 2012;35(5):798-804. doi:10.1111/j.1460-9568.2012.08013.x
247. Harris GC, Wimmer M, Aston-Jones G. A role for lateral hypothalamic orexin neurons in reward seeking. *Nature*. 2005;437(7058):556-559. doi:10.1038/nature04071
248. Narita M, Nagumo Y, Hashimoto S, et al. Direct involvement of orexinergic systems in the activation of the mesolimbic dopamine pathway and related behaviors induced by morphine. *J Neurosci*. 2006;26(2):398-405. doi:10.1523/jneurosci.2761-05.2006
249. Vittoz NM, Berridge CW. Hypocretin/orexin selectively increases dopamine efflux within the prefrontal cortex: involvement of the ventral tegmental area. *Neuropsychopharmacology*. 2006;31(2):384-395. doi:10.1038/sj.npp.1300807
250. Cummings DE, Purnell JQ, Frayo RS, Schmidova K, Wisse BE, Weigle DS. A preprandial rise in plasma ghrelin levels suggests a role in meal initiation in humans. *Diabetes*. 2001;50(8):1714-1719. doi:10.2337/diabetes.50.8.1714
251. Tschöp M, Weyer C, Tataranni PA, Devanarayan V, Ravussin E, Heiman ML. Circulating ghrelin levels are decreased in human obesity. *Diabetes*. 2001;50(4):707-709. doi:10.2337/diabetes.50.4.707
252. Overduin J, Figlewicz DP, Bennett-Jay J, Kittleson S, Cummings DE. Ghrelin increases the motivation to eat, but does not alter food palatability.

Am J Physiol Regul Integr Comp Physiol. 2012;303(3):R259-R269. doi:10.1152/ajpregu.00488.2011

253. Abizaid A, Liu ZW, Andrews ZB, et al. Ghrelin modulates the activity and synaptic input organization of midbrain dopamine neurons while promoting appetite. *J Clin Invest.* 2006;116(12):3229-3239. doi:10.1172/jci29867
254. Skibicka KP, Hansson C, Alvarez-Crespo M, Friberg PA, Dickson SL. Ghrelin directly targets the ventral tegmental area to increase food motivation. *Neuroscience.* 2011;180:129-137. doi:10.1016/j.neuroscience.2011.02.016
255. Abizaid A, Mineur YS, Roth RH, et al. Reduced locomotor responses to cocaine in ghrelin-deficient mice. *Neuroscience.* 2011;192:500-506. doi:10.1016/j.neuroscience.2011.06.001
256. Leibowitz SF, Alexander JT. Hypothalamic serotonin in control of eating behavior, meal size, and body weight. *Biol Psychiatry.* 1998;44(9):851-864. doi:10.1016/s0006-3223(98)00186-3
257. Heisler LK, Cowley MA, Tecott LH, et al. Activation of central melanocortin pathways by fenfluramine. *Science.* 2002;297(5581):609-611. doi:10.1126/science.1072327
258. Smith BK, York DA, Bray GA. Activation of hypothalamic serotonin receptors reduced intake of dietary fat and protein but not carbohydrate. *Am J Physiol.* 1999;277(3):R802-R811. doi:10.1152/ajpregu.1999.277.3.R802
259. Wurtman RJ, Wurtman JJ. Brain serotonin, carbohydrate-craving, obesity and depression. *Obes Res.* 1995;3(Suppl 4):477s-480s. doi:10.1002/j.1550-8528.1995.tb00215.x
260. Kelley AE, Bakshi VP, Haber SN, Steininger TL, Will MJ, Zhang M. Opioid modulation of taste hedonics within the ventral striatum. *Physiol Behav.* 2002;76(3):365-377. doi:10.1016/s0031-9384(02)00751-5
261. Di Marzo V, Goparaju SK, Wang L, et al. Leptin-regulated endocannabinoids are involved in maintaining food intake. *Nature.* 2001;410(6830):822-825. doi:10.1038/35071088
262. Cota D, Genghini S, Pasquali R, Pagotto U. Antagonizing the cannabinoid receptor type 1: a dual way to fight obesity. *J Endocrinol Invest.* 2003;26(10):1041-1044. doi:10.1007/bf03348205
263. Mahler SV, Smith KS, Berridge KC. Endocannabinoid hedonic hotspot for sensory pleasure: anandamide in nucleus accumbens shell enhances 'liking' of a sweet reward. *Neuropsychopharmacology.* 2007;32(11):2267-2278. doi:10.1038/sj.npp.1301376
264. Meye FJ, Trezza V, Vanderschuren LJMJ, Ramakers GMJ, Adan RAH. Neutral antagonism at the cannabinoid 1 receptor: a safer treatment for obesity. *Mol Psychiatry.* 2013;18(12):1294-1301. doi:10.1038/mp.2012.145
265. Davis C, Levitan RD, Muglia P, Bewell C, Kennedy JL. Decision-making deficits and overeating: a risk model for obesity. *Obes Res.* 2004;12(6):929-935. doi:10.1038/oby.2004.113
266. Danner UN, Ouwehand C, van Haastert NL, Hornsveld H, de Ridder DT. Decision-making impairments in women with binge eating disorder in comparison with obese and normal weight women. *Eur Eat Disord Rev.* 2012;20(1):e56-e62. doi:10.1002/erv.1098
267. Tchanturia K, Liao PC, Uher R, Lawrence N, Treasure J, Campbell IC. An investigation of decision making in anorexia nervosa using the Iowa Gambling Task and skin conductance measurements. *J Int Neuropsychol Soc.* 2007;13(4):635-641. doi:10.1017/s1355617707070798
268. Brand M, Kalbe E, Labudda K, Fujiwara E, Kessler J, Markowitsch HJ. Decision-making impairments in patients with pathological gambling. *Psychiatry Res.* 2005;133(1):91-99. doi:10.1016/j.psychres.2004.10.003
269. Brand M, Fujiwara E, Kalbe E, Steingass HP, Kessler J, Markowitsch HJ. Cognitive estimation and affective judgments in alcoholic Korsakoff patients. *J Clin Exp Neuropsychol.* 2003;25(3):324-334. doi:10.1076/jcen.25.3.324.13802
270. Carr MM, Wiedemann AA, Macdonald-Gagnon G, Potenza MN. Impulsivity and compulsivity in binge eating disorder: a systematic review of behavioral studies. *Prog Neuropsychopharmacol Biol Psychiatry.* 2021;110:110318. doi:10.1016/j.pnpbp.2021.110318
271. Rosen HJ, Gorno-Tempini ML, Goldman WP, et al. Patterns of brain atrophy in frontotemporal dementia and semantic dementia. *Neurology.* 2002;58(2):198-208. doi:10.1212/wnl.58.2.198
272. Mendez MF, Licht EA, Shapira JS. Changes in dietary or eating behavior in frontotemporal dementia versus Alzheimer's disease. *Am J Alzheimers Dis Other Demen.* 2008;23(3):280-285. doi:10.1177/1533317507313140
273. DelParigi A, Chen K, Salbe AD, et al. Successful dieters have increased neural activity in cortical areas involved in the control of behavior. *Int J Obes (Lond).* 2007;31(3):440-448. doi:10.1038/sj.ijo.0803431
274. McCaffery JM, Haley AP, Sweet LH, et al. Differential functional magnetic resonance imaging response to food pictures in successful weight-loss maintainers relative to normal-weight and obese controls. *Am J Clin Nutr.* 2009;90(4):928-934. doi:10.3945/ajcn.2009.27924
275. Uher R, Yoganathan D, Mogg A, et al. Effect of left prefrontal repetitive transcranial magnetic stimulation on food craving. *Biol Psychiatry.* 2005;58(10):840-842. doi:10.1016/j.biopsych.2005.05.043
276. Barr MS, Farzan F, Wing VC, George TP, Fitzgerald PB, Daskalakis ZJ. Repetitive transcranial magnetic stimulation and drug addiction. *Int Rev Psychiatry.* 2011;23(5):454-466. doi:10.3109/09540261.2011.618827
277. National Health and Nutrition Examination Survey 2017–March 2020 2023 Prepandemic Data Files Development of Files and Prevalence Estimates for Selected Health Outcomes. Accessed June 2, 2023. https://stacks.cdc.gov/view/cdc/106273
278. Dai H, Alsalhe TA, Chalghaf N, Riccò M, Bragazzi NL, Wu J. The global burden of disease attributable to high body mass index in 195 countries and territories, 1990-2017: an analysis of the Global Burden of Disease Study. *PLoS Med.* 2020;17(7):e1003198. doi:10.1371/journal.pmed.1003198
279. Grilo CM, White MA, Masheb RM. DSM-IV psychiatric disorder comorbidity and its correlates in binge eating disorder. *Int J Eat Disord.* 2009;42(3):228-234. doi:10.1002/eat.20599
280. Yip SW, White MA, Grilo CM, Potenza MN. An exploratory study of clinical measures associated with subsyndromal pathological gambling in patients with binge eating disorder. *J Gambl Stud.* 2011;27(2):257-270. doi:10.1007/s10899-010-9207-z
281. Hutson PH, Balodis IM, Potenza MN. Binge-eating disorder: clinical and therapeutic advances. *Pharmacol Ther.* 2018;182:15-27. doi:10.1016/j.pharmthera.2017.08.002
282. Wilding JPH, Batterham RL, Calanna S, et al. Once-weekly semaglutide in adults with overweight or obesity. *N Engl J Med.* 2021;384(11):989-1002. doi:10.1056/NEJMoa2032183
283. McElroy SL, Hudson J, Ferreira-Cornwell MC, Radewonuk J, Whitaker T, Gasior M. Lisdexamfetamine dimesylate for adults with moderate to severe binge eating disorder: results of two pivotal phase 3 randomized controlled trials. *Neuropsychopharmacology.* 2016;41(5):1251-1260. doi:10.1038/npp.2015.275
284. McElroy SL, Arnold LM, Shapira NA, et al. Topiramate in the treatment of binge eating disorder associated with obesity: a randomized, placebo-controlled trial. *Am J Psychiatry.* 2003;160(2):255-261. doi:10.1176/appi.ajp.160.2.255
285. Claudino AM, de Oliveira IR, Appolinario JC, et al. Double-blind, randomized, placebo-controlled trial of topiramate plus cognitive-behavior therapy in binge-eating disorder. *J Clin Psychiatry.* 2007;68(9):1324-1332. doi:10.4088/jcp.v68n0901
286. McElroy SL, Shapira NA, Arnold LM, et al. Topiramate in the long-term treatment of binge-eating disorder associated with obesity. *J Clin Psychiatry.* 2004;65(11):1463-1469. doi:10.4088/jcp.v65n1104
287. Grilo CM, Lydecker JA, Morgan PT, Gueorguieva R. Naltrexone + Bupropion combination for the treatment of binge-eating disorder with obesity: a randomized, controlled pilot study. *Clin Ther.* 2021;43(1):112-122.e1. doi:10.1016/j.clinthera.2020.10.010

CHAPTER

52 Gambling Disorder: Clinical Characteristics and Treatment

Jon E. Grant and Brian L. Odlaug

CHAPTER OUTLINE

- Introduction
- Epidemiology
- Assessment
- Treatment

INTRODUCTION

Gambling disorder, also called "pathologic(al) gambling," is a psychiatric disorder characterized by persistent and recurrent maladaptive patterns of gambling behavior and is associated with impaired functioning, reduced quality of life, and high rates of bankruptcy, divorce, and incarceration.[1] Defined broadly as wagering money or something of value on an event with an uncertain outcome, "gambling" and excessive gambling behaviors have been reported for millennia across cultures and have been discussed in the medical literature since the early 1800s.[2] *Disordered* gambling, however, was only recognized by the American Psychiatric Association in 1980 in the third edition of the *Diagnostic and Statistical Manual of Mental Disorders* (DSM-III).[3]

Classified in the *Diagnostic and Statistical Manual of Mental Disorders*, Fifth edition (DSM-5) as a "substance-related and addictive disorder," the diagnosis of gambling disorder necessitates that a person meets four of nine possible criteria. These criteria include (1) a preoccupation with gambling; (2) the need to gamble with higher amounts of money (tolerance); (3) has tried unsuccessfully to stop or cut back on gambling; (4) feels restless or irritable when not able to gamble; (5) gambles to escape from a mood or problems; (6) chases gambling losses; (7) lies to family, friends, and others about the amount or extent of gambling; (8) has lost or put into jeopardy a job, educational, or other opportunities due to gambling; and (9) has needed others to pay for financial obligations due to gambling losses. Further, the gambling must not be better accounted for by a manic episode. The term *problem gambling* has been used to describe forms of disordered gambling, sometimes inclusive and at other times exclusive of gambling disorder. Problem gambling, like problem drinking, is not an officially recognized disorder by the American Psychiatric Association.

Data support the conceptualization of gambling disorder as a "behavioral"—as opposed to a substance—addiction (see Chapter 51 Understanding Non-Substance Addictions). The overall concept of behavioral addiction has some scientific and clinical heuristic value but remains controversial. This is likely due to gambling disorder often being resistant to treatment, and it remains unclear whether the methods of traditional addiction treatment (group, 12-step participation, recurrence prevention, motivational enhancement, etc.) are superior, inferior, equivalent, or need to be combined with those of psychiatric treatments (medication, cognitive-behavioral therapy [CBT], psychotherapy). Far from diametrically opposed, however, evidence supports significant phenomenological, clinical, epidemiological, and biological links between gambling disorder with substance use disorders.[4,5] Indeed, issues around behavioral addiction were debated in the context of development of DSM-5[6] and ultimately led to gambling disorder shifting from its categorization in DSM-IV as an "impulse control disorder not elsewhere specified" to a DSM-5 categorization in the "substance-related and addictive disorders." Not only is substance use disorders research likely to be illustrative for gambling disorder, but the study of gambling disorder presents an opportunity to study addictive behaviors without necessarily being confounded by neurotoxicity associated with acute or chronic substance use.[7] As such, it seems increasingly important that individuals involved in the prevention and treatment of substance use disorders have a current understanding of gambling disorder and the potential for future research findings to guide prevention and treatment efforts for addiction in general. In addition, the high prevalence and adverse impact of gambling disorder among individuals with substance use disorder make it important for those in the field. Further, important clinical differences based on severity of gambling disorder are also imperative for the clinician to understand. Research examining a sample of 574 patients with gambling disorder, sorted by clinical severity, denoted that those with a moderate or severe form of gambling disorder exhibited far worse quality of life, higher depressive and anxiety-related symptoms, and increased nicotine use as compared to those in the mild gambling disorder group.[8] In order to afford more efficacious treatment to patients with gambling disorder, understanding the clinical differences that may exist among and between patients is of paramount importance.

EPIDEMIOLOGY

A range of prevalence estimates have been reported for gambling disorder depending upon the time frame of the study, the instruments used to diagnose the disorder, and the population examined. In the general population of the United States, however, only four national studies and one meta-analysis of state and regional surveys have examined prevalence estimates of gambling disorder. The first national study in 1976 noted that 0.8% of 1749 adults contacted via telephone survey had a significant gambling problem.[9] Twenty years later, the National Opinion Research Center at the University of Chicago conducted a national telephone survey (requested by the National Gambling Impact Study Commission) of 2417 adults and found a lifetime prevalence estimate of 0.8% of gambling disorder and an additional 1.3% of problem gambling.[10] Another national telephone survey of 2628 adults found that 1.3% had current gambling disorder measured by the Diagnostic Interview Schedule and 1.9% when measured by the South Oaks Gambling Screen and an additional 2.8% to 7.5% had problem gambling.[11] The National Epidemiologic Survey on Alcohol and Related Conditions (NESARC), however, found that only 0.4% of adults in a community sample met current criteria for gambling disorder.[12] A meta-analysis of 120 prevalence estimate surveys completed in North America from the late 1970s to the late 1990s found that the lifetime estimate of gambling disorder was 1.6% and of problem gambling was 3.9%, for a combined rate of 5.5% for some kind of disordered gambling[13]; however, gambling exposure may influence prevalence rates of gambling disorder.[14]

High rates of gambling disorder have been reported in racial-ethnic minority groups compared to the general population, as well as sexual minority populations, yet there is a severe poverty of research into the underlying factors that might account for these associations.[15-17] Studies have also indicated that higher rates of gambling in certain racial-ethnic minority groups may be due to different cultural norms, acculturation, and attitudes toward gambling,[18-20] as well as lower rates of social inclusivity.[21] Thus, additional research is urgently needed to understand factors contributing to increased gambling prevalence rates in these groups, to assess the efficacy of existing treatments in these subpopulations, and to explore the efficacy of culturally specific treatment options.

Other subpopulations, including military veterans, young adults, and adolescents, have also demonstrated remarkable rates of problem gambling or gambling disorder. A study of 3157 U.S. veterans noted that 2.2% met criteria for at-risk or problem gambling.[22] Young adult (18-22 years) and adolescent (14-18 years) studies have also illustrated that problem gambling is relatively common.[23] An anonymous survey study of 791 college students[24] found gambling disorder prevalence of 0.6%, while a study of 1313 adolescents showed problem gambling rates of 1.2% and at-risk gambling rates of 4%.[25] A global public health concern, similar rates of gambling disorder have been reported in the general population and subgroups of the general population of other countries.[26-30]

While troubling rates in the general population, the incidence of gambling disorder appears higher in clinical samples. In individuals seeking treatment for substance use disorders, lifetime estimates of gambling disorder range from 5% to 33%.[31-33] In studies of psychiatric inpatients, estimates of lifetime gambling disorder have ranged from 4.9% in adolescents to 6.9% in adults.[34-37]

There has been an accelerated proliferation of gambling venues over the past 10 years, particularly with greater numbers of casinos, increased online gambling opportunities, electronic sports betting, and a constant fusion of gaming/gambling opportunities.[38-40] With increased opportunity to gamble, and gambling products that allow for more bets within a shorter time period, some research suggests that we can expect greater rates of gambling disorder in the future. Physicians, therefore, will likely be seeing more individuals struggling with gambling disorder and need to be skilled in assessing and treating this disorder.

ASSESSMENT

With fairly high rates of gambling disorder based on epidemiological studies, it is important for clinicians to screen for the disorder. Although everyone should be screened for gambling disorder, it would seem particularly important in those people with histories of substance use disorders or psychiatric disorders. Gambling behavior and expenditures can be reliably measured with a timeline follow-back interview adapted from a method used for individuals who have problems with alcohol. A range of self-report and interview-based measures to screen either for gambling problems or for a gambling disorder have been developed. Many of these measures assess symptom over the past year or simply the past week. Several commonly used measures include: The Problem Gambling Severity Index (measures gambling severity but is not based on the DSM-5), the National Opinion Research Center DSM-5 Screen for Gambling Problems (NODS-GD), the Structured Clinical Interview for Pathological Gambling modified for Gambling Disorder (SCI-GD), and the Gambling Symptom Assessment Scale.[41]

Clinical Characteristics

Gambling disorder often begins in adolescence or early adulthood, with males tending to start at earlier ages.[1,12,42,43] Although prospective studies are largely lacking, gambling disorder appears to follow a trajectory similar to that of substance use disorder, with high rates in adolescent and young adult groups, lower rates in older adults, and periods of abstinence and recurrence of gambling, symptoms, or the disorder.[31] Gambling disorder can be a serious psychiatric disorder, but there is evidence that approximately one-third of individuals with gambling disorder experience natural recovery (ie, without formal treatment or attendance at Gamblers Anonymous).[44] The research on natural recovery, however, is based on retrospective reports, and there are no data regarding whether these individuals who are symptom-free for 1 year remain free of symptoms beyond that time or whether they experience a recurrence of gambling/symptoms/disorder or change addiction.

Significant clinical differences have been observed in men and women with gambling disorder.[45-50] Men with gambling disorder are more likely to be single and living alone as compared to women with the disorder.[50,51] Males with gambling disorder are also more likely to have sought treatment for DSM-IV–defined substance use, have higher rates of antisocial personality traits, and have marital consequences related to their gambling.[52] Though men seem to start gambling at earlier ages and have higher rates of gambling disorder, women, who constitute approximately 32% of those with gambling disorder in the United States, seem to progress more quickly to severe consequences than do men.[43] Women with gambling disorder are, however, more likely to recover from and to seek treatment for their gambling problem.[52]

The types of gambling preferred by men tend to be different from those preferred by women. Men with gambling disorder have higher rates of "strategic" forms of gambling, including sports betting, video poker, and blackjack. Women, on the other hand, have higher rates of "nonstrategic" gambling, such as slot machines or bingo.[53] In regard to gambling triggers, though both men and women report that advertisements trigger their urges to gamble, men tend to report gambling for reasons unrelated to their emotional state, whereas women report gambling to escape from stress or owing to depressive states.[54-57] Higher rates of sensation-seeking or "action"-seeking behavior in men have been suggested as the possible reason for this difference in gambling preference.[52,54,56,57]

Functional Impairment, Quality of Life, and Legal Difficulties

Individuals with gambling disorder suffer significant impairment in their ability to function socially and occupationally. Many individuals report intrusive thoughts and urges related to gambling that interfere with their ability to concentrate at home and work.[54,57] Work-related problems such as absenteeism, poor performance, and job loss are common.[54] The inability to control behavior about which a person has mixed feelings may lead to feelings of shame and guilt.[54] Gambling disorder is also frequently associated with marital problems[54] and diminished intimacy and trust within the family.[2] Financial difficulties (44% of those with gambling disorder report loss of savings or retirement funds and 22% report losing homes or automobiles or pawning valuables owing to gambling) often exacerbate personal and family problems.[54]

With the functional impairment that these individuals experience, it is not surprising that they also report poor quality of life. In three studies systematically evaluating quality of life, individuals with gambling disorder reported significantly poorer life satisfaction compared to general, nonclinical adult samples.[58-60]

Gambling disorder is also associated with greater medical comorbidity (eg, cardiac problems, liver disease, obesity) and increased use of medical services.[61-66] Possible reasons for the association of gambling disorder with health problems might be the sedentary nature of gambling, reduced leisure and exercise time, reduced sleep,[67,68] increased stress, and increased nicotine and alcohol consumption.[11]

Many individuals with gambling disorder report the need for psychiatric hospitalization owing to the depression, and at times suicidality they feel was brought on by their gambling losses.[54] Research on individuals in gambling treatment centers has found that 48% of individuals report having had gambling-related suicidal ideation at some time.[69] The often overwhelming financial consequences, such as bankruptcy,[70] associated with gambling disorder may also contribute to attempted or completed suicide.[71,72]

In addition to the emotional impact of problem and gambling disorder, many individuals with gambling disorder have faced legal difficulties related to their gambling. One study found that 27.3% of people with DSM-IV–defined pathological gambling had committed at least one gambling-related illegal act.[73] Problem or gambling disorder may lead people to engage in illegal behavior including embezzlement, stealing, and writing bad checks in order to either finance the gambling behavior or to compensate for past losses related to the excessive gambling.[74] Another study found high percentages of pathological gamblers endorsing prior acts of embezzlement (31%) and robbery (14%).[75]

Although gambling disorder is associated with multiple legal and functional difficulties, one caveat is that the research is based on relatively small numbers of individuals seeking treatment for gambling disorder, and, therefore, these studies may reflect the more severe cases of gambling disorder.

Co-occurring Psychiatric Disorders

Co-occurring psychiatric disorders are common in individuals with gambling disorder.[76] Frequent co-occurrence has been reported between substance use disorders (including nicotine use disorder) and gambling disorder, with the highest odds ratios generally observed between gambling and alcohol use disorder.[31,77-79] A Canadian epidemiological survey estimated that the relative risk for alcohol use disorder is increased 3.8-fold when disordered gambling is present.[80]

Among clinical samples, 52% of Gamblers Anonymous participants reported either alcohol or drug use,[81] and 35% to 63% of individuals seeking treatment for gambling disorder also screened positive for a lifetime substance use disorder,[1] rates notably higher than that found in the general population (26.6%).[82] Similarly, a study of 84 treatment-seeking individuals with gambling disorder noted lifetime rates of attention deficit hyperactivity disorder (ADHD) in 26.3% of the sample, much higher than the general population rates of 4% to 5%.[83]

Other studies clinically assessing co-occurring disorders in treatment-seeking individuals with gambling disorder have also noted high estimates of mood disorders (34%-78%).[84-86] McCormick and colleagues[84] studied 38 cases of treatment-seeking patients with gambling disorder and co-occurring major depressive disorder and found that, in 86% of cases, the gambling problem preceded the onset of depression. These findings, however, need to be interpreted with caution because the majority of these studies were derived from treatment-seeking adults with gambling disorder, which may or may not reflect non–treatment-seeking gambling disorder individuals. Yet, they also raise the question of whether co-occurring mood disorders may be secondary to gambling disorder. A twin study of self-reported family history to estimate shared genetic contributes to gambling disorder and major depression in men,[87] however, suggests a possible shared biological predisposition to the co-occurrence of the disorders.

High prevalence estimates of co-occurring anxiety disorders (28%-40%) also exist in those with gambling disorder,[82,88,89] but not all anxiety disorders are seen with equal frequency.[90] Research suggests that estimates of co-occurring generalized anxiety disorder range as high as 40% among gambling disorder patients,[77] whereas those of obsessive-compulsive disorder may be as low as 1%.[1] The relationship of obsessive-compulsive disorder to gambling disorder, however, has produced a mixed picture, with some studies reporting high estimates (17%-20%)[80,81] and other investigations generating low estimates (1%).[77] The rates of co-occurring disorders often have wide ranges, and this may be owing to lack of structured clinical interviews used in assessing for co-occurring psychiatric issues, the small sample sizes of gamblers assessed, the sample selection, and the possible heterogeneity of gambling disorder.

Significantly, fewer data are available regarding the frequencies of personality disorders in pathological gamblers. Studies have shown that estimates of any personality disorder in those with gambling disorder range from 25% to 93%.[85,90-92] Borderline (3%-70%), narcissistic (5%-57%), avoidant (5%-50%), and obsessive-compulsive (5%-59%) personality disorders are most commonly reported.[85,91-93] One of the best-studied personality disorders in gambling disorder, antisocial personality disorder, has been found in 15% to 40% of gambling disorder patients, a frequency higher than the 0.6% to 3% estimates reported for the general population.[94,95] Although multiple reasons may explain the elevated rates of co-occurring antisocial personality disorder in gambling disorder, evidence from past studies suggests a possible shared genetic vulnerability.[96]

Family History

High frequencies of psychiatric disorders are seen in the first-degree relatives of those with gambling disorder.[97] In studies of first-degree relatives of those with gambling disorder, the most common disorders were mood, anxiety, impulse control, and substance use disorders.[98,99] Studies have also found that individuals with gambling disorder report high rates of first-degree relatives with gambling problems.[100] A large sample of 517 individuals with gambling disorder found that subjects with at least one problem gambling parent were significantly more likely to have a father with an alcohol use disorder, report daily nicotine use, and have significantly worse legal and financial problems compared to the cohort without a problem gambling parent.[101]

TREATMENT

Psychologically Based Treatments

Although there is a long literature of case reports using psychodynamic psychotherapy, and psychodynamic psychotherapy is often incorporated into multimodal, eclectic, and integrated approaches to gambling disorder, there are no randomized controlled trials supporting its use.[102] Similarly, although some evidence exists that Gamblers Anonymous[103-106] and self-exclusion contracts[107-110] may be beneficial for gambling disorder, limited and conflicting data assessing the long-term efficacy for these interventions have been published.

A variety of psychosocial treatments have been examined in controlled studies for the treatment of gambling disorder.[111] Cognitive strategies have traditionally included cognitive restructuring, psychoeducation, and irrational cognition awareness training. Behavioral approaches focus on developing alternate activities to compete with reinforcers specific to gambling disorder as well as the identification of gambling triggers (see **Table 52-1** for a summary of psychotherapeutic treatments). Although no data support its use for gambling disorder, contingency management has been used successfully in the treatment of individuals with substance use disorder who also gamble and has not worsened the gambling behavior in these individuals.

Assessment of Psychologically Based Treatments

Empirical studies of CBT and using various elements CBT (ie, cognitive or behavioral therapy, motivational interviewing, and CBT workbooks) support the efficacy of using CBT for those with gambling disorder, because the majority of trials found reductions in gambling disorder symptomatology compared to the control conditions. However, these trials are insufficient to provide information about the optimal treatment duration and the level of training needed by the therapy administrator. Both brief and longer treatments have been found effective, but no study has randomized subjects into psychotherapeutic treatments of varying durations to determine the most efficacious treatment length. In addition, few studies have long-term follow-up, highlighting the need for future studies to include long-term follow-up visits to assess maintenance of therapeutic gains.

Furthermore, few studies provided a detailed description of the content of the therapy sessions or workbook and measurements of therapist adherence and competence. Inclusion of these items would aid in the interpretation, and application of study findings, for lack of therapist adherence to study protocol, may confound study results. Characteristics of individuals with gambling disorder who succeed in and do not respond to psychotherapy also need to be investigated. Possible variables that impact individual success as well as treatment adherence may include insight, desire to change, co-occurring psychological and physical conditions, and impulsivity.

TABLE 52-1 Controlled Psychological Treatment Trials

Study	Design/duration	Subjects	Outcome
Cognitive therapy			
Sylvain et al.[112]	Cognitive therapy with recurrence prevention compared to wait list/30 sessions with 6-month follow-up	40 enrolled; 14/22 in treatment group completed	36% improved on 5 variables compared to 6% on wait list
Ladouceur et al.[113]	Cognitive therapy plus recurrence prevention compared to wait list/20 sessions with 12-month follow-up	88 enrolled; 35/59 in treatment group completed	32% improved on 4 variables compared to 7% on wait list
Ladouceur et al.[114]	Group cognitive therapy plus recurrence prevention compared to wait list/10 weeks with 2-year follow-up	71 enrolled; 34/46 in treatment group completed	65% no longer met pathological gambling criteria compared to 20% for wait-list group
Behavioral therapy			
McConaghy et al.[115]	Aversion therapy compared to imaginal desensitization	20 enrolled; 20 completed	Improvement in both groups over 12 months
McConaghy et al.[116]	Imaginal relaxation vs imaginal desensitization/14 sessions over 1 week	20 enrolled	Improvement in both groups after 1 week, but therapeutic gains were not maintained by either group after 12 months.
McConaghy et al.[117]	Aversion therapy vs imaginal desensitization vs in vivo desensitization vs imaginal relaxation	120 enrolled; 63 available 2 and 9 years later	Imaginal desensitization improved at 1 month and at 9 years
Cognitive-behavioral therapy			
Echeburua et al.[118]	Stimulus control, in vivo exposure, recurrence prevention vs cognitive restructuring vs combined treatment vs wait list/6 weeks with 12 month follow-up	64 enrolled; 50 completed	At 12 months, 69% abstinence or much reduced in the first condition compared to 38% for cognitive restructuring or combined treatment
Milton et al.[119]	CBT vs CBT combined with interventions designed to improve treatment/8 sessions of manualized, individualized therapy	40 enrolled; 20 completed	At 9-month follow-up, there was no difference in outcome between treatments, though both produced clinically significant change in the amount of money spent gambling.
Melville et al.[120]	1. Group CBT with and without mapping-enhanced treatment or wait-list control/8 weeks 2. Mapping vs wait-list control/8 weeks	13 enrolled; 19 enrolled	Subjects in the CBT with mapping enhancement reported significant improvement and maintained this treatment at the 6-month follow-up.
Marceaux et al.[121]	12-step procedures vs CBT with mapping vs wait-list control/2 weekly meetings over 8 weeks	49 enrolled; 44 completed	Both treatment groups reported significant improvement at the end of treatment and at the 6-month study follow-up
Wulfert et al.[122]	Cognitive motivational behavioral therapy (CMBT) vs treatment-as-usual/3 phases of treatment	21 enrolled; 17 completed	Significant improvements were observed through a 12-month follow-up for the CMBT group.
Petry et al.[104]	Manualized CBT in individual counseling, vs CBT workbook vs Gamblers Anonymous referral/8 sessions with 1-year follow-up	231 enrolled	CBT was more effective than Gamblers Anonymous and individual counseling is more effective than workbook.
McIntosh et al.[123]	Manualized CBT vs mindfulness training vs treatment-as-usual, 3 initial psychoeducation sessions and then weekly for 4 weeks	77 randomized to the three arms	All three interventions were effective in reducing gambling severity after 7 sessions. Mindfulness and treatment-as-usual translated to better quality of life outcomes than seen in the manualized treatment group.

TABLE 52-1 Controlled Psychological Treatment Trials (*Continued*)

Study	Design/duration	Subjects	Outcome
Grant et al.[124,125]	Cue exposure with negative mood induction and imaginal desensitization with either individualized CBT or Gamblers Anonymous/6 weekly sessions	68 enrolled; 55 completed	At the end of the study, 64% of subjects receiving imaginal exposure plus the negative mood induction were able to maintain abstinence for 1 month compared to 17% of those randomly assigned to Gamblers Anonymous. At a 6-month follow-up posttreatment, 77% of subjects who had completed the therapy sessions maintained their improvement.
Carlbring and Smit[126]; Carlbring et al.[127]	Internet-based counseling vs control/4 hours over an 8-week period	66 enrolled (126); 284 enrolled (127)	Substantial improvements in gambling symptoms, depression, anxiety, and quality of life at posttreatment for the internet-based counseling group that were maintained at a 3-year posttreatment follow-up
Oei et al.[128]	Individual vs group CBT vs waitlist control/6 weeks	120 enrolled	Individual CBT treatment resulted in more efficacious outcomes at posttreatment, but both treatment conditions proved to be effective in reducing gambling behavior compared to the wait-list control group. Improvements were largely maintained at a 6-month follow-up posttreatment.
Casey et al.[129]	Internet-based CBT vs monitoring, feedback, and support vs wait-list control. CBT was delivered online, once per week for 6 weeks.	174 enrolled	Internet-based CBT and monitoring, feedback, and support groups reduced gambling severity and maintained improvement over 12-month follow-up. Internet-based CBT group showed additional improvements in gambling urges, stress, cognitions, and life satisfaction compared to the other groups.
Brief interventions and motivational interviewing			
Dickerson et al.[130]	CBT workbook vs workbook plus a single in-depth interview	29 enrolled	Both groups showed improvement at 6 months.
Diskin and Hodgins[131]	Motivational interviewing module plus a self-help workbook with the workbook and speaking to an interviewer/one 30-minute session	81 enrolled; 69 completed	Individuals receiving the workbook and motivational interviewing component reporting gambling less frequently and with less money compared to the workbook-alone group at a 1-year posttreatment follow-up
Petry et al.[132]	Brief advice, a motivational enhancement therapy (MET), MET plus workbook-oriented CBT, or a no-treatment control group/6 weeks	117 enrolled; 113 completed 9-month follow-up evaluation	All treatment conditions provided significant symptom improvement although MET had the most significant effect in reducing gambling symptoms relative to the no-treatment control group.
Hodgins et al.[133,134]	CBT workbook vs workbook plus motivational enhancement intervention via telephone vs wait list	102 enrolled; 85 available at 12 months	Rates of abstinence at 6 months did not differ between groups, though gambling frequency and money lost gambling were lower in the motivational intervention group.[135] Compared to the workbook alone, gambling subjects assigned to the motivational intervention and workbook reduced gambling throughout a 2-year follow-up period; however, 77% of the entire follow-up sample was still rated as improved at the 24-month assessment.[136]

(Continued)

TABLE 52-1 Controlled Psychological Treatment Trials (*Continued*)

Study	Design/duration	Subjects	Outcome
Hodgins and Holub[137]	Detailed recurrence prevention summary booklet mailed once or the same booklet with seven additional informational booklets mailed over the next 12 months	169 enrolled	At 12 months, groups did not differ in gambling frequency or extent of gambling losses.
Hodgins et al.[138]	Brief MI plus mailed self-help workbook vs workbook only vs wait-list control/6 weeks	314 enrolled	Significant decreases in gambling symptoms that were maintained at the 1-year follow-up were reported by the MI and the workbook only groups.
Carlbring et al.[139]	MI vs group CBT vs wait-list control/8 weeks	150 enrolled	CBT and MI groups reported significant decreases in gambling, depressive, and anxiety symptoms.
Cunningham et al.[140]	Brief personalized normative feedback vs wait-list control	209 enrolled; 146 completed 12-month follow-up	The feedback group had reductions in days gambled posttreatment and at 1 year.
Boudreault et al.[141]	Self-help treatment (including three motivational telephone interviews spread over an 11-week period) plus a cognitive-behavioral self-help workbook vs wait-list control.	62 enrolled	Relative to the waiting list, the treatment group showed a statistically significant reduction in the number of DSM-5 gambling disorder criteria met, gambling habits, and gambling consequences at Week 11.
Hodgins et al.[142]	Online version of a previously evaluated telephone-based intervention package vs a brief online normative feedback intervention.	181 enrolled	Participants in both conditions showed significant reductions in days of gambling and problem severity with no differences between conditions.
Jonas et al.[143]	Guided online program vs email counselling vs waitlist	167 enrolled	In comparison to waitlist, guided online program showed significant improvements with moderate to strong effect sizes in all outcomes.
Couples therapy			
Nilsson et al.[144]	Internet-based behavioral couples therapy vs cognitive-behavioral therapy	136 enrolled	No differences in the efficacy of internet-based behavioral couples therapy and cognitive-behavioral therapy.

Pharmacotherapy

No medication is currently approved by the US Food and Drug Administration and indicated for the treatment of gambling disorder. Twenty randomized, placebo-controlled trials of pharmacotherapy treatment in gambling disorder have been conducted, and these studies suggest that medications may be beneficial in treating gambling disorder (see **Table 52-2** for a summary of pharmacotherapeutic treatments).

Assessment of Pharmacotherapy

Due to the promising results of the double-blind trials of naltrexone and nalmefene, opioid antagonists appear to be the most promising pharmacological treatments for gambling disorder. Similar to the nalmefene, however, empiric trails of naltrexone should be conducted at additional research sites to examine the efficacy of naltrexone in varying patient populations. Results from trials investigating the glutamate modulator, *N*-acetylcysteine, and lithium suggest that these medications may also be effective, but with only one trial completed for lithium and two for *N*-acetylcysteine, additional research is needed to bolster support. Antidepressants have been the most widely examined ones with findings providing indefinite results, yet for individuals with high anxiety, escitalopram may be an effective treatment. Currently, no evidence supports the use of atypical antipsychotics.

More research is needed to determine the most effective dosage of each medication. Currently, only two studies[145,147] assessed the differential impact of various dosages. Also unevaluated is the long-term impact of these medications, with only two studies[135,150] assessing the pharmacological treatment effect for longer than 6 months. One challenge in pursuing these data is that studies historically have higher

TABLE 52-2 Controlled Pharmacotherapeutic Treatment Trials

Study	Medication	Study design	Subjects	Dosage	Outcome
Opioid antagonists					
Kim et al.[136]	Naltrexone (ReVia)	Parallel design 12 weeks with 1-week placebo lead-in	89 enrolled; 45 completed	188 mg (±96)	Naltrexone group significantly improved compared with placebo.
Grant et al.[145]	Naltrexone (ReVia)	Parallel design, 18 weeks	77 subjects	50, 100, or 150 mg/d	Compared to placebo, the naltrexone group had significantly reduced gambling urges and behavior.
Kovanen et al.[146]	Naltrexone (ReVia)	Parallel design, 20 weeks	101 enrolled	50 mg taken as-needed up to one time daily	No significant differences between treatment groups. Treatment discontinuation rate was 32%.
Grant et al.[147]	Nalmefene (Revex)	Parallel design, 16 weeks	207 enrolled; 73 completed	25, 50, or 100 mg/d	Nalmefene 25 mg and 50 mg significantly improved compared to placebo.
Grant et al.[148]	Nalmefene (Revex)	Parallel design, 16 weeks	233 enrolled	Titrated up to 5 mg/d each week until reaching a maximum dosage of 40 mg/d at week 4 through the end of the treatment period	Dosage of 40 mg/d resulted in significantly greater reductions in gambling urges and behaviors compared to placebo.
Alho et al.[149]	Intranasal Naloxone	Parallel design, 12 weeks; Naloxone used as needed; compared to placebo as needed	126 enrolled; 106 completed		Reduction in gambling urges did not differ significantly between groups
Antidepressants					
Saiz-Ruiz et al.[150]	Sertraline (Zoloft)	Parallel design, 6 months	60 enrolled; 44 completed	95 mg	Similar improvement in both groups
Hollander et al.[151]	Fluvoxamine (Luvox)	Crossover, 16 weeks with a 1-week placebo lead-in	15 enrolled; 10 completed	195 mg (±50)	Fluvoxamine superior to placebo
Blanco et al.[135]	Fluvoxamine (Luvox)	Parallel design, 6 months	32 enrolled; 13 completed	200 mg	Fluvoxamine not statistically significant from placebo
Kim et al.[152]	Paroxetine (Paxil)	Parallel design, 8 weeks with 1-week placebo lead-in	53 enrolled; 41 completed	51.7 mg (±13.1)	Paroxetine group significantly improved compared to placebo.
Grant et al.[153]	Paroxetine (Paxil)	Parallel design, 16 weeks	76 enrolled; 45 completed	50 mg (±8.3)	Paroxetine and placebo groups with comparable improvement
Grant and Potenza[154]	Escitalopram (Lexapro)	Parallel design, 8-week discontinuation from 12 week open-label	13 enrolled with co-occurring anxiety disorders	25.4 (±6.6) mg/d	Improvement in gambling and anxiety symptomology was maintained in the escitalopram group, while the placebo group reported increasing symptoms.
Black et al.[155]	Bupropion (Wellbutrin)	Parallel design, 12 weeks	39 enrolled; 22 completed	324 mg/d	Bupropion was not superior to placebo.

(Continued)

TABLE 52-2 Controlled Pharmacotherapeutic Treatment Trials (*Continued*)

Study	Medication	Study design	Subjects	Dosage	Outcome
Mood stabilizers					
de Brito et al.[156]	Topiramate (Topamax) and cognitive restructuring	Parallel design, 12 weeks	38 enrolled; 30 completed	Mean daily dose was 181 mg/d	Topiramate was superior to placebo in reducing craving to gamble and cognitive distortions.
Berlin et al.[157]	Topiramate (Topamax)	Parallel design, 14 weeks	42 enrolled	25-200 mg/d	No significant differences between groups
Hollander et al.[158]	Lithium carbonate SR (Lithobid SR)	Parallel design, 10 weeks	40 bipolar-spectrum patients enrolled; 29 completed	1170 mg (±221)	Lithium group significantly improved compared with placebo.
Glutamatergic agents					
Grant et al.[159]	*N*-acetylcysteine (NAC)	Parallel design. 6-week discontinuation from 8-week open-label	13 enrolled	1477 mg/d (±311)	83% receiving NAC were classified as responders compared to 29% on placebo.
Grant et al.[160]	*N*-acetylcysteine (NAC) as augmentation to behavioral therapy	Parallel design, 12 weeks 3-month follow-up	28 enrolled; 20 completed	12,00-3,000 mg/d	All subjects benefited from imaginal desensitization in the first 6 weeks. NAC group significantly improved on gambling symptoms over study and at 3-month follow-up compared to placebo.
Atypical antipsychotics					
Fong et al.[161]	Olanzapine (Zyprexa)	Parallel design, 7 weeks	21 enrolled	Titrated up 2.5 mg/d each week until reaching a maximum dosage of 10 mg/d at week 4 through the end of the treatment period	No significant differences between treatment groups
McElroy et al.[162]	Olanzapine (Zyprexa)	Parallel design, 12 weeks	42 enrolled	8.9 mg/d (±5.2)	No significant differences between treatment groups

rates of treatment discontinuation by the subject/patient (44%-59%).[135,150]

Understanding clinical and demographic variables may also help clinicians find the most efficacious treatments. Individuals with intense gambling urges may respond better to naltrexone,[136] and males and younger individuals with gambling disorder may respond well to fluvoxamine.[135] There are limited data concerning the efficacy of pharmacotherapy for individuals with gambling disorder and a co-occurring psychiatric disorder. Preliminary findings suggest that individuals with gambling disorder and bipolar disorder may respond best to lithium,[158] while those with co-occurring anxiety may find relief with escitalopram.[154] These findings suggest that investigating the clinical characteristics of individuals who positively respond (as well as those who do not respond) to treatment is necessary. In addition, no randomized, placebo-controlled studies have been completed comparing pharmacotherapy treatments or comparing pharmacotherapy to psychotherapy. These trials would provide insight into which individuals may respond best to a certain class of medication or psychotherapeutic treatment.

Treatment Recommendations

Gambling disorder is a common, disabling psychiatric disorder that is associated with high rates of co-occurring disorders, particularly substance use disorders, and high rates of illegal activities. Psychotherapy and pharmacotherapy have shown promise in the treatment of gambling disorder. Based on the treatment literature, the off-label use of naltrexone would appear the most promising pharmacological option for a working clinician. A selective serotonin reuptake inhibitor antidepressant used off-label may also be beneficial particularly when the individual has co-occurring depression or anxiety.

In terms of psychosocial treatments, cognitive-behavioral therapy appears promising. There are several manualized forms of this therapy. Although the stronger evidence suggests that eight sessions of CBT should be considered, a growing body of data suggests that even fewer sessions or brief interventions may be effective. With a manualized treatment, counselors with a background in addiction counseling should be able to deliver the treatment with minimal training.

Even knowing the evidence for various treatment options for gambling disorder, other factors may influence which treatment option is chosen for a particular patient. First, many clinicians are simply unaware of gambling disorder. Therefore, if a clinician is referring a patient for either medication management or psychotherapy, it may simply be difficult to find people who know how to treat the behavior. This problem can be minimized by having a list of providers who know about gambling disorder and can provide treatment. For example, if no one is available to do CBT for gambling disorder, then perhaps medication management should be attempted first.

Second, there are no clear treatment recommendations for a clinician to follow. For example, it is unclear exactly how many sessions of CBT are most helpful for gambling disorder. The exact dose of medication or duration of medication trial for optimal treatment is also unknown. These gaps in knowledge make it difficult to inform patients about what their care may entail and what expectations they may have.

Third, individuals with gambling disorder exhibit high rates of placebo response in treatment studies. Clinicians need to understand that for many patients with gambling disorder, simply talking about their problem will help substantially at first. This initial robust response, however, may cause the clinician to believe that his or her treatment approach is successful. Clinicians should carefully monitor the patient for several months and not assume they will continue to do well. Involving a family member or close friend who can assist the patient in monitoring their behavior and provide accountability may also be beneficial for some patients.

Fourth, impulsive patients do not often follow recommendations or follow-up with treatment. The treatment data consistently show that treatment discontinuation rates are high for gambling disorder. This may be owing to two factors: first, patients often believe they are doing better than in fact they are and therefore see treatment as unnecessary, and second, they do not have an instantaneous response and therefore do not stay with treatment. Both of these concerns can be minimized by providing psychoeducation about the illness, detailing the expectations of treatment, and expressing the need to stay in treatment.

In conclusion, the available data shows that gambling disorder is common, associated with a poor quality of life, and often with multiple co-occurring psychiatric and medical issues. There are several valid instruments to screen and diagnose gambling disorder and assess severity. Treatment for gambling disorder includes both psychological interventions as well as pharmacotherapy. Although current evidence-based treatment approaches for gambling disorder are promising, more work to evaluate the most effective treatments for subgroups of individuals with gambling disorder based on symptom presentation and co-occurring issues still needs to be done.

REFERENCES

1. Black DW. Clinical characteristics. In: Grant JE, Potenza MN, eds. *Gambling Disorder: A Clinical Guide to Treatment*. 2nd ed. American Psychiatric Publishing; 2021:17-38.
2. Petry NM, ed. *Pathological Gambling: Etiology, Comorbidity, and Treatment*. American Psychological Association; 2005.
3. American Psychiatric Association. *Diagnostic and Statistical Manual of Mental Disorders*. 3rd ed. (DSM-III). American Psychiatric Publishing; 1980.
4. Leeman RF, Potenza MN. Similarities and differences between pathological gambling and substance use disorders: a focus on impulsivity and compulsivity. *Psychopharmacology*. 2012;219(2):469-490.
5. Grant JE, Potenza MN, Weinstein A, Gorelick DA. Introduction to behavioral addictions. *Am J Drug Alcohol Abuse*. 2010;36(5): 233-241.
6. Holden C. Psychiatry: behavioral addictions debut in proposed DSM-V. *Science*. 2010;327(5968):935.
7. Lawrence AJ, Luty J, Bogdan NA, Sahakian BJ, Clark L. Impulsivity and response inhibition in alcohol dependence and problem gambling. *Psychopharmacology*. 2009;207(1):163-172.
8. Grant JE, Odlaug BL, Chamberlain SR. Gambling disorder, DSM-5 criteria and symptom severity. *Compr Psychiatry*. 2017;75:1-5.
9. Kallick MD, Suits T, Deilman T, et al. *A Survey of American Gambling Attitudes and Behavior*. Research report series Survey Research Center, Institute for Social Research, University of Michigan Press; 1979.
10. Gerstein D, Murphy S, Toce M, et al. *Gambling Impact and Behavior Study: Final Report to the National Gambling Impact Study Commission*. National Opinion Research Center; 1999.
11. Welte J, Barnes G, Wieczorek W. Alcohol and gambling pathology among U.S. adults: prevalence, demographic patterns and comorbidity. *J Stud Alcohol*. 2001;62(5):706-712.
12. Petry NM, Stinson FS, Grant BF. Comorbidity of DSM-IV pathological gambling and other psychiatric disorders: results from the National Epidemiologic Survey on Alcohol and Related Conditions. *J Clin Psychiatry*. 2005;66(5):564-574.
13. Shaffer HJ, Hall MN, Vander BJ. Estimating the prevalence of disordered gambling behavior in the United States and Canada: a research synthesis. *Am J Public Health*. 1999;89(9):1369-1376.
14. Rush B, Veldhuizen S, Adlaf E. Mapping the prevalence of problem gambling and its association with treatment accessibility and proximity to gambling venues. *J Gambl Issues*. 2007;20:193-214.
15. Okuda M, Liu W, Cisewski JA, Segura L, Storr CL, Martins SS. Gambling disorder and minority populations: prevalence and risk factors. *Curr Addict Rep*. 2016;3(3):280-292.
16. Richard J, Martin-Storey A, Wilkie E, Derevensky JL, Paskus T, Temcheff CE. Variations in gambling disorder symptomatology across sexual identity among college student-athletes. *J Gambl Stud*. 2019;35(4):1303-1316.
17. Broman N, Prever F, di Giacomo E, et al. Gambling, gaming, and internet behavior in a sexual minority perspective. A Cross-Sectional Study in Seven European Countries. *Front Psychol*. 2022;12:707645.
18. Alegria AA, Petry NM, Hasin DS, Liu SM, Grant BF, Blanco C. Disordered gambling among racial and ethnic groups in the US: results from the national epidemiologic survey on alcohol and related conditions. *CNS Spectr*. 2009;14(3):132-142.
19. Kong G, Tsai J, Pilver CE, Tan HS, Hoff RA, Cavallo DA. Differences in gambling problem severity and gambling and health/functioning characteristics among Asian-American and Caucasian high-school students. *Psychiatry Res*. 2013;210(3):1071-1078.
20. Raylu N. Oei TP. Role of culture in gambling and problem gambling. *Clin Psychol Rev*. 2004;23(8):1087-1114.

21. Berger M, Sarnyai Z. "More than skin deep": stress neurobiology and mental health consequences of racial discrimination. *Stress.* 2015;18(1):1-10.
22. Stefanovics EA, Potenza MN, Pietrzak RH. Gambling in a National U.S. Veteran Population: prevalence, socio-demographics, and psychiatric comorbidities. *J Gambl Stud.* 2017;33(4):1099-1120.
23. Claesdotter-Knutsson E, André F, Fridh M, Delfin C, Håkansson A, Lindström M. Gender differences and associated factors influencing problem gambling in adolescents in Sweden: cross-sectional investigation. *JMIR Pediatr Parent.* 2022;5(1):e35207.
24. Odlaug BL, Grant JE. Impulse-control disorders in a college sample: results from the self-administered Minnesota Impulse Disorders Interview (MIDI). *Prim Care Companion J Clin Psychiatry.* 2010; 12(2):
25. González-Roz A, Fernández-Hermida JR, Weidberg S, Martínez-Loredo V, Secades-Villa R. Prevalence of problem gambling among adolescents: a comparison across modes of access, gambling activities, and levels of severity. *J Gambl Stud.* 2017;33(2):371-382.
26. Wardle H, Sproston K, Orford J, et al. *British Gambling Prevalence Survey 2007.* National Center for Social Research; 2007.
27. Bakken IJ, Götestam KG, Gråwe RW, Wenzel HG, Øren A. Gambling behavior and gambling problems in Norway 2007. *Scand J Psychol.* 2009;50(4):333-339.
28. Tavares H, Carneiro E, Sanches M, et al. Gambling in Brazil: lifetime prevalences and socio-demographic correlates. *Psychiatry Res.* 2010; 180(1):35-41.
29. Romo L, Legauffre C, Genolini C, et al. Prevalence of pathological gambling in the general population around Paris: preliminary study. *Encéphale.* 2011;37(4):278-283.
30. Erbas B, Buchner UG. Pathological gambling: prevalence, diagnosis, comorbidity, and intervention in Germany. *Dtsch Arztebl Int.* 2012; 109(10):173-179.
31. Grant JE, Chamberlain SR. Gambling and substance use: comorbidity and treatment implications. *Prog Neuro-Psychopharmacol Biol Psychiatry.* 2020;99:109852.
32. Ronzitti S, Kraus SW, Decker SE, Ashrafioun L. Clinical characteristics of veterans with gambling disorders seeking pain treatment. *Addict Behav.* 2019;95:160-165.
33. ANPAA; Nalpas B, Yguel J, Fleury B, Martin S, Jarraud D, Craplet M. Pathological gambling in treatment-seeking alcoholics: a national survey in France. *Alcohol Alcohol.* 2011;46(2):156-160.
34. Grant JE, Levine L, Kim D, Potenza M. Impulse control disorders in adult psychiatric inpatients. *Am J Psychiatry.* 2005;162(11):2184-2188.
35. Grant JE, Williams KA, Potenza MN. Impulse-control disorders in adolescent psychiatric inpatients: co-occurring disorders and sex differences. *J Clin Psychiatry.* 2007;68(10):1584-1592.
36. Aragay N, Roca A, Garcia B, et al. Pathological gambling in a psychiatric sample. *Compr Psychiatry.* 2012;53(1):9-14.
37. Müller A, Rein K, Kollei I, et al. Impulse control disorders in psychiatric inpatients. *Psychiatry Res.* 2011;188(3):434-438.
38. King DL, Gainsbury SM, Delfabbro PH. Online gambling and gambling-gaming convergence. In: Grant JE, Potenza MN, eds. *Gambling Disorder: A Clinical Guide to Treatment.* 2nd ed. American Psychiatric Publishing; 2021:67-84.
39. Díaz A, Pérez L. Online gambling-related harm: findings from the study on the prevalence, behavior and characteristics of gamblers in Spain. *J Gambl Stud.* 2021;37(2):599-607.
40. Mravčík V, Chomynová P, Grohmannová K, Rous Z. Gambling products and their risk potential for gambling disorder. *Cas Lek Cesk.* 2020;159(5):196-202.
41. Stinchfield R. Screening and assessment instruments. In: Grant JE, Potenza MN, eds. *Gambling Disorder: A Clinical Guide to Treatment.* 2nd ed. American Psychiatric Publishing; 2021:135-180.
42. Ibáñez A, Blanco C, Moreryra P, Sáiz-Ruiz J. Gender differences in pathological gambling. *J Clin Psychiatry.* 2003;64(3):295-301.
43. Grant JE, Odlaug BL, Mooney ME. Telescoping phenomenon in pathological gambling: association with gender and comorbidities. *J Nerv Ment Dis.* 2012;200(11):996-998.
44. Slutske WS. Natural recovery and treatment-seeking in pathological gambling: results of two U.S. national surveys. *Am J Psychiatry.* 2006;163(2):297-302.
45. Afifi TO, Cox BJ, Martens PJ, Sareen J, Enns MW. Demographic and social variables associated with problem gambling among men and women in Canada. *Psychiatry Res.* 2010;178(2):395-400.
46. Echeburúa E, González-Ortega I, de Corral P, Polo-López R. Clinical gender differences among adult pathological gamblers seeking treatment. *J Gambl Stud.* 2011;27(2):215-227.
47. Crisp BR, Thomas SA, Jackson AC, et al. Not the same: a comparison of female and male clients seeking treatment from problem gambling counseling services. *J Gambl Stud.* 2004;20(3):283-299.
48. Jiménez-Murcia S, Granero R, Giménez M, et al. Contribution of sex on the underlying mechanism of the gambling disorder severity. *Sci Rep.* 2020;10(1):18722.
49. Dunsmuir P, Smith D, Fairweather-Schmidt AK, Riley B, Battersby M. Gender differences in temporal relationships between gambling urge and cognitions in treatment-seeking adults. *Psychiatry Res.* 2018;262:282-289.
50. Ronzitti S, Lutri V, Smith N, Clerici M, Bowden-Jones H. Gender differences in treatment-seeking British pathological gamblers. *J Behav Addict.* 2016;5(2):231-238.
51. Grant JE, Chamberlain SR. Gender differences. In: Grant JE, Potenza MN, eds. *Gambling Disorder: A Clinical Guide to Treatment.* 2nd ed. American Psychiatric Publishing; 2021:53-66.
52. Slutske WS, Blaszczynski A, Martin NG. Sex differences in the rates of recovery, treatment-seeking, and natural recovery in pathological gambling: results from an Australian community-based twin survey. *Twin Res Hum Genet.* 2009;12(5):425-432.
53. Odlaug BL, Marsch PH, Kim SW, Grant JE. Strategic versus non-strategic gambling: characteristics of pathological gamblers based on gambling preference. *Ann Clin Psychiatry.* 2011;23(2):105-112.
54. Grant JE, Kim SW. Demographic and clinical characteristics of 131 adult pathological gamblers. *J Clin Psychiatry.* 2001;62(12):957-962.
55. Vitaro F, Arseneault L, Tremblay RE. Dispositional predictors of problem gambling in male adolescents. *Am J Psychiatry.* 1997;154:1769-1770.
56. Wong G, Zane N, Saw A, Chan AK. Examining gender differences for gambling engagement and gambling problems among emerging adults. *J Gambl Stud.* 2013;29(2):171-189.
57. Pallanti S, Baldini Rossi N, Hollander E. Pathological gambling. In: Stein DJ, Hollander E, eds. *Clinical Manual of Impulse Control Disorders.* American Psychiatric Publishing; 2006:251-289.
58. Black DW, Moyer T, Schlosser S. Quality of life and family history in pathological gambling. *J Nerv Ment Disord.* 2003;191:124-126.
59. Grant JE, Kim SW. Quality of life in kleptomania and pathological gambling. *Compr Psychiatry.* 2005;46(1):34-37.
60. Mythily S, Edimansyah A, Qiu S, Munidasa W. Quality of life in pathological gamblers in a multiethnic Asian setting. *Ann Acad Med Singap.* 2011;40(6):264-268.
61. Morasco BJ, Vom Eigen KA, Petry NM. Severity of gambling is associated with physical and emotional health in urban primary care patients. *Gen Hosp Psychiatry.* 2006;28(2):94-100.
62. Morasco BJ, Petry NM. Gambling problems and health functioning in individuals receiving disability. *Disabil Rehabil.* 2006;28(10):619-623.
63. Potenza MN, Fiellin DA, Heninger GR, Rounsaville BJ, Mazure CM. Gambling: an addictive behavior with health and primary care implications. *J Gen Intern Med.* 2002;17(9):721-732.
64. Morasco BJ, Pietrzak RH, Blanco C, Grant BF, Hasin D, Petry NM. Health problems and medical utilization associated with gambling disorders: results from the National Epidemiologic Survey on Alcohol and Related Conditions. *Psychosom Med.* 2006;68(6):976-984.
65. Pietrzak RH, Morasco BJ, Blanco C, Grant BF, Petry NM. Gambling level and psychiatric and medical disorders in older adults: results from the National Epidemiologic Survey on Alcohol and Related Conditions. *Am J Geriatr Psychiatry.* 2007;15(4):301-313.
66. Grant JE, Derbyshire K, Leppink E, Chamberlain SR. Obesity and gambling: neurocognitive and clinical associations. *Acta Psychiatr Scand.* 2015;131(5):379-386.

67. Parhami I, Siani A, Rosenthal RJ, Fong TW. Pathological gambling, problem gambling and sleep complaints: an analysis of the National Comorbidity Survey: Replication (NCS-R). *J Gambl Stud.* 2013;29(2):241-253.
68. Grant JE, Chamberlain SR. Sleepiness and impulsivity: findings in non-treatment seeking young adults. *J Behav Addict.* 2018;7(3):737-742.
69. Ledgerwood DM, Petry NM. Gambling and suicidality in treatment-seeking pathological gamblers. *J Nerv Ment Disord.* 2004;192(10):711-714.
70. Grant JE, Schreiber L, Odlaug BL, Kim SW. Pathologic gambling and bankruptcy. *Compr Psychiatry.* 2010;51(2):115-120.
71. Carr MM, Ellis JD, Ledgerwood DM. Suicidality among gambling helpline callers: a consideration of the role of financial stress and conflict. *Am J Addict.* 2018;27(6):531-537.
72. Wardle H, John A, Dymond S, McManus S. Problem gambling and suicidality in England: secondary analysis of a representative cross-sectional survey. *Public Health.* 2020;184:11-16.
73. Potenza MN, Steinberg MA, McLaughlin SD, Rounsaville BJ, O'Malley SS. Illegal behaviors in problem gambling: an analysis of data from a gambling helpline. *J Am Acad Psychiatry Law.* 2000;28:389-403.
74. Adolphe A, Khatib L, van Golde C, Gainsbury SM, Blaszczynski A. Crime and gambling disorders: a systematic review. *J Gambl Stud.* 2019;35(2):395-414.
75. Ledgerwood DM, Weinstock J, Morasco BJ, Petry NM. Clinical features and treatment prognosis of pathological gamblers with and without recent gambling-related illegal behavior. *J Am Acad Psychiatry Law.* 2007;35(3):294-301.
76. Lorains FK, Cowlishaw S, Thomas SA. Prevalence of comorbid disorders in problem and pathological gambling: systematic review and meta-analysis of population surveys. *Addiction.* 2011;106(3):490-498.
77. Cunningham-Williams RM, Cottler LB, Compton WM III, Spitznagel EL. Taking chances: problem gamblers and mental health disorders—results from the St. Louis Epidemiologic Catchment Area Study. *Am J Public Health.* 1998;88(7):1093-1096.
78. Wareham JD, Potenza MN. Pathological gambling and substance use disorders. *Am J Drug Alcohol Abuse.* 2010;36(5):242-247.
79. Harries MD, Redden SA, Leppink EW, Chamberlain SR, Grant JE. Subclinical alcohol consumption and gambling disorder. *J Gambl Stud.* 2017;33(2):473-486.
80. Bland RC, Newman SC, Orn H, Stebelsky G. Epidemiology of pathological gambling in Edmonton. *Can J Psychiatr.* 1993;38(2):108-112.
81. Linden RD, Pope HG, Jonas JM. Pathological gambling and major affective disorders: preliminary findings. *J Clin Psychiatry.* 1986;47:201-203.
82. Kessler RC, McGonagle KA, Zhao S, et al. Lifetime and 12-month prevalence of DSM-III-R psychiatric disorders in the United States. Results from the National Comorbidity Survey. *Arch Gen Psychiatry.* 1994;51(1):8-19.
83. Grall-Bronnec M, Wainstein L, Augy J, et al. Attention deficit hyperactivity disorder among pathological and at-risk gamblers seeking treatment: a hidden disorder. *Eur Addict Res.* 2011;17(5):231-240.
84. McCormick RA, Russo AM, Rameriz LF, Taber JI. Affective disorders among pathological gamblers seeking treatment. *Am J Psychiatry.* 1984;141:215-218.
85. Black DW, Moyer T. Clinical features and psychiatric comorbidity of subjects with pathological gambling behavior. *Psychiatr Serv.* 1998;49:1434-1439.
86. Specker SM, Carlson GA, Christenson GA, Marcotte M. Impulse control disorders and attention deficit disorder in pathological gamblers. *Ann Clin Psychiatry.* 1995;7(4):175-179.
87. Potenza MN, Xian H, Shah K, Scherrer JF, Eisen SA. Shared genetic contributions to pathological gambling and major depression in men. *Arch Gen Psychiatry.* 2005;62(9):1015-1021.
88. Medeiros GC, Sampaio DG, Leppink EW, Chamberlain SR, Grant JE. Anxiety, gambling activity, and neurocognition: a dimensional approach to a non-treatment-seeking sample. *J Behav Addict.* 2016;5(2): 261-270.
89. Giddens JL, Stefanovics E, Pilver CE, Desai R, Potenza MN. Pathological gambling severity and co-occurring psychiatric disorders in individuals with and without anxiety disorders in a nationally representative sample. *Psychiatry Res.* 2012;199(1):58-64.
90. Specker S, Carlson G, Edmonson K, Johnson PE, Marcotte M. Psychopathology in pathological gamblers seeking treatment. *J Gambl Stud.* 1996;12:67-81.
91. Blaszczynski A, Steel Z. Personality disorders among pathological gamblers. *J Gambl Stud.* 1998;14:51-71.
92. Odlaug BL, Schreiber LR, Grant JE. Personality disorders and dimensions in pathological gambling. *J Personal Disord.* 2012;26(3):381-392.
93. Medeiros GC, Grant JE. Gambling disorder and obsessive-compulsive personality disorder: a frequent but understudied comorbidity. *J Behav Addict.* 2018;7(2):366-374.
94. Compton WM, Conway KP, Stinson FS. Prevalence, correlates, and comorbidity of DSM-IV antisocial personality syndromes and alcohol and specific drug use disorders in the United States: results from the national epidemiologic survey on alcohol and related conditions. *J Clin Psychiatry.* 2005;66(6):677-685.
95. Lenzenweger MF, Lane MC, Loranger AW, Kessler RC. DSM-IV personality disorders in the National Comorbidity Survey Replication. *Biol Psychiatry.* 2007;62(6):553-564.
96. Slutske WS, Eisen S, Xian H, et al. A twin study of the association between pathological gambling and antisocial personality disorder. *J Abnorm Psychol.* 2001;110(2):297-308.
97. Dowling NA, Francis KL, Dixon R, et al. "It Runs in Your Blood": reflections from treatment seeking gamblers on their family history of gambling. *J Gambl Stud.* 2021;37(2):689-710.
98. Black DW, Coryell WH, Crowe RR, McCormick B, Shaw MC, Allen J. A direct, controlled, blind family study of DSM-IV pathological gambling. *J Clin Psychiatry.* 2014;75(3):215-221.
99. Black DW, Monahan PO, Temkit M, Shaw M. A family study of pathologic gambling. *Psychiatry Res.* 2006;141(3):295-303.
100. Versini A, LeGauffre C, Romo L, Adès J, Gorwood P. Frequency of gambling problems among parents of pathological, versus nonpathological, casino gamblers using slot machines. *Am J Addict.* 2012;21(1):86-95.
101. Schreiber L, Odlaug BL, Kim SW, Grant JE. Characteristics of pathological gamblers with a problem gambling parent. *Am J Addict.* 2009;18(6):462-469.
102. Rosenthal RJ. Psychodynamic psychotherapy and the treatment of pathological gambling. *Brazil J Psychiatry.* 2008;30(Suppl 1):S41-S50.
103. Hodgins DC, Peden N, Cassidy E. The association between comorbidity and outcome in pathological gambling: a prospective follow-up of recent quitters. *J Gambl Stud.* 2005;21(3):255-271.
104. Petry NM, Ammerman Y, Bohl J, et al. Cognitive-behavioral therapy for pathological gamblers. *J Consult Clin Psychol.* 2006;74(3):555-567.
105. Stewart RM, Brown RI. An outcome study of gamblers anonymous. *Br J Psychiatry.* 1988;152:284-288.
106. Taber JI, McCormick RA, Ramirez LF. The prevalence and impact of major life stressors among pathological gamblers. *Int J Addict.* 1987;22(1):71-79.
107. Ladouceur R, Jacques C, Giroux I, Ferland F, Leblond J. Analysis of a casino's self-exclusion program. *J Gambl Stud.* 2000;16(4):453-460.
108. Ladouceur R, Sylvain C, Gosselin P. Self-exclusion program: a longitudinal evaluation study. *J Gambl Stud.* 2007;23(1):85-94.
109. Nelson SE, Kleschinsky JH, LaBrie RA, Kaplan S, Shaffer HJ. One decade of self exclusion: Missouri casino self-excluders four to ten years after enrollment. *J Gambl Stud.* 2010;26(1):129-144.
110. Hayer T, Meyer G. Self-exclusion as a harm minimization strategy: evidence for the casino sector from selected European countries. *J Gambl Stud.* 2011;27(4):685-700.
111. Hodgins DC, Stea JN, Grant JE. Gambling disorders. *Lancet.* 2011;378(9806):1874-1884.
112. Sylvain C, Ladouceur R, Boisvert JM. Cognitive and behavioral treatment of pathological gambling: a controlled study. *J Couns Clin Psychol.* 1997;65(5):727-732.

113. Ladouceur R, Sylvain C, Boutin C, et al. Cognitive treatment of pathological gambling. *J Nerv Ment Dis*. 2001;189(11):774-780.
114. Ladouceur R, Sylvain C, Boutin C, Lachance S, Doucet C, Leblond J. Group therapy for pathological gamblers: a cognitive approach. *Behav Res Ther*. 2003;41(5):587-596.
115. McConaghy N, Armstrong MS, Blaszczynski A, Allcock C. Controlled comparison of aversive therapy and imaginal desensitization in compulsive gambling. *Br J Psychiatry*. 1983;142:366-372.
116. McConaghy N, Armstrong MS, Blaszczynski A, Allcock C. Behavior completion versus stimulus control in compulsive gambling. Implications for behavioral assessment. *Behav Modif*. 1988;12(3):371-384.
117. McConaghy N, Blaszczynski A, Frankova A. Comparison of imaginal desensitisation with other behavioural treatments of pathological gambling: a two- to nine-year follow-up. *Br J Psychiatry*. 1991;159:390-393.
118. Echeburúa E, Baez C, Fernández-Montalvo J. Comparative effectiveness of three therapeutic modalities in psychological treatment of pathological gambling: long term outcome. *Behav Cogn Psychother*. 1996;24:51-72.
119. Milton S, Crino R, Hunt C, Prosser E. The effect of compliance-improving interventions on the cognitive-behavioural treatment of pathological gambling. *J Gambl Stud*. 2002;18(2):207-229.
120. Melville CL, Davis CS, Matzenbacher DL, Clayborne J. Node-link-mapping-enhanced group treatment for pathological gambling. *Addict Behav*. 2004;29:73-87.
121. Marceaux JC, Melville CL. Twelve-step facilitated versus mapping-enhanced cognitive-behavioral therapy for pathological gambling: a controlled study. *J Gambl Stud*. 2011;27(1):171-190.
122. Wulfert E, Blanchard EB, Freidenberg BM. Retaining pathological gamblers in cognitive behavior therapy through motivational enhancement. *Behav Modif*. 2006;30(3):315-340.
123. McIntosh CC, Crino RD, O'Neill K. Treating problem gambling samples with cognitive behavioural therapy and mindfulness-based interventions: a clinical trial. *J Gambl Stud*. 2016;32(4):1305-1325.
124. Grant JE, Donahue CB, Odlaug BL, Kim SW, Miller MJ, Petry N. Imaginal desensitisation plus motivational interviewing for pathological gambling: randomised controlled trial. *Br J Psychiatry*. 2009;195(3):266-267.
125. Grant JE, Donahue CB, Odlaug BL, Kim SW. A 6-month follow-up of imaginal desensitization plus motivational interviewing in the treatment of pathological gambling. *Ann Clin Psychiatry*. 2011;23(1):3-10.
126. Carlbring P, Smit F. Randomized trial of internet-delivered self-help with telephone support for pathological gamblers. *J Consult Clin Psychol*. 2008;76(6):1090-1094.
127. Carlbring P, Degerman N, Jonsson J, Andersson G. Internet-based treatment of pathological gambling with a three-year follow-up. *Cogn Behav Ther*. 2012;41(4):321-334.
128. Oei TP, Raylu N, Casey LM. Effectiveness of group and individual formats of a combined motivational interviewing and cognitive behavioral treatment program for problem gambling: a randomized controlled trial. *Behav Cogn Psychother*. 2010;38(2):233-238.
129. Casey LM, Oei TP, Raylu N, et al. Internet-based delivery of cognitive behaviour therapy compared to monitoring, feedback and support for problem gambling: a randomised controlled trial. *J Gambl Stud*. 2017;33(3):993-1010.
130. Dickerson M, Hinchy J, England SL. Minimal treatments and problem gamblers: a preliminary investigation. *J Gambl Stud*. 1990;6(1): 87-102.
131. Diskin KM, Hodgins DC. A randomized controlled trial of a single session motivational intervention for concerned gamblers. *Behav Res Ther*. 2009;47:382-388.
132. Petry NM, Weinstock J, Morasco BJ, Ledgerwood DM. Brief motivational interventions for college student problem gamblers. *Addiction*. 2009;104(9):1569-1578.
133. Hodgins DC, Currie S, el-Guebaly N. Motivational enhancement and self-help treatments for problem gambling. *J Couns Clin Psychol*. 2001;69(1):50-57.
134. Hodgins DC, Currie S, el-Guebaly N, Peden N. Brief motivational treatment for problem gambling: a 24-month follow-up. *Psychol Addict Behav*. 2004;18(3):293-296.
135. Blanco C, Petkova E, Ibáñez A, Sáiz-Ruiz J. A pilot placebo-controlled study of fluvoxamine for pathological gambling. *Ann Clin Psychiatry*. 2002;14(1):9-15.
136. Kim SW, Grant JE, Adson DE, Shin YC. Double-blind naltrexone and placebo comparison study in the treatment of pathological gambling. *Biol Psychiatry*. 2001;49(11):914-921.
137. Hodgins DC, Holub A. Treatment of problem gambling. In: Smith G, Hodgins DC, Williams RJ, eds. *Research and Measurement Issues in Gambling Studies*. Elsevier; 2007:371-397.
138. Hodgins DC, Currie SR, Currie G, Fick GH. Randomized trial of brief motivational treatments for pathological gamblers: more is not necessarily better. *J Consult Clin Psychol*. 2009;77(5):950-960.
139. Carlbring P, Jonsson J, Josephson H, Forsberg L. Motivational interviewing versus cognitive behavioral group therapy in the treatment of problem and pathological gambling: a randomized controlled trial. *Cogn Behav Ther*. 2010;39(2):92-103.
140. Cunningham JA, Hodgins DC, Toneatto T, Murphy M. A randomized controlled trial of personalized feedback intervention for problem gamblers. *PLoS One*. 2012;7(2):e31586.
141. Boudreault C, Giroux I, Jacques C, Goulet A, Simoneau H, Ladouceur R. Efficacy of a self-help treatment for at-risk and pathological gamblers. *J Gambl Stud*. 2018;34(2):561-580.
142. Hodgins DC, Cunningham JA, Murray R, Hagopian S. Online self-directed interventions for gambling disorder: randomized controlled trial. *J Gambl Stud*. 2019;35(2):635-651.
143. Jonas B, Leuschner F, Eiling A, Schoelen C, Soellner R, Tossmann P. Web-based intervention and email-counseling for problem gamblers: results of a randomized controlled trial. *J Gambl Stud*. 2020;36(4):1341-1358.
144. Nilsson A, Magnusson K, Carlbring P, Andersson G, Hellner C. Behavioral couples therapy versus cognitive behavioral therapy for problem gambling: a randomized controlled trial. *Addiction*. 2020;115(7):1330-1342.
145. Grant JE, Kim SW, Hartman BK. A double-blind, placebo-controlled study of the opiate antagonist, naltrexone, in the treatment of pathological gambling urges. *J Clin Psychiatry*. 2008;69(5):783-789.
146. Kovanen L, Basnet S, Castrén S, et al. A randomised, double-blind, placebo-controlled trial of As-needed Naltrexone in the treatment of pathological gambling. *Eur Addict Res*. 2016;22(2):70-79.
147. Grant JE, Potenza MN, Hollander E, et al. Multicenter investigation of the opioid antagonist nalmefene in the treatment of pathological gambling. *Am J Psychiatry*. 2006;163(2):303-312.
148. Grant JE, Odlaug BL, Potenza MN, Hollander E, Kim SW. Nalmefene in the treatment of pathological gambling: multicentre, double-blind, placebo-controlled study. *Br J Psychiatry*. 2010;197(4):330-331.
149. Alho H, Mäkelä N, Isotalo J, Toivonen L, Ollikainen J, Castrén S. Intranasal as needed naloxone in the treatment of gambling disorder: a randomised controlled trial. *Addict Behav*. 2022;125:107127.
150. Sáiz-Ruiz J, Blanco C, Ibáñez A, et al. Sertraline treatment of pathological gambling: a pilot study. *J Clin Psychiatry*. 2005;66(1):28-33.
151. Hollander E, DeCaria CM, Finkell JN, Begaz T, Wong CM, Cartwright C. A randomized double-blind fluvoxamine/placebo crossover trial in pathologic gambling. *Biol Psychiatry*. 2000;47(9):813-817.
152. Kim SW, Grant JE, Adson DE, Shin YC, Zaninelli R. A double-blind placebo-controlled study of the efficacy and safety of paroxetine in the treatment of pathological gambling. *J Clin Psychiatry*. 2002;63(6):501-507.
153. Grant JE, Kim SW, Potenza MN, et al. Paroxetine treatment of pathological gambling: a multi-centre randomized controlled trial. *Int Clin Psychopharmacol*. 2003;18(4):243-249.
154. Grant JE, Potenza MN. Escitalopram treatment of pathological gambling with co-occurring anxiety: an open-label pilot study with double-blind discontinuation. *Int Clin Psychopharmacol*. 2006;21(4):203-209.

155. Black DW, Arndt S, Coryell WH, et al. Bupropion in the treatment of pathological gambling: a randomized, double-blind, placebo-controlled, flexible-dose study. *J Clin Psychopharmacol*. 2007;27(2):143-150.
156. de Brito AM, de Almeida Pinto MG, Bronstein G, et al. Topiramate combined with cognitive restructuring for the treatment of gambling disorder: a two-center, randomized, double-blind clinical trial. *J Gambl Stud* 2017;33(1):249-263.
157. Berlin HA, Braun A, Simeon D, et al. A double-blind, placebo-controlled trial of topiramate for pathological gambling. *World J Biol Psychiatry*. 2013;14(2):121-128.
158. Hollander E, Pallanti S, Allen A, Sood E, Rossi NB. Does sustained-release lithium reduce impulsive gambling and affective instability versus placebo in pathological gamblers with bipolar spectrum disorders? *Am J Psychiatry*. 2005;162(1):137-145.
159. Grant JE, Kim SW, Odlaug BL. N-acetyl cysteine, a glutamate-modulating agent, in the treatment of pathological gambling: a pilot study. *Biol Psychiatry*. 2007;62(6):652-657.
160. Grant JE, Odlaug BL, Chamberlain SR, et al. A randomized, placebo-controlled trial of N-acetylcysteine plus imaginal desensitization for nicotine-dependent pathological gamblers. *J Clin Psychiatry*. 2014;75(1):39-45.
161. Fong T, Kalechstein A, Bernhard B, Rosenthal R, Rugle L. A double-blind, placebo-controlled trial of olanzapine for the treatment of video poker pathological gamblers. *Pharmacol Biochem Behav*. 2008;89(3):298-303.
162. McElroy SL, Nelson EB, Welge JA, Kaehler L, Keck PE Jr. Olanzapine in the treatment of pathological gambling: a negative randomized placebo-controlled trial. *J Clin Psychiatry*. 2008;69(3):433-440.
163. Kalivas PW, Peters J, Knackstedt L. Animal models and brain circuits in drug addiction. *Mol Interv*. 2006;6(6):339-344.

CHAPTER 53

Compulsive Sexual Behaviors

Timothy M. Hall, Anya Bershad, and Steven Shoptaw

CHAPTER OUTLINE

- Historical, legal, and cultural contexts
- High-volume sexual behaviors: hypersexual disorder, sexual addiction, and compulsive sexual behavior disorder
- Paraphilias and paraphilic disorders
- Pedophilia and sex with minors
- Compulsive sex in combination with substance use
- Assessment and treatment of problematic sexual behaviors
- Pharmacotherapy strategies
- Summary

A number of behaviors that are perceived as compulsive and distressing to the patient or to others, may come to clinical attention at the initiative of the individual or their partner or through involvement in the legal system. These include paraphilias and paraphilic disorders, concerns for excessive sexual desires and behaviors (high numbers of partners, excessive masturbation, compulsive pornography consumption, etc.), and the combination of compulsive sexual behavior with the use of psychoactive drugs (increasingly known as "chemsex").

Some clinicians and researchers have grouped these under labels such as "sexual addiction" and related constructs. However, significant challenges arise in extending the conceptual frame of addiction and addiction treatment to behavioral problems that do not involve substance use. Proposals for two constructs related to compulsive sexual behaviors, sexual addiction and hypersexual disorder, have been repeatedly rejected from inclusion in recent editions of the *Diagnostic and Statistical Manual of Mental Disorders* (DSM) for lack of empirical support and lack of consensus as to definition. Much of the research on these and related constructs has been limited by small sample sizes, lack of replication, and arbitrary definitions—such as deciding that seven or more orgasms per week after the age of 15 represents pathology.[1] A related construct, compulsive sexual behavior disorder (CSBD), has been included in the *International Classification of Diseases,* 11th edition (ICD-11), under impulse control disorders rather than as an addiction disorder.[2] CSBD has significant differences from substance use disorders (SUD), and needs to be distinguished from other sexual behaviors, and from discomfort around sexuality, as each has different implications for course and treatment.

In addressing the concerns of patients who report distress over their sexual behaviors or fantasies, we caution clinicians to conduct a careful biopsychosocial assessment to understand both the specific content of their sexual fantasies and behavior, (which may suggest a specific paraphilic disorder or specific internal conflicts), and the personal history and social context in which they are occurring. Such patients tend to be quite heterogeneous.[3] Labeling patients with sexual addiction or hypersexual disorder risks medicalizing problems in their primary relationships or exacerbating negative cultural or individual attitudes toward sexuality; these negative attitudes have been found to predict self-diagnosis of sexual addiction better than do objective behavioral measures of sexual frequency or of specific behaviors.[4] A premature diagnosis of "sex addiction" may also distract from identifying and treating primary mood, personality, substance use, or obsessive–compulsive disorders, or a more specific sexual disorder such as a paraphilic disorder.[3] Additionally, constructs of putative "sex addiction" have been invoked in U.S. court cases, often on questionable evidentiary bases.[5]

This chapter will use *problematic sexual behavior* as a more theory-neutral term that is closer to the clinical phenomenology, except when discussing specific diagnoses, such as CSBD. "Problematic" here is deliberately broad: patients may present because of ego-dystonic distress over the content or frequency of their fantasies or behaviors, or because their partner or family members are distressed by them, or because their behaviors have incurred legal or other disciplinary sanctions (such as violating workplace rules).

In the following, we describe some of the historical context for diagnostic categories related to problematic sexual behaviors (PSB) broadly, as well as some of the different clinical and forensic traditions that have investigated and theorized PSB. The remainder of this chapter then discusses three broad areas of PSB that have sometimes been grouped together with the concept of sexual addiction.

The closest constructs to a general sexual addiction are those characterized by high-volume sexual behaviors (HVSB): high numbers of partners, high frequency of partnered sex or masturbation, and/or high use of pornography. We use HVSB to refer to these high-volume behaviors collectively, without implying that they constitute disorders; when citing particular studies, we use the name of the construct measured in the study, such as "hypersexuality" or "sex addiction." Most studies on HVSB do not generalize directly to CSBD, as the studies on HVSB often use broader or narrower definitions or focus on frequency of behavior without assessing for functional impairment. A subset of patients with HVSB may meet criteria for the new diagnosis of CSBD, which is recognized by ICD-11 but not DSM-5-TR. CSBD is categorized as an impulse-control disorder and is defined specifically as it relates to functional impairment. The criteria for CSBD require repeated sexual activity that an individual pursues to the exclusion of other important life activities, despite adverse consequences and limited satisfaction resulting from the behaviors. The distress criterion in CSBD cannot be purely from religious or other cultural distaste for sexuality.

The second set of PSB includes the *paraphilias*, defined as intense sexual arousal to atypical sexual objects, situations, fantasies, or persons. There is great difficulty in objectively determining what counts as "atypical." In practice, those paraphilias that come to clinical attention often involve strong attractions to sexual objects, partners, and situations other than consensual sexual behavior with an adult partner. When paraphilias cause ongoing emotional distress or illegal or harmful behavior, they may rise to the level of *paraphilic disorders*.

Thirdly, we will consider the problem of compulsive sex co-occurring with use of various drugs, particularly stimulants like methamphetamine or cocaine and also club drugs such as 3,4-methylenedioxymethamphetamine (MDMA) and gamma-hydroxybutyric acid (GHB). Known in the United States since at least the 1990s by variations on *party and play* and increasingly denoted by the British slang term *chemsex*, this is a behavior that is prevalent in a significant minority of men who have sex with men (MSM), though it occurs in other populations.[6] This mixture of sex and drugs is a classical addiction embedded in a powerfully reinforcing sexual and cultural matrix, which greatly complicates standard approaches to addiction treatment.[7,8] For each of these sets of conditions, we review some of the relevant literature on prevalence, etiology, and comorbidities.

Finally, we review guidelines for treatment, necessarily based on a combination of general good clinical practice for behavioral disorders and a limited evidence base for specific PSB. Of the subtypes of PSB, treatments for paraphilic disorders have been best studied, especially libido-suppressing pharmacologic treatments for pedophilic disorder and other paraphilic disorders involving compulsions toward sexual assault. Aspects of these treatments may be considered for other PSB conditions presenting serious risk of injury, legal consequences, or psychological distress.

HISTORICAL, LEGAL, AND CULTURAL CONTEXTS

Despite definitional problems, "deviant" and compulsive sexual behaviors have been a focus of clinical attention since the early days of the modern medical and mental health professions,[9] along with speculation about their etiology[10] and attempts to change the sexual drives or behaviors. We mention this history to underscore the ways in which historical and cultural contexts shape perspectives regarding sexual behaviors and whether they require clinical attention. In different eras, a given behavior may be seen as a legal issue, a moral issue, a medical issue, or as unproblematic variation.[11] At various times, the following have all been seen as deviant forms of sexual behavior and subject to medical attention: sexual attraction to adults of the same sex, masturbation (under the term *onanism*),[12] conceiving a child outside of marriage,[13] and even the expression of sexual desire in a woman.[14] These are no longer regarded as abnormal by most medical and mental health professionals. In studying these phenomena, researchers have been more successful at documenting the wide variety of human sexual expression than in proving hypotheses about etiology. Attempts to develop cures for sexual behaviors, drives, and orientations that are seen as problematic, whether by society at large or by the individual in question, have been even less successful.

Assessing problematic and merely variant sexual behavior entails distinguishing among *sexual desires* or *orientations* (some of which may be considered *paraphilias*), *sexual behaviors* (that may or may not be motivated by a strong orientation toward a particular kind of sexual partner or sexual act), and *context* (a particular behavior may be problematic in some circumstances and not others). For instance, consensual sex between a 17-year-old and an 18-year-old may be legal in one jurisdiction but count as statutory rape in another. A man who is highly aroused by women's feet and footwear may be happy in a relationship with a woman who finds foot massages enjoyable, may be unhappy in a relationship with a woman who finds his attraction distasteful, and may come to legal or clinical attention if he attempts to satisfy his sexual desires by groping a woman's feet without her permission. It is also necessary to bear in mind that random instances of behavior do not by themselves meet criteria for a disorder. For example, a nonconsensual sexual grope may legally count as assault depending on the circumstances, but it is not sufficient for a diagnosis of frotteuristic disorder if it occurs in the absence of persistent fantasies and compelling urges about sexual groping.

Concern for equity and diversity are relevant here: sexual orientation and gender identity minorities and persons of various racial and cultural backgrounds have been purported to have higher sex drives or poorer quality relationships or otherwise problematic sexual behaviors. Such beliefs have been weaponized, for instance to deny lesbian, gay, bisexual, transgender, and queer (LGBTQ) persons custody of their children or equal rights to become foster or adoptive parents. Such beliefs have served as an invidious subtext in the engagement of social welfare agents with persons of racially and ethnically minoritized groups. Cultural anthropologists and historians have documented a wide diversity of human sexual expression and relationship structure that are compatible with healthy psychological and social functioning. At the present time in Western societies, some people are embracing a variety of identities and relationships, from asexual and graysexual to polyamorous.[15] Some forms of emergent sexuality, such as "furries" may be more common among neurodivergent persons, though initial studies do not find associations of "furry" identities with mental health problems.[16] Clinicians need to be careful not to assume that patients' sexuality is problematic merely because it is unfamiliar to the clinician.

Boundaries that define pathologic (or illegal) sexual behavior are easiest to specify when they involve children or nonconsensual aggression. Indeed, serious legal sanctions are imposed on adults who express sexual urges or fantasies involving children (child sexual abuse, child pornography) or nonconsenting adults (domestic violence/rape). Strict mandated reporting laws require clinicians to inform local authorities of domestic violence or rape, suspected child sexual abuse, or sometimes even significant potential risk for child sexual abuse. Clinicians should know and comply with their state and local legal requirements for reporting these behaviors.

HIGH-VOLUME SEXUAL BEHAVIORS: HYPERSEXUAL DISORDER, SEXUAL ADDICTION, AND COMPULSIVE SEXUAL BEHAVIOR DISORDER

Several competing sets of diagnostic criteria have been proposed to describe pathologic HVSB, reflecting different theoretical concepts. Hypersexual disorder describes a condition of recurrent and intense sexual fantasies and behaviors that cause distress, are inappropriately used to cope with stressful events or dysphoric emotional states, cannot be voluntarily curtailed, and risk or cause harm to oneself or others; this is seen as potentially related to impulse-control disorders.[17] At least two different versions of sexual addiction have been proposed, modeled after criteria sets for substance use disorders, and operationalizing analogues of tolerance (needing increased amount or intensity of stimulation over time for the same effect) and withdrawal.[18,19]

While there is no diagnosis related to HVSB in the DSM-5, the diagnosis of CSBD can be found among the Impulse Control Disorders in the ICD-11. A diagnosis of CSBD involves "a persistent pattern of failure to control intense, repetitive sexual impulses or urges resulting in repetitive sexual behavior," overlapping with some criteria for proposed hypersexual or sex addiction conditions. The ICD-11 requires that CSBD is further characterized by at least one of four domains that reflect other impulse control disorders: (1) engaging in the behavior becomes the focus of one's life to exclusion of other activities and responsibilities, (2) the individual had made numerous attempts to reduce the behavior (3) the individual engages in the behavior despite adverse consequences, (4) the individual engages in the behavior despite deriving little satisfaction from it. Beyond requiring one of these domains, a diagnosis of CSBD requires that the pattern of behavior persists beyond 6 months, and that it is not better accounted for by another mental condition—an important criterion, as we note below, as distress over sexual behavior may be a presenting complaint in mood, anxiety, personality, or post-traumatic disorders, or SUD. Finally, the pattern of behavior must result in distress or significant functional impairment. Notably, in the ICD-11 criteria for CSBD, moral distress and disapproval is not sufficient to meet the final requirement.

The relationship between what is described in the ICD-11 as "moral distress and disapproval" and the diagnosis of CSBD is a complex one. Individuals may describe themselves as "sex addicts" or use other language associated with addiction in a pejorative sense, with the intention of conveying disapproval of their own behavior. In some cases, individuals may have such feelings of disapproval for behavior that would otherwise not be considered pathological, such as a religious person believing they should not have the urge to masturbate. In fact, negative self-evaluations are often part of a clinical picture, including feeling abnormal or sick; feeling degraded, guilty, or ashamed; feeling regret, depression, or discomfort; or feeling numb, hollow, or empty.

Some studies have found that negative attitudes toward sexuality on the part of the person or of their partner predict self-identification of sexual addiction better than do objective measures of sexual acts, sexual partners, or time spent thinking about sex.[4,20] These suggest that conflicts about sexual desires and behaviors may be what lead a person or their partner to identify sexual behavior as problematic, rather than an underlying physiologic dysfunction or simple frequency of sexual behaviors. Further, views of what counts as appropriate sexual behavior vary across cultures, including differences in perception of masturbation, number of sexual partners, gender norms, and pornography. These variations may influence an individual's sense of moral disapproval, making it difficult to disentangle from the functional consequences of particular patterns of behavior. It is important to separate out and acknowledge these factors in diagnosing and treating CSBD.

The ICD-11 description of CSBD acknowledges differences in how the disorder manifests in men and women. Men are more likely than women to be diagnosed with CSBD, and men reports higher rates of sexual behaviors and higher scores on questionnaires assessing CSBD.[21] Co-morbid diagnoses of depression, anxiety, and OCD may be associated with more severe CSBD symptomatology in men than in women.[22-25] Studies have shown gender differences in the relationship between childhood adversity and hypersexuality in adults, though results remain inconclusive. One recent online survey in over 16,000 Hungarian adults showed that both male gender and a history of childhood and adolescent sexual abuse predicted hypersexuality, and that this association was stronger for men.[26] though previous studies have shown the opposite effect; that a history of childhood mistreatment predicted hypersexuality in women, but not men.[24] More research is needed to clarify differences in CSBD across the range of gender identities, and with specific diagnostic criteria rather than unreliable proxies, such as self-report of frequency of sexual behavior without the more stringent assessment of dysfunction and distress.

There is almost no data on racial or ethnic differences in prevalence or presentation of CSBD. Studies on CSBD focus largely on White/Caucasian respondents, and many do not even report racial or ethnic background in their demographic tables. A single, nationally representative sample using data from the National Survey of Sexual Health and Behavior found that respondents who identified as Black, other, or Hispanic endorsed higher rates of subjective distress about sexual impulses than did White respondents; however, the same study also found that lower income and lower educational attainment also predicted higher rates of distress,[27] suggesting possible confounds.

Neurobiology of HVSB

There exists a small literature on neurobiology relevant to CSBD, primarily among healthy males. One study used diffusion tensor imaging (DTI) to investigate structural white matter differences between patients with CSBD and healthy controls. This study showed that CSBD patients showed differences in in the superior corona radiata tract, the internal capsule tract, cerebellar tracts and occipital gyrus white matter, all of which have been implicated in OCD and addictive disorders more broadly.[25] Imaging studies have experimentally manipulated presentation of erotic and neutral stimuli among young adult male heterosexual subjects under positron emission tomography (PET) or functional magnetic resonance imaging (fMRI).[28-30] Erotic visual stimuli activate brain regions that include the right insula and claustrum (somatosensory processing and penile erection), the hypothalamus and striatum (areas of dopamine signaling), the anterior cingulate gyrus (shifting attention, repetitive behavior, endocrine and gonadal secretions), in addition to activation in the occipital cortex (visual processing).[29,30] A handful of recent studies have used fMRI to examine differences in brain responses to erotic versus monetary cues in individuals diagnosed with CSBD. One of these studies compared 29 men with CSBD to 25 healthy controls in a modified incentive delay task including both erotic and monetary stimuli. The authors reported that men with CSBD showed a stronger anticipatory response in the ventral striatum and anterior orbitofrontal cortex, a region involved in assigning incentive salience to addiction-related cues, in response to erotic stimuli.[31] Given the significant dopaminergic signaling that occurs in the striatum, Oei et al. probed the role of dopaminergic tone in sexual response by randomizing healthy males to haloperidol, levodopa or placebo. Levodopa enhanced activation in the nucleus accumbens and the dorsal anterior cingulate when participants were exposed to subconscious sexual stimuli, while haloperidol decreased activations in these areas.[32]

A role for dopamine in normal and aberrant sexual behavior has been suggested by high prevalence of impulse-control disorders emerging in response to dopamine agonist treatment among patients with Parkinson disease (PD). Among 300 patients with PD, 58 (19.3%) self-reported new-onset behavioral compulsions. Of those, 25 (43.1%) reported sexual compulsivity, and the remainder reported gambling compulsion. All those who developed sexual compulsivity were male, and all were on stable dopamine agonist therapy.[33] Preexisting histories of an impulse-control disorder (eg, substance use disorder) increased the odds of developing HVSB under dopamine agonist treatment. These findings are echoed by a more recent study systematically investigating impulsive behavior in patients with PD on dopaminergic agents. Of those receiving the target dose, 24% developed new pathologic behaviors.[34] The dopaminergic system has been shown to work together with the oxytocinergic system to mediate sexual behavior,[35] and the oxytocin system has also been implicated in CSBD. One study measured plasma levels of oxytocin, a hormone associated with social bonding, in men with CSBD and healthy controls and showed that men with CSBD had higher levels of the social bonding hormone at baseline that normalized after CBT treatment.[36]

Some of the neuroadaptations seen in substance use disorders have been reported in HVSB,[37] although other studies have failed to find similarities.[38] Case reports of brain injuries leading to sexual compulsivity later in the lifespan suggest possible neurobiologic mechanisms. Patients with brain injury in right temporal areas sometimes develop sexual compulsivity, consistent with PET studies associating these areas with male heterosexual response.[37,39]

The evidence thus far demonstrates that complex human sexual behaviors involve multiple systems and have complex neuroanatomical pathways. However, a target site or target chemical that might represent a biologic substrate for CSBD or hypersexual conditions has yet to be identified.

Psychiatric Comorbidity

Reports consistently implicate impulsivity, obsessions, and compulsivity as central issues in HVSB. Many psychiatric disorders share one or more of these features. Impulsivity is a core feature of attention-deficit hyperactivity disorder (ADHD), bipolar disorders, and SUD. In a study describing comorbid problems of 932 individuals who rated highly on measures of sexual sensation seeking and sexual compulsivity, 28% reported working compulsively, 26% reported spending compulsively, 38% reported disordered eating, and 42% reported substance use disorders.[40] High prevalence of psychiatric comorbidities is also observed in community samples of individuals who defined their behavior as sexually compulsive. In one ($N = 36$), 39% met criteria for lifetime mood disorders, 50% for lifetime anxiety disorders, and 64% for lifetime substance use disorders.[28] In another ($N = 24$, including two females), all subjects met lifetime criteria for some Axis I disorder (mood disorders, 71%; anxiety disorders, 96%). Of these, 88% met criteria for any current Axis I disorder (mood disorders, 33%; anxiety disorders, 42%), with 29% and 71% who met criteria for any current and lifetime substance use disorder, respectively, with the most frequent diagnosis involving alcohol.[29] Some data point in the other direction, finding that individuals with other psychiatric disorders have elements of HVSB. In a study of psychiatric inpatients, one-third had comorbid impulse-control disorders, with 4.4% of these having current and 4.9% lifetime prevalence of comorbid compulsive sexual behaviors.[30]

Depression

Several studies have found positive associations between depressive symptoms or diagnosis of major depressive disorder and various measures of compulsive sexual behavior, though it remains unclear whether the sexual behavior is a response or a cause of depressive symptoms, or whether depressive symptoms and compulsive sexual behavior share an underlying physiology. For instance, two studies of urban MSM, with nonprobabilistic sample sizes of 669[41] and 509,[42] respectively, found sexual compulsivity was associated with depression symptoms when controlling for a range of demographic and other risk variables.

Anxiety

Presence of anxiety symptoms and prevalence of current and lifetime anxiety disorders appear to be somewhat higher in individuals rated as having sexual addiction as compared to controls. In one study, participants recruited from 12-step self-help venues were classified into three groups based on their behavioral presentations: individuals with "sexual addiction" ($N = 32$), individuals with pathologic gambling ($N = 38$), and individuals without addiction.[43] Comparison of scores for the Symptom Check List-90-R along depression, anxiety, interpersonal sensitivity, and obsessive–compulsive subscales showed significantly higher scores for individuals in the self-identified sexual addiction group than for controls.

Attention Deficit Hyperactivity Disorder

Some retrospective reports suggest associations between ADHD during childhood and presence of HVSB. Seventy-two individuals seeking treatment for HVSB completed a variety of scales to assess symptoms of sexual compulsivity; 34% scored in the range of probable ADHD diagnosis.[44] Although retrospective reports indicate significant correlation of ADHD in samples of men with behaviors consistent with HVSB, it is also possible that childhood ADHD is a correlate of sexual behaviors in adult men who have been imprisoned. In a small imaging study, men rated as sexually compulsive made significantly more errors than did control participants in the Go-No-Go procedure, a behavioral measure that identifies impairments of inhibitory control.[45] Impulsivity has been shown to be an independent predictor of CSBD.[46] Attentional impulsivity as measured by the Barratt Impulsiveness Scale (BIS) has been shown to predict hypersexual behavior,[47] as has trait levels of sensation-seeking.[46]

Personality Disorders

One study found that 46% of a community-based sample of individuals identifying as having HVSB met criteria for any personality disorder, predominantly Cluster C disorders.[26] In a study of 403 adolescents seen in primary care settings, those rated as having three or more symptoms of Axis II diagnoses reported higher numbers of sexual partners than did those with symptoms of two or fewer Axis II diagnoses. The association was stronger in females than in males.[48] These findings underscore difficulties in separating out HVSB as a primary diagnostic entity from personality disorders. Acting out sexually is a criterion for borderline personality disorder, and may be seen in other Cluster B personality disorders, while Cluster C personality disorders may entail excessive self-criticism and guilt.[49]

PARAPHILIAS AND PARAPHILIC DISORDERS

Definitions and Diagnosis

A paraphilia is an attraction or arousal to atypical objects, persons, or situations. At one time paraphilias included phenomena from cross-dressing and frequent masturbation to foot fetishism and sexual masochism. In recent decades, "atypical" sexual desires and behaviors are more often seen as lying on a continuum from strong preferences for certain physical types of partners or situations, through harmless "kinks" that persons may include in their sexual fantasies and behaviors,[50] to paraphilias more strictly defined. Problems in drawing clear diagnostic lines among these phenomena include evolving sexual practices and attitudes in the general population,[15,51] and distinguishing between behaviors that are inherently problematic versus those that incur social stigma or are simply less common. Research indicates that merely desiring or occasionally engaging in unconventional sexual behaviors such as consensual bondage and domination, sexual sadism and masochism (BDSM) is relatively common (rates of sadistic and masochistic behavior have been reported at 5.5% and 19.2%, respectively, in a Canadian survey),[52] and is not necessarily associated with poorer mental health or psychological maladjustment.[53]

DSM-5-TR defines a paraphilia as "intense and persistent sexual interest other than sexual interest in genital stimulation or preparatory fondling with phenotypically normal, physically mature, consenting human partners."[49] Noting that "a paraphilia by itself does not necessarily justify or require clinical intervention," DSM-5-TR further distinguishes a *paraphilic disorder* as "a paraphilia that is currently causing distress or impairment to the individual or a paraphilia whose satisfaction has entailed personal harm, or risk of harm, to others."[49]

Eight specific paraphilic disorders are listed in DSM-5-TR, as well as a category for *other specific paraphilic disorder,* which would include the many historically named paraphilias, and *unspecified paraphilic disorder*, in situations where there may be insufficient information to specify but there is evidence for impairment. These specific paraphilic disorders are listed because they are relatively common (compared to other paraphilic disorders), and satisfying them is likely to entail harm or criminal activity.[49] ICD-11 has reduced the list of recognized specific paraphilic disorder even further.[54]

Distinguishing paraphilias and paraphilic disorders (both internal, enduring, mental states or predispositions) from crimes (behavior) of a sexual nature has both clinical and legal ramifications. While some persons with paraphilic disorders do commit sex crimes including sexual abuse of children and rape, a majority of these crimes are committed by persons who do not have a paraphilic disorder.[55] There is a contentious debate in many American and Canadian jurisdictions over sentencing length and appropriateness of parole or probation for persons who have been convicted of sex crimes and are also diagnosed with a paraphilic disorder. There is a need to balance concerns for public safety—recognizing that their ongoing strong desires for particular sexual acts may place them at higher risk of re-engaging in criminal activity—against obligations of fairness and justice.[56] Conversely, given that most crimes of sexual nature are not committed by persons with paraphilic disorders, a focus on paraphilic disorders can be misleading both for prevention and rehabilitation. Unfounded worries about generalized sexual addiction also feed into public support for life-long registries of persons convicted of sex crimes, which are largely unsupported by research findings and can introduce unintended negative consequences to the individual and to the community.[57]

Etiology, Development, and Prevalence of Paraphilic Disorders

Most paraphilias manifest during adolescence, though the individual may not act on them or acknowledge them at that time. Several paraphilias have been linked together in the *courtship disorder hypothesis*, which proposes that voyeurism, exhibitionism, frotteurism ("mashing" or rubbing oneself against another person, often in public), and telephone scatologia represent deviations from a psychological system that normally functions in finding and wooing a potential sexual partner.[58] DSM-5-TR groups paraphilias into two sets that are agnostic to etiology and development. Those with *anomalous activity preference* focus on atypical behaviors: the courtship disorders and the algolagnic, or pain-loving, disorders of sexual sadism and sexual masochism. Paraphilic disorders with *anomalous target preference*, on the other hand, are oriented toward targets other than adult humans; these include pedophilic disorder, fetishistic disorder, and transvestic disorder.[49]

It is difficult to ascertain prevalence of paraphilic disorders, as much of the available data come from forensic or clinical samples that are not generalizable to society at large. Additionally, many surveys ask about thoughts and fantasies, which correlate weakly with behavior and are often mediated by other personality factors such as antisocial traits or poor impulse control. For instance, one study of male undergraduates ($N = 103$) found that 95% endorsed at least one "deviant" sexual fantasy, and more than half the respondents in the same study reported occasional, individual acts that might be considered deviant, such as uninvited or nonconsensual sexual groping (44% of respondents, which counted as a frotteuristic-type behavior). However, only a minority (38%) actually carried out behavior from their specific sexual fantasies.[59] Other studies have corroborated this finding of relatively high rates of occasional fantasies along paraphilic lines, but with much lower rates of acting them out, or of the preoccupation and compulsiveness needed to meet diagnostic criteria for a paraphilic disorder.[58]

Prevalence data on the specific paraphilic disorders listed in the DSM-5-TR are also highly variable across studies. Långstrom and Seto found that in a nonclinical, nationally representative sample of nearly 2,500 Swedish adults, 11.5% of men and 3.9% of women reported at least one episode of voyeuristic behavior.[60] Other studies have reported rates of voyeuristic experience as high as nearly 35%, noting voyeuristic behavior as one that often results in interaction with law-enforcement, and the most common paraphilic disorder among men.[52] In the same Swedish sample, at least one instance of exhibitionistic behavior was reported by 4.1% of men and 3.9% of women.[60] However, Joyal and colleagues found that over 30% of their sample of over 1,000 Canadians had engaged in exhibitionistic behavior.[52] Joyal et al. also found that fetishism was the second most common paraphilic behavior, with 26.3% of their sample having engaged in at least one fetishistic behavior in their lifetime. However, behavior alone is not a formal disorder. For example, frotteuristic disorder rates are difficult to classify accurately, as much of the data label any kind of groping or nonpenetrative sexual assault as frotteurism, without evidence of whether persons engaging in these behaviors also exhibit a compulsive element, clinically significant distress, or impairment in functioning. A systematic review found that estimated prevalence rates of frotteurism varied widely across studies, ranging from 7.9% to 35%.[61]

PEDOPHILIA AND SEX WITH MINORS

The paraphilias with the largest research base and that most often come to legal attention are those that involve a predominant sexual attraction to children or adolescents. These should be distinguished from the acts of child molestation or child sexual abuse, most instances of which are not committed by persons with a predominant orientation toward minors. Additionally, they should clinically be distinguished from sexual acts between younger and slightly older adolescents or young adults who may be just on the other side of the local age of consent. Depending on the jurisdiction, these so-called "Romeo and Juliet" cases of consensual sexual behavior between individuals a few years apart in age may be legally prohibited, but they can nonetheless be age-appropriate behavior rather than evidence of a long-standing attraction to minors. For many paraphilia researchers, *pedophilia*, strictly speaking, is a long-standing attraction to prepubescent children, typically under the age of 11 or 12 or in Tanner stage 1. Sex researchers distinguish this from *hebephilia*, attraction to pubescent children, around ages 11 to 14, and *ephebophilia*, or attraction to older adolescents in Tanner stages 3 to 4. These are research categories but not currently in DSM-5-TR or ICD-11.[62]

DSM-5-TR characterizes *pedophilic disorder* as a recurrent, intense attraction to prepubescent children, generally under 13. The individual with pedophilic disorder must be at least 16 and at least 5 years older than the child. DSM-5-TR further excludes "an individual in late adolescence in an ongoing sexual relationship with a 12- or 13-year-old."[49] This does not speak to the appropriateness or inappropriateness of such a relationship, but rather recognizes that sexual exploration among adolescents does not reliably predict a lifelong, persistent attraction to children as sexual objects.

DSM-5-TR characterizes pedophilic disorder not only by the nature of sexual fantasizing (recurrent and intense) but also by interference in an individual's life, either by creating distress or interpersonal difficulty, or in the acting out of one's sexual urges. Much of the research on prevalence of pedophilic disorder focuses on sexual fantasy and urges, not always distinguishing individuals who meet DSM-5-TR criteria from those who do not. Additionally, many studies focus on criminal or clinical populations, and thus may not be generalizable to the public. These factors may contribute to overestimates of the prevalence of pedophilic disorders.

True prevalence of pedophilic disorder in the general public is unknown due to lack of large-scale epidemiologic surveys.[63] In studies examining sexual fantasy and urges, results indicate an upper limit of around 5%, though the prevalence estimates vary depending on the questions being asked.[63,64] Few studies have looked at sexual behavior involving children among nonclinical samples. Dombert and colleagues found that prevalence estimates for sexual behaviors involving children ranged from 0.04% to 5%,[65] and Mokros et al. estimate that lifetime prevalence of pedophilic disorder in males is 0.5% to 1%.[66]

Etiology of pedophilic disorder and related disorders is not well understood. Theories of developmental trauma or imprinting have been proposed, but most survivors of child sexual abuse do not grow up to have an attraction to children, and many persons with an attraction to minors were not themselves sexually abused. However, there are suggestions of distinguishing characteristics that identify men who develop pedophilic disorder. In one large forensic study, diagnosis of ADHD and more than three head injuries experienced prior to age 13 were associated with a preference for children as erotic stimuli.[67] In another study, men with pedophilic disorder ($N = 65$) completed fMRI scans, which were compared to 62 men who were nonsexual offenders. Findings showed significant reductions in white matter volume in the fiber bundles of the superior fronto-occipital fasciculus and the right arcuate in the pedophilia group. No such associations were observed in scans from the 62 men who were nonsexual offenders included as a control condition.[39] These differences are observed in fibers that connect areas of the brain that respond to sexual cues, suggesting that pedophilia may result from disruption of the networks of brain regions connected by these fibers. As noted, data were collected from a forensic setting and may not represent men in the community with an attraction to minors who do not act on those impulses. Antisocial traits have been found to predict greater likelihood of acting on paraphilic impulses, and may also be a mediating factor in paraphilic disorders involving sex with minors or nonconsenting partners. SUD may also increase likelihood of acting on paraphilic interests.[68]

Treatment of pedophilic disorder is discussed together with treatment of other PSB in the last section of this chapter.

COMPULSIVE SEX IN COMBINATION WITH SUBSTANCE USE

Sex and substance use combine some of the most powerfully reinforcing and potentially problematic behaviors known to humans. If we include alcohol in the definition, the combination goes back for millennia, while sex in combination with opioids or cannabinoids goes back at least centuries. Since about the 1970s, however, we have seen a particular intersection of stimulants (cocaine and methamphetamines), dissociatives (ketamine), and "entactogens" or "empathogens" (MDMA, GHB, etc.) with sex, particularly among MSM, though also in some other groups. This has been known in the United States under the gay slang terms "partying," "party and play," or "PnP." In the last few years, the British gay term "chemsex" has gained increasing attention in the public health literature, particularly in relation to prevention and treatment of HIV and STIs, whether through sexual acts or through shared needles, in the case of injected drugs. On a public health and sociologic level, this intersection of sex, substance use, and risk for HIV and STIs has been conceptualized as syndemic—that is, as mutually reinforcing and complexly interacting epidemics, not merely as the problem of an individual or as a single problem of a group.[6,69]

Prevalence data on compulsive sex in combination with substance use are limited, in part due to the lack of a clear consensus on how to classify this particular issue and whether it be viewed as primarily a poly-substance use disorder, primarily a compulsive sexual behavior, or both. The British-based "Chemsex Study" was one of the first quantitative publications on this topic. Of more than 1,100 respondents, around 20% reported engaging in compulsive sex in combination with substance use within the past year, and 10% within the past month.[5] Another study found that in an MSM population in London, 99% of individuals who used methamphetamine, 75% of those who used mephedrone, and 85% of those who used GBL (a prodrug for GHB) reported using the drug solely to facilitate sex, with 70% reporting having shared needles to inject drugs.[70] In a report from England, Wales, and Northern Ireland on people who inject drugs and who receive services noted a small group of women who have sex with women who reported chemsex. This remains one of the few reports of chemsex in women, a behavior that was linked to having multiple partners, male partners, and transactional sex. Though the epidemiology on chemsex may be concerning, it is impossible to extrapolate from these to prevalence numbers for a potential disorder or persistent compulsive behavior combining sex and drug use.

Compulsive sex in combination with substance use has been identified as a growing public health issue and has been linked to high rates of HIV transmission in many studies. In terms of treatment, programs such as Dean Street Clinic in London are taking a pragmatic harm-reduction approach, focusing on reducing the risk of transmission of HIV, hepatitis C, and other STIs. The program provides education about needle sharing and mitigating risks of overdose, aiming to build rapport with patients, which may ultimately result in more comprehensive treatment. In their *Lancet* article, Kirby and colleagues found that IDU among MSM involved in compulsive sex in combination with substance use increased from 30% to 70% in a single year, with 70% of people who injected drugs reporting needle sharing.[71] The authors note that individuals partaking in compulsive sex in combination with substance use often maintain professional lives and thrive financially. Nonetheless, the health consequences of compulsive sex in combination with substance use are potentially serious, with a typical episode lasting up to 72 hours and involving an average of five sexual partners. Kirby and colleagues report that 75% of those using crystal methamphetamine, GBL, or mephrodrone are HIV-positive, with 60% reportedly not taking antiretroviral treatment. Clinics serving lesbian, gay, bisexual, and transgender (LGBT) clients report difficulty in meeting demand for services related to compulsive sex in combination with substance use.

Special Populations: PSB Among MSM

We briefly address PSB among MSM in part because of the disproportionate amount of research and clinical attention paid to this population. MSM have been historically stigmatized, with their sexual behaviors often criminalized and/or medicalized. In recent years, attention has focused on various constructs of hypersexual behavior among MSM as putative mediating risk factors for HIV and other STIs. Additionally, some MSM carry significantly negative and self-critical attitudes toward their sexual desires and behaviors. MSM presenting for concerns of PSB may be at higher risk than some other persons with PSB for contracting HIV or being introduced by sexual partners to high-volume sex in the context of substance use. At the same time, they may carry excessive shame and guilt about their sexual orientation and same-sex experiences, with potentially conflicting and exacerbating messages from their MSM peers, their families and communities of origin, and their encounters with healthcare providers; these may lead them to view relatively normal MSM experiences through a lens of pathology, and may complicate efforts to access treatment for PSB, substance use disorders, mental health services, or general healthcare.

Far less research has addressed problematic sexual behaviors among other sexual and gender minorities, such as women who have sex with women, though many of the same concerns about internalized stigma apply. Transgender women are often included with MSM in studies of HVSB in context of substance use, though there are a number of differences in their experience and social contexts. There is a small and highly contentious literature on other PSB among transgender persons, the nuances of which are beyond the scope of this chapter. There is very little research on the sexual health needs of transgender men in general. All of these topics need additional research to inform better clinical care.

Studies indicate that a subgroup of MSM experience sexual behaviors that are more compulsive and more distressing than for MSM in general. Use of alcohol or drugs proximal to sex may loosen sexual safety protocols and lead to unprotected sex, which carries increased risks for HIV infection among MSM. As noted above, high volumes of sexual behavior do not necessarily constitute a disorder. Among MSM who scored one standard deviation or higher above the mean of the Sexual Compulsivity Scale,[40] qualitative interviews indicated five intrinsic explanations for sexually compulsive behaviors: negative affect, low self-esteem, needs for validation and affection, stress release, and having a high sex drive.[72] Externalizing explanations included relationship issues, the easy availability of gay sex, childhood sexual abuse, and parental conflicts/deficiencies.

Correlates of scores of sexual compulsivity and health risk behaviors are observed in several studies of MSM, particularly high numbers of sexual partners and likelihood to engage in condomless anal sex.[73] Among HIV-positive MSM in two studies, high scores on the Sexual Compulsivity Scale corresponded with older age, using methamphetamine before or during sex, going to sex venues or street corners for sex partners, low self-efficacy for condom use, low levels of self-esteem, high disinhibition, and a high number of HIV-negative or status-unknown sexual partners.[41,74] These findings are drawn from venue-based and convenience samples, which do not easily translate into prevalence of PSB in the general population of MSM. Additionally, age differences also correlate with different cultural cohorts or generations of MSM, who may have very different experiences of and attitudes toward sexuality, drug use, and HIV.[75]

Though not specifically addressing PSB, there is a growing body of work illustrating that reduction in drug use by providing evidence-based, cognitive behavioral treatments for drug use disorders corresponds with reductions in high-risk sexual behaviors. One example is *Getting Off: A Behavioral Treatment Intervention for Gay and Bisexual Methamphetamine Users,* which adapts the MATRIX Model manualized treatment for stimulant use disorders for gay- and bisexual-identified clients. This approach facilitates clients undergoing intensive outpatient treatment of their methamphetamine use disorder to enter a conversation regarding the cultural, sexual, physical, and psychological aspects of their sexual behavior. Outcomes from a randomized, controlled trial found that among gay- and bisexual-identified clients with methamphetamine use disorder, treatment-associated reductions in high-risk sexual behaviors are observed up to one year after treatment entry,[76] a finding that was replicated and effectively implemented in a community setting.[77] In a qualitative report on the experiences of the men in the initial research project, participants noted the primary mechanism driving reductions in their high-risk sexual behaviors, both in numbers of partners and in episodes of condomless anal intercourse, was treatment-associated reductions in methamphetamine use.[78]

It is difficult at present to know how best to characterize this intersection of drug use and PSB, largely though not only among cisgender MSM, transgender MSM, and transgender women. The particular role of methamphetamine in PSB among MSM has been noted since the 1990s,[70] and a focus of public health discussion since the early 2000s.[79] However, this needs to be considered in the context of a long history of moral panics about drug use among MSM,[80] including earlier concerns about a possible causal role of nitrite poppers in AIDS, which was later disproven.[81] Additionally, use of alcohol and drugs in relation to socializing and to sex has a complex history among LGBT populations[82] (see also Chapter 42). The widespread availability of drugs in sexual contexts and ongoing visibility of compulsive sex in combination with substance use also complicate the recovery process from substance use disorders for many patients from LGBTQ and other affected communities. Patients engaging in chemsex may be good candidates for preexposure prophylaxis for HIV (PrEP) and for behavioral support in staying linked to HIV care, if they are already living with HIV.

ASSESSMENT AND TREATMENT OF PROBLEMATIC SEXUAL BEHAVIORS

Assessment

Individuals who present for treatment or evaluation of PSB need careful assessment to define the presenting problem. Standard areas to review include current presentation and history of the PSB: Did something precipitate the visit? Exactly what is the patient doing, at what frequency, and under what circumstances? What are the gender(s) and ages of the partners involved with the individual? What is the development of the behavior—from childhood to present? What is the individual's experience with sexual abuse, physical abuse, and head or other physical trauma as a child? When were symptoms or distress the worst? What has helped reduce the severity of symptoms or distress in the past?

As with substance use disorders, individuals presenting for treatment of PSB may have limited motivation for treatment, particularly if referred by a partner or mandated by a court. Determining and enhancing motivation may be an important element of treatment. After seeking a thorough understanding of the chief complaint, it is important to establish whether or not there is victimization in the history. Some forms of compulsive sexual behavior (eg, child molestation) are legally reportable activities; others expose the patient to risk of arrest (eg, exhibitionism). Still others increase individual risks of infection or physical violence. All need to be empathically but carefully assessed in any extended evaluation.

In addition, careful review of ways in which PSB has impacted areas of functioning is crucial. This starts with thorough review of medical history (especially STIs), employment background and pattern, involvement with alcohol and drugs (including nicotine and cannabis) that may be used before, during, and after sexually compulsive behaviors, detailed history of legal problems (whether formally charged or convicted or not), quality of relationships with family, friends, and intimates (if any), and mental health functioning, including both diagnosable psychiatric conditions and sub-threshold mood, anxiety, and cognitive disturbances. This ancillary information provides strong indications as to whether the behaviors indicating PSB are localized or are generalized across multiple domains of functioning for the individual.

Over the past two decades, several measures have been developed, and psychometric properties established for their use in providing valid and reliable assays of PSB. Hook and colleagues provide a comprehensive review of seventeen published instruments assessing PSB.[83] Scales include self-report measures, clinician-administered measures, and a female-specific measure used in gynecologic practice and research. **Table 53-1** summarizes seven of the most commonly used assessment measures of PSB symptoms used in the literature and their psychometric properties.

When selecting a measure, it is vital to define its purpose. Screening instruments are developed to be used with large samples to identify individuals in mainstream populations who are more likely than others to have problems with PSB. By contrast, measures of specific symptoms of PSB (eg, high-volume sexual activities, paraphilia-defining behaviors) are more useful to assess severity of a disorder in cross-sectional samples and response to treatment over time in repeated measures. When assessing individuals from specific ethnic, racial, or cultural groups, it is wise to select measures that have published data describing their use within the particular group, if available.

Treatment Approaches

Treatment for individuals with PSB often occurs in the context of comorbid substance use or psychiatric disorders and in the absence of randomized controlled trials that might guide best practice. Instead, the clinician is faced with a complex task of piecing together relevant findings from psychiatric literature, small trials, and observational reports in order to arrive at an evidence-informed, bio-psycho-social approach for intervention. There is some evidence that for individuals whose PSB has strong obsessive-compulsive characteristics, medications used to treat obsessive-compulsive disorder may relieve symptoms, particularly the selective serotonin reuptake inhibitors (SSRIs).[84,85] Another source of guidance involves early literature describing normal sexual response and behavioral methods for addressing sexual dysfunction in couples.[86]

TABLE 53-1 Frequently Used Measures of Problematic Sexual Behavior

Measure	Description	Psychometrics
Sexual Addiction Screening Test (SAST)[87]	• Most popularly available assessment • 25 yes-or-no items that can be administered and scored on-line; affirmative answer = 1 point • Summed score >10 suggest need for consultation • Summed score >13 suggest need for treatment	• Internal consistency variable (α's 0.66-0.92)
Sexual Outlet Inventory[88]	• Clinician-administered scale that quantifies sexual fantasies, urges, and behaviors to distinguish unconventional (paraphilic) sexual behavior • Total sexual outlet = number of orgasms reported per week • Score ≥7 orgasms per week for at least 6 mo after age 15 defined as "*hypersexual desire*"	• Internal validity is high as number of orgasms is a proxy measure for the strength of paraphilic interests. Number of orgasms does not define paraphilic interest per se. • Strong discriminant validity. Scores of hypersexual desire identify 3% to 8% of males in national samples; 73% of men diagnosed with paraphilia disorders.[89]
Sexual Compulsivity Scale (SCS)[40]	• Used most frequently in reports of sexual addiction • 32 items answered on Likert scale ranging from 1 (not at all like me) to 4 (very much like me) • High scores not sufficient to diagnose individuals with sexual compulsivity or addiction • Also validated in African-American men.	• Internal consistency is high on this scale (α's ranging from 0.77-0.89 across gay males, heterosexual college students, and adults) • Strong discriminant validity. High scores correctly identify men with higher numbers of sexual partners, higher rates of sex risk behaviors.
Compulsive Sexual Behavior Inventory (CSBI)[90]	• Developed to measure factors of control (over sexual behaviors), abuse, and violence • Scores above the median correlated with behaviors associated with compulsive sexual behavior • Spanish-language version is available	• Strong discriminative validity: correctly identified 92% of subjects with compulsive sexual behaviors from control subjects. • Factor analysis solution replicated original two factors of control and violence.
Hypersexual Behavior Inventory (HBI)[91]	• 19-item, three-factor, self-report measure scored on a 5-point Likert (1 = Never to 5 = Very often) • Calculated summed scores ≥53 are clinically significant	• Scale items reflect concept of hypersexual disorder. • Strong internal consistency with α-coefficients ranging from 0.89 to 0.95.
Minnesota Impulsive Disorders Inventory[92]	• 4-items from compulsive sexual behavior module • Items tap: (1) whether self/others think sexual behaviors cause problems; and whether (2) repetitive sexual fantasies, (3) repetitive sexual urges, or (4) repetitive sexual behaviors are out of control or cause distress	• An answer to any one indicates PSB. • Strong face validity.
Hypersexual Disorder Screening Inventory[93]	• 7 items measuring recurrent and intense sexual fantasies, urges, and behaviors and distress and impairment in the prior 6 months. 5 items are in Criteria A, 2 times in Criteria B • Item responses are 0 (Never true) to 4 (Almost always true) • Summed scores range from 0 to 28, with higher scores indicating greater severity	• Factor analysis shows single factor. • Good reliability. • Single cutoff score of 20 significantly identifies hypersexual disorder in gay and bisexual men.

Contingency Management

There are no clinical studies applying the principles of contingency management, that is, provision of increasingly valuable reinforcers for biologic data, demonstrating elimination of PSB. One explanation for this is that there are currently no biomarkers that can reliably determine whether sexual behaviors engaged are problems. On the other hand, among those individuals in treatment for substance use, application of contingency management to reduce use of substances highly linked to PSB, especially stimulants, reliably reduces substance-related HIV-transmission behaviors.[94,95]

Behavior Therapies

Behavioral approaches for treating PSB largely adapt models that have been validated for treating substance use disorders (eg, CBT, motivational interviewing) and apply these to the problems related to PSB. Outcome reports on behavioral therapies come from open trials or case reports, which provide feasibility information but scant information about efficacy. This literature suggests that as in most behavior therapies, outpatient treatments can help a significant proportion of individuals to remain in a help-seeking process, to reduce levels of psychological distress, and to reduce behaviors related to PSB, including reductions in numbers of sexual partners, in episodes of public sex, and in combining drugs and alcohol with sex.

For individuals whose clinical distress and/or symptoms of PSB do not remit from outpatient treatments, however, considerations of referral to levels of inpatient care are appropriate. As with treatments for substance use disorders, the quality of the literature documenting outcomes for residential treatment for PSB is poor. One report showed that the majority (71%) of individuals followed over a 4-year period returned to compulsive sexual behaviors, yet most reported positive outcomes associated with retention in treatment.[96] A small literature describes integration of family therapies into inpatient and outpatient treatments for PSB, though there are no data to describe treatment outcomes.

An important clinical issue in the management of these cases is how to address the topic of the PSB with the couple and family. Female spouses/partners of men with PSB are presented as having a central role in maintaining the dysfunction of the compulsive sexual behaviors of the male. Some data describe outcomes when disclosing PSB in families. Individuals in treatment for PSB typically prefer not to disclose information to their spouses and/or children. When female spouses ($N = 63$) learned of their husbands' PSB, 75% did so by accident; few found out via planned disclosures by the husband.[97] Once the disclosure is made, however, the impact on the women was traumatic regardless of whether finding out accidentally or from a planned disclosure. Disclosures by parents with PSB ($N = 57$) to children, whether made in anger or in unplanned or forced disclosures (ie, someone threatened to tell), predictably caused upset in the children. By contrast, planned disclosures allowed for forethought about what information to tell the children and allow the discloser to acknowledge the amount of disturbance he has caused the family rather than provide accounts of his behaviors.

Part of the treatment plan will usually involve some form of behavioral treatment. There is little direction from the literature that might identify groups of patients for whom treatment works well or what might be considered for the larger group of patients who terminate early or who show only partial or wholly inadequate responses to treatment. This of course contrasts with the interests of the criminal justice system to ensure complete elimination of paraphilic behaviors for men who perpetrate sexual crimes against children or nonconsenting adults.

Cognitive Behavioral Therapy

Cognitive behavioral therapy is a general approach to treating addictive behavioral disorders that teaches patients skills to instill abstinence and to return to abstinence upon recurrence. The approach is highly didactic and involves the counselor adopting the role of a coach for the patient. The approach also is flexible and easily adapted to the needs of the clinician working with patients seeking to eliminate problem symptoms related to their sexuality and to increase sexual behaviors that are valued by the individual and their partners. CBT approaches originate from social learning theory and conceptualize compulsive sexual behaviors as being maintained both by exciting sexual experiences that initiated and sustained the compulsive behaviors and by a lack of sexual behavior experiences that are less extreme that are engaged in lieu of the compulsive behaviors. One generic CBT strategy involves identification of "triggers" (ie, persons, places, things, or internal experiences) that are specific to sexually compulsive behavior. Other skills common to CBT also are applicable, including distress tolerance (urge surfing), environmental manipulation (bans to internet access), diffusion techniques (mindfulness, meditation) and the like. An important final point in using CBT approaches is that skills that help patients to avoid problem symptoms are quickly mastered. Integrating substitution sexual behaviors that are sufficiently acceptable and reinforcing to the patient in lieu of more stimulating PSB requires most of the effort for the patient and the clinician.

There are no randomized controlled trials of CBT for PSB. There is, however, one randomized controlled trial of CBT-based HIV-prevention interventions for MSM. In MSM who completed baseline measures of sexual compulsivity along with measures of sexual risk behaviors, no differences were observed between the condition that received an HIV-prevention approach that used CBT procedures and a standard condition. Post hoc analyses of these data showed that MSM in the lowest and highest quartiles of the Sexual Compulsivity Scale reported engaging in unprotected sex with status-unknown or presumed-positive men at significantly higher rates than those in the interim quartiles.[98] The MATRIX adaptation noted above may also be helpful as a harm-reduction strategy in this population.

12-Step and Self-Help Groups

There are no controlled studies of the efficacy of 12-step self-help groups in the reduction of PSB, usually framed as "sexual addiction" or "sex and love addiction." The primary advantage to 12-step group attendance for those with PSB is that the groups are convenient and widely available. The social process of recovery, which often involves selection of a "sponsor" to provide around-the-clock assistance in managing sexual obsessions and compulsive urges, also assists affected individuals to comply with the procedures of a 12-step program of recovery. Moreover, while even the most efficacious program of psychotherapy or of medication taken for the treatment of sexual addiction eventually ends, involvement with a 12-step program for PSB can continue for many years.

Four 12-Step approaches have been adapted to assist individuals with PSB: Sexaholics Anonymous, www.sa.org; Sex Addicts Anonymous, www.saa-recovery.org; Sex and Love Addicts Anonymous, www.slaafws.org; and Sexual Compulsives Anonymous, www.sca-recovery.org. The websites listed can assist individuals seeking support in addition to ongoing psychotherapy and/or medical treatment for PSB.

Psychoanalytic Approaches

Psychoanalysis has a long interest in paraphilic and hypersexual conditions, tending to see both as particular, suboptimal responses to broader conflicts or traumas during development, often a fixation in the oral stage or a narcissistic injury.[99] The term "sexual addiction" was first used in print by Otto Fenichel in a larger discussion of sexual perversions[100]—literally deviations from normal sexual development. Kernberg discussed hypersexual aspects of borderline personality disorder; like Melanie Klein,[101] he saw them as reactions to unsatisfied oral-dependent needs and pregenital aggression.[102] Kohut and his associates[103] saw compulsive sexual behavior as providing intense stimulation to reassure the self of one's vitality and reality, defending against depression, and attempting to compensate for unmet narcissistic needs: "like all addictions, it is meant to do away with a defect in the self, to cover it, or to fill it with frantic, forever repeated activity."[104]

Psychoanalytic authors often implicitly or explicitly assume that psychoanalysis can help with PSB, either by freeing up the fixations and unconscious conflicts thought to motivate the compulsions, or by helping patients come to terms with inappropriately negative or critical attitudes toward their desires. The efficacy of psychoanalytic treatment has more often been documented with case reports than with large-scale, randomized, and/or manualized controlled trials. Moreover, psychoanalysts are likely to see PSB as part of a larger pattern of difficulties with aggression, dependency, toleration of affect, or self-esteem, among other potential causes. Like other behavioral interventions, psychoanalysis currently lacks systematic clinical trials supporting efficacy for treatment of PSB specifically.[105]

PHARMACOTHERAPY STRATEGIES

Antidepressants

One strategy for pharmacotherapy of PSB involves treatment of dysphoric mood symptoms commonly experienced during initial (and perhaps sustained) sexual abstinence. If antidepressant medications can diminish dysphoric mood symptoms, patients may be able to sustain their sexual behavior goals. However, there are no randomized, placebo-controlled trials of sexual behavior outcomes (outside of adverse experiences) for patients treated with antidepressants other than SSRIs. Instead, descriptive small and open-label trials and case reports indicate that the medications can be used safely in this group.

Selective Serotonin Reuptake Inhibitors

Treatment of PSB with SSRI antidepressants is partly based on a hypothesized underlying serotonergic dysfunction, and partly simply leveraging the well-known side effects of SSRIs on sexual function and libido. Preclinical data show serotonin depletion in the presence of testosterone greatly potentiates sexual behavior in laboratory animals. More empirically, about 60% of patients receiving SSRIs can expect to experience some form of treatment-emergent sexual dysfunction including all phases of healthy sexual response: reductions in sexual desire, difficulties with arousal, and delayed or absent orgasm. These effects appear to be related to 5-HT_2 receptor agonist effects and are not observed at the same rates in medications with primarily noradrenergic mechanisms. In some penal systems treating paraphilias, in-custody persons are given high doses of SSRIs to produce dose-dependent sexual dysfunction as a side effect, a mostly unpublished practice. SSRIs can cause hyperprolactinemia, which may reduce sexual motivation and functioning. Evidence for this suggestion comes from the only randomized, placebo-controlled trial of an SSRI for the treatment of PSB. MSM rated as having compulsive sexual behaviors who were randomly assigned to 12 weeks of citalopram (20-60 mg/d) reported significant reductions in sexual drive, in frequency of masturbation, and in viewing of pornography compared to placebo.[85]

Reports from small, open-label trials with SSRIs indicate the feasibility of a particular medication approach. In one, 17 of 24 men with paraphilias and non–paraphilia-related disorders treated with SSRIs showed sustained reductions, over a minimum of 4 weeks, in total sexual occasions.[106] Other open-label trial experiences are consistent with positive outcomes in men who present for treatment of PSB, with specifically poorer outcomes for men diagnosed with paraphilic disorders as compared to men diagnosed with nonparaphilic disorders.

On balance, there is some initial controlled evidence supporting use of the SSRI citalopram for PSB. At present, there is no evidence to support use of other types of antidepressants to target reduction in mood dysphoria as a strategy for treating PSB. When implementing this strategy in outpatient settings in individuals seeking outpatient treatment for sexual behavior disorders, effects of SSRIs on dampening libido and disrupting performance are general to all sexual behaviors, not specific to the set of sexual behaviors that cause problems for the individual. For this reason, ambivalence in the form of medication nonadherence is common.

Opioid Antagonists

Naltrexone is an opioid antagonist approved for treating alcohol and opioid use disorders. The putative mechanism of action for using naltrexone to address sexual compulsivity involves naltrexone's role in dampening the opioid-dopamine reward system, thereby reducing the euphorigenic properties of fantasy and sexual tension that are usually the initial steps in compulsive sexual behaviors.

As yet, there are no large randomized, placebo-controlled trials of opioid antagonists for PSB. An open-label trial of high-dose naltrexone (150-200 mg/d) among adolescent sexual offenders was found to reduce PSB (masturbating 3 or more times daily, reporting feelings of intrusive sexual thoughts or arousal, spending more than 30% of waking time thinking about sex) in 15 of the 21 subjects. Naltrexone was tapered and stopped in 13 of the subjects, while consent forms were being revised, resulting in an unplanned temporary abstinence of the study medication. Compulsive behaviors recurred in these participants when naltrexone dropped to 50 mg daily or lower.[107] A placebo-controlled trial of 30 MSM with high rates of methamphetamine use, binge drinking, and risky sexual behavior found that oral naltrexone 50 mg daily somewhat reduced all of these behaviors.[108] Especially for nonparaphilic disorders, naltrexone may be a reasonable candidate for evaluation in clinical trials, but the lack of data makes it premature to consider its use in clinical situations.

Hormonal Therapies for Paraphilic Disorders

Though the evidence base is still limited, pedophilic disorder, in particular, has a larger body of evidence for treatment than other PSB. Because of public safety considerations, more drastic interventions are sometimes considered for pedophilic disorder and certain forms of sadistic paraphilic disorders than for other forms of PSB.

A small number of open-label and case studies support use of androgen-blocking medications for men with paraphilic disorders that involve children or nonconsenting adults. Sometimes described as *chemical castration*, the anti-testosterone strategy is usually reserved for treating men with paraphilic disorders that involve sexual offenses involving children or violence against adults. Cyproterone acetate and depot triptorelin have approved indications for individuals with paraphilic disorders in some European nations.[109] In the absence of randomized controlled trials, reviews of observational studies and open-label trials consistently show that these medications, as well as medroxyprogesterone acetate and luteinizing hormone-releasing hormone, effectively reduce additional offenses when taken as prescribed for up to 1 year, particularly when implemented with CBT. When these men stop taking the medications, their likelihood to offend returns to baseline levels.[108]

The World Federation of Societies of Biological Psychiatry has issued guidelines for the pharmacologic treatment of paraphilic disorders.[109] However, there is a conspicuous absence of well-controlled clinical trials, in part due to reluctance to randomize forensic patients to a placebo condition. Based on the available evidence, they suggest that SSRIs at higher doses typical for obsessive-compulsive disorder may be useful. This guideline is rated as Level C evidence, or "minimal research-based evidence to support this recommendation." Adding an anti-androgen agent to SSRI treatment is also suggested, but the evidence supporting the recommendation is even lower (Level D).

SUMMARY

A number of types of compulsive or ego-dystonic sexual behavior may come to clinical attention, either at the initiative of the individual or their partner, or through involvement in the legal system. These include paraphilias and paraphilic disorders, concerns for excessive sexual desires and behaviors (high numbers of partners, compulsive masturbation, compulsive pornography consumption, etc.), and the combination of compulsive sexual behavior with the use of drugs, particularly stimulants.

For persons referred to treatment in relation to crimes of a sexual nature, it is important to keep in mind that most individuals with paraphilias do not commit sexual crimes, and a majority of sexual crimes are likely committed by individuals who do not meet criteria for a paraphilic disorder.[59,60] Patients with paraphilic disorders whose satisfaction entails sexual acts of a nonconsensual nature or involving minor children may be candidates for hormone-blocking therapies, and may be most appropriately referred to specialist programs for further evaluation and treatment. It remains that sexual orientation, including the orientation-like aspect of paraphilias, is highly resistant to directed change through any known therapies. Treatment programs thus often aim at drive-reduction for those paraphilic disorders that may entail harm to others, through SSRI antidepressants or hormone-blocking agents.[109]

Though the concept of a general sexual addiction or hypersexual disorder has a long history, it has not been supported by rigorous or replicated studies and has not so far produced evidence-based treatments. Research has been compromised by arbitrary cutoffs and lack of consensus definitions. Critics have noted frequent comorbidity of putative sexual addiction or hypersexual disorder with psychiatric disorders, particularly bipolar disorder, substance use disorders, and personality disorders. Many cases of self-diagnosed sexual addiction appear to be influenced by strongly negative attitudes toward sexuality or particular kinds of sexuality held by the individual or their partner, rather than clearly demarcated by objective measures of sexual frequency or preference for particular behaviors. Proposals for hypersexual disorder were rejected for DSM-5-TR.

Patients presenting with distress about their sexual behavior should also be carefully assessed for paraphilias or paraphilic disorders, which may have more specific treatments, though most of the evidence base is derived from forensic samples.

Patients currently seek treatment for PSB including paraphilias and HVSB at rates that are sufficient to support healthy practices and a burgeoning residential recovery industry. Many addiction clinicians are willing to seek out evidence-based (or at least evidence-informed) approaches to treating sexual behavior disorders. Yet the evidence base is generally poor, requiring clinicians to knit together bits of evidence into comprehensive bio-psycho-social approaches to PSB. At minimum, there is evidence to support use of SSRIs, with or without use of CBT. Comprehensive assessment is crucial to rule out comorbid psychiatric conditions and to evaluate psychosocial factors that may contribute to the behaviors or to the patient's discomfort with them.

ACKNOWLEDGMENTS

This chapter represents an update and revision of previous chapters in this series, most recently by Matthew Brensilver, PhD and Simone Schriger, MA from the last edition. We are indebted to Drs Brensilver and Schriger for their work and retain much of their prose in this current edition.

REFERENCES

1. Kafka MP. Hypersexual desire in males: an operational definition and clinical implications for males with paraphilias and paraphilia-related disorders. *Arch Sex Behav*. 1997;26(5):505-526.
2. World Health Organization. *International Statistical Classification of Diseases and Related Health Problems*. 11th ed. 2019.
3. Cantor JM, Klein C, Lykins A, Rullo JE, Thaler L, Walling BR. A treatment-oriented typology of self-identified hypersexuality referrals. *Arch Sex Behav*. 2013;42(5):883-893.
4. Lewczuk K, Glica A, Nowakowska I, Gola M, Grubbs JB. Evaluating pornography problems due to moral incongruence model. *J Sex Med*. 2020;17(2):300-311.
5. Ley D, Brovko JM, Reid RC. Forensic applications of "sex addiction" in US legal proceedings. *Curr Sex Health Rep*. 2015;7(2):108-116.
6. Maxwell S, Shahmanesh M, Gafos M. Chemsex behaviours among men who have sex with men: a systematic review of the literature. *Int J Drug Policy*. 2019;63:74-89.
7. Strong C, Huang P, Li CW, Ku SW, Wu HJ, Bourne A. HIV, chemsex, and the need for harm-reduction interventions to support gay, bisexual, and other men who have sex with men. *Lancet HIV*. 2022;9(10):e717-e725.
8. Halkitis PN, Singer SN. Chemsex and mental health as part of syndemic in gay and bisexual men. *Int J Drug Policy*. 2018;55:180-182.
9. Krafft-Ebing R. *Psychopathia sexualis, with especial reference to contrary sexual instinct: a medico-legal*. 7th ed. F.A. Davis; 1893.
10. Freud S. Three essays on the theory of sexuality. In: Strachey J, ed. *The Standard Edition of the Complete Psychological Works of Sigmund Freud*. Hogarth Press; 1953.
11. Downing L. Heteronormativity and repronormativity in sexological "perversion theory" and the DSM-5's "paraphilic disorder" Diagnoses. *Arch Sex Behav*. 2015;44(5):1139-1145.
12. Laqueur TW. *Solitary Sex: A Cultural History of Masturbation*. Zone Books; 2003.
13. Brumberg JJ. "Ruined" girls: changing community responses to illegitimacy in upstate New York, 1890-1920. *J Soc Hist*. 1984;18:247-272.
14. Chauncey G. From sexual inversion to homosexuality: medicine and the changing conceptualization of female deviance. *Salmagundi*. 1982;58(59):114-146.
15. Hammack PL, Frost DM, Hughes SD. Queer intimacies: a new paradigm for the study of relationship diversity. *J Sex Res*. 2019;56(4-5):556-592.
16. Reysen S, Plante CN, Chadborn D, et al. A brief report on the prevalence of self-reported mood disorders, anxiety disorders, attention-deficit/hyperactivity disorder, and autism spectrum disorder in anime, brony, and furry fandoms. *Phoenix Papers*. 2018;3(2):64-75.
17. Kafka MP. Hypersexual disorder: a proposed diagnosis for DSM-V. *Arch Sex Behav*. 2010;39(2):377-400.
18. Carnes PJ, Green BA, Merlo LJ, Polles A, Carnes S, Gold MS. PATHOS: a brief screening application for assessing sexual addiction. *J Addict Med*. 2012;6(1):29-34.
19. Goodman A. What's in a Name? Terminology for designating a syndrome of driven sexual behavior. *Sex Addict Compuls*. 2001;8(3-4):191-213.
20. Grubbs JB, Exline JJ, Pargament KI, Hook JN, Carlisle RD. Transgression as addiction: religiosity and moral disapproval as predictors of perceived addiction to pornography. *Arch Sex Behav*. 2015;44(1):125-136.
21. Levi G, Cohen C, Kaliche S, et al. Sexual addiction, compulsivity, and impulsivity among a predominantly female sample of adults who use the internet for sex. *J Behav Addict*. 2020;9(1):83-92.
22. Fuss J, Briken P, Stein DJ, Lochner C. Compulsive sexual behavior disorder in obsessive-compulsive disorder: prevalence and associated comorbidity. *J Behav Addict*. 2019;8(2):242-248.
23. Slavin MN, Blycker GR, Potenza MN, Bőthe B, Demetrovics Z, Kraus SW. Gender-related differences in associations between sexual abuse and hypersexuality. *J Sex Med*. 2020;17(10):2029-2038.
24. Castellini G, Rellini AH, Appignanesi C, et al. Deviance or Normalcy? The relationship among paraphilic thoughts and behaviors, hypersexuality, and psychopathology in a sample of university students. *J Sex Med*. 2018;15(9):1322-1335.
25. Golec K, Draps M, Stark R, Pluta A, Gola M. Aberrant orbitofrontal cortex reactivity to erotic cues in Compulsive Sexual Behavior Disorder. *J Behav Addict*. 2021;10(3):646-656.
26. Raymond NC, Coleman E, Miner MH. Psychiatric comorbidity and compulsive/impulsive traits in compulsive sexual behavior. *Compr Psychiatry*. 2003;44(5):370-380.
27. Dickenson JA, Gleason N, Coleman E, Miner MH. Prevalence of distress associated with difficulty controlling sexual urges, feelings, and behaviors in the United States. *JAMA Netw Open*. 2018;1(7):e184468.
28. Black DW, Kehrberg LL, Flumerfelt DL, Schlosser SS. Characteristics of 36 subjects reporting compulsive sexual behavior. *Am J Psychiatry*. 1997;154(2):243-249.
29. Dell'Osso B, Altamura AC, Allen A, Marazziti D, Hollander E. Epidemiologic and clinical updates on impulse control disorders: a critical review. *Eur Arch Psychiatry Clin Neurosci*. 2006;256(8):464-475.
30. Guo G, Tong Y, Xie CW, Lange LA. Dopamine transporter, gender, and number of sexual partners among young adults. *Eur J Hum Genet*. 2007;15(3):279-287.
31. Golec K, Draps M, Stark R, Pluta A, Gola M. Aberrant orbitofrontal cortex reactivity to erotic cues in Compulsive Sexual Behavior Disorder. *J Behav Addict*. 2021;10(3):646-656.
32. Oei NY, Rombouts SA, Soeter RP, van Gerven JM, Both S. Dopamine modulates reward system activity during subconscious processing of sexual stimuli. *Neuropsychopharmacology*. 2012;37(7):1729-1737.
33. Singh A, Kandimala G, Dewey RB Jr, O'Suilleabhain P. Risk factors for pathologic gambling and other compulsions among Parkinson's disease patients taking dopamine agonists. *J Clin Neurosci*. 2007;14(12):1178-1181.

34. Hassan A, Bower JH, Kumar N, et al. Dopamine agonist-triggered pathological behaviors: surveillance in the PD clinic reveals high frequencies. *Parkinsonism Relat Disord*. 2011;17(4):260-264.
35. Baskerville TA, Douglas AJ. Dopamine and oxytocin interactions underlying behaviors: potential contributions to behavioral disorders. *CNS Neurosci Ther*. 2010;16(3):e92-e123.
36. Flanagan J, Chatzittofis A, Boström ADE, et al. High plasma oxytocin levels in men with hypersexual disorder. *J Clin Endocrinol Metab*. 2022;107(5):e1816-e1822.
37. Olsen CM. Natural rewards, neuroplasticity, and non-drug addictions. *Neuropharmacology*. 2011;61(7):1109-1122.
38. Steele VR, Staley C, Fong T, Prause N. Sexual desire, not hypersexuality, is related to neurophysiological responses elicited by sexual images. *Socioaffect Neurosci Psychol*. 2013;3:20770.
39. Cantor JM, Kabani N, Christensen BK, et al. Cerebral white matter deficiencies in pedophilic men. *J Psychiatr Res*. 2008;42(3):167-183.
40. Kalichman SC, Rompa D. Sexual sensation seeking and Sexual Compulsivity Scales: reliability, validity, and predicting HIV risk behavior. *J Pers Assess*. 1995;65(3):586-601.
41. Parsons JT, Grov C, Golub SA. Sexual compulsivity, co-occurring psychosocial health problems, and HIV risk among gay and bisexual men: further evidence of a syndemic. *Am J Public Health*. 2012;102(1): 156-162.
42. Storholm ED, Satre DD, Kapadia F, Halkitis PN. Depression, compulsive sexual behavior, and sexual risk-taking among urban young gay and bisexual men: The P18 Cohort Study. *Arch Sex Behav*. 2016;45(6): 1431-1441.
43. Raviv M. Personality characteristics of sexual addicts and pathological gamblers. *J Gambl Stud*. 1993;9(1):17-30.
44. Blankenship R, Laaser M. Sexual addiction and ADHD: is there a connection? *Sex Addict Compuls*. 2004;11(1-2):7-20.
45. Miner MH, Raymond N, Mueller BA, Lloyd M, Lim KO. Preliminary investigation of the impulsive and neuroanatomical characteristics of compulsive sexual behavior. *Psychiatry Res*. 2009;174(2):146-151.
46. Castro-Calvo J, Gil-Llario MD, Giménez-García C, Gil-Juliá B, Ballester-Arnal R. Occurrence and clinical characteristics of Compulsive Sexual Behavior Disorder (CSBD): a cluster analysis in two independent community samples. *J Behav Addict*. 2020;9(2):446-468.
47. Engel J, Kessler A, Veit M, et al. Hypersexual behavior in a large online sample: Individual characteristics and signs of coercive sexual behavior. *J Behav Addict*. 2019;8(2):213-222.
48. Lavan H, Johnson JG. The association between axis I and II psychiatric symptoms and high-risk sexual behavior during adolescence. *J Personal Disord*. 2002;16(1):73-94.
49. American Psychiatric Association. *Diagnostic and Statistical Manual of Mental Disorders, Fifth Edition Text Revision (DSM-5-TR)*. American Psychiatric Association Publishing; 2022.
50. Hughes SD, Hammack PL. Narratives of the origins of kinky sexual desire held by users of a kink-oriented social networking website. *J Sex Res*. 2022;59(3):360-371.
51. Laumann EO, Gagnon JH, Michael RT, Michaels S. *The Social Organization of Sexuality: Sexual Practices in the United States*. University of Chicago Press; 1994.
52. Joyal CC, Carpentier J. The prevalence of paraphilic interests and behaviors in the general population: a provincial survey. *J Sex Res*. 2017;54(2):161-171.
53. Wismeijer AA, van Assen MA. Psychological characteristics of BDSM practitioners. *J Sex Med*. 2013;10(8):1943-1952.
54. Krueger RB, Reed GM, First MB, Marais A, Kismodi E, Briken P. Proposals for paraphilic disorders in the International Classification of Diseases and Related Health Problems, Eleventh Revision (ICD-11). *Arch Sex Behav*. 2017;46(5):1529-1545.
55. Schmidt AF, Mokros A, Banse R. Is pedophilic sexual preference continuous? A taxometric analysis based on direct and indirect measures. *Psychol Assess*. 2013;25(4):1146-1153.
56. Jackson RL, Hess DT. Evaluation for civil commitment of sex offenders: a survey of experts. *Sex Abus*. 2007;19(4):425-448.
57. Levenson J, Grady M, Leibowitz G. Grand challenges: social justice and the need for evidence-based sex offender registry reform. *J Sociol Soc Welf*. 2016;43(2):3-38.
58. Dawson SJ, Bannerman BA, Lalumiere ML. Paraphilic interests: an examination of sex differences in a nonclinical sample. *Sex Abus*. 2016;28(1):20-45.
59. Williams KM, Cooper BS, Howell TM, Yuille JC, Paulhus DL. Inferring sexually deviant behavior from corresponding fantasies: The role of personality and pornography consumption. *Crim Justice Behav*. 2009;36(2):198-222.
60. Långström N, Seto MC. Exhibitionistic and voyeuristic behavior in a swedish national population survey. *Arch Sex Behav*. 2006;35(4):427-435.
61. Johnson RS, Ostermeyer B, Sikes KA, Nelsen AJ, Coverdale JH. Prevalence and treatment of frotteurism in the community: a systematic review. *J Am Acad Psychiatry Law*. 2014;42(4):478-483.
62. Blanchard R, Lykins AD, Wherrett D, et al. Pedophilia, hebephilia, and the DSM-V. *Arch Sex Behav*. 2009;38(3):335-350.
63. Seto MC. Pedophilia. *Ann Rev Clin Psychology*. 2009;5:391-407.
64. Tenbergen G, Wittfoth M, Frieling H, et al. The neurobiology and psychology of pedophilia: recent advances and challenges. *Front Hum Neurosci*. 2015;9:344.
65. Dombert B, Schmidt AF, Banse R, et al. How common is men's self-reported sexual interest in prepubescent children? *J Sex Res*. 2016;53(2):214-223.
66. Mokros A, Osterheider M, Nitschke J. Pedophilia. Prevalence, etiology, and diagnostics. *Nervenarzt*. 2012;83(3):355-358.
67. Blanchard R, Kuban ME, Klassen P, et al. Self-reported head injuries before and after age 13 in pedophilic and nonpedophilic men referred for clinical assessment. *Arch Sex Behav*. 2003;32(6):573-581.
68. Vicenzutto A, Joyal CC, Telle É, Pham TH. Risk Factors for sexual offenses committed by men with or without a low IQ: an exploratory study. *Front Psychiatry*. 2022;13:820249.
69. Singer MC, Erickson PI, Badiane L, et al. Syndemics, sex and the city: understanding sexually transmitted diseases in social and cultural context. *Soc Sci Med*. 2006;63(8):2010-2021.
70. Reback CJ. The social construction of a gay drug: methamphetamine use among gay & bisexual males in Los Angeles. *Report for the City of Los Angeles AIDS Coordinator*. Los Angeles; 1997.
71. Kirby T, Thornber-Dunwell M. High-risk drug practices tighten grip on London gay scene. *Lancet*. 2013;381:101-102.
72. Parsons JT, Kelly BC, Bimbi DS, DiMaria L, Wainberg ML, Morgenstern J. Explanations for the origins of sexual compulsivity among gay and bisexual men. *Arch Sex Behav*. 2008;37(5):817-826.
73. Parsons JT, Bimbi DS. Intentional unprotected anal intercourse among sex who have sex with men: barebacking - from behavior to identity. *AIDS Behav*. 2007;11(2):277-287.
74. Benotsch EG, Kalichman SC, Kelly JA. Sexual compulsivity and substance use in HIV-seropositive men who have sex with men: prevalence and predictors of high-risk behaviors. *Addict Behav*. 1999;24(6):857-868.
75. Krueger EA, Holloway IW, Lightfoot M, Lin A, Hammack PL, Meyer IH. Psychological distress, felt stigma, and HIV prevention in a national probability sample of sexual minority men. *LGBT Health*. 2020;7(4):190-197.
76. Shoptaw S, Reback CJ, Peck JA, et al. Behavioral treatment approaches for methamphetamine dependence and HIV-related sexual risk behaviors among urban gay and bisexual men. *Drug Alcohol Depend*. 2005;78(2):125-134.
77. Reback CJ, Shoptaw S. Development of an evidence-based, gay-specific cognitive behavioral therapy intervention for methamphetamine-abusing gay and bisexual men. *Addict Behav*. 2014;39(8):1286-1291.
78. Reback CJ, Larkins S, Shoptaw S. Changes in the meaning of sexual risk behaviors among gay and bisexual male methamphetamine abusers before and after drug treatment. *AIDS Behav*. 2004;8(1):87-98.
79. Shoptaw S. Methamphetamine use in urban gay and bisexual populations. *Top HIV Med*. 2006;14(2):84-87.
80. Gideonse TK. Framing Samuel See: the discursive detritus of the moral panic over the "double epidemic" of methamphetamines and HIV among gay men. *Int J Drug Policy*. 2016;28:98-105.

81. Romanelli F, Smith KM, Thornton AC, Pomeroy C. Poppers: epidemiology and clinical management of inhaled nitrite abuse. *Pharmacotherapy*. 2004;24(1):69-78.
82. Race K. *Pleasure Consuming Medicine: the Queer Politics of Drugs*. Duke University Press; 2009.
83. Hook JN, Hook JP, Davis DE, Worthington EL Jr, Penberthy JK. Measuring sexual addiction and compulsivity: a critical review of instruments. *J Sex Marital Ther*. 2010;36(3):227-260.
84. Adi Y, Ashcroft D, Browne K, Beech A, Fry-Smith A, Hyde C. Clinical effectiveness and cost-consequences of selective serotonin reuptake inhibitors in the treatment of sex offenders. *Health Technol Assess*. 2002;6(28):1-66.
85. Wainberg ML, Muench F, Morgenstern J, et al. A double-blind study of citalopram versus placebo in the treatment of compulsive sexual behaviors in gay and bisexual men. *J Clin Psychiatry*. 2006;67(12):1968-1973.
86. Masters WHMV. *Human Sexual Inadequacy*. Bantam Books; 1980.
87. Carnes P. *Contrary to Love: Helping the Sexual Addict*. Hazelden; 1994.
88. Kafka MP. Successful antidepressant treatment of nonparaphilic sexual addictions and paraphilias in men. *Clin Psychiat*. 1991;52:60-65.
89. Kafka MP. Sertraline pharmacotherapy for paraphilias and paraphiliarelated disorders: an open trial. *Ann Clin Psychiatry*. 1994;6:189-195.
90. Coleman E, Miner M, Ohlerking F, Raymond N. Compulsive sexual behavior inventory: a preliminary study of reliability and validity. *J Sex Marital Ther*. 2001;27:325-332.
91. Reid RC, Garos S, Carpenter BN. Reliability, validity, and psychometric development of the Hypersexual Behavior Inventory in an outpatient sample of men. *Sexual Addiction & Compulsivity*, 2011;18(1):30-51. https://doi.org/10.1080/10720162.2011.555709
92. Odlaug BL, Grant JE. Impulse-control disorders in a college sample: results from the self-administered Minnesota Impulse Disorders Interview (MIDI). *Prim Care Companion J Clin Psychiatry*. 2010;12(2): PCC.09m00842.
93. Parsons JT, Rendina HJ, Ventuneac A, Cook KF, Grov C, Mustanski B. A psychometric investigation of the hypersexual disorder screening inventory among highly sexually active gay and bisexual men: an item response theory analysis. *J Sex Med*. 2013;10:3088-3101.
94. Menza TW, Jameson DR, Hughes JP, Colfax GN, Shoptaw S, Golden MR. Contingency management to reduce methamphetamine use and sexual risk among men who have sex with men: a randomized controlled trial. *BMC Public Health*. 2010;10:774.
95. Corsi KF, Shoptaw S, Alishahi M, Booth RE. Interventions to reduce drug use among methamphetamine users at risk for HIV. *Curr HIV/AIDS Rep*. 2019;16(1):29-36.
96. Wan M, Finlayson R, Rowles A. Sexual dependency treatment outcome study. *Sex Addict Compulsivity: J Treat Prevent*. 2000;7:77-196.
97. Steffens B, Rennie R. The traumatic nature of disclosure for wives of sexual addicts. *Sex Addict Compuls*. 2006;13:247-267.
98. Dilley JW, Loeb L, Marson K, et al. Sexual compulsiveness and change in unprotected anal intercourse: unexpected results from a randomized controlled HIV counseling intervention study. *J Acquir Immune Defic Syndr*. 2008;48(1):113-114.
99. Goodman A. *Sexual Addiction: An Integrated Approach*. International Universities Press; 1998.
100. Fenichel O. *The Psychoanalytic Theory of Neurosis*. W.W. Norton; 1945.
101. Klein M. A study of envy and gratitude. In: Mitchell J, ed. *The Selected Papers of Melanie Klein*. The Free Press; 1986 [1955]:211-229.
102. Kernberg O. Borderline personality organization. *J Am Psychoanal Assoc*. 1967;15(3):641-685.
103. Kohut H. *The Analysis of the Self: A Systematic Approach to the Psychoanalytic Treatment of Narcissistic Personality Disorders*. International Universities Press; 1971.
104. Tolpin M, Kohut H. The disorders of the self: the psychopathology of the first years of life. In: Greenspan S, Pollock G, eds. *The Course of Life*. International Universities Press; 1985.
105. Garcia FD, Assumpção AA, Malloy-diniz L, De Freitas AAC, Delavenne H, Thibaut F. A comprehensive review of psychotherapeutic treatment of sexual addiction. *J Group Addict Recovery*. 2016;11:59-71.
106. Stein DJ, Hollander E, Anthony DT, et al. Serotonergic medications for sexual obsessions, sexual addictions, and paraphilias. *J Clin Psychiatry*. 1992;53(8):267-271.
107. Ryback RS. Naltrexone in the treatment of adolescent sexual offenders. *J Clin Psychiatry*. 2004;65(7):982-986.
108. Santos GM, Coffin P, Santos D, et al. Feasibility, acceptability, and tolerability of targeted naltrexone for nondependent methamphetamine-using and binge-drinking men who have sex with men. *J Acquir Immune Defic Syndr*. 2016;72(1):21-30.
109. Thibaut F, Cosyns P, Fedoroff JP, Briken P, Goethals K, Bradford JMW. The World Federation of Societies of Biological Psychiatry (WFSBP) 2020 guidelines for the pharmacological treatment of paraphilic disorders. *World J Biol Psychiatry*. 2020;21(6):412-490.

CHAPTER

54 Disorders Associated With Technology and Social Media

Richard N. Rosenthal and Jon E. Grant

CHAPTER OUTLINE

- Introduction
- Historical perspective
- Epidemiology and comorbidity
- Diagnostic dilemmas
- Assessment
- Internet characteristics
- Treatment model
- Treatment planning
- Indications for treatment
- Pretreatment issues
- Relevant treatment research
- Summary and conclusions

INTRODUCTION

This chapter is about the use of microprocessors, their substrates, and the problems that can ensue that take the form of addictive behaviors and may be novel class of diagnosable and treatable disorders. These purported addiction disorders are supported by the microprocessors that have made all this possible and where the bulk of the activity of concern is conducted on the internet. Early on, as described below, pathological engagement with computers and videogames was described, followed by pathological engagement with the internet, or "internet addiction" once the World Wide Web made the internet broadly available and with it, the various single-user and group-interactive applications to serve as substrates for more specific classes of addictive behavior. However, people are addicted not to the microprocessors *per se*, any more than the electricity that powers their smartphones and computers, but rather to what substrates the devices provide. As such, the overall question this chapter will focus on is one of examining the validity of internet use-type disorder and/or more specific disorder substrates such as gaming, gambling, and sex or social networking.

The internet has six major uses that affect clinicians and their patients: (1) source of information on disease, diagnosis, treatments, and therapists; (2) support and self-help groups (moderated or not); (3) provision of advice, diagnosis, and counseling whereby the person being helped has not met the helper except over the internet; (4) obtaining addictive substances, both prescription and nonprescription; (5) supporting a platform for individual or group engagement in novel constructs such as social media and online gaming; and (6) enhanced opportunities for people to do things that would tend to bring them to the attention of a clinician even if they did not happen to use the internet (sex, gambling, etc.). Some of these last activities are regarded as addicting in their own right and will be discussed further.

Microprocessors are all around us, serving as prosthetic brains, guides, knowledge sources, calculators, temperature controllers, proximity alerters, and the like, a technological leap of the late 20th century that is already having profound effects on human functioning in the 21st century. Microprocessors help us manage many aspects of our lives, and we use them a lot. They can provide much stimulation, but ultimately, they do not manage our time, our motivations, and our involvements, although some applications attempt to support these things. Some of us use them too much, lose track of time while getting too involved, and become habituated to the stimulation they provide. Some of us have significant negative life consequences as a result of that level of engagement, not that different from addiction to substances, which in itself is a topic of debate.

The term "internet addiction" covers only part of the problems encountered by clinicians in patients who spend too much time using devices built around microprocessors. Consider the accident resulting from texting while driving, the gunshots exchanged over Xbox use, too many hours on the internet using a mobile phone, work impairment due to sleep deprivation after staying up too late serially binge-watching *Game of Thrones*, or a person who finds *Second Life* more real than their real life. The common denominator is the use of microprocessors in an increasingly wide variety of devices. What is clear is that the human problems that are now becoming apparent in the context of microprocessor use are related to the interaction of the novel technology and the people using it, as compared to intrinsic mental disorders that have been around for millennia, such as depression and schizophrenia, or other disorders of compulsive/impulsive behavior such as eating disorders or gambling disorder. Yet, as will be discussed below, much of the impairing use of microprocessors appears to conform, with respect to predisposing factors, cognitive function, comorbidities, and neurobiological and neuropsychological correlates, to that of substance use disorder (SUD) and other behavioral addiction. Research attention to the broad category of internet addiction has burgeoned since the American Psychiatric Association announced that it would place internet

Gaming Disorder (IGD) into Section 3, a section for disorders warranting further study, of DSM-5.[1] In fact, of the 4496 articles listed from 1996 for "internet Addiction" on PubMed (https://www.ncbi.nlm.nih.gov/pubmed) as of September 15, 2022, almost 64% have been published since 2017, almost two-thirds of which is focused on IGD over the same 5-year interval.

HISTORICAL PERSPECTIVE

The history that matters is the most recent, as the pace of change has accelerated. The internet was established in 1969 at the University of Southern California as a way of linking computers for national defense uses. Early on, computers offered opportunities to impair functioning, even in the absence of the internet. Weinberg[2] described programmers so immersed in programming they failed to properly document their work. Later, Weizenbaum[3] described the development of compulsive programmers who had lost the broad view of problem-solving and came to see problems simply as means to interact with the computer. The concept of a person with impaired computer use was described in 1992 by Kuiper,[4] who called them "space cadets," characterized as spending too much time in front of industrial or commercial computers and having too few other ambitions or interests. Once the internet became functional in the business community, it did not take long for it to become an instrument of non–work-related use in the workplace, problematic if not necessarily pathological. A survey of 224 U.S. companies by Greenfield and Davis[5] demonstrated that 60% of companies had disciplined employees about inappropriate internet use and 30% had terminated employees owing to internet behavior. Forty-seven percent of a randomly selected group of workers from the 224 companies surfed non–work-related websites more than 3 hours per week and 19% 4 or more hours per week.[5]

Specialized offers to certain customers via email began in 1973, and the first online service for people who used computers started in 1979. Use of email for therapy was documented in the 1980s, and simulated patients were developed (eg, "Eliza" and "Parry") to demonstrate typical psychopathology to those who signed on to interact with them. But widespread use of email skyrocketed in the 1990s as email programs became interoperable, and anyone was able to get and send from any of a variety of software programs. The first wave of articles about internet addiction appeared in the mid-1990s, and the Center for Internet Addiction Recovery was one of dozens of sites set up to help the addicted. A book by its founder, Kimberly Young, PsyD, provides a picture of internet addiction in the late 1990s.[6] Text and IM took off as the 21st century began with personal digital assistants (PDAs), BlackBerrys, and increasingly smart cellular telephones. By 2012, it was estimated that 94% of the American population had fixed broadband internet access, including 80% of households with download speeds as high as 100 Mbps, although about 100 million Americans were not yet subscribers where broadband is available, citing perceived lack of usefulness, lack of digital literacy, and unaffordability.[7] Modern smartphones typically include a wide variety of communication modes such as internet, email, and messaging capability as well as multiple sensor arrays and geolocation capacity over and above basic cellular telephone service. American Community Survey data from 2018 reported 91.9% of American households with at least one microprocessor-containing device for application use, including smartphones, with 85% having a broadband internet subscription.[8] Compared to 52% in 2000, by 2021, 92% of U.S. adults used the internet, including 15% who used only their smartphone for internet access.[9,10]

EPIDEMIOLOGY AND COMORBIDITY

The problem of understanding the prevalence of internet addiction and related use disorders has its origin in the lack of internationally agreed upon standardized approaches to diagnosis, the multiplicity of instruments used to assess internet-related psychopathology, and a deficit of large community-based studies. Some ground has been covered with the addition of IGD and its standardized set of criteria to the DSM-5. Cheng and Li[11] conducted a meta-analysis of 80 studies of internet addiction published between 1996 and 2012 from 31 countries and 7 world regions that used the Internet Addiction Test (IAT) or the Young Diagnostic Questionnaire and generated a global base rate estimate of 6% (but without African data) with regional differences such as 10.9% in the Middle East, 8% in North America, and 2.6% in Northern and Western Europe. However, Kuss et al.[12] conducted a systematic review of epidemiological research into the prevalence of internet addiction and found that broad regional variations in prevalence rates such as 0.8% in Italy as compared to 26.7% in Hong Kong were a consequence of differing assessments with different cutoff thresholds. Nonetheless, the authors observed that there were some replicable core symptoms across studies such as compulsive use, preoccupation/salience, and negative consequences, which should likely be included in the core criteria for the construct validity of the diagnosis.[12] A recent meta-analysis of the prevalence of internet addiction in African countries (Egypt, Ethiopia, Morocco, Nigeria, South Africa, Tanzania, and Tunisia), using the Young's 20-item Internet Addiction Test, found a pooled prevalence rate of 40.3%.[13] Rumpf et al.[14] administered the Compulsive Internet Use Scale (CIUS) (a proxy for internet addiction addressing symptoms of salience, withdrawal, loss of control, conflict, and coping with unpleasant mood) by telephone to 8130 randomly dialed German respondents (ages 14-64) who used the internet privately for at least 1 hour per day, in order to estimate internet addiction prevalence rates, finding overall 4.6% at risk for and 1% with internet addiction, increasing to 2.4% among 14- to 24-year-olds and 4% among those ages 14 to 16. The overall risk was more than doubled for those recruited with mobile-only numbers versus access to landline connections, consistent with higher mobile internet access among youth. The base prevalence of internet addiction disorder (IAD) in the German sample is consistent with other studies of IAD that surveyed the general population in the United States, 0.7%,[15] and in Norway, 1.0%.[16]

Focusing more specifically on IGD, a review by Feng et al.[17] of high-quality papers (N = 27) published from 1998 to 2016 described the prevalence of IGD-type disorders in naturally occurring convenience samples, which ranged from 0.7% to 15.7% across studies (however, 15.7% is an outlier by about 6% due to one study having used a comparatively low threshold for diagnosis) and averaging 4.7%.[17] Although the rate of internet access had increased exponentially over 15 years in the 29 countries included in the studies, the rate of IGD remained stable over the same period. A recent meta-analysis of gaming disorder internationally found an overall pooled prevalence of 3.3%.[18] Interestingly, there were not the large variations in prevalence across countries and regions as had been reported previously (eg, see Kuss et al.[12]). The higher rates of IGD among younger age groups offer the opportunity for research into primary prevention. A systematic review by Mihara and Higuchi[19] included 37 cross-sectional and 13 longitudinal studies of IGD published up to May 2017 and found prevalence rates ranging from 0.7% to 27.5%, with higher prevalence rates in younger populations as well as in males, but, as did Feng et al., found no geographic differences in prevalence.[17] In most reviews of the prevalence of internet addiction and of IGD, the differences in methodologies make it difficult to compare studies and draw conclusions.

Given the large number of IAD definitions and diagnostic assessments as well as varying prevalence rates by geographical distribution, it is not surprising that the reported comorbidity of internet-related disorders and other psychiatric disorders demonstrates a wide range of prevalence rates in different studies.[20] However, across studies, the prevalence of mental disorders in persons with IAD is increased compared to populations without IAD. For example, a Turkish cohort of 10- to 18-year-olds with IAD (N = 60) was assessed using the Turkish version of the Schedule for Affective Disorders and Schizophrenia for School-Age Children and demonstrated that 100% of the students had DSM-IV psychiatric comorbidity, including 87% with a behavioral disorder (83% ADHD, 23% oppositional defiant disorder, 15% conduct disorder), 72% with an anxiety disorder (35% social phobia [60% in girls], 23% separation anxiety, 25% OCD), 38% with a mood disorder (30% major depression, 8% dysthymia, 3% depression OS, 2% bipolar), and 7% with SUD.[21] Interestingly, as there are for SUD comorbidities, there are sex differences as most of the boys (88%) spent their internet time in gaming, whereas all of the girls spent internet time on social networking sites. This was a treatment-seeking sample and so likely to be affected by selection bias, and as such, the prevalence rates are probably inflated over base rates that might be found with an epidemiological survey.[21] Wu et al.[22] recruited a more naturalistic sample of 562 Taiwanese college students and, using structured interviews (SCID-II), compared the rates of DSM-IV personality disorders between those with and without IAD, demonstrating higher overall rates in IAD compared to non-IAD (27.4% versus 13.9%) and significantly higher risks in the IAD group of avoidant (25%), borderline (21.9%), dependent (15.6%), narcissistic (3.1%), or any personality disorder (PD) (34.4%) among women and narcissistic PD (7.3%) among men. Similarly, Zadra et al.[23] also examined the rates of personality disorders assessed by the SCID-II among a nationally representative subsample with problematic internet use (N = 168, ages 20-34 years) extracted from a large German population-based survey and demonstrated, among those (N = 71) that met 6 or more criteria for IA derived by substituting the words "internet activities" for "gaming" in the DSM-5 IGD criterion set, that 29.6% with IA and 9.3% not meeting IA criteria had at least 1 PD, significantly higher in IA for all DSM-IV personality clusters (OR = 1.72), especially Cluster C PD (anxious/avoidant) among men, supporting the authors' hypothesis that PD associated with low self-esteem and high impulsivity might increase the risk of IA. Despite different countries and age ranges, the prevalence rates of any PD among those with IA are consistent for the two studies at 27% to 30%.[22,23]

In order to ascertain a more reliable and valid estimation of relative risks, Ho et al.[24] conducted a meta-analysis examining the relationship of internet addiction and co-occurring other mental disorders from eight studies including 1641 IAD patients and 11,210 controls, which used standardized diagnostic assessments such as the IAT, the Chen Internet Addiction Scale, etc., and had sufficient data to generate effect sizes, finding positive associations between IAD and alcohol use disorder (OR = 3.04), attention deficit hyperactivity disorder (OR = 2.85), depression (OR = 2.77), and anxiety (OR = 2.70).[24] Taken all together, as with other use-type disorders, there is an increased risk of co-occurring mental disorders including personality disorders that, if clinically unaddressed, would adversely affect treatment outcomes for IAD, IGD, and other internet use disorders.[25]

Social Adaptation to Technological Change

It is important to recognize that some portion of what has been thought as problematic use of microprocessors may have to do more with social adaptation to new technology than with psychopathology. America Online's Fourth Annual Survey of people who use email found a 1-year increase in 2008 from 15% to 46% of self-described "email addicts," ie, those who check email in bed (67%), in the bathroom (59%), while driving (50%, up from 37% in 2007), and church (15%).[26] Now, these data seem quaint, given the profound integration of microprocessors into daily life in smartphones and tablets as well as desktop and laptop computers used for communications. Culture has evolved, too: in 2022, texting while driving is illegal in 48 states and the District of Columbia.

Forming new relationships with others who use computers online may have once represented eccentric or problem behavior, but the advent of internet social utilities such as social networks, commercial dating sites, special interest blogs, chats, and others has made this a mainstream activity.[27] Similarly, checking one's email before something else that you need to do is a mainstream behavior, now that internet access is ubiquitously available on wireless as well as wired and cabled devices.[27] Constant feeds of information from X (previously known as Twitter), Snapchat, Facebook, and Instagram provide a need for social adaptation that was unimagined by most in the past except science fiction authors and writers of dystopian novels.

Identity and the internet are emerging as a separate field of study due to the impact of internet-based applications and social networking sites. Participation in alternate realities offers rich material for considering identity choices and psychodynamics, although false identities and misrepresentations abound in social media such as Facebook, where there were an estimated 2.01 billion monthly active Facebook users for June 2017. *Second Life*, an online virtual reality application where one could construct a complete interactive identity capable of interpersonal and financial transactions (www.secondlife.com), at its peak, had 51 million content users,[28] and people had reported having more success in *Second Life* than in their real lives.[29] Other patients have entered therapy because of social media-based relationships gone awry.

As any assessment of addiction involves considering risk-taking behavior, it is important for clinicians to understand the current risks that the use of microprocessors offers. One can easily become a victim when participating in email and social media groups (including chat functions) wherein others are using false identities, often for a specific purpose such as sexual predation. Technology change has outstripped the legal system's ability to provide basic protections. Even where economic damages can be claimed, such as false information engendering stock price swings, prosecution has been scant. Meanwhile, there have been almost daily reports of data security breaches involving thousands of people.[30] It is also important to consider developmental vulnerability, as novel technology may carry downstream consequences for those exposed early in childhood. Parents are often limited by technological naïveté from understanding what their children may be experiencing and doing, adding a dimension of complication to the evaluation they may present. For example, in considering the potential risks of media exposure, the American Academy of Pediatrics[31] suggests no exposure to screen media at all for babies younger than 18 months except for live video chat, to avoid solo media use in children 15 months to 2 years, and to limit screen use to 1 hour per day of high-quality programming for children 2 to 5 years of age. Children below 2 years spend 2 hours per day on average with screen media, yet there is evidence of poorer word learning with "educational" on-screen media when viewing is unaccompanied.[32]

DIAGNOSTIC DILEMMAS

There has been an animated discussion of terms such as "internet addiction," "pathological computer use," "pathological internet use (PIU)," "compulsive internet use," "email addiction" (see above), and the like in the popular press, where the concept of addiction is used to describe a much less serious phenomenon than what clinicians usually mean by "addiction." With increasing use of microprocessors, the terms have progressed from being jokes to being taken seriously. In considering whether the microprocessors are a *bona fide* substrate for addictive processes, it is important to present some caveats:

- Using the computer, cell phone, or video game is not intrinsically illegal, although the media can be used for that purpose.
- Using the computer, cell phone, or video game is generally normal, prosocial, encouraged behavior.
- For many people, microprocessor use is a source of frequent high engagement that is not pathological.
- There is a learning curve to information acquisition, time management, and social behavior when people experience these new and powerful tools (eg, think about pedestrians walking in city streets holding their cell phones that block their view of oncoming traffic or listening to iPods, which attenuate their ability to hear important external auditory cues).
- Calling maladaptive microprocessor-related behavior pathological rather than, say, a bad habit may medicalize what is, in actuality, a social problem.

Unanswered questions thus arise in the context of considering whether internet addiction is a discrete disorder and whether it is an addiction or some other type of disorder:

- Are most surveys that present high rates of PIU suffering from selection bias?
- Is the term *internet addiction* overstated and overgeneralized (ie, are there too many false positives determined by current screening instruments)?
- Is it the technology or the contact or behavior that it enables something that people may become addicted to?
- Does the use of the internet as a conduit for other disorders such as pathological gambling or compulsive sexual behavior become, in itself, a substrate for addictive process?
- Is internet addiction a component of another disorder, or if a discrete disorder, does it frequently co-occur with other mental disorders?

Martin and Petry[33] debated whether non–substance-related addictions (ie, behavioral addictions) were really addiction. In this debate, Martin pointed out that addiction as a process requires transformation of basic survival-oriented drives into misdirected or overly frequent actions that leave less time for more adaptive functioning. Recent research suggests that this process is indeed seen with internet-related impairments.[34-36] A more recent debate has focused on whether internet addiction is a separate and internally consistent, though generalized, disorder or a catch-all that contains several separate but related disorders supported through internet-based activity, such as IGD[1] and proposed others related to impairing use of internet-supported gambling, pornography, and other activities.[37,38] Griffiths[39,40] conceptualizes this distinction as addiction *to* the internet and addiction *on* the internet. A similar distinction was made by Davis[41] in considering PIU, positing a generalized form and a specific form that corresponded to individual disorders accessed through the internet and related to gambling, gaming, cybersex, etc. Analysis of treatment-seeking patients at a behavioral addiction clinic supports a range of different primary substrates such as gaming, chatting, or sexual content for those seeking treatment for PIU defined as a score greater than 70 on the IAT.[42] More recently, Brand et al.[35,43] have reframed internet addiction as internet use disorder, which, as a behavioral addiction, might eventually be included in the substance-related and addictive disorders section of DSM-5 (as gambling disorder has been) and, analogous to various specific SUD, allow for specific use disorders such as IGD, internet gambling disorder, internet pornography viewing disorder, and so on. Dong and Potenza[44] proposed a cognitive-behavioral model to elucidate IGD that contained 3 components including motivational drives related to stress reduction and reward-seeking, such as enhanced reward sensitivity and decreased loss sensitivity, deficits in executive control and related response inhibition, and process that relates to the decisional balance between choosing to act on and refrain from a motivated behavior. They further hypothesized that therapeutic approaches specific to these described IGD-related deficits could be addressed with corresponding forms: cognitive-behavioral therapy (CBT) for strengthening recognition of maladaptive cognitions and improving inhibitory control; cognitive enhancement therapy to improve response inhibition, cognitive flexibility and problem-solving, and capacity for delayed gratification; and cognitive bias modification, which could address cognitive processes such as attention bias and approach bias toward internet-related cues.[44]

Brand et al.[35] have further developed their model of internet use disorders to integrate the motivational domains presented in Dong and Potenza[44] and propose that, similar to drug of choice determinations among those with SUD, among those with specific instances of internet use disorder, there will be a "first choice use" of the genre of applications supported by the internet, such as pornography/cybersex, gaming, gambling, social networking, etc. They further propose the Interaction of Person-Affect-Cognition-Execution or "I-PACE" model of specific internet use disorders that includes predisposing core characteristics of the *person* together with genetic, temperamental, personality, and psychopathological traits that render vulnerability; *affective* and *cognitive* reactivity to internal or external stimuli that render vulnerability to specific forms of stimulus, in addition to the impact of maladaptive coping strategies, attentional bias toward internet-related cues, the deficient capacity for mood regulation, and development of cue reactivity and craving; and the impact of deficient *executive* functions and/or inhibitory control on the development and maintenance of internet use disorders.[35]

Neuroimaging and Neuropsychological Correlates

Internet Addiction Disorder

Internet addiction disorder (IAD) was initially codified by Young[45] as an eight-item polythetic diagnostic set modeled on pathological gambling. Early neuroimaging research examined neural underpinnings of IAD and demonstrated altered regional cerebral activity and structural changes associated with IAD in ways generally consistent with studies of drug and behavioral addiction.[46] Positron emission tomography studies demonstrated that compared with normal individuals, those with IAD have increased glucose metabolism in the right orbitofrontal cortex, the left caudate, and the right insula and decreased metabolism in the bilateral postcentral gyrus, the left precentral gyrus, and the bilateral occipital regions[47] and, in men, decreased dorsal striatal dopamine D2 receptor availability that is inversely correlated with IAD severity, consistent with the substrates of reward deficiency hypothesized in SUD.[48] Among adolescents ($N = 18$) with IAD, Yuan and colleagues demonstrated that decreased gray matter volumes in the bilateral dorsolateral prefrontal cortex, the supplementary motor area, and the left rostral anterior cingulate cortex (rACC) as measured through voxel-based morphometry and increased white matter fractional anisotropy of the left posterior limb of the internal capsule as measured through diffusion tensor imaging were significantly correlated with the duration of internet addiction.[49] Hong et al.[50] used resting state functional magnetic resonance imaging (R-fMRI) to evaluate whole brain connectivity in adolescents with IAD and demonstrated significant and broad decrease of functional connectivity in corticostriatal circuits with the bilateral putamen being the most affected subcortical brain region. Similarly, Lin et al.[51] used R-fMRI to examine the integrity of corticostriatal circuits in adolescents with IAD compared to healthy controls and demonstrated reductions in connectivity of corticostriatal functional circuits involved in cognitive control and affective and motivation processing. Specifically, reductions in functional connectivity were found between the inferior ventral striatum and caudate head, subcallosal anterior cingulate cortex (ACC), and posterior cingulate cortex bilaterally, between the superior ventral striatum and bilateral dorsal/rostral ACC and ventral anterior thalamus, and between the dorsal caudate and dorsal/rostral ACC bilaterally as well as other regions involved in cognitive control.[51] Higher severity of IAD was significantly correlated with lower functional connectivity between the right superior ventral striatum and the dorsal caudate bilaterally.[51] R-fMRI was used to evaluate brain functional connectivity in adolescents with IAD and excessive online gaming compared to healthy controls and demonstrated between-group differences in the functional connectome, particularly between regions located in the frontal, occipital, and parietal lobes. The affected long-range and interhemispheric connections correlated with the IAD severity, and behavioral clinical assessments suggest that IAD may disrupt functional connectivity linked to behavioral impairments.[52] In addition, there appear to be differences in cortical structure between adolescents with IAD and healthy controls. Hong et al.[53] examined the thickness of orbitofrontal cortex (OFC) with MRI and found that the right lateral OFC of adolescent males with internet addiction have significantly decreased cortical thickness. These results suggest that long-term IAD may lead to structural brain changes and altered function, although a causal relationship has not yet been established. However, one might expect increased coherence in tracts carrying information about finger movement and motor imagery (posterior limb of the internal capsule) given the person-hours those deeply immersed in internet gaming spend on game play with manipulation of keyboards, mice, and/or joysticks.

In summary, internet addiction has generally been associated with structural or functional impairment in the orbitofrontal cortex, dorsolateral prefrontal cortex, anterior cingulate cortex, and posterior cingulate cortex. These regions are associated with the processing of reward, motivation, memory, and cognitive control.[54] Our understanding of the neurobiological basis of internet addiction continues to progress, with research focusing not only on a more detailed understanding of the brain's reward and inhibitory control systems but also an interplay with the brain's language system.[55-62]

Internet Gaming Disorder

Moving a step beyond IAD, recent research has examined the more particular version of IAD focusing on internet gaming. Whether IGD should be regarded as a mental health problem distinct from IAD awaits greater understanding at this time. Dong et al.[63] examined neural correlates of response inhibition using event-related functional magnetic resonance imaging (fMRI) in 24 males without SUD performing the Stroop task; among the group (N = 12) who had internet gaming-related IAD (score greater than 80 on the IAT),[64] there was greater activity in the anterior and posterior cingulate cortices, consistent with impaired inhibitory control and decreased cognitive efficiency of response inhibition processes.[63] In addition, among internet gamers with IAD, diffusion tensor imaging demonstrated abnormalities in the posterior cingulate cortex and thalamus with higher fractional anisotropy in the thalamus associated with greater severity of internet addiction.[65] More recently, a study of 41 men with IGD examined neural processes underlying impaired decision-making related to gains and losses and found that the IGD group, compared to healthy controls, showed weaker modulation for experienced risk within the bilateral dorsolateral prefrontal cortex and inferior parietal lobule for potential losses.[66] In addition, during outcome processing, the IGD group presented greater responses for the experienced reward within the ventral striatum, ventromedial prefrontal cortex, and OFC for potential gains.[66]

Recent functional neuroimaging studies have demonstrated that adolescents with IGD exhibit altered activations in the frontostriatal network, the supplemental motor area, the cingulate cortex, the insula, and the parietal lobes.[67,68] Additionally, there are alterations in functional connectivity in the resting state between multiple brain regions,[69,70] and this dysfunction is associated with greater impulsivity.[71] Other structural imaging suggests decreased gray matter volumes and altered white matter integrity in areas involved in inhibition and emotional regulation.[72-74]

More recent reviews and meta-analyses of the neuroimaging research in IGD have found that individuals with IGD, compared with healthy controls, show hyperactivation in the anterior and posterior cingulate cortices, caudate, and posterior inferior frontal gyrus; hypoactivation in the anterior inferior frontal gyrus, the posterior insula, somatomotor and somatosensory cortices; decreased loss sensitivity; enhanced reactivity to gaming cues; enhanced impulsive choice behavior; and aberrant reward-based learning. Structurally, IGD is associated with reduced gray-matter volume in the anterior cingulate, orbitofrontal, dorsolateral prefrontal, premotor cortices, and putamen.[75-77]

Exploring the Internet Addiction Disorder Construct

In considering whether internet addiction is a real disorder, an approach different from the DSM-5 polythetic approach may be useful in creating a narrow construct within which to categorize internet addiction. In a monothetic approach, all criteria must be endorsed in order to give a diagnosis, and it should have high sensitivity for diagnosing true positives. If a monothetic approach can be constructed that has good construct and predictive validity, then expanding out from that may allow a criterion set that has reasonable clinical utility in reducing false negatives. Griffiths,[78] in considering the necessary components of addiction that would subtend diagnostically both substance and behavioral addiction, identified six necessary domains based on the work of Brown[79,80] in modeling problem gambling behavior: salience, mood modification, tolerance, withdrawal symptoms, conflict, and recurrence ("relapse"). This method is interesting, and clinicians who treat patients with SUD will recognize the symptom set in their patients and thus the economy in the approach:

- Salience: The drug or behavior has gained primacy in a person's life, which can be a cognitive change, dominating the person's mental life or, behaviorally, dominating a person's activity in a compulsive fashion.
- Mood modification: The substance or behavior subjectively gives one a rewarding high or alleviates a negative mood state.
- Tolerance: The person must increase the amount or intensity of the substance or behavior in order to achieve the desired effect.
- Withdrawal symptoms: After stopping or reducing the substance or behavior, the person demonstrates either physical symptoms after or dysphoria characterized by irritability, mood lability, depressive symptoms, and so on.
- Conflict: The person has conflicts regarding the use of the substance or the behavior that manifests as either interpersonal (eg, marital strife) or intrapsychic (eg, guilt).
- Recurrence ("Relapse"): After a period of abstinence, the use or behavior is reinstated with the same intensity.

Proponents of a polythetic approach to internet addiction modeled after DSM-5 substance use disorder might point out that one of the hallmarks of the modern concept of addiction is the idea of loss of control despite negative consequences, which is embodied in several of the DSM-5 criteria and not included as one of the six necessary domains of the monothetic approach. However, compulsive behavior in the salience category accounts for the symptom of loss of control.

It may be argued that problematic internet use better fits criteria for DSM-5 disorder groups other than the substance-related disorders (ie, internet addiction). This is what was behind the differing nomenclature, such as *pathological internet use* (PIU), which is modeled after pathological gambling, which was an impulse control disorder (ICD) diagnosis in DSM-IV, but which as *gambling disorder* has been moved to the substance-related and addiction disorders in DSM-5.[1] For example, PIU has been proposed as an obsessive-compulsive disorder (OCD) spectrum disorder. However, in compulsive disorders such as OCD, the intrusive thoughts or compulsive behaviors are typically ego-dystonic, whereas in PIU, the preoccupation is ego-syntonic and pleasurable. While most patients with OCD are anxious and full of doubt and tend to avoid risk, others dispel their obsessions and resultant anxieties through compulsive internet use (CIU). Patients with unhealthy Internet use tend to underestimate risk. Shapira et al.,[81] using the Structured Clinical Interview for DSM-IV (SCID), internet use history, and a Yale-Brown Obsessive Compulsive Scale modified for internet use, examined 20 recruited volunteers or referred patients with problematic internet use characterized as uncontrollable, markedly distressing, time-consuming, or resulting in social, occupational, or financial difficulties and not solely present during hypomanic or manic symptoms. In general, the subjects had, in contrast to patients with compulsive disorders, low levels of distress and resistance to excessive internet use. Their problematic internet use symptoms were highly impulsive, with all subjects meeting DSM-IV criteria for an ICD not otherwise specified, whereas only 15% subjects met DSM-IV criteria for OCD based on their problematic internet use. However, this uncontrolled study had a small sample size and a clear selection bias, so generalizing from the results may be problematic. Nonetheless, like gambling disorder, PIU could be conceived as an ICD, and several authors have proposed this.[5,82-84] In fact, a cross-sectional association analysis of 81 subjects equally grouped into IAD, pathological gambling, and normal controls revealed that those with IAD have increased trait impulsivity comparable to those with pathological gambling and a positive correlation of trait impulsivity to IAD severity.[85] Similarly, Meerkerk et al.[86] explored personality correlates predictive of CIU, an IAD proxy, and demonstrated in a survey among 304 respondents who met the criteria (score greater than 28) on the Compulsive Internet Use Scale (CIUS)[87] that dysfunctional impulsivity (ie, rash spontaneous, including constructs of novelty seeking, sensation seeking, behavioral undercontrol, and disinhibition) was the strongest predictor of CIU compared to reward or punishment sensitivity.[86]

Hallmarks of ICD are repeated failure to resist impulses that are harmful to self or others and tension or arousal before and pleasure or relief during the act, followed by guilt or self-reproach. However, this may not necessarily be the case in patients with problematic internet use and will need to be explored with larger epidemiological studies and more refined research of potential diagnostic criteria. In addition to symptoms that overlap with impulse control disorders (eg, intense preoccupation with internet use, CIU, loss of control over online time), internet addiction also shares symptoms with behavioral addiction, such as development of euphoria, craving, and tolerance.[88] The DSM-5 workgroup had at one point been contemplating problematic internet use as a compulsive-impulsive disorder in the group of ICDs.[69] As such, it may be that the placement of what may be considered internet addiction among the DSM-IV impulse disorders was an artifact of the failure to expand the category of substance-related disorders to a broader diagnostic category that includes non–substance-related "behavioral addiction." The monothetic approach to addiction described above supplies one potential model for building that category.[78] The utility of a monothetic approach is that in requiring all symptoms to be present, if any subgroup of those with problematic internet use fits the criteria, then the high specificity should make it easier to validate as a disorder. In order to provide construct validity of the monothetic model, it remains to objectively demonstrate tolerance and perhaps physiological or neuroimaging concomitants of withdrawal that are more than reported withdrawal-related dysphoria (although dysphoria may be sufficient for a polythetic approach, as it is in pathological gambling).[89] Assuming high construct validity, if anyone has internet addiction, it is someone who meets monothetic criteria. As is, in DSM-5, IGD has been pulled from the more inclusive concept of internet addiction and placed in Section 3 with the other "Conditions for Further Study," and the placement of gambling disorder in the substance-related disorders raises the possibility of other behavioral addictions ultimately being validated as belonging to that group, modeled on "use disorders."[1] Recent work by Brand et al.[35] and others further supports this notion, and the American Society of Addiction Medicine has formally included non–substance-related behavioral patterns of pursuing reward or relief in its definition of addiction.[90]

Another approach to developing stable and valid criteria for internet addiction has been to build a bottom-up construct of most frequent symptoms from factor analysis of a group. Pratarelli and Browne[91] conducted a 94-item anonymous survey in college students (N = 524) and demonstrated the non-independent factors: internet addiction (preoccupation, external complaints, less sleep, food, exercise, and punctuality) [salience], sexual (downloading graphic sexual material), and an internet use factor (excessive use for professional, educational, gaming, shopping activities, etc.). When the data were best fit to a structural equation model, the addiction factor was primary and causal to sex and use factors rather than vice versa. Charlton[92] performed a factor analysis on 47 variables derived from the six-factor monothetic model of addiction described above,[78-80] with added items that evaluated engagement (computer apathy/engagement and computer anxiety/comfort) from data collected from a survey of 404 college and graduate students. The addiction factor loaded upon all items of the monothetic model behavioral addiction criteria supporting the construct validity of this model of computer addiction.[92] However, the engagement factor also loaded upon tolerance, euphoria, and cognitive salience, demonstrating that these factors are not unique to addiction. This suggests that high computer engagement is part of the structure of "computer (includes internet) addiction" but is not necessarily pathological in and of itself. One can be highly engaged in internet use without negative consequences. Beard and Wolf[93] describe a woman who is preoccupied by thoughts about XX; desires increased time spent in activity XX; is unsuccessful or unable to control or cut back interactions with XX; is restless, anxious, or moody when not interacting with XX; and interacts for longer periods than intended with XX. Without a defined substrate ("XX"), the symptoms seem ominous in the example above, but when it is revealed that the high engagement of this woman for her actual baby (indicated above as "XX"), it becomes readily apparent that this XX-related behavior is not at all pathological. Thus, the authors suggest that an additional requirement of impairment in a person's daily functioning (ie, jeopardized loss of relationship or work/educational opportunity, lied to significant others to conceal extent of internet involvement, or used the internet so as to escape problems or relieve dysphoria), over and above symptoms of high engagement, is necessary for a diagnosis of internet addiction.[93] This finding is paralleled in the work of Ko et al.,[94] who in establishing a criterion set for adolescent internet addiction that had high diagnostic accuracy and specificity, as well as good sensitivity, determined three main criteria: characteristic symptoms of internet addiction not dissimilar from DSM-IV substance dependence symptoms, an exclusion criterion, and functional impairment due to internet use.

Since the internet is here to stay, future work will need to differentiate the substrates of behavioral addiction from an overall diagnosis of IAD, much as SUDs are classified according to substance used, for example, alcohol, stimulants, and sedative-hypnotics. The most likely domains are static and live sexual content (frequently in the context of co-occurring stimulant and other use disorders), video gaming, and gambling/day trading and perhaps social networking/live interfacing (including chat, texting, video), shopping/auctions, netsurfing, and music/video downloading/torrenting. An interesting need for differentiating purported behavioral addiction such as "sex addiction" and those that are solely microprocessor-based will occur at some point and represents a similar problem to that of the more inclusive IAD diagnostic range and the narrower, substrate-based concepts, such as IGD. At present, only IGD is included as a proposed diagnostic category in Section 3 of DSM-5. Much as social networking is a recently invented phenomenon, there may be future internet applications that end up as new substrates for internet addiction. Inquisitive individuals are at risk for "falling down the Wiki rabbit hole" because the hypertext content links can bring one to interesting new content pages in an infinite regress, but evidence of this at a disorder level has not yet been reported. Similarly, frequent and lengthy engagement in social media apps such as TikTok have become well-known as time sinks but are only recently a documented source of potentially diagnosable microprocessor-based pathology.[95]

Recent evaluations of social network sites demonstrate that they are used for social purposes, mostly related to maintenance of already established offline networks, and there has been scant documentation of pathological use.[96] Kuss and Griffiths[96] identified interesting correlates of social networking related to increased use, such as social enhancement in extraverts with high self-esteem and social compensation in introverts with low self-esteem, as well as high narcissism and low conscientiousness. In addition, they found correlates that might signal addiction vulnerability, such as decreases in academic achievement, noninternet community participation, and relationship problems.

Substance addictions occur at high rates with other mental disorders in the population, so it would not be surprising to see a related pattern in those with behavioral addiction.[97] Carli et al.[98] conducted a systematic review of 20 studies of the correlation of PIU, as assessed by the IAT and other scales, with other psychopathology and found, among the mostly Asian cross-sectional studies, consistent and strong correlation of PIU with attention deficit hyperactivity disorder (ADHD) and depression. Among online gamers ($N = 722$) who filled out a survey questionnaire, weekly online gaming time was averaged 28.2 ± 19.7 hours and was significantly and linearly associated with severity of depression, social phobia, as well as internet addiction scores.[99]

ASSESSMENT

Talking to patients, one can discuss the intensity and impact of their use of microprocessor-containing devices and assign general risk categories based upon the information provided. A simple screening cutoff can begin to establish whether use is "normal" or unhealthy. From there, it becomes more difficult to establish what one is dealing with, owing to the lack of scientific consensus as to whether certain types of unhealthy microprocessor use rise to the level of disorders, what type of disorders they may be, and what the criteria are for those disorders. As discussed above, functional impairment is a good marker for a clinically relevant use of microprocessors.[100] Below is an attempt to broadly define various severity levels of microprocessor use.

Use: A reasonable time spent accomplishing specific goals using microprocessors, such as a Google search on "pathological computer use" or getting back your dog that strayed because the staff at the pound found the chip under his skin with your name and telephone number. Remember that high engagement does not necessarily mean pathology.

Problem use: One can conceptualize this as use with trouble in that the use is causing clinically significant impairment. The issue here is the repeated taking on of undue risk, getting oneself into legal problems, the interference with fulfilling major role obligations, or continuing the microprocessor use in spite of recurring social or interpersonal problems. These parallel the prior substance use category for the DSM-IV substance-related disorders and might present as subthreshold for DSM-5 IGD, for example, when the syndrome causes impairment but fewer than 5 of the criteria are endorsed for a 12-month period. Texting while driving is risk taking and illegal in almost all states yet emerging as more accident related in some jurisdictions than a handheld cell phone.

Use disorder: The patient experiences that they cannot get along without it. Here, the problem is the level of functioning. Can we get by without the facts so easily pulled off the internet? Can you calculate as well or as fast as your spreadsheet? Can you avoid email for a day a week, as is increasingly recommended in the popular press? As with most disorders, there may be a false sense of being in control and "able to stop any time" when, actually, one cannot.

Consistent with DSM-5 substance use disorder, a syndrome akin to substance withdrawal may become evident. Symptoms such as nervousness, aggression, agitation, insomnia, anorexia, tremulousness, and depression have been noted after microprocessor-based device deprivation. Craving, newly part of the DSM-5 criteria for SUD, has also been demonstrated in IAD[35,88] and can be purposely elicited by cues and targeted for treatment.[101,102] While one can argue that use of an exogenous substance is necessary to produce the physiological changes of true addiction, it is increasingly evident that the body and brain change in response to the environment. Whereas the brain is composed of chemicals, its final pathway of action is electrical, and input from computers increasingly taps into cerebral rhythms. Virtual reality, use of smell, more sophisticated visual and auditory inputs (eg, augmented reality), and probably other paths into the brain will increase influence on the brain. However, at least one study found surprisingly that the interactive functions of the internet are not as addictive as other functions such as salience, lack of control, or anticipation.[103] SUD can result from buying addictive substances through the internet, where enforcement has been unsuccessful against thousands of sites offering prescription drugs and a handful of sites openly offering cocaine, heroin, synthetic cannabinoids, and other illegal substances.[104]

INTERNET CHARACTERISTICS

The internet offers unique characteristics compared to other vehicles with high liability for unhealthy use and addiction,[105] including the following:

- *Always available:* 24/7, lending itself to impulsive access and marathon sessions.
- *Convenient*: No need to leave home or work (those caught playing games or downloading pornography at work are the tip of the iceberg).
- *Inexpensive*: Internet addiction was more problematic when people were paying $800 per month of access fees.[6] Costs are far lower now, supporting inexpensive access.
- *Rewarding*: Content rich, with websites consistently present, designed to increase engagement and calculated to please; increasing, mostly benign interactivity; a continuous flow of new sites that offer novelty, more and shorter (eg, TikTok) trending videos, all developed and distributed at an ever-increasing pace.
- *Controllable*: People can surf the internet wherever desired and leave at will. Of course, people with IAD usually feel they can stop at any time. Using the internet, a person can better control others' access to them, but still interact at a time and place of their choosing.
- *Validating*: One can find something that caters to one's interests and tastes, thus verifying that these are legitimate because others feel the same way. The internet is always at least nonjudgmental, unless one chooses a role-playing mode wherein negative feedback is part of the social context but positive judgments can be found readily.
- *Escapist*: Sites of interest to the individuals who have the potential of becoming addicted offer a welcoming reality in which all sex partners are attractive and interested and bets are likely to be won. Some women are attracted to the internet because they can act like men,[106] whereas introverts can act like extroverts.[107] Importantly, it is also a place where people marginalized by ethnicity, race, or gender identity may be freer to be and express themselves.

The internet provides easy access to reinforcing stimuli that may differentially support addictive processes when internet communication is anonymous and isolated from normative feedback. Powerful search engines aggregate special interest groups and provide virtual and real communities where nonmainstream behaviors and beliefs are consensually validated.[108] Given that some of the vulnerability to problem use of the internet is due to the social learning curve regarding these novel technologies and applications, some of the risks of internet addiction might be ameliorated through education and training.[109]

TREATMENT MODEL

Theory of Change

Motivation is the key to change. Similar to aspects of other use disorders, if rewards are the issue, others must be found. If obsessive-compulsive concerns are more important, efforts and medication are directed at developing different habits and thought patterns. Remission is about learning to avoid triggers for impulsive internet use, making use of social support for healthy reinforcers found in everyday life, and aligned with the quandary of abstinence in nonrestrictive eating disorders, relearning how to use microprocessors in nonpathological ways.

TREATMENT PLANNING

Evaluation—Diagnosis

Internet use disorder is not a DSM-5 diagnosis,[1] yet incidence estimates for internet addiction range from 1% to 3% of the

American population.[15] The addiction field is used to epidemics of powerfully rewarding substances that lessen in severity and become endemic. There seemed to be no end to the crack cocaine epidemic of the 1970s and 1980s—much was made of rats pressing levers to inject cocaine into their brains until they died[110]—but although that epidemic heightened in severity, it ultimately plateaued. We have had more than two decades of concern about unhealthy microprocessor use, and currently, both use and hazardous use are increasing.

The diagnostic divides are among addiction, impulse control (non–substance-based reward), and compulsive disorders. The addiction field is familiar with reward mechanisms, dopamine medication, conditioned cues, and the like. Rewards usually are related to content or specific activities, such as pornography, gambling, gaming, etc. Diagnoses related to these specific areas are well established and should be used, although, for example, pathological gambling had been classified by DSM-IV as an ICD rather than as an addiction under the substance-related disorder category, where it has now been placed in the DSM-5 as gambling disorder. There remains a population that compulsively uses devices without seeming to get much gratification. They do not feel good, but not doing it leads to feeling bad. Addiction clinicians will recognize this state of compulsive use that is frequently seen in individuals with addiction to crack cocaine using in spite of the lack of "liking" or individuals with opioid use disorder using heroin in order to "get straight" (negative reinforcement). People who use devices compulsively rearrange files, check email too often, get on mailing lists that shower them with trivia, and so on. Frequently, they meet criteria for a compulsive disorder.

Rating scales serve as diagnostic aids and, in offering objective data for feedback in motivational approaches, can help patients to realize the extent of their problems. Several are available but that from the Center for Internet Addiction Recovery, the IAT (http://netaddiction.com/Internet-addiction-test.htm), is best established, having been filled out by thousands of visitors to its website.[6] Its 20 questions are answered on a 5-point scale (with a sixth alternative: does not apply). A score of 100 is possible, with ranges of 20 to 49 indicating average online use and 50 to 79 indicating occasional or frequent problems using the internet and the "need to assess their full impact on your life." The questions explore staying on longer than intended, neglecting household chores, preferring the excitement of the internet to intimacy with one's partner, forming new relationships via the internet, others complaining about the amount of time one spends online, decreased productivity (grades, school work, job), checking email before something else one needs to do, defensiveness or secretiveness when asked about online activities, blocking out disturbing thoughts about one's life with soothing thoughts about the internet, anticipating going online, thinking life would be empty and joyless without the internet, irritability if bothered while online, losing sleep because of late-night use, preoccupation or fantasies while offline, rationalizing extra time online, attempts to reduce online time, hiding how long online, choosing online versus socializing, and depression and moodiness when offline remedied when online. Many of these items correspond to similar items in the DSM-IV-TR diagnostic categories of substance use and substance dependence.[111] The scale can be used by significant others, who usually insist on treatment for reasons common to other addiction: a sense of losing the loved one whose life has been taken over by the addiction, significant impairment in activities, and relationships, all usually minimized by the patient. Widyanto and McMurran[88] recruited 86 participants through the internet who completed a Web version of the IAT with some added items; factor analysis of the IAT revealed six factors, which showed good internal consistency and concurrent validity: salience, excessive use, neglecting work, anticipation, lack of control, and neglecting social life. More recent meta-analysis of 11 studies with 6821 participants reveals that the IAT is more reliable in college students compared to precollege students and has continent-dependent reliability in that IAT samples from Asia are more reliable than those from Europe.[112] A new scale among many others developed since the publication of DSM-5[1] attempts to improve and modernize identification of internet addiction is the Internet Disorder Scale (IDS-15), a 15-item instrument to assess IA based on a modification of the nine DSM-5 IGD.[113] Psychometric testing among 1105 participants demonstrated good construct validity and reliability and provided capability to attribute low, medium, or high risk for internet addiction in individuals based on latent profile analysis statistical techniques.[113] Finally, given the idea discussed earlier that the internet can provide a vehicle to other, process-based use disorders, Northrup et al.[114] developed the Internet Process Addiction Test (IPAT), an exploratory 26-question process addiction screening tool based on but with a broader symptom set than the IAT, which demonstrated good convergent, divergent, and concurrent validity and reliability among 270 participants, and effectively screened for pathological online Web surfing, sexual activity, video gaming, and social networking. However, each question of the 26-item set evaluates seven internet subprocess domains (eg, surfing, gaming, sexual, etc.) and is thus too lengthy for typical clinical use.

INDICATIONS FOR TREATMENT

Patients and families understand and feel impairment, so responses to the scale above and issues of morbidity and mortality can help all concerned understand indications for treatment.

Mortality

Murder and suicide have been reported after microprocessor deprivation, often manifested as an adolescent killing the depriving parent or demonstrating through suicide that life without the microprocessor is not possible. Many of these cases have occurred in South Korea where the suicide rate, the rate of suicide attempts, and the use of the internet and microprocessors are among the highest in the world.[115] One study found that among 452 South Korean adolescents, internet addiction identified by the IAT was significantly associated with depressive symptoms.[116] Lee et al.[115] examined cross-sectional data from a very large school sample of South Korean children in 7th to 12th grade (2008-2010 Korea Youth Risk Behavior Web-based Survey; $N = 221,265$) and found, compared to people who used the internet normally, potential-risk and high-risk internet users had increasing risk for both suicidal thoughts (OR = 1.49 and 1.94, respectively) and past year suicidal behavior (OR = 1.20 and 1.91, respectively) although a causal attribution is not possible. However, a systematic review suggested that more than 5 hours of daily internet use or online gaming is associated with suicidal ideation and planning, and internet interactions may inhibit revealing suicidal thoughts or plans or seeking professional help and may provide normalizing feedback about self-harm.[117]

Morbidity

Morbidity occurs at several levels. The amount of time spent with microprocessors results in necessary tasks going undone. Real-life social relationships get less time, and what may be thought to be more satisfying relationships are developed on the internet. Impairment can be difficult to tease out but, as described above, becomes a crucial component of a diagnosis over and above high engagement. The patient is not necessarily a recluse but can document that those hours spent in his room involve communicating with "friends" around the world to play *World of Warcraft*. Objective observers may rate these relationships less favorably, often reminiscent of a patient with alcohol use disorder's drinking buddies. Managing multiple identities can be taxing, and identity fragmentation occurs if one's internet persona is markedly different from one's real-life persona. Clinicians have to assess cyber relationships in detail. Some patients present as having lost touch with what is the "true" reality. Impairment may also result from physical activity of prolonged sitting in front of screens, with increased obesity and less exercise. Decreasing use of national parks, 4 million fewer golfers, and a decline in outdoor activities may be related to increasing use of microprocessors. However, inactivity is preferable to accidents that occur while multitasking. The American College of Emergency Physicians responded to increasing reports of injuries related to being hit or falling while texting in 2008 by issuing an alert against "text walking." It may seem to be common sense that people should watch where they are walking, but the number of vehicle hits, falls, and running into trees, lamp posts, and other people has become noticeable in emergency rooms across the country.

PRETREATMENT ISSUES

Motivation—Rationale for Choice of Treatment

As with most addiction, motivation prior to engagement in treatment may be scant or absent. Problems are minimalized, rationalized, or denied. A nonconfrontational discussion of impairment often helps the patient to gain perspective. This can be done using the principles of motivational interviewing, where the facts about the impact of microprocessor overuse are carefully elicited and then fed back to the patient in a nonjudgmental manner.[118] This helps the patient to use his or her native analytic capacity and values in determining that the overuse is actually problematic or impairing and helps to tip the decisional balance toward seeking help to reduce the problem.

An important way-station between internet addiction and returning to the real world is more therapeutic use of the internet and microprocessors. This is somewhat of a departure from the abstinence-oriented approach of classic addiction treatment. A mother was successful in restricting her daughter's IM from 3000 per day to 500 and then 200. Online support groups are thought to help, but a review of 38 controlled studies of illness (not just internet addiction) support groups found no robust evidence of effects, in part because most were measuring complex interventions.[119]

Selection and Preparation of Patients/Suitability

Unlike the subpopulations of individuals with substance use disorder, those with unhealthy microprocessor use are technically competent, often innovative, and well-educated,[120] which makes them more suitable as a group for clinical interventions. However, the subpopulation has been demonstrated to have high rates of current and lifetime co-occurring mental disorders, which tend to have a negative impact upon recovery.[66] Retreat into cyberspace may mask co-occurring social phobia and/or other anxiety disorders.

Therapist Characteristics

Familiarity with the internet and uses of microprocessors and technology is important for understanding patients, expressing empathy, and earning respect and credibility with patients, all of which are associated with better treatment outcomes.[121]

Treatment and Technique

Choice and Timing of Interventions

When parents or significant others are in control, taking away or restricting access to the microprocessor may increase motivation or result in destructive anger, so clinicians must expect to hear about and perhaps participate in whatever decision is made. However, similar to binge eating and other disorders of compulsive food intake, complete abstinence is usually not a feasible long-term treatment goal, as use of microprocessors is unavoidable in today's world and nonuse is associated with significant vocational and social disadvantage.

General and Stage-Specific Interventions

The general plan is reintroduction into the real world, which must be done in stages to ease transitions. It is a desensitization process, with small steps to be taken that will bring about a sense of success and increased self-esteem. Where identity issues predominate, the successful elements of the internet identity should be characterized, and there should be an open discussion of integrating these into the real-world persona. Therapy should be seen as a rewarding process that helps the patient get in real life what has been available only on the internet. This is consistent with community reinforcement principles in replacing the rewards of the used substance with more natural and socially appropriate reinforcers.[122] With compulsive patients, the therapist can take responsibility for the compulsive behavior and relieve the patient's anxiety. Medication treatment for co-occurring OCD and/or anxiety can be helpful. Clearly, treating co-occurring mood, anxiety, psychotic, and SUDs is likely to be helpful in supporting recovery from involvement of significant others and is key to supporting recovery and reintegration into the real world. Social skills training may also be helpful.

RELEVANT TREATMENT RESEARCH

Compared to research on psychosocial treatments of SUD, there has been far less relevant treatment research because funding agencies have slowly recognized the problem as deserving much attention (ie, significant clinical impact, public outcry, or political will). This has started to change. A 2017 survey of clinicaltrials.gov for internet addiction revealed only one German study of CBT-based treatment for computer gaming addiction and one nonactive CBT study of IGD and sleep disorders, whereas in September 2022, there are listed 15 recent or ongoing studies testing behavioral interventions for IGD and addiction to smartphone use or social media. The development and use of the internet are seen as an enormous technological advance. More and more material is being made available on the internet, and its legitimate use is increasing exponentially. There is strong commercial support for internet use, as the internet generates huge advertising revenues and is used to sell many products. Complaints about internet addiction can be seen as spoiling the party. The American Medical Association called in 2007 the National Institutes of Health and the Centers for Disease Control to start research programs in internet addiction, but as of 2017, no federal grant programs have as yet been announced. As such, much of the available epidemiological and treatment outcome research devoted to internet addiction has been based upon case studies and survey data, of which internet-based surveys can be driven by the motivation of the responders and thus subject to selection bias. Given the increased international attention to IGD, King et al.[123] conducted a systematic review of 30 studies mostly from China and South Korea of psychosocial interventions for IGD carried out between 2007 and 2016. The authors found, using the 25-item CONSORT statement,[124] that overall research quality was impaired due to the disparities in the definition, diagnosis, and measurement of IGD, the lack of randomized controlled studies with proper blinding of data acquisition and analysis, and unavailability of recruitment dates, sample size justification, follow-up reports on changes in gaming or internet use, and effect sizes.[123] These trends in the design and execution of international research studies continued despite the 2013 publication of DSM-5 IGD criteria and a preliminary international consensus for IGD assessment published by Petry et al. in 2014.[125] There are more than 20 instruments that have been developed to assess IGD but typically only assessed for 9 of the DSM-5 criteria, most frequently failing to assess if the patient jeopardized or lost a relationship, job, or educational or career opportunity,[125] but more recent constructs are fitted to the IGD criterion set.[126] Clearly, the research in this area is in need of standards in assessment and diagnosis with better study design and execution.

Psychologically Based Treatments

Winkler and colleagues conducted a meta-analysis of the extant treatment research for IAD, including studies with various internet-related problems, and found evidence in pre–post analyses for effective treatment of IAD, time spent online, depression, and anxiety.[127] Yeun and Han[128] conducted a meta-analysis of 37 studies to determine the effect size of prevention-oriented psychosocial interventions for internet addiction in mostly South Korean school-aged children and demonstrated, in spite of considerable variation in diagnostic approaches and predominantly nonrandomized designs, a large protective effect on the development of internet addiction as well as a large effect on self-esteem and improved self-control. Elements that weighed strongly as variables were duration of treatment exposure of more than 10 sessions, CBT, parental involvement in therapy (for children), and self-control training.[128] Yellowlees and Marks[129] suggest that given that cognitive process maintains IAD, appropriate psychotherapeutic strategies would include cognitive restructuring focused on the applications of choice, behavioral exercises, and graded exposure therapy with increasing duration of offline activity. As such, an early uncontrolled trial of CBT specifically focused upon internet addiction demonstrated efficacy in reducing pathological internet usage and improving online time management among 114 patients who were screened with the IAT.[120] Young[130] conducted a more recent noncontrolled study with 128 treatment-seeking patients screened for IAD with the IAT who were then treated with 12 weekly sessions of CBT for internet addiction (CBT-IA), a CBT-based intervention that initially uses behavior therapy to examine computer and noncomputer behavior to promote abstinence from problematic sites or applications, moves into cognitive work to identify maladaptive cognitions that serve as rationalizations and triggers, and finally works on harm reduction strategies for maintenance of gains and recurrence prevention. Most participants were able to manage their IAD symptoms effectively by the 12th session and 70% maintained this at 6 months.[130] Similarly, Wölfling et al.[131] treated 42 mostly single adult men with internet addiction (4/5 with IGD-type problems) with an integrated three-phase program with 15 group and 8 individual sessions based on CBT and demonstrated significant reductions in problem severity and negative consequences of internet use in this uncontrolled sample.[131] In a Chinese sample, Liu and colleagues conducted a study of manualized 6-session (2 hours) multifamily group therapy (MFGT) focused on strengthening adolescent-parent communication and shifting needs fulfillment away from the internet to real-life interpersonal interactions, compared to a waiting list control group in 42 adolescents and 42 parents, demonstrating in the intervention group a significant reduction in scores on the Adolescent PIU Scale and time spent on the internet both at the end of treatment and at 3-month follow-up.[132] As yet, there are no high-quality randomized controlled trials reported for psychosocial treatment of IAD as a stand-alone construct.

Focusing more specifically on treatment of specific "internet use disorders," there is some evidence from controlled trials suggesting the efficacy of psychosocial interventions for IGD and internet-related gambling. Zhang and colleagues (85) conducted a 6-week study of 40 young Chinese adults with IGD, comparing a convenience sample of those that received a weekly craving behavioral intervention (CBI) based on the cognitive behavioral model of Dong and Potenza,[44] and targeting internet gaming cue-reactive craving ($N = 23$), to a matched group that did not ($N = 17$) and found significant reductions in the CBI group on visual analogue scale (VAS) measures of cue-induced craving, durations of weekly gaming, and overall internet addiction severity.[74] Deng et al.[87] likewise targeted craving behavior in 63 Chinese college students with IGD in a quasi-experimental trial of a 6-session weekly cognitive-behavioral intervention (including identification of craving triggers and emotion regulation training, $N = 44$) compared to a convenience sample ($N = 19$) waiting list control group and found significant reductions in severity of IGD, as well as in VAS measures of current craving for online gaming at postintervention and at 3- and 6-month follow-up.[87] The change in self-reported craving accounted for a significant portion of the effect of the intervention on IGD severity at all three assessment points, and further analyses revealed that the reduction in craving was mainly attributable to amelioration in depression symptoms and shifting fulfillment of psychological needs from the internet to real-life interpersonal interactions, suggesting that craving is an important treatment target in psychosocial treatment of IGD and perhaps other internet-related disorders.[87] A study combining medications and behavioral intervention shows promise for CBT for IGD in the context of comorbid mood disorders. Kim et al.[133] tested 8-session CBT versus no behavioral intervention in Korean adolescent males ($N = 72$) with major depression and IGD-type internet addiction (based on DSM-IV substance use criteria) who were treated with bupropion and demonstrated significant reductions in online gaming time and internet addiction severity in the CBT group at study end and at 4-week follow-up, as well as a significant reduction in depression severity compared to controls.

Cognitive-behavioral–based interventions may also have applicability in treating internet gambling disorder. With internet-based behavioral addiction, it is unclear as to whether a focus on reducing pathological internet use or more specific targeting of the substrate will have more clinical efficacy. Petry and Gonzalez-Ibanez[134] conducted a secondary analysis of results from a primary study of brief interventions for problem gambling[135] where for this analysis the data from the three active intervention groups (10-15′ brief advice, 50′ motivational enhancement therapy (MET), and MET + 3 additional CBT sessions) were combined and compared to the control group (assessment only) in mostly male (more than 80%) college students with ($N = 57$) or without ($N = 60$) recent internet gambling.[134] Although at baseline the recent internet gamblers gambled more frequently and with higher stakes and had significantly more anxiety and interpersonal and school impairment than did the noninternet gamblers, the impact of the three active interventions compared to controls in significantly reducing gambling behavior over time was not different between groups, suggesting that internet-based gambling disorders are responsive to brief therapies focused on gambling behavior rather than internet behavior per se.[135] In contrast, Luquiens et al.[136] screened with a survey and recruited non–treatment-seeking problem internet gamblers on a poker website for a 6-week randomized clinical trial of three brief interventions targeting gambling behavior, emailed automated personalized feedback from individual survey scores, an emailed self-help book with an unguided CBT program, and a CBT program emailed weekly with professional guidance, versus a waiting list control group, and found that in all groups, the dropout rate was high, but study completers had significantly reduced gambling severity scores. However, the group that received the professionally guided CBT had the highest dropout rate, suggesting that CBT-type interventions may not be appropriate in internet gamblers who are not treatment seeking.[136]

Pharmacotherapy and Psychologically Based Treatments

Regarding pharmacotherapy for IAD, one study reported therapeutic success with escitalopram, a selective serotonin reuptake inhibitor antidepressant[137]; however, the active treatment phase was open label. Han et al.[138] treated males ($N = 11$) addicted to internet video gaming with sustained-release bupropion titrated to 300 mg/d over a 6-week period and compared them to healthy controls who had the same video game preference as the experimental group, but not pathologically. Not only were the total amount of time spent playing, related maladaptive behaviors, and video game craving reduced at 6 weeks and significantly correlated with the drop in time spent playing, but video cue-induced brain activity in the dorsolateral prefrontal cortex, as assessed by fMRI, was also reduced from baseline.[138] An 8-week trial of methylphenidate for ADHD (mean dose 30.5 mg/d) in Korean children ($N = 62$) examined the impact on measures of internet addiction and internet usage as well as ADHD symptoms and visual continuous performance test function and demonstrated reduced inattention and impulsivity-hyperactivity scores, as expected, as well as significantly reduced scores on hours of internet use and the Internet Addiction Scale, which was significantly correlated with the decrease in ADHD symptoms.[139] Additionally, a single case study reported, after failure of multiple antidepressant trials as well as psychosocial and self-help approaches, successful treatment of internet-based sex addiction with up to 150 mg/d of oral naltrexone when added to a baseline of sertraline 100 mg/d, which supported normalized social, occupational, and personal function.[140] Finally, Han and Renshaw[141] conducted an 8-week randomized trial of bupropion SR 300 mg/d plus weekly education for problematic internet use compared to weekly education alone in male patients ($N =$ 50, 13-45 years old) with DSM-IV major depression and severe problem internet gaming and demonstrated that in addition to significantly reduced depression severity in the medication group there was significantly reduced severity of internet addiction as well as mean online game playing time. Interestingly, in the prospective case series of recruited and treatment-seeking subjects with pathological internet use described above, there were high rates of current comorbid bipolar depression that responded to anticonvulsant treatment (with or without adjunctive antipsychotic or antidepressant agents) with both normalization of mood and moderate to marked remittance of pathological internet use.[67] However, it is important to note that if IAD follows suit with chemical addiction, then effective treatment of co-occurring other mental disorders will generally have effect sizes insufficient to treat the IAD.[142]

SUMMARY AND CONCLUSIONS

Use of microprocessors continues to increase rapidly as these are placed in a wide variety of communication and amusement devices. These devices are always available, cost little to use, and provide many rewards. About 1% of the U.S. population has unhealthy microprocessor use. These problems are likely to increase as microprocessor use and power continue to increase. While sharing many commonalities with other addiction, unhealthy microprocessor use differs in that no exogenous substance is involved and patients are technologically savvy and computer literate and are able to manipulate their identities in cyberspace.

Even without resorting to a pathology model, current societal adaptation to the use of microprocessors can, at its most extreme, be likened to the London gin epidemic, where citizens previously comfortable with a culture that drank beer and ale, frequently to intoxication, adapted poorly to a new more potent alcoholic liquid, with disastrous results in a population that was already ripe for social unrest.[143] Eventually, the culture moderated its use more globally, leaving the bulk of maladaptive and damaging alcohol-related trajectories to those with alcohol use disorders. It may be that our culture is on a similar path and in the wake of our corporate learning curve will be those for whom microprocessors provide a "substance" fulfilling its role as a substrate for a pathological use disorder.[3,15,66,140,144-146]

REFERENCES

1. American Psychiatric Association. *Diagnostic and Statistical Manual 5.* American Psychiatric Association; 2013.
2. Weinberg GM. *The Psychology of Computer Programming.* Van Nostrand Reinhold; 1971.
3. Weizenbaum J. *Computer Power and Human Reason.* Penguin; 1984.
4. Kuiper D. *Those Idiots in the Computer Room.* Macadam House; 1992.
5. Greenfield DN, Davis RA. Lost in cyberspace: the web @ work. *CyberPsychol Behav.* 2002;5(4):347-353.
6. Young K. *Caught in the Net: How to Recognize the Signs of Internet Addiction—And a Winning Strategy for Recovery.* John Wiley & Sons; 1998.
7. Federal Communications Commission. *Eighth Broadband Progress Report.* FCC 12-90, GN Docket No. 11-121. Accessed June 5, 2023. http://www.fcc.gov/reports/eighth-broadband-progress-report
8. United States Department of Commerce. American Community Survey Report Number ACS-49. *Computer and Internet Use in the United States: 2018.* Accessed August 9, 2022. https://www.census.gov/library/publications/2021/acs/acs-49.html
9. Perrin A, Duggan M. *Americans' Internet Access: 2000-2015.* Pew Research Center. Accessed August 9, 2022. InternetInternet http://www.pewInternet.org/2015/06/26/americans-Internet-access-2000-2015
10. Perrin A. *Mobile Technology and Home Broadband 2021.* Pew Research Center. Accessed August 9, 2022. https://www.pewresearch.org/Internet/2021/06/03/mobile-technology-and-home-broadband-2021/
11. Cheng C, Li AY. Internet addiction prevalence and quality of (real) life: a meta-analysis of 31 nations across seven world regions. *Cyberpsychol Behav Soc Netw.* 2014;17(12):755-760. doi:10.1089/cyber.2014.0317
12. Kuss DJ, Griffiths MD, Karila L, Billieux J. Internet addiction: a systematic review of epidemiological research for the last decade. *Curr Pharm Des.* 2014;20(25):4026-4052.
13. Endomba FT, Demina A, Meille V, et al. Prevalence of Internet addiction in Africa: a systematic review and meta-analysis. *J Behav Addict.* 2022;11(3):739-753. doi:10.1556/2006.2022.00052
14. Rumpf HJ, Vermulst AA, Bischof A, et al. Occurrence of Internet addiction in a general population sample: a latent class analysis. *Eur Addict Res.* 2014;20(4):159-166. doi:10.1159/000354321
15. Aboujaoude E, Koran LM, Gamel N, Large MD, Serpe RT. Potential markers for problematic Internet use: a telephone survey of 2,513 adults. *CNS Spectr.* 2006;11(10):750-755.
16. Bakken IJ, Wenzel HG, Götestam KG, Johansson A, Øren A. Internet addiction among Norwegian adults: a stratified probability sample study. *Scand J Psychol.* 2009;50:121-127.
17. Feng W, Ramo DE, Chan SR, Bourgeois JA. Internet gaming disorder: trends in prevalence 1998-2016. *Addict Behav.* 2017;75:17-24. doi:10.1016/j.addbeh.2017.06.010
18. Kim HS, Son G, Roh EB, et al. Prevalence of gaming disorder: a meta-analysis. *Addict Behav.* 2022;126:107183. doi:10.1016/j.addbeh.2021.107183
19. Mihara S, Higuchi S. Cross-sectional and longitudinal epidemiological studies of Internet gaming disorder: a systematic review of the literature. *Psychiatry Clin Neurosci.* 2017;71(7):425-444. doi:10.1111/pcn. 12532
20. Ko CH, Yen JY, Yen CF, Chen CS, Chen CC. The association between Internet addiction and psychiatric disorder: a review of the literature. *Eur Psychiatry.* 2012;27(1):1-8.
21. Bozkurt H, Coskun M, Ayaydin H, Adak I, Zoroglu SS. Prevalence and patterns of psychiatric disorders in referred adolescents with Internet addiction. *Psychiatry Clin Neurosci.* 2013;67(5):352-359. doi:10.1111/pcn.12065
22. Wu JY, Ko HC, Lane HY. Personality disorders in female and male college students with Internet addiction. *J Nerv Ment Dis.* 2016;204(3):221-225. doi:10.1097/NMD.0000000000000452

23. Zadra S, Bischof G, Besser B, et al. The association between Internet addiction and personality disorders in a general population-based sample. *J Behav Addict*. 2016;5(4):691-699. doi:10.1556/2006.5.2016.086
24. Ho RC, Zhang MW, Tsang TY, et al. The association between Internet addiction and psychiatric co-morbidity: a meta-analysis. *BMC Psychiatry*. 2014;14:183. doi:10.1186/1471-244X-14-183
25. Kuss DJ, Lopez-Fernandez O. Internet addiction and problematic Internet use: a systematic review of clinical research. *World J Psychiatry*. 2016;6(1):143-176. doi:10.5498/wjp.v6.i1.143
26. Gifford E. *AOL Mail Fourth Annual Email Addiction Survey*. Accessed July 30, 2008. http://corp.aol.com/press-releases/2008/07/it-s-3-am-are-you-checking-your-email-again
27. Jelenchick LA, Becker T, Moreno MA. Assessing the psychometric properties of the Internet Addiction Test (IAT) in US college students. *Psychiatry Res*. 2012;196:296-301.
28. Linden Lab Official: Live Data Feeds. Accessed July 8, 2017. http://secondlife.com/xmlhttp/secondlife.php; http://dwellonit.taterunino.net/sl-statistical-charts/
29. Au WJ. *The Making of Second Life: Notes from the New World*. Harper Collins; 2008.
30. Data Breaches, on PrivacyRights.org. Accessed March 17, 2023. https://privacyrights.org/data-breaches
31. American Academy of Pediatrics; Council on Communications and Media. Policy statement: media and young minds. *Pediatrics*. 2016;138(5):e20162591. doi:10.1542/peds.2016-2591
32. Richert RA, Robb MB, Fender JG, Wartella E. Word learning from baby videos. *Arch Pediatr Adolesc Med*. 2010;164(5):432-437. doi:10.1001/archpediatrics.2010.24
33. Martin PR, Petry NM. Are non-substance-related addictions really addictions? *Am J Addict*. 2005;14(1):1-7.
34. American Psychiatric Association (APA). *Fact Sheets: Internet Gaming Disorder*. Accessed July 19, 2017. https://www.psychiatry.org/File%20Library/Psychiatrists/Practice/DSM/APA_DSM-5-Internet-Gaming-Disorder.pdf
35. Brand M, Young KS, Laier C, Wölfling K, Potenza MN. Integrating psychological and neurobiological considerations regarding the development and maintenance of specific Internet-use disorders: an interaction of person-affect-cognition-execution (I-PACE) model. *Neurosci Biobehav Rev*. 2016;71:252-266. doi:10.1016/j.neubiorev.2016.08.033
36. Love T, Laier C, Brand M, Hatch L, Hajela R. Neuroscience of Internet pornography addiction: a review and update. *Behav Sci (Basel)*. 2015;5(3):388-433. doi:10.3390/bs5030388
37. Billieux J. Problematic mobile phone use: a literature review and a pathways model. *Curr Psychiatr Rev*. 2012;8:299-307.
38. Starcevic V. Is Internet addiction a useful concept? *Aust N Z J Psychiatry*. 2013;47:16-19.
39. Griffiths MD. Internet addiction: Internet fuels other addictions. *Stud Br Med J*. 1999;7:428-429.
40. Griffiths MD. Internet addiction—time to be taken seriously? *Addict Res*. 2000;8:413-418.
41. Davis RA. A cognitive-behavioral model of pathological Internet use. *Comput Hum Behav*. 2001;17:187-195.
42. Thorens G, Achab S, Billieux J, et al. Characteristics and treatment response of self-identified problematic Internet users in a behavioral addiction outpatient clinic. *J Behav Addict*. 2014;3(1):78-81. doi:10.1556/JBA.3.2014.008
43. Brand M, Young KS, Laier C. Prefrontal control and Internet addiction: a theoretical model and review of neuropsychological and neuroimaging findings. *Front Hum Neurosci*. 2014;8:375. doi:10.3389/fnhum.2014.00375
44. Dong G, Potenza MN. A cognitive-behavioral model of Internet gaming disorder: theoretical underpinnings and clinical implications. *J Psychiatr Res*. 2014;58:7-11. doi:10.1016/j.jpsychires.2014.07.005
45. Young K. Internet addiction: the emergence of a new clinical disorder. *CyberPsychol Behav*. 1998;1:237-244.
46. Yuan K, Qin W, Liu Y, Tian J. Internet addiction: neuroimaging findings. *Commun Integr Biol*. 2011;4(6):637-639.
47. Park HS, Kim SH, Bang SA, Yoon EJ, Choo SS, Kim SE. Altered regional cerebral glucose metabolism in Internet game overusers: a 18F-fluorodeoxyglucose positron emission tomography study. *CNS Spectr*. 2010;15(3):159-166.
48. Kim SH, Baik SH, Park CS, Kim SJ, Choi SW, Kim SE. Reduced striatal dopamine D2 receptors in people with Internet addiction. *Neuroreport*. 2011;22(8):407-411. doi:10.1097/WNR.0b013e328346e16e
49. Yuan K, Qin W, Wang G, et al. Microstructure abnormalities in adolescents with Internet addiction disorder. *PLoS One*. 2011;6:20708. doi:10.1371/journal.pone.0020708
50. Hong SB, Zalesky A, Cocchi L, et al. Decreased functional brain connectivity in adolescents with Internet addiction. *PLoS One*. 2013;8(2):e57831. doi:10.1371/journal.pone.0057831
51. Lin F, Zhou Y, Du Y, et al. Aberrant corticostriatal functional circuits in adolescents with Internet addiction disorder. *Front Hum Neurosci*. 2015;9:356. doi:10.3389/fnhum.2015.00356
52. Wee CY, Zhao Z, Yap PT, et al. Disrupted brain functional network in Internet addiction disorder: a resting-state functional magnetic resonance imaging study. *PLoS One*. 2014;9(9):e107306. doi:10.1371/journal.pone.0107306
53. Hong SB, Kim JW, Choi EJ, et al. Reduced orbitofrontal cortical thickness in male adolescents with Internet addiction. *Behav Brain Funct*. 2013;9:11. doi:10.1186/1744-9081-9-11
54. Park B, Han DH, Roh S. Neurobiological findings related to Internet use disorders. *Psychiatry Clin Neurosci*. 2017;71(7):467-478. doi:10.1111/pcn.12422
55. Zhu Y, Zhang H, Tian M. Molecular and functional imaging of Internet addiction. *Biomed Res Int*. 2015;2015:378675.
56. Sepede G, Tavino M, Santacroce R, Fiori F, Salerno RM, Di Giannantonio M. Functional magnetic resonance imaging of Internet addiction in young adults. *World J Radiol*. 2016;8(2):210-225. doi:10.4329/wjr.v8.i2.210
57. Nie J, Zhang W, Liu Y. Exploring depression, self-esteem and verbal fluency with different degrees of Internet addiction among Chinese college students. *Compr Psychiatry*. 2017;72:114-120. doi:10.1016/j.comppsych.2016.10.006
58. Wang Y, Qin Y, Li H, et al. Abnormal functional connectivity in cognitive control network, default mode network, and visual attention network in internet addiction: a Resting-State fMRI Study. *Front Neurol*. 2019;10:1006. doi:10.3389/fneur.2019.01006
59. Nie J, Zhang W, Chen J, Li W. Impaired inhibition and working memory in response to Internet-related words among adolescents with Internet addiction: a comparison with attention-deficit/hyperactivity disorder. *Psychiatry Res*. 2016;236:28-34. doi:10.1016/j.psychres.2016.01.004
60. Zhou Z, Zhou H, Zhu H. Working memory, executive function and impulsivity in Internet-addictive disorders: a comparison with pathological gambling. *Acta Neuropsychiatr*. 2016;28(2):92-100. doi:10.1017/neu.2015.54
61. Darnai G, Perlaki G, Zsidó AN, et al. Internet addiction and functional brain networks: task-related fMRI study. *Sci Rep*. 2019;9(1):15777. doi:10.1038/s41598-019-52296-1
62. Darnai G, Perlaki G, Orsi G, et al. Language processing in Internet use disorder: task-based fMRI study. *PLoS One*. 2022;17(6):e0269979. doi:10.1371/journal.pone.0269979
63. Dong G, Devito EE, Du X, Cui Z. Impaired inhibitory control in 'Internet addiction disorder': a functional magnetic resonance imaging study. *Psychiatry Res*. 2012;203:153-158. doi:10.1016/j.pscychresns.2012.02.001
64. Young K. *Internet Addiction Test*. Accessed September 15, 2022. http://netaddiction.com/Internet-addiction-test.htm
65. Dong G, DeVito E, Huang J, Du X. Diffusion tensor imaging reveals thalamus and posterior cingulate cortex abnormalities in Internet gaming addicts. *J Psychiatr Res*. 2012;46(9):1212-1216.
66. Liu L, Xue G, Potenza MN, et al. Dissociable neural processes during risky decision-making in individuals with Internet-gaming disorder. *Neuroimage Clin*. 2017;14:741-749.
67. Chen CY, Huang MF, Yen JY, et al. Brain correlates of response inhibition in Internet gaming disorder. *Psychiatry Clin Neurosci*. 2015;69:201-209.

68. Luijten M, Meerkerk GJ, Franken IH, van de Wetering BJ, Schoenmakers TM. An fMRI study of cognitive control in problem gamers. *Psychiatry Res.* 2015;231:262-268.
69. Chen CY, Yen JY, Wang PW, Liu GC, Yen CF, Ko CH. Altered functional connectivity of the insula and nucleus accumbens in Internet gaming disorder: a resting state fMRI study. *Eur Addict Res.* 2016;22(4):192-200.
70. Zhang JT, Yao YW, Li CS, et al. Altered resting-state functional connectivity of the insula in young adults with Internet gaming disorder. *Addict Biol.* 2016;21(3):743-751.
71. Ko CH, Hsieh TJ, Wang PW, et al. Altered gray matter density and disrupted functional connectivity of the amygdala in adults with Internet gaming disorder. *Prog Neuro-Psychopharmacol Biol Psychiatry.* 2015;57:185-192.
72. Du X, Qi X, Yang Y, et al. Altered structural correlates of impulsivity in adolescents with Internet gaming disorder. *Front Hum Neurosci.* 2016;10:4.
73. Jeong BS, Han DH, Kim SM, Lee SW, Renshaw PF. White matter connectivity and Internet gaming disorder. *Addict Biol.* 2016;21:732-742.
74. Yuan K, Qin W, Yu D, et al. Core brain networks interactions and cognitive control in Internet gaming disorder individuals in late adolescence/early adulthood. *Brain Struct Funct.* 2016;221:1427-1442.
75. Yao YW, Liu L, Ma SS, et al. Functional and structural neural alterations in Internet gaming disorder: a systematic review and meta-analysis. *Neurosci Biobehav Rev.* 2017;83:313-324. doi:10.1016/j.neubiorev.2017.10.029
76. Fauth-Bühler M, Mann K. Neurobiological correlates of Internet gaming disorder: similarities to pathological gambling. *Addict Behav.* 2017;64:349-356. doi:10.1016/j.addbeh.2015.11.004
77. Weinstein A, Lejoyeux M. Neurobiological mechanisms underlying Internet gaming disorder. *Dialogues Clin Neurosci.* 2020;22(2):113-126. doi:10.31887/DCNS.2020.22.2/aweinstein
78. Griffiths M. Nicotine, tobacco, and addiction. *Nature.* 1996;384:18.
79. Brown RIF. Gaming, gambling and other addictive play. In: Kerr JH, Apter MJ, eds. *Adult Play: A Reversal Theory Approach.* Swets & Zeitlinger; 1991:101-118.
80. Brown RIF. Some contributions of the study of gambling to the study of other addictions. In: Eadington WR, Cornelius JA, eds. *Gambling Behavior and Problem Gambling.* University of Nevada; 1993:241-272.
81. Shapira NA, Goldsmith TD, Keck PE Jr, Khosla UM, McElroy SL. Psychiatric features of individuals with problematic Internet use. *J Affect Disord.* 2001;66(2-3):283.
82. Young KS, Rogers RC. The relationship between depression and Internet addiction. *CyberPsychol Behav.* 1998;1:25-28.
83. Treuer T, Fabian Z, Furedi J. Internet addiction associated with features of impulse control disorder: is it a real psychiatric disorder? *J Affect Disord.* 2001;66(2-3):283.
84. Dell'Osso B, Altamura AC, Allen A, Marazziti D, Hollander E. Epidemiologic and clinical updates on impulse control disorders: a critical review. *Eur Arch Psychiatry Clin Neurosci.* 2006;256(8):464-475.
85. Lee HW, Choi JS, Shin YC, Lee JY, Jung HY, Kwon KS. Impulsivity in Internet addiction: a comparison with pathological gambling. *Cyberpsychol Behav Soc Netw.* 2012;15(7):373-377.
86. Meerkerk G-J, van den Eijnden RJJM, Franken IHA, Garretsen HFL. Is compulsive Internet use related to sensitivity to reward and punishment, and impulsivity? *Comput Hum Behav.* 2010;26:729-735.
87. Meerkerk GJ, Van Den Eijnden R, Vermulst AA, Garretsen HFL. The Compulsive Internet Use Scale (CIUS): some psychometric properties. *CyberPsychol Behav.* 2009;12:1-6.
88. Grant JE, Potenza MN, Weinstein A, Gorelick DA. Introduction to behavioral addictions. *Am J Drug Alcohol Abuse.* 2010;36:233-241.
89. Pies R. Should DSM-5 designate "Internet Addiction" a mental disorder? *Psychiatry (Edgmont).* 2009;6(2):31-37.
90. American Society of Addiction Medicine. Public Policy Statement: Definition of Addiction. Accessed July 17, 2017. http://www.asam.org/quality-practice/definition-of-addiction.
91. Pratarelli ME, Browne BL. Confirmatory factor analysis of Internet use and addiction. *CyberPsychol Behav.* 2002;5(1):53-64.
92. Charlton JP. A factor-analytic investigation of computer addiction and engagement. *Br J Psychol.* 2002;93:329-344.
93. Beard KW, Wolf EM. Modification in the proposed diagnostic criteria for Internet addiction. *CyberPsychol Behav.* 2001;4(3):377-383.
94. Ko CH, Yen JY, Chen CC, Chen SH, Yen CF. Proposed diagnostic criteria of Internet addiction for adolescents. *J Nerv Ment Dis.* 2005;193(11):728-733.
95. Sha P, Dong X. Research on adolescents regarding the indirect effect of depression, anxiety, and stress between TikTok use disorder and memory loss. *Int J Environ Res Public Health.* 2021;18(16):8820.
96. Kuss DJ, Griffiths MD. Addiction to social networks on the Internet: a literature review of empirical research. *Int J Environ Res Public Health.* 2011;8:3528-3552.
97. Grant BF, Stinson FS, Dawson DA, et al. Prevalence and co-occurrence of substance use disorders and independent mood and anxiety disorders: results from the National Epidemiologic Survey on Alcohol and Related Conditions. *Arch Gen Psychiatry.* 2004;61:807-816.
98. Carli V, Durkee T, Wasserman D, et al. The association between pathological Internet use and comorbid psychopathology: a systematic review. *Psychopathology.* 2013;46:1.
99. Wei HT, Chen MH, Huang PC, Bai YM. The association between online gaming, social phobia, and depression: an Internet survey. *BMC Psychiatry.* 2012;12(1):92.
100. Beard KW. Internet addiction: a review of current assessment techniques and potential assessment questions. *CyberPsychol Behav.* 2005;8:7-14.
101. Zhang JT, Yao YW, Potenza MN, et al. Effects of craving behavioral intervention on neural substrates of cue-induced craving in Internet gaming disorder. *Neuroimage Clin.* 2016;12:591-599.
102. Deng LY, Liu L, Xia CC, Lan J, Zhang JT, Fang XY. Craving behavior intervention in ameliorating college students' Internet game disorder: a longitudinal study. *Front Psychol.* 2017;8:526. doi:10.3389/fpsyg.2017.00526
103. Widyanto L, McMurran M. The psychometric properties of the Internet addiction test. *CyberPsychol Behav.* 2004;7(4):443-450.
104. Rosenthal RN, Solhkhah R. Club drugs and synthetic cannabinoid agonists. In: Kranzler HR, Ciraulo DA, Zindel LR, eds. *Clinical Manual of Addiction Psychopharmacology.* 2nd ed. American Psychiatric Publishing; 2013:351-386.
105. Taintor Z. Internet/computer addiction. In: Lowinson J, Ruiz P, Millman R, et al., eds. *Substance Abuse.* 4th ed. Lippincott Williams & Wilkins; 2005:540-548.
106. Grigoradis V. The casual sex revolution: how the Internet took the sting out of sleeping with strangers. *New York Mag.* 2003;13:17-20.
107. Amichai-Hamburger Y, Wainapel G, Fox S. "On the Internet no one knows I'm an introvert": extroversion, neuroticism, and Internet interaction. *CyberPsychol Behav.* 2002;5(2):125-128.
108. Griffiths M. Does Internet and computer "addiction" exist? *CyberPsychol Behav.* 2000;3:211-218.
109. Young KS, Case CJ. Internet abuse in the workplace: new trends in risk management. *CyberPsychol Behav.* 2004;7(1):105-111.
110. Bozarth MA, Wise RA. Toxicity associated with long-term intravenous heroin and cocaine self-administration in the rat. *JAMA.* 1985;254(1):81-83.
111. American Psychiatric Association. *Diagnostic and Statistical Manual of Mental Disorders.* 4th ed. Text Revision American Psychiatric Association; 2000.
112. Frangos CC, Frangos CC, Sotiropoulos I. A meta-analysis of the Reliability of Young's Internet Addiction Test. *Proceedings of the World Congress on Engineering 2012,* Vol I WCE 2012, London, UK, July 4-6, 2012.
113. Pontes HM, Griffiths MD. The development and psychometric evaluation of the Internet Disorder Scale (IDS-15). *Addict Behav.* 2017;64:261-268. doi:10.1016/j.addbeh.2015.09.003
114. Northrup JC, Lapierre C, Kirk J, Rae C. The Internet process addiction test: screening for addictions to processes facilitated by the Internet. *Behav Sci (Basel).* 2015;5(3):341-352. doi:10.3390/bs5030341

115. Lee SY, Park EC, Han KT, Kim SJ, Chun SY, Park S. The association of level of Internet use with suicidal ideation and suicide attempts in South Korean adolescents: a focus on family structure and household economic status. *Can J Psychiatr*. 2016;61(4):243-251. doi:10.1177/0706743716635550
116. Ha JH, Kim SY, Bae SC, et al. Depression and Internet addiction in adolescents. *Psychopathology*. 2007;40(6):424-430.
117. Daine K, Hawton K, Singaravelu V, Stewart A, Simkin S, Montgomery P. The power of the web: a systematic review of studies of the influence of the Internet on self-harm and suicide in young people. *PLoS One*. 2013;8(10):e77555.
118. Miller WR, Rollnick S. *Motivational Interviewing: Preparing People for Change*. 2nd ed. Guilford Press; 2002.
119. Eysenbach GP, Powell J, Englesakis M, Rizo C, Stern A. Health related virtual communities and electronic support groups: systematic effects of the effects of online peer to peer interactions. *BMJ*. 2004;328:1166-1172.
120. Young K. Cognitive behavior therapy with Internet addicts: treatment outcomes and implications. *CyberPsychol Behav*. 2007;10(5):671-679.
121. Pettinati HM, Monterosso J, Lipkin C, Volpicelli JR. Patient attitudes toward treatment predict attendance in clinical pharmacotherapy trials of alcohol and drug treatment. *Am J Addict*. 2003;12(4):324-335.
122. Higgins ST. Some potential contributions of reinforcement and consumer-demand theory to reducing cocaine use. *Addict Behav*. 1996;21:803-816.
123. King DL, Delfabbro PH, Wu AMS, et al. Treatment of Internet gaming disorder: an international systematic review and CONSORT evaluation. *Clin Psychol Rev*. 2017;54:123-133. doi:10.1016/j.cpr.2017.04.002
124. Schulz KF, Altman DG, Moher D. CONSORT 2010 statement: updated guidelines for reporting parallel group randomized trials. *Ann Intern Med*. 2010;152:1-8.
125. Petry NM, Rehbein F, Gentile DA, et al. An international consensus for assessing Internet gaming disorder using the new DSM-5 approach. *Addiction*. 2014;109(9):1399-1406. doi:10.1111/add.12457
126. Griffiths MD, van Rooij AJ, Kardefelt-Winther D, et al. Working towards an international consensus on criteria for assessing Internet gaming disorder: a critical commentary on Petry et al. (2014). *Addiction* 2016;111(1):167-175. doi:10.1111/add.13057
127. Winkler A, Dörsing B, Rief W, Shen Y, Glombiewski JA. Treatment of Internet addiction: a meta-analysis. *Clin Psychol Rev*. 2013;33(2):317-329. doi:10.1016/j.cpr.2012.12.005
128. Yeun YR, Han SJ. Effects of psychosocial interventions for school-aged children's Internet addiction, self-control and self-esteem: meta-analysis. *Healthc Inform Res*. 2016;22(3):217-230. doi:10.4258/hir.2016.22.3.217
129. Yellowlees P, Marks S. Problematic Internet use or Internet addiction? *Comput Hum Behav*. 2007;23:1447-1453.
130. Young KS. Treatment outcomes using CBT-IA with Internet-addicted patients. *J Behav Addict*. 2013;2(4):209-215. doi:10.1556/JBA.2.2013.4.3
131. Wölfling K, Beutel ME, Dreier M, Müller KW. Treatment outcomes in patients with Internet addiction: a clinical pilot study on the effects of a cognitive-behavioral therapy program. *Biomed Res Int*. 2014;2014:425924. doi:10.1155/2014/425924
132. Liu QX, Fang XY, Yan N, et al. Multi-family group therapy for adolescent Internet addiction: exploring the underlying mechanisms. *Addict Behav*. 2015;42:1-8. doi:10.1016/j.addbeh.2014.10.021
133. Kim SM, Han DH, Lee YS, Renshaw PF. Combined cognitive behavioral therapy and bupropion for the treatment of problematic on-line game play in adolescents with major depressive disorder. *Comput Hum Behav*. 2012;28:1954-1959. doi:10.1016/j.chb.2012.05.015
134. Petry NM, Gonzalez-Ibanez A. Internet gambling in problem gambling college students. *J Gambl Stud*. 2015;31(2):397-408. doi:10.1007/s10899-013-9432-3
135. Petry NM, Weinstock J, Morasco BJ, Ledgerwood DM. Brief motivational interventions for college students problem gamblers. *Addiction*. 2009;104(9):1569-1578.
136. Luquiens A, Tanguy ML, Lagadec M, Benyamina A, Aubin HJ, Reynaud M. The efficacy of three modalities of Internet-based psychotherapy for non-treatment-seeking online problem gamblers: a randomized controlled trial. *J Med Internet Res*. 2016;18(2):e36. doi:10.2196/jmir.4752
137. Dell'Osso B, Hadley S, Allen A, Baker B, Chaplin WF, Hollander E. Escitalopram in impulsive-compulsive Internet usage disorder: an open-label trial followed by a double-blind discontinuation phase. *J Clin Psychiatry*. 2008;69(3):452-456.
138. Han DH, Hwang JW, Renshaw PF. Bupropion sustained release treatment decreases craving for video games and cue-induced brain activity in patient with Internet video game addiction. *Exp Clin Psychopharmacol*. 2010;18:297-304.
139. Han DH, Lee YS, Na C, et al. The effect of methylphenidate on Internet video game play in children with attention-deficit/hyperactivity disorder. *Compr Psychiatry*. 2009;50:251-256.
140. Bostwick JM, Bucci JA. Internet sex addiction treated with naltrexone. *Mayo Clin Proc*. 2008;83(2):226-230.
141. Han DH, Renshaw PF. Bupropion in the treatment of problematic online game play in patients with major depressive disorder. *J Psychopharmacol*. 2012;26:689-696. doi:10.1177/0269881111400647
142. Rosenthal RN. Treatment of persons with dual diagnoses of substance use disorder and other psychological problems. In: McCrady BS, Epstein EE, eds. *Addictions: A Comprehensive Guidebook*. Oxford University Press; 2013:659-707.
143. Coffey TG. Beer street: gin lane. Some views of 18th-century drinking. *Q J Stud Alcohol*. 1966;27:669-692.
144. Shapira NA, Lessig MC, Goldsmith TD, et al. Problematic Internet use: proposed classification and diagnostic criteria. *Depress Anxiety*. 2003;17(4):207-216.
145. Liu CY, Kuo FY. A study of Internet addiction through the lens of the interpersonal theory. *CyberPsychol Behav*. 2007;10(6):799-804.
146. Miller MC. Questions & answers. Is "Internet addiction" a distinct mental disorder? *Harv Ment Health Lett*. 2007;24(4):8.

SECTION

7

Management of Intoxication and Withdrawal

Associate Editor: Sharon Levy
Lead Section Editor: Adam J. Gordon
Section Editors: Ana Holtey and Michael A. Incze

CHAPTER

55 Management of Intoxication and Withdrawal: General Principles

Tara M. Wright, Jeffrey S. Cluver, and Hugh Myrick

CHAPTER OUTLINE

- Introduction
- Intoxication states
- Recognizing changing drug trends
- Withdrawal states
- Special populations
- Conclusions

INTRODUCTION

Recognition of intoxication and withdrawal states is critical for the appropriate management of individuals with substance use disorders (SUD). In addition to being able to recognize the unique intoxication and withdrawal states of particular substances, the treatment of patients who are under the influence of, or experiencing withdrawal from, substances requires an understanding of many variables. These variables include an appreciation of the natural history and variants of such syndromes; a complete assessment of the patient's individual medical, psychiatric, and social issues; and knowledge of the uses and limitations of a variety of behavioral and pharmacological interventions.

While there are guidelines to identify, assess, and treat intoxication and withdrawal of many substances, therapies must be individualized to each patient's needs and adjusted to reflect the patient's response to treatment in real time. Many patients present with intoxication and withdrawal from multiple substances, requiring clinicians to manage multiple distinct intoxication and/or withdrawal syndromes simultaneously.

The number of visits to emergency departments (EDs) for management of acute intoxication or withdrawal states remains at an all-time high. Preliminary data from the Drug Abuse Warning Network (DAWN) in 2021 revealed the top five drugs involved in drug-related ED visits were alcohol (39% of all drug-related ED visits), opioids (14%), methamphetamine (11%), cannabis (10%), and cocaine (4%).[1] Fentanyl-related ED visits rose throughout 2021, peaking in the last three months of 2021. Accidental death is now the fourth leading cause of death in the United States, with drug overdose being the leading cause of accidental death.[2] Opioid use disorders are driving much of this, with overdose deaths rising steadily and a 30% jump to 68,639 deaths in 2020.[2] Overdose is often complicated by polypharmacy. DAWN preliminary findings from 2021 indicated that a significant percentage of methamphetamine-, cannabis-, cocaine-, heroin-, and fentanyl-related ED visits involved at least one other drug, while the majority of alcohol-related ED visits were due to alcohol alone.[1]

This chapter serves as an introduction to the identification and management of intoxication and withdrawal states, with the management of specific substances to be reviewed in subsequent chapters in this section.

INTOXICATION STATES

Intoxication is the result of being under the influence of, and responding to, the acute effects of alcohol or another drug. It typically includes feelings of pleasure, altered emotional responsiveness, altered perception, and impaired judgment and performance. The recognition of intoxication states is of paramount importance in the appropriate treatment of patients who have used substances. Intoxication states can range from euphoria or sedation to life-threatening emergencies when overdose occurs. Each substance has a set of signs and symptoms of intoxication, though diagnosis can be challenging because intoxication can mimic psychiatric and/or medical conditions. Identification and treatment of intoxication can lead to appropriate withdrawal management and ultimately provide an avenue for entry into SUD treatment.

Identification and Management of Intoxication

The identification of intoxication begins with the collection of patient data through history, physical examination, and laboratory screening. Of immediate concern is life-threatening intoxication or overdose. The foremost priority during the initial clinical assessment is identifying potentially life-threatening signs of overdose. If oversedation or overdose is suspected, immediate supportive care and resuscitation is necessary. This is facilitated by determining the patient's level of consciousness, which substances are involved, how much of each has been taken by the patient, and complicating medical disorders.

Information regarding the quantity and frequency of substance use is valuable for clinical decision making and can usually be provided by the patient, though acute intoxication may impede an individual's ability to provide a substance use history, and in these cases the patient's companions or family may be able to provide important collateral information. Standardized questionnaires for self-administration or use by the clinician are designed to elicit answers related to alcohol or substance use. Identifying chronic patterns of substance use may aid in subsequent referral to addiction treatment.

Toxicology screens provide valuable information regarding the type or types of substances used. Urine is the most widely used specimen because of the ease with which a sample is obtained, relatively high concentrations of drugs and metabolites, and the stability of metabolites when frozen. Drug testing can aid in the differential diagnosis when atypical symptoms are present. Such testing can be particularly helpful in cases where little clinical history is available. Having knowledge of the sensitivities, specificities, and cross-reactivities of the urine drug test being used is of vital importance to the appropriate interpretation. Knowledge of the usual duration of detectability of particular substances is important for clinical decision making. However, the duration of detectability can be significantly impacted by the amount of substance ingested, individual rates of metabolism and excretion, and hydration status. The rise in the use of synthetic or "designer" drugs can make identification of the causative substance(s) more difficult, as these substances are frequently not detected by routine toxicology testing. As well, drugs such as methadone, fentanyl, clonazepam, and others are also not detected in routine testing.

Testing for alcohol is most frequently accomplished by breathalyzer or blood alcohol levels; however, urine tests that detect alcohol metabolites are also available. Laboratory assays that measure increases in liver enzymes—such as gamma-glutamyl transferase (GGT), aspartate aminotransferase, and alanine aminotransferase—can be helpful for identifying heavy alcohol use, usually of at least several weeks duration. However, there are other causes of GGT elevation, and younger patients may not have GGT elevations even with frequent, heavy alcohol use. The percent carbohydrate-deficient transferrin (%CDT) is a more sensitive and specific indicator of heavy alcohol consumption.[3] The conjugated ethanol metabolites ethyl glucuronide (EtG) and ethyl sulfate (EtS) are other measures that can confirm or rule out recent alcohol consumption. Although EtG and EtS account for less than 0.1% of the ingested ethanol dose, they remain detectable in urine for several hours up to some days longer than ethanol depending on the amount consumed.[4] Serum-based phosphatidyl ethanol (Peth) is a biomarker that may be able to detect the presence of even a few days of heavy alcohol consumption for as long as 3 weeks after[3] and thus provides information regarding drinking pattern. Of course, these test features (eg, detection of a substance weeks after use) will complicate the identification of current toxidromes as much as they might clarify them.

RECOGNIZING CHANGING DRUG TRENDS

Local trends in prevalent withdrawal and intoxication syndromes are constantly evolving in response to a rapidly changing illicit drug supply. As many of emerging substances of interest such as illicitly manufactured fentanyl and xylazine are synthetic and may not be detected by routine drug testing, it is helpful to keep abreast of recent trends. The National Institute on Drug Abuse (NIDA) launched the National Drug Early Warning System (NDEWS) in August 2014 to create a national network for identification and monitoring of emerging drug problems. NDEWS utilizes real-time surveillance to detect early signals of potential epidemics at 18 sentinel sites across the United States.[5]

WITHDRAWAL STATES

Substance withdrawal has been defined by the American Psychiatric Association as "the development of a substance-specific maladaptive behavioral change, usually with uncomfortable physiological and cognitive consequences, that is the result of an abstinence from , or reduction in, heavy and prolonged substance use."[4] The signs and symptoms of withdrawal usually are the opposite of a substance's direct pharmacological effects. Substances in each pharmacological class produce similar withdrawal syndromes; however, the onset, duration, and intensity are variable depending on the particular agent used, the duration of use, and the degree of neuroadaptation.

Evidence for the abstinence from or reduction in use of a substance may be obtained by history or toxicology. Withdrawal may be superimposed on a medical condition or mental disorder.[4] Therefore, a thorough physical examination is necessary, including appropriate laboratory analysis of basic organ functions.

Medically supervised withdrawal is defined as the medical management of withdrawal symptoms. There are many situations in which supervised withdrawal may be medically necessary. For example, a patient has an urgent medical or psychiatric crisis that requires inpatient hospitalization where the substance used is not appropriate to continue, or a patient is entering a residential SUD treatment program, jail, or prison where the substance used is not appropriate to be administered in these settings.

Goals of Withdrawal Management

Medically managed withdrawal includes a combination of pharmacological treatments and supportive care aimed at helping individuals safely and comfortably withdraw from one or more substances. The American Society of Addiction Medicine (ASAM) lists three immediate goals for withdrawal management of alcohol and other substances: (1) "to provide a safe withdrawal from the drug(s) of dependence and enable the patient to become drug-free," (2) "to provide a withdrawal that is humane and thus protects the patient's dignity," and (3) "to prepare the patient for ongoing treatment of his or her dependence on alcohol or other drugs."[6]

Medically managed withdrawal is comprised of three essential and sequential steps: evaluation, stabilization, and fostering patient readiness for and entry into treatment.[7] It is important to distinguish withdrawal management from SUD treatment. *Substance use disorder treatment/rehabilitation* involves a constellation of ongoing therapeutic services ultimately intended to promote recovery for individuals with SUDs.[7] Withdrawal management may be the first step in this process.

Many risks are associated with withdrawal, some of which are influenced by the setting in which withdrawal management occurs. For example, in persons who are physically dependent on alcohol, abrupt, untreated abstinence may result in marked hyperautonomic signs, seizures, (which may be recurrent), withdrawal delirium, and death. Other sedative-hypnotics also can produce life-threatening withdrawal syndromes. Withdrawal from opioids and stimulants produces severe discomfort, but generally is not life-threatening in otherwise healthy individuals. Opioid and stimulant withdrawal may present an increased risk of severe harm in individuals with advanced HIV disease, advanced age, coronary artery disease, and other medical problems. Outpatients experiencing withdrawal symptoms may self-medicate with alcohol or other drugs that can interact with withdrawal medications in an additive fashion or precipitate overdose. Thus, risks are not limited to the direct withdrawal symptoms, particularly when the withdrawal management is conducted in an outpatient setting.

A caring staff, patient rapport, a supportive environment, sensitivity to cultural issues, confidentiality, and the selection of appropriate withdrawal management medications (as needed) are important components of humane withdrawal management. Clear treatment goals combined with firm boundaries and empathy from staff experienced in managing difficult behaviors that often accompany withdrawal are helpful. Enlisting supportive others (family members, friends, or employers) to assist with patient care is helpful when possible.

During withdrawal management, patients may form therapeutic relationships with treatment staff and other patients, providing an opportunity to explore alternatives to substance use. Supervised withdrawal is therefore an opportunity to offer patients information and to motivate them for longer-term treatment. Unfortunately, managed care organizations and other third-party payers often regard withdrawal management as separate from other phases of SUD treatment. In clinical practice, this separation should not exist; withdrawal management is but one component of a comprehensive treatment strategy.

General Principles of Withdrawal Management

Some procedures are specific to particular drugs, whereas others are not drug specific. General principles are presented here, whereas subsequent chapters address specific treatment protocols for each class of drugs.

There is a risk of serious adverse consequences for some patients who undergo withdrawal. An initial medical assessment is important to determine the need for medication and medical management. Such an assessment includes evaluation of predicted withdrawal severity as well as medical and psychiatric comorbidity. Although withdrawal cannot always be predicted with accuracy, the amount and duration of alcohol or other drug use, the severity of the patient's prior withdrawal experiences (if any), and the patient's medical and psychiatric history all provide helpful information. A history of complicated withdrawal makes future complicated withdrawals more likely. For example, past alcohol withdrawal seizures are a strong indicator of future alcohol withdrawal seizures.[8] Standardized withdrawal scales such as the Clinical Institute Withdrawal Assessment-Alcohol, revised (CIWA-Ar) and the Clinical Opiate Withdrawal Scale (COWS), and several other substance-specific scales help determine the stage and severity of withdrawal over time and guide medication management. However, while scales provide one piece of information, clinical reasoning remains important. For example, many patients with alcohol or opioid withdrawal do not have all of the described symptoms of the withdrawal syndromes; waiting for symptoms to occur to initiate treatment based on a CIWA or COWS score is inappropriate. Clinical judgment regarding the timing and choice of withdrawal treatment plays an important complementary role to the use of clinical algorithms.

A multimodal approach to withdrawal management is recommended. Including psychological support can help to ameliorate withdrawal and associated distress.

The duration of withdrawal management is not a clearly defined, discrete period. Because withdrawal often requires a greater intensity of services than other types of treatment, there is a practical value in defining a period during which a person is "in withdrawal." The medical management period is defined as the time during which the patient receives medications for withdrawal, even though some signs and symptoms may persist for much longer. Another way of defining the withdrawal management period is by measuring the duration of withdrawal symptoms, though this may be difficult to determine because symptoms are largely suppressed by medication.

Some patients have prolonged withdrawal symptoms or "protracted withdrawal syndrome." Symptoms may include disturbances of sleep, anxiety, irritability, mood instability, and cravings. Despite advances in the literature elucidating the neurobiology of protracted withdrawal, the optimal approach to pharmacological management remains uncertain. The protracted withdrawal syndrome is hypothesized to be a period when individuals are at a heightened risk of return to substance use.[9-11] Physicians often find it difficult to distinguish prolonged withdrawal and an underlying psychiatric disorder. The signs and symptoms of protracted withdrawal are not as predictable as acute withdrawal, which can be studied in animal models. Protracted withdrawal, on the other hand, primarily consists of distress symptoms for which there are no adequate animal models.

Ultimately, treatment of withdrawal must be individualized to the patient. The initial plan of care for withdrawal management can be adjusted to reflect the patient's response to the treatment provided. In addition, long-term aftercare planning for treatment after the withdrawal management event is vitally important.

Pharmacological Management

There are two general strategies for pharmacological management of withdrawal: suppressing withdrawal through use of a cross-tolerant medication and reducing signs and symptoms of withdrawal through alteration of another neuropharmacological process. Either or both may be used to manage withdrawal syndromes effectively. To suppress withdrawal with cross-tolerant medication, a longer-acting medication typically is used to provide a milder, controlled withdrawal. Examples include use of methadone for opioid withdrawal management and diazepam for alcohol withdrawal management. Medications that are not cross-tolerant are used to treat specific signs and symptoms of withdrawal. Examples include use of clonidine for opioid or alcohol withdrawal.

Withdrawal Management Settings

An initial assessment facilitates the selection of the appropriate level of care for withdrawal management. In determining the most appropriate setting, the practitioner matches clinical needs with the least restrictive and most cost-effective setting.[7] Withdrawal management may take place in a variety of inpatient and outpatient settings. Multiple instruments have been designed to facilitate selection of an appropriate level of care. The ASAM criteria contain detailed guidelines for matching patients to an appropriate intensity of services for withdrawal management, which can be accomplished in either inpatient or outpatient settings. Both types of settings can link patients to referrals for problems such as medical, legal, psychiatric, and family issues.

Inpatient Withdrawal Management

Inpatient withdrawal management is offered in medical hospitals, psychiatric hospitals, and medically managed residential treatment programs. It allows 24-hour supervision, observation, and support for patients who are intoxicated or experiencing withdrawal. The primary emphasis in this setting is placed on ensuring that the patient is medically stable (including the initiation and tapering of medications used for the treatment of substance withdrawal), assessing for adequate biopsychosocial stability (and quickly intervening if this is lacking), and linking the patient to appropriate inpatient and outpatient services once it is medically safe to do so.[7] Inpatient withdrawal management provides the safest setting for the treatment of substance withdrawal, because it ensures that patients will be carefully monitored and appropriately supported. Such monitoring is especially important if the patient is physically dependent on alcohol or other sedative-hypnotic drugs. Compared with outpatient withdrawal management, inpatient withdrawal management may provide better continuity of care for patients who begin treatment while in the hospital. In addition, inpatient withdrawal management separates the patient from substance-related social and environmental stimuli that might increase the risk of return to use.

Relative indications for inpatient treatment include past alcohol withdrawal seizures or delirium, pregnancy, physical dependence on multiple substances, older age, medical or psychiatric illness, or lack of a reliable support system.[12] Abnormalities of electrolytes or blood counts, infection, trauma, and the presence of structural brain lesions can be predictors of the most severe cases of withdrawal.[13,14] Inpatient care of withdrawal can be 10 to 20 times as expensive as outpatient care. Generally, therefore, it is reserved for those expected to have severe withdrawal symptoms and to require a more intensive level of care (such as patients with past severe withdrawal symptoms).

Outpatient Withdrawal Management

Outpatient withdrawal management usually is offered in community mental health centers, methadone maintenance programs, addiction treatment programs, and private clinics. Essential components to a successful outpatient withdrawal management include a positive and helpful social support network and regular accessibility to the treatment provider.[7] Medical and nursing personnel involved can evaluate and confirm that withdrawal management in the less supervised setting is safe. In outpatient treatment models, knowledgeable medical staff are available to monitor the withdrawal symptoms and are prepared to facilitate the individual's entry into treatment.[7] Advantages of outpatient withdrawal management include lower expense, less disruption for patients and less of a transition from a protected setting back to the home environment.

Emergency departments are important components of outpatient withdrawal management as they often serve as a gateway to services. Withdrawal management programs may rely on ED staff to assess and initiate treatment for patients with medical conditions or medical complications that occur during withdrawal. For social model programs, EDs often serve as a safety net for patients who need medical treatment. The ED may be the initial point of contact with the health care system for patients who have overdosed or who are experiencing a medical complication of substance use and serve as a source of case identification and referral.

Considerations for Selecting a Setting

The best setting for a given patient may be defined as the least restrictive and least expensive setting in which the goals of withdrawal management can be met. The ability to meet this standard assumes that treatment choices always are based primarily on a patient's clinical needs. A comprehensive evaluation of the patient often indicates what therapeutic goals might be achieved realistically during the time allotted for the withdrawal management process.

Patient needs drive the selection of the most appropriate setting. The severity of the withdrawal symptoms and the intensity of care required to ensure appropriate management are of primary importance. Pressures to achieve cost savings can interfere with the selection of treatment settings. Many insurance companies, managed care organizations, and other payers have adopted stringent policies that govern setting and maximum number of days per episode that are covered benefits. Such policies give insufficient weight to the complexity that affects the selection of a setting in which the patient has the greatest likelihood of achieving satisfactory management. Some persons in need of withdrawal management, for example, may not be appropriate candidates for outpatient withdrawal management because of environmental impediments such as a spouse who is using alcohol or other drugs. Such a patient may be more appropriately managed in a residential setting such as a recovery house or other substance-free environment. Panelists convened by the federal Center for Substance Abuse Treatment expressed concern that important clinical decisions often are driven by economic, rather than clinical, considerations.[6,7] They affirmed that the dominant principle in patient placement is that withdrawal management is cost-effective only if it is appropriate to the needs of the individual patient.

Use of the ASAM Criteria

Withdrawal management alone rarely constitutes adequate treatment. The provision of withdrawal management services without continuing treatment at an appropriate level of care constitutes less than optimal use of limited resources. The maintenance of abstinence can be a very difficult goal to achieve: it has been estimated that approximately 50% of patients with alcohol use disorder return to use within 3 months of withdrawal management.[15] The appropriate level of care following withdrawal is clinically determined, based on the patient's individual needs. ASAM's criteria are the most widely used and comprehensive set of guidelines for determining the appropriate level of care for a patient within the continuum of addiction services. Using the criteria, levels of treatment are differentiated based on (1) degree of direct medical management provided; (2) degree of structure, safety, and security provided; and (3) degree of treatment intensity provided.[16]

The ASAM Criteria are intended as a clinical guide for matching patients to appropriate levels of care. The criteria reflect a clinical consensus of adult and adolescent treatment specialists and incorporate the results of a comprehensive peer review by professionals in addiction treatment. They use six dimensions in the biopsychosocial assessment of individuals needing substance use services. These dimensions include acute intoxication and/or withdrawal potential; biomedical conditions and complications; emotional, behavioral, or cognitive conditions and complications; readiness to change; return to use (also referred to as "recurrence of use/disorder"), continued use, or continued problem potential; and recovery/living environment. Individual treatment plans are developed through the multidimensional assessment over five broad levels of treatment, which are based on the degree of direct medical management provided; the structure, safety, and security provided; and the intensity of treatment services provided. The five broad levels of care include early intervention, outpatient services, intensive outpatient/partial hospitalization services, residential/inpatient services, and medically managed intensive inpatient services. In between these broad levels are gradations in intensity of services.[16] The ASAM Criteria are a useful guide but not a hard and fast rule book. The full gamut of levels of treatment services may not be readily available to patients due to geographic constraints, insurance limitations, and/or patient and provider preferences for care.

Return to Use

Many individuals undergo withdrawal more than once, and some do so many times. When recently physically dependent persons return for repeat withdrawal management, their previous experiences may help them to have realistic expectations. O'Brien et al.[17] point out that compliance and return to substance use in addiction disorders are comparable to disease recurrence rates in other illnesses, such as diabetes and hypertension. Therefore, they recommend comparable long-term treatment. Return to use can happen at any time, although patients with addiction are at increased risk at certain points in their recovery. The patient who has returned to use is an appropriate candidate for withdrawal management and continued treatment, including evidence based therapies to prevent future return to use.

SPECIAL POPULATIONS

Although researchers have not yet thoroughly evaluated withdrawal strategies for certain populations, patients in several groups clearly require special consideration.

Pregnant and Nursing Women

Special concerns attend withdrawal management during pregnancy. The teratogenic effects of alcohol on a fetus are well documented. Progression to severe withdrawal from alcohol or sedative-hypnotics carries a significant mortality to mother and fetus, so early identification and management are of utmost importance. Inpatient management in collaboration with an obstetrician is recommended. Although benzodiazepines may carry risk to the fetus when given during pregnancy, the risk to both mother and fetus from untreated sedative-hypnotic withdrawal is considered greater than medically supervised use. Therefore, if medical management of withdrawal is necessary, benzodiazepines can be used judiciously.

Withdrawal from opioids can result in fetal distress, which can lead to premature labor or miscarriage. On the other hand, opioid agonist treatment, coupled with good prenatal care, is generally associated with good maternal and fetal outcomes. Methadone maintenance has historically been accepted as the standard approach to the pregnant woman with opioid use disorder; however, recent research also supports the efficacy of buprenorphine, particularly as it may reduce the harms associated with neonatal abstinence syndrome.[18,19] Both medications are classified as pregnancy category C (animal studies have shown risk to the fetus, there are no controlled studies in women, or studies in women and animals are not available). The combination product of buprenorphine/naloxone may have a similar safety profile to the mono product of buprenorphine for pregnant patients.[20] Although offspring of women on opioid agonist therapy tend to have a lower birth weight and smaller head circumference than nonexposed newborns, no developmental differences at 6 months of age have been documented. Clonidine (frequently used in opioid withdrawal management) also is a pregnancy category C medication. Opioid withdrawal management is not generally recommended due to concerns of stress for the fetus.

Federal panels recommend that all pregnant and nursing women be advised of the potential risks of drugs that are excreted in breast milk.[6,21] Nevertheless, they advise that withdrawal protocols need not be modified for nursing women unless there is specific evidence that the withdrawal medication enters the breast milk in amounts that could be harmful to the nursing infant.[6,21] These decisions are made by weighing the risks and benefits to both the mother and infant. For instance, the American Academy of Pediatrics[22] categorizes benzodiazepines as "drugs for which the effect on nursing infants is unknown but may be of concern." The addiction treatment provider can coordinate treatment decisions with an obstetrician or pediatrician in these cases.

Persons Who Are HIV Positive

A diagnosis of HIV infection does not change the indications for withdrawal medications, which can be used in HIV-positive persons in the same way they are used in uninfected patients. A federal panel advises that, if deemed appropriate, the withdrawal management process need not be altered by the presence of HIV infection.[6,23,24] However, possible drug interactions between antiretroviral agents used to treat HIV and medications used in withdrawal management require dosages to be adjusted accordingly. For instance, methadone and buprenorphine are two agents widely used in the management of opioid use disorders, both of which can have interactions with HIV medications, although methadone to a more significant degree than buprenorphine.[25]

Patients With Other Medical Conditions

Neurological Disorders

Brain-injured patients are at risk for seizures,[6] thus if a patient being managed for alcohol or other drug withdrawal becomes delirious, a workup is advised. Slower medication tapers are used in patients with seizure disorders.[6] Doses of anticonvulsant medications are stabilized before sedative-hypnotic withdrawal begins. The treatment of individuals with alcohol or other sedative dependence and past seizures is controversial largely because of challenges determining whether past convulsions were substance-related or not. In such a situation, the use of anticonvulsant agents (carbamazepine, valproate) may be considered, in combination with benzodiazepines.

Cardiovascular Disorders

Patients with cardiac disease require continued clinical assessment during withdrawal management. Underlying cardiac disease may be worsened by the symptoms of autonomic arousal (elevated blood pressure, increased pulse, and sweating) as seen in alcohol, sedative, and opioid withdrawal.[7] Because of this, it may be necessary to wean medication at a slower than normal rate and to consider use of additional medications such as beta-blockers or clonidine. Interactions between cardiac medications and the agents used to manage withdrawal management are also possible.

Hepatic or Renal Disorders

Severe liver or renal disease can slow the metabolism of both psychoactive substances and withdrawal medications. Use of shorter-acting medications and a slower taper is appropriate for such patients but requires precautions against drug accumulation and oversedation.[7]

Chronic Pain

With our current national crisis of nonmedical and unhealthy opioid use and accidental overdose, there is increased emphasis on reviewing treatment plans of noncancer patients on long term opioids, with the goal of goal of tapering when possible. However, changing treatment in context of chronic pain can certainly be complex. When taper is indicated, any patient who has taken opioids or sedative-hypnotics for a prolonged period are weaned from them gradually. Furthermore, the best outcomes often come from a multidisciplinary team, where nonpharmacological treatment is an important part of the treatment planning.[26]

Patients With Co-occurring Psychiatric Disorders

It is difficult to accurately assess underlying psychopathology in a patient who is experiencing withdrawal. Drug toxicity or psychiatric symptoms (particularly with amphetamines, cocaine, hallucinogens, or phencyclidine [PCP]) can mimic psychiatric disorders. Thorough psychiatric evaluation can be conducted after 2 to 3 weeks of abstinence. At the time patients are evaluated for withdrawal, some with underlying psychiatric disorders already may be prescribed antidepressants, antipsychotics, anxiolytics, or mood stabilizers. Although staff at some treatment programs may believe that such patients should discontinue all psychoactive medications, a federal panel has advised that this course of action may not be in the best interest of the patient.[6] Abrupt abstinence of psychotherapeutic medications may cause withdrawal symptoms or reemergence of symptoms of the underlying psychopathology. Thus, decisions about discontinuing the medication should be deferred temporarily. If, however, the patient has been misusing the prescribed medication or the psychiatric condition clearly was caused by the patient's alcohol or other drug use, the rationale for discontinuing the medication is more compelling. Individuals who use both sedative-hypnotics and alcohol pose a real challenge for withdrawal management, and generally require an inpatient setting and a prolonged period of management.

During withdrawal, some patients develop psychosis, depression, or severe anxiety. In such cases, careful evaluation of the withdrawal medication regimen is of paramount importance. Anxiety symptoms can cause an overestimation of withdrawal severity on clinical withdrawal scales and therefore result in overuse of medication. If the decompensation is the result of inadequate medication, dosing increases are appropriate. If the dose appears to be adequate, other medications can be added. Before selecting the alternative, however, it is important to consider potential side effects and interactions. If withdrawal medications are adequate and appropriate but the patient continues to decompensate, nonaddicting psychotropic medications (such as antipsychotics, anticonvulsants, or antidepressants) may be indicated for the treatment of psychoses, depression, or anxiety emerging during withdrawal. After withdrawal is completed, the patient's need for medications can be reassessed. A trial period with no medications may be indicated.

Adolescents

Adolescents in withdrawal pose somewhat different clinical issues than do adults. Patterns of use, negative consequences, context, and control of use may all be unique in adolescents in comparison to adults. Physical dependence is often not as severe in the adolescent compared with the adult, and the adolescent patient's response to withdrawal management usually is more rapid than that of the adult.[6,27,28] Inquiring about academic performance, school attendance, and disciplinary problems can be particularly important to help the clinician ascertain the adolescent's risk of a SUD. Behavioral problems may be more indirect, and careful evaluation for suicide risk is recommended. SUD, particularly when comorbid with depression, contributes to an increased rate of suicide in this age group. Adolescents in withdrawal need a structured environment that is nurturing and supportive. This is especially important because adolescents have higher rates of leaving treatment via patient-directed discharge compared to adults.[29] For hospitalized patients, adolescent-specific units are recommended. Decisions about family involvement are made on a case-by-case basis to reflect an assessment of family functioning.

Older Adults

Possible factors that may impact the treatment of intoxication and withdrawal in older adults include the increased likelihood of medical comorbidities with multiple prescribed medications and prescribing physicians, greater access to prescription medications (which may be used nonmedically), and possible impaired mobility from either social isolation or general medical conditions resulting in difficulty accessing clinic- or office-based treatment. It is essential to conduct a complete assessment and careful monitoring of the patient for co-occurring conditions, such as respiratory or cardiac disease or diabetes.[30] Older patients may take several prescription and over-the-counter medications, requiring assessment for interactions. For these reasons, withdrawal in a medically monitored or medically managed setting often is recommended. The cumulative effects of years of substance use may lead to more severe withdrawal symptoms in elderly persons.[31] The shorter-acting benzodiazepines may be of more clinical utility in this population given their lower risk of oversedation; but careful attention to emergent symptoms with tapering is warranted. It may be necessary to reduce the doses of withdrawal management medications because of older patients' slowed metabolism or coexisting medical disorders.

Persons in Criminal Justice Settings

Persons who are incarcerated or in detention in holding cells or elsewhere should be assessed for physical dependence on alcohol or other drugs because untreated withdrawal from alcohol and sedative-hypnotics can be life-threatening. Prevalence of physical dependence in these settings is higher than in the general population because an estimated 70% of people arrested for violent offenses test positive for substances. According to data from the Arrestee Drug Abuse Monitoring program in 2000, 64% of male arrestees tested positive for at least one of five illicit drugs (cocaine, opioids, cannabis, methamphetamines, and PCP), and 36% reported heavy drinking in the 30 days before arrest.[32] It is therefore critical that criminal justice and treatment staff be trained to detect signs and symptoms of SUD and to refer clients for appropriate medical treatment in cases of acute intoxication or withdrawal.[33]

Although opioid withdrawal is not life-threatening in healthy individuals, medical management is warranted. Patients who have been on opioid agonist treatment before being incarcerated should continue to receive their usual dose of medication. Opioid agonist treatment should be discontinued as gradually as possible if the jurisdiction or setting does not allow patients to receive these medications while incarcerated; however, the Americans with Disabilities Act may argue against such policies. Individuals who are on methadone maintenance may experience severe withdrawal symptoms if the medication is stopped abruptly. Indeed, methadone abstinence symptoms may persist for weeks or months and include severe vomiting and diarrhea, which can lead to complications. Pain may be severe and intractable. Withdrawal protocols need not be modified for incarcerated persons, except to the extent that state laws restrict the use of methadone or buprenorphine in criminal justice settings. In such cases, linkages with local methadone withdrawal management programs are advised.

In some carceral settings, there is an underground market for psychoactive medications. Patients may try to deceive caregivers about their physical dependence to obtain drugs for sale to others. For this reason, prison medical staff need special training in patient assessment and withdrawal management.[34]

CONCLUSIONS

The recognition and treatment of intoxication and withdrawal states represent important initial steps in the treatment of alcohol or other drug addiction. The primary goal of managing intoxication and withdrawal states is the prevention of morbidity and mortality. Whereas the treatment of intoxication often takes place in a medical setting, the treatment of withdrawal can occur in either an inpatient or an outpatient setting. Many variables must be taken into consideration in providing optimum care to patients who are undergoing treatment of withdrawal states. The ASAM Criteria can aid the clinician in matching patients to the appropriate levels of care for withdrawal management and subsequent ongoing SUD treatment.

REFERENCES

1. Substance Abuse and Mental Health Services Administration, Center for Behavioral Health Statistics and Quality (formerly the Office of Applied Studies). *Preliminary Findings from Drug-Related Emergency Department Visits, 2021.* Accessed June 5, 2023. https://store.samhsa.gov/sites/default/files/SAMHSA_Digital_Download/PEP22-07-03-001.pdf
2. Centers for Disease Control and Prevention, National Center for Health Statistics. *National Vital Statistics System—Mortality data (2020) via CDC WONDER.* Accessed June 5, 2023. http://cdc.gov/nchs/fastats/accidental-injury.htm
3. Substance Abuse and Mental Health Services Administration. The role of biomarkers in the treatment of alcohol use disorders, 2012 revision. *Spring.* 2012;11(2). Accessed June 5, 2023. https://www.niaaa.nih.gov/sites/default/files/SAMHSA-Advisory-Role-of-Biomarkers-in-the-Treatment-of-Alcohol-Use-Disorder-2012.pdf
4. American Psychiatric Association. *Diagnostic and Statistical Manual of Mental Disorders.* 5th ed. American Psychiatric Publishing; 2013.
5. National Institute of Health, National Institute of Drug Abuse, National Drug Early Warning System. *Highlights from NDEWS Sentinel Community Site 2020 Reports.* Accessed June 5, 2023. https://ndews.org/publications/site-reports
6. Center for Substance Abuse Treatment. *Detoxification from Alcohol and Other Drugs (Treatment Improvement Protocol Series, Number 19).* Substance Abuse and Mental Health Services Administration; 1995.
7. Center for Substance Abuse Treatment. *Detoxification and Substance Abuse Treatment (Treatment Improvement Protocol Series, Number 45).* Substance Abuse and Mental Health Services Administration; 2006.
8. Brown ME, Anton RF, Malcolm R, Ballenger AC. Alcohol detoxification and withdrawal seizures: clinical support for a kindling hypothesis. *Biol Psychiatry.* 1988;23:507-514.
9. Aston-Jones G, Harris GC. Brain substrates for increased drug seeking during protracted withdrawal. *Neuropharmacology.* 2004;47(suppl 1): 167-179.
10. De Sousa C, Uva M, Luminet O, et al. Distinct effects of protracted withdrawal on affect, craving, selective attention and executive functions among alcohol-dependent patients. *Alcohol Alcohol.* 2010;45(3):241-246.
11. Le Merrer J, Befort K, Gardon O, et al. Protracted abstinence from distinct drugs of abuse show regulation of a common gene network. *Addict Biol.* 2012;17(1):1-12.
12. Myrick H, Anton RF. Treatment of alcohol withdrawal. *Alcohol Health Res World.* 1998;22(1):38-43.
13. Myrick H, Anton R. Clinical management of alcohol withdrawal. *CNS Spectr.* 2000;5:22-32.
14. Eyer F, Schuster T, Felgenhauer N, et al. Risk assessment of moderate to severe alcohol withdrawal-predictors for seizures and delirium tremens in the course of withdrawal. *Alcohol Alcohol.* 2011;46(4):427-433.
15. Boothby LA, Doering RL. Acamprosate for the treatment of alcohol dependence. *Clin Ther.* 2005;27:695-614.
16. Mee-Lee D. *The ASAM Criteria; Treatment Criteria for Addictive, Substance-Related, and Co-occurring Conditions.* 3rd ed. American Society of Addiction Medicine; 2013.
17. O'Brien CP, Childress AR, McLellan AT. *Conditioning Factors May Help to Understand and Prevent Relapse in Patients Who Are Recovering from Drug Dependence (NIDA Research Monograph Number 106).* National Institute on Drug Abuse; 1991.
18. Unger A, Jagsch R, Jones H, et al. Randomized controlled trials in pregnancy: scientific and ethical aspects. Exposure to different opioid medications during pregnancy in an intra-individual comparison. *Addiction.* 2011;106(7):1355-1362.
19. Jones HE, Kaltenbach K, Heil SH, et al. Neonatal abstinence syndrome after methadone or buprenorphine exposure. *N Engl J Med.* 2010;363(24):2320-2331.
20. Mullins N, Galvin SL, Ramage M, et al. Buprenorphine and naloxone versus buprenorphine for opioid use disorder in pregnancy: a Cohort Study. *J Addict Med.* 2020;14(3):185-192.
21. Center for Substance Abuse Treatment. *Pregnant, Substance-Using Women (Treatment Improvement Protocol Series, Number 2).* Substance Abuse and Mental Health Services Administration; 1993.
22. American Academy of Pediatrics Committee on Drugs. Transfer of drugs and other chemicals into human milk. *Pediatrics.* 2001;108:776-789.
23. Center for Substance Abuse Treatment. *Treatment for HIV-Infected Alcohol and Other Drug Abusers (Treatment Improvement Protocol Series, Number 15).* Substance Abuse and Mental Health Services Administration; 1993.
24. Center for Substance Abuse Treatment. *Screening for Infectious Diseases among Substance Abusers (Treatment Improvement Protocol Series, Number 6).* Substance Abuse and Mental Health Services Administration; 1993.
25. Maas B, Kerr T, Fairbairn N, Montaner J, Wood E. Pharmacokinetic interactions between HIV antiretroviral therapy and drugs used to treat opioid dependence. *Expert Opin Drug Metab Toxicol.* 2006;2(4):533-543.
26. Center for Substance Abuse Treatment. *Managing Chronic Pain in Adults with or in Recovery from Substance Use Disorders (Treatment Improvement Protocol Series, Number 54).* Substance Abuse and Mental Health Services Administration; 2012.
27. Johnston LD, Miech RA, O'Malley PM, Bachman JG, Schulenberg JE. National press release. *Teen Use of Any Illicit Drug Other than Marijuana at New Low, Same True for Alcohol.* University of Michigan News Service. Accessed June 5, 2023. https://news.umich.edu/teen-use-of-any-illicit-drug-other-than-marijuana-at-new-low-same-true-for-alcohol/
28. Center for Substance Abuse Treatment. *Treatment of Adolescents with Substance Use Disorders (Treatment Improvement Protocol Series, Number 32).* Substance Abuse and Mental Health Services Administration; 1999.
29. Passetti LL, Godley MD, Kaminer Y. Continuing care for adolescents in treatment for substance use disorders. *Child Adolesc Psychiatr Clin N Am.* 2016;25(4):669-684.
30. Center for Substance Abuse Treatment. *Substance Abuse Among Older Adults (Treatment Improvement Protocol Series, Number 26).* Substance Abuse and Mental Health Services Administration; 2012.
31. Anton RF, Becker HC. Pharmacology and pathophysiology of alcohol withdrawal. In: Kranzler HR, ed. *Handbook of Experimental Pharmacology. Vol 114: The Pharmacology of Alcohol Abuse.* Springer; 1995:315-367.
32. Taylor BG, Fitzgerald N, Hunt D, Reardon JA, Brownstein HH. *ADAM Preliminary 2000 Findings on Drug Use & Drug Markets: Adult Male Arrestees.* U.S. Department of Justice, Office of Justice Programs, National Institute of Justice; 2001.
33. Center for Substance Abuse Treatment. *Substance Abuse Treatment for Adults in the Criminal Justice System (Treatment Improvement Protocol Series, Number 44).* Substance Abuse and Mental Health Services Administration; 2005.
34. Center for Substance Abuse Treatment. *Planning for Alcohol and Other Drug Abuse Treatment for Adults in the Criminal Justice System (Treatment Improvement Protocol Series, Number 17).* Substance Abuse and Mental Health Services Administration; 1994.

CHAPTER

56 Management of Alcohol Intoxication and Withdrawal

Alan A. Wartenberg, Hannan M. Braun, and Cara Zimmerman

CHAPTER OUTLINE

- Introduction
- Alcohol intoxication
- Hangover
- Alcohol withdrawal
- Management of alcohol withdrawal syndromes
- Common treatment issues
- Conclusions

INTRODUCTION

Management of alcohol intoxication and withdrawal is one of the clinical issues most frequently encountered by specialists in addiction medicine. Effective approaches, with a strong scientific basis, have been developed to reduce the incidence of serious complications.

ALCOHOL INTOXICATION

Clinical Picture

As blood alcohol concentration (BAC) rises so too does the clinical effect on the individual (**Table 56-1**).[1] Alcohol intoxication is defined by clinical manifestations of impairment that occur after alcohol consumption. The symptoms (significant behavioral or psychological changes due to central nervous system [CNS] effects) are reversible, specific to alcohol, and only occur in the context of recent ingestion. At a BAC between 20 and 99 mg%, loss of muscular coordination begins, and changes in mood, personality, and behavior occur. While a level of 80 mg% is considered legal intoxication in the United States, many people, particularly younger or medically/psychiatrically compromised individuals, may have significant impairment below that level. In some states, individuals below the legal drinking age are considered to be under the influence with levels of 50 mg%, with a few states having a "zero tolerance," where any detectable BAC indicates legal impairment.

As the blood alcohol level rises to the range of 100 to 199 mg%, neurological impairment occurs, accompanied by prolonged reaction time, ataxia, incoordination, and mental impairment. Acute alcohol intoxication can increase the chance of risky sex, have negative effects on witness recall, and impair witness testimony.[2-6] At a BAC of 200 to 299 mg%, obvious intoxication is present, except in those persons with marked tolerance. Nausea and vomiting and ataxia may occur. In very young and/or naive drinkers, BACs of 300 mg% may be associated with coma and death, especially when levels are reached quickly (eg, "chugging" drinks). The presence of other sedating medications or substances may result in additive or synergistic effects, increasing toxicity.

As the BAC rises to 300 to 399 mg%, hypothermia may occur, along with severe dysarthria and amnesia, with stage I anesthesia. At BAC levels between 400 and 799 mg%, the onset of alcoholic coma occurs. The precise level at which this occurs depends on tolerance; some persons experience coma at BACs of 300 mg%, whereas others do not experience it until the BAC approaches 600 mg%, depending largely on experience as well as the rapidity of reaching the peak BAC. Highly tolerant patients may be awake and conversant with levels that produce obtundation and even coma in less tolerant individuals.

BACs between 600 and 800 mg% are commonly fatal. Progressive obtundation develops, accompanied by decreases in respiration, blood pressure, and body temperature. The patient may develop urinary incontinence or retention, while reflexes are markedly decreased or absent. Death may occur from the loss of airway-protective reflexes (with subsequent airway obstruction by the flaccid tongue), from pulmonary aspiration of gastric contents, or from respiratory arrest arising from profound CNS depression.

Management

The medical management of alcohol intoxication and overdose is supportive. Studies have looked at creating a risk-stratification system for people with acute alcohol intoxication more likely to return to the ER. Risk factors include history of alcohol use disorder, being unhoused, history of incarceration, previous trauma.[7-9] The primary goal of management of alcohol intoxication is to prevent harm to the patient from severe respiratory depression and to protect the airway against aspiration. Even with very high BACs, survival is probable if the respiratory and cardiovascular systems can be supported. Attention must be paid to the potential presence of nonbeverage or surrogate alcohol (methyl alcohol, isopropyl alcohol, or ethylene glycol), as well as co-ingestion of other central nervous system depressants (eg, opioids, benzodiazepines, tricyclic antidepressants) since these intoxications may present a similar clinical picture but require different management.

Medical treatment is supportive in the alcohol-intoxicated patient. As with all patients with impaired consciousness,

TABLE 56-1 Clinical Effects of Alcohol

Blood alcohol level[a] (mg%)	Clinical manifestations
20-99	Loss of muscular coordination Changes in mood, personality, and behavior
100-199	Neurologic impairment with prolonged reaction time, ataxia, incoordination, and mental impairment
200-299	Very obvious intoxication, except in those with marked tolerance Nausea, vomiting, marked ataxia
300-399	Hypothermia, severe dysarthria, amnesia, stage I anesthesia
400-799	Onset of alcoholic coma, with precise level depending on the degree of tolerance Progressive obtundation, decreases in respiration, blood pressure, and body temperature (hypothermia) Urinary incontinence or retention, reflexes markedly decreased or absent
600-800	Often fatal because of loss of airway-protective reflexes from airway obstruction by the flaccid tongue, from pulmonary aspiration of gastric contents, or from respiratory arrest from profound central nervous system obstruction

[a]Levels of 200-300 mg%, particularly when reached quickly ("chugging"), may result in coma, aspiration, and death in nontolerant individuals, particularly adolescents and young adults. In addition, presence of other depressant drugs, even in therapeutic doses (benzodiazepines, sedative-hypnotics, opioids), may result in respiratory depression, coma, and death at lower levels of alcohol.

intravenous glucose is recommended if rapid testing of blood glucose is not immediately available, after first giving intravenous thiamine. These are of importance in alcohol intoxication as ethanol can impair gluconeogenesis, with an increased risk of hypoglycemia, and alcohol use disorder places the individual at an increased risk of thiamine deficiency. Whenever feasible, intravenous thiamine (generally 100 mg or more) should be given before glucose, particularly if glucose is given in large amounts or high concentrations.

It also is important to assess whether the patient has ingested other drugs in addition to alcohol, because these drugs may further suppress the CNS and alter the approach to treatment. Alcohol is rapidly absorbed into the bloodstream, so induction of emesis or gastric lavage is not indicated unless a substantial ingestion has occurred within the preceding 30 to 60 minutes or when other drug ingestion is suspected. Induced emesis may be useful at the scene (eg, with children at home) if it can be given within a few minutes of exposure. However, syrup of ipecac is no longer recommended, because of its toxicity if induction of emesis is unsuccessful.

Mechanical induction of emesis (ie, stimulating the gag reflex with fingers or instruments) has been discouraged because of the possibility of trauma to the upper airway. Similarly, gastric lavage is indicated only if the patient presents in the emergency department within 30 to 60 minutes after ingestion.[9] Activated charcoal does not efficiently absorb ethanol but may be given if other toxins have been ingested. More than 90% of alcohol is oxidized in the liver, and at the levels seen clinically, the rate of oxidation follows zero order kinetics; alcohol metabolism is independent of time and concentration of the drug. Elimination thus occurs at a fixed rate, with the level falling at a rate of about 20 mg/dL/h in a nontolerant individual; rates are higher in those with tolerance. In extreme cases of alcohol intoxication, hemodialysis (or peritoneal dialysis) can be used because it efficiently removes alcohol, but it is needed only rarely because supportive care usually is sufficient. Hemoperfusion and forced diuresis are not effective.

The acutely intoxicated patient may exhibit some agitation as part of the intoxication syndrome. This is best managed nonpharmacologically. Support and reassurance are helpful in dealing with agitation in an acutely intoxicated patient. On rare occasions, if pharmacological intervention is needed to manage a mildly or moderately intoxicated individual's behavior in a medical setting, intramuscular administration of a rapid-onset, short-acting benzodiazepine, such as lorazepam, alone or in combination with a neuroleptic agent such as haloperidol, can be useful. Caution must be exercised with a potential synergistic response between the alcohol already in the patient's system and an exogenously administered sedative-hypnotic, so this approach should be used only as a last resort and not in individuals with high blood alcohol levels. If such an approach is used, low doses (ie, haloperidol 1 mg with lorazepam 1 mg) are recommended.[10,11] Higher benzodiazepine doses may result in respiratory depression, vomiting, and aspiration, as well as the potential for "paradoxical" increased agitation by increasing intoxication.

There are no antidotes to alcohol that act like naloxone (an opioid antagonist) or flumazenil (a benzodiazepine/GABA antagonist). Metadoxine has been used to increase the metabolism of alcohol and shorten the period of intoxication.[12] It has been found to affect biochemical parameters and thus also may be useful in amelioration of alcoholic hepatitis with effects on early survival; however, studies have not yet demonstrated improvements in long-term clinical outcomes.

However, while a few trials with relatively few patients have shown a reduction in time to release from emergency departments, there is no strong evidence that metadoxine improves outcomes over conservative therapies, and its routine use is not recommended in acute alcohol intoxication. Modified Lvdou Gancao decoction, a traditional Chinese medicine decoction, and "a hepatocyte-mimicking antidote for alcohol intoxication" are under study in mice.[13]

HANGOVER

Hangover is a constellation of unpleasant physical and mental symptoms that occur after heavy alcohol intake.[14] Headache, malaise, diarrhea, nausea, and difficulty concentrating are the most common symptoms, often accompanied by sensitivity to light or sound, sweating, and anxiety. About 75% of individuals who drink to intoxication report experiencing a hangover at least some of the time. The primary alcohol-related morbidity in "lower-risk" drinkers is hangover. Because people who drink alcohol but do not exceed risky drinking limits make up most of the workforce, the greatest cost incurred by alcohol in the workplace is the decreased productivity caused by hangover-induced absenteeism or poor job performance. In addition to the personal discomfort, hangover increases the risk for injury and poor job performance. Patients with hangover have diminished visuospatial skills and dexterity with impairment demonstrated in pilots, automobile drivers, and skiers. There are also adverse effects on managerial skills and tasks.[15]

The pathophysiology of hangover is not completely understood. In part, it is believed to be the effect of the intermediate product of ethanol metabolism, acetaldehyde, as well as oxidative stress and inflammation.[16-19] Alcohol induces a pro-inflammatory state with release of cytokines. In addition, congeners, by-products of individual alcohol preparations found primarily in dark liquors such as brandy, whiskey, wine, and tequila, appear to play a role because they increase the frequency and severity of hangover. Clear liquors, such as rum, vodka, and gin, cause hangover less frequently.[18,19] Dehydration, electrolyte imbalance, disruption of sleep and other biological rhythms, increased physical activity while intoxicated, hypoglycemia, and the many hormonal disruptions caused by alcohol may also play contributing roles.[18-21] Patients with hangover have a diffuse slowing on electroencephalography, which may persist up to 16 hours after blood alcohol levels become undetectable.[18]

Although many interventions have been tried to alleviate hangover symptoms, to date, none has clearly demonstrated effectiveness in rigorous investigations.[18,19] Chinese publications, albeit with small samples, have found encouraging results with flat lemon–lime soda, *Plectranthus barbatus* decoctions, as well as with red ginseng.[22,23] Conservative management offers the best course of treatment, and symptoms generally resolve over 8 to 24 hours. Attentiveness to the quantity and quality of alcohol consumed can have a significant effect on preventing hangover. Asking patients about their hangover experiences offers an opportunity for education on a common cause of physical, psychiatric, and occupational consequences of drinking alcohol.

ALCOHOL WITHDRAWAL

Clinical Presentation

The relationship of heavy alcohol intake to certain syndromes has been recognized since ancient times (Hippocrates, circa 400 BCE). However, it was not until the 18th century that the clinical manifestations of alcohol withdrawal were clearly delineated. As is evident in the writings of Sutton, the vivid descriptions of severe withdrawal written at that time remain relevant today.

"It is preceded by tremors of the hands, restlessness, irregularity of thought, deficiency of memory, anxiety to be company, dreadful nocturnal dreams when the quantity of liquor through the day has been insufficient: much diminution of appetite, especially an aversion to animal food; violent vomiting in the morning and excessive perspiration from trivial causes. Confusion of thought arises to such height that objects are seen of the most hideous forms, and in positions that it is physically impossible they can be so situated; the patient generally sees flies or other insects; or pieces of money which he anxiously desires to possess…"[24]

For the most part, clinicians believed that these symptoms were a consequence of alcohol itself. It was not until the second half of the 20th century that their relationship to the start of abstinence from chronic alcohol intake—a relationship taken for granted today—was established. In 1953, Victor and Adams[25] reported their careful observations of 286 consecutive patients with DSM-IV–defined alcohol dependence admitted to an inner-city hospital, revealing the consistent relationship of abstinence from alcohol to the emergence of clinical symptoms. Their findings were supported in 1955 by a study of Isbell et al.,[26] in which 10 individuals with former opioid use disorder were given large quantities of alcohol for 7 to 8 days and then withdrawn abruptly without sedation. Over the next two decades, the concept of an alcohol withdrawal syndrome was firmly established by further animal and human studies, and diagnostic criteria based on empirical observation were developed. Today, manifestations of alcohol withdrawal are generally categorized in clinical practice as including the common alcohol withdrawal syndrome as well as the more severe manifestations of hallucinations, seizures, and delirium.

Alcohol Withdrawal Syndrome

The current understanding of the alcohol withdrawal syndrome is reflected in the diagnostic criteria of the American Psychiatric Association's *Diagnostic and Statistical Manual of Mental Disorders*, fourth and fifth editions.[27,28] In those with physiological dependence on alcohol, the clinical manifestations of alcohol withdrawal begin 6 to 24 hours after the last drink (or after marked reduction in the quantity of alcohol consumed), sometimes arising before the blood alcohol level has returned to zero. Early withdrawal signs and symptoms include anxiety, sleep disturbances, vivid dreams, anorexia, nausea, and headache. Physical signs include tachycardia, elevation of blood pressure, hyperactive reflexes, sweating, and hyperthermia. A tremor, best brought out by extension of the hands or tongue, may appear. This tremor has a rate of six to eight cycles per second and appears on electromyography to be an exaggeration of normal physiological tremor. The severity of these symptoms varies greatly among individuals, but in a majority, they are mild and transient, passing within 1 to 2 days.[27,28]

Hallucinations

In mild alcohol withdrawal, patients may experience perceptual distortions of a visual, auditory, and tactile nature. Lights may seem too bright or sounds too loud and startling. A sensation of "pins and needles" may be experienced. In more severe cases of withdrawal, these misperceptions may develop into frank hallucinations. Visual hallucinations are most common and frequently involve some type of animal life, such as seeing a dog or rodent in the room. Auditory hallucinations may begin as unformed sounds (such as clicks or buzzing) and progress to hearing voices. In contrast to the auditory hallucinations of schizophrenia, which may be of religious or political significance, these voices often are of friends or relatives and frequently are accusatory in nature. Tactile hallucinations may involve a sensation of bugs or insects crawling on the skin, known as formication. In milder cases of withdrawal, the patient's sensorium is otherwise clear, and the patient retains insight that the hallucinations are not real. In more severe withdrawal, this insight may be lost. Hallucinosis can occur in the absence of other withdrawal symptoms. They should be distinguished from the hallucinosis that can be part of delirium tremens (DTs).

Alcohol Withdrawal Seizures

Grand mal seizures are another manifestation of alcohol withdrawal. Withdrawal seizures occurred in 23% of the patients studied by Victor and Adams, in 33% of the patients in Isbell's study who drank the longest (for 48-87 days), and in 11% of placebo-treated patients who were enrolled in prospective controlled studies examining the effectiveness of benzodiazepines in symptomatic withdrawal.[29-33] Withdrawal seizures usually begin within 8 to 24 hours after the patient's last drink and may occur before the blood alcohol level has returned to zero. Most are generalized major motor seizures, occurring singly or in a burst of several seizures over a period of 1 to 6 hours. Although less than 3% of withdrawal seizures evolve into status epilepticus, alcohol withdrawal has been found to be a contributing cause in up to 15% of status epilepticus patients.[33,34] Like hallucinosis, seizures can sometimes occur with other symptoms of withdrawal minimal or absent. This is particularly the case in patients who are taking low-dose benzodiazepines, other sedatives, or adrenergic blocking agents, such as beta-blockers or alpha-2-blockers, but also can be seen in elderly or debilitated patients.

Seizures peak 24 hours after the last drink, corresponding to the peak of withdrawal-induced electroencephalogram (EEG) abnormalities, which include increased amplitude, a photo-myoclonic response, and spontaneous paroxysmal activity. These EEG abnormalities are transient, in keeping with the brevity of the convulsive attacks. Except for this brief period after withdrawal, the incidence of EEG abnormalities in patients with withdrawal seizures is not greater than in the normal population.[34] The risk of withdrawal seizures appears to be in part genetically determined and is increased in patients with past withdrawal seizures or in those who are undergoing concurrent withdrawal from benzodiazepines or other sedative-hypnotic drugs. The unhealthy use of benzodiazepines increases the likelihood of status epilepticus when withdrawing from both drugs.

There also is evidence that the risk of seizures increases as an individual undergoes repeated withdrawals.[35] This association has been described as a "kindling effect," which refers to animal studies demonstrating that repeated subcortical electrical stimulation is associated with increases in seizure susceptibility.[36] Animal studies have supported this kindling hypothesis in alcohol withdrawal, demonstrating that submitting animals to repeated alcohol withdrawal episodes increases their risk of withdrawal seizures. There is emerging evidence that this effect occurs in humans as well.[35-40]

Alcohol Withdrawal Delirium

Withdrawal is highly individualized in both severity and duration. For up to 90% of patients, withdrawal does not progress beyond the mild to moderate symptoms described previously, peaking between 24 and 36 hours and gradually subsiding. In other patients, however, manifestations can include delirium. The diagnostic criteria are delineated in the DSM-5.[28] In the classic cases of withdrawal delirium, the manifestations of withdrawal steadily worsen and progress into a severe life-threatening delirium accompanied by an autonomic storm: hence, the term delirium tremens (DTs). DTs generally appear 72 to 96 hours after the last drink. In their classic presentation, DTs are marked by all the signs and symptoms of mild withdrawal but in a much more pronounced form, with the development of marked tachycardia, tremor, diaphoresis, and fever. The patient develops global confusion and disorientation to place and time, as well as highly impaired attention (delirium). The patient may become absorbed in a separate psychic reality, often believing him- or herself to be in a location other than the hospital and misidentifies staff as personal acquaintances. Hallucinations are frequent, and the patient usually has no insight into them. Without insight, they can be extremely frightening to the patient, who may react in a way that poses a threat to the patient's or the staff's safety.

Marked psychomotor activity may develop, with severe agitation in some cases or continuous low-level motor activity in others, so that activities such as efforts to get out of bed can last for hours. Severe disruption of the normal sleep-wake cycle also is common and may be marked by the absence of clear sleep for several days. The duration of the delirium is variable but averages 2 to 3 days in most studies.[33,41] In some cases, the delirium is relatively brief, lasting only a few hours before the patient regains orientation. In other cases, the patient remains delirious for several days, with reports of periods lasting 50 days before the confusion clears.[42] Before the development of effective treatment, mortality in DTs was substantial. With the development of effective therapy, including intensive care, death from DTs is an unusual event.[33,41,43]

Because the clinical syndrome of delirium has become more carefully and broadly studied, and standard diagnostic criteria have been developed, it is becoming apparent that many cases of delirium during alcohol withdrawal occur without the autonomic storm associated with classically described DTs. Although the terms "alcohol withdrawal delirium" and "DTs" are often used interchangeably, many cases of delirium in alcohol withdrawal are mild and transient. In one retrospective chart review of 284 patients undergoing withdrawal, 20 patients were identified as meeting DSM-IV-TR criteria for alcohol withdrawal delirium, while only three had the syndrome of DTs.[43] This is an area needing further investigation, including the role that treatment with sedative-hypnotics or concurrent medical illness may play in the development of mild delirium in alcohol withdrawal.

Alcohol Withdrawal Severity Scales

Because alcohol withdrawal involves a constellation of nonspecific findings, efforts have been made to develop structured withdrawal severity assessment scales to objectively quantify the severity of withdrawal. Several such scales have been published in the literature.[44-46] The most extensively studied and best known is the Clinical Institute Withdrawal Assessment-Alcohol, or CIWA-A, and a shortened version known as the CIWA-A Revised, or Clinical Institute Withdrawal Assessment of Alcohol Scale, Revised (CIWA-Ar) (**Table 56-2**).[45,46] The CIWA-Ar has well-documented reliability, reproducibility, and validity based on comparisons with ratings of withdrawal severity by experienced clinicians.

The CIWA-Ar and similar scales require 2 to 5 minutes to complete and have proved useful in a variety of settings, including withdrawal management units, psychiatric units, medical/surgical wards, and intensive care units. Such scales allow rapid documentation of the patient's signs and symptoms and provide a simple summary score that facilitates accurate and objective communication among staff. In the case of the CIWA-Ar, a score 8 or less indicates mild withdrawal, a score of 11 to 15 moderate withdrawal, and a score more than 15 severe withdrawal. Patients consistently scoring under 8 rarely require intensive monitoring, while those with scores of 11 to 15 need monitoring at least every 2 to 4 hours, and those with scores over 15 may need a telemetry or intensive care setting.

A careful analysis of symptoms in an inpatient (ASAM level IV) withdrawal management setting, recorded using withdrawal scales found that patients with symptomatic withdrawal segregated into distinct clinical groups. Approximately 20% had no significant withdrawal symptoms.[30] Another 20% had only vegetative (physical) signs, such as tremor and sweating, but no psychological symptoms. The largest group, 40%, had both vegetative and mild to moderate psychological symptoms, primarily anxiety. The last group, about 20% of patients, had both vegetative and severe psychological symptoms with disorientation, delirium, or hallucinations. As indicated previously, relatively few patients in alcohol withdrawal experience the adrenergic and clinical manifestations of DTs. It is extremely important that staff responsible for patient assessment be adequately trained in the utilization of the CIWA-Ar. One common error is to assess the patient who is clinically intoxicated (or who has other acute medical illness), which may result in a high score because of nonspecific responses (nausea, headache, anxiety) and thus allow treatment of an already intoxicated individual (or one with another medical cause of symptoms) with benzodiazepines, with the potential for increased intoxication, respiratory depression, vomiting and aspiration, and other complications. The reverse can also be problematic, with inexperienced raters underscoring withdrawal symptoms resulting in rapidly progressing withdrawal without the balance of proper pharmacological treatment.

It is important for the responsible clinician (physician, nurse practitioner, physicians' assistant, or pharmacist) to be thoroughly familiar with the instrument and train nurses and other health professionals who will be monitoring the patients. Interobserver variability may occur and lead to inappropriate scoring (high or low) when the observers have not had adequate training in differentiating the differing anchor points given in the scoring instrument. The CIWA-Ar is not a diagnostic instrument for alcohol withdrawal, which is diagnosed based on the clinical setting, including patient history and careful examination (particularly a thorough neurological and mental status exam).

Confounding or exacerbating conditions, such as hypoglycemia, head trauma, CNS infections, other drug influences, and metabolic disturbances, must be appropriately excluded. Once the withdrawal syndrome is recognized, the CIWA-Ar can assist in determining its severity and assist in establishing the effects of treatment on its course. Clinicians utilizing such scales must understand that there may also be confounding factors present, which may increase the score (concomitant dehydration, infection, other causes of hyperautonomic signs and symptoms) or may decrease it (advanced age, use of beta-blockers or other sympatholytic drugs).

There have been several recent studies using more complex withdrawal scales, which divide withdrawal into its autonomic, psychological, and perceptual components and score them separately,[47] with a proposal to treat the autonomic component (if dominant) with adrenergic blocking agents (ie, beta-blockers), the anxiety/psychological component with benzodiazepines, and the perceptual disturbances with neuroleptic agents. Another withdrawal scale simplifies the CIWA-Ar, using fewer parameters and simpler scoring—the HAWP (Highland Alcohol Withdrawal Protocol)—with excellent results in a retrospective study.[48] An even simpler three-item scale, the AST (anxiety, sweating, tremor) produced good results but in a study with only 85 patients.[49] Larger prospective studies, including head-to-head comparisons of the performance of newer scales, including their performance in guiding treatment, against the CIWA-Ar, are needed before their widespread acceptance by clinicians.

TABLE 56-2 Clinical Institute Withdrawal Assessment of Alcohol Scale, Revised (CIWA-Ar)

Patient:______________ Date:______________ Time:________

(24-hour clock, midnight = 00:00)

Pulse or heart rate, taken for 1 min:______________ Blood pressure:______

Nausea and vomiting

Ask: "Do you feel sick to your stomach? Have you vomited?"

Observation:

0 No nausea and no vomiting
1 Mild nausea with no vomiting
2
3
4 Intermittent nausea with dry heaves
5
6
7 Constant nausea, frequent dry heaves, and vomiting

Tactile disturbances

Ask: "Do you have any itching, pin-and-needle sensations, any burning, or any numbness, or do you feel bugs crawling on or under your skin?"

Observation:

0 None
1 Very mild itching, pins and needles, burning, or numbness
2 Mild itching, pins and needles, burning, or numbness
3 Moderate itching, pins and needles, burning, or numbness
4 Moderately severe hallucinations
5 Severe hallucinations
6 Extremely severe hallucinations
7 Continuous hallucinations

Tremor

Arms extended and fingers spread apart

Observation:

0 No tremor
1 Not visible, but can be felt fingertip to fingertip
2
3
4 Moderate, with the patient's arms extended
5
6
7 Severe, even with arms not extended

Auditory disturbances

Ask: "Are you more aware of sounds around you? Are they harsh? Do they frighten you? Are you hearing anything that is disturbing to you? Are you hearing things you know are not there?"

Observation:

0 Not present
1 Very mild harshness or ability to frighten
2 Mild harshness or ability to frighten
3 Moderate harshness or ability to frighten
4 Moderately severe hallucinations
5 Severe hallucinations
6 Extremely severe hallucinations
7 Continuous hallucinations

Paroxysmal sweats

Observation:

0 No sweat visible
1 Barely perceptible sweating, palms moist
2
3
4 Beads of sweat obvious on the forehead
5
6
7 Drenching sweats

(Continued)

TABLE 56-2 Clinical Institute Withdrawal Assessment of Alcohol Scale, Revised (CIWA-Ar) *(Continued)*

Visual disturbances
Ask: "Does the light appear to be too bright? Is its color different? Does it hurt your eyes? Are you seeing anything that is disturbing to you? Are you seeing things you know are not there?"
Observation:
0 Not present
1 Very mild sensitivity
2 Mild sensitivity
3 Moderate sensitivity
4 Moderately severe hallucinations
5 Severe hallucinations
6 Extremely severe hallucinations
7 Continuous hallucinations

Anxiety
Ask: "Do you feel nervous?"
Observation:
0 No anxiety, at ease
1 Mild anxious
2
3
4 Moderately anxious, or guarded, so anxiety is inferred
5
6
7 Equivalent to acute panic states as seen in severe delirium or acute schizophrenic reactions

Headache, fullness in head
Ask: "Does your head feel different? Does it feel like there is a band around your head?"
Do not rate for dizziness or light-headedness. Otherwise, rate severity.
Observation:
0 Not present
1 Very mild
2 Mild
3 Moderate
4 Moderately severe
5 Severe
6 Very severe
7 Extremely severe

Agitation
Observation:
0 Normal activity
1 Somewhat more than normal activity
2
3
4 Moderately fidgety and restless
5
6
7 Paces back and forth during most of the interview, or constantly thrashes about

Orientation and clouding of sensorium
Ask: "What day is this? Where are you? Who am I?"
Observation:
0 Oriented and can do serial additions
1 Cannot do serial additions or is uncertain about date
2 Disoriented for date by no more than two calendar days
3 Disoriented for date by more than two calendar days
4 Disoriented for place/or person

Total CIWA-Ar score______
Rater's initials______
Maximum possible score: 67

This assessment for monitoring withdrawal symptoms requires approximately 5 minutes to administer. The maximum score is 67 (see instrument). Patients scoring less than 10 do not usually need additional medication for withdrawal.

From Sullivan JT, Sykora K, Schneiderman J, et al. Assessment of alcohol withdrawal: the revised Clinical Institute Withdrawal Assessment for Alcohol scale (CIWA-Ar). *Br J Addict.* 1989;84:1353-1357.

Predictors of Severe Withdrawal

Withdrawal scales can also contribute to appropriate triage of patients as it has been shown that high scores early in the course are predictive of the development of seizures and delirium. Those with low scores on withdrawal scales (10 or below on the CIWA-Ar) over the first 24 to 48 hours, particularly in those with such scores who have taken no benzodiazepines, have consistently been found to be at little or no risk for severe withdrawal. Other risk factors for severe withdrawal include prior DTs or withdrawal seizures. The presence of marked autonomic hyperactivity (commonly measured as elevated heart rate on admission), elevated blood alcohol level of 100 mg/dL or higher at the time of admission, serum electrolyte abnormalities, and acute medical comorbidities, particularly infection and trauma, are other clinical findings associated with an increased rate of DTs or severe withdrawal. Characteristics that have not been useful in triaging patients include the amount of daily intake, duration of heavy drinking, age, and gender, though recent regular heavy intake is a sine qua non for withdrawal risk, and longer duration of physical dependence has predicted the incidence of symptomatic withdrawal. Several rating systems have been developed combining multiple items to predict the severity of withdrawal,[47-51] but none are precise enough to be relied on exclusively. Studies have identified patients at low risk for severe withdrawal with high reliability. The clinical utility of these rating systems has not been established and requires further study. However, they may be very useful in patients where history and presentation are not typical.

Pathophysiology

Goldstein and Goldstein[52] proposed in 1961 that physical dependence develops as a cell or organism makes homeostatic adjustments to compensate for the primary effect of a drug. The primary effect of alcohol on the CNS is as a depressant. With chronic exposure, there are compensatory adjustments to this chronic depressant effect, with down-regulation of inhibitory systems and up-regulation of excitatory systems. This represents a shift from homeostasis to allostasis. With abrupt abstinence from alcohol, these relative deficiencies in inhibitory influences and relative excesses in excitatory influences are suddenly unmasked, leading to the appearance of withdrawal phenomena. The withdrawal symptoms last until the body readjusts to the absence of the alcohol and establishes a new equilibrium. Two neurotransmitter systems appear to play a central role in the development of alcohol withdrawal syndrome. Alcohol exerts its effects in part by directly or indirectly enhancing the effect of GABA, a major inhibitory neurotransmitter. GABA mediates typical sedative-hypnotic effects such as sedation, muscle relaxation, and a raised seizure threshold. Chronic alcohol intake leads to an adaptive suppression of GABA activity. A sudden relative deficiency in GABA neurotransmitter activity is produced with alcohol abstinence and is believed to contribute to the anxiety, increased psychomotor activity, and predisposition to seizures seen in withdrawal. Although alcohol enhances the effect of GABA, it inhibits the sensitivity of the autonomic adrenergic systems, with a resulting up-regulation with chronic alcohol intake. The discontinuation of alcohol leads to rebound over activity of the brain and peripheral noradrenergic systems. Increased sympathetic autonomic activity contributes to such acute manifestations as tachycardia, hypertension, tremor, diaphoresis, and anxiety.[52,53]

A second neurotransmitter, norepinephrine, also seems to be important in alcohol withdrawal presentations. Norepinephrine's metabolites are elevated in plasma, urine, and cerebral spinal fluid during withdrawal; levels of metabolites correlate significantly with the sympathetic nervous system signs of withdrawal.[54] Research has identified other neural effects of chronic alcohol intake, including effects on serotonergic systems, neuronal calcium channels, glutamate receptors, cyclic AMP systems, and the hypothalamic-pituitary-adrenal neuroendocrine axis, and these too may play a role in the pathophysiology of withdrawal. Other recent studies suggest that the glutamatergic system and NMDA (*N*-methyl-D-aspartate) dysregulation play a role in the development of CNS excitation as well, particularly seizures and delirium.[55]

Genetics

The role of genetics in alcohol withdrawal is a topic of active investigation. In animal models, the development of selectively bred strains demonstrates that severity of withdrawal and risk of seizures are strongly influenced by genotype. Investigations in humans have focused on genes regulating neurotransmitter systems. Several studies have found an association of the A9 allele, which affects central dopamine functions, with severity of alcohol withdrawal, alcohol withdrawal seizures, and DTs.[56-60] To date, no relationship with genes involved in the serotonin, GABAergic, or endorphinergic systems has been found.[60] Although these findings are not of immediate clinical use, genetic studies may shed light on basic pathophysiology and, at some point, assist in identifying high-risk individuals who may benefit from tailored therapy, including those with genetic susceptibility to specific alcohol-related organ damage, such as liver disease.

Role of Alcohol Withdrawal in Diagnostic Classification

When DSM-III-R moved to a broad definition of alcohol dependence, it removed any requirement for physiological components, tolerance, and withdrawal, for a diagnosis of alcohol dependence. This was done without intensive study of what effect would occur if neither was required for a diagnosis. DSM-IV did add a request to subtype dependence into groups with and without physiological components. Intervening studies have shown that approximately 60% of individuals meeting DSM-IV criteria for alcohol dependence report withdrawal symptoms, another 35% report tolerance without withdrawal symptoms, and only 5% report neither. Of the seven DSM-IV dependence items, withdrawal symptoms have been most strongly associated with an increased number of alcohol-related problems, higher number of drinks per occasion, and future difficulties.[61] Alternative approaches to DSM-IV have been proposed that reinstitute withdrawal as a required feature, with evidence that such approaches offer better validity and better discrimination between the dependence and abuse classifications.[61,62]

The role of withdrawal in the diagnostic taxonomy of alcohol use disorders continues to be investigated and debated. While the DSM-5 eliminates the abuse/dependence dichotomy, and instead uses substance use disorder—alcohol—based on the presence of 11 criteria (the same as the current criteria except with recurrent legal difficulties being replaced by a craving criterion),[44] and with severity indicators for absent (0-1 criterion), mild (2-3 criteria), moderate (4-5 criteria), and severe (6 or greater criteria),[28] definitions and criteria for alcohol withdrawal syndromes are not significantly different from those in the DSM-IV-TR.[27]

MANAGEMENT OF ALCOHOL WITHDRAWAL SYNDROMES

General Principles

The primary goals of the treatment of alcohol withdrawal syndromes are to first assure clinical stability of the patient and second encourage ongoing treatment (eg, rehabilitation) of a patient's alcohol use disorder. The first step in managing the patient with alcohol withdrawal is to perform an assessment for the presence of medical and psychiatric conditions. Chronic alcohol intake is associated with the development of many acute and chronic medical problems. The clinician needs to determine whether there are acute conditions that require hospital treatment or chronic conditions that may alter the approach to the management of withdrawal because they could be exacerbated significantly by the development of withdrawal or its treatment. Pertinent laboratory tests generally include complete blood count, electrolytes, magnesium, calcium, phosphate, liver enzymes, urine drug screen, pregnancy test (when appropriate), and breath or blood alcohol level. However, in patients at low risk for withdrawal requiring pharmacological intervention, and who have no history of serious medical/psychiatric problems, social setting detoxification without such laboratory studies is feasible (see section on "Social Setting" Withdrawal Management).

Others, depending on suspected co-occurring conditions, may include skin test for tuberculosis, chest x-ray, electrocardiogram, and tests for viral hepatitis, HIV, other infections, or sexually transmitted diseases. General management also involves maintaining adequate fluid balance, correction of electrolyte deficiencies, and attendance to the patient's nutritional needs. Patients in early withdrawal often are volume overloaded so that aggressive volume repletion usually is not necessary unless there have been significant fluid losses from vomiting or diarrhea. Volume status should be assessed by usual clinical signs and symptoms, as well as by laboratory means when indicated. Supportive care and reassurance from health care personnel are important elements of comfortable withdrawal management and help to facilitate continuing treatment.

Supportive nonpharmacological care is an important and useful element in the management of all patients undergoing withdrawal. Simple interventions such as reassurance, reality orientation, monitoring of signs and symptoms of withdrawal, and general nursing care are effective. There has been interest in the possible value of complementary and alternative medicine for alcohol withdrawal. Controlled trials of acupuncture have not demonstrated effectiveness,[63] whereas massage therapy did reduce alcohol withdrawal scores.[64] It is important to note that all these supportive measures do not prevent the development of major complications such as seizures and are not adequate by themselves to manage the patient with or at elevated risk for severe withdrawal or delirium, in which case pharmacological intervention is required.

Pharmacological Management of Uncomplicated Withdrawal Syndrome

The medical literature on the pharmacological management of alcohol withdrawal has been comprehensively reviewed as part of the American Society of Addiction Medicine (ASAM) evidence-based clinical practice guideline efforts.[33,41,65] This review of the evidence indicated that the cornerstone of pharmacological management of withdrawal is the use of benzodiazepines, a conclusion supported by more recent systematic reviews.[66-68]

Benzodiazepines

The major treatment goals for withdrawal delirium are to control agitation, decrease the risk of seizures, and decrease the risk of injury and death. Benzodiazepines are pharmacologically cross-tolerant with alcohol and have the similar effect of enhancing the effect of GABA-induced sedation. A specific benzodiazepine receptor site has been identified on the GABA receptor complex. It is believed that the provision of benzodiazepines alleviates the acute deficiency of GABA neurotransmitter activity that occurs with sudden abstinence from alcohol intake. Studies have consistently shown that benzodiazepines are more effective than placebo in reducing the signs and symptoms of withdrawal.

Meta-analyses of prospective placebo-controlled trials of patients admitted with symptomatic withdrawal have shown a highly significant reduction in seizures, with a risk reduction of 7.7 seizures per 100 patients treated,[33] as well as in delirium, with a risk reduction of 4.9 cases of delirium per 100 patients treated.[41] No single benzodiazepine drug has been shown to be superior to another at improving withdrawal symptoms or preventing complications of withdrawal.[68] Diazepam is often preferred due to its rapid onset, long half-life, and multiple routes of administration (ie, oral, IV, IM); however, diazepam is not preferred in cases of advanced liver disease due to active hepatic metabolites (in such cases, lorazepam is preferred, particularly for parenteral use, and lorazepam and oxazepam can be given orally).

On the other hand, pharmacological data and clinical experience suggest that longer-acting agents such as diazepam or chlordiazepoxide can pose a risk of excess sedation in some patients, including elderly persons and patients with significant liver disease (hepatic synthetic dysfunction), and in patients with chronic pulmonary disease, where prolonged respiratory depression may occur. In such patients, shorter-acting agents such as lorazepam or oxazepam may be preferable; also, these agents have the added advantage of avoiding phase I metabolism via the cytochrome P-450 system, which may be advantageous in the setting of impaired hepatic function.

Another consideration in the choice of benzodiazepine is the rapidity of onset. Certain agents with rapid onset of action (such as diazepam, alprazolam, and lorazepam) demonstrate greater potential for unhealthy use or diversion than do agents with a slower onset of action (such as chlordiazepoxide and oxazepam). This consideration may be of relevance in an outpatient setting or for patients with a past unhealthy benzodiazepine use or disorder. However, when rapid control of symptoms is needed, medications with faster onset offer an advantage, and in the context of treating withdrawal, which particularly in the outpatient setting is of short duration, the potential for unhealthy use is rarely a clinical concern.

A final consideration in the choice of benzodiazepine is cost, as these agents vary considerably in price. Given the evidence of equal efficacy, if a specific agent is available to a practitioner or program at a lower cost, cost is a legitimate factor to consider. The pharmacokinetics of different benzodiazepines should be taken into consideration depending upon the clinical circumstances, including the age and health of the patient, potential drug-drug interactions, and the stage and severity of withdrawal. Younger, healthier patients generally tolerate longer-acting drugs, which may produce a smoother course. Shorter-acting agents may be better tolerated in older, sicker patients, particularly those with hepatic insufficiency and/or pulmonary disease.

If patients are assessed for signs of oversedation prior to each dose, and when at peak levels of receiving benzodiazepine, clinically serious oversedation can be avoided, even if longer-acting agents are employed. Drug latency may also be an issue when patients present with moderate to severe withdrawal, since several commonly used drugs have longer periods between oral ingestion and peak levels, such as oxazepam (which takes 1.5-2 hours to peak) or chlordiazepoxide (1-2 hours), while diazepam may reach peak levels in 20 to 30 minutes. Since oxazepam is relatively short acting, the long latency and the rapid excretion may produce a "choppy" course; in those with hepatic disease, lorazepam may be an equally effective and safe option, with both more rapid absorption and a longer period of clinical activity. Use of oxazepam with longer dosing intervals (6-8 hours), particularly late in treatment, may result in an increase in withdrawal manifestations, including seizures.[69] There is no reason to use more than one benzodiazepine; but in some cases, adjunctive medications may be helpful (see below).

Attention to tapering doses can be important when shorter-acting agents are used as tolerance to them can develop rapidly and withdrawal from them can lead to symptoms including seizures. While physical dependence upon benzodiazepines given therapeutically is a legitimate concern, it rarely occurs unless the benzodiazepine has been prescribed for 10 to 14 days, although the author has rarely seen shorter courses leading to withdrawal.[69]

Studies have indicated that nonbenzodiazepine sedative-hypnotics (eg, barbiturates) also are effective in reducing the signs and symptoms of withdrawal and are increasingly studied. Benzodiazepines have a known margin of safety, with a lower risk of respiratory depression, as well as overall lower unhealthy use potential than the nonbenzodiazepine agents. Phenobarbital, a long-acting barbiturate that enhances GABA and suppresses glutamate activity in the CNS is used by some programs, as it has well-documented anticonvulsant activity, is inexpensive, and has low unhealthy use liability. However, as with all barbiturates, oversedation is commonly associated with both depressed consciousness and potential respiratory depression.

It is critically important to assess every patient for signs and symptoms of oversedation (sustained nystagmus, dysarthria, dysmetria, ataxia, mood lability, and depressed level of consciousness) prior to receiving additional doses and to withhold additional doses if such signs or symptoms are present. Available evidence does not show uniform benefit of phenobarbital (used alone, or in conjunction with symptom-triggered benzodiazepines) in multiple assessed outcomes: ICU admission, ED length of stay, and complications such as intubation.[70]

Chlormethiazole, an agent with benzodiazepine-like and anticonvulsant effects, while widely used elsewhere, is unavailable in the United States.

Determining the Dosing Schedule

In many studies examining the effectiveness of various medications for withdrawal, the medications were given in fixed amounts at scheduled times (such as chlordiazepoxide 50 mg every 6 hours) and were given for periods of 5 to 7 days. However, it has been shown that many patients can go through withdrawal with only minor symptoms even though they receive little or no medication.[30-32] An alternative to giving medication on a fixed schedule is known as symptom-triggered therapy.[66] In this approach, the patient is monitored using a structured assessment scale and given medication only when symptoms cross a threshold of severity. Well-designed studies have demonstrated that this approach is as effective as fixed-dose therapy but leads to the administration of significantly less medication and a significantly shorter duration of treatment.[31,32] Further research is needed to support which approach (fixed dose or symptom triggered) producing better outcomes in terms of mortality, seizure control or delirium in any setting. However, overall symptom-triggered therapy is recommended over fixed dose schedules because symptom-triggered therapy is associated with shorter length of stay and lower cumulative benzodiazepine administration.[31,65,66,71]

Symptom-triggered therapy also facilitates the delivery of large amounts of medication quickly to patients who evidence rapidly escalating withdrawal and thus reduces the risk of undertreatment that may arise with the use of fixed doses. For programs specializing in the management of addiction, use of a symptom-triggered approach with the utilization of a severity scale offers significant advantages. However, there may be situations in which the provision of fixed doses remains appropriate. For example, in patients admitted to general medical or surgical wards, the nursing staff may not have the training or experience to implement the regular use of scales to monitor patients. In certain patients, such as those with severe coronary artery disease, or those with prior histories of seizures or DT's, the clinician may wish to prevent the development of even minor symptoms of withdrawal.

Finally, because a history of past withdrawal seizures is a risk factor for seizures during a withdrawal episode, and because withdrawal seizures usually occur early in withdrawal, some practitioners administer fixed doses (or at least one single dose regardless of symptoms) to patients with a history of withdrawal seizures or who are otherwise at higher risk for symptomatic withdrawal such as those with acute medical, surgical, or psychiatric illnesses. Whenever fixed doses are given, it is very important that allowances be made to provide additional medication if the fixed dose should prove inadequate to control symptoms. In other words, despite the rationale for fixed dosing often being an inability to monitor patients frequently as is required by symptom-triggered therapy, fixed dosing does not obviate this need. For patients with a contraindication of benzodiazepines, phenobarbital may be used, though provider experience is recommended.

Loading dose therapy may also be considered, which involves monitoring the patient with CIWA-Ar scores until they reach a predetermined set point (generally 8-15) and then giving diazepam (10-20 mg), clorazepate (3.75-7.5 mg), or chlordiazepoxide (50-100 mg) on an hourly basis, evaluating the patient prior to each dose until symptoms diminish or signs of oversedation develop—sustained nystagmus, ataxia, dysarthria, mood lability, or oversedation itself (somnolence, not responsive to a normal-level voice).[72,73] The patient is then monitored for 2 to 3 hours without further medication. A front-loading regimen is recommended for patients at high risk of severe withdrawal syndrome. The average patient received three to five doses before reaching the end point, and 80% of patients were adequately treated with a single episode of loading, while an additional 10% required a second loading dose regimen within the first 24 hours. One-tenth of patients could not be successfully treated with this approach, presumably because of up-regulation of P-450 hepatic cytochrome enzymes in these patients, such that usual longer-acting benzodiazepines in effect were shorter acting in these patients.

Treatment should allow for a degree of individualization so that patients can receive large amounts of medication rapidly if needed. In all cases, medications is best administered by a route that has been shown to have reliable absorption. Therefore, the benzodiazepines are administered orally or, when necessary, intravenously. An exception is lorazepam, which has good intramuscular and sublingual absorption. In the past, intramuscular administration was commonly used. However, for most agents, intramuscular absorption is extremely variable, leading to problems when rapid control of symptoms is necessary and with delayed appearance of oversedation when large amounts are administered. Examples of some treatment regimens consistent with current recommendations are shown in **Table 56-3**.

One technique is to use fixed-dose regimens that can be loosely based on the potential for mild, moderate, or severe withdrawal and then to order as-needed (prn) doses based on the development of an arbitrary CIWA-Ar score of 10 to 15. If the CIWA-Ar does not come down to below 10 after one to two additional doses, then the patient is reassessed to determine that the medication is being given at an appropriate dose by an appropriate route and that comorbid issues are not present. If two as-needed doses fail to reduce the severity of withdrawal, reconsider the regimen, with higher standing doses and/or consideration of absorption issues and switching to a parenteral regimen. Similarly, hold orders are used to prevent administration to patients who are over sedated; if doses are withheld more than twice, reevaluate the regimen, with orders for lower standing doses. Caution should be taken to consider not continue standing protocols to taper down the dose in patients who are still requiring frequent as-needed doses. Alternatively, caution should also be taken to consider stopping the dosing completely (and not just simply reducing the dose) to patients actively manifesting toxicity; and to stop dosing until no signs of toxicity are present. Tapering off the benzodiazepines or stopping them generally is not enacted until the patient is stable and CIWA-Ar scores are consistently below 10.

Anticonvulsants

For people with contraindications to benzodiazepines, carbamazepine, gabapentin, phenobarbital, or valproic acid may be used as adjuncts.[65,73-75] Carbamazepine has been widely used in Europe for alcohol withdrawal and has been shown to be equal in efficacy to benzodiazepines for patients with mild to moderate withdrawal. Fixed, tapering doses of carbamazepine are without significant toxicity when used in 5- to 7-day protocols for alcohol withdrawal and are associated with less psychiatric distress, a faster return to work, less rebound symptoms, and reduced posttreatment drinking.[75-78] When compared with

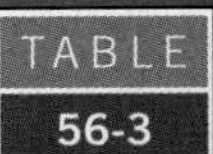

TABLE 56-3 Examples of Specific Pharmacologic Treatment Regimens

Monitoring

Monitor the patient every 4-8 h using the CIWA-Ar until the score has been below 8-10 for 24 h; use additional assessments as needed.

Symptom-triggered medication regimens

Administer one of the following medications every hour when the CIWA-Ar is >8-10:

- Chlordiazepoxide 50-100 mg
- Diazepam 10-20 mg
- Oxazepam 30-60 mg (some consider 60-120 mg to be equivalent)
- Lorazepam 2-4 mg

(Other benzodiazepines may be used at equivalent substitutions)

Repeat the CIWA-Ar 1 h after every dose to assess need for further medication.

Structured medication regimens

The physician may feel that the development of even mild to moderate withdrawal should be prevented in certain patients (eg, in a patient experiencing a myocardial infarction) and thus may order medications to be given on a predetermined schedule. One of the following regimens could be used in such a situation:

- Chlordiazepoxide 50 mg every 6 h for 4 doses and then 25 mg every 6 h for 8 doses
- Diazepam 10 mg every 6 h for 4 doses and then 5 mg every 6 h for 8 doses
- Lorazepam 2 mg every 6 h for 4 doses and then 1 mg every 6 h for 8 doses

(Other benzodiazepines may be substituted at equivalent doses—equivalency may vary secondary to hepatic/renal status)

More severe withdrawal may require starting at doses 50%-100% higher than those above, with more gradual tapering

- Carbamazepine 300-400 mg twice daily on day 1, tapering to 200 mg as single dose on day 5

It is very important that patients receiving medication on a predetermined schedule be monitored closely and that additional benzodiazepines be provided should the doses given prove inadequate

Agitation and delirium

For the patient who displays increasing agitation or hallucinations that have not responded to oral benzodiazepine, one of the following may be used:

- Haloperidol 1-5 mg intramuscularly alone or in combination with 1-5 mg of lorazepam, starting with lowest doses of both medications and increasing every 5-10 min to higher doses
- Intravenous diazepam given slowly every 5 min until the patient is lightly sedated. Begin with 5 mg for 2 doses. If needed, increase to 10 mg for 2 doses and then 20 mg every 5 min. Given the risk of respiratory depression, the patient on this regimen should be closely monitored, with equipment for respiratory support immediately available (late oversedation secondary to accumulation in fat stores may occur)

(Other phenothiazines and benzodiazepines may be substituted at equivalent doses. Because of hepatic first pass, parenteral doses are generally half that of oral doses, and oral doses twice that of parenteral)

Adapted from Mayo-Smith MF. Pharmacological management of alcohol withdrawal. A meta-analysis and evidence-based practice guideline. American Society of Addiction Medicine Working Group on Pharmacological Management of Alcohol Withdrawal. *JAMA*. 1997;278:144-151; Mayo-Smith MF, Beecher LH, Fischer TL, et al. Management of alcohol withdrawal delirium. An evidence-based practice guideline. *Arch Intern Med*. 2004;164:1405-1412.

placebo, there is significantly less use of benzodiazepines for breakthrough symptoms. Carbamazepine does not potentiate the centrally mediated respiratory depression caused by alcohol, does not inhibit learning (an important side effect of larger doses of benzodiazepines), and has no addictive potential. It has well-documented anticonvulsant activity and prevents alcohol withdrawal seizures in animal studies. One problem, however, is that rapid dose escalation is not well tolerated, and there are no trials showing seizure (and DT) prevention during withdrawal in humans.

Although the evidence base is smaller, use of tapering doses of sodium valproate could be used in similar fashion. Both medications may also be used as adjuncts to benzodiazepine-based regimens in patients who have past recurrent withdrawal seizures with prominent mood lability during withdrawal, or with concurrent benzodiazepine withdrawal. However, studies of adequate size to assess the efficacy of these agents in preventing withdrawal seizures or delirium are not yet available.[76] Carbamazepine in its oral form makes it difficult to titrate doses rapidly for the more symptomatic or rapidly worsening patient. Valproate, however, is available in parenteral form, and oral loading doses may be given. Valproate is not used in patients with liver disease or women of childbearing potential. Patients treated with carbamazepine or sodium valproate are monitored using withdrawal scales and receive benzodiazepines if severe withdrawal symptoms emerge.

While some authors are enthusiastic about anticonvulsants and recommend them for not only mild to moderate but even severe withdrawal,[76,79] the authors of a Cochrane analysis felt that evidence was insufficient to recommend their use.[77] Furthermore, since they have not been shown to prevent the most serious complications of alcohol withdrawal (seizures and DTs), they are not recommended as monotherapy without benzodiazepines in people at risk for such complications.[78,79]

The routine use of phenytoin had been advocated as a method to prevent the occurrence of withdrawal seizures. However, methodologically sound trials have shown that phenytoin is ineffective in preventing recurrent withdrawal seizures.[80,81] Moreover, studies have shown that appropriately used benzodiazepines are extremely effective in preventing withdrawal seizures and that the addition of phenytoin does not lead to improved outcomes. Its use has been largely abandoned, particularly since many patients ended up taking it chronically, and it became a common cause of phenytoin withdrawal seizures in people with alcohol use disorder.

Anticonvulsants such as gabapentin and vigabatrin show promise for use in alcohol withdrawal as they may have fewer side effects and be better tolerated.[65,82] Some studies reported success in using a combination of tiapride and levetiracetam.[82] Baclofen, a centrally acting GABA-active agent, has also been used but has its own physical dependency liability. However, until multiple replicated randomized clinical trials are reported with adequate numbers of patients, the use of these agents should be considered investigational and, if used, reserved for those with mild to moderate withdrawal in lower-risk patients who could be treated without medications or who are treated only for mild symptom control, particularly if they are being used as the sole treatment.[83-86] In addition, there is little data supporting efficacy of these agents in preventing or treating alcohol withdrawal delirium or alcohol withdrawal seizures. A conservative recommendation would be to use these agents as adjuncts in addition to benzodiazepine therapy, rather than a replacement for them. However, gabapentin has shown promise in both inpatient and outpatient settings for the treatment of mild to moderate withdrawal symptoms in selected patients.[85,86] Gabapentin, with and without naltrexone has been used in long-term treatment of AUD, but current evidence is uncertain, and it is off label at this time.[87]

Other Agents

Beta-adrenergic–blocking agents such as atenolol and propranolol, as well as centrally acting alpha-adrenergic agonists, such as clonidine, also are effective in ameliorating symptoms in patients with mild to moderate withdrawal, primarily by reducing the autonomic nervous system manifestations of withdrawal. However, these agents do not have known anticonvulsant activity, and the studies to date have not been large enough to determine their effectiveness in reducing seizures or delirium.[88] Studies on alpha blockers, such as prazosin, have been mixed.[89,90]

Beta-blockers pose a special problem in this regard because delirium is a known, albeit rare, side effect of these drugs. In addition, there is concern that selective reduction in certain manifestations of withdrawal may mask the development of other significant withdrawal symptoms and make it difficult to utilize withdrawal scales to guide treatment.[31,32,41] The author has seen many patients who were treated with beta-blockers manifest both seizures and delirium as their first symptom of alcohol withdrawal. However, they may be useful for controlling autonomic signs in people (eg, those with severe cardiac risks) for whom they could pose a danger.[91]

Neuroleptic agents, including the phenothiazines (eg, chlorpromazine, prochlorperazine) and the butyrophenones (haloperidol and droperidol), demonstrate some effectiveness in reducing the signs and symptoms of withdrawal and for a time were used extensively for that purpose.[90] However, these agents are less effective than benzodiazepines in preventing delirium and may lead to an increase in the rate of seizures. Neuroleptic agents are widely used to calm agitated patients and are useful for this purpose in the setting of alcohol withdrawal as well. They are always used in conjunction with a benzodiazepine; moreover, neuroleptic agents with less effect on the seizure threshold, such as haloperidol, are recommended.

There is limited published experience with the use of second-generation (or "atypical") antipsychotics, such as olanzapine, aripiprazole, risperidone, and others, although one small study showed that antipsychotics did not improve benzodiazepine dose requirements.[92] In addition, several authors have published a series of case reports of hospitalized patients treated with dexmedetomidine, a centrally acting alpha-2 agonist used for the treatment of alcohol withdrawal syndrome and delirium. In addition, propofol (an anesthetic agent) has also been widely used (see section Management of the Patient with Delirium). ASAM 2020 Guidelines on Alcohol Withdrawal encourage the use of dexmedetomidine to control autonomic hyperactivity and anxiety when these signs are not controlled by benzodiazepines alone.[65] There are other case reports that have used trazodone successfully for protracted delirium tremens.[93]

It has long been recognized that magnesium levels often are low during alcohol withdrawal, however, per ASAM 2020 Guidelines on Alcohol Withdrawal, there is no supporting evidence to provide magnesium for prophylaxis for alcohol withdrawal unless there is documented hypomagnesemia and hypokalemia. This is an update to ASAM's 2004 Guideline, which suggested magnesium may help with delirium.[65] In sicker and/or more debilitated patients, evaluation of phosphorus stores, particularly after refeeding, should be considered, with repletion of those with hypophosphatemia, especially less than 1 mg/dL.[65]

Ethanol

Case series describing oral or intravenous alcohol for the prevention or treatment of withdrawal symptoms continue to be published in the surgical literature, but no well-designed controlled trials evaluating the safety or relative efficacy of this approach, compared either with placebo or to benzodiazepines, have been performed.[33,41] Despite the relative lack of evidence of oral and intravenous alcohol for the management of alcohol withdrawal, several hospitals continue to use intravenous or oral alcohol in the management of alcohol withdrawal.[94-97] Intravenous alcohol infusions require close monitoring because of the potential toxicity of alcohol. Dosing for alcohol withdrawal is not clear. As a pharmacological agent ethyl alcohol has numerous adverse effects, including its well-known hepatic, gastrointestinal, and neuropathic toxicities, as well as its effects on mental status and judgment. Given the proven efficacy and safety of other agents, the use of oral or intravenous alcohol for alcohol withdrawal management is strongly discouraged—the ASAM practice guidelines recommend against its use.[33,41,65] However, the use of alcohol in the field to taper down a patient while awaiting access to medical management, such as in rural or military deployed settings where alcohol withdrawal medications are not immediately available, may be considered in rare situations.

Thiamine and Other Vitamins

A final agent with an important role in the management of patients withdrawing from alcohol is thiamine. Patients with alcohol use disorder are at risk for thiamine deficiency, which may lead to Wernicke and/or Korsakoff syndromes. Wernicke disease is an illness of acute onset characterized by the triad of mental disturbance, paralysis of eye movements, and ataxia. The ocular abnormality usually is weakness or paralysis of abduction (sixth nerve palsy), which invariably is bilateral, although rarely symmetric. It is accompanied by diplopia, strabismus, and nystagmus. The ataxia primarily affects gait and stance. Mental status changes typically involve a global confusional and apathetic state, but in some patients, a relatively disproportionate disorder of retentive memory is apparent (Korsakoff syndrome). Wernicke-Korsakoff syndrome is a neurological emergency that should be treated with the immediate parenteral administration of thiamine, with long-term thiamine, and other B vitamin replacement.[25,33,41,65]

Dosage regimens vary widely, and there is little human experimental evidence to support one regimen over another; typical dosing is 100 mg IV/IM per day for 3 to 5 days. IV or IM administration is preferred for those with poor nutritional status, malabsorption, or complicated withdrawal syndromes.[65] Delay in provision of thiamine increases the risk of permanent memory damage. In patients with clinical evidence of thiamine deficiencies, such as memory issues, high-output heart failure (beriberi), or neuropathy, thiamine and multivitamin supplementation can be prolonged and, perhaps, indefinite.

The provision of intravenous glucose solutions may exhaust a patient's reserve of B vitamins, acutely precipitating Wernicke disease. Therefore, intravenous thiamine is always given prior to glucose in the patient with alcohol use disorder if it does not delay treatment of those who are nutritionally compromised.[65] Ocular palsies may respond within hours, whereas the gait and cognitive problems of Wernicke-Korsakoff syndrome improve more slowly. As the apathy, drowsiness, and confusion recede, the patient may be left with a permanent defect in retentive memory and learning known as Korsakoff psychosis (a misnomer, as there is typically no psychosis, thus some have advocated a renaming to Korsakoff amnesia).

To reduce the risk of these sequelae, all patients presenting with alcohol withdrawal can receive thiamine at the time of initial presentation, followed by oral supplementation for several weeks. Since patients may also have other vitamin deficiencies, supplementation with B complex vitamins, including folic acid, is commonly employed. There are clinicians who believe that nutritional deficiencies play a much larger role in the pathophysiology of alcohol use disorder and alcohol withdrawal and who utilize amino acid precursors and other supplements in treatment. However, there is a great deal of controversy over this issue, and the data are inadequate to recommend use of such supplementation.

Management of the Patient After a Withdrawal Seizure

The patient who presents after experiencing a withdrawal seizure raises several management issues. It is important to recognize that not all seizures in patients with alcohol use disorder are the result of withdrawal. In epidemiological studies, the rate of epilepsy and seizures rises in parallel with the amount of an individual's alcohol intake. Patients with alcohol use disorder are at higher risk for seizures unrelated to withdrawal. A careful history of the temporal relationship of alcohol intake to the seizure should be obtained, and the diagnosis of withdrawal seizure is made only if there is a clear history of a marked decrease or cessation of drinking in the 24 to 48 hours preceding the seizure. All patients who present with their first seizure warrant a thorough neurological examination and brain imaging, with lumbar puncture and EEG also appropriate in some cases, particularly when seizures are focal, timing is inconsistent or there are focal neurological findings, nuchal rigidity, or other neck signs or fever.

Patients who are known to have a past withdrawal seizures and who present with a seizure that can be attributed clearly to withdrawal may not require a full repeat evaluation. If the seizure was generalized and without focal elements, and if a careful neurological examination reveals no evidence of focal deficits, there is no suspicion of meningitis, and there is no history of recent major head trauma; additional testing has an extremely low yield and may be safely omitted. There is a 6- to 12-hour period during which there is an increased risk of seizure. Withdrawal seizures often are multiple, with a second seizure occurring in one case out of four. For the patient who presents with a withdrawal seizure, rapid treatment is indicated to prevent further episodes. The parenteral administration of a rapidly acting benzodiazepine such as diazepam or lorazepam is effective.[64] Patients should be re-assessed at least every 1 to 2 hours during the postseizure monitoring period.[65]

Several studies have shown that phenytoin is no more effective than placebo in preventing recurrent seizures.[80,81] Initial treatment is followed by oral doses of longer-acting benzodiazepines over the ensuing 24 to 48 hours. Early studies indicated that a withdrawal seizure places the patient at increased risk for progression to DTs, so close monitoring is warranted. The period of postictal "calm" or sedation may be followed, within 12 to 24 hours, by the development of delirium, so that adequate ongoing monitoring and treatment are necessary.

Management of the Patient With Delirium

The patient who progresses to delirium raises many special management issues. Older studies showed a mortality rate of up to 30% in DTs, but with modern care, mortality has been reduced to less than 1%.[31-33,41] The principles of successful treatment involve adequate sedation and meticulous supportive medical care. Such patients require close nursing observation and supportive care that frequently necessitate admission to an intensive care unit. Careful management of fluids and electrolytes is important, given the patient's inability to manage his own intake and the presence of marked autonomic hyperactivity. Delirium often is encountered in patients admitted for acute medical problems whose alcohol use disorder was not recognized and whose withdrawal was not adequately treated.

A high index of suspicion for the development of infection—whose presenting signs may be masked by the fever, tachycardia, and confusion of the underlying delirium—is essential, as is careful management of coexisting medical conditions. Similarly, an assessment for other delirium-prone agents or withdrawal from other GABAergic agents (such as GHB, carisoprodol, etc.) is recommended. The use of cross-tolerant sedative-hypnotics has been shown to reduce mortality in DTs and is recommended.[41,98,99] However, such medications have not been shown to reverse the delirium or reduce its duration. The goal is to sedate the patient to a point of light sleep or a calm but awake state. This will control the patient's agitation, preventing behavior posing a risk to him- or herself as well as to staff, and allow staff to provide necessary supportive medical care. It is not recommended to use CIWA in patients with delirium because it relies on patient-reported symptoms. Other structured assessment scales (Confusion Assessment Method for ICU Patients [CAM-ICU], Delirium Detection Score [DDS], Richmond Agitation-Sedation Scale [RASS], or Minnesota Detoxification Scale [MINDS]) are recommended.[99]

The use of intravenous benzodiazepines with rapid onset, such as diazepam or lorazepam, has been shown to provide more rapid control of the patient's symptoms.[41,81,98,100] An example of a widely used regimen is given in **Table 56-3**. The main complication of therapy with diazepam is respiratory depression. Whenever this approach is used, providers should have equipment and personnel immediately available to provide respiratory support if needed. One advantage of diazepam is that its peak onset occurs within 5 minutes of intravenous administration. This allows the provider to deliver repeat boluses and titrate sedation quickly, with reduced likelihood of a delayed appearance of oversedation.

However, intravenous diazepam has both an "alpha" and "beta" half-life. The initial effect within 5 minutes is followed by a rapid uptake into lipid storage sites; this may result in late oversedation if several repeated boluses are used. Some clinicians prefer getting immediate control with intravenous diazepam and then (after two or three bolus doses) switching to intravenous lorazepam, which can maintain steady-state levels with bolus dosing without the high lipophilicity resulting in fat redistribution.[101] Alternatively, midazolam can be used (1- to 2-mg boluses) to attain immediate control without a beta half-life issue.[102,103] Secondary to the first-pass hepatic metabolism of benzodiazepines, intravenous doses are equivalent to half the oral dose.

Once established, delirium can be expected to last for hours, so diazepam offers another advantage in that its longer half-life helps maintain sedation with less chance of breakthrough agitation. Large doses of benzodiazepines may be needed to control the agitation of patients in DTs, with hundreds and even thousands of milligrams of diazepam or its equivalent used over the course of treatment.[42] The practitioner can use whatever amounts are needed to control the agitation while keeping in mind the possible accumulation of long-acting metabolites especially in patients with impaired hepatic function or the elderly. In addition, intravenous preparations of both lorazepam and diazepam are stabilized with propylene and polyethylene glycol, and repeated high-dose use may result in both hyponatremia and metabolic acidosis. Careful monitoring is required to prevent this complication.

The use of continuous infusions of benzodiazepines, particularly lorazepam and midazolam, has become common in most critical care units.[102,103] However, some evidence suggests that this approach is no more effective than the use of bolus treatment and is expensive. In the agitated patient, benzodiazepines can be supplemented with the addition of neuroleptic agents with less effect on seizure threshold such as haloperidol, though these medications are not used as monotherapy as they lower the seizure threshold. Newer atypical antipsychotics are also effective.

For patients in whom withdrawal is not readily controlled with oral benzodiazepines and who are beginning to demonstrate signs of agitation, intramuscular administration of a combination of lorazepam and an antipsychotic such as haloperidol often is effective in calming the patient, thus avoiding the need to use intravenous administration. Second generation atypical antipsychotics (ie, risperidone, quetiapine, etc.) have less effect on seizure threshold. Some of the very high doses used in treatment (thousands of milligrams of benzodiazepines) may in some cases represent an iatrogenic complication of producing respiratory depression requiring intubation, which then requires high-dose benzodiazepines to prevent the patient extubating themselves. Recent popularity of use of continuous infusions of the anesthetic propofol to maintain sedation has increased this problem.[103,104]

Use of high-dose intravenous benzodiazepines and propofol may lead to rapid and frequent increases of the dose and a vicious cycle of medication-induced delirium followed by further confusion upon lightening of the patient. In cases where the patient has been delirious for more than 72 hours, careful consideration should be given to this diagnosis. In such cases, since the patient is long past the peak period of seizure risk, reduction of propofol and/or benzodiazepine doses should be strongly considered, with the use of antipsychotic agents for continuing confusion or agitation. Maintenance of a sleep-like state, with easy arousal by voice, is preferable to production of deeper sedation; such deep sedation may require intubation for airway protection or ventilation, which then requires even higher doses of sedatives to prevent patients' attempts to extubate themselves or "fight" the ventilator. This may again lead to a positive feedback loop (vicious cycle) of requiring deep sedation, followed by agitation and confusion upon lightening, with reescalation of the dose and prolonged sedative treatment and extended critical care unit stays.

Several recent papers from the critical care literature have indicated that many patients requiring high-dose benzodiazepines do not need to be intubated and that their clinical course is improved if they are carefully monitored with oximetry and treated expectantly without intubation.[105-108] In addition, use of the alpha-2-blocker dexmedetomidine rather than benzodiazepine/ propofol infusions may allow successful treatment without intubation, with better clinical outcomes and shorter critical care unit stays.[108] However, a recent study of the addition of dexmedetomidine to benzodiazepine treatment showed little change in the CIWA-Ar score and an increased incidence of seizures and the need for intubation.[109] Replication and clarification of these studies may eventually alter our consultation practices with these critically ill patients.

COMMON TREATMENT ISSUES

Location of Treatment Services

As both research and clinical experience demonstrated that pharmacological therapy can significantly reduce the incidence of major complications associated with alcohol withdrawal, it became common practice to admit patients to inpatient units to provide 3 to 7 days of medication. However, such intensive—and expensive—therapy is not necessary for many patients and increasing interest has been shown in managing withdrawal on an outpatient basis. All patients presenting for management of medically significant withdrawal should undergo a comprehensive history and medical evaluation. Consideration should be given to routine laboratory evaluation, particularly a complete blood count, electrolytes, BUN/creatinine, and liver function tests. In some more debilitated patients, evaluation of phosphorus and magnesium is appropriate. Other studies are done as clinically indicated.

For patients with only mild withdrawal symptoms, no past seizures, or DTs, and no concurrent significant medical or psychiatric conditions, management on an outpatient basis is reasonable.[110] A responsible individual to help monitor at home is helpful and regular (daily if possible) clinical visits are recommended until they have been stabilized. Ready access, including transportation, to emergency medical services support a decision for outpatient management. In addition, many programs are concentrating on sharply reducing the length of stay for patients undergoing withdrawal. Patients may be treated in an observation unit or admitted for a 1-day stay. If significant withdrawal symptoms do not develop, and the withdrawal is easily controlled with little or no medication, patients can be discharged or transferred to an intensive outpatient rehabilitation program. Such programs achieve success rates comparable to inpatient/residential treatment for most patients.[110,111] Patients who experience severe withdrawal symptoms, however, need continuous close monitoring and nursing support. Loading dose treatment, as described above, is particularly suited to outpatient management.[73,74] The ASAM patient placement criteria describe specific characteristics for patients appropriate for ambulatory withdrawal management.[112]

Patients Admitted for Medical/Surgical Treatment

Studies have shown that about 20% of patients admitted to the hospital have an alcohol use disorder, and the rate among those admitted for acute trauma or for conditions related to high alcohol intake, such as head and neck cancers, is even higher. Thus, hospital admission is a frequent precipitating event for alcohol withdrawal. Universal screening for unhealthy alcohol use and withdrawal risk if excessive drinking is present at the time of hospital admission is recommended but is not yet common practice. Patients thus may develop withdrawal that goes unrecognized or becomes far advanced before being recognized and treated. Withdrawal has been shown to contribute to higher postoperative complications, mortality, and length of stay.[113-115]

Unfortunately, it is all too common to proceed with elective surgery despite knowledge of a current alcohol use disorder. Screening for unhealthy alcohol use and medically managed withdrawal as needed is recommended before proceeding with surgery.[116] Current management strategies for alcohol withdrawal rely on quantitative assessment of withdrawal severity and were developed in patients presenting specifically for alcohol withdrawal. However, signs and symptoms of withdrawal are very nonspecific, and thus, they can be difficult to differentiate from manifestations of acute medical conditions. Furthermore, critically ill patients, who may have impaired consciousness or be on ventilators, cannot provide much of the information required to assess severity of withdrawal.

Nevertheless, use of alcohol withdrawal scales in general medical/surgical patients has been studied and found to be valuable in selected patients.[116,117] Low withdrawal scales can be interpreted with confidence as indicating the absence of significant withdrawal, although patients on beta-blockers and other sympatholytic drugs may have falsely low scores. However, high scores have many causes and must be interpreted with caution. Given the frequency of alcohol use disorder in hospitalized patients, instituting standard screening, assessment, and management protocols is appropriate. Patients requiring more than small amounts of medication for withdrawal symptoms need individualized assessment by clinicians experienced in the management of withdrawal.

Alcohol Withdrawal in U.S. Jails

Another event that frequently precipitates alcohol withdrawal is arrest and incarceration. The prevalence of alcohol use disorder is higher in the correctional setting, with estimates of approximately 24%.[117] This means that unfortunately, jails have become withdrawal facilities. At the same time, only 28% of jail administrators reported that their institutions ever provided medically managed withdrawal for arrestees, despite the ruling of the U.S. Supreme Court that failure to provide proper medical care amounts to a violation of the Eighth Amendment of the U.S. Constitution proscribing cruel and unusual punishment. Overall, in 1997, 750,000 arrestees were at risk for untreated alcohol withdrawal.[118] Because progress has been slow in the intervening years, it is not surprising that inadequately treated alcohol (and other drug) withdrawal has been shown to contribute to deaths among newly arrested individuals. ASAM has issued a public policy statement on appropriate withdrawal management services for individuals incarcerated in prisons and jails, which recommends that incarcerated individuals should receive appropriate screening and medical care to manage withdrawal syndromes.[119] Though there is considerable heterogeneity in screening, a majority do include questions on current and last alcohol use.

The high-risk status of this population should be kept in mind as health care professionals encounter patients referred from jails with possible withdrawal symptoms.[118] In addition, because of the potential for polysubstance use, benzodiazepine, or other sedative-hypnotic and opioid withdrawal may also be present. Lastly, adequate provision of rehabilitative care in our prison system must be a priority since many or most of these individuals commit crimes either under the influence of these drugs or to obtain money for their drugs. With the historic criminalization of substance use, there is increasing recognition on the part of correctional system administrators and government officials and regulators that provision of alcohol and drug treatment services in the correctional system is inadequate and needs urgent remedy. Jails should thus seek to identify affected individuals, initiate treatment, and provide linkage to community-based care at the time of release.[119,120] The State of Rhode Island has developed a novel and highly progressive system for detecting substance use disorders in inmates and arranging appropriate care at admission, during their terms of incarceration and at discharge, including appropriate aftercare plans with "warm" hand-offs.[121] While this system has been largely used for those with opioid use disorder, the principles are transferrable to alcohol use disorder.

"Social Setting" Withdrawal Management

In some communities, nonmedical and nonpharmacological treatment has been made available, often associated with freestanding withdrawal management settings (so-called "public" withdrawal management programs) that offer drug-free withdrawal for patients presenting with low likelihood for moderate to severe withdrawal. In one report, these patients were monitored with the CIWA-Ar technique on a regular basis, with increased monitoring for those who scored more than 10. Patients who progressed to CIWA-Ar score of more than 15 were referred to a local hospital emergency department. In this setting, thousands of patients were safely treated without medication, and a very small number of patients required referral to a higher level of care. This was dependent, however, on accurate low-risk patient selection and well-trained staff administering the CIWA-Ar.[122,123] A review found that many such programs, when well-run, can be both clinically efficacious and cost-effective but that quality and services were highly variable.[124]

CONCLUSIONS

Successful management of alcohol withdrawal is only the first—and sometimes the most easily achieved—step toward the primary goal of treating the patient's underlying addiction to alcohol. The underlying goals of the management of alcohol intoxication and withdrawal are to assure the stability and safety of the patient and encourage ongoing treatment of their alcohol use disorder. It is important for the clinician to understand the risk factors for alcohol withdrawal as well as its pathophysiology and course. In addition, an understanding of the pharmacological principles of treatment (including assessment of those whose withdrawal is likely to respond to nonpharmacological measures, such as human contact and support) is more important than memorization of protocols. A good understanding of both the pharmacodynamics and pharmacokinetics of treatment agents supports rational choices for specific patients.

While no approach has been shown to be superior to others in the treatment of unselected patients in alcohol withdrawal, certain regimens may have advantages in specific populations in certain treatment settings. Knowledgeable about matching these treatments with patients' characteristics is helpful for physicians treating large numbers of patients with alcohol use disorders. Treatment decisions are made using clinical algorithms, which consider patients' responses to treatment, with midcourse corrections being made based on the patients' responses (or atypical and/or lack of response) to that treatment. An excellent resource is the SAMHSA Treatment Improvement Protocol (TIPs) series, which include an excellent and comprehensive review of substance use disorder and withdrawal management.[125] Updates of the TIP series can be found online.[126]

It has become increasingly common for patients to present with substance use disorders involving multiple substances, and it is not uncommon for patients to deny or minimize their use of benzodiazepines, other sedative-hypnotics, and opioids (particularly if that use is illicit). Clinicians can carefully probe for such history, utilizing information from collaterals as well as drug screening tests, and be prepared to treat the other potential withdrawal syndromes. Development of a plan to engage the patient in further treatment is a critical component of withdrawal treatment. Failure to do this increases the chance of revolving-door admissions for withdrawal management, without assisting the patient's entry into rehabilitation and recovery. Use of motivational interviewing techniques may enhance clinicians' ability to address the patient's readiness to change and facilitate entry into treatment.[127] Specific motivational techniques adapted for alcohol and other drug use disorders are available.[128,129] When feasible, engagement of family is critical and may be essential for the patient's recovery, as well as assisting the family itself.[130,131]

Lastly, treatment of alcohol intoxication and withdrawal is only the first step in assisting individuals with alcohol use disorder into recovery. Psychosocial approaches are widely used in the United States and include twelve-step facilitation, twelve-step, and other mutual-help programs (including SMART Management), cognitive-behavioral therapies, motivational interviewing, and contingency management. The effectiveness of these approaches can be significantly enhanced in many patients by specific pharmacotherapies that reduce both craving for and the use of alcohol.[132-135] These medications are vastly underutilized. I urge my colleagues to consider the use of these helpful agents in all their patients and to prescribe them when appropriate (see section 8, "Pharmacological Interventions and Other Somatic Therapies").

REFERENCES

1. Naranjo CA, Bremner KE. Behavioural correlates of alcohol intoxication. *Addiction.* 1993;88:25-35.
2. Evans JR, Schreiber-Compo N, Carol RN, et al. The impact of alcohol intoxication on witness suggestibility immediately and after a delay. *Appl Cognit Psychol.* 2019;33:358-369.
3. van Oorsouw K, Broers NJ, Sauerland M. Alcohol intoxication impairs eyewitness memory and increases suggestibility: two field studies. *Appl Cognit Psychol.* 2019;33:439-455.
4. Leone RM, Parrott DJ. Acute alcohol intoxication inhibits bystander intervention behavior for sexual aggression among men with high intent to help. *Alcohol Clin Exp Res.* 2019;43:170-179.
5. Davis KC, Gulati NK, Neilson EC, Stappenbeck CA. Men's coercive condom use resistance: the roles of sexual aggression history, alcohol intoxication, and partner condom negotiation. *Violence Against Women.* 2018;24:1349-1368.
6. Wray TB, Celio MA, Pérez AE, et al. Causal effects of alcohol intoxication on sexual risk intentions and condom negotiation skills among high-risk men who have sex with men (MSM). *AIDS Behav.* 2019;23:161-174.
7. Klein LR, Martel ML, Driver B, et al. Emergency department frequent users for acute alcohol intoxication. *West J Emerg Med.* 2018;19(2):398-402.
8. Baldassarre M, Caputo F, Pavarin RM, et al. Accesses for alcohol intoxication to the emergency department and the risk of re-hospitalization: an observational retrospective study. *Addict Behav.* 2018;77:1-6.
9. Gallagher N, Edwards FJ. The diagnosis and management of toxic alcohol poisoning in the emergency department: a review article. *Adv J Emerg Med.* 2019;3(3):28.
10. Cole J, Klein L, Martel M. Parenteral antipsychotic choice and its association with emergency department length of stay for acute agitation secondary to alcohol intoxication. *Acad Emerg Med.* 2019;26:79-84.
11. Cole J, Stang J, DeVries PA, et al. A prospective study of intramuscular droperidol or olanzapine for acute agitation in the emergency department: a natural experiment owing to drug shortages. *Ann Emerg Med.* 2021;78(2):274-286.
12. Higuera-de la Tijera F, Sevin-Caamano A, Cruz-Herrera J, et al. Treatment with metadoxine and its impact on early mortality in patients with severe alcoholic hepatitis. *Ann Hepatol.* 2014;13:343-352.
13. Xie L, Huang W, Li J, et al. The protective effects of modified Lvdou Gancao decoction on acute alcohol intoxication in mice. *J Ethnopharmacol.* 2022;282:114593.
14. Palmer E, Tyacke RM, Sastre M, et al. Alcohol hangover: underlying biochemical, inflammatory and neurochemical mechanisms. *Alcohol Alcohol.* 2019;54(3):196-203.
15. Wiese JG, Shlipak MG, Browner WS. The alcohol hangover. *Ann Intern Med.* 2000;132:897-902.
16. Janicova A, Haag F, Xu B, et al. Acute alcohol intoxication modulates monocyte subsets and their functions in a time-dependent manner in healthy volunteers. *Front Immunol.* 2021;12:652488.
17. Barney T, Vore A, Gano A, et al. The influence of central interleukin-6 on behavioral changes associated with acute alcohol intoxication in adult male rats. *Alcohol.* 2019;79:37-45.
18. Swift R, Davidson D. Alcohol hangover: mechanisms and mediators. *Alcohol Health Res World.* 1998;22:54-60.
19. Pittler MH, Verster JC, Ernst E. Interventions for preventing and treating alcohol hangover: systematic review of randomized controlled trials. *BMJ.* 2005;331:1515-1518.
20. Farokhnia M, Lee MR, Farinelli LA, et al. Pharmacological manipulation of the ghrelin system and alcohol hangover symptoms in heavy drinking individuals: is there a link? *Pharmacol Biochem Behav.* 2018;172:39-49.
21. Mackus M, Loo AJ, Garssen J, et al. The role of alcohol metabolism in the pathology of alcohol hangover. *J Clin Med.* 2020;9(11):3421.
22. Brito E, Gomes E, Falé PL, et al. Bioactivities of decoctions from *Plectranthus* species related to their traditional use on the treatment of digestive problems and alcohol intoxication. *J Ethnopharmacol.* 2018;220:147-154.
23. Lee MH, Kwak JH, Jeon G, et al. Red ginseng relieves the effects of alcohol consumption and hangover symptoms in healthy men: a randomized, crossover study. *Food Funct.* 2014;5:528-534.
24. Sutton T. *Tracts on Delirium Tremens, on Peritonitis, and on Some Other Inflammatory Affections, and on the Gout.* Thomas Underwood; 1813.
25. Victor M, Adams RD. Effect of alcohol on the nervous system. *Res Publ Assoc Res Nerv Ment Dis.* 1953;32:526-573.
26. Isbell H, Fraser HF, Wikler A, et al. An experimental study of the etiology of "rum fits" and delirium tremens. *Q J Stud Alcohol.* 1955;16:1-33.
27. American Psychiatric Association. *Diagnostic and Statistical Manual of Mental Disorders.* 4th ed. (DSM-IV-TR). American Psychiatric Association Publishing; 1997.
28. American Psychiatric Association. *Diagnostic and Statistical Manual of Mental Disorders.* 5th ed. Text Revision (DSM-5-TR). American Psychiatric Association Publishing; 2022.
29. Driessen M, Lange W, Junghanns K, et al. Proposal of a comprehensive clinical typology of alcohol withdrawal—a cluster analyses approach. *Alcohol Alcohol.* 2005;40:301-313.
30. Wetterling T, Weber B, Depfenhart M, et al. Development of a rating scale to predict severity of alcohol withdrawal syndrome. *Alcohol Alcohol.* 2006;41:611-615.
31. Saitz R, Mayo-Smith MF, Roberts MS, et al. Individualized treatment for alcohol withdrawal: a randomized double blind controlled trial. *JAMA.* 1994;272:519-523.
32. Wartenberg AA, Nirenberg TD, Liepman MR, et al. Detoxification of alcoholics: improving care by symptom triggered sedation. *Alcohol Clin Exp Res.* 1990;14:71-75.
33. Mayo-Smith MF, Cushman P, Hill AJ, et al. Pharmacological management of alcohol withdrawal: a meta-analysis and evidence-based practice guideline. *JAMA.* 1997;278:144-151.
34. Alldredge BK, Lowenstein DH. Status epilepticus related to alcohol abuse. *Epilepsia.* 1993;34:1033-1037.
35. Booth BM, Blow FC. The kindling hypothesis: further evidence from a U.S. national study of alcoholic men. *Alcohol Alcohol.* 1993;28:593-598.
36. Ballenger JC, Post RM. Kindling as a model for alcohol withdrawal syndromes. *Br J Psychiatry.* 1978;133:1-14.
37. Linnoila M, Mefford I, Nutt D, et al. NIH conference. Alcohol withdrawal and noradrenergic function. *Ann Intern Med.* 1987;107:875-889.
38. Brown ME, Anton RF, Malcolm R, et al. Alcohol detoxification and withdrawal seizures: clinical support for a kindling hypothesis. *Biol Psychiatry.* 1988;23:507-514.
39. Pinel JP. Alcohol withdrawal seizures: implications of kindling. *Pharmacol Biochem Behav.* 1980;13(Suppl 1):225-231.
40. Becker HC. The alcohol withdrawal "kindling" phenomenon: clinical and experimental findings. *Alcohol Clin Exp Res.* 1996;20(8 Suppl):121A-124A.
41. Mayo-Smith MF, Beecher LH, Fischer TL, et al. Management of alcohol withdrawal delirium: an evidence-based practice guideline. *Arch Intern Med.* 2004;164:1405-1412.
42. Wolf KM, Shaughnessy AF, Middleton DB. Prolonged delirium tremens requiring massive doses of medication. *J Am Board Fam Pract.* 1993;6:502-504.
43. Kraemer KL, Mayo-Smith MF, Calkins DR. Impact of age on the severity, course and complications of alcohol withdrawal. *Arch Intern Med.* 1997;157:2234-2241.

44. Gross M, Lewis E, Nagarajan M. An improved quantitative system for assessing the acute alcoholic psychoses and related states (TSA and SSA). In: Gross M, ed. *Alcohol Intoxication and Withdrawal: Experimental Studies.* Plenum; 1973:365-376.
45. Sullivan JT, Sykora K, Schneiderman J, et al. Assessment of alcohol withdrawal: the revised clinical institute withdrawal assessment for alcohol scale (CIWA-Ar). *Br J Addict.* 1989;84:1353-1357.
46. Stuppaeck CH, Barnas C, Falk M, et al. Assessment of the alcohol withdrawal syndrome–validity and reliability of the translated and modified Clinical Institute Withdrawal Assessment for Alcohol scale (CIWA-Ar). *Addiction.* 1994;89:1287-1292.
47. Stanley KM, Worral CL, Lunsford SL, et al. Experience with an alcohol withdrawal syndrome practice guideline in internal medicine patients. *Pharmacotherapy.* 2005;8:1073-1083.
48. Feeny C, Alter HJ, Jacobsen E, et al. A simplified protocol for the treatment of alcohol withdrawal. *J Addict Med.* 2015;9:485-490.
49. Holzman SB, Rastegar DA. AST: a simplified 3-item tool for managing alcohol withdrawal. *J Addict Med.* 2016;10:190-195.
50. Vigouroux A, Garret C, Lascarrou JB, et al. Alcohol withdrawal syndrome in ICU patients: Clinical features, management, and outcome predictors. *PLoS One.* 2021;16:e0261443.
51. Rastegar DA, Jarrell AS, Chen ES. Implementation of a protocol using the 5-item brief alcohol withdrawal scale for treatment of severe alcohol withdrawal in intensive care units. *J Intensive Care Med.* 2021;36(11):1361-1365.
52. Goldstein DB, Goldstein A. Possible role of enzyme inhibition and repression in drug tolerance and addiction. *Biochem Pharmacol.* 1961;8:48.
53. De Witte P, Pinto E, Ansseau M, et al. Alcohol and withdrawal: from animal research to clinical issues. *Neurosci Biobehav Rev.* 2003;27:189-197.
54. Hawley RJ, Major LF, Schulman EA, et al. Cerebrospinal fluid 3-methoxy-4-hydroxyphenylglycol and norepinephrine levels in alcohol withdrawal: correlations with clinical signs. *Arch Gen Psychiatry.* 1985;42:1056-1062.
55. Tsai G, Gastfriend DR, Coyle JT. The glutamatergic basis of human alcoholism. *Am J Psychiatry.* 1995;152(3):332-340.
56. Gorwood P, Limosin F, Batel P, et al. The A9 allele of the DAT gene is associated with delirium tremens and alcohol-withdrawal seizure. *Biol Psychol.* 2003;53:85-92.
57. Sander T, Harms H, Podschus J, et al. Allelic association of a dopamine transporter gene polymorphism in alcohol dependence with withdrawal seizures or delirium. *Biol Psychiatry.* 1997;41:299-304.
58. Limosin F, Loze JY, Boni C, et al. The A9 allele of the dopamine transporter gene increases the risk of visual hallucinations during alcohol withdrawal in alcoholic women. *Neurosci Lett.* 2004;362:91-94.
59. Schmidt LG, Sander T. Genetics of alcohol withdrawal. *Eur Psychiatry.* 2000;15:135-139.
60. Stickel F, Moreno C, Hampe J, Morgan MY. The genetics of alcohol dependence and alcohol-related liver disease. *J Hepatol.* 2017;66(1):195-211.
61. Schuckit MA, Danko GP, Smith TL, et al. A 5-year prospective evaluation of DSM-IV alcohol dependence with and without a physiological component. *Alcohol Clin Exp Res.* 2003;27:818-825.
62. de Bruijn C, van den Brink W, deGraf R, WAM V. The craving withdrawal model for alcoholism: towards DSM-5. Improving the discriminant validity of alcohol use disorder diagnosis. *Alcohol Alcohol.* 2005;40:308-313.
63. Grant S, Kandrack R, Motala A, et al. Acupuncture for substance use disorders: a systemic review and meta-analysis. *Drug Alcohol Depend.* 2016;163:1-15.
64. Reader M, Young R, Connor JP. Massage therapy improves the management of alcohol withdrawal syndrome. *J Altern Complement Med.* 2005;11:311-313.
65. American Society of Addiction Medicine. *The ASAM Clinical Practice Guideline on Alcohol Withdrawal Management.* ASAM; 2020.
66. Holleck JL, Merchant N, Gunderson CG. Symptom-triggered therapy for alcohol withdrawal syndrome: a systematic review and meta-analysis of randomized controlled trials. *J Gen Intern Med.* 2019;34:1018-1024.
67. Steel TL, Malte CA, Bradley KA, Hawkins EJ. Benzodiazepine treatment and hospital course of medical inpatients with alcohol withdrawal syndrome in the veterans health administration. *Mayo Clin Proc Innov Qual Outcomes.* 2022;6:126-136.
68. March KL, Twilla JD, Reaves AB, et al. Lorazepam versus chlordiazepoxide for the treatment of alcohol withdrawal syndrome and prevention of delirium tremens in general medicine ward patients. *Alcohol.* 2019;81:56-60.
69. Mayo-Smith MF, Bernard D. Late-onset seizures in alcohol withdrawal. *Alcohol Clin Exp Res.* 1995;19:656-659.
70. Nelson AC, Kehoe J, Sankoff J, et al. Benzodiazepines vs barbiturates for alcohol withdrawal: analysis of 3 different treatment protocols. *Am J Emerg Med.* 2019;37:733-736.
71. Daeppen J-B, Gache P, Landry U, et al. Symptom-triggered vs fixed-schedule doses of benzodiazepine for alcohol withdrawal: a randomized treatment trial. *Arch Intern Med.* 2002;162:1117-1121.
72. Ntais C, Pakos E, Kyzas P, et al. Benzodiazepines for alcohol withdrawal. *Cochrane Database System Rev.* 2005;3:CD005063.
73. Sellers EM, Naranjo CA, Harrison M, et al. Diazepam loading: simplified treatment of alcohol withdrawal. *Clin Pharmacol Ther.* 1983;34:822-826.
74. Tiglao SM, Meisenheimer ES, Oh RC. Alcohol withdrawal syndrome: outpatient management. *Am Fam Physician.* 2021;104:253-262.
75. Heine H. Carbamazepine as an adjunct to benzodiazepine therapy for severe alcohol withdrawal. *Crit Care Med.* 2020;48(1):476.
76. Malcolm R, Myrick H, Brady KT, Ballenger JC. Update on anticonvulsants for the treatment of alcohol withdrawal. *Am J Addictions.* 2001;10:16-23.
77. Pani PP, Trogu E, Pacini M, Maremmani I. Anticonvulsants for alcohol dependence. *Cochrane Database Syst Rev.* 2014;(2):CD008544.
78. Fargahi F, Shrestha R, Rawal H, et al. Impact of adjuvant anticonvulsant medications on benzodiazepine use and delirium in alcohol withdrawal syndrome. *Prim Care Compan CNS Disord.* 2021;23(5):20m02860.
79. Hammond CJ, Niclu MJ, Drew S, Arias AJ. Anticonvulsants for the treatment of alcohol withdrawal syndrome and alcohol use disorders. *CNS Drugs.* 2015;29:293-311.
80. Alldredge BK, Lowenstein DH, Simon RP. Placebo-controlled trial of intravenous diphenylhydantoin for short-term treatment of alcohol withdrawal seizures. *Am J Med.* 1989;87:645-648.
81. Rathlev NK, D'Onofrio G, Fish SS, et al. The lack of efficacy of phenytoin in prevention of recurrent alcohol related seizures. *Ann Emerg Med.* 1994;23:513-518.
82. Zangani C, Giordano B, Stein HC, et al. Efficacy of tiapride in the treatment of psychiatric disorders: a systematic review. *Hum Psychopharmacol.* 2022;37(5):e2842.
83. Wilming C, Alford M, Klaus L. Gabapentin use in acute alcohol withdrawal management. *Fed Pract.* 2018;35(3):40-46.
84. Levine AR, Carrasquillo L, Mueller J, et al. High-dose gabapentin for the treatment of severe alcohol withdrawal syndrome: a retrospective cohort analysis. *Pharmacotherapy.* 2019;39(9):881-888.
85. Leung J, Rakosevic DB, Allen ND, et al. Use of a gabapentin protocol for the management of alcohol withdrawal: a preliminary experience expanding from the consultation-liaison psychiatry service. *Psychosomatics.* 2018;59(5):496-505.
86. Myrick H, Malcolm R, Randall PK, et al. A double-blind trial of gabapentin versus lorazepam in the treatment of alcohol withdrawal. *Alcohol Clin Exp Res.* 2009;33(9):1582-1588.
87. Bahji A, Crockford D, El-Guebaly N. management of post-acute alcohol withdrawal: a mixed-studies scoping review. *J Stud Alcohol Drugs.* 2022;83(4):470-479.
88. Andrade C. Prazosin for alcohol use disorder: a symptom-driven approach to the choice of intervention. *J Clin Psychiatry.* 2021;82(2):21f13980.
89. Sinha R, Wemm S, Fogelman N, et al. Moderation of Prazosin's efficacy by alcohol withdrawal symptoms. *Am J Psychiatry.* 2021;178(5):447-458.

90. Zaporowska-Stachowiak I, Stachowiak-Szymczak K, Oduah MT, Sopata M. Haloperidol in palliative care: indications and risks. *Biomed Pharmacother.* 2020;132:110772.
91. Kraus ML, Gottlieb LD, Horwitz I, et al. Randomized clinical trial of atenolol in patients with alcohol withdrawal. *N Engl J Med.* 1985;313:905-909.
92. Ferreira JA, Wieruszewski PM, Cunningham DW, et al. Approach the complicated alcohol withdrawal patient. *J Intensive Care Med.* 2017;32:3-14.
93. Kathiresan P, Rao R, Narnoli S, et al. Adjuvant trazodone for management of protracted delirium tremens. *Indian J Psychol Med.* 2020;42:391-393.
94. Craft PP, Foil MB, Cunningham PR, et al. Intravenous ethanol for alcohol detoxification in trauma patients. *South Med J.* 1994;87:47-54.
95. DiPaula B, Tommasello A, Solounias B, et al. An evaluation of intravenous ethanol in hospitalized patients. *J Subst Abuse Treat.* 1998;15:437-442.
96. Smoger SH, Looney SW, Blondell RD, et al. Hospital use of ethanol survey (HUES): preliminary results. *J Addict Dis.* 2002;21:65-73.
97. Rosenbaum M, McCarty T. Alcohol prescription by surgeons in the prevention and treatment of delirium tremens: historic and current practice. *Gen Hosp Psychiatry.* 2002;24:257-259.
98. Schuckit M. Recognition and management of withdrawal delirium (delirium tremens). *N Engl J Med.* 2014;371:2109-2113.
99. Day E, Daly C. Clinical management of the alcohol withdrawal syndrome. *Addiction.* 2022;117(3):804-814.
100. D'Onofrio G, Rathlev NK, Ulrich AS, et al. Lorazepam for the prevention of recurrent seizures related to alcohol. *N Engl J Med.* 1999;340:915-919.
101. Friedman H, Greenblatt DJ, Peters GR, et al. Pharmacokinetics and pharmacodynamics of oral diazepam: effect of dose, plasma concentration, and time. *Clin Pharmacol Ther.* 1992;52:139-150.
102. Lineaweaver WC, Anderson K, Hing DN. Massive doses of midazolam infusion for delirium tremens without respiratory depression. *Crit Care Med.* 1988;16:294-295.
103. Sohraby R, Attridge RL, Hughes DW. Use of propofol-containing versus benzodiazepine regimens for alcohol withdrawal requiring mechanical ventilation. *Ann Pharmacother.* 2014;48:456-461.
104. Brotherton AL, Hamilton EP, Kloss HG, Hammond DA. Propofol for treatment of refractory alcohol withdrawal syndrome: a review of the literature. *Pharmacotherapy.* 2016;36:433-442.
105. Crispo AL, Daley MJ, Pepin JL, et al. Comparison of clinical outcomes in non-intubated patients with severe alcohol withdrawal syndrome treated with continuous-infusion sedatives: dexmedetomidine versus benzodiazepines. *Pharmacotherapy.* 2014;34(9):910-917.
106. Gershengorn HB. Not every drip needs a plumber. Continuous sedation for alcohol withdrawal syndrome may not require intubation. *Ann Am Thorac Soc.* 2016;13:162-164.
107. Stewart R, Perez R, Musial B, et al. Outcomes of patients with alcohol withdrawal syndrome treated with high-dose sedatives and deferred intubation. *Ann Am Thorac Soc.* 2016;13:248-252.
108. Ludtke KA, Stanley KS, Yount NL, Gerkin RD. Retrospective review of critically ill patients experiencing alcohol withdrawal: dexmedetomidine vs. propofol and/or lorazepam infusions. *Hosp Pharm.* 2015;50:208-213.
109. Collier TE, Farrell LB, Killian AD, Kataria VK. Effect of adjunctive dexmedetomidine in the treatment of alcohol withdrawal compared to benzodiazepine symptom-triggered therapy in critically ill patients: the EvADE study. *J Pharm Pract.* 2022;35:356-362.
110. Hayashida M, Alterman AI, McLellan T, et al. Comparative effectiveness and costs of inpatient and outpatient detoxification of patients with mild-to-moderate alcohol withdrawal syndrome. *N Engl J Med.* 1989;320:358-365.
111. Soyka M, Horak M. Outpatient alcohol detoxification: implementation efficacy and outcome effectiveness of a model project. *Eur Addict Res.* 2004;10:180-187.
112. Fishman M. *ASAM Patient Placement Criteria: Supplement for Pharmacotherapies of Alcohol Use Disorders.* Lippincott, Williams & Wilkins; 2010.
113. Spies C, Tennesen H, Andreasson S, et al. Perioperative morbidity and mortality in chronic alcoholic patients. *Alcohol Clin Exp Res.* 2001;5:164S-170S.
114. Ungur AL, Neumann T, Borchers F, Spies C, et al. Perioperative management of alcohol withdrawal syndrome. *Visc Med.* 2020;36:160-166.
115. Fernandez AC, Guetterman TC, Borsari B, et al. Gaps in alcohol screening and intervention practices in surgical healthcare: a qualitative study. *J Addict Med.* 2021;15:113-119.
116. Jaeger TM, Lohr RH, Pankratz VS. Symptom-triggered therapy for alcohol withdrawal syndrome in medical inpatients. *Mayo Clin Proc.* 2001;76:695-710.
117. Sukhenko O. Alcohol withdrawal management in adult patients in a high acuity medical surgical transitional care unit: a best practice implementation project. *JBI Database System Rev Implement Rep.* 2016;13:314-334.
118. Fazel S, Yoon IA, Hayes AJ. Substance use disorders in prisoners: an updated systematic review and meta regression analysis in recently incarcerated men and women. *Addiction.* 2017;112:1725-1739.
119. Fiscella K, Pless N, Meldrum S, et al. Benign neglect or neglected abuse: drug and alcohol withdrawal in U.S. jails. *J Law Med Ethics.* 2004;32:129-136.
120. American Society of Addiction Medicine. *Public Policy Statement on Access to Appropriate Detoxification Services for Persons Incarcerated in Prisons and Jails.* ASAM; 2005.
121. Rich JD, McKenzie M, Larney S, et.al. Methadone continuation versus forced withdrawal on incarceration in a combined US prison and jail: a randomised, open-label trial. *Lancet.* 2015;386(9991):350-359.
122. Sparadeo FR, Zwick WR, Ruggiero DA, et al. Evaluation of a social-setting detoxification program. *J Stud Alcohol Drugs.* 1982;43:1124-1127.
123. Richman A, Neumann B. Breaking the 'detox-loop' for alcoholics with social detoxification. *Drug Alcohol Depend.* 1984;13:65-73.
124. Lapham S, Hall M, Snyder J, et al. Demonstration of a mixed social/medical model detoxification program for homeless alcohol abusers. *Contemp Drug Probl.* 1996;23:301-330.
125. Center for Substance Abuse Treatment. *Detoxification and Substance Abuse Treatment.* Treatment Improvement Protocol (TIP) Series, No. 45. HHS Publication No. (SMA) 15-4131. Center for Substance Abuse Treatment; 2006.
126. National Library of Medicine. *SAMHSA/CSAT Treatment Improvement Protocols.* Accessed August 19, 2023. https://www.ncbi.nlm.nih.gov/books/NBK82999/
127. Miller WR, Rollnick S. *Motivational Interviewing: Helping People Change.* 3rd ed. Guilford Press; 2012.
128. Cole S, Bogenschutz M, Hungerford D. Motivational interviewing and psychiatry: use in addiction treatment, risky drinking and routine practice. *Focus.* 2011;9(1):42-54.
129. Veerappa A, Pendyala G, Guda C. A systems omics-based approach to decode substance use disorders and neuroadaptations. *Neurosci Biobehav Rev.* 2021;130:61-80.
130. O'Farrell TJ, Fals-Stewart W. *An Introduction to Behavioral Couples Therapy for Alcoholism: Behavioral Couples Therapy for Alcoholism and Drug Abuse.* Guilford Press; 2006:1-7.
131. McCready B, Flanagan JC. The role of the family in alcohol use disorder recovery for adults. *Alcohol Res Curr Rev.* 2021;41(1):06.
132. Haley SJ, Pinsker EA, Gerould H, et al. Patient perspective on alcohol use disorder pharmacotherapy and integration of treatment into primary care settings. *Subst Abus.* 2019;40:501-509.
133. Kranzler HR, Soyka M. Diagnosis and pharmacotherapy of alcohol use disorder: a review. *JAMA.* 2018;320:814-824.
134. Zindel LR, Kranzler HR. Pharmacotherapy of alcohol use disorders: seventy-five years of progress. *J Stud Alcohol Drugs Suppl.* 2014;75(Suppl 17):79-88.
135. Piccioni A, Tarli C, Cardone S, et al. Role of first aid in the management of acute alcohol intoxication: a narrative review. *Eur Rev Med Pharmacol Sci.* 2020;24:9121-9128.

57 Management of Sedative-Hypnotic Intoxication and Withdrawal

Steven J. Eickelberg and Adam J. Gordon

CHAPTER OUTLINE

- Introduction
- Sedative-hypnotic intoxication and overdose
- Sedative-hypnotic withdrawal
- Patient evaluation and management
- Common treatment issues
- Summary

INTRODUCTION

Sedative-hypnotics are a group of drugs that include benzodiazepines, barbiturates, nonbenzodiazepine hypnotics ("Z-drugs"), and carbamates. They are widely used to decrease anxiety and produce drowsiness facilitating sleep, and are among the most extensively prescribed medications in the United States.

Sedative-hypnotics are GABAergic agents that activate the $GABA_A$ receptor system; the main inhibitory system in the brain. They use many of the same biochemical and neurological pathways that alcohol uses; therefore, they have similar physical dependence and withdrawal characteristics, and they exhibit cross-tolerance. These stimulate the inhibitory neurotransmitters in the gamma-aminobutyric acid (GABA) receptors.[1] Although all sedatives and hypnotics have mild stimulant properties at low doses, their primary effect is to inhibit central nervous system (CNS) function. Medications in this class that are commonly associated with severe withdrawal states include methaqualone, phenobarbital, and benzodiazepines such as diazepam, lorazepam, alprazolam, and clonazepam. Sedative medications associated with less severe clinical withdrawal states include meprobamate and chlordiazepoxide. According to the 2011 data from the Drug Abuse Warning Network (DAWN), sedative-hypnotic-anxiolytics were the second most frequently reported drug class to cause an emergency department visit (34%), surpassed only by opioids. Visits due to benzodiazepines accounted for 29%. Visits to the emergency department related to alprazolam alone increased by 166% over the 7-year period from 2004 to 2011.

Barbiturates were first discovered by von Baeyer in 1864.[2] They were widely used as sedatives until benzodiazepines were introduced in the 1960s as a purported safer alternative; due to their lower potential for respiratory depression and higher therapeutic index. Today, barbiturates are still available by prescription though they are rarely used due to their relatively narrow therapeutic window.

Benzodiazepines became available in the 1960s and by 1977 they were the most prescribed medications in the world.[3] The popularity of benzodiazepine prescribing has been associated with problematic use. In 1987, the Royal College of Psychiatrists in Great Britain signaled concern regarding chronic benzodiazepine use and recommended benzodiazepine prescribing be limited to "no more than one month" stating that "consequences of long-term usage are liable to outweigh the symptomatic relief" of anxiety disorders.[4] The warning was not heeded. Between 1996 to 2013 the number of benzodiazepine prescriptions in the United States increased considerably,[5] and overdose deaths increased by a factor of 4 (from 0.58 to 3.07 deaths per 100,000 U.S. adults), Most benzodiazepine-associated deaths involved use of other substances, and overdose mortality rose at a rate faster than the percentage of individuals filling benzodiazepine prescriptions.[5] As of 2017, sedative-hypnotics were the third most commonly nonmedically used illegal drugs or prescription medications in the U.S. accounting for 2.2% of the U.S. population. Rates are similar worldwide,[6] however recent prescription trends indicate that the benzodiazepines prescribing has decreased substantially in Europe.[7] In 2016, due to the rise of morbidity associated with benzodiazepines amid the opioid epidemic, the United States Food and Drug Administration (FDA) issued a drug-safety communications associated with the concomitant use of opioid medications—including cough medications—and benzodiazepines. In 2020, the U.S. added a Food and Drug Administration (FDA) black box warning for benzodiazepine medications indicating that they have risks for unhealthy use, addiction, physical dependence, and withdrawal reactions.[8]

A study of Emergency Department visits for benzodiazepine overdose in 38 states found 23.7% increased between 2019 and 2020. Of these overdoses, 34.4% were associated with opioid use. During the same period benzodiazepine deaths increased 42.9%, including 21.8% for prescription and 519.6% for illicit benzodiazepines. During the latter part of this study (January to June 2020) most (92.7%) benzodiazepine deaths involved opioids (mainly illicitly manufactured fentanyl).[9] As such, during the period of 2019-2020 both prescription and illicit benzodiazepine deaths were characterized by high and increasing co-involvement of illegally manufactured fentanyl; a trend that was first documented in 2017-2018. Interestingly, benzodiazepine prescriptions were relatively stable during the study period.[9]

Sedative-hypnotic-anxiolytics including benzodiazepines are a major cause of overdose when used with other substances because of their synergistic effect with other agents including alcohol, opioids, antihistamines, and antipsychotics, anticonvulsants, tricyclic antidepressants, and other CNS depressants. The combination of any of these drug classes causes sedation, suppresses respiratory efforts, impairs cognition, slows response time, and increases falls. Older patients are at particularly high risk of adverse effects from combined sedative use. Eliminating concurrent use of benzodiazepines and opioids could reduce overdose risk by 15%.[10] Combination use is particularly risky for older in older patients. Due to the risk of coadministration of opioids and benzodiazepines, The Centers for Disease Control and Prevention (CDC) Guideline for Prescribing Opioids for Chronic Pain, recommends that clinicians avoid prescribing benzodiazepines with opioids whenever possible.[11] Nonetheless, the number of concurrent benzodiazepine and opioid prescriptions increased over the past decade.[12]

SEDATIVE-HYPNOTIC INTOXICATION AND OVERDOSE

Clinical Presentation

Benzodiazepines

At therapeutic doses of benzodiazepines, patients experience impairments in motor activity, immediate memory and ability to retain newly learned material and are 5 times more likely to be involved in a motor vehicle crash compared to peers.[13] The signs and symptoms of sedative-hypnotic intoxication and overdose are similar for the various medications in the class (**Table 57-1**). Patients with mild to moderate toxicity typically present with slurred speech, ataxia, and incoordination similar to alcohol intoxication.[14,15] On occasion, a paradoxical agitated confusion and delirium may occur, and this is more common in older adults. With severe intoxication, stupor and coma develop.[14]

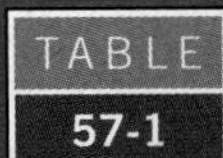

TABLE 57-1 Diagnosis of Sedative-Hypnotic Overdose

History
• Sedative-hypnotic use (ask about substance, amount, time of last use)
• Use of multiple substances
• Use multiple sources of information (family, hospital records, etc.)
• Ask about use of multiple substances
Physical examination
• Central nervous system depression
• Respiratory depression
Laboratory tests
• Rule out hypoglycemia, acidemia, and fluid and electrolyte abnormalities
• Toxicology screens for sedative-hypnotics and other substances

Benzodiazepines do not cause respiratory suppression and a lethal dose has not been established for any of the benzodiazepines. There are very few well-documented cases of death from ingestion of benzodiazepines alone. The few documented benzodiazepine-associated deaths have involved short-acting, high-potency benzodiazepines such as alprazolam and triazolam, which have higher affinities for receptors than other benzodiazepines,[16] in cases of administration of intravenous administration, or when used by patients with severe respiratory compromise. Use of cimetidine or erythromycin increases triazolam's half-life and plasma levels, thus increasing its risk of toxicity.[13] Intramuscular use of chlordiazepoxide can lead to erratic absorption, producing respiratory compromise. Despite these few exceptions, the risk of respiratory suppression from benzodiazepine alone is small.

However, combinations of benzodiazepines with *alcohol*, *barbiturates*, and/or *opioids* may lead to severe adverse consequences including coma or death. Benzodiazepine use in combination with opioids potentiates overdose possibility.[17]

Nonbenzodiazepine Sedatives

Older nonbenzodiazepine agents (eg, glutethimide, barbiturates, ethchlorvynol, methaqualone, meprobamate, chloral hydrate) directly act on $GABA_A$ receptors regardless of the presence of GABA. Their toxicity is progressive and overdose causes respiratory arrest or cardiovascular collapse. With regular use individuals may develop tolerance to therapeutic effects but not to the lethal effects such as respiratory suppression.

Barbiturates have a narrow therapeutic index (small difference between therapeutic and toxic dose that may lead life-threatening adverse drug reactions). This means that toxicity and overdose can occur with only small increases over the individual's regular intake.

Overdose with these agents may also be associated with a variety of agent-specific clinical manifestations, such as bullous skin lesions with barbiturates ("barb blisters"), details of which can be found in resources on toxicological emergencies[18] (see **Table 57-1**). In overdose, barbiturates and older sedative-hypnotics cause respiratory suppression, coma, and death.

Management

Evaluation begins with rapid assessment of the patient's airway, breathing, and circulation (ABCs of Basic Life Support). In severe cases, secure the compromised airway with an endotracheal tube (ETT) and start oxygen therapy with capnography, obtain intravenous access, and place on continuous cardiac monitoring. Patients who have been exposed to another CNS depressant and require mechanical ventilation should be admitted to a critical care unit. Gastrointestinal decontamination with activated charcoal is not advised because of the increased risk of aspiration.

Alkalization of the urine may be helpful in eliminating phenobarbital, but forced diuresis has not been shown to be helpful for any drugs in the class. In extreme cases, hemoperfusion may have a role. Measurement of serum levels can be helpful in documenting the identity and amounts of agents ingested, as well as in tracking levels over time. However, immediate clinical management is based on the patient's condition rather than serum levels.

Flumazenil is a competitive benzodiazepine receptor antagonist with very weak agonist properties at the benzodiazepine receptor.[19] It can reverse the sedative effects of benzodiazepines and may have a similar effect on ethanol, barbiturates, and some general anesthetics. It has found a role in reversing the effects of short-acting benzodiazepines, such as midazolam, after medical procedures and may be used when benzodiazepines have been ingested alone. In such settings, slow intravenous titration in amounts not exceeding 1 mg is recommended, with monitoring for the recurrence of sedation. The effects of flumazenil are short-lived, and symptoms may return in 30 to 60 minutes. Moreover, its use has been associated with seizures and cardiac arrhythmias. These adverse effects are more likely to occur when flumazenil is administered rapidly in large amounts and in patients who have ingested a sedative-hypnotic in combination with a substance capable of causing seizures, such as a tricyclic antidepressant.[20] Persons who are physically dependent on benzodiazepines are at high risk of seizures when they are given flumazenil. Flumazenil thus has not found a role as part of the standard "coma cocktail" (containing thiamine, glucose, and naloxone) because it produces a rapid benzodiazepine withdrawal. Its use in mixed overdoses or in patients who have used benzodiazepines chronically is limited because of the risk of adverse effects.

SEDATIVE-HYPNOTIC WITHDRAWAL

Overview

The use of most sedative, hypnotic, or anxiolytic agents can result in the development of physical dependence and substance use disorders. In this chapter, "dependence" is used to refer to the host's neurophysiological adaptation to regular or chronic sedative-hypnotic use (physical dependence). The definition of dependence includes adaptation to substance use that leads to an abstinence syndrome with the abrupt and, at times, tapered abstinence. The risk of dependence on benzodiazepines and Z-drugs is higher in patients with mental illness and cumulative dose.[21]

Withdrawal is tantamount to, and is defined by, the signs and symptoms contained within the abstinence syndrome. This syndrome can occur with both high- and low-dose use—even use at therapeutic levels monitored by a physician. The development of dependence to sedative-hypnotic compounds is similar across the classes of the benzodiazepines, the barbiturates, and the nonbarbiturate/nonbenzodiazepine agents. The time course and severity of the sedative-hypnotic withdrawal syndrome reflect the influences of three pharmacological factors: (1) dose, (2) duration of use, and (3) duration of medication action (Fig. 57-1), where the duration of medication action is directly related to the elimination half-life at steady-state conditions.

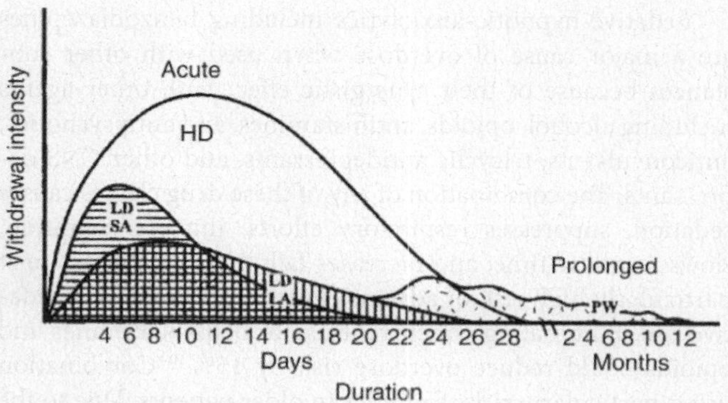

Figure 57-1. Time course of sedative-hypnotic withdrawal. Time course and potential withdrawal intensity as influenced by dose and duration of drug action. HD, high dose; LD, low or therapeutic dose; SA, short acting; LA, long acting; PW, prolonged withdrawal.

Withdrawal severity is related to dose and duration of treatment. A clinically significant withdrawal syndrome is most likely to occur after discontinuation of daily therapeutic dose (low-dose) use of a sedative-hypnotic for at least 4-6 months or, at doses that exceed 2-3 times the upper limit of recommended therapeutic use (high dose), for more than 2-3 months. However, withdrawal symptoms can occur sooner. Latency to onset of withdrawal is related to the elimination half-life.[22]

Clinical research with benzodiazepines has identified additional medication and host factors that influence the onset and severity of the withdrawal syndrome; these factors are elaborated on in the following sections.

Signs and Symptoms of Discontinuation

The spectrum of signs and symptoms that are experienced most often during the course of withdrawal are summarized in **Table 57-2**. Considerable variation exists among patients in terms of the signs and symptoms of the abstinence syndrome. Although **Figure 57-1** appears to indicate that withdrawal follows a smooth and predictable course, most patients experience significant moment-to-moment quantitative and qualitative variations in their signs and symptoms. Petursson[23] and Salzman[24] reviewed the frequency of various symptoms of benzodiazepine withdrawal. Anxiety, insomnia, restlessness, agitation, irritability, and muscle tension were very frequent. Less frequent were nausea, diaphoresis, lethargy, aches and pains, coryza, hyperacusis, blurred vision, nightmares, depression, hyperreflexia, and ataxia. Psychosis, seizures, confusion, paranoid delusions, hallucinations, and persistent tinnitus were uncommon. The areas under the curves in **Figure 57-1** outline the potential time course and withdrawal severity characteristics. The multitude of signs and symptoms outlined in **Table 57-2** illustrates that, in the absence of the knowledge that a patient is withdrawing from a sedative-hypnotic,

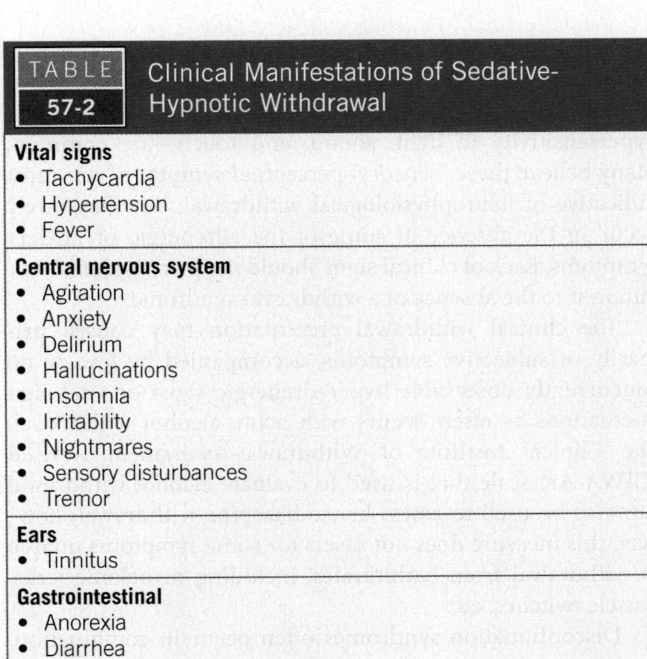

TABLE 57-2 Clinical Manifestations of Sedative-Hypnotic Withdrawal

Vital signs
• Tachycardia
• Hypertension
• Fever
Central nervous system
• Agitation
• Anxiety
• Delirium
• Hallucinations
• Insomnia
• Irritability
• Nightmares
• Sensory disturbances
• Tremor
Ears
• Tinnitus
Gastrointestinal
• Anorexia
• Diarrhea
• Nausea
High-dose (severe) withdrawal
• Seizures
• Delirium
• Death

a number of medical or psychiatric differential diagnoses would be entertained to explain the patient's condition.

Benzodiazepines

Benzodiazepine use, dependence and withdrawal are much more thoroughly researched than other classes of sedative-hypnotic compounds. Soon after chlordiazepoxide (1954) and diazepam (1963) became available commercially, clinical reports were published documenting a high-dose discontinuation withdrawal syndrome with severe characteristics (seizures, depression, delirium, psychosis).[25,26] Reports of a withdrawal syndrome after discontinuation of long-term use of benzodiazepines at therapeutic doses were published within the following decade.[27,28] It now is well established that benzodiazepine physical dependence, withdrawal, and difficulties in discontinuing chronic benzodiazepine use are influenced by multiple pharmacological and host factors (as discussed below).

Barbiturates

Reports in the medical literature evidenced an emerging awareness of barbiturate physical dependence and an abstinence syndrome as early as the 1940s. The first American article[29] directly addressing the barbiturate withdrawal syndrome was followed by a clinical study that chronicled the signs and symptoms of the barbiturate abstinence syndrome.[30] Further studies quantified, with high-dose use, the duration of barbiturate ingestion necessary for the appearance of mild, moderate, and severe withdrawal symptoms.[31,32] The first evidence that an abstinence syndrome could occur after long-term therapeutic (low-dose) barbiturate use was published nearly two decades later.[33,34]

Treatment of barbiturate withdrawal with barbiturate substitution was reported as early as 1953.[32] In 1970 and 1971, Smith and Wesson reported on a protocol that employs phenobarbital substitution, stabilization, and tapering to treat barbiturate physical dependence. Their technique is discussed later under "Sedative-Hypnotic Tolerance Testing."

Nonbarbiturate/Nonbenzodiazepine Agents

Z-drugs (zolpidem, zopiclone, and eszopiclone) were first hailed as a safer alternative to benzodiazepines to treat insomnia until increasing reports of complex sleep-related behaviors and falls in the elderly led to increased caution and regulation of their use. They achieve their hypnotic effects through preferential binding to the α_1 subunit of the $GABA_A$ receptors. They reduce sleep latency and improve sleep quality but do not significantly increase sleep duration.

Because, like benzodiazepines, they work by increasing GABA transmission at $GABA_A$ receptors, they have similar potential for nonmedical use and a withdrawal syndrome as benzodiazepines.[35] Of greatest concern is the multitude of reports documenting severe withdrawal syndromes, marked by delirium, psychosis, hallucinations, hyperthermia, cardiac arrests, and death.[36-43] Intoxication and overdose with Z-drugs present mainly as sedation and coma and are managed by supportive measures. They rarely lead to death unless they occur with polydrug use.[35]

Benzodiazepine Discontinuation

Benzodiazepine tolerance is likely due to a pharmacodynamic neuroadaptive phenomenon where GABA production is down-regulated, further exacerbating underlying psychiatric issues. In Soyka's review, he discusses signs, symptoms, and treatment of benzodiazepine withdrawal syndrome and emphasizes the symptoms of withdrawal can be divided into physical, psychological, and sensory symptoms.[7] The signs and symptoms experienced after the discontinuation of benzodiazepine use have also been described as falling into four categories: (1) symptom recurrence, (2) rebound, (3) pseudowithdrawal, and (4) true withdrawal.

Symptom recurrence is characterized by the recurrence of symptoms (such as insomnia or anxiety) for which the benzodiazepine initially was taken. The symptoms may be similar in character to the condition that existed before treatment with medication. This may occur after discontinuation, with or without the prior existence of benzodiazepine physical dependence. Reemergence of symptoms is quite common, exceeding 60% to 80% for anxiety and insomnia disorders.[44,45] Symptom recurrence can present rapidly or slowly over days to months after medication discontinuation.

This pattern can have important implications for routine reassessment of the need for continued benzodiazepine use. The need for the benzodiazepine should be reevaluated, with particular attention given to dose and duration. Because of the concern of toxicity, when the need is diminished or eliminated, so should be the benzodiazepine.

Rebound is marked by the development of symptoms, within hours to days of medication discontinuation, which are qualitatively similar (as in "symptom recurrence") to the disorder for which the benzodiazepine initially was prescribed. However, unlike symptom recurrence, the symptoms are transiently more intense than they were before drug treatment. Insomnia and anxiety disorders are the best-studied examples.[46] Rebound symptoms are of short duration and are self-limited,[45] which often distinguishes them from symptom recurrence whereby recurrence or return of the anxiety or insomnia disorder symptoms for which the medication was originally prescribed tends to remain for much longer periods, if not indefinitely until the disorder is once again treated and placed into remission.

Pseudowithdrawal may be experienced when a person, not in withdrawal, mistakenly attributes unrelated bodily sensations (such as routine anxiety, insomnia, etc.) to be due to a withdrawal syndrome. This can be a function of their anxious state, personality structure, worry about the therapeutic alliance, or other nonwithdrawal-related concerns. This effect has also been observed in study patients who either discontinued placebo medication (and thought it was the study medication), or continued benzodiazepine use but believed that the benzodiazepine had been discontinued.[47] In addition, expectations of symptoms often are influenced by concerns registered in the media or by friends or physicians.

True withdrawal is marked by the emergence of psychological and somatic signs and symptoms after the discontinuation of benzodiazepines in an individual who is physically dependent on the medication. The withdrawal syndrome can be suppressed by the reinstitution of the discontinued benzodiazepine or another cross-tolerant sedative-hypnotic. Withdrawal from benzodiazepines results from a reversal of the neuroadaptive changes in the CNS that were induced by chronic benzodiazepine use. Withdrawal reflects a relative temporal and temporary diminution of CNS GABAergic neuronal inhibition coupled with an increased glutamate response to balance the benzodiazepine-induced GABA release.

There is considerable individual variation over time among patients who discontinue benzodiazepines. The benzodiazepine withdrawal syndrome includes any of the spectrum of signs and symptoms listed in **Table 57-2**. Any combination of signs and symptoms may be experienced with varying severity throughout the initial 1-4 weeks of abstinence. None of the signs or symptoms of the abstinence syndrome are pathognomonic of benzodiazepine withdrawal. Many signs and symptoms are identical to those of anxiety or depressive disorder. Common symptoms include tremor, muscle twitching, nausea and vomiting, impaired concentration, restlessness, anxiety, anorexia, blurred vision, irritability, insomnia, sweating, and weakness. Common clinical signs include tachycardia, hypertension, hyperreflexia, mydriasis, and diaphoresis. Neuropsychiatric symptoms—including perceptual distortions and hypersensitivity to light, sound, and touch—are common. Many believe these "sensory–perceptual symptoms" are most indicative of neurophysiological withdrawal, but they rarely occur in the absence of some of the adrenergic or anxiety symptoms. Lack of clinical signs should not be considered tantamount to the absence of a withdrawal syndrome.

The clinical withdrawal presentation may consist primarily of subjective symptoms, accompanied by few or no concurrently observable hyperadrenergic signs or vital sign fluctuations as often occurs with acute alcohol withdrawal. The Clinical Institute of Withdrawal-Assessment Revised (CIWA-Ar) scale that is used to evaluate alcohol withdrawal can also be used to assess benzodiazepine withdrawal; however, this measure does not assess for some symptoms unique to withdrawal from barbiturates, including myoclonic jerks, muscle twitches, etc.

Discontinuation syndromes often occur in combination. For example, considerable overlap exists between the symptoms of recurrence in anxiety and insomnia disorders and the signs and symptoms of rebound and withdrawal. Clinical techniques that treat, minimize, and attenuate benzodiazepine abstinence symptoms also effectively alleviate rebound; however, while symptoms from withdrawal will eventually taper off as withdrawal is treated, symptoms of an underlying and separate anxiety or sleep disorder will typically return after the pharmacological treatment of sedative-hypnotic withdrawal ends. Clinicians must be attuned to the emergence or persistence of clinically important symptoms of recurrence during and after the period of acute withdrawal.

Prolonged Withdrawal/Postacute Withdrawal Syndrome

Some clinicians report,[48-50] and clinical experience confirms, that a small proportion of patients, after long-term benzodiazepine use, experience a prolonged syndrome of withdrawal. The signs and symptoms may persist for weeks to months after discontinuation. The syndrome is notable for its irregular and unpredictable day-to-day course and qualitative and quantitative differences in symptoms from both the prebenzodiazepine use state and the acute withdrawal period. It does not follow a linear pattern. Patients with prolonged withdrawal often experience slowly abating—albeit characteristic waxing and waning—symptoms of insomnia, perceptual disturbances, tremor, sensory hypersensitivities, and anxiety. These symptoms can be discouraging to patients early in recovery and are a great contributor to their return to substance use.

Role of the GABA–Benzodiazepine Receptor Complex

GABA is quantitatively the most important inhibitory neurotransmitter in the CNS.[51] It controls the state of excitability

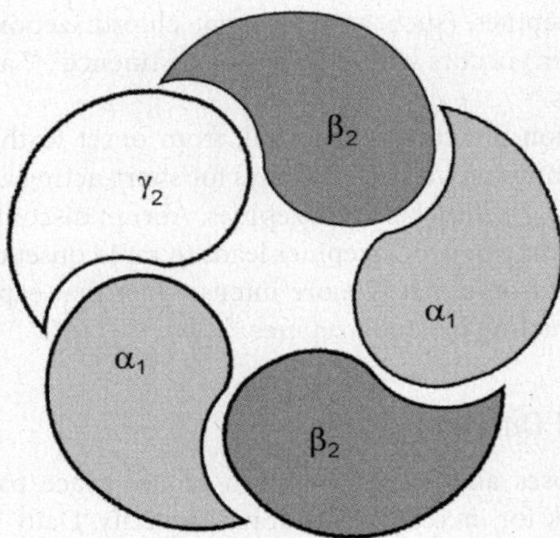

Figure 57-2. The most important and most prevalent GABA$_A$–benzodiazepine receptor in the brain is made up from α_1, β_2, and γ_2 subunits, encoded by the same cluster of genes on chromosome 5. The composition of the receptor subunits, particularly α and γ subunits, seems to determine the benzodiazepine pharmacology of the receptor, with different subtypes having different sensitivities to benzodiazepine receptor ligands. (Reproduced with permission of the Licensor through Sclear PL, Higgitt A, Fonagy P. Benzodiazepine dependence syndromes and syndromes of withdrawal. In: Hallstrom C, ed. *Benzodiazepine Dependence.* Oxford University Press; 1983:58-70.)

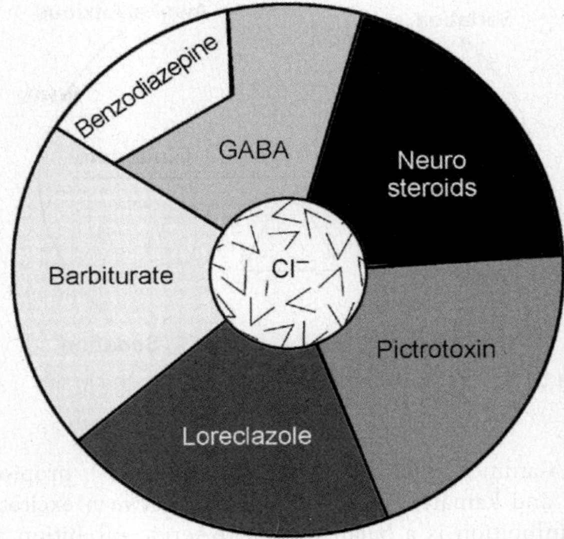

Figure 57-3. Schematic representation of the binding sites on the GABA$_A$–benzodiazepine receptor complex. Note that agonists binding to the benzodiazepine receptor site do not open the chloride channel directly, but rather augment the capacity of GABA to do so. (This is a schematic diagram and does not correspond directly to the protein subunits seen in Fig. 52-2.) (From Smith DE, Wesson DR. Benzodiazepine dependency syndromes. *J Psychoactive Drugs.* 1983;15:85-95.)

in all brain areas. GABAergic neurons are widely distributed in the CNS, with 20% to 25% of all central synapses using GABA$_A$ receptors.

GABA$_A$ receptors are made up of five protein subunits surrounding a central pore permeable to chloride ions (**Fig. 57-2**). Activating GABA$_A$ receptors opens chloride channels causing chloride influx that hyperpolarizes neurons and decreases excitability. GABA$_A$ receptors have different subtypes (isoforms) depending upon the type of protein subunits present. Different isoforms have different functions and respond to drugs differently. Receptors with two β plus a γ2 or γ3 plus two α1, α2, or α3 subunits bind to benzodiazepines. Receptors with α4, α6, γ1, and δ subunits are benzodiazepine insensitive, binding to GABA, alcohol, and some general anesthetics but not to benzodiazepines. While barbiturates and anesthetic steroids directly open chloride channels, benzodiazepines modulate the capacity of GABA and therefore need GABA to work[1,51] (**Fig. 57-3**). Neuronal inhibition results from neuronal membrane hyperpolarization secondary to the flow of chloride ions down the electrochemical gradient into the neuron.[1]

A series of studies by Miller et al.[52-55] illustrated that in a mouse model, behavioral tolerance and discontinuation syndromes are temporally associated with molecular/receptor level adaptations. The investigators reported that, as tolerance to the ataxia-inducing effects of lorazepam developed behaviorally, benzodiazepine and GABA receptors were down-regulated (through decreased receptor number, decreased GABA receptor function, and diminished protein synthesis for GABA receptors). After lorazepam was administered for 4 weeks, it was abruptly discontinued. Concurrent with signs of withdrawal, GABA receptors were up-regulated, and GABA receptor complex function was enhanced (as evidenced by greater affinity for GABA, increased affinity of the benzodiazepine receptor for benzodiazepines, increased benzodiazepine receptor number).

The rate of onset of behavioral tolerance to alprazolam and clonazepam followed by an abstinence syndrome after abrupt discontinuation was similarly computed and then compared with that of lorazepam in a subsequent report.[55] Tolerance and withdrawal developed more rapidly with alprazolam (4 days for tolerance; 2 days for withdrawal) than with lorazepam and clonazepam, which were similar (7 days for tolerance; 4 days for withdrawal).[52,53,55] However, there is no scientific evidence that there is a difference in physical dependence potential among different benzodiazepines. These studies also demonstrated that tolerance is primarily a pharmacodynamic, neuroadaptive phenomenon (brain and plasma levels remained constant throughout the period of chronic administration).

Benzodiazepines act on the GABA$_A$ receptors in the ventral tegmental area to release a surge of dopamine, which has been linked to addiction.[56] The initial change with abrupt withdrawal of a benzodiazepine is the diminished activity of the GABA$_A$–benzodiazepine receptor complex. This is paired with an excitatory system heightened by the chronic use of the benzodiazepine.

The amino acid L-glutamate is the major excitatory neurotransmitter in the CNS. Glutamate receptors have been classified into two groups: the *N*-methyl-D-aspartate (NMDA) receptors and non-NMDA receptors AMPA

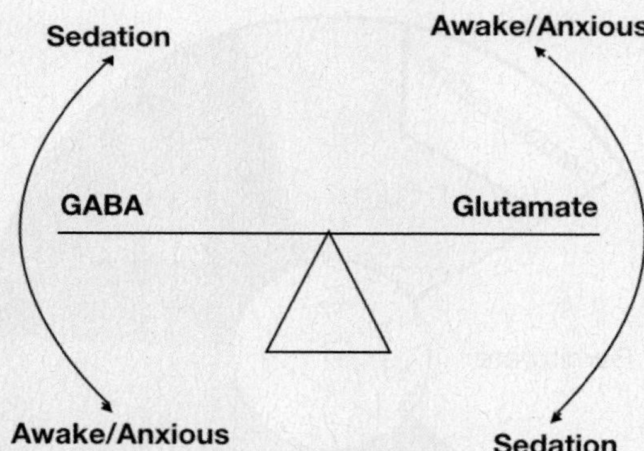

Figure 57-4. Effects of GABA and glutamate on the brain.

(alpha-amino-3-hydoxy-5-methyl-4-isoxazole propionic acid) and kainate. Neuronal plasticity between excitation and inhibition is a balance of GABAergic inhibition and glutamatergic excitation (**Fig. 57-4**).

With chronic benzodiazepine use, changes cause a new level of homeostasis. $GABA_A$ receptor expression changes with substitution of one subunits subtype for another, changing the function of the receptor and manifesting as tolerance to benzodiazepines. GABA receptors are down-regulated to maintain baseline CNS inhibitory tone without causing oversedation. By contrast glutamate-gated NMDA receptors are up-regulated. If the sedative-hypnotic is rapidly decreased or stopped, there is a great imbalance as the down-regulated GABA receptors are unable to overtake the up-regulated glutamate receptors, resulting in withdrawal manifesting as CNS excitation. This up-regulation of the CNS excitatory tone may be permanent. This may explain why successive withdrawals can progressively increase in intensity and risk for seizures, known as the kindling effect.

Pharmacological Characteristics Affecting Withdrawal

Pharmacological factors (pharmacokinetics, dose, duration, and potency) are primarily responsible for the relationship between various benzodiazepines and the differing clinical manifestations of benzodiazepine withdrawal syndrome.

Pharmacokinetics

Benzodiazepine pharmacokinetics determine the onset of discontinuation symptoms following chronic use. Abstinence is followed by declining blood levels of benzodiazepine at receptor sites, brain, blood, and peripheral tissues, with the rate of decline determined primarily by the elimination half-life. The onset, duration, and severity of the withdrawal syndrome correlate with declining serum levels of benzodiazepine.[25,52-54,57,58]

Withdrawal from short-acting benzodiazepines (such as lorazepam, oxazepam, triazolam, alprazolam, and temazepam) occurs within 24 hours of abstinence[59] and peaks in severity within 1-5 days.[59,60] Withdrawal from long-acting benzodiazepines (such as diazepam, chlordiazepoxide, and clonazepam) occurs within 5 days of abstinence[44,59] and peaks at 1-9 days.[60]

Duration of acute withdrawal, from onset to the resolution of symptoms, can be 7-21 days for short-acting and 10-28 days for long-acting benzodiazepines. Abrupt discontinuation of short-acting benzodiazepines leads to rapid onset of a withdrawal syndrome that is more intense than that experienced with long-acting benzodiazepines.[57,59,60]

Dose and Duration of Use

Higher doses and longer duration of use place patients at greater risk for increased withdrawal severity. Daily benzodiazepine use for 10 days or less can lead to transient insomnia with medication abstinence. Withdrawal syndrome following short-term (<2-3 months) low-dose therapeutic use is usually mild (with symptoms such as insomnia), and symptoms are easily managed. Vorma et al.[61] found that people with lower benzodiazepine doses and no previous withdrawal attempts were more successful with discontinuation. Withdrawal syndrome following long-term (>1 year) therapeutic (low-dose) use can present with moderate to severe symptoms (anywhere from 20% to 100% of patients, depending on dose, duration and unknown patient factors).[59,60] Discontinuation of high-dose (more than 4 or 5 times the high end of the therapeutic range for longer than 6-12 weeks) benzodiazepine use leads to at least moderate withdrawal in all patients, and severe withdrawal signs and symptoms in most patients.[62]

Use beyond 1 year may predispose patients to prolonged withdrawal sequelae but is a less important factor in the severity of acute withdrawal.[63]

Potency

Tolerance to the sedative and hypnotic effects develops most rapidly to shorter-acting, higher-potency benzodiazepines (such as triazolam and alprazolam). Withdrawal from these agents may be more intense and require more aggressive attention and longer periods of medical monitoring than is the case with other benzodiazepines.[64,65]

Host Factors Affecting Withdrawal

Host factors are implicated in patients' susceptibility to physical dependence and in the difficulty they encounter in discontinuing benzodiazepines after they become dependent. Clinically important patient factors include the following: psychiatric and medical comorbidity, use of other substances, family history of alcohol use disorder, age, sex, bariatric surgery, and pregnancy.

Psychiatric Comorbidity

The primary clinical indication for benzodiazepine use involves treatment of the highly prevalent conditions of insomnia, anxiety, thought, and mood disorders. It follows that patients with chronic psychiatric disorders who are maintained on benzodiazepines for more than 3-6 months will, become physically dependent on the benzodiazepine. Numerous benzodiazepine discontinuation studies highlight the high (40%-100%) prevalence of active concurrent psychiatric disorders seen at intake of benzodiazepine discontinuation study participants.[59,60,63,65,66] Most of these studies demonstrate a correlation between the patient's degree of psychopathology and his or her withdrawal symptom severity and difficulty in discontinuing use.

Rickels et al.[59] reported on 119 patients discontinuing long-term, therapeutic dose use. They noted a 90% prevalence of initial mental health diagnoses, including generalized anxiety disorder (44%), panic disorder (27%), depression (14%), and others (7%). Patients with greater mental health symptoms required more support and assurance. The intensity of the withdrawal syndrome was seen as partially a function of the degree of psychopathology and other personality variables.

Rickels et al.[63] also studied abrupt and tapered discontinuation of long-term, therapeutic dose benzodiazepine use. They found that 79%-84% of patients had symptoms of anxiety and/or depression at intake (primary psychiatric diagnoses included generalized anxiety disorder, panic disorder, and major depressive disorder). Patients diagnosed with more initial mental health symptoms including being easily stressed, anxious, or having personality disorders such as dependent personality disorder had significantly greater withdrawal severity. Patients with panic disorder were more vulnerable to withdrawal than patients with generalized anxiety disorder.[67]

Increased withdrawal symptoms also have been associated with high initial anxiety or depression and decreased educational level.[68] Mental health history is an important component of benzodiazepine discontinuation and clinicians are advised to observe for and be prepared to manage the emergence or reemergence of psychiatric disorders. The reduction of fear and anxiety symptoms during withdrawal was the best predictor of a patient's success for achieving and maintaining abstinence.[69]

Concurrent Use of Other Substances

Concurrent regular use of other physical dependence-producing substances increases the complexity of the benzodiazepine abstinence syndrome and the clinical management. Additional sedative-hypnotic, alcohol, opioid, and/or stimulant use contributes to a withdrawal syndrome of increased severity and a less predictable course. Opioid substance withdrawal contributes an additional cluster of signs and symptoms where the anxiety, agitation, irritability, hyperarousal, and adrenergic components of opioid and benzodiazepine withdrawal are additive, often overlap, and lead to an exacerbation of overall symptoms. Psychomotor stimulant withdrawal symptoms contribute factors from the opposite end of the withdrawal spectrum (eg, apathy, hypersomnia, and lethargy). When stimulant withdrawal is combined with sedative-hypnotic withdrawal, the clinical picture is unpredictable, with hypersomnolence and lethargy mixed with symptoms of severe agitation, depression, irritability, and somatosensory hypersensitivity. Initial hypersomnolence and lethargy can mask symptoms of benzodiazepine withdrawal, particularly involving benzodiazepines with a longer half-life.

Several factors underscore the need for clinicians to be aware of the high co-occurrence of alcohol use disorders, anxiety disorders, or benzodiazepine use disorder and their potential influence on the benzodiazepine withdrawal syndrome:

- A high percentage of people who meet criteria for alcohol dependence (DSM-III and DSM-III-R) use benzodiazepines regularly, ranging from 29%[70] to 33%[71] to 76%.[72]
- The rate of comorbid alcohol use disorders and anxiety disorders is reported to be 18%-19%.[73]
- Patients physically dependent on alcohol have a greater risk of being physically dependent on benzodiazepines.[72,74]

Exceeding 1 standard drink per day is a more significant predictor of benzodiazepine withdrawal severity than dose or half-life of the specific benzodiazepine.[63] Patients with high-dose benzodiazepine use who present for inpatient addiction treatment exhibit a high rate (70%-96%) of concurrent substance dependence (DSM-III and DSM-III-R).[65,71] DuPont[75] reported that more than 20% of patients newly admitted to inpatient addiction treatment reported using benzodiazepines at least weekly, 73% of people using heroin reported greater than weekly use, and greater than 15% of those using heroin used benzodiazepines daily.[76]

It is uncommon for a patient with substance use disorder to use a benzodiazepine as the initial or primary substance in their lifetime.[77] Instead, benzodiazepines are used in combination with other psychoactive substances. In addition, a high rate of nonprescribed benzodiazepine use in methadone maintenance clinics is supported by numerous clinical surveys. Consequently, clinicians must be aware of, and suspect, benzodiazepine use in patients with any substance use disorder. Conversely, clinicians should assess for other substance use in persons using high-dose benzodiazepines as co-occurring substance use often occurs.

Family History of Alcohol Use Disorder

Mood changes and lability associated with nonmedical benzodiazepine use (and increased propensity to develop physical dependence) have been reported after controlled clinical administration of diazepam and alprazolam in adult sons of patients with severe alcohol dependence (DSM-III-R).[72,78,79] Similar findings with alprazolam have been reported in adult daughters of patients with alcohol dependence (DSM-III-R).[80] This predisposition to use benzodiazepines nonmedically is important, because at least one study implicates a linkage of paternal history of alcohol use disorder with increased withdrawal severity in patients discontinuing alprazolam use.[64]

Concurrent Medical Conditions

Benzodiazepine withdrawal should be avoided during acute medical or surgical conditions because the physiological stress of withdrawal can adversely and unnecessarily affect the course of the medical condition. On the other hand, continued benzodiazepine use rarely has a negative effect on acute medical conditions. In an acute medical situation, the goal of therapy for a patient physically dependent on benzodiazepines is to provide adequate stabilization of the benzodiazepine dose to prevent withdrawal.

The indications for discontinuing long-term benzodiazepine use in patients with chronic medical, including mental health, conditions is important clinical knowledge, particularly when evaluating the discontinuation of benzodiazepines in patients with conditions that are significantly influenced by adrenergic and psychological stress factors (such as cardiac arrhythmia, asthma, systemic lupus erythematosus, and inflammatory bowel disease). The risks of exacerbating the medical condition through acute withdrawal or a protracted withdrawal course may outweigh the longer-term benefits of benzodiazepine discontinuation.

Patients with chronic medical conditions may experience benzodiazepine withdrawal more severely than others. During withdrawal, difficulties in managing medical conditions (diabetes, cardiovascular disease, thyroid disease, and arthritis) may emerge. However, a slower rate of tapering down the sedative-hypnotic (ie, over months or even a year) can improve the success of withdrawal management. Achieving lower doses of benzodiazepine use is an acceptable intermediate (and, in some patients, final) goal. It is important to stabilize both the patient's physical and psychological health at reduced benzodiazepine levels before proceeding with further dose reductions.

Age

Anxiolytic use peaks between the ages of 50 and 65, whereas hypnotic use is most frequent in the oldest age range.[22] Because hepatic microsomal enzyme oxidase system efficiency decreases with age, elderly patients may have elimination half-lives that are 2-5 times slower than their younger counterparts for most benzodiazepines (excepting lorazepam, temazepam, and oxazepam). The withdrawal syndrome for elderly persons who are discontinuing oxidatively metabolized benzodiazepines may be quite prolonged or approach the severity of high-dose withdrawal secondary to the pharmacokinetic factors of aging. The withdrawal course can become especially pernicious after discontinuation of long-acting benzodiazepines that are metabolized to sedative-hypnotic compounds with longer elimination half-lives (such as diazepam, chlordiazepoxide, and flurazepam). In general, younger age is associated with favorable withdrawal outcomes.[81]

Sex

Worldwide, women are prescribed benzodiazepines twice as often as men; hence, twice as many women as men are likely to become physically dependent.[82] Possibly compounding this trend are reports that female sex is a significant predictor of increased withdrawal severity in patients undergoing tapered abstinence of long-term, therapeutic benzodiazepine use.[63] However, sex has not been implicated as an influential factor in abrupt abstinence of long-term, therapeutic dose use.[60]

Bariatric Surgery

Studies show reduced serum levels of phenobarbital after Roux-en-Y gastric bypass surgery. This is significant when using phenobarbital in medically assisted withdrawal as will be later discussed. Such patients will require higher doses of phenobarbital than anticipated.[83]

Pregnancy

All classes of benzodiazepines (and phenobarbital) cross the placenta and are excreted in breast milk. Most have a pregnancy Category D rating (positive evidence of human fetal risk), but the benefits from use in pregnant women may be acceptable despite the risk. Four benzodiazepines (flurazepam, estazolam, temazepam, and quazepam) have a Category X rating (contraindicated in pregnancy). Considering the possible adverse effects to the growing fetus, it is advised to limit the number of ancillary medications used in medically assisted withdrawal. Studies on patients with epilepsy taking phenobarbital showed an increased risk of congenital abnormalities to their offspring but a later study showed that phenobarbital use in patients without epilepsy did not seem to pose a significant risk.[84] It is therefore advised to use these medications and taper down as quickly and safely as possible.

While medically assisted opioid withdrawal is contraindicated in pregnancy, sedative-hypnotic-anxiolytic withdrawal can be accomplished however only with caution and regular monitoring. Prenatal benzodiazepine use can exacerbate neonatal abstinence syndrome (NAS) in the presence of opioid use disorder and can cause seizures in the newborn. Neonatal benzodiazepine withdrawal syndrome can present as floppy infant syndrome (hypotonia, hypothermia, and suckling difficulties) or with tremors, irritability, hyperactivity, and cyanosis.[85] Severe benzodiazepine withdrawal symptoms during pregnancy can place the fetus in distress, potentially causing miscarriage, and may induce preterm labor.

PATIENT EVALUATION AND MANAGEMENT

Evaluation and Assessment

Evaluating patients for benzodiazepine abstinence and withdrawal management requires a combination of clinical, diagnostic, consultation and liaison, counseling, and pharmacological management skills. Flexibility and tolerance of ambiguities and variations during withdrawal helps clinicians support patients experiencing apprehension and anxiety effectively. Clinical evaluation and assessment of the patient typically include the following steps.

Step 1

Determine the reasons the patient or referral source is seeking evaluation of sedative-hypnotic use and/or discontinuation. Determine the medical indications for the sedative-hypnotic. If there is a referring or prescribing clinician, a discussion with that clinician regarding co-management of sedative-hypnotic treatment is recommended. Discussion with any other referring person or close family members often is helpful. Seek evidence as to whether the patient's use is improving his or her quality of life or causing a significant disability, or helping or exacerbating the original condition. Discuss the patient's expectations.

Step 2

Take a sedative-hypnotic use history, including, at a minimum, the dose, duration of use, substances used, and the patient's clinical response to sedative-hypnotic use at present and over time. Include attempts at abstinence, previous episodes of withdrawal, symptoms experienced with changing the dose, and reasons for (and responses to) increasing or decreasing the dose. Include behavioral responses to sedative-hypnotic use and adverse or toxic side effects. For persons who used sedative-hypnotics long term, determine the clinical efficacy and risks and benefits of sedative-hypnotic continuation or discontinuation.

Step 3

Elicit a detailed accounting of alcohol and other psychoactive substance use, including medical and nonmedical use, prescribed and over-the-counter medication use, current and past use, and the sequelae. In addition to prior withdrawal experiences, include prior periods of abstinence and abstinence attempts.

Step 4

Take a psychiatric history, including current and past psychiatric diagnoses, hospitalizations, suicide attempts, trauma history, prior treatment, psychotherapy, and therapists (names and locations). Ask if alcohol or other substances were used during or near the time any psychiatric diagnoses were made. Ask if the referring clinician was aware of any alcohol or other psychoactive substance use by the patient. This includes assessing for unhealthy use including substance use disorders. The Minnesota Multiphasic Personality Inventory may be helpful for the dependence subscale scores. Early taper discontinuations by patients had higher Minnesota Multiphasic Personality Inventory dependence subscale scores than did late taper discontinuations and completers of a taper.[86] Personality assessments may help identify patients who may be more suitable for attempting withdrawal. High levels of dependency, passivity, neuroticism, and harm avoidance on the Minnesota Multiphasic Personality Inventory contributed to increased withdrawal severity.[87]

Step 5

Take a family history of substance use, psychiatric, and medical disorders.

Step 6

Take a medical history of the patient, including illnesses, trauma, surgery, medications, allergies, and history of loss of consciousness, seizures, or seizure disorder. Some medications, such as beta-blockers, may mask withdrawal symptoms or limit pharmacological intervention for withdrawal.

Step 7

Take a psychosocial history, including adverse childhood experiences, current social status, and support system.

Step 8

Perform a physical and mental status examination.

Step 9

Conduct a laboratory urine drug screen for addictive substances. An alcohol breath test (if available) often is helpful in providing immediate evidence of alcohol use that was not disclosed in the history. Unfortunately, most urine drug screens test for oxazepam and therefore only screen for benzodiazepines that are metabolized to oxazepam. Such screens fail to identify alprazolam, lorazepam, and clonazepam; these must be tested for specifically if indicated. Depending on the patient's profile, a complete blood count (CBC), blood chemistry panel, liver enzymes, viral hepatitis panel, HIV test, tuberculosis test, pregnancy test, or electrocardiogram test may be indicated.

Step 10

Complete an individualized assessment, taking into account all aspects of the patient's presentation and history and, in particular, focusing on factors that would significantly influence the presence, severity, and time course of withdrawal.

Step 11

Arrive at a differential diagnosis, including a comprehensive list of diagnoses that have been considered. This greatly aids clinical management decisions as the patient's symptoms diminish, emerge, or change in character during and after abstinence from substance use.

Step 12

Determine the appropriate ASAM level of care for withdrawal management. In addition to the usual considerations for placement of any patient with the appropriate level of care for addiction treatment, patients physically dependent on alcohol and sedative-hypnotics or opioids and sedative-hypnotics may be considered for medically assisted withdrawal in an inpatient (24 hours medically monitored) or day hospital setting due to risk of sedation and overdose.

Step 13

Determine the most efficacious withdrawal management method. In addition to proven clinical and pharmacological efficacy, the method selected should be one that the clinician and clinical staff in the withdrawal management setting are comfortable with and experienced in administering.

Step 14

Obtain the patient's informed consent.

Step 15

Initiate withdrawal management. Ongoing clinician involvement is central to appropriate management of withdrawal. Subsequent to the patient assessment, develop the treatment plan, obtain informed consent from the patient, and then initiate the individualized withdrawal management approach. Monitor and flexibly manage, the dosing or withdrawal management strategy to provide the safest, most comfortable, and efficacious course of withdrawal, adjusting as necessary, to achieve optimal results. A close working relationship between the clinician and patient helps to optimize results. A written and signed withdrawal agreement can be a useful tool.

Management and Support

Strategies for discontinuation fall into two categories: minimal intervention and systematic discontinuation, both of which can include various levels of psychotherapeutic support. Minimal intervention delivers simple advice to discontinue the benzodiazepine. This can be done as part of an office visit, in a letter to the patient, or in a group setting. Several studies have investigated this tool and have found it effective in fostering benzodiazepine discontinuation. Oude Voshaar et al.[88] reviewed 29 articles and found an improved odds for discontinuation (odds ratio 2.8) by using a simple letter or group information session. After receiving a letter with advice to quit gradually, 49% (53/109) of patients using benzodiazepines did so in 30 general practice clinics and maintained abstinence for more than 2 years (mean 819 ± 100 days).[89] Cormack et al.[90] showed a two-thirds reduction in the benzodiazepine dose by using a letter advising the gradual reduction of the benzodiazepine. Minimal interventions are more effective in patients prescribed low doses of sedative-hypnotic medications.

Psychological and Psychotherapeutic Support

There are three primary goals for psychological support strategies to assist in benzodiazepine discontinuation. First, ameliorating withdrawal symptoms. Second, facilitating long-term abstinence (prevention of return to substance use) and third, treating underlying disorders (ie, anxiety, panic, insomnia, etc.).[91]

Psychological support ranges from simple support to psychoeducation, Motivational Interviewing, and Cognitive-Behavioral Therapy. To various degrees, each modality has demonstrated efficacy assisting individuals undergoing sedative-hypnotic discontinuation.[7,92] Psychoeducation begins with sharing information about physical dependence and withdrawal, the rationale behind recommendations to discontinue, the risks, benefits and alternatives to discontinuation, the anticipated clinical course of discontinuation and any recommended pharmacologic and psychological interventions. Additional psychological support includes Motivational Interviewing (MI), which can be provided by clinicians trained in MI. MI is designed to validate individuals' ambivalence while enhancing their internal motivation to change and improve outcomes.[93] Cognitive-Behavioral Therapy often plays an important role in taper/discontinuation when administered by fully trained and experienced clinicians.

A recent Cochrane review of psychosocial interventions for discontinuing benzodiazepine use (compared to pharmacologic intervention) found that CBT showed short-term benefit during the taper but not beyond. Due to the low quality of available evidence, assessment of MI was limited in this review.[94] In addition to the Cochrane Review, numerous studies demonstrate the effectiveness of CBT, adjunctive to benzodiazepine tapering, and in assisting individuals with anxiety disorders and primary insomnia (GAD,[95] Panic Disorder,[91] Primary Insomnia[96,97]).

The prognosis for individuals who discontinue long-term and/or high dose benzodiazepine use is generally good, however, those with more severe sedative-hypnotic use disorder and/or co-occurring psychiatric conditions, or SUD for other addictive substances, often require additional longer-term therapeutic approaches.[7]

Systematic Discontinuation

For patients who are physically dependent on sedative-hypnotics, there are two primary options for the withdrawal management process: tapering versus substitution and tapering. Gradual dose reduction (tapering) is the most widely used method of benzodiazepine discontinuation. The taper method is indicated for use in an outpatient ambulatory setting, patients with therapeutic dose benzodiazepine physical dependence, patients who are physically dependent only on benzodiazepines, and patients who can reliably present for regular clinical follow-up during and after withdrawal.[58,70,77,86,98-103]

Tapering

With the taper method, the patient is slowly and gradually weaned from the benzodiazepine on which he or she is physically dependent, using a fixed-dose taper schedule. This is ideal if the benzodiazepine being used is long acting. The dose is decreased on a weekly to every-other-week basis. The rate of discontinuation for patients who used benzodiazepines for the long term (>1 year) should not exceed 5-mg diazepam equivalents per week (12.5-mg chlordiazepoxide or 15-mg phenobarbital equivalents) or 10% of the current (starting) dose per week, whichever is smaller. The first 50% of the taper is usually smoother, quicker, and less symptomatic than the last 50%.[60,86] For the final 25%-35% of the taper, slow the rate or dose reduction schedule to half the previous dose reduction per week and the reduction accomplished at twice the original tapering interval. If symptoms of withdrawal occur, the dose could be increased slightly until the symptoms resolve and the subsequent taper schedule commenced at a slower rate.

Some patients may want to accelerate the reduction. This acceleration is better tolerated and can be encouraged early in the reduction.[86] In general, patients tolerate more dose reduction and with shorter intervals early in the tapering process and then require decreased dose reduction over longer intervals as the taper progresses and the dose is reduced. A common error is trying to push the taper process too quickly.[101,102]

Conduct brief office visits at least weekly to facilitate regular assessment of the patient for withdrawal symptoms, general health, taper compliance, and use of supportive therapy. Standardized advice from a prescribing clinician is an essential component.[103] Prescribe an amount sufficient only until the next visit and explain that lost, misplaced, or stolen medication will invoke a reevaluation of the current treatment plan and could lead to an alternative discontinuation paradigm and/or higher level of care. A written withdrawal agreement between the patient and clinician, signed by the patient, is strongly advised. A copy of the written schedule of daily doses, covering multiple weeks to months, may help the patient adhere to the reduction plan. A reliable support person who is in daily contact with the patient is very helpful. The patient will need to give written consent for contacting the support person.

Patients who are unable to complete a simple taper program should be reevaluated and, if indicated, an alternative withdrawal management method and/or higher level of clinical care chosen. Some patients may require a substitution and taper program or a period of hospitalization to receive more intensive monitoring and support to complete abstinence.

Substitution and Taper

Substitution and taper methods employ cross-tolerant long-acting benzodiazepines (such as chlordiazepoxide or clonazepam) or phenobarbital to substitute, at equipotent doses, for the sedative-hypnotics on which the patient is physically dependent (**Table 57-3**). Chlordiazepoxide, clonazepam, and phenobarbital are the most widely used substitution agents for several important reasons:

- At steady state, there is negligible interdose serum level variation with these medications; with tapering, there is a more gradual reduction in serum levels, reducing the risk that withdrawal symptoms will emerge.
- Each of the medications has low addictive potential (phenobarbital and chlordiazepoxide are lowest followed by clonazepam). While this point is generally accepted, there is regional variability in this potential. Phenobarbital offers the added advantage of rarely inducing behavioral disinhibition and possesses broad clinical efficacy in the management of withdrawal from all classes of sedative-hypnotic agents. Clinical experience shows that phenobarbital is most useful and effective in patients with physical

TABLE 57-3 Sedative-Hypnotic Withdrawal Substitution Dose Conversions

Substance	Dose equal to 30 mg of phenobarbital (mg)
Benzodiazepines	
Alprazolam	0.5-1
Chlordiazepoxide	25
Clonazepam	1-2
Clorazepate	7.5
Diazepam	10
Estazolam	1
Flurazepam	15
Lorazepam	2
Oxazepam	10-15
Quazepam	15
Temazepam	15
Triazolam	0.25
Barbiturates	
Pentobarbital	100
Secobarbital	100
Butalbital	100
Amobarbital	100
Phenobarbital	30
Nonbarbiturates-Nonbenzodiazepines	
Ethchlorvynol	500
Glutethimide	250
Methyprylon	200
Methaqualone	300
Meprobamate	1200
Carisoprodol	700
Chloral hydrate	500

dependence on more than one substance, in patients with high-dose dependence, and in particular in patients with unknown dose or erratic "polypharmacy" substance use. However, caution is advised to prevent over-dosing this medication.

Benzodiazepines need GABA to work. Because in chronic benzodiazepine use GABA production is down-regulated and GABA receptors are altered in expression, phenobarbital may be a better option to manage withdrawal symptoms. Barbiturates directly activate $GABA_A$ receptors, resulting in prolonging the duration that chloride channels remain open.

With impaired hepatic function or elevated liver tests, oxazepam may be a good substitute.[77] Lorazepam could be considered, but its addiction liability is higher than that of oxazepam.[76] However, if a patient is in an inpatient setting with close monitoring, one can use longer-acting agents while monitoring for sedation and adjusting dosing accordingly.

Uncomplicated Substitution and Taper

This method is used in outpatient settings for patients who are discontinuing use of short half-life benzodiazepines or for those who are unable to tolerate gradual tapering:

1. Calculate the equivalent dose of chlordiazepoxide, clonazepam, or phenobarbital using the Substitution Dose Conversion Table (**Table 57-3**). Individual variation in clinical responses to "equivalent" doses can vary, so close clinical monitoring of patient response to substitution is necessary. Adjustments to the initially calculated dose schedule are to be expected.
2. Provide the substituted medication in a divided daily dose. For chlordiazepoxide, oxazepam, or phenobarbital, give 3-4 doses per day. For clonazepam, 2-3 doses per day usually are sufficient.
3. Provide the patient with smaller as-needed (PRN) doses of the substituted medication. This will help to suppress breakthrough symptoms of withdrawal. Do this for the first 2-3 days only, and then discontinue PRN dosing. Be cautious and conservative on the amount of benzodiazepine given while being mindful that undertreatment is the main reason for treatment failure at this stage. Avoid using different types of benzodiazepines concurrently as it makes it difficult to identify the stabilizing dose and can increase a patient's risk of overdose. A rescue dose of intermediate-acting benzodiazepine (lorazepam) may be used in the setting of severe withdrawal symptoms or risk of impending seizure as a bridging dose until the long-acting medication takes effect. Do not use phenobarbital in combination with benzodiazepines in an outpatient setting.
4. Stabilize the patient on an adequate substitution dose (same dose on consecutive days without the need for regular PRN doses). This usually is accomplished within 1 week.
5. Gradually reduce the dose. The dose is decreased on a weekly to every-other-week basis, as in the simple taper model. The rate of discontinuation is 5-mg diazepam equivalents per week (or 12.5-mg chlordiazepoxide equivalents or 15-mg phenobarbital equivalents), as shown in Table 52-3, or 10% of the current (starting) dose per week. The first half of the taper usually is smoother, quicker, and less symptomatic than the latter half.
6. For the final 25%-35% of the taper, the rate, or dose reduction, should be slowed. This may be a good time to introduce ancillary medications such as gabapentin into the treatment regimen. If symptoms of withdrawal occur, hold the taper for 3-4 days to stabilize the patient, and then resume the process. Some patients may wish to accelerate the reduction. This is better tolerated early in the taper. Care should be taken not to push the taper too quickly.
7. Support the patient with short but frequent visits, as described above. Taper medication should be closely controlled by prescribing only enough medication for the time period until the next visit.

Phenobarbital Induction and Taper Protocol

Based on the Sedative-Hypnotic Tolerance Test developed by Drs Smith and Wesson,[48-50] this protocol is ideal when the degree of physical dependence is difficult to determine. Such a situation is common in high-dose, erratic-dose, nonprescribed or illegal source, "polysubstance," or alcohol plus sedative-hypnotic use. It is best done in a setting that offers 24-hour medical monitoring. Phenobarbital is used because of the adaptive changes that occur with chronic benzodiazepine use discussed previously. Also, it boasts rapid onset of action, long half-life, and ease with which signs of toxicity can be monitored:

1. A 60-mg phenobarbital dose is given orally every 2 hours PRN CIWA-Ar score greater than 15 for up to 48 hours.
2. Doses are held for signs of toxicity (intoxication), which develop in the following progression at increasing serum levels: fine lateral sustained nystagmus, coarse nystagmus, slurred speech, ataxia, and somnolence. Doses are held with the development of coarse nystagmus and slurred speech and subsequently resumed with the resolution of the signs of toxicity.
3. The patient is monitored hourly to ensure adequate dosing and to prevent oversedation. Ideally, a balance is achieved between the signs and symptoms of withdrawal and those of phenobarbital intoxication.
4. After 48 hours, the total amount of administered phenobarbital is divided by the number of days it was administered. This amount is the 24-hour stabilizing dose that was administered in the first 48 hours to stabilize the patient.
5. The taper is started after the first 48 hours of stabilization by reducing the stabilizing dose by 20%-30% every day for the first half of the taper and a gentler 10% every other day for the second half of the taper.

6. The total daily dose should be divided so that the largest dose is administered in the evening to help with sleep while avoiding sedation throughout the day.

Example of Phenobarbital Taper

If the total 48-hour dose is 600 mg, then the 24-hour stabilizing dose is 300 mg.

The initial taper dose would be 210-240 mg (correlate with clinical presentation to guide dose choice).

Taper Day	7:00	12:00	22:00	Total Dose
1	60 mg	30 mg	120 mg	210 mg
2	30 mg		120 mg	150 mg
3			120 mg	120 mg
4			90 mg	90 mg
5			90 mg	90 mg
6			60 mg	60 mg
7			60 mg	60 mg
8			30 mg	30 mg
9			30 mg	30 mg
10			15 mg	15 mg
11			15 mg	15 mg

The taper may be extended or decreased depending on patient's presentation. Patients often can be transferred from an inpatient setting to an intensive (medically monitored) outpatient program after they are stabilized and well established on the tapering portion of the protocol.

Combination Therapy Using Anticonvulsants and Phenobarbital

While acute benzodiazepine withdrawal can be managed with a combination of anticonvulsants and phenobarbital in an inpatient setting, it is falling out of favor because of adverse effects of the anticonvulsants and increased risk of medication interactions. An example of such a protocol appears here:

1. Phenobarbital is begun with a loading dose of 60 mg orally every 4 hours for 4 or 5 doses. This is followed by a maintenance dose of 60 mg 4 times per day for 2 days and then 30 mg 4 times per day for 1 or 2 days. For elderly (over 60 years of age) or in compromised health, start with a loading dose of 30 mg every 4 hours for 4-5 doses, followed by 30 mg 4 times per day for 3-4 days.
2. An anticonvulsant is started at the same time as the phenobarbital. Commonly used anticonvulsants are carbamazepine, sodium valproate/valproic acid, and gabapentin. Carbamazepine is started at 200 mg three times per day, sodium valproate/valproic acid is started at 250 mg three times per day, and gabapentin is started at 300 mg three times per day. All have similar efficacy. Gabapentin seems to have the lowest side effect profile. Anticonvulsants can be continued for 2-4 weeks after acute withdrawal management and then tapered; longer use of these agents could be considered on a case-by-case basis. Physical observation (sedation, rash) and laboratory monitoring (CBC, liver function tests [LFTs]) are indicated with use of these medications past several weeks.
3. Breakthrough withdrawal occurring in the first few days to 1 week can be effectively treated with a short course (2-3 days) of a long half-life benzodiazepine such as chlordiazepoxide (25 mg three times per day for 1 day, followed by 25 mg two times per day for 1 day, and then 25 mg one time on the third day). Breakthrough withdrawal occurring after the first week and usually when phenobarbital has stopped can be treated with a short course of low-dose phenobarbital (30-60 mg/d divided into 2-3 doses), which is then tapered over 5-7 days.

Another point of concern is that phenobarbital and carbamazepine are both strongly associated with Stevens-Johnson syndrome and their concomitant use may markedly increase this risk.

Appropriate Clinical Setting

Patients who have physical dependence on multiple substances (including sedative-hypnotics), mixed alcohol and other sedative-hypnotic use, high-dose sedative-hypnotic use, erratic behavior, incompatible/unreliable substance use histories, involvement with illegal sources, and extensive mental health issues may be best served in an inpatient facility that offers 24-hour medical monitoring.

Adjunctive Withdrawal Management Measures

Anticonvulsants

Since the 1980s, anticonvulsants have been studied and used to treat sedative-hypnotic withdrawal, especially benzodiazepine withdrawal. The use of anticonvulsants grew from the success of treating certain psychiatric disorders and the improved understanding of kindling mechanisms for withdrawal. Some anticonvulsants were also beneficial in treating mild alcohol withdrawal and cocaine intoxication. There appears to be no addiction potential with anticonvulsants, and this is a great advantage.[104]

Carbamazepine

Carbamazepine's actions have been associated with the neurotransmitters serotonin, GABA, excitatory amino acids, and glutamate.[104-107] It inhibits glutamate release. Adjunctive carbamazepine therapy is not widely used, although clinical protocols and patient selection for this method have been studied. Initial reports on small clinical trials using carbamazepine showed encouraging but mixed effectiveness and utility.[67,108-112] Pages and Ries[113] reviewed further use of carbamazepine and found it to be an effective adjunct. Schweizer et al.[111] studied 40 patients with a history of difficulty discontinuing long-term therapeutic benzodiazepines. Significantly, more patients treated with carbamazepine were benzodiazepine-free at 5 weeks. Patients receiving carbamazepine (but not the clinicians evaluating them) reported a larger reduction in withdrawal severity compared with patients taking placebo.

Ries et al.[109] and Pages and Ries[113] reported protocols for the use of carbamazepine: 600 mg/d (usually 200 mg three times per day) is used alone or in combination with a 3-day benzodiazepine taper. Chlordiazepoxide is useful because of its longer half-life and low potential for problematic use. Phenobarbital can be added PRN to this protocol for breakthrough withdrawal symptoms.

Carbamazepine is continued for a minimum of 2-3 weeks after the 3-day benzodiazepine taper is completed and can be tapered to monitor for return of withdrawal symptoms. Elderly patients who are discontinuing benzodiazepines have been treated successfully with carbamazepine at doses of 400-500 mg/d.

Adverse consequences of carbamazepine use can include gastrointestinal upset, neutropenia, thrombocytopenia, and hyponatremia, necessitating initial and ongoing laboratory evaluation and monitoring. In pregnancy, it is a risk Category D and should be avoided during the first trimester because of the risk of neural tube defects.

Sodium Valproate

Reports indicate that sodium valproate is effective in attenuating the benzodiazepine withdrawal syndrome. Valproate possesses GABAergic actions and anticonvulsant effects.[114,115] It is believed to increase brain GABA concentrations by unknown mechanisms. Valproate also may suppress NMDA and reduce l-glutamate responses.[107,114,116] Rickels et al.[117] found that although valproate did not reduce acute withdrawal severity, valproate-treated patients were 2.5 times more likely to be benzodiazepine-free at 5 weeks after taper, compared with a placebo group.

Valproate doses of 250 mg three times per day (250 mg two times per day if older than age 60) can be used in combination with a 3-day benzodiazepine taper. Chlordiazepoxide is a useful choice because of its long half-life and low addictive potential. Calculate the equivalent chlordiazepoxide dose for the amount of current benzodiazepine being discontinued. Give one-half to two-thirds of this dose spaced equally (divided in 2-3 doses) over the first day (24 hours), one-third spaced equally over the second day (second 24 hours), and 10% to 20% spaced equally over the third day (third 24 hours). Phenobarbital can be used for breakthrough withdrawal symptoms. Valproate is continued for a minimum of 2-3 weeks after the 3-day benzodiazepine taper is completed. Longer treatment may improve the proportion of patients who remain benzodiazepine-free. Valproate can be tapered to monitor for return of withdrawal symptoms.

Valproate has been used to treat anxiety. It has fewer side effects than carbamazepine. It can be used both inpatient and outpatient. For these reasons, further studies may strengthen the role of valproate in the treatment of benzodiazepine withdrawal. Side effects (including elevated LFTs, thrombocytopenia, bone marrow suppression, and pancreatitis), substance reactions (including rash and erythema multiforme), gastric upset, and behavioral changes require close monitoring. Like carbamazepine, it is a Category D drug in pregnancy, and its use in the first trimester is associated with increased risk of neural tube defects.

Gabapentin

By binding to the alpha-2/delta subunit of voltage-sensitive calcium channels, gabapentin closes N and P/Q presynaptic calcium channels, diminishing excessive neuronal activity and neurotransmitter release. It is structurally related to GABA, but there are no known direct actions on GABA or its receptors. It is useful as adjuvant therapy in alcohol and benzodiazepine withdrawal. Unlike carbamazepine and valproate, gabapentin is a pregnancy Category C medication. It still should be avoided during pregnancy but appears to be a safer option. Of note, however, its addictive potential in people with addiction has been recently recognized, which may limit some of its advantages.

Gabapentin, topiramate, and lamotrigine have been tried in several small studies. Gabapentin seems to be interchangeable with carbamazepine and with sodium valproate/valproic acid. Lamotrigine is limited by its need for a slow buildup in dose. Most of the studies using these anticonvulsants involved patients with alcohol use disorder. More studies are needed.[104,118-120]

Flumazenil

Flumazenil is useful for complications of acute intoxication with benzodiazepines as discussed earlier in this chapter. Caution must be used as it can cause marked withdrawal symptoms and seizures. Flumazenil is not useful as an adjunct to tapering. Because of its weak agonist properties, it may be useful to reduce cravings after the tapering is complete.[121] Flumazenil's antagonist properties may help prevent return to substance use, but no studies support this indication.

Propranolol

Tyrer et al.[57] demonstrated that propranolol alone does not affect the rate of successful benzodiazepine discontinuation or the incidence of withdrawal symptoms for discontinuation of chronic benzodiazepine use. However, propranolol treatment did diminish the severity of adrenergic signs and symptoms of withdrawal. Propranolol is not cross-tolerant with sedative-hypnotic medications and should not be used as the sole therapeutic agent in managing sedative-hypnotic withdrawal. It is also not known to prevent seizure as a consequence of withdrawal. Propranolol can be used, in doses of 60-120 mg/d, divided 3 or 4 times per day, as an adjunct to one of the withdrawal methods, when additional control of autonomic signs and symptoms is deemed important. However, clinicians need to be mindful that propranolol treatment will diminish some of the very symptoms and signs that are monitored to determine substitution doses. Side effects such as weight gain, sedation and depression may occur.

Clonidine

Clonidine has been shown to be ineffective in treating benzodiazepine withdrawal. Doses sufficient to decrease serum levels of norepinephrine metabolites had minimal attenuating effect on the benzodiazepine withdrawal syndrome. One significant result of this study was the demonstration that increased norepinephrine activity plays a small role in the overall benzodiazepine withdrawal syndrome. In some cases when autonomic dysregulation persists after acute withdrawal, clonidine can be used to control symptoms in the postacute withdrawal state.

Buspirone

Buspirone is a nonbenzodiazepine anxiolytic medication that is not cross-tolerant with benzodiazepines or other sedative-hypnotic medications. Schweizer and Rickels[122] and Ashton et al.[123] demonstrated that buspirone substitution in patients undergoing abrupt or gradual benzodiazepine discontinuation failed to protect against the symptoms of withdrawal.

Trazodone

Trazodone is useful augmenting agent in the management of benzodiazepine withdrawal. Trazodone decreased anxiety in benzodiazepine-tapered patients.[124] Trazodone improved patients' ability to remain benzodiazepine-free after a 4-week taper of the benzodiazepine. In one study, two-thirds of the patients treated with trazodone, compared with 31% of patients treated with placebo, were benzodiazepine-free at 5 weeks after taper.[117] Trazodone can be used to improve sleep during benzodiazepine tapering and when benzodiazepine-free. Side effects may include dry mouth, morning hangover, drowsiness, dizziness, and priapism.

Mirtazapine

Mirtazapine has been used in a similar way as trazodone and found to be useful.[125]

Cognitive-Behavioral Therapy

Two studies[126,127] demonstrate that, in patients with panic disorder, adding cognitive-behavioral therapy (CBT) to alprazolam discontinuation improved the rate of successful alprazolam discontinuation. Spiegel et al.[126] reported that patients in the combined taper and CBT groups had greater rates of abstinence from alprazolam at 6 months than did those who underwent taper alone. A cognitive group approach improved attrition rates and long-term outcomes for benzodiazepine withdrawal.[128] Oude Voshaar et al.[129] reported that adding cognitive-behavioral group therapy did not improve benzodiazepine discontinuation success.

Maintaining abstinence from benzodiazepines even in the context of recurrence of symptoms of the underlying disorder is the goal. Continue psychological treatment throughout the period of tapering. Cognitive-behavioral treatment can support the withdrawal taper and help with exacerbations of the initial disorder.[130] Of note, it is important to consider psychosocial therapy for the underlying disorder that was the indication for the benzodiazepine in the first place.

Prolonged Benzodiazepine Withdrawal

Some physicians report,[48-50] and clinical experience confirms, that a small proportion of patients, after long-term benzodiazepine use, experience a prolonged syndrome in which withdrawal signs and symptoms persist for weeks to months after discontinuation. This prolonged withdrawal syndrome is noted for its irregular and unpredictable day-to-day course and qualitative and quantitative differences in symptoms from both the prebenzodiazepine use state and the acute withdrawal period. Patients with prolonged withdrawal often experience slowly abating, albeit characteristic, waxing and waning symptoms of insomnia, perceptual disturbances, tremor, sensory hypersensitivities, and anxiety.

Smith and Wesson[48] propose that protracted symptoms reflect long-term receptor site adaptations. Higgitt and Fonagy[131] propose that a comprehensive etiological model of the prolonged syndrome includes a psychological component that can be explained through cognitive and behavioral models. They observe that many patients with persistent withdrawal symptoms resemble patients with somatization disorders. The patients often experience acute withdrawal more severely and may be "sensitized to anxiety." In addition to a potential lack of effective coping mechanisms away from benzodiazepines, such patients often possess a perceptual or cognitive style that leads to apprehensiveness, body sensation amplification and mislabeling, and misinterpretation.

Management

Before entertaining the existence of a prolonged withdrawal syndrome, rule out psychiatric conditions. A distinguishing characteristic of protracted withdrawal (as opposed to symptoms being from an underlying anxiety disorder) is the gradual diminution and eventual resolution of withdrawal symptoms; but with an underlying anxiety disorder, the symptoms tend to return as the sedative-hypnotic is tapered off.

Propranolol in doses of 10-20 mg 4 times per day often is helpful in attenuating anxiety or tremors. Extended use of anticonvulsants with eventual slow tapering should be considered. Gabapentin is well tolerated and helps relieve anxiety and insomnia. Start with 100-300 mg three times a day and increase dose every week depending on symptomatology. A higher dose in the evening to help with insomnia may be advised. Lower doses of sedating antidepressant medications—such as trazodone or mirtazapine—are helpful in treating insomnia. Frequent clinical follow-up for education, supportive psychotherapy, and regular reassurance are strongly advised. Frequent reassessment of the working diagnosis is recommended.

COMMON TREATMENT ISSUES

Treatment is indicated for nearly all patients with substance use disorders. Among persons with sedative-hypnotic physical dependence, treatment most often is indicated for those who use multiple substances, use high-doses, or patients in whom a sedative-hypnotic use disorder is diagnosed. The support, education, and recovery training available in most addiction specialty treatment programs are valuable to many patients who are physically dependent on sedative-hypnotics. On the other hand, patients with long-term, therapeutic use problems (and without a sedative-hypnotic use disorder/SUD) should not be coerced to participate in specialty programs designed to treat substance use disorder, as they often feel out of place and unable to relate to their peers.

Participation in specific components of treatment, tailored to each patient's individual needs, can be helpful and non-threatening. Patients who choose to participate in treatment often discover an immense source of support and encouragement, in addition to learning and practicing coping skills that facilitate substance discontinuation and abstinence.

Prevention

The best prevention for prescribed benzodiazepine use disorder is careful prescribing.[100,101] In England, the Committee on the Review of Medicines reported in 1980 that the hypnotic effect of benzodiazepines diminishes after 3-14 days and the anxiolytic effect diminishes after 4 months.[28] A good understanding of the mental health disorders with anxiety symptoms and their psychological and pharmacological therapies is important. Knowledge of a patient's risk factors for addiction, including his or her family's substance use disorder history is also important. Benzodiazepines are rarely the first-line treatment for any of the anxiety disorders. CBT, group therapy, relaxation therapy, stress management, structured problem solving, serotonin specific reuptake inhibitors, serotonin and norepinephrine reuptake inhibitors, tricyclic antidepressants, and buspirone are all potential options that can be employed as appropriate based on the level of severity. If used, benzodiazepines should be closely monitored for effectiveness and duration. A plan to reassess or taper the benzodiazepine when it is first given is wise. Reevaluate the need for the benzodiazepine when the initial indication has changed or the patient shows improvement.[100,132] Consider a benzodiazepine taper in the long-term management of chronic anxiety, even if only to determine whether continued treatment is required.[86]

SUMMARY

Sedative-hypnotics are among the most extensively prescribed medications in the United States. They are widely used, including in unhealthy and nonmedical ways, hence, they are the second most frequently reported drug class to cause emergency department visits, surpassed only by opioids. They utilize the same biochemical and neurological pathways as alcohol, have similar physical dependence and withdrawal characteristics, and exhibit cross-tolerance. Intoxication is characterized by impaired motor activity and immediate memory impairment and may progress to stupor and coma. Toxicity associated with older nonbenzodiazepine medications is progressive and can ultimately lead to respiratory arrest or cardiovascular collapse, while benzodiazepines and Z-drugs do not cause death unless used in combination with other CNS depressants (such as alcohol or opioids).

Sedative-hypnotic use can result in physical dependence and abrupt abstinence leads to a withdrawal syndrome that can be life-threatening. Benzodiazepine withdrawal syndromes are similar to those of alcohol. Benzodiazepine withdrawal is characterized by autonomic hyperactivity and can lead to seizures and death. Treatment of sedative-hypnotic withdrawal can be achieved by either gradual tapering of benzodiazepine or symptom-driven substitution with phenobarbital or a long-acting benzodiazepine. Other medications may have an ancillary role in treatment but are not indicated as monotherapy.

REFERENCES

1. Stahl SM, Muntner N. Anxiety disorders and anxiolytics. In: Stahl SM, ed. *Stahls Essential Psychopharmacology: Neuroscientific Basis and Practical Applications*. 4th ed. Cambridge University Press; 2013:397-403.
2. Wikipedia Contributors. *Barbiturate*. Wikipedia, The Free Encyclopedia. Accessed June 12, 2017. https://en.wikipedia.org/w/index.php?title=Barbiturate&oldid=781591812
3. Balon R, Starcevic V, Silberman E, et al. The rise and fall and rise of benzodiazepines: a return of the stigmatized and repressed. *Braz J Psychiatry*. 2020;42(3):243-244. doi:10.1590/1516-4446-2019-0773
4. Royal College of Psychiatrists. Benzodiazepines and dependence: a college statement. *Bull R Coll Psychiatrists*. 1988;12:107-108.
5. Bachhuber MA, Hennessy S, Cunningham CO, Starrels JL. Increasing benzodiazepine prescriptions and overdose mortality in the United States, 1996-2013. *Am J Public Health*. 2016;106(4):686-688. doi:10.2105/AJPH.2016.303061
6. Votaw VR, Geyer R, Rieselbach MM, McHugh RK. The epidemiology of benzodiazepine misuse: a systematic review. *Drug Alcohol Depend*. 2019;200:95-114. doi:10.1016/j.drugalcdep.2019.02.033
7. Soyka M. Treatment of benzodiazepine dependence. *N Engl J Med*. 2017;376:1147-1157.
8. U.S. Food & Drug Administration. *FDA Drug Safety Communication: FDA Requiring Boxed Warning Updated to Improve Safe Use of Benzodiazepine Drug Class*. 2020. Accessed March 27, 2023. https://www.fda.gov/media/142368/download

9. Liu S, O'Donnell J, Gladden RM, McGlone L, Chowdhury F. Trends in nonfatal and fatal overdoses involving benzodiazepines—38 States and the District of Columbia, 2019-2020. *MMWR Morb Mortal Wkly Rep.* 2021;70(34):1136-1141. doi:10.15585/mmwr.mm7034a2
10. Sun EC, Dixit A, Humphreys K, Darnall BD, Baker LC, Mackey S. Association between concurrent use of prescription opioids and benzodiazepines and overdose: retrospective analysis. *BMJ.* 2017;356:j760.
11. Dowell D, Haegerich TM, Chou R. CDC guideline for prescribing opioids for chronic pain—United States, 2016. *JAMA.* 2016;315(15):1624-1645. doi:10.1001/jama.2016.1464
12. Kao M-C, Zheng P, Mackey S. Trends in benzodiazepine prescription and coprescription with opioids in the United States, 2002-2009. *Poster presented at the annual meeting of the American Academy of Pain Medicine.* Phoenix, AZ; 2014. http://www.painmed.org/2014posters/abstract-109/
13. Gitlow S. *Substance Use Disorders: A Practical Guide.* Lippincott Williams & Wilkins; 2007:100-112.
14. Tintinalli JE, Stapczynski JS, Quan D. Benzodiazepines. In: Tintinalli JE, ed. *Tintinallis Emergency Medicine: A Comprehensive Study Guide.* 7th ed. McGraw Hill; 2011:1216-1219.
15. Latt N. Sedative hypnotics. In: Saunders JB, Conigrave KM, Latt MC, et al., eds. *Addiction Medicine (Oxford Specialist Handbooks).* Oxford University Press; 2009:167-186.
16. Litovitz T. Fatal benzodiazepine toxicity. *Am J Emerg Med.* 1987;5:472-473.
17. Jones JD, Mogali S, Comer SD. Polydrug abuse: a review of opioid and benzodiazepine combination. *Drug Alcohol Depend.* 2012;125(1-2):8-18.
18. Osborn H, Goldfrank LR. Sedative-hypnotic agents. In: Goldfrank LR, Flomenbaum NE, Lewin NA, Weisman RS, Howland MA, Hoffman RS, eds. *Goldfrank's Toxicologic Emergencies.* Appleton & Lange; 1994:787-804.
19. Howland MA. Flumazenil. In: Goldfrank LR, Flomenbaum NE, Lewin NA, Weisman RS, Howland MA, Hoffman RS, eds. *Goldfrank's Toxicologic Emergencies.* Appleton & Lange; 1994:805-810.
20. Spivey WH. Flumazenil and seizures: analysis of 43 cases. *Clin Ther.* 1992;14:292-305.
21. Guerlais M, Grall-Bronnec M, Feuillet F, Gérardin M, Jolliet P, Victorri-Vigneau C. Dependence on prescription benzodiaze-pines and Z-drugs among young to middle-aged patients in France. *Subst Use Misuse.* 2015;50:320-327.
22. Woods J, Katz J, Winger G. Benzodiazepines: use, abuse and consequences. *Pharmacol Rev.* 1992;44(2):151.
23. Petursson H. The benzodiazepine withdrawal syndrome. *Addiction.* 1994;89:1455-1459.
24. Salzman C. The benzodiazepine controversy: therapeutic effects versus dependence, withdrawal and toxicity. *Psychopharmacology.* 1997;4:279-282.
25. Hollister LE, Motzenbecker FP, Degan RO. Withdrawal reactions for chlordiazepoxide (Librium). *Psychopharmacologia.* 1961;2:63-68.
26. Essig CF. Newer sedative drugs that can cause states of intoxication and dependence of barbiturate type. *JAMA.* 1966;196(8):126-129.
27. Covi L, Park LC, Lipman RS. Factors affecting withdrawal response to certain minor tranquilizers. In: Cole JO, Wittenborn JR, eds. *Drug Abuse: Social and Pharmacological Aspects.* Charles C. Thomas; 1973:93-108.
28. Lader M. History of benzodiazepine dependence. *J Subst Abus Treat.* 1991;8:53-59.
29. Isbell H. Addiction to barbiturates and the barbiturate abstinence syndrome. *Ann Intern Med.* 1950;33:108-121.
30. Isbell H, Altschul S, Kornetsky CH, Eisenman AJ, Flanary HG, Fraser HF. Chronic barbiturate intoxication: an experimental study. *Arch Neurol Psychiatr.* 1950;64:1-28.
31. Fraser HF, Wikler A, Essig CF, Isbell H. Degree of physical dependence induced by secobarbital or phenobarbital. *JAMA.* 1958;166:126-129.
32. Isbell H, White WM. Clinical characteristics of addictions. *Am J Med.* 1953;14:558-565.
33. Covi L, Lipman RS, Pattison JH, Derogatis LR, Uhlenhuth EH. Length of treatment with anxiolytic sedatives and response to their sudden withdrawal. *Acta Psychiatr Scand.* 1973;49:51-64.
34. Epstein RS. Withdrawal symptoms from chronic use of low-dose barbiturates. *Am J Psychiatry.* 1980;137(1):107-108.
35. Gunja N. The clinical and forensic toxicology of Z-drugs. *J Med Toxicol.* 2013;9:155-162.
36. Essig CF. Addiction to nonbarbiturate sedative and tranquilizing drugs. *Clin Pharmacol Ther.* 1964;5(3):334-343.
37. Sadwin A, Glen RS. Addiction to glutethimide (Doriden). *Am J Psychiatry.* 1958;115:469-470.
38. Lloyd EA, Clark LD. Convulsions and delirium incident to glutethimide (Doriden). *Dis Nerv Syst.* 1959;20:1-3.
39. Phillips RM, Judy FR, Judy HE. Meprobamate addiction. *Northwest Med.* 1957;56:453-454.
40. Swanson LA, Okada T. Death after withdrawal of meprobamate. *JAMA.* 1963;184:780-781.
41. Flemenbaum A, Gumby B. Ethchlorvynol (Placidyl) abuse and withdrawal. *Dis Nerv Syst.* 1971;32:188-191.
42. Swartzburg M, Lieb J, Schwartz AH. Methaqualone withdrawal. *Arch Gen Psychiatry.* 1973;29:46-47.
43. Vestal R, Rumack B. Glutethimide dependence: phenobarbital treatment. *Ann Intern Med.* 1974;80:670-673.
44. Rickels K, Case WG, Downing RW, Fridman R. One-year follow-up of anxious patients treated with diazepam. *J Clin Psychopharmacol.* 1986;6:32-36.
45. Greenblatt DJ, Miller LG, Shader RI. Benzodiazepine discontinuation syndromes. *J Psychiatr Res.* 1990;24(Suppl):73-79.
46. Rickels K, Fox IL, Greenblatt DJ. Clorazepate and lorazepam: clinical improvement and rebound anxiety. *Am J Psychiatry.* 1988;145:312-317.
47. Winokur A, Rickels K. Withdrawal and pseudowithdrawal reactions from diazepam therapy. *J Clin Psychiatry.* 1981;42:442-444.
48. Smith DE, Wesson DR. Benzodiazepine dependency syndromes. *J Psychoactive Drugs.* 1983;15:85-95.
49. Smith DE, Seymour RB. Benzodiazepines. In: Miller NS, ed. *Comprehensive Handbook of Drug and Alcohol Addiction.* Marcel Dekker; 1991:405-426.
50. Landry MJ, Smith DE, McDuff DR, Baughman OL III. Benzodiazepine dependence and withdrawal: identification and medical management. *J Am Board Fam Pract.* 1992;5:167-176.
51. Nutt DJ. New insights into the role of the GABAA–benzodiazepine receptor in psychiatric disorder. *Br J Psychiatry.* 2001;179(5):390-396. doi:10.1192/bjp.179.5.390
52. Miller L, Greenblatt DJ, Barnhill JG, Shader RI. Chronic benzodiazepine administration I: tolerance is associated with benzodiazepine receptor downregulation and decreased gamma-aminobutyric acidA receptor function. *J Pharmacol Exp Ther.* 1988;246:170-176.
53. Miller L, Greenblatt DJ, Roy RB, Summer WR, Shader RI. Chronic benzodiazepine administration II: discontinuation syndrome is associated with up regulation of gamma-aminobutyric acidA receptor complex binding and function. *J Pharmacol Exp Ther.* 1988;146:177-281.
54. Miller L, Greenblatt DJ, Roy RB, Gaver A, Lopez F, Shader RI. Chronic benzodiazepine administration III: up regulation of gamma-aminobutyric acidA receptor complex binding and function associated with chronic benzodiazepine agonist administration. *J Pharmacol Exp Ther.* 1989;248:1096-1101.
55. Miller L. Chronic benzodiazepine administration: from patient to gene. *J Clin Pharmacol.* 1991;31:492-495.
56. NIDA Notes Staff. *Well-known mechanism underlies benzodiazepines' addictive properties.* NIDA Notes; 2012. Accessed January 26, 2014. http://www.drugabuse.gov/news-events/nida-notes/2012/04/well-known-mechanism-underlies-benzodiazepines-addictive-properties
57. Tyrer P, Rutherford D, Huggett T. Benzodiazepine withdrawal symptoms and propanolol. *Lancet.* 1981;1:520-522.
58. Schweizer E, Rickels K. Benzodiazepine dependence and withdrawal: a review of the syndrome and its clinical management. *Acta Psychiatr Scand.* 1998;393(Suppl):95-101.
59. Rickels K, Case WG, Schweizer E, Swenson C, Fridman RB. Low-dose dependence on chronic benzodiazepine users: a preliminary report. *Psychopharmacol Bull.* 1986;22:407-415.

60. Schweizer E, Rickels K, Case G, Greenblatt DJ. Long-term therapeutic use of benzodiazepines: effects of gradual taper. *Arch Gen Psychiatry*. 1990;47:908.
61. Vorma H, Naukkarinen HH, Sarna SJ, Kuoppasalmi KI. Predictors of benzodiazepine discontinuation in subjects manifesting complicated dependence. *Subst Use Misuse*. 2005;40:449-510.
62. Hollister LE, Bennett LL, Kimbell I Jr, Savage C, Overall JE. Diazepam in newly admitted schizophrenics. *Dis Nerv Syst*. 1961;24:746-750.
63. Rickels K, Schweizer E, Case WG, Greenblatt DJ. Long-term therapeutic use of benzodiazepines. I. Effects of abrupt discontinuation. *Arch Gen Psychiatry*. 1990;47:899-907.
64. Dickinson W, Rush PA, Radcliffe AB. Alprazolam use and dependence: a retrospective analysis of 30 cases of withdrawal. *West J Med*. 1990;152(5):604-608.
65. Malcolm R, Brady TK, Johnston AL, Cunningham M. Types of benzodiazepines abused by chemically dependent inpatients. *J Psychoactive Drugs*. 1993;25(4):315-319.
66. Romach M, Busto U, Somer GR, Kaplan HL, Sellers E. Clinical aspects of chronic use of alprazolam and lorazepam. *Am J Psychiatry*. 1995;152:1161-1167.
67. Klein RL, Colin V, Stolk J, Lenox RH. Alprazolam withdrawal in patients with panic disorder and generalized anxiety disorder: vulnerability and effect of carbamazepine. *Am J Psychiatry*. 1994;151:1760-1766.
68. Woods J, Winger G. Current benzodiazepine issues. *Psychopharmacology*. 1995;118:107-115.
69. Bruce TJ, Spiegel DA, Gregg SF, Nuzzarello A. Predictors of alprazolam discontinuation with and without cognitive behavioral therapy in panic disorder. *Am J Psychiatry*. 1995;152(8):1156-1160.
70. Busto U, Sellers E. Anxiolytics and sedative/hypnotics dependence. *Br J Addict*. 1991;86:1647-1652.
71. Busto U, Simpkins J, Sellers EM. Objective determination of benzodiazepine use and abuse in alcoholics. *Br J Addict*. 1983;78: 429-435.
72. Ciraulo DA, Barnhill JG, Greenblatt DJ, et al. Abuse liability and clinical pharmacokinetics of alprazolam in alcoholic men. *J Clin Psychiatry*. 1988;49:333-337.
73. Regier DA, Farmer ME, Raes DS, et al. Comorbidity of mental disorders with alcohol and other drug abuse. Results from the epidemiologic catchment area (ECA) study. *JAMA*. 1990;264(19):2511-2518.
74. Sellers E, Ciraulo DA, DuPont RL, et al. Alprazolam and benzodiazepine dependence. *J Clin Psychiatry*. 1993;54(Suppl 10):64-75.
75. DuPont RL. Abuse of benzodiazepines: the problems and solutions. *Am J Drug Alcohol Abuse*. 1988;14S:1-69.
76. Griffiths R, Wolf B. Relative abuse liability of different benzodiazepines in drug abusers. *J Clin Psychopharmacol*. 1990;10(4):237.
77. Smith DE, Landry M. Benzodiazepine dependency discontinuation: focus on the chemical dependency detoxification setting and benzodiazepine-polydrug abuse. *J Psychiatr Res*. 1990;24(Suppl 2):145-156.
78. Cowley DS, Roy-Byrne PP, Hommer DW, et al. Sensitivity to benzodiazepines in sons of alcoholics. *Biol Psychiatry*. 1991;29:104-112.
79. Cowley DS, Roy-Byrne PP, Gordon C, et al. Response to diazepam in sons of alcoholics. *Alcohol Clin Exp Res*. 1992;16:1057-1063.
80. Ciraulo DA, Sarid-Segal O, Knapp C, Ciraulo AM, Greenblatt DJ, Shader RI. Liability to alprazolam abuse in daughters of alcoholics. *Am J Psychiatry*. 1996;153:956-958.
81. Ashton H. Benzodiazepine withdrawal: outcome in 50 patients. *Br J Addict*. 1987;82:665-671.
82. Gabe J. Women and tranquilizer use: a case study in the social politics of health and health care. In: Hallstrom C, ed. *Benzodiazepine Dependence*. Oxford University Press; 1993:350-363.
83. Darwich AS, Henderson K, Burgin A, et al. Trends in oral drug bioavailability following bariatric surgery: examining the variable extent of impact on exposure of different drug classes. *Br J Clin Pharmacol*. 2012;74(5):774-787. doi:10.1111/j.1365-2125.2012.04284.x
84. Czeizel AE, Dudás I, Bánhidy F. Interpretation of controversial teratogenic findings of drugs such as phenobarbital. *ISRN Obstet Gynecol*. 2011;2011:1-8. doi:10.5402/2011/719675
85. Latt N. Sedative hypnotics. In: Saunders JB, Conigrave KM, Latt MC, et al., eds. *Addiction Medicine (Oxford Specialist Handbooks)*. Oxford University Press; 2009:318.
86. Rickels K, DeMartinis N, Rynn M, Mandos L. Pharmacologic strategies for discontinuing benzodiazepine treatment. *J Clin Psychopharmacol*. 1999;19(6 Suppl 2):12S-16S.
87. Schweizer E, Rickels K, DeMartinis N, Case G, García-España F. The effect of personality on withdrawal severity and taper outcome in benzodiazepine dependent patients. *Psychol Med*. 1998;28:713-720.
88. Oude Voshaar RC, Couvee JE, van Balkom AJ, Mulder PGH, Zitman FG. Strategies for discontinuing long-term benzodiazepine use. *Br J Psychiatry*. 2006;189:213-220.
89. Oude Voshaar RC, Gorgels W, Mol A, et al. Predictors of relapse after discontinuation of long-term benzodiazepine use by minimal intervention: a 2-year follow-up study. *Fam Pract*. 2003;20:370-372.
90. Cormack MA, Sweeney KG, Hughes-Jones H, Foot GA. Evaluation of a easy, cost effective strategy for cutting benzodiazepine use in general practice. *Br J Gen Pract*. 1994;44:5-8.
91. Otto MW, McHugh RK, Simon NM, Farach FJ, Worthington JJ, Pollack MH. Efficacy of CBT for benzodiazepine discontinuation in patients with panic disorder: further evaluation. *Behav Res Ther*. 2010;48(8):720-727. doi:10.1016/j.brat.2010.04.002
92. Lader M, Tylee A, Donoghue J. Withdrawing benzodiazepines in primary care. *CNS Drugs*. 2009;23:19-34.
93. Miller WR, Rollnick S. *Motivational Interviewing: Helping People Change*. 3rd ed. Guilford Press; 2012.
94. Darker CD, Sweeney BP, Barry JM, Farrell MF, Donnelly-Swi E. Psychosocial interventions for benzodiazepine harmful use, abuse or dependence. *Cochrane Database Syst Rev*. 2015;5:CD009652. doi:10.1002/14651858.CD009652.pub2
95. Gosselin P, Ladouceur R, Morin CM, Dugas MJ, Baillaregeon L. Benzodiazepine discontinuation among adults with GAD: a randomized trial of cognitive-behavioral therapy. *J Consult Clin Psychol*. 2006;74:908-919.
96. Edinger JD, Wohlgemuth WK. The significance and management of persistent primary insomnia: the past, present and future of behavioural insomnia therapies. *Sleep Med Rev*. 1999;3:101-118.
97. Morgan K, Dixon S, Mathers N, Thompson J, Tomeny M. Psychological treatment for insomnia in the regulation of long-term hypnotic use. *Health Technol Assess*. 2004;8:1-68.
98. Ashton H. Protracted withdrawal syndromes from benzodiazepines. *J Subst Abus Treat*. 1991;8:19-28.
99. Alexander B, Perry P. Detoxification from benzodiazepines: schedules and strategies. *J Subst Abus Treat*. 1991;8:9-17.
100. Higgitt AC, Lader MH, Fonagy P. Clinical management of benzodiazepine dependence. *BMJ*. 1985;291:688-690.
101. Edwards JG, Cantopher T, Olivieri S. Benzodiazepine dependence and the problems of withdrawal. *Postgrad Med J*. 1990;66(Suppl 2): S27-S35.
102. Cantopher T, Olivieri S, Cleave N, Edwards JG. Chronic benzodiazepine dependence: a comparative study of abrupt withdrawal under propranolol cover versus gradual withdrawal. *Br J Psychiatry*. 1990; 156:406-411.
103. Vicens C, Fiol F, Llobera J, et al. Withdrawal from long term benzodiazepine use: randomized trial in family practice. *Br J Gen Pract*. 2006;56:958-963.
104. Zullino DF, Khazaal Y, Hättenschwiler J, Borgeat F, Besson J. Anticonvulsant drugs in the treatment of substance withdrawal. *Drugs Today (Barc)*. 2004;40(7):603-619.
105. Granger P, Biton B, Faure C, et al. Modulation of the gamma-aminobutyric acid type A receptor by the antiepileptic drugs carbamazepine and phenytoin. *Mol Pharmacol*. 1995;47:1189-1196.
106. Elphick M, Yang D, Cowen PJ. Effects of carbamazepine on dopamine- and serotonin-mediated neuroendocrine responses. *Arch Gen Psychiatry*. 1990;47:135-140.
107. Lampe H, Bigalke H. Carbamazepine blocks NMDA-activated currents in cultured spinal cord neurons. *Neuroreport*. 1990;1:26-28.

108. Klein E, Uhde TW, Post RM. Preliminary evidence for the utility of carbamazepine in alprazolam withdrawal. *Am J Psychiatry.* 1986;143:235-236.
109. Ries RK, Roy-Byrne PP, Ward NG, Neppe V, Cullison S. Carbamazepine treatment for benzodiazepine withdrawal. *Am J Psychiatry.* 1989;146(4):536-537.
110. Garcia-Borresuerro D. Treatment of benzodiazepine withdrawal symptoms with carbamazepine. *Psychiatry Clin Neurosci.* 1990;241:145-150.
111. Schweizer E, Rickels K, Case G, Greenblatt DJ. Carbamazepine treatment in patients discontinuing long-term benzodiazepine therapy. *Arch Gen Psychiatry.* 1991;48:448.
112. Galpern W, Miller LG, Greenblatt DJ, Szabo GK, Browne TR, Shader RI. Chronic benzodiazepine administration IX. Attenuation of alprazolam discontinuation effects by carbamazepine. *Biochem Pharmacol.* 1991;42:S99-S104.
113. Pages K, Ries R. Use of anticonvulsants in benzodiazepine withdrawal. *Am J Addict.* 1998;7(3):198-204.
114. Harris J, Roache J, Thornton J. A role for valproate in the treatment of sedative-hypnotic withdrawal and for relapse prevention. *Alcohol Alcohol.* 2000;35(4):319-323.
115. Apelt S, Emrich H. Letter. *Am J Psychiatry.* 1990;147(7):950-951.
116. Zeise M, Kasparow S, Zieglgansberger W. Valproate suppresses N-methyl-d-aspartate-evoked, transient depolarizations in the rat neocortex in vitro. *Brain Res.* 1991;544:345-348.
117. Rickels K, Schweizer E, Garcia-Espana F, Case G, DeMartinis N, Greenblatt D. Trazodone and valproate in patients discontinuing long-term benzodiazepine therapy; effects on withdrawal symptoms and taper outcome. *Psychopharmacology.* 1999;141:1-5.
118. Cheseaux M, Monnat M, Zullino DF. Topiramate in benzodiazepine withdrawal. *Hum Psychopharmacol.* 2003;18:375-377.
119. White HS, Brown SD, Woodhead JH, Skeen GA, Wolf HH. Topiramate modulates GABA-evoked currents in murine cortical neurons by a nonbenzodiazepine mechanism. *Epilepsia.* 2000;41(Suppl 1):S17-S20.
120. Michopoulos I, Douzenis A, Christodoulou C, Lykouras L. Topiramate use in alprazolam addiction. *World J Biol Psychiatry.* 2006;7(4):265-267.
121. Gerra G, Zaimovic A, Giusti F, Moi G, Brewer C. Intravenous flumazenil versus oxazepam tapering in the treatment of benzodiazepine withdrawal: a randomized, placebo-controlled study. *Addict Biol.* 2002;7:385-395.
122. Schweizer E, Rickels K. Failure of buspirone to manage benzodiazepine withdrawal. *Am J Psychiatry.* 1986;143(12):1590-1592.
123. Ashton CH, Rawlins MD, Tyrer SP. A double-blind placebo-controlled study of buspirone in diazepam withdrawal in chronic benzodiazepine users. *Br J Psychiatry.* 1990;157:232-238.
124. Annsseau M, DeRoeck J. Trazodone in benzodiazepine dependence. *J Clin Psychiatry.* 1993;54(5):189-191.
125. Chandrasekaran PK. Employing mirtazapine to aid benzodiazepine withdrawal. *Singap Med J.* 2008;49(6):166-167.
126. Spiegel DA, Bruce TJ, Gregg SF, Nuzzarello A. Does cognitive behavioral therapy assist slow-taper alprazolam discontinuation in panic disorder? *Am J Psychiatry.* 1994;151:876-881.
127. Otto MN, Pollack MH, Sachs GS, Reiter SR, Meltzer-Brody S, Rosenbaum JF. Discontinuation of benzodiazepine treatment: efficacy of cognitive behavioral therapy for patients with panic disorder. *Am J Psychiatry.* 1993;150:1485-1490.
128. Higgitt AC, Golombok S, Fonagy R. Group treatment of benzodiazepine dependence. *Br J Addict.* 1987;82:517-532.
129. Oude Voshaar RC, Gorgels WJMJ, Mol AJ, et al. Tapering off long-term benzodiazepine use with or without group cognitive–behavioral therapy: three-condition, randomised controlled trial. *Br J Psychiatry.* 2003;182:498-504.
130. Spiegel DA. Psychological strategies for discontinuing benzodiazepine treatment. *J Clin Psychopharmacol.* 1999;19(6 Suppl 2):17S-22S.
131. Higgitt A, Fonagy P. Benzodiazepine dependence syndromes and syndromes of withdrawal. In: Hallstrom C, ed. *Benzodiazepine Dependence.* Oxford University Press; 1983:58-70.
132. Norman TR, Ellen SR, Burrows GD. Benzodiazepines in anxiety disorders: managing therapeutics and dependence. *Med J Aust.* 1997;167(9):490-495.

CHAPTER

58 Management of Opioid Intoxication and Withdrawal

Kenneth L. Morford, Julia M. Shi, Patrick G. O'Connor, and Jeanette M. Tetrault

CHAPTER OUTLINE

- Introduction
- Opioid intoxication and overdose
- Opioid withdrawal
- Conclusions

INTRODUCTION

Opioids are a broad category of chemical compounds that function at opioid receptors in the central nervous system and gastrointestinal tract to produce pharmacological effects and common clinical features of intoxication and withdrawal. They are classified as naturally occurring, semisynthetic, or synthetic.[1,2] Opiates refer to naturally occurring opioids derived from the opium poppy plant (*Papaver somniferum*), such as morphine and codeine. Semisynthetic opioids include diacetylmorphine (heroin), oxycodone, hydrocodone, and hydromorphone. Synthetic opioids include methadone, fentanyl, and tramadol, among others.

Opioids are further classified by their activity at mu opioid receptors as full agonists, partial agonists, and antagonists. Full agonists bind to and activate mu opioid receptors producing acute pharmacological effects, including analgesia, euphoria, sedation, respiratory depression, miosis, and reduced gastric motility.[1,3] Chronic use of opioid agonists can result in physical dependence characterized by tolerance and withdrawal.[4] Partial agonists, such as buprenorphine, bind to and activate mu opioid receptors but to a lesser degree than full agonists, resulting in a "ceiling effect" where pharmacological effects plateau despite increasing doses. Antagonists bind to mu opioid receptors but do not activate them resulting, in a blocking effect.

The most commonly encountered opioids in clinical practice include prescription opioids, such as hydrocodone, oxycodone, codeine, tramadol, buprenorphine, morphine, fentanyl, and hydromorphone.[5] While heroin has historically been the most commonly encountered nonprescribed opioid, illicitly manufactured fentanyl (IMF) and other high potency synthetic opioids have become increasingly prevalent in the United States.[6]

This chapter reviews the clinical features and management of opioid intoxication, overdose, and withdrawal. While anyone exposed to opioids is at risk of experiencing these complications, those with opioid use disorder (OUD) are especially vulnerable to opioid overdose, withdrawal, and other complications contributing to opioid-related morbidity and mortality. Thus, effective management of opioid intoxication, overdose, and withdrawal represents a critical opportunity to offer first-line medications for OUD (MOUD), including methadone, buprenorphine, and extended-release injectable naltrexone, with linkage to long-term treatment and harm reduction resources to mitigate risks of ongoing opioid use.

OPIOID INTOXICATION AND OVERDOSE

Clinical Presentation

Opioid intoxication exists on a spectrum ranging from mild-to-moderate intoxication characterized by euphoria and sedation to severe intoxication and overdose. While mild-to-moderate intoxication is not typically life-threatening, severe intoxication and overdose represent medical emergencies that may lead to death without immediate intervention[7] including administration of the opioid antagonist, naloxone. With the increasing presence of high potency synthetic opioids, such as IMF, in the drug supply globally, there has been an exponential rise in severe intoxication and overdose. In the United States in 2020, 70% of the over 38,000 drug overdose deaths reported from 28 states and the District of Columbia involved IMF.[8]

Severe opioid intoxication presents with the classic triad of respiratory depression, altered mental status, and miotic pupils.[7] While altered mental status and miosis are often present, respiratory depression is considered the cardinal feature of acute opioid intoxication and can progress to death when the respiratory rate decreases to apnea.[9] It is important to note that, compared with other opioid-related overdoses, intoxication with IMF may present with distinct symptoms including chest wall rigidity, dyskinesia, and slow or irregular heart rate.[10,11]

In addition to the cardinal features of opioid intoxication and overdose, other clinical presentations may occur. Opioid intoxication can result in other pulmonary complications besides respiratory depression, including acute lung injury related to aspiration[12] or pulmonary edema.[13] Other injuries related to acute opioid intoxication include rhabdomyolysis, myoglobinuric renal failure, and compartment syndrome from extended immobilization[14-17]; liver toxicity from contaminants or hypoxemia[18]; and seizures.[19]

Acute anterograde amnestic syndrome lasting for months has been reported with nonmedical opioid use,[20] as well as increased cardiovascular events among patients hospitalized with opioid overdose.[17,21]

Certain factors contribute to the likelihood of experiencing an opioid overdose, including an individual's level of opioid tolerance, route of administration, and the use of other substances. The development of tolerance is caused by the desensitization of the opioid receptors, whereby larger doses of opioids are required to have the same physiologic effect. Tolerance to respiratory depression may be slower to develop than tolerance to euphoric effects. This explains why overdose occurs so often, even among individuals with a long history of opioid use.[22,23] Patients who have undergone medically supervised withdrawal or those who have experienced intentional or unintentional abstinence from opioids for other reasons, such as incarceration, may be particularly susceptible to death from opioid overdose due to loss of tolerance.[24-26] Among this group, prior history of overdose and depressive symptoms are risk factors for nonfatal overdose.[27] Although injecting opioids may be the route of administration associated with the highest risk of overdose, noninjection routes are also associated with significant risk.[28]

In addition to the role of opioid tolerance in increasing the likelihood of overdose, patients who use opioids with other substances known to enhance (eg, benzodiazepines, alcohol, and other sedatives) or counteract (eg, stimulants) the opioid effect are more likely to experience overdose. The U.S. national overdose death data collected from 1999 to 2020 showed steady increases in the number of opioid-related deaths that also involved stimulants, benzodiazepines, and antidepressants.[29] More than half of all drug overdose deaths result from multiple drug overdose with opioids, alcohol, and cocaine.[30,31] Alcohol and benzodiazepine co-involvement in fatal opioid overdoses is common and associated with state-level binge drinking patterns and benzodiazepine prescribing rates.[32]

Additionally, an increasing number of published case reports describe fatal opioid overdose among opioid-naive patients who are unintentionally exposed to opioids. This may occur when individuals believe they are using stimulants (eg, cocaine or methamphetamine) or prescription medications purchased from others when in fact they are unknowingly exposed to IMF in the increasingly contaminated drug supply.[20,33] In a cross-sectional study of urine drug test (UDT) results obtained as part of routine clinical care among 1 million unique individuals across the United States from 2013 to 2017, the presence of IMF increased by 1850% in cocaine-positive UDT and by 798% in methamphetamine-positive UDT.[34] Furthermore, contamination of counterfeit pills has been linked to a sharp increase in drug overdose deaths among adolescents, especially in Indigenous American or Alaska Native and Latinx populations, between 2019 and 2020 despite decreasing rates of reported drug use.[35] Increasing IMF contamination in illicitly-sold opioid and benzodiazepine pills prompted the U.S. Drug Enforcement Administration (DEA) to warn the public of counterfeit pills that are made to look like prescription opioids such as oxycodone (Oxycontin, Percocet), hydrocodone (Vicodin), and alprazolam (Xanax); or stimulants like amphetamines (Adderall) in their "One Pill can Kill" campaign.[36]

Assessment and Diagnosis

Evaluation of opioid intoxication begins with the collection of patient data through a detailed history and physical examination (**Table 58-1**). However, in the presence of severe respiratory depression, administering naloxone and restoring pulmonary function takes precedence and should be performed immediately.[9]

When available, historical information can be obtained concerning opioid use either directly from the patient, from friends and family members, or from emergency medical service providers at the scene. Depending on the circumstances and the level of consciousness of the patient, items found with the individual at the time of overdose or intoxication can provide collateral information. These items may include pills, empty prescription bottles, needles, and other evidence of opioid use.

In addition to opioids, it is important to ask about use of other substances, in particular cocaine, methamphetamines, benzodiazepines, and alcohol.[37-39] Identification of multiple drug use has important implications for patient management. For example, identification of the co-occurrence of opioid and benzodiazepine overdose may indicate the need for additional therapy directed at managing the benzodiazepine component of the overdose.[40,41]

Physical examination of a patient with opioid intoxication may reveal CNS depression, euphoria, miosis, and respiratory depression. The clinical triad of altered mental status, depressed respiration, and miotic pupils, has a sensitivity of 92% and a specificity of 76% for the diagnosis of opioid overdose.[7] Additional evidence supports the use of clinical characteristics in the diagnosis of opioid overdose. In a study of 730 patients in Los Angeles receiving naloxone for suspected heroin overdose, the presence of one of the three clinical signs—respirations under 12 per minute, presence of pinpoint

TABLE 58-1 Diagnosis of Opioid Overdose

History[a]
• Ask about opioid use
  • Type of opioid
  • Amount
  • Time of last use
• Ask about use of other drugs or medication

Physical Examination • CNS depression • Euphoria • Pupillary size and reactivity • Respiratory depression • Chest wall rigidity (fentanyl) • Skin examination looking for signs of injection or skin and soft tissue infection

Diagnosis
• Altered level of consciousness plus one of the following:
  • Respiratory depression (respiratory rate <12/min)
  • Miotic pupils
  • Circumstantial evidence of opioid use (ie, needle tracks)

Laboratory Tests • Rule out hypoglycemia, acidemia, and fluid and electrolyte abnormalities • Toxicology screens for opioids and other drugs

[a]Use multiple sources of information (family, family, hospital records, etc.) to obtain complete history.

pupils, and circumstantial evidence of opioid use—had a sensitivity of 92% and a specificity of 76%, whereas the sensitivity of naloxone response was 88%, and specificity was 86%.[42]

The size and reactivity of the pupils should be evaluated as this may yield important information to aid in diagnostic evaluation. For example, meperidine, morphine, and propoxyphene are opioids known to paradoxically cause midpoint pupils or frank mydriasis. Examination of the skin for direct evidence of injection drug use, including needle track marks as well as skin and soft tissue infections, and the extremities for signs of compartment syndrome such as firmness, edema, and tenderness is recommended.[9]

An initial assessment includes respiratory rate, respiratory effort, and auscultation for evidence of pulmonary edema or other signs suggestive of acute lung injury. Intoxication and overdose due to IMF may produce a unique presentation known as "wooden chest syndrome," which is defined by rigidity in the respiratory muscles of the chest wall, upper airway, and diaphragm through a non-opioid mechanism.[43] This feature, along with central respiratory depression typically seen in opioid overdose, leads to a rapid and rigid respiratory depression that makes overdose with IMF particularly challenging to treat.[44]

The laboratory can also provide important information to support the evaluation of opioid intoxication. Urine toxicology testing should be performed promptly in emergency settings to detect naturally occurring and synthetic opioids. Be aware that drug testing for opiates is often limited to derivatives of the opium poppy and may not include the wider array of semisynthetic and synthetic opioids, including fentanyl, methadone, oxycodone, tramadol, and buprenorphine. Special urine testing for these substances can be ordered separately based on clinical judgement. Urine toxicology is preferred to serum toxicology because urine contains higher concentrations of opioids and their metabolites than serum. Results are usually qualitative, indicating only the presence or absence of specific substances. Even when the results of toxicological screening are not available until after acute management has been initiated, toxicology testing can support the diagnosis of opioid intoxication and may also reveal the presence of other substances not suspected on initial evaluation. Thus, toxicology testing is useful not only for acute management but also for planning care after discharge from the acute setting.[45] In addition, pooled data from UDT can facilitate real-time surveillance to alert communities about changes in local drug supplies that can be leveraged to prevent overdose deaths.[46] A serum acetaminophen concentration can be measured as part of the diagnostic workup of opioid intoxication and overdose.[9]

It is important to consider the differential diagnosis in patients presenting with symptoms of opioid intoxication. In addition to direct or additive toxicity from other substances, other causes of depressed mental status are possible, and include hypoglycemia, acidemia or other fluid and electrolyte disorders, sepsis, vitamin deficiencies including thiamine, hypoxic-ischemic encephalopathy, infectious etiologies, and complications from end-stage liver disease. Additionally, acute mental status changes from HIV-related opportunistic infections may mimic those of opioid intoxication.[47] Although HIV incidence is decreasing, outbreaks among people who inject drugs remain an important concern.[48]

Opioid intoxication and overdose also may be complicated by the effects of adulterants added to the drug supply. Along with inert substances present to add bulk, active substances—including dextromethorphan, lidocaine, veterinary medications such as xylazine, psychoactive stimulants such as eutylone, and scopolamine—may be present. It is important to note that unusual complications may develop as a result of certain adulterants. For instance, case reports of patients presenting with cutaneous necrosis, purpura, and neutropenia have been linked to levamisole, an anthelminthic, immunomodulatory, and antineoplastic medication known to be an adulterant in cocaine.[49] Xylazine, a nonopioid veterinary anesthetic and sedative, has also been increasingly detected in local drug supplies and may cause prolonged CNS depression, hypotension, bradycardia, and severe respiratory depression.[50] Cutaneous abscesses or ulceration predominantly on the extremities has also been associated with xylazine.[50] Eutylone, a psychoactive stimulant, has been detected in local opioid drug supplies leading to hypoactive delirium and agitation.[51,52] Given the ever-changing nature of the global drug supply, it is important for clinicians to pay attention to local toxicology reports and public health alerts when caring for patients presenting to emergency settings.

Management

Individuals who present with signs and symptoms of mild-to-moderate opioid intoxication without overdose can be monitored and treated supportively without naloxone administration. Supportive care measures include monitoring vital signs, including pulse oximetry, assessing level of sedation, and providing supplemental oxygen and intravenous fluids as needed.[53] In cases of suspected severe opioid intoxication resulting in overdose, institute general supportive management simultaneously with the overdose reversal agent naloxone (**Table 58-2**).[7] Adult basic life support and adult advanced cardiac life support may be needed.[54,55] The clinician must establish an adequate airway for the patient and appropriately assess and manage respiratory and cardiac function. Intravenous access is essential so that fluids and pharmacological agents can be administered as needed. Frequent monitoring of vital signs and cardiorespiratory status is needed until it is clearly established that the opioid and any other intoxicating substances have been cleared from the patient's system. The timeline for this may be variable based on individual metabolism and the respective pharmacokinetics of the substances that were used. Multiple doses of naloxone or a continuous intravenous naloxone infusion may be required in the case of intoxication or overdose with a long-acting opioid.

Among patients with opioid overdose seen in the emergency department, clinicians must determine whether patients require admission to the hospital and, if not, when they can be discharged from the emergency department. In a pre-fentanyl era study of 573 patients seen in an emergency department, a group

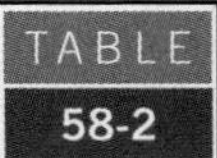

TABLE 58-2 Management of Opioid Overdose

Initial Approach
- Assessment of ventilation
  - For patients with adequate ventilation:
    - Monitor until normal level of arousal
- For patients with inadequate ventilation:
  - Naloxone hydrochloride: 0.4-0.8 mg IM/IV or 4 mg intranasal initially, repeated as necessary; consider continuous naloxone infusion if needed
  - Supportive ventilation with 100% oxygenation
  - Consider mechanical ventilation if persistent respiratory depression despite naloxone or if inadequate oxygenation
- Assessment of perfusion
- Intravenous access and fluids
- Assessment for comorbid conditions

For patients with a complete naloxone response:
- Observe for 2-3 h after response if no other complications
- Repeat naloxone if clinically significant sedation recurs and consider continuous naloxone infusion if needed
- Chest x-ray for patients with pulmonary symptoms
- Inpatient addiction medicine consultation (if available) and/or referral for substance use disorder treatment

For patients with incomplete naloxone response:
- Trial of 2-mg IM/IV dose of naloxone
- Consider multiple substance overdose or alternative diagnosis
- Once stabilized, inpatient addiction medicine consultation (if available) and/or referral for substance use disorder treatment

of investigators developed a clinical prediction rule to identify patients with opioid overdose who could be safely discharged 1 hour after naloxone administration. According to this rule, patients can be safely discharged if they can mobilize as usual, have an oxygen saturation on room air of more than 92%, have a respiratory rate greater than 10 breaths/min and fewer than 20 breaths/min, have a temperature of more than 35.0°C and less than 37.5°C, have a heart rate over 50 beats/min and under 100 beats/min, and have a Glasgow Coma Scale score of 15.[56] A 2019 study of 538 patients supports the use of this guideline to stratify patients for early discharge following naloxone administration if the threshold for oxygen saturation is set at 95%.[57] Patients with major acute medical or psychiatric comorbidities, including active suicidal ideation, may need hospitalization for further treatment. Integral components of a safe discharge plan include the absence of acute comorbidities, resolution of the symptoms of intoxication, and establishment of appropriate follow-up referrals for addiction, medical, and psychiatric care.

When managing patients with suspected opioid overdose, a complete medical assessment to evaluate for acute medical conditions and exacerbations of chronic medical conditions associated with OUD and intravenous drug use is recommended.[47,58] For example, prolonged hypoxia resulting from opioid overdose can result in rhabdomyolysis and myocardial infarction that must be treated emergently.[15-17] Other medical conditions, such as acute infection, trauma, and chronic liver disease, may have major implications for the management of a patient presenting with an opioid overdose.[58]

Pharmacological Therapies

When a patient presents with evidence of opioid overdose, immediate pharmacological therapy is indicated.[7,9] Naloxone hydrochloride, a pure opioid antagonist, can effectively reverse the CNS effects of opioid intoxication and overdose. Intranasal naloxone can be used effectively to reverse opioid overdose in both the prehospital and hospital settings.[59,60] In the hospital setting, an initial intravenous dose of 0.4 to 0.8 mg will quickly reverse neurological and cardiorespiratory depression. The onset of action of intravenously administered naloxone, as manifested by antagonism of opioid overdose, is approximately 2 minutes. While both intranasal and injectable (ie, intramuscular/intravenous) formulations of naloxone are effective in the prehospital management of opioid overdose,[61] intranasal naloxone dosed at 0.8 or 1.4 mg has been shown to be less efficient at restoring spontaneous breathing compared to 0.8 mg of intramuscular naloxone.[62,63]

Overdose with opioids that are more potent (such as fentanyl) or longer acting (such as methadone) may require higher doses of naloxone given over longer periods of time or ongoing naloxone infusion until clinical stability is established.[64] In patients who do not respond to multiple doses of naloxone, consider alternative causes of symptoms, including overdose with substances other than opioids. Of increasing concern are ultrapotent opioids, which may be less responsive to naloxone. These include carfentanil and U-47700 ("gray death," which includes a combination of fentanyl, carfentanil, and heroin).[65,66]

Another important consideration when administering naloxone is precipitating iatrogenic rapid opioid withdrawal through administration of a strong opioid antagonist. This may cause significant distress and discomfort for the patient. Administering 4mg of sublingual buprenorphine has been described to improve naloxone precipitated opioid withdrawal in a case report in the emergency department.[67] Alpha-2 adrenergic agonists and other non-opioid medications targeting specific symptoms may also be used to treat precipitated withdrawal (see section on Opioid Withdrawal). For mild to moderate opioid intoxication without overdose (ie, patient is arousable, has adequate oxygenation and stable vital signs), the patient can be monitored without naloxone to avoid precipitating withdrawal.

Research and development of naloxone has led to devices that allow for intranasal, intramuscular, and subcutaneous administration of naloxone with further development underway. In 2023, the U.S. Food and Drug Administration made intranasal naloxone available without a prescription; however, further effort is needed by policymakers, health systems, and communities to increase widespread, convenient, and low-cost access to naloxone amid the overdose crisis.[68] In the context of increasingly potent synthetic opioids in the drug supply, another important consideration is appropriate naloxone dosing to ensure adequate reversal of life-threatening overdoses while minimizing the risks of adverse effects.[69]

Follow-Up Care

Management of acute opioid overdose may represent an opportunity to engage patients with OUD into medical care, including initiation of MOUD with linkage to long-term addiction treatment. In one study of 924 individuals who use opioids in Baltimore, MD, 368 (40%) reported a history of overdose. Twenty-six percent of the patients who had experienced an overdose sought addiction treatment within 30 days after the event; the majority of those interviewed cited the overdose event as the primary catalyst for seeking treatment. Multiple "missed opportunities" were noted: 87% of overdose patients treated by emergency medical services, 74% of overdose patients treated in the emergency room, and 57% of overdose patients hospitalized reported never receiving addiction treatment information from the medical staff.[70] Moreover, a 2018 study of 17,568 individuals who experienced a nonfatal opioid overdose in Massachusetts found that only 30% received MOUD over 12 months of follow-up despite decreased mortality associated with receiving treatment with buprenorphine or methadone.[71] In light of these and similar findings, establishing ongoing addiction treatment is a major goal of patient care after treating the acute complications of overdose and related health conditions.

Once the acute overdose event has resolved, patients can be offered MOUD based on their goals and preferences. For hospitalized patients, implementation of hospital-based addiction consult services can assist with MOUD initiation and linkage to care. Addiction consult services have demonstrated efficacy in reducing length of hospital stay, hospital readmission, and increasing treatment completion for co-occurring conditions.[72-74] Similarly, initiating MOUD in the emergency department has been found to be more effective at engaging patients in addiction treatment than brief intervention and referral. In a randomized clinical trial of emergency department-initiated buprenorphine, 78% of patients with OUD who initiated buprenorphine at an urban emergency department were engaged in addiction treatment 30 days after the emergency department visit, compared with 37% in the referral group and 45% in the brief intervention group.[75] Linkage to outpatient care is critical to establish long-term MOUD treatment. Clinicians working in inpatient settings should be familiar with local opioid treatment programs providing methadone and outpatient clinicians who are willing to prescribe buprenorphine. The Substance Abuse and Mental Health Services Administration (SAMHSA) has developed an online treatment locator to help find these services.[76] Case management may also promote linkage to care from a variety of settings.[77-79] Peer recovery support services have increasingly been implemented in emergency departments and other settings to facilitate care transitions, although the effectiveness of these interventions remains inconclusive.[80] In addition to offering on site access to MOUD initiation, offering naloxone and harm reduction counseling and resources is recommended for all patients presenting with overdose.

OPIOID WITHDRAWAL

Clinical Presentation

Opioid withdrawal occurs when opioids are reduced, stopped, or displaced at the level of the mu opioid receptor in an individual who has developed physical dependence to opioids. Physical dependence develops from repeated exposure to exogenous opioids over time, resulting in neuroadaptations in the brain's reward circuity. These neuroadaptations, including mu opioid receptor desensitization, result in opioid tolerance requiring higher doses of exogenous opioids to achieve the same effects.[81,82] As opioids activate mu opioid receptors in the locus coeruleus to inhibit norepinephrine release, abstinence from exogenous opioids results in excessive norepinephrine activity causing the autonomic hyperactivity symptoms that characterize opioid withdrawal. Spontaneous opioid withdrawal occurs when opioids are abruptly reduced or stopped, while precipitated withdrawal occurs when opioid antagonists, such as naloxone or naltrexone, or the opioid partial agonist, buprenorphine, are taken in the presence of full opioid agonists leading to displacement of agonists from the mu opioid receptor.[83,84]

Clinical phenomena associated with opioid withdrawal include neurophysiological rebound in the organ systems on which opioids have their primary actions.[85] Thus, the generalized CNS suppression that occurs with opioid use is replaced by CNS hyperactivity. Neuropharmacological studies of opioid withdrawal have supported the clinical picture of CNS noradrenergic hyperactivity.[86,87] Nonopioid therapies that alter the course of opioid withdrawal (such as clonidine) are designed to decrease this hyperactivity, which occurs primarily at the locus coeruleus.[88,89] Evidence for the role of noradrenergic hyperactivity in opioid withdrawal has been provided by studies showing elevated norepinephrine metabolite levels.[90]

Withdrawal from opioids results in a specific constellation of symptoms. Early findings of opioid withdrawal may include abnormalities in vital signs, including tachycardia and hypertension. Bothersome CNS system symptoms include restlessness, irritability, and insomnia. Opioid craving also occurs in proportion to the severity of physiological withdrawal symptoms. Pupillary dilation can be marked. A variety of cutaneous and mucocutaneous symptoms including lacrimation, rhinorrhea, and piloerection (ie, "gooseflesh") can occur as well. Patients frequently report yawning and sneezing. Gastrointestinal symptoms, which initially may be mild (anorexia), can progress in moderate to severe withdrawal to include nausea, vomiting, and diarrhea.

Although some clinical features of opioid withdrawal overlap with symptoms of withdrawal from sedatives such as alcohol or benzodiazepines, opioid withdrawal is considered less likely to produce severe morbidity or mortality.[91] Seizures and death are rare, occurring typically in the setting of unattended moderate to severe withdrawal super-imposed upon preexisting underlying medical disorders that are prone to derangement from severe fluid or electrolyte loss.

However, the severe discomfort and accompanying opioid cravings that characterize opioid withdrawal often lead to continued opioid use[92] and heightened risk for overdose and other complications.

The severity of opioid withdrawal varies with the specific opioid used and the dose and duration of opioid use. Route of administration appears to be important as well. Data from one study suggests that injection opioid use is associated with significantly higher withdrawal symptom scores than inhaled opioid use for comparable heroin doses.[93] The time to onset of opioid withdrawal symptoms also depends on the half-life of the opioid being used. For example, withdrawal may begin 6 to 12 hours after the last use of heroin, but up to 72 hours after the last use of methadone.[83,85]

As with the onset of opioid withdrawal, the duration of withdrawal symptoms varies with the half-life of the opioid used and the duration of opioid use. For example, heroin withdrawal symptoms generally peak within 36 to 72 hours and may last for 7 to 10 days,[94] whereas methadone withdrawal may peak at 4 to 6 days and last for 14 to 21 days.[83] For short-acting opioids, the natural course of opioid withdrawal is generally relatively brief, but more intense and associated with a higher degree of discomfort than with equivalent doses of long-acting opioids. However, there is considerable individual variation; thus, severe early opioid withdrawal symptoms from methadone are possible, as are delayed severe heroin withdrawal symptoms.

Assessment and Diagnosis

Diagnosis of opioid withdrawal is largely based on the patient's history of opioid use and the presence of characteristic signs and symptoms of opioid withdrawal. Adulterants in the opioid supply may complicate the withdrawal picture. When initially evaluating opioid withdrawal and OUD, information about the timing and type of last opioid use, route of administration, quantity and frequency of opioid use, other substance use, and interest in initiating a medication for OUD treatment are of importance.

Several clinical tools are available to measure the severity of opioid withdrawal. One such tool is the Clinical Opiate Withdrawal Scale (COWS) (**Table 58-3**).[95] Other validated scales to assess opioid withdrawal include the 10-item Short Opioid Withdrawal Scale, which takes less than a minute to administer[96]; the 16-item Subjective Opioid Withdrawal Scale; and the 13-item Objective Opioid Withdrawal Scale.[97]

An evaluation for co-occurring medical conditions that may complicate the management of opioid withdrawal is important. The choice of pharmacotherapy used to treat acute opioid withdrawal and determination of the appropriate treatment setting (ie, inpatient versus outpatient) may be influenced by the presence and severity of a patient's underlying comorbidities.[45] Therefore, it is important for the clinician to obtain a comprehensive history, including a complete past medical and substance use history, mental health assessment, social history, and screening for social determinants of health.[98] Objective information including a physical examination and toxicology testing can detect specific findings consistent with opioid withdrawal to establish the diagnosis and identify other acute conditions. Screening for sexually transmitted infections, HIV, hepatitis C, tuberculosis, and pregnancy (if appropriate) is recommended.

Protracted opioid withdrawal, historically termed, "protracted abstinence syndrome," involves a variety of symptoms that persist beyond the typical acute withdrawal period.[99] Protracted withdrawal may include mild abnormalities in vital signs, continued craving, and ongoing sleep disturbance.[100] Despite the extensive literature on protracted opioid withdrawal, a universal definition and diagnostic criteria are lacking, making diagnosis difficult in individual patients.[101]

Management

As in the management of opioid intoxication and overdose, management of opioid withdrawal involves a combination of general supportive measures, specific pharmacological therapies, and linkage to long-term care. Be prepared to effectively treat opioid withdrawal and assure patients that their symptoms will be taken seriously as undertreated withdrawal can reduce engagement in future treatment.[102] Furthermore, many patients are unable to discontinue opioids without adequate opioid withdrawal management.[103,104]

The overall goals of managing opioid withdrawal include alleviating acute symptoms, engaging patients with OUD in treatment with first-line MOUD, and providing harm reduction education and resources to promote safer use and mitigate risks.[98] The treatment plan is guided by the patient's goals regarding their opioid use (eg, abstinence, reduced use, or ongoing opioid use) and preferences for available OUD treatment options. Thus, eliciting a patient's OUD treatment history and preferences for long-term treatment is important prior to starting opioid withdrawal management.

The decision to manage opioid withdrawal in an outpatient or inpatient setting depends on the presence of comorbid medical and psychiatric conditions, the availability of social supports (such as family members to provide monitoring and transportation), and the use of multiple substances. Access to resources for medically supervised withdrawal may also influence this decision; for example, opioid withdrawal management with methadone has been restricted in the United States by federal legislation to inpatient settings or licensed outpatient treatment programs.[105] An important exception to these restrictions is the so-called "72-hour rule" that allows clinicians outside of inpatient settings or licensed opioid treatment programs to administer methadone for opioid withdrawal for up to 72 hours in outpatient practice while arranging ongoing care.[106]

Pharmacological Therapies for Opioid Withdrawal

Several pharmacological therapies are available to treat symptoms of opioid withdrawal. These include full opioid agonists (eg, methadone), a partial agonist (eg, buprenorphine), or alpha-2 adrenergic agonists (eg, clonidine).[107] Nonopioid adjuvant medications may also be used to treat specific symptoms of opioid withdrawal. However, methadone and buprenorphine

TABLE 58-3 Clinical Opiate Withdrawal Scale

Resting pulse rate (record beats/min): *Measured after patient is sitting or lying for 1 min* 0 Pulse rate 80 or below 1 Pulse rate 81-100 2 Pulse rate 101-120 4 Pulse rate >120	GI upset (*over last half hour*): 0 No GI symptoms 1 Stomach cramps 2 Nausea or loose stool 3 Vomiting or diarrhea 5 Multiple episodes of diarrhea or vomiting
Sweating (*over past half hour not accounted for by room temperature or patient activity*): 0 No report of chills or flushing 1 Subjective report of chills or flushing 2 Flushed or observable moistness on face 3 Beads of sweat on brow or face 4 Sweat streaming off face	Tremor (*observation of outstretched hands*): 0 No tremor 1 Tremor can be felt, but not observed 2 Slight tremor observable 4 Gross tremor or muscle twitching
Restlessness (*observation during assessment*): 0 Able to sit still 1 Reports difficulty sitting still, but is able to do so 3 Frequent shifting or extraneous movements of legs/arms 5 Unable to sit still for more than a few seconds	Yawning (*observation during assessment*): 0 No yawning 1 Yawning once or twice during assessment 2 Yawning three or more times during assessment 4 Yawning several times/min
Pupil size: 0 Pupils pinned or normal size for room light 1 Pupils possibly larger than normal for room light 2 Pupils moderately dilated 5 Pupils so dilated that only the rim of the iris is visible	Anxiety or irritability: 0 None 1 Patient reports increasing irritability or anxiousness 2 Patient obviously irritable anxious 4 Patient so irritable or anxious that participation in the assessment is difficult
Bone or joint aches (*if the patient was having pain previously, only the additional component attributed to opiates withdrawal is scored*): 0 Not present 1 Mild diffuse discomfort 2 Patient reports severe diffuse aching of joints/muscles 4 Patient is rubbing joints or muscles and is unable to sit still because of discomfort	Gooseflesh skin: 0 Skin is smooth 3 Piloerection of skin can be felt or hairs standing up on arms 5 Prominent piloerection
Runny nose or tearing (*not accounted for by cold symptoms or allergies*): 0 Not present 1 Nasal stuffiness or unusually moist eyes 2 Nose running or tearing 4 Nose constantly running or tears streaming down cheeks	Total scores: Score: 5-12 = mild 13-24 = moderate 25-36 = moderately severe >36 = severe withdrawal

are considered first-line treatments for opioid withdrawal with comparable efficacy in alleviating withdrawal symptoms and completing withdrawal management over similar duration.[108]

Initiation of Medications for Opioid Use Disorder

Among patients who meet diagnostic criteria for OUD, the standard of care for managing opioid withdrawal involves initiating an opioid full agonist or partial agonist to both treat acute withdrawal symptoms and begin long-term MOUD treatment.[98] The choice of treatment should be guided by a patient's preference for and access to MOUD (eg, methadone, buprenorphine, or injectable naltrexone).[109]

For patients who prefer to start methadone or buprenorphine for ongoing MOUD treatment, the medication can be started with appropriate dose escalations to treat withdrawal symptoms and opioid cravings with the goal of achieving a therapeutic dose. Therapeutic doses can typically be reached over several days to weeks in both inpatient and outpatient settings.[98] For patients who prefer to start extended-release injectable naltrexone, opioid withdrawal should be treated with alpha-2 adrenergic agonists and other nonopioid therapies for at least 7 days until symptoms resolve and opioids are no longer detected on urine toxicology.[110] Patients who do not wish to start or cannot access long-term MOUD can be treated with tapering doses of opioid agonists (eg, methadone) or partial agonists (eg, buprenorphine) alone or in combination with alpha-2 adrenergic agonists and other adjunct medications. Harm reduction counseling, information about naloxone to prevent overdose-related mortality, and linkage to ongoing treatment is recommended for all patients.[98]

Opioid Agonists

Methadone

While methadone is considered a first-line treatment for opioid withdrawal, its availability for this indication varies internationally. In the United States, outpatient management of opioid withdrawal using methadone can only be employed by facilities licensed to dispense methadone for the treatment of OUD or through emerging applications of the 72-hour rule.[106,111] In the acute hospital setting, methadone can be used to treat opioid withdrawal and OUD without federal restriction in patients receiving medical or surgical treatment of other conditions.[112]

When choosing the initial dose of methadone, consider the potential risks of respiratory depression, sedation, and drug-drug interactions, including exposure to other QTc prolonging agents. Typically, in the inpatient setting, oral methadone is initiated at 20 to 30 mg and increased by 5 to 10 mg every 4 to 6 hours as needed for uncontrolled withdrawal symptoms.[109] The recommended maximum dose over the first 24 hours is 40 mg.[113] Subsequent dose increases can be provided in increments of 5 to 10 mg every 3 to 5 days until opioid withdrawal symptoms are adequately controlled.[98] In rare instances where hospitalized patients cannot safely tolerate oral formulations of methadone, intramuscular or intravenous methadone may be provided and dosed at half the dose of oral methadone.[114]

After a stabilizing dose has been reached, patients are ideally transitioned to long-term MOUD treatment in the outpatient setting. However, patients who prefer not to continue or cannot access ongoing methadone treatment can undergo a methadone taper prior to hospital discharge. Methadone can be tapered by 5 to 10 mg per day until discontinuation.[98] For patients receiving MOUD treatment with methadone in the outpatient setting who wish to discontinue treatment, dose tapering should be individualized and is typically more gradual, lasting as long as 6 months.[115] One study showed that even when coupled with enhanced psychosocial counseling, patients enrolled in 6-month methadone withdrawal management programs demonstrated greater illicit opioid use and greater substance-related HIV risk behaviors than patients enrolled in methadone maintenance.[116] Therefore, patients interested in discontinuing methadone treatment should be counseled on potential risks and offered alternative MOUD treatment, such as buprenorphine or extended-release injectable naltrexone.

Buprenorphine

Along with methadone, buprenorphine is considered a first-line treatment for both opioid withdrawal and OUD.

A Cochrane systematic review of 27 studies of over 3,000 participants found that buprenorphine for opioid withdrawal was superior to the alpha-2 adrenergic agonists, clonidine and lofexidine, and as effective as methadone for ameliorating withdrawal symptoms and completing withdrawal treatment.[108] It was also noted in this review that the duration of withdrawal symptoms may be significantly reduced with buprenorphine compared to methadone.[108] These findings are highlighted in a multicenter randomized clinical trial of a 13-day withdrawal management program using buprenorphine/naloxone versus clonidine. In this study of 113 inpatients and 231 outpatients, 77% of inpatients receiving buprenorphine/naloxone versus 22% of inpatients receiving clonidine and 29% of outpatients receiving buprenorphine/naloxone versus 5% of outpatients receiving clonidine achieved the combined end point of treatment retention and opioid-free urine at study completion.[117] Follow-up analysis on this population found that medication type was the single most important predictor of treatment completion and treatment success regardless of treatment setting.[118]

In order to minimize the risk of precipitated withdrawal, buprenorphine is initiated when patients have mild to moderate symptoms of opioid withdrawal.[109] A COWS score of 10 to 11 generally indicates sufficient withdrawal to safely initiate buprenorphine, although some clinicians recommend using a COWS score of 13 or higher among individuals exposed to fentanyl.[84] Sublingual buprenorphine combined with naloxone is the most common formulation used for opioid withdrawal, although buprenorphine hydrochloride formulations are also available. Buprenorphine is typically initiated at doses of 2 to 4 mg and increased every 1 to 2 hours by 2 to 4 mg as needed up to a total of 16 mg over the first 24 hours.[84,119] The dose can be further increased on a daily basis up to a recommended maximum cumulative daily dose of 24 mg.[111,120] Increasing buprenorphine doses earlier in treatment has been shown to reduce risk of returning to opioid use.[121]

In response to the increasing potency of the opioid drug supply with IMF and related challenges initiating buprenorphine for OUD, new dosing strategies have been described to initiate buprenorphine while avoiding or reducing the duration of withdrawal symptoms.[122-124] A potential mechanism for these challenges involves the lipophilic nature of fentanyl resulting in its rapid redistribution and storage in peripheral tissues and subsequent slow release back into the plasma, which produces a long-acting opioid effect despite its short duration of action.[125] Low-dose and high-dose buprenorphine initiation strategies have been proposed to overcome these challenges. Low-dose buprenorphine initiation involves starting low doses (eg, 0.5 mg/d) of the medication and gradually increasing the dose to therapeutic levels over the course of approximately 1 week (**Table 58-4**).[123,124] During this period, individuals continue to use full opioid agonists in the outpatient setting or receive full opioid agonists in the inpatient setting until the last day of the protocol; thus, they do not have to demonstrate mild-to-moderate withdrawal symptoms as recommended with traditional buprenorphine initiation.[123,124] High-dose buprenorphine initiation involves administering an initial dose of more than 12 mg and increasing the dose every 30 to 60 minutes up to a total dose of 32 mg to rapidly override opioid withdrawal symptoms and achieve a therapeutic dose.[83,126] While emerging evidence suggest these strategies are safe and effective,[126,127] traditional buprenorphine initiation remains the standard of care.

Novel extended-release buprenorphine formulations for the treatment of OUD have been developed in the form of depot injections administered every 7 days or every 28 days.[128,129] Emerging evidence has demonstrated the feasibility of

TABLE 58-4 Example Low-Dose Buprenorphine Initiation Protocol

Day	Buprenorphine dose (SL)	Full opioid agonist
1	0.5 mg once daily	Continue
2	0.5 mg twice daily	Continue
3	1 mg in morning 0.5 mg in afternoon 1 mg at night	Continue
4	2 mg twice daily	Continue
5	4 mg twice daily	Continue
6	4 mg three times daily	Continue
7	8 mg twice daily	Stop

Adapted from Cohen SM, Weimer MB, Levander XA, Peckham AM, Tetrault JM, Morford KL. Low dose initiation of buprenorphine: a narrative review and practical approach. *J Addict Med.* 2021;16(4):399-406.

administering extended-release buprenorphine during the first 24 to 72 hours of opioid withdrawal management.[130,131] However, these strategies are experimental and conflict with FDA labeling instructions for the 28-day formulation, which recommends stabilization for 7 days on a minimum of 8 mg sublingual buprenorphine before receiving the injection.[131]

Similar to methadone, patients with OUD can be continued on buprenorphine for ongoing treatment once a stabilizing dose has been reached. However, those who express a strong preference not to continue buprenorphine may be tapered by 2 to 4 mg daily until discontinuation and offered alternative MOUD options and harm reduction resources.[98]

Other Opioid Agonists

Data from observational studies and randomized clinical trials suggest that slow-release oral morphine is as effective as methadone for treating opioid withdrawal, opioid craving, or self-reported symptoms.[132,133] Initial doses are typically 30 to 60 mg and increased every 48 hours as needed to control withdrawal symptoms and suppress opioid craving up to a maximum dose of 400 mg/d.[119] Slow-release oral morphine is available as a third-line maintenance treatment for OUD in Canada[119] but is not currently approved for this indication in the United States.

Alpha-2 Adrenergic Medications

Clonidine and Lofexidine

Alpha-2 adrenergic agonists, such as clonidine and lofexidine, treat opioid withdrawal symptoms by blocking the noradrenergic hyperactivity of the locus coeruleus.[88,134] Clonidine and lofexidine are both administered orally. While lofexidine is FDA-approved for opioid withdrawal management,[135] clonidine is used off-label for this indication.

A Cochrane systematic review of 27 studies involving over 1,700 participants concluded that clonidine and lofexidine are more effective than placebo for ameliorating opioid withdrawal symptoms and completing treatment.[108] Clonidine and lofexidine also have shorter treatment durations compared to methadone.[108] Additionally, lofexidine has a better safety profile than clonidine with less associated hypotension.[108]

For the treatment of opioid withdrawal, most protocols suggest 0.1 mg of clonidine every 4 to 6 hours as needed for withdrawal discomfort on the first day, followed by an increase in clonidine by 0.1 or 0.2 mg/d, to a maximum total daily dose of 1.2 mg, with careful monitoring of blood pressure and withdrawal symptoms.[84] The average maximum daily dose is roughly 0.8 mg. Toward the end of the withdrawal management period (days 5 to 7 in heroin withdrawal management), the clonidine dose is tapered by 0.1 to 0.2 mg daily to avoid rebound hypertension, headaches, and the reemergence of withdrawal symptoms. Lofexidine is typically dosed at 0.54 mg (3 tablets) every 6 hours for a maximum daily dose of 2.88 mg (16 tablets) for up to 14 days.[84] Similar to clonidine, toward the end of the withdrawal management period, the lofexidine dose should be tapered over 2 to 4 days to discontinuation.[84]

Other Nonopioid Agents

A number of nonopioid adjuvant medications can be used for symptomatic treatment of opioid withdrawal. These medications may be used in cases where opioid agonist treatment is not available or preferred, or in combination with opioid agonists and/or alpha-2 adrenergic agonists to target specific symptoms.[84,98,111] Medications for targeted symptomatic treatment include loperamide for diarrhea, trazodone or doxepin for insomnia, acetaminophen and nonsteroidal anti-inflammatory drugs for pain, and antihistamines such as diphenhydramine and hydroxyzine for anxiety, among others.[84,98] Benzodiazepines may be considered in cases of severe anxiety,[84,111] but should be used with caution especially when combined with opioid agonists given increased risk of adverse effects.[136]

Several medications other than opioid agonists and alpha-2 adrenergic agonists have been investigated as primary or adjunctive treatments for opioid withdrawal but lack evidence to be adopted into standard practice. Memantine, a NMDA receptor antagonist, was found to have comparable efficacy to buprenorphine in improving objective signs of opioid withdrawal but not in improving subjective symptoms.[137] Tramadol, a centrally acting analgesic and variable mu-opioid agonist, has been shown to be superior to clonidine and as effective as methadone or buprenorphine for treating opioid withdrawal symptoms.[138,139] Investigations into the use of adjunctive gabapentin, an anticonvulsant, to ameliorate opioid withdrawal symptoms occurring during methadone-assisted withdrawal found that higher doses (1,600 mg) may have some efficacy.[140,141] Finally, anesthesia-assisted withdrawal management (ie, ultrarapid opioid detoxification), which involves administration of large doses of naloxone to precipitate withdrawal in an individual under general anesthesia, is not recommended due to serious risks including cardiac arrest and death.[84,142,143]

Patients may use nonprescribed treatments to self-treat opioid withdrawal. Kratom (*Mitragyna speciosa*) is a plant from Southeast Asia with stimulant and partial mu opioid agonist effects that is increasingly used for self-treatment of opioid withdrawal.[144,145] Kratom is traditionally ingested by chewing its leaves or brewing them into a tea but is more commonly available as an herbal supplement in the United States.[145] While preclinical data suggest that Kratom's main active alkaloid, mitragynine, has potential therapeutic value in treating opioid withdrawal, its safety and efficacy has not been established in humans.[146] Ibogaine is a psychoactive alkaloid derived from the rootbark of a Central African shrub, *Tabernanthe iboga*, that has been used in nonmedical settings to treat opioid withdrawal and OUD. Despite some evidence showing promise in alleviating opioid withdrawal symptoms and craving,[147] its use should be avoided due to safety concerns including risk of cardiotoxicity.[148] Cannabis is commonly used to self-treat opioid withdrawal symptoms.[149,150] Two randomized controlled trials demonstrated that dronabinol, a synthetic formulation of delta-9-tetrahydrocannabinol (THC), modestly reduced symptoms of opioid withdrawal but also produced euphoric effects and tachycardia.[151,152] While cannabis has not been rigorously investigated in humans, limited evidence suggests that cannabis may improve opioid withdrawal symptoms in some individuals while worsening symptoms in others.[150] Importantly, FDA-approved opioid agonist medications for treating opioid withdrawal and OUD are underutilized in practice and are recommended over unproven therapies.[153]

Co-Occurring Conditions

Withdrawal From Other Substances

Patients with co-occurring alcohol or benzodiazepine withdrawal in addition to opioid withdrawal often require inpatient treatment. In the case of alcohol withdrawal, validated screening instruments such as the revised clinical institute withdrawal assessment for alcohol scale (CIWA-Ar)[154] can be employed and used in conjunction with opioid withdrawal assessment tools,[155] although overlap between alcohol and opioid withdrawal symptoms may complicate the interpretation of these assessments. Recognizing unique symptoms of opioid withdrawal, such as piloerection and mydriasis, is important to assess response to opioid withdrawal management. Co-occurring withdrawal syndromes are treated concomitantly and do not preclude use of opioid agonists or partial agonists for opioid withdrawal management. Accordingly, use of benzodiazepines for treatment of alcohol or benzodiazepine withdrawal does not preclude initiation of MOUD.[156] Less severe substance withdrawal syndromes, such as those involving stimulants or nicotine, can also be appropriately managed. Although evidence to inform best practices is lacking, withdrawal from stimulants is typically managed conservatively with adequate hydration, symptomatic treatment, and a safe place to rest.[98,157] Tobacco withdrawal can be managed with nicotine replacement therapy.[158]

Acute and Chronic Pain

As opioid withdrawal itself can cause and worsen pain, it is important to appropriately address pain in conjunction with opioid withdrawal management, especially among patients with OUD who have acute or chronic pain from other sources.[159,160] Acute and chronic pain are best managed using a multimodal approach that includes a combination of nonpharmacologic treatments and nonopioid medications. In cases of severe acute pain in patients with OUD, opioid agonists may be used to provide adequate pain control but higher opioid doses are often required to account for increased opioid tolerance.[159] Patients receiving buprenorphine or methadone may also benefit from more frequent dosing (ie, dividing the total daily dose into smaller doses given BID or TID) to optimize the shorter-acting analgesic properties of these medications. For patients with chronic pain and OUD, buprenorphine has been shown to be an effective treatment for both these indications.[161,162]

Medical and Psychiatric Comorbidities

Addressing medical and psychiatric conditions that commonly occur in people with OUD is important in the course of managing opioid withdrawal.[47,58,163] Medical conditions such as acute bacterial infections, HIV, and HCV-related consequences may complicate the presentation and management. For instance, some studies suggest diminished expression of endogenous interferon-α and enhanced HCV viral replication in patients both using and withdrawing from opioids, suggesting that opioid use and withdrawal favor HCV persistence in hepatocytes.[164] Other studies suggest that intravenous drug use increases cytokine response in patients coinfected with HIV and HCV.[165] The presence of these conditions need not limit the treatment of opioid withdrawal symptoms with methadone or buprenorphine.[166-168] However, consider starting lower doses of buprenorphine in patients with severe chronic liver disease who may have decreased cytochrome P450 3A4 activity that metabolizes buprenorphine in the liver.[169] Evaluation and treatment of psychiatric conditions, including mood and anxiety disorders, is important.[163] Patients presenting with increased suicide risk or other unstable mental health conditions require psychiatric evaluation and may need inpatient psychiatric care following completion of opioid withdrawal management.

Pregnancy

Pregnancy testing is indicated in all patients of childbearing potential presenting with opioid withdrawal.[84] The recommended treatment for pregnant patients with OUD is initiation of MOUD with methadone or buprenorphine in combination with psychosocial treatment, rather than withdrawal management or psychosocial treatment alone.[84] While both of these medications have been shown to be safe and effective for treating OUD during pregnancy, buprenorphine has demonstrated improved neonatal outcomes compared with methadone.[170]

Opioid withdrawal management without initiation of MOUD is not recommended for pregnant patients given increased risk of adverse outcomes.[171,172]

Follow-Up Care

As with the management of opioid overdose, opioid withdrawal management is an important first step in the treatment of OUD. Withdrawal management alone, without plans for ongoing treatment, does not lead to optimal long term outcomes.[84] Thus, at the initiation of withdrawal management, arrangements for ongoing treatment need to be assured.

In general, withdrawal management programs focus solely on one aspect of OUD (ie, treatment of withdrawal) and often lack appropriate linkages to ongoing treatment services.[173,174] While the addition of psychosocial interventions to opioid withdrawal management have been found to improve treatment completion, opioid use during treatment, and adherence to clinic visits,[175] the most effective method of treating OUD is initiation and long-term treatment with MOUD.[120] Further research into withdrawal management-based treatments need to emphasize the importance of initiating MOUD, linkage to long-term MOUD treatment, OUD-specific counseling, and provision of harm reduction resources as part of comprehensive opioid withdrawal management in patients with OUD.

CONCLUSIONS

Familiarity with the basic pharmacological properties of opioids and their clinical manifestations is important for managing opioid intoxication, overdose, and withdrawal. Specific pharmacotherapies and treatment models can effectively manage opioid overdose and withdrawal and serve as a bridge to MOUD treatment. Management of severe opioid intoxication and overdose consists of acute supportive care and administration of naloxone to reverse the opioid effect. Among patients with OUD, an important part of comprehensive treatment is initiation of MOUD with linkage to ongoing care, along with provision of harm reduction resources and services, including overdose education and naloxone. Similarly, recognition and management of opioid withdrawal are critical among clinicians caring for patients in both inpatient and outpatient settings as withdrawal can lead to ongoing opioid use and adversely affect the management of other health conditions. Opioid withdrawal is best managed with opioid agonist medications with or without symptomatic treatment using non-opioid medications; however, the treatment plan is guided by patients' goals regarding their opioid use and preference for initiating MOUD. Ultimately, to address the opioid public health crisis, health care professionals need to be prepared to recognize and manage opioid intoxication, overdose, and withdrawal using a patient-centered approach to prevent further opioid-related harms and promote future treatment engagement.

REFERENCES

1. Trescot AM, Datta S, Lee M, Hansen H. Opioid pharmacology. *Pain Physician*. 2008;11(2 Suppl):S133-S153.
2. Nafziger AN, Barkin RL. Opioid therapy in acute and chronic pain. *J Clin Pharmacol*. 2018;58(9):1111-1122.
3. Dhaliwal A, Gupta M. *Physiology, Opioid Receptor*. StatPearls Publishing; 2022.
4. Kosten TR, George TP. The neurobiology of opioid dependence: implications for treatment. *Sci Pract Perspect*. 2002;1(1):13-20.
5. Substance Abuse and Mental Health Services Administration. *Key Substance Use and Mental Health Indicators in the United States: Results From the 2020 National Survey on Drug Use and Health*. Center for Behavioral Health Statistics and Quality, Substance Abuse and Mental Health Services Administration; 2021.
6. Pergolizzi J, Magnusson P, LeQuang JAK, Breve F. Illicitly manufactured fentanyl entering the United States. *Cureus*. 2021;13(8):e17496.
7. Sporer KA. Acute heroin overdose. *Ann Intern Med*. 1999;130(7):584.
8. Mattson CL, Kumar S, Tanz LJ, Patel P, Luo Q, Davis N. *Drug Overdose Deaths in 28 States and the District of Columbia: 2020 Data From the State Unintentional Drug Overdose Reporting System (SUDORS)*. Centers for Disease Control and Prevention, U.S. Department of Health and Human Services; 2022.
9. Boyer EW. Management of opioid analgesic overdose. *N Engl J Med*. 2012;367(2):146-155.
10. Comer SD, Cahill CM. Fentanyl: receptor pharmacology, abuse potential, and implications for treatment. *Neurosci Biobehav Rev*. 2019;106:49-57.
11. Burns G, DeRienz RT, Baker DD, Casavant M, Spiller HA. Could chest wall rigidity be a factor in rapid death from illicit fentanyl abuse? *Clin Toxicol (Phila)*. 2016;54(5):420-423.
12. Nicolakis J, Gmeiner G, Reiter C, Seltenhammer MH. Aspiration in lethal drug abuse—a consequence of opioid intoxication. *Int J Legal Med*. 2020;134(6):2121-2132.
13. Sporer KA, Dorn E. Heroin-related noncardiogenic pulmonary edema: a case series. *Chest*. 2001;120(5):1628-1632.
14. Rao SS, Mawn JG, Lobaton GO, et al. Opioid-related compartment syndrome and associated morbidity. *Injury*. 2019;50(8):1429-1432.
15. Babak K, Mohammad A, Mazaher G, Samaneh A, Fatemeh T. Clinical and laboratory findings of rhabdomyolysis in opioid overdose patients in the intensive care unit of a poisoning center in 2014 in Iran. *Epidemiol Health*. 2017;39:e2017050.
16. Kitchen SA, McCormack D, Werb D, et al. Trends and outcomes of serious complications associated with non-fatal opioid overdoses in Ontario, Canada. *Drug Alcohol Depend*. 2021;225:108830.
17. Melandri R, Re G, Lanzarini C, et al. Myocardial damage and rhabdomyolysis associated with prolonged hypoxic coma following opiate overdose. *J Toxicol Clin Toxicol*. 1996;34(2):199-203.
18. Opioids. In: *LiverTox: Clinical and Research Information on Drug-Induced Liver Injury*. National Institute of Diabetes and Digestive and Kidney Diseases; 2012.
19. Hassamal S, Miotto K, Dale W, Danovitch I. Tramadol: understanding the risk of serotonin syndrome and seizures. *Am J Med*. 2018;131(11):1382.e1-1382.e6.
20. Barash JA, Ganetsky M, Boyle KL, et al. Acute amnestic syndrome associated with fentanyl overdose. *N Engl J Med*. 2018;378(12):1157-1158.
21. Doshi R, Majmundar M, Kansara T, et al. Frequency of cardiovascular events and in-hospital mortality with opioid overdose hospitalizations. *Am J Cardiol*. 2019;124(10):1528-1533.
22. White JM, Irvine RJ. Mechanisms of fatal opioid overdose. *Addiction*. 1999;94(7):961-972.
23. Warner-Smith M, Darke S, Lynskey M, Hall W. Heroin overdose: causes and consequences. *Addiction*. 2001;96(8):1113-1125.
24. Tagliaro F, De Battisti Z, Smith FP, Marigo M. Death from heroin overdose: findings from hair analysis. *Lancet*. 1998;351(9120):1923-1925.

25. Binswanger IA, Blatchford BJ, Mueller SR, Stern MF. Mortality after prison release: opioid overdose and other causes of death, risk factors, and time trends from 1999 to 2009. *Ann Intern Med.* 2013;159(9):592-600.
26. Binswanger IA, Gordon AJ. From risk reduction to implementation: Addressing the opioid epidemic and continued challenges to our field. *Subst Abuse.* 2016;37(1):1-3.
27. Wines JD Jr, Saitz R, Horton NJ, Lloyd-Travaglini C, Samet JH. Overdose after detoxification: a prospective study. *Drug Alcohol Depend.* 2007; 89(2-3):161-169.
28. Darke S, Ross J. Fatal heroin overdoses resulting from non-injecting routes of administration, NSW, Australia, 1992-1996. *Addiction.* 2000;95(4):569-573.
29. National Institute on Drug Abuse. *Trends & Statistics: Overdose Death Rates.* Accessed June 6, 2023. https://nida.nih.gov/research-topics/trends-statistics/overdose-death-rates
30. Shah NG, Lathrop SL, Reichard RR, Landen MG. Unintentional drug overdose death trends in New Mexico, USA, 1990-2005: combinations of heroin, cocaine, prescription opioids and alcohol. *Addiction.* 2008;103(1):126-136.
31. Coffin PO, Galea S, Ahern J, Leon AC, Vlahov D, Tardiff K. Opiates, cocaine and alcohol combinations in accidental drug overdose deaths in New York City, 1990-98. *Addiction.* 2003;98(6):739-747.
32. Tori ME, Larochelle MR, Naimi TS. Alcohol or benzodiazepine co-involvement with opioid overdose deaths in the United States, 1999-2017. *JAMA Netw Open.* 2020;3(4):e202361.
33. Tomassoni AJ, Hawk KF, Jubanyik K, et al. Multiple fentanyl overdoses - New Haven, Connecticut, June 23, 2016. *MMWR Morbid Mortal Wkly Rep.* 2017;66(4):107-111.
34. LaRue L, Twillman RK, Dawson E, et al. Rate of fentanyl positivity among urine drug test results positive for cocaine or methamphetamine. *JAMA Netw Open.* 2019;2(4):e192851.
35. Friedman J, Godvin M, Shover C, Gone JP, Hansen H, Schriger D. Sharp increases in drug overdose deaths among high-school-age adolescents during the US COVID-19 epidemic and illicit fentanyl crisis. *Medrxiv.* 2021. doi:10.1101/2021.12.23.21268284
36. DEA. *One Pill Can Kill.* Accessed June 6, 2023. https://www.dea.gov/onepill
37. Gould LC. Changing patterns of multiple drug use among applicants to a multimodality drug treatment program. *Arch Gen Psychiatry.* 1974;31(3):408.
38. Burdzovic Andreas J, Lauritzen G, Nordfjaern T. Co-occurrence between mental distress and poly-drug use: a ten year prospective study of patients from substance abuse treatment. *Addict Behav.* 2015;48:71-78.
39. Jones CM, Logan J, Gladden RM, Bohm MK. Vital signs: demographic and substance use trends among heroin users—United States, 2002-2013. *MMWR Morb Mortal Wkly Rep.* 2015;64(26):719-725.
40. Dunton AW, Schwam E, Pitman V, McGrath J, Hendler J, Siegel J. Flumazenil: US clinical pharmacology studies. *Eur J Anaesthesiol Suppl.* 1988;2:81-95.
41. Sivilotti ML. Flumazenil, naloxone and the 'coma cocktail'. *Br J Clin Pharmacol.* 2016;81(3):428-436.
42. Hoffman JR, Schriger DL, Luo JS. The empiric use of naloxone in patients with altered mental status: a reappraisal. *Ann Emerg Med.* 1991;20(3):246-252.
43. Pergolizzi JV Jr, Webster LR, Vortsman E, LeQuang JA, Raffa RB. Wooden Chest syndrome: the atypical pharmacology of fentanyl overdose. *J Clin Pharm Ther.* 2021;46(6):1505-1508.
44. Torralva R, Janowsky A. Noradrenergic mechanisms in fentanyl-mediated rapid death explain failure of naloxone in the opioid crisis. *J Pharmacol Exp Ther.* 2019;371(2):453-475.
45. O'Connor PG, Samet JH, Stein MD. Management of hospitalized intravenous drug users: role of the internist. *Am J Med.* 1994;96(6): 551-558.
46. Whitley P, LaRue L, Fernandez SA, Passik SD, Dawson E, Jackson RD. Analysis of urine drug test results from substance use disorder treatment practices and overdose mortality rates, 2013-2020. *JAMA Netw Open.* 2022;5(6):e2215425.
47. O'Connor PG, Selwyn PA, Schottenfeld RS. Medical care for injection-drug users with human immunodeficiency virus infection. *N Engl J Med.* 1994;331(7):450-459.
48. Peters PJ, Pontones P, Hoover KW, et al. HIV Infection linked to injection use of oxymorphone in Indiana, 2014-2015. *N Engl J Med.* 2016;375(3):229-239.
49. Bradford M. Bilateral necrosis of earlobes and cheeks: another complication of cocaine contaminated with levamisole. *Ann Intern Med.* 2010;152(11):758.
50. Alexander RS, Canver BR, Sue KL, Morford KL. Xylazine and overdoses: trends, concerns, and recommendations. *Am J Public Health.* 2022;112(8):1212-1216.
51. Gladden RM, Chavez-Gray V, O'Donnell J, Goldberger BA. Notes from the field: overdose deaths involving eutylone (psychoactive bath salts)—United States, 2020. *MMWR Morb Mortal Wkly Rep.* 2022;71(32):1032-1034.
52. Krotulski AJ, Papsun DM, Chronister CW, et al. Eutylone intoxications—an emerging synthetic stimulant in forensic investigations. *J Anal Toxicol.* 2021;45(1):8-20.
53. Gaeta J, Bock B, Takach M. Providing a safe space and medical monitoring to prevent overdose deaths. *Health Affairs Blog.* 2016;31.
54. Merchant RM, Topjian AA, Panchal AR, et al. Part 1: executive summary: 2020 American Heart Association guidelines for cardiopulmonary resuscitation and emergency cardiovascular care. *Circulation.* 2020;142(16_Suppl_2):S337-S357.
55. Mueller SR, Walley AY, Calcaterra SL, Glanz JM, Binswanger IA. A review of opioid overdose prevention and naloxone prescribing: implications for translating community programming into clinical practice. *Subst Abus.* 2015;36(2):240-253.
56. Christenson J, Etherington J, Grafstein E, et al. Early discharge of patients with presumed opioid overdose: development of a clinical prediction rule. *Acad Emerg Med.* 2000;7(10):1110-1118.
57. Clemency BM, Eggleston W, Shaw EW, et al. Hospital observation upon reversal (hour) with naloxone: a prospective clinical prediction rule validation study. *Acad Emerg Med.* 2019;26(1):7-15.
58. Cherubin CE. The medical complications of drug addiction and the medical assessment of the intravenous drug user: 25 years later. *Ann Intern Med.* 1993;119(10):1017.
59. Sabzghabaee AM, Eizadi-Mood N, Yaraghi A, Zandifar S. Naloxone therapy in opioid overdose patients: intranasal or intravenous? A randomized clinical trial. *Arch Med Sci.* 2014;10(2):309-314.
60. Kerr D, Kelly A-M, Dietze P, Jolley D, Barger B. Randomized controlled trial comparing the effectiveness and safety of intranasal and intramuscular naloxone for the treatment of suspected heroin overdose. *Addiction.* 2009;104(12):2067-2074.
61. Yousefifard M, Vazirizadeh-Mahabadi MH, Neishaboori AM, et al. Intranasal versus intramuscular/intravenous naloxone for pre-hospital opioid overdose: a systematic review and meta-analysis. *Adv J Emerg Med.* 2020;4(2):e27.
62. Skulberg AK, Tylleskär I, Valberg M, et al. Comparison of intranasal and intramuscular naloxone in opioid overdoses managed by ambulance staff: a double-dummy, randomised, controlled trial. *Addiction.* 2022;117(6):1658-1667.
63. Dietze P, Jauncey M, Salmon A, et al. Effect of intranasal vs intramuscular naloxone on opioid overdose: a randomized clinical trial. *JAMA Netw Open.* 2019;2(11):e1914977.
64. LoVecchio F, Pizon A, Riley B, Sami A, D'Incognito C. Onset of symptoms after methadone overdose. *Am J Emerg Med.* 2007;25(1):57-59.
65. Eriksson O, Antoni G. [^{11}C]Carfentanil binds preferentially to μ-opioid receptor subtype 1 compared to subtype 2. *Mol Imaging.* 2015;14(9):7290.2015.00019.
66. O'Malley PA. "Gray Death"-the trojan horse of the opioid epidemic: historical, clinical, and safety evidence for the clinical nurse specialist. *Clin Nurse Spec.* 2017;31(6):304-308.
67. Chhabra N, Aks SE. Treatment of acute naloxone-precipitated opioid withdrawal with buprenorphine. *Am J Emerg Med.* 2020;38(3):691.e3-691.e4.

68. Evoy KE, Hill LG, Davis CS. Considering the potential benefits of over-the-counter naloxone. *Integr Pharm Res Pract*. 2021;10:13-21.
69. Rzasa Lynn R, Galinkin JL. Naloxone dosage for opioid reversal: current evidence and clinical implications. *Ther Adv Drug Saf*. 2018;9(1):63-88.
70. Pollini RA, McCall L, Mehta SH, Vlahov D, Strathdee SA. Non-fatal overdose and subsequent drug treatment among injection drug users. *Drug Alcohol Depend*. 2006;83(2):104-110.
71. Larochelle MR, Bernson D, Land T, et al. Medication for opioid use disorder after nonfatal opioid overdose and association with mortality: a cohort study. *Ann Intern Med*. 2018;169(3):137-145.
72. Calcaterra SL, Martin M, Bottner R, et al. Management of opioid use disorder and associated conditions among hospitalized adults: a consensus statement from the Society of Hospital Medicine. *J Hosp Med*. 2022;17(9):744-756.
73. Weinstein ZM, Wakeman SE, Nolan S. Inpatient addiction consult service: expertise for hospitalized patients with complex addiction problems. *Med Clin North Am*. 2018;102(4):587-601.
74. Englander H, Dobbertin K, Lind BK, et al. Inpatient addiction medicine consultation and post-hospital substance use disorder treatment engagement: a propensity-matched analysis. *J Gen Intern Med*. 2019;34(12):2796-2803.
75. D'Onofrio G, O'Connor PG, Pantalon MV, et al. Emergency department-initiated buprenorphine/naloxone treatment for opioid dependence: a randomized clinical trial. *JAMA*. 2015;313(16):1636-1644.
76. SAMHSA. *Medication-Assisted Treatment Services Locators*. Accessed September 8, 2022. https://www.samhsa.gov/medication-assisted-treatment/find-treatment
77. Hesse M, Vanderplasschen W, Rapp RC, Broekaert E, Fridell M. Case management for persons with substance use disorders. *Cochrane Database Syst Rev*. 2007;(4):CD006265.
78. Rapp RC, Van Den Noortgate W, Broekaert E, Vanderplasschen W. The efficacy of case management with persons who have substance abuse problems: a three-level meta-analysis of outcomes. *J Consult Clin Psychol*. 2014;82(4):605-618.
79. Vanderplasschen W, Rapp RC, De Maeyer J, Van Den Noortgate W. A meta-analysis of the efficacy of case management for substance use disorders: a recovery perspective. *Front Psychiatry*. 2019;10:186.
80. Gormley MA, Pericot-Valverde I, Diaz L, et al. Effectiveness of peer recovery support services on stages of the opioid use disorder treatment cascade: a systematic review. *Drug Alcohol Depend*. 2021;229(Pt B):109123.
81. Williams JT, Ingram SL, Henderson G, et al. Regulation of μ-opioid receptors: desensitization, phosphorylation, internalization, and tolerance. *Pharmacol Rev*. 2013;65(1):223-254.
82. Volkow ND, Koob GF, McLellan AT. Neurobiologic advances from the brain disease model of addiction. *N Engl J Med*. 2016;374(4):363-371.
83. Herring AA, Perrone J, Nelson LS. Managing opioid withdrawal in the emergency department with buprenorphine. *Ann Emerg Med*. 2019;73(5):481-487.
84. The ASAM National Practice Guideline for the Treatment of Opioid Use Disorder: 2020 Focused Update. *J Addict Med*. 2020;14(2S Suppl 1):1-91.
85. Kosten TR, Baxter LE. Review article: effective management of opioid withdrawal symptoms: a gateway to opioid dependence treatment. *Am J Addict*. 2019;28(2):55-62.
86. Gunne L-M. Noradrenaline and adrenaline in the rat brain during acute and chronic morphine administration and during withdrawal. *Nature*. 1959;184(4703):1950-1951.
87. Mazei-Robison MS, Nestler EJ. Opiate-induced molecular and cellular plasticity of ventral tegmental area and locus coeruleus catecholamine neurons. *Cold Spring Harb Perspect Med*. 2012;2(7):a012070.
88. Aghajanian GK. Tolerance of locus coeruleus neurones to morphine and suppression of withdrawal response by clonidine. *Nature*. 1978;276(5684):186-188.
89. Gold M, Redmond DE, Kleber H. Clonidine blocks acute opiate-withdrawal symptoms. *Lancet*. 1978;312(8090):599-602.
90. Crawley JN, Laverty R, Roth RH. Clonidine reversal of increased norepinephrine metabolite levels during morphine withdrawal. *Eur J Pharmacol*. 1979;57(2-3):247-250.
91. Long D, Long B, Koyfman A. The emergency medicine management of severe alcohol withdrawal. *Am J Emerg Med*. 2017;35(7):1005-1011.
92. Cicero TJ, Ellis MS. The prescription opioid epidemic: a review of qualitative studies on the progression from initial use to abuse. *Dialogues Clin Neurosci*. 2017;19(3):259-269.
93. Smolka M, Schmidt LG. The influence of heroin dose and route of administration on the severity of the opiate withdrawal syndrome. *Addiction*. 1999;94(8):1191-1198.
94. Kosten TR, O'Connor PG. Management of drug and alcohol withdrawal. *N Engl J Med*. 2003;348(18):1786-1795.
95. Wesson DR, Ling W. The Clinical Opiate Withdrawal Scale (COWS). *J Psychoactive Drugs*. 2003;35(2):253-259.
96. Gossop M. The development of a short opiate withdrawal scale (SOWS). *Addict Behav*. 1990;15(5):487-490.
97. Handelsman L, Cochrane KJ, Aronson MJ, Ness R, Rubinstein KJ, Kanof PD. Two new rating scales for opiate withdrawal. *Am J Drug Alcohol Abuse*. 1987;13(3):293-308.
98. Torres-Lockhart KE, Lu TY, Weimer MB, Stein MR, Cunningham CO. Clinical management of opioid withdrawal. *Addiction*. 2022;117(9):2540-2550.
99. Schuckit MA. Opiates and other analgesics. In: *Drug and Alcohol Abuse*. Springer; 1989:118-142.
100. Lai Wen H, Ho WKK, Wen PYC. Comparison of the effectiveness of different opioid peptides in suppressing heroin withdrawal. *Eur J Pharmacol*. 1984;100(2):155-162.
101. Satel SL, Kosten TR, Schuckit MA, Fischman MW. Should protracted withdrawal from drugs be included in DSM-IV? *Am J Psychiatry*. 1993;150(5):695-704.
102. Mitchell SG, Kelly SM, Brown BS, et al. Incarceration and opioid withdrawal: the experiences of methadone patients and out-of-treatment heroin users. *J Psychoactive Drugs*. 2009;41(2):145-152.
103. Mattick RP, Kimber J, Breen C, Davoli M. Buprenorphine maintenance versus placebo or methadone maintenance for opioid dependence. *Cochrane Database Syst Rev*. 2014;(2):CD002207.
104. Jarvis BP, Holtyn AF, Subramaniam S, et al. Extended-release injectable naltrexone for opioid use disorder: a systematic review. *Addiction*. 2018;113(7):1188-1209.
105. Substance Abuse and Mental Health Services Administration. *Federal Guidelines for Opioid Treatment Programs*. SAMHSA; 2015.
106. Taylor JL, Laks J, Christine PJ, et al. Bridge clinic implementation of "72-hour rule" methadone for opioid withdrawal management: Impact on opioid treatment program linkage and retention in care. *Drug Alcohol Depend*. 2022;236:109497. doi: 10.1016/j.drugalcdep.2022.109497
107. O'Connor PG, Fiellin DA. Pharmacologic treatment of heroin-dependent patients. *Ann Intern Med*. 2000;133(1):40.
108. Gowing L, Ali R, White JM, Mbewe D. Buprenorphine for managing opioid withdrawal. *Cochrane Database Syst Rev*. 2017;2(2):CD002025.
109. Calcaterra SL, Bottner R, Martin M, et al. Management of opioid use disorder, opioid withdrawal, and opioid overdose prevention in hospitalized adults: a systematic review of existing guidelines. *J Hosp Med*. 2022;17(9):679-692.
110. Lee JD, Nunes EV Jr, Novo P, et al. Comparative effectiveness of extended-release naltrexone versus buprenorphine-naloxone for opioid relapse prevention (X:BOT): a multicentre, open-label, randomised controlled trial. *Lancet*. 2018;391(10118):309-318.
111. Kampman K, Jarvis M. American Society of Addiction Medicine (ASAM) National Practice Guideline for the use of medications in the treatment of addiction involving opioid use. *J Addict Med*. 2015;9(5):358-367.
112. Code of Federal Regulations 1306.07. *Administering or Dispensing of Narcotic Drugs*. 2022.
113. Chou R, Cruciani RA, Fiellin DA, et al. Methadone safety: a clinical practice guideline from the American Pain Society and College on Problems of Drug Dependence, in collaboration with the Heart Rhythm Society. *J Pain*. 2014;15(4):321-337.

114. González-Barboteo J, Porta-Sales J, Sánchez D, Tuca A, Gómez-Batiste X. Conversion from parenteral to oral methadone. *J Pain Palliat Care Pharmacother*. 2008;22(3):200-205.
115. Margolin A, Kosten T, Miller N. *Opioid Detoxification and Maintenance with Blocking Agents*. Marcel Dekker, Inc; 1991.
116. Sees KL, Delucchi KL, Masson C, et al. Methadone maintenance vs 180-day psychosocially enriched detoxification for treatment of opioid dependence. *JAMA*. 2000;283(10):1303.
117. Ling W, Amass L, Shoptaw S, et al. A multi-center randomized trial of buprenorphine-naloxone versus clonidine for opioid detoxification: findings from the National Institute on Drug Abuse Clinical Trials Network. *Addiction*. 2005;100(8):1090-1100.
118. Ziedonis DM, Amass L, Steinberg M, et al. Predictors of outcome for short-term medically supervised opioid withdrawal during a randomized, multicenter trial of buprenorphine-naloxone and clonidine in the NIDA clinical trials network drug and alcohol dependence. *Drug Alcohol Depend*. 2009;99(1-3):28-36.
119. British Columbia Centre on Substance Use and BC Ministry of Health. *A Guideline for the Clinical Management of Opioid Use Disorder*; 2017.
120. Substance Abuse and Mental Health Services Administration. *Medications for Opioid Use Disorder: For Healthcare and Addiction Professionals, Policymakers, Patients, and Families*. SAMHSA; 2018.
121. Rudolph KE, Shulman M, Fishman M, Díaz I, Rotrosen J, Nunes EV. Association between dynamic dose increases of buprenorphine for treatment of opioid use disorder and risk of relapse. *Addiction*. 2022;117(3):637-645.
122. Greenwald MK, Herring AA, Perrone J, Nelson LS, Azar P. A neuro-pharmacological model to explain buprenorphine induction challenges. *Ann Emerg Med*. 2022;80(6):509-524.
123. Bhatraju EP, Klein JW, Hall AN, et al. Low dose buprenorphine induction with full agonist overlap in hospitalized patients with opioid use disorder: a retrospective cohort study. *J Addict Med*. 2022;16(4): 461-465.
124. Cohen SM, Weimer MB, Levander XA, Peckham AM, Tetrault JM, Morford KL. Low dose initiation of buprenorphine: a narrative review and practical approach. *J Addict Med*. 2021;16(4):399-406.
125. Shearer D, Young S, Fairbairn S, Brar R. Challenges with buprenorphine inductions in the context of the fentanyl overdose crisis: a case series. *Drug Alcohol Rev*. 2022;41(2):444-448.
126. Herring AA, Vosooghi AA, Luftig J, et al. High-dose buprenorphine induction in the emergency department for treatment of opioid use disorder. *JAMA Netw Open*. 2021;4(7):e2117128.
127. Spreen LA, Dittmar EN, Quirk KC, Smith MA. Buprenorphine initiation strategies for opioid use disorder and pain management: a systematic review. *Pharmacotherapy*. 2022;42(5):411-427.
128. Haight BR, Learned SM, Laffont CM, et al. Efficacy and safety of a monthly buprenorphine depot injection for opioid use disorder: a multicentre, randomised, double-blind, placebo-controlled, phase 3 trial. *Lancet*. 2019;393(10173):778-790.
129. Lofwall MR, Walsh SL, Nunes EV, et al. Weekly and monthly subcutaneous buprenorphine depot formulations vs daily sublingual buprenorphine with naloxone for treatment of opioid use disorder: a randomized clinical trial. *JAMA Intern Med*. 2018;178(6):764-773.
130. Mariani JJ, Mahony AL, Iqbal MN, Luo SX, Naqvi NH, Levin FR. Case series: rapid induction onto long acting buprenorphine injection for high potency synthetic opioid users. *Am J Addict*. 2020;29(4):345-348.
131. Mariani JJ, Mahony AL, Podell SC, et al. Open-label trial of a single-day induction onto buprenorphine extended-release injection for users of heroin and fentanyl. *Am J Addict*. 2021;30(5):470-476.
132. Kastelic A, Dubajic G, Strbad E. Slow-release oral morphine for maintenance treatment of opioid addicts intolerant to methadone or with inadequate withdrawal suppression. *Addiction*. 2008;103(11):1837-1846.
133. Madlung-Kratzer E, Spitzer B, Brosch R, Dunkel D, Haring C. A double-blind, randomized, parallel group study to compare the efficacy, safety and tolerability of slow-release oral morphine versus methadone in opioid-dependent in-patients willing to undergo detoxification. *Addiction*. 2009;104(9):1549-1557.
134. Gowing L, Farrell M, Ali R, White J. Alpha$_2$-adrenergic agonists for the management of opioid withdrawal. *Cochrane Database Syst Rev*. 2004;(4):CD002024.
135. Doughty B, Morgenson D, Brooks T. Lofexidine: a newly FDA-approved, nonopioid treatment for opioid withdrawal. *Ann Pharmacother*. 2019;53(7):746-753.
136. Crotty K, Freedman KI, Kampman KM. Executive summary of the focused update of the ASAM National Practice Guideline for the Treatment of Opioid Use Disorder. *J Addict Med*. 2020;14(2):99-112.
137. Jain MDK, Jain PFCR, Dhawan MDA. A double-blind, double-dummy, randomized controlled study of memantine versus buprenorphine in naloxone-precipitated acute withdrawal in heroin addicts. *J Opioid Manag*. 2018;7(1):11-20.
138. Dunn KE, Tompkins DA, Bigelow GE, Strain EC. Efficacy of tramadol extended-release for opioid withdrawal: a randomized clinical trial. *JAMA Psychiatry*. 2017;74(9):885-893.
139. Zarghami M, Masoum B, Shiran M-R. Tramadol versus methadone for treatment of opiate withdrawal: a double-blind, randomized, clinical trial. *J Addict Dis*. 2012;31(2):112-117.
140. Kheirabadi GR, Ranjkesh M, Maracy MR, Salehi M. Effect of add-on gabapentin on opioid withdrawal symptoms in opium-dependent patients. *Addiction*. 2008;103(9):1495-1499.
141. Salehi M, Kheirabadi GR, Maracy MR, Ranjkesh M. Importance of gabapentin dose in treatment of opioid withdrawal. *J Clin Psychopharmacol*. 2011;31(5):593-596.
142. Hamilton RJ, Olmedo RE, Shah S, et al. Complications of ultrarapid opioid detoxification with subcutaneous naltrexone pellets. *Acad Emerg Med*. 2002;9(1):63-68.
143. Gowing L, Ali R, White JM. Opioid antagonists under heavy sedation or anaesthesia for opioid withdrawal. *Cochrane Database Syst Rev*. 2010;(1):CD002022.
144. Prozialeck WC, Avery BA, Boyer EW, et al. Kratom policy: the challenge of balancing therapeutic potential with public safety. *Int J Drug Policy*. 2019;70:70-77.
145. Prozialeck WC, Jivan JK, Andurkar SV. Pharmacology of kratom: an emerging botanical agent with stimulant, analgesic and opioid-like effects. *J Am Osteopath Assoc*. 2012;112(12):792-799.
146. Harun N, Kamaruzaman NA, Sofian ZM, Hassan Z. Mini review: potential therapeutic values of mitragynine as an opioid substitution therapy. *Neurosci Lett*. 2022;773:136500.
147. Malcolm BJ, Polanco M, Barsuglia JP. Changes in withdrawal and craving scores in participants undergoing opioid detoxification utilizing ibogaine. *J Psychoactive Drugs*. 2018;50(3):256-265.
148. Knuijver T, Schellekens A, Belgers M, et al. Safety of ibogaine administration in detoxification of opioid-dependent individuals: a descriptive open-label observational study. *Addiction*. 2022;117(1):118-128.
149. Meacham MC, Nobles AL, Tompkins DA, Thrul J. "I got a bunch of weed to help me through the withdrawals": naturalistic cannabis use reported in online opioid and opioid recovery community discussion forums. *PLoS One*. 2022;17(2):e0263583.
150. Bergeria CL, Huhn AS, Dunn KE. The impact of naturalistic cannabis use on self-reported opioid withdrawal. *J Subst Abuse Treat*. 2020;113:108005.
151. Bisaga A, Sullivan MA, Glass A, et al. The effects of dronabinol during detoxification and the initiation of treatment with extended release naltrexone. *Drug Alcohol Depend*. 2015;154:38-45.
152. Lofwall MR, Babalonis S, Nuzzo PA, Elayi SC, Walsh SL. Opioid withdrawal suppression efficacy of oral dronabinol in opioid dependent humans. *Drug Alcohol Depend*. 2016;164:143-150.
153. Humphreys K, Saitz R. Should physicians recommend replacing opioids with cannabis? *JAMA*. 2019;321(7):639-640.
154. Sullivan JT, Sykora K, Schneiderman J, Naranjo CA, Sellers EM. Assessment of alcohol withdrawal: the revised clinical institute withdrawal assessment for alcohol scale (CIWA-Ar). *Br J Addict*. 1989;84(11):1353-1357.
155. Lindsay DL, Freedman K, Jarvis M, et al. Executive summary of the American Society of Addiction Medicine (ASAM) clinical practice guideline on alcohol withdrawal management. *J Addict Med*. 2020;14(5):376-392.

156. Drug Safety Communications. *FDA Urges Caution About Withholding Opioid Addiction Medications Whom Patients Taking Benzodiazepines or CNS Depressants: Careful Medication Management Can Reduce Risks* [press release]; 2017.
157. Pennay AE, Lee NK. Putting the call out for more research: the poor evidence base for treating methamphetamine withdrawal. *Drug Alcohol Rev*. 2011;30(2):216-222.
158. Hartmann-Boyce J, Chepkin SC, Ye W, Bullen C, Lancaster T. Nicotine replacement therapy versus control for smoking cessation. *Cochrane Database Syst Rev*. 2018;5(5):CD000146.
159. Alford DP, Compton P, Samet JH. Acute pain management for patients receiving maintenance methadone or buprenorphine therapy. *Ann Intern Med*. 2006;144(2):127-134.
160. Hser YI, Mooney LJ, Saxon AJ, Miotto K, Bell DS. Chronic pain among patients with opioid use disorder: results from electronic health records data. *J Subst Abuse Treat*. 2017;77:26-30.
161. Oldfield BJ, Edens EL, Agnoli A, et al. Multimodal treatment options, including rotating to buprenorphine, within a multidisciplinary pain clinic for patients on risky opioid regimens: a quality improvement study. *Pain Med*. 2018;19(suppl_1):S38-S45.
162. Cote J, Montgomery L. Sublingual buprenorphine as an analgesic in chronic pain: a systematic review. *Pain Med*. 2014;15(7):1171-1178.
163. Substance Abuse and Mental Health Services Administration. *Substance Use Treatment for Persons with Co-Occurring Disorders*. SAMHSA; 2020.
164. Wang C-Q, Li Y, Douglas SD, et al. Morphine withdrawal enhances hepatitis C virus replicon expression, *Am J Pathol*. 2005;167(5):1333-1340.
165. Jackson AH, Shader RI. Guidelines for the withdrawal of narcotic and general depressant drugs. *Dis Nerv Syst*. 1973;34(3):162-166.
166. Tetrault JM, Tate JP, Edelman EJ, et al. Hepatic safety of buprenorphine in HIV-infected and uninfected patients with opioid use disorder: the role of HCV-infection. *J Subst Abuse Treat*. 2016;68:62-67.
167. Gourevitch MN, Friedland GH. Interactions between methadone and medications used to treat HIV infection: a review. *Mt Sinai J Med*. 2000;67(5-6):429-436.
168. McCance-Katz EF. Treatment of opioid dependence and coinfection with HIV and hepatitis C virus in opioid-dependent patients: the importance of drug interactions between opioids and antiretroviral agents. *Clin Infect Dis*. 2005;41(Suppl 1):S89-S95.
169. Elkader A, Sproule B. Buprenorphine: clinical pharmacokinetics in the treatment of opioid dependence. *Clin Pharmacokinet*. 2005;44(7):661-680.
170. Jones HE, Kaltenbach K, Heil SH, et al. Neonatal abstinence syndrome after methadone or buprenorphine exposure. *N Engl J Med*. 2010; 363(24):2320-2331.
171. Terplan M, Laird HJ, Hand DJ, et al. Opioid detoxification during pregnancy: a systematic review. *Obstet Gynecol*. 2018;131(5):803-814.
172. Wang MJ, Kuper SG, Sims B, et al. Opioid detoxification in pregnancy: systematic review and meta-analysis of perinatal outcomes. *Am J Perinatol*. 2019;36(6):581-587.
173. O'Connor PG. Methods of detoxification and their role in treating patients with opioid dependence. *JAMA*. 2005;294(8):961-963.
174. Zhu H, Wu LT. National trends and characteristics of inpatient detoxification for drug use disorders in the United States. *BMC Public Health*. 2018;18(1):1073.
175. Amato L, Minozzi S, Davoli M, Vecchi S, Ferri MF, Mayet S. Psychosocial and pharmacological treatments versus pharmacological treatments for opioid detoxification. *Cochrane Database of Syst Rev*. 2008;(3):CD005031.

59 Management of Stimulant, Hallucinogen, Cannabis, Phencyclidine, and Other Drug Intoxication and Withdrawal

Jeffery N. Wilkins, David A. Gorelick, Itai Danovitch, Nicholas Athanasiou, and Steven Allen

CHAPTER OUTLINE

- Introduction
- Stimulants
- Hallucinogens
- Cannabis
- Dissociative anesthetics
- Inhalants
- Kratom
- Club drugs
- MDMA ("ecstasy")
- Gamma-hydroxybutyrate
- Psychoactive herbs
- Flunitrazepam
- Withdrawal from multiple drugs
- Population-specific considerations

INTRODUCTION

This chapter reviews the treatment of acute intoxication and withdrawal states associated with the use of stimulants such as cocaine and amphetamine-type stimulants (ATS); hallucinogens such as lysergic acid diethylamide (LSD); cannabis; dissociative anesthetics such as phencyclidine (PCP), ketamine, and dextromethorphan (DXM); kratom; "club drugs" such as 3,4-methylenedioxymethamphetamine (MDMA or "ecstasy") and gamma-hydroxybutyrate (GHB); and psychoactive plant materials referred to as herbals. It also reviews withdrawal from multiple substances. Psychiatric and medical complications are considered separately because they often are treated differently and in different settings (eg, in psychiatric versus medical emergency departments). Not all of the substances reviewed here have clinically distinct intoxication or withdrawal syndromes nor are there pharmacological treatments for all such syndromes.

Successful treatment of acute intoxication, overdose, or withdrawal can facilitate entry into addiction treatment by reducing uncomfortable withdrawal symptoms that negatively reinforce taking an illicit substance. Even when successful, these early stages of treatment often are followed by return to substance use, with patients potentially reentering a "revolving door" of repeated withdrawal management programs. Short-term treatment of acute intoxication or withdrawal does not obviate the need for long-term treatment of the substance use disorder.

Pharmacological treatment of drug intoxication and overdose generally follows one of three approaches including; increasing the clearance of drugs from the body, either by increasing catabolism or by increasing excretion, or both;[1] blockade of the neuronal site to which the drug binds to exert its effect (as through the use of naloxone to block the mu-opioid receptor in the treatment of opiate overdose); and counteracting effects of the drug through alternative neuropharmacological action.

Pharmacological treatment of any drug withdrawal syndrome generally follows one of the two approaches: suppression by a cross-tolerant medication from the same pharmacological class—usually a longer-acting one to provide a milder, albeit longer, withdrawal—and/or reducing the signs and symptoms of withdrawal by targeting the neurochemical or receptor systems that mediate withdrawal (as in the use of clonidine, a nonopioid medication, to treat opioid withdrawal syndrome).[2]

The application of these pharmacological treatment approaches to the drugs reviewed in this chapter is limited. There may be no practical method for altering drug clearance (as with cannabis) or no specific drug receptor sites may have been identified. Even when a receptor site has been identified, there may not be a clinically useful antagonist. Finally, current understanding of the neuropharmacological processes that mediate intoxication or withdrawal may be too limited to suggest appropriate pharmacological interventions. Thus, clinical stabilization, supportive management, and palliation of symptoms remain the mainstays of treatment.

STIMULANTS

Stimulant Intoxication

The acute psychological and medical effects of cocaine, amphetamines, and other stimulants are attributable principally to increases in catecholamine neurotransmitter activity. Enhanced catecholamine activity occurs through blockade of the presynaptic neurotransmitter reuptake pumps (as by cocaine) or by presynaptic release of catecholamines (as by amphetamines).[3] Resulting stimulation of the corticomesolimbic dopaminergic brain reward circuit mediates the psychological effects of stimulants. The resulting stimulation of the sympathetic nervous system leads to peripheral vasoconstriction (with organ ischemia), increased heart rate, and lowered seizure threshold, among other adverse effects. **Table 59-1** lists acute medical complications of stimulant intoxication.

Blockade of presynaptic catecholamine reuptake sites or postsynaptic receptors should, in principle, be an effective treatment for stimulant intoxication. Several medications have attenuated the acute subjective effects of stimulants in phase I human laboratory studies, but none has been evaluated clinically.

Another method for treating stimulant intoxication might be to decrease drug availability in the central nervous system (CNS) by binding it peripherally with antidrug antibodies or by increasing its catabolism with catalytic antibodies or with the endogenous cocaine-metabolizing enzyme butyrylcholinesterase (BChE, E.C. 3.1.1.8) or other esterases.[1] Treatment with a genetically enhanced bacterial cocaine esterase (IV)[4] or BChE (conjugated to albumin: sc)[5] significantly reduced the acute subjective and cardiovascular effects of an IV cocaine challenge in phase I studies.

Table 59-2 gives an overview of treatment for the acute psychiatric and medical complications of stimulant intoxication.

TABLE 59-1 Acute Medical Complications Associated With Stimulant Intoxication

Organ system	Physical effects
Head, ears, eyes, nose, throat	Pupil dilation; headache; bruxism
Pulmonary[a]	Hyperventilation, dyspnea; cough; chest pain; wheezing; hemoptysis; acute exacerbation of asthma; barotrauma (pneumothorax, pneumomediastinum); pulmonary edema
Cardiovascular	Tachycardia; palpitations; increased blood pressure; arrhythmia; chest pain; myocardial ischemia or infarction; ruptured aneurysm; cardiogenic shock
Neurologic	Headache; agitation; psychosis; tremor, hyperreflexia; small muscle twitching; tics; stereotyped movements; myoclonus; seizures; cerebral hemorrhage or infarct (stroke); cerebral edema
Gastrointestinal	Nausea, vomiting; mesenteric ischemia; bowel infarction or perforation
Renal	Diuresis; myoglobinuria; acute renal failure
Body temperature	Mild fever; malignant hyperthermia
Others	Rhabdomyolysis

[a]All pulmonary complications except hyperventilation and pulmonary edema come primarily from the smoked route of administration.

From Docherty JR, Alsufanyi HA. Pharmacology of drugs used as stimulants. *J Clin Pharmacol.* 2021;61(S2):S53-S69; Ciccarone D, Shoptaw S. Understanding stimulant use and use disorders in a new era. *Med Clin N Am.* 2022;106:81-97; Richards JR, Wang CG, Fontenette RW, et al. Rhabdomyolysis, methamphetamine, amphetamine and MDMA use: associated factors and risks. *J Dual Diagn.* 2020;16(4):429-437; Kim ST, Park T. Acute and chronic effects of cocaine on cardiovascular health. *Int J Mol Sci.* 2019;20:584; Lappin JM, Sara GE. Psychostimulant use and the brain. *Addiction.* 2019;114:2065-2077; Tseng W, Sutter ME, Albertson TE. Stimulants and the lung: review of literature. *Clin Rev Allergy Immunol.* 2014;46(1):82-100.

Psychological and Behavioral Effects of Stimulant Intoxication

The initial effects of stimulant intoxication include increased energy, alertness, and sociability, elation, euphoria, and decreased fatigue, need for sleep, and appetite.[6,7] At this stage, treatment may not be sought or needed. With high dose or repeated use, stimulant intoxication usually progresses to unwanted effects such as anxiety, irritability, interpersonal sensitivity, hypervigilance, suspiciousness, grandiosity, impaired judgment, stereotyped behavior, and psychotic symptoms such as paranoia and hallucinations. Up to three-quarters of persons who use stimulants report paranoia or psychotic symptoms associated with their use, although the contribution of acute versus chronic stimulant exposure is unclear,[8] and findings may reflect selection bias among these persons who come to attention of clinicians. Persons who use stimulants typically remain alert and oriented, but the intoxicated state may impair judgment, cognition, and attention.

Patients with stimulant-induced psychoses may closely resemble those with acute schizophrenia and may be misdiagnosed as such.[8] Cocaine-induced psychosis may differ from acute schizophrenic psychosis in having less thought disorder and less bizarre delusions and fewer negative symptoms such as alogia and inattention. Stimulant-induced hallucinations may be auditory, visual, or somatosensory.[8,9] Tactile hallucinations are especially typical of stimulant psychosis, such as the sensation of something crawling under the skin (formication). Specific genetic variations may account for some differences in individual vulnerability to stimulant-induced psychosis.[10] Panic reactions are common and may evolve into a panic disorder. This may be exacerbated by anxiety elicited by the physiological symptoms commonly associated with stimulant use, such as palpitations and hyperventilation.

Very severe stimulant intoxication may produce an excited delirium or organic brain syndrome that can be fatal.[11] Such patients should be evaluated promptly for an acute neurological lesion (eg, intracranial bleeding) or a preexisting neuropsychiatric condition and be treated aggressively.

Management of Psychological and Behavioral Effects of Stimulant Intoxication

The initial clinical evaluation includes a substance use history and toxicology testing to confirm stimulant intoxication. As

TABLE 59-2 Treatment of Acute Stimulant Intoxication

Clinical problem	Moderate syndrome	Severe syndrome
Anxiety; agitation	Provide reassurance; place in a quiet, nonthreatening environment	Diazepam (10-30 mg PO, 2-10 mg IM, IV) or lorazepam (2-4 mg PO, IM, IV); may repeat every 1-3 h
Paranoia; psychosis	Place in a quiet, nonthreatening environment; benzodiazepines for sedation	High-potency antipsychotic (eg, haloperidol) or second-generation antipsychotic
Hyperthermia	Monitor body temperature; place in a cool room	If temperature is >102 °F (oral), use external cooling with cold water, ice packs, hypothermic blanket; if >106 °F, use internal cooling; epigastric lavage with iced saline
Seizures	Diazepam (2-20 mg IV, <5 mg/min) or lorazepam (2-8 mg)	For status epilepticus: IV diazepam or phenytoin (15-20 mg/kg IV, <150 mg/min) or phenobarbital (25-50 mg IV)
Hypertension	Monitor blood pressure closely; benzodiazepines for sedation. Generally avoid beta-adrenergic antagonists (ie, "beta-blockers")	If diastolic is >120 for 15 min, give phentolamine (2-10 mg IV over 10 min)
Cardiac arrhythmia	Monitor electrocardiogram, vital signs; benzodiazepines for sedation	As appropriate for specific rhythm, based on advanced cardiac life-support criteria
Myocardial infarction	Benzodiazepines for sedation; supplemental oxygen; sublingual nitroglycerin for vasodilation; aspirin for anticlotting; morphine for pain	Give nitrates IV for coronary artery dilation; phentolamine (2-10 mg IV) to control blood pressure; thrombolysis, angioplasty (if clot is confirmed and no hemorrhage)
Rhabdomyolysis	IV hydration to maintain urine output >2 mL/kg/h	Force diuresis with aggressive intravenous hydration
Increased urinary drug excretion	Cranberry juice (8 oz tid) or ammonium chloride (500 mg PO every 3-4 h) until urine pH is <6.6 (if renal and hepatic function are normal)	Same as for moderate intoxication
Recent (few hours) oral drug ingestion	Activated charcoal orally or gastric lavage via nasogastric tube (if patient is awake and cooperative)	Gastric lavage via nasogastric tube after endotracheal intubation (if patient is unconscious)

Source: From Isoardi KZ, Fayles S, Harris K, et al. Methamphetamine presentations to an emergency department: management and complications. *Emerg Med Australasia*. 2019;31:593-599.

the patient's condition permits, further evaluation can rule out other potential medical (hyperthyroidism, hypoglycemia)[12] or neuropsychiatric (panic or bipolar affective disorder) conditions. The initial treatment approach is nonpharmacological.[13,14] The patient can be observed in a quiet environment with minimal sensory stimulation to avoid exacerbating symptoms. Treatment staff are encouraged to interact in a calm and confident manner, using the "ART" approach: *A*cceptance of the patient's immediate needs (such as pain relief or use of the bathroom), *R*eassurance that the condition is due to the drug and likely will dissipate within a few hours, and "*T*alk down" to provide reality orientation and avoid hostility. Explaining procedures to the patient before initiation is highly recommended. Avoid physical restraints to control agitation or violent behavior unless absolutely necessary, as the use of restraints can increase the risk of hyperthermia and rhabdomyolysis, with resulting severe medical complications.[15]

If medication is needed, most experts prefer benzodiazepines (such as diazepam [10-30 mg PO or 2-10 mg IM or IV] or lorazepam [2-4 mg PO or 1-2 mg IM or IV]) over antipsychotics to control severe agitation, anxiety, or psychotic symptoms,[10,13,16] although there are very few controlled clinical trials.[16] Parenteral benzodiazepine dosing may be repeated every 5 to 10 minutes until light sedation is achieved. Benzodiazepines protect against the CNS and cardiovascular toxicities of stimulants, whereas antipsychotics may worsen the sympathomimetic and cardiovascular effects, lower the seizure threshold, increase the risk of hyperthermia, or precipitate extrapyramidal reactions. Additionally, the anticholinergic activity of many antipsychotics may contribute to delirium and hyperthermia by impairing heat dissipation from sweating, with the greatest risk associated with first-generation antipsychotics such as chlorpromazine.

Hospitalization until the episode has resolved is recommended for psychotic or agitated patients who have not responded to initial treatment. Resolution usually occurs within a few days if no more stimulants are consumed. Psychiatric symptoms that persist beyond a few days suggest an etiology other than stimulant use.[9] Transient psychotic symptoms during periods of abstinence ("flashbacks") have been reported among persons who use methamphetamine.[17]

Physical Effects of Stimulant Intoxication

Mild stimulant intoxication may be accompanied by a range of self-limiting physiological effects such as restlessness, sinus tachycardia, hyperventilation, mydriasis, bruxism, headache, diaphoresis, or tremor. These do not usually bring the individual to medical attention or require treatment. Higher doses or repeated use are associated with more serious medical events, including ischemic colitis, acute coronary syndrome (unstable angina or myocardial infarction, usually resulting in chest pain), cardiac tachyarrhythmia, hypertension, seizures, stroke, hyperthermia, or rhabdomyolysis.[3,14,18-22] Acute medical complications associated with acute stimulant intoxication are summarized in **Table 59-1**.

Stimulant use is high on the list of possible diagnoses for any younger patient presenting with one of these events, especially in the absence of other risk factors.[20] Urine or blood samples for toxicological analysis can be obtained to determine what drugs, if any, are in the patient's system. Even if an adequate history has been obtained, the patient or those providing collateral information may not know the actual content of illegal drugs. Stimulant use within the preceding 96 hours or a positive toxicology test is highly suggestive of active stimulant intoxication in the context of typical symptoms. The blood cocaine concentration has little prognostic significance.[23]

Nontraumatic chest pain is a common presenting symptom among persons who use stimulants seeking acute medical care. The differential diagnosis includes acute coronary syndrome, acute aortic dissection, pneumothorax or pneumomediastinum (especially in those who have smoked the drug), endocarditis (especially among people who inject drugs), pneumonia, pulmonary embolus, myocarditis or cardiomyopathy, or musculoskeletal pain after a seizure.[3,20] About 1% to 6% of patients with cocaine-associated chest pain and up to one-fourth of those with methamphetamine-associated chest pain will have an acute myocardial infarction.[24] The risk for infarction is greatest during the first 1 to 3 hours after cocaine use and then declines rapidly.[24] Concurrent use of multiple stimulants (eg, cocaine and methamphetamine) or of cocaine and alcohol (which produces cocaethylene) may enhance cardiotoxicity, whereas concurrent use of opioids (such as "speedballing") may mask the diagnosis.[25]

Patients who present with nontraumatic stimulant-associated chest pain usually can be observed for 9 to 12 hours while undergoing evaluation.[26] Delayed complications are rare, so resolution of symptoms with a negative evaluation warrants discharge. Patients who have persistent chest pain despite standard treatment, hypotension, congestive heart failure, or cardiac arrhythmia require hospitalization for further evaluation and treatment. Even patients with confirmed acute myocardial infarction have a favorable prognosis, particularly if they are relatively young and in good underlying health.[24]

Rhabdomyolysis may be due to a direct effect of the drug, hyperthermia, excessive muscle activity, or trauma.[19] The usual symptoms of myalgia and muscle tenderness and swelling often are absent in rhabdomyolysis associated with stimulants. The diagnosis is suggested by a plasma CK level greater than five times normal (with other tissue sources such as brain and cardiac ruled out) and a urine dipstick positive for heme, the nonprotein component of hemoglobin, but without red blood cells (indicating free myoglobin [or hemoglobin] in the urine).

Management of Medical Effects of Stimulant Intoxication

The first priority in the management of severe acute stimulant intoxication is maintenance of basic life-support functions. Vital signs, hydration status, and neurological status should be monitored closely.

Treat severe hypertension (eg, diastolic blood pressure >120) that lasts more than 15 minutes promptly to avoid CNS hemorrhage. Hypertension or tachycardia that does not respond to sedation alone may be treated with an alpha-adrenergic blocker such as phentolamine. Beta-adrenergic blockers such as propranolol or esmolol should be used with caution because of the risk of unopposed alpha-adrenergic stimulation by the stimulant, resulting in vasoconstriction and worsening hypertension,[22] although recent evidence suggests they are safe.[27] Calcium channel blockers may reduce vasospasm, but their role remains unclear; calcium channel blockers enhance CNS toxicity in animal studies, have inconsistent effects in case series, and should be avoided in patients with heart block or heart failure. Dexmedetomidine, an α_2-adrenergic receptor agonist, has shown promise in ameliorating the acute cardiovascular effects of severe cocaine intoxication, as well as providing sedation.[26] Benzodiazepines in sedative doses are the initial treatment of choice for both acute cardiovascular and CNS toxicity from stimulants.[26,28] Intravenous benzodiazepines (diazepam 0.15 mg/kg IV [5 mg/min] or lorazepam 0.1 mg/kg [up to 4 mg] over 2 minutes, repeated as needed) are recommended to control seizures stemming from stimulant intoxication.[26,28]

Rhabdomyolysis should be treated vigorously with intravenous fluid to maintain a urine output of more than 2 mL/kg/h to avoid myoglobinuric renal failure. Maintenance of urine pH over 5.6 with sodium bicarbonate (1 mmol/kg IV) helps to prevent the dissociation and precipitation of myoglobin.

Treatment of cocaine-induced cardiac tachyarrhythmias begins with correction of any exacerbating conditions such as myocardial ischemia, hypoxia, electrolyte abnormalities, or acid-base disturbance.[26] Standard arrhythmia management is usually appropriate.[29]

The treatment of stimulant-associated acute coronary syndrome largely resembles that for the non–drug-associated syndrome.[26,28] Initial treatment includes oxygen, benzodiazepine for sedation, morphine for pain, sublingual nitroglycerin for vasodilation, and aspirin for antiplatelet action, while evaluation is continuing. Further treatment can include phentolamine or intravenous nitrates (10 µg/kg/min) to lower blood pressure and reverse coronary artery vasoconstriction. The role of calcium channel blockers is not well-defined. They may be useful in patients who have not responded to benzodiazepines and nitroglycerin.

Excretion of amphetamine can be increased by acidifying the urine to pH less than 6.6 (as with 500 mg of oral ammonium chloride every 3-4 hours), which inhibits renal reabsorption of amphetamine.[30] The actual clinical usefulness of this maneuver is uncertain. Acidification is contraindicated in the presence of myoglobinuria, if renal or hepatic function is abnormal, or in overdose situations, when plasma acidification may compromise cardiovascular function.

Stimulant Withdrawal

Abrupt abstinence from regular stimulant use generates a withdrawal syndrome comprised of depression, irritability, fatigue, difficulty concentrating, anhedonia, increased drug craving, increased appetite, and hypersomnolence.[31] Increased dreaming may occur because of increased REM sleep.[32] Symptoms typically peak in 2 to 3 days (commonly termed the "crash") and resolve within 1 to 2 weeks without treatment. Some individuals experience more protracted withdrawal, with mild depression and cognitive impairment lasting a month or more. This is more common with ATS than with cocaine withdrawal, possibly because of the longer half-life of the former. Recent cannabis use, but not alcohol or tobacco use, is associated with increased severity of cocaine withdrawal.[33]

Physical Effects of Stimulant Withdrawal

Medical effects of stimulant withdrawal include headache, nonspecific musculoskeletal pain, dental pain, tremor, and chills.[31] These are usually self-limiting and do not require medical treatment. Myocardial ischemia has been observed during the first week of cocaine withdrawal,[34] possibly because of coronary vasospasm. Hospitalization for stimulant withdrawal is rarely indicated on medical grounds and has not been shown to improve the short-term outcome for stimulant use disorder.[31]

Management of Stimulant Withdrawal

The stimulant withdrawal syndrome has been hypothesized to result from down-regulation of brain dopamine activity due to chronic stimulant exposure.[35] This so-called dopamine deficiency hypothesis of withdrawal, while not consistently supported by clinical studies, has generated the use of dopamine agonists to treat cocaine withdrawal, most commonly bromocriptine and amantadine. However, these medications have not proven to be effective in large randomized controlled clinical trials (RCTs),[31,36] nor are they approved for the treatment of stimulant withdrawal by the U.S. Food and Drug Administration (FDA).

Small RCTs found that mirtazapine and modafinil provided no benefit in the treatment of cocaine or methamphetamine withdrawal.[31,36] A recent open-label case series involving 10 adults admitted for inpatient treatment of methamphetamine use disorder found that lisdexamfetamine (a long-acting prodrug of amphetamine) significantly reduced withdrawal symptoms over the first 5 days.[37] A sham-controlled RCT found that repetitive transcranial magnetic stimulation (TrMS) (10 Hz directed at the left dorsolateral prefrontal cortex) significantly reduced withdrawal symptoms in 48 men admitted for inpatient treatment of methamphetamine use disorder.

Psychological symptoms of stimulant withdrawal are best treated supportively with rest, exercise, and a healthy diet.[31] Short-acting benzodiazepines such as lorazepam may be helpful in selected patients who develop agitation or sleep disturbance. Severe or persistent (>2-3 weeks) depression may require antidepressant treatment and psychiatric admission. The risk of recurrence of substance use is high during the early withdrawal period, in part because drug craving is easily triggered by encounters with drug-associated stimuli. Medications may be useful in stimulant intoxication and/or withdrawal. However, after any stimulant withdrawal symptoms are addressed, it is imperative to prevent long-term recurrence of stimulant use through psychosocial treatments. These treatments include supportive therapy, cognitive-behavioral therapy, relapse prevention therapy, and contingency management.

HALLUCINOGENS

Hallucinogen Intoxication

Hallucinogens (also termed "psychedelics") are a chemically heterogenous category that have in common the ability to change or distort sensory perceptions in a clear sensorium.[38] Most hallucinogens fall into one of two chemical groups (see Chapter 18, "The Pharmacology of Hallucinogens"). Indolealkylamine hallucinogens (including LSD, psilocybin, or *N,N*-dimethyltryptamine) are structurally related to serotonin; phenylethylamine hallucinogens (including 3,4,5-trimethoxyphenethylamine [mescaline], 3,5-dimeth oxy-4-methylamphetamine [DOM, STP]) are structurally related to norepinephrine. Two other substances that produce psychedelic-type effects are covered elsewhere in this chapter. 3,4-Methylenedioxymethamphetamine (MDMA, "ecstasy") has characteristics of both a hallucinogen and a stimulant (see also Chapter 18). PCP and its close analog ketamine as well as dextrorphan (from dextromethorphan) are dissociative anesthetics that are taken for their euphoric effects (see Chapter 19, "The Pharmacology of Dissociatives").

Psychological and Behavioral Effects of Hallucinogen Intoxication

The acute psychological and behavioral effects of hallucinogen intoxication are summarized in **Table 59-3**. The subjective experience is influenced greatly by set and setting, that is, the expectations and personality of the person who uses hallucinogens, coupled with the environmental and social conditions of use. Mood can vary from euphoria and feelings of spiritual insight to depression, anxiety, and terror.[39-42]

TABLE 59-3 Acute Psychological and Behavioral Effects of Intoxication With LSD, Cannabis, MDMA, or Kratom

Effects	LSD	Cannabis	MDMA	Kratom
"Abnormal" overall behavior and appearance	XX	X	X	XX
Disoriented to person, place, time, or situation	XX	None	None	X/XX
Impaired memory	X	XX	X	XX
Inappropriate affect	XXX	X	XX	X/XX
Depressed mood	XX	X	X	XXX
Overly elated mood	XXX	XX	XXX	XX
Confused, disorganized thinking	XX	XX	X	XX
Hallucinations	XXX	X	X	XX
Delusions	X/XXX	XXX	?	XX
Bizarre behavior	XXX	X	?	XX
Suicidal or danger to self	XX	XX	?	XXX
Homicidal or danger to others	XX	X	X	X
Poor judgment	X/XXX	XXX	XX	XX/XXX

Relative weighting: X, mild; XX, moderate; XXX, marked; /, common/rare; ?, unknown; MDMA, 3,4-methylenedioxymethamphetamine.

Source: From Brust, JCM. Neurologic complications of illicit drug abuse. *Continuum.* 2014;20:642-656; Edland-Gryt M, Sandberg S, Pedersen W. From ecstasy to MDMA: recreational drug use, symbolic boundaries, and drug trends. *Int J Drug Policy.* 2017;50:1-8; Gorelick DA. Kratom: substance of abuse or therapeutic plant? *Psychiatric Clin North Am.* 2022;45(3):415-430.

Perception usually is intensified and distorted, with alterations in the sense of time, space, and body boundaries. While illusions (visual and auditory distortions of reality perception) are common, true hallucinations (perceptions that do not have any basis in reality) are not. Synesthesia, a blending of the senses wherein colors are heard and sounds are seen, is a common perceptual distortion. Cognitive function may range from clarity to confusion and disorientation, although reality testing usually remains intact.

A "bad trip" usually takes the form of an anxiety attack or panic reaction, with the person feeling out of control.[39,40] An experience of depersonalization may precipitate the fear of losing one's mind permanently. Panic reactions are more common in those who have limited experience with hallucinogens, but previous "positive" experiences provide no protection against an adverse reaction. While higher doses are associated with more intense experiences, adverse reactions are less a function of dose than of context and environment. Hallucinogens may trigger a transient psychosis even in persons who are psychologically normal; however, a true psychotic episode is rare. Hallucinogen-induced psychosis may resemble acute paranoid schizophrenia. The two usually can be distinguished because patients with schizophrenia tend to have auditory (rather than visual) hallucinations and a history of prior mental illness. Persons who use hallucinogens, unlike patients with schizophrenia, usually retain at least partial insight that their symptoms are drug related. Hallucinogen use can trigger or exacerbate psychotic disorders[43] or result in persisting or delayed symptoms (so-called hallucinogen persisting perception disorder).[44] The specific risk factors for these adverse outcomes are poorly understood.

Hallucinogen ingestion may result in life-threatening intoxication that is characterized by delusions, hallucinations, agitation, confusion, paranoia, and inadvertent suicide attempts (eg, attempts to fly or perform other impossible activities). Acute LSD intoxication may last up to 12 hours, with little evidence of acute tolerance.

Physical Effects of Hallucinogen Intoxication

Acute medical complications of hallucinogen intoxication are summarized in **Table 59-4**. Sympathomimetic effects are common, particularly pupillary dilation, hyperreflexia, piloerection, tachycardia, and increases in blood pressure. Dizziness, paresthesias, headache, nausea, or tremor may occur. Monitor body temperature and treat elevation promptly. Dry skin, increased muscle tone, agitation, and seizures are warning signs of a potential hyperthermic crisis.

Oral LSD is rapidly absorbed, thus ipecac-induced vomiting or gastric lavage usually is not helpful and may exacerbate the patient's psychological distress. There is no evidence that LSD binds to charcoal. Gastric lavage may be useful in psilocybin ingestion or when there is doubt as to the identity of the ingested mushrooms.

Management of Hallucinogen Intoxication

Initial treatment is supportive. Place the patient in a quiet environment with minimal sensory stimulation and observe for unintended self-injury (as the result of delusions or hallucinations) or suicide attempts. The presence of a familiar person usually is comforting. Unless the patient presents in an acutely agitated or threatening state, physical restraints

TABLE 59-4 Acute Physical Complications of Intoxication With LSD, MDMA, Cannabis, or PCP

Organ system	LSD	MDMA	Cannabis	PCP (stage I)	PCP (stage II)	PCP (stage III)
Head, eyes, ears, nose, throat	Pupil dilation	Bruxism; headache; trismus; dry mouth	Pupil constriction; conjunctival injection; headache	Horizontal nystagmus; lid reflex lost; variable pupil size; laryngeal/pharyngeal reflexes hyperactive; ↑ tearing; ↑ saliva	Corneal reflex lost; disconjugate gaze; pupils in midposition and reactive; laryngeal/pharyngeal reflexes diminished; ↑ tearing; ↑ saliva	"Eyes open" coma; pupil dilation; laryngeal/pharyngeal reflexes absent; ↑ tearing; ↑ saliva
Skin	Piloerection; diaphoresis	Diaphoresis; flushing		Diaphoresis; flushing	Diaphoresis; flushing	Diaphoresis; flushing
Pulmonary			Mild tachypnea	Moderate tachypnea	Periodic breathing; apnea; pneumonia; edema	
Cardiovascular	↑ HR; ↑ BP	↑ HR; ↑ BP (rarely, ↓ BP)	↑ HR, ↓ BP, orthostatic hypotension	Mildly ↑ HR, BP	Moderately ↑ HR, BP	Greatly ↑ HR, BP; high-output cardiac failure
Neurologic	Hyperreflexia; tremors; seizures	Tremor; trismus; ↑ muscle tone	Tremor; ↓ coordination; ataxia	Conscious; muscle rigidity; repetitive movements; hyperreflexia	Stupor to mild coma; tonic-clonic seizures; deep pain response intact; muscle rigidity; muscle twitching	Deep coma; tonic-clonic seizures; stroke; deep pain response absent; generalized myoclonus, opisthotonus, or decerebrate posturing; deep tendon reflexes absent
Gastrointestinal	Nausea; vomiting	Nausea; ↓ appetite	↑ Appetite	Nausea; vomiting	Protracted vomiting	
Renal	Urinary retention	Acute renal failure	Urinary retention	Acute renal failure		
Body temperature	↑ or ↓	↑ (possible malignant hyperthermia)		Mild ↑	Moderate ↑	Possible malignant hyperthermia
Others		Rhabdomyolysis		Rhabdomyolysis		

MDMA, 3,4-methylenedioxymethamphetamine; PCP, phencyclidine, HR, heart rate; BP, blood pressure.

Source: From Noble MJ, Hedberg K, Hendrickson RG. Acute cannabis toxicity. *Clin Toxicol (Phila).* 2019;57:735-742; Mion G, Villevieille T. Ketamine pharmacology: an update (pharmacodynamics and molecular aspects, recent findings). *CNS Neurosci Ther.* 2013;19:370-380; Hardaway R, Schweitzer J, Suzuki J. Hallucinogen use disorders. *Child Adolesc Psychiatric Clin N Am.* 2016;25:489-496; Davies N, English W, Grundlingh J. MDMA toxicity: management of acute and life-threatening presentations. *Br J Nursing.* 2018;27:616-622.

are contraindicated because they may exacerbate anxiety and increase the risk of rhabdomyolysis associated with muscle rigidity or spasms. The use of any of a variety of physical restraints for nonviolent, non–self-destructive behaviors and soft restraints in combination with muscle massage and individualized counseling may be helpful.

The "talk down" or reassurance techniques may be helpful. The clinician, in a concerned and nonjudgmental manner, discusses the patient's anxiety reaction, stressing that the drug's effects are temporary and that the patient will recover completely.

For patients who do not respond to reassurance alone, oral benzodiazepines such as lorazepam (1-2 mg) or diazepam (2-10 mg) are the medications of choice. When oral medication is too slow, or the patient will not take oral medication, intramuscular lorazepam (2 mg, repeated hourly as needed) may be effective. If benzodiazepines are insufficient, a high-potency antipsychotic such as haloperidol (0.25-10 mg per dose) may be helpful. The role of second-generation antipsychotics in this situation remains unclear, but 5-HT_{2A} receptor antagonism may be a useful property.[38-40] Phenothiazines should be avoided because they are associated with poor outcomes.

Patients usually recover sufficiently after several hours and may be released into the care of a responsible relative or friend. Psychosis that does not resolve within 1 or 2 days makes ingestion of a longer-acting drug such as PCP or dioxymethamphetamine (DOM) more likely. Symptoms that persist beyond a few days raise the strong likelihood of a preexisting or concurrent psychiatric or neurological condition. Psychiatric problems that last more than a month are likely related to preexisting psychopathology.

Treatment for severe hallucinogen intoxication generally follows the guidelines for simple intoxication: isolate the patient, provide safety monitoring, and minimize sensory input until effects of the drug have worn off. Reassurance that the experience will abate as the drug is metabolized also may be helpful. Pharmacological treatment is not necessary in most cases and may confuse the clinical picture. If medication is needed, neuroleptic agents such as haloperidol (0.25-10 mg per dose), risperidone (0.25-4 mg per dose), or olanzapine (1.25-20 mg per dose) may be useful in attenuating agitation.

Hallucinogen Withdrawal

Withdrawal symptoms, including fatigue, irritability, and anhedonia, are reported by about 10% of persons who use hallucinogens. There is no evidence to suggest a clinically significant hallucinogen withdrawal syndrome,[38] and such a syndrome is not recognized in the DSM-5.[45] The rapid development of tolerance (within 3-4 days) may explain in part why use of LSD-like drugs generally is intermittent. There is no role for medication in the treatment of hallucinogen withdrawal.

Some persons who use hallucinogens describe experiencing flashbacks, vivid memories, or brief recurrences of intoxication-like sensory experiences days to months after their last use. This syndrome is diagnosed as "hallucinogen persisting perception disorder" in DSM-5 and is not truly a withdrawal syndrome.[44,45] There is no broadly effective medication for the treatment of hallucinogen persisting perception disorder.[46] The α_2-adrenergic receptor agonists clonidine and lofexidine, benzodiazepines, and antipsychotics have shown some efficacy in case series.[46] Selective serotonin reuptake inhibitors (SSRIs) show mixed results, with some patients worsening.

CANNABIS

Cannabis Intoxication

The major psychological and physiological effects of cannabis (marijuana) are mediated by the interaction of delta-9-tetrahydrocannabinol (THC), the primary intoxicating compound in the *Cannabis* plant,[47] with specific cannabinoid (CB1) receptors on neuronal membranes. The regional distribution of CB1 receptors in the human brain is consistent with the known psychoactive effects of cannabis.[48] Other cannabinoids found in the plant (eg, cannabidiol, cannabinol) do not produce these typical intoxicating effects.[47] In animal and human studies, acute THC effects are reduced or blocked by CB1 receptor antagonists.[49] (More information about the pharmacology of cannabis and endocannabinoids can be found in Chapter 17, "The Pharmacology of Cannabinoids.")

Psychological and Behavioral Effects of Cannabis Intoxication

The initial psychological effects of cannabis intoxication include relaxation, euphoria, slowed time perception, altered (often intensified) sensory perception, increased awareness of the environment, impaired concentration, anterograde amnesia, motor incoordination, and increased appetite.[50,51] Psychological set, environmental factors, and prior experience with the drug can substantially influence the quality of the experience. Higher doses, repeated use, or a stressful setting are associated with adverse effects such as hypervigilance, anxiety, paranoia, derealization/depersonalization, altered time sense, acute panic, hallucinations, psychosis, or delirium.[51,52] Acute cannabis-associated psychosis can be difficult to distinguish from schizophrenic psychosis other than by its transient time course.[53] Cannabis-associated psychosis may be more likely to exhibit derealization/depersonalization experiences and visual—rather than auditory-hallucinations.[53] Preexisting psychopathology increases the risk of more severe adverse events such as panic attack or psychosis.[53] Table 56-3 summarizes the acute adverse psychological effects of cannabis intoxication.

Physical Effects of Cannabis Intoxication

The acute physiological effects of cannabis intoxication include conjunctival injection due to vasodilation, tachycardia (sometimes with palpitations), orthostatic hypotension, and dry mouth (see Table 56-4). Neurological effects include poor motor coordination, head jerks, and impairment of smooth pursuit eye movements.[50,51,54] These generally are mild, self-limiting, and do not require medical treatment.[55] Overdose from cannabis is usually not life threatening, though children are increasingly being exposed. Such exposures to large doses of THC in edible products may require ICU level support for treatment of sedation. Intravenous use of cannabis, although rare, can be associated with cardiovascular shock and renal failure.[56]

Management of Cannabis Intoxication

Adverse effects of cannabis intoxication tend to be self-limited and often can be managed without medication. The patient can be kept in a quiet environment and offered supportive reassurance.[51,54] No medication is approved by the U.S. FDA (or any other national regulatory authority) as a specific treatment of cannabis intoxication.[57] If immediate pharmacological intervention is needed to control severe agitation or anxiety, benzodiazepines are preferred to antipsychotics, although there are no controlled studies to confirm this. Psychosis usually responds to low doses of second-generation antipsychotics,[58] which are preferred to haloperidol because of lower incidence of side-effects.

The selective cannabinoid CB1 receptor antagonist/inverse agonist rimonabant (developed for weight loss) blocked the acute psychological and cardiovascular effects of smoked cannabis in human laboratory studies.[49] However, rimonabant and several similar medications were withdrawn from the market and from clinical development in 2008 because of psychiatric side effects.

Cannabis Withdrawal

Acute cannabis withdrawal is a distinct clinical syndrome reported by up to one-third of those with regular cannabis use in the community and approximately 40% of those seeking treatment for cannabis use disorder.[59] Its diagnostic criteria are listed in the DSM-5. Symptoms are primarily psychological, including irritability, anxiety, depression, restlessness, anorexia, insomnia, and disturbed sleep.[60] Much less common are physiological symptoms such as gastrointestinal distress, diaphoresis, chills, nausea, shakiness, muscle twitches, and increased blood pressure. The syndrome is usually mild, rarely requiring medical treatment, but may impair some normal activities of daily life. Supportive medication treatment may be warranted in the treatment of cannabis use disorders because withdrawal symptoms can serve as negative reinforcement for return to use among those trying to maintain abstinence.[60]

Management of Cannabis Withdrawal

Cannabis withdrawal rarely requires treatment for intrinsic medical or psychiatric reasons, although treatment might be warranted in some cases in patients with major psychiatric comorbidity.[61] No medication is approved by the U.S. FDA (or any national regulatory authority) for the specific treatment of cannabis withdrawal.[57,61] In controlled clinical trials involving treatment-seeking adults with moderate-severe cannabis use disorder, dronabinol (oral synthetic THC, 30, 40, or 60 mg daily), gabapentin (1,200 mg daily in divided doses), and nabiximols (1:1 mixture of THC + cannabidiol as a sublingual spray, not available in the United States) significantly reduced cannabis withdrawal symptoms.[61] For sleep disturbance associated with cannabis withdrawal, small clinical trials suggest that short-term use of zolpidem (12.5 mg extended release at bedtime) or nitrazepam (10 mg at bedtime) may be helpful[57]; however, they should be closely monitored as they also have risk for unhealthy use or SUD.

DISSOCIATIVE ANESTHETICS

Phencyclidine, Ketamine, and Dextromethorphan Intoxication

PCP, ketamine, and dextromethorphan are dissociative anesthetics.[62,63] Dextromethorphan (DXM) is widely available as an antitussive in over-the-counter cough and cold medicines, though at the recommended antitussive dose of 15 to 30 mg every 6 to 8 hours, clinically significant psychoactive reactions are rare.[64,65] Ketamine has received considerable attention in recent years because of its ability, at subanesthetic doses, to rapidly treat depression[66] and various pain syndromes.[67] These three dissociative agents have been used for decades and new psychoactive analogs frequently appear on the illegal drug market.[63] Both PCP and ketamine are controlled substances in the United States: PCP in Schedule II and ketamine is Schedule III. DXM is not controlled.

The main effects of PCP and ketamine are mediated by their action as noncompetitive antagonists of the NMDA glutamate excitatory amino acid neurotransmitter receptor.[62,63] In addition to NMDA antagonism, DXM has activity at the sigma receptor, which likely contributes to its therapeutic effects as a cough suppressant.[64,68] See Chapter 19 for more information about the pharmacology of dissociative anesthetics.

Psychological and Behavioral Effects of Dissociative Anesthetic Intoxication

Dissociative anesthetics produce a range of intoxicated states that can be grouped into three stages: stage I, conscious with psychological effects but mild or absent physiological effects; stage II, stuporous or in a light coma yet responsive to pain; and stage III, comatose and unresponsive to pain. Table 56-3 summarizes the acute psychological and behavioral effects of PCP intoxication and overdose. The time course of psychological effects is highly variable and unpredictable, so that even a recovering patient should be kept under observation until all symptoms have resolved (typically at least 12 hours).[69,70] Patients may "emerge" from one stage of intoxication to the next; that is, a patient in stage II or III may enter stage I and become agitated and delirious.[69,70] Similarly, a conscious patient in stage I may suddenly become comatose. The entire clinical episode may require up to 6 weeks to resolve.

The psychiatric manifestations of stage I intoxication can resemble a variety of psychiatric syndromes, making differential diagnosis difficult in the absence of toxicology results or a history of recent PCP, ketamine, or DXM intake. Common syndromes seen in treatment settings include delirium, psychosis without delirium, catatonia, hypomania with euphoria, and depression with lethargy. Agitated or bizarre behavior, with increased risk of violence, can occur with any psychiatric presentation.[69,70] Because of the analgesic effect of PCP, patients may not report the existence of even serious injuries (which may be self-inflicted).

TABLE 59-5 Psychological and Behavioral Effects of Dextromethorphan Intoxication

Plateau	Dose (mg)	Behavioral effects
First	100-200	Mild stimulation
Second	200-400	Euphoria and hallucinations Distorted visual perceptions
Third	300-600	Loss of motor coordination Disorientation
Fourth	500–1,500	Depersonalization Dissociative sedation
Toxicity	Variable	Hyperexcitability, lethargy, ataxia, diaphoresis, hypertension, and nystagmus

Source: From Silva AR, Dinis-Oliveira RA. Pharmacokinetics and pharmacodynamics of dextromethorphan: clinical and forensic aspects. *Drug Metab Rev.* 2020;52(2):258-282.

Clinically significant psychological and behavioral effects of DXM can be grouped into four dose-dependent plateaus (**Table 59-5**).

Physical Effects of Dissociative Anesthetic Intoxication

Mild (stage 1) intoxication is associated with few serious medical complications (see **Table 59-4**). Common medical effects at this stage include nystagmus (especially horizontal), tachycardia, increased blood pressure, ataxia, dysarthria, numbness, increased salivation, and hyperreflexia. Higher stages are associated with severe medical effects, including hypertension, stroke, cardiac failure, seizures, rhabdomyolysis, acute renal failure, coma, and death.

The acute effects of ketamine tend to be less severe and of shorter duration than those of PCP, possibly due to its shorter half-life.[66] Nystagmus occurs less often than with PCP.[66]

Management of Psychological and Behavioral Effects of Dissociative Anesthetic Intoxication

Treatment of intoxication with dissociative anesthetics is largely supportive and aimed at controlling or reversing specific signs and symptoms. No clinically useful antagonist is currently available. A small, pilot RCT in surgical patients found that the anticonvulsant lamotrigine (300 mg daily), which inhibits glutamate release, reduced the postoperative psychological effects of the ketamine anesthetic.[71] Mild stage I intoxication is best treated without medication. The patient can be isolated in a quiet room with unobtrusive observation and minimal external stimuli. Frequent or intrusive contact or aggressive medical intervention may worsen symptoms. Because reality testing is impaired, the use of reassuring, reality-oriented communication ("talking down") often does not work with such patients and may exacerbate their condition. Benzodiazepines can be used if medication is needed to control severe anxiety, agitation, or psychotic behavior.

If benzodiazepines are insufficient to control psychosis, second-generation antipsychotics, such as risperidone or olanzapine, may be used.[72] They are less likely to produce anticholinergic or cardiovascular side effects that may exacerbate PCP's own anticholinergic and cardiovascular effects than high-potency first-generation antipsychotics, such as haloperidol or droperidol. No clinical trials have directly compared the efficacy and safety of first- versus second-generation antipsychotics or of benzodiazepines versus antipsychotics.

Management of Physical Effects of Dissociative Anesthetic Intoxication

The mild physical effects commonly associated with stage I intoxication usually do not need specific medical treatment.

Tachycardia and hypertension can be treated with adrenergic blockers such as labetalol or calcium channel blockers such as verapamil, although there are no controlled trials to substantiate their efficacy.

Stage II and III intoxications are medical emergencies that require treatment in a comprehensive medical setting to maintain life-support functions until the drug has been eliminated from the body. **Tables 59-6** and **59-7** summarize medical treatment for acute PCP intoxication. Activated charcoal may be helpful and gastric lavage more likely will be helpful in Stage III but also possibly in Stage II. Dialysis is not helpful because these agents have a large volume of distribution.

DXM toxicity may result from the other ingredients found in cough or cold preparations (eg, acetaminophen, pseudoephedrine, phenylephrine, guaifenesin, antihistamines).[68] Considering the possibility of acetaminophen or other concomitant toxicities as part of the evaluation and treatment of patients with suspected DXM is recommended.

Dissociative Anesthetic Withdrawal

Although a dissociative anesthetic withdrawal syndrome is not recognized in the DSM-5-TR,[45] some persons using PCP report symptoms after stopping use, including depression, anxiety, irritability, hypersomnolence, diaphoresis, and tremor. It is not clear to what extent these represent a true withdrawal syndrome. Abstinence from DXM use has been associated with craving, dysphoria, and insomnia. Tricyclic antidepressants such as desipramine may reduce the psychological symptoms associated with discontinuation of PCP use, but there is no evidence that such treatment improves the outcome of PCP addiction.[73] The efficacy of SSRIs, which may be less likely to exacerbate the anticholinergic and cardiovascular effects of PCP if there is a return to use, is unknown.

Prolonged Psychiatric Sequelae

Hallucinogens and dissociative anesthetics (PCP, ketamine, and dextromethorphan) have the potential to trigger psychiatric sequelae that last beyond the period of acute intoxication, including prolonged states of anxiety, depression, psychosis, and cognitive dysfunction. The risk of a prolonged psychiatric

TABLE 59-6 Procedures for Managing Acute PCP Intoxication

Procedure	Stage I	Stage II	Stage III
Monitor level of consciousness	Yes	Yes	Yes
Monitor vital signs	Yes	Yes	Yes
Collect blood and urine samples for toxicology	Yes	Yes	Yes
Lower body temperature	Loosen clothing	Sponging, ice packs	Sponging, ice packs
Catheterize urinary bladder	No	Yes	Yes
Gastric lavage	No	Sometimes	Yes
Oral suctioning	Rarely	Gently, as needed	Yes
Tracheal suctioning	No	Sometimes	Yes
Insert nasogastric tube	No	Sometimes	Yes
Neuromuscular blockade and mechanical ventilation	No	Sometimes	Sometimes

Source: From Dominici P, Kopec K, Manur R, Khalid A, Damiron K, Rowden A. Phencyclidine intoxication case series study. *J Med Toxicol.* 2015;11(3): 321-325.

reaction appears to depend on several factors: the patient's premorbid psychopathology, the number of prior exposures to the drug, and past use of multiple drugs.[44,72] Prolonged reactions occasionally are reported in apparently well-adjusted individuals with no obvious risk factors.

Treatment of prolonged anxiety or depression usually is psychosocial but may involve medication if symptoms become sufficiently severe. Treatment of prolonged psychosis essentially follows guidelines for treatment of chronic functional psychosis. Patients may present with wide-ranging symptoms: apathy, insomnia, hypomania, dissociative states, formal thought disorder, hallucinations, delusions, and paranoia. An observation period of at least several days with no or minimal medication (such as sedatives) is helpful to ensure an accurate diagnosis.

The term "flashback" (hallucinogen persisting perception disorder in the DSM-5) is given to brief episodes often lasting a few seconds in which perceptual aspects of a previous hallucinogenic drug experience are unexpectedly reexperienced

TABLE 59-7 Medications for Treating Acute PCP Intoxication

Medication	Stage I conscious	Stage II stuporous to unconscious; deep pain response intact	Stage III unconscious; unresponsive to deep pain
Syrup of ipecac	Not indicated	Not indicated	Not indicated
Activated charcoal	Not indicated	If needed	50-150 g initially, then 30-40 g every 6-8 h
Diazepam	For agitation: 10-30 mg orally or 2.5 IV, up to 25 mg total	For muscle rigidity: same dosage, IM or IV, as for agitation in stage I	For muscle rigidity: same as for stage II. For status epilepticus: 5-10 mg IV to 30 mg total
Lorazepam	For agitation: 2-4 mg IM as needed	Not indicated	Not indicated
Haloperidol	For psychosis: 5-10 mg	Not indicated	Not indicated
Ascorbic acid	Not indicated	For urine pH < 5.5: 0.5-1.5 g every 4-6 hours as needed	As for stage II
Hydralazine	Not indicated	For hypertension: 5-10 mg IV	For hypertension: 10-20 mg IV
Propranolol	Not indicated	For hypertension: 1 mg IV every 30 min as needed up to 8 mg total	As for stage II
Furosemide	Not indicated	For increased urinary PCP output: 20-40 mg IV every 6 h	As for stage II
Aminophylline	Not indicated	For bronchospasm: 250 mg IV	As for stage II

From Milhorn TH. Diagnosis and management of phencyclidine intoxication. *Am Fam Phys.* 1991;43(4):1293-1302.

after acute intoxication has resolved. Flashbacks are associated principally with LSD, although they can occur after use of other hallucinogens, MDMA, PCP, and, occasionally, cannabis.[44] Flashbacks can precipitate considerable anxiety, particularly if the original drug experience had negative overtones. Reexperience of perceptual effects may be accompanied by somatic and emotional components of the original experience. Flashbacks may occur spontaneously or be triggered by stress, exercise, another drug (such as cannabis), or a situation reminiscent of the original drug experience.

Flashbacks usually are brief and self-limiting. Treatment may involve no more than alleviating anxiety with supportive reassurance. Over time, flashbacks tend to decrease in frequency, duration, and intensity, as long as no further hallucinogens are taken.[44]

There have been no RCTs of pharmacological treatment for flashbacks.[44] Small case series suggest that naltrexone, clonidine, and lamotrigine may be helpful (see Chapter 66, "Pharmacological Interventions for Other Drugs and Multiple Drug Use Disorders" for more information).

Prolonged psychiatric sequelae also include dissociative drug-induced cognitive deficits and depressed mood. For example, a number of studies have demonstrated ketamine-induced cognitive dysfunction[73-77]; depressed mood has also been identified in persons with active ketamine use.[76,77] Conversely, one study found no compelling evidence of long-term ketamine-induced changes in cognitive function,[78] while another[79] proposed that a lower level of education in persons who use ketamine contributed to the apparent ketamine-induced cognitive impairment. A recent study of 100 persons with current or past ketamine use in Hong Kong,[78] controlled for level of education, demonstrated cognitive dysfunction. Deficits were measured in cognition and moto speed, visual and verbal memory and executive function persons with current use (N = 49) but not use in past 30 days (N = 51).[78] Significant increases in depression (Beck Depression Inventory) were found in 72% of the persons with current ketamine use.[78] The above studies collectively suggest that repeated ketamine use produces cognitive deficits as well as depressed mood in the majority of persons actively using ketamine, though not in those who had prior use[79]; the issue of reversibility remains unclear. Recent neuroimaging studies of persons chronically using ketamine found reduced frontal gray matter volume[80] and bilateral frontal and left temporoparietal white matter abnormalities.[81]

INHALANTS

Inhalant Intoxication

Inhalants are a chemically heterogeneous group of volatile substances chemicals that can be inhaled at room temperature for psychoactive effect.[82,83] Psychoactive inhalants fall into three chemical classes: hydrocarbons (found in glue, fuel, paint, aerosol propellant, and other products), nitrites, and nitrous oxide (see Chapter 20, "The Pharmacology of Inhalants"). Inhalant intoxication produces initial euphoria or "rush," followed by lightheadedness, excitability, and perceptual changes.[82,83] Significant mood changes or cognitive impairment are rare. Higher doses or more prolonged exposure may cause dizziness, slurred speech, and motor incoordination, followed by drowsiness and headache. Intoxicated persons rarely seek medical attention, in part because exposure tends to be self-limited and the duration of effect from a single exposure is usually only a few minutes.

Even a single episode of inhalant use can result in sudden death.[84] Inhalant-induced brain neurotoxicity, especially to the white matter, as well as kidney, heart, and nerve damage, may complicate the clinical presentation of acute inhalant intoxication.[83]

There is no specific treatment for inhalant intoxication.[83] The patient is assessed, stabilized, and monitored in accordance with their clinical condition, with special attention to cardiopulmonary status and hydration. Inhalants may sensitize the myocardium, so pressor medications and bronchodilators are relatively contraindicated.

Inhalant Withdrawal

Inhalant withdrawal is not a recognized clinical syndrome in the DSM-5 but is recognized in ICD-11.[83] A 2001-2002 population-based, cross-sectional survey of U.S. residents found that almost half (47.8%) of these meeting putative DSM-IV criteria for inhalant dependence reported at least three clinically significant symptoms of inhalant withdrawal.[85] Ten percent of respondents reported using inhalants to avoid inhalant withdrawal, suggesting that withdrawal can serve as negative reinforcement for inhalant use. Common inhalant withdrawal symptoms include depressed mood, fatigue, anxiety, difficulty concentrating, tachycardia, diaphoresis, muscle trembling or twitching, increased tearing and nasal secretions, headache, nausea and vomiting, and craving for inhalants.[83,85] There is no specific treatment for inhalant withdrawal; case reports suggest that high-potency benzodiazepines (eg, clonazepam) may reduce severe anxiety, agitation, and insomnia.[83]

KRATOM

Kratom is the common term for the *Mitragyna speciosa* tree and its products.[86] Its major active compounds are the alkaloids mitragynine and 7-hydroxymitragynine, which are agonists at the μ-opioid receptor. Kratom use is associated with cardiac-related morbidities including cardiac arrest, elevated blood pressure, prolonged QT interval, and tachycardia.[87] In addition, 152 unintentional kratom use-involved deaths occurred from 2011 to 2017. In these deaths fentanyl co-occurred in 65.1% and heroin in 32.9% of postmortem toxicology; in 7 of the 152 deaths, kratom was the only substance detected by the postmortem toxicology.[88]

Kratom Intoxication

Kratom intoxication typically presents with opioid-like signs and symptom, including sedation, pupil constriction (miosis), respiratory depression, sweating, dry mouth, and nausea.[86] Most cases are mild and self-limiting, requiring only supportive care. In more severe cases, treatment with naloxone, a mu-opioid receptor antagonist, is usually, but not always, effective.[86] However, naloxone has not been systematically studied and no medication is FDA-approved to treat kratom intoxication.

Kratom Withdrawal

Kratom withdrawal is common within 5 to 48 hours of abrupt abstinence from long-term, daily use.[86] Such individuals usually present with signs and symptoms typical of opioid-like withdrawal, including restlessness, irritability, pupil dilation (mydriasis), rhinorrhea, lacrimation, and sweating.[86] Individuals using kratom product doses of less than 5 g daily usually experience mild withdrawal and do well with several days of symptomatic treatment, such as tapering doses of an alpha-adrenergic agonist such as clonidine or lofexidine. Individuals using higher kratom doses (>5 g daily) usually experience more severe withdrawal. Such severe cases, whether adults or neonates, need medical detoxification with tapering doses of an opioid agonist such as buprenorphine as described in the management of kratom dependence that includes both initiation and maintenance of buprenorphine.[89]

CLUB DRUGS

"Club drugs" are a pharmacologically heterogeneous group of drugs associated with a youth subculture that revolves around late-night dance parties known as "raves" or "trances."[90] The illicit use of these substances was popularized in this setting because of their perceived ability to enhance the sensory experience and allow outside of such social settings as well. Common club drugs include MDMA, gamma-hydroxybutyrate (GHB), and flunitrazepam, which are described separately below. Pharmacological interactions from the concurrent use of multiple club drugs substantially increase the risk of toxicity.

MDMA ("ECSTASY")

"Ecstasy" is the common street name for MDMA (see Chapter 18). Related amphetamine analogs such as 3,4-methylenedioxyethylamphetamine ("eve"); 3,4-methylenedioxyamphetamine; and *N*-methyl-1-(3,4-methylenedioxyphenyl)-2-butanamine are also sold illicitly (see Chapter 23, "Novel Psychoactive Substances"). The effects of MDMA are those of a stimulant combined with a mild hallucinogen.[91,92] "Herbal ecstasy" often refers to preparations containing the stimulant ephedrine.

MDMA often is taken concurrently with other drugs, such as LSD (a combination called "candy flipping"), for enhanced effect. "Stacking" is the practice of taking multiple MDMA doses over a short period, often alternating with other drugs to enhance the experience. Menthol, camphor, or ephedrine may be applied to the nasal mucosa or chest wall to enhance the drug experience.[91]

MDMA has good oral bioavailability and readily crosses the blood-brain barrier.[91,92] The onset of action is within 30 minutes; peak plasma concentrations are achieved in 1 to 3 hours.[93] The elimination half-life is 7 to 8 hours. Because MDMA is a weak acid, this is delayed to 16 to 31 hours with alkaline urine. MDMA is metabolized by several hepatic microsomal enzymes, chiefly CYP2D6.

Individuals who are genetically deficient in CYP2D6 (up to 10% of those of European ancestry) are theoretically at increased risk of developing MDMA toxicity,[94] although this is not well established clinically.

MDMA has nonlinear pharmacokinetics because the higher-affinity metabolizing enzymes become saturated at relatively low drug concentrations.[94] This results in disproportionately large increases in drug plasma concentrations in response to small increases in dose[93] and may account for the poor correlation between plasma concentration and toxicity. However, psychological effects may not increase proportionally with plasma concentrations, suggesting acute tolerance.[91] A major MDMA metabolite is 3,4-methylenedioxyamphetamine (MDA), which also is pharmacologically active and has a longer elimination half-life of 16 to 38 hours.

MDMA Intoxication

Most signs and symptoms of MDMA intoxication are not specific to MDMA but resemble those of stimulants or hallucinogens. MDMA is not detected by many routine toxicology screening tests, although toxicology testing may be positive for amphetamines, which are byproducts of MDMA metabolism.[92,93] Thus, the diagnosis of MDMA intoxication is most commonly made by clinical history and/or analysis of unused drug.

Gastric lavage with activated charcoal may be helpful within the first hour after ingestion, especially if other drugs also have been taken.[95] Induced emesis is not recommended. Acidification of urine would quicken MDMA elimination but usually is contraindicated because it increases the risk of metabolic acidosis, thereby exacerbating renal toxicity from rhabdomyolysis.

Psychological and Behavioral Effects of MDMA Intoxication

Low to moderate oral doses of MDMA (50-150 mg) typically produce an intense initial effect (known as "coming on" or "rush"), especially if taken on an empty stomach, that may last 30 to 45 minutes.[93,95] Reported effects include increased wakefulness and energy, euphoria, increased sexual desire and satisfaction, heightened sensory perception, sociability, and increased empathy and sense of closeness to others.[93,95] The initial phase is followed by several hours of less intense experience ("plateau"), during which repetitive dancing is common. Persons using MDMA often start to "come down" 3 to 6 hours after ingestion.[92]

At higher doses, effects include hyperactivity, fatigue, insomnia, anxiety, agitation, impaired decision-making, flight of ideas, hallucinations, depersonalization, "derealization," and bizarre or reckless behavior.[93,95,96] Some persons develop panic attacks, brief psychotic episodes, or delirium, which usually resolve rapidly as the drug effect wears off. Initial treatment is the same as for hallucinogen intoxication: placement in a quiet, reassuring environment, with observation to reduce the risk of unintended self-injury. Physical restraints are contraindicated because they may exacerbate anxiety and increase the risk of rhabdomyolysis. If severe or persisting symptoms require medication, benzodiazepines are preferred. Avoid antipsychotics as much as possible because they increase the risk of hyperthermia and seizures. A high-potency antipsychotic such as haloperidol can be used if necessary. A few persons who use MDMA may develop persisting depression or recurrent psychotic symptoms or panic attacks requiring psychiatric treatment.

Physical Effects of MDMA Intoxication

The acute physiological effects of MDMA at low to moderate doses resemble those of a stimulant: increased muscle tension, jaw clenching, tooth grinding (bruxism), restlessness, insomnia, ataxia, headache, nausea, decreased appetite, dry mouth, dilated pupils, and increased heart rate and blood pressure.[93,95,96] Doses higher than 200 mg are associated with life-threatening toxicities. The most dangerous is hyperthermia, which results from a combination of direct thermogenic effects of the drug (probably via adrenergic mechanisms), increased physical activity (as through vigorous dancing), warm environment (as in a crowded, poorly ventilated dance club), and disruption of thermoregulation by the drug, often exacerbated by dehydration. The syndrome may resemble that of severe heatstroke. The high body temperature may cause rhabdomyolysis, liver damage, renal failure, or disseminated intravascular coagulation. Treatment is based on early recognition, close monitoring of serum creatine kinase levels to detect rhabdomyolysis, and reversal of the hyperthermia. Core body temperatures over 102 °F call for urgent measures such as ice water sponging, gastric or bladder lavage with cool liquids, and intravenous infusion of chilled saline. Muscle paralysis with intubation may be required for refractory, ongoing rhabdomyolysis. Rhabdomyolysis treatment includes vigorous hydration and alkalinization of the urine to minimize myoglobin precipitation in the renal tubules.

Benzodiazepines help control both the hyperthermia and agitation. Antipsychotics should be avoided because they interfere with heat dissipation and lower the seizure threshold. Case series suggest that intravenous dantrolene can be helpful.[97] Because of similarities between MDMA toxicity and the serotonin syndrome,[98] serotonin antagonists such as methysergide and cyproheptadine have been used successfully.

Acute hepatic toxicity from MDMA may be related to metabolism into reactive intermediaries that deplete hepatic glutathione, resulting in cell death. The clinical picture can vary from a mild hepatitis that resolves spontaneously over several weeks to fulminant liver failure requiring transplantation. Liver toxicity may be exacerbated by hyperthermia.

Acute cardiovascular toxicity from MDMA is the result of increased catecholamine activity. This may cause severe hypertension, tachycardia, and cardiac arrhythmia. The preferred treatment is an adrenergic antagonist with both alpha- and beta-blocking activities, combined with a vasodilator such as nitroglycerin or nitroprusside if needed to control blood pressure. A pure beta-adrenergic blocker should be avoided because of the remaining unopposed alpha-adrenergic stimulation, resulting in vasoconstriction and worsening hypertension. Hypertensive crisis unresponsive to mixed adrenergic blockers and vasodilators is treated with an alpha-adrenergic antagonist such as phentolamine. Cardiac ischemia or arrhythmia can be treated by standard clinical protocols.

In addition to direct MDMA-mediated neurotoxicity, acute toxicity can result from hyponatremia ("water intoxication"), which may cause seizures and intracranial fluid shifts that compress the brain stem into the foramen magnum.[99] The hyponatremia is caused by loss of sodium in sweat (as during vigorous dancing in a warm environment) and hemodilution from drinking large amounts of water and the antidiuretic effect of MDMA. The conservative initial treatment is fluid restriction. Profound hyponatremia can be treated with hypertonic saline solution. Intravenous benzodiazepines are used to control seizures.

MDMA Withdrawal

Symptoms during the first few days after MDMA use may resemble a mild form of stimulant withdrawal or "crash," with depression, anxiety, fatigue, and difficulty concentrating. These usually resolve without treatment. Prevalence of withdrawal was 1% in a convenience sample of 214 Australian MDMA users.[100]

Physical Effects of MDMA Withdrawal

There is no evidence of a physically prominent or distinctive withdrawal syndrome associated with MDMA that would require specific pharmacological treatment. Persons withdrawing from MDMA may complain of muscle pain and stiffness in the jaw, neck, lower back, and limbs for the first 2 to 3 days after use, which may be the result of MDMA-induced muscle tension and the vigorous dancing often associated with MDMA use.

GAMMA-HYDROXYBUTYRATE

Gamma-hydroxybutyrate (GHB) (sometimes termed "liquid ecstasy") is a naturally occurring metabolite of the neurotransmitter gamma-aminobutyric acid (GABA) that also functions as an agonist at the $GABA_B$ receptor.[101,102] It is approved for the treatment of narcolepsy (sodium oxybate, a Schedule III controlled substance) and is also used recreationally. GHB became popular in the late 1980s, marketed in health food stores as a nutritional supplement for body building and other putative health effects. Use of GHB increased beyond the supplement market, in part because of its reputed euphoric, aphrodisiac, disinhibitory, and amnestic effects. GHB's short duration of action, minimal "hangover" effects, and difficulty in detection by standard drug screens contributed to its popularity. The legal precursors gamma-butyrolactone (GBL, an industrial solvent found in floor strippers and some household products) and 1,4-butanediol (1,4-BD), which are readily metabolized to GHB in the body, are also used recreationally,[101] as are structural analogs such as β-phenyl-GABA (phenibut), developed in the Soviet Union as a sedative/anxiolytic and now readily available in the United States and Europe as a nutritional supplement.[103]

GHB is taken orally as a liquid or in a powder mixed into drinks. A typical dose is one to three teaspoons or capfuls, though variations in concentration make it challenging to determine the actual dosage of GHB in recreational preparations. GHB is rapidly absorbed from the gastrointestinal tract and readily crosses the blood-brain barrier. Effects begin within 15 minutes of ingestion and last 2 to 4 hours.[101,102] The blood elimination half-life is about 30 minutes, largely because of rapid redistribution into other tissues.

GHB Intoxication

The diagnosis of GHB intoxication is based on clinical suspicion, a history of drug ingestion, or analysis of unused drug. The signs and symptoms of GHB intoxication are not specific and are difficult to differentiate from other CNS depressants. GHB is not detected by routine drug toxicology assays.

There is no proven antidote for GHB intoxication. Naloxone and flumazenil have reversed some GHB effects in small case series[102] but their use is considered experimental. Gastric lavage usually is not helpful because of rapid gastrointestinal absorption, but activated charcoal may be.

Psychological and Behavioral Effects of GHB Intoxication

Acute effects of GHB at low oral doses (<20 mg/kg) include relaxation, euphoria, sedation, disinhibition, sociability, and anterograde amnesia,[101,102,104] which contribute to GHB's use in drug-facilitated sexual assault.[105] Higher doses produce somnolence, confusion, and hallucinations.[102,104] Unintended overdose may occur because of GHB's very steep dose-response curve, narrow therapeutic index, and the great variability in potency of illicit preparations. Persons using GHB for the first time often underestimate its potency. The effects are prolonged and intensified when taken with other CNS depressants, such as alcohol. Patients recovering from acute GHB intoxication may wake up abruptly with a clear sensorium or may go through a brief period of agitation and combativeness.

Physical Effects of GHB Intoxication

Low to moderate oral doses of GHB may cause headache, dizziness, ataxia, hypotonia, and vomiting. Higher doses (>30 mg/kg) may cause incontinence, myoclonic movements, bradycardia, hypotension, hypothermia, generalized tonic-clonic seizures, and coma.[102,104] Concurrent ingestion of other drugs, including alcohol, substantially increases the severity of GHB intoxication.[105] Most patients with pure GHB intoxication recover completely within several hours with supportive care and do not require intubation. However, death may result from respiratory depression, and intubation and mechanical ventilation may be indicated in severe cases.

GHB Withdrawal

Abstinence from chronic GHB, GBL, or phenibut use leads to a withdrawal syndrome resembling that of sedative-hypnotic withdrawal, presumably mediated by unopposed excitation in the neurotransmitter systems ordinarily inhibited by $GABA_B$ receptors.[102] Anxiety, restlessness, insomnia, tremor, nystagmus, tachycardia, and hypertension usually appear 2 to 12 hours after the last dose.[102,103,106] Mild symptoms usually resolve gradually over 1 to 2 weeks. More severe withdrawal may present with delirium and/or seizures, which may resemble delirium tremens.[102,103,107]

Published case series indicate that GHB withdrawal can be successfully managed using tapering doses of a long-acting benzodiazepine,[108] GHB itself,[109] or baclofen.[110] Severe cases may require high doses and/or parenteral administration. Because of the unpredictability of GHB withdrawal and vulnerability to severe complications such as delirium and seizures, withdrawal management is best undertaken in a hospital setting. Mild withdrawal syndromes may be managed in an outpatient setting with close supervision.[108]

PSYCHOACTIVE HERBS

Herbs are plants used for medicinal, culinary, or spiritual purposes. Many herbs contain psychoactive compounds with stimulant, anxiogenic, anxiolytic, hallucinogenic, euphoric, or dissociative effects.[111] These properties have long been recognized in many indigenous cultures.

The psychoactive profile of herbs, combined with the fact that production, sale, and purchase of most herbs are largely unregulated, has contributed to a growing market for their recreational use. Internet distribution of herbs makes them widely available to minors. The perception that herbs are safer than illegal drugs, coupled with the absence of clearly established dosing parameters, and lack of drug testing contributes to their unhealthy use. Routine toxicology screens do not detect many of these substances, so that identifying specific intoxication syndromes may be challenging. Accurate diagnosis may rest on collateral information from family, friends, and first responders, in addition to a thorough clinical examination.

Intoxication

Herbs prone to misuse often contain multiple psychoactive compounds, so that intoxication syndromes may not fit neatly into distinctive classifications. For clarity, these herbs may be categorized as predominantly hallucinogenic or stimulating. **Table 59-8** describes basic characteristics of some of the most common herbs being used in unhealthy ways.

Hallucinogenic herbs achieve their psychotomimetic effects principally through activity at serotonergic or cholinergic receptors. Stimulating herbs generally augment the activity of norepinephrine or dopamine. Thus, the manifestations and management of intoxication syndromes for this varied group of substances generally follow that for hallucinogen or stimulant intoxication.

TABLE 59-8 Commonly Misused Psychoactive Herbs

Herb	Street names	Predominant psychoactive compound	Predominant mechanism of action	Typical duration of action	Dosage at which toxicity becomes more prominent
Salvia divinorum	Magic mint; sallyD; salvia	Salvinorin A	Kappa opioid agonist	15 min	>500 μg
Toxicity/adverse effects: Psychosis, fear, anxiety, panic, irritability, uncontrollable laughter, headaches, respiratory tract irritation, diaphoresis			Reported indigenous medicinal usages: anti-inflammatory, analgesia, tonic effects, drug addiction, and treatment for various GI and neurological ailments		
Myristica fragrans	Nutmeg	Myristicin, elemicin, safrole	MAO inhibition, serotonergic	24-72 h	>20 g (5 teaspoons)
Toxicity/adverse effects: hallucinations, delirium, agitation, tachycardia, hypertension, facial flushing, blurred vision, xerostomia, blurred vision, hepatotoxicity, neurotoxicity, and carcinogen			Reported indigenous medicinal usages: analgesic, anti-inflammatory, antithrombotic, blood purification, antiparasitic, antiepileptic, antiarthritic, antidiarrheal, improved digestion, stimulant, aphrodisiac, and treatment for edema and beriberi		
Lophophora williamsii	Peyote; buttons; mescal	Mescaline	Serotonergic; dopaminergic	1-12 h	400-500 mg (6-12 buttons)
Toxicity/adverse effects: psychosis, depression, anxiety, fear, violent behaviors, suicidal tendencies, skin reactions, paresthesia, impaired vision, mydriasis, GI issues, autonomic instability, dyspnea, nephrotoxicity			Reported indigenous medicinal usages: analgesia, antipyretic, antimicrobial, antidiabetic, and increased empathy		
Psilocybe mushrooms	Magic mushrooms, shrooms	Psilocybin, psilocin	Serotonergic	2-6 h	>50 mg (>5 g mushrooms)
Toxicity/adverse effects: hallucinations, headaches, mydriasis, diaphoresis, hyperthermia, chills, tachycardia, abdominal pain, imbalance			Reported indigenous medicinal usages: antidepressant and anxiolytic effects		
Amanita muscaria	Fly agaric	Ibotenic acid, muscimol	Glutamatergic; GABAergic	0.5-3 h	(100 g dried mushrooms)
Toxicity/adverse effects: hallucinations, disorientation, depersonalization, agitation, CNS depression, respiratory failure, nausea, vomiting, diarrhea, cramping, restlessness, tremor, incoordination, and ataxia			Reported indigenous medicinal usages: antiepileptic, antioxidant, insecticidal, treatment for ringworm		
Ayahuasca (mixture of various plants)	Huasca, yage, brew, daime	DMT + MAO inhibitor	Serotonergic; anticholinergic	20-60 min	Varies
Toxicity/adverse effects: paranoia, fear, anxiety, nausea, vomiting, mydriasis, disequilibrium, coma, death			Reported indigenous medicinal usages: antidepressant, increased open-mindedness, reduced materialistic values, tonic effects, analgesia, antioxidant, antimicrobial		
Ipomoea violacea	Morning glory	LSA	Serotonergic	6-10 h	3-6 g (25-200 seeds)
Toxicity/adverse effects: hallucinations, disassociations, depression, memory loss, anorexia, hypertension, polyuria, diarrhea, hyporeflexia, coma, death			Reported indigenous medicinal usages: diuretic, laxative, expectorant, antitussive, treatment for indigestion and headaches		
Argyreia nervosa	Hawaiian baby	LSA	Serotonergic	6-10 h	3-6 g (5-10 seeds)
Toxicity/adverse effects: psychosis, dissociation, anxiety, mood swings, psychomotor agitation, impaired memory, nausea, vomiting, headache, dizziness, tachycardia			Reported indigenous medicinal usages: analgesia, anti-inflammatory, antimicrobial, aphrodisiac, diuretic, antidiabetic, tonic effects, hepato-protection, and treatment for rheumatism, gonorrhea, ulcers, and neurological diseases		

TABLE 59-8 Commonly Misused Psychoactive Herbs (*Continued*)

Herb	Street names	Predominant psychoactive compound	Predominant mechanism of action	Typical duration of action	Dosage at which toxicity becomes more prominent
Datura stramonium	Jimsonweed, locoweed, stinkweed	Atropine, scopolamine, hyoscyamine	Anticholinergic	1 h to several days	Varies
Toxicity/adverse effects: narrow therapeutic window, psychosis, agitation, anticholinergic toxicity and delirium, amnesia, decreased thermo-regulation, hypoventilation, convulsions, coma			Reported indigenous medicinal usages: antirheumatic, antiemetic, analgesia, sleep aid, sedation for agitation, antispasmodic treatment for asthma and bronchitis		
Ephedra species	Ma huang, herbal ecstasy	Ephedrine, pseudoephedrine	Sympathomimetic	6 h	>8 mg at one time, or >100 mg
Toxicity/adverse effects: psychosis, agitation, anxiety, restlessness, insomnia, urinary retention, hypertension, tachycardia, palpitations, arrhythmias, acute myocardial infarction, cardiac arrest, sudden death			Reported indigenous medicinal usages: anti-inflammatory, antimicrobial, antioxidant, antipyretic, antitussive, diuretic, anti-obesity, antidiabetes, anticancer, and treatment of asthma, cold, flu, nasal congestion, headache		
Pausinystalia yohimbe	Yohimbine	Yohimbine	Adrenergic, serotonergic	3-4 h	>35 mg
Toxicity/adverse effects: hallucinations, dissociations, agitation, anxiety, dizziness, hypertension, tachycardia, arrhythmias, tremor, GI distress			Reported indigenous medicinal usages: erectile dysfunction, weight loss, psychostimulant, enhanced athletic performance, antidiuretic		
Catha edulis	Khat; qat	Cathinone, cathine	Sympathomimetic	1-4 h	>100 mg
Toxicity/adverse effects: psychosis, aggressive and violent behaviors, depression, insomnia, anorexia, headaches, autonomic instability, increased risk for myocardial infarction, esophagitis and gastritis, hepatotoxicity, hyperthermia, sexual dysfunction			Reported indigenous medicinal usages: analgesic, antimicrobial, anti-asthma, weight loss, psychostimulant/increased alertness, tonic effects, antitussive, and treatment of GERD, GI issues, erectile dysfunction, gonorrhea, influenza		
Areca catechu	Betel nut	Arecoline	Cholinergic	2-17 min	Varies
Toxicity/adverse effects: severe EPS, asthma, increased risk for myocardial infarction, GI side effects, carcinogenic (increased risk for oral, esophageal and uterine cancers), fertility issues, symptoms of abstinence syndrome			Reported indigenous medicinal usages: stress reduction, sense of wellbeing, sweetens breath, antimicrobial/antiparasitic, antipyretic, antihypertensive, antidiarrheal, digestive aid, treatment for hernia, urinary stones, edema, and beriberi		
Mitragyna speciosa (Kratom)	Thang, Kakuam, Thom, Ketum, Biak	Mitragynine, 7-hydroxymitraginine	Opioid	2-17 min	Varies
Toxicity/adverse effects: nausea, constipation, erectile dysfunction, sleep dysregulation, anorexia, hyperpigmentation, pruritis, hair loss, hypothyroidism, hepatoxicity, acute respiratory distress syndrome, seizure, coma, opioid-like withdrawal symptoms			Reported indigenous medicinal usages: analgesia, antidiarrheal, anti-inflammatory, antitussive, antihypertensive, increased energy/alertness, antidepressant, treatment for opioid withdrawal and addiction		

DMT, *N,N*-dimethyltryptamine; GABA, γ-aminobutyric acid; LSA, lysergic acid amide; MA, methamphetamine; MAO, monoamine oxidase.

Sources: From Gonçalves J, Luís Â, Gallardo E, Duarte AP. Psychoactive substances of natural origin: toxicological aspects, therapeutic properties and analysis in biological samples. *Molecules.* 2021;26(5):1397. doi:10.3390/molecules26051397

Management of Psychological, Behavioral, and Medical Effects

Management of intoxication with hallucinogenic herbs is largely supportive because most symptoms, including psychosis, are self-limited. The goal is to maintain safety, preventing patients from physically harming themselves or others. A quiet environment, with calm counseling and guidance, often avoids the need for pharmacological interventions. Medications with anticholinergic properties, such as many first-generation antipsychotics, are best avoided to minimize exacerbating substance-induced delirium. Avoid physical restraints because they increase psychological distress and may contribute to rhabdomyolysis. Patients who are agitated, in severe panic, or having distressing psychotic symptoms may be treated with benzodiazepines (eg, lorazepam 2 mg PO/IM every 1-2 hours as needed, titrated to mild sedation). In cases where predisposing factors or heavy chronic use contributes to prolonged psychotic symptoms, antipsychotic agents may be useful.

Management of intoxication with stimulant herbs is similar to that with hallucinogenic herbs, except that the former are more likely to generate hyperexcitable, agitated, and psychotic states. Patients with unstable vital signs should be closely monitored, including cardiac function, blood pressure, and body temperature. Beta-adrenergic blockers are generally avoided due to concern about unopposed alpha-adrenergic activity.

There are no specific antidotes to intoxication with psychoactive herbs, with two exceptions. Intoxication with herbs having anticholinergic activity (eg, jimsonweed) has been successfully treated with physostigmine, a short-acting acetylcholinesterase inhibitor. Severe intoxication with herbs having cholinergic activity (eg, betel nut) can be treated with atropine, a cholinergic antagonist.

Withdrawal

Most persons withdrawing from psychoactive herbs do not consume large enough amounts for long enough periods to develop physical dependence or a withdrawal syndrome. Some persons who use khat and betel nuts do experience a withdrawal syndrome, often including irritability, fatigue, and rhinorrhea.[111] Protracted withdrawal symptoms (eg, psychosis, depression, anxiety) should be treated symptomatically while the patient is evaluated for an underlying psychiatric disorder.

FLUNITRAZEPAM

Flunitrazepam (also known as "roofies" or the "date rape pill") is a potent, fast-acting benzodiazepine that frequently causes anterograde amnesia.[90] It is legally manufactured and marketed in South America but is illegal in the United States and Canada because of its common association with drug-facilitated sexual assault ("date rape").[105,112] Flunitrazepam is difficult to detect with routine toxicology screens because of the low concentration needed for pharmacological effects and its short half-life.

Flunitrazepam Intoxication

Flunitrazepam intoxication resembles intoxication with other benzodiazepines and features sedation, disinhibition, anterograde amnesia, confusion, ataxia, bradycardia, hypotension, and respiratory depression.[90] Overdose, alone or concurrently with alcohol, can be lethal.[90] When respiratory depression or circulatory compromise is severe, the benzodiazepine antagonist flumazenil may be used, albeit cautiously. Flumazenil precipitates acute withdrawal in patients who are physically dependent on benzodiazepines and lowers the seizure threshold, thus increasing the risk of withdrawal seizures. Flumazenil is effective for about 20 minutes, so that repeated dosing is necessary to avoid resedation by flunitrazepam.

Flunitrazepam Withdrawal

A typical sedative-hypnotic withdrawal syndrome can develop after abstinence from chronic flunitrazepam use.[90] Withdrawal symptoms can develop up to 36 hours after the last dose and include anxiety, restlessness, tremors, headache, insomnia, and paresthesias. Treatment of withdrawal involves supportive measures and substitution with cross-tolerant medications such as lorazepam or clonazepam, followed by gradual tapering.

WITHDRAWAL FROM MULTIPLE DRUGS

Multiple Sedative-Hypnotics

Withdrawal from multiple sedative-hypnotic agents, including alcohol, is best managed in the same way as withdrawal from a single drug: by using tapering dosages of a single, longer-acting sedative-hypnotic such as diazepam or clonazepam. The time course of withdrawal from multiple sedative-hypnotics is less predictable than from single drugs; for example, there may be a bimodal time course of symptomatology if one drug is short acting and the other is longer acting. The rate at which the dose is tapered usually should not exceed 10% per day. Successful withdrawal is facilitated by use of an anticonvulsant such as carbamazepine,[113] although such use has not been evaluated in multiple drug withdrawal.

Sedative-Hypnotics With Other Drugs

In the pharmacological management of patients withdrawing from both sedative-hypnotics and CNS stimulants, it is preferable to treat the sedative-hypnotic withdrawal first because this poses the greatest complexity and medical risk. For concurrent withdrawal from sedative-hypnotics and opioids, concurrent pharmacological treatment is recommended.[113] The patient may be stabilized on an opioid (preferably oral methadone, although codeine can be used if methadone is not available) at the same time that the sedative-hypnotic dose is tapered by 10% per day. After the sedative-hypnotic withdrawal is completed, opioid withdrawal can begin. Clonidine has been suggested as adjunctive treatment for mixed sedative-hypnotic and opiate withdrawal because it can alleviate withdrawal symptoms from both drug classes, but this has not been evaluated systematically.

POPULATION-SPECIFIC CONSIDERATIONS

Neonates

Neonatal drug exposure is a substantial public health problem. Many addictive drugs are readily transferred from the maternal circulation across the placenta to the fetus. Thus, perinatal drug use by the mother raises the possibility of drug intoxication or withdrawal in the newborn.[114-116] Obtaining an accurate maternal drug use history for the period preceding delivery is essential. Meconium is the most accurate substrate for neonatal toxicology through the third to fourth day of life, but such testing is not widely available.

Neonatal signs and symptoms of drug intoxication or withdrawal often are nonspecific, including sedation, irritability, restlessness, hypertonia, hyperreflexia, tremors, poor feeding, abnormal sleep patterns, respiratory difficulty, and seizures. Stimulants (such as cocaine), cannabis, LSD, and PCP all have been associated with a neonatal withdrawal syndrome, although one that usually is less intense than opioid withdrawal.[117]

Perinatal use of stimulants by the mother is associated with either bradycardia or tachycardia in the newborn.[118]

The additive cardiovascular effects of the stimulant exposure and the normal catecholamine surge during labor may cause fetal distress and retard delivery.[116] These cardiac effects usually resolve as the drug is eliminated from the body. Neonatal stimulant intoxication is associated with irritability, tremors, hyperactivity, abnormal movements, excessive sucking, and high-pitched and excessive crying for 1 to 2 days, followed by a period of lethargy and hyporeactivity.[119]

Treatment of newborns exposed to nonopioid drugs is largely supportive, with avoidance of overstimulation. Pharmacological treatment should be used cautiously because it has its own potential for morbidity. Phenobarbital is the preferred medication for newborns with nonopioid drug withdrawal who do require pharmacological treatment, as when seizures are a factor. A loading dose of 5 mg/kg/d is given until withdrawal is controlled, with adjustments of 10% to 20% every 2 to 3 days based on the response. Phenobarbital has a long half-life, so plasma concentrations should be checked periodically to avoid drug accumulation and overtreatment.

Older Adults

Rates of illicit drug use by the elderly are low but increasing.[120] There are few published data on the treatment of drug intoxication or withdrawal in this age group. The elderly may be more susceptible to confusion and disorientation during withdrawal and to medication-induced delirium. The recommended dosing approach is "start low and go slow"; that is, start medication to treat withdrawal or intoxication at a lower dose, and increase the dose in smaller increments than would be used in younger individuals.

Adolescents

Adolescence is the most common age of onset for illegal drug use,[121] and the developing adolescent brain may be especially vulnerable to the neurobiological effects of drugs.[122] Adolescents experience symptoms of drug withdrawal similar to those in adults, including physical symptoms. There are few published data on the treatment of drug intoxication or withdrawal in adolescents.[123,124]

Women

Women often differ from men in their response to psychoactive drugs and to substance use disorder treatment,[125] but there has been little systematic study of gender differences in the treatment of drug intoxication and withdrawal. Limited anecdotal evidence suggests that pharmacological treatment for women is similar to that for men, taking into account possible gender differences in medication pharmacokinetics. Two topics requiring further research are the influence of the menstrual cycle on intoxication and withdrawal and their treatment and the effects of intoxication and withdrawal and their treatment on pregnancy and the fetus.

REFERENCES

1. Gorelick DA. Pharmacokinetic strategies for treatment of drug overdose and addiction. *Future Med Chem.* 2012;4(2):227-243.
2. Diaper AM, Law FD, Melichar JK. Pharmacological strategies for detoxification. *Br J Clin Pharmacol.* 2014;77(2):302-314.
3. Docherty JR, Alsufanyi HA. Pharmacology of drugs used as stimulants. *J Clin Pharmacol.* 2021;61(S2):S53-S69.
4. Nasser AF, Fudala PJ, Zheng B, Liu Y, Heidbreder C. A randomized, double-blind, placebo-controlled trial of RBP-8000 in cocaine abusers: pharmacokinetic profile of rbp-8000 and cocaine and effects of RBP-8000 on cocaine-induced physiological effects. *J Addict Dis.* 2014;33(4):289-302.
5. Shram MJ, Cohen-Barak O, Chakraborty B, et al. Assessment of pharmacokinetic and pharmacodynamic interactions between albumin-fused mutated butyrylcholinesterase and intravenously administered cocaine in recreational cocaine users. *J Clin Psychopharmacol.* 2015;35(4):396-405.
6. Roque Bravo R, Faria AC, Brito-da-Costa AM, et al. Cocaine: an updated review on chemistry, detection, biokinetics, and pharmacotoxicological aspects including abuse patterns. *Toxins.* 2022;14:278.
7. Ciccarone D, Shoptaw S. Understanding stimulant use and use disorders in a new era. *Med Clin N Am.* 2022;106:81-97.
8. Tang Y, Martin NL, Cotes RO. Cocaine-induced psychotic disorders: presentation, mechanism, and management. *J Dual Diagn.* 2014;10(2):98-105.
9. Voce A, Calabria B, Burns R, et al. A systematic review of the symptom profile and course of methamphetamine-associated psychosis. *Subst Use Misuse.* 2019;54(4):549-559.
10. Chiang M, Lombardi D, Du J, et al. Methamphetamine-associated psychosis: clinical presentation, biological basis, and treatment options. *Hum Psychopharmacol Clin Exp.* 2019;34:e2710.
11. Plush T, Shakespeare W, Jacobs D, Ladi L, Sethi S, Gasperino J. Cocaine-induced agitated delirium: a case report and review. *J Intensive Care Med.* 2015;30(1):49-57.
12. McKee J, Brahm N. Medical mimic: differential diagnostic considerations for psychiatric symptoms. *Ment Health Clin.* 2016;6(6):289-296.
13. Pasha AK, Chowdhury A, Sadiq S, Fairbanks J, Sinha S. Substance use disorders: diagnosis and management for hospitalists. *J Commun Hosp Intern Med Perspect.* 2020;10(2):117-126.
14. Isoardi KZ, Fayles S, Harris K, Finch CJ, Page CB. Methamphetamine presentations to an emergency department: management and complications. *Emerg Med Australas.* 2019;31:593-599.
15. Mohr WK, Petti TA, Mohr BD. Adverse effects associated with physical restraint. *Can J Psychiatry.* 2003;48(5):330-337.
16. Bramness JG, Rognli EB. Psychosis induced by amphetamines. *Curr Opin Psychiatry.* 2016;29:236-241.
17. Yui K, Goto K, Ikemoto S. The role of noradrenergic and dopaminergic hyperactivity in the development of spontaneous recurrence of methamphetamine psychosis and susceptibility to episode recurrence. *Ann N Y Acad Sci.* 2004;1025:296-306.
18. Pendergraft WF III, Herlitz LC, Thornley-Brown D, Rosner M, Niles JL. Nephrototoxic effects of common and emerging drug of abuse. *Clin J Am Soc Nephrol.* 2014;9(11):1996-2005.
19. Richards JR, Wang CG, Fontenette RW, Stuart RP, McMahon KF, Turnipseed SD. Rhabdomyolysis, methamphetamine, amphetamine and MDMA use: associated factors and risks. *J Dual Diagn.* 2020;16(4):429-437.
20. Kim ST, Park T. Acute and chronic effects of cocaine on cardiovascular health. *Int J Mol Sci.* 2019;20:584.
21. Lappin JM, Sara GE. Psychostimulant use and the brain. *Addiction.* 2019;114:2065-2077.
22. Tseng W, Sutter ME, Albertson TE. Stimulants and the lung: review of literature. *Clin Rev Allergy Immunol.* 2014;46(1):82-100.
23. Blaho K, Logan B, Winbery S, Park L, Schwilke E. Blood cocaine and metabolite concentrations, clinical findings, and outcome of patients presenting to an ED. *Am J Emerg Med.* 2000;18(5):593-598.
24. Almeida I, Miranda H, Santos H, Santos M, Paula S, Chin J. Cocaine-associated myocardial infarction: features of diagnosis and treatment. *J Electrocardiol.* 2021;67:11-12.

25. Attaran R, Ragavan D, Probst A. Cocaine-related myocardial infarction: concomitant heroin use can cloud the picture. *Eur J Emerg Med.* 2005;12: 199-201.
26. Richards JR, Garber D, Laurin EG, et al. Treatment of cocaine cardiovascular toxicity: a systematic review. *Clin Toxicol.* 2016;54(5): 345-364.
27. Wilson T, Pitcher I, Bach P. Avoidance of β-blockers in patients who use stimulants is not supported by good evidence. *CMAJ.* 2022;194:E127-E128.
28. Richards JR, Albertson TE, Derlet RW, Lange RA, Olson KR, Horowitz BZ. Treatment of toxicity from amphetamines, related derivatives, and analogues: a systematic clinical review. *Drug Alcohol Depend.* 2015;150:1-15.
29. Hsue PY, McManus D, Selby V, et al. Cardiac arrest in patients who smoke crack cocaine. *Am J Cardiol.* 2007;99:822-824.
30. Huang W, Czuba LC, Isoherranen N. Mechanistic PBPK modeling of urine pH effect on renal and systemic disposition of methamphetamine and amphetamine. *J Pharmacol Exp Ther.* 2020;373:488-501.
31. Li MJ, Shoptaw SJ. Clinical management of psychostimulant withdrawal: review of the evidence. *Addiction.* 2023;118(4):750-765.
32. Garcia AN, Salloum IM. Polysomnographic sleep disturbances in nicotine, caffeine, alcohol, cocaine, opioid, and cannabis use: a focused review. *Am J Addict.* 2015;24(7):590-598.
33. Viola TW, Sanvicente-Vieira B, Kluwe-Schiavon B, et al. Association between recent cannabis consumption and withdrawal-related symptoms during early abstinence among females with smoked cocaine use disorder. *J Addict Med.* 2020;14:e37-e43.
34. Nademanee K, Gorelick DA, Josephson MA, et al. Myocardial ischemia during cocaine withdrawal. *Ann Intern Med.* 1989;111:376-380.
35. Solinas M, Belujon P, Fernagut PO, Jaber M, Thiriet N. Dopamine and addiction: what have we learned from 40 years of research. *J Neural Transm (Vienna).* 2019;126(4):481-516.
36. Acheson LS, Williams BH, Farrell M, McKetin R, Ezard N, Siefried KJ. Pharmacological treatment for methamphetamine withdrawal: a systematic review and meta-analysis of randomised controlled trials. *Drug Alcohol Rev.* 2023;42:7-19.
37. Acheson LS, Ezard N, Lintzeris N, et al. Lisdexamfetamine for the treatment of acute methamphetamine withdrawal: a pilot feasibility and safety trial. *Drug Alcohol Depend.* 2022;241:109692.
38. Nichols DE. Psychedelics. *Pharmacol Rev.* 2016;68:264-355.
39. Hardaway R, Schweitzer J, Suzuki J. Hallucinogen use disorders. *Child Adolesc Psychiatric Clin N Am.* 2016;25:489-496.
40. Li C, Tang MHY, Chong YK, Chan TYC, Mak TWL. Lysergic acid diethylamide-associated intoxication in Hong Kong: a case series. *Hong Kong Med J.* 2019;25:323-325.
41. Malaca S, Lo Faro AF, Tamborra A, Pichini S, Busardò FP, Huestis MA. Toxicology and analysis of psychoactive tryptamines. *Int J Mol Sci.* 2020;21:9279.
42. Dinis-Oliveira RJ, Pereira CL, da Silva DD. Pharmacokinetic and pharmacodynamic aspects of peyote and mescaline: clinical and forensic repercussions. *Curr Molec Pharmacol.* 2019;12:184-194.
43. Starzer MSK, Nordentoft M, Hjorthoj C. Rates and predictors of conversion to schizophrenia or bipolar disorder following substance-induced psychosis. *Am J Psychiatry.* 2018;175:343-350.
44. Doyle MA, Ling S, Liu LMW, et al. Hallucinogen persisting perceptual disorder: a scoping review covering frequency, risk factors, prevention, and treatment. *Expert Opin Drug Saf.* 2022;21(6):733-743.
45. American Psychiatric Association. *Diagnostic and Statistical Manual of Mental Disorders.* 5th ed., text revision. American Psychiatric Association Publishing; 2022.
46. Skryabin VK, Vinnokova M, Nenastieva A, Alekseyuk V. Hallucinogen persisting perception disorder. *J Addict Dis.* 2018;37:268-278.
47. Radwan MH, Chandra S, Gul S, ElSohly MA. Cannabinoids, phenolics, terpenes, and alkaloids of *Cannabis. Molecules.* 2021;26:2774.
48. Lu H-C, Mackie K. Review of the endocannabinoid system. *Biol Psychiatry Cogn Sci Neuroimaging.* 2021;6:607-615.
49. Huestis MA, Boyd SJ, Heishman SJ, et al. Single and multiple doses of rimonabant antagonize acute effects of smoked cannabis in male cannabis users. *Psychopharmacology (Berl).* 2007;194:505-515.
50. Curran HV, Freeman TP, Mokrysz C, Lewis DA, Morgan CJ, Parsons LH. Keep off the grass? Cannabis, cognition and addiction. *Nat Rev Neurosci.* 2016;17(5):293-306.
51. Wong KU, Baum CR. Acute cannabis toxicity. *Pediatr Emerg Care.* 2019;35:799-804.
52. Hindley G, Beck K, Borgan F, et al. Psychiatric symptoms caused by cannabis constituents: a systematic review and meta-analysis. *Lancet Psychiatry.* 2020;7:344-353.
53. Fiorentini A, Cantu F, Crisanti C, Cereda G, Oldani L, Brambilla P. Substance-induced psychoses: an updated literature review. *Front Psychiatry.* 2021;12:694863.
54. Noble MJ, Hedberg K, Hendrickson RG. Acute cannabis toxicity. *Clin Toxicol (Phila).* 2019;57:735-742.
55. Fridell M, Backstrom M, Hesse M, Krantz P, Perrin S, Nyhlén A. Prediction of psychiatric comorbidity on premature death in a cohort of patients with substance use disorders: a 42-year follow-up. *BMC Psychiatry.* 2019;19:150.
56. King AB, Cowen DL. Effect of intravenous injection of marihuana. *JAMA.* 1969;210:724-725.
57. Gorelick DA. Pharmacological treatment of cannabis-related disorders: a narrative review. *Curr Pharm Des.* 2016;22(42):6409-6419.
58. Crippa JAS, Derenusson GN, Chagas MHN, et al. Pharmacological interventions in the treatment of acute effects of cannabis: a systematic review of the literature. *Harm Reduction J.* 2012;9:7.
59. Bahji A, Gorelick DA. Factors associated with past-year and lifetime prevalence of cannabis withdrawal: an updated systematic review and meta-analysis. *Can J Addict.* 2022;13(3):14-25.
60. Bonnet U, Preuss UW. The cannabis withdrawal syndrome: current insights. *Subst Abuse Rehabil.* 2017;8:9.
61. Connor JP, Stjepanović D, Budney AJ, Le Foll B, Hall WD. Clinical management of cannabis withdrawal. *Addiction.* 2022;117(7): 2075-2095.
62. Lodge D, Mercier MS. Ketamine and phencyclidine: the good, the bad and the unexpected. *Br J Pharmacol.* 2015;172(17):4254-4276.
63. Morris H, Wallach J. From PCP to MXE: a comprehensive review of the non-medical use of dissociative drugs. *Drug Test Anal.* 2014;6(7-8): 614-632.
64. Silva AR, Dinis-Oliveira RA. Pharmacokinetics and pharmacodynamics of dextromethorphan: clinical and forensic aspects. *Drug Metab Rev.* 2020;52(2):258-282.
65. Williams JF, Kokotailo PK. Abuse of proprietary (over-the-counter) drugs. *Adolesc Med Clin.* 2006;7:733-750.
66. Kritzer MD, Mischel NA, Young JR, et al. Ketamine for treatment of mood disorders and suicidality: a narrative review of recent progress. *Ann Clin Psychiatry.* 2022;34(1):33-43.
67. Duncan C, Riley B. BET 2: low-dose ketamine for acute pain in the ED. *Emerg Med J.* 2016;33(12):892-893.
68. Shawn Bates ML, Trujillo ML. Use and abuse of dissociative and psychedelic drugs in adolescence. *Pharmacol Biochem Behav.* 2021;203:173129.
69. Dominici P, Kopec K, Manur R, Khalid A, Damiron K, Rowden A. Phencyclidine intoxication case series study. *J Med Toxicol.* 2015;11(3):321-325.
70. Bertron JL, Seto M, Lindsley CW. DARK classics in chemical neuroscience: phencyclidine (PCP). *ACS Chem Neurosci.* 2018;9:2459-2474.
71. Maheshwari K, Bakal O, Xuan P, et al. Lamotrigine for reducing ketamine-induced psychological disturbances: a pilot randomized and blinded trial. *J Clin Anesth.* 2021;68:110074.
72. Carls KA, Ruehter VL. An evaluation of phencyclidine (PCP) psychosis: a retrospective analysis at a state facility. *Am J Drug Alcohol Abuse.* 2006;32:673-678.
73. Morgan CJA, Monaghan L, Curran HV. Beyond the K-hole: a 3-year longitudinal investigation of the cognitive and subjective effects of

ketamine in recreational users who have substantially reduced their use of the drug. *Addiction.* 2004;99:1450-1461.
74. Morgan CJA, Curran HV, Valerie C. Acute and chronic effects of ketamine upon human memory: a review. *Psychopharmacology (Berl).* 2006;188:408-424.
75. Morgan CJA, Muetzelfeldt L, Curran HV. Ketamine use, cognition and psychological wellbeing: a comparison of frequent, infrequent and ex-users with polydrug and non-using controls. *Addiction.* 2009;104:77-87.
76. Morgan CJA, Muetzelfeldt L, Curran HV. Consequences of chronic ketamine self-administration upon neurocognitive function and psychological wellbeing: a 1-year longitudinal study. *Addiction.* 2010;105:121-133.
77. Tang WK, Liang HJ, Lau CG, Ungvari GS. Relationship between cognitive impairment and depressive symptoms in current ketamine users. *J Stud Alcohol Drugs.* 2013;74:460-468.
78. Latvala A, Castaneda AE, Perälä J, et al. Cognitive functioning in substance abuse and dependence: a population-based study of young adults. *Addiction.* 2009;104:1558-1568.
79. Morgan CJA, Curran HV. The Independent Scientific Committee on Drugs (ISCD). Ketamine use: a review. Addiction. 2012;107:27-38.
80. Liao Y, Tang J, Corlett PR. Reduced dorsal prefrontal gray matter after chronic ketamine use. *Biol Psychiatry.* 2011;69:42-48.
81. Liao Y, Tang J, Ma M. Frontal white matter abnormalities following chronic ketamine use: a diffusion tensor imaging study. *Brain.* 2010;133:2115-2122.
82. Cojanu AI. Inhalant abuse: the wolf in sheep's clothing. *Am J Psychiatry Residents' J.* 2018;2-14.
83. Cruz SL, Bowen SE. The last two decades on preclinical and clinical research on inhalant effects. *Neurotoxicol Teratol.* 2021;87:106999.
84. Alunni V, Gaillard Y, Castier F, Piercecchi-Marti M-D, Quatrehomme G. Death from butane inhalation abuse in teenagers: two new cases studies and review of the literature. *J Forensic Sci.* 2018;63:330-335.
85. Perron BE, Glass JE, Ahmedani BK, Vaughn MG, Roberts DE, Wu L-T. The prevalence and clinical significance of inhalant withdrawal symptoms among a national sample. *Subst Abuse Rehabil.* 2011;2:69-76.
86. Gorelick DA. Kratom: substance of abuse or therapeutic plant? *Psychiatric Clin North Am.* 2022;45(3):415-430.
87. Striley CW, Hoeflich CC, Viegas AT, et al. Health effects associated with kratom (*Mitragyna speciosa*) and polysubstance use: a narrative review. *Subst Abuse.* 2022;16:11782218221095873.
88. Olsen EO, O'Donnell J, Mattson CL, Schier JG, Wilson N. Notes from the field: unintentional drug overdose deaths with kratom detected-27 states, July 2016-December 2017. *MMWR Morb Mortal Wkly Rep.* 2019;68(14):326-327.
89. Lei J, Butz A, Valentino N. Management of kratom dependence with buprenorphine/naloxone in a veteran population. *Subst Abus.* 2021;42(4):497-502.
90. Williams JF, Lundahl LH. Focus on adolescent use of club drugs and "other" substances. *Pediatr Clin North Am.* 2019;66(6):1121-1134.
91. Liechti M. Novel psychoactive substances (designer drugs): overview and pharmacology of modulators of monoamine signaling. *Swiss Med Wkly.* 2015;145:w14043.
92. Farre M, Tomillero A, Perez-Mana C, et al. Human pharmacology of 3,4-methylenedioxymethamphetamine (MDMA, ecstasy) after repeated doses taken 4 h apart. *Eur Neuropsychopharmacol.* 2015;25(10):1637-1649.
93. Mead J, Parrott A. Mephadrone and MDMA: a comparative review. *Brain Res.* 1735;2020:146740.
94. Rietjens SJ, Hondebrink L, Westerink RHS, Meulenbelt J. Pharmacokinetics and pharmacodynamics of 3,4-methylenedioxymethamphetamine (MDMA): interindividual differences due to polymorphisms and drug–drug interactions. *Crit Rev Toxicol.* 2012;42:854-876.
95. Davies N, English W, Grundlingh J. MDMA toxicity: management of acute and life-threatening presentations. *Br J Nursing.* 2018;27:616-622.
96. Noseda R, Schmid Y, Scholz I, et al. MDAM-related presentations to the emergency departments of the European Drug Emergencies Network plus (Euro-DEN Plus) over the four-year period 2014-2017. *Clin Toxicol.* 2021;59:131-137.
97. Nikoomanesh K, Phan AT, Choi J, Arabian S, Neeki MM. Dantrolene administration in the management of the prehospital patient with methylenedioxymethamphetamine overdose: a case series and literature review. *Case Rep Crit Care.* 2022;2022:5346792.
98. Makunts T, Jerome L, Abagyan R, de Boer A. Reported cases of serotonin syndrome in MDMA users in FAERS database. *Front Psychiatry.* 2022;12:824288.
99. Elkattaway S, Mowafy A, Younes I, Tucktuck M, Agresti J. Methylenedioxymethamphetamine (MDMA)-induced hyponatremia: case report and literature review. *Cureus.* 2021;13:e15223.
100. McKetin R, Copeland J, Norberg MM, Bruno R, Hides L, Khawar L. The effect of the ecstasy 'come-down' on the diagnosis of ecstasy dependence. *Drug Alcohol Depend.* 2014;139:26-32.
101. Tay E, Lo WKW, Murnion B. Current insights on the impact of gamma-hydroxybutyrate (GJB) abuse. *Subst Abuse Rehabil.* 2022;13:13-23.
102. Marinelli E, Beck R, Malvasi A, Faro AFL, Zaami S. Gamma-hydroxybutyrate abuse: pharmacology and poisoning and withdrawal management. *Arh Hig Rada Toksikol.* 2020;71:19-26.
103. Jouney EA. Phenibut (β-phenyl-γ-aminobutyric acid): an easily obtainable "dietary supplement" with propensities for physical dependence and addiction. *Curr Psychiatry Rep.* 2019;21:23.
104. Miro O, Galicia M, Dargan P, et al. Intoxication by gamma hydroxybutyrate and related analogues: clinical characteristics and comparison between pure intoxication and that combined with other substances of abuse. *Toxicol Lett.* 2017;277:84-91.
105. Grela A, Gautam L, Cole MD. A multifactorial critical appraisal of substances found in drug facilitated sexual assault cases. *Forensic Sci Int.* 2018;292:50-60.
106. Kamal RM, van Noorden MS, Franzek E, Dijkstra BA, Loonen AJ, De Jong CA. The neurobiological mechanisms of gamma-hydroxybutyrate dependence and withdrawal and their clinical relevance: a review. *Neuropsychobiology.* 2016;73:65-80.
107. Cappetta M, Murnion BP. Inpatient management of gamma-hydroxybutyrate withdrawal. *Australas Psychiatry.* 2019;27(3):284-287.
108. Kamal RM, van Noorden MS, Wannet W, Beurmanjer H, Dijkstra BA, Schellekens A. Pharmacological treatment in gamma-hydroxybutyrate (GHB) and gamma-butyrolactone (GBL) dependence: detoxification and relapse prevention. *CNS Drugs.* 2017;31(1):51-64.
109. Wolf CJH, Beurmanjer H, Dijkstra BAG, et al. Characterization of the GHB withdrawal syndrome. *J Clin Med.* 2021;10:2333.
110. Kamal RM, Floyd CN, Wood DN, Dargan PI. Baclofen in gamma-hydroxybutyrate withdrawal: patterns of use and online availability. *Eur J Clin Pharamcol.* 2018;74:349-356.
111. Goncalves J, Luis A, Gallardo E, Duarte AP. Psychoactive substances of natural origin: toxicological aspects, therapeutic properties and analysis in biological samples. *Molecules.* 2021;26:1397.
112. Busardo FP, Vari MR, di Trana A, Malaca S, Carlier J, di Luca NM. Drug-facilitated sexual assaults (DFSA): a serious underestimated issue. *Eur Rev Med Pharmacol Sci.* 2019;23:10577-10587.
113. Zullino DF, Khazaal Y, Hättenschwiler J, Borgeat F, Besson J. Anticonvulsant drugs in the treatment of substance withdrawal. *Drugs Today (Barc).* 2004;40:603-619.
114. Kuschel C. Managing drug withdrawal in the newborn infant. *Semin Fetal Neonatal Med.* 2007;12:127-133.
115. Patrick SW, Barfield WD, Poindexter BB; Committee On Fetus And Newborn, Committee on Substance Use and Prevention. Neonatal opioid withdrawal syndrome. *Pediatrics.* 2020;146(5):e2020029074.
116. Rayburn WF. Maternal and fetal effects from substance use. *Clin Perinatol.* 2007;34:559-571.
117. Jansson LM, Patrick SW. Neonatal abstinence syndrome. *Pediatr Clin North Am.* 2019;66(2):353-367.
118. Smith LM, Lagasse LL, Derauf C, et al. Prenatal methamphetamine use and neonatal neurobehavioral outcome. *Neurotoxicol Teratol.* 2008;30(1):20-28.
119. Chomchai C, Na Manorom N, Watanarungsan P, Yossuck P, Chomchai S. Methamphetamine abuse during pregnancy and its health impact on

neonates born at Siriraj Hospital, Bangkok, Thailand. *Southeast Asian J Trop Med Public Health.* 2004;35(1):228-231.
120. Simoni-Wastila L, Yang HK. Psychoactive drug abuse in older adults. *Am J Geriatr Pharmacother.* 2006;4(4):380-394.
121. Kessler RC, Amminger GP, Aguilar-Gaxiola S, Alonso J, Lee S, Ustün TB. Age of onset of mental disorders: a review of recent literature. *Curr Opin Psychiatry.* 2007;20:359-364.
122. Schepis TS, Adinoff B, Rao U. Neurobiological processes in adolescent addictive disorders. *Am J Addict.* 2008;17:6-23.
123. Winters KC, Botzet AM, Fahnhorst T. Advances in adolescent substance abuse treatment. *Curr Psychiatry Rep.* 2011;13:416-421.
124. D'Amico EJ, Parast L, Meredith LS, Ewing B, Shadel WG, Stein BD. Screening in primary care: what is the best way to identify at-risk youth for substance use? *Pediatrics.* 2016;138(6):e20161717.
125. Becker JB, Chartoff E. Sex differences in neural mechanisms mediating reward and addiction. *Neuropsychopharm Rev.* 2019;44:166-183.

SECTION

8

Pharmacological Interventions and Other Somatic Therapies

Associate Editor: Andrew J. Saxon
Lead Section Editor: Maria Gabriela Garcia Vassallo
Section Editors: Smita Das and Amy J. Kennedy

CHAPTER

60 Pharmacological Interventions for Alcohol Use Disorder

Norah Essali, Hugh Myrick, and Andrew J. Saxon

CHAPTER OUTLINE

- Introduction
- Medications used to reduce or stop drinking
- Medications to treat co-occurring psychiatric symptoms or disorders in patients with alcohol use disorder
- Utilization of pharmacotherapy in the treatment of alcohol use disorder
- Summary and conclusions

INTRODUCTION

There were over 140,000 deaths, attributable to excessive alcohol use, annually, from 2015 to 2019. Each year, there was a total of 3.6 million years of potential life lost due to these deaths[1] Most recent national statistics estimate that 14.5 million people, above the age of 12, meet criteria for alcohol use disorder (AUD) with less than 10% of them receiving any treatment.[2] The first medication to treat AUD, disulfiram, was approved in 1949 and yet, in 2020, less than 6% of individuals who received care for AUD were treated with a U.S. Food and Drug Administration (FDA) approved medication.[3] These data show substantial underutilization of these pharmacological interventions that have been shown to reduce return to use risk, improve retention in treatment, and reduce health care costs associated with AUD.[4] Medications used to treat substance use disorders, including AUD, have been shown to restore in part the upregulation of impulse and reward circuitry and down regulation of cognitive control, which occur with these disorders and lead to compulsive substance use despite negative consequences.[5] In this chapter, we selectively review the literature on the use of medications to reduce drinking or prevent return to use in those with alcohol use above recommended limits with a focus of the chapter on developments of current interest to the clinician or that are likely to yield important clinical advances in the future.

The first main approach to the use of medications in the treatment of individuals with AUD involves direct efforts to reduce or stop drinking behavior by producing adverse effects when alcohol is consumed or by modifying the neurotransmitter systems that mediate alcohol reinforcement. **Table 60-1** lists the four medications or formulations that use this approach and are approved by the FDA for the treatment of AUD. The table also shows the year of FDA approval, the presumed mechanism of action, and the approved dosage for each. The medications are discussed individually in the sections that follow. The second main approach to the treatment of AUD involves the treatment of persistent psychiatric symptoms, which aims to stop or reduce drinking by modifying the motivation to use alcohol to "self-medicate" such symptoms. Medications for which this rationale underlies their use in the treatment of AUD are discussed in the latter part of this chapter.

In guiding patients in choosing a medication to help them manage excessive alcohol use, clinicians must personalize treatment recommendations to fit with patient determined outcomes. For some patients, complete abstinence from alcohol will be the goal, while others may express desire to merely moderate their drinking. Both goals are acceptable as many health outcomes improve significantly with the reduction of heavy drinking.[6]

MEDICATIONS USED TO REDUCE OR STOP DRINKING

Several neurotransmitter systems appear to influence the reinforcing or discriminative stimulus effects of ethanol: endogenous opioids; catecholamines, especially dopamine; serotonin (5-HT); and excitatory amino acids (eg, glutamate).[7,8] Although these systems function interactively to influence drinking behavior, many of the medications that have been employed to treat AUD affect neurotransmitter systems relatively selectively. Consequently, these systems are discussed individually here.

Opioidergic Agents

Naltrexone and, to a lesser extent, nalmefene, both of which are opioid antagonists with no intrinsic agonist properties, have been studied for the treatment of AUD. In 1984, naltrexone was approved by the FDA for the treatment of (pre-DSM-5) opioid dependence; in 1994, it was approved for the treatment of (pre-DSM-5) alcohol dependence. Nalmefene is approved in the United States as a parenteral formulation for the acute reversal of opioid effects. As we discuss these medications below, we'll be using the terms (from the DSM-5) AUD or (pre-DSM-5) alcohol dependence, depending on the terminology and diagnostic criteria used in the referenced studies.

Naltrexone

The approval by the FDA of naltrexone for alcohol dependence was based on the results of two single-site studies, which

TABLE 60-1 Medications Approved by the U.S. Food and Drug Administration for the Treatment of Alcohol Dependence

Medication	Year Approved	Description
Disulfiram	1949	Aversive medication; after ingestion, alcohol consumption leads to a variety of aversive symptoms. Approved dosage is 250-500 mg/d.
Naltrexone	1994	Orally bioavailable opioid antagonist that decreases the reinforcing effects of alcohol. Most robust effects clinically are to reduce risk of heavy drinking. Approved dosage is 50 mg/d.
Acamprosate	2004	GABA receptor agonist and NMDA receptor modulator. Most robust effects clinically are to maintain abstinence. Approved dosage is 666 mg three times daily.
Long-acting naltrexone	2006	Injectable formulation that produces detectable plasma concentrations for 30 days. May help to improve adherence compared to oral formulation. Approved dosage is 380 mg/mo.

showed it to be efficacious in the prevention of return to heavy drinking.[9,10] In a 12-week trial in a sample of veterans with alcohol dependence, Volpicelli et al.[9] found naltrexone to be well tolerated and to result in significantly less craving for alcohol and fewer drinking days than placebo. Among patients who drank, naltrexone also limited the progression from initial sampling of alcohol to return to heavy drinking, presumably because of their experiencing less euphoric effects of alcohol, suggesting that naltrexone blocked the endogenous opioid system's contribution to alcohol's "priming effect."[11]

The efficacy of combining naltrexone with either supportive or cognitive-behavioral therapy (CBT) in patients with alcohol dependence was studied by O'Malley et al.[10] This 12-week trial showed the medication to be well tolerated and to be superior to placebo in increasing the rate of abstinence and reducing the number of drinking days and return to use events and the severity of alcohol-related problems. There was an interaction effect of medication and therapy. The cumulative rate of abstinence was highest for patients treated with naltrexone and supportive therapy. However, for patients who drank, those who received naltrexone and coping skills therapy were least likely to return to heavy drinking.

Analysis of the potential mediating variables in these effects showed that naltrexone reduced craving for alcohol, alcohol's reinforcing properties, the experience of intoxication, and the chances of continued drinking following a brief period of drinking.[11] During a 6-month, posttreatment follow-up period, the effects of naltrexone diminished gradually over time, suggesting that patients may benefit from treatment with naltrexone for longer than 12 weeks.[12]

Many, but not all, subsequent studies of naltrexone have provided support for its use in alcohol treatment. The literature on naltrexone treatment of AUD has been reviewed in detail in a number of meta-analyses. The meta-analyses that included the largest number of studies[13,14,15] show a clear advantage for naltrexone over placebo on several drinking outcomes.

A network meta-analysis of 54 RCTs found naltrexone to be effective in reducing heavy drinking days and promoting abstinence when compared to placebo.[13]

A Cochrane systematic review included 50 RCTs investigating the effect of naltrexone versus placebo on drinking outcomes with (N = 7,793). They concluded that naltrexone reduced the risk of heavy drinking, drinking days, heavy drinking days, consumed amount of alcohol, and the alcohol consumption biomarker, gamma-glutamyl transferase. Naltrexone was not found to effectively prevent return to any drinking.[14]

The meta-analysis of Jonas et al.[15] included 44 placebo-controlled trials of naltrexone (N = 2,347). The number needed to treat to prevent any return to any alcohol drinking was 20 and the number needed to treat to prevent return to heavy drinking was 12.

Follow-up studies of patients treated with naltrexone or placebo for 12 weeks[12,16] or 4 months[17] have shown that the medication group differences are no longer significant at post-treatment follow-up. These findings suggest that treatment with naltrexone is warranted for longer than 4 months, though the optimal duration of treatment is unknown.

An alternate approach to the use of naltrexone based on its efficacy in reducing the risk of heavy drinking among patients who continue to drink was evaluated in a study that compared the effects of naltrexone 50 mg with those of placebo in an 8-week study of unhealthy drinking.[18] In this study, patients were randomly assigned to receive study medication either daily or for use targeted to situations identified by the patients as being high risk for heavy drinking (with the number of tablets available for use by patients in the targeted conditions decreasing over the course of the trial). Irrespective of whether they received naltrexone or placebo, patients who were trained and encouraged to use targeted treatment showed a reduced likelihood of any drinking. There was also a 19% reduction in the likelihood of heavy drinking with naltrexone treatment, suggesting that naltrexone may be useful in reducing heavy drinking, among patients who want to reduce their drinking to safe levels.

Targeted naltrexone was also used by Heinala et al.,[19] who compared it with placebo, paired with either coping skills or supportive therapy. During an initial 12 weeks of treatment, this study showed an advantage for naltrexone in preventing return to heavy drinking but only when combined with coping skills therapy. During a subsequent 20-week period, subjects were told to use the medication only when they craved alcohol (ie, targeted treatment). The beneficial effect of naltrexone on the risk of return to use was generally sustained during the period of targeted treatment. Based on these findings, it appears that targeted medication administration may be useful both for the initial treatment of unhealthy drinking and for maintenance of the beneficial effects of an initial period of daily naltrexone.

O'Malley et al.[20] conducted a sequence of randomized trials in which subjects with alcohol dependence were first treated with 10 weeks of open-label naltrexone 50 mg, combined with either CBT or primary care management (PCM; a less intensive, supportive approach). Treatment responders from the PCM group and from the CBT group continued in separate 24-week, placebo-controlled studies of maintenance naltrexone. No difference was observed with respect to persistent heavy drinking, with more than 80% of both groups having a positive outcome. However, the percentage of days abstinent declined more over time for the PCM group. In the follow-up studies, there was a greater maintenance response for naltrexone than placebo when combined with PCM, but the advantage for naltrexone did not reach significance when combined with CBT. These findings suggest that the beneficial effects of treatment with naltrexone can be maintained during an extended period using either a more intensive, skills-oriented treatment (ie, CBT) or a less intensive, supportive treatment combined with continued naltrexone administration.

Since naltrexone only targets certain aspects of AUD (ie, reduced alcohol reinforcement or cue-induced craving), there has been an interest in combining it with medications that might influence other signs/symptoms of AUD. Symptoms often seen after alcohol abstinence are difficulty sleeping, anxiety, irritability, decreased concentration, and depressed mood. This constellation of symptoms has been called protracted withdrawal. If not addressed, the symptoms of protracted withdrawal are thought to lead to return to alcohol use (ie, negative reinforcement). The anticonvulsant gabapentin may help reduce these symptoms. As such, naltrexone has been evaluated in combination with gabapentin to determine if the combination was superior to naltrexone alone and/or placebo in decreasing alcohol use.

Anton et al.[21] conducted a 16-week clinical trial of 150 subjects with alcohol dependence who were randomly assigned to naltrexone 50 mg/d alone for 16 weeks (N = 50), naltrexone 50 mg/d with gabapentin up to 1,200 mg/d for the first 6 weeks (N = 50), or double placebo (N = 50). All study patients received a combined behavioral intervention that combined CBT, motivation enhancement, and twelve-step facilitation techniques. The results indicated that during the first 6 weeks, when gabapentin was combined with naltrexone, the combination group had a longer interval to heavy drinking than did the naltrexone alone group (which was similar to placebo), had fewer heavy drinking days than did the naltrexone alone group (which had more than did the placebo group), and had fewer drinks per drinking day than did the naltrexone alone group and the placebo group. The findings in the combination group faded over the remaining weeks of the study. There was some suggestion that the combination may work best in individuals who had previously experienced alcohol withdrawal. The investigators hypothesized that the lack of efficacy for naltrexone versus placebo may have been due to the robust psychosocial intervention.[17]

Poor adherence to oral naltrexone has been shown to reduce the potential benefits of the medication.[22] This generated interest in the development and evaluation of long-acting injectable formulations of the medication. The rationale behind this approach is that monthly, compared with daily, administration would improve medication adherence and that parenteral administration would increase bioavailability by avoiding first-pass metabolism.

Two dosage strengths of a second formulation were evaluated over 6 months of treatment in combination with a low-intensity psychosocial intervention in more than 600 individuals with AUD who received 6 monthly injections of either long-acting naltrexone (380 mg or 190 mg) or matching volumes of placebo.[23] Abstinence from alcohol was not required for study participation. The medication and the injections were well tolerated. Compared with placebo, treatment with the 380-mg naltrexone formulation reduced the event rate of heavy drinking by 25%, a statistically significant effect. The 17% reduction in the rate of heavy drinking produced by the 190-mg formulation did not reach statistical significance. Based on these findings, the FDA approved long-acting naltrexone for monthly administration at a dosage of 380 mg. Because the analysis also showed that the most robust effects of the medication were seen in patients who were abstinent (by choice) for at least a week before randomization, the package insert states that the medication should be used only in individuals with AUD who are abstinent at treatment initiation. However, abstinence should not be a requirement for initiating treatment with long-acting naltrexone, as patients can still experience reduction in heavy drinking days without requiring a lead in period of abstinence.[23,24]

In a meta-analysis of 7 RCTs (N =1,500) of adults with AUD receiving treatment in outpatient clinics, long-acting naltrexone was compared to placebo in its effect on alcohol consumption. Long-acting naltrexone was found to significantly reduce drinking and heavy drinking days per month. Additionally, treatment duration of more than 3 months was found to be significantly associated with a reduction of heavy drinking days per month.[24]

Clinical Considerations in the Use of Naltrexone

The clinical use of naltrexone is relatively straightforward. The medication can be prescribed with or without psychosocial treatment. Liver function tests (LFTs) should be checked at baseline and within several weeks after initiating treatment. Prescribing should be avoided in the context of acute liver injury or severe impairment. Naltrexone can be started in patients with mild liver impairment, where liver function tests are no higher than 3 times the upper limit of normal range. Ongoing monitoring is required only if symptoms warrant it because the consistent effect of naltrexone in studies of AUD has been to decrease liver enzyme concentrations.

Oral naltrexone should be administered initially at a dosage of 25 mg/d to minimize adverse effects. The dosage can then be increased in 25-mg increments every 3 to 7 days to a maximum dosage of 150 mg/d using desire to drink or another symptom that the patient identifies as reflective of risk of return to heavy drinking. It should be noted, however, that there is no clear evidence that a higher dosage is more efficacious than is the FDA-approved dosage of 50 mg/d. Nausea and other gastrointestinal symptoms are most common early in treatment, as are neuropsychiatric symptoms (eg, headache, dizziness, lightheadedness, weakness), and are usually transient. Delaying or avoiding a dosage increase can be used to address more persistent adverse events. In a few patients flu-like symptoms occur, and the patient may not be willing to consider options other than discontinuation.

Long-acting naltrexone is only available as a 380-mg dose, which should be administered as a deep intramuscular injection in the upper, outer quadrant of the gluteal muscle of the buttock every 4 weeks. With repeated administrations, the injection should be alternated to the side contralateral to the immediately preceding injection. The medication is approved for use in patients who are abstinent from alcohol and who are also receiving psychosocial treatment. The precise length of the period of abstinence is not specified, and there is no evidence of any risk of consuming alcohol with naltrexone. Adverse effects with this formulation are similar to those of the oral medication, though pain and inflammation at the injection site may also occur. Local interventions, such as warm compresses, and nonsteroidal anti-inflammatory medications can be used to treat such injection site reactions.

Nalmefene

Nalmefene has also been evaluated as a treatment for AUD. As with naltrexone, nalmefene is an opioid antagonist without agonist properties. Nalmefene's affinity for the μ- and κ-opioid receptors is similar to that of naltrexone, though its affinity for the δ-opioid receptor is greater than that of naltrexone.[25] A pilot study of nalmefene 40 mg/d showed it to be superior to both 10 mg/d of the medication and placebo in the prevention of return to heavy drinking in patients with alcohol dependence.[26] A subsequent study showed no difference between nalmefene 20 or 80 mg/d. However, when combined, the nalmefene-treated subjects reported significantly less heavy drinking than did the placebo group.[27] A 12-week, multisite, dose-ranging study compared placebo with 5, 20, or 40 mg of nalmefene in a sample of recently abstinent outpatients with alcohol dependence.[28] In this study, all subjects showed a reduction in self-reported heavy drinking days and on biological measures of drinking, with no difference between the active medication and placebo groups on these measures. Targeted nalmefene (where subjects were encouraged to use 10 to 40 mg of the medication when they believed drinking to be imminent) was combined with a minimal psychosocial intervention in a multicenter, placebo-controlled, randomized trial.[29] Nalmefene was superior to placebo in reducing heavy drinking days, very heavy drinking days, and drinks per drinking day and in increasing abstinent days. Further, after 28 weeks of treatment, when a subgroup of nalmefene-treated subjects was randomized to a withdrawal extension, patients assigned to receive placebo were more likely to return to heavier drinking. Nalmefene was approved for reduction of alcohol use by the European Medicines Agency in 2013 at a dosage of 18 mg/d as needed when the patient perceives a risk of alcohol consumption.

Summary

There is an abundance of evidence demonstrating the efficacy of opioid antagonists (particularly naltrexone) for the treatment of AUD. These are safe medications that can be used to assist patients in achieving complete abstinence from alcohol or reduction in heavy drinking days. Naltrexone can be used as targeted treatment, on days with potential increased risk of drinking, if patients are having difficulty with daily adherence or with tolerating it. Patients who have a family history of AUD, early age of drinking onset, or who have co-occurring use of substances other than alcohol, may have a better clinical response to naltrexone.[30] Long-acting naltrexone should be considered when adherence to medication is challenging. Treatment with it can be initiated even if patients are not abstinent, and outcomes are likely to improve with longer duration of treatment.

Acamprosate

Acamprosate (calcium acetyl homotaurinate) is an amino acid derivative that increases gamma-aminobutyric acid (GABA) neurotransmission and has complex effects on excitatory amino acid (ie, glutamate) neurotransmission, which is most likely the effect that is important for its therapeutic effects in AUD. Acamprosate was first shown in a single-site study to be twice as effective as placebo in reducing the rate at which patients with alcohol dependence returned to drinking.[31] The medication has been studied extensively in Europe, and three of the European studies provided the basis for the approval of acamprosate by the FDA for clinical use in the United States.[32]

A meta-analysis of 35 RCTs investigating acamprosate's utility in treating AUD concluded that it was effective in reducing heavy drinking as well as promoting abstinence from alcohol.[13] A meta-analysis of continuous abstinence showed also significant advantage for acamprosate over placebo, and although the effects were modest, they increased progressively as treatment duration increased from 3 to 6 and then to 12 months.[33]

In a study that has implications for the use of acamprosate in combination with disulfiram, a multicenter trial was conducted in which patients were randomly assigned to receive acamprosate or placebo, with stratification for those who voluntarily were using disulfiram. Acamprosate was found to be superior to placebo on measures of total abstinence and on cumulative abstinent days.[34] The group treated with acamprosate and disulfiram showed a significantly greater percentage of abstinent days than did any of the other three groups. However, because the design was not fully randomized, more rigorous studies of this combination therapy are needed to evaluate the validity of these findings.

Studies in more than 4,000 patients in Europe provided evidence of a beneficial effect of acamprosate in the prevention of return to drinking and in the reduction of drinking in those who return to use. However, two multicenter trials conducted in the United States, the first being a multicenter trial of two active dosages of acamprosate[35] and the second being the COMBINE (Combining Medications and Behavioral Interventions for Alcoholism) study,[17] the largest alcohol treatment trial to date (described in the following section), failed to show an advantage of acamprosate over placebo on an intent-to-treat basis. This raises the question of the factors that distinguish alcohol pharmacotherapy trials in Europe from those in the United States. Differences in features of study design (eg, European studies required a lengthier period of abstinence) and of the samples studied (eg, European subjects drank more heavily) may explain these discrepant findings.

Clinical Considerations in the Use of Acamprosate

Acamprosate is FDA approved at a dosage of 1,998 mg/d (ie, two 333-mg capsules three times per day) in patients who are abstinent from alcohol and receiving psychosocial treatment. The most common adverse effects of the drug are generally mild and transient and include gastrointestinal (eg, diarrhea, bloating) and dermatological (eg, pruritus) complaints. In contrast to disulfiram and naltrexone, which are metabolized in the liver, acamprosate is excreted unmetabolized, so that renal function is the rate-limiting factor in the drug's elimination. Evaluation of renal function prior to initiation of the drug is warranted, particularly in individuals who have a history or are otherwise at risk of renal disease and in the elderly.

Studies Comparing Acamprosate With Naltrexone and the Two Medications Combined

Two placebo-controlled studies have directly compared treatment with acamprosate, naltrexone, and acamprosate and naltrexone combined. In the first study, a 12-week trial in 160 patients, all three active medication groups (naltrexone, acamprosate, and the two medications combined) were significantly more efficacious than was placebo.[36] In that study, although the rate of return to use of participants in the combined medication group was significantly lower than that in either the placebo or acamprosate groups, it was not statistically better than naltrexone alone.

The COMBINE study, a 4-month, multicenter, placebo-controlled study conducted at 11 sites in the United States, compared naltrexone, acamprosate, and their combination in a sample of nearly 1,400 abstinent individuals with alcohol-dependence. The design of the study was complex, insofar as two different behavioral interventions (medical management or an intensive behavioral treatment) were combined with naltrexone (100 mg/d), acamprosate (3 g/d), naltrexone and acamprosate, or placebo, so that eight groups received study medication. Further, to evaluate the effects of placebo treatment, a ninth group, which received an intensive behavioral treatment but no medication, was also included. Overall, when receiving treatment, subjects significantly increased the percentage of abstinent days. Groups receiving naltrexone and medical management; intensive behavioral treatment, medical management, and placebo; and naltrexone, intensive behavioral treatment, and medical management had a significantly greater percentage of days abstinent than the group receiving placebo and medical management. Naltrexone also reduced the risk of heavy drinking days in the group receiving medical management but not intensive psychotherapy. In addition to showing a modest advantage for the use of either naltrexone or intensive behavioral treatment, it is noteworthy that the study failed to show an advantage for acamprosate over placebo, either alone or when added to naltrexone, on any of the drinking outcomes. The study also showed evidence of a placebo response among individuals receiving the intensive behavioral intervention, in that those who received neither an active nor a placebo medication showed significantly less improvement than those who were treated with placebo.

Alcohol-Sensitizing Agents

Alcohol-sensitizing agents alter the body's response to alcohol, thereby making its ingestion unpleasant or toxic. Disulfiram is the only alcohol-sensitizing medication approved in the United States for the treatment of AUD and that is used clinically. Consequently, we focus on that agent here.

Disulfiram inhibits the enzyme aldehyde dehydrogenase, which catalyzes the oxidation of acetaldehyde to acetic acid. The ingestion of alcohol while this enzyme is inhibited elevates the blood acetaldehyde concentration, resulting in the disulfiram-ethanol reaction (DER). Symptoms and signs of the DER include warmness and flushing of the skin, especially that of the upper chest and face; increased heart rate; palpitations; and decreased blood pressure. They may also include nausea, vomiting, shortness of breath, sweating, dizziness, blurred vision, and confusion. Most DERs are self-limited, lasting about 30 minutes. Occasionally, the DER may be severe, with marked tachycardia, hypotension, or bradycardia; rarely, it may result in cardiovascular collapse, congestive failure, and convulsions. The intensity of the DER varies both with the dose of disulfiram and the volume of alcohol ingested. It should be noted that some patients may show a complete absence of a DER while others may have a severe reaction even with small quantities of alcohol.[37] Although severe reactions are usually associated with high doses of disulfiram (over 500 mg/d), combined with more than 2 oz of alcohol, deaths have occurred with lower dosage and after a single drink.[38,39]

The largest and most methodologically sound study of disulfiram was a multicenter trial conducted by the Veterans Administration Cooperative Studies Group. In that 1-year study, more than 600 male patients with alcohol dependence were randomly assigned to receive either 1 mg of disulfiram per day, 250 mg/d or an inactive placebo.[40] Patients assigned to the two disulfiram groups were told they were receiving the medication, but neither patients nor staff knew the dosage. Results showed that greater adherence with the medication regimen (in all three groups) was associated with a greater likelihood of complete abstinence. Among patients who resumed drinking, those in the group receiving 250 mg of disulfiram reported significantly fewer drinking days than did patients in either of the other two groups. Based on these findings, it appears that disulfiram may be helpful in reducing the frequency of drinking in men who continue to drink, though given the large number of statistical analyses, it is possible that this finding arose by chance. Similarly, a systematic review of 11 randomized controlled trials (N = 1,527) concluded that supervised administration of disulfiram improved short-term abstinence, prolonged days until return to drinking, and reduced the number of drinking days.[41]

In taking these results into consideration, and given disulfiram's aversive mechanism of action, this medication will likely be most clinically effective in a patient whose goal is complete abstinence from alcohol and who agrees to supervised treatment.[42] Specific behavioral efforts to enhance adherence to disulfiram (as well as other medications for the treatment of alcohol use disorder) include contracting with the patient and a significant other to work together to ensure adherence and the provision to the patient of incentives, regular reminders and other information, and behavioral training and social support.[43]

During shared decision-making with the patient on selecting disulfiram, clinicians should make patients aware of the potential hazards of the medication. This includes recommending avoidance of over-the-counter preparations that contain alcohol (eg, mouthwash) and substances that can interact with disulfiram and the potential for a DER to be precipitated by alcohol used in food preparation. Patients should also do a patch test for any topical products that may contain alcohol (eg, sanitizer, perfume). The administration of disulfiram to anyone who does not agree to use it, does not seek to be abstinent from alcohol, has not attained at least 48 hours of abstinence prior to first administration, or has any psychological or medical contraindications is not recommended. Given its potential to produce serious adverse effects when combined with alcohol, disulfiram cannot be recommended for use as part of a moderation approach to alcohol treatment.

Pharmacology and Clinical Use of Disulfiram

Disulfiram is administered and is almost completely absorbed orally. Because it binds irreversibly to aldehyde dehydrogenase, renewed enzyme activity requires the synthesis of new enzyme, so that the potential exists for a DER to occur at least 2 weeks from the last ingestion of disulfiram. Consequently, alcohol should be avoided during this period.

Disulfiram commonly produces a variety of adverse effects, including drowsiness, lethargy, and fatigue.[44] Although more serious adverse effects, such as optic neuritis, peripheral neuropathy, and hepatotoxicity occur rarely, patients treated with disulfiram should be monitored regularly for visual changes and symptoms of peripheral neuropathy and the medication should be discontinued if they appear. Further, the patient's liver enzymes should be monitored every 3 months to identify hepatotoxic effects, which may also warrant discontinuation of the medication. Psychiatric effects of disulfiram, though uncommon and probably occur only at higher dosages of the drug, may occur due to disulfiram's inhibition of a variety of enzymes in addition to aldehyde dehydrogenase. For example, disulfiram inhibits dopamine beta-hydroxylase, which increases dopamine concentrations, which in turn can exacerbate psychotic symptoms in patients with schizophrenia and rarely result in psychotic or depressive symptoms among individuals without a psychotic disorder. Such symptoms should also lead to the discontinuation of the medication.

There is a correlation between the risk of most adverse effects and dosage, although the risk of hepatic injury does not appear to be related to dose. This concern about dosage-related adverse events has resulted in the daily dosage prescribed in the United States being limited to 250 to 500 mg/d.

GABAergic Agents

There is growing interest in the use of GABAergic medications for the treatment of AUD, although currently none are FDA approved for this indication. Although these medications have different mechanisms of action, it is likely that they exert beneficial effects in AUD through their actions as glutamate antagonists and GABA agonists, helping to normalize the abnormal activity in these neurotransmitter systems seen following chronic heavy drinking. Medications in this group include topiramate, gabapentin, pregabalin, and baclofen.

Topiramate

Topiramate was initially studied in a single-site, 12-week, placebo-controlled trial, with the dosage gradually increased over 8 weeks to a maximum of 300 mg/d. Topiramate-treated patients showed significantly greater reductions than did placebo-treated patients in drinks per day, drinks per drinking day, drinking days, heavy drinking days, and γ-glutamyl transpeptidase levels.[45] Based on these findings, a subsequent multicenter study was conducted,[46] which showed many of the same effects on drinking as the single-site study, though topiramate was not as well tolerated as it was in the initial trial. The authors interpreted these findings to reflect the more rapid dose titration (to a maximum of 300 mg/d, but over 6 weeks). Topiramate's effect on the above reported drinking outcomes was also reported in a meta-analysis of 7 RCTs (N = 1,125).[47] A subsequent network meta-analysis of 12 RCTs concluded that topiramate had a moderate effect size for abstinence though it was not significantly better than oral naltrexone or acamprosate. It was also twice as likely as placebo to cause significant adverse effects leading to discontinuation.[13] The most common adverse effect of topiramate compared to placebo is numbness and tingling (which is secondary to the commonly observed metabolic acidosis produced by the antagonism by topiramate of carbonic anhydrase), with other common side effects including a change in the sense of taste, tiredness/sleepiness, fatigue, dizziness, loss of appetite, nausea, diarrhea, weight decrease, and difficulty concentrating, with memory, and in word finding. Of clinical concern also are suicidal thoughts or actions, which have been reported uncommonly but at a frequency greater than that seen with placebo treatment. Other adverse effects of topiramate that are less likely to occur but potentially serious are renal calculi and acute secondary glaucoma. Topiramate is also category D in pregnancy and is associated with oral clefts in exposed infants.

These findings provide clear support for the efficacy of this anticonvulsant for the treatment of AUD and suggest that the use of topiramate for this purpose should include a slowly increasing dosage. Additional research focusing on the optimal rate of dosage increase and the minimal dosage that is efficacious in AUD is warranted. In regard to precision medicine, a randomized, controlled, double-blind trial of topiramate 200 mg/d versus placebo showed a robust effect of topiramate on number of heavy drinking days, but in a subsample of Americans of European descent, this effect was accounted for almost entirely by a single nucleotide polymorphism in the gene coding for one of the subunits of the kainate type of glutamate receptor.[48] This finding requires replication in a larger prospective study before it would be clinically applicable.

Gabapentin and Pregabalin

Gabapentin is FDA approved for the adjunctive treatment of partial seizures and postherpetic neuralgia. It is a structural analog of the inhibitory neurotransmitter γ-aminobutyric acid (GABA) and is hypothesized to work via blocking voltage-dependent calcium channels and modulating excitatory neurotransmitter release.[49] Its off-label use to treat AUD was initially demonstrated in three randomized clinical trials ($N = 231$) concluding that gabapentin reduced heavy drinking, increased abstinence, improved sleep, and reduced acute/protracted withdrawal syndromes.[50,51] A dose-related effect on abstinence rate, no heavy drinking, cravings, mood and sleep was found. These effects were more pronounced in the gabapentin 1,800-mg group (abstinence: NNT = 8; no heavy drinking: NNT = 5).[52] A subsequent multicenter RCT of ($N = 346$) patients with AUD used an extended-release formulation, gabapentin enacarbil and found no significant difference compared to placebo in any outcomes; percent of no heavy drinking days, subjects abstinent, days abstinent, heavy drinking days, drinks per week, drinks per drinking day, alcohol craving, alcohol-related consequences, sleep problems, smoking, and depression/anxiety symptoms.[53] The use of gabapentin's prodrug in this trial and differences in pharmacokinetics may explain this outcome. A meta-analysis of 7 RCTs, including the above negative study, reported on gabapentin's effect on 6 AUD treatment-related outcomes; complete abstinence, relapse to heavy drinking, percent days abstinent, percent heavy drinking days, drinks per day, and gamma-glutamyl transferase (GGT) concentration. It concluded that, despite effect sizes trending favorably for gabapentin over placebo, only reduction in percent of heavy drinking days was significant, highlighting a need to more clearly define gabapentin's role in AUD treatment.[54] This role may include treating patients with AUD who are also experiencing withdrawal symptoms as exemplified in a RCT of ($N = 96$) patients with AUD, who also met criteria for alcohol withdrawal, randomized to receive gabapentin (1,200 mg/d) versus placebo.[55] The gabapentin arm was found to have fewer heavy drinking days (NNT = 5.4) and more total abstinence (NNT = 6.2). These effects were even more pronounced in the high alcohol withdrawal group ($N = 45$) in terms of heavy drinking days (NNT = 3.1) and total abstinence (NNT = 2.7). The group with low alcohol withdrawal showed no difference between gabapentin and placebo on these outcomes.

Pregabalin is structurally similar to gabapentin and exerts its effect via similar action at voltage-gated calcium channels. Pregabalin is thought to have some pharmacokinetic and pharmacodynamic advantages over gabapentin, including more binding affinity at its target, more potency, more bioavailability, and better absorption.[56] Pregabalin has been studied for treatment of AUD as well. A 3-month double-blind RCT compared pregabalin 150 mg to placebo in ($N = 100$) patients with AUD. Pregabalin was found to be superior in treatment retention, reducing total alcohol consumption, reducing heavy drinking days, and increasing abstinent days. Pregabalin did not differ from placebo in terms of its effect on cravings, depression, anxiety, or GGT activity.[57] Similar outcomes were reported in an open-label, 8-week long, study of ($N = 18$) participants with AUD, who were titrated to 600 mg/d. However, 80% of participants reported adverse events with 11% dropping out.[58] Since this was not an RCT, more studies are needed to determine the optimal dose of pregabalin for AUD, but these results suggest lower doses will likely be better tolerated while maintaining effectiveness.

Baclofen

This GABA-B receptor agonist has been approved as an antispasmodic for more than 30 years and has recently been studied as a treatment for AUD, although is not FDA approved for such treatment. In a small trial, Addolorato et al.[59] randomly assigned recently abstinent individuals with alcohol dependence to receive up to 30 mg/d of the medication or placebo divided into three daily doses. The medication was well tolerated, and the baclofen-treated group was more likely to remain abstinent over the 1-month treatment period (also showing a greater number of cumulative abstinence days) than was the placebo group. Another study by these investigators[60] evaluated the efficacy of baclofen in a sample of 84 patients with alcohol dependence with liver cirrhosis. Baclofen-treated patients were significantly more likely than placebo-treated patients to maintain abstinence (71% versus 29%), with a concomitant doubling of abstinence days in the baclofen group. The medication was well tolerated, and the baclofen group showed a nonsignificant lower rate of study dropout than did the placebo group (14% versus 31%). Subsequent studies have shown contradictory findings. A flexible dosing double-blind randomized trial with 56 participants found significantly higher total abstinence rates and abstinence duration among participant who received active medication (mean dose in the active baclofen group = 180 mg [SD = 86.9]/day).[61] However, a larger multicenter randomized, double-blind trial with 151 participants compared a high-dose baclofen group (mean = 93.6 [SD = 40.3]/day) to 30 mg/d and placebo groups and saw no differences between groups in any measure of alcohol use while also noting frequent adverse events in the high-dose group.[62] Another multicenter randomized, double-blind trial among 180 U.S. military veterans similarly found no effect of baclofen 30 mg/d compared to placebo on any alcohol use outcomes.[63]

A Cochrane review of 12 RCTs concluded that there was no significant difference between baclofen and placebo with regards to AUD treatment outcomes.[64] Since baclofen has demonstrated safety and efficacy in reducing drinking in patients with alcohol-related liver disease,[60,65] there has been continued interest in delineating moderators of its potential benefit in treating AUD. An RCT of (N = 120) participants with AUD, randomized to receive baclofen 30mg or 90mg or placebo, showed that baclofen reduced heavy drinking days (−13.6 days) and increased abstinent days (+12.9 days) over the 16-week trial period; 90 mg showed greater efficacy. However, they also found a moderating effect of sex, with men benefitting from and tolerating 90 mg, while women benefited only from 30 mg and did not tolerate 90 mg.[66]

Taken together, current evidence suggests that higher doses of baclofen may result in positive outcomes in treatment of AUD and that it can be a potential treatment in patients with alcohol-related liver disease.

Serotonergic Agents

Ondansetron

Ondansetron is a 5-HT receptor antagonist approved for the treatment of chemotherapy-induced and postoperative nausea. Using a subtyping approach, Johnson et al.[67] found that ondansetron selectively reduced drinking among patients with early onset of unhealthy drinking (ie, before age 25; early-onset patients with alcohol dependence). Specifically, ondansetron was superior to placebo on the proportion of days abstinent and on the intensity of alcohol intake. In contrast, late-onset patients with alcohol dependence showed effects of ondansetron on drinking behavior that were comparable to those of placebo. In a subsequent 8-week, open-label study of ondansetron, early-onset patients with alcohol dependence had a significantly greater decrease in drinks per day, drinks per drinking day, and alcohol-related problems than did late-onset patients with alcohol dependence.[68] Furthermore, a prospective double-blind trial of ondansetron in which participants were randomized based upon polymorphisms in the gene coding for the serotonin transporter showed a positive response in participants with the polymorphisms.[69] A retrospective analysis of the same data showed that polymorphisms in the genes coding for serotonin 5-HT3 receptor subtypes also predicted outcome.[70]

Psychedelics

There has been re-ignited interest in the use of psychedelics in a variety of psychiatric and substance use disorders. Certain serotonergic psychedelics have evidence of variable strength investigating their potential benefit in treating AUD. A small open label trial in (N = 10) participants with AUD that combined 2 doses of psilocybin with a 12-session psychosocial intervention found that percent drinking days and heavy drinking days were significantly reduced, as compared to prior to treatment. These improvements were sustained throughout the 36-week follow-up period. It was also noted to reduce drinking consequences, cravings, self-efficacy, and mood with no notable adverse effects.[71] A larger randomized, double-blind trial (N = 95) used a similar design with diphenhydramine as the control condition, 12 psychotherapy sessions and two medication sessions at 4 and 8 weeks. Compared to control, psilocybin treatment reduced percent of heavy drinking days and mean daily alcohol consumption over the 32 study weeks.[72] A meta-analysis of 6 RCTs (N = 536), investigating lysergic acid diethylamide's (LSD) use in AUD treatment, found a single dose of LSD to have a beneficial effect on unhealthy alcohol use (NNT = 6) until 6 months post treatment. It was also found to increase total abstinence (NNT = 7) after a single dose until 3 months posttreatment.[73]

More modern-day trials and replication studies are needed to evaluate whether there is a clearer role for serotonergic agents in the treatment of heavy drinking or AUD in individuals differentiated by AUD subtype or genotype.

Alpha Adrenergic Antagonists

There is growing interest in targeting autonomic and stress response systems in AUD treatment, using adrenergic antagonists, such as prazosin and doxazosin. A randomized, double-blind, controlled trial of (N = 40) participants with AUD, compared prazosin 16 mg/d with placebo. Participants were exposed to cues related to stress, alcohol, and relaxation. Alcohol cravings, anxiety, heart rate, and ACTH levels were checked at baseline and after the cues. Prazosin reduced stress and cue-induced alcohol cravings as well as alcohol and stress cue-induced anxiety. It lowered basal cortisol and ACTH levels as well. This effect was only observed in those without a lifetime anxiety disorder.[74] This normalization of autonomic stress response may improve alcohol cravings and drinking outcomes. This was highlighted in a two-part study where patients with AUD, with varying degrees of alcohol withdrawal, initially underwent functional magnetic resonance imaging then were randomized to a 12-week trial, comparing prazosin to placebo, with regards to their effects on neural circuit stress response and subsequent heavy drinking outcomes. Part 1 of the study identified greater disruption in response to stress and alcohol cues in the medial prefrontal cortex and striatum in patients with high alcohol withdrawal symptoms, with a subsequent increase in heavy drinking days. In part 2, prazosin reversed this identified stress response, when compared with placebo, in turn leading to fewer drinking days during the 12-week treatment period.[75] Another RCT on (N = 90) participants with AUD compared prazosin 16 mg/d (divided in TID dosing) to placebo with regards to effect on number of drinks per week, number of drinking days per week, and number of heavy drinking days per week. Participants with PTSD were excluded in order to isolate prazosin's effect on AUD. Eighty participants were able to complete the dose titration period. Prazosin decreased the number of heavy drinking days and the number of drinks per week, more rapidly than placebo, over the 12-week trial period. Prazosin had no effect on the number of drinking days per week.[76]

Another study of (N = 36) participants with AUD, that also excluded PTSD, found no difference between prazosin and placebo in reduction of drinking. However, in a post-hoc analyses, prazosin was found to increase the rate of reduction in the number of drinks per week in a subgroup of participants who were able to adhere to and tolerate the medication, A larger effect was also observed in participants with higher baseline diastolic blood pressure.[77] An additional 12-week, double-blind RCT of prazosin versus placebo (N = 100) found that in the subset of participants with high levels of alcohol withdrawal, participants treated with prazosin had significantly fewer drinking days and heavy drinking days than did those treated with placebo, but this effect was not observed among the subset with low alcohol withdrawal.[78]

Thus, tolerability concerns may be contributing to this variation in study outcomes, or, as with gabapentin as described above, prazosin may be most efficacious among individuals with high levels of alcohol withdrawal.

Doxazosin differs from prazosin with its longer half-life, allowing for once-a-day dosing and improved adherence, slower onset of action, and lower risk of hypotensive side effects. In a double-blind RCT of (N = 41) participants with AUD, 16 mg/d of doxazosin did not differ from placebo in its effect on drinks per week and heavy drinking days per week. However, family history was found to be a moderator of effect with doxazosin reducing drinking in participants with a high family history density of AUD.[79] Further analyses from this study found higher baseline diastolic blood pressure predicted a significant effect of doxazosin in reducing heavy drinking days and drinks per week.[80]

These studies support the hypothesis of potential benefit from alpha antagonists in treating AUD and warrant more research. Investigating precision medicine approaches such as baseline stress reactivity, blood pressure, and family history and potential genetic markers mediating response, may enhance our understanding of the role of these agents in AUD treatment.

Other Agents

Varenicline

Research is ongoing to identify new treatment targets for management of AUD. Varenicline, a partial agonist of $\alpha 4\beta 2$ nicotinic acetylcholine receptors and full agonist of $\alpha 7$ nicotinic acetylcholine receptors, is FDA approved for helping people to stop smoking. Given its central action in the ventral tegmental area, it may affect dopamine activity, which, in turn, could explain its potential utility in AUD treatment. A meta-analysis of ten studies (N = 731) found varenicline to significantly decrease cravings for alcohol, but it had no significant effect on other drinking outcomes.[81] In an RCT of (N = 200) participants with AUD, varenicline was found to reduce both alcohol consumption and cravings.[82] Its investigators explored potential moderators of response to varenicline and suggested it may be more effective in patients with less severe AUD (ie, patients with less alcohol-related consequences), of older age (>45 years), longer drinking time (>28 years), who preferred a goal of nonabstinence, and those who reduced their cigarette consumption due to treatment with varenicline.[83]

N-acetylcysteine

N-acetylcysteine (NAC) is a derivative of the amino acid L-cysteine. It is FDA approved for its hepatoprotective use in acetaminophen overdose and as a mucolytic. There is growing interest in its utility in treating substance use disorders as it has been shown to modulate glutamate transmission, which has been implicated in craving and withdrawal states. It has shown promise in treating cocaine, cannabis, opioid, and nicotine use disorders.[84] Its effect on alcohol consumption was observed in an RCT with (N = 302) participants randomized to treatment with NAC (600 mg BID) or placebo for cannabis use disorder. Compared to placebo, the NAC group had increased odds of abstinence, fewer drinks per week, and fewer drinking days per week. This was not correlated to changes in cannabis consumption.[85] These findings highlight the need to investigate the effect of NAC on alcohol use further in studies focused on AUD.

MEDICATIONS TO TREAT CO-OCCURRING PSYCHIATRIC SYMPTOMS OR DISORDERS IN PATIENTS WITH ALCOHOL USE DISORDER

Although most patients with AUD report a reduction in mood or anxiety symptoms following acute withdrawal, for some these symptoms may persist for months. Even among patients without substantial symptoms of alcohol withdrawal, persistent, low-level mood or anxiety symptoms may develop, a condition that has been called "postacute withdrawal." In a substantial minority of patients, these symptoms may reflect diagnosable psychiatric disorders. Although medications (eg, serotonin reuptake inhibitors) are often prescribed during the post withdrawal period in hopes of relieving these symptoms, there is no good evidence that the treatment of persistent or subacute withdrawal symptoms that do not meet diagnostic criteria for a co-occurring psychiatric disorder results in better outcome in patients with AUD.

Many of the early studies of the efficacy of medications to treat mood disturbances targeted symptoms of depression and anxiety in unselected groups of patients with AUD after withdrawal. These and other methodological limitations in these studies make the failure to demonstrate an advantage over control conditions through reductions in either psychiatric symptoms or drinking behavior difficult to interpret.[86] Community studies have shown high rates of co-occurrence of psychiatric disorders in individuals with AUD.[87,88] Further, the majority of such individuals who seek treatment meet lifetime criteria for one or more psychiatric disorders in addition to AUD, most commonly mood disorders, other substance use disorders, antisocial personality disorder, and anxiety disorders.[74,75]

Antidepressants, benzodiazepines, and other anxiolytics, antipsychotics, and lithium have been used to treat anxiety and depression in the post withdrawal state. Although, in general, the indications for use of these medications in patients with AUD are similar to those for patients with psychiatric illness who do not have AUD, careful differential diagnosis is warranted to identify patients for whom the symptoms can be ascribed to substance use. Further, the choice of medications should take into account the increased potential for adverse effects when prescribed to individuals who are actively drinking heavily. Adverse effects can result from pharmacodynamic interactions with medical disorders that commonly occur in the course of AUD, as well as from pharmacokinetic interactions with medications prescribed to treat these disorders.[89]

Antidepressant Treatment of Unipolar Depression and Alcohol Use Disorder

Most of the studies in a meta-analysis that included 14 prospective, parallel-group, double-blind, randomized, placebo-controlled trials of antidepressants for a co-occurring substance use disorder and unipolar depression focused on alcohol dependence.[90] Eight studies (six of which were in patients with alcohol dependence) showed a significant or near-significant advantage for the active medication over placebo in reducing symptoms of depression. The pooled effect size on the standardized difference between means on the Hamilton Depression Rating Scale was 0.38 (95% CI 0.18 to 0.58), a small to moderate effect. Studies with a placebo response rate of more than 25% showed no advantage for the active medication, whereas those with a smaller placebo response rate yielded effects in the moderate to large range. Allowing a week of abstinence to transpire before making a diagnosis of depression predicted a better antidepressant response. In contrast, a larger proportion of women in the study sample, the use of serotonin reuptake inhibitors (versus tricyclic or other antidepressants), and a concurrent psychosocial intervention were associated with a poorer medication response. Studies that showed a moderate effect of the medication on depression scores also showed moderate reductions in substance use, whereas smaller effects on depressive symptoms were associated with no beneficial effects on substance use.

Subsequent to this analysis, there have been studies of pharmacotherapy for co-occurring alcohol dependence and depression. A multicenter trial compared sertraline versus placebo in 328 patients with co-occurring major depressive disorder and alcohol dependence.[91] After a 1-week, single-blind, placebo lead-in period, patients were randomly assigned to receive 10 weeks of treatment with sertraline or placebo. Randomization was stratified, based on whether initially elevated depression scores declined with abstinence from heavy drinking. Both depressive symptoms and alcohol consumption decreased substantially over time in both groups, with no reliable medication group differences on depressive symptoms or drinking behavior in either group. The high placebo response rate may have contributed to the null findings.

An elegant clinical trial randomly assigned participants with co-occurring major depression and alcohol dependence, in double-blind fashion, to one of four treatment conditions: (1) sertraline 200 mg/d (N = 40), (2) naltrexone 100 mg/d (N = 49), (3) the combination of sertraline 200 mg/d and naltrexone 100 mg/d (N = 42), and (4) double placebo (N = 39). Over 14 weeks, the combination treatment group had a significantly higher abstinence rate and a significantly longer mean time to relapse to heavy drinking than did the other three groups. The combination group also had higher, though not statistically significantly higher, rates of depression remission with fewer serious adverse events than did the other three groups. The findings from this study, absent any contraindications, encourage the combination of naltrexone and sertraline for the treatment of patients with co-occurring AUD and depression.[92] If patients already had a therapeutic trial of sertraline and found it ineffective or intolerable, it is reasonable to consider an alternative antidepressant.

In summary, there is evidence that most episodes of post withdrawal depression will remit without specific treatment if abstinence from alcohol is maintained for a period of days or weeks.[93,94] Starting new medications during this period should be minimized given this transient nature of substance induced depression. This will avoid the risks and confounding effects of polypharmacy. However, depression that persists a month out from last alcohol use requires a careful assessment for a separate but co-occurring depressive disorder that may warrant treatment; including psychotherapy, medication, or both. Serotonin reuptake inhibitors and other antidepressants approved after the tricyclic antidepressants have become the first-line treatment of depression because they have a favorable adverse event profile. These medications have significantly less of the anticholinergic, hypotensive, or sedative effects of the tricyclic antidepressants, nor do they, with the possible exception of citalopram, have the adverse cardiovascular effects, which in overdose can be lethal. However, serotonin reuptake inhibitors can exacerbate the tremor, anxiety, and insomnia often experienced by patients with physiological dependence on alcohol who have been recently withdrawn from alcohol and may slightly increase the risk of gastrointestinal bleeding (particularly in combination with nonsteroidal anti-inflammatory drugs or aspirin).

Mood Stabilizer Treatment of Bipolar Disorder and Alcohol Use Disorder

Bipolar disorder co-occurs commonly with AUD. The presence of comorbid AUD is associated with an increased rate of mixed or dysphoric mania and rapid cycling, as well as greater bipolar symptom severity, suicidality, and aggression.[95] However, controlled trials of medication to treat these co-occurring disorders are difficult to conduct. A placebo-controlled trial of divalproex sodium in bipolar patients with alcohol dependence taking lithium showed that the drug significantly decreased the proportion of heavy drinking days (corroborated by a decrease in the concentration of gamma-glutamyl transpeptidase), whereas manic and depressive symptoms improved equally in both groups.[96]

Treatment of Co-occurring Anxiety Disorders and Alcohol Use Disorder

Benzodiazepines and Other Anxiolytics

Benzodiazepines are widely used and generally considered to be acceptable treatment for acute alcohol withdrawal. The relative merits of the use of benzodiazepines in patients with alcohol and other substance use disorders during the post withdrawal period for the management of anxiety or insomnia have been debated in the medical literature.[97,98]

Early return to use, which commonly disrupts alcohol rehabilitation, can result from protracted withdrawal-related symptoms (eg, anxiety, depression, insomnia). This highlights the importance of addressing these symptoms in early abstinence to prevent relapse.

Short-term use of benzodiazepines to address anxiety must be weighed against the risk both of overdose, unhealthy use including addiction, physical dependence, and diversion on benzodiazepines. Although these medications alone are comparatively safe, even in overdose, their combination with other brain depressants (including alcohol) can be lethal. Although there is little doubt that individuals with AUD are more vulnerable to develop physical dependence on the benzodiazepines than is the average person, the potential for developing a sedative hypnotic use disorder may be lower than is generally believed.[99,100] However, physiological dependence on both alcohol and benzodiazepines may increase depressive symptoms,[93] and co-occurring alcohol and benzodiazepine use disorders may be more difficult to treat than is AUD alone.[101]

Buspirone, a nonbenzodiazepine anxiolytic, exerts its effects largely via its partial agonist activity at serotonergic auto receptors. Although comparable in efficacy to diazepam in the relief of anxiety and associated depression in outpatients with moderate-to-severe anxiety,[102,103] buspirone is less sedating than is diazepam or clorazepate, does not interact with alcohol to impair psychomotor skills, and does not have substance use disorder liability.[104,105] This pharmacological profile makes buspirone more suitable than benzodiazepines to treat anxiety symptoms among patients with alcohol dependence. In contrast to benzodiazepines, however, buspirone does not have acute anxiolytic effects, is not useful in the treatment of alcohol withdrawal, and is not useful for treating the insomnia that is commonly reported by patients with AUD during acute and protracted withdrawal.

Results from three of four placebo-controlled, double-blind trials of buspirone to treat anxiety symptoms among patients with AUD have shown the drug to be superior to placebo in increasing treatment retention and reducing anxiety symptoms and measures of drinking.[106,107] Although buspirone appears to be useful in the treatment of anxiety symptoms in patients with AUD, it has not been possible to identify clinical features that differentiate individuals for whom buspirone may be most efficacious from those who are not responsive to the medication.

UTILIZATION OF PHARMACOTHERAPY IN THE TREATMENT OF ALCOHOL USE DISORDER

Despite data suggesting efficacy, the use of medications that have been FDA approved for treatment of AUD remains very limited. The lack of robust utilization can be found in large organizations such as the Veterans Health Administration as well as other public and private entities.[108,109] This limited use is evident even in clinicians who have been trained to treat AUD—addiction physicians. A survey of nearly 1,400 members of the American Society of Addiction Medicine and the American Academy of Addiction Psychiatry[110] showed that they prescribed disulfiram to only 9% of their patients with alcohol dependence, and naltrexone was prescribed only slightly more frequently (ie, to 13% of patients). In contrast, antidepressants were prescribed to 44% of patients with AUD. Although nearly all these physicians had heard of disulfiram and naltrexone, their self-reported level of knowledge of these medications was much lower than that for antidepressants and benzodiazepines. Additionally, primary care physicians, who represent the clinicians most likely to diagnose AUD, were found to be unfamiliar with approved pharmacotherapies.[111] Clearly, additional education is needed to improve awareness among treatment professionals as well as patients.

SUMMARY AND CONCLUSIONS

As evidence has accumulated showing that a growing number of medications are efficacious for the treatment of AUD, the therapeutic options available to physicians in treating these patients have increased. Because all three medications that are FDA approved for the treatment of AUD have demonstrated efficacy in some patients, these medications should be considered a first-line treatment in patients with AUD. They can be used in combination with behavioral treatment, depending on availability and patient preference. Given limited data on how to choose which of the efficacious medications is appropriate for any given patient, the choice can be made collaboratively with the patient.

The treatment of psychiatric symptoms that co-occur with AUD, which can augment efforts at addressing alcohol use that is above recommended limits, has been studied in some detail. However, the literature remains mixed with respect to the efficacy of specific interventions. Anxiolytics, such as buspirone, and antidepressants with benign side effect profiles, such as serotonin reuptake inhibitors, may reduce alcohol intake and warrant careful evaluation in the treatment of anxious and depressed patients with AUD. However, even if medications that are prescribed to patients with AUD with persistent co-occurring mood and anxiety symptoms, they will not necessarily reduce alcohol consumption after moderate to severe AUD develops. This is likely to hold true even if pathological mood states were important in the initiation of heavy drinking.[68,112] That is, the neuroadaptive changes and the complex learning that characterize AUD[113] are not likely to resolve because one major contributing factor is brought under control. The challenge for practitioners treating AUD is to combine efficacious medications with empirically based psychological interventions and self-help group participation for those patients willing and able to incorporate these elements into their treatment.

The use of medications in patients who are actively participating in self-help groups may be particularly challenging. Although members of abstinence-oriented groups such as Alcoholics Anonymous may be willing to work with physicians when they prescribe disulfiram, the use of which is supportive of their goal of total abstinence, they may be less supportive of other medications that aim to reduce drinking and its associated medical, psychological, and social harm. Nonetheless, clinicians should support patients, as allowing patients to choose their treatment goals increases their odds of success.[114]

Future research should investigate the safety and efficacy of medications to treat AUD, with adequate statistical power, in women, in different ethnic/racial groups, and in adolescent and geriatric samples.

REFERENCES

1. Centers for Disease Control and Prevention. Alcohol Related Disease Impact (ARDI) Application. Accessed June 7, 2023. www.cdc.gov/ARDI
2. Substance Abuse and Mental Health Services Administration. Center for Behavioral Health Statistics and Quality. *1999 to 2020 National Survey on Drug Use and Health (NSDUH) Small Area Estimation Dataset: State Small Area Estimates, by Survey Year, Outcome, State, and Age Group, NSDUH Methodological Report*. SAMHSA; 2021.
3. Substance Abuse and Mental Health Services Administration. National Survey of Substance Abuse Treatment Services (N-SSATS): 2020. Data on Substance Abuse Treatment Facilities. SAMHSA; 2021.
4. Baser O, Chalk M, Rawson R, Gastfriend DR. Alcohol dependence treatments: comprehensive healthcare costs, utilization outcomes, and pharmacotherapy persistence. *Am J Manag Care.* 2011;17 Suppl 8: S222-S234.
5. Cabrera EA, Wiers CE, Lindgren E, Miller G, Volkow ND, Wang GJ. Neuroimaging the effectiveness of substance use disorder treatments. *J Neuroimmune Pharmacol.* 2016;11(3):408-433. doi:10.1007/s11481-016-9680-y
6. Witkiewitz K, Kranzler HR, Hallgren KA, et al. Drinking risk level reductions associated with improvements in physical health and quality of life among individuals with alcohol use disorder. *Alcohol Clin Exp Res.* 2018;42(12):2453-2465.
7. Heilig M, Egli M. Pharmacological treatment of alcohol dependence: target symptoms and target mechanisms. *Pharmacol Ther.* 2006;111: 855-876.
8. Oslin DW, Leong SH, Lynch KG, et al. Naltrexone vs placebo for the treatment of alcohol dependence a randomized clinical trial. *JAMA Psychiat.* 2015;72:430-437.
9. Volpicelli JR, Alterman AI, Hayashida M, O'Brien CP. Naltrexone in the treatment of alcohol dependence. *Arch Gen Psychiatry.* 1992;49: 876-880.
10. O'Malley SS, Jaffe AJ, Chang G, Schottenfeld RS, Meyer RE, Rounsaville B. Naltrexone and coping skills therapy for alcohol dependence. A controlled study. *Arch Gen Psychiatry.* 1992;49:881-887.
11. Volpicelli JR, Watson NT, King AC, Sherman CE, O'Brien CP. Effect of naltrexone on alcohol "high" in alcoholics. *Am J Psychiatry.* 1995;152: 613-615.
12. O'Malley SS, Jaffe AJ, Chang G, et al. Six-month follow-up of naltrexone and psychotherapy for alcohol dependence. *Arch Gen Psychiatry.* 1996;53:217-224.
13. Bahji A, Bach P, Danilewitz M, et al. Pharmacotherapies for adults with alcohol use disorders: a systematic review and network meta-analysis. *J Addict Med.* 2022;16(6):630-638. doi:10.1097/ADM.0000000000000992
14. Rösner S, Hackl-Herrwerth A, Leucht S, Vecchi S, Srisurapanont M, Soyka M. Opioid antagonists for alcohol dependence. *Cochrane Database Syst Rev.* 2010;12:CD001867. doi:10.1002/14651858.CD001867.pub3
15. Jonas DE, Amick HR, Feltner C, et al. Pharmacotherapy for adults with alcohol use disorders in outpatient settings a systematic review and meta-analysis. *JAMA.* 2014;311:1889-1900.
16. Anton RF, Moak DH, Latham PK, et al. Posttreatment results of combining naltrexone with cognitive-behavior therapy for the treatment of alcoholism. *J Clin Psychopharmacol.* 2001;21:72-77.
17. Anton RF, O'Malley SS, Ciraulo DA, et al. Combined pharmacotherapies and behavioral interventions for alcohol dependence: the COMBINE study: a randomized controlled trial. *JAMA.* 2006;295:2003-2017.
18. Kranzler HR, Armeli S, Tennen H, et al. Targeted naltrexone for early problem drinkers. *J Clin Psychopharmacol.* 2003;23:294-304.
19. Heinala P, Alho H, Kiianmaa K, Lönnqvist J, Kuoppasalmi K, Sinclair JD. Targeted use of naltrexone without prior detoxification in the treatment of alcohol dependence: a factorial double-blind, placebo-controlled trial. *J Clin Psychopharmacol.* 2001;21:287-292.
20. O'Malley SS, Rounsaville BJ, Farren C, et al. Initial and maintenance naltrexone treatment for alcohol dependence using primary care vs. specialty care: a nested sequence of 3 randomized trials. *Arch Intern Med.* 2003;163:1695-1704.
21. Anton RF, Myrick H, Wright TM, et al. Gabapentin combined with naltrexone for the treatment of alcohol dependence. *Am J Psychiatry.* 2011;168(7):709-717.
22. Volpicelli JR, Rhines KC, Rhines JS, et al. Naltrexone and alcohol dependence. Role of subject compliance. *Arch Gen Psychiatry.* 1997;54:737-742.
23. Garbutt JC, Kranzler HR, O'Malley SS, et al. Efficacy and tolerability of long-acting injectable naltrexone for alcohol dependence: a randomized controlled trial. *JAMA.* 2005;293(13):1617-1625.
24. Murphy CE IV, Wang RC, Montoy JC, Whittaker E, Raven M. Effect of extended-release naltrexone on alcohol consumption: a systematic review and meta-analysis. *Addiction.* 2022;117(2):271-281. doi:10.1111/add.15572
25. Emmerson PJ, Liu MR, Woods JH, Medzihradsky F. Binding affinity and selectivity of opioids at mu, delta and kappa receptors in monkey brain membranes. *J Pharmacol Exp Ther.* 1994;271:1630-1637.

26. Mason BJ, Ritvo EC, Morgan RO, et al. A double-blind, placebo-controlled pilot study to evaluate the efficacy and safety of oral nalmefene HCl for alcohol dependence. *Alcohol Clin Exp Res.* 1994;18:1162-1167.
27. Mason BJ, Salvato FR, Williams LD, Ritvo EC, Cutler RB. A double-blind, placebo-controlled study of oral nalmefene for alcohol dependence. *Arch Gen Psychiatry.* 1999;56:719-724.
28. Anton RF, Pettinati H, Zweben A, et al. A multi-site dose ranging study of nalmefene in the treatment of alcohol dependence. *J Clin Psychopharmacol.* 2004;24:421-428.
29. Karhuvaara S, Simojoki K, Virta A, et al. Targeted nalmefene with simple medical management in the treatment of heavy drinkers: a randomized double-blind placebo-controlled multicenter study. *Alcohol Clin Exp Res.* 2007;31:1179-1187.
30. Rubio G, Ponce G, Rodriguez-Jiménez R, Jiménez-Arriero MA, Hoenicka J, Palomo T. Clinical predictors of response to naltrexone in alcoholic patients: who benefits most from treatment with naltrexone? *Alcohol*. 2005;40(3):227-233.
31. Lhuintre JP, Daoust M, Moore ND, et al. Ability of calcium bis acetyl homotaurine, a GABA agonist, to prevent relapse in weaned alcoholics. *Lancet.* 1985;1:1014-1016.
32. Kranzler HR, Gage A. Acamprosate efficacy in alcohol-dependent patients: reanalysis of results from 3 pivotal trials. *Am J Addict.* 2008;17:70-76.
33. Chick J, Lehert P, Landron F. Does acamprosate improve reduction of drinking as well as aiding abstinence? *J Psychopharmacol.* 2003;17:397-402.
34. Besson J, Aeby F, Kasas A, Lehert P, Potgieter A. Combined efficacy of acamprosate and disulfiram in the treatment of alcoholism: a controlled study. *Alcohol Clin Exp Res.* 1998;22:573-579.
35. Mason BJ, Goodman AM, Chabac S, Lehert P. Effect of oral acamprosate on abstinence in patients with alcohol dependence in a double-blind, placebo-controlled trial: the role of patient motivation. *J Psychiatr Res.* 2006;40:383-393.
36. Kiefer F, Jahn H, Tarnaske T, et al. Comparing and combining naltrexone and acamprosate in relapse prevention of alcoholism: a double-blind, placebo-controlled study. *Arch Gen Psychiatry.* 2003;60:92-99.
37. Mutschler J, Grosshans M, Soyka M, Rösner S. Current findings and mechanisms of action of disulfiram in the treatment of alcohol dependence. *Pharmacopsychiatry.* 2016;49(4):137-141. doi:10.1055/s-0042-103592
38. Lindros KO, Stowell A, Pikkarainen P, Salaspuro M. The disulfiram (Antabuse)-alcohol reaction in male alcoholics: its efficient management by 4-methylpyrazole. *Alcohol Clin Exp Res.* 1981;5:528-530.
39. Favazza AR, Martin P. Chemotherapy of delirium tremens: a survey of physicians' preferences. *Am J Psychiatry.* 1974;131:1031-1033.
40. Fuller RK, Branchey L, Brightwell DR, et al. Disulfiram treatment of alcoholism. A veterans administration cooperative study. *JAMA.* 1986;256:1449-1455.
41. Jørgensen CH, Pedersen B, Tønnesen H. The efficacy of disulfiram for the treatment of alcohol use disorder. *Alcohol Clin Exp Res.* 2011;35(10):1749-1758. doi:10.1111/j.1530-0277.2011.01523.x
42. Brewer C, Meyers RJ, Johnsen J. Does disulfiram help to prevent relapse in alcohol abuse? *CNS Drugs.* 2000;14:329-341.
43. Allen JP, Litten RZ. Techniques to enhance compliance with disulfiram. *Alcohol Clin Exp Res.* 1992;16:1035-1041.
44. Chick J. Safety issues concerning the use of disulfiram in treating alcohol dependence. *Drug Saf.* 1999;20:427-435.
45. Johnson BA, Ait-Daoud N, Bowden CL, et al. Oral topiramate for treatment of alcohol dependence: a randomised controlled trial. *Lancet.* 2003;361:1677-1685.
46. Johnson BA, Rosenthal N, Capece JA, et al. Topiramate for treating alcohol dependence: a randomized controlled trial. *JAMA.* 2007;298:1641-1651.
47. Blodgett JC, Del Re AC, Maisel NC, Finney JW. A meta-analysis of topiramate's effects for individuals with alcohol use disorders. *Alcohol Clin Exp Res.* 2014;38(6):1481-1488. doi:10.1111/acer.12411
48. Kranzler HR, Covault J, Feinn R, et al. Topiramate treatment for heavy drinkers: moderation by a GRIK1 polymorphism. *Am J Psychiatry.* 2014;171:445-452.
49. Sills GJ. The mechanisms of action of gabapentin and pregabalin. *Curr Opin Pharmacol.* 2006;6(1):108-113. doi:10.1016/j.coph.2005.11.003
50. Brower KJ, Kim HM, Strobbe S, Karam-Hage MA, Consens F, Zucker RA. A randomized double-blind pilot trial of gabapentin versus placebo to treat alcohol dependence and comorbid insomnia. *Alcohol Clin Exp Res.* 2008;32(8):1429-1438.
51. Furieri FA, Nakamura-Palacios EM. Gabapentin reduces alcohol consumption and craving: a randomized, double-blind, placebo-controlled trial. *J Clin Psychiatry.* 2007;68(11):1691-1700.
52. Mason BJ, Quello S, Goodell V, Shadan F, Kyle M, Begovic A. Gabapentin treatment for alcohol dependence: a randomized clinical trial. *JAMA Intern Med.* 2014;174(1):70-77.
53. Falk DE, Ryan ML, Fertig JB, et al. Gabapentin enacarbil extended-release for alcohol use disorder: a randomized, double-blind, placebo-controlled, multisite trial assessing efficacy and safety. *Alcohol Clin Exp Res.* 2019;43(1):158-169. doi:10.1111/acer.13917
54. Kranzler HR, Feinn R, Morris P, Hartwell EE. A meta-analysis of the efficacy of gabapentin for treating alcohol use disorder. *Addiction.* 2019;114(9):1547-1555. doi:10.1111/add.14655
55. Anton RF, Latham P, Voronin K, et al. Efficacy of gabapentin for the treatment of alcohol use disorder in patients with alcohol withdrawal symptoms: a randomized clinical trial. *JAMA Intern Med.* 2020;180(5):728-736. doi:10.1001/jamainternmed.2020.0249
56. Bockbrader HN, Wesche D, Miller R, Chapel S, Janiczek N, Burger P. A comparison of the pharmacokinetics and pharmacodynamics of pregabalin and gabapentin. *Clin Pharmacokinetics.* 2010;49(10):661-669.
57. Krupitsky EM, Rybakova KV, Skurat EP, Semenova NV, Neznanov NG. Dvoĭnoe slepoe randomizirovannoe platsebo-kontroliruemoe issledovanie éffektivnosti i bezopasnosti primeneniia pregabalina dlia stabilizatsii remissii sindroma zavisimosti ot alkogolia [A double blind placebo controlled randomized clinical trial of the efficacy and safety of pregabalin in induction of remission in patients with alcohol dependence]. *Zh Nevrol Psikhiatr Im S Korsakova.* 2020;120(1):33-43. Russian. doi:10.17116/jnevro202012001133
58. Mariani JJ, Pavlicova M, Choi CJ, et al. An open-label pilot study of pregabalin pharmacotherapy for alcohol use disorder. *Am J Drug Alcohol Abuse.* 2021;47(4):467-475. doi:10.1080/00952990.2021.1901105
59. Addolorato G, Caputo F, Capristo E, et al. Baclofen efficacy in reducing alcohol craving and intake: a preliminary double-blind randomized controlled study. *Alcohol Alcohol.* 2002;37:504-508.
60. Addolorato G, Leggio L, Ferrulli A, et al. Effectiveness and safety of baclofen for maintenance of alcohol abstinence in alcohol-dependent patients with liver cirrhosis: randomised, double-blind controlled study. *Lancet.* 2007;370:1915-1922.
61. Müller CA, Geisel PP, Higl V, et al. High dose baclofen for the treatment of alcohol dependence (BACLAD study): a randomized, placebo-controlled trial. *Eur Neuropsychopharmacol.* 2015;25:1167-1177.
62. Beraha EM, Salemink E, Goudriaan AE, et al. Efficacy and safety of high-dose baclofen for the treatment of alcohol dependence: a multicenter, randomized, double-blind controlled trial. *Eur Neuropsychopharmacol.* 2016;26:1950-1959.
63. Hauser P, Fuller B, Ho SB, Thuras P, Kern S, Dieperink E. The safety and efficacy of baclofen to reduce alcohol use in veterans with chronic Hepatitis C: a randomized clinical trial. *Addiction.* 2017;112:1173-1183. doi:10.1111/add.13787
64. Minozzi S, Saulle R, Rösner S. Baclofen for alcohol use disorder. *Cochrane Database Syst Rev.* 2018;11(11):CD012557. doi:10.1002/14651858.CD012557.pub2
65. Morley KC, Baillie A, Fraser I, et al. Baclofen in the treatment of alcohol dependence with or without liver disease: multisite, randomised, double-blind, placebo-controlled trial. *Br J Psychiatry.* 2018;212(6):362-369. doi:10.1192/bjp.2018.13
66. Garbutt JC, Kampov-Polevoy AB, Pedersen C, et al. Efficacy and tolerability of baclofen in a U.S. community population with alcohol use disorder: a dose-response, randomized, controlled trial. *Neuropsychopharmacology.* 2021;46(13):2250-2256. doi:10.1038/s41386-021-01055-w

67. Johnson BA, Roache JD, Javors MA, et al. Ondansetron for reduction of drinking among biologically predisposed alcoholic patients: a randomized controlled trial. *JAMA.* 2000;284:963-971.
68. Kranzler HR, Pierucci-Lagha A, Feinn R, Hernandez-Avila C. Effects of ondansetron in early versus late-onset alcoholics: a prospective study. *Alcohol Clin Exp Res.* 2003;27(7):1150-1155.
69. Johnson BA, Ait-Daoud N, Seneviratne C, et al. Pharmacogenetic approach at the serotonin transporter gene as a method of reducing the severity of alcohol drinking. *Am J Psychiatry.* 2011;168:265-275.
70. Johnson BA, Seneviratne C, Wang XQ, Ait-Daoud N, Li MD. Determination of genotype combinations that can predict the outcome of the treatment of alcohol dependence using the 5-HT(3) antagonist ondansetron. *Am J Psychiatry.* 2013;170:1020-1031.
71. Bogenschutz MP, Forcehimes AA, Pommy JA, Wilcox CE, Barbosa PC, Strassman RJ. Psilocybin-assisted treatment for alcohol dependence: a proof-of-concept study. *J Psychopharmacol.* 2015;29(3):289-299. doi:10.1177/0269881114565144
72. Bogenschutz MP, Ross S, Bhatt S, et al. Percentage of heavy drinking days following psilocybin-assisted psychotherapy vs placebo in the treatment of adult patients with alcohol use disorder: a randomized clinical trial. *JAMA Psychiatry.* 2022;2022:e222096. doi:10.1001/jamapsychiatry.2022.2096 Erratum in: *JAMA Psychiatry.* 2022;79(11):1141
73. Krebs TS, Johansen PØ. Lysergic acid diethylamide (LSD) for alcoholism: meta-analysis of randomized controlled trials. *J Psychopharmacol.* 2012;26(7):994-1002. doi:10.1177/0269881112439253
74. Milivojevic V, Angarita GA, Hermes G, Sinha R, Fox HC. Effects of prazosin on provoked alcohol craving and autonomic and neuroendocrine response to stress in alcohol use disorder. *Alcohol Clin Exp Res.* 2020;44(7):1488-1496. doi:10.1111/acer.14378
75. Sinha R, Fogelman N, Wemm S, Angarita G, Seo D, Hermes G. Alcohol withdrawal symptoms predict corticostriatal dysfunction that is reversed by prazosin treatment in alcohol use disorder. *Addict Biol.* 2022;27(2):e13116. doi:10.1111/adb.13116
76. Simpson TL, Saxon AJ, Stappenbeck C, et al. Double-blind randomized clinical trial of prazosin for alcohol use disorder. *Am J Psychiatry.* 2018;175(12):1216-1224. doi:10.1176/appi.ajp.2018.17080913
77. Wilcox CE, Tonigan JS, Bogenschutz MP, Clifford J, Bigelow R, Simpson T. A randomized, placebo-controlled, clinical trial of prazosin for the treatment of alcohol use disorder. *J Addict Med.* 2018;12(5):339-345. doi:10.1097/ADM.0000000000000413
78. Sinha R, Wemm S, Fogelman N, et al. Moderation of prazosin's efficacy by alcohol withdrawal symptoms. *Am J Psychiatry.* 2021;178(5):447-458. doi:10.1176/appi.ajp.2020.20050609
79. Kenna GA, Haass-Koffler CL, Zywiak WH, et al. Role of the α1 blocker doxazosin in alcoholism: a proof-of-concept randomized controlled trial. *Addict Biol.* 2016;21(4):904-914. doi:10.1111/adb.12275
80. Haass-Koffler CL, Goodyear K, Zywiak WH, et al. Higher pretreatment blood pressure is associated with greater alcohol drinking reduction in alcohol-dependent individuals treated with doxazosin. *Drug Alcohol Depend.* 2017;177:23-28. doi:10.1016/j.drugalcdep.2017.03.016
81. Gandhi KD, Mansukhani MP, Karpyak VM, Schneekloth TD, Wang Z, Kolla BP. The impact of varenicline on alcohol consumption in subjects with alcohol use disorders: systematic review and meta-analyses. *J Clin Psychiatry.* 2020;81(2) 19r12924: doi:10.4088/JCP.19r12924
82. Litten RZ, Ryan ML, Fertig JB, et al. A double-blind, placebo-controlled trial assessing the efficacy of varenicline tartrate for alcohol dependence. *J Addict Med.* 2013;7(4):277-286. doi:10.1097/ADM.0b013e31829623f4
83. Falk DE, Castle IJ, Ryan M, Fertig J, Litten RZ. Moderators of varenicline treatment effects in a double-blind, placebo-controlled trial for alcohol dependence: an exploratory analysis. *J Addict Med.* 2015;9(4):296-303. doi:10.1097/ADM.0000000000000133
84. Smaga I, Frankowska M, Filip M. N-acetylcysteine in substance use disorder: a lesson from preclinical and clinical research. *Pharmacol Rep.* 2021;73(5):1205-1219. doi:10.1007/s43440-021-00283-7
85. Squeglia LM, Tomko RL, Baker NL, McClure EA, Book GA, Gray KM. The effect of N-acetylcysteine on alcohol use during a cannabis cessation trial. *Drug Alcohol Depend.* 2018;185:17-22. doi:10.1016/j.drugalcdep.2017.12.005
86. Ciraulo DA, Jaffe JH. Tricyclic antidepressants in the treatment of depression associated with alcoholism. *J Clin Psychopharmacol.* 1981;1:146-150.
87. Regier DA, Farmer ME, Rae DS, et al. Comorbidity of mental disorders with alcohol and other drug abuse. Results from the Epidemiologic Catchment Area (ECA) study. *JAMA.* 1990;264:2511-2518.
88. Grant BF, Dawson DA, Stinson FS, et al. The 12-month prevalence and trends in DSM-IV alcohol abuse and dependence: United States, 1991-1992 and 2001-2002. *Drug Alcohol Depend.* 2004;74:223-234.
89. Sullivan L, O'Connor P. Medical disorders in substance abuse patients. In: Kranzler H, Tinsley J, eds. *Dual Diagnosis and Psychiatric Treatment: Substance Abuse and Comorbid Disorders.* 2nd ed. Marcel Dekker; 2004:515-553.
90. Nunes EV, Levin FR. Treatment of depression in patients with alcohol or other drug dependence: a meta-analysis. *JAMA.* 2004;291:1887-1896.
91. Kranzler HR, Mueller T, Cornelius J, et al. Sertraline treatment of co-occurring alcohol dependence and major depression. *J Clin Psychopharmacol.* 2006;26:13-20.
92. Pettinati HM, Oslin DW, Kampman KM, et al. A double-blind, placebo-controlled trial combining sertraline and naltrexone for treating co-occurring depression and alcohol dependence. *Am J Psychiatry.* 2010;167(6):668–675.
93. Schuckit M. Alcoholic patients with secondary depression. *Am J Psychiatry.* 1983;140:711-714.
94. Brown SA, Schuckit MA. Changes in depression among abstinent alcoholics. *J Stud Alcohol.* 1988;49:412-417.
95. Frye MA, Salloum IM. Bipolar disorder and comorbid alcoholism: prevalence rate and treatment considerations. *Bipolar Disord.* 2006;8:677-685.
96. Salloum IM, Cornelius JR, Daley DC, Kirisci L, Himmelhoch JM, Thase ME. Efficacy of valproate maintenance in patients with bipolar disorder and alcoholism: a double-blind placebo-controlled study. *Arch Gen Psychiatry.* 2005;62(1):37-45.
97. Ciraulo DA, Nace EP. Benzodiazepine treatment of anxiety or insomnia in substance abuse patients. *Am J Addict.* 2000;9:276-279. discussion 280–284
98. Posternak MA, Mueller TI. Assessing the risks and benefits of benzodiazepines for anxiety disorders in patients with a history of substance abuse or dependence. *Am J Addict.* 2001;10:48-68.
99. Bliding A. The abuse potential of benzodiazepines with special reference to oxazepam. *Acta Psychiatr Scand Suppl.* 1978;274:111-116.
100. Ciraulo DA, Barnhill JG, Jaffe JH, Ciraulo AM, Tarmey MF. Intravenous pharmacokinetics of 2-hydroxyimipramine in alcoholics and normal controls. *J Stud Alcohol.* 1990;51:366-372.
101. Sokolow L, Welte J, Hynes G, Lyons J. Multiple substance use by alcoholics. *Br J Addict.* 1981;76:147-158.
102. Goldberg HL, Finnerty RJ. Comparative efficacy of tofisopam and placebo. *Am J Psychiatry.* 1979;136:196-199.
103. Jacobson AF, Dominguez RA, Goldstein BJ, Steinbook RM. Comparison of buspirone and diazepam in generalized anxiety disorder. *Pharmacotherapy.* 1985;5:290-296.
104. Seppälä T, Aranko K, Mattila MJ, Shrotriya RC. Effects of alcohol on buspirone and lorazepam actions. *Clin Pharmacol Ther.* 1982;32:201-207.
105. Mattila MJ, Aranko K, Seppala T. Acute effects of buspirone and alcohol on psychomotor skills. *J Clin Psychiatry.* 1982;43:56-61.
106. Griffith JD, Jasinski DR, Casten GP, McKinney GR. Investigation of the abuse liability of buspirone in alcohol-dependent patients. *Am J Med.* 1986;80:30-35.
107. Bruno F. Buspirone in the treatment of alcoholic patients. *Psychopathology.* 1989;22(Suppl 1):49-59.
108. Harris HS, Kivlahan DR, Bowe T, Humphreys KN. Pharmacotherapy of alcohol use disorders in the Veterans Health Administration. *Psychiatr Serv.* 2010;61(4):392-398.

109. Roman PM, Abraham AJ, Knudsen HK. Using medication-assisted treatment for substance use disorders: evidence of barriers and facilitators of implementation. *Addict Behav.* 2011;36(6):584-589.

110. Mark TL, Kranzler HR, Song X, Bransberger P, Poole VH, Crosse S. Physicians' opinions about medications to treat alcoholism. *Addiction.* 2003;98:617-626.

111. Mark TL, Kassed CA, Vandivort-Warren R, Levit KR, Kranzler HR. Alcohol and opioid dependence medications prescription trends, overall and by physician specialty. *Drug Alcohol Depend.* 2009;99:345-349.

112. Meyer RE. How to understand the relationship between psychopathology and addictive disorders: another example of the chicken and the egg. In: Meyer RE, ed. *Psychopathology and Addictive Disorders.* Guilford Press; 1986:3-16.

113. Edwards G, Gross MM. Alcohol dependence: provisional description of a clinical syndrome. *Br Med J.* 1976;1:1058-1061.

114. van Amsterdam J, van den Brink W. Reduced-risk drinking as a viable treatment goal in problematic alcohol use and alcohol dependence. *J Psychopharmacol.* 2013;27(11):987-997. doi:10.1177/0269881113495320

CHAPTER

61 Pharmacological Interventions for Sedative-Hypnotic Use Disorder

Alyssa Braxton, Jeffrey S. Cluver, Tara M. Wright, and Hugh Myrick

CHAPTER OUTLINE

- Introduction
- Pharmacology
- Definitions
- Use of sedative-hypnotic medications
- Indications for pharmacological interventions
- Treatment setting
- Treatment of co-occurring disorders
- Conclusions and future directions

INTRODUCTION

Sedative-hypnotic agents have historically been utilized for their ability to mitigate anxiety and induce sleep. Most of the medications in this class have a mechanism of action in the central nervous system (CNS) that leads to their anxiolytic and sleep-inducing properties. Prior to 1900, agents such as chloral hydrate, bromide, paraldehyde, and sulfur were used. The first barbiturate, barbital, was introduced in 1903 and was popularized due to its predictable ability to induce sleep and decrease anxiety. Phenobarbital was introduced in 1912, which proved to have additional anticonvulsant properties. Despite safety issues including its narrow therapeutic index, tolerance, and drug interactions, phenobarbital proved to be a popular medication, and thousands of derivative compounds were developed.

The first benzodiazepine, chlordiazepoxide, was synthesized in 1957. With similar properties to barbiturates, the relative safety and tolerability of the benzodiazepines has led to their widespread and lasting use.

A more recent addition to the sedative-hypnotic class of medications includes imidazopyridine derivatives (such as zolpidem), zaleplon, and eszopiclone. These medications are chemically distinct from benzodiazepines, but they also bind to the gamma-aminobutyric acid (GABA) receptor at the omega subunit. It has been reported that the behavioral and subjective effects (including subject-rated measures related to addiction potential) of these newer compounds (zolpidem, zaleplon, and eszopiclone) are similar to benzodiazepines, in both individuals with and without a history of substance use disorders.[1,2]

In 2018, the National Survey on Drug Use and Health (NSDUH) added reports for tranquilizers and sedatives, which provided more insight to their use. It is estimated 5.4 million people aged 12 or older engaged in unhealthy use of prescription benzodiazepines in 2018, which corresponds to 2.0% of the population. Additionally, the correlating quantity of prescribed tablets more than tripled and the rate of overdose involving benzodiazepines increased more than fourfold.[3,4]

Table 61-1, lists sedative-hypnotics currently available in the United States. The pharmacological effects of benzodiazepines and other sedative-hypnotics lend themselves to unhealthy use, either as a mono product or in conjunction with other substances.[5] When used in combination with other substances, benzodiazepines may enhance the effects of the other substances, mediate unpleasant side effects, or help manage withdrawal from other substances. Additionally, alone or when used with other CNS depressants, benzodiazepines and sedative-hypnotics can lead to respiratory depression, coma, and death. In this chapter, we focus on the management of individuals with sedative, hypnotic, or anxiolytic use disorder.

PHARMACOLOGY

The effects of benzodiazepines and other sedative-hypnotics are mediated by their binding to the GABA receptor. GABA receptors are distributed widely throughout the brain and bind GABA, the major inhibitory neurotransmitter in the CNS. There are specific receptor subunits that are allosterically bound to the GABA receptor, and these medications act as agonists by increasing the ability of the inhibitory neurotransmitter GABA to bind to and activate the GABA-A receptor. When an agonist such as a benzodiazepine or barbiturate binds to the GABA receptor, the receptor opens its chloride channels, leading to neuronal excitability. Clinically, this leads to the effects of decreased anxiety, increased sedation, muscle relaxation, and increased seizure threshold. The toxic effects of these compounds are caused by excessive opening of chloride channels and can lead to respiratory depression. Barbiturates increase GABA-A activity by increasing the duration of chloride channel opening whereas benzodiazepines affect GABA-A activity by increasing the frequency of chloride channel opening. The imidazopyridine derivatives zolpidem and zaleplon bind with high affinity at the type I benzodiazepine recognition site on the GABA-A receptor omega subunit. Among the sedative-hypnotic agents, there are important differences in the onset of activity, half-life of the medication, presence of active metabolites, and specificity of the clinical effects. Benzodiazepines cannot be divided based on anxiolytic versus hypnotic effects.[2] Modest evidence suggests that benzodiazepines with a shorter half-life have a higher rate of sedative hypnotic use disorder.[3]

TABLE 61-1 Classes of Sedative-Hypnotic Drugs: Drug Classes, Nonproprietary Names, and Trade Names

Benzodiazepines	Barbiturates	Miscellaneous
Alprazolam (Xanax)	Amobarbital (Amytal)	Chloral hydrate (Noctec, others)
Chlordiazepoxide (Librium, others)	Aprobarbital (Alurate)	Carisoprodol (Soma)
Clonazepam (Klonopin, others)	Butabarbital (Butisol Sodium, others)	Cyclobenzaprine (Flexeril)
Clorazepate (Tranxene, others)	Butalbital	Eszopiclone (Lunesta)
Diazepam (Valium, others)	Mephobarbital (Mebaral)	Ethchlorvynol (Placidyl)
Flurazepam HCl (Dalmane, others)	Pentobarbital (Nembutal)	Ethinamate (Valmid)
Lorazepam (Ativan, others)	Phenobarbital (Luminal Sodium, others)	Glutethimide (Doriden, others)
Oxazepam (Serax, others)	Secobarbital (Seconal Sodium)	Meprobamate (Miltown, others)
Temazepam (Restoril, others)	Talbutal (Lotusate)	Methyprylon (Noludar)
Triazolam (Halcion)		Paraldehyde (Paral)
		Zaleplon (Sonata)
		Zolpidem (Ambien)

While benzodiazepines and other sedative-hypnotics are agonists at the GABA receptor, there are also GABA receptor antagonists (such as beta-carboline) that bind to the receptor and cause the chloride channels to close. GABA receptor antagonists can cause increased anxiety and lower the seizure threshold. Flumazenil is an antagonist compound with a high affinity for the GABA receptor. This medication was developed and marketed to reverse the effects of benzodiazepines, including sedation and respiratory depression. Further information regarding pharmacology is found in section 2 of this textbook.

DEFINITIONS

Physical dependence can be defined as an altered homeostasis at several levels of drug effect and activity. Examples of physical dependence include tolerance and withdrawal. Discontinuation of the drug in this state leads to symptoms resulting from a disruption of this homeostasis. *Tolerance* can be defined as a decreased pharmacological effect after repeated or prolonged exposure to the substance so that higher doses are needed to achieve the same initial clinical effects. Physical dependence and tolerance develop with prolonged and repeated use of benzodiazepines and other sedative-hypnotics. The nonmedical use of prescription medications, defined as the use of prescription medications, whether obtained by prescription or otherwise, other than in the manner, for the reasons, or time period prescribed or by a person for whom the medication was not prescribed, may lead to the development of a substance use disorder (SUD). SUD is defined by the *Diagnostic and Statistical Manual of Mental Disorders* (DSM-5) criteria as a maladaptive pattern of substance use leading to clinically significant impairment or distress, defined by meeting multiple specified criteria within a 12-month period. Drugs with reinforcing properties, such as the ability to produce euphoria, reduce unpleasant sensations, or induce other positive subjective experiences, are more likely to lead to a SUD. The onset of physical dependence should not be equated with or imply the presence of a SUD, although the two often coexist. Similarly, the misuse of a medication does not directly imply a SUD, as may be the case in patients with severe anxiety disorders who do not achieve relief with their initially prescribed doses.

USE OF SEDATIVE-HYPNOTIC MEDICATIONS

Benzodiazepines have largely replaced barbiturates and other sedative-hypnotics in clinical settings due to their preferred pharmacological and safety profile.

Laboratory studies involving rats and nonhuman primates demonstrate that many sedative-hypnotics are self-administered, although the benzodiazepines appear to be less reinforcing than barbiturates.[6] While there have been human studies that have demonstrated the reinforcing effects of the benzodiazepines, there are notable differences among the compounds, which correlate with the agents' onset of action. Lorazepam, alprazolam, and diazepam all appear to have a greater potential for nonmedical use, likely based on their inherent lipophilic properties, and therefore more rapid onset of action. It is also important to note that other human studies have demonstrated that benzodiazepines do not have reinforcing effects in most individuals,[7] thus suggesting that some individuals may have a vulnerability that leads to nonmedical use.

According to NSDUH 2018, 14.8% of adult responders reported lifetime benzodiazepine unhealthy use, and 7.9% reported unhealthy use of sedatives.[4] The nonmedical use of benzodiazepines and sedative-hypnotics is commonly seen in individuals with other substance use disorders.[8] In this context, sedative-hypnotics are often used to enhance the effects of other drugs and alleviate unpleasant side effects from use or withdrawal of other substances. Many patients who develop benzodiazepine and sedative-hypnotic use disorders were initially treated for sleep and anxiety disorders. Individuals seeking treatment for anxiety disorders, sleep disorders, and depression are at higher risk for developing sedative-hypnotic use disorder if they have a history of SUDs. A family history of SUDs also places an individual at higher risk for developing a SUD. The issue of alcohol use disorder warrants special caution because of the potential for dangerous interactions. The assumption that all individuals with alcohol use disorder have a propensity for nonmedical use of benzodiazepines or invariably developing a use disorder has been challenged,[9] but the use of these medications should be closely monitored in this population.

Deciding whether a benzodiazepine or other sedative-hypnotic should be used on a long-term basis is important to consider early in the treatment course. In general, if there is a clear diagnosis, benefit from the treatment, minimal side effects, and no evidence of nonmedical or unhealthy use or a SUD, then the medication could be continued.[10] Sedative-hypnotics are commonly recommended for the shortest timeframe possible, and these medications are often seen as short-term therapies that should be discontinued as soon as the clinical situation permits.

INDICATIONS FOR PHARMACOLOGICAL INTERVENTIONS

In general, there are two clear indications for pharmacological intervention in individuals who are taking benzodiazepines and other sedative-hypnotics: (1) during intoxication and (2) during withdrawal. In a state of intoxication, a patient may require monitoring and even intervention to ensure a safe recovery. In patients experiencing acute withdrawal, pharmacological management is often recommended due to the risk of dangerous sequelae, including seizures and sedative withdrawal delirium.

Management of Intoxication and Overdose

The signs and symptoms of benzodiazepine and sedative-hypnotic intoxication are very similar to those of alcohol intoxication, including slowed mentation, slurred speech, and ataxia. Severe intoxication can lead to respiratory depression, coma, and death, which most commonly occurs when combined with other CNS depressants. The management of acute intoxication is mostly supportive with special attention to airway management as respiratory depression is the most likely cause of death in overdose. In overdose, it is also critical to know what other psychoactive agents (especially CNS depressants) may have been acutely or chronically taken.

Flumazenil can be used in the case of benzodiazepine intoxication and overdose, but its use is limited by the risk of precipitating withdrawal symptoms, including seizures. Flumazenil can be considered in patients who have confirmed or suspected benzodiazepine toxicity, who have lost consciousness or are at risk of losing consciousness, and who may require intubation. Flumazenil should be avoided in patients who have recently used medications or substances that lower the seizure threshold, in patients with known or suspected epilepsy, and in patients who have developed physiologic dependence on benzodiazepines. Because of the risk of adverse events related to the administration of flumazenil, it should be administered in the lowest possible doses for the shortest period required and in a medical setting where resuscitation equipment and appropriately trained health care personnel are present. In cases of severe toxicity, multiple doses of flumazenil may be required for longer acting agents.[11-14]

Withdrawal

Withdrawal symptoms are most often seen in patients with physiologic dependence after abruptly discontinuing benzodiazepines or other sedative-hypnotics.[15] Withdrawal may be precipitated unintentionally when an individual stops taking a prescribed medication or is unable to obtain the sedative-hypnotic from illicit sources. Withdrawal may also be inadvertently initiated by a provider due to concerns of unhealthy use, psychological dependence, or other SUDs. In some cases, the decision is made to stop benzodiazepines because of side effects, such as memory impairment, fall risks, or behavioral problems. Individuals are more likely to develop withdrawal symptoms when they have been taking high doses of sedative-hypnotics or taking low or moderate doses for a prolonged period.[16]

While withdrawal symptoms are similar to those seen in alcohol withdrawal (**Tables 61-2** and **61-3**), the signs and symptoms of withdrawal manifest in a somewhat idiosyncratic manner in each patient. Individual traits such as age and medical conditions and the unique pharmacological properties of each medication[17] all impact the types and severity of the withdrawal symptoms that are experienced. The onset and duration of withdrawal symptoms depend on the intrinsic pharmacokinetic properties (eg, half-life) of the agent itself as well as extrinsic factors that impact the metabolism and effective half-life of the agent, such as the inhibition or induction of cytochrome P-450 enzymes, patient age, and preexisting liver disease. The half-life of the medication and its active metabolites are of particular importance, especially when discussing the onset of withdrawal symptoms. Withdrawal from medications with short half-lives usually begins within 12 to 24 hours

TABLE 61-2 Sedative-Hypnotic Withdrawal Symptoms

Mild	Moderate	Severe
• Anxiety • Insomnia • Dizziness • Headache • Anorexia • Perceptual hyperacusis • Irritability • Agitation	• Panic • Decreased concentration • Tremor • Sweating • Palpitations • Perceptual distortions • Muscle fasciculations • Muscle aches • GI upset • Insomnia • Elevated vital signs • Depression	• Hypothermia • Vital sign instability • Muscle fasciculations • Seizures • Delirium • Psychosis

TABLE 61-3 Benzodiazepine Equivalency

Benzodiazepine	Approximate equivalent oral dose
Alprazolam	0.5 mg
Chlordiazepoxide	10 mg
Clonazepam	0.25 mg
Diazepam	5 mg
Flurazepam	30 mg
Lorazepam	1 mg
Oxazepam	15 mg
Temazepam	30 mg
Triazolam	0.25 mg

From: Chouinard G. Issues in the Clinical Use of Benzodiazepines: Potency, Withdrawal and Rebound. *J Clin Psychiatry*. 2004;65 Suppl 5: 7-12.

and reaches peak intensity within 1 to 3 days. With longer-acting agents, withdrawal symptoms may begin later and not peak until 4 to 7 days after discontinuation. Symptoms may then continue for several more days or even weeks, depending on the half-life the of drug. Advanced liver disease may lead to significantly prolonged half-lives and reduced elimination rates for benzodiazepines requiring oxidative metabolism prior to glucuronidation (eg, diazepam, clonazepam, chlordiazepoxide, and alprazolam) due to the impairment of the oxidative process. Impairment of the oxidative process and resulting prolongation of the half-lives of these benzodiazepines may also occur due to advanced age.[18,19] As one example of cytochrome P-450 enzyme effects, norfluoxetine (a metabolite of fluoxetine) may lead to the inhibition of the liver microsomal system responsible for alprazolam metabolism, resulting in clinically significant changes in the half-life and clearance of this benzodiazepine.[20] Lorazepam, oxazepam, and temazepam avoid phase I metabolism via cytochrome P-450 enzymes and are conjugated directly in phase II metabolism; as such they are often the preferred agents in situations where there are concerns about liver function, age, and medication interactions.

It has been estimated that up to 50% of those who take benzodiazepines on a regular basis will experience clinically significant signs of withdrawal with sudden discontinuation.[21] The duration and intensity of use necessary to cause withdrawal symptoms is unclear. Some sources suggest that it may take as little as 4 to 6 weeks,[22] while rebound insomnia has been seen after just 2 weeks of daily drug use.[23]

Another common occurrence during withdrawal is the reemergence of symptoms of anxiety and insomnia, which has been found to occur in 60% to 80% of patients physiologically dependent on benzodiazepines who were initially treated for these disorders.[24-28] Initially, these reemergence symptoms are perceived to be more severe and intense than the original symptoms but within several weeks return to pretreatment levels.

Management of Withdrawal

The decision to discontinue or taper sedative-hypnotic medications should be discussed at length with patients with education provided about the reasons for discontinuation, the signs and symptoms that are likely to be experienced, and the risks and benefits of the available withdrawal strategies. There are several strategies that may be employed in the management of sedative-hypnotic withdrawal. The approach with the most data to support its safety and efficacy includes slowly tapering a medication over a prolonged period in efforts to minimize withdrawal symptoms. One benefit of this strategy is that it can be safely completed in an outpatient setting. Modest evidence exists to support more acute and rapid medically supervised withdrawals, similar to the approach taken in alcohol withdrawal treatment, though this is generally not as well tolerated as a prolonged taper.[29] The latter approach requires close observation and monitoring and should only be undertaken in a closely supervised setting. There is conflicting evidence on the use of certain anticonvulsants (eg, valproic acid, carbamazepine) for the treatment of alcohol withdrawal, indicating there may be a role for the use of similar agents in the treatment of sedative-hypnotic withdrawal.[29-31] However, importantly, there is no evidence suggesting their use will prevent a more severe withdrawal course, including seizures and delirium tremens, especially in high-risk patients. The use of phenobarbital in the setting of an acute medically supervised withdrawal has also been studied, though the evidence to support this treatment is limited and somewhat dated. Flumazenil has also been studied for use in the management of benzodiazepine withdrawal.

Benzodiazepine Taper

The approach with the most data to support its safety and efficacy is a taper that uses decreasing doses of the currently used medication over the course of 4 to 12 weeks.[32-34] This approach is useful in cases of long-term use and physical dependence when there is not an urgent need to abruptly discontinue the current medication. While this method may be utilized in cases of unhealthy use and use disorder, this approach must be used with caution in such a context because it would provide the patient with continued doses of the medication for a period of weeks to months—creating risk for worsening of SUD or diversion. For this strategy to be effective, the patient must be able to follow complex dosing regimens and adhere to regular follow-up appointments. It is recommended that as lower doses are achieved, the dose reduction at each stage be more modest, especially if medications with a short half-life are prescribed. More frequent dosing intervals can also be used in the later stages to help prevent the emergence of any withdrawal symptoms.

There is an increased likelihood of withdrawal symptoms with medications with a short half-life, even during prolonged tapers. Another withdrawal management strategy involves conversion of the therapeutic agent to an equivalent dose of a longer acting medication, and then a gradual reduction in the dose of the latter, using the principles described above. Agents such as clonazepam[35] and chlordiazepoxide are especially good choices given their long half-lives and slower onset of action and therefore relatively lower addiction and diversion potential.

Short-acting benzodiazepines, like the triazolobenzodiazepines alprazolam and triazolam, warrant special consideration as they can be particularly difficult to taper. Traditionally, these medications have been thought to have a higher binding affinity at a subpopulation of benzodiazepine GABA receptors that are not targeted by other benzodiazepines.[36] There is limited evidence to support that longer acting, benzodiazepines may not have fully effective cross-tolerance. Therefore, they may be less effective when used for tapering and withdrawal management and result in breakthrough withdrawal symptoms. There are case reports that suggest that clonazepam can be used effectively for the treatment of triazolobenzodiazepine withdrawal,[35] while others have reported distinct withdrawal symptoms with alprazolam.[24,37]

A Cochrane review found that cognitive-behavioral therapy interventions provided some short-term benefit when combined with a medication taper, though this benefit did not extend past 3 months. Additionally, motivational interviewing combined with a taper did not provide any additional benefit.[38]

Anticonvulsants

Another strategy for the treatment of withdrawal is the use of anticonvulsants, with an emphasis on the data that supports the use of carbamazepine. This anticonvulsant has been shown to be as effective as oxazepam in the treatment of alcohol withdrawal,[39] and two open-label studies also demonstrated the effectiveness of this agent in the management of complicated benzodiazepine withdrawal. One multisite, placebo-controlled study suggested that carbamazepine could also be effective for the treatment of alprazolam withdrawal, but the findings were limited by a high dropout rate. Based on these small initial studies, the suggested dosing of carbamazepine is in the range of 200 mg three times a day for 7 to 10 days.[40,41] A follow up Cochrane review from 2018 found little evidence to support the use of anticonvulsants during benzodiazepine taper.[42] Many of these studies excluded patients at risk for severe withdrawal, including seizures and delirium tremens, and as such these agents should be used with caution in more complicated populations at risk.

Phenobarbital

Smith and Wesson[43,44] elucidated a protocol for utilizing phenobarbital for medically supervised withdrawal by converting patients from other sedative-hypnotics to equivalent phenobarbital doses. The starting daily dose of phenobarbital should be based on the patient's drug use during the previous month. In cases when this is not known, a pentobarbital challenge test[43] can be used to determine the starting dose. The maximum starting dose is 500 mg daily, in divided doses, three times a day, and then tapered by 30 mg a day. Signs of phenobarbital intoxication are similar to those seen with other sedative-hypnotics and include slurred speech, ataxia, and nystagmus. If signs and symptoms of intoxication are present, then the total daily dose should be decreased by 50% or more and the patient reassessed at frequent intervals until the intoxication resolves. This strategy has limitations due to the narrow therapeutic index of phenobarbital compared to benzodiazepines.

Flumazenil

Another treatment strategy for managing benzodiazepine withdrawal that has been studied involves the use of flumazenil.[45-50] The data on the use of flumazenil are limited but published reports and studies suggest that parenteral and subcutaneous flumazenil may be effective in the management of benzodiazepine withdrawal. While flumazenil is generally thought of as a pure antagonist, it acts as a partial agonist with weak affinity at the benzodiazepine receptor site. Explanations for flumazenil's potential efficacy in the treatment of withdrawal symptoms include flumazenil-induced changes in receptor sensitivity and binding affinity, though the exact mechanism of action in ameliorating withdrawal symptoms is not clear.[51,52] Flumazenil was also shown to precipitate severe panic attacks in a trial which may limit utilization.[53] Additional factors that may limit the use of this strategy include the method of intravenous administration of the medication and increased risk of seizures.

Protracted Withdrawal Symptoms

In addition to experiencing the initial symptoms of benzodiazepine/sedative withdrawal, many patients report longer lasting residual symptoms in the days and weeks following the discontinuation of the medication used to manage the withdrawal. Because of the lack of literature and unclear delineation between acute and protracted withdrawal, this syndrome has not been included in the DSM. Benzodiazepine protracted withdrawal may be difficult to diagnose due to possibility of symptom rebound or reemergence.[54] Prolonged or protracted withdrawal symptoms may include anxiety; sensitivity to light, sound, and touch, restlessness, anxiety; insomnia; dysphoria; depression; fatigue; low energy; and tinnitus.[24,25] In contrast to symptom reemergence, protracted withdrawal symptoms often wax and wane and slowly resolve with continued abstinence. Although there is some debate as to the validity of the "protracted abstinence syndrome," these residual symptoms are thought to persist for weeks to months and, in some cases, even years. Smith and Wesson[28] suggest that receptor-mediated changes lead to worsening of withdrawal symptoms when patients are tapered from the remaining low-dose medication. There are no definitive pharmacological options for the treatment of protracted benzodiazepine withdrawal symptoms; this is a subject that needs further investigation and understanding. Pharmacological strategies with antidepressants, antihistamines, alpha adrenergic agents, anticonvulsants, buspirone, melatonin, and others have been described, but there is not an evidence base to support the use of a particular agent or strategy.[55-59]

TREATMENT SETTING

While discussing the pharmacological strategy for the treatment of withdrawal with patients, a decision must also be made regarding the setting in which the withdrawal will be treated. While inpatient treatment is often optimal because of the close observation and controlled environment, this is often not feasible due to limited accessibility to inpatient resources and cost considerations. Therefore, inpatient treatment of withdrawal should be limited to cases in which the patient is medically compromised or a high risk of the patient developing severe symptoms, such as seizures. This may be the case in patients who have been taking high doses of sedative-hypnotics for a long period of time, and who require a rapid withdrawal or abrupt discontinuation of the medication. Medically supervised withdrawal on an inpatient basis may also be appropriate if the patient has been taking multiple sedative-hypnotics or has physiologic dependence on alcohol. Patients who have a history of experiencing severe withdrawal when they have previously stopped using sedative-hypnotics are also at high risk for having their withdrawal complicated by serious side effects.

Medically supervised outpatient withdrawal is reasonable if the patient does not appear to be at risk for severe withdrawal, especially if the method of slowly reducing the sedative-hypnotic dose can be utilized. If outpatient management is undertaken, the patient should be given clear instructions and close follow-up appointments. If a gradual dose reduction approach is employed, it is recommended that the patient be seen each time there is a dose reduction. If this is not possible, then there should be a mechanism by which the patient can access the provider to address any questions or concerns. It is preferable for the patient to have some level of supervision by friends or family, but this is not always possible. Urine drug screens and clinical and laboratory assessments for the use of alcohol should be utilized to monitor for complications that could arise from the concomitant use of other sedating substances.

TREATMENT OF CO-OCCURRING DISORDERS

Currently, there is no long-term medication to treat sedative-hypnotic use disorder. Medically supervised withdrawal should not be seen as definitive treatment in the case of sedative-hypnotic use disorder. This is the first step in the management of patients who often have other SUDs, anxiety and sleep disorders, and other co-occurring medical and psychiatric disorders. In the case of other SUDs, a treatment plan should include co-occurring medically supervised withdrawal from other substances and SUD treatment in an appropriate setting. When treating patients with underlying anxiety and sleep disorders, other pharmacological and psychotherapeutic treatments, particularly cognitive-behavioral therapy, should be initiated to counter any reemerging symptoms that may be experienced following withdrawal, which may help to reduce the risk of recurrence of use or the disorder.[60-62] Other co-occurring psychiatric disorders should also be addressed during, or soon after, withdrawal. Failure to stabilize anxiety, sleep, or other co-occurring conditions will likely lead to higher rates of resumed use due to patient discomfort, limited compliance, and inability to effectively engage in the early stages of rehabilitative treatment. Although there are clear evidenced based recommendations for sedative withdrawal, additional research on pharmacotherapy and treatment options for management of sedative hypnotic use disorder after acute withdrawal is needed.

CONCLUSIONS AND FUTURE DIRECTIONS

Sedative-hypnotic medications have been used for many years for a variety of disorders and symptoms. Today, benzodiazepines are by far the most commonly used sedative-hypnotics, and their use is widespread. The appropriate use of benzodiazepines requires a clear understanding of the medications, an accurate diagnosis and treatment plan, and close monitoring. Most individuals who use sedative-hypnotic medications take their medications as prescribed and do not manifest nonmedical use or develop a SUD. Physical dependence may be unavoidable in cases of prolonged use; therefore, benzodiazepines should be prescribed for the shortest period of time that is clinically reasonable. Potential withdrawal signs and symptoms should be initially discussed with patients before treatment with this class of medications is initiated. Prescribers must be aware of the risks inherent in prescribing benzodiazepines and other sedative-hypnotics, but they should be careful not to withhold treatment when appropriate. If providers and patients are well informed and openly discuss the risks and benefits of these medications, and they are prescribed at therapeutic doses, sedative-hypnotics can be used safely and effectively for the treatment of a number of otherwise disabling conditions.

Sedative-hypnotics continue to be widely prescribed, and while these medications are relatively safe when taken alone, their use in conjunction with opioids is receiving increased attention. The risk of death in the context of concurrent sedative-hypnotic and opioid use has led to renewed debate and discussion about the overall efficacy and safety of the sedative-hypnotic medications, and in many cases, it precipitates a more urgent need to address issues related to overdose and withdrawal. Pharmacological strategies to manage intoxication and withdrawal are limited in their scope, and the evidence base to support newer strategies and manage protracted withdrawal symptoms needs to be expanded so that patients and prescribers have more options at their disposal.

REFERENCES

1. Rush CR, Frey JM, Griffiths RR. Zaleplon and triazolam in humans: acute behavioral effects and abuse potential. *Psychopharmacology (Berl).* 1999;145:39-51.
2. Rush CR, Griffiths RR. Zolpidem, triazolam, and temazepam: behavioral and subject-related effects in normal volunteers. *J Clin Psychopharmacol.* 1996;16:146-157.
3. Bachhuber M, Hennessey S, Cunningham CO, Starrels JL. Increasing benzodiazepine prescriptions and overdose mortality in the United States 1996-2013. *Am J Public Health.* 2016;106:686-688.
4. Substance Abuse and Mental Health Services Administration. *Key substance use and mental health indicators in the United State: results from the 2017 National Survey on drug use and health.* SAMHSA; 2018.
5. Sokya M. Treatment of benzodiazepine dependence. *N Engl J Med.* 2017;376:1147-1157.
6. Griffiths RR, Sannerud CA. Abuse and dependence on benzodiazepines and other anxiolytic/sedative drugs. In: Meltzer HY, Coyle JT, eds. *Psychopharmacology: The Third Generation of Progress.* 2nd ed. Raven Press; 1987:1535-1541.
7. Chutuape MA, de Wit H. Relationship between subjective effects and drug preferences: ethanol and diazepam. *Drug Alcohol Depend.* 1994;34:243-251.
8. Malcolm R, Brady KT, Johnson AL, Cunningham M. Types of benzodiazepines abused by chemically dependent inpatients. *J Psychoactive Drugs.* 1993;25:315-319.
9. Ciraulo DA, Sands BF, Shader RI. Critical review of liability for benzodiazepine abuse among alcoholics. *Am J Psychiatry.* 1988;145: 1501-1506.
10. O'Brien CP. Benzodiazepine use, abuse, and dependence. *J Clin Psychiatry.* 2005;66(Suppl 2):28-33.
11. Veiraiah A, Dyas J, Cooper G, Routledge PA, Thompson JP. Flumazenil use in benzodiazepine overdose in the UK: a retrospective survey of NPIS data. *Emerg Med J.* 2012;29:565-569.
12. National Institute for Health and Care Excellence, Clinical Guidelines, CG 16. *Self-Harm: The Short-Term Physical and Psychological Management and Secondary Prevention of Self-Harm in Primary and Secondary Care.* NICE; 2004.
13. Weinbroum A, Rudick V, Sorkine P, Szold O, Rudick V. Use of flumazenil in the treatment of drug overdose: a double-blind and open clinical study in 110 patients. *Crit Care Med.* 1996;24:199-206.
14. Weinbroum AA, Flaishon R, Sorkine P, Szold O, Rudick V. A risk-benefit assessment of flumazenil in the management of benzodiazepine overdose. *Drug Saf.* 1997;17:181-196.
15. Pertussen H. The benzodiazepine withdrawal syndrome. *Addiction.* 1994;89:1455-1459.
16. MacKinnon GL, Parker WA. Benzodiazepine withdrawal syndrome: a literature review and evaluation. *Am J Drug Alcohol Abuse.* 1982;9: 19-33.
17. Greenblatt DJ, Miller LG, Shader RI. Benzodiazepine discontinuation syndromes. *J Psychiatr Res.* 1990;24(Suppl 2):73-79.
18. Wolf B, Griffiths RR. Physical dependence on benzodiazepines: differences within the class. *Drug Alcohol Depend.* 1991;29:153-156.
19. Chouinard G, Lefko-Singh K, Teboul E. Metabolism of anxiolytics and hypnotics: benzodiazepines, buspirone, zopiclone, and zolpidem. *Cell Mol Neurobiol.* 1999;19:533-552.
20. Mandrioli R, Mercolini L, Raggi MA. Benzodiazepine metabolism: an analytical perspective. *Curr Drug Metab.* 2008;9:827-844.
21. Bixler EO, Kales JD, Kales A, Jacoby JA, Soldatos CR. Rebound insomnia and elimination half-life: assessment of individual subject response. *J Clin Pharmacol.* 1985;25:115-124.
22. Denis C, Fatséas M, Lavie E, Auriacombe M. Pharmacological interventions for benzodiazepine mono-dependence management in outpatient settings. *Cochrane Database Syst Rev.* 2006;3:CD005194.
23. Alexander B, Perry PJ. Detoxification from benzodiazepines: schedules and strategies. *J Subst Abuse Treat.* 1991;8:9-17.
24. Fontaine R, Chouinard G, Annable L. Rebound anxiety in anxious patients after abrupt withdrawal of benzodiazepine treatment. *Am J Psychiatry.* 1984;141:848-852.
25. Noyes R, Garvey MJ, Cook B, Suelzer M. Controlled discontinuation of benzodiazepine treatment for patients with panic disorder. *Am J Psychiatry.* 1991;148:517-523.
26. Pecknold JC. Discontinuation reactions to alprazolam in panic disorder. *J Psychiatr Res.* 1993;27(Suppl 1):155-170.
27. Lader M, Tylee A, Donoghue J. Withdrawing benzodiazepines in primary care. *CNS Drugs.* 2009;23:19-34.
28. Smith DE, Wesson DR. Benzodiazepines and other sedative-hypnotics. In: Galanter M, Kleber H, eds. *American Psychiatric Press Textbook of Substance Abuse Treatment.* 1st ed. American Psychiatric Press; 1995.
29. Lader M. Drug development optimization—benzodiazepines. *Agents Actions Suppl.* 1990;29:59-69.
30. Busto U, Fornazzari L, Naranjo CA. Protracted tinnitus after discontinuation of long-term therapeutic use of benzodiazepines. *J Clin Psychopharmacol.* 1988;8:359-362.
31. Tyrer P. Benzodiazepine dependence: a shadowy diagnosis. *Biochem Soc Symp.* 1993;59:107-119.
32. Voshaar RC, Couvee JE, van Balkom AJ, Mulder PGH, Zitman FG. Strategies for discontinuing long-term benzodiazepine use: meta-analysis. *Br J Psychiatry.* 2006;189:213-220.
33. Denis C, Fatseas M, Lavie E, Auriacombe M. Pharmacologic interventions for benzodiazepine mono-dependence management in outpatient settings. *Cochrane Database Syst Rev.* 2006;(3):CD005194.
34. Herman JB, Rosenblum JF, Brotman AW. The alprazolam to clonazepam switch for the treatment of panic disorder. *J Clin Psychopharmacol.* 1987;7:175-178.
35. Brown JL, Hauges KJ. A review of alprazolam withdrawal. *Drug Intell Clin Pharm.* 1986;20:837-884.
36. Rashi K, Patrissi G, Cook B. Alprazolam found to have serious side effects. *Psychiatr News.* 1988;23:14.
37. Darker CD, Sweeney BP, Barry JM, Farrell MF, Donnelly-Swift E. Psychosocial interventions for benzodiazepine harmful use, abuse or dependence. *Cochrane Database Syst Rev.* 2015;(5):CD009652. doi:10.1002/14651858.CD009652.pub2
38. Malcolm R, Ballenger JC, Sturgis E, Anton R. A double blind controlled trial of carbamazepine in alcohol withdrawal. *Am J Psychiatry.* 1989;146:617-621.
39. Klein E, Uhde TW, Post RM. Preliminary evidence for the utility of carbamazepine in alprazolam withdrawal. *Am J Psychiatry.* 1986;143: 235-236.
40. Ries RK, Roy-Byrne PP, Ward NG, Neppe V, Cullison S. Carbamazepine treatment for benzodiazepine withdrawal. *Am J Psychiatry.* 1989;146: 536-537.
41. Baandrup L, Ebdrup BH, Rasmussen JØ, Lindschou J, Gluud C, Glenthøj BY. Pharmacological Interventions for benzodiazepine discontinuation in chronic benzodiazepine uses. *Cochrane Database Syst Rev.* 2018;(3):CD011481.
42. Smith D, Wesson D. A new method for treatment of barbiturate dependence. *JAMA.* 1970;213:294-295.
43. Smith D, Wesson D. A phenobarbital technique for withdrawal of barbiturate abuse. *Arch Gen Psychiatry.* 1971;24:56-60.
44. Jackson AH, Shader RI. Guidelines for the withdrawal of narcotic and general depressant drugs. *Dis Nerv Syst.* 1973;34:162.
45. Gerra G, Zaimovic A, Giusti F, Moi G, Brewer C. Intravenous flumazenil versus oxazepam tapering in the treatment of benzodiazepine withdrawal: a randomized, placebo-controlled study. *Addict Biol.* 2002;7:385-395.
46. Quaglio G, Pattaro C, Gerra G, et al. High dose benzodiazepine dependence: description of 29 patients treated with flumazenil infusion and stabilized with clonazepam. *Psychiatry Res.* 2012;198(3):457-462.
47. Hulse G, O'Neill G, Morris N, Bennett K, Norman A, Hood S. Withdrawal and psychological sequelae, and patients satisfaction associated with subcutaneous flumazenil infusion for the management of benzodiazepine withdrawal—a case series. *J Psychopharmacol.* 2013;27(2):222-227.

48. Hood S, O'Neil G, Hulse G. The role of flumazenil in the treatment of benzodiazepine dependence: physiological and psychological profiles. *J Psychopharmacol.* 2009;23:401-409.
49. Hood SD, Norman A, Hince DA, Melichar JK, Hulse GK. Benzodiazepine dependence and its treatment with low dose flumazenil. *Br J Clin Pharmacol.* 2014;77(2):285-294.
50. Faccini M, Leone R, Opri S, et al. Slow subcutaneous infusion of flumazenil for the treatment of long-term, high-dose benzodiazepine users: a review of 214 cases. *J Psychopharmacol.* 2016;30:1047-1053.
51. Nutt DJ, Costello MJ. Rapid induction of lorazepam dependence and reversal with flumazenil. *Life Sci.* 1988;43:1045-1053.
52. Gonsalves SF, Gallagher DW. Spontaneous and Ro 15-1788-induced reversal of subsensitivity to GABA following chronic benzodiazepines. *Eur J Pharmacol.* 1985;110:163-170.
53. Parr JM, Kavanagh DJ, Cahill L, Mitchell G, Young RM. Effectiveness of current treatment approaches for benzodiazepine discontinuation: a meta-analysis. *Addiction.* 2009;104(1):13-24.
54. Smith DE, Wesson DR. Benzodiazepines and other sedative-hypnotics. In: Galanter M, Kleber HD, eds. *The American Psychiatric Press Textbook of Substance Abuse Treatment.* American Psychiatric Association; 1994.
55. Morton S, Lader M. Buspirone treatment as an aid to benzodiazepine withdrawal. *J Psychopharmacol.* 1995;9:331-335.
56. Ashton H. Protracted withdrawal syndromes from benzodiazepines. *J Subst Abuse Treat.* 1991;8:19-28.
57. Udelman HD, Udelman DL. Concurrent use of buspirone in anxious patients during withdrawal from alprazolam therapy. *J Clin Psychiatry.* 1990;51(Suppl):46-50.
58. Fyer AJ, Liebowitz MR, Gorman JM, et al. Effects of clonidine on alprazolam discontinuation in panic attacks: a pilot study. *J Clin Psychopharmacol.* 1988;8:270-274.
59. Banndrup L, Fasmar OB, Glenthøj BY, Jennum PJ. Circadian rest-activity rhythms during benzodiazepine tapering covered by melatonin versus placebo add-on: data derived from a randomized clinical trial. *BMC Psychiatry.* 2016;16:348.
60. Spiegel DA, Bruce TJ, Gregg SF, Nuzzarello A. Does cognitive behavior therapy assist slow-taper alprazolam discontinuation in panic disorder? *Am J Psychiatry.* 1994;151:876-881.
61. Spiegel DA. Psychological strategies for discontinuing benzodiazepine treatment. *J Clin Psychopharmacol.* 1999;19(6 Suppl 2):17-22.
62. Otto MW, McHugh RK, Simon NM, Farach FJ, Worthington JJ, Pollack MH. Efficacy of CBT for benzodiazepine discontinuation in patients with panic disorder: further evaluation. *Behav Res Ther.* 2010;48: 720-727.

CHAPTER

62 Pharmacological Treatment for Opioid Use Disorder

David Kan and Joan E. Zweben

CHAPTER OUTLINE

- Introduction
- History and context of opioid agonist treatment
- Modern understandings of opioid use disorder
- Overview of pharmacologic interventions
- Opioid withdrawal symptoms and medically supervised withdrawal
- Treatments for opioid use disorder
- Special issues in ongoing medication treatment
- Patients with co-occurring psychiatric disorders
- The opioid treatment system
- Conclusion

INTRODUCTION

In 2020, 2.7 million American adults had an opioid use disorder (OUD) related to any opioid, and 691,000 related to heroin.[1] Shulgin predicted in 1975 that it was a matter of "when" not "if" novel synthetic opioids like fentanyl would displace heroin as the majority illicit opioid.[2] The United States finds itself in the third wave of opioid overdoses.[3] Prescription opioid overdose deaths increased in the 1990s, and heroin overdoses began increasing in 2010. Synthetic opioids, particularly illicitly manufactured fentanyl began in 2013 with fentanyl overdose deaths exceeding other opioids beginning in 2017.[4]

Of the estimated 2.7 million persons with OUD in the United States in 2020, approximately 409,000 were enrolled in federally licensed programs offering opioid agonist treatment (OAT).[5] The 1,460 specially licensed opioid treatment programs (OTPs) in the United States offer counseling, testing, and pharmacotherapy using methadone (and buprenorphine and naltrexone in certain facilities), with daily dispensing or strictly regulated take-home medication for selected patients.[6] In 2021, there were almost 100,000 prescribers authorized to prescribe buprenorphine for OUD under the DATA 2000 Act.[7] From 2017 to 2018, 50% of all buprenorphine prescriptions came from less than 5% of waivered prescribers.[8] In 2020, 798,000 total individuals in the United States received some form of medication for opioid use disorder (MOUD).[1] This chapter focuses on OAT in the context of the licensed methadone OTP and office-based buprenorphine for OUD treatment, which has been supported by the World Health Organization (WHO), the Surgeon General, the Office of National Drug Control Policy (ONDCP), the National Governors Association, the National Institute on Drug Abuse (NIDA), and the U.S. Department of Health and Human Services (HHS).[9-11]

HISTORY AND CONTEXT OF OPIOID AGONIST TREATMENT

Dole and Nyswander demonstrated the feasibility and efficacy of opioid agonist pharmacotherapy using methadone in the 1960s,[12] but some negative attitudes toward OAT have stemmed from the misguided perception of OAT as "just substituting one addicting drug for another."[13] However, OAT is not simple substitution but provides stabilization or correction of neuroadaptations to chronic opioid exposure.[14] OAT provides cross-tolerance and blockade of the opioid system[15,16] and is associated with decreased mortality, reduced illicit drug use, reduced seroconversion to human immunodeficiency virus (HIV), reduced criminal activity, and increased engagement in socially productive activities.[17-22] Nevertheless, U.S. regulatory requirements continue to stigmatize OAT and create barriers to providing treatment.[23] Provider stigma is influenced by a lack of training and abstinent treatment preferences.[13] Physicians sometimes refuse to treat a patient who discloses that he or she is receiving OAT.[13] Occasionally, patients are told that they must withdraw from OAT to receive treatment for other medical conditions. A physician may withhold medication needed for symptomatic relief, thus causing unnecessary discomfort and pain. Many patients with OUD enter OAT with great ambivalence and want to discontinue OAT, which is consistent with the short-term treatment that many practitioners, policy makers, and regulators seem to favor. However, studies demonstrate that only 10% to 20% of patients who quickly discontinue OAT are able to remain abstinent,[18,24-27] which is similar to most chronic medical conditions that also require ongoing medication.

MODERN UNDERSTANDINGS OF OPIOID USE DISORDER

Medication has demonstrated efficacy in the treatment for OUD, but biologic, psychosocial, and cultural variables also impact OUD and may need attention. Prior to the discovery of the opioid receptor system, Dole and Nyswander[28] conceptualized OUD as a "metabolic disease," a view that won

Dr Dole the Albert Lasker Clinical Medicine Research Award in 1988.[14] He wrote in the *Journal of the American Medical Association*[15]:

It is postulated that the high rate of relapse of addicts after detoxification from heroin use is due to persistent derangement of the endogenous ligand narcotic receptor system and that methadone in an adequate daily dose compensates for this defect.... The treatment, therefore, is corrective but not curative for severely addicted persons. A major challenge for future research is to identify the specific defect in receptor function and to repair it. Meanwhile, methadone maintenance provides a safe and effective way to normalize the function of otherwise intractable opiate addicts.

In Dole's view, the persistent receptor dysfunction is the result of chronic opioid use, leading to downregulation of the modulating system and possibly also to suppression of the endogenous ligands. Goldstein[16] supported the concept of a genetic and metabolic disease and suggested that genetic influence carries an exceptional vulnerability to the disease in the presence of certain environmental influences. Kreek[29] and others suggested that multiple genes may account for different degrees of vulnerability to developing addiction.[30-34]

Positron emission tomography of cerebral metabolism in patients with OUD compared with patients withdrawn from methadone and in sustained remission suggests that methadone treatment at least partly normalizes cerebral glucose metabolism.[35] Magnetic resonance spectroscopy comparing patients receiving methadone with different elapsed treatment times showed a nearly normal phosphorus metabolism profile in those patients who had been in long-term OAT, suggesting resumption of predisease reactivity at the neurochemical level over time.[36]

OVERVIEW OF PHARMACOLOGIC INTERVENTIONS

The principal medications used to treat OUD are the opioid μ-receptor antagonist, naltrexone; the full agonists methadone, heroin, slow release oral morphine and hydromorphone; the partial agonist buprenorphine; and the nonopioid α_2-adrenergic agonists clonidine and lofexidine used for opioid withdrawal.

Opioid Antagonists

Naltrexone is a long-acting, orally and parenterally effective, predominantly μ-opioid antagonist that provides complete blockade of μ-opioid receptors when the oral formulation is taken at least three times a week for a total weekly dose of about 350 mg.[37] Because the reinforcing properties of opioids are blocked, naltrexone is theoretically an ideal agent in the treatment of patients with OUD who can successfully complete withdrawal and maintain abstinence from opioids.

Naloxone is a short-acting, intranasal, and parenterally effective μ-opioid antagonist that reverses acute opioid overdose.

Opioid Full and Partial Agonists

Methadone

Methadone is an orally active, long-acting synthetic opioid. Increasing doses of methadone reduce withdrawal symptoms and drug craving. Effective methadone doses ranging from 80 to 120 mg/d also produce a resistance to the effects of injected heroin, hydromorphone, and methadone. The term *agonist blockade* was coined to describe this phenomenon.

Levo-Alpha-Acetylmethadol

Levo-alpha-acetylmethadol (LAAM) is the α-acetyl congener of methadone. Its principal difference from methadone is its longer half-life and its conversion to the active metabolites norLAAM and dinorLAAM. It is approved by the U.S. Food and Drug Administration (FDA) for treatment in OTPs but is no longer marketed owing to low demand in the wake of reports of an association with cardiac arrhythmias (torsade de pointes [TdP]).

Buprenorphine

Buprenorphine is a high-affinity μ-opioid partial agonist and κ-opioid antagonist that the FDA approved as a pharmacotherapy for OUD in October 2002.[38,39] Despite its higher unit-dose cost compared to methadone, buprenorphine has expanded access to OUD treatment due its availability through office-based practice. This could reduce the disparity between the number of individuals with OUD and the number of available treatment slots and facilitate general medical care of such individuals.[40-42]

Heroin and Hydromorphone

Heroin and hydromorphone are short-acting μ-opioid agonists. Heroin is classified as a Schedule I drug by the Drug Enforcement Administration (DEA). Routes of administration include insufflation, smoking, and injection. Although illegal in the United States, heroin treatment has been used in select patients and jurisdictions internationally to treat OUD. Studies of heroin treatment demonstrated reduced illicit heroin use, health status improvements, increasing employment, and decreased crime.[43-46] Importantly, heroin treatment is typically reserved for individuals who have trialed first-line MOUD and did not find the treatment effective.[45] Hydromorphone is a Schedule II medication. A randomized controlled trial indicated that it is also effective for individuals for whom methadone treatment was ineffective.[47]

Slow Release Oral Morphine

Another μ-opioid agonist, slow release oral morphine, although not approved to treat OUD in the United States, has demonstrated efficacy in retaining patients in treatment and reducing heroin use in other countries.[48]

Nonopioids: α-Adrenergic Agents

Clonidine

Clonidine is a centrally acting α_2-adrenergic receptor agonist. It decreases adrenergic neurotransmission from the locus coeruleus through feedback inhibition. Clonidine is FDA approved for the treatment of hypertension but is used off label for the medical management of opioid withdrawal. Many of the autonomic symptoms of opioid withdrawal result from the loss of opioid suppression of the locus coeruleus system during opioid withdrawal.[14] Side effects of sedation and hypotension limit the use of clonidine in opioid withdrawal. Combining clonidine with buprenorphine for treatment of OUD can reduce opioid craving and use compared to buprenorphine combined with placebo.[49]

Lofexidine

Lofexidine is a centrally acting α_2-adrenergic agonist that preferentially binds the α_{2a} receptor FDA approved in the United States for the medical management of opioid withdrawal. It is associated with less hypotension than is clonidine. The high price of lofexidine in the United States means it has limited clinical uptake.[50]

OPIOID WITHDRAWAL SYMPTOMS AND MEDICALLY SUPERVISED WITHDRAWAL

The opioid withdrawal syndrome (OWS) is characterized by two phases[51]: a relatively brief initial phase in which patients with physiologic dependence on opioids experience acute withdrawal followed by a protracted withdrawal syndrome. Current pharmacologic strategies are designed to address these two distinct phases, acute withdrawal, and protracted withdrawal. The acute withdrawal syndrome lasts from 5 to 14 days and consists of a wide range of symptoms. Symptoms include gastrointestinal distress (such as diarrhea and vomiting), disturbances in thermal regulation including piloerection, pupillary dilatation, insomnia, muscle pain, joint pain, marked anxiety, tremor, yawning, sneezing, rhinorrhea, lacrimation, and dysphoria.[52] Mu-opioid receptors in the GI system contribute to GI distress. In addition, three major brain regions and circuits undergo changes with continued opioid exposure and contribute to OWS. First, changes in the mesolimbic reward circuits cause opioid craving, compulsive use, and depression in OWS. Insomnia in OWS is caused by the ascending reticular activating system (RAS). The locus coeruleus (LC) which also projects to the RAS is responsible for many physical symptoms of withdrawal. Acute opioid use suppresses norepinepinephrine production in the LC leading to drowsiness, reduced blood pressure, respiration, and muscle tone. Chronic use of opioids causes adaptation of the LC. Abrupt opioid reduction or discontinuation results in hyperactivity of the LC due to neuroadaptation lasting days to weeks.

Although these symptoms generally are not life-threatening, the acute withdrawal syndrome causes marked discomfort, often prompting continuation of opioid use, even in the absence of any opioid-associated euphoria. Longer-term, protracted withdrawal symptoms are discussed in this chapter under long-term treatments. Medically supervised withdrawal without MOUD results in high rates of return to opioid use and overdose risk.[53-55] An essential point is that medically managed withdrawal from opioids is not considered treatment for OUD, and the vast majority of patients return to use after withdrawal without continued medication treatment.[56-62]

Medically supervised withdrawal is discussed briefly next and in greater detail in Section 7 of this textbook.

Opioid Agonists and Partial Agonists

Opioid-based medically supervised withdrawal is based on the principle of cross-tolerance, in which one opioid is replaced with another that is then tapered. Methadone is often used because it has a long half-life and can be administered once daily. Withdrawal is usually managed with initial dosages of methadone in the range of 15 to 30 mg/d.[63] Although this dosage is generally adequate to control symptoms in many individuals who use opioids, additional methadone may be given as needed based on clinical findings. However, a simple conversion based on morphine equivalents should not be utilized, as methadone's complex pharmacokinetics and long half-life lead to interperson variability and may increase the risk of overdose. Thus, any methadone dose over about 40 mg daily, if needed, should involve careful and slow dosage increases over at least several days to eliminate withdrawal symptoms and opioid craving.

In acute medical settings, the dosage can be maintained through the 2nd or 3rd day after the peak dose is attained, and then, the methadone can be slowly tapered by about 10% to 15% per day. Although in the United States a licensed physician can perform supervised methadone withdrawal in an inpatient medical setting when the primary reason for hospital admission is not OUD, longer-term, outpatient withdrawal using methadone must be performed in a federally licensed OTP.

Buprenorphine can also be used for medically managed opioid withdrawal. Buprenorphine's slow dissociation from μ-opioid receptors results in a long duration of action, and it also has milder withdrawal signs and symptoms on discontinuation than full agonists,[56,57,64-67] making it useful for medically supervised withdrawal from opioids. The extant literature contains various findings on the length of a buprenorphine taper with limited evidence favoring a more rapid taper[38] and some supporting a more prolonged taper.[68] On the basis of current knowledge, the recommended clinical approach is to stabilize the patient within a day on a dose of buprenorphine that suppresses most withdrawal signs and symptoms. The optimum dose of buprenorphine for acute inpatient opioid withdrawal has not been determined and typically ranges from 8 to 16 mg/24 hours. The dosage can then be tapered over a time frame as brief as 3 days or extending for weeks or even months depending upon patient and clinician goals and preferences.

A meta-analysis compared different strategies to manage opioid withdrawal such as buprenorphine,[69] methadone, α_2-adrenergic agonists, other symptomatic medications, and placebo demonstrated buprenorphine had a moderate effect size in producing lower withdrawal score relative to clonidine and lofexidine. While no significant difference was observed in the incidence of adverse effects, dropout due to adverse effects may be more likely with clonidine. Overall conclusions were that buprenorphine more effectively controlled withdrawal signs and symptoms than did clonidine or lofexidine. There was no difference between buprenorphine and methadone in terms of average treatment duration or treatment completion rates.

Nonopioid Medication Treatments

Clonidine

Early clinical studies demonstrated that clonidine diminished withdrawal symptoms in patients who were withdrawn from methadone.[70,71] Clonidine seems to be most effective in suppressing autonomic signs and symptoms of opioid withdrawal but is less effective for subjective withdrawal symptoms.[72] Initial daily doses of up to 1.2 mg per 24 hours in divided doses are commonly suggested. For example, a regimen of 0.1 to 0.2 mg every 4 hours has been used in two clinical trials for heroin withdrawal, with careful monitoring of blood pressure. Because it may be less effective in managing subjective withdrawal symptoms, adjuvant therapy (nonsteroidal anti-inflammatory drugs [NSAIDs] for myalgia, benzodiazepines for insomnia, medications for diarrhea, and antiemetics) may be needed.[60,73] Multiple studies have described clonidine's use in medically assisted withdrawal.[60,74]

Lofexidine and Other α_2-Adrenergic Agonists

The use of clonidine in the management of opioid withdrawal has been hampered by limited long-term efficacy and side effects including sedation and hypotension. This in turn has led to the investigation of the effectiveness of other α_2-adrenergic agonists—lofexidine, guanfacine, and guanabenz acetate—in the management of opioid withdrawal, to find a drug that has clonidine's capacity to manage the signs and symptoms of opioid withdrawal but with fewer side effects.

Lofexidine, a centrally acting α_2-adrenergic agonist, has, after clonidine, been the most used and investigated α_2-adrenergic treatment for opioid withdrawal.

Lofexidine treatment is typically initiated at 0.18 mg twice daily, increasing daily by 0.18 to 0.36 mg.[75] The package insert of the approved product suggests 0.54 mg qid (twelve 0.18-mg tablets per day) with a maximum daily dose of 2.88 mg (16 tablets per day).[76] Doses required to decrease withdrawal symptoms, however, vary for each patient depending on the amount, frequency, and duration of opioid used. In randomized trials, lofexidine was found superior to placebo and generally equivalent to clonidine in reducing signs and symptoms of opioid withdrawal. It appeared to cause less hypotension than clonidine. Lofexidine was somewhat less useful than methadone at managing signs and symptoms of withdrawal.[74,77-83] The most common adverse event with lofexidine was somnolence, and hypotension was also reported. Overall, lofexidine has a decreased incidence and severity of side effects compared with clonidine.

The high cost of lofexidine has inhibited uptake of the medication in the United States.[84]

Medication Combinations, Rapid and Ultrarapid Opioid Withdrawal

Because most opioid and nonopioid approaches to medically supervised withdrawal require a prolonged timeframe of a week or more, "rapid" and "ultrarapid" opioid withdrawal protocols have been attempted.[85,86] These "rapid" protocols use an opioid antagonist (eg, naloxone or naltrexone) to cause an accelerated withdrawal response, with the goal of completing the withdrawal portion in shorter periods from 8 days to as little as 2 or 3 days. In addition to an opioid antagonist, rapid approaches use pharmacotherapies (eg, clonidine and sedation procedures) in an attempt to minimize the acute withdrawal symptoms experienced when opioid antagonists are administered. These methods for transition to naltrexone in less than 7 to 10 days from physiologic opioid dependence have shown efficacy in a multisite study[87] but are not in widespread use. Ultrarapid methods are similar in pharmacologic approach to the rapid method, use general anesthesia and complete the procedure in several hours, and are associated with life-threatening adverse events. Ultrarapid withdrawal management was not found to be superior in long-term efficacy to the use of buprenorphine or clonidine in a 2006 review and therefore was not deemed to justify the risks of general anesthesia.[88]

TREATMENTS FOR OPIOID USE DISORDER

Clinical Issues in Ongoing Pharmacotherapy

Goals of Pharmacotherapy of OUD

The first, last, and most enduring goal of MOUD is fatal overdose prevention. In 2021, more than 107,000 people died of drug overdose in the United States. 75% of those overdose deaths involved opioids.[89] MOUD reduces the risk of fatal overdose by 80%. There is no chance for recovery after overdose death.

Kreek[29,90] outlined the goals of treatment and the properties of desirable opioid agonist medications as follows:

1. Prevention or reduction of withdrawal symptoms
2. Prevention or reduction of opioid craving

3. Prevention of return to use of addictive opioids
4. Restoration to or toward normalcy of any physiologic function disrupted by chronic opioid use

Notably, like other medical conditions, the goals are focused on controlling signs and symptoms of the condition rather than discontinuation of medication treatment. This helps to provide a useful framework when patients, clinicians, and policymakers inquire as to the appropriate length of pharmacotherapy.

Profile of Potential Medications to Treat OUD

Ideal characteristics of potential medications can be defined as follows:

1. Such medications are effective.
2. They have a long biologic half-life (>24 hours).
3. They have minimal side effects during chronic administration.
4. They are safe (ie, they lack true toxic or serious adverse effects).
5. They are efficacious for a substantial proportion of persons with the disorder. Methadone and buprenorphine are agonists, and naltrexone is an antagonist generally exhibiting these characteristics, although methadone does have capacity to cause serious and even fatal overdoses.

Opioid Physical Dependence and Protracted Withdrawal Syndrome

Himmelsbach,[90] reporting on 21 prisoners physiologically dependent on morphine, observed that "physical recovery requires not less than 6 months of total abstinence." Martin and Jasinski[51] reported in a subsequent study that the period of protracted withdrawal (PW) persisted for 6 months or more after completely stopping opioids and that it was associated with "altered physiologic function." They found decreased blood pressure, decreased heart rate and body temperature, miosis, and a decreased sensitivity of the respiratory center to carbon dioxide, beginning about 6 weeks after withdrawal and persisting for 26 to 30 or more weeks. They also found increased sedimentation rates (which persisted for months) and electroencephalograph (EEG) changes. Martin and Jasinski[51] postulated a relationship between the PA syndrome and return to substance use. In another study, Shi et al.[91] also studied PW symptoms in individuals who formerly used heroin, comparing those who were not receiving medication and those receiving methadone after similar lengths of heroin abstinence. Seventy individuals who had formerly used heroin were included in one of four groups: in days 15 to 45 of short-term methadone treatment (MT), in months 5 to 6 of MT (long-term MT), no opioids for 15 to 45 days after methadone-assisted heroin withdrawal (short-term post methadone), and no opioids for 5 to 6 months after methadone-assisted heroin withdrawal (long-term post methadone). Analysis of PW symptoms during the study allowed the investigators to conclude that long-term methadone treatment reduces PW symptoms of heroin abstinence and cue-induced craving.

The concept of PW has been controversial[92] but remains a useful model for scientific hypothesis testing and development of new therapeutic approaches.[93] As Dole pointed out, since methadone continues physical dependence, PW may remain a problem later if medically supervised withdrawal from methadone is undertaken. In addition to biologic considerations, psychosocial concomitants of OUD also necessitate longer, more specialized adjunct treatments for these and additional problems.

Treatment Using Methadone

Continued Illicit Opioid Use Versus Methadone Treatment

The person with OUD who is actively using nonprescribed short-acting opioids typically experiences rapid and wide swings from a brief pleasure usually characterized by relief of withdrawal symptoms, sedation, fading into a period of normalcy and alertness, which can be described as the "comfort zone." This period is uniformly followed by the beginnings of subjective withdrawal, which soon develops into the full objective withdrawal syndrome typical of OUD. This cycle is particularly evident in the patient who engages in injection or inhalation of potent short-acting opioids such as heroin. A full cycle from "sick" (withdrawal) to "high" (intoxication) to "normal" (alert, comfortable) to "sick" (withdrawal) can occur repeatedly throughout the day (**Fig. 62-1**). The sensation of the "rush" is associated with a very rapid increase in blood levels. The pleasure is experienced during the time that drug levels remain above the therapeutic window (**Fig. 62-2**). OATs, such as methadone or buprenorphine regularly administered at steady state, are present at levels sufficient to maintain alertness without craving or drug preoccupation (comfort zone or therapeutic window) throughout the dosing interval—usually 24 hours.

With each administration of methadone, there is a gradual rise in blood level, reaching a peak at 3 to 4 hours. Typically, the peak level is less than two times the trough level. There is

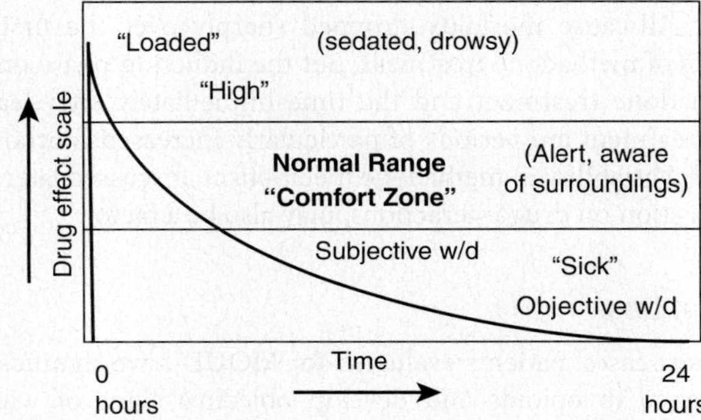

Figure 62-1. Heroin-simulated 24-hour dose-response.

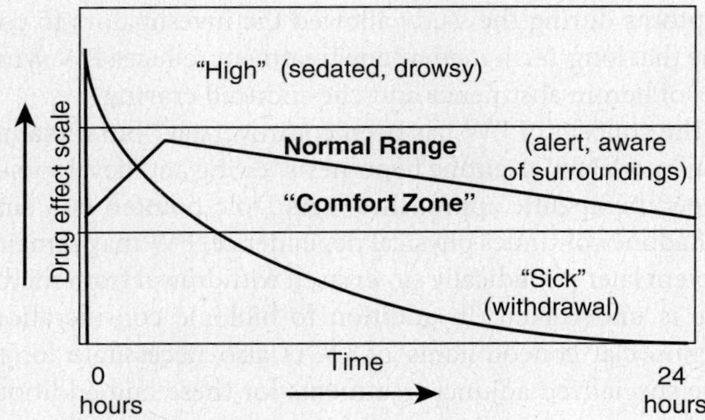

Figure 62-2. Methadone 24 hours at steady state.

a gradual decline over the rest of the 24-hour period, back to the trough level. When the patient is on a therapeutic dose at steady state and with development of sufficient tolerance, at no time does the rate or extent of change in blood levels cause a sensation of being intoxicated or result in withdrawal symptoms.

Methadone Induction

Before the fentanyl era, most patients stabilized at 80 to 120 mg/d of methadone.[20] There has not been rigorous study of optimal doses in the fentanyl era, but experienced clinicians are noting that methadone doses higher than 120 mg/d are needed to stabilize patients using fentanyl. Although adequate doses of methadone are needed to provide stability and increase retention in treatment,[94] the starting dose must be much lower, and the eventual steady state is reached slowly over many days to weeks. The first several doses require careful evaluation and adjustment. This phase is called *induction*. Even though methadone treatment has been shown to reduce mortality, including overdose mortality,[95,96] several studies have reported deaths during the first 10 to 14 days of treatment, particularly when induction doses are high and particularly if the patient is also ingesting sedatives.[97-101] About 42% of drug-related deaths during treatment occurred during the first week of methadone OAT.[102] In one study, patients were reported to be 6.7 times more likely to die during induction as compared to untreated individuals using heroin.[99] The mean induction dose was more than 50 mg among those who had died. All-cause mortality dropped sharply over the first 4 weeks of methadone treatment, but the induction phase onto methadone treatment and the time immediately after leaving treatment are periods of particularly increased mortality risk.[22] Variability in methadone metabolism, discussed later in the section on drug interactions, may also be a factor.

Initial Dose

In most cases, patients evaluated for MOUD have significant tolerance to opioids and develop objective signs of withdrawal as evidence of current opioid physical dependence. The response to the initial dose of agonist medication provides valuable information about tolerance levels and the target "therapeutic window." Significant relief during peak methadone effect (2-4 hours) indicates that the dose is in the range of the established level of tolerance and may not require further escalation. The absence of relief suggests that the dose is well short of the therapeutic window. Additional methadone can be provided when withdrawal symptoms persist during peak methadone levels. Twenty-four hours after their first methadone dose patients are usually uncomfortable as tissue saturation has not occurred. If they were comfortable during the first 4 to 12 hours after their dose, they probably need more time at the same dose and not a higher daily dose. Under federal regulations, the initial dose of methadone is no more than 30 mg and may be lower in patients with lower or zero tolerance (eg, resumed use after a significant period of abstinence, use of lower-potency opioids such as hydrocodone or codeine, people who smoke opium, or those released from incarceration). Identification of level of tolerance is the principal task of the initial medical assessment after confirming the diagnosis of OUD. An additional dose of 10 mg of methadone may be administered on day 1 of dosing if documentation is present that withdrawal is inadequately suppressed with the initial 30-mg dose. A total dose of no more than 40 mg may be given on the first treatment day unless the program physician documents in the patient's record that 40 mg did not suppress opioid abstinence symptoms.

Stabilization and Steady State

After the initial dose, the induction phase allows for subsequent careful adjustments of the dose to achieve elimination of drug craving and prevention of withdrawal while avoiding the risk of intoxication or overdose associated with accumulation of methadone.[103,104] The induction phase can be considered to last until the patient has attained a methadone dose that meets the four goals outlined above. The safe and effective introduction of methadone requires an understanding of steady-state pharmacologic principles. In general, steady-state levels are reached after a drug is administered for four to five half-lives (methadone has an average half-life of 24-36 hours). The clinical significance is that, with daily dosing, a significant portion of the previous dose remains in tissue stores, resulting in increased peak-and-trough methadone levels after the second and subsequent doses. Thus, the blood levels of methadone increase daily, even without an increase in dose. The rate of increase levels off as steady state is achieved at four to five half-lives, that is, 3 to 7 days (**Fig. 62-3**). Further dose changes every 3 to 7 days may be needed to achieve the maintenance dose. Dose adjustments can be done in 5- to 10-mg increments for highly tolerant patients. Liquid medication allows dose adjustments by smaller increments for less tolerant patients.[105]

Duration and Dose

A patient's optimal dose and duration of treatment are individualized clinical decisions. There is no scientific or clinical

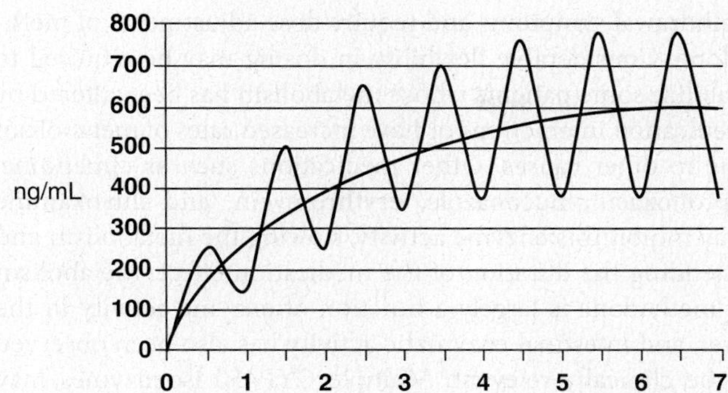

Figure 62-3. Steady-state simulation—maintenance pharmacology attained after four to five half-times, 1 dose/half-life.

basis for an arbitrary dose ceiling on methadone, although QT prolongation is dose dependent and has been seen in the electrocardiograms of patients receiving high doses of methadone.[104] Methadone doses of 80 to 100 mg have greater benefits than doses below 50 mg in patients with physiologic dependence on heroin.[106-108] (We do not yet have sufficient data to know how well patients with physiologic dependence on fentanyl respond to typical methadone titration schedules or typical daily doses.) For most patients receiving methadone, a long-term approach is most appropriate. Based on an extensive review of the research literature on the prognosis of patients who have been withdrawn from methadone, as well as the safety of continued treatment, the American Society of Addiction Medicine supports the principle that methadone treatment is most effective as a long-term modality.[109]

The known risks of discontinuing methadone treatment, with predictable return to use of injected heroin or fentanyl use, become increasingly critical when viewed in the context of overdose and the HIV and hepatitis C virus (HCV) prevalence among people who inject drugs. These risks, when combined with the proven safety and efficacy of long-term methadone treatment, suggest that long-term—even indefinite—methadone treatment is appropriate and even essential for a significant proportion of eligible patients. Methadone treatment is therefore a treatment of a chronic medical disorder, with the goal of achieving control of the opioid use disorder and avoiding the consequences of the untreated disease.[110] Treatment should be continued as long as the patient continues to benefit, wishes to continue, remains at risk of resumed opioid use or other substance use, and suffers no significant adverse effects and as long as continued treatment is indicated in the professional judgment of the physician.[111] Patients receiving methadone do at times seek to discontinue treatment for nonmedical but very real and practical reasons (eg, transportation or scheduling difficulties) and to escape continued disruption of their lives associated with the burdensome restrictions, regulations, and structure of the treatment delivery system. Post COVID-19 regulations permit clinic attendance just once a month with take-home doses for the other days for stable patients with over 90 days in treatment. Prior to the COVID-19 pandemic, patients had to complete 2 years in treatment to obtain a 1-month supply of methadone. A review of liberalized take-home dosing to comply with public-health recommendations showed a 28% decrease in methadone-related overdose death over time.[112] For patients who attempt withdrawal, it is important for practitioners to provide encouragement along with the best medical and supportive treatment available, without fostering unrealistic expectations or unnecessary guilt, and to provide a means for rapid readmission to methadone treatment in the event of resumed use or impending return to the use of opioids.[109]

Techniques to Ensure Adequacy of Dose

In most cases, clinical observation and patient reporting are adequate to make appropriate dose determinations. For cases in which patients continue to report withdrawal symptoms at doses above 120 mg/d evaluation of methadone blood levels may be indicated.

Procedure for Obtaining Blood Levels

Peak blood levels should be drawn at three (2-4) hours after a dose and trough levels at 24 hours, once said dose has been stable for at least 5 days, to allow tissue store equilibration. Patients already on a divided dose, such as every 12 hours, should have 2- to 3-hour and 12-hour specimens. A trough level alone is of little clinical value unless it is extremely low or very high. Blood levels are interpreted in the context of a clinical presentation for which the laboratory values can supplement clinical judgment. The peak level at 2 to 4 hours should be no more than twice the trough level. A peak-to-trough ratio of two or less is ideal (peak/trough = ratio). Ratios greater than two suggest rapid metabolism. The rate of change is of greater clinical significance than the actual levels. For example, a patient with a 24-hour level of 350 ng/mL after a peak of 1,225 ng/mL (1,225/350 = 3.5, indicating rapid metabolism) may be experiencing early opioid withdrawal, whereas a patient with a trough of 150 ng/mL and a peak of 250 ng/mL (250/150 = 1.7, indicating a normal metabolism) may be quite comfortable. No particular blood level should be considered "therapeutic" outside of the clinical context.

Recent research supports measuring methadone-metabolite ratios (MMR) to assess the metabolism rate of methadone.[113] Advantages of MMR include requiring only one blood draw and MMR can be done at any point during the induction process to precisely characterize metabolism rates. The research needs to be reproduced before becoming standard assessment. Blood draws may generate cue induced cravings for patients with a history of injection drugs, and venous access may be compromised from scaring and venous collapse. It is reasonable to consider MMR to measure metabolism rate in patients who are reluctant to submit to blood draws due to poor vasculature, cue-induced cravings, and concerns for multiple blood draws.

Observed Doses and Take-Home Medication

Patient stability reduces need for daily visits. Patients with improved functional status who meet specified criteria set out in U.S. federal regulations can receive take-home medications. The criteria include adherence to treatment, stability of home environment, involvement in productive activity, abstinence from illicit substance use, and resolution of any legal problems. The former guidelines governing methadone treatment allow patients to take home up to six doses a week after 9 months, 2 weeks of medication after the first year, and 30-day doses after the 2nd year of treatment (42 CFR 8.12). The guidelines created during COVID-19 permit OTPs to grant 14 days of take-home medications to less stable patients, if the clinic deems the patient can safely handle take-home medications, and 28 days of take-home for stable patients.[114] SAMHSA has recently updated regulations to make COVID-19-era take-home permanent.[115]

Monthly observed dosing at the OTP, with take home doses for the month, is as close as most patients receiving methadone come to receiving their medication in a fashion like that in other well-controlled medical conditions. Methadone medical maintenance (MMM) and office-based opioid treatment (OBOT) with methadone remain a rarity in the United States. Advocacy and legislative efforts are underway to expand access to MMM and methadone OBOT as of the writing of this chapter.

Methadone Medical Maintenance

MMM, designed for "stable, recovered" patients on methadone, is an effort to release the patient from attendance in an OTP by allowing a physician who is affiliated with the clinic, but in office practice, to prescribe or administer methadone. In April 2000, the CSAT circulated draft guidelines describing medical maintenance. These guidelines were developed after more than 10 years of pilot projects and showed that this approach to care works and that it improves the quality of life for patients.[116] A 2001 study randomly assigning patients to either office- or OTP-based methadone showed no difference in clinical outcomes and improved patient and physician satisfaction.[117]

For those who are attempting to receive ongoing treatment in a different setting rather than from the effects of daily medication, medical maintenance could be an acceptable solution. Current regulations require a federal waiver for medical maintenance; however, as of 2022, MMM is still rarely used.

Methadone-Medication Interactions

Clinical experience suggests that concomitant medications can either induce or inhibit cytochrome (CY) CYP450 activity on methadone metabolism.[118] Drugs that stimulate or induce CYP450 activity can precipitate opioid withdrawal by accelerating metabolism, thus shortening duration and diminishing intensity of the effect of methadone. For example, addition of ethyl alcohol, rifampicin, phenytoin, carbamazepine, phenobarbital, nevirapine, or efavirenz may result in the onset of withdrawal symptoms and require dose adjustments of methadone. Considerable flexibility in dosing may be required to stabilize some patients whose metabolism has been altered by medication interactions or have increased rates of metabolism due to other causes. Other medications such as cimetidine, ciprofloxacin, fluconazole, erythromycin, and fluvoxamine may inhibit this enzyme activity, slowing the metabolism and extending the duration of the medication effect. Metabolism of methadone is largely a function of enzyme activity in the liver, and intestinal enzymatic activity has also been observed to be clinically relevant. Multiple CYP450 isoenzymes may affect methadone metabolism in vivo.[119] Liver 3A4 activity in vitro is shown to influence methadone metabolism.[120] Methadone exists as a racemic mixture of *R* and *S* isomers. Genetic variability in CYP2D6 activity may affect clinical status by affecting metabolism of the *R*-methadone isomer[121-123] and may also affect toxicity.[124] Enzymatic activity of intestinal CYP2B6 is stereoselective and may be important in clinical effects and drug interactions.[125] A 17-fold variability between patients in their methadone metabolism is shown, mostly due to activity of various CYP450 enzymes.[126] Due to variability in methadone metabolism, it is important for clinicians to focus on functional outcomes rather than absolute dose amounts when determining the appropriateness of treatment.

Methadone and QT Interval

Several case series have been published showing that methadone treatment is associated with prolongation of the QT interval on the electrocardiogram and possible consequent cardiac arrhythmia (torsade des pointes or TdP).[127,128] In 2006, the FDA published a boxed warning that included QT interval prolongation and the risk of arrhythmia.

In vitro study of human ether-à-go-go–related gene potassium channels (hERG K^+) confirms that methadone at therapeutic doses can affect cardiac conduction.[129] Genomics of CYP2B6 were shown to be associated with QT interval, and in vitro studies suggest that most of this prolongation is due to the nontherapeutic *S*-methadone enantiomer.[130] Interviews of patients receiving methadone treatment found an association between longer QT and retrospective self-report of syncopal episodes.[131] Several studies look at QT interval in the methadone clinic setting.[132-134] However, there are no clear data to guide any intervention. Some clinics are offering cardiograms and are screening patients for cardiac risk. Risk-benefit discussion with patients includes a review of other medications that might contribute additional cardiac risk, eliciting a history of structural heart disease, unexplained syncopal episodes, or familial prolonged QT syndrome. All of these conditions may heighten the risk for TdP and may warrant ECG screening. In general, it is considered almost certain that resumed use of uncontrolled opioid use is riskier than the rare occurrence of an arrhythmia. However, coordination of care with outside physicians to monitor the use of other medications or transfer to buprenorphine treatment might in some cases be indicated.[135] Hospitalized patients receiving methadone may have particularly high risk of TdP.[135] The Center for Substance Abuse Treatment (CSAT) convened a consensus panel on this topic, and the final iteration of the consensus panel's recommendations include risk assessment and ECG screening, patient and staff education about cardiac risk, and informed consent.[136,137] However, this advice was not based upon solid evidence of preventing deaths and did not include a cost-benefit assessment. Thus, the support of the panel for this viewpoint was not unanimous. Feasibility of offering QT screening on-site in the OTP has been shown in several studies,[136,138] but substantial barriers remain including cost, staff time, and access to cardiologists to read the tracings. It has not become standard of care to do routine ECG screening in licensed OTPs.

Benzodiazepines and OAT Including Methadone

The potentially lethal combination of benzodiazepines with OAT is important to address in patients who have concomitant benzodiazepine use or benzodiazepine use disorder. For patients with therapeutic sources of benzodiazepines, careful coordination with prescribers is indicated. Alternate treatments for insomnia or anxiety may be possible. Abrupt abstinence from high doses of benzodiazepines may require medically supervised withdrawal due to the risk of withdrawal seizures. Reported rates of nonprescribed benzodiazepine use among methadone-treated patients are between 24.9% and 50.6%.[139] Benzodiazepine testing should be a routine in OTPs.[140] A recent retrospective chart review of 278 OAT patients showed patients prescribed benzodiazepines had longer treatment retention and lower mortality than patients who never received benzodiazepine prescriptions. However, mortality significantly increased once patients receiving benzodiazepines left treatment.[141] The greatest concern with benzodiazepine use and OUD is withholding MOUD due to concomitant benzodiazepine use.[142]

Medical Monitoring of Methadone

The initial pharmacologic rationale for long-term methadone maintenance was its ability to relieve the PW syndrome and to block heroin euphoria.[54,143] No serious side effects are associated with continued methadone use[144] with the exception of hypogonadism in men, sleep apnea,[145] and risk of QT prolongation with exceedingly rare but potential subsequent progression to TdP.[136] Minor side effects, such as constipation, excess sweating, peripheral edema, drowsiness, weight gain and decreased sexual interest and performance, have been noted. In addition, neuroendocrine studies have shown normalization of stress hormone responses and reproductive functioning after several months of stabilization on methadone.[146]

Buprenorphine Treatment

In October 2002, the FDA approved two sublingual formulations of buprenorphine for treatment of DSM-IV opioid dependence. In the initial FDA-approved formulation, a combination of buprenorphine and naloxone in a 4:1 ratio was designed to discourage injected diversion and misuse. There are now four FDA-approved buprenorphine/naloxone products for the treatment of OUD that are administered sublingually or through buccal administration. The originally approved formulation had a buprenorphine:naloxone ratio of 4:1. Current formulations range from buprenorphine:naloxone from 7:1 to 3.88:1. Newer formulations were approved based upon demonstrating the production of equivalent serum levels of buprenorphine compared with the 4:1 product. Technologies deployed to allow for lower doses of buprenorphine include saliva pH modification to enhance buprenorphine absorption. Naloxone is an opioid antagonist that is not significantly bioavailable when taken sublingually or when swallowed. When injected into individuals actively using opioids who are blinded, the buprenorphine/naloxone combination was not judged to be desirable or to be different from the antagonist in the first hour after injection.[147,148] In our opinion, the necessity for a naloxone and BUP-NLX combination to prevent misuse is controversial. Buprenorphine binds tighter than naloxone to the mu receptor.[149-151] Furthermore, the addition of naloxone may increase overdose risk upon treatment cessation.[152-155]

Pharmacology of Sublingual/Buccal Buprenorphine

Buprenorphine has slow onset and long duration of action, conferring similar benefits as discussed earlier for methadone. As a partial mu agonist, buprenorphine has a maximal dose-effect ceiling that is well below significant respiratory depression for most patients. This safety profile led to its DEA Schedule III, allowing office-based use under the restrictions of the Drug Addiction Treatment Act of 2000.[156]

Pharmacology of Injectable Buprenorphine

Extended-release (XR) injectable buprenorphine was approved and released in the United States in March 2018. BUP-XR is a buprenorphine-only product administered subcutaneously in the skin overlying the abdomen. BUP-XR is available in 300-mg and 100-mg doses to be given once monthly. One 12-week study of BUP-XR showed blockade of drug liking effects of intramuscular hydromorphone after two injections of BUP-XR.[157] A 24-week study with BUP-XR administered at 300 mg on months 1 and 2 followed by administration of four 100-mg doses monthly demonstrated superiority to placebo producing more illicit opioid-free weeks.[158] In both studies, patients receiving BUP-XR were stabilized on 8 to 24 mg of sublingual buprenorphine prior to receiving BUP-XR. Serum levels of BUP-XR were comparable to sublingual buprenorphine doses usually used to treat OUD. BUP-XR has detectable serum levels for up to 1 year after six injections.

A recent study examined the effects of BUP-XR over an 18-month study period. Longer duration of use BUP-XR was associated with higher abstinence. Sixty percent of patients had stable or improved outcomes at 6-, 12-, and 18-month assessments. Forty-seven percent of patients showed self-reported sustained opioid abstinence for the full 18-month study period.[159] The BUP-XR study allowed for flexible dosing and the majority of patients remained on BUP-XR 300 mg monthly.

A second BUP-XR preparation (CAM2038) is approved, and European and FDA approval is anticipated.[160] Differences between the first approved BUP-XR include 1 week and 1 month dosing. The binder is different and the injection can be given in multiple sites due to less fluid volume. The peak serum level of buprenorphine is comparable to the first BUP-XR preparation. However, the trough of the second is approximately 10% that first.

Initiation and Precipitated Withdrawal

Buprenorphine has strong receptor affinity. Relative to a displaced full agonist, its activity can be felt as the rapid onset of (relative) opioid withdrawal by the patient unless the first dose is clinically well timed. The first dose should be given when the patient is already in mild to moderate opioid withdrawal. When opioid withdrawal is present, the onset of activity will be felt as agonist, with relief of withdrawal. In contrast to methadone, induction doses are not set by regulation, though clinical guidelines and physician training courses recommend 2-4 mg of sublingual buprenorphine/naloxone as a first dose, with first-day maximum of 8 mg.[161] There are no serious safety concerns with going higher than 8 mg on day 1 if necessary to relieve withdrawal symptoms or craving.[162] Higher initiation doses were associated with better engagement in ongoing care.[163,164]

Setting

The majority of published studies have conducted buprenorphine inductions with supervised dosing. The advantages of supervised dosing include attenuation of withdrawal symptoms under medical supervision. However, observed inductions require significant staff time and monitoring. Observed induction logistics are seen as a barrier to buprenorphine prescribing.[165] There is a growing practice and body of evidence that supports the feasibility and safety of unobserved or "home" inductions particularly from office-based practices.[166]

Low-Dose Buprenorphine Initiation

Use of buprenorphine in the setting of fentanyl use disorder has attracted substantial attention. Fentanyl is a short-acting, high-potency opioid. Fentanyl binds to plasma protein and is stored in adipose tissue creating a depot-type effect for people who use it regularly.[167] The depot effect raises concern for precipitated withdrawal.

Low-dose buprenorphine is used to spare patients from OWS. It can be utilized for people who are currently taking illegal or prescribed opioids. Considerations in use of low-dose buprenorphine initiation include patient selection, specific dose titration schedule, and timeline for removing the full agonist.[168,169] A recent review showed alternative low-dose models being effective for patients who are withdrawal-averse, on opioids for chronic pain, high-dose methadone, and people who use fentanyl.[170] Schedules for low dose vary, but a common one is to titrate upward gradually from a dose of 0.5 mg buprenorphine on day 1 to 4 mg buprenorphine TID on day 7 with subsequent discontinuation of the full agonist opioid and further up titration of buprenorphine as indicated.[171]

Buprenorphine Dose Adjustment

The dose of buprenorphine can be titrated over the first 3 days or more rapidly to control withdrawal. Average daily doses are 16 to 24 mg. One labeled imaging study showed mu-opioid receptors to be approximately 90% occupied depending upon the brain region at doses of 16 mg/d of sublingual solution.[172] Because of the partial agonist ceiling effect, no additional benefit is expected in doses above 32 mg/d, although this theoretical precept has not been empirically studied. Sublingual buprenorphine/naloxone is usually prescribed as a single daily dose. Some patients, especially those who have chronic pain in addition to OUD prefer to divide their daily dose, which is also an acceptable dosing strategy.

Buprenorphine-Medication Interactions

Compared to methadone, buprenorphine may confer advantages when certain HIV medications are used[173] and in cases of QT prolongation with methadone.[134,174] The presence of an active metabolite—norbuprenorphine—and strong affinity for the mu opioid receptor make this medication less dependent than methadone on blood level and tissue stores.

Federal Regulations and Sublingual Buprenorphine

When dispensed in the OTP, sublingual buprenorphine/naloxone is subject to the same regulations as methadone, except for the time in treatment requirements, as explained below. When prescribed in the office-based setting, there are certain restrictions set forth in the Drug Addiction Treatment Act of 2000. This law provides for a waiver to the 1914 Harrison Act that forbids prescription of a "narcotic" to a person with an addiction. However, the DATA 2000 requirements were repealed in December 2022. All DEA-licensed prescribers who are authorized to prescribe Schedule III medications can now prescribe buprenorphine with no caps on the number of patients treated. The DATA 2000 restrictions did not apply when buprenorphine or buprenorphine/naloxone are dispensed at clinics under their OTP license. In those cases, the same federal regulatory restrictions apply to both buprenorphine and methadone except that the time-in-treatment regulations that apply to take-home doses of methadone no longer apply for buprenorphine so that decisions about the number of buprenorphine take-home doses given are determined purely based on patient stability and not on how long the patient has been in treatment. Alternate-day or thrice-weekly dosing is an option for the buprenorphine-maintained patient who is not stable enough to have take-home doses.[175,176]

Diversion and Nonmedical Use of Buprenorphine

An early and limited investigation of the effects of DATA 2000 was carried out in 2005. No serious adverse events were found by the introduction of sublingual buprenorphine/naloxone in the office-based setting. That study showed that most of the patients treated with buprenorphine listed prescription pain relievers as their primary opioid of nonmedical use.[177] In view of the increase in nonmedical use of prescription opioids, it is hoped that buprenorphine/naloxone may provide a timely treatment for those who struggling with OUD who might not otherwise seek out an OTP.

In many locations when buprenorphine treatment has been introduced, there has been diversion and nonmedical use of the medication, including injected use.[178,179] As the clinical use of buprenorphine has increased since 2002, so have reports of diversion. One study in the United States showed that diverted buprenorphine/naloxone is being used mostly for relief of withdrawal and rarely as a primary drug of misuse.[180] A more recent study found that diversion increased as treatment with buprenorphine became more available, though not as steeply as full agonists.[181] In areas of higher prescribing of buprenorphine, most treatment seekers have already tried the medication, having used it nonprescribed for relief of withdrawal or during times when the preferred opioid of misuse is not available.[182] Buprenorphine diversion suggests a lack of OUD treatment availability.[183] An Australian study that interviewed patients who were found to be diverting doses given under observation at pharmacies found that discarding it, saving it for another time, or giving the dose to someone else were cited as reasons for not taking an observed dose.[184,185] Buprenorphine has two- to threefold lower rates of drug diversion reports compared with methadone and other full agonist opioids.[183,186,187] Guidelines for agonist treatment recommend monitoring for diversion with urine testing or pill counts and adding observed dosing or shortening time span between prescriptions when diversion is suspected. A long-acting buprenorphine formulation such as the XR injection is also an option.

Patient Selection

Increasing evidence supports low-barrier buprenorphine intervention.[188-190] Low-barrier buprenorphine increases treatment engagement in unhoused people who inject drugs with medical, psychiatric, and co-occurring other drug use.[189] Buprenorphine services to Syringe Service Programs (SSP) have been shown to be safe and effective.[191,192] One SSP study showed that the majority of patients could start MOUD on the same day and most patients were Medicare/Medicaid recipients.[192]

SPECIAL ISSUES IN ONGOING MEDICATION TREATMENT

Comparative Efficacy of Buprenorphine Versus Methadone: Choice Between Methadone and Buprenorphine

The clinical issue of choosing between pharmacotherapy options or matching patients to buprenorphine versus methadone maintenance continues to be an open question that is actively investigated.

Though both medications have been shown to be comparable in various outcomes[193-196] systematic reviews suggest that methadone and buprenorphine are roughly equivalent in reducing opioid use with methadone demonstrating slightly better rates of treatment retention.[197,198] In the United States, site of care and level of care, local availability, or cost may determine which medication is applicable for a given patient. A blinded study showed that a "stepped" approach of starting patients on buprenorphine and transferring those who did not stabilize onto methadone had identical outcomes to directly admitting patients to methadone treatment.[199]

Buprenorphine may confer less cardiac risk,[131,174] although no prospective studies have been carried out. A randomized prospective liver safety study showed no liver damage produced by either medication.[200]

Opioid Agonist Treatment during Pregnancy

Use of nonprescribed opioids during pregnancy is a growing concern in the United States and internationally and is often associated with adverse consequences for both the mother and her infant, especially prematurity and low birth weight.[201-209] From 1999 to 2014, the rate of maternal OUD increased from 1.5 to 6.5 per 1000 deliveries.[210] The current literature suggests that children of women with OUD might be at risk for poor outcomes not only because of opioid drug exposure but also because of concomitant alcohol and tobacco exposure and numerous factors related to the caregiving environment.[205,210,211] Treatment options studied include methadone or buprenorphine,[212,213] antagonist maintenance[214] (ie, naltrexone), and medication-assisted withdrawal.[215] Methadone has been the recommended standard of care over no treatment or medication-assisted withdrawal. This is based on longer durations of maternal drug abstinence, better obstetrical care compliance, avoidance of associated risk behaviors, reductions in fetal illicit drug exposure, and enhanced neonatal outcomes.[212] In comparison to infants born to mothers using heroin, infants born to mothers treated with methadone have increased fetal growth, reduced fetal mortality, and decreased risk of HIV infection.[204,216] Moreover, for pregnant women under conditions where nonmedication and methadone treatment were both available, methadone is associated with longer treatment retention[217,218] and less resumed use.[216] Studies examining the consequences of prenatal methadone exposure on later development have produced inconsistent results[219-225] that could be due to confounding factors and are complicated by study attrition.[225] Overall, methadone treatment in pregnancy does not appear to be associated with developmental or cognitive impairments.[219-225]

Nevertheless, methadone use at effective clinical doses during pregnancy may be avoided by some practitioners due to concerns over the associated Neonatal Opioid Withdrawal Syndrome (NOWS). Although newborns of women receiving methadone may experience NOWS, these are readily treated without consequences.[225] Furthermore, dose is not a reliable proxy for fetal exposure since the fetus is not exposed to the maternal dose but to the maternal serum level, which is largely determined by individual patient pharmacogenomics and pharmacokinetics.[226] (See discussion below in NOWS subheading.) Hence, pregnant women should receive appropriate methadone doses to treat OUD.[227] There have been 31 published reports of buprenorphine exposure during pregnancy that were reviewed and summarized by Jones et al.[227] Overall, the pregnancies were uneventful, without physical teratogenic effects and with low rates of prematurity, suggesting that buprenorphine is relatively safe and effective in this population. Conclusions from data on the prenatal exposure to buprenorphine are limited by methodologic challenges (eg, varied dose ranges, lengths of exposure, care settings). Many reports omitted information regarding concomitant substance use and prescribed medications that could impact the expression of NOWS. The Maternal Opioid Treatment: Human Experimental Research (MOTHER) study was a large multisite clinical trial enrolling a diverse sample of pregnant women with DSM-IV opioid dependence into both methadone and buprenorphine treatment.[198] The methadone group had better retention (the most important variable in drug treatment outcomes): treatment was discontinued by 18% of methadone patients and 33% of buprenorphine patients. However, infants born to mothers in the buprenorphine group required less morphine, had a shorter hospital stay, and had a shorter duration of treatment for the NOWS.[198] There were no differences between groups in other primary or secondary outcomes or in the rates of maternal or neonatal adverse events. The authors conclude that buprenorphine is an alternative to methadone for the treatment of OUD during pregnancy. While buprenorphine appears to be associated with reduced severity of NOWS, methadone dosing was done as a single daily dose in the MOTHER study, rather than the divided dosing dictated by pharmacokinetic science and clinical studies[228] More research is needed into optimal dosing of both medications. Dosing that does not address the variability in drug elimination between mothers or that limits maternal dose to an arbitrary limit (the MOTHER study set a dose limit of 140 mg/d that is below the needs of many rapid metabolizing mothers) ignores the risk of protracted and/or episodic stressful maternal-fetal withdrawal and potential adverse effects on neonatal health[229]

Clinicians should also take into account the possibility of reduced adherence and the ceiling effect of buprenorphine compared with methadone. It is unknown how many buprenorphine practices provide the intensity of medical monitoring needed by pregnant women. Methadone regulations require intensive clinic attendance, monitored dosing, a counselor, and an actively involved prescriber who meets regularly with the patient. The higher rate of treatment discontinuation in the buprenorphine group raises issues of optimal induction onto buprenorphine and retention as an issue for future exploration.

Comparison studies have been done in specific clinical areas. Prospective, randomized, and blinded studies during pregnancy and the perinatal period show that both methadone and buprenorphine are safe, with methadone associated with more severe NOWS.[198,230-232] In addition, a cohort study of several thousand pregnant women and their neonates exposed to either methadone or buprenorphine showed that buprenorphine treatment was associated with lower rates of neonatal complications than was methadone, whereas maternal complications did not differ between the two medications.[233]

Methadone dosing in pregnancy is complicated by the clinical need to respond to the altered metabolism caused by pregnancy-related induction of the key metabolic enzymes, which convert the active medication to an inactive metabolite.[234] The variable timing and rate of enzyme induction during gestation dictates that dose increases are likely to be required at any stage of pregnancy to minimize maternal/fetal withdrawal symptoms, and divided doses are routinely needed to manage the reduced half-life of the medication.[228] Further, divided dosing eliminates or minimizes fetal physiologic abnormalities seen with single-dose methadone treatment.[235,236] Pharmacokinetic science should be the basis for dosing to minimize withdrawal stress by maintaining a stable level of mu receptor occupancy in both maternal and fetal brain.[229] Methadone trough serum levels provide an objective window on both maternal metabolism and fetal exposure. This information can document the need for dose increases and reduce anxiety about adverse effects of increased doses on the fetus. It is not uncommon to see the methadone dose go up and the serum level go down or remain constant.[228] Further, serum levels postpartum can be helpful for clinical safety to monitor the reversal of enzyme induction and a rise in serum levels, which can pose problems of oversedation, higher than normal amounts of methadone entering breast milk, and maternal dependence on unnecessarily high serum levels. Most women will need dose decreases in the early postpartum period.

Buprenorphine is converted to three active metabolites: norbuprenorphine and the glucuronide conjugates of the parent and norbuprenorphine.[237] Therefore, serum levels are likely to remain more constant than methadone and require less frequent dose adjustments. However, accelerated metabolic effects can also affect buprenorphine metabolite levels, and dose increases and divided dosing are likely needed for optimal maternal/fetal mu receptor occupancy, as with methadone.[238]

The treating clinician should partner with an obstetrician and neonatologist in the management of a pregnancy in the context of OUD. Consultants may lack understanding of the nature of addiction and the special issues related to maternal/fetal OUD, leading to negative physician-patient interactions and maternal stress and shame.[229] Pregnant women are especially reassured to know that their clinicians communicate and agree on a treatment plan.

Neonatal Opioid Withdrawal Syndrome

NOWS is an important outcome for OAT in pregnancy. Although the scoring systems used to assess NOWS treatment efficacy vary across reports (eg, Finnegan[239] or modifications of this scale and Lipsitz[240]), the literature suggests that buprenorphine is associated with NOWS, half the cases of which require pharmacotherapy. The pregnancy, birth, and NOWS outcomes are confounded by other drug use in 86% of the reports. Although considerable individual variability exists, the NOWS timing observed to date has an apparent onset within the first 12 to 48 hours, peaks within approximately 66 to 96 hours, and lasts about 120 to 168 hours. The exception to this has been the few infants who were reported to exhibit withdrawal signs for 6 to 10 weeks after delivery.[241,242] These cases may represent protracted withdrawal, as seen with adults, or neonatal ill health related to adverse pregnancy events beyond simple opioid exposure, such as illicit drug use and long-term effects of chronic intrauterine withdrawal stress. To date, only one report has found a correlation between buprenorphine dose and the severity of the NOWS.[243] Other reports[230,244,245] have reported no correlation.

Research has demonstrated that NOWS is not managed consistently after delivery.[246] Across studies, there is often insufficient detail regarding medication used to treat ensuing NOWS as well as the criteria for initiation, maintenance, and weaning of NOWS medication. Sublingual buprenorphine shows promise in one placebo-controlled trial in significantly reducing length of hospitalization for NOWS when compared to oral morphine[247] There is likely major overuse of Neonatal Intensive Care Units for uncomplicated withdrawal leading to unnecessary maternal/fetal separations at a time critical for bonding. A rooming-in model of care where the mother and fetus are not separated and where the mother is an active part of NOWS management has been shown to reduce NOWS symptoms and length of hospitalization.[248] The OTP clinician should explain the advantage of rooming-in to the mother and encourage her to discuss this option with her doctors.

Intrauterine Abstinence Syndrome

Intrauterine abstinence syndrome (IAS) has received little attention until recently.[249] Maternal and fetal withdrawal usually coincide, and the fetus is at risk of seizures, hyperactivity, and catecholamine excess. This increases fetal oxygen consumption and risk for asphyxia. Because of these risks, medically supervised withdrawal from opioids during pregnancy is not recommended.[250] Increasing evidence shows unfavorable intrauterine conditions affect developing systems and produce epigenetic changes associated with adult disease and long-term behavioral abnormalities.[251,252] While fetal demise is not a common outcome with maternal opioid withdrawal during pregnancy,[253] resumed use exposes the fetus to erratic drug levels and to episodic withdrawal. The ASAM and the American College of Gynecology jointly recommend against the practice of medically supervised withdrawal because of the high risk of resumed substance use.[254] OAT with partial or full agonists should be offered to all female patients with OUD when pregnancy is discovered for the health of the mother and developing fetus no matter the determination to continue or terminate the pregnancy.

Interactions of Opioid Agonist Treatment and Human Immunodeficiency Virus and Acquired Immunodeficiency Syndrome Pharmacotherapy

The introduction of new antiretroviral agents and antiretroviral therapy (ART) created a new therapeutic era for patients with HIV infection but also has introduced new complexities related to potential toxicities and interactions. Preclinical studies of ART and opioids indicate that drug interactions may occur as methadone and buprenorphine are both primarily metabolized by hepatic cytochrome CYP4503A4.[120,255] A number of antiretroviral medications have been shown in preclinical studies to inhibit or induce the activity of this same enzyme.

Methadone has been associated with several clinically important adverse drug interactions with ART. Significant drug-drug interactions between methadone and antiretroviral medications include potential for opioid withdrawal symptoms with efavirenz, nevirapine, lopinavir/ritonavir, and rilpivirine while methadone levels may be increased as a result of inhibition of methadone metabolism with delavirdine, although this medication is rarely used for the treatment of HIV infection at this time. Medications known to inhibit CYP3A4 have been used as a means of enhancing the plasma concentrations of other HIV medications. These include ritonavir and cobicistat, but neither has a clinically significant effect on methadone metabolism. Antiviral medications for the treatment of hepatitis C including, boceprevir, sofosbuvir, and telaprevir have no significant drug interactions with methadone.[256]

Antiretroviral medications that induce methadone metabolism present a risk for methadone toxicity if discontinued without concurrent tapering of methadone dose that had been increased to assure therapeutic effect of methadone while treatment with the inducing medication occurred.[183] It has been recommended that after the medication that is inducing CYP4503A enzymes is stopped, the methadone dose should be tapered over 1 to 2 weeks to reestablish the previous therapeutic dose of methadone (ie, that dose on which the patient was stable before starting the antiretroviral medication that induced methadone metabolism).[6]

Buprenorphine has been studied in combination with antiretroviral medications more recently. To date, reductions in buprenorphine concentrations resulting from drug interactions have not been associated with opioid withdrawal. Further, a review[173] regarding specific interactions between buprenorphine and ART found that drug interactions between buprenorphine/naloxone and HIV medications are less likely than with methadone.

Methadone-to-Buprenorphine Transfer

Some patients will be transferred from methadone to buprenorphine. This clinical decision may be driven by several possible factors. First, there is the unique pharmacology of buprenorphine, leading to its more favorable safety profile and longer duration of action (thus permitting thrice-weekly dosing) relative to methadone.[66,257-259] Second, buprenorphine may engender less fear of stigma than methadone.[260] Third, owing to its availability in office-based primary care—outside standard OTPs[59,77,261]—buprenorphine is more accessible over a wide geographic area. It also may be more appropriate as an early intervention strategy for those with short OUD histories (eg, adolescents) or with less physical dependence. However, if a patient is stable on methadone, the advisability of transfer to buprenorphine requires careful scrutiny of the factors motivating the request. Furthermore, transferring patients from a long-acting agonist such as methadone to buprenorphine without producing significant withdrawal discomfort, attrition, or resumed drug use has been shown to be more challenging than transfer from a short-acting opioid.

Research on transfer from methadone to buprenorphine is limited. These studies support an important role for methadone dose and interval between methadone and buprenorphine administration in determining precipitated withdrawal symptoms. Four studies examined the effect of time interval between the last methadone dose and the initial buprenorphine dose.[262-265] Most subjects received methadone at 30 mg/d. Buprenorphine has a lower risk of precipitating withdrawal the greater the time between the last methadone dose and the first buprenorphine dose.[262,263,265-268] Buprenorphine transitions from methadone doses of 30 mg/d are generally well tolerated.[269] Buprenorphine induction from methadone doses of 60 mg/d risks increasing opioid withdrawal symptom.[265] Two additional studies[266,268] showed mild withdrawal with buprenorphine initiation from methadone, but withdrawal severity was not correlated with methadone dose. Five studies have directly examined a full medication transfer.[266,268,270,271] Precipitated withdrawal was not consistently seen with the transition from methadone to buprenorphine. Some patients were not adequately treated with buprenorphine. If a patient experiences precipitated withdrawal with the initial buprenorphine dose, additional doses of buprenorphine are not likely to worsen withdrawal and may produce greater comfort.[272] Lofexidine may assist in the transition from methadone doses of 30 to 70 mg to buprenorphine.[273]

Owing to variable designs and individual differences among volunteers, a single recommended protocol is not currently available. In the absence of large clinical trials, the Provider Clinical Support System (PCSS) guidance (PCSS 2013) recommends tapering to 20 or 30 mg of methadone, waiting a minimum of 48 to 72 hours after last methadone dose, obtaining a COWS of 15 to quantify withdrawal, and starting buprenorphine at 2 mg, continuing to dose until the patient is comfortable at up to 32 mg on day 1. If withdrawal is precipitated, management with ancillary medications is advised. Discomfort may persist for up to 96 hours, but usually after 3 to 5 days, the patient will be stable and comfortable.

Novel approaches have been studied including using a transdermal fentanyl bridge[274], short-acting opioid agonist[275], and buprenorphine low dose initiation[276-279]. Novel strategies are largely limited to case-reports, and large RCTs are lacking.

In addition to clarifying the best strategy for minimizing symptoms during the transfer, clinical trials are needed to answer questions concerning short- and long-term clinical outcomes after methadone-to-buprenorphine transfer. A related relevant clinical need is identification of profiles and genetics of patients responding differentially to methadone versus buprenorphine (pharmacotherapy treatment matching).

Buprenorphine in Agonist-to-Antagonist Treatment

A number of strategies have been tried to transition patients from buprenorphine to treatment with the antagonist naltrexone. No specific protocol has emerged as the optimal way to effect the transfer. This procedure can be accomplished within the span of a few days, but precipitated withdrawal can occur. Often, α_2 adrenergic and other ancillary medications are needed to manage precipitated withdrawal. There should be good justification, even if just patient preference, for using naltrexone in this situation when patients could be stabilized on buprenorphine or methadone much more easily.

Naltrexone Treatment

The theoretical value of the opioid antagonist, naltrexone, is tempered by clinical reality, as reflected in retention rates of only 20% to 30% over 6 months. Multiple factors account for such poor retention.[144] Opioid antagonists, unlike methadone and buprenorphine, do not provide cross-tolerance. Therefore, if antagonists are stopped, there is no immediate reminder in the form of withdrawal. In addition, craving for opioids may continue during naltrexone treatment. A meta-analysis did not provide strong support for oral naltrexone treatment of OUD.[280] Nevertheless, for certain highly motivated subsamples of patients with OUD (such as healthcare professionals, business executives, or probation referrals) for whom there is an external incentive to comply with oral naltrexone therapy and to remain opioid abstinent, oral naltrexone has been very effective.[281-284] Improved adherence has also been reported in programs that include psychosocial therapy,[285,286] including contingency management.[287,288]

Clinically, oral naltrexone is initiated after withdrawal from opioids. There should be at least a 5- to 7-day opioid-free period for the short-acting opioids and a 7- to 10-day period for the long-acting agents. This does not apply to withdrawal treatments using the naltrexone-clonidine combination. The first dosage of naltrexone may be preceded by a naloxone challenge test to assure the absence of precipitated withdrawal prior to administering naltrexone. Naloxone challenges can utilize intranasal, subcutaneous, intravenous, and intramuscular naloxone. The initial dose of naltrexone used generally is 25 mg on the first day, followed by 50 mg daily or an equivalent of 350 mg weekly, divided into three doses (100, 100, and 150 mg). The principal reason for the reduced dose on day 1 is the potential for gastrointestinal side effects, such as nausea and vomiting. This occurs in about 10% of patients taking naltrexone. In most cases, gastrointestinal upset is relatively mild and transient, but in some cases, it may be so severe as to cause discontinuation of the naltrexone. Oral naltrexone also has infrequent potential to cause transaminitis; however, 50 mg daily has been given safely to individuals with OUD.[289] Transaminitis, in the rare instances it occurs, appears to be limited in extent in that it resolves when naltrexone is discontinued and does not progress to liver failure. The enzyme dihydrodiol dehydrogenase appears to catalyze the metabolism of naltrexone to the active metabolite, 6β-naltrexol. When administered orally, naltrexone has an average plasma half-life of 4 hours, whereas 6β-naltrexol has an average half-life of 13 hours after oral administration of the parent drug. In summary, though oral naltrexone has not lived up to expectations, for selected, motivated patients with OUD, it may represent a very effective form of maintenance pharmacotherapy.

Extended-release formulations of naltrexone (by implant and by depot injection) have been investigated. An extended-release formulation of naltrexone (XR-NTX) injected once monthly (every 4 weeks), found safe and well tolerated by participants in studies of treatment for alcohol use disorder,[290-292] was approved for OUD by the FDA in 2010. The medication has peak drug concentrations occurring at 2 hours and again at 2 to 3 days, remaining at therapeutic levels through 30 days. The recommended dose of 380 mg of extended-release naltrexone resulted in minimal and mild adverse events. The most common adverse events associated with XR-NTX in clinical trials were nausea, vomiting, headache, dizziness, and injection site reactions. It can also reduce opioid tolerance, which can increase the potential for overdose if opioids are used following cessation of long-term naltrexone treatment. In preliminary studies of sustained-release naltrexone in participants with physiologic dependence on opioids, Comer et al.[293-295] found that 384-mg XR-NTX was able to block the reinforcing, subjective, and physiologic effects of up to 25-mg heroin and provided therapeutic plasma levels for approximately 30 days.[293-295] At this dose, naltrexone also resulted in better than 80% retention in treatment at 6 weeks versus 40% for placebo.[295] Adverse events were minimal and limited to local injection site responses.[296] A trial of XR-NTX in patients with DSM-IV opioid dependence was reported by Krupitsky.[297,298] This randomized, placebo-controlled, double-blind trial of XR-NTX was conducted in Russia, where agonist therapy is not available.[297,298] Participants received monthly intramuscular injections of XR-NTX 380 mg ($N = 126$) or placebo ($N = 124$) for 4 months with 12 biweekly counseling sessions. The number of weeks of confirmed abstinence (based on rate of opioid-negative urine drug tests and self-report during weeks 5-24) was the primary outcome. In the XR-NTX group, 90% were abstinent versus 35% for placebo ($p = 0.0002$). The XR-NTX participants also had more opioid-free days, greater retention, and reduced craving compared to no change in the placebo group. No XR-NTX participants died, overdosed, or ended participation due to severe adverse events associated with the study protocol. A more recent open-label randomized trial in the United States among criminal-legal–involved individuals with OUD showed that XR-NTX was superior to treatment as usual in preventing return to opioid use.[299]

XR-NTX was compared to daily sublingual buprenorphine in two studies.[299,300] A 12-week open-label randomized clinical trial of 159 subjects showed XR-NTX was noninferior to daily sublingual BUP-NLX in measures of treatment retention, total number of opioid-negative urine drug screens, and use of heroin and other illicit opioids.[300] A 24-week open-label randomized controlled comparative effectiveness study of 570 subjects showed that XR-NTX was not successfully initiated in 28% of subjects compared with nonsuccessful initiation in 6% of BUP-NLX subjects. Outcomes of opioid-negative urine samples and opioid abstinent days favored BUP-NLX in an intent to treat analysis but were similar in the per-protocol population (those who started the assigned medication). Self-reported opioid cravings was less with XR-NTX than with BUP-NLX initially, but these converged by week 24. Five fatal overdoses occurred with two in the XR-NTX group and three in the BUP-NLX group. These studies demonstrate that XR-NTX has a role in the treatment of OUD, but getting patients onto XR-NTX is a challenge.

XR-NTX helps patient retention but does not reduce rates of overdose and opioid related morbidity compared with OAT like buprenorphine and methadone.[194,301]

Other implant formulations of depot naltrexone are being studied; several international implant studies are reviewed by Krupitsky and Blokhina[297]. The most studied is a single-dose Australian naltrexone implant. A double-blind, placebo-controlled, randomized clinical trial showed the effectiveness of this formulation in comparison with oral naltrexone.[82] In comparison with the oral formulation, naltrexone implants (not XR-NTX) showed significantly higher abstinence rates and better treatment outcomes at 12 months.[302-305]

According to unpublished data from a registry trial of XR-NTX for OUD,[306] 30% of patients dropped out before receiving their first XR-NTX injection. Seventy-six percent of 403 patients treated with XR-NTX dropped out in the first 6 months. Over 90% of patients were treatment failures during the duration of the study itself. Three patients died from overdose within 21, 55, and 115 days of their last dose of XR-NTX. Only 8.5% of patients discontinued XR-NTX because treatment goals were met. This registry study raises serious questions about the safety and long-term efficacy of XR-NTX.

Another study observed the majority of overdose deaths post XR-NTX occurred within 2 months of treatment discontinuation.[154] Overdose death is associated with discontinuation of all MOUD.

Pain Management in Patients Receiving Opioid Agonist Treatment

Patients on OAT with pain require special consideration because of their baseline maintenance opioid. They will be tolerant to additional opioids, and if nonopioid approaches are not effective, they may need higher and more frequent doses of opioids to manage their pain.

Methadone and Acute Pain Management

In cases of acute pain associated with surgery, trauma, or dental work, the physicians or dentists involved often—incorrectly—assume that usual daily dose of methadone will relieve any ensuing pain from the injury or procedure. Several points should be kept in mind. First, single daily doses of methadone may be effective in treating OUD, but multiple daily doses may be required for analgesia. Second, long-term use of methadone and possibly buprenorphine is associated with hyperalgesia.[307,308] Tolerance and hyperalgesia combined means that patients in OAT who require opioids for acute pain management may need very high doses of opioids. However, high-potency NSAIDs and nonopioid analgesics can also be considered as primary or adjunctive medications in the management for acute pain. Mixed agonist-antagonists (pentazocine, butorphanol, nalbuphine) and partial agonists (buprenorphine) must not be used in patients receiving methadone as they will precipitate an opioid withdrawal syndrome. Meperidine should be avoided because of the risk of seizures at the higher doses required to produce analgesia in patients receiving methadone.

In summary, for patients receiving methadone who require opioids for acute pain management, (1) continue methadone without interruption and use nonopioid pain treatments whenever possible; split dosing of methadone may be considered to optimize analgesic effect (2) provide adequate individualized doses of opioid agonists, which must be titrated to the desired analgesic or functional effect; and (3) doses should be given more frequently and on a fixed schedule rather than "as needed for pain." Although not thoroughly documented, it is probably best to choose agonists different from those previously misused.

Buprenorphine and Acute Pain Management

Buprenorphine has a ceiling on respiratory depression. The ceiling on analgesia is controversial. Management of acute pain (eg, postsurgical pain) remains a persistent fear of patients and clinicians. A small case series reported on five patients receiving buprenorphine through seven major surgeries. Postoperative pain was adequately controlled using full agonist opioids by patient report and physician assessment while maintaining buprenorphine.[309] Patients can be managed for acute pain on buprenorphine OAT.[310] Patients should continue buprenorphine and further receive a multimodal analgesic approach. Care coordination and an individualized approach with shared-decision-making increases the likelihood of success in acute pain management. Several guidelines emphasize regional anesthesia and nonopioid adjuncts,[310,311] but patients remaining on buprenorphine who need full agonist opioids for optimal acute pain control can receive them if needed. Few current guidelines or research recommend discontinuation or reduction of buprenorphine OAT to manage acute pain.

Chronic Pain in Patients Receiving OAT

More than 30% of patients receiving OAT report chronic, severe pain.[312] Compared to those who primarily use heroin, patients admitted to the OTP for prescription opioid use disorder may have higher prevalence of pain.[187,313] The historical separation of pain treatment from addiction treatment in American medicine gets in the way of properly caring for patients with chronic pain who are receiving OAT. The OTP and office-based clinician can sometimes bridge this gap by coordinating care with the patient's primary care or pain specialist. For example, in a patient with chronic noncancer pain who is able to comply with the regulatory criteria for take-home medication, the OTP physician can order a divided dose of methadone, and the outside physician can prescribe short-acting rescue medication. This might improve baseline pain control without the need for multiple sources of long-acting medication. Nonopioid pharmacologic strategies and nonpharmacologic interventions for chronic pain should typically be attempted before or in addition to relying solely on opioid medications to manage chronic pain.

Improving Treatment Access Through Emergency Departments

A randomized clinical trial tested the efficacy of various treatments for emergency department (ED) care for the treatment of OUD. Three hundred and twenty-nine patients with opioid use disorder were enrolled. One hundred and four patients were randomized to a referral only, 111 patients were assigned to a brief intervention group, and 114 were assigned to receive buprenorphine and connection with a buprenorphine prescriber. Doses of buprenorphine were 8 mg on day 1 and 16 mg on days 2 and 3. Thirty-four percent of all subjects were seeking treatment for OUD, and 8.8% presented with an overdose. The primary outcome at 30 days showed that 78% of patients who received buprenorphine were receiving formal addiction treatment, while only 37% in the referral group and 45% of patients in the brief intervention group were receiving such treatment.[314] The DEA allows for daily dispensing (not prescription) of any opioid medication for up to 72 hours to treat

OUD while arranging for more definitive treatment, and since 2022 clinicians can request an exception from DEA to dispense all 72 hour's worth of medication at a single time.

Overdose Education and Naloxone Distribution

Overdose education and naloxone distribution (OEND) is a service that has demonstrated efficacy and is addressed in detail in the chapter on harm reduction. OEND traditionally has been relegated to syringe services programs. OEND in programs that serve high-risk individuals have served to reduce overdose death rates in heroin-using populations. In a study of 2,500 injection drug using participants from 2010 to 2013, 702 overdose reversals were reported.[315] All individuals using opioids and some who are prescribed opioids are at risk for accidental overdose. Federal, state, and local governments have made efforts to increase the distribution of naloxone. It is recommended that all patients who are using opioids have access to FDA-approved parenteral or intranasal naloxone reversal devices. It is further recommended that peers and family members of persons using opioids receive training on overdose identification and instruction on naloxone use. Many states have increased access to naloxone by removing physician prescribing requirements and allowing pharmacists to dispense naloxone.

PATIENTS WITH CO-OCCURRING PSYCHIATRIC DISORDERS

The high rate of co-occurring psychiatric and substance use disorders obligates treatment providers to equip themselves to address both problems. It can be difficult to differentiate substance-induced disorders from independent conditions at intake, but it is noteworthy that symptoms can diminish rapidly upon initiation of methadone, especially within the first month. Nonetheless, many patients will remain with psychiatric conditions that need to be addressed.

In an important early study, Woody and colleagues[316] found that low-severity patients benefited from both drug counseling (focused on current life problems) and psychotherapy (employing supportive-expressive and cognitive-behavioral approaches). Patients with high levels of psychiatric symptoms were lower in all areas of pretreatment functioning, but the addition of psychotherapy by professionally trained therapists did maximize their improvement in many areas.

Major depression and persistent depressive disorder (dysthymia) are common co-occurring disorders in the treatment-seeking population[1,317] especially for women.[318] Psychosocial stress and the discomforts of withdrawal may contribute to temporarily low mood as well. Life crises and depressive symptoms posed a substantial risk of resumed use, which lessened for those who remained in treatment.[319]

Anxiety disorders also are common, with symptoms abating with a combination of an adequate methadone dose and the provision of counseling or psychotherapy over a period of time.[320] Posttraumatic stress disorder (PTSD) is common in patients receiving methadone, and though it may be associated with greater drug use disorder severity, PTSD does not necessarily worsen the outcome of substance use disorder treatment.[321] However, both traumatic events and a resurgence of PTSD symptoms are associated with increased risk of treatment interruption.[322]

Sleep disorders are often overlooked and appear to be common in those with psychiatric disorders, chronic pain, and benzodiazepine misuse and in those whose methadone dose is high.[323] Schizophrenia is relatively uncommon in patients receiving MOUD,[324] though most programs have some patients with the disorder. Based on historical references and clinical observations, some clinicians have proposed that opioids have antipsychotic properties.[325] Clinicians have described a subgroup of patients, who appear calmed and stabilized by the medication; when their doses drop, they become disorganized.

It is common to find reports of personality disorders, particularly antisocial personality disorder, among individuals who have OUD. Effective treatments are being developed, even for this difficult group. Ball studied patients on methadone with at least one personality disorder who were receiving two different forms of psychotherapy and who showed significant reductions in various severity indicators, including psychiatric symptoms and psychosocial impairment.[326]

Although neither heroin nor methadone has been found to be neurotoxic, several factors among some patients with OUD can increase the likelihood of cognitive impairment. These include overdose, concomitant hazardous alcohol use, and traumatic brain injury. Deficits in information processing may also result in difficulty following instructions and problem solving.[327] However, significant improvement in concentration and executive functions after 8 to 10 weeks of treatment have been reported in both methadone and buprenorphine groups.[328]

A 2016 systematic review of medication use and the risk of vehicle collisions concluded that both methadone and buprenorphine are among 15 medications associated with increased risk.[329] However, a 2014 comprehensive review indicated that although opioids induced some impairment of driving ability, this is less than other psychotropic agents or drugs of misuse. These authors note that impulsivity, sensation seeking, low-risk perception, antisocial behavior, and comorbid psychiatric and neurologic disorders also play a role. They suggest that the risk for impaired driving is likely less for patients stabilized on opioid medications.[330]

THE OPIOID TREATMENT SYSTEM

Treatment clinics specializing in people who use opioids were developed in the 1960s in response to the heroin epidemic following World War II. Because of the controversies and stigma, this treatment modality was under close scrutiny and was accompanied by research efforts that have continued for decades. Researchers found the clinics fertile ground due to the ease of patient recruitment and so there is an extensive research base documenting safety and efficacy. It has been demonstrated that MMT reduces or eliminates the use of heroin, and reduces the death rates and criminality associated with heroin use. Because clinics required regular attendance, they provide an opportunity to address infectious diseases such as HIV and hepatitis. Research documents the improvements in patient health and social productivity.[331]

Because of the stigma and fears of diversion, OTPs were required to have a tight structure around the medication and to provide counseling to foster a comprehensive rehabilitative effort. In recent years, they have expanded considerably. As of this writing, there are now almost 2,000 opioid treatment programs, treating over 600,000 patients (personal communication, Mark Parrino, 12-22-2022). Pressures from the fentanyl epidemic are continuing to encourage expansion.

In many OTPs, psychosocial interventions are provided by counselors, who range widely in educational level and professional training. The counselor's task is to identify and address specific problems in the areas of drug use, physical health, interpersonal relationships (including family interaction), psychological problems, and educational or vocational goals.[332] Short- and long-term treatment plans provide structure for the counseling sessions and a tool by which to monitor the patient's progress and quality of care. The counselor often serves as a case manager as well, initiating screening for medication and other program services; attending to issues concerning program rules, privileges, and policies; and providing links to other agencies. Clinics that have access to professionally trained staff may offer psychotherapy to selected patients. Typically, this access is found in programs involved in research or professional training. Barriers to utilization include negative attitudes on the part of patients, providers, and community members. Burdensome restrictions on take home medications top the list of patient objections. The COVID-19 and fentanyl epidemics have led to the loosening of many regulations and patients have welcomed these changes.

The embrace of a medication-only strategy by persons in leadership positions has heightened concerns that the structure and services offered by OTPs will receive significantly reduced funding. This can be expected to lead to more treatment discontinuation.[333]

CONCLUSION

The emergence of the coronavirus in 2020 and epidemic of fentanyl overdose deaths have brought both great challenges and opportunities. The search for powerful interventions has led to the revision of regulations that served as barriers to care. In December 2022, the elimination of the requirement of an X-waiver to prescribe buprenorphine and the elimination of a cap on the number of patients that a physician can treat significantly increased treatment options.[334] Mobile units are expanding. Greater availability of telehealth appointments and revision of take-home regulations for methadone patients are two major accomplishments. Clinicians have long sought greater flexibility to respond to a variety of patient needs, as well as to validate patient accomplishments by offering greater freedoms.

In the legal system, there has been increased expansion of opioid medications into prisons. The Federal Bureau of Prisons is implementing MOUD in all prisons. Some states are doing the same. While improving access to medications is a considerable accomplishment, funding for case management and counseling services is inadequate. People with opioid use disorder have multiple needs: housing, co-occurring disorders (depression, anxiety disorders, PTSD), basic medical care. Some in leadership positions have devalued psychosocial intervention, eliciting concerns from those in the trenches. Most who work in the field can agree on the importance of reducing death rates, but the devaluing of psychosocial intervention is of major concern. Medication alone buys time but the discontinuation rates are high. Basic counseling improves retention for both Medicaid and commercially insured patients.[331,332]

The NIH HEAL Initiative (Helping to End Addiction Long Term Initiative) is "an aggressive, trans-agency effort to speed scientific solutions to stem the national opioid public health crisis." Hundreds of researchers nationwide have focused on improving prevention and treatment for unhealthy opioid use including addiction, and understanding, managing, and treating pain. Annual reports describe these efforts in detail (https://heal.nih.gov/). It is likely that this large-scale effort will continue to bear fruit over a long period of time.

At the time of this writing, many challenges remain:

1. Not every state has the Medicaid expansion, or alternative funding sources to address the needs of individuals who use opioids.
2. State regulations may not permit the greater flexibility offered by the federal government.
3. Workforce challenges have grown more severe. This includes physicians, nurses, nurse practitioners, physician associates, counselors/case managers. This holds back expansion.
4. More research is needed to clarify the distinctive features of fentanyl, for example, choice of medications, appropriate dosing schedules, community level prevention efforts, etc.
5. The devaluation of training about addiction is likely to reduce the effectiveness of medication interventions by failing to address factors that allow patients to preserve their gains.

The current opioid epidemic represents unprecedented challenges that will continue to engage addiction medicine specialists for a long time. Maintaining and expanding access to treatment are crucial to meet this challenging public health threat.

REFERENCES

1. SAMHSA. *Substance Use Disorder for Specific Substances in Past Year: Among People Aged 12 or Older; by Age Group, Numbers in Thousands, 2019 and 2020*. Accessed October 26, 2023. https://www.samhsa.gov/data/sites/default/files/reports/rpt35323/NSDUHDetailedTabs2020v25/NSDUHDetailedTabs2020v25/NSDUHDetTabs5-1pe2020.pdf
2. Shulgin AT. Drugs of abuse in the future. *Clin Toxicol.* 1975;8(4):405-456. doi:10.3109/15563657508990076
3. Centers for Disease Control and Prevention. *Overdose Death Rates Involving Opioids, by Type, United States, 1999-2020*. 2021.
4. Centers for Disease Control and Prevention. *CDC WONDER*. Accessed May 25, 2018. https://wonder.cdc.gov/
5. SAMHSA. *Opioid Treatment Program Directory*. 2022.
6. Parrino M. *The Opioid Crisis—Urgent Need for Timely Action*. American Association for the Treatment of Opioid Dependence; 2016.
7. Spetz J, Hailer L, Gay C, et al. Changes in US clinician waivers to prescribe buprenorphine management for opioid use disorder during the COVID-19 pandemic and after relaxation of training requirements. *JAMA Netw Open.* 2022;5(5):e225996. doi:10.1001/jamanetworkopen.2022.5996
8. Stein BD, Saloner B, Schuler MS, Gurvey J, Sorbero M, Gordon AJ. Concentration of patient care among buprenorphine-prescribing clinicians in the US. *JAMA.* 2021;325(21):2206-2208. doi:10.1001/jama.2021.4469
9. Rettig RA, Yarmolinsky A. *Federal Regulation of Methadone Treatment*. National Academy Press; 1995.
10. NIH Consensus Statement. *Effective Medical Treatment of Opiate Addiction*. National Institutes of Health; 1997:1-38.
11. WHO. *Guidelines for the Psychosocially Assisted Pharmacological Treatment of Opioid Dependence*. World Health Organization; 2009:134. Accessed October 26, 2023. https://www.ncbi.nlm.nih.gov/books/NBK143185/
12. Dole VP, Nyswander MM. A medical treatment for diacetylmorphine (heroin) addiction. *J Am Med Assoc.* 1965;193(8):646-650.
13. Madden EF, Prevedel S, Light T, Sulzer SH. Intervention stigma toward medications for opioid use disorder: a systematic review. *Subst Use Misuse.* 2021;56(14):2181-2201. doi:10.1080/10826084.2021.1975749
14. Nestler EJ. Molecular mechanisms of drug addiction. *J Neurosci.* 1992;12(7):2439. Erratum in *J Neurosci* 1992;12(8).
15. Dole V. Implication of methadone maintenance for theories of narcotic addiction. *J Am Med Assoc.* 1988;260:3025-3029.
16. Goldstein A. Heroin addiction: neurobiology, pharmacology, and policy. *J Psychoactive Drugs.* 1991;23(2):123-134.
17. Ball JC, Lange WR, Myers CP, Friedman SR. Reducing the risk of AIDS through methadone maintenance treatment. *J Health Soc Behav.* 1988;29:214-226.
18. Ball J, Ross A. *The Effectiveness of Methadone Maintenance Treatment*. Springer-Verlag; 1991.
19. Gronbladh L, Ohlund L, Gunne L. Mortality in heroin addiction: impact of methadone treatment. *Acta Psychiatr Scand.* 1990;82(3):223-227.
20. Joseph H, Stancliff S, Langrod J. Methadone maintenance treatment (MMT): a review of historical and clinical issues. *Mt Sinai J Med.* 2000;65(5-6):347-364.
21. Mattick RP, Breen C, Kimber J, Davoli M. Buprenorphine maintenance versus placebo or methadone maintenance for opioid dependence. *Cochrane Database Syst Rev.* 2014;2:CD002207.
22. Sordo L, Barrio G, Bravo MJ, et al. Mortality risk during and after opioid substitution treatment: systematic review and meta-analysis of cohort studies. *BMJ.* 2017;357:j1550.
23. Zweben JE, Payte JT. Methadone maintenance in the treatment of opioid dependence: a current perspective. *West J Med.* 1990;152(5):588-599.
24. AT ML. Patient characteristics associated with outcome. In: Cooper J, Altman F, Brown BS, Czechowicz D, eds. *Research on the Treatment of Narcotic Addiction*. US Department of Health and Human Services; 1983:500-529.
25. Magura S, Rosenblum A. Leaving methadone treatment: lessons learned, lessons forgotten, lessons ignored. *Mt Sinai J Med.* 2001;68(1):62-74.
26. Mattick R. Methadone maintenance therapy versus no opioid replacement therapy for opioid dependence. *Cochrane Database Syst Rev.* 2009;3:CD002209.
27. O'Connor P. Methods of detoxification and their role in treating patients with opioid dependence. *JAMA.* 2005;294(8):961-963.
28. Dole V, Nyswander M. Heroin addiction. A metabolic disease. *Arch Intern Med.* 1967;20:19-24.
29. Kreek MJ, Brien CP, Jaffee JH, York NY. Rationale for maintenance pharmacotherapy of opiate dependence. In: O'Brien CP, Jaffe JH, eds. *Addictive States*. Raven Press; 1992:205-230.
30. Pickens RW. *Genetic and other risk factors in opiate addiction. Paper presented at: Effective medical treatment of heroin addiction*; November 17, 1997 William H. Natcher Conference Center National Institutes of Health Bethesda, MD.
31. Merikangas KR, Stolar M, Stevens DE, et al. Familial transmission of substance use disorders. *Arch Gen Psychiatry.* 1998;55:973-979.
32. Tsuang MT, Lyons MJ, Meyer JM, et al. Co-occurrence of abuse of different drugs in men. *Arch Gen Psychiatry.* 1998;55:967-972.
33. Kreek M. Methadone-related opioid agonist pharmacotherapy for heroin addiction. History, recent molecular and neurochemical research and future in mainstream medicine. *Ann NY Acad Sci.* 2000;909:186-216.
34. Gelernter J, Panhuysen C, Wilcox M, et al. Genomewide linkage scan for opioid dependence and related traits. *Am J Hum Genet.* 2006;78(5):759-769.
35. Galynker II, Watras-Ganz S, Miner C, et al. Cerebral metabolism in opiate-dependent subjects: effects of methadone maintenance. *Mt Sinai J Med.* 2000;67(5-6):381-387.
36. Kaufman M, Pollack M, Villafuerte R, et al. Cerebral phosphorus metabolite abnormalities in opiate-dependent polydrug users in methadone maintenance treatment. *Psychiatry Res.* 1999;90(3):143-152.
37. Kosten TR, Kleber HD. Strategies to improve compliance with narcotic antagonists. *The Am J Drug Alcohol Abuse.* 1984;10(2):249-266.
38. Ling W, Rawson RA, Compton MA. Substitution pharmacotherapies for opioid addiction: from methadone to LAAM and buprenorphine. *J Psychoactive Drugs.* 1994;26(2):119-128.
39. Walsh SL, Chausmer AE, Strain EC, Bigelow GE. Evaluation of the mu and kappa opioid actions of butorphanol in humans through differential naltrexone blockade. *Psychopharmacology (Berl).* 2008;196(1):143-155.
40. NIH consensus panel recommends expanding access to and improving methadone treatment programs for heroin addiction. *Eur Addict Res.* 1999;5(1):50-51.
41. Lewis DC. Access to narcotic addiction treatment and medical care: prospects for the expansion of methadone maintenance treatment. *J Addict Dis.* 1999;18(2):5-21.
42. Rounsaville BJ, Kosten TR. Treatment for opioid dependence: quality and access. *JAMA.* 2000;283(10):1337-1339.
43. Perneger TV, Giner F, del Rio M, Mino A. Randomised trial of heroin maintenance programme for addicts who fail in conventional drug treatments. *BMJ.* 1998;317(7150):13-18.
44. Uchtenhagen AA. Heroin maintenance treatment: from idea to research to practice. *Drug Alcohol Rev.* 2011;30(2):130-137.
45. Rehm J, Gschwend P, Steffen T, Gutzwiller F, Dobler-Mikola A, Uchtenhagen A. Feasibility, safety, and efficacy of injectable heroin prescription for refractory opioid addicts: a follow-up study. *Lancet.* 2001;358(9291):1417-1420.
46. MLF M, Wilthagen EA, Oviedo-Joekes E, et al. The suitability of oral diacetylmorphine in treatment-refractory patients with heroin dependence: a scoping review. *Drug Alcohol Depend.* 2021;227:108984. doi:10.1016/j.drugalcdep.2021.108984
47. Oviedo-Joekes E, Guh D, Brissette S, et al. Hydromorphone compared with diacetylmorphine for long-term opioid dependence: a randomized clinical trial. *JAMA Psychiatry.* 2016;73(5):447-455.
48. Klimas J, Gorfinkel L, Giacomuzzi SM, et al. Slow release oral morphine versus methadone for the treatment of opioid use disorder. *BMJ Open.* 2019;9(4):e025799. doi:10.1136/bmjopen-2018-025799

49. Kowalczyk WJ, Phillips KA, Jobes ML, et al. Clonidine maintenance prolongs opioid abstinence and decouples stress from craving in daily life: a randomized controlled trial with ecological momentary assessment. *Am J Psychiatry.* 2015;172(8):760-767.
50. Goodrx.com. Lucymera Prices; 2022.
51. Martin WR, Jasinski DR. Physiological parameters of morphine dependence in man—tolerance, early abstinence, protracted abstinence. *J Psychiatr Res.* 1969;7(1):9-17.
52. Kosten TR, Baxter LE. Review article: Effective management of opioid withdrawal symptoms: a gateway to opioid dependence treatment. *Am J Addict.* 2019;28(2):55-62. doi:10.1111/ajad.12862
53. Stein MD, Flori JN, Risi MM, Conti MT, Anderson BJ, Bailey GL. Overdose history is associated with post-detoxification treatment preference for persons with opioid use disorder. *Subst Abus.* 2017;38(4):389-393.
54. Dole VP. Narcotic addiction, physical dependence and relapse. *N Engl J Med.* 1972;286(18):988-992.
55. Buresh M, Stern R, Rastegar D. Treatment of opioid use disorder in primary care. *BMJ.* 2021;373:n784. doi:10.1136/bmj.n784
56. Amass L, Bickel WK, Higgins ST, Hughes JR. A preliminary investigation of outcome following gradual or rapid buprenorphine detoxification. *J Addict Dis.* 1994;13(3):33-45.
57. Cheskin LJ, Fudala PJ, Johnson RE. A controlled comparison of buprenorphine and clonidine for acute detoxification from opioids. *Drug Alcohol Depend.* 1994;36(2):115-121.
58. Bickel WK, Stitzer ML, Bigelow GE, Liebson IA, Jasinski DR, Johnson RE. A clinical trial of buprenorphine: comparison with methadone in the detoxification of heroin addicts. *Clin Pharmacol Ther.* 1988;43(1): 72-78.
59. Nigam AK, Ray R, Tripathi BM. Buprenorphine in opiate withdrawal: a comparison with clonidine. *J Subst Abuse Treat.* 1993;10(4):391-394.
60. O'Connor PG, Carroll KM, Shi JM, Schottenfeld RS, Kosten TR, Rounsaville BJ. Three methods of opioid detoxification in a primary care setting. A randomized trial. *Ann Intern Med.* 1997;127(7):526-530.
61. Ling W, Amass L, Shoptaw S, et al. A multi-center randomized trial of buprenorphine–naloxone versus clonidine for opioid detoxification: findings from the National Institute on Drug Abuse Clinical Trials Network. *Addiction.* 2005;100(8):1090-1100.
62. Oreskovich MR, Saxon AJ, Ellis ML, Malte CA, Reoux JP, Knox PC. A double-blind, double-dummy, randomized, prospective pilot study of the partial mu opiate agonist, buprenorphine, for acute detoxification from heroin. *Drug Alcohol Depend.* 2005;77(1):71-79.
63. Fultz JM, Senay EC. Guidelines for the management of hospitalized narcotics addicts. *Ann Intern Med.* 1975;82(6):815-818.
64. Jasinski DR, Pevnick JS, Griffith JD. Human pharmacology and abuse potential of the analgesic buprenorphine: a potential agent for treating narcotic addiction. *Arch Gen Psychiatry.* 1978;35(4):501-516.
65. Seow SS, Quigley AJ, Ilett KF, et al. Buprenorphine: a new maintenance opiate? *Med J Aust.* 1986;144(8):407-411.
66. Fudala PJ, Jaffe JH, Dax EM, Johnson RE. Use of buprenorphine in the treatment of opioid addiction. II. Physiologic and behavioral effects of daily and alternate-day administration and abrupt withdrawal. *Clin Pharmacol Ther.* 1990;47(4):525-534.
67. Greenwald M, Johanson C-E, Bueller J, et al. Buprenorphine duration of action: mu-opioid receptor availability and pharmacokinetic and behavioral indices. *Biol Psychiatry.* 2007;61(1):101-110.
68. Sigmon SC, Dunn KE, Saulsgiver K, et al. A randomized, double-blind evaluation of buprenorphine taper duration in primary prescription opioid abusers. *JAMA Psychiatry.* 2013;70(12):1347-1354. doi:10.1001/jamapsychiatry.2013.2216
69. Gowing L, Ali R, White JM, Mbewe D. Buprenorphine for managing opioid withdrawal. *Cochrane Database Syst Rev.* 2017;2(2):CD002025. doi:10.1002/14651858.CD002025.pub5
70. Charney DS, Sternberg DE, Kleber HD, Heninger GR, Redmond DE. The clinical use of clonidine in abrupt withdrawal from methadone. Effects on blood pressure and specific signs and symptoms. *Arch Gen Psychiatry.* 1981;38(11):1273-1277.
71. Kleber HD, Riordan CE, Rounsaville B, et al. Clonidine in outpatient detoxification from methadone maintenance. *Arch Gen Psychiatry.* 1985;42(4):391-394.
72. Rosen MI, McMahon TJ, Hameedi FA, et al. Effect of clonidine pretreatment on naloxone-precipitated opiate withdrawal. *J Pharmacol Exp Ther.* 1996;276(3):1128-1135.
73. Connor PG, Waugh ME, Carroll KM, J. Primary care-based ambulatory opioid detoxification: the results of a clinical trial. *Intern Med.* 1995;10(5):255-260.
74. McCann MJ, Miotto K, Rawson RA, Huber A, Shoptaw S, Ling W. Outpatient non-opioid detoxification for opioid withdrawal. Who is likely to benefit? *Am J Addict.* 1997;6(3):218-223.
75. Stotts AL, Dodrill CL, Kosten TR. Opioid dependence treatment: options in pharmacotherapy. *Expert Opin Pharmacother.* 2009;10(11):1727-1740.
76. FDA. Lofexidine Package Insert. 2018.
77. Bearn J, Gossop M, Strang J. Randomised double-blind comparison of lofexidine and methadone in the in-patient treatment of opiate withdrawal. *Drug Alcohol Depend.* 1996;43(1-2):87-91.
78. Kahn A, Mumford JP, Rogers GA, Beckford H. Double-blind study of lofexidine and clonidine in the detoxification of opiate addicts in hospital. *Drug Alcohol Depend.* 1997;44(1):57-61.
79. Lin SK, Strang J, Su LW, Tsai CJ, Hu WH. Double-blind randomised controlled trial of lofexidine versus clonidine in the treatment of heroin withdrawal. *Drug Alcohol Depend.* 1997;48(2):127-133.
80. Bearn J, Gossop M, Strang J. Accelerated lofexidine treatment regimen compared with conventional lofexidine and methadone treatment for in-patient opiate detoxification. *Drug Alcohol Depend.* 1998;50(3):227-232.
81. Yu E, Miotto K, Akerele E. A phase 3 placebo-controlled, double-blind, multi-site trial of the alpha-2-adrenergic agonist, lofexidine, for opioid withdrawal. *Drug Alcohol Depend.* 2008;97(1-2):158-168.
82. Gowing L, Farrell M, Ali R, White JM. Alpha2-adrenergic agonists for the management of opioid withdrawal. *Cochrane Database Syst Rev.* 2009;2:CD002024.
83. Gish EC, Miller JL, Honey BL, Johnson PN. Lofexidine, an ^{79}2-receptor agonist for opioid detoxification. *Ann Pharmacother.* 2010;44(2):343-351.
84. Renfro ML, Loera LJ, Tirado CF, Hill LG. Lofexidine for acute opioid withdrawal: a clinical case series. *Ment Health Clin.* 2020;10(5):259-263. doi:10.9740/mhc.2020.09.259
85. Connor P, Kosten TR. Rapid and ultrarapid opioid detoxification techniques. *JAMA.* 1998;279(3):229-234.
86. Collins ED, Kleber HD, Whittington RA, Heitler NE. Anesthesia-assisted vs buprenorphine- or clonidine-assisted heroin detoxification and naltrexone induction: a randomized trial. *JAMA.* 2005;294(8):903-913.
87. Sullivan M, Bisaga A, Pavlicova M, et al. Long-acting injectable naltrexone induction: a randomized trial of outpatient opioid detoxification with naltrexone versus buprenorphine. *Am J Psychiatry.* 2017;174(5):459-467. doi:10.1176/appi.ajp.2016.16050548
88. Gowing LR, Ali RL. The place of detoxification in treatment of opioid dependence. *Curr Opin Psychiatry.* 2006;19(3):266-270.
89. National Institute on Drug Abuse. Percentage of overdose deaths involving methadone declined between January 2019 and. *NIDA Research Monograph.* August 2021;2022.
90. Himmelsbach CK. Clinical studies of drug addiction: physical dependence, withdrawal and recovery. *Arch Intern Med.* 1942;69:766-772.
91. Shi J, Zhao L-Y, Epstein DH, Zhang X-L, Lu L. Long-term methadone maintenance reduces protracted symptoms of heroin abstinence and cue-induced craving in Chinese heroin abusers. *Pharmacol Biochem Behav.* 2007;87(1):141-145.
92. Satel SL, Kosten TR, Schuckit MA, Fischman MW. Should protracted withdrawal from drugs be included in DSM-IV? *Am J Psychiatry.* 1993;150(5):695-704.
93. Stine SM, Kosten TR. Reduction of opiate withdrawal-like symptoms by cocaine abuse during methadone and buprenorphine maintenance. *Am J Drug Alcohol Abuse.* 1994;20(4):445-458.
94. Caplehorn JR, Dalton MS, Cluff MC, Petrenas AM. Retention in methadone maintenance and heroin addicts' risk of death. *Addiction.* 1994;89(2):203-209.

95. Fugelstad A, Rajs J, Böttiger M, Gerhardsson de Verdier M. Mortality among HIV-infected intravenous drug addicts in Stockholm in relation to methadone treatment. *Addiction.* 1995;90(5):711-716.
96. Langendam MW, van Brussel GH, Coutinho RA, van Ameijden EJ. The impact of harm-reduction-based methadone treatment on mortality among heroin users. *Am J Public Health.* 2001;91(5):774-780.
97. Wu CH, Henry JA. Deaths of heroin addicts starting on methadone maintenance. *Lancet.* 1990;335(8686):424.
98. Drummer OH, Opeskin K, Syrjanen M, Cordner SM. Methadone toxicity causing death in ten subjects starting on a methadone maintenance program. *Am J Forensic Med Pathol.* 1992;13(4):346-350.
99. Caplehorn JR, Drummer OH. Mortality associated with New South Wales methadone programs in 1994: lives lost and saved. *Med J Aust.* 1999;170(3):104-109.
100. Vormfelde SV, Poser W. Death attributed to methadone. *Pharmacopsychiatry.* 2001;34(6):217-222.
101. Wagner-Servais D, Erkens M. Methadone-related deaths associated with faulty induction procedures. *Addict.* 2003;2(3):57-67.
102. Zador D, Sunjic S. Deaths in methadone maintenance treatment in New South Wales, Australia 1990-1995. *Addiction.* 2000;95(1):77-84.
103. Payte JT, Khuri ET, Parrino M. *Principles of Methadone Dose Determination.* 1993.
104. Kaufman J, Payte JT, McLellan AT, Rettig RA, Yarmolinski A. *Treatment Standards and Optimal Treatment.* Institute of Medicine Federal Regulation of Methadone Treatment. National Academy Press; 1995:185-216.
105. Buresh M, Nahvi S, Steiger S, Weinstein ZM. Adapting methadone inductions to the fentanyl era. *J Subst Abuse Treat.* 2022;141:108832. doi:10.1016/j.jsat.2022.108832
106. Caplehorn JR, Bell J, Kleinbaum DG, Gebski VJ. Methadone dose and heroin use during maintenance treatment. *Addiction.* 1993;88(1):119-124.
107. Strain EC, Bigelow GE, Liebson IA, Stitzer ML. Moderate- vs high-dose methadone in the treatment of opioid dependence: a randomized trial. *JAMA.* 1999;281(11):1000-1005.
108. Amato L, Davoli M, Perucci CA, Ferri M, Faggiano F, Mattick RP. An overview of systematic reviews of the effectiveness of opiate maintenance therapies: available evidence to inform clinical practice and research. *J Subst Abuse Treat.* 2005;28(4):321-329.
109. ASAM. *American Society of Addiction Medicine Policy Statement on Methadone Treatment.* American Society of Addiction Medicine; 1991.
110. Hser YI, Grella CE, Hubbard RL, et al. An evaluation of drug treatments for adolescents in 4 US cities. *Arch Gen Psychiatry.* 2001;58(7):689-695.
111. Payte JT, Khuri ET, Parrino MW. *Treatment Duration and Patient Retention.* 1993.
112. Jones CM, Compton WM, Han B, Baldwin G, Volkow ND. Methadone-involved overdose deaths in the US before and after federal policy changes expanding take-home methadone doses from opioid treatment programs. *JAMA Psychiatry.* 2022;79(9):932-934. doi:10.1001/jamapsychiatry.2022.1776
113. McCarthy JJ, Graas J, Leamon MH, Ward C, Vasti EJ, Fassbender C. The use of the methadone/metabolite ratio (MMR) to identify an individual metabolic phenotype and assess risks of poor response and adverse effects: towards scientific methadone dosing. *J Addict Med.* 2020;14(5):431-436. doi:10.1097/adm.0000000000000620
114. SAMHSA. *Methadone Take-Home Flexibilities Extension Guidance.* 2020.
115. SAMHSA. *Code of Federal Register.* 2022.
116. Salsitz EA, Joseph H, Frank B, et al. Methadone medical maintenance (MMM): treating chronic opioid dependence in private medical practice—a summary report (1983-1998). *Mt Sinai J Med.* 2000;67(5-6):388-397.
117. Fiellin DA, O'Connor PG, Chawarski M, Pakes JP, Pantalon MV, Schottenfeld RS. Methadone maintenance in primary care: a randomized controlled trial. *JAMA.* 2001;286(14):1724-1731.
118. Grudzinskas CV, Woosley RL, Payte TJ, et al. The documented role of pharmacogenetic: in the identification and administration of new medications for treating drug abuse. *NIDA Res Monogr.* 1996;162:60-63.
119. Kharasch ED, Hoffer C, Whittington D, Sheffels P. Role of hepatic and intestinal cytochrome P450 3A and 2B6 in the metabolism, disposition, and miotic effects of methadone. *Clin Pharmacol Ther.* 2004;76(3):250-269.
120. Moody DE, Alburges ME, Parker RJ, Collins JM, Strong JM. The involvement of cytochrome P450 3A4 in the N-demethylation of L-alpha-acetylmethadol (LAAM), norLAAM, and methadone. *Drug Metab Dispos.* 1997;25(12):1347-1353.
121. Eap CB, Broly F, Mino A, et al. Cytochrome P450 2D6 genotype and methadone steady-state concentrations. *J Clin Psychopharmacol.* 2001;21(2):229-234.
122. PerezdelosCobos J, Sinol N, Trujols J. Association of CYP2D6 ultrarapid metabolizer genotype with deficient patient satisfaction regarding methadone maintenance treatment. *Drug Alcohol Depend.* 2007;89(2-3):190-194.
123. Kharasch ED, Regina KJ, Blood J, Friedel C. Methadone pharmacogenetics: CYP2B6 polymorphisms determine plasma concentrations, clearance, and metabolism. *Anesthesiology.* 2015;123(5):1142-1153.
124. Wong SH, Wagner MA, Jentzen JM, et al. Pharmacogenomics as an aspect of molecular autopsy for forensic pathology/toxicology: does genotyping CYP 2D6 serve as an adjunct for certifying methadone toxicity? *J Forensic Sci.* 2003;48(6):1406-1415.
125. Totah RA, Allen KE, Sheffels P, Whittington D, Kharasch ED. Enantiomeric metabolic interactions and stereoselective human methadone metabolism. *J Pharmacol Exp Ther.* 2007;321(1):389-399.
126. Eap CB, Buclin T, Baumann P. Interindividual variability of the clinical pharmacokinetics of methadone: implications for the treatment of opioid dependence. *Clin Pharmacokinet.* 2002;41(14):1153-1193.
127. Krantz MJ, Lewkowiez L, Hays H, Woodroffe MA, Robertson AD, Mehler PS. Torsade de pointes associated with very-high-dose methadone. *Ann Intern Med.* 2002;137(6):501-504.
128. Walker PW, Klein D, Kasza L. High dose methadone and ventricular arrhythmias: a report of three cases. *Pain.* 2003;103(3):321-324.
129. Katchman AN, McGroary KA, Kilborn MJ, et al. Influence of opioid agonists on cardiac human ether-a-go-go-related gene K(+) currents. *J Pharmacol Exp Ther.* 2002;303(2):688-694.
130. Eap CB, Crettol S, Rougier JS, et al. Stereoselective block of hERG channel by (S)-methadone and QT interval prolongation in CYP2B6 slow metabolizers. *Clin Pharmacol Ther.* 2007;81(5):719-728.
131. Fanoe S, Hvidt C, Ege P, Jensen GB. Syncope and QT prolongation among patients treated with methadone for heroin dependence in the city of Copenhagen. *Heart.* 2007;93(9):1051-1055.
132. Martell BA, Arnsten JH, Krantz MJ, Gourevitch MN. Impact of methadone treatment on cardiac repolarization and conduction in opioid users. *Am J Cardiol.* 2005;95(7):915-918.
133. Peles E, Bodner G, Kreek MJ, Rados V, Adelson M. Corrected-QT intervals as related to methadone dose and serum level in methadone maintenance treatment (MMT) patients: a cross-sectional study. *Addiction.* 2007;102(2):289-300.
134. Wedam EF, Bigelow GE, Johnson RE, Nuzzo PA, Haigney MCP. QT-interval effects of methadone, levomethadyl, and buprenorphine in a randomized trial. *Arch Intern Med.* 2007;167(22):2469-2475.
135. Krantz MJ, Rowan SB, Schmittner J, Bucher BB. Physician awareness of the cardiac effects of methadone: results of a national survey. *J Addict Dis.* 2007;26(4):79-85.
136. Krantz MJ, Martin J, Stimmel B, Mehta D, Haigney MCP. QTc interval screening in methadone treatment. *Ann Intern Med.* 2009;150(6):387-395.
137. Martin JA, Campbell A, Killip T, et al. QT interval screening in methadone maintenance treatment: report of a SAMHSA expert panel. *J Addict Dis.* 2011;30(4):283-306.
138. Fareed A, Vayalapalli S, Byrd-Sellers J, et al. Onsite QTc interval screening for patients in methadone maintenance treatment. *J Addict Dis.* 2010;29(1):15-22.
139. Gelkopf M, Bleich A, Hayward R, Bodner G, Adelson M. Characteristics of benzodiazepine abuse in methadone maintenance treatment patients: a 1 year prospective study in an Israeli clinic. *Drug Alcohol Depend.* 1999;55(1-2):63-68.

140. AATOD. *Guidelines for Addressing Benzodiazepine Use in Opioid Treatment Programs (OTPs)*. Accessed July 18, 2017. http://www.aatod.org/guidelines-for-addressing-benzodiazepine-use-in-opioid-treatment-programs-otps
141. Bakker A. Benzodiazepine maintenance in opiate substitution treatment: good or bad? A retrospective primary care case-note review. *Psychopharmacology.* 2016;31(1):62-66.
142. Ford BR, Bart G, Grahan B, Shearer RD, Winkelman TNA. Associations between polysubstance use patterns and receipt of medications for opioid use disorder among adults in treatment for opioid use disorder. *J Addict Med.* 2021;15(2):159-162. doi:10.1097/adm.0000000000000726
143. Kosten TR. Current pharmacotherapies for opioid dependence. *Psychopharmacol Bull.* 1990;26(1):69-74.
144. Kleber HD. Treatment of narcotic addicts. *Psychiatr Med.* 1987;3:389-418.
145. Wang D, Teichtahl H, Drummer O, et al. Central sleep apnea in stable methadone maintenance treatment patients. *Chest.* 2005;128(3): 1348-1356.
146. Kreek MJ, Lowinson JH, Ruiz P, Baltimore MD. Medical management of methadone-maintained patients. In: Lowinson JH, Ruiz P, eds. *Substance Abuse Clinical Problems and Perspectives*. Williams & Wilkins; 1981: 660-673.
147. Mendelson J, Jones RT, Fernandez I, Welm S, Melby AK, Baggott MJ. Buprenorphine and naloxone interactions in opiate-dependent volunteers. *Clin Pharmacol Ther.* 1996;60(1):105-114.
148. Mendelson J, Jones RT, Welm S, et al. Buprenorphine and naloxone combinations: the effects of three dose ratios in morphine-stabilized, opiate-dependent volunteers. *Psychopharmacology.* 1999;141(1):37-46.
149. Volpe DA, McMahon Tobin GA, Mellon RD, et al. Uniform assessment and ranking of opioid μ receptor binding constants for selected opioid drugs. *Regul Toxicol Pharmacol.* 2011;59(3):385-390. doi:10.1016/j.yrtph.2010.12.007
150. Lee KO, Akil H, Woods JH, Traynor JR. Differential binding properties of oripavines at cloned mu- and delta-opioid receptors. *Eur J Pharmacol.* 1999;378(3):323-330. doi:10.1016/s0014-2999(99)00460-4
151. Neilan CL, Husbands SM, Breeden S, et al. Characterization of the complex morphinan derivative BU72 as a high efficacy, long-lasting mu-opioid receptor agonist. *Eur J Pharmacol.* 2004;499(1-2):107-116. doi:10.1016/j.ejphar.2004.07.097
152. Tempel A, Gardner EL, Zukin RS. Neurochemical and functional correlates of naltrexone-induced opiate receptor up-regulation. *J Pharmacol Exp Ther.* 1985;232(2):439-444.
153. Tang AH, Collins RJ. Enhanced analgesic effects of morphine after chronic administration of naloxone in the rat. *Eur J Pharmacol.* 1978;47(4):473-474. doi:10.1016/0014-2999(78)90131-0
154. Unterwald EM, Anton B, To T, Lam H, Evans CJ. Quantitative immunolocalization of mu opioid receptors: regulation by naltrexone. *Neuroscience.* 1998;85(3):897-905. doi:10.1016/s0306-4522(97)00659-3
155. Blazes CK, Morrow JD. Reconsidering the usefulness of adding naloxone to buprenorphine. *Front Psychiatry.* 2020;11:549272. doi:10.3389/fpsyt.2020.549272
156. United States Congress. *Drug Addiction Treatment Act of 2000*. 2000.
157. Nasser AF, Greenwald MK, Vince B, et al. Sustained-release buprenorphine (RBP-6000) blocks the effects of opioid challenge with hydromorphone in subjects with opioid use disorder. *J Clin Psychopharmacol.* 2016;36(1):18-26. doi:10.1097/jcp.0000000000000434
158. Indivior Inc. Treatment seeking participants with opioid use disorders assessing tolerability of depot injections of buprenorphine. *Clinical Trials Network.* Accessed May 25, 2018. https://clinicaltrials.gov/ct2/show/NCT02357901
159. Boyett B, Nadipelli VR, Solem CT, Chilcoat H, Bickel WK, Ling W. Continued posttrial benefits of buprenorphine extended release: RECOVER study findings. *J Addict Med.* 2022; doi:10.1097/adm.0000000000001070
160. Ling W, Shoptaw S, Goodman-Meza D. Depot buprenorphine injection in the management of opioid use disorder: from development to implementation. *Subst Abuse Rehabil.* 2019;10:69-78. doi:10.2147/sar.S155843
161. Fiellin DA, Kleber H, Trumble-Hejduk JG, McLellan AT, Kosten TR. Consensus statement on office-based treatment of opioid dependence using buprenorphine. *J Subst Abuse Treat.* 2004;27(2):153-159.
162. Herring AA, Vosooghi AA, Luftig J, et al. High-dose buprenorphine induction in the emergency department for treatment of opioid use disorder. *JAMA Netw Open.* 2021;4(7):e2117128-e2117128. doi:10.1001/jamanetworkopen.2021.17128
163. Leonardi C, Hanna N, Laurenzi P, Fagetti R; Group IDAC. Multi-centre observational study of buprenorphine use in 32 Italian drug addiction centres. *Drug Alcohol Depend.* 2008;94(1-3):125-132.
164. Meinhofer A, Williams AR, Johnson P, Schackman BR, Bao Y. Prescribing decisions at buprenorphine treatment initiation: do they matter for treatment discontinuation and adverse opioid-related events? *J Subst Abuse Treat.* 2019;105:37-43. doi:10.1016/j.jsat.2019.07.010
165. Walley AY, Alperen JK, Cheng DM, et al. Office-based management of opioid dependence with buprenorphine: clinical practices and barriers. *J Gen Intern Med.* 2008;23(9):1393-1398.
166. Lee JD, Vocci F, Fiellin DA. Unobserved "home" induction onto buprenorphine. *J Addict Med.* 2014;8(5):299-308.
167. Bista SR, Haywood A, Hardy J, Lobb M, Tapuni A, Norris R. Protein binding of fentanyl and its metabolite nor-fentanyl in human plasma, albumin and α-1 acid glycoprotein. *Xenobiotica.* 2015;45(3):207-212. doi:10.3109/00498254.2014.971093
168. Cohen SM, Weimer MB, Levander XA, Peckham AM, Tetrault JM, Morford KL. Low dose initiation of buprenorphine: a narrative review and practical approach. *J Addict Med.* 2022;16(4):399-406. doi:10.1097/adm.0000000000000945
169. Spreen LA, Dittmar EN, Quirk KC, Smith MA. Buprenorphine initiation strategies for opioid use disorder and pain management: a systematic review. *Pharmacotherapy.* 2022;42(5):411-427. doi:10.1002/phar.2676
170. Ahmed S, Bhivandkar S, Lonergan BB, Suzuki J. Microinduction of buprenorphine/naloxone: a review of the literature. *Am J Addict.* 2021;30(4):305-315. doi:10.1111/ajad.13135
171. Robbins JL, Englander H, Gregg J. Buprenorphine microdose induction for the management of prescription opioid dependence. *J Am Board Fam Med.* 2021;34(Suppl):S141-S146. doi:10.3122/jabfm.2021.S1.200236
172. Zubieta J, Greenwald MK, Lombardi U, et al. Buprenorphine-induced changes in mu-opioid receptor availability in male heroin-dependent volunteers: a preliminary study. *Neuropsychopharmacology.* 2000;23(3):326-334.
173. Bruce RD, McCance-Katz E, Kharasch ED, et al. Pharmacokinetic interactions between buprenorphine and antiretroviral medications. *Clin Infect Dis.* 2006;43(Suppl 4):S216–S223.
174. Krantz MJ, Garcia JA, Mehler PS. Effects of buprenorphine on cardiac repolarization in a patient with methadone-related torsade de pointes. *Pharmacotherapy.* 2005;25(4):611-614.
175. Amass L, Kamien JB, Mikulich SK. Efficacy of daily and alternate-day dosing regimens with the combination buprenorphine–naloxone tablet. *Drug Alcohol Depend.* 2000;58(1-2):143-152.
176. Amass L, Kamien JB, Mikulich SK. Thrice-weekly supervised dosing with the combination buprenorphine–naloxone tablet is preferred to daily supervised dosing by opioid-dependent humans. *Drug Alcohol Depend.* 2001;61(2):173-181.
177. Kissin W, McLeod C, Sonnefeld J, Stanton A. Experiences of a national sample of qualified addiction specialists who have and have not prescribed buprenorphine for opioid dependence. *J Addict Dis.* 2006;25(4):91-103.
178. Hakansson A, Medvedeo A, Andersson M, Berglund M. Buprenorphine misuse among heroin and amphetamine users in Malmo, Sweden: purpose of misuse and route of administration. *Eur Addict Res.* 2007;13(4):207-215.
179. Aitken CK, Higgs PG, Hellard ME. Buprenorphine injection in Melbourne. *Australia—an update. Drug Alcohol Rev.* 2008;27(2):197-199.
180. Cicero TJ, Surratt HL, Inciardi J. Use and misuse of buprenorphine in the management of opioid addiction. *J Opioid Manag.* 2007;3(6):302-308.
181. Johanson C, Arfken C, Menza S. Diversion and abuse of buprenorphine: findings from national surveys of treatment patients and physicians. *Drug Alcohol Depend.* 2012;1-3.

182. Monte AA, Mandell T, Wilford BB, Tennyson J, Boyer EW. Diversion of buprenorphine/naloxone coformulated tablets in a region with high prescribing prevalence. *J Addict Dis.* 2009;28(3):226-231.
183. Lofwall MR, Walsh SL. A review of buprenorphine diversion and misuse: the current evidence base and experiences from around the world. *J Addict Med.* 2014;8(5):315-326. doi:10.1097/ADM.0000000000000045
184. Winstock AR, Lea T, Jackson AP. Methods and motivations for buprenorphine diversion from public opioid substitution treatment clinics. *J Addict Dis.* 2009;28(1):57-63.
185. Winstock AR, Lea T, Sheridan J. What is diversion of supervised buprenorphine and how common is it? *J Addict Dis.* 2009;28(3): 269-278.
186. Schneider MF, Bailey JE, Cicero TJ, et al. Integrating nine prescription opioid analgesics and/or four signal detection systems to summarize statewide prescription drug abuse in the United States in 2007. *Pharmacoepidemiol Drug Saf.* 2009;18(9):778-790.
187. Rosenblum A, Parrino M, Schnoll SH, et al. Prescription opioid abuse among enrollees into methadone maintenance treatment. *Drug Alcohol Depend.* 2007;90(1):64-71.
188. Mackey K, Veazie S, Anderson J, Bourne D, Peterson K. Barriers and facilitators to the use of medications for opioid use disorder: a rapid review. *J Gen Intern Med.* 2020;35(Suppl 3):954-963. doi:10.1007/s11606-020-06257-4
189. Carter J, Zevin B, Lum PJ. Low barrier buprenorphine treatment for persons experiencing homelessness and injecting heroin in San Francisco. *Addict Sci Clin Pract.* 2019;14(1):20. doi:10.1186/s13722-019-0149-1
190. Buchheit BM, Wheelock H, Lee A, Brandt K, Gregg J. Low-barrier buprenorphine during the COVID-19 pandemic: a rapid transition to on-demand telemedicine with wide-ranging effects. *J Subst Abuse Treat.* 2021;131:108444. doi:10.1016/j.jsat.2021.108444
191. Jakubowski A, Norton BL, Hayes BT, et al. Low-threshold buprenorphine treatment in a syringe services program: program description and outcomes. *J Addict Med.* 2022;16(4):447-453. doi:10.1097/adm.0000000000000934
192. Lambdin BH, Kan D, Kral AH. Improving equity and access to buprenorphine treatment through telemedicine at syringe services programs. *Subst Abuse Treat Prev Policy.* 2022;17(1):51. doi:10.1186/s13011-022-00483-1
193. Hser YI, Evans E, Huang D, et al. Long-term outcomes after randomization to buprenorphine/naloxone versus methadone in a multi-site trial. *Addiction.* 2016;111(4):695-705. doi:10.1111/add.13238
194. Wakeman SE, Larochelle MR, Ameli O, et al. Comparative effectiveness of different treatment pathways for opioid use disorder. *JAMA Netw Open.* 2020;3(2):e1920622-e1920622. doi:10.1001/jamanetworkopen.2019.20622
195. Ling W, Wesson DR, Charuvastra C, Klett CJ. A controlled trial comparing buprenorphine and methadone maintenance in opioid dependence. *Arch Gen Psychiatry.* 1996;53(5):401-407.
196. Jones HE, Tuten M. Specialty treatment for women. In: Strain EC, Stitzer M, eds. *Methadone Treatment for Opioid Dependence.* Johns Hopkins University Press; 2006:455–484.
197. Mattick R, Kimber J, Breen C, et al. Buprenorphine maintenance versus placebo or methadone maintenance for opioid dependence. *Cochrane Database Syst Rev.* 2014;6(2):CD002207.
198. Jones HE, Kaltenbach K, Heil SH, et al. Neonatal abstinence syndrome after methadone or buprenorphine exposure. *N Engl J Med.* 2010;363(24):2320-2331.
199. Kakko J, Grönbladh L, Svanborg KD, et al. A stepped care strategy using buprenorphine and methadone versus conventional methadone maintenance in heroin dependence: a randomized controlled trial. *Am J Psychiatry.* 2007;164(5):797-803.
200. Saxon AJ, Ling W, Hillhouse M, et al. Buprenorphine/naloxone and methadone effects on laboratory indices of liver health: a randomized trial. *Drug Alcohol Depend.* 2013;128(1-2):71-76.
201. Glass L, Evans HE. Narcotic withdrawal in the newborn. *Am Fam Physician.* 1972;6(1):75-78.
202. Naeye RL, Blanc W, Leblanc W, Khatamee MA. Fetal complications of maternal heroin addiction: abnormal growth, infections, and episodes of stress. *J Pediatr.* 1973;83(6):1055-1061.
203. Connaughton JF, Reeser D, Schut J, Finnegan LP. Perinatal addiction: outcome and management. *Am J Obstet Gynecol.* 1977;129(6):679-686.
204. Kandall SR, Albin S, Gartner LM, Lee KS, Eidelman A, Lowinson J. The narcotic-dependent mother: fetal and neonatal consequences. *Early Hum Dev.* 1977;1(2):159-169.
205. Kaltenbach K, Finnegan L. *Exposed to Methadone In Utero: Cognitive Ability in Preschool Years.* Vol. 81. NIDA Research Monograph; 1988.
206. Hulse GK, Milne E, English DR, Holman CD. The relationship between maternal use of heroin and methadone and infant birth weight. *Addiction.* 1997;92(11):1571-1579.
207. Alroomi LG. Maternal narcotic abuse and the newborn. *Arch Dis Child.* 1998;63:81-83.
208. Berghella V, Lim PJ, Hill MK, Cherpes J, Chennat J, Kaltenbach K. Maternal methadone dose and neonatal withdrawal. *Am J Obstet Gynecol.* 2003;189(2):312-317.
209. Messinger DS, Bauer CR, Das A, et al. The maternal lifestyle study: cognitive, motor, and behavioral outcomes of cocaine-exposed and opiate-exposed infants through three years of age. *Pediatrics.* 2004;113(6):1677-1685.
210. Kuehn B. Opioid use disorder during pregnancy. *JAMA.* 2018;320(12):1232-1232. doi:10.1001/jama.2018.13546
211. Lester BM, Andreozzi L, Appiah L. Substance use during pregnancy: time for policy to catch up with research. *Harm Reduc J.* 2004;1(1):5.
212. Kaltenbach K, Berghella V, Finnegan L. Opioid dependence during pregnancy. Effects and management. *Obstet Gynecol Clin North Am.* 1998;25(1):139-151.
213. Jones HE, Tuten M, Strain EC, Stitzer M, Baltimore MD. *Specialty Treatment for Women.* Vol 20062006.
214. Hulse G, O'Neil G. Using naltrexone implants in the management of the pregnant heroin user. *Aust N Z J Obstet Gynaecol.* 2002;42(5):569-573.
215. Dashe JS, Jackson GL, Olscher DA, Zane EH, Wendel GD. Opioid detoxification in pregnancy. *Obstet Gynecol.* 1998;92(5):854-858.
216. Finnegan LP. Treatment issues for opioid-dependent women during the perinatal period. *J Psychoactive Drugs.* 1991;23(2):191-201.
217. Finnegan LP, Kaltenbach K. Neonatal abstinence syndrome. In: Hoekelman RA, Friedman SB, Nelson NM, et al., eds. *Primary Pediatric Care.* 2nd ed. Mosby; 1992:1367–1378.
218. Jones HE, Haug N, Silverman K, Stitzer M, Svikis D. The effectiveness of incentives in enhancing treatment attendance and drug abstinence in methadone-maintained pregnant women. *Drug Alcohol Depend.* 2001;61(3):297-306.
219. Strauss ME, Starr RH, Ostrea EM, Chavez CJ, Stryker JC. Behavioural concomitants of prenatal addiction to narcotics. *J Pediatr.* 1976;89(5): 842-846.
220. Wilson GS, Desmond MM, Wait RB. Follow-up of methadone-treated and untreated narcotic-dependent women and their infants: health, developmental, and social implications. *J Pediatr.* 1981;98(5):716-722.
221. Rosen TS, Johnson HL. Children of methadone-maintained mothers: follow-up to 18 months of age. *J Pediatr.* 1982;101(2):192-196.
222. Rosen TS, Johnson HL. *Long Term Effects of Prenatal Methadone Maintenance.* Vol. 59 NIDA Research Monograph; 1985:73-83.
223. Chasnoff IJ, Schnoll SH, Burns WJ, Burns K. Maternal nonnarcotic substance abuse during pregnancy: effects on infant development. *Neurobehav Toxicol Teratol.* 1984;6(4):277-280.
224. Kaltenbach K, Finnegan LP. Developmental outcome of infants exposed to methadone in utero: a longitudinal study. *Pediatr Res. 57.* 1986;20.
225. Kaltenbach K. Exposure to opiates: behavioral outcomes in preschool and school age children. In: Wetherington CL, Smeriglio VL, Finnegan LP, eds. *Behavioral Studies of Drug-Exposed Offspring: Methodological Issues in Human and Animal Research.* 164 DHHS National Institute on Drug Abuse; 1996:230-241.
226. McCarthy JJ, Vasti EJ, Leamon MH, Graas J, Ward C, Fassbender C. The use of serum methadone/metabolite ratios to monitor changing perinatal pharmacokinetics. *J Addict Med.* 2018;12(3):241-246. doi:10.1097/adm.0000000000000398

227. Jones HE, Martin PR, Heil SH, et al. Treatment of opioid-dependent pregnant women: clinical and research issues. *J Subst Abuse Treat.* 2008;35(3):245-259.
228. McCarthy JJ, Leamon MH, Willits NH, Salo R. The effect of methadone dose regimen on neonatal abstinence syndrome. *J Addict Med.* 2015;9(2):105-110. doi:10.1097/adm.0000000000000099
229. McCarthy JJ, Leamon MH, Finnegan LP, Fassbender C. Opioid dependence and pregnancy: minimizing stress on the fetal brain. *Am J Obstet Gynecol.* 2017;216(3):226-231. doi:10.1016/j.ajog.2016.10.003
230. Lejeune C, Simmat-Durand L, Gourarier L, Aubisson S. Groupe d'Etudes Grossesse et Addictions. Prospective multicenter observational study of 260 infants born to 259 opiate-dependent mothers on methadone or high-dose buprenorphine substitution. *Drug Alcohol Depend.* 2006;82(3):250-257.
231. Lacroix I, Berrebi A, Garipuy D, et al. Buprenorphine versus methadone in pregnant opioid-dependent women: a prospective multicenter study. *Eur J Clin Pharmacol.* 2011;67(10):1053-1059.
232. Gaalema DE, Scott TL, Heil SH, et al. Differences in the profile of neonatal abstinence syndrome signs in methadone- versus buprenorphine-exposed neonates. *Addiction.* 2012;107(Suppl 1):53-62.
233. Suarez EA, Huybrechts KF, Straub L, et al. Buprenorphine versus methadone for opioid use disorder in pregnancy. *N Eng J Med.* 2022;387(22):2033-2044. doi:10.1056/NEJMoa2203318
234. Bogen DL, Perel JM, Helsel JC, et al. Pharmacologic evidence to support clinical decision making for peripartum methadone treatment. *Psychopharmacology (Berl).* 2013;225(2):441-451. doi:10.1007/s00213-012-2833-7
235. Jansson LM, Dipietro JA, Velez M, Elko A, Knauer H, Kivlighan KT. Maternal methadone dosing schedule and fetal neurobehaviour. *J Matern Fetal Neonatal Med.* 2009;22(1):29-35. doi:10.1080/14767050802452291
236. Wittmann BK, Segal S. A comparison of the effects of single- and split-dose methadone administration on the fetus: ultrasound evaluation. *Int J Addict.* 1991;26(2):213-218. doi:10.3109/10826089109053183
237. Brown SM, Holtzman M, Kim T, Kharasch ED. Buprenorphine metabolites, buprenorphine-3-glucuronide and norbuprenorphine-3-glucuronide, are biologically active. *Anesthesiology.* 2011;115(6):1251-1260. doi:10.1097/ALN.0b013e318238fea0
238. Kacinko SL, Jones HE, Johnson RE, Choo RE, Huestis MA. Correlations of maternal buprenorphine dose, buprenorphine, and metabolite concentrations in meconium with neonatal outcomes. *Clin Pharmacol Ther.* 2008;84(5):604-612. doi:10.1038/clpt.2008.156
239. Finnegan LP, Connaughton JF, Kron RE. Neonatal abstinence syndrome: assessment and management. *Addict Dis.* 1975;2(1):141-158.
240. Lipsitz PJ. A proposed narcotic withdrawal score for use with newborn infants. A pragmatic evaluation of its efficacy. *Clin Pediatr (Phila).* 1975;14(6):592-594.
241. Hudak ML, Tan RC. Neonatal drug withdrawal. *Pediatrics.* 2012;129(2):e540-e560.
242. Desmond MM, Wilson GS. Neonatal abstinence syndrome: recognition and diagnosis. *Addict Dis.* 1975;2(1-2):113-121.
243. Marquet P, Lavignasse P, Gaulier JM, Kintz P, Totowa NJ. Case study of neonates born to mothers undergoing buprenorphine maintenance treatment. In: Kintz P, Marquet P, eds. *Buprenorphine Therapy of Opiate Addiction.* Humana Press; 2002:123-135.
244. Jones HE, Johnson RE, Jasinski DR, et al. Buprenorphine versus methadone in the treatment of pregnant opioid-dependent patients: effects on the neonatal abstinence syndrome. *Drug Alcohol Depend.* 2005;79(1):1-10.
245. Fischer G, Ortner R, Rohrmeister K, et al. Methadone versus buprenorphine in pregnant addicts: a double-blind, double-dummy comparison study. *Addiction.* 2006;101(2):275-281.
246. Patrick SW, Kaplan HC, Passarella M, Davis MM, Lorch SA. Variation in treatment of neonatal abstinence syndrome in US children's hospitals, 2004-2011. *J Perinatol.* 2014;34:867-872.
247. Kraft WK, Adeniyi-Jones SC, Chervoneva I, et al. Buprenorphine for the treatment of the neonatal abstinence syndrome. *N Engl J Med.* 2017;376(24):2341-2348.
248. MacMillan KDL, Rendon CP, Verma K, Riblet N, Washer DB, Volpe HA. Association of rooming-in with outcomes for neonatal abstinence syndrome: a systematic review and meta-analysis. *JAMA Pediatr.* 2018;172(4):345-351. doi:10.1001/jamapediatrics.2017.5195
249. McCarthy JJ. Intrauterine abstinence syndrome (IAS) during buprenorphine inductions and methadone tapers: can we assure the safety of the fetus? *J Matern Fetal Neonatal Med.* 2012;25(2):109-112.
250. Kenner C, Lott JW. *Comprehensive Neonatal Care: An Interdisciplinary Approach.* 4th ed. Saunders; 2007.
251. Barker DJP, Hanson MA. Altered regional blood flow in the fetus: the origins of cardiovascular disease? *Acta Paediatrica.* 2004;93(12):1559-1560.
252. Jansson LM, DiPietro JA, Elko A, Velez M. Infant autonomic functioning and neonatal abstinence syndrome. *Drug Alcohol Depend.* 2010;109(1-3):198-204.
253. Bell J, Towers CV, Hennessy MD, Heitzman C, Smith B, Chattin K. Detoxification from opiate drugs during pregnancy. *Am J Obstet Gynecol.* 2016;215(3): 374.e1-6.
254. ACOG Committee on Health Care for Underserved Women; American Society of Addiction Medicine. ACOG Committee Opinion No. 524: Opioid abuse, dependence, and addiction in pregnancy. *Obstet Gynecol.* 2012;119(5):1070-1076.
255. Iribarne C, Picart D, Dréano Y, Bail JP, Berthou F. Involvement of cytochrome P450 3A4 in N-dealkylation of buprenorphine in human liver microsomes. *Life Sci.* 1997;60(22):1953-1964.
256. Bruce RD, Moody DE, Altice FL, Gourevitch MN, Friedland GH. A review of pharmacological interactions between HIV or hepatitis C virus medications and opioid agonist therapy: implications and management for clinical practice. *Expert Rev Clin Pharmacol.* 2013;6(3):249-269. doi:10.1586/ecp.13.18
257. Bickel WK, Amass L, Crean JP, Badger GJ. Buprenorphine dosing every 1, 2, or 3 days in opioid-dependent patients. *Psychopharmacology.* 1999;146(2):111-118.
258. Petry NM, Bickel WK, Badger GJ. A comparison of four buprenorphine dosing regimens in the treatment of opioid dependence. *Clin Pharmacol Ther.* 1999;66(3):306-314.
259. Schottenfeld RS, Pakes J, O'Connor P, Chawarski M, Oliveto A, Kosten TR. Thrice-weekly versus daily buprenorphine maintenance. *Biol Psychiatry.* 2000;47(12):1072-1079.
260. Helmus TC, Downey KK, Arfken CL, Henderson MJ, Schuster CR. Novelty seeking as a predictor of treatment retention for heroin dependent cocaine users. *Drug Alcohol Depend.* 2001;61(3):287-295.
261. Amass L, Ling W, Freese TE, et al. Bringing buprenorphine–naloxone detoxification to community treatment providers: the NIDA Clinical Trials Network field experience. *Am J Addict.* 2004;13(Suppl 1):S42-S66.
262. Preston KL, Bigelow GE, Liebson IA. Buprenorphine and naloxone alone and in combination in opioid-dependent humans. *Psychopharmacology.* 1988;94(4):484-490.
263. Strain EC, Preston KL, Liebson IA, Bigelow GE. Acute effects of buprenorphine, hydromorphone and naloxone in methadone-maintained volunteers. *J Pharmacol Exp Ther.* 1992;261(3):985-993.
264. Strain EC, Preston KL, Liebson IA, Bigelow GE. Buprenorphine effects in methadone-maintained volunteers: effects at two hours after methadone. *J Pharmacol Exp Ther.* 1995;272(2):628-638.
265. Walsh SL, June HL, Schuh KJ, Preston KL, Bigelow GE, Stitzer ML. Effects of buprenorphine and methadone in methadone-maintained subjects. *Psychopharmacology.* 1995;119(3):268-276.
266. Kosten TR, Kleber HD. Buprenorphine detoxification from opioid dependence: a pilot study. *Life Sci.* 1988;42(6):635-641.
267. Hartel D, Ball JC, Ross A. Cocaine use, inadequate methadone dose increase risk of AIDS for IV drug users in treatment. In: Ball JC, Ross A, eds. *The Effectiveness of Methadone Maintenance Treatment.* Vol. 5(1) Springer-Verlag; 1991:1989-1990.
268. Banys P, Clark HW, Tusel DJ, et al. An open trial of low dose buprenorphine in treating methadone withdrawal. *J Subst Abuse Treat.* 1994;11(1):9-15.

269. Glasper A, Reed LJ, de Wet CJ, Gossop M, Bearn J. Induction of patients with moderately severe methadone dependence onto buprenorphine. *Addict Biol.* 2005;10(2):149-155.
270. Lukas SE, Jasinski DR, Johnson RE. Electroencephalographic and behavioral correlates of buprenorphine administration. *Clin Pharmacol Ther.* 1984;36(1):127-132.
271. Levin FR, Fischman MW, Connerney I, Foltin RW. A protocol to switch high-dose, methadone-maintained subjects to buprenorphine. *Am J Addict.* 1997;6(2):105-116.
272. Rosado J, Walsh SL, Bigelow GE, Strain EC. Sublingual buprenorphine/naloxone precipitated withdrawal in subjects maintained on 100 mg of daily methadone. *Drug Alcohol Depend.* 2007;90(2-3):261-269.
273. Breen CL, Harris SJ, Lintzeris N, et al. Cessation of methadone maintenance treatment using buprenorphine: transfer from methadone to buprenorphine and subsequent buprenorphine reductions. *Drug Alcohol Depend.* 2003;71(1):49-55.
274. Azar P, Nikoo M, Miles I. Methadone to buprenorphine/naloxone induction without withdrawal utilizing transdermal fentanyl bridge in an inpatient setting-Azar method. *Am J Addict.* 2018;27(8):601-604. doi:10.1111/ajad.12809
275. Callan J, Pytell J, Ross J, Rastegar DA. Transition from methadone to buprenorphine using a short-acting agonist bridge in the inpatient setting: a case study. *J Addict Med.* 2020;14(5):e274-e276. doi:10.1097/adm.0000000000000623
276. Terasaki D, Smith C, Calcaterra SL. Transitioning hospitalized patients with opioid use disorder from methadone to buprenorphine without a period of opioid abstinence using a microdosing protocol. *Pharmacotherapy.* 2019;39(10):1023-1029. doi:10.1002/phar.2313
277. Anderson C, Cooley R, Patil D. Transitioning from high-dose methadone to buprenorphine using a microdosing approach: unique considerations at ASAM Level 3 facilities. *J Addict Med.* 2022; doi:10.1097/adm.0000000000001085
278. De Aquino JP, Fairgrieve C, Klaire S, Garcia-Vassallo G. Rapid transition from methadone to buprenorphine utilizing a micro-dosing protocol in the outpatient veteran affairs setting. *J Addict Med.* 2020;14(5):e271-e273. doi:10.1097/adm.0000000000000618
279. Menard S, Jhawar A. Microdose induction of buprenorphine-naloxone in a patient using high dose methadone: a case report. *Ment Health Clin.* 2021;11(6):369-372. doi:10.9740/mhc.2021.11.369
280. Minozzi S, Amato L, Vecchi S, Davoli M, Kirchmayer U, Verster A. Oral naltrexone maintenance treatment for opioid dependence. *Cochrane Database Syst Rev.* 2006;1:CD001333.
281. Brahen LS, Henderson RK, Capone T, Kordal N. Naltrexone treatment in a jail work-release program. *J Clin Psychiatry.* 1984;45(9 Pt 2):49-52.
282. Ling W, Wesson DR. Naltrexone treatment for addicted health-care professionals: a collaborative private practice experience. *J Clin Psychiatry.* 1984;45(9 Pt 2):46-48.
283. Washton AM, Gold MS, Pottash AC. *Addicted Physicians and Business Executives.* Vol. 55 NIDA Research Monograph; 1984:185-190.
284. Cornish JW, Metzger D, Woody GE, et al. Naltrexone pharmacotherapy for opioid dependent federal probationers. *J Subst Abuse Treat.* 1997;14(6):529-534.
285. Anton RF, Hogan I, Jalali B, Riordan CE, Kleber HD. Multiple family therapy and naltrexone in the treatment of opiate dependence. *Drug Alcohol Depend.* 1981;8(2):157-168.
286. Resnick RB, Washton AM, Stone-Washton N. *Psychotherapy and Naltrexone in Opioid Dependence.* Vol. 34 NIDA Research Monograph; 1981:109-115.
287. Preston KL, Silverman K, Umbricht A, DeJesus A, Montoya ID, Schuster CR. Improvement in naltrexone treatment compliance with contingency management. *Drug Alcohol Depend.* 1999;54(2):127-135.
288. Carroll KM, Ball SA, Nich C, et al. Targeting behavioral therapies to enhance naltrexone treatment of opioid dependence: efficacy of contingency management and significant other involvement. *Arch Gen Psychiatry.* 2001;58(8):755-761.
289. Brahen LS, Capone TJ, Capone DM. Naltrexone: lack of effect on hepatic enzymes. *J Clin Pharmacol.* 1988;28(1):64-70.
290. Johnson BA, Ait-Daoud N, Aubin H-J, et al. A pilot evaluation of the safety and tolerability of repeat dose administration of long-acting injectable naltrexone (Vivitrex) in patients with alcohol dependence. *Alcohol Clin Exp Res.* 2004;28(9):1356-1361.
291. Garbutt JC, Kranzler HR, O'Malley SS, et al. Efficacy and tolerability of long-acting injectable naltrexone for alcohol dependence: a randomized controlled trial. *JAMA.* 2005;293(13):1617-1625.
292. Roozen HG, de Waart R, van den Brink W. Efficacy and tolerability of naltrexone in the treatment of alcohol dependence: oral versus injectable delivery. *Eur Addict Res.* 2007;13(4):201-206.
293. Comer SD, Collins ED, Kleber HD, Nuwayser ES, Kerrigan JH, Fischman MW. Depot naltrexone: long-lasting antagonism of the effects of heroin in humans. *Psychopharmacology (Berl).* 2002;159(4):351-360.
294. Comer SD, Sullivan MA, Walker EA. Comparison of intravenous buprenorphine and methadone self-administration by recently detoxified heroin-dependent individuals. *J Pharmacol Exp Ther.* 2005;315(3):1320-1330.
295. Comer SD, Sullivan MA, Yu E, et al. Injectable, sustained-release naltrexone for the treatment of opioid dependence: a randomized, placebo-controlled trial. *Arch Gen Psychiatry.* 2006;63(2):210-218.
296. Carreño JE, Alvarez CE, Narciso GIS, Bascarán MT, Díaz M, Bobes J. Maintenance treatment with depot opioid antagonists in subcutaneous implants: an alternative in the treatment of opioid dependence. *Addict Biol.* 2003;8(4):429-438.
297. Krupitsky EM, Blokhina EA. Long-acting depot formulations of naltrexone for heroin dependence: a review. *Curr Opin Psychiatry.* 2010;23(3):210-214.
298. Krupitsky EM, Zvartau EE, Masalov DV, et al. Naltrexone for heroin dependence treatment in St Petersburg. *Russia. J Subst Abuse Treat.* 2004;26(4):285-294.
299. Lee JD, Nunes EV Jr, Novo P, et al. Comparative effectiveness of extended-release naltrexone versus buprenorphine-naloxone for opioid relapse prevention (X:BOT): a multicentre, open-label, randomised controlled trial. *Lancet.* 2018;391(10118):309-318. doi:10.1016/S0140-6736(17)32812-X
300. Tanum L, Solli K, Latif Z, et al. Effectiveness of injectable extended-release naltrexone vs daily buprenorphine-naloxone for opioid dependence: a randomized clinical noninferiority trial. *JAMA Psychiatry.* 2017;74(12):1197-1205. doi:10.1001/jamapsychiatry.2017.3206
301. Morgan JR, Schackman BR, Weinstein ZM, Walley AY, Linas BP. Overdose following initiation of naltrexone and buprenorphine medication treatment for opioid use disorder in a United States commercially insured cohort. *Drug Alcohol Depend.* 2019;200:34-39.
302. Hulse GK, Arnold-Reed DE, O'Neil G, Chan CT, Hansson R, O'Neil P. Blood naltrexone and 6-beta-naltrexol levels following naltrexone implant: comparing two naltrexone implants. *Addict Biol.* 2004;9(1):59-65.
303. Hulse GK, Arnold-Reed DE, O'Neil G, Chan CT, Hansson RC. Achieving long-term continuous blood naltrexone and 6-beta-naltrexol coverage following sequential naltrexone implants. *Addict Biol.* 2004;9(1):67-72.
304. Olsen L, Christophersen AS, Frogopsahl G, Waal H, Mørland J. Plasma concentrations during naltrexone implant treatment of opiate-dependent patients. *Br J Clin Pharmacol.* 2004;58(2):219-222.
305. Colquhoun R, Tan DYK, Hull S. A comparison of oral and implant naltrexone outcomes at 12 months. *J Opioid Manag.* 2005;1(5):249-256.
306. Vocci F. *Extended-Release Naltrexone (XR-NTX) Opioid Dependence Registry: Clinical And Functional Effectiveness.* 2014 ASAM National Meeting 2014:33.
307. Compton MA, McCaffrey M. Controlling pain: treating acute pain in addicted patients. *Nursing.* 2001;17.
308. Compton P, Charuvastra VC, Ling W. Pain intolerance in opioid-maintained former opiate addicts: effect of long-acting maintenance agent. *Drug Alcohol Depend.* 2001;63(2):139-146.
309. Kornfeld H, Manfredi L. Effectiveness of full agonist opioids in patients stabilized on buprenorphine undergoing major surgery: a case series. *Am J Ther.* 2010;17(5):523-528.
310. Buresh M, Ratner J, Zgierska A, Gordin V, Alvanzo A. Treating perioperative and acute pain in patients on buprenorphine: narrative literature review and practice recommendations. *J Gen Intern Med.* 2020;35(12):3635-3643. doi:10.1007/s11606-020-06115-3

311. Warner NS, Warner MA, Cunningham JL, et al. A practical approach for the management of the mixed opioid agonist-antagonist buprenorphine during acute pain and surgery. *Mayo Clin Proc.* 2020;95(6):1253-1267. doi:10.1016/j.mayocp.2019.10.007
312. Rosenblum A, Joseph H, Fong C, Kipnis S, Cleland C, Portenoy RK. Prevalence and characteristics of chronic pain among chemically dependent patients in methadone maintenance and residential treatment facilities. *JAMA.* 2003;289(18):2370-2378.
313. Brands B, Blake J, Sproule B, Gourlay D, Busto U. Prescription opioid abuse in patients presenting for methadone maintenance treatment. *Drug Alcohol Depend.* 2004;73(2):199-207.
314. D'Onofrio G, Chawarski MC, O'Connor PG, et al. Emergency department-initiated buprenorphine for opioid dependence with continuation in primary care: outcomes during and after intervention. *J Gen Intern Med.* 2017;32(6):660-666. doi:10.1007/s11606-017-3993-2
315. Rowe C, Santos G-M, Vittinghoff E, Wheeler E, Davidson P, Coffin PO. Predictors of participant engagement and naloxone utilization in a community-based naloxone distribution program. *Addiction.* 2015;110(8):1301-1310.
316. Woody GE, Luborsky L, McLellan AT, et al. Psychotherapy for opiate addicts. Does it help? *Arch Gen Psychiatry.* 1983;40(6):639-645.
317. Rounsaville BJ, Kleber HD. Untreated opiate addicts: how do they differ from those seeking treatment? *Arch Gen Psychiatry.* 1985;42:1072-1077.
318. Peles E, Schreiber S, Naumovsky Y, Adelson M. Depression in methadone maintenance treatment patients: rate and risk factors. *J Affect Disord.* 2007;99(1-3):213-220.
319. Kosten TR, Rounsaville BJ, Kleber HD. A 2.5 year follow-up of depression, life crises, and treatment effects on abstinence among opioid addicts. *Arch Gen Psychiatry.* 1986;43:733-738.
320. Musselman DL, Kell MJ. Prevalence and improvement in psychopathology in opioid dependent patients participating in methadone maintenance. *J Addict Dis.* 1995;14(3):67-82.
321. Trafton JA, Minkel J, Humphreys K. Opioid substitution treatment reduces substance use equivalently in patients with and without posttraumatic stress disorder. *J Stud Alcohol.* 2006;67(2):228-235.
322. Peirce JM, Brooner RK, King VL, Kidorf MS. Effect of traumatic event reexposure and PTSD on substance use disorder treatment response. *Drug Alcohol Depend.* 2016;158:126-131.
323. Peles E, Schreiber S, Adelson M. Variables associated with perceived sleep disorders in methadone maintenance treatment (MMT) patients. *Drug Alcohol Depend.* 2006;82(2):103-110.
324. Rounsaville BJ, Weissman MM, Wilber CH, Kleber HD. The heterogeneity of psychiatric diagnosis in treated opiate addicts. *Arch Gen Psychiatry.* 1982;39:161-169.
325. Verebey K. *Opioids in Mental Illness: Theories, Clinical Observations, and Treatment Possibilities.* Annals of the New York Academy of Sciences; 1982:398.
326. Ball SA. Comparing individual therapies for personality disordered opioid dependent patients. *J Personal Disord.* 2007;21(3):305-321.
327. Darke S, Sims J, McDonald S, Wickes W. Cognitive impairment among methadone maintenance patients. *Addiction.* 2000;95(5):687-695.
328. Soyka M, Lieb M, Kagerer S, et al. Cognitive functioning during methadone and buprenorphine treatment: results of a randomized clinical trial. *J Clin Psychopharmacol.* 2008;28(6):699-703.
329. Rudisill TM, Zhu M, Kelley GA, Pilkerton C, Rudisill BR. Medication use and the risk of motor vehicle collisions among licensed drivers: a systematic review. *Accid Anal Prev.* 2016;96:255-270.
330. Soyka M. Opioids and traffic safety—focus on buprenorphine. *Pharmacopsychiatry.* 2014;47(1):7-17.
331. Eren K, Schuster J, Herschell A, et al. Association of counseling and psychotherapy on retention in medication for addiction treatment within a large medicaid population. *J Addict Med.* 2022;16(3):346-353.
332. Busch AB, Greenfield SF, Reif S, Normand ST, Huskamp HA. Outpatient care for opioid use disorder among the commercially insured: Use of medication and psychosocial treatment. *J Subst Abuse Treat.* 2020;115.
333. Joseph H, Stancliff S, Langrod J. Methadone maintenance treatment (MMT): a review of historical and clinical issues. *Mt Sinai J Med.* 2000;67(5-6):347-364.
334. HR2617, *The Consolidated Appropriations Act*, 2023.

Sidebar

Medical Director Stewardship of Opioid Treatment Programs

Kenneth B. Stoller

GENERAL REQUIREMENTS AND ORGANIZATIONAL ROLE

It is important to first note that federal and state statutes and regulations, guidelines, best practices, accreditation standards, payer requirements, and company policies governing Opioid Treatment Programs (OTPs) often change. In fact, at present, the federal regulations regarding OTPs are under consideration for change as state and federal COVID-era allowances are expiring, getting extended, or being made permanent in some fashion through regulatory revision. Although the general concepts described below will largely persist over time, specifics may change requiring OTP leaders must remain informed about how such changes may require operational modifications to maintain ongoing compliance.

Federal Definition

Although specific duties of an OTP medical director may differ from one program setting to another, in all cases the role is grounded in federal regulation and guidelines. The OTP medical director role is defined in 42 CFR Part 8, the federal regulation governing OTP creation and operations. It states "Medical director means a physician, licensed to practice medicine in the jurisdiction in which the opioid treatment program is located, who assumes responsibility for administering all medical services performed by the program, either by performing them directly or by delegating specific responsibility to authorized program physicians and health care professionals functioning under the medical director's direct supervision." It goes on to explain that "The medical director shall assume responsibility for administering all medical services performed by the OTP. In addition, the medical director shall be responsible for ensuring that the OTP complies with all applicable Federal, State, and local laws and regulations." The Substance Abuse and Mental Health Services Administration (SAMHSA) is the federal body that issued these regulations; SAMHSA describes their expectations of how their regulations are best satisfied by OTPs in their published OTP guidelines, the latest version of which was issued in 2015. These Federal Guidelines for Opioid Treatment Programs advise that the medical director is responsible for monitoring and supervising all medical and nursing services and assures that all medical, psychiatric, nursing, pharmacy, toxicology, and other services are conducted in compliance with regulations.

As to which physicians may serve in this role, the SAMHSA OTP guidelines state that the medical director should (1) have completed an accredited residency training program and (2) have at least one year of experience practicing in either addiction medicine or addiction psychiatry, adding that there is a *preference* for physicians who are board certified in both their own primary medical specialty and either addiction psychiatry or addiction medicine. Beyond that, SAMHSA urges OTP medical directors to complete the training which until recently was required to obtain a waiver to prescribe buprenorphine (as per the Drug Addiction Treatment Act of 2000—DATA 2000), even though provision of buprenorphine through the OTP involves physician ordering and staff dispensing, and not pharmacy prescribing. Some of these duties of the medical director overlap with duties of the OTP "program sponsor," another obligatory role in every OTP; and in fact it is allowable for the medical director to also serve as the program sponsor. The program sponsor is the role described in federal OTP regulations who is responsible for OTP operation and who assumes responsibility for all its employees. If and when a change in medical director occurs, SAMHSA requires formal notification (by the program sponsor, through its SAMHSA/CSAT Opioid Treatment Program Extranet within 3 weeks of this change).

State-Specific Regulations

It is important to note here that states may write into their own regulations additional rules governing OTPs, including those involving the role of medical director. For example, some states have imposed more stringent criteria regarding the training, certification and/or experience of physicians who can serve as an OTP medical director, such as *requiring* specialty board certification in addiction treatment. Since doing so may significantly limit the pool of qualified physicians interested and able to fill this role, those states may implement rules allowing "interim" medical directors while they seek out the necessary additional credentials, or there may be an allowance specified for a practice-based alternative pathway. Another area of potential divergence between state and federal rules involves time physically spent in the OTP. The SAMHSA guidelines specify that "The medical director should be present at the program a sufficient number of hours to assure regulatory compliance and carry out those duties specifically assigned to the medical director by regulation." However, some states choose to impose more rigid requirements, specifying particular numbers of hours or percent effort based on patient census. For these reasons, it is critical that the OTP medical director maintain a high level of current knowledge about both federal and state regulations.

Delegated Responsibilities

While the OTP medical director is responsible for ensuring that a wide range of operations meet regulatory and best practice expectations, it is not necessary that they directly provide or oversee all such services. Many aspects can be provided by other health care professionals including other physicians, advanced practice nurses (nurse practitioners), physician assistants, or advanced-practice pharmacists. The OTP leadership must ensure that the duties performed by any such professional are consistent with the allowable scope of services for that licensure in the state where the OTP is sited and that their licensure remains up to date and unrestricted. For example, SAMHSA has determined that in order to fully manage methadone or buprenorphine pharmacotherapy within an OTP, an advance practice nurse or physician assistant ("mid-level" practitioners) must be covered under an approved state and SAMHSA "mid-level exemption request" covering that OTP for up to 3 years at a time. However, in states where such professionals are not permitted to order or prescribe controlled substances, an exemption will not be granted covering that licensure type. Whatever the subject matter, when there exist both state and federal regulations covering the same aspect of OTP practice, the more restrictive rule must be followed.

Medical Director in Program Structure

Organizationally, the OTP medical director usually reports upward to the program director, program sponsor, and/or chief medical officer, depending on the program and larger corporate structure for multiprogram entities. Some companies have regional medical directors who directly supervise program-based OTP medical directors. Positions that report *upward* to the OTP medical director typically include other program physicians, advanced practice nurses and pharmacists, and senior clinical/counseling staff. Alternatively, some programs may have counseling staff reporting flow upward to a clinical manager/director and/or on to a chief clinical officer. The size and organization of the program and umbrella organization determine these variations, as may the nature of the medical director's training and experience. For example, a medical director who is a psychiatrist may be considered more appropriate to oversee the program counseling services than a physician not as abundantly trained in behavioral health care. OTP nursing staff may directly report to the medical director, to other program physicians or advance practitioners, or to a senior nurse. In summary, given differences in program and corporate structures, the specific nature of the OTP medical director role may vary. When the role is more limited, requiring less than full-time effort in any one OTP, it is not uncommon for OTP medical directors to function in this role across multiple OTPs, whether in the same company or across different entities, as an experienced OTP medical director may be a valuable rare commodity in some geographic areas.

RESPONSIBILITIES

Program Leadership

The OTP medical director collaborates with the program director (who often serves as the program sponsor) and other program leaders (administrative and clinical) to form an effective program leadership group. The medical director works with human resources to hire, evaluate, manage, discipline, and terminate the medical staff, including program physicians, advance practice professionals (nurse practitioners, physician assistants), and nursing staff. In some programs this may also include clinical/counseling staff. The medical director provides oversight to their reportees, which may include providing clinical and/or administrative supervision, ensuring staff are adequately trained (with documented competency) for their varying activities, and ensuring that they maintain the necessary credentials and licensure. The medical director often completes annual performance evaluations for their reportees and works with the program director and/or the human resources department to address difficulties in job performance or professionalism among their staff.

Medical Policies and Procedures

The medical director ensures that policies and procedures are written, implemented and followed, in order to achieve compliance with numerous oversight bodies and to deliver high quality of care. Such policies reflect requirements and regulations issued by the following nonexhaustive list of entities:

- SAMHSA OTP regulations and guidelines.
- Drug Enforcement Administration (DEA) regulations covering "Narcotic Treatment Programs (NTPs)" (note different nomenclature versus SAMHSA) as well as related regulations such as those published covering NTP remote fixed site and mobile treatment units.
- State and local behavioral health authority regulations.
- Accreditation body standards—most typically one of the following: The Joint Commission (TJC), Commission on Accreditation of Rehabilitation Facilities (CARF), Council on Accreditation (COA), and less commonly, the state behavioral health agency itself (currently an option in Missouri and Washington states).
- State controlled dangerous substance administration regulations.
- Payer-specific requirements (eg, CMS/Medicare or the state Medicaid office).
- Grant funding agencies (federal, state or local government, private grantors).
- For hospital-based OTPs, hospital policies and procedures and CMS conditions of participation.
- For larger companies, corporate policies and procedures.
- Best clinical practices based on field guidelines and medical literature.

The subject matter of OTP policies and procedures for which the medical director tends to be instrumental in formulating, educating, and ensuring ongoing compliance often include:

- Medication provision through the OTP dispensary.
  - Nurse and/or pharmacist dose preparation and dispensing.
  - Narcotic storage, destruction and recordkeeping.
  - Emergency ("business continuity") contingency plans.
  - Diversion control.
- Other medical service provision
  - Scope and mission of the OTP.
  - Medical assessment of new patients.
    - Medical treatment (if offered).
    - Hepatitis, HIV and tuberculosis risk assessment.
  - Mental health assessment and treatment (if offered).
    - Regardless, should include suicide risk assessment and risk mitigation.
  - Clinic health and safety protocols (eg, COVID-related).
  - Dispensary handling of medication for co-occurring physical and behavioral health conditions (eg, hepatitis or HIV antivirals, antipsychotics, disulfiram) if directly observed therapy is offered.
  - Harm reduction services (eg, naloxone, fentanyl test strips, referral to syringe services programs).
- Depending on organizational structure, nonmedical clinical activities (counseling).

Direct Clinic Service Activities

As mentioned above, the extent to which a particular OTP medical director might provide direct care to patients can greatly vary. Some spend most of their effort supervising delegates such as program physicians, nurse practitioners and physician assistants who provide all direct services. Others may be the only medical provider in the program and spend most of their time providing direct care. Regardless, the OTP medical director should be familiar with the logistics of service provision and be prepared to fill in should workforce issues arise. The following are some domains of service provision that the medical director either provides or oversees:

- New patient assessment
  - ☐ Obtain and/or confirm diagnosis of opioid use disorder.
  - ☐ Determine medical appropriateness for OTP admission.
  - ☐ Educate the patient on medication options, determine which to use, obtain informed consent.
  - ☐ Determine whether an urgent medical admission is needed for alcohol/sedative medically supervised withdrawal, medical instability, suicidality, etc.
  - ☐ Perform a comprehensive medical history and physical.
  - ☐ Order and review admission laboratory assessments.
  - ☐ Write medication induction orders.
- Ongoing patient care
  - ☐ Write nonurgent orders for changes to medication dose or clinic reporting schedule.
  - ☐ Be available to nursing staff in person or telephonically for immediate issues that arise at the medication dispensary. Examples include:
    - Determine whether an impaired patient should be dosed.
    - Address urgent needs for dose adjustment or take-home changes.
    - Assess patients for timely medical, mental health, or addiction medication needs.
    - Assess and address possible medical or mental health emergencies.
  - ☐ Participate in and sign patient treatment plans.
    - Formulate strategies for optimizing care of co-occurring substance use disorder, medical, mental health, chronic pain, and social problems.
  - ☐ Coordinate care with external medical providers (primary care, behavioral health, specialty medical care).
  - ☐ Query the state prescription drug monitoring program (PDMP) or review query performed by a delegate. Communicate with prescribers of controlled substances after obtaining patient release of information.

Interface With External Agencies

The OTP medical director is a primary contact for many external entities involved in the delivery of OTP-based services, including:

DEA

The OTP medical director is the primary contact for interactions with the DEA. The medical director should be present for (typically triennial) unannounced OTP inspections performed by the DEA. When issues or questions are brought up by DEA, or when the program has questions regarding how DEA rules should be interpreted, or when medication security events occur, it is typically the OTP medical director who directs communication. The medical director reports to the DEA (via DEA form 106) whenever there is a loss or theft of controlled substances. Given these responsibilities, the medical director may have the opportunity to develop productive working relationships with staff and leadership from the local or regional DEA office.

SAMHSA

The medical director interacts as needed with another federal oversight agency, SAMHSA's Department of Pharmacotherapeutics (DPT). The medical director, or an assigned delegate, enters exception requests in the SAMHSA OTP extranet. Examples of when this is necessary include if patients require more take-homes than permitted by regulation (for patient travel or, for an entire clinic, for extreme weather closures), or for new admissions not meeting regulatory requirements such as those having less than 1 year documented opioid use disorder, or minors not already failing two detoxification attempts. The medical director, with the program sponsor, also requests an exemption from the DPT to allow advance practice providers to function in the same manner as program physicians.

Accreditation Body

Each program is required to maintain OTP-specific accreditation per federal regulation 42 CFR part 8. The medical director, as part of the OTP leadership group, keeps track of communications from their accreditation body describing changes to its standards, and ensures ongoing compliance with all standards and leads efforts regarding standards covering medical treatments. The medical director also plays a pivotal role in triennial accreditation surveys and in the drafting and monitoring of any necessary corrective action plans following those surveys.

State and Local Oversight Authorities

Along with other leadership group members, the medical director interfaces with behavioral health, controlled substances, and Medicaid authorities within state and local governments. It is important to keep apprised of regulatory changes—many were instituted as allowances during COVID-19 to facilitate treatment continuity. The medical director can advocate for sensible regulations, system configurations, and state Medicaid payment structures to better align state and local rules with conditions that facilitate best medical practices. The medical director may choose to attend local/state meetings involving the treatment system, particularly those specifically related to OTP-based medical care. The medical director is the primary point of contact for the State Opioid Treatment Authority (SOTA), the SAMHSA-mandated state position charged with overseeing OTP operations. Communication with the SOTA is required when changes are made to OTP days/hours of operation, special clinic closures, concerning occurrences (such as theft/loss of narcotics), establishment of new clinics or dosing units, or system problems (such as a health care entity refusing to serve individuals receiving methadone treatment or addressing a complaint regarding their OTP). This relationship between the SOTA and the OTP medical director became particularly important during the COVID-19 pandemic, given the SOTA's role in requesting blanket take-home exemptions from SAMHSA (allowing for more liberal issuance of take-home doses by OTPs), obtaining personal protective equipment and naloxone supplies for the state's OTPs, and providing guidance and assistance when OTPs had to navigate emergencies such as staffing crises when dispensary nurses all contracted COVID-19.

Payers

Although routine issues can typically be managed by other OTP staff (billing, counseling), at times the OTP medical director may need to communicate with payers to resolve problems or facilitate contracting.

Provider Associations

In advocating for optimal federal, state, and local governmental statutes and regulations, as well as health plan payment systems, it is helpful for OTP leaders, including medical directors, to be active in a local provider association—such as state chapter of the American Association for the Treatment of Opioid Dependence (AATOD) the American Academy of Addiction Psychiatry (AAAP), or the American Society of Addiction Medicine (ASAM). Additionally, having colleagues within such associations practicing in similar programs and treating patients with the same disorder can provide clinical support for the less experienced medical director, ranging from formal clinical mentorship to "curbside consults" when desired.

Miscellaneous Duties

The following are additional functions that the OTP medical director or assigned delegate, may perform:

- Determine the need for clinic closure and special take-home doses when serious weather events are forecast.
- Determine logistics as to when more medication (methadone, buprenorphine) needs to be ordered from distributors and how much to order.
- Ordering medication (using DEA form 222 for methadone). Per DEA rules, this may be done by a delegate only when a "power of attorney" specific for each delegate has been assigned and documented by the medical director.
- Ensuring that data are collected for quality improvement, such as treatment retention, toxicology results and patient satisfaction surveys.
- Other reporting requirements that may be set down by oversight authorities, such as:
  - Reporting of cases of diseases (such as COVID-19).
  - Reporting of patient deaths and other critical incidents, to local and/or state authorities.
- Maintain an order with the clinic's external laboratory for routine (urine) toxicology testing.

In summary, the OTP medical director plays a pivotal role in the routine operation of the program—providing oversight to, and in many cases direct delivery of, medical services to OTP patients. In so doing, the medical director must not only maintain productive relationships with clinical and administrative staff within the program but also with entities outside the OTP. This includes but is not limited to oversight, accreditation, and reimbursement entities, as well as provider associations. Before becoming an OTP medical director, the individual should become well-familiarized with the numerous sets of statutes, regulations, guidelines, policies, and standards that govern OTP operation and should keep apprised of revisions. Some of those national resources can be found online as follows:

- 42 CFR part 8 for regulations governing OTPs: https://www.ecfr.gov/current/title-42/chapter-I/subchapter-A/part-8?toc=1
- 42 CFR part 2 for regulations governing confidentiality of SUD treatment records: https://www.ecfr.gov/current/title-42/chapter-I/subchapter-A/part-2
- SAMHSA Federal Guidelines for Opioid Treatment Programs and Treatment capitalize Improvement Protocol (TIP) 63—both at the SAMHSA Store: https://store.samhsa.gov/
- SAMHSA's website with links to statutes, regulations and guidelines, including recent guidance letters to the field: https://www.samhsa.gov/medication-assisted-treatment/statutes-regulations-guidelines
- SAMHSA's OTP Extranet: https://otp-extranet.samhsa.gov/ HYPERLINK "https://store.samhsa.gov/product/Federal-Guidelines-for-Opioid-Treatment-Programs/PEP15-FEDGUIDEOTP"
- DEA regulations for NTPs can be found by entering "Narcotic Treatment Program" in the search field at: https://www.ecfr.gov/current/title-21/. DEA's NTP manual (a guide to its NTP regulations), revised in 2022: https://www.deadiversion.usdoj.gov/GDP/(DEA-DC-056)(EO-DEA169)_NTP_manual_Final.pdf
- US Health and Human Services OTP resources: https://www.hhs.gov/opioids/treatment/resources-opioid-treatment-providers/index.html

CHAPTER

63 Special Issues in Office-Based Opioid Treatment (OBOT)

Amy J. Kennedy and Andrew J. Saxon

CHAPTER OUTLINE

- Introduction
- Epidemiologic and regulatory issues
- Research issues
- Clinical issues
- Conclusions

INTRODUCTION

Current interest in office-based approaches for the treatment of opioid use disorder (OUD) springs in part from a recognition that the numbers and needs of individuals with this disorder continue to overwhelm the capacity of the traditional, program-based treatment system. In the United States, these traditional, program-based, federally licensed opioid treatment programs (OTPs) typically provide methadone and sometimes buprenorphine pharmacotherapy but are typically fewer in numbers and found less often outside of urban areas; whereas office-based opioid treatment (OBOT) is limited to buprenorphine only but is present in greater numbers and wider settings throughout the United States Many individuals with OUD cannot gain access to medication for opioid use disorder (MOUD), which is the most effective intervention yet devised for this disorder.[1] Meanwhile, indicators of opioid-related health care costs and criminal justice contacts continue to surge,[2,3] as does the number of opioid-related deaths.[4] Many individuals with OUD have unique and serious medical and psychiatric conditions that program-based treatment systems alone cannot always address, and which contribute to morbidity and mortality.[1] OBOT offers one potential avenue and has made substantial inroads in the drive to ameliorate this unsatisfactory situation.

In addition to referencing research on office-based treatment from France and the United Kingdom, this chapter reviews some of the historic and regulatory events that shaped the current treatment system in the United States and account for some of the ongoing gaps in services for individuals with OUD. Office-based treatment effectively fills some of these gaps, in part because office-based treatment encompasses two distinct treatment paradigms. First, OBOT offers a less structured, more flexible, and more personalized form of intervention for people with OUD who have succeeded in the traditional treatment system of opioid agonist clinics licensed by the Center for Substance Abuse Treatment of the Substance Abuse and Mental Health Services Administration but who need to continue in pharmacotherapy. Second, OBOT provides an alternative route of entry into treatment for individuals with OUD who, for a variety of reasons, have not accessed adequate treatment or wish to reengage in treatment after not achieving their goals in the traditional treatment system.

A summary of the evidence for the benefits of transferring selected, stable methadone-treated patients into office-based settings precedes a synopsis of efforts to apply and evaluate the office-based approach for less stable patients newly entering treatment. Results of these investigations of office-based treatment then guide a discussion of clinical issues pertinent to conducting office-based treatment with patients who have OUD. Finally, this chapter will briefly touch on changes to regulatory issues regarding office-based treatment of OUD during the COVID-19 pandemic.

EPIDEMIOLOGIC AND REGULATORY ISSUES

During the first few years of the 21st century, the purity of heroin sold in the United States continued to increase, while the price decreased.[5] Heroin-related emergency department visits increased from 33,900 in 1990 to 258,482 in 2011.[6] Heroin-related overdose deaths more than tripled between 2010 and 2014 rising to 3.4 per 100,000 individuals in the United States.[7] Overdose accounts for only half the overall observed mortality in people who use heroin, who exhibit mortality rates 6 to 20 times greater than those of age-matched populations.[8,9]

The past decades have also seen a surge in the illicit use of and problems with prescription opioid medications. Emergency department visits related to nonmedical use of opioid analgesics increased from 168,379 in 2005 to 366,181 in 2011.[10] Large numbers of overdoses on prescription opioids have also been noted.[7] In 2015, 3.78 million people in the United States inappropriately used prescription opioids in the past month.[11]

More recently, the United States has seen a significant increase in the illicit use of synthetic opioids, such as fentanyl. Fentanyl, a pharmaceutically developed opioid that is over 50 to 100 times stronger than morphine, has become widely used across the country's illicit substance market.[12] Its high potency has led to an increase in substance overdose deaths; more than 100,000 individuals died of a substance overdose in 2021, an increase in over 28% from the previous year.[7] A significant number of these deaths were from synthetic opioids (primarily fentanyl).

Despite these trends, most individuals with OUD cannot access adequate treatment services. In 2020, 2.7 million Americans were living with an OUD, but only 29.5% received medication treatment.[13] These data reflect a circumstance that has been prevalent throughout the past 100 years. The mobilization of OBOT as a response to this public health problem does not represent a true innovation but rather a return to a once commonly used strategy. Thousands of untreated individuals with OUD also worried society in the early part of the 20th century. Before the Harrison Narcotic Act was enacted in 1914 (see Chapter 35, "Addiction Medicine in America: Its Birth, Early History, and Current Status (1750-2022)"), physicians prescribed MOUD. Although controversy raged then as it does now surrounding treatment of individuals with OUD, many experts of that generation recognized the likelihood that patients with OUD would resume opioid use after enforced withdrawal. At the time, physicians in many areas of the country viewed opioid addiction as a medical disorder that could be managed from their outpatient offices and treated with prescribed medications such as full agonist opioids.

Most physicians caring for people with OUD practiced responsibly. A minority of physicians allowed their practice to become conduits for controlled substances out of a profit motive without always providing adequate medical care. Due to a small number of reports brought on by this type of inappropriate prescribing, concerns about the safety and efficacy of prescribing MOUD increased in the medical profession as well as among regulators and the general public. In 1919, the US Supreme Court ruled that the Harrison Act disallowed such physician prescribing to individuals with OUD for "maintenance" purposes.[14] This decision effectively ended the first era of OBOT.

This shift in policy left patients without access to MOUD. Municipalities responded by creating publicly funded and administered opioid agonist treatment clinics.[15] For example, when New York City experienced one of its waves of heroin addiction after World War I, a clinic under the auspices of the city health department treated 8000 patients with prescribed heroin.[16] These pioneer efforts at agonist pharmacotherapy ended within a few years when the Narcotic Division of the Federal Prohibition Unit shut down these clinics as violators of the Harrison Act.[15] Thus, from the 1920s onward, physicians were actively discouraged from treating individuals with OUD, and medical schools did not train physicians on the management of OUD. In essence, OUD was reconceptualized as a criminal legal issue rather than a medical condition. Convicted violators of the federal narcotics laws caused an overload in the federal penal system, so the Congress established "federal narcotics hospitals" at Lexington, KY, and Forth Worth, TX, in the 1930s. Despite high rates of disease recurrence, these isolated facilities remained the only treatment option for individuals with OUD until the advent of methadone maintenance 30 years later.[15]

The separation of OUD treatment from the general practice of medicine was exaggerated in the 1970s when opioid agonist therapy, in the form of methadone maintenance, once again was permitted in licensed treatment programs (OTPs). Federal methadone regulations (21 CFR Part 291) disseminated in 1972, and the Narcotic Addict Treatment Act of 1974 mandated a closed distribution system for methadone, with special licensing by both federal and state authorities. These regulations effectively made it illegal for physicians not associated with a licensed program to treat patients with OUD with agonist pharmacotherapy in an office setting. Until 2003, private physicians were required to obtain additional registration from the US Drug Enforcement Administration, annual certification by the US Department of Health and Human Services, and approval by state drug authorities to provide MOUD.[16] A small number of physicians around the country have been able and willing to negotiate this bureaucratic maze. As a result, the only option for patients who desired MOUD was to enroll in a specialized, licensed OTP. Once again, most practicing physicians had zero training or experience in treating people with OUD.

The disconnect between mainstream medicine and treatment for OUD led to some unfortunate consequences. OUD causes considerable medical morbidity because of drug effects and injection routes of administration.[17] Medical problems common in people who use illicit opioids include infectious diseases such as pneumonia, tuberculosis, endocarditis, as well as sexually transmitted diseases,[18] soft tissue infections,[19] bone and joint infections,[20] central nervous system infections,[21] and viral hepatitis.[22] particularly hepatitis C.[23] In addition, HIV infection poses a considerable problem among people who inject drugs (PWID). [22,24] Within the last decade, there have been several outbreaks of HIV among PWID both nationally and globally, highlighting a need for improved access to safe injection equipment and public health messaging.[25,26] Noninfectious problems also typically occur in the lungs,[27] the central and peripheral nervous systems,[21] the vascular system,[19] and the musculoskeletal system.[19] Licensed opioid agonist treatment programs often lack the resources to provide comprehensive medical care,[16] with the result that co-occurring medical disorders may be unattended, delaying care and driving up its ultimate cost. The economic burden to society in the United States from nonmedical prescription opioid use alone was $78.5 billion in 2013 with $28.9 billion of that total consumed by health care costs.[2]

Similarly, a high prevalence of co-occurring psychiatric disorders, particularly mood and anxiety disorders, is seen among patients with OUD,[28,29] and OTPs typically don't provide treatment for these co-occurring conditions.[16] Bridging the gap between general medical practice and OUD treatment would allow providers to simultaneously care for these chronic conditions.

Many patients interested in MOUD and willing to enroll in OTPs cannot overcome the barriers to entry. Geography creates an impossible hurdle for some. One state (Wyoming) does not offer licensed OTPs. In states that do offer programs, the licensed clinics, by virtue of economic necessity and neighborhood acceptance, tend to be located primarily in urban settings.[16,30] Even within larger metropolitan areas, specific neighborhoods or communities can oppose licensed clinics.[16,31] A few patients who reside in states or communities without OTPs or in rural areas invest considerable effort in traveling to other states or cities to obtain treatment; most who cannot afford the time or cost simply must forgo it.[30]

Inadequate treatment capacity creates another barrier for potential patients who live within reasonable proximity to an OTP.[32] Many clinics have waiting lists that discourage potential patients from even attempting entry.[33] Many more potential patients lack the financial resources to pay for their treatment.[33] Although OBOT does not necessarily cost less than treatment in an OTP, insurance companies and managed care organizations frequently reimburse at least some of the expense of physician office visits, particularly if co-occurring conditions are addressed.[32]

Finally, the rigid structure of licensed OTPs, with the potential to be recognized and stigmatized by passersby, waiting lines for medication administration, rigid attendance policies, and lack of privacy, deters some potential patients.[34]

Many of the latter concerns impact patients who have achieved their goals of recovery on opioid agonist treatment. Many have ceased illicit substance use and many are employed with additional family responsibilities.[32,35] To make their schedules accommodate frequent clinic visits with waits for medication, to hold up their travel plans to obtain regulatory approval, and to bring them to a locale where patients with active substance use congregate may undermine rather than support their recovery.[32,35] In addition, many of them have already derived maximum benefit from counseling and other services available at OTPs. Implementing a step-down approach and transferring stable patients out of a restrictive clinical setting while continuing their MOUD would facilitate reallocation of clinic resources to patients who most need them.

Four important developments altered the landscape of opioid agonist treatment in the United States. First, since 2001, stable, long-term patients in licensed OTPs can obtain medication for longer than 1 week. Second, the Children's Health Act of 2000, signed into law in October 2000, included a provision waiving the requirements of the Narcotic Addict Treatment Act to permit qualified physicians to dispense or prescribe schedule III, IV, or V narcotic drugs or combinations of such drugs that are approved by the Food and Drug Administration (FDA) for the treatment of OUD. This change, termed the *Drug Addiction Treatment Act* (DATA), allows qualified physicians to prescribe certain opioid agonist medications in an office-based setting. Third, in October 2002, the FDA approved buprenorphine and buprenorphine + naloxone for the treatment of Diagnostic and Statistical Manual-IV (DSM-IV) opioid dependence (now called OUD in DSM-5). These medications were placed in schedule III and are available for use in OBOT. Fourth, the more recent developments in regulations regarding OUD treatment occurred in March of 2020 at the start of the COVID-19 Pandemic. The Substance Abuse and Mental Health Service Administration (SAMHSA) in conjunction with the DEA, expanded access to OUD services by relaxing certain requirements regarding prescribing and dispensing of MOUD during the COVID-19 pandemic. Under the emergency provision, DATA 2000 waivered practitioners (both within and outside of an OTP) were allowed to prescribe buprenorphine for OUD over telemedicine/telephone services, waiving the requirement for an in-person examination. Additionally, in early 2021, the Health and Human Services (HHS) administration issued new practice guidelines for OUD, removing the requirements to complete an 8-hour training course to obtain a DEA X waiver to prescribe buprenorphine for prescribers who intend to treat 30 or fewer patients at any one time.

Although recent developments increased access to MOUD, the current U.S. treatment system cannot accommodate all the individuals with OUD who want or need treatment. A century ago, OBOT had some success in the United States in meeting the needs of people with OUD. The current reemergence of OBOT has also helped remove geographic, social, and regulatory barriers and made MOUD more widely available. Due to the historical divide between OUD treatment and general medical practice, offering provider education and training in the management of OUD has been necessary and will continue to be needed. Considerable data, described in detail in the subsequent text, offer instruction to providers.

RESEARCH ISSUES

Research Related to Stable, Long-Term Patients in Office-Based Practice

Several studies have demonstrated the overall safety and utility of transferring stable patients enrolled in licensed OTPs into an office-based (OBOT) setting (**Table 63-1**). The concept of transferring stable patients receiving methadone for OUD to office-based practice originated with Novick et al.[40,41] of New York City, who have utilized this step-down approach since 1983 and have documented their findings in several reports over the years. While countries outside of the United States prescribe methadone for OUD from an office-based setting, the United States requires special exemption for treatment outside of a licensed OTP.

Overall, data suggest patients who have achieved some degree of stability on methadone for the management of OUD within OTPs may transfer successfully to office-based care (OBOT). In addition, those patients who resume use of illicit substances in OBOT or are unable to meet clinic expectations can return to licensed OTPs without undue harm. The controlled studies also suggest that return to use or other problems in previously stable patients in office-based practice occur at rates no greater than those of similarly stable patients who remain in OTP care.

Research Related to Patients Entering Directly into Office-Based Practice

Although policies and attitudes in the United States had, until 2000, steered practitioners away from bringing unstable

TABLE 63-1 Studies of Stable Methadone-Treated Patients Transferred to OBO

Author, year	Method	Requirements for entry	*N*	Methadone dose (take-home)	Protocol retention	Use of illicit opioids	Use of Other illicit substances
Schwartz et al.[33]	Naturalistic program evaluation	Employment; 5 y on methadone; 5 year no illicit use	21	Mean = 71.4 mg (28 day supply)	71.4% over 12 years	None	2/21-1 cocaine-positive urinanalysis;1/21-1 positive barb urinalysis
Salsitz et al.[36]	Naturalistic program evaluation	Employment; 4-5 year on methadone; 3 y no illicit use	158	Mean = 60 mg (30-d supply)	83.5%; median retention = 13.8 year	None	15/158 excessive cocaine use
Merrill et al.[37]	Naturalistic program evaluation	1 year on methadone; 1 year no illicit use; responsible with take-home medications	30	Mean = 63 mg (30 day supply)	93.3% 12 month	445 of 449 (99%) of collected specimens negative; type of positive not specified	445 of 449 (99%) of collected specimens negative; type of positive not specified
Senay et al.[38]	Randomized clinical trial: medical maintenance vs control	Employment; 1 year on methadone; 6 month no illicit use	130	N/A (14 day supply)	73% reached 1 year for both conditions	2 experimental; 1 control	14 experimental; 8 control
Fiellin et al.[39]	Randomized clinical trial: office-based vs clinic treatment	Stable income, >1 year on methadone; 1 year free of illicit opioid use; no dependence on other substances	22 office; 24 standard	Mean = 69 mg office (7 day supply); mean = 70 mg standard (2- to 7-day supply)	82% office; 79% standard over 6 months	55% office; 42% standard	Cocaine use: 27% office; 25% standard
King et al., 2006	Randomized clinical trial: office-based vs monthly clinic pickup vs clinic	Employment; 1 year on methadone; 1 year free of illicit substance use; 2 years of no problems	32 office; 33 monthly pickup; 27 routine clinic care	Mean = 65 mg (28 day supply vs 3 to 7 day supply)	92% office; 79% monthly clinic; 82% routine clinic over 12 months	0.4% office; 2.3% monthly clinic; 1.3% routine clinic; type of substance not specified	0.4% office; 2.3% monthly clinic; 1.3% routine clinic; type of substance not specified

individuals with OUD directly into OBOT, other countries have, out of necessity and an innovative spirit, embraced this concept early on (Table 63-2).

For example, in Scotland, most patients are prescribed methadone for OUD in general practitioners' offices and pick up their medication in community pharmacies where methadone is dispensed.[42,57-60] These general practitioners receive training specific to this endeavor.[42] A 1-year follow-up of 204 patients with OUD who entered such a paradigm in 1996 has been reported by Hutchinson et al.[42] A total of 58 general practitioners provided treatment to patients with OUD. The study report does not specify the frequency or content of office visits, so practitioners presumably arranged their interventions on an individualized basis. The report also does not explicitly mention the frequency with which methadone doses were taken under observation, but it implies that this occurred on a daily or near-daily basis. Methadone dose levels are reported only for the 50 subjects who remained in continuous treatment for 12 months and who completed follow-up interviews. These subjects began at an average dose of 43 mg and increased to an average dose of 65 mg at 12 months. Follow-up interviews at 12 months were completed with 119 subjects (58.3%). Predictors of failure at follow-up included sex work, unstable living arrangements, higher proportion of substance-using associates, higher daily drug expenditures, a higher level of benzodiazepine use, and a higher proportion of income from unofficial sources. Among the 119 subjects followed up, 50 (42.4%) remained continuously on methadone for 12 months, 34 (28.8%) interrupted treatment and then resumed methadone treatment, and 35 stopped methadone treatment. In the group who stopped treatment, 39% did so because of imprisonment, 33% did so because they were taking other substances or behaving inappropriately in the pharmacy, and 27% left voluntarily because they disliked the program. In one analysis, the researchers imputed missing data for follow-up misses by carrying forward their baseline values. In this analysis, daily opioid injection use for the entire cohort declined from 80% at baseline to 43% at 12 months, the mean daily amount spent on illicit substances declined from £63 to £38, and the mean number of acquisitive crimes in the preceding month declined from 18 to 11. Another analysis that examined subjects followed up at 12 months compared 50 subjects who remained continuously on methadone with 57 subjects who interrupted methadone treatment during the first 6 months. Only 2% of those who remained continuously on methadone reported daily opioid injection use at 12 months as compared with 21% of those with interrupted treatment. Continuous treatment subjects were spending a daily mean of £4 on illicit substances at 12 months, compared with £16 for those with interrupted treatment. Continuous treatment subjects committed a mean of three acquisitive crimes in the preceding month, compared with five for those with interrupted treatment.

England also has had a policy since the 1980s encouraging individuals with OUD to receive methadone treatment outside of an OTP by general practitioners.[43] A nonrandomized comparison study evaluated subjects who began methadone in 1995, either in an OTP ($N = 297$) or with a general practitioner ($N = 155$). Training required for general practitioners was not described. At baseline, the two groups were similar in regard to illicit substance use except that the OTP group had greater use of amphetamines. The mean initial methadone dose was 51 mg (standard deviation [SD] = 18.7) for the general practitioner group and 48 mg (SD = 19.1) for OTP care. General practitioners prescribed less than daily dispensing for 43% of their patients, while OTP clinics allowed less than daily dispensing for only 25% of their patients. Only 14% of general practitioners required that methadone administration (at retail pharmacies) be supervised. Frequency of office visits with general practitioners was not described. Follow-up at 6 months was achieved with 76% of the original sample.

At 6 months, 66% of general practitioner patients and 60% of OTP clinic patients remained in treatment. In both groups, heroin use was reduced, on average, from more than 19 days per month at baseline to fewer than 10 days per month at follow-up; there was no significant difference between groups. All other substance use was reduced significantly and similarly for both groups. Drug injection use decreased among the general practitioner group from 53% to 41% and among the OTP care group from 66% to 53%. Non–drug-related crime fell among both groups but significantly more so among the general practitioner group.

France did not offer agonist pharmacotherapy to individuals with OUD until the introduction of methadone at OTPs in 1995.[44] Shortly thereafter, buprenorphine became available in France for the treatment of OUD, and general practitioners, regardless of their training, gained permission to prescribe it for this indication.[44,61] General practitioners in France can prescribe up to 28 days' supply of take-home medications and a maximum daily buprenorphine dose of 16 mg. As of 2004, about 65,000 patients per year had received buprenorphine in this office-based paradigm.[62] A nonrandomized comparison study examined outcomes for patients with OUD in France who were treated with buprenorphine by general practitioners ($N = 32$), compared with patients treated with buprenorphine at OTPs ($N = 37$).[44] The general practitioners had a fixed frequency of consultations, although the report does not specify the frequency. General practitioners performed urine testing weekly, required cannabis abstinence, and could arrange psychosocial services but did not necessarily have such services available. The OTPs had a variable frequency of consultations, had no systematic frequency of urine testing, did not require cannabis abstinence, but had psychosocial services directly available. Subjects self-selected their own treatment settings.

The two groups differed at baseline on important variables. The patients treated in the OTPs were older, less likely to be employed, had more polydrug use, experienced many more episodes of overdose, and were more likely to inject heroin. Doses of buprenorphine (5.9 mg/d for the general practitioner group versus 6.6 mg/d in the addiction center group) were relatively low in both groups. Treatment retention at 180 days was about 70% in the general practitioner group and about

TABLE 63-2 Studies of Patients Admitted Directly to Office-Based Opioid Treatment

Author, year	Method	Requirements for entry	N	Medication dose (take-home)	Protocol retention	Use of illicit opioids	Use of other illicit substances
Hutchinson et al.[42]	Naturalistic program evaluation	Opioid dependence	204	Methadone: mean initial dose = 43 mg	42.4% of 119 followed up at 12 months	2% daily heroin for subjects in continuous treatment	0% daily benzodiazepine for subjects in continuous treatment
Gossop et al.[43]	Nonrandomized comparison: GP office vs clinic	Opioid dependence	155-GP; 297 clinic	Methadone: mean initial dose = 51 mg (GP) or 48 mg (clinic)	6 month: 66% GP; 60% clinic	<10 d heroin use per month, both groups	Reduced significantly and equally for both groups
Vignau and Brunelle[44]	Nonrandomized comparison: GP office vs clinic	Opioid dependence	32-GP; 37 clinic	Buprenorphine: mean = 5.9 mg/d (GP) or 6.6 mg/d (clinic)	6 month:70% GP; 60% clinic	N/A	N/A
O'Connor et al.[45]	Randomized clinical trial: primary care clinic vs drug clinic treatment	Opioid dependence	23 in each condition	Buprenorphine: 22 mg Mon/Wed; 40 mg Fri	12 wk: 78% primary care; 52% drug clinic	63% positive UAs primary care; 85% drug clinic	33% cocaine-positive UAs both conditions
Fudala et al.[46]	Randomized clinical trial: buprenorphine vs buprenorphine + naloxone vs placebo	Opioid dependence	326 randomized subjects	Buprenorphine: 16 mg/d vs buprenorphine + naloxone 16/4 mg/d vs placebo (on weekends or holidays)	4 week: buprenorphine 86%; buprenorphine + naloxone 82%; placebo 75%	% negative urine specimens: buprenorphine 20.7%; buprenorphine + naloxone 17.8%; placebo 5.8%	Cocaine 40%-45%; benzodiazepines, 10%; no significant differences across groups
Walsh, 2007	Naturalistic study	Opioid dependence	582	Buprenorphine + naloxone: 2/0.5 mg/d to 24/6 mg/d (weekly to every 4 weeks)	62% at 16 weeks; 32% at 52 weeks	29.6% UAs positive at 3 months, 23.6% at 6 months, 19.0% at 12 months	Not reported
Fiellin et al.[47]	Randomized clinical trial: standard medical management with once vs thrice weekly buprenorphine + naloxone dispensing vs enhanced medical management with thrice weekly dispensing	Opioid dependence	166 randomized subjects	Buprenorphine + naloxone: 16/4 to 24/6 mg/d (once or thrice weekly dispensing)	39%-48% retention at 24 weeks with no significant difference across groups	40%-44% negative urine specimens with no difference across groups	71.1%-75.5% negative specimens for cocaine with no difference across groups
Alford et al.[48]	Retrospective chart review	Opioid dependence	41 housed, 44 homeless	Buprenorphine: dose not given (1 to 4 week supply of take-homes)	Mean = 9 month both groups	4% positive urines both groups at 12 months	8% positive urines both groups at 12 months
Magura et al.[49]	Retrospective chart review	Receiving buprenorphine in 1 of 6 offices in New York City	86	Buprenorphine: median dose = 15 mg	Median = 8 months	8% estimated to be using at data collection end point	16% estimated using at data collection end point

Mintzer et al.[50]	Chart abstraction	Receiving buprenorphine + naloxone in 1 of 3 primary care practices in Boston	99	Buprenorphine + naloxone: mean dose = 15.4 mg/d	Abstinent patients mean = 169 days; nonabstinent mean = 62 days	54% judged abstinent at 6 months	54% judged abstinent at 6 months
Fiellin et al.[51]	Naturalistic follow-up	Stable completion of randomized clinical trial of buprenorphine + naloxone for opioid dependence	53	Buprenorphine + naloxone: 16 mg to 24 mg/d	37.7% completed 2 years	91% opioid free	96% cocaine free; 98% benzodiazepine free
Parran et al.[52]	Retrospective chart review with telephone interviews	Opioid dependence	176 chart review; 110 completed interview	Buprenorphine + naloxone: 12/3 mg to 16/4 mg/d	85/110 (77%) remained on buprenorphine + naloxone when contacted 18-48 months after induction	13% using heroin at time of interview	7% using cocaine at time of interview
Alford et al.[53]	Cohort study in primary care using nurse care managers	Opioid dependence	382	Buprenorphine + naloxone: 8/2 mg to 16/4 mg/d	169/382 (44.2%) remained in treatment for 1 year	Of 169 remaining in treatment 12 months, 91% not using illicit opioids	Of 169 remaining in treatment 12 months, 91% not using cocaine
Fiellin et al.[54]	Prospective, nonrandomized, open-label study	Opioid dependence and HIV infection	303	Buprenorphine-naloxone: median dose = 16 mg/4 mg	49% retained at 12 months	42.4% among 49% retained (*N* = 191) during final 3 months	38.7% stimulants, 11.5% sedatives; among 49% retained (*N* = 191) during final 3 months
Fiellin et al.[55]	24-wk randomized clinical trial: physician management vs physician management plus cognitive-behavioral therapy	Opioid dependence	141	Buprenorphine-naloxone: 16 mg/4 mg	39%-45% at 24 weeks with no significant difference between treatment conditions	Mean = 0.4 d per week during second half of maintenance period with no significant difference between treatment conditions	Significant reduction in cocaine use with no significant difference between treatment conditions
Fiellin et al.[56]	14-wk randomized clinical trial: buprenorphine maintenance vs taper	Prescription opioid dependence	113	Buprenorphine-naloxone mean dose = 15.0 mg/3.0 mg	11% for taper condition; 66% for maintenance conditions	Opioid negative urine samples: 35.2% in taper condition; 53.2% in maintenance condition	Not reported

60% in the OTP group. Addiction Severity Index scores improved similarly for both groups from baseline to 90 days.

The first U.S. study to evaluate a quasi–office-based approach to individuals with OUD just entering treatment also used buprenorphine as an agonist pharmacotherapeutic agent.[45] Potential subjects with other substance or alcohol use disorders, recent cocaine use, or complex medical or co-occurring psychiatric disorders were excluded. Subjects were assigned randomly to receive 12 weeks of buprenorphine pharmacotherapy, either in a primary care setting or in a OTP setting that typically provided methadone treatment. The primary care setting was housed in a clinic designed to manage the primary care needs of people who use substances and patients with psychiatric disorders. Physicians in the primary care setting relied on a manual-guided clinical management protocol. Subjects assigned to the primary care setting ($N = 23$) received an initial 1-hour visit with a primary care provider, who recorded a substance use and medical history, created a treatment plan, made a referral to group psychotherapy, and prescribed buprenorphine. The subjects then saw their primary care provider in weekly 20-minute sessions. Group therapy conducted by a primary care nurse practitioner occurred weekly for 50 minutes, with a self-help focus on promoting abstinence.

Subjects assigned to OTP settings ($N = 23$) received a standard set of services, including individualized substance use disorder counseling and weekly relapse prevention group therapy. In both settings, subjects attended 5 days during week 1, with a buprenorphine dose escalation beginning at 2 mg and doubling daily until the dose reached 32 mg on day 5. From weeks 2 through 12, subjects attended clinic three times a week and received observed buprenorphine doses of 22 mg on Mondays and Wednesdays and 40 mg on Fridays. Thus, this study avoided prescribing take-home medications. Subjects in both settings provided urine specimens three times a week. Patients were withdrawn from the study for missing three consecutive medication doses or if they were unable to attend group therapy. Successful completion of 12 weeks of treatment was observed for 78% of the subjects in primary care, compared with 52% of the subjects in specialty care. Urine specimens were positive for opioids in 63% of primary care subjects, compared with 85% of OTP subjects. Primary care subjects showed a decreasing trend of opioid-positive specimens over time, whereas OTP subjects did not. Roughly a third of urine specimens in both groups tested positive for cocaine.[45]

This study lends some support to the notion that treatment-seeking patients with OUD can derive as much benefit from treatment in an office-based setting as from an OTP setting. Nevertheless, the researchers themselves properly note several aspects of the study design that limit its applicability to a true office-based setting. The primary care setting in this study required many more visits and more observed medication administration than would be practical in a typical office-based practice. The clinic used for the primary care setting had much more familiarity and expertise with patients who use substances than would most office-based settings. The study excluded patients with the medical and psychiatric complications commonly seen in treatment seekers with OUD.

Another, much larger U.S. study also examined a quasi–office-based approach for patients with OUD just entering treatment.[46] This study differed from the others in that it did not compare an office-based with an OTP approach but rather compared different medication strategies within a quasi–office-based setting. In this randomized, double-blind, placebo-controlled, multicenter trial, 326 subjects were randomly assigned to receive (1) buprenorphine 16 mg/d, (2) buprenorphine 16 mg + naloxone 4 mg/d, or (3) placebo. Medication was administered in office-based settings affiliated with Veterans Affairs Medical Centers. Subjects received their doses 5 days a week, with take-home medications given for weekends and holidays. The trial was terminated early because of the demonstrated efficacy of buprenorphine + naloxone compared with placebo. Subjects treated with either buprenorphine alone or buprenorphine + naloxone had a greater proportion of urine specimens that were negative for opiates than did the subjects given placebo. The rate of adverse events was manageable and comparable between the two active treatments.

One of the largest studies yet conducted of office-based treatment, A Multicenter Safety Trial of Buprenorphine + Naloxone for the Treatment of Opiate Dependence, consisted of an uncontrolled, naturalistic investigation that examined outcomes for 582 individuals with OUD newly entering office-based treatment. Patients were not excluded for psychiatric or medical problems (other than pregnancy, because buprenorphine + naloxone was not then approved for use in pregnant patients) if the treating physician could manage the problems on her or his own or by appropriate referral. Patients were treated by 38 physicians in seven states with buprenorphine + naloxone, in doses ranging from 2 mg/0.5 mg to 24 mg/6 mg/d. Medications were dispensed by institutional and community pharmacies. Physicians and pharmacists involved in the study received at least 8 hours of training in the pharmacology of buprenorphine + naloxone and issues pertinent to office-based treatment of OUD. Treatment lasted up to a year. Patients were seen by the physicians at least twice in the first week of treatment, at least weekly during weeks 2 through 12 of treatment, at least biweekly from weeks 13 to 26, and monthly thereafter until week 52. For stable patients, medication dispensing followed a pattern similar to the office visits, so that in the final 6 months of treatment, patients could have monthly medication pickups. Urine toxicology screens were obtained onsite at each office visit. Return to use prevention counseling was available and encouraged but not required. Patients who became stable early in treatment had the option to taper the dose of buprenorphine + naloxone between weeks 7 and 9 and to complete treatment at that time.

Most patients (97.6%) successfully initiated treatment with the buprenorphine-naloxone combination. Most patients received 4 mg (22%), 8 mg (33%), or 16 mg (18%) on their first day. The most common stabilizing doses prescribed to patients were 8 mg (11%), 16 mg (26%), and 24 mg (29%). The 16-week completion/retention rate was 362 (62%), with

189 patients (32.5%) completing either a supervised withdrawal or 52 full weeks of treatment. Patients demonstrated a significant decrease in percent of opioid-positive urines over time. There was significant improvement in composite scores for drug, legal, and family/social domains of the Addiction Severity Index. A significant reduction in HIV risk behavior was also seen (R. Walsh, personal communication, 2007). Four subsequent smaller uncontrolled studies of patients treated for OUD with buprenorphine + naloxone showed outcomes quite similar to those found in the multicenter safety study.[48-50,63]

As mandated by the Drug Addiction Treatment Act, SAMHSA conducted a 3-year evaluation of the impact of buprenorphine availability between 2002 and 2005.[64] Among the data sources used for this evaluation were surveys of 959 addiction medicine specialists (80% response rate), surveys of 1837 physicians who had obtained a waiver to prescribe buprenorphine (86% response rate), and telephone interviews with 433 buprenorphine-treated patients recruited through prescribing physicians' offices or clinics. The results showed that about half the patients receiving buprenorphine had never previously received opioid agonist treatment. More than half the patients surveyed did not use heroin and were consuming prescription opioids. Both the patients and the physicians overwhelmingly believed that buprenorphine was effective. At 6 months after treatment initiation, more than 70% of patients remained in treatment or had completed treatment, and 81% were abstinent from nonprescribed opioids. Increases in employment and decreases in criminal activity occurred among the patient group. MOUD became available in geographic locations previously not served.

All these early evaluations of direct entry to office-based treatment for OUD support its viability as a treatment option and show its acceptance by patients, physicians, and pharmacists. Treatment retention in these office-based investigations did not fall markedly below—nor did illicit opioid use rise strikingly above—rates reported in recent clinic-based investigations of opioid agonist treatment, even though the European studies discussed here used doses of agonist medications that currently would be considered less than optimal.

Recent years have witnessed a considerable increase in reports in the literature regarding OBOT with buprenorphine. Five will be highlighted here because of data they provide on longer-term outcomes, on effects of this intervention in impoverished populations, on individuals with co-occurring OUD and HIV infection, and on the impact of additional behavioral treatment given in addition to basic physician management.

One study of longer-term outcomes arose as an extension of a randomized controlled trial.[63] The controlled trial enrolled and randomized 166 patients to one of three treatments over 24 weeks: (1) standard medical management with once weekly buprenorphine + naloxone dispensing, (2) standard medical management with thrice weekly buprenorphine + naloxone dispensing, and (3) enhanced medical management with thrice weekly buprenorphine + naloxone dispensing. Standard medical management involved brief, manual-guided, medically focused counseling (20 minutes); enhanced management used similar techniques, but each session was extended (45 minutes). The mean maintenance buprenorphine dose was 17.5 mg. All three treatments had statistically indistinguishable outcomes and so showed no advantage for extended counseling or more frequent buprenorphine + naloxone dispensing. Of the 166 patients randomized in the trial, 53 (32%) achieved at least 9 consecutive weeks free of illicit opioid use. These patients were enrolled in a long-term study.[51] Thirty-seven and a half percent of patients remained in treatment for at least 2 years beyond the original 24 weeks, and 24.5% remained 3 years or longer. Of 1106 urine toxicology specimens provided, 91% were negative for illicit opioids.

A second study of longer-term outcomes included 176 patients with OUD from both high and low socioeconomic status started on buprenorphine + naloxone in the office setting with buprenorphine doses of 12 to 16 mg/d, although all were also enrolled in intensive outpatient treatment.[52] Data were collected via retrospective chart review and cross-sectional phone interviews conducted 18 to 42 months after starting the medication. Among the 110 patients (67%) who completed the interview, 77% remained continuously on buprenorphine + naloxone. Patients who continued buprenorphine + naloxone were significantly less likely to have used heroin or any substance and to be employed at both baseline and follow-up. High socioeconomic status patients were more likely to be employed at baseline but not at follow-up. Low socioeconomic status patients were more likely to remain continuously on buprenorphine + naloxone but also more likely to have substance use at follow-up.

An examination of 408 patients with OUD treated with buprenorphine + naloxone at doses of 8 mg/2 mg/d or 16 mg/4 mg/d in a primary care setting using nurse care managers showed that of 382 who could be evaluated, 187 (49%) remained successfully in treatment for 1 year, and 9 (2.4%) were stable for at least 6 months and successfully tapered off medication.[53] Among those who completed 1 year, 91% were no longer using opioids or cocaine based upon urine toxicology testing. Predictors of success in a multivariate analysis were White, older age, and prior nonprescribed use of buprenorphine.

Among 303 patients with OUD and HIV infection treated in HIV primary care clinics with buprenorphine + naloxone at a median dose (buprenorphine) of 16 mg/d over 1 year in a prospective, multisite, clinical demonstration project, 49% remained on buprenorphine + naloxone for the entire year.[54] Rates of illicit substance use decreased from 84% at baseline to 42% among patients retained for the full year. This study demonstrates both the feasibility and effectiveness of integrating office-based opioid treatment into HIV care.

A question often arises concerning how much behavioral or psychosocial intervention is needed in addition to basic physician office management for patients receiving buprenorphine for OUD. To address this point, 141 such patients treated in a primary care clinic were randomly assigned to receive either physician management alone or physician management with an added 12-week course of manual-guided cognitive-behavioral treatment for substance use disorders.[55] Illicit opioid use decreased significantly and equivalently in both groups, and both had equivalent study retention over 24 weeks. Two other studies, though not conducted in office-based settings, found similarly that the addition of substance use counseling[65] or the addition of cognitive-behavioral therapy and/or contingency management[66] to physician management alone did not produce superior outcomes. Thus, current evidence suggests that while adding behavioral interventions to physician management of OUD with buprenorphine may have benefit for unmeasured outcomes such as interpersonal functioning or promoting productive activities, it is unlikely to have much additional effect on reduction of illicit opioid use or treatment retention.

Whether patients in OBOT should continue on medication for OUD or be tapered is another question that frequently comes up. One study examined this topic by randomly assigning 113 patients with DSM-IV prescription opioid dependence to 14 weeks of continuous buprenorphine treatment or 6 weeks of stabilization followed by a 3-week taper and the offer of naltrexone treatment. Patients in the group who continued buprenorphine treatment had far less illicit opioid use and much greater rates of completing the 14-week study.[56] Another study, not conducted in an office-based setting, also found very low success rates with a buprenorphine taper.[65] Therefore, current evidence argues buprenorphine should be continued for the first several months of treatment at the least.

CLINICAL ISSUES

OBOT has increased considerably in the past few years, and the body of evidence reviewed offers ideas and recommendations relevant to clinical practice in this setting. As mentioned earlier in this chapter, it makes sense to divide this discussion into two segments: one most pertinent to care of long-term, stable patients transferred from a licensed OTP and one focused on management of patients who are admitted de novo to an office-based setting.

Patients Transferred From OTP

Identifying patients who will continue to successfully meet their goals once transferred to an OBOT setting is a key element of this paradigm. A comparison of the various studies discussed earlier gives rise to the expected impression that more stringent selection criteria with more required time and stability in OTP treatment led to better success after transfer to office-based treatment. When several years of treatment and stability are required,[33,36] patients exhibit no illicit opioid use and minimal other substance use and most remain in the protocol for many years. Within the group of subjects in the study by Salsitz et al.,[36] more episodes of methadone treatment and longer time in treatment were associated with a greater likelihood of continued success in OBOT. When less stringent selection criteria are used,[39,67] illicit substance use is more likely to manifest in the office-based setting.

Successful patient transfer from OTP to OBOT will also depend on how resumed substance use is managed in a step-down setting such as OBOT. The programs thus far reported in the literature and reviewed here tolerated very little use before initiating transfer of the patient back to OTP care. Since patients in OBOT may have a larger quantities of take-home methadone doses, this conservative approach toward resumed substance use makes sense. Nevertheless, the controlled studies indicate that substance use did not differ based on treatment in office-based versus OTP care.[68]

What remains unknown is whether patients transferred to OBOT who resume substance use will continue to deteriorate in OBOT and benefit from a transfer to a higher level of care such as an OTP, or whether such episodes of return to use could be managed as effectively within an office-based setting, presuming a practical mechanism exists to limit the number of take-home doses of methadone provided until stability is regained. The report by Salsitz et al.[36] described the need for termination of 15 patients with serious use of cocaine who could not be treated within private practice, but it does not specify what measures might be taken within an office-based setting to address this type of situation. The stepped care intensification procedure used in the study by King et al.[68] offered one model for managing resumed substance use in office-based settings that does not preclude rapid return to office-based care. Future studies could help to answer this question through controlled trials that randomly assign office-based patients with resumed substance use either to stay in office-based care or transfer back to a higher level of care such as an OTP.

Further, office-based practitioners have different levels of risk tolerance and experience managing episodes of resumed use. Those less experienced may choose to transfer the patient to a higher level of care, while others may choose to increase monitoring and/or support by increased number of office visits, a referral to counseling or self-help groups, or an increase in the methadone dose.

Concerns about return to use lead directly to a consideration of techniques for monitoring stable patients in OBOT. All the studies described used urine toxicology screening, which would be a common practice in licensed OTPs. Apart from the study by Senay et al.,[38] these studies typically collected monthly urine samples often in a nonrandom fashion. In the study by Fiellin et al.,[39] subjects who provided positive urine samples were required to provide a second sample within the following week. The study by King et al.[68] used a monthly, random medication callback schedule that also required subjects to give a random urine sample. Rates of illicit substance use were lower in this study than in the study by Fiellin et al.,[39] even though the subject populations appear to be relatively similar. Despite the dangers of comparing results across different studies, these observations lead to speculation that the random nature of the callback procedures in the King et al.[68] study may have deterred some illicit substance use. Although the regular and frequent callback procedure used in that study might prove somewhat cumbersome in a purely clinical setting, the data argue for physicians who provide MOUD in an office-based setting to institute some type of callback procedure. The office-based subjects in the King et al.[68] study were highly satisfied with their treatment, even though the callback procedures meant that they had to visit their physician's office twice rather than once a month. A callback procedure may also help minimize the risk of nonmedical use of medication or diversion.

A monitoring plan for patients on MOUD that would be practical in OBOT would involve nonrandom urine samples at the time of scheduled office visits; unscheduled callbacks if any clinical evidence of instability arises, with medication checks and provision of random urine samples; and a very quick callback after any positive results to obtain a repeat sample within a few days. The latter part of the plan recommends the provider use a laboratory with a rapid turnaround and respond to positive test results as soon as possible. Alternatively, with the technology to conduct onsite urine testing now readily available, OBOT with that capacity could detect resumed substance use at the time of the office visit. A more frequent medication pickup schedule could be instituted immediately, along with plans to return for repeat urine monitoring.

The clinical management of methadone pharmacotherapy encompasses another major consideration, ongoing dose changes. A substantial number of subjects in the investigation by Salsitz et al.[36] required methadone dose changes. Providers who treat patients with methadone in OBOT will need to remain alert to the need for alterations in medication dose. Methadone plasma concentrations can change over time in response to a variety of somewhat unpredictable environmental factors, and such changes could lead to variations in clinical medication effects.[67,69] Thus, providers should frequently inquire about symptoms such as rhinorrhea, lacrimation, chills, nausea, diarrhea, muscle aches, and insomnia and assess whether these symptoms could be related to opioid withdrawal. They should assess for ongoing triggers and cravings. If such symptoms are occurring, an increase in the methadone dose should be considered. Similarly, providers should ask about possible methadone side effects (such as constipation, excess sedation, or lowered libido) and offer alternatives to address them. In the absence of serious side effects or serious risk of resumed use, patient's wishes about dose changes often serve as the best guide to clinical decision-making.[70]

Psychosocial interventions form another potentially valuable element of OBOT for transferred patients. It would be expected, in general, that such interventions would be brief and might be minimal or unnecessary for the highly stable, long-term patients seen in the studies by Salsitz et al.[36] and Schwartz et al.[33] In the context of an office visit, it would be desirable for the provider to ask about the patient's substance and alcohol use and cravings; how the patient is doing at work and/or with family or childcare responsibilities, financial and housing circumstances; about psychiatric and medical status; and about use of leisure time. In most cases, long-term patients will indicate in a few words that they have maintained stability in these areas of their lives. If a patient acknowledges some problem or added stress, a few moments to delineate the scope of the difficulty, express concern, and empathy, and provide support, advice, and encouragement may suffice to assist the patient in coping with mild or moderate distress. If the problem seems more severe, the office-based provider must either arrange more frequent sessions with the patient or have ready access to referral to counseling resources. Some of the office-based paradigms described earlier[37,68] had ongoing arrangements for temporary intensification of counseling services at the OTP.

Patients Newly Engaging in OBOT

The clinical management of unstable newly engaged OBOT patients with OUD poses challenges that are both distinct and similar to challenges associated with stable patients. Patients who enter directly into OBOT exhibit marked reductions in substance use, risk behavior, and criminality; also, they have higher rates of patients discontinuing treatment and using substances when compared to stable patients. Even in the study by O'Connor et al.,[45] which excluded subjects with recent cocaine use or serious psychiatric or medical problems, rates of patients discontinuing treatment and using substances were substantial. Apart from that study, most investigations of direct entry into OBOT have applied no exclusions to admission, so little direct scientific information exists to guide patient selection. To a certain extent, patient selection for direct entry into OBOT must rely on the specific areas of expertise and clinical skills of the treating provider. Through thorough assessment, including a complete history and physical examination, the provider should ascertain whether they can comfortably manage—either by direct care or by adequate referral networks—the combination of substance use problems, general medical problems, psychiatric problems, and life crises likely to arise in the treatment of each patient. Providers should refer patients who are not good candidates for their practice settings to licensed OTPs. Although the current evidence suggests that many patients who enter directly into OBOT treatment have a smooth course, many remain unstable for some time.

As with stable, transferred patients, identifying appropriate monitoring strategies will help patients newly engaged in OBOT reach their treatment goals. Again, no clear scientific data are currently available to guide precise techniques or monitoring schedules. Urine toxicology testing and medication callbacks if indicated, coupled with regular clinical evaluation, likely will continue to serve as the mainstays of monitoring. As telemedicine services become more prominent in the COVID-19 era, new monitoring practices will need be standardized as well.

The ability to modify medication-dispensing schedules provide an additional mechanism for increased monitoring for those who benefit from closer follow up. Monitoring and dispensing schedules will vary much more for newly entering patients, with more intensity of services expected initially, later decreasing as indicators of stability appear. Such indicators would include reaching established treatment plan goals, attending scheduled office visits, taking medication as prescribed, decrease or abstinence of substance use, involvement in daily routines and activities, supportive interpersonal relationships, and the absence of criminal legal involvement. As such signs of stability appear, medication dispensing can be liberalized from once a week to biweekly, or monthly, with an appropriate number of take-home doses. The frequency of scheduled office visits, urine testing, and medication callbacks can be adjusted in a similar fashion. If signs of instability reappear, any or all of these monitoring techniques can be readjusted for greater frequency.

As in the treatment of stable, transferred patients, careful titration of pharmacotherapy of newly entering patients can contribute to their stability. The provider needs considerable skill to prescribe buprenorphine, particularly in view of its potential to precipitate opioid withdrawal during induction of patients with high levels of physical dependence.[71-73] This characteristic of buprenorphine generally dictates initiation of pharmacotherapy at low doses, followed by dose escalation as soon as the patient demonstrates medication tolerance. Throughout the course of treatment, as in the care of transferred patients, the provider will need to be alert to the signs and symptoms described earlier and be ready to adjust the dose.

The potential for medication diversion should be considered as changes in frequency and dose are incorporated into patients' treatment plans. The presence of illicit methadone and buprenorphine in the community lets us know that some diversion is indeed occurring. Scant firm data exist on the frequency, or the patient characteristics and behaviors associated with diversion, though self-reports suggest that 18% to 28% of patients in treatment with methadone or buprenorphine have diverted or received diverted medications.[74] Not responding to medication callbacks or recurring requests for early refills may offer some warning signs. A negative urine test for methadone metabolite or buprenorphine or its metabolite norbuprenorphine also suggests possible diversion. Other more subtle but certainly not pathognomonic signs might be a sudden unexplained increase in disposable income or a sudden request for a dose increase in a previously stable patient without clear clinical explanation. Providers should discuss with patients at the onset of treatment safety concerns surrounding prescribed opioid medications including the importance of safely handling and storing their medication. Patients should be aware that monitoring is incorporated into their care as a means to promote safety and evaluate treatment response. If safety concerns arise, and OBOT is unable to increase monitoring, providers may consider transferring the person to a higher level of care such as an OTP.

Psychosocial treatments may be even more important to patients who are newly entering OBOT than to stable patients who already have received regular counseling at an OTP. Scant scientific data are available to provide reliable instruction as to the optimal modality or frequency of psychosocial treatments for these patients. The uncontrolled studies conducted in Britain did not evaluate the variety of psychosocial treatments prescribed by providers. The study by O'Connor et al.[45] used weekly provider visits and weekly group therapy—an intensity of psychosocial services that might not be available or reimbursable in most clinical settings. Studies of various intensities of psychosocial services in licensed methadone programs[75-77] do offer some illumination on this point: patients who receive minimal psychosocial services do not fare as well as do those who receive moderate or high levels of services; however, the lower cost-effectiveness of more intensive services may nullify any slight advantage they hold over moderate services.[77,78] One controlled study of the efficacy of weekly extended medical management counseling (45-minute sessions) compared to weekly standard medical management counseling (20-minute sessions) added to buprenorphine + naloxone treatment, as noted above, found no advantage from the extended counseling.[47] As noted above, recent evidence suggests that high-quality medical management may be sufficient for many newly entering patients.[55,65,66] For patients struggling to reach their treatment goals, additional psychosocial services could be offered and integrated. One convenient way to provide free psychosocial services is by referral to mutual help groups in the community. Sometimes such groups are not supportive of pharmacotherapy for OUD, so it behooves the provider to assist patients in locating groups that will not stigmatize them for taking appropriately prescribed medications. Many of the studies summarized here used some form of brief provider training before the provider engaged in OBOT. As with many aspects of OBOT, little empirical evidence exists to specify the optimal training method. Practicing providers have limited amounts of time in their schedules for training, so a brief course might be most feasible. At present, providers in the United States are eligible to prescribe office-based buprenorphine for OUD to thirty or fewer patients at any one time after submitting a written notice of intent for an X-waiver to the SAMHSA. To prescribe buprenorphine to greater than 30 concurrent patients, physicians must complete 8 hours of formal training, and physician assistants and nurse practitioners are eligible with 24 hours of formal training. Expert consensus suggests that appropriate training should consist of most of the following topics: (1) overview of OUD and rationale for agonist treatment; (2) legislation permitting office-based treatment; (3) general opioid pharmacology; (4) pharmacology of buprenorphine and buprenorphine + naloxone; (5) efficacy and safety of buprenorphine; (6) clinical use of buprenorphine, including induction, stabilization, and withdrawal; (7) patient assessment and selection; (8) office management, including treatment agreements, urine testing, record keeping, and confidentiality; (9) co-occurring psychiatric and medical disorders; (10) psychosocial treatments; and (11) special populations, including adolescents, pregnancy, and patients with pain.

CONCLUSIONS

Patients with OUD clearly need medical treatment, which has not always been readily available. In recent decades, the system has tried to meet the challenge by providing MOUD at licensed OTPs. This approach has greatly improved the outcomes and lives of many patients but has failed to accommodate many others because of inadequate capacity and because, for some individuals, attendance at such a program creates undue hardships. Robust peer reviewed scientific data now show that transfer of patients who have 1 or 2 years of demonstrated stability in a licensed OTP to OBOT leads to outcomes comparable to those obtained if the patients had continued at a licensed clinic. If such patients become unstable in OBOT, they can be transferred safely back to clinic care.

OBOT is oftentimes more accessible leaving patients with more time to pursue activities that support their recovery. Moreover, transferring patients to OBOT opens treatment slots in the licensed OTP to previously untreated patients. Now that many thousands of patients have been treated in office settings, the appropriate management techniques (including patient selection, monitoring, and pharmacotherapy) have been reasonably well established.

Studies of OBOT of patients with OUD newly entering treatment likewise suggest that such care is reasonable for many such patients and that their short-term outcomes appear nearly equivalent to those achieved with similar patients in traditional licensed programs. More can still be learned about optimal management techniques in office-based treatment via additional rigorous research.

As more knowledge has accrued about office-based treatment of OUD, and as it has become a more widespread practice, some positive "ripple effects" have ensued. The "treatment gap" has narrowed somewhat as more patients who live in a variety of locations and with varying needs have gained access to MOUD. The medical and addiction treatment systems have taken small steps toward reintegration. With these efforts, ideally co-occurring medical and psychiatric issues will be attended to more fully, and providers may become more willing to address other substance use disorders in addition to OUD. Society in general may benefit from reductions in crime and its associated costs, from an increased engagement in the workforce by previously unemployable individuals, and, possibly, from an overall decline in health care expenditures shifted from acute care for the medical sequelae of untreated OUD.

Concerning Veterans and Office-Based Treatment of Opioid Use Disorder

Office-based treatment with buprenorphine has seen rapid uptake for veterans with opioid use disorder (OUD) treated by the Department of Veterans Affairs. The number of veterans receiving buprenorphine increased from 300 at 27 facilities in 2004 to 6147 in 118 facilities in 2010.[79] Unfortunately, consistent with the nationwide epidemic of OUD described in this chapter, the number of veterans with OUD receiving care at the VA increased by 45% during that same interval so that the proportion of veterans with OUD getting medication for OUD had not gone above 27%.[79] In 2016, the number of VA patients receiving buprenorphine rose again to 12,525 but still represented only 20.9% of those diagnosed with OUD. An additional 4045 (6.8% of those with OUD) received naltrexone. In 2017, this number had risen to 35%.[80] In 2018 the VA launched a national initiative, Stepped Care for Opioid Use Disorder Train the Trainer (SCOUTT) which intended to increase treatment for OUD in primary care, pain clinics, and general mental health. By the third quarter of fiscal year 2022 an upward trajectory in OUD treatment continued to be evident. Of 59,563 patients diagnosed with OUD across the VA nationally, 27,431 (46.6%) were receiving some form of MOUD at that time. Though a treatment gap still exists in the VA, as it does elsewhere, and more widespread implementation of buprenorphine treatment is still needed, the VA is far ahead of most other health care systems in making MOUD available.[81]

REFERENCES

1. National Consensus Development Panel on Effective Medical Treatment of Opiate Addiction (Consensus Development Panel). Effective medical treatment of opiate addiction. *JAMA*. 1998;280(22):136-143.
2. Florence CS, Zhou C, Luo F, Xu L. The economic burden of prescription opioid overdose, abuse, and dependence in the United States, 2013. *Med Care*. 2016;54(10):901-906.
3. Oderda GM, Lake J, Rudell K, Roland CL, Masters ET. Economic burden of prescription opioid misuse and abuse: a systematic review. *J Pain Palliat Care Pharmacother*. 2015;29(4):388-400.
4. Center for Disease Control/National Center for Health Statistics. *Drug Overdose Deaths in the U.S. Top 100,000 Annually*. Accessed June 20, 2022. https://www.cdc.gov/nchs/pressroom/nchs_press_releases/2021/20211117.htm.
5. U.S. Department of Justice National Drug Intelligence Center. *National Drug Threat Assessment 2011*. Product No. 2011-Q0317-001. U.S. Department of Justice National Drug Intelligence Center; 2011.
6. Substance Abuse and Mental Health Services Administration. Accessed October 21, 2016. http://www.samhsa.gov/data/emergency-department-data-dawn/reports?tab=26
7. Rudd RA, Aleshire N, Zibbell JE, Gladden RM. Increases in drug and opioid overdose deaths in the United States, 2000-2014. *MMWR Morb Mortal Wkly Rep*. 2016;64(50-51):1378-1382.
8. Substance Abuse and Mental Health Services Administration. *Drug Abuse Warning Network, 2009: Area Profiles of Drug-Related Mortality*. HHS Publication No. (SMA) 11-4639, DAWN Series D-24. SAMHSA; 2011.
9. Darke S, Zador D. Fatal heroin "overdose": a review. *Addiction*. 1996;91(12):1765-1772.
10. Office of National Drug Control Policy. *Arrestee Drug Abuse Monitoring (ADAM II) 2010 Annual Report*. Vol. 2011 ONDCP, Executive Office of the President:29-31.
11. Crane EH. *The CBHSQ Report: Emergency Department Visits Involving Narcotic Pain Relievers*. Substance Abuse and Mental Health Services Administration, Center for Behavioral Health Statistics and Quality; 2015.

12. Drug Enforcement Administration (DEA): 2020 National Drug Threat Assessment. March 2021. Accessed June 20, 2022. https://www.dea.gov/sites/default/files/2021-02/DIR-008-21%202020%20National%20Drug%20Threat%20Assessment_WEB.pdf
13. Center for Behavioral Health Statistics and Quality. *2020 National Survey on Drug Use and Health: Detailed Tables.* Substance Abuse and Mental Health Services Administration; 2022.
14. Substance Abuse and Mental Health Services Administration, Center for Behavioral Health Statistics and Quality. *Treatment Episode Data Set (TEDS): 2004-2014.* National Admissions to Substance Abuse Treatment Services. BHSIS Series S-84, HHS Publication No. (SMA) 16-4986. SAMHSA; 2016.
15. Musto DF. *The American Disease.* Oxford University Press; 1987.
16. Wren CS. Holding an uneasy line in the long war on heroin: methadone emerged in city now debating it. *New York Times.* October 3, 1998.
17. Cooper JR. Including narcotic addiction treatment in an office-based practice. *JAMA.* 1995;273(20):1619-1620.
18. Cushman P. The major medical sequelae of opioid addiction. *Drug Alcohol Depend.* 1980;5:239-254.
19. Haverkos HW, Lange WR. Serious infections other than human immunodeficiency virus among intravenous drug abusers. *J Infect Dis.* 1990;161:894-902.
20. Makower RM, Pennycock AG, Moulton C. Intravenous drug abusers attending an inner city accident and emergency department. *Arch Emerg Med.* 1992;9:32-39.
21. Chandrasekar PH, Narula AP. Bone and joint infections in intravenous drug abusers. *Rev Infect Dis.* 1986;6:904-911.
22. Rubin AM. Neurologic complications of intravenous drug abuse. *Hosp Pract.* 1987;22:279-288.
23. Chamot E, de Saussure PH, Hirschel B, Déglon JJ, Perrin LH. Incidence of hepatitis C, hepatitis B and HIV infections among drug users in a methadone maintenance programme. *AIDS.* 1992;6:430-431.
24. Dieperink E, Willenbring M, Ho SB. Neuropsychiatric symptoms associated with hepatitis C and interferon alpha: a review. *Am J Psychiatry.* 2000;157:867-876.
25. Des Jarlais DC, Sypsa V, Feelemyer J, et al. HIV outbreaks among people who inject drugs in Europe, North America, and Israel. *Lancet HIV.* 2020;7(6):e434-e442. doi:10.1016/S2352-3018(20)30082-5
26. Strathdee SA, Kuo I, El-Bassel N, Hodder S, Smith LR, Springer SA. Preventing HIV outbreaks among people who inject drugs in the United States: plus ça change, plus ça même chose. *AIDS.* 2020;34(14):1997-2005. doi:10.1097/QAD.0000000000002673
27. Selwyn PA, Alcabes P, Hartel D. Clinical manifestations and predictors of disease progression in drug users with human immunodeficiency virus infection. *N Engl J Med.* 1992;327:1697-1703.
28. O'Donnell AE, Pappas LS. Pulmonary complications of intravenous drug abuse, experience at an inner city hospital. *Chest.* 1988;94:251-253.
29. Brooner RK, King VL, Kidorf M, Schmidt CW Jr, Bigelow GE. Psychiatric and substance use comorbidity among treatment-seeking opioid abusers. *Arch Gen Psychiatry.* 1997;54(1):71-80.
30. Mason BJ, Kocsis JH, Melia D, et al. Psychiatric comorbidity in methadone maintained patients. *J Addict Dis.* 1998;17(3):75-89.
31. Wren CS. Ex-addicts find methadone more elusive than heroin. *New York Times.* February 2, 1997.
32. Roane KR. Legislation for those with a methadone clinic next door. *New York Times.* April 6, 1997.
33. Schwartz RP, Brooner RK, Montoya ID, Currens M, Hayes M. A 12-year follow-up of a methadone medical maintenance program. *Am J Addict.* 1999;8(4):293-299.
34. Modie N. More heroin addicts may be offered treatment. *Seattle Post-Intelligencer.* December 8; 1999.
35. Hunt DE, Lipton DS, Goldsmith DS, Strug DL, Spunt B. "It takes your heart": the image of methadone maintenance in the addict world and its effect on recruitment into treatment. *Int J Addict.* 1985;20(11-12):1751-1771.
36. Salsitz EA, Joseph H, Fran B, et al. Methadone medical maintenance (MMM): treating chronic opioid dependence in private medical practice—a summary report (1983-1998). *Mt Sinai J Med.* 2000;67(5-6):388-397.
37. Merrill JO, Jackson TR, Schulman BA, et al. Methadone medical maintenance in primary care. An implementation evaluation. *J Gen Intern Med.* 2005;20(4):344-349.
38. Senay EC, Barthwell AG, Marks R, Bokos P, Gillman D, White R. Medical maintenance: a pilot study. *J Addict Dis.* 1993;12(4):59-76.
39. Fiellin DA, O'Connor PG, Chawarski M, Pakes JP, Pantalon MV, Shottenfeld RS. Methadone maintenance in primary care: a randomized controlled trial. *JAMA.* 2001;286:1724-1731.
40. Novick DM, Joseph H. Medical maintenance: the treatment of chronic opiate dependence in general medical practice. *J Subst Abuse Treat.* 1991;8(4):233-239.
41. Novick DM, Joseph H, Salsitz EA, et al. Outcomes of treatment of socially rehabilitated methadone maintenance patients in physicians' offices (medical maintenance): follow-up at three and a half to nine and a fourth years. *J Gen Intern Med.* 1994;9(3):127-130.
42. Hutchinson SJ, Taylor A, Gruer L, et al. One-year follow-up of opiate injectors treated with oral methadone in a GP-centred programme. *Addiction.* 2000;95(7):1055-1068.
43. Gossop M, Marsden J, Stewart D, Lehmann P, Strang J. Methadone treatment practices and outcome for opiate addicts treated in drug clinics and in general practice: results from the National Treatment Outcome Research Study. *Br J Gen Pract.* 1999;49(438):31-34.
44. Vignau J, Brunelle E. Differences between general practitioner- and addiction-centre-prescribed buprenorphine substitution therapy in France. *Eur Addict Res.* 1998;4(Suppl 1):24-28.
45. O'Connor PG, Oliveto AH, Shi JM, et al. A randomized trial of buprenorphine maintenance for heroin dependence in a primary care clinic for substance users versus a methadone clinic. *Am J Med.* 1998;105(2):100-105.
46. Fudala PJ, Bridge TP, Herbert S, et al. Office-based treatment of opiate addiction with a sublingual-tablet formulation of buprenorphine and naloxone. *N Engl J Med.* 2003;349(10):949-958.
47. Fiellin DA, Pantalon MV, Chawarski MC, et al. Counseling plus buprenorphine–naloxone maintenance therapy for opioid dependence. *N Engl J Med.* 2006;355(4):365-374.
48. Alford DP, LaBelle CT, Richardson JM, et al. Treating homeless opioid dependent patients with buprenorphine in an office-based setting. *J Gen Intern Med.* 2007;22(2):171-176.
49. Magura S, Lee SJ, Salsitz EA, et al. Outcomes of buprenorphine maintenance in office-based practice. *J Addict Dis.* 2007;26(2):13-23.
50. Mintzer IL, Eisenberg M, Terra M, MacVane C, Himmelstein DU, Woolhandler S. Treating opioid addiction with buprenorphine–naloxone in community-based primary care settings. *Ann Fam Med.* 2007;5(2):146-150.
51. Fiellin DA, Moore BA, Sullivan LE, et al. Long-term treatment with buprenorphine/naloxone in primary care: results at 2-5 years. *Am J Addict.* 2008;17:116-120.
52. Parran TV, Adelman CA, Merkin B, et al. Long-term outcomes of office-based buprenorphine/naloxone maintenance therapy. *Drug Alcohol Depend.* 2010;106:56-60.
53. Alford DP, LaBelle CT, Kretsch N, et al. Collaborative care of opioid-addicted patients in primary care using buprenorphine: five-year experience. *Arch Intern Med.* 2011;171:425-431.
54. Fiellin DA, Weiss L, Botsko M, et al. Drug treatment outcomes among HIV-infected opioid-dependent patients receiving buprenorphine/naloxone. *J Acquir Immune Defic Syndr.* 2011;56(Suppl 1):S33-S38.
55. Fiellin DA, Barry DT, Sullivan LE, et al. A randomized trial of cognitive behavioral therapy in primary care-based buprenorphine. *Am J Med.* 2013;126(1):74. e11-e17.
56. Fiellin DA, Schottenfeld RS, Cutter CJ, Moore BA, Barry DT, O'Connor PG. Primary care-based buprenorphine taper vs maintenance therapy for prescription opioid dependence: a randomized clinical trial. *JAMA Intern Med.* 2014;174(12):1947-1954.
57. Gruer L, Wilson P, Scott R, et al. General practitioner centered scheme for treatment of opiate dependent drug injectors in Glasgow. *BMJ.* 1997;314(7096):1730-1735.
58. Peters AD, Reid MM. Methadone treatment in the Scottish context: outcomes of a community-based service for drug users in Lothian. *Drug Alcohol Depend.* 1998;50(1):47-55.

59. Weinrich M, Stuart M. Provision of methadone treatment in primary care medical practices: review of the Scottish experience and implications for U.S. policy. *JAMA*. 2000;283(10):1343-1348.
60. Wilson P, Watson R, Ralston GE. Methadone maintenance in general practice: patients, workload, and outcomes. *BMJ*. 1994;309(6955):641-644.
61. Moatti JP, Souville M, Escaffre N, Obadia Y. French general practitioners' attitudes toward maintenance drug abuse treatment with buprenorphine. *Addiction*. 1998;93(10):1567-1575.
62. Auriacombe M, Fatseas M, Dubernet J, Daulouède JP, Tignol J. French field experience with buprenorphine. *Am J Addict*. 2004;13 (Suppl 1):S17-S28.
63. Stein MD, Cioe P, Friedmann PD. Buprenorphine retention in primary care. *J Gen Intern Med*. 2005;20(11):1038-1041.
64. *Center for Substance Abuse Treatment. The SAMHSA Evaluation of the Impact of the DATA Waiver Program*. Westat; 2006.
65. Weiss RD, Potter JS, Fiellin DA, et al. Adjunctive counseling during brief and extended buprenorphine–naloxone treatment for prescription opioid dependence: a 2-phase randomized controlled trial. *Arch Gen Psychiatry*. 2011;68(12):1238-1246.
66. Ling W, Hillhouse M, Ang A, Jenkins J, Fahey J. Comparison of behavioral treatment conditions in buprenorphine maintenance. *Addiction*. 2013;108(10):1788-1798.
67. Eap CB, Bertschy G, Baumann P, Finkbeiner T, Gastpar M, Scherbaum N. High interindividual variability of methadone enantiomer blood levels to dose ratios. *Arch Gen Psychiatry*. 1998;55(1):89-90.
68. King VL, Stoller KB, Hayes M, et al. A multicenter randomized evaluation of methadone medical maintenance. *Drug Alcohol Depend*. 2002;65(2):137-148.
69. Rostami-Hodjegan A, Wolff K, Hay AW, Raistrick D, Calvert R, Tucker GT. Population pharmacokinetics of methadone in opiate users: characterization of time-dependent changes. *Br J Clin Pharmacol*. 1999;48(1):43-52.
70. Maddux JF, Desmond DP, Vogtsberger KN. Patient-regulated methadone dose and optional counseling in methadone maintenance. *Am J Addict*. 1995;4(1):18-32.
71. Jacobs EA, Bickel WK. Precipitated withdrawal in an opioid-dependent outpatient receiving alternate-day buprenorphine dosing. *Addiction*. 1999;94(1):140-141.
72. Strain EC, Preston KL, Liebson IA, Bigelow GE. Buprenorphine effects in methadone-maintained volunteers: effects at two hours after methadone. *J Pharmacol Exp Ther*. 1995;272(2):628-638.
73. Walsh SL, Preston KL, Bigelow GE, Stitzer ML. Acute administration of buprenorphine in humans: partial agonist and blockade effects. *J Pharmacol Exp Ther*. 1995;274(1):361-372.
74. Lofwall MR, Walsh SL. Buprenorphine diversion and misuse in outpatient practice. *J Addict Med*. 2014;8(5):327-332.
75. Avants SK, Margolin A, Sindelar JL, et al. Day treatment versus enhanced standard methadone services for opioid-dependent patients: a comparison of clinical efficacy and cost. *Am J Psychiatry*. 1999;156(1):27-33.
76. Calsyn DA, Wells EA, Saxon AJ, et al. Contingency management of urinalysis results and intensity of counseling services have an interactive impact on methadone maintenance treatment outcome. *J Addict Dis*. 1994;13(3):47-63.
77. McLellan AT, Arndt IO, Metzger DS, Woody GE, O'Brien CP. The effects of psychosocial services in substance abuse treatment. *JAMA*. 1993;269(15):1953-1959.
78. Kraft MK, Rothbard AB, Hadley TR, McLellan AT, Asch DA. Are supplementary services provided during methadone maintenance really cost-effective? *Am J Psychiatry*. 1997;154(9):1214-1219.
79. Oliva EM, Gordon AJ, Harris AHS, et al. Trends in opioid agonist therapy in the Veterans Health Administration: is supply keeping up with demand? *Am J Drug Alcohol Abuse*. 2013;39(2):103-107.
80. Wyse JJ, Gordon AJ, Dobscha SK, et al. Medications for opioid use disorder in the Department of Veterans Affairs (VA) health care system: historical perspective, lessons learned, and next steps. *Subst Abus*. 2018;39(2):139-144. doi:10.1080/08897077.2018.1452327
81. Hawkins EJ, Malte CA, Gordon AJ, et al. Accessibility to medication for opioid use disorder after interventions to improve prescribing among nonaddiction clinics in the U.S. *Veterans Health Care System. JAMA Netw Open*. 2021;4(12):e2137238.

CHAPTER

64 Pharmacological Treatment of Stimulant Use Disorders

David A. Gorelick and Jeffery N. Wilkins

CHAPTER OUTLINE

- Introduction
- Cocaine use disorder
- Choice of medication
- Amphetamine-type stimulants use disorder
- Special treatment situations
- Future prospects
- Conclusions

INTRODUCTION

Stimulants such as cocaine and amphetamine-type stimulants (ATS; amphetamine, methamphetamine, methylphenidate) are the fifth most widely used psychoactive substances, after alcohol, tobacco, caffeine, and cannabis. In 2016, an estimated 5.8 million people (15-64 years old) worldwide had a cocaine use disorder (CUD), a 39.7% increase from 1990; an estimated 5.0 million people had an ATS use disorder (ATSUD), a 22.5% increase from 1990 (based on *Diagnostic and Statistical Manual of Mental Disorders*, 4th ed. [DSM-IV] and *International Classification of Diseases*, 10th ed. [ICD-10] diagnostic criteria).[1] In the United States in 2020, an estimated 1.3 million people (12 years and older) had a CUD, and 5.5 million had a stimulant use disorder (StUD) other than cocaine (DSM-5 diagnostic criteria).[2,3] In 2019, 330,000 patients reporting cocaine, amphetamines, or other stimulants as their primary substance use problem were admitted to publicly funded and/or licensed addiction treatment programs in the United States.[4] In 2021, an estimated 1.13 million U.S. emergency department visits were related to methamphetamine or cocaine use, representing almost one-sixth (15.73%) of all substance-related visits.[5] In 2019, there were 15,883 overdose deaths with cocaine involvement (three-quarters [75.5%] with opioid co-involvement) in the U.S. and 16,667 overdose deaths with involvement of other psychostimulants (about half [53.3%] with opioid co-involvement).[6] These were 8.9% and 28.2% increases, respectively, from 2018. Despite this demonstrated clinical need, there is no well-established, broadly effective pharmacotherapy for StUD. Interest in pharmacological treatment remains high because of the disappointingly low success rates of current psychosocial treatments.[7,8]

This chapter reviews the current state of pharmacological treatment for cocaine and ATS use disorders, including choice of medication and medications for use in special treatment situations, such as patients with two concurrent substance use disorders (SUDs) or psychiatric comorbidity. The focus is on outpatient randomized, placebo-controlled, double-blind clinical trials (RCTs), rather than open-label cases series, human laboratory studies or animal models. (See Chapter 14, "The Pharmacology of Stimulants" for more information). Proof of efficacy and safety from replicated, well-designed, adequately powered RCTs should be a key prerequisite for adopting any new medication into clinical practice.

Cocaine and ATS use disorders are considered separately. Pharmacological treatment of other StUDs such as khat and synthetic cathinones ("bath salts") is not covered, as we are not aware of any published RCTs on this topic. The extent to which findings related to cocaine can be extrapolated to other stimulants remains unknown.

Goals of Treatment

The goals of pharmacological treatment of StUD are the same as for any other treatment modality, that is, to help patients abstain from use and regain control of their lives. The behavioral mechanisms by which medication achieves these goals are poorly understood and can vary across patients and medications. In theory, medication could shift the balance of reinforcement away from stimulant use in favor of other behaviors through one or more of five behavioral mechanisms (see **Table 64-1**).

Because psychosocial factors are important in engaging these mechanisms, as well as promoting treatment and medication adherence, pharmacological treatment is best delivered combined with a psychosocial treatment component. Psychosocial treatment alone, especially contingency management, can be effective in promoting stimulant abstinence.[7-9] Limited evidence suggests that concurrent contingency management treatment enhances the efficacy of pharmacological treatment for StUD,[10] especially if reinforcement is directed at stimulant use itself, rather than treatment adherence.[11] A meta-analysis of four published RCTs found no benefit of adding cognitive-behavioral therapy (CBT) to usual care plus medication in reducing cocaine use during the treatment period but a modest beneficial effect (Hodges g [SE] 0.76 [0.30]) at post-treatment follow-up.[12] The addition of CBT was less effective than adding contingency management (Hodges g -0.61 [0.21]).

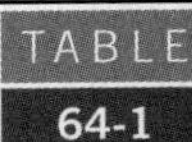

TABLE 64-1 Behavioral Mechanisms for Treating Stimulant Use Disorders

1. Reducing or eliminating the positive reinforcement from using the stimulant (eg, by reducing the euphoria or "high")
2. Reducing or eliminating a subjective state (such as "craving") that predisposes to taking the stimulant
3. Reducing or eliminating negative reinforcement from stimulant withdrawal (as by reducing withdrawal-associated dysphoria)
4. Making stimulant use aversive
5. Increasing the positive reinforcement obtained from non–stimulant-taking behaviors

Pharmacological Mechanisms

Four pharmacological approaches are potentially useful in the treatment of StUD disorder (see **Table 64-2**).[13-15] Most current research focuses on long-acting cross-tolerant stimulants and reducing or blocking stimulant actions, either directly at its neuronal binding site (true pharmacological antagonism) or indirectly by otherwise reducing reinforcing effects.

See Chapter 14, "The Pharmacology of Stimulants" for more information about mechanisms of action of stimulants.

COCAINE USE DISORDER

No medication is approved for the treatment of CUD by the U.S. Food and Drug Administration or any other national regulatory authority.[7,16] Many RCTs have one or more methodological deficiencies (see **Table 64-3**), which limit the strength of evidence that they provide.[16] Overall, 12 medications have low- to moderate-quality evidence of efficacy (see **Table 64-4**); no medication has high-quality evidence of efficacy (eg, an adequately powered phase III RCT).

CHOICE OF MEDICATION

Antidepressants

A systematic review and meta-analysis of published RCTs found at least moderate strength of evidence that antidepressants as a class (including tricyclics, selective serotonin

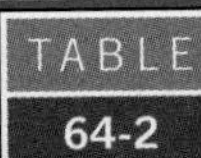

TABLE 64-2 Pharmacological Mechanisms for Treating Stimulant Use Disorders

1. Cross-tolerant stimulant (analogous to methadone or buprenorphine treatment of opioid use disorder)
2. Antagonist medication that blocks the binding of the stimulant at its site of action (true pharmacological antagonism, analogous to naltrexone treatment of opioid use disorder)
3. Medication that functionally antagonizes the effects of the stimulant (as by reducing its reinforcing effects or craving)
4. Alteration of stimulant pharmacokinetics so that less drug reaches or remains at its site(s) of action in the brain[15]

Source: From Gorelick DA, Gardner EL, Xi ZX. Agents in development for the management of cocaine abuse. *Drugs.* 2004;64(14):1547-1573.

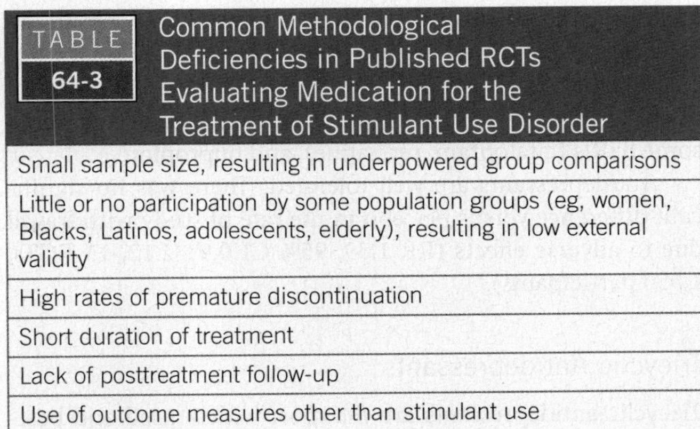

TABLE 64-3 Common Methodological Deficiencies in Published RCTs Evaluating Medication for the Treatment of Stimulant Use Disorder

Small sample size, resulting in underpowered group comparisons
Little or no participation by some population groups (eg, women, Blacks, Latinos, adolescents, elderly), resulting in low external validity
High rates of premature discontinuation
Short duration of treatment
Lack of posttreatment follow-up
Use of outcome measures other than stimulant use (eg, craving, mood)
Use of subjective outcome measures, such as self-report, rather than objectively assessed stimulant use

RCT, randomized, double-blind, placebo-controlled clinical trial.

reuptake inhibitors [SSRIs], serotonin–norepinephrine uptake inhibitors [SNRIs], bupropion, mirtazapine, and nefazodone) were no more effective than placebo in terms of retention in treatment (relative risk [RR] 0.95, 95% CI 0.87-1.03, based on 33 RCTs, 2,918 participants), achieving at least 3 weeks of

TABLE 64-4 Medications With Evidence of Efficacy for the Treatment of Cocaine Use Disorder

Medication	Outcome measure	Type of evidence
Low-quality evidence		
Buprenorphine (history of opioid use disorder)[67]	↓ use	1 RCT
Disulfiram (men with specific genotypes)[36-40]	↓ use	5 RCTs
Doxazosin[89,90]	↓ use, cont abst ≥ 2 weeks	2 RCTs
Naltrexone[65,66]	↓ use	2 RCTs
Ondansetron (specific genotypes)[51,52]	↓ use, ↑ retention in tx	2 RCTs
Moderate-quality evidence		
Amphetamines—long-acting formulations[8,17,72]	↓ use, cont abst ≥ 3 weeks	5 RCTs
Bupropion[17]	cont abst ≥ 3 weeks	2 RCTs
Desipramine (mild CUD)[16,17]	cont abst ≥ 3 weeks	5 RCTs
Modafinil[73]	Achieve abstinence	6 U.S. RCTs
SSRIs—citalopram[24,25] Sertraline[17]	↓ use 2 consecutive cocaine-negative urine samples	2 RCTs 2 RCTs
Topiramate[17]	cont abst ≥ 3 weeks	2 RCTs

Cont abst, continuous abstinence confirmed by urine samples negative for cocaine metabolites; CUD, cocaine use disorder; RCT, randomized, double-blind, placebo-controlled clinical trial; SSRI, selective serotonin reuptake inhibitor antidepressant; tx, treatment; cocaine use assessed in terms of urine testing for cocaine metabolites.

continuous abstinence (RR 1.27, 95% CI 0.99-1.63, ten RCTs, 1,226 participants), or use of cocaine (RR 1.05, 95% CI 0.91-1.21, six RCTs, 405 participants.[17] However, there was evidence of efficacy for a few specific types of antidepressants: tricyclics, some SSRIs (citalopram, sertraline), and bupropion.

Antidepressants are well tolerated. There was no significant difference versus placebo in the rate of study withdrawal due to adverse effects (RR 1.39, 95% CI 0.91-2.12, 15 RCTs, 1,550 participants).[17]

Tricyclic Antidepressants

Tricyclic antidepressants are the most widely used and best-studied class of medications for the treatment of CUD.[16] Their pharmacological mechanism of action is to increase biogenic amine neurotransmitter activity in synapses, primarily by inhibiting presynaptic neurotransmitter reuptake pumps. A meta-analysis of published RCTs (all but two with desipramine) at antidepressant doses found no advantage over placebo for retention in treatment (RR 1.00, 95% CI 0.85-1.18, 15 RCTs, 1,141 participants) and cocaine use (RR 0.85, 95% CI 0.34-2.11, 2 RCTs, 37 participants), but a significant advantage in achieving at least 3 weeks of continuous abstinence (RR 1.55, 95% CI 1.10-2.17, 5 RCTs, 367 participants).[17] This advantage over placebo disappeared when the analysis was limited to participants with moderate-to-severe CUD (RR 1.41, 95% CI 0.93-2.14, 3 RCTs, 234 participants), suggesting that the therapeutic effect is not very robust.

Differences in patient characteristics, concomitant treatment, and desipramine plasma concentrations may account for some of the variability in the efficacy of desipramine. For example, patients with depression[18] and without antisocial personality disorder[19] may respond best to desipramine. Patients with co-occurring CUD and opioid use disorder (OUD) may do better on desipramine if their opioid use is treated with buprenorphine rather than methadone or if they receive contingency management treatment along with medication.[20] There is low-quality evidence that patients with steady-state desipramine plasma concentrations above 200 ng/mL have poorer outcomes,[21] with better outcomes at concentrations around 125 ng/mL.[20]

Tricyclic antidepressants are well tolerated. There was no significant difference versus placebo in the rate of study withdrawal due to adverse effects (RR 1.24, 95% CI 0.64-2.43, 5 RCTs, 381 participants).[17] However, patients who return to cocaine use while still on antidepressant medications could, in theory, be at increased risk of cardiovascular side effects. Both cocaine and the tricyclics have quinidine-like membrane effects that, when superimposed, could lead to cardiac arrhythmias. The concurrent administration of cocaine and desipramine (blood concentrations above 100 ng/mL) to research volunteers has produced additive increases in heart rate and blood pressure.[22]

Selective Serotonin Reuptake Inhibitors

SSRI antidepressants have attracted interest because of the role of serotonin and its receptors in modulating dopaminergic brain reward circuits and the behavioral effects of cocaine[23] (see Chapter 14, "The Pharmacology of Stimulants"). A systematic review and meta-analysis of published RCTs (fluoxetine, paroxetine, and sertraline) found no significant advantage over placebo in retention in treatment (relative risk RR 0.99, 95% CI 0.70-1.41, 9 studies, 660 participants).[17] No studies evaluated cocaine use or continuous abstinence. Two RCTs that evaluated sertraline in 133 participants who had achieved abstinence found a significant reduction in return to use, defined as two consecutive urine drug tests positive for cocaine (RR 0.74, 95% CI 0.57-0.96).[17] Citalopram (20 mg or 40 mg daily) significantly reduced cocaine use in two small RCTs (183 total participants).[24,25]

SSRIs are not well tolerated. Participants receiving an SSRI were significantly more likely to withdraw from a study due to an adverse event than were those receiving placebo (RR 3.55, 95% CI 1.11-11.34, 3 RCTs, 251 participants).[17]

Serotonin-Norepinephrine Reuptake Inhibitors

Nefazodone (2 RCTs, 279 participants)[26,27] and venlafaxine (2 RCTs, 170 participants)[28,29] which block both serotonin and norepinephrine reuptake, were not effective; 1 RCT with each medication involved participants with comorbid depression. Mirtazapine, which increases brain serotonin and norepinephrine activity by blocking autoregulatory α_2-adrenergic and 5-HT_2 receptors, was not effective in one small RCT (24 participants) involving participants with comorbid depression.[30]

Monoamine Oxidase Inhibitors

The rationale for use of MAO inhibitors lies in their effect of increasing brain levels of biogenic amine neurotransmitters by inhibiting a major catabolic enzyme for those neurotransmitters. Selegiline, FDA-approved for the treatment of Parkinson disease and, in the transdermal form, for treatment of depression, is fairly selective for MAO type B (the predominant type in the brain) at recommended doses (10 mg/day or 12 mg/day). A multisite, controlled clinical trial using selegiline administered via a skin patch found no evidence for efficacy in treatment of DSM-IV cocaine dependence.[31]

Other Antidepressants

The norepinephrine reuptake inhibitor atomoxetine, FDA-approved for the treatment of attention deficit hyperactivity disorder (ADHD), showed no efficacy in a small controlled clinical trial.[32]

Bupropion is a weak inhibitor of monoamine reuptake that is also FDA-approved for abstinence from cigarette smoking. A meta-analysis of two published RCTs found bupropion significantly better than placebo in promoting at least 3 weeks of sustained abstinence (RR 1.63, 95% CI 1.03-2.59, 176 participants), but no significant effect on overall cocaine use or retention in treatment.[17]

Dopamine Agonists (Antiparkinson Agents)

A variety of direct and indirect dopamine agonist medications have been evaluated, based on the dopamine depletion hypothesis of cocaine addiction. Dopamine agonists, by stimulating synaptic dopamine activity, would ameliorate the effects of decreased dopamine activity caused by abstinence from cocaine use, including anhedonia, anergia, depression, and cocaine craving.

A meta-analysis of published RCTs found that dopamine receptor agonists as a class (direct agonists [bromocriptine, pergolide, pramipexole, cabergoline, hydergine], indirect agonists [amantadine], and the amino acid dopamine precursor L-DOPA [sometimes combined with the peripheral dopa-decarboxylase inhibitor carbidopa]), compared to placebo, did not improve treatment retention (RR 1.04, 95% CI 0.94-1.14, 20 RCTs, 1,656 participants) or increase the proportion of participants achieving at least 3 weeks of continuous abstinence (RR 1.12, 95% CI 0.85-1.47, 11 RCTs, 731 participants).[17] A separate meta-analysis of published clinical trials (of any design) found no effect on cocaine use (RR 1.55, 95% CI 0.80-3.00, 10 RCTs, 645 participants).[8] L-Tyrosine, the amino acid precursor of L-dopa, was not effective in reducing cocaine use in one small RCT.[33]

Disulfiram

Disulfiram can be considered a functional dopamine agonist because it blocks the conversion of dopamine to norepinephrine by the enzyme dopamine-β-hydroxylase, thereby increasing dopamine concentration.[34] A meta-analysis of published RCTs found that disulfiram, compared to placebo, slightly worsened treatment retention (RR 0.90, 95% CI 0.83-0.99, 7 RCTs, 704 participants) and provided no benefit for cocaine use (RR 0.95, 95% CI 0.64-1.39, 4 RCTs, 440 participants) or achievement of at least 3 weeks of continuous abstinence (RR 0.96, 95% CI 0.63-1.45, 3 RCTs, 296 participants).[17]

There is evidence of efficacy in some genetic and gender subgroups of individuals with CUD. One RCT that found disulfiram efficacious overall found no efficacy in participants with a dopamine-β-hydroxylase gene allele that results in low enzyme activity.[35] Four other small RCTs in patients also receiving methadone to treat comorbid OUD found no disulfiram efficacy overall, but did find significant efficacy in subgroups with functional variants in the ankyrin repeat and kinase domain-containing 1 (*ANKK1*),[36] dopamine D_2 receptor (*DRD2*) genes,[36] dopamine transporter gene,[37] α_{1A}-adrenoreceptor (*ADRA1A*) gene,[38] and δ-opioid receptor gene.[39]

Gender also influences the treatment response to disulfiram. An analysis of pooled data from 434 participants in five published RCTs found that disulfiram was less effective in women than in men in treatment retention and reducing cocaine use.[40] There was no such gender difference in response to behavioral treatments.

Although disulfiram is well tolerated in clinical trials, where subjects are carefully screened for medical and psychiatric comorbidity and closely monitored, questions have been raised about its safety in routine clinical practice.[41] Human laboratory studies give conflicting results on the safety of the cocaine-disulfiram interaction,[42] although one study found no clinically significant adverse effects from even the triple interaction of cocaine-alcohol-disulfiram.[43] Disulfiram may increase plasma concentrations of cocaine by inhibiting the cocaine-metabolizing enzyme butyrylcholinesterase.[42] A 12-week RCT with nepicastat, a dopamine β-hydroxylase inhibitor that does not have significant pharmacological interactions with cocaine,[44] also found the medication no different from placebo in reducing cocaine use.[45]

Serotonergic Agents

Buspirone and gepirone are primarily 5-HT_{1A} receptor agonists used to treat generalized anxiety disorder. Single RCTs found neither effective in improving retention or reducing cocaine use.[46,47]

Ritanserin, a 5-HT_{2A} receptor antagonist developed as an antidepressant, was no better than placebo in reducing cocaine use in two RCTs.[48,49]

Lorcaserin, a 5-HT_{2C} receptor antagonist previously FDA-approved for weight loss but removed from the market by FDA in 2020 because of cancer risk, did not significantly reduce proportion of cocaine-positive urine samples in one RCT, although self-reported cocaine was significantly reduced.[50]

Ondansetron, a 5-HT_3 receptor antagonist approved for the treatment of nausea and vomiting, significantly improved retention and reduced cocaine use in a small RCT (63 participants) at the highest dose (4 mg twice daily) but not at lower doses (0.25 and 1.0 mg twice daily).[51] A subsequent larger RCT (108 participants) found no beneficial effect of ondansetron (4 mg twice daily).[52] Post hoc analysis found that ondansetron significantly reduced cocaine use in a subgroup of participants with a specific single nucleotide polymorphism (SNP) in the gene for the serotonin 5-HT_{3A} receptor.

Cholinergic Agents

Cholinergic agents have been studied because they influence cocaine reward in animal models and human laboratory studies.[53] Small RCTs with muscarinic cholinergic receptor antagonists yielded inconsistent results. Biperiden (2 mg tid) significantly reduced cocaine use in one RCT,[54] while mecamylamine did not reduce cocaine use in another RCT.[55]

Varenicline, a partial agonist at α4β2 nicotinic cholinergic receptors FDA-approved for helping smoking abstinence, had no significant effect on treatment retention or cocaine use in 3 RCTs (224 total participants).[17,56] Increasing brain cholinergic activity nonspecifically with the cholinesterase inhibitors donepezil[57] or galantamine[58-60] had no significant effect on cocaine use in 3 of 4 small RCTs (261 total participants).

Opioid Receptor Ligands

μ-Opioid receptor (mOR) antagonists have been evaluated as treatments for CUD because of the role of brain mORs in cocaine use. Those who use cocaine on a chronic basis have a decreased response to mOR agonists compared to those who do not use cocaine,[61] and elevated mOR binding potential in brain regions that mediate reward sensitivity is associated with increased cocaine craving,[62] increased rate of recurrence of cocaine use after enforced abstinence,[63] and greater cocaine use during outpatient treatment.[64] These findings suggest that blockade of μ-opioid receptors might reduce cocaine craving and use. Two small RCTs found that naltrexone (50 mg daily) significantly reduced cocaine use compared to placebo,[65,66] but only in those receiving cognitive-behavioral therapy and not already abstinent when starting treatment.

Buprenorphine, a partial mOR agonist and κ-opioid receptor antagonist FDA-approved for the treatment of OUD, has been studied for the treatment of CUD. The rationale is twofold: a RCT showed efficacy in treating patients with concurrent CUD and OUD (see Concurrent Opioid Use Disorder below) and activation of κ-opioid receptors by the endogenous agonist prodynorphin mediates cocaine self-administration in animals.[67] An RCT gave 302 participants with current moderate-severe CUD and past or current OUD intramuscular extended-release naltrexone every 4 weeks plus sublingual buprenorphine (4 mg or 16 mg) or placebo daily for 8 weeks, making buprenorphine act functionally as a pure κ-opioid receptor antagonist.[67] Buprenorphine-16 mg (but not 4 mg) significantly reduced the proportion of cocaine-positive urine samples over the last 4 weeks of treatment (OR 1.71, $p = 0.022$), but did not alter self-reported cocaine use, the proportion of participants achieving complete abstinence, or treatment retention. A post hoc secondary analysis found that 16 mg buprenorphine preferentially reduced cocaine use in participants with one of two genetic variations (SNPs) in the prodynorphin gene, while the 4 mg dose had no significant effect in either genotype.[68]

Stimulants

Stimulant medications have been evaluated to implement the agonist substitution approach, analogous to methadone treatment of OUD or nicotine treatment of tobacco use disorder. Advantages include use of the medically safer oral route of administration (vs injected or smoked cocaine), use of pure medication of known potency (thus avoiding adulterant effects or inadvertent overdose), provision by a medical professional as part of a comprehensive treatment regimen, and use of a medication with slower onset (less euphoria) and longer duration (eg, daily dosing) of action (thus avoiding "rush"/"crash" cycling).[69]

A meta-analysis of published RCTs found that stimulants as a class (including amphetamines, lisdexamfetamine, methylphenidate, modafinil, and mazindol) were significantly better than placebo in promoting at least 3 weeks of sustained abstinence (RR 1.36, 95% CI 1.05-1.77, 14 RCTs, 1,549 participants) but did not increase the proportion of cocaine-free urine samples among those who did not achieve sustained abstinence (standardized mean difference 0.16, 95% CI −0.02-0.33, 8 RCTs, 526 participants) nor improve treatment retention (RR 1.00, 95% CI 0.93-1.06, 24 RCTs, 2,205 participants).[17] A separate meta-analysis found that stimulants as a class significantly increased the overall proportion of cocaine-free urine samples (standardized mean difference 5.24, 95% CI 0.97-9.51, 11 RCTs, 921 participants).[70] Among specific stimulants, only dexamphetamine (RR 1.98, 95% CI 1.12-3.52, 3 RCTs, 154 participants) and mixed amphetamine salts (3.63, 95% CI 1.15-11.48, 1 RCT, 176 participants) were significantly better than placebo in promoting at least 3 weeks of sustained abstinence.[71] Another RCT not included in the meta-analyses also found that sustained release D-amphetamine significantly reduced cocaine use over a 12-week treatment period (mean difference in number of days of cocaine use 16.7, 95% CI 3.1-28.4).[72]

A separate meta-analysis of 6 published RCTs involving 669 participants that were conducted in the U.S. (excluding one French RCT with 27 participants) found that modafinil significantly increased the proportion of participants achieving abstinence (RR 1.440, 95% CI 1.027-2.020) but did not affect treatment retention (RR 1.086, 95% CI 0.940-1.142).[73]

Antipsychotics

Older ("first-generation") antipsychotics, which are potent dopamine receptor antagonists (chiefly D_2 [postsynaptic] subtype), do not significantly alter cocaine craving or use, as evidenced by clinical experience with patients with schizophrenia who use cocaine while receiving chronic antipsychotic treatment.[74] Newer ("second-generation") antipsychotics, which have a broader spectrum of receptor binding (including dopamine D_1 and serotonin receptors), are not more effective. A meta-analysis of published RCTs found that newer antipsychotics as a class (aripiprazole, olanzapine, quetiapine, risperidone) reduced treatment dropout (RR 0.75, 95% CI 0.57-0.97, 8 RCTs, 397 participants) but did not significantly reduce proportion of subjects achieving at least 3 weeks of continuous abstinence (RR 1.30, 95% CI 0.73-2.32, 3 RCTs, 139 participants) or number of participants using cocaine during treatment (RR 1.02, 95% CI 0.65-1.62, 2 RCTs, 91 participants).[17] An RCT (not included in the meta-analysis) in 18 individuals who had achieved 2 weeks of continuous cocaine abstinence with contingency management found that aripiprazole had no significant effect on rates of recurrence of use.[75]

Caution is advised when prescribing antipsychotic medication to individuals using cocaine. Cocaine use is associated with significantly increased risk of developing neuroleptic malignant syndrome[76] and antipsychotic-induced extra-pyramidal movement disorders such as akathisia, Parkinsonism, and acute dystonia, especially in individuals with schizophrenia.[77,78] This vulnerability may be related to the reduced brain dopamine activity found in individuals who use cocaine.[79]

Anticonvulsants

Anticonvulsants might be effective in the treatment of CUD because they decrease the response to cocaine in the dopaminergic cortico-mesolimbic brain reward circuit by either increasing inhibitory GABA activity, decreasing excitatory glutamate activity, or both (eg, topiramate).[80]

A meta-analysis of published RCTs found that anticonvulsants as a class (carbamazepine, gabapentin, lamotrigine, phenytoin, tiagabine, topiramate, and vigabatrin) had no significant effect on rate of premature departure from treatment (RR 0.95, 95% CI 0.86-1.05, 17 RCTs, 1,695 participants) or cocaine use (RR 0.92, 95% CI 0.84-1.02, 9 RCTs, 867 participants).[17] When considered individually, no anticonvulsant except topiramate showed any significant benefit over placebo. A separate meta-analysis found that topiramate significantly increased the proportion of subjects achieving continuous abstinence for at least 3 weeks (RR 2.43, 95% CI 1.31-4.53, 2 RCTs, 210 participants) but did not improve treatment retention.[17] A secondary analysis of one RCT (142 participants) found that higher impulsivity was associated with better response to topiramate.[81] Valproate was not effective in one RCT (32 participants) not included in the meta-analysis.[82]

Baclofen, an antispasmodic rather than anticonvulsant, increases GABA activity by acting as an agonist at $GABA_B$ receptors. Two RCTs (230 total participants) found no evidence that baclofen improved treatment retention or reduced cocaine use.[17]

Nutritional Supplements and Herbal Products

Nutritional Supplements

Nutritional supplements have been widely promoted in the addiction treatment field, encouraged by their freedom from the regulations imposed on prescription medications and their perceived safety and absence of side effects. Small RCTs found no benefit from the combination of tyrosine and tryptophan (1 g each daily),[83] L-tryptophan,[84] L-carnitine (500 mg/day) plus coenzyme Q10 (200 mg/day),[82] magnesium L-aspartate (732 mg daily), an easily absorbed form of magnesium,[85] or citicoline, a dietary supplement that enhances phospholipid turnover.[17]

Herbal Products

Various herbal and plant-derived products have been touted as treatments for SUD, but very few have undergone rigorous clinical evaluation. Ibogaine is an indole alkaloid found in the root bark of the West African shrub *Tabernanthe iboga* that acts on several different neurotransmitter systems, including glutamate (*N*-methyl-D-aspartate [NMDA] type), κ- and μ-opioid, $5\text{-}HT_2$, $5\text{-}HT_3$, α3β4 nicotinic, and sigma-2 receptors; the 5-HT transporter; and alters the brain expression of substance P and brain-derived neurotrophic factor [BDNF].[87] In open-label case reports and case series, ibogaine suppresses cocaine (and opioid and alcohol) withdrawal and craving for several months after a single oral dose.[87] However, no RCTs have been conducted, in part because of cases of cardiac arrhythmia (especially Q-T interval prolongation and ventricular fibrillation) and sudden death, probably due to ibogaine's inhibition of hERG potassium channels.[87]

A small RCT (26 participants) found *Ginkgo biloba* (120 mg/day for 8 weeks) of no benefit in reducing return to substance use in participants already abstinent from cocaine at the start of treatment.[88]

Adrenergic Receptor Antagonists

Small RCTs of adrenergic receptor antagonists have generated mixed results. Two small RCTs (35 and 76 participants) found that doxazosin (8 mg daily), an α_1-adrenergic receptor antagonist FDA-approved for treatment of hypertension, significantly reduced cocaine use[89,90] and the proportion of participants achieving at least 2 weeks of continuous abstinence[89] but only when rapidly titrated to the target dose over 2 or 4 weeks. The response to doxazosin was enhanced in participants with genetic variants in the α_1-adrenergic receptor[91] or with variants that reduce activity of dopamine-β-hydroxylase,[90] the enzyme that converts dopamine to norepinephrine. In contrast, the β-adrenergic receptor antagonist propranolol[92] and the combined α_1- and β-adrenergic receptor antagonist carvedilol[93] had no significant effect on cocaine use in small RCTs.

Cannabinoids

Cannabidiol, a phytocannabinoid that is FDA-approved to treat some forms of intractable childhood epilepsy, has been evaluated as a treatment for CUD based on its reduction of cocaine reinforcement in animal models.[94] However, a recent RCT in 78 participants who had achieved cocaine abstinence over 10 days of hospitalization found that oral cannabidiol (800 mg daily) did not significantly alter the risk of return to use of cocaine use after discharge (hazard ratio 1.20, CI 0.65-2.20).[95]

Glutamatergic Agents

Neither riluzole, an inhibitor of glutamate release[28]; memantine, an NMDA glutamate receptor antagonist,[17] nor *N*-acetylcysteine, which increases brain glutamate levels,[17] were effective in small RCTs.

Other Medications

A wide variety of other medications have been evaluated for the treatment of CUD[17] but found no better than placebo in (usually small-scale) RCTs. These include amlodipine, a calcium channel blocker used to treat hypertension[96]; hydergine, an agonist at dopamine and serotonin receptors and antagonist at α-adrenergic receptors that stimulates blood flow[17]; pentoxifylline, a phosphodiesterase inhibitor[28]; celecoxib, a nonsteroidal anti-inflammatory drug[17]; reserpine,[17] and dehydroepiandrosterone (DHEA), an endogenous steroid precursor of androstenedione, itself a precursor of androgenic and estrogenic hormones.[97] DHEA is also a sigma-1 receptor agonist.

Medication Combinations

Concurrent use of two different medications is evaluated in the hope that such combinations will enhance efficacy while minimizing side effects by acting through different mechanisms.[98] Some RCTs of medication combinations show efficacy compared with placebo, but very few RCT's compare the individual medications against the combination. Thus, it remains unknown whether efficacy resides in an individual medication or the combination or whether a beneficial combination effect is additive or synergistic. For example, the combination of topiramate and extended-release mixed amphetamine salts significantly reduced cocaine use among frequent cocaine users in two RCTs,[99,100] but the individual medications were not evaluated. In the few RCTs where individual medications are evaluated, the combination is sometimes better and sometimes worse than the individual medication.[98]

Other Physical Treatments

Acupuncture is an ancient Chinese treatment that involves mechanical (needles), thermal (moxibustion), or electrical (electroacupuncture) stimulation of specific points on the body surface.[86] The mechanism of action is unknown; speculation has included stimulation of endogenous opioid systems. A meta-analysis of seven published clinical trials involving 1,433 participants did not find a significant benefit of active acupuncture over sham treatment.[86]

Two methods for noninvasive neuromodulation of brain activity have been studied as treatment for CUD: transcranial magnetic stimulation (TMS) and transcranial direct current stimulation (tDCS)[101] (see also Chapter 68, "Neuromodulation for Substance Use Disorders"). TMS alters the firing of brain neurons by rapidly alternating magnetic fields generated by electromagnetic coils placed on the scalp. High-frequency repetitive TMS (rTMS), which stimulates neuronal firing, is FDA-approved as treatment for major depressive disorder, obsessive-compulsive disorder, and tobacco use disorder (cigarette smoking) (see Chapter 68). Several human laboratory studies and small, short-term RCTs found that rTMS (usually high frequency [10-15 Hz]) directed at the prefrontal cortex reduced cocaine craving and use.[102] However, two recent RCTs involving a total of 142 participants that targeted 15 Hz rTMS at the left dorsolateral prefrontal cortex found no significant effect on cocaine craving or use over 3 or 14 weeks.[103,104]

tDCS involves sending low-amplitude direct electrical current into the brain via scalp electrodes.[101] tDCS reduced self-reported cocaine craving in two small, sham-controlled human laboratory studies.[101,105]

AMPHETAMINE-TYPE STIMULANTS USE DISORDER

Many of the medications evaluated for the treatment of CUD have been studied for the treatment of amphetamine-type stimulants (ATS) use disorder (ATSUD), often for the same pharmacological rationale.[106] No medication has robust evidence for efficacy; none is approved for treatment of ATSUD by the FDA or any other national regulatory authority.

Stimulants

Meta-analyses of published RCTs found that stimulants as a class (D-amphetamine, methamphetamine, methylphenidate, modafinil) were not significantly better than placebo in reducing proportion of amphetamine-positive urine samples (mean difference −0.26, 95% CI −0.85-0.33, 7 RCTs, 473 participants)[107] or promoting at least 2-3 weeks of sustained abstinence (relative risk 0.89, 95% CI 0.62-1.27, 3 RCTs, 305 participants).[70] No individual stimulant was significantly effective when evaluated separately.

Two recent studies, not included in the meta-analysis, suggest efficacy for lisdexamfetamine, a pro-drug that is hydrolyzed to D-amphetamine after ingestion. Lisdexamfetamine has a pharmacokinetic profile similar to that of sustained release amphetamine and is FDA-approved to treat ADHD in adults and for binge eating disorder. A small open-label clinical trial found that lisdexamfetamine (escalating doses up to 250 mg daily over 2 weeks) reduced median days of methamphetamine use by 38% in 16 adults with methamphetamine dependence (ICD-10).[108] A retrospective cohort study of Swedish nation-wide health registries found that treatment with lisdexamfetamine was significantly associated with decreased hospitalization for SUD treatment (adjusted hazard ratio 0.82, 95% CI 0.72-0.94) among individuals with amphetamine or methamphetamine use disorder.[109] No other stimulant medication (amphetamine, methylphenidate, modafinil, atomoxetine) was associated with a significant change in hospitalization.

Anti-Convulsants

Single RCTs of topiramate, gabapentin, and baclofen found no evidence of efficacy.[107]

Opioid Antagonists

A meta-analysis of published RCTs found that the μ-opioid receptor antagonist naltrexone (oral immediate or sustained release or subcutaneous implant formulations) had no significant effect on proportion of amphetamine-free urine samples (RR 1.05, 95% CI 0.92-1.18, 3 RCTs) or retention in treatment (RR 1.11, 95% CI 0,88-1.41, 4 RCTs).[107] A single small RCT found that oral naltrexone combined with *N*-acetylcysteine was also not effective in reducing methamphetamine use.[110] A large (403 participants), 12-week RCT found that naltrexone (380 mg im every 3 weeks) plus bupropion (450 mg oral extended release daily) significantly increased the proportion of participants with at least 75% methamphetamine-free urine samples over the last 2 weeks of treatment (13.6% versus 2.5%).[111]

Anti-Depressants

Three anti-depressants have been studied for the treatment of ATSUD, with none showing efficacy. A meta-analysis of published RCTs found that bupropion had no significant effect on achieving abstinence (RR 1.12, 95% CI 0.54-2.33, 3 RCTs) or treatment retention (RR 1.10, 95% CI 0.73-1,67, 4 RCTs).[112] A meta-analysis of 2 published RCTs involving 180 participants found that mirtazapine had no significant effect on methamphetamine use (RR 0.81, 95% CI 0.63-1.03) or treatment retention (RR 1.01, 95% CI 0.91-1.12).[113] Sertraline had no efficacy in a single RCT.[107]

Antipsychotics

Two published RCTs involving a combined 153 participants found no evidence of efficacy for aripiprazole.[107]

Other Medications

Riluzole, a glutamatergic agent that is FDA-approved for the treatment of amyotrophic lateral sclerosis, significantly reduced the proportion of methamphetamine-positive urine samples at the end of a 12-week RCT (5% vs 45%, respectively, $p = 0.004$).[114] Medications not showing efficacy in the treatment of ATSUD in single RCTs include atomoxetine (selective norepinephrine reuptake inhibitor), citicoline (dietary supplement that enhances phospholipid turnover), ondansetron (5-HT_3 receptor antagonist), and varenicline (partial agonist at $\alpha4\beta2$ nicotinic cholinergic receptors).[107]

Other Physical Treatments

We are not aware of any published RCTs studying acupuncture[115] or noninvasive brain neuromodulation methods (eg, TMS)[101,116] as treatment for ATSUD that evaluated actual ATS use (as opposed to craving, withdrawal, or mood).

SPECIAL TREATMENT SITUATIONS

Concurrent Substance Use Disorders

Concurrent Opioid Use Disorder

Concurrent opioid use, including opioid use disorder (OUD), is a common clinical problem among individuals with CUD. About one-third of community-dwelling individuals with current cocaine use have comorbid OUD,[117] and about one-third of patients in treatment for OUD have a comorbid StUD.[118,119] Three different pharmacological approaches have been used for the treatment of dual cocaine and opioid use disorders among individuals receiving treatment with methadone: adjustment of methadone dose, treatment with a different opioid medication (buprenorphine or naltrexone), and addition of medication targeting the CUD.

Higher methadone doses (>60 mg daily) are associated with less cocaine use in many[120] but not all[121,122] studies. There is a significant association between reduction in opioid use and reduction in cocaine use; the adequacy of the methadone dose in suppressing opioid craving and withdrawal symptoms may be more important than the actual methadone dosage in mediating reduction in cocaine use.[121,122] Increasing the methadone dose as a contingency in response to cocaine use can be effective in reducing cocaine use; more so than decreasing the methadone dose.[123]

Buprenorphine reduces both cocaine and opioid use in RCTs involving patients with concurrent OUD and CUD, but only at higher buprenorphine doses (16-32 mg daily sublingually).[124,125] Making buprenorphine dosing partially dependent on cocaine-free urine samples can also reduce cocaine use in patients with OUD.[126] In one head-to-head RCT, methadone was significantly better than buprenorphine in reducing cocaine use.[125] A retrospective review of insurance claims found buprenorphine better than naltrexone in reducing cocaine use.[127]

Many of the nonopioid medications for the treatment of CUD that are mentioned above were evaluated in patients receiving methadone or buprenorphine treatment for OUD. A meta-analysis of 34 published RCTs involving 22 different medications found no evidence of efficacy in patients with OUD.[128] Anti-depressants (desipramine, fluoxetine, bupropion) (RR [for dropout] 1.22, 95% CI 1.05-1.41, 10 RCTs, 1,006 participants) and disulfiram (RR 0.86, 95 % CI 0.77-0.95, 6 RCTs, 605 participants) significantly worsened treatment retention. However, the meta-analysis did not directly compare participants with and without comorbid OUD, so the influence of this comorbidity on treatment outcome remains unclear. Topiramate significantly reduced cocaine use in two RCTs involving patients without comorbid OUD[17] but was not effective in two other RCTs involving participants with comorbid OUD,[129] suggesting a negative interaction between the efficacy of topiramate and OUD.

Alcohol Use Disorder

About three-quarters of community-dwelling individuals with current CUD engage in binge drinking of alcohol; about one-third have alcohol use disorder (AUD).[117] Alcohol use by patients with CUD is associated with poorer treatment outcome.[130]

Two medications used in the treatment of AUD have been studied in the treatment of patients with concurrent CUD and AUD. Disulfiram substantially decreased both cocaine and alcohol use in two of three RCTs.[131-133] Naltrexone substantially decreased both cocaine and alcohol use at 150 mg daily,[133,134] but not at 50 mg daily[135-137] or 100 mg daily, the doses more typically used in treatment of AUD or OUD. Naltrexone was not effective when given as a monthly extended-release injection.[138] Combined treatment with both disulfiram (250 mg daily) and naltrexone (100 mg daily) significantly improved abstinence from cocaine and alcohol in one RCT.[133]

One RCT found no significant effect of topiramate compared to placebo in reducing cocaine or alcohol use in outpatients with comorbid CUD and AUD, although topiramate-treated participants had better treatment retention and were more likely to be abstinent from cocaine during the final 3 weeks of the 13-week trial.[139]

Psychiatric Comorbidity

About one-third of community-dwelling adults with current CUD report having a depression or anxiety syndrome.[140] About half of treatment-seeking individuals with CUD have a current psychiatric comorbidity.[141] Psychiatric comorbidity is associated with poorer treatment outcome.[142] Despite these high rates of comorbidity, there are relatively few RCTs evaluating pharmacological treatment of this patient population.[143]

Depression

About one-fifth of community-dwelling individuals with current CUD report a major depressive episode within the prior year.[117] Antidepressants vary in their efficacy for reducing cocaine use among patients with comorbid major depression.[144] Sertraline (200 mg daily) significantly reduced cocaine use in one RCT.[145] Other SSRIs, tricyclics, bupropion, mirtazapine, venlafaxine, and nefazodone are not consistently effective. All anti-depressants significantly reduce depressive symptoms.[144]

Bipolar Disorder

Up to 30% of the general population with a StUD have a comorbid bipolar disorder.[146] Both anticonvulsant "mood stabilizers" and second-generation antipsychotics[147] have been used to treat comorbid bipolar disorder and CUD but there are few RCTs.[148,149] Citicoline significantly reduced cocaine use in two RCTs and methamphetamine use in one RCT. Lamotrigine reduced methamphetamine use in one RCT but did not improve mood. Risperidone and quetiapine both reduced cocaine and methamphetamine use when added to standard pharmacotherapy in a randomized, double-blind trial, but there was no placebo group to validate efficacy. Valproate and divalproex have not been evaluated in RCTs.

Bupropion, as an add-on to mood stabilizers, significantly reduced both cocaine use and depression symptoms, without inducing mania, in a small (12 participants), randomized, open-label clinical trial.[150]

Attention Deficit Hyperactivity Disorder

A meta-analysis of 9 published studies found that adult patients with attention deficit hyperactivity disorder (ADHD) had an estimated 10.0% (95% CI 8%-13%) lifetime prevalence of CUD.[151] Conversely, about 20% of adults with prescription StUD or CUD have ADHD.[152,153] Stimulant medications, which are the mainstay of ADHD treatment, have been evaluated for the treatment of comorbid StUD.[154] Mixed amphetamine salts (extended-release formulation) significantly reduced cocaine use in one RCT, while methylphenidate (either immediate or sustained release [SR] formulations) had no significant effect on cocaine use. Methylphenidate (SR formulation) significantly reduced methamphetamine use in one RCT but not in another. Bupropion (SR formulation) had no significant effect on cocaine use in one RCT.[154]

Schizophrenia

The prevalence of schizophrenia spectrum disorders among patients in treatment for CUD is about 1%,[155] roughly comparable to that in the general population. Conversely, the prevalence of CUD among individuals with schizophrenia averages 7% across studies, with a range of 4% to 12%.[156] Clinical experience suggests that antipsychotics, at doses that are often effective in the treatment of schizophrenia, are not generally effective in reducing cocaine use.[157,158] Several head-to-head RCTs found clozapine better than other antipsychotics in reducing cocaine use, with no significant differences among other antipsychotics.[159,160] However, the absence of a placebo group in these RCTs precludes assessing absolute efficacy.

Use of cocaine or amphetamines can exacerbate or provoke antipsychotic-induced movement disorders[77,78] and increase vulnerability to the neuroleptic malignant syndrome.[76]

Medical Comorbidity

Few studies have directly evaluated the safety and efficacy of medications for the treatment of StUD in patients with significant medical comorbidity, in part because such patients are excluded from many clinical trials for safety and ethical reasons. Limited clinical studies suggest that buprenorphine[161] and most anticonvulsants,[162] anti-depressants,[163] and anti-psychotics[163] can be safely given to patients receiving anti-retroviral treatment for HIV/AIDS. Drug-drug pharmacokinetic interactions may alter the plasma concentrations of bupropion and several other psychoactive medications, but these interactions are rarely clinically significant.[163] Buprenorphine may be safely given to patients with viral hepatitis.[161]

Gender-Specific Issues

Women tend to be excluded from or underrepresented in many clinical trials of pharmacotherapy for StUD,[164] in part because of concern, embodied in former FDA regulations, over risk to the fetus and neonate should a female subject become pregnant. Thus, there is a substantial lack of information about gender-specific issues of pharmacotherapy in general and the pharmacotherapy of StUD in particular.[40,165] This situation should improve in the future because current FDA and National Institutes of Health regulations require appropriate representation of women in clinical trials. Very few published RCTs have compared the effects of pharmacotherapy in men versus women; all do so post hoc rather than by prospective randomization.[165] Secondary analysis of an aggregate sample of 434 participants in five RCTs found that women had a poorer response to disulfiram than did men but a similar response to the behavioral treatment.[40] Single RCTs of modafinil and naltrexone also found that women had a poorer response than men to the treatment medication.[40] The reasons for these differences in medication response remain unclear, but may include gender differences in medication pharmacokinetics or pharmacodynamics (eg, resulting in different achieved plasma concentrations or adverse effects), hormonal interactions, or baseline characteristics that influence treatment outcome.

Two independent RCTs indirectly compared the effect of progesterone in men or women with CUD. In men, oral progesterone (100-300 mg twice daily) modestly but significantly increased cocaine use over a 10-week treatment period.[166] In postpartum (within 12 weeks of delivery) women, oral progesterone (25-100 mg daily) significantly reduced cocaine use over a 12-week treatment period.[167] The substantial difference in progesterone dosage makes it difficult to interpret the difference in outcome.

We are not aware of any published clinical studies evaluating pharmacotherapy for StUD in transgender participants.

Age

Adolescents (12-17 years old) and the elderly (65 years or older) are usually excluded from RCTs to evaluate pharmacological treatment for StUD—the former for legal and ethical (informed consent) considerations; the latter for safety concerns. We are not aware of any published RCTs that evaluated treatment medications for StUD alone in either age group.[168-170]

FUTURE PROSPECTS

Future progress in pharmacological treatment for StUD may come from two approaches: development of new medications with novel or more selective mechanisms of action and improved patient-treatment matching, that is, personalized medicine.

New medications or repurposing of existing medication should evolve from an improved understanding of the neuropharmacology of StUD and animal studies of the interactions of cocaine with novel compounds.[171] For example, a single intravenous infusion of ketamine significantly increased cocaine abstinence over the 5-week RCT.[172] Atypical presynaptic dopamine transporter ligands that may act as functional cocaine "antagonists,"[173] selective dopamine D_3 receptor partial agonists/antagonists that attenuate the rewarding effects of cocaine in animal studies,[173] and targeting the network of proteins and protein-protein interactions that mediate cocaine's actions on presynaptic biogenic amine neurotransmitter transporters[174,175] all hold promise. The endogenous cannabinoid (endocannabinoid) brain neurotransmitter system modulates the dopaminergic reward system.[176] Blockade of cannabinoid CB_1 receptors inhibits return to cocaine self-administration after abstinence in animals.[177] Therefore, CB_1 receptor neutral antagonists or inverse agonists have therapeutic potential if they become available for clinical research, although this will require compounds without the psychiatric side effects seen with previously available agents such as rimonabant.[178]

The failure of the pharmacodynamic approach to show consistent efficacy in the treatment of StUD has prompted interest in pharmacokinetic approaches that prevent ingested stimulants from entering the brain and/or enhance their elimination from the body.[15,179] The former approach could be implemented by active or passive immunization to produce binding antibodies that form a drug-antibody complex too large to cross the blood-brain barrier. The latter approach could be implemented for CUD by administration of an enzyme (eg, butyrylcholinesterase [BChE, EC 3.1.1.8]) that catalyzes cocaine hydrolysis or by immunization with a catalytic antibody.

These pharmacokinetic approaches show promise in early clinical trials. An anti-cocaine vaccine (ie, active immunization against cocaine) significantly reduced cocaine use in a phase II RCT among the one-third of participants who mounted a substantial antibody response but only during the first 8 weeks of treatment.[180] Further work is needed to increase the consistency of the antibody response, lengthen the duration of effect, and evaluate combination treatments; for example, an immediately active treatment to promptly reduce cocaine effects until vaccine-induced antibodies reach effective concentrations.[15] Several anti-methamphetamine vaccines are currently undergoing phase I human laboratory study.[179]

Parenteral treatment with a genetically enhanced bacterial cocaine esterase (IV)[181] or with genetically enhanced BChE conjugated to albumin to increase half-life (TV-1380; sc)[182] significantly reduced the acute subjective and cardiovascular effects of an IV cocaine challenge in two human laboratory studies. In a phase II RCT, TV-1380 (IM weekly) significantly increased the proportion of cocaine-free urine samples over the last 8 weeks of the 12-week treatment period; there was no difference in proportion of participants achieving 3 weeks of continuous abstinence.[183] These enhanced cocaine-metabolizing enzymes could serve as a bridge treatment for vaccination until effective anti-cocaine antibody concentrations were achieved.

Personalized medicine, in the form of pharmacogenomics, offers another approach to improving treatment for StUD, by identifying subsets of patients, based on their genetic characteristics, who are more likely to respond better to a specific treatment than does the typical patient. Early phase II studies identified 3 medications and the anti-cocaine vaccine whose efficacy was influenced by genetic variation in 8 different genes (**Table 64-5**).

TABLE 64-5 Medications With Genetic Influence on Efficacy for Treatment of Cocaine Use Disorder

Medication	Gene
Buprenorphine	Prodynorphin[68]
Disulfiram	ANKK1[36] Dopamine D2 receptor[36] Dopamine transporter[37] α_{1a}-adrenergic receptor[38] δ-opioid receptor[39]
Doxazosin	α_1-adrenergic receptor[91] dopamine-β-hydroxlase[90]
Anti-cocaine vaccine	dopamine-β-hydroxlase[185]

ANKK1, ankyrin repeat and kinase domain containing 1.

CONCLUSIONS

The evidence base for effectiveness of pharmacological treatment of StUD is relatively weak. Many clinical trials are underpowered because of small sample size and have limited internal validity because of high premature discontinuation rates (40% or more in many studies). Thus, no medication is approved by the FDA or any national regulatory authority for this indication.

For the treatment of CUD, there is medium-quality evidence, based on at least two adequately powered RCTs or a meta-analysis, for antidepressants such as desipramine (in patients with mild CUD), the SSRIs citalopram and sertraline, and bupropion, stimulants such as sustained release amphetamines and modafinil, and the anti-convulsant topiramate. There is low-quality evidence to support use of opioid receptor ligands (buprenorphine [in those with a history of OUD], naltrexone), disulfiram (in men with specific responsive genotypes), doxazosin, and ondansetron. For the treatment of ATSUD, there is low-quality evidence for the use of riluzole.

There is even less evidence to guide the treatment of patients with StUD and comorbid SUDs or other psychiatric comorbidity. Disulfiram and naltrexone have low-quality evidence for efficacy in patients with comorbid AUD. High-dose buprenorphine or methadone have low-quality evidence for efficacy in patients with comorbid OUD. Several antidepressants (eg, desipramine, sertraline, venlafaxine) have low-quality evidence for reducing both depression symptoms and cocaine use in patients with mild CUD. Bupropion, citicoline, and lamotrigine have at least low-quality evidence for reducing stimulant use in patients with comorbid bipolar disorder. Clozapine has moderate-quality evidence for being better than other antipsychotics in reducing stimulant use in patients with comorbid schizophrenia, although there is no evidence regarding its absolute efficacy.

More sophisticated patient-treatment matching could enhance the efficacy of current medications by taking into account both patient characteristics that can influence treatment response (eg, severity of dependence, withdrawal status, psychiatric comorbidity, concomitant medications, or genotype) and characteristics of the psychosocial treatment, which should always accompany pharmacological treatment. Several studies show that contingency management and CBT, or their combination, are most effective in enhancing the response to medication.

Improved understanding of the neurobiology of StUD should lead to identification of new treatment targets and development of more effective medications, possibly by specific manipulation of dopaminergic or endocannabinoid systems or by a pharmacokinetic mechanism. Adoption of any medication into clinical practice should be guided by acceptable scientific proof of efficacy and safety, based on data from replicated, well-designed, adequately powered RCTs. Clinicians should also keep in mind the distinctions between efficacy (how well treatment works in a carefully selected research population getting close attention) and effectiveness (how well treatment works in a heterogeneous population in a realistic clinical environment) and between a statistically significant and clinically meaningful treatment effect.[184]

REFERENCES

1. Global Burden of Disease 2016 Alcohol and Drug Use Collaborators. The global burden of disease attributable to alcohol and drug use in 195 countries and territories, 1990–2016: a systematic analysis for the Global Burden of Disease Study 2016. *Lancet Psychiatry*. 2018;5:987-1012.
2. Compton WM, Dawson DA, Goldstein RB, Grant BF. Crosswalk between DSM-IV dependence and DSM-5 substance use disorders for opioids, cannabis, cocaine and alcohol. *Drug Alcohol Depend.* 2013;132(1-2):387-390.
3. Center for Behavioral Health Statistics and Quality. *Results from the 2020 National Survey on Drug Use and Health: Detailed Tables*. Substance Abuse and Mental Health Services Administration; 2021. Accessed January 21, 2022. https://www.samhsa.gov/data/
4. Center for Behavioral Health Statistics and Quality. *Treatment Episode Data Set (TEDS): 2019. Admissions to and Discharges from Publicly Funded Substance Use Treatment*. Substance Abuse and Mental Health Services Administration; 2021.
5. Substance Abuse and Mental Health Services Administration. *Preliminary Findings from Drug-Related Emergency Department Visits, 2021*. Drug Abuse Warning Network (HHS Publication No. PEP22-07-03-001). Center for Behavioral Health Statistics and Quality, SAMHSA; 2022. Accessed June 1, 2022. https://www.samhsa.gov/data/
6. Kariisa M, Seth P, Scholl L, et al. Trends in drug overdose deaths involving cocaine and psychostimulants with abuse potential among racial and ethnic groups – United States, 2004–2019. *Drug Alcohol Depend.* 2021;227:109001.
7. Ronsley C, Nolan S, Knight R, Hayashi K, et al. Treatment of stimulant use disorder: a systematic review of reviews. *PLoS ONE*. 2020;15(6):e0234809.
8. Bentzley BS, Han SS, Neuner S, et al. Comparison of treatments for cocaine use disorder among adults. A systematic review and meta-analysis. *JAMA Netw Open.* 2021;4(5):e218049.
9. Crescenzo F, Ciabattini M, D'Alò GL, et al. Comparative efficacy and acceptability of psychosocial interventions for individuals with cocaine and amphetamine addiction: a systematic review and network meta-analysis. *PLoS Med.* 2018;15(12):e1002715.
10. Tardelli VS, Pádua do Lagoa MP, Mendez M, et al. Contingency management with pharmacologic treatment for stimulant use disorders: a review. *Behav Res Ther.* 2018;111:57-63.

11. Schmitz JM, Lindsay JA, Stotts AL, Green CE, Moeller FG. Contingency management and levodopa-carbidopa for cocaine treatment: a comparison of three behavioral targets. *Exp Clin Psychopharmacology.* 2010;18(3):238-244.
12. Ray LA, Meredith LR, Kiluk BD, et al. Combined pharmacotherapy and cognitive behavioral therapy for adults with alcohol or substance use disorder. A systematic review and meta-analysis. *JAMA Netw Open.* 2020;3(6):e208279.
13. Gorelick DA, Gardner EL, Xi ZX. Agents in development for the management of cocaine abuse. *Drugs.* 2004;64(14):1547-1573.
14. Howell LL, Kimmel HL. Monoamine transporters and psychostimulant addiction. *Biochem Pharmacol.* 2008;75(1):196-217.
15. Gorelick DA. Pharmacokinetic strategies for treatment of drug overdose and addiction. *Future Med Chem.* 2012;4(2):227-243.
16. Brandt L, Chao T, Comer SD, et al. Pharmacotherapeutic strategies for treating cocaine use disorder—what do we have to offer? *Addiction.* 2020;116:694-710.
17. Chan B, Kondo K, Freeman M, et al. Pharmacotherapy for cocaine use disorder—a systematic review and meta-analysis. *J Gen Intern Med.* 2019;34(12):2858-2873.
18. Ziedonis DM, Kosten TR. Pharmacotherapy improves treatment outcome in depressed cocaine addicts. *J Psychoactive Drugs.* 1991; 23(4):417-425.
19. Arndt IO, McLellan AT, Dorozynsky L, Woody GE, O'Brien CP. Desipramine treatment for cocaine dependence. Role of antisocial personality disorder. *J Nerv Ment Dis.* 1994;182(3):151-156.
20. Kosten T, Oliveto A, Feingold A, et al. Desipramine and contingency management for cocaine and opiate dependence in buprenorphine maintained patients. *Drug Alcohol Depend.* 2003;70(3):315-325.
21. Khalsa ME, Gawin FH, Rawson R, et al. *A Desipramine Ceiling in Cocaine Abusers. College on Problems of Drug Dependence, 1992.* National Institute on Drug Abuse; 1993:18.
22. Fischman MW, Foltin RW, Nestadt G, Pearlson GD. Effects of desipramine maintenance on cocaine self-administration by humans. *J Pharmacol Exp Ther.* 1990;253(2):760-770.
23. Li Y, Simmler LD, Van Zessen R, et al. Synaptic mechanism underlying serotonin modulation of transition to cocaine addiction. *Science.* 2021;373:1252-1256.
24. Moeller FG, Schmitz JM, Steinberg JL, et al. Citalopram combined with behavioral therapy reduces cocaine use: a double-blind, placebo-controlled trial. *Am J Drug Alcohol Abuse.* 2007;33:367-378.
25. Suchting R, Green CE, de Dios C, et al. Citalopram for treatment of cocaine use disorder: a Bayesian drop-the-loser randomized clinical trial. *Drug Alcohol Depend.* 2021;228:109054.
26. Ciraulo DA, Knapp C, Rotrosen J, et al. Nefazodone treatment of cocaine dependence with comorbid depressive symptoms. *Addiction.* 2005;100(Suppl 1):23-31.
27. Passos SR, Camacho LA, Lopes CS, dos Santos MA. Nefazodone in out-patient treatment of inhaled cocaine dependence: a randomized double-blind placebo-controlled trial. *Addiction.* 2005;100(4):489-494.
28. Ciraulo DA, Sarid-Segal O, Knapp CM, et al. Efficacy screening trials of paroxetine, pentoxifylline, riluzole, pramipexole and venlafaxine in cocaine dependence. *Addiction.* 2005;100(suppl 1):12-22.
29. Raby WN, Rubin EA, Garawi F, et al. A randomized, double-blind, placebo-controlled trial of venlafaxine for the treatment of depressed cocaine-dependent patients. *Am J Addiction.* 2014;23:68-75.
30. Afshar M, Knapp CM, Sarid-Segal O, et al. The efficacy of mirtazapine in the treatment of cocaine dependence with comorbid depression. *Am J Drug Alcohol Depend.* 2012;8:181-186.
31. Elkashef A, Fudala PJ, Gorgon L, et al. Double-blind, placebo-controlled trial of selegiline transdermal system (STS) for the treatment of cocaine dependence. *Drug Alcohol Depend.* 2006;85(3):191-197.
32. Walsh SL, Middleton LS, Wong CJ, et al. Atomoxetine does not alter cocaine use in cocaine dependent individuals: double blind randomized trial. *Drug Alcohol Depend.* 2013;130(1-3):150-157.
33. Thomas HM, Campbell J, Laster L, et al. *Efficacy of Two Doses of Tyrosine in Retaining Crack Cocaine Abusers in Outpatient Treatment. College on Problems of Drug Dependence 1995.* National Institute on Drug Abuse; 1996:148.
34. Gaval-Cruz M, Weinshenker D. Mechanisms of disulfiram-induced cocaine abstinence: antabuse and cocaine relapse. *Mol Interv.* 2009; 9(4):175-187.
35. Kosten TR, Wu G, Huang W, et al. Pharmacogenetic randomized trial for cocaine abuse: disulfiram and dopamine beta-hydroxylase. *Biol Psychiatry.* 2013;73(3):219-224.
36. Spellicy CJ, Kosten TR, Hamon SC, Harding MJ, Nielsen DA. ANKK1 and DRD2 pharmacogenetics of disulfiram treatment for cocaine abuse. *Pharmacogenet Genomics.* 2013;23(7):333-340.
37. Kampangkaew JP, Spellicy CJ, Nielsen EM, et al. Pharmacogenetic role of dopamine transporter (SLC6A3) variation on response to disulfiram treatment for cocaine addiction. *Am J Addict.* 2019;28:311-317.
38. Shorter D, Nielsen DA, Huang W, Harding MJ, Hamon SC, Kosten TR. Pharmacogenetic randomized trial for cocaine abuse: disulfiram and alpha1A-adrenoceptor gene variation. *Eur Neuropsychopharmacol.* 2013;23(11):1401-1407.
39. Thomas PS Jr, Nielsen EM, Spellicy CJ, et al. The *OPRD1* rs678849 variant influences outcome of disulfiram treatment for cocaine dependency in methadone-maintained patients. *Psychiatr Genet.* 2021;31:88-94.
40. DeVito EE, Babuscio TA, Nich C, Ball SA, Carroll KM. Gender differences in clinical outcomes for cocaine dependence: randomized clinical trials of behavioral therapy and disulfiram. *Drug Alcohol Depend.* 2014;145:156-167.
41. Malcolm R, Olive MF, Lechner W. The safety of disulfiram for the treatment of alcohol and cocaine dependence in randomized clinical trials: guidance for clinical practice. *Expert Opin Drug Saf.* 2008;7(4):459-472.
42. Haile CN, de la Garza IIR, Mahoney JJ III, et al. The impact of disulfiram treatment on the reinforcing effects of cocaine: a randomized clinical trial. *PLoS One.* 2012;7(11):e47702.
43. Roache JD, Kahn R, Newton TF, et al. A double-blind, placebo-controlled assessment of the safety of potential interactions between intravenous cocaine, ethanol, and oral disulfiram. *Drug Alcohol Depend.* 2011;119(1-2):37-45.
44. De La Garza R II, Bubar MJ, Carbone CL, et al. Evaluation of the dopamine beta-hydroxylase (DβH) inhibitor nepicastat in participants who meet criteria for cocaine use disorder. *Prog Neuropsychopharmacol Biol Psychiatry.* 2015;59:40-48.
45. U.S. National Library of Medicine. *A Multi-Center Trial of Nepicastat for Cocaine Dependence.* ClinicalTrials.gov. 2017; NCT01704196. Accessed August 2, 2022. www.clinicaltrials.gov
46. Winhusen TM, Kropp F, Lindblad R, et al. Multisite, randomized, double-blind, placebo-controlled pilot clinical trial to evaluate the efficacy of buspirone as a relapse-prevention treatment for cocaine dependence. *J Clin Psychiatry.* 2014;75(7):757-764.
47. Jenkins SW, Warfield NA, Blaine JD, et al. A pilot trial of gepirone vs. placebo in the treatment of cocaine dependency. *Psychopharmacol Bull.* 1992;28(1):21-26.
48. Cornish JW, Maany I, Fudala PJ, Ehrman RN, Robbins SJ, O'Brien CP. A randomized, double-blind, placebo-controlled study of ritanserin pharmacotherapy for cocaine dependence. *Drug Alcohol Depend.* 2001;61(2):183-189.
49. Johnson BA, Chen YR, Swann AC, et al. Ritanserin in the treatment of cocaine dependence. *Biol Psychiatry.* 1997;42(10):932-940.
50. Santos G-M, Ikeda J, Coffin P, et al. Pilot study of extended-release lorcarserin for cocaine use disorder in men who sleep with men: a double-blind, placebo-controlled randomized trial. *PLoS One.* 2021;16(7):me0254724.
51. Johnson BA, Roache JD, Ait-Daoud N, et al. A preliminary randomized, double-blind, placebo-controlled study of the safety and efficacy of ondansetron in the treatment of cocaine dependence. *Drug Alcohol Depend.* 2006;84(3):256-263.
52. Blevins D, Seneviratne C, Wang X-Q, et al. A randomized, double-blind, placebo-controlled trial of ondansetron for the treatment of cocaine use disorder with post hoc pharmacogenetic analysis. *Drug Alcohol Depend.* 2021;228:109074.

53. Grasing K. A threshold model for opposing actions of acetylcholine on reward behavior: molecular mechanisms and implications for treatment of substance abuse disorders. *Behav Brain Res.* 2016;312:148-162.
54. Dieckmann LH, Ramos AC, Silva EA, et al. Effects of biperiden on the treatment of cocaine/crack addiction: a randomised, double-blind, placebo-controlled trial. *Eur Neuropsychopharmacol.* 2014;24(8):1196-1202.
55. Reid MS, Angrist B, Baker SA, et al. A placebo controlled, double-blind study of mecamylamine treatment for cocaine dependence in patients enrolled in an opiate replacement program. *Subst Abuse.* 2005;26(2):5-14.
56. Lynch KG, Plebani J, Spratt K, et al. Varenicline for the treatment of cocaine dependence. *J Addict Med.* 2022;16(2):157-163.
57. Winhusen TM, Somoza EC, Harrer JM, et al. A placebo-controlled screening trial of tiagabine, sertraline and donepezil as cocaine dependence treatments. *Addiction.* 2005;100(suppl 1):68-77.
58. Sofuoglu M, Carroll KM. Effects of galantamine on cocaine use in chronic cocaine users. *Am J Addict.* 2011;20(3):302-303.
59. Carroll KM, Nich C, DeVito EE, et al. Galantamine and computerized cognitive behavioral therapy for cocaine dependence: a randomized clinical trial. *J Clin Psychiatry.* 2018;79(1):17m11669.
60. DeVito EE, Carroll KM, Babuscio T, et al. Randomized placebo-controlled trial of galantamine in individuals with cocaine use disorder. *J Subst Abuse Treatment.* 2019;107:29-37.
61. Minkowski CP, Epstein D, Frost JJ, Gorelick DA. Differential response to IV carfentanil in chronic cocaine users and healthy controls. *Addict Biol.* 2012;17(1):149-155.
62. Gorelick DA, Kim YK, Bencherif B, et al. Imaging brain mu-opioid receptors in abstinent cocaine users: time course and relation to cocaine craving. *Biol Psychiatry.* 2005;57(12):1573-1582.
63. Gorelick DA, Kim YK, Bencherif B, et al. Brain mu-opioid receptor binding: relationship to relapse to cocaine use after monitored abstinence. *Psychopharmacology (Berl).* 2008;200(4):475-486.
64. Ghitza UE, Preston KL, Epstein DH, et al. Brain mu-opioid receptor binding predicts treatment outcome in cocaine-abusing outpatients. *Biol Psychiatry.* 2010;68(8):697-703.
65. Schmitz JM, Stotts AL, Rhoades HM, Grabowski J. Naltrexone and relapse prevention treatment for cocaine-dependent patients. *Addict Behav.* 2001;26(2):167-180.
66. Schmitz JM, Green CE, Stotts AL, et al. A two-phased screening paradigm for evaluating candidate medications for cocaine cessation or relapse prevention: modafinil, levodopa-carbidopa, naltrexone. *Drug Alcohol Depend.* 2014;136:100-107.
67. Ling W, Hillhouse MP, Saxon AJ, et al. Buprenorphine + naloxone plus naltrexone for the treatment of cocaine dependence: the Cocaine Use Reduction with Buprenorphine (CURB) study. *Addiction.* 2016; 111(8):1416-1427.
68. Nielsen DA, Walker R, Graham DP, et al. Moderation of buprenorphine therapy for cocaine dependence efficacy by variation in the *Prodynorphin* gene. *Eur J Clin Pharmacol.* 2022;78:965-973.
69. Gorelick DA. The rate hypothesis and agonist substitution approaches to cocaine abuse treatment. *Adv Pharmacol.* 1998;42:995-997.
70. Tardelli VS, Bisaga A, Arcadepani FB, et al. Prescription psychostimulants for the treatment of stimulant use disorder: a systematic review and meta-analysis. *Psychopharmacology.* 2020;237:2233-2255.
71. Castells X, Cunill R, Perez-Mana C, et al. Psychostimulant drugs for cocaine dependence. *Cochrane Database Syst Rev.* 2016;9:CD007380.
72. Nuijten M, Blanken P, van de Wetering B, Nuijen B, van den Brink W, Hendriks VM. Sustained-release dexamfetamine in the treatment of chronic cocaine-dependent patients on heroin-assisted treatment: a randomised, double-blind, placebo-controlled trial. *Lancet.* 2016;387(10034):2226-2234.
73. Sangroula D, Motiwala F, Wagle B, et al. Modafinil treatment of cocaine dependence: a systematic review and meta-analysis. *Subst Use Misuse.* 2017;52(10):1292-1306.
74. Green AI, Noordsy DL, Brunette MF, et al. Substance abuse and schizophrenia: Pharmacotherapeutic intervention. *J Subst Abuse Treatment.* 2008;34:61-71.
75. Moran LM, Phillips KA, Kowalczyk WJ, et al. Aripiprazole for cocaine abstinence: a randomized-controlled trial with ecological momentary assessment. *Behav Pharmacol.* 2017;28(1):63-73.
76. Akpaffiong MJ, Ruiz P. Neuroleptic malignant syndrome: a complication of neuroleptics and cocaine abuse. *Psychiatr Q.* 1991;62(4):299-309.
77. Potvin S, Blancet P, Stip E. Substance abuse is associated with increased extrapyramidal symptoms in schizophrenia: a meta-analysis. *Schiz Res.* 2009;113:181-188.
78. Cenci D, Carbone MG, Callegari C, et al. Psychomotor symptoms in chronic cocaine users: an interpretive model. *Int J Environ Res Public Health.* 2022;19:1897.
79. Ashok AH, Mizuno Y, Volkow ND, Howes OD. Association of stimulant use with dopaminergic alterations in users of cocaine, amphetamine, or methamphetamine. A systematic review and meta-analysis. *JAMA Psychiatry.* 2017;74(5):511-519.
80. Manhapra A, Chakraborty A, Arias AJ. Topiramate pharmacotherapy for alcohol use disorder and other addictions: a narrative review. *J Addict Med.* 2019;13:7-22.
81. Blevins D, Wang X-Q, Sharma S, et al. Impulsiveness as a predictor of topiramate response for cocaine use disorder. *Am J Addiction.* 2019;28:71-76.
82. Reid MS, Casadonte P, Baker S, et al. A placebo-controlled screening trial of olanzapine, valproate, and coenzyme Q10/L-carnitine for the treatment of cocaine dependence. *Addiction.* 2005;100(suppl 1):43-57.
83. Chadwick MJ, Gregory DL, Wendling G. A double-blind amino acids, L-tryptophan and L-tyrosine, and placebo study with cocaine-dependent subjects in an inpatient chemical dependency treatment center. *Am J Drug Alcohol Abuse.* 1990;16(3-4):275-286.
84. Jones HE, Johnson RE, Bigelow GE, Silverman K, Mudric T, Strain EC. Safety and efficacy of L-tryptophan and behavioral incentives for treatment of cocaine dependence: a randomized clinical trial. *Am J Addict.* 2004;13(5):421-437.
85. Margolin A, Kantak K, Copenhaver M, Avants SK. A preliminary, controlled investigation of magnesium L-aspartate hydrochloride for illicit cocaine and opiate use in methadone-maintained patients. *J Addict Dis.* 2003;22(2):49-61.
86. White A. Trials of acupuncture for drug dependence: a recommendation for hypotheses based on the literature. *Acupunct Med.* 2013;31(3):297-304.
87. Vorobyeva N, Kozlova AA. Three naturally-occurring psychedelics and their significance in the treatment of mental health disorders. *Frontiers Pharmacol.* 2022;13:927984.
88. Kampman K, Majewska MD, Tourian K, et al. A pilot trial of piracetam and ginkgo biloba for the treatment of cocaine dependence. *Addict Behav.* 2003;28(3):437-448.
89. Shorter D, Lindsay JA, Kosten TR. The alpha-1 adrenergic antagonist doxazosin for treatment of cocaine dependence: a pilot study. *Drug Alcohol Depend.* 2013;131(1-2):66-70.
90. Zhang X, Nielsen DA, Domingo CB, et al. Pharmacogenetics of *Dopamine β-Hydroxylase* in cocaine dependence therapy with doxazosin. *Addiction Biol.* 2019;24:531-538.
91. Shorter DI, Zhang X, Domingo CB, et al. Doxazosin treatment in cocaine use disorder: pharmacogenetic response based on an *alpha-1 adrenoreceptor subtype D* genetic variant. *Am J Drug Alcohol Abuse.* 2020;46(2):184-193.
92. Kampman KM, Dackis C, Lynch KG, et al. A double-blind, placebo-controlled trial of amantadine, propranolol, and their combination for the treatment of cocaine dependence in patients with severe cocaine withdrawal symptoms. *Drug Alcohol Depend.* 2006;85(2):129-137.
93. Sofuoglu M, Poling J, Babuscio T, et al. Carvedilol does not reduce cocaine use in methadone-maintained cocaine users. *J Subst Abuse Treat.* 2017;73:63-69.
94. Rodrigues LA, Caroba MES, Taba FK, et al. Evaluation of the potential use of cannabidiol in the treatment of cocaine use disorder: a systematic review. *Pharmacol Biochem Behav.* 2020;196:172982.
95. Mongeau-Perusse V, Brissette S, Bruneau J, et al. Cannabidiol as a treatment for craving and relapse in individuals with cocaine use disorder: a randomized, placebo-controlled trial. *Addiction.* 2021;116:2431-2442.

96. Malcolm R, LaRowe S, Cochran K, et al. A controlled trial of amlodipine for cocaine dependence: a negative report. *J Subst Abuse Treat.* 2005;28(2):197-204.
97. Shoptaw S, Majewska MD, Wilkins J, Twitchell G, Yang X, Ling W. Participants receiving dehydroepiandrosterone during treatment for cocaine dependence show high rates of cocaine use in a placebo-controlled pilot study. *Exp Clin Psychopharmacol.* 2004;12(2):126-135.
98. Stoops WW, Rush CR. Combination pharmacotherapies for stimulant use disorder: a review of clinical findings and recommendations for future research. *Expert Rev Clin Pharmacol.* 2014;7(3):363-374.
99. Mariani JJ, Pavlicova M, Bisaga A, Nunes EV, Brooks DJ, Levin FR. Extended-release mixed amphetamine salts and topiramate for cocaine dependence: a randomized controlled trial. *Biol Psychiatry.* 2012;72(11):950-956.
100. Levin FR, Mariani JJ, Pavlicova M, et al. Extended release mixed amphetamine salts and topiramate for cocaine dependence: a randomized clinical replication trial with frequent users. *Drug Alcohol Depend.* 2020;206:107700.
101. Mahoney JJ III, Hanlon CA, Marshalek PJ, et al. Transcranial magnetic stimulation, deep brain stimulation, and other forms of neuromodulation for substance use disorders: review of modalities and implications for treatment. *J Neurol Sci.* 2020;418:117149.
102. Antonelli M, Fattore L, Sestito L, et al. Transcranial magnetic stimulation: a review about its efficacy in the treatment of alcohol, tobacco, and cocaine addiction. *Addict Behav.* 2021;14:106760.
103. Lolli F, Salimova M, Scarpino M, et al. A randomized, double-blind, sham-controlled, study of left prefrontal cortex 15 Hz repetitive transcranial magnetic stimulation in cocaine consumption and craving. *PLoS One.* 2021;16(11):e0259860.
104. Martinotti G, Pettorruso M, Montemitro C, et al. Repetitive transcranial magnetic stimulation in treatment-seeking subjects with cocaine use disorder: a randomized, double-blind, sham-controlled trial. *Progr Neuropsychopharmacol Biol Psychiatry.* 2022;116:110513.
105. Gaudreault P-O, Sharma A, Datta A, et al. A double-blind, sham-controlled phae I clinical trial of tDCS of the dorsolateral prefrontal cortex in cocaine inpatients: craving, sleepiness, and contemplation to change. *Eur J Neurosci.* 2021;53:3212-3230.
106. Cao DN, Shi JJ, Hao W, Wu N, Li J. Advances and challenges in pharmacotherapeutics for amphetamine-type stimulants addiction. *Eur J Pharmacol.* 2016;780:129-135.
107. Chan B, Freeman M, Kondo K, et al. Pharmacotherapy for methamphetamine-amphetamine use disorder—a systematic review and meta-analysis. *Addiction.* 2019;114:2122-2136.
108. Ezard N, Clifford B, Dunlop A, et al. Safety and tolerability of oral lisdexamfetamine in adults with methamphetamine dependence: a phase-2 dose-escalation study. *BMJ Open.* 2021;11:e044696.
109. Heikkinen M, Taipale H, Tanskanen A, et al. Association of pharmacological treatments and hospitalization and death in individuals with amphetamine use disorders in a Swedish nationwide cohort of 13 965 patients. *JAMA Psychiatry.* 2023;80(1):31-39.
110. Grant JE, Odlaug BL, Kim SW. A double-blind, placebo-controlled study of *N*-acetyl cysteine plus naltrexone for methamphetamine dependence. *Eur Neuropsychopharmacol.* 2010;20(11):823-828.
111. Trivedi MH, Walker R, Ling W, et al. Bupropion and naltrexone in methamphetamine use disorder. *N Engl J Med.* 2021;384(2):140-153. doi:10.1056/NEJMoa2020214
112. Bhatt M, Zielinski L, Baker-Beal L, et al. Efficacy and safety of psychostimulants for amphetamine and methamphetamine use disorders: a systematic review and meta-analysis. *Syst Rev.* 2016;5:189.
113. Naji L, Dennis B, Rosic T, et al. Mirtazapine for the treatment of amphetamine and methamphetamine use disorder: a systematic review and meta-analysis. *Drug Alcohol Depend.* 2022;232:109295.
114. Farahzahdi M-H, Moazen-Zadeh E, Razaghi E, et al. Riluzole for treatment of men with methamphetamine dependence: a randomized, double-blind, placebo-controlled clinical trial. *J Psychopharmacol.* 2019;33(3):305-315.
115. Sun H-Q, Chen H-M, Yang F-D, et al. Epidemiological trends and the advancement of treatments of amphetamine-type stimulants (ATS) in China. *Am J Addict.* 2014;23:313-317.
116. Zhang JJQ, Fong KNK, Ouyang R-G, Siu AMH, Kranz GS. Effects of repetitive transcranial magnetic stimulation (rTMS) on craving and substance consumption in patients with substance dependence: a systematic review and meta-analysis. *Addiction.* 2019;114:2137-2149.
117. Mustaquim D, Jones CM, Compton WM. Trends and correlates of cocaine use among adults in the United States, 2006-2019. *Addictive Behav.* 2021;120:106950.
118. Lin LA, Bohnert ASB, Blow FC, et al. Polysubstance use and association with opioid use disorder treatment in the US Veterans Health Administration. *Addiction.* 2020;116:96-104.
119. Mahoney JJ III, Winstanley EL, Lander LR, et al. High prevalence of substance use in individuals with opioid use disorder. *Addict Behav.* 2021;114:106752.
120. Peles E, Kreek MJ, Kellogg S, Adelson M. High methadone dose significantly reduces cocaine use in methadone maintenance treatment (MMT) patients. *J Addict Dis.* 2006;25(1):43-50.
121. Baumeister M, Vogel M, Dursteler-MacFarland KM, et al. Association between methadone dose and concomitant cocaine use in methadone maintenance treatment: a register-based study. *Subst Abuse Treatment Prevent Policy.* 2014;9:46.
122. Heikman PK, Muhonen LH, Ohanpera IA. Polydrug abuse among opioid maintenance treatment patients is related to inadequate dose of maintenance treatment medicine. *BMC Psychiatry.* 2017;17:245.
123. Stine SM, Freeman M, Burns B. Effect of methadone dose on cocaine abuse in a methadone program. *Am J Addict.* 1992;1(4):294-303.
124. Montoya ID, Gorelick DA, Preston KL, et al. Randomized trial of buprenorphine for treatment of concurrent opiate and cocaine dependence. *Clin Pharmacol Ther.* 2004;75(1):34-48.
125. Schottenfeld RS, Chawarski MC, Pakes JR, Pantalon MV, Carroll KM, Kosten TR. Methadone versus buprenorphine with contingency management or performance feedback for cocaine and opioid dependence. *Am J Psychiatry.* 2005;162(2):340-349.
126. Gross A, Marsch LA, Badger GJ, Bickel WK. A comparison between low-magnitude voucher and buprenorphine medication contingencies in promoting abstinence from opioids and cocaine. *Exp Clin Psychopharmacol.* 2006;14(2):148-156.
127. Xu KY, Mintz CM, Presnall N, et al. Comparative effectiveness of buprenorphine and naltrexone in opioid use disorder and co-occurring polysubstance use. *JAMA Netw Open.* 2022;5(5):e2211363.
128. Chan B, Freeman M, Ayers C, et al. A systematic review and meta-analysis of medications for stimulant use disorders in patients with co-occurring opioid use disorders. *Drug Alcohol Depend.* 2020;216:108193.
129. Prince V, Bowling KC. Topiramate in the treatment of cocaine use disorder. *Am J Health-Syst Pharm.* 2018;75:e13-e22.
130. Carroll KM, Nich C, Ball SA, McCance E, Rounsavile BJ. Treatment of cocaine and alcohol dependence with psychotherapy and disulfiram. *Addiction.* 1998;93(5):713-727.
131. Carroll KM, Nich C, Ball SA, McCance E, Frankforter TL, Rounsaville BJ. One-year follow-up of disulfiram and psychotherapy for cocaine-alcohol users: sustained effects of treatment. *Addiction.* 2000;95(9):1335-1349.
132. Higgins ST, Budney AJ, Bickel WK, Hughes JR, Foerg F. Disulfiram therapy in patients abusing cocaine and alcohol. *Am J Psychiatry.* 1993;150(4):675-676.
133. Pettinati HM, Kampman KM, Lynch KG, et al. A double blind, placebo-controlled trial that combines disulfiram and naltrexone for treating co-occurring cocaine and alcohol dependence. *Addict Behav.* 2008;33(5):651-667.
134. Oslin DW, Pettinati HM, Volpicelli JR, Wolf AL, Kampman KM, O'Brien CP. The effects of naltrexone on alcohol and cocaine use in dually addicted patients. *J Subst Abuse Treat.* 1999;16(2):163-167.
135. Carroll KM, Ziedonis D, O'Malley S, et al. Pharmacologic interventions for alcohol- and cocaine-abusing individuals. *Am J Addict.* 1993; 2(1):77-79.

136. Hersh D, Van Kirk JR, Kranzler HR. Naltrexone treatment of comorbid alcohol and cocaine use disorders. *Psychopharmacology (Berl).* 1998;139(1-2):44-52.
137. Schmitz JM, Stotts AL, Sayre SL, DeLaune KA, Grabowski J. Treatment of cocaine-alcohol dependence with naltrexone and relapse prevention therapy. *Am J Addict.* 2004;13(4):333-341.
138. Pettinati HM, Kampman KM, Lynch KG, et al. A pilot trial of injectable, extended-release naltrexone for the treatment of co-occurring cocaine and alcohol dependence. *Am J Addict.* 2014;23(6):591-597.
139. Kampman KM, Pettinati HM, Lynch KG, Spratt K, Wierzbicki MR, O'Brien CP. A double-blind, placebo-controlled trial of topiramate for the treatment of comorbid cocaine and alcohol dependence. *Drug Alcohol Depend.* 2013;133(1):94-99.
140. Kandel DB, Huang F-Y, Davies M. Comorbidity between patterns of substance use dependence and psychiatric syndromes. *Drug Alcohol Depend.* 2001;204:233-241.
141. Ford JD, Gelernter J, DeVoe JS, et al. Association of psychiatric and substance use disorder comorbidity with cocaine dependence severity and treatment utilization in cocaine-dependent individuals. *Drug Alcohol Depend.* 2009;99(1-3):193-203.
142. Gonzalez-Saiz F, Vergara-Moragues E, Verdejo-Garcia A, Fernandez-Calderon F, Lozano OM. Impact of psychiatric comorbidity on the in-treatment outcomes of cocaine-dependent patients in therapeutic communities. *Subst Abuse.* 2014;35(2):133-140.
143. Murthy P, Mahadevan J, Chand PK. Treatment of substance use disorders with severe co-occurring mental health disorders. *Curr Opin Psychiatry.* 2019;32:293-299.
144. Torrens M, Tirado-Munoz J, Fonseca F, et al. Clinical practice guideline on pharmacological and psychological management of adult patients with depression and a comorbid substance use disorder. *Addiciones.* 2022;34(2):128-141.
145. Mancino MJ, McGaugh J, Chopra MP, et al. Clinical efficacy of sertraline alone and augmented with gabapentin in recently abstinent cocaine-dependent patients with depressive symptoms. *J Clin Psychopharmacol.* 2014;34(2):234-239.
146. Hunt GE, Malhi GS, Cleary M, et al. Comorbidity of bipolar and substance use disorders in national surveys of general populations, 1990=2015: systematic review and meta-analysis. *J Affect Disorders.* 2016;206:321-330.
147. Spede G, Lorusso M, Spano MC, et al. Efficacy and safety of atypical antipsychotics in bipolar disorder with comorbid substance dependence: a systematic review. *Clin Neuropharmacol.* 2018;41:181-191.
148. Preuss UW, Shaeffer M, Born C, et al. Bipolar disorder and comorbid use of illicit substances. *Medicina.* 2021;57:1256.
149. Gonzalex-Pinto A, Goikolea JM, Zorrilla I, et al. Clinical practice guideline on pharmacological and psychological management of adult patients with bipolar disorder and comorbid substance use. *Addiciones.* 2022;34(2):142-156.
150. Sepede G, Di Lorio G, Lupi M, et al. Bupropion as an add-on therapy in depressed bipolar disorder type I patients with comorbid cocaine dependence. *Clin Neuropharmacol.* 2014;37(1):17-21.
151. Oliva F, Mangiopane C, Nibbio G, et al. Prevalence of cocaine use and cocaine use disorder among adult patients with attention deficit/hyperactivity disorder: a systematic review and meta-analysis. *J Psychiatr Res.* 2021;143:587-598.
152. Willens T, Zulauf C, Martelon MK, et al. Nonmedical stimulant use in college students: Association with attention deficit/hyperactivity disorder and other disorders. *J Clin Psychiatry.* 2016;77(7):940-947.
153. de Los Cobos JP, Sinol N, Puerta C, et al. Features and prevalence of patients with probable adult attention deficit hyperactivity disorder who request treatment for cocaine use disorders. *Psychiatry Res.* 2011;185:205-211.
154. Cook J, Lloyd-Jones M, Arunogiri S, et al. Managing attention deficit hyperactivity disorder in adults using illicit stimulants: a systematic review. *Aust N Z J Psychiatry.* 2017;51(9):876-885.
155. Libuy N, de Angel V, Ibanez C, et al. The relative prevalence of schizophrenia among cannabis and cocaine users attending addiction services. *Schizophrenia Res.* 2018;194:13-17.
156. Hunt GE, Large MM, Cleary M, et al. Prevalence of comorbid substance use in schizophrenia spectrum disorders in community and clinical settings, 1990-2017: systematic review and meta-analysis. *Drug Alcohol Depend.* 2018;191:243-258.
157. Ackerman SC, Brunette MF, Noordsy DL, et al. Pharmacotherapy of co-occurring schizophrenia and substance use disorders. *Curr Addict Rep.* 2014;1:251-260.
158. Azorin J-M, Simon N, Adida M, et al. Pharmacological treatment of schizophrenia with comorbid substance use disorder. *Expert Opin Pharmacother.* 2016;17(2):231-253.
159. Krause M, Huhn M, Schneider-Thoma J, et al. Efficacy, acceptability and tolerability of antipsychotics in patients with schizophrenia and comorbid substance use. A systematic review and meta-analysis. *Eur Neuropsychopharmacol.* 2019;29:32-45.
160. Arranz B, Garriga M, Garcia-Rizo C, et al. Clozapine in patients with schizophrenia and a comorbid substance use disorder: a systematic review. *Eur Neuropsychopharmacol.* 2018;28:227-242.
161. Soyka M. New developments in the management of opioid dependence—focus on sublingual buprenorphine-naloxone. *Subst Abuse Rehabil.* 2015;6:1-14.
162. American Academy of Neurology. Antiepileptic drug selection for people with HIV/AIDS. *Continuum.* 2015;21(6):1766-1767.
163. Hill L, Lee KC. Pharmacotherapy considerations in patients with HIV and psychiatric disorders: focus on antidepressants and antipsychotics. *Ann Pharmacother.* 2013;47:75-89.
164. Gorelick DA, Montoya ID, Johnson EO. Sociodemographic representation in published studies of cocaine abuse pharmacotherapy. *Drug Alcohol Depend.* 1998;49(2):89-93.
165. McKee SA, McRae-Clark AL. Consideration of sex and gender differences in addiction medication response. *Biol Sex Diff.* 2022;13(1):34.
166. Sofuoglu M, Poling J, Gonzalez G, et al. Progesterone effects on cocaine use in male cocaine users maintained on methadone: a randomized, double-blind, pilot study. *Exp Clin Psychopharmacol.* 2007;15(5):453-460.
167. Yonkers KA, Forray A, Nich C, et al. Progesterone reduces cocaine use in postpartum women with a cocaine use disorder: a randomized, double-blind study. *Lancet Psychiatry.* 2014;1(5):360-367.
168. Stockings E, Hall WE, Lynskey M, et al. Prevention, early intervention, harm reduction, and treatment of substance use in young people. *Lancet Psychiatry.* 2016;3:280-296.
169. Tampi RR, Chhatlani A, Ahmad H, et al. Substance use disorders among older adults: a review of randomized controlled pharmacotherapy trials. *World J Psychiatry.* 2019;9(5):78-82.
170. Yarnell SC. Cocaine abuse in later life: a case series and review of the literature. *Prim Care Companion CNS Disord.* 2015;17(2):10.4088.
171. Czoty PW, Stoops WW, Rush CR. Evaluation of the "Pipeline" for development of medications for cocaine use disorder: a review of translational preclinical, human laboratory, and clinical trial research. *Pharmacol Rev.* 2016;68(3):533-562.
172. Dakwar E, Nunes EV, Hart CL, et al. A single ketamine infusion combined with mindfulness-based behavioral modification to treat cocaine dependence: a randomized clinical trial. *Am J Psychiatry.* 2019;176:923-930.
173. Newman AH, Ku T, Jordan CJ, et al. New drugs, old targets: tweaking the dopamine system to treat psychostimulant use disorders. *Annu Rev Pharmacol Toxicol.* 2021;61:609-628.
174. Feng H, Gao K, Chen D, et al. Machine learning analysis of cocaine addiction informed by DAT, SERT, and NET-based interactome networks. *J Chem Theory Comput.* 2022;18:2703-2719.
175. Gao K, Chen D, Robison AJ, et al. Proteome-informed machine learning studies of cocaine addiction. *J Phys Chem Lett.* 2021;12:11122-11134.
176. Spanagel R. Cannabinoids and the endocannabinoid system in reward processing and addiction: from mechanisms to interventions. *Dialogues Clin Neurosci.* 2020;22(3):241-250.
177. Galaz E, Z-X XI. Potential of cannabinoid receptor ligands as treatment for substance use disorders. *CNS Drugs.* 2019;33(10):1001-1030.
178. Le Foll B, Gorelick DA, Goldberg SR. The future of endocannabinoid-oriented clinical research after CB1 antagonists. *Psychopharmacology (Berl).* 2009;205(1):171-174.

179. Vasiliu O. Current trends and perspectives in the immune therapy for substance use disorders. *Front Psychiatry.* 2022;19:882491.
180. Kosten TR, Domingo CB, Shorter D, et al. Vaccine for cocaine dependence: a randomized double-blind placebo-controlled efficacy trial. *Drug Alcohol Depend.* 2014;140:42-47.
181. Nasser AF, Fudala PJ, Zheng B, Liu Y, Heidbreder C. A randomized, double-blind, placebo-controlled trial of RBP-8000 in cocaine abusers: pharmacokinetic profile of rbp- cocaine and effects of RBP-8000 on cocaine-induced physiological effects. *J Addict Dis.* 2014;33(4):289-302.
182. Shram MJ, Cohen-Barak O, Chakraborty B, et al. Assessment of pharmacokinetic and pharmacodynamic interactions between albumin-fused mutated butyrylcholinesterase and intravenously administered cocaine in recreational cocaine users. *J Clin Psychopharmacol.* 2015;35(4):396-405.
183. Gilgun-Sherki Y, Eliaz RE, McCann DJ, et al. Placebo-controlled evaluation of a bioengineered, cocaine-metabolizing fusion protein, TV-1380 (AlbuBChE), in the treatment of cocaine dependence. *Drug Alcohol Depend.* 2016;166:13-20.
184. Miller WR, Manuel JK. How large must a treatment effect be before it matters to practitioners? An estimation method and demonstration. *Drug Alcohol Rev.* 2008;27(5):524-528.
185. Kosten TR, Dominog CB, Hamon SC, Nielsen DA. *DBH* gene as predictor of response in a cocaine vaccine clinical trial. *Neurosci Lett.* 2013;541:29-33.

CHAPTER

65

Pharmacological Interventions for Nicotine and Tobacco Use

Randi M. Williams, Frank T. Leone, and Robert Schnoll

CHAPTER OUTLINE

- Introduction
- Neurobiology of nicotine/tobacco use disorder
- Assessing and addressing nicotine/tobacco use within addiction treatment
- Pharmacotherapies for nicotine/tobacco use
- Methods to optimize pharmacotherapies for nicotine/tobacco use
- Electronic drug delivery devices
- Recurrence of use: Causes and treatments
- Treating tobacco use in underserved communities
- Conclusions

INTRODUCTION

Tobacco use remains the leading cause of premature death in the United States, responsible for close to 500,000 deaths each year and at least one-third of all cancer deaths.[1] The annual global toll of tobacco-related mortality exceeds 7 million.[2] While a range of new tobacco products have emerged in the marketplace, by far, the leading form of tobacco consumption remains the traditional cigarette. Over the past decade or so, the development and broader use of treatments for tobacco use, an increased awareness of the harmful effects of tobacco use, and the expanded implementation of effective tobacco control policies have led to a steady decrease in the overall rate of tobacco use in the United States.[3] Unfortunately, though the prevalence has dropped to less than 14%, close to 35 million Americans still smoke, with 300 Americans under the age of 18 becoming daily tobacco users every day.[3,4] Further, the rates of tobacco use can be 2 to 3 times higher in subpopulations in the United States such as those with co-occurring psychiatric conditions, including substance use disorders.[5]

Nevertheless, surveys of people who currently smoke in the United States consistently show that almost 70% express a high level of motivation to quit, and more than half of these people make a serious quit attempt every year.[6] Providing these individuals with access to appropriate counseling and U.S. Food and Drug Administration (FDA)–approved medications and ensuring proper use is critical to increasing the success of a quit attempt and further reducing the overall rates of tobacco use in the United States.[7]

In this chapter, we briefly review the underlying neurobiology of nicotine/tobacco use disorder to help understand the mechanisms through which pharmacotherapies can help people quit smoking. We then discuss the importance of addressing tobacco use in the context of treatment for other substance use disorders. Next, we review the latest scientific data on the efficacy of the seven FDA-approved pharmacotherapies for tobacco use and discuss the latest research on methods to optimize the efficacy of these medications. We then discuss the research regarding use of electronic drug delivery devices (EDDDs), including electronic cigarettes, as a treatment for tobacco use. This chapter ends with a discussion of the leading causes and potential treatments for recurrence of use and the need for treatments for two subpopulations who report very high levels of tobacco use and disproportionate rates of tobacco-related morbidity and mortality: those with a serious mental illness (SMI) and those from minority racial and sexual orientation groups. A summary is provided to close this chapter.

NEUROBIOLOGY OF NICOTINE/TOBACCO USE DISORDER

Nicotine/tobacco use disorder is the result of nicotine's distorting influence on complex signaling pathways within a variety of neurotransmitter and regulatory systems of the central nervous system.[8] With repeated administration, nicotine alters complex systems of homeostatic control within the brain's cholinergic, GABA-ergic (γ-aminobutyric acid), glutamatergic, peptidergic (including endogenous opioids), serotonergic, dopaminergic and catecholaminergic systems, and can distort the stress management function of glucocorticoids within the hypothalamic-pituitary-adrenal axis.[9-14] Nicotine acts as an exogenous ligand for the nicotinic acetylcholine receptors (nAChR) located in all areas of the mammalian brain, with the main locus of addiction concentrated within the structures making up the mesolimbic system.[15,16]

Critical to basic survival functions of the organism, the mesolimbic system acts like a "prediction machine," assessing the survival relevance of incoming sensory inputs, imbuing them with corresponding salience based on past experience, and recruiting areas of the brain charged with responding appropriately.[17] The mesolimbic system "activates" the organism, producing a generalized appetitive state and motivating goal-directed behaviors aimed at resolving the challenge to survival. Mesolimbic activation also influences cognition by activating prefrontal and fronto-orbital areas of the cortex, constricting the universe of available ideas to those aimed at overcoming obstacles to gratification, and creating the emotional context within which decision-making occurs.[18,19]

A key component of the mesolimbic system is a collection of neurons at the base of the midbrain called the ventral tegmental area (VTA). Nicotine binds to a number of nAChR subtypes on dopaminergic cell bodies projecting from the VTA to a variety of target regions responsible for motivational control, including the amygdala, the hippocampus, and the nucleus accumbens (NAC).[20,21] Rapid delivery of nicotine[22,23] to this region causes a shift in VTA neuronal firing patterns from tonic to burst firing, leading to increased levels of dopamine in the NAC, reinforcing the operant association between stimulus and response, and perpetuating nicotine use along with its linked behaviors.[24,25] Chronic administration of nicotine increases the incentive salience of otherwise irrelevant sensory inputs, distorting the balance of motivational control until survival "drive" pressure dominates any restraint signaling, making nicotine use ineluctable.[26] In this manner, nicotine's ability to compel learned behaviors despite negative consequences makes nicotine use disorder both more rapidly developed and more difficult to control than heroin use disorder, despite the relatively benign social perceptions of the smoking behavior.[27,28] The neurobiology of nicotine's impact on the human brain is discussed in greater detail in Section 2 of this textbook.

In the presence of conditioned stimuli, forced nicotine abstinence results in a withdrawal syndrome characterized by anxiety, irritability and a strong drive to resume nicotine use.[29-31] Anhedonia, defined as the inability to experience pleasure from normally rewarding stimuli and a common feature of depression, can also occur following nicotine abstinence, particularly among those with a preexisting history of mood disorders.[32-34] It has been postulated that this effect may arise from some combination of loss of anticipatory excitement and interrupted reward processing.[35] Taken together, these resulting symptoms of ill-being prompted by abstinence might be imagined as the survival system's defensive posture, creating an emotional load that is relieved by nicotine administration.

ASSESSING AND ADDRESSING NICOTINE/ TOBACCO USE WITHIN ADDICTION TREATMENT

The prevalence of nicotine/tobacco use disorder among patients being treated for substance use disorders (SUD) is quite high, with more than three-quarters using tobacco in the form of cigarettes, 15% as EDDDs, and 10% using multiple forms of tobacco at the time of treatment.[36,37] Despite prevailing assumptions to the contrary, patients report high levels of interest in making a quit attempt and respond to pharmacotherapy with relative effects similar to those experienced by the general population.[38-40] The majority of patients report making a quit attempt (of more than 24 hours) in the year preceding treatment, however confidence in their ability to achieve *unsupported* abstinence is low.[41] Several studies and a meta-analytic review have concluded that patients who receive DSM-IV–defined nicotine/tobacco dependence treatment during addiction treatment have better overall SUD treatment outcomes compared with those who do not.[42] Treating tobacco use during SUD treatment has no deleterious effect on recovery outcomes.[43] Conversely, continued smoking following SUD treatment significantly increases the odds of recurrence of their nontobacco substance use[44-46] and reduces the probability of achieving long term abstinence.[47] Among patients who have developed opioid use disorder in response to noncancer pain syndromes, continued tobacco use is a recognized risk factor for accidental overdose deaths, emergency department visits, and inpatient hospitalizations.[48]

Persistent cultural attitudes about the "trivial" nature of tobacco use relative to the dramatic harms of SUD (eg, "One thing at a time") form an important emotional barrier to change[49] and ignore both the shared psychosocial and phenomenological mechanisms of addiction among co-occurring SUDs,[50] as well as Nobel-winning insights into the synergistic effects of nicotine exposure in producing other substance use disorders.[51,52] In one study, though there was an association between a patient's expressed desire for help in quitting and receiving tobacco related services, many who wanted help did not receive it.[53] As many as 15% of nonsmoking patients who enter SUD treatment facilities begin smoking during their treatment period.[54] Thirty percent of patients engaged in opioid use disorder treatment smoke more after entering their program.[41] Though tobacco use is routinely documented in SUD treatment records, a diagnosis of nicotine dependence is made in only a small proportion of patients.[55] In one important study, implementing a tobacco-free policy and offering tobacco services in a residential treatment setting to patients admitted for SUDs other than tobacco was associated with greater interest in and receipt of tobacco pharmacotherapies without any resulting increases in irregular or AMA discharges.[56]

When integrating nicotine/tobacco treatment into SUD treatment workflow, the first critical step is to ensure systems are in place to identify current nicotine use among patients engaged in therapy (ie, the "Ask").[57] Systems designed to increase the rate of assessment and documentation of tobacco use status markedly increase the rate at which clinicians intervene (OR 3.1; 95% CI 2.2-4.2).[57] Identifying tobacco use status also increases the likelihood that patients will achieve abstinence (OR 2.0; 95% CI 0.8-4.8). Actionable scripts for identifying tobacco use disorder use nonjudgmental language, validate the client's a priori concern over the perceived impact on recovery, and frame treatment as part of effective recovery work—not as an optional adjunct (ie, the "Advise").[58] The national experience of SUD providers suggests integration of tobacco treatment objectives into SUD treatment systems is feasible and well-accepted (ie, the "Assist").[59]

PHARMACOTHERAPIES FOR NICOTINE/TOBACCO USE

The U.S. FDA has approved seven medications for the treatment of tobacco use; two nonnicotine medications and five nicotine replacement therapies (NRTs), including the transdermal patch, gum, lozenge, inhaler, and nasal spray (see Table 65-1). Though frequently imagined as therapeutically equivalent, there are clinically important distinctions within this class based on both mechanism of action and pharmacokinetics. For example, the transdermal nicotine patch produces a slow and steady increase in nicotine over several hours, whereas the other four NRTs provide faster peak concentrations of nicotine that more quickly dissipate.[63] Varenicline is a nicotinic-cholinergic receptor partial agonist felt to blunt the reinforcing effects of nicotine, while bupropion is a monocyclic antidepressant with nAChR antagonist properties that exerts its complex effect by increasing concentrations of norepinephrine and dopamine.[64,65]

Nicotine Replacement Therapies

All NRTs treat tobacco use by directly alleviating symptoms of abstinence-induced nicotine withdrawal and craving, including cue-induced craving,[66] despite variation in pharmacokinetic profiles across the NRT formulations.[67,68] Overall, the safety and efficacy of NRTs have been well-demonstrated, with meta-analyses indicating that NRTs yield 6-month quit rates of about 25%.[57,60] While response rates are more modest for those with co-occurring SUD, NRTs are more effective than no treatment for this subpopulation.[69] Further, while very little evidence suggests differential efficacy between the NRT formulations, several studies indicate that combining NRTs—especially the transdermal patch with an acute-dosing NRT like the gum or lozenge—can significantly increase quit rates, compared to the use of a single NRT.[7,65,67] Moreover, while the evidence supporting the potential for increased efficacy from extended duration of treatment with NRT remains equivocal,[70] meta-analyses indicate modestly improved rates of nicotine abstinence when NRT is used for an extended period of time *prior* to a designated quit day, commonly referred to as preloading.[7]

Nicotine Gum

This was one of the first NRTs developed and is available both by prescription and over-the-counter (OTC). Nicotine gum has a very favorable safety profile and is available in two doses

TABLE 65-1 FDA-Approved Medications for Tobacco Dependence

Medication	Recommended duration and dosea	Odds ratio[a] (95% CI) Number of studies	Considerations
Nicotine gum	Up to[b] 12 weeks; 2 mg (for those who smoke < 25 cigarettes per day; 4 mg (for those who smoke > 25 cigarettes per day	1.49 (1.40-1.60) 56 trials	Addresses cue-elicited craving and affordable; lower compliance
Nicotine patch	Up to 10 weeks; dose duration (7, 14, 21 mg) varies by cigarettes per day	1.64 (1.53-1.75) 51 trials	Better compliance, few side effects, affordable; does not address cue-elicited craving
Nicotine spray	Up to 6 mo; 8-40 sprays per day	2.02 (1.49-2.73) 4 trials	Rapid nicotine absorption and addresses cue-elicited craving; higher side effects and poor adherence
Nicotine inhaler	Up to 6 mo; 6-16 cartridges per day	1.90 (1.36-2.67) 4 trials	Address cue-elicited craving; higher side effects and poor adherence
Nicotine lozenge	Up to 12 weeks; 2 mg (for those who smoke their first cigarette >30 min after waking) and 4 mg (for those who smoke their first cigarette <30 min of waking)	1.52 (1.32-1.74) 8 trials	Address cue-elicited craving and affordable; lower compliance
Bupropion	12-24 weeks; 300 mg/d; 150 mg/d for 3 d then 300 mg/d from day 4 to end of treatment	1.85 (1.63-2.10) 36 trials	More contraindications and more expensive; can mitigate abstinence-induced weight gain
Varenicline	12-24 weeks; 2 mg/d; 0.5 mg for days 1-3, 0.5 mg twice daily for 4 d, and 1 mg twice daily from day 8 to end of treatment	2.24 (2.06-2.43) 27 trials	Well-tolerated; reduces withdrawal and reinforcing effects of nicotine; can cause nausea

[a]6-month or greater point-prevalence quit rates, biochemically verified, from Hartmann-Boyce et al.[60] and Cahill et al.[61,62]

[b]While typical recommendations for treatment duration are reported here, clinicians are encouraged to use judgement when determining the personalized treatment plans for individual patients. For patients who continue to display the compulsion to smoke, extended duration pharmacotherapy may be indicated.

(2 and 4 mg) and in a variety of flavors. While it can alleviate cue-induced craving,[71] the gum provides far less nicotine at far slower rates than tobacco, rendering it nonaddictive.[67,72] Importantly, the efficacy of gum is often limited by improper use; chewing the gum continuously rather than "parking" it against the oral mucosa reduces absorption of nicotine, reduces impact and increases the risk of gastrointestinal side effects. Some individuals who smoke are unable to use this NRT because of dental issues and adherence to recommended use can be very low.[73] The efficacy of nicotine gum can be significantly increased if combined with another NRT compared to using this medication as a monotherapy.[7]

The Nicotine Lozenge

Like nicotine gum, the nicotine lozenge is available by prescription and OTC, and comes in two doses (2 and 4 mg) and a variety of flavors. The lozenge has minimal side effects and can effectively mitigate cue-induced craving.[74] The level of nicotine replacement achieved with proper lozenge use is similar to that of the gum,[75] however adherence with this formulation is often poor given the chalky taste of the binding agents.[76] Specifying use of the mini-lozenge formulation can sometimes overcome this obstacle to adherence. As with nicotine gum, the efficacy of the nicotine lozenge can be significantly increased if it is combined with another NRT.[7]

Nicotine Nasal Spray

Available only by prescription, nicotine nasal spray provides significantly faster nicotine delivery through absorption via the nasal mucosa.[77] Although not as pharmacologically efficient as tobacco use,[67] nicotine nasal spray effectively reduces nicotine craving.[78] In addition, combining the nicotine spray with the patch may increase quit rates compared to using the patch alone.[79] However, the nasal spray's side effect profile, including notable nasal and throat irritation, is relatively worse than other NRTs and is associated with higher treatment discontinuation.[7]

The Nicotine Inhaler

Like the spray, the nicotine inhaler is also only available by prescription. The inhaler effectively reduces craving[80] and can significantly increase quit rates when combined with the nicotine patch.[81] For some patients, the appeal of the inhaler is its ability to mimic the repetitive behaviors of smoking. However, reproducing the cigarette's nicotine delivery is challenging, with studies showing that use of the inhaler yields 50% to 70% of the nicotine concentrations compared to tobacco use, with levels dependent on adequate puff volume and frequency.[82] Side effects of frequent and vigorous puffing, such as cough or mouth and throat irritation, may present barriers to the use of this NRT.[82]

The Nicotine Patch

The transdermal nicotine patch supplies steady-state delivery of medication over the course of 24 hours.[67,83] Contrary to popular concerns, the nicotine patch has a very favorable side effect profile, with skin irritation at the site of application being most common. When irritation does occur, it is most frequently due to nicotine's direct degranulation of skin mast cells and not a true allergic reaction. This occurrence need not be treatment limiting and can be managed with steroid or antihistamine cream skin preconditioning, or even oral antihistamines. The patch is available in three strengths (7, 14, and 21 mg), with the manufacturer recommending dose selection based on number of cigarettes smoked per day. However, highly physically dependent patients can compensate their smoking technique to maximize nicotine absorption and are therefore more likely to benefit from starting on the 21 mg dose regardless of the reported number of cigarettes consumed. Concern over the possibility of overdose is excessive, resulting in frequent under-dosing and compromised effectiveness.[84] Patients using the patch are often advised to stepdown the dose over the course of treatment, although there is limited evidence supporting this dose-reduction approach.[83] A notable advantage of the nicotine patch is its ease of use, which leads to greater compliance compared to other NRT formulations.[85] In contrast, one disadvantage for the nicotine patch relative to other NRT formulations is that it does not mitigate cue-induced craving to the same extent as acute dosing NRTs like the lozenge or gum.[86,87] This limitation has stimulated several clinical trials that evaluated variability in efficacy between the nicotine patch and the combination of the nicotine patch with an acute-dosing NRT, with recent meta-analyses concluding that the patch plus acute dosing NRT (eg, gum lozenge) significantly increases quit rates compared to the patch alone.[7,88]

Bupropion

Bupropion was first marketed as an antidepressant, but post-marketing surveillance studies found that it was also associated with increasing rates of stopping smoking.[89] Subsequent placebo-controlled randomized clinical trials showed bupropion to be effective as a medication for tobacco use and equal in efficacy to NRT.[7] The mechanisms through which bupropion affects tobacco use are thought to involve the inhibition of dopamine and norepinephrine reuptake in the NUC, which reduces abstinence-induced symptoms of withdrawal.[90] When used to treat tobacco use disorder, bupropion is formulated as sustained or extended release, although a recent study indicated no significant difference in efficacy between the two.[91] For both formulations, treatment is initiated with the 150 mg total dose and gradually increased to 300 mg total. Treatment duration is at least 3 months.

At higher therapeutic doses, bupropion can decrease seizure threshold and increase the risk for seizures, and so it is contraindicated for those who have a seizure disorder or a condition that increases the risk for seizures. The most common side effects from bupropion include insomnia, headache, agitation, and dry mouth.[90] In addition, in 2009, the FDA placed a black box warning on bupropion because of reports that the medication increased the risk for adverse psychiatric reactions.[92] In 2016, the findings from a large clinical that was specifically designed to evaluate the safety of bupropion (and varenicline) for individuals who smoke with and without co-occurring psychiatric disorders showed that bupropion was safe (and effective) for both populations, leading to a removal of the black box warning.[40] Subsequent evaluations with subgroups of people who smoke with co-occurring psychiatric conditions such as major depressive disorder[93] and schizophrenia[94] indicated that bupropion was safe and efficacious for these individuals, although there are limited data on the efficacy of bupropion for individuals with co-occurring SUD.[69] Additionally, a potential advantage of using bupropion to quit smoking is that it may prevent weight gain following abstinence from tobacco, which is a leading cause of return to smoking.[95]

Several approaches have been examined as strategies to enhance the efficacy of bupropion.[96] Adding NRT to bupropion failed to reliably result in increased quit rates, compared to bupropion alone.[61] Also, there is little evidence to support the significant extension of therapy duration, although this question has not been adequately studied.[97] Preloading bupropion for 3 weeks (versus one) prior to a quit attempt significantly increased nicotine abstinence rates in one small study.[98]

Varenicline

As the most recently developed FDA-approved medication for tobacco use, varenicline is a partial agonist of the α4ß2 (and α6ß6) nicotinic acetylcholine receptor, thought to reduce smoking-related reward and abstinence-induced withdrawal symptoms by preventing nicotine's agonist activity while partially stimulating dopamine release.[99,100] Varenicline also acts as an agonist to α7 nicotinic receptors, which alter the reinforcing capacity of salient stimuli[101] and can reduce adverse psychological and cognitive effects from quitting smoking.[99,102-105] Varenicline is available in two doses, 0.5 mg and 1.0 mg, and is prescribed twice daily for 12 weeks, using an initial one-week dose run-up phase. The manufacturer suggests a run-up schedule of 0.5 mg daily on days 1-3, 0.5 mg twice daily on days 4-7, and 1 mg twice daily until the end of treatment.

Several meta-analyses show that varenicline is an efficacious medication for tobacco use,[62,96] even among individuals with co-occurring SUD.[69] Evidence suggests that varenicline is more effective than bupropion[7] and monotherapy with NRT[62] but equally effective when compared to combination NRT.[61] Further, although counterintuitive to the proposed pharmacologic mechanisms, combining varenicline with an NRT appears to improve abstinence rates over varenicline alone.[106] There is also some evidence that combining varenicline with bupropion is more effective than varenicline alone but the data are limited.[64,106] Overall, leading advocacy organizations conclude that either varenicline or combination NRT should be considered as the most effective treatment approach.[107]

Varenicline can produce side effects that can lead to the discontinuation of treatment, namely nausea and vomiting, headaches, and insomnia.[108] In addition, as with bupropion, the FDA required a black box warning for varenicline concerning potential neuropsychiatric risks associated with the medication. However, the cumulative evidence indicates that early concerns over the safety of varenicline were unsubstantiated, and varenicline is a safe medication to treat tobacco use.[109,110] Less severe but more common side effects such as nausea or sleeplessness can be mitigated with simple behavioral strategies, including taking the medication on a full stomach or taking the evening dose several hours before bedtime, respectively. In 2022, the manufacturer recalled the global supply of varenicline due to elevated levels of N-nitroso-varenicline in several production lots. N-nitroso-varenicline may increase cancer risk if exposure exceeds the acceptable limit of 37 ng/d over a long period of time.[111] A generic form of varenicline is now available, alleviating this safety concern.

The EAGLES trial[40] demonstrated the safety and efficacy of varenicline for individuals who smoke with and without co-occurring psychiatric disorders, leading to the removal of the black box warning. Secondary analyses of data from this trial indicated that varenicline is safe for people with major depressive disorder[93] and schizophrenia.[94] Similarly, early reports suggested a potential increased risk for adverse cardiovascular side effects.[112] In a randomized trial testing varenicline among individuals with cardiovascular disease, treatment with varenicline did not increase risk for adverse cardiovascular outcomes,[113] a finding that has now been supported by a more recent meta-analysis involving 38 trials of varenicline.[114]

The efficacy of varenicline may be enhanced with the addition of NRT.[106] Further, extending the duration of treatment with varenicline may increase long-term efficacy.[70] Likewise, there are some data to suggest that extending the use of varenicline prior to the quit day (ie, preloading for five weeks versus one week) may improve the medication's efficacy.[115,116]

METHODS TO OPTIMIZE PHARMACOTHERAPIES FOR NICOTINE/TOBACCO USE

As described above, combining medications, extending medications, and using the medications for a longer time frame prior to making a quit attempt may improve quit rates. Below, we discuss several additional strategies to improve the efficacy of pharmacotherapies for tobacco use, including the use of adjunctive behavioral counseling, improving medication adherence, and tailoring the selection of medications based on genetic information.

Behavioral Counseling

Perhaps the most impactful method to improve the efficacy of medications for tobacco use is to include a behavioral intervention as well. Behavioral interventions are designed to help individuals who smoke prepare for quitting, develop problem-solving skills to avoid return to use, and build motivation and confidence. Notably, medications are effective for people who smoke who are unmotivated/unwilling to make a quit attempt (eg, so behavioral counseling to promote willingness to quit should not be seen as a prerequisite to the provision of pharmacotherapy).[117,118] Behavioral interventions are based on divergent conceptual theories and models (eg, social-cognitive theory, transtheoretical model), use varied formats (eg, in-person, telephone), and range in intensity and duration.[95] Behavioral interventions that use cognitive-behavioral therapy (eg, focus on coping skills, beliefs, and self-efficacy) have the most support,[119] but other models such as acceptance and commitment therapy,[120] behavioral activation therapy,[121] and contingency management[122] have also received support from randomized clinical trials, albeit to a lesser extent and with less consistency.

Meta-analyses conclude that behavioral counseling for tobacco use improves quit rates, compared to minimal contact or no treatment.[123] Moreover, the inclusion of behavioral counseling with any pharmacotherapy significantly improves outcomes (by upward of 10% to 20%), compared to the use of pharmacotherapy alone,[60] and the effects are greater with more intense behavioral interventions (eg, more sessions).[95] Importantly, the efficacy of behavioral counseling for tobacco use is the same whether delivered in-person or by telephone,[60] which has provided support for the continued use of the national tobacco use quit-line. Among individuals who smoke with co-occurring SUD, behavioral interventions for smoking have limited effectiveness when provided without pharmacotherapy, but there is some support for contingency management in this subpopulation.[69]

Behavioral interventions can be costly and can have limited reach. In order to overcome barriers to the delivery of behavioral interventions, Web-based, smart-phone, and text-based platforms such as those offered for free through the National Quitline (1-800-QUIT-NOW), have emerged that facilitate treatment. The ubiquity of cell and smartphones, the low maintenance and dissemination costs, and the ability to reach diverse and under-served populations of people who smoke has made the use of digital interventions more popular.[124] While the diversity of content and format of digital intervention as well as their rapid and routine evolution makes it challenging to evaluate the efficacy of these interventions, recent national guidelines have recommend their use in clinical contexts.[125] Meta-analytic studies suggests that Web-based interventions can improve quit rates, compared to no treatment.[126-128] However, the effects of Web-based interventions may be dependent on how interactive they are, with more static forms yielding a much lower impact on smoking rates.[127,129] Likewise, text messaging-based abstinence interventions have grown in popularity over the years and meta-analytic studies indicate that they can be effective for reducing smoking rates, compared to no treatment.[95,126,130] More recent advances in this area have used smartphone apps to deliver behavioral interventions for smoking.[131] To date, while there is some evidence that smartphone apps can effectively reduce smoking rates,[132] meta-analyses of studies that have tested smartphone apps for tobacco abstinence have not found them to be effective.[130,133] It should be noted, however, that very few smoking abstinence apps have been rigorously evaluated, new smoking abstinence apps are emerging regularly, and there is substantial variability in format and content of apps. Thus, the impact of this approach to deliver behavioral interventions for tobacco use remains inconclusive.

Adherence

There is a growing literature that adherence to tobacco use disorder medication is a critical determinant of treatment efficacy. Reviews show that rates of nonadherence for varenicline (ie, taking <80% of medication) and the nicotine patch (ie, using the patch <5/6 days/week) are very high (approximately 50%), which significantly undermines treatment effectiveness.[134] In one study, 55% of patients receiving varenicline in a primary care setting were adherent, and quit rates were nearly doubled for these patients versus those who were non- or partially adherent.[135] Likewise, other studies have reported that only 45% of individuals using the nicotine patch are adherent,[136] and in another study quit rates among those who were adherent to the patch were almost three times higher versus those who were nonadherent.[137] Unfortunately, there has been remarkably little attention paid to the development and evaluation of interventions to address tobacco use medication adherence.

One meta-analysis that included ten studies testing adherence and problem-solving techniques found moderate evidence of effect of interventions on medication adherence rates.[138] Interventions that tried to increase adherence by focusing on pragmatic solutions to reasons for nonadherence (eg, using pill boxes or reminder notes) may be more effective.[138] A recent study tested adherence counseling, automated adherence calls, and electronic medication monitoring and feedback to promote NRT adherence.[139] The electronic monitoring condition, which involved a dispenser that recorded NRT use and problem-solving counseling for those who showed low adherence, yielded a significant increase in adherence. Clinicians should monitor adherence to pharmacotherapy and support patients in understanding and overcoming barriers to adherence if the benefits of these treatments are to be fully realized.

Personalizing the Selection of Pharmacotherapy Based on Rate of Nicotine Metabolism

Over the past two decades, landmark advances in our understanding of the human genome have led to subgroup-specific treatment tailoring for several medical conditions, in an effort to improve response rates and lower toxicities.[140,141] We now have this potential for nicotine/tobacco use disorder treatment.[142] Rooted in an understanding of the neurobiology of tobacco use, scientists have evaluated variation in nicotinic receptors (eg, *CHRNA5*), nicotine metabolizing genes (*CYP2A6*), dopaminergic genes (eg, *ANKK1*, *DRD2*), serotonergic genes (eg, *5-HTTLPR*), and genes regulating the opioid pathway (eg, *OPRM1* gene) as potential moderators of response to pharmacotherapies for nicotine/tobacco use disorder with variable findings.[143-145] However, consistent and accumulating evidence suggests that variation in the rate at which people metabolize nicotine, as measured by the nicotine metabolite ratio (NMR), may be a reliable and valid way of personalizing treatment for tobacco use in order to optimize efficacy.[146,147]

The NMR is calculated by identifying the ratio of two primary nicotine metabolites derived from smoking (3′hydroxycotinine [3HC]/cotinine). The NMR is a valid marker of *CYP2A6* gene variants across varying racial and ethnic groups but has the added benefit of also capturing environmental influences on nicotine clearance (eg, age, hormonal factors, race, gender, rate of smoking, and use of menthol cigarettes).[146,147] It has strong test-retest and between labs reliability and is independent of time-since-last-cigarette. NMR assessment does not present the same potential ethical challenges inherent to *CYP2A6* genotyping, is simpler and cheaper to perform, and employs procedures familiar to routine clinical practice.[148]

The association between the NMR and response to treatments for tobacco use has been examined in numerous studies, including most recently a multisite, prospectively stratified, double-blind randomized clinical trial.[149] Collectively, these studies support a personalized treatment model for optimizing treatment response and minimizing treatment side effects: provide slow metabolizers of nicotine with the nicotine patch and fast metabolizers of nicotine with varenicline.[147] Among slow metabolizers of nicotine there is little difference in the number-needed-to-treat (NNT) to yield one person successful in quitting (10.3 for patch versus 8.1 for varenicline), but NNT is significantly different for fast metabolizers of nicotine (26 for patch versus 4.9 for varenicline).[149] While slow metabolizers of nicotine do not appear to benefit significantly more from varenicline relative to nicotine patch, they do experience more side-effects on varenicline—a balance potentially favoring use of nicotine patch in this group.

While the use of the NMR to optimize pharmacotherapies for tobacco use shows promise, the translation of this treatment model into clinical practice and real-world settings remains a challenge. One study showed that integrating a personalized treatment model guided by the NMR yields high rates of NMR-matched medication prescribing (84%) and strong endorsement among people who smoke (approximately 90%).[150] Nevertheless, studies are needed to address potential patient, clinician, and system barriers to the integration of NMR testing to optimize tobacco use treatment, including potential concerns from people who smoke (eg, discrimination, stigma), clinicians (eg, coordinating sample collection, analysis, and feedback), and health systems (eg, costs, treatment delivery). The integration of the NMR to personalize the selection of treatment for tobacco use may also serve to address the substantial under-prescribing and under-use of pharmacotherapies for tobacco by providing clinicians with a novel treatment model and by addressing the concerns of people who smoke about treatment effectiveness and safety,

ELECTRONIC DRUG DELIVERY DEVICES

In August 2006, the first electronic cigarette was introduced into the US market. Soon after, the electronic cigarette evolved into a variety of devices, which are today more inclusively referred to as electronic drug delivery devices (EDDDs). As well, opinions regarding both the safety and efficacy of EDDDs in reducing the health impact of nicotine/tobacco use disorder began to quickly harden within the lay community notwithstanding the lack of empiric data.[151] Despite the established efficacy of pharmacologic agents approved for the treatment of tobacco use disorder and the lack of evidence in support of EDDDs as a clinical intervention, a significant number of clinicians have recommended EDDDs as a means of helping their patients stop smoking.[152-154] As a result, in the United States, EDDDs have been used more often than FDA-approved therapies by individuals trying to control their tobacco use disorder.[155]

A recent network meta-analysis failed to identify any advantage to using EDDDs to treat tobacco use disorder compared to standard varenicline monotherapy.[107] In contrast to popular assumptions however, the analysis identified that the odds of adverse events with EDDDs use was threefold higher than the comparator varenicline. There are limited clinical trial data supporting the use of EDDDs, and few studies have been judged to be at low risk of bias.[156] Significant differences in the chosen comparator continue to plague estimates of clinical effect; studies estimating the effect of pharmacotherapy typically use dummy medications and/or placebo as controls, whereas studies evaluating the effect of EDDDs often use open-label designs susceptible to performance bias.[157] In addition, pharmacotherapy trials often use discontinuation of the smoking behavior as the primary outcome, whereas EDDD studies often rely on simple substitution in delivery mechanism (ie, a switch in delivery may indicate continuation of addiction, whereas abstinence does not).

The overall health consequences of EDDDs use have become increasingly suspect.[158-161] Longer term health risks are largely unstudied. Though often compared to conventional cigarettes, EDDDs appear to carry their own unique risk profile.[162] The device uses a mixture of organic flavorants, nicotine and humectants such as propylene glycol, drawn across a heating element to facilitate the hydrogen bonding necessary to forming the visible aerosol giving the appearance of smoke. Both in vitro and in vivo studies suggest exposure to ultra-fine particles in the aerosol can lead to adverse cardiovascular effects, hemodynamic hyper-reactivity and oxidative stress after a single vaping instance in otherwise naive subjects.[163] At the population level, youth EDDD use was associated with increased odds of subsequent cigarette smoking after adjusting for behavioral, demographic and psychosocial risk factors.[164] Though EDDDs may someday find a place in the clinical armamentarium, perhaps especially in the management of specific behavioral phenotypes, they have not yet risen to the level of certainty in either safety or efficacy to warrant transitioning away from available evidence-based approaches.

RECURRENCE OF USE: CAUSES AND TREATMENTS

The majority of individuals who smoke report a willingness to quit, and more than half make a quit attempt annually.[165] However, the complex biopsychosocial aspects of nicotine addiction make the disorder a chronic recurring condition, with individuals making repeated abstinence attempts over a lifetime.[166] While evidence-based interventions like the pharmacological treatments discussed in this chapter are effective in supporting long-term quit rates compared to control interventions, research trials often document a progressive decline in abstinence rates over time due to recurrence of use. Individuals making an abstinence attempt often experience a temporary return to the smoking behavior, with many returning to a priori smoking patterns within 3 months.[64] There are several risk factors associated with an elevated risk for return to use, including personal variables such as age at initiation and weight gain during abstinence, social variables such as living or working with individuals who smoke, psychological covariates such as depression or stress/anxiety, and physiologic parameters such as level of nicotine physical dependence.[167] In this section we discuss two leading causes of return to nicotine use, weight gain and symptoms of nicotine withdrawal, and review strategies to help prevent relapse using pharmacotherapy.

Personal Risk Factor: Weight Gain

When individuals who smoke are asked about concerns with quitting, many attribute their continued cigarette smoking to an effort to control body weight.[168,169] In addition to individuals' perceptions about smoking-related weight control, a meta-analysis that included 62 studies found that stopping smoking is associated with increased body weight (mean of 4-5 kg) after 12 months of abstinence, and most weight gain occurs within the first 3 months of quitting.[170] Proposed mechanisms for abstinence-related weight gain include decreased metabolic rate and increased caloric intake. Nicotine acts as an appetite suppressant,[171] and when someone is abstaining from smoking a common withdrawal symptom is increased appetite. Abstinence activates instinctive drive outputs in the mesolimbic system, producing a generalized appetitive state that is modestly gratified by concentrated carbohydrates.[172] Though only a minority of people gain excessive weight following an abstinence attempt,[173] clinicians can help control weight gain most effectively by aggressively attending to nicotine withdrawal and appropriately utilizing pharmacologic interventions for tobacco use disorder. Nicotine replacement, bupropion and varenicline have all been shown to limit postabstinence weight gain.[95]

There have been several behavioral and pharmacological studies conducted to address postabstinence weight gain.[174] While there has been some evidence of short-term success in using weight management medications (eg, naltrexone) to address postabstinence weight gain, there are limited data on the long-term impact following discontinuation of the medication as well as sustained abstinence.[174] Additionally, some pharmacotherapies for tobacco use disorder may also be used to limit weight gain, although the effects are modest. Compared to placebo, small reductions in weight gain were observed at the end of 12 weeks of treatment with varenicline (−0.41 kg), NRT (−0.45 kg), and bupropion (−1.12 kg)[174]; however, these positive effects also lessen after pharmacotherapy treatment ends. In a randomized controlled clinical trial evaluating the efficacy and safety of varenicline and bupropion combination therapy versus varenicline alone, weight changes were measured as a secondary study endpoint.[175] Among those participants meeting criteria for prolonged abstinence defined as abstinent at the end of treatment (12 weeks), the weight gain from baseline to 12-week follow-up was significantly less in the combination therapy with varenicline and bupropion group versus the monotherapy group (1.1 kg [95% CI 0.5-1.7] versus 2.5 kg [95% CI 2.0-3.0]; $p<0.001$). However, no significant group difference were observed at the 26- and 52-week follow-up assessments. Additional studies are needed to determine the most effective interventions to prevent postabstinence weight gain, but the medications discussed above could be helpful in limiting weight gain and improving smoking abstinence rates in individuals concerned about gaining weight postabstinence.

Physiological Risk Factor: Symptoms of Nicotine Withdrawal

Due to the physiological mechanisms of nicotine addiction, withdrawal and cravings, including cue-induced cravings, are highly related to return to use. Individuals are at highest risk for a slip in the first week when symptoms of nicotine withdrawal are strongest.[176] Severity of nicotine use disorder is also a predictor of smoking abstinence success.[177,178] Individuals who have high levels of nicotine use disorder may be more likely to experience strong withdrawal symptoms and be susceptible to return to use. Using pharmacotherapy is one strategy for helping to prevent recurrence of use in addition to skills-based approaches and other behavioral interventions. Individuals at risk for return to use can benefit from pharmacotherapy, including a higher dosage when initiating treatment to stop smoking to prevent initial slips,[179] extended use of medications to aid stopping smoking,[180] and prescribing medications to those who have achieved abstinence to prevent return to use.[181] These strategies can be individually tailored to the individual's smoking behavior as discussed in Section "Methods to Optimize Pharmacotherapies for Nicotine/Tobacco Use" above.

In a recent Cochrane review of relapse prevention interventions for stopping smoking, the authors assessed whether behavioral and pharmacological interventions reduced the proportion of people who returned to use.[182] Of the 81 studies included in the review, 12 studies focus on trials that randomized individuals who were abstaining from smoking. A few of the pharmacotherapy interventions showed promise in helping to prevent recurrence of use including nicotine gum and varenicline treatment. The analysis did not support bupropion for prevention of nicotine use, with estimated effect sizes accompanied by wide confidence intervals. The review of the behavioral interventions did not detect an effect in preventing return to use, and the study concluded that the current evidence does not support the use of behavioral treatments to help prevent return to use.

TREATING TOBACCO USE IN UNDERSERVED COMMUNITIES

Disparities in tobacco-related morbidity and mortality exist among subpopulations who report higher levels of tobacco use, who smoke for longer periods, and who are less likely to achieve abstinence. These subpopulations are more vulnerable to the risks of tobacco use and include those with a serious mental illness (SMI), those from minority racial and sexual orientation groups, people living with HIV, and those with lower socioeconomic status (eg, education, income).[1] In this section, we describe differences in smoking patterns and in utilization of evidence-based tobacco use disorder treatments among these subpopulations. Increasing both treatment access and utilization are necessary prerequisites to addressing the disproportionate rates of initiation, use, and abstinence that ultimately result in disparities in tobacco-related morbidity and mortality.

Tobacco-Related Disparities

The tobacco industry has aggressively targeted some subgroups of the population more than others, making these subgroups more vulnerable to exposure to tobacco products and the risks of tobacco use.[183] In addition to aggressive marketing, the availability of tobacco products as well as price promotions are greater in communities of color.[184] Communities of color tend to have more tobacco retailers, which contributes to greater tobacco advertising exposure and marketing. In April 2021, the Food and Drug Administration announced that it is pursuing a policy to ban menthol flavoring in cigars and cigarettes.[185] The decision aims to address the health disparities faced by communities of color, low-income populations, and members of the LGBTQ+ community who have historically been targeted by this market and are more likely to use menthol tobacco products.

People with SMI smoke at rates almost twice as high as the general population (41% versus 22.5%), with higher rates among people diagnosed with depression, bipolar disorder, or schizophrenia.[186] Despite smoking fewer cigarettes per day on average and initiating smoking at older ages compared to Whites, Black/African American individuals are more likely to die from tobacco-related diseases.[187] Individuals who identify as lesbian, gay, bisexual, transgender (LGBTQ+) are 1.5 to 2.5 times more likely to smoke cigarettes than individuals who identify as heterosexual.[188,189]

Treatment Access and Utilization

Despite being at greater risk of tobacco exposure and its associated risks, the percentage of people who report that they want to quit is similar across many subpopulations.[165] However, there are differences in the success of quit attempts. Certain groups are less likely to receive advice to quit from a health care provider and less likely to use evidence-based abstinence treatments, including pharmacotherapy.[190] Using over 10 years of data from the U.S. Department of Health and Human Services Medical Expenditure Panel Survey (MEPS), a large nationally representative study found lower rates of self-reported receipt of advice to quit and lower prescription medication use for quitting among men, younger adults, uninsured individuals, racial and ethnic minority groups, and those without smoking-associated comorbidities.[191] The study's findings align with previous studies including the National Health Interview Survey study that found that 60.2% of White patients reported receiving advice to quit from their provider compared to 55.7% of Black/African American, 42.2% of Latinx, 38.1% of American Indian/Alaska Native, and 34.2% of Asian respondents.[165] In addition to differential delivery of tobacco use disorder advice and medications within the health care setting, other factors may contribute to the underuse of pharmacotherapy among certain subgroups.[192] Clinicians may be less likely to prescribe abstinence medications to individuals who smoke fewer cigarettes per day (eg, Black individuals who smoke).[193] Other factors include receiving limited information about medications, attitudes and beliefs regarding abstinence medications, and barriers to access (eg, cost). Subpopulations (eg, racial and ethnic minority groups, adults with SMI) have been historically underrepresented in pharmacotherapy clinical trials.

Only recently, studies have been conducted to assess the efficacy of medications to aid smoking abstinence in these groups. Systematic reviews and meta-analyses conducted to evaluate the effectiveness of pharmacotherapy for tobacco use disorder in adults with SMI suggest that bupropion and varenicline are effective.[194-196] Systematic reviews focusing on racial and ethnic minority populations have also recommended pharmacotherapy for smoking abstinence.[197,198] In a large randomized clinical trial of 500 Black/African American adults who were currently smoking, participants were randomized (3:2 ratio) to receive varenicline versus placebo for 12 weeks in addition to receiving 6 sessions of culturally relevant individualized behavioral counseling.[199] The study found significantly higher 7-day point prevalence smoking abstinence at week 26 among those receiving varenicline (15.7%) compared to the placebo (6.5%; p = 0.002). Among individuals who smoked fewer cigarettes per day (1-10 cigarettes per day), those in the varenicline study arm were also were more likely to quit compared to placebo by the end of treatment (week 12; 22.1% versus 8.5%). Importantly, there were no reports of serious adverse events among this subgroup. This evidence supports the need for clinicians to equitably offer pharmacotherapy to individuals who want to quit.

CONCLUSIONS

In this chapter, our goals were to provide a rationale for the provision of FDA-approved medications for tobacco use and to provide the reader with the information necessary to effectively treat tobacco use, particularly in the context of treating people with SUDs. Understanding the neurobiology of nicotine/tobacco use disorder has helped to develop medications for treating tobacco use disorder; the seven FDA-approved medications have a well-established efficacy and safety record, even when used in patients with co-occurring psychiatric conditions. Varenicline or combination NRT yield the strongest impact on abstinence attempts. In contrast, data remain insufficient to support the use of EDDDs in the treatment of tobacco use disorder. The efficacy of FDA-approved medications for tobacco use may be enhanced by ensuring the concurrent provision of behavioral treatments, increasing medication adherence, or tailoring the selection of medications based on the individuals' rate of nicotine metabolism. Reducing the probability for return to use following abstinence may be associated with weight gain and symptoms of withdrawal, which may be treated with varenicline or nicotine gum.

Although the rates of tobacco use overall have been steadily decreasing over the past several decades, tobacco use continues to be a significant public health issue, especially among specific under-resourced communities, including people with co-occurring SUDs. Further, use of nicotine in EDDDs has been expanding significantly. Using the information presented in this chapter may help ensure optimal treatment for tobacco use in this community, thereby improving the overall well-being of these individuals.

REFERENCES

1. National Center for Chronic Disease Prevention and Health Promotion (U.S.) Office on Smoking and Health. *The Health Consequences of Smoking—50 Years of Progress: A Report of the Surgeon General.* Centers for Disease Control and Prevention (U.S.); 2014. Accessed June 9, 2022. http://www.ncbi.nlm.nih.gov/books/NBK179276/
2. World Health Organization. *WHO Report on the Global Tobacco Epidemic, 2017: Monitoring Tobacco Use and Prevention Policies.* World Health Organization; 2017. Accessed June 9, 2022. https://apps.who.int/iris/handle/10665/255874
3. Creamer MR, Wang TW, Babb S, et al. Tobacco product use and cessation indicators among adults—United States, 2018. *MMWR Morb Mortal Wkly Rep.* 2019;68(45):1013-1019. doi:10.15585/mmwr.mm6845a2
4. 2017 NSDUH Annual National Report. CBHSQ Data. Accessed June 9, 2022. https://www.samhsa.gov/data/report/2017-nsduh-annual-national-report
5. Fornaro M, Carvalho AF, De Prisco M, et al. The prevalence, odds, predictors, and management of tobacco use disorder or nicotine dependence among people with severe mental illness: systematic review and meta-analysis. *Neurosci Biobehav Rev.* 2022;132:289-303. doi:10.1016/j.neubiorev.2021.11.039
6. Babb S, Malarcher A, Schauer G, Asman K, Jamal A. Quitting smoking among adults—United States, 2000-2015. *MMWR Morb Mortal Wkly Rep.* 2017;65(52):1457-1464. doi:10.15585/mmwr.mm6552a1
7. Livingstone-Banks J, Lindson N, Hartmann-Boyce J, Aveyard P. Effects of interventions to combat tobacco addiction: Cochrane update of 2019 and 2020 reviews. *Addiction.* 2022;117(6). doi:10.1111/add.15769
8. Koob GF, Volkow ND. Neurobiology of addiction: a neurocircuitry analysis. *Lancet Psychiatry.* 2016;3(8):760-773. doi:10.1016/S2215-0366(16)00104-8
9. Kalivas PW. Neurotransmitter regulation of dopamine neurons in the ventral tegmental area. *Brain Res Rev.* 1993;18(1):75-113. doi:10.1016/0165-0173(93)90008-N
10. Sesack SR, Pickel VM. Prefrontal cortical efferents in the rat synapse on unlabeled neuronal targets of catecholamine terminals in the nucleus accumbens septi and on dopamine neurons in the ventral tegmental area. *J Comp Neurol.* 1992;320(2):145-160. doi:10.1002/cne.903200202
11. Jones IW, Wonnacott S. Precise localization of α7 nicotinic acetylcholine receptors on glutamatergic axon terminals in the rat ventral tegmental area. *J Neurosci.* 2004;24(50):11244-11252. doi:10.1523/JNEUROSCI.3009-04.2004
12. George TP, Weinberger AH. Monoamine oxidase inhibition for tobacco pharmacotherapy. *Clin Pharmacol Ther.* 2008;83(4):619-621. doi:10.1038/sj.clpt.6100474
13. Dhatt RK, Gudehithlu KP, Wemlinger TA, Tejwani GA, Neff NH, Hadjiconstantinou M. Preproenkephalin mRNA and methionine-enkephalin content are increased in mouse striatum after treatment with nicotine. *J Neurochem.* 1995;64(4):1878-1883. doi:10.1046/j.1471-4159.1995.64041878.x
14. Davenport KE, Houdi AA, Van Loon GR. Nicotine protects against μ-opioid receptor antagonism by β-funaltrexamine: evidence for nicotine-induced release of endogenous opioids in brain. *Neurosci Lett.* 1990;113(1):40-46. doi:10.1016/0304-3940(90)90491-Q
15. Clarke PBS. Mesolimbic dopamine activation—the key to nicotine reinforcement? In: *Ciba Foundation Symposium 152—The Biology of Nicotine Dependence.* John Wiley & Sons, Ltd; 2007:153-168. doi:10.1002/9780470513965.ch9
16. U.S. Dept of Health and Human Services. Neurobiology of nicotine addiction. *Smoking Cessation: A Report of the Surgeon General;* 2020:125-129. Accessed July 14, 2020. https://www.cdc.gov/tobacco/data_statistics/sgr/2020-smoking-cessation/index.html
17. Leone FT, Evers-Casey S. Developing a rational approach to tobacco use treatment in pulmonary practice. *Clin Pulm Med.* 2012;19(2):53-61. doi:10.1097/CPM.0b013e318247cada
18. Alcaro A, Huber R, Panksepp J. Behavioral functions of the mesolimbic dopaminergic system: an affective neuroethological perspective. *Brain Res Rev.* 2007;56(2):283-321. doi:10.1016/j.brainresrev.2007.07.014
19. Rao TS, Correa LD, Adams P, Santori EM, Sacaan AI. Pharmacological characterization of dopamine, norepinephrine and serotonin release in the rat prefrontal cortex by neuronal nicotinic acetylcholine receptor agonists. *Brain Res.* 2003;990(1):203-208. doi:10.1016/S0006-8993(03)03532-7
20. Mansvelder HD, Keath JR, McGehee DS. Synaptic mechanisms underlie nicotine-induced excitability of brain reward areas. *Neuron.* 2002;33(6):905-919.
21. Azam L, Winzer-Serhan UH, Chen Y, Leslie FM. Expression of neuronal nicotinic acetylcholine receptor subunit mRNAs within midbrain dopamine neurons. *J Comp Neurol.* 2002;444(3):260-274. doi:10.1002/cne.10138
22. Benowitz NL, Hukkanen J, Jacob P. Nicotine chemistry, metabolism, kinetics and biomarkers. *Handb Exp Pharmacol.* 2009;192:29-60. doi:10.1007/978-3-540-69248-5_2
23. Henningfield JE, Stapleton JM, Benowitz NL, Grayson RF, London ED. Higher levels of nicotine in arterial than in venous blood after cigarette smoking. *Drug Alcohol Depend.* 1993;33(1):23-29.
24. Rice ME, Cragg SJ. Nicotine amplifies reward-related dopamine signals in striatum. *Nat Neurosci.* 2004;7(6):583-584. doi:10.1038/nn1244
25. Nestler EJ. Is there a common molecular pathway for addiction? *Nat Neurosci.* 2005;8(11):1445-1449. doi:10.1038/nn1578
26. Brunzell DH, Picciotto MR. Molecular mechanisms underlying the motivational effects of nicotine. *Nebr Symp Motiv.* 2009;55:17-30. doi:10.1007/978-0-387-78748-0_3
27. Kozlowski LT, Wilkinson DA, Skinner W, Kent C, Franklin T, Pope M. Comparing tobacco cigarette dependence with other drug dependencies: greater or equal "difficulty quitting" and "urges to use," but less "pleasure" from cigarettes. *JAMA.* 1989;261(6):898-901. doi:10.1001/jama.1989.03420060114043
28. Rubinstein ML, Luks TL, Moscicki AB, Dryden W, Rait MA, Simpson GV. Smoking-related cue-induced brain activation in adolescent light smokers. *J Adolesc Health.* 2011;48(1):7-12. doi:10.1016/j.jadohealth.2010.09.016

29. Hughes JR, Hatsukami D. Signs and symptoms of tobacco withdrawal. *Arch Gen Psychiatry*. 1986;43(3):289-294.
30. Piper ME, Schlam TR, Cook JW, et al. Tobacco withdrawal components and their relations with cessation success. *Psychopharmacology (Berl)*. 2011;216(4):569-578. doi:10.1007/s00213-011-2250-3
31. Javitz HS, Swan GE, Lerman C. The dynamics of the urge-to-smoke following smoking cessation via pharmacotherapy. *Addiction*. 2011;106(10):1835-1845. doi:10.1111/j.1360-0443.2011.03495.x
32. Epping-Jordan MP, Watkins SS, Koob GF, Markou A. Dramatic decreases in brain reward function during nicotine withdrawal. *Nature*. 1998;393(6680):76-79. doi:10.1038/30001
33. Cook JW, Piper ME, Leventhal AM, Schlam TR, Fiore MC, Baker TB. Anhedonia as a component of the tobacco withdrawal syndrome. *J Abnorm Psychol*. 2015;124(1):215-225. doi:10.1037/abn0000016
34. Bacher I, Houle S, Xu X, et al. Monoamine oxidase A binding in the prefrontal and anterior cingulate cortices during acute withdrawal from heavy cigarette smoking. *Arch Gen Psychiatry*. 2011;68(8):817-826. doi:10.1001/archgenpsychiatry.2011.82
35. Bruijnzeel AW. Reward processing and smoking. *Nicotine Tob Res*. 2017;19(6):661-662. doi:10.1093/ntr/ntw303
36. Guydish J, Yip D, Le T, Gubner NR, Delucchi K, Roman P. Smoking-related outcomes and associations with tobacco-free policy in addiction treatment, 2015-2016. *Drug Alcohol Depend*. 2017;179:355-361. doi:10.1016/j.drugalcdep.2017.06.041
37. Poirier MF, Canceil O, Baylé F, et al. Prevalence of smoking in psychiatric patients. *Prog Neuropsychopharmacol Biol Psychiatry*. 2002;26(3):529-537. doi:10.1016/S0278-5846(01)00304-9
38. Nahvi S, Richter K, Li X, Modali L, Arnsten J. Cigarette smoking and interest in quitting in methadone maintenance patients. *Addict Behav*. 2006;31(11):2127-2134. doi:10.1016/j.addbeh.2006.01.006
39. Richter KP, McCool RM, Okuyemi KS, Mayo MS, Ahluwalia JS. Patients' views on smoking cessation and tobacco harm reduction during drug treatment. *Nicotine Tob Res*. 2002;4(Suppl 2):S175-S182. doi:10.1080/1462220021000032735
40. Anthenelli RM, Benowitz NL, West R, et al. Neuropsychiatric safety and efficacy of varenicline, bupropion, and nicotine patch in smokers with and without psychiatric disorders (EAGLES): a double-blind, randomised, placebo-controlled clinical trial. *Lancet*. 2016;387(10037):2507-2520. doi:10.1016/S0140-6736(16)30272-0
41. McClure EA, Acquavita SP, Dunn KE, Stoller KB, Stitzer ML. Characterizing smoking, cessation services, and quit interest across outpatient substance abuse treatment modalities. *J Subst Abuse Treat*. 2014;46(2):194-201. doi:10.1016/j.jsat.2013.07.009
42. Prochaska JJ, Delucchi K, Hall SM. A meta-analysis of smoking cessation interventions with individuals in substance abuse treatment or recovery. *J Consult Clin Psychol*. 2004;72(6):1144-1156.
43. Das S, Hickman NJ, Prochaska JJ. Treating smoking in adults with co-occurring acute psychiatric and addictive disorders. *J Addict Med*. 2017;11(4):273-279. doi:10.1097/ADM.0000000000000320
44. Weinberger AH, Platt J, Esan H, Galea S, Erlich D, Goodwin RD. Cigarette smoking is associated with increased risk of substance use disorder relapse: a nationally representative, prospective longitudinal investigation. *J Clin Psychiatry*. 2017;78(2):e152-e160. doi:10.4088/JCP.15m10062
45. Kohn CS, Tsoh JY, Weisner CM. Changes in smoking status among substance abusers: baseline characteristics and abstinence from alcohol and drugs at 12-month follow-up. *Drug Alcohol Depend*. 2003;69(1):61-71. doi:10.1016/S0376-8716(02)00256-9
46. Satre DD, Kohn CS, Weisner C. Cigarette smoking and long-term alcohol and drug treatment outcomes: a telephone follow-up at five years. *Am J Addict*. 2007;16(1):32-37. doi:10.1080/10550490601077825
47. Tsoh JY, Chi FW, Mertens JR, Weisner CM. Stopping smoking during first year of substance use treatment predicted 9-year alcohol and drug treatment outcomes. *Drug Alcohol Depend*. 2011;114(2):110-118. doi:10.1016/j.drugalcdep.2010.09.008
48. John WS, Wu LT. Chronic non-cancer pain among adults with substance use disorders: prevalence, characteristics, and association with opioid overdose and healthcare utilization. *Drug Alcohol Depend*. 2020;209:107902. doi:10.1016/j.drugalcdep.2020.107902
49. Prochaska JJ. Failure to treat tobacco use in mental health and addiction treatment settings: a form of harm reduction? *Drug Alcohol Depend*. 2010;110(3):177-182. doi:10.1016/j.drugalcdep.2010.03.002
50. Kotyuk E, Magi A, Eisinger A, et al. Co-occurrences of substance use and other potentially addictive behaviors: epidemiological results from the psychological and genetic factors of the addictive behaviors (PGA) Study. *J Behav Addict*. 2020;9(2):272-288. doi:10.1556/2006.2020.00033
51. Kandel ER, Kandel DB. A molecular basis for nicotine as a gateway drug. *N Engl J Med*. 2014;371(10):932-943. doi:10.1056/NEJMsa1405092
52. Levine A, Huang Y, Drisaldi B, et al. Molecular mechanism for a gateway drug: epigenetic changes initiated by nicotine prime gene expression by cocaine. *Sci Transl Med*. 2011;3(107):107ra109. doi:10.1126/scitranslmed.3003062
53. Guydish J, Kapiten K, Le T, Campbell B, Pinsker E, Delucchi K. Tobacco use and tobacco services in California substance use treatment programs. *Drug Alcohol Depend*. 2020;214:108173. doi:10.1016/j.drugalcdep.2020.108173
54. Friend KB, Pagano ME. Smoking initiation among nonsmokers during and following treatment for alcohol use disorders. *J Subst Abuse Treat*. 2004;26(3):219-224. doi:10.1016/S0740-5472(04)00003-0
55. Peterson AL, Hryshko-Mullen AS, Cortez Y. Assessment and diagnosis of nicotine dependence in mental health settings. *Am J Addict*. 2003;12(3):192-197. doi:10.1080/10550490390201795
56. Hemmy Asamsama O, Miller SC, Silvestri MM, Bonanno C, Krondilou K. Impact of implementing a tobacco and recreational nicotine-free policy and enhanced treatments on programmatic and patient-level outcomes within a residential substance use disorder treatment program. *J Subst Abuse Treat*. 2019;107:44-49. doi:10.1016/j.jsat.2019.09.004
57. Fiore M, Jaén C, Baker T, et al. *Treating Tobacco Use and Dependence: 2008 Update Clinical Practice Guideline*. U.S. Department of Health and Human Services. Public Health Service; 2008.
58. Leone FT, Evers-Casey S. Behavioral interventions in tobacco dependence. *Prim Care*. 2009;36(3):489-507. doi:10.1016/j.pop.2009.04.002
59. Marynak K, VanFrank B, Tetlow S, et al. Tobacco cessation interventions and smoke-free policies in mental health and substance abuse treatment facilities—United States, 2016. *MMWR Morb Mortal Wkly Rep*. 2018;67(18):519-523. doi:10.15585/mmwr.mm6718a3
60. Hartmann-Boyce J, Chepkin SC, Ye W, Bullen C, Lancaster T. Nicotine replacement therapy versus control for smoking cessation. *Cochrane Database Syst Rev*. 2018;5:CD000146. doi:10.1002/14651858.CD000146.pub5
61. Cahill K, Stevens S, Perera R, Lancaster T. Pharmacological interventions for smoking cessation: an overview and network meta-analysis. *Cochrane Database Syst Rev*. 2013;5:CD009329. doi:10.1002/14651858.CD009329.pub2
62. Cahill K, Lindson-Hawley N, Thomas KH, Fanshawe TR, Lancaster T. Nicotine receptor partial agonists for smoking cessation. *Cochrane Database Syst Rev*. 2016;5:CD006103. doi:10.1002/14651858.CD006103.pub7
63. Le Houezec J. Role of nicotine pharmacokinetics in nicotine addiction and nicotine replacement therapy: a review. *Int J Tuberc Lung Dis*. 2003;7(9):811-819.
64. Rigotti NA, Kruse GR, Livingstone-Banks J, Hartmann-Boyce J. Treatment of tobacco smoking: a review. *JAMA*. 2022;327(6):566-577. doi:10.1001/jama.2022.0395
65. Slemmer JE, Martin BR, Damaj MI. Bupropion is a nicotinic antagonist. *J Pharmacol Exp Ther*. 2000;295(1):321-327.
66. Ferguson SG, Shiffman S. The relevance and treatment of cue-induced cravings in tobacco dependence. *J Subst Abuse Treat*. 2009;36(3):235-243. doi:10.1016/j.jsat.2008.06.005
67. Fant RV, Owen LL, Henningfield JE. Nicotine replacement therapy. *Prim Care*. 1999;26(3):633-652. doi:10.1016/s0095-4543(05)70121-4
68. Germovsek E, Hansson A, Kjellsson MC, et al. Relating nicotine plasma concentration to momentary craving across four nicotine replacement therapy formulations. *Clin Pharmacol Ther*. 2020;107(1):238-245. doi:10.1002/cpt.1595

69. Vlad C, Arnsten JH, Nahvi S. Achieving smoking cessation among persons with opioid use disorder. *CNS Drugs*. 2020;34(4):367-387. doi:10.1007/s40263-020-00701-z
70. Murray RL, Zhang YQ, Ross S, et al. Extended duration treatment of tobacco dependence: a systematic review. *Ann Am Thorac Soc*. 2022;19(8):1390-1403. doi:10.1513/AnnalsATS.202110-1140OC
71. Shiffman S, Shadel WG, Niaura R, et al. Efficacy of acute administration of nicotine gum in relief of cue-provoked cigarette craving. *Psychopharmacology (Berl)*. 2003;166(4):343-350. doi:10.1007/s00213-002-1338-1
72. Scherer G, Mütze J, Pluym N, Scherer M. Assessment of nicotine delivery and uptake in users of various tobacco/nicotine products. *Curr Res Toxicol*. 2022;3:100067. doi:10.1016/j.crtox.2022.100067
73. Okuyemi KS, Zheng H, Guo H, Ahluwalia JS. Predictors of adherence to nicotine gum and counseling among African-American light smokers. *J Gen Intern Med*. 2010;25(9):969-976. doi:10.1007/s11606-010-1386-x
74. Shiffman S. Effect of nicotine lozenges on affective smoking withdrawal symptoms: secondary analysis of a randomized, double-blind, placebo-controlled clinical trial. *Clin Ther*. 2008;30(8):1461-1475. doi:10.1016/j.clinthera.2008.07.019
75. Choi JH, Dresler CM, Norton MR, Strahs KR. Pharmacokinetics of a nicotine polacrilex lozenge. *Nicotine Tob Res*. 2003;5(5):635-644. doi:10.1080/1462220031000158690
76. Shiffman S, Dresler CM, Hajek P, Gilburt SJA, Targett DA, Strahs KR. Efficacy of a nicotine lozenge for smoking cessation. *Arch Intern Med*. 2002;162(11):1267-1276. doi:10.1001/archinte.162.11.1267
77. Schneider NG, Olmstead R, Nilsson F, Mody FV, Franzon M, Doan K. Efficacy of a nicotine inhaler in smoking cessation: a double-blind, placebo-controlled trial. *Addiction*. 1996;91(9):1293-1306.
78. Hurt RD, Offord KP, Croghan IT, et al. Temporal effects of nicotine nasal spray and gum on nicotine withdrawal symptoms. *Psychopharmacology (Berl)*. 1998;140(1):98-104. doi:10.1007/s002130050744
79. Blondal T, Gudmundsson LJ, Olafsdottir I, Gustavsson G, Westin A. Nicotine nasal spray with nicotine patch for smoking cessation: randomised trial with six year follow up. *BMJ*. 1999;318(7179):285-288. doi:10.1136/bmj.318.7179.285
80. Schneider NG, Lunell E, Olmstead RE, Fagerström KO. Clinical pharmacokinetics of nasal nicotine delivery. A review and comparison to other nicotine systems. *Clin Pharmacokinet*. 1996;31(1):65-80. doi:10.2165/00003088-199631010-00005
81. Caldwell BO, Crane J. Combination nicotine metered dose inhaler and nicotine patch for smoking cessation: a randomized controlled trial. *Nicotine Tob Res*. 2016;18(10):1944-1951. doi:10.1093/ntr/ntw093
82. Schneider NG, Olmstead RE, Franzon MA, Lunell E. The nicotine inhaler: clinical pharmacokinetics and comparison with other nicotine treatments. *Clin Pharmacokinet*. 2001;40(9):661-684. doi:10.2165/00003088-200140090-00003
83. Shiffman S, Fant RV, Buchhalter AR, Gitchell JG, Henningfield JE. Nicotine delivery systems. *Expert Opin Drug Deliv*. 2005;2(3):563-577. doi:10.1517/17425247.2.3.563
84. Shiffman S, Ferguson SG, Hellebusch SJ. Physicians' counseling of patients when prescribing nicotine replacement therapy. *Addict Behav*. 2007;32(4):728-739. doi:10.1016/j.addbeh.2006.06.021
85. Hajek P, West R, Foulds J, Nilsson F, Burrows S, Meadow A. Randomized comparative trial of nicotine polacrilex, a transdermal patch, nasal spray, and an inhaler. *Arch Intern Med*. 1999;159(17):2033-2038. doi:10.1001/archinte.159.17.2033
86. Tiffany ST, Cox LS, Elash CA. Effects of transdermal nicotine patches on abstinence-induced and cue-elicited craving in cigarette smokers. *J Consult Clin Psychol*. 2000;68(2):233-240. doi:10.1037//0022-006x.68.2.233
87. Waters AJ, Shiffman S, Sayette MA, Paty JA, Gwaltney CJ, Balabanis MH. Cue-provoked craving and nicotine replacement therapy in smoking cessation. *J Consult Clin Psychol*. 2004;72(6):1136-1143. doi:10.1037/0022-006X.72.6.1136
88. Lindson N, Chepkin SC, Ye W, Fanshawe TR, Bullen C, Hartmann-Boyce J. Different doses, durations and modes of delivery of nicotine replacement therapy for smoking cessation. *Cochrane Database Syst Rev*. 2019;4:CD013308. doi:10.1002/14651858.CD013308
89. Ferry L, Johnston JA. Efficacy and safety of bupropion SR for smoking cessation: data from clinical trials and five years of postmarketing experience. *Int J Clin Pract*. 2003;57(3):224-230.
90. Huecker MR, Smiley A, Saadabadi A. Bupropion. In: *StatPearls*. StatPearls Publishing; 2022. Accessed June 9, 2022. http://www.ncbi.nlm.nih.gov/books/NBK470212/
91. Robinson JD, Karam-Hage M, Kypriotakis G, et al. Bupropion XL and SR have similar effectiveness and adverse event profiles when used to treat smoking among patients at a comprehensive cancer center. *Am J Addict*. 2022;31(3):236-241. doi:10.1111/ajad.13282
92. Shah D, Shah A, Tan X, Sambamoorthi U. Trends in utilization of smoking cessation agents before and after the passage of FDA boxed warning in the United States. *Drug Alcohol Depend*. 2017;177:187-193. doi:10.1016/j.drugalcdep.2017.03.021
93. Cinciripini PM, Kypriotakis G, Green C, et al. The effects of varenicline, bupropion, nicotine patch, and placebo on smoking cessation among smokers with major depression: a randomized clinical trial. *Depress Anxiety*. 2022;39(5):429-440. doi:10.1002/da.23259
94. Evins AE, West R, Benowitz NL, et al. Efficacy and safety of pharmacotherapeutic smoking cessation aids in schizophrenia spectrum disorders: subgroup analysis of EAGLES. *Psychiatr Serv Wash DC*. 2021;72(1):7-15. doi:10.1176/appi.ps.202000032
95. Hartmann-Boyce J, Theodoulou A, Farley A, et al. Interventions for preventing weight gain after smoking cessation. *Cochrane Database Syst Rev*. 2021;10:CD006219. doi:10.1002/14651858.CD006219.pub4
96. Howes S, Hartmann-Boyce J, Livingstone-Banks J, Hong B, Lindson N. Antidepressants for smoking cessation. *Cochrane Database Syst Rev*. 2020;4:CD000031. doi:10.1002/14651858.CD000031.pub5
97. Killen JD, Fortmann SP, Murphy GM, et al. Extended treatment with bupropion SR for cigarette smoking cessation. *J Consult Clin Psychol*. 2006;74(2):286-294. doi:10.1037/0022-006X.74.2.286
98. Hawk LW, Ashare RL, Rhodes JD, Oliver JA, Cummings KM, Mahoney MC. Does extended pre quit bupropion aid in extinguishing smoking behavior? *Nicotine Tob Res*. 2015;17(11):1377-1384. doi:10.1093/ntr/ntu347
99. Rollema H, Hajós M, Seymour PA, et al. Preclinical pharmacology of the alpha4beta2 nAChR partial agonist varenicline related to effects on reward, mood and cognition. *Biochem Pharmacol*. 2009;78(7):813-824. doi:10.1016/j.bcp.2009.05.033
100. Tonstad S, Arons C, Rollema H, et al. Varenicline: mode of action, efficacy, safety and accumulated experience salient for clinical populations. *Curr Med Res Opin*. 2020;36(5):713-730. doi:10.1080/03007995.2020.1729708
101. Mihalak KB, Carroll FI, Luetje CW. Varenicline is a partial agonist at alpha4beta2 and a full agonist at alpha7 neuronal nicotinic receptors. *Mol Pharmacol*. 2006;70(3):801-805. doi:10.1124/mol.106.025130
102. Patterson F, Jepson C, Strasser AA, et al. Varenicline improves mood and cognition during smoking abstinence. *Biol Psychiatry*. 2009;65(2):144-149. doi:10.1016/j.biopsych.2008.08.028
103. Philip NS, Carpenter LL, Tyrka AR, Whiteley LB, Price LH. Varenicline augmentation in depressed smokers: an 8-week, open-label study. *J Clin Psychiatry*. 2009;70(7):1026-1031. doi:10.4088/jcp.08m04441
104. Smith RC, Lindenmayer JP, Davis JM, et al. Cognitive and antismoking effects of varenicline in patients with schizophrenia or schizoaffective disorder. *Schizophr Res*. 2009;110(1-3):149-155. doi:10.1016/j.schres.2009.02.001
105. Sofuoglu M, Herman AI, Mooney M, Waters AJ. Varenicline attenuates some of the subjective and physiological effects of intravenous nicotine in humans. *Psychopharmacology (Berl)*. 2009;207(1):153-162. doi:10.1007/s00213-009-1643-z
106. Guo K, Wang S, Shang X, et al. The effect of Varenicline and bupropion on smoking cessation: a network meta-analysis of 20 randomized controlled trials. *Addict Behav*. 2022;131:107329. doi:10.1016/j.addbeh.2022.107329
107. Leone FT, Zhang Y, Evers-Casey S, et al. Initiating pharmacologic treatment in tobacco-dependent adults. an official American Thoracic Society Clinical Practice Guideline. *Am J Respir Crit Care Med*. 2020;202(2):e5-e31. doi:10.1164/rccm.202005-1982ST

108. Drovandi AD, Chen CC, Glass BD. Adverse effects cause varenicline discontinuation: a meta-analysis. *Curr Drug Saf.* 2016;11(1):78-85. doi:10.2174/1574886311207040282
109. Thomas KH, Dalili MN, López-López JA, et al. Comparative clinical effectiveness and safety of tobacco cessation pharmacotherapies and electronic cigarettes: a systematic review and network meta-analysis of randomized controlled trials. *Addiction.* 2022;117(4):861-876. doi:10.1111/add.15675
110. Leone FT, Schnoll RA. Reframing the varenicline question: have anecdotes and emotional filters clouded our decision making? *Lancet Respir Med.* 2015;3(10):736-737.
111. U.S. Food and Drug Administration. *Laboratory analysis of varenicline products.* Accessed June 9, 2022. https://www.fda.gov/drugs/drug-safety-and-availability/laboratory-analysis-varenicline-products
112. Singh JA, Sloan JA, Atherton PJ, et al. Preferred roles in treatment decision making among patients with cancer: a pooled analysis of studies using the Control Preferences Scale. *Am J Manag Care.* 2010;16(9):688-696.
113. Rigotti NA, Pipe AL, Benowitz NL, Arteaga C, Garza D, Tonstad S. Efficacy and safety of varenicline for smoking cessation in patients with cardiovascular disease: a randomized trial. *Circulation.* 2010;121(2):221-229. doi:10.1161/CIRCULATIONAHA.109.869008
114. Sterling LH, Windle SB, Filion KB, Touma L, Eisenberg MJ. Varenicline and adverse cardiovascular events: a systematic review and meta-analysis of randomized controlled trials. *J Am Heart Assoc.* 2016;5(2):e002849. doi:10.1161/JAHA.115.002849
115. Hawk LW, Ashare RL, Lohnes SF, et al. The effects of extended pre-quit varenicline treatment on smoking behavior and short-term abstinence: a randomized clinical trial. *Clin Pharmacol Ther.* 2012;91(2):172-180. doi:10.1038/clpt.2011.317
116. Lawson SC, Gass JC, Cooper RK, et al. The impact of three weeks of pre-quit varenicline on reinforcing value and craving for cigarettes in a laboratory choice procedure. *Psychopharmacology (Berl).* 2021;238(2):599-609. doi:10.1007/s00213-020-05713-7
117. Carpenter MJ, Wahlquist AE, Dahne J, et al. Nicotine replacement therapy sampling for smoking cessation within primary care: results from a pragmatic cluster randomized clinical trial. *Addiction.* 2020;115(7):1358-1367. doi:10.1111/add.14953
118. Ebbert JO, Hughes JR, West RJ, et al. Effect of varenicline on smoking cessation through smoking reduction: a randomized clinical trial. *JAMA.* 2015;313(7):687-694. doi:10.1001/jama.2015.280
119. Vinci C. Cognitive behavioral and mindfulness-based interventions for smoking cessation: a review of the recent literature. *Curr Oncol Rep.* 2020;22(6):58. doi:10.1007/s11912-020-00915-w
120. McClure JB, Bricker J, Mull K, Heffner JL. Comparative effectiveness of group-delivered acceptance and commitment therapy versus cognitive behavioral therapy for smoking cessation: a randomized controlled trial. *Nicotine Tob Res.* 2020;22(3):354-362. doi:10.1093/ntr/nty268
121. Martínez-Vispo C, Rodríguez-Cano R, López-Durán A, Senra C, Fernández Del Río E, Becoña E. Cognitive-behavioral treatment with behavioral activation for smoking cessation: randomized controlled trial. *PloS One.* 2019;14(4):e0214252. doi:10.1371/journal.pone.0214252
122. Notley C, Gentry S, Livingstone-Banks J, Bauld L, Perera R, Hartmann-Boyce J. Incentives for smoking cessation. *Cochrane Database Syst Rev.* 2019;7:CD004307. doi:10.1002/14651858.CD004307.pub6
123. Lancaster T, Stead LF. Individual behavioural counselling for smoking cessation. *Cochrane Database Syst Rev.* 2017;3:CD001292. doi:10.1002/14651858.CD001292.pub3
124. United States Public Health Service Office of the Surgeon General, National Center for Chronic Disease Prevention and Health Promotion (U.S.) Office on Smoking and Health. *Smoking Cessation: A Report of the Surgeon General.* U.S. Department of Health and Human Services; 2020. Accessed June 9, 2022. http://www.ncbi.nlm.nih.gov/books/NBK555591/
125. U.S. Preventive Services Task Force, Krist AH, Davidson KW, et al. Interventions for tobacco smoking cessation in adults, including pregnant persons: us preventive services task force recommendation statement. *JAMA.* 2021;325(3):265-279. doi:10.1001/jama.2020.25019
126. Do HP, Tran BX, Le Pham Q, et al. Which eHealth interventions are most effective for smoking cessation? A systematic review. *Patient Prefer Adherence.* 2018;12:2065-2084. doi:10.2147/PPA.S169397
127. Graham AL, Carpenter KM, Cha S, et al. Systematic review and meta-analysis of Internet interventions for smoking cessation among adults. *Subst Abuse Rehabil.* 2016;7:55-69. doi:10.2147/SAR.S101660
128. Taylor GMJ, Dalili MN, Semwal M, Civljak M, Sheikh A, Car J. Internet-based interventions for smoking cessation. *Cochrane Database Syst Rev.* 2017;9:CD007078. doi:10.1002/14651858.CD007078.pub5
129. McCrabb S, Baker AL, Attia J, et al. Internet-based programs incorporating behavior change techniques are associated with increased smoking cessation in the general population: a systematic review and meta-analysis. *Ann Behav Med.* 2019;53(2):180-195. doi:10.1093/abm/kay026
130. Whittaker R, McRobbie H, Bullen C, Rodgers A, Gu Y, Dobson R. Mobile phone text messaging and app-based interventions for smoking cessation. *Cochrane Database Syst Rev.* 2019;10:CD006611. doi:10.1002/14651858.CD006611.pub5
131. Barroso-Hurtado M, Suárez-Castro D, Martínez-Vispo C, Becoña E, López-Durán A. Smoking cessation apps: a systematic review of format, outcomes, and features. *Int J Environ Res Public Health.* 2021;18(21):11664. doi:10.3390/ijerph182111664
132. Bricker JB, Watson NL, Mull KE, Sullivan BM, Heffner JL. Efficacy of smartphone applications for smoking cessation: a randomized clinical trial. *JAMA Intern Med.* 2020;180(11):1472-1480. doi:10.1001/jamainternmed.2020.4055
133. Cobos-Campos R, de Lafuente AS, Apiñaniz A, Parraza N, Llanos IP, Orive G. Effectiveness of mobile applications to quit smoking: systematic review and meta-analysis. *Tob Prev Cessat.* 2020;6:62. doi:10.18332/tpc/127770
134. Pacek LR, McClernon FJ, Bosworth HB. Adherence to pharmacological smoking cessation interventions: a literature review and synthesis of correlates and barriers. *Nicotine Tob Res.* 2018;20(10):1163-1172. doi:10.1093/ntr/ntx210
135. Liberman JN, Lichtenfeld MJ, Galaznik A, et al. Adherence to varenicline and associated smoking cessation in a community-based patient setting. *J Manag Care Pharm.* 2013;19(2):125-131. doi:10.18553/jmcp.2013.19.2.125
136. Baker TB, Piper ME, Stein JH, et al. Effects of nicotine patch vs varenicline vs combination nicotine replacement therapy on smoking cessation at 26 weeks: a randomized clinical trial. *JAMA.* 2016;315(4):371-379. doi:10.1001/jama.2015.19284
137. Handschin J, Hitsman B, Blazekovic S, et al. Factors associated with adherence to transdermal nicotine patches within a smoking cessation effectiveness trial. *J Smok Cessat.* 2018;13(1):33-43. doi:10.1017/jsc.2017.2
138. Hollands GJ, Naughton F, Farley A, Lindson N, Aveyard P. Interventions to increase adherence to medications for tobacco dependence. *Cochrane Database Syst Rev.* 2019;8:CD009164. doi:10.1002/14651858.CD009164.pub3
139. Schlam TR, Cook JW, Baker TB, et al. Can we increase smokers' adherence to nicotine replacement therapy and does this help them quit? *Psychopharmacology (Berl).* 2018;235(7):2065-2075. doi:10.1007/s00213-018-4903-y
140. Feero WG, Guttmacher AE, Collins FS. Genomic medicine—an updated primer. *N Engl J Med.* 2010;362(21):2001-2011. doi:10.1056/NEJMra0907175
141. Patel J, Abd T, Blumenthal RS, Nasir K, Superko HR. Genetics and personalized medicine—a role in statin therapy? *Curr Atheroscler Rep.* 2014;16(1):384. doi:10.1007/s11883-013-0384-y
142. Bierut LJ, Tyndale RF. Preparing the way: exploiting genomic medicine to stop smoking. *Trends Mol Med.* 2018;24(2):187-196. doi:10.1016/j.molmed.2017.12.001
143. Panagiotou OA, Schuit E, Munafò MR, Bennett DA, Bergen AW, David SP. Smoking cessation pharmacotherapy based on genetically-informed biomarkers: what is the evidence? *Nicotine Tob Res.* 2019;21(9):1289-1293. doi:10.1093/ntr/ntz009

144. Saccone NL, Baurley JW, Bergen AW, et al. The value of biosamples in smoking cessation trials: a review of genetic, metabolomic, and epigenetic findings. *Nicotine Tob Res*. 2018;20(4):403-413. doi:10.1093/ntr/ntx096
145. Schuit E, Panagiotou OA, Munafò MR, Bennett DA, Bergen AW, David SP. Pharmacotherapy for smoking cessation: effects by subgroup defined by genetically informed biomarkers. *Cochrane Database Syst Rev*. 2021;11:CD011823. doi:10.1002/14651858.CD011823.pub3
146. Perez-Paramo YX, Lazarus P. Pharmacogenetics factors influencing smoking cessation success; the importance of nicotine metabolism. *Expert Opin Drug Metab Toxicol*. 2021;17(3):333-349. doi:10.1080/17425255.2021.1863948
147. Siegel SD, Lerman C, Flitter A, Schnoll RA. The use of the nicotine metabolite ratio as a biomarker to personalize smoking cessation treatment: current evidence and future directions. *Cancer Prev Res (Phila)*. 2020;13(3):261-272. doi:10.1158/1940-6207.CAPR-19-0259
148. Allenby CE, Boylan KA, Lerman C, Falcone M. Precision medicine for tobacco dependence: development and validation of the nicotine metabolite ratio. *J Neuroimmune Pharmacol*. 2016;11(3):471-483. doi:10.1007/s11481-016-9656-y
149. Lerman C, Schnoll RA, Hawk LW, et al. Use of the nicotine metabolite ratio as a genetically informed biomarker of response to nicotine patch or varenicline for smoking cessation: a randomised, double-blind placebo-controlled trial. *Lancet Respir Med*. 2015;3(2):131-138. doi:10.1016/S2213-2600(14)70294-2
150. Wells QS, Freiberg MS, Greevy RA, et al. Nicotine metabolism-informed care for smoking cessation: a pilot precision RCT. *Nicotine Tob Res*. 2018;20(12):1489-1496. doi:10.1093/ntr/ntx235
151. Leone FT, Douglas IS. The emergence of e-cigarettes: a triumph of wishful thinking over science. *Ann Am Thorac Soc*. 2014;11(2):216-219. doi:10.1513/AnnalsATS.201312-428ED
152. Kandra KL, Ranney LM, Lee JGL, Goldstein AO. Physicians' attitudes and use of e-cigarettes as cessation devices, North Carolina, 2013. Bullen C, ed. *PLoS One*. 2014;9(7):e103462. doi:10.1371/journal.pone.0103462
153. Steinberg MB, Giovenco DP, Delnevo CD. Patient–physician communication regarding electronic cigarettes. *Prev Med Rep*. 2015;2:96-98. doi:10.1016/j.pmedr.2015.01.006
154. Baldassarri SR, Chupp GL, Leone FT, Warren GW, Toll BA. Practice patterns and perceptions of chest health care providers on electronic cigarette use: an in-depth discussion and report of survey results. *J Smok Cessat*. 2018;13(2):72-77. doi:10.1017/jsc.2017.6
155. Benmarhnia T, Pierce JP, Leas E, et al. Can e-cigarettes and pharmaceutical aids increase smoking cessation and reduce cigarette consumption? Findings from a nationally representative cohort of American smokers. *Am J Epidemiol*. 2018;187(11):2397-2404. doi:10.1093/aje/kwy129
156. Hartmann-Boyce J, McRobbie H, Butler AR, et al. Electronic cigarettes for smoking cessation. *Cochrane Database Syst Rev*. 2021;(9):CD010216. doi:10.1002/14651858.CD010216.pub6
157. Kalkhoran S, Glantz SA. E-cigarettes and smoking cessation in real-world and clinical settings: a systematic review and meta-analysis. *Lancet Respir Med*. 2016;4(2):116-128. doi:10.1016/S2213-2600(15)00521-4
158. Li D, Sundar IK, McIntosh S, et al. Association of smoking and electronic cigarette use with wheezing and related respiratory symptoms in adults: cross-sectional results from the Population Assessment of Tobacco and Health (PATH) study, wave 2. *Tob Control*. 2020;29(2):140-147. doi:10.1136/tobaccocontrol-2018-054694
159. Wang JB, Olgin JE, Nah G, et al. Cigarette and e-cigarette dual use and risk of cardiopulmonary symptoms in the Health eHeart Study. *PLoS One*. 2018;13(7):e0198681. doi:10.1371/journal.pone.0198681
160. Hedman L, Backman H, Stridsman C, et al. Association of electronic cigarette use with smoking habits, demographic factors, and respiratory symptoms. *JAMA Netw Open*. 2018;1(3):e180789. doi:10.1001/jamanetworkopen.2018.0789
161. Bhatta DN, Glantz SA. Electronic cigarette use and myocardial infarction among adults in the us population assessment of tobacco and health. *J Am Heart Assoc*. 2019;8(12):e012317. doi:10.1161/JAHA.119.012317
162. Leone FT, Carlsen KH, Chooljian D, et al. Recommendations for the appropriate structure, communication, and investigation of tobacco harm reduction claims. an official American Thoracic Society policy statement. *Am J Respir Crit Care Med*. 2018;198(8):e90-e105. doi:10.1164/rccm.201808-1443ST
163. Chatterjee S, Caporale A, Tao JQ, et al. Acute e-cig inhalation impacts vascular health: a study in smoking naïve subjects. *Am J Physiol Heart Circ Physiol*. 2020;320(1):H144-H158. doi:10.1152/ajpheart.00628.2020
164. Soneji S, Barrington-Trimis JL, Wills TA, et al. Association between initial use of e-cigarettes and subsequent cigarette smoking among adolescents and young adults: a systematic review and meta-analysis. *JAMA Pediatr*. 2017;171(8):788-797. doi:10.1001/jamapediatrics.2017.1488
165. Babb S. Quitting smoking among adults—United States, 2000-2015. *MMWR Morb Mortal Wkly Rep*. 2017;65. doi:10.15585/mmwr.mm6552a1
166. Chaiton M, Diemert L, Cohen JE, et al. Estimating the number of quit attempts it takes to quit smoking successfully in a longitudinal cohort of smokers. *BMJ Open*. 2016;6(6):e011045. doi:10.1136/bmjopen-2016-011045
167. Caponnetto P, Polosa R. Common predictors of smoking cessation in clinical practice. *Respir Med*. 2008;102(8):1182-1192. doi:10.1016/j.rmed.2008.02.017
168. Audrain-McGovern J, Benowitz NL. Cigarette smoking, nicotine, and body weight. *Clin Pharmacol Ther*. 2011;90(1):164-168. doi:10.1038/clpt.2011.105
169. Pisinger C, Jorgensen T. Weight concerns and smoking in a general population: the Inter99 study. *Prev Med*. 2007;44(4):283-289. doi:10.1016/j.ypmed.2006.11.014
170. Aubin HJ, Farley A, Lycett D, Lahmek P, Aveyard P. Weight gain in smokers after quitting cigarettes: meta-analysis. *BMJ*. 2012;345:e4439. doi:10.1136/bmj.e4439
171. Filozof C, Fernández Pinilla MC, Fernández-Cruz A. Smoking cessation and weight gain. *Obes Rev*. 2004;5(2):95-103. doi:10.1111/j.1467-789X.2004.00131.x
172. Berlin I, Vorspan F, Warot D, Manéglier B, Spreux-Varoquaux O. Effect of glucose on tobacco craving. Is it mediated by tryptophan and serotonin? *Psychopharmacology (Berl)*. 2005;178(1):27-34. doi:10.1007/s00213-004-1980-x
173. Williamson DF, Madans J, Anda RF, Kleinman JC, Giovino GA, Byers T. Smoking cessation and severity of weight gain in a national cohort. *N Engl J Med*. 1991;324(11):739-745. doi:10.1056/NEJM199103143241106
174. Farley AC, Hajek P, Lycett D, Aveyard P. Interventions for preventing weight gain after smoking cessation. *Cochrane Database Syst Rev*. 2012;1:CD006219. doi:10.1002/14651858.CD006219.pub3
175. Ebbert JO, Hatsukami DK, Croghan IT, et al. Combination varenicline and bupropion SR for tobacco-dependence treatment in cigarette smokers: a randomized trial. *JAMA*. 2014;311(2):155-163. doi:10.1001/jama.2013.283185
176. Hughes JR, Keely J, Naud S. Shape of the relapse curve and long-term abstinence among untreated smokers. *Addiction*. 2004;99(1):29-38. doi:10.1111/j.1360-0443.2004.00540.x
177. Hymowitz N, Cummings KM, Hyland A, Lynn WR, Pechacek TF, Hartwell TD. Predictors of smoking cessation in a cohort of adult smokers followed for five years. *Tob Control*. 1997;6(suppl 2):S57. doi:10.1136/tc.6.suppl_2.S57
178. Khuder SA, Dayal HH, Mutgi AB. Age at smoking onset and its effect on smoking cessation. *Addict Behav*. 1999;24(5):673-677. doi:10.1016/S0306-4603(98)00113-0
179. Dale LC, Glover ED, Sachs DPL, et al. Bupropion for smoking cessation: predictors of successful outcome. *Chest*. 2001;119(5):1357-1364. doi:10.1378/chest.119.5.1357
180. Segan CJ, Borland R. Does extended telephone callback counselling prevent smoking relapse? *Health Educ Res*. 2011;26(2):336-347. doi:10.1093/her/cyr009
181. Schnoll RA, Goelz PM, Veluz-Wilkins A, et al. Long-term nicotine replacement therapy: a randomized clinical trial. *JAMA Intern Med*. 2015;175(4):504-511. doi:10.1001/jamainternmed.2014.8313

182. Livingstone-Banks J, Norris E, Hartmann-Boyce J, et al. Relapse prevention interventions for smoking cessation. *Cochrane Database Syst Rev*. 2019;10:CD003999. doi:10.1002/14651858.CD003999.pub6
183. Healthy People 2030. *The Role of the Media in Promoting and Reducing Tobacco Use*. Accessed June 9, 2022. https://health.gov/healthypeople/tools-action/browse-evidence-based-resources/role-media-promoting-and-reducing-tobacco-use
184. Lee JGL, Henriksen L, Rose SW, Moreland-Russell S, Ribisl KM. A systematic review of neighborhood disparities in point-of-sale tobacco marketing. *Am J Public Health*. 2015;105(9):e8-e18. doi:10.2105/AJPH.2015.302777
185. U.S. Food and Drug Administration. *FDA Proposes Rules Prohibiting Menthol Cigarettes and Flavored Cigars to Prevent Youth Initiation, Significantly Reduce Tobacco-Related Disease and Death*. Accessed June 9, 2022. https://www.fda.gov/news-events/press-announcements/fda-proposes-rules-prohibiting-menthol-cigarettes-and-flavored-cigars-prevent-youth-initiation
186. Lawrence D, Mitrou F, Zubrick SR. Smoking and mental illness: results from population surveys in Australia and the United States. *BMC Public Health*. 2009;9:285. doi:10.1186/1471-2458-9-285
187. Cornelius ME, Loretan CG, Wang TW, Jamal A, Homa DM. Tobacco product use among adults—United States, 2020. *MMWR Morb Mortal Wkly Rep*. 2022;71(11):397-405. doi:10.15585/mmwr.mm7111a1
188. CDC. Smoking & tobacco use. *LGBTQ+ People and Commercial Tobacco: Health Disparities and Ways to Advance Health Equity*. Centers for Disease Control and Prevention. Accessed June 9, 2022. https://www.cdc.gov/tobacco/disparities/lgbt/index.htm
189. Ryan H, Wortley PM, Easton A, Pederson L, Greenwood G. Smoking among lesbians, gays, and bisexuals: a review of the literature. *Am J Prev Med*. 2001;21(2):142-149. doi:10.1016/s0749-3797(01)00331-2
190. Fu SS, Burgess D, van Ryn M, Hatsukami DK, Solomon J, Joseph AM. Views on smoking cessation methods in ethnic minority communities: a qualitative investigation. *Prev Med*. 2007;44(3):235-240. doi:10.1016/j.ypmed.2006.11.002
191. National Trends in Cessation Counseling, Prescription Medication Use, and Associated Costs Among U.S. Adult Cigarette Smokers. *JAMA Netw Open*. Accessed June 9, 2022. https://jamanetwork.com/journals/jamanetworkopen/fullarticle/2734073?utm_campaign=articlePDF&utm_medium=articlePDFlink&utm_source=articlePDF&utm_content=jamanetworkopen.2020.12164
192. Hooper MW, Payne M, Parkinson KA. Tobacco cessation pharmacotherapy use among racial/ethnic minorities in the United States: considerations for primary care. *Fam Med Community Health*. 2017;5(3):193-203. doi:10.15212/FMCH.2017.0138
193. Cokkinides VE, Ward E, Jemal A, Thun MJ. Under-use of smoking-cessation treatments: results from the National Health Interview Survey, 2000. *Am J Prev Med*. 2005;28(1):119-122. doi:10.1016/j.amepre.2004.09.007
194. Roberts E, Eden Evins A, McNeill A, Robson D. Efficacy and tolerability of pharmacotherapy for smoking cessation in adults with serious mental illness: a systematic review and network meta-analysis. *Addiction*. 2016;111(4):599-612. doi:10.1111/add.13236
195. Wu Q, Gilbody S, Peckham E, Brabyn S, Parrott S. Varenicline for smoking cessation and reduction in people with severe mental illnesses: systematic review and meta-analysis. *Addiction*. 2016;111(9):1554-1567. doi:10.1111/add.13415
196. Peckham E, Brabyn S, Cook L, Tew G, Gilbody S. Smoking cessation in severe mental ill health: what works? An updated systematic review and meta-analysis. *BMC Psychiatry*. 2017;17(1):252. doi:10.1186/s12888-017-1419-7
197. Cox LS, Okuyemi K, Choi WS, Ahluwalia JS. A review of tobacco use treatments in U.S. ethnic minority populations. *Am J Health Promot*. 2011;25(5 Suppl):S11-S30. doi:10.4278/ajhp.100610-LIT-177
198. Robles GI, Singh-Franco D, Ghin HL. A review of the efficacy of smoking-cessation pharmacotherapies in nonwhite populations. *Clin Ther*. 2008;30(5):800-812. doi:10.1016/j.clinthera.2008.05.010
199. Cox LS, Nollen NL, Mayo MS, et al. Effect of varenicline added to counseling on smoking cessation among African American daily smokers: the Kick It at Swope IV Randomized Clinical Trial. *JAMA*. 2022;327(22):2201-2209. doi:10.1001/jama.2022.8274

CHAPTER

66

Pharmacological Interventions for Other Substances and Multiple Substance Use Disorders

Jeffery N. Wilkins, Mark Hrymoc, Manjit Bhandal, and David A. Gorelick

CHAPTER OUTLINE

- Introduction
- Cannabis
- Anabolic androgenic steroids
- Dissociatives
- Inhalants
- Nicotine (tobacco) with other substances
- Opioids with other substances
- Hallucinogens
- Kratom
- Conclusions

INTRODUCTION

This chapter focuses on pharmacological therapies for single substance use disorders (SUDs), such as cannabis (marijuana), anabolic steroids, phencyclidine (PCP) and ketamine, inhalants, hallucinogens, and kratom, as well as the following mixed substance use disorders—nicotine (tobacco) with other substances (alcohol, opioids, cocaine), opioids with other substances (alcohol, cocaine), and cocaine with PCP. In many cases, the pharmacological treatments described are experimental or based on weak evidence, in that they lack controlled clinical trials to support their use. Thus, the mainstay of treatment for these substance use disorders is psychosocial modalities (see section 9, "Psychologically Based Interventions").

CANNABIS

There is currently no well-established role for pharmacotherapy in the short- or long-term treatment of cannabis use disorder (CUD); no medication is approved for this indication by the U.S. Food and Drug Administration (FDA) or any other national regulatory body.[1,2] Further complicating treatment for CUD is the absence of federal or state regulation of the potency of cannabis products[3] and the significant rise in the potency of cannabis products over the past two decades.[4] Some cannabis waxes and oils ("concentrates")[5] and liquids for vaporization in electronic drug delivery devices ("e-cigarettes")[6] have concentrations of the chief euphorigenic cannabinoid delta-9 tetrahydrocannabinol (Δ9-THC) as high as 90%.

A 2019 Cochrane review of randomized controlled clinical trials (RCT) published between 2004 and 2019 evaluated 21 RCTs (45 reports), involving 1,755 study participants (909 active medication, 846 placebo) who received eight different classes of active medications.[7] (See **Table 66-1** for the main findings.)

More recent studies not included in the Cochrane review found that the nicotinic cholinergic receptor partial agonist varenicline (up to 1 mg bid for 6 weeks) significantly reduced cannabis use in adults[29] and the cannabinoid cannabidiol (CBD) (400 mg orally twice daily for 4 weeks of synthetic formulation) significantly reduced cannabis use in adults.[30] A subsequent study of nabiximols showed reduced cannabis use with sublingual (oromucosal spray) doses up to 113.4 mg THC/105 mg CBD daily for 12 weeks or a mean (SD) dose of 47.5 [25.7] mg THC/44.0 [23.8] mg CBD.[31] Nabiximols is not available in the United States but is approved in Canada and several European countries for treatment of muscle spasticity associated with multiple sclerosis. In contrast to studies with cannabidiol, either alone or in combination with THC, neither synthetic THC alone (dronabinol, 20 mg orally twice daily for 8 weeks)[26] nor the synthetic THC analogue nabilone (2 mg orally daily for 10 weeks)[32] significantly reduce cannabis use in adults.

ANABOLIC ANDROGENIC STEROIDS

We are not aware of any published clinical trials evaluating treatment of unhealthy use of anabolic androgenic steroids. A recent scoping review[33] identified 11 case reports and one case series involving a total of 15 adult patients treated with antipsychotic medications, selective serotonin reuptake inhibitor (SSRI) antidepressants, lithium, or clonidine. There were no clear indications of efficacy, as treatment outcome was often not well assessed and some patients withdrew from treatment early. Thus, there is no established medication for the treatment of unhealthy anabolic androgenic steroid use. See Chapter 21, "The Pharmacology of Anabolic–Androgenic Steroids."

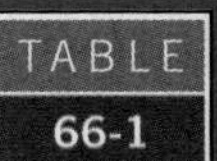

TABLE 66-1 Main Findings of 2019 Cochrane Review of Pharmacotherapy for Cannabis Dependence

- **Δ9-THC preparations**: No change in cannabis use vs placebo
  - risk ratio (RR) 0.98, 95% confidence interval (CI) 0.64 to 1.52; 305 participants for 3 medication preparations: dronabinol, dronabinol plus lofexidine and nabiximols, a cannabis extract containing a 1:1 ratio of Δ^9-THC and cannabidiol[8,9]; moderate-quality evidence
- **Selective serotonin reuptake inhibitor (SSRI) antidepressants**[10-12]: no change in cannabis use vs placebo
- **Mixed action antidepressants**[13-15]: no change in cannabis use vs placebo
- **Anticonvulsants and mood stabilizers** (divalproex sodium, gabapentin, lithium, topiramate)[16-19]: no change in cannabis use vs placebo
- **Bupropion** (atypical antidepressant bupropion): no change in cannabis use vs placebo[20]
- **Buspirone** (anxiolytic): no change in cannabis use vs placebo[21,22]
- **Atomoxetine** (selective noradrenaline reuptake inhibitor atomoxetine): no change in cannabis use vs placebo[23]
- ***N*-acetylcysteine**: no change in cannabis use vs placebo[24,25]
- **Δ^9-THC preparations** (dronabinol, nabiximols): qualitative reductions of intensity of withdrawal symptoms[8,9,25,27]
- **Gabapentin, atomoxetine, oxytocin**: available evidence insufficient for estimates of effectiveness
- **Gabapentin,[17] oxytocin,[28] and *N*-acetylcysteine**[24,25]: evidence base is weak, but these medications are worth further investigation

From Nielsen S, Gowing L, Sabioni P, Le Foll B. Pharmacotherapies for cannabis dependence. *Cochrane Database Syst Rev.* 2019;1(1):CD008940. doi:10.1002/14651858.CD008940.pub3

DISSOCIATIVES

Phencyclidine (PCP) and ketamine are synthetic dissociative anesthetics that act as antagonists of the *N*-methyl-D-aspartate (NMDA) receptor.[34,35] Dextromethorphan (DXM) and its major active metabolite dextrorphan (DXO) are also NMDA receptor antagonists and interact with several other receptors as well.[36] The NMDA receptor is a G protein-coupled ionotropic glutamate receptor (see Chapter 19, "The Pharmacology of Dissociatives"). PCP gained popularity as a substance of unhealthy use in the 1960s and no longer is legally available in the United States.[34] Ketamine, a synthetic analogue of PCP, is still legally available as an anesthetic and is also subject to unhealthy use.[35] Dextromethorphan is widely available as an ingredient in over-the-counter cough medications.[36] At higher than recommended doses, it has psychoactive effects such as euphoria and sedation, which can promote unhealthy use. There is very little published experience with pharmacological treatment of PCP or ketamine unhealthy use.[35,37] Both the tricyclic antidepressant desipramine and the anxiolytic buspirone have significantly improved psychological symptoms such as depression in small outpatient controlled clinical trials, but neither medication significantly reduced PCP use.[38,39] A case report found that oral naltrexone (50 mg daily) produced complete abstinence from ketamine over 12 months in an adult with ketamine dependence (DSM-IV criteria).[40] There is almost no published literature on pharmacological treatment of unhealthy DXM use. Two published case reports suggest that naltrexone (100 mg orally daily), with or without gabapentin, decreases DXM use in those with unhealthy use.[41,42]

PCP in Combination With Cocaine or Cannabis

PCP is often smoked with cocaine ("space basing") or cannabis ("primos"). There is very little literature on the treatment of these co-occurring substance use disorders. No clinical trial has shown any medication to be effective. In a double-blind study of 20 people chronically using PCP/cocaine, desipramine (200 mg/d) significantly reduced withdrawal symptoms but had no significant effect on actual drug use.[43]

INHALANTS

Inhalants are a heterogeneous group of volatile substances that include adhesives, aerosols, solvents, anesthetics (including nitrous oxide), gasoline, cleaning agents, and nitrites[44] (see Chapter 20, "The Pharmacology of Inhalants"). Because these agents are marketed legally for commercial and household purposes, they generally are inexpensive and readily available. Many individuals who receive treatment for neurobehavioral and physical health problems related to inhalant use have co-occurring psychiatric and substance use disorders, typically involving alcohol and cannabis, which can complicate treatment. There is little published experience with pharmacological treatment and few placebo-controlled clinical trials.[45] Case reports suggest possible benefit from buspirone, lamotrigine, risperidone, haloperidol, or carbamazepine. Pharmacological treatment of associated or comorbid psychiatric conditions may be effective (eg, antipsychotics for psychosis).

NICOTINE (TOBACCO) WITH OTHER SUBSTANCES

There is substantial comorbidity between tobacco use disorder and other SUDs. Among U.S. adults with a DSM-5–defined tobacco (nicotine) use disorder, 18% have a current nonalcohol SUD and an odds ratio of 3.2 (95% CI 2.91-3.45) for having another SUD compared with those without tobacco use disorder, after adjusting for other psychiatric disorders and sociodemographic characteristics.[46] SUDs in this study included sedative/tranquilizer, cannabis, amphetamine, cocaine, nonheroin opioid, heroin, hallucinogen, and solvent/inhalant use disorders.

Past-month self-reported tobacco cigarette smoking prevalence declined among U.S. adults with comorbid SUD from

46.5% in 2006 to 35.8% in 2019 (average annual change of −1.7% (95% CI, −2.8 to −0.6; p = 0.002).[47] This was a lower rate of decline than in those without comorbid SUD. Cigarette smoking prevalence declined significantly in each demographic subgroup (age, sex, race, and ethnicity), except for Indigenous American/Alaska Natives.

Tobacco and Alcohol

Varenicline, which is FDA approved for helping people to stop cigarette smoking, reduced both heavy alcohol use and cigarette smoking in two RCTs[48,49] but reduced only cigarette smoking in a third RCT.[50] Varenicline was more effective alone (45.1% stopped smoking) than when combined with naltrexone (26.5% abstinence rate).[48]

A recent small (44 adults with comorbid tobacco use disorder and AUD), 12-week RCT found that varenicline plus nicotine patch, compared with placebo plus nicotine patch, significantly increased rates of stopping smoking during the last four weeks of the trial (44.3% versus 27.9%, respectively; odds ratio 2.20; 95% CI, 1.01-4.80; p = 0.047).[51] The treatment groups did not differ significantly in alcohol use measures.

Tobacco and Opioids

The prevalence of current (past-year) cigarette smoking in the U.S. is significantly higher among adults with current opioid use disorder (OUD) (about two-thirds) than in those without OUD (about one-fifth).[52,53] The prevalence of smoking is higher among primary care outpatients with than without OUD (90% versus 42%, respectively)[54] and among persons with OUD who are not in OUD treatment (92%-95%).[55] Persons with chronic pain appropriately taking prescription opioid analgesics are nearly twice as likely to smoke as persons without opioid analgesic prescriptions.[56]

Tobacco abstinence rates achieved by FDA-approved medications for tobacco use such as nicotine replacement therapy (NRT), bupropion, and varenicline among individuals with OUD who smoke tobacco and who are in treatment for OUD are approximately one-quarter of the rates achieved among individuals without OUD who smoke tobacco, in part because of poor treatment adherence.[55] Adding intensive psychosocial treatment (motivational enhancement, cognitive behavioral therapy) does not significantly improve long-term abstinence rates.[57]

Tobacco and Stimulants

Adults who use stimulants have very high rates of tobacco cigarette smoking: 70% to 80% among those using cocaine and 90% among those using methamphetamine.[58] Reduced tobacco cigarette smoking among those in treatment for cocaine use disorder (CoUD) is associated with better treatment outcomes for CUD, although the same benefit is not always found among those in treatment for methamphetamine use disorder.[59] These findings suggest the importance of offering treatment for tobacco use disorder to patients with stimulant use disorder. We are not aware of any clinical studies of pharmacological treatment for comorbid tobacco and stimulant use disorders.

OPIOIDS WITH OTHER SUBSTANCES

Opioids and Alcohol

Up to one-third of adults with OUD also have AUD; such comorbidity is especially common in patients taking opioid analgesics for chronic pain[56,60-63] Among patients with OUD (three-quarters with heroin use) admitted to U.S. publicly funded SUD treatment programs in 2019, about one-eighth (12.5%) reported having a problem with alcohol use.[64] Comorbid AUD is often associated with poorer treatment outcome in patients with OUD receiving opioid agonist treatment.[61,62] These findings support the importance of effective pharmacotherapy for comorbid OUD and AUD.

Opioid agonist maintenance treatment for OUD has inconsistent effects on comorbid AUD, with some studies showing decreased alcohol intake and others showing no effect or increased alcohol use.[61-63] Limited observational data suggest that buprenorphine may be more effective than methadone in reducing alcohol use among patients with OUD receiving opioid agonist maintenance treatment.[61] Naltrexone, a mu-opioid receptor antagonist FDA-approved to treat both OUD and AUD, has been suggested as a treatment for the comorbid disorders,[62] but does not appear superior to opioid agonists in reducing alcohol use.[63] Disulfiram, FDA-approved for the treatment of AUD, has been evaluated in patients with OUD receiving opioid agonist maintenance treatment (chiefly methadone).[65-67] Reductions in alcohol use are significant in studies that administer disulfiram under contingency management conditions (thus enhancing treatment adherence) but are inconsistent in other studies. Disulfiram is generally well tolerated, but some patients experience significant side-effects.

Opioids and Stimulants

Up to 80% of U.S. adults with an opioid use disorder (OUD) have a lifetime history of stimulant use (cocaine, amphetamines, and/or prescription stimulants).[68] Among people currently (past-year) using opioids, at least 10% are also currently using cocaine.[69] Use of stimulants is high even among adults in treatment for OUD, with usage rates as high as 50%.[70,71] About one-third of patients in treatment for OUD have a comorbid stimulant use disorder.[72,73] Among patients with OUD (three-quarters with heroin use) admitted to U.S. publicly funded SUD treatment programs in 2019, more than one-third (38.4%) reported having a problem with stimulant use.[62] Stimulant use by patients in OUD treatment is associated with poorer treatment adherence,[74] retention,[75] and outcome,[71,75-77] so effective treatment of both comorbid disorders is clinically important.

Three different pharmacological approaches have been used for the treatment of dual OUD and stimulant use disorder among individuals receiving treatment with opioid agonists: adjustment of methadone dose, treatment with a different opioid medication (buprenorphine or naltrexone), and addition of medication targeting the stimulant use disorder. Higher methadone doses (>60 mg daily) are associated with less cocaine use in many,[78] but not all,[79,80] studies. The adequacy of the methadone dose in suppressing opioid craving and withdrawal symptoms may be more important than the actual methadone dosage in mediating reduction in cocaine use.[79,80] Buprenorphine reduces both opioid and cocaine use in RCTs involving patients with concurrent OUD and CoUD but only at higher buprenorphine doses (16-32 mg daily sublingually).[81,82] Single studies suggest that methadone is better than buprenorphine[82] and buprenorphine better than naltrexone in reducing cocaine use.[83] No nonopioid medication has shown efficacy in the treatment of patients with dual OUD and stimulant use disorder.[84-86] (See Chapter 64, "Pharmacological Treatment of Stimulant Use Disorders" for more information on pharmacological treatment of comorbid OUD and stimulant use disorder.)

HALLUCINOGENS

Hallucinogens are a varied group of plant-derived alkaloids and synthetic compounds that have in common the ability to produce sensory, perceptual, and cognitive changes without impairing attention or level of consciousness (ie, with a clear sensorium)[87] (see Chapter 18, "The Pharmacology of Hallucinogens"). They include compounds that influence serotonergic neurotransmission, such as LSD, psilocybin, and DMT, and those that influence catecholaminergic neurotransmission, such as mescaline and amphetamine analogues like 3,4-methylenedioxy-*N*-methamphetamine (MDMA, "ecstasy").

There is currently no proven pharmacological treatment for hallucinogen use disorder, nor are we aware of any published clinical trials of pharmacological treatment. A case report found that topiramate (200 mg daily) was associated with three months of abstinence in a young adult with a 4-year history of frequent MDMA use.[88] Retrospective case reports suggest that adults with depression taking monoamine oxidase inhibitors (such as phenelzine) or SSRI antidepressants (specifically fluoxetine, sertraline, and paroxetine) experience reduced acute psychological effects of LSD, whereas those taking tricyclic antidepressants (imipramine, desipramine) or lithium experience enhanced LSD effects.[89] In double-blind, placebo-controlled human laboratory studies, pretreatment with the 5-$HT_{2A/C}$ receptor antagonist ketanserin[90] or the SSRI antidepressant escitalopram[91] significantly attenuates the acute psychological effects of LSD or psilocybin, respectively. These findings suggest that medications affecting monoaminergic neurotransmission are a promising area for development of pharmacological treatments for hallucinogen use disorder.

LSD use is associated with perceptual abnormalities, such as illusions, distortions, and hallucinations, persisting or recurring intermittently for long periods (up to years) after the last LSD use. When these abnormalities occur after a period of normal perceptual functioning, they are termed flashbacks,[92] defined as hallucinogen persisting perception disorder (HPPD) in DSM-5.[93] Case reports and small case series suggest that naltrexone, clonidine, reboxetine, benzodiazepines, and lamotrigine can be helpful in the treatment of HPDD, while second-generation antipsychotics and SSRI antidepressants show mixed results.[92] Risperidone is beneficial at low doses (≤ 1 mg/d) but may worsen symptoms at higher doses. Sertraline and fluoxetine are the SSRIs most often found beneficial.

KRATOM

Kratom is the common term for the *Mitragyna speciosa* tree (native to Southeast Asia) and its products,[94] Its major active compounds are the alkaloids mitragynine and 7-hydroxymitragynine, which are agonists at the μ-opioid receptor. Kratom has prominent opioid-like effects, especially with chronic or high-dose use. While there is no approved pharmacological treatment for kratom use disorder, case series suggest that long-term treatment with buprenorphine is effective in weaning patients off kratom use and maintaining long-term abstinence.[95]

CONCLUSIONS

This chapter reviewed approaches to pharmacological treatment of single SUDs involving cannabis, anabolic androgenic steroids, dissociatives inhalants, hallucinogens, or kratom, as well as comorbid SUDs involving nicotine (tobacco), PCP, or opioids with other substances such as alcohol and stimulants. There are no FDA-approved medications for these disorders; in most cases, there is little or no published literature to guide the choice of pharmacological treatment and no clinical trials to support the efficacy of any treatment. The current mainstay of treatment for these substance use disorders is psychosocial intervention. When the use of pharmacological treatments is considered (eg, due to severe behavioral disturbances or treatment resistance), the clinician must rely almost exclusively on their own experience and clinical judgment, with very little help from the medical or scientific literature. Careful consideration must be given that any potential gains from use of such pharmacotherapies not be outweighed by the many and varied potential short- and long-term side effects of their use.

Future research is needed to identify effective new pharmacotherapies that enhance the treatment of these substance use disorders and of co-occurring substance use disorders, especially their combination with tobacco and alcohol use disorders. Effective treatments may come from medications or new treatment modalities that influence multiple classes of substances, such as noninvasive brain stimulation, for example, transcranial magnetic stimulation.

REFERENCES

1. Gorelick DA. Pharmacological treatment of cannabis-related disorders: a narrative review. *Curr Pharm Des.* 2016;22(42):6409-6419.
2. Kondo KK, Morasco BJ, Nugent SM, et al. Pharmacotherapy for the treatment of cannabis use disorder: a systematic review. *Ann Intern Med.* 2020;172(6):398-412. doi:10.7326/M19-1105
3. Shover CL, Humphreys K. Six policy lessons relevant to cannabis legalization. *Am J Drug Alcohol Abuse.* 2019;45(6):698-706.
4. Freeman TP, Craft S, Wilson J, et al. Changes in delta-9-tetrahydrocannabinol (THC) and cannabidiol (CBD) concentrations in cannabis over time: systematic review and meta-analysis. *Addiction.* 2021;116(5):1000-1010.
5. Matheson J, Le Foll B. Cannabis legalization and acute harm from high potency cannabis products: a narrative review and recommendations for public health. *Front Psychiatry.* 2020;11:591979.
6. Meehan-Atrash J, Rahman I. Cannabis vaping: existing and emerging modalities, chemistry, and pulmonary toxicology. *Chem Res Toxicol.* 2021;34(10):2169-2179.
7. Nielsen S, Gowing L, Sabioni P, Le Foll B. Pharmacotherapies for cannabis dependence. *Cochrane Database Syst Rev.* 2019;1:CD008940. doi:10.1002/14651858.CD008940.pub3
8. Allsop DJ, Copeland J, Lintzeris N, et al. Nabiximols as an agonist replacement therapy during cannabis withdrawal: a randomized clinical trial. *JAMA Psychiatry.* 2014;71(3):281-291.
9. Trigo JM, Soliman A, Quilty LC, et al. Nabiximols combined with motivational enhancement/cognitive behavioral therapy for the treatment of cannabis dependence: a pilot randomized clinical trial. *PLoS One.* 2018;13:e0190768.
10. Cornelius JR, Bukstein OG, Douaihy AB, et al. Double-blind fluoxetine trial in comorbid MDD- CUD youth and young adults. *Drug Alcohol Depend.* 2010;112(1-2):39-45.
11. Weinstein AM, Miller H, Bluvstein I, Rapoport E, et al. Treatment of cannabis dependence using escitalopram in combination with cognitive-behavior therapy: a double-blind placebo-controlled study. *Am J Drug Alcohol Abuse.* 2014;40(1):16-22.
12. McRae-Clark AL, Baker NL, Gray KM, Killeen T, Hartwell KJ, Simonian SJ. Vilazodone for cannabis dependence: a randomized, controlled pilot trial. *Am J Addict.* 2016;25(1):69-75.
13. Carpenter KM, McDowell D, Brooks DJ, Cheng WY, Levin FR. A preliminary trial: double-blind comparison of nefazodone, bupropion-SR, and placebo in the treatment of cannabis dependence. *Am J Addict.* 2009;18(1):53-64.
14. Frewen A, Montebello ME, Baillie A, Rea F. Effects of mirtazapine on withdrawal from dependent cannabis use. *69th Annual Scientific Meeting of the College on Problems of Drug Dependence; 2007 June 16-21; Quebec City, Canada*; 2007:21.
15. Levin FR, Mariani J, Brooks DJ, et al. A randomized double-blind, placebo-controlled trial of venlafaxine-extended release for co-occurring cannabis dependence and depressive disorders. *Addiction.* 2013;108(6):1084-1094.
16. Levin FR, McDowell D, Evans SM, et al. Pharmacotherapy for marijuana dependence: a double-blind, placebo-controlled pilot study of divalproex sodium. *Am J Addict.* 2004;13:21-32.
17. Mason BJ, Crean R, Goodell V, et al. A proof-of-concept randomized controlled study of gabapentin: effects on cannabis use, withdrawal and executive function deficits in cannabis-dependent adults. *Neuropsychopharmacology.* 2012;37:1689-1698.
18. Johnston J, Lintzeris N, Allsop DJ, et al. Lithium carbonate in the management of cannabis withdrawal: a randomized placebo-controlled trial in an inpatient setting. *Psychopharmacology.* 2014;231(24):4623-4636.
19. Miranda R Jr, Treloar H, Blanchard A, et al. Topiramate and motivational enhancement therapy for cannabis use among youth: a randomized placebo-controlled pilot study. *Addict Biol.* 2017;22:779-790.
20. Penetar DM, Looby AR, Ryan ET, Maywalt MA, Lukas SE. Bupropion reduces some of the symptoms of marihuana withdrawal in chronic marihuana users: a pilot study. *Subst Abuse.* 2012;6:63-71.
21. McRae-Clark AL, Carter RE, Killeen TK, et al. A placebo-controlled trial of buspirone for the treatment of marijuana dependence. *Drug Alcohol Depend.* 2009;105:132-138.
22. McRae-Clark AL, Baker NL, Gray KM, et al. Buspirone treatment of cannabis dependence: a randomized, placebo-controlled trial. *Drug Alcohol Depend.* 2015;156:29-37.
23. McRae-Clark AL, Carter RE, Killeen TK, Carpenter MJ, White KG, Brady KT. A placebo-controlled trial of atomoxetine in marijuana-dependent individuals with attention deficit hyperactivity disorder. *Am J Addict.* 2010;19(6):481-489.
24. Gray KM, Carpenter MJ, Baker NL, et al. A double-blind randomized controlled trial of N-acetylcysteine in cannabis-dependent adolescents. *Am J Psychiatry.* 2012;169:805-812.
25. Gray KM, Sonne SC, McClure EA, et al. A randomized placebo-controlled trial of N-acetylcysteine for cannabis use disorder in adults. *Drug Alcohol Depend.* 2017;177:249-257.
26. Levin FR, Mariani JJ, Brooks DJ, Pavlicova M, Cheng W, Nunes EV. Dronabinol for the treatment of cannabis dependence: a randomized, double-blind, placebo-controlled trial. *Drug Alcohol Depend.* 2011; 116(1-3):142-150.
27. Levin FR, Mariani JJ, Pavlicova M, et al. Dronabinol and lofexidine for cannabis use disorder: a randomized, double-blind, placebo-controlled trial. *Drug Alcohol Depend.* 2016;159:53-60.
28. Sherman BJ, Baker NL, McRae-Clark AL. Effect of oxytocin pretreatment on cannabis outcomes in a brief motivational intervention. *Psychiatry Res.* 2017;249:318-320.
29. McRae-Clark AL, Kevin M, Gray KM, et al. Varenicline as a treatment for cannabis use disorder: a placebo-controlled pilot trial. *Drug Alcohol Depend.* 2021;229:109111.
30. Freeman TP, Hindocha C, Baio G, et al. Cannabidiol for the treatment of cannabis use disorder: a phase 2a, double-blind, placebo-controlled, randomised, adaptive Bayesian trial. *Lancet Psychiatry.* 2020;7:865-874.
31. Lintzeris N, Bhardwaj A, Mills L, et al. Nabiximols for the treatment of cannabis dependence: a randomized clinical trial. *JAMA Intern Med.* 2019;179(9):1242-1253.
32. Hill KP, Palastro MD, Gruber SA, et al. Nabilone pharmacotherapy for cannabis dependence: A randomized controlled pilot study. *Am J Addictions.* 2017;26:795-801.
33. Bates G, Van Hout MC, JTW T, McVeigh J. Treatments for people who use anabolic androgenic steroids: a scoping review. *Harm Reduct J.* 2019;16(1):1-15.
34. Bertron JL, Seto M, Lindsley CW. DARK classics in chemical neuroscience: phencyclidine (PCP). *ACS Chem Neurosci.* 2018;9:2459-2474.
35. Lodge D, Mercier MS. Ketamine and phencyclidine: the good, the bad and the unexpected. *Br J Pharmacol.* 2015;172:4254-4276.
36. Silva AR, Dinis-Oliveira J. Pharmacokinetics and pharmacodynamics of dextromethorphan: clinical and forensic aspects. *Drug Metab Rev.* 2020;52:258-282.
37. Liu Y, Lina D, Wua B, Zhou W. Ketamine abuse potential and use disorder. *Brain Res Bull.* 2016;126:68-73.
38. Giannini AJ, Malone DA, Giannini MC, Price WA, Loiselle RH. Treatment of depression in chronic cocaine and phencyclidine abuse with desipramine. *J Clin Pharmacol.* 1986;26:211-214.
39. Giannini AJ, Loiselle RH, Graham BH. Behavioral response to buspirone in cocaine and phencyclidine withdrawal. *J Subst Abuse Treat.* 1993;10:523-527.
40. Garg A, Sinha P, Kumar P, Prakash O. Use of naltrexone in ketamine dependence. *Addict Behav.* 2014;39:1215-1216.
41. Miller SC. Treatment of dextromethorphan dependence with naltrexone. *Addict Disord Treat.* 2005;4:145-148.
42. Ledwos N, Andreiev A, Costa T, Chopra N, George TP. Successful treatment of dextromethorphan use disorder with combined naltrexone and gabapentin: a case report. *Am J Drug Alcohol Abuse.* 2023;49(2):266-267. doi:10.1080/00952990.2023.2175323
43. Giannini AJ, Loiselle RH, Giannini MC. Space-based abstinence: alleviation of withdrawal symptoms in combinative cocaine-phencyclidine abuse. *Clin Toxicol.* 1987;25:493-500.

44. Cojanu AI. Inhalant abuse: the wolf in sheep's clothing. *Am J Psychiatry Residents' J.* 2018;13(2):7-9.
45. Konghom S, Verachai V, Srisurapanont M, et al. Treatment for inhalant dependence and abuse. *Cochrane Database Syst Rev.* 2010;12:CD007537.
46. Chou SP, Goldstein RB, Smith SM, et al. The Epidemiology of DSM-5 nicotine use disorder: results from the National Epidemiologic Survey on Alcohol and Related Conditions-III. *J Clin Psychiatry.* 2016;77(10):1404-1412.
47. Han B, Volkow ND, Blanco C, Tipperman D, Einstein EB, Compton WM. Trends in prevalence of cigarette smoking among US adults with major depression or substance use disorders, 2006-2019. *JAMA.* 2022;327(16):1566-1576.
48. Ray LA, Green R, Enders C, et al. Efficacy of combining varenicline and naltrexone for smoking cessation and drinking reduction: a randomized clinical trial. *Am J Psychiatry.* 2021;178:818-828.
49. O'Malley SS, Zweben A, Fucito LM, et al. Effect of varenicline combined with medical management on alcohol use disorder with comorbid cigarette smoking: a randomized clinical trial. *JAMA Psychiatry.* 2018;75:129-138.
50. Haeny AM, Gueorguieva R, Montgomery L, et al. The effect of varenicline on smoking and drinking outcomes among Black and White adults with alcohol use disorder and co-occurring cigarette smoking: a secondary analysis of two clinical trials. *Addict Behav.* 2021;122:106970.
51. King A, Vena A, de Wit H, Grant JE, Cao D. Effect of combination treatment with varenicline and nicotine patch on smoking cessation among smokers who drink heavily: a randomized clinical trial. *JAMA Netw Open.* 2022;5(3):e220951.
52. Parker MA, Stigmon SC, Villanti AC. Higher smoking prevalence among United States adults with co-occurring affective and drug use diagnoses. *Addict Behav.* 2019;99:106112.
53. Parker MA, Weinberger AH, Villanti AC. Quit ratios for cigarette smoking among individuals with opioid misuse and opioid use disorder in the United States. *Drug Alcohol Depend.* 2020;214:108164.
54. John WS, Zhu H, Mannelli P, et al. Prevalence and pattern of opioid misuse and opioid use disorder among primary care patients who use tobacco. *Drug Alcohol Depend.* 2019;194:468-475.
55. Vlad C, Arnsten JH, Nahvi S. Achieving smoking cessation among persons with opioid use disorder. *CNS Drugs.* 2020;34(4):367-387.
56. Witkiewitz K, Vowles KE. Alcohol and opioid use, co-use, and chronic pain in the context of the opioid epidemic: a critical review. *Alcohol Clin Exp Res.* 2018;42(3):478-488.
57. Hall SM, Humfleet GL, Gasper JJ, Delucchi KL, Hersh DF, Guydish JR. Cigarette smoking cessation intervention for buprenorphine treatment patients. *Nicotine Tob Res.* 2018;20(5):628-635.
58. McPherson S, Orr M, Lederhos C, et al. Decreases in smoking during treatment for methamphetamine-use disorders: preliminary evidence. *Behav Pharmacol.* 2018;29:370-374.
59. Winhusen TM, Kropp F, Theobald J, Lewis DF. Achieving smoking abstinence is associated with decreased cocaine use in cocaine-dependent patients receiving smoking-cessation treatment. *Drug Alcohol Depend.* 2014;134:391-395.
60. Winstanley EL, Stover AN, Feinberg J. Concurrent alcohol and opioid use among harm reduction clients. *Addict Behav.* 2020;100:106027. doi:10.1016/j.addbeh.2019.06.016
61. Soyka M. Alcohol use disorders in opioid maintenance therapy: prevalence, clinical correlates and treatment. *Eur Addict Res.* 2015; 21:78-87.
62. Hood LE, Leyrer-Jackson JM, Olive MF. Pharmacotherapeutic management of co-morbid alcohol and opioid use. *Expert Opin Pharmacother.* 2020;21(7):823-839.
63. Roche JD, Pavlicova M, Campbell A, et al. Is extended release naltrexone superior to buprenorphine-naloxone in reducing drinking among outpatients receiving treatment for opioid use disorder? A secondary analysis of the CTN X:BOT trial. *Alcohol Clin Exp Res.* 2021;45:2569-2578.
64. Substance Abuse and Mental Health Services Administration, Center for Behavioral Health Statistics and Quality. *Treatment Episode Data Set (TEDS): 2019. Admissions to and Discharges From Publicly Funded Substance Use Treatment.* SAMHSA; 2021.
65. Specka M, Heilmann M, Lieb B, Scherbaum N. Use of disulfiram for alcohol relapse prevention in patients in opioid maintenance treatment. *Clin Neuropharmacol.* 2014;37(6):161-165.
66. Bickel WK, Marion I, Lowinson JH. The treatment of alcoholic methadone patients: a review. *J Subst Abuse Treat.* 1987;4(1):15-19.
67. Bickel WK, Rizzuto P, Zielony RD, et al. Combined behavioral and pharmacological treatment of alcoholic methadone patients. *J Subst Abuse.* 1988;1(2):161-171.
68. Ellis MS, Kasper ZA, Scroggins S. Shifting Pathways of stimulant use among individuals with opioid use disorder: a retrospective analysis of the last thirty years. *Front Psychiatry.* 2021;12:786056.
69. Leeman RF, Sun Q, Bogart D, et al. Comparisons of cocaine-only, opioid-only, and users of both substances in the national epidemiologic survey on alcohol and related conditions (NESARC). *Subst Use Misuse.* 2016;51(5):553-564.
70. Lopez AM, Dhatt Z, Howe M, et al. Co-use of methamphetamine and opioids among people in treatment in Oregon: a qualitative examination of interrelated structural, community, and individual-level factors. *Int J Drug Policy.* 2021;91:103098.
71. McNeil R, Puri N, Boyd J, Mayer S, Hayashi K, Small W. Understanding concurrent stimulant use among people on methadone: a qualitative study. *Drug Alcohol Rev.* 2020;39(3):209-215.
72. Lin LA, Bohnert ASB, Blow FC, et al. Polysubstance use and association with opioid use disorder treatment in the U.S. Veterans Health Administration. *Addiction.* 2021;116:96-104.
73. Mahoney JJ III, Winstanley EL, Lander LR, et al. High prevalence of substance use in individuals with opioid use disorder. *Addict Behav.* 2021;114:106752.
74. Roux P, Lions C, Michel L, et al. Predictors of non-adherence to methadone maintenance treatment in opioid-dependent individuals: implications for clinicians. *Curr Pharm Des.* 2014;20(25):4097-4105.
75. Proctor SL, Copeland AL, Kopak AM, Hoffmann NG, Herschman PL, Polukhina N. Predictors of patient retention in methadone maintenance treatment. *Psychol Addict Behav.* 2015;29(4):906-917.
76. Roux P, Lions C, Vilotich A, et al. Correlates of cocaine use during methadone treatment: implications for screening and clinical management (ANRS Methaville study). *Harm Reduct J.* 2016;13:12.
77. Frost MC, Lampert H, Tsui JI, Iles-Shih MD, Williams EC. The impact of methamphetamine/ amphetamine use on receipt and outcomes of medications for opioid use disorder: a systematic review. *Addict Sci Clin Pract.* 2021;16:62.
78. Peles E, Kreek MJ, Kellogg S, Adelson M. High methadone dose significantly reduces cocaine use in methadone maintenance treatment (MMT) patients. *J Addict Dis.* 2006;25(1):43-50.
79. Baumeister M, Vogel M, Dursteler-MacFarland KM, et al. Association between methadone dose and concomitant cocaine use in methadone maintenance treatment: a register-based study. *Subst Abuse Treat Prev Policy.* 2014;9:46.
80. Heikman PK, Muhonen LH, Ohanpera IA. Polydrug abuse among opioid maintenance treatment patients is related to inadequate dose of maintenance treatment medicine. *BMC Psychiatry.* 2017;17:245.
81. Montoya ID, Gorelick DA, Preston KL, et al. Randomized trial of buprenorphine for treatment of concurrent opiate and cocaine dependence. *Clin Pharmacol Ther.* 2004;75(1):34-48.
82. Schottenfeld RS, Chawarski MC, Pakes JR, Pantalon MV, Carroll KM, Kosten TR. Methadone versus buprenorphine with contingency management or performance feedback for cocaine and opioid dependence. *Am J Psychiatry.* 2005;162(2):340-349.
83. Xu KY, Mintz CM, Presnall N, Beirut LJ, Grucza RA. Comparative effectiveness associated with buprenorphine and naltrexone in opioid use disorder and co-occurring polysubstance use. *JAMA Netw Open.* 2022;5(5):e2211363.
84. Chan B, Freeman M, Ayers C, et al. A systematic review and meta-analysis of medications for stimulant use disorders in patients with co-occurring opioid use disorders. *Drug Alcohol Depend.* 2020;216:108193.

85. Prince V, Bowling KC. Topiramate in the treatment of cocaine use disorder. *Am J Health Syst Pharm.* 2018;75:e13-e22.
86. DeVito EE, Poling J, Babuscio T, Nich C, Carroll KM, Sofuoglu M. Modafinil does not reduce cocaine use in methadone-maintained individuals. *Drug Alcohol Depend Rep.* 2022;2:100032.
87. Nichols DE. Psychedelics. *Pharmacol Rev.* 2016;68(2):264-355.
88. Akhondzadeh S, Hampa AD. Topiramate prevents ecstasy consumption: a case report. *Fundam Clin Pharmacol.* 2005;19(5):601-602.
89. Bonson KR, Murphy DL. Alterations in responses to LSD in humans associated with chronic administration of tricyclic antidepressants, monoamine oxidase inhibitors or lithium. *Behav Brain Res.* 1996;73:229-233.
90. Becker AM, Klaiber A, Holze F, et al. Ketanserin reverses the acute response to LSD in a randomized, double-blind, placebo-controlled, crossover study in healthy participants. *Int J Neuropsychopharmacol.* 2023;26:97-106.
91. Becker AM, Holze F, Grandinetti T, et al. Acute effects of psilocybin after escitalopram or placebo pretreatment in a randomized, double-blind, placebo-controlled, crossover study in healthy subjects. *Clin Pharmacol Ther.* 2021;111:886-895.
92. Doyle MA, Ling S, Lui LMW, et al. Hallucinogen persisting perceptual disorder: a scoping review covering frequency, risk factors, prevention, and treatment. *Expert Opin Drug Saf.* 2022;21(6):733-743.
93. American Psychiatric Association. *Diagnostic and Statistical Manual of Mental Disorders: 5th ed, Text Revision (DSM-5-TR).* American Psychiatric Association Publishing; 2022.
94. Gorelick DA. Kratom: Substance of abuse or therapeutic plant? *Psychiatric Clin North Am.* 2022;45(3):415-430.
95. Weiss MD, Douglas HE. Treatment of kratom withdrawal and dependence with buprenorphine/naloxone: a case series and systematic literature review. *J Addict Med.* 2021;15:167-172.

CHAPTER

67

Complementary and Integrative Interventions for Substance Use Disorders

Ripal Shah and David Spiegel

CHAPTER OUTLINE

- Introduction
- Botanical remedies with antiaddictive potential
- Plant-based psychedelic compounds
- Transcutaneous electrical acupuncture stimulation as a noninvasive alternative therapy for unhealthy alcohol and substance use
- Opioid withdrawal management with transcutaneous electrical acupuncture stimulation
- Prevention of craving and resumed use of opioids
- Acupuncture and unhealthy alcohol use
- Hypnosis
- Conclusions

INTRODUCTION

Addiction is a complex process with physiological, behavioral, psychological, and social components, resulting in a treatment plan that is often multifaceted. Approaches to substance use disorders can be conceptualized as falling along a spectrum: prevention of the onset of use, prevention of complications and harm reduction, prevention of resumed use (and the craving that leads to resumed use), and treatment of acute symptoms of toxicity. Historically, much medical attention has been directed toward managing the sequelae of acute abstinence (withdrawal), and there exists a burgeoning world of academic and private centers working to advance the therapies that address acute withdrawal. However, resumed use, which may be precipitated by withdrawal and/or craving even after prolonged abstinence, poses the most difficult therapeutic challenge. In view of the ongoing opioid epidemic in the United States and worldwide, the complexity of substance use disorders (SUD), and the logistical concerns associated with effective treatments, it is conceivable that select complementary therapies may have significant impact on reducing the burden of disease of SUD. This chapter reviews plant-based (botanical) medicines, as well as noningested evidence-based therapies as complementary and integrative interventions for the management of SUD.

As is often the case with complementary and integrative techniques, study sample sizes can be quite small in comparison to the robust randomized controlled trials that the scientific community of the Western medicine world is accustomed to. While integrative medicine is gaining more of a following in the United States, large scale rigorous studies in humans are still necessary in order to improve generalizability of these treatments to larger populations to best allow for complementary treatment options to be widely and safely adopted in standard practice. Nonetheless, much of the research outlined in this chapter provides important preliminary insights into the possible eventual impact of these treatments and provides a foundation from which to better understand the potential for future research in this field.

BOTANICAL REMEDIES WITH ANTIADDICTIVE POTENTIAL

Opioids

Herbal remedies, which usually consist of a complex mixture of herbs, have been used in China for thousands of years in an effort to treat human disease. Poppy has been known in China for 12 centuries and for its medicinal use for nine centuries. Opiates, alkaloids derived from poppy, effectively activate the endogenous opioid system in the body. This activation produces many cardiovascular, endocrine, immune, and neuropsychological effects including euphoria, analgesia, and addiction. It has been clear that the effects of opioids are mediated through interaction with specific opioid receptors. Moreover, studies of the binding of various related opioid compounds in the brain indicate the existence of at least three opioid receptor types such as μ, κ, and δ (with multiple subtypes).[1] Since the rewarding effects of opioids are mediated primarily through action at μ-opioid receptors, interference with actions at these receptors presents a rational strategy for developing medications for the treatment of opioid use disorder (OUD).[2,3] Specifically, medications that block activation of μ-opioid receptors (eg, naltrexone) might reduce drug-seeking behavior.[1,3,4]

It is estimated that smoking opium for recreational purposes was practiced throughout China by the middle of the 19th century. The quantity of opium imported into China rose from 5,000 chests in 1820 to 16,000 in 1830, 20,000 in 1838, and 70,000 in 1858. After more than a century of aggressive opium distribution by European powers, with half the Chinese population (nearly that of the U.S. population today) presumed to be physiologically dependent, China finally determined to give up opium, which ultimately led to the "Opium Wars." During this period, Chinese herbal remedies were developed for treating addiction or relieving the withdrawal syndrome.

The Chinese remedies developed during the Opium Wars era were combinations of more than a dozen herbs; thus, a mixture of herbs may well represent a multitargeted approach, perhaps acting on opioid receptors that would have the benefit of improved overall efficacy at reducing or relieving the withdrawal syndrome, combined with reduced toxicity. However, it is necessary to isolate and characterize the bioactive compounds, as well as elucidate the mechanism of actions for further development of safe and complementary natural medications for OUDs. Few remedies from the ancient world have undergone scientific testing involving randomized and controlled experimentation.

NPI-025

Yukunja-tang YGT (also known as NPI-025), otherwise called Liu Jin Zi Tang in China and Rikkunshito in Japan, and used clinically in Hong Kong, is a herbal medicine consisting of five herbs (Qiang Huo, Gou Teng, Chun Xiong, Fu Zi, and Yan Hu Suo). After the cloning of the mouse κ-opioid receptor,[5,6] the μ, δ, and κ receptors of several species were cloned (for reviews, see[7,8]). These cloned opioid receptors provide excellent tools for pharmacological screening of botanical remedies for SUDs. When subjected to bioactivity guided fractionation, NPI-025 showed potent opioid receptor binding activities to μ, κ, D1 and D2 subtypes of dopamine receptors and is now frequently used for OUD treatment in China.[9,10] The alkaloids, such as L-tetrahydropalmatine (L-THP) isolated from one of the components (Yuan Hu), also show potent opioid receptor–binding activities.[11] These studies provide significant scientific basis for better understanding these plant products and important evidence for further development of such natural products.

Yang et al.[9] observed NPI-025 effects among 300 individuals with OUD over a 10-year period from 1975 to 1985 and reported that NPI-025 significantly was associated with reduced withdrawal symptoms (−48%) compared to individuals with OUD without treatment. Follow-up visits of many patients 1 to 3 years after treatment suggested that the use of NPI-025 may have been associated with overcoming craving for opioids.

Cocaine and Methamphetamine

Dopamine Receptors and Pharmacological Actions of L-THP

Despite extensive research for new approaches, there is currently no effective pharmacotherapy for cocaine or methamphetamine addiction.[12-14] *Corydalis yanhusuo* is one of the five Chinese medicinal plants in NPI-025. Chemical fractionation resulted in the isolation and characterization of L-tetrahydropalmatine (L-THP) (**Fig. 67-1**) as one of the bioactive components. Optical resolution or chemical synthesis resulted in pure L-THP, which is the active compound with significant binding activities to D1 and D5 dopamine receptors.

Some effects of L-THP on cocaine and methamphetamine self-administration have been demonstrated,[15,16] suggesting potential, but not yet proven, clinical utility. Cocaine binds differentially to the dopamine, serotonin, and norepinephrine transporter proteins and directly prevents the reuptake of dopamine, serotonin, and norepinephrine into presynaptic neurons[17-19]; this inhibition of reuptake by cocaine subsequently elevates the synaptic concentrations of each of these neurotransmitters, thus potentially reducing craving for cocaine and methamphetamine but also possibly causing reward, reinforcement, and addiction.

Two types of dopamine receptors, D1 class and D2 class, mediate dopamine neurotransmission. The D1 class includes both D1 and D5 receptors, while the D2 class includes D2, D3, and D4 receptors.[20] There is a high-density distribution of D1 and D2 receptors in the striatum, which is relevant to the pharmacology of cocaine. Recent preclinical studies suggest that drugs, like L-THP that are selective for D1 or D2 receptors may reduce some aspects of cocaine self-administration[21,22] or ethanol self-administration.[23] Though both selective D1 and D2 receptor agonists can reduce cocaine self-administration, these agents can also mimic the discriminative stimulus produced by cocaine and stimulate locomotor activity[24-26]; therefore, there is a risk that these drugs may also have potential for unhealthy use and addiction, and would not be useful in practice for cocaine use disorder treatment. However, plant-derived L-THP has both D1 receptor agonist and D2 receptor antagonist actions. Its effects on cocaine and methamphetamine addiction are suggested.[15,16] One mechanism is that L-THP appears to suppress the expression of stimulant-induced conditioned place preference (CPP). L-THP could also block the discrimination behavior for methamphetamine and the reestablishment after its extinction. Interestingly, it has been reported that L-THP suppresses the craving/resumed use for cocaine in addiction. Thus, L-THP may have potential as a novel natural option for inhibiting the craving/resumed use of the psychostimulants addiction including cocaine and methamphetamine.

L-THP and L-isocorypalmine, a demethylated analog of L-THP, are two interesting compounds isolated from *C. yanhusuo*. An in vitro experiment demonstrated that both L-THP

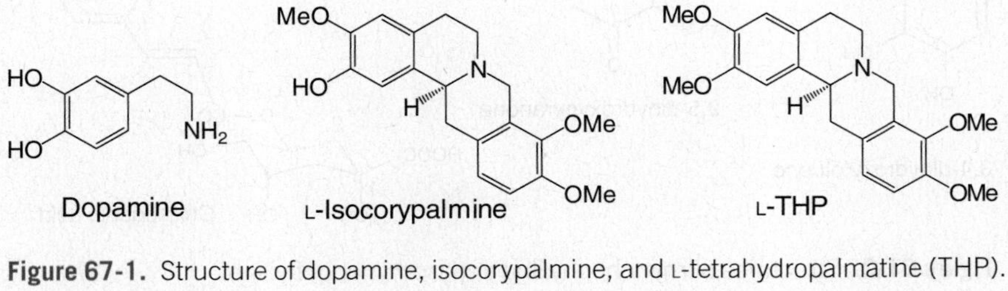

Figure 67-1. Structure of dopamine, isocorypalmine, and L-tetrahydropalmatine (THP).

and L-isocorypalmine have affinity toward D1 and D5 receptors. In the functional assay, L-isocorypalmine is more potent than L-THP as D1 and D5 partial agonists. It is interesting to note that the partial skeleton of both L-THP and isocorypalmine resembles the dopamine molecule (see **Fig. 67-1**) with a different number of methoxy groups attached.

These bioactive compounds derived from fractionation and in vitro screening may provide a better understanding of the mechanism of action of NPI-025 as a whole.

LEK-8829

Though selective D1 receptor agonists or D2 receptor antagonists might modulate cocaine-induced behavior,[27] they also can come with severe side effects such as dysrhythmias, tachycardia, hypertension, seizures, necrotic ischemia, and extremity cyanosis in some rare cases, appropriately preventing them from becoming useful therapeutic agents. Indeed, preliminary clinical studies have not provided promising results.[28,29] Because of the limited success of these selective compounds, interest has turned to medications that may have dual actions. In particular, a medication that stimulates D1 receptors and blocks D2 receptors may have the right profile to become a promising treatment for cocaine or substance use. A recent study of one such compound, an ergoline derivative (LEK-8829) with D1 agonistic and D2 antagonist characteristics, attenuated reinstatement of cocaine seeking induced by cocaine-priming injections and diminished cocaine intake in cocaine self-administration sessions.[30] Thus, it has a better profile than selective D1 receptor agonists alone for inhibiting cocaine self-administration. Furthermore, LEK-8829 reduced cocaine reinstatement behavior and did not induce reinstatement of cocaine use. The combined results suggest that the strategy of using compounds with dual D1 receptor agonist/D2 receptor antagonist properties to treat SUDs may be worth pursuing.

Uncaria rhynchophylla

Uncaria rhynchophylla is an important traditional Chinese medicine used in the treatment of pain, infantile convulsions, headaches, dizziness, hypertension, and rheumatoid arthritis. *U. rhynchophylla* is another ingredient in NPI-025.[9] In order to clarify the mechanism of action, 12 compounds have been isolated by solvent extraction, followed by silica gel fractionation and Toyopearl HW-40, MCI gel column chromatography. Two major alkaloids, rhynchophylline and isorhynchophylline (**Fig. 67-2**), have been identified as potential/unproven antiaddictive compounds with moderate binding activity for dopamine receptors $[^3H]$DIP rMOR and $[^3H]$DIP mDOR. The clinical significance of these findings is not clear.

Alcohol

Reduction of Alcohol Consumption by the Extract of *Pueraria lobata*

Isoflavone compounds naturally occurring in the root of the kudzu plant (*Pueraria lobata*) have been used historically to treat alcohol-related problems.[31] Early work by Overstreet et al.[32,33] showed that the herbal formula NPI-028, which contains *P. lobata*, reduced acute alcohol consumption in two strains of alcohol-preferring rats when administered parenterally (0.25-1 g/kg i.p.) or orally (1 and 1.5 g/kg) without affecting water intake. Daily treatment with 1 g/kg i.p. for 5 days also was effective, as was 0.18 to 0.75 g/kg i.p. in African vervet monkeys. Several studies have systematically explored the ability of three major isoflavones of kudzu root—daidzin, daidzein, and puerarin—to reduce alcohol consumption in animals and humans. The effects of the isoflavones singly on alcohol consumption also have been studied. Keung and Vallee[34] showed that daidzin reduced consumption by 50% in Syrian golden hamsters. Heyman et al.[35] showed a dose-related decrease in

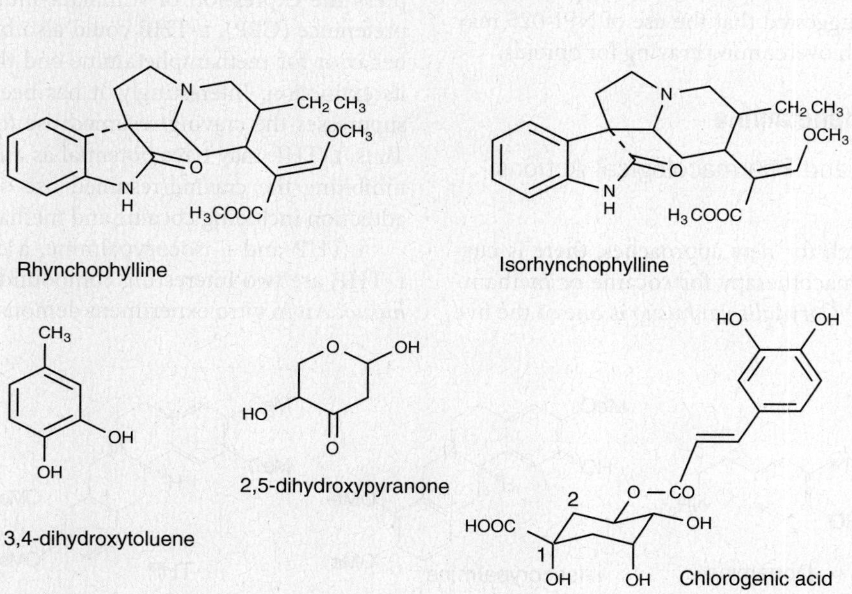

Rhynchophylline

Isorhynchophylline

3,4-dihydroxytoluene

2,5-dihydroxypyranone

Chlorogenic acid

Figure 67-2. Structures of rhynchophylline and isorhynchophylline.

alcohol-reinforced lever pressing by daidzin in rats. Puerarin was effective in two studies: Lin et al.[36,37] showed a 40% reduction of intake in female alcohol-preferring rats given 100 mg/kg/d for 7 days mixed in food and a 65% reduction at 300 mg/kg/d. In the same study, daidzin and daidzein 100 mg/kg/d reduced consumption to 75% and 50%. Benlhabib et al.[38] showed a 50% suppression of intake in rats by puerarin 50 mg/kg.

In humans, Lukas et al.[39] studied the effects of a kudzu root extract that contained 25% isoflavones (19% puerarin, 4% daidzin, 2% daidzein) in individuals who drink alcohol heavily. Three grams of the extract (750 mg total isoflavones) was administered for one week before a 1.5-hour afternoon drinking session in 21 people. In comparison to drinking following the placebo week, there was a significant reduction in beer consumption in addition to several significant changes in drinking topography, including an increase in the number of sips taken to finish a beer and an increase in the latency to open subsequent beers. In a second study, where the same extract was administered for four weeks in an outpatient setting, Lukas et al.[39] found a significant reduction in intake during weeks two through four, though the study just had 20 participants. Building on these encouraging results, Penetar et al. repeated the in-laboratory afternoon drinking session paradigm in 10 adults through a double-blind placebo-controlled cross-sectional study using the single isoflavone puerarin, and found that participants consumed on average 3.5 (±0.6) beers after placebo and 2.4 (±0.4) after puerarin.[40] None of the puerarin subjects (N = 10) drank five or six beers, while three of the same 10 subjects given placebo drank five, and one drank all six.[41] These studies demonstrate that puerarin may reduce alcohol consumption in humans. However, the mechanism of action of puerarin remains to be elucidated, and any potential utility for treatment of alcohol use disorder outside of laboratory settings remain to be confirmed.

PLANT-BASED PSYCHEDELIC COMPOUNDS

Perhaps the most controversial botanicals being studied for the treatment of substance use disorders are psychedelics (hallucinogens and dissociatives). While some psychedelic compounds are made synthetically (MDMA, psilocin), many still fall under the domain of plant-based therapies. Nonetheless, use of select plant-based psychedelic compounds have been shown to be associated with lower rates of substance use disorders.[42]

Psilocybin, a psychoactive compound found in "magic" mushrooms (hence the slang term "shrooms"), turns into psilocin upon ingestion and has been studied in abstinence from alcohol use and nicotine use.[43] Because of psilocin's agonism of the serotonin 2A receptor, there are potentially many therapeutic benefits of this compound in SUDs.[44]

In a double-blind randomized clinical trial (N = 93), the percentage of heavy drinking days for patients with alcohol use disorder (AUDs) during 32 weeks of follow-up was much lower in those receiving two sessions of psilocybin-assisted treatment compared to those receiving two sessions with an active placebo (diphenhydramine), which only added to recent and historical evidence suggesting high success rates when using classic psychedelics in addition to psychotherapy in the treatment of SUDs.[45]

A study on the use of psilocybin in conjunction with CBT for stopping smoking showed much higher rates of abstinence after 6 months, than those who received CBT alone.[46] Please refer to **Chapter 18** for more information on psilocybin.

MDMA-like compounds have been found in plants such as sassafras (in the form of MDA). Given promising studies on synthetic MDMA and alcohol use disorder, there is a hypothesis that plant based forms of this compound may also decrease alcohol use. Please refer to **Chapter 18** for more information on MDMA.

Ibogaine, a naturally occurring psychoactive substance extracted from an African plant, has been studied for opiate use disorder and withdrawal.

Ketamine, a synthetic compound, has been studied for alcohol and opiate use disorder. Given its complex receptor affinity profile, it is unlikely that a combination of plants will work similarly to ketamine. Please refer to **Chapter 19** for more information on ketamine.

Notably, the research on these compounds for the treatment of SUDs is still ongoing, and there is considerably more left to learn about how to integrate these approaches into treatment safely and effectively. Currently, there are no FDA approved hallucinogens for the treatments of SUDs.

TRANSCUTANEOUS ELECTRICAL ACUPUNCTURE STIMULATION AS A NONINVASIVE ALTERNATIVE THERAPY FOR UNHEALTHY ALCOHOL AND SUBSTANCE USE

In a serendipitous observation in 1972, Dr H. L. Wen in Hong Kong noted that electroacupuncture relieved a patient's withdrawal from opium.[47] Dr Wen and Dr Cheung at the Kwong Wah Hospital[47] subsequently reported that, in a study of 40 individuals addicted to heroin and/or opium, acupuncture combined with electrical stimulation was effective in relieving withdrawal. This method was later adopted in many clinical settings in Western countries, including the Lincoln Hospital in New York. However, the body acupuncture points originally used by Wen and Cheung on the arm and hand were gradually omitted, with only auricular acupuncture being used,[48] and electrical stimulation also was omitted, leaving only needles staying in situ. Whether these two omissions will affect therapeutic efficacy deserves further investigation.

The discovery of morphine-like substances (endorphins) in the mammalian brain[49] had a great impact on acupuncture research. It was soon made clear that acupuncture-induced analgesia (manual needling) can be blocked by the narcotic antagonist naloxone, suggesting the involvement of endogenous opioid substances.[50] In animal experiments, manual acupuncture or acupuncture combined with electrical stimulation (electroacupuncture, or EA) was shown to accelerate the production and release of endorphins that can interact with different kinds of opioid receptors to ease pain.[51] It was further clarified that endorphins are, in fact, a group of neuropeptides possessing different characteristics. Among these neuropeptides, β-endorphin and enkephalin are primarily agonists at μ- and δ-opioid receptors, whereas dynorphin is an agonist at κ receptors.[52] Interestingly, electrical stimulation of different frequencies can induce the release of different kinds of endorphins. For example, low-frequency (2-4 Hz) EA accelerates the release of enkephalins to interact with μ and δ receptors, whereas high-frequency (100 Hz) EA accelerates the release of dynorphin to interact with κ receptors.[53] These findings strengthen the scientific basis of this ancient healing art and point the way to its use in areas beyond pain control.

It is natural to hypothesize that if acupuncture can release endogenous opioids in the brain to ease pain, it might relieve withdrawal symptoms. In fact, the first observation made by Wen in 1972 was that in attempting to use acupuncture for reducing surgical pain, he incidentally found that it ameliorated the opioid withdrawal syndrome. This hypothesis was tested in morphine-addicted rats. Withdrawal signs were significantly reduced by high-frequency (100 Hz) EA administered on the hind limb acupoints St 36 and Sp 6.[54] This effect was much greater than that induced by low-frequency (2 Hz) stimulation. On the basis of these results, EA was applied to individuals with heroin use disorder and obtained very promising results. However, it was inconvenient for patients to go to the clinic for treatment several times a day. As a result, they missed sessions, which affects the therapeutic outcome. One possible solution was to have patients treat themselves by using acupoint stimulation without a needle but still under the control of a physician. To overcome this problem, a team in China led by Ji-Sheng Han developed a constant current electrical stimulator: Han's Acupoint Nerve Stimulator (HANS).

Experiments in the rat using HANS showed that electrical stimulation applied at the surface of the skin over acupoints can produce an analgesic effect similar to that produced by EA.[55] Satisfactory results were obtained using this transcutaneous electrical acupoint stimulation (TEAS) by HANS for the treatment of heroin withdrawal syndrome in humans.[56] In summary, the results observed in humans were in line with the findings obtained in rats: low-frequency HANS is more effective than high-frequency HANS in suppressing the morphine-induced CPP. When a control group was set up using the TEAS equipment and skin electrodes placed on the same acupoints but with the output leads of the stimulator disconnected,[56] the method was shown to suppress CPP, an animal model of craving for morphine in rats.[57] Subsequent human studies revealed that this form of stimulation could indeed suppress craving in patients with opioid use disorders.

According to another study by Da Ma et al.,[58] the activation of dynorphin gene expression in the central nervous system of rats through electroacupuncture at 100 Hz can result in improved production and release of dynorphin in the spinal cord, leading to a significant reduction in withdrawal syndrome in rats with morphine dependence. On the other hand, electroacupuncture at 2 Hz can activate the gene expression of enkephalin and beta endorphin in the brain of rats, the increase of which leads to decreases in the CPP induced by morphine. When a combination of 2 Hz and 100 Hz electroacupuncture is applied (alternating every three seconds), it not only inhibits the withdrawal syndrome in rats with morphine dependence, but also inhibits the CPP induced by morphine. These findings have also been preliminarily verified in humans.

OPIOID WITHDRAWAL MANAGEMENT WITH TRANSCUTANEOUS ELECTRICAL ACUPUNCTURE STIMULATION

Animal Studies

Systematic studies have revealed that the mechanism of acupuncture analgesia is attributed mainly to the increased release of endogenous opioid peptides in the central nervous system (CNS).[51] A rational extrapolation would be that the activation of the endogenous opioid system by acupuncture should ease opioid withdrawal symptoms.

Transauricular electrostimulation was reported to suppress the naloxone-induced morphine withdrawal syndrome in mice[59] and rats.[60] Auriacombe et al.[61] demonstrated that transcutaneous electro nerve stimulation with an intermittent high-frequency current effectively attenuated signs in the rat after abrupt cessation of morphine; the mechanism remains obscure. Based on the findings that low-frequency EA (2 Hz) accelerated the release of β-endorphin and enkephalin in the CNS, whereas high-frequency EA (100 Hz) accelerated the release of dynorphin[53,62] in the spinal cord, the effect of EA was tested in naloxone-precipitated morphine withdrawal in the rat. Because the effect of 2 Hz EA is to accelerate the release of the morphine-like opioid peptides enkephalin and endorphin, it was predicted that 2 Hz would be more effective than 100 Hz in replacing morphine and ameliorating the abstinence syndrome. However, 2 Hz was only marginally effective in reducing two of five withdrawal signs, whereas 100 Hz suppressed all five signs.[54]

Human Studies

To observe the effect of TEAS on the withdrawal syndrome in patients with opioid use disorders, the method was applied for 30 minutes once a day for 10 days in an addiction treatment center.[56] In addition to a standard questionnaire, two objective parameters were measured—heart rate and body weight.

Single Treatment

To observe the immediate effect on heart rate, the two pairs of output leads were placed on four acupoints in the upper extremities: one pair at *Hegu* (LI4) on the dorsum of the hand

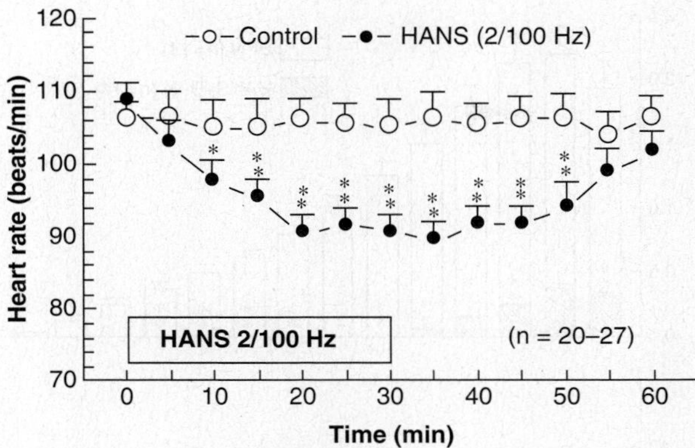

Figure 67-3. Effects of 2/100 Hz electric stimulation (HANS) on the heart rate of individuals with opioid use disorder during episodes of withdrawal. *,** represent $p < 0.05$ and $p < 0.01$, respectively, compared with control groups. (Reprinted from Han JS, Trachtenberg AI, Lowinson JH. Acupuncture. In: Lowinson JH, Ruiz P, Millman RB, Langrod JG, eds. *Substance Abuse: A Comprehensive Textbook.* Lippincott Williams & Wilkins; 2004: 743-782, with permission.)

and on the palmar aspect of the hand opposite to LI4 *Laogon* (P-8), to complete the circuit, and the other pair at *Neiguan* (PC6) on the palmar side of the forearm two inches above the palmar groove between the two tendons and *Waiguan* (TE5) on the opposite side of PC6. A dense-and-disperse (DD) mode of stimulation was administered, with 2 Hz alternating automatically with 100 Hz, each lasting 3 seconds. This mode was shown to release four of the opioid peptides in the CNS,[53] thus producing maximal therapeutic effect. The control group received the same placement of electrodes, which were disconnected from the circuitry. The average heart rate of the abstinent individuals was 109 beats per minute before treatment. DD stimulation for 30 minutes reduced the heart rate significantly, as shown in **Figure 67-3**. Reduction occurred within the first 5 to 10 minutes, continued for 20 minutes, and plateaued at 90 per minute in the last 10 minutes. The aftereffect remained for 20 minutes, after which the heart rate began to return to the original level.[63]

Multiple Treatments

To observe the cumulative effect of multiple daily treatments with TEAS, 117 individuals with opioid use disorder were divided randomly into four groups. Three groups received TEAS of 2 Hz (constant frequency), 100 Hz (constant frequency), or 2/100 Hz (2 Hz alternating with 100 Hz, DD mode). The control group received mock stimulation, where the skin electrodes were placed on the points and connected to the stimulator with blinking signals but with the electric circuitry disconnected. The treatment was applied for 30 minutes a day over 10 consecutive days. Heart rate was measured with an electrocardiogram before and immediately after the TEAS stimulation. **Figure 67-4** shows the results. In the 2-Hz group, for example, on the first day of observation, the heart rate averaged 110, which dropped to 90 immediately after the TEAS treatment ($p < 0.01$). On the second day, the heart rate averaged 102 and then fell to 91 after TEAS ($p < 0.01$). This trend continued for days 3 and 4. On day 5, there was no significant difference before and after the treatment (91 versus 89), suggesting that the rate had returned to "normal."[56] In the three TEAS groups, 100 Hz produced a slightly better result than 2 Hz. In the 2/100 Hz group, the after-TEAS rate reached an even lower level (72 beats). Also, the 2/100 Hz returned to "normal" in day 4, which was 1 day earlier than the fixed frequency groups (day 5). In the control group ($N = 30$) receiving mock TEAS, the rate did not come down to 100 until the 8th day of treatment. These results suggest that repeated daily EA treatment is effective in reducing tachycardia in individuals with opioid use disorder, with an order of DD >100 Hz >2 Hz (see **Fig. 67-3**).

Body weight was also affected. The age of the patients ranged from 17 to 35, and their average weight was only 49 to 51 kg. In the control group receiving mock TEAS, weight declined by 1 kg at the end of the first week, probably owing to the presence of withdrawal distress. In the TEAS groups, weight had increased significantly after four days of treatment

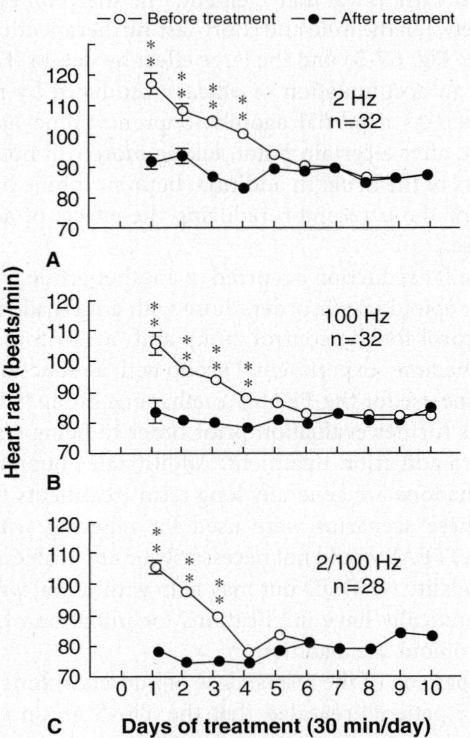

Figure 67-4. Changes of heart rate before and after treatment by TEAS administered every day: A normalization of the heart rate was obtained by day 4 **(C)** or day 5 **(A and B)**. ** $p < 0.01$ compared with after treatment (ANOVA). (Reprinted from Han JS, Trachtenberg AI, Lowinson JH. Acupuncture. In: Lowinson JH, Ruiz P, Millman RB, Langrod JG, eds. *Substance Abuse: A Comprehensive Textbook.* Lippincott Williams & Wilkins; 2004:743-782, with permission.)

and continued to increase thereafter. By day 10, the TEAS groups weighed 5 kg more than the control group. This 10% increase was apparently due to reduced withdrawal symptoms and increased food and water intake. Though the DD mode was significantly better than the fixed frequency mode in reducing tachycardia, weight change did not differ among the three TEAS groups, suggesting that the mechanisms modulating heart rate and body weight may not be identical.[56]

In clinical practice, opioid withdrawal symptoms could be reduced but not abolished by the TEAS treatment, especially in those cases with a history of heroin use for more than five years. To obtain a quantitative estimate of the efficacy of TEAS[64] (a) TEAS was applied on the acupoints *Hegu/Laogong, Neiguan/Waiguan*, and *Xingjian/Sanyinjiao*. Buprenorphine (BPN, i.m.) was used as a supplement to TEAS when the patient experienced a specified degree of withdrawal distress and was given immediately upon request. The purpose of this arrangement was to maintain a comfortable withdrawal management procedure without any withdrawal syndrome. In this study, 28 individuals with opioid use disorder were randomly divided into BPN only and TEAS + BPN groups. **Figure 67-5A** shows the results. The group receiving TEAS required only 8% of the BPN required by the group not receiving TEAS. This can be taken as a quantitative estimate of the effect of TEAS for opioid withdrawal management. The sharp difference observed between the mild and short-lasting therapeutic effect on day 1 (see **Fig. 67-3**) and the large effect by day 14 (**Fig. 67-5**) suggests an accumulation of efficacy produced by repetitive treatments. As a partial agonist, buprenorphine has a ceiling effect; after a certain point, taking more will not increase the effects of the drug. In addition, buprenorphine has a high affinity for the μ receptor, reducing the effects of additional opioid use.

A similar reduction occurred in another group of individuals with opioid use disorder, those with a methadone reduction protocol for the control group and "a TEAS (2/100 Hz) plus methadone" experimental group with a reduction of 75% methadone use for the TEAS + methadone group.[65] This finding needs further evaluation prior order to being considered a standard addiction treatment. Additionally, buprenorphine and methadone are generally long term treatments for OUD, but in these scenarios were used for relieving withdrawal. Therefore, TEAS would not necessarily be applicable as a treatment modality for OUD but may help with initial withdrawal and theoretically have implications for initiation of medications for opioid use disorder.

Comparison of the rescue dose of buprenorphine requested by the patients revealed that the TEAS group requested much less buprenorphine than that in the control group. This is in line with previous research showing that TEAS can reduce the dose of methadone and increase the retention time of methadone maintenance. Since the premature departure rate of patients in methadone maintenance programs was reported to be as high as 63% in China, if TEAS can prolong the retention of methadone maintenance, it may well contribute to the prevention of resumed use of heroin. This is also supported

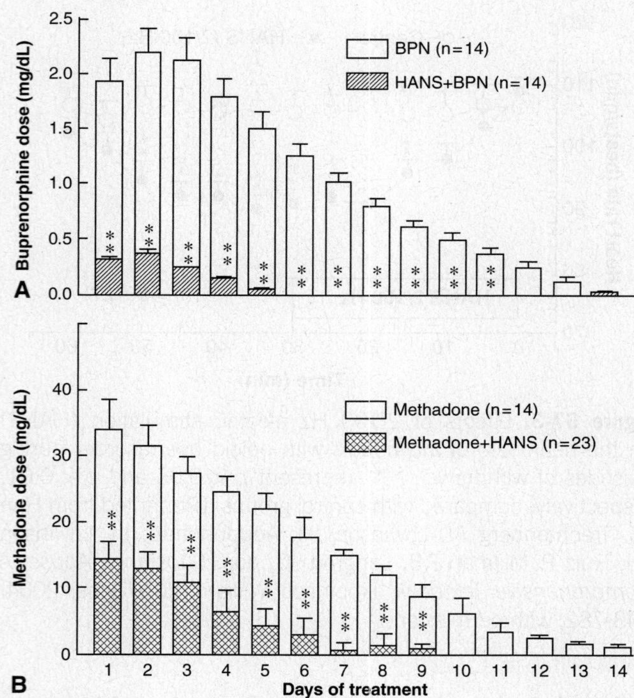

Figure 67-5. Influence of 2/100 Hz electric simulation (HANS) on the requirement of BPN **(A)** or methadone **(A, B)** for heroin withdrawal management. ** $p < 0.01$ compared with the corresponding control group. (Reprinted from Han JS, Trachtenberg AI, Lowinson JH. Acupuncture. In: Lowinson JH, Ruiz P, Millman RB, Langrod JG, eds. *Substance Abuse: A Comprehensive Textbook*. Lippincott Williams & Wilkins; 2004:743-782, with permission.)

by a paper by Meade et al., showing that people with OUD treated with TEAS are less likely to use illicit substances after their discharge from the hospital and reported to have greater improvements in pain interference and physical health.[66,67]

PREVENTION OF CRAVING AND RESUMED USE OF OPIOIDS

SUD is a chronic and recurrent condition. Resumed use after prolonged substance-free periods is common amongst people with SUD who may experience ongoing cravings and protracted withdrawal. Recently, electrical acupuncture has been shown to reduce craving and postpone or prevent resumed use.[57]

Animal Studies

Several animal procedures have been proposed to model craving.[67] Conditioned Place Preference (CPP) has been frequently used.[68] The drug (unconditioned stimulus) is given in one chamber of a two- or three-chamber apparatus, thereby becoming associated with the environmental stimuli unique to that chamber (color, floor texture, etc.). After repeated

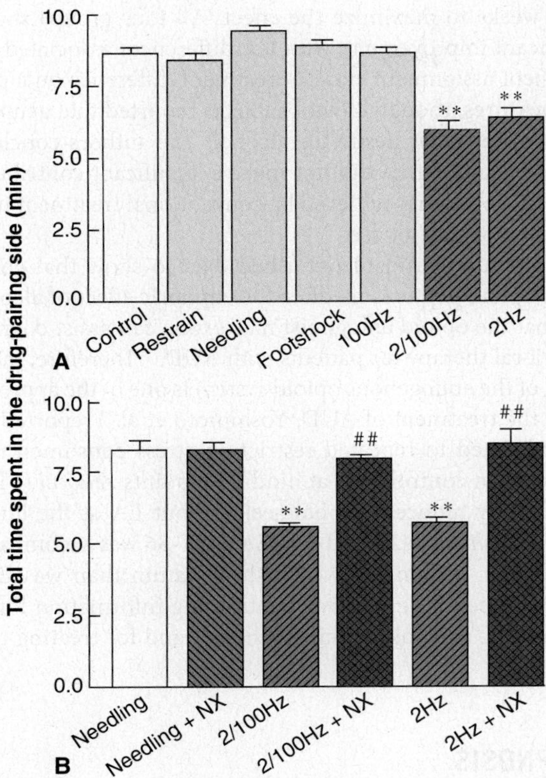

Figure 67-6. A. Effects of electroacupuncture on 4 mg/kg morphine-induced CPP (N = 11-12). ** $p < 0.01$, compared with four control groups as well as the group treated with 100-Hz stimulation. **B.** Naloxone blockade of the inhibitory effect of electroacupuncture on morphine-induced CPP (n = 9-0). ** $p < 0.01$, compared with the needling control group. ## $p < 0.01$, compared with their corresponding naloxone-treated group. (Reprinted from Han JS, Trachtenberg AI, Lowinson JH. Acupuncture. In: Lowinson JH, Ruiz P, Millman RB, Langrod JG, eds. *Substance Abuse: A Comprehensive Textbook*. Lippincott Williams & Wilkins; 2004:743-782, with permission.)

pairings, the rat will spend more time in the chamber associated with drug. The ratio between the times spent in drug-associated and vehicle-associated areas is assumed to reflect the degree of craving. CPP has been regarded as a relatively pure measure of psychic dependence in that the preference for the drug-associated chamber can be demonstrated when the rat is in the undrugged condition and free of withdrawal symptoms. Experiments were done to determine whether acupuncture could suppress the expression of CPP.

Wang et al.[57] were among the first to explore the effect of EA on morphine CPP in the rat. They found that 2 Hz and 2/100 Hz significantly suppressed CPP but that 100 Hz did not (**Fig. 67-6**A). Since the effect of EA can be reversed by a dose of the opioid receptor antagonist naloxone (**Fig. 67-6**B) that is sufficient to block μ and δ but not κ receptors, it was concluded that the effect of EA is mediated by endogenously released μ- and δ-opioid agonists, most likely endorphins and enkephalins, to ease craving for exogenous opioid (in this case, morphine). Another issue deserving attention is that the effect of EA was demonstrable 12 hours after application. Acupuncture-induced analgesia usually disappears within one hour. Thus, EA might sensitize endogenous opioid circuits to produce a continuous release of opioid peptides, resulting in a long-lasting effect.

In the everyday life of those with SUD, craving and resumed use can be triggered by stress or by a very small dose of opioid. This phenomenon can be reproduced in the rat CPP model. Wang et al.[57] reported that morphine-induced CPP disappeared after a 9-day extinction period and was reinstated by foot shock stress or by a small dose of morphine or amphetamine. Reinstated CPP could be reversed by 2 Hz or 2/100 Hz EA, an effect easily reversed by naloxone.[69] However, the mechanisms of EA suppression of morphine CPP may involve different neural pathways.

Human Study of Cravings

To obtain a quantitative estimate of suppression of craving in response to acupuncture or related techniques, a visual analogue scale (VAS) in individuals with OUD at least 1 month after withdrawal management was used. The scale for the VAS is 100 mm long: 0 is equal to no craving and 100 is equal to the most severe craving imaginable. One hundred seventeen subjects were assigned randomly into four groups. Three groups received TEAS at 2 Hz, 100 Hz, or 2/100 Hz. Self-adhesive skin electrodes were placed on four acupoints: *Hegu* and *Laogong* (palmar side of the *Hegu* point) on the left (or right) hand to complete the circuit and *Neiguan* and *Weiguan* on the right (or left) arm to complete the circuit. The intensity was increased from threshold on the first day to two or three times threshold on the following days. The mock TEAS control group was processed like the other groups except that the intensity was minimal (at threshold stimulation for 3 minutes, followed by 1 mA thereafter). The results, shown in **Figure 67-7**, indicate a slow decline of the VAS in the mock TEAS group and a parallel slow

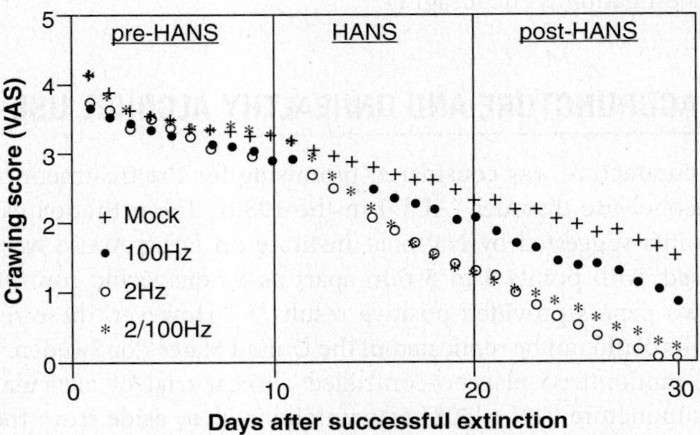

Figure 67-7. Effects of HANS on craving scores in individuals with opioid use disorder (n = 29-30 in each group). HANS of 2 Hz and 2/100 Hz accelerated the decay of craving scores during the 10-day treatment period. (Reprinted from Han JS, Trachtenberg AI, Lowinson JH. Acupuncture. In: Lowinson JH, Ruiz P, Millman RB, Langrod JG, eds. *Substance Abuse: A Comprehensive Textbook*. Lippincott Williams & Wilkins; 2004:743-782, with permission.)

decline in 100 Hz group, in contrast with a dramatic decline in the 2 Hz and 2/100 Hz groups. In summary, the results in humans coincided with the results in rats—that low frequency is more effective than high frequency in reducing craving for opioids.[69]

On the basis of the experimental effects of TEAS described earlier, the subjects were encouraged to take with them a portable TEAS unit when they were discharged from the withdrawal management center. The purpose was to ameliorate the protracted withdrawal syndrome and to suppress the craving induced by environmental cues. At least one 30-minute session before going to bed was recommended to facilitate sleep, as was use whenever they encountered a cue. It was found that the anticraving effect usually appears within 20 minutes. As per Zhong et al., although the use of single session of EA or HANS is effective in reducing opiate withdrawal, it is recommended for use three times a day in the first 5 days, two times a day in the next five days and at least once a day for the rest of the time for a total of 2 weeks. The session applied immediately before sleep is critical since this could facilitate a good sleep.[70]

HANS treatment was offered at a rehabilitation center of Peking University for free. As an alternative, people could buy a unit of the device at an affordable cost and apply HANS at home under the staff's continuing supervision. A follow-up study was conducted on a group of 56 subjects who used HANS at home. Using monthly urine test as an outcome criterion, the recurrence rates at 3, 6, 9, and 12 months were 50.0%, 71.4%, 80.4%, and 83.9%, respectively. Those showing negative urine tests for 12 or 24 consecutive months were given a naloxone test (0.4 mg subcutaneously twice at a 15-minute interval) to further confirm their heroin-free status. Compared with the 94% recurrence rate at 6 months and more than 98% recurrence rate at 1 year in the majority of the reports on heroin addiction (without methadone maintenance), an 83.9% recurrence rate (16.1% success rate) at 1 year in the present investigation is encouraging.[71]

ACUPUNCTURE AND UNHEALTHY ALCOHOL USE

Acupuncture was considered promising for the treatment of alcohol use disorder (AUD) in the 1980s. The orthodox ear points suggested by National Institute on Drug Abuse were used, with points 3 to 5 mm apart as a nonspecific control. Two papers provided positive results.[72,73] However, these results could not be replicated in the United States[74] or Sweden.[75] A randomized placebo-controlled clinical trial of auricular acupuncture[76] (N = 503) was unique in that, aside from the "specific" ear acupuncture group, "nonspecific" ear acupuncture group, and conventional treatment group, there was a symptom-based acupuncture group for which the acupuncturists were not constrained to the four ear points stipulated for the other acupuncture groups, and the point prescription could be changed from day to day according to the patients' discomfort. Six treatments per week were given for as long as three weeks to maximize the effect. All four groups showed significant improvement, with few differences associated with treatment assignment and no treatment difference on alcohol use measures, though 49% of subjects reported that acupuncture reduced their desire for alcohol. The authors concluded that ear acupuncture did not make a significant contribution over and above that achieved by conventional treatment in the reduction of alcohol use.

There are abundant published data to show that endogenous opioid peptides mediate the euphoric effect of alcohol[77] and that the opioid antagonist naltrexone can assist cognitive behavioral therapy for patients with AUD.[78] Therefore, modulation of the endogenous opioid system is one of the approaches for the treatment of AUD. Yoshimoto et al.[79] reported that rats subjected to repeated restriction stress consumed more alcohol than controls. EA at hind limb points *Zusanli* (ST-36) significantly reduced alcohol seeking, but EA at the lumbar point *Shenshu* (BL-23) did not. EA at ST-36 was accompanied by a higher dopamine level in the striatum than was EA at BL-23. These findings provide intriguing information for understanding alcohol-drinking behavior and for treating those with AUD.

HYPNOSIS

Hypnosis is a complementary approach that has been proven effective for numerous indications including stopping nicotine use. It has been widely promoted as a method for aiding stopping smoking by improving the ability to focus on a treatment program by increasing concentration, for example in order to weaken underlying impulses or desire to smoke, or to strengthen the motivation to stop.[80] Many different clinical hypnosis techniques have been employed, but the most frequently used approaches are variants of the "one session, three point" method developed by Spiegel.[81] This method attempts to modify patients' perceptions of smoking by using the potential of hypnosis to induce deep concentration while disrupting customary assumptions about the need to smoke.[82] During the session the person who smokes is instructed that: (1) for my body, smoking is a poison, (2) I need my body to live, and (3) I owe my body respect and protection.[83] This approach provides immediate positive reinforcement by helping people who smoke to focus on what they are for rather than what they are against. It also includes training in self-hypnosis, which some posit may be as effective as undergoing hypnosis by a therapist.[84] Self-hypnosis can be used at will by the patient whenever they have an urge to smoke. Also, compliance may be higher and costs lower because only one session with a trained clinician is required. A single session of training in self-hypnosis for stopping smoking results in 23% of participants maintaining 2 years of abstinence from nicotine, and this effect may even be minimized since all nonresponders were counted as having resumed smoking.[85] In other studies, this method is associated with 6-month abstinence rates of between 20% and 35%.[81] Barnes et al. examined 14 studies on the use of hypnosis for stopping smoking, and the results of six studies (totaling 957 people), showed no statistically significant difference supporting the idea that hypnosis helped people quit smoking more than attention-matched behavioral interventions, such as psychotherapy, when delivered over the same amount of time.[86] Therefore hypnosis may be equally effective to behavioral interventions. However, one small study of 40 participants did show a statistically significant benefit of hypnosis compared to no intervention.[86] When tested as an adjunctive treatment, five studies led to a pooled result of a statistically significant benefit of hypnosis.[86]

Many older studies on hypnosis for stopping smoking show great variability in quit rates (4%-88%) 6 months after treatment.[83] Interpretation of these studies is complicated by the many different hypnosis regimens used and the variation in number and frequency of treatments.[87] Since hypnosis is often used as an aid to stopping smoking, larger trials may further establish its benefits, particularly if approaches to hypnosis can be standardized and clearly defined. Studies that highlight comparisons of hypnosis with no or minimal treatment, as well as comparisons with active interventions, can be particularly helpful, ideally matching for therapist contact time.[82]

CONCLUSIONS

In view of the current opioid epidemic in the United States and the lack of effective remediation, there is an urgent need to develop safe, cost-effective, accessible, and efficacious additional therapies for treating SUDs. Traditional Chinese medicines have been used in the treatment of human disease for more than 2,000 years. It is estimated that roughly one-half of current pharmaceuticals originally were procured from plants.[88] Examples include foxglove leaf (digitalis), belladonna tops (atropine), poppy herb (morphine), white willow tree bark (salicin), and cinchona bark (quinine). Modern drugs developed from plant products include warfarin from coumarin anticoagulants found in sweet clover silage, ergotamine from ergot alkaloids of a fungus that infects rye grass, antineoplastic vincristine from the vinca alkaloid fractions of the rosy periwinkle, the anticancer drug paclitaxel from pacific yew tree, and antimalarial artemisinin from Qingdao.[89] It is therefore reasonable that medication development for unhealthy drug and alcohol use could seek active isolates from traditional herbal remedies.

That said, many believe that a combination of medicinal plants with synergistic effects is a better approach. Though it is difficult to prove the synergism of multicomponent herbal remedies, the concept of a multitargeted approach is familiar to Western medicine as it is the basis of chemotherapy for most cancers and seen in highly active retroviral therapy for HIV. It is also conceivable that a multitargeted approach would improve the overall outcomes in SUD cases and reduce effects of unwanted toxicity. Human diseases, including SUDs, are highly complex and the efficacy of a single chemical entity targeting one disease site or receptor is often limited. On the other hand, Chung et al.[90] reported multicomponent natural products with good in vitro binding activities may have been used successfully to treat psychosis.

Although acupuncture and related acupoint therapies are most commonly recognized for analgesic effect, their medical applications extend beyond pain treatment. Though alternative therapies may provide new treatments for existing drug treatments, rigorous studies to evaluate both the risks and the benefits of such treatments are needed. Biological investigations that couple in vitro and in vivo pharmacological models to characterize the mechanism of action and the possibility of synergistic effects of components are crucial to further the development of successful complementary and alternative therapies for SUDs and related conditions.

ACKNOWLEDGEMENTS

The authors would like to thank David Y. W. Lee, for his tremendous contributions to this chapter in the prior editions of the book, which provided the frame for this updated chapter.

REFERENCES

1. Shippenberg TS, Chefer VI, Zapata A, Heidbreder CA. Modulation of the behavioral and neurochemical effects of psychostimulants by kappa-opioid receptor systems. *Ann N Y Acad Sci.* 2001;937:50-73.
2. Kreek MJ. Cocaine, dopamine and the endogenous opioid system. *J Addict Dis.* 1996;15(4):73-96.
3. Kreek MJ, LaForge KS, Butelman E. Pharmacotherapy of addictions. *Nat Rev Drug Discov.* 2002;1(9):710-726.
4. Schenk S, Partridge B, Shippenberg TS. U69593, a kappa-opioid agonist, decreases cocaine self-administration and decreases cocaine-produced drug-seeking. *Psychopharmacology (Berl).* 1999;144(4):339-346.
5. Kieffer BL, Befort K, Gavériaux-Ruff C, Hirth CG. The delta-opioid receptor: isolation of a cDNA by expression cloning and pharmacological characterization. *Proc Natl Acad Sci U S A.* 1992;89(24):12048-12052.
6. Evans CJ, Keith DE Jr, Morrison H, Magendzo K, Edwards RH. Cloning of a delta opioid receptor by functional expression. *Science.* 1992;258(5090):1952-1955.
7. Kieffer BL. Recent advances in molecular recognition and signal transduction of active peptides: receptors for opioid peptides. *Cell Mol Neurobiol.* 1995;15(6):615-635.
8. Knapp RJ, Malatynska E, Collins N, et al. Molecular biology and pharmacology of cloned opioid receptors. *FASEB J.* 1995;9(7):516-525.
9. Yang MMP, Yeun RCF, Kwok JSL. Effect of certain Chinese herbs on drug addiction. In: Chang HM, Yeung HW, Tso W-W, Koo A, eds. *Advances in Chinese Medicinal Materials Research.* World Scientific Publishing; 1985:147-158.
10. Yang MMP, Yuen RCF, Kok SH. Experimental studies on the effects of certain Chinese herbs on morphine withdrawal syndrome in rats. *J Am Coll Trad Chin Med.* 1983;2:3-24.
11. Ma Z, Xu W, Liu-Chen LY, Lee DYW. Novel coumarin glycoside and phenethyl vanillate from *Notopterygium forbesii* and their binding affinities for opioid and dopamine receptors. *Bioorg Med Chem.* 2008;16:3231-3236.
12. Gottschalk PC, Jacobsen LK, Kosten TR. Current concepts in pharmacotherapy of substance abuse. *Curr Psychiatry Rep.* 1999;1(2):172-178.
13. de Lima MS, de Oliveira Soares BG, Reisser AA, Farrell M. Pharmacological treatment of cocaine dependence: a systematic review. *Addiction.* 2002;97(8):931-949.

14. Majewska MD. Cocaine addiction as a neurological disorder: implications for treatment. *NIDA Res Monogr.* 1996;163:1-26.
15. Luo J, Ren Y, Zhu R, et al. The effect of l-tetrahydropalmatine on cocaine-induced conditioned place preference. *Chin J Drug Depend.* 2003;12(3):177-179.
16. Ren Y, Zhang K. Effect of L-tetrahydropalmatine on discrimination of methamphetamine in rats. *Chin J Drug Depend.* 2002;9(2):108-110.
17. Heikkila RE, Orlansky H, Cohen G. Studies on the distinction between uptake inhibition and release of (3H)dopamine in rat brain tissue slices. *Biochem Pharmacol.* 1975;24(8):847-852.
18. Reith ME, Meisler BE, Sershen H, Lajtha A. Structural requirements for cocaine congeners to interact with dopamine and serotonin uptake sites in mouse brain and to induce stereotyped behavior. *Biochem Pharmacol.* 1986;35(7):1123-1129.
19. Ritz MC, Lamb RJ, Goldberg SR, Kuhar MJ. Cocaine receptors on dopamine transporters are related to self-administration of cocaine. *Science.* 1987;237(4819):1219-1223.
20. Sibley DR, Monsma FJ Jr. Molecular biology of dopamine receptors. *Trends Pharmacol Sci.* 1992;13(2):61-69.
21. Koob GF. Animal models of craving for ethanol. *Addiction.* 2000; 95(Suppl 2):S73-S81.
22. Everitt BJ, Dickinson A, Robbins TW. The neuropsychological basis of addictive behaviour. *Brain Res Brain Res Rev.* 2001;36(2-3):129-138.
23. Silvestre JS, O'Neill MF, Fernandez AG, Palacios JM. Effects of a range of dopamine receptor agonists and antagonists on ethanol intake in the rat. *Eur J Pharmacol.* 1996;318(23):257-265.
24. Callahan PM, Appel JB, Cunningham KA. Dopamine D1 and D2 mediation of the discriminative stimulus properties of d-amphetamine and cocaine. *Psychopharmacology (Berl).* 1991;103(1):50-55.
25. Caine SB, Negus SS, Mello NK, Bergman J. Effects of dopamine D(1-like) and D(2-like) agonists in rats that self-administer cocaine. *J Pharmacol Exp Ther.* 1999;291(1):353-360.
26. Self DW, Barnhart WJ, Lehman DA, Nestler EJ. Opposite modulation of cocaine-seeking behavior by D1- and D2-like dopamine receptor agonists. *Science.* 1996;271(5255):1586-1589.
27. Platt DM, Rowlett JK, Spealman RD. Behavioral effects of cocaine and dopaminergic strategies for preclinical medication development. *Psychopharmacology (Berl).* 2002;163(3-4):265-282.
28. Haney M, Collins ED, Ward AS, Foltin RW, Fischman MW. Effect of a selective dopamine D1 agonist (ABT–431) on smoked cocaine self-administration in humans. *Psychopharmacology (Berl).* 1999;143(1):102-110.
29. Berger SP, Hall S, Mickalian JD, et al. Haloperidol antagonism of cue-elicited cocaine craving. *Lancet.* 1996;l347(9000):504-508.
30. Milivojevic N, Krisch I, Sket D, Zivin M. The dopamine D1 receptor agonist and D2 receptor antagonist LEK-8829 attenuates reinstatement of cocaine-seeking in rats. *Naunyn Schmiedebergs Arch Pharmacol.* 2004;369(6):576-582.
31. Lu L, Liu Y, Zhu W, et al. Traditional medicine in the treatment of drug addiction. *Am J Drug Alcohol Abuse.* 2009;35:1-11.
32. Overstreet DH, Lee YW, Rezvani AH, Pei YH, Criswell HE, Janowsky DS. Suppression of alcohol intake after administration of the Chinese herbal medicine, NPI-028, and its derivatives. *Alcohol Clin Exp Res.* 1996;20:221-227.
33. Overstreet DH, Lee DYW, Chen YT, et al. The Chinese herbal medicine NPI-028 suppresses alcohol intake in alcohol-preferring rats and monkeys without inducing taste aversion. *J Perfusion.* 1998;11:381-383.
34. Keung WM, Vallee BL. Daidzin and daidzein suppress free-choice ethanol intake by Syrian golden hamsters. *Proc Natl Acad Sci U S A.* 1993;90:10008-10012.
35. Heyman GM, Keung WM, Vallee BL. Daidzin decreases ethanol consumption in rats. *Alcohol Clin Exp Res.* 1996;20:1083-1087.
36. Lin RC, Guthrie S, Xie CY, et al. Isoflavonoid compounds extracted from *Pueraria lobata* suppress alcohol preference in a pharmacogenetic rat model of alcoholism. *Alcohol Clin Exp Res.* 1996;20:659-663.
37. Lin RC, Li TK. Effects of isoflavones on alcohol pharmacokinetics and alcohol-drinking behavior in rats. *Am J Clin Nutr.* 1998;68(6 Suppl):1512S-1515S.
38. Benlhabib E, Baker JI, Keyler DE, Singh AK. Effects of purified puerarin on voluntary alcohol intake and alcohol withdrawal symptoms in P rats receiving free access to water and alcohol. *J Med Food.* 2004;7:180-186.
39. Lukas SE, Penetar D, Berko J, et al. An extract of the Chinese herbal root kudzu reduces alcohol drinking by heavy drinkers in a naturalistic setting. *Alcohol Clin Exp Res.* 2005;29:756-762.
40. Penetar DM, Toto LH, Farmer SL, et al. The isoflavone puerarin reduces alcohol intake in heavy drinkers: a pilot study. *Drug Alcohol Depend.* 2012;126:251-256.
41. Lukas SE, Penetar D, Su Z, et al. A standardized Kudzu extract (NPI-031) reduces alcohol consumption in non treatment seeking male heavy drinkers. *Psychopharmacology (Berl).* 2013;226:65-73.
42. Jones G, Lipson J, Nock MK. Associations between classic psychedelics and nicotine dependence in a nationally representative sample. *Sci Rep.* 2022;12(1):10578. doi:10.1038/s41598-022-14809-3
43. Bogenschutz MP. It's time to take psilocybin seriously as a possible treatment for substance use disorders. *Am J Drug Alcohol Abuse.* 2017;43(1):4-6. doi:10.1080/00952990.2016.1200060
44. Johnson MW. Classic psychedelics in addiction treatment: the case for psilocybin in tobacco smoking cessation. *Curr Top Behav Neurosci.* 2022;56:213-227. doi:10.1007/7854_2022_327
45. Bogenschutz MP, Ross S, Bhatt S, et al. Percentage of heavy drinking days following psilocybin-assisted psychotherapy vs placebo in the treatment of adult patients with alcohol use disorder: a randomized clinical trial. *JAMA Psychiatry.* 2022;79(10):953-962. doi:10.1001/jamapsychiatry.2022.2096
46. Johnson MW, Garcia-Romeu A, Griffiths RR. Long-term follow-up of psilocybin-facilitated smoking cessation. *Am J Drug Alcohol Abuse.* 2017;43(1):55-60. doi:10.3109/00952990.2016.1170135. Erratum in: *Am J Drug Alcohol Abuse.* 2017;43(1):127.
47. Wen HL, Cheung SYC. Treatment of drug addiction by acupuncture and electrical stimulation. *Asian J Med.* 1973;9:138-141.
48. McLellan AT, Grossman DS, Blaine JD, Haverkos HW. Acupuncture treatment for drug abuse: a technical review. *J Subst Abuse Treat.* 1993;10(6):569-576.
49. Hughes J, Smith TW, Kosterlitz HW, Fothergill LA, Morgan BA, Morris HR. Identification of two related pentapeptides from the brain with potent opiate agonist activity. *Nature.* 1975;258(5536):577-580.
50. Mayer DJ, Price DD, Rafii A. Antagonism of acupuncture analgesia in man by the narcotic antagonist naloxone. *Brain Res.* 1977;121(2):368-372.
51. Han JS, Terenius L. Neurochemical basis of acupuncture analgesia. *Annu Rev Pharmacol Toxicol.* 1982;22:193-220.
52. Herz A, ed. *Handbook of Experimental Pharmacology.* Vol. 104/I. Springer-Verlag; 1993.
53. Han JS, Wang Q. Mobilization of specific neuropeptides by peripheral stimulation of different frequencies. *News Physiol Sci.* 1992;7:176-180.
54. Han JS, Zhang RL. Suppression of morphine abstinence syndrome by body electroacupuncture of different frequencies in rats. *Drug Alcohol Depend.* 1993;31(2):169-175.
55. Wang JQ, Mao L, Han JS. Comparison of the antinociceptive effects induced by electroacupuncture and transcutaneous electrical nerve stimulation in the rat. *Int J Neurosci.* 1992;65(1-4):117-129.
56. Wu LZ, Cui CL, Han JS. Han's acupoint nerve stimulator for the treatment of opiate withdrawal syndrome. *Chin J Pain Med.* 1995;1:30-35.
57. Wang B, Luo F, Xia YQ, et al. Peripheral electric stimulation inhibits morphine-induced place preference in rats. *Neuroreport.* 2000;11(5):1017-1020.
58. Ma D, Han J-S, Diao Q-H, et al. Transcutaneous electrical acupoint stimulation for the treatment of withdrawal syndrome in heroin addicts. *Pain Med.* 2015;16(5):839-848. doi:10.1111/pme.12738
59. Choy YM, Tso WW, Fung KP, et al. Suppression of narcotic withdrawals and plasma ACTH by auricular electroacupuncture. *Biochem Biophys Res Commun.* 1978;82(1):305-309.
60. Ng LK, Douthitt TC, Thoa NB, Albert CA. Modification of morphine-withdrawal syndrome in rats following transauricular electrostimulation: an experimental paradigm for auricular electroacupuncture. *Biol Psychiatry.* 1975;10(5):575-580.

61. Auriacombe M, Tignol J, Le Moal M, Stinus L. Transcutaneous electrical stimulation with Limoge current potentiates morphine analgesia and attenuates opiate abstinence syndrome. *Biol Psychiatry.* 1990;28(8):650-656.
62. Han JS, Chen XH, Sun SL, et al. Effect of low- and high-frequency TENS on Met-enkephalin-Arg-Phe and dynorphin A immunoreactivity in human lumbar CSF. *Pain.* 1991;47(3):295-298.
63. Wu LZ, Cui CL, Han JS. Effect of Han's acupoint nerve stimulator (HANS) on the heart rate of 75 inpatients during heroin withdrawal. *Chin J Pain Med.* 1996;2:98-102.
64. Wu LZ, Cui CL, Han JS. Treatment on heroin addicts by 4 channel Han's Acupoint Nerve Stimulator (HANS). *J Beijing Med Univ.* 1999;31:239-242.
65. Wu LZ, Cui CL, Han JS. Reduction of methadone dosage and relief of depression and anxiety by 2/100 Hz TENS for heroin detoxification. *Chin J Drug Depend.* 2001;10:124-126.
66. Meade CS, Lukas SE, McDonald LJ, et al. A randomized trial of transcutaneous electric acupoint stimulation as adjunctive treatment for opioid detoxification. *J Subst Abuse Treat.* 2010;38(1):12-21. doi:10.1016/j.jsat.2009.05.010
67. Markou A, Weiss F, Gold LH, Caine SB, Schulteis G, Koob GF. Animal models of drug craving. *Psychopharmacology (Berl).* 1993;112(2-3): 163-182.
68. Bardo MT, Bevins RA. Conditioned place preference: what does it add to our preclinical understanding of drug reward? *Psychopharmacology (Berl).* 2000;153(1):31-43.
69. Wang B, Zhang B, Ge X, Luo F, Han J. Inhibition by peripheral electric stimulation of the reinstatement of morphine-induced place preference in rats and drug-craving in heroin addicts. *Beijing Da Xue Xue Bao Yi Xue Ban.* 2003;35(3):241-247.
70. Zhong F, Wu L-Z, Han J-S. Suppression of cue-induced heroin craving and cue-reactivity by single-trial transcutaneous electrical nerve stimulation at 2 Hz. *Addict Biol.* 2006;11:184-189. doi:10.1111/j.1369-1600.2006.00020.x
71. Han J. Acupuncture: neuropeptide release produced by electrical stimulation of different frequencies. *Trends Neurosci.* 2003;26(1):17-22. doi:10.1016/S0166-2236(02)00006-1
72. Bullock ML, Umen AJ, Culliton PD, Olander RT. Acupuncture treatment of alcoholic recidivism: a pilot study. *Alcohol Clin Exp Res.* 1987;11(3):292-295.
73. Bullock ML, Culliton PD, Olander RT. Controlled trial of acupuncture for severe recidivist alcoholism. *Lancet.* 1989;1(8652):1435-1439.
74. Worner TM, Zeller B, Schwarz H, Zwas F, Lyon D. Acupuncture fails to improve treatment outcome in alcoholics. *Drug Alcohol Depend.* 1992;30(2):169-173.
75. Sapir-Weise R, Berglund M, Frank A, Kristenson H. Acupuncture in alcoholism treatment: a randomized out-patient study. *Alcohol Alcohol.* 1999;34(4):629-635.
76. Bullock ML, Kiresuk TJ, Sherman RE, et al. A large randomized placebo controlled study of auricular acupuncture for alcohol dependence. *J Subst Abuse Treat.* 2002;22(2):71-77.
77. Olive MF, Koenig HN, Nannini MA, Hodge CW. Stimulation of endorphin neurotransmission in the nucleus accumbens by ethanol, cocaine, and amphetamine. *J Neurosci.* 2001;21(23):RC184.
78. Anton RF, Moak DH, Waid LR, Latham PK, Malcolm RJ, Dia JK. Naltrexone and cognitive behavioral therapy for the treatment of outpatient alcoholics: results of a placebo-controlled trial. *Am J Psychiatry.* 1999;156(11):1758-1764.
79. Yoshimoto K, Kato B, Sakai K, Shibata M, Yano T, Yasuhara M. Electroacupuncture stimulation suppresses the increase in alcohol-drinking behavior in restricted rats. *Alcohol Clin Exp Res.* 2001;25(Suppl 6):63S-68S.
80. Taylor D, Paton C, Kerwin R. *The Maudsley Prescribing Guidelines.* 9th ed. Informa Healthcare; 2007.
81. Spiegel D, Frischholz EJ, Fleiss JL, Spiegel H. Predictors of smoking abstinence following a single-session restructuring intervention with self-hypnosis. *Am J Psychiatry.* 1993;150:1090-1097.
82. Faerman A, Spiegel D. Shared cognitive mechanisms of hypnotizability with executive functioning and information salience. *Sci Rep.* 2021;11(1):5704. doi:10.1038/s41598-021-84954-8
83. Spiegel H. A single treatment method to stop smoking using ancillary self-hypnosis. *Int J Clin Exp Hypn.* 1970;18:235-250.
84. Katz NW. Hypnosis and the addictions: a critical review. *Addict Behav.* 1980;5:41-47.
85. Spiegel D. Tranceformations: hypnosis in brain and body. *Depress Anxiety.* 2013;30(4):342-352.
86. Barnes J, McRobbie H, Dong CY, Walker N, Hartmann-Boyce J. Hypnotherapy for smoking cessation. *Cochrane Database Syst Rev.* 2019;6(6):CD001008. doi:10.1002/14651858.CD001008.pub3
87. Holroyd J. Hypnosis treatment for smoking: an evaluative review. *Int J Clin Exp Hypn.* 1980;28:341-357.
88. Fugh-Berman A. Clinical trials of herbs. *Prim Care.* 1997;24(4):889-903.
89. Clark AM. Natural products as a resource for new drugs. *Pharm Res.* 1996;13(8):1133-1144.
90. Chung IW, Kim YS, Ahn JS, et al. Pharmacologic profile of natural products used to treat psychotic illnesses. *Psychopharmacol Bull.* 1995;31(1):139-145.

CHAPTER

68

Neuromodulation for Substance Use Disorders

Colleen A. Hanlon, Kaitlin R. Kinney, Miranda P. Ramirez, and Michael J. Wesley

CHAPTER OUTLINE

- Introduction
- Brain regions that contribute to addiction and are primary neuromodulation targets
- Transcranial magnetic stimulation for addiction
- Other promising neuromodulation techniques for addiction
- Conclusions

INTRODUCTION

Neuromodulation is the process by which electrical, chemical, and mechanical interventions can impact nervous system functioning.[1] With a growing appreciation for multimodal and individualized treatment strategies in medicine, neuromodulation has gained popularity as a brain-based approach for treating a wide range of neurological and psychiatric conditions. Unlike pharmacological interventions that often come with off-target effects that can be poorly tolerated, neuromodulation techniques can be highly focal and may be better tailored to a patient's individual needs.

Substance use disorder (SUD) is characterized by a cluster of cognitive, behavioral, and physiological symptoms indicating that the individual continues to use the substance despite significant substance-related problems.[2] These include clusters of impaired control, social impairment, risky use, and pharmacological changes within the brain. These relate to changes in brain circuitry that may persist beyond detoxification, and especially in those with severe SUD. Since the neural circuits involved in SUD have been well mapped,[3] there is promise that neuromodulation of the brain physiology underlying the expression SUD may promote disease remission and minimize the harms of substance use. This possibility was highlighted in 2020 with the first FDA cleared neural circuit based therapeutic for treatment in the addiction space (transcranial magnetic stimulation for the treatment of nicotine use disorder)[4]—likely the first of many.

In this chapter, we introduce primary brain regions and neural circuits associated with SUD. We discuss the ability of neuromodulation to augment or change physiology in targeted regions in an effort to affect SUD. Based on our current state of knowledge in the neuromodulation field and the application of neuromodulation for psychiatric treatment, we emphasize effects related to the preoccupation/anticipation (eg, craving) stage of the medical disease of addiction and focus on transcranial magnetic stimulation (TMS) as a primary neuromodulation modality. Finally, we touch on mechanisms of action, common targets, and efficacy of additional neuromodulation modalities that show promise for SUD treatment.

BRAIN REGIONS THAT CONTRIBUTE TO ADDICTION AND ARE PRIMARY NEUROMODULATION TARGETS

A seminal paper by Koob and Volkow describes addiction as a process with three stages: (1) binge/intoxication, (2) withdrawal/negative affect, and (3) preoccupation/anticipation (eg, craving). It is worth noting that each of these stages of the addiction cycle may engage relevant brain regions differently (see Figure 5 in reference[5] for illustration) and therefore may benefit from different neuromodulation approaches. It is also important to state that focusing on the networks involved in craving and resisting drug cues represent only one portion of the addiction cycle. **Figure 68-1** lists key brain regions implicated in SUD that are major neuromodulation targets. For a more detailed description of the neurotransmitter circuitry linked to SUD please refer to sections 1 and 2 of this textbook, among others.

Striatum

The striatum refers to the caudate, putamen, and nucleus accumbens (NAcc). It is likely the most widely recognized hub involved in the addictive process due to its involvement in reward processing, information integration, and action planning. The ventral striatum, specifically the NAcc, receives afferent dopaminergic projections from the ventral tegmental area (VTA) and is particularly important for reward processing. While dopamine is not a particularly abundant neurotransmitter (relative to the major excitatory transmitter, glutamate or the major inhibitory transmitter, GABA, for example), it is a critical signaling mechanism for reward, prediction, and learning. Consistent with preclinical studies described in previous chapters, human brain imaging studies have demonstrated that NAcc activity is positively correlated with anticipation of a drug reward, but activity decreases during the drug-induced high itself.[6,7]

From a neuromodulation perspective, direct modulation of the NAcc is difficult. The NAcc is located deep within the human brain, close to the midline, and is only 1.4 cm × 0.7 cm,[8] slightly smaller than an average peanut. By comparison, the

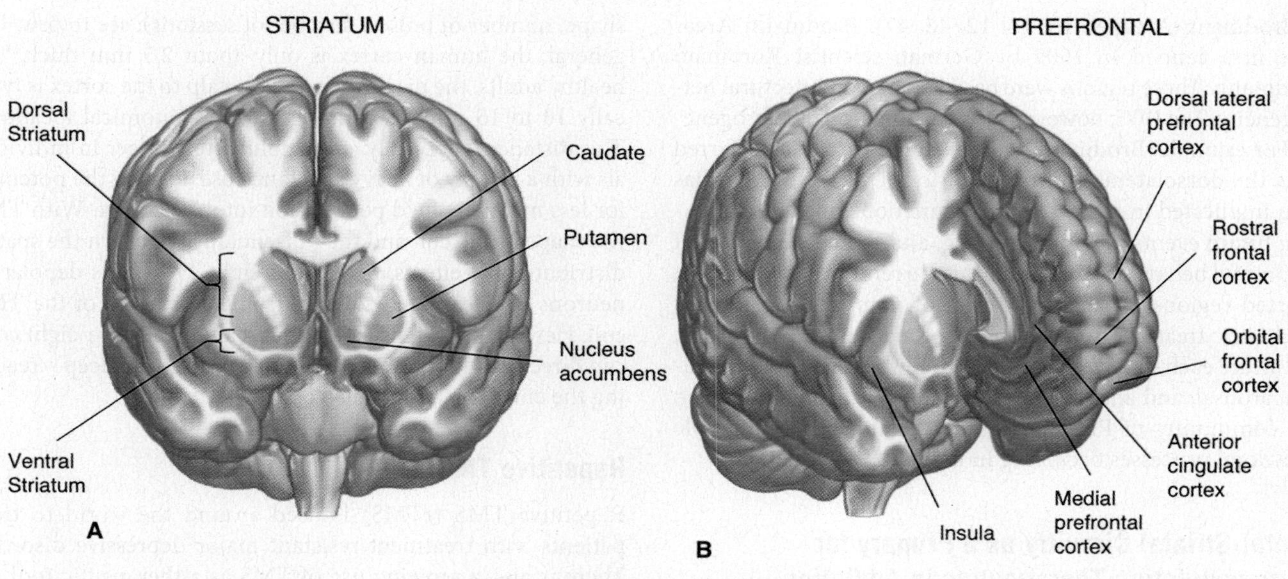

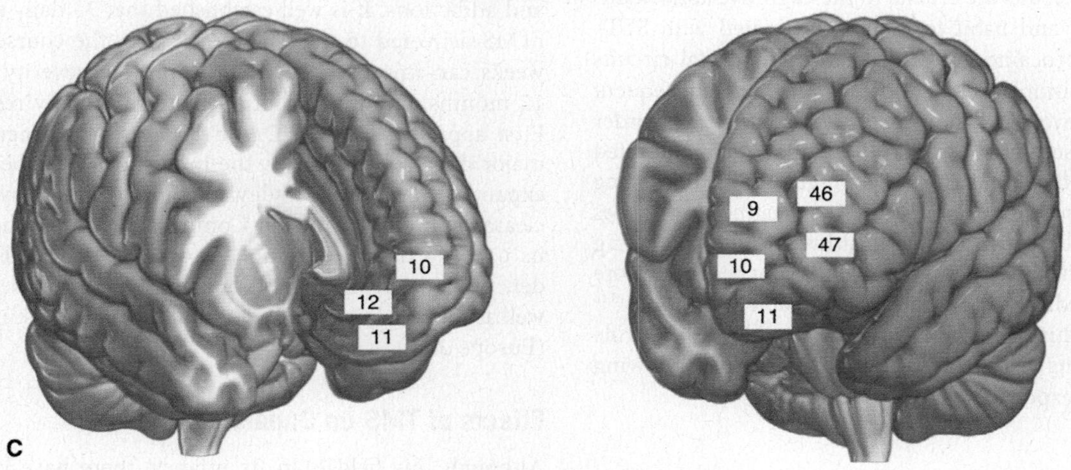

Figure 68-1. Brain regions that contribute to addiction and are primary neuromodulation targets. **A.** The striatum includes dorsal and ventral portions. The ventral striatum is synonymous with the nucleus accumbens (NAcc) whereas the dorsal striatum refers to the caudate and putamen. The prefrontal cortex (PFC) is comprised of several targets presented by **(B)** cortical region name and **(C)** Brodmann Area convention.

intracranial volume of an average adult is approximately 1,200 cubic centimeters, about the size of an average cantaloupe. In general, targets farther from the scalp are more difficult to modulate directly. That is because the major stimulation modalities (eg, electric, magnetic, and ultrasonic) disperse with distance. The dorsal striatum is above the NAcc and farther from the midline. It includes the caudate and putamen, which are larger than the NAcc and positioned closer to the skull making them more feasible for targeting, but this is still difficult with existing noninvasive neuromodulation technology.

Modulating the Striatum Via Cortical Projections

We have two possible approaches for modulating the striatum: direct invasive techniques (eg, with deep brain stimulation from a cannula or wire) or indirect noninvasive techniques that target connected neural regions that are closer to the skull (eg, with TMS). For example, the striatum receives abundant inputs from the prefrontal cortex[9] and frontal-striatal connections have been highly implicated in drug taking behavior. It is feasible, then, to modulate striatal-linked drug taking behavior by modulating the prefrontal cortical regions that project to the striatum. This is envisioned as using the cortex as a "window" for accessing deeper brain structures. Indeed, this is a common theoretical model used in the development of TMS protocols for a variety of neuropsychiatric disorders.

Prefrontal Cortex

The prefrontal cortex (PFC) is located anterior to the precentral gyrus. It is often divided into six discrete areas (known as Brodmann Areas 9, 10, 11, 12, 46, 47). Brodmann Areas were first defined in 1909 by German scientist Korbinian Brodmann. These regions were based on cytoarchitectural heterogeneity. The PFC, however, also has functional heterogeneity. For example, Brodmann Areas 9 and 46 are often referred to as the dorsolateral prefrontal cortex (DLPFC), which has been implicated in many executive functions, including planning future events, decision making, and the coordination of purposeful behavior.[10] The DLPFC is currently one of the most targeted regions in the application of neuromodulation for psychiatric treatment. Additional Brodmann Areas 10, 11, 12, and 47 are each involved in aspects of reward signaling, valuation, arousal, and affective or emotional processing. Together, this community of PFC regions contributes to the multiple behavioral processes occurring in individuals with SUD.[11]

Frontal-Striatal Circuitry as a Primary for Neuromodulation Therapeutics in Addiction

Frontal-striatal circuits are crucial to the cognitive abnormalities, impulsivity, and habit formation associated with SUD. For example, in cocaine use disorder frontal-striatal circuits mediate the volitional seeking of cocaine and subsequent learning, which eventually becomes more habitual as disorder severity progresses.[12] Preclinical studies have demonstrated that the mesolimbic dopamine system regulates the rewarding and reinforcing properties of cocaine. As drug use progresses from use to maladaptive and unhealthy use, the rewarding properties become less salient, and drug taking becomes more reflective of conditioned responses and habit formation.[13,14] Engagement of this circuitry appears to also play a large role in the mechanisms that forecast a return to drug use following context and cue exposure.

TRANSCRANIAL MAGNETIC STIMULATION FOR ADDICTION

TMS is a noninvasive form of brain stimulation that induces a depolarization of neurons through electromagnetic induction. Although a comprehensive review of studies that have demonstrated the principles of TMS is beyond the scope of this chapter, prior behavioral, electrophysiological, and neuroimaging work in this area is well described and summarized in several review articles.[15-19] Most of our knowledge regarding the basic physiological effects of TMS applied to the brain is from studies in the motor system. When applied over the hand knob of the primary motor cortex, a single, transient TMS pulse can induce a reliable contraction of the contralateral hand that is proportional to the amplitude of the induced electrical field.[20] The amplitude of this motor evoked potential (MEP) in the contralateral hand has been manipulated pharmacologically to reveal primary effects related to voltage gated sodium channels and glutamate,[21,22] for example.

Many factors can influence the effects of a given TMS protocol (eg, frequency, amplitude, cortical location, coil shape, number of pulses, number of sessions); see review.[23] In general, the human cortex is only about 2.5 mm thick.[24] In healthy adults, the distance from the scalp to the cortex is typically 10 to 15 mm (depending on the anatomical location). This distance is typically a few millimeters larger in individuals with a history of heavy substance use, leaving the potential for less magnetic field penetration into the cortex. With TMS the shape of the coil and the pulse intensity govern the spatial distribution of effects. Flat figure-eight TMS coils depolarize neurons approximately 20 mm from the surface of the TMS coil. Hesed coil designs (H-coil) and angular figure-eight coils can directly modulate regions as far as 6 to 8 mm deep—reaching the cingulate and insula cortices.

Repetitive TMS

Repetitive TMS (rTMS) is used around the world to treat patients with treatment-resistant major depressive disorder. There is also a growing use of TMS as a therapeutic tool for obsessive compulsive disorder, anxious depression, headache and addictions. It is well established that 30 daily sessions of rTMS delivered to the left DLPFC over the course of 6 to 8 weeks can improve depression symptom severity for up to 12 months among individuals that are initially responsive.[25] First approved by the FDA in 2008 as a treatment tool for major depressive disorder, the indications have been rapidly expanding. Several TMS device manufacturers have received clearance by the European Commission and/or the FDA for its use as a therapeutic tool for obsessive compulsive disorder, anxious depression, headache, pain (Europe only); as well as tobacco/nicotine (FDA and Europe) and stimulant use (Europe only).

Effects of TMS on Dopamine

Although this field is in its infancy, there have been some important strides made utilizing positron emission tomography (PET) to assess for the impact of TMS on dopamine release.[25-35] In the motor cortex, high frequency TMS tends to reduce [(11)C]raclopride D2/D3 receptor antagonist binding, suggesting a TMS-induced increase in dopamine release. In healthy controls, 10 Hz rTMS to the left DLPFC decreased dopamine receptor availability in the left dorsal caudate,[31] left subgenual and pregenual anterior cingulate cortex (ACC) and the left medial orbital frontal cortex (OFC),[32] but there was no effect following right DLPFC stimulation. One study stimulated the medial prefrontal cortex (MPFC) of 24 healthy controls and reported a reduction in dopamine receptor binding potential in the bilateral dorsal putamen and the bilateral dorsal and ventral globus pallidus—indicating TMS induced increases in dopamine.[36] Another study using an H-coil to modulate the bilateral inferior PFC and insula in a small group of eight healthy individuals demonstrated that 1 Hz rTMS increased [^{11}C]-(+)-PHNO dopamine radiotracer binding, suggesting a decrease in dopamine levels in the substantia nigra and the sensorimotor striatum.[37] Together these data suggest that there are frequency dependent effects of rTMS on dopamine release, wherein 10 Hz and faster stimulation protocols (eg, theta burst stimulation) induce dopamine release in the striatum and low frequency stimulation decreases dopamine release.

Application of TMS to SUDs

While a full discussion of the state of the field is beyond the scope of this introductory chapter, there are multiple review articles describing the current state of the field.[38-42] As mentioned above, in 2020, the FDA cleared the H4 Deep TMS coil for nicotine/tobacco use disorder. This coil has an electric field that intersects the bilateral inferior PFC, medial PFC, and the anterior insula—all brain regions that are involved in drug taking and return to use. This approval was based on data from a multisite, double-blind, sham-controlled study wherein 10 Hz TMS was delivered for 15 sessions over the course of 3 to 4 weeks. TMS efficacy was comparable to medications, such as varenicline and bupropion, yet had very few side effects. This was an important milestone for the neuromodulation field and the addiction treatment field as it is the first indication that the FDA acknowledges that SUDs are neural circuit-based diseases and that neural circuit-based medical devices can be safe and effective treatment options.

It is naive, however, to think there will be a single "optimal" TMS protocol to treat SUDs. As the field develops, it will be guided by questions like these: (1) What cortical location should we target to maximally affect the circuitry we are interested in changing and (2) what neuromodulation protocol should we choose to directionally impact a given outcome? Neuroimaging guided TMS has been recommended as a strategy for isolating structural and functional targets within an individual to improve TMS efficacy.[43,44] Additionally, some individuals may benefit the most from a treatment strategy that amplifies their executive control circuitry (eg, 10 Hz DLPFC stimulation), while others may benefit the most from a strategy that attenuates limbic circuitry involved in drug craving (eg, 1 Hz MPFC/frontal pole stimulation). Before moving forward with expensive and slow multisite clinical trials investigating the efficacy of rTMS as a viable treatment tool for addiction, however, it is useful to explore the cortical targets and combinations of frequencies that may help to maximize treatment impact.

TMS to the DLPFC

To date nearly all the rTMS studies in addiction have targeted the same neural region—the DLPFC.[45-52] These data are supported by previous findings suggesting that rTMS to the DLPFC can modulate craving, and that anatomical integrity and functional connectivity of the insula are important for craving.[53,54] A greater understanding of the direct physiological effects of this neuromodulation tool and protocol may allow us to improve the efficacy and expand treatment to other SUD categories. For example, there have not been any studies to date that have measured changes in dopamine following TMS in individuals with cocaine use disorder. This is an open area of research that would provide vital information about the biological mechanisms of TMS interventions in individuals with SUDs.

TMS to the MPFC

The primary cortical inputs to the ventral striatum are the medial and orbital prefrontal cortices. Given that the ventral striatum is one of the primary brain regions involved in processing drug-associated reward, it seems that targeting the MPFC would be a more direct method to modulate ventral striatal activity than DLPFC stimulation. Since craving for cocaine is associated with an increase in activity in the striatum (eg, fMRI BOLD [blood oxygen level dependent] signal), it is reasonable to pursue an LTD/long-term depression-like rTMS protocol over the MPFC to attenuate activity in this neural circuit. Single pulses of TMS to the MPFC in healthy individuals leads to an increase in BOLD signal in the ventral striatum,[55] a phenomenon that is dependent upon both the gray matter volume within the scope of the electric field and the white matter integrity between the site of stimulation and the striatum.[56]

Martinez and colleagues demonstrated that 10 Hz TMS delivered to the dorsal MPFC/cingulate (H7 coil) decreased cocaine self-administration in a pilot study of 18 individuals with CUD (cocaine use disorder) on an inpatient research unit. Cocaine self administration sessions were conducted before rTMS (baseline), after 4 rTMS sessions (week 1), and after 13 rTMS sessions (week 3). Individuals received 10 Hz, 1Hz, or sham TMS (one session/day, three weeks). For each self-administration session, participants received a "priming" dose of smoked cocaine (12 mg). Following the priming dose, participants were presented with the choice between smoked cocaine (12 mg) and money ($5) nine times during each session. At baseline, participants chose cocaine over money approximately 50% of the time. After 13 sessions of rTMS, individuals who received 10 Hz stimulation only chose cocaine 1.8 of the nine times (20%), while the group that received 1 Hz rTMS chose cocaine over money 61% of the time, and the group that received sham rTMS remained stable at 52% of the time. This decrease after 13 sessions was significantly greater than the change observed after only four sessions of active 10 Hz rTMS to the left DLPFC ($t = 4.0$, $p = 0.001$).[57]

As an initial proof of principle, we conducted a clinical trial evaluating the effect of 10 sessions of MPFC rTMS on cue-reactivity and drug use among treatment-seeking people with CUD (ClinicalTrials.gov: NCT03238859). Treatment-seeking individuals with CUD were invited to enroll in this single site, double-blind, sham controlled TMS trial, which included randomized assignment and longitudinal MRI scanning for a 3-month period. MPFC TMS was delivered three times/week for 10 sessions. Each treatment session consisted of 3,600 pulses (110% resting motor threshold). Brain reactivity to cocaine cues was acquired at baseline, after 1 month (the conclusion of the TMS intervention), and at 2- and 3-month follow ups. A summary of the trial design, retention and brain imaging data is shown in **Figure 68-2**. These preliminary data

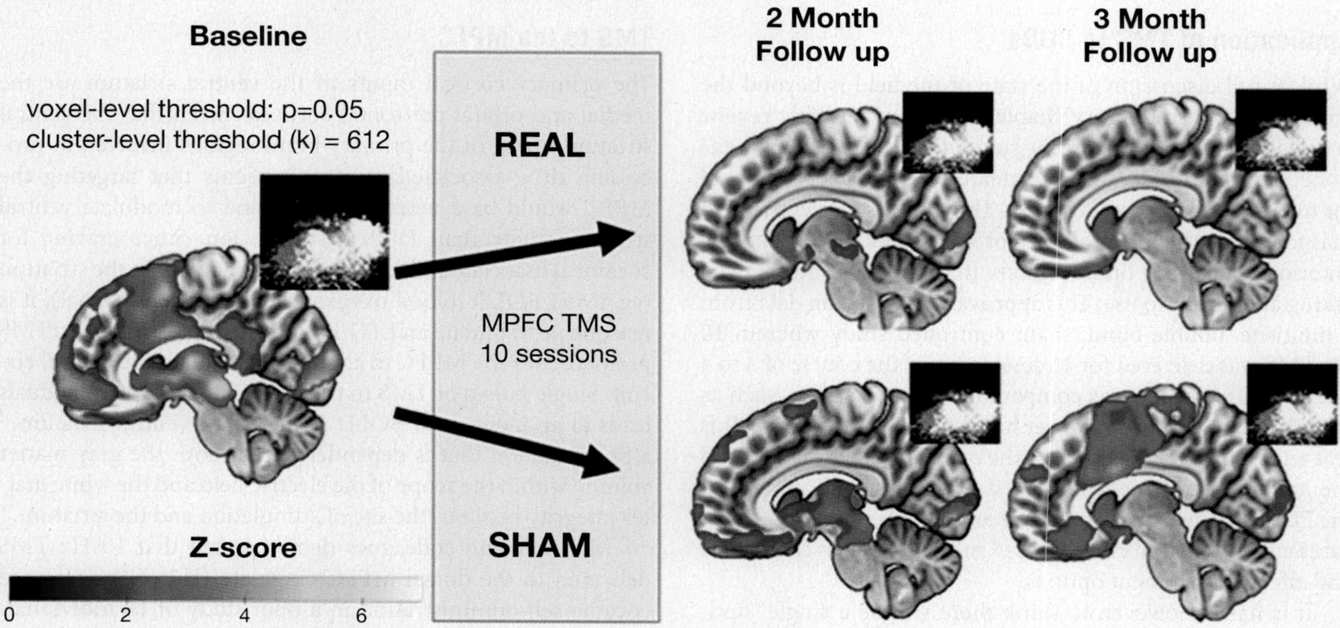

Figure 68-2. A double-blinded sham-controlled clinical trial was conducted to evaluate the efficacy of 10 days of mPFC TMS as a tool to decrease cocaine cue reactivity and decrease brain reactivity to cues in 33 treatment-seeking individuals with CUD. MPFC TMS was delivered three times/week for 10 sessions (figure of eight coil, left frontal pole, 3,600 pulses/session, cTBS, 110% RMT). Functional MRI was acquired while participants viewed cocaine and neutral cues (*top*). Real TMS increased the odds of remaining enrolled in the treatment program (OR: 1.43) and decreased striatal reactivity to cocaine cues.

suggest that mPFC TMS is feasible, well tolerated by the participants, and demonstrate the high fidelity of the sham. The fMRI data indicate that mPFC TMS decreases cocaine cue reactivity in frontal and striatal areas. Notably, 100% of these participants also smoked tobacco cigarettes regularly (which is common among people who use cocaine). Although the effect of mPFC TMS on cigarette smoking rates was not captured in this pilot study, the results of the prior studies suggest that mPFC TMS may also be attenuating smoking rates and cue reactivity in these people who use cocaine.

Alcohol use disorder (AUD) also appears to benefit from TMS to the MPFC. Two relatively large studies were published in 2021 and 2022, which demonstrated that TMS delivered to the left frontal pole (MPFC, 3,600 pulses, theta burst, 10 sessions[58]) and TMS delivered to the dorsal MPFC/cingulate via the deep TMS H7 coil (3,000 pulses, 10 Hz, 15 sessions[59]) both decrease heavy drinking days in individuals with AUD for up to 3 months. The electric field distribution of the H7 coil (FDA cleared for obsessive compulsive disorder) and the H4 coil (FDA cleared for treating tobacco use disorder) also overlaps with a region of the MPFC that has been associated with relapse prediction for people with tobacco use disorder as well as individuals with risky drinking.[60]

Considered together, this body of work indicates that: (1) the mPFC is a transdiagnostically relevant brain stimulation target for disorders of cue-reactivity, (2) a single session of mPFC TMS can decrease brain reactivity to multiple classes of drug cues, and (3) multiple days of mPFC TMS is a feasible, well-tolerated intervention for CUD and AUD. These data add to the growing evidence that the mPFC TMS may be an efficacious target to modulate cocaine use and brain activity associated with cocaine cues.

TMS With Cognitive Therapy

In the first applications of rTMS for neuropsychiatric disorders, treatment was performed at rest and in the absence of other forms of intervention.[61,62] Today, there is a growing interest in how to improve the therapeutic effects of rTMS. The principle that a neural circuit is more "plastic" or primed when it is engaged during stimulation has offered the field of rTMS a potential solution to increase treatment efficacy and longevity.[63] In clinical depression and posttraumatic stress disorder (PTSD) studies, combining modified cognitive-behavioral therapy (CBT) protocols with high frequency DLPFC stimulation have shown both feasibility and promise.[64-66] Combined rTMS and behavioral therapy is now in the early stages of being evaluated for SUD.[67] Independently, CBT is well established as a therapeutic approach to prevent relapse in SUDs by having patients identify and correct maladaptive behaviors.

This form of therapy has been shown to be effective for AUD, and people with DSM-IV cannabis dependence and cocaine dependence.[68] Cognitive therapies such as CBT engage executive and inhibitory control circuitry involving brain regions like the DLPFC and ACC.[69] Although several other behavioral interventions have been explored for SUD, cognitive therapies are unique in their ability to enhance the engagement of networks being explored as potential rTMS targets.[42] In a study of tobacco/nicotine use disorder relapse prevention, 29 participants were given eight Forever Free (FF) relapse prevention booklets to read during and between sessions of 20 Hz DLPFC stimulation.[67] Results showed that combining evidence-based self-help with rTMS treatment can significantly increase abstinence rates and reduce relapse. One question that remains in combining cognitive therapies with rTMS treatment is the impact of their temporal relationship. The timing of the therapies can be delivered concurrently, sequentially, or interleaved; however, a consensus on the best ordering has yet to be determined.[70]

TMS and Pharmacotherapy

A full discussion of this can be found elsewhere,[71] but we will highlight main components here. Much of the promise of rTMS stems from its characterization as a circuit-based tool, in contrast to the effective, but systemic nature of pharmacological agents. Furthermore, rTMS is being developed as a treatment specifically for SUDs, which currently lack FDA-approved medications. Despite this posture, there may be untapped potential in the combination of these tools. Blending the circuit-specific effects of TMS with the more established knowledge of medications may lead to larger or more durable effects on plasticity in the circuit of interest.

Final Thoughts on TMS as an Intervention for Addiction

Before pursuing large expensive clinical trials exploring rTMS (and other promising neuromodulation modalities) as a potential stand-alone or adjunct therapy for SUD, it is critical to determine whether it is safe and tolerable in treatment-engaged individuals and feasible for impacting targeted clinical endpoints. Selective modulation of frontal-striatal circuits involved in limbic and executive control may be an innovative and useful treatment strategy to prevent cue-associated relapse in individuals with SUD. Clinical rTMS is growing in acceptance and use, with more than 700 machines in the United States and emerging insurance reimbursement. The data presented in this chapter demonstrate that while most of the efforts for rTMS in addiction have been focused on increasing activity in the DLPFC, focusing on decreasing activity in the MPFC and NAcc may also be a feasible and fruitful target to consider. It seems plausible that either increasing neural firing in the executive control circuit (perhaps via high frequency TMS in the DLPFC) or decreasing firing in the limbic circuit in the presence of drug context and cues (perhaps via low frequency TMS in the MPFC) are both valuable strategies to pursue.

OTHER PROMISING NEUROMODULATION TECHNIQUES FOR ADDICTION

Transcranial Direct Current Stimulation

Transcranial direct current stimulation (tDCS) is a noninvasive form of neuromodulation where low-amplitude direct currents are applied directly to the scalp via electrodes to stimulate two parallel brain regions.[72,73] tDCS is not currently FDA approved for any indication and the literature regarding its potential efficacy is mixed. While some studies have shown promise in tDCS as a treatment of psychiatric disorders, researchers have failed to demonstrate efficacy above and beyond that of standard pharmacological treatments.[74] Inconsistency in study design, such as not having a sufficient number of stimulation sessions and small sample sizes,[75,76] likely contribute to null findings. Regardless, tDCS has been shown to modify behavior, improve learning, and improve inhibition[77,78] and continues to be explored in the treatment of psychiatric disorders. Though modest, tDCS has been shown to improve depressive symptoms in patients with bipolar depression[79] and to reduce anxiety symptoms when combined with cognitive tasks.

tDCS has also been explored for the treatment of SUD in small studies. For example, anodal tDCS to both the right and left DLPFC has been shown to reduce cue-induced nicotine craving and smoking behavior.[80,81] Furthermore, both left cathodal/right anodal and left anodal/right cathodal combined stimulation reduced alcohol craving compared to sham.[82] Anodal tDCS targeting the left DLPFC in treatment seeking individuals reduced cue-induced alcohol craving and emotional symptoms (eg, anxiety, depression) compared to sham but was associated with a trend toward greater relapse.[83] In a sample of 36 individuals with cocaine use disorder, sessions of tDCS to the DLPFC (left cathodal/right anodal) significantly reduced cocaine craving when compared to sham.[84] In 25 people who use cannabis chronically (≥3 days/week for ≥3 years), right anodal/left cathodal applied to the DLPFC reduced cannabis craving compared to sham stimulation.[85]

Focused Ultrasound

Transcranial focused ultrasound (FUS) uses sound waves to manipulate brain function. An advantage of sonification is that the signal does not decay with distance as quickly as magnetic energy, and it is not impeded by alterations in tissue density as in electrical stimulation. This results in the capability to target subcortical brain structures in a manner that is more effective than electrical or magnetic approaches (eg, TDCS or TMS).[86] A specific form of FUS called low intensity focused ultrasound (LIFU) is being pursued as a potential therapeutic approach for several neurologic and psychiatric conditions.

Through low intensity stimulation it is possible to create transient functional disruption in deep brain structures without pathological changes on histological examination.[87] While LIFU is not yet approved for therapeutic use in any neuropsychiatric condition, it is worth noting given the spatial resolution and ability to target subcortical regions linked to addiction.

Deep Brain Stimulation

Deep brain stimulation (DBS) involves a surgical procedure where electrodes are placed into specific brain regions and stimulated through implanted pulse generators.[88] DBS is FDA approved for treatment for patients with a variety of neurological disorders (eg, Parkinson disease, essential tremor, etc.). Though DBS has not been investigated extensively in human SUD, case studies have reported that stimulation to the NAcc reduced the consumption of various substances, such as alcohol, nicotine, and heroin. One case reported an individual who underwent the NAcc DBS procedure and abstained from drug use during active DBS for the first 2.5 years and remained drug free for 3.5 years following DBS removal with no relapse at a 6-year follow-up with notable improvements in memory, IQ, and emotional status.[89] Another case study showed two individuals with treatment refractory heroin use disorder who achieved complete heroin abstinence (apart from a single incident) at 2-year follow-up.[90] In a study of five participants with treatment-resistant AUD who received DBS of the NAcc, all reported a complete loss of alcohol craving up to eight years following DBS implantation; two patients remained abstinent for several years, and three showed a marked reduction of alcohol consumption.[91] Another case study reported that DBS of the NAcc reduced OCD-related symptoms, providing additional support for DBS's efficacy in SUD treatment given the compulsive nature of some drug-taking behavior.[92-95] In addition to the NAcc, several other brain regions have been recommended as potential targets for DBS aimed to treat addiction, including several deep regions and the MPFC.[96]

CONCLUSIONS

In summary, this chapter provides insight into the utility of neuromodulation tools as useful therapeutic options for SUDs. Many of the challenges facing development of efficacious pharmacotherapies could be ameliorated with neuromodulation to specific neural circuits in a functionally relevant manner. Through the continued refinement of neuromodulation technologies and approaches, in the next decade we will be rigorously evaluating this possibility. Just as a patient with cancer is given a multidimensional cancer treatment plan including chemotherapy, tumor resection, and behavioral counselling, treatment plans for individuals with SUD could be equally as comprehensive. In this vision for the future, providers will not only rely on pharmaceutical and behavioral interventions alone, but will also utilize neuromodulation to treat specific neural circuit dysfunctions to further enhance addiction treatment outcomes.

REFERENCES

1. Cole RC, Okine DN, Yeager BE, Narayanan NS. Neuromodulation of cognition in Parkinson's disease. In: Narayanan NS, Albin RL, eds. *Progress in Brain Research*. Elsevier; 2022:435-455.
2. *Diagnostic and Statistical Manual of Mental Disorders*. 5th ed. American Psychiatric Association Publishing; 2013:591-643.
3. Koob GF. Dynamics of neuronal circuits in addiction: reward, antireward, and emotional memory. *Pharmacopsychiatry*. 2009;42(Suppl 1):S32-S41.
4. *BrainsWay Receives FDA Clearance for Smoking Addiction in Adults*. Accessed August 16, 2023. https://www.globenewswire.com/news-release/2020/08/24/2082476/0/en/BrainsWay-Receives-FDA-Clearance-for-Smoking-Addiction-in-Adults.html
5. Koob GF, Volkow ND. Neurocircuitry of addiction. *Neuropsychopharmacology*. 2010;35(1):217-238.
6. Breiter HC, Gollub RL, Weisskoff RM, et al. Acute effects of cocaine on human brain activity and emotion. *Neuron*. 1997;19(3):591-611.
7. Risinger RC, Salmeron BJ, Ross TJ, et al. Neural correlates of high and craving during cocaine self-administration using BOLD fMRI. *Neuroimage*. 2005;26(4):1097-1108.
8. Neto LL, Oliveira E, Correia F, Ferreira AG. The human nucleus accumbens: where is it? A stereotactic, anatomical and magnetic resonance imaging study. *Neuromodulation*. 2008;11(1):13-22.
9. Haber SN, Knutson B. The reward circuit: linking primate anatomy and human imaging. *Neuropsychopharmacology*. 2010;35(1):4-26.
10. Miller EK, Cohen JD. An integrative theory of prefrontal cortex function. *Annu Rev Neurosci*. 2001;24:167-202.
11. Jones DT, Graff-Radford J. Executive dysfunction and the prefrontal cortex. *Continuum (Minneap Minn)*. 2021;27(6):1586-1601.
12. Goldstein RZ, Volkow ND. Drug addiction and its underlying neurobiological basis: neuroimaging evidence for the involvement of the frontal cortex. *Am J Psychiatry*. 2002;159(10):1642-1652.
13. Porrino LJ, Lyons D, Smith HR, Daunais JB, Nader MA. Cocaine self-administration produces a progressive involvement of limbic, association, and sensorimotor striatal domains. *J Neurosci*. 2004;24(14):3554-3562.
14. Everitt BJ, Robbins TW. Neural systems of reinforcement for drug addiction: from actions to habits to compulsion. *Nat Neurosci*. 2005;8(11):1481-1489.
15. Daskalakis ZJ, Levinson AJ, Fitzgerald PB. Repetitive transcranial magnetic stimulation for major depressive disorder: a review. *Can J Psychiatry*. 2008;53(9):555-566.
16. Hoogendam JM, Ramakers GM, Di Lazzaro V. Physiology of repetitive transcranial magnetic stimulation of the human brain. *Brain Stimul*. 2010;3(2):95-118.
17. Thickbroom GW. Transcranial magnetic stimulation and synaptic plasticity: experimental framework and human models. *Exp Brain Res*. 2007;180(4):583-593.
18. Ziemann U. Transcranial magnetic stimulation at the interface with other techniques: a powerful tool for studying the human cortex. *Neuroscientist*. 2011;17(4):368-381.
19. Barker AT. An introduction to the basic principles of magnetic nerve stimulation. *J Clin Neurophysiol*. 1991;8(1):26-37.
20. Barker AT, Freeston IL, Jabinous R, Jarratt JA. Clinical evaluation of conduction time measurements in central motor pathways using magnetic stimulation of human brain. *Lancet*. 1986;1(8493):1325-1326.
21. Ziemann U, Rothwell JC. I-waves in motor cortex. *J Clin Neurophysiol*. 2000;17(4):397-405.
22. Di Lazzaro V, Ziemann U, Lemon RN. State of the art: physiology of transcranial motor cortex stimulation. *Brain Stimul*. 2008;1(4):345-362.
23. Fitzgerald PB, Fountain S, Daskalakis ZJ. A comprehensive review of the effects of rTMS on motor cortical excitability and inhibition. *Clin Neurophysiol*. 2006;117(12):2584-2596.

24. Fischl B, Dale AM. Measuring the thickness of the human cerebral cortex from magnetic resonance images. *Proc Natl Acad Sci U S A.* 2000;97(20):11050-11055.
25. George MS. Transcranial magnetic stimulation for the treatment of depression. *Expert Rev Neurother.* 2010;10(11):1761-1772.
26. Lamusuo S, Hirvonen J, Lindholm P, et al. Neurotransmitters behind pain relief with transcranial magnetic stimulation—positron emission tomography evidence for release of endogenous opioids. *Eur J Pain.* 2017;21(9):1505-1515.
27. Strafella AP, Paus T, Fraraccio M, Dagher A. Striatal dopamine release induced by repetitive transcranial magnetic stimulation of the human motor cortex. *Brain.* 2003;126(Pt 12):2609-2615.
28. Ohnishi T, Hayashi T, Okabe S, et al. Endogenous dopamine release induced by repetitive transcranial magnetic stimulation over the primary motor cortex: an [11C]raclopride positron emission tomography study in anesthetized macaque monkeys. *Biol Psychiatry.* 2004;55(5):484-489.
29. Kim JY, Chung EJ, Lee WY, et al. Therapeutic effect of repetitive transcranial magnetic stimulation in Parkinson's disease: analysis of [11C] raclopride PET study. *Mov Disord.* 2008;23(2):207-211.
30. Strafella AP, Ko JH, Grant J, Fraraccio M, Monchi O. Corticostriatal functional interactions in Parkinson's disease: a rTMS/[11C]raclopride PET study. *Eur J Neurosci.* 2005;22(11):2946-2952.
31. Strafella AP, Paus T, Barrett J, Dagher A. Repetitive transcranial magnetic stimulation of the human prefrontal cortex induces dopamine release in the caudate nucleus. *J Neurosci.* 2001;21(15):RC157.
32. Cho SS, Strafella AP. rTMS of the left dorsolateral prefrontal cortex modulates dopamine release in the ipsilateral anterior cingulate cortex and orbitofrontal cortex. *PLoS One.* 2009;4(8):e6725.
33. Kuroda Y, Motohashi N, Ito H, et al. Effects of repetitive transcranial magnetic stimulation on [11C]raclopride binding and cognitive function in patients with depression. *J Affect Disord.* 2006;95(1-3): 35-42.
34. Kuroda Y, Motohashi N, Ito H, et al. Chronic repetitive transcranial magnetic stimulation failed to change dopamine synthesis rate: preliminary L-[beta-11C]DOPA positron emission tomography study in patients with depression. *Psychiatry Clin Neurosci.* 2010;64(6):659-662.
35. Ko JH, Monchi O, Ptito A, Bloomfield P, Houle S, Strafella AP. Theta burst stimulation-induced inhibition of dorsolateral prefrontal cortex reveals hemispheric asymmetry in striatal dopamine release during a set-shifting task: a TMS-[(11)C]raclopride PET study. *Eur J Neurosci.* 2008;28(10):2147-2155.
36. Cho SS, Koshimori Y, Aminian K, et al. Investing in the future: stimulation of the medial prefrontal cortex reduces discounting of delayed rewards. *Neuropsychopharmacology.* 2015;40(3):546-553.
37. Malik S, Jacobs M, Cho S-S, et al. Deep TMS of the insula using the H-coil modulates dopamine release: a crossover [(11)C] PHNO-PET pilot trial in healthy humans. *Brain Imaging Behav.* 2018;12(5):1306-1317.
38. Bellamoli E, Manganotti P, Schwartz RP, Rimondo C, Gomma M, Serpelloni G. rTMS in the treatment of drug addiction: an update about human studies. *Behav Neurol.* 2014;2014:815215.
39. Feil J, Zangen A. Brain stimulation in the study and treatment of addiction. *Neurosci Biobehav Rev.* 2010;34(4):559-574.
40. Gorelick DA, Zangen A, George MS. Transcranial magnetic stimulation in the treatment of substance addiction. *Ann N Y Acad Sci.* 2014;1327:79-93.
41. Wing VC, Barr MS, Wass CE, et al. Brain stimulation methods to treat tobacco addiction. *Brain Stimul.* 2013;6(3):221-230.
42. Hanlon CA, Dowdle LT, Austelle CW, et al. What goes up, can come down: novel brain stimulation paradigms may attenuate craving and craving-related neural circuitry in substance dependent individuals. *Brain Res.* 2015;1628(Pt A):199-209.
43. Sandrini M, Umilta C, Rusconi E. The use of transcranial magnetic stimulation in cognitive neuroscience: a new synthesis of methodological issues. *Neurosci Biobehav Rev.* 2011;35(3):516-536.
44. Luber BM, Davis S, Bernhardt E, et al. Using neuroimaging to individualize TMS treatment for depression: toward a new paradigm for imaging-guided intervention. *Neuroimage.* 2017;148:1-7.
45. Eichhammer P, Johann M, Kharraz A, et al. High-frequency repetitive transcranial magnetic stimulation decreases cigarette smoking. *J Clin Psychiatry.* 2003;64(8):951-953.
46. Li X, Hartwell KJ, Owens M, et al. Repetitive transcranial magnetic stimulation of the dorsolateral prefrontal cortex reduces nicotine cue craving. *Biol Psychiatry.* 2013;73(8):714-720.
47. Pripfl J, Tomova L, Riecansky I, Lamm C. Transcranial magnetic stimulation of the left dorsolateral prefrontal cortex decreases cue-induced nicotine craving and EEG delta power. *Brain Stimul.* 2014;7(2):226-233.
48. Herremans SC, Baeken C, Vanderbruggen N, et al. No influence of one right-sided prefrontal HF-rTMS session on alcohol craving in recently detoxified alcohol-dependent patients: results of a naturalistic study. *Drug Alcohol Depend.* 2012;120(1-3):209-213.
49. Höppner J, Broese T, Wendler L, Berger C, Thome J. Repetitive transcranial magnetic stimulation (rTMS) for treatment of alcohol dependence. *World J Biol Psychiatry.* 2011;12(Suppl 1):57-62.
50. Mishra BR, Nizamie SH, Das B, Praharaj SK. Efficacy of repetitive transcranial magnetic stimulation in alcohol dependence: a sham-controlled study. *Addiction.* 2010;105(1):49-55.
51. Camprodon JA, Martínez-Raga J, Alonso-Alonso M, Shih M-C, Pascual-Leone A. One session of high frequency repetitive transcranial magnetic stimulation (rTMS) to the right prefrontal cortex transiently reduces cocaine craving. *Drug Alcohol Depend.* 2007;86(1):91-94.
52. Politi E, Fauci E, Santoro A, Smeraldi E. Daily sessions of transcranial magnetic stimulation to the left prefrontal cortex gradually reduce cocaine craving. *Am J Addict.* 2008;17(4):345-346.
53. Moran-Santa Maria MM, Hartwell KJ, Hanlon CA, et al. Right anterior insula connectivity is important for cue-induced craving in nicotine-dependent smokers. *Addict Biol.* 2015;20(2):407-414.
54. Naqvi NH, Gaznick N, Tranel D, Bechara A. The insula: a critical neural substrate for craving and drug seeking under conflict and risk. *Ann N Y Acad Sci.* 2014;1316:53-70.
55. Hanlon CA, Canterberry M, Taylor JJ, et al. Probing the frontostriatal loops involved in executive and limbic processing via interleaved TMS and functional MRI at two prefrontal locations: a pilot study. *PLoS One.* 2013;8(7):e67917.
56. Kearney-Ramos TE, Lench DH, Hoffmann M, et al. Gray and white matter integrity influence TMS signal propagation: a multimodal evaluation in cocaine-dependent individuals. *Sci Rep.* 2018;8(1):3253.
57. Martinez D, Urban N, Grassetti A, et al. Transcranial magnetic stimulation of medial prefrontal and cingulate cortices reduces cocaine self-administration: a pilot study. *Front Psychiatry.* 20189:80.
58. McCalley DM, Hanlon CA. Regionally specific gray matter volume is lower in alcohol use disorder: implications for noninvasive brain stimulation treatment. *Alcohol Clin Exp Res.* 2021;45(8):1672-1683.
59. Harel M, Perini I, Kämpe R, et al. Repetitive transcranial magnetic stimulation in alcohol dependence: a randomized, double-blind, sham-controlled proof-of-concept trial targeting the medial prefrontal and anterior cingulate cortices. *Biol Psychiatry.* 2022;91(12):1061-1069.
60. Joutsa J, Moussawi K, Siddiqi SH, et al. Brain lesions disrupting addiction map to a common human brain circuit. *Nat Med.* 2022;28(6):1249-1255.
61. Tsagaris KZ, Labar DR, Edwards DJ. A framework for combining rTMS with behavioral therapy. *Front Syst Neurosci.* 2016;10:82.
62. George MS, Lisanby SH, Avery D, et al. Daily left prefrontal transcranial magnetic stimulation therapy for major depressive disorder: a sham-controlled randomized trial. *Arch Gen Psychiatry.* 2010;67(5):507-516.
63. Vedeniapin A, Cheng L, George MS. Feasibility of simultaneous cognitive behavioral therapy and left prefrontal rTMS for treatment resistant depression. *Brain Stimul.* 2010;3(4):207-210.
64. Donse L, Padberg F, Sack AT, Rush AJ, Arns M. Simultaneous rTMS and psychotherapy in major depressive disorder: clinical outcomes and predictors from a large naturalistic study. *Brain Stimul.* 2018;11(2):337-345.
65. Vedeniapin A, Cheng L, George MS. Feasibility of simultaneous cognitive behavioral therapy (CBT) and left prefrontal rTMS for treatment resistant depression. *Brain Stimul.* 2010;3(4):207-210.

66. Kozel FA, Motes MA, Didehbani N, et al. Repetitive TMS to augment cognitive processing therapy in combat veterans of recent conflicts with PTSD: a randomized clinical trial. *J Affect Disord.* 2018;229:506-514.
67. Sheffer CE, Bickel WK, Brandon TH, et al. Preventing relapse to smoking with transcranial magnetic stimulation: feasibility and potential efficacy. *Drug Alcohol Depend.* 2018;182:8-18.
68. Carroll KM, Onken LS. Behavioral therapies for drug abuse. *Am J Psychiatry.* 2005;162(8):1452-1460.
69. Beauregard M. Functional neuroimaging studies of the effects of psychotherapy. *Dialogues Clin Neurosci.* 2014;16(1):75-81.
70. Huerta PT, Volpe BT. Transcranial magnetic stimulation, synaptic plasticity and network oscillations. *J NeuroEng Rehabil.* 2009;6:7.
71. Hanlon CA, Dowdle LT, Henderson JS. Modulating neural circuits with transcranial magnetic stimulation: implications for addiction treatment development. *Pharmacol Rev.* 2018;70(3):661-683.
72. Thair H, Holloway AL, Newport R, Smith AD. Transcranial Direct Current Stimulation (tDCS): a beginner's guide for design and implementation. *Front Neurosci.* 2017;11:641.
73. Benwell CS, Learmonth G, Miniussi C, Harvey M, Thut G. Non-linear effects of transcranial direct current stimulation as a function of individual baseline performance: evidence from biparietal tDCS influence on lateralized attention bias. *Cortex.* 2015;69:152-165.
74. Brunoni AR, Moffa AH, Sampaio-Junior B, et al. trial of electrical direct-current therapy versus escitalopram for depression. *N Engl J Med.* 2017;376(26):2523-2533.
75. Berryhill ME, Peterson DJ, Jones KT, Stephens JA. Hits and misses: leveraging tDCS to advance cognitive research. *Front Psychol.* 2014;5:800.
76. Li LM, Uehara K, Hanakawa T. The contribution of interindividual factors to variability of response in transcranial direct current stimulation studies. *Front Cell Neurosci.* 2015;9:181.
77. Coffman BA, Clark VP, Parasuraman R. Battery powered thought: enhancement of attention, learning, and memory in healthy adults using transcranial direct current stimulation. *Neuroimage.* 2014;85(Pt 3): 895-908.
78. Parasuraman R, McKinley RA. Using noninvasive brain stimulation to accelerate learning and enhance human performance. *Hum Factors.* 2014;56(5):816-824.
79. Herrera-Melendez AL, Bajbouj M, Aust S. Application of transcranial direct current stimulation in psychiatry. *Neuropsychobiology.* 2020; 79(6):372-383.
80. Fregni F, Liguori P, Fecteau S, Nitsche MA, Pascual-Leone A, Boggio PS. Cortical stimulation of the prefrontal cortex with transcranial direct current stimulation reduces cue-provoked smoking craving: a randomized, sham-controlled study. *J Clin Psychiatry.* 2008;69(1):32-40.
81. Boggio PS, Liguori P, Sultani S, Rezende L, Fecteau S, Fregni F. Cumulative priming effects of cortical stimulation on smoking cue-induced craving. *Neurosci Lett.* 2009;463(1):82-86.
82. Boggio PS, Sultani S, Fecteau S, et al. Prefrontal cortex modulation using transcranial DC stimulation reduces alcohol craving: a double-blind, sham-controlled study. *Drug Alcohol Depend.* 2008;92(1-3):55-60.
83. da Silva MC, Conti CL, Klauss J, et al. Behavioral effects of transcranial direct current stimulation (tDCS) induced dorsolateral prefrontal cortex plasticity in alcohol dependence. *J Physiol Paris.* 2013;107(6):493-502.
84. Batista EK, Klauss J, Fregni F, Nitsche MA, Nakamura-Palacios EM. A randomized placebo-controlled trial of targeted prefrontal cortex modulation with bilateral tDCS in patients with crack-cocaine dependence. *Int J Neuropsychopharmacol.* 2015;18(12):pyv066.
85. Boggio PS, Zaghi S, Villani AB, Fecteau S, Pascual-Leone A, Fregni F. Modulation of risk-taking in marijuana users by transcranial direct current stimulation (tDCS) of the dorsolateral prefrontal cortex (DLPFC). *Drug Alcohol Depend.* 2010;112(3):220-225.
86. di Biase L, Falato E, Di Lazzaro V. Transcranial Focused Ultrasound (tFUS) and Transcranial Unfocused Ultrasound (tUS) neuromodulation: from theoretical principles to stimulation practices. *Front Neurol.* 2019;10:549.
87. Darrow DP. Focused ultrasound for neuromodulation. *Neurotherapeutics.* 2019;16(1):88-99.
88. Hardesty DE, Sackeim HA. Deep brain stimulation in movement and psychiatric disorders. *Biol Psychiatry.* 2007;61(7):831-835.
89. Zhou H, Xu J, Jiang J. Deep brain stimulation of nucleus accumbens on heroin-seeking behaviors: a case report. *Biol Psychiatry.* 2011;69(11): e41-e42.
90. Kuhn J, Möller M, Treppmann JF, et al. Deep brain stimulation of the nucleus accumbens and its usefulness in severe opioid addiction. *Mol Psychiatry.* 2014;19(2):145-146.
91. Müller UJ, Sturm V, Voges J, et al. Nucleus accumbens deep brain stimulation for alcohol addiction—safety and clinical long-term results of a pilot trial. *Pharmacopsychiatry.* 2016;49(4):170-173.
92. Kuhn J, Lenartz D, Mai JK, et al. Deep brain stimulation of the nucleus accumbens and the internal capsule in therapeutically refractory Tourette-syndrome. *J Neurol.* 2007;254(7):963-965.
93. Denys D, Mantione M, Figee M, et al. Deep brain stimulation of the nucleus accumbens for treatment-refractory obsessive-compulsive disorder. *Arch Gen Psychiatry.* 2010;67(10):1061-1068.
94. Grant JE, Odlaug BL, Chamberlain SR. Neurocognitive response to deep brain stimulation for obsessive-compulsive disorder: a case report. *Am J Psychiatry.* 2011;168(12):1338-1339.
95. Sachdev PS, Cannon E, Coyne TJ, Silburn P. Bilateral deep brain stimulation of the nucleus accumbens for comorbid obsessive compulsive disorder and Tourette's syndrome. *BMJ Case Rep.* 2012;2012:bcr2012006579.
96. Luigjes J, van den Brink W, Feenstra M, et al. Deep brain stimulation in addiction: a review of potential brain targets. *Mol Psychiatry.* 2012;17(6):572-583.

Psychologically Based Interventions

Associate Editor: Richard N. Rosenthal
Lead Section Editor: Antoine Douaihy
Section Editors: Dennis C. Daley and Eric L. Garland

CHAPTER

69 Enhancing Motivation to Change

James O. Prochaska and Janice M. Prochaska

CHAPTER OUTLINE

- Introduction
- The stages of change
- Using the stages of change model to catalyze motivation
- Multiple domains of well-being: From suffering or struggling to thriving
- Conclusions

INTRODUCTION

What motivates people to take action? The answer to this key question depends on what type of action is to be taken. What moves people to start therapy? What motivates them to continue therapy? What moves people to progress in therapy or to continue to progress after therapy?

Answers to these questions can provide better alternatives to one of the field's most pressing concerns: What types of therapeutic interventions would have the greatest effect on the entire population at risk for or experiencing addiction?

What motivates people to change? The answer to this question depends in part on where they start. What motivates people to begin thinking about change can be different from what motivates them to begin preparing to take action. Once people are prepared, different forces can move them to take action. Once action is taken, what motivates people to maintain that action? Conversely, what causes people to return to their addictive behaviors? Fortunately, the answers to this complex set of questions may be simpler, or at least more systematic, than are the questions themselves. To appreciate the answers, it is helpful to begin with the authors' model of change.[1-4]

THE STAGES OF CHANGE

Change is a process that unfolds over time through a series of stages: precontemplation, contemplation, preparation, action, maintenance, and termination.

Precontemplation (not ready) is a stage in which the individual does not intend to take action in the foreseeable future (usually measured as the next 6 months). Individuals may be at this stage because they are uninformed or underinformed about the consequences of a given behavior. Or they may have tried to change a number of times and become demoralized about their ability to do so. Individuals in both categories tend to avoid reading, talking, or thinking about their high-risk behaviors. In other theories, such individuals are characterized as "resistant" or "unmotivated" or "not ready" for therapy or health promotion programs. In fact, traditional treatment programs were not ready for such individuals and were not motivated to match their needs.

Individuals who are in the precontemplation stage typically underestimate the benefits of change and overestimate its costs but are unaware that they are making such mistakes. If they are not conscious of making such mistakes, it is difficult for them to change. As a result, many remain in the precontemplation stage for years, with considerable resulting harm to their bodies, themselves, and others. There appears to be no inherent motivation for people to progress from one stage to the next. The stages are not like stages of human development, in which children have inherent motivation to progress from crawling to walking, even though crawling works very well and even though learning to walk can be painful and embarrassing. Instead, two major forces can move people to progress.

The first is *developmental events*. In the author's research, the mean age of people who smoke tobacco who reach long-term maintenance is 39 years. Those who have passed 39 recognize it as an age to reevaluate how one has been living and whether one wants to die from that lifestyle or whether one wants to enhance the quality and quantity of the second half of life. The other naturally occurring force is *environmental events*. A favorite example is a couple who both smoked heavily. Their dog of many years died of lung cancer. This death eventually moved the wife to quit smoking. The husband bought a new dog. So, even the same events can be processed differently by different people.

A common belief is that people with substance use disorders (SUD) must "hit bottom" before they are motivated to change. So family, friends, and physicians wait helplessly for a crisis to occur. But how often do people turn 39 or have a dog die? When individuals show the first signs of a serious physical illness, such as cancer or cardiovascular disease, those around them usually become mobilized to help them seek early intervention. Evidence shows that early interventions often are life- saving, and so it would not be acceptable to wait for such a patient to "hit bottom." In opposition to such a passive stance, a third force that has been created to help patients with addiction progress beyond the precontemplation stage is called *planned interventions*.

Contemplation (getting ready) is a stage in which individuals intend to take action within the ensuing 6 months. Such persons are more aware of the benefits of changing, but also are acutely aware of the costs. When addicted persons begin to seriously contemplate giving up favorite substances, their awareness of the costs of changing can increase. There is no free change. This balance between the costs and benefits of change can produce profound ambivalence, which may reflect a type of love-hate relationship with an addictive substance, and thus can keep an individual stuck at the contemplation stage for long periods of time. This phenomenon often is characterized as "chronic contemplation" or "behavioral procrastination." Such individuals are not ready for traditional action-oriented programs.

Preparation (ready) is a stage in which individuals intend to take action in the immediate future (usually measured as the ensuing month). Such persons typically have taken some significant action within the preceding year. They generally have a plan of action, such as participating in a recovery group, consulting a counselor, talking to a physician, buying a self-help book, or relying on a self-change approach. It is these individuals who should be recruited for action-oriented treatment programs.

Action (doing the healthy behavior) is a stage in which individuals have made specific, overt modifications in their lifestyle within the preceding 6 months. Because action is observable, behavior change often has been equated with action. But in the transtheoretical model (TTM), action is only one of six stages.[3] In this model, not all modifications of behavior count as action. An individual must attain a criterion that scientists and professionals agree is sufficient to reduce the risk of disease. In smoking tobacco for example, for the vast majority of consequences, only total abstinence counts. With alcohol use disorders, many believe that only total abstinence can be effective, whereas others accept controlled drinking as an effective action.

Maintenance (keeping up the healthy behavior) is a stage in which individuals are working to prevent recurrence of use but do not need to apply change processes as frequently as one would in the action stage. Such persons are less tempted and are increasingly confident that they can sustain the changes made. Temptation and self-efficacy data suggest that maintenance lasts from 6 months to about 5 years. One of the common reasons for early return to use is that individuals are not well prepared for the prolonged effort needed to progress to maintenance. Many persons think the worst will be over in a few weeks or a few months. If, as a result, they ease up on their efforts too early, they are at great risk.

To prepare such individuals for what is to come, they should be encouraged to think of overcoming a SUD as running a marathon rather than a sprint. They may have wanted to enter the Boston Marathon, but they know they would not succeed without preparation and so would not enter the race. With some preparation, they might compete for several miles but still would fail to finish the race. Only those who are well prepared could maintain their efforts mile after mile. Using the Boston Marathon metaphor, people know they have to be well prepared if they are to survive Heartbreak Hill, which runners encounter at about mile 20. What is the behavioral equivalent of Heartbreak Hill? The best evidence available suggests that most return to use occurs at times of emotional distress. It is in the presence of depression, anxiety, anger, boredom, loneliness, stress, and distress that humans are at their emotional and psychological weak point.

How does the average person cope with troubling times? They drink more, eat more, smoke more, and take more substances to cope with distress.[4] It is not surprising, therefore, that persons struggling to overcome a SUD will be at greatest risk when they face distress without their substance of choice. Although emotional distress cannot be prevented, return to use can be prevented if patients have been prepared to cope with distress without falling back on addictive substances.

If so many Americans rely on oral consumptive behavior as a way to manage their emotions, what is the healthiest oral behavior they could use? Talking with others about one's distress is a means of seeking support that can help prevent recurrence of their illness. Another healthy alternative is exercise. Physical activity helps manage moods, stress, and distress. Also, 150 minutes per week of exercise can provide a recovering person with more than 70 health and mental health benefits.[4]

Exercise of a medically appropriate level thus should be prescribed to all sedentary patients with a SUD. A third healthy alternative is some form of deep relaxation, such as meditation, yoga, prayer, massage, or deep muscle relaxation. Letting the stress and distress drift away from one's muscles and one's mind helps the patient move forward at the most tempting of times.

Helping patient populations to not smoke, eat healthy, exercise, and manage stress effectively has recently been recommended by three federal agencies that have major responsibilities for SUD and mental illness. The Substance Abuse and Mental Health Agency (SAMSHA),[5] the National Institutes of Health (NIH),[6] and the Center for Medicare and Medicaid Innovation (CMMI)[7] have concluded that these health risk behaviors are major causes of chronic diseases and disabilities and premature death in almost all populations. But populations with severe mental illness (SMI) and SUD die an average of 10 years earlier. The latest recovery movement also recommends such holistic health care, in part, because any commitment to enhance health can be motivators that can begin the recovery process.[8]

Termination is a stage at which individuals have zero temptation and 100% self-efficacy. No matter whether they are depressed, anxious, bored, lonely, angry, or stressed, such persons are certain that they will not return to their old unhealthy habits as a method of coping. It is as if they never acquired the habit in the first place. In a study of people who formerly smoked and people with alcohol use disorders, fewer than 20% of each group had reached the stage of no temptation and total self-efficacy.[9] The latest recovery movement also recognizes that many people want to be recovered so that they can dedicate their time and resources to enhancing other aspects of their health and well-being.[8] Although the ideal is to be cured or totally recovered, it is important to recognize that, for many patients, a more realistic expectation is a lifetime of maintenance.

USING THE STAGES OF CHANGE MODEL TO CATALYZE MOTIVATION

The stages of change model can be applied to identify ways to motivate more patients at each phase of planned interventions for the SUD. The five phases are recruitment, retention, progress, process, and outcomes.

Recruitment

Too few studies have paid attention to the fact that professional treatment programs recruit or reach too few persons with SUDs. Across all diagnoses in the *Diagnostic and Statistical Manual of Mental Disorders*, 5th edition,[10] fewer than 25% of persons with SUDs enter professional treatment in their lifetimes. With tobacco/nicotine use disorder, the deadliest of use disorders, fewer than 10% ever participate in a professional treatment program.

Given that SUDs are among the costliest of contemporary conditions, it is crucial to motivate many more persons to participate in appropriate treatment. These conditions are costly to the individuals with addiction, their families and friends, their employers, their communities, and their health care systems. Health professionals no longer can treat addiction just on a case basis; instead, they must develop programs that can reach persons with a SUD on a population basis.

How can more people with SUDs be motivated to seek the appropriate help? By changing both paradigms and practices. There are two paradigms that need to be changed. The first is an action-oriented paradigm that construes behavior change as an event that can occur quickly, immediately, discretely, and dramatically. Treatment programs that are designed to have patients immediately quit using substances are implicitly or explicitly designed for the portion of the population in the preparation stage.

The problem is that, with most unhealthy behaviors, fewer than 20% of the affected population are prepared to take action. Among people who smoke (the vast majority of which have tobacco/nicotine use disorder) in the United States, for example, about 40% are in the precontemplation stage, 40% in the contemplation stage, and 20% in the preparation stage.[11] Among college students with alcohol use disorder, about 85% are in the precontemplation stage, 10% in the contemplation stage, and 5% in the preparation stage.[12]

When only action-oriented interventions are offered, less than 20% of the at-risk population is being recruited. To meet the needs of the entire addicted population, interventions must meet the needs of the 40% in the precontemplation and the 40% in the contemplation stages.

By offering stage-matched interventions and applying proactive or outreach recruitment methods in three large-scale clinical trials, the author and others have been able to motivate 80% to 90% of people who smoke tobacco to enter a treatment program.[13,14] Comparable participation rates were generated with college students with at-risk alcohol use, even though 75% were in the precontemplation stage.[12] These results represent a quantum increase in our ability to move many more people to take the action of starting therapy.

The second paradigm change that is required is movement from a passive-reactive approach to a proactive approach. Most professionals have been trained to be passive-reactive: to passively wait for patients to seek their services and then to react. The problem with this approach is that most persons with SUDs never seek such services.

The passive-reactive paradigm is designed to serve populations with acute conditions. The pain, distress, or discomfort of such conditions can motivate patients to seek the services of health professionals. But the major killers today are chronic lifestyle disorders such as SUDs. To treat the SUDs seriously, professionals must learn how to reach out to entire populations and offer them stage-matched treatments.

There are a growing number of national disease management and disease prevention companies who train health professionals in these new paradigms. Nurses, counselors, and health coaches have been trained to proactively reach out by telephone to interact at each stage of change with entire patient and employee populations with unhealthy behaviors including smoking tobacco, hazardous alcohol use, and obesity. With the major movement toward integrated care in patient-centered medical homes, providers on multidisciplinary teams are being trained in how to deliver such stage-based interventions within primary care and other medical settings.

Historically, the established wisdom was that therapists should not address tobacco use disorders with mental health patients.[15] The tobacco industry supported this perspective with ads and reports targeting mental health professionals. In the Clinical Guideline for the Treatment of Tobacco, there were no evidence-based treatments for people with co-occurring tobacco use disorder and mental health disorders, even though they consume over 40% of all cigarettes in the United States.[16] One unsupported bias that was encouraged was that such patients could not be motivated to quit, in part, because they used nicotine to self-medicate their co-occurring psychiatric disorder.

Two studies using computer-tailored TTM interventions (CTIs) provided evidence that such assumptions were invalid. In the first study, people who smoked tobacco engaged in depression clinics were proactively recruited to a randomized clinical trial (RCT) for such CTIs. The results were clear. The treatment group had long-term quit rates of about 25%, which were significantly higher than the controls (19%) and were essentially identical to people who smoked but did not have co-occurring without mental illness. Furthermore, the treatment group had as good results with depression that were comparable to controls, indicating that stopping smoking did not interfere with depression treatments.

The second study was with patients hospitalized for acute episodes of serious mental illness (SMI). People who smoked tobacco were proactively recruited to an RCT comparing a TTM-based CTI to controls. The treatment group had a long-term abstinence rate (20%) that was not as high as most populations (25%) but was 2.5 times greater than controls (8%).[15] What was particularly striking was that over the next 12 months, the treatment group had significantly fewer rehospitalizations than controls. Rather than stopping smoking resulting in decreasing motivation with mental health treatments, with depression, there was no apparent effect, and with SMIs, the group that stopped smoking actually did better.

In the face of this evidence, there may be several answers to the question: What can move a majority of people to enter a professional treatment program for an addiction? One is the availability of professionals who are motivated and prepared to proactively reach out to entire populations and offer them interventions that match whatever stage of change they are in.

Retention

What motivates patients to continue in therapy? Or conversely, what moves clients to terminate counseling quickly and prematurely, as judged by their counselors? A meta-analysis of 125 studies found that nearly 50% of clients drop out of treatment.[17] Across studies, there were few consistent predictors of premature termination. Although SUD, minority status, and lower education predicted a higher percentage of people prematurely leaving treatment, these variables did not account for much of the variance.

Studies are available on people who prematurely leave treatment from a stage model perspective on SUD, obesity, and a broad spectrum of psychiatric disorders. These studies found that stage-related variables were more reliable predictors than were demographics, type of problem, severity of problem, and other problem-related variables. Figure 66-1 presents the stage profiles of three groups of patients with a broad spectrum of psychiatric disorders.[18] In that study, the investigators were able to predict 93% of the three groups: premature terminators, early but appropriate terminators, and those who continued in therapy.[18] **Figure 69-1** shows that the before-therapy profile of the entire group who dropped out quickly and prematurely (40%) was a profile of persons in the precontemplation stage. The 20% who finished quickly but appropriately had a profile of patients who were in the action stage at the time they entered therapy. Those who continued in long-term treatment were a mixed group, with most in the contemplation stage.

The lesson is clear: Persons in the precontemplation stage cannot be treated as if they are starting in the same place as those in the action stage. If they are pressured to take action when they are not prepared, they simply will leave therapy. For patients in the action stage who enter therapy, what would be an appropriate approach? One alternative would be to provide return to use prevention strategies. But would return to use prevention strategies make any sense with the 40% of patients who enter in the precontemplation stage? What might be a good match for them? Experience suggests an early treatment departure prevention approach, because such patients are likely to leave early if they are not helped to continue.

With patients who begin therapy in the precontemplation stage, it is useful for the therapist to share key concerns: "I'm concerned that therapy may not have a chance to make a significant difference in your life, because you may be tempted to leave early." The therapist then can explore whether the patient has been pressured to enter therapy. How do such patients react when someone tries to pressure or coerce them into quitting an addiction when they are not ready? Can they tell the therapist if they feel pressured or coerced? It is only feasible to encourage them to take steps when they are most ready to succeed.

Patients in treatment for SUDs were assessed on their perceptions of the pros and cons of therapy and whether they were in therapy because of coercion or by choice.[19] Patients in precontemplation perceived the cons of therapy as higher than the pros and that they were in therapy more out of coercion than by choice. Patients in action, on the other hand, had the opposite pattern: pros were greater than cons and choice greater than coercion. These patterns were only found when raw scores were standardized to control for ease of responding, with it being harder to endorse cons and coercions. These results indicate that such standardized

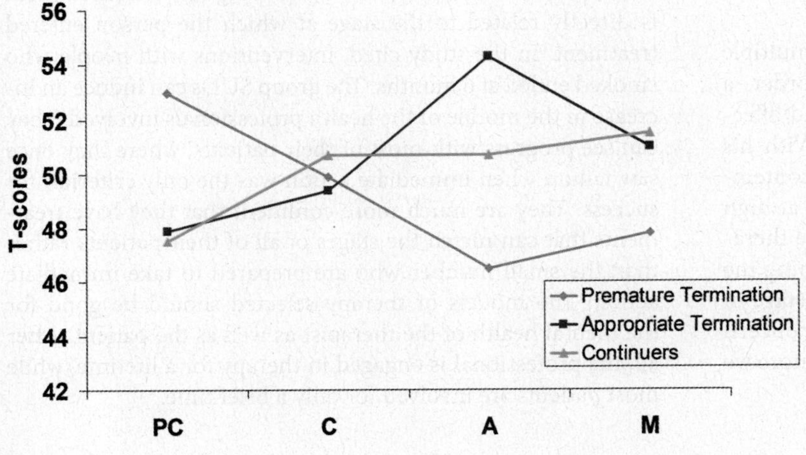

Figure 69-1. Pretherapy stage profiles for premature terminators and continuers. PC, precontemplation; C, contemplation; A, action; M, management. (From Brogan ME, Prochaska JO, Prochaska JM. Predicting termination and continuation status in psychotherapy using the Transtheoretical Model. *Psychotherapy*. 1999;36:105-113.)

perspectives are likely revealing implicit cognitions rather than rational choices. These patterns help to explain why patients in precontemplation are so likely to terminate quickly from SUD clinics.

The patterns also suggest that as people progress from precontemplation, they are likely to transform coercion into personal choice as motivators driving their engagement in treatment and their changes in their SUD. A large study in the U.S. Air Force supports this interpretation. Wanting a tobacco-free Air Force, all enlisted people had to be fully nicotine free for 6 weeks of basic training. Random urine samples were drawn, and the consequence of any sign of cotinine was severe—the entire 6 weeks of basic training had to be repeated. Such coercion produced immediate and essentially absolute abstinence for 6 weeks.[20] But at 12-month follow-up, the nicotine use rates were remarkable at 123%, meaning that there were 23% more enlisted people using tobacco than when they joined.

To reduce such recurrence of use, 7,000 people who smoked were given a 45-minute intervention that involved the discussion of the important pros or benefits of staying quit. This was seen as a return to use prevention program, but in TTM terms, we shall soon see that it would be the first principle (raise the pros) to help people in precontemplation to progress. As it turned out, this intervention had no significant impact on preventing return to use in the total treatment group compared to the 30,000 controls. But, people in the precontemplation group who were intending to return to smoking as soon as basic training ended were four times more likely to be quit at 12 months, and enlisted people of color were five times more likely to stay quit. With precontemplators who would be likely to feel particularly coerced, this brief but matched treatment was likely to have helped them progress to choosing to stay quit even after they were fully free to smoke.

Here is a brief case illustration of a therapist sharing his concern with a patient in precontemplation:

Case Illustration

An artist in his late thirties started therapy with multiple problems, including a chronic cocaine use disorder, a troubled marriage, career at risk of collapsing, and affective problems with depression and aggression. With his help, we are able to assess that he was in the precontemplation stage, and his therapist knew that he was at high risk for terminating treatment prematurely. So, the therapist shared his concern: "I appreciate you are helping me to understand that you are currently in the initial stage of change that we call precontemplation. Our first concern needs to be that you might drop out of treatment before we have a chance to make a significant difference in your life. What pressures were there for you to come to therapy?"

"My wife threatened to leave if I didn't show up," he responded. "If you feel me pressuring you to do something you are not ready to do, would you let me know?" the therapist asked. "You will know!" he snapped.

"How will I know?"

Because I will get angry as hell!" the patient said.

"That's O.K. I can work with that. What I can't work with is you not coming back."

"That's cool," he said.

The author and others have conducted four studies with stage-matched interventions in which retention rates of persons entering interventions in the precontemplation stage can be examined. When treatment is matched to stage, persons in the precontemplation stage will remain in treatment at the same rates as those who start in the preparation stage.[13,14] This result was consistent in clinical trials in which patients were recruited proactively (the therapist reached out with an offer of help) as well as in trials in which patients were recruited reactively (they asked for help). What motivates people to continue in therapy? Receiving treatments that match their stage of readiness to change.

Another strategy is to begin therapy with a single session of motivational interviewing. Connors et al.[21] found that a single session reduced premature treatment departure from their 12-session alcohol treatment program from 75% to 50%. A session of role induction designed to prepare people for what to expect from therapy made no difference, even though, clinically, it has been most widely used to try to prevent premature treatment discontinuation.

Progress

What moves people to progress in therapy and to continue to progress after therapy? **Figure 69-2** presents an example of what is called the *stage effect*. The stage effect predicts that the amount of successful action taken during and after treatment is directly related to the stage at which the person entered treatment. In the study cited, interventions with people who smoked ended at 6 months. The group SUDs can induce an increase in the morale of the health professionals involved. They can see progress with most of their patients, where they once saw failure when immediate action was the only criterion for success. They are much more confident that they have treatments that can match the stages of all of their patients rather than the small number who are prepared to take immediate action. The models of therapy selected should be good for the mental health of the therapist as well as the patient. After all, the professional is engaged in therapy for a lifetime, while most patients are involved for only a brief time.

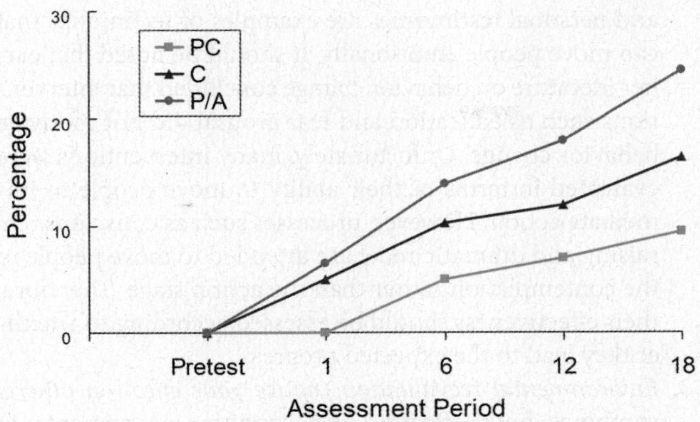

Figure 69-2. Percentage of people smoking who maintained abstinence over 18 months. Groups were in the following stages at the time they went into treatment: precontemplation (PC), contemplation (C), and preparation (P/A) ($N = 570$).

As health care organizations move to briefer and briefer therapies for SUD and other disorders, there is a danger that most health professionals will feel pressured to produce immediate action. If this pressure is transferred to patients who are not prepared for such action, most patients will not be reached or not retained in treatment. A majority of patients can be helped to progress in treatment through relatively brief encounters, but only if realistic goals are set for both patient and therapist. Otherwise, there is a risk of demoralizing and demotivating both patient and therapist. Given the vast public health needs described above, another misuse of the model is for health care organizations or health professionals to limit treatment only to patients who are prepared to take immediate action.

Process

To help motivate patients to progress from one stage to the next, it is necessary to know the principles and processes of change that can produce such progress.

Principle 1

The benefits for changing must increase if patients are to progress beyond precontemplation. In a review of 12 studies, all showed that the perceived benefits were higher in the contemplation than in the precontemplation stage.[22,23] This pattern held true across 12 behaviors: use of cocaine, smoking, delinquency, obesity, inconsistent condom use, unsafe sex, sedentary lifestyles, high-fat diets, sun exposure, radon testing, mammography screening, and physicians practicing behavioral medicine.

A technique that can be used in population-based programs involves asking a patient in the precontemplation stage to describe all the benefits of a change such as quitting smoking or starting to exercise. Most persons can list four or five. The therapist can let the patient know that there are 8 to 10 times that number and challenge the patient to double or triple the list for the next meeting. If the patient's list of benefits of stopping tobacco use begins to indicate many more motives, such as a healthier heart, healthier lungs, more energy, healthier immune system, better moods, less stress, and enhanced self-esteem, they will be more motivated to begin to seriously contemplate such a change.

Principle 2

The "cons" of changing must decrease if patients are to progress from contemplation to action. In 12 of 12 studies, the author found that the perceived costs of changing were lower in the action than in the contemplation stage.[23]

Principle 3

The relative weight assigned to benefits and costs must cross over before a patient will be prepared to take action. In 12 of 12 studies, the costs of changing were assessed as higher than the rewards in the precontemplation stage, but in 11 of 12, the rewards were assessed as higher than the costs in the action stage. The sole exception involved quitting cocaine. In that study, a large percentage of treatment was delivered to inpatients. We interpret this exception to mean that the actions of these patients may have been more under the social control of residential care than under their self-control. At a minimum, their pattern would not bode well for immediate discharge. It should be noted that, if raw scores are used to assess these patterns, it would appear that the rewards for changing are seen as greater than the costs, even by persons in the precontemplation stage. It is only when standardized scores are used that clear patterns emerge, with the costs of changing always perceived as greater than the rewards. This suggests that, compared with their peers at other stages of change, persons in the precontemplation stage underestimate the rewards and overestimate the costs of change.

Principle 4

The strong principle of progress holds that to progress from precontemplation to effective action, the rewards for changing must increase by one standard deviation (SD).[23]

Principle 5

The weak principle of progress holds that to progress from contemplation to effective action, the perceived costs of changing must decrease by one-half SD. Because the perceived benefits for changing must increase twice as much as the perceived costs decrease, twice as much emphasis must be placed on the benefits than the costs of changing.

In a recent meta-analysis of nearly 140 studies on 48 behaviors, the pros of changing increased by exactly 1.00 SD, whereas the cons decreased by 0.54 SD.[24] Such principles can produce much more sensitive assessments to guide interventions, giving therapists and patients feedback for when therapeutic efforts are producing progress and when they are failing. Together, they can modify methods if movement is needed for the patient to become adequately prepared for action.

Principle 6

It is important to match particular processes of change with specific stages of change. **Table 69-1** presents the empirical integration found between processes and stages of change. Guided by this integration, the following processes would be applied to patients in various stages of change:

1. *Consciousness raising (get the facts)* involves increased awareness of the causes, consequences, and responses to a particular problem. Interventions that can increase awareness include observations, confrontations, interpretations, feedback, and education. Some techniques, such as confrontation, pose considerable risk in terms of retention and are not recommended as highly as motivational enhancement methods such as personal feedback about the current and long-term consequences of continuing the addictive behavior. Increasing the costs of not changing is the corollary of raising the rewards for changing. So, consciousness raising should be designed to increase the perceived rewards for changing.
2. *Dramatic relief (pay attention to feelings)* involves emotional arousal about one's current behavior and the relief that can come from changing. Fear, inspiration, guilt, and hope are some of the emotions that can move persons to contemplate changing. Psychodrama, role-playing, grieving, and personal testimonies are examples of techniques that can move people emotionally. It should be noted that earlier literature on behavior change concluded that interventions such as education and fear arousal did not motivate behavior change. Unfortunately, many interventions were evaluated in terms of their ability to move people to immediate action. However, processes such as consciousness raising and dramatic relief are intended to move people to the contemplation rather than the action stage. Therefore, their effectiveness should be assessed according to whether they lead to the expected progress.
3. *Environmental reevaluation (notice your effect on others)* combines both affective and cognitive assessments of how addiction affects one's social environment and how changing would affect that environment. Empathy training, values clarification, and family or network interventions can facilitate such reevaluation. For example, a brief media intervention aimed at a person who smokes in precontemplation might involve an image of a man clearly in grief saying, "I always feared that my smoking would lead to an early death. I always worried that my smoking would cause lung cancer. But I never imagined it would happen to my wife." Beneath his grieving face appears this statistic: "50,000 deaths per year are caused by passive smoking." In 30 seconds, this message achieves consciousness raising, dramatic relief, and environmental reevaluation.
4. *Self-reevaluation (create a new self-image)* combines both cognitive and affective assessments of an image of one's self free from addiction. Imagery, healthier role models, and values clarification are techniques that can move individuals in this type of intervention. Clinically, patients first look back and reevaluate how they have lived as individuals with an addiction. As they progress into the

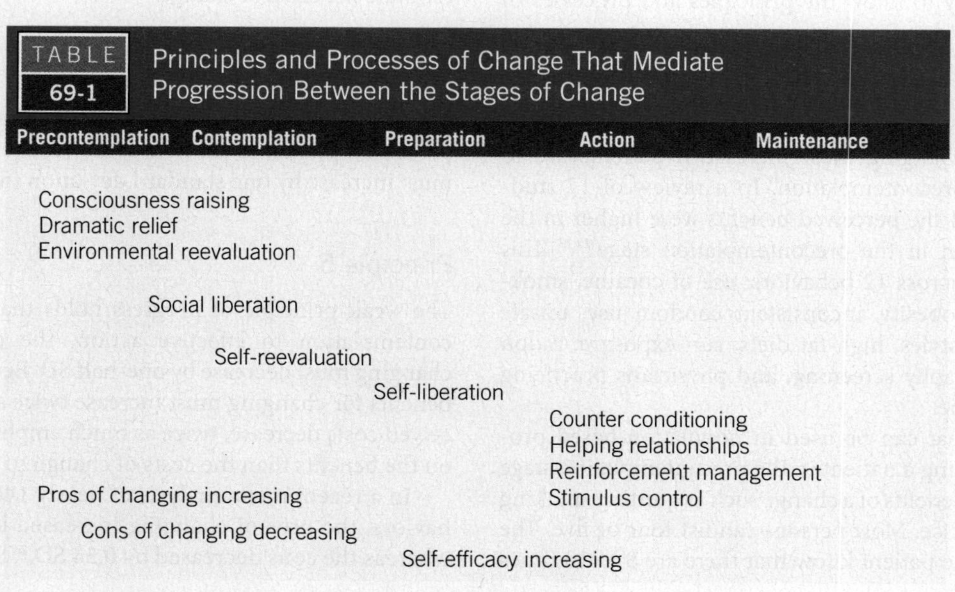

TABLE 69-1 Principles and Processes of Change That Mediate Progression Between the Stages of Change

Precontemplation	Contemplation	Preparation	Action	Maintenance
Consciousness raising Dramatic relief Environmental reevaluation				
	Social liberation			
	Self-reevaluation			
		Self-liberation		
			Counter conditioning Helping relationships Reinforcement management Stimulus control	
Pros of changing increasing				
	Cons of changing decreasing			
		Self-efficacy increasing		

preparation stage, they begin to develop a focus on the future as they imagine how life could be if they were free of addiction.

5. *Self-liberation (make a commitment)* involves both the belief that one can change and the commitment and recommitment to act on that belief. Techniques that can enhance such willpower include public rather than private commitments. Motivational research also suggests that individuals who have only one choice are not as motivated as if they have two choices.[25] Three choices are even better, but four choices do not seem to enhance motivation. Wherever possible, then, patients should be given three of the best choices for applying each process. With stopping smoking, for example, there are at least three good choices: using nicotine replacement therapy to taper nicotine under medical supervision, using nicotine fading (self-taper), and using FDA-approved medications to reduce return to use (varenicline, bupropion), or combinations thereof. Asking patients to choose which alternative they believe would be most effective for them and which they would be most committed to can enhance their motivation and their self-liberation.
6. *Counter conditioning (use substitutes)* requires the learning of healthier behaviors that can substitute for addictive behaviors. Counter conditioning techniques tend to be quite specific to a particular behavior. They include desensitization, assertion, and cognitive counters to irrational self-statements that can elicit distress.
7. *Reinforcement management (use rewards)* involves the systematic use of reinforcements and punishments for taking steps in a particular direction. Because successful self-changers rely much more on reinforcement than punishment, it is useful to emphasize reinforcements for progressing rather than punishments for regressing. Contingency contracts, overt and covert reinforcements, and group recognition are methods of increasing reinforcement and incentives that increase the probability that healthier responses will be repeated. To prepare patients for the longer term, they should be taught to rely more on self-reinforcements than on social reinforcements. Clinical experience shows that many patients expect much more reinforcement and recognition from others than they actually receive. Relatives and friends may take action for granted. Average acquaintances typically generate only a few positive consequences early in the action stage. Self-reinforcements obviously are much more under self-control and can be given more quickly and consistently when temptations to return to use are resisted.
8. *Stimulus control (mange your environment)* involves modifying the environment to increase cues that prompt healthy responses and decrease cues that lead to relapse. Avoidance, environmental reengineering (such as removing substances and paraphernalia), and attending self-help groups can provide stimuli that elicit healthy responses and reduce the risk of return to addiction-related behaviors.
9. *Helping relationships (get support)* combine caring, openness, trust, and acceptance, as well as support for changing. Rapport building, a therapeutic alliance, counselor calls, buddy systems, sponsors, and self-help groups can be excellent resources for social support. If patients become dependent on such support to maintain change, the support will need to be carefully faded, lest termination of therapy becomes a condition for return to use.
10. *Social liberation (notice the public effort)* is the process by which changes in society increase the options and opportunities to have healthier and happier lives freer from addiction. Social networks are examples of a dramatic increase in being able to participate in positive interactions free from pressures to rely on substance use.

Competing theories of therapy have implicitly or explicitly advocated alternative processes of enhancing motivation for change. Is it ideas or emotions that move people? Is it values, decisions, or dedication? Do contingencies incentivize humans, or is behavior determined by environmental conditions or habits? Or is it the therapeutic relationship that is the common healer across all therapeutic modalities?

The answer to each of these questions is "yes." Therapeutic processes originating from competing theories can be compatible when they are combined in a stage-matched paradigm. With patients in earlier stages of change, motivation can be enhanced through more experiential processes that produce healthier cognitions, emotions, evaluations, decisions, and commitments. In later stages, it is possible to build on such solid preparation and motivation by emphasizing more behavioral processes that can help condition healthier habits, reinforce these habits, and provide physical and social environments that support healthier lifestyles freer from addiction.

It is important to know that Velicer et al. found that there were no significant differences in outcomes across gender, race, and ethnicity subgroups. There were significant and small effect sizes for age and education groups.[26] Along equity issues, presently Community Health Clinics are finding a marked difference between insured and uninsured patients.

Outcomes

What is the result when all of these principles and processes of change are combined to help patients and entire populations move toward action on their SUD? A series of clinical trials applying stage-matched interventions offers lessons about the future of behavioral health care generally and treatment of SUDs specifically.

TTM-based approaches result in increased participation and engagement because they appeal to the whole population rather than the minority ready to take action. TTM research across many behaviors and populations have demonstrated repeatedly that only a minority of any at risk group are in preparation typically 20% with 40% in precontemplation and 40% contemplation.[27] Yet, most behavior change messaging and treatments are action-oriented and assume readiness to participate in action-oriented programs. Such methods engage mostly the 20% or so of people who are ready to take action and misserve the majority of at-risk people who are not prepared to take action. TTM-based programs often achieve greater than 80% participation.[14,28] TTM approaches engage whole populations those in precontemplation, contemplation, preparation, action and maintenance because they are perceived as more respectful, relevant, engaging, and appealing, thereby reducing resistance and reactance among early-stage individuals.

TTM-based approaches can dramatically increase rates of behavior change. While action-oriented programs may do well to help those ready to change, their impact is limited to the small percentage (20%) of people who are ready to take action. By using a stage approach, one not only increases participation, one also increases the likelihood that individuals will eventually take action. Research demonstrates that helping participants move forward at least one stage of change (such as moving from precontemplation to contemplation) can as much as double the likelihood that they will move to the action stage in the next 6 months. Helping them to move two stages can triple their chances of taking action.[14]

TTM-based approaches have greater impacts. A large body of literature supports the increased impacts of stage matched programs over action oriented and one size fits all interventions. Meta-analyses conclude that tailoring treatments on TTM constructs produces greater impacts than tailoring on most constructs of other behavior change theories.[29,30] TTM-based treatments have been found effective across dozens of behaviors and populations. And have been found to surpass the average outcomes of other behavior change programs identified as benchmarks by a national task force.[31]

TTM-based approaches impact multiple risks. Several randomized clinical trials of TTM based interventions have demonstrated the ability to impact multiple risks, even risks that were not specifically treated.[32,33] We call this transfer effect from a treatment to a nontreated behavior. This phenomenon reflects the synergy of TTM programs. This research includes areas such as adherence to antihypertension and lipid-lowering medication, weight management, obesity prevention, and prenatal care.[34-38] Through this research, the phenomena of coaction have been described as the increased probability that individuals who adopt one health behavior will adopt another health behavior. For example, in a randomized clinical trial of a TTM-tailored weight management intervention for overweight adults, the treatment group demonstrated a 2.5 to 5.2 increased likelihood of success on a second behavior. The control group demonstrated a 1.2 to 2.6 increase likelihood of success on a second behavior.[36] Given the vast differences in probability of additional behavior change between successful changers in the treatment group compared to control, it can be concluded that this is not a naturally occurring phenomenon. This is another example of synergy, where more changes are produced than are treated. Similar findings from other multiple behavior trials cumulate evidence that coaction occurs more in groups receiving TTM-tailored behavior change treatments. It can be hypothesized that by teaching individuals strategies that support the change process, they then apply those strategies successfully to other areas.

Most recent research looks at participation incentives versus outcome incentives. The outcome financial incentives significantly increased the rates of people stopping smoking over the participation incentive group and for the assessment only groups. However, outcome incentives plus nonincentivized TTM treatment participation quit at an unprecedented rate.[39]

Most relevantly the TTM is being applied to changing long term care by embedding equity, diversity, and inclusion in long-term research in Canada. The TTM offers the framework for planning and enacting individual, organizational, and system level changes addressing structural barriers, engaging diverse knowledge users, addressing intersectionality data collection and changing demographic composition.[40]

MULTIPLE DOMAINS OF WELL-BEING: FROM SUFFERING OR STRUGGLING TO THRIVING

Motivated by a "risky test" philosophy of science,[41] we keep raising the bar to have increasing impacts with vulnerable populations, such as moving from changing a single behavior to a riskier goal of changing multiple risk behaviors. A recent challenge has been to simultaneously enhance multiple domains of well-being, for example, physical, emotional, social, and work well-being. A project with 4000 participants from 39 states who had an average of almost four chronic conditions and almost four risk behaviors, with 40% obese, 35% overweight, and 0% exercising adequately or managing stress effectively was conducted. A majority had poor diets, were or had been people who regularly smoked, and had problems with depression.[42]

Compared to national norms, this population with 59% women, a mean age of 48 and 48% unemployment, had much lower scores on each domain of well-being. Most striking was that a majority were suffering or struggling and only a minority were thriving. The only time this pattern was seen in the United States was with the economic crash of 2008.[43]

With random assignment, one group received telephonic TTM CTI coaching with exercise as the primary target and stress management as secondary. A second group received a CTI with stress management as the primary behavior and exercise as a secondary behavior. Compared to a third control group, both treatment groups produced more multiple behavior change than do controls and more improvement on multiple domains of well-being. In all comparisons, the telephonic coaching that spent most of the time on exercise produced more positive changes than the CTI that treated stress management primarily and exercise secondarily.

What was most rewarding to the investigators was that the majority of both treatment groups but not the control group had progressed from suffering or struggling to thriving. These results led us to produce a follow-up book to *Changing for Good*,[3] which for over 25 years has been a guide for many addiction counselors. The new book, titled, *Changing to Thrive*[4] is designed to help both professionals, their patients, and other populations to reduce multiple risk behaviors, enhance multiple domains of well-being, and progress from suffering or struggling to thriving.

CONCLUSIONS

It seems clear that the future of SUD programs lies in stage-matched, proactive, interactive interventions. Much greater effects can be generated through the use of proactive programs because participation rates are increased, even if efficacy rates are lower.

Results with multiple behavior interventions using some type of TTM tailoring and proactive recruitment have found as good effects as when smoking alone is treated. The results with the other treated behaviors were even better. If these results continue to be replicated, therapeutic programs will be able to produce unprecedented effects on entire populations. To do so will require scientific and professional shifts: (1) from an action paradigm to a stage paradigm; (2) from reactive to proactive recruitment; (3) from expecting participants to match the needs of programs to having programs match the needs of patients; (4) from single to multiple behavior interventions; (5) from clinic-based to population-based programs that apply individualized and interactive intervention strategies; and (6) reducing multiple problem behaviors to enhance multiple domains of well-being to help vulnerable populations to progress from suffering or struggling to thriving.

REFERENCES

1. Prochaska JO, DiClemente CC. Stages and processes of self-change of smoking: toward an integrative model of change. *J Consult Clin Psychol.* 1983;51:390-395.
2. Prochaska JO, DiClemente CC, Norcross JC. In search of how people change: applications to the addictive behaviors. *Am Psychol.* 1992;47:1102-1114.
3. Prochaska JO, Norcross JC, DiClemente CC. *Changing for Good.* William Morrow; 1994.
4. Prochaska JO, Prochaska JM. *Changing to Thrive: Overcome the Top Risks to Lasting Health and Happiness.* Hazelden Publishing; 2016.
5. SAMSHA. *Substance Abuse and Mental Health Services Administration.* RUSC Committee, Recovery and Recovery Support. Accessed June 9, 2023. https://www.samhsa.gov/recovery
6. National Institutes of Health (NIH) Strategic Coordination. Science of Behavior Change, Meeting Report, Common Fund. Accessed June 9, 2023. https://commonfund.nih.gov/behaviorchange/meetings/sobc061509/report
7. CMS. *Resources for Integrated Care.* https://www.ResourcesForIntegratedCare.com
8. White W. The rhetoric of recovery advocacy: an essay on the power of language. In: White W, ed. *Let's Go Make Some History: Chronicles of the New Addiction Recovery Advocacy Movement.* Johnson Institute and Faces and Voices of Recovery; 2006:37-76.
9. Snow MG, Prochaska JO, Rossi JS. Stages of change for smoking cessation among former problem drinkers: a cross-sectional analysis. *J Subst Abuse.* 1992;4:107-116.
10. American Psychiatric Association. *Diagnostic and Statistical Manual of Mental Disorders.* 4th ed. (DSM-IV). American Psychiatric Press; 1994.
11. Velicer WF, Fava JL, Prochaska JO, Abrams DB, Emmons KM, Pierce JP. Distribution of smokers by stage in three representative samples. *Prev Med.* 1995;24:401-411.
12. Laforge RG, Gomes SO, Cottrill SD, et al. Baseline results of proactive telephone recruitment of college drinkers in the College-Based Alcohol Risk Reduction (C-BARR) trial [Abstract]. *Alcohol Clin Exp Res.* 2001;25(5):147A.
13. Prochaska JO, Velicer WF, Fava JL, et al. Counselor and stimulus control enhancements of a stage-matched expert system for smokers in a managed care setting. *Prev Med.* 2000;32:39-46.
14. Prochaska JO, Velicer WF, Fava JL, Rossi JS, Tsoh JY. Evaluating a population-based recruitment approach and a stage-based expert system intervention for smoking cessation. *Addict Behav.* 2002;26:583-602.
15. Prochaska JJ, Hall SE, Delucchi K, Hall SM. Efficacy of initiating tobacco dependence treatment in inpatient psychiatry: a randomized controlled trial. *Am J Public Health.* 2014;104(8):1557-1565.
16. Fiore MC, Jaén CR, Baker TB, et al. *Treating Tobacco Use and Dependence: 2008 Update. Clinical Practice Guideline.* U.S. Department of Health and Human Services: Public Health Service; 2008.
17. Wierzbicki M, Pekarik G. A meta-analysis of psychotherapy dropout. *Prof Psychol Res Pr.* 1993;29:190-195.
18. Brogan ME, Prochaska JO, Prochaska JM. Predicting termination and continuation status in psychotherapy using the transtheoretical model. *Psychotherapy.* 1999;36:105-113.
19. Tsoh J. *Stages of change, drop-outs and outcome in substance abuse treatment.* Dissertation. University of Rhode Island; 1995.
20. Klesges R, Sherrill-Mittleman S, Ebbert JO, Talcott GW, Debon M. Tobacco use harm reduction, elimination, and escalation in a large military cohort. *Am J Public Health.* 2010;100(12):2487-2492.
21. Connors G, Walitzer K, Dermen K. Preparing clients for alcoholism treatment: effects on treatment participation and outcomes. *J Consult Clin Psychol.* 2002;70:1161-1169.
22. Prochaska JO, Velicer WF, Rossi JS, et al. Stages of change and decisional balance for twelve problem behaviors. *Health Psychol.* 1994;13:39-46.
23. Prochaska JO. Strong and weak principles for progressing from precontemplation to action based on twelve problem behaviors. *Health Psychol.* 1994;13:47-51.
24. Hall KL, Rossi JS. Meta-analytic examination of the strong and weak principles across 48 health behaviors. *Prev Med.* 2008;46(3):266-274.
25. Miller WR. Motivation for treatment: a review with special emphasis on alcoholism. *Psychol Bull.* 1985;98:84-107.
26. Velicer WF, Redding CA, Sun X, Prochaska JO. Demographic variables, smoking variables, and outcome across five studies. *Health Psychol.* 2007;26(3):278-287.
27. Wewers ME, Stillman FA, Hartman AM, Shopland DR. Distribution of daily smokers by stage of change: current Population Survey results. *Prev Med.* 2003;36(6):710-720. doi:10.1016/s0091-7435(03)00044-6
28. Prochaska JO, Norcross JC, Saul SF. Generating psychotherapy breakthroughs: transtheoretical strategies from population health psychology. *Am Psychol.* 2020;75(7):996-1010. doi:10.1037/amp0000568
29. Krebs P, Prochaska JO, Rossi JS. A meta-analysis of computer-tailored interventions for health behavior change. *Prev Med.* 2010;51:214-221.
30. Noar S, Benac C, Harris M. Does tailoring matter? Meta-analytic review of tailored print health behavior change interventions. *Psychol Bull.* 2007;133:673-693.
31. Johnson JL, Prochaska JO, Paiva AL, Fernandez AC, DeWees SL, Prochaska JM. Advancing bodies of evidence for population-based health promotion programs: randomized controlled trials and case studies. *Popul Health Manag.* 2013;16:373-380. doi:10.1089/pop.2012.0094
32. Johnson SS, Paiva AL, Mauriello L, Prochaska JO, Redding C, Velicer WF. Coaction in multiple behavior change interventions: consistency across multiple studies on weight management and obesity prevention. *Health Psychol.* 2014;13:475-480.
33. Johnson S, Evers K. Advances in multiple behavior change. *Am J Health Promot.* 2015;29(4):TAHP6-TAHP8.

34. Johnson SS, Driskell MM, Johnson J, Prochaska JM, Zwick W, Prochaska JO. Efficacy of a transtheoretical model-based expert system for antihypertensive adherence. *Dis Manage.* 2006;9:291-301.
35. Johnson SS, Driskel MM, Johnson JL, et al. Transtheoretical model intervention for adherence to lipid-lowering drugs. *Dis Manage.* 2006;9:102-114.
36. Johnson SS, Paiva AL, Cummins CO, et al. Transtheoretical model-based multiple behavior intervention for weight management: effectiveness on a population basis. *Prev Med.* 2008;46:238-246. doi:10.1016/j.ypmed.2007.09.010
37. Mauriello LM, Ciavatta MM, Paiva AL, et al. Results of a multi-media multiple behavior obesity prevention program for adolescents. *Prev Med.* 2010;51:451-456. doi:10.1016/j.ypmed.2010.08.004
38. Mauriello LM, Van Marter DF, Umanzor CD, Castle PH, de Aguiar EL. Using mHealth to deliver behavior change interventions within prenatal care at community health centers. *Am J Health Promot.* 2016;30:554-562. doi:10.4278/ajhp.140530-QUAN-248
39. Prochaska JO, Paiva AL, Redding CA, et al. In search of breakthroughs in population cessation via participation incentives or outcome incentives. *Under review.*
40. Finnegan HA, Daari L, Jaiswal A, et al. Changing care: applying the transtheoretical model of change to embed equity, diversity, and inclusion in long-term care research in Canada. *Societies.* 2022;12(3):87.
41. Prochaska JO, Wright JA, Velicer WF. Evaluating theories of health behavior change: A hierarchy of criteria applied to the transtheoretical model. *Appl Psychol Intern Rev.* 2008;57(4):561-588.
42. Prochaska JO, Evers KE, Castle PH, et al. Enhancing multiple domains of well-being by decreasing multiple health risk behaviors: a randomized clinical trial. *Popul Health Manag.* 2012;15:1-11.
43. Gallup-Healthways. Well-Being Index. Accessed June 9, 2023. https://ia800501.us.archive.org/33/items/SubjectiveWell-beingScienceOfHappiness/Gallup-healthwaysWell-beingIndex.pdf

CHAPTER

70

Motivational Interviewing

Cassandra L. Boness, Antoine Douaihy, and Karen S. Ingersoll

CHAPTER OUTLINE

- Motivational interviewing "spirit"
- Motivational interviewing skills
- Motivational interviewing processes and stages of change
- Motivational interviewing as an evidence-based approach for substance use disorders
- Combining motivational interviewing with other therapeutic modalities
- Patient profiles and response to motivational interviewing in substance use disorder treatment
- Motivational interviewing and social justice
- Conclusion
- Chapter summary

Motivational interviewing (MI) describes "a collaborative conversation style for strengthening a person's own motivation and commitment to change."[1] MI is a brief, patient-centered approach that engages people in conversations about change. MI is based on the assumption that the client or patient holds the key to successful change. MI practitioners assume that ambivalence, or uncertainty about a specific behavior change, is a normal part of the change process.[1,2] MI may be useful in any medical condition where behavior plays a role. MI is especially relevant in addiction medicine to help patients reduce or abstain from substance use and improve overall wellbeing. MI helps to meet a patient where they are in the change process without creating discord in the interaction. The MI approach may therefore be especially useful when talking to patients about their substance use and related harms because individuals who use substances or have a substance use disorder (SUD) often face stigma and judgment, particularly from health care practitioners.[3,4] While there is no true theory of MI, Miller and Rose[5] described the basis of its efficacy as arising from the combination of relational and technical behaviors of the therapist.

MOTIVATIONAL INTERVIEWING "SPIRIT"

MI can be described by its spirit, skills, and processes. The spirit, or way of being, in MI involves four key elements including, partnership, acceptance, compassion, and evocation (PACE). Partnership, or collaboration, involves coming alongside a patient, holding them as an equal and as the expert on their behaviors and experiences while working together toward change. Acceptance, or absolute worth, is the assumption that each patient should be valued and respected as an individual that is capable of change and potential. Recognizing a person's absolute worth requires an acceptance of the patient as they are currently, curiosity about their values and beliefs, and the active resistance of any urge to judge them. When patients are accepted, they learn to accept themselves, and this can free them up to make changes consistent with the life they want to live.[2] Acceptance also includes autonomy support, which involves acknowledging a patient's right to self-determination and recognizing that patients can make the best decisions for themselves. Compassion describes the intention to act in a kind and generous manner with the goal of alleviating suffering and promoting the wellbeing of others.[6] Evocation is a process that is used in MI to explore a patient's experience and perspectives related to change and elicit and strengthen their own intrinsic motivation to change.

It is important to understand how the MI spirit compares with traditional medical interactions. In traditional medical interactions, the physician's goal may be to instruct a patient on how to change their substance use. Here, the physician is positioned as expert and the patient is positioned as a passive recipient of such expertise. In these interactions, there is a tendency for the physician to engage in the "righting reflex" or to set the patient on the "right" path. In a MI-consistent interaction, the goal may instead be to guide the patient in a way that resolves ambivalence and strengthens motivation to change, only providing instruction or information with permission from the patient. The MI spirit can be an abrupt shift for practitioners who are accustomed to a directing communication style in which the practitioner may try to "fix" the patient with their expert knowledge or expertise.[2]

The "righting reflex" may be especially strong when it comes to working with patients who express goals related to harm reduction, moderation, or nonabstinence from substances. The predominant medical model of addiction tends to frame it as a "brain disease" characterized by its chronic and relapsing nature as well as compulsive drug seeking and use,[7] suggesting abstinence from the substance as the only plausible treatment approach. However, this perspective is challenged by research suggesting that most people recover from SUDs without treatment[8,9] and people can experience improvements in health and wellbeing even without being fully abstinent from a substance.[10] Indeed, even small reductions in use can improve a person's psychosocial functioning. Thus, the brain disease model may not be accurate for all people[11] and, as a result, abstinence might not be the only path to recovery from a SUD. It is therefore important to consider how one's training related to the etiology and maintenance of addiction may influence what is seen as an "acceptable" treatment goal or treatment outcome and how that may show up in encounters with patients (eg, as a righting reflex).

MOTIVATIONAL INTERVIEWING SKILLS

The core MI skills include open-ended questions, affirmations, reflections, and summaries (OARS; **Table 70-1**). Open-ended questions are questions that encourage a patient to expand upon their thoughts, behaviors, or emotions. Open-ended questions stand in comparison to closed-ended questions, which can usually be answered with a yes, no, or single word answer. Open-ended questions leave the door open for a patient to respond and elaborate, whereas close-ended questions tend to close the door to elaboration. Affirmations are used strategically to acknowledge a patient's personal strengths or efforts toward change. Reflections, or reflective listening, requires actively listening to a patient and subsequently responding with a statement that reflects meaning or emotion, clarifies the person's thoughts and emotions, and communicates that you are listening, engaged, and understand what was said. Summaries are an opportunity to show that we understand the patient, with strategic emphasis on key points (such as change talk) in the conversation and, at times, to transition to a new focus in the conversation. Together, these MI skills are used to facilitate the four key processes of MI. Those interested in learning more about the MI "toolbox," or additional skills to be used in MI encounters, could refer to Miller and Rollnick,[1] Douaihy, Kelly, and Gold,[2] or Ingersoll.[12]

TABLE 70-1 OARS Skills and Examples

Skill	Example
Open-ended questions	How might your life be different if you were to change your opioid use?
Affirmations	You have really thought a lot about whether you need to change your substance use.
Reflections	It really upsets you that your family is trying to force you to stop using heroin.
Summaries	You really don't see your substance use as a problem and it provides you with a way to relax and let loose with your friends. At the same time, it does concern you that your family is worried about you, and you find it especially painful when they criticize your substance use. You're only here today because your primary care physician recommended you come talk to me to hear what kind of options we might have available to help you manage your substance use.

MOTIVATIONAL INTERVIEWING PROCESSES AND STAGES OF CHANGE

Four Processes

The four motivational interviewing processes one may move through during motivational interviewing includes engaging, focusing, evoking, and planning.[1] Engaging is the task of establishing a collaborative partnership, through use of the MI spirit and skills, with a patient. Engaging begins at the very first encounter. Focusing is the collaborative task of identifying, developing, and maintaining a specific direction related to change. Evoking involves eliciting a patient's motivations and arguments in favor of change, the specific expression of which is known as "change talk." For example, evoking might include asking the patient, "How might reducing your substance use positively impact your life?" When change talk is evoked, it is typically expressed as preparation or mobilization language in the categories of *desire* to change, *ability* to change, *reasons* for change, *need* to change, *commitment* to change, *activation* toward change, and *taking steps* toward change (nicknamed "DARN CAT"; **Table 70-2**). The final step involves planning and this includes developing and refining a patient's commitment to change through a specific action plan.[1,2]

Engaging, focusing, evoking, and planning build upon one another such that engaging is the foundation upon which focusing is built, and so forth. By engaging and building rapport and trust with a patient, this will allow them to focus their attention on the behaviors they would like to

TABLE 70-2 Types of Change Talk

Change talk type	Example
Desire	I would like to change my alcohol use.
Ability	I can probably cut back by one drink a day.
Reasons	I would perform better at work if I reduced my drinking.
Need	I have to reduce my drinking, or my partner will pursue separation.
Commitment	I intend to only drink low alcohol content beverages when I go out with friends after work.
Activation	I am ready to do what it takes to reduce my drinking.
Taking Steps	When I drank last night, I only had two instead of my usual three drinks.

change. Through a focus on the specific behavior that they desire to change, reasons for change can be evoked and, thus, commitment to change can be strengthened. This prepares the patient for the final process of planning where specific and actionable steps toward change can be described and implemented. Although these processes tend to build on one another, it is important to remember that change is rarely linear and a truly collaborative and guiding style may at times require moving to an earlier process to keep the patient engaged in the interaction.[2]

Conceptualizing Patient Change

A key part of determining which MI process(es) is most relevant in each interaction, and it can be helpful to think about which stage of the change the patient is in currently. Because change occurs on a continuum, a person can be at any given point along the continuum and can move through the continuum at different rates, moving forward toward change, or backward from change. This can be conceptualized as levels of readiness for change,[13-16] or could be segmented into stages, as in Prochaska and DiClemente's transtheoretical model, colloquially known as the stages of change model.[17,18] This model describes five stages along the continuum of change: precontemplation, contemplation, preparation, action, and maintenance (**Fig. 70-1**).

A patient in precontemplation may not recognize a particular behavior as problematic and therefore is unlikely to seek treatment for the behavior. These patients may be encountered in an addiction medicine setting because they present for a related problem, such as in the ER for a lesion or alcohol-related injury, or through a referral, legal sanction, or insistence of a loved one. Individuals in the precontemplation stage may make statements such as, "I perform better when I am high than when I am sober." The contemplation stage of change tends to be characterized by ambivalence about behavior change. The patient may express reasons for and against change, using both change and sustain (maintaining the status quo) talk. For example, "I hate the way drinking makes me feel but I can't imagine my life without it." The preparation stage of change is characterized by a commitment to change and is typically identified by change talk (DARN CAT). For example, "I *need* to reduce my use in order to function better at my job." The action stage of change is characterized by a belief in one's ability to change and clear, actionable steps toward such change. For example, "Last night I had three drinks instead of my usual four." Individuals in the action stage of change may be considering and testing different strategies to implement their behavior change goals and may present with questions about their options or additional services. Finally, the maintenance stage of change is characterized by an individual's attempts to uphold their behavior change. It is important to remember and normalize that individuals in the maintenance stage of change may return to earlier stages and that this is both typical and expected rather than some indication of failure.

One of the most challenging aspects of practicing MI is deciding when and how to transition from the evoking

Stages Along the Continuum of Change

	Precontemplation	Contemplation	Preparation	Action	Maintenance
Description	Patient has not considered changing their behavior	Patient may be stuck in ambivalence	Patient demonstrates commitment talk	Patient may express intermittent ambivalence still	
MI-Response	Use curiosity and express neutrality (neither approving nor disapproving) of the specific behavior	Elicit values, develop discrepancies between behavior and values, reflect change talk	Brainstorm to elicit and produce a menu of options through which change can occur	Affirm the patient and return to the MI skills to address ambivalence as needed	

Figure 70-1. Stages of change and MI-consistent responses to each stage. (Adapted from Douaihy AB, Kelly TM, Gold MA, eds. *Motivational Interviewing: A Guide for Medical Trainees.* Oxford University Press; 2014.)

process, specifically building motivation and strengthening change talk, to the planning process or moving from "why" make the change to "how" to make the change.[19] This shift is intimately tied to change talk. That is, when the patient begins to express progressively stronger change talk, which can occur at various points along the readiness to change continuum but may be most common in the contemplation and preparation stages, this may be one indication that it is time to shift to the planning process. Although this shift to planning may sound straightforward, it is actually one of the later stages of learning MI and requires great skillfulness.[20]

MOTIVATIONAL INTERVIEWING AS AN EVIDENCE-BASED APPROACH FOR SUBSTANCE USE DISORDERS

A wealth of research supports motivational interviewing in the treatment of heavy or harmful substance use and SUDs for adolescents and adults across a variety of treatment settings.[21-23] However, it is worth noting that effect sizes tend to vary, sometimes greatly, across different substances, specific trials, and type of comparison group (eg, treatment as usual or minimal treatment versus comparable treatment).[24] One hypothesized reason for the heterogeneity in MI effect sizes is lack of specification and monitoring of MI's active ingredients.[24] As such, there are ongoing efforts to better understand MI's mechanisms of behavior change in order to maximize treatment outcomes.[25] Notably, efforts are currently underway to systematically evaluate MI as an evidence-based treatment for substance use disorders per the American Psychological Association's Society for Clinical Psychology evidence-based treatment guidelines.[26,27]

MI can be applied by professionals from a range of training backgrounds across a variety of settings with roughly the same effectiveness in outcomes.[28] Although MI can be effectively practiced by a range of professionals, this does not necessarily mean that practicing MI is straightforward or simple. Indeed, acquisition of the motivational interviewing style and skills is thought to proceed through eight, roughly additive developmental stages with their own specific tasks. These include, understanding the spirit of MI, patient-centered counseling through reflective listening, recognizing and reinforcing change talk, strengthening change talk, responding to sustain talk and rolling with resistance, developing a change plan, consolidating commitment language, and incorporating other therapeutic modalities.[20] It is unlikely that the MI trainee can self-guide themselves through these steps successfully with independence. Instead, feedback and coaching from other MI practitioners is needed for the acquisition and maintenance of MI skills.[29]

Thorough training is important given the MI practitioner's skillfulness and techniques (eg, the use of reflective listening) predict increased change talk, which is in turn related to better behavioral outcomes among patients with SUDs.[30-32] For addiction medicine physicians that wish to learn more about applying MI in medical settings or to specific clinical scenarios (eg, substance use in pregnancy), we suggest Douaihy and colleagues.[2]

COMBINING MOTIVATIONAL INTERVIEWING WITH OTHER THERAPEUTIC MODALITIES

Although MI is often examined in isolation for the purpose of clinical trials, MI was not initially intended to exist in isolation or serve as a long-term therapeutic approach. This is especially true in the treatment of SUDs, which are often best treated by psychological treatments and medication. MI, instead, has typically been used toward the goal of engaging the patient in a collaborative discussion and increasing their readiness to change.[33,34] The MI spirit may also be engaged during the course of providing other interventions (eg, through the use of neutrality and compassion).

Indeed, MI can be, and is often, a precursor to, or integrated with other treatment approaches such as medication and other therapeutic modalities such as personalized feedback, cognitive-behavioral therapy, mindfulness-based interventions, or contingency management.[35] The combination of MI with other treatment modalities is supported by research suggesting that MI may enhance engagement in or outcomes of other interventions such as residential treatment.[34,36] Outside of other behavioral treatment approaches, MI has also been combined with medication and pharmacotherapy, specifically antidepressants,[37] as a way to improve the likelihood that patients take medication as prescribed. This strongly suggests that MI may also be useful in discussing medication for SUDs.

PATIENT PROFILES AND RESPONSE TO MOTIVATIONAL INTERVIEWING IN SUBSTANCE USE DISORDER TREATMENT

An important question to consider is *what type of patient might benefit most from MI?* Although there is not a clear answer to this question to date and may differ by the type of substance,[24] there is preliminary evidence to suggest which patients might benefit most from MI on the basis of their unique features and identities including the severity of substance use, degree of ambivalence about changing one's substance use, and racial or ethnic identity.

Severity of Substance Use

Individuals who use substances at heavier amounts may benefit most from MI. For example, in a sample of adolescents presenting to an emergency department following an alcohol-related event, those adolescents with more problematic alcohol use at baseline reported significantly greater improvements in alcohol-related outcomes following MI compared to those with less problematic use.[38] Similar results have been found among adolescents who use cannabis heavily.[39]

Degree of Ambivalence

Recent evidence suggests that MI for substance use may be most effective for individuals who express a high degree of ambivalence, evidenced by equal ratios of change talk to sustain talk, early on in a single MI session.[40] The same study found that individuals who expressed readiness to change, and thus less ambivalence, early on in a single MI session exhibited a decrease in the percentage of change talk over the course of the session, suggesting MI was counterproductive for those already committed to behavior change. Thus, a high degree of ambivalence about changing one's substance use may be one indicator for the application of MI and a low degree of ambivalence about changing one's use may indicate that other interventions such as relapse prevention are more appropriate when people are ready for change.

Patients From Marginalized Racial and Ethnic Backgrounds

Although some evidence suggests that MI is more effective among those who identify with racially or ethnically marginalized groups when compared to those who do not identify with these groups,[41,42] other research has found no differences in MI effect sizes on the basis of racial or ethnic identity.[43] Despite this mixed evidence on racial or ethnic differences in response to traditional MI, MI treatment response may be better for culturally adapted MI interventions (CAMIs) compared to standard MI among patients from marginalized racial and ethnic backgrounds,[44-46] and this may be especially true for individuals who experience more discrimination.[47]

MOTIVATIONAL INTERVIEWING AND SOCIAL JUSTICE

Individuals with SUDs experience significant stigma and marginalization in their day-to-day lives, especially in health care settings.[3,4] Individuals with SUDs who are also marginalized in other ways, perhaps as a result of their racial or ethnic identity, sexual orientation, socioeconomic status, or other psychopathology, experience additional oppression and stigma.[48] This is sometimes known as "multiple marginalization" or "intersectional stigma." Motivational interviewing is well-suited for working with individuals with SUDs who experience multiple marginalization and oppression through its focus on compassion, respect for all persons, justice, acceptance, and collaboration as well as the eschewing of coercion.[6] Approaches such as Macro MI embrace the traditional spirt of MI but also shift the focus from the individual (micro) level (eg, individual well-being) to the structural (macro) level (eg, social justice, liberation) to include additional foci such as activism, community organizing, and peer support. Although fully addressing multiple marginalization is likely best achieved through structural and institutional reform (eg, housing, universal health care, reproductive rights, decriminalization), which is deserving of a book itself, addiction medicine practitioners can play a small part in reducing stigma and marginalization by embodying these values in their practice.

Clinical Case Example A

The following case example describes an addiction medicine physician's first encounter with a 58-year-old cisgender male referred for medication for alcohol use disorder by his primary care physician after screening positive for hazardous alcohol use at an annual exam.

PHYSICIAN: Hello, Mr Z, my name is Dr S, and I am the addiction medicine physician here at our clinic.

PATIENT: Hi, it's nice to meet you, Dr S.

PHYSICIAN: It's my understanding that you were referred to our clinic by your primary care physician. What is your understanding of why you were referred to us? [Information provision; open-ended question]

PATIENT: Well… I'm not sure, to be honest. I went in for a check-up and the doctor asked me a few questions about my alcohol use. He said I was drinking at unsafe levels, and it would be best for me to come talk with you.

PHYSICIAN: Your primary care physician was concerned about how much you're drinking and suggested you come chat with us. How do you feel about the amount you're drinking? [Reflection; open-ended evocative question]

PATIENT: I mean, I guess I do drink a lot sometimes but it's just something I do to relax, and it never really causes me problems.

PHYSICIAN: Drinking sometimes helps you unwind. Your primary care physician was concerned about the amount you're drinking specifically. How much would you say you are currently drinking? [Reflection; closed-ended question]

PATIENT: I probably have about 4 beers a day after work and sometimes more on the weekend when I'm visiting with friends.

PHYSICIAN: Ok, so about 4, or sometimes more, drinks a day, which is about 28 to 35 drinks a week. Does that sound right? [Reflection; closed-ended question]

PATIENT: That seems about right.

PHYSICIAN: Ok. Help me understand what you were hoping to get out of today's visit. [Open-ended question]

PATIENT: I guess I want you to tell me if I really am drinking too much or not.

PHYSICIAN: Would it be OK if I told you a little bit about what I know about safe levels of drinking? [Asking permission]

PATIENT: That would be fine.

PHYSICIAN: Ok. Well, we typically consider more than 14 drinks a week for men to be risky. What I mean by risky is that men who drink more than 14 drinks a week tend to be at increased risk for other health problems. What do you think about that? [Providing information; eliciting]

PATIENT: Well, I didn't know that. I am drinking more than that each week.

PHYSICIAN: How are you feeling about that? [Open-ended question]

PATIENT: I guess it's a bit concerning. I thought I was just letting loose, but I am getting older, and I want to live long enough to enjoy my retirement and time with my family.

PHYSICIAN: You're worried that any consequences of your drinking might interfere with things you plan to do in the future. [Reflection]

PATIENT: Exactly... but I've been drinking like this for 20 years without problems.

PHYSICIAN: So, if I'm understanding correctly, you came here today hoping to learn more about your drinking and whether it is potentially harmful. You've been drinking at about the same amount for the last 20 or so years without many consequences. At the same time, you're a bit concerned that your drinking does exceed these recommended limits and you're especially worried that the consequences of your drinking might put your future life plans at risk. Where does that leave you? [Summary; open-ended question]

PATIENT: Well, I guess my primary care doc was right that I should probably consider cutting back a bit.

PHYSICIAN: You're thinking it might be worth coming up with a plan for cutting down. [Reflection]

PATIENT: Yeah.

PHYSICIAN: How would you feel about discussing some of the options we have available for helping patients cut down on their alcohol use? [Asking permission as an open-ended question]

PATIENT: I'd be open to that.

PHYSICIAN: [Delivers information about psychological treatments, community and peer support, and medications available to the patient]... What do you think? [Providing information; eliciting]

PATIENT: Thank you. I think I'd be open to trying the medication you mentioned to help with my cravings and maybe also talking with the peer support specialists who work here.

[Physician moves into MI-consistent discussion about medication-specific information and facilitates an introduction to the peer support specialist. A follow-up appointment is also made.]

Clinical Case Example B

The following case example describes an encounter with an 18-year-old transgender woman who was hospitalized following a vehicle crash that occurred while she was driving under the influence of several substances.

PHYSICIAN: Hello, Ms L, my name is Dr S, and I am the addiction medicine physician here on our unit.

PATIENT: Hi.

PHYSICIAN: What's your understanding of why you're in the hospital? [Open-ended question]

PATIENT: You tell me.

PHYSICIAN: You're not sure what happened. [Reflection]

PATIENT: I remember everything that happened.

PHYSICIAN: Ah... so you do recall the events that led to the hospitalization. [Reflection]

PATIENT: I remember enough.

PHYSICIAN: Would it be OK if I tell you what the admission note here says? [Asking permission]

PATIENT: I guess.

PHYSICIAN: Ok... well, this note is from the emergency department last night. It says here that you were brought in by the police after crashing your vehicle into a tree... [Sharing information]

PATIENT: Guess so.

PHYSICIAN: The note also says that you were fairly confused when you arrived. How are you feeling now? [Open-ended question]

PATIENT: My head hurts, but I feel fine enough.

PHYSICIAN: You're feeling better. Great. I can send the nurse in here when I'm done to see if we can do anything to help with your head. What do you think caused your confusion last night? [Reflection; open-ended question]

PATIENT: You tell me, you're the doctor.

PHYSICIAN: Well, there could be several explanations for your confusion. It's possible you hit your head during the accident and became disoriented. Some of the lab tests we gathered last night suggested you might have been using substances, which can also cause confusion. What are your thoughts? [Providing information; open-ended question]

PATIENT: It could have been either of those things.

PHYSICIAN: You believe it's possible that you hit your head or had been using substances. What types of substances do you typically use? [Reflection; open-ended question]

PATIENT: Usually just cannabis but last night I went to a party and used other things.

PHYSICIAN: Something you don't typically use. [Reflection]

PATIENT: Yeah.

PHYSICIAN: What else was going on last night at this party? [Open-ended question]

PATIENT: Some of my friends were just being jerks.

PHYSICIAN: You had a conflict with your friends. [Reflection]

PATIENT: Sort of... my friends were just picking on me and what I chose to wear to the party. Next thing I knew, I left the party and got into my car. I remember pulling away but then not much else until the cops pulled me out of my car.

PHYSICIAN: You don't remember crashing. [Reflection]

PATIENT: No... just being put into the back of the police car.

PHYSICIAN: That's scary. [Reflection]

PATIENT: It was.

PHYSICIAN: Has anything like that ever happened to you before? [Closed-ended question]

PATIENT: Like what?

PHYSICIAN: Where you've been using substances other than cannabis and you lose parts of your day or night? [Clarifying]

PATIENT: Yeah, it happens to me sometimes but nothing bad usually happens.

PHYSICIAN: You black out sometimes and are usually able to keep yourself safe when that happens. [Reflection]

PATIENT: Sure, I mean it never feels good, but I don't usually crash my car and get brought to the hospital by the cops.

PHYSICIAN: This time was different. [Reflection]

PATIENT: Seems so.

PHYSICIAN: How are you typically able to keep yourself safe when you black out? [Open-ended question]

PATIENT: Well... usually I don't drive to parties. I usually don't even go to parties because my friends are jerks and I usually just end up upset when I spend time with them. I usually stay in my room at home and go to work. That's it.

PHYSICIAN: Spending time with those people tends to be a trigger. [Reflection]

PATIENT: Yes, I should have known better.

PHYSICIAN: You're wishing you had made a different choice. [Reflection]

PATIENT: Yeah.

PHYSICIAN: What else helps to keep you safe when you're using?

PATIENT: Well, usually I just stick to cannabis but this time I also took some pills someone gave me. I think that's what caught up to me.

PHYSICIAN: Ah, you took some pills. [Reflection]

PATIENT: Exactly. That never ends up well for me.

PHYSICIAN: How confident do you feel that you could avoid using pills like those again in the future? With 0 being not at all confident, and 100 being totally confident. [Open-ended question; assessing self-efficacy to change]

PATIENT: Like... a 20.

PHYSICIAN: Why a 20 and not a 10? [Open-ended question]

PATIENT: Well, in the past I've been able to just say no. It usually helps when I avoid parties, but I often have a hard time saying no to those because I want those people to like me. They all take pills.

PHYSICIAN: Sometimes the desire to be liked leads to decisions that cause problems for you. At the same time, you've been successful in saying no to other substances in the past. [Reflection; emphasizing past successes]

PATIENT: Yeah, I guess.

PHYSICIAN: I appreciate you being willing to talk with me today. I expect I'll see you a few more times before you are discharged. Would it be OK if next time we talk a bit more about strategies you might use to help keep yourself safe? [Affirmation; asking permission]

PATIENT: Like more medications?

PHYSICIAN: Well, medication is one option but there are several others as well. [Providing information]

PATIENT: Ok, yeah, that would be fine.

PHYSICIAN: Ok, see you soon.

CONCLUSION

MI is a collaborative, patient-centered approach that is especially useful when working with patients that use substances. Through the MI spirit, skills, and processes, practitioners can tailor their conversation to the patient's interest in or readiness for change about changing their substance use, creating a supportive and judgment-free environment to explore their substance use and consider behavior change.

CHAPTER SUMMARY

This chapter describes the core components of MI including the spirit, skills, and processes. MI is an evidence-based approach that can be implemented by a range of health care practitioners and may be especially useful for engaging patients in conversations about their substance use, even during a brief encounter. Although gaining mastery in MI is not simple, addiction medicine practitioners can practice the techniques described here to move toward MI-consistent conversation with their patients to create a supportive environment that is free of judgment and increases the likelihood of behavior change.

REFERENCES

1. Miller WR, Rollnick S. *Motivational Interviewing: Helping People Change*. 3rd ed. Guilford Press; 2013.
2. Douaihy AB, Kelly TM, Gold MA, eds. *Motivational Interviewing: A Guide for Medical Trainees*. Oxford University Press; 2014.
3. Weiss L, McCoy K, Kluger M, Finkelstein R. Access to and use of health care: perceptions and experiences among people who use heroin and cocaine. *Addict Res Theory*. 2004;12(2):155-165. doi:10.1080/1606635031000155099
4. Hammarlund RA, Crapanzano KA, Luce L, Mulligan LA, Ward KM. Review of the effects of self-stigma and perceived social stigma on the treatment-seeking decisions of individuals with drug- and alcohol-use disorders. *Subst Abuse Rehabil*. 2018;9:115-136. doi:10.2147/SAR.S183256
5. Miller WR, Rose GS. Toward a theory of motivational interviewing. *Am Psychol*. 2009;64(6):527-537. doi:10.1037/a0016830
6. Miller WR. Motivational interviewing and social justice. *Motiv Interviewing Train Res Implement Pract*. 2013;1(2):15-18. doi:10.5195/MITRIP.2013.32
7. Leshner AI. Addiction is a brain disease, and it matters. *Science*. 1997;278(5335):45-47. doi:10.1126/science.278.5335.45
8. Tucker J. Epidemiology of recovery from alcohol use disorder. *Alcohol Res Curr Rev*. 2020;40(3):02. doi:10.35946/arcr.v40.3.02
9. Sobell LC, Cunningham JA, Sobell MB. Recovery from alcohol problems with and without treatment: prevalence in two population surveys. *Am J Public Health*. 1996;86(7):966-972. doi:10.2105/AJPH.86.7.966
10. Witkiewitz K, Tucker JA. Abstinence not required: expanding the definition of recovery from alcohol use disorder. *Alcohol Clin Exp Res*. 2020;44(1):36-40. doi:10.1111/acer.14235
11. Pickard H. Is addiction a brain disease? A plea for agnosticism and heterogeneity. *Psychopharmacology (Berl)*. 2022;239(4):993-1007. doi:10.1007/s00213-021-06013-4
12. Ingersoll KS. Motivational interviewing for substance use disorders. *UpToDate*. Accessed June 9, 2023. https://www.uptodate.com/contents/motivational-interviewing-for-substance-use-disorders#!
13. Heather N, Rollnick S, Bell A. Predictive validity of the Readiness to Change Questionnaire. *Addiction*. 1993;88(12):1667-1677. doi:10.1111/j.1360-0443.1993.tb02042.x
14. Engle DE, Arkowitz H. Ambivalence in psychotherapy: facilitating readiness to change. *Guilford Press*. 2006;xiv:240.
15. Budd RJ, Rollnick S. The structure of the Readiness to Change Questionnaire: a test of Prochaska & DiClemente's transtheoretical model. *Br J Health Psychol*. 1996;1(4):365-376. doi:10.1111/j.2044-8287.1996.tb00517.x
16. Emmons KM, Rollnick S. Motivational interviewing in health care settings: opportunities and limitations. *Am J Prev Med*. 2001;20(1):68-74. doi:10.1016/S0749-3797(00)00254-3
17. Prochaska JO, DiClemente CC. *The Transtheoretical Approach: Crossing Traditional Boundaries of Therapy*. Krieger Pub; 1994.
18. DiClemente CC, Prochaska JO. Toward a comprehensive, transtheoretical model of change. In: Miller WR, Heather N, eds. *Treating Addictive Behaviors*. Springer; 1998:3-24. doi:10.1007/978-1-4899-1934-2_1
19. Resnicow K, McMaster F. Motivational interviewing: moving from why to how with autonomy support. *Int J Behav Nutr Phys Act*. 2012;9(1):19. doi:10.1186/1479-5868-9-19
20. Miller WR, Moyers TB. Eight stages in learning motivational interviewing. *J Teach Addict*. 2006;5(1):3-17. doi:10.1300/J188v05n01_02
21. Jensen CD, Cushing CC, Aylward BS, Craig JT, Sorell DM, Steele RG. Effectiveness of motivational interviewing interventions for adolescent substance use behavior change: a meta-analytic review. *J Consult Clin Psychol*. 2011;79(4):433-440. doi:10.1037/a0023992
22. Barnett E, Sussman S, Smith C, Rohrbach LA, Spruijt-Metz D. Motivational Interviewing for adolescent substance use: a review of the literature. *Addict Behav*. 2012;37(12):1325-1334. doi:10.1016/j.addbeh.2012.07.001
23. VanBuskirk KA, Wetherell JL. Motivational interviewing with primary care populations: a systematic review and meta-analysis. *J Behav Med*. 2014;37(4):768-780. doi:10.1007/s10865-013-9527-4
24. DiClemente CC, Corno CM, Graydon MM, Wiprovnick AE, Knoblach DJ. Motivational interviewing, enhancement, and brief interventions over the last decade: a review of reviews of efficacy and effectiveness. *Psychol Addict Behav*. 2017;31(8):862-887. doi:10.1037/adb0000318
25. Magill M, Hallgren KA. Mechanisms of behavior change in motivational interviewing: do we understand how MI works? *Curr Opin Psychol*. 2019;30:1-5. doi:10.1016/j.copsyc.2018.12.010
26. Boness CL, Votaw V, Schwebel FJ, Moniz-Lewis DIK, McHugh RK, Witkiewitz K. An evaluation of cognitive behavioral therapy for substance use: an application of tolin's criteria for empirically supported treatments. Open Science Framework. 2022; doi:10.31219/osf.io/rbx8s
27. Boness CL, Hershenberg R, Grasso D, et al. The society of clinical psychology's manual for the evaluation of psychological treatments using the tolin criteria. Open Science Framework. 2021; doi:10.31219/osf.io/8hcsz
28. Rubak S, Sandbaek A, Lauritzen T, Christensen B. Motivational interviewing: a systematic review and meta-analysis. *Br J Gen Pract*. 2005;55(513):305-312.
29. Schwalbe CS, Oh HY, Zweben A. Sustaining motivational interviewing: a meta-analysis of training studies. *Addiction*. 2014;109(8):1287-1294. doi:10.1111/add.12558
30. Barnett E, Spruijt-Metz D, Moyers TB, et al. Bidirectional relationships between client and counselor speech: The importance of reframing. *Psychol Addict Behav*. 2014;28(4):1212-1219. doi:10.1037/a0036227
31. Moyers TB, Martin T, Houck JM, Christopher PJ, Tonigan JS. From in-session behaviors to drinking outcomes: A causal chain for motivational interviewing. *J Consult Clin Psychol*. 2009;77(6):1113-1124. doi:10.1037/a0017189
32. Gaume J, Bertholet N, Faouzi M, Gmel G, Daeppen JB. Counselor motivational interviewing skills and young adult change talk articulation during brief motivational interventions. *J Subst Abuse Treat*. 2010;39(3):272-281. doi:10.1016/j.jsat.2010.06.010
33. Miller WR. *Combined Behavioral Intervention Manual: A Clinical Research Guide for Therapists Treating People with Alcohol Abuse and Dependence*. U.S. Department of Health and Human Services, National Institutes of Health, National Institute on Alcohol Abuse and Alcoholism; 2004.
34. Bien TH, Miller WR, Tonigan JS. Brief interventions for alcohol problems: a review. *Addiction*. 1993;88(3):315-336. doi:10.1111/j.1360-0443.1993.tb00820.x
35. Moyers TB, Houck J. Combining motivational interviewing with cognitive-behavioral treatments for substance abuse: lessons from the COMBINE research project. *Cogn Behav Pract*. 2011;18(1):38-45. doi:10.1016/j.cbpra.2009.09.005
36. Brown JM, Miller WR. Impact of motivational interviewing on participation and outcome in residential alcoholism treatment. *Psychol Addict Behav*. 1993;7(4):211-218. doi:10.1037/0893-164X.7.4.211
37. Balán IC, Moyers TB, Lewis-Fernández R. Motivational pharmacotherapy: combining motivational interviewing and antidepressant therapy to improve treatment adherence. *Psychiatry Interpers Biol Process*. 2013;76(3):203-209. doi:10.1521/psyc.2013.76.3.203
38. Spirito A, Monti PM, Barnett NP, et al. A randomized clinical trial of a brief motivational intervention for alcohol-positive adolescents treated in an emergency department. *J Pediatr*. 2004;145(3):396-402. doi:10.1016/j.jpeds.2004.04.057
39. de Gee EA, Verdurmen JEE, Bransen E, de Jonge JM, Schippers GM. A randomized controlled trial of a brief motivational enhancement for non-treatment-seeking adolescent cannabis users. *J Subst Abuse Treat*. 2014;47(3):181-188. doi:10.1016/j.jsat.2014.05.001

40. Forman DP, Moyers TB, Houck JM. What can clients tell us about whether to use motivational interviewing? An analysis of early-session ambivalent language. *J Subst Abuse Treat.* 2022;132:108642. doi:10.1016/j.jsat.2021.108642
41. Clair M, Stein LAR, Soenksen S, Martin RA, Lebeau R, Golembeske C. Ethnicity as a moderator of motivational interviewing for incarcerated adolescents after release. *J Subst Abuse Treat.* 2013;45(4):370-375. doi:10.1016/j.jsat.2013.05.006
42. Hettema J, Steele J, Miller WR. Motivational interviewing. *Annu Rev Clin Psychol.* 2005;1(1):91-111. doi:10.1146/annurev.clinpsy.1.102803.143833
43. Lundahl BW, Kunz C, Brownell C, Tollefson D, Burke BL. A meta-analysis of motivational interviewing: twenty-five years of empirical studies. *Res Soc Work Pract.* 2010;20(2):137-160. doi:10.1177/1049731509347850
44. Lee CS, Colby SM, Magill M, Almeida J, Tavares T, Rohsenow DJ. A randomized controlled trial of culturally adapted motivational interviewing for Hispanic heavy drinkers: theory of adaptation and study protocol. *Contemp Clin Trials.* 2016;50:193-200. doi:10.1016/j.cct.2016.08.013
45. Lee CS, López SR, Colby SM, et al. Culturally adapted motivational interviewing for latino heavy drinkers: results from a randomized clinical trial. *J Ethn Subst Abuse.* 2013;12(4):356-373. doi:10.1080/15332640.2013.836730
46. Venner KL, Hernandez-Vallant A, Hirchak KA, Herron JL. A scoping review of cultural adaptations of substance use disorder treatments across Latinx communities: guidance for future research and practice. *J Subst Abuse Treat.* 2022;137:108716. doi:10.1016/j.jsat.2021.108716
47. Lee CS, Colby SM, Rohsenow DJ, et al. A randomized controlled trial of motivational interviewing tailored for heavy drinking Latinxs. *J Consult Clin Psychol.* 2019;87(9):815-830. doi:10.1037/ccp0000428
48. Kelly LM, Shepherd BF, Becker SJ. Elevated risk of substance use disorder and suicidal ideation among Black and Hispanic lesbian, gay, and bisexual adults. *Drug Alcohol Depend.* 2021;226:108848. doi:10.1016/j.drugalcdep.2021.108848

CHAPTER

71 Group Therapies

Dennis C. Daley, Antoine Douaihy, and Roger D. Weiss

CHAPTER OUTLINE

- Introduction
- Goals of group therapies
- Organization of group therapies
- Empirical validation of group therapies
- Group therapies for co-occurring psychiatric and substance use disorders
- Survey of group therapists
- Limitations of group therapies
- Conclusions

INTRODUCTION

Group therapies are used widely in the treatment of substance use disorders (SUDs), gambling and co-occurring psychiatric disorders (CODs). These are often the main form of treatment used in SUD treatment programs. Group therapies include milieu, psychoeducational recovery, coping skills, family, and therapy or problem-solving groups.[1,2] This chapter provides an overview of goals and types of group therapies used to treat SUDs or CODs, a discussion of studies examining the effectiveness of group therapies for SUDs and their limitations, and training and supervision issues for group leaders.

Groups aim to promote recovery and may address physical, lifestyle, psychological, behavioral, emotional, cognitive, family, interpersonal, social, spiritual, financial issues, depending on the type and goals of the specific group (see **Table 71-1**).[3-20] Group therapies also are widely used in the treatment of specific populations including women[21,22]; individuals with alcohol use disorders[23]; persons in the legal system[24,25]; those with cannabis use disorders[26] or cocaine or methamphetamine use disorders[3-5,27]; and families.[1,2,4,28-30] Furthermore, cognitive-behavioral group therapy (CBGT) is a promising treatment approach for gambling disorders.[31]

GOALS OF GROUP THERAPIES

The long-term goals of treatment are to help the individual with the SUD to achieve and maintain abstinence or reduction and improve the quality of life. Short-term goals are to evaluate and reduce substance use, become motivated to change, address problems caused or worsened by the SUD, and improve functioning. Group therapies help patients achieve these goals by creating a milieu in which group members can bond with each other, thus reducing the stigma associated with addiction.[1] The specific ways in which groups can help achieve this include providing education on addiction, recovery, and relapse; resolving ambivalence and enhancing motivation to change; evoking hope and optimism for change; providing an opportunity to give and receive feedback from peers; teaching recovery skills to manage the SUD; addressing problems resulting from the SUD; providing a context in which the group member can identify with others and give and receive support; creating an experience of positive membership in a recovery-oriented group in which feelings, thoughts, and conflicts can be freely expressed; preparing the patient for involvement in long-term recovery; and facilitating the patient's interest in participating in mutual support programs in addition to treatment groups.[3,4] Group members learn how those with SUDs think, feel, and act, including the manipulations, schemes, and diversions they sometimes use to rationalize their substance use and other maladaptive behaviors.[6]

ORGANIZATION OF GROUP THERAPIES

Group therapies vary in their theoretical underpinnings, structure, format, rules, number and duration of sessions, clinical focus, size, types of patients accepted, goals or requirements for abstinence, approach to the group model, relative focus on content or process, and roles of the group leader. An effective group leader should have the same important therapeutic skills as a good individual therapist such as listening skills, empathy, and therapeutic alliance. A client-centered empathic style is crucial in group therapy. However, scientific evidence has shown that poor outcomes are associated with a confrontational group leader.[32] Self-awareness and monitoring are important components of successful dynamics in group therapy. Yalom[33] described four basic leadership qualities that were associated with positive treatment outcomes: acceptance; caring; meaning attribution; and executive function. So, clearly the group leader characteristics matter, particularly being empathic, encouraging a nonjudgmental and collaborative relationship, and genuinely complements rather than denigrates or diminishes another person.[34] Many recovery-oriented groups are structured and content-focused and depend on the leader to facilitate interactive discussions of educational material with specific objectives and clinical or recovery issues to cover in each session. These groups can accommodate larger numbers of patients than can therapy groups. Models include psychoeducational,[12,35] motivational cognitive-behavioral,- cognitive therapy,[36,37] stages of change,[38] recovery and self-help groups,[13] or family groups.[4,30]

Therapy groups usually are limited to 6 to 10 persons, with the content of discussions determined by the participants. Leaders facilitate members' exploration of problems and sharing of support and feedback. Although some groups incorporate principles and information from mutual support programs such as Alcoholics Anonymous (AA), Narcotics Anonymous (NA), or Self-Management and Recovery Training (SMART Recovery), therapy groups differ in their focus on exploration of psychological, interpersonal, social, spiritual, and intrapersonal issues. A large multisite study of outpatient treatment for cocaine addiction[39] offered 24 weekly group counseling sessions, over a period of 6 months of active treatment in addition to individual or brief case management sessions. The Matrix Model offered 8 early recovery skills, 32 relapse prevention, and 36 social support group sessions (for 76 total group sessions) over 6+ months combined with individual and family sessions.[4,28]

Orienting Patients to Groups

Patients can be prepared for group programs so they understand the goals and structure of groups they will attend, potential benefits, and what is expected from their participation. Clinicians can describe the types and formats of the groups offered and how these differ from AA, NA, SMART Recovery, or other recovery meetings in the community. Patients can be encouraged to express their anxieties about groups or raise questions during this preparation session. The clinician can focus on how groups can help patients increase self-awareness, gain knowledge of their disorder(s), and learn coping skills to meet the challenges of recovery. Patients can also be told that they will receive support and feedback from other group members and to self-disclose their struggles, feelings, and thoughts so that they learn to let others help them. Patients can be told the importance of being on time for group sessions, attending all sessions, and talk about any desire to drop out before they decide to do so. Finally, patients can be assured that if they cannot engage in the groups due to a relapse, the clinician or team will help them find a level of care that can help them stabilize.

Types of Group Therapies

Many of the problems or issues addressed in different models of group treatment are similar (**Table 71-1**). The specific issues or problems addressed depend on the treatment model and number of sessions offered.

Groups usually fall into one of the following categories.[4,12,15,16]

Milieu Groups

These are offered in residential and hospital programs and involve a meeting to start and/or end the day. A morning group reviews the day's schedule and issues pertinent to the community of patients and asks each patient to state a goal for the day or reflect on a recovery or inspirational reading. An evening wrap-up group reviews the day's activities and provides participants a chance to discuss their experiences and what they learned.

Psychoeducational Recovery Groups

These are structured groups that provide information about SUD and recovery and help patients learn strategies to cope with recovery challenges such as cravings, motivation changes, social pressure to use, boredom, anger, other negative emotions, sober relationships, and assessing the impact of SUDs on the family. Many use a curriculum for each session with a specific topic (eg, managing anxiety), objectives, and content areas to cover.[2,4,11-13,15,17,18,22] Ambulatory programs start with a "check-in" process in which patients briefly share their recovery status, level of motivation, cravings for substances, or other issue determined by the specific group. Many groups end with patients sharing something they learned or a recovery issue they will focus on between sessions.

Coping Skill Groups

These help patients develop or improve intrapersonal and interpersonal skills. They may teach problem-solving methods, stress management, or relapse prevention (RP) strategies. RP groups help patients identify and manage early signs of relapse, identify, and manage high-risk factors, or learn how to intervene early with a lapse or relapse.

Therapy or Counseling Groups (Also Called Problem-Solving or Process Groups)

In these groups, participants identify problems, conflicts, or struggles to work on during the session. Any of the issues in Table 64-1 may be discussed. These issues focus on raising self-awareness more than on education or skill development although participants learn many things and are exposed to coping strategies that others use to manage the challenges of recovery from an SUD.

Specialized Groups

These may be based on developmental stage (adolescents, young adults, adults, older adults), gender, different clinical populations (women, patients involved in the criminal justice system, patients with co-occurring psychiatric illness), or groups addressing specific issues (parenting issues, anger or mood management, relapse prevention, or trauma).

More extensive discussions of group approaches for addiction, such as interactional group therapy,[34,40] modified dynamic group therapy,[29,41] cognitive or cognitive-behavioral therapy,[12,22,35,42,43] psychoeducational and problem-solving therapy,[39,44] skills training therapy,[23] recovery stage–specific group therapy,[6,9,37,45] relapse prevention therapy,[4,6,11,12] or mindfulness-based approaches[46,47] can be found in texts elsewhere.

Format of Group Sessions

Group sessions usually last 60 to 90 minutes. Groups can be limited to a specific number of sessions in which all participants start the group together or be open ended so that new patients can be continuously added to the group.

TABLE 71-1 Issues Commonly Addressed in Recovery Groups

Physical/lifestyle issues	Lapse/relapse interruption
Tolerance, physical withdrawal, and the need for withdrawal management	Spirituality
Craving management	Meditation and prayer
Medications for addiction and for co-occurring disorders (including naloxone for reversing opioid overdoses)	**Understanding addiction and recovery**
Medical problems including pain issues	Understanding addiction (etiology, symptoms, effects)
Good health care and dental habits	Effects of specific substances (eg, alcohol, cocaine, cannabis)
Pregnancy and substance use or addiction, neonatal abstinence syndrome, fetal alcohol syndrome	Acceptance of addiction
HIV/AIDS, hepatitis C virus, and hepatitis B virus	Stages of change
Sexuality issues	Motivation to change and motivational struggles such as ambivalence
Exercise, rest, relaxation, and nutrition in recovery	Tips for quitting alcohol or drug use
Types and purposes of treatment	Pros and cons of change
Defining personal goals/values	Pros and cons of abstinence
Seeking employment	Denial and other defenses
Managing money	Phases of recovery and domains of recovery (physical, psychological, family, social, spiritual)
Structuring time, using schedules, and keeping busy	Risky behaviors (such as sharing needles and equipment)
Engaging in non–substance-using activities	Other nonsubstance addiction (gambling, sex, eating, spending, internet, etc.)
Achieving balance in life	Positive outcomes based on clinical trials, surveys of individuals and families in recovery, and membership surveys of AA, NA, and Al-Anon
Regular use of recovery tools in daily life	
Psychological/behavioral/spiritual issues	**Family/interpersonal/social issues**
Understanding and identifying feelings and their connections to relapse	Effects of addiction on family and interpersonal relationships
Changing thoughts and beliefs	Role of the family, concerned significant others in treatment/recovery
Managing anxiety	Resolving marital or family conflicts
Managing boredom	Making amends to family or others
Managing depression	Managing high-risk people, places, and events
Managing feelings of emptiness	Engaging in healthy leisure interests
Reducing shame and guilt	Addressing social life and relationship conflicts
Grief and loss issues	Resisting social pressures to drink alcohol or use other drugs
Trauma	Presenting a history of addiction disorders to the employer
Positive emotions (gratitude, compassion, forgiveness, love)	Facing versus avoiding interpersonal conflicts
Mindfulness	Learning to ask for help and support
Self-esteem	Love and intimacy
Self-defeating and therapy-sabotaging behaviors	Mutual support programs in recovery (12-step and non–12-step programs)
Psychiatric comorbidities	The 12 steps (overview or focus on specific steps)
Relapse and personal growth	Sponsorship
High-risk factors or dangerous situations for relapse	Recovery tools
Relapse warning signs	Recovery clubs
Relapse setups	

Treatment programs vary in the frequency of group sessions as well as whether individual and/or family sessions are also provided as part of a total "program." For example, the Matrix Model[4] offered individual and family sessions in addition to their extensive group program. In our multisite trial of treatment for cocaine addiction,[37] 24 group sessions were provided to all study participants over 6 months. Three-fourths of patients also received up to 42 individual sessions over 9 months. In our study called STAGE-12 (Stimulant Groups to Engage in 12-Step Programs), participants received five weekly group sessions in addition to three individual sessions over an 8-week period while participating in a structured ambulatory intensive outpatient program.[3] The Washton[45] structured outpatient model involved group therapy two to four times each week in combination with weekly individual counseling sessions. These examples show the diversity of treatment programs utilizing groups with patients who have SUDs.

Interventions of Group Leaders

A group can have different designs. It can be led by one individual, co-led by 2 facilitators, or led by a primary facilitator with the presence of a secondary facilitator. Two cofacilitators could complement each other's skills and expertise, provide different social roles, and guide difficult and challenging sessions. Group leaders may use a combination of any of the following:

- *Educational presentations* in which members are provided information about substances and their effects, causes and symptoms of SUDs, treatments, recovery, relapse, family issues, medical issues such as HIV or hepatitis C, co-occurring psychiatric illness, and other issues that may be specific to the group members (eg, women's issues, LGBTQIA+ issues). Interactive discussions can engage members in meaningful discussions of content, so they relate information reviewed to their personal situations.
- *Brief stories* to illustrate an issue or point discussed. Stories can be told by the group leader, guest presenter, or group members to illustrate success or failure in dealing with specific issues or challenges of recovery discussed.
- *Guest presenters with expertise in specific areas* such as a psychiatrist, psychologist, or therapist on mental health issues; pharmacist on effects of drugs; physician, nurse, or other health professional on medical issues; religious professional on spiritual issues; social worker on family issues or community resources; or recovering persons to share their stories.
- *Video or audio* to provide information or hopeful stories of recovery. These should be brief and used to stimulate discussion of SUDs and recovery issues.
- *Workbooks, journals, or worksheets* in which patients share answers to questions about their SUDs or CODs, their recovery, or specific issues discussed by the group (eg, managing anger; reducing boredom; dealing with high-risk people). These client workbooks can be used as facilitator guides. Surveys completed by 300+ patients in our treatment programs showed that the majority found workbooks useful in learning information and coping strategies to deal with their SUDs or CODs. Comments to open-ended questions had a 4:1 ratio of positive (eg, "helped me accept the need for long-term help; helped make me motivated to recover; taught me ways to cope with urges or cravings") to negative (eg, "need better preparation on how to use workbooks; material was redundant"). In addition, 41 staff members completed surveys and 8 were interviewed by an addiction fellow for their input. Results showed that staff from all disciplines routinely use workbooks and find them very useful or useful with patients. Over 80% used four or more workbooks with patients in the past year. Staff also shared positive responses to open-ended questions. Only a few staff did not use workbooks and stated they preferred focusing on "therapy" issues rather than education or coping skills.[48]
- *Readings* on recovery or other related topics. These can be assigned to the group or specific members.
- *Visual handouts* to provide information and stimulate discussion. We use a diagram of the brain to show the areas involved in decision-making, emotions, and memory. We elicit examples of members of struggles in recovery associated with different areas of the brain.
- *PowerPoint slides* show visual examples of the effects of substances or SUDs or recovery. Or these can be used to illustrate ways to think about recovery. For example, showing pictures of drugs and the works can be used to discuss how these trigger cravings to use.
- *Behavioral assignments.* Group members can be asked to complete assignments related to the group topic reviewed in structured recovery sessions. For example, if the group topic is understanding and managing depression, members can be instructed to keep a daily calendar in which they rate their mood so they can see changes between group sessions.
- *In vivo role-plays.* These address interpersonal problems such as dealing with a conflict, resisting pressure to engage in risky sex or substance use, or helping a group member practice asking a member of AA or NA to serve as his sponsor. Role-plays can include dyads or triads or use multiple people. Follow-up discussions can focus on the interpersonal interaction observed, thoughts and feelings the issue illustrated generates, and behavioral options to manage the problem that is the focus of the role-play.
- *Monodramas to externalize a problem, conflict, or recovery issue.* For example, a member can be asked to create a dialogue between his "healthy recovering self" and his "unhealthy addicted self." Or a member can be asked to imagine his craving for drugs, sitting on a chair and trying to convince him to get high. This member goes back and forth between being the craving and the person in recovery with a focus on building confidence to resist giving in to the craving despite how strong or convincing it is during the role-play. Other members coach this person if they feel vulnerable to letting a conflict lead to poor decisions.
- *Creative media* (arts, crafts, media) *or other health lifestyle strategies* (meditation, yoga, exercise). These not only aid recovery but also help members improve their overall health and the quality of their lives.

Phase 1: Recovery Group Sessions

In the NIDA Collaborative Cocaine Treatment Study, in which three of the authors participated, patients attended 90-minute recovery group sessions each week for 12 weeks.[40,43,44] Each session focused on a specific topic relevant to early or middle recovery. At every session, patients were encouraged to abstain from all substances, seek and use a sponsor, participate in mutual support groups, and use the "tools" of recovery (eg, talking about versus acting on strong cravings, reaching out for support, and the like). Patients were encouraged to socialize with each other before the start of the session while the group leader administered a breathalyzer test. Each session began with a check-in (10-20 minutes), in which patients briefly reported any substance use, strong cravings, or "close calls." This was followed by a discussion of the topic for the session (40-60 minutes). Each session provided materials from a workbook with information about the topic and questions for members to relate the material to their lives. During discussions, patients were encouraged to ask questions, share experiences related to the material, give each other feedback, and identify strategies to manage the issues discussed.

Each session ended with a brief review of patients' plans for the coming week (10-15 minutes). Patients discussed mutual support meetings and other steps they would in their recovery. Patients recited the Serenity Prayer of AA/NA to end the meeting. Topics of phase 1 included (these topics are similar to those offered in other group models) understanding addiction, the recovery process, social and interpersonal issues in recovery, cravings, mutual support programs, recovery support systems, managing emotions, relapse issues (warning signs or high-risk factors or intervention early in a lapse or relapse), and using recovery tools to maintain change over time.

Phase 2: Problem-Solving (Therapy) Groups

Phase 2 groups met for 90 minutes weekly for 12 sessions. The goals were to help patients identify, prioritize, and discuss problems in recovery and identify strategies to manage these. Patients gave and received support and feedback from each other. After the check-in period, participants were asked to identify a problem or recovery issue for discussion. Often, more than one member would identify a similar problem or issue. The issues and problems reviewed in the phase 1 groups were revisited frequently. Common issues discussed include struggles with motivation to change or remain abstinent; obsessions or compulsions or close calls to use; lapses or relapses; boredom, anxiety, anger, depression, or other emotions; concerns with mutual support programs, the twelve steps, or a sponsor; interpersonal problems; social pressures to use substances; financial, job, and lifestyle problems; other addiction; and spirituality. At the end of each session, patients stated their plans for the coming week in terms of meetings or other steps to aid their recovery or resolve a problem.

Group Process Issues

Counselors had to attend to the group process to keep the group focused and productive. This required counselors to engage quiet members in discussions and facilitate their self-disclosure and to limit or redirect members who talked too much and dominated discussions, listened poorly, or used the group for individual therapy. Counselors kept the group from going off on unrelated tangents or talking in generalities, balanced the discussions between problems and coping strategies, facilitated group members' sharing of support and feedback, and addressed impasses or problems in the group. In phase 1 groups, the counselor had to ensure that the curriculum for each session was covered.

Obstacles to Group Therapy

Researchers who have written about group treatments identify problems that create obstacles to group treatment. Washton[6] reports the following problems among members of therapy groups: lateness and absenteeism, intoxication, hostility and chronic complaining, silence and lack of participation, terse and superficial presentations, factual reporting and focusing on externals, proselytizing, and hiding behind AA, and playing co-therapist. Because the problems affect the group, the leader must have strategies to address any that arise during a group session. For example, if a member consistently rejects the advice or feedback of other members, the leader can point out this pattern and engage the group in a discussion of why this is occurring. The members whose help and support are rejected can be asked to talk about what this feels like so that the member who rejects it is aware of the impact this behavior has on others.

Family Psychoeducational Workshops

Family psychoeducation workshops (FPWs) aim to educate the family, provide support, help reduce the family's burden, increase helpful behaviors, decrease unhelpful behaviors, and provide hope.[4,28-30] FPWs are semi structured sessions with multiple families and members with SUDs present. Families are encouraged to share their questions, concerns, and feelings.

Strong affect often is present in these workshops, and some sharing of emotion is necessary. However, encouraging families to share their emotions too much can be counterproductive, so education and support are the main areas of focus. Thus, the group leader must be careful not to allow the group to become a venue for sharing deep-seated emotions. Interactive discussion is encouraged because it increases participants' understanding of addiction and recovery. The specific material covered in FPWs depends on the amount of time available. The following topics and issues may be discussed:

- *An overview of substance use and SUDs:* current trends in substance use, prevalence, types, causes, and symptoms of SUDs.
- *Effects of SUDs:* on the individual with the SUD, the family system, and family members, including children.
- *An overview of treatment and helpful resources:* programs and interventions (including medications) and resources for the affected individual are discussed. These include professional services and community resources such as mutual support programs.
- *Overview of recovery:* the recovery process and biopsychosocial-spiritual issues that may be addressed.

- *How the family can help:* behaviors for the family to avoid and behaviors that are helpful in supporting recovery of the member with the SUD.
- *Family recovery:* how the family member can recover from the adverse effects of an SUD. What they can do to help themselves rather than solely focus on the impaired family member.
- *Mutual support programs:* for individuals with SUDs and family members. How these programs can help family members and how to access them (eg, Al-Anon, Nar-Anon, NAMI for psychiatric illness).
- *Relapse:* warning signs, high-risk factors, how the family can be involved in relapse prevention plans, and how to deal with setbacks.

In the NIDA Collaborative Cocaine Treatment Study,[37,39] we offered a single 2-hour FPW during the first month of treatment. The purpose of the session was to educate families about the study; seek their help in supporting the patients' compliance with treatment; and provide education about addiction, recovery, effects on the family, and community resources available to the family. The Matrix program offered a group "family education" curriculum to supplement individual and group sessions for program participants.[4] This involves 12 sessions that focused on issues of concern for the family such as triggers and cravings for substances, recovery, alcohol and drugs, relapse, family issues in recovery, rebuilding trust, recovery challenges for families, and communication issues. However, not all treatment programs or group approaches incorporate sessions or focus on family issues. The role of interpersonal processes and social support is a critical component of relapse prevention.[49] This underscores the value of involving family members in supporting the patient's recovery efforts through their participation in sessions.

Group Motivational Interviewing

One of the major challenges of incorporating motivational interviewing (MI) in group format—group motivational interviewing (GMI)— is ensuring that the spirit, processes, skills, and strategies are translated and delivered effectively with fidelity.[50,51] When facilitating GMI, clinicians are expected to create a safe empathic and nonconfrontational atmosphere aligned with the elements of MI spirit such as partnership, autonomy respect, compassion, evocation, and acceptance among group members. The focus of the GMI leaders is to use strategies to facilitate evoking and supporting group members' change talk statements (Desire, Ability, Reasons and Need: DARN) and commitment language that favors change, while helping members explore and resolve ambivalence for change. An advantage of GMI is that the leaders encourage group members to express how they connect and relate to each other's change talk and to open up about their value system and motivations for change. This process where group members mutually "cull for change talk" is referred to as *relatedness*.[52,53] The efficacy of GMI remains unclear. In a recent study, Santa Ana et al. developed a 4-session, GMI intervention for veterans who had alcohol use and co-occurring psychiatric disorders and found that it outperformed the treatment control condition on measures of alcohol use, outpatient treatment engagement, and 12-step group attendance over 3 months.[54] This study supports the implementation of a brief GMI that could help facilitate early treatment engagement and maybe cost-effective compared to individually based intervention.

EMPIRICAL VALIDATION OF GROUP THERAPIES

Despite the widespread use of group therapies in addiction treatment, controlled trials of group interventions are limited, and many studies report results from "programs" that involve multiple components (ie, individual plus group, multiple types of group treatments, or group plus other services). In a review of the group treatment of addiction literature, Sobell and Sobell[42] found only five studies that compared the same cognitive-behavioral intervention in both individual and group formats. All studies found both types of treatment to be effective, but none showed a significant difference in outcomes of patients receiving individual versus group treatment suggesting that group is as effective as individual treatment.

Weiss et al.[55] reviewed 24 prospective treatment outcome studies comparing group therapy with one or more treatment conditions. The results of the studies were mixed, varying on the nature of the research design, the population studied, and the format of treatment (content, intensity, and length). The findings showed three important patterns: additional specialized group therapy can enhance the effectiveness of "treatment as usual," no differences were found between group and individual modalities, and no single type of group therapy demonstrated any consistent superiority in efficacy. The content of the group (whether skill based or interpersonal) did not make a difference. The authors concluded that the most notable finding of that study was the paucity of research on this topic. However, researchers and clinicians agree on the importance of group therapies, and groups remain one of the principal modalities of treatment in most SUD or COD treatment programs.

Lopez et al.[56] reviewed 50 studies that reported on the efficacy of group treatment for SUDs. They identified several types of effective group models. These include Cognitive–Behavioral Therapy, Dialectical Behavior Therapy, Seeking Safety, and Contingency Management groups. They also found that group therapy plus pharmacotherapy was effective in reducing illicit opioid use.

Several effective group treatments have been developed and implemented for women with SUDs, many of whom also had mood, anxiety, or other psychiatric issues.[21,56-60] A randomized controlled trial of a Women's Recovery Group (WRG) demonstrated significant reductions of alcohol and drug use and improvements in anxiety, depression, and general mental health symptoms at 6 and 9 months posttreatment.[59] Compared to a mixed-gender control group treatment condition, women in the WRG endorsed feeling safe, embracing all aspects of the self, having their needs met, and feeling intimacy, empathy, and honesty in group sessions.[21] These sessions focused on issues common in other group therapies for SUDs and also on issues specific to women and their recovery such as caretaking, substance use through the lifecycle, substance use and reproductive health, women and their partners including violence and abuse, and psychiatric issues such as anxiety, depression, or eating disorders.

Najavits' Seeking Safety (SS) is a present-focused coping skills program that addresses substance use and trauma. It is one of the best-established integrated treatments for co-occurring PTSD and SUD,[22] a manualized CBT model. A meta-analysis on controlled studies of Seeking Safety by Lenz, Henesy, and Callender[61] found medium effect sizes for decreasing PTSD symptoms and modest effects for decreasing SUD symptoms. A recent study compared Seeking Safety program for co-occurring PTSD and SUDs to another cognitive behavioral treatment (Relapse Prevention Training) and to treatment as usual (TAU). The results showed decreases in PTSD severity that were comparable in all three conditions. The SS group improved more on depression and emotion regulation than TAU alone and The Relapse Prevention group improved more on alcohol and drug use than TAU alone.[62] SS helps patients attain safety in relationships, thinking, behavior, and emotions by addressing both substance use and trauma issues in an integrated way. Cognitive, behavioral, interpersonal, and case management strategies are used in SS to address these issues. SS was initially developed for women in groups but later was implemented with men, in individual sessions, and in mental health as well as SUDs programs.[22,60]

Adherence to Group Sessions and Treatment Discontinuation

Most randomized clinical trials showed significant reductions in drug use, improved health, and reduced social pathology.[63] Patients who comply with sessions and attend enough sessions show better outcomes than do those who discontinue prematurely. However, two of the major problems in the treatment of SUDs and CODs are poor adherence with session attendance or medications and early termination.[64] Integrated supportive group therapy in a randomized trial has shown a differential effect on treatment retention in subjects with severe mental disorders and SUDs.[65] We used a contingency management (CM) intervention for patients in an intensive outpatient program (IOP) in which patients earned rewards (draws from a fishbowl to choose small, medium, or large prizes) for attending an IOP 3-hour session. Patients receiving the CM intervention ($N = 88$) attended 16.2 program days compared to 9.9 days that the controls ($N = 72$) attended.[66]

Reasons for Treatment Discontinuation

In the NIDA Collaborative Cocaine Treatment Study,[37] the reasons patients cited most commonly for discontinuation were time problems (42.7%); recurrence of use or the desire to use (30.7%); not finding group helpful (29.3%); wanting a different treatment, such as individual therapy (30.7%); improvement in the problem (18.7%); other unspecified reasons (18.7%); unwillingness to participate in treatment (16%); and need for hospitalization (13.3%).

Limitations of Research

Although evidence suggests that group treatments are effective for SUDs, limitations to the research conducted on group treatments arise from two sources: variations in content and differences in process. Also, discontinuation rates are higher among patients in groups compared to individual therapy.

A level of interaction and complexity must be taken into consideration, over and above the content of the intervention and the counselor's skill in conducting it. Very often, group programs are evaluated rather than a single-group intervention. For example, studies of intensive outpatient programs often evaluate a comprehensive program that involves several different types of groups that together make up the intensive outpatient program. Some studies of group treatments were conducted on patients who first participated in an intensive residential program or concurrent treatment program, making it difficult to determine the impact of the group or other factors on patient outcome. Therefore, it is unclear how much each type of group contributes to outcome. In addition, studies sometimes involve a combination of group and individual treatments, making it difficult to determine how much each intervention contributes to the outcome.

The discrepancy between the widespread clinical application of group therapy and the limited research stems from the inherent difficulties in conducting meaningful research on group therapy.[49] Since group treatment is the most common psychosocial intervention offered, more research is clearly needed to study both the efficacy and effectiveness of group interventions.

GROUP THERAPIES FOR CO-OCCURRING PSYCHIATRIC AND SUBSTANCE USE DISORDERS

Epidemiological and clinical studies document high rates of co-occurring psychiatric and SUDs.[16-18,67,68] Research supports the use of group treatments for patients with CODs, including those with chronic and persistent mental disorders.[16,18,21,22,69-71] Several investigators have developed and tested integrated interventions in clinical trials using manual-driven group treatments.[63]

The Najavits' Seeking Safety (SS) model mentioned previously involves 24 weekly group sessions, divided into "units" dealing with problems frequently encountered.[17,22,72,73] Education is provided on trauma or posttraumatic stress disorder (PTSD) and SUDs, community resources, and mutual aid programs. Specific units focus on behavioral, communication, relationship, cognitive issues, and the importance of ongoing support following program completion. When the group treatment contract is signed, an interview is conducted with each patient before he or she enters the group, and ways to benefit from this treatment are reviewed. An individual HIV counseling session is provided to each patient within the first 3 weeks of treatment, at which time an HIV risk assessment is completed and education and counseling on HIV issues are provided. Homework assignments and action techniques such as role-play are used throughout this protocol. SS has been used in numerous programs in the United States and other countries. Its efficacy and effectiveness are supported by some clinical trials[21] but not others.[56]

A randomized clinical trial evaluated the efficacy of a 12-session CBGT for DSM-defined alcohol-dependent males with co-occurring interpersonal violence.[71] Results showed a significant difference between participants in the integrated approach (SUD-domestic violence) versus the twelve-step facilitation group on alcohol use outcomes. The group assigned to substance use-domestic violence reported using alcohol significantly fewer days as compared with the twelve-step facilitation group. Regarding physical violence, there was a trend for participants in the SUD-domestic violence condition to achieve a greater reduction in the frequency of violent behaviors across time compared with individuals in the twelve-step facilitation group.[74]

Weiss et al. developed and tested an integrated cognitive-behavioral group treatment (IGT) for bipolar patients with SUDs.[75] This involved a 20-week randomized controlled trial ($N = 62$) with 3 months of posttreatment follow-up, to compare the efficacy of IGT versus an active addiction treatment, group drug counseling (GDC), an adaptation of the model used in the NIDA Collaborative Cocaine Treatment Study.[37,39] Both IGT and GDC are manual-driven treatments that involve 20 weekly group sessions of 1 hour each. IGT focuses on issues pertinent to substance use and bipolar illness, whereas GDC focuses solely on SUD. GDC patients address psychiatric issues in separate sessions with a mental health professional. All patients in the study also received medications for their bipolar illness. Patients in both conditions improved, but IGT was more successful at reducing substance use despite more subclinical mood symptoms. A briefer, revised version of IGT with 12 group sessions also favored IGT, with nearly three times as many patients attaining abstinence throughout treatment. Moreover, more than twice as many IGT patients experienced a "good clinical outcome," defined as abstinence and the absence of any mood episode during the last month of treatment.[71]

In a quality improvement study of 117 patients who participated in an integrated COD-intensive outpatient program developed by two of the authors (DD and AD),[15] there was a steady weekly decrease in mean scores for the Beck Anxiety Inventory, Beck Depression Inventory, and Addiction Severity Index from baseline to week 4. The mean rating of both Beck Anxiety Inventory and Beck Depression Inventory scores declined from "moderate" to "mild" by week 4, and the mean Addiction Severity Index scored was 58% lower at week 4 than at baseline.[15] A review of studies assessing group interventions for patients with SUDs and psychotic disorders concluded that the most encouraging interventions include assertive outreach, integration within the treatment setting, motivational interviewing, and follow-up longer than 1 year to attain clinically significant reductions in substance use over time.[76]

Short-term results from a randomized controlled trial among people with psychotic disorders, which used group MI and CBT within a harm minimization paradigm over six 90-minute sessions, showed that compared to a control group that received a single hour-long session of education regarding drug use, the MI/CBT group intervention condition did significantly better in terms of reductions in global psychopathology, drug use, severity of DSM-IV–defined dependence, and, in addition, a lower rate of hospitalization at 3 months after intervention.[77]

Bradley et al.[78] evaluated an open-ended outpatient group intervention (in the context of a service evaluation project with clinicians administered ratings), incorporating the features reported in the previous study,[74] consisting of MI and CBT, among patients with psychosis and SUDs. This group intervention was conducted in a rural setting and with groups led by clinicians from mental health and drug and alcohol services, including coleaders who were not originators of the intervention model. Compared with baseline, the group intervention was associated with significant improvements in substance use, symptomatology, treatment noncompliance, and overall functioning.

Group MI in a nonrandomized but sequentially assigned study showed promising results when added to standard treatment for psychiatric inpatients with CODs, leading to improved treatment outcomes. Of those patients who attended aftercare and who used substances, those who participated in group MI were more adherent to treatment sessions, used less alcohol, and engaged in less binge drinking at follow-up compared with those in the control group.[79]

The Need for Physician Input and Support

Physicians can play a significant role in providing input into group program development and supporting and facilitating patients' participation in groups. First, physicians can suggest specific topics for recovery groups and/or conduct a group. For example, in one of the first author's ambulatory programs, a physician developed and conducted a group on "addiction and the brain" and created a curriculum for clinicians to use when they conducted this session. Some treatment programs use physicians to present groups on topics such as medical aspects of addiction, medications that can support recovery, causes of addiction or mental illness, and other relevant topics that can tap the expertise of the physician. Patients often respond very favorably to the "doctor" who conducts a group session, and they often have many questions to ask the physician. Second, physicians can educate, encourage, and persuade patients to participate in treatment groups as part of their overall treatment program. It is helpful for clinical staff to give patients a consistent message about the value of group treatments.

The physician can use his or her status as a healer to help the patient decide to participate and not underestimate his or her influence, given the power of even brief interventions on substance behaviors.[80] Third, the physician can monitor and discuss the patient's group participation. This allows the physician to identify and resolve any barriers related to the patient's continued participation, to understand the reasons for poor adherence or early dropout, and to help the patient re-engage in group. Fourth, the physician can collaborate with group therapists about patients' clinical status or problems with adherence. A physician may also see a patient for management of withdrawal, for management of a COD, or for medication management. If, during such a visit, the physician learns that the patient is not adhering to the plan to attend or participate actively in treatment groups, the physician can facilitate a discussion with the group leader or even hold a joint meeting with the patient and group therapist to try to resolve the problem. The physician or the psychiatrist can also cofacilitate a group session with the group leader. Again, the message the patient receives from this collaboration is that the group is an important part of the overall treatment plan and is valued by the physician.

SURVEY OF GROUP THERAPISTS

We conducted a confidential online survey of 89 staff members employed in addiction Community Treatment Programs that were part of NIDA's Clinical Trials Network, a national research group.[81,82] Our goal was to gather information about current practices of therapists in conducting groups as well as training needs. The majority of respondents were therapists or counselors with a master's or bachelor's degree (86.4%). The majority (63.2%) had more than 5 years of clinical experience in addiction treatment programs. The settings in which they provided group services were diverse and covered the continuum of care including outpatient clinics (43.2%), short-term (<30 days) residential treatment programs (27.3%), intensive outpatient programs providing up to 10 hours of clinical services per week (26.1%), specialized narcotic addiction programs providing opioid maintenance therapies (23.9%), long-term residential (>30 days) or therapeutic community programs (15.9%), withdrawal management units in rehabilitation programs or medical hospitals (12.5%), partial hospital programs providing over 10 hours of clinical services per week (10.2%), or psychiatric hospitals (6.8%). In a typical week, therapists provided an average of 10 hours in structured recovery or psychoeducational groups (2.5 hours), therapy groups (2.2 hours), coping skills or relapse prevention groups (1.9 hours), milieu groups (1.9 hours), expressive arts groups (0.8 hours), and family groups (0.7 hours).

Counselor Training

To provide effective group treatment, it is necessary for therapists to be familiar with and skillful in SUD treatment and group therapy. Ongoing training and supervision help to keep counselors abreast of current developments in the field and enthusiastic about their work.

The knowledge base to provide competent treatment for SUDs involves understanding effects of substances as well as the medical, psychological, social, family, and spiritual consequences of SUDs. Other areas of knowledge needed include the recovery process, causes and effects of relapse, and the strategies for recovering persons to manage the SUD and reduce relapse risk. The clinician should also be familiar with AA or NA and other 12-step programs and with alternative mutual support programs and online resources. Counselors need to have experience in counseling individuals because situations arise that require the group counselor to intervene with an individual member. Conducting groups thus involve an additional level of complexity compared with working with individuals, in that the group leader must be able to understand and respond to individual as well as group dynamics or group process issues simultaneously.

Counselors also need an understanding of stages of groups and the "group process," which refers to the attitudes and interaction of the group members and leader. The group leader should be familiar with group interventions and how to deal with problem situations that are common in groups. Intervention skills include active listening, clarification and questioning, information giving, summarization, encouraging and supporting, modeling, eliciting feedback, and addressing problems that commonly arise in group (eg, a member who dominates the group, resistant members who are reluctant to participate, a member who tries to assume the role of the leader, mutually hostile members, insensitive feedback, and members who challenge the leader).

Counselor Supervision

Supervision is important, yet it often is overlooked or provided in a less than optimal manner. The group counselor should have access to someone who has experience and expertise in the field, to whom the counselor can bring any problems as they emerge. It also is important to communicate that supervision is not primarily about evaluation of the counselor's work but rather an opportunity for the counselor to air problems, hone his or her skills, and continue to learn. In one of our (DD and AD) ambulatory clinics, we provided monthly group consultation to all group leaders in a group format so they could learn from each other. These sessions often focused more on group process issues and patient behaviors in group than on specific content.

Therapists in the NIDA Cocaine Collaborative Study protocol received weekly and then biweekly supervision by telephone from a supervisor who viewed videos of sessions conducted and rated with an adherence scale. Because this study was for comparative research, adherence to the counseling approach was of utmost importance. An adherence scale provides specific operational definitions of desired interventions. These definitions make it clear to counselors what interventions should be incorporated into their work and make it easy for supervisors to point out strengths and deficiencies when giving feedback.

Adherence scales associated with a treatment manual can be a useful tool for both research and clinical purposes, in that they allow researchers to assess whether therapists are following the specified treatment manual. They are helpful in showing that treatments can be differentiated from one another and in assessing the extent to which counselors incorporate techniques from other treatments. Moreover, they are useful clinically in training and supervision of a model of treatment.

Counselor Satisfaction

It is important that counselors feel satisfied with the group services they are providing and with the clinical environment in which they work. When counselors are dissatisfied, burnout, indifferent treatment, and departures from appropriate counseling behavior often result. Dissatisfied counselors also tend to feel less positive about their work and to express less confidence in their patients' ability to achieve recovery; such feelings can undermine the patients' own perception of their ability to recover. Therefore, access to group supervision and consultation and training programs are important for counselors conducting groups.

LIMITATIONS OF GROUP THERAPIES

Although groups offer many benefits, they also have limitations. One of the most common is an overemphasis on group treatment with little or no individual treatment. As part of an ongoing quality improvement effort, the first author met with small focus groups of patients (totaling more than 1,000 over several years) in a broad range of addiction and COD treatment programs to inquire about what they liked and disliked about treatment. He also met with patients from other treatment programs as part of evaluating their programs and making recommendations. Programs with minimal groups were often viewed by patients as lacking in opportunities for learning about their disorders and ways to cope. Patients also report getting bored when they have too much time on their hands while in an inpatient or residential program that does not offer many treatment groups or that does not use homework assignments to aid their recovery (eg, keeping written journals, completing reading or workbook assignments).

Although most patients participating in group treatments were able to articulate benefits of the group, a consistent criticism heard over many years has been a concern that they did not receive any or enough individual therapy. Patients often reported that there were certain types of problems or issues that they would not discuss in group sessions and that they preferred the privacy and confidentiality afforded by an individual counseling or therapy session.

Examples that patients reported of the personal problems difficult to disclose in group sessions included experiences as a victim or perpetrator of violence, sexual abuse, child abuse, some types of deviant behaviors, the presence of certain psychiatric symptoms, and conflicts related to sexual identity or behaviors. In addition to difficulties disclosing such traumas, it may be difficult to perform exposure therapy or cognitive processing of traumas in a group format given the need for personalization of treatment. Confidentiality issues were cited as another reason for reluctance to disclose personal information in some group sessions. This was particularly true of patients who participated in a group session in which another member was from the same neighborhood or shared mutual friends. Patients who had difficulty with assertiveness or disclosing personal problems reported that it was easy for them to blend into the background in a group. Although this felt "safe," the patients recognized that this feeling led to less-than-optimal gain from group therapy. Some patients described attending group sessions in which the leader did not control participants who talked too much or who listened poorly to others or leaders who did not engage quiet members in group discussions. Social anxiety or phobias are common among patients with SUDs.[83] Daley and Salloum[84] administered the Davidson Brief Social Phobia questionnaire to 128 outpatients with CODs and found that more than one-third reported high levels of social anxiety and avoidance behavior. Patients reported high levels of anxiety about speaking at AA or NA meetings or in group therapy. Because of social anxiety, patients may choose to limit participation in group discussions, miss group sessions, or drop out prematurely. They often do so without discussing their reasons with a therapist, counselor, or sponsor.

CONCLUSIONS

The research literature and clinical experience suggest several points that are important to an understanding of group therapies for SUDs and CODs. First, group therapies play a critical role in treatment of these disorders and should be supported by all clinicians, regardless of whether they provide group sessions themselves. Second, different group therapies can be used, depending on a given patient's progress in relation to the stages of change and the treatment context. Third, a combination of group and individual treatment is optimal. This issue is important because group therapy is the primary and often sole modality offered by some SUD treatment programs. Fourth, integrated group interventions that focus on both addiction and psychiatric issues are the preferred approach for patients with CODs. Fifth, staff training and ongoing supervision can enhance the effectiveness of group therapies. Sixth, patients who participate in group therapies often benefit from medications, so the benefits can be discussed in group sessions.[85] Seventh, mutual support programs and group therapies are different in their purpose and structure. Group therapies can encourage attendance at mutual support programs, provide education, and explore experiences and resistances. Therapy groups are designed to explore psychological, personal, and interpersonal issues in a safe environment in which self-disclosure, self-awareness, and self-change are encouraged and valued. Eighth, treatment personnel must be sensitive to the fact that SUDs are debilitating and chronic conditions for many patients. As with other chronic disorders, more severe SUDs require ongoing management. Group therapy is an approach to initiating and continuing this process to the maintenance phase of recovery. Ninth, group leaders can utilize recovery materials to aid patient learning of information and coping skills. Our surveys of over 300 patients in multiple treatment programs show that patients rate using recovery workbooks as very helpful in learning information and coping skills.[48] They are able to identify numerous ways in which these materials aid their recovery. Finally, leaders can improve group services by eliciting feedback from patients, both in group sessions and with the use of written evaluations. For example, a group leader could say to members "I am interested in knowing what you like and do not like about our group. Can we discuss what you find helpful, what you think is unhelpful, and suggestions to improve our group?" Alternatively, a group leader could have members anonymously complete a brief questionnaire in which they rate the group sessions in terms of information learned, coping strategies learned, self-awareness gained, or other areas, depending on the type and purpose of the group.

Group therapy is one of the most common therapeutic approaches in SUD treatment settings. Clinical supervision and formal training in specific group processes and dynamics, as well as evidence-based SUD group therapies are needed. Strong empirical data showed that group therapy is cost effective and produces patient outcomes comparable to individual therapy in SUD treatment acceptance, retention, reductions in frequency of use, abstinence rates, and psychological symptoms and distress.[86,87]

REFERENCES

1. U.S. Department of Health and Human Services. *Substance Abuse Treatment: Group Therapy. A Treatment Improvement Protocol TIP 41.* U.S. DHHS; 2005.
2. Daley DC, Douaihy A. *Group Treatments of Addiction: Counseling Strategies for Recovery and Therapy Groups.* Daley Publications; 2011.
3. Daley DC, Baker MAS, Donovan DM, Hodgkins CG, Perl H. A combined group and individual 12-step facilitative intervention targeting stimulant abuse in the NIDA Clinical Trials Network: STAGE-12. *J Groups Addict Recover.* 2011;6:228-244.
4. Rawson RA, Obert JL, McCann MJ, et al. *The Matrix Model: Intensive Outpatient Alcohol and Drug Treatment.* Hazelden; 2005.
5. McAuliffe WE, Albert J. *Clean Start: An Outpatient Program for Initiating Cocaine Recovery.* Guilford Press; 1992.
6. Washton AM. Outpatient group therapy at different stages of substance abuse treatment: preparation, initial abstinence, and relapse prevention. In: Brook DW, Spitz HI, eds. *Group Psychotherapy of Substance Abuse.* Haworth Medical Press; 2002:99-1194.
7. Daley DC, Douaihy A. *Managing Substance Use Disorder.* 3rd ed. Practitioner Guide. Oxford University Press; 2019.
8. Schmitz JM, Oswald LM, Jacks SD, Rustin T, Rhoades HM, Grabowski J. Relapse prevention treatment for cocaine dependence: group vs. individual format. *Addict Behav.* 1997;22(3):405-418.
9. Washton AM. Group therapy for substance abuse: a clinician's guide to doing what works. In: Coombs R, ed. *Addiction Recovery Tools.* Sage Publications; 2001:239-256.
10. Reilly PM, Shropshire MS. Anger management group treatment for cocaine dependence: preliminary outcomes. *Am J Drug Alcohol Abuse.* 2000;26(2):161-177.
11. Bowen S, Chawla N, Marlatt GA. *Mindfulness-Based Relapse Prevention for Addictive Behaviors.* Guilford Press; 2011.
12. Daley DC, Douaihy A. *Relapse Prevention Counseling: Clinical Strategies to Guide Addiction Recovery and Reduce Relapse.* PESI Publishing & Media; 2015.
13. National Institute on Drug Abuse. *Recovery Training and Self-help.* Department of Health and Human Services; 1994.
14. Substance Abuse and Mental Health Services Administration. *Substance Abuse Relapse Prevention for Older Adults: A Group Treatment Approach.* DHHS Pub No (SMA) 05-4053. SAMHSA; 2005.
15. Daley DC, Douaihy A. *Co-occurring Disorders Counseling Manual: Integrated Treatment for Substance Use and Psychiatric Disorders.* 4th ed. Daley Publications; 2022.
16. Daley DC, Moss HB. *Dual Disorders: Counseling Clients with Chemical Dependency and Mental Illness.* 3rd ed. Hazelden; 2002.
17. Najavits LM, Weiss RD, Liese BS. Group cognitive-behavioral therapy for women with PTSD and substance use disorder. *J Subst Abuse Treat.* 1995;13(1):13-22.
18. Mueser KT, Noordsy DL, Drake RE, Smith LF. *Integrated Treatment for Dual Disorders; A Guide to Effective Practice.* Guilford Press; 2002.
19. Rosenthal RN. Group treatments for schizophrenic substance abusers. In: Brook DW, Spitz HI, eds. *The Group Psychotherapy of Substance Abuse.* The Haworth Press; 2002.
20. Weiss RD, Connery HS. *Integrated Group Therapy for Bipolar Disorder and Substance Abuse.* Guilford Press; 2011.
21. Greenfield SF. *Treating Women with Substance Use Disorders.* Guilford Press; 2016.
22. *Seeking Safety.* Substance Abuse and Mental Health Services Administration. National Registry of Evidence-based Programs and Practices. Accessed October 14, 2016. https://www.samhsa.gov/resource/dbhis/seeking-safety
23. Monti PM, Abrams DB, Kadden RM, et al. *Treating Alcohol Dependence.* Guilford Press; 1989.
24. Peters RH, Hills HA. Community treatment and supervision strategies for offenders with co-occurring disorders: what works? In: Latessa E, ed. *Strategic Solutions: The International Community Corrections Association Examines Substance Abuse.* American Correctional Association; 1999:81-137.
25. Gorski TT, Kelly JM. *Counselor's Manual for Relapse Prevention with Chemically Dependent Criminal Offenders.* Substance Abuse and Mental Health Services Administration; 1996.
26. Roffman RA, Stephens RS, Simpson EE. Relapse prevention with adult chronic marijuana smokers. In: Daley DC, ed. *Relapse: Conceptual, Research and Clinical Perspectives.* Haworth Press; 1988:241-257.
27. Gottheil E, Weinstein SP, Sterling RC, Lundy A, Serota RD. A randomized controlled study of the effectiveness of intensive outpatient treatment for cocaine dependence. *Psychiatr Serv.* 1998;49(6):782-787.
28. Obert JL, McCann MJ, Marinelli-Casey P, et al. The matrix model of outpatient stimulant abuse treatment: history and description. *J Psychoactive Drugs.* 2000;32(2):157-164.
29. Vannicelli M. Group psychotherapy with substance abusers and family members. In: Washton AM, ed. *Psychotherapy and Substance Abuse: A Practitioner's Handbook.* Guilford Press; 1995:337-356.
30. Daley DC, Douaihy A. *A Family Guide to Coping with Substance Use Disorders.* Oxford University Press; 2019.
31. Carlbring P, Jonsson J, Josephson H, Forsberg L. Motivational Interviewing versus cognitive behavioral group therapy in the treatment of problem and pathological gambling: a randomized controlled trial. *Cogn Behav Ther.* 2010;39(2):92-103.
32. Liberman MA, Yalom ID, Miles MD. *Encounter Groups: First Facts.* Basic Books; 1973.
33. Yalom ID. *The Theory and Practice of Group Psychotherapy.* Basic Books; 1995.
34. Miller WR, Rollnick S. *Motivational Interviewing: Preparing People to Change Addictive Behavior.* Guilford Press; 1991.

35. Daley DC. A psychoeducational approach to relapse prevention. In: Daley DC, ed. *Relapse: Conceptual, Research and Clinical Perspectives*. Haworth Press; 1988:105-124.
36. Wenzel A, Liese BS, Beck AT, Friedman-Wheeler DG. *Group Cognitive Therapy for Addictions*. Guilford Press; 2012.
37. Crits-Christoph P, Siqueland L, Blaine J, et al. The National Institute on Drug Abuse Collaborative Cocaine Treatment Study: rationale and methods. *Arch Gen Psychiatry*. 1997;54:721-726.
38. Valasquez MM, Maurer GG, Crouch C. *Group Treatment for Substance Abuse: A Stages-of-Change Therapy Manual*. Guilford Press; 2001.
39. Daley DC, Mercer D, Carpenter G. *Group Drug Counseling for Cocaine Dependence*. Therapy Manuals for Addiction, Manual 4. National Institute on Drug Abuse; 2002.
40. Flores PJ. *Group Psychotherapy with Addicted Populations*. Haworth Press; 1988.
41. Khantzian EJ, Halliday KS, McAuliffe WE. *Addiction and the Vulnerable Self: Modified Dynamic Group Therapy for Substance Abusers*. Guilford Press; 1990.
42. Sobell LC, Sobell MB. *Group Therapy for Substance use Disorders: A Motivational Cognitive-Behavioral Approach*. Guilford Press; 2011.
43. Daley DC, Mercer D, Carpenter G. *Group Drug Counseling Manual*. Learning Publications; 1988.
44. Daley DC. *Group Addiction Counseling: Participant Workbook*. 3rd ed. Daley Recovery Publications; 2022.
45. Washton AM. Structured outpatient group treatment. In: Lowinson JH, Ruiz P, Millman RB, et al., eds. *Substance Abuse: A Comprehensive Textbook*. 3rd ed. Lippincott Williams & Wilkins; 1997:440-447.
46. Bowen S, Witkiewitz K, Clifasefi SL, et al. Relative efficacy of mindfulness-based relapse prevention, standard relapse prevention, and treatment as usual for substance use disorders: a randomized clinical trial. *JAMA Psychiatry*. 2014;71(5):547-556.
47. Garland EL, Hanley AW, Nakamura Y, et al. Mindfulness-oriented recovery enhancement vs supportive group therapy for co-occurring opioid misuse and chronic pain in primary care: a randomized clinical trial. *JAMA Intern Med*. 2022;182(4):407-417.
48. Daley DC. *Patient Evaluation of Recovery Workbooks*. Unpublished data from quality improvement study; 2007.
49. Stanton M. Relapse prevention needs more emphasis on interpersonal factors. *Am Psychol*. 2005;60(4):340-341.
50. Miller WR, Rollnick S. *Motivational Interviewing: Helping People Change*. 3rd ed. Guilford Press; 2013.
51. Wagner CC, Ingersoll KS. *Motivational Interviewing in Groups*. Applications of Motivational Interviewing. Guilford Press; 2013.
52. Martino S, Santa Ana EJ. Motivational interviewing groups for dually diagnosed patients. In: Wagner CC, Ingersoll KS, eds. *Motivational Interviewing in Groups*. Guilford Press; 2013:297-313.
53. Shorey RC, Martino S, Lamb KE, LaRowe SD, Santa Ana EJ. Change talk and relatedness in group motivational interviewing: a pilot study. *J Subst Abuse Treat*. 2015;51:75-81.
54. Santa Ana EJ, LaRowe SD, Gebregziabher M, et al. Randomized controlled trial of group motivational interviewing for veterans with substance use disorders. *Drug Alcohol Depend*. 2021;223:108716.
55. Weiss RD, Jaffee WB, de Menil VP, Cogley CB. Group therapy for substance use disorders: what do we know? *Harv Rev Psychiatry*. 2004;12:339-350.
56. Lopez G, Orchowski LM, Reddy MK, Nargiso J, Johnson JE. A review of research-supported group treatments for drug use disorders. *Subst Abuse Treat Prev Policy*. 2021;16(51):1-21. doi:10.1186/s13011-021-00371-0
57. Hien DA, Wells EA, Jiang H, et al. Multisite randomized trial of behavioral interventions for women with co-occurring PTSD and substance use disorders. *J Consult Clin Psychol*. 2009;77(4):607-619.
58. Greenfield SF, Brooks AJ, Gordon SM, et al. Substance abuse treatment, entry, retention, and outcome in women: a review of the literature. *Drug Alcohol Depend*. 2007;86:1-21.
59. Greenfield SF, Trucco EM, McHugh RK, Lincoln M, Gallop RJ. The Women's Recovery Group Study: a stage I trial of women-focused group therapy for substance use disorders versus mixed-gender group drug counseling. *Drug Alcohol Depend*. 2007;90:39-47.
60. Najavits LM, Rosier M, Nolan AL, Freeman MC. A new gender-based model for women's recovery from substance use disorder: results of a pilot study. *Am J Drug Alcohol Abuse*. 2007;33(1):5-11.
61. Lenz AS, Henesy R, Callender K. Effectiveness of Seeking Safety for co-occurring posttraumatic stress disorder and substance use. *J Couns Dev*. 2016;94(1):51-61.
62. Schäfer I, Lotzin A, Hiller P, et al. A multisite randomized controlled trial of Seeking Safety vs. Relapse Prevention Training for women with co-occurring posttraumatic stress disorder and substance use disorders. *Eur J Psychotraumatol*. 2019;10(1):1577092.
63. McLellan AT, Lewis DC, O'Brien CP, Kleber HD. Drug dependence, a chronic medical illness: implications for treatment, insurance, and outcomes evaluation. *JAMA*. 2000;284(13):1689-1695.
64. Daley DC, Zuckoff A. *Improving Treatment Compliance: Counseling and System Strategies for Substance Use and Dual Disorders*. Hazelden; 1999.
65. Hellerstein DJ, Rosenthal RN, Miner CR. A prospective study of integrated outpatient treatment for substance-abusing schizophrenic patients. *Am J Addict*. 1995;4:33-42.
66. Kelly TM, Daley DC, Douaihy AB. Contingency management for patients with dual disorders in an intensive outpatient treatment for addiction. *J Dual Diagnosis*. 2014;10(3):108-117.
67. Robins LN, Regier DA. *Psychiatric Disorders in America*. Free Press; 1991.
68. Kessler RC, McGonagle KA, Zhao S, et al. Lifetime and 12-month prevalence of DSM-IIIR psychiatric disorders in the United States. Results from the National Comorbidity Survey. *Arch Gen Psychiatry*. 1994;41:8-19.
69. Minkoff K, Drake RE. *Dual Diagnosis of Major Mental Illness and Substance Disorder*. Jossey-Bass; 1991.
70. Montrose K, Daley DC. *Celebrating Small Victories: A Counselor's Manual for Treating Chronic Mental Illness and Substance Abuse*. Hazelden; 1995.
71. Weiss RD, Giffin ML, Jaffee WB, et al. A "community friendly" version of integrated group therapy for patients with bipolar disorder and substance dependence: a randomized controlled trial. *Drug Alcohol Depend*. 2009;104:212-219.
72. Najavits LM, Weiss RD, Shaw SR. A clinical profile of women with posttraumatic stress disorder and substance dependence. *Psychol Addict Behav*. 1998;13(2):98-104.
73. Najavits LM, Weiss RD. "Seeking safety" outcome of a new cognitive-behavioral psychotherapy for women with posttraumatic stress disorder and substance dependence. *J Trauma Stress*. 1998;11:437-456.
74. Eaton CJ, Mandel DL, Hunkele KA, Nich C, Rounsaville BJ, Carroll KM. A cognitive behavioral therapy for alcohol-dependent domestic violence offenders: an integrated substance abuse-domestic violence treatment approach (SADV). *Am J Addict*. 2007;16(1):24-31.
75. Weiss RD, Griffin ML, Kolodziej ME, et al. A randomized trial of integrated group therapy versus group drug counseling for patients with bipolar disorders and substance dependence. *Am J Psychiatry*. 2007;164:100-107.
76. Drake R, Mercer-McFadden C, Mueser KT. Review of integrated mental health and substance abuse treatment for patients with dual diagnosis. *Schizophr Bull*. 1998;24:589-608.
77. James W, Preston NJ, Koh G, Spencer C, Kisley SR, Castle DJ. A group intervention which assists patients with dual diagnosis reduces their drug use: a randomized controlled trial. *Psychol Med*. 2004;34:983-990.
78. Bradley AC, Baker A, Lewin TJ. Group intervention for co-existing psychosis and substance use disorders in rural Australia: outcomes over 3 years. *Aust N Z J Psychiatry*. 2007;41(6):501-508.
79. Santa Ana EJ, Wulfert E, Nietert PJ. Efficacy of group motivational interviewing for psychiatric inpatients with chemical dependence. *J Consult Clin Psychol*. 2007;75(5):816-822.
80. Fleming MF, Mundt MP, French MT, Manwell LB, Stauffacher EA, Barry KL. Brief physician advice for problem drinkers: long-term efficacy and benefit cost-analysis. *Alcohol Clin Exp Res*. 2002;26(1):36-43.
81. National Institute on Drug Abuse (NIDA). *Clinical Trials Network: Forging Partnerships to Improve the Quality of Drug Abuse Treatment Throughout the Nation*. U.S. Department of Health and Human Services; 2010.

82. Daley DC. *Group Treatment of Substance Use Disorders: Survey of Community Providers*. Unpublished data from quality improvement study; 2011.
83. Myrick H, Brady KT. Social phobia in cocaine-dependent individuals. *Am J Addict*. 1997;6(2):99-104.
84. Daley DC, Salloum IM. *Social Anxiety Among Dual Diagnosis Outpatients*. Unpublished data from quality improvement study; 1996.
85. National Institute on Drug Abuse (NIDA). *Principles of Drug Addiction Treatment: A Research-based Guide*. 3rd ed, rev. ed. NIDA; 2018.
86. Lo Coco G, Melchiori F, Oieni V, et al. Group treatment for substance use disorder in adults: a systematic review and meta-analysis of randomized-controlled trials. *J Subst Abuse Treat*. 2019;99:104-116.
87. Olmstead TA, Graff FS, Ames-Sikora A, McCrady BS, Gaba A, Epstein EE. Cost-effectiveness of individual versus group female-specific cognitive behavioral therapy for alcohol use disorder. *J Subst Abuse Treat*. 2019;100:1-7.

CHAPTER

72 Individual Treatment

Edward V. Nunes and Kenneth M. Carpenter

CHAPTER OUTLINE

- Introduction
- History of psychotherapy for substance use disorders
- Developing behavioral therapies for substance use disorders: the technology model and science of behavior change
- Common elements of effective behavioral therapies
- Overview of evidence-based psychotherapies for substance use disorders
- Role of significant others in treatment of substance use disorders
- Combining individual psychotherapy with other modalities: group therapy and medications
- Differential therapeutics: how to match patients with therapies
- Virtual therapy and computer-delivered technology-based interventions
- Technology transfer: how to effectively train clinicians to deliver evidence-based psychotherapies

INTRODUCTION

This chapter introduces behavioral and psychotherapeutic treatments for substance use disorders (SUDs), typically delivered on an individual basis between therapist and patient, many of which are covered in detail in subsequent chapters. The chapter describes the technology model for the development of novel interventions and for testing their effectiveness through clinical trials, summaries of contemporary therapy methods that have evidence supporting their effectiveness, and common elements shared by effective behavioral and psychotherapeutic therapies for SUD. Challenges of implementing evidence-based treatments widely across real-world treatment systems are discussed, and the advent of technology-based treatments in part as an effort to bridge the implementation gap. It is hoped that the chapter provides a foundation enabling readers to critically evaluate the various therapies currently available for treating SUDs in terms of their supporting evidence, selecting the most appropriate psychotherapeutic approach for a given patient, and understanding what is necessary to deliver these treatments effectively.

HISTORY OF PSYCHOTHERAPY FOR SUBSTANCE USE DISORDERS

Psychoanalysis, founded in the late 19th century by Viennese psychiatrist Sigmund Freud, is based on the premise that mental life is both conscious and unconscious and that early life experiences have a powerful psychological influence on the individual throughout the life span. The goal of psychoanalysis, or the broader family of psychodynamic psychotherapies, is to increase awareness and understanding of unconscious patterns of thought and feeling and, by making them conscious, to correct the overt symptoms. A central focus is the transference, namely the relationship, thoughts, and feelings that the patient develops toward the therapist, and how this reflects conflicts in the patient's life. Manual-guided psychodynamic or transference-based therapies have been developed and rigorously tested and shown effectiveness for other psychiatric disorders, such as borderline personality disorder or some of the anxiety disorders,[1-3] disorders that have substantial comorbidity with SUDs. However, there has been little rigorous research testing of psychodynamic psychotherapies for SUD per se with the exception of Supportive Expressive Therapy (see below). Clinical experience has not found psychoanalysis particularly helpful for treating SUDs. Limitations[4] include that psychodynamic approaches do not focus predominantly on overt symptoms such as substance use. In contrast, therapies with demonstrated effectiveness directly address substance use and related symptoms and behaviors and typically provide concrete coping strategies. A psychodynamic therapist typically maintains therapeutic "neutrality," which stands in contrast to the relatively supportive and directive stance that characterizes most contemporary, evidence-based psychotherapies targeting SUD. Psychodynamic approaches tend to arouse anxiety and other painful affects, which could act as stressors and promote return to substance use in vulnerable individuals. That said, the focus of psychoanalysis on early trauma is consistent with the established role of stress, trauma, and adverse childhood experiences on risk for substance and other mental disorders.

In the mid-20th century, self-help approaches emerged. The first of these, Alcoholics Anonymous (AA)[5] was founded in 1935 by two "alcoholics" (Dr Bob and Bill W). AA borrowed the principle of spiritual values in daily living from the Oxford Group, a non–alcohol-based fellowship,[6] and the concept of alcoholism as an illness of mind, emotions, and body from the first private "drying out hospital" in New York

City (Towns Hospital), where Bill W. began his own recovery.[7] AA offered the Twelve Steps,[5] which, in many ways, resemble a treatment plan (ie, need for problem recognition, commitment to abstinence and change, and focus on changing "character defects"). The 12-step "program" focuses on drinking as the identified problem behavior and abstinence as the goal. It provides a structured pathway, including a variety of concrete coping skills, thus anticipating many of the features of contemporary, evidence-based psychotherapies. Although AA is a group-based approach, "sponsorship"[8] bears a resemblance to counseling per se, including adoption of a nonjudgmental stance, encouragement, education, advice on how to sustain sobriety, and support for socialization within the context of a long-term relationship. During the 1950s and 1960s, related self-help approaches for addressing SUD emerged. An Addicts Anonymous meeting was held at the U.S. Public Health Hospital in Lexington, Kentucky, in 1947, 12 years after the first AA meeting. Now known as Narcotics Anonymous, NA today has evolved into a viable resource for patients struggling with substance use problems.[9]

Residential treatment programs began to emerge in the mid-20th century. The classic "Minnesota Model" of treatment for SUDs, which first appeared in 1949, was based on a simple 5-point recovery plan: (1) behave responsibly, (2) attend lectures on the 12 steps, (3) talk with other patients, (4) make your bed, and (5) stay sober; conspicuously, absent from the original model was any sort of counseling or therapy.[10]

In 1958, the first therapeutic community (TC) (Synanon) was established. TCs seek to rehabilitate individuals with SUD through long-term stays in residential programs that employ a hierarchical model with treatment stages corresponding to gradually increasing levels of personal and social responsibility. (See Chapter 76 "Therapeutic Communities and Modified Therapeutic Communities for Co-occurring Mental and Substance Use Disorders" of this textbook to learn more about TC-based treatment.) In this self-help approach, the community is the primary agent of change.[11] Thus, at first, there was little involvement of professionally delivered psychotherapy. Over the recent decades, residential treatment models have evolved to include professional psychotherapeutic and medical treatment in addition to self-help.

Provisions for "substance abuse counseling" were written into legislation to fund community mental health centers, antipoverty programs, and criminal justice diversion beginning in the 1960s. Concurrently, health insurance companies began paying for treatment for SUDs. These factors resulted in a dramatic increase in the number of patients with SUD who accessed treatment.[12] However, while treatment (including counseling) was readily available, the interventions were poorly defined and delivered mostly by counselors whose primary credential was their own recovery. Meanwhile, the field of behavioral pharmacology showed that alcohol and drugs serve as reinforcers, ushering in the conceptualization of SUD according to classical learning theory. The discovery of the brain reward system and its role in the addictive phenomena established a biological basis for SUD.[13] Psychotherapeutic and behavioral approaches to SUD subsequently have drawn heavily from classical learning theory, cognitive psychology, and social learning theory.

In the 1980s, researchers began adapting and testing psychotherapies originally developed to treat psychiatric problems such as depression and anxiety for use with patients with SUD.[4,12] Thus, cognitive-behavioral therapy (CBT) for depression[14] was a forerunner of a broad family of therapies for SUD including cognitive-behavioral relapse prevention[15,16] and coping skills therapies.[17] The community reinforcement approach (CRA)[18] and Contingency Management (CM) techniques for treating SUD[19] grew out of applications of classical behavioral theory and the use of principles of reinforcement to create a context that can support alternative nonsubstance using behaviors. Motivational interviewing (MI) evolved, in part, from client centered approaches to counseling and social psychological theories of interpersonal influence and social learning.[20,21]

DEVELOPING BEHAVIORAL THERAPIES FOR SUBSTANCE USE DISORDERS: THE TECHNOLOGY MODEL AND SCIENCE OF BEHAVIOR CHANGE

Beginning in the 1970s, consensus emerged that behavioral/psychotherapies, just like medication treatments, should be based on rigorous evidence from randomized clinical trials,[22] and steps needed to specify a psychotherapy and test their effectiveness were elaborated: development of a treatment manual, describing the treatment in detail; prescribing methods for training and supervising therapists; specifying methods for monitoring and assuring accurate delivery of the treatment.[23] Early landmark studies applying these principles to SUDs include those of Woody et al.[24,25] focusing on psychotherapy for methadone maintenance patients; Project MATCH,[26,27] which contrasted motivational enhancement therapy (MET),[28] cognitive-behavioral coping skills therapy,[29] and twelve-step facilitation (TSF) for treatment of alcohol dependence[30]; and the National Institute on Drug Abuse (NIDA) Collaborative Cocaine Study,[31] which randomized patients with cocaine use disorders to either supportive-expressive (SE) psychotherapy or cognitive therapy (CT) (delivered by professional psychotherapists) or manual-guided drug counseling (delivered by experienced counselors working at substance treatment programs). All participants received group drug counseling (GDC), and a fourth randomized condition consisted of GDC plus brief case management sessions, intended as a control condition.

The NIDA Behavioral Therapies Development Program, launched in the 1990s with a series of Program Announcements that have been continuously renewed since (eg PA-16-073; PA-16-074; PA-16-072), elaborated the features of those landmark studies (treatment manual, training methods, methods for measuring therapist skill and fidelity to the treatment technique, etc.) into the "technology model" for developing and testing behavioral treatments.[32-34] In addition, it outlined a stage model for developing treatments, beginning with early-stage pilot work, and moving through controlled trials for efficacy, and studies of effectiveness and implementation in real world, community-based treatment settings.[35-38] Importantly, it provided the opportunity to obtain funding to conduct formative and pilot work at the initial stages of development of a therapy. The NIH Science of Behavior Change (SOBC) Common Fund Program, has expanded this approach across NIH institutes and disease areas, recognizing that treatment for diverse illnesses involves challenges, such as adherence to medication or lifestyle change, that call for behavioral interventions.[39,40]

Table 72-1 summarizes the stage model elaborated by the NIH SOBC. Stage 0 represents basic behavioral science work testing a theory of mechanism of behavior change to be applied to a disorder such as SUD. Stage I, initial formative work, involves developing a treatment manual specifying how to deliver the treatment, methods for training clinicians and measuring fidelity to the treatment (are clinicians delivering the treatment as specified), small uncontrolled pilot trials (Stage Ia) with qualitative work gathering patients' and clinicians' responses to treatment as well as quantitative measurement outcomes, and small controlled trials (Stage Ib) to begin formal testing of efficacy. Stage I is roughly analogous to Phase 1 in pharmacotherapy studies. Stage II is efficacy testing in tightly controlled randomized trials, usually conducted in research settings, and is roughly analogous to Phase 2 in pharmacotherapy trials. Stages III and IV examine effectiveness where the treatment is moved into community-based treatment settings, delivered by community-based clinicians. Stage V examines implementation—once the treatment has been found efficacious and effective, what happens when you attempt to implement it in community treatment settings without the support of research teams typically in place in controlled trials.

An important feature the Technology Model/Science of Behavior Change initiative is the emphasis on basic behavioral science and specification and measurement of behavioral mechanisms. **Figure 72-1** illustrates and provides examples of the role of behavioral mechanisms as mediators of the effect of a treatment. The notion is that treatments should be designed from the outset based on one or more mechanistic theories grounded in basic science, corresponding to Stage 0 (see **Table 72-1**). Subsequent clinical trials, especially in Stages I and II, should measure the mechanistic targets to determine whether the treatment is working as intended and to inform further therapy development work. For example, a cognitive-behavioral therapy may provide exercises and strategies to improve cognitive control over impulsive decisions to use drugs. Trials, then, should include proximal outcome measures tapping cognitive control, such as neuropsychological or behavioral economic tasks or neuroimaging, and test whether these outcomes mediate the impact of treatment on the ultimate outcome of substance use.

Possible patterns of outcome in the schema (see **Fig. 72-1**) have differing implications for treatment development. If the treatment impacts the target, and this mediates a beneficial effect on substance outcome, this supports the underlying theory and encourages further work in the same direction. If the treatment does not improve substance use, and does not impact the mechanistic target, then perhaps more work is needed on how to design the treatment to impact the target. If the treatment impacts the target, but fails to improve substance use outcome, either a more potent effect on the target is needed, or perhaps that mechanism is not promising. The schematic in **Figure 72-1** also recognizes that nonspecific elements of behavioral therapy, such as Therapeutic Alliance, often explain much of the effect of the therapy on the intended outcome. Put another way, a therapy may work for reasons not directly related to its behavioral mechanistic theory. In this instance, the therapy would show a beneficial effect on substance use outcome, but either a weak or null effect on the proximal, mechanistic outcome, or the mechanistic outcome is only weakly associated with substance outcome. This would suggest focusing further development on aspects of the therapy that impact those other mechanisms.

Clinical Implications: The Science of Behavior Change approach has clinical implications as well. If a clinician is working with a patient applying a particular behavioral therapy, they can observe whether the hypothesized mechanistic target is moving. In the example of a cognitive-behavioral treatment, Is the patient recognizing and exerting more control over cravings and impulsive decisions toward substance use? If not, perhaps the approach needs to be adjusted, maybe double down on control strategies, or shift gears to a different approach such as a focus on motivation.

Large Clinical Trials: In 1999, NIDA established the Clinical Trials Network (CTN), a nationwide network of research centers and associated treatment programs dedicated to testing new treatments through multisite trials in real-world treatment settings (ie, mainly Stage III and IV work). Trials with large sample sizes across multiple community-based treatment programs are needed both to test effectiveness and to understand how a treatment works when moved into a real-world treatment setting, as this is critical to demonstrating the potential public health impact of a treatment. Since its inception, the CTN has completed over 30 multisite studies. A number of these studies have focused on behavioral interventions, including those testing the effectiveness of Motivational Interviewing,[41,42] Contingency Management,[43,44] Brief Strategic Family Therapy,[45] Seeking Safety,[46] 12-Step Facilitation,[47] and Drug Counseling in the setting of buprenorphine treatment for prescription opioid use disorder[48] and computer-delivered Community Reinforcement Approach with Contingency Management.[49]

Implementation: Once a therapy has been determined to be effective, the next step is dissemination throughout the larger addiction treatment community. The delay between demonstration of effectiveness and widespread implementation is typically over 10 years and involves the challenges of so-called technology transfer.[50] Treatment manuals and didactic sessions (eg, lectures or workshops) may increase awareness and knowledge of new therapeutic methods, but generally do not change practice. Rather, for new therapy methods to be

TABLE 72-1 Stage Model for the Development of Behavioral Therapies

Stage	Question to be answered	Activities and benchmarks
Stage 0: Basic science	Are there basic brain or behavioral mechanisms that can be applied to developing a therapy?	• Basic neuroscience or behavioral studies in animal models or the human laboratory, identifying mechanisms and measurable targets, such as behavioral assays, neuropsychological tests, psychophysiological measures, or brain imaging.
Stage I: Preliminary therapy development	Is the new therapy feasible and promising?	• Conceptualize the treatment design and its theoretical basis, including translation from basic behavioral science to clinical application. • Write a treatment manual, which describes the therapy in detail and serves as the guide for therapists delivering the therapy. • Develop and test instruments for measuring accurate delivery of the therapy (fidelity). • Develop methods for training and certifying therapists' competence to deliver the therapy and methods of ongoing supervision to support fidelity and minimize drift. • Stage Ia trial: Usually small, uncontrolled pilot trial to explore feasibility and preliminary indicators of efficacy. • Stage Ib trial: Often a small, randomized controlled trial to further explore feasibility and obtain a first estimate of effect size. • Explore outcome measures reflecting the underlying basic or behavioral mechanisms of treatment effect. • Revise the treatment manual and training materials, based on the findings of Stage Ia and/or Ib trials. • Decision point with options: (1) Continue Phase I work, (2) move to Phase II or III, or (3) abandon the effort.
Stage II: Efficacy	How does the new therapy work under ideal conditions?	• Conduct rigorous, adequately powered randomized controlled trial to test the efficacy of the intervention under relatively ideal conditions, using the training, monitoring, and supervision methods developed in Stage I. • Select control condition with emphasis on internal validity (generally with control for professional attention). • Clinical research or tertiary care setting. • Intervention delivered by closely supervised research clinicians. • Careful selection of sample. • Explore mechanisms of effect through moderator and mediator analyses. • Revise the treatment manual and training materials, based on the findings. • Decision point with options: (1) proceed to Stage III if evidence of efficacy is clear, or (2) return to Stage I or II if more development work or testing is needed.
Stage III-IV: Effectiveness	How does the new therapy work in real-world clinical settings?	• Conduct a controlled effectiveness trial in real-world, community-based treatment settings. • Community-based treatment settings and their clinicians deliver the intervention. • Adapt training and supervision methods for community-based settings and clinicians. • Control condition usually some variation on TAU, so that the trial addresses the question of what if the new intervention is added to or substituted for the treatment that is currently delivered as standard practice. • Less selected sample, more representative of patients who actually present to community-based treatment settings (more comorbidity, etc.). • Health economic analysis (cost-effectiveness).
Stage V: Implementation	How to achieve widespread adoption of new treatments into standard practice across the treatment system?	• Address the challenges of technology transfer and the barriers to implementation. • Develop training methods for clinicians that involve not only didactics, but also supervised practice with feedback and coaching. • Address barriers at the levels of treatment systems, such as reimbursement and other incentives.

Adapted from National Institute on Drug Abuse. *Behavioral & Integrative Treatment Development Program.* 2013:NIDA Pub Number: PA-13-077.

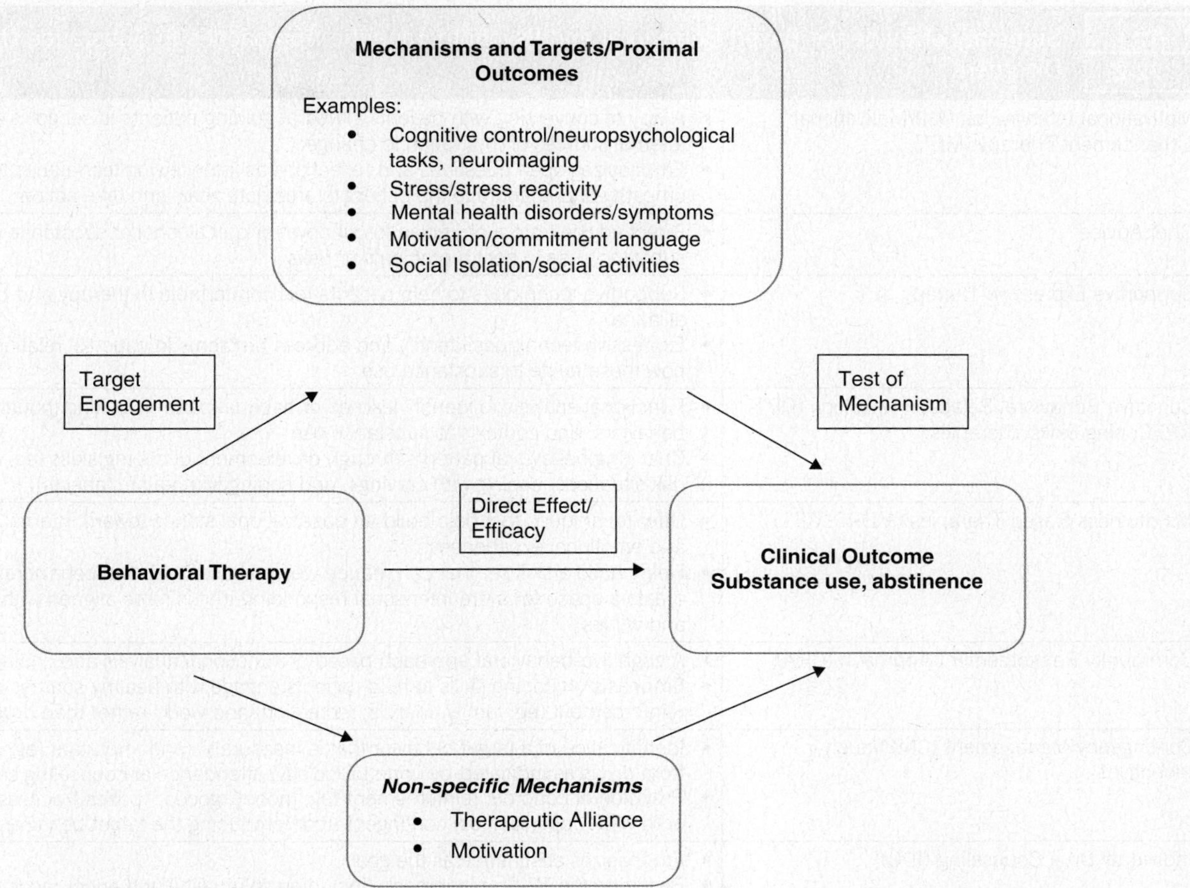

Figure 72-1. Development of Behavioral Therapies for Substance Use Disorders: Basic Behavioral Mechanisms as Targets of Therapy and Mediators of Clinical Outcome. (Adapted from Nielsen L, Riddle M, King JW. NIH science of behavior change implementation team. the NIH science of behavior change program: transforming the science through a focus on mechanisms of change. *Behav Res Ther.* 2018;101:3-11.)

implemented, clinicians need training that involves practice with feedback and coaching.[51] Barriers at the level of treatment systems, including reimbursement and other incentives, also need to be overcome.

COMMON ELEMENTS OF EFFECTIVE BEHAVIORAL THERAPIES

A number of the behavioral or psychotherapeutic treatment approaches for SUDs that have evidence of efficacy and/or effectiveness from clinical trials are summarized in **Table 72-2**. Treatment specific processes of change have yet to be clearly supported in systematic reviews of SUD interventions.[52,53] Thus, the empirical evidence to date and consideration of similarities and differences between these approaches suggests a set of common elements that may underlie successful treatments for SUD[4]:

- Focusing directly on substance use
- Enhancing motivation to change
- Building coping skills (eg, strategies for: managing cravings; saying "no" when tempted by others to use substances; managing boredom and using free time constructively; reaching out to members of one's support network when needed)
- Changing reinforcement contingencies
- Managing painful moods
- Improving interpersonal functioning
- Fostering a treatment alliance

Focusing Directly on Substance Use

Effective behavioral and psychotherapeutic approaches for SUD generally maintain an overt focus on stopping or reducing substance use. Even when the immediate focus of a session may be outside of substance use, the underlying agenda is always the substance problem. For example, in Motivational

TABLE 72-2 Summary of Evidence-Based Behavioral and Psychotherapeutic Approaches to Substance Use Disorders

Approach	Description
Motivational Interviewing (MI)/Motivational Enhancement Therapy (MET)	• A way of conversing with patients aimed at guiding patients to set goals and build internal sources of motivation to change • Emphasizes open questions and reflections as interviewing techniques to build empathy and encourage the patient to articulate goals and take action
Brief Advice	• Direct advice from a physician to cut down or quit alcohol or substance use, relating substance use to health problems or risks
Supportive Expressive Therapy	• Supportive techniques to help patients feel comfortable in therapy and build treatment alliance • Expressive techniques identify and address problems in patients' relationships and how these relate to substance use
Cognitive-Behavioral Relapse Prevention (CBT-RP)/Coping Skills Therapies	• Functional analysis to identify learned or habitual patterns linking thoughts, feelings, behaviors, and contexts to substance use • Changing behavioral patterns through development of coping skills (eg, avoiding high risk situations, coping with cravings, and coping with painful affects)
Mindfulness-Based Therapies (MBRP; ACT)	• Offer techniques that help build an observational stance toward internal psychological and emotional experiences. • Helps build a skill set that can reduce well-practiced habitual behavioral reactions and create a space for more intentional responding that is more aligned with desired goals and values.
Community Reinforcement Approach (CRA)	• A cognitive-behavioral approach based on functional analysis and coping skills • Emphasis on coping skills to help patients engage with healthy sources of reinforcement (eg, family, friends, recreation, and work) rather than drug reinforcers
Contingency Management (CM)/Voucher Incentives	• Identification of a target behavior that is measurable and important (eg, abstinence from drugs as indicated by urine toxicology; attendance at counseling sessions) • Provision of concrete reinforcement (eg, money, goods, "prizes," access to privileges or to work opportunities) contingent upon producing the target behavior
Individual Drug Counseling (IDC)	• Emphasizes abstinence as the goal • Based on the 12-Step approach (including spirituality) and encourages 12-Step meeting attendance • Coping skills to address problems in maintaining abstinence and drug-free lifestyle
12-Step Facilitation (TSF)	• Gives therapists tools and strategies to encourage their patients to engage in 12-Step groups (eg, AA and NA) • Emphasizes acceptance of the need for abstinence • Emphasizes giving oneself over to the 12-Step group, and provides education and support around 12-Step attendance
Medical Management	• Emphasizes abstinence as goal • Emphasizes and supports adherence to medication, as well as adherence to behavioral aspects of treatment plan such as AA attendance
Approaches Involving Significant Others and Families	
Network Therapy (NT)	• Includes a group of family and significant others as partners in supporting the treatment plan (eg, monitoring adherence to medication or behavioral interventions, helping with practice of coping skills)
Community Reinforcement and Family Training (CRAFT)	• Trains concerned family members to use communication skills and the principles of reinforcement to engage in treatment and succeed in treatment—for example, using positive reinforcement to encourage treatment participation, and letting the individual experience the negative consequences of substance use without inadvertently supporting continued substance use
Family Therapies	• The identified patient's substance use disorder is viewed within the context of his/her family system • Intervention focuses at the level of the family system, with all family members participating, to return the family system to a healthy mode of functioning

Interviewing (MI), the therapist may "roll with resistance" and change the subject to something else (eg, job functioning, family relationships), but the agenda is to increase the patient's awareness and understanding of how substance use may be affecting his/her functioning in those areas and to help him/her circle back to a direct focus on the substance problem. Likewise, in cognitive-behavioral relapse prevention or the Community Reinforcement Approach (CRA), a session might be focused on managing painful affects or conflict in relationships, but the reason is that these represent stresses that are likely to engender substance use.

Enhancing Motivation to Reduce/Stop Substance Use and Adhere to a Treatment Plan

Addiction is fundamentally a disorder of motivation. Addictive substances interact with the brain reward system and function as positive reinforcers, creating a natural drive to partake. Clinically, this manifests as cravings and repetitive use. Conversely, patients present to treatment because of the adverse consequences of substance use, which create the wish to cut down or quit. These opposing desires to both use and quit create a state of ambivalence, which is typical of patients seeking treatment for SUDs. This manifests as efforts to reduce substance use, punctuated by cravings, brief or even prolonged recurrence of use, and/or fluctuating engagement with treatment. For example, patients may miss treatment sessions, fail to carry follow through with parts of the treatment plan (eg, homework), or avoid discussing substance use during sessions. They also may express the wish to cut down or control their substance use without stopping altogether; that is, they may seek to continue to enjoy the positive effects of substances, while minimizing the adverse consequences. Any psychotherapeutic or behavioral approach to treating a SUD must address these variations. Motivational Interviewing provides guidance on the interpersonal stance and a way for conversations with patients to enhance their own motivation to quit substance use. MI can be viewed as a fundamental skill, which clinicians can implement any time motivation for treatment wavers. (For a more detailed look at MI, see Chapter 69, "Enhancing Motivation to Change" and Chapter 70, "Motivational Interviewing.") Other approaches, such as Individual Drug Counseling (IDC) or Medical Management (MM), provide direct advice from the therapist to quit, which can be powerful when coming from someone who is respected as an expert. In IDC, the therapist helps the patient learn strategies to abstain from substances and make positive changes in self and lifestyle. Contingency Management strategies, where concrete rewards or punishments are established contingent upon substance use (or treatment participation, etc.), can enhance external motivation in the absence of internal motivation to change. Cognitive-behavioral approaches, such as Relapse Prevention or Community Reinforcement Approach (CRA), seek to render more salient the adverse consequences of substance use on the one hand and alternative sources of satisfaction and reward on the other, which, in turn, should have an impact on patients' decisions to use versus abstain. Thus, while MI is most directly focused on motivation to change substance use behavior, other therapies for SUD also have the capacity to evoke motivation, albeit by different methods and means.

Coping Skills to Avoid Substance Use and Change Lifestyle

Whether patients are struggling to achieve initial abstinence, avoid return to use, or effect other lifestyle changes that will improve their prospects for a long-term recovery, they generally need to be taught skills and strategies to achieve these ends. Alcoholics Anonymous (AA) and other 12-step groups can be viewed as conveying such skills (eg, practicing acceptance, maintaining focus on abstinence, avoiding "people, places, and things" associated with use, wariness of strong emotions, taking "a day at a time"). Cognitive-behavioral approaches and Individual Drug Counseling (IDC) focus specifically on skills building, providing practice, both in role-plays within sessions and through homework assignments between sessions. Similarly, CRA focuses on building social, recreational, and occupational skills, again through practice and homework.

Changing Reinforcement Contingencies

Addictive substances function as reinforcers, becoming increasingly salient and predominant as a SUD progresses. As a patient's behavior increasingly falls under the control of the substance, more time is spent seeking out and using the substance while normal or healthy sources of reinforcement are displaced, such as family, friends, recreation, work, and even food and sex. Thus, an effort to reconnect a patient with his or her former sources of healthy reinforcement may help to combat the reinforcement value of substances, resulting in reductions in substance use. When a patient with a SUD achieves abstinence, this often leaves a gap, since important areas (ie, family, friends, work, and recreation) have been forsaken during extended periods of substance use. To reduce the likelihood of return to use, such patients need to literally rebuild their lives by reestablishing their networks of family and friends. To this end, MI focuses on what a patient values in life and how substance use conflicts with those values; for instance, if family relationships are important to a patient, but substance use has contributed to the patient becoming alienated from his/her significant others, this discrepancy could be a focus of MI. CRA specifically emphasizes engagement in healthy social and recreational activities and relationships and teaches skills (eg, conflict resolution) to foster growth in those areas. CM provides concrete monetary rewards for avoiding substance use, often in conjunction with CRA.

Managing Painful Emotions and Stress

Stress is a risk factor for the development and progression of substance use and use disorders; furthermore, painful emotions and moods can contribute to return to use.

Thus, patients with SUD need to learn to recognize, label, and tolerate painful feelings as part of the recovery process. Supportive Expressive (SE) therapy focuses on helping patients to feel comfortable recognizing and expressing their feelings and understanding the relationship between their emotions, substance use, and problematic relationships. MI stresses the fostering of empathy; patients are encouraged to experience and share their feelings, which are reflected back by the clinician so that the patient feels understood. Cognitive-behavioral approaches, such as Relapse Prevention, Community Reinforcement Approach (CRA), or Dialectical Behavior Therapy (DBT),[54] teach explicit skills for tolerating and managing strong emotions similar to those conveyed by versions of CBT developed to treat depression or anxiety disorders. AA and systematized 12-step approaches like Individual Drug Counseling (IDC) also recognize and label the role of strong emotions in substance use and recurrence of use, encourage sharing and discussion of feelings at meetings, and provide coping skills (eg, the concepts of acceptance and serenity) to help deal with problematic emotions.

Improving Interpersonal Functioning and Social Support

Individuals with SUD have often damaged or lost contact with positive social networks (eg, divorce, alienation from family and friends, loss of connection to social groups and activities). Remaining relationships tend to revolve around others who also are unstable in recovery or actively using (eg, "drug buddies"). Absence of positive social support can interfere with efforts to recover from SUDs. To enhance interpersonal functioning and improve support, CRA places an emphasis on social skills building by helping patients rebuild and reengage in their social networks. When CRA is combined with CM, patients are encouraged to spend the monetary rewards they earn by engaging in social activities with family or friends.[55] The functional analysis component of cognitive-behavioral approaches often identifies social settings that promote substance use, affording the clinician an opportunity to teach skills to avoid those particular situations and substitute healthy ones instead. MI seeks to help patients become more aware of the relationships they have damaged/lost but would like to reestablish, and to foster self-efficacy to reengage. Approaches like Network Therapy that involve the family in a supportive way provide an in vivo opportunity for relationship repair work to begin. For some individuals, attendance at 12-step mutual aid meetings such as Alcoholics Anonymous (AA), Narcotics Anonymous (NA) (or Cocaine Anonymous) (and sponsored events) can provide community and become an important part of their social life; individual treatments that encourage the 12-step approach (eg, Twelve Step Facilitation [TSF], Individual Drug Counseling [IDC]) likewise are promoting development of a support network as one of the main objectives.

Fostering the Treatment Alliance

Treatment alliance refers to the collaborative relationship that develops between the patient and therapist. It is measured from both the patient's and therapist's perspectives using questionnaires such as the Helping Alliance Questionnaire–II (HAq-II).[56] Alliance is composed of three components—that is, shared goals, tasks, and emotional bonds.[57,58] A common mediator of effectiveness of treatments across a wide range of therapies and disorders,[59] treatment alliance affects treatment retention, completion, and outcomes among patients with SUD.[60] In addition, therapist empathy, a component of therapeutic alliance,[61] accounts for differences in treatment outcome among individuals seeking help for their SUD.[62,63] While all psychotherapies acknowledge the importance of a good therapeutic relationship, some focus more intently on this element, namely, those that are more emotionally based (ie, SE therapy and MI). Nevertheless, across therapies for SUDs, it is necessary for the clinician to monitor the extent to which the patient is engaged in the therapy and to address therapeutic lapses in a nonjudgmental fashion. Clinicians also need to monitor their own level of alliance, which may falter if the patient's outcome is not going well.[64]

OVERVIEW OF EVIDENCE-BASED PSYCHOTHERAPIES FOR SUBSTANCE USE DISORDERS

This section provides an overview of many of the individual treatments for SUD that have evidence of efficacy or effectiveness from substantial controlled clinical trials (see **Table 72-2**). Most of these approaches are covered in detail in other chapters here in Section 9 and Section 10 of this volume. Treatment manuals and training materials are available from SAMHSA (search Treatment Improvement Protocol (TIP) at https://store.samhsa.gov), as well as therapy manuals from NIDA and NIAAA.

Motivational Interviewing and Motivational Enhancement Therapy

Motivational Interviewing is a way of approaching and talking to patients that is designed to increase their commitment to reducing or stopping substance use based on tapping the patient's intrinsic motivation for change and taking the steps necessary to do so.[20,21] MI can be viewed as an essential therapeutic skill, to be employed during the initial contact and evaluation of a patient and redeployed periodically whenever a patient's motivation wavers during treatment. MI can be used either as a stand-alone intervention or as a prelude to another treatment such as CBT. MI is founded on guiding principles, called the "spirit" of MI, namely, collaboration, evocation, and respect for the autonomy of the patient. The formulation of MI also includes acceptance of the patient for who he or she is and empathy as an essential stance of the therapist.[21] Collaboration means that the clinician avoids taking on the role of an authority figure (eg, teacher, expert) but rather creates a sense of partnership with the patient. Evocation means that the clinician makes an effort, partly through the concerted use of open questions, reflective listening, summarizing, and affirming, to invite the patient to talk about his or her life and what he or she values. By expressing genuine curiosity and openness to the patient's experience and values, the clinician builds and communicates empathy. Respect for autonomy means that the clinician makes it clear that the patient is making the decisions about whether and how to change; additionally, the clinician supports the patient's self-efficacy to change. However, MI is not simply an empathic, exploratory interview. It is intentional and directional, seeking to guide the patient toward change. MI is not a sales technique in the sense of trying to sell the patient on what the therapist or others may want. However, in common with a good salesman, a therapist practicing MI tries to understand and draw out what the patient most values in order to help the patient find the outcome that will be most valuable and useful to him/her.

MI prescribes a set of interviewing skills, which include open questions, reflections, affirmations, summarizations, and avoidance of statements that run counter to MI principles (eg, avoiding confrontation, argumentation, or unsolicited advice). Simple reflections are statements made by the therapist that reflect back to patient what the therapist has been hearing—as a way for the therapist to check with the patient that he or she has understood what has been said; reflections convey genuine interest and curiosity, thus building empathy. Complex reflections go beyond simply reflecting, by also expressing some level of inference—that is, by probing for things the patient may not have said directly and thus gently moving the patient toward change. Another tactical strategy, "developing discrepancy," consists of trying to help the patient become more aware of divergence between the things he or she values, their current behavior, and the impact substance use may have on attaining these things. Reliable measures of MI therapist behaviors have been developed—for example, motivational interviewing training instrument or MITI,[65,66] which can be used to rate the skill of clinicians and provide feedback to them as part of supervision. Thus, MI has the fundamental features of therapy technology, namely, treatment manuals (the Miller and Rollnick texts and other training materials), as well as a reliable method for measuring performance and for training and supervising clinicians.

MI therapists also are trained to recognize, elicit, and respond to "change talk." Change talk consists of statements by the patient that reflect one or more of desire, ability, reasons, need, and commitment (DARN-C) to change their substance using behavior. An instrument to measure DARN-C statements by patients has been developed and can be used to help train clinicians to recognize change talk. In particular, commitment talk, a clear expression of intent to do something to change—for example, "I have set my quit date for tomorrow," has been shown to be a strong predictor of good outcome among patients with SUD.[67] Hence, an important tactic is for the therapist to recognize and reinforce change talk whenever it occurs. While MI represents a style of interviewing that may take the interview in a variety of directions depending on what the patient brings to the session, Motivational Enhancement Therapy (MET) is a manual-guided approach that is more structured and includes giving patients feedback on their substance use behaviors and other structured activities aimed at enhancing motivation.

Motivational interviewing approaches (both MI and MET) have been shown to be effective in multiple randomized trials for a wide range of substance problems and related health behaviors.[21,68] The evidence is stronger for nicotine and alcohol use disorders though less consistent for substance use disorders.[32,42] The mixed results found for some populations suggest what may seem self-evident, namely, that a single or limited set of MI or MET sessions may be insufficient to effect much change, particularly among patients with more severe SUDs, comorbidity, or disorganization. This suggests the strategy of combining MI or MET within a larger treatment plan, including other evidence-based approaches. For more on enhancing motivation to change, see Chapter 69, "Enhancing Motivation to Change" and Chapter 70, "Motivational Interviewing."

Brief Advice

Any encounter between a clinician and a patient represents an opportunity for therapeutic effect. While not an elaborate psychotherapy method, brief advice from a clinician, such as a physician, has been shown to be beneficial in influencing patients to reduce alcohol use,[69,70] and thus is important to include in this overview of individual psychotherapeutic interventions. In a busy clinical setting, with limited time for encounters with patients, brief advice has obvious advantages. In some respects, brief advice seems a polar opposite to MI. MI instructs clinicians to avoid the role of expert or authority figure, to forego giving direct advice, and to take a more collaborative and exploratory approach. However, clinicians (particularly physicians) command respect in our society. Thus, simple advice from a physician is likely to be salient, and the evidence suggests it can be beneficial in reducing substance use. Brief advice also can be reconciled with, and understood within, the context of the theory of MI. MI does not necessarily proscribe advice giving; rather, it recommends that advice giving needs to be done in the context of an empathic relationship. One concrete strategy of MI is to ask for a patient's permission before giving advice—for example, "Would it be OK with you if I let you know what I'm thinking about your drinking?" This maintains the collaborative nature of the interaction and respects the patient's autonomy, by asking the patient's permission.

Supportive-Expressive Therapy

As previously noted, in the early years of psychotherapy development, psychoanalytic therapy was attempted with patients with SUD with limited success. Going forward, treatment development went in a more behavioral direction, with few dynamically oriented interventions for SUD being systematized—that is, with treatment manuals, methods of training, and measuring therapist performance. One exception was supportive-expressive therapy. SE psychotherapy[71] is a time-limited therapy that was adapted for use with patients with both cocaine and heroin (opioid) use disorder. It represents an effort to apply psychoanalytic and psychodynamic principles in a systematic way to the problem of SUD. Substance use and efforts to quit are viewed in relation to the patient's relationships and intrapsychic world. The patterns that are identified are viewed either as triggers for return to use or as linked to avoidance of appropriate actions needed to achieve sobriety, rather than as direct causes of SUD. Emphasis is placed on development and maintenance of the therapeutic alliance. SE has two main components. The first employs supportive techniques to assist patients in feeling comfortable discussing their feelings and life experiences while addressing the role that substances have played with regard to problematic feelings and behaviors. In this phase, the therapist focuses on developing a helping relationship with the patient and on identifying and bolstering the patient's strengths and areas of competence. The second component involves the use of expressive techniques to help the patient understand and work through relationship issues. To achieve this goal, the therapist employs reflective listening, evaluative understanding, and responding to identify problematic patterns in relationships with others. SE helps patients explore the meanings they attach to their SUD and address their relationship problems more directly, thus allowing them to develop better solutions to life problems than substance use.

The SE treatment model for SUD is based on Luborsky's standard SE model[71]; however, a more detailed treatment manual is available, which includes adaptations specifically for cocaine users.[72] These adaptations were made when SE was employed in the Collaborative Cocaine Study, described below.

Clinical trials testing the effectiveness of SE among patients with SUD have generated mixed results, with some evidence of efficacy. In the NIDA Collaborative Cocaine Treatment Study,[31] patients received group therapy (ie, group drug counseling [GDC]); three of four study groups also got individual psychotherapy—that is, SE therapy, Individual Drug Counseling (IDC), or cognitive therapy (CT). SE (plus group therapy) was associated with reduced cocaine use but was not superior to the control group, which received group therapy only. Furthermore, IDC produced significantly greater abstinence from cocaine than either SE therapy or CT.[31] Among patients with opioid use disorder maintained on methadone pharmacotherapy, those with high psychopathology who received 6 months of SE therapy or CBT in addition to traditional substance use counseling achieved better outcomes than did those receiving substance use counseling only, although substance use counseling was beneficial for those with lower levels of psychopathology.[24] A second study found that clients in three methadone clinics who received SE required lower doses of methadone than did those receiving standard substance use counseling; not only did they maintain their gains after 6 months of treatment, they also continued to improve compared to those receiving substance use counseling only.[25]

Cognitive-Behavioral Approaches: Relapse Prevention and Coping Skills Therapies

Cognitive-behavioral relapse prevention and related approaches are based on the premise that the development and continuation of substance use is a learning process.[15-17] Accordingly, the therapy is founded on a "functional analysis," where the sequences of thoughts, feelings, behaviors, and circumstances that lead to substance use for a given patient are reviewed and understood. The therapist then introduces coping skills to promote the unlearning of these maladaptive patterns and to substitute more adaptive patterns that will oppose and prevent substance use. This is a structured, time-limited (usually 8-12 weeks in duration), goal-oriented treatment, which can be flexibly adapted for a variety of individual obstacles, skill deficits, settings, and formats. Specific foci of CBTs include recognizing triggers that lead to substance use (eg, places, persons, or particular emotions), avoiding high-risk situations, and coping with cravings. Skills that are taught and rehearsed include drug refusal skills (literally, how to respond when someone asks the patient to use substances), decisional delay (putting off a decision to use for a brief period—eg, 20 minutes during which time the desire often goes away), and talking oneself through cravings. Patients also are taught to recognize, tolerate, and counteract painful feelings (eg, sadness or worry), much along the lines of skills conveyed in CBTs for depression or anxiety disorders. In addition to role-plays during sessions, patients typically are given homework and instructed to practice skills in real life between sessions.

Cognitive-behavioral relapse prevention and related approaches, such as coping skills therapies, have extensive evidence from clinical trials supporting efficacy among patients with DSM-IV–defined nicotine-, alcohol-,[73] and cocaine-dependence.[74] One interesting feature of cognitive-behavioral approaches is that the outcome data often show a "sleeper effect," namely, that the beneficial effect on substance use builds over time after the treatment has been completed; that is, at long-term follow-ups, the treated group often continues to evidence further reductions in substance use, while control group does not.[74,75] This suggests that, as intended, the patients have learned skills that must be exercised and practiced to sustain a beneficial effect, even after treatment had ended. Chapter 80 "Relapse Prevention: Clinical Models and Intervention Strategies" explores prevention of return to use and further discussion of cognitive-behavioral approaches to treatment of SUDs.

Community Reinforcement Approach

Community Reinforcement Approach (CRA) is a cognitive-behavioral approach that places greater emphasis on examining the reinforcers in a patient's life and helps the patient to reengage and reconnect with healthy sources of reinforcement (eg, family, friends, work, and recreation).[18] The theory is that this will interfere with and replace substance-seeking behaviors, which are under the control of reinforcement by the drugs or alcohol. CRA involves teaching patients to conduct a functional analysis so that they can better understand their drug use and problem solve ways to decrease the probability of substance use going forward. Other key skills include self-management planning and drug refusal skills, much like in other CBT approaches. Another component of CRA involves encouraging patients to engage in healthy sources of reinforcement to include vocational and recreational activities, as well as positive relationships. CRA often has been combined with CM in which voucher-based rewards are used to enhance abstinence.[55] These two approaches seem synergistic, as the vouchers provide concrete rewards within the therapy, while the CRA attempts to foster rewards within the patient's life outside of therapy.

Contingency Management

CM seeks to directly harness the principles of reinforcement and behavior modification by making concrete rewards or punishments contingent upon some key target behavior.[76] The target behavior usually has been abstinence from substances as confirmed by urine testing, but other targets (eg, attendance at therapeutic activities) also can be reinforced. The basic principle is that contingent rewards or punishments will help reduce the likelihood of substance use and help patients achieve and sustain abstinence. The key principles of this approach, derived from theory of learning and behavior modification, include the following: (1) the target behavior needs to be well defined and measurable and (2) the reinforcement should be well defined, delivered as immediately as possible upon production of the target behavior, and be as salient (or valuable) to the patient as possible. CM has been applied effectively for drugs such as cocaine, heroin, and cannabis, where use over the last several days can be readily detected in urine.[43,44,77-79] Alcohol can be detected in blood, urine, or breath but washes out of the system quickly. Thus, while CM with rewards contingent on negative breath testing has some evidence of efficacy,[80] false negatives are more likely, defeating the requirement for accurate detection of use. Recently, ethyl glucuronide (EtG), a metabolite of alcohol that is longer lasting, has been used successfully as the basis for a CM intervention for alcohol use disorder.[81] In addition to toxicology results, treatment plan adherence (eg, carrying out verifiable homework assignments, attendance at groups) is readily verifiable and also has been tested in clinical trials[82,83]; this may be a more natural application of CM when adapted to community-based practice.[84] Similar examples of incentives for program participation can be seen in the business world, an example being frequent flyer miles offered to airline passengers.

When employing CM based on results of urine testing, direct observation of urine collection is ideal in order to avoid patients adulterating or substituting specimens. However, while direct observation typically has been employed in efficacy trials, this can be a barrier in community-based treatment where bathrooms often are too small to accommodate both patient and observer, where same-sex staff may be unavailable to conduct observation, and/or where clinic staff may be too embarrassed to observe patients urinating. To overcome these obstacles, many urine collection systems now incorporate tests for detecting falsification based on temperature or concentration. Another caveat when using results from urine testing to determine whether or not to reinforce a patient who is on a CM protocol is to make sure that the urine testing method will in fact detect the drugs that are the target of the intervention.

Contingent reinforcement can consist of rewards such as vouchers that are exchangeable for actual dollar amounts contingent on negative urines[85,86] or access to a workplace where wages can be earned[87] or punishments to include loss of methadone take-home privileges or threat of arrest and incarceration—an incentive often inherent in drug courts and other alternative sentencing programs. Principles of learning suggest that positive reinforcement tends to produce behaviors that are more durable and generalizable beyond the immediate context. Hence, many of the most successful CM treatments have worked with rewards, often on an escalating schedule, where the magnitude of the reward increases with each consecutive negative urine; this procedure is intended to shape prolonged periods of abstinence on the theory that sustained abstinence is the most valuable clinical outcome.

Principles of learning also suggest that the impact of a reinforcer will be proportional to its magnitude; thus, it is not surprising that larger monetary rewards produce more abstinence.[88] This has led to one of the key barriers to widespread implementation of CM, namely, the problem of how to finance the rewards. Typical reinforcement schedules in clinical trials have allowed patients to earn around $1,000 for 3 months of sustained abstinence. In response to this problem, Petry et al. developed a lower-cost voucher regimen that involves rewarding patients not with set monetary vouchers but rather with opportunities to engage in a sort of lottery where what is earned are draws from a "fish bowl;" only some draws yield prizes, most of small magnitude, with a few of larger magnitude, whereas other draws simply yield praise ("good job"). This "fish bowl" model has shown strong evidence of both efficacy and effectiveness in community-based treatment settings.[44,89]

Among psychotherapeutic and behavioral treatments for SUDs, CM has shown the most consistent and strongest evidence of efficacy compared to control conditions, at least during treatment.[78] Response tends to be bimodal; however, some patients (usually around 50% of the sample) rapidly achieve and sustain abstinence, whereas the remainder produce little or no abstinence and earn few or no vouchers at all. This raises one immediate question for future research, which is how to better understand which patients will respond to incentives and how to better help those who fail to respond. Another limitation of CM is that its impact tends to wear off, at least partially, when the treatment ends and contingencies are no longer in force meaning that some (but not all) successful patients will return to use.[75] CM often has been combined with other treatment methods. As previously noted, CRA, with its emphasis on fostering reinforcers in a patient's environment, most commonly has been combined with CM. This approach (CRA + CM), originally pioneered by Higgins,[55] has proven to be one of the most effective and consistently replicated treatments for substance use disorders. Chapter 73, "Contingency Management and the Community Reinforcement Approach," presents a broader explication of the CRA + CM approach.

Individual Drug Counseling

Although substance use counseling was readily accessible to patients entering treatment for SUD in the 1970s, its active ingredients and efficacy were unclear. In an effort to learn more about "what good counselors do," Woody et al.[24,31,90] studied them, both in outpatient drug-free and methadone maintenance clinics. This early work contributed to the development of Individual Drug Counseling (IDC), one of the first science-based treatments for SUD. The IDC manual was developed for use in the Collaborative Cocaine Study and is available as part of the "Therapy Manuals for Drug Addiction" series.[91] The first section of the manual is devoted to discussing the contribution of the 12-step approach to the IDC model. An overview of IDC, including a comparison to other approaches to treating SUDs, is provided. The IDC approach includes assessing the patient's status prior to initiating treatment; recommendations include using the Addiction Severity Index,[92] along with urine toxicology to ascertain abstinence. The role of the counselor, including developing alliance and proscribed behaviors (ie, those that should not occur during treatment), is described. The phases of treatment include (1) treatment initiation (targeting denial and ambivalence); (2) early abstinence (which focuses on advice for avoiding recurrence of use, such as "people, places, and things"), cravings, dealing with high-risk situations and resisting social pressure to use substances (all reminiscent of cognitive-behavioral approaches), and 12-step meeting attendance; (3) maintaining abstinence by addressing the potential for return to use, dealing with relationships while in recovery, living a drug-free lifestyle (eg, employment, constructive use of leisure time), encouraging spirituality, dealing with character defects, handling negative emotions, addressing other addictions; (4) advanced recovery (sustaining gains and addressing issues or problems that arise); (5) dealing with specific problems, including recurrence of use; (6) counselor characteristics and training; and (7) counselor supervision. The IDC intervention incorporates the essential elements of the 12-step approach, while also addressing the important issue of intervention fidelity, thus allowing IDC to be compared with other evidence-based interventions for SUDs.

The efficacy of IDC was demonstrated in the NIDA-funded Collaborative Cocaine Treatment Study[31] in which patients treated by substance use counselors who were trained and supervised according to the IDC manual produced superior rates of cocaine abstinence at follow-up compared to those who were treated with either CT or SE therapy administered by professional therapists; all patients also received group therapy. The results surprised the investigators as IDC had been designed to be the control condition, with the hypothesis that the CT and SE interventions would be superior. The results show that high-quality substance use counseling delivered by trained clinicians, 12-step meeting attendance, and a commitment to abstinence can make for an effective therapy.

As noted above, secondary analyses of the NIDA-funded Collaborative Cocaine Treatment Study among methadone-maintained patients in the sample suggested better outcomes for IDC among those with less co-occurring psychopathology, while those with more psychopathology CT or SE produced better outcomes.[25] This suggests a patient-treatment matching strategy where more psychologically focused treatments, or practitioners with more psychological training and orientation, might be considered for patients with higher levels of psychopathology in addition to the target addiction.

Twelve-Step Facilitation

Twelve-Step Facilitation (TSF) therapy[30] is characterized as a guided approach to facilitating early recovery and is intended to give clinicians a tool to help their patients engage productively in AA or other 12-step groups. Clinical trials testing TSF are the closest of any research studies to testing the effectiveness of 12-step participation itself. TSF is an individual treatment that, by design, is brief (12-15 sessions) and structured. Like IDC, it is based on the principles of the 12-step program. The therapy focuses on two general goals, acceptance of the need for abstinence and surrender, which includes a willingness to engage in the 12-step fellowship as a means to achieving sobriety. These principles include acknowledging that addiction is incurable and that willpower is insufficient to achieve and sustain abstinence. In this model, it is considered necessary to surrender to the "group conscience." The act of surrender also involves acknowledging that 12-step programs have helped millions of people to achieve and sustain sobriety and that the best chances at recovery come through following the 12-step path. Hope for recovery comes through recognition of loss of control and by having faith in a "higher power" (such as God or even the 12-step group). In this way, recovery is seen as a process of spiritual renewal. TSF counselors assess patients' substance use, advocate for abstinence, explain basic 12-step concepts, and actively support and facilitate involvement in AA/NA. Counselors also discuss 12-step reading and share resources with their patients. For more on 12-Step approaches, see also Section 10, "Mutual Help: Twelve Step and Other Recovery Programs."

The TSF manual incorporates material originally developed for Project MATCH, a clinical trial focusing on patient-treatment matching and funded by NIAAA. Project MATCH included two independent (but parallel) study arms, with patients recruited from both outpatient and aftercare programs and randomly assigned to TSF, CBT, or MET. When the data from Project MATCH were analyzed, only 1 of 16 of the hypothesized patient-treatment matches was confirmed, challenging the idea that patient characteristics could be used to assign patients to alcohol treatments. Patients in all three treatments evidenced substantial improvements in their drinking behavior (from baseline) on the two primary outcome measures—percentage of days abstinent and number if drinks consumed on drinking days, with improvements maintained across the 3-year follow-up period.[27] However, when examining total abstinence, which had been specified as a secondary outcome, patients who received TSF were significantly more likely to be abstinent at all follow-up points compared to those receiving CBT or MET; the magnitude of this difference was substantial, about 10 percentage points, and was evident across the entire 3-year follow-up period. Thus, the intervention that focused most on abstinence (TSF), and encouraged a long-term therapeutic effort (AA meetings) was more likely to produce long-term abstinence in this landmark study.

Recently, TSF was adapted for stimulant use disorders (cocaine or methamphetamine), and found to increase the likelihood of abstinence at the end of active treatment compared to TAU and to increase 12-step meeting participation,[47] and 12-step meeting attendance was associated with better substance use outcomes.[93] The advantage on abstinence diminished over long-term follow-up after the TSF intervention ended. It may be that the idea that behavioral interventions for SUD can be delivered as short-term, time-limited interventions is flawed, and that long-term interventions are needed for what is a chronic recurring disorder. A treatment like TSF could be continued indefinitely, perhaps with a lower frequency of sessions.

Medical Management

Manual-guided Medical Management (MM) interventions originally were developed to provide physicians who were treating patients in pharmacotherapy trials with a standard, well-specified set of goals and talking points to cover during clinic visits. This represented an effort to systematize what good prescribing physicians do during medication visits, analogous to the effort in IDC to define what good substance use counselors do. Typically, clinicians are asked to systematically address symptoms, side effects, and medication adherence and to troubleshoot any problems in an empathic, supportive, nonjudgmental manner. In the setting of clinical trials for SUDs, MM interventions, in addition to focusing on medication adherence, monitoring side effects, and troubleshooting problems with adherence, also focus on abstinence as a goal and trouble-shooting problems achieving or sustaining abstinence, sometimes recommending 12-step participation. In clinical trials examining combinations of medications with psychotherapies, MM interventions have sometimes been used as control conditions. For example, an intervention called compliance enhancement therapy (K. Carroll and S. O'Malley, *unpublished treatment manual*, 1996) was used as the control condition in clinical trials, which showed that more elaborate behavioral interventions (eg, CM; significant other involvement) improved adherence with naltrexone treatment for DSM-IV defined opioid dependence.[94,95] In another landmark study, the NIAAA-funded COMBINE,[96] participants were randomly assigned to an enhanced behavioral therapy including aspects of MI and CBT or a Medication Management control called BRENDA,[97] and also randomized to placebo, naltrexone, or acamprosate. While the expectation was that the enhanced behavioral therapy would improve the outcome of medication treatment, there was no main effect for therapy type; if anything, the best drinking outcomes were observed among patients who received medication management (BRENDA) plus naltrexone. Patients who seek to enter a medication trial probably are more favorably inclined to medication and may be less interested in psychotherapy. However, the results of this trial also could be interpreted as showing that the most essential elements of successful treatment for SUD may involve encouraging a commitment to abstinence and treatment adherence. See Chapter 83 "Medical Management Techniques and Collaborative Care: Integrating Behavioral With Pharmacological Interventions" for more detail on MM.

Mindfulness-Based Therapies

Contemplative and meditative practices from Eastern religious traditions such as Buddhism have formed the foundation for what has become a family of mindfulness-based therapies that have considerable evidence of efficacy from Stage II trials. Mindfulness meditation, for example, involves quiet focus on a sensory experience such as breathing, while monitoring thoughts and feelings that arise. Evidence suggests regular practice of this type cultivates reduction of emotional reactivity to distressing thoughts or feelings and engenders cognitive control, which can work against responding to stress or craving by using substances and in favor of alternative, healthy behavioral repertoires. Evidence from measures of affect and cognition, autonomic measures, and fMRI, support this mechanistic formulation.[98] Mindfulness-Based Stress Reduction and Mindfulness-Based Cognitive Therapy were developed, incorporating mindfulness techniques to help reduce distress in mood or anxiety disorders.

Mindfulness-Based Relapse Prevention and Mindfulness-Oriented Recovery Enhancement (MORE) have extended this approach to address the cognitive and behavioral processes experienced when stepping away from substance use and enjoy considerable evidence of efficacy across a range of substances. They lend themselves to combination with other treatment approaches and settings (eg, outpatient, inpatient, or residential treatment). As with other therapies covered in this chapter, challenges include adequate training of therapists to deliver mindfulness-based therapies with fidelity and the need for more Phase III and IV trials to examine effectiveness in real world treatment settings in the hands of community-based clinicians.[98] For more on mindfulness-based treatment approaches, see Chapter 81, "Mindfulness-Based Treatments of Addiction."

Acceptance and Commitment Therapy

Traditional cognitive-behavioral therapy approaches emphasize techniques to control, avoid, or alter painful thoughts and feelings. Acceptance and Commitment Therapy (ACT)[99] is a newer treatment model, based on behavioral formulations of language and cognition,[100] that in a sense turns this way of relating to thoughts and feelings on its head. ACT strives to increase psychological flexibility by incorporating techniques of mindfulness, emphasizing mindful awareness, the acceptance of painful or difficult feelings when in the service of moving toward what a patient values, and committing to action to make changes that are in line with those values, rather than avoiding such action when it may evoke painful or difficult feelings.[101] The emphasis on value guided actions has echoes of the probing for fundamental values emphasized in Motivational Interviewing. The utility of acceptance and committed action processes aligns with the Serenity Prayer, an often cited perspective in Alcohol Anonymous ("God grant me the serenity to accept the things I cannot change, courage to change the things I can, and the wisdom to know the difference."). ACT was originally developed to address health behavior change broadly, such as management of chronic pain, depression, or anxiety, which often co-occur with substance use disorders. ACT has also shown evidence of efficacy for nicotine use disorder[101] and alcohol use disorder.[102]

ROLE OF SIGNIFICANT OTHERS IN TREATMENT OF SUBSTANCE USE DISORDERS

Several individual therapies for SUD involve family and significant others in the treatment in some way. For example, 12-step approaches ask members to "make amends" to family and friends who have been wronged, offer opportunities for significant others to attend "open meetings" with the patient, and provide family support through the 12-step family programs (eg, Al-Anon). CRA encourages patients to reengage with significant others as part of the effort to restore healthy sources of reinforcement. CRA also provides for more direct involvement of family members, for example, by having them monitor medication ingestion. Early work on CRA[103] outlined a strategy for disulfiram monitoring in which the patient, significant other, and therapist all agree that the patient will take his/her medication in the presence of the significant other every day, at a scheduled time. The significant other then thanks the patient for his/her adherence, providing social reinforcement. If the patient refuses to take the medication, the significant other simply informs the therapist, and the matter is taken up at the next visit. Thus, the treatment remains focused on the patient with the SUD, but the significant other plays a concrete role designed to enhance the patient's chances for success.

Network Therapy

In the 1990s, Galanter[104] developed Network Therapy in an effort to harness the therapeutic potential of concerned significant others. In Network Therapy, the therapist employs tools of MI and cognitive-behavioral relapse prevention, but the unique aspect is that one or more significant others is directly involved in the treatment, also attending the therapy sessions. In contrast to family systems therapies, where there is an effort to diagnose and repair dysfunctional family systems, Network Therapy has more concrete goals. The significant others mainly are asked to support the patient's treatment, for example, by understanding the treatment and its goals, helping with homework assignments (eg, practicing relapse prevention skills), delivering social reinforcers contingent on abstinence or treatment adherence (eg, a gift, meal, night out), and/or monitoring medication taking. During treatment sessions, the therapist seeks to support the integrity of the network by keeping patient and significant others motivated, by improving communication, and by diffusing any tension that may arise. Such tension is common and can function as a stressor that promotes recurrence of use. Network Therapy has been tested and found to be effective as an adjunct to buprenorphine treatment for DSM-IV–defined opioid dependence[105]; aspects of Network Therapy also have shown promise in promoting adherence to naltrexone treatment for opioid dependence.[106] For more information about Network Therapy, see Chapter 75 "Network Therapy."

Community Reinforcement and Family Training Model

In contrast to Network Therapy, where the family is involved in the treatment in a mainly supportive role, Community Reinforcement and Family Training (CRAFT) trains the family to be an instrument of therapeutic change. Specifically, CRAFT teaches significant others behavioral and communication strategies that can increase the chances their treatment-refusing loved ones engage in treatment.[107,108] Unlike in planned "interventions," where stakeholders (generally with assistance from a clinician experienced with interventions) confront the person with the SUD with the goal of convincing him/her to go immediately to treatment, the CRAFT model steers away from confrontation. Instead, family and friends are taught to identify contexts in which substance use occurs, to make use of positive reinforcers, and to let the person with a SUD experience the natural negative consequences of substance use without inadvertently supporting ongoing substance use. Studies have suggested up to 70% of significant others using CRAFT can induce patients who are not interested in seeking help to engage in treatment,[109] while also improving their own emotional functioning, even if the individual with the SUD does not enter treatment.

Family Therapies

In family therapies, the patient is the family unit. While an individual's SUD may be the identified source of problems (the "identified patient"), there is an expectation that all family members will need to make changes to effect, support, and sustain positive changes in functioning within the family unit as a whole. Several family therapies for families dealing with a substance using family member have been tested and shown to have evidence of efficacy in controlled clinical trials.[108-114] However, such family therapies have not been widely adopted in clinical practice. Barriers to implementation of family interventions in routine community-based treatment include the fact that these treatments often require a relatively high level of training and sophistication on the part of therapists, lengthy therapy sessions, and cooperation on the part of family members who often are reticent to participate.[115] A recent large-scale effectiveness trial of Brief Strategic Family Therapy (BSFT), conducted by the NIDA-funded CTN, found limited effects of family therapy on short-term outcomes (eg, adolescent drug use). In this trial, BSFT was delivered by community-based therapists who were new to the method, although carefully trained and supervised during the study.[45] This study highlights potential difficulties associated with transporting family systems therapy into broad clinical use. However, the study did yield some interesting findings. BSFT was associated with reductions in parental drinking and drug use, and the benefit of BSFT on adolescent drug use was greater when parents were drinking or taking drugs at baseline.[116] BSFT was also associated with better outcome for adolescents in both drug use and functioning over long term (3- to 7-year follow-up).[117] The latter suggests that family therapy is an approach that can have a durable effect long after the intervention has been completed. More work is needed on how to successfully implement family therapy approaches in the context of routine community-based treatment for SUD."[118] For more on family therapies and involvement of significant others in treatment, see Chapter 78, "Family Involvement in Addiction, Treatment, and Recovery."

COMBINING INDIVIDUAL PSYCHOTHERAPY WITH OTHER MODALITIES: GROUP THERAPY AND MEDICATIONS

Group Therapy

It is common for patients with SUD who are receiving individual treatment also to be engaged in other interventions. The predominant treatment modality in most treatment programs is group therapy, even though there is limited evidence from clinical trials as to its effectiveness. One reason for the popularity of group therapy is its lower cost, because multiple patients can be treated simultaneously by a single therapist. In the Collaborative Cocaine Treatment Study,[31] all patients received Group Drug Counseling (GDC) as the background treatment; those who also received IDC had better outcomes compared to those receiving GDC only. Thus, in this trial, individual treatment provided additional therapeutic benefits beyond those conveyed by group treatment alone. Similarly, a recently completed NIDA-funded study in the Clinical Trials Network (CTN) demonstrated the efficacy, among patients with stimulant use disorders, of a TSF intervention that consisted of a combination of group and individual formats (see above).[47] Thus, combining group therapy and individual therapy may produce enhanced outcomes and therefore should be considered. More evidence is needed to guide clinicians regarding which combinations of individual and group treatments are most effect and for which SUDs. Chapter 71 "Group Therapies" further explores the research and clinical basis for the use of group therapies in the treatment of SUDs.

Individual Therapy and Medications for Substance Use Disorders

Several effective medications are available for treating SUDs, particularly for alcohol use disorder (eg, disulfiram, naltrexone, acamprosate, others) and opioid use disorder (methadone, buprenorphine, injection naltrexone). Yet, these medications remain underutilized. Individual treatment sessions are a natural setting in which the potential benefits of medications could be discussed, encouraged, and supported; however, nonphysicians may not be knowledgeable or comfortable enough to have this conversation with their patients. In addition, many drug treatment programs have limited medication options available to them (eg, only methadone for opioid use disorder). Another limitation is that many "unique" combinations of individual treatments and medications simply have not been tested, despite each treatment having shown evidence of efficacy as a stand-alone intervention. That said, several of the psychotherapies that have been reviewed in this chapter have been tested in combination with certain medications (eg, SE therapy with methadone,[24,25] Network Therapy with buprenorphine,[105] Medical Management or a combined motivational and cognitive-behavioral intervention in combination with naltrexone or acamprosate,[96] and Contingency Management plus Community Reinforcement Approach in combination with buprenorphine.[119])

Carroll, Kosten, and Rounsaville[120] reviewed a number of potential synergistic combinations between behavioral or psychotherapy and medication treatments, which may be considered during treatment planning. Their paper not only provides a roadmap of potential hypotheses to test in clinical trials but also can be used as a framework when tailoring treatment for a patient where pharmacotherapy is planned. These potential combinations and their rationales are summarized in **Table 72-3**. As can be seen in **Table 72-3**, there are several possible logical combinations, some of which already have been tested in clinical trials; other promising combinations also are suggested. While adherence to treatment is a general problem in the treatment of SUD, adherence to medications is a particular problem. Even agonist treatments like methadone or buprenorphine, which are inherently reinforcing, are accompanied by substantial dropout rates. However, MI could be employed to decrease ambivalence about medication taking. CM could identify medication ingestion as the target behavior and provide rewards contingent on ingestion. Following the CRA approach, or Network Therapy, family members

TABLE 72-3 Rationales for Combining Medications With Behavioral Therapies

Problem/issue	Characteristic of medication	Characteristic of behavioral therapy	Examples
Medication adherence	Medication is effective, but adherence is limited	Behavioral therapy focus on securing medication adherence	Network Therapy + buprenorphine[96]; MM plus naltrexone[30]; disulfiram plus medication monitoring
Abstinence induction	Medication works best for patients who are abstinent at baseline	Behavioral therapy focus on initial abstinence	Injection naltrexone for alcohol dependence
Prevention of recurrent substance use	Medication works to initiate abstinence	Behavioral therapy focus on prevention of return to substance use	Relapse prevention therapy after an inpatient withdrawal management
Adherence to behavioral therapy	Medication effective, keeps patients in treatment	Behavioral therapy requires good adherence	SE therapy and methadone maintenance[24,25]; CRA and buprenorphine[110]
Cognitive enhancement	Medication enhances attention or memory	Behavioral therapy is cognitively demanding	Stimulant medication plus CBT

Adapted from: Carroll KM, Kosten TR, Rounsaville BJ. Choosing a behavioral therapy platform for pharmacotherapy of substance users. *Drug Alcohol Depend.* 2004;75(2):123-134.

could be enlisted in helping to monitor medication ingestion to improve adherence. Return to substance use after discontinuation of medications is common, and several therapies, including cognitive-behavioral relapse prevention therapy and TSF, focus specifically on this problem. Cognitive enhancement is a relatively unexplored area, but neuropsychological deficits are common among patients with SUD[121] and have been shown to predict dropout from cognitive-behavioral relapse prevention.[122] Thus, medications to improve attention and reduce impulsivity, such as those used to treat attention deficit disorder (ADHD), might be considered in conjunction with CBT-RP. For example, one substantial placebo-controlled trial among patients with ADHD who were receiving a version of CBT, showed that extended release mixed amphetamine salts (Adderall XR) increased abstinence compared to placebo.[123] Further discussion of convergent and complimentary strategies for combining medication and behavioral treatments can be found in Chapter 83, "Medical Management Techniques and Collaborative Care: Integrating Behavioral with Pharmacological Interventions." Considerable work needs to be done in this area. Further, the only medications addressed in that chapter are those designed specifically to address SUD. Additionally, medications for psychiatric disorders like depression and anxiety should be considered as possible adjuncts to individual psychotherapy since unstable mood states and co-occurring mental disorders also can destabilize patients and contribute to substance use and recurrence of use.

DIFFERENTIAL THERAPEUTICS: HOW TO MATCH PATIENTS WITH THERAPIES

As in much of mental health therapeutics, choosing the best treatment for a given patient with a SUD remains more art than science in many instances. Most of the research studies testing individual treatments for SUD tests efficacy or effectiveness against a control condition. Moderator analyses, examining patient characteristics that predict good response to a specific treatment, are usually exploratory. One exception was Project MATCH,[26,27] which specifically sought to generate information on matching of DSM-IV–defined alcohol-dependent patients to one of three individual treatments (MET, cognitive-behavioral relapse prevention, or TSF) based on a broad panel of baseline characteristics. As previously noted, only one of the prespecified matching hypotheses was supported by the data, although several secondary matching factors were identified. For example, MET was found to be particularly effective, compared to the other treatments, for angry patients. Angry patients may be irritated by being told what to do as in more directive therapies and, conversely, may be more responsive to the collaborative, person-centered approach of MET. In contrast, TSF was found to be particularly effective for patients whose social networks included other people who use substances, which makes sense, given that 12-step participation encourages access to a substance-free social network.

In the absence of strong indicators for matching patients to specific treatments, a sensible approach is to make a best guess as to where to start, and then be prepared to switch interventions if the initial effort fails. For example, should an MET approach fail, one might consider switching to a more directive approach, such as TSF. Unfortunately, clinicians (and treatment programs) tend to offer just one or only a few predominant treatment methods in a "one-size-fits-all" approach. Clinicians or programs may ascribe strongly to a particular theoretical orientation, have limited training in other approaches, and/or lack confidence in their ability to deliver alternative therapies beyond those with which they are most familiar. Many patients will fail to respond to the initial treatment to which they are assigned and thus will require recalibration. Clinicians should be prepared to deliver alternative interventions themselves or else refer their patients to other therapists who have different repertoires. Future research should examine adaptive approaches that regularly measure progress and provide opportunities for patients to switch treatments when the first treatment tried is not working. For this to occur, treatment programs must regularly assess for change among their clientele and must foster expertise among their clinicians in a wider range of approaches, so that patients will have more treatment options available to them should these be needed.

VIRTUAL THERAPY AND COMPUTER-DELIVERED TECHNOLOGY-BASED INTERVENTIONS

Over the past decade, technology has played an increasingly important role in treatment of SUD. This includes evidence-based interventions that are conducted remotely via Skype, FaceTime, telephonic or videoconferencing methodology. These telemedicine approaches expanded dramatically during the COVID-19 pandemic and have been well accepted. Treatments delivered by computer, tablet, or smartphone in the absence of a clinician are also expanding. One advantage of all technology-assisted interventions is their potential to get more patients engaged in care. It is well documented that a large proportion of patients with SUD do not seek out or otherwise engage in treatment. The reasons for this are speculative, but likely include low motivation to change, stigma, high cost, and/or limited availability of services. Technology-assisted interventions can help to overcome these barriers by making treatment more accessible. In the case of virtual therapy, the treatment comes to patients in rural and other underserved areas where services are lacking.[124] Although clinical trials comparing outcomes for patients receiving virtual versus face-to-face therapy are lacking, a study of patients with alcohol use disorders who participated in an 8-week group-based videoconferencing intervention[125] demonstrated feasibility and acceptability with 14 of 18 patients (78%) attending at least four sessions—an attendance rate similar to what has been reported for face-to-face treatment. Patients liked the approach and found the treatment to be credible with 82% stating they would recommend it to a family member or friend. Evidence for efficacy was demonstrated in a Brazilian study[126] in which 524 people who used cannabis received a Brief Motivational Intervention (BMI) by telephone or reference materials. At 6-month follow-up, 73% of those in the BMI group were abstinent versus 59% of the control group although there was no significant difference found for motivation for change. While Health Insurance Portability and Accountability Act (HIPAA) compliance and cross-state practice restrictions (including licensure) must be considered when employing telemedicine, most can be resolved if clinicians are thoughtful when establishing their on-line practices.

In the case of computer-delivered interventions, patients who are not yet ready to seek out treatment may still be willing to complete a screening tool anonymously through the web, including those that provide feedback and/or advice to change. Furthermore, to the extent that behavioral therapies, such as those reviewed in this chapter, can be automated, or portions of the therapies automated, this lowers barriers to implementation. If an intervention, such a cognitive-behavioral intervention, can be delivered through a computer, or an app on a phone, then clinicians at a treatment program can prescribe the intervention and monitor patient participation. But the clinicians do not have to be trained and supervised in how to deliver the intervention, and do not need to spend the extra time delivering the intervention. This potentially lowers costs and conserves clinicians' time for managing issues unique to each individual patient, while the computer delivers some of the routine behavioral programming.

Prominent examples of such interventions supported by evidence of effectiveness from controlled trials include (1) a computer-delivered version of Cognitive-Behavioral Relapse Prevention for SUDs, CBT4CBT, which is delivered as seven 30- to 40-minute interactive, computer-delivered modules[127]; and (2) a web-based version of Community Reinforcement Approach plus Contingency Management, developed as the "Therapeutic Education System," which combines computer-delivered CRA counseling with a system for tracking target behaviors and rewards of a contingency management regimen.[49,128] Other types of interventions take advantage of the ability of a smartphone to deliver text messages with therapeutic content.[129] Smartphones and wearable devices can gather data from patients in real time (so-called ecological momentary assessment), which can be put to therapeutic purposes. DynamiCare uses the smartphone camera to directly monitor saliva drug testing and deliver rewards contingent on abstinence, or directly monitor medication taking.[130]

Although there is great potential among these emerging technology-based interventions, an important caveat is that many interventions and apps, although developed and marketed, do not have adequate empirical evidence to support their efficacy.[131] Another barrier to implementation of technology-based interventions has been funding. The interventions have costs, and mechanisms for treatment programs to bill third parties and recover those costs have been problematic. Technology-delivered therapies for SUD are discussed further in Chapter 82, "Digital Health Interventions for Substance Use Disorders: The State of the Science."

TECHNOLOGY TRANSFER: HOW TO EFFECTIVELY TRAIN CLINICIANS TO DELIVER EVIDENCE-BASED PSYCHOTHERAPIES

As the preceding review suggests, a number of different individual psychotherapy and behavioral therapy approaches for the SUD have been developed, which have proven effective in clinical trials. Yet, these treatments are not widely used in the community-based treatment system.[132] Technology transfer refers to the process of taking a new technology, evidence-based psychotherapy in our case, and getting it into widespread use in the community. People and systems resist new technologies. Clinicians are no different. A fundamental precept of technology transfer is that clinicians need encouragement, feedback, and supervision in order to learn and successfully use new psychotherapeutic skills. Clinical trials among physicians have repeatedly shown that traditional methods of introducing new treatments (journal articles, lectures, and didactic symposia or workshops) may increase knowledge but do not get physicians to actually practice the new methods. Rather, what is effective in promoting use of new treatments are training methods that include feedback and supervision.[133-137] This is the reason, for example, that pharmaceutical companies invest heavily in sales forces of well-educated representatives, who visit physicians and engage in "academic detailing"—that is, teaching physicians about their new medical product while also getting physicians to talk about their caseloads, try out the new treatment, and obtain feedback. The representative serves as a champion and coach for the new treatment.

Unfortunately, in the field of SUDs, most training takes the form of conferences and workshops. This stands in contrast to the clinical trials of psychotherapies, where clinicians are trained on a treatment manual and receive regular measurement of their performance along with supervision sessions to help them hone and maintain their skills. Studies of methods for training community-based clinicians in MI have tended to confirm the lack of effectiveness of didactic workshops alone[135-137]; when skill at MI interviewing was measured at follow-up points after workshop training, some improvement in knowledge can be observed, but little improvement in actual skill. However, in these training trials, clinicians who received ongoing feedback and supervision after the workshop did evidence increases in skill over time.

These findings suggest that efforts to disseminate new psychotherapies and other treatments for SUD into the treatment community should shift focus from didactic exercises to clinical supervision. During initial training (eg, psychology or social work graduate school and internship or physicians' clinical clerkships and residency training), clinicians usually meet regularly with supervisors to go over cases and may even interview patients with supervisors present. Audio and video recording are common. However, this type of supervision often ceases once a clinician graduates and gets a job in a treatment program. Programs and their clinicians are under increasing pressure to see more patients and generate corresponding revenue; putting time aside for supervision sacrifices time that could be spent seeing patients. However, given the likely effect of supervision on quality of care, this probably is an investment worth making. Thus, treatment programs should be encouraged to set aside time for clinical supervision intended to introduce, build, and maintain new clinical skills. A related problem is how to make enough expert supervisors available to clinical programs and how to fund staff training and ongoing supervision efforts. Most psychotherapies have a small cadre of "experts" and certainly do not have anything like the large pharmaceutical companies that are able to fund, train, and deploy extensive sales forces. The NIH Institutes and SAMHSA have recognized this problem over the last several decades and have begun funding research on dissemination, as well as dissemination efforts themselves. Examples of these efforts include the Addiction Technology Transfer Centers (ATTCs) (http://www.attcnetwork.org) and the Blending Initiatives (http://www.drugabuse.gov/blending-initiative) that have developed and disseminated training materials for interventions found effective in studies by the CTN. Mandates from government and third-party payers for delivery of evidence-based treatment also have created incentives for programs to adopt new treatment approaches. Technology-delivered therapies, reviewed in the previous section also have the potential to surmount barriers to implementation. The therapies reviewed in this chapter have the potential to improve the public health by improving the quality of care for patients with SUDs across the treatment system. However, in order for this impact to be realized, widespread adoption of these treatments will be needed, along with research to develop innovative methods of dissemination for promising treatments.

ACKNOWLEDGMENTS

This chapter is dedicated to the memories of the late Drs Bruce Rounsaville and Kathleen Carroll previous authors of this chapter. Based at Yale where they directed programs in psychotherapy development and research training, their contributions to the field of psychotherapy research are extensive, dating back more than 30 years, including work in developing and validating CBT and other behavioral treatments for substance use disorders and for the "stage model" of psychotherapy development, described in this chapter. We are grateful for their leadership and groundbreaking work in this field.

REFERENCES

1. Doering S, Hörz S, Rentrop M, et al. Transference-focused psychotherapy v. treatment by community psychotherapists for borderline personality disorder: randomized controlled trial. *Br J Psychiatry.* 2010;196(5):389-395.
2. Clarkin JF, Levy KN, Lenzenweger MF, Kernberg OF. Evaluating three treatments for borderline personality disorder: a multiwave study. *Am J Psychiatry.* 2007;164(6):922-928.
3. Milrod B, Chambless DL, Gallop R, et al. Psychotherapies for panic disorder: a tale of two sites. *J Clin Psychiatry.* 2016;77(7):927-935.
4. Rounsaville BJ, Carroll KM, Back SE. Behavioral interventions: individual psychotherapy. In: Ries RK, Fiellin DA, Miller SC, Saitz R, eds. *Principles of Addiction Medicine.* 4th ed. Lippincott Williams & Wilkins; 2009.
5. Alcoholics Anonymous. Accessed June 9, 2023. http://www.aa.org
6. Pittman BAA. *The Way It Began.* Glen Abbey Books; 1988.
7. Hartigan F, Bill W. *A Biography of Alcoholics Anonymous Cofounder Bill Wilson.* 1st ed. St Martin's Press; 2000:50-53.
8. Alcoholics Anonymous. *Questions and Answers on Sponsorship.* Accessed June 9, 2023. http://www.aa.org/pdf/products/p-15_Q&AonSpon.pdf
9. White W, Budnick C, Pickard B. Narcotics anonymous: its history and culture. *Counselor.* 2011;12(2):22-27.
10. Hazelden. *The Minnesota Model.* Accessed June 9, 2023. http://www.hazelden.org/web/public/minnesotamodel.page
11. National Institute on Drug Abuse. *Therapeutic Community.* National Institute on Drug Abuse; 2002 NIH Pub Number: 02-4877.

12. White W. *Slaying The Dragon: The History of Addiction Treatment and Recovery in America*. Chestnut Health Systems; 1998.
13. Volkow ND, Li TK. Drug addiction: the neurobiology of behavior gone awry. In: Ries RK, Fiellin DA, Miller SC, Saitz R, eds. *Principles of Addiction Medicine*. 4th ed. Lippincott Williams & Wilkins; 2009.
14. Beck AT. The evolution of the cognitive model of depression and its neurobiological correlates. *Am J Psychiatry*. 2008;165(8):969-977.
15. Carroll KM, Rounsaville BJ, Keller DS. Relapse prevention strategies for the treatment of cocaine abuse. *Am J Drug Alcohol Abuse*. 1991;17(3):249-265.
16. Larimer ME, Palmer RS, Marlatt GA. Relapse prevention: an overview of Marlatt's cognitive-behavioral model. *Alcohol Res Health*. 1999;23(2):151-160.
17. Longabaugh R, Morgenstern J. Cognitive-behavioral coping-skills therapy for alcohol dependence. Current status and future directions. *Alcohol Res Health*. 1999;23(2):78-85.
18. Smith JE, Meyers RJ, Miller WR. The community reinforcement approach to the treatment of substance use disorders. *Am J Addict*. 2001;10(Suppl):51-59.
19. Stitzer M, Petry N. Contingency management for treatment of substance abuse. *Annu Rev Clin Psychol*. 2006;2:411-434.
20. Miller WR, Rollnick S, Conforti K. *Motivational Interviewing: Preparing People for Change*. 2nd ed. Guilford Publications Inc; 2002.
21. Miller WR, Rollnick S. *Motivational Interviewing: Helping People Change (Applications of Motivational Interviewing)*. 3rd ed. Guilford Publications Inc; 2013.
22. Cochrane AL. *Effectiveness and Efficiency: Random Reflections on Health Services*. Royal Society of Medicine Press Ltd; 1972:1999.
23. Chambless DL, Hollon SD. Defining empirically supported therapies. *J Consult Clin Psychol*. 1998;66(1):7-18.
24. Woody GE, Luborsky L, McLellan AT, et al. Psychotherapy for opiate addicts: does it help? *Arch Gen Psychiatry*. 1983;40:639-645.
25. Woody GE, McLellan AT, Luborsky L, O'Brien CP. Sociopathy and psychotherapy outcome. *Arch Gen Psychiatry*. 1985;42(11):1081-1086.
26. Project MATCH Research Group. Matching alcoholism treatments to client heterogeneity: project MATCH post treatment drinking outcomes. *J Stud Alcohol Drugs*. 1997;58(1):7-29.
27. Project MATCH Research Group. Matching alcoholism treatments to client heterogeneity: project MATCH three-year drinking outcomes. *Alcohol Clin Exp Res*. 1998;22(6):1300-1311.
28. Miller WR, Zweben A, DiClemente CC, et al. *Motivational Enhancement Therapy Manual: A Clinical Research Guide for Therapists Treating Individuals with Alcohol Abuse and Dependence*. National Institute on Alcohol Abuse and Alcoholism; 1994.
29. Kadden R, Carroll KM, Donovan D, et al. *Cognitive-Behavioral Coping Skills Therapy Manual: A Clinical Research Guide for Therapists Treating Individuals with Alcohol Abuse and Dependence*. National Institute on Alcohol Abuse and Alcoholism; 1992.
30. Nowinski J, Baker S, Carroll KM. *Twelve-step Facilitation Therapy Manual: A Clinical Research Guide for Therapists Treating Individuals with Alcohol Abuse and Dependence*. National Institute on Alcohol Abuse and Alcoholism; 1992.
31. Crits-Christoph P, Siqueland L, Blaine J, et al. Psychosocial treatments for cocaine dependence: National Institute on Drug Abuse Collaborative Cocaine Treatment Study. *Arch Gen Psychiatry*. 1999;56(6):493-502.
32. Carroll KM, Onken LS. Behavioral therapies for drug abuse. *Am J Psychiatry*. 2005;162:1452-1460.
33. Waskow IE. Specification of the technique variable in the NIMH Treatment of Depression Collaborative Research Program. In: Williams JBW, Spitzer RL, eds. *Psychotherapy Research: Where Are We and Where Should We Go?* Guilford Press; 1984:150-159.
34. Docherty JP. Implications of the technological model of psychotherapy. In: Williams JBW, Spitzer RL, eds. *Psychotherapy Research: Where Are We and Where Should We Go?* Guilford Press; 1984:139-149.
35. National Institutes of Health. *Development of Theoretically-based Psychosocial Therapies for Drug Dependence*. NIH Guides; 1992 21(34):Part II.
36. Rounsaville BJ, Carroll KM, Onken LS. A stage model of behavioral therapies development: getting started and moving on from Stage I. *Clin Psychol Sci Pract*. 2001;8(2):133-142.
37. National Institute on Drug Abuse. *Behavioral & Integrative Treatment Development Program*. 2013: NIDA Pub Number: PA-13-077.
38. Nunes EV, Ball S, Booth R, et al. Multisite effectiveness trials of treatments for substance abuse and co-occurring problems: have we chosen the best designs? *J Subst Abuse Treat*. 2010;38(Suppl 1):S97-S112.
39. Nielsen L, Riddle M, King JW, et al. The NIH Science of Behavior Change Program: transforming the science through a focus on mechanisms of change. *Behav Res Ther*. 2018;101:3-11.
40. Onken LS, Carroll KM, Shoham V, Cuthbert BN, Riddle M. Reenvisioning clinical science: unifying the discipline to improve the public health. *Clin Psychol Sci*. 2014;2(1):22-34.
41. Carroll KM, Ball SA, Nich C, et al. Motivational interviewing to improve treatment engagement and outcome in individuals seeking treatment for substance abuse: a multisite effectiveness study. National Institute on Drug Abuse Clinical Trials Network. *Drug Alcohol Depend*. 2006;81(3):301-312.
42. Ball SA, Martino S, Nich C, et al. Site matters: multisite randomized trial of motivational enhancement therapy in community drug abuse clinics. National Institute on Drug Abuse Clinical Trials Network. *J Consult Clin Psychol*. 2007;75(4):556-567.
43. Petry NM, Peirce JM, Stitzer ML, et al. Effect of prize-based incentives on outcomes in stimulant abusers in outpatient psychosocial treatment programs: a national drug abuse treatment clinical trials network study. *Arch Gen Psychiatry*. 2005;62(10):1148-1156.
44. Peirce JM, Petry NM, Stitzer ML, et al. Effects of lower-cost incentives on stimulant abstinence in methadone maintenance treatment: a National Drug Abuse Treatment Clinical Trials Network study. *Arch Gen Psychiatry*. 2006;63(2):201-208.
45. Robbins MS, Feaster DJ, Horigian VE, et al. Brief strategic family therapy versus treatment as usual: results of a multisite randomized trial for substance using adolescents. *J Consult Clin Psychol*. 2011;79(6):713-727.
46. Hien DA, Jiang H, Campbell AN, et al. Do treatment improvements in PTSD severity affect substance use outcomes? A secondary analysis from a randomized clinical trial in NIDA's Clinical Trials Network. *Am J Psychiatry*. 2010;167(1):95-101.
47. Donovan DM, Daley DC, Brigham GS, et al. Stimulant abuser groups to engage in 12-step: a multisite trial in the National Institute on Drug Abuse Clinical Trials Network. *J Subst Abuse Treat*. 2013;44(1):103-114.
48. Weiss RD, Potter JS, Fiellin DA, et al. Adjunctive counseling during brief and extended buprenorphine-naloxone treatment for prescription opioid dependence: a 2-phase randomized controlled trial. *Arch Gen Psychiatry*. 2011;68(12):1238-1246.
49. Campbell AN, Nunes EV, Matthews AG, et al. Internet-delivered treatment for substance abuse: a multisite randomized controlled trial. *Am J Psychiatry*. 2014;171(6):683-690.
50. Morris ZS, Wooding S, Grant J. The answer is 17 years, what is the question: understanding lag times in translational research. *J R Soc Med*. 2011;104:510-520.
51. Miller WR, Sorensen JL, Selzer JA, Brigham GS. Disseminating evidence-based practices in substance abuse treatment: a review with suggestions. *J Subst Abuse Treat*. 2006;31(1):25-39.
52. Morgenstern J, Longabaugh R. Cognitive-behavioral treatment for alcohol dependence: a review of evidence for its hypothesized mechanisms of action. *Addiction*. 2000;95(10):1475-1490.
53. Magill M, Tonigan JS, Kiluk B, Ray L, Walthers J, Carroll K. The search for mechanisms of cognitive behavioral therapy for alcohol or other drug use disorders: a systematic review. *Behav Res Ther*. 2020;131:103648.
54. Linehan MM, McDavid JD, Brown MZ, Sayrs JHR, Gallop RJ. Olanzapine plus dialectical behavior therapy for women with high irritability who meet criteria for borderline personality disorder: a double-blind, placebo-controlled pilot study. *J Clin Psychiatry*. 2008;69(6):999-1005.
55. Higgins ST, Sigmon SC, Wong CJ, et al. Community reinforcement therapy for cocaine-dependent outpatients. *Arch Gen Psychiatry*. 2003;60(10):1043-1052.

56. Luborsky L, Barber JP, Siqueland L, et al. The revised helping alliance questionnaire (HAq-II): psychometric properties. *J Psychother Pract Res.* 1996;5(3):260-271.
57. Bordin ES. The generalizability of the psychoanalytic concept of the working alliance. *Psychol Psychother.* 1979;16:252-260.
58. Horvath AO. The alliance in context: accomplishments, challenges, and future directions. *Psychotherapy (Chic).* 2006;43:258-263.
59. Meier PS, Barrowclough C, Donmall MC. The role of therapeutic alliance in the treatment of substance misuse: a critical review of the literature. *Addiction.* 2005;100(3):304-316.
60. Carroll KM, Nich C, Rounsaville BJ. Contribution of the therapeutic alliance to outcome in active versus control psychotherapies. *J Consult Clin Psychol.* 1997;65:510-514.
61. Baldwin SA, Wampold BE, Imel ZE. Untangling the alliance-outcome correlation: exploring the relative importance of therapist and patient variability in the alliance. *J Consult Clin Psychol.* 2007;75(6):842-852.
62. Moyers TB, Miller WR. Is low therapist empathy toxic? *Psychol Addict Behav.* 2013;27(3):878-884.
63. Moyers TB, Houck J, Rice SL, Longabaugh R, Miller WR. Therapist empathy, combined behavioral intervention, and alcohol outcomes in the COMBINE research project. *J Consult Clin Psychol.* 2016;84(3):221-229.
64. Bethea A, Acosta MC, Haller DL. Patient versus therapist alliance: whose perception matters? *J Subst Abuse Treat.* 2008;35:174-183.
65. Moyers TB, Martin T, Manuel JK, Hendrickson SML, Miller WR. Assessing competence in the use of motivational interviewing. *J Subst Abuse Treat.* 2005;28(1):19-26.
66. Moyers TB, Martin T, Manual JK, Miller WR, Ernst D. *Revised Global Scales: Motivational Interviewing Treatment Integrity 3.1.1 (MITI 3.1.1).* University of New Mexico Center on Alcoholism, Substance Abuse and Addictions; 2010.
67. Amrhein PC, Miller WR, Yahne CE, Palmer M, Fulcher L. Client commitment language during motivational interviewing predicts drug use outcomes. *J Consult Clin Psychol.* 2003;71:862-878.
68. Hettema J, Steele J, Miller WR. Motivational interviewing. *Annu Rev Clin Psychol.* 2005;1:91-111.
69. Bien TH, Miller WR, Tonigan JS. Brief interventions for alcohol problems: a review. *Addiction.* 1993;88:315-335.
70. Wilk AI, Jensen NM, Havighurst TC. Meta-analysis of randomized controlled trials addressing brief interventions in heavy alcohol drinkers. *J Gen Intern Med.* 1997;12:274-283.
71. Luborsky L. *Principles of Psychoanalytic Psychotherapy: A Manual for Supportive-expressive (SE) Treatment.* Basic Books; 1984.
72. Mark D, Luborsky L. *A Manual for the Use of Supportive-Expressive Psychotherapy in the Treatment of Cocaine Abuse.* University of Pennsylvania; 1992.
73. O'Malley SS, Jaffe AJ, Chang G, Schottenfeld RS, Meyer RE, Rounsaville B. Naltrexone and coping skills therapy for alcohol dependence: a controlled study. *Arch Gen Psychiatry.* 1992;49(11):881-887.
74. Carroll KM, Rounsaville BJ, Nich C, Gordon LT, Wirtz PW, Gawin F. One-year follow-up of psychotherapy and pharmacotherapy for cocaine dependence. Delayed emergence of psychotherapy effects. *Arch Gen Psychiatry.* 1994;51(12):989-997.
75. Rawson RA, Huber A, McCann M, et al. A comparison of contingency management and cognitive-behavioral approaches during methadone maintenance treatment for cocaine dependence. *Arch Gen Psychiatry.* 2002;59(9):817-824.
76. Kellogg SH, Stitzer ML, Petry NM, et al. *Contingency Management: Foundations and Principles.* Accessed February 24, 2013. https://attcnetwork.org/sites/default/files/2021-01/Kellog-Stitzer.pdf
77. Higgins ST, Wong CJ, Badger GJ, Ogden DE, Dantona RL. Contingent reinforcement increases cocaine abstinence during outpatient treatment and 1 year of follow-up. *J Consult Clin Psychol.* 2000;68:64-72.
78. Lussier JP, Heil SH, Mongeon JA, Badger GJ, Higgns ST. A meta-analysis of voucher-based reinforcement therapy for substance use disorders. *Addiction.* 2006;101(2):192-203.
79. Prendergast M, Podus D, Finney J, Greenwell L, Roll J. Contingency management for treatment of substance use disorders: a meta-analysis. *Addiction.* 2006;101(11):1546-1560.
80. Petry NM, Martin B, Cooney JL, Kranzler HR. Give them prizes, and they will come: contingency management for treatment of alcohol dependence. *J Consult Clin Psychol.* 2000;68(2):250-257.
81. McDonell MG, Leickly E, McPherson S, et al. A randomized controlled trial of ethyl glucuronide-based contingency management for outpatients with co-occurring alcohol use disorders and serious mental illness. *Am J Psychiatry.* 2017;174(4):370-377.
82. Iguchi MY, Belding MA, Morral AR, Lamb RJ, Husband SD. Reinforcing operants other than abstinence in drug abuse treatment: an effective alternative for reducing drug use. *J Consult Clin Psychol.* 1997;65(3):421-428.
83. Carpenter KM, Smith JL, Aharonovich E, Nunes EV. Developing therapies for depression in drug dependence: results of a stage 1 therapy study. *Am J Drug Alcohol Abuse.* 2008;34(5):642-652.
84. Kellogg SH, Burns M, Coleman P, Stitzer M, Wale JB, Kreek MJ. Something of value: the introduction of contingency management interventions into the New York City Health and Hospital Addiction Treatment Service. *J Subst Abuse Treat.* 2005;28(1):57-65.
85. Petry NM. A comprehensive guide for the application of contingency management procedures in standard clinic settings. *Drug Alcohol Depend.* 2000;58:9-25.
86. Silverman K, Higgins ST, Brooner RK, et al. Sustained cocaine abstinence in methadone maintenance patients through voucher-based reinforcement therapy. *Arch Gen Psychiatry.* 1996;53(5):409-415.
87. Silverman K, Svikis D, Wong CJ, Hampton J, Stitzer ML, Bigelow GE. A reinforcement-based therapeutic workplace for the treatment of drug abuse: three-year abstinence outcomes. *Exp Clin Psychopharmacol.* 2002;10(3):228-240.
88. Higgins ST, Heil SH, Dantona R, Donham R, Matthews M, Badger GJ. Effects of varying the monetary value of voucher-based incentives on abstinence achieved during and following treatment among cocaine-dependent outpatients. *Addiction.* 2007;102(2):271-281.
89. Petry NM. Contingency management treatments. *Br J Psychiatry.* 2006;189:97-98.
90. Woody GE, McLellan AT, Luborsky L, O'Brien CP. Psychotherapy in community methadone programs: a validation study. *Am J Psychiatry.* 1995;152(9):1302-1308.
91. Mercer DE, Woody GE. *Therapy Manuals for Drug Abuse: Manual 3.* National Institute on Drug Abuse; 1999.
92. McLellan AT, Luborsky L, Woody GE, O'Brien CP. An improved diagnostic instrument for substance abuse patients: the Addiction Severity Index. *J Nerv Ment Dis.* 1980;168:26-33.
93. Wells EA, Donovan DM, Daley DC, et al. Is level of exposure to a 12-step facilitation therapy associated with treatment outcome? *J Subst Abuse Treat.* 2014;47(4):265-274.
94. Carroll KM, Ball SA, Nich C, et al. Targeting behavioral therapies to enhance naltrexone treatment of opioid dependence: efficacy of contingency management and significant other involvement. *Arch Gen Psychiatry.* 2001;58(8):755-761.
95. Nunes EV, Rothenberg JL, Sullivan MA, Carpenter KM, Kleber HD. Behavioral therapy to augment oral naltrexone for opioid dependence: a ceiling on effectiveness? *Am J Drug Alcohol Abuse.* 2006;32(4):503-517.
96. Anton RF, O'Malley SS, Ciraulo DA, et al. Combined pharmacotherapies and behavioral interventions for alcohol dependence: the COMBINE study: a randomized controlled trial. *JAMA.* 2006;295(17):2003-2017.
97. Volpicelli JR, Pettinati HM, McLellan AT, et al. *Combining Medication and Psychosocial Treatments for Addictions: The BRENDA Approach.* Guilford Press; 2001.
98. Garland EL, Howard MO. Mindfulness-based treatment of addiction: current state of the field and envisioning the next wave of research. *Addict Sci Clin Pract.* 2018;13(1):14.
99. Hayes SC, Strosahl KD, Wilson KG. *Acceptance and Commitment Therapy: An Experiential Approach to Behavior Change.* Guilford Press; 1999.

100. Hayes SC, Barnes-Holmes D, Roche B, eds. *Relational frame theory: A post-Skinnerian account of human language and cognition.* Kluwer Academic/Plenum; 2001.
101. Zhang CQ, Leeming E, Smith P, Chung PK, Hagger MS, Hayes SC. Acceptance and commitment therapy for health behavior change: a contextually-driven approach. *Front Psychol.* 2018;11(8):2350.
102. Byrne SP, Haber P, Baillie A, Costa DSJ, Fogliati V, Morley K. Systematic reviews of mindfulness and acceptance and commitment therapy for alcohol use disorder: should we be using third wave therapies? *Alcohol Alcohol.* 2019;54(2):159-166.
103. Hunt GM, Azrin NH. A community-reinforcement approach to alcoholism. *Behav Res Ther.* 1973;11(1):91-104.
104. Galanter M. Network therapy for addiction: a model for office practice. *Am J Psychiatry.* 1993;150(1):28-36.
105. Galanter M, Dermatis H, Glickman L, et al. Network therapy: decreased secondary opioid use during buprenorphine maintenance. *J Subst Abuse Treat.* 2004;26(4):313-318.
106. Brooks AC, Comer SD, Sullivan MA, et al. Long-acting injectable versus oral naltrexone maintenance therapy with psychosocial intervention for heroin dependence: a quasi-experiment. *J Clin Psychiatry.* 2010;71(10):1371-1378.
107. Meyers RJ, Miller WR, Hill DE, Tonigan JS. Community reinforcement and family training (CRAFT): engaging unmotivated drug users in treatment. *J Subst Abuse.* 1998;10(3):291-308.
108. O'Farrell TJ, Clements K. Review of outcome research on marital and family therapy in treatment for alcoholism. *J Marital Fam Ther.* 2012;38(1):122-144.
109. Archer M, Harwood H, Stevelink S, Rafferty L, Greenberg N. Community reinforcement and family training and rates of treatment entry: a systematic review. *Addiction.* 2020;115(6):1024-1037.
110. Henggeler SW, Sheidow AJ. Empirically supported family-based treatments for conduct disorder and delinquency in adolescents. *J Marital Fam Ther.* 2012;38(1):30-58.
111. Santisteban DA, Coatsworth JD, Perez-Vidal A, et al. Efficacy of brief strategic family therapy in modifying Hispanic adolescent behavior problems and substance use. *J Fam Psychol.* 2003;17(1):121-133.
112. Santisteban DA, Suarez-Morales L, Robbins MS, Szapocznik J. Brief strategic family therapy: lessons learned in efficacy research and challenges to blending research and practice. *Fam Process.* 2006;45(2):259-271.
113. Hogue A, Liddle HA. Family-based treatment for adolescent substance abuse: controlled trials and new horizons in services research. *J Fam Ther.* 2009;31(2):126-154.
114. Henderson CE, Dakof GA, Greenbaum PE, Liddle HA. Effectiveness of multidimensional family therapy with higher severity substance-abusing adolescents: report from two randomized controlled trials. *J Consult Clin Psychol.* 2010;78(6):885-897.
115. Smith JE, Meyers RJ. *Motivating Substance Abusers to Enter Treatment: Working with Family Members.* Guilford Press; 2004.
116. Horigian VE, Feaster DJ, Brincks A, Robbins MS, Perez MA, Szapocznik J. The effects of Brief Strategic Family Therapy (BSFT) on parent substance use and the association between parent and adolescent substance use. *Addict Behav.* 2015;42:44-50.
117. Horigian VE, Feaster DJ, Robbins MS, et al. A cross-sectional assessment of the long term effects of brief strategic family therapy for adolescent substance use. *Am J Addict.* 2015;24(7):637-645.
118. Horigian VE, Anderson AR, Szapocznik J. Family-based treatments for adolescent substance use. *Child Adolesc Psychiatr Clin N Am.* 2016;25(4):603-628.
119. Bickel WK, Amass L, Higgins ST, Badger GJ, Esch RA. Effects of adding behavioral treatment to opioid detoxification with buprenorphine. *J Consult Clin Psychol.* 1997;65(5):803-810.
120. Carroll KM, Kosten TR, Rounsaville BJ. Choosing a behavioral therapy platform for pharmacotherapy of substance users. *Drug Alcohol Depend.* 2004;75(2):123-134.
121. Bates ME, Bowden SC, Barry D. Neurocognitive impairment associated with alcohol use disorders: implications for treatment. *Exp Clin Psychopharmacol.* 2002;10:193-212.
122. Aharonovich E, Nunes E, Hasin D. Cognitive impairment, retention and abstinence among cocaine abusers in cognitive-behavioral treatment. *Drug Alcohol Depend.* 2003;71:207-211.
123. Levin FR, Mariani JJ, Specker S, et al. Extended-release mixed amphetamine salts vs placebo for comorbid adult attention-deficit/hyperactivity disorder and cocaine use disorder: a randomized clinical trial. *JAMA Psychiat.* 2015;72(6):593-602.
124. Benavides-Viello S, Strode A, Sherrran BC. Using technology in the delivery of mental health and substance abuse treatment in rural communities: a review. *J Behav Health Serv Res.* 2013;40(1):111-120.
125. Frueh BC, Henderson S, Myrick H. Telehealth service delivery for persons with alcoholism. *J Telemed Telecare.* 2005;11(7):372-375.
126. Fernandez S, Ferigolo M, Benchaya MC, et al. Brief motivational intervention and telemedicine: a new perspective of treatment to marijuana users. *Addict Behav.* 2010;35(8):750-755.
127. Carroll KM, Kiluk BD, Nich C, et al. Computer-assisted delivery of cognitive-behavioral therapy: efficacy and durability of CBT4CBT among cocaine-dependent individuals maintained on methadone. *Am J Psychiatry.* 2014;171(4):436-444.
128. Bickel WK, Marsch LA, Buchhalter AR, Badger GJ. Computerized behavior therapy for opioid-dependent outpatients: a randomized controlled trial. *Exp Clin Psychopharmacol.* 2008;16(2):132-143.
129. Whittaker R, McRobbie H, Bullen C, Rodgers A, Gu Y. Mobile phone-based interventions for smoking cessation. *Cochrane Database Syst Rev.* 2016;4:CD006611.
130. Hammond AS, Sweeney MM, Chikosi TU, Stitzer ML. Digital delivery of a contingency management intervention for substance use disorder: a feasibility study with DynamiCare Health. *J Subst Abuse Treat.* 2021;126:108425.
131. Kiluk BD, Sugarman DE, Nich C, et al. A methodological analysis of randomized clinical trials of computer-assisted therapies for psychiatric disorders: toward improved standards for an emerging field. *Am J Psychiatry.* 2011;168(8):790-799.
132. Institute of Medicine of the National Academies. *Statement on Quality of Care: National Roundtable on Health Care Quality—The Urgent Need to Improve Health Care Quality.* National Academy Press; 1998.
133. Grol R. Improving the quality of medical care: building bridges among professional pride, payer profit, and patient satisfaction. *JAMA.* 2001;286:2578-2585.
134. Grol R, Grimshaw J. From best evidence to best practice: effective implementation of change in patients' care. *Lancet.* 2003;362:1225-1230.
135. Miller WR, Mount KA. A small study of training in motivational interviewing: does one workshop change clinician and client behavior? *Behav Cogn Psychother.* 2001;29:457-471.
136. Moyers TB, Manual JK, Wilson PG, Hendrickson SML, Talcott W, Durand P. A randomized trial investigating training in motivational interviewing for behavioral health providers. *Behav Cogn Psychother.* 2008;36:149-162.
137. Smith JL, Carpenter KM, Amrhein PC, et al. Training substance abuse clinicians in motivational interviewing using live supervision via teleconferencing. *J Consult Clin Psychol.* 2012;80(3):450-464.

CHAPTER

73

Contingency Management and the Community Reinforcement Approach

Sarah H. Heil, Tyler G. Erath, Roxanne F. Harfmann, and Stephen T. Higgins

CHAPTER OUTLINE

- Historical perspective
- Treatment model
- Treatment planning
- Pretreatment issues
- Treatment and technique
- Empirical support
- Conclusions

Contingency-management (CM) interventions and community reinforcement approach (CRA) therapy for treating substance use disorders (SUDs) are based in the conceptual framework of learning and conditioning theory. Especially fundamental to these treatment approaches is operant conditioning, which is the study of how systematically applied environmental consequences increase (ie, reinforce) or decrease (ie, punish) the frequency and patterning of voluntary behavior.[1] The approaches are also informed by the disciplines of behavioral pharmacology regarding the fundamental role of the reinforcing effects of substances in promoting SUDs and behavioral economics regarding the potential role of systematic biases in how humans make choices in complex environments and how they may increase the likelihood of SUDs and other health problems.[2]

In this chapter, we describe how SUDs are conceptualized within such a theoretical framework, describe the treatments, and review controlled studies on the efficacy of CM and CRA in the treatment of SUDs. These interventions have been researched most extensively with regard to treating alcohol, cocaine, and opioid use disorder, each of which is addressed in this chapter. Over time, CM and CRA have been extended to other forms of SUDs and to special populations.[2,3] These and other advances are reviewed as well. The review is restricted to controlled studies published in peer-reviewed journals unless otherwise noted.

HISTORICAL PERSPECTIVE

Studying and conceptualizing SUDs within an operant conditioning framework began in earnest in the 1960s and early 1970s.[4] Convergent evidence from studies conducted with laboratory animals residing in highly controlled experimental chambers, humans with SUDs residing in medically supervised hospital settings, and humans seeking treatment for SUDs demonstrated the operant nature of drug use. In the studies with laboratory animals, for example, subjects fitted with intravenous catheters readily learned arbitrary behavioral responses such as pressing a lever or pulling a chain when the only consequence for doing so was the delivery of an injection of a drug that can promote unhealthy use (eg, morphine or cocaine). Effects were pharmacologically specific in that injections of drugs that humans rarely use in unhealthy ways (eg, chlorpromazine) or saline failed to generate or maintain responding. In some instances, the reinforcing effects of drugs like morphine and cocaine were so robust that they promoted in these laboratory animals the dangerous extremes in consumption characteristic of humans with SUDs. Monkeys given unconstrained opportunities to self-administer intravenous cocaine, for example, would consume the drug to the exclusion of basic sustenance, and barring experimenter intervention, to the point of death.[5] Substitute saline for the cocaine and the animals would readily discontinue giving themselves injections (ie, responding extinguished). A robust body of evidence demonstrated that the drugs that humans commonly use in an unhealthy manner function as unconditioned positive reinforcers much as food, water, and sex do.[4]

The residential studies of humans with SUDs often examined the sensitivity of drug use to systematically administered environmental consequences. An elegant series of studies demonstrated the operant nature of alcohol use among those with severe alcohol use disorders.[6] In this programmatic series of studies, participants resided on an inpatient unit where they were permitted to purchase and consume alcoholic drinks. Abstinence from voluntary drinking increased when (1) access to an alternative reinforcer (enriched environment) was made available contingent on doing so, (2) monetary reinforcement was provided contingent on abstinence from drinking, (3) the amount of work required to obtain drinks was increased, or (4) brief periods of social isolation were imposed contingent upon drinking. The studies provided strong evidence that even among individuals with severe SUDs, drug use was sensitive to environmental consequences.

Initial studies with treatment seekers typically involved small-sample demonstrations that systematically applied consequences could improve treatment outcome. In a controlled case study, for example, breath samples were collected twice weekly on a quasi-random schedule from a male with severe alcohol use disorder.[7] Baseline observations demonstrated a high rate of drinking. During the intervention period, the patient received a $3.00 coupon book contingent on randomly scheduled alcohol-negative breath samples. Coupons could be exchanged for goods at a hospital commissary. After a discernible increase in the rate of negative breath tests during the period of contingent coupon delivery, the contingency was removed, and booklets were delivered independent of breath results. Under that condition, the frequency of negative specimens decreased toward baseline levels. Reimposing the contingency again increased the frequency of alcohol-negative breath results. Around this same time, several studies were reported suggesting that allowing participants to earn back monetary deposits contingent on objective verification of smoking abstinence improved outcomes among those trying to quit cigarette smoking.[8,9] These studies illustrated the clinical implications of the emerging body of evidence supporting the operant nature of SUDs.

Such studies provided the empirical foundation for a conceptual model, wherein drug use is considered a normal, learned behavior that falls along a continuum ranging from little use and few problems to excessive use and many untoward effects.[4,10] The same principles of learning and conditioning are assumed to operate across this continuum. Within this framework, all physically intact humans are considered to possess the necessary neurobiological systems to experience drug-produced reinforcement and hence to develop drug use and SUDs. Genetic or acquired characteristics (eg, family history of alcohol use disorder, other psychiatric disorders) are recognized as factors that affect the probability of developing SUDs but are not deemed to be necessary for the problem to emerge.

TREATMENT MODEL

Within an operant conceptual framework, reinforcement derived from drug use and the associated lifestyle is deemed to have monopolized the behavioral repertoire of the person with addiction. Treatments developed within this framework are designed to reorganize the user's environment to systematically increase the rate of reinforcement obtained while abstinent from drug use and reduce or eliminate the rate of reinforcement obtained through drug use and associated activities. Primary emphasis is placed on decreasing drug use by systematically increasing the availability and frequency of alternative reinforcing activities either through relatively contrived sources of reinforcement as in CM interventions or more naturalistic sources as in CRA therapy.[2,11] Additionally, arranging the environment so that aversive events or the loss of reinforcing events (ie, punishment) occur as a consequence of drug use also can decrease drug use. As with reinforcement, such aversive procedures can involve relatively contrived (eg, forfeiture of a large-value incentive) or more naturalistic (eg, suspension from work) consequences. This distinction between CM and CRA with regard to the former's relying primarily on contrived contingencies and the latter's relying primarily on naturalistic contingencies will become clearer when the treatments are described in greater detail later. By *contrived*, we mean a set of contingencies that are put in place explicitly and exclusively for therapeutic purposes (eg, earning vouchers exchangeable for retail items contingent on cocaine-negative urine toxicology results). By *naturalistic*, we mean a set of contingencies that are already operating in the natural environment for nontherapeutic purposes but can be used to support the therapeutic process (eg, teaching a spouse to deliver praise when a patient avoids bars and to withhold praise or express disapproval for going to bars).

Some treatments, such as the CRA + vouchers treatment for cocaine use disorder,[12,13] are designed to deliver contrived consequences during the initial treatment period, with a transition to more naturalistic sources later in treatment. The rationale for that sequence is that the lifestyle of the patient is often so disrupted upon treatment entry that it is largely devoid of effective alternative sources of reinforcement that can compete with the reinforcement derived from drug use. Contrived sources of alternative reinforcement delivered through CM are designed to promote initial abstinence, thereby allowing time for therapists and patient to work toward reestablishing more naturalistic alternatives (eg, job, stable family life, participation in self-help, and other social groups that reinforce abstinence). Of course, it is these naturalistic alternatives that eventually will need to sustain long-term abstinence once the contrived reinforcers are discontinued.

Also important to recognize is that for any number of reasons, some patients may have behavioral repertoires that are too limited to recruit sufficient sources of naturalistic reinforcement to effectively compete with drug use. As such, these patients will need some form of maintenance treatment involving contrived reinforcement contingencies in order to sustain long-term abstinence, as is widely recognized with individuals with opioid use disorder who often need maintenance pharmacotherapy to sustain long-term abstinence from illicit drug use. Others may need lifelong participation in self-help programs in order to succeed. Such programs might be deemed as falling somewhere around the midpoint on the continuum of contrived versus naturalistic sources of alternative reinforcement.[11] The following discussion illustrates how this general strategy is implemented in CM and CRA interventions.

TREATMENT PLANNING

A thorough patient evaluation is an essential first step in effective clinical management of SUDs and that certainly holds true when using CM and CRA interventions. The assessment framework used in the CRA + vouchers treatment for cocaine use disorder[13] is relatively generic and can be readily applied to other types of SUDs by substituting information specific to cocaine use with pertinent information on whatever other type of SUD is the presenting problem.

Every effort is made to schedule an intake assessment interview as soon as possible after initial patient contact with the clinic. Scheduling the interview within 24 hours of clinic contact significantly reduces attrition between the initial clinic contact and assessment interview, which is a substantial problem among those with SUDs.[14] Some patients cannot come into the clinic within 24 hours, so secondary plans are made to get them in as soon as is practicable.

TABLE 73-1 Instruments Used in an Intake Assessment to Obtain Detailed Information From Patients With Cocaine Use Disorder

Instrument	Comments
Brief demographics questionnaire	Locally developed instrument that collects information such as current address and phone number, as well as the number of someone who will always know the client's whereabouts, which are important for during-treatment outreach efforts should the client stop coming to scheduled therapy sessions or need to be contacted for other reasons.
Stages of Change Readiness and Treatment Eagerness Scale (SOCRATES)[15]	Provides information on clients' perception of the severity of their drug use problems and their readiness to engage in behavior to reduce their use. Versions of the SOCRATES that refer to specific substances (eg, cocaine, alcohol, and other drug use) can be used, as the patient's motivation to reduce substance use is often drug-specific.
Adapted cocaine dependency self-test[16]	Collects information on the type of adverse effects from cocaine use that patients have experienced, which can be useful in helping patients problem solve regarding the pros and cons of cocaine use as part of efforts to promote and sustain motivation for change during the course of treatment.
Michigan Alcoholism Screening Test (MAST)[17]	Brief alcoholism screening instrument.
Beck Depression Inventory (BDI)[18]	Screens for depressive symptoms.
Symptom Checklist-90-Revised (SCL-90-R)[19]	Screens for psychiatric symptoms more broadly and is helpful in determining whether a more in-depth psychiatric evaluation is warranted.
Semistructured drug history interview	Locally developed instrument that collects information on current and past substance use, including detailed information regarding the duration, severity, and pattern of the patient's drug use, with recent use assessed using the timeline follow-back technique.[20]
Addiction Severity Index (ASI)[21]	Quantitative, time-based assessment of problem severity in the following areas: alcohol use, drug use, and employment, medical, legal, family, social, and psychological functioning.
Practical needs assessment questionnaire	Locally developed instrument that determines whether the patient has any pressing needs or crises that may interfere with initial treatment engagement (eg, housing, legal, transportation, or childcare).

Detailed information is collected on drug use, treatment readiness, psychiatric functioning, employment/vocational status, recreational interests, current social supports, family and social problems, and legal issues. **Table 73-1** is a list of instruments[15-21] that can be used to obtain such information, listed in the order in which they are typically administered. If it appears that a medication is indicated, the first steps are taken after the initial intake assessment toward implementing the relevant medical protocols. With the cocaine use disorder population, a regimen of clinic-monitored disulfiram therapy can be used to address problem drinking, which also reduces cocaine use.[22] As the prevalence of opioid use has grown, clinic-monitored naltrexone therapy may be increasingly indicated.

PRETREATMENT ISSUES

Motivation

Within an operant framework, motivation is not thought of as a characteristic of the patient per se but rather as a product of current and past reinforcement contingencies tempered by potential individual differences in delay discounting, educational attainment, and other matters that may influence behavioral choice.[2,10] The overarching focus of the interventions is to directly ensure the availability of sufficient reinforcement to promote and sustain therapeutic change. Following, we discuss how that is accomplished.

Rationale for Choice of Treatment

The historical and conceptual background information described previously provides the overarching rationale for the use of CM and CRA interventions. CM and CRA have the potential to be useful with virtually any type of SUD. There is no minimal or maximal intensity or duration of CM or CRA, and thus there is a great deal of flexibility in terms of adapting them to particular forms of SUDs and special populations.

Selection and Preparation of Patients

As noted, we know of no particular type of SUD patient for whom CM or CRA is contraindicated. Both interventions require a detailed and careful patient orientation. With CM, it is quite common to have patients sign a written contract stipulating all aspects of the CM arrangement so as to avoid any confusion about the contingencies. Brief tests (eg, a true/false quiz) are also commonly administered to ensure that patients understand the contingencies. The vocabulary and other information contained in the contract and tests should be prepared with the potential intellectual limitations of the patient population in mind and plans to surmount potential individual difficulties. For example, reading problems are common among patients with SUDs, and certain patients may need to have written materials read aloud to them.

Therapist Characteristics

Therapists typically do not manage CM programs owing to the detailed record keeping involved and the need to biochemically verify abstinence, though there are exceptions. Thus, this section largely pertains to characteristics of CRA therapists. CRA is a manual based intervention, which minimizes the influence of therapist characteristics on outcome. In the series of studies examining CRA + vouchers treatment of cocaine use disorder, for example, there have not been any significant therapist effects on outcome noted.

To implement CRA effectively, therapists need to be directive but also flexible, which we believe facilitates treatment retention and progress toward achieving treatment goals. Particularly in the early stages of treatment, therapists try to work around patient schedules and generally make participation in treatment convenient to the patient. Therapists try to be flexible with regard to tardiness to sessions, early departure from sessions, and the time of day that sessions are scheduled and will meet with patients outside the office if necessary. With especially difficult patients, improvements in these areas can be worked on as part of the treatment plan. CRA therapists must exhibit appropriate empathy and good listening skills. They need to convey a sincere understanding of the patient's situation and its inherent difficulties. Throughout treatment, therapists avoid making value judgments and, instead, exhibit genuine empathy and consideration for the difficult challenges that patients face.

CRA requires that therapists and patients develop an active, make-it-happen attitude throughout treatment. Therapists must have good organizational skills, which are important to developing, implementing, monitoring, and adapting treatment plans. Problem-solving skills also are important. Within ethical boundaries, therapists must be committed to doing what it takes to facilitate lifestyle changes on the part of patients. For example, therapists often accompany patients to appointments or job interviews. They initiate recreational activities with patients and schedule sessions at different times of day to accomplish specific goals. They have patients make phone calls from their office. They search newspapers and online postings for job possibilities or ideas for healthy recreational activities in which patients might be able to participate. Without question, the amount of direct support that CRA therapists provide to patients can represent a rather significant departure from more traditional forms of SUD counseling. However, in CRA, these therapeutic efforts are deemed to be very important for at least three reasons. First, while patients may have the aptitude, they may simply lack certain skills to accomplish important tasks (eg, effective job searching). Second, early in treatment, patients may lack the requisite reinforcement history (ie, motivation) with certain healthy activities (eg, attending the local YMCA) to carry through on assigned tasks in the absence of the therapist being present to prompt the response and provide social reinforcement for completing the task. Third, patients may lack the necessary material resources (eg, transportation or materials for résumé preparation) to complete a task in a timely manner. CRA therapists are committed to overcoming such deficiencies in skills, motivation, or resources to facilitate patient movement in the direction of a healthier, non-drug-using lifestyle.

TREATMENT AND TECHNIQUE

In this section, the basic elements of CM and CRA interventions are described using the CRA + vouchers treatment for cocaine use disorder for illustration purposes.

Contingency Management

The efficacy of CM interventions is very much dependent on how they are structured and implemented. A brief description of a voucher-based CM intervention is described below, followed by an outline of 10 features of CM interventions that are important to their efficacy.[23]

In the voucher-based CM program, patients sign a written contract stipulating all aspects of the CM interventions. Vouchers exchangeable for retail items are earned contingent on cocaine-negative results in thrice-weekly urine toxicology testing (Monday, Wednesday, and Friday). The program is 12 weeks in duration. The first cocaine-negative specimen earns a voucher worth $2.50 in purchasing power. The value of each subsequent consecutive cocaine-negative specimen increases by $1.25. The equivalent of a $10 bonus is provided for every three consecutive cocaine-negative specimens. The intent of the escalating magnitude of reinforcement and bonuses is to reinforce continuous cocaine abstinence. A cocaine-positive specimen or failure to submit a scheduled specimen resets the value of vouchers back to the initial $2.50 value. This reset feature is designed to punish relapse to cocaine use after a period of sustained abstinence, with the intensity of the punishment tied directly to the length of sustained abstinence that would be broken. In order to provide patients with a reason to continue abstaining from drug use after a reset, submission of five consecutive cocaine-negative specimens after a cocaine-positive specimen returns the value to where it was prior to the reset. Vouchers cannot be lost once earned. If someone is continuously abstinent throughout the 12-week intervention, total earnings would be $997.50. However, because most patients are unable to sustain abstinence throughout the intervention, the average earned is usually about half that maximal amount.

The voucher CM intervention contains most of the 10 features important to effective CM. First, as was noted, the details of the intervention are carefully explained to patients in the form of a written contract prior to beginning treatment. Second, the response being targeted by the CM intervention—cocaine abstinence—is defined in objective terms (cocaine-negative urine toxicology results). Third, the methods for verifying that the target response occurred are well specified and objective (urine toxicology testing). Fourth, the schedule for monitoring progress is well specified (each Monday, Wednesday, and Friday). Fifth, the schedule is designed to include frequent opportunities for patients to experience the programmed consequences (thrice weekly). Sixth, the duration of the intervention is stipulated in advance (12 weeks). Seventh, the intervention is focused on a single target (cocaine abstinence). CM interventions that focus on a single target tend to produce larger treatment effects on average than those that try to modify multiple targets (eg, abstinence from multiple substances).[24] Eighth, the consequences that will follow success and failure to emit the target response are clear (carefully detailed voucher reinforcement schedule). Ninth, there is minimal delay in delivering designated consequences (urine specimens are analyzed on-site, and the vouchers earned are delivered immediately after testing). Delivering the consequence on the same day that occurrence of the target response is verified produces larger treatment effects than delivering the consequence at a later time.[24] Tenth, the magnitude of reinforcement that can be earned is relatively substantial (maximal total earnings = $997.50). Larger value incentives produce larger treatment effects on average.[24]

Community Reinforcement Approach

The CRA component of the CRA + vouchers treatment is implemented in twice weekly 1-hour counseling sessions for 12 weeks and then once weekly during the subsequent 12 weeks. It has seven elements. First, patients are instructed in how to recognize antecedents and consequences of their cocaine use; that is, how to functionally analyze their cocaine use. They are also instructed in how to use that information to reduce the probability of using cocaine. A twofold message is conveyed to the patient: (1) his/her cocaine use is orderly behavior that is more likely to occur under certain circumstances than others, and (2) by learning to identify the circumstances that affect one's cocaine use, plans can be developed and implemented to reduce the likelihood of future cocaine use. In conjunction with functional analysis, patients are taught self-management plans for using the information revealed in the functional analyses to decrease the chances of future cocaine use. Patients are counseled to restructure their daily activities in order to minimize contact with known antecedents of cocaine use, to find alternatives to the positive consequences of cocaine use, and to make explicit the negative consequences of cocaine use.

Second, developing a new social network that will support a healthier lifestyle and getting involved with recreational activities that are enjoyable and do not involve cocaine or other drug use is addressed with all patients. Systematically developing and maintaining contacts with "safe" social networks and participation in "safe" recreational activities remains a high priority throughout treatment for the vast majority of patients. Specific treatment goals are set, and weekly progress on specific goals is monitored. Clearly, plans for developing healthy social networks and recreational activities must be individualized depending on the circumstances, skills and interests of the patient. For those patients who are willing to participate, self-help groups (Alcoholics or Narcotics Anonymous) can be an effective way to develop a new network of associates who will support a sober lifestyle.

Third, various other forms of individualized skills training are provided, usually to address some specific skill deficit that may directly or indirectly influence a patient's risk for cocaine use (eg, time management, problem solving, assertiveness training, social skills training, and mood management). For example, essential to success with the self-management skills and social/recreational goals discussed is some level of time-management skills. As another example, protocols on controlling depression are implemented with those patients whose depression continues after discontinuing cocaine use.[25,26]

Fourth, unemployed patients are offered Job Club, which is an efficacious method for assisting chronically unemployed individuals obtain employment.[27] The majority of patients who seek treatment for cocaine use disorder are unemployed, so this is a service that can be offered to many patients. For others, assistance is provided in pursuing educational goals or new career paths.

Fifth, patients with romantic partners who do not engage in unhealthy drug use are offered behavioral couples therapy, which is an intervention designed to teach couples positive communication skills and how to negotiate reciprocal contracts for desired changes in each other's behavior.[28] Relationship counseling tends to be delivered across eight sessions, with the first four sessions taking place across consecutive weeks and the next four delivered on alternating weeks.

Sixth, human immunodeficiency virus/acquired immunodeficiency syndrome (HIV/AIDS) and hepatitis C virus (HCV) education is provided to all clients in the early stages of treatment, along with counseling directed at addressing any specific needs or risk behavior of the individual patient.[29] The potential for acquiring HIV/AIDS and HCV from sharing injection equipment and through sexual activity is addressed with all patients. This involves at least two sessions. First, patients complete an HIV/AIDS and HCV knowledge test. They next watch and discuss a video on HIV/AIDS with their therapist. Patients are also provided HIV/AIDS and HCV prevention pamphlets and free condoms if desired. The HIV/AIDS and HCV knowledge test is repeated and any remaining errors discussed and resolved. Last, patients are given information about testing for HIV and hepatitis B and C and are encouraged to get tested. Those interested in being tested are assisted in scheduling an appointment to do so.

Seventh, as noted previously, all who meet diagnostic criteria for alcohol use disorder or report that alcohol use is involved in their use of cocaine are offered disulfiram therapy, which is an integral part of the CRA treatment for alcohol use disorder.[30] Patients generally ingest a 250-mg daily dose under clinic staff observation on urinalysis test days and, when possible, under the observation of a significant other (SO) on the other days. Disulfiram therapy is only effective when implemented with procedures to monitor compliance with the recommended dosing regimen. Having an SO monitor compliance on nonclinic days can work well if an appropriate person is available to do so at the frequency needed. When that is not possible, clients can ingest a larger dose (500 mg) on days when they report to the clinic and skip dosing on the intervening days.

Use of other substances is also discouraged in CRA therapy. Anyone who meets criteria for physical dependence on opioids is referred for methadone or buprenorphine therapy. Cannabis abstinence is recommended because of problems associated with its use and because the literature is mixed on whether the use of cannabis interferes with achieving abstinence from other drugs. Abstinence from nicotine/tobacco use is also recommended and there is evidence suggesting that nicotine/tobacco treatment can be successfully integrated into simultaneous treatment for other SUDs and may improve treatment outcomes for those other substances.[31] As important, patients are never dismissed or refused treatment owing to other drug use.

Upon completion of the 24 weeks of treatment, patients are encouraged to participate in 6 months of aftercare, which involves at least once-monthly brief therapy sessions and urine toxicology screening. More frequent clinic contact is recommended if the therapist or patients deem it necessary.

EMPIRICAL SUPPORT

Community Reinforcement Approach + Vouchers

A major reason why this intervention garnered significant interest was its efficacy with cocaine use disorder. At a time when most clinical trials investigating treatments for cocaine use disorder were consistently producing negative outcomes, a series of controlled trials examining this intervention produced reliably positive outcomes.[12,32-37]

The initial two trials involved comparisons of this combined treatment to standard outpatient SUD counseling.[12,32] The first trial was 12 weeks in duration, and 28 outpatients with cocaine use disorder were assigned as consecutive admissions to their respective treatment conditions.[12] The second trial was 24 weeks in duration, and 38 patients with cocaine use disorder were randomly assigned to the same two treatment conditions.[32] Outcomes in both trials were significantly better among those treated with the CRA + voucher treatment than standard SUD counseling. In the randomized trial, for example, 58% of patients assigned to CRA + vouchers completed the recommended 24 weeks of treatment compared to 11% of those assigned to SUD counseling. Regarding cocaine use, 68% of those assigned to CRA + vouchers were objectively verified to have achieved 8 or more weeks of continuous cocaine abstinence as compared to only 11% of those treated with SUD counseling.

Other trials examined the CRA + vouchers treatment with other SUDs, using different modalities, and in other settings. One trial tested whether the CRA + vouchers treatment could improve what are usually poor outcomes with opioid withdrawal.[38] Those assigned to CRA + vouchers were more likely to complete a buprenorphine dose taper protocol and achieved greater periods of biochemically confirmed abstinence from illicit opioid use. A number of later trials have examined a version of this intervention, wherein CRA was delivered primarily via an interactive, computer-based program known as the Therapeutic Education System.[39-41] In the seminal study, retention was comparable but biochemically confirmed abstinence from opioids and cocaine was significantly higher among patients receiving buprenorphine assigned to therapist-delivered CRA + voucher and computer-assisted CRA + vouchers as compared to standard counseling, with no differences between therapist-delivered and computer-assisted CRA conditions.[39] A randomized controlled trial with cocaine use disorder patients conducted in Spain using CRA plus a variation of the voucher intervention reported positive improvements in retention and cocaine abstinence as compared to standard care during 6 months of treatment, with effects on cocaine remaining discernible through 6 months of posttreatment follow-up.[42,43] Together, these trials help demonstrate the generality of the CRA + vouchers intervention across drug classes, modalities, and to communities outside the United States.

Additional trials dismantled the CRA + vouchers intervention to examine the contribution of each component. A randomized trial designed to isolate the contribution of voucher-based CM was conducted with 40 outpatients with cocaine use disorder who were assigned to receive CRA with or without vouchers.[33] Average (± standard error of the mean) duration of continuous cocaine abstinence across 24 weeks of treatment in the two groups was 11.7 ± 2.0 weeks in the voucher group versus 6.0 ± 1.5 weeks in the no-voucher group (**Fig. 73-1**) and a separate report documented continued differences between conditions posttreatment.[34] Subsequent trials testing specific parameters of the voucher part of the intervention also demonstrated the importance of the contingency[35] and of voucher magnitude.[36]

Another randomized clinical trial was conducted to isolate the contributions of CRA.[37] One hundred outpatients with cocaine use disorder were randomly assigned to receive the CRA + vouchers treatment or the vouchers component only. Vouchers were in place for 12 weeks, CRA for 24 weeks, and patients were assessed at least every 3 months for 2 years after treatment entry. Patients treated with CRA + vouchers were better retained in treatment, used cocaine at a lower frequency during treatment but not follow-up, and reported a lower frequency of drinking to intoxication during treatment and follow-up as compared with patients treated with vouchers only. Patients treated with CRA + vouchers also reported a higher frequency of days of paid employment during treatment and 6 months of posttreatment follow-up, decreased depressive symptoms during treatment only, and fewer hospitalizations and legal problems during follow-up. The results provided a strong case that CRA contributed in numerous ways to the positive outcomes observed during treatment and posttreatment follow-up with the CRA + vouchers treatment.

Contingency Management Interventions

Initial Contingency Management Studies

Up to this point in the chapter, the emphasis has been on the combination treatment of CRA + vouchers, but voucher-based CM as a standalone treatment for SUDs has received a lot of

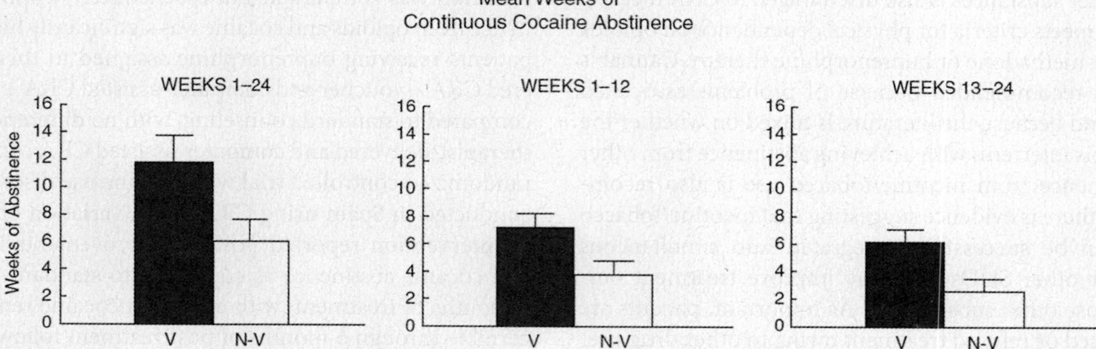

Figure 73-1. Mean durations of continuous cocaine abstinence. Mean durations of continuous cocaine abstinence documented via urinalysis testing in each treatment group during weeks 1-24, 1-12, and 13-24 of treatment. V and N-V indicate the voucher and no-voucher groups, respectively. Error bars represent + standard error of the mean. (Reproduced with permission from Higgins ST, Budney AJ, Bickel WK, et al. Incentives improve outcome in outpatient behavioral treatment of cocaine dependence. *Arch Gen Psychiatry.* 1994;51:568-576. Copyright © 1994. American Medical Association. All rights reserved.)

scientific attention. One of the first studies in this area tested the efficacy of voucher-based incentives to promote cocaine abstinence among 37 patients receiving methadone to treat opioid use disorder.[44] Though medications for opioid use disorder like methadone and buprenorphine are effective at eliminating the use of illicit opioids, a subset of patients continues using other nonopioid drugs. During the 12-week study, subjects in the experimental group received vouchers exchangeable for retail items contingent on cocaine-negative urinalysis tests. A matched control group received the vouchers independent of urinalysis results. Both groups received a standard form of outpatient SUD counseling. Cocaine use was substantially reduced in the experimental group but remained relatively unchanged in the control group (**Fig. 73-2**). Use of opioids also decreased during the voucher period in the contingent compared to the noncontingent conditions even though the contingency was exclusively on cocaine use. This was the first study to demonstrate the efficacy of voucher-based incentives to promote cocaine abstinence among people living in urban areas, as all prior trials conducted with voucher-based incentives (usually combined with CRA) took place in a clinic located in relatively rural Vermont.[12,32-37] Later randomized trials further demonstrated the efficacy of this approach in decreasing cocaine use among people living in urban areas.[45-47]

The significance and importance of this work has become more apparent in recent years as psychomotor stimulant use among people with opioid use disorder increased dramatically. For example, methamphetamine use among people entering treatment for opioid use disorder in the United States increased 85% between 2011 and 2018.[48] There is concern that this surge in use could undermine the considerable progress made in curtailing the current opioid crisis using medications for opioid use disorder. Our group recently completed a systematic review and meta-analysis of the effects of contingency management on stimulant use, as well as polysubstance use, illicit opioid use, tobacco cigarette smoking, therapy attendance, and medication adherence, among people receiving medications for opioid use disorder.[49] Seventy-four reports involving more than 10,000 patients published between 1984 and 2019 met inclusion criteria for narrative review; 60 of these reports involving 7,000 patients were included in meta-analyses. Twenty-two studies tested the efficacy of contingency management for increasing abstinence from psychomotor stimulant use, with 18 (82%) reporting significant increases in abstinence at end-of-treatment assessment. Participants were treated with methadone in all but 1 study. The mean (SD) contingency

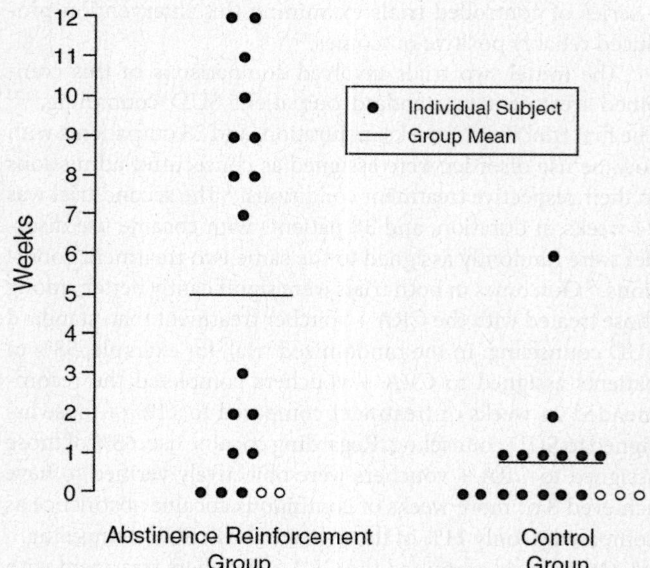

Figure 73-2. Longest duration of sustained cocaine abstinence. Longest duration of sustained cocaine abstinence achieved during the 12-week voucher condition. Each data point indicates data from an individual subject and the lines represent group means. Subjects in the reinforcement and control conditions are displayed in the left and right columns, respectively. *Open circles* represent early study drop outs. (Reproduced with permission from Silverman K, Higgins ST, Brooner RK, et al. Sustained cocaine abstinence in methadone maintenance patients through voucher-based reinforcement therapy. *Arch Gen Psychiatry.* 1996;53:409-415. Copyright © 1996. American Medical Association. All rights reserved.)

management duration was 17.2 (13.8) weeks, and the mean (SD) maximum daily earnings was $14.51 ($11.94). There was sufficient information to calculate effect sizes for 18 of 22 studies and contingency management was associated with an overall medium-large effect size on psychomotor stimulant abstinence compared with controls at the end-of-treatment assessment. Medium-large mean effect sizes were also observed for cigarette use, illicit opioid use, and medication adherence, while small-medium mean effect sizes were evident for polysubstance use and therapy attendance. Collapsing across abstinence and adherence categories, contingency management was associated with medium effect sizes for abstinence and treatment adherence compared with controls.

Growth of the Contingency Management Literature

The large number of studies included in the review in the prior section is illustrative of the tremendous interest in CM over the years. A PubMed search of contingency management and SUDs today returns more than 900 publications, nearly double the number since the last edition of this chapter. The large literature has made robust systematic reviews and meta-analyses possible, which have made plain the efficacy of this treatment approach and furthered our understanding of it. For example, our group conducted the first meta-analysis of the voucher-based CM literature comprising 40 controlled studies published in peer-reviewed journals from January 1991 (when the voucher model was introduced) to March 2004 (13.25 years).[24] There was overwhelming evidence of the efficacy of this treatment approach for increasing abstinence from drug use and retention in treatment across a wide range of different types of SUDs, with overall effect sizes in the moderate range. The review also examined potential moderators of treatment efficacy. Of seven moderators tested, two were significant: incentive magnitude and delay in delivering incentives, with higher magnitudes and shorter delays both increasing effect size.

In the last edition of this chapter, we highlighted efforts in this sizeable literature to extend CM to special populations, to investigate longer-term outcomes, and to integrate CM into community clinics because we believed these topics were especially important to the further development of this approach in research and clinical settings. In the next sections, we revisit these three important areas.

Extending Contingency Management to Special Populations

Special populations continue to be an area where CM has a niche, perhaps because CM has been demonstrated to be among the most effective treatments at promoting abstinence in these populations. One of the best examples of this is the use of voucher-based reinforcement of abstinence among pregnant cigarette smokers. The last two Cochrane reviews focused on incentives for smoking have included pregnant people. The most recent, published in 2019, included seven trials, all published since 2000.[50] The review supported the efficacy of incentives based on biochemically-verified abstinence in late pregnancy and the longest follow-up outcomes reported, which was 24 weeks postpartum in the majority of trials. Overall, late-pregnancy outcomes were based on 1,244 women (645 treated with incentives and 599 without incentives). Those treated with incentives had 2.79 (95% CI: 2.10-3.72) greater odds of abstaining from smoking than controls. With regard to longest follow-up outcomes reported, those treated with incentives had 2.38 (95% CI: 1.54-3.69) greater odds of abstaining from smoking than controls. This has been a dramatic advance given that efforts to develop efficacious nicotine/tobacco treatment interventions for this population have been ongoing since the mid 1980s, with little to show for it.

One of the efficacy trials in the Cochrane review[51] also provided data for the first econometric analysis of this approach, showing financial incentives to be highly cost effective.[52] Cost effectiveness is an area where CM and other treatment development research for SUDs has historically been lacking, and in the previous edition of this chapter, we called for more work in this area. Subsequently, our group conducted our fifth and most recent randomized trial of financial incentives for tobacco/nicotine abstinence during pregnancy and postpartum, including assessment of economic impacts.[53,54] One hundred and sixty-nine women who smoked were assigned to best practices only (BP) or BP plus financial incentives (BP+FI) for smoking abstinence; incentives remained available through 12 weeks postpartum. A third condition included 80 who never smoked (NS) sociodemographically-matched to women who smoked. Outcomes included 7-day point-prevalence abstinence assessed antepartum through 1 year postpartum, birth and other infant outcomes during first year of life, as well as economic impacts. Reliability and external validity of trial results were also assessed using pooled results from the current and the four prior controlled trials coupled with data on maternal-smoking status and birth outcomes for all 2019 singleton live births in the state of Vermont. Compared to BP, BP+FI significantly increased abstinence in early and late pregnancy and through 12 weeks postpartum although not 24 or 48 weeks postpartum (Fig. 73-3). There was a significant effect of trial condition on small for gestational age (SGA) deliveries, with percent SGA deliveries greatest in BP, intermediate in BP+FI, and lowest in NS. Reliability analyses supported the efficacy of financial incentives for increasing abstinence antepartum and postpartum and decreasing SGA deliveries; external-validity analyses supported relationships between antepartum abstinence and decreased SGA risk. Each dollar invested in BP+FI versus BP yielded an estimated $12.00 in economic benefits, demonstrating clear cost-effectiveness from a societal perspective.

Our group has also completed two trials testing the efficacy of using a smartphone-based app to deliver financial incentives for stopping smoking during pregnancy. The first technology-based CM intervention was developed nearly 20 years ago and relied on laptop computers with Internet connectivity.[55] Since then, there have been many advances in technology-based CM, including improvements in information processing that

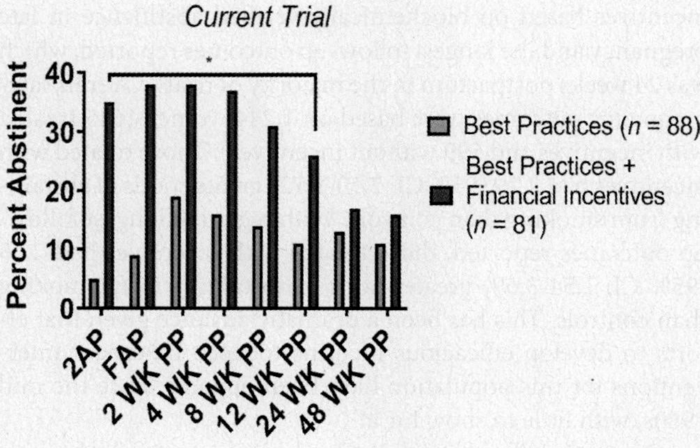

Figure 73-3. Seven-day point-prevalence smoking abstinence. Percent of participants documented smoking abstinent via urinalysis testing in each treatment group at each assessment. *Shaded* and *solid bars* indicate the Best Practices and Best Practices + Financial Incentives conditions, respectively. *Error bars* represent + standard error of the mean. *Asterisks* represent assessments where abstinence was significantly greater in Best Practices + Financial Incentives compared to Best Practices. (Reprinted from Higgins ST, Nighbor TD, Kurti AN, et al. Randomized controlled trial examining the efficacy of adding financial incentives to best practices for smoking cessation among pregnant and newly postpartum women. *Prev Med.* 2022;165:107012. Copyright 2022, with permission from Elsevier.)

have extended the reach of CM nationwide; advances in sensor technology that make it possible to detect drug use with mobile phones; and software upgrades that mean all aspects of technology-based CM (ie, monitoring, reinforcer delivery, user authentication) can now be automated.[56] We took advantage of many of these advances in our first study of this intervention delivered using a smartphone app.[57] Sixty pregnant women who smoke were recruited from more than 30 states, primarily via Facebook. Participants were assigned to one of two treatments. One group received BP treatment. The other received BP+FI delivered via an app. More specifically, participants submitted videos of themselves conducing breath carbon monoxide and salivary cotinine tests using the app. When these samples indicated that they had not been smoking, money was added to a debit card given to participants by the study. Participants could earn incentives throughout pregnancy and for the first 12 weeks postpartum.

Consistent with prior clinic-based studies, participants receiving BP+FI had nearly three times greater odds of abstaining from smoking than the BP condition at a late-pregnancy assessment. Higher rates of abstinence were maintained well into the postpartum period, although differences between groups declined around the time the incentives ended. These results were subsequently replicated with 90 pregnant women recruited from 33 states.[58] In addition, two randomized feasibility studies using a similar app have shown promise for reducing nicotine vaping among young adults[59] and decreasing alcohol use among adults with moderate or severe alcohol use disorder.[60]

Investigating Longer-Term Outcomes of Contingency Management

From early in the development of the voucher-based CM approach to the treatment of cocaine use disorder, there has been interest in longer-term outcomes. While treatment effects often decrease once any type of treatment ends, the durability of CM's effects has been questioned more than many other approaches and in the previous edition of this chapter, we called for more to be done to rigorously assess longer-term outcomes. A recent meta-analysis assessed for the first time the long-term efficacy of CM for stimulant, opioid, or polysubstance abstinence based on urine toxicology testing up to a year after the CM intervention ended.[61] Twenty-three reports involving more than 3,000 patients published between 1997 and 2015 met inclusion criteria for the meta-analysis. The mean (SD) contingency management duration was 14.5 (8.9) weeks, and the mean maximum magnitude of reinforcement was $914.46. Participants who received CM had a 22% greater likelihood of abstinence at a median of 24 weeks after treatment ended than participants receiving comparison treatments (OR = 1.2, 95% CI 1.01-1.44), a number of which were robust, high intensity treatments, including specific protocol-based evidence-based treatments (eg, cognitive-behavioral therapy), and intensive outpatient treatment. Eighteen moderators were tested, including age, race, gender, length of follow-up, substance(s) used, and whether participants were receiving medication for opioid use disorder. The only significant factor was treatment duration, with longer treatment duration associated with better long-term outcomes.

Extending Contingency Management Into the Community

Although decades of research have demonstrated the effectiveness of CM for a myriad of substance use disorders, its implementation in real-world settings has been limited to date. Two major exceptions to this were the adoption of CM as an intensive outpatient treatment for illicit SUDs by the United Kingdom's National Institute for Health and Care Excellence in 2007[62] and an initiative within the U.S. Veterans Health Administration that started in 2011. The VA initiative aimed primarily at veterans with stimulant use disorders and provided funds for CM costs and regional training for their providers. From 2011 to 2014, more than 200 providers from 129 programs were trained in CM. Training workshops were designed to provide background knowledge about CM, address barriers to CM, provide education about how to design CM protocols that adhere to efficacious parameters, and role play CM delivery.[63,64] Abstinence-based CM targeting a single drug (cocaine or methamphetamine, depending on regional prevalence) or single drug class (eg, all stimulants) was emphasized, though attendance and other behavioral targets were discussed. A "standard" protocol was offered, which reinforced stimulant abstinence using prize CM, a variation of voucher-based CM that is typically arranged in such a way that average incentive earnings are lower than in many of the voucher-based CM interventions described earlier in this chapter and therefore typically produces proportionally less abstinence. Providers also engaged with CM experts pre- and postimplementation on coaching calls that aimed to prevent protocol deviations from research-based parameters that might undermine CM's efficacy. By the end of 2018, 126 (98%) of programs had implemented CM, with 107 targeting abstinence and 19 targeting attendance. An average of two clinicians (range = 1-9) per program were delivering CM to a median of 17 clients (range = 1-136 patients). These clients attended a median 14 sessions and submitted 95% negative samples.[65]

More recently, a number of states in the United States have shown interest in expanding access to CM. For example, statewide implementation of CM is currently set to begin in California in late 2022. The program will be implemented in SUD specialty care programs wherein Medi-Cal patients will take part in a 24-week outpatient program and 6 months of follow-up recovery support. Within this program, individuals with stimulant use disorder can earn up to \$599 for providing negative urine samples (≥\$600 would have required clinics to report the payments as nonemployee compensation under California tax law). Incentives will be earned on an escalating schedule and delivered as gift cards that can be used in various retail stores.[66] Interest in CM is likely to increase further given that the Biden-Harris Administration included expanding access to CM in their 2021 drug policy priorities.[67]

Much can be learned from the VA's implementation of CM and recent and ongoing studies by implementation scientists will also teach us how best to implement CM in community clinics that are more heterogeneous than those in the VA. For example, in some of the first work in this area, researchers tested a state-of-the-art multi-component training strategy consisting of didactic training in CM, specialized training focused on the change process, and nine months of support from a technology transfer specialist and an in-house innovation champion. Fifteen methadone clinics were assigned to either the multi-component training (N = 7 clinics with 39 consenting providers) or didactic training only (N = 8 clinics with 21 consenting providers). Odds of adopting CM over the next year were 13.2 times greater in the multi-component training strategy condition than the didactic training only condition.[68] However, it took many months for the multi-component strategy to demonstrate a significant advantage over didactic training only and the differences between conditions started to decrease once active support ended.[68-70] These same researchers are currently testing the multi-component strategy against the multi-component strategy enhanced with Pay-for-Performance and Implementation & Sustainment Facilitation to try to improve and sustain implementation outcomes.[71]

Conclusions

There remains no question that CM interventions are efficacious. Though the promise of CM interventions for treating SUDs across a broad range of substances, populations, and settings is clear, more research is needed (1) to further explore the potential benefits of CM interventions among vulnerable groups like pregnant and postpartum women as well as adolescents and young adults and patients with co-occurring psychiatric disorders; (2) to develop procedures that extend abstinence even longer; and (3) to develop evidence-based implementation strategies that maintain the efficacy of this approach. Advances in these areas should assist in efforts to disseminate this approach to more treatment settings. More generally, readers interested in CM may also be interested in a supplement and two special issues of *Preventive Medicine* (Supplement to Volume 55 published in 2012, Volume 92 published in 2016, and a volume to be published in 2023) dedicated in whole in part to the use of financial incentives to promote better health more broadly that includes reviews on their use in treating SUDs but also a wide range of other health-related behavior problems.

Community Reinforcement Approach

CRA was developed and most extensively researched in the treatment of alcohol use disorder. Subsequently, CRA has been extended to the treatment of cocaine and opioid use disorder in adults, adolescents with SUDs, and families of treatment-resistant patients with SUDs. Each of those applications is addressed in more detail below.

Initial Community Reinforcement Approach Study

The seminal CRA study was conducted with 16 men admitted to a rural state hospital for treatment of alcohol use disorder.[72] These men were divided into eight matched pairs. Pair members were randomly assigned to receive CRA plus standard hospital care or standard care alone. Standard hospital care consisted of 25 one-hour didactic sessions involving lectures on Alcoholics Anonymous, alcohol use disorder, and related medical problems. CRA was designed to rearrange and improve the quality of the reinforcers obtained by patients through their vocational, family, social, and recreational activities. The goal was for these reinforcers to be available and of high quality when the patient was sober and unavailable when drinking resumed. Plans for rearranging these reinforcers were individualized to conform to each patient's unique situation. During the 6-month follow-up period after hospital discharge, time spent drinking was 14% for participants in CRA versus 79% for those in standard treatment (**Fig. 73-4**). Those treated with CRA had superior outcomes on a number of other outcome measures as well.

Further Developing the Community Reinforcement Approach

After publication of the seminal study, CRA was subsequently expanded to include disulfiram therapy, with monitoring by an SO to ensure medication adherence. Additionally, counseling directed at crises resolution was added, as was a "buddy"

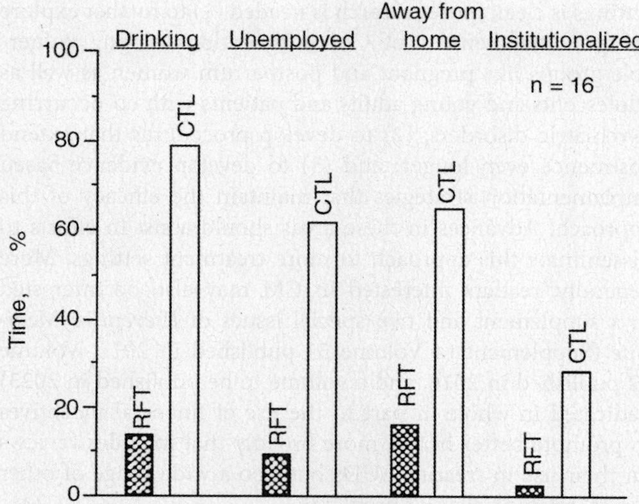

Figure 73-4. Comparison of CRA and control groups on key dependent measures. Comparison of the CRA and control groups on key dependent measures during the 6 months of follow-up after hospital discharge: mean percentage of time spent drinking, unemployed, away from home, and institutionalized. (Reprinted from Hunt GM, Azrin NH. A community-reinforcement approach to alcoholism. *Behav Res Ther.* 1973;11(1): 91-104. Copyright 1973, with permission from Elsevier.)

system in which individuals in the participant's neighborhood volunteered to be available to give assistance with practical issues such as repairing cars and the like and a switch from individual to group counseling to reduce cost. This revised intervention was investigated in a study where 20 matched pairs of men hospitalized for the treatment of alcohol use disorder were randomly assigned to receive this "improved" CRA or standard hospital care.[73] Standard care included advice to take disulfiram but no steps to ensure medication compliance. During the 6 months after hospital discharge, outcomes achieved with CRA were superior to standard care in terms of percent time spent drinking (2% versus 55%), time unemployed (20% versus 56%), time away from family (7% versus 67%), and time institutionalized (0% versus 45%). The CRA group spent 90% or more of the time abstinent during a 2-year follow-up period; comparable data were not reported for the standard treatment group.

Another study completed as part of the original CRA series examined the effects of adding the social club previously described to a standard regimen of outpatient counseling.[74] The club was designed to have the social atmosphere of a tavern but without alcohol. Individuals had to be abstinent to attend. Forty male and female participants with alcohol use disorder were randomly assigned to a group that was encouraged to attend the social club or to a control group that was not. At 3-month follow-up, drinking in the social-club group decreased from a baseline average of 4.67 oz of alcohol consumed daily to 0.85 oz, whereas in the control group, values were 3.56 and 3.32 oz, respectively. Greater improvements in the social-club group than control group were also observed in ratings of behavioral impairment and time spent in heavy-drinking situations.

Azrin et al.[75] also completed a study dissociating the effects of monitored disulfiram therapy from the other aspects of CRA. In a parallel-groups design, 43 male and female outpatients with alcohol use disorder were randomly assigned to receive usual care plus disulfiram therapy without adherence support, usual care plus disulfiram therapy involving SOs to support adherence, or CRA in combination with disulfiram therapy and significant-other support. CRA in combination with disulfiram and adherence procedures produced the greatest reductions in drinking, disulfiram in combination with adherence procedures but without CRA produced intermediate results, and the usual care plus disulfiram therapy without adherence support produced the poorest outcome. Interestingly, married patients did equally well with the full CRA treatment or disulfiram plus adherence procedures alone. Only unmarried subjects appeared to need CRA treatment plus monitored disulfiram to achieve abstinence. This was the first full report on the efficacy of CRA with less-impaired outpatients. With these less impaired individuals, treatment group differences were noted on measures of drinking only, whereas in the prior studies with more severe hospitalized patients, differences also were discerned on measures of time institutionalized and employed.

Developing the Community Reinforcement Approach as a Treatment for Illicit Drug Use Disorders

Studies on the use of CRA to treat cocaine use disorders represented, to our knowledge, the first reports on the use of CRA from investigators who were not part of the original investigative team of Azrin et al. As was mentioned, these studies examined a treatment involving CRA in combination with voucher-based CM (CRA + vouchers) and in one trial, experimentally isolated the contribution of CRA to outcomes produced by the combined intervention.[37] In another trial,[76] 180 methadone maintenance patients were randomly assigned to CRA or SUD counseling. More patients treated with CRA than SUD counseling achieved 3 weeks of biochemically-verified abstinence from illicit opioid use (89% versus 78%). No other significant differences were reported. Considered together, these trials are encouraging that CRA can improve outcomes among patients with cocaine or opioid use disorders.

Extending the Community Reinforcement Approach to Special Populations

CRA has been successfully extended to at least two special subpopulations, adolescents and people experiencing homelessness. The first study with adolescents involved 26 individuals randomly assigned to CRA or supportive counseling.[77] The intervention had three major components: stimulus control, urge control, and social control/contracting. The stimulus control component involved assisting youth in identifying safe and risky situations for substance use and therapist-assisted problem solving regarding how to increase the amount of time spent in the former and decrease time spent in the latter. Urge control involved teaching youth to recognize the early internal events that were precursors to drug use and how to interrupt them with alternative activities that are incompatible with drug use. Social control/contracting focused on involving parents in providing youth with opportunities to engage in safe activities contingent on youth compliance with activities that are incompatible with substance use. Abstinence from drug use in the CRA condition ranged between 27% and 73% across the 6-month study period as compared to 9% in the supportive counseling condition. Measures of attendance at school and employment, family relationships, and depression were also better in the CRA as compared to the supportive counseling condition.

Adolescent CRA (A-CRA) therapy was compared to motivational enhancement therapy plus CBT (MET/CBT) and multidimensional family therapy (MDFT) in a multi-site trial conducted with 300 adolescent cannabis users.[78] Therapy was approximately 3 months in duration, and patients were followed up for 1 year. Across that time period, overall percent of patients in recovery was somewhat higher among patients treated with CRA than MET/CBT and MDFT (34%, 23%, and 19%, respectively). That difference was not statistically significant overall, though it was at several of the individual sites.

The use of CRA with individuals experiencing homelessness was examined in two studies involving adults with alcohol use disorder[79] and youth.[80] In the study with adults, 106 people experiencing homelessness with alcohol use disorder were randomly assigned to CRA or standard treatment at a large day shelter. Those treated with CRA showed greater improvement on measures of drinking across five assessments conducted over a 1-year period (**Fig. 73-5**). Both conditions showed marked improvement in employment and housing stability. In the study with youth, 180 individuals between 14 and 22 years who attended an urban community drop-in center were randomly assigned to receive adolescent CRA or usual care. Substance use decreased during a 6-month study period among a larger proportion of those treated with CRA than usual care (37% versus 17%) as did depression scores (40% versus 23%) and measures of social stability increased more among those treated with CRA than usual care (58% versus 13%).

Evidence supporting the efficacy of CRA with adolescents has been sufficiently positive to warrant large-scale dissemination and implementation efforts throughout the United States. One study of some of these efforts aimed to characterize levels of A-CRA implementation in 84 programs across 27 states who received federal funding to implement the treatment and to determine whether programs continued to offer the treatment in the years after implementation funding ended.[81] Initial analyses suggest that even after a lengthy period of implementation support, programs found it challenging to sustain delivery of A-CRA longer-term, and that one important contributor to sustainment was successful implementation during the initial funding phase.[82]

Extending the Community Reinforcement Approach to Assist Relatives of Treatment-Resistant Persons with Substance Use Disorders

As part of the original series of studies on CRA, Sisson and Azrin[83] adapted CRA for use with the SOs of treatment-resistant patients with alcohol use disorder. Twelve SOs were randomly assigned to receive either the CRA intervention or a standard program involving group instruction about alcohol and the disease model of alcoholism. The CRA intervention included education about alcohol problems, information and discussion of the positive consequences of not drinking, assistance in involving the patient with alcohol use disorder in healthy activities, increasing the involvement of the SO in social and recreational activities, and training in how to respond to drinking episodes (including dangerous situations) and how

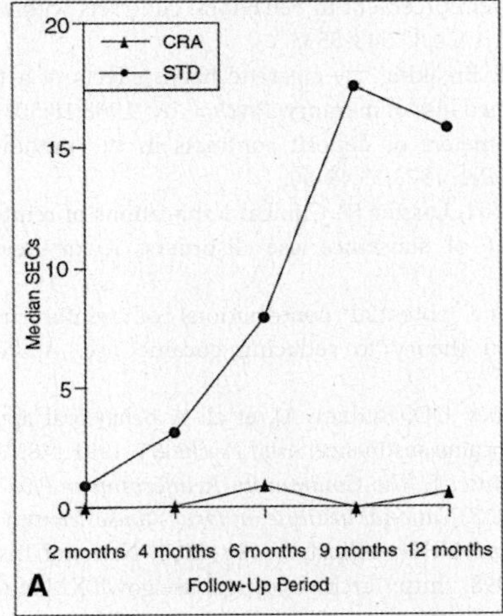

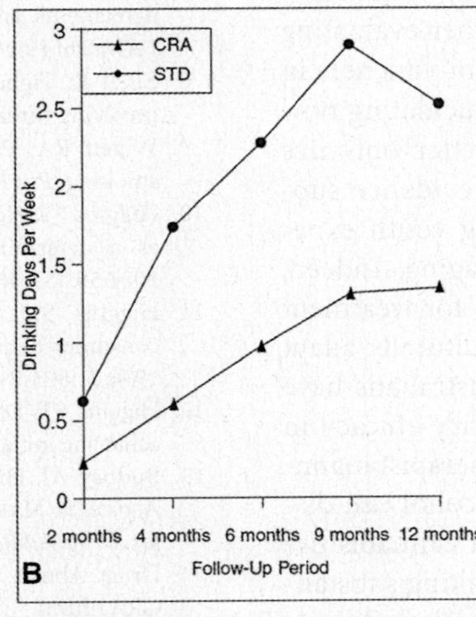

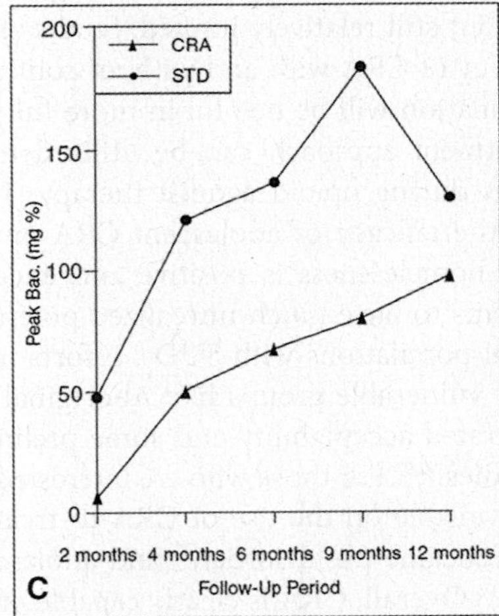

Figure 73-5. Comparison of CRA and standard treatment groups on key dependent measures. Comparison of the CRA and standard treatment groups on standard ethanol content **(A)**, drinking days per week **(B)**, and peak blood alcohol concentration **(C)**. (Reprinted from Smith JE, Meyers RJ, Delaney HD. The community reinforcement approach with homeless alcohol-dependent individuals. *J Consult Clin Psychol.* 1998;66:541-548, with permission.)

to recommend treatment entry to the family member with alcohol use disorder. In the control group, none of the patients with alcohol use disorder entered treatment over the next 3 months, and their drinking remained unchanged. In the CRA group, six of seven patients with alcohol use disorder entered treatment, and average drinking decreased from 24 days per month at pretreatment to fewer than five.

Subsequent controlled trials have consistently supported the efficacy of CRA in assisting concerned SOs (CSOs) to get unmotivated individuals with alcohol use disorders and individuals with illicit SUDs to enter treatment. The treatment has come to be referred to as community reinforcement and family training (CRAFT). A systematic review and meta-analysis of CRAFT identified six studies (including Sisson and Azrin[83]) involving nearly 500 SOs of patients using alcohol and/or drugs where CRAFT was compared to a control/comparison condition.[84] In most of these studies, CRAFT was delivered in individual sessions and treatment for the patient was provided by or linked directly to the same team providing the CRAFT intervention. CRAFT was more than twice as effective on treatment entry rates than control/comparison conditions (RR = 2.35, 95% CI = 1.77-3.12).

Conclusions

Considered together, the evidence supporting the efficacy of CRA is quite robust. No fewer than seven systematic reviews and one meta-analysis confirm this conclusion.[3,85-91] The evidence is strong in support of CRA's efficacy in treating alcohol use disorder, even when the clinical situation is complicated by homelessness. The evidence is also quite strong regarding the efficacy of CRA combined with voucher-based CM for outpatient treatment of cocaine use disorder. Experimental evidence demonstrates that CRA and voucher-based CM each contribute significantly to the positive outcomes achieved with that intervention. The evidence in support of CRA plus vouchers or CRA alone in the treatment of opioid use disorders is positive but still relatively limited. Studies further evaluating the efficacy of CRA with and without contingent vouchers in this population will be helpful in more fully elucidating how this treatment approach can be utilized to better optimize outcomes during opioid agonist therapy. The evidence supporting the efficacy of adolescent CRA among youth experiencing homelessness is positive and encouraging. Indeed, CRA seems to have much unrealized potential for treatment of special populations with SUDs. Efforts to culturally adapt CRA for vulnerable groups like Aboriginal Australians have demonstrated acceptability and some preliminary efficacy in early studies.[92,93] For those who are interested, therapist manuals are available on the use of CRA to treat alcohol use disorders,[94] cocaine use disorder,[13] and adolescent cannabis use disorder.[95] Overall, CRA is clearly capable of making substantive contributions to the development of evidence-based treatments for a wide range of different types of SUDs, populations, problems, and settings.

CONCLUSIONS

This chapter has reviewed how within an operant framework drug use is considered a normal, learned behavior that can be fruitfully conceptualized to fall along a continuum ranging from light use with no problems to heavy use with many untoward effects. The same basic learning processes are assumed to operate across the drug-use continuum. Treatment strategies based on this conceptual framework look to weaken the reinforcement obtained from drug use and related activities and to enhance the material and social reinforcement obtained from other sources, especially from participation in activities deemed to be incompatible with a drug-using lifestyle. CM and CRA procedures are based on this general strategy and are efficacious in treating alcohol, cocaine, opioid, and other types of SUDs. CM and CRA offer no "magic bullets" for the treatment of these disorders and, as discussed, much more remains to be learned about each of them. Those limitations notwithstanding, CM and CRA offer a range of empirically based and effective strategies for treating some of the most challenging populations and daunting aspects of SUDs.

REFERENCES

1. Mazur JE. *Learning and Behavior*. 8th ed. Routledge; 2016.
2. Higgins ST, Silverman K, Sigmon SC, Naito NA. Incentives and health: an introduction. *Prev Med*. 2012;55(Suppl 1):S2-S6.
3. Meyers RJ, Roozen HG, Smith JE. The community reinforcement approach: an update of the evidence. *Alcohol Res Health*. 2011;33:380-388.
4. Schuster CR, Thompson T. Self-administration of and behavioral dependence on drugs. *Ann Rev Pharmacol*. 1969;9:483-502.
5. Aigner TG, Balster RL. Choice behavior in rhesus monkeys: cocaine versus food. *Science*. 1978;201:434-435.
6. Bigelow GE, Griffiths R, Liebson I. Experimental models for the modification of human drug self-administration: methodological developments in the study of ethanol self-administration by alcoholics. *Fed Proc*. 1975;34:1785-1792.
7. Miller PM, Hersen M, Eisler RM. Relative effectiveness of instructions, agreements, and reinforcement in behavioral contracts with alcoholics. *J Abnorm Psychol*. 1974;83:548-553.
8. Elliot R, Tighe T. Breaking the cigarette habit: effects of a technique involving threatened loss of memory. *Psychol Rec*. 1968;18:503-513.
9. Winett RA. Parameters of deposit contracts in the modification of smoking. *Psychol Rec*. 1973;23:49-60.
10. Higgins ST, Heil SH, Lussier JP. Clinical implications of reinforcement as a determinant of substance use disorders. *Annu Rev Psychol*. 2004;55:431-461.
11. Higgins ST. Some potential contributions of reinforcement and consumer-demand theory to reducing cocaine use. *Addict Behav*. 1996;21:803-816.
12. Higgins ST, Delaney DD, Budney AJ, et al. A behavioral approach to achieving initial cocaine abstinence. *Am J Psychiatry*. 1991;148:1218-1224.
13. Budney AJ, Higgins ST. *The Community Reinforcement Plus Vouchers Approach: Manual 2. National Institute on Drug Abuse Therapy Manuals for Drug Addiction*. NIH publication #98-4308. National Institute on Drug Abuse; 1998. http://archives.drugabuse.gov/TXManuals/CRA/CRA1.html
14. Festinger DS, Lamb RJ, Kirby KC, Marlowe DB. The accelerated intake: a method for increasing initial attendance to outpatient cocaine treatment. *J Appl Behav Anal*. 1996;29:387-389.

15. Miller WR, Tonigan JS. Assessing drinkers' motivation to change: the Stages of Change Readiness and Treatment Eagerness Scale (SOCRATES). *Psychol Addict Behav.* 1996;10:81-89.
16. Washton AM, Stone NS, Hendrickson EC. Cocaine abuse. In: Donovan DM, Marlatt GA, eds. *Assessment of Addictive Behavior.* Guilford Press; 1988:364-389.
17. Selzer ML. The Michigan Alcoholism Screening Test: the quest for a new diagnostic instrument. *Am J Psychiatry.* 1971;127:1653-1658.
18. Beck AT, Steer RA, Ball R, Ranieri W. Comparison of Beck Depression Inventories-IA and -II in psychiatric outpatients. *J Pers Assess.* 1996;67:588-597.
19. Derogatis LR. Misuse of the symptom checklist 90. *Arch Gen Psychiatry.* 1983;40:1152-1153.
20. Sobell LC, Sobell MB. Timeline follow-back: a technique for assessing self-reported alcohol consumption. In: Litten RZ, Allen JP, eds. *Measuring Alcohol Consumption: Psychosocial and Biochemical Methods.* Humana Press; 1992:41-72.
21. McLellan AT, Cacciola J, Alterman AI, Rikoon SH, Carise D. The Addiction Severity Index at 25: origins, contributions, and transitions. *Am J Addict.* 2006;15:113-124.
22. Carroll KM, Nich C, Ball SA, McCance E, Rounsaville BJ. Treatment of cocaine and alcohol dependence with psychotherapy and disulfiram. *Addiction.* 1998;93:713-728.
23. Higgins ST, Silverman K. Contingency management. In: Galanter M, Kleber HD, eds. *Textbook of Substance Abuse Treatment.* 4th ed. The American Psychiatric Press; 2008:387-399.
24. Lussier JP, Heil SH, Mongeon JA, Badger GJ, Higgins ST. A meta-analysis of voucher-based reinforcement therapy for substance use disorders. *Addiction.* 2006;101:192-203.
25. Lewinsohn PM, Munoz RF, Youngren MA, et al. *Control Your Depression.* Simon & Schuster; 1986.
26. Munoz RF, Miranda J. *Individual Therapy Manual for Cognitive Behavioral Treatment for Depression.* RAND Corporation; 2000.
27. Azrin NH, Besalel VA. *Job Club Counselor's Manual.* University Park Press; 1980.
28. O'Farrel TJ, Fals-Stewart W. Alcohol abuse. In: Sprenkle DH, ed. *Effectiveness Research in Marriage and Family Therapy.* American Association for Marriage and Family Therapy; 2002:123-161.
29. Dunn KE, Saulsgiver KA, Patrick ME, Heil SH, Higgins ST, Sigmon SC. Characterizing and improving HIV and hepatitis knowledge among primary prescription opioid abusers. *Drug Alcohol Depend.* 2013;133:625-632.
30. Smith JE, Meyers RJ. The community reinforcement approach. In: Hester R, Miller W, eds. *Handbook of Alcoholism Treatment Approaches: Effective Alternatives.* 2nd ed. Allyn & Bacon; 1995.
31. Knudsen HK. Implementation of smoking cessation treatment in substance use disorder treatment settings: a review. *Am J Drug Alcohol Abuse.* 2016;17:1-11.
32. Higgins ST, Budney AJ, Bickel WK, Hughes JR, Foerg F, Badger G. Achieving cocaine abstinence with a behavioral approach. *Am J Psychiatry.* 1993;150:763-769.
33. Higgins ST, Budney AJ, Bickel WK, Foerg F, Donham R, Badger GJ. Incentives improve outcome in outpatient behavioral treatment of cocaine dependence. *Arch Gen Psychiatry.* 1994;51:568-576.
34. Higgins ST, Budney AJ, Bickel WK, Badger GJ, Foerg FE, Ogden D. Outpatient behavioral treatment for cocaine dependence: one-year outcome. *Exp Clin Psychopharmacol.* 1995;3:205-212.
35. Higgins ST, Wong CJ, Badger GJ, Ogden DE, Dantona RL. Contingent reinforcement increases cocaine abstinence during outpatient treatment and 1-year of follow-up. *J Consult Clin Psychol.* 2000;68:64-72.
36. Higgins ST, Heil SH, Dantona RL, Donham R, Matthews M, Badger GJ. Effects of varying the monetary value of voucher-based incentives on abstinence achieved during and following treatment among cocaine-dependent outpatients. *Addiction.* 2007;102:271-281.
37. Higgins ST, Sigmon SC, Wong CJ, et al. Community reinforcement therapy for cocaine-dependent outpatients. *Arch Gen Psychiatry.* 2003;60:1043-1052.
38. Bickel WK, Amass L, Higgins ST, Badger GJ, Esch RA. Effects of adding behavioral treatment to opioid detoxification with buprenorphine. *J Consult Clin Psychol.* 1997;65:803-810.
39. Bickel WK, Marsch LA, Buchhalter AR, Badger GJ. Computerized behavior therapy for opioid-dependent outpatients: a randomized controlled trial. *Exp Clin Psychopharmacol.* 2008;16:132-143.
40. Christensen DR, Landes RD, Jackson L, et al. Adding an internet-delivered treatment to an efficacious treatment package for opioid dependence. *J Consult Clin Psychol.* 2014;82:964-972.
41. Campbell AN, Nunes EV, Matthews AG, et al. Internet-delivered treatment for substance abuse: a multisite randomized controlled trial. *Am J Psychiatry.* 2014;171:683-690.
42. Secades-Villa R, Garcia-Rodriguez O, Rodriguez AH, et al. Community reinforcement approach plus vouchers for cocaine dependence treatment. *Addicciones.* 2007;19:51-57.
43. Secades-Villa R, Garcia-Rodriguez O, Garcia-Fernandez G, et al. Community reinforcement approach plus vouchers among cocaine-dependent outpatients: twelve-month outcomes. *Psychol Addict Behav.* 2011;25:174-179.
44. Silverman K, Higgins ST, Brooner RK, et al. Sustained cocaine abstinence in methadone maintenance patients through voucher-based reinforcement therapy. *Arch Gen Psychiatry.* 1996;53:409-415.
45. Silverman K, Preston KL, Stitzer ML, et al. Treatment of cocaine abuse in methadone maintenance patients. In: Higgins ST, Katz JL, eds. *Cocaine Abuse Research: Pharmacology, Behavior, and Clinical Application.* Academic Press; 1998:363-388.
46. Silverman K, Chutuape MA, Bigelow GE, Stitzer ML. Voucher-based reinforcement of cocaine abstinence in treatment-resistant methadone patients: effects of reinforcer magnitude. *Psychopharmacology.* 1999;146:128-138.
47. Kirby KC, Marlowe DB, Festinger DS, Lamb RJ, Platt JJ. Schedule of voucher delivery influences initiation of cocaine abstinence. *J Consult Clin Psychol.* 1998;66:761-767.
48. Cicero TJ, Ellis MS, Kasper ZA. Polysubstance use: a broader understanding of substance use during the opioid crisis. *Am J Public Health.* 2020;110:244-250.
49. Bolívar HA, Klemperer EM, Coleman SRM, DeSarno M, Skelly JM, Higgins ST. Contingency management for patients receiving medication for opioid use disorder: a systematic review and meta-analysis. *JAMA Psychiatry.* 2021;78:1092-1102.
50. Notley C, Gentry S, Livingstone-Banks J, Bauld L, Perera R, Hartmann-Boyce J. Incentives for smoking cessation. *Cochrane Database Syst Rev.* 2019;7:CD004307.
51. Tappin D, Bauld L, Purves D, et al. Financial incentives for smoking cessation in pregnancy: randomised controlled trial. *BMJ.* 2015; 350:h134.
52. Boyd KA, Briggs AH, Bauld L, et al. Are financial incentives cost-effective to support smoking cessation during pregnancy? *Addiction.* 2016;111:360-370.
53. Higgins ST, Nighbor TD, Kurti AN, et al. Randomized controlled trial examining the efficacy of adding financial incentives to best practices for smoking cessation among pregnant and newly postpartum women. *Prev Med.* 2022;165:107012.
54. Shepard DS, Slade EP, Nighbor TD, et al. Economic analysis of financial incentives for smoking cessation during pregnancy and postpartum. *Prev Med.* 2022;165:107079.
55. Dallery J, Glenn IM. Effects of an internet-based voucher reinforcement program for smoking abstinence: a feasibility study. *J Appl Behav Anal.* 2005;38:349-357.
56. Dallery J, Raiff BR, Grabinski MJ, Marsch LA. Technology-based contingency management in the treatment of substance-use disorders. *Perspect Behav Sci.* 2019;42:445-464.
57. Kurti AN, Tang K, Bolivar HA, et al. Smartphone-based financial incentives to promote smoking cessation during pregnancy: a pilot study. *Prev Med.* 2020;140:106201.
58. Kurti AN, Nighbor TD, Tang K, et al. Effect of smartphone-based financial incentives on peripartum smoking among pregnant individuals: a randomized clinical trial. *JAMA Netw Open.* 2022;5:e2211889.

59. Palmer AM, Tomko RL, Squeglia LM, et al. A pilot feasibility study of a behavioral intervention for nicotine vaping cessation among young adults delivered via telehealth. *Drug Alcohol Depend.* 2022;232:109311.
60. Hammond AS, Sweeney MM, Chikosi TU, Stitzer ML. Digital delivery of a contingency management intervention for substance use disorder: a feasibility study with DynamiCare Health. *J Subst Abuse Treat.* 2021;126:108425.
61. Ginley MK, Pfund RA, Rash CJ, Zajac K. Long-term efficacy of contingency management treatment based on objective indicators of abstinence from illicit substance use up to 1 year following treatment: a meta-analysis. *J Consult Clin Psychol.* 2021;89:58-71.
62. Pilling S, Strang J, Gerada C, NICE. Psychosocial interventions and opioid detoxification for drug misuse: summary of NICE guidance. *BMJ.* 2007;335:203-205.
63. Petry NM, DePhilippis D, Rash CJ, Drapkin M, McKay JR. Nationwide dissemination of contingency management: the Veterans Administration initiative. *Am J Addict.* 2014;23:205-210.
64. Rash CJ, DePhilippis D, McKay JR, Drapkin M, Petry NM. Training workshops positively impact beliefs about contingency management in a nationwide dissemination effort. *J Subst Abuse Treat.* 2013;45:306-312.
65. DePhilippis D, Petry NM, Bonn-Miller MO, Rosenbach SB, McKay JR. The national implementation of contingency management (CM) in the Department of Veterans Affairs: attendance at CM sessions and substance use outcomes. *Drug Alcohol Depend.* 2018;185:367-373.
66. Hernandez-Delgado H. *Treating Stimulant Use Disorder: CalAIM's Contingency Management Pilot.* Accessed June 12, 2023. https://www.chcf.org/wp-content/uploads/2022/05/TreatingStimulantUseDisorderCalAIMsContingencyMgmtPilot.pdf
67. The White House. *Biden-Harris Administration Announces First-Year Drug Policy Priorities.* 2021. Accessed June 12, 2023. https://www.whitehouse.gov/ondcp/briefing-room/2021/04/01/biden-harris-administration-announces-first-year-drug-policy-priorities/
68. Becker SJ, Squires DD, Stron DR, Barnett NP, Monti PM, Petry NM. Training opioid addiction treatment providers to adopt contingency management: a prospective pilot trial of a comprehensive implementation science approach. *Subst Abus.* 2016;37:134-140.
69. Becker SJ, Kelly LM, Kang AW, Escobar KI, Squires DD. Factors associated with contingency management adoption among opioid treatment providers receiving a comprehensive implementation strategy. *Subst Abus.* 2019;40:56-60.
70. Helseth SA, Janssen T, Scott K, Squires DD, Becker SJ. Training community-based treatment providers to implement contingency management for opioid addiction: time to and frequency of adoption. *J Subst Abuse Treat.* 2018;95:26-34.
71. Becker SJ, Murphy CM, Hartzler B, et al. Project MIMIC (Maximizing Implementation of Motivational Incentives in Clinics): a cluster-randomized type 3 hybrid effectiveness-implementation trial. *Addict Sci Clin Pract.* 2021;16:61.
72. Hunt GM, Azrin NH. A community-reinforcement approach to alcoholism. *Behav Res Ther.* 1973;11:91-104.
73. Azrin NH. Improvements in the community-reinforcement approach to alcoholism. *Behav Res Ther.* 1976;14:339-348.
74. Mallams JH, Godley MD, Hall GM, Meyers RJ. A social-systems approach to resocializing alcoholics in the community. *J Stud Alcohol.* 1982;43:1115-1123.
75. Azrin NH, Sisson RW, Meyers R, Godley M. Alcoholism treatment by disulfiram and community reinforcement therapy. *J Behav Ther Exp Psychiatry.* 1982;13:105-112.
76. Abbott PJ, Weller SB, Delaney HD, Moore BA. Community reinforcement approach in the treatment of opiate addicts. *Am J Drug Alcohol Abuse.* 1998;24:17-30.
77. Azrin NH, Donohue B, Besalel VA, et al. Youth drug abuse treatment: a controlled outcome study. *J Child Adolesc Subst Abuse.* 1994;3:1-16.
78. Dennis M, Godley SH, Diamond G, et al. The cannabis youth treatment (CYT) study: main findings from two randomized trials. *J Subst Abuse Treat.* 2004;27:197-213.
79. Smith JE, Meyers RJ, Delaney HD. The community reinforcement approach with homeless alcohol-dependent individuals. *J Consult Clin Psychol.* 1998;66:541-548.
80. Slesnick N, Prestopnik JL, Meyers RJ, Glassman M. Treatment outcome for street-living, homeless youth. *Addict Behav.* 2007;32:1237-1251.
81. Hunter SB, Ayer L, Han B, Garner BR, Godley SH. Examining the sustainment of the Adolescent-Community Reinforcement Approach in community addiction treatment settings: protocol for a longitudinal mixed method study. *Implement Sci.* 2014;9:104.
82. Hunter SB, Han B, Slaughter ME, Godley SH, Garner BR. Predicting evidence-based treatment sustainment: results from a longitudinal study of the Adolescent-Community Reinforcement Approach. *Implement Sci.* 2017;12:75.
83. Sisson RW, Azrin AH. Family-member involvement to initiate and promote treatment of problem drinkers. *J Behav Ther Exp Psychiatry.* 1986;17:15-21.
84. Archer M, Harwood H, Stevelink S, Rafferty L, Greenberg N. Community reinforcement and family training and rates of treatment entry: a systematic review. *Addiction.* 2019;115:1024-1037.
85. Holder H, Longabaugh R, Miller WR, Rubonis AV. The cost effectiveness of treatment for alcoholism: a first approximation. *J Stud Alcohol.* 1991;52:517-540.
86. Miller WR, Brown RK, Simpson TL, et al. What works? A methodological analysis of the alcohol treatment outcome literature. In: Hester RK, Miller WR, eds. *Handbook of Alcoholism Treatment Approaches: Effective Alternatives.* 2nd ed. Allyn and Bacon; 1995:12-44.
87. Finney JW, Monahan SC. The cost-effectiveness of treatment for alcoholism: a second approximation. *J Stud Alcohol.* 1996;57:229-243.
88. Milller WR, Andrews NR, Wilbourne P, et al. A wealth of alternatives: effective treatments for alcohol problems. In: Miller WR, Heather N, eds. *Treating Addictive Behaviors: Processes of Change.* 2nd ed. Plenum Press; 1998:203-216.
89. Miller WR, Wilbourne PL, Hettema JE. What works? A summary of alcohol treatment outcome research. In: Hester RK, Miller WR, eds. *Handbook of Alcoholism Treatment Approaches: Effective Alternatives.* 3rd ed. Allyn and Bacon; 2003:13-63.
90. Roozen GH, Boulogne JJ, van Tulder MW, van den Brink W, De Jong CAJ, Kerkhof AJFM. A systematic review of the effectiveness of the community reinforcement approach in alcohol, cocaine and opioid addiction. *Drug Alcohol Depend.* 2004;74:1-13.
91. Miller WR, Zweben J, Johnson WR. Evidence-based treatment: why, what, where, when, and how? *J Subst Abuse Treat.* 2005;29:267-276.
92. Calabria B, Clifford A, Shakeshaft A, Allan J, Bliss D, Doran C. The acceptability to Aboriginal Australians of a family-based intervention to reduce alcohol-related harms. *Drug Alcohol Rev.* 2013;32:328-332.
93. Calabria B, Shakeshaft AP, Clifford A, et al. Reducing drug and alcohol use and improving well-being for Indigenous and non-Indigenous Australians using the Community Reinforcement Approach: a feasibility and acceptability study. *Int J Psychol.* 2020;55(Suppl 1):88-95.
94. Meyers RJ, Smith JE. *Clinical Guide to Alcohol Treatment: The Community Reinforcement Approach.* Guilford Press; 1995.
95. Godley SH, Meyers RJ, Smith JE, et al. *The Adolescent Community Reinforcement Approach (ACRA) for Adolescent Cannabis Users.* Center for Substance Abuse Treatment; 2001.

CHAPTER

74

Behavioral Interventions for Tobacco Use Disorder

Joanna M. Streck, Angela Wangari Walter, Rachel L. Rosen, and Elyse R. Park

CHAPTER OUTLINE

- Introduction
- Chapter overview
- History of treatments for tobacco use disorder
- Treatment model
- Treatment planning
- Treatment and techniques
- Abstinence stage interventions
- Other intensive interventions for tobacco use disorder
- TUD treatment considerations for systematically excluded populations
- Novel treatment approach in development
- Novel methods of intervention delivery
- Summary and conclusions

INTRODUCTION

Tobacco smoking is the leading cause of preventable death in the United States, resulting in over 480,000 deaths each year (ie, about 1 in 5 deaths),[1] with almost one-third of all deaths from cancer attributable to smoking.[2] Costs of medical care and lost productivity due to smoking-related disability are estimated at over $289 billion per year.[1] Following significant public health efforts, cigarette smoking among adults in the United States has declined from a peak of 42.4% in 1965[1] to 13% in 2020.[3,4] Whereas cigarette smoking has declined in the past decade in the United States, the sale and consumption of alternative tobacco and nicotine products (eg, electronic drug delivery devices [EDDD] such as electronic cigarettes) has increased.[3-5]

According to the *Diagnostic and Statistical Manual of Mental Disorders*, nicotine/tobacco use disorder (TUD; formerly referred to as "tobacco abuse" and "tobacco dependence") is a clinical diagnosis given to individuals demonstrating a problematic pattern of nicotine/tobacco use leading to clinically significant impairment or distress manifested by at least 2 of 11 symptoms experienced in the past 12 months (ie, tobacco taken in larger amounts or over a longer period than was intended, persistent desire or unsuccessful efforts to cut down or control tobacco use, a great deal of time spent in activities necessary to obtain or use tobacco, craving or strong desire or urge to use, recurrent use leading to failure to fulfill major role obligations, continued use despite recurrent problems from use, important activities given up because of use, recurrent use in situations when use is physically hazardous, continued use despite knowledge of physical or psychological problems from use, nicotine tolerance, nicotine withdrawal).[6] According to national estimates (2012-2013), about 20% of the adult population meets criteria for TUD.[7]

Many individuals who smoke or have TUD are aware of the risks associated with smoking and the possible benefits of quitting,[8-10] with about two-thirds expressing interest in quitting and about 55% attempting to quit smoking each year.[4,11] However, only about 7.5% of those attempting to quit remain abstinent for 6 months or more in the past year.[5,12] Rates of success are much higher for those engaged in more intensive TUD treatments (eg, FDA-approved pharmacotherapy and longer duration behavioral treatments), ranging from about 15% to 30% abstinent.[13] Nevertheless, even in those receiving more intensive treatments, return to use rates are high once treatment ends, and multiple quit attempts are often needed before individuals are successful in quitting and sustaining abstinence.[14] Thus, TUD is considered a chronic recurring condition with a need for longitudinal treatment approaches that consider periods of abstinence and periods of return to smoking.[15,16]

Individuals with behavioral health conditions such as psychiatric and substance use disorders (SUDs) face higher rates of tobacco smoking and have less success in quitting smoking compared to the general population, even when using existing evidence-based behavioral and pharmacological treatments. For example, recent estimates suggest 36% of individuals with SUDs and over 70% of individuals with serious mental illness reported current cigarette smoking.[4,17-20] Additionally, there are racial disparities observed in smoking prevalence and quit rates with Indigenous Americans and Alaska Natives having the highest rates of tobacco smoking and Black/African Americans consistently having the lowest success rate in lifetime quitting compared to any other racial/ethnic group.[21-23]

Clinicians play a crucial role in assessing nicotine/tobacco use and TUD, encouraging all patients to quit, and providing ongoing assistance for patients attempting to quit and for those who may return to tobacco use throughout the course of behavioral interventions.[1,24-26]

CHAPTER OVERVIEW

In this chapter, we describe a variety of behavioral interventions that can improve remission rates for nicotine/tobacco use and TUD. We begin by briefly reviewing the history of treatment of TUD before outlining some general theories of behavior change. We then discuss treatment planning and techniques for working with individuals who intend to quit smoking in the near future and those who do not. We conclude by reviewing considerations for working with specific subpopulations of individuals who face disparities in tobacco use and TUD. In discussing behavioral interventions, we focus primarily on traditional tobacco smoking (eg, cigarette smoking) among adults where research and clinical applications have been most well developed. With the rise of use of nicotine and tobacco products in the past decade, such as EDDDs, this area of research is less well developed though scientific efforts are underway to develop interventions that address EDDD abstinence.[27]

There are few theoretical reasons to expect that behavioral principles for tobacco smoking do not apply equally well to adolescents, although the context of treatment dissemination may require modification[28] and consideration should be given to adolescents' cognitive and social developmental stage.[29] The literature on adolescent treatment of tobacco smoking is less well-developed relative to adults, but evidence suggests that cognitive-behavioral, motivational and contingency management-based interventions are effective for adolescents.[29-33] Nevertheless, success rates for some tobacco abstinence interventions appear lower compared to adults.[29,33,34] Additionally, EDDD use is the most common tobacco product used by youth and thus there have been growing concerns about youth EDDD use including the potential for the impaired brain maturation from exposure, development of TUD, as well as transition from EDDD use to traditional tobacco cigarette use among youth.[32,33,35] However, there is little work available on evidence-based treatments, including behavioral treatments, for EDDD abstinence in youth.[36-38] For a thorough review of substance use and treatment considerations among youth and adolescents refer to Section 14, and for more information about nicotine pharmacology and EDDDs please refer to Chapter 22, "Electronic Drug Delivery Devices."

HISTORY OF TREATMENTS FOR TOBACCO USE DISORDER

Historical records indicate that as early as the mid-1800s, accounts of TUD were reported. Nineteenth century antitobacco organizations branded "tobaccoism" (ie, habitual tobacco use, now known generally as TUD or tobacco addiction) a disease that can cause a range of ailments from insanity to cancer.[39,40] During this period, cigarettes were considered narcotics because they appeared to have addictive qualities. Despite these early reports of the negative effects of tobacco use, pervasive efforts to develop and disseminate treatments designed to help people who smoked to quit did not come into favor until after the 1960s. At that time, the medical community reached a consensus that smoking is a principal etiologic factor in the development of several harmful conditions, including cancer.[41]

Earlier reports, prior to 1990, estimated that most (>90%) people who previously smoked and who successfully quit smoking did not use any formal treatment program.[42] However, the awareness of TUD as a medical disease, and the paucity of medications and therapies available to treat TUD provide some contextual explanation. More recent estimates indicate that approximately 30% of people who smoke are using some form of assistance when trying to quit,[43-48] which coincides with the advancement and dissemination of treatment methods including health care provider advice to use treatments for TUD. Initial treatment efforts mainly involved physicians using unsystematic methods to advise their patients to quit smoking. However, with the medical and scientific community's evolution in understanding regular smoking not being a "habit" or volitional, but rather an "addiction,"[49] more substantial, standardized interventions have been developed. For example, early research led to the development of nicotine gum as the first FDA-approved pharmacologic treatment for TUD in 1984. This was followed by FDA approval of transdermal nicotine patches and nicotine nasal spray, and more recently bupropion and varenicline.

With regard to behavioral interventions, systematic study of the factors that increase treatment efficacy (eg, treatment approach and content, components of intervention, length of sessions, number of sessions, type of practitioner) started in the 1970s and 1980s.[50] Early interventions varied markedly in their approach from systematic brief advice[51] to aversive-smoking strategies (eg, rapid smoking[52]). More recently, behavioral interventions have focused on enhancing commitment in individuals with TUD toward initiating and maintaining abstinence,[53-55] engagement in exercise,[56] skill building techniques to increase individual coping resources,[57] and acceptance and mindfulness-based practices to increase resilience to withdrawal-related and other affective distress.[58-66] These behavioral strategies are reviewed in detail in subsequent sections of this chapter.

In addition to content changes, the modality of treatment has also transformed with advancement in technology. While traditionally, behavioral treatments were exclusively delivered face-to-face between the provider and patient or in group formats, technology-based interventions delivered through telephones (eg, telephone counseling or text messaging), computers (eg, video, internet-based), and smartphone applications[67] have increased in prevalence.[68-72] Future scientific, medical, and technologic developments will likely continue to change the landscape of behavioral interventions for TUD, particularly in the era of COVID-19, potentially increasing their effectiveness as well as their impact on public health. These novel intervention delivery methods are reviewed at the end of the chapter.

TREATMENT MODEL

Theory of Change

The treatment model we rely on in this chapter is based on a theory of change that proposes that in order for individuals to change their behavior they must (1) be motivated or ready (eg, perceived confidence plus importance in quitting smoking) to change and (2) have the skills to execute the change in behavior effectively.[73,74]

Motivation

Motivation (or readiness) to change a behavior is defined as the desire and intention to discontinue an old behavior and initiate a new behavior. Readiness to change is thought to lie along a continuum ranging from very low motivation (ie, no desire to change) to moderate motivation (ie, some interest in changing but no current intentions) to very high motivation (ie, firm intention to change). This conceptualization of motivation is also consistent with the stages of change model, which suggests that individuals who smoke move between one of five stages of change: precontemplation (ie, not planning to quit for at least 6 months), contemplation (ie, planning to quit within the next 6 months but not the next 30 days), preparation (ie, planning to quit in the next 30 days and made an attempt to quit within the last year), action (ie, quit smoking within the past 6 months), and maintenance (ie, quit smoking more than 6 months ago).[75,76] Some have critiqued stage-based theories of change for prescriptiveness, and it is important use to a patient-centered framework and consider the whole patient in treatment including integrating their social context (eg, socioeconomic status) and tailoring treatment to the patient's unique needs.

Psychological theories such as the Theory of Planned Behavior argue that people are motivated to cease behaviors that yield low reward and high risk, whereas they are motivated to initiate behaviors that yield high reward and low risk.[73,77] Accordingly, motivation to change is thought to be determined by cognitive processes involved in weighing the personal pros versus cons of persisting with the old behavior and weighing the personal pros versus cons of initiating the new behavior. Motivation will be greater if (1) the cons of the old behavior and the pros of the new behavior are *high* and (2) the pros of the old behavior and the cons of the new behavior are *low*.

Motivation is dynamic as it can vary within an individual across time and circumstances (presumably due to changes in the accessibility, salience, and strength of beliefs regarding the relevance of benefits and costs of smoking versus quitting). Based on this framework, behavioral change occurs when there is a transformation in an individual's internal beliefs toward greater cons for the old behavior and pros for the new behavior and/or lesser pros for the old behavior and cons for the new behavior. When this shift is sufficiently large, an intention to change will occur. In addition, a particular benefit that is especially salient to a given individual may have a larger impact on overall motivation than the other pros and cons (eg, an individual who is hospitalized for a smoking-related illness and sees the immediate benefits of quitting smoking). Furthermore, the personal relevance of certain pros or cons for a particular individual may change in response to new circumstances and external influences (eg, learning that you have developed lung cancer, your spouse demands that you quit). Therefore, external influences that help individuals who smoke shift their beliefs regarding the pros and cons of smoking versus quitting may enhance motivation and ultimately result in their initiating an abstinence attempt.

Skills-Based Behavioral Treatments

According to behavioral theories of behavior change, once an intention to change a behavior has been formed, specific skills are required in order for the individual to effectively initiate and maintain the new behavior. Therefore, the acquisition or use of new skills is likely to be necessary to promote persistence of the new behavior. When stopping nicotine/tobacco use, various factors make it difficult to initiate and maintain the new behavior of abstinence, these include nicotine withdrawal, cravings, stress, triggers/stimuli in the environment that tempt people to smoke (eg, ashtrays, lighters, living with other individuals who smoke), negative mood states, missing the pleasure of smoking, and boredom. Especially among individuals making their first quit attempt, these barriers are novel, and these individuals may not know strategies that could help them to maintain abstinence in the face of these barriers. Accordingly, learning "nonsmoking skills" can be helpful to prevent these barriers from impeding abstinence. For example, learning strategies of how to anticipate and manage situations that are high risk (eg, running into my friend who I used to smoke with) may provide individuals with skills necessary to maintain their new behavior (ie, abstinence) without going back to their old behavior (ie, smoking).

Theoretical Framework for Behavioral Treatments

Social learning theory provides a useful framework for conceptualizing behavioral treatment of TUD[78]; this theory has also been extended to treatment of other substances such as alcohol where similar processes may operate (eg, see social learning theory applications for alcohol use disorder[79]). In this model, smoking and/or other nicotine use is viewed as a learned behavior acquired through classical and operant conditioning, modeling, and other cognitive processes.[80] Through repeated pairings over time, various external and interoceptive stimuli, for example, drinking coffee, feeling stressed, celebrating at a party,[81] come to be associated with smoking behavior. These stimuli or *antecedents* can then trigger an urge to smoke. Once the individual smokes a cigarette (the *behavior*), they experience the negative reinforcement *consequences* (eg, relief of nicotine withdrawal, causing an experience of relaxation), increasing the likelihood of future smoking, as research suggests that behavior that is reinforced is repeated. Individuals with TUD also develop certain expectations about the effects of smoking, which in turn influence smoking behavior. Positive outcome expectancies (eg, "smoking will relax me") increase the likelihood of continued smoking, whereas negative outcome expectancies (eg, "smoking increases my risk of heart disease") increase the likelihood of quitting especially if the negative outcome expectancy is perceived to be a more immediate proximal health threat.

The general rationale of behavioral treatment is that through skills training, the automatic chain of events (Antecedent → Behavior → Consequences) leading to smoking can be disrupted, and smoking behavior can be replaced with alternative nonsmoking behaviors. The learning of nonsmoking skills occurs through a series of success experiences. As individuals with TUD become more proficient in these skills, their self-efficacy for quitting increases; thereby increasing the likelihood of sustained smoking abstinence in the future. This general theory provides the core of most intensive behavioral TUD treatment programs.

TREATMENT PLANNING

Clinicians typically initiate counseling with patients who smoke through one of two distinct pathways: (1) clinicians may identify them through routine clinical practice in a variety of settings and advise these patients to quit or (2) such patients may approach clinicians with an interest in quitting smoking and seek specific assistance in doing so. In each of these contexts, the methods of behavioral counseling for those who want to quit would be similar. For those who are not ready to quit, methods for moving patients toward initiating a quit attempt and for continuing to assess readiness to quit are indicated (see Motivational Interviewing section). Each of these methods is detailed in the section below entitled Treatment and Technique. A simple set of brief procedures for working with patients who smoke is to follow what has been termed the 5 A's model of intervention: *Ask* patients whether they use tobacco; *Advise* all patients to quit; *Assess* willingness to make a quit attempt; *Assist* patients in making a quit attempt; and *Arrange* follow-up contacts to help prevent recurrence of smoking.[13] In **Figure 74-1**, we also provide a general schematic for treatment planning with patients who smoke. The figure provides different steps for those who are interested and those who are not interested in quitting smoking in the near future. It also highlights the need for continued assessment of smoking status at each stage of intervention and the dynamic nature of interest in quitting.

The first step in effectively treating TUD for any clinician is to ask all patients about tobacco use.[12] Clinicians can ask whether patients had ever smoked, when they last smoked a cigarette, and the typical number of cigarettes they currently smoke per day. Although not a focus of this chapter, screening questions should also be framed to capture all other forms of nicotine (chewing tobacco, snus, EDDDs, synthetic nicotine sources, etc.). Recent research indicates that while a majority of physicians do ask about smoking status and advise patients to quit smoking,[82,83] clinicians do not consistently refer patients to tobacco treatment.[84-87] Further, there are disparities in screening and referring for tobacco treatment with certain groups less likely to receive abstinence assistance including those without health insurance (versus with private health insurance), those in Southern and Western United States geographic regions (versus Northern) and those that do not have a usual place for care (versus those that have one or more places to receive preventive care).[88] The enactment of procedures and systems that routinely identify and document smoking status in health care settings is critical, resulting in increased rates of TUD interventions being delivered by clinicians and increased TUD remission rates by patients at follow-up.[13,89-92] Possible methods of documentation and identification of individuals who smoke or use tobacco include expanded vital sign sheets that incorporate tobacco use status along with blood pressure, pulse, and temperature, and integration of tobacco use assessment and referral into electronic health records.[89]

The second step in treating TUD is to provide clear advice to quit smoking. Individuals with TUD report that physician advice to quit smoking is often an important factor in their deciding to make a quit attempt[93,94] and clinical trials have found that brief advice (<3 minutes) by a clinician to quit smoking increases the odds of abstinence compared to the absence of such advice.[13] Therefore, individuals with TUD should be provided at least a brief intervention at each office visit. Advice is most effective if it is clear ("It is very important for you to quit smoking"), strong ("Quitting smoking is one of the most important things you can do to improve and protect your health"), and personalized ("Smoking increases the risk of heart attacks, which is especially important for you given your family history of heart disease and your high blood pressure").

The third step in treating TUD is to assess readiness to quit smoking among those who are actively smoking. It is also important to provide positive reinforcement to those who have quit smoking and to continue to assess smoking status in those patients at later follow-ups as intervention may be needed to address return to smoking or recurrence of symptoms. Patients present with differing levels of motivation for quitting smoking, and intervention should be based upon patients' readiness to change. As noted above, readiness to change can be viewed as a continuum ranging from being entirely not ready to quit to being actively involved in quitting.[95] In this regard, motivation is not a static trait but a state that fluctuates over time.[96] It is therefore crucial to assess and monitor readiness to quit smoking with all patients who continue to smoke. Doing so can allow a clinician to provide appropriate assistance with quitting smoking at a time in which a given individual with TUD is expressing a willingness to make a quit attempt.

For many clinicians it may be helpful to conceptualize readiness to change among individuals with TUD as falling into three discrete stages of change: precontemplation, contemplation, and preparation.[97] Individuals at the precontemplation stage are not considering stopping smoking in the foreseeable future. Individuals in the contemplation stage are considering making a quit attempt within the next 6 months but have not yet made a firm commitment to change.[98,99] For individuals who smoke in either the precontemplation or contemplation stages (ie, those who are not planning to quit for at least 30 days and who have not made a recent attempt to quit), intervention should be aimed at increasing motivation using methods outlined later in this chapter. Clinicians also should clearly state that they are ready to provide assistance with

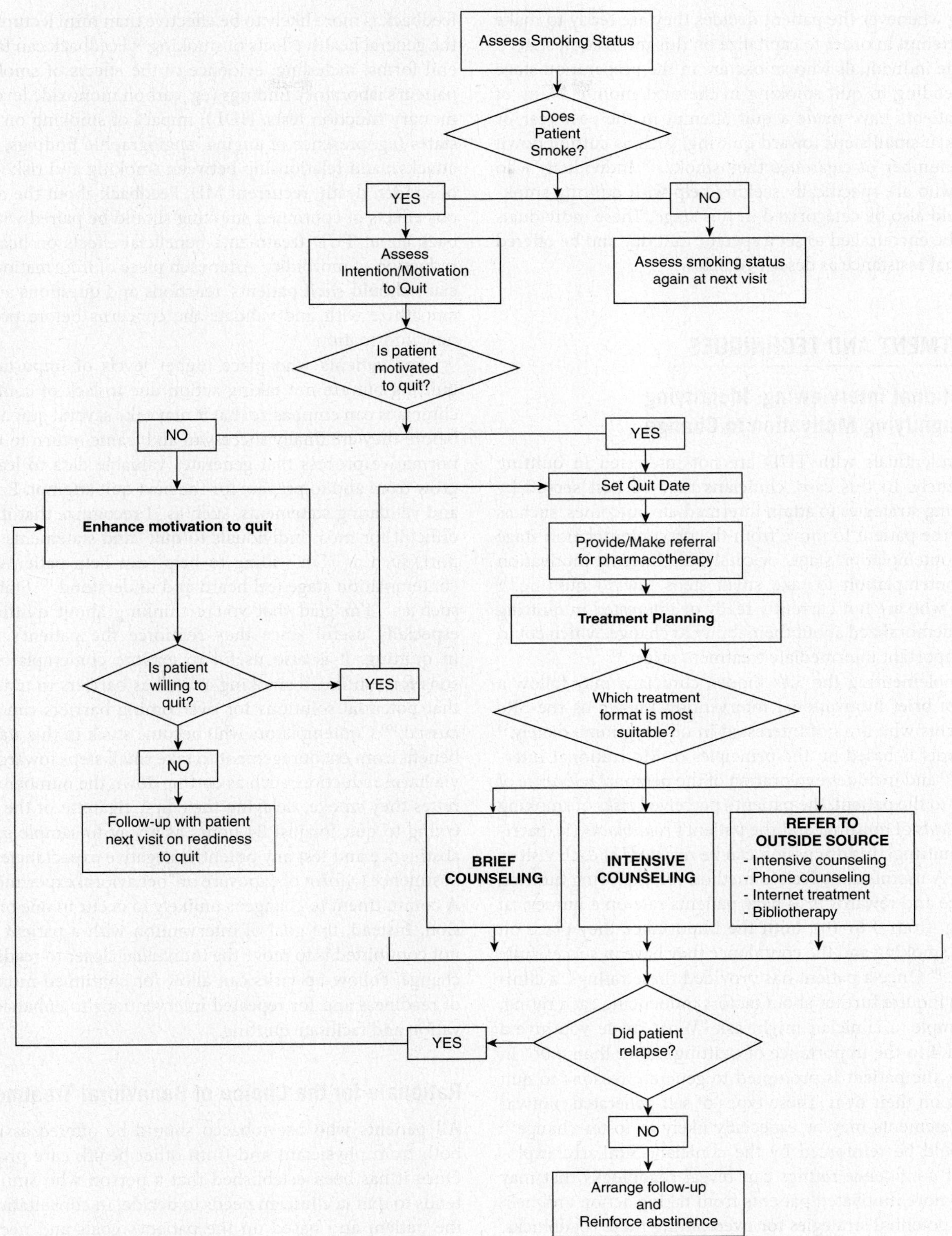

Figure 74-1. Schematic for treating cigarette smoking.

quitting whenever the patient decides they are ready to make a quit attempt in order to capitalize on this motivation state.

Some individuals who smoke are in the preparation stage and intending to quit smoking in the next month. Many of these patients have made a quit attempt in the past year or have taken small steps toward quitting, such as cutting down on the number of cigarettes they smoke.[100] Individuals who smoke who are specifically seeking help with quitting smoking would also be categorized in this stage. These individuals should be encouraged to set a specific quit day and be offered additional assistance as described below.

TREATMENT AND TECHNIQUES

Motivational Interviewing: Identifying and Magnifying Motivation to Change

Many individuals with TUD are not interested in quitting immediately. In this case, clinicians may be best served by developing strategies to attain intermediate outcomes, such as helping the patient to move from the precontemplation stage to the contemplation stage, or catalyzing internal motivation from contemplation to take small steps toward quitting.[100] Patients who are not currently ready or interested in quitting may be demoralized about their ability to change, which could be an important intermediate treatment target.[100]

Complementing the 5A's model, clinicians may follow a model of brief motivational intervention known as the 5R's for patients who are not interested in quitting immediately.[13] This model is based on the principles of Motivational Interviewing[53] and includes exploration of the personal *relevance* of quitting to the patient, the patient's perceived *risks* of smoking and *rewards* of quitting, and the patient's *roadblocks* (ie, barriers) to quitting; this discussion can be *reviewed* at each visit as needed. A useful and effective method for exploring quitting relevance and rewards is to have patients rate on a numerical scale (eg, from 0 to 10), both the importance they place on quitting smoking and the confidence they have in successfully quitting.[101] Once a patient has provided these ratings, a clinician can inquire further about factors influencing each rating. For example, a clinician might ask "What made you give a rating of 4 to the importance of quitting rather than a 0?" In this way, the patient is prompted to generate reasons to quit smoking on their own. These types of self-generated motivational statements may be especially likely to foster change[102] and should be reinforced by the clinician. Similarly, exploration of confidence ratings can reveal roadblocks that may prevent more motivated patients from taking action and help identify potential strategies for overcoming these roadblocks. For example, a clinician might ask, "Why is your confidence a 6 and not a 4?" and then "What would have to happen for your confidence to go from a 6 to an 8?"

For patients who have low importance ratings, personalized information and feedback can raise awareness of the ways in which smoking is affecting their health. Such personalized feedback is more likely to be effective than mini lectures about the general health effects of smoking.[53] Feedback can take several forms, including: evidence of the effects of smoking on patient's laboratory findings (eg, carbon monoxide levels, pulmonary function tests, HDL); impact of smoking on disease states (eg, presence of angina, angiographic findings, asthma attacks); and relationship between smoking and risk (eg, risk of sudden death, recurrent MI). Feedback about the deleterious effects of continued smoking should be paired with feedback about TUD treatment's beneficial effects on health and reduction of morbidity. After each piece of information, clinicians should elicit patients' reactions and questions and then empathize with and validate the concerns before providing new information.

For patients who place higher levels of importance on quitting but are not taking action due to lack of confidence, clinicians can emphasize that it may take several quit attempts before they are finally successful and frame return to use as a normative process that generates valuable data to learn and grow from and to prepare for the next quit attempt. Empathic and validating statements, such as "I recognize that it's really difficult for most individuals to quit" and statements of support, such as "I'm willing to help" can help patients in the contemplation stage feel heard and understood.[100] Statements such as, "I'm glad that you're thinking about quitting" are especially useful since they reinforce the patient's interest in quitting. It is also useful to explore contemplators' reasons for continued smoking as well as barriers to quitting so that potential solutions for overcoming barriers can be discussed.[100] Contemplators who become stuck in this stage may benefit from encouragement to take small steps toward action via harm reduction, such as cutting down the number of cigarettes they smoke, delaying their first cigarette of the day, or trying to quit for just 24 hours as a way to sample smoking abstinence and test any potential negative expectancies about abstinence (a form of exposure or "behavioral experiment").[100] A commitment to change is unlikely to occur in one brief session. Instead, the goal of intervention with a patient who is not committed is to move the individual closer to readiness to change. Follow-up visits can allow for continued monitoring of readiness and for repeated interventions to enhance motivation and facilitate quitting.

Rationale for the Choice of Behavioral Treatments

All patients who use tobacco should be offered assistance, both from physicians and from other health care providers. Once it has been established that a person who smokes intends to quit, a clinician needs to decide, in consultation with the patient and based on the patient's goals and needs, the nature of the assistance that will be provided. Interventions delivered by multiple types of providers increase the likelihood of stopping smoking, suggesting that treatment interventions should be delivered by as many clinicians and types of clinicians as feasible.[13] There is also a strong dose-response relationship between the intensity of treatment contact and treatment outcome.[13] It has been shown that relatively intensive interventions involving 4 or more sessions lasting 10 or more minutes of duration produce higher rates of smoking abstinence than brief interventions. However, there are a number of obstacles to using these more intensive interventions. First, in many settings, clinician time to deliver extended interventions is simply not available. Clinicians also may not possess the relevant training and experience to conduct such interventions. Patients, too, may be reluctant to commit to coming to counseling on a regular basis. For these reasons, brief clinical interventions with appropriate referral to pharmacotherapy and other resources are often most readily implemented in many clinical settings.

Brief Clinical Interventions

The primary component of a brief clinical intervention for tobacco use is helping the patient create a plan of action for quitting. An important step is to review past quit attempts to identify strategies that were successful and to highlight potential obstacles to success. Central to the quit plan is setting a target quit date, ideally within 2 weeks. Setting this quit date allows patients to plan for quitting and to obtain the necessary support for quitting. Patients should be advised to smoke their last cigarette on the night before their quit date so that they wake up nonsmoking. It is important to stress that quitting smoking means avoiding smoking completely (not even a puff), as even one puff of a cigarette can lead to further smoking.

As part of a plan to quit smoking, patients should be encouraged to tell their family and friends about their quit date and to elicit support from these people. For those who live with other individuals who smoke in their household, this might necessitate asking these individuals to refrain from smoking in the house or in front of them and consider cleaning the house to remove any scent of tobacco. Patients also should make sure that they have eliminated all nicotine/tobacco products and associated cues, such as ashtrays and cigarette lighters. Finally, patients should be encouraged to think about their potential triggers for smoking and consider the situations in which they might be likely to return to smoking. Once situations have been identified, the clinician can discuss with the patient potential strategies for handling those high-risk situations.

Additional assistance can be provided in the form of self-help groups such as Nicotine Anonymous and self-help materials or "bibliotherapy." Self-help is an important tool that enhances the capacity of the health care provider to provide information and advice. Print and online materials are available through agencies such as the National Cancer Institute, Public Health Service (PHS), American Cancer Society, American Heart Association, American Lung Association, and the Office on Smoking and Health. A second option is to refer patients to state-funded quitlines. Quitlines are now available in all 50 states. Quitlines often offer 3 to 6 sessions of proactive counseling (ie, the quitline counselor calls the patient to deliver counseling according to the quitline's protocol), and many offer free nicotine replacement therapy for participants. Proactive telephone counseling has been found to be both efficacious and effective.[13,68,103] See **Table 74-1** below for a list of selected TUD resources for patients.

Finally, except where special circumstances exist, all patients willing to quit should be offered pharmacotherapy along with an explanation that such medication can reduce withdrawal symptoms and cravings and increase success rates.[13] First-line pharmacotherapies include nicotine replacement therapies (gum, inhaler, nasal spray, lozenge, or patch), varenicline, and bupropion SR (see Section 8 of this textbook).

TABLE 74-1 Smoking Abstinence Self-help and Other Resources for Patients

Resource	Link to resource
Self-help counseling resources	
Nicotine Anonymous • 12-step program for tobacco use disorder offering virtual and in person meetings	Website: https://www.nicotine-anonymous.org/
Smokefree.Gov • Government website with instructions on quitting smoking and the Smokefree Texting support program and mobile apps to help quit	Website: https://smokefree.gov/; https://smokefree.gov/tools-tips/text-programs
BecomeAnEx.Gov/Mayo Clinic • Web-based resources for quitting smoking and staying quit including access to a community of individuals who formerly smoked	Website: https://www.becomeanex.org/decide-to-quit/
NCI's Clearing the Air booklet • Booklet for preparing to quit and support staying quit	Bibliotherapy resource: https://smokefree.gov/sites/default/files/pdf/clearing-the-air-accessible.pdf Website: https://www.cancer.gov/about-cancer/causes-prevention/risk/tobacco/help-quitting-fact-sheet
Helping a loved one who smokes	
Smokefree.Gov	https://smokefree.gov/help-others-quit/how-to-support-someone-quitting; https://smokefree.gov/help-others-quit/how-to-support-someone-quitting
State quitlines (live telephone counseling + often medication)	Phone: 1–800–QUIT–NOW (1–800–784–8669) NCI's quitline: 1–877–44U–QUIT (1–877–448–7848)

Follow-up

For individuals with TUD who are attempting to quit, providers should schedule a specific time to connect immediately after quit day to reinforce successes and trouble-shoot difficulties, including use and potential side effects of medication. Follow-up contacts also provide an opportunity to work with patients who have only briefly returned to smoking. Clinicians can empathize with patients about the difficulty in maintaining abstinence, help patients view a brief slip as a learning experience that is part of the normal process of quitting, and encourage patients to continue their efforts to quit.

Intensive Clinical Interventions

Intensive clinical interventions involve many of the same components used in brief interventions. However, they add additional components and go into greater depth in specific areas, such as managing stress and coping with high-risk situations. These intensive interventions would be likely to be administered primarily by individuals who specialize in treating TUD. As noted above, more intensive counseling (longer duration sessions and more sessions) tends to produce higher abstinence rates, although evidence for increasing improvements in abstinence rates beyond 90 minutes of total counseling time is lacking.[13] Many of these intensive interventions may be delivered in group settings to increase economy of delivery and also to enhance the social support provided by other patients attempting to quit. While a description of an intensive group behavioral intervention is provided below, more detailed accounts of this intensive intervention are also available.[104]

Preparing for Quitting

We recommend a preparation period prior to quitting smoking, the length of which can vary according to program needs. There are three key objectives for this period. First, patients' motivation to quit and commitment to the program should be clarified and reinforced. Second, a target quit day should be clearly established to allow patients the time to prepare and develop coping strategies for quitting smoking. Third, patients should self-monitor their daily smoking behavior to begin to learn about their smoking triggers (ie, antecedents).

Enhancing Motivation in Patients Who Are Quitting

Even after patients express an intent to quit smoking in the near future, it remains important for clinicians to work to enhance and maintain motivation and commitment to quitting. Being motivated to quit is strongly associated with making a quit attempt.[105] However, a specific commitment to quitting, which can be distinguished from a general desire to quit, has been shown to be a robust predictor of TUD treatment outcome.[106] Individuals with TUD may be ambivalent about the prospect of quitting for a variety of reasons. While acknowledging reasons for quitting, they may have negative expectations and fears about the discomfort of quitting, feel that they are attached to smoking and that they are giving up a friend, lack confidence or hope in their ability to quit, and continue to question whether the health risks could ever really impact them (especially those which are not immediate/proximal). This may be especially true of patients who may have tried in the past to quit and failed (a majority of people who smoke). Acknowledging this ambivalence without directly challenging it can help diffuse some of its power to undermine commitment and to meet the patient where they are at in a patient-centered manner. For example, clinicians can use double-sided reflective statements to highlight both sides of ambivalence[53] (eg, "On the one hand, you find that smoking helps you relax and serves as a reward for a hard day's work, and on the other hand, you know that it is costing you a lot of money, has made it harder for you to be physically active, and is greatly raising your risk of having a heart attack").

For many individuals who smoke, the expected short-term benefits of smoking (eg, "smoking calms my nerves") override the more distal, negative consequences (eg, potentially life-threatening illnesses). The challenge is to move individuals with TUD from general acceptance of potential negative consequences ("Smoking is dangerous to health") to personalized acceptance ("Smoking is dangerous to my *own* health").[107] Encouraging individuals who smoke to consider their cough, for example, or other *current* physical symptoms is one way to make negative consequences more personally salient and immediate. A concurrent focus on the health benefits of quitting may be especially effective in motivating and sustaining efforts to quit smoking.[108] A useful approach to enhance motivation involves having patients write down their specific, personalized reasons for wanting to stop smoking and for wanting to continue smoking. Listing reasons to continue smoking may seem contradictory but can help patients identify likely barriers to quitting. A recently developed treatment grounded in acceptance and commitment therapy approach involves helping individuals who smoke focus on how stopping smoking is consistent with their most salient life values[62] (see Novel Treatments section below for details). As mentioned previously, motivation for quitting smoking needs to be monitored throughout treatment for potential setbacks.

Self-monitoring of Smoking Behavior

The first phase of intensive TUD treatments often involves self-monitoring. Keeping a written record of cigarettes smoked can help increase knowledge about the factors cueing and maintaining smoking behavior. Self-monitoring also interrupts the automatic smoking reflex, encouraging patients to think about every cigarette they smoke and why they smoke it. Often, even without instruction to do so, this procedure of awareness training reduces the number of cigarettes smoked per day.[109] Preprinted cards or "wrap sheets" (wrapped around cigarette pack as a visual cue) can be given to patients to record the time of day and the situation in which each cigarette is smoked (eg, "talking on the phone") with this information ideally recorded prior to the patient smoking the cigarette. Assessment of mood at the time of each cigarette also can be useful. The situational notations allow patients to identify antecedents that trigger their smoking.

Patients may find self-monitoring of their smoking behavior inconvenient. It is important that clinicians present the rationale for self-monitoring clearly and follow through at all sessions by reviewing wrap sheets with patients to highlight the relevance of the information in their quitting efforts. For example, it is useful to ask each patient what they learned about their smoking behavior and its patterns over the course of a typical week; specifically, what moods were common triggers of smoking, during which times of the day did they smoke most often, and which people or events typically triggered their smoking. For those who have trouble remembering to use the wrap sheet, visual or other cues can be recommended (eg, setting daily reminders to track in your cell phone). Modifications can also be made to the wrap sheet based on patient's needs and to reduce inconvenience such as using notes in cell phone to self-monitor or using notes on your computer versus a physical paper wrap sheet. It may also be helpful to share with patients that self-monitoring is a common component of behavioral treatment for most other SUDs and psychiatric disorders (eg, depression).

ABSTINENCE STAGE INTERVENTIONS

Self-management

Self-management (sometimes termed self-control or stimulus control) procedures are a critical component of behavioral smoking interventions. They refer to strategies intended to rearrange environmental cues that "trigger" smoking or to alter the consequences of smoking. Using their wrap sheets, patients develop a list of trigger situations. They then begin to intervene in these situations to break up the smoking behavior chain (situation–urge–smoke) by utilizing one of three general strategies: (1) avoid the trigger situation, (2) alter or change the trigger situation, and (3) use an alternative or substitute in place of the cigarette. Examples of avoiding trigger situations include foregoing a coffee break at work with other individuals who smoke and avoiding social situations involving alcohol. Altering a trigger situation might involve drinking tea or juice in the morning instead of coffee. Alternatives or substitutes for smoking behavior (ideally that are behaviors that are incompatible with smoking) can be used in conjunction with avoiding or altering trigger situations or in situations that cannot be avoided or altered. Possible alternatives include eating sugarless candy or gum, cut-up vegetables such as carrot or celery sticks, toothpicks, relaxation techniques in stressful situations, or activities such as needlework that keep hands busy. Patients should choose strategies they think will work for them and then try out different approaches, rejecting those that are not useful until they have successfully managed all or most trigger situations without smoking.

Social Support

Positive social support both within (eg, from the clinician) and outside of treatment has been shown to increase abstinence.[13,110,111] Social support can be a source of motivation for quitting and of positive reinforcement for maintaining abstinence. Social support also may provide a buffer against stressful life events that might precipitate a recurrence of smoking. Clinicians should encourage patients' efforts at stopping smoking, communicate care and concern for their well-being, and encourage open discussion about their experiences during quitting. Encouraging patients to access social support outside of treatment also may be helpful; this might include making specific requests to friends and family members about steps they can take to support patients' abstinence efforts, and building nonsmoking peer networks comprised of nonsmoking friends and family and those who may be supportive of patient's nonsmoking goals.

Maintenance

Since many patients who initially quit resume smoking within several months of treatment termination,[12] maintenance treatment is a critical issue.[112] The most commonly used behavioral maintenance strategies are based on the Relapse Prevention (RP) model,[74] the main components of which are described below. Research on the effectiveness of RP components has been mixed[113] with RP treatments generally outperforming no-treatment controls, but rarely outperforming credible alternative treatments.[112,114] A notable exception is a study by Stevens and Hollis,[115] in which RP booster sessions produced higher abstinence rates than both social support and no treatment controls. Also, Hall et al.[116] found that extended treatment involving an additional 44 weeks of medication, 9 monthly counseling sessions, and between-session check-up telephone calls resulted in better outcomes than an 8-week protocol. Mounting evidence suggests that extending behavioral treatment and pharmacotherapy improves smoking outcomes.[117,118] Self-help RP materials that are available at no cost via www.smokefree.gov also have been shown to decrease recurrence of use significantly among individuals who recently quit smoking.[119,120]

Identifying and Coping With High-Risk Situations for Return to Smoking

Relapse Prevention theory[74] proposes that the ability to cope with "high-risk" situations for return to use determines an individual's probability of maintaining abstinence. High-risk situations often involve at least one of the following elements: negative moods, positive moods, social situations involving alcohol, and being in the presence of other people who smoke. To help patients identify high-risk situations, a clinician can ask, "If you were to slip and smoke a cigarette after quit day, in what situation would it be?" For each high-risk situation, patients can develop a set of strategies for managing the situation without smoking. They should be reminded that these high-risk situations are functionally similar to the trigger situations they have previously addressed and that they can apply similar self-management strategies (ie, avoid, alter, or use a substitute), as well as other problem-solving skills.

Managing Slips

When patients experience a slip to smoking, they often progress to further smoking and recurrence of disease (ie, full return to regular patterns of smoking). Preventing slips is the best way to achieve smoking abstinence, however this is not possible for many patients given challenges in quitting and staying quit. In the event that a slip happens, a few steps can be taken to manage the slip and regain abstinence. First, a slip is an important time for clinicians to assess motivation or commitment to quitting. Has motivation changed or is the patient ambivalent about quitting? Does the patient support the goal of quitting completely or do they believe that occasional cigarettes are unlikely to be harmful? If motivation has changed, then use of the motivational interventions described above is appropriate. On the other hand, if motivation remains high, then it is important for the clinician and the patient to review the circumstances of the slip to figure out what conditions allowed that brief use to occur. For example, potentially the patient may identify additional "high-risk" situations and can plan for managing these in the future. The lessons learned from the period of brief use are reviewed, and plans for avoiding similar episodes in the future can then be made. These plans often involve application of the coping strategies described above. Additionally, it is very important for clinicians to repeatedly normalize slips as a part of the quitting process and an opportunity to learn and grow from in addition to employing other principles from cognitive therapy such as cognitive restructuring to identify and challenge negative automatic thoughts that may prevent attempting to quit again (eg, "I smoked a cigarette and slipped up, which means I failed and will never quit again").

Lifestyle Change

It is also important for patients with TUD to work to manage general life stress and maintain an overall healthy lifestyle to support smoking abstinence and general wellness. Indeed, stress is a commonly reported barrier to quitting smoking.[121-123] Clinicians can encourage patients to be aware of stress-related symptoms that they experience as a trigger to smoke, and to use behavioral strategies to manage stress such as deep breathing, guided imagery, progressive muscle relaxation, or brief meditation. If the patient is experiencing nicotine withdrawal symptoms that are contributing to the feelings of stress, nicotine replacement therapy (NRT) may be added or adjusted (see Section 8 on pharmacotherapy). Additionally, Marlatt and Gordon[74] discuss the importance of increasing participation in activities that are incompatible with smoking and are a source of pleasure. Patients are encouraged to set aside time as often as possible (ideally, on a daily basis) for this purpose. It is, in this context, clinicians could encourage patients to engage in some type of regular physical activity that the patient finds enjoyable. Indeed, research has consistently demonstrated that engaging in physical exercise reduces craving and withdrawal symptoms in individuals with TUD.[56,124] Some exercise-based interventions for nicotine/tobacco have produced positive results, for example, reference,[125] and research in this area is continuing to grow.[126-128]

OTHER INTENSIVE INTERVENTIONS FOR TOBACCO USE DISORDER

Contingency Management

Contingency management (CM) is a behavioral treatment approach whereby tangible incentives (eg, cash or vouchers) are provided contingent on biochemical evidence of smoking abstinence.[129,130] Contingency management has been demonstrated to be a highly efficacious approach for treating TUD as well as for treating other SUDs (eg, opioid use). CM produces the highest TUD abstinence rates during treatment and has been found to be the most efficacious behavioral treatment for TUD in many underserved populations including those with SUDs who also smoke cigarettes. However, CM is resource intensive and current work is underway to improve the implementation and dissemination of CM in less resourced clinical settings including advocacy for payer coverage (eg, Medicaid) of CM. Contingency management for TUD would for example entail rigorous biochemical monitoring where a patient's urine or saliva samples were monitored weekly, and incentives would be provided contingent on the biochemical result demonstrating smoking abstinence. The larger goal of this approach is to facilitate temporary abstinence from TUD with incentives in order to allow patients to engage with non-SUD reinforcers to support longer term abstinence once incentives are removed. While CM is a highly efficacious treatment modality, treatment effects are not maintained once incentives are removed[129] and thus work is ongoing to test interventions to sustain abstinence beyond the incentivized period.

TUD TREATMENT CONSIDERATIONS FOR SYSTEMATICALLY EXCLUDED POPULATIONS

Racial and Ethnic Subgroups

Black and African Americans

African Americans experience a disproportionate burden of tobacco-related morbidity and mortality.[131,132] The current prevalence of tobacco product use among Black and African Americans (14.4%) is higher than the general population (13.3%).[4] Black and African Americans also have longer smoking histories and have the lowest success in quitting among all racial and ethnic groups.[21,22,133-135] Research has shown that culturally responsive and tailored interventions that include culturally relevant images, language and communication styles, improve tobacco abstinence outcomes for this population.[136-138] For example, culturally specific group-based cognitive-behavior TUD treatment has resulted in higher quit rates and greater adherence to nicotine replace therapy,[136] and greater 7-day point prevalence abstinence[138] among Black and African Americans who smoke. Additionally, culturally specific print content gains more interest than standard materials,[137] and culturally specific tobacco intervention delivered via video-text messages has shown to increase utilization of nicotine replacement therapy among African American adults.[138,139]

Hispanics/Latinos

Hispanics/Latinos are among the largest ethnic groups in the United States.[140] Overall, Hispanics/Latinos smoke at a lower rate (8%) than the general population (13.3%)[3] and tend to smoke fewer cigarettes per day than other groups[141]; however, a higher prevalence of smoking is observed among men, certain subgroups, and within medically underserved communities.[142-144] Furthermore, smoking is a primary contributing risk factor to the leading causes of death among Hispanics/Latinos.[145] Hispanics/Latinos are less likely than other racial groups to be screened for tobacco use or advised to quit,[126,142,146,147] and have lower rates of abstinence than individuals identifying as non-Hispanic White.[21,148] Another study that evaluated the effect of preferred language and cultural specificity in a written TUD intervention found that when participants received the intervention in their preferred language, intended utilization was greater, participants reported smoking fewer cigarettes per day at 2-week follow-up and were more likely to report quitting smoking at 2-week follow-up.[149] Pilot research utilizing culturally and linguistically adapted TUD text messaging has shown uptake and greater adherence to nicotine replacement therapy among Latinos who smoke.[150]

Indigenous American

Although results of the largest RCT to date conducted with Indigenous Americans who smoke[151] suggest that a culturally specific program may be beneficial, more TUD intervention research is needed for this subgroup.

Other Population Subgroups

Additional intervention research is needed for population subgroups such as persons identifying as lesbian, gay, bisexual, or transgender, and persons with disabilities, that have a high prevalence of cigarette smoking and difficulty quitting.[23,49] Much of the TUD research to date has examined behavioral treatments for TUD among predominantly non-Hispanic White samples, thus overall, more research is needed on efficacious TUD treatments for systematically excluded populations.

Individuals With Co-occurring Substance Use Disorders

Individuals with co-occurring substance use disorders (SUDs) have higher prevalence of TUD and less success in quitting smoking.[18,152] All individuals with TUD should be routinely screened for SUDs and those with active untreated SUDs should be offered/referred to SUD treatment. This is especially important given the overwhelming evidence of a bidirectional relationship between SUDs and tobacco use such that substance use increases use of tobacco and decreases success in quitting smoking. Correspondingly, treating SUDs improves tobacco abstinence rates.[131,132] Although individuals with SUDs have lower rates of abstinence success compared to the general population, they should still be offered current first-line TUD treatments.

The majority of research on this topic has focused on TUD for individuals with alcohol use disorder. For example, alcohol use is involved in about 25% of all brief recurrences of smoking,[153-155] and up to 40% of brief recurrences of smoking among people who drink heavily.[156] The risk of smoking is four times higher on days when moderate drinking occurs (1-3 drinks for women and 1-4 drinks for men) compared to days when no drinking occurs, and heavy drinking (4+ drinks in a day for women, 5+ drinks for men) doubles the risk of brief recurrences of smoking compared to moderate drinking.[156] Heavy alcohol use is one risk factor that commonly co-occurs with smoking[157-159] and impedes treatment efforts.[160] Alcohol consumption is the third leading cause of death in the United States,[161] and excessive drinking results in numerous well-documented health, mental health, and social problems.[162] The combined effects of excessive drinking and smoking are enormous. For example, smoking and heavy drinking combine to produce especially negative consequences on brain morphology and function,[163-166] and smoking negates any possible cardioprotective effects of regular drinking.[167,168] Furthermore, a multiplicative effect operates when smoking is combined with heavy drinking, conferring markedly greater risk for oral, pharyngeal, laryngeal, and esophageal cancers relative to just smoking, just drinking, or neither smoking nor drinking.[2,169-171] Abstinence from smoking,[169,170] as well as abstinence from drinking,[172] can significantly reduce cancer risk.

A recent clinical trial found that incorporating a brief alcohol intervention for heavy drinking patients who also smoke led to significantly lower levels of drinking and increased the odds of smoking abstinence.[173] However, both effects were relatively small. Another trial involving callers to a quitline who drank heavily demonstrated that those who received a brief alcohol intervention in addition to TUD counseling achieved higher smoking abstinence rates compared to those who received TUD counseling alone. There were no group differences in heavy drinking outcomes, but other analyses suggested that the difference in smoking outcomes may have been attributable to reduced heavy drinking.[174] More research in this area is needed, but it appears that conducting brief alcohol interventions in conjunction with nicotine/tobacco treatment with people who drink excessively is feasible and may benefit both behaviors. The NIAAA Clinician's Guide provides a set of strategies for conducting brief interventions for people who drink heavily.[175] Heavy drinking is defined as either 4+ or 5+ drinks for women and men, respectively, or drinking 8+/15+ drinks per week for women and men, respectively. Steps for brief alcohol intervention include assessing alcohol use and problems, providing clear advice to reduce drinking to those who are drinking at medically unsafe levels, assessing readiness to change drinking, and helping patients set drinking goals and make plans for achieving those goals. It is also important to educate patients that any alcohol use and especially heavy drinking greatly increases the odds of recurrence of smoking. Stressing that avoiding heavy drinking may increase the odds of quitting smoking successfully is one way of using motivation to quit smoking to encourage changes in heavy drinking as well.

There is a growing body of work examining behavioral treatments for TUD among those with other SUDs. Of all of the substance use disorders, opioid use disorder (OUD) appears to be associated with the highest smoking rates and the least success in quitting, particularly for those with OUD not in OUD treatment and actively using nonprescribed opioids.[129,176,177] Several hypotheses have been posited to explain the high rates of smoking and poor abstinence outcomes in this population including evidence of neurobiological and clinical interactions between opioids and nicotine such that opioid administration leads to dose-dependent increases in smoking and shared cues (eg, urges) between the two substances particularly around the period of peak medication treatment for opioid use disorder effects, higher levels of nicotine use disorder, nicotine withdrawal discomfort and co-occurring psychiatric symptoms, and finally, lower adherence to behavioral and pharmacological treatments.[177-179] All individuals with OUD should be offered TUD treatment. Of note, individuals in OUD treatment (eg, receiving medication treatment for OUD) are potentially good candidates for TUD interventions as they are significantly less likely to die of their OUD and to experience OUD-related negative consequences.[180,181] However, individuals not in OUD treatment who express interest in quitting tobacco smoking should also be offered TUD treatment and could potentially benefit from concurrent OUD and TUD treatment, though research is still ongoing to determine the optimal timing of TUD treatment for individuals with OUD and other SUDs in relation to their SUD treatment. In terms of TUD treatment approaches in this population, CM is the most effective treatment for TUD in those with OUD stable in their OUD treatment while other behavioral treatments, particularly when offered in the absence of pharmacotherapy, appear suboptimal for those with OUD.[177] More research is sorely needed to identify effective behavioral treatments for those with OUD and other SUDs. Unfortunately, individuals with SUDs face additional unique social-environmental barriers to quitting smoking in that many SUD treatment staff smoke cigarettes, hold misconceptions about smoking (eg, quitting smoking would be "too much" for a patient in SUD treatment to take on) and there is high social acceptability of smoking in SUD treatment, which has been found to be associated with less receipt of abstinence services by patients with SUDs.[182-185]

Psychiatric Populations

Individuals with psychiatric disorders are almost twice as likely to smoke as those without a psychiatric disorder.[5,18,186] They also smoke more cigarettes per day, and are less likely to quit.[186] Psychotic disorders, mood disorders, anxiety disorders, and attention deficit hyperactivity disorder are among the most common psychiatric problems among people who smoke.[187] Despite the high prevalence of smoking in this population, evidence from routine practice indicates there are low rates of identification and treatment of TUD among patients treated by psychiatrists[82] and psychologists.[95] Similar to individuals with SUD, this disparity may be a result of perceptions that patients are unmotivated to quit, limited provider time, concerns about possible harms associated with quitting smoking on other psychiatric symptoms, and limited provider training on treating TUD in psychiatric patients.[82,185,188,189]

Evidence suggests that psychological interventions such as motivational interviewing and cognitive-behavioral therapy are effective in treating TUD in psychiatric patients.[190] Consistent with recommendations in the Clinical Practice Guidelines for Treating Tobacco Use,[24] the general treatment strategies outlined earlier in the chapter may be the most appropriate methods of reducing smoking rates among psychiatric patients. However, certain clinical characteristics of psychiatric patients and contextual factors present only in psychiatric settings should be taken into account when applying behavioral treatments for smoking.

In comparison to psychiatric patients without TUD, psychiatric patients with TUD are more likely to have sociodemographic risk factors that could in lead to poorer smoking outcomes including being divorced or separated, disabled, and uninsured, and have fewer years of education.[191,192] Psychiatric patients who smoke have lower global functioning, poorer psychiatric treatment adherence relative to psychiatric patients who do not smoke.[191] Thus, patients with co-occurring TUD and other psychiatric disorders may be encountering severe and complex psychosocial problems, which should be considered by clinicians. Despite this, there is mounting evidence that individuals who smoke with mental illness are motivated to quit[193] and are capable of quitting with use of evidence-based treatment approaches.[190,194] Thus, psychiatric patients who smoke (even those with greater levels of psychosocial problems) would benefit from being offered TUD treatment.

Another clinical characteristic that may differ in those with versus without co-occurring psychiatric problems is nicotine withdrawal. Evidence suggests that individuals with TUD with co-occurring mental health diagnoses are more likely to experience nicotine withdrawal symptoms when discontinuing tobacco use.[195] Further, increased severity of withdrawal symptoms and physiological dependence may explain the relationship between psychological distress and difficulty quitting smoking.[195] Together, these findings suggest that psychiatric patients may potentially benefit from increased assessment and treatment to buffer the effects of nicotine withdrawal. Despite risk of more severe withdrawal in the short-term, evidence demonstrates that nicotine/tobacco abstinence does not worsen, and in fact improves, psychiatric functioning over the long-term.[190,196] Psychiatric patients also are more likely to experience cognitive problems, as disorders such as major depression and psychosis often present with disturbances in memory, concentration, and thinking.[6] Nonetheless, studies have demonstrated[190] and current guidelines[24] recommend that evidence-based treatments, such as those that use skill-building and motivational enhancement techniques can be applied to psychiatric patients including those with psychotic disorders,[197,198] though modifications should be made to meet the needs of this population. Modifications may include (1) ensuring that cognitive processing demands do not exceed patients' capacity; (2) using devices for remembering, such as notices, schedules, and diaries, and for organizing and monitoring the correct order of task behaviors; (3) prompting or using supportive reminder cues, which may be more appropriate than teaching skills or imparting information; and (4) considering the social and financial limitations of individuals with severe mental illness when designing potential rewards and alternate behaviors and strategies to smoking.[199-201]

A major contextual issue specific to the inpatient psychiatric setting that should be considered when planning TUD treatment is the smoking policy of the psychiatric treatment program. Although evidence from hospitals that have implemented smoking bans does not support notions that patients' psychiatric status will deteriorate after discontinuing tobacco use,[202,203] it is important to consult with inpatient staff when implementing a TUD treatment. If there is resistance, education should be provided regarding how the benefits of TUD services offered in this setting outweigh risks, including that less smoking may enable lower doses of psychiatric medications and fewer side effects (due to tobacco's effects on inducing hepatic enzymes). Relatedly, if cigarettes are used as reinforcers in a psychiatric treatment program, it is important to work with staff to develop alternative noncigarette reinforcers that can be used to promote healthy behaviors.

Addressing and Co-occurring Tobacco and Psychiatric Problems

Increasingly, attention has been paid to the important roles mood and anxiety symptoms play in impeding efforts at smoking abstinence. Cigarette smoking is disproportionately higher among people with depression than among people in the general U.S. population.[18,204,205] In 2017, nearly a quarter of those with depression also smoked tobacco, compared to only 15.6% in those without depression.[206] Data from a nationally representative sample of adults in the United States indicated that quit ratios were consistently lower among individuals with past-year depression who smoke compared to those without depression.[206] A number of studies have shown that having current elevated depressive symptoms, for example, references[207,208] or significant affective distress at the beginning of treatment[209,210] and after quitting[211-213] predicts poor treatment outcomes. Additional evidence suggests that adults with anxiety disorders have higher rates of cigarette smoking than those without anxiety[214,215] and lower rates of successful abstinence.[216]

Given high rates of co-occurring TUD and psychiatric problems, there have been efforts to develop targeted interventions for this population. For example, Brown et al. developed a TUD treatment[217] that incorporates cognitive-behavioral therapy for depression and found that this was particularly efficacious for patients with co-occurring smoking and recurrent major depressive disorder (MDD), even when equating for therapist contact time. Subsequent analyses of pooled data from three studies of Hall et al.[218-220] revealed that people with co-occurring smoking and recurrent MDD who received cognitive-behavioral depression skills training were 2.4 times more likely to be abstinent at 12-month follow-up compared to people with co-occurring smoking and recurrent MDD who received the control conditions.[221] Thus, evidence suggests that adding a depression management component to standard TUD treatment is efficacious for people who smoke with a history of recurrent MDD, although the mechanism by which this effect is achieved does not appear to be through the reduction of depressive symptoms. Behavioral activation,[222] an efficacious treatment approach for depression in which individuals are assisted with increasing the frequency of positively reinforcing activities in their lives that are consistent with their goals and values, has also been shown to improve treatment outcomes among adults with TUD and depression.[223]

Emotional vulnerability factors, such as distress intolerance (ie, perceived inability to tolerate emotional distress) and anxiety sensitivity (ie, fear of anxiety-related symptoms) were identified as possible mechanisms to explain the relationship between high rates of smoking among adults with emotional disorders. Subsequently, a theoretical model was proposed to explain the relationship between emotional disorders and smoking.[224] Specifically, this model proposes that transdiagnostic vulnerability factors, such as anhedonia (ie, decreased experience of pleasure), distress tolerance, and anxiety sensitivity, which underlie emotional disorders, such as depression and anxiety, amplify the perceived reinforcing effects of smoking on affect and contribute to smoking onset, maintenance, and abstinence.[224] Research on targeted interventions for transdiagnostic vulnerabilities and smoking is emerging. To date, novel interventions for anxiety sensitivity[224] and distress intolerance[58] among adults with TUD have shown promise for smoking abstinence.

NOVEL TREATMENT APPROACH IN DEVELOPMENT

Acceptance and Commitment and Mind-Body Therapies

Emerging work suggests that some components of Acceptance and Commitment Therapy (ACT) may be useful to incorporate in behavioral TUD treatments.[225] ACT is a third-wave newer behavioral treatment derived from mindfulness- and exposure-based therapies. Individuals are encouraged to be open and willing to experience any thoughts and feelings that arise and experience them without judgement and to use life values (eg, health, relationships) to guide behavior (rather than avoidance or reduction of distress and discomfort with the latter being the goal of CBT-based treatments).[226] Research suggests that an individual's willingness and ability to tolerate discomfort (eg, "negative" thoughts and feelings, cravings) can help promote positive TUD outcomes.[227-229] These findings have led to the testing of incorporation of novel, acceptance-based coping strategies into intensive clinical interventions.[57-61,63-65,228,230,231] Mindfulness interventions for tobacco use focused on decoupling associations between cravings and smoking have also been used increasingly in TUD treatment. More research is needed prior to broad dissemination of these approaches or prior to recommending these treatments as stand-alone approaches to TUD treatment. Indeed, there is limited evidence that mindfulness interventions are effective as standalone treatment for smoking. According to a 2022 Cochrane review, individuals who received mindfulness training were no more likely to quit smoking than individuals who received intensity-matched TUD treatments or no support.[232] Mindfulness interventions showed benefits (eg, stress reduction) as a complementary treatment to be added with existing TUD treatments mentioned earlier in the chapter[233] and is a useful skill for clinicians to have in their toolkit.

NOVEL METHODS OF INTERVENTION DELIVERY

Telephone counseling via tobacco quitlines is now available around the world[234] and has well-established efficacy in enhancing abstinence success.[68] Technology-based modalities may be more cost-effective[235] and may have the potential for reaching a wider range of individuals with TUD who may not have otherwise had access to treatment (eg, rural and poor populations). Therefore, technology-based interventions may ultimately have a high overall impact on public health (ie, number of patients able to achieve TUD remission) than more intensive, face-to-face treatments.[236] Evidence for the efficacy of other technology-based interventions is increasing,[69-72] and this area of research continues to expand rapidly particularly in light of the increased use of these and interest in these modalities during the COVID-19 pandemic.[237]

Text messaging interventions for example involve mobile phone text messaging of personalized TUD support through automated motivational messages. Messages can suggest behavioral changes and provide positive feedback, and in some cases also allow patients to request additional assistance as needed. Several randomized trials have found that text messaging is effective for short- and long-term abstinence. In a 2019 meta-analysis, automated text-based interventions increased 6-month abstinence compared with minimal support.[238] Furthermore, the addition of text messaging to another existing evidence-based TUD intervention was more effective than the existing intervention alone, suggesting additive effects of text messaging support.

Mobile TUD applications (apps) on smart phones have also proliferated and have the potential to be useful as behavioral therapy tools; however, studies of TUD apps have determined there is often low adherence to clinical practice guidelines.[239-242]

Several types of behavioral interventions through mobile phones are being studied, including short video clips and cognitive-behavioral tips to quit smoking; however, rigorous studies of the long-term effects of mobile phone apps on smoking abstinence have not yet been conducted.[238,243,244]

SUMMARY AND CONCLUSIONS

Treating TUD is a high priority for improving public health. Behavioral interventions increase abstinence rates and should be regularly applied in a range of settings including primary care settings, addiction treatment settings, and psychiatric settings. Combining behavioral interventions with pharmacotherapy produces the highest rates of success during treatment. Nonetheless, rates of sustained abstinence are relatively low even when the most intensive interventions are applied, and return to use is common when treatment ends. Therefore, multiple attempts at quitting are often needed, and clinicians should continue to follow up with patients who have made a quit attempt in order to reinforce abstinence, encourage new quit attempts and offer continued treatment for those who have returned to use, and normalize the recovery process. Disparities in smoking and quitting tobacco persist with certain groups less likely to quit smoking even when using effective treatments (eg, those with co-occurring SUD and psychiatric disorders). Although there is empirical support for specific behavioral interventions to target specific co-occurring issues with smoking, such as current heavy drinking and a history of recurrent MDD among those who smoke cigarettes, more research in this area is needed across a larger array of comorbidities and risk factors to determine whether such targeted interventions can substantially improve overall quit rates in these historically excluded and underserved populations. Additionally, as the tobacco product landscape changes and novel nicotine and tobacco products emerge on the marketplace (eg, EDDDs), additional research is needed to develop effective abstinence interventions for individuals who use these products and want to quit. Regardless, clinicians should offer behavioral treatment to all individuals who use tobacco and take a patient-centered approach to tailor their treatment approach to individual's stage of change and specific treatment goals.

REFERENCES

1. National Center for Chronic Disease Prevention and Health Promotion (U.S.) Office on Smoking and Health. *The Health Consequences of Smoking—50 Years of Progress: A Report of the Surgeon General.* Centers for Disease Control and Prevention (U.S.). Accessed August 30, 2022. http://www.ncbi.nlm.nih.gov/books/NBK179276/
2. American Cancer Society. *Cancer Facts & Figures 2016.* American Cancer Society; 2016.
3. Current Cigarette Smoking Among Adults—United States, 2011. Published online November 9, 2012. https://www.cdc.gov/mmwr/preview/mmwrhtml/mm6144a2.htm
4. Cornelius ME, Wang TW, Jamal A, Loretan CG, Neff LJ. Tobacco product use among adults—United States, 2019. *MMWR Morb Mortal Wkly Rep.* 2020;69(46):1736-1742. doi:10.15585/mmwr.mm6946a4
5. Creamer MR, Wang TW, Babb S, et al. Tobacco product use and cessation indicators among adults—United States, 2018. *MMWR Morb Mortal Wkly Rep.* 2019;68(45):1013-1019. doi:10.15585/mmwr.mm6845a2
6. American Psychiatric Association. *Diagnostic and Statistical Manual of Mental Disorders.* DSM-5-TR. American Psychiatric Association Publishing; 2022. doi:10.1176/appi.books.9780890425787
7. Chou SP, Goldstein RB, Smith SM, et al. The epidemiology of DSM-5 nicotine use disorder: results from the National Epidemiologic Survey on Alcohol and Related Conditions-III. *J Clin Psychiatry.* 2016;77(10):1404-1412. doi:10.4088/JCP.15m10114
8. Centers for Disease Control. Smokers' beliefs about the health benefits of smoking cessation—20 U.S. Communities, 1989. *Morb Mortal Wkly Rep.* 1990;39(38):653-656. https://www.cdc.gov/mmwr/preview/mmwrhtml/00001779.htm
9. Ahluwalia IB, Smith T, Arrazola RA, et al. Current tobacco smoking, quit attempts, and knowledge about smoking risks among persons aged ≥15 years—Global Adult Tobacco Survey, 28 Countries, 2008-2016. *MMWR Morb Mortal Wkly Rep.* 2018;67(38):1072-1076. doi:10.15585/mmwr.mm6738a7
10. Babb S, Malarcher A, Schauer G, Asman K, Jamal A. Quitting smoking among adults—United States, 2000-2015. *MMWR Morb Mortal Wkly Rep.* 2017;65(52):1457-1464. doi:10.15585/mmwr.mm6552a1
11. Lavinghouze SR, Malarcher A, Jama A, Neff L, Debrot K, Whalen L. Trends in quit attempts among adult cigarette smokers—United States, 2001-2013. *MMWR Morb Mortal Wkly Rep.* 2015;64(40):1129-1135. doi:10.15585/mmwr.mm6440a1
12. Hughes JR, Keely J, Naud S. Shape of the relapse curve and long-term abstinence among untreated smokers. *Addiction.* 2004;99(1):29-38. doi:10.1111/j.1360-0443.2004.00540.x
13. Fiore MC, Jaén CR, Baker TB, et al. *Treating Tobacco Use and Dependence: 2008 Update. Clinical Practice Guideline.* U.S. Department of Health and Human Services. Public Health Service; 2008.
14. Chaiton M, Diemert L, Cohen JE, et al. Estimating the number of quit attempts it takes to quit smoking successfully in a longitudinal cohort of smokers. *BMJ Open.* 2016;6(6):e011045. doi:10.1136/bmjopen-2016-011045
15. Steinberg MB, Schmelzer AC, Richardson DL, Foulds J. The case for treating tobacco dependence as a chronic disease. *Ann Intern Med.* 2008;148(7):554-556. doi:10.7326/0003-4819-148-7-200804010-00012
16. Bernstein SL, Toll BA. Ask about smoking, not quitting: a chronic disease approach to assessing and treating tobacco use. *Addict Sci Clin Pract.* 2019;14(1):29. doi:10.1186/s13722-019-0159-z
17. Han B, Volkow ND, Blanco C, Tipperman D, Einstein EB, Compton WM. Trends in prevalence of cigarette smoking among us adults with major depression or substance use disorders, 2006-2019. *JAMA.* 2022;327(16):1566. doi:10.1001/jama.2022.4790
18. Lasser K, Boyd JW, Woolhandler S, Himmelstein DU, McCormick D, Bor DH. Smoking and mental illness: a population-based prevalence study. *JAMA.* 2000;284(20):2606. doi:10.1001/jama.284.20.2606
19. Ziedonis D, Hitsman B, Beckham JC, et al. Tobacco use and cessation in psychiatric disorders: National Institute of Mental Health report. *Nicotine Tob Res.* 2008;10(12):1691-1715. doi:10.1080/14622200802443569
20. Heffner JL, Strawn JR, DelBello MP, Strakowski SM, Anthenelli RM. The co-occurrence of cigarette smoking and bipolar disorder: phenomenology and treatment considerations: cigarette smoking and bipolar disorder. *Bipolar Disord.* 2011;13(5-6):439-453. doi:10.1111/j.1399-5618.2011.00943.x
21. Trinidad DR, Pérez-Stable EJ, White MM, Emery SL, Messer K. A nationwide analysis of us racial/ethnic disparities in smoking behaviors, smoking cessation, and cessation-related factors. *Am J Public Health.* 2011;101(4):699-706. doi:10.2105/AJPH.2010.191668
22. U.S. Department of Health and Human Services. *Office of Disease Prevention and Health Promotion.* Healthy People; 2030. Accessed June 12, 2023. https://health.gov/healthypeople
23. Wang TW, Asman K, Gentzke AS, et al. Tobacco product use among adults—United States, 2017. *MMWR Morb Mortal Wkly Rep.* 2018;67(44):1225-1232. doi:10.15585/mmwr.mm6744a2
24. A clinical practice guideline treating tobacco use and dependence 2008 update. A U.S. Public Health Service report. *Am J Prev Med.* 2008;35(2):158-176. doi:10.1016/j.amepre.2008.04.009
25. Cunningham P. Patient engagement during medical visits and smoking cessation counseling. *JAMA Intern Med.* 2014;174(8):1291. doi:10.1001/jamainternmed.2014.2170
26. Wackowski OA, Bover Manderski MT, Delnevo CD. Smokers' sources of e-cigarette awareness and risk information. *Prev Med Rep.* 2015;2:906-910. doi:10.1016/j.pmedr.2015.10.006
27. Graham AL, Amato MS, Cha S, Jacobs MA, Bottcher MM, Papandonatos GD. Effectiveness of a vaping cessation text message program among young adult e-cigarette users: a randomized clinical trial. *JAMA Intern Med.* 2021;181(7):923. doi:10.1001/jamainternmed.2021.1793
28. McVea KLSP. Evidence for clinical smoking cessation for adolescents. *Health Psychol.* 2006;25(5):558-562. doi:10.1037/0278-6133.25.5.558
29. Curry SJ, Mermelstein RJ, Sporer AK. Therapy for specific problems: youth tobacco cessation. *Annu Rev Psychol.* 2009;60(1):229-255. doi:10.1146/annurev.psych.60.110707.163659
30. Curry SJ, Mermelstein RJ, Emery SL, et al. A national evaluation of community-based youth cessation programs: end of program and twelve-month outcomes. *Am J Community Psychol.* 2013;51(1-2):15-29. doi:10.1007/s10464-012-9496-8
31. Cavallo DA, Cooney JL, Duhig AM, et al. Combining cognitive behavioral therapy with contingency management for smoking cessation in adolescent smokers: a preliminary comparison of two different CBT formats. *Am J Addict.* 2007;16(6):468-474. doi:10.1080/10550490701641173
32. Simon P, Kong G, Cavallo DA, Krishnan-Sarin S. Update of adolescent smoking cessation interventions: 2009-2014. *Curr Addict Rep.* 2015;2(1):15-23. doi:10.1007/s40429-015-0040-4
33. Stanton A, Grimshaw G. Tobacco cessation interventions for young people. *Cochrane Database Syst Rev.* 2013;8:CD003289. doi:10.1002/14651858.CD003289.pub5
34. Sussman S, Sun P, Dent CW. A meta-analysis of teen cigarette smoking cessation. *Health Psychol.* 2006;25(5):549-557. doi:10.1037/0278-6133.25.5.549
35. Becker TD, Rice TR. Youth vaping: a review and update on global epidemiology, physical and behavioral health risks, and clinical considerations. *Eur J Pediatr.* 2022;181(2):453-462. doi:10.1007/s00431-021-04220-x
36. Bold K, Kong G, Cavallo D, Davis D, Jackson A, Krishnan-Sarin S. School-based e-cigarette cessation programs: what do youth want? *Addict Behav.* 2022;125:107167. doi:10.1016/j.addbeh.2021.107167
37. Gaiha SM, Halpern-Felsher B. Stemming the tide of youth e-cigarette use: promising progress in the development and evaluation of e-cigarette

prevention and cessation programs. *Addict Behav*. 2021;120:106960. doi:10.1016/j.addbeh.2021.106960
38. Berg CJ, Krishnan N, Graham AL, Abroms LC. A synthesis of the literature to inform vaping cessation interventions for young adults. *Addict Behav*. 2021;119:106898. doi:10.1016/j.addbeh.2021.106898
39. Burnham JC. American physicians and tobacco use: two Surgeons General, 1929 and 1964. *Bull Hist Med*. 1989;63(1):1-31.
40. Tate C. *Cigarette Wars: The Triumph of "The Little White Slaver"*. Oxford University Press; 1999.
41. U.S. Department of Health Education, and Welfare. *Smoking and Health: Report of the Advisory Committee of the Surgeon General of the Public Health Service*. U.S. DHEW; 1964.
42. U.S. Department of Health and Human Services. *Reducing the Health Consequences of Smoking: 25 Years of Progress. A Report of the Surgeon General*. U.S. Department of Health and Human Services, Public Health Service, Centers for Disease Control, National Center for Chronic Disease Prevention and Health Promotion, Office on Smoking and Health; 1989. DHHS Publication No. (CDC) 89-8411.
43. Solberg LI, Boyle RG, Davidson G, Magnan S, Link Carlson C, Alesci NL. Aids to quitting tobacco use: how important are they outside controlled trials? *Prev Med*. 2001;33(1):53-58. doi:10.1006/pmed.2001.0853
44. Willemsen MC, Wiebing M, van Emst A, Zeeman G. Helping smokers to decide on the use of efficacious smoking cessation methods: a randomized controlled trial of a decision aid. *Addiction*. 2006;101(3):441-449. doi:10.1111/j.1360-0443.2006.01349.x
45. Hung WT, Dunlop SM, Perez D, Cotter T. Use and perceived helpfulness of smoking cessation methods: results from a population survey of recent quitters. *BMC Public Health*. 2011;11:592. doi:10.1186/1471-2458-11-592
46. Shiffman S, Brockwell SE, Pillitteri JL, Gitchell JG. Use of smoking-cessation treatments in the United States. *Am J Prev Med*. 2008;34(2):102-111. doi:10.1016/j.amepre.2007.09.033
47. Caraballo RS, Shafer PR, Patel D, Davis KC, McAfee TA. Quit methods used by us adult cigarette smokers, 2014-2016. *Prev Chronic Dis*. 2017;14:E32. doi:10.5888/pcd14.160600
48. Zhu S, Melcer T, Sun J, Rosbrook B, Pierce JP. Smoking cessation with and without assistance: a population-based analysis. *Am J Prev Med*. 2000;18(4):305-311. doi:10.1016/s0749-3797(00)00124-0
49. U.S. Department of Health and Human Services. *Reducing Tobacco Use: A Report of the Surgeon General*. CDC, National Center for Chronic Disease Prevention and Health Promotion, Office on Smoking and Health; 2000.
50. Kottke TE. Attributes of successful smoking cessation interventions in medical practice: a meta-analysis of 39 controlled trials. *JAMA*. 1988;259(19):2882. doi:10.1001/jama.1988.03720190050031
51. Cummings SR, Coates TJ, Richard RJ, et al. Training physicians in counseling about smoking cessation. A randomized trial of the "Quit for Life" program. *Ann Intern Med*. 1989;110(8):640-647. doi:10.7326/0003-4819-110-8-640
52. Lando HA. A comparison of excessive and rapid smoking in the modification of chronic smoking behavior. *J Consult Clin Psychol*. 1975;43(3):350-355. doi:10.1037/h0076741
53. Miller WR, Rollnick S. *Motivational Interviewing: Preparing People for Change*. 2nd ed. Guilford Press; 2002.
54. Hettema JE, Hendricks PS. Motivational interviewing for smoking cessation: a meta-analytic review. *J Consult Clin Psychol*. 2010;78(6):868-884. doi:10.1037/a0021498
55. Heckman CJ, Egleston BL, Hofmann MT. Efficacy of motivational interviewing for smoking cessation: a systematic review and meta-analysis. *Tob Control*. 2010;19(5):410-416. doi:10.1136/tc.2009.033175
56. Ussher MH, Taylor A, Faulkner G. Exercise interventions for smoking cessation. *Cochrane Database Syst Rev*. 2008;4:CD002295. doi:10.1002/14651858.CD002295.pub3
57. Shiffman S, Kassel J, Gwaltney C, McChargue D. Relapse prevention for smoking. In: Marlatt GA, Donovan DM, eds. *Relapse Prevention: Maintenance Strategies in the Treatment of Addictive Behaviors*. Guilford Press; 2005:92-129.
58. Bricker JB, Mull KE, Kientz JA, et al. Randomized, controlled pilot trial of a smartphone app for smoking cessation using acceptance and commitment therapy. *Drug Alcohol Depend*. 2014;143:87-94. doi:10.1016/j.drugalcdep.2014.07.006
59. Brown RA, Reed KMP, Bloom EL, et al. Development and preliminary randomized controlled trial of a distress tolerance treatment for smokers with a history of early lapse. *Nicotine Tob Res*. 2013;15(12):2005-2015. doi:10.1093/ntr/ntt093
60. Bricker J, Wyszynski C, Comstock B, Heffner JL. Pilot randomized controlled trial of web-based acceptance and commitment therapy for smoking cessation. *Nicotine Tob Res*. 2013;15(10):1756-1764. doi:10.1093/ntr/ntt056
61. Bricker JB, Bush T, Zbikowski SM, Mercer LD, Heffner JL. Randomized trial of telephone-delivered acceptance and commitment therapy versus cognitive behavioral therapy for smoking cessation: a pilot study. *Nicotine Tob Res*. 2014;16(11):1446-1454. doi:10.1093/ntr/ntu102
62. Brown RA, Palm KM, Strong DR, et al. Distress tolerance treatment for early-lapse smokers: rationale, program description, and preliminary findings. *Behav Modif*. 2008;32(3):302-332. doi:10.1177/0145445507309024
63. Gifford EV, Kohlenberg BS, Hayes SC, et al. Acceptance-based treatment for smoking cessation. *Behav Ther*. 2004;35:689-705.
64. Brewer JA, Mallik S, Babuscio TA, et al. Mindfulness training for smoking cessation: results from a randomized controlled trial. *Drug Alcohol Depend*. 2011;119(1-2):72-80. doi:10.1016/j.drugalcdep.2011.05.027
65. Bricker JB, Mann SL, Marek PM, Liu J, Peterson AV. Telephone-delivered acceptance and commitment therapy for adult smoking cessation: a feasibility study. *Nicotine Tob Res*. 2010;12(4):454-458. doi:10.1093/ntr/ntq002
66. Gifford EV, Kohlenberg BS, Hayes SC, et al. Does acceptance and relationship focused behavior therapy contribute to bupropion outcomes? A randomized controlled trial of functional analytic psychotherapy and acceptance and commitment therapy for smoking cessation. *Behav Ther*. 2011;42(4):700-715. doi:10.1016/j.beth.2011.03.002
67. Ubhi HK, Michie S, Kotz D, van Schayck OCP, Selladurai A, West R. Characterising smoking cessation smartphone applications in terms of behaviour change techniques, engagement and ease-of-use features. *Transl Behav Med*. 2016;6(3):410-417. doi:10.1007/s13142-015-0352-x
68. Stead LF, Hartmann-Boyce J, Perera R, Lancaster T. Telephone counselling for smoking cessation. *Cochrane Database Syst Rev*. 2013;8:CD002850. doi:10.1002/14651858.CD002850.pub3
69. Graham AL, Carpenter KM, Cha S, et al. Systematic review and meta-analysis of Internet interventions for smoking cessation among adults. *Subst Abuse Rehabil*. 2016;7:55-69. doi:10.2147/SAR.S101660
70. Spohr SA, Nandy R, Gandhiraj D, Vemulapalli A, Anne S, Walters ST. Efficacy of SMS text message interventions for smoking cessation: a meta-analysis. *J Subst Abuse Treat*. 2015;56:1-10. doi:10.1016/j.jsat.2015.01.011
71. Ybarra ML, Jiang Y, Free C, Abroms LC, Whittaker R. Participant-level meta-analysis of mobile phone-based interventions for smoking cessation across different countries. *Prev Med*. 2016;89:90-97. doi:10.1016/j.ypmed.2016.05.002
72. Scott-Sheldon LAJ, Lantini R, Jennings EG, et al. Text messaging-based interventions for smoking cessation: a systematic review and meta-analysis. *JMIR Mhealth Uhealth*. 2016;4(2):e49. doi:10.2196/mhealth.5436
73. Azjen I. From intentions to actions: a theory of planned behavior. In: Kuhl J, Beckman J, eds. *Action-Control: From Cognition to Behavior*. Springer; 1985.
74. Marlatt GA, Gordon JR. *Relapse Prevention: Maintenance Strategies in the Treatment of Addictive Behaviors*. Guilford Press; 1985.
75. DiClemente CC, Schlundt D, Gemmell L. Readiness and stages of change in addiction treatment. *Am J Addict*. 2004;13(2):103-119. doi:10.1080/10550490490435777
76. Norcross JC, Krebs PM, Prochaska JO. Stages of change. *J Clin Psychol*. 2011;67(2):143-154. doi:10.1002/jclp.20758

77. Ajzen I, Fishbein M. *Understanding Attitudes and Predicting Social Behavior*. Prentice-Hall; 2002.
78. Bandura A. Self-efficacy: toward a unifying theory of behavioral change. *Psychol Rev*. 1977;84(2):191-215. doi:10.1037//0033-295x.84.2.191
79. Abrams DB, Niaura RS. Social learning theory. In: Blane HT, Leonard KE, eds. *Psychological Theories of Drinking and Alcoholism*. Guilford Press; 1987:131-178.
80. Bandura A. *Social Foundations of Thought and Action: A Social Cognitive Theory*. Prentice-Hall; 1986.
81. Niaura RS, Rohsenow DJ, Binkoff JA, Monti PM, Pedraza M, Abrams DB. Relevance of cue reactivity to understanding alcohol and smoking relapse. *J Abnorm Psychol*. 1988;97(2):133-152. doi:10.1037//0021-843x.97.2.133
82. American Legacy Foundation. *Physician Behavior and Practice Patterns Related to Smoking Cessation*. Association of American Medical Colleges; 2007.
83. National Institutes of Health. *Clinicians' Advice to Quit Smoking*. Accessed August 31, 2022. https://progressreport.cancer.gov/prevention/clinicians_advice#:~:text=In%202018%20to%202019%2C%2069.5,that%20doctor%20to%20quit%20smoking
84. Ferketich AK, Khan Y, Wewers ME. Are physicians asking about tobacco use and assisting with cessation? Results from the 2001-2004 national ambulatory medical care survey (NAMCS). *Prev Med*. 2006;43(6):472-476. doi:10.1016/j.ypmed.2006.07.009
85. Stevens VJ, Solberg LI, Quinn VP, et al. Relationship between tobacco control policies and the delivery of smoking cessation services in nonprofit HMOs. *J Natl Cancer Inst Monogr*. 2005;35:75-80. doi:10.1093/jncimonographs/lgi042
86. Price SN, Studts JL, Hamann HA. Tobacco use assessment and treatment in cancer patients: a scoping review of oncology care clinician adherence to clinical practice guidelines in the U.S. *Oncologist*. 2019;24(2):229-238. doi:10.1634/theoncologist.2018-0246
87. Kruger J, O'Halloran A, Rosenthal A. Assessment of compliance with U.S. Public Health Service Clinical Practice Guideline for tobacco by primary care physicians. *Harm Reduct J*. 2015;12(1):7. doi:10.1186/s12954-015-0044-3
88. Maki KG, Volk RJ. Disparities in receipt of smoking cessation assistance within the U.S. *JAMA Netw Open*. 2022;5(6):e2215681. doi:10.1001/jamanetworkopen.2022.15681
89. Boyle R, Solberg L, Fiore M. Use of electronic health records to support smoking cessation. *Cochrane Database Syst Rev*. 2014;12:CD008743. doi:10.1002/14651858.CD008743.pub3
90. Adsit RT, Fox BM, Tsiolis T, et al. Using the electronic health record to connect primary care patients to evidence-based telephonic tobacco quitline services: a closed-loop demonstration project. *Transl Behav Med*. 2014;4(3):324-332. doi:10.1007/s13142-014-0259-y
91. Lindholm C, Adsit R, Bain P, et al. A demonstration project for using the electronic health record to identify and treat tobacco users. *WMJ*. 2010;109(6):335-340.
92. Greenwood DA, Parise CA, MacAller TA, et al. Utilizing clinical support staff and electronic health records to increase tobacco use documentation and referrals to a state quitline. *J Vasc Nurs*. 2012;30(4):107-111. doi:10.1016/j.jvn.2012.04.001
93. Ockene JK, Hosmer DW, Williams JW, Goldberg RJ, Ockene IS, Raia TJ. Factors related to patient smoking status. *Am J Public Health*. 1987;77(3):356-357. doi:10.2105/ajph.77.3.356
94. Pederson LL. Compliance with physician advice to quit smoking: a review of the literature. *Prev Med*. 1982;11(1):71-84. doi:10.1016/0091-7435(82)90006-8
95. Biener L, Abrams DB. The contemplation ladder: validation of a measure of readiness to consider smoking cessation. *Health Psychol*. 1991;10(5):360-365. doi:10.1037/0278-6133.10.5.360
96. Herzog T, Pokhrel P, Kawamoto CT. Short-term fluctuations in motivation to quit smoking in a sample of smokers in Hawaii. *Subst Use Misuse*. 2015;50(2):236-241. doi:10.3109/10826084.2014.966846
97. Prochaska JO, DiClemente CC. Stages and processes of self-change of smoking: toward an integrative model of change. *J Consult Clin Psychol*. 1983;51(3):390-395. doi:10.1037//0022-006x.51.3.390
98. Sun X, Prochaska JO, Velicer WF, Laforge RG. Transtheoretical principles and processes for quitting smoking: a 24-month comparison of a representative sample of quitters, relapsers, and non-quitters. *Addict Behav*. 2007;32(12):2707-2726. doi:10.1016/j.addbeh.2007.04.005
99. Velicer WF, Fava JL, Prochaska JO, Abrams DB, Emmons KM, Pierce JP. Distribution of smokers by stage in three representative samples. *Prev Med*. 1995;24(4):401-411. doi:10.1006/pmed.1995.1065
100. Prochaska JO, Goldstein MG. Process of smoking cessation. Implications for clinicians. *Clin Chest Med*. 1991;12(4):727-735.
101. Rollnick S, Mason P, Butler C. *Health Behaviour Change: A Guide for Practitioners*. Churchill Livingstone; 2007.
102. Apodaca TR, Longabaugh R. Mechanisms of change in motivational interviewing: a review and preliminary evaluation of the evidence. *Addiction*. 2009;104(5):705-715. doi:10.1111/j.1360-0443.2009.02527.x
103. Pan W. Proactive telephone counseling as an adjunct to minimal intervention for smoking cessation: a meta-analysis. *Health Educ Res*. 2006;21(3):416-427. doi:10.1093/her/cyl040
104. Abrams DB. *The Tobacco Dependence Treatment Handbook: A Guide to Best Practices*. Guilford Press; 2007.
105. Hummel K, Candel MJJM, Nagelhout GE, et al. Construct and predictive validity of three measures of intention to quit smoking: findings from the International Tobacco Control (ITC) Netherlands Survey. *Nicotine Tob Res*. 2018;20(9):1101-1108. doi:10.1093/ntr/ntx092
106. Kahler CW, Lachance HR, Strong DR, Ramsey SE, Monti PM, Brown RA. The commitment to quitting smoking scale: initial validation in a smoking cessation trial for heavy social drinkers. *Addict Behav*. 2007;32(10):2420-2424. doi:10.1016/j.addbeh.2007.04.002
107. Rosenstock IM. The health belief model and preventive health behavior. *Health Educ Monogr*. 1974;2(4):354-386. doi:10.1177/109019817400200405
108. Brown RA, Emmons KM. *The Clinical Management of Nicotine Dependence*. https://link.springer.com/chapter/10.1007/978-1-4613-9112-8_9
109. Mermelstein R, Cohen S, Lichtenstein E, Baer JS, Kamarck T. Social support and smoking cessation and maintenance. *J Consult Clin Psychol*. 1986;54(4):447-453. doi:10.1037//0022-006x.54.4.447
110. Soulakova JN, Tang CY, Leonardo SA, Taliaferro LA. Motivational benefits of social support and behavioural interventions for smoking cessation. *J Smok Cessat*. 2018;13(4):216-226. doi:10.1017/jsc.2017.26
111. Hunt WA, Bespalec DA. An evaluation of current methods of modifying smoking behavior. *J Clin Psychol*. 1974;30(4):431-438. doi:10.1002/1097-4679(197410)30:4<431::aid-jclp2270300402>3.0.co;2-5
112. Carroll KM. Relapse prevention as a psychosocial treatment: a review of controlled clinical trials. *Exp Clin Psychopharmacol*. 1996;4(1):46-54. doi:10.1037/1064-1297.4.1.46
113. Collins SE, Witkiewitz K, Kirouac M, Marlatt GA. Preventing relapse following smoking cessation. *Curr Cardiovasc Risk Rep*. 2010;4(6):421-428. doi:10.1007/s12170-010-0124-6
114. Ockene JK, Emmons KM, Mermelstein RJ, et al. Relapse and maintenance issues for smoking cessation. *Health Psychol*. 2000;19(1S):17-31. doi:10.1037/0278-6133.19.suppl1.17
115. Stevens VJ, Hollis JF. Preventing smoking relapse, using an individually tailored skills-training technique. *J Consult Clin Psychol*. 1989;57(3):420-424. doi:10.1037//0022-006x.57.3.420
116. Hall SM, Humfleet GL, Reus VI, Muñoz RF, Cullen J. Extended nortriptyline and psychological treatment for cigarette smoking. *Am J Psychiatry*. 2004;161(11):2100-2107. doi:10.1176/appi.ajp.161.11.2100
117. Baker TB, Piper ME, Smith SS, Bolt DM, Stein JH, Fiore MC. Effects of combined varenicline with nicotine patch and of extended treatment duration on smoking cessation: a randomized clinical trial. *JAMA*. 2021;326(15):1485. doi:10.1001/jama.2021.15333
118. Brandon TH, Simmons VN, Sutton SK, et al. Extended self-help for smoking cessation: a randomized controlled trial. *Am J Prev Med*. 2016;51(1):54-62. doi:10.1016/j.amepre.2015.12.016
119. Brandon TH, Collins BN, Juliano LM, Lazev AB. Preventing relapse among former smokers: a comparison of minimal interventions through telephone and mail. *J Consult Clin Psychol*. 2000;68(1):103-113. doi:10.1037//0022-006x.68.1.103

120. Brandon TH, Meade CD, Herzog TA, Chirikos TN, Webb MS, Cantor AB. Efficacy and cost-effectiveness of a minimal intervention to prevent smoking relapse: dismantling the effects of amount of content versus contact. *J Consult Clin Psychol.* 2004;72(5):797-808. doi:10.1037/0022-006X.72.5.797
121. Streck JM, Luberto CM, Muzikansky A, et al. Examining the effects of stress and psychological distress on smoking abstinence in cancer patients. *Prev Med Rep.* 2021;23:101402. doi:10.1016/j.pmedr.2021.101402
122. Hajek P, Taylor T, McRobbie H. The effect of stopping smoking on perceived stress levels: smoking cessation and stress. *Addiction.* 2010;105(8):1466-1471. doi:10.1111/j.1360-0443.2010.02979.x
123. Parrott AC. Smoking cessation leads to reduced stress, but why? *Int J Addict.* 1995;30(11):1509-1516. doi:10.3109/10826089509055846
124. Taylor AH, Ussher MH, Faulkner G. The acute effects of exercise on cigarette cravings, withdrawal symptoms, affect and smoking behaviour: a systematic review. *Addiction.* 2007;102(4):534-543. doi:10.1111/j.1360-0443.2006.01739.x
125. Marcus BH, Albrecht AE, King TK, et al. The efficacy of exercise as an aid for smoking cessation in women: a randomized controlled trial. *Arch Intern Med.* 1999;159(11):1229-1234. doi:10.1001/archinte.159.11.1229
126. Lopez-Quintero C, Crum RM, Neumark YD. Racial/ethnic disparities in report of physician-provided smoking cessation advice: analysis of the 2000 National Health Interview Survey. *Am J Public Health.* 2006;96(12):2235-2239. doi:10.2105/AJPH.2005.071035
127. Abrantes AM, Bloom EL, Strong DR, et al. A preliminary randomized controlled trial of a behavioral exercise intervention for smoking cessation. *Nicotine Tob Res.* 2014;16(8):1094-1103. doi:10.1093/ntr/ntu036
128. Ussher MH, Faulkner GEJ, Angus K, Hartmann-Boyce J, Taylor AH. Exercise interventions for smoking cessation. *Cochrane Database Syst Rev.* 2019;2019(10):Cochrane Tobacco Addiction Group, ed. doi:10.1002/14651858.CD002295.pub6
129. Bolívar HA, Klemperer EM, Coleman SRM, DeSarno M, Skelly JM, Higgins ST. Contingency management for patients receiving medication for opioid use disorder: a systematic review and meta-analysis. *JAMA Psychiatry.* 2021;78(10):1092. doi:10.1001/jamapsychiatry.2021.1969
130. Higgins ST, Silverman K. Contingency management. In: Galanter M, Kleber HD, eds. *The American Psychiatric Publishing Textbook of Substance Abuse Treatment.* American Psychiatric Publishing, Inc; 2008:387-399.
131. Prochaska JJ, Delucchi K, Hall SM. A meta-analysis of smoking cessation interventions with individuals in substance abuse treatment or recovery. *J Consult Clin Psychol.* 2004;72(6):1144-1156. doi:10.1037/0022-006X.72.6.1144
132. McKelvey K, Thrul J, Ramo D. Impact of quitting smoking and smoking cessation treatment on substance use outcomes: an updated and narrative review. *Addict Behav.* 2017;65:161-170. doi:10.1016/j.addbeh.2016.10.012
133. Holford TR, Levy DT, Meza R. Comparison of smoking history patterns among African American and White cohorts in the United States Born 1890 to 1990. *Nicotine Tob Res.* 2016;18(Suppl 1):S16-S29. doi:10.1093/ntr/ntv274
134. Nollen NL, Ahluwalia JS, Sanderson Cox L, et al. Assessment of racial differences in pharmacotherapy efficacy for smoking cessation: secondary analysis of the EAGLES randomized clinical trial. *JAMA Netw Open.* 2021;4(1):e2032053. doi:10.1001/jamanetworkopen.2020.32053
135. Jones MR, Joshu CE, Navas-Acien A, Platz EA. Racial/ethnic differences in duration of smoking among former smokers in the National Health and Nutrition Examination Surveys (NHANES). *Nicotine Tob Res.* 2018;20(3):303-311. doi:10.1093/ntr/ntw326
136. Matthews AK, Sánchez-Johnsen L, King A. Development of a culturally targeted smoking cessation intervention for African American smokers. *J Community Health.* 2009;34(6):480-492. doi:10.1007/s10900-009-9181-5
137. Webb MS. Culturally specific interventions for African American smokers: an efficacy experiment. *J Natl Med Assoc.* 2009;101(9):927-935. doi:10.1016/s0027-9684(15)31041-5
138. Webb Hooper M, Antoni MH, Okuyemi K, Dietz NA, Resnicow K. Randomized controlled trial of group-based culturally specific cognitive behavioral therapy among African American Smokers. *Nicotine Tob Res.* 2017;19(3):333-341. doi:10.1093/ntr/ntw181
139. Webb Hooper M, Miller DB, Saldivar E, et al. Randomized controlled trial testing a video-text tobacco cessation intervention among economically disadvantaged African American adults. *Psychol Addict Behav.* 2021;35(7):769-777. doi:10.1037/adb0000691
140. U.S. Census Bureau. Facts for Features: Hispanic Heritage Month, 2016—Sept. 15-Oct. 15, 2016. Accessed June 12, 2023. https://www.census.gov/newsroom/facts-for-features/2016/cb16-ff16.html
141. Cokkinides VE, Halpern MT, Barbeau EM, Ward E, Thun MJ. Racial and ethnic disparities in smoking-cessation interventions: analysis of the 2005 National Health Interview Survey. *Am J Prev Med.* 2008;34(5):404-412. doi:10.1016/j.amepre.2008.02.003
142. Centers for Disease Control and Prevention. *Vital Signs: Current Cigarette Smoking Among Adults Aged ≥18 Years—United States, 2009.* CDC; 2010. Accessed June 12, 2023. https://www.cdc.gov/mmwr/preview/mmwrhtml/mm5935a3.htm
143. Báezconde-Garbanati L, Beebe LA, Pérez-Stable EJ. Building capacity to address tobacco-related disparities among American Indian and Hispanic/Latino communities: conceptual and systemic considerations. *Addiction.* 2007;102(Suppl 2):112-122. doi:10.1111/j.1360-0443.2007.01962.x
144. Pérez-Stable EJ, Ramirez A, Villareal R, et al. Cigarette smoking behavior among us latino men and women from different countries of origin. *Am J Public Health.* 2001;91(9):1424-1430. doi:10.2105/AJPH.91.9.1424
145. Heron M. Deaths: leading causes for 2008. *Natl Vital Stat Rep.* 2012;60(6):1-94.
146. Sonnenfeld N, Schappert SM, Lin SX. Racial and ethnic differences in delivery of tobacco-cessation services. *Am J Prev Med.* 2009;36(1):21-28. doi:10.1016/j.amepre.2008.09.028
147. Houston TK, Scarinci IC, Person SD, Greene PG. Patient smoking cessation advice by health care providers: the role of ethnicity, socioeconomic status, and health. *Am J Public Health.* 2005;95(6):1056-1061. doi:10.2105/AJPH.2004.039909
148. Webb MS, Rodríguez-Esquivel D, Baker EA. Smoking cessation interventions among Hispanics in the United States: a systematic review and mini meta-analysis. *Am J Health Promot.* 2010;25(2):109-118. doi:10.4278/ajhp.090123-LIT-25
149. Rodríguez Esquivel D, Webb Hooper M, Baker EA, McNutt MD. Culturally specific versus standard smoking cessation messages targeting Hispanics: an experiment. *Psychol Addict Behav.* 2015;29(2):283-289. doi:10.1037/adb0000044
150. Cartujano-Barrera F, Sanderson Cox L, Arana-Chicas E, et al. Feasibility and acceptability of a culturally- and linguistically-adapted smoking cessation text messaging intervention for Latino smokers. *Front Public Health.* 2020;8:269. doi:10.3389/fpubh.2020.00269
151. Choi WS, Beebe LA, Nazir N, et al. All nations breath of life: a randomized trial of smoking cessation for American Indians. *Am J Prev Med.* 2016;51(5):743-751. doi:10.1016/j.amepre.2016.05.021
152. Guydish J, Passalacqua E, Pagano A, et al. An international systematic review of smoking prevalence in addiction treatment: smoking prevalence in addiction treatment. *Addiction.* 2016;111(2):220-230. doi:10.1111/add.13099
153. Baer JS, Lichtenstein E. Classification and prediction of smoking relapse episodes: an exploration of individual differences. *J Consult Clin Psychol.* 1988;56(1):104-110. doi:10.1037//0022-006x.56.1.104
154. Borland R. Slip-ups and relapse in attempts to quit smoking. *Addict Behav.* 1990;15(3):235-245. doi:10.1016/0306-4603(90)90066-7
155. Shiffman S. Relapse following smoking cessation: a situational analysis. *J Consult Clin Psychol.* 1982;50(1):71-86. doi:10.1037//0022-006x.50.1.71
156. Kahler CW, Spillane NS, Metrik J. Alcohol use and initial smoking lapses among heavy drinkers in smoking cessation treatment. *Nicotine Tob Res.* 2010;12(7):781-785. doi:10.1093/ntr/ntq083

157. Kahler CW, Strong DR, Papandonatos GD, et al. Cigarette smoking and the lifetime alcohol involvement continuum. *Drug Alcohol Depend.* 2008;93(1-2):111-120. doi:10.1016/j.drugalcdep.2007.09.004
158. Dawson DA. Drinking as a risk factor for sustained smoking. *Drug Alcohol Depend.* 2000;59(3):235-249. doi:10.1016/s0376-8716(99)00130-1
159. Ockene JK, Adams A. Screening and intervention for smoking and alcohol use in primary care settings: similarities, differences, gaps, and challenges. In: Fertig JB, Allen JP, eds. *Alcohol and Tobacco: From Basic Science to Clinical Practice*. National Institutes of Health; 1995:281-294.
160. Murray RP, Istvan JA, Voelker HT, Rigdon MA, Wallace MD. Level of involvement with alcohol and success at smoking cessation in the lung health study. *J Stud Alcohol.* 1995;56(1):74-82. doi:10.15288/jsa.1995.56.74
161. Mokdad AH, Marks JS, Stroup DF, Gerberding JL. Actual causes of death in the United States, 2000. *JAMA*. 2004;291(10):1238-1245. doi:10.1001/jama.291.10.1238
162. NIAAA. *Ninth Special Report to the U.S. Congress on Alcohol and Health.* U.S. Department of Health and Human Services; 1997.
163. Durazzo TC, Gazdzinski S, Banys P, Meyerhoff DJ. Cigarette smoking exacerbates chronic alcohol-induced brain damage: a preliminary metabolite imaging study. *Alcohol Clin Exp Res.* 2004;28(12):1849-1860. doi:10.1097/01.alc.0000148112.92525.ac
164. Gazdzinski S, Durazzo TC, Studholme C, Song E, Banys P, Meyerhoff DJ. Quantitative brain MRI in alcohol dependence: preliminary evidence for effects of concurrent chronic cigarette smoking on regional brain volumes. *Alcohol Clin Exp Res.* 2005;29(8):1484-1495. doi:10.1097/01.alc.0000175018.72488.61
165. Durazzo TC, Rothlind JC, Gazdzinski S, Banys P, Meyerhoff DJ. A comparison of neurocognitive function in nonsmoking and chronically smoking short-term abstinent alcoholics. *Alcohol.* 2006;39(1):1-11. doi:10.1016/j.alcohol.2006.06.006
166. Durazzo TC, Cardenas VA, Studholme C, Weiner MW, Meyerhoff DJ. Non-treatment-seeking heavy drinkers: effects of chronic cigarette smoking on brain structure. *Drug Alcohol Depend.* 2007;87(1):76-82. doi:10.1016/j.drugalcdep.2006.08.003
167. Ebbert JO, Janney CA, Sellers TA, Folsom AR, Cerhan JR. The association of alcohol consumption with coronary heart disease mortality and cancer incidence varies by smoking history. *J Gen Intern Med.* 2005;20(1):14-20. doi:10.1111/j.1525-1497.2005.40129.x
168. Schröder H, Marrugat J, Elosua R, Covas MI. Tobacco and alcohol consumption: impact on other cardiovascular and cancer risk factors in a southern European Mediterranean population. *Br J Nutr.* 2002;88(3):273-281. doi:10.1079/BJN2002655
169. Tuyns AJ, Estève J, Raymond L, et al. Cancer of the larynx/hypopharynx, tobacco and alcohol: IARC international case-control study in Turin and Varese (Italy), Zaragoza and Navarra (Spain), Geneva (Switzerland) and Calvados (France). *Int J Cancer.* 1988;41(4):483-491. doi:10.1002/ijc.2910410403
170. Blot WJ, McLaughlin JK, Winn DM, et al. Smoking and drinking in relation to oral and pharyngeal cancer. *Cancer Res.* 1988;48(11):3282-3287.
171. Zambon P, Talamini R, La Vecchia C, et al. Smoking, type of alcoholic beverage and squamous-cell oesophageal cancer in northern Italy. *Int J Cancer.* 2000;86(1):144-149. doi:10.1002/(sici)1097-0215(20000401)86:1<144::aid-ijc23>3.0.co;2-b
172. Bosetti C, Franceschi S, Levi F, Negri E, Talamini R, La Vecchia C. Smoking and drinking cessation and the risk of oesophageal cancer. *Br J Cancer.* 2000;83(5):689-691. doi:10.1054/bjoc.2000.1274
173. Kahler CW, Metrik J, LaChance HR, et al. Addressing heavy drinking in smoking cessation treatment: a randomized clinical trial. *J Consult Clin Psychol.* 2008;76(5):852-862. doi:10.1037/a0012717
174. Toll BA, Martino S, O'Malley SS, et al. A randomized trial for hazardous drinking and smoking cessation for callers to a quitline. *J Consult Clin Psychol.* 2015;83(3):445-454. doi:10.1037/a0038183
175. National Institute on Alcohol Abuse and Alcoholism. *Helping Patients Who Drink Too Much: A Clinician's Guide.* U.S. Department of Health and Human Services; 2005.
176. Sigmon SC, Miller ME, Meyer AC, et al. Financial incentives to promote extended smoking abstinence in opioid-maintained patients: a randomized trial: promoting extended smoking abstinence in opioid-dependent patients. *Addiction.* 2016;111(5):903-912. doi:10.1111/add.13264
177. Vlad C, Arnsten JH, Nahvi S. Achieving smoking cessation among persons with opioid use disorder. *CNS Drugs.* 2020;34(4):367-387. doi:10.1007/s40263-020-00701-z
178. Miller ME, Sigmon SC. Are pharmacotherapies ineffective in opioid-dependent smokers? reflections on the scientific literature and future directions: Table 1. *Nicotine Tob Res.* 2015;17(8):955-959. doi:10.1093/ntr/ntv030
179. Parker MA, Streck JM, Sigmon SC. Associations between opioid and nicotine dependence in nationally representative samples of United States adult daily smokers. *Drug Alcohol Depend.* 2018;186:167-170. doi:10.1016/j.drugalcdep.2018.01.024
180. Mattick RP, Breen C, Kimber J, Davoli M. Buprenorphine maintenance versus placebo or methadone maintenance for opioid dependence. *Cochrane Database Syst Rev.* 2014;2:CD002207. Cochrane Drugs and Alcohol Group, ed. doi:10.1002/14651858.CD002207.pub4
181. Stotts AL, Dodrill CL, Kosten TR. Opioid dependence treatment: options in pharmacotherapy. *Expert Opin Pharmacother.* 2009;10(11):1727-1740. doi:10.1517/14656560903037168
182. Marynak K, VanFrank B, Tetlow S, et al. Tobacco cessation interventions and smoke-free policies in mental health and substance abuse treatment facilities—United States, 2016. *MMWR Morb Mortal Wkly Rep.* 2018;67(18):519-523. doi:10.15585/mmwr.mm6718a3
183. Cohn A, Elmasry H, Niaura R. Facility-level, state, and financial factors associated with changes in the provision of smoking cessation services in U.S. substance abuse treatment facilities: Results from the National Survey of Substance Abuse Treatment Services 2006 to 2012. *J Subst Abuse Treat.* 2017(77):107-114. doi:10.1016/j.jsat.2017.03.014
184. Guydish J, Le T, Hosakote S, et al. Tobacco use among substance use disorder (SUD) treatment staff is associated with tobacco-related services received by clients. *J Subst Abuse Treat.* 2022;132:108496. doi:10.1016/j.jsat.2021.108496
185. Sheals K, Tombor I, McNeill A, Shahab L. A mixed-method systematic review and meta-analysis of mental health professionals' attitudes toward smoking and smoking cessation among people with mental illnesses. *Addiction.* 2016;111(9):1536-1553. doi:10.1111/add.13387
186. Streck JM, Weinberger AH, Pacek LR, Gbedemah M, Goodwin RD. Cigarette smoking quit rates among persons with serious psychological distress in the United States from 2008 to 2016: are mental health disparities in cigarette use increasing? *Nicotine Tob Res.* 2020;22(1):130-134.
187. Williams JM, Ziedonis D. Addressing tobacco among individuals with a mental illness or an addiction. *Addict Behav.* 2004;29(6):1067-1083. doi:10.1016/j.addbeh.2004.03.009
188. Prochaska JJ, Fromont SC, Louie AK, Jacobs MH, Hall SM. Training in tobacco treatments in psychiatry: a national survey of psychiatry residency training directors. *Acad Psychiatry.* 2006;30(5):372-378. doi:10.1176/appi.ap.30.5.372
189. Fuller BE, Guydish J, Tsoh J, et al. Attitudes toward the integration of smoking cessation treatment into drug abuse clinics. *J Subst Abuse Treat.* 2007;32(1):53-60. doi:10.1016/j.jsat.2006.06.011
190. Lightfoot K, Panagiotaki G, Nobes G. Effectiveness of psychological interventions for smoking cessation in adults with mental health problems: a systematic review. *Br J Health Psychol.* 2020;25(3):615-638. doi:10.1111/bjhp.12431
191. Montoya ID, Herbeck DM, Svikis DS, Pincus HA. Identification and treatment of patients with nicotine problems in routine clinical psychiatry practice. *Am J Addict.* 2005;14(5):441-454. doi:10.1080/10550490500247123
192. Gfroerer J, Dube SR, King BA, Garrett BE, Babb S, McAfee T. Vital signs: current cigarette smoking among adults aged ≥18 years with mental illness—United States, 2009-2011. *MMWR Morbid Mortal Wkly Rep.* 2013;62(5):81-87.

193. Siru R, Hulse GK, Tait RJ. Assessing motivation to quit smoking in people with mental illness: a review. *Addiction*. 2009;104(5):719-733. doi:10.1111/j.1360-0443.2009.02545.x
194. Hitsman B, Moss TG, Montoya ID, George TP. Treatment of tobacco dependence in mental health and addictive disorders. *Can J Psychiatry*. 2009;54(6):368-378. doi:10.1177/070674370905400604
195. Smith PH, Homish GG, Giovino GA, Kozlowski LT. Cigarette smoking and mental illness: a study of nicotine withdrawal. *Am J Public Health*. 2014;104(2):e127-e133. doi:10.2105/AJPH.2013.301502
196. Taylor GM, Lindson N, Farley A, et al. Smoking cessation for improving mental health. *Cochrane Database Syst Rev*. 2021;3:CD013522. doi:10.1002/14651858.CD013522.pub2
197. Steinberg ML, Williams JM, Stahl NF, Budsock PD, Cooperman NA. An adaptation of motivational interviewing increases quit attempts in smokers with serious mental illness. *Nicotine Tob Res*. 2016;18(3):243-250. doi:10.1093/ntr/ntv043
198. Brown RA, Minami H, Hecht J, et al. Sustained care smoking cessation intervention for individuals hospitalized for psychiatric disorders: the Helping HAND 3 randomized clinical trial. *JAMA Psychiatry*. 2021;78(8):839. doi:10.1001/jamapsychiatry.2021.0707
199. Ziedonis DM, George TP. Schizophrenia and nicotine use: report of a pilot smoking cessation program and review of neurobiological and clinical issues. *Schizophr Bull*. 1997;23(2):247-254. doi:10.1093/schbul/23.2.247
200. Addington J. Group treatment for smoking cessation among persons with schizophrenia. *Psychiatr Serv Wash DC*. 1998;49(7):925-928. doi:10.1176/ps.49.7.925
201. Washington A, Moll S, Pawlick J. *Smokebusters: An Approach to Help People with Mental Illness Move Closer to a Smoke-Free Lifestyle*. Community Social and Vocational Rehabilitation Foundation; 1997.
202. Jochelson K. Smoke-free legislation and mental health units: the challenges ahead. *Br J Psychiatry*. 2006;189:479-480. doi:10.1192/bjp.bp.106.029942
203. Asamsama OH, Miller SC, Silvestri MM, Bonanno C, Krondilou K. Impact of implementing a tobacco and recreational nicotine-free policy and enhanced treatments on programmatic and patient-level outcomes within a residential substance use disorder treatment program. *J Sub Abuse Treat*. 2019;107:44-49. doi:doi.org/10.1016/j.jsat.2019.09.004
204. Grant BF, Hasin DS, Chou SP, Stinson FS, Dawson DA. Nicotine dependence and psychiatric disorders in the united states: results from the national epidemiologic survey on alcohol and related conditions. *Arch Gen Psychiatry*. 2004;61(11):1107. doi:10.1001/archpsyc.61.11.1107
205. Pratt LA, Brody DJ. Depression and smoking in the U.S. household population aged 20 and over, 2005-2008. *NCHS Data Brief*. 2010;34:1-8.
206. Weinberger AH, Chaiton MO, Zhu J, Wall MM, Hasin DS, Goodwin RD. Trends in the prevalence of current, daily, and nondaily cigarette smoking and quit ratios by depression status in the U.S.: 2005-2017. *Am J Prev Med*. 2020;58(5):691-698. doi:10.1016/j.amepre.2019.12.023
207. Cinciripini PM, Wetter DW, Fouladi RT, et al. The effects of depressed mood on smoking cessation: mediation by postcessation self-efficacy. *J Consult Clin Psychol*. 2003;71(2):292-301. doi:10.1037/0022-006x.71.2.292
208. Niaura R, Britt DM, Shadel WG, Goldstein M, Abrams D, Brown R. Symptoms of depression and survival experience among three samples of smokers trying to quit. *Psychol Addict Behav*. 2001;15(1):13-17. doi:10.1037/0893-164x.15.1.13
209. Kinnunen T, Doherty K, Militello FS, Garvey AJ. Depression and smoking cessation: characteristics of depressed smokers and effects of nicotine replacement. *J Consult Clin Psychol*. 1996;64(4):791-798. doi:10.1037/0022-006X.64.4.791
210. Berlin I, Covey LS. Pre-cessation depressive mood predicts failure to quit smoking: the role of coping and personality traits. *Addiction*. 2006;101(12):1814-1821. doi:10.1111/j.1360-0443.2006.01616.x
211. Covey LS, Glassman AH, Stetner F. Depression and depressive symptoms in smoking cessation. *Compr Psychiatry*. 1990;31(4):350-354. doi:10.1016/0010-440x(90)90042-q
212. Ginsberg D, Hall SM, Reus VI, Muñoz RF. Mood and depression diagnosis in smoking cessation. *Exp Clin Psychopharmacol*. 1995;3(4):389-395.
213. West RJ, Hajek P, Belcher M. Severity of withdrawal symptoms as a predictor of outcome of an attempt to quit smoking. *Psychol Med*. 1989;19(4):981-985. doi:10.1017/s0033291700005705
214. Moylan S, Jacka FN, Pasco JA, Berk M. Cigarette smoking, nicotine dependence and anxiety disorders: a systematic review of population-based, epidemiological studies. *BMC Med*. 2012;10(1):123. doi:10.1186/1741-7015-10-123
215. Garey L, Olofsson H, Garza T, Shepherd JM, Smit T, Zvolensky MJ. The role of anxiety in smoking onset, severity, and cessation-related outcomes: a review of recent literature. *Curr Psychiatry Rep*. 2020;22(8):38. doi:10.1007/s11920-020-01160-5
216. Piper ME, Smith SS, Schlam TR, et al. Psychiatric disorders in smokers seeking treatment for tobacco dependence: relations with tobacco dependence and cessation. *J Consult Clin Psychol*. 2010;78(1):13-23. doi:10.1037/a0018065
217. Brown RA, Kahler CW, Niaura R, et al. Cognitive-behavioral treatment for depression in smoking cessation. *J Consult Clin Psychol*. 2001;69(3):471-480. doi:10.1037//0022-006x.69.3.471
218. Hall SM, Muñoz RF, Reus VI. Cognitive-behavioral intervention increases abstinence rates for depressive-history smokers. *J Consult Clin Psychol*. 1994;62(1):141-146. doi:10.1037//0022-006x.62.1.141
219. Hall SM, Reus VI, Muñoz RF, et al. Nortriptyline and cognitive-behavioral therapy in the treatment of cigarette smoking. *Arch Gen Psychiatry*. 1998;55(8):683-690. doi:10.1001/archpsyc.55.8.683
220. Hall SM, Muñoz RF, Reus VI, et al. Mood management and nicotine gum in smoking treatment: a therapeutic contact and placebo-controlled study. *J Consult Clin Psychol*. 1996;64(5):1003-1009. doi:10.1037//0022-006x.64.5.1003
221. Haas AL, Muñoz RF, Humfleet GL, Reus VI, Hall SM. Influences of mood, depression history, and treatment modality on outcomes in smoking cessation. *J Consult Clin Psychol*. 2004;72(4):563-570. doi:10.1037/0022-006X.72.4.563
222. Lejuez CW, Hopko DR, Hopko SD. A brief behavioral activation treatment for depression. *Treatment manual. Behav Modif*. 2001;25(2):255-286. doi:10.1177/0145445501252005
223. MacPherson L, Tull MT, Matusiewicz AK, et al. Randomized controlled trial of behavioral activation smoking cessation treatment for smokers with elevated depressive symptoms. *J Consult Clin Psychol*. 2010;78(1):55-61. doi:10.1037/a0017939
224. Leventhal AM, Zvolensky MJ. Anxiety, depression, and cigarette smoking: a transdiagnostic vulnerability framework to understanding emotion–smoking comorbidity. *Psychol Bull*. 2015;141(1):176-212. doi:10.1037/bul0000003
225. Mak YW, Leung DYP, Loke AY. Effectiveness of an individual acceptance and commitment therapy for smoking cessation, delivered face-to-face and by telephone to adults recruited in primary health care settings: a randomized controlled trial. *BMC Public Health*. 2020;20(1):1719. doi:10.1186/s12889-020-09820-0
226. Hayes SC, Luoma JB, Bond FW, Masuda A, Lillis J. Acceptance and commitment therapy: model, processes and outcomes. *Behav Res Ther*. 2006;44(1):1-25. doi:10.1016/j.brat.2005.06.006
227. Brown RA, Lejuez CW, Strong DR, et al. A prospective examination of distress tolerance and early smoking lapse in adult self-quitters. *Nicotine Tob Res*. 2009;11(5):493-502. doi:10.1093/ntr/ntp041
228. Brown RA, Lejuez CW, Kahler CW, Strong DR. Distress tolerance and duration of past smoking cessation attempts. *J Abnorm Psychol*. 2002;111(1):180-185.
229. Brandon TH, Herzog TA, Juliano LM, Irvin JE, Lazev AB, Simmons VN. Pretreatment task persistence predicts smoking cessation outcome. *J Abnorm Psychol*. 2003;112(3):448-456. doi:10.1037/0021-843x.112.3.448
230. Hernández-López M, Luciano MC, Bricker JB, Roales-Nieto JG, Montesinos F. Acceptance and commitment therapy for smoking cessation: a preliminary study of its effectiveness in comparison with cognitive behavioral therapy. *Psychol Addict Behav*. 2009;23(4):723-730. doi:10.1037/a0017632
231. Davis JM, Fleming MF, Bonus KA, Baker TB. A pilot study on mindfulness based stress reduction for smokers. *BMC Complement Altern Med*. 2007;7:2. doi:10.1186/1472-6882-7-2

232. Jackson S, Brown J, Norris E, Livingstone-Banks J, Hayes E, Lindson N. Mindfulness for smoking cessation. *Cochrane Database Syst Rev.* 2022;2022(4):Cochrane Tobacco Addiction Group, ed. doi:10.1002/14651858.CD013696.pub2

233. Khanna S, Greeson JM. A narrative review of yoga and mindfulness as complementary therapies for addiction. *Complement Ther Med.* 2013;21(3):244-252. doi:10.1016/j.ctim.2013.01.008

234. Anderson CM, Zhu SH. Tobacco quitlines: looking back and looking ahead. *Tob Control.* 2007;16(Suppl 1):i81-i86. doi:10.1136/tc.2007.020701

235. Parker DR, Windsor RA, Roberts MB, et al. Feasibility, cost, and cost-effectiveness of a telephone-based motivational intervention for underserved pregnant smokers. *Nicotine Tob Res.* 2007;9(10):1043-1051. doi:10.1080/14622200701591617

236. Glasgow RE, Vogt TM, Boles SM. Evaluating the public health impact of health promotion interventions: the RE-AIM framework. *Am J Public Health.* 1999;89(9):1322-1327. doi:10.2105/ajph.89.9.1322

237. El-Toukhy S. Insights From the SmokeFree.gov initiative regarding the use of smoking cessation digital platforms during the COVID-19 pandemic: cross-sectional trends analysis study. *J Med Internet Res.* 2021;23(3):e24593. doi:10.2196/24593

238. Whittaker R, McRobbie H, Bullen C, Rodgers A, Gu Y, Dobson R. Mobile phone text messaging and app-based interventions for smoking cessation. *Cochrane Database Syst Rev.* 2019;10:CD006611. doi:10.1002/14651858.CD006611.pub5

239. Abroms LC, Padmanabhan N, Thaweethai L, Phillips T. iPhone apps for smoking cessation: a content analysis. *Am J Prev Med.* 2011;40(3):279-285. doi:10.1016/j.amepre.2010.10.032

240. Cheng F, Xu J, Su C, Fu X, Bricker J. Content analysis of smartphone apps for smoking cessation in China: empirical study. *JMIR Mhealth Uhealth.* 2017;5(7):e93. doi:10.2196/mhealth.7462

241. Thornton L, Quinn C, Birrell L, et al. Free smoking cessation mobile apps available in Australia: a quality review and content analysis. *Aust N Z J Public Health.* 2017;41(6):625-630. doi:10.1111/1753-6405.12688

242. Formagini TDB, Ervilha RR, Machado NM, de Andrade BABB, Gomide HP, Ronzani TM. A review of smartphone apps for smoking cessation available in Portuguese. *Cad Saude Publica.* 2017;33(2):e00178215. doi:10.1590/0102-311X00178215

243. Regmi K, Kassim N, Ahmad N, Tuah N. Effectiveness of mobile apps for smoking cessation: α review. *Tob Prev Cessat.* 2017;3:12. doi:10.18332/tpc/70088

244. Dar R. Effect of real-time monitoring and notification of smoking episodes on smoking reduction: a pilot study of a novel smoking cessation app. *Nicotine Tob Res.* 2018;20(12):1515-1518. doi:10.1093/ntr/ntx223

CHAPTER

75 Network Therapy

Marc Galanter

CHAPTER OUTLINE

- Introduction
- The network therapy technique
- Cognitive-behavioral therapy and social support
- A longer course
- Research on network therapy
- Adaptations of network therapy treatment
- Community-based family involvement
- Principles of network treatment

INTRODUCTION

Psychotherapy for people with substance use disorders (SUDs) presents unique problems for the office-based practitioner. Among these is the ever-present vulnerability to recurrence of substance use and high rates of patients discontinuing treatment. In order to address this problem, we can consider how engaging the input of people close to a person with an addiction can help in achieving a stable recovery. To understand this option, it is first important to understand that certain conditioned drug-seeking behaviors may be extinguished if appropriate aversive stimuli are interposed after triggers to drug use are presented.

It is important to help the patient recall relevant conditioned stimuli in a psychotherapeutic context, whereby the person with alcohol or other SUD may become aware of the sequence of circumstances that can precipitate a return to use (or return to SUD symptoms/criteria, etc.).[1] Once this is done, the patient's own distress at the course of the addictive process, generated by the patient's own motivation for escaping the addictive pattern, may be mobilized. This motivational distress then serves as an aversive stimulus. The implicit assumption behind this therapeutic approach is that the patient in question wants to alter his or her pattern of drug use and that the recognition of a particular stimulus as a conditioned component of addiction will then allow the patient, in effect, to initiate the extinction process. If a patient is committed to achieving abstinence from an addictive drug such as alcohol or cocaine but is in jeopardy of occasional slips, this cognitive labeling can facilitate consolidation of an abstinent adaptation.

As we shall see, the input of people close to the patient can help to reveal triggers to drug use that may not have been apparent to the patient. Such an approach is less valuable in the context of (1) a lack of motivation for abstinence, (2) fragile social supports, or (3) compulsive substance use unmanageable by the patient in the patient's usual social settings. A higher level of care such as residential or inpatient hospitalization, or opioid agonist therapy (eg, methadone or buprenorphine), may be necessary in such cases because ambulatory stabilization through psychotherapeutic support is often not feasible, even with the support of family and close peers. On the other hand, for willing patients, or ones whom family and friends have convinced to cooperate, the network approach can be most valuable.

THE NETWORK THERAPY TECHNIQUE

This approach can be useful in addressing a broad range of patients with SUD characterized by the following clinical hallmarks of the disease of addiction. When they initiate consumption of their addictive agent, be it alcohol, cocaine, opioids, or depressant drugs, they frequently cannot limit that consumption to a reasonable and predictable level; this phenomenon has been termed *loss of control* by clinicians who treat persons with SUDs.[2] Second, they have consistently attempted to stop using the drug for varying periods of time but have returned to it, despite a specific intent to avoid it.

This treatment approach is not necessary for those patients who can learn to set limits on their use of alcohol or drugs; their substance use may be treated as a behavioral symptom in a more traditional psychotherapeutic fashion, nor is this approach directed at those patients for whom the addictive pattern is most unmanageable, such as addicted people with unusual destabilizing circumstances such as homelessness, severe personality disorders, or psychosis. These patients may need special supportive care such as inpatient withdrawal management or long-term residential treatment.

Key Elements

Two key elements are introduced into the network therapy (NT) technique. The first is a cognitive-behavioral approach to prevention of return to substance use (or gambling), which has been considered valuable in addiction treatment.[3,4] Emphasis in this approach is placed on triggers to use and behavioral techniques on managing them, in preference to exploring underlying psychodynamic issues.

Second, support of the patient's natural social network is engaged in treatment. Peer support in Alcoholics Anonymous (AA) and Narcotics Anonymous (NA) has long been shown to be an effective vehicle for promoting abstinence, and the idea of the therapist intervening with family and friends in starting treatment was employed in one of the early ambulatory techniques specific to addiction.[5] The involvement of spouses[6] has since been shown to be effective in enhancing the outcome of professional therapy.

COGNITIVE-BEHAVIORAL THERAPY AND SOCIAL SUPPORT

Cognitive-Behavioral Therapy

Cognitive-behavioral therapy (CBT) for treatment has been shown to be effective for a wide variety of SUDs, including alcohol,[7] cannabis,[8] and cocaine.[9] It is premised on the original findings by Wikler[10] on conditioning models of drug seeking in heroin-addicted subjects.

The CBT approach is goal oriented and focuses on current circumstances in the patient's life. In NT, reference both in individual and conjoint sessions can be made to salient past experiences. CBT sessions are typically structured, so, for example, patients begin each network session with a recounting of recent events directly relevant to their addiction and recovery. This is followed by active participation and interaction of the therapist, patient, and network members in response to the patient's report. CBT emphasizes psychoeducation in the context of prevention of return to use, so that circumstances, thoughts, and interpersonal situations that have historically precipitated substance use are identified, and the patients (and network members as well) are taught to anticipate where such triggers can precipitate substance use.

The process of guided recall is particularly important because it allows the therapist to both individualize sessions with the patient alone and have network sessions—in conjunction with network members along with the patient—to guide the patient to recognize a sequence of conditioned stimuli (triggers) that play a role in drug seeking. Such triggers may not initially be apparent to the patient or network members but, with encouragement and prompting, can emerge over the course of an exploration of the circumstances that have led, either in the past or in a recent "slip," to substance use.

Social Support

This issue has been studied in a variety of data sets in relation to the recovery from SUDs. For example, in the Project MATCH, three modalities, 12-step facilitation, motivational enhancement, and cognitive-behavioral approaches, were compared. In a secondary analysis of findings from this multisite study, it was found[11] that certain aspects of social support were most predictive of abstinence outcomes. Two social network characteristics that had a positive effect on outcome were the size of the supportive social network in the person's life and the number of members who were abstainers (or persons recovering from an alcohol use disorder [AUD]). Having network members who do not have substance-related problems is important to a long-term clinical outcome. As a matter of fact, a large number of network members, when their participation is effectively maintained over time, can counter a variety of circumstances that may undermine a patient's abstinence. Additionally, they can provide varied aspects of support relative to the patient's experience in recovery. And indeed, they should be free of substance-related problems. Of interest in this context, it has been reported that men are more typically encouraged by their wives to seek help, whereas women are more often encouraged by mothers, siblings, and children.[12]

Contrast With Other Approaches

The contrast between NT and interpersonal group therapy, on the other hand, highlights the nature of NT itself. The interpersonal model[13] posits that the SUD reflects problems of relationship. NT, on the other hand, assumes that once an addiction or SUD is established, it will continue, even if interpersonal issues are resolved, and therefore, NT is not directed at resolved relational issues as such. Such issues, do, however, generally improve once abstinence is established.

On the other hand, NT does bear relation to relapse prevention treatment[14] as it embodies a forward-looking approach to anticipate potential triggers for return to use. It can also be similar to some approaches to couples therapy, such as the Behavioral Couples Therapy model[6] in that the spouse is encouraged to support behaviors that reinforce abstinence in both modalities.

Relapse prevention is a term used in literature to describe a specific clinical model of treatment. Variations of this approach are aimed to reduce the risk of a patient returning to substance (or gambling) use after a period of change, or what Marlatt refers to as a "breakdown or setback" in an attempt to change substance use behaviors. Many definitions of the term "relapse" exist and in recent years, "recurrence" of DSM-5 symptoms of a substance use disorder or "return to substance use" following a period of recovery has replaced the term relapse and are preferred current terminology when not referring to the specific RP intervention and its terminology.

Community Reinforcement

A community reinforcement and family training (CRAFT) program includes many aspects of treatment that were employed in NT. The CRAFT approach was developed to encourage patients with AUD to enter therapy and reduce drinking, in part by eliciting support of concerned others as well as to enhance satisfaction with life among members of the patient's social network who were concerned about his or her drinking. As in NT, the CRAFT program includes a functional analysis of the patient's substance use, that is to say, understanding the substance use with respect to its antecedents and consequences. Like NT, it also serves to minimize reciprocal blaming and defensiveness among the concerned significant others and to promote a patient's sobriety-oriented activities.

Initial Encounter: Starting a Social Network

So how does one go about developing NT? The patient should be asked to bring his or her spouse or a close friend or confidante to the first session. Patients with AUDs often dislike certain things they hear when they first come for treatment and may deny or rationalize, even if they have voluntarily sought help. Because of their denial of the problem, a significant other is essential both to history taking and to implementing a viable treatment plan. A close relative or spouse can often cut through the denial in a way that an unfamiliar therapist cannot and can therefore be invaluable in setting a standard of realism in dealing with the addiction.

Some patients make clear that they wish to come to the initial session on their own. This is often associated with their desire to preserve the option of continued substance use and is born out of the fear that an alliance will be established independent of them being able to prevent this. Although a delay may be tolerated for a session or two, it should be stated unambiguously at the outset that effective treatment can be undertaken only on the basis of a therapeutic alliance built around the addiction issue that includes the support of significant others and that it is expected that a network of close friends and/or relatives will be brought in within a session or two at the most.

The weight of clinical experience supports the view that abstinence is the most practical goal to propose to the addicted person for his or her rehabilitation.[15,16] For abstinence to be expected, however, the therapist should assure the provision of necessary social supports for the patient. Let us consider how a long-term support network is initiated for this purpose, beginning with availability of the therapist, significant others, and a self-help group.

In the first place, the therapist should be available for consultation on the phone and should indicate to the patient that the therapist wants to be called if problems arise. This makes the therapist's commitment clear and sets the tone for a "team effort." It begins to undercut one reason for return to use, the patient's sense of being on their own if unable to manage the situation. The astute therapist, however, will assure that he or she does not spend excessive time on the telephone or in emergency sessions. The patient will therefore develop a support network that can handle the majority of problems involved in day-to-day assistance. This generally will leave the therapist to respond only to occasional questions of interpreting the terms of the understanding among himself or herself, the patient, and support network members. If there is a question about the ability of the patient and network to manage the period between the initial sessions, the first few scheduled sessions may be arranged at intervals of only 1 to 3 days. In any case, frequent appointments should be scheduled at the outset if a pharmacological withdrawal management with benzodiazepines is indicated, so that the patient need never manage more than a few days' medication at a time.

What is most essential, however, is that the network be forged into a working group to provide necessary support for the patient between the initial sessions. Membership ranges from one to several persons close to the patient. Larger networks have been used by Speck[17] in treating patients with schizophrenia. Contacts between network members at this stage typically include telephone calls (at the therapist's or patient's initiative), dinner arrangements, and social encounters and should be preplanned to a fair extent during the joint session. These encounters are most often undertaken at the time when alcohol or drug use is likely to occur. In planning together, however, it should be made clear to network members that relatively little unusual effort will be required for the long term, and that after the patient is stabilized, their participation will amount to little more than attendance at infrequent meetings with the patient and therapist. This is reassuring to those network members who are unable to make a major time commitment to the patient as well as to those patients who do not want to be placed in a dependent position.

Defining the Network's Membership

Once the patient has come for an appointment, establishing a network is a task undertaken with active collaboration of patient and therapist. The two, aided by those parties who join the network initially, must search for the right balance of members. However, the therapist must carefully promote the choice of appropriate network members; just as the platoon leader selects those who will go into combat. The network will be crucial in determining the balance of the therapy. This process is not without problems, and the therapist must think in a strategic fashion of the interactions that may take place among network members. The following case illustrates the nature of their task.

A 25-year-old graduate student had been using cocaine since high school, in part drawing from funds from his affluent family, who lived in a remote city. At two points in the process of establishing his support network, the reactions of his live-in girlfriend, who worked with us from the outset, were particularly important. Both he and she agreed to bring in his 19-year-old sister, a freshman at a nearby college. He then mentioned a "friend" of his, apparently a woman whom he had apparently found attractive, even though there was no history of an overt romantic involvement. The expression on his girlfriend's face suggested that she did not like this idea, although she offered no rationale for excluding this potential rival. However, the idea of having to rely for assistance solely on two women who might see each other as competitors was unappealing. The therapist therefore finessed the idea of the "friend," and both she and the patient moved on to evaluating the patient's uncle, whom he initially preferred to exclude, despite the fact that his girlfriend thought him appropriate. It later turned out (as expected) that the uncle was perceived as a potentially disapproving representative of the parental generation.

The therapist encouraged the patient to accept the uncle as a network member nonetheless, so as to round out the range of relationships within the group and did spell out my rationale for his inclusion. The uncle did turn out to be caring and supportive, particularly after he was helped to understand the nature of the addictive process.

Defining the Network's Task

As conceived here, the therapist's relationship to the network is like that of a task-oriented team leader, rather than that of a family therapist oriented toward insight. The network is established to implement a straightforward task, that of aiding the therapist in sustaining the patient's abstinence. It must be directed with the same clarity of purpose that a task force is directed in any effective organization. Competing and alternative goals must be suppressed or at least prevented from interfering with the primary task.

Unlike family members involved in traditional family therapy, network members are not led to expect symptom relief for themselves or self-realization. This prevents the development of competing goals for the network's meetings. It also assures the members protection from having their own motives scrutinized and thereby supports their continuing involvement without the threat of an assault on their psychological defenses. Because network members have—kindly—volunteered to participate, their motives must not be impugned. Their constructive behavior should be commended. It is useful to acknowledge appreciation for the contribution they are making to the therapy. There is always a counterproductive tendency on their part to minimize the value of their contribution. The network must, therefore, be structured as an effective working group with high morale. This is not always easy.

A 45-year-old single woman served as an executive in a large family-held business—except when her alcohol problem led her into protracted binges. Her father, brother, and sister were prepared to banish her from the business but decided first to seek consultation. Because they had initiated the contact, they were included in the initial network and indeed were very helpful in stabilizing the patient. Unfortunately, however, the father was a domineering figure who intruded in all aspects of the business, evoking angry outbursts from his children. The children typically reacted with petulance, provoking him in return. The situation came to a head when both of the patient's siblings angrily petitioned the therapist to exclude the father from the network, 2 months into the treatment. This presented a problem because the father's control over the business made his involvement important to securing the patient's compliance. The patient's return to use was still a real possibility. This potentially coercive role, however, was an issue that the group could not easily deal with. The therapist decided to support the father's membership in the group, pointing out the constructive role he had played in getting the therapy started. It seemed necessary to support the earnestness of his concern for his daughter, rather than the children's dismay at their father's (very real) obstinacy. It was clear to the therapist that the father could not deal with a situation in which he was not accorded sufficient respect and that there was no real place in this network for addressing the father's character pathology directly. The hubbub did, in fact, quiet down with time. The children became less provocative themselves, as the group responded to the therapists' pleas for civil behavior.

The Use of Alcoholics Anonymous

Use of self-help modalities is desirable whenever possible. For the person defined by AA as an "alcoholic," certainly, participation in AA is strongly encouraged. Groups such as Narcotics Anonymous, Pills Anonymous, Nicotine Anonymous, and Cocaine Anonymous are modeled after AA and play a similarly useful role for those with SUDs. One approach is to tell the patient that he or she is expected to attend at least two AA meetings a week for at least 1 month, so as to become familiar with the program. If after a month the patient is quite reluctant to continue and other aspects of the treatment are going well, the patient's nonparticipation may have to be accepted. Network members can attend Twelve Step meetings with the patient if he/she wants them to come. Alternatively, the patient can be educated about other mutual aid programs that are non-Twelve Step related (SMART Recovery, Women for Sobriety, Secular Organizations for Sobriety, etc.).

Some patients are more easily convinced to attend AA meetings; others may be less adherent. The therapist should mobilize the support network as appropriate, so as to continue pressure for the patient's involvement with AA for a reasonable trial. It may take a considerable period of time, but ultimately a patient may experience something of a conversion, wherein the patient adopts the group ethos and expresses a deep commitment to abstinence, a measure of commitment rarely observed in patients who undergo psychotherapy alone. When this occurs, the therapist may assume a more passive role in monitoring the patient's abstinence and keep an eye on the patient's ongoing involvement in AA. Should a network member solicit advice for treatment referral, the clinician can provide referral.

Use of Pharmacotherapy in the Network Format

For the patient with AUD, disulfiram or other pharmacotherapy may be of marginal use in assuring abstinence when used in a traditional counseling context[18] but becomes much more valuable when carefully integrated into work with the patient and network, particularly when the medication is taken under observation. A similar circumstance applies to the use of other pharmacotherapies for other substance use disorders. In the case of alcohol, it is a good idea to use the initial telephone contact to engage the patient's agreement to abstain from alcohol for the day immediately prior to the first session. The therapist then has the option of prescribing or administering disulfiram at that time. For a patient who is earnest about seeking assistance for alcoholism, this is often not difficult, if some time is spent on the phone making plans to avoid a drinking context during that period. If it is not feasible to undertake this on the phone, it may be addressed in the first session. Such planning with the patient almost always involves organizing time with significant others and therefore serves as a basis for developing the patient's support network.

The administration of disulfiram under observation is a treatment option that is easily adapted to work with social networks. A patient who takes disulfiram and who agrees to be observed by a responsible party while taking it will not miss his or her dose without the observer's knowing and is significantly less likely to drink. This may take a measure of persuasion and, above all, the therapist's commitment that such an approach can be reasonable and helpful.

Disulfiram typically is initiated with a dose of 500 mg and then reduced to 250 mg daily. It is taken every morning when the urge to drink is generally the least. Particulars of administration in the context of treatment have been described.[19]

If the patient returns to use, access to their close relations may be helpful in terms of re-initiating contact.

How can the support network be used to deal with recurrences of alcohol use when in fact the patient's prior association with these same persons did not prevent him or her from drinking? The following example illustrates how this may be done when social resources are limited. In this case, a specific format was defined with the network to monitor a patient's compliance with a disulfiram regimen.

A 33-year-old public relations executive had moved to New York from a remote city 3 years before coming to treatment. She had no long-standing close relationships in the city, a circumstance not uncommon for a single woman with an AUD in a setting removed from her origins. She presented with a 10-year history of heavy drinking that had increased in severity since her arrival, no doubt associated with her social isolation. Although she consumed a bottle of wine each night and additional hard liquor, she was able to get to work regularly. Six months before the outset of treatment, she attended AA meetings for two weeks and had been abstinent during that time. She had then returned to alcohol use, though, and became disillusioned about the possibility of maintaining abstinence. At the outset of treatment, it was necessary to reassure her that alcohol use was in large part a function of not having established sufficient outside supports (including more sound relationships within AA) and of having seen herself as failed after only one slip. However, there was basis for real concern as to whether she would do any better now if the same formula was reinstituted in the absence of sufficient, reliable supports, which she did not seem to have. Together the therapist and she came up with the idea of bringing in an old friend whom she saw occasionally and whom she felt she could trust. They made the following arrangement with her friend. The patient came to sessions twice a week. She would see her friend once each weekend. On each of these thrice-weekly occasions, she would be observed taking disulfiram, so that even if she missed a daily dose in between it would make it significantly less likely for her to resume drinking on a regular basis undetected. The interpersonal support inherent in this arrangement, bolstered by conjoint meetings with her and her friend, also allowed her to return to AA with a sense of confidence in her ability to maintain abstinence.

Format for Medication Observation by the Network

1. Take the medication every morning in front of a network member.
2. Take the pill so that that person can observe you swallowing them.
3. Have the observer write down the time of day the pills were taken on a list prepared by the therapist.
4. The observer brings the list in to the therapist's office at each network session.
5. The observer leaves a message on the therapist's answering machine on any day in which the patient had not taken the pills in a way that ingestion was not clearly observed.

Meeting Arrangements

At the outset of therapy, it is important to see the patient with the group on a weekly basis for at least the first month. Unstable circumstances demand more frequent contacts with the network. Sessions can be tapered off to biweekly and then to monthly intervals after a time.

To sustain the continuing commitment of the group, particularly that between the therapist and the network members, network sessions should be held every 3 months or so for the duration of the individual therapy. Once the patient has stabilized, the meetings tend less to address day-to-day issues. They may begin with the patient's recounting of the drug situation. Reflections on the patient's progress and goals, or sometimes on relations among the network members, then may be discussed. In any case, it is essential that network members contact the therapist if they are concerned about the patient's possible use of alcohol or drugs and that the therapist contact the network members if the therapist becomes concerned about a potential return to use.

Adapting Individual Therapy to the Network Treatment

As noted previously, network sessions are scheduled on a weekly basis at the outset of treatment. This is likely to compromise the number of individual contacts. Indeed, if sessions are held once a week, the patient may not be seen individually for a period of time. The patient may perceive this as a deprivation unless the individual therapy is presented as an opportunity for further growth predicated on achieving stable abstinence assured through work with the network.

When the individual therapy does begin, the traditional objectives of therapy must be arranged so as to accommodate the goals of the SUD treatment. For insight-oriented therapy, clarification of unconscious motivations is a primary objective; for supportive therapy, the bolstering of established constructive defenses is primary. In the therapeutic context that is described here, however, the following objectives are given precedence.

Of first importance is the need to address exposure to drugs including alcohol or exposure to cues or stressors that might precipitate alcohol or drug use. Both patient and therapist should be sensitive to this matter and explore these situations as they arise. Second, a stable social context in an appropriate social environment—one conducive to abstinence with minimal disruption of life circumstances—should be supported. Considerations of minor disruptions in place of residence, friends, or job need not be a primary issue for the patient with a personality disorder or neurosis, but they cannot go untended here. For a considerable period of time, the patient is highly vulnerable to exacerbations of their addiction and, in some respects, must be viewed with the considerable caution with which one treats the recently compensated psychotic.

Finally, after these priorities have been attended to, psychological conflicts that the patient must resolve, relative to his or her own growth, are considered. As the therapy continues, these come to assume a more prominent role. In the earlier phases, they are likely to reflect directly issues associated with previous drug use. Later, however, as the issue of addiction becomes less compelling from day to day, the context of the treatment increasingly will come to resemble the traditional psychotherapeutic context. Given the optimism generated by an initial victory over the addictive process, the patient will be in an excellent position to move forward in therapy with a positive view of his or her future.

A LONGER COURSE

The following case description illustrates how a network was engaged in treating a patient in long-term care for his addiction.

A 22-year-old man left a message on the therapist's answering machine asking if he could make an appointment. When called back, he said he wanted help to address his heroin use. He said, "I gotta get clean." In response to a few questions, he described himself as a 30-year-old, single artist who clearly had aspirations to achieve wider recognition. He had been using heroin intranasally on and off for 3 years, but for the past 6 months was "sniffing" large doses at least twice a day.

At the initial encounter, given concern about his reliability, the therapist asked to engage collateral support for the patient. He asked if they could both speak on the phone with a friend or a close family member of his who could be a resource for him until the next session. Although he was somewhat wary, he agreed to their calling a cousin with whom he had a close relationship, and who had repeatedly expressed concern over his drug use. The three agreed that the cousin would meet him for dinner right before the next scheduled session and come with him to that appointment.

The patient appeared with his cousin 4 days later. He was somewhat tremulous and reported that he and a friend, also addicted to heroin, had decided to "detoxify" themselves abruptly with some naltrexone that his friend had acquired. They supported each other, suffering miserably over the intervening days.

This patient was a good candidate for network therapy and for treatment with buprenorphine. His network was constituted of three people: his cousin, a close friend, and an uncle 20 years his senior, whom he viewed as a mentor and friend. For the first 3 weeks, individual and network sessions were alternated in each week. Over the subsequent weeks, the frequency of network meetings was decreased relative to the therapist's sense of the patient's stability in treatment. After 6 months, the network members came to a session only once every month or two.

A second component of the treatment was to provide protection from a return to heroin/opioids by having the patient take oral naltrexone, an opioid antagonist, which blocks the effect of an agonist, heroin or otherwise, such as hydrocodone. It was arranged that he would take two 50 mg pills twice weekly (Monday, Wednesday), and three on a third occasion (Friday). He would do this in front of his cousin, who lived only one block away from him. This naltrexone regimen was continued over the course of the ensuing 10 months, and after that on the patient's own recognizance.

At the outset of treatment, the therapist had stipulated that the patient was not to use cannabis, alcohol, or other drugs, explaining to him and the network how any of these could lead to a return to use. He was also expected to give a urine sample for toxicology at random times in order to assure abstinence from drugs. The patient did indeed say at one point in the treatment that he felt supported in avoiding cannabis by virtue of the fact that he did not want to have a positive urine toxicology.

The therapist had often discussed with the patient his vulnerability to alcoholism given his family history. Alcohol was a blight on his family, as his father always drank heavily every evening, making him very uncomfortable during his occasional visits home. After three months in treatment, however, the patient said that he had "never bargained for not drinking at all" and that he didn't quite see himself as abstinent from alcohol for the long term. As the therapist and he discussed this, they agreed that it was best that he stay abstinent for at least a year, and toward the end of that time, his options could be discussed. The issue was also discussed with the network members, who were wary of the patient embarking on something other than total abstinence, but the therapist pointed out that a test of drinking was, "better during treatment than afterward." This was discussed at some length, and the patient implemented a diary of his drinking, limited to no more than two beers a day, and no wine or hard liquor.

At one point during the subsequent treatment, tragedy befell the family, as the patient's younger brother, who also drank in an unhealthy manner, had an auto accident while intoxicated and was gravely injured. After this, the patient had continued to keep his drinking diary, but a month after his brother's accident, he decided that he was better off remaining abstinent, and decided to do so. He did indeed maintain abstinence over a year of subsequent ongoing psychotherapy for general adaptive issues and reported being abstinent 3 years after that.

RESEARCH ON NETWORK THERAPY

Network therapy is included under the American Psychiatric Association (APA) Practice Guidelines[20] for SUDs as an approach to facilitating adherence to a treatment plan. The Substance Abuse and Mental Health Services Administration as one of its Treatment Improvement Protocol TIP 39 SUD treatment and family therapy approaches.[21] To date, five studies have demonstrated its effectiveness in treatment and training. Each addressed the technique's validation from a different perspective: a trial in office management, studies of its effectiveness in the training of psychiatric residents and of counselors who work with people with cocaine use disorder, an evaluation of acceptance of the network approach in an internet technology transfer course, and a trial evaluating the impact of NT relative to medication management in people with opioid (heroin) use disorder inducted on to buprenorphine. In addition, NT components that have been adapted and combined with other psychosocial treatments to treat patients with OUD or AUDs are described below.

An Office-Based Clinical Trial

A chart review was conducted on a series of 60 patients with SUDs, with follow-up appointments scheduled through the period of treatment and up to 1 year thereafter.[22] For 27 patients, the primary drug was alcohol; for 23, it was cocaine; for 6, it was opioids; for 3, it was cannabis; and for 1, it was nicotine. In all but eight of the patients, networks were fully established. Of the 60 patients, 46 experienced full improvement (ie, abstinence for at least 6 months) or major improvement (ie, a marked decline in unhealthy drug use). The study demonstrated the viability of establishing networks and applying them in the practitioner's treatment setting. It also served as a basis for the ensuing developmental research supported by the National Institute on Drug Abuse.

Treatment by Psychiatry Residents

We developed and implemented a NT training sequence in the New York University psychiatric residency program and then evaluated the clinical outcome of a group of patients with cocaine use disorder (CUD) treated by the residents. The psychiatric residency was chosen because of the growing importance of clinical training in the management of addiction in outpatient care in residency programs, in line with the standards set for specialty certification.

A training manual was prepared on the network technique, defining the specifics of the treatment in a manner allowing for uniformity in practice. It was developed for use as a training tool and then as a guide for the residents during the treatment phase. NT video segments drawn from a library of 130 videoed sessions were used to illustrate typical therapy situations. A NT rating scale was developed to assess the technique's application, with items emphasizing key aspects of treatment.[23] The scale was evaluated for its reliability in distinguishing between two contrasting addiction therapies, NT and systemic family therapy, both presented to faculty and residents on video. The internal consistency of responses for each of the techniques was high for both the faculty and the resident samples, and both groups consistently distinguished the two modalities. The scale was then used by clinical supervisors as a didactic aid for training and monitoring therapist adherence to the study treatment manual.

We trained 3rd-year psychiatry residents to apply the NT approach, with an emphasis placed on distinctions in technique between the treatment of addiction and of other major mental illness or personality disorder. The residents then worked with a sample of 47 people with CUD. Once treatment was initiated, 77% of the subjects did establish a network, that is, bring in at least one member for a network session. In fact, 1.47 collaterals on average attended any given network session, across all the subjects and sessions. This is notable, because compliance after initial screening was not necessarily assured. Almost all of those who completed a 24-week regimen (15 of 17) produced urines negative for cocaine in their last three toxicologies. On the other hand, only a minority of those who attended the first week but who did not complete the sequence (4 of 18) met this outcome criterion.[24] The residents, inexperienced in drug treatment, achieved results similar to those reported for experienced professionals.[25,26] These comparisons supported the feasibility of successful training of psychiatry residents naive to addiction treatment and the efficacy of the treatment in their hands.

To better understand the role of therapeutic alliance in NT, Glazer et al.[27] reviewed videoed network sessions on 21 out of the 47 people with CUD and rated them on level of patient-therapist alliance using the PENN Helping Alliance Rating Scale and the Working Alliance Inventory. The tapes that were selected to be rated were those that represented the participants' first videoed NT session. Results showed a significant positive correlation between therapeutic alliance and outcomes as measured by the percentage of cocaine-free urine toxicology screens and by eight consecutive cocaine-free urines.

Treatment by Addiction Counselors

This study was conducted in a community-based addiction treatment clinic, and the NT training sequence was essentially the same as the one applied to the psychiatry residents.[28] A cohort of 10 patients with CUD received treatment at the community program with a format that included NT, along with the clinic's usual package of modalities, and an additional 20 patients with CUD received treatment as usual and served as control subjects. The NT was found to enhance the outcome of the experimental patients. Of 107 urinalyses conducted on the NT patients, 88% were negative, but only 66% of the 82 urine samples from the control subjects were negative, a significantly lower proportion. The mean retention in treatment was 13.9 weeks for the network patients, reflecting a trend toward greater retention than the 10.7 weeks for control subjects.

The results of this study supported the feasibility of transferring the network technology into community-based settings with the potential for enhancing outcomes. Addiction counselors working in a typical outpatient rehabilitation setting were able to learn and then incorporate NT into their largely 12-step–oriented treatment regimens without undue difficulty and with improved outcome.

Use of the Internet

We studied ways in which psychiatrists and other professionals could be offered training by a distance learning method using the internet, a medium that offers the advantage of not being fixed in either time or location. An advertisement was placed in *Psychiatric News*, the newspaper of the APA, offering an internet course combining NT with the use of naltrexone for the treatment of alcoholism.

The sequence of material presented on the internet was divided into three didactic "sessions," followed by a set of questions, with a hypertext link to download relevant references and a certificate of completion. The course took about 2 hours for the student to complete. Our assessment was based on 679 sequential counts, representing 240 unique respondents who went beyond the introductory Web page.[29] Of these respondents, 154 were psychiatrists, who responded positively to the course. A majority responded "a good deal" or "very much" (a score of 3 or 4 on a four-point scale) to the following statements: "It helped me understand the management of alcoholism treatment" (56%), "It helped me learn to use family or friends in network treatment for alcoholism" (75%), and "It improved my ability to use naltrexone in treating alcoholism" (64%). The four studies described in this section support the use of NT as an effective treatment for SUD. They are especially encouraging given the relative ease with which different types of clinicians were engaged and trained in the network approach. Because the approach combines a number of well-established clinical techniques that can be adapted to delivery in typical clinical settings, it is apparently suitable for use by general clinicians and addiction specialists.

Network Therapy in Buprenorphine Maintenance

Galanter et al.[30] evaluated the impact of NT relative to a control condition (medical management [MM]) among 66 patients who were inducted on to buprenorphine for 16 weeks and then tapered to zero dose. NT resulted in a greater percentage of opioid-free urines than did MM (65% versus 45%). By the end of treatment, NT patients were more likely to experience a positive outcome relative to secondary heroin use (50% versus 23%). The use of NT in office practice may enhance the effectiveness of eliminating secondary heroin use during buprenorphine treatment.

ADAPTATIONS OF NETWORK THERAPY TREATMENT

Rothenberg et al.[31] adapted NT and combined it with Relapse Prevention (RP) and a voucher reinforcement system in the treatment of patients with OUD who were enrolled in a 6-month course of treatment with naltrexone referred to as behavioral naltrexone therapy. The NT component involved one significant other who could monitor adherence to naltrexone. In addition to the patient receiving vouchers for each day of abstinence and each pill taken, the network member was reinforced with a voucher for each pill recorded as monitored. The primary treatment outcome was retention in treatment. Patients who used methadone at baseline did more poorly than those using only heroin as demonstrated in the retention rates: 39% versus 65% and 0% versus 31%, respectively, at 1 month and 6 months.

Copello et al.[32] combined elements of NT with social aspects of the community reinforcement approach and RP referred to as social behavior and network therapy (SBNT) in the treatment of persons with alcohol-drinking problems. A number of social skills training strategies are incorporated into the treatment especially those involving social competence in relation to the development of positive social support for change in alcohol use. Every individual involved in treatment is considered a client in his/her own right, and the person with alcohol problems is referred to as the focal client. The core element of the approach is mobilizing the support of the network even though this may involve network sessions that are conducted in the absence of the focal client. In their initial feasibility study with 33 clients, there were two cases in which sessions were held with network members in the absence of the focal client and, in both cases, reengagement of the focal client in treatment was achieved. Out of the 33 clients enrolled in the study, 23 formed a network with the mean number of network members = 1.82 and the mean number of network sessions = 5.24. In a multisite, randomized, controlled trial of 742 clients with unhealthy alcohol use, the United Kingdom Alcohol Treatment Trial (UKATT) research team[33] compared SBNT to motivational enhancement therapy (MET). Both treatment groups exhibited similar reductions in alcohol consumption and unhealthy alcohol-related behaviors and improvement in mental functioning over a 12-month period. Attending more sessions was associated with a better outcome, and SBNT patients with greater motivation to change and those with more negative short-term expectancies were more likely to attend.[34]

Additional studies involving the UKATT study sample were conducted assessing (1) cost-effectiveness,[35] (2) client–treatment matching effects,[36] (3) clients' perceptions of change in alcohol-drinking behaviors,[37] and drinking goal preference.[38] The UKATT team evaluated the cost-effectiveness of SBNT relative to MET. SBNT resulted in a fivefold cost savings in health, social, and criminal justice service expenditures and was similar to cost-effectiveness estimates obtained for MET. The UKATT research team[36] tested a priori hypotheses concerning client–treatment matching effects similar to those tested in Project MATCH. The findings were consistent with Project MATCH in that no hypothesized matching effects were significant. Orford et al.[37] interviewed a subset of clients (N = 397) who participated in this trial to assess their views concerning whether any positive changes in drinking behavior had occurred and to what they attributed those changes. At 3 months after randomization to treatment, SBNT clients made more social attributions (eg, involvement of others in supporting behavior change), and MET clients made more motivational attributions (eg, awareness of the consequences of drinking). Patients who initially stated a preference for abstinence showed a better outcome than those stating a preference for nonabstinence. This was true both at 3- and 12-month follow-up.[38]

Copello et al.[39] adapted SBNT for persons presenting with unhealthy drug use. Of 31 clients enrolled in the study, 23 received SBNT and had outcomes data available at 3-month follow-up. Reductions in the amount of heroin used per day and increases in family cohesion and family satisfaction were documented. Open-ended interviews with clients, network members, and therapists were conducted in a qualitative investigation of respondents' perceptions of SBNT.[40] Major themes that emerged from analysis of the interview responses included the value of SBNT in (1) increasing network support for reducing drug use, (2) promoting open and honest communication between clients and network members about drug use, and (3) increasing network members' understanding of drugs and the focal person's behavior. Williamson et al.[40] suggest that these features of SBNT may be more prominent when the problem is one of illicit drug use than when the problem involves alcohol use.

COMMUNITY-BASED FAMILY INVOLVEMENT

The nature of the involvement of families in community-based recovery programs is difficult to evaluate, given the diversity of such programs and differences in the nature of the families' roles. Nonetheless, documentation of clinical experiences can be helpful in generating an understanding of such options. Articles describing the following clinical programs can be helpful in this regard. Two studies reported on in-depth interviews characterizing such programs, and a third examined the rates of patients' program completion relative to family participation.

An interview with a small number of family members who had undergone a family intervention program in Malaysia characterized themes that emerged from their experience. They related to the therapeutic alliance between counselor and family members, and behaviors within the program that interviewees found helpful.[41] More systematic measurements on larger programs with documentation of relevant items can be useful in parsing out such themes.

A similar assessment was made on families of persons treated for an overdose in one of their members. It revealed that clinicians were often unaware how the families were involved with the patients. Outcomes were better when families and clinicians worked together to develop a shared treatment plan and had similar perspectives on unhealthy drug use. The study also underlined the importance of some clinicians being unaware of family contacts with patients and did not communicate with them.[42] As indicated here, clinicians are often unaware at all of family involvement with their patients. This underlines the importance of clinicians being aware of the nature of families' involvement and addressing the role it should play in the treatment planning.

A third study described results of relative completion rates for 274 patients admitted to a residential addiction treatment program. Patients were divided into two groups, one having family or significant others actively involved in the 7-day family program, and the other did not have them involved. This study describes how completion rates were greater for the former group.[43] It would be useful for studies such as this to provide description of the family programs applied.

PRINCIPLES OF NETWORK TREATMENT

Start a Network as soon as Possible

- It is important to see the person with unhealthy alcohol or drug use promptly, because the window of opportunity for openness to treatment is generally brief. A week's delay can result in a person's reverting back to substance use or losing motivation.
- If the person is married, engage the spouse early on, preferably at the time of the first phone call. Point out that addiction is a family problem.
- In the initial interview, frame the exchange so that a good case is built for the grave consequences of the patient's

addiction, and do this before the patient can introduce his or her system of denial. That way you are not putting the spouse or other network members in the awkward position of having to contradict a close relation.

- Start arranging for a network to be assembled as soon as possible, generally involving a number of the patient's family or close friends.
- From the very first meeting, you should consider how to ensure sobriety until the next meeting, and plan that with the network.
- Include people who are close to the patient, have a longstanding relationship with the patient, and are trusted. Avoid members with unhealthy substance use. Avoid superiors and subordinates at work.
- Make sure that the mood of meetings is trusting and free of recrimination. Avoid letting the patient or the network members feel guilty or angry in meetings. Explain issues of conflict in terms of the problems presented by addiction; do not get into personality conflicts.
- A feeling of teamwork should be promoted, with no psychologizing or impugning members' motives.
- Meet as frequently as necessary to ensure abstinence.
- The network should have no agenda other than to support the patient's abstinence but as abstinence is stabilized, the network can help the patient plan for a new drug-free adaptation. It is not there to work on family relations or help other members with their problems although it may do this indirectly.
- Maintaining abstinence: The patient and the network members should report at the outset of each session any exposure of the patient to alcohol and drugs. The patient and network members should be instructed on the nature of the return of use or symptoms and plan with the therapist how to sustain abstinence.
- The therapist does whatever is necessary to secure stability of the membership if the patient is having trouble doing so.
- Securing future behavior: The therapist should combine any and all modalities necessary to ensure the patient's stability, such as a stable, drug-free residence, the avoidance of substance-using friends, attendance at 12-step meetings, pharmacotherapies, and observed urinalysis.
- Patients can be expected to go to meetings of AA or related groups at least two to three times, with follow-up discussion in therapy.
- If patients have reservations about these meetings, try to help them understand how to deal with those reservations. Issues such as social anxiety should be explored if they make a patient reluctant to participate.

Nonetheless, issues may arise among network members, which should be addressed. Adverse effects of the SUD on family members are frequently a problem that merits being attendees, as individual members may manifest disorders such as anxiety or depression. In such circumstances, referral for a network member to an outside health professional may be warranted, as may be referral to a related program for mutual aid, such as Nar-Anon or Al-Anon.

REFERENCES

1. Galanter M. Cognitive labeling: psychotherapy for alcohol and drug abuse: an approach based on learning theory. *J Psychiatr Treat Eval*. 1983;5:551-556.
2. Jellinek EM. *The Disease Concept of Alcoholism*. Hillhouse; 1963.
3. Marlatt GA, Gordon J. *Relapse Prevention: Maintenance Strategies in the Treatment of Addictive Behaviors*. 2nd ed. Guilford Press; 2004.
4. Beck AT, Wright FD, Newman CF, et al. *Cognitive Therapy of Substance Abuse*. Guilford Press; 1993.
5. Johnson VE. *Intervention: How to Help Someone Who Doesn't Want Help*. Johnson Institute; 1986.
6. McCrady BS. Treating alcohol problems with couple therapy. *J Clin Psychol*. 2012;68(5):514-525.
7. Morgenstern J, Longabaugh R. Cognitive-behavioral treatment for alcohol dependence: a review of the evidence for its hypothesized mechanisms of action. *Addiction*. 2000;95:1475-1490.
8. Stephens RS, Babor TF, Kadden R, Miller M; Marijuana Treatment Project Research Group. The Marijuana Treatment Project: rationale, design, and participant characteristics. *Addiction*. 2002;94:109-124.
9. Carroll KM. *A Cognitive-Behavioral Approach: Treating Cocaine Addiction*. National Institute on Drug Abuse; 1998.
10. Wikler A. Dynamics of drug dependence: implications of a conditioning theory for research and treatment. *Arch Gen Psychiatry*. 1973;28:611-616.
11. Zywiak WH, Wirtz PW. Decomposing the relationships between pretreatment social network characteristics and alcohol treatment outcome. *J Stud Alcohol*. 2002;63(1):114-121.
12. Beckman LJ, Amaro H. Personal and social difficulties faced by women and men entering alcoholism treatment. *J Stud Alcohol*. 1986;47:135-145.
13. Yalom ID, Leszcz M. *The Theory and Practice of Group Psychotherapy*. 5th ed. Basic Books; 2005.
14. Marlatt GA, Carlini-Marlatt B. Harm reduction: a pragmatic approach for alcohol-related problems. In: Fearnow-Kenny M, Wyrick DL, eds. *Alcohol Use and Prevention: A Resource for College Students*. Tanglewood Research; 2005:61-70.
15. Helzer JE, Robins LN, Taylor JR, et al. The extent of long-term drinking among alcoholics discharged from medical and psychiatric facilities. *N Engl J Med*. 1985;312:1678-1682.
16. Gitlow SE, Peyser HS, eds. *Alcoholism: A Practical Treatment Guide*. Grune & Stratton; 1980.
17. Speck R. Psychotherapy of the social network of a schizophrenic family. *Fam Process*. 1967;6:208.
18. Fuller R, Branchey L, Brightwell DR, et al. Disulfiram treatment of alcoholism. A Veterans Administration cooperative study. *JAMA*. 1986; 256:1449-1455.
19. Galanter M. Network therapy for addiction: a model for office practice. *Am J Psychiatry*. 1993;150:28-36.
20. American Psychiatric Association. Practice guidelines for the treatment of patients with substance use disorders: alcohol, cocaine, opioids. *Am J Psychiatry*. 1995;152(Suppl 11):1-59.
21. Center for Substance Abuse Treatment. *Substance Abuse Treatment and Family Therapy*. Treatment Improvement Protocol (TIP) Series, No. 39. DHHS Publication No. (SMA) 05-4006. Substance Abuse and Mental Health Services Administration; 2004.
22. Galanter M. Network therapy for substance abuse: a clinical trial. *Psychotherapy*. 1993;30:251-258.
23. Keller D, Galanter M, Weinberg S. Validation of a scale for network therapy: a technique for systematic use of peer and family support in addiction treatment. *Am J Drug Alcohol Abuse*. 1997;23:115-127.
24. Galanter M, Dermatis H, Keller D, Trujillo M. Network therapy for cocaine abuse: use of family and peer supports. *Am J Addict*. 2002;11:161-166.
25. Carroll KM, Rounsaville BJ, Gordon LT, et al. Psychotherapy and pharmacotherapy for ambulatory cocaine abusers. *Arch Gen Psychiatry*. 1994;51:177-187.
26. Higgins ST, Budney AJ, Bickel WK, et al. Achieving cocaine abstinence with a behavioral approach. *Am J Psychiatry*. 1993;150:763-769.
27. Glazer SS, Galanter M, Megwinoff O, Dermatis H, Keller DS. The role of therapeutic alliance in network therapy: a family and peer support-based treatment for cocaine abuse. *Subst Abus*. 2003;24(2):93-100.

28. Keller D, Galanter M, Dermatis H. Technology transfer of network therapy to community-based addiction counselors. *J Subst Abuse Treat.* 1999;16:183-189.
29. Galanter M, Keller DS, Dermatis H. Using the Internet for clinical training: a course on network therapy. *Psychiatr Serv.* 1997;48:999-1000.
30. Galanter M, Dermatis H, Glickman L, et al. Network therapy: decreased secondary opioid use during buprenorphine maintenance. *J Subst Abuse Treat.* 2004;26:313-318.
31. Rothenberg JL, Sullivan MA, Church SH, et al. Behavioral naltrexone therapy: an integrated treatment for opiate dependence. *J Subst Abuse Treat.* 2002;23:351-360.
32. Copello A, Orford J, Hodgson R, et al. Social behaviour and network therapy: basic principles and early experiences. *Addict Behav.* 2002;27:345-366.
33. UKATT Research Team. Effectiveness of treatment for alcohol problems: findings of the randomised UK alcohol treatment trial (UKATT). *BMJ.* 2005;331:541-543.
34. Dale V, Coulton S, Godfrey C, et al. Exploring treatment attendance and its relationship to outcome in a randomized controlled trial of treatment for alcohol problems: secondary analysis of the UK alcohol treatment trial (UKATT). *Alcohol Alcohol.* 2011;46:592-599.
35. UKATT Research Team. Cost effectiveness of treatment for alcohol problems: findings of the randomised UK alcohol treatment trial (UKATT). *BMJ.* 2005;331:544-549.
36. UKATT Research Team. UK Alcohol Treatment Trial: client-treatment matching effects. *Addiction.* 2008;103:228-238.
37. Orford J, Hodgson R, Copello A, Wilton S, Slegg G; UKATT Research Team. To what factors do clients attribute change? Content analysis of follow-up interview with clients of the UK Alcohol Treatment Trial. *J Subst Abuse Treat.* 2009;36:49-58.
38. Adamson S, Heather N, Morton V, Raistrick D; UKATT Research Team. Initial preference for drinking goal in the treatment of alcohol problems: II. Treatment outcomes. *Alcohol Alcohol.* 2010;45:136-142.
39. Copello A, Williamson E, Orford J, Day E. Implementing and evaluating social behaviour and network therapy in drug treatment practice in the UK: a feasibility study. *Addict Behav.* 2006;31:802-810.
40. Williamson E, Smith M, Orford J, Copello A, Day E. Social behavior and network therapy for drug problems: evidence of benefits and challenges. *Addict Disord Treat.* 2007;6:167-179.
41. Baharudin DF, Hussin AHM, Sumari M, Mohamed S, Zakaria MZ, Sawai RP. Family intervention for the treatment and rehabilitation of drug addiction. *J Subst Use.* 2013;19(4):301-306.
42. Stumbo SP, Yarborough BJH, Janoff SL, Yarborough MT, McCarty D, Green CA. A qualitative analysis of family involvement in prescribed opioid medication monitoring among individuals who have experienced opioid overdoses. *Subst Abus.* 2016;37(1):96-103.
43. McPherson C, Boyne H, Willis R. The role of family in residential treatment patient retention. *Int J Ment Health Addict.* 2017;15:933-941.

CHAPTER 76

Therapeutic Communities and Modified Therapeutic Communities for Co-occurring Mental and Substance Use Disorders

George De Leon and Stanley Sacks

CHAPTER OUTLINE

- Introduction
- Part I: Traditional therapeutic communities
- Part II: Modified therapeutic community for persons with co-occurring mental and substance use disorders

INTRODUCTION

Drug-free residential programs for substance use disorders (SUDs) appeared a decade later than did therapeutic communities (TCs) in psychiatric hospitals pioneered by Maxwell Jones and others in the United Kingdom. The term therapeutic community evolved in these hospital settings, although the two models arose independently. The TC for SUDs emerged in the 1960s as a self-help alternative to existing conventional treatments.

Those recovering from alcohol and other SUDs were its first participant developers. Although its modern antecedents can be traced to Alcoholics Anonymous and Synanon, the TC prototype is ancient, existing in all forms of communal healing and support. Contemporary TCs are sophisticated human services institutions. Today, the label therapeutic community is generic, describing a variety of short- and long-term residential and nonresidential programs that serve a wide spectrum of individuals with SUDs.

Although the TC model has been widely adapted for different populations and settings, it is the traditional long-term residential prototype for has documented effectiveness for SUDs. Part I of this chapter details the theory, method and model of the traditional TC. Part II summarizes the adaptation and modifications of the traditional TC for individuals with co-occurring mental and SUDs.

PART I: TRADITIONAL THERAPEUTIC COMMUNITIES

Traditional TCs[1] are similar to each other in structure, staffing pattern, perspective, and treatment regimen although they differ in size (30 to several hundred beds in a facility) and client demography. Staffs are composed of TC-trained clinicians, with and without recovery experiences, and other human service professionals who provide medical, mental health, vocational, educational, family counseling, fiscal, administrative, and legal services. The recommended planned duration of stay of long-term TCs has gradually decreased across the years from 15-24 months to 9-12 months.

The TC Perspective

The TC perspective or theory shapes its program model and its unique approach, community as method. The perspective consists of four interrelated views of the SUD, the individual, the recovery process, and of healthy living.

View of the Disorder

Substance use disorder is viewed as a disorder of the whole person, affecting some or all areas of functioning. Cognitive and behavioral problems are evident, as are mood disturbances. Thinking may be unrealistic or disorganized; values are confused, nonexistent, or antisocial. Frequently there are deficits in verbal, reading, writing, and marketable skills. Moral or even spiritual issues, whether expressed in existential or psychological terms, are apparent. Thus, from the TC perspective, the problem stems from the individual, not the drug. Substance use is a symptom, not the essence of the disorder.

View of the Person

In TCs, individuals are distinguished in terms of psychological dysfunction and social deficits rather than according to drug use patterns. In many TC residents, vocational and educational problems are marked; middle-class, mainstream values are either missing or not sought. Usually these residents emerge from a socially disadvantaged sector. The poor employment and educational histories of a number of people who use substances who enter publicly funded treatment in general are documented in the sociodemographic research literature,[2] particularly TCs.[3] Their TC experience is better termed habilitation, that is, development of a socially productive, and conventional lifestyle for the first time. Among residents from more advantaged backgrounds, the term rehabilitation is more suitable, which emphasizes a return to a lifestyle previously lived, known, and perhaps rejected.

Regardless of differences in social background, drug preference or psychological problems, however, most individuals admitted to TCs share clinical characteristics that reflect immaturity and antisocial dimensions (see **Table 76-1**). Whether they are antecedents or consequences these characteristics are commonly observed to correlate with serious substance involvement. More important, in TCs, a positive change in these characteristics is considered to be essential for stable recovery.

View of Recovery

In the TC perspective, recovery involves a change in lifestyle as well as in social and personal identity. Thus, the primary psychological goal of treatment is to change the negative patterns of behavior, thinking, and feeling; the main social goal is to develop the skills, attitudes, and values of a responsible drug-free lifestyle. Stable recovery, however, depends on a successful integration of these social and psychological goals. Behavioral change is unstable without insight, and insight is insufficient without felt experience. Several key assumptions underlie the recovery process in the TC.

Motivation

Recovery depends on pressures to change, positive and negative. Some individuals seek help, driven by stressful external pressures; others are moved by more intrinsic factors. For all, however, remaining in treatment requires continued internal motivation to change. Therefore, elements of the treatment approach are designed to sustain motivation or to enable detection of early signs of premature termination.

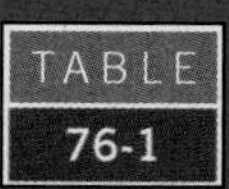

TABLE 76-1 Typical Behavioral, Cognitive, and Emotional Characteristics of People With Substance Use Disorders in Therapeutic Communities[a]

Characteristics
Low tolerance for all forms of discomfort and delay of gratification
Problems with authority
Inability to manage feelings (particularly hostility, guilt, and anxiety)
Poor impulse control (particularly sexual or aggressive impulses)
Poor judgment and reality testing concerning consequences of actions
Unrealistic self-appraisal regarding discrepancies between personal resources and aspirations
Prominence of lying, manipulation, and deception as coping behaviors
Personal and social irresponsibility (eg, inconsistency or failures in meeting obligations)
Marked deficits in learning and in marketable and communication skills that predispose the individual to drug use

[a]A fuller description of the social psychological profiles or TC residents drawn from clinical assessment and relevant research studies is contained in De Leon 2000, chapter 4.

Self-Help and Mutual Self-Help

Strictly speaking, treatment is not provided; rather, it is made available to the individual in the TC through its staff and peers and the daily regimen of work, groups, meetings, seminars, and recreation. However, the effectiveness of these elements depends on the individual, who must fully engage in the treatment regimen. In self-help recovery, the individual makes the main contribution to the change process. In mutual self-help, the principal messages of recovery, personal growth, and "right living" are mediated by peers through confrontation and sharing in groups, by example as role models, and as supportive encouraging friends in daily interactions.

Social Learning

A lifestyle change occurs in a social context. Negative behavioral patterns, attitudes, and roles were not acquired in isolation, nor can they be altered in isolation. This assumption is the basis for the use of a peer community to facilitate recovery. A socially responsible role is learned by acting the role within a community of similar others.

View of Right Living

TCs adhere to certain precepts, values, and a social perspective that guide and reinforce recovery. For example, there are community sanctions to address antisocial behaviors and attitudes: the negative values of the street, jails, or negative peers; and irresponsible or exploitative sexual conduct. Positive values are emphasized as being essential to social learning and personal growth. These values include truth and honesty (in word and deed), a work ethic, self-reliance, earned rewards and achievement, personal accountability, responsible concern (being one's brother's or sister's keeper), social manners, and community involvement. The precepts of right living are constantly reinforced in various formal and informal ways (eg, signs, seminars, in groups and community meetings).

The TC Approach: Community as Method

The TC approach can be summarized in the phrase "community as method." Theoretical writings offer a definition of "community as method" as *the purposive use of the community to teach individuals to use the community to change themselves.*[1]

The fundamental assumption underlying community as method is that individuals obtain maximum therapeutic and educational impact when they engage in and learn to use all of the diverse elements of the community as the tools for self-change. Thus, community-as-method means that the community itself provides a *context* for social learning. Its membership establishes *expectations* or standards of participation in the community. It continually *assesses* how individuals are meeting these expectations and *responds* to them with strategies that promote continued participation.

The TC for addictions has evolved a unique social learning approach captured in the phrase "community as method." The latter, however, contains familiar elements and practices that are supported by abundant behavioral and social-psychological research outside TCs, for example, peer tutoring, goal attainment, behavior modification. Similarly, behavioral training and social learning *principles* are evident, for example, social role training, vicarious learning, social reinforcement. As discussed elsewhere, these principles are *naturalistically mediated* within the context of community living.[1]

The diverse elements and activities of the community can be organized in terms of the TC program model, specific methods, and the program stages that facilitate the process of change.

The TC Program Model

The TC program model is its social and psychological environment. Each component of the environment reflects an understanding of the TC perspective and each is used to transmit community teachings, promote affiliation, and self-change. The key components of the program model are summarized in terms of its social organization, work, peer and staff roles.

TC Structure/Social Organization

The social organization of a TC consists of a relatively small staff complemented by a large base of residents or peers at junior, intermediate, and senior levels. This vertical structure arranges relationships of mutual responsibility to others at various levels in the program. The daily operation of the community itself is the task of the residents, who work together under staff supervision. The broad range of resident job assignments illustrates the extent of the self-help process. Residents perform all house services (eg, cooking, cleaning, kitchen service, minor repair); serve as apprentices; run all departments; and conduct house meetings, certain seminars, and peer encounter groups.

The TC is managed by the staff that monitor and evaluate client status, supervise resident groups, assign and supervise resident jobs, and oversee house operations. The staff conduct therapeutic groups (other than peer encounter groups) using a variety of approaches from behavioral to psychodynamic as suitable to the issue, provide individual counseling, organize social and recreational projects, and confer with significant others. They make all decisions about resident status, discipline, promotion, transfers, discharges, furloughs, and treatment planning.

Work as Education and Therapy

Work and job changes have clinical relevance for substance-using patients in TCs, most of whom have not successfully negotiated the social and occupational world of the larger society. Vertical job movements carry the obvious rewards of status and privilege. However, lateral job changes are more frequent and permit exposure to all aspects of the community. In addition to skill development, the primary clinical aim of job functions is to facilitate personal change in behaviors, attitudes and values.

Peers as Role Models

TC participants who demonstrate the expected behaviors and reflect the values and teachings of the community are viewed as role models. Thus, all peers and staff are expected to be role models. TCs require multiple role models in order to maintain the integrity of the community and ensure the spread of positive social learning effects.

Staff as Rational Authorities

Staff facilitates community as method, as role models, counselors, and particularly as rational authorities. In their management and clinical functions, staff as rational authorities provide the reasons for their decisions and explain the meaning of consequences. Staff exercise their authority to teach, guide, and correct rather than to punish or control.

Therapeutic Community Methods

In the TC, all activities, planned (eg, groups, meetings) and unplanned (eg, interpersonal and social interactions) facilitate recovery and right living. However, planned activities are viewed as interventions or methods, designed to impact both individuals and the general community in specific ways. They can be organized in accordance with their primary purpose, therapeutic-educational change, community enhancement, and community and clinical management.

Therapeutic-Educative Activities (Groups-Counseling)

Therapeutic-educative activities consist of various group processes and individual counseling. They increase communication and interpersonal skills, bring about examination of behavior and attitudes, and offer instruction in alternative modes of behavior. The main groups include encounters, probes, and tutorials. These differ somewhat in format and objectives, but all have the common goal of fostering trust, personal disclosure, intimacy, and peer solidarity to facilitate therapeutic change.

Encounters are the cornerstone of group process in the TC. The term encounter is generic, describing a variety of activity forms that use confrontational (face-to-face) and supportive procedures as their main approach. The basic encounter group is a peer-led group composed of a changing composition of 12 to 20 community residents; it meets 1 to 3 times weekly, usually for 2 hours, with an additional 30-minute period for snacking and socializing following each group. The primary objective of each encounter is to heighten individual awareness of specific attitudes or behavioral patterns that should be modified.

Probes are staff-led groups that originally were conducted as needed to obtain in-depth clinical information on residents for purposes of problem identification and treatment planning. They have evolved into regularly scheduled therapy groups of 60 to 90 minutes duration consisting of 12 to 20 residents. For example, weekly or biweekly staff caseload groups consist of the same composition of peers who mutually monitor ongoing clinical progress. These groups address individual problems of program adjustment as well as trauma issues related to substance use, (eg, violence, sexual abuse, abandonment). In contrast with the behavioral focus of encounters, probe/therapy groups emphasize sharing and the empathy to foster self-disclosure.

Marathons are extended therapy groups conducted by staff as needed to initiate resolution of traumatic life experiences. The intimacy, safety, and bonding in the marathon setting facilitate emotional processing ("working through") of significant life events identified in individual counseling, probe/caseload, or other groups. The use of marathons has sharply declined commensurate with the decreases in planned duration of residential stay.

Tutorials are regularly scheduled groups that are primarily directed toward skills training (eg, management of the department or the reception desk; training in the use of group tools). Tutorials now include cognitive-behavioral groups using manualized curricula for targeted clinical areas such as trauma, relapse prevention, criminal thinking, and anger management. Two examples of manuals in common usage are *Thinking for a Change* (mostly in prison TCs) and *Seeking Safety* in community-based and prison-based TCs.

Other groups that convene regularly or, as needed, supplement the main groups. These vary in focus, format, and composition. For example, dormitory, or departmental encounter groups may address issues of operating the community or resident conflict resolution. Special theme groups may use tutorial and caseload formats to address domestic violence, re-entry issues (eg, work, family reconciliation), gender, ethnic, age-specific, or health issues. In addition, sensitivity training, and psychodrama are implemented to varying extents. These activities were conducted by invited experts as needed. As with marathons, however, the frequency of these groups has declined significantly commensurate with shorter planned durations of treatment.

One-to-one counseling balances the needs of the individual with those of the community. Peer exchange is ongoing and is the most consistent form of informal counseling in TCs. Staff counseling sessions may be formal or informal and are usually conducted as needed. The focus of staff counseling is to address issues that may impede clinical progress and to facilitate the individual's adjustment to and constructive use of the peer community. The counseling approach is nontraditional in its emphasis on facilitating program adjustment, retention, and treatment planning. However, for special populations and contemporary modified TCs, traditional staff counseling is more typical.[1]

Community Enhancement Activities (Meetings)

Community enhancement activities include the four main facility-wide meetings: the morning meeting, the seminar, the house meeting that meet daily, and the general meeting, (which is called when needed). Though different in format and specific purpose, all meetings have the common objective of strengthening community cohesion. The purpose of the morning meeting is motivational, to instill a positive attitude in the community at the beginning of the day. This meeting is particularly relevant for residents in TCs most of whom have never adapted to the routine of an ordinary day. Led by resident teams, morning meetings occur daily for 30 minutes and utilize a plan of songs, dance, music, games skits, and inspirational words to achieve its objective.

The afternoon seminar is viewed as a community meeting since it includes all the residents in the program (subsets of all residents are groups). Residents conduct most seminars, although some are presented by staff members or less frequently by outside speakers. Seminar topics directly or indirectly relate to the TC perspective including themes of personal growth, recovery, and right-living concepts (eg, self-reliance, maturity, relationships). However, topics may include special knowledge themes (eg, such as the brain and addiction, preparing for reentry, family genealogy). The educational format of the seminar focuses on impacting conceptual and communication skills.

House meetings take place nightly after dinner, usually last 30 to 45 minutes, and are coordinated by senior residents. The main aim of these meetings is to transact community business (eg, departmental reports, special announcements, phase changes, introduction of new residents, disciplinary issues, etc.), although they also have a clinical objective. In this forum, social pressure through public acknowledgment of positive or negative behaviors is judiciously applied to facilitate both community and individual change.

General meetings are called when needed usually to address negative behavior, attitudes, or incidents in the facility. All residents and staff members are assembled at any time and for an indefinite duration. Conducted by staff and selected senior residents they are designed to identify problem individuals or conditions or to reaffirm motivation and reinforce positive behavior and attitudes in the community.

Community enhancement meetings also include a variety of informal activities. These may be rituals and traditions, and celebrations (eg, birthdays, graduations, program phase changes), ceremonies (eg, those relating to general and cultural holidays), and memorial observances for deceased residents, family members of residents, and staff members.

Community and Clinical Management Elements

Community and clinical management elements maintain the physical and psychological safety of the environment and ensure that resident life is orderly and productive. They protect the community as a whole and strengthen it as a context for social learning. The main elements are staff managed and include privileges, disciplinary sanctions, surveillance (as described below), and urine testing.

Privileges

In the TC, privileges are explicit rewards that reinforce the value of positive/desired change and overall clinical progress. Staff members deliver all privileges, which may range from telephone use and letter writing early in treatment to overnight furloughs later in treatment. Successful movement through each stage earns privileges that grant wider personal latitude and increased self-responsibility. Displays of inappropriate behavior or negative attitude can result in loss of privileges, which can be regained through demonstrated improvement. The privilege system in the TC teaches that productive participation or membership in a family or a community is based on an earning process.

Disciplinary Sanctions

TCs have their own specific rules and regulations that guide the behavior of residents and the management of facilities. The explicit purpose of these rules is to ensure the safety and health of the community. However, their implicit aim is to train and teach residents through consequential learning.

The code of rules may be organized into three levels of severity or strictness reflecting their importance to the health and safety of the community: Cardinal rules (such as no drug use, violence or threat of violence); major rules (such as stealing or vandalizing); and house rules (such as respect for authority, no displays of street code behaviors). Disciplinary actions may also be delivered for resident's persistent failure in meeting community expectations. Examples are nonparticipation in community activities or repeated displays of negative attitudes toward the program.

Delivered by staff members, the disciplinary sanction employed relates to the severity of the infraction. For example, these may range from written assignments, job demotions, or loss of privileges to administrative discharge. The sanction is usually a written contract with the resident. These agreements make explicit the behaviors addressed, nature, and duration of the consequences. Although contracts may be perceived as punitive, their basic purpose is to promote a learning experience by compelling residents to attend to their own conduct, to reflect on their own motivation, and to consider alternative forms of acting under similar situations.

An evolutionary change in TCs is the abandonment of questionable learning experiences (eg, shaved heads, stocking caps, wearing signs). These were once rationalized as useful strategies for some clients in addressing the immaturity and social deviancy features of their disorder. Since the early 1980s such practices are excluded in the practice standards of contemporary TCs. It should be noted that while unnecessary and appropriately renounced, there is no compelling statistical or clinical evidence that such practices resulted in harmful outcomes. (Author observation: No publications on this issue, only the absence of validated reports in the literature.)

Surveillance

The TC's most comprehensive method for assessing the overall physical and psychological status of the residential community is the house run. Several times a day, staff members and selected senior residents walk through the entire facility, examining its overall condition. House runs provide global snapshot impressions of the facility: its cleanliness, planned routines, and safety procedures. They also illuminate the overall morale and psychological tone of the community in the attitudes and social functioning of individual residents and peer groups. Most TCs implement unannounced random urine testing or incident-related urine-testing procedures. When urine tests are positive for drugs, the action taken depends on several factors (eg, the substance used, the resident's time and status in the program, the resident's history of drug and other infractions, and the locus and condition of use). Positive urines initiate a disciplinary action or learning experience that includes exploration of conditions precipitating the infraction.

Peer Confrontation: Verbal Affirmations and Correctives

In the TC, verbal affirmations and correctives are the main ways that peers engage in community management. These verbal interactions illustrate examples of peer confrontation in that they provide face-to-face feedback to members as to whether they are meeting community expectations concerning program participation, recovery and right living. Correctives aim to raise the individual's awareness of behaviors and attitudes that require changing. Correctives range in severity from mild reminders ("pull ups") to stern conversations ("verbal reprimands"). Affirmations aim to encourage or reinforce positive clinical change or personal growth and provide the crucial balance to verbal correctives and staff disciplinary sanctions.

Peer confrontations are intended to facilitate learning for those delivering as well as receiving them. Observing, affirming, reminding, and correcting others reciprocally reinforce self-learning through practice, rehearsal, or role modeling. Thus, verbal affirmations and correctives are quintessential examples of the principle of mutual self-help.

The Program Stages and Phases

Recovery in the TC is a developmental process, one that occurs in a social learning setting. The developmental process itself can be understood as a passage through stages of learning. The learning that occurs at each stage facilitates change at the next, and each change reflects movement toward the goals of recovery. Three major program stages characterize change in long-term residential TCs: orientation-induction, primary treatment, and re-entry.

Stage 1: Orientation-Induction (0-60 Days)

The main goal of stage 1 is to provide new residents with a formal orientation to the TC. The aim of orientation in the initial phase of residence is for the individual to be assimilated into the community through full participation and involvement in all of its activities. Formal seminars and informal peer instruction focus on dissemination of information and instruction concerning program philosophy, rules, house regulations, and community expectations as to participation in the program meetings and group activities.

Stage 2: Primary Treatment (2-12 Months)

The stage of primary treatment consists of three sub phases that roughly correlate with time in the program (2-4, 5-8, and 9-12 months). The daily therapeutic-educational regimen of meetings, groups, job assignments, and peer and staff counseling remains the same throughout the year of primary treatment. However, progress is reflected at the end of each phase in terms of explicit behavioral indicators (eg, resident "sets an example" by month 8) and more broadly in terms of three interrelated dimensions of change: community status (role model), development or maturity, and overall psychological adjustment. Progress in this stage and throughout is informally assessed by staff with input from peers and in recent years with clinical scales.[4]

Stage 3: Re-entry (13-24 Months)

Re-entry is the stage at which the individual must strengthen skills for autonomous decision-making and the capacity for self-management and must rely less on rational authorities or a well-formed peer network. The main objective of the early re-entry phase (13-18 months) is to prepare for separation from the TC. Particular emphasis is placed on life-skills seminars, which provide training for living outside the community Plans are developed for long-term psychological, educational, housing, and vocational objectives. Clients may be attending school or holding full-time jobs, either within or outside the TC while still living in the facility (see above).

The objective of the later re-entry phase (18-24 months) is successful separation from the TC. Clients have a "live-out" status; they hold full-time jobs or attend school full time, and they maintain their own households, usually with live-out peers. They may participate in Alcoholics Anonymous or Narcotics Anonymous or attend family or individual therapy sessions. Contact with the TC is gradually reduced to weekly telephone calls and monthly visits with a primary counselor.

Graduation

Completion marks the end of active program involvement. Graduation itself, however, is an annual event conducted in the facility for individuals who have completed the program, usually 1 year after their residence is over. Thus, the TC experience is preparation rather than a cure. Residence in the program facilitates a process of change that must continue throughout life, and what is gained in treatment are tools to guide the individual on a path of continued change. Completion, or graduation, therefore, is not an end but a beginning.

Aftercare

TCs have always acknowledged the client's efforts to maintain sobriety and a positive lifestyle beyond graduation. Until recently, long-term TCs addressed key clinical and life adjustment issues of aftercare during the re-entry stages of the 2-year program. However, funding pressures have resulted in shorter planned durations of residential treatment and the stages and phases therein. This has underscored the necessity for aftercare resources to address both continuing primary treatment as well as re-entry issues. Thus, many contemporary TCs offer postresidential aftercare treatment and social services within their systems, such as intensive day treatment and step-down outpatient ambulatory treatment, or through linkages with outside agencies.

Criteria for Residential TC Treatment

Traditional TCs maintain an open-door policy with respect to admission for residential treatment. This understandably results in a wide range of treatment candidates, not all of who are equally ready for, suited for, or motivated to face the demands of the residential regimen. Relatively few are excluded, because the TC policy is to accept individuals who are mandated to or elect residential treatment, regardless of the reasons influencing their choice.

The general consideration concerning suitability for the TC is risk—the extent to which clients present a management burden to the staff or pose a threat to the security and health of the treatment community. Thus, specific exclusionary criteria most often include histories of arson, suicide attempts, and serious psychiatric disorders. Psychiatric exclusion is usually based on documented history of psychiatric hospitalizations or evidence of psychotic symptoms on interview (eg, frank delusions, thought disorder, hallucinations, confused orientation, signs of a serious affective disorder). However, psychotropic medication is more widely used in TCs to accommodate increasing numbers of admissions with co-occurring conditions. Clients taking medication for medical conditions can be admitted, as can disabled individuals or persons who require prosthetics, providing these individuals can participate fully in the program.

Physical examinations and laboratory workups (blood and urine profiles) are performed after admission. Because of concern about communicable disease in a residential setting, some TCs require tests for conditions such as tuberculosis, and hepatitis to be performed before clients enter the facility or at least within the first weeks of admission. Policies and practices concerning testing for human immunodeficiency virus (HIV) and management of acquired immune deficiency syndrome (AIDS) and hepatitis C emphasize voluntary testing with counseling, special education seminars on health management and sexual practices, and special support groups for residents who are HIV positive or who have a clinical diagnosis of AIDS or hepatitis C.

Research: The Effectiveness of Traditional Therapeutic Communities

Over the past five decades, a considerable scientific knowledge base has developed from follow-up studies on thousands of individuals treated in TCs worldwide. The main findings and conclusions have been briefly summarized from multiple sources of outcome research including multi-program field effectiveness studies, single program-controlled studies, meta-analytic statistical surveys, and cost-benefit studies. The most extensive body of research bearing on the effectiveness of TC programs has amassed from field evaluations. These studies have been conducted by different research teams across different eras (1969-2000), have accounted for more than 5,000 admissions to community-based TCs in North America, and have employed similar methodologies (eg, assessment instruments, longitudinal designs [followed 1-12 years post-treatment], and statistical analyses).

Results from four major national multimodality, multi-year evaluations[5-8] and three notable uncontrolled "case studies" of single community-based TC programs[9-12] have yielded similar, consistent findings with respect to profiles, outcomes, and retention.[5-12] Specifically, all of these studies have demonstrated:

1. That TC admissions typically have high severity of substance use, social deviance, and psychological symptoms.
2. TC participants evidence significant decreases in measures of substance use, criminality, and psychological symptoms and consistent increases in employment and/or educational involvement. In studies that utilize a composite index of favorable or successful outcome over 60% of the intent to treat samples (dropouts and completions combined) show most favorable or favorable outcomes.
3. That reductions in substance use, criminality, and increase in employment are related to time spent in treatment. Those who complete TC treatment show the best outcomes; among dropouts, retention is highly correlated with outcomes.

The striking replications across studies (often within percentage points on some variables) leave little doubt as to the reliability of the main conclusions. Namely, there is a consistent relationship between retention in treatment and positive post-treatment outcomes in TCs (**Fig. 76-1**). Similar conclusions are obtained with the smaller number of controlled and comparative studies involving TC programs. With few exceptions,

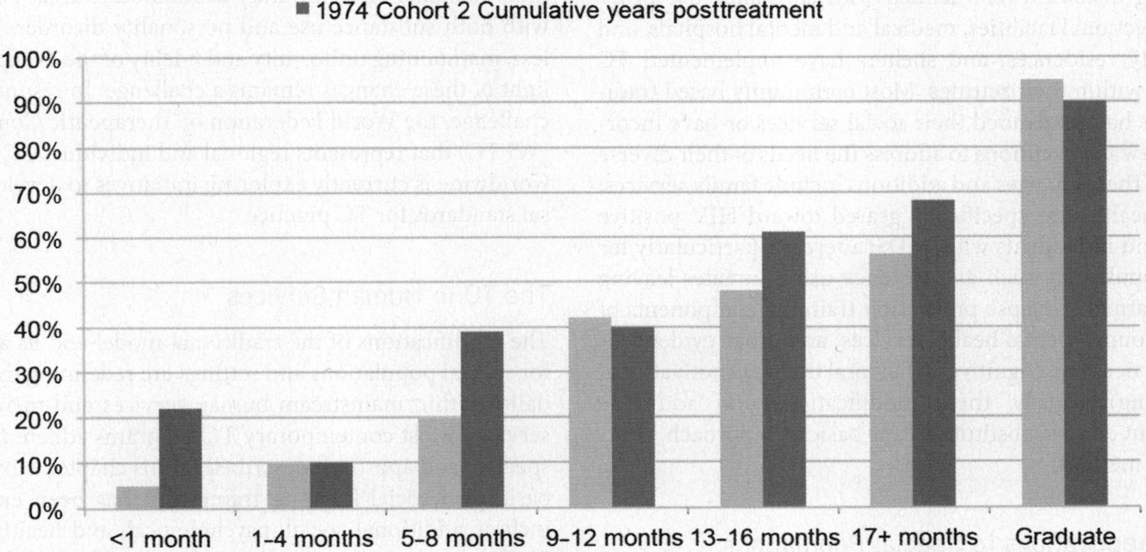

Figure 76-1. Relationship between time in treatment and posttreatment outcomes. Success (defined as no drug use and no criminal activity) through all years of follow-up for primary abusers. (Adapted from De Leon G. *The Therapeutic Community: Study of Effectiveness.* National Institute on Drug Abuse Treatment Research Monograph Series (DHHS Publication No. ADM 84-1286). National Institute on Drug Abuse; 1984.)

in the studies with a bona fide non-TC comparison condition (eg, generic substance use treatment programs in residential settings for adolescents or in prison-based samples), the TCs showed significantly better outcomes, as specified in #2 above, than the comparison condition. Finally, the main findings from five published cost-benefit evaluations involving TC programs report a significant and positive cost-benefit outcome for TCs. That is, the TC shows relatively higher benefits with regard to reductions in costs associated with criminal activity and gains in employment.[13]

Overall, the weight of the research evidence from multiple sources (multi-program field effectiveness studies, single program-controlled studies, meta-analytic statistical surveys, and cost-benefit studies) is compelling in supporting the hypothesis that the TC is an effective and cost-effective treatment for certain subgroups of people with SUDs, particularly those who present with serious co-occurring social and psychological problems in addition.

The Evolution of the TC: Modifications and Applications

The traditional TC model described in this chapter is actually the prototype of a variety of TC-oriented programs. Today, the TC modality consists of a wide range of programs serving a diversity of patients who use a variety of drugs and present with complex social and psychological problems in addition to their substance use. Client differences as well as clinical requirements and funding realities have encouraged the development of modified residential TC programs with shorter planned durations of stay (3, 6, and 12 months) as well as TC-oriented day treatment and outpatient ambulatory models.[14]

Having become overwhelmed with substance use problems, correctional facilities, medical and mental hospitals, and community residences, and shelters have implemented TC programs within their settings. Most community based traditional TCs have expanded their social services or have incorporated new interventions to address the needs of their diverse residents. These changes and additions include family services; primary health care specifically geared toward HIV positive patients and individuals with AIDS; aftercare, particularly for special populations such as substance using inmates leaving prison treatment; relapse prevention training; components of 12-step groups; mental health services, and other evidenced-based practices (eg, cognitive-behavioral therapy, motivational interviewing). Mostly, these modifications and additions enhance but do not substitute for the basic TC approach, community as method.

Current Applications to Special Populations

An important sign of the evolution of the TC is its application to special populations with substance use problems (eg, adolescents, those with co-occurring substance use and other mental disorders [COD], criminal justice clients, women with children, methadone maintained patients) and special settings (eg, prisons, shelters, psychiatric hospitals). Research provides impressive evidence for the effectiveness and cost benefits of modified TCs for special populations. Modifications in practices and in program elements for special populations and settings center on the treatment goals and planned duration of treatment, flexibility of the program structure to accommodate individual differences, and in the intensity of peer interactions. Special services and interventions are integrated into the program as supplemental to the primary TC treatment. Part II of this chapter provides a description of the modified TC for persons with co-occurring mental and SUDs.

The TC Worldwide

In the past 50 years, the TC for SUDs launched in North America has been adapted worldwide with programs implemented on every continent, in 65 countries and throughout the United States. These programs reflect cultural and societal differences (eg, influences of religion, the prominence of the family, political orientation). To a considerable extent, however, many retain the basic perspective, approach, and elements of the standard TC. A European research literature documents the effectiveness and cost benefits for these programs.[15] Similar conclusions are obtained in outcome studies of TC programs in Peru and Thailand[16,17] and Australia[18]; TCs worldwide are also undergoing the evolutionary changes described above including modifications for special populations and particularly adapting to fiscal pressures to reduce time in residential treatment. Another notable development is the rapprochement between the substance use disorder TC and the psychiatric TC pioneered by Maxwell Jones that has been prominent in Europe. Both of these TC approaches share many of the common elements of community as method to treat populations with both substance use and personality disorder. Nevertheless, maintaining uniformity and fidelity of the TC approach in light of these changes remains a challenge. In response to this challenge, the World Federation of Therapeutic Communities (WFTC) that represents regional and individual TC programs worldwide is currently exploring initiatives to develop universal standards for TC practice.

The TC in Human Services

The modifications of the traditional model and its adaptation for special populations and settings are redefining the TC modality within mainstream human services and mental health services. Most contemporary TC programs adhere to the perspective and approach described in this chapter. However, the basic peer/social-learning framework has been enlarged to include additional social, psychological, and health services. Staffing compositions have been altered, reflecting the fact that traditional professionals—correctional, mental health, medical and educational, family, and child care specialists; social workers; and case managers—serve along with experientially trained TC professionals. Indeed, the cross-fertilization of personnel and methods between traditional TCs and mental health and human services portends the evolution of a new TC: a generic treatment model applicable to a broad range of populations for whom affiliation with a self-help community is the foundation for effecting the process of individual change.

PART II: MODIFIED THERAPEUTIC COMMUNITY FOR PERSONS WITH CO-OCCURRING MENTAL AND SUBSTANCE USE DISORDERS

The demonstrated improvement in psychological well-being[9,10,19,20] and self-concept[21] following traditional TC treatment provided the rationale for modifying the TC to respond to the multiple needs of individuals with co-occurring substance use and mental disorders. As TCs began adapting to clients with co-occurring substance use and mental disorders (then known as "dual disorders," among other terms; today, commonly called "co-occurring disorders"), three models emerged: an "inclusive" model, in which community-based TCs admitted a small number of clients with co-occurring disorders, often developing a specialized track within the program for such clients; an "ancillary service" model, in which clients with co-occurring disorders functioned within the traditional TC, and received enriched mental health services concomitant to their TC programming; and an "exclusive" or "stand-alone" model designed specifically for co-occurring disorders. This latter model, wherein the treatment environment and most of its accompanying interventions are modified to incorporate features that address both substance use and psychiatric symptoms, treats both disorders as equally important.[22]

Over time, TCs adapted to changing needs and populations, to different settings, and to advances in research and practice. In the early and mid-1990s, the modified TC (typically abbreviated as "MTC"), described here, was developed from the theoretical framework of the traditional TC model, as detailed in the definitive text, *The Therapeutic Community: Theory, Model & Method*,[1] adapted to treat individuals with co-occurring disorders.[22-26] The use of "modified TC," or "MTC," in this report is intended *to capture those adaptations of the TC model designed to serve substance-using individuals with co-occurring mental disorders, most of which were* ***serious*** *(ie, schizophrenia and other psychotic disorders, bipolar disorders and major depression) mental disorders.*[25]

Description of the Modified TC Program

TC Principles and Methods

The TC principles and methods of particular relevance to co-occurring disorders include:

- a highly structured daily regimen,
- coping with life's challenges with personal responsibility and self-help; using the peer community as the healing agent within a strategy of "community-as-method" (the community provides both the context for and mechanism of change),
- assigning role models and guides from within the peer group,
- viewing change as a gradual, developmental process, wherein clients advance through stages of treatment; emphasizing work and self-reliance through the development of vocational and independent living skills, and
- adopting prosocial values within healthy social networks to sustain recovery.

The TC Stage and Phase Treatment Process for Co-occurring Disorders

The treatment process involves stages and phases as adapted for persons with co-occurring disorders. The four stages are admission and engagement (Stage One), primary treatment (Stage Two), live-in re-entry (Stage Three), and live-out re-entry (Stage Four). The first three stages mark the residential portion of the program; the fourth stage takes place in a supported housing apartment complex. The stage and phase format, which is both clinically relevant and potent, is widely accepted in the drug treatment and mental health fields. The format allows gradual progress, rewarding improvement with increased independence and responsibility. The client is given a clear road map for progression through the program, with explicit program expectations, and an outline of program and client goals, objectives, methods, and outcomes. Broad criteria are supplied for movement from one stage to the next, and the clinical decision-making process is informed on matters such as increased responsibility, needed supervision, and discharge.

The stage and phase format for clients with co-occurring disorders differs from other formulations as follows:

i. more time and effort are spent on engaging and stabilizing the client in the community,
ii. the rate of program movement is individualized to take into account developmental level, diagnostic differences, and variability in rates of learning (clients sometimes return to an earlier phases to solidify gains before progressing), and
iii. phase criteria have sufficient flexibility to allow even low-functioning clients to move through the program system.

Other Modifications

The MTC model retains, but reshapes, most of the central elements, structure, and processes of the traditional TC, so as to accommodate the many needs that accompany co-occurring disorders, particularly, psychiatric symptoms, cognitive deficits and reduced level of functioning. (A complete description of the MTC for clients with co-occurring disorders, including treatment manuals and guides to implementation for implementation guidance, can be found elsewhere.[22-24,26]) **A key alteration is the change from encounter group to conflict resolution group.** As compared to a standard encounter group, the conflict resolution group has shorter duration, reduced intensity of interaction, more emphasis on instruction, and increased modeling by staff and more experienced clients. The conflict resolution group focuses on personal conflicts, conflicts between people, and conflicts in relation to an individual's performance of program tasks and activities. The goals of this group are the same as those of a standard encounter group; specifically, to identify and modify self-defeating patterns of thinking, feeling, and behaving, and to facilitate self-discovery through personal disclosure and direct interpersonal interaction.

Other alterations in the modified TC for co-occurring disorders include:

- more flexibility in program activities,
- shorter duration of various activities,
- less confrontation and intensity of interpersonal interaction,
- greater emphasis on orientation and instruction in programming and planning,
- fewer sanctions and greater opportunity for corrective learning experiences,
- more explicit affirmation for achievements,
- greater sensitivity to individual differences, and
- greater responsiveness to the special developmental needs of the clients.

To summarize, three key alterations were made in designing the modified TC program for co-occurring disorders: increased flexibility; decreased intensity; and greater individualization. Still, the MTC, like all TC programs, promotes a culture wherein self-help advances learning and promotes change, both in themselves and in others. In other words, the community becomes the agent of healing. Thus, this variant of the TC also shares certain features with the psychiatric (Democratic) TC that emerged in England and elsewhere in Europe.

Interventions

The basic MTC program, delivered over a planned stay of 12 months, is a highly structured, comprehensive residential program that consisted of multiple interventions organized in four areas: (1) *Community Enhancement*—to facilitate the individual's assimilation into the community and reaffirm the individual's commitment to recovery (eg, Morning meeting, Orientation Seminars, General Meetings); (2) *Therapeutic/Educative*—to promote self-expression, divert acting-out behavior, and resolve personal and social issues (eg, Individual Counseling, Dual Recovery Classes, Conflict Resolution Groups); (3) *Community and Clinical Management*—to maintain the physical and psychological safety of the environment and ensure that residential life is orderly and productive (eg, Program Policies, Social Learning Consequences); and (4) *Work/Vocational*—to promote positive work attitudes and develop work skills (eg, Peer Work Hierarchy, Vocational Counseling).

All program activities and interactions, singly and in combination, are designed to produce change. Implementation of the groups and activities listed in **Table 76-2** are necessary to establish the TC community. Although each intervention has specific individual functions, all share community, therapeutic, and educational purposes.

Research

A systematic series of studies has established an evidence base for the MTC model. A study, employing a quasi-experimental design, conducted in a drug treatment setting with clients showing evidence of co-occurring disorders found that those who received ancillary MTC programming achieved more positive mental health outcomes during treatment (significantly greater reductions in symptoms of depression) than those who received standard TC services.[27] A study with a quasi-experimental design of a long-term (1 year), fully developed, modified TC for people who were homeless and has co-occurring mental and substance use disorders found significantly more positive outcomes for MTC clients on measures of drug use and employment 1-year posttreatment than were obtained for their counterparts receiving the standard care typically provided to people who were homeless and using drugs,[28] pointing both to the adaptability of the TC to the needs of particular clients and the importance of making these types of adjustments to programming. Economic analysis of this MTC treatment reported $5 of benefit for every dollar spent on MTC treatment.[29] Another randomized controlled study evaluated a *Modified Therapeutic Community Aftercare* program for a population triply diagnosed with HIV/AIDS, a substance use disorder, and a mental disorder. Results indicated that MTC aftercare can help to maintain, or even enhance treatment gains achieved during residential treatment.[26]

Subsequently, the MTC has been introduced in prisons to address the complex needs of people with legal offenses as well as co-occurring mental health and SUDs,[30] and has shown significant reductions in reincarceration rates,[31] and substance use[32] for clients randomly assigned to the MTC compared to those receiving standard mental health treatment services. In another prison study, another intent-to-treat analysis 12 months after release from prison showed that participants randomly assigned to a Re-Entry Modified TC (RMTC) after prison treatment were significantly less likely to be reincarcerated than those assigned to a Parole Supervision and Case Management condition (19% versus 38%), The study found the greatest reduction in recidivism for participants who received modified TC treatment in both in-prison and postprison settings. These findings support the RMTC as a stand-alone intervention, and provide initial evidence for integrated MTC programs in prison and in aftercare for offenders with COD.[33]

In a single investigator meta-analysis of four studies[34,35] (shown in **Fig. 76-2**), the MTC produced significantly greater improvements in five domains; substance use (odds ratio = 0.65), mental health (odds ratio = 0.68), crime (odds ratio = 0.66), employment (odds ratio = 0.40), and housing (odds ratio = 0.63)—only HIV-risk behavior failed to show significant treatment effects (ie, odds ratio = 1.01).[36] (A single investigator (or research team) application of meta-analytic tools is not

TABLE 76-2 Residential Interventions

Community enhancement	
Morning meetings	to increase motivation for the day's activities and to create a positive family atmosphere
Concept seminars	to review the concept of the day
General interest seminars	to provide information in areas of general interest (eg, current events)
Program-related seminars	to address issues of particular relevance (eg, homelessness, AIDS prevention, psychotropic medication)
Orientation seminars	to orient new members and to introduce all new activities
Evening meetings	to review house business for the day, to outline plans for the next day, and to monitor the emotional tone of the house
General meetings	to provide a public review of critical events
Therapeutic/educative	
Individual counseling	to incorporate both traditional mental health and unique modified TC goals and methods
Psychoeducational classes	are predominant, in a format to facilitate learning among persons with co-occurring disorders, and to include topics such as entitlements/money management, positive relationship skills training, triple trouble group, and feelings management
Conflict resolution groups	are modified encounter groups designed specifically for persons with co-occurring disorders
Gender-specific groups	to combine features of "discussion groups" and therapy groups focusing on gender-based issues
Community and clinical management	
Policies	to form a system of rules and regulations to maintain the physical and psychological safety of the environment, ensuring that resident life is orderly and productive, strengthening the community as a context for social learning
Social learning consequence	to prescribe a set of required behaviors as a response to unacceptable behavior, designed to enhance individual and community learning by transforming negative events into learning opportunities
Vocational	
Peer work hierarchy	a rotating assignment of residents to jobs necessary to the day-to-day functioning of the facility, serving to diversify and develop clients' work skills and experience
World of work	a psychoeducational class providing instruction in applications and interviews, time and attendance, relationships with others at work, employers' expectations, discipline, promotion, etc.
Recovery and world of work	a psychoeducational class that addresses issues of mental illness, addiction, etc. in a work context
Peer advocate training	a program for suitable clients offering role model, group facilitator, and individual counseling training
Work performance evaluations	to provide regular, systematic feedback on work performance
Job selection and placement	individual counseling after 6 months to establish direction and to determine future employment

Adapted from Sacks S, Sacks JY, De Leon G. Treatment for MICAs: design and implementation of the modified TC. *J Psychoactive Drugs.* 1999;31(1):19-30.

intended by itself to provide a definitive determination of the effectiveness of a particular approach.)

Future research should emphasize independent replications, clinical trials, multiple outcome domains and other meta-analyses. Nonetheless, findings from this research synthesis hold considerable clinical relevance since individuals with co-occurring disorders are typically perceived to have multifaceted needs requiring multidimensional interventions.[26] Given the need for research-based approaches, program and policy planners should consider the MTC when designing programs for individuals with co-occurring disorders.

Finally, the modified TC has been listed on the *National Registry of Effective Programs and Practice* since 2008.[37] The goal of the registry is to encourage the use of evidence-based based interventions.

Also, a recent review concluded that the "MTC approach has, to date, accumulated sufficient support to encourage

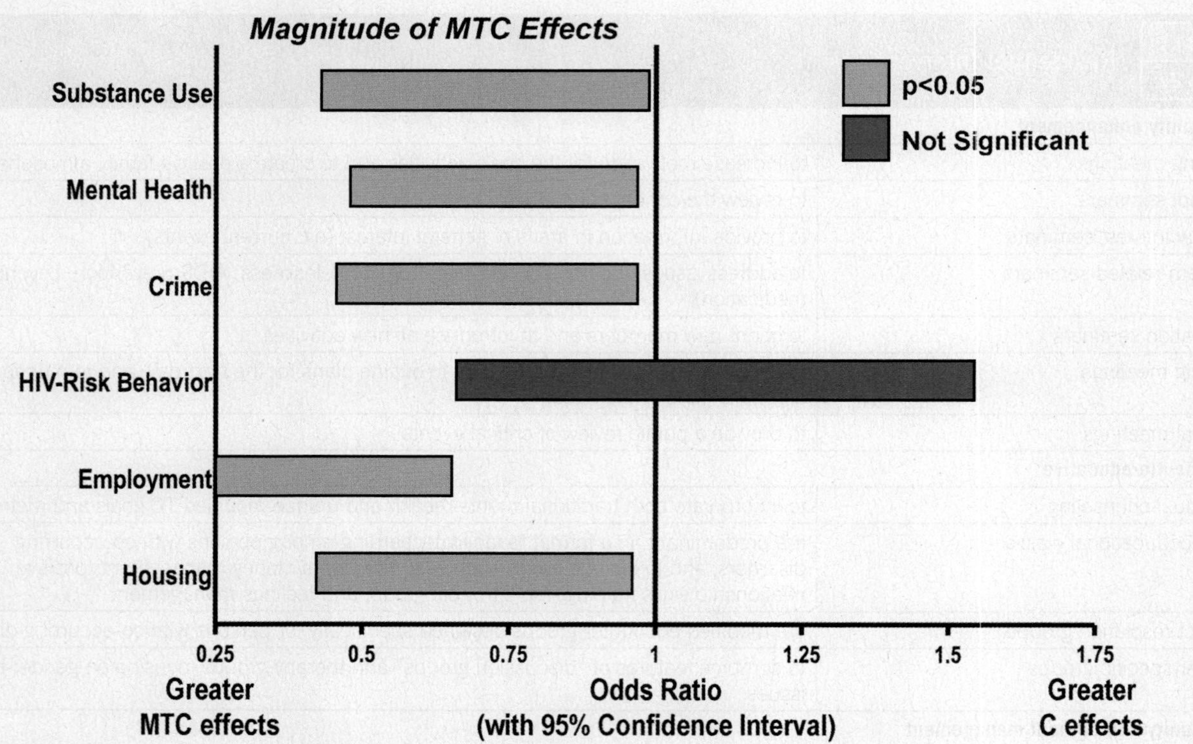

Figure 76-2. Single investigator meta-analysis of four MTC studies.

policy and program planners to consider its application for persons with co-occurring disorders in a variety of settings."[37(p. 202)]

Future Directions

Continuity of Care

Rationale

The evidence available suggests that co-occurring substance use and mental disorders, especially serious mental disorders, have chronic features that require extended residential treatment followed by period of community-based support (ie, continuing care) to solidify the successes achieved with MTC. Continuity of care implies coordination of care as clients move across different service systems, and is characterized by three features: *consistency* among primary treatment activities and ancillary services; *seamless transitions* across levels of care (eg, from residential to outpatient treatment); and *coordination* of present with past treatment episodes. Because both substance use and mental disorders are typically chronic conditions, continuity of care is critical; the challenge in any system of care is to institute mechanisms to ensure that all individuals with co-occurring disorders experience the benefits of continuity of care.

MTC Residential Aftercare Models

In examining continuity of care, Sacks and colleagues[38] conducted a series of studies among special populations of persons with co-occurring disorders; the co-occurring population in one of these studies was people who were homeless,[39] and in another was people with legal violations.[40] The MTC aftercare programs in these two studies retained the core features of the MTC but added elements specific to the co-occurring disorders population being treated and that were necessary for reintegration with mainstream living.

The aftercare program in the study of people who were homeless and with co-occurring disorders was conducted in a supported housing facility and consisted of community meetings (held in the supported housing facility), with continued treatment and support groups held in an associated day treatment program (located outside the supported housing facility). In addition to co-occurring disorders treatment and support, this aftercare program emphasized housing and employment.[39]

In a study of people with legal violations and co-occurring disorders,[30,31] the aftercare program, which was housed in a Community Corrections apartment-like facility, consisted of community and peer support meetings with certain treatment services provided at local community treatment facilities. Along with co-occurring disorders treatment and support, this aftercare program incorporated elements related to criminal thinking and behavior, as well as employment.[26] In general, quasi-experimental studies suggest that aftercare programs sustained the gains of the more intensive residential MTC facilities.[31,35,36,39]

Modified TC Outpatient Models

Despite the fact that outpatient SUD programs often may not be equipped to provide services for mental conditions, let alone the accompanying health and social problems, many of the clients who enter these programs have a diagnosable co-occurring mental disorder. Sacks and colleagues developed an outpatient MTC model, the *Dual Assessment & Recovery Track* (DART), for persons with co-occurring substance use and mental disorders. A study of the model's effectiveness demonstrated that, compared to the control condition, the DART group had significantly better outcomes on measures of psychological symptoms as well as on a key measure of housing stability (ie, "lived where paid rent"), which indicated that the DART group had acquired more stable housing.[35] The MTC features of this program were designed: to strengthen identification with the community (ie, community meetings); to teach clients about mental illness in a *Psycho-Educational Seminar*[40-42]; to assist clients to cope with trauma within the context of addictions and recovery using the *Trauma-Informed Addictions Treatment* approach[43-45]; and to expand clients' ability to negotiate health and social services agencies using case management skills, imparted through a *Case Management* component.[46-48]

The Medically Integrated Therapeutic Community

The Affordable Care Act afforded an opportunity for the continued adaptation and growth of the MTC model, which is ideally suited for alterations to support integration with primary care services. The rationale for such an approach is based on the fact that the conceptual framework of the MTC (and the TC) endorses a view of "whole person" treatment that is compatible with holistic, person-centered medicine, and the model has been modified in the past to suit special populations, retaining core TC principles while adding interventions to accommodate particular services. Further, the central feature of TC methods (ie, "Community-as-Method," wherein the community of patients becomes the healing agent) can be naturally extended to include SUD, mental health, and primary care services. In fact, the residential MTC model already encompasses much of this integration in its existing provision of services. In requiring an onsite psychiatrist to prescribe and monitor psychotropic medication, the MTC for co-occurring disorders sets the stage for additional integration. Furthermore, the MTC requires integrated team planning and coordination of both residential and aftercare services.

In developing the *Medically Integrated Therapeutic Community*, the following service components are recommended for inclusion:

1. Integrated primary and behavioral care becomes the agency's primary focus, and is so stated in the mission or service statement.
2. A welcoming social and interpersonal environment for patients with medical problems is evident.
3. Routine screening and assessment for medical problems is established.
4. Teams develop integrated treatment plans.
5. Medical conditions are considered in the process of planning for discharge or during a postacute stabilization phase.
6. Onsite staff have medical expertise and prescribing authority.
7. All program staff members have basic training in life support, infectious diseases and infection on control, and patient privacy/confidentiality, according to a formal agency plan.

Finally, in the articulation of its services, each program will need to determine the extent of medical services to be provided, the use of referral resources and their broader relationship with the medical community.

Summary

To summarize, over the past 20 years, an MTC model has been articulated for persons with co-occurring mental and substance use disorders, and a series of studies has established a research base for the model. The *National Registry of Effective Programs and Practices* (NREPP) recognizes and lists the MTC model.[37] The proposed development of the "*Medically Integrated Therapeutic Community*" (MITC) represents a natural evolution for the MTC model, one that promises to improve health care through the integration of mental health, substance use disorder, and primary care services.

REFERENCES

1. De Leon G. *The Therapeutic Community: Theory, Model and Method.* Springer Publishers; 2000.
2. Platt JJ. *Heroin Addiction: Theory, Research and Treatment.* Vol. 1. 2nd ed. Krieger Publishing Company; 1986.
3. De Leon G. *The Therapeutic Community: Study of Effectiveness.* National Institute on Drug Abuse Treatment Research Monograph Series (DHHS Publication No. ADM 84-1286). National Institute on Drug Abuse; 1984.
4. Kressel D, De Leon G, Palij M, Rubin G. Measuring client clinical progress in therapeutic community treatment: the client assessment inventory, client assessment summary and staff assessment summary. *J Subst Abuse Treat.* 2000;19(3):267-272.
5. Simpson DD, Sells SB. Effectiveness of treatment for drug abuse: an overview of the DARP research program. *Adv Alcohol Subst Abuse.* 1982;2:7-29.
6. Hubbard RL, Marsden ME, Rachal JV, Harwood HJ, Cavanaugh ER, Ginzburg HM. *Drug Abuse Treatment: A National Study of Effectiveness.* University of North Carolina Press; 1989.
7. U.S. Department of Health and Human Services (SAMHSA, CSAT). *Preliminary Report: The Persistent Effects of Substance Abuse Treatment One Year Later.* National Treatment Improvement Evaluation Study (NTIES); 1996.
8. Simpson DD, Curry S. Drug abuse treatment outcome study (DATOS). *Psychol Addict Behav.* 1997;11(4):211-337.
9. De Leon G, Wexler H, Jainchill N. The therapeutic community: success and improvement rates five years after treatment. *Int J Addict.* 1982;17(4):703-747.
10. De Leon G, Jainchill N. Male and female drug abusers: social and psychological status 2 years after treatment in a therapeutic community. *Am J Drug Alcohol Abuse.* 1981;8(4):465-497.
11. Barr, H. Outcomes in drug abuse treatment in two modalities. In: De Leon G, Zeigenfuss JT, eds. *Therapeutic Communities for Addictions.* Charles C. Thomas Publications; 1986:97-108.

Disclaimer: The content is solely the responsibility of the authors and does not necessarily represent the official views of the Department of Health & Human Services (DHHS), SAMHSA, CSAT, or the National Institutes of Health (NIH), NIDA.

12. Holland S. Evaluating community-based treatment programs: a model for strengthening inferences about effectiveness. *Int J Ther Commun.* 1983;4(4):285-306.
13. De Leon G. Is the therapeutic community an evidence based treatment? What the evidence says. *Ther Commun.* 2010;31(2):104-175.
14. De Leon G, ed. *Community as Method: Therapeutic Communities for Special Populations and Special Settings.* Greenwood; 1997.
15. Vanderplasschen W, Colbert K, Autrique M, et al. Therapeutic communities for addictions: a review of their effectiveness from a recovery-oriented perspective. *ScientificWorldJournal.* 2013;2013:427817. doi:10.1155/2013/427817
16. Johnson K, Pan Z, Young L, et al. Therapeutic community drug treatment success in Peru: a follow-up outcome study. *Subst Abuse Treat Prev Policy.* 2008;3:26.
17. Johnson KW, Young L, Pan T, Zimmerman RS, Vanderhoff KJ. *Therapeutic Communities (TC) Drug Treatment Success in Thailand: A Follow-up Study.* Research Monograph. U.S. Department of State's Bureau of International Narcotics and Law Enforcement Affairs Pacific Institute for Research and Evaluation—Louisville Center; 2007.
18. Pitts J, Yates R. Cost benefits of therapeutic community programming: results of a self-funded study. *Int J Ther Commun.* 2010;31(2):129-144.
19. Jainchill N, De Leon G. Therapeutic community research: recent studies of psychopathology and retention. In: Buhringer G, Platt JJ, eds. *Drug Addiction Treatment Research: German and American Perspectives.* Krieger Publications; 1992:367-388.
20. Sacks S, De Leon G. Modified therapeutic communities for dual disorders: Evaluation overview. *Proceedings of Therapeutic Communities of America 1992 Planning Conference, Paradigms: Past, Present and Future;* December 6-9, 1992. Chantilly, VA.
21. Biase DV, Sullivan AP, Wheeler B. Daytop miniversity—phase 2—college training in a therapeutic community: development of self-concept among drug free addict/abusers. In: De Leon G, Ziegenfuss JT, eds. *Therapeutic Community for Addictions: Readings in Theory, Research, and Practice.* Charles C. Thomas Publishing; 1986:121-130.
22. Sacks S, Sacks JY, De Leon G. Treatment for MICAs: design and implementation of the modified TC. *J Psychoactive Drugs.* 1999;31(1):19-30.
23. De Leon G. Modified therapeutic communities for co-occurring substance abuse and psychiatric disorders. In: Solomon J, Zimberg S, Shollar E, eds. *Dual Diagnosis: Evaluation, Treatment, and Training and Program Development.* Plenum Publishing Corporation; 1993: 137-156.
24. Sacks S, De Leon G, Bernhardt AI, Sacks JY. A modified therapeutic community for homeless MICA clients. In: De Leon G, ed. *Community-As-Method: Therapeutic Communities for Special Populations and Special Settings.* Greenwood Publishing Group, Inc; 1997.
25. Sacks S, Sacks JY, De Leon G, Bernhardt AI, Staines GL. Modified therapeutic community for mentally Ill chemical "abusers": background; influences; program description; preliminary findings. *Subst Use Misuse.* 1997;32(9):1217-1259.
26. Sacks S, De Leon G, Bernhardt AI, Sacks J. *Modified Therapeutic Community for Homeless MICA Individuals: A Treatment Manual (Revised).* Center for Mental Health Services (CMHS)/Center for Substance Abuse Treatment (CSAT) Grant #1UD3 SM/TI51558-01. NDRI; 1998.
27. Rahav M, Rivera JJ, Nuttbrock L, et al. Characteristics and treatment of homeless, mentally ill chemical-abusing men. *J Psychoactive Drugs.* 1995;21(1):93-103.
28. De Leon G, Sacks S, Staines GL, McKendrick K. Modified therapeutic community for homeless MICAs: treatment outcomes. *Am J Drug Alcohol Abuse.* 2000;26(3):461-480. doi:10.1081/ADA-100100256
29. French MT, McCollister KE, Sacks S, McKendrick K, De Leon G. Benefit-cost analysis of a modified TC for mentally ill chemical abusers. *Eval Prog Plan.* 2002;25(2):137-148. doi:10.1016/S0149-7189(02)00006-X
30. Sacks S, Sacks JY, Stommel J. Modified TC for MICA inmates in correctional settings: a program description. *Correct Today.* 2003; October:90-99.
31. Sacks S, Sacks J, McKendrick K, Banks S, Stommel J. Modified TC for MICA offenders: crime outcomes. *Behav Sci Law.* 2004;22:477-501. doi:10.1002/bsl.599
32. Sullivan CJ, McKendrick K, Sacks S, Banks S. Modified therapeutic community treatment for offenders with MICA disorders: substance use outcomes. *Am J Drug Alcohol Abuse.* 2007;33(6):823-832. doi:10.1080/00952990701653800
33. Sacks S, Chaple M, Sacks JY, McKendrick K, Cleland CM. Randomized trial of a re-entry modified therapeutic community for offenders with co-occurring disorders: crime outcomes. *J Subst Abuse Treat.* 2012;42(3):247-259.
34. Sacks S, McKendrick K, Vazan P, Sacks JY. Modified TC aftercare for triply diagnosed clients with HIV/AIDS and co-occurring mental and substance use disorders. *AIDS Care.* 2011;23(12):1676-1686. doi:10.1080/09540121.2011.582075
35. Sacks S, McKendrick K, Sacks JY, Banks S, Harle M. Enhanced outpatient treatment for co-occurring disorders: main outcomes. *J Subst Abuse Treat.* 2008;34(1):48-60. doi:10.1016/j.jsat.2007.01.009
36. Sacks S, McKendrick K, Sacks JY, Cleland C. Modified therapeutic community for co-occurring disorders: single investigator meta-analysis. *Subst Abuse.* 2010;31(3):146-161. doi:10.1080/08897077.2010.495662
37. National Registry of Evidence-based Programs and Practices (NREPP). *Intervention Summary: Modified Therapeutic Community for Persons with Co-Occurring Disorders.* U.S. Department of Health & Human Services (DHHS), Substance Abuse & Mental Health Services Administration (SAMHSA); 2009. Updated 2010. Accessed November 28, 2012. https://peerta.acf.hhs.gov/content/national-registry-evidence-based-programs-and-practices-nrepp-0
38. Sacks S, Banks S, McKendrick K, Sacks JY. Modified therapeutic community for co-occurring disorders: a summary of four studies. *J Subst Abuse Treat.* 2008;34(1):112-122. doi:10.1016/j.jsat.2007.02.008
39. Sacks S, De Leon G, McKendrick K, Brown B, Sacks JY. TC-oriented supported housing for homeless MICAs. *J Psychoactive Drugs.* 2003;35(3):355-366.
40. Jerrell JM, Ridgely MS. Impact of robustness of program implementation on outcomes of clients in dual diagnosis programs. *Psychiatr Serv.* 1999;50:109-112.
41. Sciacca K. New initiatives in the treatment of the chronic patient with alcohol/substance abuse problems. *TIE Lines.* 1987-1988;4(3):5-6. Accessed June 13, 2023. http://users.erols.com/ksciacca/newinit.htm
42. Sciacca K. An integrated treatment approach for severely mentally ill individuals with substance disorders. In: Minkoff K, Drake RE, eds. *Dual Diagnosis of Major Mental Illness and Substance Disorder.* Jossey-Bass Inc; 1992:69-84.
43. Harris M, Fallot R. Using trauma theory to design service systems. *New Directions for Mental Health Services,* Number 89. Jossey Bass; 2001.
44. Harris M, Fallot R, Holzapfel A, Mitchell C, Singleton K, Wolfson R. *Trauma-Informed Addictions Treatment.* Community Connections, Inc; 2001.
45. Sacks S, Sacks JY. *Dual Assessment & Recovery Track (DART) for Co-occurring Disorders—Treatment Manual.* Grant 5 KD1 TI12553 Substance Abuse & Mental Health Services Administration (SAMHSA)/Center for Substance Abuse Treatment (CSAT) TI 00-002 (FDA No. 93.230). *Grants for Evaluation of Outpatient Treatment Models for Persons with Co-Occurring Substance Abuse & Mental Health Disorders* (*Co-Occurring Disorders Study*). Center for the Integration of Research & Practice (CIRP), National Development & Research Institutes, Inc. (NDRI); 2005.
46. Brown BS, Farrell E, Voskuhl TC. Case management. In: Brown BS, Farrell E, Voskuhl TC, eds. *Manual for the Friends Care Program—A Program of Aftercare Services for Clients Referred from the Criminal Justice System (Revised).* Friends Research Institute; 1999:31-48.
47. Brown BS, O'Grady KE, Battjes RJ, Farrell EV. Factors associated with treatment outcomes in an aftercare population. *Am J Addict.* 2004;13:447-480.
48. Brown BS, O'Grady KE, Battjes RJ, Farrell EV, Smith MP, Nurco DN. Effectiveness of a stand-alone aftercare program for drug-involved offenders. *J Subst Abuse Treat.* 2001;21:185-192.

CHAPTER

77 Aversion Therapies

Hanne Tonnesen, P. Joseph Frawley, and Richard Montgomery

CHAPTER OUTLINE

- Aversion therapy as part of a multimodality treatment program
- Principles of conditioning and taste aversion
- Uses of aversion therapy
- Effect of aversion on craving for alcohol
- Functional MRI studies of substance use disorders and aversion and craving
- Effect of aversion on cocaine craving
- Need for further research

AVERSION THERAPY AS PART OF A MULTIMODALITY TREATMENT PROGRAM

Aversion therapy, or counterconditioning, is a useful tool in the treatment of alcohol and other substance use disorders (SUDs). Its goal is to reduce or eliminate the "hedonic memory" or craving for a drug and to simultaneously develop a distaste and avoidance response to the substance. Unlike punishments (jail, firings, fines, divorce, hangovers, cirrhosis, and the like), which often are delayed in time from the use episode, aversion therapy relies on the immediate association of the sight, smell, taste, and act of using the substance with an unpleasant or "aversive" experience. This treatment was not designed to appeal to the logical part of the individual's brain, which often is all too aware of the negative consequences of substance use, but to the part of the brain where emotional attachments are made or broken through experienced associations of pleasure or discomfort.

The net result of a series of aversion therapy treatments is an attenuated level of craving for the primary substance; uncontrolled craving is the variable that shifts consumption-reward feedback cycles into an ungoverned state, or "addiction." It takes a lot of mental energy to fight active craving. Through removing much of the conscious effort to resist craving, the patient is able to engage more fully in all other concurrent treatment modalities, which are a heavily emphasized as part of a multimodal treatment. Aversion therapy provides a means of achieving control over injurious behavior for a period of time, during which alternative and more rewarding modes of response can be established and strengthened.[1] It was first reported by Benjamin Rush, a physician, in 1789.[2]

It is important not to confuse aversion with punishment. In punishment, it is the individual who receives the negative consequences; whereas in aversion therapy, the negative consequences are only paired with the act of using the drug. This has a very important benefit to self-esteem. Self-esteem is rebuilt by separating the drug from the self.[3]

In populations that do not have chronic problems with alcohol, hangovers have been cited as a significant reason to cut down or stop drinking.[4] However, the hangover is delayed in time from the actual use of alcohol; thus, for the person with an alcohol use disorder, who drinks for the immediate euphoric effects of alcohol, a hangover often is ineffective in producing aversion because it is delayed in time from use of the substance whose immediate effect was experienced as pleasant or euphoric. Moreover, the discomfort of a hangover, though logically understood to be the result of drinking, is blamed on "drinking too much" (weakness) rather than drinking at all (disease). Even worse, alcohol may be used to cure the withdrawal ("hair of the dog"), which ensures that emotionally the patient perceives the alcohol as a solution, not a problem. Also termed negative reinforcement, this is seen with nicotine use disorder and other SUDs. In addition to the time differential between when someone initially consumes alcohol and later experiences a hangover, there is the factor of being intoxicated versus sober during the formation of the aversion. During treatment, aversion therapy patients are experiencing noxious physical status at a time when they are completely sober—not while experiencing the intoxicating effects of their primary substance. Thus, the aversion is effectively and optimally established during a state of relative physiologic and cognitive equilibrium.

Contrary to popular belief, disulfiram is not an aversion treatment. In aversion therapy for alcohol use disorder (AUD), alcohol is not absorbed into the system.[3] If disulfiram had been developed today, it would probably be categorized as a designer drug.[5] When ethyl alcohol is taken into the system, it is first converted to acetaldehyde before next going to acetic acid. Disulfiram causes nausea, flushing and systemic vasodilation by competitively blocking the conversion of acetaldehyde to acetic acid, resulting in high levels of acetaldehyde, which is toxic. With disulfiram, alcohol must be absorbed, and metabolism begun for it to produce its toxic effect.[6] Today, disulfiram is not a standalone drug, but part of a multi-modal rehabilitation program in line with other pharmaceutical therapy. Aversion relies on safe but uncomfortable experiences that can be repeated, whereas disulfiram reactions can be life-threatening, even in healthy persons. For this reason, patients today are no longer given alcohol at the same time that they are prescribed disulfiram. As a result, they have not actually experienced a disulfiram reaction. Thus, disulfiram does not change the way the patient feels about alcohol. He or she may fear the consequence of drinking, just as he or she fears being arrested for drinking and driving; nevertheless, he or she still retains the euphoric recall of past episodes of drinking alcohol and hence the craving for the alcohol itself. Aversion works to reduce cravings for alcohol or drugs by recording new negative experiences with the drug while the patient is sober, and not in an intoxicated or physiologically compromised state or hungover.[7,8] While there are many patient characteristics that influence the likelihood of return to use, in those patients that do return to use, there is an association between the strength of the conditioned aversion and time to return to use.[9] This increased time can allow other multimodal aspects of treatment to have more opportunity to take hold.

There is some evidence that presenting patients when sober with how they look when undergoing delirium tremens (DTs) will help reduce recurrence of drinking. Mihai et al.[9] conducted a randomized controlled study whereby persons with AUD who had gone through DTs were randomly assigned to watch the video of themself in DTs and then have a psychiatrist explain the videos to them, or to a control group who did not have this intervention. Watching the DT video significantly reduced alcohol recurrence rates after the first month (0 versus 20%), 2 months (13.3% versus 46.67%) and 3 months (26.67% versus 53.33%).

In fact, spontaneous aversions are common (eg, developing an aversion to onion soup by getting a stomach flu at the same time as eating the soup), because the capacity to develop aversions is a biological defense mechanism. DeSilva and Rachman[10] published a study of 125 students and hospital employees, 105 (84%) of whom had a history of natural aversions. There was an average of 3.5 aversions per person (women more than men), and 70.1% had been present since childhood.

PRINCIPLES OF CONDITIONING AND TASTE AVERSION

Ivan Pavlov noted that the repetitive pairing of a bell with food soon led to a "conditioned response" in dogs, who salivated at the sound of the bell alone, even with no food present. This type of pairing or training is called classical conditioning. Taste aversion is a natural biological defense, which has been developed in animals to avoid re-ingesting foods/materials that caused nausea. Nausea-induced learned aversions to ingested substances constitute the strongest conditioned reactions that humans normally acquire.[11,12] Burrhus Skinner expounded on the observation that the nervous system is so constructed that organisms will reduce or avoid behavior that is consistently paired with negative consequences and will increase behavior that is rewarded. This type of learning is called operant conditioning. Both types of learning can be shown to occur in addiction.[13] Aversion therapy uses the above principles in reversing the drug-rewarded learning and conditioned reflex to seek drugs. The development of an aversion can be very specific. Inadequate treatment can occur when aversion is developed only to one type of alcoholic beverage.[14,15] In professional alcohol addiction treatment, for example, 50% of trials may be with the patient's favorite brand or type of liquor, but the other trials include a range of alcoholic beverages.[3,16] Repetition is an essential part of training and conditioning.[17] Adequate trials are needed to develop an aversion[18] and to maintain and reinforce it to prevent extinction.[18,19] People with SUDs already have been conditioned by the drug prior to entry into treatment. Studies have shown that people with an AUD increase the number of swallows and amount of salivation in response to the sight of alcohol, as compared to people without the disorder.[20] Studies of people with tobacco/nicotine use disorder seeking to permanently stop their use show that those who are least likely to be successful in this aim have a much larger conditioned drop in pulse (presumably to compensate for the increase in pulse rate caused by smoking nicotine) when presented with a cigarette.[21] People with a cocaine use disorder experience progressively steeper drops in skin temperature and increased galvanic skin response (a sign of arousal) when viewing progressively more intense and explicit pictures of cocaine use. These responses can be shown to decay in strength as time away from the drug increases. The presence of these phenomena suggests that one of the consequences of SUDs is that the brain becomes conditioned to drink or use drugs in the presence of certain stimuli. This may contribute to the sensation of physical craving experienced by the person. The availability of drugs such as heroin or cocaine in the environment also influences craving.[22-24] This brain change is at the core of SUDs.

USES OF AVERSION THERAPY

Aversion Therapy for Alcohol Use Disorder

Nausea Aversion

Smith[3] has reported on the induction of nausea as an aversion technique. Before a typical treatment session, the patient is kept fasting except for clear liquids for 6 hours, which reduces the risk of solid stomach contents being aspirated. After informed consent about the procedure is obtained, the patient is escorted to a small treatment room that has bookcases filled with bottles of various alcoholic beverages and wall hangings of alcohol-related advertising. This provides needed visual cues related to drinking alcohol. After the patient sits in a comfortable chair in front of a large emesis basin. The patient is given an oral dose of emetine. Prior to the expected onset of emesis (5 to 8 minutes), the patient drinks two 10-oz glasses of lightly salted warm water (to counteract electrolyte loss), which creates a bolus of easily vomited fluid. The clinician doing the procedure pours a drink of the patient's preferred alcoholic beverage, diluting it 1:1 with warm water, and presents it to the patient just prior to the expected onset of nausea. The patient smells the drink, takes a small mouthful to swish around, and then spits it out into the basin. The "sniff, swish, and spit" procedure provides a differentiated visual, olfactory, and gustatory experience that will be linked to the patient's preferred beverage before the aversive stimulus of nausea begins. After nausea and vomiting begin, the patient can then "sniff, swish, and swallow" the preferred beverage mixture, but it stays down for only a short time, with little absorption, before it is vomited up. This first phase of intensive conditioning, which lasts 20 to 30 minutes, is followed by a second, longer phase back in the hospital room, where the preferred alcohol-containing beverage, which contains an oral dose of emetine, is drunk after another 30 minutes. This precipitates residual nausea for up to 3 hours duration. Five treatments are given on an every other day basis to a typical patient over 10 days.

Faradic Aversion Therapy for Alcohol

For a faradic session, Smith[3] reports that a pair of electrodes is placed 2 inches apart on the forearm of the patient's dominant hand. An electro-stimulus machine provides 1 to 20 mA of direct current through the electrodes, and the therapist begins test stimuli in increasing amplitude to determine the stimulus that the patient will experience as aversive but not unduly painful. This must be done on each session as there is wide variation by day within and between patients that requires individual thresholds be set for each patient on each day. The intervention pairs the visual, olfactory, and gustatory stimuli of alcoholic beverages with the predetermined amplitude of electrostimulation that the patient will find aversive. The clinician directs the patient to pour some of a bottled alcoholic beverage into a glass and to taste it but not to swallow it. During this forced-choice phase, from reaching for the bottle to tasting the drink, the onset of the aversive stimulus occurs at random intervals, with varying numbers (from 1 up to 8) of aversive stimuli among trials. A free-choice phase of 10 supplemental trials provides negative reinforcement, such that if the patient selects a nonalcoholic choice such as fruit juice, the aversive stimulus is removed. The clinician monitors the patient's compliance with the directive that he or she must not swallow any alcohol at any time during the treatment session. Sessions last 20 to 45 minutes, depending on the individual patient. After the aversion conditioning session in the treatment room, the patient returns to his or her room, listens to a relaxation tape, makes a list of positive changes with sobriety, and contrasts them with the negative consequences of continued use (**Table 77-1**).

TABLE 77-1 Percent Abstinence From Alcohol During Specified Follow-Up Periods

Follow-up period	Aversion (%)	Match (%)	*p* Value x^2, 1 df
0-6 mo	85	72	0.01
0-12 mo	79	67	0.05

From Smith JW, Frawley PJ, Polissar L. Six- and twelve-month abstinence rates in inpatients with alcohol use disorder treated with either faradic aversion or chemical aversion compared with matched inpatients from a treatment registry. *J Addict Dis.* 1997;16(1):5-24.

Covert Sensitization

Elkins[25,26] has published on the use of covert sensitization to demonstrate that conditioned nausea responses can be trained in patients with AUD, through the use of imagination and verbal suggestion without the use of an emetic drug. In covert sensitization, patients are helped to imagine personally relevant drinking scenes that emphasize the motivational, sensory, and behavioral precursors and concomitants of alcohol ingestion. The drinking scenes then are paired repeatedly with verbally induced nausea. Most cooperative participants can learn to experience genuine and intense nausea reactions by focusing on the therapist's noxious verbal suggestions; these suggestions prompt recipients to remember and recreate prior feelings and thoughts that have been prominent in their former nausea experiences. Such verbally induced nausea is designated as demand nausea. Repeated presentations of the drinking scenes (ie, conditioned stimulus or CS) followed by episodes of verbally induced demand nausea (ie, unconditioned stimulus or US) can, over extended conditioning trials, produce conditioned aversions to alcohol in a majority of participants. Elkins[25] described behavioral and psychophysical indices that can be used to define an individual subject's transition from demand nausea to conditioned nausea, the goal of treatment. Conditioned nausea is nausea as an automatic consequence of the patient's focusing on a drinking scene without any attempted therapist or self-induction of nausea. Fifty-two patients were entered. Thirty-three were able to develop verbally induced nausea after imagined drinking scenes. It took an average of four CS-US pairings over an average of 1.8 sessions to develop this demand nausea. Of these patients, 23 were able to develop conditioned nausea to either the desire for alcohol or other alcohol-related physical stimuli. It took an average of 13.43 scenes over 4.83 sessions for them to develop conditioned aversion. Of note, the 10 patients who did not develop conditioned nausea had the same number of training sessions compared to those who did (11.79 versus 11.64) but had more scenes (48.48 versus 37.82). Those who developed conditioned nausea had the same number of training sessions compared to those who did (11.79 versus 11.64) but had more scenes (48.48 versus 37.82). Those who developed conditioned nausea had an average of 13.74 months of total abstinence as compared to 4.52 months for those who failed to progress beyond the demand nausea stage of treatment ($p < 0.05$). Elkins suggests that some patients are biologically resistant to developing conditioned nausea to alcohol, despite the ability to develop demand nausea to verbal prompting.

Covert Sensitization is now only used in an abbreviated form, and as an adjunct to chemical counter-conditioning when there is difficulty with either establishing an adequate level of nausea, vomiting, and subsequent aversion, or when aversion is established but inconsistent among different varieties of alcohol or other substances. It is also used in faradic counter-conditioning when aversion is suboptimal, or established but inconsistent among different varieties of alcohol or other substances. Notable also is that barriers to establishing aversion are often correlated with a patient's profession or trade. For example, patients who work at heights such as in high-rise construction, and patients who work in maritime jobs such as offshore fishing, often have a high tolerance for the dosage range of ipecac and difficulty achieving nausea. In these cases, ipecac is often augmented with naltrexone or a longer ipecac pre-medication time prior to going into the treatment room. Further, pro re nata (PRN) or scheduled medications that can secondarily attenuate nausea, such as diphenhydramine or vitamin B-6, can be discontinued.

Aversion Therapy as a Treatment for Tobacco/Nicotine Use Disorder

Sachs[27,28] reviewed treatments available as of 1986 and 1991 and concluded that programs that use rapid smoking aversion or satiation had superior outcomes. Rapid smoking or satiation involves smoking cigarettes with inhalations every 6 seconds. Sessions last an average of 15 minutes, and the subject smoker smokes an average of five cigarettes during that session.[29] The treatment sessions are usually daily for 5 days with a tapering frequency of booster treatments after that. When compared to the physical effects of normally paced smoking, patients undergoing rapid smoking experience increased burning in the lungs, palpitations, facial flush, headache and feeling faint or weak.[30] Hall et al.[31] and Lando[32] reported in separate studies that the best results were reported by programs in which aversion was combined with several other modalities, including "relapse prevention" (RP, a specific form of therapy), relaxation training, written exercises, contract management, booster sessions of aversion and group support. Hall et al.[33] found that skills training (cue-produced relaxation training, commitment-enhanced training, and RP training) were more effective than the type of aversive smoking on outcome. Conversely, in a study of 18 patients with cardiopulmonary disease, Hall et al.[29] reported that those in a waiting list control group had no abstinence as compared with those treated with satiation aversion, 50% of whom achieved 2-year abstinence. Their study of 18 patients with cardiopulmonary disease who underwent satiation treatment also found no myocardial ischemia or significant arrhythmia in this group. Five patients with ischemic changes on the treadmill did not experience changes during satiation treatment.

Much of the research on aversion therapy as a treatment for tobacco/nicotine use disorder has focused on improved outcomes with aversive smoking (puffing or inhaling smoke from the cigarettes in a rapid manner to induce nicotine toxicity, often including nausea).[34] Though nicotine is taken into the system during this treatment, the aversion developed to smoking is adequate to prevent recurrence despite the transient presence of nicotine in the bloodstream during treatment. However, a Cochrane review of 25 trials of aversion therapy for smoking reported that "the existing studies provide insufficient evidence to determine the efficacy of rapid smoking, or whether there is a dose response to aversive stimulation. Milder versions of aversive smoking seem to lack specific efficacy. Rapid smoking is an unproven method with sufficient indications of promise to warrant evaluation using modern rigorous methodology."[35]

Faradic aversion (mild electrical stimulus applied to the forearm) has been used commercially for tobacco/nicotine use disorder since 1972.[36] With faradic aversion, the smoke is not inhaled but merely puffed. Inhaling during faradic aversion may lead to early recurrence of smoking.[37] One advantage of this form of treatment is that less medically sophisticated staff can supervise the administration of the treatment. In both forms of treatment, patients personally administer the aversive agent (rapid smoking or electrical stimulus) to themselves, while the therapist serves as a coach. In the case of faradic aversion, each time a patient brings a cigarette toward his or her lips, a mild electrical stimulus is administered automatically by a 9-V battery. The stimulus is activated by a string attached to the smoker's wrist. The therapist also instructs the patient in RP methods and behavior changes that help maintain abstinence and achieve comfort during the initial period after stopping smoking. Smith[36] contacted 59% of 556 patients treated with this method in a commercial program and found that 52% had achieved continuous abstinence at 1 year.

Aversion Therapy for Cannabis Use Disorder

The spontaneous recovery rate from cannabis use disorder is not known and, like that for alcohol and nicotine, probably depends on multiple factors. Both chemical counter-conditioning and faradic counter-conditioning are used for cannabis use disorder. Strains of cannabis that have 0% THC content are used in treatment to enhance olfactory authenticity. The protocol for aversion is similar to that of the treatment for alcohol, except that it uses a variety of bongs, vape pens, drug paraphernalia, and visual imagery. A one-year abstinence rate of 84% was reported after five days of treatment, combined with three weekly group sessions on self-management techniques.[38]

Aversion Therapy for Stimulant Use Disorder (Cocaine and Methamphetamine)

The spontaneous recovery rate from stimulant use disorders involving cocaine or methamphetamine is not known.[39] Frawley and Smith[40] reported the use of chemical aversion for the treatment of cocaine use disorder. In this treatment, an artificial cocaine substitute called Articaine was developed from tetracaine, mannitol, and quinine. Patients snorted this substance and paired it with nausea induced by emetine. Of those so treated, 56% were continuously abstinent and 78% currently abstinent (ie, for the prior 30 days) at 6 months after treatment; at 18 months, 38% were continuously abstinent and 75% currently abstinent. For those treated for both alcohol and cocaine, 70% were continuously and currently abstinent from cocaine at 6 months, 50% were continuously abstinent, and 80% were currently abstinent at 18 months after treatment. Frawley and Smith[41] reported a 53% 1-year continuous abstinence rate in 156 patients with cocaine dependence treated with aversion. This was based on a 73% follow-up rate. Outcomes for chemical and faradic aversion were not significantly different. The report also compared patients with both alcohol and cocaine use disorders who were treated with aversion to alcohol only with a later group when aversion was available for cocaine also. The addition of the aversion for cocaine produced statistically significantly improved abstinence rate for cocaine in this population. The increase in cocaine abstinence in the later group compared to the first (55% versus 88%) is greater than the decrease on follow-up from the first to the second group (84% versus 64%). Because of the lower follow-up rate in the second study, this research needs replication. Elkins et al. reported a well-designed experimental evaluation of three aversion therapy treatments for cocaine use disorder. Volunteer participants satisfied the stringent medical criteria that must be met for participation in emetic therapy, the most physically demanding treatment. The additional two experimental treatments were faradic therapy and covert sensitization therapy. Participants were randomly assigned to one of the three aversion therapy groups or to one of the two control conditions—milieu treatment or relaxation therapy. Milieu therapy was the baseline control treatment that was received by all participants. Emetic and faradic therapy participants used realistic placebo cocaine products during their assigned aversion interventions. The covert sensitization subjects imagined cocaine usage in conjunction with verbal nausea induction. The placebo cocaine products included simulated "rocks" of crack cocaine, simulated snortable cocaine, and Psychem, an essence that contains oils that mimic the odor of street cocaine. Each "rock" of smokeable placebo cocaine was prepared from benzocaine, baking soda, and water. Snortable placebo cocaine consisted of 97% mannitol, 1% quinine, and 2% tetracaine in powder form. The quinine was added to simulate the bitter aspect of cocaine, and the tetracaine was added to mimic the "nose-deadening" anesthetic properties of snorted cocaine. All efforts were made to provide paraphernalia for snorting and smoking the placebo cocaine that resembled each patient's customary paraphernalia. All aversion therapy sessions were completed without any serious side effects. Posttreatment abstinence performance was rigorously tracked during a 6-month follow-up period through telephone queries of the participants and their designated collateral contacts and via in-person contacts that included urine drug screens. Patients lost during follow-up were classified as if they had a recurrence of use. The 57.9% 6-month follow-up abstinence finding for the emetic therapy recipients significantly exceeded the 26.5% 6-month abstinence finding for the milieu control participants. These emetic therapy data are quite encouraging and are consistent with the reported 56% 6-month abstinence rate from the previously discussed clinical trial of emetic therapy for DSM-IV–defined cocaine dependence.[40] Covert sensitization produced a significant therapeutic benefit, but its effect did not extend beyond 3 months after treatment. The second major positive outcome is found in the emetic therapy participants uniquely reported total loss of cravings for cocaine by the end of treatment (discussed in more detail in section "Effect of Aversion on Cocaine Craving," below).

There is some literature on the ability of disulfiram to reduce cocaine use.[42] Various mechanisms are proposed. The major effect is thought to be the ability of disulfiram to block Dopamine beta-hydroxylase, an enzyme that coverts dopamine to norepinephrine. Norepinephrine is thought to enhance the effect of cocaine. As such, disulfiram would not be an aversive therapy.

Aversion Therapy for Opioid Use Disorder (Heroin and Prescription Opioids)

Copemann[43] employed a unique approach to aversion therapy by pairing aversive stimuli to cognitive images of heroin use. Patients were asked to verbalize only after they had conjured up a strong mental image. A second part of the treatment asked subjects to conjure images of socially appropriate behavior, involving employment, education, or nondrug entertainment. Latency to verbalization was measured. Copemann found that, at baseline, subjects could rapidly conjure up positive thoughts about heroin use but had significant delays in conjuring up thoughts about rewarding nondrug activities. Subjects were in a halfway house for heroin-addicted patients and received group therapy in conjunction with relaxation therapy in addition to the aversion treatment. A faradic stimulator was used. Once subjects had conjured up drug images, faradic aversion was applied. At other times, they were given 15 seconds to conjure images of nondrug socially appropriate behavior to prevent aversion from being applied. With this training over an average of 15 sessions (range, 5 to 25), latency for drug-related images increased, while that for socially appropriate images decreased. Thirty of 50 patients completed the treatment, and, at 24 months, 80% (24 of 30) were reported to be drug-free.

In the counter-conditioning treatment pathway, naltrexone is started either in daily tablet form or monthly injectable-suspension form with recommended use for at least six months following discharge. Additionally, all patients with opioid use disorder leave the hospital with prescriptions for nasal Narcan for use in opioid overdose. A novel counter-conditioning treatment for opioid use disorder first developed by Merchant (personal communication, 2008) has been evolved to address the surge in use of OxyContin and counterfeit oxycodone equivalents in recent years ("blue" fentanyl-based tablets). Following verification of completion of opioid withdrawal with a series of four small 12.5 mg challenge-response doses of naltrexone, the patient then begins a daily dose of 50 mg of naltrexone. The patient is then able to consume actual oxycodone in their preferred manner of smoking, insufflating, or swallowing during their counter-conditioning treatment sessions with typically significantly reduced euphoric, analgesic, or otherwise effects of the opioid. This treatment capitalizes on the ability of naltrexone to competitively block the effects of opioids at the receptor level.

Elkins presented four case reports in 2013 of patients with opioid use disorder meeting the DSM-4 criteria for heroin dependence at admission, successfully treated with aversion therapy utilizing covert sensitization in conjunction with emetic treatment.[44] These patients entered treatment with strong Desire-Aversion Scale (DAS)-confirmed heroin and opioid pill cravings and left with strong aversions. Ages ranged from 19 to 33, two males and two females. One smoked pills and heroin, one smoked pills but also smoked and injected heroin, one smoked opioids but injected heroin, and one had a AUD, who also injected heroin. Each had developed strong aversions during their initial treatment and had maintained those aversions when they returned for their reinforcement aversions and not experienced opioid cravings since being discharged. Follow ups were done 7 to 12 months after completion of treatment and patients reported continued abstinence at the follow up visit. Importantly, however, more rigorous trials are needed in which patients could be randomly assigned to different treatments.

Use of Reinforcement (Booster) Aversion Treatments

Smith and Frawley[45] followed up at 1 year on 437 patients of 600 patients (73%) treated with chemical and faradic aversion for alcohol, marijuana, or cocaine (**Table 77-2**). One-year complete abstinence rates for alcohol for those who did not return for any reinforcements ($N = 51$) was 29.4%; for one booster aversion treatment ($N = 93$), the abstinence rate was 50.5%; with two booster aversions ($N = 273$) the abstinence rate was 68.5%; and for more than two boosters ($N = 10$), the abstinence rate was 80%. Wiens and Menustik[46] reported that the use of reinforcement aversion treatments (or recaps) was associated with improvement in abstinence at 1 year after treatment: no recaps, 24%; 1 recap, 21%; 2 recaps, 40%; 3 recaps, 27%; 4 recaps, 64%; 5 recaps, 72%; and 6 recaps, 99%. Of note, 144 of 385 (38%) patients received the 6 recaps.

Use of Support Programs and 12-Step Meetings After Receiving Aversion Therapy

Smith and Frawley[19] found no association between the use of support groups during the period of being at risk for return to use and the status of urges to drink. There was an insignificant trend toward more urges with greater support group use (**Table 77-3**). However, there was an association between use of reinforcements and urge to drink. Seventy-six and one-half percent of those who used no reinforcements ($N = 51$) reported urges to drink, while 54.8% of those who had one reinforcement ($N = 93$) and 49.8% of those who had at least two reinforcements ($N = 283$) reported urges ($p < 0.01$).

TABLE 77-2 One-Year Total Abstinence Rates: Use of Reinforcements and Follow-Up Support

Condition	1	2	3	4
Number of patients	79	65	116	167
Support group use	No	Yes	No	Yes
Reinforcements	<2	<2	>2	>2
Total abstinence (%)	34.2	52.3	58.6	74.3

Reprinted from Smith JW, Frawley PJ. Treatment outcome of 600 patients with substance use disorder treated in a multimodal inpatient program including aversion therapy and pentothal interviews. *J Subst Abuse Treat.* 1993;10:359-369, with permission.

TABLE 77-3 Patients With Urges: Association Between Support Group Attendance and 1-Year Abstinence

	Frequency of support group attendance			
	>1/wk	1/wk	<1/wk	*p* value
AA no. of patients	25	17	29	–
Total abstinence (%)	20	35	66	<0.01
Schick no. of patients	8	30	24	–
Total abstinence (%)	38	50	63	NS

Reprinted from Smith JW, Frawley PJ. Treatment outcome of 600 patients with substance use disorders treated in a multimodal inpatient program including aversion therapy and pentothal interviews. *J Subst Abuse Treat.* 1993;10:359-369, with permission.

EFFECT OF AVERSION ON CRAVING FOR ALCOHOL

A detailed review of chemical aversion therapy, its rationale, and comparison with other treatments for AUD has been presented by Howard et al.[47] They emphasize that patients are able to develop an aversion to alcohol as demonstrated by autonomic markers and patient report and that there is an association between the strength of the aversion and abstinence from alcohol. Elkins[2] notes that a variety of researchers have reported that some patients do not seem to develop aversions. Patients who report that aversion therapy greatly reduced their urges have the best outcome. Smith and Frawley[19] found that at follow-up, patients who reported the loss of all urges to drink after aversion treatment ($N = 165$) had a total abstinence rate at 1 year from alcohol of 89.7%. Those who reported only the loss of uncontrollable urges ($N = 183$) had an abstinence rate of 56.8%. Those who reported that they still had urges had an abstinence rate of 6.3%. Nurses providing aversion therapy use a Likert scale, which ranges from −5 for high craving to +5 strong aversion based upon the patient's physical and emotional reaction to seeing, smelling, and tasting their favorite drinks. As can be seen in **Figure 77-1**, which averaged the responses of 10 patients who completed all five of the aversion sessions and both reinforcement treatments, there is a progression from craving to aversion over the course of the treatment, which is maintained at one and three months when the patients return for treatment.

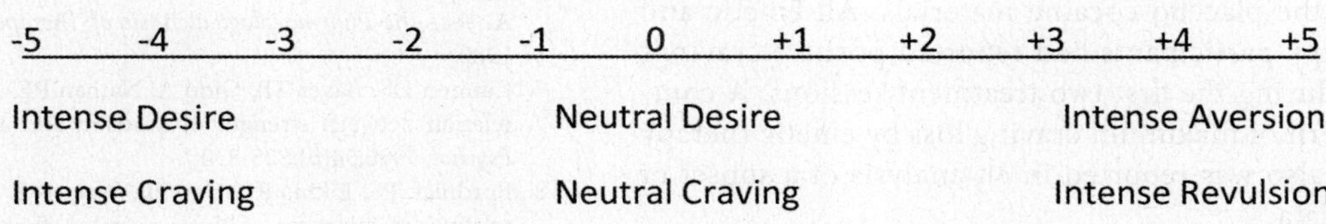

	Pre	Post	Date	Treatment Nurse
Treatment # 1	-2	1		
Treatment # 2	0	2		
Treatment # 3	2	3		
Treatment # 4	3	5		
Treatment # 5	5	5		
Treatment # 6 Recap # 1, 30 days post d/c	5	5		
Treatment # 7 Recap # 2,90 days post d/c	5	5		

Figure 77-1. These values reflect median pretreatment and posttreatment data from 10 patients who had cravings, who underwent chemical counterconditioning treatments for alcohol and who returned for their 90-day booster treatment. (Courtesy of Elkins, R.L.)

FUNCTIONAL MRI STUDIES OF SUBSTANCE USE DISORDERS AND AVERSION AND CRAVING

Thirteen adult patients with AUD were recruited by hospital clinicians to serve as subjects in a neuroimaging study. Subjects had functional MRI studies before and after chemical aversion therapy for alcohol.[48] During the fMRI, 10-minute sessions patients would be given suggestions to self-generate mental images of drinking their favorite alcoholic beverage and then alternate to a session of self-generated mental images of pleasant non–alcohol related settings such as relaxing scenes by a beach but without the presence of alcohol. A total of 5 cycles were done during the 10 minutes of fMRI scanning (see **Table 77-4**).

The fMRI studies showed that after treatment there were significant reductions in cue related activity in the occipital cortex, $p < 0.05$.[49] At one year follow-up patients had a 69% total abstinence rate for at least a year after treatment.[48]

Studies have shown that the activity of different brain areas at fMRI depends on study design, genotypes, medications, and ways in which the alcohol stimulus is presented. Goodyear recommends that studies standardize the stimuli by using taste (even different tastes depending on the drinker's preferences), smell, visual and psychological stimuli to stimulate craving and then to use fMRI to measure those differences.[49]

TABLE 77-4 Alcohol Craving Scale

	Mean pretreatment	Mean post 4 aversion treatments	*p* Value
Wants alcohol	4.46	0.00	<0.005
Crave alcohol	3.85	0.00	<0.005
Alcohol Craving Questionnaire	33.09	14.91	<0.01

Patient's ratings/responses to subjective graphic rating scale questions before and after treatment (3 questions).

EFFECT OF AVERSION ON COCAINE CRAVING

Ninety-seven participants within the relaxation training, covert sensitization, faradic treatment, and emetic therapy conditions of the Elkins et al. study provided pre- and postsession subjective ratings of cocaine cravings. The emetic therapy and faradic therapy participants all reported positive cue-induced cravings for cocaine upon their initial exposure to the placebo cocaine materials. All emetic and faradic therapy participants had reported positive cravings for cocaine during the first two treatment sessions. A comparable pattern of maximum craving loss by emetic therapy participants also was reported in an analysis of a subset of the present data.[8]

NEED FOR FURTHER RESEARCH

Aversion therapy has not been studied extensively despite the initial positive results.[19,27,38,41,43] Today it will probably not be ethically approved to have a control group not receiving treatment. Instead, aversion therapy should be compared to state-of-the-art treatment.

Research is needed in sizable, randomized designs using standardized outcome measurements and methods for cravings and aversions. In addition, nested interviews and major cohort studies would add to the research area of aversion therapy. Furthermore, the effects of social media/virtual treatment platforms on aversion have not been studied.

Future studies should incorporate bidirectional scales that measure maximum craving at one extreme and maximum revulsion at the other extreme with a neutral zero-craving midscale region as shown in **Figure 77-1**. The dynamically expanding field of brain imaging research is likely to provide the greatest near-term advancements in our basic understanding and possible clinical applications of cue-induced brain changes that occur during the emetic therapy-induced transition from alcohol and other drug cravings to revulsions and may be appropriate at some time to measure brain changes resulting from treatment that predict long term sobriety. Elkins[2] noted that a variety of researchers have reported that some patients do not seem to develop aversions. This indicates the need for identifications of biological indices to separate conditionable and nonconditionable potential emetic therapy recipients. Additionally, studies of the two groups may support the development of relevant pharmacological or nutritional interventions to increase the nausea-based conditionability of the nonconditional patients.

REFERENCES

1. Bandura A. *Principles of Behavior Modification*. Holt, Rinehart and Winston; 1969:509.
2. Elkins RL. An appraisal of chemical aversion (emetic therapy) approaches to alcoholism treatment. *Behav Res Ther.* 1991;29(3):387-413.
3. Smith JW. Treatment of alcoholism in aversion conditioning hospitals. In: Pattison EM, Kaufman E, eds. *Encyclopedic Handbook of Alcoholism.* Gardner Press; 1982:874-884.
4. Smith C, Bookner S, Dreher F. *Effects of Alcohol Intoxication and Hangovers on Subsequent Drinking.* NIDA Research Monograph 90. National Institute on Drug Abuse; 1988:366.
5. Ray LA, Meredith LR, Kiluk BD, Walthers J, Carroll KM, Magill M. Combined pharmacotherapy and cognitive behavioral therapy for adults with alcohol or substance use disorders: a systematic review and meta-analysis. *JAMA Netw Open.* 2020;3(6):e208279. doi:10.1001/jamanetworkopen.2020.8279
6. Ritchie JM. The aliphatic alcohols. In: Gilman AG, Goodman LS, Gilman A, eds. *The Pharmacological Basis of Therapeutics.* 6th ed. Macmillan; 1980.
7. Cannon DS, Baker TB, Gino A, Nathan PE. Alcohol-aversion therapy: relation between strength of aversion and abstinence. *J Consult Clin Psychol.* 1986;54(6):825-830.
8. Bordnick PS, Elkins RL, Orr TE, Walters P, Thyer BA. Evaluating the relative effectiveness of three aversion therapies designed to reduce craving among cocaine abusers. *Behav Interv.* 2004;19:1-24.
9. Mihai A, Damsa C, Allen M, Baleydier B, Lazignac C, Heinz A. Viewing videotape of themselves while experiencing delirium tremens could reduce the relapse rate in alcohol-dependent patients. *Addiction.* 2007;102:226-231.
10. deSilva P, Rachman S. Human food aversions: nature and acquisition. *J Consult Clin Psychol.* 1987;25(6):457-468.
11. Garcia J, Ervin FR, Koelling RA. Learning with prolonged delay of reinforcement. *Psychon Sci.* 1966;5:121-122.
12. Garcia J, McGowan BK, Ervin FR, Koelling RA. Cues: their relative effectiveness as a function of the reinforcer. *Science.* 1968;160:784-795.
13. Hoeschen LE. The pharmacokinetics and pharmacodynamics of alcohol and drugs of addiction. In: Miller NS, ed. *Comprehensive Handbook of Drug and Alcohol Addiction.* Marcel Dekker; 1991:745-746.
14. Lemere F, Voegtlin WL. Conditioned reflex therapy of alcoholic addiction: specificity of conditioning against chronic alcoholism. *Cal West Med.* 1940;53(6):1-4.
15. Quinn JT, Henbest R. Partial failure of generalization in alcoholics following aversion therapy. *Q J Stud Alcohol.* 1967;28:70-75.
16. Lemere F, Voegtlin WL, Broz WR, O'Hollaren P, Tupper WE. The conditioned reflex treatment of chronic alcoholism: VIII. A review of six years' experience with this treatment of 1,526 patients. *JAMA.* 1942;120(4):269-271. doi:10.1001/jama.1942.02830390019005
17. Robbins SJ, Schwartz B, Wasserman EA. *Psychology of Learning and Behavior.* 5th ed. W.W. Norton & Co; 2001.
18. Voegtlin WL, Lemere F, Broz WR, O'Hollaren P. Conditioned reflex therapy of chronic alcoholism: IV. A preliminary report on the value of reinforcement. *Q J Stud Alcohol.* 1941;2(3):505-511.
19. Smith JW, Frawley PJ, Polissar L. Six- and twelve-month abstinence rates in inpatient alcoholics treated with aversion therapy compared with matched inpatients from a treatment registry. *Alcohol Clin Exp Res.* 1991;15(5):862-870.
20. Pomerleau OF, Fertig J, Baker L, Cooney N. Reactivity to alcohol cue in alcoholics and non-alcoholics: implications for a stimulus control analysis of drinking. *Addict Behav.* 1983;8:1-10.
21. Niaura R, Abrams D, Demuth B, Pinto R, Monti P. Responses to smoking-related stimuli and early relapse to smoking. *Addict Behav.* 1989;14:419-428.
22. Sherman JE, Zinser MC, Sideroff SI, Baker TB. Subjective dimensions of heroin urges: influence of heroin-related and affectively related stimuli. *Addict Behav.* 1989;14:611-623.
23. Weddington WW, Brown BS, Haertzen CA, et al. Changes in mood, craving, and sleep during short-term abstinence reported by male cocaine addicts. *Arch Gen Psychiatry.* 1990;47:861-868.
24. Gawin FH, Kleber HD. Abstinence symptomatology and psychiatric diagnosis in cocaine abusers. *Arch Gen Psychiatry.* 1986;43:107-113.
25. Elkins RL. Covert sensitization treatment of alcoholism: contributions of successful conditioning to subsequent abstinence maintenance. *Addict Behav.* 1980;5:67-89.
26. Elkins RL. Aversion therapy for alcoholism: chemical, electrical, or verbal imagery? *Int J Addict.* 1975;10(2):157-209.
27. Sachs DPL. Advances in smoking cessation treatment. *Curr Pulmonol.* 1991;12:139-198.
28. Sachs DPL. Cigarette smoking: health effects and cessation strategies. *Clin Geriatr Med.* 1986;2(2):337-363.

29. Hall RG, Sachs DPL, Hall SM, Benowitz NL. Two-year efficacy and safety of rapid smoking therapy in patients with cardiac and pulmonary disease. *J Consult Clin Psychol.* 1984;52(4):574-581.
30. Glasgow RE, Lichtenstein E, Beaver C, O'Neill K. Subjective reactions to rapid and normal pace aversive smoking. *Addict Behav.* 1981;6:53-59.
31. Hall S, Tunstall C, Rugg D, Jones RT, Benowitz N. Nicotine gum and behavioral treatment in smoking cessation. *J Consult Clin Psychol.* 1985;53(2):256-258.
32. Lando HA. Successful treatment of smokers with a broad-spectrum behavioral approach. *J Consult Clin Psychol.* 1977;45(3):361-366.
33. Hall SM, Rugg D, Tunstall C, Jones RT. Preventing relapse to cigarette smoking by behavioral skill training. *J Consult Clin Psychol.* 1984;52(3):372-382.
34. Erickson LM, Tiffany ST, Martin EM, Baker TB. Aversive smoking therapies: a conditioning analysis of therapeutic effectiveness. *Behav Res Ther.* 1983;21(60):595-611.
35. Hajek P, Stead LF. Aversive smoking for smoking cessation. *Cochrane Database Syst Rev.* 2004;2001(3):CD000546. doi:10.1002/14651858.CD000546.pub2
36. Smith JW. Long-term outcome of clients treated in a commercial stop smoking program. *J Subst Abuse Treat.* 1988;5:33-36.
37. Berecz JM. Reduction of cigarette smoking through self-administered aversion conditioning: a new treatment model with implications for public health. *Soc Sci Med.* 1972;6:57-66.
38. Smith JW, Schmeling G, Knowles PL. A marijuana smoking cessation clinical trial utilizing THC-free marijuana, aversion therapy, and self-management counseling. *J Subst Abuse Treat.* 1988;5(2):89-98.
39. Rawson RA, Obert JL, McCann MJ, et al. In: Harris LS, ed. *Cocaine Treatment Outcome: Cocaine Use Following Inpatient, Outpatient and No Treatment (NIDA Research Monograph 67).* National Institute on Drug Abuse; 1986:271-277.
40. Frawley PJ, Smith JW. Chemical aversion therapy in the treatment of cocaine dependence as part of a multimodal treatment program: treatment outcome. *J Subst Abuse Treat.* 1990;7:21-29.
41. Frawley PJ, Smith JW. One-year follow-up after multimodal inpatient treatment for cocaine and methamphetamine dependence. *J Subst Abuse Treat.* 1992;9(4):271-286.
42. Gaval-Cruz M, Weinshenker D. Mechanisms of disulfiram-induced cocaine abstinence: antabuse and cocaine relapse. *Mol Interv.* 2009;9(4):175-187. doi:10.1124/mi.9.4.6
43. Copemann CD. Drug addiction: II. An aversive counterconditioning technique for treatment. *Psychol Rep.* 1976;38:1271-1281.
44. Elkins R, Beck D, Dandala K. *Hypnotically-guided counter conditioning for heroin dependence: case reports of anti-craving benefits and abstinence outcomes. Poster presented at: Society for Clinical & Experimental Hypnosis's 64th Annual Scientific Session;* October 4-6, 2013. Berkeley.
45. Smith JW, Frawley PJ. Treatment outcome of 600 chemically dependent patients treated in a multimodal inpatient program including aversion therapy and pentothal interviews. *J Subst Abuse Treat.* 1993;10:359-369.
46. Wiens AN, Menustik CA. Treatment outcome and patient characteristics in an aversion therapy program for alcoholism. *Am Psychol.* 1983;38(10):1089-1096.
47. Howard MO, Elkins RL, Rimmele C, Smith JW. Chemical aversion treatment for alcohol dependence. *Drug Alcohol Depend.* 1991;29:107-143.
48. Elkins RL, Richards TL, Nielsen R, Repass R, Stahlbrand H, Hoffmann HG. The neurobiological mechanism of chemical aversion (Emetic) therapy for alcohol use disorder: an fMRI study. *Front Behav Neurosci.* 2017;11:182. doi:10.3389/fnbeh.2017.00182
49. Goodyear K. Multisensory environments to measure craving during functional magnetic resonance imaging. *Alcohol Alcohol.* 2019;54(3):193-195.

CHAPTER

78 Family Involvement in Addiction, Treatment, and Recovery

Julianne C. Flanagan and Brandi C. Fink

CHAPTER OUTLINE

- Introduction
- Biopsychosocial model explaining the role of family members in addiction and recovery
- Effective screening and identification of substance use disorders
- Evidence-based couple and family treatments for substance use disorder
- Family psychoeducation and 12-step program engagement
- Couple and family modalities for adults
- Family approaches with adolescents
- Population-specific considerations
- Summary

INTRODUCTION

Partners and family members play an important role in the etiology, course, and treatment of substance use disorders (SUDs). It is vital, therefore, to address relationship and family issues with every patient who has, or might possibly have, SUD. Learning about the relational aspects contributing to SUD and related treatment outcomes is useful for providers from various disciplines, as evidenced by the following:

- SUDs are highly prevalent in the United States, and their impact may include significant morbidity and mortality.
- SUD etiology and course correlates with familial, environmental, and genetic factors and heavily cluster within families; therefore, individuals diagnosed with SUD incur an increased likelihood of family history of SUD. These factors require consideration when developing and adapting a patient's treatment and recovery needs.
- It is often difficult for patients, family members, and clinicians to identify, assess, and diagnose SUD. Equally difficult is the task of staying current on the patient's recurrence/remission/recovery status and treatment activities. Family members are often in a position to assist treatment engagement and recovery, but family-related obstacles may also prevent adaptive support utilization and recovery.
- Incorporating family education and evidence-based couple and family therapies into SUD treatment has substantial therapeutic value for patients and family members.
- Several efficacious couple and family intervention modalities are available to help patients and family members make sustainable adaptive changes during the recovery process.

BIOPSYCHOSOCIAL MODEL EXPLAINING THE ROLE OF FAMILY MEMBERS IN ADDICTION AND RECOVERY

Approximately 8% to 13% of the United States general population will experience a SUD during their lifetime, with alcohol being the most prevalent and commonly diagnosed SUD. Rates of past-year SUD approximate 14.5%. Substance use is also most likely to initiate in late adolescence or early adulthood but can emerge at any age and is likely to persist if untreated. Substance use including use of nicotine, alcohol, and other drugs, confers a substantially increased risk of physical injury and illness regardless of age of onset. Mental health challenges such as depression, anxiety, and posttraumatic stress disorder (PTSD) are also highly co-occurring with non-medical substance use and SUD and may result from or become exacerbated by episodes of negative substance-related sequelae.

The extant literature is clear that alcohol and drug use as well as associated problems have a significant and mutually causal relationship with social and family functioning. For example, a national survey was conducted in the United Kingdom (ie, the Survey of Life in Recovery for Families[1]; *N* = 1,565). The duration of SUD among participants in this study was 14.1 years and the majority of those with SUD (78.8%) had engaged in formal treatment at some point in their lifetime. Most participants endorsed having an alcohol use disorder (62.6%) as well as drug use disorders (67.7 illicit drugs; 34.8% prescription medications; 7.3% other drugs). This study found that engaging in a program of recovery conveyed substantial benefits. Many participants reported a reduction in financial debt (20.1%) and an improvement in their ability to pay household expenses (36.4%). Approximately two-thirds of participants reported a reduction in family violence (66.9%), and specifically a reduction in their own violence perpetration (66.2%), as well as a reduction in arrests (60%), incarceration (64.7%), and DUI charges (69.8%). Approximately one-third of participants also reported having returned to substance use at some point in their life (33.2%), which they perceived to have negative impacts on the gains they had achieved with treatment.

In a separate line of literature, the partner influence hypothesis explains that close significant others, and romantic partners specifically, might enter into or develop a "drinking partnership," in which they reinforce and maintain one another's drinking patterns, even when the patterns are maladaptive for their health, occupational, or relational functioning.[2-5] For example, a recent meta-analysis of 17 studies focused on different-sex couples ($N = 10{,}553$ dyads) found within-dyad associations between partners' drinking.[6] This meta-analysis also found that the effect of women's drinking on men's drinking was slightly greater than the effect of men's drinking on women's drinking. Similarly, interpersonal verbal, physical, and sexual violence victimization is a prominent risk factor for substance use, and use of violence is a prevalent negative outcome associated with alcohol and drug use. Current conceptual models such as the I-cubed model of aggression indicate that both cognitive and emotion regulation abilities under intoxication are diminished.[7] When intoxication interacts with aggressogenic stable personality characteristics or mental health symptoms, interpersonal violence is more likely to occur, particularly with alcohol.[8] Similar effects are observed with substances other than alcohol but with varying outcomes and myriad individual differences influencing such outcomes.[9] Relatedly, findings emerged from the international Life in Recovery Surveys that included participants from the United States, United Kingdom, Canada, and Australia. Some notable findings among participants in the United States indicated that engaging in recovery had conveyed a 450% reduction in experiencing violence perpetration or victimization; a 600% reduction in having children removed from the home due to abuse or neglect; a 110% increase in regaining child custody for those who did not have custody of their children due to their SUD. Participants also indicated a 50% increase in engaging in positive family activities.[1]

Identifying emerging alcohol and drug use is particularly important for clinical care across settings.[10] If substance use and SUDs remain unassessed, co-occurring physical and mental health concerns such as depression, anxiety, morbidity, and suicidality, may also remain unrecognized and untreated. It is equally important to identify family-focused risk and protective factors in the transition from use to SUD. For example, childhood trauma, family conflict including violence, relationship dissolution are all stressful life experiences that might inform substance use trajectories. Conversely, adaptive support and functioning can facilitate resilience. Such information is essential to effective treatment motivation, planning, and engagement.

SUDs are best understood as chronic health conditions with a biopsychosocial etiology,[11] and applying this framework to assessment and intervention can help clinicians maximize their effectiveness. With respect to such etiology, families contribute unique "bio," "psycho," and "social" influences on the development of SUD within the family. Factors such as family history density of SUD, substance use among family members and peers, and attitudes toward alcohol and drug use in family and social networks can facilitate early age of first use, emergence of alcohol and drug related problems, and early onset of SUD. Maladaptive couple and family functioning are known salient risk factors for recurrence of use and can interrupt adaptive treatment seeking and engagement. Conversely, adaptive family relationships are associated with reduced rates of alcohol and drug experimentation in adolescents, leading to lower rates of SUD in young adulthood.[6] The family-focused biopsychosocial contributions to SUD etiology, course, and treatment are briefly outlined and described below.

Biological Factors

Familial *bio*logical risk factors vary. Some biological risk factors include substance-specific genetic predisposition that convey numerous risks for SUD such as individual differences in the metabolism of alcohol and drugs.[12-15] For example, in a sample of over 5 million participants examining 11 different psychiatric conditions in first- through fifth-degree relatives, family genetic risk scores were among the strongest pertaining to alcohol and drug use disorders.[16] Similarly, family history density of alcohol use disorder is a well-established risk factor for individuals of varying demographic backgrounds.[17] Meta-analyses indicate that the degree of heritability is estimated at 50%.[18]

Psychological Factors

Couple and familial *psycho*logical risk factors are vast and varied.[19] Some established risk factors include parental modeling of substance use and positive attitudes toward alcohol and drug use,[20] having a parent or caregiver with a substance use disorder,[21] experiencing childhood adversity, abuse, and neglect,[22] sibling substance use,[21,23-25] and poor parental monitoring of children.[26] There is mounting evidence that adverse childhood experiences lead to a wide variety of adult adverse health outcomes and are a strong risk factor for substance use and SUD.[27-29]

Social Factors

Familial *socio*logical risk factors include the community in which the family resides and associated community substance use controls and laws[30] and whether one lives in a rural versus and urban setting[31] with differing levels of drug availability. For example, tobacco retailer density and proximity are known predictors of adult tobacco use behavior.[32] Similarly, stricter policies regulating youth alcohol access and consequences are inversely associated with recent drinking.[33] Social influences regarding substance use, both presently and in one's early life, are also known to subsequently impact the onset and course of SUD and treatment. For example, women who live with a male partner who engages in heavy drinking are more likely to drink heavily themselves.[34] Conversely, women who separate from, or divorce, partners who have an SUD subsequently reduce their own drinking or drug use and are more likely to seek treatment. Peers, family members, and romantic partners also play an important role in discouraging risky substance use and reducing the risk for SUD by facilitating adaptive substance-free recreation and treatment seeking and recovery.

The research investigating the role of relationship functioning and substance use in same-sex couples is in its nascence. Much of the work conducted thus far has occurred through the lens of how relationship dynamics and substance use affect the risk for HIV transmission,[35] intimate partner violence[36-38] or other negative health outcomes.

A separate line of SUD prevention research suggests that tobacco and alcohol use are two early steps in an adolescent's progression to drug use.[39] Exposure to drinking, smoking, and drug use in the home provides behavioral role modeling, tacit approval, and ease of access to drugs, all of which encourage early use. In contrast, children whose parents pursue treatment and engage a program of recovery have a reduced likelihood of developing substance use disorder themselves. For example, in early exploration of the topic, Moos and Billings[40] found that latency-age sons of recovering veterans with alcohol use disorder performed better at home and in school as compared with both sons of actively drinking veterans with alcohol use disorders and sons of veterans without alcohol use disorders. The improvement in functioning in these youth is certainly related to improvements in parenting behaviors, such as improved parental monitoring and more positively balanced parent-child interactions. Conversely, children who are exposed to adverse experiences during childhood have substantially greater medical and mental health morbidities and poorer outcomes on multiple domains of functioning.[41,42] This is likely the result of the disruptions that parental SUDs cause to effective parenting. Some commonly co-occurring conditions include depression, anxiety, oppositional defiant disorder, externalizing behaviors, and academic problems. Indeed, it is possible that the benefits conveyed by adaptive treatment seeking and engagement may outweigh the risks posed by substance use disorder occurrence, which further underscores the need for accessible, cost-effective, and efficacious individual and family treatment.

As an individual's nonmedical use of substances and accepting attitudes towards substance use expands, it severely stresses family and partner relationships. Substance use, craving, and possible withdrawal symptoms may interfere with both family and occupational responsibilities. As SUD progresses in severity, the amount and quality of time spent together in adaptive, nonsubstance related activities might diminish. Over time, an individual with a substance use disorder may experience, and develop supporting cognition, that functioning in various settings without substances is increasingly difficult. Family members may likewise incorporate substance-accommodating behavior into their lives and might become discouraged that the substance use disorder can be effectively treated. Some accommodating behaviors include supplying alcohol or drugs and may do so despite misgivings in order to avoid the unpleasantness of their loved one's withdrawal symptoms. For example, a family member may purchase alcohol or cigarettes in order to avoid a loved one's irritability or illness due to withdrawal.

Cultural Factors

Although a comprehensive discussion of cultural factors in the prevention as well as the emergence of substance use problems is beyond the scope of this chapter, there are a few notable cultural factors to which one must be sensitive in understanding and working with families from different cultures. The "healthy immigrant" or immigration paradox is a phenomenon whereby first-generation immigrants are at a reduced risk for the development of a substance use or other behavioral health disorder.[43,44] It is widely understood that levels of acculturation and acculturation stress are risk factors for the emergence of substance use among immigrant youth from a range of racial and ethnic backgrounds. Of particular relevance to our discussion in this chapter is the acculturation-gap distress hypothesis,[45] which states that parent-child cultural conflict that arises from parent-child cultural differences put youth at risk for the development of substance use disorders. This phenomenon has been studies well in Latinx and Hispanic youth[46] and appears to be a process present in other immigrant populations as well.[47]

Just as there are general familial risk factors present for the development of substance use disorders in immigrant youth and youth from diverse racial and ethnic backgrounds, there are also important general protective factors that families convey as well. For example, family protective factors include good parental monitoring,[26,48] family cohesion,[49] meaningful family communication, and family rules against substance use.[50,51]

While the contemporary thinking of prevention science is that effective interventions should be tailored to the particular communities of focus,[52] there is evidence that interventions that focus on general principles and the similarities in protective and risk factors are at least as effective as those tailored to particular racial and ethnic groups.[53-56] For example, interventions that focus on increasing parental competencies, parental monitoring, parental involvement,[48,57-59] family rules against substance use,[51] and youth developmental needs, like improving family interactions, have been shown to be as effective as interventions specifically tailored to the particular racial and ethnic groups in preventing youth substance use.[60]

One final note about treatment access and racial and ethnic minority populations, studies of Latinx and Hispanic individuals have consistently reported an underutilization of behavioral health and substance use services. While much of this underutilization of treatment services by Hispanic individuals has been attributed to workforce shortages,[61] shortages of behavioral health facilities,[62] and shortages of services in one's native language, recent data suggest that underutilization may also be due to the reliance on supportive familial, social networks, folk healers and religious-oriented services.[63,64] Because of this, when these patients do present for treatment, efforts to bolster the skills to better access familial and social networks may be particularly advantageous for these individuals.

EFFECTIVE SCREENING AND IDENTIFICATION OF SUBSTANCE USE DISORDERS

Effective, judgement-free, and evidence-based screening and diagnostic assessment are essential components of SUD identification, psychoeducation, treatment engagement, and treatment-planning. Factors such as socioeconomic background, country of origin, possible cognitive or learning challenges, gender identity and pronoun preferences, English language proficiency with spoken and written word, and race and ethnic self-identification (and related cultural norms) should always be considered in this process. Age and developmental stage are also essential considerations. A detailed review of screening tools for SUDs is found in this textbook in Section 4 "Diagnosis, Assessment, and Early Intervention Treatment" and also in Section 14 "Children and Adolescents." A family-specific assessment is outlined below.

Family History Density

Family history density (FHD)[65] can be assessed either dichotomously (yes/no)[66] or via a more comprehensive scoring method that considers both the number and type (first, second degree) of relatives with known or possible SUD.[67] Some measures include the FH Density assessment[65] and the Family Expression of Alcoholism measure,[68] as well as the family history subscale of the Addiction Severity Index (ASI).[69]

EVIDENCE-BASED COUPLE AND FAMILY TREATMENTS FOR SUBSTANCE USE DISORDER

The full range of treatments that individuals or families may require to address the family consequences of addiction and co-occurring issues in each family member is beyond the scope of this chapter, but the most comprehensive review possible is provided here. It is important for clinicians to be aware that, in addition to formal treatment programs, a broad range of treatment resources are available to help patients engage in the process.

Overall, partner and family-involved interventions that employ cognitive behavioral techniques to (1) reinforce reductions in alcohol consumption, (2) enhance family members' skills to facilitate recovery (eg, communication), and (3) enhance family functioning have garnered a strong and sustained evidence base.[70,71] Even brief integration of concerned significant others into individual treatment is likely to convey benefit. For example, when patients in the COMBINE study ($N = 776$) had a family member attend at least one alcohol treatment session, they evidenced fewer drinking days at 16-week treatment completion.[72] Other evidence suggests that couples therapies for AUD commonly outperform individual treatment modalities.[71] Additional promising data has emerged in support of family-based contingency management to improve aftercare[73] and medication adherence.[74] Behaviors such as reinforcing sobriety and adaptive help-seeking, adaptively communicating requests for changes in drinking behavior, decreasing negative or controlling behaviors that are antecedents to drinking, and setting boundaries to allow the drinker to experience the natural negative sequelae of drinking are all fruitful.[75] However, these adaptive behaviors often become eroded during the stressful course of AUD and thus require motivation and guidance for patients and family members to learn and implement effectively. Over time, improvements in family functioning and drinking reductions can be mutually reinforcing; drinking reductions may result in more positive family functioning, which in turn may increase the likelihood of sustained recovery. Similar patterns exist with regard to family (including peer) influences on drinking behavior among populations with salient social network cohesion such as active-duty military service members and Veteran populations.[76-79]

Meta-analyses and reviews of studies on family-oriented treatment approaches have shown superior rates of engagement, positive treatment outcome, and participation in aftercare when compared to individual-oriented care.[80,81] Notably, the most recent update from three prior meta-analyses conducted in 2000, 2004, and 2014 favored family therapy over individual counseling or therapy, peer group therapy, and family psychoeducation.[70,81] It was effective for both adolescents and adults, and in enhancing pharmacotherapy for opioid use disorder, including methadone. It also promoted higher treatment retention, which improves outcome.

Motivational Interviewing

Likelihood of substance-related change behavior can be enhanced by using motivational interviewing techniques.[82] Motivational interviewing offers the opportunity to assess barriers and facilitate change by using an array of possible stage-specific goals and outcomes. Motivational interviewing has been conceptualized to apply to an individual, using their current level of readiness to change as a guide to treatment planning and engagement. Engaging family members in motivational interviewing approaches is also indicated for some individuals with SUD. When observing the situation from a family systems perspective, it is possible that different members of the family will present in different stages of readiness to change. When integrating partners or family members into SUD treatment that is primarily comprised of individual and/or group modalities, concerns regarding privacy and confidentiality should be addressed at the outset such that all parties are informed regarding confidentiality practices and limitations and questions or concerns can be adequately addressed.

Engaging Family Members During Inpatient Treatment

In hospital inpatient settings, scheduling rounds to coincide with family visits might provide an opportunity to discuss the reason(s) frankly and openly for the hospitalization and may naturally lead to dialogue about treatment engagement for the underlying condition(s) including SUD. During such discussion, families have the opportunity to share their experiences and learn the experiences, concerns, and perspectives of the family member with SUD. Conjoint sessions provide clinicians with uniquely valuable opportunities to receive additional information about substance use behaviors and family functioning that may not have been shared previously. For example, clinicians can facilitate discussions regarding how SUD and related sequelae has influenced the patient's adult and child family members as a unit and as individuals. The clinician can then refer or provide "warm handoffs" to a couple and family therapist with skills in addiction treatment to facilitate engagement with individual and/or family treatment and recovery support systems.[83]

Community Reinforcement and Family Training

Community reinforcement and family training (CRAFT)[84-87] is used to train concerned significant others (CSOs) to positively reinforce abstinence, reduced substance use, and recovery behaviors while negatively reinforcing continuing substance use. The CRAFT procedure, when tested in a randomized controlled trial with 130 CSOs of people who engage in problematic drinking, found that 64% of their Identified Patients (IPs) engaged in treatment for alcohol use disorder, while the Johnson Institute Intervention engaged only 30%, and Al-Anon facilitation, only 13%.[86] The strategies involved in Al-Anon facilitation reflect the dominant themes of Al-Anon: disengage from the behavior associated with alcohol use disorder (stop enabling), abandon hope of influencing the drinking behavior, and take care of oneself. With regard to the CSOs, 89% of CRAFT participants and 95% of those attending Al-Anon completed their assigned sessions; in contrast, only 53% of those using the Johnson Intervention completed their sessions, mostly due to being intimidated by the coercive nature of the family confrontation. A trial using CRAFT and CRAFT plus group aftercare with persons who use illegal drugs engaged 59% and 77% of IPs, compared to 17% and 29% in the Al-Anon condition.[88] The CSOs in these trials seemed to derive substantial benefit (in pre-post comparisons of levels of depression and anger as well as relationship characteristics such as happiness, cohesion, and conflict) from whatever treatment condition they were assigned, regardless of IP outcomes. It is important to realize that the IP may suffer from co-occurring mental health conditions such as depression, anxiety, posttraumatic stress, or others. It may be necessary to refer the IP to an addiction-trained prescriber or practitioner as not all mental health condition require medications so the other disorders can also be addressed.

FAMILY PSYCHOEDUCATION AND 12-STEP PROGRAM ENGAGEMENT

Psychoeducation

Providing information and addressing questions about genetic influences and familial transmission of SUDs, the impact of growing up amongst family members and/or caregivers with SUD, and the role of 12-step programs (AA, NA, etc.) and other mutual support groups in enhancing and supporting one's recovery as well as significant others (Al-Anon, Adult Children of Alcoholics, Families Anonymous, etc.). Family or couples therapy may be offered to individual families, as indicated, focusing on either recovery only or on broader issues that trouble the family. Single parents whose children are symptomatic or who have been removed by a child protective services agency may be provided parenting education, parent-child therapy, and/or reunification therapy. Families with domestic violence may undergo communication and problem-solving training and/or anger management training. Some modalities offer variants of empirically tested cognitive behavioral treatments designed specifically to promote abstinence while improving family function (see detailed discussion of ABCT and BCT protocols below). While most alcohol and drug treatment programs offer family-oriented components, there can be wide variation in attendance policies and degree of family involvement.

Bibliotherapy

Providing self-guided reading materials related to families and addiction is often beneficial, regardless of whether more formal treatments are in progress.[89,90] Materials from Al-Anon are quite useful, as are a number of self-help books and addiction memoirs that discuss family involvement. For individuals or families who are willing, referral to individual or family counseling or psychoeducational sessions can be extraordinarily helpful. In making such a referral, the physician needs to communicate with the therapist regarding the family illness and the consequences that led to the referral; otherwise, individuals, and even whole families, can participate in counseling for long periods of time without ever disclosing the presence of the underlying SUD. It is as necessary to assess the therapist's knowledge, experience, and skill in working with families who suffer from SUDs as it is to assess the family's motivation for change and ability to engage in active treatment. It is helpful also to communicate to both the therapist and the family your commitment to working as a member of the team and to assure them that all medical issues will be addressed properly and promptly during the treatment process. It is important to recognize that partners and close family members also may suffer from other mental health conditions such as mood disorders, PTSD, SUD, which are treatable. Their ability to engage with SUD-focused recovery with their loved one may be hindered by these conditions unless they too are adequately treated. Fortunately, most of the evidence-based treatments described here are suitable for treating dyads in which both members have SUD.

Mutual Support Groups

Mutual support and 12-step programs have demonstrated promising efficacy for many participants of varying backgrounds.[91,92] Options including Women for Sobriety, Al-Anon Family, Nar-Anon Family, Alateen, Alatot, and Families Anonymous are available in every part of the country. Contact information generally can be found in the telephone book, on the internet, or from local addiction treatment professionals. Most such groups are organized around the principles and steps of Alcoholics Anonymous (AA), but focus on the recovery tasks (ie, engaging social support systems, individual supportive counseling, learning and improving skills such as communication and boundary setting) of the family member who is experiencing pain from another's SUD. A recent survey conducted among Al-Anon members ($N = 13{,}395$) found that most Al-Anon participants identify as women and began attending as a result of a professional (ie, treatment provider) referral. Longevity of engagement for some participants, particularly those with more severe or chronically relapsing AUD, can exceeds 14 years. At the same time, nearly one-third (29%) of participants endorsed having a mental health condition diagnosis such as depression, anxiety, or PTSD and the majority of participants with a diagnosis (78%) had engaged in mental health treatment themselves. Many participants also reported that their parents had lived with an SUD (58%) and that they had experienced physical, sexual, emotional, or verbal abuse in their lifetime (56%). Participants in this survey were highly enthusiastic about the benefits of Al-Anon, with the vast majority attributing improvements in their emotional health (93%), mental health (88%), and home and/or occupational life (83%), to the program.

COUPLE AND FAMILY MODALITIES FOR ADULTS

Alcohol Behavioral Couple Therapy

Alcohol behavioral couple therapy (ABCT)[93] is a 12-week, manualized, cognitive-behavioral treatment developed for romantic couples that has demonstrated efficacy in reducing alcohol consumption, enhancing relationship functioning, and improving partners' skills to facilitate reductions in drinking.[94,95] Core activities involve a harm-reduction approach (ie, abstinence is encouraged but not required) and include normative feedback, communication skills, managing urges, and other activities. Target engagement of family-focused mechanisms of drinking reductions has also been supported in the research testing ABCT. For example, reductions in drinking among men in one ABCT trial was associated with increases in partner coping, conflict resolution, and support behaviors. Men's abstinence and drinking severity six months after ABCT treatment was predicted by greater pretreatment relationship quality,[96] and higher relationship satisfaction is associated with better ABCT completion.[97] Among women, higher relationship satisfaction is associated with fewer drinking urges overall and greater reduction in drinking urges during ABCT.[98]

Brief Family-Involved Treatment

In a recent NIH-sponsored pilot study, three core components of ABCT were distilled to create a brief adaptation of ABCT (Brief Family Involved Treatment; B-FIT[99]). B-FIT includes (1) increasing family support for drinking change, (2) increasing positive and decreasing negative family exchanges, and (3) improving communication. While this pilot study supported preliminary feasibility, acceptability, and efficacy in drinking outcomes, large-scale trials are warranted to identify possible modifications and to test its efficacy in real-world treatment settings. Whether specific to the B-FIT model or other modalities, there is a large and growing need for brief dyadic and family treatments to be tested for efficacy as both adjunct and standalone treatment protocols.

Behavioral Couples Therapy

Behavioral couples therapy (BCT)[100] is a 12 to 20 session treatment with a strong evidence base derived from numerous rigorous trials.[100-102] BCT is designed for romantic partners with SUD. Although originally designed for couples in which only one partner has SUD, its efficacy has been supported in settings where both partners have a SUD. It has also shown encouraging effects to safely reduce intimate partner violence as well.[103] It is distinct from ABCT in that it emphasizes abstinence rather than harm reduction. Toward that end, BCT utilizes a *recovery contract* to clearly set out the goals of treatment and the conditions that would indicate a return to use or of symptoms. Partners learn to go over the recovery contract together daily, with a *trust discussion* in which the partner with SUD verbalizes his/her intent to remain sober and receives verbal reinforcement for doing so. Urges and triggers to use are discussed openly but arguing about past or future recurrences of use is avoided or deferred to therapy sessions. Medications to assist in maintaining sobriety are taken in the presence of the partner, regular urine drug screens are performed to provide evidence of adherence, and progress is recorded on a calendar. Return to use may be identified by either partner and must be interrupted as soon as possible, in a manner specified in the recovery contract.

Once continuing abstinence is maintained, the focus for the therapy shifts to improving the dyadic relationship. Increasing positive emotion and behavior in the relationship are achieved through three strategies: (1) acknowledging positive behaviors and reinforcing progress ("catch your partner doing something nice"); (2) planning shared experiences that are mutually rewarding (reintroduction of leisure time activities that had been neglected or supplanted by the addiction behaviors and fighting); (3) completing *Caring Day* assignments (encouragement of partners to initiate special acts of caring for one another). Communication is improved by developing good listening skills; directly expressing feelings; planning daily times to communicate about feelings, events, and problems without employing aggression or passivity; and using assertive negotiation skills in satisfying desires and needs.

Efficacy of BCT has been supported for alcohol use disorder and for drug use disorder by two early meta-analyses.[80,104] There was a moderate effect size, and a robust advantage was indicated over individual-oriented treatments in the following areas: frequency and duration of abstinence, happiness in relationships, decreased number of separations, reduction of domestic violence, benefits to the children of the couple, improved adherence to recovery medications, and a 5:1 benefit to cost ratio. Despite ample efficacy evidence for various family SUD treatments,[105] there is much room to improve uptake and implementation of evidence-based modalities.[106] One study found that less than 25% of clinicians ($N = 325$) had used ABCT in the 14 months following formal training in the modality.[107] Qualitative research has revealed several obstacles such as time burden and needing to schedule both parties to present in-person to clinic simultaneously.[108,109] Indeed, poor uptake of these modalities persists, which in turn prevents patient access. This line of research, including barriers and facilitators to uptake urgently warrants extension to couples and families with more complex SUDs (eg, prescription opioid use disorder, multiple SUDs), families with diverse identities related to race, ethnicity, nationality and English proficiency, socioeconomic resources, gender identity, and sexual orientation.

FAMILY APPROACHES WITH ADOLESCENTS

Families with adolescents who require SUD treatment present special considerations given the complex interplay of adolescent development, substance use, and family dynamics. Regardless of specific modality, recent research evidences support for several shared components that have been associated with effective change behavior.[110]

Behavioral Exchange Systems Training

Toumbourou and colleagues[111] conducted an evaluation of the behavioral exchange systems training (BEST) program, which is an 8-week parent group that supports and assists parents in coping with their adolescent's substance use. Parents participating in the BEST program showed reductions in mental health symptoms and increases in satisfaction and assertive parenting behaviors. McGillicuddy and colleagues[112] developed a coping skills training program for parents of substance-using adolescents that was associated with improved parental coping, family communication, and parental reports of their own functioning.

Brief Strategic Family Therapy

Brief strategic family therapy (BSFT)[113] was been developed to address not only drug use behavior but also the host of other behavioral problems that cluster with drug use such as oppositional defiance, underachievement and lack of interest in school, aggression and delinquency, risky sexual behaviors, and disinterest in pro-social behaviors.[114] In this approach, a phone call from a concerned parent immediately leads to the scheduling of an initial family visit. In a randomized controlled trial among Hispanic youth, BSFT engaged 93% of families compared to 42% using the usual approach.[115] Further, 77% of the BSFT assigned families remained engaged in treatment for at least eight sessions compared to only 25% of the control families. It is well known that adolescents exposed to unstructured group therapy approaches often actually get worse, as they tend to imitate one another's pathological attitudes and behaviors; in contrast, this family therapy approach helps immensely in improving outcomes: cannabis use was reduced by 75%, association with antisocial peers dropped by 58%, and acting out improved by 42%, all substantially better than the control group therapy condition.[116] However, BSFT has also received critiques related to fidelity obstacles that may be used to inform more effective translation to health care settings.[117]

Multidimensional Family Therapy

Multidimensional family therapy (MFT)[87] is a manualized, evidenced based intervention that addresses expectations related to substance use, the role of parental addiction, and prevention of family recurrence of use. MFT has demonstrated significant but moderate efficacy in several randomized controlled trials as well as a recent meta-analysis.[118-120] This model uses both individual and family sessions to address the myriad of issues within the addiction-affected family. In a three-condition randomized controlled trial, MDFT outperformed adolescent group therapy and family psychoeducation in reducing alcohol and cannabis use (54% versus 18% and 24%).[121] Another study, comparing MDFT with adolescent group therapy, showed that MDFT was superior in reducing externalizing symptoms and peer delinquency, and in improving family cohesion and school behavior.[122] These teens showed a 71% decrease in drinking alcohol, compared to an 18% *increase* in those attending group therapy. One study using MDFT with higher-severity substance using adolescents found better outcomes among those with the most severe drug use and those with co-occurring psychiatric disorders.[123]

Multisystemic Therapy

Multisystemic therapy[124] is a modality developed for juvenile offenders that has been shown to be effective in reducing substance use. This approach analyzes the symptomatic behavior in its environmental context, maintains an optimistic attitude, and empowers parents and caregivers to influence youth to take progressively more responsibility for their behavior. Treatment may occur at home, in schools, and elsewhere in the youth's environment. Its efficacy is supported by numerous clinical trials, including trials with juvenile offenders who use substances.[125-128] One primary goal of MST is to prevent out-of-home placement. Some studies demonstrate outcomes including 100% retention for 2 months and 98% for the full 4 months of the program. The cost of treatment was offset by the saved costs of out-of-home placement and hospitalizations. Clinical benefits were evident at 4- and 14-year follow-ups. In the drug court study, enhancement with MST reduced positive urine drug screens from 70% to 28%. However, a recent review and meta-analysis also indicates that findings are more robust in the United States as compared to other high-income countries. Findings also indicate that outcomes specific to youth substance use are less strong than treatment effects on other outcomes such as delinquency and parent and family functioning.[129]

POPULATION-SPECIFIC CONSIDERATIONS

Considerations for Older Adults

Given recent age-related demographic changes in the United States shifting towards longer life spans, there is an expected increase in the number of older adults experiencing SUD.[96] Family therapy approaches for adult children and their parents engaging in unhealthy substance use will become increasingly important. The current U.S. life expectancy has steadily increased over recent decades and currently rests at approximately 78.9 years.[130] Binge drinking, heavy alcohol use, and other recreational and nonmedical prescription drug use are prevalent among older Americans. For example, binge drinking among persons aged 65 or older in 2020 was 9.8% while illegal drug use was 7.9%.[131]

SUDs in older people are underrecognized due to multiple factors including failure to identify symptoms, attribution of symptoms to the aging process or disease, ageism, lack of knowledge about screening, and clinician discomfort with the topic of SUD.[132,133] In addition, older individuals are more likely to use prescription drugs from multiple sources and may combine them with tobacco and alcohol. For example, one recent study indicated that in a sample of adults seeking treatment for alcohol use disorder ($N = 258$), 30% also used benzodiazepines nonmedically, which is a potentially lethal combination.[134] Nonmedical benzodiazepine and opioid use is associated with increased risk of suicide among older adults,[135] and cannabis use is also increasing among older adults.[136] Although the prescribed doses of individual medications may not be excessive, interactions among them may cause episodes of intoxication, memory loss, accidents and falls, impaired driving, and mood instability. Indeed, co-use of alcohol and benzodiazepines are implicated in opioid-related overdose deaths in the United States.

Screening and Assessment

Tools that were developed for younger populations are occasionally insufficient or inappropriate for older adults,[137] and some of the DSM-5 criteria for alcohol use disorder may not apply well to older people.[138] Age-appropriate tools, such as the AUDIT and the Michigan Alcoholism Screening Test—Geriatric version, improve accuracy in detection among older adults.[139] Family involvement can play a crucial role in helping the clinician to identify patterns of substance use, substance-related negative health sequelae, and SUD, as family members frequently have additional information to contribute about the older person's life, such as whether there have been any changes in behavior or circumstances, including alterations in mood, new or worsening illness, or recent loss.

Family Treatment Modalities

Recent reviews of family approaches to the treatment of alcohol-related problems among older adults show that this is an understudied area,[140] especially in terms of access to family therapy and outcomes research, but a few treatment approaches have been evaluated with the older population. The Consensus Panel of the Treatment Improvement Protocols (TIPs) developed by the Substance Abuse and Mental Health Services Administration (SAMHSA) within the U.S. Department of Health and Human Services recommends that with this population, the least intensive treatment options should be explored first. Brief intervention is the recommended first step, supplemented or followed by intervention and motivational counseling.[141]

Brief Intervention

A brief intervention such as personalized normative feedback by a health care provider may be sufficient,[142] either by reducing the dose of harmful drugs or discontinuing them altogether. The health care provider may gradually modify the prescription regimen, consolidating multiple medications with similar functions into one, and when possible, substituting safer, nonaddictive alternative medications. Providers will find partnering with family very helpful, both in assessing the extent of functional impairment, as well as in monitoring adherence and improvements in function as changes are made. If this brief intervention is not sufficient, family involvement may help move a patient toward more intensive (though costly) specialized treatment. If additional intervention seems necessary to facilitate entry into an inpatient or outpatient treatment program, family and significant other cooperation will be vital.

Despite advances in family interventions, there is a lack of empirical validation of family therapies oriented specifically toward older adults. The TIP Consensus Panel's recommendations on treatment of the older person with an alcohol use disorder include the following:

1. Age-specific group treatment that is supportive and nonconfrontational and aims to build or rebuild the patient's self-esteem, as well as train significant others to use a more supportive and effective communication style instead of maladaptive communication approaches.
2. A focus on coping with depression, loneliness, and loss (eg, death of spouse and friends, retirement) by generating ways to reintegrate the person into the family and community.

3. A focus on rebuilding the client's social support network, including the family.
4. Pace and content of treatment appropriate for the older person.
5. Staff members who are interested and experienced in working with older adults.
6. Linkage with medical services, services for the aging, and other appropriate institutions in order to facilitate referral into and out of treatment, as well as support case management.

Considerations for Military Members and Veterans

Those who have served in the U.S. Armed Forces incur particularly high risk of SUD, and AUD in particular. For example, the lifetime prevalence of AUD among veterans is double that of the general population.[143-145] Alcohol problems commonly emerge during active duty service and persist following separation.[146-148] Veterans also incur more severe and persistent AUD with more lengthy and complex treatment courses. For example, compared to veterans without AUD, veterans with AUD have 2 to 4 times greater odds of having a mood and anxiety disorder, 10 times greater likelihood of having a co-occurring drug use disorder, and 4 times greater odds of making a suicide attempt during their lifetime.[145] Much as in the civilian population, SUDs cause significant distress and impairment in military members and veterans.

Support for Family Treatment at VA

Although service members and veterans face unique, but addressable, obstacles to accessing evidence-based family SUD treatment, the VA enthusiastically supports family involvement in veteran health care. The VA MISSION Act of 2018 provided unprecedented treatment access to family members and caregivers. The VA Office of Mental Health Services also provides clinicians with formal training in evidence-based family treatment modalities. VA's commitment to family engagement is also exemplified through the national rollout of Integrative Behavioral Couple Therapy (IBCT) and Coaching into Care, which provides education and support to family members who aim to help veterans gain access to mental health care. However, neither of these programs was designed or tested to reduce nonmedical substance use or to treat SUD.

Impact of Co-Occurring Mental Health Diagnoses Among Veterans

SUDs are often associated with co-occurring psychiatric disorders and can both cause, and result from, co-occurring disorders. Trauma exposure before and during service may result in debilitating psychiatric symptoms and the development of PTSD; however, PTSD may be triggered by situations of helplessness that may be otherwise unrelated to combat. Family members, particularly the partners of returning soldiers, may find that the changes in their loved one difficult to understand and manage, as PTSD is characterized by avoidance of sharing emotions and of discussing the traumatic events. Spousal bewilderment over what to do in such situations may be a focus of early family treatment. While there are effective treatments for PTSD, a common response of many returning veterans is to isolate and rely on intoxicants to suppress anxiety. Therefore, addiction treatment often must be combined with PTSD treatment, and partner involvement is critical. Multiple family therapy groups can also be very helpful in addressing some of these challenges.[149,150] While PTSD often leads to avoidance of discussing painful memories, especially with partners who might be frightened by the content of such memories, these groups allow men and women to find peers who understand and support them by virtue of their common experiences.

Impact of Military Occupational Stressors and Sexual Trauma

Sexual harassment and assaults frequently occur in military settings and are directed toward individuals of any gender identity. Alcohol use is strongly implicated in sexual assault perpetration and increases risk for victimization.[151] Substance use is also a well-established sequelae of sexual assault victimization among service members and veterans as well as civilians.[144,152] Stressors associated with occupational demands such as deployment also presents challenges related to childcare, less time spent together as a couple or family, and more serious challenges such as intimate partner violence, which is highly prevalent among active duty service members and veterans than civilians, also increases risk for substance use.[153]

Military families often have different social constructs and stressors compared to average civilian families, even after active duty has ended. On the return home, possibly having experienced traumatic brain injury, other physical injury, chronic pain, addiction, disability, or PTSD and also facing relationship problems, difficulty finding a civilian job, and the reality of having missed parts of one's children's early years, the soldier's adjustment back to civilian life can be quite challenging. Traumatic brain injuries, in particular, are associated with increased risk of intimate partner violence,[154] and mild traumatic brain injury in military populations has been prospectively associated with increased incidence of SUDs.[155] A study of family reintegration following deployment offers data demonstrating the correlations among deployment, family reintegration difficulties, and alcohol use. Nearly 20% of returning service people experienced moderate to severe family reintegration difficulties, and the majority of individuals experienced trouble in at least one part of their lives. Both predeployment as well as postdeployment alcohol use were positively correlated with poor family reintegration. Postdeployment alcohol use predicted reintegration difficulties much more strongly than depressive and PTSD symptoms.[156] Fischer and colleagues examined the preferences regarding family-based treatment for veterans suffering from PTSD. Veterans, as well as families of veterans, emphasized the importance of family involvement when dealing with reintegration difficulties.[157]

Family-based treatment also offers an opportunity to identify substance use and SUDs in other family members. Partners of service members are subject to a constellation of psychosocial stressors as they progress through their lives. In a cross-sectional study of 242 veteran couples, use of substances by the intimate partner explained 20% (alcohol) and 13% (drugs) of the variance in the association with veteran SUD, compared to only 2% each for PTSD, antisocial personality disorder, and depression.[158] This underscores the importance of assessing and treating the couple or family together, as the veteran who is treated individually and then returns home to a partner engaged in unhealthy substance use may be subject to cue-triggered craving, easy access to substances in the home, and urges to join in, especially if the substance use previously constituted a shared activity leading to mutual satisfaction and intimacy.

Several family-oriented treatment approaches are pertinent to this population. One recent pilot trial examined the preliminary efficacy of a brief (4-session) web-based intervention for military partners who were concerned about their veteran's drinking (N = 12). Outcomes were promising and supported feasibility and acceptability.[76] BCT is identified as an effective treatment for SUDs among veterans that encourages teamwork and behavioral modification to help reduce substance use. Both couples and family therapy address concerns that are related to continued substance use. For example, family behaviors may promote substance use, especially if other family members have disorders. Instances like these make it very difficult for the patient to sustain sobriety. With engagement, family members can become integral parts in the treatment process. Efficacy has also been demonstrated in conjoint relapse prevention therapy as demonstrated by Maisto and colleagues. They present data from veteran populations that support the use of dyadic treatment with subsequent relapse prevention interventions. Patients engaged in relapse prevention interventions showed the same substance use recurrence rates; however, duration of return to use was significantly shorter.[159] Similarly, pilot examinations of an integrated, dyadic treatment to address PTSD and substance use disorders simultaneously have shown promise.[160]

Considerations for Pregnant Women

Perinatal drug and alcohol use is a problem that affects all socioeconomic levels and significantly contributes to increased medical and psychiatric complications for both mother and child. About 15% of pregnancies are complicated by substance use, with up to 20% of pregnant patients reporting past month alcohol use.[161] Although the most commonly used substance is tobacco, ingestion of alcohol, cannabis, opioids, sedatives, and stimulants is not uncommon. Alcohol has been implicated in the teratological Fetal Alcohol Effects spectrum, characterized by serious health problems and mental handicaps. However, there are still many misconceptions, held both by professional and lay people, about alcohol use among pregnant women, and there is a need to involve families in efforts to detect and treat addiction in pregnant and postpartum women.

Women planning to become pregnant may try to abstain from substances or may attempt to quit using as soon as they discover they are pregnant; therefore, pregnancy may present an ideal opportunity for treatment, enhanced by a patient's added motivation to change due to concern for their unborn child.[162] The most commonly used substance, tobacco, can be addressed easily as a part of routine prenatal care. Abstinence from smoking during pregnancy is beneficial to the developing fetus and reduces the risk of recurrence of use later. The presence of tobacco use during pregnancy also may be an indicator of other substance use. Approaching the tobacco issue first may be a relatively nonthreatening first step in establishing a therapeutic alliance. If the pregnancy is welcomed, a desire to protect the baby may support adherence to recommendations of abstinence and ongoing addiction care, as needed. It is possible that prepregnancy patterns of substance use may unintentionally be continued well into the first trimester period of greatest teratogenic risk or longer.

When substance use reductions and abstinence is established early in pregnancy, the mother and family may be less concerned than if it is not; nevertheless, recovery efforts should be strongly encouraged and supported *throughout* the pregnancy and during postpartum. Family involvement in evidence-based treatments described above as well as other options including Al-Anon and family-oriented psychoeducation can increase the likelihood of positive health outcomes for mother and child, especially if there are brief or more enduring returns to substance use. For those with poor natural support systems, more intensive or longer-term treatments may be indicated to provide adequate support and scaffolding during the transition to parenthood or following the birth of another child.

For women who have developed a SUD with opioid drugs, the standard of care has become opioid maintenance, especially after the 5th month during which meconium production begins. Effective, nonjudgmental screening and openly discussing pain management is a critical concern during pregnancy and postpartum.[163] Initiation of methadone or buprenorphine maintenance will curb the craving to use opioids and help prevent reinforcement from incidents of substance use. Furthermore, the duration of action of these two medications is long, reducing the likelihood that the mother and fetus will experience intermittent episodes of opioid withdrawal, triggering meconium release into the amniotic fluid. Two large randomized clinical trials comparing methadone with buprenorphine during pregnancy have shown a high rate of continued participation in recovery, a low rate of return to substance use, and manageable postnatal withdrawal in the infants.[164] However, some women and their families may resist taking such medications during pregnancy for fear that it will harm the developing fetus. Relapses may lead to use of short-acting opioids that can produce several episodes of withdrawal every day. Thus, working with mothers and family supports regarding the risks and benefits of pharmacotherapy for opioid use disorder is important.

For those with an alcohol use disorder, medications used to support recovery such as acamprosate, naltrexone, or disulfiram may be helpful. Likewise, medications may be offered to help with management of co-occurring anxiety, depression, bipolar disorder, or other psychiatric disorders, but they should be selected carefully, and the risks explained thoroughly. Education of the patient and her significant others might facilitate improved treatment engagement similar to other populations, but this is an understudied area of the literature.

It is worth noting that the immediate postpartum period is a time of high risk for return to substance use, as substance use may no longer perceived as being harmful to the offspring. It is also a very stressful time, especially for inexperienced mothers learning to manage an infant's care needs. Intimate partner violence may initiate or increase during this time. A postpartum mood disorder also may develop. Involvement in 12-step recovery support groups and interventions described earlier is critical to success in managing stress and either initiating or maintaining sobriety. Although support from family or others can mitigate the stress to some extent, awareness of the risks can facilitate early recognition of relapse and prompt referral for care.

SUMMARY

Effective, evidence-supported screening, assessment, motivational enhancement, referral, intervention services, recovery monitoring, and training in prevention of future substance use are imperative. Family members and partners play a crucial role in substance use disorder etiology, course, and treatment trajectories. Current literature indicates that dyadic and family-oriented approaches enhance engagement in treatment, facilitate treatment completion to ensure an adequate dose is received, and sustained participation in aftercare. However, even well-intentioned family members also may actively or passively interfere with treatment and recovery without inclusion in the care team and without developing adaptive individual skills to participate. Various effective family therapy approaches have demonstrated enhanced success rates in treating substance use disorders and simultaneously improving domains of family functioning. Improved access to evidence-based family-oriented care for SUDs is recommended across treatment venues to optimize efficacy and reduce overall costs to the community.

It is recommended that treatment providers provide warm handoffs to help patients and their partners and/or family members engage in evidence-based therapies with qualified clinicians with training in such modalities. In addition, micro-interventions to aid the motivation to engage in evidence-based therapies include encouraging the patient to observe the effects of their SUD on family members and family functioning. The following are not yet evidence-based, but rather informal approaches to communicating with patients and family members. It may be beneficial to inquire about the forms of support that the patient would prefer from family members, and about family members' willingness and availability to consider participating in one or more aspects of their recovery program. Providing information about the vast array of family-engaged treatment and recovery-supportive options, including bibliotherapy and online options such as Faces and Voices of Recovery, and Partnership for Drug-Free Kids, might be helpful. When family members are available and willing to engage in recovery and treatment options, clinicians might begin by querying them about their views of the severity of their loved one's SUD, the impacts it has had on them and their children, their hopes and preferences for their loved one's recovery, and ways in which they can provide instrumental support.

ACKNOWLEDGEMENT

We would like to acknowledge the contributions of the authors of the most recent prior version of this chapter: Kathleen A. Gross, Maritza E. Lagos, Elmira Yessengaliyeva, Matthew M. LaCasse, and Michael R. Liepman (deceased). The primary updates focused on the addition of new scientific literature available since the last version of the chapter.

REFERENCES

1. Andersson C, Best D, Irving J, et al. *Understanding Recovery From a Family Perspective: A Survey of Life in Recovery for Families.* The Helena Kennedy Centre for International Justice; 2018.
2. Mushquash AR, Stewart SH, Sherry SB, Mackinnon P, Antony MM, Sherry DL. Heavy episodic drinking among dating partners: a longitudinal actor–partner interdependence model. *Psychol Addict Behav.* 2013;27(1):178.
3. Windle M, Windle RC. A prospective study of alcohol use among middle-aged adults and marital partner influences on drinking. *J Stud Alcohol Drugs.* 2014;75(4):546-556.
4. Bartel SJ, Sherry SB, Molnar DS, et al. Do romantic partners influence each other's heavy episodic drinking? Support for the partner influence hypothesis in a three-year longitudinal study. *Addict Behav.* 2017;69:55-58.
5. Homish GG, Leonard KE. The drinking partnership and marital satisfaction: the longitudinal influence of discrepant drinking. *J Consult Clin Psychol.* 2007;75(1):43.
6. Muyingo L, Smith MM, Sherry SB, McEachern E, Leonard KE, Stewart SH. Relationships on the rocks: a meta-analysis of romantic partner effects on alcohol use. *Psychol Addict Behav.* 2020;34(6):629.
7. Finkel EJ, Hall AN. The I3 model: a metatheoretical framework for understanding aggression. *Curr Opin Psychol.* 2018;19:125-130.
8. Parrott DJ, Eckhardt CI. Effects of alcohol on human aggression. *Curr Opin Psychol.* 2018;19:1-5.
9. Tomlinson MF, Brown M, Hoaken P. Recreational drug use and human aggressive behavior: a comprehensive review since 2003. *Aggress Violent Behav.* 2016;27:9-29.
10. Volkow ND, Han B, Einstein EB, Compton WM. Prevalence of substance use disorders by time since first substance use among young people in the U.S. *JAMA Pediatrics.* 2021;175(6):640-643.
11. MacKillop J, Ray LA. The etiology of addiction: a contemporary biopsychosocial approach. In: MacKillop J, Kenna GA, Leggio L, Ray LA, eds. *Integrating Psychological and Pharmacological Treatments for Addictive Disorders: An Evidence-Based Guide.* Routledge; 2017:32-53.

12. Tawa EA, Hall SD, Lohoff FW. Overview of the genetics of alcohol use disorder. *Alcohol Alcohol.* 2016;51(5):507-514.
13. Young-Wolff KC, Enoch M, Prescott CA. The influence of gene–environment interactions on alcohol consumption and alcohol use disorders: a comprehensive review. *Clin Psychol Rev.* 2011;31(5):800-816.
14. Johnson EC, Sanchez-Roige S, Acion L, et al. Polygenic contributions to alcohol use and alcohol use disorders across population-based and clinically ascertained samples. *Psychol Med.* 2021;51(7):1147-1156.
15. Bierut LJ. Genetic vulnerability and susceptibility to substance dependence. *Neuron.* 2011;69:618-627.
16. Kendler KS, Ohlsson H, Sundquist J, Sundquist K. The patterns of family genetic risk scores for eleven major psychiatric and substance use disorders in a Swedish national sample. *Transl Psychiatry.* 2021;11(1):1-8.
17. Pandey G, Seay MJ, Meyers JL, et al. Density and dichotomous family history measures of alcohol use disorder as predictors of behavioral and neural phenotypes: a comparative study across gender and race/ethnicity. *Alcohol Clin Exp Res.* 2020;44(3):697-710.
18. Verhulst B, Neale MC, Kendler KS. The heritability of alcohol use disorders: a meta-analysis of twin and adoption studies. *Psychol Med.* 2015;45(5):1061-1072.
19. Sánchez-Queija I, Oliva A, Parra Á, Camacho C. Longitudinal analysis of the role of family functioning in substance use. *J Child Fam Stud.* 2016;25(1):232-240.
20. Ryan SM, Jorm AF, Lubman DI. Parenting factors associated with reduced adolescent alcohol use: a systematic review of longitudinal studies. *Aus N Z J Psychiatry.* 2010;44(9):774-783.
21. Farmer RF, Kosty DB, Seeley JR, Gau JM, Klein DN. Family aggregation of substance use disorders: substance specific, nonspecific, and intrafamilial sources of risk. *J Stud Alcohol Drugs.* 2019;80(4):462-471.
22. Yoon D, Kobulsky JM, Yoon M, Park J, Yoon S, Arias LN. Racial differences in early adolescent substance use: child abuse types and family/peer substance use as predictors. *J Ethn Subst Abus.* 2022;1-18.
23. Widom CS, White HR, Czaja SJ, Marmorstein NR. Long-term effects of child abuse and neglect on alcohol use and excessive drinking in middle adulthood. *J Studies Alcohol Drugs.* 2007;68(3):317-326.
24. Kendler KS, Ohlsson H, Sundqusit K, Sundquist J. Within-family environmental transmission of drug abuse: a Swedish national study. *JAMA Psychiatry.* 2013;70:235-242.
25. Whiteman SD, Jensen AC, Maggs JL. Similarities in adolescent siblings' substance use: testing competing pathways of influence. *J Stud Alcohol Drugs.* 2013;74:104-113.
26. Fulkerson JA, Pasch KE, Perry CL, Komro K. Relationships between alcohol-related informal social control, parental monitoring and adolescent problem behaviors among racially diverse urban youth. *J Community Health.* 2008;33(6):425-433.
27. Wilsnack RW, Wilsnack SC, Gmel G, Kantor LW. Gender differences in binge drinking: prevalence, predictors, and consequences. *Alcohol Res.* 2018;39(1):57-76.
28. Brown DW, Anda RF, Tiemeier H, et al. Adverse childhood experiences and the risk of premature mortality. *Am J Prev Med.* 2009;37(5):389-396.
29. Leza L, Siria S, López-Goñi JJ, et al. Adverse childhood experiences (ACEs) and substance use disorder (SUD): a scoping review. *Drug Alcohol Depend.* 2021;221:108563.
30. McGue M, Elkins I, Iacono WG. Genetic and environmental influences on adolescent substance use and abuse. *Am J Med Genet.* 2000;96(5):671-677.
31. Legrand LN, Keyes M, McGue M, Iacono WG, Krueger RF. Rural environments reduce the genetic influence on adolescent substance use and rule-breaking behavior. *Psychol Med.* 2008;38(9):1341-1350.
32. Lee J, Kong AY, Sewell KB, et al. Associations of tobacco retailer density and proximity with adult tobacco use behaviours and health outcomes: a meta-analysis. *Tob Control.* 2021;31(e2):e189-e200.
33. White V, Azar D, Faulkner A, et al. Adolescents' alcohol use and strength of policy relating to youth access, trading hours and driving under the influence: findings from Australia. *Addiction.* 2018;113(6):1030-1042.
34. Levitt A, Cooper ML. Daily alcohol use and romantic relationship functioning: evidence of bidirectional, gender-, and context-specific effects. *Personal Soc Psychol Bull.* 2010;36(12):1706-1722.
35. Mimiaga MJ, Suarez N, Garofalo R, et al. Relationship dynamics in the context of binge drinking and polydrug use among same-sex male couples in Atlanta, Boston, and Chicago. *Arch Sex Behav.* 2019;48(4):1171-1184.
36. Veldhuis CB, Porsch LM, Bochicchio LA, et al. The Chicago health and life experiences of women couples study: protocol for a study of stress, hazardous drinking, and intimate partner aggression among sexual minority women and their partners. *JMIR Res Protoc.* 2021;10(10):e28080.
37. Rostad WL, Clayton HB, Estefan LF, Johns MM. Substance use and disparities in teen dating violence victimization by sexual identity among high school students. *Prev Sci.* 2020;21(3):398-407.
38. Wu E, El-Bassel N, McVinney LD, et al. The association between substance use and intimate partner violence within Black male same-sex relationships. *J Interpers Violence.* 2015;30(5):762-781.
39. Reed ZE, Wootton RE, Munafò MR. Using Mendelian randomization to explore the gateway hypothesis: possible causal effects of smoking initiation and alcohol consumption on substance use outcomes. *Addiction.* 2022;117(3):741-750.
40. Moos RH, Billings AG. Children of alcoholics during the recovery process: alcoholic and matched control families. *Addict Behav.* 1982;7(2):155-163.
41. Scully C, McLaughlin J, Fitzgerald A. The relationship between adverse childhood experiences, family functioning, and mental health problems among children and adolescents: a systematic review. *J Fam Ther.* 2020;42(2):291-316.
42. Balistreri KS, Alvira-Hammond M. Adverse childhood experiences, family functioning and adolescent health and emotional well-being. *Public Health.* 2016;132:72-78.
43. Alegría M, Canino G, Shrout PE, et al. Prevalence of mental illness in immigrant and non-immigrant U.S. Latino groups. *Am J Psychiatry.* 2008;165(3):359-369.
44. Alegría M, Mulvaney-Day N, Woo M, Torres M, Gao S, Oddo V. Correlates of past-year mental health service use among Latinos: results from the National Latino and Asian American Study. *Am J Public Health.* 2007;97(1):76-83.
45. Telzer EH. Expanding the acculturation gap-distress model: an integrative review of research. *Hum Dev.* 2010;53:313-340.
46. Szapocznik J, Kurtines WM. Family psychology and cultural diversity: opportunities for theory, research, and application. *Am Psychologist.* 1993;48(4):400.
47. Fang L, Schinke SP. Alcohol use among Asian American adolescent girls: the impact of immigrant generation status and family relationships. *J Ethn Subst Abus.* 2011;10(4):275-294.
48. Cruz RA, King KM, Mechammil M, Bámaca-Colbert M, Robins RW. Mexican-origin youth substance use trajectories: associations with cultural and family factors. *Dev Psychol.* 2018;54(1):111.
49. Doherty EE, Green KM, Reisinger HS, Ensminger ME. Long-term patterns of drug use among an urban African-American cohort: the role of gender and family. *J Urban Health.* 2008;85(2):250-267.
50. Brody GH, Chen Y, Kogan SM, et al. Family-centered program deters substance use, conduct problems, and depressive symptoms in black adolescents. *Pediatrics.* 2012;129(1):108-115.
51. Fang L, Barnes-Ceeney K, Schinke SP. Substance use behavior among early-adolescent Asian American girls: the impact of psychological and family factors. *Women Health.* 2011;51(7):623-642.
52. Hawkins JD, Catalano RF, Arthur MW. Promoting science-based prevention in communities. *Addict Behav.* 2002;27(6):951-976.
53. Botvin GJ, Epstein JA, Schinke SP, Diaz T. Predictors of cigarette smoking among inner-city minority youth. *J Dev Behav Pediatr.* 1994;15(2):67-73.
54. Johnson CA, Unger JB, Ritt-Olson A, et al. Smoking prevention for ethnically diverse adolescents: 2-year outcomes of a multicultural, school-based smoking prevention curriculum in Southern California. *Prev Med.* 2005;40(6):842-852.
55. Komro KA, Perry CL, Veblen-Mortenson S, et al. Cross-cultural adaptation and evaluation of a home-based program for alcohol use prevention among urban youth: the "Slick Tracy Home Team Program". *J Prim Prev.* 2006;27(2):135-154.

56. Unger A, Jung E, Winklbaur B, Fischer G. Gender issues in the pharmacotherapy of opioid-addicted women: buprenorphine. *J Addict Dis.* 2010;29(2):217-230.
57. Lochman JE, Wells KC. The Coping Power program at the middle-school transition: universal and indicated prevention effects. *Psychol Addict Behav.* 2002;16(4S):S40.
58. Molgaard VK, Spoth R. The Strengthening Families Program for young adolescents: overview and outcomes. *Resid Treat Child Youth.* 2001;18(3):15-29.
59. Schinke SP, Schwinn TM, Fang L. Longitudinal outcomes of an alcohol abuse prevention program for urban adolescents. *J Adolesc Health.* 2010;46(5):451-457.
60. Elliott DS, Mihalic S. Issues in disseminating and replicating effective prevention programs. *Prev Sci.* 2004;5(1):47-53.
61. Vega WA, Lopez SR. Priority issues in Latino mental health services research. *Ment Health Serv Res.* 2001;3(4):189-200.
62. Cabassa LJ, Zayas LH, Hansen MC. Latino adults' access to mental health care: a review of epidemiological studies. *Admin Pol Ment Health.* 2006;33(3):316-330.
63. Kane MN, Williams MR. Perceptions of South Florida Hispanic and Anglo Catholics: from whom would they seek help? *J Relig Health.* 2000;39(2):107-122.
64. Loera S, Muñoz LM, Nott E, et al. Call the curandero: improving mental health services for Mexican immigrants. *Where Reflection & Practice Meet the Changing Nature of Social Work: Towards Global Practice*; 2009.
65. Stoltenberg SF, Mudd SA, Blow FC, Hill EM. Evaluating measures of family history of alcoholism: density versus dichotomy. *Addiction.* 1998;93(10):1511-1520.
66. Schuckit MA, Smith TL. An 8-year follow-up of 450 sons of alcoholic and control subjects. *Arch Gen Psychiatry.* 1996;53(3):202-210.
67. Cservenka A. Neurobiological phenotypes associated with a family history of alcoholism. *Drug Alcohol Depend.* 2016;158:8-21.
68. Zucker RA, Ellis DA, Fitzgerald HE. Developmental evidence for at least two alcoholisms: i. biopsychosocial variation among pathways into symptomatic difficulty. *Ann N Y Acad Sci.* 1994;708(1):134-146.
69. McLellan AT, Kushner H, Metzger D, et al. The fifth edition of the Addiction Severity Index. *J Subst Abus Treat.* 1992;9(3):199-213.
70. Carr A. Couple therapy, family therapy and systemic interventions for adult-focused problems: the current evidence base. *J Fam Ther.* 2019;41(4):492-536.
71. Dutra L, Stathopoulou G, Basden SL, Leyro TM, Powers MB, Otto MW. A meta-analytic review of psychosocial interventions for substance use disorders. *Am J Psychiatry.* 2008;165:179-187.
72. Hunter-Reel D, Witkiewitz K, Zweben A. Does session attendance by a supportive significant other predict outcomes in individual treatment for alcohol use disorders? *Alcohol Clin Exp Res.* 2012;36(7):1237-1243.
73. Ossip-Klein DJ, Rychtarik RG. Behavioral contracts between alcoholics and family members: Improving aftercare participation and maintaining sobriety after inpatient alcoholism treatment. In: O'Farrell TJ, ed. *Treating Alcohol Problems: Marital and Family Interventions.* Guilford Press; 1993:281-304.
74. Azrin NH, Sisson RW, Meyers R, Godley M. Alcoholism treatment by disulfiram and community reinforcement therapy. *J Behav Ther Exp Psychiatry.* 1982;13(2):105-112.
75. Meyers RJ, Wolfe BI. *Get Your Loved One Sober. Alternatives to Nagging, Pleading, and Threatening.* Hazelden; 2004.
76. Osilla KC, Pedersen ER, Tolpadi A, Howard SS, Phillips JL, Gore KL. The feasibility of a web intervention for military and veteran spouses concerned about their partner's alcohol misuse. *J Behav Health Serv Res.* 2018;45(1):57-73.
77. Rodriguez LM, Neighbors C, Osilla KC, Trail TE. The longitudinal effects of military spouses' concern and behaviors over partner drinking on relationship functioning. *Alcohol.* 2019;76:29-36.
78. Rodriguez LM, Osilla KC, Trail TE, Gore KL, Pedersen ER. Alcohol use among concerned partners of heavy drinking service members and veterans. *J Marital Fam Ther.* 2018;44(2):277-291.
79. Goodell E, Johnson RM, Latkin CA, Homish DL, Homish GG. Risk and protective effects of social networks on alcohol use problems among Army Reserve and National Guard soldiers. *Addict Behav.* 2020;103:106244.
80. Ripley JS, Cunion A, Noble N. Alcohol abuse in marriage and family contexts: relational pathways to recovery. *Alcohol Treat Q.* 2006;24(1-2):171-184.
81. Stanton MD, Shadish WR. Outcome, attrition, and family–couples treatment for drug abuse: a meta-analysis and review of the controlled, comparative studies. *Psychol Bull.* 1997;122(2):170.
82. Miller WR, Rollnick S. *Motivational Interviewing: Preparing People for Change.* 2nd ed. Guilford Press; 2002.
83. Liepman MR, Flachier R, Tareen RS. Family behavior loop mapping: a technique to analyze the grip addictive disorders have on families and to help them recover. *Alcohol Treat Q.* 2008;26(1-2):59-80.
84. Smith JE, Meyers RJ, Austin JL. Working with family members to engage treatment-refusing drinkers: the CRAFT program. *Alcohol Treat Q.* 2008;26(1-2):169-193.
85. Kirby KC, Marlowe DB, Festinger DS, Garvey KA, La Monaca V. Community reinforcement training for family and significant others of drug abusers: a unilateral intervention to increase treatment entry of drug users. *Drug Alcohol Depend.* 1999;56(1):85-96.
86. Miller WR, Meyers RJ, Tonigan JS. Engaging the unmotivated in treatment for alcohol problems: a comparison of three strategies for intervention through family members. *J Consult Clin Psychol.* 1999;67(5):688.
87. Bischof G, Iwen J, Freyer-Adam J, Rumpf HJ. Efficacy of the community reinforcement and family training for concerned significant others of treatment-refusing individuals with alcohol dependence: a randomized controlled trial. *Drug Alcohol Depend.* 2016;163:179-185.
88. Meyers RJ, Miller WR, Smith JE, Tonigan JS. A randomized trial of two methods for engaging treatment-refusing drug users through concerned significant others. *J Consult Clin Psychol.* 2002;70(5):1182.
89. Humphreys K, Wing S, McCarty D, et al. Self-help organizations for alcohol and drug problems: toward evidence-based practice and policy. *J Subst Abus Treat.* 2004;26(3):151-158.
90. Johansson M, Sinadinovic K, Hammarberg A, et al. Web-based self-help for problematic alcohol use: a large naturalistic study. *Int J Behav Med.* 2017;24(5):749-759.
91. Kelly JF, Abry A, Ferri M, Humphreys K. Alcoholics anonymous and 12-step facilitation treatments for alcohol use disorder: a distillation of a 2020 Cochrane review for clinicians and policy makers. *Alcohol Alcohol.* 2020;55(6):641-651.
92. Zemore SE, Lui C, Mericle A, Hemberg J, Kaskutas LA. A longitudinal study of the comparative efficacy of Women for Sobriety, LifeRing, SMART Recovery, and 12-step groups for those with AUD. *J Subst Abus Treat.* 2018;88:18-26.
93. McCrady BS, Epstein EE. *Overcoming Alcohol Problems: A Couples-Focused Program.* Oxford University Press; 2008.
94. McCrady BS, Epstein EE, Cook S, Jensen N, Hildebrandt T. A randomized trial of individual and couple behavioral alcohol treatment for women. *J Consult Clin Psychol.* 2009;77:243-256.
95. McCrady BS, Epstein EE, Hallgren KA, Cook S, Jensen NK. Women with alcohol dependence: a randomized trial of couple versus individual plus couple therapy. *Psychol Addict Behav.* 2016;30(3):287.
96. McCrady BS, Hayaki J, Epstein EE, Hirsch LS. Testing hypothesized predictors of change in conjoint behavioral alcoholism treatment for men. *Alcohol Clin Exp Res.* 2002;26(4):463-470.
97. Graff FS, Morgan TJ, Epstein EE, et al. Engagement and retention in outpatient alcoholism treatment for women. *Am J Addict.* 2009;18(4):277-288.
98. Owens MD, Hallgren KA, Ladd BO, Rynes K, McCrady BS, Epstein E. Associations between relationship satisfaction and drinking urges for women in alcohol behavioral couples and individual therapy. *Alcohol Treat Q.* 2013;31(4):415-430.
99. McCrady BS, Tonigan JS, Fink BC, et al. A randomized pilot trial of brief family-involved treatment for alcohol use disorder: treatment outcomes. *Psychol Addict Behav.* 2023. doi:10.1037/adb0000912.

100. O'Farrell TJ, Schein AZ. Behavioral couples therapy for alcoholism and drug abuse. *J Fam Psychother*. 2011;22(3):193-215.
101. Schumm JA, O'Farrell TJ, Kahler CW, Murphy MM, Muchowski P. A randomized clinical trial of behavioral couples therapy versus individually based treatment for women with alcohol dependence. *J Consult Clin Psychol*. 2014;82(6):993-1004.
102. Schumm JA, O'Farrell TJ, Andreas JB. Behavioral couples therapy when both partners have a current alcohol use disorder. *Alcohol Treat Q*. 2012;30(4):407-421.
103. O'Farrell TJ, Fals-Stewart W, Murphy M, Murphy CM. Partner violence before and after individually based alcoholism treatment for male alcoholic patients. *J Consult Clin Psychol*. 2003;71(1):92.
104. Edwards ME, Steinglass P. Family therapy treatment outcomes for alcoholism. *J Marital Family Ther*. 1995;21(4):475-509.
105. McCrady BS, Flanagan JC. The role of the family in alcohol use disorder recovery for adults. *Alcohol Res*. 2021;41(1):06.
106. Schonbrun YC, Stuart GL, Wetle T, Glynn TR, Titelius EN, Strong D. Mental health experts' perspectives on barriers to dissemination of couples treatment for alcohol use disorders. *Psychol Serv*. 2012;9(1):64.
107. Houck JM, Forcehimes AA, Davis M, Bogenschutz MP. Qualitative and quantitative feedback following workshop training in evidence-based practices: a dissemination study. *Prof Psychol Res Pr*. 2016;47(6):413-417.
108. McCrady BS, Epstein EE, Cook S, Jensen NK, Ladd BO. What do women want? Alcohol treatment choices, treatment entry and retention. *Psychol Addict Behav*. 2011;25(3):521-529.
109. McCrady BS, Wilson A, Fink B, Borders A, Muñoz R, Fokas K. A consumer's eye view of family-involved alcohol treatment. *Alcohol Treat Q*. 2019;37(1):43-59.
110. Hogue A, Bobek M, Dauber S, Henderson CE, Mclead BD, Southam-Gerow MA. Core elements of family therapy for adolescent behavior problems: empirical distillation of three manualized treatments. *J Clin Child Adolesc Psychol*. 2019;48(1):29-41.
111. Toumbourou JW, Blyth A, Bamberg J, Forer D. Early impact of the BEST intervention for parents stressed by adolescent substance abuse. *J Community Appl Soc Psychol*. 2001;11(4):291-304.
112. McGillicuddy NB, Rychtarik RG, Duquette JA, Morsheimer ET. Development of a skill training program for parents of substance-abusing adolescents. *J Subst Abus Treat*. 2001;20(1):59-68.
113. Szapocznik J, Schwartz SJ, Muir JA, Brown CH. Brief strategic family therapy: an intervention to reduce adolescent risk behavior. *Couple Family Psychol*. 2012;1(2):134.
114. Briones E, Robbins MS, Szapocznik J. Brief strategic family therapy: engagement and treatment. *Alcohol Treat Q*. 2008;26(1-2):81-103.
115. Santisteban DA, Coatsworth JD, Perez-Vidal A, et al. Efficacy of brief strategic family therapy in modifying Hispanic adolescent behavior problems and substance use. *J Fam Psychol*. 2003;17(1):121.
116. Szapocznik J, Williams RA. Brief strategic family therapy: twenty-five years of interplay among theory, research and practice in adolescent behavior problems and drug abuse. *Clin Child Fam Psychol Rev*. 2000;3(2):117-134.
117. Lebensohn-Chialvo F, Rohrbaugh MJ, Hasler BP. Fidelity failures in brief strategic family therapy for adolescent drug abuse: a clinical analysis. *Fam Process*. 2019;58(2):305-317.
118. van der Pol TM, Hoeve M, Noom MJ, et al. Research review: the effectiveness of multidimensional family therapy in treating adolescents with multiple behavior problems—a meta-analysis. *J Child Psychol Psychiatry*. 2017;58(5):532-545.
119. Liddle HA, Dakof GA, Turner RM, Henderson CE, Greenbaum PE. Treating adolescent drug abuse: a randomized trial comparing multidimensional family therapy and cognitive behavior therapy. *Addiction*. 2008;103(10):1660-1670.
120. Filges T, Andersen D, Jørgensen AK. Effects of multidimensional family therapy (MDFT) on nonopioid drug abuse: a systematic review and meta-analysis. *Res Soc Work Pract*. 2018;28(1):68-83.
121. Liddle HA, Dakof GA, Parker K, Diamond GS, Barrett K, Tejeda M. Multidimensional family therapy for adolescent drug abuse: results of a randomized clinical trial. *Am J Drug Alcohol Abuse*. 2001;27(4):651-688.
122. Liddle HA, Rowe CL, Dakof GA, Ungaro RA, Henderson CE. Early intervention for adolescent substance abuse: pretreatment to posttreatment outcomes of a randomized clinical trial comparing multidimensional family therapy and peer group treatment. *J Psychoactive Drugs*. 2004;36(1):49-63.
123. Henderson CE, Dakof GA, Greenbaum PE, Liddle HA. Effectiveness of multidimensional family therapy with higher severity substance-abusing adolescents: report from two randomized controlled trials. *J Consult Clin Psychol*. 2010;78(6):885.
124. Henggeler SW. Multisystemic therapy: an overview of clinical procedures, outcomes, and policy implications. *Child Psychol Psychiatry Rev*. 1999;4(1):2-10.
125. Henggeler SW, Halliday-Boykins CA, Cunningham PB, Randall J, Shapiro SB, Chapman JE. Juvenile drug court: enhancing outcomes by integrating evidence-based treatments. *J Consult Clin Psychol*. 2006;74(1):42.
126. Baglivio MT, Jackowski K, Greenwald MA, Wolff KT. Comparison of multisystemic therapy and functional family therapy effectiveness: a multiyear statewide propensity score matching analysis of juvenile offenders. *Crim Justice Behav*. 2014;41(9):1033-1056.
127. Fonagy P, Butler S, Cottrell D, et al. Multisystemic therapy compared with management as usual for adolescents at risk of offending: the START II RCT. *Health Services Delivery Res*. 2020;8(23):1-114.
128. Markham A. A review following systematic principles of multisystemic therapy for antisocial behavior in adolescents aged 10-17 years. *Adolesc Res Rev*. 2018;3(1):67-93.
129. Littell JH, Pigott TD, Nilsen KH, et al. Multisystemic Therapy® for social, emotional, and behavioural problems in youth age 10 to 17: an updated systematic review and meta-analysis. *Campbell Syst Rev*. 2021;17(4):e1158.
130. Woolf SH, Schoomaker H. Life expectancy and mortality rates in the United States, 1959-2017. *JAMA*. 2019;322(20):1996-2016.
131. Substance Abuse and Mental Health Services Administration. *Results From the 2020 National Survey on Drug Use and Health: Summary of National Findings*. HHS Publication No (SMA) 13-4795; 2021.
132. Barry KL, Blow FC, Oslin DW. Substance abuse in older adults: review and recommendations for education and practice in medical settings. *Subst Abus*. 2002;23(S1):105-131.
133. Lehmann SW, Fingerhood M. Substance-use disorders in later life. *N Engl J Med*. 2018;379(24):2351-2360.
134. McHugh RK, Votaw VR, Taghian NR, Griffin ML, Weiss RD. Benzodiazepine misuse in adults with alcohol use disorder: prevalence, motives and patterns of use. *J Subst Abus Treat*. 2020;117:108061.
135. Schepis TS, Simoni-Wastila L, McCabe SE. Prescription opioid and benzodiazepine misuse is associated with suicidal ideation in older adults. *Int J Geriat Psychiatry*. 2019;34(1):122-129.
136. Han BH, Sherman S, Mauro PM, Martins SS, Rotenberg J, Palamr JJ. Demographic trends among older cannabis users in the United States, 2006-13. *Addiction*. 2017;112(3):516-525.
137. Sarkar S, Sood E, Bhad R, et al. Validated scales for substance use disorders in the geriatric population: a scoping review. *J Geriatr Mental Health*. 2021;8(2):70.
138. Kuerbis A. Substance use among older adults: an update on prevalence, etiology, assessment, and intervention. *Gerontology*. 2020;66(3):249-258.
139. Blow FC, Brower KJ, Schulenberg JE, Demo-Dananberg LM, Young JP, Beresford TP. The Michigan alcoholism screening test-geriatric version (MAST-G): a new elderly-specific screening instrument. *Alcohol Clin Exp Res*. 1992;16(2):372.
140. Stelle C, Scott J. Alcohol abuse by older family members: a family systems analysis of assessment and intervention. *Alcohol Treat Q*. 2007;25:43-63.
141. Blow FC, Barry KL. Substance misuse and abuse in older adults: what do we need to know to help? *Generations*. 2014;38(3):53-67.
142. Curry SJ, Krist AH, Owens DK, et al. Screening and behavioral counseling interventions to reduce unhealthy alcohol use in adolescents and adults: U.S. Preventive Services Task Force recommendation statement. *JAMA*. 2018;320(18):1899-1909.
143. Calhoun PS, Elter JR, Jones ER, Kudler H, Straits-Tröster K. Hazardous alcohol use and receipt of risk-reduction counseling among U.S. veterans of the wars in Iraq and Afghanistan. *J Clin Psychiatry*. 2008;69(11):1686-1693.

144. Straus E, Norman SB, Pietrzak RH. Determinants of new-onset alcohol use disorder in U.S. military veterans: results from the National Health and Resilience in Veterans Study. *Addict Behav*. 2020;105:106313.
145. Fuehrlein BS, Mota N, Arias AJ, et al. The burden of alcohol use disorders in U.S. military veterans: results from the National Health and Resilience in Veterans Study. *Addiction*. 2016;111(10):1786-1794.
146. Jacobson IG, Ryan M, Hooper TI, et al. Alcohol use and alcohol-related problems before and after military combat deployment. *JAMA*. 2008;300(6):663-675.
147. Milliken CS, Auchterlonie JL, Hoge CW. Longitudinal assessment of mental health problems among active and reserve component soldiers returning from the Iraq war. *JAMA*. 2007;298(18):2141-2148.
148. Bray RM, Brown JM, Williams J. Trends in binge and heavy drinking, alcohol-related problems, and combat exposure in the U.S. military. *Subst Use Misuse*. 2013;48(10):799-810.
149. Fredman SJ, Macdonald A, Monson CM, et al. Intensive, multi-couple group therapy for PTSD: a nonrandomized pilot study with military and veteran dyads. *Behav Ther*. 2020;51(5):700-714.
150. Monson CM, Fredman SJ, Macdonald A, Pukay-Martin ND, Resick PA, Schnurr PP. Effect of cognitive-behavioral couple therapy for ptsd: a randomized controlled trial. *JAMA*. 2012;308(7):700-709.
151. Gidycz CA, Wyatt J, Galbreath NW, et al. Sexual assault prevention in the military: key issues and recommendations. *Mil Psychol*. 2018;30(3): 240-251.
152. Goldberg SB, Livingston WS, Blais RK, et al. A positive screen for military sexual trauma is associated with greater risk for substance use disorders in women veterans. *Psychol Addict Behav*. 2019;33(5):477-483.
153. Banducci AN, McCaughey VK, Gradus JL, Street AE. The associations between deployment experiences, PTSD, and alcohol use among male and female veterans. *Addict Behav*. 2019;98:106032.
154. Farrer TJ, Frost RB, Hedges DW. Prevalence of traumatic brain injury in intimate partner violence offenders compared to the general population: a meta-analysis. *Trauma Violence Abuse*. 2012;13(2):77-82.
155. Miller SC, Baktash SH, Webb TS, et al. Risk for addiction-related disorders following mild traumatic brain injury in a large cohort of active-duty U.S. airmen. *Am J Psychiatry*. 2013;170(4):383-390.
156. Balderrama-Durbin C, Cigrang JA, Osborne LJ, et al. Coming home: a prospective study of family reintegration following deployment to a war zone. *Psychol Serv*. 2015;12(3):213-221.
157. Fischer EP, Sherman M, McSweeney JC, Pyne JM, Owen RR, Dixon LB. Perspectives of family and veterans on family programs to support reintegration of returning veterans with posttraumatic stress disorder. *Psychol Serv*. 2015;12(3):187-198.
158. Miller MW, Reardon AF, Wolf EJ, Prince LB, Hein CL. Alcohol and drug abuse among U.S. veterans: comparing associations with intimate partner substance abuse and veteran psychopathology. *J Trauma Stress*. 2013;26(1):71-76.
159. Maisto SA, McKay JR, O'Farrell TJ. Relapse precipitants and behavioral marital therapy. *Addict Behav*. 1995;20(3):383-393.
160. Schumm JA, Monson CM, O'Farrell TJ, Gustin NG, Chard KM. Couple treatment for alcohol use disorder and posttraumatic stress disorder: pilot results from U.S. military veterans and their partners. *J Trauma Stress*. 2015;28(3):247-252.
161. England LJ, Bennett C, Denny CH, et al. Alcohol use and co-use of other substances among pregnant females aged 12-44 years-United States, 2015-2018. *MMWR Morb Mortal Wkly Rep*. 2020;69(31):1009-1014.
162. Steele S, Osorio R, Page LM. Substance misuse in pregnancy. *Obstet Gynaecol Repro Med*. 2020;30(11):347-355.
163. Ecker J, Abuhamad A, Hill W, et al. Substance use disorders in pregnancy: clinical, ethical, and research imperatives of the opioid epidemic: a report of a joint workshop of the Society for Maternal-Fetal Medicine, American College of Obstetricians and Gynecologists, and American Society of Addiction Medicine. *Am J Obstet Gynecol*. 2019;221(1): B5-B28.
164. Terplan M, Laird HJ, Hand DJ, et al. Opioid detoxification during pregnancy: a systematic review. *Obstet Gynecol*. 2018;131(5):803-814.

CHAPTER 79

Twelve-Step Facilitation Approaches

Antoine Douaihy, Dennis M. Donovan, and Dennis C. Daley

CHAPTER OUTLINE

- Introduction
- Historical perspective
- Treatment model
- Theory of change
- Treatment planning and evaluation
- Indications for treatment
- Pretreatment issues
- Research studies
- Summary and conclusions

INTRODUCTION

Of the behavioral therapies described in this volume, Twelve-Step facilitation (TSF) is perhaps unique in that it is an approach that had its roots in traditional clinical practice and was then codified and moved into clinical research, as opposed to a scientifically developed treatment then transferred to clinical practice. TSF therapy[1] is a manual-guided treatment that was developed for use in Project MATCH, a major multisite trial of behavioral treatments for alcohol use disorders (formerly as "alcohol abuse" and "alcohol dependence"). TSF was developed specifically to approximate the style of counseling commonly used in treatment programs throughout the United States. Thus, its content was intended to be consistent with active involvement in Twelve-Step recovery programs, such as Alcoholics Anonymous (AA), and with a treatment goal of abstinence from all psychoactive substances. Since its introduction in 1992, utilization and empirical support for this approach has shown steadily. This chapter describes its historical roots, summarizes its use in clinical practice, and briefly reviews the empirical data regarding its use with patients with substance use disorders (SUDs).

HISTORICAL PERSPECTIVE

For many years, treatment based on or related to the Twelve Steps of AA was widely practiced in the clinical community, particularly residential and 90-day programs. In many ways, mutual support and 12-Step-oriented groups formed the foundation of SUDs treatment in the United States and played major formative roles in the philosophies of some of the most influential treatment centers and programs, including the Hazelden Foundation, the Betty Ford Center, and many more programs using the Minnesota Model and similar approaches. Although there were differences across programs, in general they had two related foci: emphasis on abstinence from all psychoactive substances and encouraging mutual support group attendance. Although AA has been challenging to study systematically[2] and the quality of research on the effectiveness of self-help approaches has been variable,[3] the bulk of the evidence suggests that attendance at mutual support groups is associated with better outcomes.[4,5]

Recognizing that mutual support programs represent an important, broadly available, and inexpensive resource, the defining feature of TSF is to encourage meaningful, long-term involvement with AA and other mutual support groups. Because of the importance of including an approach that was representative of the dominant model of clinical practice in Project MATCH,[6] and the need for a clear, structured description of these approaches that could be used in a large research protocol, the Project MATCH Steering Committee asked Joe Nowinski, and Stu Baker, two clinical experts, to collaborate with Yale group (Kathleen Carroll)[7] to develop the TSF manual, which was done in close collaboration with experts from the Hazelden Foundation.[6,8] After its initial evaluation in Project MATCH, TSF and closely related approaches have been evaluated in several subsequent trials and have extended to populations other than those with alcohol use disorders.[9,10]

TREATMENT MODEL

TSF is a highly structured, individual, manual-guided approach delivered by a practitioner (usually a therapist) over the course of 12 to 24 weeks, intended to contrast with cognitive-behavioral therpy (CBT) and motivational interviewing (MI). It is a counseling method that invokes 12-Step recovery philosophy and facilitates engagement and active involvement in mutual support groups, in contrast to the development of specific coping skills as done in CBT or MI. As described in the manual,[1] it consists of a set of core topics (assessment and overview, acceptance, surrender, and getting active in 12-step support groups), which are to be covered with all patients; a set of elective topics, which can be selected to tailor the treatment to different individuals ("people, places, and things" that may be associated with increased use of or return to substance use; review of a genogram; enabling, managing emotions: "hungry, angry, lonely, or tired [HALT]," which reflect emotions associated with high risk of return to use); as well as guidelines for conjoint sessions with family members. While based on the principles of AA, TSF is not itself a 12-step support group, not equivalent to AA/NA referral, and is not equivalent to "treatment as usual."

TSF sessions follow a common format. Each session begins with a careful review of the previous week and mutual support group attendance, as well as review of the patient's recovery journal and reactions to any AA-related readings that may have been assigned. Next, the TSF therapist introduces the "recovery topic" for the week from the set of core and elective sessions, to which the bulk of the session is devoted. Finally, sessions end with assignment of the patient's recovery tasks for the weeks (specific mutual support meetings and activities to attend, readings, and other tasks).

TSF assumes that alcohol use disorder and other SUDs are progressive diseases of mind, body, and spirit, for which the only effective remedy is abstinence from mood-altering substances, "*one day at a time*." TSF adheres to the concepts set forth in the Twelve Steps and Twelve Traditions.[11] The core essential features of TSF include the following:

- Taking a thorough alcohol and substance use history, identifying positive and negative consequences of substance use, and giving feedback as groundwork to Step 1.
- Providing education about Steps 1, 2, and 3 of AA, as well as explanation of the disease concept of alcohol use disorder (old terminology used "alcoholism") and addiction.
- Exploring discrepancies between the patient's stated goals and actions in terms of denial.
- Identifying "people, places, and things" that could trigger substance use and identification of "people, places, and things" that support recovery.
- Encouraging patients to actively work the "Twelve Steps" as the primary goal of treatment.
- Supporting the point of view that the best chance of abstinence and health is to accept loss of control and the need to reach out to the fellowship of AA (or NA or CA).

THEORY OF CHANGE

As with AA, which grew out of the experiences of a group of men as they struggled with severe alcohol use disorder, TSF has historic, rather than theoretic, foundations. In TSF, change is thought to occur through building a meaningful relationship with the fellowship of AA and in following the Twelve Steps of AA. Several authors have pointed out similarities between the processes of change in AA and those of other effective behavioral therapies.[12,13] McCrady[13] noted that the key change principles of AA include changing reference groups through group affiliation, articulating a clear treatment goal through commitment to abstinence, and emphasizing spirituality and intra- and interpersonal change. The TSF theory of change is, essentially, the process of the Twelve Steps, as the individual moves from acceptance of "alcoholism" or "addiction" and the need for complete abstinence, through the need for affiliation with others and with a Higher Power, to recognizing and making amends to others. Hence, TSF makes no commitment to a particular causal model of addiction; emphasis is placed on the core concepts of loss of control and denial, and two themes are emphasized.

- Spirituality: Belief in a "power greater than ourselves," which is defined individually, by each person, and represents faith and hope for recovery.
- Pragmatism: Belief in doing "what works" for the individual, meaning doing whatever it takes in order to avoid taking the first drink.

TREATMENT PLANNING AND EVALUATION

A thorough evaluation of the individual's alcohol and drug use history is an essential feature of TSF, and in fact, dominates much of the first session and may extend into several sessions. The goal is to begin the breakdown of the patient's "denial system." The comprehensive alcohol and drug history is taken in a particular format to do this, highlighting progressive loss of control over alcohol and drugs, and covering age, substances used (amount and frequency), positive and negative consequences of use, and major life events.

Therapists introduce this section by advising the patient that completing this history will help them begin to make sense of what has happened in their life in relation to their use of alcohol or drugs and is used as a means for preparing for Step 1 (admitting powerlessness and acknowledging unmanageability). The TSF therapist begins with the age of earliest use, outside the home, and then progresses by looking at different time periods. Typically, the TSF therapist would ask about a period 3 years after the initial use and then ask about subsequent periods of time in 5-year intervals. For example, if a patient was 28 years old, who started using cannabis at age 12, the TSF therapist would start at 12, then go to age 15, then to age 20 (or late teens), and then to age 25 (or early 20s). Finally, the TSF therapist would ask about the past year to get a sense of current use patterns and issues. At each age, the TSF therapist would ask about each of the categories. As this is done, patterns usually emerge. The TSF therapist pays particular attention to any increase in the amount and frequency of use and periods of time that the patient abstained from use or attempted to control their use. This information is used to highlight loss of control over alcohol or drugs, which is the hallmark of addiction in TSF.

The TSF therapist also explores positive and negative consequences of substance use. Typically, the relationship with alcohol and drugs starts out very positively with tremendous enjoyment by the patient. However, as use increases in amount and frequency, there is invariably an increase in negative consequences (eg, spending too much money, problems at work, problems at home, legal problems). These negative consequences are evidence of the "unmanageability" referred to in the first step. Examining major life events at different ages helps to place the patient's relationship with alcohol and drugs in perspective.

TSF recognizes that substance use takes place in a social and environmental context and is not an isolated behavior.

After the alcohol and drug use history is completed, the TSF therapist asks the patient to react to what they have observed. For some, this is the first time they have looked at the big picture of how alcohol or substance use has affected their life. The practitioner then underlines evidence of unmanageability by pointing out negative consequences from their SUD in the following areas:

Physical: Health problems, accidents, or injuries the patient may have experienced.

Legal: Arrests, difficulties with child protection agencies, civil problems, lawsuits, etc.

Social: Loss of friends, family relationship problems, lack of supportive relationships, and lack of social skills.

Sexual: Changes in sexual functioning, positive and negative, trading sex for drugs.

Psychological: Depression, anxiety, shame, and guilt about using despite the intention to remain abstinent.

Financial: Loss of job, effects on job performance, income used to buy drugs or alcohol, and indebtedness.

Finally, the TSF practitioner asks about loss of control over alcohol or drug use. This includes behaviors such as repeated failed attempts to stop or control use, using alone, preoccupation with drugs or alcohol, and substance substitution. Using the evidence offered by the patient, usually the only logical conclusion is that the patient is a person with an alcohol use disorder or a SUD.

The TSF therapist then describes addiction as follows. Alcohol or other SUD is a disease that is chronic (the patient will remain as a person with addiction for the remainder of their life), is progressive, and, if left untreated, can be fatal. Because of the nature of the disease, once a person becomes addicted, he or she can never return to safe use of mood-altering substances. The progressive nature of the disease is noted in the patient's history of increasing losses and problems and increasing amounts and frequency of use over time. It is emphasized, however, that alcohol and drug use disorders are treatable. The therapist emphasizes that what has worked best for most is to abstain from all mood-altering substances, one day at a time. To learn how to do this and to gain support to do this task, the TSF therapist then recommends that the patient makes use of 12-Step recovery programs such as AA, NA, or CA. This leads naturally and easily into contracting with the patient about participating in TSF therapy and beginning to attend mutual support group meetings.

INDICATIONS FOR TREATMENT

In general, TSF therapy is intended for alcohol and drug users at the higher end of severity—that is, those who meet criteria for severe alcohol and drug use disorder. As described previously, the assumption is that the patient is coming to treatment after incurring significant consequences of substance use and being unable to control or stop use on their own and thus would meet formal *Diagnostic and Statistical Manual of Mental Disorders* criteria for severe SUD. Thus, TSF is not intended for those who are at the earlier stage of a use disorder or are "at risk." However, contrary to expectations (and a Project MATCH a priori hypothesis), the level of alcohol involvement did not predict differential response to TSF in Project MATCH.[14]

Similarly, although it was predicted that several patient characteristics (gender, psychiatric severity, conceptual level, and motivation) would be associated with poorer response to TSF compared with CBT and MI, the primary matching hypotheses in Project MATCH did not receive strong empirical support. Thus, the data from Project MATCH suggested that TSF was generally appropriate for a wide range of individuals with alcohol use disorders; that is, there were few strong contraindications for TSF found in that dataset.

PRETREATMENT ISSUES

Motivation

In TSF, motivation, especially lack thereof, is generally interpreted in terms of denial. The goal of treatment is to engage the patient's interest in voluntarily committing to this TSF program. Hence, approaches that use excessive pressure, threat, or coercion toward this are likely to elicit a false commitment from the patient at best. In TSF, the therapist is advised to take a direct, nonjudgmental, and educative approach to confrontation of denial. The history of substance use, along with symptomatology (eg, tolerance) and an understanding of the process of addiction, is relied on consistently as the basis for directly confronting patients with their current situation. The therapist attempts to highlight denial in a direct yet supportive and empathetic way.

Therapist Characteristics

In Project MATCH and the other research studies that have evaluated this approach, TSF has been implemented primarily by master's-level therapists with substantial experience in and commitment to 12-Step programs as a therapeutic intervention, who also had extensive experience treating a broad range of people with SUD. Because the therapist training period for these clinical trials was brief, it was important to select therapists who already had a high level of expertise and experience in this approach and thus could achieve optimal levels of adherence and competence rapidly. However, a much broader range of therapists can, with appropriate training and supervision, implement this treatment effectively.

In TSF, the therapists use their therapeutic skills to help the patient overcome barriers to becoming actively involved in 12-Step recovery programs. Skills such as active listening, accurate empathy, problem solving, feedback, and confrontation all have a place in this therapy. A critically important role is to be an educator about 12-Step programs and knowledgeable about local meetings, types of meetings, and guidance and advice about how best to access the resources of 12-Step programs. This may be based on and supplemented by the wisdom found in recovering literature, slogans, or the stories of others in recovery. Last, the therapist provides empathy and a sense of hope for the patient through communicating an understanding of the struggles of early recovery.

TSF requires an active, supportive, and involved presence by the therapist in sessions. Good TSF appears almost conversational in tone. A good session involves give and take interaction between the therapist and the patient. The session, however, is quite focused. The therapist takes an active part in keeping the focus of the session on recovery. Some therapists begin their sessions by asking the patient, "How has your recovery week been?" When faced with the day-to-day struggles of the patient, the therapist refers the patient back to the use of Twelve-Step program tools. For example, the therapist frequently suggests also talking a problem over with a sponsor or peer, as well as talk about the issue at a meeting.

Last, an effective TSF therapist uses confrontation constructively. The technique of *confrontation* here means to bring that which has been passively kept out of awareness or consciously avoided, into awareness, by a frank, nonjudgmental and respectful therapeutically, as compared to the common usage of the term where activity is often in the context of negative emotion and critical. The TSF therapist is careful to confront the patient's behavior as it relates to his or her addiction (ie, denial and avoidance) rather than the person. This means separating the person from the disease and communicating that the patient is a "good person" who has a disease (addiction) that leads him or her to act in ways that are hurtful toward himself or herself and others.

RESEARCH STUDIES

For many years, treatments based on the Twelve Steps of AA and Cocaine Anonymous were widely used and had a great deal of popular support in the treatment community, but until recently have had very little empirical support from controlled clinical trials.[15-17] However, several rigorous randomized clinical trials have been done that have found strong support for the efficacy of well-defined, manualized, 12-Step-oriented treatments. TSF therapies lead to an increased involvement in community mutual aid programs like AA and NA. According to a recent population study by Kelly and colleagues, more people recovering from a SUD participate in mutual aid programs (45%) compared to professional treatment (28%) or medication treatment (9%). This finding shows how prevalent mutual aid programs are in recovery from all types of SUDs.[18]

For example, in Project MATCH,[19,20] the largest randomized trial of treatments for alcoholism conducted to date, TSF was not significantly different in effectiveness from CBT and motivational enhancement therapy (MET), two forms of treatment with strong records of empirical support. Moreover, where there were differences in the outcomes of some variables (eg, rates of complete abstinence and negative consequences of drinking), these tended to favor the TSF approach over CBT and MET.[19-22] TSF has also been associated with higher rates of self-help involvement,[23-26] which in turn has been associated with better drinking and drug use outcomes.[5,24,27,28]

TSF has also been found to be effective with people with nonalcohol SUD. In a clinical trial of disulfiram and psychotherapy with subjects with severe cocaine and alcohol-use disorders, TSF was found to be comparable in effectiveness to CBT in reducing cocaine and alcohol use; moreover, both TSF and CBT were found to be significantly more effective than a supportive psychotherapy clinical management control condition.[29] The effects of TSF in this study were also durable and associated with good outcome up to 1 year after patients completed the 12-week treatment program.[30] These findings were similar to those of Wells et al.,[31] who demonstrated that TSF was comparable in effectiveness to CBT in a randomized controlled trial of persons with a SUD in a group setting. Finally, Ouimette et al.,[32] in a nonrandomized trial, evaluated the effectiveness of 12-Step and CBT approaches in 15 Veterans Affairs programs in a sample of 3,018 subjects. Both types of treatment programs were equally effective in reducing substance use and improving most other areas of functioning at 1 year; moreover, patients in the 12-Step-oriented programs had somewhat higher rates of abstinence.

The STAGE-12 intervention (Stimulant Abuser Groups to Engage in 12-Step) used in the NIDA Clinical Trial Network (CTN0031) was evaluated in patients with stimulant use disorders. It is a manualized intervention incorporating individual and group components and combines elements of TSF and intensive referral to help facilitate involvement in 12-Step meetings.[33] A multisite randomized controlled trial, with assessments at baseline, mid-treatment, end of treatment, and 3- and 6-month postrandomization follow-ups (FUs) evaluated the effectiveness of the 8-week combined group plus individual 12-Step facilitative STAGE-12 intervention on stimulant drug use, 12-Step meeting attendance and service in intensive outpatient substance treatment programs. The results indicated that, in comparison those in Treatment as Usual, individuals in STAGE-12 had higher rates of self-reported abstinence from stimulant use during the active phase of treatment; a significant reduction on the Addiction Severity Index Drug Composite scores from baseline through the 3-month follow-up period; and both higher rates of 12-Step meeting attendance and engagement in more 12-Step related activities throughout both the active treatment phase and the entire 6-month FU period.[34] Among those receiving the STAGE-12 intervention, higher rates of individual and group therapy session attendance were associated with higher odds of self-reported and urine-verified abstinence from stimulant drugs, as well as greater 12-Step group attendance and related activities.[35] This latter finding about 12-Step attendance is of note in that Humphreys and colleagues have found that greater attendance at and involvement in 12-Step mutual help meetings by individuals with SUDs was predictive of reduced use of and problems related to illicit drugs and alcohol.[36]

Despite emerging support for the efficacy of TSF, it has proven challenging to disseminate TSF and other empirically validated treatments to the clinical community. Many clinicians have limited access to comprehensive training in TSF or other empirically validated therapies.[37] Although workshops in some empirically supported therapies are more available recently, training sessions are usually quite brief (eg, workshops of several hours duration) and hence unlikely to produce lasting change in the clinician's ability to implement new therapies.[38] Moreover, it should not be assumed that counselors, even those espousing a 12-Step model, can implement TSF without training. Although based on standard counseling models, TSF differs from it in several ways. These include its high emphasis on therapist support, discouragement of aggressive "confrontation of denial" and therapist self-disclosure, and highly focused and structured format.

In this context, Sholomskas and Carroll completed a randomized training trial in which predominantly bachelor's- and master's-level counselors were randomly assigned to one of the two training conditions: either the TSF manual[1] or a computer-assisted training method.[39] Pre- to posttraining data indicated that the clinicians' ability to implement TSF, as assessed by independent ratings of adherence and skill for five key TSF interventions, was significantly higher after training for those assigned to the computer-assisted training method than for those who were assigned to the manual-only training condition. Those who were assigned to the computerized training condition also evidenced greater gains in a knowledge test assessing familiarity with concepts presented in the TSF manual. Moreover, no significant effects of the clinicians' self-reported recovery status were seen on adherence, competence, or knowledge scores.[39]

SUMMARY AND CONCLUSIONS

TSF is a professionally delivered, individual, manualized therapy that is grounded in the principles and Twelve Steps of AA. It is important to note, however, that TSF has no official relationship with, or sanction from, any 12-Step program. AA does not sponsor or conduct research on alcohol or drug treatment and does not endorse any treatment programs. While intended to be consistent with 12-Step principles, it is important to note that TSF was designed for delivery in research protocols and in clinical settings, and it is an addition to the repertoire of behavioral therapies for SUDs. With that as its basis, TSF received comparatively strong empirical support in Project MATCH, one of the largest alcohol treatment trials ever conducted in the United States, and support is emerging for its use with other patient groups as well.

ACKNOWLEDGMENTS

This chapter represents an update and revision of previous chapters in this series, most recently by Dr Kathleen Carroll in the last edition. As a leading addiction researcher and educator, Dr Carroll conducted numerous clinical trials and disseminated information about evidenced-based treatments to the addiction treatment community. Her contributions were substantial.

REFERENCES

1. Nowinski J, Baker S, Carroll KM. *Twelve-Step Facilitation Therapy Manual: A Clinical Research Guide for Therapists Treating Individuals With Alcohol Abuse and Dependence.* NIAAA; 1992.
2. Humphreys K. The trials of Alcoholics Anonymous. *Addiction.* 2006;101:617-618.
3. Ferri M, Amato L, Davoli M. Alcoholics Anonymous and other 12-step programmes for alcohol dependence. *Cochrane Database Syst Rev.* 2008;3:1-25.
4. Humphreys K. *Circles of Recovery: Self-Help Organizations for Addictions.* Cambridge University Press; 2004.
5. Humphreys K, Wing S, McCarty D, et al. Self-help organizations for alcohol and drug problems: toward evidence-based practice and policy. *J Subst Abus Treat.* 2004;26:151-158.
6. Donovan D, Kadden R, DiClemente CC, et al. Issues in the selection and development of therapies in alcoholism treatment matching. *J Stud Alcohol Suppl.* 1994;12:138-148.
7. Connors GJ, Tonigan JS, Miller WR. A longitudinal model of intake symptomatology, AA participation and outcome: retrospective study of the project MATCH outpatient and aftercare samples. *J Stud Alcohol.* 2001;62(6):817-825.
8. Carroll KM, Kadden R, Donovan D, Zweben A, Rounsaville BJ. Implementing treatment and protecting the validity of the independent variable in treatment matching studies. *J Stud Alcohol Suppl.* 1994;12:149-155.
9. Donovan DM, Ingalsbe MH, Benbow J, Daley DC. 12-Step interventions and mutual support programs for substance use disorders: an overview. *Soc Work Public Health.* 2013;28(3-4):313-332.
10. Donovan DM, Floyd AS. Facilitating involvement in Twelve-Step programs. In: Galanter M, Kaskutas LA, eds. *Recent Developments in Alcoholism.* Vol. 18. Springer; 2008:303-320.
11. Alcoholic Anonymous World Services. *Alcoholics Anonymous-Big Book.* 4th ed. Alcoholic Anonymous World Services; 2002.
12. Longabaugh R, Donovan DM, Karno MP, McCrady BS, Morgenstern J, Tonigan JS. Active ingredients: how and why evidence-based alcohol behavioral treatment interventions work. *Alcohol Clin Exp Res.* 2005;29:235-247.
13. McCrady BS. Alcoholics Anonymous and behavior therapy: can habits be treated as diseases? Can diseases be treated as habits? *J Consult Clin Psychol.* 1994;62(6):1159-1166.
14. Babor TF, Del Boca FK, eds. *Treatment Matching in Alcoholism.* Cambridge University Press; 2003.
15. Morgenstern J, Labouvie E, McCrady BS, Kahler CW, Frey RM. Affiliation with Alcoholics Anonymous after treatment: a study of its therapeutic effects and mechanisms of action. *J Consult Clin Psychol.* 1997;65:768-777.
16. Miller WR, Brown JM, Simpson TL, et al. What works? A methodological analysis of the alcohol treatment literature. In: Hester RK, Miller WR, eds. *Handbook of Alcoholism Treatment Approaches: Effective Alternatives.* Allyn & Bacon; 1995:12-44.
17. Tonigan JS, Toscova R, Miller WR. Meta-analysis of the literature on Alcoholics Anonymous: sample and study characteristics that moderate findings. *J Stud Alcohol.* 1996;57:65-72.
18. Kelly JF, Bergman B, Hoeppner B, et al. Prevalence, pathways and predictors of recovery from drug and alcohol problems in the U.S. population. *Drug Alcohol Depend.* 2017;181:162-169.
19. Project MATCH Research Group. Matching alcohol treatments to client heterogeneity: project MATCH posttreatment drinking outcomes. *J Stud Alcohol.* 1997;58:7-29.
20. Project MATCH Research Group. Project MATCH secondary a priori hypotheses. *Addiction.* 1997;92:1671-1698.

21. Project MATCH Research Group. Matching alcoholism treatments to client heterogeneity: project MATCH three-year drinking outcomes. *Alcohol Clin Exp Res*. 1998;22:1300-1311.
22. Project MATCH Research Group. Matching alcoholism treatments to client heterogeneity: treatment main effects and matching effects on drinking during treatment. *J Stud Alcohol*. 1998;59:631-639.
23. Bogenschutz MP, Tonigan JS, Miller WR. Examining the effects of alcoholism typology and AA attendance on self-efficacy as a mechanism of change. *J Stud Alcohol*. 2006;67(4):562-567.
24. Carroll KM, Nuro KF. One size can't fit all: a stage model for psychotherapy manual development. *Clin Psychol Sci Pract*. 2002;9:396-406.
25. Weiss RD, Griffin ML, Gallop RJ, et al. The effect of 12-step self-help group attendance and participation on drug use outcomes among cocaine-dependent patients. *Drug Alcohol Depend*. 2005;77:177-184.
26. Weiss RD, Griffin ML, Najavits LM, et al. Self-help activities in cocaine dependent patients entering treatment: results from the NIDA collaborative cocaine treatment study. *Drug Alcohol Depend*. 1996;43:79-86.
27. Brown TG, Seraganian P, Tremblay J, Annis H. Process and outcome changes with relapse prevention versus 12-Step aftercare programs for substance abusers. *Addiction*. 2002;97:677-689.
28. Owen PL, Slaymaker V, Tonigan JS, et al. Participation in alcoholics anonymous: intended and unintended change mechanisms. *Alcohol Clin Exp Res*. 2003;27(3):524-532.
29. Carroll KM, Nich C, Ball SA, McCance E, Rounsaville BJ. Treatment of cocaine and alcohol dependence with psychotherapy and disulfiram. *Addiction*. 1998;93:713-728.
30. Carroll KM, Nich C, Ball SA, Frankforter TL, Rounsaville BJ. One year follow-up of disulfiram and psychotherapy for cocaine-alcohol abusers: sustained effects of treatment. *Addiction*. 2000;95:1335-1349.
31. Wells EA, Peterson PL, Gainey RR, Hawkins JD, Catalano RF. Outpatient treatment for cocaine abuse: a controlled comparison of relapse prevention and twelve-step approaches. *Am J Drug Alcohol Abuse*. 1994;20:1-17.
32. Ouimette PC, Finney JW, Moos RH. Twelve-step and cognitive behavioral treatment for substance abuse: a comparison of treatment effectiveness. *J Consult Clin Psychol*. 1997;65:230-240.
33. Daley DC, Baker S, Donovan DM, Hodgkins CG, Perl H. A combined group and individual 12-step facilitative intervention targeting stimulant abuse in the NIDA Clinical Trials Network: stage-12. *J Groups Addict Recover*. 2011;6(3):228-244.
34. Donovan DM, Daley DC, Brigham GS, et al. Stimulant abuser groups to engage in 12-Step: a multisite trial in the National Institute on Drug Abuse Clinical Trials Network. *J Subst Abus Treat*. 2013;44:103-114.
35. Wells EA, Donovan DM, Daley DC, et al. Is level of exposure to a 12-step facilitation therapy associated with treatment outcome? *J Subst Abus Treat*. 2014;47(4):265-274.
36. Humphreys K, Barreto NB, Alessi SM, et al. Impact of 12 step mutual help groups on drug use disorder patients across six clinical trials. *Drug Alcohol Depend*. 2020;215:108213. doi:10.1016/j.drugalcdep.2020.108213.
37. Institute of Medicine. *Bridging the Gap Between Practice and Research: Forging Partnerships with Community-Based Drug and Alcohol Treatment*. National Academy Press; 1998.
38. Walters ST, Matson SA, Baer JS, Ziedonis DM. Effectiveness of workshop training for psychosocial addiction treatments: a systematic review. *J Subst Abus Treat*. 2005;29:283-293.
39. Sholomskas DE, Carroll KM. One small step for manuals: computer-assisted training in twelve-step facilitation. *J Stud Alcohol*. 2006;67:939-945.

CHAPTER

80 Relapse Prevention: Clinical Models and Intervention Strategies

Antoine Douaihy, Dennis C. Daley, and Dennis M. Donovan

CHAPTER OUTLINE

- Introduction
- Lapse, relapse, and recovery
- Treatment outcome studies
- Effectiveness and efficacy of recurrence prevention
- Relapse replication and extension project
- Determinants of relapse
- Models of relapse prevention
- Prevention of recurrence for co-occurring disorders
- Conclusions

INTRODUCTION

Note to readers: Relapse prevention (RP) is a term used in the literature to describe a specific clinical model or treatment. Variations of this approach are aimed to reduce the risk of a patient returning to substance (or gambling or other addictive behaviors) use after a period of change, or what Marlatt refers to as a "breakdown or setback" in an attempt to change substance use behaviors. Many definitions of the term "relapse" exist and in recent years, however, "recurrence of disease" or "of (DSM-5) symptoms" of a substance use disorder or "return to (substance) use" following a period of recovery have replaced the term relapse and are preferred current terminology when not referring to the specific RP intervention and its terminology.

Longitudinal studies demonstrate that the treatment of substance use disorders (SUDs) is associated with major reductions in substance use, related problems, and societal costs.[1,2] Epidemiological studies of people with lifetime DSM-IV-TR substance dependence suggest that 58% eventually enter sustained recovery (ie, no symptoms for the past year).[3] Of the people who eventually achieved a state of sustained recovery, the majority managed to do so after participating in treatment.[4]

According to a recent population study, most people with a SUD recover without professional help.[5] However, those with more significant substance problems benefit from treatment. Many suffer from a long-lasting chronic condition, whereby they cycle through episodes of lapse (brief return to, or recurrence of, use and/or of symptoms of SUD/addiction/gambling disorder), relapse (a lengthier and more sustained recurrence), treatment reentry, and recovery.[6]

For example, 12-month recurrence rates following alcohol or nicotine abstinence attempts range from 80% to 95%, and evidence suggests comparable trajectories of recurrence of disease or use across various classes of substance use.[7] High rates of recurrence have led many researchers to conceptualize addiction as a "chronic relapsing illness"[8] and understand relapse prevention (RP) as an iterative process of change rather than as a full inoculation against recurrence.[9] Numerous approaches and models have been suggested to explain this process.

A review paper described the development, adaptation, and dissemination of RP over the past 30 years.[10] Highlighted in that review, the pioneering work of Alan Marlatt and his colleagues, initiated in the early 1970s, revolutionized the understanding of addiction and said that "relapse" need not be inevitable. RP was originally described as an aftercare program for individuals receiving treatment for an alcohol use disorder[11]; it was later used to encompass any cognitive-behavioral skills that address variables and risk factors predicting recurrence of use, high-risk situations, and effective coping strategies to assist individuals in maintaining desired behavioral changes. RP strategies have been incorporated into treatment programs throughout the continuum of care, and are described in treatment manuals.[12-14]

This chapter summarizes the major tenets of RP including the concepts of "lapse," "relapse," and "recovery." It provides a summary of the empirical support of RP (efficacy and effectiveness of RP), determinants of relapse, models of RP, and a review of the conceptualization of relapse as a dynamic process. We also present highlights of RP assessment and intervention strategies representing the most common principles espoused in the RP models. An overview of RP for co-occurring disorders is discussed.

LAPSE, RELAPSE, AND RECOVERY

Relapse has been described as a discrete phenomenon and as a process of behavior change.[15] Marlatt identified a *lapse* as the initial episode of use of a substance after a period of abstinence, a *relapse* as a continued use after the initial slip, "a breakdown or setback in the person's attempt to change or modify any target behavior," and a *prolapse* as a behavior that is consistent with getting back on track in the direction of positive behavior change.[11,16,17] Multiple meanings have emerged to describe the concept of relapse, including: daily use for a specific number of sequential days such as hazardous drinking, a consequence of substance use resulting in the need for subsequent treatment,[18] an "unfolding process in which the resumption of substance use is the last event in a long series of maladaptive responses to internal or external stressors or stimuli,"[19] a continuous process defined by a series of transgressive behaviors,[20] and a complex multidimensional composite index of outcome that takes into account the different aspects of return to the addictive behavior, goes beyond the binary classification of abstinence-relapse, and fits better into the concept of "harm reduction" in some programs that have nonabstinence goals.[21,22]

The definition of relapse has a significant impact on the conceptual and clinical approach to assessment. The ways in which clinicians quantify and qualify relapse (better termed "recurrence of use or disease") determine how they will respond to the patient's substance use behaviors. If a patient is involved in a treatment program that identifies *any drinking* behavior such as one drink after a period of abstinence as a "relapse," it is more probable for him or her to engage in heavier drinking behavior, which is explained by the phenomenon of the "abstinence violation effect" (eg, self-blame and loss of perceived control that individuals often experience after the violation of self-imposed rules).[15,16] However, if the same patient is receiving treatment in a program that does not convey that this behavior (one drink) is a "relapse," it is more probable for him or her to have an increased awareness of his or her reactions to drinking and may be less vulnerable to the abstinence violation effect. "Lapse" and "relapse" may also be defined according to the individual's goals for change. If abstinence is a goal, then a drink may be considered as a "lapse"; but if the individual maintains harm reduction goals, then a "lapse" may be defined as harmful consequence of drinking behavior. However, it is in part because of these many varied definitions of the term, and it's artificial creation of a binary outcome that "relapse" and the associated terms above are being slowly replaced by my more medically precise and less potentially stigmatizing terms such as "recurrence" of disease, symptoms, or of a substance (or gambling, etc.).

A brief recurrence of use or symptoms (previously referred to as "lapse") does not necessarily herald permanence in people who use tobacco or cocaine.[22,23] The different rates of recurrence vary between studies and across substances, but "relapse is the rule" not the exception as stated by De Leon[24] in a review of addiction treatment outcome research. It has become clearer to think of "relapse" as both a dichotomous outcome and a dynamic process involving a series of prior related events, immediate precipitants, and related consequences as predictors of return to use or of disease recurrence interfering with behavior change.[25-27] The process has been studied in many types of addiction,[17,28-30] and it may be highly similar across the different substances.[31,32] Therefore, a dynamic assessment model is necessary to gain a clearer picture of the process and would potentially capture all the elements of disease recurrence and their dynamic interactions across time and in the moment of crisis.[18,30,32]

Recovery is defined as a long-term and ongoing process rather than an end point.[33] There are many pathways to recovery.[34] It remains anything but linear and smooth and the outcome anything but predictable.[34] Specific areas of change during the process of recovery may include physical, psychological, spiritual, behavioral, interpersonal, sociocultural, familial, and financial.[26,35] Recovery tasks and areas of clinical focus are contingent on the stage or phase of recovery the individual is in.[36,37] Recovery and recurrence are mediated by the severity and damage caused by the SUD, the presence of co-occurring psychiatric or medical illness, and the individual's coping skills, motivation, and support system. Although some individuals achieve full recovery, others achieve only partial recovery.[38] The latter group is at risk for multiple recurrences over time, yet still can benefit from the cumulative effects of multiple treatments. One study identified predictors of long-term stable recovery from heroin addiction based on 242 people with heroin addiction who have been followed for more than 30 years. The study findings showed that in addition to early intervention to address heroin addiction, increasing self-efficacy and addressing psychological problems are likely to enhance the odds of maintaining long-term stable recovery.[39]

Recovering from SUD involves gaining information, increasing self-awareness, developing skills for sober living, and following a program of change.[26] The program of change may also incorporate psychotherapy, pharmacotherapy, case management, participation in self-help groups including 12-step programs, and self-management approaches. As recovery progresses, patients rely more on themselves after initially using their support system, with the goal of improving their overall quality of life. Flynn et al.[40] studied a group of people who use opioids 5 years after treatment and compared those who were in recovery and those who were not. The subjects in recovery were more likely to benefit from family and friends as a support group and were more likely to agree that their social network did not include people with SUDs. The subjects in recovery were four times more likely to perceive themselves as improving their overall personal growth and ability to lead a fulfilling life.

TREATMENT OUTCOME STUDIES

Despite advances in treatment, recurrence rates are still high.[41-44] Substantial research provides good evidence that treatment can be successful, but treatment is not always followed by positive treatment outcomes.[45] Multiple variables including amount of drug use at treatment entry, treatment retention and completion, and frequency of participation in 12-step program before and throughout treatment have been found to predict treatment outcome.[46] Research continues to attempt to differentiate predictors of in-treatment performance and posttreatment outcomes; for example, a study examined the utility of individual SUD treatment characteristics for predicting in-treatment performance and posttreatment outcomes over a 1-year period in the Methamphetamine Treatment Project.[47] The most consistent finding is that pre-treatment methamphetamine use predicted in-treatment performance and posttreatment outcomes, emphasizing the importance of assessing individual and in-treatment characteristics in the development of appropriate treatment plans.[47] Another review exploring gender differences in SUD recurrence showed that, for women, marriage and marital stress were risk factors for recurrence of alcohol use, and, among men, marriage lowered risk for disease recurrence.[48] In contrast to the lack of gender differences in rates of recurrence of alcohol use, this review showed that women appear less likely to experience recurrence of use to substance use relative to men. Women experiencing a recurrence of substance use appear to be more sensitive to negative affect and interpersonal problems. Men, in contrast, may be more likely to have positive experiences prior to recurrence of use.[48]

Even though retention and treatment dosage may predict better outcomes for a given episode of care,[49] multiple episodes of care can also be a marker for individuals who have not been responsive to prior treatment and hence have a worse prognosis.[46,50] Multiple episodes of care seem to be the norm.[51] Treatment episodes may have a cumulative effect on the recovery process.[52] Scott et al.[1] demonstrated the need to adopt a chronic versus acute care model for substance use that helps better identify targets of interventions designed to shorten the cycle of recurrence.

Early studies and reviews of the outcome literature reported rates of recurrence of more than 70% among patients with SUDs participating in treatment.[53,54] Miller and Hester[53] reviewed more than 500 alcoholism outcome studies and reported that three-fourths of subjects experience a recurrence of alcohol use within 1 year. McLellan et al.[3] reviewed more than a hundred clinical trials of SUD treatments and reported that most studies showed significant reductions in substance use, improved personal heath, and reduced social pathology. In addition, they noted that in 1-year-postdischarge follow-up studies, 40% to 60% of individuals discharged from treatment were continuously abstinent, and 15% to 30% had not used substances addictively. Those positive outcomes are similar to those seen with other chronic medical illnesses such as diabetes type 2, hypertension, and asthma. Also, as with other chronic disorders, persons with SUDs have difficulty adhering to treatment, sometimes may discontinue their treatment early, and may experience a recurrence of substance use. Numerous publications of the U.S. Government clinical studies, surveys of individuals in recovery in the United States, United Kingdom, Canada, and Australia, and membership surveys of Alcoholics Anonymous and Narcotics Anonymous show significant improvements of individuals with SUDs who received treatment and participated in mutual aid programs. Improvements include reduced rates of substance use, reduced medical costs, reduced rates of criminal behaviors, improved medical health and health care behaviors, improved psychological functioning, improved employment rates, improved family relationships and more community involvement, financial improvements, and reduced suicidal thoughts and behaviors.[33,34,55-58] Patients who remain in treatment the longest generally have the best outcomes.[59,60]

There is a large body of research-based evidence related to the outcomes of RP treatment and its related mindfulness-based application that supports continued use of the RP Model more than 30 years after it was conceptualized by G. Alan Marlatt. Mindfulness-Based Relapse Prevention (MBRP), a group-based psychosocial intervention, integrates evidence-based practices to decrease the probability and severity of recurrence for patients in SUD aftercare.[61,62] The program incorporates a number of specific components of RP, such as common antecedents of recurrence,[27] and mindfulness-based stress reduction that increases awareness and exposure to emotional and cognitive experience.

EFFECTIVENESS AND EFFICACY OF RECURRENCE PREVENTION

Several studies have evaluated the effectiveness and efficacy of RP approaches for SUDs. Chaney et al.[63] provided the first randomized trial of RP techniques in an inpatient population of people with unhealthy alcohol use. The authors concluded that these peoples' "responses to situations that present a high risk of relapse could be improved through training."

Carroll[64] reviewed randomized controlled trials on the effectiveness of RP among people who smoke (12 studies), individuals with alcohol use disorders (6 studies), individuals with cocaine use disorders (3 studies), individuals with opioid use disorders (1 study), and other individuals with other SUDs (2 studies), using the RP strategies that explicitly cited the work of Marlatt and Gordon.[11] The review examined the relative effectiveness of RP compared with no-treatment controls, attention controls, and an active treatment (interpersonal therapy [IPT], supportive therapy). Carroll concluded that there was evidence for the effectiveness of RP compared with no-treatment controls, particularly in the area of tobacco/nicotine treatment. Carroll found less consistent evidence of effectiveness when RP was compared with discussion control groups or to another active treatment. Results from the analysis also indicate that RP may be particularly promising in reducing the severity of recurrences when they occur, in enhancing durability of treatment effects, and for patients who demonstrate higher levels of impairment across multiple dimensions (psychopathology and addiction severity).

Several studies showed sustained main effects for RP, suggesting that RP may provide continued improvement over a longer period (indicating a "delayed emergence effect" or "sleeper effect"), whereas the effects of other treatments may only be short lived.[65-67] These findings of delayed effects of RP suggest a learning curve, in which there is a higher likelihood of brief use immediately after treatment but learning new coping skills leads to a decreased probability of a more permanent return to use over time. Polivy and Herman[68] emphasized the problem of learning new behaviors and demonstrated that 90% of individuals who attempt to change their behavior struggle with brief periods of return to use and do not achieve change on their first attempt.

Project MATCH is a multisite study sponsored by the National Institute on Alcohol Abuse and Alcoholism that compared three different treatments for 1,726 patients diagnosed with DSM-III-R alcohol abuse or alcohol dependence.[69] Patients were randomly assigned to cognitive-behavioral coping skills therapy (CBT), motivational enhancement therapy (MET), and 12-step facilitation therapy (TSF), all of which were delivered over a 12-week period. Patients in all three conditions demonstrated significant improvements from pretreatment through the 1-year posttreatment follow-up. Surprisingly, no statistically significant differences were found in outcome by type of treatment, and no matching hypotheses were confirmed. Another large study involved 3,018 substance using patients receiving services at 15 Veteran Affairs Medical Centers across the country.[70] Conducted in a naturalistic setting, participants were not randomly assigned to group conditions. Similar to the Project MATCH results, patients in all three conditions (TSF, CBT, or a combination of both) performed equally well at 1-year follow-up. The study used an all-male sample. The study extends MATCH results by illustrating that comparative treatment effectiveness between 12-step and CBT holds across all SUDs all in addition to alcohol.

There have been two meta-analyses of RP. Irvin et al.[71] evaluated the efficacy of Marlatt-based RP across SUDs in a meta-analytic review based on 26 studies representing a sample of 9,504 participants. The authors found a significant overall effect size for reduction in substance use and a much larger effect for improving psychosocial adjustment. Treatment effects were strongest for alcohol and polysubstance use and weaker for tobacco/nicotine use, but all three were significant. The results indicate that certain characteristics of alcohol use are particularly amenable to the RP model. The analysis showed that individual, group, and marital modalities were equally effective.

Randomized trials of RP for tobacco/nicotine showed that additional supportive elements such as stress management, emotion regulation techniques, and abstinence "resource renewal" might be needed in addition to RP in a tobacco/nicotine intervention.[28,72] Research should focus more on improving and modifying RP techniques in the context of other substances such as cocaine and opioids. The most recent meta-analysis focused solely on smoking cigarettes[73] and included 42 studies of controlled trials with at least 6 months of follow-up, most of which used skills-training approaches. Although odd ratios were generally positive, they were small, and no significant effects were found for relapse prevention interventions. These findings are in contrast with the strong meta-analytic evidence for the efficacy of interventions consistent with RP for tobacco/nicotine use reported in the U.S. Public Health Service's Clinical Practice Guideline.[74] These disparate findings may be the result of the analysis using more conservative strategy in evaluating outcomes, and most interventions were low intensity, and the included studies were not limited to Marlatt-based interventions.

Self-help RP interventions have been most commonly used in the area of tobacco/nicotine treatment. Brandon et al.[75,76] conducted two randomized controlled trials of self-help RP intervention for people who used to smoke tobacco who had quit on their own before study enrollment. The first study found that eight RP booklets (based on the principles of GA Marlatt) mailed to those who self-quit over the course of 1-year reduced recurrence of use by two-thirds among those who recently quit. The follow-up study indicated that efficacy was due to the content of the booklets rather than to the frequency of contact made with participants via the repeated mailings, and the intervention was cost-effective relative to other public health interventions.

Randomized controlled trials support the reported efficacy of combined CBT-like therapies and naltrexone for people with DSM-IV-TR alcohol dependence.[77] The Effect of Combined Pharmacotherapies and Behavioral Interventions study suggested that medical management of a patient with alcohol dependence via a physician providing treatment with naltrexone and basic advice and information is as effective as CBT. The trial enrolled 1,383 subjects with alcohol dependence and randomly assigned them to one of eight groups that include naltrexone, acamprosate, or both of the drugs, with or without what was identified as a cognitive-behavioral intervention (CBI). One group received the CBI alone, without placebo. The patients who received a medication received medical management that was fairly rigorous (nine appointments over 16 weeks), during which a physician or a nurse discussed the patient's diagnosis and progress and suggested attendance to Alcoholics Anonymous (AA). Those who got the CBI received up to 20 sessions, which was comparable with a streamlined version of outpatient alcoholism treatment. Subjects receiving medical management with naltrexone, CBI, or both fared better on drinking outcomes, whereas acamprosate showed no evidence of efficacy, with or without CBI. Describing it more from a clinical perspective, the percentage of subjects with a good clinical outcome were 58% for those who received only medical management and placebo, 74% for those who received medical management with naltrexone only, 74% for those who received medical management with naltrexone and CBI, and 71% for those who received medical management with placebo and CBI. The subjects were also followed for a year after the 16-week treatment, and although the patterns of efficacy remained much the same, there was appreciable falloff for all groups. However, there was also a sleeper effect shown for CBI during the initial phases of the follow-up period.[78-81] Maude-Griffin et al.[82] randomized 128 people who used cocaine to either CBT or TSF to test several a priori matching hypotheses. Treatment was delivered in both group and individual sessions. Results suggested that CBT was more effective than TSF overall. CBT was differentially effective for individuals with depression, whereas TSF was more effective for participants with low levels of abstract reasoning skills. A total of 121 individuals meeting the DSM-IV-TR criteria for current cocaine dependence were randomized using a randomized, placebo-controlled, double-masked (for medication condition), factorial (2 × 2) design with four treatment conditions: disulfiram plus CBT, disulfiram plus IPT, placebo plus CBT, and placebo plus IPT.[83] The findings from this study have showed that patients assigned to CBT reduced their cocaine use significantly more than those assigned to IPT, and patients assigned to disulfiram reduced their cocaine use significantly more than those assigned to placebo. Effects of CBT plus placebo were comparable to those of the CBT-disulfiram combination.

The literature evaluating the efficacy and effectiveness of RP with stimulant using patients has been nearly all conducted with those who use cocaine. Some data support the view that the response to RP treatment is quite comparable between people with DSM-IV cocaine dependence and those with methamphetamine dependence.[84] Rawson et al.[85] conducted a multisite study with people with DSM-IV methamphetamine dependence to assess the effectiveness of the Matrix treatment protocol[11,67,85] versus "treatment as usual" in eight community treatment organizations. A total of 978 people with methamphetamine dependence were randomly assigned to outpatient treatment with either the Matrix 16-week protocol or the treatment approach that was routinely used by the eight treatment organizations. The study provided support for the superior treatment response of the Matrix approach in people with methamphetamine dependence. These gains were not significantly different at posttreatment follow-up (ie, not sustained). Clearly, the Matrix treatment approach has positive empirical evidence for treating methamphetamine dependence when compared to a group of community treatment protocols.

Rawson et al.[67] recently compared group CBT, voucher contingency management (CM), and a CBT/CM in combination with standard methadone maintenance treatment for methadone maintenance patients who were using cocaine. During the acute phase of treatment, the CM group had significantly better cocaine use outcomes. However, during the follow-up period, a CBT sleeper effect emerged again, where the CBT group had better outcomes at the 26- and 52-week follow-up than did the CM group. Another study in the context of intensive methadone maintenance showed best 1-year outcomes for the CBT and CM combination.[86] No difference has been found in group versus individually delivered CBT/RP.[87,88]

The empirical evidence on testing RP strategies for DSM-IV-TR cannabis dependence (12 studies) has also sometimes added other treatment components such as aversion training, MET, contingency reinforcement, and case management. A multisite study involving 450 people with cannabis dependence demonstrated that a nine-session individual approach that integrated CBT and motivational interviewing (MI) was more effective than a two-session MI approach, which in turn was more effective than a delayed-treatment control.[89] The relatively modest long-term outcomes reported in the trials conducted thus far suggest that intervention protocols need to be developed to effectively meet the needs of this population. There are no efficacy studies evaluating RP specifically for dissociative, hallucinogens, inhalants, and steroid use disorders.[90]

Several studies included spouses in the RP intervention.[91,92] A recent study evaluated conjoint treatments in 90 men with unhealthy alcohol use and their female partners. The subjects were randomly assigned to one of the three outpatient conjoint treatments: alcohol behavioral couples therapy (ABCT), ABCT with RP techniques (RP/ABCT),[11] or ABCT with interventions encouraging AA involvement (AA/ABCT). Couples were followed 18 months after treatment. Across the three treatment approaches, subjects who provided follow-up data-maintained abstinence on almost 80% of days during follow-up, with no difference in drinking or marital happiness outcomes between groups. In the RP/ABCT treatment, attendance at posttreatment booster sessions was related to posttreatment abstinence. AA attendance was positively related to abstinence during follow-up treatment in both concurrent and time-lagged analyses.[93] Despite strong evidence for efficacy of psychosocial treatments for alcohol use disorders, aggregate rates of continuous abstinence are well below 50%, and recurrences of use are more common than abstinence, indicating the need for more efforts to develop efficacious treatments.[94]

To date, based on many meta-analyses, other studies, and narrative reviews, RP is currently identified as an evidence-based program by the U.S. SAMHSA National Registry of Evidence-Based Programs and Practices.[95] So, despite several limitations to studies on RP, the literature generally favors the efficacy and effectiveness of RP and shows that RP strategies especially as a component of a multimodal treatment approach enhance the recovery of individuals with SUDs.

RELAPSE REPLICATION AND EXTENSION PROJECT

In a series of studies led by the National Institute on Alcohol Abuse and Alcoholism called the "Relapse Replication Extension Project" (RREP), aspects of RP including Marlatt's taxonomy for relapse determinants were explored. The RREP focused on the identification of high-risk situations, and several studies in it showed that the taxonomy had minimal ability to predict drinking outcomes.[96,97] While many of the RREP findings are quite supportive of the original RP model,[17] other data in the RREP raised significant methodological issues concerning the predictive validity of Marlatt's[98] relapse taxonomy model and coding system.[97,99] Based on the findings, a major reconceptualization and expansion of the relapse taxonomy was recommended.[100,101] Longabaugh et al.[99] suggested a revision of the taxonomy categories to include greater distinction between inter- and intrapersonal determinants of relapse. A new reconceptualization of cognitive-behavioral model of recurrence of use that focuses on the dynamic interactions between multiple risk factors and situational determinants was proposed and will be discussed later.[32]

DETERMINANTS OF RELAPSE

Marlatt et al.[17] developed a taxonomy of high-risk situations that included three hierarchically arranged levels of categories used in the classification of relapse episodes. The first level distinguishes between the intrapersonal and interpersonal precipitants of relapse. The second level consists of eight subdivisions including five within the intrapersonal category and three within the interpersonal category. The third level of the taxonomy provides a more detailed inspection of five of the eight level two subdivisions. This classification scheme has been found useful in other countries[102,103] and is supported by prospective studies.[104,105] It also has been used as the basis of research protocols,[106] treatment protocols,[107] and patient recovery guides.[108,109] In this section, we review the most commonly identified "relapse" determinants based on Marlatt's relapse taxonomy.

Intrapersonal Determinants

Self-Efficacy

Self-efficacy refers to individuals' beliefs in their capabilities to organize and carry out specific courses of action to attain some goal or situation-specific task.[110] These beliefs have great influence on self-regulation and the quality of human functioning because they shape the goals individuals set for themselves, the persistence in reaching those goals, and the effectiveness of problem-solving activities.[111] Individuals' sense of efficacy is the result of their cognitive processing from many sources of efficacy information.[111] This construct is intimately related to the individual's coping abilities and reflects the degree of confidence that the individual has about being confronted with a high-risk situation and successfully avoiding a recurrence of use, however brief. The patient's personal belief in his or her ability to control his or her substance use is a reliable predictor of recurrence of use immediately after treatment[112,113] and over long-term outcomes.[114] In general, self-efficacy is a predictor of outcomes across all types of addiction, including gambling and various substances.[115] Low levels of self-efficacy are predictive of recurrence of use.[116] Shiffman et al.[117] found that baseline self-efficacy was as predictive of the first use of smoked tobacco as daily measures of self-efficacy, explaining the stability of self-efficacy during abstinence. More evidence from a daily monitoring study showed decreases in self-efficacy preceded a first use on the following day and daily variation in self-efficacy predicted transitions from first use to heavier use.[112] Given the relationship between self-efficacy and recurrence of sustained use, self-efficacy should be thoroughly assessed during treatment and appropriately targeted for interventions.

Outcome Expectancies

A factor enhancing the likelihood of recurrence of use is the set of cognitive expectancies that individuals develop about the expected outcomes associated with behaviors relating to their addiction or SUD. Such expectancies are known as outcome expectancies.[118] Underlying motives for engaging in behaviors relating to addiction include a desire to both change one's mood and to increase sociability.[119] Individuals who developed an addiction typically have developed a set of expectancies that anticipate positive outcomes from engaging in the behavior, serving as a source of motivation to engage in it. Such outcome expectancies are shaped by an individual's past direct and indirect experience with the behaviors related to the addiction, including vicarious learning through the modeling they see early on displayed by parents and later by peers.[120] Jones et al.[121] reported that although expectancies are strongly related to outcome, there is little evidence that targeting expectancies in treatment leads to changes in posttreatment consumption. There is a possibility that expectancies influence outcome via their relationship with other disease recurrence predictors. In fact, outcome expectancies may be influencing substance use behavior via the relationship between negative emotional states and beliefs about substances relieving negative affect, particularly among treatment-seeking individuals.[122,123] When individuals endorse positive outcome expectancies at the beginning of treatment, some evidence supports the use of an intervention to challenge expectancies.[124]

Craving

Although craving has been implicated in general in the process of recurrence of use or disease, its role in alcohol recurrence remains controversial, because studies examining the relationship of craving to recurrence of use have yielded equivocal results.[125] Multiple and often conflicting theories, definitions, and measurements have plagued the study of craving. Craving has been described as a cognitive experience focused on the desire to use a substance and is often highly related to expectancies for the desired effect of the substance, whereas an urge has been defined as the behavioral intention or impulse to use a substance or gambling. One common finding is that craving is a poor predictor of recurrence of use.[126,127] Lower spirituality upon admission into SUD treatment, weaker alcohol refusal self-efficacy, and higher self-reported levels of depression differentiated subjects with craving (from those without craving). Patients who crave alcohol in residential treatment may be at higher risk for recurrence of alcohol use and identified by intake assessments of self-efficacy, depression, and spirituality.[128] Another study demonstrated that stress-induced cocaine craving is predictive of recurrence of cocaine use outcomes.[129] Mindfulness and meditation may provide a useful antidote to the experience of craving.[130,131] The heightened state of present-focused awareness that is encouraged by meditation may directly counteract the conditioned automatic response to use alcohol in response to cravings and urges. In addition, the use of anticraving medications, which is described later, can pharmacologically reduce the experience of craving.

Motivation

An important element in determining the likelihood of recurrence of use is the individual's commitment to or motivation for self-improvement.[132] The motivation may relate to the recurrence of use process in two distinct ways: the motivation for positive behavior change and the motivation to engage in the problematic behavior. Motivation is judged with regard to a particular action or outcome. The transtheoretical model of the stages of change, precontemplation, contemplation, preparation, action, and maintenance, are measured in relation to a specific behavior or goal.[133] Precontemplation represents the lowest level of readiness to change. A person's level of motivation (eg, desire, self-efficacy, readiness, problem recognition) is action specific. A person might be quite motivated for change but not for treatment. People who use multiple substances commonly show levels of motivation that are different depending on the drug. The most common motivational obstacle to early help seeking is ambivalence. The ambivalence toward change is highly related to self-efficacy and outcome expectancies. Baer et al.[9] indicated that an analysis of recurrence of use needs to examine the interaction between commitment and coping skills. Even well-developed coping abilities will not prevent disease recurrence if the individual's commitment to remain abstinent is low; conversely, strong commitment may be insufficient in the absence of adequate coping skills. Interventions that focus on addressing ambivalence (decisional balance) may increase intrinsic motivation by allowing patients to explore their own values and how they differ from their actual behavioral choices. MI is a collaborative person-centered form of guiding to elicit and strengthen motivation for change.[134] MI has demonstrated efficacy for reducing alcohol consumption and frequency of drinking in this population. Rohsenow et al.[135] evaluated the effectiveness of MET and group coping skills in individuals with cocaine use disorders and showed that the motivational intervention had better substance use outcomes with individuals having a low level of initial motivation to change when compared with those with higher levels of initial motivation. Thus, it is important to assess commitment and motivation to change and understand that motivation for change is composed of multiple dimensions that are at best modestly inter-correlated. Interventions designed to enhance commitment to change should be a component of any RP approach.

Coping

Based on the cognitive-behavioral model of recurrence of use, the most critical predictor of recurrence is the individual's ability to utilize adequate coping strategies in dealing with high-risk situations. The assessment of coping in general[136] and more specifically in relation to recurrence is very challenging.[137,138] A number of different dimensions of coping need to be considered in the assessment process.[18] Coping has been shown to be a critical predictor of substance use treatment outcomes and is often the strongest predictor of behavioral slips of substance use in the moment.[139-141] Moos and Holahan[136] highlighted the distinction between approach and avoidance coping. Approach coping may involve attempts to accept, confront, and reframe, as a means of coping, whereas avoidance coping may include distraction from cues or engaging in other activities. Chung et al.[142] predicted 12-month treatment outcomes in patients with alcohol use disorder by focusing on the distinction between the behavioral and cognitive components of approach and avoidance coping. Results suggested that avoidance coping, particularly cognitive avoidance coping, was predictive of fewer alcohol ("alcohol problem severity" and "alcohol dependence symptoms"), interpersonal, and psychological problems at the 12-month follow-up. Behavioral approach coping also predicted decreased alcohol problem severity at 12-month follow-up. Coping appears to be a dynamic process.[31] The dynamic interaction between coping, self-efficacy, and motivation explains alcohol treatment outcomes.[143,144] Coping may be also experienced as inaction. Inaction has been understood as the acceptance of substance cues,[143] which can be described as "letting go" and not acting on an urge. This view is consistent with the Buddhist notion of skillful means.[145] The focus is not about "doing what is right," but rather the goal is "just do." An example of that coping strategy is the use of "urge surfing."[146] In this strategy, the patient is first taught to label internal sensations and cognitive preoccupation as an urge and to foster an attitude of detachment from the urge. The focus is on identifying and accepting the urge, not attempting to fight it. In a study on the effectiveness of a mindfulness meditation technique of the Vipassana tradition in reducing substance use in an incarcerated population, participants reported that accepting the "here and now," "staying in the moment," and being mindful of the urges were helpful coping strategies.[147]

Emotional States

Studies have reported a strong link between negative affect and recurrence of substance use.[148,149] Baker et al.[150] identified negative affect as the primary motive for drug use. Excessive substance use is motivated by affective regulation, both positive and negative. Furthermore, substance use is often reinforcing for patients, leading the individual to engage in future substance use. Oftentimes, substance use provides negative reinforcement via the amelioration of an unpleasant affective state, such as physical withdrawal symptoms.[150] Thus, clinicians should incorporate strategies to decrease and manage negative emotional states as a part of the RP approach.

Interpersonal Determinants

Stanton[151] reviewed the research on the role of social support in brief slips of substance use and provided an overview of interpersonal dynamics as a high-risk situation for recurrence of sustained use. However, the relationship between interpersonal factors and recurrence of use is not well understood.[93,152] Functional social support or the level of emotional support is highly predictive of long-term abstinence across several addictions.[153-155] The social support network size, the perceived quality of social support, and the level of support from non-substance using people have also been shown to predict recurrence of sustained use.[154,155] Negative social support in the form of interpersonal conflict and social pressure to use substances has been related to an increased risk of sustained return to use.[156] Behavioral marital therapy, which incorporates partner support in treatment goals, has been described as one of the top three empirically supported treatment methods for alcohol problems.[157,158]

MODELS OF RELAPSE PREVENTION

As discussed previously, most of the RP interventions have a multicomponent character. Studies of treatment interventions such as MET, CM, individual and group counseling approaches, and case management typically have included RP modules.[12,13] Psychopharmacological interventions combined with RP are evaluated as a part of an overall treatment strategy to reduce risk for recurrence of use and improve abstinence rates.[77] Various models of RP are described in the literature, and many of these have been adapted for use in clinical trials. There are summaries of various RP models[17,108] in the literature. RP models include the following:

- Marlatt and Gordon's cognitive-behavioral approach.[12,157]
- Annis' cognitive-behavioral approach,[159] which incorporates concepts of Marlatt's model with Bandura's self-efficacy theory.
- Daley's psychoeducational approach,[12,25] which adapted Marlatt's classification of relapse precipitants to a treatment protocol that can be used in individual or group sessions.
- Gorski's neurological impairment model, which incorporates elements from the disease model of addiction and relapse, as well as Marlatt's model.[160]
- Zackon, McAuliffe, and Chien's recovery training and self-help model.[161]
- The Matrix neurobehavioral model of treatment of Rawson et al., which includes RP as a central component of treatment.[162-164]
- Washton's intensive outpatient model,[36,37] which includes significant attention to RP during the third phase of treatment.
- The coping/social skills-training model of Monti et al.,[165] which served as the basis of the cognitive-behavioral therapy in Project MATCH.
- The cue extinction (CE) model developed by Childress et al.[19]

The Cognitive-Behavioral Model of Relapse

Drawing from the taxonomy of high-risk situations, Marlatt proposed the first cognitive-behavioral model of the relapse process.[11] As shown in **Figure 80-1**, the model centers on the individual's response to high-risk situations. The components include the interaction between the person (affect, coping, self-efficacy, outcome expectancies) and environmental risk factors such as social influences, cue exposure, and access to substance. If the individual lacks an adequate coping response or confidence to deal with the situation (low self-efficacy), the tendency is "to give in to temptation." The "decision" to use or not is then mediated by the individual's outcome expectancies for the initial effects of using the substance. The combination of being unable to cope effectively in a high-risk situation and positive outcome expectancies greatly increases the probability that an initial substance use will occur. Whether the first use is followed by a recurrence to sustained use depends in part on the person's attributions as to the cause of return to use and the reactions associated with its occurrence. Individuals who decide to use the substance may be vulnerable to the abstinence violation effect. Persons who experience intense abstinence violation effect such as conflict and self-blame after a initial use

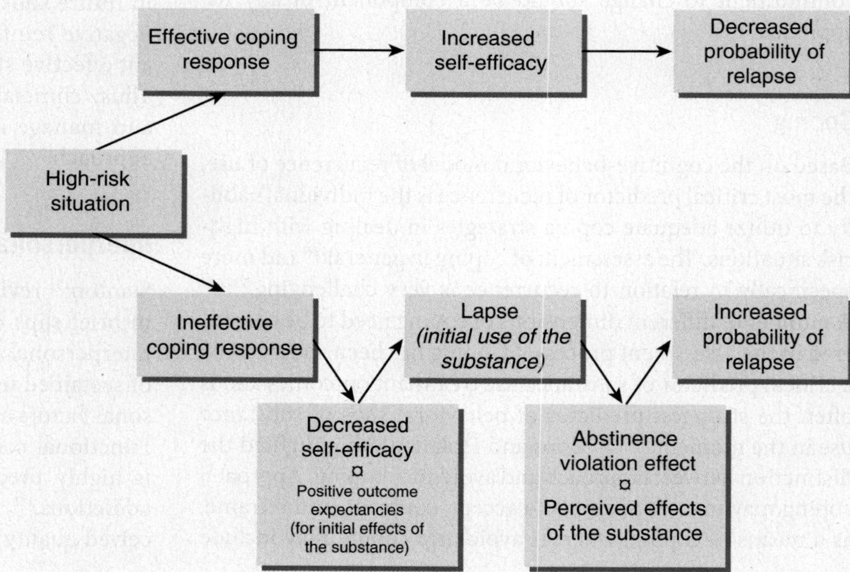

Figure 80-1. Cognitive-behavioral model of relapse/disease recurrence.

go through a motivation crisis (demoralization) that undermines their commitment to abstinence goals. The initial use is more likely to lead to sustained use if the person views it as an irreparable failure. The individual's restorative coping abilities to deal with the negative consequences and emotions, the reaction of friends and family, and the individual's commitment to return to abstinence or moderation/harm reduction should be considered.

The Cognitive-Behavioral Model of Relapse, Revised

Based on previous descriptions of "relapse" as complex process, Witkiewitz and Marlatt[32] proposed a dynamic model of the relapse process. This model incorporates the temporal dynamic relationships between cognitive (self-efficacy, outcome expectancies, motivation, craving, abstinence violation effect), behavioral (coping strategies), affective (emotional states), and physical (withdrawal) processes, leading up to, and during, a high-risk situation. In every situation, an individual is faced with the challenge of balancing multiple cues and possible consequences. According to the model, the interrelationship between these processes is contextual, but the driving force behind the processes may be traced back to an individual's vulnerability to recurrence of sustained use. As shown in Figure 80-2, this model allows for several configurations of distal and proximal relapse risks. Distal risks (solid lines) are defined as stable predispositions that increase an individual's vulnerability to lapse (years of dependence, family history, social support, and comorbid psychopathology), whereas proximal risks (dotted lines) are immediate precipitants that actualize the statistical probability of a lapse. Connected boxes are hypothesized to be related through reciprocal causation (eg, coping skills influence drinking behavior and, in turn, drinking influences coping).[166] These feedback loops (indicated by double-headed arrows) allow for the bidirectional interaction between cognitions and lapse, as well as affect and lapse. Coping is shown as directly interrelated with lapse. The difference between a feedback loop and interrelatedness in the model is primarily a consideration of the distinction between the tonic and the phasic processes. The large striped circle in Figure 80-2 indicates the role of contextual factors, with situational cues (eg, walking by the liquor store) moderating the relationship between risk factors and substance use behavior.[143] The source of support for the model comes from clinical anecdotes and recent empirical studies on the complexity of substance use behavior.[30,32,167-171] Recognizing the complexity of the disease recurrence process may help clinicians see the importance of a comprehensive assessment of multiple domains related to relapse.[18] The consideration of how the factors in the domains may interact within a high-risk situation and how changes in proximal risk factors can alter behavior leading up to high-risk situations will enable patients to continually assess their own vulnerability to disease recurrence.

Clinical Relapse Prevention Interventions to Reduce Risk for Initial Use or Sustained Use

This section describes practical RP clinical interventions that reflect the models of RP discussed earlier and approaches of

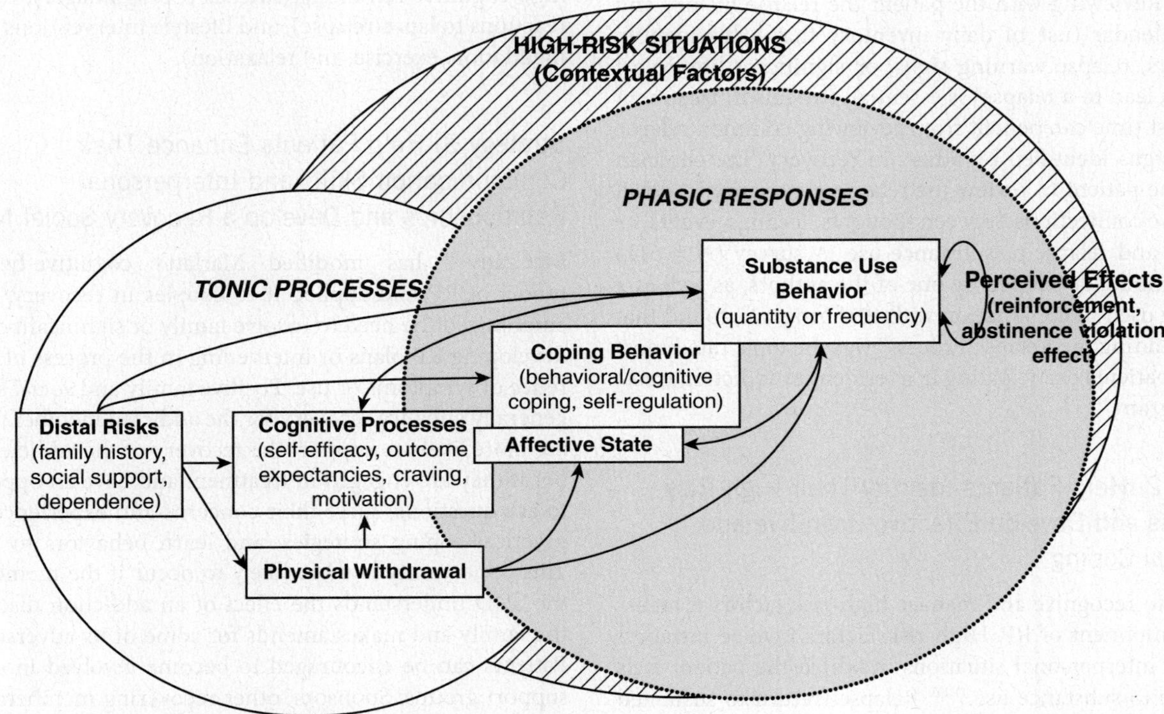

Figure 80-2. Dynamic model of relapse/disease recurrence.

numerous clinicians and researchers who have developed specific models of RP or written patient-oriented RP recovery materials. The literature emphasizes individualizing RP strategies, considering the patient's level of motivation, severity of substance use, ego functioning, and sociocultural environment. These RP interventions can be provided in individual or group sessions (many RP programs were designed for small groups of participants).[12,19,37,172,173] The most recent version of the counselor's manual detailing the clinical interventions has incorporated the theoretical bases of RP as discussed above.[12,174]

The use of experiential learning or action techniques such as role-playing or behavioral rehearsal, metaphors, monodramas, psychodrama, bibliotherapy, use of workbooks, a daily inventory, interactive videos, and homework assignments makes learning an active experience for the patient. Such techniques enhance self-awareness, decrease defensiveness, facilitate acquisition, and practice of coping skills, and encourage behavioral change.[8,19,38,108,109,161]

Strategy 1: Help Patients Understand Relapse as a Process and Not an Event, and Learn to Identify Warning Signs

The understanding of addiction as a chronic cyclical condition often involving many transitions between lapse, relapse, and recovery helps the patient look at relapse as a process occurring in certain context and understand that early warning signs often precede initial return to use. Attitudinal, emotional, cognitive, and behavioral changes seem to occur days, weeks, and even longer before resuming the use of substances.[25] Warning signs can be conceptualized as links in a relapse chain.[26,35] Reviewing with the patient the relapse history and relapse calendar (use of daily inventory that helps identify risk factors, relapse warning signs, or significant life events that could lead to a relapse) is essential. Patients in treatment for the first time can benefit from reviewing common relapse warning signs identified by others in recovery. The clinician can ask the patient to review the relapse experience in detail to learn the connections between thoughts, feelings, events, or situations and relapse to substance use. A survey (N = 511) of an RP model developed by one of the authors, as well as a workbook used in conjunction with that program, found that "Understanding the Relapse Process" was the topic rated most useful by patients participating in a residential addiction treatment program.[175]

Strategy 2: Help Patients Identify Their High-Risk Situations and Develop Effective Cognitive and Behavioral Coping

The need to recognize and manage high-risk factors is an essential component of RP. High-risk factors involve intrapersonal and interpersonal situations in which the patient feels vulnerable to substance use.[11,176] Relapse (return to sustained use) is more likely to occur as the result of lack of coping skills than the high-risk situation itself, so the clinician should assess the patient's coping style to identify targets for an intervention.[103,177] A person "heading for a relapse" usually makes a number of mini-decisions over time, each of which brings the person closer to creating a high-risk situation or giving in. These choices are called "apparently irrelevant decisions," and they need to be identified and addressed with patients to decrease risk for use. The meaning of specific high-risk factors also varies among patients. RP strategies and interventions therefore need to consider the nuances of each patient's high-risk factors. For example, two patients identified depression as a serious risk for return to use. In the first case, depression was described as the rather common and normal feeling experienced when the patient realized that his drug addiction caused serious problems in his relationships with his wife and children. Getting his family involved in his treatment, facilitating their attendance at self-help meetings, and helping him make amends to them and spend time with them led to improvement in his mood. In the second case, the patient's depression worsened significantly the longer she was sober from alcohol. Although she felt that some of the behavioral and cognitive strategies explored in therapy were helpful in improving her mood, it was not until she took an antidepressant that she experienced the full benefits of treatment. Both of these patients reported that an improved mood was a significant factor in their ability to prevent a subsequent return to use and to addiction. Marlatt,[178] for example, suggested that in addition to teaching patients "specific" RP skills to deal with high-risk factors, the clinician also should use "global" approaches such as problem-solving or skills-training strategies (such as behavioral rehearsal, covert modeling, and assertiveness training), cognitive reframing (such as coping imagery, reframing reactions to lapse/relapse), and lifestyle interventions (such as meditation, exercise, and relaxation).

Strategy 3: Help Patients Enhance Their Communication Skills and Interpersonal Relationships and Develop a Recovery Social Network

McCrady[179] has modified Marlatt's cognitive-behavioral model of RP and applied it to couples in recovery. Daley[175] emphasized the need to involve family or significant others in developing RP plans or intervening in the process of a recurrence of symptoms or use. Positive family and social supports generally enhance recovery for the addicted member. Families are more likely to support the recovery of the addicted member if they are engaged in treatment and have an opportunity to ask questions, share their concerns and experiences, learn practical coping strategies, and learn behaviors to avoid.[180] This opportunity is more likely to occur if the member with the SUD understands the effect of an addiction disorder on the family and makes amends for some of its adverse effects. Patients can be encouraged to become involved in self-help support groups. Sponsors, other recovering members of self-help groups, personal friends, and employers can become part of an individual's RP network. The following are some suggested steps for helping patients develop an RP network. First, the patient needs to identify whom to include in or exclude from this network. Others who engage in using substances, harbor strong negative feelings toward the recovering person, or who generally are not supportive of recovery usually should be excluded. The patient then can determine how and when to ask for support or help. Behavioral rehearsal can help the patient practice ways to make specific requests for support. Rehearsal also helps to increase confidence and clarify thoughts and feelings about reaching out for help. Rehearsal can help to clarify the patient's ambivalence about asking for help or support from others. This process helps the patient better understand how the person being asked for support can respond, thus preparing the patient for potentially negative responses from others.

Some patients find it helpful to put their action plan into writing. The action plan can address the following issues: how to communicate about and deal with warning signs and high-risk situations, how to interrupt initial use from progressing to sustained use, how to intervene if use occurs, and the importance of exploring all the details of initial or sustained use after the patient is stable so that it can be used as a learning experience.

Strategy 4: Help Patients Reduce, Identify, and Manage Negative Emotional States

Negative affective states, such as depression and anxiety, are factors in a substantial number of recurrences of use.[105] Zackon[181] believed that persons with a SUD frequently experience recurrence of use as a result of joylessness in their lives. Shiffman et al.,[138] found that coping responses for high-risk situations were less effective for people who smoked tobacco and also had depression. Other negative affective states associated with recurrence include anger and boredom.[35] The acronym HALT, frequently cited by members of AA, Narcotics Anonymous (NA), and Crystal Meth Anonymous (CMA), speaks to this important issue of negative affect when it warns not to become too *h*ungry, too *a*ngry, too *l*onely, or too *t*ired. Interventions that help patients develop appropriate coping skills for managing negative emotional states depend on the issues and needs of the individual.

Strategy 5: Help Patients Identify and Manage Cravings and Cues That Precede Cravings

A strong desire or craving for a substance can be triggered by exposure to environmental or internal cues associated with prior use. Cues such as the sight or smell of the substance can trigger cravings that are evidenced in increased thoughts of using and physiological changes (eg, anxiety). The concept of craving is not clearly defined across autonomic, behavioral, or subjective domains. Further, trials looking at craving and recurrence of use may be measuring different aspects of the phenomenon.[127] What is clear is that craving has clinical meaning. Cue Exposure (CE) treatment[182] is one method used to help patients identify drug use triggers and master or learn to control the conditioned response to those triggers. This treatment differs from the traditional focus on "avoiding people, places, and things" and instead involves exposing the patient to specific cues associated with substance use. CE aims to enhance behavioral and cognitive coping skills as well as the patient's confidence in his or her ability to resist the desire to use. Systematic relaxation, behavioral alternatives, visual imagery, and cognitive interventions are used in CE. Several studies have validated CE.[182,183] The clinician can provide information about cues and how they trigger cravings for alcohol or other drugs. Monitoring and recording cravings, associated thoughts, and outcomes in a daily log or journal can help patients become more vigilant and prepare them to cope when they occur. Cognitive interventions include changing thoughts about the craving or desire to use, challenging euphoric recall, talking oneself through the craving, thinking beyond the high by identifying negative consequences of using (immediate and delayed) and positive benefits of not using, using 12-step recovery slogans, and delaying the decision to use. Behavioral interventions include avoiding, leaving, or changing situations that trigger or worsen a craving; redirecting activities or becoming involved in pleasant activities; obtaining help or support from others by admitting and talking about cravings and hearing how others have survived them; attending self-help support group meetings; or taking medications that reduce craving and increase confidence in the ability to cope.

As discussed earlier, Marlatt and his colleagues developed a new approach to the treatment of addiction, MBRP, an outpatient program that integrates skills from cognitive-behavioral RP and training in mindfulness meditation practices.[184] The overall goal of MBRP is to develop awareness and nonjudgmental acceptance of thoughts, sensations, and emotional states, through the practice of mindfulness meditation, and to practice these skills as a coping strategy in the face of high-risk trigger situations for recurrence of use.[26] Between-session practice and therapeutic alliance appear to be important factors in the initial increases in mindfulness after mindfulness-based treatments.[185] One example of how mindfulness meditation can be helpful in preventing disease or use recurrence is known as "urge surfing."[143] The patient is instructed to "detach" from his or her craving by externalizing and labeling it. Similar to a surfer who must learn to ride the waves so as not to get wiped out, the patient imagines "riding the crest" of an urge or craving, maintaining balance until the crest has finally broken and the wave of feeling subsides. The process of incorporating a mindfulness practice and learning to accept and tolerate urges fits well within RP therapy.[186]

Strategy 6: Help Patients Identify and Challenge Cognitive Distortions

Marlatt[178] observed "the patient's cognitive errors and distortions may increase the probability that an initial slip will develop into a total relapse." Twelve-step programs refer to these patterns as "stinking thinking" and suggest that recovering persons need to alter their thinking if they are to remain alcohol and drug free. Teaching patients to identify their negative thinking patterns or cognitive errors (eg, black-and-white thinking, overgeneralizing, catastrophizing, jumping to conclusions) and to evaluate how these affect recovery and recurrence of use is one strategy. Patients then can be taught to use counter thoughts to challenge their thinking errors or specific negative thoughts. One way to achieve this is to have the patient discuss or write down specific substance or gambling use–related thoughts (eg, "I will never use alcohol or drugs again," "I can control my use of alcohol or other drugs," "a few drinks, tokes, pills, lines will not hurt," "recovery is not happening fast enough," "I need alcohol or other drugs to have fun," and "my problem is cured") and challenge them to and address them to minimize the risk of disease recurrence.[34] Many of the 12-step slogans were devised to help people with SUDs alter their thinking and survive desires to use substances. Slogans such as "this too will pass," "let go and let God," and "one day at a time" have helped many patients manage thoughts of using.

Strategy 7: Help Patients Work Toward a More Balanced Lifestyle

In addition to identifying and managing intrapersonal and interpersonal high-risk factors, patients can benefit from global changes to restore or achieve balance in their lives.[178] Development of a healthy lifestyle is seen as important in reducing stress that makes the patient less vulnerable to disease recurrence or substance use. Lifestyle can be assessed by evaluating patterns of daily activities, sources of stress, stressful life events, daily hassles and uplifts, the balance between "wants" (activities engaged in for pleasure or self-fulfillment) and "shoulds" (external demands), health, exercise and relaxation patterns, interpersonal activities, and religious beliefs.[178] Working with patients to develop positive habits or substitute indulgences (such as jogging, meditation, relaxation, exercise, hobbies, or creative tasks) for an addiction disorder can help balance their lifestyles.[187] Patients with a need for greater adventure or action may become involved in more challenging activities.[35]

Strategy 8: Consider the Use of Medications in Combination With Psychosocial Treatments

In the treatment of substance use and gambling disorders, there are two goals for the use of medications: to help patients attain an initial period of abstinence after treating withdrawal syndromes and to assist patients with disease remission. There is now a range of medications available for some of the major classes of addictive substances. None of the medications approved for treating DSM-IV-TR alcohol dependence has proven effective without some form of concurrent behavioral therapy. The best use of medications may be in combination with one another and with psychosocial interventions. For example, treatment with both acamprosate and naltrexone has been shown to be efficacious in reducing risk for alcohol use and is safe.[188,189] Furthermore, studies show that individuals who experience recurrence of use while on these medications still drink a lot less, which presumably means fewer negative consequences. It was hypothesized that naltrexone would specifically attenuate reward craving and acamprosate would diminish relief craving. Naltrexone seems more indicated in programs geared to controlled consumption (harm reduction) because it has been shown to reduce the recurrence of heavy alcohol use but was not associated with a significant change in the abstinence rate, whereas acamprosate seems especially useful in a therapeutic approach targeted at achieving abstinence because it appears to be associated with a significant improvement in abstinence rates.[190] The old concept of total abstinence as the only goal to treat alcohol use disorder stemmed from two sources: AA and the use of medications such as disulfiram, which makes a person feel sick when she or he drinks (aversive response to alcohol). A survey of AA members' attitudes about taking a medication to help prevent alcohol use recurrence yielded an interesting finding. Only 17% of the 277 AA members surveyed believed they should *not* take a medication; more than 50% of the sample thought medication that helped reduce drinking was a good idea.[191] Although many patients may benefit from the use of available medications for the treatment of alcohol use disorders, their treatment effects are moderate at best, and some individuals fail to respond. This to some degree reflects the heterogeneous nature of the patients and possibly of the illness itself. Clearly, in the treatment of patients with alcohol use disorders, one size does not fit all. At present, no medication is U.S. Food and Drug Administration approved for the treatment of stimulant use disorders. Three types of U.S. Food and Drug Administration-approved medications are available to treat nicotine use disorders: sustained-release bupropion, nicotine replacement therapies, and varenicline. Research showed that the combined effects of the pharmacological and behavioral treatment are additive.[192] Medications can be of major benefit in preventing recurrence of use in opioid use disorders. These medications can provide antagonism to the reinforcing effects of opioid drugs and can provide stable replacement for drug use. These medications include opioid agonist agents such as methadone, a partial agonist, buprenorphine, and an opioid antagonist such as naltrexone. Despite some clinical trials with good outcomes, medications are still under prescribed by physicians.

Strategy 9: Facilitate the Transition Between Levels of Care for Patients Completing Residential or Hospital-Based Inpatient Treatment Programs, or Structured Partial Hospital or Intensive Outpatient Programs

Patients can make significant gains in residential or DT programs only to have the gains negated because of failure to adhere to ongoing outpatient or aftercare treatment. Interventions used to enhance treatment entry and adherence that also lower the risk for recurrence of use include providing a single session of motivational therapy before discharge from residential or intensive treatment, using telephone or mail reminders of initial treatment appointments, and providing reinforcers for appropriate participation in treatment activities or for providing drug-free urine tests.[193] In a quality improvement survey, the authors found that a single motivational therapy session provided to hospitalized psychiatric patients with comorbid SUDs led to a nearly twofold increase in the show rate for the initial outpatient appointment.[194] Patients who complied with their initial appointment had a reduced risk of treatment discontinuation and subsequent psychiatric or substance use recurrence.

Strategy 10: Incorporate Strategies to Improve Adherence to Treatment and Medications

Numerous studies and reports show that patients who are retained in treatment show better outcomes, including lower use recurrence rates, than those who discontinue their treatment early.[59,60] Many clinical and systems strategies have been shown to improve adherence to treatment among patients with SUDs and co-occurring disorders.[194]

PREVENTION OF RECURRENCE FOR CO-OCCURRING DISORDERS

Individuals with severe mental illness and SUDs have increased vulnerability for recurrence because of many challenges including cognitive and social skills deficits and psychosocial issues. There is a significantly high rate of co-occurring mood and anxiety disorders with SUDs.[195] For example, co-occurring posttraumatic stress disorder (PTSD) and SUD is common and associated with poorer treatment outcomes than found with SUD only.[196,197] Recent evidence suggests that patients with unremitted PTSD are at greater risk than those with remitted PTSD for continued SUD problems and that improvement in PTSD symptoms strongly associated with improvement in alcohol-related symptoms than is the inverse relationship.[198] Many CBI and other interventions such as mindfulness-based approach targeting this population have been associated with reductions in substance use.[199,200] In addition, pharmacological interventions have been demonstrated to improve outcomes for patients with comorbid depression, bipolar disorder, and SUDs.[195,201,202]

CONCLUSIONS

Recurrence of use or disease (historically termed "relapse") is a major challenge in the treatment of addiction. The dynamic model of relapse acknowledges the complexity and unpredictable nature of substance use behavior after the commitment to abstinence or a harm reduction goal. An adequate assessment model must be sufficiently comprehensive to include theoretically relevant variables from each of the domains of relapse and different levels of potential predictors. Clinical RP strategies can be used throughout the continuum of care and be integrated with other treatment modalities such as MI and CM, pharmacotherapy, spirituality, mindfulness-based, 12-step mutual support groups, and family-based interventions. Several areas for future research, including examining the dynamic interplay of disease recurrence factors, will add to the understanding of recurrence of substance or gambling use and how to prevent it as well as the dynamic models of treatment outcomes, extensions of RP to incorporate mindfulness, research on the mechanisms of the process of intentional behavior change and natural recovery, the role of genetic influences on treatment response and disease recurrence, and neurobiological determinants of the disease recurrence process using innovative neuroimaging modalities.

REFERENCES

1. Scott CK, Foss MA, Dennis ML. Pathways in the relapse–treatment–recovery cycle over 3 years. *J Subst Abus Treat*. 2005;28:S63-S72.
2. Salomé HJ, French MT, Miller M, McLellan AT. Estimating the client costs of addiction treatment: first findings from the Client DATCAP. *Drug Alcohol Depend*. 2003;71:195-206.
3. McLellan AT, Lewis DC, O'Brien CP, Kleber HD. Drug dependence, a chronic medical illness: implications for treatment, insurance, and outcomes evaluation. *JAMA*. 2000;284:1689-1695.
4. Cunningham JA, Lin E, Ross HE, Walsh GW. Factors associated with untreated remissions from alcohol abuse or dependence. *Addict Behav*. 2000;25:317-321.
5. Kelly JF, Bergman B, Hoeppner B, et al. Prevalence, pathways and predictors of recovery from drug and alcohol problems in the U.S. population. *Drug Alcohol Depend*. 2017;181:162-169.
6. Annglin MD, Hser YI, Grella CE, et al. Drug treatment careers: conceptual overview and clinical, research, and policy implications. In: Tims F, Leukefeld C, Platt J, eds. *Relapse and Recovery in Addictions*. Yale University Press; 2001:18-39.
7. Hendershot C, Witkiewitz K, George W, Marlatt AG. Relapse prevention for addictive behaviors. *Subst Abuse Treat Prev Policy*. 2011;6:17.
8. Dimeff LA, Marlatt GA. Relapse prevention. In: Hester R, Miller W, eds. *Handbook of Alcoholism Treatment Approaches*. 2nd ed. Allyn & Bacon; 1995:176-194.
9. Baer JS, Kivlahan DR, Donovan DM. Integrating skills training and motivational therapies: implications for the treatment of substance dependence. *J Subst Abus Treat*. 1999;17(1-2):15-23.
10. Donovan D, Witkiewitz K. Relapse prevention: from radical idea to common practice. *Addict Res Theory*. 2012;20(3):204-217.
11. Marlatt GA, Gordon JR, eds. *Relapse Prevention: Maintenance Strategies in the Treatment of Addiction Behaviors*. Guilford Press; 1985.
12. Daley DC, Douaihy A. *Relapse Prevention Counseling: Clinical Strategies to Guide Addiction Recovery and Reduce Relapse*. PESI Publishing & Media; 2015.
13. National Institute on Drug Abuse (NIDA). *Group Drug Counseling for Cocaine Dependence: The Cocaine Collaborative Model*. NIDA, National Institutes of Health; 2001.
14. Rawson RA, Obert JL, McCann MJ, et al. *The Matrix Modal of Intensive Outpatient Alcohol and Drug Treatment*. Hazelden; 2005.
15. Miller WR. What is a relapse? Fifty ways to leave the wagon. *Addiction*. 1996;91:S15-S27.
16. Marlatt GA. Relapse prevention: theoretical rationale and overview model. In: Marlatt GA, Gordon G, eds. *Relapse Prevention: A Self-Control Strategy for the Maintenance of Behavioral Change*. Guilford Press; 1985:3-70.

17. Marlatt GA. Taxonomy of high-risk situations for alcohol relapse: evolution and development of a cognitive-behavioral model. *Addiction*. 1986;91:S37-S49.
18. Donovan DM. Assessment issues and domains in the prediction of relapse. *Addiction*. 1996;91:S29-S36.
19. National Institute on Drug Abuse (NIDA). *Cue Extinction Techniques: IDA Technology Transfer Package*. NIDA, National Institutes of Health; 1993.
20. Larimar ME, Palmer RS, Marlatt GA. Relapse prevention: an overview of Marlatt's cognitive behavioral model. *Alcohol Res Health*. 1999;23(2): 151-161.
21. Marlatt GA, Witkiewitz K. Harm reduction approaches to alcohol use: health promotion, prevention, treatment. *Addict Behav*. 2002;27: 867-886.
22. Zweben A, Cisler RA. Clinical and methodological utility of a composite outcome measure for alcohol treatment research. *Alcohol Clin Exp Res*. 2003;27:1680-1685.
23. Milby JB, Schumacher JE, Vuchinich RE, et al. Transitions during effective treatment for cocaine-abusing homeless persons: establishing abstinence, lapse, and relapse, and reestablishing abstinence. *Psychol Addict Behav*. 2004;18:250-256.
24. De Leon G. Cocaine abusers in therapeutic community treatment. In: Tims FM, Leukefeld CG, eds. *Cocaine Treatment: Research and Clinical Perspectives*. NIDA Research Monograph 135, NIH Publication No. 93-3639. Advances in Cocaine Treatment. NIDA Technical Review Meeting, Bethesda, MD; 1993:163-189.
25. Daley DC, Marlatt GA. Relapse prevention. In: Lowinson JH, Ruiz P, Millman RB, et al., eds. *Substance Abuse: A Comprehensive Textbook*. 4th ed. Lippincott Williams & Wilkins; 2005:772-785.
26. Daley DC, Marlatt GA. *Overcoming Your Alcohol and Drug Problem: Effective Recovery Strategies. Therapist Guide*. 2nd ed. Oxford University Press; 2006.
27. Wang SJ, Winchell CJ, McCormick CG, Nevius SE, O'Neill RT. Short of complete abstinence: an analysis exploration of multiple drinking episodes in alcoholism treatment trials. *Alcohol Clin Exp Res*. 2002;26:1803-1809.
28. Piasecki TM, Fiore MC, McCarthy DE, Baker TB. Have we lost our way? The need for dynamic formulations of smoking relapse proneness. *Addiction*. 2002;97(9):1093-1108.
29. Moore BA, Budney AJ. Relapse in outpatient treatment for marijuana dependence. *J Subst Abus Treat*. 2003;25(2):85-89.
30. Hufford MH, Witkiewitz K, Shields AL, et al. Applying nonlinear dynamics to the prediction of alcohol use disorder treatment outcomes. *J Abnorm Psychol*. 2003;112:219-227.
31. Marlatt GA, Witkiewitz K. Relapse prevention for drug and alcohol problems. In: Marlatt GA, Donovan D, eds. *Relapse Prevention*. 2nd ed. Guilford Press; 2005:1-44.
32. Witkiewitz K, Marlatt GA. Relapse prevention for alcohol and drug problems: that was Zen, this is Tao. *Am Psychol*. 2004;59:224-235.
33. Dimeff AA, Marlatt GA. Preventing relapse and maintaining change in addictive behaviors. *Clin Psychol Sci Pract*. 1998;5:513-525.
34. Daley DC. Pathways to recovery from substance use disorders. *Counselor*. 2019;6:16-18. 23
35. Daley DC, Douaihy A. *Managing Substance Use Disorder: Practitioner Guide*. 3rd ed. Oxford University Press; 2019.
36. Washton AM. Group therapy: a clinician's guide to doing what works. In: Coombs R, ed. *Addiction Recovery Tools: A Practical Handbook*. Sage Publications; 2001.
37. Washton AM. Outpatient groups at different stages of substance abuse treatment: preparation, initial abstinence, and relapse prevention. In: Brook DW, Spitz HI, eds. *The Group Therapy of Substance Abuse*. Haworth Medical Publishing; 2002.
38. Gorski TT, Kelly JM. *Counselor's Manual for Relapse Prevention with Chemically Dependent Criminal Offenders*. Substance Abuse and Mental Health Services Administration; 1996.
39. Hser YI. Predicting long-term stable recovery from heroin addiction: findings from a 33 year follow-up study. *J Addict Dis*. 2007;26(1):51-60.
40. Flynn PM, Joe GW, Broome KM, Simpson DD, Brown BS. Recovery from opioid addiction in DATOS. *J Subst Abus Treat*. 2003;25:177-186.
41. Hughes JR, Keely J, Naud S. Shape of the relapse curve and long-term abstinence among untreated smokers. *Addiction*. 2004;99:29-38.
42. Medioni J, Berlin I, Mallet A. Increased risk of relapse after stopping nicotine replacement therapies: a mathematical modeling approach. *Addiction*. 2005;100:247-254.
43. Shah NG, Galai N, Celentano DD, Vlahov D, Strathdee SA. Longitudinal predictors of injection cessation and subsequent relapse among a cohort of injection drug users in Baltimore, MD, 1988-2000. *Drug Alcohol Depend*. 2006;83:147-156.
44. Fleury MJ, Djouini A, Huynh C, et al. Remission from substance use disorders: a systematic review and meta-analysis. *Drug Alcohol Depend*. 2016;168:293-306.
45. Rawson RA, The Methamphetamine Treatment Project Corporate Authors. A multi-site comparison of psychosocial approaches for the treatment of methamphetamine dependence. *Addiction*. 2004;99: 708-717.
46. Hser YI, Joshi V, Anglin MD, Fletcher B. Predicting post-treatment cocaine abstinence for first-time admissions and treatment repeaters. *Am J Public Health*. 1999;89:666-671.
47. Hillhouse MP, Marinelli P, Gonzales R, Ang A, Rawson RA; The Methamphetamine Treatment Project Corporate Authors. Predicting in-treatment performance and post-treatment outcomes in methamphetamine users. *Addiction*. 2007;102(Suppl 1):84-95.
48. Walitzer KS, Dearing R. Gender differences in alcohol and substance use relapse. *Clin Psychol Rev*. 2006;26:128-148.
49. Simpson DD, Joe GW, Broome KM. A national 5-year follow-up of treatment outcomes for cocaine dependence. *Arch Gen Psychiatry*. 2002;59:538-544.
50. Hser YI, Hoffman V, Grella CE, Anglin MD. A 33-year follow-up of narcotics addicts. *Arch Gen Psychiatry*. 2001;58:503-508.
51. Dennis ML, Scott CK, Funk R, Foss MA. The duration and correlates of addiction treatment careers. *J Subst Abus Treat*. 2005;28:S51-S62.
52. Hser YI, Anglin MD, Grella C, Alongshore D, Prendergast ML. Drug treatment careers: a conceptual framework and existing research findings. *J Subst Abus Treat*. 1997;14:543-558.
53. Miller W, Hester R. Treating the problem drinker: modern approaches. *The Addictive Behaviors Treatment of Alcoholism, Drug Abuse, Smoking and Obesity*. Pergamon Press; 1980.
54. Catalano R, Howard M, Hawkins J, et al. *Relapse in the Addictions: Rates, Determinants, and Promising Prevention Strategies. 1988 Surgeon General's Report on Health Consequences of Smoking*. Office of Smoking and Health, Department of Health and Human Services; 1988.
55. Center for Substance Abuse Treatment (CSAT). Treatment succeeds in fighting crime. *Substance Abuse Brief*. CSAT, SAMHSA; 2000.
56. Center for Substance Abuse Treatment (CSAT). Substance abuse treatment reduces family dysfunction, improves productivity. *Substance Abuse Brief*. CSAT, SAMHSA; 2000.
57. Center for Substance Abuse Treatment (CSAT). Treatment cuts medical costs. *Substance Abuse Brief*. CSAT, SAMHSA; 2000.
58. McQuaid RJ, Malik A, Moussouni K, Baydack N, Stargardter M, Morrisey M. *Life in Recovery from Addiction in Canada*. Canadian Centre on Substance Use and Addiction; 2017.
59. Simon Onken L, Blaine JD, Boren JJ, eds. *Beyond the Therapeutic Alliance: Keeping the Drug Dependent Individual in Treatment*. NIDA Research Monograph 165. NIDA, National Institutes of Health; 1997.
60. National Institute on Drug Abuse (NIDA). Study sheds new light on the state of drug abuse treatment nationwide. *NIDA Notes*. 1997;12(5):1-8.
61. Bowen S, Chawla N, Marlatt GA. *Mindfulness-Based Relapse Prevention for Addictive Behaviors: A Clinician's Guide*. Guilford Press; 2010.
62. Bowen S, Witkiewitz K, Clifasefi SL, et al. Relative efficacy of mindfulness-based relapse prevention, standard relapse prevention, and treatment as usual for substance use disorders: a randomized clinical trial. *JAMA Psychiatry*. 2014;71(5):547-556.
63. Chaney ER, O'Leary MR, Marlatt GA. Skill training with alcoholics. *J Consult Clin Psychol*. 1978;46:1092-1104.

64. Carroll KM. Relapse prevention as a psychosocial treatment: a review of controlled clinical trials. *Exp Clin Psychopharmacol.* 1996;4:46-54.
65. Goldstein MG, Niaura R, Follick MJ, Abrams DB. Effects of behavioral skills training and schedule of nicotine gum administration on smoking cessation. *Am J Psychiatry.* 1989;146:56-60.
66. Carroll KM, Rounsaville BJ, Nich C, Gordon LT, Wirtz PW, Gawin F. One-year follow-up of psychotherapy and pharmacotherapy for cocaine dependence. Delayed emergence of psychotherapy effects. *Arch Gen Psychiatry.* 1994;51:989-997.
67. Rawson R, McCann M, Flammino F, et al. A comparison of contingency management and cognitive-behavioral approaches for cocaine and methamphetamine-dependent individuals. *Arch Gen Psychiatry.* 2002; 59:817-824.
68. Polivy J, Herman CP. If at first you don't succeed: false hopes of self-change. *Am Psychol.* 2002;109:74-86.
69. Project MATCH Research Group. Matching alcoholism treatment to client heterogeneity: post treatment drinking outcomes. *J Stud Alcohol.* 1997;58:7-29.
70. Ouimette PC, Finney JW, Moos RH. 12-Step and cognitive behavioral treatment for substance abuse: a comparison of treatment effectiveness. *J Consult Clin Psychol.* 1997;65:230-240.
71. Irvin JE, Bowers CA, Dunn ME, Wang MC. Efficacy of relapse prevention: a meta-analytic review. *J Consult Clin Psychol.* 1999;67:563-570.
72. Hajek P, Stead LF, West R, Jarvis M, Lancaster T. Relapse prevention interventions for smoking cessation. *Cochrane Database Syst Rev.* 2005;1:CD003999.
73. Lancaster T, Hajek P, Stead L, West R, Jarvis MJ. Prevention of relapse after quitting smoking: a systematic review of trials. *Arch Intern Med.* 2006;166:828-835.
74. Fiore MC, Bailey WC, Cohen SJ, et al. *Treating Tobacco Use and Dependence: Clinical Practice Guideline.* U.S. Department of Health and Human Services, Public Health Service; 2000.
75. Brandon TH, Collin BN, Juliano LM, Lazev AB. Preventing relapse among former smokers: a comparison of minimal interventions through telephone and mail. *J Consult Clin Psychol.* 2000;68(1):103-113.
76. Brandon TH, Meade CD, Herzog S, Chirikos TN, Webb MS, Cantor AB. Efficacy and cost-effectiveness of a minimal intervention to prevent smoking relapse: dismantling the effects of amount of content versus contact. *J Consult Clin Psychol.* 2004;72(5):797-808.
77. Anton RF, Moak DH, Latham P, et al. Naltrexone combined with either cognitive behavioral or motivational enhancement therapy for alcohol dependence. *J Clin Psychopharmacol.* 2005;25:349-357.
78. Anton RF, O'Malley SS, Ciraulo DA, et al. Combined pharmacotherapies and behavioral interventions for alcohol dependence. *JAMA.* 2006; 295:2003-2017.
79. The COMBINE Study Group. Testing combined pharmacotherapies and behavioral interventions for alcohol dependence (the COMIBINE study): rationale and methods. *Alcohol Clin Exp Res.* 2003;27:1107-1122.
80. The COMBINE Study Group. Testing combined pharmacotherapies and behavioral interventions for alcohol dependence (the COMIBINE study): a pilot feasibility study. *Alcohol Clin Exp Res.* 2003;27:1123-1131.
81. Donovan DM, Anton RF, Miller WR, et al. Combined pharmacotherapies and behavioral interventions for alcohol dependence (The COMBINE Study). Examination of posttreatment drinking outcomes. *J Stud Alcohol Drugs.* 2008;69(1):5-13.
82. Maude-Griffin PM, Hohenstein JM, Humfleet GL, Reilly PM, Tusel DJ, Hall SM. Superior efficacy of cognitive-behavioral therapy for crack cocaine abusers: main and matching effects. *J Consult Clin Psychol.* 1998;66:832-837.
83. Carroll KM, Fenton LR, Ball S, et al. Efficacy of disulfiram and cognitive-behavioral therapy for cocaine-dependent outpatients. *Arch Gen Psychiatry.* 2004;64:264-272.
84. Rawson RA, Huber A, Brethen PB, et al. Methamphetamine and cocaine users: differences in characteristics and treatment retention. *J Psychoactive Drugs.* 2000;32:233-238.
85. Rawson RA, Obert JL, McCann MJ, et al. *The Neurobehavioral Treatment Manual.* Matrix; 1989.
86. Epstein DE, Hawkins WF, Covi L, Umbricht A, Preston KL. Cognitive behavioral therapy plus contingency management for cocaine use: findings during treatment and across 12-month follow-up. *Psychol Addict Behav.* 2003;17:73-82.
87. Schmitz JM, Oswald LM, Jacks SM, Rustin T, Rhoades HM, Grabowski J. Relapse prevention treatment for cocaine dependence: group versus individual format. *Addict Behav.* 1997;22:405-418.
88. Marques AC, Formigoni ML. Comparison of individual and group cognitive behavioral therapy for alcohol and/or drug dependent patients. *Addiction.* 2001;96:832-837.
89. MTP Research Group. Brief treatments for cannabis dependence: findings from a randomized multi-site trial. *J Consult Clin Psychol.* 2004;72:455-466.
90. Kilmer JR, Cronce JM, Paler RS. Relapse prevention for abuse of club drugs, hallucinogens, inhalants, and steroids. In: Marlatt GA, Donovan D, eds. *Relapse Prevention.* 2nd ed. Guilford Press; 2005:208-247.
91. Maisto SA, McKay JR, O'Farrell TJ. Relapse precipitants and behavioral marital therapy. *Addict Behav.* 1995;20(3):383-393.
92. O'Farrell TJ, Choquette KA, Cutter HS, Brown ED, McCourt WF. Behavioral marital therapy with and without additional couples relapse prevention sessions for alcoholics and their wives. *J Stud Alcohol.* 1993;54:652-666.
93. McCrady BS, Epstein EE, Kahler CW. Alcoholics Anonymous and relapse prevention as maintenance strategies after conjoint behavioral alcohol treatment for men: 18-month outcomes. *J Consult Clin Psychol.* 2004;72:870-878.
94. McCrady BS, Nathan PE. Technique factors in treating substance use disorders. In: Castonguay LG, Beutler LE, eds. *Principles of Therapeutic Change That Work.* Oxford Series in Clinical Psychology. Oxford University Press; 2005.
95. National Registry of Evidence-based Programs and Practices. Accessed September 7, 2011. http://nrepp.-samhsa.gov
96. Maisto SA, Connors GJ, Zwyiak WH. Construct validation analyses on the Marlatt typology of relapse precipitants. *Addiction.* 1996;91:89-98.
97. Stout RL, Longabaugh R, Rubin R. Predictive validity of Marlatt's taxonomy versus a more general relapse code. *Addiction.* 1996;91: 99-110.
98. Marlatt GA. Craving for alcohol, loss of control, and relapse: a cognitive-behavioral analysis. In: Nathan PE, Marlatt GA, Loberg T, eds. *New Directions in Behavioral Research and Treatment.* Rutgers Center of Alcohol Studies; 1978:271-314.
99. Longabaugh R, Rubin A, Stout RL, Zywiak WH, Lowman C. The reliability of Marlatt's taxonomy for classifying relapses. *Addiction.* 1996;91:73-88.
100. Donovan DM. Marlatt's classification of relapse precipitants: is the emperor still wearing clothes? *Addiction.* 1996;91:S131-S137.
101. Kadden R. Is Marlatt's taxonomy reliable or valid? *Addiction.* 1996;91:139-146.
102. Sandahl C. Determinants of relapse among alcoholics: a cross-cultural replication study. *Int J Addict.* 1984;19:833-848.
103. Annis H. A relapse prevention model for treatment of alcoholics. In: Miller W, Heather N, eds. *Treating Addictive Behaviors: Processes of Change.* Plenum Books; 1986.
104. Miller WR, Westerberg VS, Harris RJ, Tonigan JS. What predicts relapse? Prospective testing of antecedent models. *Addiction.* 1996;91:S155-S171.
105. Hodgins DC, Guebaly N, Armstrong S. Prospective and retrospective reports of mood states before relapse to substance use. *J Consult Clin Psychol.* 1995;63:400-407.
106. Carroll KM, Rounsaville BJ, Gawin FH. A comparative trial of psychotherapies for ambulatory cocaine abusers: relapse prevention and interpersonal psychotherapy. *Am J Drug Alcohol Abuse.* 1991;17:229-249.
107. Daley DC, ed. *Relapse: Conceptual, Research and Clinical Perspectives.* Haworth Medical Publishing; 1989.
108. Daley DC. *Relapse Prevention: Treatment Alternatives and Counseling Aids.* Human Services Institute; 1988.
109. Daley DC, Ross JR. *Relapse Prevention Workbook for Sexually Compulsive Behavior.* Learning Publications; 2000.

110. Bandura A. Self-efficacy: toward a unifying theory of behavioral change. *Psychol Rev*. 1977;84:191-215.
111. Bandura A. *Self-Efficacy: The Exercise of Control*. Freeman; 1997.
112. Gwaltney CJ, Shiffman S, Balabanis MH, Paty JA. Dynamic self-efficacy and outcome expectancies: prediction of smoking lapse and relapse. *J Abnorm Psychol*. 2005;114(4):661-675.
113. Demell R, Rist F. Prediction of treatment outcome in a clinical sample of problem drinkers: self-efficacy and coping style. *Addict Disord Treat*. 2005;4(1):5-10.
114. Maisto SA, Clifford PR, Longabaugh R, Beattie M. The relationship between abstinence for one year following pretreatment assessment and alcohol use and other functioning at 2 years in individuals presenting for alcohol treatment. *J Stud Alcohol*. 2002;63(4):397-403.
115. Sklar SM, Annis HM, Turner NE. Development and validation of the drug-taking confidence questionnaire: a measure of coping self-efficacy. *Addict Behav*. 1997;22:655-670.
116. Monti PM, Rohsenow DJ, Swift RM, et al. Naltrexone and cue exposure with coping and communication skills training for alcoholics: treatment process and 1-year outcomes. *Alcohol Clin Exp Res*. 2001;25:1634-1647.
117. Shiffman S, Balabanis M, Paty J, et al. Dynamic effects of self-efficacy on smoking lapse and relapse. *Health Psychol*. 2000;19:315-323.
118. Oei TPS, Baldwin AR. Expectancy theory: a two-process model of alcohol use and abuse. *J Stud Alcohol*. 1994;55(5):525-534.
119. Smith DE, Seymour RB. The nature of addiction. In: Coombs RH, ed. *Handbook of Addictive Behaviors: A Practical Guide to Diagnosis and Treatment*. Wiley; 2004:3-30.
120. Sale E, Sambrano S, Springer JF, et al. Risk, protection, and substance use in adolescents: a multisite trial. *J Drug Addict*. 2003;33(1):91-105.
121. Jones BT, Corbin W, Fromme K. A review of expectancy theory and alcohol consumption. *Addiction*. 2001;96:57-72.
122. Abrams K, Kushner MG. The moderating effects of tension reduction alcohol outcome expectancies on placebo responding in individuals with social phobia. *Addict Behav*. 2004;29(6):1221-1224.
123. Demmel R, Nicolai J, Gregorzik S. Alcohol expectancies and current mood state in social drinkers. *Addict Behav*. 2006;31(5):859-867.
124. Corbin WR, McNair LD, Carter JA. Evaluation of a treatment appropriate cognitive intervention for challenging alcohol outcome expectancies. *Addict Behav*. 2001;26(4):475-488.
125. Rohsenow DJ, Monti PM. Does urge to drink predict relapse after treatment? *Alcohol Res Health*. 1999;23:225-232.
126. Tiffany ST, Carter BL, Singleton EG. Challenges in the manipulation, assessment, and interpretation of craving relevant variables. *Addiction*. 2000;95:177-187.
127. Drummond DC, Litten RZ, Lowman C, Hunt WA. Craving research: future directions. *Addiction*. 2000;95(Suppl 2):131-137.
128. Gordon SM, Sterling R, Siatkowski C, Raively K, Weinstein S, Hill PC. Inpatient desire to drink as a predictor of relapse to alcohol use following treatment. *Am J Addict*. 2006;15:242-245.
129. Sinha R, Garcia M, Paliwal P, Kreek MJ, Rounsaville BJ. Stress-induced cocaine craving and hypothalamic-pituitary-adrenal responses are predictive of cocaine relapse outcomes. *Arch Gen Psychiatry*. 2006;63:324-331.
130. Marlatt GA, Ostafin BD. Being mindful of automaticity in addiction: a clinical perspective. In: Weirs RW, Stacy AW, eds. *Handbook of Implicit Cognition and Addiction*. Sage Publications, Inc; 2006:489-495.
131. Witkiewitz K, Marlatt GA, Walker D. Mindfulness based relapse prevention for alcohol and substance use disorders: the meditative tortoise wins the race. *J Cogn Psychother*. 2006;19(3):211-228.
132. Donovan DM, Rosengren DB. Motivation for behavior change and treatment among substance abusers. In: Tucker JA, Donovan DM, Marlatt GA, eds. *Changing Addictive Behavior: Bridging Clinical and Public Health Strategies*. Guilford Press; 1999:127-159.
133. Prochaska JO, DiClementa CC. *The Transtheoretical Approach: Crossing the Traditional Boundaries of Therapy*. Krieger; 1984.
134. Miller WR, Rollnick S. Ten things that motivational interviewing is not. *Behav Cogn Psychother*. 2009;37:129-140.
135. Rohsenow DJ, Monti PM, Martin RA, et al. Motivational enhancement and coping skills training for cocaine abusers: effects on substance use outcomes. *Addiction*. 2004;99(7):862-874.
136. Moos RH, Holahan CJ. Dispositional and contextual perspectives on coping: toward an integrative framework. *J Clin Psychol*. 2003;59:1387-1403.
137. Shiffman S. Maintenance and relapse: coping with temptation. In: Nirenberg TD, Maisto SA, eds. *Developments in the Assessment and Treatment of Addictive Behaviors*. Ablex; 1987:352-385.
138. Shiffman S. Conceptual issues in the study of relapse. In: Gossop M, ed. *Relapse and Addictive Behaviour*. Tavistock/Routledge; 1989:149-179.
139. Carels RA, Douglass OM, Cacciapaglia HM, O'Brien WH. An ecological momentary assessment of relapse crises in dieting. *J Consult Clin Psychol*. 2004;72(2):341-348.
140. Maisto SA, Zywiak WH, Connors GJ. Course of functioning one year following admission for treatment of alcohol use disorders. *Addict Behav*. 2006;31(1):69-79.
141. Moser AE, Annis HM. The role of coping in relapse crisis outcome: a prospective study of treated alcoholics. *Addiction*. 1996;91:1101-1114.
142. Chung T, Langenbucher J, Labouvie E, Pandina RJ, Moos RH. Changes in alcoholic patients' coping responses predict 12-month treatment outcomes. *J Consult Clin Psychol*. 2001;69:92-100.
143. Litt MD, Cooney NL, Morse P. Reactivity to alcohol-related stimuli in the laboratory and in the field: predictors of craving in treated alcoholics. *Addiction*. 2000;95:889-900.
144. Litt MD, Kadden RM, Cooney NL, et al. Coping skills and treatment outcomes in cognitive-behavioral and interactional group therapy for alcoholism. *J Consult Clin Psychol*. 2003;71:118-128.
145. Marlatt GA. Buddhist philosophy and the treatment of addictive behaviors. *Cogn Behav Pract*. 2002;9:44-49.
146. Marlatt GA, Kristellar J. Mindfulness and meditation. In: Miller WR, ed. *Integrating Spirituality in Treatment: Resources for Practitioners*. American Psychological Association Books; 1999:67-84.
147. Marlatt GA, Witkiewitz K, Dillworth T, et al. Vipassana meditation as a treatment for alcohol and drug use disorders. In: Hayes SC, Follette VM, Linehan MM, eds. *Mindfulness and Acceptance: Expanding the Cognitive-Behavioral Tradition*. Guilford Press; 2004:261-287.
148. Cooney NL, Litt MD, Morse PA, Bauer LO, Gaupp L. Alcohol cue reactivity, negative mood reactivity, and relapse in treated alcoholic men. *J Abnorm Psychol*. 1997;106:243-250.
149. Shiffman S, Paty JA, Gnys M, Kassel JA, Hickcox M. First lapses to smoking: within subject analysis of real time reports. *J Consult Clin Psychol*. 1996;2:366-379.
150. Baker TB, Piper ME, McCarthy DE, Majeskie MR, Fiore MC. Addiction motivation reformulated: an affective processing model of negative reinforcement. *Psychol Bull*. 2004;111:33-51.
151. Stanton M. Relapse prevention needs more emphasis on interpersonal factors. *Am Psychol*. 2005;60:340-349.
152. Armeli S, Todd M, Mohr C. A daily process approach to individual differences in stress-related alcohol use. *J Pers*. 2005;73(6):1657-1686.
153. Beattie MC, Longabaugh R. General and alcohol-specific social support following treatment. *Addict Behav*. 1999;24:593-606.
154. Dobkin PL, Civita M, Paraherakis A, Gill K. The role of functional social support in treatment retention and outcomes among outpatient adult substance abusers. *Addiction*. 2002;97:347-356.
155. McMahon RC. Personality, stress, and social support in cocaine relapse prediction. *J Subst Abus Treat*. 2001;21:77-87.
156. Annis H, Davis CS. Self-efficacy and the prevention of alcoholic relapse: initial findings from a treatment trial. In: Baker TB, Cannon DS, eds. *Assessment and Treatment of Addictive Disorders*. Praeger; 1988:88-112.
157. Winters J, Fals-Stewart W, O'Farrell TJ, Birchler GR, Kelley ML. Behavioral couples therapy for female substance-abusing patients: effects on substance use and relationship adjustment. *J Consult Clin Psychol*. 2002;70:344-355.
158. Finney JW, Monahan SC. The cost-effectiveness of treatment for alcoholism: a second approximation. *J Stud Alcohol*. 1999;52:517-540.
159. Annis H. A cognitive-social learning approach to relapse: pharmacotherapy and relapse prevention counseling. *Alcohol Alcohol*. 1991;1(Suppl):527-530.

160. Marlatt GA, Barrett K, Daley DC. Relapse prevention. In: Galanter M, Kleber HD, eds. *Textbook of Substance Abuse*. 2nd ed. American Psychiatric Press; 1999.
161. National Institute on Drug Abuse (NIDA). *Recovery Training and Self-Help*. 2nd ed. NIDA, National Institutes of Health; 1994.
162. Rawson RA, Shoptaw SJ, Obert JL, et al. An intensive outpatient approach for cocaine abuse treatment: the Matrix Model. *J Subst Abus Treat*. 1995;12:117-127.
163. Shoptaw S, Reback CJ, Frosch DL, Rawson RA. Stimulant abuse treatment as HIV prevention. *J Addict Dis*. 1998;17:19-32.
164. Obert JL, McCann MJ, Marinelli-Casey P, et al. The matrix model of outpatient stimulant abuse treatment: history and description. *J Psychoactive Drugs*. 2000;32:157-164.
165. Monti PM, Rohsenow DJ, Rubonis AV, et al. Cue exposure with coping skills treatment for male alcoholics: a preliminary investigation. *J Consult Clin Psychol*. 1993;61:1011-1019.
166. Gossop M, Stewart D, Browne N, Marsden J. Factors associated with abstinence, lapse or relapse to heroin use after residential treatment: protective effect of coping responses. *Addiction*. 2002;97:1259-1267.
167. Boker SM, Graham JS. Dynamical systems analysis of adolescent substance abuse. *Multivar Behav Res*. 1998;33(4):479-507.
168. Warran K, Hawkins RC, Sprott JC. Substance abuse as a dynamical disease: evidence and clinical implications of nonlinearity in a time series of daily alcohol consumption. *Addict Behav*. 2005;28:369-374.
169. Burgess ES, Brown RA, Kahler CW, et al. Patterns of change in depressive symptoms during smoking cessation: who's at risk for relapse? *J Consult Clin Psychol*. 2002;70:356-361.
170. Cinciripini P, Cinciripini L, Wallfisch A, Haque W, Van Vunakis H. Behavior therapy and transdermal nicotine patch: effects on cessation outcome, affect, and coping. *J Consult Clin Psychol*. 1996;64:314-323.
171. Witkiewitz K, Marlatt GA. Modeling the complexity of post-treatment drinking: it is a rocky road to relapse. *Clin Psychol Rev*. 2007;27:724-738.
172. Monti P, Adams D, Kadden R, et al. *Treating Alcohol Dependence*. Guilford Press; 1989.
173. Daley DC. Substance use disorders. In: Daley DC, Salloum IM, eds. *A Clinician's Guide to Mental Illness*. McGraw Hill/Hazelden; 2001.
174. Daley DC, Douaihy A. *Relapse Prevention Counseling: Strategies to Aid Recovery from Addiction and Reduce Relapse Risk*. Daley Publications; 2011.
175. Daley DC. Five perspectives on relapse in chemical dependency. *J Chem Depend Treat*. 1989;2:3-26.
176. Daley DC, Marlatt GA. *Overcoming Your Alcohol or Drug Problem: Therapist Guide*. 2nd ed. Oxford University Press; 2006.
177. Marlatt GA. Relapse prevention: theoretical rationale and overview of the model. In: Marlatt GA, Gordon JR, eds. *Relapse Prevention*. Guilford Press; 1985:108-250.
178. Marlatt GA. Cognitive factors in the relapse process. In: Marlatt GA, Gordon J, eds. *Relapse Prevention: A Self-Control Strategy for the Maintenance of Behavior Change*. Guilford Press; 1985:128-200.
179. McCrady BS. Relapse prevention: a couple's therapy perspective. In: O'Farrell TJ, ed. *Treating Alcohol Problems: Marital and Family Interventions*. Guilford Press; 1989:165-182.
180. Daley DC, Douaihy A. *A Family Guide to Coping With Substance Use Disorders*. Oxford University Press; 2019.
181. Zackon F. Relapse and "re-joyment": observations and reflections. *J Chem Depend Treat*. 1989;2(2):67-80.
182. McCusker CG, Brown K. Cue-exposure to alcohol-associated stimuli reduces autonomic reactivity, but not craving and anxiety, independent drinkers. *Alcohol Alcohol*. 1995;30(3):319-327.
183. Staiger PK, Greeley JD, Wallace SD. Alcohol exposure therapy: generalization and changes in responsivity. *Drug Alcohol Depend*. 1999;57(1):29-40.
184. Bowen S, Vieten C. A compassionate approach to the treatment of addictive behaviors: the contributions of Alan Marlatt to the field of mindfulness-based interventions. *Addict Res Theory*. 2012;20(3):243-249.
185. Bowen S, Kurz AS. Between-session practice and therapeutic alliance as predictors of mindfulness after mindfulness-based relapse prevention. *J Clin Psychol*. 2012;68(3):236-245.
186. Witkiewitz K, Bowen S, Douglas H, Hsu SH. Mindfulness-based relapse prevention for substance craving. *Addict Behav*. 2013;38:1563-1571.
187. O'Connell DF, Alexander CN. *Self-Recovery: Treating Addictions Using Transcendental Meditation and Maharishi Ayurveda*. Haworth Press; 1994.
188. Mann K, Lehert P, Morgan MY. The efficacy of acamprosate in the maintenance in alcohol-dependent individuals: results of a meta-analysis. *Alcohol Clin Exp Res*. 2004;28:51-63.
189. Kiefer F, Wiedemann K. Combined therapy: what does acamprosate and naltrexone combination tell us? *Alcohol Alcohol*. 2004;39:542-547.
190. Bouza C, Magro A, Muñoz A, Amate JM. Efficacy and safety of naltrexone and acamprosate in the treatment of alcohol dependence. *Addiction*. 2004;99(7):811-828.
191. Rychtarik RG, Connors GJ, Dermen KH, Stasiewicz PR. Alcoholics anonymous and the use of medications to prevent relapse: an anonymous survey of member attitudes. *J Stud Alcohol*. 2000;61:134-138.
192. Hughes JR. Combining behavioral therapy and pharmacotherapy for smoking cessation: an update. *NIDA Res Monogr*. 1995;150:92-109.
193. Higgins ST, Silverman K, eds. *Motivating Behavior Change Among Illicit Drug Abusers: Research on Contingency Management*. American Psychological Association; 1999.
194. Daley DC, Zuckoff A. *Improving Treatment Compliance: Counseling and System Strategies for Substance Use and Dual Disorders*. Hazelden; 1999.
195. Bradizza CM, Stasiewicz PR, Paas ND. Relapse to alcohol and drug use among individuals diagnosed with co-occurring mental health and substance use disorders: a review. *Clin Psychol Rev*. 2006;26:162-178.
196. Kaysen D, Simpson T, Dillworth T, Larimer ME, Gutner C, Resick PA. Alcohol problems and posttraumatic stress disorder in female crime victims. *J Trauma Stress*. 2006;19(3):399-403.
197. Ouimette PC, Gima K, Moos RH, Finney JW. A comparative evaluation of substance abuse treatment IV. The effect of comorbid psychiatric diagnoses on amount of treatment, continuing care, and 1-year outcomes. *Alcohol Clin Exp Res*. 1999;23(3):552-557.
198. Back SE, Brady KT, Sonne SC, Verduin ML. Symptom improvement in co-occurring PTSD and alcohol dependence. *J Nerv Ment Dis*. 2006;194:690-696.
199. Simpson TL, Kaysen D, Bowen S, et al. PTSD symptoms, substance use, and Vipassana meditation among incarcerated individuals. *J Trauma Stress*. 2007;20(3):239-249.
200. Najavits LM. Treatment of PTSD and substance abuse: clinical guidelines for implementing seeking safety. *Alcohol Treat Q*. 2004;22:43-62.
201. Cornelius JR, Salloum IM, Ehler JG, et al. Fluoxetine in depressed alcoholics: a double-blind, placebo-controlled trial. *Arch Gen Psychiatry*. 1997;54:700-705.
202. Salloum IM, Cornelius JR, Daley DC, Kirisci L, Himmelhoch M, Thase ME. Efficacy of valproate maintenance in patients with bipolar disorder and alcoholism. *Arch Gen Psychiatry*. 2005;62:37-45.

CHAPTER

81

Mindfulness-Based Treatment of Addiction

Eric L. Garland and Anna Parisi

CHAPTER OUTLINE

- Introduction
- Operationalizing the construct of mindfulness
- Mindfulness-based interventions for addiction
- Efficacy of MBIs for addiction
- Therapeutic mechanisms of mindfulness as treatment for addiction
- Clinical strategies for treating addiction with mindfulness
- Future directions for implementing mindfulness as a treatment for addiction
- Conclusion

INTRODUCTION

The neuroscience of addiction has provided novel insights regarding the mechanisms underpinning the development and maintenance of addiction. Increasingly, this body of research suggests that addiction is characterized by a chronic, relapsing cycle of behavioral escalation propelled by dysregulated neurocognitive processes governing motivation, hedonic experience, habit formation, and executive functioning.[1] To disrupt this cycle, there is a critical need for interventions that directly target the pathophysiological processes underlying addiction.

In light of their putative neurocognitive mechanisms of action,[2] a rapidly expanding body of literature suggests that mindfulness-based interventions (MBIs) may hold special promise as treatments for addiction. Over the past decade, multiple randomized controlled trials (RCTs) have provided evidence for the beneficial effects of MBIs in the treatment of alcohol,[3] stimulant,[4] opioid,[5] tobacco,[6] and other substance use disorders (SUDs),[7] as well as behavioral addictions.[8] More recently, research on MBIs for addiction has expanded to focus on elucidating the cognitive, affective, and neurobiological mechanisms underlying the effects of these interventions.

In this chapter, we first operationalize the construct of mindfulness and discuss how it may be applied in addiction treatment. Next, we review evidence for the efficacy and mechanisms of MBIs for addiction. Finally, we provide recommendations to inform future research and intervention efforts.

OPERATIONALIZING THE CONSTRUCT OF MINDFULNESS

The concept of mindfulness is rooted in Indo–Sino–Tibetan contemplative traditions dating back over 2,500 years. However, only within the past 30 years has mindfulness become a major focus of clinical research and practice. The past several decades have witnessed exponential growth in research on mindfulness.[9] In this growing body of literature, mindfulness is conceptualized as a state, a trait, and a practice.

The *state* of mindfulness is characterized by meta-awareness of present-moment thoughts, emotions, and sensations, without judgment or reactivity.[10,11] This state may be evoked by various mindfulness meditation *practices*, which typically involve two primary elements: focused attention and open monitoring.[12] Focused attention entails intentionally directing one's attention to the object of mindfulness; detecting cognitive, emotional, or sensory distractions that arise during attentional engagement with the meditative object; and then disengaging from these distractions by re-orienting attention back towards the chosen object. The breath is commonly used as an object of focus, although other interoceptive (eg, body sensations) and exteroceptive stimuli (eg, a candle flame, the sound of running water), thoughts, or even emotions can serve as the object of mindfulness. The cultivation of attentional control in this manner is thought to create a foundation for the more advanced practice of open monitoring, during which ambient attention is directed towards the field of awareness itself while encompassing the thoughts, emotions, and sensations that arise and cease within this field.[12] Focused attention and open monitoring are often integrated within a single meditation session, although both types of practices engage distinct cognitive processes crucial to self-regulating of behaviors that subserving addiction, including inhibitory control, attention regulation, emotion regulation, and metacognition.[13]

Over time, engaging in meditation practices that evoke the state of mindfulness may enhance the *trait* of mindfulness.[14,15] Thus, MBIs appear to operate through a *state-by-trait interaction*.[16] That is, repeatedly eliciting the state of mindfulness may accrue into durable increases in trait (or dispositional mindfulness), the propensity to exhibit mindful qualities in daily life including: the tendency to observe interoceptive and exteroceptive events; describe emotional states; act with awareness rather than automaticity; and exhibit nonjudgmental and nonreactive responses to distressing thoughts and emotions.[17] Although trait mindfulness is normally distributed in meditation-naive populations,[17] it is enhanced by MBIs, whose therapeutic effects are mediated by increases in trait mindfulness.[18,19]

As such, MBIs aim to cultivate trait mindfulness through practices that induce state mindfulness. Insofar as trait mindfulness is characterized by an increased capacity for self-regulation and self-awareness, it may provide an important buffer against the automatized, habit-based processes that drive addiction.[19-22] Indeed, individuals with higher levels of trait mindfulness exhibit greater cognitive control[23] and are better able to regulate attentional and autonomic responses to addiction-related cues.[24-26] Moreover, studies have observed a negative association between trait mindfulness and drug craving,[27] as well as substance use behaviors.[28,29]

MINDFULNESS-BASED INTERVENTIONS FOR ADDICTION

The integration of mindfulness practices into behavioral intervention programs began in the early 1980s with the development of mindfulness-based stress seduction (MBSR).[30] Initially developed for the treatment of chronic pain, evidence of MBSR's therapeutic benefits for mood and anxiety symptoms encouraged the development of other standardized mindfulness training programs, such as Mindfulness Based Cognitive Therapy (MBCT).[31] These first-generation MBIs influenced the development of some of the most prominent contemporary MBIs for addiction, including mindfulness-based relapse prevention (MBRP)[32] and Mindfulness-Oriented Recovery Enhancement (MORE).[5]

Emulating the structure established by first-generation MBIs, contemporary MBIs for addiction are typically implemented via a multi-week, group therapy format. Trained clinicians provide guided mindfulness meditation practices and debriefing, psychoeducational material, and experiential exercises designed to illustrate and reinforce novel didactic content. Participants are assigned homework to practice mindfulness skills in everyday life and asked to monitor symptoms (eg, craving, stress, negative affect, anhedonia, pain) that contribute to addictive behavior. Despite these commonalities, MBIs for addiction may be distinguished from first-generation MBIs by their use of tailored techniques designed to target pathogenic mechanisms undergirding addictive behaviors.

In that regard, mindfulness practices can be used to de-automatize substance use responses and strengthen self-regulation of addictive behaviors. For example, in MORE, participants learn to practice mindfulness of craving by bringing a piece of chocolate to their nose and lips without eating it, and to notice any sensations, thoughts, or emotions that arise. Participants are invited to become aware of any urges to eat the chocolate, which are analogized to cravings for addictive substances. The clinician then guides the participant to use mindfulness to deconstruct the experience craving into its constituent sensorial, affective, and cognitive subcomponents. That is, participants are instructed to practice mindfulness to "zoom in" and decompose cravings into their constituent sensations (eg, tightness, vibration, heat), noticing their center, periphery, and permeability (versus solidity). By cultivating meta-awareness of craving in this way, participants can recognize the insubstantial and transitory nature of craving, as well as to recognize their own agency over the craving experience.[33]

Building upon such formal mindfulness of craving techniques taught in MBI sessions, participants may also be instructed to practice three minutes of mindfulness before engaging in drug use or an addictive behavior. For instance, a patient who uses opioids in a manner other than prescribed (ie, nonmedical opioid use) could be instructed to stop before taking their next dose, and asked to cultivate mindfulness of thoughts, emotions, and body sensations while holding the opioid pill bottle. Similarly, a person preparing to quit smoking tobacco might practice mindfulness before they remove a cigarette from the pack. In this way, cultivating mindfulness in the context of everyday life may disrupt automatic substance use habits and help individuals re-evaluate their motivation for substance use in the moments prior to engaging in the addictive behavior.

EFFICACY OF MBIs FOR ADDICTION

Several large-scale clinical trials ($n \geq 250$) demonstrate the long-term efficacy of MBIs for addictive behavior.[5,7] These results have been bolstered by systematic reviews and meta-analyses. Li and colleagues[34] conducted a meta-analysis of 34 RCTs of MBIs designed to target substance use behaviors. Results from this review found greater reductions in substance use ($SMD = -0.33$, 95% CI [-0.88, -0.14]) and craving ($SMD = -0.68$, 95% CI [-1.11, -0.25]) at posttreatment and follow-up assessments for MBIs relative to comparison conditions. A subsequent meta-analysis by Goldberg et al. reviewed 142 RCTs examining the efficacy of MBIs for psychiatric disorders, including 26 that specifically focused on addiction, smoking tobacco, and weight/eating-related disorders. The authors found that MBIs were superior to active control conditions for improving outcomes in patients with SUDs.[35] In a more recent systematic review, Garland et al. found evidence that MBIs reduce opioid use.[36] However, authors have noted the presence of significant heterogeneity across this body of studies. Exploration of this heterogeneity via subgroup analyses indicated that MORE was associated with larger effects than other MBIs for substance use, craving, stress, and mindfulness measures.[34] Moreover, random effects meta-regressions revealed significantly larger effect sizes among samples comprised entirely of men compared to all-women or mixed-gender samples, suggesting that the effects of MBIs on craving, stress, and mindfulness measures may differ systematically as a function of gender identity.[34] That said, well-powered trials are needed to draw firm conclusions about whether gender moderates mindfulness-based treatment response.

THERAPEUTIC MECHANISMS OF MINDFULNESS AS TREATMENT FOR ADDICTION

The growth in research on MBIs for addiction has facilitated investigation of the therapeutic mechanisms underlying their beneficial effects on craving and substance use. In that regard, Garland, Froeliger, and Howard[2,37] posited that MBIs may be conceptualized as form of cognitive training to remediate and strengthen the neurocognitive processes that have become dysregulated during the process of addiction. Seen in this light, focused attention and open monitoring meditation practices may exercise prefrontal and parietal brain networks underlying metacognitive awareness, attention regulation, and inhibitory control that have been compromised by recurrent drug seeking and use. By strengthening functional connectivity between top-down prefrontal networks and bottom-up limbic-striatal brain circuitry (see **Fig. 81-1**) involved in reward processing and motivation, MBIs may augment a "domain general" neurocognitive resource that can broadly be applied to modulate a variety of mechanisms implicated in addiction.[2] Evidence for these mechanisms (see **Fig. 81-2**) is detailed below.

Strengthening Cognitive Control

Long-term exposure to psychoactive substances is associated with impairments in top-down frontal executive brain circuitry subserving a range of cognitive control functions, including self-control over automatic habits, decision-making, and response inhibition.[38] Hypothetically, mindfulness may rehabilitate compromised executive function by strengthening prefrontally-mediated cognitive control networks, and thereby potentially enhance self-control over substance use.

Mounting evidence supports the salutary effects of mindfulness on executive functioning. For example, a quasi-experimental study found that individuals with alcohol and other SUDs who participated in a combined goal management and mindfulness training intervention demonstrated significant improvements in working memory, selective attention/response inhibition, and decision-making skills relative to those participating in treatment-as-usual.[39] These findings were replicated by a subsequent RCT of this intervention, which found that combined goal management and mindfulness training was associated with improvements in executive functioning as measured by laboratory-based tasks and ecologically valid measures.[40]

Among individuals with tobacco use disorder (TUD), an MBI for abstinence of tobacco use was shown to improve concentration relative to TAU, which predicted improved abstinence from smoking following treatment.[41] Another RCT found that two weeks of mindfulness training was associated with reductions in smoking, coupled with increases in resting-state activity in cognitive control regions including the anterior cingulate and prefrontal cortices.[42] Similar results have been observed for individuals with nonmedical opioid use who were treated with MORE. For example, RCTs have found that participants in MORE exhibit increases in heart rate variability (HRV), an autonomic marker of self-regulatory capacity,[43] as well as increased frontal midline theta oscillations (see **Fig. 81-3**), a mechanism of cognitive control,[44] during mindfulness meditation, both of which mediate the effect of MORE on reducing opioid use.[45,46]

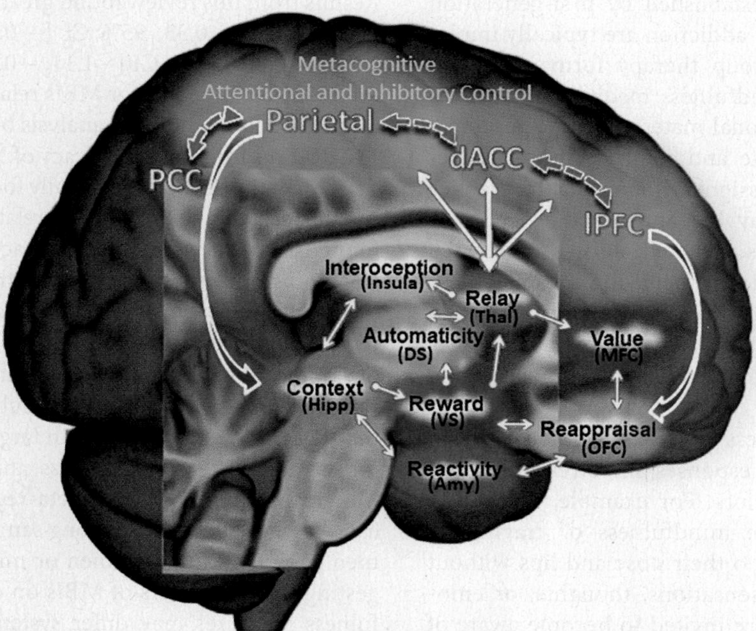

Figure 81-1. Putative brain circuitry involved in mindfulness as a treatment for addiction. (From Garland EL, Froeliger B, Howard MO. Mindfulness training targets neurocognitive mechanisms of addiction at the attention-appraisal-emotion interface. *Front Psychiatry.* 2013;4. Accessed September 27, 2017. https://www.ncbi.nlm.nih.gov/pmc/articles/PMC3887509/)

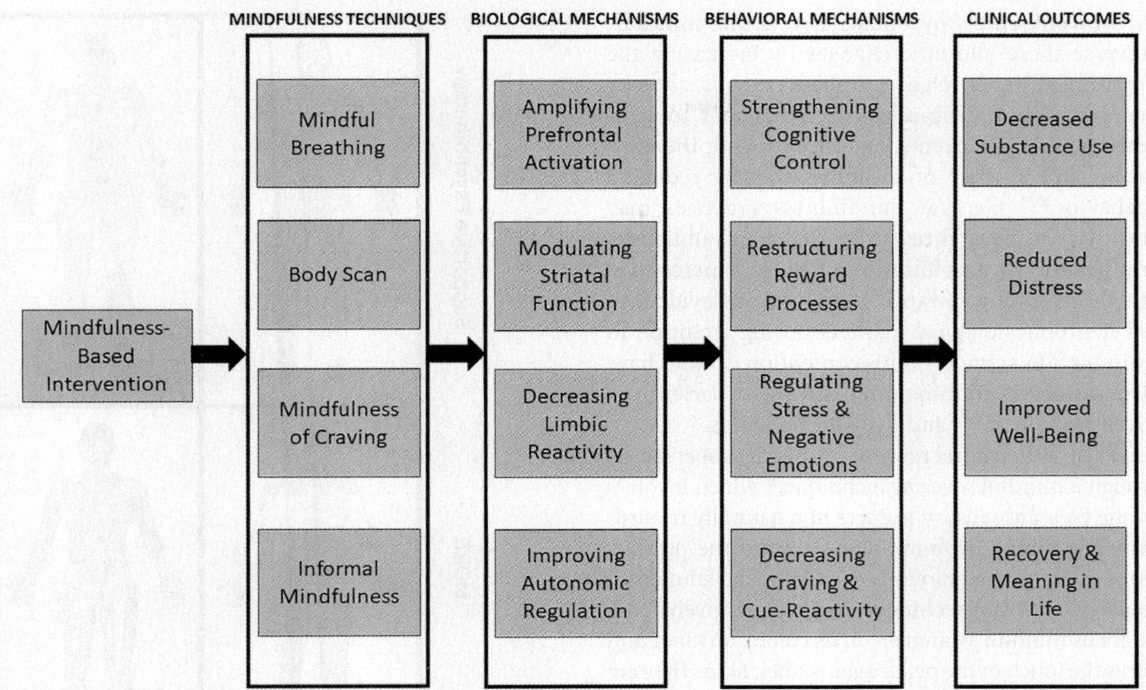

Figure 81-2. Therapeutic mechanisms of action for mindfulness-based interventions for addiction. (From Garland EL, Howard MO. Mindfulness-based treatment of addiction: current state of the field and envisioning the next wave of research. *Addict Sci Clin Pract.* 2018;13:14. Accessed September 27, 2017. https://ascpjournal.biomedcentral.com/articles/10.1186/s13722-018-0115-3)

Restructuring Reward Processes

Deficits in natural reward processing represent a significant challenge in the therapeutic rehabilitation of individuals with SUDs. Recurrent substance use is associated with neuroplastic modifications to brain circuits subserving stress and reward, such that individuals become increasingly insensitive to natural rewards while becoming sensitized to stress and aversive experiences.[47-49] As a result of these changes, the desire to seek and consume substances becomes a central motivational drive that occurs at the expense of pursuing natural rewards.

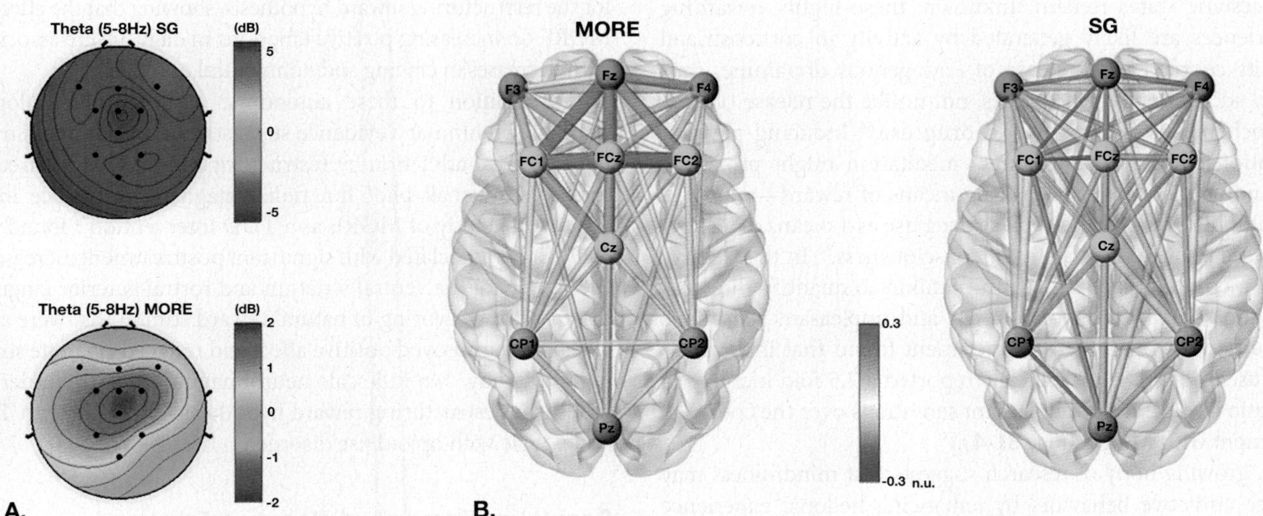

Figure 81-3. In a randomized mechanistic study of individuals who use opioids, mindfulness-oriented recovery enhancement (MORE) significantly increased frontal midline theta EEG power **(A)** and coherence **(B)** relative to supportive group (SG) therapy. Frontal midline theta power was significantly associated with reduced opioid use following treatment with MORE. (From Hudak J, Hanley AW, Marchand WR, Nakamura Y, Yabko B, Garland EL. Endogenous theta stimulation during meditation predicts reduced opioid dosing following treatment with Mindfulness-Oriented Recovery Enhancement. *Neuropsychopharmacology.* 2021;46(4):836-843.)

The *restructuring reward hypothesis* asserts that mindfulness may reverse these allostatic changes by increasing the salience of natural rewards relative to drug rewards, thereby shifting over-valuation of drug-related rewards back to valuing the healthy objects and events that once brought the individual pleasure and a sense of meaning, thereby reducing addictive behavior.[50,51] General mindfulness practices may increase sensitivity to natural rewards[52] (ie, social affiliation, food, natural beauty) by amplification of sensory-perceptual contact with the naturally rewarding stimulus, as evidenced by increased neurophysiological markers during attention to emotional stimuli.[53] In support of this contention, studies have shown that mindfulness training increases the experience of reward derived from food[54,55] and daily life activities.[56]

However, in MORE, natural reward processing is specifically targeted through a mindful *savoring* technique,[33] which involves attending to the pleasant sensory features of a naturally rewarding stimulus while tuning meta-awareness toward the pleasurable sensations and positive emotions elicited by the stimulus.[51] As one example of a savoring technique, participants given a rose and asked to focus mindful awareness on its colors, textures, and scent, as well as the touch of the petals against their skin. They are then instructed to turn their attention inward to notice how their mind and body are responding to this experience. When positive emotions or pleasant sensations arise, the clinician guides participants to use mindfulness to savor and absorb these experiences "like water seeping into soil." After learning this technique, MORE participants are asked to practice mindful savoring with other pleasant objects and experiences that occur in their daily lives as a means of training the reward system.

Relatedly, mindfulness meditation may evoke pleasurable body sensations,[57,58] and in the deepest of meditative states, elicit experiences of bliss or even ecstasy.[59-63] Though the neurobiological mediators of meditation-induced hedonic pleasure and ecstatic states remain unknown, these highly rewarding experiences are likely generated by activity in corticostriatal circuits coupled with release of endogenous dopamine, cannabinoid, and opioid molecules, not unlike the release of such neurochemicals in response to drug use.[64] Inducing pleasant sensations through mindfulness meditation might provide a safe, nonaddictive, and non-drug means of reward—a kind of "natural high" that could replace drug use as a means of achieving pleasurable altered states of consciousness.[51] In that regard, using a computerized sensation manikin to quantify the location and spatial extent of pleasant and unpleasant sensations in the body, a randomized experiment found that individuals who used opioids nonmedically reported a 7.5 fold increase in the ratio of pleasant to unpleasant sensations over the course of treatment with MORE (**Fig. 81-4**).[65]

A growing body of research suggests that mindfulness may reduce addictive behaviors by enhancing hedonic experience and positive emotion. Several randomized controlled mechanistic studies demonstrate that MORE enhances autonomic and neurophysiological responses (see **Fig. 81-5**) to natural reward stimuli[66-69] that were in turn associated with decreases in anhedonia,[68] opioid craving[66,69] and nonmedical opioid use,[70] providing support for the restructuring reward hypothesis.

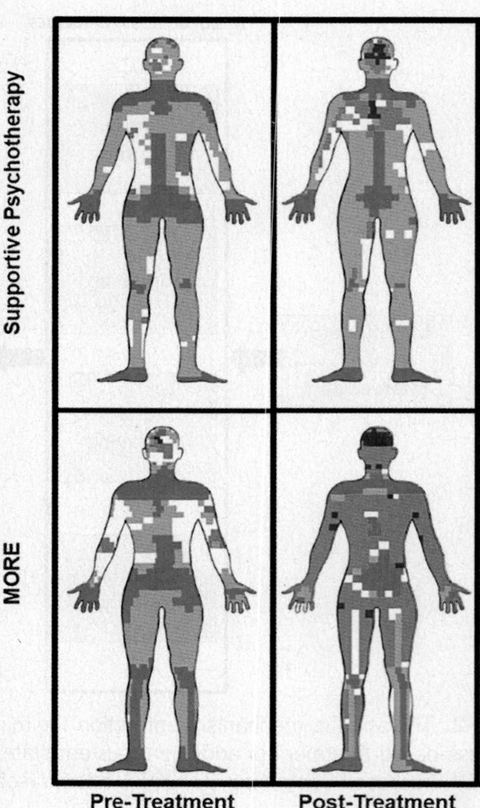

Figure 81-4. Mindfulness-oriented recovery enhancement (MORE) produced significant increases in pleasant body sensations in a sample of opioid users. (Modified from Garland EL. Mindful positive emotion regulation as a treatment for addiction: from hedonic pleasure to self-transcendent meaning. *Curr Opin Behav Sci.* 2021;39:168-177.)

Ecological momentary assessment data provide additional support for the restructuring reward hypothesis, showing that the effects of MORE on increasing positive emotions in daily life are associated with decreases in craving and nonmedical opioid use.[71,72]

In addition to these autonomic and neurophysiological findings, preliminary evidence suggests that mindfulness training may treat addiction by restructuring brain reward circuitry function. A small pilot functional magnetic resonance imaging (fMRI) study of MORE as a TUD intervention[73] found that MORE was associated with significant posttreatment increases in the activity of the ventral striatum and rostral anterior cingulate cortex during savoring of natural reward stimuli that were associated with improved positive affect and reduced cigarette smoking. Currently, two full-scale neuroimaging trials are underway to test the restructuring reward hypothesis in people with TUD and people with opioid use disorder.

Regulating Stress and Negative Emotions

Stress and negative emotions are common precipitants of substance use and relapse and have been shown to impair cognitive control over habitual addictive behaviors.[48,74-76] MBIs may attenuate the impact of stress and negative emotions in the context of addiction.[77-80] In that regard, meta-analyses demonstrate decreases

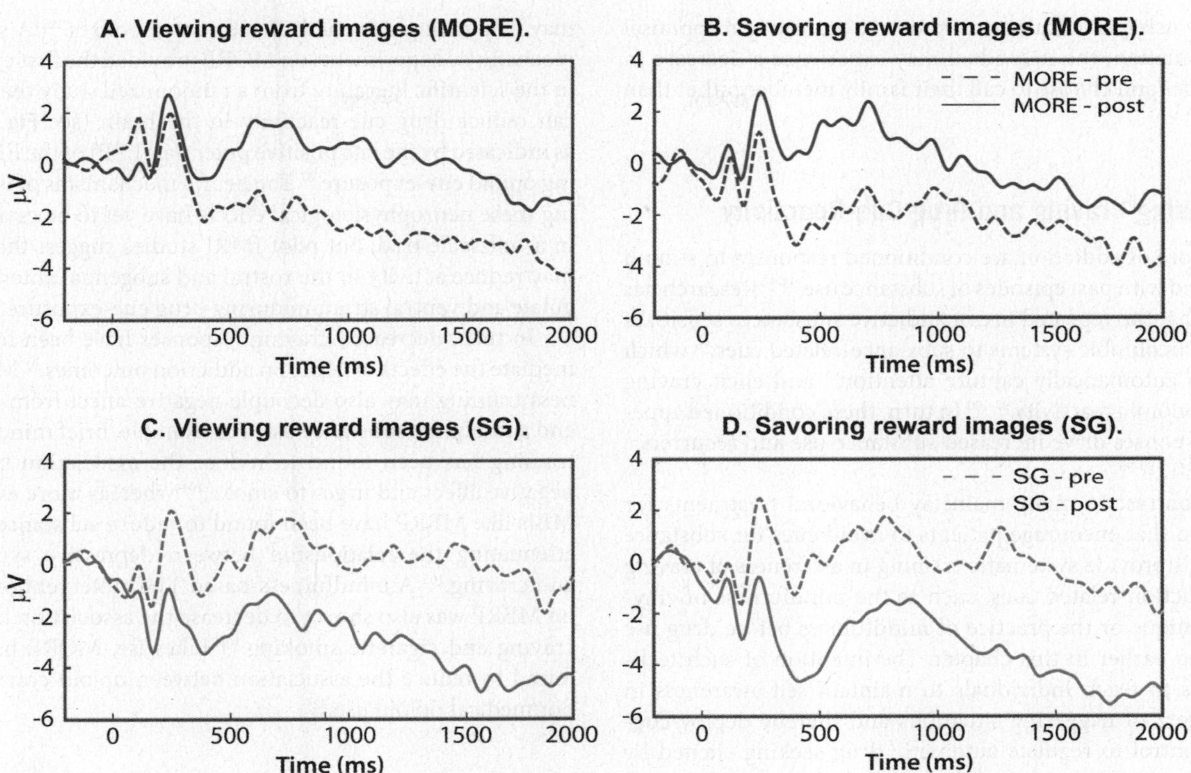

Figure 81-5. Relative to a supportive group (SG) therapy control condition, mindfulness-oriented recovery enhancement (MORE) significantly increased the late positive potential of the EEG during viewing and savoring of natural reward images in a sample of individuals who used opioids nonmedically. (From Garland EL, Fix ST, Hudak JP, et al. Mindfulness-Oriented Recovery Enhancement remediates anhedonia in chronic opioid use by enhancing neurophysiological responses during savoring of natural rewards. *Psychol Med.* 2023; 53(5):2085-2094. doi:10.1017/S0033291721003834)

in self-reported stress and improvements in adaptive regulation of negative emotions following MBIs.[81] Among individuals who use tobacco and opioids nonmedically, specifically, MBIs have been shown decrease stress and negative emotions,[5,72,82] enhance emotion regulation strategies including reappraisal,[82,83] and increase activity in the ACC and PFC[73,84]—brain regions associated with enhanced emotion regulatory capacity.

With respect to stress, experiments examining HRV are an important source of mechanistic evidence for the impact of MBIs.[85] HRV reflects parasympathetic regulation of heart rate by the central autonomic network, and as such, research examining HRV provides insight into the way in which mindfulness regulates physiological reactivity and recovery from stress.[43] In general, studies have generally supported the notion that MBIs improve stress reactivity and regulation in individuals who use substances, as indicated by the effects of mindfulness on HRV during experimental stress induction procedures.[3,86-88] Beyond autonomic measures, research has also shown that stress biomarkers, including saliva and hair cortisol, decrease following mindfulness training.[89,90] Moreover, a RCT of an MBI for TUD found reduced amygdala and insula activation during stress exposure relative to an active control condition, which predicted decreases in smoking three months after the intervention.[91] However, to better understand the stress-regulatory impact of MBIs, additional mechanistic studies are needed.

The salutary effects of MBIs on stress and emotion regulation may arise from their focus on cultivating awareness and acceptance of negative affective states and their ability to facilitate reappraisal of stressful life experiences. In that regard, the Mindfulness-to-Meaning Theory proposes that mindfulness regulates stress and negative emotions by fostering interoceptive awareness of the stress reaction and promoting reappraisals of the meaning of the stressor and the context in which it occurs.[92] For instance, an individual in recovery from AUD who has gotten into an argument with a family member may use mindfulness to become aware that they are angry and notice the physiological and cognitive reactions associated with this emotion, such as sensations of tightness in their chest and judgments about the other person (eg, "They never listen to me! They don't care about what I want."). During this process, the individual may also become aware that they are having an urge to drink "to calm myself down." Practicing mindfulness may allow the individual to disengage from these negative appraisals while broadening their attentional scope to encompass previously unattended information that promotes novel ways of appraising the stressor context. As a result, the individual may come to realize "I know this person is going through a difficult time. Maybe they are distracted and don't realize how they are coming across. I should talk to them about this, and I need to be sober for this conversation."

Thus, by using mindfulness to promote a positive reappraisal of the situation, the individual may experience a decrease in their anger and choose to call their family member rather than drink.

Decreasing Craving and Drug Cue-Reactivity

At the core of addiction are conditioned responses to stimuli associated with past episodes of substance use.[93-95] Research has shown that the repeated use of addictive substances sensitizes mesocorticolimbic systems to substance-related cues,[96] which come to automatically capture attention[97] and elicit craving and autonomic reactivity.[98-100] In turn, these conditioned appetitive responses drive increased substance use and recurrence of the SUD.[93-95]

In contrast to many mainstay behavioral treatments for addiction that encourage patients to avoid cues for substance use, MBIs provide systematic training in awareness of craving and addiction-related cues, such as the mindfulness of craving technique or the practice of mindfulness before drug use described earlier in this chapter. The intention of such techniques is to teach individuals to maintain self-awareness in the context of triggering situations and thereby deploy cognitive control to regulate automatic drug seeking elicited by addiction cue-exposure. In this regard, clinical and laboratory studies have shown that MBIs reduce subjective cue-elicited craving while decreasing attentional and autonomic indices of drug cue-reactivity.[69,70,101] In a small but provocative randomized study, MORE was shown to decrease cue-elicited opioid craving and reduce conditioned salivary responses to in vivo opioid cue-exposure, suggesting that mindfulness may help extinguish conditioned cue-responses.[102] A series of mechanistic experiments on MORE provided the first evidence in the scientific literature from a randomized study that a MBI can reduce drug cue-reactivity in the brain (see **Fig. 81-6**), as indicated by the late positive potential (LPP) of the EEG during opioid cue-exposure.[67] The neural mechanisms of underlying these neurophysiological effects have yet to be established in a full-scale trial, but pilot fMRI studies suggest that MBIs may reduce activity in the rostral and subgenual anterior cingulate and ventral striatum during drug cue-exposure.[73,103]

In turn, decreased craving responses have been found to mediate the effects of MBIs on addiction outcomes.[41] Mindfulness training may also decouple negative affect from craving and subsequent substance use. For example, brief mindfulness training has been found to reduce the association between negative affect and urges to smoke,[104] whereas more extensive MBIs like MBRP have been found to reduce substance use by attenuating the relationship between depressive symptoms and craving.[105] A mindfulness-based TUD intervention based on MBRP was also shown to decrease the association between craving and cigarette smoking.[106] Likewise, MORE has been found to reduce the association between opioid craving and nonmedical opioid use.[82]

CLINICAL STRATEGIES FOR TREATING ADDICTION WITH MINDFULNESS

In light of the aforementioned mechanistic findings, a number of strategies for treating addiction with mindfulness can be derived. First, therapists can frame mindfulness as a form

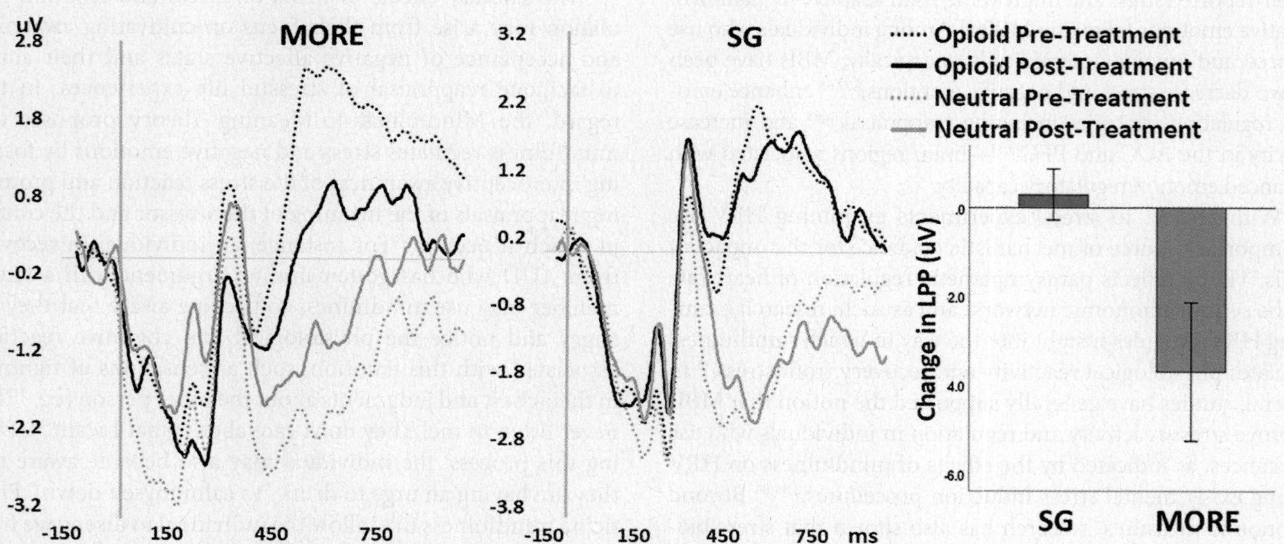

Figure 81-6. In a randomized trial of people who used opioids nonmedically, mindfulness-oriented recovery enhancement (MORE) reduced opioid cue-reactivity, as indicated by the late positive potential of the EEG, to a significantly greater extent than supportive group (SG) therapy. Following treatment with MORE, EEG amplitude in response opioid cues decreased to levels approaching those elicited by neutral cues, indicating that opioid cues became, in effect, more neutral. (Reprinted with permission of AAAS from Garland EL, Atchley RM, Hanley AW, Zubieta JK, Froeliger B. Mindfulness-Oriented Recovery Enhancement remediates hedonic dysregulation in opioid users: neural and affective evidence of target engagement. *Sci Adv.* 2019;5(10):eaax1569. © The Authors, some rights reserved; exclusive licensee AAAS. Distributed under a CC BY-NC 4.0 License (http://creativecommons.org/licenses/by-nc/4.0/))

of "mental training," not unlike weight training or endurance exercise, where repeated mindfulness practice yields increases in "inner strength" and self-control over addictive behaviors by strengthening neural function in the prefrontal cortex. This sort of framing may be useful in demystifying mindfulness, increasing its acceptability. As a corollary to this notion, mindfulness practice is often challenging, especially in the context of high levels of distress or cognitive impairments—both of which are common in people with SUDs. If patients express difficulty practicing mindfulness for long periods of time (eg, 30+ minutes), mindfulness practice may be done in smaller increments. This "chunking" of mindfulness practice requirements may make mindfulness more accessible to a broader range of patients. It is also imperative to explain the concept of mindfulness to the patient to dispel any myths that might serve as barriers to practice. For instance, many patients have the expectation that mindfulness involves an unwavering focus of attention on the breath, and then when their minds begin to wander, they assume that they have failed and that "mindfulness doesn't work." In actuality, mindfulness involves the entire process of attending to a meditative object (eg, the breath), noticing when the mind has wandered, acknowledging and accepting the mind wandering, and then returning the focus of the attention back to the object. This entire arc from focusing attention on the object of mindfulness to cultivating meta-awareness of mind wandering and then returning back to the focused attention on the object should be defined as a "loop of mindfulness." Then, when patients report noticing mind wandering, this can be reframed as part of the practice of mindfulness.

Another key strategy involves recognition that mindfulness may first increase awareness of craving, and then provide a means of regulating craving. According to cognitive processing models of craving, over time addictive behaviors become automatized, driven by impulses outside of conscious awareness.[107,108] Mindfulness may provide a means of deautomatization, reinvesting behaviors that have been rendered automatic and unconscious through repetition with conscious awareness.[109] Informal mindfulness practice during simple, daily life activities that are usually executed without thinking (eg, washing dishes, taking a shower, brushing one's teeth) may increase the capacity for self-monitoring, increasing meta-awareness of when one slips into automatized motor habits. As such, this type of practice might increase the likelihood of a patient with SUD becoming aware when they slip into automatic addictive habits triggered by "people, places, and things." Further, mindfulness may increase awareness of cravings that might usually be ignored or suppressed by a patient in recovery from addiction—an important first step in learning to regulate craving. In that regard, a study found that patients treated with MORE as an adjunct to methadone treatment reported significantly more instances of craving that patients undergoing methadone treatment as usual; yet these same patients reported significant decreases in the intensity of cravings as well as a significantly greater increase in self-control over craving.[72]

Finally, given indications that mindfulness amplifies natural reward processing while decreasing reactivity to drug-related rewards, mindfulness can be used to help people with SUDs restore a sense of value to activities and relationships they once found meaningful prior to developing addiction. Moreover, because mindfulness can elicit internal reward responses such as the positive emotions and pleasant body sensations produced during meditation, it may provide a "natural high" as an alternative to the high sought about through drug use. While patients should be cautioned to not become attached to such pleasant internal states (lest they become yet a new source of craving), it can be empowering to suggest that if the patient is able to endogenously produce reward through mindfulness meditation, they no longer need to seek exogenous rewards from outside themselves through substance use, pathological gambling, etc.

FUTURE DIRECTIONS FOR IMPLEMENTING MINDFULNESS AS A TREATMENT FOR ADDICTION

Multiple RCTs have provided an empirical foundation for the efficacy and mechanisms of MBIs for addiction treatment in research settings. However, positive findings from clinical trials are not always consistently replicated when interventions are delivered in community-based settings.[110] Consequently, real-world effectiveness trials are now needed to examine MBIs in addiction treatment contexts using methods that address the methodological limitations observed in meta-analyses of these interventions. Specifically, there is a need for longitudinal designs with follow-up periods of at least 1 year, triangulation of self-reported outcomes with biochemical verification of substance use, and probability sampling designs to enhance generalizability to a wider-array of clinical populations.

To guide the continued refinement of MBIs and optimize their potential efficacy, *mediation* studies are needed—particularly those that employ innovative imaging technologies to examine the neural mechanisms of MBIs for addiction treatment. For example, fully-powered, randomized studies using fMRI are needed to test basic mechanistic assumptions and novel hypotheses regarding how MBIs facilitate improvements in addiction-related outcomes. Moreover, molecular neuroimaging (eg, positron emission tomography) allows for high-resolution mapping of the brain in vivo and should be employed to understand the effects of MBIs on neurotransmitters and neuropeptides that contribute to addictive behavior. Neuroimaging techniques with a high temporal resolution like electroencephalography (EEG) or magnetoencephalography could be used to learn more about how mindfulness training modulates the dynamic time course of neural responses to drug cues.

Diverse Clinical Populations

Marginalized populations, including racial/ethnic minorities; lesbian, gay, bisexual, and transgender and socio-economically disadvantaged individuals are disproportionately affected by structural inequalities that harm their well-being and place them at heightened risk for psychological and physical health issues.[111,112] Moreover, these populations are underrepresented in studies examining the efficacy and effectiveness of MBIs[113] including those developed to address addiction.[114] Thus, the efficacy and acceptability of MBIs for these populations is unclear.

A recent systematic review of 22 RCTs delivered to samples primarily comprised of people of color found that MBIs were modestly superior to active (g = 0.11, 95% CI = [0.04, 0.18], p = .002) and inactive (g = 0.26, 95%CI = [0.07,0.45], p = .007) control conditions—effects that were smaller in magnitude compared to previous large-scale meta-analyses of MBI RCTs.[35,115,116] To ensure that MBIs for addiction are culturally appropriate, accessible, and inclusive, empirical investigations are needed to examine the treatment *moderators* of these interventions and learn more about the populations for whom MBIs work most optimally to improve addiction-related outcomes. We do not yet know who is likely to respond, or not to respond, to MBI. Moreover, culturally-tailored adaptations of MBIs may be necessary to increase the uptake of mindfulness in diverse populations. Investigation is also warranted to identify populations who may be at heightened risk for adverse effects. Such evidence would indicate a need for treatment adaptions to enhance the safety and efficacy of MBIs for diverse populations.

Treatment Combinations and Sequencing

Although the majority of studies examining MBIs for addiction have evaluated their delivery as stand-alone interventions, many community-based addiction treatment programs provide multiple interventions concurrently. It is not yet known whether delivering MBIs as part of a comprehensive treatment package impacts clinical outcomes. In addition, multimodal addiction treatment programs might be optimized by adjusting the timing when MBIs are introduced in the intervention sequence. To maximize treatment outcomes, should mindfulness be introduced as a harm reduction strategy, during substance withdrawal management, an inpatient addiction treatment program, an intensive outpatient program, or during long-term recovery? Any of these applications could be potentially useful, but systematic investigation of these various options is needed. How might mindfulness outcomes be optimized by combining mindfulness with other interventions? For example, motivational interviewing delivered prior to MBIs may increase motivation and engagement in these interventions. Conversely, delivering MBIs prior to motivational enhancement therapies could increase their therapeutic potential by enhancing awareness of the adverse consequences of addiction, thereby bolstering motivational enhancement.

Similarly, determining optimal sequencing of MBIs vis-à-vis addiction pharmacotherapy is also of value given the demonstrated effectiveness of medications for opioid use disorders.[117] In that regard, a pilot RCT demonstrated that adding MORE to methadone treatment significantly improves addiction treatment outcomes beyond methadone treatment as usual[118]; a recently completed larger RCT replicated these outcomes, with results forthcoming. Whether MBIs can improve outcomes among people treated with buprenorphine or naltrexone remains to be seen. Other adjunctive interventions, including psychopharmacological agents, computer-based cognitive remediation, neurofeedback, neurostimulation, virtual reality, and psychedelics administered prior to, during, or following MBI might also improve outcomes, but the ideal intervention package and sequence remains unknown. The use of these technologies could also be explored to enhance the accessibility and feasibility of these interventions for marginalized populations that face barriers to care access.[114] Research examining treatment sequencing should employ the multiphase optimization strategy, as well as sequential multiple assignment randomized trials, to determine the optimal sequencing of MBIs within addiction treatment programs.[119]

Dose-Response Relationships

The beneficial effects of MBIs are commonly assumed to accrue with practice over time, suggesting that greater "doses" of MBIs are associated with greater responses to treatment. However, supporting evidence for the existence of a dose–response relationship is mixed, with a recent meta-analysis finding nonsignificant dose-response relationships between MBIs and clinical outcomes in nonaddicted populations.[120] The eight-week format of MBSR has become the canonical standard among MBIs, including those developed for addiction.[121] Yet the time demands of extended weekly sessions and the closed group format of most MBIs may hinder the feasibility of these interventions among individuals with SUDs, particularly given the ubiquity of brief inpatient stays and rolling admissions. Moreover, research has shown that brief MBIs are associated with significant improvements in psychological health, pain, and addictive behaviors.[42,104,122,123] Pushing the boundaries of brevity, a recent RCT found that a single 15-minute mindfulness practice reduced opioid use four weeks later.[124] Consequently, determining the minimum dose needed to produce clinical benefits is a critical area for future research.

Although brief interventions are becoming increasingly valued throughout healthcare and addictions treatment, given the chronic recurring nature of addiction, it is plausible that mindfulness may be most effective when used daily as part of a broader recovery lifestyle. Addiction recovery has been conceptualized as an experience involving not only sustained abstinence in the frequency and quantity of drug use, but the development of a healthy, productive, and meaningful life in which vulnerability to drug-related problems is recognized and managed on an ongoing basis.[125] Moreover, the neuroplastic changes induced by mindfulness practice may require long-term, recurrent practice to manifest, particularly for individuals with extensive histories of addictive behavior. The standard 8-week MBI format may be optimized by periodic booster sessions delivered to maintain and strengthen the gains generated during initial exposure to mindfulness practice. One might envision a mindfulness-based peer support approach, in which graduates of clinician-led 8-week MBIs could continue to meet on a regular basis for months (or years) to practice mindfulness meditation as a group and experience supportive social interactions, not unlike those provided by twelve-step fellowships. Indeed, mindfulness-based twelve-step meetings do exist in multiple communities around the United States and internationally, though their outcomes have yet to be studied in any controlled research trials. Concomitantly, MBIs may be wholly congruent with Step 11, increasing conscious contact with a higher power "through prayer and meditation." In that regard, in the largest neuroscientific study of mindfulness as a treatment for addiction to date ($N = 165$), MORE was found to increase experiences of self-transcendence, the sense of being connected to something greater than the self. Increases in self-transcendence during meditation were associated with increases in frontal midline theta EEG activity that in turn mediated the effect of MORE on reduced nonmedical opioid use.[126]

Dissemination and Implementation Challenges

To bridge the gap from research to practice, MBI implementation issues must be addressed. First, the financial and training requirements for many MBIs represent a significant obstacle for clinicians who might otherwise be interested in delivering these interventions and may inhibit their adoption and implementation into community-based practice.[110] Most MBI programs mandate that clinicians have extensive personal mindfulness practice experience, but how much practice is actually needed to be an effective mindfulness therapist? Also, what level of professional education is necessary and sufficient to implement a MBI for addiction? MBRP and MORE are typically delivered by licensed clinicians, whereas MBSR may be provided by people who are not trained healthcare providers. Given the clinical complexity and co-occurring psychiatric disorders common to SUDs, it is likely that well-trained, graduate-level providers are needed to deliver MBIs effectively in addictions treatment. But, can mindfulness be delivered effectively by paraprofessionals or peer support specialists? To date, no best practice guidelines exist detailing the training and supervision requirements and processes for MBI therapists or the extent of personal mindfulness practice required for effective implementation of MBIs in a clinical setting.

Relatedly, quality control is also an important issue for widespread dissemination of MBIs. Though it is becoming more common for behavioral health clinicians in the addictions treatment field to offer mindfulness-based therapy for their patients, no licensing or accreditation bodies exist to verify their training in evidence-based MBIs, and quality may vary widely. Monitoring therapist competence and adherence to intervention content is vital to the successful implementation of MBIs in clinical practice. In that regard, validated therapist fidelity measures exist for both MBRP[127] and MORE.[128] It is important for such instruments to be used during the rollout of MBIs in clinical contexts to improve clinician training and supervision, and maximize MBI treatment outcomes.

Intervention acceptability is another key factor for intervention dissemination, attendance, and adoption.[129] Investigations in this area may lead to more informed decisions regarding the implementation of these interventions. For example, MBI participants who experience immediate benefits may be more likely to establish and maintain a regular practice outside of group sessions. In contrast, those who experience no benefits or even adverse effects may be likely to discontinue participation. Therapeutic alliance (bolstered by techniques including reinforcement and motivational enhancement) may also influence the acceptability of MBIs for addiction—for example, it is possible that participants may be more likely to adhere to treatment when they are positively reinforced by their clinician for initial mindfulness efforts. In that regard, MORE leverages social-behavioral learning principles including positive reinforcement, therapeutic expectancy, shaping, and successive approximation to maximize patient engagement and motivate mindfulness practice. Whether this facilitation approach is superior to the nondirective style employed in MBRP remains to be seen.

Finally, the pathway to reimbursement for MBIs remains unclear. At present, many practitioners offer mindfulness training for private pay, whereas others bill MBIs using the same standard group and individual psychotherapy procedure codes that might be used for other therapeutic approaches like cognitive–behavioral therapy or motivational interviewing. Some health care providers currently receive reimbursement for MBIs when they are billed as group medical visits in primary care. Whether Medicaid (and Medicare) will ultimately cover MBIs remains an issue of great importance, given that many people with SUDs rely on social safety net programs for treatment and recovery services.

CONCLUSION

The past decade has witnessed a proliferation of increasingly rigorous research on the application of mindfulness as a treatment for addiction. Accumulating evidence suggests that MBIs effectively reduce craving and substance use by enhancing top-down executive control over bottom-up motivation and reward functions. Paralleling this growth in research, interest in mindfulness among addiction treatment providers has increased significantly. As such, there is a great need to develop effective approaches to disseminate and implement MBIs in the context of community-based addictions treatment. In light of rigorous RCTs and meta-analyses demonstrating therapeutic effects of MBIs in people with SUDs, now is the time to integrate mindfulness into the armamentarium of addiction medicine.

REFERENCES

1. Koob GF, Volkow ND. Neurobiology of addiction: a neurocircuitry analysis. *Lancet Psychiatry*. 2016;3(8):760-773. doi:10.1016/S2215-0366(16)00104-8
2. Garland EL, Froeliger B, Howard MO. Mindfulness training targets neurocognitive mechanisms of addiction at the attention-appraisal-emotion interface. *Front Psychiatry*. 2013;4. Accessed September 27, 2017. https://www.ncbi.nlm.nih.gov/pmc/articles/PMC3887509/

3. Garland EL, Gaylord SA, Boettiger CA, Howard MO. Mindfulness training modifies cognitive, affective, and physiological mechanisms implicated in alcohol dependence: results of a randomized controlled pilot trial. *J Psychoactive Drugs*. 2010;42(2):177-192.
4. Glasner-Edwards S, Mooney LJ, Ang A, et al. Mindfulness based relapse prevention for stimulant dependent adults: a pilot randomized clinical trial. *Mindfulness*. 2017;8(1):126-135. doi:10.1007/s12671-016-0586-9
5. Garland EL, Hanley AW, Nakamura Y, et al. Mindfulness-oriented recovery enhancement vs supportive group therapy for co-occurring opioid misuse and chronic pain in primary care: a randomized clinical trial. *JAMA Intern Med*. 2022;182(4):407-417.
6. Brewer JA, Mallik S, Babuscio TA, et al. Mindfulness training for smoking cessation: results from a randomized controlled trial. *Drug Alcohol Depend*. 2011;119:72-80.
7. Bowen S, Witkiewitz K, Clifasefi SL, et al. Relative efficacy of mindfulness-based relapse prevention, standard relapse prevention, and treatment as usual for substance use disorders: a randomized clinical trial. *JAMA Psychiatry*. 2014;71(5):547-556.
8. Li W, Garland EL, McGovern P, O'Brien JE, Tronnier C, Howard MO. Mindfulness-oriented recovery enhancement for Internet gaming disorder in U.S. adults: a stage I randomized controlled trial. *Psychol Addict Behav*. 2017;31(4):393.
9. Baminiwatta A, Solangaarachchi I. Trends and developments in mindfulness research over 55 years: a bibliometric analysis of publications indexed in web of science. *Mindfulness (N Y)*. 2021;12(9):2099-2116. doi:10.1007/s12671-021-01681-x
10. Brown KW, Ryan RM. The benefits of being present: mindfulness and its role in psychological well-being. *J Pers Soc Psychol*. 2003;84(4):822-848. doi:10.1037/0022-3514.84.4.822
11. Friese M, Hofmann W. State mindfulness, self-regulation, and emotional experience in everyday life. *Motiv Sci*. 2016;2. doi:10.1037/mot0000027
12. Lutz A, Slagter HA, Dunne JD, Davidson RJ. Attention regulation and monitoring in meditation. *Trends Cogn Sci*. 2008;12(4):163-169. doi:10.1016/j.tics.2008.01.005
13. Vago DR, Silbersweig DA. Self-awareness, self-regulation, and self-transcendence (S-ART): a framework for understanding the neurobiological mechanisms of mindfulness. *Front Hum Neurosci*. 2012;6. Accessed October 8, 2017. https://www.ncbi.nlm.nih.gov/pmc/articles/PMC3480633/
14. Tang YY, Hölzel BK, Posner MI. The neuroscience of mindfulness meditation. *Nat Rev Neurosci*. 2015;16(4):213-225.
15. Kiken LG, Garland EL, Bluth K, Palsson OS, Gaylord SA. From a state to a trait: trajectories of state mindfulness in meditation during intervention predict changes in trait mindfulness. *Personal Individ Differ*. 2015;81:41-46.
16. Davidson RJ. Empirical explorations of mindfulness: conceptual and methodological conundrums. *Emot Wash DC*. 2010;10(1):8-11. doi:10.1037/a0018480
17. Baer RA, Smith GT, Hopkins J, Krietemeyer J, Toney L. Using self-report assessment methods to explore facets of mindfulness. *Assessment*. 2006;13(1):27-45. doi:10.1177/1073191105283504
18. Carmody J, Baer RA. Relationships between mindfulness practice and levels of mindfulness, medical and psychological symptoms and well-being in a mindfulness-based stress reduction program. *J Behav Med*. 2008;31(1):23-33. doi:10.1007/s10865-007-9130-7
19. Gu J, Strauss C, Bond R, Cavanagh K. How do mindfulness-based cognitive therapy and mindfulness-based stress reduction improve mental health and wellbeing? A systematic review and meta-analysis of mediation studies. *Clin Psychol Rev*. 2015;37:1-12. doi:10.1016/j.cpr.2015.01.006
20. Brown KW, Ryan RM, Creswell JD. Mindfulness: theoretical foundations and evidence for its salutary effects. *Psychol Inq*. 2007;18(4):211-237. doi:10.1080/10478400701598298
21. Tomlinson ER, Yousaf O, Vittersø AD, Jones L. Dispositional mindfulness and psychological health: a systematic review. *Mindfulness*. 2018;9(1):23-43. doi:10.1007/s12671-017-0762-6
22. Kang Y, Gruber J, Gray JR. Mindfulness: deautomatization of cognitive and emotional life. In: Ie A, Ngnoumen CT, Langer EJ, eds. *Wiley Blackwell Handbook of Mindfulness*. Wiley; 2014:168-185.
23. Anicha CL, Ode S, Moeller SK, Robinson MD. Toward a cognitive view of trait mindfulness: distinct cognitive skills predict Its observing and nonreactivity Facets. *J Pers*. 2012;80(2):255-285. doi:10.1111/j.1467-6494.2011.00722.x
24. Garland EL. Trait mindfulness predicts attentional and autonomic regulation of alcohol cue-reactivity. *J Psychophysiol*. 2011;25(4):180-189. doi:10.1027/0269-8803/a000060
25. Garland EL, Boettiger CA, Gaylord S, Chanon VW, Howard MO. Mindfulness is inversely associated with alcohol attentional bias among recovering alcohol-dependent adults. *Cogn Ther Res*. 2012;36(5):441-450.
26. Baker AK, Garland EL. Autonomic and affective mediators of the relationship between mindfulness and opioid craving among chronic pain patients. *Exp Clin Psychopharmacol*. 2019;27(1):55-63. doi:10.1037/pha0000225
27. Garland EL, Roberts-Lewis A, Kelley K, Tronnier C, Hanley A. Cognitive and affective mechanisms linking trait mindfulness to craving among individuals in addiction recovery. *Subst Use Misuse*. 2014;49(5):525-535.
28. Karyadi KA, VanderVeen JD, Cyders MA. A meta-analysis of the relationship between trait mindfulness and substance use behaviors. *Drug Alcohol Depend*. 2014;143:1-10. doi:10.1016/j.drugalcdep.2014.07.014
29. Priddy SE, Hanley AW, Riquino MR, Platt KA, Baker AK, Garland EL. Dispositional mindfulness and prescription opioid misuse among chronic pain patients: craving and attention to positive information as mediating mechanisms. *Drug Alcohol Depend*. 2018;188:86-93. doi:10.1016/j.drugalcdep.2018.03.040
30. Kabat-Zinn J. An outpatient program in behavioral medicine for chronic pain patients based on the practice of mindfulness meditation: theoretical considerations and preliminary results. *Gen Hosp Psychiatry*. 1982;4(1):33-47. doi:10.1016/0163-8343(82)90026-3
31. Segal ZV, Teasdale JD, Williams JMG. Mindfulness-based cognitive therapy: theoretical rationale and empirical status. In: Hayes SC, Follette VM, Linehan MM, eds. *Mindfulness and Acceptance: Expanding the Cognitive-Behavioral Tradition*. Guilford Press; 2004:45-65.
32. Bowen S, Chawla N, Grow J, Marlatt G. *Mindfulness-Based Relapse Prevention for Addictive Behaviors*. Guilford Press; 2010.
33. Garland EL. *Mindfulness-Oriented Recovery Enhancement for Addiction, Stress, and Pain*. NASW Press; 2013.
34. Li W, Howard MO, Garland EL, McGovern P, Lazar M. Mindfulness treatment for substance misuse: a systematic review and meta-analysis. *J Subst Abus Treat*. 2017;75:62-96. doi:10.1016/j.jsat.2017.01.008
35. Goldberg SB, Tucker RP, Greene PA, et al. Mindfulness-based interventions for psychiatric disorders: a systematic review and meta-analysis. *Clin Psychol Rev*. 2018;59:52-60. doi:10.1016/j.cpr.2017.10.011
36. Garland EL, Brintz CE, Hanley AW, et al. Mind-body therapies for opioid-treated pain: a systematic review and meta-analysis. *JAMA Intern Med*. 2020;180(1):91-105.
37. Garland EL, Howard MO. Mindfulness-based treatment of addiction: current state of the field and envisioning the next wave of research. *Addict Sci Clin Pract*. 2018;13. doi:10.1186/s13722-018-0115-3
38. Goldstein RZ, Volkow ND. Dysfunction of the prefrontal cortex in addiction: neuroimaging findings and clinical implications. *Nat Rev Neurosci*. 2011;12(11):652-669.
39. Alfonso JP, Caracuel A, Delgado-Pastor LC, Verdejo-García A. Combined goal management training and mindfulness meditation improve executive functions and decision-making performance in abstinent polysubstance abusers. *Drug Alcohol Depend*. 2011;117(1):78-81. doi:10.1016/j.drugalcdep.2010.12.025
40. Valls-Serrano C, Caracuel A, Verdejo-Garcia A. Goal management training and mindfulness meditation improve executive functions and transfer to ecological tasks of daily life in polysubstance users enrolled in therapeutic community treatment. *Drug Alcohol Depend*. 2016;165:9-14. doi:10.1016/j.drugalcdep.2016.04.040
41. Spears CA, Hedeker D, Li L, et al. Mechanisms underlying mindfulness-based addiction treatment versus cognitive behavioral therapy and usual care for smoking cessation. *J Consult Clin Psychol*. 2017;85(11):1029-1040. doi:10.1037/ccp0000229

42. Tang YY, Tang R, Posner MI. Brief meditation training induces smoking reduction. *Proc Natl Acad Sci U S A*. 2013;110(34):13971-13975. doi:10.1073/pnas.1311887110
43. Holzman JB, Bridgett DJ. Heart rate variability indices as bio-markers of top-down self-regulatory mechanisms: a meta-analytic review. *Neurosci Biobehav Rev*. 2017;74:233-255. doi:10.1016/j.neubiorev.2016.12.032
44. Cavanagh JF, Frank MJ. Frontal theta as a mechanism for cognitive control. *Trends Cogn Sci*. 2014;18(8):414-421.
45. Hudak J, Hanley AW, Marchand WR, Nakamura Y, Yabko B, Garland EL. Endogenous theta stimulation during meditation predicts reduced opioid dosing following treatment with Mindfulness-Oriented Recovery Enhancement. *Neuropsychopharmacology*. 2021;46(4):836-843.
46. Garland EL, Hudak J, Hanley AW, Nakamura Y. Mindfulness-oriented recovery enhancement reduces opioid dose in primary care by strengthening autonomic regulation during meditation. *Am Psychol*. 2020;75(6):840.
47. Garland EL, Froeliger B, Zeidan F, Partin K, Howard MO. The downward spiral of chronic pain, prescription opioid misuse, and addiction: cognitive, affective, and neuropsychopharmacologic pathways. *Neurosci Biobehav Rev*. 2013;37(10):2597-2607.
48. Koob GF. A role for brain stress systems in addiction. *Neuron*. 2008;59(1):11-34.
49. Shurman J, Koob GF, Gutstein HB. Opioids, pain, the brain, and hyperkatifeia: a framework for the rational use of opioids for pain. *Pain Med Malden Mass*. 2010;11(7):1092-1098. doi:10.1111/j.1526-4637.2010.00881.x
50. Garland EL. Restructuring reward processing with mindfulness-oriented recovery enhancement: novel therapeutic mechanisms to remediate hedonic dysregulation in addiction, stress, and pain. *Ann N Y Acad Sci*. 2016;1373(1):25-37.
51. Garland EL. Mindful positive emotion regulation as a treatment for addiction: from hedonic pleasure to self-transcendent meaning. *Curr Opin Behav Sci*. 2021;39:168-177.
52. Arch JJ, Brown KW, Goodman RJ, Della Porta MD, Kiken LG, Tillman S. Enjoying food without caloric cost: the impact of brief mindfulness on laboratory eating outcomes. *Behav Res Ther*. 2016;79:23-34. doi:10.1016/j.brat.2016.02.002
53. Egan RP, Hill KE, Foti D. Differential effects of state and trait mindfulness on the late positive potential. *Emotion*. 2018;18(8):1128-1141. doi:10.1037/emo0000383
54. Hong PY, Lishner DA, Han KH, Huss EA. The positive impact of mindful eating on expectations of food liking. *Mindfulness*. 2011;2(2):103-113.
55. Hong PY, Lishner DA, Han KH. Mindfulness and eating: an experiment examining the effect of mindful raisin eating on the enjoyment of sampled food. *Mindfulness*. 2014;5(1):80-87.
56. Geschwind N, Peeters F, Drukker M, van Os J, Wichers M. Mindfulness training increases momentary positive emotions and reward experience in adults vulnerable to depression: a randomized controlled trial. *J Consult Clin Psychol*. 2011;79(5):618.
57. Garland EL, Baker AK, Larsen P, et al. Randomized controlled trial of brief mindfulness training and hypnotic suggestion for acute pain relief in the hospital setting. *J Gen Intern Med*. 2017;32(10):1106-1113. doi:10.1007/s11606-017-4116-9
58. Dambrun M, Berniard A, Didelot T, et al. Unified consciousness and the effect of body scan meditation on happiness: alteration of inner-body experience and feeling of harmony as central processes. *Mindfulness*. 2019;10(8):153-1544. doi:10.1007/s12671-019-01104-y
59. Hagerty MR, Isaacs J, Brasington L, Shupe L, Fetz EE, Cramer SC. Case study of ecstatic meditation: fMRI and EEG evidence of self-stimulating a reward system. *Neural Plast*. 2013;2013: doi:10.1155/2013/653572
60. Garland EL, Fredrickson BL. Positive psychological states in the arc from mindfulness to self-transcendence: extensions of the Mindfulness-to-Meaning Theory and applications to addiction and chronic pain treatment. *Curr Opin Psychol*. 2019;28:184-191. doi:10.1016/j.copsyc.2019.01.004
61. Dyczkowski MS. *The Doctrine of Vibration: An Analysis of the Doctrines and Practices Associated with Kashmir Shaivism*. SUNY Press; 1987.
62. Sharp PE. Meditation-induced bliss viewed as release from conditioned neural (thought) patterns that block reward signals in the brain pleasure center. *Relig Brain Behav*. 2014;4(3):202-229.
63. Hanley AW, Nakamura Y, Garland EL. The Nondual Awareness Dimensional Assessment (NADA): new tools to assess nondual traits and states of consciousness occurring within and beyond the context of meditation. *Psychol Assess*. 2018;30(12):1625.
64. Spagnolo PA, Kimes A, Schwandt ML, et al. Striatal dopamine release in response to morphine: a [11C]raclopride positron emission tomography study in healthy men. *Biol Psychiatry*. 2019;86(5):356-364. doi:10.1016/j.biopsych.2019.03.965
65. Hanley AW, Garland EL. Mapping the affective dimension of embodiment with the sensation manikin: validation among chronic pain patients and modification by mindfulness-oriented recovery enhancement. *Psychosom Med*. 2019;81(7):612. doi:10.1097/PSY.0000000000000725
66. Garland EL, Froeliger B, Howard MO. Neurophysiological evidence for remediation of reward processing deficits in chronic pain and opioid misuse following treatment with Mindfulness-Oriented Recovery Enhancement: exploratory ERP findings from a pilot RCT. *J Behav Med*. 2015;38(2):327-336. doi:10.1007/s10865-014-9607-0
67. Garland EL, Atchley RM, Hanley AW, Zubieta JK, Froeliger B. Mindfulness-oriented recovery enhancement remediates hedonic dysregulation in opioid users: neural and affective evidence of target engagement. *Sci Adv*. 2019;5(10):eaax1569.
68. Garland EL, Fix S, Hudak J, et al. Mindfulness-oriented recovery enhancement remediates anhedonia in chronic opioid use by enhancing neurophysiological responses during savoring of natural reward. *Psychol Med*. 2023;53(5):2085-2094. doi:10.1017/S0033291721003834
69. Garland EL, Froeliger B, Howard MO. Effects of mindfulness-oriented recovery enhancement on reward responsiveness and opioid cue-reactivity. *Psychopharmacology*. 2014;231(16):3229-3238. doi:10.1007/s00213-014-3504-7
70. Garland EL, Howard MO, Zubieta JK, Froeliger B. Restructuring hedonic dysregulation in chronic pain and prescription opioid misuse: effects of mindfulness-oriented recovery enhancement on responsiveness to drug cues and natural rewards. *Psychother Psychosom*. 2017;86(2):111-112.
71. Garland EL, Bryan CJ, Finan PH, et al. Pain, hedonic regulation, and opioid misuse: modulation of momentary experience by mindfulness-oriented recovery enhancement in opioid-treated chronic pain patients. *Drug Alcohol Depend*. 2017;173:S65-S72.
72. Garland EL, Hanley AW, Kline A, Cooperman NA. Mindfulness-oriented recovery enhancement reduces opioid craving among individuals with opioid use disorder and chronic pain in medication assisted treatment: ecological momentary assessments from a stage 1 randomized controlled trial. *Drug Alcohol Depend*. 2019;203(1):61-65.
73. Froeliger B, Mathew AR, McConnell PA, et al. Restructuring reward mechanisms in nicotine addiction: A pilot fMRI study of mindfulness-oriented recovery enhancement for cigarette smokers. *Evid Based Complement Alternat Med*. 2017;2017:e7018014. doi:10.1155/2017/7018014
74. Garland E, Bell S, Atchley R, Froeliger B. Emotion dysregulation in addiction. In: Beauchaine TP, Crowell SE, eds. *The Oxford Handbook of Emotion Dysregulation*. Oxford University Press; 2019.
75. Kober H. Emotion regulation in substance use disorders. In: Gross JJ, ed. *Handbook of Emotion Regulation*. 2nd ed. Guilford Press; 2014:428-446.
76. Schwabe L, Dickinson A, Wolf OT. Stress, habits, and drug addiction: a psychoneuroendocrinological perspective. *Exp Clin Psychopharmacol*. 2011;19(1):53.
77. Chambers R, Gullone E, Allen NB. Mindful emotion regulation: an integrative review. *Clin Psychol Rev*. 2009;29(6):560-572. doi:10.1016/j.cpr.2009.06.005
78. Eberth J, Sedlmeier P. The effects of mindfulness meditation: a meta-analysis. *Mindfulness*. 2012;3(3):174-189. doi:10.1007/s12671-012-0101-x
79. Farb NAS, Anderson AK, Irving JA, Segal ZV. Mindfulness interventions and emotion regulation. In: Gross JJ, ed. *Handbook of Emotion Regulation*. 2nd ed. The Guilford Press; 2014:548-567.

80. Hölzel BK, Lazar SW, Gard T, Schuman-Olivier Z, Vago DR, Ott U. How does mindfulness meditation work? proposing mechanisms of action from a conceptual and neural perspective. *Perspect Psychol Sci.* 2011;6(6):537-559. doi:10.1177/1745691611419671
81. Goyal M, Singh S, Sibinga EM, et al. Meditation programs for psychological stress and well-being: a systematic review and meta-analysis. *JAMA Intern Med.* 2014;174(3):357-368.
82. Garland EL, Manusov EG, Froeliger B, Kelly A, Williams JM, Howard MO. Mindfulness-oriented recovery enhancement for chronic pain and prescription opioid misuse: results from an early-stage randomized controlled trial. *J Consult Clin Psychol.* 2014;82(3):448.
83. Roberts RL, Ledermann K, Garland EL. Mindfulness-oriented recovery enhancement improves negative emotion regulation among opioid-treated chronic pain patients by increasing interoceptive awareness. *J Psychosom Res.* 2022;152:110677. doi:10.1016/j.jpsychores.2021.110677
84. Tang YY, Tang R, Posner MI. Mindfulness meditation improves emotion regulation and reduces drug abuse. *Drug Alcohol Depend.* 2016;163:S13-S18. doi:10.1016/j.drugalcdep.2015.11.041
85. Thayer JF, Hansen AL, Psychol E, Johnsen BH. Heart rate variability, prefrontal neural function, and cognitive performance: the neurovisceral integration perspective on self-regulation, adaptation, and health. *Ann Behav Med.* 2009;37(2):141-153.
86. Brewer JA, Sinha R, Chen JA, et al. Mindfulness training and stress reactivity in substance abuse: results from a randomized, controlled stage I pilot study. *Subst Abuse.* 2009;30(4):306-317. doi:10.1080/08897070903250241
87. Carroll H, Lustyk MKB. Mindfulness-based relapse prevention for substance use disorders: effects on cardiac vagal control and craving Under stress. *Mindfulness.* 2018;9:488-499. doi:10.1007/s12671-017-0791-1
88. Paz R, Zvielli A, Goldstein P, Bernstein A. Brief mindfulness training de-couples the anxiogenic effects of distress intolerance on reactivity to and recovery from stress among deprived smokers. *Behav Res Ther.* 2017;95:117-127. doi:10.1016/j.brat.2017.05.017
89. Goldberg SB, Manley AR, Smith SS, et al. Hair cortisol as a biomarker of stress in mindfulness training for smokers. *J Altern Complement Med.* 2014;20(8):630-634.
90. Marcus MT, Fine PM, Moeller FG, et al. Change in stress levels following mindfulness-based stress reduction in a therapeutic community. *Addict Disord Their Treat.* 2003;2(3):63.
91. Kober H, Brewer JA, Height KL, Sinha R. Neural stress reactivity relates to smoking outcomes and differentiates between mindfulness and cognitive-behavioral treatments. *NeuroImage.* 2017;151:4-13.
92. Garland EL, Farb NA, Goldin PR, Fredrickson BL. Mindfulness broadens awareness and builds eudaimonic meaning: a process model of mindful positive emotion regulation. *Psychol Inq.* 2015;26(4):293-314. doi:10.1080/1047840X.2015.1064294
93. Garland EL, Franken I, Howard M. Cue-elicited heart rate variability and attentional bias predict alcohol relapse following treatment. *Psychopharmacology.* 2012;222(1):17-26.
94. Garland EL, Howard MO. Opioid attentional bias and cue-elicited craving predict future risk of prescription opioid misuse among chronic pain patients. *Drug Alcohol Depend.* 2014;144:283-287. doi:10.1016/j.drugalcdep.2014.09.014
95. Wasan AD, Ross EL, Michna E, et al. Craving of prescription opioids in patients with chronic pain: a longitudinal outcomes trial. *J Pain.* 2012;13(2):146-154. doi:10.1016/j.jpain.2011.10.010
96. Robinson T, Berridge KC. The neural basis of drug craving: an incentive-sensitization theory of addiction. *Brain Res Rev.* 1993;18(3):247-291. doi:10.1016/0165-0173(93)90013-P
97. Field M, Cox W. Attentional bias in addictive behaviors: a review of its development, causes, and consequences. *Drug Alcohol Depend.* 2008;97(1-2):1-20. doi:10.1016/j.drugalcdep.2008.03.030
98. Berger SP, Reid MS, Delucchi K, et al. Haloperidol antagonism of cue-elicited cocaine craving. *Lancet.* 1996;347(9000):504-508.
99. McRae-Clark AL, Carter RE, Price KL, et al. Stress-and cue-elicited craving and reactivity in marijuana-dependent individuals. *Psychopharmacology.* 2011;218(1):49-58.
100. Sayette MA, Martin CS, Wertz JM, Shiffman S, Perrott MA. A multi-dimensional analysis of cue-elicited craving in heavy smokers and tobacco chippers. *Addiction.* 2001;96(10):1419-1432.
101. Garland EL, Baker AK, Howard MO. Mindfulness-oriented recovery enhancement reduces opioid attentional bias among prescription opioid-treated chronic pain patients. *J Soc Soc Work Res.* 2017;8(4):493-509. doi:10.1086/694324
102. Hanley AW, Garland EL. Salivary measurement and mindfulness-based modulation of prescription opioid cue-reactivity. *Drug Alcohol Depend.* 2020;217:108351. doi:10.1016/j.drugalcdep.2020.108351
103. Westbrook C, Creswell JD, Tabibnia G, Julson E, Kober H, Tindle HA. Mindful attention reduces neural and self-reported cue-induced craving in smokers. *Soc Cogn Affect Neurosci.* 2011;8(1):73-84.
104. Bowen S, Marlatt A. Surfing the urge: brief mindfulness-based intervention for college student smokers. *Psychol Addict Behav.* 2009;23(4):666-671. doi:10.1037/a0017127
105. Witkiewitz K, Bowen S. Depression, craving, and substance use following a randomized trial of mindfulness-based relapse prevention. *J Consult Clin Psychol.* 2010;78(3):362.
106. Elwafi HM, Witkiewitz K, Mallik S, Thornhill TA IV, Brewer JA. Mindfulness training for smoking cessation: moderation of the relationship between craving and cigarette use. *Drug Alcohol Depend.* 2013;130(1):222-229.
107. Tiffany ST. A cognitive model of drug urges and drug-use behavior: role of automatic and nonautomatic processes. *Psychol Rev.* 1990;97:147-168.
108. Tiffany ST. Cognitive concepts of craving. *Alcohol Res Health.* 1999;23:215-224.
109. Deikman AJ. Deautomatization and the mystic experience. *Psychiatry.* 1966;29:324-388.
110. Wilson AD, Roos CR, Robinson CS, et al. Mindfulness-based interventions for addictive behaviors: implementation issues on the road ahead. *Psychol Addict Behav.* 2017;31(8):888.
111. Chatterjee S, Biswas P, Guria RT. LGBTQ care at the time of COVID-19. *Diabetes Metab Syndr.* 2020;14(6):1757-1758. doi:10.1016/j.dsx.2020.09.001
112. Wildeman C, Wang EA. Mass incarceration, public health, and widening inequality in the USA. *Lancet.* 2017;389(10077):1464-1474. doi:10.1016/S0140-6736(17)30259-3
113. Waldron EM, Hong S, Moskowitz JT, Burnett-Zeigler I. A systematic review of the demographic characteristics of participants in us-based randomized controlled trials of mindfulness-based interventions. *Mindfulness.* 2018;9(6):1671-1692. doi:10.1007/s12671-018-0920-5
114. Spears CA. Mindfulness-based interventions for addictions among diverse and underserved populations. *Curr Opin Psychol.* 2019;30:11-16. doi:10.1016/j.copsyc.2018.12.012
115. Khoury B, Lecomte T, Fortin G, et al. Mindfulness-based therapy: a comprehensive meta-analysis. *Clin Psychol Rev.* 2013;33(6):763-771. doi:10.1016/j.cpr.2013.05.005
116. Sun S, Goldberg SB, Loucks EB, Brewer JA. Mindfulness-based interventions among people of color: a systematic review and meta-analysis. *Psychother Res.* 2022;32(3):277-290. doi:10.1080/10503307.2021.1937369
117. Volkow ND, Frieden TR, Hyde PS, Cha SS. Medication-assisted therapies—tackling the opioid-overdose epidemic. *N Engl J Med.* 2014;370(22):2063-2066.
118. Cooperman NA, Hanley AW, Kline A, Garland EL. A pilot randomized clinical trial of mindfulness-oriented recovery enhancement as an adjunct to methadone treatment for people with opioid use disorder and chronic pain: impact on illicit drug use, health, and well-being. *J Subst Abus Treat.* 2021;127:108468. doi:10.1016/j.jsat.2021.108468
119. Collins LM, Murphy SA, Strecher V. The multiphase optimization strategy (MOST) and the sequential multiple assignment randomized trial (SMART): new methods for more potent eHealth interventions. *Am J Prev Med.* 2007;32(5):S112-S118.
120. Strohmaier S. The relationship between doses of mindfulness-based programs and depression, anxiety, stress, and mindfulness: a dose-response meta-regression of randomized controlled trials. *Mindfulness.* 2020;11(6):1315-1335. doi:10.1007/s12671-020-01319-4

121. Demarzo M, Montero-Marin J, Puebla-Guedea M, et al. Efficacy of 8- and 4-session mindfulness-based interventions in a non-clinical population: a controlled study. *Front Psychol.* 2017;8:1343. doi:10.3389/fpsyg.2017.01343
122. Strohmaier S, Jones FW, Cane JE. Effects of length of mindfulness practice on mindfulness, depression, anxiety, and stress: a randomized controlled experiment. *Mindfulness.* 2021;12(1):198-214. doi:10.1007/s12671-020-01512-5
123. Hanley AW, Gililland J, Erickson J, et al. Brief preoperative mind–body therapies for total joint arthroplasty patients: a randomized controlled trial. *Pain.* 2021;162(6):1749-1757.
124. Hanley AW, Gililland J, Garland EL. To be mindful of the breath or pain: comparing two brief preoperative mindfulness techniques for total joint arthroplasty patients. *J Consult Clin Psychol.* 2021;89(7):590-600. doi:10.1037/ccp0000657
125. White WL. Addiction recovery: its definition and conceptual boundaries. *J Subst Abus Treat.* 2007;33(3):229-241. doi:10.1016/j.jsat.2007.04.015
126. Garland EL, Hanley AW, Hudak J, Nakamura Y, Froeliger B. Mindfulness-induced endogenous theta stimulation occasions self-transcendence and inhibits addictive behavior. *Sci Adv.* 2022;8(41):1-9. doi:10.1126/sciadv.abo4455
127. Chawla N, Collins S, Bowen S, et al. The mindfulness-based relapse prevention adherence and competence scale: development, interrater reliability, and validity. *Psychother Res.* 2010;20(4):388-397. doi:10.1080/10503300903544257
128. Hanley AW, Garland EL. The Mindfulness-Oriented Recovery Enhancement Fidelity Measure (MORE-FM): development and validation of a new tool to assess therapist adherence and competence. *J Evid-Based Soc Work.* 2021;18(3):308-322.
129. Bautista T, James D, Amaro H. Acceptability of mindfulness-based interventions for substance use disorder: a systematic review. *Complement Ther Clin Pract.* 2019;35:201-207. doi:10.1016/j.ctcp.2019.02.012

CHAPTER

82

Digital Health Interventions for Substance Use Disorders: The State of the Science

Smita Das

CHAPTER OUTLINE

- Evolution of digital health interventions in the past 5 years
- Digital therapeutics for substance use disorders
- Mobile applications or apps or stand-alone websites
- Telehealth (with focus on OUD)
- Newer digital technologies
- Integration into practice
- Future opportunities and responsible digital health

EVOLUTION OF DIGITAL HEALTH INTERVENTIONS IN THE PAST 5 YEARS

Since the previous publication of this chapter 5 years ago in 2018, there have been considerable advances and changes in the space of digital mental health. Previously, there was a growing body of evidence around the emerging potential of digital health. Since then, in part due to the SARS-CoV-2 or COVID-19 pandemic, digital technology has revolutionized the delivery of care as well as digital resources available in the field of substance use disorders (SUD). This includes previously discussed mobile therapeutic tools, emerging wearable devices and digital therapeutics. Newer areas in this field that have been impactful are machine learning, telehealth and leveraging technology for team-based care. While mobile phone adoption has increased, digital health interventions also include computers, tablets and measurement devices. This area of science is increasingly being referred to as "digital health."[1]

The International Telecommunications Union (ITU) of the United Nations reports that nearly two-thirds of the world's population uses the internet, representing a 17% increase since 2019 and demonstrating the impacts of the pandemic.[2] In developed countries, that proportion is 90%. The ITU also reports that in almost half of the countries for which data are available for the 2018 to 2020 timeframe, more than 90% of the population owned a mobile phone. A recent review examining smartphone usage and attitudes in the literature reported that mobile phone ownership among the population with SUD from 2013 to 2019 ranged from 83% to 94%, while smartphone ownership ranged from 57% to 94%.[3] In the literature, baby boomers (>52 years of age) were less likely compared to Generation X and millennials to own a mobile phone with app capability, so digital innovations will need to keep that in mind. The review notes that in previous studies, 79% to 96% of individuals with SUDs had phones with text messaging capabilities and between 61% and 68% of individuals used their mobile phones to access the internet.

Given the ubiquity of technology worldwide combined with the impacts of the pandemic, access to internet or technology-based interventions, care tools and self-care has gained traction and continues to grow. For substance use specifically, the illness is intertwined with daily activities and life, so activities related to and impacts of use are important to acknowledge and treat in those settings in real time. For example, being able to log use of a substance as it happens is not only helpful for measurement-based care, but also may influence behavior as it makes the activity more mindful. Or having access to a plan to prevent recurrence of use at one's fingertips may truly change the course of their recovery. The DSM-5-TR classifies SUDs according to the impact on someone's life and functioning, so it follows that during everyday life technology could have impact, rather than just in the confines of a medical office.[4] Being able to observe, discuss and influence choices made during everyday activities in real-time arguably constitutes the "single greatest opportunity to improve health and reduce premature deaths" in the United States.[5] Indeed, technology could help affect the "5000-hour problem"—that even patients with multiple chronic diseases only spend a few hours a year in front of a doctor, and during the 5,000+ other waking hours of that year, their doctor neither knows what they are doing nor has effective tools to support them in the management of their chronic diseases.[6]

Another concept to consider in delivery of technology-based interventions is mechanism. It has been suggested that the mechanisms (the theoretical bases) employed in digital interventions are generally the same as traditional modalities (self-efficacy, motivation, refusal skills, etc.). However, the research into this area and a priori declaration of mechanisms in studies is limited. A 2018 review investigating behavior change techniques (BCTs) in 41 studies of digital interventions for reducing alcohol consumption identified that the interventions used a mean of 9.1 BCTs.[7] Behavior substitution, problem solving, and credible source were most effective in reducing alcohol use. Most trials used feedback as well (though less effective at reducing alcohol use). Other BCTs used less were control theory, goal setting and self-monitoring. Interestingly this study notes that several of these well validated approaches in traditional settings were less employed in digital interventions for alcohol.

Whether digital interventions are similar in content and efficacy to traditional (in person) care (discussed in this chapter) or not, there remains another impetus to continue to research: access. Stigma is already high when it comes to seeking care and less than 1% of people with an SUD who did not receive substance use treatment at a specialty facility felt they needed treatment and made an effort to get treatment.[8] Offering another avenue to access care is vital with growing rates of substance use and SUDs. And, even if stigma were not an issue, the SUD clinician workforce cannot meet the population-level needs for SUD. Further, even if the SUD clinician workforce were to be dramatically expanded, the workforce could never be sufficiently scalable to meet the full needs of the population or to offer anytime/anywhere care. The challenge of having an insufficient workforce to meet need at scale is becoming an increasing problem in the United States, where drug overdoses (particularly from opioids) have dramatically spiked in recent years, especially during the COVID-19 pandemic.[9]

There are four main categories of digital health we will consider in this chapter. The first is what had been summarized in the previous edition: digital therapeutics also referred to as DTx. DTx are mobile, Web, or other software-based platforms or devices that deliver effective treatments for medical conditions or diseases but do not include general wellness apps or telehealth that provide remote access to a clinician.[10] Rather, they are evidence-based software that can complement or even replace prescription drugs for managing certain health conditions.[11] Further, DTx are medical treatments that can make medical claims, receive regulatory authorization and reimbursement. Developers can apply for Food and Drug Administration (FDA) clearance to be considered prescription digital therapeutics. As of 2022, there are also pieces of legislation to cover access to digital therapeutics in Medicare and Medicaid.[12]

The second category to be discussed are applications or mobile applications not subject to regulatory review of digital therapeutics. These may range from self-monitoring apps to apps that supplement care. We will review evidence for standalone apps as well as guided apps.

The third category includes technology to deliver standard care. While not revolutionary, telemedicine applied to SUD at scale has the potential to increase reach and access of services. The way this care is delivered needs to be adapted to account for the virtual world. From drug screens to groups, telemedicine delivery of traditional clinic services such as medication visits and intensive outpatient programs (IOP) deserves some attention.

A fourth section will address emerging areas in digital health such as social media, chatbots, peer support/groups, wearables and virtual reality.

As noted in the introductory paragraph, digital health has seen major gains and developments since the publication of the previous edition of this text. With the developments over the past 5 years, this chapter will now shift to include more meta-analyses and reviews as opposed to single site studies. Discussion of effect sizes will be common, where values of 0.20, 0.50, and 0.80 for Cohens d (also known as SMD or standard mean difference) and Hedges g are commonly considered to be indicative of small, medium, and large effects when comparing interventions. Targets of interest in these comparisons are decrease in substance use and retention in treatment. We will note defining characteristics of quality digital health so that users and health care entities can better evaluate them for consideration in practice. It is also important to note that with increased technology adoption, globalization and the COVID-19 pandemic, digital health will continue to shift rapidly. This chapter will attempt to capture the current transitory state of the field. After discussing the aforementioned categories of digital health, the chapter will close with potential future directions as well as ethical and safety considerations when evaluating the future of digital health and SUD.

DIGITAL THERAPEUTICS FOR SUBSTANCE USE DISORDERS

Digital therapeutics, also referred to as DTx are evidence-based software that can complement or even replace prescription drugs for managing certain health conditions.[11] With FDA clearance, they can make medical claims, receive regulatory authorization and reimbursement. Authors from NIDA (National Institute of Drug Abuse) and the FDA support the development of safe and effective DTx for SUDs, noting they "offer unique treatment options and can deliver interventions with fidelity and state-of-the-art practices."[10]

To be cleared by the FDA, a DTx develop must complete trials to demonstrate at least equivalence of existing products or modalities or de novo value and safety. Aside from FDA clearance, DTx are different from general apps because they require RCTs as part of the clearance, are disease specific, offered by prescription and are subject to regulatory oversight.[10] DTx can either be software as a medical device (SaMD—separate from hardware) or mobile medical applications (MMAs—for a medical device or can transform a platform into a medical device).

Only two SUD DTx have applied for and received FDA clearance as a prescription DTx and readily able to integrate into practice for patients interested in using a digital resource to complement care: reSET, a 90-day program for treating SUDs; and reSET-O, an 84-day program to treat opioid use disorder (OUD), which are based on TES or Therapeutic Education System (TES).[13] TES is an internet-delivered behavioral intervention that includes motivational incentives and serves as a clinician-extender in the treatment of SUDs.[14] Due to the small number of DTx available, there are no meta-analyses available but the trials required for FDA approval are presented.

The initial DTx cleared by the FDA in 2017 was reSET, which is intended to use with outpatient therapy to treat alcohol, cocaine, cannabis, and stimulant SUDs (not OUD)[15] using CRA or Community Reinforcement Approach. reSET is a patient mobile application (app) with a clinician interface delivering cognitive-behavioral therapy through 61 modules (30 min of treatment each) plus quizzes. The DTx is intended to be used with outpatient therapy and in addition to a contingency management (CM). The FDA reviewed data from a multisite, unblinded, 12-week clinical trial of 399 patients who received either treatment as usual or the addition of a desktop-based version of reSET. There was a statistically significant increase in adherence to abstinence for the patients with alcohol, cocaine, cannabis, and stimulant SUD in those who used reSET (40.3%), compared with patients who did not (17.6%) ($p = 0.0004$). It was not effective for OUD.

In another iteration of reSET, known as reSET-O, which the FDA cleared in 2018, the developers did focus on opioids[16] but added in buprenorphine treatment.[17] The FDA reviewed data from a multi-site, unblinded, controlled 12-week clinical trial of 170 patients who received supervised buprenorphine treatment paired with a behavior therapy program, either with or without the addition of a desktop-based version of reSET-O for use in the clinic. While reSET-O did not decrease illegal drug use, there was a statistically significant increase in retention in a treatment program for 12 weeks for the patients who used the desktop computer version of the reSET-O program (82.4%) compared to those who did not (68.4%) ($p = 0.02$).

Of note, the research settings had many resources that may not always be in place including CM, 30 minutes of face-to-face counseling every other week and 3 times a week urine testing. A review of adjunct digital therapeutics for SUD discusses reSET-O and two other commonly compared programs that do not have FDA clearance. This review was completed by the Clinical and Economic Review's Midwest Comparative Effectiveness Public Advisory Council, an independent appraisal committees convened by Institute for Clinical and Economic Review to engage in the public deliberation of the evidence on clinical and cost-effectiveness of health care interventions.[18] The first of the two other mentioned programs uses digital CBT with a program that enhances patient communication with addiction experts, peer support groups, and counselors. The second program is a CBT + CM app with substance use screening results, Bluetooth-enabled breathalyzer for alcohol testing, drug saliva testing, and appointment monitoring and reminders. As noted previously, retention (long term, defined as 6 months to 2 years) was a major outcome of interest; the review authors reported that data were limited with respect to retention. The authors do cite the above-mentioned reSET-O studies but are not confident in the results proving an effect on retention given the nature of the studies. For the other two therapeutics, the authors cite one study for each, but they were unable to comment on retention. In a cost effectiveness analysis, the panel only had data for reSET-O and estimated that cost per quality-adjusted life-year (QALY) ranged from approximately $50,000 to $500,000 per QALY depending on parameters uses. This panel was tasked with reviewing the report and voting on the state of the evidence; they voted 10 to 3 that the clinical evidence was not adequate to demonstrate greater net health benefit for reSET-O compared with best supportive care and 13 to 0 that the evidence was not adequate to demonstrate greater net health benefit for either the other 2 apps compared with best supportive care. Ultimately the panel recommended that due to the overwhelming value of MAT (medications for addictions treatment), digital technologies must be carefully studied/implemented if used, so as to not negatively interfere with proven interventions; RCTs and better methodologies in development studies should be required.

Due to the cost associated with developing and gaining clearance for digital therapeutics, combined with the friction of getting payers to reimburse for and providers to prescribe DTx, there has not been widespread adoption of these tools in practice as of the writing of this chapter. Simultaneously, more easily accessible apps are available to users (described more in later parts of the chapter). The American Medical Association and Centers for Medicare and Medicaid Services have put forth codes for "prescription digital behavioral therapy," which could make it easier to get coverage moving forward.[12,19,20]

MOBILE APPLICATIONS OR APPS OR STAND-ALONE WEBSITES

Mobile applications or apps are generally pieces of software one can download directly on to a mobile device. It has been estimated that over 10,000 such mental health apps exist but the quality is not always guaranteed.[21] In 2017, one report noted that there were over 318,000 health apps available on top app stores worldwide with more than 200 health apps being added each day.[22] A 2019 review identified 93 apps with over 10,000 installs targeting anxiety, depression, or emotional well-being. However, these apps had only 4% median daily active users, indicating possible low utility in practice.[23] The medians of app 15-day and 30-day retention rates were 3.9% and 3.3% respectively. Therefore, while there are many apps, the engagement and retention may be limited. A 2020 review found 1,009 apps related to wellness and stress.[24] Only 2.08% (21/1,009) were supported by original research publications, with a total of 25 efficacy studies and 10 feasibility studies (but 8 efficacy studies were from one vendor). In a recent meta-review looking at digital interventions for all mental illness, 304 met the criteria for study inclusion and interestingly a majority (52%) of research involved the treatment of SUDs.[25] Also included in this section are stand-alone websites, predecessors to mobile apps. Finally, there is some mixing of stand-alone app studies (unguided) and guided studies; they are sometimes combined in reviews and efforts will be made to mention them when any studies in this section have guided interventions.

A 2019 review and meta-analysis of stand-alone mental health apps reported that in 3 apps aimed to help people quit smoking and 3 alcohol app studies the effects of the apps were small compared to control for smoking, there was no significant effects for alcohol and no significant difference when pooled.[26] The authors discuss the merits of guided interventions (versus purely stand-alone) to possibly increase efficacy. There is also the factor of adherence, which may be less in stand-alone apps; it may be that the apps are not effective because they are not used as intended. The authors close noting that knowledge on how to design effective mental health apps is in infancy.

Another systematic review looked at apps to reduce tobacco ($N = 6$), alcohol ($N = 11$), illegal drug use ($N = 1$) or a combination ($N = 1$).[27] Comparison groups were very diverse, ranging from assessment only, or Web-based/text-based extractions of the app contents without interaction or waitlist. Only 6 of the 20 apps reported significant reductions in substance use at post or follow-up compared with a comparison condition, with small to moderate effect sizes; 3 of those were low quality studies. The authors conclude that the trials are not well powered and follow up times are insufficient. They also emphasize study preregistration, adhering to guidelines and using theoretical models to guide design.

Cognitive-behavioral therapy (CBT) is the most well-known evidence-based approach to treat alcohol use disorder, often combined with motivational approaches, CRA and mindfulness. A 2019 meta-analysis examining CBT-based interventions (those identified as CBT or containing key elements of CBT, such as coping skills training) that have been programmed to be delivered through a computer (eg, Web-based program) or mobile device (eg, mobile app) without guidance identified 15 studies where controls were assessment, treatment as usual, psychoeducational reading and waitlist.[28] Studies comparing technology provided CBT (CBT tech) to minimal or no treatment found small positive effect at early follow up, but were nonsignificant at late follow up, notable since CBT often demonstrates impacts over time as patients implement skills. Studies comparing CBT tech to treatment as usual showed no significant differences. CBT tech added to treatment as usual was helpful at both follow up times compared to just treatment as usual. Finally, no difference was found between CBT tech versus therapist delivered, but notably the statistic (not significant) was negative for CBT tech. All effect sizes mentioned were small, with the largest ($g = 0.3$) being for added CBT tech to treatment as usual. The studies were heterogeneous in design. Most of the included studies incorporated MI/ME (motivational interviewing/motivation enhancement) into therapy and were not just CBT. Content varied with some having as few as 4 modules up to 62. Notably in the program with 62 exercises each would take 3 to 10 minutes to complete, which is distinctly different from a traditional CBT session. Adherence, engagement and exposure were also low for the majority of programs, which users could access at their will. Reach on the other hand was huge for the interventions with the average RCT enrolling 656, with the largest being nearly 8,000 people and with diverse populations. The authors conclude that while the effect sizes were small, the potential reach and potential effect of these interventions warrants more research. They also note that their review does not suggest these models should replace in-person or established services, as there have been few well-controlled comparisons thus far.

A 2017 Cochrane review investigated digital interventions for alcohol with personalized advice compared to no treatment or face to face intervention among community settings like workplaces, colleges, clinics and internet users.[29] The authors aimed to assess the effectiveness and cost-effectiveness of digital interventions for reducing hazardous and harmful alcohol consumption, alcohol-related problems, or both, in people living in the community compared to no treatment or face-to-face brief interventions. They also were interested in what behavior change components were most important as well as what therapies were used in development of the program. To be included in the study, an intervention must provide tailored feedback based on the amount someone drinks including suggestions to cut down. Control groups may have been provided with general (nontailored interventions). The review included 41 studies (42 comparisons, 19,241 participants) and found that most people reported drinking less (on the order of 23 g of alcohol or 1.6 standard drinks) if they received advice about alcohol from a computer or mobile device compared to people who did not get this advice (studies were moderate quality). (As time to follow up increased, differences in groups diminished.) There was not enough data to differentiate the efficacy of computers, telephone or internet advice, but trusted virtual sources such as doctors were more helpful as were specific recommendations. Only 5 studies compared digital advice (computers or mobile) to face-to-face conversations with doctors and nurses and there were little to no differences detected. The authors reported the most common BCTs were feedback on behavior (85.7%, $N = 36$), social comparison (81.0%, $N = 34$), information about social and environmental consequences (71.4%, $N = 30$) feedback on outcomes of behavior (69.0%, $N = 29$) and social support (64.3%, $N = 27$). Interventions had an average 9 BCTs with the most effective being, in an adjusted model, behavior substitution, problem solving and credible source. While the most common theories cited were Motivational Interviewing Theory (7/20), Transtheoretical Model (6/20) and Social Norms Theory (6/20), over half of the interventions[21] had no theory mentioned. There was also no intentionally used theory to guide recruitment.

The authors conclude that from a public health perspective, despite the small effect, with the low cost and wide reach of digital inventions, more research and work in the area is warranted. Further, digital advice was not found to be significantly different from face-to-face, but more data and studies are needed to prove out thus low-cost solution. Interestingly, other BCTs, which were not as prevalent in the interventions, such as self-monitoring, goal setting and review of behavioral/outcome goals, have great efficacy in traditional settings and should be implemented/studied in digital. Overall, the authors suggest that digital interventions are considered alongside face-to-face interventions as part of a strategy for addressing hazardous alcohol consumption and there is moderate-quality evidence that digital interactions may reduce alcohol use compared to no treatment.

Following this review, another literature review sought to look solely at mobile applications and alcohol consumption.[30] They identified 19 unique apps in 21 studies (11 that were no longer available in app stores); 7 were for youth and 12 for adults. For young people, the efficacy was inconclusive with only 2 out of 5 RCTs finding any significant reduction in alcohol consumption. For adults the results were more promising but still not convincing with 7 out of 12 finding reductions in alcohol and 1 finding a significant increase. The authors note that while there are hundreds of alcohol apps available, even for the apps reported in peer reviewed literature, the evidence is underwhelming and in infancy. Nonetheless, they also mention the potential in offering some intervention versus no intervention.

Mobile Applications or Websites Reviews With Guided Components

A 2018 review investigated internet-based alcohol interventions (iAIs as noted in the paper, both guided and unguided) with the aim of commenting on whether usually underrepresented groups benefit (women and older people), groups with varying levels of alcohol use benefit and whether guided or unguided are more effective.[31] Using an individual patient data meta-analysis (IPDMA) with author collaboration to boost the number of participants studied and statistical power, they identified 183 papers, 24 of which were eligible, 19 of which chose to participate. There were 26 comparisons made, 19 of which were for unguided interventions. The main outcome of interest was standard units (SU) of alcohol use postintervention with a secondary outcome of treatment response (drinking 14 SUs [females] or 21 SUs [males]) at varying times of follow up. Of the total of 14,198 enrolled participants, 8,095 provided postintervention outcome data (mean age 40.7 [SD = 13.2], 47.6% women, mean weekly SU level at baseline was 38.1 [SD = 26.9]). Studies were considered relatively high quality based on Cochrane Collaboration risk-of-bias assessment tool. Controls were largely psychoeducational material, assessment only and waitlist controls (WLC). Compared to controls, iAI participants had a significant difference in mean weekly alcohol reduction (5 SUs) and treatment response. Women had a less robust reduction in drinks than men and participants over 55-year-old had a better treatment response than those who are younger. Guided interventions and therapeutic principal interventions (versus just personalized normative feedback) were also more helpful. Interestingly, WLC studies had a greater effect size, which may be related to participants delaying changes in alcohol use. A conventional meta-analysis was also done and only showed small significant difference in mean weekly SUs at the first follow-up in favor of iAI participants as compared with controls (Hedges' $g = 0.26$, 95% CI 0.17-0.34, $p < 0.001$). The authors suggest that the IPDMA method provided greater power and some insights into how iAI can be a helpful first step for many people. And they note that not all treatment participants benefited from iAIs, so more research is needed to understand which people such interventions work for and in what contexts.

Cannabis use rates are increasing, and digital interventions may reach more people than the small percent who currently seek treatment. A 2018 review and metanalysis related to cannabis investigated prevention versus treatment.[32] 30 studies were in the review (10 prevention—4 guided/6 unguided and 20 treatment—8 guided/12 unguided) and 21 for the meta-analysis (6 prevention and 15 treatment). The age of participants was 12 to 20 years, 61% female, with attrition ranging from 1.5% to 55%. Comparison in the digital prevention groups were either prevention as usual or assessment only and comparisons for the treatment group were largely education and assessment only. The quality of studies was low based on the Cochrane risk-of-bias tool. Prevention programs were associated with a reduction in cannabis use at posttreatment (immediate; $g=0.33$; 95% CI 0.13 to 0.54 and follow up 3 to 12 months later; $g=0.22$; 95% CI 0.12 to 0.33, $p=0.001$). Digital treatment programs were mildly significant ($g=0.12$; 95% CI 0.02 to 0.22) at post treatment but not at follow up ($p = 0.1$). Subgroup analyses did not show significant differences between groups like number of sessions, recruitment strategy/location, guided/unguided, intervention type (MI, personalized normative feedback [PNF], MI+CBT or solution focused), or analysis type. There were some trends though, for example, multi-session interventions, such as those combining CBT with MI, produced higher effect sizes than single session using PNF, MI, something that has been noted in alcohol interventions as well. While the quality of studies and effect sizes are low, because of the impact on prevention and potentially reaching a large number of people, the authors note that there is promise. However future research should preserve randomization and blinding more as well as institute further clinical rigor.

A 2017 systematic review of internet inventions (versus TAU, MI, brief intervention or psychoeducation) for illegal drug use identified 17 studies, 9 of which were added on to guided care.[33] The approaches included CRA largely for people who used opioid, whereas CBT was the main treatment for people who used stimulants. The overall effect of the intervention was significant but modest (Hedge's $g = 0.301$, $p < 0.001$). People who used opioids and people who used any illegal substance had a small but significant effect whereas those who used stimulants did not benefit. Further analysis found that guided interventions were more effective, validated outcomes (toxicology) versus self-report was more effective and clinic-based technology was also more effective than school or home. The authors conclude that the effectiveness was small but promising and more research is needed.

A 2021 review of apps to help people quit smoking identified 6,016 studies, narrowing to 24 apps, some of which were standalone general apps and others which combined face-to-face intervention with the app.[34] Of these, only 8 studies reported significant differences between treatment and other intervention. And only 6 (3 of each kind) were considered high quality studies (but only half showed differences in outcomes). While there was not superiority of the digital interventions, many were just as effective as the control groups. The control groups ranged from self-help material, text messaging service and other waitlist design studies compared pre/post-treatment. In the control condition studies, abstinence rates ranged from 36% to 100% in the digital treatments arms. In the before and after (waitlist), abstinence rates ranged between 12.5% and 51.5% during treatment. Especially for stand-alone apps, there is an opportunity to function at least as well as no intervention as most individuals get very little support with stopping smoking to begin with. Notably, seven of the studies targeted more complex groups who smoke and need more assistance and attention, including people with co-occurring other mental disorders and homeless populations. Also, several studies were pilots, which often don't have sufficient sample size to power significant findings. Finally, a concerning finding was that most studies did not adequately describe their apps, mentioned in several other reviews, but especially highlighted by these authors. The authors were able to extract components of interest including carbon monoxide (CO) monitoring, setting a quit date, ecological momentary assessment (EMA—sampling of subjects' current behaviors and experiences in real time), smoking self-report, mindfulness content, ACT content from their analysis of components of interventions.

Not discussed in this section are apps to help with parallel areas of SUDs. For example, pain management is very relevant to the field and a number of digital approaches (software and hardware) are being evaluated.[35] Another area of research and development is on public health approaches such as overdose surveillance through technology.[36]

TELEHEALTH (WITH FOCUS ON OUD)

Telemedicine was already growing in popularity before the COVID-19 pandemic. Data from prior to the pandemic from the Veterans Health Administration (VHA), for example, showed that tele-buprenorphine increased from 2.29% of buprenorphine patients in FY2012 (N = 187) to 7.96% (N = 1,352) in FY2019 in VHA veterans nationally.[37] A separate study looking at VHA data from 2008 to 2017 found that treatment discontinuation from buprenorphine was lower for the telemedicine group.[38]

COVID-19 drastically shifted systems. Prior to the pandemic, less than 1% of mental health and SUD outpatient care was via telehealth based on national data.[39] That increased to 40% of mental health and substance use outpatient visits and 11% of other visits (during the March-August 2020 period).

Furthermore, regulatory exceptions took place. At the start of COVID-19, to reduce transmission of the virus, federal restrictions on mOUD (medications for Opioid Use Disorder) were loosened. These include Substance Abuse and Mental Health Services Administration (SAMHSA) granting flexibility for patients in OTPs (Opioid Treatment Programs) to receive a 28-day supply of take-home medications via state request. For less stable patients, the state could request up to 14 days.[40] The DEA (Drug Enforcement Agency) waived the in-person requirement for buprenorphine prescribing via telemedicine.[41] Unfortunately despite all of this, from 2019 to 2020, overdose rates increased by 30% and again by 15% in 2021.[9]

A scoping review of innovation to meet the needs of COVID-19 conditions identified 25 studies, mostly commentary or program descriptions.[42] 16 of these studies included telemedicine as an innovation. This ranged from basic video or phone sessions for care, distributing phones to help patient with limited access, building sanitized phone booths for socially distanced calls, naloxone education online, text messaging to connect to young people and shifting to virtual groups. Of course, in this review was a discussion of take-home dosing increasing and how variable the use of those relaxed regulations were. Other challenges presented were related to technology access, toxicology testing and how best to integrate care.

In 2018, The American Telemedicine Association (ATA) and The American Psychiatric Association (APA) developed best practices for video-based telehealth.[43] These include practical recommendations from administrative issues, legal and regulatory, emergencies, technical considerations, clinical considerations and special populations (eg, child/adolescent) recommendations. In order to help clinicians learn more about options with telehealth for SUD specifically during the COVID-19 pandemic, an article summarized best practices in addiction, which range from sections on assessment to testing and subsequent visits.[44] They also provide guidance for buprenorphine teleprescribing, which under the current public health emergency, extended as of this writing, is permitted federally and in many states. Also, with respect to logistics, telehealth reimbursement versus in person visits is a topic to consider when there are parity discussions. Regardless, telehealth is expanding and all health care providers must be versed in its delivery.

A review of telemedicine for SUD summarized the evidence for medication and psychotherapy use. It included 13 publications about 12 studies, including 7 RCTs that were described for tobacco (N = 3), alcohol (N = 5) and opioid (N = 5).[45] The nicotine studies were centered on psychoeducation and counseling with medications. For alcohol there was only a psychotherapy study and for OUD, it was telepsychotherapy to accompany methadone; in three of the studies (nonrandomized), evaluation and buprenorphine prescribing was delivered via telemedicine at clinic sites. Overwhelmingly, telemedicine outcomes in studies with comparison groups didn't find differences compared to in-person or phone or usual care. However, there were noticeable effects on retention and some studies reported high satisfaction with telemedicine. Overall, the reviewers cannot recommend telemedicine over conventional treatments, but in resource strained places where evidence-based treatments are not readily available, telemedicine is promising. Aftercare and IOP telemedicine are also gaining traction related to COVID-19 but research is still limited to single site studies.

NEWER DIGITAL TECHNOLOGIES

Technology is rapidly evolving, and new concepts and ideas are introduced into health every day. This section will not cover all possible digital solutions but will focus on some that have been discussed more widely in scientific literature; in contrast to the majority of the chapter, this section will rely on single study data, as opposed to reviews, given the scarcity of studies.

Social Media

A relatively new and unresearched area is in social media and use of social media for good in SUD treatment. While social media is often cited as a negative influence on mental health, especially with young people, there is a function for it to do good for patients.[46] A survey of adults with Alcohol Use Disorder who use social media found that exposure to peer pro-drinking posts was negatively associated with intentions to seek treatment, whereas exposures to peer alcohol-related negative consequences posts AND peer posts about positive experiences with treatment/recovery were positively associated with treatment-seeking intention.[47] While a single study, other applications of this theoretical model in mental health contribute to a need for research into how to utilize the approach for SUDs.

TikTok is a relatively new social media platform increasing in popularity for showing brief videos recorded by people who use them. A recent study examined 82 of the most liked TikTok videos related to attempts to cut down on or abstain from substances and/or strengthen SUD recovery; these videos had 2 million views and 325,000 "likes" on average; the videos shared themes of a journey from active SUD to recovery, recovery milestones and recurrences of use.[48] This is potentially a wide reaching way to engage people in the community among a population where less than 1% of people with an SUD who did not receive substance use treatment at a specialty facility felt they needed treatment and made an effort to get treatment.[8]

In addition to having an influencing affect, social media platforms such as Facebook or X(previously known as Twitter) have been increasingly studied for treating SUDs. A 2018 review on social media interventions for tobacco smoking identified seven studies between 2014 and 2018 ($N = 9{,}755$) using Facebook ($N = 4$) and X(previously known as Twitter) ($N = 2$) to report on feasibility, acceptability, usability, or smoking related outcomes, four of which were RCTs.[49] The interventions involved tailored content, targeted reminders and moderated discussions. Most of the studies examining quit outcomes did find that the treatment groups smoked less at follow up. Active participation, for example posting comments or liking, may be associated with improved outcomes. Length of study ranged from 30 to 365 days and retention in the studies range from 35% to 84%. While the review authors acknowledge the feasibility of the interventions, they note that future rigorous trials are necessary to establish effectiveness, evaluate the costs/sustainability of these programs, and determine whether these programs can reach vulnerable populations who smoke more.

Chatbots

Chatbots are pieces of software or hardware that can converse with users without a human facilitator using machine learning and artificial intelligence.[50] Only one qualitative review from 2019 describes 14 early chatbots in mental health, none of which were specific to substance use, but one focused on healthy lifestyle in women ($N = 61$), which did help people who used them to significantly decrease alcohol consumption. While commercial and noncommercial chatbots exist, the amount of research has been insufficient for review data. These bots tend to provide warm and friendly messages based on the user, similar to reflections in motivational interviewing.

Peer Support

Millions of Americans use peer support groups or organizations like Alcoholics Anonymous (AA) or SMART recovery. In fact a recent Cochrane Review determined that AA/TSF (Twelve Step Facilitation, a manualized, professional psychosocial intervention to promote initial and continuing engagement in AA, see Chapter 79) were more effective than other established treatments, such as CBT, for increasing abstinence.[51] With the COVID-19 pandemic, there was a rise in digital recovery support services. These digital options are generally free, leverage peer-to-peer connection, online video recovery support meetings, discussion boards and chat rooms. While quantitative data from these services in the pandemic are not available, literature reviews have posed concerns that it may be more challenging to complete elements of TSF (finding a sponsor, disclosure, picking up on cues) via video. There may be challenges around access to technology and privacy, especially for groups that have "anonymity" as a core element. However, having online options increases accessibility overall. A summary of early guidance on virtual peer support notes organizations with compiled lists of free, social-online links with include, but are not limited to[52]:

- The Grayken Center for Addiction at the Boston Medical Center (https://www.bmc.org/addiction/covid-19-recovery-resources)
- The American Society of Addiction Medicine (https://www.asam.org/quality-care/clinical-recommendations/covid/promoting-support-group-attendance)
- The National Institute on Drug Abuse (https://www.usa.gov/substance-abuse)
- Google's Recover Together (https://recovertogether.withgoogle.com/)
- The Recovery Research Institute (https://www.recoveryanswers.org/media/digital-recovery-support-online-and-mobile-resources/)

Wearables and Tracking

Wearables and tracking are a relatively new area of research. The greatest investment has been in substance detection. A systematic review of 32 studies on transdermal alcohol sensors (often compared to SCRAM devices) found lack of consistency with respect to accuracy.[53] Overall, true comparisons were not possible due to flaws in the studies, but do point to an area to continue research. While not a sensor or a wearable, the use of a mobile phone can support digital phenotyping. Digital phenotyping or behavioral sensing uses passively collected, real-time data from a mobile phone (eg, GPS tracking, social patterns, typing patterns) to inform clinical assessment, predict changes in clinical status, and deliver on-demand interventions in a scalable, cost-effective manner.[54] For SUDs, this can help with prevention and intervention (eg, when a person is close to a triggering location like bar), or detect return to use, for example with a smartwatch detecting heart rate, detect overdose risk and more.

Virtual Reality

Virtual reality (VR) is a new area of research when it comes to digital interventions that uses computer-generated simulation of a three-dimensional environment using social equipment such as head mounted displaces (HMD). Most research in the field has to do with VRET or VR exposure therapy, where a user is introduced to the anxiety inducing stimuli gradually and then able to be conditioned to reduce their response. Similarly, in SUDs, patients can be confronted with the substance, paraphernalia associated with use, or other stressors and work toward not craving or using the substance through exposure-based extinction of cue-induced responses.[55] A 2021 systematic review aimed to evaluate the diagnostic/prognostic value of VR-induced cue-reactivity for the clinical assessment of patients with SUDs (19 studies) and the effectiveness of VR-delivered treatment in patients (17 studies).[56] They used the International Working Group Recommendations for Methodology of Virtual Reality Clinical Trials in Healthcare to assess quality.[57] Focusing on treatment studies, half used VRET (for alcohol tobacco and gambling). Participants were exposed to cues like a lighter or a cigarette in a typical virtual environment like a cafe. The environments were mostly visual and auditory although two included olfactory or haptic stimuli. The outcome was craving or urge to use (gamble in one case). Of the studies, 4 found null results and 2 reported negative results. Five found a reduction in craving. Of the 10 studies looking at substance use as an outcome, 6 reported reductions, 2 found no change, 2 found increased use and 1 was mixed. One study for example found a negative effect of VR compared to standard CBT on tobacco use disorder. Study quality was overall low with many limitations. The authors conclude that future research should correct methodological shortcomings of existing studies through scientific rigor, including better preregistered outcomes, investigating severity of SUD, accounting for multiple interventions and testing in representative clinical populations. Ultimately, VR is too early in its development for widespread clinical implementation until more is known. An adjacent area of technology development is gamification, which also needs more research.

INTEGRATION INTO PRACTICE

With all of the solutions presented, it is important to comment on how to choose which solutions to use in practice. First, it is important that the resource is evidence-based (a topic outlined throughout this chapter) and safe (outlined in the next section). Second, it is important to consider if the patient will use the solution. Items to consider include accessibility, cost, usability, how engaging the solution is, and how interactive it is. An app that requires a user to log in of own volition may be less engaging than an app that provides reminders. Another point about use is whether a patient is already interested in a solution—if they are invested in a solution and excited, then employing motivational interviewing and seizing the opportunity to add a resource to their treatment can have the most impact.

It is also of utmost importance to recognize that in most cases, a digital solution is not sufficient for treatment of a SUD. For a person who does not have an SUD and is looking for a community or monitoring, only using an app may be sufficient, but working with a professional (physician, peer support) is essential for those with SUDs. Some of the solutions like digital therapeutics and of course telemedicine integrate technology with human support. Similarly, since support is important, using solutions with communities for family/friend portals can reinforce progress. At the same time, for a patient unwilling to engage in interactive treatment or unable to access it, it is reasonable from a harm-reduction standpoint to consider a digital solution as a stand alone solution.

FUTURE OPPORTUNITIES AND RESPONSIBLE DIGITAL HEALTH

In summary, there have been unprecedented rates of growth and innovation for digital solutions in the field of substance use and SUDs. While the growth has been fast, the research has been limited. Importantly, while most of the effect sizes and findings were minimally in favor of digital interventions, rarely were the digital interventions harmful. This combined with generally positive impacts on retention and the potential to reach a greater number of people who often don't seek treatment could impact public health. We know, for example from research relating to helping people stop smoking tobacco, that the level of exposure to advice to quit is related to success rates.[58] Applying this to digital tools could add one more exposure to help someone in their journey. Notably, in many reviews, control groups also fared well—if a patient is getting some attention to the idea of quitting, the salience of quitting may increase in the face of incentive salience of the drug. That is, any intervention (even assessments asking about quit goals), is better than the standard of care in many cases, which is often no attention being given to substance use. Many reviewers also recommend that digital approaches at this stage should supplement, rather than replace care. This also raises the point that often guided-interventions performed better than unguided, and facility-based interventions may also fare better. Overall, research must continue in this field, with some considerations to firm our understanding of interventions.

These resources must be backed by scientific evidence. For example, a review of apps for bipolar disorder found that of those reviewed, one recommended drinking liquor before bed and another listed bipolar disorder as contagious.[59] In SUDs, use of evidence-based treatments is still lacking in many traditional settings and digital interventions can certainly increase the risk of misinformation or unsafe practices. Aside from platforms that seek FDA clearance, there are no universal regulatory practices in place to prevent apps from being available on appstores or websites. In 2019, the APA compiled guidance on how to evaluate apps; patients in crisis may not consider these factors.[60]

There exist common issues with several of the cited studies in the field of digital solutions for SUD. First, many of the reviews note unclear theoretical foundations or behavioral change theories in the digital interventions. There are well established theories and approaches in SUDs, from stages of change to motivational interviewing to cognitive-behavioral therapy that are proven elements of theory, but a limited number of studies define their approaches a priori; rather many study designs implement interventions without discussion of a theoretical basis,[61] and, when there are theoretical foundations mentioned, it is hard to piece together, which contributed most to outcomes. Alternatively, it may be that the theoretical approach is inherently different for digital approaches, in which case that should be further researched.

Other issues with studies thus far have to do with design. Aside from the obvious suggestions to have more true RCTs, many of the analyses are insufficiently powered and follow up times are also insufficient. We need more partnership between science and development. As of 2020, there were 13 trials in the U.S. National Drug Abuse Treatment Clinical Trials Network in the space of digital interventions: (1) digital SUD screening and/or assessment ($N = 6$), (2) digital therapeutics ($N = 2$), (3) telehealth ($N = 2$), (4) EMA and passive sensing technologies ($N = 2$), and (5) social media platforms ($N = 1$).[62] There are certainly more opportunities to engage in the research to increase the reach of science-based SUD service delivery models according to the Clinical Trials Network.

With respect to logistics, some applications or solutions do not stay on the market long. When reviewers sought to access apps in studies, often they were obsolete. Investment in digital solutions needs to be longer term to (1) assess for efficacy, (2) iteratively improve and (3) be accessible. Accessibility is important—is the digital solution available to the population most in need? This barrier has to do with access to technology as well as the infrequency of patient centered design. The studies in the reviews in this chapter are largely from the United States and Europe; generalizability may be limited and more needs to be understood about how geography, language, etc. may affect the uptake and efficacy of a solution.

As noted above, one positive outcome of several digital approaches was increased retention. In SUD treatment, engagement and retention are important. The longer someone is retained in treatment, the more likely they will have sustained outcomes, in both traditional and digital settings. A 2018 review using Cochrane methodology sought to understand factors that make online substance intervention engaging.[63] Using 15 studies identified, five engagement strategies were identified and ranked by frequency of use: tailoring (47% of studies), reminders (email) and social support (40% of studies) and delivery strategies (33% of studies) were most frequent. The most frequent tailoring was with readiness to quit, self-efficacy, and barriers to quit, and tailoring overall was the most promising for engagement. These findings can help shape future interventions to increase adoption.

Interestingly, while several reviews and meta-analyses do discuss substance use outcomes and targets in treatments, the number of interventions for patients with SUD and co-occurring other mental disorders is relatively low. A 2018 review on comorbid depression and SUD examined 6 studies and found promising results but could not comment on long term effectiveness, noting that data were limited and larger studies are needed before digital mental health care is standard practice.[64]

Finally, how scalable and implementable a solution is will impact how effective it is. A highly expensive and complex intervention delivered by an expert to one person may not impact public health compared to a screening and brief intervention model in the waiting room of an ER. Similarly, a digital solution needs to be both high quality and also accessible.

As the field of digital health for SUD evolves rapidly, it is imperative to consider the ethical and safety responsibilities of providing care. There are multiple layers to this. On the most basic level, state and federal regulations must be respected. For example, the Ryan Haight Online Pharmacy Consumer Protection Act of 2008 was intended to prevent the illegal distribution and dispensing of controlled substances by means of the internet.[65] It required at least one in person medical evaluation to dispense controlled substances. During the pandemic, these requirements were temporary paused at the federal level under a Public Health Emergency status, with various state adjustments. It is important to continue to provide care, keeping in mind safety, ethics and putting the patient first, given the uncertain path of the pandemic. Equitable care is also important. Throughout this chapter there has been mention of groups that are not reached by some technologies, for example people who are older or don't have access to technology; if more care is offered virtually, it has to be done thoughtfully to reach all people in need. On another level, patient data must be protected and preserved. Everything from who has access to the data, to maintaining technology security standards, to preventing unauthorized access, to extreme cases of selling data, is important.[66] Transparency of policies is also vital. All the digital tools mentioned in this chapter should be clear about their data policies and safeguard protected health information.

To close, digital mental health is rapidly evolving. Future editions of this text will likely have new modalities not discussed here and much of this data will be dated. As research and development moves forward, more data accounting for trial design, sufficient power, theoretical bases and applicable populations will be important to consider. Further, ethics, safety and privacy must be front and center. While digital interventions have the potential to increase access and reach, it is imperative to center them on science and evidence-based approaches. Notably, the null results in the studies where both treatment and control groups improve, make it clear that any attention given to SUD is a step in the right direction for a field that is underserved.

DISCLOSURE

The author is affiliated with Lyra Health. Lyra Health offers a behavioral health benefit to companies through which employees and dependents have access to video based therapy, behavioral health coaching, and medication management consultations.

REFERENCES

1. Bhavnani SP, Narula J, Sengupta PP. Mobile technology and the digitization of healthcare. *Eur Heart J*. 2016;37(18):1428-1438.
2. ITU Statistics. Accessed 15 June, 2023. https://www.itu.int:443/en/ITU-D/Statistics/Pages/stat/default.aspx
3. Hsu M, Martin B, Ahmed S, Torous J, Suzuki J. Smartphone ownership, smartphone utilization, and interest in using mental health apps to address substance use disorders: literature review and cross-sectional survey study across two sites. *JMIR Form Res*. 2022;6(7):e38684.
4. *Diagnostic and Statistical Manual of Mental Disorders*. 5th ed. Text Revision (DSM-5-TR™). American Psychiatric Association; 2022.
5. Schroeder SA. Shattuck Lecture. We can do better--improving the health of the American people. *N Engl J Med*. 2007;357(12):1221-1228.
6. Asch DA, Muller RW, Volpp KG. Automated hovering in health care--watching over the 5000 hours. *N Engl J Med*. 2012;367(1):1-3.
7. Garnett CV, Crane D, Brown J, et al. Behavior change techniques used in digital behavior change interventions to reduce excessive alcohol consumption: a meta-regression. *Ann Behav Med*. 2018;52(6):530-543.
8. Substance Abuse and Mental Health Services Administration. *Key Substance Use and Mental Health Indicators in the United States: Results from the 2020 National Survey on Drug Use and Health*. SAMHSA; 2021:114. (HHS Publication No. PEP21-07-01-003, NSDUH Series H-56). Accessed June 15, 2023. https://www.samhsa.gov/data/
9. National Center for Health Statistics. *U.S. Overdose Deaths In 2021 Increased Half as Much as in 2020 - But Are Still Up 15%*. Accessed June 15, 2023. https://www.cdc.gov/nchs/pressroom/nchs_press_releases/2022/202205.htm
10. Aklin WM, Walton KM, Antkowiak P. Digital therapeutics for substance use disorders: research priorities and clinical validation. *Drug Alcohol Depend*. 2021;229(Pt A):109120.
11. Lougheed T. How "digital therapeutics" differ from traditional health and wellness apps. *CMAJ*. 2019;191(43):E1200-E1201.
12. Capito SM. *S.3791 - 117th Congress (2021-2022): Access to Prescription Digital Therapeutics Act of 2022*. Accessed June 15, 2023. https://www.congress.gov/bill/117th-congress/senate-bill/3791
13. New York State Psychiatric Institute. *NIDA-CTN-0044: Web-delivery of Evidence-Based, Psychosocial Treatment for Substance Use Disorders Using the Therapeutic Education System (TES)* Report No: NCT01104805. Accessed June 15, 2023. https://clinicaltrials.gov/ct2/show/NCT01104805
14. Campbell ANC, Miele GM, Nunes EV, McCrimmon S, Ghitza UE. Web-based, psychosocial treatment for substance use disorders in community treatment settings. *Psychol Serv*. 2012;9(2):212-214.
15. U.S. Food and Drug Administration. *FDA Permits Marketing of Mobile Medical Application for Substance Use Disorder*. Accessed June 15, 2023. https://www.fda.gov/news-events/press-announcements/fda-permits-marketing-mobile-medical-application-substance-use-disorder
16. Christensen DR, Landes RD, Jackson L, et al. Adding an Internet-delivered treatment to an efficacious treatment package for opioid dependence. *J Consult Clin Psychol*. 2014;82(6):964-972.
17. U.S. Food and Drug Administration. *FDA Clears Mobile Medical App to Help Those With Opioid Use Disorder Stay in Recovery Programs*. Accessed June 15, 2023. https://www.fda.gov/news-events/press-announcements/fda-clears-mobile-medical-app-help-those-opioid-use-disorder-stay-recovery-programs
18. Tice JA, Whittington MD, Campbell JD, Pearson SD. The effectiveness and value of digital health technologies as an adjunct to medication-assisted therapy for opioid use disorder. *J Manag Care Spec Pharm*. 2021;27(4):528-532.
19. American Medical Association. *6 New Digital Health CPT Codes That you Should Know About*. Accessed June 15, 2023. https://www.ama-assn.org/practice-management/cpt/6-new-digital-health-cpt-codes-you-should-know-about
20. Cenetrs for Medicare and Medicaid Services. *HCPCS Quarterly Update*. Accessed June 15, 2023. https://www.cms.gov/Medicare/Coding/HCPCSReleaseCodeSets/HCPCS-Quarterly-Update
21. Torous J, Roberts LW. Needed innovation in digital health and smartphone applications for mental health: transparency and trust. *JAMA Psychiatry*. 2017;74(5):437-438.
22. IQVIA. *The Growing Value of Digital Health*. Accessed June 15, 2023. https://www.iqvia.com/insights/the-iqvia-institute/reports/the-growing-value-of-digital-health
23. Baumel A, Muench F, Edan S, Kane JM. Objective user engagement with mental health apps: systematic search and panel-based usage analysis. *J Med Internet Res*. 2019;21(9):e14567.
24. Lau N, O'Daffer A, Colt S, et al. Android and iPhone mobile apps for psychosocial wellness and stress management: systematic search in app stores and literature review. *JMIR Mhealth Uhealth*. 2020;8(5):e17798.
25. Philippe TJ, Sikder N, Jackson A, et al. Digital health interventions for delivery of mental health care: systematic and comprehensive meta-review. *JMIR Ment Health*. 2022;9(5):e35159.
26. Weisel KK, Fuhrmann LM, Berking M, Baumeister H, Cuijpers P, Ebert DD. Standalone smartphone apps for mental health—a systematic review and meta-analysis. *NPJ Digit Med*. 2019;2:118.
27. Staiger PK, O'Donnell R, Liknaitzky P, Bush R, Milward J. Mobile apps to reduce tobacco, alcohol, and illicit drug use: systematic review of the first decade. *J Med Internet Res*. 2020;22(11):e17156.
28. Kiluk BD, Ray LA, Walthers J, Bernstein M, Tonigan JS, Magill M. Technology-delivered cognitive-behavioral interventions for alcohol use: a meta-analysis. *Alcohol Clin Exp Res*. 2019;43(11):2285-2295.
29. Kaner EF, Beyer FR, Garnett C, et al. Personalised digital interventions for reducing hazardous and harmful alcohol consumption in community-dwelling populations. *Cochrane Database Syst Rev*. 2017;2017(9):CD011479.
30. Colbert S, Thornton L, Richmond R. Smartphone apps for managing alcohol consumption: a literature review. *Addict Sci Clin Pract*. 2020;15:17.
31. Riper H, Hoogendoorn A, Cuijpers P, et al. Effectiveness and treatment moderators of Internet interventions for adult problem drinking: an individual patient data meta-analysis of 19 randomised controlled trials. *PLoS Med*. 2018;15(12):e1002714.
32. Boumparis N, Loheide-Niesmann L, Blankers M, et al. Short- and long-term effects of digital prevention and treatment interventions for cannabis use reduction: a systematic review and meta-analysis. *Drug Alcohol Depend*. 2019;200:82-94.
33. Boumparis N, Karyotaki E, Schaub MP, Cuijpers P, Riper H. Internet interventions for adult illicit substance users: a meta-analysis. *Addiction*. 2017;112(9):1521-1532.
34. Barroso-Hurtado M, Suárez-Castro D, Martínez-Vispo C, Becoña E, López-Durán A. Smoking cessation apps: a systematic review of format, outcomes, and features. *Int J Environ Res Public Health*. 2021;18(21):11664.

35. Nicholl BI, Sandal LF, Stochkendahl MJ, et al. Digital support interventions for the self-management of low back pain: a systematic review. *J Med Internet Res.* 2017;19(5):e179.
36. Claborn K, Creech S, Conway FN, et al. Development of a digital platform to improve community response to overdose and prevention among harm reduction organizations. *Harm Reduct J.* 2022;19(1):62.
37. Lin LA, Fortney JC, Bohnert ASB, Coughlin LN, Zhang L, Piette JD. Comparing telemedicine to in-person buprenorphine treatment in U.S. veterans with opioid use disorder. *J Subst Abus Treat.* 2022;133:108492.
38. Vakkalanka JP, Lund BC, Ward MM, et al. Telehealth utilization is associated with lower risk of discontinuation of buprenorphine: a retrospective cohort study of U.S. veterans. *J Gen Intern Med.* 2022;37(7):1610-1618.
39. Lo J, Panchal N. *Telehealth Has Played an Outsized Role Meeting Mental Health Needs During the COVID-19 Pandemic*; Mar 15 BFMP, 2022. Accessed June 15, 2023. https://www.kff.org/coronavirus-covid-19/issue-brief/telehealth-has-played-an-outsized-role-meeting-mental-health-needs-during-the-covid-19-pandemic/
40. Opioid Treatment Program (OTP) Guidance. Accessed June 15, 2023. https://www.samhsa.gov/sites/default/files/otp-guidance-20200316.pdf
41. Davis CS, Samuels EA. Opioid policy changes during the COVID-19 pandemic - and beyond. *J Addict Med.* 2020;14(4):e4-e5.
42. Krawczyk N, Fawole A, Yang J, Tofighi B. Early innovations in opioid use disorder treatment and harm reduction during the COVID-19 pandemic: a scoping review. *Addict Sci Clin Pract.* 2021;16:68.
43. Shore JH, Yellowlees P, Caudill R, et al. Best practices in videoconferencing-based telemental health April 2018. *Telemed J E Health.* 2018;24(11):827-832.
44. Oesterle TS, Kolla B, Risma CJ, et al. Substance use disorders and telehealth in the COVID-19 pandemic era: a new outlook. *Mayo Clin Proc.* 2020;95(12):2709-2718.
45. Lin LA, Casteel D, Shigekawa E, Weyrich MS, Roby DH, McMenamin SB. Telemedicine-delivered treatment interventions for substance use disorders: a systematic review. *J Subst Abus Treat.* 2019;101:38-49.
46. Liu M, Kamper-DeMarco KE, Zhang J, Xiao J, Dong D, Xue P. Time spent on social media and risk of depression in adolescents: a dose-response meta-analysis. *Int J Environ Res Public Health.* 2022;19(9):5164.
47. Russell AM, Ou TS, Bergman BG, Massey PM, Barry AE, Lin HC. Associations between heavy drinker's alcohol-related social media exposures and personal beliefs and attitudes regarding alcohol treatment. *Addict Behav Rep.* 2022;15:100434.
48. Russell AM, Bergman BG, Colditz JB, Kelly JF, Milaham PJ, Massey PM. Using TikTok in recovery from substance use disorder. *Drug Alcohol Depend.* 2021;229(Pt A):109147.
49. Naslund JA, Kim SJ, Aschbrenner KA, et al. Systematic review of social media interventions for smoking cessation. *Addict Behav.* 2017;73:81-93.
50. Vaidyam AN, Wisniewski H, Halamka JD, Kashavan MS, Torous JB. Chatbots and conversational agents in mental health: a review of the psychiatric landscape. *Can J Psychiatr.* 2019;64(7):456-464.
51. Kelly JF, Humphreys K, Ferri M. Alcoholics Anonymous and other 12-step programs for alcohol use disorder. *Cochrane Database Syst Rev.* 2020;3:CD012880.
52. Bergman BG, Kelly JF. Online digital recovery support services: an overview of the science and their potential to help individuals with substance use disorder during COVID-19 and beyond. *J Subst Abus Treat.* 2021;120:108152.
53. Brobbin E, Deluca P, Hemrage S, Drummond C. Accuracy of wearable transdermal alcohol sensors: systematic review. *J Med Internet Res.* 2022;24(4):e35178.
54. Mohr DC, Shilton K, Hotopf M. Digital phenotyping, behavioral sensing, or personal sensing: names and transparency in the digital age. *NPJ Digit Med.* 2020;3:45.
55. Carter BL, Tiffany ST. Meta-analysis of cue-reactivity in addiction research. *Addiction.* 1999;94(3):327-340.
56. Langener S, Van Der Nagel J, van Manen J, et al. Clinical relevance of immersive virtual reality in the assessment and treatment of addictive disorders: a systematic review and future perspective. *J Clin Med* 2021;10(16):3658.
57. Birckhead B, Khalil C, Liu X, et al. Recommendations for methodology of virtual reality clinical trials in health care by an international working group: iterative study. *JMIR Ment Health.* 2019;6(1):e11973.
58. Tobacco Use and Dependence Guideline Panel. *Treating Tobacco Use and Dependence: 2008 Update.* U.S. Department of Health and Human Services; 2008.
59. Nicholas J, Larsen ME, Proudfoot J, Christensen H. Mobile apps for bipolar disorder: a systematic review of features and content quality. *J Med Internet Res.* 2015;17(8):e198.
60. Lagan S, Emerson MR, King D, et al. Mental health app evaluation: updating the American Psychiatric Association's framework through a stakeholder-engaged workshop. *Psychiatr Serv.* 2021;72(9):1095-1098.
61. National Institute on Drug Abuse. *Principles of Effective Treatment.* Accessed August 10, 2022. https://archives.nida.nih.gov/publications/principles-drug-addiction-treatment-research-based-guide-third-edition
62. Marsch LA, Campbell A, Campbell C, et al. The application of digital health to the assessment and treatment of substance use disorders: the past, current, and future role of the National Drug Abuse Treatment Clinical Trials Network. *J Subst Abus Treat.* 2020;112(Suppl):4-11.
63. Milward J, Drummond C, Fincham-Campbell S, Deluca P. What makes online substance-use interventions engaging? A systematic review and narrative synthesis. *Digit Health.* 2018;4:2055207617743354.
64. Holmes NA, van Agteren JE, Dorstyn DS. A systematic review of technology-assisted interventions for co-morbid depression and substance use. *J Telemed Telecare* 2019;25(3):131-141.
65. Federal Register. *Implementation of the Ryan Haight Online Pharmacy Consumer Protection Act of 2008.* Accessed June 15, 2023. https://www.federalregister.gov/documents/2009/04/06/E9-7698/implementation-of-the-ryan-haight-online-pharmacy-consumer-protection-act-of-2008
66. LaMonica HM, Roberts AE, Lee GY, Davenport TA, Hickie IB. Privacy practices of health information technologies: privacy policy risk assessment study and proposed guidelines. *J Med Internet Res.* 2021;23(9):e26317.

CHAPTER

83

Medical Management Techniques and Collaborative Care: Integrating Behavioral With Pharmacological Interventions

Richard N. Rosenthal, Richard K. Ries, and Joan E. Zweben

CHAPTER OUTLINE

- Introduction
- Overview of issues and approaches
- Collaborative care with counselors and psychotherapists

INTRODUCTION

Many professionals who prescribe medicines for addiction or other medications, such as psychotropics, as part of addiction treatment, are faced with the question of what sort of evidence base exists for the "talking part" of what they do, as well as how best to do this. Independent of the impact of pharmacotherapies, several types of brief psychosocial intervention have been established as effective in treatment of substance use disorders (SUDs), with meta-analyses demonstrating low-moderate to high-moderate effect sizes depending on the specific substance disorder or treatment type.[1,2] For busy physicians who treat patients with addiction, this may present somewhat of a quandary, especially if that clinician is in a solo practice, is not trained to deliver psychotherapy, or does not typically provide those services in the course of daily clinical practice. For physicians who work with or in addiction treatment programs, given current cost constraints, effective interdisciplinary teamwork that can coordinate psychosocial treatments with medical care often makes the difference between a first-rate program and an average one.

One of the great strengths of the addiction field has been its evolution of a multidisciplinary approach and teamwork. Today, with the movement in primary care to patient-centered medical homes that encompass multiple clinical disciplines and care coordination, the decades of team approaches to addiction care appear prescient. Though a physician who works in a program with multiple components is an essential part of the health care team, clinicians who offer psychosocial interventions also play a major role. Thus, there are various combinations of individually administered and collaborative psychosocial approaches that physicians may use in addressing the treatment of SUDs, with or without co-occurring psychiatric disorders.

This chapter is divided in two sections. The first section provides an overview of the issues and approach for the addiction medicine physician regarding the integration of brief psychosocial interventions with medication treatment for addiction. Then begins a discussion of a basic psychosocial intervention that clinicians can and should be implementing with all patients. The term "brief" in this context most usually refers to the total number of sessions but in this chapter may also refer to the relatively "brief" amount of time that a prescribing clinician has in the context of a 15- to 30-minute medication management session. Such sessions are often of short duration due to large caseloads, limits on insurance or other benefit coverage, or that patients may be getting most of their psychosocial treatment through a structured addiction program and/or peer support through 12-step or other mutual aid programs. Section 1 further explicates the evidence base for the various psychotherapeutic interventions for SUD (many of which are found more fully discussed in this volume) and presents principles for integrating brief but more differentiated behavioral interventions into medication management sessions.

The second section focuses on the clinician who is engaged in coordinating addiction and psychosocial treatment services on behalf of patients with substance use as well as with co-occurring psychiatric disorders. It addresses key elements affecting how physicians in office-based practice, through teamwork and coordination, become adept at integrating services that are not provided at the office site. Finally, good supervision or collaboration is time-consuming and requires strong facilitation skills at the leadership level. When treatment providers are in conflict, patients suffer. This section also describes a variety of common situations and dilemmas and offers practical options for handling them.

OVERVIEW OF ISSUES AND APPROACHES

Clinical Skills Any Clinician Should Use

Engagement

Since the outcome of addiction treatment has been related to the time spent in treatment,[3,4] techniques that maximize treatment engagement and retention are likely to promote better outcomes. The underlying clinical approaches to treating patients with co-occurring SUD and other mental disorders are also active for those with SUD alone. Clinicians can use these basic techniques, which use clinical skills to achieve a specific outcome, manage intoxication, develop a therapeutic alliance, and facilitate patients' engagement in or adherence to psychosocial or medical treatment. In order to facilitate the accomplishment of these goals, clinicians can learn specific techniques such as motivational interviewing (MI), cognitive-behavioral recurrence of use prevention, 12-step facilitation, supportive psychotherapy, acceptance and commitment therapy (ACT), and contingency management (CM).[5,6]

One technique likely to sustain engagement and retention in treatment is to facilitate the therapeutic alliance through psychological support. Observational studies suggest that psychological support is among the most prominent and necessary components of management of addicted patients, especially those with more severe SUDs.[7] As such, clinicians, even very busy ones, should focus special attention in supporting the development of a therapeutic alliance with the patient. Alliance building is one of the core tactical techniques of supportive therapy and uses several straightforward approaches accessible to clinicians who may not have had any formal psychotherapy training: expression of interest, expression of empathy, expression of understanding, and repairing a misalliance.[8] For example, interest is expressed by the clinician's bringing in his or her knowledge of the patient into the conversation. In assessing primary care quality, more whole-person knowledge (medical history, home/work/school responsibilities, health concerns, values, and beliefs) of the patient by the clinician predicts lower drug and alcohol addiction severity scores on the addiction severity index and lower odds of subsequent substance use in recently primary care patients who have recently completed withdrawal management.[9] It is also important that the clinician is aware that asking too many questions of some patients, especially repetitively asking "why?" questions, can be experienced as intrusive or even an attack, which is off-putting to patients and reduces the likelihood of engagement. Information is best garnered by what, when, where, and how questions, but with monitoring patient comfort in this process, if the patient does not return, such "interrogation" information is not doing the patient or clinician much good. On the other hand, when a patient describes multiple "failures" at recovery, it may be helpful to ask, "Why do you think this keeps happening? What did you learn from that episode, about your future needs in treatment?"

For patients who lack insight that their substance use is problematic, motivational enhancement strategies (described below) have proved beneficial.[10-13] The therapist identifies where the patient is on the continuum of readiness to change and makes reflective statements matched to his or her current stage in order to elicit intrinsic motivation from the patient.[14]

Expression of accurate empathy has a long history as an important psychotherapeutic technique and corresponds to the concept of "reflective listening" used in MI,[15] as well as the "E" for empathy in the BRENDA therapy for the Penn clinical trials of SUD pharmacotherapies.[16] Empathy, which is more than simple care or concern, is expressed by the clinician relating his or her own internal emotional experience (without inappropriate self-disclosure) to corroborate that of the patient; for example, "It must've felt terrible to come back after your last heavy drinking episode and find out your intoxicated behavior was so scary that she'd changed the locks." The clinician can express his or her understanding by simply stating that he or she "gets" what the patient is communicating and sometimes paraphrasing what the patient has said. This demonstrates his or her alignment with the patient in an empathic way, which helps the patient to feel "in sync" with the clinician.

Misalliances occur in all human relationships, and addiction treatment is certainly no exception. However, when patients in SUD treatment get frustrated or resentful about the treatment, they frequently discontinue treatment participation, change to another provider, return to actively engaging in their addiction (via returning to substance use or gambling), or enact elements of each, any of which typically has a negative impact on outcome. The willingness of the clinician to entertain a patient's grievances, whether factually based or the result of misunderstanding, is a powerful interpersonal reinforcer for patients who may have relatively little experience of a nonjudgmental person willing to listen. Trust (including the experience of the clinician as the patient's agent) is also a factor associated with a lower risk of substance use in abstinent SUD patients in primary care.[9] In dealing with the patient's negative sentiments or concerns, it is a useful strategy to first start with practical issues related to the current situation, and if the misalliance is not resolved with careful evaluation and response to the actual facts and the patient's experience of them, the clinician can only then tactfully move to discussion of possible problems in the relationship between the patient and the clinician.[8] The clinician can clarify the facts or address incorrect assumptions to help support the patient in having more accurate perceptions and assumptions.

Example:

Clinician: "Hi, how have you been doing since your last visit?"

Patient: "Well, it seems that the main thing you want is that I keep taking my meds so it will help the pharmacy budget. Do you get kickbacks or something?"

Clinician: "Wow, it sounds like you are frustrated with something. We've discussed this before—medications are only a part of what addiction treatment and recovery are all about. First, the simple answer to your question is no; I don't get any kickbacks. That would actually be illegal." (Patient frowns.) "I was wondering whether you have other concerns regarding the medication so we can have a conversation about it and hear your thoughts."

Patient: "Um, uh, I threw my naltrexone away 2 weeks ago because my friend told me that it was bad stuff and addicting, and then I used again briefly last week. So, I guess you doctors might be right… Anyway, you guys have it so easy."

Clinician: "So you listened to your friend, threw the medications away, and started using again. Is that accurate?"

Patient: "Yeah."

Clinician: "Ok. I wanted to be clear that I understood you. Now, I don't understand what you mean when you say 'you guys have it so easy'?"

Patient: "I don't know, look, I'm just, I don't know…(annoyed)… I know I screwed up, but I guess I'm waiting for the other shoe to drop, and you kick me out of treatment" (looks away).

Clinician: "So to me, it sounds like you're upset with your going back to using and angry at yourself that stopping your medications may have been part of that. Perhaps, it's more comfortable for you to be angry at me and at the treatment? I appreciate your being honest with me about how you feel. You were concerned that I will be angry with you and not understand your struggles."

Patient: (Shrugs) "Been there, done that."

Clinician: "You've had negative treatment experiences in the past, and it feels like you are concerned that this will happen again in working together?"

Patient: "Right."

Clinician: "I would appreciate if you can share with me about any conflicts and concerns about our working relationship. I am here to listen and we can discuss it openly. But, have I done anything specific in our work together that made you feel this way? Your insights are very central to ensuring we do a good job in helping you."

Patient: "Hmmm….well, no major concerns."

Clinician: "So, going forward, I need to be mindful of your concern that I'll be unhelpful to you, as you have experienced that with other providers."

Patient: "Huh….well, yes" (turns and gives clinician full eye contact).

Clinician: "What can we do together to help get things back on track? I'll help in any reasonable way I can …do you want to restart the naltrexone?"

Patient: "You mean I could try it again even though I threw the last bottle away?"

Clinician: "Sure, we can restart it. This stuff can happen as part of recovery. How do you feel about exploring what also led up to your going back to using and how you are dealing with it in your groups and 12-step meetings?"

Clinical attention to patient treatment satisfaction is associated with better attendance at outpatient visits for SUD.[17]

Motivational Interviewing

Motivational interviewing is detailed in Chapter 70 of this textbook but, in short, it is a very well-researched and evidence-based technique for interacting with patients in such a way as to enhance better communication, engagement, and motivation to change. Compared to a traditional paternalistic and prescriptive approach to the patient's maladaptive choices around substance use, MI encourages internally driven change through a collaborative effort that elicits, through the use of clinical feedback, the patient's own recovery-oriented thoughts and feelings (intrinsic motivation), thus promoting and supporting the patient's sense of autonomy. It is strongly suggested that clinicians read the Chapter 69 of this ASAM textbook on "Enhancing Motivation to Change," and for more detailed information, read the online version of the Center for Substance Abuse Treatment Improvement Protocols TIP 35,[18] which is focused on the MI overview and application, and TIP 42 Chapter 5,[19] which addresses using MI with patients who have co-occurring mental disorders in addition to SUD. In addition to the standard supportive stance with the patient, the motivational interviewer further explores the patient's ambivalence about change and addresses any discord in the therapeutic relationship. This would be in the service of tipping the patient's "decisional balance" toward higher motivation toward treatment engagement and reducing substance use. The clinician would have continued to explore and clarify exactly what the patient was feeling, what the patient wanted to call that feeling, and why they were having it, by restating the patient's concerns, supplying statements of empathy, and asking for clarification:

Clinician: "You sound angry."

Patient: "No, I don't get angry, but I am frustrated."

Clinician: "Tell me about your frustration."

Patient: "Well, it just seems that nothing I do works, and I used again last week."

Clinician: "Going back to using is not unusual for most people and you are frustrated with yourself for having this setback."

Patient: "I thought you would be angry at me."

Clinician: "No, I am not angry with you, I am concerned about you and would like to brainstorm together so we can figure out what changes you want to make and how we can facilitate that."

Behavioral Therapies in the Context of Withdrawal Management

It is well described that the rates of recurrence of substance use or SUDs after withdrawal management are quite high.[20] Only about 20% to 50% of patients receive postwithdrawal management treatment for SUD, yet engagement in follow-up treatment increases the time to a second admission for withdrawal management.[21] Systematic review has demonstrated that over and above pharmacologic withdrawal management for opioid use disorder (OUD), psychosocial treatments such as CM or SUD counseling offered in addition demonstrate beneficial effects in terms of completion of treatment (relative risk [RR] 1.68), use of opioids (RR 0.82), follow-up abstinence (RR 2.43), and compliance with clinic visits (RR 0.48).[22] During outpatient opioid withdrawal management, relapse to opioid use is not uncommon,[23,24] but CM improves treatment retention and reduces symptom complaints.[25]

It is important to remind clinicians that withdrawal management is not a treatment for SUDs per se but rather is medical stabilization and an opportunity to engage patients in the work of recovery. Thus, it appears sensible to provide some form of effective psychosocial intervention in addition to pharmacotherapy of substance withdrawal, and clearly, this is useful with OUD. Given that the exposure to treatment during inpatient withdrawal management is relatively brief and that the most important outcome for those in withdrawal management programs is continued engagement in treatment, MI is probably the modality of therapy that best matches the needs of the patient during the period of treatment.[26] With outpatient withdrawal management, given the generally longer duration of treatment as compared to inpatient withdrawal management, MI with boosters to support continued motivation for treatment engagement, plus some form of contingency management (CM), is a sensible approach to treatment. It is important to recognize that CM-provided incentives do not necessarily have to be in the form of monetary rewards but can be anything that the patients value, offering an opportunity for clinicians' or patients' creativity. For example, in one outpatient SUD clinic, the clinical staff pooled their collections of hotel soaps, shampoos, and conditioners garnered from their vacations and conferences and had a sufficient volume of prizes to run a fishbowl-type CM program for the patients.

Medication Adherence

Medications do not work unless one takes them. It is estimated that the overall adherence to medication regimens for general medical disorders such as hypertension, diabetes, and asthma is between 40% and 60%, with factors such as low socioeconomic status, lack of family and social supports, or significant psychiatric comorbidity associated with the lowest percentages.[27] It would be surprising if adherence rates for unsupervised addiction medications were higher, and they are not. In a 12-week randomized controlled trial (RCT) of naltrexone versus placebo for DSM-IV alcohol dependence in a clinic setting with 98 subjects, the medication showed only modest effects in reducing alcohol drinking, but the subjects who were highly compliant with taking medication had high naltrexone treatment efficacy on a range of measures.[28] Similarly, in the VA Cooperative Study, a randomized placebo-controlled trial of disulfiram for DSM-III alcohol dependence in 605 subjects showed no difference in the intention-to-treat sample in abstinence rates from placebo or from an inactive dose of disulfiram. Yet, in a subgroup with high adherence to medication, there were clear improvements in abstinence rates.[29]

Thus, improved medication adherence could improve the efficacy of pharmacological interventions for SUD, and it makes sense to propose behavioral interventions that might foster improved medication adherence.[30] The basic rationale and monitoring strategies that nonprescribing clinicians can implement to foster and manage medication adherence are listed in **Table 83-1**.

Various factors have been identified that adversely affect patients' adherence to a medication regimen. Some of these factors, both intrinsic to patients and external to them, are co-occurring mental disorders, medication side effects, long waiting times, and inadequate understanding of the proposed treatment.[32] For short-term pharmacotherapeutic interventions, counseling, written materials, and personal phone support may be helpful.[33] In general, interventions that are effective in increasing long-term medication adherence, albeit modestly, include providing information, counseling, reminders, self-monitoring, reinforcement, family therapy, additional supervision or attention, and higher convenience of care.[34]

TABLE 83-1 Medication Adherence Has an Important Relationship to Treatment Outcome

Reasons for non-adherence	Ambivalence, precontemplation state, attitudes and feelings, side effects, poor social support, low self-efficacy, impulsivity, 1° and 2° cognitive problems[31]
Non prescriber (eg, counselor) role	Periodic inquiry, exploring charged issues, keeping physician informed
Non prescriber queries	"How often have you taken your medication in the past xxx (days, weeks, months)?" If the patient stopped medication, the non-prescriber can ask "why do you think you decided to stop your medicine? How did this affect your recovery?"
Adherence	"Sometimes people forget their medications… how often does this happen to you?"
Effectiveness	"How well do you think your medications are working?" "What do you notice?" "Here's what I notice."
Side effects	" Are you having any side effects from the medication?" (if yes) "What are they?" "Have you told your physician?" "Do you need help talking to the doc?"

Reid et al.[35] conducted a RCT with 40 subjects with DSM-IV alcohol dependence of four to six individual sessions of usual medical care versus a compliance therapy for acamprosate consisting of exploration of the patient's beliefs and ambivalence about alcohol use disorder and the nature of medication and psychosocial treatment; addressing the patient's concerns, symptoms, and side effects; supporting patient's evaluation of benefits and consequences of sobriety versus a return to drinking; and supporting self-efficacy and continued treatment engagement. Post hoc analyses of the group that attended at least 50% of the compliance groups found that they demonstrated significantly more days on acamprosate and more days to an extended relapse (3 or more days of more than five drinks) than the usual care group. Therefore, psychosocial interventions specifically aimed at supporting medication adherence appear to have clinical impact; however, a common concern in both the acamprosate and the disulfiram studies is that better results may not be caused by better adherence, but rather, a common other trait results in both better adherence and better addiction treatment outcome. Of course, adherence to medication can't be supported if it is not prescribed in the first place, so given the traditional under-prescribing of evidence-based medications for say, AUD, it behooves prescribing clinicians to educate other clinicians treating substance use disorders (eg, counselors) about the role of these medications, so they can proactively support their patients' engagement in discussions about their potential value in their recovery.

Network Therapy has as one of its main foci to enlist the aid of the patient's supportive others to assist in optimizing patient adherence with medications. An 18-week RCT of Network Therapy or medication management in patients with DSM-IV–defined OUD receiving daily buprenorphine/naltrexone (16 mg) demonstrated higher abstinence rates in the Network Therapy group.[36]

Sometimes, strategies designed to promote medication adherence do not demonstrate the magnitude of effects due to patient characteristics or due to loss of impact over time. Naltrexone would seem to be a tailor-made medication for patients with OUD; however, adherence rates with oral preparations are very poor. Preston et al.[37] conducted a 3-month randomized clinical trial in patients with DSM-IV opioid dependence who completed withdrawal management ($N = 58$) using CM voucher incentives for adherence to naltrexone versus random vouchers independent of adherence versus giving no vouchers. Those getting the contingent vouchers had better treatment retention and a higher number of naltrexone doses taken than either control group. Behavioral naltrexone therapy (BNT) was a therapy specifically developed to improve retention on oral naltrexone by adding elements of CM as above, MI and CBT, and a significant other for monitoring medication adherence similar to Network Therapy.[38] However, in a 6-month, randomized, controlled trial (RCT) in patients with OUD (heroin), BNT ($N = 36$) improved retention in treatment compared to standard medical management (MM), but overall treatment discontinuation was very high (>75%), and there was no between-group difference in the subjects who were very adherent (ie, >70% of doses) with the medications.[39]

Medical Management

Medical management (MM) is a manualized intervention that is a composite of several different psychosocial interventions focusing upon medication compliance and psychosocial treatment engagement and adherence, all of which were integrated for use in the Project COMBINE study.[40] The MM intervention is semi-structured and brief in duration (about nine sessions) and, for each session (about 20 minutes after the initial 40-minute session), suitable for delivery in a primary care environment by a medical professional and, with some adaptation, could focus upon medications other than that used in COMBINE and on SUD other than alcohol use disorder.[41] The manual is available for hard copy order or online (http://pubs.niaaa.nih.gov/publications/combine/) and is highly recommended as probably the most clinically useful, evidence-based practice manual available to the addiction clinician who combines medications and psychosocial interventions in typical office visits. The initial intervention has several components, each of which has evidence supporting its use—using targeted feedback of medical information and individualized advice, the intervention motivates the patient toward medication adherence and reduction in harmful substance use, educates the patient about the need for medication, and offers referral to support groups, such as AA. Brief interventions have a substantial evidence base, and brief motivational interviewing-type interventions have been demonstrated as more effective than traditional advice giving in the treatment of SUDs, with small to moderate effect sizes.[42-44] Giving the patient self-help materials and supporting involvement in mutual self-help groups, each has support in the research literature.[45-47] In Project COMBINE, the most expensive multisite trial that NIAAA has performed to date, which evaluated the effect of both psychosocial therapy and medications (acamprosate and naltrexone), this relatively brief but well-rounded biopsychosocial therapy accounted for the bulk of positive treatment outcome whether the patients took active or placebo medications. Thus, MM is a model that the busy clinician can use, whether using medications as part of treatment or not. Further, as mentioned above, though not yet tested, it is likely that the MM strategy and structure of sessions would also allow for better adherence to both psychosocial and psychiatric medication interventions, and thus outcomes, for those with substance use and co-occurring psychiatric disorders.

The intrinsic themes of MM are educating the patient about the disorder and its specific personal impact; advising the patient about the nature of the treatment, the specific rationale for the medication, and the importance of medication adherence; and recovery support in the form of discussion and advice for implementing medication adherence and alcohol or drug abstinence strategies.[48] The initial MM visit takes place after comprehensive clinical evaluation and lasts 40 to 60 minutes. In many cases in clinical practice, this may be shortly after the initial evaluation, but it is optimal to have an interval within which the clinician can compile the relevant medical information necessary for the initial feedback to the patient. In the case of alcohol problems, these data will typically include blood pressure, liver enzymes, other significant lab findings (eg, urine or blood), findings on physical exam, recent alcohol intake (days, amount/day), self-reported alcohol problems, and description of specific alcohol use disorder symptoms.[49] The MM manual offers a Clinician Report (form A-1) that offers a concise format in which to record the salient data. The clinician reviews the results of the evaluation with the patient, first focusing on the medical data and then moving to a review of the symptoms of alcohol use disorder that the patient endorsed. Any medical concerns of the patient are addressed. The intent is to link the patient's use of alcohol in this case to each biopsychosocial consequence that has been identified. Having done so and answering his or her questions, the patient is then given information about alcohol use disorder in a clear, nonthreatening, and supportive manner and advised to stop drinking.

Framing the problem as a routine medical one and offering a friendly "can-do" attitude about treatment and recovery support the patient in not feeling impugned by the clinician, since patients with SUD are frequently full of shame or hopelessness about their drinking. Communicating a judgmental attitude is likely to engender more resistance to treatment engagement. The clinician advises the patient about the rationale and use of pharmacotherapy as an important medical strategy in assisting recovery. The patient is then instructed about how to take the medicine, and potential side effects are discussed in advance so as to minimize their contribution to nonadherence.[48] The clinician also discusses the rationale of checking the patient's adherence with medication at each subsequent session. The patient's past patterns of medication adherence are evaluated and discussed, so that the patient and clinician together can elaborate a specific plan to assist the patient in remaining adherent with the regimen. The MM manual appendix has a Medication Compliance Plan (form A-13) that can assist the clinician in formalizing the plan with a patient. Finally, the patient is given education and encouragement for attendance at support groups such as AA and is given brochures and other written materials that have source information on medications, alcohol use disorder, and recovery groups. Time is given to the patient to raise questions about the diagnosis or treatment plan.[49]

In each of the subsequent visits, which typically range from 15 to 25 minutes, the clinician checks the patient in terms of medical status, appropriate laboratory data, vital signs, and weight and evaluates the blood alcohol concentration. Then, the question about drinking status is asked, focusing upon how the patient coped: with difficulty or ease, the strength of the desire to drink, or, in the case of continued drinking, what was the context of use. If the patient is abstinent, other problems, such as an increase in other substance use, are evaluated.

Since patients often stop medications when they feel better, it is important that the patient is instructed that even if he or she is doing well in treatment and is abstinent, that is not the time to stop the medication. Another intervention motivates the patient to agree to talk with the physician, counselor, sponsor or other confidante *prior* to making a decision to stop taking medication. Anticipatory guidance and even role playing the interchange in the session may help the patient feel more comfortable expressing the desire to stop the medicine, and to then elicit feedback. The patient should be given positive feedback for medication adherence, and the positive health and lifestyle impact of abstinence are reiterated.

If the desire to drink has reduced but the patient is still drinking, that reduction is reinforced as a first step toward change. A nonjudgmental attitude is key in supporting that change may occur slowly, that there may be ups and downs along the way, and that continuing attempts are associated with success. Any positive step, however small, in reduction in use or craving is given positive feedback, and consistent with supportive therapy, the clinician looks for opportunities to provide appropriate, data-based praise.[8] If it is earlier in treatment and the patient is continuing to drink but adherent to the medication, it is important that the patient is told that the medication has not yet had sufficient time to work completely. If the patient confirms adherence with the medications at the prescribed dose and frequency of oral naltrexone or acamprosate, and at least 2 to 3 weeks has passed with no alteration in drinking pattern, then the prescribing clinician should evaluate the medication dose, and if the dose is optimal, consider nonresponse to that medication with plans for another class of pharmacotherapy. With certain anticonvulsant medications, such as topiramate, because the optimal dose requires many weeks of titration, the length of time to decide whether the medication effect is clinically sufficient must be similarly extended. In addition, the patient is encouraged to attend mutual support groups. In determining the patient's context of use, the patient can be advised to avoid "people, places, and things" associated with use or to substitute a different healthy pleasure at the time when use usually occurs.

Clinician: "So, how have you been doing over the past week?"

Patient: "I'm taking the naltrexone, but it makes me a little jittery and queasy after I take it."

Clinician: "We discussed that it might do that. Is it severe enough to make you want to stop?"

Patient: "No, It's not too bad. I just distract myself, and it gets better as the day goes on. I'm using the plan we talked about!"

Clinician: "Well, it's really good that you are able to continue on it, and usually, those side effects tend to go away over time. Any effects on your desire to drink?"

Patient: "I think so, maybe a little. I hadn't really thought about it. I still get pretty strong urges at times, but I think maybe they're less frequent."

Clinician: "Changes in your desire to drink may be an early sign of a change for you. How well were you able to keep from drinking?"

Patient: "I'm still drinking, but I think it's less than twice this week—Wednesday and yesterday—I started and basically had had enough after two drinks. That's not regular for me. Actually, I didn't even finished the second one yesterday. Funny, I don't know why, I just lost interest!"

Clinician: "Well, you've only been on the medication for a week, and we know it takes time to fully kick in. How have you been doing with your AA involvement?"

Patient: "I went to a meeting on the day after I saw you; then I started drinking again and sort of figured "what the hey?"

Clinician: "You know that 'what the hey' attitude frequently comes with the experience of going back to using almost automatically. One of the benefits of going to meetings is that it offers social support for abstinence. Listening to all those stories and folks succeeding in their recovery can really help motivate and support you in your own recovery."

Patient: "I know, I think I need to plan it out in advance, so I know where I'm supposed to go. That way, it'll be easier to get to the meetings."

Clinician: "That's an excellent way to anticipate problems in getting support for yourself by planning properly. Can we review? In spite of it giving you some uncomfortable feelings, you are sticking with the medications and coping with unpleasant effects according to your plan, which demonstrates your commitment. And though you briefly relapsed, your alcohol intake has diminished somewhat... All in all, I'd say that you made major progress. You are making better plans to get to AA meetings—in fact, let's talk about what specific meeting you are going to go to next, where it is, and what you will say when you get there."

The patient who is abstinent but not taking medications as prescribed is given positive feedback for not drinking, and the general benefits of abstinence are reinforced. The reasons for the nonadherence (eg, side effects, forgetting, misinformation) are explored with the patient, and the clinician presents the patient with the information that over time the risks of return to use are reduced by the medication. The compliance plan is amended with strategies addressing the reasons for nonadherence.

The patient who is nonadherent to medications and is drinking but motivated to stop is encouraged to engage in treatment more fully. The medical rationale for treatment that was explained in the initial MM visit is repeated. As above, the reasons for nonadherence with medication are explored, and the compliance plan is amended with strategies addressing the reasons for nonadherence.

Strategies to Integrate Medication Treatment and Behavioral Therapies

There is not yet a wealth of empirical data to support the concept, and there clearly has not been a great deal of positive results for attempts at elucidating the beneficial effects of treatment matching.[47,50] Nonetheless, since no singular treatment is a "slam dunk," it is still clinically sensible to have an approach to any return to substance use that places as many barriers as practicable of differing content and strategy in the way of the person with an addiction struggling with craving and opportunities to use. This means that both external and internal structures can be brought to bear in this process and that a combination of different interventions, whether psychosocial or pharmacological, may have *convergent* or *complementary* effects on the inhibition of recurrence. In the context of providing an appropriate behavioral therapy platform for use in pharmacotherapy trials, Carroll et al.[51] described the available empirically supported and well-operationalized behavioral therapies as having a range of possible targets such as enhancing medication adherence, reducing attrition, addressing co-occurring problems, promoting abstinence, and targeting specific weaknesses of the pharmacological agent.

Poldrugo[52] conceptualized the impact of pharmacotherapy for SUDs, in this case, alcohol use disorder, as biologically enhancing mechanisms of either external or internal control. For example, disulfiram, as an aversive agent, would be considered as supportive of external control. Medications that purportedly affected the endogenous reward system, such as neuromodulators like acamprosate, or inhibitors of substance-induced reward, like naltrexone, would be considered enhancers of mechanisms of internal control. So, in constructing a combination medication and psychosocial intervention for alcohol use disorder, one could consider aligning psychosocial interventions that either augment the control impact of the medication or offer a complementary control locus. Expanding the concept along similar lines, Mattson and Litten[53] described four strategies for combining medications and behavioral therapies in alcohol use disorder, probably the addiction domain best researched for treatment matching and combining behavioral therapy with medication: (1) targeting the same drinking behavior with both the medication and behavioral intervention; (2) medications and therapy each targeting one of two different drinking behaviors; (3) targeting a drinking behavior and a secondary problem that creates a context for drinking or impairs recovery, such as co-occurring mental illness, family problems, or comorbid medical disorders; and (4) adding to a medication regimen a behavioral therapy specifically targeting medication adherence or treatment retention, which was discussed above. The other strategies will be discussed below, in the context not only of alcohol use disorder but also with other SUDs.

Using Matching Data to Facilitate Integration

In a recent post hoc analysis of Project MATCH data, DSM-IV–defined alcohol-dependent patients with social networks supportive of drinking had better short-term outcomes if they were assigned to 12-step facilitation (TSF).[54] This has face validity as a convergent strategy in that TSF attempts to reduce social support for drinking behavior through linkage with the pro abstinence social support found in AA. Patient characteristics may also interact with the effectiveness of certain types of behavioral intervention. In another Project MATCH data reanalysis using growth mixture modeling, individuals with lower self-efficacy who received cognitive–behavioral therapy (CBT) drank far less frequently than did those with low self-efficacy who received motivational enhancement therapy (MET).[55] This also has face validity in that CBT attempts to increase the patient's self-efficacy related to abstinence.[56] Certain character traits may also have negative impact in the context of specific therapies. For example, across Project MATCH therapies (CBT, MET, and TSF), patients with DSM-IV alcohol dependence ($N = 141$) treated in a more confrontative and directive therapy who had moderate to high trait reactance (the tendency to resist relinquishing control) had worse 1-year alcohol outcomes than those with low trait reactance, but especially so in the MET group.[57]

Convergent Strategies

Naltrexone has been demonstrated in meta-analyses to be a medication effective in the treatment of alcohol use disorder with the greatest effect on reduction in relapse to heavy drinking, modulated either by reductions in cue-induced reward or by reducing the rewarding effects of alcohol, or both.[58-61] Work by Myrick et al.[62] demonstrated that naltrexone reduces alcohol cue-induced brain activation. Therefore, with naltrexone therapy in alcohol use disorder, one could use a complementary behavioral intervention strategy that supported non-initiation of drinking or a convergent one that increased the likelihood of a slip remaining a slip (a drink or two) rather than becoming a return to regular use or to heavy drinking. Similarly, the craving reduction aspect of naltrexone could be paired as a convergent strategy with the craving attenuating effects of CBT or cue extinction therapy.

In randomized trials of a convergent strategy, Balldin et al.[63] and Heinälä et al.[64] found that CBT focused on coping with a slip produced better reductions in return to heavy drinking than abstinence-focused supportive therapy when paired with naltrexone. In contrast, O'Malley et al.[65] in a four-cell randomized comparison ($N = 97$) of naltrexone versus placebo, and also CBT versus supportive therapy, demonstrated better cumulative alcohol abstinence rates in the naltrexone-treated patients who were given supportive therapy as compared to CBT. However, taking into consideration that the main effect of naltrexone is reduction in return to heavy drinking, the O'Malley et al. study also demonstrated this in the CBT group compared to the group receiving supportive therapy. Anton et al.[66] tested naltrexone against placebo in a 12-week RCT in 131 detoxified outpatients with alcohol dependence who were offered weekly CBT. The group treated with naltrexone had fewer subjects who returned to use, a longer time to return to heavy drinking, fewer drinks per drinking day, and higher percentage of days abstinent. Interestingly, the naltrexone-treated group appeared to make better use of CBT—they had more resistance to alcohol-treated thoughts and urges as measured on the Obsessive Compulsive Drinking Scale. More recently, Anton et al.[67] completed a 12-week RCT testing of naltrexone versus placebo, combined with either CBT or MET in 120 outpatient subjects with alcohol dependence. Again, subjects receiving CBT and naltrexone had significantly fewer returns to heavy drinking (OR = 0.40) than the other groups, and those that did had a longer time to subsequent return to use. It is hypothesized that CBT offers specific skills to deal with craving, high-risk situations, and family conflict that may be a more complete adjunct to the effects of naltrexone than MET provides. Thus, taken together, it is reasonable to provide CBT and naltrexone in combination as a convergent strategy to decrease return to heavy drinking in patients with alcohol use disorder.

Complementary Strategies

Stanton and Shadish[68] demonstrated in a meta-analysis of randomized trials that compared to individual and peer group therapy, family and couples therapies have significantly better impact on recovery from SUD. As a complementary strategy, behavioral couples therapy (BCT), a well-researched and effective behavioral intervention, can provide elements of increased social support for the patient's efforts to change and contingency for sobriety, while disulfiram can assist the maintenance of sobriety through deterrence.[69] Meta-analysis of BCT studies demonstrates its superiority over individual interventions for SUDs at treatment follow-up on frequency of use, consequences of use, and relationship satisfaction.[70] As one part of BCT, the couple enters into a disulfiram contract, an agreement that stipulates that the spouse observes and records on a calendar the patient taking the daily disulfiram dose, and the patient and spouse then thank each other for their efforts and refrain from arguments or discussions about the patient's drinking behavior.[71] The structured way of relating around the patient's use of sobriety-supporting medications helps to reduce relationship dysfunction in the couple, which is seen as a major driver of substance use.

In a variant of BCT, Fals-Stewart and O'Farrell[72] used naltrexone contracting with 124 men with opioid dependence and the family members they lived within a randomized 24-week trial of behavioral family contracting (BFC) and individual therapy versus individual therapy alone. The BFC patients took more doses of naltrexone, were more compliant with scheduled sessions, and had longer continuous abstinence and more opioid and other illicit drug abstinence during and for the year after treatment. They also had fewer drug-related, legal, and family problems at 1-year follow-up. In this example of complementary strategies, BFC increased medication adherence and provided social support for continuing opioid abstinence, while naltrexone blocked the rewarding effects of opioids. Since the effects of BCT tend to fade over time, as couples tend to regress back toward dysfunctional relating, a study of booster sessions provided to couples after the main treatment had ended supported the maintenance of treatment gains.[73]

Other psychosocial interventions may introduce similar convergent factors or complementary factors other than increasing social support or reducing return to use potential that have equivalent impact as CBT in the context of naltrexone. Latt et al.[74] demonstrated in an RCT ($N = 107$) that naltrexone with adjunctive medical advice in a primary care setting was effective in reducing the return to heavy drinking by about 50% irrespective of whether it was accompanied by counseling and supportive therapy. Similarly, in a comparison of CBT and primary care management in 197 subjects with alcohol dependence treated with naltrexone, O'Malley et al.[75] found that the primary care intervention (including referral to and support of AA attendance, medication issues and adherence support, and clinical advice) had similar impact over 10 weeks on reducing return to heavy drinking as did CBT. However, the CBT group was better at maintaining days of abstinence over time.

The interaction of bupropion and CM is another complementary strategy, where the bupropion may affect subjective negative mood and cognitive symptoms post cocaine withdrawal and the CM reinforces retention in treatment and rewards abstinence. Poling et al.[76] conducted a 25-week, double-blind RCT in methadone-maintained patients with DSM-IV cocaine dependence ($N = 106$) with four cells: CM that gave vouchers for negative cocaine urine screens and abstinence-related activities and medication placebo, CM and bupropion 300 mg/d, control vouchers for giving urine specimens and placebo medication, or control vouchers and bupropion. Although bupropion had independent effects upon cocaine use over the 12 weeks, results demonstrated that bupropion plus CM significantly improved cocaine outcomes relative to bupropion alone.

Sometimes, reasonable complementary strategies do not work synergistically, perhaps as one of the interventions is more robust. Disulfiram is hypothesized to reduce cocaine use through direct impact on neurotransmitter metabolism, reducing the pleasurable effects of cocaine, whereas CBT supports maintenance of abstinence through cognitive restructuring in the form of functional analysis and new skills acquisition.[77,78] CBT was tested by Carroll et al.[79] against interpersonal psychotherapy (IPT) in a four-cell (disulfiram/CBT, disulfiram/IPT, placebo/CBT, placebo/IPT) 12-week comparison with disulfiram versus placebo in 121 patients with cocaine dependence. Cocaine use was reduced significantly in the disulfiram group and in the CBT group compared to the IPT group in the context of placebo, but there was no difference between therapies in the context of disulfiram. The effects of the disulfiram on cocaine use were greatest in subjects who were abstinent from alcohol or without alcohol dependence at baseline, suggesting that the effects of disulfiram are not moderated by its effect on alcohol use.

Other Strategies

Combination strategies can also target the SUD and in addition attempt to treat co-occurring mental or medical disorders. It is clear that both disorders need to be targeted independently, although there may be some convergent effects in treating the co-occurring disorder. For example, depression and depressive symptoms have an adverse effect upon recovery from SUD. Although it has been reasonable to test a parsimonious treatment such as an SSRI to attempt to treat both the depression and the SUD, meta-analysis of this strategy has demonstrated that (with one exception below) antidepressant medications are efficacious for the treatment of depression in patients with SUD but that other interventions are necessary for treating the SUD.[80] For example, Stein et al.[81] conducted an RCT of citalopram plus 8 sessions of CBT for depression compared to an assessment control condition in 109 people who were actively injecting drugs with a DSM-IV mood disorder spectrum diagnosis and a Hamilton Rating Scale for Depression score greater than 13. At follow-up, more than twice the patients receiving the intervention were in remission of the depression, but there was no impact on heroin or cocaine use. In addition to the lack of evidence that treating other co-occurring mental disorders is clinically effective for SUD, some interventions for mental disorders can have adverse impact on SUD. Recent data have suggested that a subset of patients with alcohol use disorder, type A (later onset), may respond differentially to SSRI treatment compared to placebo with reductions in drinking but that type B (early onset, prior to age 25) patients with alcohol use disorder may actually do worse.[40,82]

Patients treated with methadone maintenance often have problems in multiple life dimensions other than SUD, and some of these are likely to respond to psychosocial interventions that may also promote abstinence from opioids. Specific gains in psychosocial therapy of methadone-maintained patients tend to be related to the type of therapy (eg, supportive–expressive, CBT) the patient is exposed to over and in addition to counseling alone and the impact of psychiatric symptoms.[83] The improvement in psychological functioning is correlated with better overall functioning, including SUD; thus, it is sensible to provide behavioral therapies to patients on methadone who have psychiatric symptoms.[84]

Principles for Care Integration

There are no research data to demonstrate whether convergent or complementary strategies have more robust effects. In the spirit of constructing multiple obstacles to relapse, clinical practice often engages multiple strategies that may be both convergent and complementary. It is likely that there will be individual patient characteristics such as genetics, addiction severity, co-occurring disorders, and drug of choice that will impact what the optimal combination of medications and psychosocial interventions will be. As such, a stage-wise approach to recovery may help to guide the clinician in choosing an appropriate mix of medication and therapy. The clinician can determine what the important tasks are for this stage in treatment. For example, in establishing abstinence, there are several acute issues that typically need to be dealt with: negative mood states and craving, conditioned cues, access to substances, and immersion in contexts supportive of substance use. Thus, one could pick treatments based upon the impact in those various domains, for example, reducing social isolation and offering social support for sobriety with mutual self-help groups and TSF, BCT, or Network Therapy, supporting treatment engagement with MI, supporting cognitive and coping skills functioning in early recovery with CBT/relapse prevention and/or improving baseline cognitive deficits with appropriate medications, reducing alcohol craving with naltrexone and opioid craving with buprenorphine or methadone, supporting self-efficacy and resilience for craving and negative states with CBT, and reducing substance use with CM and supporting alcohol abstinence with disulfiram or acamprosate. Fortunately, in most cases, appropriately applied interventions are not usually mutually exclusive, but on occasion, this occurs (eg, disulfiram and moderation management).

COLLABORATIVE CARE WITH COUNSELORS AND PSYCHOTHERAPISTS

Psychosocial interventions typically are provided by practitioners from a variety of disciplines, ranging from noncredentialed counselors and patient navigators (frequently peers in recovery) to licensed psychologists, social workers, licensed professional mental health counselors, registered nurses and nurse practitioners, marriage, family, and child counselors, and certified recovery peer advocates and peer support specialists, as well as pharmacists. Such practitioners differ widely in their attitudes, preparation, and skills; however, the trend within many states has been to create a group of licensed professional counselors with standardized training and credentials that will slowly become the predominant form of addiction counseling as noncredentialed counselors age out of the workforce. Addiction treatment personnel also vary in the degree to which they are accustomed to working with physicians and other medical personnel. Understanding the background and orientation of specific staff can enhance communication and teamwork.

Counselors

In most states, treatment programs that are not certified, licensed, or accredited are ineligible to receive state or federal funding; thus, most state-approved addiction treatment programs require addiction counselors to meet certain competency standards established by state boards or other certification bodies such as the International Certification and Reciprocity Consortium or the Association for Addiction Professionals (NAADAC).[85] Although most states have moved toward credentialing counselors, noncredentialed counselors have been integrated into treatment teams on inpatient units since the 1950s when the Minnesota Model was developed by Hazelden and Wilmar.[86] Before that time, alcoholism was seen as a psychological vulnerability to be treated on mental health units; however, this theoretical framework failed to produce effective treatment. Collaboration by the leaders of Hazelden and Wilmar led to an adaptation of the principles of AA to create a new model within hospital-based treatment. The blended approaches of Wilmar and Hazelden produced the Minnesota Model, which was the prototype of the 28-day inpatient program. Proponents of the model refined their treatment practices and restructured institutional relationships to emphasize collaboration between professional staff and noncredentialed recovering persons. By 1954, counselors without professional degrees shared both responsibility and decision-making authority.

Therapeutic communities (TCs), which developed and expanded in the 1960s, historically relied on recovering noncredentialed staff.[87-90] Some of these gifted clinicians and managers subsequently were hired into the private, insurance-funded treatment system, to which they brought their perspective on the importance of developing a culture that supports recovery. Their appreciation of the need to strengthen environmental or micro-community forces to foster change added an important dimension to the developing professional addiction care model, which presumed that professional services were the primary factor in promoting change.

Currently, nonlicensed, recovering personnel are found in short-term, Minnesota Model, addiction or so-called "chemical dependency" inpatient programs, as peer counselors in co-occurring disorder programs and in community-based addiction treatment programs. They also predominate in TCs that integrate 12-step elements into their conceptual model. Some counselors return to school and obtain graduate degrees and licenses, building the cadre of professionals in recovery.

Like licensed staff members, noncredentialed counselors vary widely in talent, experience, and skill. Some have little training, except for occasional in-service training sessions. Others have completed comprehensive credentialing programs and are far more sophisticated than some licensed staff. For example, certificate programs (often attached to universities) may require 200 to 300 hours of course work plus supervised field placement experience. However, many programs still use the 12-step perspective as a sole orientation and do not include important evidence-based or alternative approaches, including FDA-approved medications for SUDs. The current emphasis on incorporating evidence-based approaches exerts a growing influence on these certificate programs.

Some counselors have superb skills, as their "street savvy" and personal experience in recovery can produce a highly sophisticated clinician. Others, however, may have rigid, non–patient-centered concepts of recovery ("what worked for me will work for you") and have difficulty tolerating the ambiguities of complex clinical populations, such as those with co-occurring psychiatric disorders, who may need extended time or harm reduction approaches on the path toward abstinence. Harm reduction approaches are increasingly available in the community and may be effective as engagement strategies, as damage control, or as sufficient intervention for mild to moderate problems.[91] These complex patients have always been in the addiction treatment system and are well documented in the epidemiological literature[92] but were not recognized as such, due to lack of training, skills, professional diagnostic evaluation, and program ideology, and so had typically poor outcomes including discontinuation or termination. In short, physicians should draw conclusions about the skill level of the counselors with whom they work from direct observation, not from inferences based on the presence or absence of credentials.

At their best, such counselors, as peers, can present powerful role models, a contribution deeply valued by addicted patients, especially those in early recovery.

Licensed Providers

Within addiction treatment settings, one finds licensed professionals, some of whom are recovering, others who are not. Though most such professionals have basic clinical skills, as with any clinician, their ability and comfort in adapting those skills to the addicted patient population may vary greatly. The rigidities of some licensed professionals arise from devotion to theoretical models in which they have extensive training, in addition to their own personality traits. Physicians should be cautious about drawing conclusions from the presence of academic credentials and professional licenses. Graduate schools of nursing, psychology, medicine, and social work may fail to integrate sufficient training in the assessment and treatment of addiction into their core curricula. This is in spite of the fact that patients with whom graduates will work frequently have SUDs. Often, such training is provided as an elective (if at all) or in a course mandated by the increasing number of states that require an introductory course for initial licensure or license renewal. Other programs offer extensive training through extension courses or specialized training institutes, and some graduate programs offer addiction treatment as a subspecialty. However, nonphysician health professionals can improve their ability to diagnose and manage SUDs by obtaining additional addiction training and certification, leading to a Certified Addictions RN, Licensed Chemical Dependency

Counselor, Certified Tobacco Treatment Specialist, or Masters in Addiction Studies. Physicians should never assume that a professional is knowledgeable in this area, or that a professional in recovery with "lived experience" is more effective than one who is not in recovery. Professionals may underestimate their own lack of knowledge, preferring to believe that the models they acquired in training can be adapted to treating addiction with little modification or that specialized knowledge about treatment of SUDs is unnecessary.

Clinical experience alone may tell little about qualifications. A therapist may say, "I've been seeing alcohol and drug users for 20 years." Many psychotherapists have evolved comfortable practice styles whose content bears little relation to those supported by the evidence base or to the experience of addiction specialists. The comfort level of these therapists is sustained because they do not track their patients who drop out of treatment and so do not incorporate those rates and the reasons for those rates as quality feedback into their clinical practice. As such, they have no objective means of monitoring patient progress in becoming alcohol-free and drug-free. This process is also found in many freestanding drug treatment centers, where the failure of the patient to adhere to the strict rules leading to dropout or premature discharge is explained as "he hasn't reached his bottom," compared to the reality that the patient has an untreated co-occurring mental disorder that impairs his abilities to participate in groups, speak coherently, control affect and impulse, etc. Patients frequently report concealing or minimizing their alcohol and drug use during psychotherapy, so this is of clinical importance. In selecting good therapists for referral, physicians should look for evidence of recent systematic training, through either conferences or course work. Such evidence increases the likelihood that the therapist will be familiar with sound treatment practices.

Tensions can occur between addiction recovering and nonrecovering staff and between those with and without professional training and licenses. Passions can run high, and clinicians can use basic addiction treatment concepts to express disapproval or to discredit one's colleagues. The concepts of enabling and codependency in particular have been used to disparage colleagues who take certain positions. They often are used to discourage appropriate forms of helping and to terminate treatment prematurely. Time in treatment is correlated significantly with positive outcomes in a large number of treatment outcome studies.[93-96] Thus, engagement and retention of patients in treatment are paramount. Terminating patients for manifesting symptoms of their psychiatric or addictive disorder is simply not supported by research. Physicians also may struggle in dealing with this phenomenon, although other chronic diseases such as asthma, diabetes, and hypertension have compliance rates comparable to those of addiction treatment.[27,97] Physicians may need to be the voice of reason, preventing premature termination of the patient's treatment while avoiding colluding with patient behaviors that have a negative impact on their or others' course of treatment or on the overall recovery environment.

Physicians in leadership roles should establish weekly in-service training sessions that address both basic and specialized topics. A multidisciplinary team can develop a shared language and will become knowledgeable about integrating the treatment of addiction, psychiatric, and other medical disorders. Some excellent training materials are available at no charge (eg, downloadable Treatment Improvement Protocols published by the federal government's Center for Substance Abuse Treatment [http://www.ncbi.nlm.nih.gov/books/NBK82999/]).[98] These materials can be used to organize on-site training sessions. Securing continuing education credits for each discipline of the staff enhances participation and commitment to a high-quality training sequence.

The National Addiction Technology Transfer Center (https://attcnetwork.org/centers/global-attc/about-attc-network) offers a comprehensive list of institutions offering a certificate, associate, bachelor, master, and/or doctoral program in SUDs. Also included in this directory are institutions offering a concentration, specialty, or minor in the addiction field. It also offers licensing and certification requirements by state and organization.

Collaboration With Psychotherapists in the Community

The diversity of psychotherapists in the community can make effective collaboration even more challenging.

The programmatic approach to addiction treatment typically is highly structured, with multiple behavioral expectations. More traditional psychodynamically-oriented therapists may have difficulty incorporating behavioral commitments, as their treatment style tends to be more patient and process driven, whereas cognitive-behavioral therapists (who are directive and offer a structured approach to treatment) or those with MI experience (who are comfortable being directive) or with a supportive orientation[8] may more easily adapt to working with an addiction medicine physician. Therapists and counselors in addiction treatment are active and directive, whereas the treatment style of private practice psychotherapists may be more or less compatible with addiction treatment styles. In a recovery-oriented psychotherapy model, the therapist focuses his or her activity according to the tasks faced by the recovering person. These tasks can be conceptualized as recognizing the negative consequences of substance use, making a commitment to abstinence, becoming abstinent and getting sober, and shaping lifestyle transitions to support a comfortable and satisfying sobriety.[99]

Addiction treatment often includes breath and urine testing if resources permit, whereas general psychotherapists without addiction training rarely arrange for such testing, and many consider it invasive and abhorrent. These differences pose an adaptive challenge to the physician who is arranging for treatment of patients with co-occurring substance use and other mental disorders.

Most programmatic outpatient addiction treatment is abstinence oriented, although medical center-based or medical center-affiliated programs have tended to integrate newer, evidence-based more harm reduction treatments into their protocols that can use MI techniques to engage and support patients at various stages of change. Although abstinence is a frequent goal of clinicians for their patients, their patients may access SUD treatment without a commitment to or understanding of why abstinence could be a goal. Harm reduction strategies can serve as a treatment engagement strategy or be implemented as a clinical endpoint, but the context is the same willingness to work with the patient at where their current recovery stage determines their initial goals to be. That stated, there will be variation in what the patient considers success, for example ranging from elimination of heavy drinking episodes and associated harm to complete abstinence. In all cases, a clear structure and patient accountability support clinical progress.[91] This model is the usual in primary care treatments of hypertension, diabetes, and other chronic diseases with outcomes varying around patients' understanding, motivation, commitment and, of course, the nature and degree of illness.

Pharmacotherapy Support From Nonphysicians

Recovering patients who have conditions that require psychotropic or other medications have clinical needs that have historically been out of the scope of practice of addiction treatment programs, and more traditional programs have slowly incorporated on-site or referral for pharmacotherapy for either addiction or other mental disorders.[100] However, in more recent years, the use of pharmacotherapy in conjunction with addiction treatment appears to be picking up, especially with support of professional counseling organizations and nationally known private recovery systems. The use of drugs with a high addiction liability, such as benzodiazepines or opioids, may precipitate a return to the primary substance. Patients who present for treatment may be taking medications prescribed by physicians who are not trained in addiction medicine. In settings wherein physicians see patients only when specific problems emerge, counselors should use a screening tool that incorporates warning signals (such as prescriptions for benzodiazepines or opioids for pain) that warrant a physician review.

Recovering patients may have complex feelings and attitudes toward medications that need to be understood and addressed. Many define recovery as living a comfortable and responsible lifestyle without the use of psychoactive drugs. However, some disorders require psychiatric medications for appropriate treatment, such as antipsychotic agents for schizophrenia or mood stabilizers for bipolar disorder without which risk for return to substance use is increased. Family members or 12-step program participants may criticize the patient or pressure them for discontinuation of medication, generating conflict that undermines treatment. Because physicians often lack adequate time to deal with such issues, these tasks should be delegated specifically to other members of the treatment team. Such providers may need additional training to handle medication issues. Family psychoeducation about addiction and co-occurring psychiatric disorders can be helpful in aligning family members to the treatment team and the goals of treatment.[5]

Collaborating to Achieve Patients' Treatment Adherence

As discussed above, adherence to treatment recommendations is a key factor in successful treatment outcomes. Hence, physicians should monitor how well the treatment team attends to this issue. As compliance with medication regimens is far from perfect, even in well-educated middle-class patients who do not have a stigmatized illness, addicted patients, who often have additional psychiatric and medical disorders, have difficulty in this area. As with other patients, carefully eliciting patient concerns and objections is worthwhile. Many behavioral strategies yield poor results because no one took the time to identify the actual obstacles to adherence. Sympathetic, reflective listening, combined with well-timed doses of information, can improve medication adherence significantly. Collaborative models utilizing pharmacists as part of the treatment team have been shown both useful and effective.[101]

Physicians can help counselors and psychotherapists to understand and explore these issues in their counseling sessions with patients. Nonphysicians vary considerably in their attitudes and education about medication. Time spent on educating therapists usually yields multiple benefits. Certain forms of resistance occur frequently.[102] Patients on psychotropic medications often feel ashamed and guilty, believing that they have failed if they cannot master their illness by themselves. For persons who are in recovery, there are added layers of difficulty. Taking a medication to feel better is highly charged, as many link this motive inextricably with their substance use. Even in the case of medications such as antidepressants, which produce no feelings of euphoria or "high," such guilt can persist. Some patients report they feel they are "cheating," even though their depression precipitated multiple relapses during the time it was untreated.

Rejecting a recommendation for medication may reflect the "all-or-none" thinking characteristic of the person with an SUD. The same patient who at one time consumed every available substance becomes horrified at the idea of "putting something foreign in my body" or "relying on drugs." With respect to disulfiram, Banys[103] notes that many patients disdainfully describe it as a "crutch." Even though these are the same patients who used alcohol as a "crutch" for years, they are paradoxically fastidious about this one. Medications such as disulfiram or naltrexone can provide an invaluable (and lifesaving) opportunity to alter behavior patterns; however, patients who use these medications may feel unable to take credit for their achievements. Reliance on the medication can undermine the sense of mastery that ultimately promotes lasting sobriety; for others, it becomes an intermediate stage while recovery concepts are internalized and mastered. Thus, it is important to handle this issue carefully and specifically to each patient when such treatment adjuncts are used.

Medication is not a substitute for the work of recovery, which requires developing more adaptive (ie, less relapse-prone) coping skills. Medications can, however, offer a stabilizing influence on experience and behavior as SUD patients reduce harm and move toward maintaining abstinence. One marker of recovery in the context of medication treatment that is useful for clinicians to monitor is the evidence of the patient's transitioning toward more traditionally meaningful and normative reinforcers, such as:

- new or revitalized interpersonal relationships with people who don't use alcohol or use drugs nonmedically,
- achievement of gainful employment or renewed educational pursuits,
- re-engagement into family networks when clinically appropriate, and
- exploration or engagement in health-promoting, creative and/or recreational pastimes.

For example, a patient taking disulfiram can be asked to keep a daily journal describing situations that would have been hazardous if he or she were not on the medication. The patient then can be asked what behaviors need to be strengthened (often assertive behaviors) to create safety even in the absence of medication. Washton and Zweben[91] offer a collaborative, problem-solving set of queries with patients that improves patient self-knowledge of risk factors and helps clarify and support steps they can take to discontinue disulfiram treatment and still maintain abstinence (**Table 83-2**).

The decision to discontinue can be implemented once the patient has developed coping skills for the high-risk situations previously identified. However, for some patients with high risk of return to use with major consequences, use of medications over a long period is clinically appropriate.

Adherence with medication regimens can be monitored through refill requests. Many states now have prescription monitoring programs for controlled substances, where prescribers of a controlled substance must check a database to make sure the patient is not obtaining the same or similar medications elsewhere, or receiving other potentially unsafe medications; with some states also recording state authorized cannabis used as treatment. Patients who are adhering to their regimens typically initiate contact with their physicians for refills before the existing supplies expire. Prescribing sufficient doses for a long period deprives the physician of this potential warning signal. Communication with other treatment staff is essential when noncompliance is suspected. Discontinuation of psychotropic medication often is a harbinger of return to substance use, as distressing psychiatric symptoms begin to reemerge. It may also be an indicator that a return to substance use already has occurred.

It is important to train counselors to follow up on adherence issues and to make sure they know when to contact the physician directly. TIP 42 has good recommendations on this.[19] Once counselors are "onboard" with the concepts and recovery utility of pharmacotherapies, it is important for them to identify medication side effects that influence adherence,

TABLE 83-2 Monitoring Recovery Skills Prior to Discontinuing Disulfiram

Topics	Ask the patient
Episodes where disulfiram made a difference	to identify high-risk situations that didn't become drinking episodes because they were taking disulfiram. What do they think put them at risk?
Where disulfiram gave protection against substance use, but the patient needs better adaptive skills in its absence	are there behaviors that still need to be addressed to reduce their risk for return to substance use once they discontinue disulfiram? If so, what do they plan to change? (Focus on refusal skills and strategies the patient can use to cope with situational stress.)
Where the patient anticipates behavioral change in order to cope with risk, prior to setting a d/c date for disulfiram	what goals must they achieve before they commit to a medication d/c date. In the first 3 months off disulfiram, what do they foresee that will be challenging, and what help will they need to have or changes in behavior they will need to make to reduce their risk for recurrence of use?
Where disulfiram may again need to protect against return to use of the substance	what they anticipate will be specific early markers that indicate restarting disulfiram is the best option to head off a recurrence of use. How might you engage your significant other to support this?

Used with permission of Guilford Press, from Washton AM, Zweben JE. *Treating Alcohol and Drug Problems in Psychotherapy Practice: Doing What Works.* 2nd ed. Guilford Press; in press, permission conveyed through Copyright Clearance Center, Inc.

discuss them with the patient, and facilitate a plan to coordinate with the physician. As stated above, counselors should also discuss the need for the patient to contact the physician or counselor (or a confidant) before making a unilateral decision to stop taking their medication. For example, Johnson et al.[104] have documented that patients with bipolar disorder are more likely to be consistent about medications that reduce the severity of their depressive episodes and do not cause weight gain or cognitive effects. Supporting the patient in a problem-solving process with the physician is an important role for the counselor.

In prescribing medications to address withdrawal phenomena, physicians need to communicate to nonphysician therapists what to expect and what might constitute warning signs of impending problems. For example, the therapist may not be aware that a patient given a 3-day supply of chlordiazepoxide for alcohol withdrawal by an addiction specialist also may have obtained a month's supply of diazepam from his or her family physician for "back spasm" and thus be in a high-risk situation. Patients who are drinking and using may skip their prescribed medication because they fear their interaction with drugs and alcohol. Physicians should provide guidance to therapists about whether to encourage adherence to medication during these episodes, based on the preferable scenarios. As therapists spend considerable time with their patients, they are in a good position to detect developing problems and initiate communication with the physician or clinician responsible for coordinating care.

The physician needs to discuss with the patient and other members of the treatment team the indications for discontinuing medications and the process by which such discontinuation should occur. Many patients with prescriptions for disulfiram report that they have not had discussions with their physicians on this topic. Physicians should clarify that disulfiram is a tool to allow other accomplishments to take place. The patient needs to review his or her progress with the program staff, a private therapist, or the prescribing physician before discontinuing medication. Patients who are taking antidepressants may go into denial about their psychiatric disorder once they feel better and thus discontinue use of the medication prematurely. The physician needs to educate both patients and nonphysician therapists about the dangers of psychiatric and addiction relapse that attend such a decision.

Control issues are common. Some patients will accept the need for prescribed medications but will tinker with frequency and dose, much as they did with their illicit substances. Some may operate on the assumption that if one pill is good, three are better and escalate their dose of medications even though [that] drug is not usually considered capable of providing a "high." Drug mixing is another common practice. "Surrendering control of medication use to your physician" is a concept that can be proven useful; under such a scenario, any deviation from the prescribed regimen is the subject of inquiry. Patients who are engaged in serious self-examination may spontaneously report such behavior as a residual part of their addictive pattern.

The encouraging news is that collaborative care models have a significant impact on engagement in SUD treatment with improved outcomes in primary care settings. In a federally qualified health center, the SUMMIT RCT of collaborative care provided a population-based management approach including measurement-based care and integrated addiction expertise supporting a six-session brief MI/CBT psychotherapy treatment and/or sublingual buprenorphine/naloxone treatment for OUD or long-acting injectable naltrexone treatment for alcohol use disorder or OUD and, compared to treatment as usual, demonstrated more than doubled SUD treatment engagement (39.0% versus 16.8%, $p < 0.001$) and greater alcohol or illicit opioid abstinence at 6 months (32.8% versus 22.3%, $p = 0.03$).[105]

REFERENCES

1. Dutra L, Stathopoulou G, Basden SL, Leyro TM, Powers MB, Otto MW. A meta-analytic review of psychosocial interventions for substance use disorders. *Am J Psychiatry*. 2008;165:179-187.
2. Miller WR, Wilbourne PL. Mesa Grande: a methodological analysis of clinical trials of treatments for alcohol use disorders. *Addiction*. 2002;97:265-277.
3. Greenfield L, Fountain D. Influence of time in treatment and follow-up duration on methadone treatment outcomes. *J Psychopathol Behav Assess*. 2000;22:353-364.
4. French MT, Zarkin GA, Hubbard RL, Rachal JV. The effects of time in drug abuse treatment and employment on posttreatment drug use and criminal activity. *Am J Drug Alcohol Abuse*. 1993;19:19-33.
5. Rosenthal RN. Basic treatment techniques for persons with substance use disorders and co-occurring mental disorders. In: Sowers WE, HL MQ, Feldman JM, et al., eds. *American Association for Community Psychiatry Textbook of Community Psychiatry*. 2nd ed. Springer Nature; 2022.
6. Osaji J, Ojimba C, Ahmed S. The use of acceptance and commitment therapy in substance use disorders: a review of literature. *J Clin Med Res*. 2020;12(10):629-633. doi:10.14740/jocmr4311
7. Nalpas B, Matelak F, Martin S, Boulze I, Balmes J-L, Crouzet C. Clinical management methods for out-patients with alcohol dependence. *Subst Abuse Treat Prev Policy*. 2006;1(1):5.
8. Rosenthal RN, Urmanche AA, Muran JC. Techniques of individual supportive psychotherapy. In: Crisp H, Gabbard GO, eds. *The American Psychiatric Publishing Textbook of Psychotherapeutic Treatments in Psychiatry*. 2nd ed. American Psychiatric Publishing; 2022.
9. Kim TW, Samet JH, Cheng DM, Winter MR, Safran DG, Saitz R. Primary care quality and addiction severity: a prospective cohort study. *Health Serv Res*. 2007;42(2):755-772.
10. Miller WR. *Enhancing Motivation for Change in Substance Abuse Treatment*. Vol. 35. U.S. Department of Health and Human Services; 1999.
11. Miller WR, Page AC. Warm turkey: other routes to abstinence. *J Subst Abus Treat*. 1991;8:227-232.
12. Miller WR, Rollnick S. *Motivational Interviewing: Preparing People to Change Addictive Behavior*. Guilford Press; 1991.
13. Miller WR, Zweben A, DiClemente CC, et al. *Motivational Enhancement Therapy Manual*. National Institute on Drug Abuse; 1994.
14. Prochaska JO, DiClemente CC, Norcross JC. In search of how people change: applications to addictive behaviors. *Am Psychol*. 1992;47:1102-1114.
15. Rogers CR. *Client-Centered Therapy*. Houghton-Mifflin; 1951.
16. Pettinati HM, Volpicelli JR, Pierce JD Jr, O'Brien CP. Improving naltrexone response: an intervention for medical practitioners to enhance medication compliance in alcohol dependent patients. *J Addict Dis*. 2000;19:71-83.
17. Pettinati HM, Monterosso J, Lipkin C, Volpicelli JR. Patient attitudes toward treatment predict attendance in clinical pharmacotherapy trials of alcohol and drug treatment. *Am J Addict*. 2003;12(4):324-335.
18. U.S. DHHS Center for Substance Abuse Treatment. *Enhancing Motivation for Change in Substance Abuse Treatment*. Treatment Improvement Protocol (TIP) Series, No. 35. Substance Abuse and Mental Health Services Administration; 1999. Accessed June 15, 2023. http://www.ncbi.nlm.nih.gov/books/NBK64967/
19. U.S. DHHS Center for Substance Abuse Treatment. *Substance Abuse Treatment for Persons with Co-Occurring Disorders*. Treatment Improvement Protocol (TIP) Series, No. 42. Substance Abuse and Mental Health Services Administration; 2005. Accessed June 15, 2023. http://www.ncbi.nlm.nih.gov/books/NBK64197/
20. Day E, Ison J, Strang J. Inpatient versus other settings for detoxification for opioid dependence. *Cochrane Database Syst Rev*. 2005;2:CD004580.
21. Mark TL, Vandivort-Warren R, Montejano LB. Factors affecting detoxification readmission: analysis of public sector data from three states. *J Subst Abus Treat*. 2006;31(4):439-445.
22. Amato L, Minozzi S, Davoli M, Vecchi S, Ferri MM, Mayet S. Psychosocial and pharmacological treatments versus pharmacological treatments for opioid detoxification. *Cochrane Database Syst Rev*. 2008;3:CD005031.
23. Iguchi MY, Stitzer ML. Predictors of opiate drug abuse during a 90-day methadone detoxification. *Am J Drug Alcohol Abuse*. 1991;17(3):279-294.
24. Sees KL, Delucchi KL, Masson C, et al. Methadone maintenance vs 180-day psychosocially enriched detoxification for treatment of opioid dependence: a randomized controlled trial. *JAMA*. 2000;283(10):1303-1310.

25. McCaul ME, Stitzer ML, Bigelow GE, Liebson IA. Contingency management interventions: effects on treatment outcome during methadone detoxification. *J Appl Behav Anal.* 1984;17(1):35-43.
26. Soyka M, Horak M. Outpatient alcohol detoxification: implementation efficacy and outcome effectiveness of a model project. *Eur Addict Res.* 2004;10(4):180-187.
27. McLellan AT, Lewis DC, O'Brien CP, Kleber HD. Drug dependence, a chronic medical illness: implications for treatment, insurance, and outcomes evaluation. *JAMA.* 2000;284(13):1689-1695.
28. Volpicelli JR, Rhines KC, Rhines JS, Volpicelli LA, Alterman AI, O'Brien CP. Naltrexone and alcohol dependence. Role of subject compliance. *Arch Gen Psychiatry.* 1997;54(8):737-742.
29. Fuller RK, Branchey L, Brightwell DR, et al. Disulfiram treatment of alcoholism: a Veterans Administration cooperative study. *JAMA.* 1986;256:1449-1455.
30. O'Malley SS, Carroll KM. Psychotherapeutic considerations in pharmacological trials. *Alcohol Clin Exp Res.* 1996;20(S7):17A-22A.
31. Selby MJ, Azrin RL. Neuropsychological functioning in drug abusers. *Drug Alcohol Depend.* 1998;50(1):39-45.
32. Rohsenow DJ, Colby SM, Monti PM, et al. Predictors of compliance with naltrexone among alcoholics. *Alcohol Clin Exp Res.* 2000;24(10):1542-1549.
33. Haynes RB, Ackloo E, Sahota N, McDonald HP, Yao X. Interventions for enhancing medication adherence. *Cochrane Database Syst Rev.* 2008;2:CD000011. doi:10.1002/14651858.CD000011.pub3
34. McDonald HP, Garg AX, Haynes RB. Interventions to enhance patient adherence to medication prescriptions: scientific review. *JAMA.* 2002;288(22):2868-2879. Review. Erratum in: *JAMA* 2003; 25;289(24):3242.
35. Reid SC, Teesson M, Sannibale C, Matsuda M, Haber PS. The efficacy of compliance therapy in pharmacotherapy for alcohol dependence: a randomized controlled trial. *J Stud Alcohol.* 2005;66(6):833-841.
36. Galanter M, Dermatis H, Glickman L, et al. Network therapy: decreased secondary opioid use during buprenorphine maintenance. *J Subst Abus Treat.* 2004;26:313-318.
37. Preston KL, Silverman K, Umbricht A, DeJesus A, Montoya ID, Schuster CR. Improvement in naltrexone treatment compliance with contingency management. *Drug Alcohol Depend.* 1999;54:127-135.
38. Rothenberg JL, Sullivan MA, Church SH, et al. Behavioral naltrexone therapy: an integrated treatment for opiate dependence. *J Subst Abus Treat.* 2002;23(4):351-360.
39. Nunes EV, Rothenberg JL, Sullivan MA, Carpenter KM, Kleber HD. Behavioral therapy to augment oral naltrexone for opioid dependence: a ceiling on effectiveness? *Am J Drug Alcohol Abuse.* 2006;32(4): 503-517.
40. Pettinati HM, Volpicelli JR, Kranzler HR, Luck G, Rukstalis MR, Cnaan A. Sertraline treatment for alcohol dependence: interactive effects of medication and alcoholic subtype. *Alcohol Clin Exp Res.* 2000;24(7):1041-1049.
41. Fiellin DA, Reid MC, O'Connor PG. New therapies for alcohol problems: application to primary care. *Am J Med.* 2000;108(3):227-237.
42. Burke BL, Arkowitz H, Menchola M. The efficacy of motivational interviewing: a meta-analysis of controlled clinical trials. *J Consult Clin Psychol.* 2003;71(5):843-861.
43. Rubak S, Sandbæk A, Lauritzen T, Bo C. Motivational interviewing: a systematic review and meta-analysis. *Br J Gen Pract.* 2005; 55(513):305-312.
44. Vasilaki EI, Hosier SG, Cox WM. The efficacy of motivational interviewing as a brief intervention for excessive drinking: a meta-analytic review. *Alcohol Alcohol.* 2006;41(3):328-335.
45. Apodaca TR, Miller WR. A meta-analysis of the effectiveness of bibliotherapy for alcohol problems. *J Clin Psychol.* 2003;59(3):289-304.
46. Nowinski J, Baker S, Carroll K. *Twelve-Step Facilitation Therapy Manual: A Clinical Research Guide for Therapists Treating Individuals with Alcohol Abuse and Dependence.* Project MATCH Monograph Series. Vol 1. DHHS Publication No. (ADM) 92-1893. National Institute on Alcohol Abuse and Alcoholism; 1992.
47. Project MATCH Research Group. Matching alcoholism treatments to client heterogeneity: treatment main effects and matching effects on drinking during treatment. *J Stud Alcohol.* 1998;59:631-639.
48. Pettinati HM, Weiss RD, Dundon W, et al. A structured approach to medical management: a psychosocial intervention to support pharmacotherapy in the treatment of alcohol dependence. *J Stud Alcohol Suppl.* 2005;15:170-178.
49. Pettinati HM, Weiss RD, Dundon W, et al. *Medical Management Treatment Manual: A Clinical Research Guide for Medically Trained Clinicians Providing Pharmacotherapy as Part of the Treatment for Alcohol Dependence.* COMBINE Monograph Series. Vol 2. DHHS Publication No. (NIH) 04-5289. NIAAA; 2004.
50. UKATT Research Team. UK alcohol treatment trial: client-treatment matching effects. *Addiction.* 2008;103(2):228-238.
51. Carroll KM, Kosten TR, Rounsaville BJ. Choosing a behavioral therapy platform for pharmacotherapy of substance users. *Drug Alcohol Depend.* 2004;75(2):123-134.
52. Poldrugo F. Integration of pharmacotherapies in the existing programs for the treatment of alcoholics: an international perspective. *J Addict Dis.* 1997;16(4):65-82.
53. Mattson ME, Litten RZ. Combining treatments for alcoholism: why and how? *J Stud Alcohol Suppl.* 2005;15:8-16; discussion 16-17.
54. Wu J, Witkiewitz K. Network support for drinking: an application of multiple groups growth mixture modeling to examine client-treatment matching. *J Stud Alcohol Drugs.* 2008;69(1):21-29.
55. Witkiewitz K, van der Maas HL, Hufford MR, Marlatt GA. Nonnormality and divergence in posttreatment alcohol use: reexamining the Project MATCH data "another way". *J Abnorm Psychol.* 2007;116(2):378-394.
56. Kadden R, Carroll KM, Donovan D, et al. *Cognitive-Behavioral Coping Skills Therapy Manual: A Clinical Research Guide for Therapists Treating Individuals with Alcohol Abuse and Dependence.* NIAAA Project MATCH Monograph Series. Vol 3. DHHS Pub. No. (ADM) 92-1895. National Institute on Alcohol Abuse and Alcoholism; 1992.
57. Karno MP, Longabaugh R. Less directiveness by therapists improves drinking outcomes of reactant clients in alcoholism treatment. *J Consult Clin Psychol.* 2005;73(2):262-267.
58. Bouza C, Angeles M, Muñoz A, Amate JM. Efficacy and safety of naltrexone and acamprosate in the treatment of alcohol dependence: a systematic review. *Addiction.* 2004;99:811-828.
59. Rosenthal RN. Current and future drug therapies for alcohol dependence. *J Clin Psychopharmacol.* 2006;26(Suppl 1):S20-S29.
60. Rösner S, Leucht S, Lehert P, Soyka M. Acamprosate supports abstinence, naltrexone prevents excessive drinking: evidence from a meta-analysis with unreported outcomes. *J Psychopharmacol.* 2008;22(1):11-23.
61. Srisurapanont M, Jarusuraisin N. Naltrexone for the treatment of alcoholism: a meta-analysis of randomized controlled trials. *Int J Neuropsychopharmacol.* 2005;8(2):267-280.
62. Myrick H, Anton RF, Li X, Henderson S, Randall PK, Voronin K. Effect of naltrexone and ondansetron on alcohol cue-induced activation of the ventral striatum in alcohol-dependent people. *Arch Gen Psychiatry.* 2008;65(4):466-475.
63. Balldin J, Berglund M, Borg S, et al. A 6-month controlled naltrexone study: combined effect with cognitive behavioral therapy in outpatient treatment of alcohol dependence. *Alcohol Clin Exp Res.* 2003;27(7):1142-1149.
64. Heinälä P, Alho H, Kiianmaa K, Lönnqvist J, Kuoppasalmi K, Sinclair JD. Targeted use of naltrexone without prior detoxification in the treatment of alcohol dependence: a factorial double-blind, placebo-controlled trial. *J Clin Psychopharmacol.* 2001;21(3):287-292.
65. O'Malley SS, Jaffe AJ, Chang G, Shottenfeld RS, Meyer RE, Rounsaville B. Naltrexone and coping skills therapy for alcohol dependence. A controlled study. *Arch Gen Psychiatry.* 1992;49(11):881-887.
66. Anton RF, Moak DH, Waid LR, Latham PK, Malcolm RJ, Dias JK. Naltrexone and cognitive behavioral therapy for the treatment of outpatient alcoholics: results of a placebo-controlled trial. *Am J Psychiatry.* 1999;156(11):1758-1764.

67. Anton RF, Moak DH, Latham P, et al. Naltrexone combined with either cognitive behavioral or motivational enhancement therapy for alcohol dependence. *J Clin Psychopharmacol*. 2005;25(4):349-357.
68. Stanton MD, Shadish WR. Outcome, attrition, and family-couple treatment for drug abuse: a meta-analysis and review of the controlled, comparative studies. *Psychol Bull*. 1997;122:170-191.
69. Azrin NH, Sisson RW, Meyers R, Godley M. Alcoholism treatment by disulfiram and community reinforcement therapy. *J Behav Ther Exp Psychiatry*. 1982;13(2):105-112.
70. Powers MB, Vedel E, Emmelkamp PM. Behavioral couples therapy (BCT) for alcohol and drug use disorders: a meta-analysis. *Clin Psychol Rev*. 2008;28(6):952-962.
71. O'Farrell TJ, Bayog RD. Antabuse contracts for married alcoholics and their spouses: a method to maintain antabuse ingestion and decrease conflict about drinking. *J Subst Abus Treat*. 1986;3(1):1-8.
72. Fals-Stewart W, O'Farrell TJ. Behavioral family counseling and naltrexone compliance for male opioid-dependent patients. *J Consult Clin Psychol*. 2003;71(3):432-442.
73. O'Farrell TJ, Choquette KA, Cutter HS, Brown ED, McCourt WF. Behavioral marital therapy with and without additional couples relapse prevention sessions for alcoholics and their wives. *J Stud Alcohol*. 1993;54(6):652-666.
74. Latt NC, Jurd S, Houseman J, Wutzke SE. Naltrexone in alcohol dependence: a randomised controlled trial of effectiveness in a standard clinical setting. *Med J Aust*. 2002;176(11):530-534.
75. O'Malley SS, Rounsaville BJ, Farren C, et al. Initial and maintenance naltrexone treatment for alcohol dependence using primary care vs specialty care: a nested sequence of 3 randomized trials. *Arch Intern Med*. 2003;163(14):1695-1704.
76. Poling J, Oliveto A, Petry N, et al. Six-month trial of bupropion with contingency management for cocaine dependence in a methadone-maintained population. *Arch Gen Psychiatry*. 2006;63(2):219-228.
77. Baker JR, Jatlow P, McCance-Katz EF. Disulfiram effects on responses to intravenous cocaine administration. *Drug Alcohol Depend*. 2007;87(2-3): 202-219.
78. McCance-Katz EF, Kosten TR, Jatlow P. Chronic disulfiram treatment effects on intranasal cocaine administration: initial results. *Biol Psychiatry*. 1998;43(7):540-543.
79. Carroll KM, Fenton LR, Ball SA, et al. Efficacy of disulfiram and cognitive behavior therapy in cocaine-dependent outpatients: a randomized placebo-controlled trial. *Arch Gen Psychiatry*. 2004;61(3):264-272.
80. Nunes EV, Levin FR. Treatment of depression in patients with alcohol or other drug dependence: a meta-analysis. *JAMA*. 2004;291(15):1887-1896.
81. Stein MD, Solomon DA, Herman DS, et al. Pharmacotherapy plus psychotherapy for treatment of depression in active injection drug users. *Arch Gen Psychiatry*. 2004;61(2):152-159.
82. Kranzler HR, Burleson JA, Brown J, Babor TF. Fluoxetine treatment seems to reduce the beneficial effects of cognitive-behavioral therapy in type B alcoholics. *Alcohol Clin Exp Res*. 1996;20(9):1534-1541.
83. Woody GE, Luborsky L, McLellan AT, et al. Psychotherapy for opiate addicts. *NIDA Res Monogr*. 1983;43:59-70.
84. McLellan AT, Luborsky L, Woody GE, O'Brien CP, Kron R. Are the "addiction-related" problems of substance abusers really related? *J Nerv Ment Dis*. 1981;169(4):232-239.
85. U.S. DHHS Center for Substance Abuse Treatment. *A National Review of State Alcohol and Drug Treatment Programs and Certification Standards for Substance Abuse Counselors and Prevention Professionals*. Substance Abuse and Mental Health Services Administration; 2005. http://www.hhs.gov/partnerships/resources/fbci_counselor_standards.pdf.
86. McElrath D. The Minnesota model. *J Psychoactive Drugs*. 1997; 29(2):141-144.
87. Deitch DA. The treatment of drug abuse in the therapeutic community: historical influences, current considerations, future outlook. *Drug Abuse in America: Problem in Perspective*. Vol. Vol IV Treatment and rehabilitation. National Commission on Marijuana and Drug Abuse; 1973: 158-175.
88. DeLeon G. The therapeutic community: toward a general theory and model. In: Tims FM, DeLeon G, Jainchill N, eds. *Therapeutic Community: Advances in Research and Application*. NIDA Research Monograph 144. National Institute on Drug Abuse; 1994.
89. DeLeon G. Residential therapeutic communities in the mainstream: diversity and issues. *J Psychoactive Drugs*. 1995;27:13-15.
90. DeLeon G. *The Therapeutic Community: Theory, Model, and Method*. Springer Publishing Company; 2000.
91. Washton AM, Zweben JE. *Treating Alcohol and Drug Problems in Psychotherapy Practice: Doing What Works*. 2nd ed. Guilford Press; 2022.
92. Rosenthal RN, Nunes EV, Le Fauve C. Implications of epidemiological data for identifying persons with substance use and other mental disorders. *Am J Addict*. 2012;21:97-103.
93. Gerstein DR, Harwood HJ. *Treating Drug Problems*. Vol. 1. National Academy Press; 1990.
94. Gerstein DR. Outcome research: drug abuse. In: Galanter M, Kleber HD, eds. *Textbook of Substance Abuse Treatment*. American Psychiatric Press; 1994:45-64.
95. Hubbard RL, Marsden ME, Rachal JV. *Drug Abuse Treatment: A National Study of Effectiveness*. University of North Carolina Press; 1989.
96. Simpson DD, Curry SJ, eds. *Drug Abuse Treatment Outcome Study*. Vol. 11. Educational Publishing Foundation; 1997.
97. McLellan AT, Metzger DS, Alterman AI, et al. Is addiction treatment "worth it?" Public health expectations, policy-based comparisons. In: Lewis D, ed. *The Macy Conference on Medical Education*. The Josiah Macy Foundation Press; 1995.
98. Center for Substance Abuse Treatment. *Managing Depressive Symptoms in Substance Abuse Clients during Early Recovery*. Treatment Improvement Protocol (TIP) Series, No. 48. Substance Abuse and Mental Health Services Administration; 2008. Accessed June 18, 2023. http://www.ncbi.nlm.nih.gov/books/NBK64057
99. Zweben JE. Recovery oriented psychotherapy: a model for addiction treatment. *Psychotherapy*. 1993;30(2):259-268.
100. Ducharme LJ, Knudsen HK, Roman PM. Trends in the adoption of medications for alcohol dependence. *J Clin Psychopharmacol*. 2006;26(Suppl 1):S13-S19.
101. Lagisetty P, Smith A, Antoku D, et al. A physician-pharmacist collaborative care model to prevent opioid misuse. *Am J Health Syst Pharm*. 2020;77(10):771-780. doi:10.1093/ajhp/zxaa060
102. Zweben JE, Smith DE. Considerations in using psychotropic medication with dual diagnosis patients in recovery. *J Psychoactive Drugs*. 1989;21(2):221-229.
103. Banys P. The clinical use of disulfiram (Antabuse): a review. *J Psychoactive Drugs*. 1988;20:243-261.
104. Johnson FR, Ozdemir S, Manjunath R, Hauber AB, Burch SP, Thompson TR. Factors that affect adherence to bipolar disorder treatments: a stated-preference approach. *Med Care*. 2007;45(6):545-552.
105. Watkins KE, Ober AJ, Lamp K, et al. Collaborative care for opioid and alcohol use disorders in primary care. The SUMMIT randomized clinical trial. *JAMA Intern Med*. 2017;177(10):1480-1488. doi:10.1001/jamainternmed.2017.3947

BIBLIOGRAPHY

Barth J, Critchley J, Bengel J. Psychosocial interventions for smoking cessation in patients with coronary heart disease. *Cochrane Database Syst Rev*. 2008;1:CD006886.

Burke BL, Arkowitz H, Menchola M. The efficacy of motivational interviewing: a meta-analysis of controlled clinical trials. *J Consult Clin Psychol*. 2003;71(5):843-861.

Carroll KM, Fenton LR, Ball SA, et al. Efficacy of disulfiram and cognitive behavior therapy in cocaine-dependent outpatients: a randomized placebo-controlled trial. *Arch Gen Psychiatry*. 2004;61(3):264-272.

Clark LT. Improving compliance and increasing control of hypertension: needs of special hypertensive populations. *Am Heart J*. 1991;121:664-669.

Fals-Stewart W, O'Farrell TJ, Birchler GR. Behavioral couples therapy for substance abuse: rationale, methods, and findings. *Sci Pract Perspect.* 2004;2(2):30-41.

Karno MP, Longabaugh R. Does matching matter? Examining matches and mismatches between patient attributes and therapy techniques in alcoholism treatment. *Addiction*. 2007;102(4):587-596.

Markowitz JC, Kocsis JH, Christos P, et al. Pilot study of interpersonal psychotherapy versus supportive psychotherapy for dysthymic patients with secondary alcohol abuse or dependence. *J Nerv Ment Dis.* 2008;196(6):468-474.

Miller R, Rollnick S. *Motivational Interviewing: Preparing People to Change Addictive Behavior*. Guilford Press; 1992.

Prochaska JJ, Delucchi K, Hall SM. A meta-analysis of smoking cessation interventions with individuals in substance abuse treatment or recovery. *J Consult Clin Psychol.* 2004;72(6):1144-1156.

Project MATCH Research Group. Matching alcoholism treatments to client heterogeneity: project MATCH posttreatment drinking outcomes. *J Stud Alcohol.* 1997;58:7-29.

Reid SC, Teesson M, Sannibale C, Matsuda M, Haber PS. The efficacy of compliance therapy in pharmacotherapy for alcohol dependence: a randomized controlled trial. *J Stud Alcohol.* 2005;66(6):833-841.

Robles E, Stitzer ML, Strain EC, Bigelow GE, Silverman K. Voucher-based reinforcement of opiate abstinence during methadone detoxification. *Drug Alcohol Depend.* 2002;65(2):179-189.

U.S. DHHS Center for Substance Abuse Treatment. *Enhancing Motivation for Change in Substance Abuse Treatment.* Treatment Improvement Protocol (TIP) Series, No. 35. Substance Abuse and Mental Health Services Administration; 1999. Accessed June 18, 2023. http://www.ncbi.nlm.nih.gov/books/NBK64967

U.S. DHHS Center for Substance Abuse Treatment. *Substance Abuse Treatment for Persons With Co-Occurring Disorders.* Treatment Improvement Protocol (TIP) Series, No. 42. Substance Abuse and Mental Health Services Administration; 2005. Accessed June 18, 2023. http://www.ncbi.nlm.nih.gov/books/NBK64197

SECTION

10

Mutual Help: Twelve Step and Other Programs in Addiction Recovery

Associate Editor: Richard N. Rosenthal
Lead Section Editor: Richard K. Ries

CHAPTER

84 Twelve-Step and Other Programs in Addiction Recovery

Edgar P. Nace

CHAPTER OUTLINE

- Introduction
- Alcoholics anonymous
- Other 12-step programs
- Other non–12-step recovery groups
- The effects of the COVID-19 pandemic
- Clinician facilitation of 12-step participation
- Outcome studies
- Why are 12-step programs effective?
- Conclusion

INTRODUCTION

This chapter describes the structure and usefulness of 12-step programs and other programs. Emphasis is placed on Alcoholics Anonymous (AA) as it is the progenitor of all subsequent 12-step programs. The history of AA is described to express the complex and varied background to 12-step programs. AA is a fellowship of men and women who offer their hope, strength, and experience to anyone desiring to not drink. Meetings are held at various times throughout the day and evening. There are speaker meetings, step discussion meetings, women's meetings, and other formats. Participation is anonymous, there is no cost, and questions are not asked of newcomers. Participants are not told what to do but learn what worked for experienced members.

That 12-step programs have been beneficial to most of their participants as they attempt to overcome substance use disorders and that they have been lifesaving for some is well recognized. Empirical support exists for the effectiveness of 12-step programs, although controversy and divergent interpretations will be found (see Chapter 85). The continuing expansion of such programs and the endorsement of 12-step programs by medical and judicial systems lend further support to their credibility. In this chapter, the clinician is encouraged to learn about 12-step programs and urged to educate and encourage patients about this readily available therapeutic modality.

ALCOHOLICS ANONYMOUS

AA is an organization that has a single purpose: "to carry its message to the alcoholic who still suffers."[1] In 2021, AA membership was estimated to be 1,967,613 members with 120,455 registered groups.[2] AA does not engage in fund-raising or lobbying; it endorses no causes and does not promote itself. It is interested in the person having a problem with alcohol, not the "disease of alcoholism" per se or a formal diagnosis such as alcohol use disorder. AA will decline outside contributions and does not provide treatment or educational services. Personal anonymity is a guiding principle.

AA refers to itself as a "fellowship." A fellowship is a "mutual association of persons on equal and friendly terms; a mutual sharing, as of experience, activity, or interest."[3] There are no dues, but a collection is commonly taken at meetings to assure that AA remains self-supporting and not dependent on outside funds. There are no age or educational requirements. All are welcome based on a desire to stop drinking. Admitting that one is an "alcoholic" is not necessary, nor will AA attempt to proffer a diagnosis on an attendee. It is left to each participant to decide whether or not he or she is an "alcoholic." While the term "alcoholic" is commonly used and accepted among AA attendees, it is increasingly not a favored term to be used by clinicians as it is not "person first" language, and may be viewed by some as a potentially stigmatizing term. Instead, clinicians may consider alternative terms such as "person with alcohol use disorder" or "addiction" or "alcoholism."

The Program

To "work" the AA program means to study the 12 steps (**Table 84-1**) and to follow the directions contained within these steps. In addition, AA members and AA groups will respect and adhere to the 12 traditions (**Table 84-2**). The person with an alcohol use disorder (AUD) learns the steps and traditions and how to follow the same by attending AA meetings, reading AA literature, and working with a sponsor. Working the 12 steps and adhering to the 12 traditions lead to the possibilities listed in the 12 promises (**Table 84-3**).[4]

AA meetings may be "open" or "closed." Closed meetings are for those who consider themselves an "alcoholic" per AA (or as "a person with alcohol use disorder" as medical professionals would refer to them) or are questioning whether they might have this disease. Open meetings are for anyone interested in attending a meeting. For example, when medical students are required to attend an AA meeting as part of their training in psychiatry, they will be taken to an open meeting. If a person with AUD did not wish to be seen at an AA meeting except by other people with this disease, she/he would attend only closed meetings. A meeting is usually 1 hour in duration and may be followed by informal socializing. A "speakers" meeting will

TABLE 84-1 12 Steps

1. We admitted we were powerless over alcohol—that our lives had become unmanageable.
2. Came to believe that a power greater than ourselves could restore us to sanity.
3. Made a decision to turn our will and our lives over to the care of God as we understood Him.
4. Made a searching and fearless moral inventory of ourselves.
5. Admitted to God, to ourselves, and to another human being the exact nature of our wrongs.
6. We are entirely ready to have God remove all these defects of character.
7. Humbly asked Him to remove our shortcomings.
8. Made a list of all persons we had harmed and became willing to make amends to them all.
9. Made direct amends to such people wherever possible, except when to do so would injure them or others.
10. Continued to take personal inventory and when we were wrong promptly admitted it.
11. Sought through prayer and meditation to improve our conscious contact with God, as we understood Him, praying only for knowledge of His will for us and the power to carry that out.
12. Having had a spiritual awakening as the result of these steps, we tried to carry this message to alcoholics and to practice these principles in all our affairs.

TABLE 84-2 12 Traditions

1. Our common welfare should come first; personal recovery depends upon AA unity.
2. For our group purpose, there is but one ultimate authority—a loving God as He may express Himself in our group conscience. Our leaders are but trusted servants; they do not govern.
3. The only requirement for AA membership is a desire to stop drinking.
4. Each group should be autonomous except in matters affecting other groups or AA as a whole.
5. Each group has but one primary purpose—to carry its message to the alcoholic who still suffers.
6. An AA group ought never endorse, finance, or lend the AA name to any related facility or outside enterprise, lest problems of money, property, and prestige divert us from our primary purpose.
7. Every AA group ought to be fully self-supporting, declining outside contributions.
8. Alcoholics Anonymous should remain forever nonprofessional, but our service centers may employ special workers.
9. AA, as such, ought never be organized; but we may create service boards or committees directly responsible to those they serve.
10. Alcoholics Anonymous has no opinion on outside issues; hence, the AA name ought never be drawn into public controversy.
11. Our public relations policy is based on attraction rather than promotion; we need always maintain personal anonymity at the level of press, radio, and films.
12. Anonymity is the spiritual foundation of all our traditions, ever reminding us to place principles before personalities.

TABLE 84-3 12 Promises

1. We are going to know a new freedom and a new happiness.
2. We will not regret the past or wish to shut the door on it.
3. We will comprehend the word serenity.
4. We will know peace.
5. No matter how far down the scale we have gone, we will see how our experience can benefit others.
6. That feeling of uselessness and self-pity will disappear.
7. We will lose interest in selfish things and gain interest in our fellows.
8. Self-seeking will slip away.
9. Our whole attitude and outlook in life will change.
10. Fear of people and economic insecurity will leave us.
11. We will intuitively know how to handle situations that used to baffle us.
12. We will suddenly realize that God is doing for us what we could not do for ourselves.

consist of a member telling her story—emphasizing "what it was like" (the drinking experience), "what happened" (the process of recognizing the consequences of drinking and doing something about it), and "what it is like now" (how life has changed since beginning recovery from alcoholism). Step meetings will focus on one of the 12 steps in a discussion format. Discussion meetings are those where a topic is picked (eg, "gratitude") and the group shares thoughts and experiences of the same.

Each group is autonomous. A small collection is commonly taken, but groups are cautious not to let a till be built up as that can lead to conflict over how to use the money. Instead, the collection is spent on coffee, on purchases of the book *Alcoholics Anonymous*, or on other AA literature. Today, it is common for the leader of any group to initial a proof of an attendance form for an attendee who may be required to document his or her attendance for the court, for a professional organization, or for any other reason.

An issue that many groups may confront is whether to include persons who attend because of a substance use disorder (SUD) rather than an AUD. Some AA members and some groups will believe that those with a SUD (other than alcohol) would be better served in similar 12-step programs such as Narcotics Anonymous (NA) or Cocaine Anonymous (CA). If a new person arrives at an AA meeting and indicates that his or her problem is heroin or cocaine or pills, occasionally that person will be advised to attend other 12-step meetings such as those mentioned above. This can be awkward or embarrassing and occurs infrequently. Since clinical wisdom typically advises those with drug problems to avoid alcohol as well, the person who uses drugs can fit into AA based on his or her desire not to drink (even if alcohol was not the problem). Most new members will attend several different groups in order to find one where they feel most comfortable (a "home group"). It is not unusual to hear persons say as they struggle to get comfortable with AA that they hear the same thing over and over again, that one person talks too much, or that they cannot identify with those in the meeting ("I've never been in jail,"

"I'm better educated," etc.). With time, such individuals may see that they do have a common bond with those who are different from them in terms of life experiences as they recognize that they all share the struggle to not drink. A good attitude toward meetings was expressed by a recovering counselor with AUD who when asked "Hey, how was the meeting last night" would respond "It was great; I didn't drink the whole time I was there."

Most AA groups will have people who serve as the "group conscience." This is a committee of sorts that will address group problems should they occur. An example would be the member who took money from the collection basket for personal use. This action, noticed by another member, took the issue to those who comprise the group conscience. The member who took the money would be confronted and asked to make amends—that is, confess, apologize, and return the money to the group. This direct process usually proves to be satisfactory. The group conscience might also determine when and how to spend whatever monies have accrued.

Sponsorship

Sponsorship may be seen to derive from Steps 5 and 12 (see Table 81-1). A sponsor is an experienced AA member with sustained sobriety. How long should one be sober before serving as a sponsor? There is no fixed rule as to length of sobriety, but most AA members would expect at least 1 year of continuous sobriety and preferably 2 years. It is not expected that all AA members will eventually be a sponsor for another AA member. It is expected that those who sponsor other members remain committed to attending meetings, read AA literature, and be available to meet with those they sponsor. AA estimates that 82% of members are sponsored.[5] Sponsors are more likely to be older than those sponsored and are more likely to be married and/or be parents and be religious/spiritual compared to those who do not serve as sponsors. The details of one's substance use do not distinguish those who sponsor or those who seek sponsoring.[6]

New members to AA, as well as members who have relapsed or been without a sponsor for a prolonged period of time, are encouraged to ask for a sponsor. The sponsor offers a helping hand and serves as a mentor. He or she guides the person being sponsored in understanding the 12 steps and typically goes over each step with the person being sponsored. A very specific function of a sponsor is to have the member make "a searching and fearless moral inventory" of himself or herself (Step 4). The person being sponsored then admits "to God, to ourselves, and to another human being (the sponsor, usually) the exact nature of our wrongs" (Step 5). Sponsors often have their member do the steps over again or review specific steps or read selected passages from *Alcoholics Anonymous* (referred to informally as the "Big Book"). Some sponsors will ask to be called each day to review the day's activities. Other sponsors are less intense but most will meet their member at a meeting on a regular basis. The relationship is informal, and styles of sponsoring vary. An AA rule of thumb is to have a same-sex sponsor; however with increased attention to diversity, this issue is in flux. The neophyte to AA need not hesitate to ask someone to be a sponsor out of fear of being a burden, as those who sponsor feel that they benefit from the relationship—"you keep it (abstinence) by giving it away." Further, the new member need not look for the perfect person to be his or her sponsor nor be looking for the best friend he or she might find. Certainly, the member will want to ask a person to be a sponsor because the member respects how the prospective sponsor works the program and because he or she feels some general compatibility. Having a sponsor is a major part of working the program and has priority over the "personality" of the sponsor.

Predecessors to Alcoholics Anonymous

June 10, 1935, is the founding date of *Alcoholics Anonymous*. That date is the last day that Dr Bob Smith took a drink—a beer to steady his nerves before surgery. Dr Bob and Bill Wilson had met in Bob's hometown of Akron, Ohio, in May 1935, and became the cofounders of AA.[7] Their unplanned yet fateful meeting would spur the formation of the most successful self-help movement known. However, for at least the 100 years prior to the founding of AA, various grassroots efforts had emerged to address the disease of alcoholism. Their brilliant yet brief efforts failed and are historically obscure. Nevertheless, as we shall see, these efforts laid a foundation upon which AA would grow.

Nearly 100 years before the founding of AA, the Washingtonian Total Abstinence Society was formed in 1840 in Baltimore, Maryland. Six men, members of a drinking club, decided after hearing a lecture on temperance to quit the club and form the Washingtonian society. They initially held private meetings, met nightly because they had been drinking nightly, and invited local people with alcoholism to attend. Later, they held public meetings as interest in their society was growing, assessed dues, and formed committees to recruit others struggling with alcohol.[8] In 1841, a branch for women was formed—the Martha Washington Society.[9] The Washingtonians grew rapidly but did not develop a central organization, became divided over the issue of alcohol prohibition, and began to fade away by the end of the decade. AA is similar in that mutual self-help, personal shared commitment, and a religious/spiritual foundation are utilized. AA has wisely avoided political concerns (eg, the prohibition issue) and, unlike the Washingtonians, does not rely on charismatic speakers to carry the message, nor does AA assess dues.

Following on the heels of the Washingtonians was the Independent Order of Good Templars, founded in 1851. A pledge of abstinence was required, and expulsion could be expected if the pledge was not kept. Many other fraternal temperance societies and reform clubs formed during the 19th century and emphasized anonymity; a principle later adopted by AA.

Early in the 20th century, numerous mutual aid societies to help people with AUD flourished at least for a while. They included, for example, the United Order of Ex-Boozers, the Keeley Leagues, the Emmanuel Clinic, and the Oxford Group.[7] The Oxford Group, also now out of existence, was a direct predecessor of *Alcoholics Anonymous*. The Oxford Group considered spiritual growth as the solution to many of mankind's problems. "Four absolutes"—absolute honesty, absolute purity, absolute unselfishness, and absolute love—were necessary as well as the "five Cs," confidence, confession, conviction, conversion, and continuance, for spiritual change to occur.

Founded in the early 1900s, the Oxford Group strove to recapture the fervor of 1st-century Christianity. The group was not founded to specifically help people with AUD, but under the leadership of Episcopal priest Reverend Sam Shoemaker, it became active with such people in New York City.[7] Shoemaker's church, Calvary Episcopal, was the headquarters of the Oxford Group in New York City where a seminal figure in the early days of AA found a spiritual home. This figure was Roland H. who was from a wealthy Connecticut family and had suffered from a chronic alcohol use disorder and who had exhausted his family's financial resources. Roland H. went to Zurich for analysis with Carl Jung and subsequently returned to New York confident that he had been cured. He promptly was intoxicated again, returned to Jung, and was told that psychiatry and medicine could do nothing for him, but there was hope, however uncertain, of a spiritual experience that might release him from drink. While visiting with Jung, Roland H. joined the Oxford Group, which was very active in Europe. Apparently, he had a conversion experience, returned to New York, and began to share his experience with others with AUD.[10] Using his experience with the Oxford Group, Roland H. encountered an old friend, Edwin Thatcher (a.k.a. Ebby), who in 1934 was about to be committed to a state institution. Ebby responded to Roland H.'s outreach and attended Oxford Group activities. This led to a period of sobriety for Ebby, which was accompanied by friendship from the Oxford Group.

It must be apparent now to anyone familiar with AA that a nascent process of one person with AUD reaching out to another was in effect. Ebby had a friend, the hopeless Bill Wilson who had AUD. Kurtz[10] describes Ebby's outreach to Bill wherein they sat at Bill's kitchen table in Brooklyn as Ebby describes that he is not "on the wagon" but that he has religion and is a changed person. Bill, drinking, offers Ebby the same but is turned down. Ebby explained to Bill the impact of the Oxford Group, its origins on the Princeton campus, and its spread to Oxford and beyond. Bill was apparently embarrassed, if not feeling betrayed, by his friend's display of religion and the resulting change. Thomsen[11] reports that Bill had heard of the group but considered them too zealous for Christ, too rich, and too social. According to Thomsen, Ebby sensed Bill's discomfort with talk of God and began to use the term "another power" or "higher power."[11(p209)] This watering down of religious terms may have influenced current language of AA, which uses the phrase "higher power" in addition to referencing God.

The Birth of Alcoholics Anonymous

Bill Wilson continued drinking, and Ebby continued to visit and brought other Oxford Group members with him. Bill finally went to an Oxford Group meeting, was intoxicated, and spoke but does not remember what he said.[11] Bill, fearing brain damage, checked himself into Towns Hospital where he had been detoxified several times in the past. William D. Silkworth was a neurologist who took care of Bill and who had a reputation for helping people with AUD—an estimated 50,000 over the course of his medical career. During this hospital stay, Bill was depressed and resistant to the notion of a "higher power." Bill described that during that stay in Towns Hospital, he had cried out in despair, experienced the room lit up with a white light, and felt ecstatic. He asked Dr Silkworth if this was the effect of brain damage, and Silkworth reassured him that it was not.[10] Bill then returned to the Oxford meetings sober and with his wife. Encouraged by Reverend Mr Shoemaker and counseled by Dr Silkworth, Bill shared his drinking experiences with others with this same disease after the Oxford meetings and began to sense that one such person talking to another in a nonjudgmental manner was a tool or a dynamic that helped him stay alcohol-free. Over the next 6 months, Bill fervently told his story to other people with AUD. He stayed sober, but they did not.

Bill, discouraged, returned to his work as a stockbroker. A proxy fight took him to Akron, Ohio, in May 1935. The proxy fight was lost, and Bill found himself alone in Akron on a Saturday afternoon. He wanted to drink and headed toward the hotel bar but became very anxious over what he was about to do. Providentially, he went back to the lobby and called a minister, Reverend Walter Tunks, who was listed on the church directory. Tunks provided names of people Bill might talk to. He reached Henrietta Seiberling, a member of the local Oxford Group and who was the daughter-in-law of the president of Goodyear Tire. She, who did not have alcoholism herself, had been trying to help a local surgeon who was in her Oxford Group and invited Bill to her house the next day to meet Dr Bob Smith.

Dr Bob Smith had been through numerous treatments and was considered hopeless. He apparently looked poorly, and Bill planned that the meeting would be brief. Bill talked about his past broken promises and his failures related to his disease. He did not talk down to Dr Smith but reviewed his treatments and his visits from Ebby. Kurtz[10] described the conversation: "This stranger from New York didn't preach; he offered no 'you must's' or even 'let's us's.' He had simply told the dreary but fascinating facts about himself, about his own drinking."

Bill thanked Bob for hearing him out and knew now he (Bill) was not going to take a drink. Bob, while listening to Bill, would say "Yes, that's like me, that's just like me." Bill remained sober thereafter, but Bob went to a medical convention in Atlantic City and returned intoxicated to Akron. With Bill's help and the help of Dr Bob's wife, Bob acquired lasting sobriety on June 10, 1935. That date is considered the founding of *Alcoholics Anonymous.*

The Growth of Alcoholics Anonymous

The identity of AA gradually took shape beginning in the late 1930s. Initially, AA meetings were held within the structure of the Oxford Group. But the Oxford Group wanted publicity and AA did not. The Oxford Group was protestant and many coming to AA were Catholic. The Oxford Group was zealous about their beliefs, and AA wanted to accept all comers, believers or not. AA was able to form its own identity by 1939 when the book *Alcoholics Anonymous* was written by Bill Wilson.[11] The book—*Alcoholics Anonymous*—remains the "bible" of AA, and every member is encouraged to read it. Its reviews when first published were discouraging—"no scientific merit or interest."

There were about 100 members when AA officially adopted the name "Alcoholics Anonymous" in 1939. Articles in popular magazines such as the Saturday Evening Post helped with publicity, and growth began to rapidly take place. As sales and membership increased, AA wisely curbed dissension and conflict by committing itself "to corporate poverty, group authority rather than personal authority and leadership, and the lowest level of organization necessary to carry AA's message of recovery."[7]

When Dr Bob Smith, cofounder of AA, died in 1950, there were about 90,000 members. A 2014 survey by AA's General Service Office estimated nearly 2 million members and over 120,000 groups worldwide. This survey reported the average age of members was 50 years and members attended an average of 2.5 meetings a week. 57% of members report being referred to AA by a physician or a mental health practitioner and 58% received some form of treatment or counseling after starting AA. The average length of sobriety for those surveyed was 10 years.[5]

OTHER 12-STEP PROGRAMS

Narcotics Anonymous

NA is the second largest 12-step program focused on SUDs. NA grew out of AA in Los Angeles in the late 1940s and follows the format of AA with its 12 steps and 12 traditions. NA substituted the word "addiction" for alcohol, removing drug-specific references. NA is open to all people with SUDs without regard to the type of drug or combination of drugs.[12]

NA's basic text published in 1976, *Narcotics Anonymous*, describes the purpose of NA as follows:

"NA is a nonprofit fellowship or society of men and women for whom drugs had become a major problem. We … meet regularly to help each other stay clean. … We are not interested in what or how much you used … but only in what you want to do about your problem and how we can help."[13] The organization encompassed over 2,900 weekly meetings by the mid-1980s and has continued to grow.[12] As of May 2018, the organization reported nearly 70,000 weekly meetings in 144 countries. NA members are likely, on the average, to be younger than AA members. NA, in its 2018 survey, reports that 1% are under age 21, 14% are ages 21 to 30, 70% are aged 31 to 60, and 15% are over age 60.[14]

Cocaine Anonymous

CA began in Los Angeles in 1982. CA is adapted from the AA program and follows the 12-step model. It is open to all individuals who want to stop using cocaine as well as all other addictive substances. CA literature is available in French and Spanish as well as English. Its first book was published in 1996: *Hope, Faith, and Courage: Stories from the Fellowship of Cocaine Anonymous*. As of 1996, membership was estimated to be 30,000 members in 2,000 groups.[15] The 2018 Membership Survey indicates that almost half (49.7%) the members are ages 25 to 44 years old. 35.1% of members have completed some form of post-high school education.[16]

Marijuana Anonymous

Marijuana Anonymous (MA) was founded in June 1989 and is based on the 12-step program of Alcoholics Anonymous.[17] MA is for those who experience cannabis as controlling their lives. The organization's website states: "We lose interest in all else; our dreams go up in smoke. Ours is a progressive illness often leading us to addiction to other drugs, including alcohol. Our lives, our thinking, and our desires center around marijuana—scoring it, dealing it, and finding ways to stay high."[17] MA meetings are far fewer in number than the older 12-step programs but can be found in most urban areas and can be accessed online. The average age of MA attendees is 36 years and the average weekly attendance is three meetings per week according to a recent survey.[18] Before coming to MA, 61% of members receive some form of treatment or counseling related to their use of cannabis. Attitudes about cannabis use lean toward legalization in some circles, and "medical marijuana" (better termed "cannabis as medicine") is available in several states. The impact of legalization on rates of cannabis use disorder are addressed in several other chapters in this textbook. Potentially, MA could become more prominent in countering pathological use.

Nicotine Anonymous

Nicotine Anonymous (NicA), formerly Smokers Anonymous, was founded in the early 1980s and is modeled on AA. Nicotine Anonymous, as with other 12-step programs, emphasizes that the user is neither unique nor alone.[19] They emphasize the importance of sharing experiences and reaching out to sponsors, for example, their slogan—"to postpone it, phone it."[20] They welcome all those seeking freedom from nicotine use, regardless of form.

Gamblers Anonymous

Gambling disorder was included in the *Diagnostic and Statistical Manual of Mental Disorders*, 5th edition (DSM-5).[21] It is part of the "substance-related and addictive disorders" section as a "non-substance-related disorder." Decades before gambling disorder became an official diagnosis, those inflicted by "gambling addiction" found a way to organize their own "self-help" organization: Gamblers Anonymous. As with substance use disorders, a 12-step approach is seen as helpful to those with gambling addiction.

Gamblers Anonymous had its first meeting September 13, 1957, in Los Angeles, California. The prelude to this formal beginning was the experience of two men who had been meeting with each other since January of 1957, encouraging each other to avoid relapses. They used spiritual principles that they understood had helped others struggling with compulsive behaviors. These principles included honesty, humility, kindness, and generosity.[22]

Gamblers Anonymous follows a 12-step program nearly identical to that of Alcoholics Anonymous. The person who gambles compulsively is seen to be in the grip of a progressive illness where one bet is the same as one drink to a person with alcoholism—the start of a progressive destructive process. The only requirement for attendance is a desire to stop gambling. This starts with conceding fully that they are compulsive gamblers, out of control over betting, and in need of bringing about a change within themselves.[23]

Al-Anon and Alateen

Al-Anon is an international fellowship of friends or relatives of people with AUD who have been impacted by another's drinking. They share their experience, strength, and hope and follow their own 12-step format. Al-Anon is not family or group therapy and does not provide counseling in any formal sense. Alateen grew out of Al-Anon and is for teenagers ages 13 to 17 although the age range may vary by group. An Alateen meeting is sponsored by Al-Anon members; adults do not attend except for a few Al-Anon sponsors.

Al-Anon was founded in 1951 by Lois Wilson who was the wife of AA cofounder Bill Wilson. In "Lois's Story,"[24] Lois Wilson describes her own unhappiness even after her husband became sober. She realized that much of her life had been directed toward helping Bill get sober and that now she had to develop her own spiritual life.

Al-Anon meetings will focus not on the person with alcoholism but on their family member or friend who tolerates unhealthy alcohol use, or who indulges in excessive caretaking, and who may have developed low self-esteem because he or she thought he or she should be able to help the person with AUD stop or control alcohol use. Al-Anon members will learn that they did not cause the alcoholism and cannot cure it or control it but are affected by it and, therefore, need help for themselves.

Al-Anon members in the United States are mostly women. A 2021 survey by Al-Anon reported 90% of members were identified as white, 86% were female, and 48.9% joined Al-Anon due to a romantic partner's alcohol use. Eighty-two percent reported that their mental health was improved since attending Al-Anon.[25]

OTHER NON–12-STEP RECOVERY GROUPS

SMART Recovery

In 1985, Rational Recovery was founded; it was the forerunner to what is now Smart Recovery.[26] Rational Recovery's first meeting took place in a hospital in Cambridge, MA, in 1990. In 1994, the board of Rational Recovery Self Help, Inc voted to change the name to SMART Recovery (Self-Management And Recovery Training). A full chronology of SMART Recovery has been compiled by Shari Allwood and William White and can be downloaded from www.smartrecovery.org.

SMART Recovery offers tools and techniques to implement its four-point program, which involves: (1) building and maintaining motivation; (2) coping with urges; (3) managing thoughts, feelings, and behaviors; (4) living a balanced life.

Reliance on self-empowerment is emphasized, rather than commitment to a spiritual orientation, although each participant is encouraged to use what is found helpful. Online meetings, as well as face-to-face meetings, are available, and the organization states that it is committed to evolving as more scientific knowledge becomes available.

Women for Sobriety

Women for Sobriety, founded in 1976, is an abstinence-based program. Although physical recovery is claimed to be the same for both sexes, Women for Sobriety asserts that the psychological recovery is different for women. A 13-point program of affirmations is to be utilized daily in order to remove negative thinking and to develop a sense of self. The organization claims to have a worldwide presence and states that hundreds of meetings are held daily. Their website is www.womenforsobriety.org.[27]

Secular Organizations for Sobriety

A nonprofit group founded in 1985, Secular Organizations for Sobriety, is directed at those who wish to avoid a religious or spiritual approach to recovery, such as might be expected in traditional 12-step programs. Information on where to find meetings, products related to the organization, and meeting locations can be found on the website www.sossobriety.org.[28]

THE EFFECTS OF THE COVID-19 PANDEMIC

The COVID-19 pandemic led to 12-step meetings largely being conducted virtually rather than in traditional person to person settings. Many persons who attend 12-step meetings are likely more vulnerable to complications from COVID-19 due to histories of having a SUD and/or smoking tobacco.[29] Thus, the shift to virtual meetings, compatible with social distancing and stay-at home orders, made sense but raised the question as to whether the effectiveness or impact of 12-Step fellowships was compromised. The welcoming atmosphere, collegiality, and informal support wouldn't be as clearly experienced virtually.

Trepte et al.[30] studied "life satisfaction" with social support received offline and online. Social support received offline related to greater life satisfaction than support received online. However, focused online support forums addressing specific diseases have been found to increase well-being and life satisfaction.[31]

A study on the effectiveness of virtual meetings for 12-Step programs by Galanter et al.[32] yielded data on over 2,100 members of Narcotics Anonymous (NA). The participants reported attending more virtual meetings (average 4.13) in the past week than face to face pre-COVID meetings (average 3.35). 64.9% of participants considered virtual meetings to be as good or better than face-to-face meetings and 41.8% believed that virtual meetings were as good or better than face-to-face meetings for maintaining newcomers' abstinence. These findings are encouraging as virtual meetings were well-attended and the majority of participants endorsed their effectiveness.

CLINICIAN FACILITATION OF 12-STEP PARTICIPATION

Physicians and other clinicians would do well to inform patients of the existence, format, and benefits of participating in a 12-step or other self-help programs. This obligation is based on empirical evidence that AA participation (and by extension use of other 12-step programs) and engagement/commitment to AA are consistent predictors of positive outcomes for those patients.[33] Even attendance at AA (apart from "commitment") produces modest yet positive results.[34]

Should AA or other 12-step programs be recommended for only certain individuals? There is no basis to restrict recommendations to participate in 12-step programs based on individual demographics or characteristics. Strickler et al.[35] found that patients referred to self-help groups while in formal treatment programs are significantly more likely to attend after completing the program and that race, employment status, marital status, and education did not affect who followed through with 12-step participation.

However, some patients, for example, those with a social anxiety disorder, may find it difficult to engage in a 12-step setting although it should not be assumed that anxiety states preclude participation. The patient with a severe mood disorder or a psychotic disorder may not be able to participate until stabilization or remission is accomplished. Today, there are AA meetings for persons with an additional psychiatric disorder such as bipolar disorder, schizophrenia, etc. These groups are sensitive to "coexisting psychiatric disorder" concerns. AA does not diagnose or offer medical advice. Twelve-step programs are not "against" prescribed medications for members. This is true for maintenance medications including buprenorphine and methadone. The pamphlet "The AA Member–Medications & Other Drugs" (available from Alcoholics Anonymous World Services, Inc., 475 Riverside Drive, New York, NY 10115. Also https://www.aa.org/aa-member-medications-and-other-drugs) explains the AA position and emphasizes to AA members that they be honest with their physicians about their alcoholism and any use of drugs as well as how medications may be affecting them.[36]

Practical Information and Advice for Your Patients

1. Offer a brief explanation of 12-step programs. For example, they are a fellowship of men and women who offer their hope, strength, and experience to anyone desiring not to drink or do drugs. There is no cost, the meetings are at various times throughout the day or evening, participation is anonymous, questions are not asked of a newcomer, and there are different formats—for example, women's meetings, speaker meetings, step discussion meetings, and so forth.
2. After your patient has attended 12-step meetings, ask what they have heard, whether it has been helpful, and whether or not there are aspects of the program that they do not understand or agree with. Try to discern whether your treatment approach and advice to the patient are in synchrony with what they are learning in the 12-step program. If you find contradictions or conflict between your treatment approach and what the patient is reporting from AA, try to resolve and explain any possible differences. Occasionally, an AA member may advise that one not take certain medications. AA as an organization offers no opinion on medical matters, so it may be necessary to review with a patient the rationale for your course of treatment that an AA member (not AA itself) finds objectionable. Obviously, this requires tact and patience. It is important that the patient see that he/she can benefit from your medical input as well as what the 12-step program has to offer.

Countering Objections

The clinician encouraging a substance using patient to attend a 12-step program can expect to counter objections, reasons, or excuses as to why this recommendation is objectionable. Resistance to attending may be based on the following:

1. Fear of stigma. To attend confers an identity of having a "problem" and thereby the potential stigmatizing effect. That one may feel stigmatized or, in fact, be stigmatized by others is not uncommon. But the patient may be reassured that if others learn of his or her "problem" but see that it is being effectively addressed (as may occur through 12-step participation), the issue of stigma typically is replaced by respect for this positive change.

2. "I can't identify with them." A patient may go to a 12-step meeting and feel out of place not on the basis of the substance experience that brought him or her there but on the characteristics of the group itself. The usual recommendation is that a person try several different meetings and eventually find a "home group" where he or she is most comfortable on the basis of the people he or she has met or where the meeting is located. It is recognized that in some instances, a woman may be most comfortable in an all-female group and a professional more comfortable in groups with people of similar daily experiences.

OUTCOME STUDIES

Support for encouraging AA (and by extension other 12-step programs) is found in several large studies. Please also see Chapter 85 in this textbook. Project MATCH compared patients with AUD randomly assigned to cognitive-behavioral therapy (CBT), motivational treatment (MT), and 12-step facilitation (TSF). TSF is a professionally led group therapy, which points patients to 12-step participation. In the outpatient arm of this study, TSF patients had significantly higher rates of abstinence at 1- and 3-year follow-ups.[37,38] AA participation for those in the other treatment arms—CBT and MT—also predicted abstinence. A large Veterans Administration study found that at 1 year and at 18 months, those whose aftercare was only AA or another 12-step program had abstinence rates twice those who did not attend any 12-step program.[39] The rate of abstinence for the 12-step participants was approximately 45%, whereas for the nonparticipants, it was just under 25%. Further, the number of meetings attended functions in a dose-response relationship. Fifty or more meetings attended in months 9 to 12 in a 1-year follow-up resulted in higher rates of abstinence (about 60%) compared to 1 to 19 meetings (30%).[40] Addiction is well known to be a chronic illness that requires monitoring over time to assess outcomes. In that regard, AA attendance on a regular basis for at least 27 weeks in a given year has been found to yield to 70% abstinence by year 16 of follow-up.[41]

For those interested in detailed accounts of follow-up studies, see Ferri et al.[42]

WHY ARE 12-STEP PROGRAMS EFFECTIVE?

No one answer or variable is known to explain why any one individual benefits from 12-step participation. There are, however, several dynamics that may account for or explain, at least in part, why benefit ensues.

1. Group dynamics clearly are in effect in 12-step meetings. Elements of group process include hope, information, learning, catharsis, and universality.[43] Universality refers to feeling connected to others' experiences and the value for others of one's own experience. Catharsis follows from being allowed to speak without condemnation. Group cohesiveness, which includes a sense of belonging, predicts continued engagement and increased rates of abstinence for those who experience "cohesion" at meetings.[44]
2. Growth of the self: the self can be thought of as the collection of ideas we have about ourselves including our motivations, feelings, and ideas as they are expressed in and formed by relationship to others and by the choices we make.[45] The maturing or growth of the "self" is a potentially vital aspect of 12-step participation and possibly occurs by virtue of the following:
   a. Improved self-governance. Self-governance refers to the capacity to sense oneself as an autonomous being capable of taking charge of one's life yet in need, interdependently, of relationship with others. It differs from what are called the executive functions of the ego (planning, initiating, correcting, and completing behavior) as it acknowledges interdependence between self and others. A sharing of control with others is implied, which is particularly apt for the person with alcoholism who has lost control over alcohol consumption. Acceptance of supportive, caring interaction with others provides a counterbalance to the drive to drink through a "borrowing" of self-governance from the group.[46] As a result, self-care skills are improved as the individual internalizes from the group the values of impulse control, anticipation of consequences, and good judgment.
   b. Self-awareness. Persons with SUDs not infrequently have undeveloped skills in recognizing, regulating, or tolerating affect.[47] Fear of painful emotions or difficulty tolerating emotional pain is resolved by the immediate gratification of a drug. Further, some will have poor stress management skills and seek immediate gratification from substances. The 12 steps emphasize reflection (see Table 81-1), and the 12 promises (see Table 81-3) include "we will comprehend the word serenity" and "we will know peace." Thus, participants learn from the experiences of others that change is possible and are asked to take to heart AA slogans such as "easy does it," "one day at a time," and "live and let live."
   c. Self-deflation. Early students of alcoholism[48] recognized that defiance and grandiosity would stand in the way of accepting "powerlessness" over alcohol (or other drugs). An overvaluation on self-sufficiency and counter-dependent attitudes may form if one has experienced early empathic failures and thereby compensate by only relying on oneself.[49] Therefore, it may be a struggle to accept the "powerlessness" required in Step 1 and the turning of will and "our lives over to the care of God as we understood him" (see Table 81-1). Twelve-step programs counter narcissistic (self-sufficient) attitudes by emphasizing humility, service, and acceptance of vulnerability.[10] Acquisition of these attitudes may lead to fulfillment of the 12-step promise: "Self-seeking will slip away."[4]

3. Experiencing empathy. The person with a SUD is used to feeling ashamed or debased. How differently he or she is treated at a 12-step meeting: others understand what the person has been through and what struggles lie ahead; the person feels protected in this environment; his or her experience is valued not criticized as it might be useful to someone else; demands to change are not made, but one is encouraged to "keep coming back"; and the attraction of drugs or alcohol is openly acknowledged but linked with the understanding that "we couldn't handle it."[50]
4. Spirituality. 12-step programs emphasize spirituality rather than a specific religious creed. Reference to God occurs throughout the 12 steps and the 12 traditions, but an emphasis is put on each individual's understanding of "higher power." But how is spirituality manifested in the context of a 12-step program? Spirituality may be experienced as a release from the compulsion to use substances. This "release" may occur slowly or, in some instances, suddenly and is experienced as having been "given" rather than being achieved. From a decrease in the compulsion to use substances emerges a feeling of gratitude, which promotes thankfulness for what one has rather than what one does not have. Humility is part of spirituality and accompanies acceptance of being "powerless" over alcohol (or drugs). Further, a sense of forgiveness likely occurs and can be a powerful incentive for continuing constructive changes. Steps 5 to 10 imply a seeking of forgiveness as one honestly addresses behaviors connected to the addicted state or which have been embedded in one's character. Emmonds[51] has empirically demonstrated that goals that have religious significance promote personality integration and help to resolve the pernicious effects of mental conflict.

The above-proposed mechanisms as to why 12-step programs change persons' lives are, of course, incomplete. Many in AA or other 12-step programs would explain the benefits simply from their having "worked the steps." This may be as sufficient an explanation as we need and certainly is the most practical.

CONCLUSION

Understanding 12-step programs, as well as programs that are not 12-step based, will allow physicians as well as other clinicians to confidently recommend these programs to patients in need.

Referral requires no variables to be considered beyond the desire to be free from alcohol or drugs. No cost is incurred by the patient beyond the expenditure of time. Age, gender, ethnicity, education, or status will not limit the potential utility of active participation. Resistance to and objections about 12-step programs can be expected. A calm encouraging stance will usually overcome initial fears or concerns. Participation in a 12-step program does not conflict with or replace other clinical interventions such as medicine, psychotherapy, or commitment to a religious preference.

As careful consideration of the costs of medical care continues to grow, we welcome volunteer, supportive entities with demonstrated records of accomplishment and acceptance such as 12-step programs.

REFERENCES

1. Alcoholics Anonymous. *Twelve Steps and Twelve Traditions.* Alcoholics Anonymous World Services; 1978.
2. Alcoholics Anonymous. *Estimated Worldwide A.A. Individual and Group Membership.* Alcoholics World Services, Inc. Accessed June 6, 2022. https://www.aa.org/sites/default/files/literature/smf-132_Estimated_Membership_EN_1221.pdf
3. Webster N, Mckechnie JL. *Webster's New Twentieth Century Dictionary of the English Language, Unabridged: Based upon the Broad Foundations Laid down by Noah Webster.* 2nd ed. William Collins Publishers; 1980.
4. Alcoholics Anonymous. *Alcoholics Anonymous: The Story of How Many Thousands of Men and Women Have Recovered from Alcoholism.* 4th ed. Alcoholics Anonymous World Services; 2001.
5. Alcoholics Anonymous. *Alcoholics Anonymous 2014 Membership Survey.* Alcoholics Anonymous World Services, Inc. Accessed June 6, 2022. https://www.aa.org/sites/default/files/literature/assets/p-48_membershipsurvey.pdf
6. Young LB. Alcoholics Anonymous sponsorship: characteristics of sponsored and sponsoring members. *Alcohol Treat Q.* 2012;30(1):52-66. doi:10.1080/07347324.2012.635553
7. White WL. *Slaying the Dragon: The History of Addiction Treatment and Recovery in America.* Chestnut Health Systems/Lighthouse Institute; 1998.
8. Tyrrell IR. *Sobering Up: From Temperance to Prohibition in Antebellum America, 1800-1860.* Greenwood Press; 1979.
9. Maxwell MA. The Washingtonian movement. *Q J Stud Alcohol.* 1950;11(3):410-451. doi:10.15288/qjsa.1950.11.410
10. Kurtz E. *Not-God: A History of Alcoholics Anonymous.* Hazelden Educational Services; 1979.
11. Thomsen R. *Bill W.* Hamilton; 1975.
12. Narcotics Anonymous World Services, Inc. *Information about NA.* Narcotics Anonymous World Services, Inc; 2018. Accessed June 13, 2022. https://www.na.org/admin/include/spaw2/uploads/pdf/PR/2302_2018.pdf
13. Narcotics Anonymous. *NA White Booklet, Narcotics Anonymous.* Narcotics Anonymous World Services, Inc; 1976. Accessed June 13, 2022. https://na.org/admin/include/spaw2/uploads/pdf/litfiles/us_english/Booklet/NA%20White%20Booklet.pdf
14. Narcotics Anonymous. *Membership Survey.* Narcotics Anonymous World Services, Inc. Accessed June 6, 2023. https://www.na.org/admin/include/spaw2/uploads/pdf/pr/2301_MS_2018.pdf
15. Cocaine Anonymous. *Cocaine Anonymous Fact File.* Cocaine Anonymous World Services, Inc. Accessed November 21, 2013. http://ca.org
16. Cocaine Anonymous. Cocaine Anonymous Public Information Fact File. Cocaine Anonymous World Services, Inc. Accessed June 13, 2022. https://pi.ca.org/fact-file-survey
17. Marijuana Anonymous. *Why Marijuana Anonymous?* Marijuana Anonymous World Services, Inc. Accessed June 13, 2022. https://marijuana-anonymous.org/wp-content/uploads/p05-en-ltr_201711.pdf
18. Marijuana Anonymous. *Marijuana Anonymous 2021 Membership Survey.* Marijuana Anonymous World Services, Inc. Accessed June 13, 2022. https://marijuana-anonymous.org/wp-content/uploads/2021-MA-Member-Survey-final-without-crop-marks.pdf
19. Nicotine Anonymous. *Introducing Nicotine Anonymous.* Accessed June 13, 2022. https://www.nicotine-anonymous.org/introducing-nicotine-anonymous
20. Nicotine Anonymous. *Nicotine Anonymous Slogans To Help Us Be Happy, Joyous and Free Living Without Nicotine.* Accessed June 13, 2022. https://www.nicotine-anonymous.org/nicotine-anonymous-slogans-to-help-us-be-happy-joyous-and-free

21. American Psychiatric Association. *Diagnostic and Statistical Manual of Mental Disorders*. 5th ed. American Psychiatric Association; 2013.
22. Gamblers Anonymous. *History*. Accessed June 16, 2022. http://www.gamblersanonymous.org/ga/content/history
23. Gamblers Anonymous. *About Us*. Accessed June 16, 2022. http://www.gamblersanonymous.org/ga/content/about-us
24. Al-Anon Family Group. Lois's story. *How Al-Anon Works for Families and Friends of Alcoholics*. Al-Anon Family Groups; 1995.
25. Al-Anon Family Groups. *2021 Membership Survey Results*. Accessed June 6, 2022. https://al-anon.org/pdf/2021-MembershipSurvey.pdf
26. SMART Recovery. Accessed June 16, 2022. https://www.smartrecovery.org
27. Humphreys K, Kaskutas LA. World views of alcoholics anonymous, women for sobriety, and adult children of alcoholics/Al-Anon Mutual Help Groups. *Addict Res*. 1995;3(3):231-243. doi:10.3109/16066359509005240
28. Secular Organization for Sobriety. Accessed June 16, 2022. https://www.sossobriety.org
29. Volkow ND. Collision of the COVID-19 and Addiction Epidemics. *Ann Intern Med*. 2020;173(1): doi:10.7326/M20-1212
30. Trepte S, Dienlin T, Reinecke L. Influence of social support received in online and offline contexts on satisfaction with social support and satisfaction with life: a longitudinal study. *Media Psychol*. 2014;18(1): 74-105. doi:10.1080/15213269.2013.838904
31. Miller SM. The effect of frequency and type of internet use on perceived social support and sense of well-being in individuals with spinal cord injury. *Rehabil Counseling Bull*. 2008;51(3):148-158. doi:10.1177/0034355207311315
32. Galanter M, White WL, Hunter B. Virtual twelve step meeting attendance during the COVID-19 period: a study of members of narcotics anonymous. *J Addict Med*. 2022;16(2):e81-e86. doi:10.1097/ADM.0000000000000852
33. Weiss RD, Griffin ML, Gallop R, et al. Self-help group attendance and participation among cocaine dependent patients. *Drug Alcohol Depend*. 2000;60(2):169-177. doi:10.1016/s0376-8716(99)00154-4
34. Forcehimes AA, Tonigan JS. Self-efficacy as a factor in abstinence from alcohol/other drug abuse: a meta-analysis. *Alcohol Treat Q*. 2008;26(4):480-489. doi:10.1080/07347320802347145
35. Strickler GK, Reif S, Horgan CM, Acevedo A. The relationship between substance abuse performance measures and mutual-help group participation after treatment. *Alcohol Treat Q*. 2012;30(2):190-210. doi:10.1080/07347324.2012.663305
36. Alcoholics Anonymous. *The A.A. Member—Medications and Other Drugs*. Alcoholics Anonymous World Services. Accessed June 16, 2022. https://www.aa.org/aa-member-medications-and-other-drugs
37. Project MATCH Research Group. Matching alcoholism treatments to client heterogeneity: Project MATCH posttreatment drinking outcomes. *J Stud Alcohol*. 1997;58(1):7-29. doi:10.15288/jsa.1997.58.7
38. Project MATCH Research Group. Matching alcoholism treatments to client heterogeneity: Project MATCH Three-Year Drinking Outcomes. *Alcohol Clin Exp Res*. 1998;22(6):1300-1311. doi:10.1111/j.1530-0277.1998.tb03912.x
39. Kaskutas LA. Alcoholics Anonymous effectiveness: faith meets science. *J Addict Dis*. 2009;28(2):145-157. doi:10.1080/10550880902772464
40. Ouimette PC, Moos RH, Finney JW. Influence of outpatient treatment and 12-step group involvement on one-year substance abuse treatment outcomes. *J Stud Alcohol*. 1998;59(5):513-522. doi:10.15288/jsa.1998.59.513
41. Moos RH, Moos BS. Participation in treatment and Alcoholics Anonymous: a 16-year follow-up of initially untreated individuals. *J Clin Psychol*. 2006;62(6):735-750. doi:10.1002/jclp.20259
42. Ferri M, Amato L, Davoli M. Alcoholics Anonymous and other 12-step programs for alcohol dependence. *Cochrane Database Syst Rev*. 2006;(3):CD005032. doi:10.1002/14651858.cd005032.pub2
43. Yalom ID. *The Theory and Practice of Group Psychotherapy*. Basic Books; 1975.
44. Rice SL, Tonigan JS. Impressions of Alcoholics Anonymous (AA) group cohesion: a case for a nonspecific factor predicting later AA attendance. *Alcohol Treat Q*. 2012;30(1):40-51. doi:10.1080/07347324.2012.635550
45. Vitz PC, Felch SM. *The Self: Beyond the Postmodern Crisis*. Isi Books; 2006.
46. Mack J. Alcoholism, AA, the governance of self. In: Bean MH, Zinberg NE, eds. *Dynamic Approaches to the Understanding and Treatment of Alcoholism*. Free Press; 1981:128-162.
47. Khantzian EJ, Mack JE. Alcoholics anonymous and contemporary psychodynamic theory. In: Galanter M, ed. *Recent Developments in Alcoholism*. Plenum Press; 1989:67-89.
48. Tiebout HM. Surrender versus compliance in therapy; with special reference to alcoholism. *Q J Stud Alcohol*. 1953;14(1):58-68. doi:10.15288/qjsa.1953.14.058
49. Kohut H. *The Restoration of the Self*. The University Of Chicago Press; 1977.
50. Bean MH. Alcoholics Anonymous: AA. *Psychiatr Ann*. 1975;5(2):3-64.
51. Emmons RA. *The Psychology of Ultimate Concerns: Motivation and Spirituality in Personality*. Guilford Press; 1999.

CHAPTER

85 Recent Research Into Twelve-Step Programs

John F. Kelly

CHAPTER OUTLINE

- Introduction
- Utilization of AA
- Factors associated with successful affiliation with AA
- AA and population subgroups
- The effectiveness of AA and treatments based on AA
- Mechanisms of change in AA
- Future directions
- Conclusions

INTRODUCTION

The term, "Twelve-Step program," is a broad one encompassing several types of professionally delivered clinical interventions as well as the network of nonprofessional peer-led community-based addiction recovery support and relapse prevention efforts provided through in-person or online meetings and based on the 12-step principles and practices of Alcoholics Anonymous (AA). Professional 12-step programs include a variety of residential treatments that are based either entirely, or in part, on intensive immersion in the 12-step philosophy, principles, and practices emanating from AA in an attempt to foster ongoing community-based 12-step meeting participation postdischarge. Clinically delivered 12-step programming also operates through outpatient treatments ("Twelve-Step Facilitations [TSFs]") that aim to introduce, facilitate, and monitor, patients' community-based AA participation during outpatient care as a means of helping patients maintain and enhance treatment gains and prevent relapse after the professionally delivered outpatient treatment has ended.

Twelve-step philosophy and practices are based on the notion that alcohol and other drug (AOD) disorders are clinical conditions susceptible to relapse over the long-term.[1,2] Thus, 12-step programs implicitly advocate for continued, even life-long, involvement over time in 12-step fellowships to achieve long-term stable remission and enhanced quality of life as explicated in AA's "Twelve Promises."[1(p83)] Some advantages of AA and similar mutual-help organizations is their ease of accessibility in person and online—particularly at times of high-relapse risk when professional care is often unavailable (eg, evenings, weekends, holidays)—provision of flexible recovery support "on demand" between formal meetings (through phone/text) through the large social network of recovering peers; and its free nature (any monetary contributions are optional and voluntary).

Beginning in 1935, AA was designed to address severe alcohol addiction.[1,3] As other drug epidemics emerged during subsequent decades, similar fellowships based on AA's 12-step template emerged and grew, focusing on opioids (Narcotics Anonymous), cocaine (Cocaine Anonymous), cannabis (Marijuana Anonymous), and methamphetamine (Crystal Meth Anonymous). Perhaps through its longevity and the predominance of alcohol use disorder relative to other types of less prevalent substance use disorders (SUDs), AA has remained by far the largest of these 12-step organizations and has received the majority of scientific scrutiny from an empirical research standpoint.

AA remains the largest freely available addiction recovery support service for in the United States and globally. Worldwide, there are an estimated 123,000 groups and more than 2 million members.[4] The formal structure of AA is similar across nations, though there is some variability in emphasis on different parts of the AA program, and differences in the demography of membership are apparent, depending on the cultural context in which AA occurs.[5] Though most addiction professionals have some familiarity with AA and other mutual-help groups based on 12-step principles, professionals' scientific knowledge about AA often is more limited.

The past 30 years, in particular, have seen an explosion of research on AA and on treatments designed to facilitate involvement in AA. Despite earlier skepticism about the possibility of conducting research on AA,[6] researchers have used a range of methodologies, including randomized clinical trials (RCTs) and meta-analyses, rigorously conducted longitudinal studies of treatment-seeking and non–treatment-seeking populations, epidemiologic surveys, and smaller qualitative studies using ethnographic methodology. The more recent dramatic growth in this research followed from a request in 1990 from the Institute of Medicine (now National Academy of Medicine) of the National Academy of Sciences[7] for more research on AA and related professional 12-step treatments, and on understanding AA's mechanisms. Subsequently, a flurry of RCTs, quasi-experimental, and controlled prospective observational studies emerged funded by the U.S. National Institutes of Health (NIH) and the Department of Veterans Affairs (VA). These have produced a coherent and largely consistent set of findings supporting the clinical and public health utility of a variety of clinical and community-based 12-step programs, while also uncovering many of AA's mechanisms of action, and demonstrating strong potential for health care cost-benefits related to clinical linkage of addiction patients with AA.[8-10] This chapter reviews the research on AA addressing several major topics, including patterns of utilization of AA, the unique experiences and views of AA among specific population groups, the effectiveness of AA and treatments designed to facilitate AA involvement, and mechanisms of change associated with involvement with AA and other 12-step programs. The chapter concludes with methodologic comments and directions for future research.

UTILIZATION OF AA

AA members enter the program by a number of routes, including self-referral or referral by family or friends, referral from treatment centers, or through coercion from the legal system, employers, or the social welfare system.

Population Studies

Population surveys provide information on utilization of AA in the general and alcohol problem populations. Using data from the National Epidemiologic Survey on Alcohol and Related Conditions (NESARC), Dawson et al.[11] reported that AA attendance among respondents with a history of DSM-IV alcohol dependence was 20.1%. Additional analyses of NESARC data[12] found, among persons who had developed alcohol dependence at least a year before the survey, that 25.5% had sought treatment. Among those seeking assistance, 88.9% attended a community-based 12-step program (eg, AA), including 12.1% who attended only a 12-step program, and 66.7% who attended both formal treatment and a community-based 12-step program.

Help-Seeking Populations

A different perspective on the utilization of AA is provided by studies of patterns of help seeking among individuals seeking assistance for an alcohol problem. Dawson et al.,[12] also using NESARC data, reported that among individuals with DSM-IV alcohol dependence who sought help, 78.5% had used AA and other 12-step programs (11.7% using only AA, 66.8% using AA in combination with formal treatment), compared to 88.7% who used professional services (21.9% using only professional treatment, 66.8% using treatment in combination with AA). In a 16-year longitudinal study, Timko et al.[13] examined treatment utilization among individuals with alcohol use disorder who first contacted an information and referral center or who underwent alcohol withdrawal management. One year later, 75% had sought treatment: 18% had attended only AA or another mutual-help group (24% of help seekers), 25% had sought only outpatient treatment (33% of help seekers), and 32% had sought only inpatient/residential treatment (43% of help seekers). AA involvement was high among treatment seekers, with two-thirds of outpatients and inpatients also attending AA. By the time of an 8-year follow-up,[14] 17% still had sought no treatment and 14% had attended only AA. The majority (53%) participated in both formal treatment and AA. Study participants who attended AA (either AA alone or in conjunction with treatment) showed a pattern of remarkably steady and consistent involvement over time: 66 to 91 meetings in the first year, 68 to 97 meetings per year in the subsequent 2 years, 63 to 71 meetings per year in years 4 to 8, and 46 to 52 meetings per year in years 9 to 16.[15]

Mandated Populations

Though there has been considerable controversy about the current legal system practice of mandating individuals to attend AA, little research has examined the actual process of their referral to AA. Speiglman[16] selected four counties in California that varied in the degree to which they used presentencing screening strategies to deal with people who had repeatedly offended through the use of driving under the influence (DUI) statutes. Two of the four counties referred cases to AA, referring 37% to 40% of cases. People who had offended and were represented by private attorneys were more likely to be referred to AA than those who had public representation. However, among those also mandated to parole or to participation in probation-defined treatment, the vast majority (88% to 97%) were required to attend AA. Frequency of attendance also was specified and typically involved two to three required meetings per week. Mandating attendance at AA requires the cooperation of the AA groups that the person attends. Information at the AA website indicates that

> ...some groups, with the consent of the prospective member, have the AA group secretary sign or initial a slip that has been furnished by the court together with a self-addressed court envelope. The referred person supplies identification and mails the slip back to the court as proof of attendance. Other groups cooperate in different ways. There is no set procedure. The nature and extent of any group's involvement in this process [of verifying attendance] is entirely up to the individual group.[17]

Recent qualitative research[18] explored the views of mandated AA attendance among African American participants in a drug court program. Participants expressed negative opinions about the required frequency of attendance and that the culture of AA, which encourages public sharing, was incompatible with their cultural values about privacy.

Patterns of Utilization of AA

Both cross-sectional and longitudinal studies provide information about patterns of utilization of AA. Data from the Epidemiologic Catchment Area Study[19] suggest that individuals who attend AA or other mutual-help groups make about twice as many visits to meetings as to professional treatment. Persons with DSM-IV defined alcohol dependence who attend AA averaged 44.8 visits/person/year, or just under one meeting per week. Data from Timko and Moos' 16-year longitudinal study also showed variability in AA utilization. In the first year of help seeking, 24.9% attended AA for more than

26 weeks, 19.1% attended for 9 to 26 weeks, and 14.3% attended for only 1 to 8 weeks.[20] Regular attendance was remarkably stable over time—in years 4 to 8, 28% had attended AA for more than 26 weeks. However, infrequent attendance dropped off, with only 8.1% of the sample attending for fewer than 26 weeks.

Kaskutas et al.[21] reported on 7-year longitudinal patterns of AA attendance in a treatment-seeking population. The *low*-attendance group participated in AA during treatment but was attending fewer than five meetings at follow-up points. The *medium*-attendance group reported attending AA an average of once a week during follow-up. The *high*-attendance groups attended AA an average of four times per week during the first year and then gradually reduced their attendance. Kaskutas et al. also identified a *descending*-attendance group that had very high attendance initially but then had dropped off sharply in attendance. Abstinence rates were highest for the two groups still attending AA fairly regularly, were somewhat lower for the group that had declined in attendance, and were lowest for the group that discontinued attendance after the first year.[22] Two long-term studies of adolescents treated initially at roughly age 16 years old on average, and followed across 7 years[23] and 8 years[24] into young adulthood, found similarly high initial rates of participation during and post-treatment discharge that diminished steadily and quite rapidly over follow-up.

Mäkelä[25] studied anniversary announcements published in a Finnish AA newsletter to track AA membership over time. Over 3 consecutive years, he found that the probability of remaining sober and involved with AA was about 67% for those with 1 year of sobriety, 85% for those with 2 to 5 years of sobriety, and 90% for those with more than 5 years of sobriety.

Summary

Data derived from a number of different methodologies converge in suggesting clearly different patterns of involvement with AA—those who initially are actively involved but taper off over time, those with a steady level of involvement, and those who have a more variable or less engaged type of involvement. Data also suggest that consistent involvement is associated with better outcomes.

FACTORS ASSOCIATED WITH SUCCESSFUL AFFILIATION WITH AA

Despite the diversity of the membership of AA, research shows that certain factors are associated with more successful affiliation with AA. Research to identify characteristics of those more likely to affiliate with AA does not imply that individuals without those characteristics will not affiliate. Over time, a body of single studies has accrued about a wide range of characteristics found to be predictive of affiliation with AA, including male gender,[26] more serious alcohol problems,[14,27-29] greater commitment to abstinence,[29] more social support to stop drinking,[30] less support from and more stress in marriage/intimate relationships,[31] fewer psychological problems such as depression or poor self-esteem,[13] use of a more avoidant style for coping with problems,[31] and having a greater desire to find meaning in life.[32] Most findings, however, are supported by only one recent study, with the exception of greater severity of DSM-IV defined alcohol dependence[33,34] and greater commitment to abstinence, which have been found to be robust predictors of affiliation across multiple studies. Findings are contradictory for some variables, such as education, where affiliation is predicted by greater education among Whites but less education among Hispanic Americans, or marital status, where unmarried status predicts affiliation among Hispanics,[27] but being married generally is predictive of affiliation in population surveys.

The personal characteristic of spirituality, religiosity, or purpose in life has been examined in a series of studies. Professionals and the public alike believe that individuals who are more religious will be more successful in AA because of the intrinsically spiritual nature of the recovery program. An older survey found that program directors in Department of Veterans Affairs (VA) facilities were less likely to refer a patient to AA if the individual was an atheist.[35] Winzelberg and Humphreys[36] looked at the relationships among clinician referral to 12-step groups, client religiosity, group attendance, and client outcomes. They too found that professionals were less likely to refer patients to 12-step groups if the patients engaged in fewer religious behaviors. However, though more frequent religious behaviors predicted 12-step meeting attendance, clinician referral to such groups increased attendance regardless of religiosity. They also found that attendance at 12-step groups predicted better outcomes, regardless of religiousness. Tonigan et al.[37] examined religious beliefs and AA affiliation among patients in Project MATCH. They found that clients assigned to twelve-step facilitation (TSF) treatment were most likely to report increased belief in God, but clients who described themselves as atheists or agnostics generally were less likely to attend AA, even if assigned to TSF treatment, compared to clients who were spiritual or religious in their beliefs. Similar to Winzelberg and Humphreys, Tonigan et al. found that AA attendance was positively associated with outcomes regardless of religious beliefs. More recently, Krentzman et al.[34] examined baseline characteristics of individuals who had successfully maintained abstinence for a year or more during a 3-year follow-up period. Those abstinent individuals who considered themselves to be members of AA (compared to non-AA members) were more likely to have been raised in a religious tradition and to endorse a belief in God.

Co-occurrence of psychiatric disorders is another patient characteristic that could affect AA affiliation. In an early study, Tomasson and Vaglum[38] determined that the presence or absence of most co-occurring disorders was unrelated to AA attendance in an aftercare sample of people with alcohol use disorder, though the presence of co-occurring disorders was associated with higher rates of professional help seeking. Schizophrenia, however, was the one diagnosis associated with lower rates of attendance. In a more recent review of the literature on co-occurrence and AA involvement, Bogenschutz[39] also concluded that patients with co-occurring psychiatric disorders attended AA at about the same rate as other patients, though attendance was lower for those with psychotic disorder diagnoses.[40] He also noted the added benefit of 12-step programs that are specialized for those with co-occurring disorders (eg, Dual Recovery Anonymous; Double Trouble in Recovery) and that mechanisms of change associated with success in AA, such as enhanced self-efficacy and greater social support, are similar for those with and without co-occurring disorders. Tonigan and colleagues conducted a meta-analysis that included 22 studies and over 8,000 patients finding higher rates of AA participation among those with co-occurring psychiatric disorders, as well as superior outcomes for patients with co-occurring psychiatric disorders attending AA compared to those not attending. Moser et al.[41] examined AA attendance among individuals with social anxiety and found that higher social anxiety was associated with less AA involvement. In contrast, Timko and colleagues[42] in a 2-year follow-up study of AA participation among patients with a variety of co-occurring disorders, including social anxiety disorder, found that social anxiety had no effect on rates of participation and those with higher social anxiety benefitted more from AA participation than those without social anxiety disorder.

Summary

Data generally support the view of AA as a program that attracts a diverse membership. However, those with more severe alcohol problems and those with a greater commitment to change are more likely to affiliate. Patient religiosity affects clinicians' referrals to AA, and patients with agnostic and atheist beliefs may attend fewer meetings, but patients who go to AA increase their spirituality regardless of their initial beliefs. Patients with co-occurring psychiatric disorders also affiliate with AA at high rates, though those with a psychotic spectrum diagnosis are somewhat less likely to attend and may do better in 12-step "dual-diagnosis"-specific fellowships, such as Double Trouble in Recovery, where benefits have been shown.[43]

AA AND POPULATION SUBGROUPS

Two contrasting views of AA lead to different predictions about AA and different population subgroups. One perspective suggests that AA is a program of recovery for a person first and foremost with an alcohol use disorder and that this common experience should supersede any other type of individual demographic or clinical history difference. An alternative perspective is that, because AA was developed by educated, middle-aged, White, severely addicted men, its fit for less-educated, young or older persons, persons of color, women, or less severely addicted individuals is likely to vary. Reflecting AA's flexibility and freedom regarding how each AA meeting can operate[44] many "special interest" group meetings that cater to specific subpopulations (eg, women, gay men and lesbians, young people, and certain racial/ethnic groups) are common.[4] The growth and maintenance of these groups suggest such additional subgroups are useful as they attract and engage individuals having additional significant identity and life-context concerns that can affect recovery stability. AA's own triennial surveys have found an increase in the proportion of women in AA from about 22% in 1968 to about 38%, leveling off starting in 1989.[45] The average age of AA members responding to AA's triennial survey has increased to about 50 years of age,[45] and the triennial survey data as well as observation of AA meetings reveal a broad diversity among the membership in age and occupational status, but less racial/ethnic diversity.

Women

Several controlled and qualitative studies have examined women and AA. Recent studies in the United States[46] and Sweden[47] have found similar rates of AA attendance in men and women, and the 2014 AA triennial survey reports that about 38% of members responding to the survey were women, rates comparable to the rates of women with DSM-IV alcohol dependence in the general population. Likewise, no substantive gender difference was found in Twelve-Step Facilitation treatment compliance and engagement in Project MATCH,[48] despite the fact that it was believed that women might find TSF less appealing, perhaps because of its emphasis on "powerlessness" (although this emphasis only pertains to the drug itself not other societal aspects of disempowerment).

Women may have different reasons than men for affiliating with AA, however. For example, Kaskutas[49] studied women attending Women for Sobriety (WFS) meetings, approximately 25% of whom also attended AA. The women attended AA for reasons somewhat different from those for attending WFS: AA was cited as the program most crucial to their staying sober, though the fellowship, support, sharing, and spirituality in AA all were cited as important as well. The women perceived WFS as most valuable for the nurturing atmosphere, involvement with an all-women's program, and exposure to positive female role models.

In a comprehensive review of the scientific literature on women and AA, Ullman et al.[50] examined issues related to help seeking, affiliation, and outcomes for women in AA; potential moderators of women's affiliation with AA; and issues unique to women. They concluded that women may perceive more barriers to utilizing AA, particularly in terms of access, child care, and a sense of stigma about their alcohol use disorder, but that there was little evidence of gender differences in actual help seeking from or affiliation with AA. Women may use AA differently from men, as they attend more meetings but may be less likely to have a sponsor. Bodin[47] also found that women were more likely than men to call other AA members for help, to have experienced a spiritual awakening, and to have read AA literature; in other words to be more involved with the AA program.

Ullman et al.'s review[50] also found that AA attendance and affiliation generally are related to better outcomes among women; several studies suggest that AA is more related to positive outcomes in women than men, but some find no differences. Several individual variables may affect the likelihood that women will attend or affiliate with AA. For example, younger women are more likely to attend AA meetings; Black women are more likely to attend than Hispanic/Latinx women. Work on sexual minorities is very limited and does not lend itself to clear conclusions although qualitative studies suggest that lesbian women may view AA as heterosexist.

There also may be aspects of AA that make it less appealing to women. In Kaskutas'[49] research, she found that the women in the sample reported reasons why they did not attend AA, including a feeling that they did not fit in; a perception that AA is too punitive and focused on shame and guilt; disagreement with program principles related to powerlessness, surrender, and reliance on a higher power; and a perception that AA is male dominated. Another survey of 55 women attending AA[51] found that half the women had experienced "thirteenth stepping," in which they felt sexually targeted by men in the program. Such experience was less common among women who attended at least some women-only AA meetings.

Cultural, Racial, and Ethnic Subgroups

The most recent triennial survey[4] reported under-representation among the AA membership in all racial/ethnic categories, with membership including only 3% Hispanics, 4% Blacks, 1% Indigenous Americans, and 1% Asians. Research on involvement in AA by cultural, racial, and ethnic subgroups is limited. Older data reported by Caetano[27] from a national survey showed that, in general, Hispanics, African Americans, and Whites tended to endorse equally the basic tenets of the disease model. All groups held fairly positive views of AA (meaning that they would be more likely to recommend it than any other treatment modality). Some variability was noted in support for AA, with 97% of Hispanics, 94% of Whites, 87% of African Americans, and 76% of Asian Americans recommending AA as a resource. More recent research[52] utilizing data from three national alcohol surveys showed that Hispanics with lifetime DSM-IV alcohol dependence were less likely to have used AA than White samples (18% of males and 9.7% of females). Within the Hispanic sample, several factors were associated with lower utilization, including being female, older, Spanish speaking, and having fewer social pressures, legal consequences, or dependence symptoms Recently, a new group has been formed for Latinos, the 4th and 5th Step Group (Grupos de Cuarto y Quinto Paso, of CQ), which uses the AA 12-Steps and 12 Traditions, but focuses largely on steps 4 and 5. An ethnographic study[53] of CQ found notable adaptations from traditional AA meetings that are tailored to Latino culture and traditions. To date, efficacy studies of CQ have not been reported, but it may provide a culturally attractive alternative to traditional AA. Tonigan et al.[54] reported on a subsample of Project MATCH participants from Albuquerque, NM. They found that though Hispanics attended fewer AA meetings, they reported being equally or more committed to AA than Whites (as evidenced by working the steps, having or being a sponsor, and celebrating AA birthdays) and higher in "God consciousness." AA involvement predicted better drinking outcomes in both Hispanics and Whites.

Kaskutas et al.[55] examined previous self-help group participation among African American and White treatment seekers. African Americans more frequently reported prior Narcotics Anonymous (NA) or Cocaine Anonymous (CA) exposure, with a trend toward more previous AA exposure. Of those who had been exposed to AA in the past, more African Americans (76%) than Whites (55%) said they had gone to AA as a part of prior treatment, whereas more Whites had gone to AA through other referrals or on their own. Active participation was equivalent for both groups, as measured by mean AA affiliation scale scores. However, analysis of the individual items from the affiliation scale revealed differential types of participation. African Americans were more likely than Whites to identify themselves as AA members (64% versus 54%), to say they had a spiritual awakening through AA (38% versus 27%), and to have done service at an AA meeting recently (48% versus 37%). African Americans were less likely than Whites to have a sponsor currently (14% versus 23%) and less likely to have read AA literature recently (67% versus 77%). These patterns held true after controlling for prior treatment and exposure to AA during treatment. More recent research on AA utilization in a longitudinal sample[56] found that the association between AA attendance and abstinence was similar between Whites and Blacks but that this relationship was stronger for Whites than Blacks. Blacks with alcohol use disorders were more likely than Whites to be abstinent without AA, largely due to their higher levels of religiosity[57] and their "drier" social networks.

Research on AA affiliation and Indigenous American populations is very limited. In a study of help seeking among two Indigenous American reservation populations, Beals et al.[58] found that 38.9% of those with an alcohol or other drug (AOD) disorder had sought treatment; within this group, 39% had used a 12-step group. Several factors were correlated with 12-step use, including having an alcohol but not other drug problem, being from a Northern Plains rather than Southwest tribe, having a higher level of education, having a high level of spirituality, and having greater identification with White than Indigenous culture. Despite the substantial level of AA involvement reported by Beals, a small sample study of Indigenous American participants in Project MATCH had better outcomes with motivational enhancement therapy (MET) than TSF.[59]

Age-Specific Groups

There is some hesitancy about involving adolescents in AA because of their developmental status[60] and concern that adolescent SUD are, in some cases, age-limited phenomena. However, several studies have suggested a strong association between AA/NA involvement and abstinence in adolescents, similar to that found in adults. (These studies are reviewed in the section "The Effectiveness of AA and Treatments Based on AA.") Research to date has focused on adolescents in inpatient treatment programs, arguably the population with the most severe problems. Hohman and LeCroy[61] examined a sample of adolescents who had completed inpatient treatment and reported that about 44% had participated in AA. Kelly et al.[62] found that adolescents were more likely to attend if the AA groups they attended had more age peers. They also found[63] that the severity of the adolescent's alcohol use disorder was correlated positively with motivation to attend AA. Treatment providers view AA involvement as important for adolescents.[64] Adolescents themselves report positively on the group processes in AA such as the sense of universality of experience, received support, and the sense of hope that the program provided them. However, many adolescents report boredom or a sense that the program was not a good fit for them as reasons to discontinue attendance.[65]

Research has examined perceptions of AA in young adult populations (ie, 18- to 24-year olds). In systematic qualitative studies,[66,67] young adults reported that the sense of belonging, group cohesiveness, hope, and emotional support were important experiences for them in why they liked AA. Similar to adolescents, though, some young adults cited low interest as well as low motivation for recovery as reasons to discontinue use. Some young adults also had a negative view of the emphasis in AA on powerless and on a higher power.

Individuals With Co-occurring Psychiatric Disorders

Research on persons with SUDs and other co-occurring psychiatric disorders has been focused primarily on a comparison of the substance use, psychiatric, and other life outcomes of those with multiple diagnoses compared to those with SUDs alone. Recent research also supports understanding of those with co-occurring psychiatric disorders (CPD) in AA. As noted previously, utilization of AA and benefits appear to be similar among SUD-only and CPD diagnosed young adults.[68] In contrast, veterans with co-occurring depressive disorders appear to have more difficult in sustaining involvement in 12-step groups[69] and may benefit less.[70] In a comprehensive review of the literature on 12-step involvement among CPD patients, Aase et al.[71] found that participation in AA and other 12-step programs was associated with positive substance use outcomes for individuals with co-occurring psychiatric diagnoses, although results were more variable for measures of psychological functioning. In addition, they found that increases in self-efficacy and the social support received in 12-step groups that had a dual focus on recovery and psychiatric disorders mediated the relationship between group involvement and positive outcomes. They also found that 12-step attendance was particularly high for homeless individuals with CPD. In looking at specific aspects of involvement with AA, Polcin and Zemore[72] found that higher psychiatric severity was associated with lower levels of spirituality and less working the 12 steps or serving as a sponsor.

An important implication of the presence of co-occurring disorders is the need for prescription medications. The subject of medication use by AA members is a particularly important one, given that medications play a large role in mental health treatment, but there are thoughtful cautions raised in the core AA literature about the use of psychoactive drugs.[73] In an anonymous survey, Rychtarik et al.[74] assessed AA members' attitudes toward the use of medication, either to prevent relapse or to treat other disorders (medications included antidepressants, pain medications, anxiolytics, lithium, antipsychotics, naltrexone, and disulfiram). The majority (53%) of the sample thought that use of medications to prevent relapse was either a good idea or might be a good idea, 17% reported that they did not like the idea of medication and believed the individual should not take it, and 12% said they would recommend that another member discontinue medication use. About 29% said they had been encouraged to stop taking any type of medication, and an additional 20% had heard of others who had been encouraged to discontinue use. Of those who were encouraged to stop medication use, 31% actually stopped.

Swift et al.[75] predicted that persons with more prior AA exposure would be less likely to take naltrexone for DSM-IV defined alcohol dependence. They reported that in a treatment-seeking sample, willingness to take naltrexone was unrelated to frequency of past AA meetings attended, and, surprisingly, having an AA sponsor was positively related to willingness to take medications, albeit modestly. Studies of AA members' perceptions and practices support the counterintuitive idea that AA exposure has a negligible effect on the use of medications for an alcohol use disorder. Tonigan and Kelly,[76] for example, reported that AA affiliation was unrelated to attitudes about the use of medications for alcohol use disorder. It seems that though negative messages may be voiced by some members in AA about the use of medications, AA exposure in itself does not deter medication compliance.

Gay Men, Lesbian, and Bisexual Individuals

Research on the experience of gay men and lesbians in relation to AA is quite limited. One ethnographic study[77] recruited lesbians who had been in recovery for at least 1 year. All respondents were familiar with AA; 74% were actively involved. Hall identified three sources of tension for the lesbians in AA. First, they reported a tension between a sense of assimilation and a sense of differentiation. The women said they felt that AA was a program in which people of very different backgrounds could relate because of their common concerns, but at times, they viewed AA as a white, male, heterosexist organization. Second, they said they understood the value of the authority of AA as a prescription for sobriety but at times viewed AA more as a program that provided a set of tools for recovery. The perceived sexist older language in the AA literature[1,3,44] and the lack of focus on lesbian issues made following the program prescriptively a difficult task. Finally, the women said they experienced tension between the strongly individual focus of AA and their perception of the importance of examining issues in a cultural context.

Summary

It appears that individuals from minority groups (eg, women, gay men and lesbians, and racial/ethnic minorities) have a mixed experience in AA, seeing particular value in the support for sobriety but also having a different set of experiences with AA, some of which are somewhat negative. That said, there is much to be learned from research in these areas as the existing published studies are few and most consisted of secondary analyses on small samples.

THE EFFECTIVENESS OF AA AND TREATMENTS BASED ON AA

Answering the apparently simple question "Does AA work?" has historically been challenge but new and more rigorous evidence during the past 30 years has been able to shed light on this. That said, there are numerous levels and types of "evidence" beyond RCTs, that can be viewed in concert to assess whether the evidence base produces the evidentiary hallmarks of "consistency" and "coherence"[78] in addition to efficacy and effectiveness in determining whether a health intervention works.

One simple piece of observational evidence is to look at the success of AA as an organization. The broad dissemination of the program around the world and the large membership suggest that AA has been enormously successful in attracting persons to AA as a program of recovery for almost 100 years. The AA triennial surveys also point to the substantial proportion of abstaining, long-term members, as do Mäkelä's studies[25] of stability of sobriety in AA. More challenging questions, however, such as, "How effective is AA *in comparison* to other treatments for alcohol use disorder?" "Is AA involvement *necessary* to successful resolution of alcohol problems?" "Does AA *lead to* better outcomes or is it simply a correlate?" "What are the most effective strategies to *engage* individuals with AA?" Research to answer these questions has used several different methodologies: (1) randomized clinical trials (RCTs) comparing AA or treatments designed to clinically facilitate AA involvement to other types of alcohol treatment, (2) naturalistic studies of treatments designed to engage individuals with AA, (3) studies examining the unique contribution of AA to the prediction of outcomes in clinical and nonclinical samples, and (4) studies of effective approaches to engaging patients in AA. Review of these four lines of evidence provides some answers to questions about the relative effectiveness of AA.

Randomized Clinical Trials

RCTs in which persons are randomly assigned to different treatment conditions are considered the most rigorous experimental tests of therapeutic effectiveness because, when of sufficient size, can effectively rule out alternative explanations of cause and effect that might be attributable to other factors, such as differences in clinical severity or demographics, for example.

As noted previously, as a result of the request from the IOM[7] dozens of moderate to large RCTs of treatments based on 12-step principles have been reported over the past several years. These were recently summarized and reviewed systematically through the Cochrane Library of systematic reviews in a meta-analysis.[10]

The Cochrane review system is considered to be the "gold standard" for scientific transparency and rigor and is the database to which national governments and health care systems look in order to inform health care decisions. The review by Kelly and colleagues[10,79] included 27 clinical trial results reported across 36 published reports (ie, some trials reported on more than follow-up) and included one purely economic study and four other trials that examined economic health care cost savings analyses. The review included almost 11,000 broad-ranging, clinical patients (eg severe inpatients, less severe outpatients, patients with co-occurring psychiatric disorders, young adults, women, and veterans), from various settings (hospitals, community clinics, inpatient, outpatient, residential and withdrawal management), treated by numerous types of clinicians (counselors, psychiatrists, psychologists, peers, and social workers) from various geographic locations (from all across the United States and internationally). All major international databases were searched and any published study in any language that reported any type of clinical or quality of life outcome was included in the review provided it compared to some kind of AA/TSF type treatment to another type of active psychosocial treatment for alcohol use disorder and was longitudinal. Patients with co-occurring psychiatric disorders or other co-occurring SUDs were included. Outcomes were reported through 3 years following receipt of the initial AA/TSF or other types of clinical intervention (most often CBTs). Findings from the review revealed that patients receiving an AA/TSF therapy or linkage intervention performed at least as well on every reported outcome (ie, addiction severity, drinks per drinking day/percent days heavy drinking, alcohol consequences, percent days abstinent, longest average period of abstinence) as other clinical interventions (eg, CBTs, METs) and was substantially better at helping patients achieve continuous abstinence and remission.[10] In fact, patients assigned to receive an AA/TSF intervention had, on average, 20% to 60% higher rates of continuous abstinence relative to other clinical treatments in the most rigorous, manual guided clinical RCTs. Also, economic analyses found that patients receiving AA/TSF interventions also had much lower health care utilization while being simultaneously able to achieve these higher rates of continuous abstinence and remission resulting in a $10,000 lower health care cost (in 2018 US dollars) over a 2-year period than patients receiving CBT treatments.[10] As noted in the review findings, these findings should be viewed as conservative estimates of the potential clinical and public health value of AA/TSF interventions given that that the other treatment conditions to which patients were randomly assigned could not completely prevent patients in those conditions (eg, CBT) who elected to attend AA from attending, and many did elect to attend. Also of note, was that when included studies had conducted the extra analytic step to test why the AA/TSF intervention produced better outcomes than comparison treatment conditions[80-82] it was found that it was because patients in the AA/TSF condition were more involved in AA posttreatment, thereby enhancing outcomes.[10]

Thus, when high-quality RCTs are aggregated quantitatively and examined systematically in meta-analyses, AA/TSF is shown to be helpful—particularly so if continuous abstinence and remission are the therapeutic goals—and it also reduces health care costs. Some of the studies included in the review are described below in a little more detail.

One of the most prominent and visible RCTs included in the Cochrane review mentioned above was Project MATCH.[32,83-85] This RCT was designed to study the interactions between specific patient characteristics (eg, gender, severity of alcohol addiction) and one of three structured 12-week outpatient individually delivered treatments: Twelve-Step Facilitation (TSF), Motivational Enhancement Therapy (MET), or cognitive-behavioral therapy (CBT). Participants were 1,726 persons with diagnosed DSM-IV alcohol abuse or dependence (952 outpatients and 774 "aftercare" patients—who had undergone withdrawal management and an inpatient stay prior to enrollment in the outpatient trial and thus were more clinically severe) who were recruited from among 4,481 patients screened at 9 participating clinical research units in the United States. Participants were assessed thoroughly and then randomly assigned to one of the three treatments. Clinicians were nested within treatments, received extensive training prior to the study, and were carefully supervised throughout. Consequently, clinical competence and adherence was uniformly high reflecting high treatment fidelity and quality.

Treatment was delivered over a 3-month period. Individuals assigned to TSF or CBT could receive up to 12 manual-guided treatment sessions, whereas MET participants received up to four treatment sessions over the same 12-week period. All participants were followed up for 15 months from baseline, with research contacts scheduled every 3 months. Participants in the outpatient arm of the study were contacted again 39 months after the initial baseline evaluation, and their functioning during the preceding 3 months was assessed. Though Project MATCH was not designed specifically to study the main effects of the three study treatments, some treatment main effects did emerge.

During treatment,[84] patients in the outpatient arm of the study were much more likely to maintain abstinence or moderate drinking if they received CBT or TSF rather than MET (41% versus 28%). One year after treatment, patients in the three treatments had roughly comparable outcomes in the percentage of days that they were abstinent and the mean number of drinks consumed per day.[32] Two variables favored the TSF treatment: patients who were randomly assigned to the TSF treatment condition were up to 60% more likely to have maintained continuous abstinence and were less likely to have returned to heavy drinking after treatment. At the 3-year follow-up of the outpatient arm of the study, few significant differences among the three treatment conditions were noted, but, as at the 1-year follow-up, patients assigned to the TSF treatment condition were substantially more likely to have been abstinent during the 3 months prior to the 3-year follow-up. Also, compared to patients who had participated in CBT, TSF subjects had a significantly greater percentage of abstinent days during the preceding 3 months.[85]

Several significant client-treatment matching effects were found. During treatment, no client-treatment match affected drinking.[84] However, during the first year after treatment, patients who had low levels of psychiatric symptoms had more days of abstinence if they had received the TSF rather than the CBT treatment[32] (patients with high psychiatric symptoms showed no difference between TSF and CBT). Aftercare patients with higher levels of alcohol dependence also had better outcomes with TSF. In contrast, patients who were low in DSM-IV alcohol dependence had better outcomes with CBT.[85] A second important matching finding emerged at 3 years: Outpatients (n = 774) whose social networks were highly supportive of alcohol use at treatment intake had much better outcomes if they received TSF rather than MET treatment.[82]

Litt et al.[86] tested an individually delivered AA/TSF-based network support intervention designed to help patients with DSM-IV defined alcohol dependence change their social network to be supportive of abstinence. Two years after treatment, patients randomly assigned to receive the 12-step oriented network support intervention had better alcohol use outcomes, as well as greater AA attendance and involvement. Similarly, an RCT by Walitzer et al.[80] found that patients randomly assigned to receive individually delivered CBT alone, or one of two types of AA/TSF treatments, one of which was more client-centered and one being more therapist directed, found that alcohol use disorder patients assigned to the more directive AA/TSF intervention where AA participation was prescribed and more of the treatment content was centered on AA, patients were more involved in AA and had 10% to 20% better alcohol outcomes in the year following treatment.

Kaskutas et al.[87] developed and tested one of the few group-delivered AA/TSF interventions, called Making Alcoholics Anonymous Easier (MAAEZ), to enhance patients' connection with AA, led by clinicians who also were themselves experienced with AA. Using a quasi-experimental design, they found that patients who participated in the MAAEZ groups were more likely to be abstinent from alcohol and other drugs during and in the year following treatment.

Another RCT with couples found equal alcohol outcomes effects when adding an AA/TSF component to therapy. McCrady et al. studied the impact of adding AA to alcohol-focused behavioral couples therapy (ABCT). Participants assigned to the combined AA/ABCT treatment were significantly more likely to attend AA meetings during treatment,[88] but AA involvement did not result in better drinking outcomes at either 6 or 18 months after treatment.[88,89]

Naturalistic Studies of Treatments Based on Twelve-Step Principles

In contrast to RCTs, which typically include strict experimental controls to maximize internal validity, naturalistic study designs evaluate existing treatment programs and patient populations. Experimental controls are lacking, but the inclusion of a broader sample and the evaluation of extant treatments provide information complementary to that obtained from RCTs. In the largest comparative study of 12-step–based treatments, Moos et al.[90] studied 3,698 male veterans being treated at 1 of 15 VA treatment units. The treatment units were classified as 12-step oriented, CBT oriented, or eclectic. No patient was excluded from the study, and 97% of the patients were followed up successfully 1 year after treatment. Overall, patients showed significant decreases in alcohol use, symptoms of DSM-IV defined alcohol dependence, and psychological problems, and improved in social functioning. Patients who participated in 12-step–oriented treatment were about 1.5 times more likely to be abstinent than CBT patients.[91] Patients from both types of programs, however (CBT or 12-step), were more likely to be employed than patients whose treatment was more eclectic in focus. Patient-treatment matching also was examined in the VA study,[92] but there was no evidence that specific patient characteristics predicted differential response to either 12-step–oriented or CBT. In the year after treatment, patients from the 12-step–oriented programs attended significantly more mutual-help groups than patients from the CBT programs and had significantly fewer outpatient visits and inpatient treatment days. Subsequent costs of treatment were 64% higher for patients who had not participated in a 12-step–oriented treatment unit and the clinical outcomes not as good.[8]

Single-group evaluations of treatments based on 12-step principles and practices typically have studied inpatient treatment programs. Most studies have focused on private treatment centers, whose populations can be more socially stable than patients in public treatment programs. The largest study of this type[93] reported that 67% to 75% of participants reported abstinence 6 months after treatment and 60% to 68% abstinent rates at a 12-month follow-up. However, study attrition was substantial, and the investigators estimated that abstinence rates would have been 56% to 65% at 6 months and 34% to 42% at 12 months if patients lost to follow-up were considered to have relapsed (ie, in "intent to treat" analysis). An evaluation of 1,083 patients treated at the Hazelden Foundation treatment program[94] reported that at 6 months after discharge, 59% of patients said they had not used alcohol or drugs since discharge; at the 12-month follow-up, 53% said they had not used alcohol or drugs since discharge. Follow-up rates were better than 70%. If patients lost to follow-up are included as treatment failures, adjusted rates of continuous abstinence were 45% at 6 months and 37% at 12 months—results very comparable to those reported by Hoffmann and Miller.[93]

AA Involvement and the Prediction of Treatment Outcomes

Many studies have examined the contribution of AA attendance and involvement to the successful resolution of a drinking problem. One of the most consistent and robust findings is that there is a positive correlation between AA attendance and drinking outcomes. Studies of treatment populations in the 1990s[94-96] found that patients who attended AA were significantly more likely to be abstinent 1 year after treatment than were those who did not attend AA. Analyses of Project MATCH data by treatment site also found that AA attendance correlated positively with drinking outcomes for all sites irrespective of which clinical treatment they were assigned to.[97] More recent studies have reported longer-term follow-ups, with similar results. For example, a 3-year follow-up of participants in a study of posttreatment telephone case monitoring found that mutual help group involvement in years 1 and 2 of follow-up was associated with more abstinence in years 2 and 3 of the study.[98] Similar results from a 5-year follow-up by Gossop et al.[99] found a positive association between AA/NA attendance and abstinence from opiates and alcohol but not from stimulants. More recently, Chi et al.[100] examined 7-year outcomes in a sample of adolescents with SUDs with and without co-occurring psychiatric disorders. Similar to the adult literature, they found strong associations between AA participation and positive outcomes, regardless of comorbidity status; and an 8-year follow-up study by Kelly et al.[24] found that participation in AA/NA early posttreatment in the first 6 months was associated with higher abstinence and remission at 6- and 8-year follow-ups and for every AA/NA meeting attended across the entire 8-year follow-up adolescents/young adults gained an addiction abstinence of 2 days.

Four studies specifically examined the causal relationship between AA attendance and outcomes. In a series of concurrent and time-lagged analyses, McCrady et al.[89] found that AA attendance predicted subsequent abstinence throughout 18 months of posttreatment follow-up but that abstinence did not predict AA attendance, thus suggesting a causal relationship between AA attendance and positive outcomes of treatment. Similarly, McKellar et al.[101] reported that the level of AA affiliation 1 year after treatment predicted lower levels of alcohol-related problems 2 years after treatment but that the converse was not the case. In analyses of the Project MATCH data, Magura et al.[102] used an advanced quantitative technique, cross-lagged regression panel analysis, to test whether AA attendance in the Project MATCH sample directly predicted abstinence. Also testing the opposite direction of causality (ie, did abstinence predict AA attendance), they established a clear predictive relationship between AA attendance and subsequent abstinence.

Humphreys et al.[103] used data from six RCTs that included a condition to enhance AA involvement to isolate the incremental change in AA attendance attributable to the AA enhancement treatment condition. With the exception of the Project MATCH aftercare group, which already had very high rates of AA involvement prior to study entry, they established that the interventions to enhance AA involvement led directly to increases in AA involvement, which, in turn, predicted better alcohol use outcomes.

Studies of non–treatment-seeking populations have found that AA involvement was one of a handful of significant predictors of long-term (>5 years) abstinence. Follow-ups 8[14,104] and 16 years[15] after initial study recruitment of individuals who had presented to an information and referral center or received withdrawal management found that AA attendance was significantly correlated with less alcohol consumption, less intoxication, more abstinence, and fewer symptoms of alcohol dependence or alcohol-related problems. Non–treatment-seeking people who used alcohol who had been involved with AA were more likely to have positive long-term outcomes than those who had received no treatment. Compared to those who received treatment without AA, those who attended AA alone were more likely to be abstinent up to 3 years after initial contact, but outcomes were equivalent at the 8-year follow-up. Outcomes were comparable for persons who attended treatment alone or who combined treatment with AA. Findings from NESARC[12] are remarkably similar. They found that individuals involved with treatment and 12-step programs were almost twice as likely to have successful outcomes as those involved with formal treatment alone. An 11-year longitudinal study of people who drank alcohol with consequent problems also found an association between AA attendance and better alcohol use outcomes.[104]

Engaging Patients With AA

Three recent studies examined methods to engage patients in AA. Kahler et al.[105] randomly assigned patients in withdrawal management to a brief advice condition or to a Motivational Enhancement Therapy (MET) intervention focused on AA participation (MET-12). They found that MET-12 resulted in better outcomes than advice for patients who had no prior experience with AA, but that the more simple advice condition was more effective for those with past AA experience. The results suggest that it may be confusing for patients already positively oriented toward AA to be asked to examine their perceptions of the value of AA. As noted above, Walitzer and colleagues[80] compared an MET AA/TSF approach to a more directive approach to facilitate AA involvement and found that the directive approach was significantly more effective at increasing AA attendance and involvement and led to more positive drinking outcomes than either the MET approach or the CBT-alone approach. In contrast, Blondell et al.[106] randomly assigned patients undergoing withdrawal management to treatment as usual, MET, or a peer-delivered TSF. Treatment initiation was similar across interventions 30 days later, but by 90 days after withdrawal management, the peer TSF was significantly less effective than MET at getting patients to seek additional care.

Summary

The research literature suggests that involvement with AA is clearly associated with positive outcomes and that AA involvement leads to positive outcomes, rather than simply being a correlate. An accumulating body of literature suggests that treatment programs (inpatient and outpatient) based on 12-step principles may be more successful in effecting total abstinence and remission over time and may be more cost-effective than other treatment models. The literature on methods to engage individuals with AA is limited, but findings suggest that methods for engagement may need to vary depending on the individual's past experience with the program and that simple, directive, methods can be effective.

Given the immense increase in online mutual-help resources (especially during the era of transmittable viral diseases such as via COVID-19), including online AA meetings, more research is needed to understand how the increased accessibility may result in more frequent meeting attendance within persons, or greater numbers of individuals being able to access and try groups like AA more easily across persons. Other important research questions pertain to the extent to which the degree and nature of involvement online differs from that in-person, and whether any such observed differences may affect ultimate therapeutic outcomes in any meaningful way (either positive or negative) and for whom. For example, online participation may be just as helpful for those individuals who are merely continuing their established group social connections initially made at in-person meetings; but online participation may be less engaging and helpful for brand new members seeking recovery who are trying to make those social connections via an online platform in more of a social vacuum. Specifically, increased online accessibility could be a double-edged sword. On the one hand, whereas the lower threshold for attendance (eg, clicking on a mouse at the kitchen table instead of finding a baby sitter, leaving the house, and driving for 20 minutes) could mean more people can sample AA meetings, the lack of social intimacy and connection that may be obtained from the in-person encounter (eg, through the handshakes, hugs, coffee, and natural conversations that occur prior to, and following, formal meetings), may mean that these same individuals may prematurely conclude that AA is not of value, because they have not experienced the more holistic and multisensory meeting context. Future research is needed to begin to answer these types of "telemedicine/telerecovery" versus "in-person" questions.

MECHANISMS OF CHANGE IN AA

With empirical evidence that AA is beneficial for many people with alcohol-related problems, investigators have begun to understand why AA is beneficial. This line of research necessarily involves three integrated aims, and it is important to keep them distinct.

First, investigators are seeking to identify the active ingredients of AA that mobilize behavior change. Such catalysts may include prescribed behaviors such as sponsorship, reading core AA literature, and AA step work, but may also include less formal or more subtle processes, such as frequency and nature of social support offered through AA participation. Second, actual active ingredients must produce changes that enhance the probability of successfully changing behavior (eg, they in turn produce enhancements in abstinence self-efficacy, relapse prevention coping skills, maintaining or enhancing commitment to sobriety). And, third, mobilized changes in an individual (eg, increases in abstinence self-efficacy) must predict later reductions in alcohol use.

Active Ingredients

Of the three aims to study why AA is beneficial, investigators have focused most directly on identifying the active ingredients of AA. Historically, the AA meeting has been considered the "dose," and frequency of AA meeting attendance thus indicated the intensity of the dose.[107] This monolithic view of AA has yielded to a multidimensional perspective, one that first distinguished between physical exposure and engagement in prescribed AA behaviors. Although data suggest that attendance is related to outcomes,[22,108] Montgomery et al.[109] made an important distinction between AA *attendance* and AA *involvement*, which included, in addition to attendance, the degree of involvement with various aspects of AA, such as participation during meetings, having a sponsor, leading meetings, working specific steps, or helping others (ie, doing 12-step work). They reported that AA involvement and attendance were moderately correlated (0.45); however, involvement, not attendance, correlated with posttreatment reductions in harmful alcohol consumption ($r = -0.44$) in a sample of patients in an inpatient 12-step treatment program. Similar results have been reported in other samples.[110]

Using Project MATCH data, Tonigan et al.[111] examined the nature of participants' experience with AA. As in other research, there was a positive correlation between AA-related actions and the degree to which patients were abstinent. Tonigan et al. anticipated that there would be two aspects of experience with AA—a subjective dimension and a behavioral dimension. Statistically, however, experiences with AA seemed to reflect one major dimension rather than two. Greater participation was reflected in a combination of factors: a spiritual awakening, God consciousness, the perception that attending AA meetings was helpful, actually attending AA meetings, being involved with other AA-related practices, and completing more steps. They also found that participation in AA during treatment and in the first 6 months after treatment predicted better drinking outcomes in the second 6 months after treatment.[111] In later work, however, Greenfield and Tonigan[112] found evidence for two factors in AA involvement—behavioral step work and spiritual step work. Of the two, spiritual step work predicted later abstinence, but behavioral step work did not. Weiss et al.[113] reported similar findings about the importance of commitment to 12-step practices, with the important distinction that they were investigating 12-step–related benefit among 487 cocaine-dependent adults. In addition to receiving 24 weeks of behavioral counseling, these patients were encouraged to attend 12-step programs. Findings indicated that frequency of 12-step attendance did not predict later substance use but that a composite measure reflecting engagement in 12-step programs was significantly and positively associated with increased abstinence. Most recently, Zemore et al.[114] reported that both attendance and specific 12-step activities mediated the impact of AA on outcomes.

Research tends to support the importance of many of the prescribed AA-related behaviors for abstinence seen as important by AA members (eg, having a sponsor, service work). Research has consistently identified having or being a sponsor as important to success in AA. Pagano et al.,[115] for example, in a reexamination of the Project MATCH dataset, reported that being an AA sponsor led to a significant reduction in the probability of relapse at 1 year (eg, 60% relapse among sponsors versus 78% relapse for nonsponsors); however, it was relatively rare in this sample for a participant to be a sponsor (8%; n = 120), suggesting the desirability of encouraging this behavior more often during the treatment experience. Further, investigating whether type of SUD (ie, DSM-IV alcohol dependence, drug dependence, or both alcohol and drug dependence) moderated the relative benefits of 12-step meeting attendance and prescribed behaviors, Witbrodt and Kaskutas[116] found that of seven specific measured AA behaviors, only having a sponsor predicted positive outcome across substance categories. Secondary benefits of sponsorship have been reported by Witbrodt et al.[22] Specifically, in a 5-year study of 349 alcohol-dependent adults, they reported that sponsorship and frequency of AA attendance were positively associated such that high and medium AA attendees at 5 years had three times the rates of being sponsors as the individuals who had low or declining rates of AA attendance. More recent research has continued to support the strong association between having a sponsor and positive drinking outcomes.[22,108,117-120]

Research on sponsorship has begun to examine the characteristics and behaviors of sponsors. Based on qualitative analyses, Stevens et al.[121,122] reported that personal engagement with AA, trustworthiness, and confidentiality were seen as key to being a successful sponsor. The sponsee's experience of a strong "therapeutic" alliance with their sponsor has been found to an important predictor of abstinence in adolescent populations.[123]

Other AA program behaviors also appear to predict later improvements, even after statistically controlling for AA fellowship behaviors such as AA attendance. Tonigan and Miller,[124] for example, reported that the specific number of AA steps completed at 3-year follow-up and alcohol consumed at 10-year follow-up were significantly and negatively related; Pagano et al.[115] also found a relationship between number of steps worked and successful abstinence. Further, Tonigan and Miller[125] reported that commitment to and understanding of the 12 steps were significantly and positively predictive of 1-year abstinence. Some research has suggested that specific steps are most associated with later abstinence, particularly Steps 4, 5, and 11.[124]

Less easily classified, AA fellowship behaviors also have been identified as potential candidates to understand what mobilizes mechanisms of change. Essentially, this body of research has focused on the benefits of social support and network support for abstinence provided through AA participation. Involvement in mutual-help groups, for example, may influence the *nature* of an addicted individual's social network. Humphreys and Noke[126] followed male SUD inpatients after treatment and examined AA, NA, or CA participation and social network outcomes. They found that greater group participation predicted both better quality of general friendship and less support of substance use by friends at follow-up. Individuals involved significantly in 12-step groups (involved in at least two of three 12-step activities measured) actually increased the size of their friendship networks by an average of 16%; those *not* significantly involved in 12-step groups showed no change in the size of their friendship networks. The greater increase in social network size was attributable to the fact that those significantly more involved in 12-step groups increased their number of friends in 12-step programs, not because those less involved with 12-step groups lost friends. Humphreys and Noke[126] also found that those who had networks composed almost entirely of 12-step members experienced better friendship quality than did others who held social networks composed of almost no 12-step members.

Evidence suggests that the benefits of social networks supportive of abstinence in 12-step programs may vary temporally. In particular, Witbrodt and Kaskutas[116] reported that, for adults with DSM-III-R alcohol dependence, network support for abstinence was significantly predictive of abstinence at 6 months but not at 12-month follow-up. The reverse situation was found for individuals with DSM-III-R drug dependence in whom the benefits of social support were unrelated to 6-month abstinence but significantly and positively related to 12-month abstinence rates. The exact reasons for this reversal effect are unclear, but it may be related to unintended stimulus cues encouraging illicit drug use during early efforts to achieve abstinence. Also intriguing is the finding that the magnitude of benefit associated with social support for abstinence is different between support provided by 12-step members and support from others.[127] Specifically, at 30- and 90-day follow-up interviews, abstinence rates were twice as high for AA members who reported AA member social support compared to those of AA members reporting social support for abstinence from non-AA sources. Combined, both temporal and social support characteristics appear to moderate the benefit of social support for abstinence, with early AA member support most beneficial for alcohol-dependent individuals.

Research has also found that changes in social networks directly mediate the relationship between AA attendance and alcohol use outcomes. Using Project MATCH data, Stout et al.[128] and Kelly et al.[129,130] found that AA attendance led to decreases in pro-drinking social ties and drinking-related activities and increases in pro-abstinent social ties and greater engagement in abstinent-related activities. Both reductions in pro-drinking ties and increases in pro-abstinent ties partially explained the relationship between AA attendance and better alcohol use outcomes. Subbaraman and Kaskutas[131] looked beyond the nature of the social network to the experience of receiving social support for abstinence and found that support for sobriety at 6 months mediated the positive impact of the MAAEZ intervention on 12-month drinking outcomes.

Given the importance of social network variables in alcohol treatment outcome in general and AA in particular, recent studies have focused on the role formal treatment can play in facilitating AA-related social network benefit. Litt et al.,[81] for instance, designed a treatment to enhance network support through either AA or other social resources such as families and social activities. The network support therapy significantly increased AA involvement and more general support for abstinence from members of their social network. Similar to other studies, both network support and AA involvement correlated positively with treatment outcomes.

Treatment outcome research suggests that social variables also may function as moderators of the relationship between 12-step participation and outcome. Though the Project MATCH studies are reviewed elsewhere in this chapter, one study by Longabaugh et al.[82] is of particular interest here. In examining the effects of matching patient characteristics with specific treatment modalities, Longabaugh et al. found that TSF treatment, which aimed to involve patients in AA, was more effective than MET for individuals who had social networks that were supportive of alcohol use at treatment intake. Those with low support for drinking had similar outcomes, regardless of treatment type. The investigators also found that AA participation mediated the interaction between treatment type and network support for alcohol use. In other words, TSF treatment emphasized AA involvement and thus helped to create improved social networks, which in turn predicted better alcohol use outcomes. This was especially true for those individuals who had networks that supported their active alcohol use.

What Do the AA Active Ingredients Influence?

Spirituality

Of course, from AA's own perspective, the chief and central mechanism through which recovery is purported to be achieved is through what it calls a "spiritual awakening" (eg, Step 12: "Having had a spiritual awakening as a result of these steps…"; "The truth is we have had deep and effective spiritual experiences…"[1,132,133] Spiritual development therefore seems an ideal candidate to be a central AA change mechanism.

In cross-sectional and longitudinal studies that have employed dozens of different psychometrically validated measures of spirituality and religiosity (eg, religious beliefs and behavior,[134] spiritual coping questionnaire,[135] brief measure of religiosity and spirituality,[136] daily spiritual experiences[137]), two findings have been reported consistently: (1) AA program and fellowship behaviors are significantly and positively associated with measures of spirituality and religiosity and

(2) the endorsement of spiritual and religious practices increases in amplitude with longer periods of AA affiliation.[76,109,138-140] Based upon a sample (n = 123) of alcohol-dependent adults, for example, Robinson et al.[138] provided estimates of the magnitude of spirituality/religiosity before and after gains among AA-exposed adults in the first 6 months after outpatient treatment. Pre- to postchanges were largest for the measures that inventoried spiritual and religious *practices*, for example, prayer and other private religious practices,[141] while pre- to postchanges in measures of spiritual and religious values, beliefs, and meaning were minimal (eg, d = 10).

Evidence is mixed about the relative importance of spiritual/religious changes for explaining greater abstinence among AA members. In a 3-year follow-up of adults who used substances who received private and public treatment, for instance, Kaskutas et al.[127] reported that about equal proportions of abstinent adults reported having or not having a spiritual awakening as a result of AA participation. Robinson et al.[138] provided the most compelling evidence that increased spirituality accounts for AA-related benefit. They reported that the average before and after increase in daily spiritual experiences enhanced the odds of reduced heavy drinking at 6 months by 12% after *controlling* for changes in AA involvement. More recent analyses[141,142] support Robinson's earlier findings. In one set of analyses of the Project MATCH dataset,[130] Kelly et al. tested multiple potential mediators of the effects of AA on outcomes and found that increases in spirituality/religiosity were mediators only for the portion of the sample that entered Project MATCH after completing an inpatient treatment program. Additional analyses[143] suggested that AA attendance did lead to increases in spiritual practices, which partially mediated the relationship between AA and outcomes. In the few cases wherein religious and spiritual measures did "significantly" predict later abstinence, the actual magnitude of these relationships was small and was not clinically meaningful.[143] Spirituality, however, may offer secondary benefit. Specifically, Christo and Franey[144] found that, although neither spiritual beliefs nor believing in addiction as a disease predicted drug use outcomes, both predicted NA attendance, which was related to reduced drug use. Clearly, there is strong evidence that the greater use of the active ingredients of AA (eg, working the 12 steps) produces, on average, increased spirituality. Whether such increases account for later improvement, however, is open to question at this time.

Cognitive Shifts

Several studies have investigated "AA-specific" cognitive mechanisms in 12-step therapy, arguably replicating the mechanisms of change in community-based AA. Morgenstern and Bates,[145] for example, reported that some cognitive shifts promoted by 12-step therapists predicted later improvement (eg, powerlessness over alcohol), but others did not. Further, Tonigan[146] reported that therapist emphasis on complete abstinence was stronger in 12-step therapy relative to motivational enhancement and cognitive-behavioral therapies but that this differential emphasis did not explain higher rates of complete abstinence of TSF clients at 1-year follow-up.[32] Likewise, using a composite measure of 12-step beliefs, Finney et al.[147,148] found modest increases in AA-related cognitions during 12-step treatment, but such changes did not explain later abstinence rates. In general, then, we find that cognitive shifts congruent with AA ideology can be successfully mobilized in 12-step therapy but that the relative importance of these shifts in accounting for increased abstinence is mixed at best.

In contrast, the study of one "nonspecific" therapeutic mechanism in AA has yielded consistent positive findings. Eleven studies have shown, for example, that frequency of AA meeting attendance is associated with gains in abstinence self-efficacy and, in turn, that these gains partially explain AA benefit.[5,29,138,149-152] Meta-analytic work[153] further shows that the actual magnitude of the temporal path from AA attendance to self-efficacy gains is, on average, about r = 0.21 (SD = 0.08), though there was significant variability in this estimate across studies (range, r = 0.11-0.31). Likewise, these studies also reported positive (r = 0.33) but significantly different estimates of the utility of self-efficacy in explaining AA-related abstinence (range, r = 0.06-0.45). Whether significant variation in the magnitude of relationships was the result of different sample characteristics or in AA practices is speculative because the measure used across these studies to define AA participation, AA meeting attendance, was unfortunately a composite indicator of both AA program and fellowship behaviors.

Psychological Variables

Recent research has begun to examine the mediational role of four psychological variables (impulsivity, attachment style, depression and narcissism) in attempting to explain the impact of AA involvement on drinking outcomes. In two longitudinal studies, Blonigen et al.[154,155] examined the impact of AA involvement on impulsivity. They found that impulsivity decreased in the first year after study involvement, that longer participation in AA during the 16-year longitudinal study was associated with greater decreases in impulsivity, and that decreased impulsivity was associated with fewer drinking problems.

A second psychological construct, psychological attachment, has been examined in cross-sectional and longitudinal analyses of a naturalistic study of patterns of AA involvement and outcomes. In the first of two studies, Smith and Tonigan[156] assessed interpersonal attachment styles of individuals attending AA and found that AA participation was corrected with higher secure attachment and lower avoidant and anxious attachment. In subsequent longitudinal analyses, Jenkins and Tonigan[157] found that attachment avoidance but not attachment anxiety was related to less frequent AA attendance and use of AA behaviors but was unrelated to drinking outcomes.

Third, Kelly et al.[158] have begun to examine changes in depression as a possible mediator of the relationship between AA and drinking outcomes. In lagged analyses using the Project MATCH dataset, the investigators found that depression decreased during treatment, that AA attendance was associated with decreases in depression, and that changes in depression partially mediated the relationship between AA attendance and drinking outcomes. However, because depression and drinking both decreased during treatment, it may be that the impact of depression as a mediator is accounted for directly by changes in drinking, ie, that a proportion of depression is alcohol-induced.

Tonigan et al.[159] tested the concept in the 12-step literature that persons with AUDs have pathological levels of selfishness, and that one mechanism of change in AA is decreases in selfishness. Using a measure of pathological narcissism, they found no changes in pathological narcissism across a 9-month period, and no mediating relationship between narcissism and drinking outcomes.

Of note, the mechanisms of behavior change through which AA confers recovery benefits appears to differ among different participants. A number of analyses[130,160,161] have found the way that AA helps more severely addicted individuals versus less severely addicted individuals, women versus men, and young people versus older people all may differ. Specifically, in studies where multiple mediators are examined simultaneously, among more severely addicted patients, AA appears to aid recovery my mobilizing a number of therapeutic factors (eg, abstinence self-efficacy; social network changes) including spirituality, but among less severely addicted AA participants, AA does not confer therapeutic relapse prevention benefits through enhancing spirituality.[130] Also, similarly for women and men, although women tend to show equal recovery benefits from AA participation compared to men, women tend to benefit to a much greater extent from AA's ability to enhance women's ability to cope with negative affect (depression, anxiety, anger etc.) without drinking whereas men are shown to benefit much more from AA's ability to boost their ability to cope with high risk social situations where alcohol may be present (eg, at social sporting events) without relapsing. For younger adults (18-29 years old) compared to older adults (30+ years old), it has been found that whereas each age group derives similar overall relapse prevention therapeutic benefits from AA participation, younger adults benefit much more from AA's ability to help them shed people who use alcohol heavily/use drug from their social networks, whereas among older AA participants, AA helps them drop these negative influences but also adopt positive recovering friends.[161] This set of findings suggest that, similar the psychotherapy mechanisms literature[162] rather than thinking about "how AA works" it might be more apt to think about how individuals *make* AA work for them. Depending on particular characteristics, life-context, and life-stage challenges, individuals seeking recovery are able to utilize different aspects of AA to help them cope with the particular challenges facing them in their lives at any particular phase of their recovery and life-course.[163]

Summary

AA-related benefit occurs because of a tapestry of social interactions, prescribed behaviors, and mobilized psychological processes. There is strong evidence that social support for abstinence in 12-step programs is an important element accounting for 12-step–related benefit, but evidence also indicates that the nature and temporal benefits associated with such support are complex and are only beginning to be understood. Likewise, consistent support is found for the benefit of two AA-prescribed behaviors: AA meeting attendance and engagement in the AA program by having, and being, an AA sponsor. Because sponsorship is a vital prerequisite for working the 12 steps, an important outstanding question is whether sponsorship per se predicts positive outcome or, alternatively, whether being guided through the 12 steps by a sponsor accounts for AA-related benefit. Changes in spirituality or religious/spiritual practices appear to be an important mechanism by which AA exerts a positive impact of outcomes. Contrary to conventional wisdom, cognitive shifts that appear to account for AA-related benefit are not AA specific. Though changes in many beliefs and values occur among AA-exposed individuals, such changes do not seem to have a direct, and definitive, effect explaining reduced drinking. AA works through multiple mechanisms simultaneously and similar to the psychotherapy mechanisms literature more broadly, AA participants utilize the available multifaceted components of AA in different ways to help meet diverse and dynamic needs related to life contexts and life stage.

FUTURE DIRECTIONS

Research on AA has become increasingly sophisticated over the past 30 years, and a body of accrued knowledge provides a richer and more articulated research-based picture of AA than was available previously. However, there are important research and conceptual issues not well addressed in the current body of literature.

AA as a Single Entity

The formal program of AA is relatively invariant, but there is substantial variation in the practice of the AA program (eg, the fellowship[108,164,165]). Typically, AA-focused research disregards such variation and treats AA as a monolithic and static entity. This research practice makes several assumptions, ones that probably are not valid. Specifically, (1) the "dose" of AA is fixed and invariant across meetings regardless of meeting type (eg, speaker, closed, open discussion), size, and membership characteristics; (2) AA group social dynamics do not influence the generation, transmission, or reception of the "dose" of AA; (3) AA social context itself does not account for alcohol use outcomes, directly or indirectly; (4) AA social context and individual characteristics do not interact in accounting for sustaining AA membership or drinking outcome; and (5) the importance of AA social context in accounting for AA-related benefit is temporally invariant (eg, the "unit benefit" of one AA meeting was the same for AA members regardless of length of membership). Though these assumptions have some utility in research, they may also shackle the continued development of AA-related research and seriously erode the application of evidence-based findings in clinical settings.

Understanding Utilization of and Affiliation With AA

Data from AA's triennial surveys and studies of persons in 12-step–oriented treatment indicate that the majority of individuals who try AA do not continue or affiliate. Despite a large body of research directed toward trying to understand what drives initial and sustained involvement with AA, we still have a very incomplete picture of why some individuals affiliate with AA and thrive while others either avoid AA completely or do not stay with the program or benefit. Given that there are few individual characteristics that are consistent predictors of AA involvement and affiliation, research needs to look elsewhere. One untapped area of research is the possibility of key events or experiences that define affiliation or disaffiliation with AA. Qualitative and narrative analysis methodologies could be brought to bear in understanding these processes.

Population Subgroups

The population of the United States is increasingly diverse in race and ethnicity, a diversity that is not well represented in AA. In other ways, though, the membership of AA is diverse—in age, socioeconomic status, and gender. The research literature, however, provides little information about the experience, utilization, and barriers to use of AA for different groups. Data are particularly scant for older adults, LGBT populations, persons of color, and persons mandated to attend AA. Culturally informed research methodologies, such as community-based participatory research, may be needed to access populations with limited involvement with AA.

CONCLUSIONS

This chapter has reviewed a substantial body of research on AA and other 12-step-based clinical interventions and programs. AA remains the most commonly sought source of help for alcohol and other drug problems in the United States with 6% to 10% of the population having attended an AA meeting, with that rate doubling or tripling among those with alcohol problems. Individuals continue to be mandated to attend AA through the legal system, but such practices may not be appropriate for some groups, and also may raise civil liberties questions about the separation of church and state. When individuals seek help voluntarily, a substantial proportion uses AA either as their sole source of assistance or in conjunction with formal treatment. Typically, individuals become actively involved in AA for several months, attending meetings about twice a week. There is, however, considerable variability in patterns of affiliation, with some individuals becoming increasingly committed over time and others gradually slipping away from the program. Longer-term involvement is less common, but those who stay with AA for more than a year are very likely to continue their involvement for many years.

Like alcohol use disorder itself, AA is highly heterogeneous and it is difficult to draw generalizations about who is most or least likely to affiliate. There is little evidence of problems with affiliation among specific subpopulations, but some minor concerns about aspects of the AA program have been documented among some women and African Americans. It may be that the presence of tailored meeting types within AA (eg, men's and women's specific meetings) and modifications of meetings at the local level can effectively address these concerns. Overall, data suggest that individuals who have more severe alcohol problems, more concerns about their alcohol use, a greater commitment to staying abstinent, less support from a spouse, a social network supportive of continued harmful and hazardous alcohol use, a history of turning to others for support, and a greater desire to find meaning in their lives may be most likely to affiliate with AA.

In terms of clarifying the efficacy of 12-step–related clinical treatments as well as AA's ability to confer relapse prevention and remission benefits over time, the past 30 years has seen a very large volume of high quality and rigorously conducted clinical trial and other research emerge. Findings from this body of research indicate that when AA and related 12-step clinical facilitation treatment studies are subjected to the same rigorous scientific evaluation standards as any other clinical interventions, AA/12-step treatments are shown to perform at least as well on all outcomes, except for continuous abstinence and remission, where AA/12-step treatments are shown to outperform other psychosocial interventions. Research also demonstrates that clinical implementation of AA/12-step clinical models of care for alcohol use disorder, in particular, is likely not only to boost rates of long-term remission but also to substantially reduce health care costs. A sophisticated and scientifically rigorous body of research on the mechanisms of behavior change through which AA participation itself is shown to confer recovery-related benefits, indicates that the reason why AA-facilitation treatments are able to achieve these better outcomes over the long-term is because they facilitate and prescribe active participation in AA and, in doing so, are more likely actually to engage patients with the AA organization. In turn, ongoing AA participation is shown subsequently to mobilize the same kinds of therapeutic factors that are mobilized by formal clinical interventions such as CBT; that is, by boosting relapse prevention coping skills, abstinence self-efficacy, recovery motivation; decreasing craving and impulsivity; facilitating recovery-promoting changes in patients' social networks; but is able to do this over the long-term for free in the communities in which people live and work. AA's (and similar groups) availability, easy accessibility (in person and online), flexibility, and demonstrated empirical effectiveness and cost-effectiveness in enhancing recovery, makes AA and similar organizations significant public health allies in helping to ameliorate the health and economic burdens associated with alcohol and other drug use disorders.

ACKNOWLEDGMENT

This chapter represents an update and revision of previous chapters in this series, most recently by Barbara S. McCrady from the last edition. We are indebted to Dr McCrady for her work and retain much of her prose in this current edition.

REFERENCES

1. Alcoholics Anonymous. *Alcoholics Anonymous: The Story of How Thousands of Men and Women have Recovered from Alcoholism*. 4th ed. Alcoholics Anonymous World Services; 2001.
2. Kelly JF. The protective wall of human community: the new evidence on the clinical and public health utility of twelve-step mutual-help organizations and related treatments. *Psychiatr Clin North Am*. 2022; 45(3):557-575.
3. Alcoholics Anonymous. *Alcoholics Anonymous: The Story of How Many Thousands of Men and Women Have Recovered from Alcoholism*. 1st ed. Alcoholics Anonymous World Services; 1939.
4. Alcoholics Anonymous. Estimated Worldwide AA Individual and Group Membership. Accessed June 19, 2023. https://www.aa.org/aa-around-the-world
5. Mäkelä K, Arminen I, Bloomfield K, et al. *Alcoholics Anonymous as a Mutual-Help Movement*. University of Wisconsin Press; 1996.
6. McCrady BS, Miller WR. *Research on Alcoholics Anonymous: Opportunities and Alternatives*. Rutgers Center of Alcohol Studies; 1993.
7. Institute of Medicine. *Broadening the Base of Treatment for Alcohol Problems*. National Academy Press; 1990.
8. Humphreys K, Moos R. Can encouraging substance abuse patients to participate in self-help groups reduce demand for health care? A quasi-experimental study. *Alcohol Clin Exp Res*. 2001;25(5):711-716.
9. Humphreys K, Moos RH. Encouraging posttreatment self-help group involvement to reduce demand for continuing care services: two-year clinical and utilization outcomes. *Alcohol Clin Exp Res*. 2007;31(1):64-68.
10. Kelly JF, Humphreys K, Ferri M. Alcoholics Anonymous and other 12-step programs for alcohol use disorder. *Cochrane Database Syst Rev*. 2020;3(3):CD012880.
11. Dawson DA, Grant BF, Stinson FS, Chou PS. Estimating the effect of help-seeking on achieving recovery from alcohol dependence. *Addiction*. 2006;101(6):824-834.
12. Dawson DA, Grant BF, Stinson FS, Chou PS, Huang B, Ruan WJ. Recovery from DSM-IV alcohol dependence: United States, 2001-2002. *Addiction*. 2005;100(3):281-292.
13. Timko C, Finney JW, Moos RH, Moos BS, Steinbaum DP. The process of treatment selection among previously untreated help-seeking problem drinkers. *J Subst Abus*. 1993;5(3):203-220.
14. Timko C, Moos RH, Finney JW, Lesar MD. Long-term outcomes of alcohol use disorders: comparing untreated individuals with those in alcoholics anonymous and formal treatment. *J Stud Alcohol*. 2000;61(4):529-540.
15. Moos RH, Moos BS. Paths of entry into alcoholics anonymous: consequences for participation and remission. *Alcohol Clin Exp Res*. 2005;29(10):1858-1868.
16. Speiglman R. Mandated AA attendance for recidivist drinking drivers: ideology, organization, and California criminal justice practices. *Addiction*. 1994;89(7):859-868.
17. Alcoholics Anonymous. Information on Alcoholics Anonymous. Accessed February 15, 2023. https://www.aa.org/information-alcoholics-anonymous.
18. Gallagher JR. African American participants' views on racial disparities in drug court outcomes. *J Soc Work Pract Addict*. 2013;13(2):143-162.
19. Narrow WE, Regier DA, Rae DS, Manderscheid RW, Locke BZ. Use of services by persons with mental and addictive disorders. Findings from the National Institute of Mental Health Epidemiologic Catchment Area Program. *Arch Gen Psychiatry*. 1993;50(2):95-107.
20. Moos RH, Moos BS. Participation in treatment and Alcoholics Anonymous: a 16-year follow-up of initially untreated individuals. *J Clin Psychol*. 2006;62(6):735-750.
21. Kaskutas LA, Bond J, Avalos LA. 7-year trajectories of Alcoholics Anonymous attendance and associations with treatment. *Addict Behav*. 2009;34(12):1029-1035.
22. Witbrodt J, Kaskutas L, Bond J, Delucchi K. Does sponsorship improve outcomes above Alcoholics Anonymous attendance? A latent class growth curve analysis. *Addiction*. 2012;107(2):301-311.
23. Chi FW, Campbell CI, Sterling S, Weisner C. Twelve-Step attendance trajectories over 7 years among adolescents entering substance use treatment in an integrated health plan. *Addiction*. 2012;107(5):933-942.
24. Kelly JF, Brown SA, Abrantes A, Kahler CW, Myers M. Social recovery model: an 8-year investigation of adolescent 12-step group involvement following inpatient treatment. *Alcohol Clin Exp Res*. 2008;32(8):1468-1478.
25. Mäkelä K. Rates of attrition among the membership of Alcoholics Anonymous in Finland. *J Stud Alcohol*. 1994;55(1):91-95.
26. Room R, Greenfield T. Alcoholics anonymous, other 12-step movements and psychotherapy in the U.S. population, 1990. *Addiction*. 1993;88(4): 555-562.
27. Caetano R. Ethnic minority groups and Alcoholics Anonymous: a review. In: BS MC, Miller WR, eds. *Research on Alcoholics Anonymous: Opportunities and Alternatives*. Rutgers Center of Alcohol Studies; 1993:209-232.
28. Morgenstern J, Labouvie E, McCrady BS, Kahler CW, Frey RM. Affiliation with Alcoholics Anonymous after treatment: a study of its therapeutic effects and mechanisms of action. *J Consult Clin Psychol*. 1997;65(5): 768-777.
29. Tonigan JS, Bogenschutz MP, Miller WR. Is alcoholism typology a predictor of both Alcoholics Anonymous affiliation and disaffiliation after treatment? *J Subst Abus Treat*. 2006;30(4):323-330.
30. Hasin DS, Grant BF. AA and other helpseeking for alcohol problems: former drinkers in the U.S. general population. *J Subst Abus*. 1995; 7(3):281-292.
31. Humphreys K, Finney JW, Moos RH. Applying a stress and coping framework to research on mutual help organizations. *J Community Psychol*. 1994;22(4):312-327.
32. Project MATCH Research Group. Matching alcoholism treatments to client heterogeneity: Project MATCH posttreatment drinking outcomes. *J Stud Alcohol*. 1997;58(1):7-29.
33. Morey LC, Hopwood CJ. An IRT-based measure of alcohol trait severity and the role of traitedness in trait validity: a reanalysis of Project MATCH data. *Drug Alcohol Depend*. 2009;105(3):177-184.
34. Krentzman AR, Robinson EA, Perron BE, Cranford JA. Predictors of membership in Alcoholics Anonymous in a sample of successfully remitted alcoholics. *J Psychoactive Drugs*. 2011;43(1):20-26.
35. Humphreys K. Clinicians' referral and matching of substance abuse patients to self-help groups after treatment. *Psychiatr Serv*. 1997;48(11):1445-1449.
36. Winzelberg A, Humphreys K. Should patients' religiosity influence clinicians' referral to 12-step self-help groups? Evidence from a study of 3,018 male substance abuse patients. *J Consult Clin Psychol*. 1999; 67(5):790-794.
37. Tonigan JS, Miller WR, Schermer C. Atheists, agnostics and Alcoholics Anonymous. *J Stud Alcohol*. 2002;63(5):534-541.
38. Tómasson K, Vaglum P. Psychiatric co-morbidity and aftercare among alcoholics: a prospective study of a nationwide representative sample. *Addiction*. 1998;93(3):423-431.
39. Bogenschutz MP. 12-step approaches for the dually diagnosed: mechanisms of change. *Alcohol Clin Exp Res*. 2007;31(10 Suppl):64s-66s.
40. Jordan LC, Davidson WS, Herman SE, BootsMiller BJ. Involvement in 12-step programs among persons with dual diagnoses. *Psychiatr Serv*. 2002;53(7):894-896.

41. Moser J, Turk C, Glover J. The relationship between participation in Alcoholics Anonymous and social anxiety. *Psi Chi J Psychological Res.* 2015;20:97-101.
42. Timko C, Cronkite RC, McKellar J, Zemore S, Moos RH. Dually diagnosed patients' benefits of mutual-help groups and the role of social anxiety. *J Subst Abus Treat.* 2013;44(2):216-223.
43. Magura S, Rosenblum A, Villano CL, Vogel HS, Fong C, Betzler T. Dual-focus mutual aid for co-occurring disorders: a quasi-experimental outcome evaluation study. *Am J Drug Alcohol Abuse.* 2008;34(1):61-74.
44. Alcoholics Anonymous. *Twelve Steps and Twelve Traditions.* Alcoholics Anonymous World Services; 1952.
45. Alcoholics Anonymous. 2014 Membership Survey. Accessed June 19, 2023. http://www.aa.org/assets/en_US/p-48_membershipsurvey.pdf
46. Timko C, Finney JW, Moos RH. The 8-year course of alcohol abuse: gender differences in social context and coping. *Alcohol Clin Exp Res.* 2005;29(4):612-621.
47. Bodin M. Gender aspects of affiliation with Alcoholics Anonymous after treatment. *Contemp Drug Prob.* 2006;33(1):123-141.
48. Delboca FK, Mattson ME. The gender matching hypothesis. In: Longabaugh R, Wirtz PW, eds. *Project MATCH Hypotheses: Results and Causal Chain Analyses.* Project MATCH Monograph Series. National Institute on Alcohol Abuse and Alcoholism; 2002:223-238.
49. Kaskutas LA. What do women get out of self-help? Their reasons for attending Women for Sobriety and Alcoholics Anonymous. *J Subst Abus Treat.* 1994;11(3):185-195.
50. Ullman SE, Najdowski CJ, Adams EB. Women, Alcoholics Anonymous, and related mutual aid groups: review and recommendations for research. *Alcohol Treat Q.* 2012;30(4):443-486.
51. Bogart CJ, Pearce CE. "13th-Stepping": why Alcoholics Anonymous is not always a safe place for women. *J Addict Nurs.* 2003;14(1):43-47.
52. Zemore SE, Mulia N, Yu Y, Borges G, Greenfield TK. Gender, acculturation, and other barriers to alcohol treatment utilization among Latinos in three National Alcohol Surveys. *J Subst Abus Treat.* 2009;36(4):446-456.
53. Garcia A, Anderson B, Humphreys K. Fourth and fifth step groups: a new and growing self-help organization for underserved Latinos with substance use disorders. *Alcohol Treat Q.* 2015;33(2):235-243.
54. Tonigan JS, Miller WR, Juarez P, Villanueva M. Utilization of AA by Hispanic and non-Hispanic white clients receiving outpatient alcohol treatment. *J Stud Alcohol.* 2002;63(2):215-218.
55. Kaskutas LA, Weisner C, Lee M, Humphreys K. Alcoholics anonymous affiliation at treatment intake among white and black Americans. *J Stud Alcohol.* 1999;60(6):810-816.
56. Avalos LA, Mulia N. Formal and informal substance use treatment utilization and alcohol abstinence over seven years: is the relationship different for blacks and whites? *Drug Alcohol Depend.* 2012;121(1-2): 73-80.
57. Kelly JF, Eddie D. The role of spirituality and religiousness in aiding recovery from alcohol and other drug problems: an investigation in a National U.S. Sample. *Psycholog Relig Spiritual.* 2020;12(1):116-123.
58. Beals J, Novins DK, Spicer P, Whitesell NR, Mitchell CM, Manson SM. Help seeking for substance use problems in two American Indian reservation populations. *Psychiatr Serv.* 2006;57(4):512-520.
59. Villanueva M, Tonigan JS, Miller WR. Response of Native American clients to three treatment methods for alcohol dependence. *J Ethn Subst Abus.* 2007;6(2):41-48.
60. Kelly JF, Myers MG. Adolescents' participation in Alcoholics Anonymous and Narcotics Anonymous: review, implications and future directions. *J Psychoactive Drugs.* 2007;39(3):259-269.
61. Hohman M, LeCroy CW. Predictors of adolescent A. A affiliation. *Adolescence.* 1996;31(122):339-352.
62. Kelly JF, Myers MG, Brown SA. The effects of age composition of 12-step groups on adolescent 12-step participation and substance use outcome. *J Child Adolesc Subst Abuse.* 2005;15(1):63-72.
63. Kelly JF, Myers MG, Brown SA. Do adolescents affiliate with 12-step groups? A multivariate process model of effects. *J Stud Alcohol.* 2002;63(3):293-304.
64. Kelly JF, Yeterian J, Myers MG. Treatment staff referrals, participation expectations, and perceived benefits and barriers to adolescent involvement in 12-step groups. *Alcohol Treat Q.* 2008;26(4).
65. Kelly JF, Myers MG, Rodolico J. What do adolescents exposed to Alcoholics Anonymous think about 12-step groups? *Subst Abus.* 2008;29(2):53-62.
66. Labbe AK, Slaymaker V, Kelly JF. Toward enhancing 12-step facilitation among young people: a systematic qualitative investigation of young adults' 12-step experiences. *Subst Abus.* 2014;35(4):399-407.
67. Kingston S, Knight E, Williams J, Gordon H. How do young adults view 12-step programs? A qualitative study. *J Addict Dis.* 2015;34(4):311-322.
68. Bergman BG, Greene MC, Hoeppner BB, Slaymaker V, Kelly JF. Psychiatric comorbidity and 12-step participation: a longitudinal investigation of treated young adults. *Alcohol Clin Exp Res.* 2014;38(2):501-510.
69. Worley MJ, Tate SR, McQuaid JR, Granholm EL, Brown SA. 12-step affiliation and attendance following treatment for comorbid substance dependence and depression: a latent growth curve mediation model. *Subst Abus.* 2013;34(1):43-50.
70. Kelly JF, McKellar JD, Moos R. Major depression in patients with substance use disorders: relationship to 12-Step self-help involvement and substance use outcomes. *Addiction.* 2003;98(4):499-508.
71. Aase DM, Jason LA, Robinson WL. 12-step participation among dually-diagnosed individuals: a review of individual and contextual factors. *Clin Psychol Rev.* 2008;28(7):1235-1248.
72. Polcin DL, Zemore S. Psychiatric severity and spirituality, helping, and participation in alcoholics anonymous during recovery. *Am J Drug Alcohol Abuse.* 2004;30(3):577-592.
73. Alcoholics Anonymous World Services. *The AA Member—Medications and Other Drugs.* Alcoholics Anonymous World Services; 2006.
74. Rychtarik RG, Connors GJ, Dermen KH, Stasiewicz PR. Alcoholics Anonymous and the use of medications to prevent relapse: an anonymous survey of member attitudes. *J Stud Alcohol.* 2000;61(1): 134-138.
75. Swift RM, Duncan D, Nirenberg T, Femino J. Alcoholic patients' experience and attitudes on pharmacotherapy for alcoholism. *J Addict Dis.* 1998;17(3):35-47.
76. Tonigan JS, Kelly JF. Beliefs about AA and the use of medications: a comparison of three groups of AA-exposed alcohol dependent persons. *Alcohol Treat Q.* 2004;22(2):67-78.
77. Hall JM. The experiences of lesbians in Alcoholics Anonymous. *West J Nurs Res.* 1994;16(5):556-576.
78. Hill AB. The environment and disease: association or causation? *Proc R Soc Med.* 1965;58(5):295-300.
79. Kelly JF, Abry A, Ferri M, Humphreys K. Alcoholics Anonymous and 12-step facilitation treatments for alcohol use disorder: a distillation of a 2020 Cochrane review for clinicians and policy makers. *Alcohol Alcohol.* 2020;55(6):641-651.
80. Walitzer KS, Dermen KH, Barrick C. Facilitating involvement in Alcoholics Anonymous during out-patient treatment: a randomized clinical trial. *Addiction.* 2009;104(3):391-401.
81. Litt MD, Kadden RM, Kabela-Cormier E, Petry N. Changing network support for drinking: initial findings from the network support project. *J Consult Clin Psychol.* 2007;75(4):542-555.
82. Longabaugh R, Wirtz PW, Zweben A, Stout RL. Network support for drinking, Alcoholics Anonymous and long-term matching effects. *Addiction.* 1998;93(9):1313-1333.
83. Project MATCH Research Group. Project MATCH secondary a priori hypotheses. *Addiction.* 1997;92(12):1671-1698.
84. Project MATCH Research Group. Matching alcoholism treatments to client heterogeneity: treatment main effects and matching effects on drinking during treatment. *J Stud Alcohol.* 1998;59(6):631-639.
85. Project MATCH Research Group. Matching alcoholism treatments to client heterogeneity: Project MATCH three-year drinking outcomes. *Alcohol Clin Exp Res.* 1998;22(6):1300-1311.
86. Litt MD, Kadden RM, Kabela-Cormier E, Petry NM. Changing network support for drinking: network support project 2-year follow-up. *J Consult Clin Psychol.* 2009;77(2):229-242.

87. Kaskutas LA, Subbaraman MS, Witbrodt J, Zemore SE. Effectiveness of Making Alcoholics Anonymous Easier: a group format 12-step facilitation approach. *J Subst Abus Treat.* 2009;37(3):228-239.
88. McCrady BS, Epstein EE, Hirsch LS. Maintaining change after conjoint behavioral alcohol treatment for men: outcomes at 6 months. *Addiction.* 1999;94(9):1381-1396.
89. McCrady BS, Epstein EE, Kahler CW. Alcoholics anonymous and relapse prevention as maintenance strategies after conjoint behavioral alcohol treatment for men: 18-month outcomes. *J Consult Clin Psychol.* 2004;72(5):870-878.
90. Moos RH, Finney JW, Ouimette PC, Suchinsky RT. A comparative evaluation of substance abuse treatment: I. Treatment orientation, amount of care, and 1-year outcomes. *Alcohol Clin Exp Res.* 1999;23(3): 529-536.
91. Ouimette PC, Finney JW, Moos RH. Twelve-step and cognitive-behavioral treatment for substance abuse: a comparison of treatment effectiveness. *J Consult Clin Psychol.* 1997;65(2):230-240.
92. Ouimette PC, Finney JW, Gima K, Moos RH. A comparative evaluation of substance abuse treatment III. Examining mechanisms underlying patient-treatment matching hypotheses for 12-step and cognitive-behavioral treatments for substance abuse. *Alcohol Clin Exp Res.* 1999;23(3):545-551.
93. Hoffmann N, Miller N. Treatment outcomes for abstinence based programs. *Psychiatr Ann.* 1992;22:402-408.
94. Stinchfield R, Owen P. Hazelden's model of treatment and its outcome. *Addict Behav.* 1998;23(5):669-683.
95. Fortney J, Booth B, Zhang M, Humphrey J, Wiseman E. Controlling for selection bias in the evaluation of Alcoholics Anonymous as aftercare treatment. *J Stud Alcohol.* 1998;59(6):690-697.
96. Johnsen E, Herringer LG. A note on the utilization of common support activities and relapse following substance abuse treatment. *J Psychol.* 1993;127(1):73-77.
97. Tonigan JS. Benefits of Alcoholics Anonymous attendance: replication of findings between clinical research sites in Project MATCH. *Alcohol Treat Q.* 2001;19(1):67-77.
98. Kelly JF, Stout R, Zywiak W, Schneider R. A 3-year study of addiction mutual-help group participation following intensive outpatient treatment. *Alcohol Clin Exp Res.* 2006;30(8):1381-1392.
99. Gossop M, Stewart D, Marsden J. Attendance at Narcotics Anonymous and Alcoholics Anonymous meetings, frequency of attendance and substance use outcomes after residential treatment for drug dependence: a 5-year follow-up study. *Addiction.* 2008;103(1):119-125.
100. Chi FW, Sterling S, Campbell CI, Weisner C. 12-step participation and outcomes over 7 years among adolescent substance use patients with and without psychiatric comorbidity. *Subst Abus.* 2013;34(1):33-42.
101. McKellar J, Stewart E, Humphreys K. Alcoholics anonymous involvement and positive alcohol-related outcomes: cause, consequence, or just a correlate? A prospective 2-year study of 2,319 alcohol-dependent men. *J Consult Clin Psychol.* 2003;71(2):302-308.
102. Magura S, Cleland CM, Tonigan JS. Evaluating Alcoholics Anonymous's effect on drinking in Project MATCH using cross-lagged regression panel analysis. *J Stud Alcohol Drugs.* 2013;74(3):378-385.
103. Humphreys K, Blodgett JC, Wagner TH. Estimating the efficacy of Alcoholics Anonymous without self-selection bias: an instrumental variables re-analysis of randomized clinical trials. *Alcohol Clin Exp Res.* 2014;38(11):2688-2694.
104. Delucchi KL, Kaskutas LA. Following problem drinkers over eleven years: understanding changes in alcohol consumption. *J Stud Alcohol Drugs.* 2010;71(6):831-836.
105. Kahler CW, Read JP, Ramsey SE, Stuart GL, McCrady BS, Brown RA. Motivational enhancement for 12-step involvement among patients undergoing alcohol detoxification. *J Consult Clin Psychol.* 2004;72(4):736-741.
106. Blondell RD, Frydrych LM, Jaanimagi U, et al. A randomized trial of two behavioral interventions to improve outcomes following inpatient detoxification for alcohol dependence. *J Addict Dis.* 2011;30(2):136-148.
107. Emrick CD, Tonigan JS, Montgomery H, Little L. Alcoholics Anonymous: what is currently known? In: BS MC, Miller WR, eds. *Research on Alcoholics Anonymous: Opportunities and Alternatives.* Rutgers Center on Alcohol Studies; 1993:41-76.
108. Tonigan JS, Rice SL. Is it beneficial to have an alcoholics anonymous sponsor? *Psychol Addict Behav.* 2010;24(3):397-403.
109. Montgomery HA, Miller WR, Tonigan JS. Does Alcoholics Anonymous involvement predict treatment outcome? *J Subst Abus Treat.* 1995;12(4): 241-246.
110. Majer JM, Jason LA, Aase DM, Droege JR, Ferrari JR. Categorical 12-step involvement and continuous abstinence at 2 years. *J Subst Abus Treat.* 2013;44(1):46-51.
111. Tonigan JS, Miller WR, Connors GJ. Project MATCH client impressions about Alcoholics Anonymous: measurement issues and relationship treatment outcome. *Alcohol Treat Q.* 2000;18(1):25-41.
112. Greenfield BL, Tonigan JS. The general alcoholics anonymous tools of recovery: the adoption of 12-step practices and beliefs. *Psychol Addict Behav.* 2013;27(3):553-561.
113. Weiss RD, Griffin ML, Najavits LM, et al. Self-help activities in cocaine dependent patients entering treatment: results from NIDA collaborative cocaine treatment study. *Drug Alcohol Depend.* 1996;43(1-2):79-86.
114. Zemore SE, Subbaraman M, Tonigan JS. Involvement in 12-step activities and treatment outcomes. *Subst Abus.* 2013;34(1):60-69.
115. Pagano ME, Friend KB, Tonigan JS, Stout R. Sponsoring others in Alcoholics Anonymous and avoiding a drink in the first year following treatment: findings from Project MATCH. *J Stud Alcohol.* 2004;65: 766-773.
116. Witbrodt J, Kaskutas LA. Does diagnosis matter? Differential effects of 12-step participation and social networks on abstinence. *Am J Drug Alcohol Abuse.* 2005;31(4):685-707.
117. Gomes K, Hart KE. Adherence to recovery practices prescribed by Alcoholics Anonymous: benefits to sustained abstinence and subjective quality of life. *Alcohol Treat Q.* 2009;27(2):223-235.
118. Kingree JB, Thompson M. Participation in Alcoholics Anonymous and post-treatment abstinence from alcohol and other drugs. *Addict Behav.* 2011;36(8):882-885.
119. Pagano ME, Zemore SE, Onder CC, Stout RL. Predictors of initial AA-related helping: findings from project MATCH. *J Stud Alcohol Drugs.* 2009;70(1):117-125.
120. Subbaraman MS, Kaskutas LA, Zemore S. Sponsorship and service as mediators of the effects of Making Alcoholics Anonymous Easier (MAAEZ), a 12-step facilitation intervention. *Drug Alcohol Depend.* 2011;116(1-3):117-124.
121. Stevens EB, Jason LA. An exploratory investigation of important qualities and characteristics of Alcoholics Anonymous sponsors. *Alcohol Treat Q.* 2015;33(4):367-384.
122. Stevens EB, Jason LA. Evaluating alcoholics anonymous sponsor attributes using conjoint analysis. *Addict Behav.* 2015;51:12-17.
123. Kelly JF, Greene MC, Bergman BG. Recovery benefits of the "therapeutic alliance" among 12-step mutual-help organization attendees and their sponsors. *Drug Alcohol Depend.* 2016;162:64-71.
124. Tonigan JS, Miller WR. AA practicing subtypes: are there multiple AA fellowships? *Alcohol Clin Exp Res.* 2005;295(suppl):384.
125. Tonigan JS, Miller WR. The relative importance of pretreatment characteristics in predicting AA participation 10 years after treatment. *Alcohol Clin Exp Res.* 2004;285(suppl):135.
126. Humphreys K, Noke JM. The influence of posttreatment mutual help group participation on the friendship networks of substance abuse patients. *Am J Community Psychol.* 1997;25(1):1-16.
127. Kaskutas LA, Bond J, Humphreys K. Social networks as mediators of the effect of Alcoholics Anonymous. *Addiction.* 2002;97(7):891-900.
128. Stout RL, Kelly JF, Magill M, Pagano ME. Association between social influences and drinking outcomes across three years. *J Stud Alcohol Drugs.* 2012;73(3):489-497.
129. Kelly JF, Stout RL, Magill M, Tonigan JS. The role of Alcoholics Anonymous in mobilizing adaptive social network changes: a prospective lagged mediational analysis. *Drug Alcohol Depend.* 2011;114(2-3):119-126.

130. Kelly JF, Hoeppner B, Stout RL, Pagano M. Determining the relative importance of the mechanisms of behavior change within Alcoholics Anonymous: a multiple mediator analysis. *Addiction.* 2012;107(2): 289-299.
131. Subbaraman MS, Kaskutas LA. Social support and comfort in AA as mediators of "Making AA easier" (MAAEZ), a 12-step facilitation intervention. *Psychol Addict Behav.* 2012;26(4):759-765.
132. Alcoholics Anonymous World Services. *Alcoholics Anonymous.* 4th ed. Alcoholics Anonymous World Services; 1992.
133. Alcoholics Anonymous World Services. *Twelve Steps and Twelve Traditions.* Alcoholics Anonymous World Services; 1981.
134. Connors GJ, Tonigan JS, Miller WR. A measure of religious background and behavior for use in behavior change research. *Psychol Addict Behav.* 1996;10(2):90-96.
135. Pargament KI, Kennell J, Hathaway W, Grevengoed N, Newman J, Jones W. Religion and the problem-solving process: three styles of coping. *J Sci Study Relig.* 1988;27(1):90-104.
136. Fetzer Institute. *Multidimensional Measurement of Religiousness/Spirituality for Use in Health Research.* John E. Fetzer Institute; 1999.
137. Underwood LG, Teresi JA. The daily spiritual experience scale: development, theoretical description, reliability, exploratory factor analysis, and preliminary construct validity using health-related data. *Ann Behav Med.* 2002;24(1):22-33.
138. Robinson EA, Cranford JA, Webb JR, Brower KJ. Six-month changes in spirituality, religiousness, and heavy drinking in a treatment-seeking sample. *J Stud Alcohol Drugs.* 2007;68(2):282-290.
139. Connors GJ, Tonigan JS, Miller WR. A longitudinal model of intake symptomatology, AA participation and outcome: retrospective study of the project MATCH outpatient and aftercare samples. *J Stud Alcohol.* 2001;62(6):817-825.
140. Tonigan JS, McCallion EA, Frohe T, Pearson MR. Lifetime Alcoholics Anonymous attendance as a predictor of spiritual gains in the Relapse Replication and Extension Project (RREP). *Psychol Addict Behav.* 2017;31(1):54-60.
141. Krentzman AR, Cranford JA, Robinson EA. Multiple dimensions of spirituality in recovery: a lagged mediational analysis of Alcoholics Anonymous' principal theoretical mechanism of behavior change. *Subst Abus.* 2013;34(1):20-32.
142. Tonigan JS, Rynes KN, McCrady BS. Spirituality as a change mechanism in 12-step programs: a replication, extension, and refinement. *Subst Use Misuse.* 2013;48(12):1161-1173.
143. Kelly JF, Stout RL, Magill M, Tonigan JS, Pagano ME. Spirituality in recovery: a lagged mediational analysis of alcoholics anonymous' principal theoretical mechanism of behavior change. *Alcohol Clin Exp Res.* 2011;35(3):454-463.
144. Christo G, Franey C. Drug users' spiritual beliefs, locus of control and the disease concept in relation to Narcotics Anonymous attendance and six-month outcomes. *Drug Alcohol Depend.* 1995;38(1):51-56.
145. Morgenstern J, Bates ME. Effects of executive function impairment on change processes and substance use outcomes in 12-step treatment. *J Stud Alcohol.* 1999;60(6):846-855.
146. Tonigan JS. Examination of the active ingredients of twelve-step facilitation (TSF) in the Project MATCH outpatient sample. *Alcohol Clin Exp Res.* 2005;29(2):240-241.
147. Finney JW, Noyes CA, Coutts AI, Moos RH. Evaluating substance abuse treatment process models: I. Changes on proximal outcome variables during 12-step and cognitive-behavioral treatment. *J Stud Alcohol.* 1998;59(4):371-380.
148. Finney JW, Moos RH, Humphreys K. A comparative evaluation of substance abuse treatment: II. Linking proximal outcomes of 12-step and cognitive-behavioral treatment to substance use outcomes. *Alcohol Clin Exp Res.* 1999;23(3):537-544.
149. Kelly JF, Myers MG, Brown SA. A multivariate process model of adolescent 12-step attendance and substance use outcome following inpatient treatment. *Psychol Addict Behav.* 2000;14(4):376-389.
150. Brown TG, Seraganian P, Tremblay J, Annis H. Process and outcome changes with relapse prevention versus 12-Step aftercare programs for substance abusers. *Addiction.* 2002;97(6):677-689.
151. Demmel R, Rist F. Prediction of treatment outcome in a clinical sample of problem drinkers: self-efficacy and coping style. *Addict Disord Treat.* 2005;4(1):5-10.
152. Magura S, Laudet AB, Mahmood D, Rosenblum A, Vogel HS, Knight EL. Role of self-help processes in achieving abstinence among dually diagnosed persons. *Addict Behav.* 2003;28(3):399-413.
153. Forcehimes AA, Tonigan JS. Self-efficacy as a factor in abstinence from alcohol/other drug abuse: a meta-analysis. *Alcohol Treat Q.* 2008;26(4):480-489.
154. Blonigen DM, Timko C, Finney JW, Moos BS, Moos RH. Alcoholics Anonymous attendance, decreases in impulsivity and drinking and psychosocial outcomes over 16 years: moderated-mediation from a developmental perspective. *Addiction.* 2011;106(12):2167-2177.
155. Blonigen DM, Timko C, Moos BS, Moos RH. Treatment, alcoholics anonymous, and 16-year changes in impulsivity and legal problems among men and women with alcohol use disorders. *J Stud Alcohol Drugs.* 2009;70(5):714-725.
156. Smith BW, Tonigan JS. Alcoholics Anonymous benefit and social attachment. *Alcohol Treat Q.* 2009;27(2):164-173.
157. Jenkins CO, Tonigan JS. Attachment avoidance and anxiety as predictors of 12-step group engagement. *J Stud Alcohol Drugs.* 2011;72(5):854-863.
158. Kelly JF, Stout RL, Magill M, Tonigan JS, Pagano ME. Mechanisms of behavior change in alcoholics anonymous: does Alcoholics Anonymous lead to better alcohol use outcomes by reducing depression symptoms? *Addiction.* 2010;105(4):626-636.
159. Tonigan JS, Rynes K, Toscova R, Hagler K. Do changes in selfishness explain 12-step benefit? A prospective lagged analysis. *Subst Abus.* 2013;34(1):13-19.
160. Kelly JF, Hoeppner BB. Does Alcoholics Anonymous work differently for men and women? A moderated multiple-mediation analysis in a large clinical sample. *Drug Alcohol Depend.* 2013;130(1-3):186-193.
161. Hoeppner BB, Hoeppner SS, Kelly JF. Do young people benefit from AA as much, and in the same ways, as adult aged 30+? A moderated multiple mediation analysis. *Drug Alcohol Depend.* 2014;143:181-188.
162. Bohart AC, Tallman K. *Clients Make Therapy Work: The Process of Active Self-healing.* American Psychological Association; 1999.
163. Kelly JF. Is Alcoholics Anonymous religious, spiritual, neither? Findings from 25 years of mechanisms of behavior change research. *Addiction.* 2017;112(6):929-936.
164. Horstmann MJ, Tonigan JS. Faith development in Alcoholics Anonymous (AA). *Alcohol Treat Q.* 2000;18(4):75-84.
165. Tonigan JS, Ashcroft F, Miller WR. AA group dynamics and 12-step activity. *J Stud Alcohol.* 1995;56(6):616-621.

CHAPTER

86

Spirituality in the Recovery Process

Marc Galanter

CHAPTER OUTLINE

- What is spirituality?
- AA as a spiritual recovery movement
- Conceptualizing addiction and recovery
- Recovery capital
- Spiritually grounded recovery in AA
- Neurobiology
- AA in the professional context

WHAT IS SPIRITUALITY?

Dictionaries define spirituality with phrases like "concerned with or affecting the soul," "not tangible or material," or "pertaining to God."[1] More broadly, it consists of the nonmaterial issues that give a person meaning and purpose in life; these not only can be found in a person's religious orientation but can also be seen in their ethnic heritage, altruism, humanism, or naturalism. Spirituality infuses some alternative medical therapies that are not grounded in empirical science but have gained popularity because they address symptoms like anxiety or depression. Given the prominence of Alcoholics Anonymous (AA) and related 12-step groups, it can play an important role in the rehabilitation of people with substance use disorders (SUDs).

The issue of spirituality is prominent within contemporary culture, as evidenced in a probability sampling of American adults, among whom 95% of respondents reply positively when asked if they believe in "God or a universal spirit." Responses to a follow-up question survey suggest that this belief affects the daily lives of the majority (51%) of those sampled, who indicated that they had talked to someone about God or some aspect of their faith or spirituality within the previous 24 hours.[2]

AA AS A SPIRITUAL RECOVERY MOVEMENT

How does spirituality relate to recovery from addiction? There is a parallel between the way attitudes are transformed in intensely zealous groups and the way the denial of illness and the self-defeating behaviors of people with SUD may be reversed through induction into 12-step groups like AA.

Members of the lay public may conclude that certain health care issues are inadequately addressed by the medical community, particularly when doctors are not sufficiently attentive to the emotional burden that an illness produces. When mutually supportive groups of laymen coalesce to implement a response to this perceived deficit, they may form a spiritual recovery movement,[3] one premised on achieving remission based on beliefs independent of evidence-based medicine. Such movements may ascribe their effectiveness to higher metaphysical or nonmaterial forces and claim to offer relief from illness.

AA can be considered as a highly successful example of a spiritual recovery movement, as such movements have three primary characteristics. They (1) claim to provide relief from disease; (2) operate outside the modalities of established empirical medicine; and (3) ascribe their effectiveness to higher metaphysical powers. The appeal of such movements in the contemporary period is due in part to the fact that physicians tend not to attend the spiritual or emotional concerns of their patients.[4]

Clearly, the attitudes and behavioral norms that AA espouses are much more in conformity with the values of the larger culture than those of zealous religious sects. The expectation of avoiding intoxication in AA, normative in our culture, illustrates this. People who are highly distressed over the consequences of their addiction are therefore candidates to respond to the strong ideological orientation of AA toward recovery and are operantly reinforced by the relief produced by affiliation with the group's ideology and behavioral norms, all related to abstinence and a spiritually grounded lifestyle. Significantly, AA generates distress in its members by pressing them to give up their use of addictive substances and the behaviors associated with them, but the distress associated with this conflict is relieved if they sustain affiliation and cleave to the group.

CONCEPTUALIZING ADDICTION AND RECOVERY

Two empirically grounded perspectives have played a material role in framing how we conceptualize recovery. One derived from a model of psychopathology modeled on the work of Emil Kraeplin.[5] He framed an approach that now characterizes the contemporary medical model for mental disorders, categorizing disease entities diagnosed on the basis of explicit and discrete symptoms. This approach is evident in the development of criteria for SUDs employed in recent editions of the symptom-based *Diagnostic and Statistical Manual of Mental Disorders*.[6] From this perspective, a state of remission, colloquially called recovery in rehabilitation circles, can take place with the resolution of the specific symptoms listed as diagnostic criteria. A second perspective on recovery derives from behavioral psychology, whose model of stimulus-response sequences has led to the ordering of experience around discrete phenomena that can be observed by a researcher or clinician. From this perspective, recovery can also be defined in terms of observable, measurable responses to substance use, lending credence to recovery as a process defined in behavioral terms.

Both perspectives are well suited to the study of psychopathology and have lent the addiction field approaches to studying addiction as a disorder, one that is compatible with research approaches employing experimental controls that are used in the physical and biological sciences. Both have, therefore, had heuristic value in promoting a research field that has yielded many advances in addiction treatment. There is a third perspective, however, that is defined on the basis of reports from people with SUDs of their own subjective experience. These experiences are not directly observable by the clinician, but are available only as reported through the prism of the person's own introspection and reflection. This model is more difficult to subject to measurement, but instruments are being developed that can be applied for its study, as will be discussed below. This approach is inherent in the spiritually oriented psychology of Carl Jung,[7] who had a direct influence on Bill W.'s framing of the Alcoholics Anonymous ethos.[8] William James,[9] often described as the father of American psychology, also discussed mental phenomena in terms of subjectively experienced mystical or spiritual experience. (In fact, he wrote that "the drunken consciousness is one bit of the mystic consciousness [p. 378].") The need for spiritual redemption was vital in the writings of Viktor Frankl, who wrote "Man's Search for Meaning,"[10] and has recently been espoused with regard to psychotherapy by William Miller.[11]

RECOVERY CAPITAL

This third perspective is related to the model of spiritually grounded recovery we discuss here, insofar as it emphasizes the achievement of meaningful or positive experiences, rather than a focus on observable, dysfunctional behaviors. This aspect of securing sustained recovery is included under the concept of "recovery capital." That describes the resources that people with addiction disorders can draw on. The term has been defined by the World Health Organization[12] as the internal and external resources available to an individual to promote a sustained recovery, including peer-based and culturally related support for discovering "meaning and purpose in life." In this respect, achieving an enhanced spiritual orientation can provide increased recovery capital, and the enhanced ability to sustain recovery from SUDs.

SPIRITUALLY GROUNDED RECOVERY IN AA

The relative role of spiritual experience in the 12-step recovery process has been investigated from a variety of perspectives, generally in relation to patients' experience in AA. Zemore[13] followed up a large sample of people who used substances 1 year after inpatient treatment and found that increases in spirituality contributed to the increment in total abstinence associated with 12-step involvement. Variations in the Twelve Step format are described below under Spirituality Without Theism. Our own experience is compatible with these findings, as we have found in multiple settings[14-16] that spirituality is integral to recovery in 12-step groups. This was particularly evident among long-term members.

The AA "program of recovery" is mentioned in numerous places in the Big Book, *Alcoholics Anonymous*,[17] and is associated there with terms such as "spiritual experience" and "spiritual awakening" and with working AA's Twelve Steps. Four of the steps include the word God, which is qualified "as we understood Him." Some clarity is lent to this latter phrase in the Big Book where it is pointed out that "with few exceptions, our members find that they have tapped an unsuspected inner resource, which they presently identify with their own conception of a Power greater than themselves" (p. 569-570). Flexibility on the issue of theistic belief is also made clear in one chapter that addresses any person with alcoholism "who feels he is an atheist or agnostic," encouraging their membership as well. The text points out for these members that even "We Agnostics ... had to face the fact that we must find a spiritual basis for life" (p. 44) in order to achieve recovery, implying therein the fellowship's distinction between spirituality and theistic religion.

Spirituality among long-term members is likely instrumental in sustaining the integrity of the fellowship itself. The prominence of spiritually committed long-term members at meetings and their availability to serve in the sponsorship role create readily available models for earnestly held sobriety. They serve as role models for believing commitment to the 12-step spiritual ethos to help newcomers achieve stabilization in membership. Nonetheless, some people attending NA meetings may find it hard to identify with the spiritual orientation of long-term members.

A spiritually grounded definition of recovery, however, can be useful as well. Such a concept relates to the importance of nondemographic subject factors, originally proposed as "quality of life" issues[18]—among which spirituality can be considered. In this context, a series of suitable criteria for "diagnosing" addiction could be developed. They could then be used to assess the spiritual aspect of recovery associated with the 12-step experience. Resolution of these issues could be considered as important to the spiritual aspect of recovery from addiction. A series of criteria could include items such as:

- Loss of sense of purpose due to excessive substance use.
- A feeling of inadequate social support because of one's addiction.
- Continued use of a substance while experiencing moral qualms over its consumption.
- Loss of the will to resist temptation when the substance is available.

Another aspect of the DSM format can be considered as well. The manual stipulates "course specifiers" of remission such as "on agonist therapy" and "in a controlled environment."

These are included because they are explanatory to the clinician. To them could be added "fully engaged in a program of Twelve-Step recovery," which would be equally explanatory to many clinicians. This option is supported by the outcome literature on AA overall, and in relation to medication assisted treatment as well.[19]

A methodology for defining recovery based on measurements like these may not have the same appeal to biomedically oriented clinicians as does the conventional symptom-based approach, as these measurements are based on self-report of the person's subjective state. Furthermore, the enthusiasm of newfound recovery may yield a Hawthorne effect. The biomedical format currently applied in diagnosis derives from the school of Kraeplin and subsequent investigators like those who developed the Feighner criteria[20] in the 1970s and then in the ensuing DSM system. Spiritual variables, however, have a lineage as well, from William James, Carl Jung, and Bill W.

Spirituality Without Theism

The AA Agnostica website has become a resource for people in Twelve-Step recovery who value the support and the fidelity that the fellowship provides its members but are not prepared to accept its commitment to a God, even if it is "*as we understood Him*." The website includes a citation from the book, *Alcoholics Anonymous Comes of Age*[21]: "We must remember that AA's steps are suggestions only. A belief in them is not at all a requirement for membership among us." The Agnostica website then lists a number of modified versions of the Steps, for example, "We came to believe and accept that we needed strengths beyond our awareness and resources" rather than "a Power greater than ourselves…"

The issue of agnosticism in AA is not a new one. As early as 1938, one member objected to God-related terminology in the Steps, and they were modified accordingly by adding the phrase "as we understood Him," and the mentions of God in the Steps were reduced from six to four, and the Seventh Step—"Humbly asked him to remove our shortcomings"—was modified by removing the phrase "on our knees." A chapter, "We Agnostics," was also added.

A key for validating the nontheistic AA groups can also be seen in the Twelve Traditions, AA's governing philosophy, which states that "the only requirement for AA membership is a desire to stop drinking" and no mention of accepting a Higher Power. *A History of Agnostic Groups in AA*[22] is available as an e-book.

While some members have gone the opposite way of liberalization, introducing the Lord's prayer in meetings, others have adopted a Buddhist outlook on the Steps. Unlike the Biblical prophets, Buddha is not seen as speaking for a supernatural creator, but rather leading people to a "right way of living." The AA General Service Conference has tried to define boundaries of the spirituality it espouses, and its policies were recently spelled out in one of its leaflets under the heading, *Many Paths to Spirituality*: "Many of us came to rely on a 'Higher Power', whether it was the collective power of A.A., the A.A. group itself, or some other entity, concept or being that helped us to stay sober… Many of us come from different belief systems and cultures, yet there has always been plenty of latitude in A.A. for members to practice whatever belief works best for them."[23]

NEUROBIOLOGY

There is a body of empirical study that suggests that there may be certain brain regions associated with spiritual (on related religions) experiences, as distinct from regions unrelated to spirituality.[24] This can be useful in considering the interface between the experience of spirituality and SUDs, as related neurobiological phenomena. The evidence emerging from such studies is preliminary, and based on studies with methodological constraints, but may be useful in characterizing this interface. In one illustrative study, subjects were engaged in guided imagery to achieve stress relaxation. Neural findings related to one of the conditions that was spiritually oriented in the study were found to be associated with a distinctive functional neural network.[25] The pattern of spiritual experience observed in this latter study was considered by the investigators to be useful for future study on a role of spirituality in recovery from compulsive behaviors.

Craving is a key aspect of SUD. Neurophysiologically related studies of experimentally induced subjective responses may reflect on circumstances that generate craving. They may relate to either modifying or suppressing sensory input. Schienle and colleagues[26] monitored resting state functional activity of religious subjects who believed in the healing aspects of visits to Lourdes. The subjects were asked to describe the sensations experienced with sacred water labeled as originating in Lourdes. Their responses to tap water labeled as coming from Lourdes were compared to those for tap water with no such label. The former samples generated a distinct pattern of subjective sensations associated with neurophysiologically related measurements. In another study, responses were compared to pain stimulation where religious subjects were exposed to either religious or neutral stimuli. Analgesic responses associated with religious imagery were compared to responses to neutral imagery, and the two neurophysiologically measured patterns were distinguishable on functional magnetic resonance.[27]

Findings related to spiritual aspects of personal prayer can also be informative. Recitation of prayer by self-identified religious subjects was found in one study to generate specific patterns of neural activation suggestive of related cognitive processes.[28] In another study, a distinction between formalized and improvised prayer was observed in respective patterns of neural response.[29] In one experimental setting, long term AA members were presented with alcohol related stimuli. They experienced lower craving responses with a distinct neural response pattern when reciting Twelve Step-related prayer, as compared to when they recited neutral text passages.[30]

Neural patterns associated with affect may be considered to reflect on the correlates of the subjective experience, such as craving, as illustrated in two studies on persons with genetically based risk for depression. Miller and colleagues[31] studied individuals at high familial risk for developing depressive illness. They found that a relationship between higher importance of religiosity/spirituality among subjects was related to greater cortical thickness, which they reported to be associated with lower risk of depressive illness. Similarly, Panier et al.[32] followed up on EEG patterns over 5 to 10 years on subjects at familial risk for depressive disorders and found that the personal importance of religiosity/spirituality was associated with a lesser incidence of future depression.

Each of such studies, respectively, may not be considered suggestive of biologically based association of spirituality and its relationship with SUDs. As a group, however, they suggest that further investigation along the lines presented here may be useful for understanding neural mechanisms operating in this domain.

AA IN THE PROFESSIONAL CONTEXT

The spiritually oriented 12-step approach has been integrated into professional treatment in some settings where it serves as the overriding philosophy of an entire program or, in others, where it is one aspect of a multimodal eclectic approach. The Minnesota Model for treatment, typically located in an isolated institutional setting, is characterized by an intensive inpatient stay during which a primary goal of treatment is to acculturate patients to acceptance of the philosophy of AA and to continue with AA attendance after discharge.[33] Although a variety of exercises are included during the stay, this approach has been criticized as dogmatic because of its sole reliance on the 12-step approach. The outcome of this model, however, has been shown to yield positive results in a survey of patients discharged from one such setting (Hazelden, in Center City, MN),[34] but randomization of patients treated in Minnesota Model facilities with those treated by means of an alternative approach is needed.

A more eclectic option is illustrated in the integration of 12-step groups into a general psychiatric facility for the treatment of patients diagnosed with co-occurring major mental illness and SUDs. The importance of spirituality in such a highly compromised population was evidenced in our studies[35] in which such patients ranked spiritual issues like belief in God and inner peace higher than tangible benefits like social service support and outpatient treatment. One inherent advantage of this format is that it benefits from the introduction of an inspirational approach to patients who, as Goffman[36] has pointed out, have become "degraded" by stigmatization due to their psychiatric disorders.

In summary, spirituality is a matter of personal meaning that is widely accepted. It is also central to the recovery process from addiction for many members of Twelve-Step fellowships. The fellowship of AA, in fact, can be considered a movement developed in relation to people's spiritual needs. Although spirituality is subjectively experienced, it can be assessed systematically in given individuals by employing currently available empirical techniques. By such means, an important aspect of addiction recovery can be defined and studied.

REFERENCES

1. Morris W, ed. *The American Heritage Dictionary of the English Language*. American Heritage Publishing Co. Inc, and Houghton Mifflin Company; 1970.
2. Gallup GH. *Religion in America 2002*. Princeton Religious Research Center; 2002.
3. Galanter M. Spiritual recovery movements and contemporary medical care. *Psychiatry*. 1997;60:236-248.
4. Galanter M. *Spirituality and the Healthy Mind: Science, Therapy and the Need for Personal Meaning*. Oxford University Press; 2005.
5. Kraeplin E. *Clinical Psychiatry: A Textbook for Students and Physicians*. Macmillan; 1902.
6. American Psychiatric Association. *Diagnostic and Statistical Manual of Mental Disorders*. 4th ed. Text Revision. American Psychiatric Association; 2000.
7. Jung C. Instinct and unconscious. In: Read H, Fordham M, Adler G, et al., eds. *The Collected Works of C.B. Jung*. Princeton University Press; 1978.
8. Cheever S. *My name is Bill: Bill Wilson—His Life and the Creation of Alcoholics Anonymous*. Simon & Schuster; 2004.
9. James W. *The Varieties of Religious Experience*. Modern Library; 1929.
10. Frankl V. *Man's Search for Meaning*. 3rd ed. Touchstone, Simon & Schuster; 1984.
11. Miller WR, ed. *Integrating Spirituality into Treatment*. American Psychological Association; 1999.
12. The United Nations Office on Drugs and Crime. *International Standards for the Treatment of Drug Use Disorders 2017*. Accessed May 10, 2020. https://www.who.int/publications/i/item/international-standards-for-the-treatment-of-drug-use-disorders
13. Zemore SE. A role for spiritual change in the benefits of 12-Step involvement. *Alcohol Clin Exp Res*. 2007;31:76S-79S.
14. Galanter M, Dermatis H, Stanievich J, Santucci C. Physicians in long-term recovery who are members of Alcoholics Anonymous. *Am J Addict*. 2013;22:323-328.
15. Galanter M, Dermatis H, Santucci C. Young people in alcoholics anonymous: the role of spiritual orientation and AA member affiliation. *J Addict Dis*. 2012;31:173-182.
16. Galanter M, Dermatis H, Post S, Sampson C. Spirituality-based recovery from drug addiction in the twelve-step fellowship of narcotics anonymous. *J Addict Med*. 2013;7:189-195.
17. Alcoholics Anonymous World Services. *Alcoholics Anonymous: The Story of How Many Thousands of Men and Women Have Recovered from Alcoholism*. Alcoholics Anonymous Publishing Inc; 1955.
18. Campbell A, Converse PE, Rogers WL. *The Quality of American Life*. Russell Sage Foundation; 1976.
19. Monico LB. Buprenorphine treatment and 12-step meeting attendance: conflicts, compatibilities, and patient outcomes. *J Subst Abuse Treat*. 2015;57:89-95.
20. Feighner JP, Robins E, Guze SB, Woodruff RA Jr, Winokur G, Munoz R. Diagnostic criteria for use in psychiatric research. *Arch Gen Psychiatry*. 1972;26:57-63.
21. Alcoholics Anonymous. *Alcoholics Anonymous Comes of Age*. Alcoholics Anonymous Publishing; 1957.
22. Roger C. *A History of Agnostic Groups in AA*. AA Agnostica; 2012.
23. Alcoholics Anonymous World Services. *Many Paths to Spirituality*. Alcoholics Anonymous Publishing; 2014.
24. Rim JI, Ojeda JC, Svob C, et al. Current understanding of religion, spirituality, and their neurobiological correlates. *Harv Rev Psychiatry*. 2019;27(5):303-316.

25. McClintock CH, Worhunsky PD, Xu J, et al. Spiritual experiences are related to engagement of a ventral frontotemporal functional brain network: implications for prevention and treatment of behavioral and substance addictions. *J Behav Addict*. 2019;8(4):678-691.
26. Schienle A, Gremsl A, Wabnegger A. Placebo effects in the context of religious beliefs and practices: a resting-state functional connectivity study. *Front Behav Neurosci*. 2021;15:653359.
27. Wiech K, Farias M, Kahane G, et al. An fMRI study measuring analgesia enhanced by religion as a belief system. *Pain*. 2008;139(2):467-476.
28. Azari NP, Nickel J, Wunderlich G, et al. Neural correlates of religious experience. *Eur J Neurosci*. 2001;13(8):1649-1652.
29. Schjøedt U, Stødkilde-Jørgensen H, Geertz AW, Roepstorff A. Highly religious participants recruit areas of social cognition in personal prayer. *Soc Cogn Affect Neurosci*. 2009;4(2):199-207.
30. Galanter M, Josipovic Z, Dermatis H, Weber J, Millard MA. An initial fMRI study on neural correlates of prayer in members of Alcoholics Anonymous. *Am J Drug Alcohol Abuse*. 2017;43:44-54.
31. Miller L, Bansal R, Wickramaratne P, et al. Neuroanatomical correlates of religiosity and spirituality: a study in adults at high and low familial risk for depression. *JAMA Psychiatry*. 2014;71(2):128-135.
32. Panier LYX, Bruder GE, Svob C, et al. Predicting depression symptoms in families at risk for depression: interrelations of posterior EEG alpha and religion/spirituality. *J Affect Disord*. 2020;274:969-976.
33. Cook CCH. The Minnesota Model in the management of drug and alcohol dependency: miracle, method or myth? Part II: evidence and conclusions. *Br J Addict*. 1988;83:735-748.
34. Stinchfield R, Owen P. Hazelden's model of treatment and its outcome. *Addict Behav*. 1998;23:669-683.
35. Galanter M, Dermatis H, Bunt G, Williams C, Trujillo M, Steinke P. Assessment of spirituality and its relevance to addiction treatment. *J Subst Abuse Treat*. 2007;33:257-264.
36. Goffman E. *Stigma*. Simon & Schuster; 1963.

SECTION

11

Medical Disorders and Complications of Addiction

Associate Editor: Sarah E. Wakeman
Lead Section Editor: Darius A. Rastegar
Section Editors: Anika Alvanzo and Paula Lum

CHAPTER

87 Medical Care of Patients With Unhealthy Substance Use

Darius A. Rastegar

CHAPTER OUTLINE

- Introduction
- Primary and preventive care
- Substance use and treatment of other medical conditions
- Care during hospitalization
- Older adults
- Medical complications related to substance use
- Conclusions

INTRODUCTION

Persons with unhealthy substance use often do not receive regular health care and their care can be fragmented. As a result, they may miss opportunities to receive primary and preventive health care. In addition to the direct effects of intoxication, overdose, and withdrawal, substances can affect every body system. Unhealthy substance use may also be associated with behaviors that place individuals at risk of complications that are not a direct consequence of the substance used.

Regular health care can improve the health of persons who use substances and can be accessed at general medical or addiction treatment sites. This introductory chapter reviews primary and preventive care, care during medical or surgical hospitalization and complications in older adults. This is followed by an overview of the wide range of health complications associated with substance use, focusing on the most common and serious, by organ system, substance, and route of use. The following chapters in this section provide more detailed discussion of medical complications.

PRIMARY AND PREVENTIVE CARE

Preventive care for healthy adults and issues specific to persons with unhealthy substance use are presented herein because any health care contact is an opportunity for patients to obtain routine and preventive care. While substance use care and primary care have traditionally been segregated from one another, there is growing evidence that integration can improve substance use and general medical outcomes. Integration has many potential benefits, including improved prevention, identification and management of chronic conditions, coordination of other health care services, and providing substance use disorder treatment and recovery support.[1] Chapter 48 of this textbook "Linking Addiction Treatment with Other Medical and Psychiatric Treatment Systems" covers linkage of addiction treatment with other medical and psychiatric treatment systems.

Historically, preventive health care meant a thorough periodic evaluation focused on examination and testing. Despite the fact that many in the general public, including physicians, tend to believe in extensive checkups "to make sure everything is OK," preventive care expert panels recommend targeted evaluations based on age and other risk factors. The rationale for this is based on the notion that time and resources are limited and, perhaps more importantly, the recognition that recommended preventive care can result not only in benefit but in harm (eg, a perforated colon from a colonoscopy). In addition, some preventive testing predicted to offer health benefit has been shown to offer no benefit when evaluated in clinical trials (eg, screening exercise stress testing in asymptomatic individuals) or to result in "overdiagnosis": identification of conditions without clinical significance that must nonetheless be addressed (eg, breast or prostate premalignancy or early malignancies that would never manifest clinically). The approach presented here follows a targeted strategy based on the known effectiveness of interventions. Though disagreements exist among organizations (and their guidelines) regarding some details, most agree on which diseases should be identified during their preclinical stages.

Medical History

The medical history in a person who uses substances should include the categories of assessment employed for all patients, such as *current complaints* and the *history of present illness*, *allergies*, *systems review* (including any symptoms of conditions that could be related to substance use), *medications* (including over-the-counter and alternative products [including cannabinoids used as treatment]), and *past medical and surgical history*. Questions regarding past history should address hospitalizations and any medical conditions (eg, cardiovascular, pulmonary, hepatic, renal, or neurological diseases and specific illnesses such as cellulitis, pneumonia, hepatitis) that are associated with substance use and might not be volunteered by the patient without direct questions. The *social and family history* is of particular importance. Queries should be made to understand the current living, work, and financial situation, support system, and travel history.

When gathering a history, the clinician must be mindful of the fact that many patients have experienced trauma in the form of violence, abuse, neglect or stigma and that these experiences are associated with mental disorders and substance use disorders (SUDs). A trauma-informed approach can help to mitigate these harms; one way of formulating this approach is the four "R's": *realizing* the widespread impact of trauma, including its role in SUDs, *recognizing* the signs and symptoms of trauma, *responding* by integrating knowledge about trauma into policies, procedures and practices and actively *resisting* re-traumatization.[2]

In an asymptomatic person who uses substances, in addition to a thorough alcohol, tobacco, and other drug use history, historical items relevant to preventive care become more of the focus. These assessments should include a review of sexual practices, including condom and contraceptive use; dental care; diet; physical activity; falls; use of seatbelts when in vehicles; use of helmets when riding a bicycle or motorcycle; presence of a firearm and smoke detector in the household; and opioid overdose education and naloxone distribution for households where opioids are used or kept. These assessments are recommended because they can lead to counseling interventions. Screening for depression and anxiety, assessment of sexual practices, intention to conceive a child, and behavior that might lead to injury—including intimate partner violence (IPV) screening of all persons of childbearing age and being alert for signs of IPV in others—are particularly important. Such patients should be asked specifically about substance use before operating a motor vehicle, riding with intoxicated drivers, and sexual encounters.

In addition, a thorough history must include past immunizations or chemoprophylaxis (eg, for tuberculosis). People with heavy alcohol use are at risk of folate deficiency; this is of particular importance for persons of childbearing age, because of the risk of fetal neural tube defects. Additional history can determine if the patient belongs to a high-risk group that would indicate additional preventive interventions. For example, patients should be asked about chronic medical illnesses, whether they have housing instability, live or have lived in an institutional setting, contact with active cases of tuberculosis, recency of immigration, cardiovascular risk factors (smoking, cholesterol elevation, family history of heart disease, and diabetes), history or family history of cancer, travel patterns, receipt of blood products, drug injection, food insecurity and occupation.

Physical Examination

Physical examination on an initial encounter should at the minimum address body systems related to any reported symptoms; some clinicians may choose to perform a comprehensive examination.

Vital Signs and Measurements

In asymptomatic persons, height, weight, and blood pressure and pulse assessments should be performed. The height and weight should be used to determine the body mass index and assess nutritional status. Pulse oximetry can be useful for symptomatic patients or those with chronic lung disease.

Skin

Skin examination can reveal signs of injection drug use, the facial wrinkles associated with tobacco use, or the palmar erythema associated with alcohol-related liver disease. For patients who are injecting drugs, it can be helpful to ask them where they inject because it may be in locations that may not otherwise be examined (eg, the groin or buttocks).

Head, Eyes, Ears, Nose, and Throat

On examination of the oral cavity, clinicians should be alert to the possibility that people who smoke or drink heavily may have premalignant and malignant oral cavity lesions to which they are particularly susceptible, synergistically. Tobacco-stained teeth can serve as a focus for discussion. The oral examination may also find tooth decay associated with methamphetamine use.

Chest/Cardiovascular

Particular attention should be paid to auscultation for cardiac murmurs that may be evidence of past valvular damage from injection drug use. Cardiac auscultation can also detect the irregular heartbeat of atrial fibrillation, which may be associated with alcohol use.

Abdomen

Examination of the liver is advisable, if only to draw attention to the many possible complications of alcohol and other drug use. Asymptomatic persons can have the small hard liver of cirrhosis or the enlarged liver of chronic viral or alcohol-related hepatitis. People who smoke tobacco may have a palpable aortic aneurysm.

Breast

There is no evidence that routine breast examination for adult women (including transgender women receiving gender-affirming hormone therapy) reduces breast cancer mortality though it does lead to further assessments and biopsies. Most masses detected in young women will be benign but may require investigation once detected to rule out malignancy.

Genitalia

Testicular examination and rectal and prostate examinations for males (to screen for cancers) are recommended by some specialty organizations though their value is uncertain at best (they miss most cancers and most abnormalities detected are not cancer).

For females, a pelvic examination without testing (eg, for cervical cancer) is not routinely indicated, unless an individual is describing symptoms or recent exposures, which may increase the risk of sexually transmitted infections.

Lymph Nodes

Persons who use substances should have the cervical, axillary, supraclavicular, and inguinal lymph node regions examined for lymphadenopathy. Tuberculosis, chancroid, syphilis, and HIV are more common in persons with unhealthy substance use who present with lymphadenopathy. Supraclavicular adenopathy can be the presenting sign of lung or gastrointestinal cancers in people who smoke tobacco.

Neurologic

Brief cognitive assessments can be useful particularly in veterans and the elderly in whom traumatic brain injury or mild cognitive impairment or dementia may need management and may be complicated by substance use.

Screening Tests

Table 87-1 provides a summary of selected preventive measures recommended by the U.S. Preventive Services Task Force (USPSTF). Updates and additional details can be accessed at www.USPreventiveServicesTaskForce.org.

Because people with unhealthy substance use are at risk for many medical illnesses, by various mechanisms, across organ systems and because some tests are widely available and relatively inexpensive, it is reasonable for them to have a complete blood count, blood glucose, serum creatinine, liver enzymes, and urinalysis at least once and at regular intervals guided by risks and symptoms.

Routine preventive care for all includes tests for cardiovascular risk. All males aged 35 years and older and females and younger adults at increased cardiovascular risk (eg, smoking) should be screened with serum total cholesterol and high-density lipoprotein. A fasting lipid profile could identify hypertriglyceridemia, which is associated with heavy drinking and can cause pancreatitis. Primary prevention in high-risk patients with hyperlipidemia can decrease the risk of heart

TABLE 87-1 Summary of Select Preventative Care Measures Recommended by the U.S. Preventive Services Task Force[a]

Condition (Method)	Interval	Population
Cancer and other disease screening		
Breast cancer (mammogram)	Every 2 y	Females aged 50-74 y
Cervical cancer (cervical cytology or HPV testing)	Every 3-5 y	Females aged 21-65 y
Colorectal cancer (stool test or direct visualization)	Every 1-10 y	All adults aged 45-75
Lung cancer (low-dose computed tomography)	Yearly	All adults aged 50-80 with ≥20 pack-year history and currently smoke or have quit within 15 y
Abdominal aortic aneurysm (ultrasonography)	One time	Males aged 65-75 who ever smoked
Screening for infection		
Chlamydia and Gonorrhea		All sexually active females aged 24 or younger and females 25 y or older at increased risk
Hepatitis B		All persons at increased risk, all pregnant persons
Hepatitis C		All adults aged 18-79
HIV		Adolescents and adults aged 15-65, all pregnant persons
Syphilis		All persons at increased risk, all pregnant persons
Latent TB		All persons at increased risk
Screening/counseling		
Tobacco		All adults, pregnant persons
Unhealthy alcohol use		All adults aged 18 y or older
Unhealthy drug use		All adults aged 18 y or older

[a]Refer to guidelines for updates and further details.

Source: From U.S. Preventive Services Task Force Recommendation Topics. Accessed April 1, 2022. https://www.uspreventiveservicestaskforce.org/uspstf/recommendation-topics

disease and death. Online risk calculators (eg, https://static.heart.org/riskcalc/app/index.html#!/baseline-risk) can help guide the decision on when to recommend treatment.

Hematological testing for preventive purposes includes a hemoglobin and a mean corpuscular volume (MCV). An unsuspected anemia or pancytopenia may be found in persons with alcohol use disorder or HIV.

Sexually Transmitted Infections

The USPSTF and CDC recommend screening females aged 24 and younger who are sexually active and older female patients at high risk for chlamydia with urine or vaginal swab and gonorrhea with vaginal culture or urine or vaginal swab. The CDC recommends that male patients who practice receptive anal intercourse and oral sex should have testing at sites of contact and that rectal testing for chlamydia be considered for female patients based on sexual behaviors and exposures. For transgender and gender diverse persons, the CDC recommends screening based on anatomy and sexual behaviors/exposures.[3]

The USPSTF and CDC recommend that all pregnant people, all people aged 15 to 65 years, and any others at high risk (men who have sex with men, injection drug use, other sexually transmitted infections) be tested for HIV.

The CDC recommends syphilis testing for all pregnant people, men who have sex with men and others at high risk based on risk behaviors and local epidemiology. Testing for syphilis involves a combination of treponemal and nontreponemal tests; the traditional algorithm is to perform a nontreponemal test (eg, RPR or VDRL) first followed by a treponemal test to confirm. Some laboratories use a "reverse sequence algorithm" with a treponemal immunoassay followed by a nontreponemal test and titer.

Other Infectious Diseases

Screening for latent tuberculosis is recommended for high-risk individuals, including: those with household contacts or recent exposure to an active case, mycobacteriology laboratory personnel, immigrants from high-burden countries, and residents (and employees) of high-risk congregate settings. Interferon gamma release assay (IGRA) testing, (which measures release in response to antigens representing *Mycobacterium tuberculosis*), is preferred. Skin testing is an acceptable alternative and preferred in immune suppression. IGRAs have advantages for testing people unlikely to return for reading skin test results and for those who received bacille Calmette-Guérin (BCG) vaccination. In the case of a positive test, a chest radiograph should be performed. Provided the radiograph is not consistent with active tuberculosis, prophylactic pharmacotherapy for latent TB infection should be considered.[4]

People who inject drugs (PWID), those with unhealthy alcohol use, and persons with multiple sexual partners or high-risk sexual activity should have the prothrombin international normalized ratio (INR), the serum bilirubin, the transaminases (aspartate aminotransferase [AST] and alanine aminotransferase [ALT]), and the serum albumin and alkaline phosphatase checked as screening tests for chronic hepatitis and cirrhosis (and the serum albumin for nutritional status). Abnormal liver enzymes, INR, or serum bilirubin tests should be followed by hepatitis B (surface antigen/antibody and core antibody) and hepatitis C antibody testing.

The CDC recommends testing at least once for hepatitis C virus regardless of risk factors for persons aged 18 or older and all pregnant people during each pregnancy and periodic testing for all with any history of injecting drugs or other risks, including sharing drug paraphernalia.[5] The CDC recommends hepatitis B virus screening for populations at increased risk, including individuals with household contacts or sexual partners with hepatitis B virus infection, men who have sex with men, persons with injection drug use, and individuals with HCV or HIV.[6] Hepatitis B-vaccinated individuals should have the hepatitis B surface antibody determined to assess current seroprotection. PWID and those who practice anal intercourse and who are not from endemic areas should be tested for immunity to hepatitis A virus.

Cancer Screening

People who smoke are at higher risk of cervical cancer. All female patients who have had sexual intercourse should have a cervical cytology (Papanicolaou smear) performed every 3 years starting at age 21 to detect the premalignant lesions of cervical cancer, stopping at age 65 unless prior screening has not been adequate or the person is at high risk. Human papillomavirus (HPV) testing has become part of cervical cancer testing protocols for those between 30 and 65 years and can be used to extend the screening interval to every 5 years.[7] Similarly, for persons living with HIV, screening for anal cancer and treating early lesions may help prevent progression to cancer.[8]

The USPSTF recommends annual screening for lung cancer with low-dose computed tomography (LDCT) in adults aged 50 to 80 years who have a 20 pack-year smoking history and currently smoke (or have within 15 years), provided life expectancy is not limited and they would be willing and able to have curative lung surgery.[9]

Biennial mammography should be offered to women aged 50 to 74, with the benefit being a possible small decrease in breast cancer mortality. Screening prior to age 50 should be individualized based on patient risks, preferences, and values after discussing risks and benefits of screening.[10] For transgender women who are taking hormonal therapy, some recommend considering screening mammography every 2 years, beginning at age 50 and after at least 5 to 10 years of feminizing hormone use.[11]

Prostate cancer screening remains controversial. The serum prostate-specific antigen (PSA) test is recommended by some specialty organizations, but many other groups (eg, generalist physician organizations) do not. For male patients aged 55 to 69 years, the USPSTF recommends that the decision to undergo periodic PSA testing be individualized and performed only after a discussion of the benefits (small reduction in the chance of death from prostate cancer) and risks (need for further testing, overdiagnosis and overtreatment, complications of treatment). The USPTF recommends against screening men aged 70 years and older.[12] The decision to perform prostate cancer screening in transgender women should be based on guidelines for nontransgender men.

Colorectal cancer screening is not controversial. Colorectal cancer mortality can be decreased in adults aged 45 years and older (younger for those with risk factors or familial disease) by a variety of approaches. Screening is not recommended after age 75. Current recommended approaches include various stool-based testing, flexible sigmoidoscopy, CT colonography, or colonoscopy with intervals depending on the type of test and the results. Abnormalities on tests other than colonoscopy should be followed by a direct examination of the complete colon.[13]

Testing for Other Conditions

Male patients between ages 65 and 75 who ever smoked should be screened for abdominal aortic aneurysm with ultrasonography once.[14] Older adults (aged 65 or older) should consider thyroid function testing (serum thyroid-stimulating hormone) because abnormalities are common, difficult to recognize clinically, and easily treatable. They should also consider vision and hearing testing, as impairments are associated with a lower quality of life.[15]

Bone mineral density (BMD) testing should be done in female patients aged 65 and older and in younger female patients with increased risk of osteoporosis.[16] Current smoking and drinking 3 or more units per day are both risk factors. Risk can be determined using an online risk calculator (www.sheffield.ac.uk/FRAX). Although not included in the FRAX risk score, methadone maintenance treatment is also associated with low BMD[17] and may be another reason to do testing. Some groups also recommend osteoporosis screening for all persons with HIV aged 50 and older.[18]

Preventive Counseling

All persons with SUD should be counseled that, in addition to their addiction specialty care, they should engage in regular primary and preventive health care with a primary care clinician. In addition, because psychiatric illness is so common in patients with SUD, linkage to mental health care should be offered when appropriate.

Although the benefit is thought to be small, patients should be counseled about healthy dietary habits and physical activity. All sexually active adolescents and adults with past sexually transmitted infections or multiple sexual partners or non-monogamous relationships (or in groups with high prevalence) should be counseled about safer sexual practices (abstinence, condom use, and preexposure prophylaxis for HIV). The counseling should be high intensity (eg, multiple sessions). PWID should be educated about safer injection practices and educated regarding naloxone and overdose prevention. Given the contamination of the drug supply with illicitly manufactured fentanyl, any person using nonprescription drugs should be counseled about universal fentanyl precautions, including drug checking when available, overdose education, and naloxone. People who smoke drugs should be counseled about safer smoking practices. Persons of childbearing age and their partners should be counseled about contraceptive options.

Persons who store or carry weapons should be reminded of gun safety, especially if there are children in the home; moreover, in patients with unhealthy substance use, this can be of particular importance if there are concurrent issues with impulsive behavior or risk for suicide (eg, heavy alcohol use is a risk factor). All patients may be advised about seat belt and helmet use. Referrals for both regular eye and dental care should be routine. Preventive advice about safe lifting may help prevent low back injury.

Immunizations

Table 87-2 provides a summary of select immunizations for adults recommended by the CDC.[19] Detailed updated

TABLE 87-2 Summary of Select Vaccinations Recommended for Adults[a]

Vaccination	Doses/interval	Populations/selected indications
Influenza	Yearly	All adults
Tetanus diphtheria, pertussis (Tdap or Td)	1 dose Tdap, then Td or Tdap booster every 10 y	All adults All adults with wounds if more than 5 y since last booster
Zoster recombinant	2 doses	Age 50 or older
Pneumococcal (PCV15, PCV20, PPSV23)	1 or 2 doses depending on vaccine	Age 65 or older All adults with HIV infection, chronic liver disease, cigarette smoking, alcohol use disorder
Hepatitis A	2 or 3 doses depending on vaccine	All adults with injection drug use, HIV infection, chronic liver/ lung disease, homelessness
Hepatitis B	2 or 3 doses depending on vaccine	All adults with injection drug use, HIV infection, chronic liver disease, incarceration
Human papillomavirus (HPV)	2 or 3 doses depending on age or condition	All adults through 26 y, depending on vaccinations received during adolescence. Some adults aged 27-45 y

[a]See CDC guidelines for updated recommendations and further details.

Adapted from CDC. *Recommended Adult Immunization Schedule for Ages 19 Years or Older, United States, 2021*. https://www.cdc.gov/vaccines/schedules/hcp/imz/adult.html

recommendations are published by the CDC at http://www.cdc.gov/vaccines/schedules/hcp/index.html.

Injection drug use is a risk factor for tetanus.[20] Tetanus toxoid is recommended every 10 years for everyone; to provide protection for pertussis, the Tdap version should be given at least once when a booster is due or prior to having close contact with a baby or work as a health care professional and may be repeated once as a booster after age 65.

Hepatitis B vaccination (a series of two or three injections depending on the formulation) is indicated for PWID, health care workers, persons with hepatitis C, sexually-active individuals who are not involved in long-term monogamous relationships, and any adult seeking protection from infection. Hepatitis A vaccination (two injections) is indicated for travelers, those with chronic liver disease, those who practice anal intercourse, and PWID, when not already immune (hepatitis A IgG negative).

Pneumococcal vaccination should be administered to all persons aged 65 years and older and others at high risk including those with chronic pulmonary/liver/kidney disease, HIV infection or other immunocompromising conditions. Cigarette smoking and alcohol use disorder are also indications for the vaccine, and many practitioners believe other SUDs are another reasonable indication. The 20-valent pneumococcal conjugate vaccine (PCV20) can be given one time; an alternative is the 15-valent version (PCV15) followed by the pneumococcal polysaccharide (PPSV23) at least 1 year later.

Smoking and other substance use is associated with an increased risk for other respiratory infections. Influenza vaccination should be given yearly to all persons, particularly those with cardiopulmonary disease, older adults and those living in group settings. Individuals who smoke and have SUDs are also at increased risk for severe COVID-19 infection and should be targeted for vaccination.

Varicella vaccine is recommended for all adults without immunity; zoster vaccine for all older people (aged 50 or older), regardless of prior episodes of herpes zoster. HPV vaccine is recommended for everyone up to age 26 and the CDC also recommends offering HPV vaccine to some adults age 27 to 45 based on shared clinical decision making. Meningococcal vaccine should be offered to high risk groups, including military recruits, those with complement deficiency, asplenia or HIV, or being part of a community with a disease outbreak.

When childhood vaccinations are unknown, consideration should be given to a primary series for polio; measles, mumps, and rubella; and varicella. Many adults will have immunity to these, but if unknown, testing is warranted, given that many persons with unhealthy substance use may be in group living situations, sometimes with children and young adults, in which measles and varicella can spread easily.

Chemoprophylaxis

Persons of childbearing age who are trying to conceive or who are sexually active and not using contraception should take folate supplement daily to prevent fetal neural tube defects. Because of the risk of thiamine, vitamin D, pyridoxine, niacin, riboflavin, zinc, and folic acid deficiency in people with heavy alcohol use, other substance use disorders and those with deficient diets, a daily multivitamin including vitamin D, thiamine, and folic acid can be recommended. Because magnesium deficiency is common in people with chronic alcohol use, replacement by encouraging the use of foods with high magnesium content (such as peanuts) or a magnesium supplement (magnesium oxide tablets or magnesium hydroxide-containing antacids) is recommended.

In addition to assuring adequate vitamin and mineral intake and encouraging weightbearing exercise, bisphosphonates, parathyroid hormone, estrogen, and raloxifene may be used for the prevention of fractures in patients with osteoporosis. Risks for osteoporosis are higher in people with alcohol use disorders and some other persons with unhealthy substance use, but the interaction between estrogens and estrogen receptor modulators and alcohol on breast cancer is not clear, and the side effects of the drugs in people who drink heavily (eg, bisphosphonates and esophageal irritation) and those with liver disease are not well characterized.

Another form of chemoprophylaxis is to prescribe intranasal or intramuscular naloxone to people who use illicit drugs or are prescribed opioids—and their significant others—to treat overdose. In addition to prescription of naloxone, patients and their significant others should be educated regarding how to use the medication, to call for emergency services and to provide first aid if needed (including rescue breathing and chest compressions).

A recent addition to chemoprophylaxis relevant to patients with unhealthy substance use is preexposure prophylaxis for the prevention of HIV infection (PrEP). A once-daily dose of tenofovir and emtricitabine has been shown to be effective and is recommended for high-risk individuals, including those who inject drugs, particularly those with recent use and those who share injection equipment.[21] Adherence is critical, as is counseling on other risk reduction methods, and testing for HIV infection should be done every 3 months. An intramuscular injection of cabotegravir given every 2 months was approved by the FDA in 2021, which may improve PrEP uptake and adherence in at-risk populations. Postexposure prophylaxis (PEP) may also be considered within 72 hours after sharing syringes or other injection equipment or engaging in high-risk sex with someone who has or might have HIV. Further information and guidance can be found on the CDC website (https://www.cdc.gov/hiv/clinicians/prevention/index.html).

SUBSTANCE USE AND TREATMENT OF OTHER MEDICAL CONDITIONS

In addition to the medical complications outlined later in this chapter, it is important to note that persons with unhealthy substance use suffer from the same medical conditions as other persons, but substance use can affect the disease course and interfere with their management. Treatment adherence can be a problem in patients with and without unhealthy substance use, but it takes on particular importance with the management of chronic medical illnesses.

Cardiovascular diseases are the most common cause of death in the United States. Coronary artery disease is particularly common in persons with substance use because of concomitant tobacco use. The diagnosis of hypertension can be problematic in persons with SUD. A single elevated blood pressure should not be equated with the diagnosis of hypertension, because this can be due to pain, withdrawal, or intoxication, depending on the substance used. Alcohol (and other drugs, such as stimulants) can elevate blood pressure. Ideally, hypertension should be diagnosed after at least three blood pressure measurements (130/80 or higher) during prolonged abstinence. Nevertheless, though a diagnosis of hypertension should not be made during withdrawal or in an emergency setting (unless end-organ damage is evident), persistently elevated blood pressure in a patient who drinks or uses other drugs regularly should be managed as hypertension to prevent complications. Treatment of hypertension is the same as in persons without unhealthy substance use, in that attention to medication adherence for an asymptomatic condition is important, lifestyle modification can help, and many medications are available. Though diuretics are inexpensive and effective, they can be somewhat riskier in people with alcohol use disorders because of the adverse effects on potassium balance.

Diabetes may be more difficult to manage in persons with unhealthy substance use, not only because of difficulty with adherence but also due to more irregular eating patterns, food insecurity and limited access to healthy food in disadvantaged neighborhoods. Another factor to consider are the effects of alcohol and other drugs on glucose metabolism. People who drink heavily are more prone to prolonged and severe hypoglycemia from the sulfonylurea agents often used to treat type 2 diabetes. Metformin should be used with caution in patients with hepatic impairment or those at risk for lactic acidosis.

In addition to having etiological roles in cancers, substance use can lead to difficulties in cancer management. Renal, hepatic, or cardiac consequences of substance use can limit the choice of chemotherapeutic agents. Pulmonary complications of combustible tobacco use may limit surgical options. Finally, pain management can be complicated by ongoing or past substance use.

Although substance use can complicate the treatment of other conditions, it should not be used as an excuse to not offer needed treatment to individuals with unhealthy substance use. For example, hepatitis C treatment adherence is somewhat lower among individuals with active alcohol or other substance use, but treatment success rates are nonetheless very high.[22]

CARE DURING HOSPITALIZATION

Individuals with unhealthy substance use are at increased risk for hospitalization, increased length of stay, and readmission.[23] During a medical hospitalization, three areas deserve particular attention: management of substance withdrawal, pain, and common comorbidities. Treatment (including brief interventions) and withdrawal and pain management are addressed elsewhere in this textbook, but several points are relevant to medical hospitalizations specifically. Hospitalization is an opportunity to engage individuals in long-term treatment and strong consideration should be given to initiating treatment for addiction in the hospital and assuring its seamless continuation after discharge. Addiction consult services can help with assessments of addiction severity, treatment initiation, and linkage to follow up SUD care that may reduce readmission and postdischarge mortality.[24,25]

Withdrawal

Persons whose regular substance or medication use has led to physiologic dependence are at risk for withdrawal when hospitalized. Symptom management should be planned before withdrawal symptoms appear and treated promptly, given that untreated withdrawal is a major reason for self-directed discharges from the hospital.[26] Persons not yet symptomatic with alcohol withdrawal but with past alcohol-related seizures or concomitant acute medical or surgical conditions (which increase the risk of withdrawal) may benefit from proactive treatment before they develop severe withdrawal.[27] Because the symptoms of withdrawal may overlap with systemic symptoms of infection, heart disease, or neurological conditions, treatment for withdrawal should proceed while investigations to identify other treatable medical disorders continue. Though symptom-triggered treatment using standardized withdrawal scales is the standard of care, the information these scales provide should be considered in the context of the coexisting medical illness. Opioid and other drug withdrawal should be identified and managed pharmacologically. Patients who already are in treatment for SUD should have their treating clinician or program contacted when they are hospitalized, so that any ongoing treatment, such as medications for opioid use disorder, can be continued. Similarly, addiction treatment providers should communicate directly with hospital clinicians to facilitate appropriate treatment continuation and care coordination. Recognition and treatment of substance withdrawal syndromes are discussed in more detail in Section 7 of this textbook.

For patients with opioid use disorder who are admitted for treatment of other conditions and are experiencing or at risk for withdrawal, there are a number of treatment options. However, it is important to keep in mind that acute withdrawal management alone is not adequate OUD treatment; patients should be offered ongoing opioid agonist treatment and advised that this is the safest and most effective option for most.[28] Methadone can be administered as a taper or can be initiated and uptitrated if maintenance is the ultimate goal, provided that the patient can be connected with a licensed opioid treatment program on discharge. Buprenorphine is a reasonable alternative and is generally more easily accessible. Both medications can be utilized during hospitalization for a medical condition and do not require the facility being licensed as an opioid treatment program. When deciding on the best treatment, the patient's disposition at discharge should be anticipated. Short-acting opioids can be administered for discomfort while a long-term plan is being worked out.[29] Coordination of care to the outpatient setting, including provision of a bridge prescription for buprenorphine when needed, is key to ensure a smooth transition for the patient.

In addition to providing comfort and helping to prevent the more serious complications of withdrawal, treatment of withdrawal minimizes autonomic symptoms that can worsen a patient's medical condition (such as tachycardia during a myocardial infarction) and helps the patient continue with and complete treatment for the medical condition that prompted hospitalization. For further details, see Section 7 of this textbook.

Pain

Pain management often becomes an issue during medical hospitalization of patients with unhealthy substance use. Hospital clinicians and staff may fear that providing pain control with opioids to a patient with opioid use disorder may worsen their addiction.[30] This management style generally results in inadequate pain management and frustration for patient and clinicians alike,[31] as well as premature or self-directed discharges.[26]

In the case of persons with opioid use disorder, adequate pain control with opioids can be achieved only with substantially higher doses of opioids (above those required for maintenance treatment or to prevent withdrawal), with careful reassessment of the dose effect and timing to make appropriate adjustments. Once an effective dose is determined, pain medications given on a regular schedule (with holding parameters for sedation and respiratory depression) rather than as needed may prevent unfortunate scenarios in which the patient must request pain medication to relieve uncontrolled symptoms and is labelled as "drug seeking." Similar principles apply for patients on opioid agonist treatment.[32] These issues are discussed in greater detail in Section 13 of this textbook.

Co-Occurring Medical Issues

While patients are hospitalized, several co-occurring medical issues should be considered. First, because psychiatric co-occurring disorders are common (in particular, posttraumatic stress disorder, anxiety, and depression), attention to behavioral issues is important. Hospital staff members should take extra care to explain hospital procedures. Patients should be assured that their medical, psychiatric, and substance-related symptoms and pain will be attended to. Discussing withdrawal and pain treatment plans with the patient can help avoid later problems and disagreements and help allay the fears and preconceptions patients may have about clinicians. Screening for coexisting medical disorders (such as HIV and hepatitis) during a medical hospitalization should be considered because the acute care setting may provide the only medical care received by the patient. Treatment for coexisting medical and psychiatric conditions should be made available.

Perioperative Care

Several issues arise in the perioperative period with people with unhealthy substance use. First, it is essential to assess (through history and drug testing) what substances have been used. Second, attention to and treatment of withdrawal symptoms can avert development of signs such as tachycardia and hypertension, which may complicate interpretation of assessments and operative and anesthetic treatments. Third, the anesthesiologist must be informed of any recent substance use because of potential interactions (eg, the potentiation of sedative and anesthetic drugs). Finally, anesthesia and pain management generally require much higher doses than usual in patients with opioid tolerance. Nutritional issues often require attention in persons with unhealthy substance use undergoing surgery, as wound healing may be impaired. Further details may be found in Chapter 99 of this textbook "Perioperative Management of Patients with Substance Use Disorders."

OLDER ADULTS

Substance use can lead to additional consequences in older adults.[33] This is due to a number of factors, including declines in cognitive and physical reserve, changes in body composition and metabolism, co-existing health conditions and interactions with prescribed medications. Often, substance use is a contributor to an illness or condition rather than the sole cause. For example, hip fracture, a leading cause of death in older adults, can result from an increased propensity to fall related to alcohol or other substance use and to osteopenia. Older adults are more susceptible to injury from motor vehicle crashes, even more so when alcohol and other substances are used. Medications (such as antidepressants, warfarin, phenytoin, aspirin, and acetaminophen) are less effective or can be harmful when taken with alcohol.

Older adults are more susceptible than younger individuals to the chronic brain-damaging effects of alcohol, benzodiazepines, and amphetamine-type stimulants, including cognitive deficits, and are less likely to recover completely from those effects. For this reason, the U.S. National Institute on Alcohol Abuse and Alcoholism (NIAAA) recommends lower drinking limits for older adults than younger adults.

In addition to greater susceptibility, alcohol and other substances can cause many consequences in older adults that may be misdiagnosed. The tremor of alcohol or sedative withdrawal may be diagnosed as Parkinson disease or an essential tremor. Dementia, malnutrition, self-neglect, functional decline, sleep problems, and anxiety or depression all may be attributed to "normal" aging when the true cause is alcohol or other substance use. Similarly, cardiovascular disease and congestive heart failure are common in older adults; alcohol or stimulants as the cause of cardiomyopathy or exacerbations of congestive heart failure may be overlooked. Fractures, seizures, and cerebellar degeneration may be misattributed to other "medical" causes when alcohol is a key contributor.

Alcohol can contribute to the worsening of chronic illness (such as hypertension), interference with medication adherence and side effects, incontinence, fatigue, neuropathy, sexual dysfunction, and pneumonia. Other drug use can lead to similar consequences in the elderly—confusion, falls, and interference with activities of daily living. While rates of illicit drug use tend to be lower among older adults than younger adults, there are many "baby boomers" who began use when they were younger and rates are increasing. As with younger adults, cannabis is the most commonly-used illicit drug. Older adults are more susceptible to its deleterious effects on memory, coordination and driving and the increased risks of injury and delirium.[34]

Many older adults are prescribed psychoactive medications, including benzodiazepines and opioids; taking these medications as prescribed—or taking more than was intended or for purposes other than intended (nonmedical use)—can lead to physical, functional, and psychosocial impairments.

The effects of smoking are of great significance in older adults because smoking-related diseases often appear with aging and can be exacerbated by continued smoking. Examples include coronary artery disease and COPD.

MEDICAL COMPLICATIONS RELATED TO SUBSTANCE USE

Medical complications associated with unhealthy substance use may be due to drug-specific effects, methods of administration, adulterants or contaminants in or vehicles for drugs used, behaviors associated with substance use, or common co-occurring issues (Table 87-3). In this portion of the chapter, common and important medical consequences of substance use are reviewed and organized by substance and then by organ system or clinical area. More details can be found in the subsequent chapters in this section of the textbook.

It is important to keep in mind that there are various levels of evidence to support the association between the use

TABLE 87-3 Select Medical Disorders Associated With Substance Use

Category	Disorder (substance)
Head and neck	Parotid enlargement (alcohol); head and neck cancer (alcohol, tobacco, betel nut); cataracts (tobacco); macular degeneration (tobacco); septal erosion/perforation (cocaine); corneal ulcerations (cocaine); vision loss (methanol, nitrites); periodontal disease (tobacco, stimulants, cannabis)
Pulmonary	Aspiration pneumonia (alcohol); tuberculosis (alcohol, tobacco); respiratory infections (tobacco); chronic obstructive lung disease (tobacco); lung cancer (tobacco); pulmonary edema (opioids); bronchoconstriction (stimulants); alveolar hemorrhage (stimulants); pulmonary hypertension (stimulants); bronchitis (tobacco, cannabis)
Cardiovascular	Cardiomyopathy (alcohol, stimulants); atrial fibrillation (alcohol); hypertension (alcohol); coronary artery disease (tobacco); myocardial infarction (tobacco, stimulants, MDMA); peripheral vascular disease (tobacco, stimulants); aortic aneurysm (tobacco); aortic dissection (stimulants); endocarditis (injection drug use); arrhythmia (stimulants); ventricular arrhythmia (organic compounds)
Gastrointestinal	Pancreatitis (alcohol); gastritis/gastric ulcers (alcohol, tobacco); esophageal stricture (alcohol); esophageal/gastric/pancreatic/colorectal cancer (tobacco); gastroesophageal reflux (alcohol); constipation (opioids); ischemic colitis (stimulants); hyperemesis (cannabis)
Hepatic	Hepatitis (alcohol, MDMA); viral hepatitis (injection drug use); cirrhosis (alcohol)
Renal/electrolyte	Hyponatremia (alcohol, MDMA); hypokalemia (alcohol); hypomagnesemia (alcohol); hypophosphatemia (alcohol); renovascular disease (tobacco, stimulants); acute kidney injury (stimulants, synthetic cannabinoids, toluene); chronic kidney disease (tobacco, stimulants); renal cell carcinoma (tobacco); metabolic acidosis (alcohol, methanol)
Genitourinary	Testicular atrophy (alcohol); testicular germ cell tumors (cannabis); erectile dysfunction (tobacco)
Musculoskeletal	Traumatic injures (alcohol, stimulants); gout (alcohol); rheumatoid arthritis (tobacco); rhabdomyolysis (stimulants, MDMA, PCP); low bone mineral density (cannabis)
Skin/breast	Premature aging of the skin (tobacco); breast cancer (alcohol); burns (tobacco, inhalants)
Neurologic	Seizures (alcohol, stimulants, PCP); memory impairment (alcohol, organic compounds); ataxia (alcohol, organic compounds); peripheral neuropathy (alcohol, organic compounds, nitrous oxide); stroke (tobacco, stimulants, MDMA); Parkinson disease (methamphetamine)
Hematologic	Anemia (alcohol, nitrous oxide); thrombocytopenia (alcohol); methemoglobinemia (nitrites)
Endocrine	Hypertriglyceridemia (alcohol); type II diabetes (tobacco); hypogonadism (opioids); adrenal insufficiency (opioids); Graves disease (tobacco)
Reproductive	Amenorrhea (alcohol, opioids); fetal alcohol spectrum disorders (alcohol); infertility (tobacco); premature birth (tobacco, stimulants, cannabis); low birth weight (tobacco, stimulants, cannabis); neonatal abstinence syndrome (opioids)

of specific substances and medical complications, and that association supports—but does not prove—causation. Therapeutic interventions and the impact of exposures are best tested in randomized controlled trials that compare two similar populations, one of which has received the treatment or exposure and the other that has not. However, for obvious reasons, we cannot evaluate potentially harmful substances in this way. Our understanding of medical consequences often begins with physiology and observations of cases where individuals using specific substances experienced a medical complication. Stronger evidence can be obtained through observational studies. One way to do this is through *case-control* studies that compare persons with an illness with those who do not have the illness and collect information about substance use and other factors that may have contributed. Another way is to conduct a *cohort study*, which follows a group of patients over time to assess outcomes and their association with substance use and other factors prospectively (or retrospectively). Observational studies are limited by the potential that the groups compared are different in other ways that influence the outcome (*confounders*). For example, individuals with alcohol use disorder often smoke tobacco, and as a result, suffer from many of the complications of tobacco use disproportionately when compared to the general population. These studies can try to take into account known determinants of outcomes, but cannot account for factors that were not measured or considered (*residual confounders*).

Complications Related to Alcohol Use

Alcohol effects almost every organ system of the body; female patients are more susceptible at lower doses because of more absorption (less gastric alcohol dehydrogenase), less first-pass metabolism of alcohol, and lower average body weight. Though some studies have found lower-risk drinking (compared with abstinence or higher levels or drinking) is associated with a lower risk of mortality,[35] this association may be entirely due to other factors.[36] Nevertheless, alcohol is major contributor to morbidity and mortality worldwide.[37]

Cardiovascular

Observational studies have found a lower risk of cardiovascular mortality at low levels of drinking, but these findings may be due to unmeasured confounders, because moderate drinking is associated with other healthy behaviors. A recent analysis, using a technique called "mendelian randomization" to minimize confounding, found an increased risk for cardiovascular disease that rises with the level of drinking and begins at low levels.[38] It is clear that higher levels of alcohol use have detrimental effects on the cardiovascular system, including increased risk of hypertension, cardiac arrhythmias (especially atrial fibrillation), and cardiomyopathy.[39]

In addition to the transient blood pressure elevation seen during withdrawal, alcohol use, particularly heavy drinking (about 2 or more standard drinks/day), is associated with hypertension, which can lead to cardiac, renal, and vascular damage.

Long-term regular heavy drinking can lead to cardiomyopathy and heart failure. Treatment consists of alcohol abstinence or moderation (which can lead to an increase in the left ventricular ejection fraction[40]) and standard heart failure treatments, including heart transplant. Cardiomyopathy may lead to ventricular dysrhythmias requiring antiarrhythmic therapy or implantation of an automatic implantable cardioverter-defibrillator (AICD) to decrease the risk of sudden death. Anticoagulation may be indicated when there is a ventricular thrombosis, but the risk-benefit balance often is unclear, particularly when the patient continues to drink heavily.

Atrial fibrillation can occur as a consequence of alcohol use or withdrawal ("holiday heart") and usually resolves spontaneously. Among individuals with a history of atrial fibrillation, abstinence from alcohol reduces the risk of recurrent arrhythmia.[41]

Liver

Alcohol is one of the most common causes of liver disease worldwide.[42] Alcohol use can lead to hepatitis ranging in severity from asymptomatic elevation of hepatic transaminases to critical illness with hepatic failure. In alcohol-related hepatitis, aspartate aminotransferase (AST) usually is higher than alanine aminotransferase (ALT); a higher ALT suggests another or a concomitant etiology, such as viral hepatitis. Hepatic steatosis can cause elevations in serum transaminases, and may be (but is not always) related to alcohol use. Though liver biopsy is the gold standard, metabolic dysfunction-associated steatohepatitis is often diagnosed clinically when serology for hepatitis B and hepatitis C is negative, the abnormality persists with abstinence, and ultrasound examination is consistent with the diagnosis.

Classic alcohol-related hepatitis presents with fever, leukocytosis, right upper quadrant pain and tenderness, and elevations of the AST out of proportion to ALT. Risk factors for alcohol-related hepatitis include genetic factors, obesity, female sex, malnutrition, and concomitant hepatitis C infection.[43] Management consists of abstinence from alcohol as well as supportive care, with attention to fluid and electrolyte balance, vitamin K for coagulopathy, clotting factor replacement when there is active bleeding and coagulopathy, and attention to volume and mental status. Patients with coagulopathy, hyperbilirubinemia, and hepatic encephalopathy are at high risk of death. Corticosteroids have been shown to decrease mortality in selected severe cases. In general, before giving steroids, active infection should be excluded. In addition, efficacy is not known for patients with concomitant pancreatitis, gastrointestinal bleeding, or renal failure. For life-threatening cases of alcohol-related hepatitis, liver transplantation is sometimes the only option to prevent death.[44]

Cirrhosis can develop in people who drink heavily and regularly over time either as a consequence of recurrent alcohol-related hepatitis, co-occurring hepatitis C, or, simply, chronic heavy use.[45] An increase in the incidence of cirrhosis can be detected in populations drinking 3 standard drinks per day compared with people who do not drink, though heavier amounts are more commonly associated with the condition and not everyone who drinks heavily develops liver disease. Cirrhosis may lead to hypoalbuminemia, coagulopathy, and hyperbilirubinemia. Hepatocellular carcinoma (HCC) can occur, and the risk of HCC is increased when hepatitis C is also present. Some recommend screening for HCC by ultrasound and/or serum alpha-fetoprotein because HCC can be cured if detected early, though this is based primarily on observational data.[46] Complications of cirrhosis portend a poor prognosis; these include hepatic encephalopathy, esophageal or gastric variceal bleeding, ascites and spontaneous bacterial peritonitis, volume overload and edema, and hepatorenal syndrome. When cirrhosis and alcohol-related hepatitis coexist, the prognosis is poor, particularly when drinking continues. End-stage liver disease can be treated with liver transplantation. Patients receiving transplants because of alcohol-related liver disease have similar survival to those with other causes of liver failure.[47] Many liver transplantation programs require defined periods of abstinence from alcohol and other substances—often 6 months—before patients will be evaluated for this extensive surgery and scarce resource. Assessing risk of recurrence of heavy alcohol use without requiring an arbitrary period of abstinence is an alternative approach.[48] Early transplantation for acute alcohol-related hepatitis without requiring a period of abstinence has been increasingly studied and shows similar 2-year survival rates compared to traditional delayed transplantation.[49]

Renal and Metabolic

Renal and metabolic consequences of alcohol use are often seen in acute care settings. Cirrhosis can be complicated by hepatorenal syndrome. Chronic renal insufficiency may be seen in persons who ingest home-distilled alcohol made with lead equipment ("moonshine"). Acute renal failure from rhabdomyolysis can occur after alcohol intoxication (or immobilization during obtundation from any sedating substance). Fluid and electrolyte abnormalities are very common in people with heavy alcohol use who present for medical care. Many will be volume depleted from vomiting, diarrhea, and diuresis. Volume repletion is best accomplished orally when possible, and with intravenous fluids and electrolytes when necessary.

Patients can present with metabolic acidosis due to varying etiologies. The first step is to distinguish between a nonanion gap and an anion gap acidosis. If an anion gap is not present, diarrhea is the most common cause in people with heavy alcohol use. If an anion gap is present, the differential diagnosis is broad, but lactic acidosis (from sepsis, injury, severe pancreatitis, or after convulsion), ketoacidosis, and ingestion of ethylene glycol or methanol should be considered. To rule this out, in addition to the history, the measured serum osmolality should be compared with the calculated osmolality (accounting for the serum ethanol in the calculation). If no osmolar gap is present, ingestions are unlikely. If a gap is present, testing for these ingestions should be done, though levels are usually not available in time to assist with acute management. These ingestions require prompt treatment with fomepizole, hemodialysis, or parenteral ethanol to prevent blindness or death.

Ketoacidosis can also occur in people with alcohol use disorders, typically in the setting of heavy alcohol use followed by nausea and vomiting.[50] The glucose concentration can be high, normal, or low, and the urine ketones can be negative (although serum ketones should be positive). The treatment is volume expansion with 5% dextrose in normal saline (preceded by thiamine). In the absence of ketones or an osmolar gap, lactic acidosis is the next most serious diagnosis to consider, mainly because it can be the only clue to an unrecognized coexisting problem (eg, myocardial infarction or recent convulsion).

Alcohol use is associated with a number of electrolyte abnormalities.[51] Malnourished people with heavy alcohol use can develop hypophosphatemia that may be unmasked or exacerbated when dextrose is given, leading to severe hypophosphatemia that requires treatment. Hypomagnesemia is common, as a result of diuretic use, hypokalemia, and reversible hypoparathyroidism resulting from impaired parathyroid hormone release when the magnesium cofactor is deficient. The latter condition also leads to hypocalcemia, which does not respond to calcium replacement; rather, it requires magnesium repletion. The hypokalemia often seen in people with heavy alcohol use with hyperaldosteronism from volume depletion and diuretic use cannot be corrected until magnesium is replaced. Serum levels do not reflect total body magnesium stores, so empiric replacement is the best approach. Oral replacement of magnesium and phosphate is possible, but may be limited by inability to take food by mouth or the presence of diarrhea (which worsens the deficiencies). Intravenous replacement, with cardiac monitoring in the case of severe hypophosphatemia, may be necessary. Hyperglycemia can be seen in people with chronic heavy alcohol use as a result of pancreatic insufficiency. Hypoglycemia can be seen with end-stage cirrhosis; this is due to depleted glycogen stores and is a very poor prognostic sign.

Gastrointestinal

Alcohol effects the gastrointestinal tract from the mouth to the anus.[52] Alcohol is associated with gastrointestinal reflux disease. Alcohol is directly toxic to the gastric mucosa leading to gastritis, which can be asymptomatic or present as epigastric burning, nausea, vomiting, or hematemesis (coffee-ground emesis). Repeated vomiting can lead to a Mallory-Weiss tears and hematemesis. Alcohol can lead to stomatitis, esophagitis, duodenitis, esophageal cancer, and gastric cancer. Endoscopy is warranted for persistent reflux symptoms or epigastric pain, despite adequate pharmacological treatment, particularly if weight loss is present, if patients are aged 40 years or older, or if they smoke cigarettes.

Alcohol use is a common cause of pancreatitis, which typically presents as epigastric pain, sometimes radiating to the back.[53] The serum lipase (or amylase) level often is elevated unless there has been chronic pancreatic damage. In people with regular and heavy alcohol consumption, amylase may also be elevated because of chronic parotitis. Abdominal computed tomography is the most sensitive and specific test for pancreatitis, but it is not routinely indicated unless the presentation is atypical, fever is present, or the patient does not improve as expected. Severity can range from mild epigastric pain after eating, with some nausea, to a life-threatening condition complicated by acidosis, adult respiratory distress syndrome, and hypovolemia. Standard therapy includes volume repletion and pain control by using opioids parenterally. When acute episodes resolve, a return to drinking can lead to recurrent episodes and ultimately to chronic pancreatitis, with loss of pancreatic exocrine function. Greasy stools from malabsorption, hyperglycemia and diabetes may result. The prognosis is markedly worse with any ongoing alcohol consumption. Oral pancreatic enzyme supplementation with meals then is indicated, although pain management may be difficult. Serum amylase and lipase often are normal, although calcifications may be seen on radiographs.

Respiratory

Alcohol intoxication can lead to respiratory depression and aspiration, resulting in a chemical or infectious pneumonia. Tachypnea can be the result of pulmonary infection, respiratory alkalosis of liver disease or sepsis, alcohol withdrawal, or compensation for a metabolic acidosis.

Neurologic

Alcohol can affect the neurologic system in a number of different ways—directly or indirectly.[54] Intoxication can lead to head trauma and intracranial hemorrhage—particularly subdural hematoma—which can be confused with intoxication. Imaging of the brain is indicated when there are signs of significant head trauma and abnormal mental status, or signs of focal neurological deficits, or when neurological symptoms do not resolve with declining alcohol levels.

Lower-risk drinking may decrease the risk for ischemic stroke, but heavy drinking increases the risk for ischemic and hemorrhagic stroke, with a stronger association for hemorrhagic strokes.[55]

Cognitive impairment may be caused acutely by Wernicke-Korsakoff disease due to thiamine deficiency, presenting with confusion, ataxia, or nystagmus. This can develop into Korsakoff syndrome, a memory impairment classically characterized by confabulation. More commonly, chronic alcohol consumption is associated with a nonspecific dementia and volume loss on brain imaging. Alcoholic cerebellar dysfunction results in ataxia and incoordination and often is irreversible.

Alcohol-related peripheral neuropathy may be caused by vitamin deficiency, nerve compression, or direct ethanol toxicity on nerves. The classic presentation of alcohol-related polyneuropathy is of sensory disturbance, including burning, pain, and numbness in a stocking-glove distribution.

Withdrawal seizures and alcohol withdrawal delirium are major and well-known neurological consequences of heavy drinking. These direct medical consequences of alcohol withdrawal (hyperautonomic states, seizures, and delirium) are covered in detail elsewhere in this book (Section 7). In addition to withdrawal seizures, alcohol can lower the seizure threshold in patients with epilepsy, and seizures may be the presenting sign of an intracranial hemorrhage.

Infectious Diseases

People with unhealthy alcohol use are at increased risk of infections because of impaired structural gastrointestinal and respiratory tract defense mechanisms as well as impaired immune system; concomitant liver disease further increases this risk.[56] Pneumonia is more common in people with excessive alcohol use, partly because of the association with aspiration; moreover, unhealthy alcohol use increases the risk of mortality and hospital length of stay. Concomitant smoking increases the risk further by impairing the mucociliary elevator.

Tuberculosis is a consideration when symptoms are chronic, weight loss is present, and upper lobe infiltrates appear on the chest x-ray, particularly in people with alcohol use disorders who are experiencing homelessness, have immigrated from a country where the disease is endemic, are known to have a previous positive tuberculin skin test, or have had contact with an active case.

Individuals with alcohol-related cirrhosis with ascites can develop spontaneous bacterial peritonitis. Symptoms may include only fever or abdominal discomfort or encephalopathy. Abdominal tenderness may be minimal or absent. Diagnosis is made by paracentesis, which should be done when there is any clinical suspicion. Spontaneous bacterial empyema can occur when pleural effusion is present.

Sexually transmitted infections, including HIV, are more common in people with unhealthy alcohol use, in part because of sexual risk-taking behavior. Updated treatment guidelines can be found at the CDC website (www.cdc.gov/std/treatment-guidelines).

Sleep

Sleep-related problems are common among individuals with unhealthy alcohol use.[57] While alcohol may help initiate sleep, the sleep quality is poorer and more fragmented. Alcohol increases the risk of obstructive sleep apnea and worsens the disease because of its depressant effects on respiration and relaxation of the upper airway. Alcohol can increase the risk of periodic limb movements of sleep. Persons in recovery may resume drinking because of intolerable insomnia. Treatment of insomnia involves attention to sleep hygiene as well as pharmacotherapy with medications with a low or no risk of physiologic dependence.

Injury/Trauma

Alcohol can interfere with balance and coordination, thus predisposing to injury. It also interferes with judgment, and some individuals who drink heavily already have a predisposition to risk taking. Heavy episodic (sometimes called *binge*) drinking (ie, >4 standard drinks on an occasion for men and >3 for women) poses a particular risk of injury and accidents. Patients who present to emergency departments and trauma centers with serious injuries are far more likely than others to have used alcohol recently. Although the evidence from randomized trials is limited and mixed at best, the high frequency of injury in persons with heavy alcohol use suggests that facilities where such persons are seen for health care (ie, emergency departments and trauma centers) should routinely identify patients with heavy drinking and refer those with alcohol-related disorders for treatment in order to prevent additional injury. Moreover, addiction specialists should be attuned to the high rates of injury (both past trauma and the risk of future injury) when counseling people with alcohol use disorders. Injury can be a motivating factor for discontinuing alcohol use or a focus of counseling to prevent future injuries.

Endocrinologic

Alcohol causes sexual dysfunction and hypogonadism through direct effects on the testes and secondary effects in chronic liver disease, in which gynecomastia may also be seen. Alcohol increases the high-density lipoprotein fraction of cholesterol; however, it also increases serum triglycerides, which can lead to heart disease, hepatic steatosis, and pancreatitis. Low-risk drinking is associated with a reduced risk of developing type 2 diabetes mellitus, but heavier drinking increases the risk.[58]

Fetal, Neonatal, and Infant

Use of alcohol during pregnancy, even in amounts considered to be low risk in nonpregnant adults, can lead to neurobehavioral deficits in children. Fetal alcohol spectrum disorders are a group of conditions that can occur when persons are exposed to alcohol before birth. Clinical manifestations include craniofacial abnormalities, neurological abnormalities, and growth retardation. Affected individuals may have some or all of the manifestations and disabilities persist into adulthood. Because no safe amount of alcohol during pregnancy has been identified and there is no treatment for the effects of alcohol on the fetus, abstinence is recommended during pregnancy.

Hematologic

Alcohol has various effects on blood cells through different mechanisms. In addition to the iron deficiency anemia that can result from gastrointestinal hemorrhage or chronic blood loss (from variceal bleeding, gastritis, Mallory-Weiss tears, coexisting ulcers, esophagitis, or gastrointestinal cancers), excessive alcohol use can lead to pancytopenia (leukopenia, thrombocytopenia, and anemia) from alcohol's direct toxic effects on the bone marrow. Splenic sequestration as a result of the splenomegaly associated with cirrhosis and portal hypertension also can cause pancytopenia. People with chronic alcohol use often have not only leukopenia but also an impaired white blood cell response to infection. Thrombocytopenia can lead to serious bleeding (eg, as a result of trauma or varices), when the platelet count is below 50,000 platelets per microliter of blood.

Folate deficiency can result in a megaloblastic anemia. However, the MCV, often used to assist in the differential diagnosis of anemia, can be misleadingly normal because iron deficiency lowers the MCV and hemolytic anemias related to liver disease with reticulocytosis or megaloblastic processes simultaneously increases it. The treatment recommendation for bone marrow suppression is abstinence; for iron deficiency, it is identification of the cause and iron replacement; and for folate deficiency, it is folate (after testing for and treating concomitant vitamin B_{12} deficiency). Anemias can also be the result of abnormal red blood cell membranes in patients with cirrhosis (ie, spur and burr cell anemia).

Coagulopathy (manifested as easy bleeding and ecchymoses), confirmed by elevation of the prothrombin INR and prolongation of the partial thromboplastin time, usually is a result of chronic liver disease, though a trial of vitamin K replacement is warranted.

Oncologic

Alcohol is a known carcinogen and is associated with an increased risk for a number of cancers.[59] These include malignancies of the oral cavity, pharynx, larynx, breast, liver, pancreas, prostate, esophagus, stomach, colon, and rectum. Though most of these cancers are associated with heavy alcohol use, often in association with smoking, the increased risk of some of the cancers is detectable in large populations at lower levels in a linear, dose-response fashion starting with any consumption. For example, breast cancer risk increases with consumption of 1 or 2 standard drinks/day on average.

Musculoskeletal

Musculoskeletal consequences can occur from the chronic heavy use of alcohol. Intoxication may result in the individual remaining in one position for prolonged periods of time, potentially leading to compression nerve palsies, rhabdomyolysis and compartment syndrome—a surgical emergency that requires fasciotomy along with debridement of necrotic tissue.

Hyperuricemia and gout are more common in persons with heavy alcohol use. Gout classically presents as podagra: an edematous, exquisitely painful, erythematous great toe. Treatment is with colchicine, using caution in renal or hepatic insufficiency, or indomethacin, using caution in the presence of gastritis or renal insufficiency. A brief course of corticosteroids may be a safer choice for the person with an alcohol use disorder. Chronic treatment in the setting of renal disease, tophaceous gout, or polyarticular gout is typically with medications that lower uric acid levels, such as allopurinol or febuxostat.

Though light alcohol use can be associated with an increase in bone density (either because of alcohol's effect on estrogens or other hormones or because of lifestyle factors associated with increased bone density), chronic heavy consumption is associated with reductions in bone density. Heavy alcohol use increases the risk of skeletal fracture.[60] This is likely due to a combination of low bone mass and increased risk for falls. Heavy alcohol use can also lead to osteonecrosis of the bone, such as that at the femoral head.

Vitamin Deficiencies

Chronic heavy alcohol consumption may lead to vitamin deficiencies because of malabsorption and reduced dietary intake. Alcohol has been associated with deficiencies of fat-soluble vitamins when there is malabsorption because of pancreatic disease and also with deficiencies of thiamine, pyridoxine, niacin, riboflavin, vitamin D, and zinc. Symptoms commonly attributed to alcohol use may be due to vitamin deficiency. For example, thiamine deficiency can cause confusion and ataxia, whereas diarrhea, abdominal discomfort, amnesia, anxiety, insomnia, nausea, seizure, and ataxia may be the result of pellagra (niacin deficiency). A clue to the diagnosis of pellagra is the coexistence of glossitis and rash in sun-exposed areas, but these more specific features may be absent. Vitamin replacement is safe and should be done empirically when there is suspicion of deficiency.

Perioperative

Heavy alcohol consumption is a risk factor for postoperative complications. In the perioperative period, attention must be given to identifying a risk of withdrawal, managing withdrawal, and managing pain. Elective surgery can be an opportune time to try to achieve abstinence, both as treatment for alcohol use disorder and prevention of perioperative morbidity.[61]

Complications Related to Tobacco Use

Tobacco use increases the risk of death while significantly contributing to medical problems and lowering quality of life. Smoking tobacco has the largest worldwide impact on morbidity and mortality of any substance.[62] An analysis of data from the Nurse's Health Study offers further insight into the health impact of smoking.[63] In this study:

- When compared to those who never smoked, people currently smoking had an increased risk of overall mortality (adjusted hazard ratio [aHR]: 2.8), as did people who formerly smoked (aHR: 1.2).
- There was a graded relationship between the number of cigarettes smoked and mortality among people currently smoking; compared to people who never smoked, those who smoked 1 to 14 cigarettes/day had an aHR of 2.0, while those who smoked 35 or more per day had an aHR of 4.4.
- Those who started smoking at an earlier age (≤17) had an increased risk of mortality, particularly from lung cancer and COPD, compared to those who started later.
- The overall mortality for people who formerly smoked declined significantly within the first 5 years after quitting and approached the level of never smoking after 20 years. Mortality from vascular disease declined more rapidly than other causes; in contrast, the risk of lung cancer declined slowly and was still significantly higher than never smoking 30 years after quitting.

Though nicotine withdrawal is not life-threatening, it can interfere with psychosocial functioning and the craving can complicate treatment for other medical illnesses (eg, causing patients to leave the hospital in order to smoke). Nicotine replacement should be provided for medically-ill patients with tobacco use disorder who are hospitalized. Bupropion and varenicline are alternatives.

Cardiovascular

Smoking is one of the most important risk factors for atherosclerosis.[64] People who smoke are at higher risk of myocardial infarction (MI) and sudden death, as well as cerebrovascular disease and stroke. Smoking is also is an important risk factor for peripheral vascular disease, which leads to intermittent claudication, pain, and loss of limb. The risk of heart disease and peripheral vascular disease and stroke morbidity and mortality decrease soon after stopping smoking. The risks also extend to others with second-hand exposure to tobacco smoke.

Renal

The renal consequences of tobacco use are limited primarily to the effects of atherosclerosis of the renal arteries, which can lead to ischemic renal failure and hypertension from renal artery stenosis.

Gastrointestinal

Smoking is a cause of gastric and duodenal ulcers and interferes with ulcer healing. Smoking can cause and exacerbate gastroesophageal reflux disease. These diseases may require pharmacotherapy with histamine type 2 receptor antagonists, proton pump inhibitors, or antibiotics for *Helicobacter pylori*.

Respiratory

Chronic obstructive pulmonary disease (COPD) is a leading cause of morbidity and mortality worldwide and smoking tobacco is an important cause of this condition, particularly in high-income countries like the United States.[65] Smoking is also the leading cause of lung cancer. The risks of both of these mortal diagnoses can be lowered with smoking abstinence. Stopping smoking can slow the steady decline in pulmonary function seen in COPD. Smoking is also associated with pulmonary hypertension, interstitial lung disease, and pneumothorax.

Neurologic

Tobacco use is associated with cerebrovascular disease and ischemic and hemorrhagic stroke. Atherosclerotic disease can involve small vessels and result in cognitive deficits.

Aside from the potential effects of nicotine-containing electronic cigarettes on attention, mood, cognition, and impulse control, concentrated nicotine liquid can lead to severe acute neurological toxicity in children who ingest it. Further details about nicotine and electronic cigarettes can be found in Section 2, and further details regarding neurological issues may be found in this section.

Infections

Smoking has direct detrimental effects on the respiratory tract and increases the risk of upper and lower respiratory tract infections, including acute and chronic bronchitis, influenza, pneumonia and tuberculosis.[66] These risks decrease with abstinence from smoking.

Sleep

Nicotine use has detrimental effects on sleep, including increasing the time it takes to fall asleep (sleep latency), increasing sleep fragmentation and reducing sleep efficiency.[67] Nicotine withdrawal is associated with insomnia, resulting in daytime sleepiness.

Injury

Combustible tobacco use can lead to house fires, smoke inhalation, and death, as well as other accidental deaths. Smoking in medically-ill patients using oxygen has resulted in burns and fires. Electronic cigarette devices have also ignited and even exploded, resulting in serious injury.

Endocrinologic

Smoking increases the risk of thyroid disorders, particularly Graves disease (hyperthyroidism), but also toxic nodular goiter and hypothyroidism.[68] Smoking and nicotine increase insulin resistance and risk of type II diabetes, as well as complications from diabetes.[69] Estrogen is decreased in males and females who smoke, as is sperm count and function in men. Smoking is one of the leading causes of erectile dysfunction, mainly because of atherosclerosis. Smoking is also associated with osteopenia, osteoporosis, and fractures.

Fetal, Neonatal, and Infant

Tobacco use during pregnancy is associated with low birth weight, spontaneous abortion, and perinatal mortality. Nicotine in electronic cigarettes also appears to be associated with sudden infant death and other maternal and fetal consequences. The risks of sudden infant death syndrome and neurodevelopmental impairment are increased with cigarette use, though studies have had difficulty separating the effects of tobacco, alcohol, nutrition, and social environment.

Oncologic

Smoking is associated with a number of cancers, including oral cavity, larynx, lung, esophagus, bladder, kidney, pancreas, stomach, and cervix.[70] People who smoke who have one smoking-related cancer are at higher risk for a second one. These risks decrease with abstinence, but persist for many years. Smokeless tobacco use is associated with oral, esophageal, and pancreatic cancer.[71]

Perioperative

Smoking increases the risk of postoperative pulmonary complications and is associated with impaired wound healing.[72] Smoking abstinence before elective surgery is advisable and some surgeons require abstinence from all forms of nicotine before performing elective surgeries. It should be noted that nicotine replacement therapy (NRT) is an important tool in helping individuals stop using tobacco and that available evidence does not indicate that NRT increases surgical complications.[73,74]

Complications Related to Opioids, Stimulants, and Injection Drug Use

The complications of opioids and stimulants may be related to the route of administration. Injection and inhalation of drugs have particular consequences. In addition to route of administration, these drugs have unique organ system complications.

Injection Drug Use

Skin and soft tissue infections (SSTI) are common in people who inject drugs (PWID), usually caused by staphylococci and streptococci. Treatment for minor bacterial infections may include an oral antibiotic chosen based on current guidelines and local epidemiology. Intravenous antibiotics such as vancomycin may be used for more severe infections or infections that do not respond to first-line treatment. Purulent SSTIs are often caused by *Staphylococcus aureus* and drainable abscesses should undergo surgical incision and drainage in addition to empiric treatment with antibiotics that provide coverage for methicillin-resistant *Staphylococcus aureus* (MRSA), which are common among PWID. One must be aware of local epidemiology and practices because there have been reports of unusual pathogens (eg, *Pseudomonas aeruginosa* and *Serratia* species) and polymicrobial infections from use of saliva to prepare the injection. Furthermore, patients sometimes use antibiotics obtained without prescription, which places them at risk of infection with resistant organisms. Soft tissue infections can progress to become serious and life-threatening if necrotizing fasciitis develops or if there is significant local ischemia. Intravenous injection can result in septic thrombophlebitis. Arterial injection can lead to embolus, digital ischemia, and infection. Repeated intravenous and subcutaneous injection can lead to venous valvular damage in the extremities, marked by leg ulcers, edema, and a propensity to deep vein thrombosis.

Injection drug use can spread blood-borne pathogens when needles or other equipment are shared; these include HIV, hepatitis B, and hepatitis C. Hepatitis B usually clears spontaneously but can develop into chronic infection, while hepatitis C usually develops into a chronic infection (in the absence of treatment). HIV infection almost invariably leads to chronic illness. Hepatitis B and C can lead to cirrhosis and its sequelae, including hepatocellular carcinoma and death; untreated HIV can lead to opportunistic infections and death. Hepatitis B can be managed with antiviral drugs or prevented by immunization. Hepatitis C is largely curable now with 2 to 3 months of antiviral treatment. HIV can be managed with combinations of two or three antiretroviral drugs often delivered in one-pill daily formulations or, since 2021, with extended-release, intramuscular injections every 1 or 2 months. These treatments should not be withheld from people who use substances, though HIV treatment outcomes are improved if substance use disorders are addressed concurrently.[75]

One of the most serious infectious consequences of injection drug use is bacterial endocarditis. In PWID, fever is an indication for hospitalization, empiric antibiotics, and infectious work up. Other deep-seated infections can include septic arthritis in unusual locations (sternoclavicular or sacroiliac joints), spinal epidural or vertebral infections, osteomyelitis, or meningitis. A significant proportion of PWID with fever and no identifiable cause will have an unrecognized serious illness, most often endocarditis and missing this diagnosis can be fatal. A cardiac murmur may or may not be present. The classic "textbook" signs of subacute bacterial endocarditis, most of which are immunological phenomena, often are not present in PWID, who often present with right-sided (eg, tricuspid valve) endocarditis. Therefore, blood cultures should be taken and close observation (often in the hospital) instituted; antibiotics should be given empirically while awaiting culture results. If endocarditis is diagnosed, treatment is with bactericidal antibiotics for 4 to 6 weeks. Selected uncomplicated cases may be treated with shorter courses or oral antibiotics. Mycotic aneurysms; endophthalmitis; congestive heart failure; brain, spleen, or myocardial abscesses and emboli; renal failure from interstitial nephritis; pulmonary septic emboli with effusions; stroke; and heart block can complicate the course. Patients who have multiple emboli or hemodynamic decompensation may require surgical intervention and valve replacement. Surgery indications are the same as for those without SUD, and should not be withheld only because of substance use.

In addition to infectious complications, drug injection has been associated with pulmonary or hepatic talc granulomatosis from injected crushed tablets containing talc, pulmonary hypertension from granulomatous disease or stimulated-related vasoconstriction, needle embolization, pneumothorax or hemothorax from injection into large central veins gone awry, and pulmonary emphysema. Cerebral infarction has resulted from injection of crushed tablets (intravenously and via inadvertent intra-arterial injection).

Injection drug use can also lead to renal complications. Amyloidosis and nephrotic syndrome can occur because of chronic skin infections. Hepatitis C infection can lead to glomerulonephritis. Untreated HIV infection can lead to nephropathy.

Complications can also arise from adulterants mixed with the intended psychoactive drug that could range from quinine or atropine or other cardiovascular medications (eg, diltiazem), to local anesthetics, veterinary anesthetics (eg, xylazine), to acetaminophen, caffeine and other stimulants, antipsychotics, or antihistamines. These adulterants can lead to toxic effects known to be associated with the individual drugs (eg, hepatic failure for acetaminophen, vasculitis for levamisole, dysrhythmias from lidocaine or quinine).

In addition to adulterants that are deliberately combined with other drugs, inadvertent contaminants may lead to infectious complications with drug use. One example of this is *Clostridium* species in black tar heroin leading to wound botulism.[76] Another is heroin contaminated with anthrax leading to cutaneous and soft tissue infection after injection use or respiratory, gastrointestinal or systemic infection after inhaled use.[77]

Complications of injection drug use can be mitigated by a number of harm reduction measures, including providing patients with sterile equipment, safer consumption (or supervised injection or overdose prevention) facilities and teaching safe injection practices.

Respiratory

Opioid overdose can lead to respiratory depression and death. Atelectasis can develop, as can aspiration and chemical pneumonitis. Opioid use can lead to bronchospasm, as a result of stimulation of histamine release, and pulmonary edema in the setting of overdose. Stimulant use can lead to pulmonary hemorrhage, edema, hypertension, emphysema, interstitial fibrosis, and hypersensitivity pneumonitis. Pulmonary hypertension has also been associated with stimulant use.

Cocaine use can also lead to nasal septal perforation and sinusitis when used intranasally and epiglottitis, upper airway obstruction, and hemoptysis when smoked, primarily from irritant and vasoconstrictive effects.

Cardiovascular

Some of the most serious complications of stimulant use are related to their effects on the heart and blood vessels. Both cocaine and methamphetamine use have been associated with severe hypertension, cardiac dysrhythmias, angina, myocardial infarction, sudden death, and stroke. Chest pain often occurs during or after stimulant use, but most persons evaluated in emergency departments with chest pain and stimulant use do not have myocardial infarction. Nonetheless, heart attacks do occur and are thought to be related to coronary vasospasm, in situ thrombosis, or the accelerated development of atherosclerosis (or underlying atherosclerotic coronary artery disease, eg, from smoking). Cardiomyopathy can occur either as a consequence of ischemic damage or possibly direct toxicity.[78]

Gastrointestinal

Opioids slow gastrointestinal transit and chronic opioid use causes constipation; in contrast to respiratory depression, this is not a side effect to which individuals develop a tolerance. Stimulant use has been associated with ischemic colitis, which can present with abdominal pain constipation or diarrhea and gastrointestinal bleeding[79] and may require surgical intervention.[80]

Renal and Metabolic

Aside from the previously discussed infectious and injection-related renal complications, any drug that leads to sedation with intoxication or overdose (such as opioids) can lead to muscle compression and rhabdomyolysis and acute renal failure.

Rhabdomyolysis can be seen with amphetamine and cocaine use. Stimulant use has been associated with hyperthermia, accelerated hypertension and renal failure, hypertensive nephrosclerosis, thrombotic microangiopathy, and renal infarction.

Neuropsychiatric

Stimulant use is associated with a number of neuropsychiatric complications, including agitation, psychosis, tremor, hyperkinetic and stereotypical movements, and cognitive impairment.[81,82] Cocaine and methamphetamine use have been associated with hemorrhagic and ischemic strokes. Stimulant use, particularly cocaine, is associated with seizures. Methamphetamine (but not cocaine) use has been associated with an increased risk of Parkinson disease.

Sleep

Stimulants, including caffeine, can suppress sleep, which often is an intended effect and withdrawal may result in hypersomnolence. Many persons with SUD also experience sleep disturbances; this can be due to the drug used, other behaviors, or comorbid psychiatric conditions. Sleep problems can contribute to the desire to use drugs to promote sleep. In fact, opioids help with restless leg syndrome and periodic movements of sleep, something a person with an opioid use disorder may have discovered in the course of illicit use.

Endocrinologic

Opioids can impair gonadotropin release. Clinically, men may have impaired sperm motility, and women may have menstrual and ovulatory irregularities. This mechanism may explain the osteopenia seen in people with opioid use disorder, though etiology is likely multifactorial.

Cutaneous

Cocaine is sometimes adulterated with levamisole, an anti-helminthic drug that can cause complications including purpuric rash and cutaneous necrosis with a predilection for the extremities, ears, nose and malar regions of the cheeks.[83] In addition to cutaneous infections from injection drug use, use of some drugs, including methamphetamines, is associated with skin-picking behaviors that can lead to skin infections.[84]

Fetal, Neonatal, and Infant

No clear teratogenic effects of opioids are known. Though many studies have been conducted, studies that did find effects often did not control for the effects of important confounders such as nutrition, alcohol, and tobacco use. However, opioid exposure in utero can lead to the neonatal abstinence or neonatal opioid withdrawal syndrome. Stimulant use by pregnant persons has been associated with some adverse perinatal outcomes including preterm delivery and low birth weight.[85]

Complications Related to Cannabinoids and Other Drugs

Most of the morbidity and mortality related to substance use is the consequence of tobacco, alcohol, opioid, stimulant, and injection drug use. Other drugs—including cannabinoids, hallucinogens, inhalants—tend to have less impact on health, but are associated with some medical complications.

Respiratory

Similar to tobacco, cannabis smoking can lead to respiratory symptoms including cough and mucus production, but does not seem to lead to chronic obstructive lung disease.[86] There have been cases of lung injury associated with cannabinoid use through vaping; studies suggest that vitamin E acetate, an additive in vaping products, may be the culprit.[87] Smoking cannabis has also been associated with spontaneous pneumothorax.[88]

Inhalants can lead to methemoglobinemia, tracheobronchitis, asphyxiation, and hypersensitivity pneumonitis. Nitrous oxide can cause respiratory depression and hypoxemia.

Cardiovascular

Exposure to tetrahydrocannabinol (THC), which is found in cannabis, is associated with an increase in heart rate and blood pressure, but has not been shown convincingly to increase the risk for adverse cardiovascular outcomes such as myocardial infarction or arrhythmia.[89] Psychedelic drugs such as psilocybin and lysergic acid diethylamide (LSD) can also transiently increase blood pressure and heart rate.[90] Drugs with anticholinergic effects (muscle relaxants, antihistamines, and antidepressants) cause tachycardia and can cause dysrhythmias with intoxication or overdose. Inhalants (volatile fluorocarbons) can cause dysrhythmias and this is thought to be the cause of cases of sudden death associated with their use.[91]

Gastrointestinal

Cannabis use may be associated with a hyperemesis syndrome that is characterized by cyclic nausea and vomiting with abdominal pain, often relieved with hot showers or baths.[92] Synthetic cannabinoid use may be complicated by abdominal pain, nausea, and vomiting.[93] Nausea and vomiting are also common with use of some psychedelic drugs such as ayahuasca.[94]

There have been case reports of ecstasy (MDMA) and phencyclidine (PCP) use causing liver failure. Androgenic steroids can cause hepatic toxicity.

Renal and Metabolic

Any drug that leads to sedation with intoxication or overdose (such as phencyclidine or synthetic cannabinoids) can lead to muscle compression and rhabdomyolysis and to acute renal failure.

3,4-Methylenedioxymethamphetamine (MDMA or "ecstasy") use can lead to hyponatremia when people drink excess water to prevent the hypovolemia associated with use of this drug. Toluene inhalation can lead to metabolic acidosis.

Neurologic

Inhalation of organic compounds acutely causes a variety of neurologic sequelae, including ataxia, tremor, and encephalopathy; regular use may lead to irreversible cognitive or motor deficits.[95]

Neuropathy (including plexopathies and Guillain-Barré syndrome) may be caused by compression neuropathy related to any drug use, inhalation of organic solvents including glue, and combined system degeneration from vitamin B_{12} deficiency induced by nitrous oxide use.

Injury

Cannabis use impairs psychomotor skills and is associated with motor vehicle crashes, especially fatal collisions.[96] Inhalant use may lead to burns, either from ignition of flammable compounds or thermal injury from compressed compounds (eg, computer duster spray).

Endocrinologic

Cannabinoids have multiple effects on the endocrine system; the most clinically significant are a reduced risk of type II diabetes and decrease in bone density.[97] Anabolic steroids also have significant effects, including virilization in women and testicular atrophy in men.

Fetal, Neonatal, and Infant

Cannabis use among pregnant person has been associated with increased risk of preterm birth, stillbirth, and small for gestational age,[98] although some findings should be interpreted with caution due to the risk of confounders like tobacco use and poverty.[99] Inhaled toluene appears to cause an embryopathy, and other inhalants have been associated with various effects, some similar to fetal alcohol syndrome.[100]

Hematologic

Synthetic cannabinoids are sometimes adulterated with long-acting vitamin K antagonist rodenticides that can lead to serious bleeding complications requiring very high doses of vitamin K for reversal of coagulopathy.[101]

Amyl nitrate, isobutyl nitrate, and other "poppers" can cause methemoglobinemia. The arterial partial pressure of oxygen is normal, the saturation is low, and cyanosis is present. The condition can be diagnosed by measuring serum methemoglobin and treated with methylene blue.

Vitamin Deficiencies

Nitrous oxide use is a well-known cause of vitamin B_{12} deficiency, which may lead to symptoms of myeloneuropathy including limb numbness, limb weakness, and unsteady gait.[102]

CONCLUSIONS

Persons with unhealthy substance use often do not receive adequate medical care. A medical, psychiatric, or addiction health care visit is an opportunity to provide symptom-oriented as well as preventive care or to link individuals to primary and preventive health care services. Routine health care of the person with unhealthy substance use should take into account the higher risk of specific conditions. This warrants a targeted approach to the conditions for which the patient is at risk and the risks of which can be ameliorated or reduced through safer use. During hospitalization for medical or surgical reasons, special attention must be directed toward management of intoxication and withdrawal and adequate symptom control, including craving, for people with SUD. Persons with unhealthy substance use are at risk of a large number of specific acute and chronic medical illnesses in almost every organ system. Further, the management of unrelated but common medical illnesses is complicated by substance use, its effect on medication adherence, and the direct consequences of the substances, contaminants or adulterants, and routes of administration. Older adults often suffer from a number of chronic disorders including addiction; beyond worsening the common chronic diseases of aging, substance use can further impair functional status. The subsequent chapters in this section delve into the medical complications of substance use by organ systems in greater detail.

ACKNOWLEDGMENT

An earlier version of this chapter was written by Richard Saitz. The chapter was edited by Paula Lum.

REFERENCES

1. Friedmann PD, Saitz R, Samet JH. Management of adults recovering from alcohol or other drug problems: relapse prevention in primary care. *JAMA.* 1998;279(15):1227-1231.
2. Substance Abuse and Mental Health Services Administration. *SAMHSA's Concept of Trauma and Guidance for Trauma-Informed Approach.* HHS Publication No. (SMA) 14-884. SAMHSA; 2014.
3. Walensky RP, Houry D, Jernigan DB, et al. Sexually transmitted infection treatment guidelines, 2021. *MMWR Recomm Rep.* 2021;70(4):1-192.
4. Lewinsohn DM, Leonard MK, LoBue PA, et al. Official American Thoracic Society/Infectious Diseases Society of America/Centers for Disease Control and Prevention Clinical Practice Guidelines: diagnosis of tuberculosis in adults and children. *Clin Infect Dis.* 2017;64(2):e1-e33.
5. Schillie S, Wester C, Osborne M, Wesolowski L, Ryerson AB. CDC recommendations for hepatitis C screening among adults—United States, 2020. *MMWR Recomm Rep.* 2020;69:1-17.
6. Weinbaum CM, Williams I, Mast EE, et al. Recommendations for identification and public health management of persons with chronic hepatitis B virus infection. *MMWR Recomm Rep.* 2008;57:1-20.
7. Curry SJ, Krist AH, Owens DK, et al. Screening for cervical cancer: U.S. Preventive Services Task Force recommendation statement. *JAMA.* 2018;320(7):674-686.
8. Palefsky JM, Lee JY, Jay N, et al. Treatment of anal high-grade squamous intraepithelial lesions to prevent anal cancer. *N Engl J Med.* 2022;386(24):2273-2282.
9. Krist AH, Davidson KW, Mangione CM, et al. Screening for lung cancer: U.S. Preventive Services Task Force recommendation statement. *JAMA.* 2021;325(10):962-970.
10. Siu AL; U.S. Preventive Services Task Force. Screening for breast cancer: U.S. Preventive Services Task Force recommendation statement. *Ann Intern Med.* 2016;164(4):279-296.
11. Deutsch MB. *Screening for Breast Cancer in Transgender Women.* UCSF Transgender Care & Treatment Guidelines. Accessed June 10, 2022. https://transcare.ucsf.edu/guidelines/breast-cancer-women
12. Grossman DC, Curry SJ, Owens DK, et al. Screening for prostate cancer: U.S. Preventive Services Task Force recommendation statement. *JAMA.* 2018;319(18):1901-1913.
13. Davidson KW, Barry MJ, Mangione CM, et al. Screening for colorectal cancer: U.S. Preventive Services Task Force recommendation statement. *JAMA.* 2021;325(19):1965-1977.
14. Owens DK, Davidson KW, Krist AH, et al. Screening for abdominal aortic aneurysm: U.S. Preventive Services Task Force recommendation statement. *JAMA.* 2019;322(22):2211-2218.
15. Tseng YC, Liu SHY, Lou MF, Huang GS. Quality of life in older adults with sensory impairments: a systematic review. *Qual Life Res.* 2018;27(8):1957-1971.
16. Curry SJ, Krist AH, Owens DK, et al. Screening for osteoporosis to prevent fractures: U.S. Preventive Services Task Force recommendation statement. *JAMA.* 2018;319(24):2521-2531.
17. Kim TW, Alford DP, Malabanan A, Holick MF, Samet JH. Low bone density in patients receiving methadone maintenance treatment. *Drug Alcohol Depend.* 2006;85:258-262.
18. Aberg JA, Gallant JE, Ghanem KG, et al. Primary care guidelines for the management of persons infected with HIV: 2013 update by the HIV Medicine Association of the Infectious Disease Society of America. *Clin Infect Dis.* 2014;58(1):1-10.
19. Freedman MS, Ault K, Bernstein H. Advisory committee on immunization practices recommended immunization schedule for adults aged 19 years or older—United States, 2021. *MMWR Morb Mortal Wkly Rep.* 2021;70(6):193-196.
20. Beeching NJ, Crowcroft NS. Tetanus in injecting drug users. *BMJ.* 2005;330(7485):208-209.
21. Centers for Disease Control and Prevention: U.S. Public Health Service: Preexposure prophylaxis for the prevention of HIV infection in the United States—2021 Update: a clinical practice guideline. Accessed June 19, 2023. https://www.cdc.gov/hiv/pdf/risk/prep/cdc-hiv-prep-guidelines-2021.pdf
22. Cunningham EB, Hajarizadeh B, Amin J, et al. Adherence to once-daily and twice-daily direct-acting antiviral treatment for hepatitis C infection among people with recent injection drug use or current opioid agonist therapy. *Clin Infect Dis.* 2020;71(7):e115-e124.
23. Rowell-Cunsolo TL, Liu J, Hu G, Larson E. Length of hospitalization and hospital readmissions among patients with substance use disorders in New York City, NY, USA. *Drug Alcohol Depend.* 2020;212:107987.
24. Wakeman SE, Kane M, Powell E, Howard S, Shaw C, Regan S. Impact of inpatient addiction consultation on hospital readmission. *J Gen Intern Med.* 2021;36(7):2162-2163.
25. Wilson JD, Dunn SCA, Roy P, Joseph E, Klipp S, Liebschutz J. Inpatient addiction medicine consultation service impact on post-discharge patient mortality: a propensity matched analysis. *J Gen Intern Med.* 2022;37(10):2521-2525.
26. Simon R, Snow R, Wakeman S. Understanding why patients with substance use disorders leave the hospital against medical advice: a qualitative study. *Subst Abus.* 2020;41(4):519-525.
27. ASAM Alcohol Withdrawal Guideline Committee. The ASAM clinical practice guideline on alcohol withdrawal management. *J Addict Med.* 2020;14(3S Suppl 1):1-72.
28. Crotty K, Freedman KI, Kampman KM. Executive summary of the focused update of the ASAM National Practice Guideline for the treatment of opioid use disorder. *J Addict Med.* 2020;14(2):99-112.
29. Kleinman RA, Wakeman SE. Treating opioid withdrawal in the hospital: a role for short-acting opioids. *Ann Intern Med.* 2022;175(2):283-284.
30. Thakrar AP. Short-acting opioids for hospitalized patients with opioid use disorder. *JAMA Intern Med.* 2022;182(3):247-248.
31. Merrill JO, Rhodes LA, Deyo RA, Marlatt GA, Bradley KA. Mutual mistrust in the medical care of drug users: the keys to the "narc" cabinet. *J Gen Inter Med.* 2022;17(5):327-333.
32. Agin-Liebes G, Huhn AS, Strain EC, et al. Methadone maintenance patients lack analgesic response to a cumulative intravenous dose of 32 mg of hydromorphone. *Drug Alcohol Depend.* 2021;226:108869.
33. Lehmann SW, Fingerhood MI. Substance-use disorders in later life. *N Engl J Med.* 2018;379:2351-2360.
34. Solomon HV, Greenstein AP, DeLisi LE. Cannabis use in older adults: a perspective. *Harv Rev Psychiatry.* 2021;29(3):225-233.
35. DiCastelnouvo A, Costanzo S, Bagnardi V, Donati MB, Iacoviello L, de Gaetano G. Alcohol dosing and total mortality in men and women: an updated meta-analysis of 34 prospective studies. *Arch Intern Med.* 2006;166:2437-2445.
36. Stockwell T, Zhao J, Panwar S, Roemer A, Naimi T, Chikritzhs T. Do "moderate" drinkers have reduced mortality risk? A systematic review and meta-analysis of alcohol consumption and all-cause mortality. *J Stud Alcohol Drugs.* 2016;77(2):185-198.
37. Whiteford HA, Degenhardt L, Rehm J, et al. Global burden of disease attributable to mental and substance use disorders: findings from the Global Burden of Disease Study 2010. *Lancet.* 2013;382(9904):1575-1586.
38. Biddinger KJ, Emdin CA, Haas ME, et al. Association of habitual alcohol intake with risk of cardiovascular disease. *JAMA Netw Open.* 2022;5(3):e223849.
39. Day E, Rudd JHF. Alcohol use disorders and the heart. *Addiction.* 2019;114(9):1670-1678.
40. Nicolás JM, Fernández-Solà J, Estruch R, et al. The effect of controlled drinking in alcoholic cardiomyopathy. *Ann Intern Med.* 2002;136(3):192-200.

41. Voskoboinik A, Kalman JM, De Silva A, et al. Alcohol abstinence in drinkers with atrial fibrillation. *N Engl J Med.* 2020;382:20-28.
42. Singal AK, Mathurin P. Diagnosis and treatment of alcohol-associated liver disease: a review. *JAMA.* 2021;326(2):165-176.
43. Hosseini N, Shor J, Szabo G. Alcoholic hepatitis: a review. *Alcohol Alcohol.* 2019;54(4):408-416.
44. Im GY, Cameron AM, Lucey MR. Liver transplantation for alcoholic hepatitis. *J Hepatol.* 2019;70(2):328-334.
45. Ginès P, Krag A, Albraldes JG, Solà E, Fabrellas N, Kamath PS. Liver cirrhosis. *Lancet.* 2021;398:1359-1376.
46. Singal AG, Pillai A, Tiro J. Early detection, curative treatment, and survival rates for hepatocellular carcinoma surveillance in patients with cirrhosis: a meta-analysis. *PLoS Med.* 2014;11(4):e1001624.
47. Jain A, Reyes J, Kashyap R, et al. Long-term survival after liver transplantation in 4,000 consecutive patients at a single center. *Ann Surg.* 2000;232(4):490-500.
48. Herrick-Reynolds KM, Punchhi G, Greenberg RS, et al. Evaluation of early vs standard liver transplant for alcohol-associated liver disease. *JAMA Surg.* 2021;156(11):1026-1034.
49. Louvet A, Labreuche J, Moreno C, et al. Early liver transplantation for severe alcohol-related hepatitis not responding to medical treatment: a prospective-controlled study. *Lancet Gastroenterol Hepatol.* 2022;7(5):421-425.
50. Long B, Lentz S, Gottlieb M. Alcoholic ketoacidosis: etiologies, evaluation, and management. *J Emerg Med.* 2021;61(6):658-665.
51. Vamvakas S, Teschner M, Bahner U, Heidland A. Alcohol abuse: potential role in electrolyte disturbances and kidney diseases. *Clin Nephrol.* 1998;49(4):205-213.
52. Haber PS, Kortt NC. Alcohol use disorder and the gut. *Addiction.* 2021;116(3):658-667.
53. Lankisch PG, Apte M, Banks PA. Acute pancreatitis. *Lancet.* 2015;386:85-96.
54. Hammoud N, Jimenez-Shahed J. Chronic neurologic effects of alcohol. *Clin Liver Dis.* 2019;23(1):141-155.
55. Larsson SC, Wallin A, Wolk A, Markus HS. Differing associations of alcohol consumption with different stroke types: a systematic review and meta-analysis. *BMC Med.* 2016;14(1):178.
56. Molina PE, Happel KI, Zhang P, Kolls JK, Nelson S. Focus on: alcohol and the immune system. *Alcohol Res Health.* 2010;33:97-108.
57. Chakrovorty S, Chaudhary NS, Brower KJ. Alcohol dependence and its relationship with insomnia and other sleep disorders. *Alcohol Clin Exp Res.* 2016;40(11):2271-2282.
58. Knott C, Bell S, Britton A. Alcohol consumption and the risk of type 2 diabetes: a systematic review and dose-response meta-analysis of more than 1.9 million individuals from 38 observational studies. *Diabetes Care.* 2015;38(9):1804-1812.
59. Boffetta P, Hashibe M. Alcohol and cancer. *Lancet Oncol.* 2006;7(2):149-156.
60. Maurel DB, Boisseau N, Benhamou CL, Jaffre C. Alcohol and bone: review of dose effects and mechanisms. *Osteoporosis Int.* 2012;23(1):1-16.
61. Oppedal K, Moller AM, Pederson B, Tonnesen H. Preoperative alcohol cessation prior to elective surgery. *Cochrane Database Syst Rev.* 2012;(7):CD008343.
62. Peacock A, Leung J, Larney S, et al. Global statistics on alcohol, tobacco and illicit drug use: 2017 status report. *Addiction.* 2018;113(10):1905-1926.
63. Kenfield SA, Stampfer MJ, Rosner BA, Colditz GA. Smoking and smoking cessation in relation to mortality in women. *JAMA.* 2008;299:2037-2047.
64. Greenland P, Knoll MD, Stamler J. Major risk factors as antecedents of fatal and nonfatal coronary heart disease events. *JAMA.* 2003;290(7):891-897.
65. Mannino DM, Buist AS. Global burden of COPD: risk factors, prevalence, and future trends. *Lancet.* 2007;370(9589):765-773.
66. Arcavi L, Benowitz NL. Cigarette smoking and infection. *Arch Intern Med.* 2004;164(20):2206-2216.
67. Jaehne A, Loessl B, Bárkai Z, Riemann D, Hornyak M. Effects of nicotine on sleep during consumption, withdrawal and replacement therapy. *Sleep Med Rev.* 2009;13(5):363-377.
68. Vestergaard P, Renjmark L, Weeke J, et al. Smoking as a risk factor for Grave's disease, toxic nodular goiter, and autoimmune hypothyroidism. *Thyroid.* 2002;12(1):69-75.
69. Sliwinska-Mosson M, Milnerowicz H. The impact of smoking on the development of diabetes and its complications. *Diab Vasc Dis Res.* 2017;14(4):265-276.
70. Sasco AJ, Secretan MB, Straif K. Tobacco smoking and cancer: a brief review of recent epidemiological evidence. *Lung Cancer.* 2004;45(Suppl 2):S3-S9.
71. Boffetta P, Hecht S, Gray N, et al. Smokeless tobacco and cancer. *Lancet Oncol.* 2008;9(7):667-675.
72. Sorensen LT. Wound healing and infection in surgery: the pathophysiological impact of smoking, smoking cessation and nicotine replacement therapy: a systematic review. *Ann Surg.* 2012;255(6):1069-1089.
73. Nolan MB, Warner DO. Safety and efficacy of nicotine replacement therapy in the perioperative period: a narrative review. *Mayo Clin Proc.* 2015;90(11):1553-1561.
74. Stefan MS, Pack Q, Shieh MS, et al. The association of nicotine replacement therapy with outcomes among smokers hospitalized for a major surgical procedure. *Chest.* 2020;157(5):1354-1361.
75. Altice FL, Kamarulzaman A, Soriano VV, Schechter M, Friedland GH. Treatment of medical, psychiatric, and substance-use comorbidities in people infected with HIV who use drugs. *Lancet.* 2010;376(9738):367-387.
76. Raza N, Dhital S, Espinoza VE, et al. Wound botulism in black tar heroin injecting users: a case series. *J Investig Med High Impact Case Rep.* 2021;9:23247096211028078.
77. Zasada AA. Injectional anthrax in human: a new face of the old disease. *Adv Clin Exp Med.* 2018;27(4):553-558.
78. Arenas DJ, Beltran S, Zhou S, Goldberg LR. Cocaine, cardiomyopathy, and heart failure: a systematic review and meta-analysis. *Sci Rep.* 2020;10(1):19795.
79. Prakash MD, Tangalakis K, Antonipillai J, Stojanovska L, Nurgali K, Apostolopoulos. Methamphetamine: effects on the brain, gut and immune system. *Pharmacol Res.* 2017;120:60-67.
80. Costa AV, Zhunus A, Hafeez R, Gupta A. Cocaine-induced mesenteric ischemia requiring small bowel resection. *BMJ Case Rep.* 2021;14(1):e238593.
81. Asser A, Taba P. Psychostimulants and movement disorders. *Front Neurol.* 2015;6:75.
82. Lappin JM, Sara GE. Psychostimulant use and the brain. *Addiction.* 2019;114(11):2065-2077.
83. Roberts JA, Chevez-Barrios P. Levamisole-induced vasculitis: a characteristic cutaneous vasculitis associated with levamisole adulterated cocaine. *Arch Pathol Lab Med.* 2015;139(8):1058-1061.
84. Cohen AL, Shuler C, McAllister S, et al. Methamphetamine use and methicillin-resistant *Staphylococcus aureus* skin infections. *Emerg Infect Dis.* 2007;13(11):1707-1713.
85. Smid MC, Metz TD, Gordon AJ. Stimulant use in pregnancy: an under-recognized epidemic among pregnant women. *Clin Obstet Gynecol.* 2019;62(1):168-184.
86. Gracie K, Hancox RJ. Cannabis use disorder and the lungs. *Addiction.* 2021;116(1):182-190.
87. Mikosz CA, Danielson M, Anderson KN, et al. Characteristics of patients experiencing rehospitalization or death after hospital discharge in a nationwide outbreak of E-cigarette, or vaping, product use-associated lung injury—United States, 2019. *MMWR Morb Mortal Wkly Rep.* 2020;68:1183-1188.
88. Wakefield CJ, Seder CW, Arndt AT, Giessen N, Liptay MJ, Karush JM. Cannabis use is associated with recurrence after primary spontaneous pneumothorax. *Front Surg.* 2021;8:668588.
89. Page RL, Allen LA, Kloner RA, et al. Medical marijuana, recreational cannabis, and cardiovascular health: a scientific statement from the American Heart Association. *Circulation.* 2020;10(8):e131-e151.
90. Holze F, Ley L, Muller F, et al. Direct comparison of the acute effects of lysergic acid diethylamide and psilocybin in a double-blind placebo-controlled study in healthy subjects. *Neuropsychopharmacology.* 2022;47(6):1180-1187.

91. Bass M. Sudden sniffing death. *JAMA*. 1970;212(12):2017-2079.
92. Sorensen CJ, DeSanto K, Borgelt L, Phillips KT, Monte AA. Cannabinoid hyperemesis syndrome: diagnosis, pathophysiology, and treatment—a systematic review. *J Med Toxicol.* 2017;13(1):71-87.
93. Hakiman D, Benson AA, Khoury T, et al. Gastrointestinal manifestations of synthetic cannabinoids: a retrospective cohort study. *BMC Gastroenterol.* 2021;21(1):274.
94. Bender D, Hellerstein DJ. Assessing the risk-benefit profile of classical psychedelics: a clinical review of second-wave psychedelic research. *Psychopharmacol (Berl).* 2022;239:1907-1932.
95. Tormoehlen LM, Tekulve KJ, Nanagas KA. Hydrocarbon toxicity: a review. *Clin Toxicol (Phila).* 2014;52(5):479-489.
96. Asbridge M, Hayden JA, Cartwright JL. Acute cannabis consumption and motor vehicle collision risk: a systematic review of observational studies and meta-analysis. *BMJ.* 2012;344:e536.
97. Meah F, Lundholm M, Emanuele N, et al. The effects of cannabis and cannabinoids on the endocrine system. *Rev Endocr Metab Disord.* 2022;23(3):401-420.
98. Marijuana use during pregnancy and lactation. Committee Opinion No. 722. American College of Obstetricians and Gynecologists. *Obstet Gynecol.* 2017;130:e205-e209.
99. Corsi DJ, Walsh L, Weiss D, et al. Association between self-reported prenatal cannabis use and maternal, perinatal, and neonatal outcomes. *JAMA.* 2019;322:145-152.
100. Ford JB, Sutter ME, Owen KP, Albertson TE. Volatile substance misuse: an updated review of toxicity and treatment. *Clin Rev Allergy Immmunol.* 2014;46(1):19-33.
101. Bahouth MN, Kraus P, Dane K, et al. Synthetic cannabinoid-associated coagulopathy secondary to long-acting anticoagulant rodenticides: observational case series and management recommendations. *Medicine (Baltimore).* 2019;98:e17015.
102. Lan SY, Kuo CY, Chou CC, et al. Recreational nitrous oxide abuse related subacute combined degeneration of the spinal cord in adolescents—a case series and literature review. *Brain Dev.* 2019;41(5):428-435.

CHAPTER

88 Cardiovascular Disorders Related to Substance Use

Andi Shahu, Steven E. Pfau, and Samit M. Shah

CHAPTER OUTLINE

- Introduction
- Alcohol
- Tobacco/nicotine
- Cocaine
- Amphetamines
- Opioids
- Cannabinoids
- Conclusion

INTRODUCTION

Diseases of the heart and blood vessels account for substantial medical morbidity and mortality worldwide. Lifetime risk for coronary heart disease alone at age 40 approaches 50% for men and 33% for women in the United States.[1] While use of some substances may rarely precipitate uncommon cardiovascular conditions—cocaine use causing aortic dissection, for example—substance use may contribute to the pathogenesis of common cardiovascular conditions (**Table 88-1**). The most common cardiovascular diseases in Western society—hypertension, coronary artery disease (CAD), atrial fibrillation (AF), heart failure, and stroke—have important associations with the use of both alcohol and nicotine (eg, through cigarette smoking). As a general practitioner, a specialist in addiction medicine, or a cardiovascular specialist, it is important to understand the implications of these relationships as treatment of a common cardiac condition (eg, hypertension) may require recognizing and addressing disordered substance use (eg, alcohol). Similarly, addressing substance use requires recognition of risk for common cardiac diseases. Here, we explore the relationship of substance use with the development and clinical manifestations of cardiovascular disease.

ALCOHOL

Clinical heart disease related to alcohol use is an old observation, familiar to physicians for over a century. The term "alcoholic heart disease" was first used by William MacKenzie in 1902.[2] The manifestations of alcohol-related heart disease depend in large part on the amount and duration of exposure.[3] Alcohol adversely impacts cardiovascular health, and recent data suggests that alcohol use independently increases the risk of developing common cardiovascular conditions—AF, myocardial infarction, and heart failure, with a similar effect to more commonly-recognized risk factors such as obesity or hypertension.[4] Alcohol use and related disorders are a group of conditions that may be defined by a variety of parameters and consequences of alcohol consumption,[5] and specific threshold amounts may be relatively crude descriptors. An association between relatively low amounts of alcohol, also called "lower risk" or "moderate" alcohol consumption, and protection from cardiovascular diseases has been observed,[6,7] with heterogeneous associations between the amount of alcohol intake and heart disease.[8] The complexity comes not only from the possible mix of benefits and risks but also from the strong likelihood that benefits observed in epidemiological studies may not exist (may not be casual associations). For the purpose of definitions used in this discussion, drinking no more than 3 standard (14 g) drinks in a day or 7 drinks a week for women (and those over 65 years old) and drinking no more than 4 drinks in a day or 14 drinks a week for men are considered lower-risk drinking.

Direct Effects

Ingestion of even a single small dose of alcohol has acute effects on the circulatory system. Because ethanol and its metabolites, acetaldehyde and acetate, also have adrenergic and vasodilatory effects,[9,10] the direct myocardial depressant actions of ethanol may be obscured when cardiac "pump" function is assessed after ethanol administration. Cardiac output usually increases after alcohol ingestion in healthy subjects, reflecting the changes in heart rate and peripheral resistance[11,12]; by contrast, a more sensitive index of cardiac function, such as left ventricular (LV) ejection fraction, generally worsens.[12-14]

Previously, nutritional factors were considered to be primary in the development of cardiac dysfunction in patients with chronic heavy alcohol ingestion. It is now generally accepted that direct effects of alcohol on the myocardium are responsible for clinical effects.[14] A number of metabolic abnormalities associated with the presence of alcohol may contribute to acute depression of myocardial contractility. Ethanol reduces the amplitude, duration, and rate of rise of the myocardial transmembrane action potential, an effect related directly to the reduction in contractile force.[15] Acetaldehyde, a metabolite of alcohol produced by alcohol dehydrogenase in the liver, also has direct myocardial depressant effects.[16] Additionally, there are likely genetic factors that predispose to the development of cardiac dysfunction. For example, polymorphisms of the gene for angiotensin converting enzyme have been associated with the development of

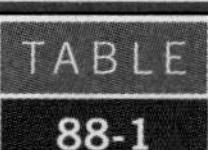

TABLE 88-1 Salient Cardiovascular Effects of Alcohol and Other Drugs

Alcohol
Hemodynamics
Myocardial depression
Increased cardiac output (heart rate increases and/or peripheral resistance decreases)
Increased skin and splanchnic blood flow
Decreased brain and pancreatic blood flow
Disorders
Dilated cardiomyopathy (sometimes with marked increase of LV wall thickness)
Systemic hypertension
Arrhythmias, especially atrial fibrillation
Increased risk of stroke
Sudden death

Nicotine
Hemodynamics
Increased heart rate and blood pressure
Coronary vasoconstriction
Cerebral vasospasm
Disorders
Worsens angina pectoris
Increases risk for acute coronary syndromes
Promotes atherogenesis

Cocaine
Hemodynamics
Increases heart rate
Increases blood pressure
Myocardial depressant
Vasoconstrictor
Promotes thrombosis
Promotes atherogenesis
Disorders
Atypical chest pain syndrome
Worsens angina pectoris
Promotes acute MI
LV hypertrophy and dilatation (myocarditis/cardiomyopathy)
Arrhythmias
Hypertension, systemic
Stroke
Sudden death

Opioids
Hemodynamics
Lower heart rate
Lower blood pressure
Vasodilation
Disorders
Injection-related endocarditis
LV hypertrophy and dilation (myocarditis/cardiomyopathy)
Arrhythmias
Stroke

Amphetamines
Hemodynamics
Increase blood pressure
Increase heart rate (with sharp increases of blood pressure may have reflex slowing)
Promote thrombosis
Disorders
Promote acute MI
LV hypertrophy and dilation (myocarditis/cardiomyopathy)
Arrhythmias
Stroke
Sudden death

Cannabis
Hemodynamics
Increases heart rate
Variable effect on blood pressure
Vasodilation
Increases cardiac output (heart rate increases and/or peripheral resistance decreases)
Disorders
Worsens angina pectoris and promotes acute coronary syndromes
Promotes atherosclerosis
Stroke

cardiomyopathy in men with alcohol use disorders (AUD).[17] Chronic activation of the renin-angiotensin system is present in people with AUD,[18] and animal models indicate that this may contribute to the development of cardiomyopathy.[19]

Alcohol-Related Cardiomyopathy

Because alcohol can have toxic effects on cardiac myocytes, chronic heavy alcohol consumption can result in a cardiomyopathy that is characterized by four-chamber cardiac enlargement, loss of LV systolic function, and the development of typical symptoms of congestive heart failure: dyspnea on exertion, orthopnea, and nocturnal dyspnea.[20] Historically, this syndrome has been described with the term "alcoholic cardiomyopathy," but this outdated term stigmatizes the victims of alcohol-related heart disease. Both the fields of Addiction Medicine and Cardiovascular Medicine have moved towards the term "alcohol-related cardiomyopathy," which will be used throughout the rest of this section.

In Western societies, alcohol-related cardiomyopathy is second only to ischemia as a cause of secondary dilated cardiomyopathies.[21,22] Worldwide, as many as one-third to one-half of cases of dilated cardiomyopathy may be attributable to alcohol use.[23] AUD remains very common in the United States, affecting as much as 29% of the population.[24]

The likelihood of developing clinical cardiomyopathy correlates with the mean daily alcohol intake and duration of drinking,[25] but the proportion of people with AUD who develop overt cardiomyopathy is difficult to estimate. Recent data suggest that the incidence among people with heavy alcohol use may be 1% to 2%, with up to 36% of nonischemic cardiomyopathies potentially attributable to alcohol use.[26] Men develop alcohol-related cardiomyopathy more often than women, primarily because men drink alcohol more frequently and in greater amounts.[27] Differences in alcohol metabolism between women and men, however, may explain the observation that women develop cardiomyopathy at lower levels of drinking.[28,29] The relationship between alcohol-related cardiomyopathy and liver disease due to alcohol is debated: some studies suggest that cardiomyopathy is more likely to occur in patients with cirrhosis due to alcohol,[30] and the coexistence of both entities portends a worse prognosis than cardiomyopathy alone.[31] Others suggest that overt alcohol-related liver disease and cardiomyopathy rarely coexist, but rather a separate entity of cirrhotic cardiomyopathy may be present.[21] Cirrhotic cardiomyopathy is less well defined but is characterized by high cardiac output at rest and a blunted cardiac response to stress.[32]

Patients with AUD begin to manifest abnormalities of cardiac function even before clinical symptoms of heart failure are apparent. A variety of echocardiographic abnormalities have been described in people with AUD without apparent heart disease.[33] Asymptomatic LV dysfunction is present in as many as one-third of patients with AUD,[34] and they may have increased wall thickness, LV mass, and LV systolic and diastolic volumes before there is a decrease in ejection fraction.[35,36] Similarly, cardiac performance with exercise can be impaired in people with AUD, even when resting ejection fraction is normal.[37] Autopsy studies also confirm a high incidence of findings of cardiomyopathy in people with AUD who had no clinical heart disease.[38]

The signs and symptoms of alcohol-related cardiomyopathy are not unique and the history is primary in establishing the diagnosis. Chronic and prolonged alcohol use, usually 80 to 90 g of alcohol daily or more for at least 5 years, is of primary importance.[39] In the United States, ischemia is the most common cause of cardiomyopathy,[40] so it must be excluded. This can be difficult, given that patients who present with cardiomyopathy may also have important risk factors for atherosclerosis, such as hypertension, elevated cholesterol, and tobacco use. Additionally, AUD itself is also a risk factor for ischemic heart disease.[41,42] Prior myocardial infarction (MI), chest discomfort, or evidence of ischemia or infarction on the electrocardiogram must move the clinician to rule out ischemic cardiomyopathy first.

The echocardiogram is the standard first step in the evaluation of new cardiomyopathy. Four-chamber enlargement is typically seen with alcohol-related cardiomyopathy, with either normal or increased wall thickness.[43] Cardiac magnetic resonance imaging (MRI) is also a useful technique in structural heart disease, with increasing utility in the evaluation of various cardiomyopathies,[44] but abnormalities of cardiac MRI specific to alcohol-related cardiomyopathy have not been defined.[45,46] Ultimately, the diagnosis of alcohol-related cardiomyopathy is one of exclusion, established only after more common conditions such as ischemic cardiomyopathy are no longer likely.

The prognosis in alcohol-related cardiomyopathy is correlated strongly with continued use of alcohol. When detected early and treated with alcohol abstinence and standard medical therapy, the prognosis may be better than in other dilated cardiomyopathies. This may be explained in large part by improvement in LV function with abstinence.[46-48] However, with continued alcohol use, the prognosis is as poor or worse than in other nonischemic dilated cardiomyopathies.[49] As many as 19% of patients who experience sudden cardiac death in the absence of ischemic heart disease have alcohol-related cardiomyopathy,[50] second only to obesity-related cardiomyopathy. Without complete abstinence, 4-year mortality approaches 50%.[51] Therefore, treatment should focus first on helping the patient achieve abstinence.

For patients who develop clinical signs of heart failure, standard medical therapies may be used. Historically, this has included loop diuretics (furosemide, torsemide, bumetanide), which have been shown to reduce hospitalization and improve symptoms but do not improve mortality.[52] For patients with AUD who develop heart failure with reduced ejection fraction (HFrEF, ie, LV ejection fraction less than 40%), as for all other patients who develop clinical heart failure with systolic dysfunction, four classes of medications are recommended as the cornerstone of guideline directed medical therapy: angiotensin converting enzyme inhibitors (eg, lisinopril), angiotensin II receptor blockers (eg, losartan), or angiotensin II receptor blocker neprolysin inhibitor (ie, sacubitril-valsartan), mineralocorticoids (eg, spironolactone), beta blockers (eg, metoprolol, carvedilol, bisoprolol), and sodium-glucose cotransporter 2 inhibitors (eg, empagliflozin, dapagliflozin).[53] Patients with HFrEF and an LVEF less than or equal to 35% have also been shown to have a higher incidence of sudden cardiac death, typically from fatal arrhythmias. For patients with AUD who fall into this category, are able to adhere with therapy and have a meaningful life expectancy of at least 1 year, implantation of a device such as an implantable cardioverter defibrillator, may help reduce the incidence of sudden cardiac death.[52]

More advanced therapies, such as LV assist devices and cardiac transplantation, require a high level of patient treatment adherence and social support and necessarily demand complex decision-making[54]; these therapies can be applicable to patients with alcohol-related cardiomyopathy as long as the patient is able to demonstrate abstinence. Although there are no data available specific to heart transplantation, in liver transplantation, the majority of transplant recipients remain abstinent.[55]

Heart Failure

The data on the association between alcohol use and outcomes for patients with heart failure is mixed, with some studies finding better outcomes with low-moderate consumption. An early retrospective study suggested an decreased risk of hospitalization for CHF in patients who engaged in "light to moderate" alcohol consumption.[56] However, subsequent observational studies suggested that patients with light to moderate drinking may have a higher baseline functional status than those who abstained. Accordingly, a prospective observational study of over 2,000 elderly patients showed that subjects who consumed 30 to 600 mL of alcohol in the preceding month were less likely to be hospitalized than patients who consumed lower quantities of alcohol.[57] A secondary analysis of the Survival and Ventricular Enlargement (SAVE) trial, which enrolled survivors of acute myocardial infarction, showed a lower unadjusted risk of heart failure in people who reported drinking light to moderate amounts (1-10 drinks/week). However, this effect was no longer significant after controlling for baseline medical comorbidities, confirming that individuals who abstained from alcohol were more medically ill at baseline.[58] In a retrospective analysis of patients at a single large Veteran's Administration medical center, over 35% of patients with known heart failure continued to use alcohol and this was a strong predictor of multiple heart failure-related hospital admissions.[59] Regardless of any ambiguity with "low to moderate" risk drinking, heavy alcohol consumption (>6 drinks/day) is strongly associated with an increased risk of developing clinically evident heart failure in older adults.[60] The 2013 American College of Cardiology Foundation/American Heart Association Guideline for the Management of Heart Failure lists excessive alcohol consumption as a common factor that may precipitate decompensated CHF and the recommendation is to counsel patients appropriately.[61]

Hypertension

Alcohol use, especially heavy use, is associated with hypertension[62] and may be responsible for as much as 16% of the global burden of hypertensive disease.[63] While some observational studies have suggested cardiovascular benefit from relatively low alcohol intake, the relationship between alcohol use and cardiovascular disease relies in large part on self-reporting of intake, which may be inaccurate[64]; more important methodologically are the many favorable lifestyle factors associated with both low alcohol consumption and cardiovascular health that are difficult or even impossible to adjust for adequately in analyses.[65]

The mechanisms by which alcohol raises blood pressure are through direct sympathetic vasomotor effects and secondary mechanisms, such as worsened sleep apnea.[66] Regular consumption of one or more drinks a day for men (and more than 2 for women) is associated with increased blood pressure, and the degree of increase is dose dependent.[64,67] The elevation in blood pressure is accompanied by the expected rise in hypertension-related cardiovascular morbidity and mortality. Although there is some debate regarding the possible benefits of red wine, the hypertensive effects of alcohol are consistent regardless of source.[68] In hypertensive individuals, the sympathetic and hemodynamic responses to alcohol are accentuated when compared to normotensive individuals.[69] Alcohol can be an important factor in hypertension that is refractory to standard therapy[66]; this is associated with an increased risk of cardiovascular complications.[70,71] Reduction of alcohol consumption is associated with significant decreases in blood pressure in hypertensive patients.[72,73] In patients being treated for hypertension, guidelines recommend limiting alcohol consumption to 2 drinks per day.[74]

Atrial Fibrillation and Other Arrhythmias

Atrial fibrillation is the most common clinical arrhythmia in adults, with a lifetime risk of 1 in 4 for men and women over the age of 40.[75] Prevalence is highly age-dependent and increases from 1% in patients under 60 years of age to 18% in patients older than 85.[76] After age, the next two most important risk factors are hypertension and CAD. Other risk factors include heart failure, congenital heart disease, valvular heart disease, hypertrophic cardiomyopathy, family history, obesity, chronic kidney disease, diabetes, hyperthyroidism, sleep apnea, increased birth weight, pericardial fat, and autonomic dysfunction.[75,77]

Alcohol use has also been associated with an increased risk for the development of AF. "Holiday Heart" is a term that has historically been applied to AF that occurs after binge drinking and implies the absence of other heart disease.[78] From a pathophysiological basis, alcohol can trigger AF by direct effects on myocytes and ion channels, autonomic modulation by increasing adrenergic tone, and by decreasing the atrial effective refractory period.[79] Though previous studies suggested that low-risk levels of alcohol use are benign, more recent studies have shown that even low daily alcohol intake is associated with increased incidence of AF.[80-83] Heavy alcohol use is significantly associated with incidence of AF.[13,82] Because of early structural abnormalities that occur in the heart with chronic heavy alcohol use, alterations in cardiac function with acute ingestion,[13] and associations between alcohol and coronary heart disease, hypertension, and cardiomyopathy, the occurrence of AF in patients with any level of alcohol use must be considered as a potential harbinger of significant heart disease. AF in the setting of alcohol use must be evaluated in the same manner as new-onset AF occurring in any other context: a full history and physical exam, 12-lead electrocardiogram, echocardiogram, and blood tests for renal, thyroid, and liver function.[84]

In addition to AF, heavy alcohol consumption has also been linked to sinus tachycardia and ventricular arrhythmias. Studies have shown that patients with alcohol-related cardiomyopathy have a higher risk of ventricular tachycardia, ventricular fibrillation, or sudden death compared to those who stopped drinking.[85] A study based on a national database of 7600 in patients with alcohol-related cardiomyopathy showed that 33% suffered an arrhythmia, with AF occurring in 22%, ventricular tachycardia in 10%, atrial flutter in 5%, and ventricular fibrillation in 2%.[86] A more recent study of 3,028 participants from the 2015 Munich Octoberfest found that alcohol use was associated with a variety of sinus, atrial and ventricular arrhythmias.[87] Thus, the proarrhythmic effects of alcohol ingestion are common and can be life-threatening in susceptible patients.

Coronary Artery Disease and Stroke

The relationship between alcohol use and CAD is complex. Low to moderate alcohol consumption may be protective when compared to those who abstain.[88] In patients with established CAD, studies have suggested that both cardiovascular mortality and all-cause mortality are lower with low to moderate alcohol intake, with the dose–response curve indicating benefit between 5 and 26 g/day.[89] However, there is no agreed-upon amount of alcohol that is considered "safe" with regard to lowering cardiovascular risk.[20]

The evidence for the beneficial effect of alcohol at low consumption levels has been debated, due to the lack of robust epidemiological data, the potential bias of self-reporting of intake, the likely overwhelming influence of uncontrolled confounding (low use being associated with more physical activity, higher income, positive health behaviors) and lack of long-term randomized controlled trials.[90] Studies from the U.S. and U.K. continue to support this point of view,[65,91] but studies from China and India indicate there may be different relationships in different genetic or ethnic groups.[92,93] There are reasonable biological mechanisms to support a protective effect of alcohol though these generally do not account for the magnitude of benefit in observational studies.[90,94] In addition to favorably affecting lipid profiles, low to "moderate" alcohol consumption has been associated with improved insulin sensitivity and decreased incidence of type 2 diabetes.[95-97] There may also be particular advantages to red wine over other forms of alcohol because of the presence of polyphenols, tannins, and flavonoids, which have been associated with favorable effects on lipids, platelet function, endothelial function, and inflammatory parameters.[98]

The epidemiological evidence for increasing CAD risk with heavy alcohol use has also been consistent, leading to the so-called J-shaped curve of alcohol-related cardiovascular risk.[99-102] The prevalence of coronary artery calcium on CT is a marker for coronary atherosclerosis in asymptomatic patients and is predictive of risk of incident MI and cardiovascular mortality. Studies have consistently failed to demonstrate a J-shaped relationship between coronary artery calcification and alcohol intake, but heavy alcohol use is associated with the highest risk.[103-106] Progression of coronary calcification over a 2- to 4-year period is increased with heavy alcohol consumption,[105] with incident coronary events occurring most often in those with the highest alcohol intake, independent of coronary calcification. These data suggest that protection from coronary events is not through prevention of atherosclerosis but, if there is any, through mechanisms that promote the clinical manifestations of atherosclerosis such as thrombosis. The mechanism of higher clinical events in people with the heaviest alcohol use is less clear.

Consumption of moderate amounts of alcohol is also associated with a lower risk of stroke, although the data are less robust than that for CAD. Low to moderate alcohol use is associated with a lower risk of ischemic stroke and a higher risk of hemorrhagic stroke and may be explained by antithrombotic properties of alcohol.[107,108] The increased risk of stroke with heavy alcohol use is consistent across many studies, with an increased relative risk of total, ischemic, and hemorrhagic stroke of approximately 1.6.[108] Similar to coronary disease, some have suggested a J-shaped curve to the risk relationship where people who don't drink have a greater risk of stroke than those who consume light quantities.[109] A retrospective cohort analysis of the Swedish Twin Registry showed that consumption of more than two drinks of alcohol per day before the age of 60 increased the risk of stroke by 34% compared to lighter drinking. Heavy alcohol intake shortened the time to stroke by 5 years and was more significant a risk factor for stroke than hypertension or diabetes mellitus in patients younger than age 75.[110]

TOBACCO/NICOTINE

Nicotine use is common, with the most common route of use being cigarette smoking. An estimated 13% of the U.S. adult population smoked tobacco in 2020 (>30 million people). While nicotine has direct and immediate effects on the cardiovascular system, the specific role of nicotine in cigarette-related heart disease is debated.

Hemodynamic Effects

Within minutes of a nicotine dose, either by tobacco smoking or by direct administration, both heart rate and blood pressure rise.[111,112] These hemodynamic changes are accompanied by increases in plasma epinephrine and norepinephrine.[113] Nicotine exerts its adrenergic actions mainly by release of norepinephrine from nerve terminals and release of epinephrine from the adrenal medulla.[114]

Arrythmia

Nicotine use, both acute and chronic, has also been implicated as a risk factor for cardiac arrhythmias, especially AF.[115,116] In both animal models and cell culture, nicotine can alter atrial structure, with increased fibrosis and increased likelihood of AF and other arrhythmias.[117-120] However, in human studies of stable cardiac disease or those hospitalized with acute coronary syndrome, there is no evidence of an increase in cardiac arrhythmias attributable to nicotine replacement therapy.[121,122] It is likely that while nicotine administration to otherwise healthy hearts may be arrhythmogenic, there is net benefit and overall decreased events when nicotine administration replaces cigarette smoking, which is highly associated with both supraventricular and ventricular arrhythmias.[123]

Coronary Artery Disease

The development and progression of atherosclerosis require arterial (especially endothelial) injury, recruitment of leukocytes, and adherence and activation of platelets.[124,125] Clinical manifestations often are the result of alterations in the arterial microenvironment that favor thrombosis at the site of plaque.[126,127] In patients who smoke traditional cigarettes, it appears that the role of nicotine in both atherogenesis and atherothrombosis is relatively small and other components of cigarette smoke play more important roles.[128,129] Cigarette smoke is a complex mixture of chemicals, many of which have been closely associated with a direct role in coronary atherosclerosis and its clinical manifestations.[130] Endothelial injury and dysfunction occur early with smoking, with impaired nitric oxide production and endothelium-dependent vasodilatation.[131,132] Markers of endothelial injury are apparent within 20 minutes of smoking cigarettes.[133] People who smoke have increased markers of endothelial cell activation and evidence for increased adhesion and migration of leukocytes into the artery wall.[134-136] Chronic smoking alters platelet function, with evidence of increased aggregation when stimulated compared to those who don't smoke.[137] Finally, soluble plasma proteins such as fibrinogen are increased in people who smoke; elevated fibrinogen is among the strongest acquired cardiovascular risk factors. Particulate matter inhalation, through either air pollution or cigarette smoke, has also been demonstrated to be proinflammatory and contribute to atherogenesis.[130]

The importance of cigarette smoking as a risk factor for atherosclerotic vascular disease cannot be overemphasized. Cigarette smoking is an important risk factor for virtually every clinical manifestation of atherosclerosis, including the presence and progression of CAD, carotid disease, peripheral vascular disease including abdominal aortic aneurysm, thoracic aortic plaque burden, ischemic stroke, and particularly the incidence of acute MI.[138-140] Notably, children raised in homes where one or both parents smoke are at substantially elevated risk of developing carotid atherosclerotic plaque later in life, suggesting that the irreversible cardiovascular effects of cigarette smoke occur even with secondhand exposure.[141]

Stopping smoking is a public heath priority. Mandatory smoking prohibition programs (such as indoor smoking bans or workplace smoking restrictions) have consistently been shown to decrease hospitalization rates for acute MI.[142-145] Stopping smoking is associated with a rapid decline in the risk for acute MI, approaching the level of nonsmoking after 2-3 years.[146] Implementation of a nonsmoking policy in hospitals has been shown to decrease the incidence of myocardial infarction during hospital stays.[147] Stopping smoking also reduces to the risk of congestive heart failure or death after a period of 15 years. However, people who previously smoked heavily remain at elevated risk of CAD (up to 20 years later), peripheral artery disease (up to 30 years later), heart failure (for those with >32 pack-years) or death but at lower risk than people who continue to smoke.[139,148]

Electronic Drug Delivery Devices

Electronic Drug Delivery Devices (EDDDs) deliver atomized nicotine-containing liquid as an aerosol (colloquially referred to as a "vapor"), typically in a flavored propylene glycol base.[149] EDDDs have rapidly grown in popularity as an alternative to conventional cigarettes. Centers for Disease Control (CDC) data show that more than 8 million adults and more than 3.6 million middle and high school students in the U.S. used EDDDs in 2018. In young adults, use of EDDD now surpasses the use of all tobacco products.[150] The highest rate of EDDD use is among people who currently and formerly smoke, with relatively low rates of use among people who don't smoke.[151] However, among those 18 to 24 years old, at least 40% had never smoked regular cigarettes prior to using EDDDs, suggesting that EDDDs may increasingly be the initial exposure to nicotine in young people. In the U.S., youth are also more likely than adults to use EDDDs, with increased concern that the introduction of numerous varieties of flavored EDDDs and targeted advertising as possible reasons for the rapid uptake among young people.[152,153]

From a cardiovascular perspective, the most concerning constituents of EDDD aerosol are nicotine, carbonyls, and particulates. The amount of nicotine delivered in each "puff" is highly variable and depends on the characteristics of each device.[154] The simulated amount of nicotine in individual puffs ranges from 0 to 35 μg, and it is estimated that it would take several puffs to deliver the 1 mg of nicotine that is typically delivered from a conventional cigarette.[154] In a 2013 laboratory study of nicotine exposure in people who use EDDDs, plasma nicotine concentration after a 12-hour abstinence period increased to 10 ng/mL within 5 minutes of the first puff and peaked at 16.3 ng/mL after 1 hour of ad lib use.[155] These levels are comparatively lower than in people who smoke conventional cigarettes and similar to the effect of low-dose nicotine-containing gum, but newer EDDDs such as "heat-not-burn" devices have been shown to deliver 84% of the nicotine content of cigarettes.[156-158] Before 2013, most EDDD nicotine strength varied from 0.05% to 1.5%. During 2013 to 2018, EDDDs with higher nicotine levels (>5%) increased considerably in unit share, and average nicotine strength rose from 2.1% to 4.3%. From 2017 to 2022, sales of EDDDs with the highest levels of nicotine (5% or greater) have risen drastically, and the price of EDDDs with high nicotine levels has either decreased or not changed while those with lower nicotine levels became more expensive, suggesting the amount of nicotine delivered per EDDD may increase over time and over a broader segment of people who use them.[159] People who formerly smoked as well as patients with known cardiovascular disease who are maintained on therapeutic doses of non-EDDD nicotine replacement therapy have not been shown to have adverse outcomes.[160,161]

EDDD fluid typically contains a solvent base such as glycerin or propylene glycol, nicotine, and flavors or other additives. At the high temperatures required for atomization, the solvent base reacts to form toxic compounds. For example, propylene glycol undergoes thermal degradation and can generate propylene oxide, a class 2B carcinogen. Both glycerin and propylene glycol have been shown to generate formaldehyde, acetaldehyde, acrolein, and acetone.[162,163] While these compounds are known irritants with established systemic toxicity, their direct effect on cardiovascular health is unknown. The aerosol also contains ultrafine particles, many of which are heavy metals, that are capable of reaching the alveolar membrane and subsequently the circulatory system.[154] These compounds can cause local respiratory toxicity and enter the blood stream. The particle size and number in EDDD aerosol is comparable to that of conventional cigarettes (120-165 nm), and direct or secondhand exposure to ultrafine particles has been associated with increased cardiovascular mortality.[164] In fact, exposure to particles smaller than 2.5 μm has been associated with increased risk of myocardial infarction, stroke, arrhythmia, and heart failure exacerbation in multiple cohort studies.[165] The pathophysiological mechanisms for these effects are numerous and include a systemic inflammatory response, oxidative stress, altered platelet function, higher systemic blood pressure, and endothelial dysfunction.[166-170] Based on laboratory studies, physiological observations, and population-level studies, exposure to ultrafine particles in EDDDs likely has an adverse effect on cardiovascular health. As a result, experts have advised that EDDDs not be labeled as "safe" for use from a cardiovascular perspective, though data on cardiovascular outcomes as a result of EDDD use, particularly in adolescent or young adult populations, is still very limited.[171]

COCAINE

Cocaine is a local anesthetic with potent sympathomimetic actions. The adrenergic effects are the result of blocking presynaptic norepinephrine and dopamine reuptake, thereby making more catecholamines available at postsynaptic receptors, stimulating the sympathetic nervous system, and enhancing the effects of endogenous catecholamines.[172-175] As a local anesthetic, cocaine inhibits transmembrane sodium flux during electrical excitation, producing a delay in the upstroke and amplitude of the myocardial action potential; this action diminishes intracellular calcium indirectly (making less sodium available for sodium-calcium exchange).[176] Thus, depending on the dosage and the clinical or experimental conditions, cocaine may produce seemingly contradictory effects, reflecting whether the sympathomimetic or the local anesthetic actions are predominant.[177]

Hemodynamic Effects

The illicit use of cocaine has been associated with a wide variety of cardiovascular complications. Cocaine use accounts for many substance-related emergency department visits,[178] many of these for complaints of chest pain. In addition to chest pain, other conditions such as acute MI, aortic dissection, stroke, heart failure, and sudden cardiac death have all been associated with cocaine use.[179] A high proportion of asymptomatic individuals who use cocaine, especially those over the age of 40, have MRI evidence of ischemia-related fibrosis on cardiac MRI or LV dysfunction by echocardiography.[180,181] Cocaine can alter hemodynamics, arterial muscular tone, and both cellular and humoral parameters of coagulation—all factors that conspire to produce the observed cardiovascular pathology.

Acute hemodynamic effects of cocaine administration include elevation in heart rate, systolic blood pressure, diastolic blood pressure, and mean arterial pressure.[182] Repeated use results in the development of tolerance, with limited hemodynamic responses to increasing doses and serum concentrations.[183] Animal data indicate that inhibition of norepinephrine and dopamine reabsorption raises serum concentrations, leading to increased sympathetic stimulation[184]; this is presumed to be the primary mechanism of hemodynamic alterations in humans. In the coronary arteries of human subjects, cocaine use results in vasoconstriction, an effect that may be accentuated by the presence of atherosclerosis and cigarette smoking.[185-188]

Coronary Artery Disease

Cocaine affects all three components of the normal system of hemostasis: blood cells, soluble plasma proteins, and the vessel wall (particularly the endothelium). Cocaine shifts the balance of this tightly regulated system toward arterial thrombus formation, particularly in the presence of atherosclerosis. Platelets are of primary importance in both physiological and pathological arterial thrombus formation,[127,189] and activation of platelets is apparent in both chronic use and after acute ingestion.[190-192] Monocyte-platelet aggregates, soluble CD40 ligand, neutrophil-activating peptide-2, and regulated on activation, normal T cells expressed and secreted—all indicators of platelet activation—are higher at baseline in chronic cocaine use.[190] These effects are completely reversed following 4 weeks of abstinence, indicating specific effects of the drug on the platelets rather than an effect of some other cocaine-induced vascular process. However, at least some measures of platelet reactivity are not altered by direct exposure of platelets in vitro to doses of cocaine similar to plasma levels obtained with illicit use, indicating an indirect mechanism such as catecholamines.[192] Evidence for acute endothelial dysfunction related to direct exposure to cocaine exists in cultured human aortic endothelial cells, with increases in endothelin-1 and decreases in nitric oxide production and endothelial nitric oxide synthase expression. Finally, levels of soluble plasma proteins such as fibrinogen and von Willebrand factor are increased in individuals with chronic cocaine use.[193] These markers are associated with increased long-term risk for cardiovascular disease and predict short-term risk in those with acute coronary syndromes.[194]

Although some have suggested that cocaine use accelerates the atherosclerotic process, it is difficult to separate cocaine from other major environmental, genetic, and behavioral factors that confound this relationship in those who use cocaine, for example, cigarettes, alcohol, and hypertension.[195] The development and progression of atherosclerosis necessarily proceed through three related steps: arterial injury, inflammatory cell recruitment, and platelet adhesion and activation.[124] Cocaine directly (in the case of elevation of blood pressure) or indirectly (by increased cigarette use while using cocaine) impacts all three of these pathological processes.

Cocaine levels peak in the bloodstream at different times depending upon method of ingestion, ranging from 3 minutes with smoking to 40 to 60 minutes with intranasal administration.[178] Cocaine metabolites are hemodynamically active and can persist at detectable levels for 48 hours after a single dose. Concomitant use of alcohol can slow the clearance of metabolites as well as produce additional active metabolites such as cocaethylene, which is associated with an increased risk of cardiac arrest.[196,197] In general, presentation with cardiovascular symptoms occurs early after cocaine use, with a markedly elevated risk of cocaine-related MI within the first 24 hours.[198]

Cocaine-related chest pain is the most frequent cardiovascular presentation associated with cocaine use, an outcome often attributed to the supply/demand imbalance in coronary arteries resulting from use.[199] The incidence of acute MI in this group of patients is relatively low, however, with reports ranging from 0.7% to 6%.[200,201] Still, as the demographic of cocaine shifts to an older population with a high proportion of other CAD risk factors, the diagnosis must be considered carefully. Compared to individuals who do not use cocaine, risk stratification tools such as the TIMI risk score are not clinically useful in the setting of cocaine use, as more than half of cardiovascular events occur in patients with a TIMI risk score of less than 1.[202] Similarly, stress testing and coronary CT angiography rarely lead to identification of significant CAD among people with cocaine-associated chest pain.[203] Similar to conventional (non–cocaine-related) MI, measurement of troponin maintains a high level of sensitivity and specificity, though serum troponin levels are typically higher in patients who use cocaine versus those who do not.[204] The high index of suspicion with poor discriminatory power of conventional risk stratification tools leads to frequent utilization of observation units and hospital admission in patients with cocaine-associated chest pain.[205] It appears that observation with serial measurement of electrocardiograms (ECGs) and serum troponin levels is the best compromise of cost and sensitivity when evaluating patients with this clinical presentation.[206] During the observation period, both benzodiazepines and nitroglycerin, which may have an anxiolytic effect and counteract coronary-induced vasoconstriction, respectively, have been shown to alleviate symptoms.[207,208]

When MI in the context of cocaine use does occur, the treatment approach differs from non–cocaine-associated infarction in several important aspects. Similar to patients who are not using cocaine, patients with ST-segment elevations on ECG should receive coronary angiography.[199] Whether ST-segment elevation is present or not, if myocardial infarction is identified, antiplatelet therapy with aspirin and an inhibitor of the platelet P2Y12 receptor (ie, ticagrelor, clopidogrel or prasugrel) is a cornerstone of current infarction management.[209] Given the evidence for platelet activation by cocaine, antiplatelet therapy with aspirin or P2Y12 inhibitors is thought to be beneficial, and most experts agree with following standard treatment algorithms for antiplatelet therapy in these patients.[210] Registry data have shown that patients who suffer acute coronary syndromes in the setting of cocaine use are typically younger than cocaine-negative patients (50 versus 64 years) and typically have fewer conventional risk factors for cardiovascular disease. Individuals with cocaine use are more likely to suffer ST-elevation myocardial infarction and present to the hospital with congestive heart failure or cardiogenic shock. They are also more likely to undergo coronary angiography but less likely to undergo percutaneous intervention with a drug-eluting stent (due to the recommendation for 1 year of strict medication adherence to dual antiplatelet therapy).[211]

Beta-adrenergic receptor blockers are a class of medications that have demonstrated mortality benefit in clinical trials when administered in the setting of acute MI.[212] In the setting of recent cocaine use, the possibility of precipitating arterial vasoconstriction by unopposed alpha-receptor stimulation raises concern about administration of beta-blockers in cocaine-related infarction. Arterial vasoconstriction in response to beta-blockers in the context of cocaine appears to be corroborated by two small studies in humans without acute infarction.[186,213] More recent data suggest that this may not be as concerning as previously thought both for patients with an acute coronary syndrome as well as for patients presenting with more stable chest pain. In two recent studies, each including over 300 subjects with cocaine-associated chest pain, the effect of beta-blocker administration to patients who were subsequently found to have drug testing consistent with cocaine use was examined with regard to blood pressure and clinical outcome.[214,215] In fact, people who had received beta-blockers had lower blood pressure and lower rate of MI, and in one study, there was a trend toward decreased post-discharge mortality.[215] One randomized study of a combined alpha- and beta-blocker (labetalol) showed similar blood pressure reduction compared to diltiazem with no in-hospital adverse events.[195] Still, though studies have suggested that unopposed alpha-receptor stimulation resulting from beta-blocker use in these patients is rare,[216] the most recent American Heart Association (AHA)/American College of Cardiology (ACC) practice guidelines to address cocaine-related chest pain/acute coronary syndrome, published in 2008, do not endorse beta-blockers in early management and give a class IIIC recommendation to the use beta-blockers in patients with acute coronary syndromes and active cocaine use.[210,217] Other, more recent AHA/ACC consensus guidelines have provided a weak recommendation for consideration of a combined alpha and beta-blocking agent such as labetalol for treatment of hypertension and tachycardia in patients with myocardial infarction.

Reperfusion therapy, by systemic thrombolytics or primary angioplasty with stent placement, is the standard of care of ST-segment elevation MI because of demonstrated mortality benefit in large clinical trials.[218] Primary angioplasty with stenting has improved MI outcomes across many demographic groups,[219] but patients who use cocaine have an increased risk for stent thrombosis,[220] a platelet-mediated event. Presumably, this observation can be attributed to both the activation of platelets by ongoing cocaine use and the possible lack of adherence to prescribed dual antiplatelet therapy.

Aortic Dissection

Cocaine use has been associated with aortic dissection. The proportion of aortic dissection related to cocaine ranges from 0.5% to 37% depending upon the population studied.[221-223] Cocaine-related dissection tends to occur more frequently in young, hypertensive subjects.[224] Cocaine use may accelerate the progression of atherosclerosis, and the presence of other traditional atherosclerosis risk factors such as hypertension and cigarette smoking contributes to the arterial pathology that predisposes to dissection.[225] In addition, shear stress of the aorta from sudden and significant elevations in blood pressure resulting from cocaine use is thought to contribute to the pathophysiology of aortic dissection in this patient population. Treatment is similar as in other patients with aortic dissection—precise and careful blood pressure management with a goal systolic blood pressure of 100 to 120 mm Hg, and surgical intervention if indicated.[226]

Stroke

Cocaine has been associated with both ischemic stroke and intracerebral hemorrhage, with approximately equal frequency. Hemorrhage appears to be more frequent in individuals with current use, while ischemic stroke and transient ischemic attack are more common in patients with past cocaine use. Most strokes occur within 6 to 24 hours of using cocaine and individuals who smoke crack cocaine are at an increased risk of stroke compared to those with intranasal use.[227] The mechanisms of stroke in cocaine use are not entirely clear, but severe vasospasm, in either normal or atherosclerotic arteries, is implicated from animal studies and observations in patients. Decrease in cerebral blood flow is observed in human research participants after a single intravenous dose of cocaine.[228] Consistent with the effects of cocaine on platelet activation, platelet-rich thrombi have been observed after fatal cerebral infarcts in individuals with chronic cocaine use.[229] Large artery atherosclerotic disease is the most common finding in ischemic stroke, consistent with the hypothesis that cocaine use accelerates atherosclerotic vascular disease.

Cardiomyopathy

Cocaine use has also been associated with LV dysfunction and cardiomyopathy, including dilated cardiomyopathy, catecholamine-related heart failure, stress cardiomyopathy, and myocarditis.[230] Often in patients with cocaine use and LV dysfunction, ischemic heart disease may concurrently be present, making the etiology of the cardiomyopathy multifactorial. In patients with heart failure with a reduced ejection fraction (HFrEF) that has been attributed to cocaine use, abstinence from cocaine has been shown to result in improvement in LV ejection fraction.[231] In patients with HFrEF who develop clinical signs of heart failure, standard medication therapy is similar to that for other patients with HFrEF (see discussion on alcohol-related cardiomyopathy earlier in this chapter). In one notable variation, beta-blockers are sometimes avoided in this population due to the concern about unopposed alpha-receptor stimulation, though if a beta-blocker is to be used to reduce cardiac remodeling, carvedilol is preferred due to its combined alpha- and beta-blocking effects.[232]

AMPHETAMINES

Amphetamines (a contraction of alpha-methylphenethylamine) are a group of synthetic compounds used for both medical and nonmedical purposes. Amphetamines have a common β-phenylethylamine chemical structure, which they share with catecholamines; the differences in their chemical composition determine their modes of action, relative potency, and sympathomimetic properties.[233] Though these substances differ in their central nervous system and peripheral effects, as a group, they act by stimulating the sympathetic nervous system, by displacing catecholamines or interfering with reuptake from their storage sites, by blocking the actions of monoamine oxidase inhibition, and/or by direct adrenergic actions.[233] Amphetamines and their derivatives such as methamphetamine include medications used in the treatment of attention deficit hyperactivity disorder and traumatic brain injury. Other derivatives are used only nonmedically and include mephedrone/methylenedioxypyrovalerone (MDPV or "bath salts"), 3,4-methylenedioxymethamphetamine (MDMA or "ecstasy"), and methyldiethanolamine (MDEA or "eve").

Hemodynamic Effects

Amphetamines produce a dose-dependent elevation of blood pressure and increase of heart rate.[234,235] The magnitude of the changes reflects their relative α_1-adrenergic (elevate blood pressure with reflex slowing of heart rate) and β_1-adrenergic (enhance cardiac contractility and increase heart rate) effects. When amphetamines are taken parenterally, the peak vasopressor effects are evident within a half hour, whereas when taken by mouth, they are observed within 1 to 2 hours.[235,236] Under experimental conditions, amphetamines increase systolic and diastolic blood pressure in healthy subjects by 30 and 20 mm Hg, respectively. The blood pressure elevations dissipate over 3 to 4 hours. Though for MDMA and methylphenidate an increase in heart rate (20 beats/min) parallels their blood pressure changes, for amphetamine and methamphetamine, only modest heart rate changes are initially observed, with the magnitude of the heart rate changes actually having an inverse relation to the blood pressure changes. Three to four hours after the administration of amphetamine, methamphetamine, or methylphenidate, as the blood pressure elevations dissipate and the reflex baroreceptor response is attenuated, further heart rate increases ensue (a total change of as many as 20-30 beats/min) that may persist above baseline for 10 hours.[235]

Coronary Artery Disease, Stroke, Valvular Heart Disease

Cardiovascular disease is the second leading cause of death for patients who overdose on methamphetamines.[237] The most common presentation in patients seen in the emergency department after recent amphetamine use is tachycardia and hypertension.[238] The presence of early CAD may be related to chronic amphetamine use.[239] Although the evidence is not as compelling as for cocaine, posthumous studies have found a higher incidence of CAD in patients who used amphetamines.[240] Amphetamine-related stimulants are reported to be associated with acute MI and may be associated with a worse prognosis.[241,242] Amphetamines may cause myocardial ischemia by several mechanisms, including focal or diffuse vasospasm, increased myocardial demand on preexisting coronary disease, structural and electrical cardiac remodeling and increased platelet reactivity.[242] Amphetamine use has been associated with acute myocardial infarction in adolescents as well, possibly as a result of rapid increases in blood pressure and coronary vasospasm.[243]

Similarly, ischemic and hemorrhagic stroke have been associated with amphetamine use.[244] Phenylpropanolamine, a stimulant used as a decongestant and appetite suppressant, was removed from over-the-counter sale by the FDA in the United States because of a strong association with an increased risk for hemorrhagic stroke, especially in young women.[245]

Some amphetamine derivatives developed as appetite suppressants (such as fenfluramine) are strong serotonin receptor (especially the 5-HT_{2B} receptor) agonists and were removed from the market after evidence linking them to the development of a specific form of valvular heart disease previously associated with serotonin-secreting carcinoid tumors; similar lesions have been described in illicit amphetamine use.[246,247]

Cardiomyopathy

Cardiomyopathy has also been associated with amphetamine use.[248-250] As many as 5% of patients presenting to emergency rooms in the United States with decompensated heart failure may have chronic stimulant use.[251] Concentric hypertrophy is a common finding in individuals with methamphetamine use and may precede the development of heart failure.[239,252] In general, patients tend to be younger and have more severe depression of LV function when compared to patients presenting with other forms of nonischemic myopathy.[248] Both animal models and human pathological data suggest that direct toxicity to myocytes can occur with chronic amphetamine exposure.[253,254] Contraction band necrosis, a myocyte injury pattern seen in exposure to high levels of catecholamines, may be present.[135] Treatment options for patients in this population would be similar to those of patients with alcohol or cocaine use and concurrent or resulting cardiomyopathy.

OPIOIDS

From a strictly cardiovascular perspective, opioids have significant therapeutic value. The hemodynamic effects of lowering heart rate and blood pressure, as well as decreasing preload, combined with their analgesic and anxiolytic properties, have made morphine a cornerstone of guideline-directed treatment of myocardial infarction and acute pulmonary edema.[255] Data also support that patients with acute myocardial infarction do not experience adverse cardiovascular outcomes as a result of opioid use, though other data suggest that morphine use may adversely reduce therapeutic efficacy of P2Y12 receptor antagonists such as clopidogrel.[256]

In the United States, deaths from drug overdose have dramatically increased in the past decade to about 70,000 per year as of 2018, with two thirds of these occurring as a result of opioid use.[257] Due to the rise in opioid-related overdoses and deaths, the American Heart Association has recently updated its guidelines for adult basic and advanced life support for both health care professionals and laypeople to including management of patients with opioid overdose.[258,259]

Endocarditis

Injection drug use has been associated with a number of cardiovascular consequences, particularly infective endocarditis, which is important because of the extremely high morbidity and mortality and associated costs of treatment. It is estimated that in 2007 as many as 21 million people worldwide injected drugs. It is difficult to estimate the incidence of injection-related endocarditis, but the number of hospitalizations for this diagnosis have dramatically risen in the United States since 2010 as a result of the opioid epidemic.[260,261] The demographics of infectious endocarditis related to injection drug use are changing and there have been significant increases in endocarditis-related hospital admissions in young people between the age of 15 and 34 years old, with the greatest impact on White women.[262]

Injection drug use associated infectious endocarditis is characterized by several features that distinguish this entity from other causes. First, the right heart valves, especially the tricuspid valve, are more commonly involved.[263] While less than 10% of endocarditis in individuals without injection drug use is right-sided, as much as 75% of endocarditis in individuals with injection drug use involves the right heart valves.[264] The mechanisms may be related to direct toxicity to the right-sided valve structures by the injected drugs or contaminants.[263] Left-sided endocarditis in those who use drugs may be associated with a worse prognosis.[265] Second, polymicrobial infections and endocarditis due to fungal pathogens are much more common in those who use injection drugs.[266] Polymicrobial endocarditis is much more likely to require surgery and carries a higher mortality than single-organism infections.[266] Fungal endocarditis mortality ranges from 37% to 80%, even with aggressive surgical and medical therapy.[267,268] Finally, because patients with opioid use disorder have a high likelihood of continued use if left untreated, recurrent endocarditis is common. Recurrence of endocarditis after valve replacement surgery carries a worse prognosis compared to native valve endocarditis.[269]

Heart Disease and Stroke

Opioids have not been demonstrated to have direct toxic effects on myocytes or other components of the heart, a fact underscored by the general lack of abnormalities in cardiac dimension and structure in individuals with heroin use.[270] However, there is some evidence that prescription opioid use may be a risk factor for cardiovascular disease, myocardial infarction and death related to CAD though the pathophysiology behind this association is not well understood.[271-273] However, other studies have not found an association between prescription drug use and incidence of coronary heart disease.[274] Though patients with infective endocarditis resulting from injection drug use are at risk, data on association between overall opioid use and hemorrhagic or ischemic stroke are inconsistent, with some studies suggesting no relationship between these variables, while others have suggested a possible association between opioid use and hemorrhagic stroke. The greatest and most concerning adverse cardiac event associated with opioid use remains the increased incidence in cardiac arrest as a result of overdoses.

Prolonged QT

Studies have also shown an association between opioid use and arrhythmia.[275] The most commonly cited opioid in this regard is methadone, which is used to treat opioid use disorder and chronic pain. Methadone and other opioids can lead to prolongation of the QT interval on ECG via changes in cardiac repolarization, which can increase the risk of ventricular arrhythmias such as Torsades de Pointes, leading to sudden cardiac death, particularly if the patient is concurrently taking other medications that interact with methadone.[276] Anywhere between 5% and 30% of patients with methadone may experience QT prolongation, in particular as the dose of methadone increases to 120 mg or higher, though significant ventricular arrhythmias such as Torsades de Pointes are rare.[277-279] Patients on higher doses of methadone should receive regular ECGs to monitor their QT interval. If the QT interval is prolonged above 500 ms, consultation with a cardiologist may be indicated. Most patients on methadone who are found to have QT-interval prolongation should remain on methadone as the risks of discontinuation (eg, overdose) may outweigh the benefit with regard to reducing arrhythmic risk.[280] Consultation with a pharmacist may be helpful to identify other medications that may cause QT prolongation. The other commonly used agent for treatment of opioid use disorder, buprenorphine, on the other hand, has not been associated with prolonged QT or cardiac arrhythmias.

Finally, naloxone (in particular the intravenous formulation), which is typically administered to revive people who overdose on opioids can, rarely, cause pulmonary edema from increased volume in the pulmonary vasculature, possibly as a result of a catecholamine surge.[281]

CANNABINOIDS

Cannabis increases heart rate and cardiac output.[282] The effects on the cardiovascular system are likely mediated through sympathetic activation.[283] With continued use, tolerance develops, blunting the cardiovascular changes observed.[282] However, in the past decade, the concentration of the key psychoactive derivative tetrahydrocannabinol (THC) has increased in cannabis, and utilization of synthetic cannabinoid products has also increased, raising concern about the possible cardiovascular effects of these products.[284]

Cannabis is most commonly used through smoking the dried plant, but may also be directly ingested. At least two types of cannabis receptors have been identified (CB1 and CB2) and exist on a variety of tissues, including those that play a role in the development of atherosclerosis: endothelial cells, leukocytes, vascular smooth muscle cells, and platelets.[285-288] Cannabis smoke has been shown to impair endothelial function and reduce flow mediated arterial dilatation in humans, as well as increasing oxidative stress, inflammation and even atherosclerosis in animal models.[289]

Observational data suggest a temporal relationship between smoking of cannabis and the onset of acute MI and worsened outcome of MI, particularly in women and young adults.[290-293] However, population-based studies have not consistently shown increased risk of mortality associated with cannabis use.[294-297] Data are limited as most studies are observational, retrospective and do not include extended follow-up. Similar to cigarette smoking, components of cannabis smoke could predispose to atherosclerosis, as inhaled particulates are associated with vascular inflammation and the development of atherosclerosis.[298] Cannabis use has also been temporally associated with stroke in adults as well as children, with a 17% increase in risk of acute ischemic stroke in young adults after cannabis use.[299,300] The mechanism of cerebrovascular events is potentially due to cerebral vasospasm, oxidative stress and transient intracranial arterial stenosis.[301-303] The vasoactive effect of cannabis has been suggested in the coronary arteries as well, as there are documented reports of slow contrast flow on coronary angiograms of patients who have suffered ventricular arrhythmias after using cannabis.[304] In patients with known CAD, cannabis use has been shown to decrease myocardial oxygen delivery, increase myocardial oxygen demand, and decrease the time to develop angina during exercise.[305,306] Moreover, smoking cannabis has also been associated with peripheral arterial disease and associated vasculitis, though this data is somewhat controversial.[299] Some studies have attempted to establish a possible association between cannabis use and heart failure, though a clear relationship has not been established. Finally, though cannabis use has not been specifically associated with ECG abnormalities, some studies have shown a possible greater burden of arrythmias in people who use cannabis.[307,308]

Synthetic cannabinoids known by the street names K2, Spice, and Black Mamba are "designer drug" compounds that are synthesized to have higher binding affinity to the CB1 cannabinoid receptor than the THC found in naturally-grown cannabis.[309] These were initially designed as research tools, but illicit use has been increasing. In 2012, there were 28,531 emergency department visits for synthetic cannabinoid use and over 40% of patients have reported adverse cardiovascular effects.[310,311] There have been multiple reports of myocardial ischemia by electrocardiographic changes or serum biomarkers in children and adults who have used synthetic cannabinoids.[312,313] In several cases, coronary angiography did not show obstructive atherosclerotic lesions, and the mechanism has been hypothesized to be increased myocardial oxygen demand with impaired oxygen carrying capacity, increased inflammation and possibly systemic hypotension due to increased parasympathetic activity.[314] However, in one report, a 39-year-old man presented with a cardiac arrest and was found to have an acute thrombotic occlusion of the ostial left anterior descending coronary artery.[315] Despite electrocardiographic and biomarker evidence of myocardial infarction, most reported patients have shown normal LV function by echocardiography.[316] Notably, case reports of ischemic stroke in individuals with synthetic cannabinoid use have demonstrated acute thrombotic occlusion in the intracranial vessels suggestive of thromboembolic events.[317,318] The underlying mechanism for these clinical syndromes remains unclear, but synthetic cannabinoids have been associated with significant cardiovascular morbidity in particular as the THC content of these products has increased.[284,311] Clinicians should remain vigilant when treating patients who are at risk for using these substances.

CONCLUSION

In summary, both short-term and chronic use of common addictive substances have myriad effects on the circulatory system. The development and progression of several cardiac diseases are related to exposure to these substances, and substance use disorder is strongly linked to poor cardiovascular outcomes. Alcohol, opioids, cannabis and stimulants are frequently used by patients with some of the most common medical conditions—hypertension, dyslipidemia and CAD—thereby increasing the potential for harmful cardiovascular events. As a result, the cardiovascular effects of addictive substances will be encountered by pediatric and adult general practitioners, addiction medicine clinicians, and specialists in nearly every field.

REFERENCES

1. Lloyd-Jones DM, Wang TJ, Leip EP, et al. Lifetime risk for development of atrial fibrillation: the Framingham Heart Study. *Circulation.* 2004;110(9):1042-1046. doi:10.1161/01.CIR.0000140263.20897.42
2. George A, Figueredo VM. Alcoholic cardiomyopathy: a review. *J Card Fail.* 2011;17(10):844-849. doi:10.1016/j.cardfail.2011.05.008
3. Piano MR. Alcohol's effects on the cardiovascular system. *Alcohol Res.* 2017;38(2):219-241. https://www.ncbi.nlm.nih.gov/pubmed/28988575
4. Whitman IR, Agarwal V, Nah G, et al. Alcohol abuse and cardiac disease. *J Am Coll Cardiol.* 2017;69(1):13-24. doi:10.1016/j.jacc.2016.10.048
5. Reid MC, Fiellin DA, O'Connor PG. Hazardous and harmful alcohol consumption in primary care. *Arch Intern Med.* 1999;159(15):1681-1689. doi:10.1001/archinte.159.15.1681
6. Malinski MK, Sesso HD, Lopez-Jimenez F, Buring JE, Gaziano JM. Alcohol consumption and cardiovascular disease mortality in hypertensive men. *Arch Intern Med.* 2004;164(6):623-628. doi:10.1001/archinte.164.6.623
7. Costanzo S, Di Castelnuovo A, Donati MB, Iacoviello L, de Gaetano G. Alcohol consumption and mortality in patients with cardiovascular disease: a meta-analysis. *J Am Coll Cardiol.* 2010;55(13):1339-1347. doi:10.1016/j.jacc.2010.01.006
8. Bell S, Daskalopoulou M, Rapsomaniki E, et al. Association between clinically recorded alcohol consumption and initial presentation of 12 cardiovascular diseases: population based cohort study using linked health records. *BMJ.* 2017;356:j909. doi:10.1136/bmj.j909
9. Kelbaek H, Gjorup T, Hartling OJ, Marving J, Christensen NJ, Godtfredsen J. Left ventricular function during alcohol intoxication and autonomic nervous blockade. *Am J Cardiol.* 1987;59(6):685-688. http://www.ncbi.nlm.nih.gov/pubmed/3825913
10. Altura BM, Altura BT. Microvascular and vascular smooth muscle actions of ethanol, acetaldehyde, and acetate. *Fed Proc.* 1982;41(8):2447-2451. http://www.ncbi.nlm.nih.gov/pubmed/7044829
11. Riff DP, Jain AC, Doyle JT. Acute hemodynamic effects of ethanol on normal human volunteers. *Am Heart J.* 1969;78(5):592-597. http://www.ncbi.nlm.nih.gov/pubmed/5348743
12. Blomqvist G, Saltin B, Mitchell JH. Acute effects of ethanol ingestion on the response to submaximal and maximal exercise in man. *Circulation.* 1970;42(3):463-470. http://www.ncbi.nlm.nih.gov/pubmed/5451231
13. Kelbaek H, Gjorup T, Brynjolf I, Christensen NJ, Godtfredsen J. Acute effects of alcohol on left ventricular function in healthy subjects at rest and during upright exercise. *Am J Cardiol.* 1985;55(1):164-167. https://www.ncbi.nlm.nih.gov/pubmed/3966376
14. Patel VB, Why HJ, Richardson PJ, Preedy VR. The effects of alcohol on the heart. *Adverse Drug React Toxicol Rev.* 1997;16(1):15-43. http://www.ncbi.nlm.nih.gov/pubmed/9192055
15. Williams ES, Mirro MJ, Bailey JC. Electrophysiological effects of ethanol, acetaldehyde, and acetate on cardiac tissues from dog and guinea pig. *Circ Res.* 1980;47(3):473-478. http://www.ncbi.nlm.nih.gov/pubmed/7408127
16. Lange RA, Hillis LD. Cardiovascular complications of cocaine use. *N Engl J Med.* 2001;345(5):351-358. doi:10.1056/NEJM200108023450507
17. Fernandez-Sola J, Nicolas JM, Oriola J, et al. Angiotensin-converting enzyme gene polymorphism is associated with vulnerability to alcoholic cardiomyopathy. *Ann Intern Med.* 2002;137(5 Part 1):321-326. http://www.ncbi.nlm.nih.gov/pubmed/12204015
18. Okuno F, Arai M, Ishii H, et al. Mild but prolonged elevation of serum angiotensin converting enzyme (ACE) activity in alcoholics. *Alcohol.* 1986;3(6):357-359. http://www.ncbi.nlm.nih.gov/pubmed/3028446
19. Cheng CP, Cheng HJ, Cunningham C, et al. Angiotensin II type 1 receptor blockade prevents alcoholic cardiomyopathy. *Circulation.* 2006;114(3):226-236. doi:10.1161/CIRCULATIONAHA.105.596494
20. Day E, Rudd JHF. Alcohol use disorders and the heart. *Addiction.* 2019;114(9):1670-1678. doi:10.1111/add.14703
21. Ripoll C, Yotti R, Bermejo J, Banares R. The heart in liver transplantation. *J Hepatol.* 2011;54(4):810-822. doi:10.1016/j.jhep.2010.11.003

22. Piano MR. Alcoholic cardiomyopathy: incidence, clinical characteristics, and pathophysiology. *Chest.* 2002;121(5):1638-1650. http://www.ncbi.nlm.nih.gov/pubmed/12006456
23. Regan TJ. Alcoholic cardiomyopathy. *Prog Cardiovasc Dis.* 1984; 27(3):141-152. http://www.ncbi.nlm.nih.gov/pubmed/6093193
24. Reus VI, Fochtmann LJ, Bukstein O, et al. The American Psychiatric Association Practice Guideline for the pharmacological treatment of patients with alcohol use disorder. *Am J Psychiatry.* 2018;175(1):86-90. doi:10.1176/appi.ajp.2017.1750101
25. Kajander OA, Kupari M, Laippala P, et al. Dose dependent but non-linear effects of alcohol on the left and right ventricle. *Heart.* 2001;86(4):417-423. http://www.ncbi.nlm.nih.gov/pubmed/11559683
26. Shaaban A, Gangwani MK, Pendela VS, Vindhyal MR. *Alcoholic Cardiomyopathy.* StatPearls Publishing; 2022. Accessed June 20, 2023. https://www.ncbi.nlm.nih.gov/books/NBK513322/
27. Hasin DS, Stinson FS, Ogburn E, Grant BF. Prevalence, correlates, disability, and comorbidity of DSM-IV alcohol abuse and dependence in the United States: results from the National Epidemiologic Survey on Alcohol and Related Conditions. *Arch Gen Psychiatry.* 2007;64(7):830-842. doi:10.1001/archpsyc.64.7.830.
28. Rubin E, Urbano-Marquez A. Alcoholic cardiomyopathy. *Alcohol Clin Exp Res.* 1994;18(1):111-114. http://www.ncbi.nlm.nih.gov/pubmed/8198205
29. Fernandez-Solà J, Estruch R, Nicolás JM, et al. Comparison of alcoholic cardiomyopathy in women versus men. *Am J Cardiol.* 1997;80(4):481-485. http://www.ncbi.nlm.nih.gov/pubmed/9285662
30. Estruch R, Fernandez-Solà J, Sacanella E, Pare C, Rubin E, Urbano-Marquez A. Relationship between cardiomyopathy and liver disease in chronic alcoholism. *Hepatology.* 1995;22(2):532-538. http://www.ncbi.nlm.nih.gov/pubmed/7635421
31. Henriksen JH, Moller S. Cardiac and systemic haemodynamic complications of liver cirrhosis. *Scand Cardiovasc J.* 2009;43(4):218-225. doi:10.1080/14017430802691528
32. Moller S, Henriksen JH. Cirrhotic cardiomyopathy. *J Hepatol.* 2010;53(1):179-190. doi:10.1016/j.jhep.2010.02.023
33. Mathews EC Jr, Gardin JM, Henry WL, et al. Echocardiographic abnormalities in chronic alcoholics with and without overt congestive heart failure. *Am J Cardiol.* 1981;47(3):570-578. http://www.ncbi.nlm.nih.gov/pubmed/6451168
34. Urbano-Marquez A, Estruch R, Fernandez-Solà J, Nicolás JM, Pare JC, Rubin E. The greater risk of alcoholic cardiomyopathy and myopathy in women compared with men. *JAMA.* 1995;274(2):149-154. http://www.ncbi.nlm.nih.gov/pubmed/7596003
35. Lazarevic AM, Nakatani S, Neskovic AN, et al. Early changes in left ventricular function in chronic asymptomatic alcoholics: relation to the duration of heavy drinking. *J Am Coll Cardiol.* 2000;35(6):1599-1606. http://www.ncbi.nlm.nih.gov/pubmed/10807466
36. Gonçalves A, Jhund PS, Claggett B, et al. Relationship between alcohol consumption and cardiac structure and function in the elderly: the Atherosclerosis Risk In Communities Study. *Circ Cardiovasc Imaging.* 2015;8(6). doi:10.1161/CIRCIMAGING.114.002846
37. Kelbaek H, Eriksen J, Brynjolf I, et al. Cardiac performance in patients with asymptomatic alcoholic cirrhosis of the liver. *Am J Cardiol.* 1984;54(7):852-855. http://www.ncbi.nlm.nih.gov/pubmed/6486037
38. Davidson DM. Cardiovascular effects of alcohol. *West J Med.* 1989;151(4):430-439. http://www.ncbi.nlm.nih.gov/pubmed/2686174
39. McKenna CJ, Codd MB, McCann HA, Sugrue DD. Alcohol consumption and idiopathic dilated cardiomyopathy: a case control study. *Am Heart J.* 1998;135(5 Pt 1):833-837. http://www.ncbi.nlm.nih.gov/pubmed/9588413
40. Ho KK, Anderson KM, Kannel WB, Grossman W, Levy D. Survival after the onset of congestive heart failure in Framingham Heart Study Subjects. *Circulation.* 1993;88(1):107-115.
41. Corrao G, Rubbiati L, Bagnardi V, Zambon A, Poikolainen K. Alcohol and coronary heart disease: a meta-analysis. *Addiction.* 2000;95(10):1505-1523. http://www.ncbi.nlm.nih.gov/pubmed/11070527
42. Britton KA, Gaziano JM, Sesso HD, Djousse L. Relation of alcohol consumption and coronary heart disease in hypertensive male physicians (from the Physicians' Health Study). *Am J Cardiol.* 2009;104(7):932-935. doi:10.1016/j.amjcard.2009.05.036
43. Tayal U, Gregson J, Buchan R, et al. Moderate excess alcohol consumption and adverse cardiac remodelling in dilated cardiomyopathy. *Heart.* 2022;108(8):619-625. doi:10.1136/heartjnl-2021-319418
44. Dickerson JA, Raman SV, Baker PM, Leier CV. Relationship of cardiac magnetic resonance imaging and myocardial biopsy in the evaluation of nonischemic cardiomyopathy. *Congest Heart Fail.* 2013;19(1):29-38. doi:10.1111/chf.12003
45. Shehata ML, Turkbey EB, Vogel-Claussen J, Bluemke DA. Role of cardiac magnetic resonance imaging in assessment of nonischemic cardiomyopathies. *Top Magn Reson Imaging.* 2008;19(1):43-57. doi:10.1097/RMR.0b013e31816fcb22
46. La Vecchia LL, Bedogni F, Bozzola L, Bevilacqua P, Ometto R, Vincenzi M. Prediction of recovery after abstinence in alcoholic cardiomyopathy: role of hemodynamic and morphometric parameters. *Clin Cardiol.* 1996;19(1):45-50. http://www.ncbi.nlm.nih.gov/pubmed/8903537
47. Guillo P, Mansourati J, Maheu B, et al. Long-term prognosis in patients with alcoholic cardiomyopathy and severe heart failure after total abstinence. *Am J Cardiol.* 1997;79(9):1276-1278. http://www.ncbi.nlm.nih.gov/pubmed/9164905
48. Nicolás JM, Fernandez-Solà J, Estruch R, et al. The effect of controlled drinking in alcoholic cardiomyopathy. *Ann Intern Med.* 2002;136(3): 192-200. http://www.ncbi.nlm.nih.gov/pubmed/11827495
49. Fauchier L, Babuty D, Poret P, et al. Comparison of long-term outcome of alcoholic and idiopathic dilated cardiomyopathy. *Eur Heart J.* 2000;21(4):306-314. doi:10.1053/euhj.1999.1761
50. Hookana E, Junttila MJ, Puurunen VP, et al. Causes of nonischemic sudden cardiac death in the current era. *Heart Rhythm.* 2011;8(10): 1570-1575. doi:10.1016/j.hrthm.2011.06.031
51. Laonigro I, Correale M, Di Biase M, Altomare E. Alcohol abuse and heart failure. *Eur J Heart Fail.* 2009;11(5):453-462. doi:10.1093/eurjhf/hfp037
52. Faselis C, Arundel C, Patel S, et al. Loop diuretic prescription and 30-day outcomes in older patients with heart failure. *J Am Coll Cardiol.* 2020;76(6):669-679. doi:10.1016/j.jacc.2020.06.022
53. Heidenreich PA, Bozkurt B, Aguilar D, et al. 2022 AHA/ACC/HFSA Guideline for the management of heart failure: executive summary: a report of the American College of Cardiology/American Heart Association Joint Committee on Clinical Practice Guidelines. *J Am Coll Cardiol.* 2022;79(17):1757-1780. doi:10.1016/j.jacc.2021.12.011
54. Allen LA, Stevenson LW, Grady KL, et al. Decision making in advanced heart failure: a scientific statement from the American Heart Association. *Circulation.* 2012;125(15):1928-1952. doi:10.1161/CIR.0b013e31824f2173
55. Dew MA, DiMartini AF, Steel J, et al. Meta-analysis of risk for relapse to substance use after transplantation of the liver or other solid organs. *Liver Transpl.* 2008;14(2):159-172. doi:10.1002/lt.21278
56. Cooper HA, Exner DV, Domanski MJ. Light-to-moderate alcohol consumption and prognosis in patients with left ventricular systolic dysfunction. *J Am Coll Cardiol.* 2000;35(7):1753-1759. http://www.ncbi.nlm.nih.gov/pubmed/10841221
57. Abramson JL, Williams SA, Krumholz HM, Vaccarino V. Moderate alcohol consumption and risk of heart failure among older persons. *JAMA.* 2001;285(15):1971-1977. https://www.ncbi.nlm.nih.gov/pubmed/11308433
58. Aguilar D, Skali H, Moye LA, et al. Alcohol consumption and prognosis in patients with left ventricular systolic dysfunction after a myocardial infarction. *J Am Coll Cardiol.* 2004;43(11):2015-2021. doi:10.1016/j.jacc.2004.01.042
59. Evangelista LS, Doering LV, Dracup K. Usefulness of a history of tobacco and alcohol use in predicting multiple heart failure readmissions among veterans. *Am J Cardiol.* 2000;86(12):1339-1342. https://www.ncbi.nlm.nih.gov/pubmed/11113409

60. Wannamethee SG, Whincup PH, Lennon L, Papacosta O, Shaper AG. Alcohol consumption and risk of incident heart failure in older men: a prospective cohort study. *Open Heart.* 2015;2(1):e000266. doi:10.1136/openhrt-2015-000266
61. Yancy CW, Jessup M, Bozkurt B, et al. 2013 ACCF/AHA guideline for the management of heart failure: a report of the American College of Cardiology Foundation/American Heart Association Task Force on Practice Guidelines. *J Am Coll Cardiol.* 2013;62(16):e147-e239. doi:10.1016/j.jacc.2013.05.019
62. Puddey IB, Mori TA, Barden AE, Beilin LJ. Alcohol and hypertension-new insights and lingering controversies. *Curr Hypertens Rep.* 2019;21(10):79. doi:10.1007/s11906-019-0984-1
63. Rehm J, Room R, Monteiro M, et al. Alcohol as a risk factor for global burden of disease. *Eur Addict Res.* 2003;9(4):157-164. doi:10.1159/000072222
64. Beilin LJ, Puddey IB. Alcohol and hypertension: an update. *Hypertension.* 2006;47(6):1035-1038. doi:10.1161/01.HYP.0000218586.21932.3c
65. Biddinger KJ, Emdin CA, Haas ME, et al. Association of habitual alcohol intake with risk of cardiovascular disease. *JAMA Netw Open.* 2022;5(3):e223849. doi:10.1001/jamanetworkopen.2022.3849
66. Sarafidis PA, Bakris GL. Resistant hypertension: an overview of evaluation and treatment. *J Am Coll Cardiol.* 2008;52(22):1749-1757. doi:10.1016/j.jacc.2008.08.036
67. Abdel-Rahman AR, Merrill RH, Wooles WR. Effect of acute ethanol administration on the baroreceptor reflex control of heart rate in normotensive human volunteers. *Clin Sci (Lond).* 1987;72(1):113-122. http://www.ncbi.nlm.nih.gov/pubmed/3802717
68. Zilkens RR, Burke V, Hodgson JM, Barden A, Beilin LJ, Puddey IB. Red wine and beer elevate blood pressure in normotensive men. *Hypertension.* 2005;45(5):874-879. doi:10.1161/01.HYP.0000164639.83623.76
69. Hering D, Kucharska W, Kara T, Somers VK, Narkiewicz K. Potentiated sympathetic and hemodynamic responses to alcohol in hypertensive vs. normotensive individuals. *J Hypertens.* 2011;29(3):537-541. doi:10.1097/HJH.0b013e328342b2a9
70. Pierdomenico SD, Lapenna D, Bucci A, et al. Cardiovascular outcome in treated hypertensive patients with responder, masked, false resistant, and true resistant hypertension. *Am J Hypertens.* 2005;18(11):1422-1428. doi:10.1016/j.amjhyper.2005.05.014
71. Daugherty SL, Powers JD, Magid DJ, et al. Incidence and prognosis of resistant hypertension in hypertensive patients. *Circulation.* 2012;125(13):1635-1642. doi:10.1161/CIRCULATIONAHA.111.068064
72. Xin X, He J, Frontini MG, Ogden LG, Motsamai OI, Whelton PK. Effects of alcohol reduction on blood pressure: a meta-analysis of randomized controlled trials. *Hypertension.* 2001;38(5):1112-1117. http://www.ncbi.nlm.nih.gov/pubmed/11711507
73. McFadden CB, Brensinger CM, Berlin JA, Townsend RR. Systematic review of the effect of daily alcohol intake on blood pressure. *Am J Hypertens.* 2005;18(2 Pt 1):276-286. doi:10.1016/j.amjhyper.2004.07.020
74. Chobanian AV, Bakris GL, Black HR, et al. Seventh report of the Joint National Committee on prevention, detection, evaluation, and treatment of high blood pressure. *Hypertension.* 2003;42(6):1206-1252. doi:10.1161/01.HYP.0000107251.49515.c2
75. Magnani JW, Rienstra M, Lin H, et al. Atrial fibrillation: current knowledge and future directions in epidemiology and genomics. *Circulation.* 2011;124(18):1982-1993. doi:10.1161/CIRCULATIONAHA.111.039677
76. Heeringa J, van der Kuip DA, Hofman A, et al. Prevalence, incidence and lifetime risk of atrial fibrillation: the Rotterdam study. *Eur Heart J.* 2006;27(8):949-953. doi:10.1093/eurheartj/ehi825
77. Schoonderwoerd BA, Smit MD, Pen L, Van Gelder IC. New risk factors for atrial fibrillation: causes of 'not-so-lone atrial fibrillation'. *Europace.* 2008;10(6):668-673. doi:10.1093/europace/eun124
78. Ettinger PO, Wu CF, De La Cruz C Jr, Weisse AB, Ahmed SS, Regan TJ. Arrhythmias and the "Holiday Heart": alcohol-associated cardiac rhythm disorders. *Am Heart J.* 1978;95(5):555-562. https://www.ncbi.nlm.nih.gov/pubmed/636996
79. Voskoboinik A, Prabhu S, Ling LH, Kalman JM, Kistler PM. Alcohol and atrial fibrillation: a sobering review. *J Am Coll Cardiol.* 2016;68(23):2567-2576. doi:10.1016/j.jacc.2016.08.074
80. Djousse L, Levy D, Benjamin EJ, et al. Long-term alcohol consumption and the risk of atrial fibrillation in the Framingham Study. *Am J Cardiol.* 2004;93(6):710-713. doi:10.1016/j.amjcard.2003.12.004
81. Csengeri D, Sprunker NA, Di Castelnuovo A, et al. Alcohol consumption, cardiac biomarkers, and risk of atrial fibrillation and adverse outcomes. *Eur Heart J.* 2021;42(12):1170-1177. doi:10.1093/eurheartj/ehaa953
82. Mukamal KJ, Psaty BM, Rautaharju PM, et al. Alcohol consumption and risk and prognosis of atrial fibrillation among older adults: the Cardiovascular Health Study. *Am Heart J.* 2007;153(2):260-266. doi:10.1016/j.ahj.2006.10.039
83. Kodama S, Saito K, Tanaka S, et al. Alcohol consumption and risk of atrial fibrillation: a meta-analysis. *J Am Coll Cardiol.* 2011;57(4):427-436. doi:10.1016/j.jacc.2010.08.641
84. Fuster V, Ryden LE, Cannom DS, et al. ACC/AHA/ESC 2006 Guidelines for the Management of Patients with Atrial Fibrillation: a report of the American College of Cardiology/American Heart Association Task Force on Practice Guidelines and the European Society of Cardiology Committee for Practice Guidelines (Writing Committee to Revise the 2001 Guidelines for the Management of Patients With Atrial Fibrillation): developed in collaboration with the European Heart Rhythm Association and the Heart Rhythm Society. *Circulation.* 2006;114(7):e257-e354. doi:10.1161/CIRCULATIONAHA.106.177292
85. Fauchier L. Alcoholic cardiomyopathy and ventricular arrhythmias. *Chest.* 2003;123(4):1320. http://www.ncbi.nlm.nih.gov/pubmed/12684336
86. Harikrishnan P, Gupta T, Kolte D, et al. Burden of arrhythmias in patients with alcoholic cardiomyopathy: findings from the nationwide inpatient sample 2003-2011. *J Am Coll Cardiol.* 2015;65(10, Supplement):A297. doi:10.1016/S0735-1097(15)60297-2
87. Tonino PA, Fearon WF, De Bruyne B, et al. Angiographic versus functional severity of coronary artery stenoses in the FAME study fractional flow reserve versus angiography in multivessel evaluation. *J Am Coll Cardiol.* 2010;55(25):2816-2821. doi:10.1016/j.jacc.2009.11.096
88. Song RJ, Nguyen XT, Quaden R, et al. Alcohol consumption and risk of coronary artery disease (from the Million Veteran Program). *Am J Cardiol.* 2018;121(10):1162-1168. doi:10.1016/j.amjcard.2018.01.042
89. Roerecke M, Rehm J. Alcohol consumption, drinking patterns, and ischemic heart disease: a narrative review of meta-analyses and a systematic review and meta-analysis of the impact of heavy drinking occasions on risk for moderate drinkers. *BMC Med.* 2014;12:182. doi:10.1186/s12916-014-0182-6
90. Klatsky AL. Alcohol and cardiovascular mortality: common sense and scientific truth. *J Am Coll Cardiol.* 2010;55(13):1336-1338. doi:10.1016/j.jacc.2009.10.057
91. Mukamal KJ, Chen CM, Rao SR, Breslow RA. Alcohol consumption and cardiovascular mortality among U.S. adults, 1987 to 2002. *J Am Coll Cardiol.* 2010;55(13):1328-1335. doi:10.1016/j.jacc.2009.10.056
92. Zhou X, Li C, Xu W, Hong X, Chen J. Relation of alcohol consumption to angiographically proved coronary artery disease in chinese men. *Am J Cardiol.* 2010;106(8):1101-1103. doi:10.1016/j.amjcard.2010.06.012
93. Roy A, Prabhakaran D, Jeemon P, et al. Impact of alcohol on coronary heart disease in Indian men. *Atherosclerosis.* 2010;210(2):531-535. doi:10.1016/j.atherosclerosis.2010.02.033
94. Booyse FM, Parks DA. Moderate wine and alcohol consumption: beneficial effects on cardiovascular disease. *Thromb Haemost.* 2001;86(2):517-528. http://www.ncbi.nlm.nih.gov/pubmed/11521997
95. Gaziano JM, Buring JE, Breslow JL, et al. Moderate alcohol intake, increased levels of high-density lipoprotein and its subfractions, and decreased risk of myocardial infarction. *N Engl J Med.* 1993;329(25):1829-1834. doi:10.1056/NEJM199312163292501
96. Davies MJ, Baer DJ, Judd JT, Brown ED, Campbell WS, Taylor PR. Effects of moderate alcohol intake on fasting insulin and glucose concentrations and insulin sensitivity in postmenopausal women: a randomized controlled trial. *JAMA.* 2002;287(19):2559-2562. http://www.ncbi.nlm.nih.gov/pubmed/12020337

97. Baliunas DO, Taylor BJ, Irving H, et al. Alcohol as a risk factor for type 2 diabetes: a systematic review and meta-analysis. *Diabetes Care.* 2009;32(11):2123-2132. doi:10.2337/dc09-0227
98. Di Minno MN, Franchini M, Russolillo A, Lupoli R, Iervolino S, Di Minno G. Alcohol dosing and the heart: updating clinical evidence. *Semin Thromb Hemost.* 2011;37(8):875-884. doi:10.1055/s-0031-1297366
99. Mostofsky E, Chahal HS, Mukamal KJ, Rimm EB, Mittleman MA. Alcohol and immediate risk of cardiovascular events: a systematic review and dose-response meta-analysis. *Circulation.* 2016;133(10): 979-987. doi:10.1161/CIRCULATIONAHA.115.019743
100. Castelnuovo DA, Rotondo S, Iacoviello L, Donati MB, Gaetano DG. Meta-analysis of wine and beer consumption in relation to vascular risk. *Circulation.* 2002;105(24):2836-2844. http://www.ncbi.nlm.nih.gov/pubmed/12070110
101. White IR, Altmann DR, Nanchahal K. Alcohol consumption and mortality: modelling risks for men and women at different ages. *BMJ.* 2002;325(7357):191. http://www.ncbi.nlm.nih.gov/pubmed/12142306
102. Di Castelnuovo A, Costanzo S, Bagnardi V, Donati MB, Iacoviello L, de Gaetano G. Alcohol dosing and total mortality in men and women: an updated meta-analysis of 34 prospective studies. *Arch Intern Med.* 2006;166(22):2437-2445. doi:10.1001/archinte.166.22.2437
103. Yang T, Doherty TM, Wong ND, Detrano RC. Alcohol consumption, coronary calcium, and coronary heart disease events. *Am J Cardiol.* 1999;84(7):802-806. http://www.ncbi.nlm.nih.gov/pubmed/10513777
104. Pletcher MJ, Varosy P, Kiefe CI, Lewis CE, Sidney S, Hulley SB. Alcohol consumption, binge drinking, and early coronary calcification: findings from the Coronary Artery Risk Development in Young Adults (CARDIA) Study. *Am J Epidemiol.* 2005;161(5):423-433. doi:10.1093/aje/kwi062
105. McClelland RL, Bild DE, Burke GL, Mukamal KJ, Lima JA, Kronmal RA. Alcohol and coronary artery calcium prevalence, incidence, and progression: results from the Multi-Ethnic Study of Atherosclerosis (MESA). *Am J Clin Nutr.* 2008;88(6):1593-1601. doi:10.3945/ajcn.2008.26420
106. Vliegenthart R, Oei HH, van den Elzen AP, et al. Alcohol consumption and coronary calcification in a general population. *Arch Intern Med.* 2004;164(21):2355-2360. doi:10.1001/archinte.164.21.2355
107. Ronksley PE, Brien SE, Turner BJ, Mukamal KJ, Ghali WA. Association of alcohol consumption with selected cardiovascular disease outcomes: a systematic review and meta-analysis. *BMJ.* 2011;342:d671. doi:10.1136/bmj.d671
108. Reynolds K, Lewis B, Nolen JD, Kinney GL, Sathya B, He J. Alcohol consumption and risk of stroke: a meta-analysis. *JAMA.* 2003;289(5): 579-588. http://www.ncbi.nlm.nih.gov/pubmed/12578491
109. Zhang C, Qin YY, Chen Q, et al. Alcohol intake and risk of stroke: a dose-response meta-analysis of prospective studies. *Int J Cardiol.* 2014;174(3):669-677. doi:10.1016/j.ijcard.2014.04.225
110. Kadlecova P, Andel R, Mikulik R, Handing EP, Pedersen NL. Alcohol consumption at midlife and risk of stroke during 43 years of follow-up: cohort and twin analyses. *Stroke.* 2015;46(3):627-633. doi:10.1161/STROKEAHA.114.006724
111. Cryer PE, Haymond MW, Santiago JV, Shah SD. Norepinephrine and epinephrine release and adrenergic mediation of smoking-associated hemodynamic and metabolic events. *N Engl J Med.* 1976;295(11):573-577. doi:10.1056/NEJM197609092951101
112. Benowitz NL, Jacob P III, Jones RT, Rosenberg J. Interindividual variability in the metabolism and cardiovascular effects of nicotine in man. *J Pharmacol Exp Ther.* 1982;221(2):368-372. http://www.ncbi.nlm.nih.gov/pubmed/7077531
113. Grassi G, Seravalle G, Calhoun DA, et al. Mechanisms responsible for sympathetic activation by cigarette smoking in humans. *Circulation.* 1994;90(1):248-253. http://www.ncbi.nlm.nih.gov/pubmed/8026005
114. Benowitz NL, Gourlay SG. Cardiovascular toxicity of nicotine: implications for nicotine replacement therapy. *J Am Coll Cardiol.* 1997;29(7):1422-1431. http://www.ncbi.nlm.nih.gov/pubmed/9180099
115. Stewart PM, Catterall JR. Chronic nicotine ingestion and atrial fibrillation. *Br Heart J.* 1985;54(2):222-223. http://www.ncbi.nlm.nih.gov/pubmed/4015933
116. Rigotti NA, Eagle KA. Atrial fibrillation while chewing nicotine gum. *JAMA.* 1986;255(8):1018. http://www.ncbi.nlm.nih.gov/pubmed/3945010
117. Shao XM, Lopez-Valdes HE, Liang J, Feldman JL. Inhaled nicotine equivalent to cigarette smoking disrupts systemic and uterine hemodynamics and induces cardiac arrhythmia in pregnant rats. *Sci Rep.* 2017;7(1):16974. doi:10.1038/s41598-017-17301-5
118. Mehta MC, Jain AC, Mehta A, Billie M. Cardiac arrhythmias following intravenous nicotine: experimental study in dogs. *J Cardiovasc Pharmacol Ther.* 1997;2(4):291-298. doi:10.1054/jcpt.1997.0291
119. Miyauchi M, Qu Z, Miyauchi Y, et al. Chronic nicotine in hearts with healed ventricular myocardial infarction promotes atrial flutter that resembles typical human atrial flutter. *Am J Physiol Heart Circ Physiol.* 2005;288(6):H2878-H2886. doi:10.1152/ajpheart.01165.2004
120. Wang H, Shi H, Wang Z. Nicotine depresses the functions of multiple cardiac potassium channels. *Life Sci.* 1999;65(12):PL143-PL149. https://www.ncbi.nlm.nih.gov/pubmed/10503950
121. Joseph AM, Norman SM, Ferry LH, et al. The safety of transdermal nicotine as an aid to smoking cessation in patients with cardiac disease. *N Engl J Med.* 1996;335(24):1792-1798. doi:10.1056/NEJM199612123352402
122. Woolf KJ, Zabad MN, Post JM, McNitt S, Williams GC, Bisognano JD. Effect of nicotine replacement therapy on cardiovascular outcomes after acute coronary syndromes. *Am J Cardiol.* 2012;110(7):968-970. doi:10.1016/j.amjcard.2012.05.028
123. D'Alessandro A, Boeckelmann I, Hammwhoner M, Goette A. Nicotine, cigarette smoking and cardiac arrhythmia: an overview. *Eur J Prev Cardiol.* 2012;19(3):297-305. http://www.ncbi.nlm.nih.gov/pubmed/22779085
124. Ross R. Atherosclerosis--an inflammatory disease. *N Engl J Med.* 1999;340(2):115-126. doi:10.1056/NEJM199901143400207
125. Ross R. The pathogenesis of atherosclerosis: a perspective for the 1990s. *Nature.* 1993;362(6423):801-809. doi:10.1038/362801a0
126. Ruberg FL, Loscalzo J. Prothrombotic determinants of coronary atherothrombosis. *Vasc Med.* 2003;7(4):289-299. http://www.ncbi.nlm.nih.gov/pubmed/12710845
127. Lippi G, Franchini M, Targher G. Arterial thrombus formation in cardiovascular disease. *Nat Rev Cardiol.* 2011;8(9):502-512. doi:10.1038/nrcardio.2011.91
128. Ambrose JA, Barua RS. The pathophysiology of cigarette smoking and cardiovascular disease: an update. *J Am Coll Cardiol.* 2004;43(10): 1731-1737. doi:10.1016/j.jacc.2003.12.047
129. Blann AD, Steele C, McCollum CN. The influence of smoking and of oral and transdermal nicotine on blood pressure, and haematology and coagulation indices. *Thromb Haemost.* 1997;78(3):1093-1096. http://www.ncbi.nlm.nih.gov/pubmed/9308759
130. Talhout R, Schulz T, Florek E, van Benthem J, Wester P, Opperhuizen A. Hazardous compounds in tobacco smoke. *Int J Environ Res Public Health.* 2011;8(2):613-628. doi:10.3390/ijerph8020613
131. Kugiyama K, Yasue H, Ohgushi M, et al. Deficiency in nitric oxide bioactivity in epicardial coronary arteries of cigarette smokers. *J Am Coll Cardiol.* 1996;28(5):1161-1167. doi:10.1016/S0735-1097(96)00325-7
132. Barua RS, Ambrose JA, Eales-Reynolds LJ, DeVoe MC, Zervas JG, Saha DC. Dysfunctional endothelial nitric oxide biosynthesis in healthy smokers with impaired endothelium-dependent vasodilatation. *Circulation.* 2001;104(16):1905-1910. http://www.ncbi.nlm.nih.gov/pubmed/11602492
133. Blann AD, Kirkpatrick U, Devine C, Naser S, McCollum CN. The influence of acute smoking on leucocytes, platelets and the endothelium. *Atherosclerosis.* 1998;141(1):133-139. http://www.ncbi.nlm.nih.gov/pubmed/9863546
134. Bermudez EA, Rifai N, Buring JE, Manson JE, Ridker PM. Relation between markers of systemic vascular inflammation and smoking in women. *Am J Cardiol.* 2002;89(9):1117-1119. http://www.ncbi.nlm.nih.gov/pubmed/11988205
135. Adams MR, Jessup W, Celermajer DS. Cigarette smoking is associated with increased human monocyte adhesion to endothelial cells:

reversibility with oral L-arginine but not vitamin C. *J Am Coll Cardiol.* 1997;29(3):491-497. http://www.ncbi.nlm.nih.gov/pubmed/9060883

136. Golbidi S, Edvinsson L, Laher I. Smoking and endothelial dysfunction. *Curr Vasc Pharmacol.* 2020;18(1):1-11. doi:10.2174/1573403X14666180913120015
137. Rival J, Riddle JM, Stein PD. Effects of chronic smoking on platelet function. *Thromb Res.* 1987;45(1):75-85. http://www.ncbi.nlm.nih.gov/pubmed/2951895
138. Yusuf S, Hawken S, Ounpuu S, et al. Effect of potentially modifiable risk factors associated with myocardial infarction in 52 countries (the INTERHEART study): case-control study. *Lancet.* 2004;364(9438):937-952. doi:10.1016/S0140-6736(04)17018-9
139. Ding N, Sang Y, Chen J, et al. Cigarette smoking, smoking cessation, and long-term risk of 3 major atherosclerotic diseases. *J Am Coll Cardiol.* 2019;74(4):498-507. doi:10.1016/j.jacc.2019.05.049
140. Wolf PA, D'Agostino RB, Kannel WB, Bonita R, Belanger AJ. Cigarette smoking as a risk factor for stroke. *The Framingham Study. JAMA.* 1988;259(7):1025-1029. http://www.ncbi.nlm.nih.gov/pubmed/3339799
141. West HW, Juonala M, Gall SL, et al. Exposure to parental smoking in childhood is associated with increased risk of carotid atherosclerotic plaque in adulthood: the Cardiovascular Risk in Young Finns Study. *Circulation.* 2015;131(14):1239-1246. doi:10.1161/CIRCULATIONAHA.114.013485
142. Pell JP, Haw S, Cobbe S, et al. Smoke-free legislation and hospitalizations for acute coronary syndrome. *N Engl J Med.* 2008;359(5):482-491. doi:10.1056/NEJMsa0706740
143. Juster HR, Loomis BR, Hinman TM, et al. Declines in hospital admissions for acute myocardial infarction in New York state after implementation of a comprehensive smoking ban. *Am J Public Health.* 2007;97(11):2035-2039. doi:10.2105/AJPH.2006.099994
144. Bartecchi C, Alsever RN, Nevin-Woods C, et al. Reduction in the incidence of acute myocardial infarction associated with a citywide smoking ordinance. *Circulation.* 2006;114(14):1490-1496. doi:10.1161/CIRCULATIONAHA.106.615245
145. Bruintjes G, Bartelson BB, Hurst P, Levinson AH, Hokanson JE, Krantz MJ. Reduction in acute myocardial infarction hospitalization after implementation of a smoking ordinance. *Am J Med.* 2011;124(7):647-654. doi:10.1016/j.amjmed.2011.02.022
146. Gordon T, Kannel WB, McGee D, Dawber TR. Death and coronary attacks in men after giving up cigarette smoking. A report from the Framingham study. *Lancet.* 1974;2(7893):1345-1348. http://www.ncbi.nlm.nih.gov/pubmed/4143310
147. Morito N, Miura SI, Yano M, Hitaka Y, Nishikawa H, Saku K. Association between a ban on smoking in a hospital and the in-hospital onset of acute myocardial infarction. *Cardiol Res.* 2015;6(3):278-282. doi:10.14740/cr404e
148. Ahmed AA, Patel K, Nyaku MA, et al. Risk of heart failure and death after prolonged smoking cessation: role of amount and duration of prior smoking. *Circ Heart Fail.* 2015;8(4):694-701. doi:10.1161/CIRCHEARTFAILURE.114.001885
149. Abbasi J. FDA extends authority to e-cigarettes: implications for smoking cessation? *JAMA.* 2016;316(6):572-574. doi:10.1001/jama.2016.8568
150. Syamlal G, Jamal A, King BA, Mazurek JM. Electronic cigarette use among working adults - United States, 2014. *MMWR Morbid Mortal Wkly Rep.* 2016;65(22):557-561. doi:10.15585/mmwr.mm6522a1
151. Choi K, Forster JL. Beliefs and experimentation with electronic cigarettes: a prospective analysis among young adults. *Am J Prev Med.* 2014;46(2):175-178. doi:10.1016/j.amepre.2013.10.007
152. Kreitzberg DS, Pasch KE, Marti CN, Loukas A, Perry CL. Bidirectional associations between young adults' reported exposure to e-cigarette marketing and e-cigarette use. *Addiction.* 2019;114(10):1834-1841. doi:10.1111/add.14710
153. Pokhrel P, Kawamoto CT, Pagano I, Herzog TA. Trajectories of e-cigarette advertising exposure, e-cigarette use and cigarette smoking in a sample of young adults from Hawaii. *Addiction.* 2022;117(7):2015-2026. doi:10.1111/add.15815
154. Grana R, Benowitz N, Glantz SA. E-cigarettes: a scientific review. *Circulation.* 2014;129(19):1972-1986. doi:10.1161/CIRCULATIONAHA.114.007667
155. Vansickel AR, Eissenberg T. Electronic cigarettes: effective nicotine delivery after acute administration. *Nicotine Tob Res.* 2013;15(1):267-270. doi:10.1093/ntr/ntr316
156. Russell MA, Wilson C, Patel UA, Feyerabend C, Cole PV. Plasma nicotine levels after smoking cigarettes with high, medium, and low nicotine yields. *BMJ.* 1975;2(5968):414-416. https://www.ncbi.nlm.nih.gov/pubmed/1168517
157. Russell MA, Feyerabend C, Cole PV. Plasma nicotine levels after cigarette smoking and chewing nicotine gum. *BMJ.* 1976;1(6017):1043-1046. https://www.ncbi.nlm.nih.gov/pubmed/1268547
158. Auer R, Concha-Lozano N, Jacot-Sadowski I, Cornuz J, Berthet A. Heat-not-burn tobacco cigarettes: smoke by any other name. *JAMA Intern Med.* 2017;177(7):1050-1052. doi:10.1001/jamainternmed.2017.1419
159. Ali FRM, Seaman EL, Crane E, Schillo B, King BA. Trends in U.S. e-cigarette sales and prices by nicotine strength, overall and by product and flavor type, 2017-2022. *Nicotine Tob Res.* 2022. doi:10.1093/ntr/ntac284
160. Murray RP, Bailey WC, Daniels K, et al. Safety of nicotine polacrilex gum used by 3,094 participants in the Lung Health Study. Lung Health Study Research Group. 1996;109(2):438-445. https://www.ncbi.nlm.nih.gov/pubmed/8620719
161. Hubbard R, Lewis S, Smith C, et al. Use of nicotine replacement therapy and the risk of acute myocardial infarction, stroke, and death. *Tob Control.* 2005;14(6):416-421. doi:10.1136/tc.2005.011387
162. Kosmider L, Sobczak A, Fik M, et al. Carbonyl compounds in electronic cigarette vapors: effects of nicotine solvent and battery output voltage. *Nicotine Tob Res.* 2014;16(10):1319-1326. doi:10.1093/ntr/ntu078
163. Goniewicz ML, Knysak J, Gawron M, et al. Levels of selected carcinogens and toxicants in vapour from electronic cigarettes. *Tob Control.* 2014;23(2):133-139. doi:10.1136/tobaccocontrol-2012-050859
164. Pope CA, Burnett RT, Krewski D, et al. Cardiovascular mortality and exposure to airborne fine particulate matter and cigarette smoke: shape of the exposure-response relationship. *Circulation.* 2009;120(11):941-948. doi:10.1161/CIRCULATIONAHA.109.857888
165. Brook RD, Rajagopalan S, Pope CA, et al. Particulate matter air pollution and cardiovascular disease: an update to the scientific statement from the American Heart Association. *Circulation.* 2010;121(21):2331-2378. doi:10.1161/CIR.0b013e3181dbece1
166. Munzel T, Hahad O, Kuntic M, Keaney JF, Deanfield JE, Daiber A. Effects of tobacco cigarettes, e-cigarettes, and waterpipe smoking on endothelial function and clinical outcomes. *Eur Heart J.* 2020;41(41):4057-4070. doi:10.1093/eurheartj/ehaa460
167. Zeka A, Sullivan JR, Vokonas PS, Sparrow D, Schwartz J. Inflammatory markers and particulate air pollution: characterizing the pathway to disease. *Int J Epidemiol.* 2006;35(5):1347-1354. doi:10.1093/ije/dyl132
168. Bräuner EV, Forchhammer L, Møller P, et al. Exposure to ultrafine particles from ambient air and oxidative stress-induced DNA damage. *Environ Health Perspect.* 2007;115(8):1177-1182. doi:10.1289/ehp.9984
169. Rudez G, Janssen NA, Kilinc E, et al. Effects of ambient air pollution on hemostasis and inflammation. *Environ Health Perspect.* 2009;117(6):995-1001. doi:10.1289/ehp.0800437
170. Dvonch JT, Kannan S, Schulz AJ, et al. Acute effects of ambient particulate matter on blood pressure: differential effects across urban communities. *Hypertension.* 2009;53(5):853-859. doi:10.1161/HYPERTENSIONAHA.108.123877
171. Skotsimara G, Antonopoulos AS, Oikonomou E, et al. Cardiovascular effects of electronic cigarettes: a systematic review and meta-analysis. *Eur J Prev Cardiol.* 2019;26(11):1219-1228. doi:10.1177/2047487319832975
172. Kloner RA, Hale S, Alker K, Rezkalla S. The effects of acute and chronic cocaine use on the heart. *Circulation.* 1992;85(2):407-419. http://www.ncbi.nlm.nih.gov/pubmed/1346509
173. Pitts WR, Lange RA, Cigarroa JE, Hillis LD. Cocaine-induced myocardial ischemia and infarction: pathophysiology, recognition, and management. *Prog Cardiovasc Dis.* 1997;40(1):65-76. http://www.ncbi.nlm.nih.gov/pubmed/9247556

174. Trendelenburg U. The effect of cocaine on the pacemaker of isolated guinea-pig atria. *J Pharmacol Exp Ther.* 1968;161(2):222-231. http://www.ncbi.nlm.nih.gov/pubmed/5652849
175. Greenberg R, Innes IR. The role of bound calcium in supersensitivity induced by cocaine. *Br J Pharmacol.* 1976;57(3):329-334. http://www.ncbi.nlm.nih.gov/pubmed/823996
176. Gilman AG, Goodman LS, Rall TW, Murad F. *The Pharmacologic Basis of Therapeutics.* 7th ed. Pergamon Press; 1990.
177. Egashira K, Morgan KG, Morgan JP. Effects of cocaine on excitation-contraction coupling of aortic smooth muscle from the ferret. *J Clin Invest.* 1991;87(4):1322-1328. doi:10.1172/JCI115135
178. Finkel JB, Marhefka GD. Rethinking cocaine-associated chest pain and acute coronary syndromes. *Mayo Clin Proc.* 2011;86(12):1198-1207. doi:10.4065/mcp.2011.0338
179. Basso C, Marra MP, Thiene G. Cocaine and the heart: more than just coronary disease. *Heart.* 2011;97(24):1995-1996. doi:10.1136/heartjnl-2011-300736
180. Paraschin K, Guerra De Andrade A, Rodrigues Parga J. Assessment of myocardial infarction by CT angiography and cardiovascular MRI in patients with cocaine-associated chest pain: a pilot study. *Br J Radiol.* 2012;85(1015):e274-e278. doi:10.1259/bjr/52001979
181. Aquaro GD, Gabutti A, Meini M, et al. Silent myocardial damage in cocaine addicts. *Heart.* 2011;97(24):2056-2062. doi:10.1136/hrt.2011.226977
182. Resnick RB, Kestenbaum RS, Schwartz LK. Acute systemic effects of cocaine in man: a controlled study by intranasal and intravenous routes. *Science.* 1977;195(4279):696-698. http://www.ncbi.nlm.nih.gov/pubmed/841307
183. Fischman MW, Schuster CR, Javaid J, Hatano Y, Davis J. Acute tolerance development to the cardiovascular and subjective effects of cocaine. *J Pharmacol Exp Ther.* 1985;235(3):677-682. http://www.ncbi.nlm.nih.gov/pubmed/4078729
184. Whitby LG, Hertting G, Axelrod J. Effect of cocaine on the disposition of noradrenaline labelled with tritium. *Nature.* 1960;187:604-605. http://www.ncbi.nlm.nih.gov/pubmed/13844323
185. Brogan WC III, Lange RA, Kim AS, Moliterno DJ, Hillis LD. Alleviation of cocaine-induced coronary vasoconstriction by nitroglycerin. *J Am Coll Cardiol.* 1991;18(2):581-586. http://www.ncbi.nlm.nih.gov/pubmed/1906905
186. Boehrer JD, Moliterno DJ, Willard JE, Hillis LD, Lange RA. Influence of labetalol on cocaine-induced coronary vasoconstriction in humans. *Am J Med.* 1993;94(6):608-610. http://www.ncbi.nlm.nih.gov/pubmed/8506886
187. Flores ED, Lange RA, Cigarroa RG, Hillis LD. Effect of cocaine on coronary artery dimensions in atherosclerotic coronary artery disease: enhanced vasoconstriction at sites of significant stenoses. *J Am Coll Cardiol.* 1990;16(1):74-79. http://www.ncbi.nlm.nih.gov/pubmed/2358608
188. Moliterno DJ, Willard JE, Lange RA, et al. Coronary-artery vasoconstriction induced by cocaine, cigarette smoking, or both. *N Engl J Med.* 1994;330(7):454-459. doi:10.1056/NEJM199402173300702
189. Pradhan L, Mondal D, Chandra S, Ali M, Agrawal KC. Molecular analysis of cocaine-induced endothelial dysfunction: role of endothelin-1 and nitric oxide. *Cardiovasc Toxicol.* 2008;8(4):161-171. doi:10.1007/s12012-008-9025-z
190. Pereira J, Saez CG, Pallavicini J, et al. Platelet activation in chronic cocaine users: effect of short term abstinence. *Platelets.* 2011;22(8):596-601. doi:10.3109/09537104.2011.578181
191. Heesch CM, Wilhelm CR, Ristich J, Adnane J, Bontempo FA, Wagner WR. Cocaine activates platelets and increases the formation of circulating platelet containing microaggregates in humans. *Heart.* 2000;83(6):688-695. http://www.ncbi.nlm.nih.gov/pubmed/10814631
192. Rinder HM, Ault KA, Jatlow PI, Kosten TR, Smith BR. Platelet alpha-granule release in cocaine users. *Circulation.* 1994;90(3):1162-1167. http://www.ncbi.nlm.nih.gov/pubmed/7522132
193. Siegel AJ, Mendelson JH, Sholar MB, et al. Effect of cocaine usage on C-reactive protein, von Willebrand factor, and fibrinogen. *Am J Cardiol.* 2002;89(9):1133-1135. http://www.ncbi.nlm.nih.gov/pubmed/11988210
194. Stec JJ, Silbershatz H, Tofler GH, et al. Association of fibrinogen with cardiovascular risk factors and cardiovascular disease in the Framingham Offspring Population. *Circulation.* 2000;102(14):1634-1638. http://www.ncbi.nlm.nih.gov/pubmed/11015340
195. Kolodgie FD, Virmani R, Cornhill JF, Herderick EE, Smialek J. Increase in atherosclerosis and adventitial mast cells in cocaine abusers: an alternative mechanism of cocaine-associated coronary vasospasm and thrombosis. *J Am Coll Cardiol.* 1991;17(7):1553-1560. http://www.ncbi.nlm.nih.gov/pubmed/2033185
196. Wilson LD, Malik M, Willson H. Cocaine and ethanol: combined effects on coronary artery blood flow and myocardial function in dogs. *Acad Emerg Med.* 2009;16(7):646-655. doi:10.1111/j.1553-2712.2009.00443.x
197. Shastry S, Manoochehri O, Richardson LD, Manini AF. Cocaethylene cardiotoxicity in emergency department patients with acute drug overdose. *Acad Emerg Med.* 2023;30(2):82-88. doi:10.1111/acem.14584
198. Mittleman MA, Mintzer D, Maclure M, Tofler GH, Sherwood JB, Muller JE. Triggering of myocardial infarction by cocaine. *Circulation.* 1999;99(21):2737-2741. http://www.ncbi.nlm.nih.gov/pubmed/10351966
199. Havakuk O, Rezkalla SH, Kloner RA. The cardiovascular effects of cocaine. *J Am Coll Cardiol.* 2017;70(1):101-113. doi:10.1016/j.jacc.2017.05.014
200. Feldman JA, Fish SS, Beshansky JR, Griffith JL, Woolard RH, Selker HP. Acute cardiac ischemia in patients with cocaine-associated complaints: results of a multicenter trial. *Ann Emerg Med.* 2000;36(5):469-476. doi:10.1067/mem.2000.110994
201. Hollander JE, Hoffman RS, Gennis P, et al. Prospective multicenter evaluation of cocaine-associated chest pain. Cocaine Associated Chest Pain (COCHPA) Study Group. *Acad Emerg Med.* 1994;1(4):330-339. http://www.ncbi.nlm.nih.gov/pubmed/7614278
202. Chase M, Brown AM, Robey JL, et al. Application of the TIMI risk score in ED patients with cocaine-associated chest pain. *Am J Emerg Med.* 2007;25(9):1015-1018. doi:10.1016/j.ajem.2007.03.004
203. Dribben WH, Kirk MA, Trippi JA, Cordell WH. A pilot study to assess the safety of dobutamine stress echocardiography in the emergency department evaluation of cocaine-associated chest pain. *Ann Emerg Med.* 2001;38(1):42-48. doi:10.1067/mem.2001.115623
204. Riley ED, Hsue PY, Vittinghoff E, et al. Higher prevalence of detectable troponin I among cocaine-users without known cardiovascular disease. *Drug Alcohol Depend.* 2017;172:88-93. doi:10.1016/j.drugalcdep.2016.11.039
205. Gitter MJ, Goldsmith SR, Dunbar DN, Sharkey SW. Cocaine and chest pain: clinical features and outcome of patients hospitalized to rule out myocardial infarction. *Ann Intern Med.* 1991;115(4):277-282. http://www.ncbi.nlm.nih.gov/pubmed/1854111
206. Weber JE, Shofer FS, Larkin GL, Kalaria AS, Hollander JE. Validation of a brief observation period for patients with cocaine-associated chest pain. *N Engl J Med.* 2003;348(6):510-517. doi:10.1056/NEJMoa022206
207. Schwartz BG, Rezkalla S, Kloner RA. Cardiovascular effects of cocaine. *Circulation.* 2010;122(24):2558-2569. doi:10.1161/CIRCULATIONAHA.110.940569
208. Baumann BM, Perrone J, Hornig SE, Shofer FS, Hollander JE. Randomized, double-blind, placebo-controlled trial of diazepam, nitroglycerin, or both for treatment of patients with potential cocaine-associated acute coronary syndromes. *Acad Emerg Med.* 2000;7(8):878-885. http://www.ncbi.nlm.nih.gov/pubmed/10958127
209. Jneid H, Anderson JL, Wright RS, et al. 2012 ACCF/AHA focused update of the guideline for the management of patients with unstable angina/Non-ST-elevation myocardial infarction (updating the 2007 guideline and replacing the 2011 focused update): a report of the American College of Cardiology Foundation/American Heart Association Task Force on practice guidelines. *Circulation.* 2012;126(7):875-910. doi:10.1161/CIR.0b013e318256f1e0

210. Anderson JL, Adams CD, Antman EM, et al. ACC/AHA 2007 guidelines for the management of patients with unstable angina/non-ST-Elevation myocardial infarction: a report of the American College of Cardiology/American Heart Association Task Force on Practice Guidelines (Writing Committee to Revise the 2002 Guidelines for the Management of Patients With Unstable Angina/Non-ST-Elevation Myocardial Infarction) developed in collaboration with the American College of Emergency Physicians, the Society for Cardiovascular Angiography and Interventions, and the Society of Thoracic Surgeons endorsed by the American Association of Cardiovascular and Pulmonary Rehabilitation and the Society for Academic Emergency Medicine. *J Am Coll Cardiol.* 2007;50(7):e1-e157. doi:10.1016/j.jacc.2007.02.013
211. Gupta N, Washam JB, Mountantonakis SE, et al. Characteristics, management, and outcomes of cocaine-positive patients with acute coronary syndrome (from the National Cardiovascular Data Registry). *Am J Cardiol.* 2014;113(5):749-756. doi:10.1016/j.amjcard.2013.11.023
212. Wright RS, Anderson JL, Adams CD, et al. 2011 ACCF/AHA focused update of the Guidelines for the Management of Patients with Unstable Angina/Non-ST-Elevation Myocardial Infarction (updating the 2007 guideline): a report of the American College of Cardiology Foundation/American Heart Association Task Force on Practice Guidelines developed in collaboration with the American College of Emergency Physicians, Society for Cardiovascular Angiography and Interventions, and Society of Thoracic Surgeons. *J Am Coll Cardiol.* 2011;57(19):1920-1959. doi:10.1016/j.jacc.2011.02.009
213. Lange RA, Cigarroa RG, Flores ED, et al. Potentiation of cocaine-induced coronary vasoconstriction by beta-adrenergic blockade. *Ann Intern Med.* 1990;112(12):897-903. http://www.ncbi.nlm.nih.gov/pubmed/1971166
214. Dattilo PB, Hailpern SM, Fearon K, Sohal D, Nordin C. Beta-blockers are associated with reduced risk of myocardial infarction after cocaine use. *Ann Emerg Med.* 2008;51(2):117-125. doi:10.1016/j.annemergmed.2007.04.015
215. Rangel C, Shu RG, Lazar LD, Vittinghoff E, Hsue PY, Marcus GM. Beta-blockers for chest pain associated with recent cocaine use. *Arch Intern Med.* 2010;170(10):874-879. doi:10.1001/archinternmed.2010.115
216. Richards JR, Hollander JE, Ramoska EA, et al. β-blockers, cocaine, and the unopposed α-stimulation phenomenon. *J Cardiovasc Pharmacol Ther.* 2017;22(3):239-249. doi:10.1177/1074248416681644
217. Amsterdam EA, Wenger NK, Brindis RG, et al. 2014 AHA/ACC guideline for the management of patients with non-ST-elevation acute coronary syndromes: a report of the American College of Cardiology/American Heart Association Task Force on Practice Guidelines. *J Am Coll Cardiol.* 2014;64(24):e139-e228. doi:10.1016/j.jacc.2014.09.017
218. Jernberg T, Johanson P, Held C, Svennblad B, Lindback J, Wallentin L. Association between adoption of evidence-based treatment and survival for patients with ST-elevation myocardial infarction. *JAMA.* 2011;305(16):1677-1684. doi:10.1001/jama.2011.522
219. Newell MC, Henry JT, Henry TD, et al. Impact of age on treatment and outcomes in ST-elevation myocardial infarction. *Am Heart J.* 2011;161(4):664-672. doi:10.1016/j.ahj.2010.12.018
220. Karlsson G, Rehman J, Kalaria V, Breall JA. Increased incidence of stent thrombosis in patients with cocaine use. *Catheter Cardiovasc Interv.* 2007;69(7):955-958. doi:10.1002/ccd.21151
221. Daniel JC, Huynh TT, Zhou W, et al. Acute aortic dissection associated with use of cocaine. *J Vasc Surg.* 2007;46(3):427-433. doi:10.1016/j.jvs.2007.05.040
222. Prakash SK, Haden-Pinneri K, Milewicz DM. Susceptibility to acute thoracic aortic dissections in patients dying outside the hospital: an autopsy study. *Am Heart J.* 2011;162(3):474-479. doi:10.1016/j.ahj.2011.06.020
223. Hsue PY, Salinas CL, Bolger AF, Benowitz NL, Waters DD. Acute aortic dissection related to crack cocaine. *Circulation.* 2002;105(13):1592-1595. http://www.ncbi.nlm.nih.gov/pubmed/11927528
224. Eagle KA, Isselbacher EM, DeSanctis RW. Cocaine-related aortic dissection in perspective. *Circulation.* 2002;105(13):1529-1530.
225. Roll JM, Higgins ST, Tidey J. Cocaine use can increase cigarette smoking: evidence from laboratory and naturalistic settings. *Exp Clin Psychopharmacol.* 1997;5(3):263-268.
226. Singh A, Khaja A, Alpert MA. Cocaine and aortic dissection. *Vasc Med.* 2010;15(2):127-133. doi:10.1177/1358863X09358749
227. Cheng YC, Ryan KA, Qadwai SA, et al. Cocaine use and risk of ischemic stroke in young adults. *Stroke.* 2016;47(4):918-922. doi:10.1161/STROKEAHA.115.011417
228. Wallace EA, Wisniewski G, Zubal G, et al. Acute cocaine effects on absolute cerebral blood flow. *Psychopharmacology (Berl).* 1996;128(1):17-20. http://www.ncbi.nlm.nih.gov/pubmed/8944401
229. Kolodgie FD, Farb A, Virmani R. Pathobiological determinants of cocaine-associated cardiovascular syndromes. *Hum Pathol.* 1995;26(6):583-586. http://www.ncbi.nlm.nih.gov/pubmed/7774885
230. Barison A, Aimo A, Emdin M. Cocaine and methamphetamine use and hospitalization for acute heart failure: epidemiological evidence from a nationwide dataset. *Int J Cardiol.* 2021;333:141-142. doi:10.1016/j.ijcard.2021.02.076
231. Willens HJ, Chakko SC, Kessler KM. Cardiovascular manifestations of cocaine abuse. A case of recurrent dilated cardiomyopathy. *Chest.* 1994;106(2):594-600. doi:10.1378/chest.106.2.594
232. Grubb AF, Greene SJ, Fudim M, Dewald T, Mentz RJ. Drugs of abuse and heart failure. *J Card Fail.* 2021;27(11):1260-1275. doi:10.1016/j.cardfail.2021.05.023
233. Cruickshank CC, Dyer KR. A review of the clinical pharmacology of methamphetamine. *Addiction.* 2009;104(7):1085-1099. doi:10.1111/j.1360-0443.2009.02564.x
234. Schindler CW, Thorndike EB, Suzuki M, Rice KC, Baumann MH. Pharmacological mechanisms underlying the cardiovascular effects of the "bath salt" constituent 3,4-methylenedioxypyrovalerone (MDPV). *Br J Pharmacol.* 2016;173(24):3492-3501. doi:10.1111/bph.13640
235. Martin WR, Sloan JW, Sapira JD, Jasinski DR. Physiologic, subjective, and behavioral effects of amphetamine, methamphetamine, ephedrine, phenmetrazine, and methylphenidate in man. *Clin Pharmacol Ther.* 1971;12(2):245-258. http://www.ncbi.nlm.nih.gov/pubmed/5554941
236. Mas M, Farre M, de la Torre R, et al. Cardiovascular and neuroendocrine effects and pharmacokinetics of 3, 4-methylenedioxymethamphetamine in humans. *J Pharmacol Exp Ther.* 1999;290(1):136-145. http://www.ncbi.nlm.nih.gov/pubmed/10381769
237. Kevil CG, Goeders NE, Woolard MD, et al. Methamphetamine use and cardiovascular disease. *Arterioscler Thromb Vasc Biol.* 2019;39(9):1739-1746. doi:10.1161/ATVBAHA.119.312461
238. Gray SD, Fatovich DM, McCoubrie DL, Daly FF. Amphetamine-related presentations to an inner-city tertiary emergency department: a prospective evaluation. *Med J Aust.* 2007;186(7):336-339. http://www.ncbi.nlm.nih.gov/pubmed/17407428
239. Karch SB, Stephens BG, Ho CH. Methamphetamine-related deaths in San Francisco: demographic, pathologic, and toxicologic profiles. *J Forensic Sci.* 1999;44(2):359-368. http://www.ncbi.nlm.nih.gov/pubmed/10097363
240. Darke S, Duflou J, Kaye S. Prevalence and nature of cardiovascular disease in methamphetamine-related death: a national study. *Drug Alcohol Depend.* 2017;179:174-179. doi:10.1016/j.drugalcdep.2017.07.001
241. Turnipseed SD, Richards JR, Kirk JD, Diercks DB, Amsterdam EA. Frequency of acute coronary syndrome in patients presenting to the emergency department with chest pain after methamphetamine use. *J Emerg Med.* 2003;24(4):369-373. http://www.ncbi.nlm.nih.gov/pubmed/12745036
242. Ali WM, Al Habib KF, Al-Motarreb A, et al. Acute coronary syndrome and khat herbal amphetamine use: an observational report. *Circulation.* 2011;124(24):2681-2689. doi:10.1161/CIRCULATIONAHA.111.039768
243. Ramphul K, Mejias SG, Joynauth J. Cocaine, amphetamine, and cannabis use increases the risk of acute myocardial infarction in teenagers. *Am J Cardiol.* 2019;123(2):354. doi:10.1016/j.amjcard.2018.10.019
244. Westover AN, McBride S, Haley RW. Stroke in young adults who abuse amphetamines or cocaine: a population-based study of hospitalized patients. *Arch Gen Psychiatry.* 2007;64(4):495-502. doi:10.1001/archpsyc.64.4.495
245. Kernan WN, Viscoli CM, Brass LM, et al. Phenylpropanolamine and the risk of hemorrhagic stroke. *N Engl J Med.* 2000;343(25):1826-1832. doi:10.1056/NEJM200012213432501

246. Setola V, Hufeisen SJ, Grande-Allen KJ, et al. 3,4-methylenedioxymethamphetamine (MDMA, "Ecstasy") induces fenfluramine-like proliferative actions on human cardiac valvular interstitial cells in vitro. *Mol Pharmacol.* 2003;63(6):1223-1229. doi:10.1124/mol.63.6.1223
247. Connolly HM, Crary JL, McGoon MD, et al. Valvular heart disease associated with fenfluramine-phentermine. *N Engl J Med.* 1997;337(9):581-588. doi:10.1056/NEJM199708283370901
248. Yeo KK, Wijetunga M, Ito H, et al. The association of methamphetamine use and cardiomyopathy in young patients. *Am J Med.* 2007;120(2):165-171. doi:10.1016/j.amjmed.2006.01.024
249. Hong R, Matsuyama E, Nur K. Cardiomyopathy associated with the smoking of crystal methamphetamine. *JAMA.* 1991;265(9):1152-1154. http://www.ncbi.nlm.nih.gov/pubmed/1996001
250. Wijetunga M, Seto T, Lindsay J, Schatz I. Crystal methamphetamine-associated cardiomyopathy: tip of the iceberg? *J Toxicol Clin Toxicol.* 2003;41(7):981-986. http://www.ncbi.nlm.nih.gov/pubmed/14705845
251. Diercks DB, Fonarow GC, Kirk JD, et al. Illicit stimulant use in a United States heart failure population presenting to the emergency department (from the Acute Decompensated Heart Failure National Registry Emergency Module). *Am J Cardiol.* 2008;102(9):1216-1219. doi:10.1016/j.amjcard.2008.06.045
252. Karch SB. The unique histology of methamphetamine cardiomyopathy: a case report. *Forensic Sci Int.* 2011;212(1-3):e1-e4. doi:10.1016/j.forsciint.2011.04.028
253. He SY, Matoba R, Fujitani N, Sodesaki K, Onishi S. Cardiac muscle lesions associated with chronic administration of methamphetamine in rats. *Am J Forensic Med Pathol.* 1996;17(2):155-162. http://www.ncbi.nlm.nih.gov/pubmed/8727293
254. Maeno Y, Iwasa M, Inoue H, Koyama H, Matoba R, Nagao M. Direct effects of methamphetamine on hypertrophy and microtubules in cultured adult rat ventricular myocytes. *Forensic Sci Int.* 2000;113(1-3):239-243. http://www.ncbi.nlm.nih.gov/pubmed/10978632
255. Gulati M, Levy PD, Mukherjee D, et al. 2021 AHA/ACC/ASE/CHEST/SAEM/SCCT/SCMR Guideline for the Evaluation and Diagnosis of Chest Pain: executive summary: a report of the American College of Cardiology/American Heart Association Joint Committee on Clinical Practice Guidelines. *Circulation.* 2021;144(22):e368-e454. doi:10.1161/CIR.0000000000001030
256. Bonin M, Mewton N, Roubille F, et al. Effect and safety of morphine use in acute anterior ST-segment elevation myocardial infarction. *J Am Heart Assoc.* 2018;7(4):e006833. doi:10.1161/JAHA.117.006833
257. Mattson CL, Tanz LJ, Quinn K, Kariisa M, Patel P, Davis NL. Trends and geographic patterns in drug and synthetic opioid overdose deaths - United States, 2013-2019. *MMWR Morb Mortal Wkly Rep.* 2021;70(6):202-207. doi:10.15585/mmwr.mm7006a4
258. Panchal AR, Bartos JA, Cabanas JG, et al. Part 3: Adult basic and advanced life support: 2020 American Heart Association guidelines for cardiopulmonary resuscitation and emergency cardiovascular care. *Circulation.* 2020;142(16_suppl_2):S366-S468. doi:10.1161/CIR.0000000000000916
259. Dezfulian C, Orkin AM, Maron BA, et al. Opioid-associated out-of-hospital cardiac arrest: distinctive clinical features and implications for health care and public responses: a scientific statement from the American Heart Association. *Circulation.* 2021;143(16):e836-e870. doi:10.1161/CIR.0000000000000958
260. Mathers BM, Degenhardt L, Phillips B, et al. Global epidemiology of injecting drug use and HIV among people who inject drugs: a systematic review. *Lancet.* 2008;372(9651):1733-1745. doi:10.1016/S0140-6736(08)61311-2
261. Cooper HL, Brady JE, Ciccarone D, Tempalski B, Gostnell K, Friedman SR. Nationwide increase in the number of hospitalizations for illicit injection drug use-related infective endocarditis. *Clin Infect Dis.* 2007;45(9):1200-1203. doi:10.1086/522176
262. Wurcel AG, Anderson JE, Chui KK, et al. Increasing infectious endocarditis admissions among young people who inject drugs. *Open Forum Infect Dis.* 2016;3(3):ofw157. doi:10.1093/ofid/ofw157
263. Frontera JA, Gradon JD. Right-side endocarditis in injection drug users: review of proposed mechanisms of pathogenesis. *Clin Infect Dis.* 2000;30(2):374-379. doi:10.1086/313664
264. Chambers HF, Korzeniowski OM, Sande MA. *Staphylococcus aureus* endocarditis: clinical manifestations in addicts and nonaddicts. *Medicine (Baltimore).* 1983;62(3):170-177. http://www.ncbi.nlm.nih.gov/pubmed/6843356
265. DeWitt DE, Paauw DS. Endocarditis in injection drug users. *Am Fam Physician.* 1996;53(6):2045-2049. http://www.ncbi.nlm.nih.gov/pubmed/8623717
266. Sousa C, Botelho C, Rodrigues D, Azeredo J, Oliveira R. Infective endocarditis in intravenous drug abusers: an update. *Eur J Clin Microbiol Infect Dis.* 2012;31(11):2905-2910. doi:10.1007/s10096-012-1675-x
267. Baddley JW, Benjamin DK Jr, Patel M, et al. Candida infective endocarditis. *Eur J Clin Microbiol Infect Dis.* 2008;27(7):519-529. doi:10.1007/s10096-008-0466-x
268. Lefort A, Chartier L, Sendid B, et al. Diagnosis, management and outcome of *Candida* endocarditis. *Clin Microbiol Infect.* 2012;18(4):E99-E109. doi:10.1111/j.1469-0691.2012.03764.x
269. Habib G, Thuny F, Avierinos JF. Prosthetic valve endocarditis: current approach and therapeutic options. *Prog Cardiovasc Dis.* 2008;50(4):274-281. doi:10.1016/j.pcad.2007.10.007
270. Pons-Llado G, Carreras F, Borras X, et al. Findings on Doppler echocardiography in asymptomatic intravenous heroin users. *Am J Cardiol.* 1992;69(3):238-241. http://www.ncbi.nlm.nih.gov/pubmed/1731465
271. Carman WJ, Su S, Cook SF, Wurzelmann JI, McAfee A. Coronary heart disease outcomes among chronic opioid and cyclooxygenase-2 users compared with a general population cohort. *Pharmacoepidemiol Drug Saf.* 2011;20(7):754-762. doi:10.1002/pds.2131
272. Li L, Setoguchi S, Cabral H, Jick S. Opioid use for noncancer pain and risk of fracture in adults: a nested case-control study using the general practice research database. *Am J Epidemiol.* 2013;178(4):559-569. doi:10.1093/aje/kwt013
273. Singleton JH, Abner EL, Akpunonu PD, Kucharska-Newton AM. Association of nonacute opioid use and cardiovascular diseases: a scoping review of the literature. *J Am Heart Assoc.* 2021;10(13):e021260. doi:10.1161/JAHA.121.021260
274. Khodneva Y, Muntner P, Kertesz S, Kissela B, Safford MM. Prescription opioid use and risk of coronary heart disease, stroke, and cardiovascular death among adults from a prospective cohort (REGARDS Study). *Pain Med.* 2016;17(3):444-455. doi:10.1111/pme.12916
275. Lentine KL, Lam NN, Xiao H, et al. Associations of pre-transplant prescription narcotic use with clinical complications after kidney transplantation. *Am J Nephrol.* 2015;41(2):165-176. doi:10.1159/000377685
276. Behzadi M, Joukar S, Beik A. Opioids and cardiac arrhythmia: a literature review. *Med Princ Pract.* 2018;27(5):401-414. doi:10.1159/000492616
277. Wedam EF, Bigelow GE, Johnson RE, Nuzzo PA, Haigney MC. QT-interval effects of methadone, levomethadyl, and buprenorphine in a randomized trial. *Arch Intern Med.* 2007;167(22):2469-2475. doi:10.1001/archinte.167.22.2469
278. van den Beuken-van Everdingen MH, Geurts JW, Patijn J. Prolonged QT interval by methadone: relevance for daily practice? A prospective study in patients with cancer and noncancer pain. *J Opioid Manag.* 2013;9(4):263-267. doi:10.5055/jom.2013.0167
279. Pearson EC, Woosley RL. QT prolongation and torsades de pointes among methadone users: reports to the FDA spontaneous reporting system. *Pharmacoepidemiol Drug Saf.* 2005;14(11):747-753. doi:10.1002/pds.1112
280. Anchersen K, Clausen T, Gossop M, Hansteen V, Waal H. Prevalence and clinical relevance of corrected QT interval prolongation during methadone and buprenorphine treatment: a mortality assessment study. *Addiction.* 2009;104(6):993-999. doi:10.1111/j.1360-0443.2009.02549.x
281. Elkattawy S, Alyacoub R, Ejikeme C, Noori MAM, Remolina C. Naloxone induced pulmonary edema. *J Community Hosp Intern Med Perspect.* 2021;11(1):139-142. doi:10.1080/20009666.2020.1854417
282. Tashkin DP, Levisman JA, Abbasi AS, Shapiro BJ, Ellis NM. Short-term effects of smoked marihuana on left ventricular function in man. *Chest.* 1977;72(1):20-26. http://www.ncbi.nlm.nih.gov/pubmed/326498

283. Beaconsfield P, Ginsburg J, Rainsbury R. Marihuana smoking. Cardiovascular effects in man and possible mechanisms. *N Engl J Med.* 1972;287(5):209-212. doi:10.1056/NEJM197208032870501
284. Pacher P, Steffens S, Hasko G, Schindler TH, Kunos G. Cardiovascular effects of marijuana and synthetic cannabinoids: the good, the bad, and the ugly. *Nat Rev Cardiol.* 2018;15(3):151-166. doi:10.1038/nrcardio.2017.130
285. Liu J, Gao B, Mirshahi F, et al. Functional CB1 cannabinoid receptors in human vascular endothelial cells. *Biochem J.* 2000;346(Pt 3):835-840. http://www.ncbi.nlm.nih.gov/pubmed/10698714
286. Han KH, Lim S, Ryu J, et al. CB1 and CB2 cannabinoid receptors differentially regulate the production of reactive oxygen species by macrophages. *Cardiovasc Res.* 2009;84(3):378-386. doi:10.1093/cvr/cvp240
287. Rajesh M, Mukhopadhyay P, Batkai S, et al. CB2-receptor stimulation attenuates TNF-alpha-induced human endothelial cell activation, transendothelial migration of monocytes, and monocyte-endothelial adhesion. *Am J Physiol Heart Circ Physiol.* 2007;293(4):H2210-H2218. doi:10.1152/ajpheart.00688.2007
288. Deusch E, Kress HG, Kraft B, Kozek-Langenecker SA. The procoagulatory effects of delta-9-tetrahydrocannabinol in human platelets. *Anesth Analg.* 2004;99(4):1127-1130. doi:10.1213/01.ANE.0000131505.03006.74
289. Wei TT, Chandy M, Nishiga M, et al. Cannabinoid receptor 1 antagonist genistein attenuates marijuana-induced vascular inflammation. *Cell.* 2022;185(13):2387-2389. doi:10.1016/j.cell.2022.06.006
290. Desai R, Patel U, Sharma S, et al. Recreational marijuana use and acute myocardial infarction: insights from nationwide inpatient sample in the united states. *Cureus.* 2017;9(11):e1816. doi:10.7759/cureus.1816
291. DeFilippis EM, Singh A, Divakaran S, et al. Cocaine and marijuana use among young adults with myocardial infarction. *J Am Coll Cardiol.* 2018;71(22):2540-2551. doi:10.1016/j.jacc.2018.02.047
292. Mittleman MA, Lewis RA, Maclure M, Sherwood JB, Muller JE. Triggering myocardial infarction by marijuana. *Circulation.* 2001;103(23):2805-2809.
293. Mukamal KJ, Maclure M, Muller JE, Mittleman MA. An exploratory prospective study of marijuana use and mortality following acute myocardial infarction. *Am Heart J.* 2008;155(3):465-470. doi:10.1016/j.ahj.2007.10.049
294. Sidney S, Beck JE, Tekawa IS, Quesenberry CP, Friedman GD. Marijuana use and mortality. *Am J Public Health.* 1997;87(4):585-590.
295. Calabria B, Degenhardt L, Hall W, Lynskey M. Does cannabis use increase the risk of death? Systematic review of epidemiological evidence on adverse effects of cannabis use. *Drug Alcohol Rev.* 2010;29(3):318-330. doi:10.1111/j.1465-3362.2009.00149.x
296. Pradhan RR, Pradhan SR, Mandal S, Pradhan DR. A systematic review of marijuana use and outcomes in patients with myocardial infarction. *Cureus.* 2018;10(9):e3333. doi:10.7759/cureus.3333
297. Chami T, Kim CH. Cannabis abuse and elevated risk of myocardial infarction in the young: a population-based study. *Mayo Clin Proc.* 2019;94(8):1647-1649. doi:10.1016/j.mayocp.2019.05.008
298. Polichetti G, Cocco S, Spinali A, Trimarco V, Nunziata A. Effects of particulate matter (PM(10), PM(2.5) and PM(1)) on the cardiovascular system. *Toxicology.* 2009;261(1-2):1-8. doi:10.1016/j.tox.2009.04.035
299. Page RL 2nd, Allen LA, Kloner RA, et al. Medical marijuana, recreational cannabis, and cardiovascular health: a scientific statement from the American Heart Association. *Circulation.* 2020;142(10):e131-e152. doi:10.1161/CIR.0000000000000883
300. Rumalla K, Reddy AY, Mittal MK. Recreational marijuana use and acute ischemic stroke: a population-based analysis of hospitalized patients in the United States. *J Neurol Sci.* 2016;364:191-196. doi:10.1016/j.jns.2016.01.066
301. Zachariah SB. Stroke after heavy marijuana smoking. *Stroke.* 1991;22(3):406-409. https://www.ncbi.nlm.nih.gov/pubmed/2003312
302. Geller T, Loftis L, Brink DS. Cerebellar infarction in adolescent males associated with acute marijuana use. *Pediatrics.* 2004;113(4):e365-e370. https://www.ncbi.nlm.nih.gov/pubmed/15060269
303. Wolff V, Zinchenko I, Quenardelle V, Rouyer O, Geny B. Characteristics and prognosis of ischemic stroke in young cannabis users compared with non-cannabis users. *J Am Coll Cardiol.* 2015;66(18):2052-2053. doi:10.1016/j.jacc.2015.08.867
304. Rezkalla SH, Sharma P, Kloner RA. Coronary no-flow and ventricular tachycardia associated with habitual marijuana use. *Ann Emerg Med.* 2003;42(3):365-369. doi:10.1067/mem.2003.297
305. Thomas G, Kloner RA, Rezkalla S. Adverse cardiovascular, cerebrovascular, and peripheral vascular effects of marijuana inhalation: what cardiologists need to know. *Am J Cardiol.* 2014;113(1):187-190. doi:10.1016/j.amjcard.2013.09.042
306. Gottschalk LA, Aronow WS, Prakash R. Effect of marijuana and placebo-marijuana smoking on psychological state and on psychophysiological cardiovascular functioning in anginal patients. *Biol Psychiatry.* 1977;12(2):255-266.
307. Harding BN, Austin TR, Floyd JS, Smith BM, Szklo M, Heckbert SR. Self-reported marijuana use and cardiac arrhythmias (from the Multiethnic Study of Atherosclerosis). *Am J Cardiol.* 2022;177:48-52. doi:10.1016/j.amjcard.2022.05.004
308. Desai R, Thakkar S, Patel HP, et al. Higher odds and rising trends in arrhythmia among young cannabis users with comorbid depression. *Eur J Intern Med.* 2020;80:24-28. doi:10.1016/j.ejim.2020.04.048
309. Castaneto MS, Gorelick DA, Desrosiers NA, Hartman RL, Pirard S, Huestis MA. Synthetic cannabinoids: epidemiology, pharmacodynamics, and clinical implications. *Drug Alcohol Depend.* 2014;144:12-41. doi:10.1016/j.drugalcdep.2014.08.005
310. Forrester MB, Kleinschmidt K, Schwarz E, Young A. Synthetic cannabinoid and marijuana exposures reported to poison centers. *Hum Exp Toxicol.* 2012;31(10):1006-1011. doi:10.1177/0960327111421945
311. Monte AA, Bronstein AC, Cao DJ, et al. An outbreak of exposure to a novel synthetic cannabinoid. *N Engl J Med.* 2014;370(4):389-390. doi:10.1056/NEJMc1313655
312. Clark BC, Georgekutty J, Berul CI. Myocardial ischemia secondary to synthetic cannabinoid (K2) use in pediatric patients. *J Pediatr.* 2015;167(3):757-761.e1. doi:10.1016/j.jpeds.2015.06.001
313. McKeever RG, Vearrier D, Jacobs D, LaSala G, Okaneku J, Greenberg MI. K2--not the spice of life; synthetic cannabinoids and ST elevation myocardial infarction: a case report. *J Med Toxicol.* 2015;11(1):129-131. doi:10.1007/s13181-014-0424-1
314. Alfulaij N, Meiners F, Michalek J, Small-Howard AL, Turner HC, Stokes AJ. Cannabinoids, the heart of the matter. *J Am Heart Assoc.* 2018;7(14):e009099. doi:10.1161/JAHA.118.009099
315. McIlroy G, Ford L, Khan JM. Acute myocardial infarction, associated with the use of a synthetic adamantyl-cannabinoid: a case report. *BMC Pharmacol Toxicol.* 2016;17:2. doi:10.1186/s40360-016-0045-1
316. Mir A, Obafemi A, Young A, Kane C. Myocardial infarction associated with use of the synthetic cannabinoid K2. *Pediatrics.* 2011;128(6):e1622-e1627. doi:10.1542/peds.2010-3823
317. Freeman MJ, Rose DZ, Myers MA, Gooch CL, Bozeman AC, Burgin WS. Ischemic stroke after use of the synthetic marijuana "spice". *Neurology.* 2013;81(24):2090-2093. doi:10.1212/01.wnl.0000437297.05570.a2
318. Raheemullah A, Laurence TN. Repeated thrombosis after synthetic cannabinoid use. *J Emerg Med.* 2016;51(5):540-543. doi:10.1016/j.jemermed.2016.06.015

CHAPTER

89 Liver Disorders Related to Substance Use

Paul S. Haber and Emily Nash

CHAPTER OUTLINE

- Introduction
- Alcohol-associated liver disease
- Viral hepatitis
- Other modes of transmission
- Summary

INTRODUCTION

The liver is commonly affected by regular or heavy alcohol or other substance use. This may be the result of direct toxicity, metabolic or immunological damage initiated by drug use, or infections acquired through drug use. Hospitalization and mortality are rising, particularly amongst younger individuals, women and Indigenous American/Alaskan Native individuals[1] accentuating existing disparity between different population groups in the burden of liver diseases. This chapter describes the more common liver diseases associated with use of alcohol and other drugs with a clinical emphasis (**Table 89-1**).

ALCOHOL-ASSOCIATED LIVER DISEASE

Alcohol-associated liver disease (AALD) is one of the major causes of chronic liver disease in Western countries.[2] The complex pathogenesis of AaLD and the apparent ability of some individuals to drink large amounts of alcohol without overt harm continue to challenge our understanding of this disorder. Once alcohol-related injury has been initiated, it may progress rapidly if alcohol intake persists, demanding early detection of this form of liver disease. Treatment of alcohol use disorder is one of few effective strategies to assist patients in recovery from alcohol-associated liver diseases. Early detection of heavy alcohol use and organ damage followed by specific management strategies can also improve patient outcomes.

The terms alcohol-associated or alcohol-related liver disease are preferred to "alcoholic liver disease" preferencing a person-centered approach and recognizing the stigma associated with the term "alcoholic."[3]

Epidemiology

Chronic liver disease and cirrhosis comprised the 11th most common cause of death in the United States in 2019, with 44,358 deaths of which 54% were attributable to AaLD.[4] Over the past three decades, the prevalence of chronic hepatitis B has remained stable, hepatitis C has decreased twofold and metabolic-associated fatty liver disease (MAFLD) has substantially increased.[2] This changing epidemiology has been attributed to the global obesity epidemic and the success of antiviral therapy for suppression of hepatitis B and cure of hepatitis C.[2] The prevalence of AALD has increased over time, and particularly recently due to increased alcohol consumption during the COVID-19 pandemic.[5] Among those with liver disease, the mortality is higher in those with comorbid substance use disorder.[1] In 2020, AaLD overtook hepatitis C as the leading indication for liver transplant in the United States[6] due to an increase in the prevalence of AaLD,[5,7] expansion of AaLD transplant criteria to include alcohol-associated hepatitis,[8,9] and direct-acting antiviral therapy reducing the need for transplantation in patients with hepatitis C.[6] MAFLD is predicted by some to emerge as the leading indication for liver transplantation in the Western World.[10]

Risk Factors for Alcohol-Associated Liver Disease

AaLD represents a spectrum from alcohol-associated steatosis to cirrhosis, and only a subset of patients consuming potentially harmful levels of alcohol will develop advanced liver disease. Recognized risk factors for progression of AaLD include modifiable factors such as the pattern of alcohol consumption and nutrition and nonmodifiable factors such as sex, genetic polymorphisms, and exposure to toxins.

Amount of Alcohol Consumed

The prevalence of AaLD and associated mortality mirror the population level of alcohol consumption. A rise or fall in national per capita intake is followed by a variable lag before the benefit or adverse effects are seen clinically.[11]

Reversible fatty liver may be observed after a single heavy drinking episode, but epidemiological data suggest progression to cirrhosis requires daily intake of 50 g or more over several years.[12] However, only 10% of heavy drinkers will ever develop cirrhosis.[13] Data also show that long-term consumption of even 10 g of alcohol daily in females portends an increased risk of cirrhosis.[12]

Sex

Female individuals are at greater risk of developing AaLD for a given level of alcohol consumption.[14] Differences in weight,

TABLE 89-1 Associations Between Drugs and Liver Disease

Hepatic drug toxicity	Alcohol MDMA Cocaine Methamphetamine Phencyclidine Androgenic steroids Kava
Toxic interactions with other drugs	Alcohol plus MDMA Alcohol plus cocaine (cocaethylene) Alcohol plus acetaminophen
Systemic effect of drugs leading to liver injury	Hyper- and hypothermia Shock Rhabdomyolysis
Infectious complications	Viral hepatitis: A to D, particularly B and C Bacteria: SBE, septicemia
Coinjected material	Talc (hepatic granulomas)

MDMA, 3,4-methylenedioxymethamphetamine; SBE, subacute bacterial endocarditis

body composition, gastric alcohol dehydrogenase (ADH) activity (accounting, in part, for first-pass alcohol metabolism), hepatic alcohol metabolic rate, and liver mass per kilogram of body weight result in a higher relative alcohol dose in female individuals compared to male individuals drinking the same amount. This is reflected in a higher blood alcohol level for a given amount of alcohol.[15,16] Female individuals have a higher alcohol metabolism rate than male individuals due to testosterone-mediated downregulation of hepatic ADH[17] and a higher liver mass per kilogram of body weight.[18] There is also a sex difference in endotoxin-induced Kupffer cell activation in alcohol-associated liver injury.[19,20]

Genetic Factors

Genetic factors may contribute to development of alcohol use disorder, to the progression of liver disease or to both processes. There is substantial heritability in the development of alcohol use disorder, with twin studies showing about 50% heritability.[21] These are considered further in Chapters 1 and 24. A genetic susceptibility to the development and progression of AaLD has been evident for years, with studies showing higher rates in monozygotic twins compared to dizygotic twins.[22,23] Gene association studies have identified numerous candidate predictors of AaLD including oxidative stress (manganese superoxide dismutase [MnSOD], glutathione *S*-transferase [GST], hemochromatosis [HFE], hepatic lipid storage genes, peroxisome proliferator–activated receptor-γ [PPARγ]), fibrosis (matrix metalloproteinases [MMP3]), and tissue growth factor α and β, but these studies have been limited in quality with inconsistent results.[13]

Large scale Genome-Wide Association Studies (GWAS) have confirmed a strong association with a polymorphism (rs738409) of palatine-like phospholipase domain-containing protein 3 (PNPLA3) and progression of AaLD.[24,25] PNPLA3 encodes adiponutrin, a lipid hydrolase. The rs738409 variant leads to increased fat accumulation. Two other gene loci have been identified as risk factors for the development of advanced AaLD: transmembrane 6 superfamily member 2 (TM6SF2) and membrane-bound *O*-acetyltransferase domain-containing protein 7 (MBOAT7) (24). Both PNPLA3 and TM6SF2 have also been linked to increased risk of developing hepatocellular carcinoma (HCC) in AaLD.[26] Most recently, a genetic risk score combined with the presence or absence of diabetes mellitus has identified up to 10-fold elevated risk of cirrhosis amongst people with risky alcohol use (**Table 89-2**).

Obesity and Metabolic-Associated Fatty Liver Disease

In the United States, 41.9% of adults are obese, including 9.2% with severe obesity and 19.7% of youth are obese.[27] MAFLD, formerly known as nonalcoholic fatty liver disease (NAFLD), is one of the most common causes of chronic liver disease, with a rising prevalence in the United States.[2] NAFLD describes hepatic steatosis in the absence of significant alcohol intake, viral hepatitis, or autoimmune disease. However, a diagnosis of MAFLD is based on the presence of metabolic dysfunction rather than the absence of other conditions. MAFLD is diagnosed when hepatic steatosis is detected on imaging, pathology or histopathology in the presence of obesity or type 2 diabetes mellitus, or where hepatic steatosis is identified in an individual with a normal weight and no diabetes, but with two or more metabolic abnormalities present (including increased waist circumference, hypertension, hypertriglyceridemia, hypercholesterolemia, or impaired glucose tolerance).[28] Staufer found that one in four of those diagnosed with apparently non–alcohol-related fatty liver disease have biomarker evidence of harmful alcohol use.[29] An increasing proportion of individuals have coexisting AaLD and MAFLD and modification of all contributing risk factors is important to limit progression of chronic liver disease.[30]

MAFLD resembles AaLD with respect to the pathological appearance of liver tissue and certain mechanisms of injury including genetic associations such as with PNPLA3.[21,31] There is both experimental and clinical evidence of an alcohol-obesity interaction in the liver. Alcohol-fed rats develop more severe liver disease if given a high-fat diet.[32] In patients who have a

TABLE 89-2 Risk of Alcohol-Related Cirrhosis by Diabetes Status and PRS Score

	Genetic risk score	
	Low risk (<0)	**High risk (>0.7)**
Diabetes absent	1	3-fold
Diabetes present	3-fold	Over 10-fold

Source: Whitfield JB, Schwantes-An T-H, Darlay R, et al. A genetic risk score and diabetes predict development of alcohol-related cirrhosis in drinkers. *J Hepatol*. 2022;76(2):275-282. doi:10.1016/j.jhep.2021.10.005

history of heavy alcohol consumption, high BMI amplifies the harmful effect of alcohol on the liver and contributes to liver disease incidence and mortality,[33] including higher short term mortality in alcohol-associated hepatitis.[33,34]

Chronic Viral Hepatitis

Chronic viral hepatitis, particularly hepatitis C virus (HCV), is more common in people with alcohol use disorder.[35,36] This association may be explained by an increased prevalence of injection drug use. The combined hepatotoxic effect of HCV and alcohol contributes to an increased risk of advanced liver disease.[36] This is due to alcohol increasing the viral replication of HCV and attenuating the immune response to HCV.[36] Similarly, alcohol leads to rapid progression of liver disease in patients with hepatitis B virus (HBV), in particular the development of hepatocellular carcinoma. This is partly attributed to alcohol promoting persistence of chronic HBV.[37]

Ingestion of Hepatotoxins

Chronic alcohol consumption is associated with a range of drug interactions that may alter drug effects or increase the risk of liver injury. Chronic alcohol consumption increases the hepatotoxicity of compounds including acetaminophen, industrial solvents, anesthetic gases, isoniazid, phenylbutazone, and cocaine. Cytochrome P-450 2E1 (CYP2E1) oxidizes ethanol and is induced by chronic alcohol consumption. CYP2E1 has an extraordinary capacity to activate many xenobiotics (environmental chemicals, such as pesticides) to highly toxic metabolites. Alcohol use disorder is associated with increased severity of acute hepatic injury secondary to acetaminophen poisoning,[38] potentially within otherwise low risk doses (up to 4 g/day).[39] It is likely that the enhanced hepatotoxicity of acetaminophen after chronic ethanol consumption is caused by increased microsomal production of the toxic metabolite (*N*-acetyl-*p*-benzoquinoneimine) via CYP2E1. Conversely, acute ingestion of alcohol appears to be protective in acetaminophen poisoning, due to competitive inhibition of microsomal oxidative metabolism.[38,40]

Nutrition

Nutritional impairment is universally present in patients with AaLD and correlates with the severity of the disease. Nonetheless, Lieber and DeCarli[41] showed in the baboon model that experimental alcohol administration leads to progressive liver injury, including cirrhosis, even in the presence of an otherwise nutritionally adequate diet.

Nutritional disorders may accelerate progression of AaLD. Protein deficiency is a recognized cause for fatty liver owing to impaired synthesis of apoprotein required to export lipid from hepatocytes. Choline deficiency is associated with hepatic fibrosis. Alcohol is associated with hyperzincuria, and zinc deficiency markedly impairs hepatic regeneration.

Pathogenesis of AaLD

The pathogenesis of AaLD results from interactions between the toxin (alcohol), and host metabolic, immunological, necroinflammatory, and regenerative responses.[42] In brief, ethanol metabolism within the liver generates hepatotoxic metabolites, leading to oxidative stress and subsequent inflammation and liver injury.[43] This, in association with endotoxin-mediated activation of the innate immune system and cytokine production, leads to progressive fibrogenesis. Long-term alcohol consumption inhibits the regenerative capacity of the liver via an altered transmission of growth signals.[44]

Ethanol is metabolized via several pathways. The primary oxidative metabolite is acetaldehyde, which is known to affect many aspects of normal cellular functioning, including DNA repair and fibrogenesis.[45,46] CYP2E1 is inducible by continuing ingestion of ethanol,[47] generating reactive oxygen species (ROS).[48] Endotoxin is a toxic lipopolysaccharide (LPS) present in the cell wall of all gram-negative bacteria. Circulating endotoxin levels are increased in patients with alcohol-associated hepatitis.[49] This pathway of injury may be partly explained by variations in the gut microbiome. Patients with alcohol use disorder may have a higher percentage of colonic *Proteobacteria*, associated with greater LPS production.[50]

Progressive liver fibrosis underlies advanced AaLD. The major source of hepatic collagen is hepatic stellate cells (HSC).[51] TGF-β1 is released primarily by macrophages and is the most potent profibrogenic liver cytokine. Abstinence from alcohol[52] allows resolution of early hepatic fibrosis. During regression of fibrosis, HSCs contribute to matrix degradation and undergo apoptosis and/or revert to a quiescent state.[53]

Clinical Features of AaLD

AaLD is typically asymptomatic until advanced disease is established. This paucity of symptoms may delay detection of unhealthy alcohol use and/or underlying liver disease until late complications occur. AaLD is a spectrum of disease, which can be grouped into three clinicopathological entities, but these frequently coexist:

1. *Alcohol-associated fatty liver or steatosis* is often asymptomatic and self-limited and may be completely reversible with a period of abstinence. It may be observed after several days of heavy drinking or in long-term drinking and may present with anorexia, nausea, and right upper quadrant discomfort. The liver is enlarged (sometimes massively, with a span of 25-30 cm) and is soft or firm and may be tender, without signs of chronic liver disease.
2. *Alcohol-associated hepatitis* is classically defined by the symptoms and signs of hepatitis in association with heavy alcohol use and often presents on a background of chronic liver disease. Alcohol-associated hepatitis presents as a spectrum from mild to severe. Milder forms are most common, but severe cases, when present, carry a high short-term mortality.[54] Common clinical features include

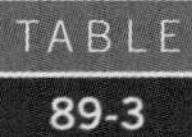

TABLE 89-3 Scores to Assess Short-Term Prognosis of Alcohol-Associated Hepatitis

Maddrey Discriminant Function (MDF) (modified version)
1. Serum bilirubin (mg/dL). Convert results expressed in mol/L to mg/dL by dividing by 17.1 2. Patient and control prothrombin time (PT) (seconds) MDF = 4.6 × ($PT_{patient}$ − $PT_{control}$) + Bilirubin (mg/dL) (eg, PT 16s, control PT 12s, Bili 250 µmol/L yields MDF of 33) Scores above 32 indicate high risk of inhospital mortality. https://www.mdcalc.com/calc/56/maddreys-discriminant-function-alcoholic-hepatitis
MELD (Model for End-Stage Liver Disease)
MELD score = 0.957 × Ln (creatinine mg/dL) +0.378 × Ln (bilirubin mg/dL) +1.120 × Ln (INR) +0.643; Multiply the score by 10 and round to the nearest whole number. https://www.mdcalc.com/calc/78/meld-score-model-end-stage-liver-disease-12-older

If MELD>11, the MELD-Na is a better predictor of mortality.

Data from Kamath PS. *Meld Na (UNOS/OPTN): Stratifies Severity of End-Stage Liver Disease, for Transplant Planning.* MDCalc. https://www.mdcalc.com/calc/78/meld-score-model-end-stage-liver-disease-12-older

rapid onset of jaundice, anorexia, right upper quadrant pain, fever, ascites, and proximal muscle loss. The liver may be enlarged and tender.[55] Severe cases may be complicated by hepatic encephalopathy and other features of liver failure. Neutrophilia is found in severe cases and may reflect the degree of hepatitis but should prompt a search for a septic focus, which is a common complication. The severity of alcohol-associated hepatitis can be assessed using objective rating scales such as the Maddrey Discriminant Function (MDF) or the Model for End-Stage Liver Disease (MELD).[56] These scales correlate closely with each other, and both give an indication of prognosis used to guide specific treatments (**Table 89-3**). Patients may have few signs of chronic liver disease at first presentation, but a majority with progressive disease will develop signs of cirrhosis. Unlike viral or toxic hepatitis, alcohol-associated hepatitis evolves more slowly, and recovery may take many months after abstinence has been achieved.

3. *Alcohol-associated cirrhosis* may be asymptomatic but typically presents with complications such as portal hypertension leading to variceal bleeding, ascites, liver failure, recurrent infections due to impaired immune function, or HCC. Occasionally anorexia, nausea, weight loss, and general malaise are present. Patients with hepatic encephalopathy may initially report reversal of circadian sleep–wake cycle as well as altered cognition. Alcohol-associated cirrhosis is a recognized risk factor for HCC[57] with an incidence of about 1.5% per year.[58] The risk increases with male sex, increasing age, duration of alcohol intake, diabetes, and the presence of other chronic liver diseases.[59] Six-monthly surveillance for HCC is recommended in all patients with cirrhosis.[60]

Diagnosis and Assessment of Severity of Alcohol-Associated Liver Disease

The diagnosis of AaLD rests on the history of prolonged heavy alcohol ingestion (usually >100 g of alcohol daily for >20 years) with a compatible clinical and laboratory picture.[61] The risk of liver disease increases according to daily alcohol use, but at lower levels of use, other factors are likely to be present. Clinical features of chronic liver disease include decreased muscle mass, palmar erythema, presence of spider nevi, nail changes, loss of body hair in males and hirsutism in women, gynecomastia, testicular atrophy, splenomegaly, and caput medusa, indicating portal hypertension. In decompensated disease, there may be jaundice, encephalopathy with or without asterixis, petechial hemorrhage or ecchymoses, and ascites. Clinicians are increasingly aware of the entity of minimal hepatic encephalopathy with subtly impaired cognitive function without overt asterixis.[62] Deranged liver function tests are a sensitive marker for AaLD. However, they are not specific as similar abnormalities may be observed in other liver diseases, and in patients treated with certain medications such as anticonvulsants.

The γ-glutamyl transpeptidase (γGT) level is the dominant abnormality in the liver tests.[63] The transaminases are only moderately elevated and levels above 500 U/L suggest an additional disorder such as acetaminophen ingestion, viral hepatitis, or liver ischemia. The aspartate aminotransferase (AST) exceeds the alanine aminotransferase (ALT) level in most cases, and a ratio of 2:1 AST/ALT is typical.[64] AST is a mitochondrial enzyme and alcohol selectively injures mitochondria. If the ALT exceeds the AST, other causes for hepatocellular injury should be excluded.

As the severity of liver disease increases and cirrhosis develops, INR levels increase, albumin decreases, bilirubin rises, and serum globulin concentrations rise. Thrombocytopenia may result from direct bone marrow suppression by the toxic effect of alcohol, splenic sequestration of platelets in association with portal hypertension and splenomegaly, and from reduced hepatic thrombopoietin synthesis, which affects thrombopoiesis in bone marrow. Macrocytic anemia with spur cells is seen in the most severe cases. These features are also seen in severe alcohol-associated hepatitis. Liver failure from these conditions can lead to hypoglycemia due to loss of glycogen stores and failure of gluconeogenesis. Undiagnosed, this can be fatal.

Imaging of the abdomen with ultrasound, computed tomography (CT), or magnetic resonance imaging (MRI) has a role in establishing the presence of chronic liver disease and its complications (steatosis, portal hypertension, HCC). Transient elastography (TE) is a rapid, noninvasive test to estimate the degree of liver fibrosis. In AaLD, TE is an accurate test to diagnose fibrosis, and sensitivity and specificity are highest for severe fibrosis (F3) and cirrhosis (F4).[65] Liver stiffness can be mildly elevated with active alcohol use due to inflammation and increased portal vein flow.[66] Accordingly, TE is a useful test to rule out F3 or F4 fibrosis in AaLD.

Once cirrhosis is suspected, it is important to determine whether clinically significant portal hypertension (CSPH) is present, which can be diagnosed noninvasively with TE. If CSPH is ruled out (liver stiffness measurement (LSM) of ≤15 kPa on TE and platelet count ≥150 × 10^9/L), gastroscopy is not indicated. If CSPH is present (LSM ≥25 kPa; LSM 20-25 kPa and platelet count <150 × 10^9/L; or LSM 15-20 kPa and platelet count <110 × 10^9/L), nonselective beta-blockade is indicated in the compensated patient for prevention of decompensating events (ascites, variceal bleeding, or hepatic encephalopathy). Carvedilol is the beta blocker of choice as compared to propranolol; it is better tolerated and more effective at reducing portal pressures and decompensation. Screening gastroscopy with prophylactic variceal banding has a role in patients that fall outside the diagnostic criteria, or in those that have contraindications or intolerance to beta blockers.[67]

Liver biopsy is now less often performed owing to improvements in noninvasive evaluation. Biopsy is also subject to sampling error,[68] and the use of the procedure is restricted now to those patients with complex or incompletely understood disease and in those being considered for liver transplantation. Challenges to percutaneous liver biopsy include ascites, obesity and coagulopathy, but these can be overcome with the transjugular approach.[69]

Treatment of Alcohol-Associated Liver Disease

Treatment of Causative Factors

The treatment of AaLD centers on achieving abstinence from alcohol, which limits progression of the disease and improves survival.[70] Medical treatment for AUD in this setting is associated with reduced progression of AaLD[71] leading to advocacy to make integrated care for these disorders more widely available.[72] The improvement in γGT with abstinence is so consistent that it falls with an apparent half-life of 26 days.[73] Failure to achieve biochemical improvement may suggest continuing alcohol consumption or occasionally coexisting liver disease. Advanced cirrhosis may be partially reversible following abstinence with some patients making striking improvements, often returning to compensated cirrhosis. In practice, for patients with AaLD, it is never too late to stop drinking.

The first issue is to define if there is a threshold level that a patient with AaLD can drink. Those with severe alcohol use disorder or severe liver disease should be given clear advice to remain abstinent long term. However, patients with only minor abnormalities in liver function tests without any evidence of cirrhosis may be able to return to moderate consumption. A typical recommendation is a 6-week period of abstinence followed by repeat liver tests. If these normalize and the patient wishes to resume drinking, consumption at lower risk levels can be resumed with close monitoring of liver function tests. Continuing follow-up in a primary care setting is important, as the major causes of death in mild AaLD are extrahepatic problems related to alcohol use such as suicide. Another problem for the generalist clinician is that many patients with alcohol use disorder decline referral to a specialist treatment service. This places clinical responsibility on primary care clinicians to develop brief counseling skills including motivational interviewing, and clinical skills to treat unhealthy alcohol use. At a minimum, primary care clinicians can provide feedback concerning medical progress, which may influence drinking behavior.

Pharmacotherapies to address alcohol use disorder are addressed in Chapter 60 and must be used with particular caution in the presence of advanced liver disease. Disulfiram may be considered in mild liver disease with close monitoring of liver tests for the first few months but is contraindicated in advanced liver disease owing to recognized hepatotoxicity. Acamprosate has a favorable safety profile with regard to the liver and has been studied in Child-Pugh class A and B disease.[74] While it has not been studied in advanced cirrhosis, the drug does not accumulate even in severe liver disease, as it is excreted unchanged in the urine. Severe decompensated (Child-Pugh C) cirrhosis is a contraindication to acamprosate and it may exacerbate encephalopathy.

Naltrexone is associated with dose-dependent hepatotoxicity (typically at supratherapeutic doses of 300 mg/day), but reactions are unlikely at the standard dose of 50 mg/day. Two studies showed improvements in liver function tests, with no cases of clinically evident hepatotoxicity, indicating the therapeutic effect to reduce alcohol consumption exceeded the potential hepatotoxic effect,[75] even in those with HCV or HIV on medications that may raise liver enzymes.[76] Close monitoring of liver function tests (at least monthly) is recommended particularly in those with decompensated cirrhosis (Child-Pugh B or C) where limited evidence suggests the drug may be well tolerated.[75] The long-acting depot naltrexone product similarly does not appear to induce hepatotoxicity.[77] Nalmefene has been approved for use in Europe but not in the United States and although not studied in AaLD, hepatotoxicity has not been reported to date.

Topiramate is an anticonvulsant that potentiates GABA-A activity and inhibits glutamate activity. It is currently used as an off-label treatment option for patients with AaLD, given proven efficacy in the treatment of alcohol use disorder,[78] limited hepatic metabolism and exceedingly rare reports of drug-induced hepatotoxicity. However, it has not been studied in AaLD populations.[79]

Two trials of baclofen in AaLD showed this drug is safe and effective when taken as prescribed.[80,81] Baclofen is mostly renally excreted and does not cause liver toxicity, but there are a number of other risks including excess sedation, exacerbation of encephalopathy, misuse, withdrawal, and overdose. Accordingly, baclofen may be considered as second-line treatment in specialist services for AaLD.[82]

Managing Acute Alcohol-Associated Hepatitis

The management of patients with alcohol-associated hepatitis includes treatment of alcohol withdrawal, nutritional support and hydration, and, in selected cases, pharmacotherapy and liver transplantation. Treatment for patients with mild-moderate alcohol-associated hepatitis should focus on maintaining abstinence. General supportive care such as nutritional support and hydration is indicated. Nutritional support with parenteral and enteral feeding improves nutritional status but does not improve survival.[83]

Pharmacotherapy is indicated for severe alcohol-associated hepatitis (MDF ≥ 32, **Table 89-3**). A meta-analysis showed an improved 28-day mortality rate in this subgroup treated with glucocorticoids compared to placebo.[84] Pharmacotherapy appears to have no benefit in mild-moderate disease.[84,85] The 2019 American Association for the Study of Liver Diseases (AASLD) practice guidelines (https://www.aasld.org/practice-guidelines/alcohol-associated-liver-disease) recommend oral prednisolone 40 mg once daily, provided no contraindication to corticosteroids exists.[3] The Lille score should be calculated at day 7 and treatment only continued for 28 days total if the patient has shown a response (<0.45). Pentoxifylline is no longer recommended.[86] Other agents have not shown any consistent survival benefit when compared with either placebo or corticosteroids. *N*-acetyl cysteine appeared promising in one study[87] but not in another.[88] Currently, there are many trials underway exploring the therapeutic role of other molecules in alcohol-associated hepatitis. These include bovine colostrum, amoxicillin and clavulanic acid, anakinra, obeticholic acid, selonsertib, emricasan, metadoxine, IL-22, G-CSF, and fecal microbiota transplant.[89] Liver transplantation in alcohol-associated hepatitis is a relatively new option, reserved for highly selected steroid nonresponders who meet medical, psychiatric and social criteria (see below).

Treatment of Alcohol-Associated Cirrhosis

Currently, the only effective treatments for AaLD are to maintain abstinence from alcohol or undergo liver transplantation. Trials of metadoxine, propylthiouracil, colchicine, androgenic-anabolic steroids, *S*-adenosylmethionine, and polyenylphosphatidylcholine have not shown consistent benefit.[3]

Patients with cirrhosis should be advised to follow a high-energy, high-protein diet, as advised by the European Society for Clinical Nutrition and Metabolism.[90] Protein restriction should be avoided as this can impair hepatic recovery.[91] All patients should undergo screening for clinically significant portal hypertension and HCC.[67] Patients who present with signs of hepatocellular insufficiency or portal hypertension should be evaluated by a gastroenterologist or hepatologist.

Liver Transplant

Liver transplantation is an accepted treatment option for carefully selected individuals with advanced liver disease who have stopped drinking, but few patients with end-stage AaLD receive transplants. The procedure remains controversial despite years of experience because of inherent stigma about alcohol use disorder, leading to ethical concerns about allocation of the scarce supply of donor livers to individuals with what some still perceive as a "self-induced disease." However, the 5-year survival after transplantation for AaLD is comparable to that of patients without alcohol use disorder.[92] The rate of rejection may be lower than for non-AaLD.[93] Resumption of alcohol consumption remains the major concern and occurs in between 30% and 50% of survivors.[94,95] Of those who return to drinking, one-third develop life-threatening alcohol-related morbidity such as pancreatitis, recurrent AaLD, and nonadherence with immune suppression resulting in graft rejection.[96] These outcomes are comparable to the post-transplantation recurrence rate of other liver diseases. The rate of recurrent, problematic alcohol consumption is lower than that generally observed after treatment of AUD. This may be due to careful case selection for transplantation and/or the intensity of treatment by the transplant team.[97] Treatment for substance use disorders pre- and posttransplant decreases the risk of recurrence significantly.[98]

Psychosocial evaluation seeks to stratify patients by their risk of return to alcohol use. An objective and valid assessment method is highly desirable but has not been devised. An ideal candidate for transplant will be motivated to achieve abstinence once learning the diagnosis of advanced liver disease, will have demonstrated sustained abstinence despite access to alcohol and adequate health to drink, will have supportive family members available to assist their preparation for the transplant and recovery thereafter, and will have had no other significant, untreated mental health issues.[99,100] Individualized assessment remains critical, and while duration of abstinence pretransplant is a poor predictor of outcome, most centers still somewhat arbitrarily aim for a minimum of 6 months of abstinence before surgery. Long-term 10-year survival is 63%, which is satisfactory, but inferior to that of other liver diseases.[101] More research is needed to identify the optimal selection criteria and peri- and posttransplant AUD supports needed to maximize long-term outcomes.

Alcohol-associated hepatitis has traditionally been a contraindication to liver transplant as the diagnosis implies recent alcohol ingestion. However, there is now evidence that early transplantation for life-threatening alcohol-associated hepatitis, in carefully selected patients, is effective and outcomes match those undertaken for non–alcohol-related disease.[100] Indeed, outcomes in highly selected patients are superior than management without transplantation.[102]

Equity of access to liver transplantation remains a challenge. Disparity of access may be related to differences in disease prevalence, access to care, willingness to refer to a transplant center, ability to travel to a center, or likelihood to be listed. Alcohol etiology for liver disease, female sex and racial background (Black Americans) all adversely influence transplantation likelihood.[103] In addition, neighborhood poverty and health insurance status influenced likelihood to be transplanted.[104] Even amongst pediatric transplantation, equity issues have been identified.[105]

VIRAL HEPATITIS

Hepatitis A

Hepatitis A is a ribonucleic acid (RNA) virus that is transmitted by fecal-oral contamination. In developing countries, almost all children develop IgG antibodies by the age of 10, the acute infection resulting in clinically inapparent or mild hepatitis. With improving hygiene, the seroprevalence has fallen so that adults in the developed world are now generally susceptible to hepatitis A virus (HAV). The clinical consequences of HAV infection become increasingly severe with advancing age so that hepatitis A is now less common but often more severe than in the past. The illness does not persist as a chronic infection. Parenteral transmission of hepatitis A has been described but is rare owing to the short period of viremia.[106]

The prevalence of hepatitis A IgG antibodies is high among people who inject drugs (PWID) and incarcerated people.[107] Hepatitis A outbreaks may occur in prison, and vaccination of seronegative individuals on incarceration is recommended.

Prevention of HAV infection is achieved by hygienic precautions to prevent fecal-oral contamination, administration of immunoglobulin to household contacts of cases, and active immunization to those at risk. Hepatitis A vaccine is given as two doses by intramuscular injection and is safe and effective.

Hepatitis B

Epidemiology

An estimated 296 million people worldwide were chronically infected with the hepatitis B virus (HBV) in 2019.[108] It is readily transmitted among PWID. Sexual exposure and injecting drug use are now the most common associations of hepatitis B infection acquired in adults in Western societies. In many Western countries, more new diagnoses of HBV occur in people who have migrated from countries of medium to high HBV prevalence than in those born in the country.

Transmission

HBV is highly infectious via blood and bodily fluids. Perinatal transmission remains the most common route in high-prevalence countries. Transmission typically occurs in utero or at the time of birth and is reduced by passive immunization of the infant and antiviral therapy of the mother in the third trimester.[109] Breastfeeding does not appear to increase the risk of transmission and can be encouraged.[109] In low-prevalence countries, transmission is predominantly via injection of drugs and sexual routes.[110] The risk of transmission increases with increasing duration and frequency of drug use and with the practice of sharing drug preparation equipment.[111]

Virology

HBV is a hepadnavirus consisting of partly double-stranded DNA. Multiple mutant forms of the virus exist, the most common of which are in the precore and basal core regions. The mutation in the precore region decreases transcription of the hepatitis B e antigen (HBeAg) but does not affect the replication ability of the virus.[112] Mutations involving the surface antigen of the virus lead to forms of the virus that can be more difficult to detect by standard assays.[113] Many infections with the HBV virus are not detected by standard assays and these are known as occult HBV infection. HCV, for example, suppresses HBV replication and may lead to a failure to recognize dual virus infection.[114] Infection with HBV is associated with the production of a nuclear covalently closed circular (ccc) DNA, a template of the virus that allows infection to persist even in those who apparently clear the infection and develop hepatitis B surface antibodies (anti-HBs), hepatitis B core antibodies (anti-HBc), and hepatitis B e antibodies (anti-HBe).

Outcome of Infection with HBV

Vertical transmission of HBV or horizontal transmission in early childhood results in a high percentage of chronic HBV infection. Over 90% of those infected early in life remain infected as the immune system fails to clear the virus. Infection in adult life is associated with an effective immune response, and clearance of serological markers occurs in 90% to 95% of cases.

Diagnosis

Testing for hepatitis B surface antigen (HBsAg), anti-HBs, and anti-HBc should be performed in at-risk individuals, and seronegative persons should be offered vaccination (**Table 89-4**).[115] Acute and chronic hepatitis B are diagnosed by serological tests (HBsAg, anti-HBs, anti-HBc, HBeAg, and anti-HBe) and HBV DNA testing. The hallmark of infection is the presence of HBsAg positivity. In combination, these assays allow one to define the phase of the infection, risk of HCC, and need for treatment.

Acute Hepatitis B

The incubation period of HBV infection is 6 weeks to 6 months, and is not influenced by the mode of transmission.

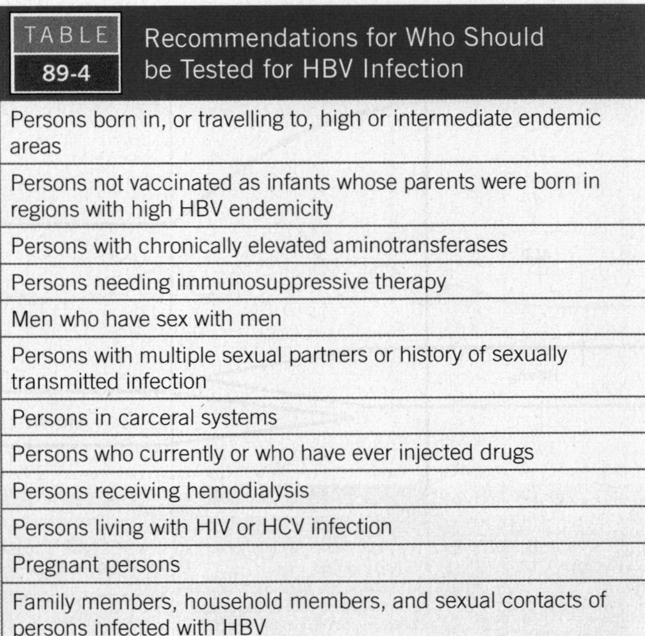

TABLE 89-4 Recommendations for Who Should be Tested for HBV Infection

Recommendations for Who Should be Tested for HBV Infection
Persons born in, or travelling to, high or intermediate endemic areas
Persons not vaccinated as infants whose parents were born in regions with high HBV endemicity
Persons with chronically elevated aminotransferases
Persons needing immunosuppressive therapy
Men who have sex with men
Persons with multiple sexual partners or history of sexually transmitted infection
Persons in carceral systems
Persons who currently or who have ever injected drugs
Persons receiving hemodialysis
Persons living with HIV or HCV infection
Pregnant persons
Family members, household members, and sexual contacts of persons infected with HBV

Acute hepatitis B may be preceded by a transient serum sickness prodrome, with polyarthralgia, fever, malaise, urticaria, and proteinuria.[116] The acute illness is characterized by anorexia, nausea, and sometimes vomiting with malaise, jaundice, pale stools, and dark urine. The infection is frequently subclinical. Acute hepatitis B is usually self-limiting and treatment is supportive. Antiviral treatment can be considered if the disease is severe or protracted.

Chronic Hepatitis B

Chronic hepatitis B infection is associated with progressive inflammation, which leads to the histological changes of hepatic fibrosis, cirrhosis, and HCC. Disease severity is increased by a variety of factors common in populations with substance use: duration of infection, male sex, origin from countries of high HBV prevalence, coinfection with other hepatitis viruses or HIV, use of alcohol or other drugs, obesity and diabetes. Chronic HBV infection is a more aggressive liver disease than is chronic HCV infection, and 40% of males and 15% of females with perinatally acquired chronic HBV will eventually die of liver failure or cirrhosis without treatment.[117]

Liver injury is not always apparent in the chronically infected individual, and the disease is now recognized to pass through a series of phases (**Fig. 89-1**). Inflammation, when present, is the result of a cell-mediated response to infected hepatocytes. In chronic disease, a series of hepatitis flares in the immune clearance, or immune escape phases may precede viral clearance and recovery. These flares vary in severity from subclinical to life-threatening.

Patients with chronic HBV should be assessed and the phase of the disease and the HBV DNA level documented. Patients in the immune clearance or immune escape phases of the disease (with abnormal ALT levels) or those with clinical evidence of liver disease should be referred for specialist assessment and consideration of antiviral therapy. Patients with chronic HBV should be offered regular screening for HCC, as the risk is increased in all infected patients but especially in those with cirrhosis. The 2018 AASLD guidelines recommend 6 monthly abdominal ultrasound with or without alpha-fetoprotein levels.[60]

Treatment of Chronic Hepatitis B

The treatment goals in chronic hepatitis B are to suppress HBV DNA and to achieve loss of HBsAg and HBeAg (in patients who were initially HBeAg positive). Generally, patients in the immune clearance and immune escape phases of infection are candidates for therapy. Treatment is also now considered for patients with high HBV DNA as a strategy to reduce risk of HCC. Patients are best managed by referral to a specialist service for initial assessment and treatment planning. Ongoing monitoring and prescribing of antiviral agents are now undertaken by a range of suitably trained health care providers including primary care clinicians in a number of jurisdictions. The most current U.S. clinical guidelines are available at https://www.aasld.org/practice-guidelines.

A liver biopsy is no longer regarded as a compulsory requirement preceding treatment initiation. Ultrasound-based transient elastography is increasingly available in most centers to provide noninvasive estimation of fibrosis and to reduce the need for biopsy. Other noninvasive measures of liver fibrosis include the AST to Platelet Ratio Index (APRI) (https://www.mdcalc.com/calc/3094/ast-platelet-ratio-index-apri)

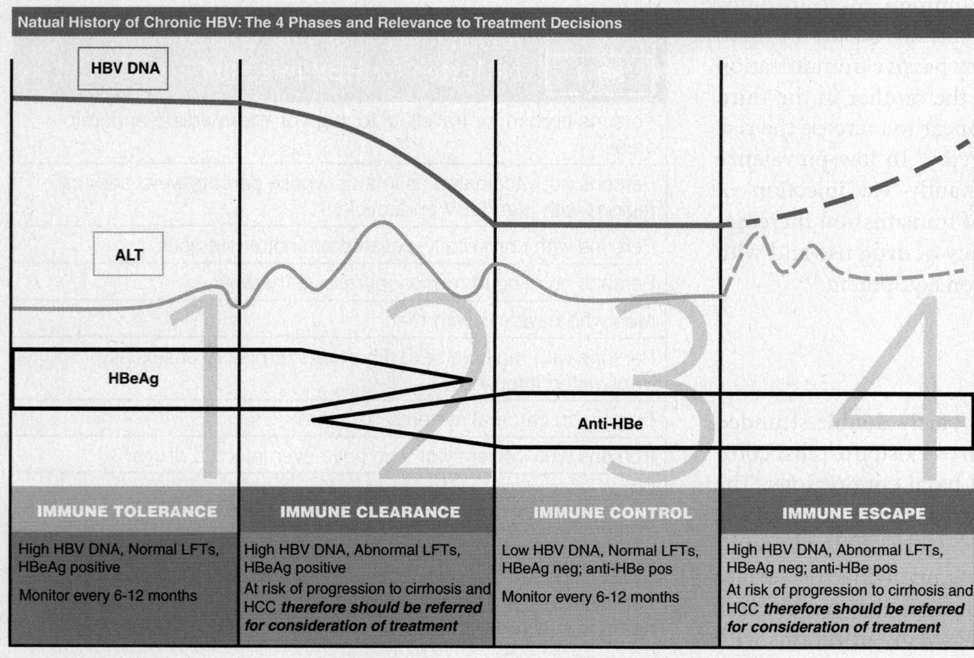

Figure 89-1. The four stages of chronic hepatitis B infection and relevance to treatment decisions.

and FIB-4 (https://www.mdcalc.com/calc/2200/fibrosis-4-fib-4-index-liver-fibrosis). The APRI score is calculated using the formula (AST in U/L)/(AST upper limit of normal in U/L)/(platelets in 10^9/L). A score of more than 1.0 is suggestive of cirrhosis.[118] FIB-4 score is calculated using the formula (age in years × AST in U/L)/([platelets in 10^9/L] × [ALT in U/L]$^{1/2}$). Scores of less than 1.45 and more than 3.25 suggest the absence and presence of advanced fibrosis, respectively.[119]

Current First-Line Therapies for Treatment-Naive Hepatitis B

- Entecavir (ETV)—a nucleoside analogue with a high barrier to resistance (<2% at 6 years in treatment-naive patients). Lamivudine-resistant strains develop resistance to entecavir more readily, and the drug should not be the first choice in this group of patients.
- Tenofovir disoproxil fumarate (TDF)—a nucleotide analogue with a high barrier to resistance (<1% at 5 years). This drug should be the first choice in those with lamivudine-resistant strains. This is the drug of choice in pregnancy.
- Tenofovir alafenamide (TAF)—prodrug of TDF. Associated with similar efficacy but less renal and bone abnormalities, including acute renal failure and hypophosphatemia, compared to TDF. If these side effects occur with TDF, TAF or entecavir should be substituted.
- Pegylated interferon-alpha (PEG-IFN-α) does have significant side effects but has a defined 1-year duration of therapy and the possibility of HBsAg clearance. PEG-IFN-α can be useful in selected younger patients, particularly women who are intending to get pregnant. A response is more likely in HBeAg-positive patients with high ALT and low HBV DNA viral load. PEG-IFN-α should not be used in patients with HBV-related Child-Pugh B or C cirrhosis, as it may induce a flare of hepatitis and lead to further hepatic decompensation.[115]

Treatment of active chronic hepatitis B is of value in those patients with active liver inflammation and in those with very high viral load. Treatment is cost effective in several settings. Loss of HBeAg has been associated with improvements in liver histology and clinical outcome, but patients remain infected and infectious.

Oral antiviral agents are now more frequently used than interferon products owing to greater patient acceptability and high viral resistance barriers. Both entecavir and tenofovir produce a rapid and marked fall in viral load in the majority of patients. These agents are continued for prolonged periods as dictated by the viral response. Viral clearance from serum is the goal of therapy with subsequent seroconversion from HBeAg positivity to anti-HBe status. In a small percentage, HBsAg loss occurs. Attempts to stop treatment are appropriate when the patient has had 12 months of normal liver enzymes after seroconversion to anti-HBe status. In those fortunate to have HBsAg clearance, antivirals may be ceased. Patients with HBV requiring treatment are best managed by referral to units with a special interest in HBV management.

Immunosuppressive drugs such as cancer chemotherapies are associated with increased HBV viral load and flares of hepatitis such that prophylactic treatment is indicated. Immune reconstitution may follow successful HIV antiretroviral therapy, leading to hepatitis flare and HBV medications should be continued and disease status monitored closely. Successful HCV treatment may also be associated with HBV reactivation.

Hepatitis C Virus

Virology

Hepatitis C virus (HCV) is an RNA virus from the flavivirus family and was identified in 1989.[120] It has a single open reading frame that generates a large viral polyprotein, which is ligated by viral polymerases to produce structural and nonstructural viral proteins. HCV antibodies in the blood reliably indicate exposure to the virus, but these antibodies provide little protection against infection. To identify ongoing infection, HCV RNA testing is required. Despite extensive research,[121] there remains no effective vaccine.

There are seven genotypes of the virus,[122] which are further divided into subtypes (eg, a, b, c). The distribution of genotypes varies worldwide. Genotype 1 is the most prevalent worldwide and predominates in the United States, Latin America, Europe, and Australasia, followed by genotypes 2 and 3. Genotype 3 is most common is India and Pakistan; genotype 4 predominates in the Middle East and Egypt; genotype 5 is localized to South Africa, genotype 6 to Hong Kong, and genotype 7 to Central Africa.[123] Coinfection with more than one genotype occurs infrequently.

Epidemiology

HCV infection is a major public health problem with an estimated 57 million people with viremic HCV infections worldwide at the beginning of 2020[124] (**Fig. 89-2**). HCV prevalence varies greatly, with the lowest estimates in most Western nations (<2%). HCV remains a leading indication for liver transplantation and it is projected that despite new treatment, the number of people with advanced liver disease and associated HCC will continue to increase for some years.[125] A rise in the incidence of HCV in the United States over the past decade has been observed particularly in younger adults, and at least partly attributed to the opioid crisis.[126]

Transmission

Injecting Drug Use

HCV is a blood-borne virus, and in the United States, Europe, and Australia, the most common risk factor for transmission is injection drug use (IDU) (**Table 89-5**). Other associations include homelessness, incarceration in the past year, and high frequency injection drug use.[127] Infection control interven-

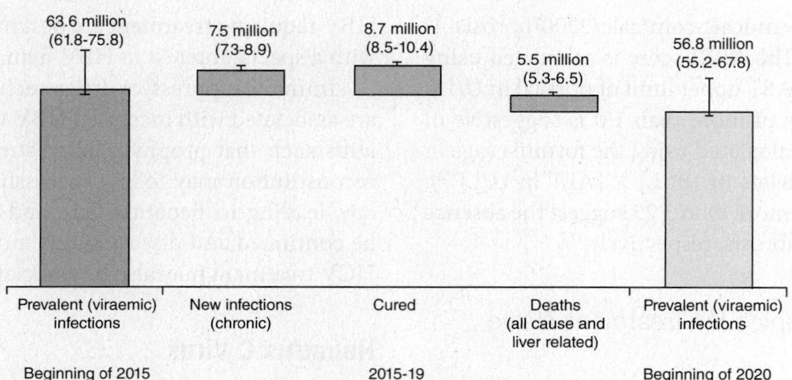

Figure 89-2. Worldwide prevalence of hepatitis C. The introduction of highly effective antiviral treatment has only modestly reduced HCV prevalence internationally. (Source: The Polaris Observatory HCV Collaborators. Global change in Hepatitis C prevalence and cascade of care between 2015 and 2020: a modelling study. *Lancet.* 2022;7(5):396-415.)

tions such as syringe service programs have had variable success in modifying HCV transmission. However, there has been a marked decrease in HCV transmission amongst PWID due to the uptake of widespread testing and unrestricted access to direct-acting antivirals (DAAs) in Australia since 2016. The proportion of PWID with HCV in Australia who have undergone treatment increased from 3% in 2015 to 47% in 2019. Additionally, among those who had undergone treatment, the proportion who had cleared the virus increased from 27% in 2015 to 88% in 2019.[128]

TABLE 89-5 Risk Factors for Hepatitis C

High risk
• Sharing contaminated drug-injecting equipment: 90% who share are infected after 10 years • Regular or large volume transfusions of blood products prior to 1990 • Incarceration: due to the high prevalence of injecting drug use, and possibly other high-risk events among individuals in carceral systems
Moderate risk
• Body piercing and tattooing: using contaminated equipment • Perinatal: occurs in about 5% if mother is RNA positive
Low risk
• Small-volume blood transfusion prior to 1990 • Sharing toothbrushes, razors, etc. • Healthcare worker, needlestick, or sharps injury • Birth or medical procedure in a country of high HCV prevalence • Drug use via snorting straws
Very low risk
• Sexual activity: few well-documented cases. The presence of genital ulcerative STDs and/or traumatic sexual practices may increase the risk. Outbreaks in HIV-positive men who have sex with men. • Blood transfusion/blood products after 1990
No evidence of increased risk
• Household and casual contacts of people with hepatitis C

OTHER MODES OF TRANSMISSION

Sexual transmission is rare. The risk of transmission among monogamous heterosexual couples is as low as 1/190,000 sexual encounters.[129] Sexual transmission is more common among HIV-positive men who have sex with men.[130]

Vertical transmission occurs in approximately 5% of HCV RNA-positive birthing people and is twice as common in those with HIV coinfection.[131] Transmission does not occur if HCV RNA is undetectable at birth.[132] Breastfeeding can be recommended provided the nipple is not cracked or bleeding. HCV antibody testing of infants should be deferred for 18 months as maternal HCV Ab is detectable until this time in healthy infants. HCV RNA testing at 3 months provides the earliest indication of transmission, but the majority of infants at risk are not tested in accordance with these guidelines.

The introduction of screening blood donors for HCV infection has markedly reduced, but not eliminated, the risk of transmission from the use of blood products in the United States.[133] Healthcare and laboratory staff handling blood and blood products are at risk of contracting hepatitis C. Estimates for the risk of transmission from an HCV RNA-positive needlestick injury range from 0% to 7%.[134] Nosocomial transmission of hepatitis C continues to be reported rarely in a variety of clinical settings.

Systematic review has confirmed an association between tattooing and hepatitis C infection, even after adjusting for confounders such as a history of IDU.[135] High rates (10%-30%) of HCV positivity have been observed in patients with alcohol use disorder.[136,137] Alcohol intoxication may promote high-risk behavior such as injection drug use and hence risk of HCV acquisition. Intranasal cocaine use has been associated with HCV infection. Sharing of nasal insufflation equipment can theoretically transmit the virus as cocaine use causes denuding and bleeding of the nasal mucus membranes, and HCV RNA can be detected in nasal secretions.[136]

Hepatitis C in Special Populations

Individuals In Carceral Systems

The prevalence of hepatitis C in incarcerated individuals is high, largely due to the criminalization of drug use. Globally, the prevalence of HCV in incarcerated individuals is 17.7%, with the highest reported prevalence of 28.4% in Australia and Oceania.[138] Imprisonment has been reported to be associated with hepatitis C even after adjusting for IDU[139] potentially related to transmission from poor hygiene and physical violence.[140] Tattooing using unsterilized equipment may also play a role.[141] Measures that may limit the spread of HCV in the community are frequently not available to individuals in carceral systems, including opioid agonist treatment and sterile injecting equipment.

People Born in Countries of High Hepatitis C Prevalence

In Mediterranean, Eastern European, Asian, South American, and African countries, the prevalence of hepatitis C is much higher than in the United States. The Egyptian hepatitis C epidemic has been related to mass inoculations for schistosomiasis.[142] The prevalence of hepatitis C virus in Egypt has been reduced dramatically from 10% to 0.38% in the past decade, following the introduction of free testing and treatment.[143]

Outcome of Infection With HCV

Infection with HCV is associated with a high rate of chronic infection. Around one third of patients clear the virus spontaneously usually within 12 months of infection. Interestingly, some infants born to HCV-positive mothers demonstrate a transient viremia, which may clear without the production of HCV Ab.[144]

Clinical Manifestations

Primary Infection

Primary infection with HCV is typically subclinical, but mild hepatitis may occur. Fulminant hepatitis is rare. Peak viremia occurs in the pre-acute or early in the acute phase (weeks 2 to 3), and antibodies appear as early as 4 weeks (average 6 to 8 weeks). Clinically evident hepatitis reflects a significant immune response to the virus and may be associated with a higher rate of viral clearance than subclinical infection. Female sex, HBV coinfection, absence of HIV coinfection, younger age, genotype 1 infection, the absence of injecting drug use and the IL28B gene are other independent factors associated with higher rates of spontaneous clearance. A number of exposed seronegative individuals have evidence of T-cell immunity to HCV, demonstrating both infection and viral elimination without detectable antibodies.[145]

Chronic Infection

Most patients infected with hepatitis C do not clear the virus and become chronically infected. Liver injury predominantly results from immune damage to infected liver cells. After 30 years of chronic infection, about 25% will develop cirrhosis. Progression to cirrhosis is associated with duration of disease, age over 40 at the time of infection, alcohol consumption (even at low levels), coinfection with HBV and/or HIV, obesity, insulin resistance, diabetes, and male sex.[146] The route of transmission and viral titer do not appear to play a role. Even untreated, the vast majority of HCV-infected individuals will not die of the disease.

The majority of chronic hepatitis C infections are asymptomatic; however, nonspecific symptoms may include fatigue, arthralgia, weakness, and weight loss.[147] Symptoms and signs of decompensated cirrhosis are common to all etiologies of chronic liver disease and not specific for hepatitis C. A number of extrahepatic conditions are associated with chronic hepatitis C including essential mixed cryoglobulinemia, renal disease (membranoproliferative or membranous glomerulonephritis), autoimmune thyroid disease, diabetes mellitus, and a number of cutaneous diseases including sporadic porphyria cutanea tarda, lichen planus, and leukocytoclastic vasculitis. Symptoms of chronic hepatitis C without cirrhosis do not correlate well with disease activity or severity, but they can have a major impact on quality of life. The mechanisms leading to the widely variable symptomatology of HCV infection are poorly understood. Some neurological symptoms such as fatigue and altered mood may reflect the presence of the HCV in the CNS.[148]

Diagnosis

The measurement of HCV antibodies is the most appropriate test for screening populations for HCV exposure (**Table 89-6**). A positive HCV Ab result should be followed by HCV RNA testing. A positive hepatitis C RNA test indicates the presence of active infection. A positive antibody combined with a negative RNA indicates clearance of HCV infection, either spontaneously or with treatment. In a patient who has not undergone treatment, a second negative HCV RNA at 3 to 6 months is reassurance that the virus has been cleared. Genotyping and viral load determination are available, but less relevant in the era of pan-genotypic treatment (see **Table 89-6**).

Management Issues

Access to Health Care and Hepatitis C Information for People Who Inject Drugs

PWID often lack access to health care for many complex reasons.[149] In dealing with a stigmatized problem such as HCV infection, it is important to provide culturally appropriate written material that matches the educational level of the patient, as many cannot discuss their illness with others. Many outreach clinics have been established in syringe service programs, in opioid treatment programs, and in prisons.[150] These provide diagnostic evaluation, build a therapeutic relationship to facilitate referral for full evaluation of antiviral therapy along with other substance use disorder treatments, as well as offering DAA treatment onsite. Primary care clinicians, addiction medicine clinicians, or other healthcare workers can also

TABLE 89-6 Interpretation of Serological Markers for Viral Hepatitis

	Interpretation	Comments
Hepatitis A		
IgG	Past infection	Persists for life
IgM	Recent infection	Generally indicates acute hepatitis but may persist 18 months after recovery
Hepatitis B		
Hepatitis B surface antigen (HBsAg)	Current infection	Positive in both acute and chronic hepatitis B Marker of infectivity
Antibody to hepatitis B surface antigen (anti-HBs)	Immunity (either after infection or vaccination)	Antibody titers >10 IU/L correlate with protection
Hepatitis B core antigen	Not found in peripheral blood	Present in liver tissue
Antibody to hepatitis B core (anti-HBc)	IgG: past exposure to HBV	Anti-HBc + anti-HBs = past infection with recovery; anti-HBc + HBsAg = chronic HBV infection
	IgM: (high titer) acute hepatitis B, (low titer) active chronic hepatitis B	Distinguishes acute from chronic HBV In chronic HBV, low-level titer correlates with ALT level and immune response (some laboratories report all low titer antibodies as negative)
Hepatitis B e-antigen (HBeAg)	Acute hepatitis B	Marker of infectivity in variety of settings
	Chronic active hepatitis B	Correlates with HBV DNA
Hepatitis B viral DNA (HBV DNA)	Infectivity, active viral replication	Detection by PCR is the most sensitive marker of HBV infection HBV DNA without HBeAg indicates infection with mutant HBV Levels useful to monitor antiviral therapy
Antibody to hepatitis B e-antigen (anti-HBe)	Convalescence after acute HBV Marker of lower infectivity	May be associated with active disease, usually with a lower viral load. Less responsive to antiviral therapy
Hepatitis C		
Hepatitis C antibody	Positive result indicates exposure to HCV Negative result does not exclude infection if transmission is within 3 months; in rare cases, HCV infections occur without antibody response	Positive result in person without any risk factor is more likely to be a false-positive test (confirm this by negative PCR or recombinant immunoblot assay (RIBA) Positive HCV antibody does not distinguish past infection from current infection Transplacental passage of HCV antibody makes antibody test an unreliable marker of infantile infection for 18 months
Hepatitis C viral RNA (HCV RNA)	Positive: confirms antibody result indicating HCV infection	
Hepatitis C viral load	High: >8 × 10^5 copies per mL	High viral load associated with poorer response to therapy
Hepatitis C genotype	1-6	Pangenotypic therapies reduce the need for testing genotype. Genotype is still relevant for retreatment in people with cirrhosis.
Hepatitis D (delta)		
IgG	Past and/or present infection	
IgM	Recent or chronic infection	
Hepatitis D viral RNA (HDV RNA)	Current viremia	

HAV, hepatitis A virus; HBV, hepatitis B virus; HCV, hepatitis C virus; PCR, polymerase chain reaction (sensitive molecular diagnostic procedure that can detect minute amounts of specific DNA or RNA).

engage HCV-infected patients to help overcome barriers to treatment, and clinical guidelines can assist them to provide appropriate management: see https://www.hcvguidelines.org/unique-populations/pwid. Evidence suggests high rates of HCV cure with DAAs in these cohorts despite barriers, substance use disorders and other comorbidities.[151]

Pre- and Posttest Counseling Issues

A diagnosis of hepatitis C often engenders a high level of anxiety, disproportionate to the medical risk, but reflecting continuing stigma of this diagnosis. Adequate time and privacy should be set aside for discussing HCV testing and for obtaining informed consent for the testing process. The results of

HCV testing should be given in person including the natural history of the disease, the symptomatology, and privacy issues. Accurate, nonjudgmental language helps to build the patient's trust. Patients may be fearful of transmitting HCV to others and can be reassured accordingly. It may take several consultations for the patient and their close family and friends to fully understand the disease process.

Assessing the Severity of the Disease

Symptoms, including lethargy, do not correlate with the severity of liver disease. A normal ALT level does not exclude active infection or cirrhosis. Liver biopsy is no longer considered essential before commencing treatment for HCV infection, and its role is diminishing rapidly. Noninvasive approaches can define the extent of hepatic fibrosis using blood tests or devices such as transient elastography[152] or the APRI or FIB-4 scores as described above.

Hepatitis A and B Vaccination

When there is no evidence of immunity, vaccination is indicated in those at risk of infection to reduce the risk of further liver injury. Chronic coinfection with multiple hepatitis viruses is associated with accelerated progression to cirrhosis.[146] Hepatitis B vaccination should be offered, and patients with HCV respond well, albeit with lower titers, compared to uninfected controls.

Alcohol

Alcohol interacts adversely with chronic HCV in several ways. It is widely accepted that daily intake of more than 40 g[153] is associated with accelerated progression of fibrosis; however, there is evidence to suggest this may occur even with modest intake (<20 g daily).[154] Adherence to treatment may be reduced in patients who drink alcohol, but cure rates are equal to patients who do not drink alcohol when treatment is completed.[155] The risk of developing HCC in patients with chronic HCV is increased with concurrent ingestion of alcohol.[156] Complete abstinence is recommended for patients with HCV-related cirrhosis or concurrent alcohol use disorder.

Dietary Guidelines

There is no published evidence to support any specific diet in unselected people with HCV. Hepatic steatosis is a feature of hepatitis C, and obesity and type 2 diabetes mellitus are associated with hepatitis C and accelerated progression of fibrosis.[146] Vitamin D deficiency is associated with increased fibrosis in the liver in HCV-infected individuals. Caffeine consumption may be associated with milder liver injury.[157]

Management of Risk Factors

The presence of HCV infection may increase motivation to participate in substance use disorder treatment, particularly if the patient is seeking antiviral therapy. Avoidance of injection drug use is the preferred option, when possible. There is no clinical evidence that methadone or buprenorphine maintenance therapy impairs treatment response, and opioid agonist treatment is encouraged, when indicated, if HCV treatment is contemplated.[74,158] Ongoing injection use is not a contraindication to treatment.[159] Indeed, treatment of PWID may reduce viral transmission. Evidence-based harm reduction and addiction treatment should be offered, as described elsewhere in this volume.

Antiviral Treatment

HCV treatment has rapidly evolved from the early days of subcutaneous interferon (IFN) monotherapy, which achieved response rates of just 10% to current pangenotypic DAAs with excellent tolerance and efficacy over 95%. Consequently, the World Health Organization (WHO) has set a target to eliminate HCV as a major public health threat by 2030 but progress towards this goal internationally is limited.[160]

The main goal of antiviral therapy is sustained virologic response (SVR), defined as HCV RNA clearance 12 weeks after treatment completion. SVR is associated with a 97% to 100% chance of being HCV RNA negative over 5 years of follow-up and can therefore be considered a cure.[161] SVR is associated with decreased all-cause mortality and cirrhosis,[162] and improved psychological wellbeing and self-care and reductions in shame related to HCV and substance use.[163] As in other liver diseases, some patients with cirrhosis who clear the virus may experience partial reversal of fibrosis. The risk of HCC in HCV-infected patients appears to be confined to those with cirrhosis or advanced fibrosis and is reduced by successful treatment. The general approach for acute HCV is to repeat HCV viral load in 12 weeks to check for spontaneous clearance before consideration of antiviral treatment.

Direct-Acting Antivirals

A number of highly efficacious and well-tolerated oral DAAs are available. The choice and duration of treatment depend on a number of factors: presence or absence of cirrhosis, past treatment history, viral load, availability, and less importantly, genotype.

- *NS3/4A protease inhibitors* inhibit the NS3/4A serine protease, involved in HCV posttranslational processing and replication. NS3/4A protease inhibitors including grazoprevir, paritaprevir, simeprevir, and glecaprevir are available within combination regimens.
- *NS5A inhibitors:* The NS5A protein is involved in viral replication and assembly of the HCV virion. NS5A inhibitors in general have anti-HCV activity across all genotypes. Daclatasvir, elbasvir, ombitasvir, velpatasvir, ledipasvir, and pibrentasvir are available within combination regimens.
- *NS5B inhibitors:* NS5B is an RNA-dependent RNA polymerase involved in posttranslational processing and is required for HCV replication. NS5B protein structure is highly conserved across all genotypes resulting in pangenotypic activity of inhibitors.[164] Sofosbuvir and dasabuvir are available.

Standard of Care HCV Treatment Regimens

Two options for pangenotypic first-line treatment of HCV without cirrhosis are one tablet of co-formulated sofosbuvir (400 mg) and velpatasvir (100 mg) once daily for a duration of 12 weeks or three tablets of co-formulated glecaprevir (300 mg) and pibrentasvir (120 mg) taken once daily with food for a duration of 8 weeks. For treatment of those with cirrhosis or retreatment of nonresponders, clinicians are encouraged to check the most recent treatment guidelines created by the AASLD and Infectious Diseases Society of America (IDSA) at http://www.hcvguidelines.org.[158] Genotype is only important in limited circumstances such as retreatment of patients with cirrhosis.

Treatment During Pregnancy

All pregnant persons should be tested for HCV at the start of each pregnancy. Treatment of HCV during pregnancy was not possible with past treatments due to teratogenicity, toxicity and side effects. A small phase 1 trial of 12 weeks of ledipasvir/sofosbuvir treatment in 15 pregnant women with genotype 1 HCV infection initiated between 23 and 24 weeks' gestation showed 100% SVR and no early safety concern, but further safety and efficacy data from large-scale clinical trials are needed before DAA treatment can be recommended in pregnancy.[165] Treatment before planned pregnancy is recommended. Frequently updated guidelines created by the AASLD and IDSA for peripartum screening, treatment, monitoring, and breastfeeding can be found here: https://www.hcvguidelines.org/unique-populations/pregnancy.

Hepatocellular Carcinoma

It is currently recommended that patients with HCV and cirrhosis undergo screening with upper abdominal ultrasound with or without serum alpha-fetoprotein (AFP) every 6 months. If abnormalities are found, more extensive evaluation should be undertaken in a specialist liver center. Small primary liver cancers can be resected or treated by local therapies. Patients with cirrhosis and HCC are considered for transplantation if the size and number of tumors is within recognized criteria with no extrahepatic spread or vascular invasion. Current AASLD guidelines are available from https://www.aasld.org/practice-guidelines/management-hepatocellular-carcinoma.

Liver Transplantation

Hepatitis C was previously the leading indication for liver transplantation, but widespread adoption of DAA treatment is reducing the burden of advanced HCV.[166] Patients with cirrhosis should be considered for transplantation if they develop decompensation such as variceal bleeding, ascites, or hepatic encephalopathy as life expectancy is limited without transplantation. In general, transplantation is indicated if patient has a MELD score of 15 or more; certain patients may warrant transplantation at lower MELD scores, such as those with severe portal hypertension or HCC. Treatment of HCV with DAAs can be considered in patients with decompensated cirrhosis prior to transplantation. Otherwise, the HCV recurrence rate after transplantation is almost 100%. Survival after transplantation for HCV-related liver disease is equivalent to that of patients transplanted with other forms of liver disease.[167] Methadone treatment for opioid use disorder is not considered a contraindication for transplantation,[168] but careful individualized assessment is required and opioid use is associated with increased mortality.[169] There is a significant risk of return to opioid use after transplantation in part due to analgesia for surgery and its complications. Particular care in opioid prescribing is recommended according to principles described in Section 13, and coordination with an addiction medicine specialist is highly encouraged.

Cannabis is commonly used after liver transplantation for relief of symptoms or as a safer alternative to alcohol. Notwithstanding concerns regarding drug-drug interactions and potential for *Aspergillus* infection in the immunosuppressed patient, a retrospective study found no adverse impact on survival.[170]

Hepatitis D

The delta agent is a viral RNA particle that cannot replicate without HBV coinfection.[171] It requires HBsAg to allow entry into the hepatocyte. Outbreaks of delta virus coinfection with hepatitis B have occurred among PWID and were associated with high mortality. Control of hepatitis B by vaccination will limit the spread of HDV. The diagnosis is by rising titers of IgG antibody or IgM antibody (**Table 89-6**). HDV RNA can be assayed, and it may be useful in some circumstances to identify current infection. Delta infection should be considered in any HBV-positive patient with new clinical features of hepatitis. HBV and delta hepatitis coinfection respond poorly to interferon treatment. Addressing the primary HBV infection with entecavir or tenofovir is appropriate and will improve outcome in a majority of patients. A new antiviral, bulevirtide, has been shown to reduce HDV RNA levels but these rebounded after cessation of treatment.[172] Further investigation of this and other antiviral drugs is underway.

Hepatic Toxicity Associated With Other Drug Use

Cocaine and Other Stimulants

Cocaine-induced hepatic injury appears to be uncommon,[173] accounting for around 1% of fulminant hepatic failure. Most cases occur in association with systemic heat-shock–like features of cocaine toxicity such as hyperthermia, rhabdomyolysis, hypoxia, and hypotension.[174] In experimental animals, cocaine hepatotoxicity is readily demonstrated and is both time and dose dependent.[175]

The clinical presentation of cocaine-associated hepatitis is characterized by a marked increase in serum aminotransferase activities beginning within a few hours of drug ingestion associated with the systemic features of cocaine toxicity listed earlier. Rhabdomyolysis may account for some of the increase in transaminases, as AST and ALT are both present in muscle. The liver biopsy shows coagulative hepatic necrosis typically in a centrilobular distribution, extending to panlobular necrosis in extreme cases. Micro- and macrovesicular steatosis may be present, consistent with involvement of mitochondria in hepatic injury. Clinically, viral and other causes of hepatitis should be excluded.

The mechanism of hepatic injury is thought to involve *hepatic ischemia* and/or *toxic oxidative metabolites*. Hepatic ischemia is a likely mechanism as cocaine is a powerful vasoconstrictor resulting in organ damage from impaired systemic perfusion. The pericentral location of hepatic necrosis supports this concept. Evidence supporting a role for toxic oxidative metabolites comes from experimental animal models in which hepatotoxicity has been prevented by inhibition of enzymes metabolizing cocaine or in animals genetically unable to metabolize cocaine.[176] Usually, more than 90% of cocaine is hydrolyzed by plasma pseudocholinesterase.[177] The remainder is metabolized by cytochrome P-450 isoenzymes, including CYP3A1. The hepatotoxic metabolite of cocaine has not been identified with certainty, but the oxidative metabolites of *N*-hydroxynorcocaine may generate reactive alkylating species. The severity of liver toxicity is correlated to the extent of cocaine oxidation by hepatic cytochrome P-450, which is increased by inducers of the cytochrome P-450 system such as phenobarbital and ethanol and reduced by P-450 inhibitors such as cimetidine. Pretreatment of experimental animals with cimetidine or cysteine protects against cocaine toxicity and provides additional evidence in support of the metabolic theory of toxicity, but pretreatment is not an appropriate approach in humans. In the mouse, chronic cocaine administration induces P-450 3A and may increase the risk of hepatotoxicity.[178] Inhibition or deficiency of pseudocholinesterase increases hepatotoxicity by diverting drug toward the P-450 pathway, and induction of pseudocholinesterase may lessen toxicity. No specific therapy has been shown to be effective, but *N*-acetylcysteine may be considered.

Cocaine is commonly taken with alcohol, and hepatic carboxylesterase generates ethylcocaine (cocaethylene),[179] which may be more toxic than cocaine as evidenced by a lower LD50.[180] Indeed, a large clinical series found increased liver disease among people with alcohol use disorder using cocaine compared to those not using cocaine.[181]

3,4-Methylenedioxymethamphetamine (MDMA, "Ecstasy") has been associated with fulminant liver failure requiring liver transplantation.[182] There are two clinical syndromes.[175] One is similar to cocaine hepatitis and presents shortly after ingestion with systemic toxicity accompanied by severe liver injury. The other presents days to weeks after ingestion with jaundice and pruritus and may proceed to fulminant liver failure. Biochemically, marked hyperbilirubinemia is noted with a disproportionate increase in AST as compared to ALT. The severity of hepatic dysfunction does not appear to be dose-related.[183]

Severe liver injury is a rare complication of MDMA use, suggesting that other factors may contribute to liver injury such as hyperthermia and volume depletion. Those who suffer from hepatic dysfunction with rhabdomyolysis and hyperpyrexia may have an abnormality of muscle metabolism similar to that seen in malignant hyperthermia syndrome. An immunological mode of liver injury has been proposed on the basis that rechallenge with MDMA has produced greater liver damage in the absence of hyperthermia, and liver biopsy features suggest an autoimmune hepatitis-like injury that resolved spontaneously on withdrawal of the drug.[184]

The differential diagnosis of a patient with grossly elevated transaminases includes acute viral hepatitis, toxin ingestion, and ischemia. Unexplained liver test abnormalities particularly in young adults with hepatomegaly should prompt inquiry into illicit drug use and toxicological evaluation. A false negative drug screen may result from delayed presentation or that the substance is not included on the assay. Meticulous supportive care should be employed, with rigorous rehydration and active cooling measures.[184] Early discussion of cases with fulminant liver failure with a liver transplant unit is advised.

Methamphetamine and amphetamine: Amphetamine is less strongly associated with liver disease reflecting that not all members of this drug class are the same when toxicity is considered.[185] Prescribed amphetamine use for ADHD is not generally associated with abnormal liver enzymes.

Other Agents

The synthetic stimulants (cathinones, "bath salts") have been linked to liver injury with mechanisms similar to those described for MDMA above.[186] A few cases of liver failure associated with malignant hyperthermia have been reported after phencyclidine use.[187] In experimental animals, liver toxicity has been demonstrated without hyperthermia.

Khat ingestion has also been linked uncommonly to life-threatening liver injury.[188,189] In addition, an association with chronic liver disease has been reported that was dose related and statistically independent of alcohol exposure or chronic hepatitis virus infection. The mechanism and significance remains to be explored. It appears appropriate to monitor liver tests and recommend abstinence from khat use in the presence of significantly abnormal findings or other evidence of chronic liver disease.[190]

Kava is an intoxicating beverage made from the root of the Kava plant and is widely used amongst Pacific Islanders including Hawaii. Hepatotoxicity is increasingly recognized and although rare, it may lead to fulminant liver failure requiring transplantation or death.[189] Kava should be considered in cases of unexplained liver injury connected to the communities where this substance is used. Kava products have been withdrawn from the United States, Australia and elsewhere as a consequence.

Kratom is a plant found in Southeast Asia and Africa whose leaves may be chewed, smoked or made into a bitter and intoxicating tea. Several case reports have identified hepatotoxicity amongst users[191] but this does appear rare.[189]

Cannabis

Cannabis use has been long regarded as relatively safe for the liver. A concern has risen that cannabis use may accentuate other hepatic insults and not serve as an "innocent bystander."[170] Regular cannabis use was linked to steatosis and progression of fibrosis in HCV[192] but the most recent evidence suggests cannabis use does not affect outcome of HCV or its treatment.[170] There are comparable experimental data with respect to alcohol-associated liver disease (AaLD). The CB1 receptor is upregulated in human AaLD and contributes to liver injury,[193] and CB1 knockout diminishes experimental hepatotoxicity of alcohol.[194] However, there is a paucity of clinical data regarding the effect of cannabis use on AaLD, which is a concern given use of these substances commonly coexists. Cannabinoid receptor antagonists have undergone investigation as treatments for alcohol-associated and metabolic-associated steatohepatitis,[193] but recent research questions the role of the CB1 pathway in this disorder.[195]

Opioids

Currently, there are no studies that demonstrate hepatotoxicity from pure preparations of opioid agonists. There is strong evidence that the opioid agonists methadone and buprenorphine can safely be prescribed without risk of hepatotoxicity.[76,196] Antagonists such as naltrexone can cause a minor elevation of liver enzymes in a small percentage of patients, discussed under AaLD earlier in this chapter, but severe liver disease is not described. Patients commencing naltrexone should have liver tests monitored and treatment suspended if enzymes continue to rise after 2 to 3 weeks.

Sedatives

Regularly prescribed benzodiazepine use is not associated with liver damage. Elevation of γ-glutamyl transpeptidase (γGT) associated with barbiturate therapy reflects microsomal induction and metabolism of other drugs but is not pathologically significant per se.

Androgenic/Anabolic Steroids

Androgenic steroids are commonly used by athletes and others seeking to build muscle mass. Products may be taken in dietary supplements or by injection. Steroids particularly 17α-alkylated androgens can produce cholestasis, toxic hepatitis, and hepatic adenomas and carcinomas[197] thought to be via oxidative stress.[198] Most reports are of small numbers of cases, but these make it imperative that individuals who use these drugs are warned of potentially life-threatening consequences. Products purchased via the Internet may contain a range of contaminants that complicate the picture of organ and specifically liver damage.

Toxicity From Coinjected Materials

It is often suspected that other materials may contribute substantially to toxicity after injecting illicit drugs, but this problem appears to be uncommon.

Injection of drugs intended for oral ingestion may lead to accumulation of talc in a dose-dependent fashion at several sites, particularly the lung and liver.[173] Talc liver is inconsequential clinically.[199] A series of 70 liver biopsies from PWID with chronic hepatitis was examined under polarizing microscopy, revealing talc particles in two-thirds with no granulomas.[200]

SUMMARY

As the major site of drug metabolism and elimination, the liver is affected by a broad range of substances whether licit or illicit, taken sporadically or habitually. Alcohol remains the most common and most serious cause of substance-related liver disease. Worldwide, the burden of this disease continues to rise. Along with other direct toxins, abstinence from use is linked to improvement of liver disease and potentially to its complete resolution. There is no specific medical therapy for alcohol-related liver injury, so achieving abstinence from alcohol remains the cornerstone of treatment. Chronic viral hepatitis is commonly seen in people who inject drugs and, while the burden of these diseases is high, new and highly effective antiviral drugs are reducing the impact of chronic hepatitis B and C. Consequently, alcohol has regained its invidious position as the leading indicator for liver transplantation in the U.S. Opioids are generally safe for the liver and in particular methadone and buprenorphine treatment are not associated with liver injury. Sporadic liver toxicity is encountered with a number of other substances including stimulants particularly cocaine and MDMA, kava and androgenic steroids.

REFERENCES

1. Desai AP, Greene M, Nephew LD, et al. Contemporary trends in hospitalizations for comorbid chronic liver disease and substance use disorders. *Clin Transl Gastroenterol.* 2021;12(6):e00372. doi:10.14309/ctg.0000000000000372
2. Younossi ZM, Stepanova M, Younossi Y, et al. Epidemiology of chronic liver diseases in the USA in the past three decades. *Gut.* 2020;69(3):564-568. doi:10.1136/gutjnl-2019-318813
3. Crabb DW, Im GY, Szabo G, Mellinger JL, Lucey MR. Diagnosis and treatment of alcohol-associated liver diseases: 2019 practice guidance from the American Association for the Study of Liver Diseases. *Hepatology.* 2020;71(1):306-333. doi:10.1002/hep.30866
4. Xu J, Murphy SL, Kochanek KD, Arias E. Deaths: final data for 2019. *National Vital Statistics Reports.* 2021;70(8).
5. Cholankeril G, Goli K, Rana A, et al. Impact of COVID-19 pandemic on liver transplantation and alcohol-associated liver disease in the USA. *Hepatology.* 2021;74(6):3316-3329. doi:10.1002/hep.32067
6. Kwong AJ, Ebel NH, Kim WR, et al. OPTN SRTR 2020 annual data report: liver. *Am J Transplant.* 2022;22(Suppl 2):204-309. doi:10.1111/ajt.16978
7. Moon AM, Yang JY, Barritt AS, Bataller R, Peery AF. Rising mortality from alcohol-associated liver disease in the United States in the 21st century. *Am J Gastroenterol.* 2020;115(1):79-87. doi:10.14309/ajg.0000000000000442

8. Bittermann T, Mahmud N, Abt P. Trends in liver transplantation for acute alcohol-associated hepatitis during the COVID-19 pandemic in the US. *JAMA Netw Open.* 2021;4(7):e2118713. doi:10.1001/jamanetworkopen.2021.18713
9. Herrick-Reynolds KM, Punchhi G, Greenberg RS, et al. Evaluation of early vs standard liver transplant for alcohol-associated liver disease. *JAMA Surg.* 2021;156(11):1026-1034. doi:10.1001/jamasurg.2021.3748
10. JPG E, Asgharpour A. Evaluation of liver transplant candidates with non-alcoholic steatohepatitis. *Transl Gastroenterol Hepatol.* 2022;7:24. doi:10.21037/tgh.2020.03.04
11. Holmes J, Meier PS, Booth A, Guo Y, Brennan A. The temporal relationship between per capita alcohol consumption and harm: a systematic review of time lag specifications in aggregate time series analyses. *Drug Alcohol Depend.* 2021;123(1-3):7-14. doi:10.1016/j.drugalcdep.2011.12.005
12. Roerecke M, Vafaei A, OSM H, et al. Alcohol consumption and risk of liver cirrhosis: a systematic review and meta-analysis. *Am J Gastroenterol.* 2019;114(10):1574-1586. doi:10.14309/ajg.0000000000000340
13. Stickel F, Hampe J. Genetic determinants of alcoholic liver disease. *Gut.* 2021;61(1):150-159. doi:10.1136/gutjnl-2011-301239
14. Raynard B, Balian A, Fallik D, et al. Risk factors of fibrosis in alcohol-induced liver disease. *Hepatology.* 2002;35(3):635-638. doi:10.1053/jhep.2002.31782
15. Crabb DW. First pass metabolism of ethanol: gastric or hepatic, mountain or molehill? *Hepatology.* 1997;25(5):1292-1294. doi:10.1002/hep.510250543
16. Frezza M, di Padova C, Pozzato G, Terpin M, Baraona E, Lieber CS. High blood alcohol levels in women. The role of decreased gastric alcohol dehydrogenase activity and first-pass metabolism. *N Engl J Med.* 1990;322(2):95-99. doi:10.1056/nejm199001113220205
17. Teschke R, Wiese B. Sex-dependency of hepatic alcohol metabolizing enzymes. *J Endocrinol Invest.* 1982;5(4):243-250. doi:10.1007/bf03348330
18. Kwo PY, Ramchandani VA, O'Connor S, et al. Gender differences in alcohol metabolism: relationship to liver volume and effect of adjusting for body mass. *Gastroenterology.* 1998;115(6):1552-1557. doi:10.1016/s0016-5085(98)70035-6
19. Iimuro Y, Frankenberg MV, Arteel GE, Bradford BU, Wall CA, Thurman RG. Female rats exhibit greater susceptibility to early alcohol-induced liver injury than males. *Am J Physiol.* 1997;272(5 Pt 1):G1186-G1194. doi:10.1152/ajpgi.1997.272.5.G1186
20. Kono H, Wheeler MD, Rusyn I, et al. Gender differences in early alcohol-induced liver injury: role of CD14, NF-κB, and TNF-α. *Am J Physiol Gastrointest Liver Physiol.* 2000;278(4):G652-G661. doi:10.1152/ajpgi.2000.278.4.G652
21. Anstee QM, Daly AK, Day CP. Genetics of alcoholic and nonalcoholic fatty liver disease. *Semin Liver Dis.* 2011;31(2):128-146.
22. Hrubec Z, Omenn GS. Evidence of genetic predisposition to alcoholic cirrhosis and psychosis: twin concordances for alcoholism and its biological end points by zygosity among male veterans. *Alcohol Clin Exp Res.* 1981;5(2):207-215. doi:10.1111/j.1530-0277.1981.tb04890.x
23. Reed T, Page WF, Viken RJ, Christian JC. Genetic predisposition to organ-specific endpoints of alcoholism. *Alcohol Clin Exp Res.* 1996;20(9):1528-1533. doi:10.1111/j.1530-0277.1996.tb01695.x
24. Buch S, Stickel F, Trepo E, et al. A genome-wide association study confirms PNPLA3 and identifies TM6SF2 and MBOAT7 as risk loci for alcohol-related cirrhosis. *Nat Genet.* 2015;47(12):1443-1448. doi:10.1038/ng.3417
25. Schwantes-An T-H, Darlay R, Mathurin P, et al. Genome-wide association study and meta-analysis on alcohol-associated liver cirrhosis identifies genetic risk factors. *Hepatology.* 2021;73(5):1920-1931. doi:10.1002/hep.31535
26. Falleti E, Cussigh A, Cmet S, Fabris C, Toniutto P. PNPLA3 rs738409 and TM6SF2 rs58542926 variants increase the risk of hepatocellular carcinoma in alcoholic cirrhosis. *Dig Liver Dis.* 2016;48(1):69-75. doi:10.1016/j.dld.2015.09.009
27. Stierman B, Afful J, Carroll MD, et al. National Center for Health Statistics (U.S.). National Health and Nutrition Examination Survey 2017–March 2020 Prepandemic Data Files Development of Files and Prevalence Estimates for Selected Health Outcomes. National Health Statistics. NHSR No. 158. Accessed June 14, 2021. https://stacks.cdc.gov/view/cdc/106273
28. Eslam M, Newsome PN, Sarin SK, et al. A new definition for metabolic dysfunction-associated fatty liver disease: an international expert consensus statement. *J Hepatol.* 2020;73(1):202-209. doi:10.1016/j.jhep.2020.03.039
29. Staufer K, Huber-Schonauer U, Strebinger G, et al. Ethyl glucuronide in hair detects a high rate of harmful alcohol consumption in presumed non-alcoholic fatty liver disease. *J Hepatol.* 2022;77(4):918-930. doi:10.1016/j.jhep.2022.04.040
30. Eslam M, Sanyal AJ, George J; International Consensus Panel. MAFLD: a consensus-driven proposed nomenclature for metabolic associated fatty liver disease. *Gastroenterology.* 2020;158(7):1999-2014 e1991. doi:10.1053/j.gastro.2019.11.312
31. Ogden CL, Carroll MD, Fryar CD, Flegal KM. Prevalence of obesity among adults and youth: United States, 2011-2014. *NCHS Data Brief.* 2015;219:1-8.
32. Tsukamoto H, Towner SJ, Ciofalo LM, French SW. Ethanol-induced liver fibrosis in rats fed high fat diet. *Hepatology.* 1986;6(5):814-822. doi:10.1002/hep.1840060503
33. Inan-Eroglu E, Huang BH, Ahmadi MN, Johnson N, El-Omar EM, Stamatakis E. Joint associations of adiposity and alcohol consumption with liver disease-related morbidity and mortality risk: findings from the UK Biobank. *Eur J Clin Nutr.* 2022;76(1):74-83. doi:10.1038/s41430-021-00923-4
34. Parker R, Kim SJ, Im GY, et al. Obesity in acute alcoholic hepatitis increases morbidity and mortality. *EBioMedicine.* 2019;45:511-518. doi:10.1016/j.ebiom.2019.03.046
35. Llamosas-Falcon L, Shield KD, Gelovany M, Manthey J, Rehm J. Alcohol use disorders and the risk of progression of liver disease in people with hepatitis C virus infection - a systematic review. *Subst Abuse Treat Prev Policy.* 2020;15(1):45. doi:10.1186/s13011-020-00287-1
36. Novo-Veleiro I, Alvela-Suarez L, Chamorro AJ, Gonzalez-Sarmiento R, Laso FJ, Marcos M. Alcoholic liver disease and hepatitis C virus infection. *World J Gastroenterol.* 2016;22(4):1411-1420. doi:10.3748/wjg.v22.i4.1411
37. Ganesan M, Eikenberry A, Poluektova LY, Kharbanda KK, Osna NA. Role of alcohol in pathogenesis of hepatitis B virus infection. *World J Gastroenterol.* 2020;26(9):883-903. doi:10.3748/wjg.v26.i9.883
38. Schmidt LE, Dalhoff K, Poulsen HE. Acute versus chronic alcohol consumption in acetaminophen-induced hepatotoxicity. *Hepatology.* 2002;35(4):876-882. doi:10.1053/jhep.2002.32148
39. Black M. Acetaminophen hepatotoxicity. *Annu Rev Med.* 1984;35:577-593. doi:10.1146/annurev.me.35.020184.003045
40. Prescott LF. Paracetamol, alcohol and the liver. *Br J Clin Pharmacol.* 2000;49(4):291-301. doi:10.1046/j.1365-2125.2000.00167.x
41. Lieber CS, DeCarli L, Rubin E. Sequential production of fatty liver, hepatitis, and cirrhosis in sub-human primates fed ethanol with adequate diets. *Proc Natl Acad Sci U S A. 1975*;72(2):437-441. doi:10.1073/pnas.72.2.437
42. Schnabl B, Arteel GE, Stickel F, et al. Liver specific, systemic and genetic contributors to alcohol-related liver disease progression. *Z Gastroenterol.* 2022;60(1):36-44. doi:10.1055/a-1714-9330
43. Ambade A, Mandrekar P. Oxidative stress and inflammation: essential partners in alcoholic liver disease. *Int J Hepatol.* 2012;2012:853175. doi:10.1155/2012/853175
44. Mohr L, Tanaka S, Wands JR. Ethanol inhibits hepatocyte proliferation in insulin receptor substrate 1 transgenic mice. *Gastroenterology.* 1998;115(6):1558-1565. doi:10.1016/s0016-5085(98)70036-8
45. Mello T, Ceni E, Surrenti C, Galli A. Alcohol induced hepatic fibrosis: role of acetaldehyde. *Mol Aspects Med.* 2008;29(1-2):17-21. doi:10.1016/j.mam.2007.10.001
46. Svegliati-Baroni G, Ridolfi F, Di Sario A, et al. Intracellular signaling pathways involved in acetaldehyde-induced collagen and fibronectin gene expression in human hepatic stellate cells. *Hepatology.* 2001;33(5):1130-1140. doi:10.1053/jhep.2001.23788

47. Lu Y, Cederbaum AI. CYP2E1 and oxidative liver injury by alcohol. *Free Radic Biol Med.* 2008;44(5):723-738. doi:10.1016/j.freeradbiomed.2007.11.004
48. Cederbaum AI. Cytochrome P450 2E1-dependent oxidant stress and upregulation of anti-oxidant defense in liver cells. *J Gastroenterol Hepatol.* 2006;21(Suppl 3):S22-S25. doi:10.1111/j.1440-1746.2006.04595.x
49. Fujimoto M, Uemura M, Nakatani Y, et al. Plasma endotoxin and serum cytokine levels in patients with alcoholic hepatitis: relation to severity of liver disturbance. *Alcohol Clin Exp Res.* 2000;24(4 Suppl):48s-54s.
50. Mutlu EA, Gillevet PM, Rangwala H. Colonic microbiome is altered in alcoholism. *Am J Physiol Gastrointest Liver Physiol.* 2021;302(9):G966-G978. doi:10.1152/ajpgi.00380.2011
51. Friedman SL. Seminars in medicine of the Beth Israel Hospital, Boston. The cellular basis of hepatic fibrosis. Mechanisms and treatment strategies. *N Engl J Med.* 1993;328(25):1828-1835. doi:10.1056/nejm199306243282508
52. Parés A, Caballería J, Bruguera M, Torres M, Rodés J. Histological course of alcoholic hepatitis. Influence of abstinence, sex and extent of hepatic damage. *J Hepatol.* 1986;2(1):33-42. doi:10.1016/s0168-8278(86)80006-x
53. Kisseleva T, Cong M, Paik Y, et al. Myofibroblasts revert to an inactive phenotype during regression of liver fibrosis. *Proc Natl Acad Sci U S A.* 2021;109(24):9448-9453. doi:10.1073/pnas.1201840109
54. Yu CH, Xu CF, Ye H, Li L, Li YM. Early mortality of alcoholic hepatitis: a review of data from placebo-controlled clinical trials. *World J Gastroenterol.* 2010;16(19):2435-2439. doi:10.3748/wjg.v16.i19.2435
55. Mathurin P, Lucey MR. Management of alcoholic hepatitis. *J Hepatol.* 2012;56(Suppl 1):S39-S45. doi:10.1016/s0168-8278(12)60005-1
56. Mitra A, Myers L, Ahn J. Assessing the severity and prognosis of alcoholic hepatitis. *Clin Liver Dis.* 2021;25(3):585-593. doi:10.1016/j.cld.2021.03.004
57. Joshi K, Kohli A, Manch R, Gish R. Alcoholic liver disease: high risk or low risk for developing hepatocellular carcinoma? *Clin Liver Dis.* 2016;20(3):563-580. doi:10.1016/j.cld.2016.02.012
58. Lee K, Choi GH, Jang ES, Jeong SH, Kim JW. A scoring system for predicting hepatocellular carcinoma risk in alcoholic cirrhosis. *Sci Rep.* 2022;12(1):1717. doi:10.1038/s41598-022-05196-w
59. Jepsen P, Kraglund F, West J, Villadsen GE, Sorensen HT, Vilstrup H. Risk of hepatocellular carcinoma in Danish outpatients with alcohol-related cirrhosis. *J Hepatol.* 2020;73(5):1030-1036. doi:10.1016/j.jhep.2020.05.043
60. Marrero JA, Kulik LM, Sirlin CB, et al. Diagnosis, Staging, and Management of Hepatocellular Carcinoma: 2018 Practice Guidance by the American Association for the Study of Liver Diseases. *Hepatology.* 2018;68(2):723-750. doi:10.1002/hep.29913
61. Mendenhall CL, Moritz TE, Roselle GA, et al. A study of oral nutritional support with oxandrolone in malnourished patients with alcoholic hepatitis: results of a Department of Veterans Affairs cooperative study. *Hepatology.* 1993;17(4):564-576. doi:10.1002/hep.1840170407
62. Bajaj JS, Pinkerton SD, Sanyal AJ, Heuman DM. Diagnosis and treatment of minimal hepatic encephalopathy to prevent motor vehicle accidents: a cost-effectiveness analysis. *Hepatology.* 2012;55(4):1164-1171. doi:10.1002/hep.25507
63. Moussavian SN, Becker RC, Piepmeyer JL, Mezey E, Bozian RC. Serum gamma-glutamyl transpeptidase and chronic alcoholism. Influence of alcohol ingestion and liver disease. *Dig Dis Sci.* 1985;30(3):211-214. doi:10.1007/bf01347885
64. Cohen JA, Kaplan MM. The SGOT/SGPT ratio—an indicator of alcoholic liver disease. *Dig Dis Sci.* 1979;24(11):835-838. doi:10.1007/bf01324898
65. Pavlov CS, Casazza G, Nikolova D, Tsochatzis E, Gluud C. Systematic review with meta-analysis: diagnostic accuracy of transient elastography for staging of fibrosis in people with alcoholic liver disease. *Aliment Pharmacol Ther.* 2016;43(5):575-585. doi:10.1111/apt.13524
66. Gianni E, Forte P, Galli V, Razzolini G, Bardazzi G, Annese V. Prospective evaluation of liver stiffness using transient elastography in alcoholic patients following abstinence. *Alcohol Alcohol.* 2017;52(1):42-47. doi:10.1093/alcalc/agw053
67. de Franchis R, Bosch J, Garcia-Tsao G, Reiberger T, Ripoll C; Baveno VIIFaculty. Baveno VII—renewing consensus in portal hypertension. *J Hepatol.* 2022;76(4):959-974. doi:10.1016/j.jhep.2021.12.022
68. Ratziu V, Charlotte F, Heurtier A, et al. Sampling variability of liver biopsy in nonalcoholic fatty liver disease. *Gastroenterology.* 2005;128(7):1898-1906. doi:10.1053/j.gastro.2005.03.084
69. Neuberger J, Patel J, Caldwell H, et al. Guidelines on the use of liver biopsy in clinical practice from the British Society of Gastroenterology, the Royal College of Radiologists and the Royal College of Pathology. *Gut.* 2020;69(8):1382-1403. doi:10.1136/gutjnl-2020-321299
70. Lackner C, Spindelboeck W, Haybaeck J, et al. Histological parameters and alcohol abstinence determine long-term prognosis in patients with alcoholic liver disease. *J Hepatol.* 2017;66(3):610-618. doi:10.1016/j.jhep.2016.11.011
71. AGL V, JES S, Fomin V, et al. Incidence and progression of alcohol-associated liver disease after medical therapy for alcohol use disorder. *JAMA Netw Open.* 2022;5(5):e2213014. doi:10.1001/jamanetworkopen.2022.13014
72. Leggio L, Jung MK. The need for integrating addiction medicine and hepatology. *JAMA Netw Open.* 2022;5(5):e2213022. doi:10.1001/jamanetworkopen.2022.13022
73. Orrego H, Blake JE, Israel Y. Relationship between gamma-glutamyl transpeptidase and mean urinary alcohol levels in alcoholics while drinking and after alcohol withdrawal. *Alcohol Clin Exp Res.* 1985;9(1):10-13. doi:10.1111/j.1530-0277.1985.tb05038.x
74. Delgrange T, Khater J, Capron D, Duron B, Capron JP. Effect of acute administration of acamprosate on the risk of encephalopathy and on arterial pressure in patients with alcoholic cirrhosis. *Gastroenterol Clin Biol.* 1992;16(8-9):687-691.
75. Ayyala D, Bottyan T, Tien C, et al. Naltrexone for alcohol use disorder: Hepatic safety in patients with and without liver disease. *Hepatol Commun.* 2022;6(12):3433-3442. doi:10.1002/hep4.2080
76. Tetrault JM, Tate JP, KA MG, et al. Hepatic safety and antiretroviral effectiveness in HIV-infected patients receiving naltrexone. *Alcohol Clin Exp Res.* 2012;36(2):318-324. doi:10.1111/j.1530-0277.2011.01601.x
77. Mitchell MC, Memisoglu A, Silverman BL. Hepatic safety of injectable extended-release naltrexone in patients with chronic hepatitis C and HIV infection. *J Stud Alcohol Drugs.* 2012;73(6):991-997. doi:10.15288/jsad.2012.73.991
78. Jonas DE, Amick HR, Feltner C, et al. Pharmacotherapy for adults with alcohol use disorders in outpatient settings: a systematic review and meta-analysis. *JAMA.* 2014;311(18):1889-1900. doi:10.1001/jama.2014.3628
79. Addolorato G, Mirijello A, Leggio L, Ferrulli A, Landolfi R. Management of alcohol dependence in patients with liver disease. *CNS Drugs.* 2013;27(4):287-299. doi:10.1007/s40263-013-0043-4
80. Addolorato G, Leggio L, Ferrulli A, et al. Effectiveness and safety of baclofen for maintenance of alcohol abstinence in alcohol-dependent patients with liver cirrhosis: randomised, double-blind controlled study. *Lancet.* 2007;370(9603):1915-1922. doi:10.1016/S0140-6736(07)61814-5
81. Morley KC, Baillie A, Fraser I, et al. Baclofen in the treatment of alcohol dependence with or without liver disease: multisite, randomised, double-blind, placebo-controlled trial. *Br J Psychiatry.* 2018;212(6):362-369. doi:10.1192/bjp.2018.13
82. Haber PS, Riordan BC, Winter DT, et al. New Australian guidelines for the treatment of alcohol problems: an overview of recommendations. *Med J Aust.* 2021;215(Suppl 7):S3-S32. doi:10.5694/mja2.51254
83. Stickel F, Hoehn B, Schuppan D, Seitz HK. Review article: nutritional therapy in alcoholic liver disease. *Aliment Pharmacol Ther.* 2003;18(4):357-373. doi:10.1046/j.1365-2036.2003.01660.x
84. Mathurin P, O'Grady J, Carithers RL, et al. Corticosteroids improve short-term survival in patients with severe alcoholic hepatitis: meta-analysis of individual patient data. *Gut.* 2011;60(2):255-260. doi:10.1136/gut.2010.224097
85. Rambaldi A, Saconato HH, Christensen E, Thorlund K, Wetterslev J, Gluud C. Systematic review: glucocorticosteroids for alcoholic

hepatitis—a Cochrane Hepato-Biliary Group systematic review with meta-analyses and trial sequential analyses of randomized clinical trials. *Aliment Pharmacol Ther.* 2008;27(12):1167-1178. doi:10.1111/j.1365-2036.2008.03685.x

86. Thursz MR, Richardson P, Allison M, et al. Prednisolone or pentoxifylline for alcoholic hepatitis. *N Engl J Med.* 2015;372(17):1619-1628. doi:10.1056/NEJMoa1412278
87. Nguyen-Khac E, Thevenot T, Piquet MA, et al. Glucocorticoids plus N-acetylcysteine in severe alcoholic hepatitis. *N Engl J Med.* 2011;365(19):1781-1789. doi:10.1056/NEJMoa1101214
88. Thursz M, Morgan TR. Treatment of severe alcoholic hepatitis. *Gastroenterology.* 2016;150(8):1823-1834. doi:10.1053/j.gastro.2016.02.074
89. Singal AK, Shah VH. Current trials and novel therapeutic targets for alcoholic hepatitis. *J Hepatol.* 2019;70(2):305-313. doi:10.1016/j.jhep.2018.10.026
90. Plauth M, Cabré E, Riggio O, et al. ESPEN Guidelines on enteral nutrition: liver disease. *Clin Nutr.* 2006;25(2):285-294. doi:10.1016/j.clnu.2006.01.018
91. Bémeur C, Desjardins P, Butterworth RF. Role of nutrition in the management of hepatic encephalopathy in end-stage liver failure. *J Nutr Metab.* 2010;2010:489823. doi:10.1155/2010/489823
92. Wiesner RH, Lombardero M, Lake JR, Everhart J, Detre KM. Liver transplantation for end-stage alcoholic liver disease: an assessment of outcomes. *Liver Transpl Surg.* 1997;3(3):231-239. doi:10.1002/lt.500030307
93. Van Thiel DH, Bonet H, Gavaler J, Wright HI. Effect of alcohol use on allograft rejection rates after liver transplantation for alcoholic liver disease. *Alcohol Clin Exp Res.* 1995;19(5):1151-1155. doi:10.1111/j.1530-0277.1995.tb01594.x
94. DiMartini A, Day N, Dew MA, et al. Alcohol consumption patterns and predictors of use following liver transplantation for alcoholic liver disease. *Liver Transpl.* 2006;12(5):813-820. doi:10.1002/lt.20688
95. Faure S, Herrero A, Jung B, et al. Excessive alcohol consumption after liver transplantation impacts on long-term survival, whatever the primary indication. *J Hepatol.* 2012;57(2):306-312. doi:10.1016/j.jhep.2012.03.014
96. Lim J, Curry MP, Sundaram V. Risk factors and outcomes associated with alcohol relapse after liver transplantation. *World J Hepatol.* 2017;9(17):771-780. doi:10.4254/wjh.v9.i17.771
97. Vaillant GE. The natural history of alcoholism and its relationship to liver transplantation. *Liver Transpl Surg.* 1997;3(3):304-310. doi:10.1002/lt.500030318
98. Rodrigue JR, Hanto DW, Curry MP. Substance abuse treatment and its association with relapse to alcohol use after liver transplantation. *Liver Transpl.* 2013;19(12):1387-1395. doi:10.1002/lt.23747
99. Lucey MR. Liver transplantation in patients with alcoholic liver disease. *Liver Transpl.* 2011;17(7):751-759. doi:10.1002/lt.22330
100. Singal AK, Bashar H, Anand BS, Jampana SC, Singal V, Kuo YF. Outcomes after liver transplantation for alcoholic hepatitis are similar to alcoholic cirrhosis: exploratory analysis from the UNOS database. *Hepatology.* 2012;55(5):1398-1405. doi:10.1002/hep.25544
101. Lee BP, Vittinghoff E, Dodge JL, Cullaro G, Terrault NA. National trends and long-term outcomes of liver transplant for alcohol-associated liver disease in the United States. *JAMA Intern Med.* 2019;179(3):340-348. doi:10.1001/jamainternmed.2018.6536
102. Louvet A, Labreuche J, Moreno C, et al. Early liver transplantation for severe alcohol-related hepatitis not responding to medical treatment: a prospective controlled study. *Lancet Gastroenterol Hepatol.* 2022;7(5):416-425. doi:10.1016/S2468-1253(21)00430-1
103. Kaplan A, Wahid N, Fortune BE, et al. Black patients and women have reduced access to liver transplantation for alcohol associated liver disease. *Liver Transpl.* 2023;29(3):259-267. doi:10.1002/lt.26544
104. Mohamed KA, Ghabril M, Desai A, et al. Neighborhood poverty is associated with failure to be waitlisted and death during liver transplantation evaluation. *Liver Transpl.* 2022;28(9):1441-1453. doi:10.1002/lt.26473
105. Ebel NH, Lai JC, Bucuvalas JC, Wadhwani SI. A review of racial, socioeconomic, and geographic disparities in pediatric liver transplantation. *Liver Transpl.* 2022;28(9):1520-1528. doi:10.1002/lt.26437
106. Hollinger FB, Khan NC, Oefinger PE, et al. Posttransfusion hepatitis type A. *JAMA.* 1983;250(17):2313-2317. doi:10.1001/jama.1983.03340170039025
107. Tennant F, Moll D. Seroprevalence of hepatitis A, B, C, and D markers and liver function abnormalities in intravenous heroin addicts. *J Addict Dis.* 1995;14(3):35-49. doi:10.1300/J069v14n03_03
108. World Health Organization. (2022). *Criteria for Validation of Elimination of Viral Hepatitis B and C: Report of Seven Country Pilots.* Accessed August 18, 2023. https://www.who.int/publications/i/item/9789240055292
109. World Health Organization. (2015). *Guidelines for the Prevention, Care and Treatment of Persons with Chronic Hepatitis B Infection.* Accessed August 18, 2023. https://www.who.int/publications/i/item/9789241549059
110. Iqbal K, Klevens RM, Kainer MA, et al. Epidemiology of acute hepatitis B in the United States from population-based surveillance, 2006-2011. *Clin Infect Dis.* 2015;61(4):584-592. doi:10.1093/cid/civ332
111. Bialek SR, Bower WA, Mottram K, et al. Risk factors for hepatitis B in an outbreak of hepatitis B and D among injection drug users. *J Urban Health.* 2005;82(3):468-478. doi:10.1093/jurban/jti094
112. Okamoto H, Tsuda F, Akahane Y, et al. Hepatitis B virus with mutations in the core promoter for an e antigen-negative phenotype in carriers with antibody to e antigen. *J Virol.* 1994;68(12):8102-8110. doi:10.1128/jvi.68.12.8102-8110.1994
113. Huang CH, Yuan Q, Chen PJ, et al. Influence of mutations in hepatitis B virus surface protein on viral antigenicity and phenotype in occult HBV strains from blood donors. *J Hepatol.* 2012;57(4):720-729. doi:10.1016/j.jhep.2012.05.009
114. Raimondo G, Pollicino T, Romanò L, Zanetti AR. A 2010 update on occult hepatitis B infection. *Pathol Biol (Paris).* 2010;58(4):254-257. doi:10.1016/j.patbio.2010.02.003
115. Terrault NA, ASF L, BJ MM, et al. Update on prevention, diagnosis, and treatment of chronic hepatitis B: AASLD 2018 hepatitis B guidance. *Hepatology.* 2018;67(4):1560-1599. doi:10.1002/hep.29800
116. Sherlock S, Dooley J. *Diseases of the Liver and Biliary System.* Blackwell Publishing; 1997.
117. Beasley RP, Hwang LY, Lin CC, Chien CS. Hepatocellular carcinoma and hepatitis B virus. A prospective study of 22,707 men in Taiwan. *Lancet.* 1981;2(8256):1129-1133. doi:10.1016/s0140-6736(81)90585-7
118. Lin ZH, Xin YN, Dong QJ, et al. Performance of the aspartate aminotransferase-to-platelet ratio index for the staging of hepatitis C-related fibrosis: an updated meta-analysis. *Hepatology.* 2011;53(3):726-736. doi:10.1002/hep.24105
119. Sterling RK, Lissen E, Clumeck N, et al. Development of a simple noninvasive index to predict significant fibrosis in patients with HIV/HCV coinfection. *Hepatology.* 2006;43(6):1317-1325. doi:10.1002/hep.21178
120. Choo QL, Kuo G, Weiner AJ, Overby LR, Bradley DW, Houghton M. Isolation of a cDNA clone derived from a blood-borne non-A, non-B viral hepatitis genome. *Science.* 1989;244(4902):359-362. doi:10.1126/science.2523562
121. Page K, Melia MT, Veenhuis RT, et al. Randomized trial of a vaccine regimen to prevent chronic HCV infection. *N Engl J Med.* 2021;384(6):541-549. doi:10.1056/NEJMoa2023345
122. Smith DB, Bukh J, Kuiken C, et al. Expanded classification of hepatitis C virus into 7 genotypes and 67 subtypes: updated criteria and genotype assignment web resource. *Hepatology.* 2014;59(1):318-327. doi:10.1002/hep.26744
123. Messina JP, Humphreys I, Flaxman A, et al. Global distribution and prevalence of hepatitis C virus genotypes. *Hepatology.* 2015;61(1):77-87. doi:10.1002/hep.27259
124. Polaris Observatory, HCV Collaborators. Global change in hepatitis C virus prevalence and cascade of care between 2015 and 2020: a modelling study. *Lancet Gastroenterol Hepatol.* 2022;7(5):396-415. doi:10.1016/S2468-1253(21)00472-6
125. Baumert TF, Jühling F, Ono A, Hoshida Y. Hepatitis C-related hepatocellular carcinoma in the era of new generation antivirals. *BMC Med.* 2017;15(1):52. doi:10.1186/s12916-017-0815-7

126. Holtzman D, Asher AK, Schillie S. The changing epidemiology of hepatitis C virus infection in the United States during the years 2010 to 2018. *Am J Public Health.* 2021;111(5):949-955. doi:10.2105/AJPH.2020.306149
127. Valerio H, Alavi M, Silk D, et al. Progress towards elimination of hepatitis C infection among people who inject drugs in Australia: the ETHOS Engage Study. *Clin Infect Dis.* 2021;73(1):e69-e78. doi:10.1093/cid/ciaa571
128. Iversen J, Dore GJ, Starr M, et al. Estimating the consensus hepatitis C cascade of care among people who inject drugs in Australia: pre and post availability of direct acting antiviral therapy. *Int J Drug Policy.* 2020;83:102837. doi:10.1016/j.drugpo.2020.102837
129. Terrault NA, Dodge JL, Murphy EL, et al. Sexual transmission of hepatitis C virus among monogamous heterosexual couples: the HCV partners study. *Hepatology.* 2013;57(3):881-889. doi:10.1002/hep.26164
130. Danta M, Brown D, Bhagani S, et al. Recent epidemic of acute hepatitis C virus in HIV-positive men who have sex with men linked to high-risk sexual behaviours. *Aids.* 2017;21(8):983-991. doi:10.1097/QAD.0b013e3281053a0c
131. Zanetti AR, Tanzi E, Paccagnini S, et al. Mother-to-infant transmission of hepatitis C virus. Lombardy Study Group on Vertical HCV Transmission. *Lancet.* 1995;345(8945):289-291. doi:10.1016/s0140-6736(95)90277-5
132. Conte D, Fraquelli M, Prati D, Colucci A, Minola E. Prevalence and clinical course of chronic hepatitis C virus (HCV) infection and rate of HCV vertical transmission in a cohort of 15,250 pregnant women. *Hepatology.* 2000;31(3):751-755. doi:10.1002/hep.510310328
133. Dodd RY, Crowder LA, Haynes JM, et al. Screening blood donors for HIV, HCV, and HBV at the American Red Cross: 10-year trends in prevalence, incidence, and residual risk, 2007 to 2016. *Transfus Med Rev.* 2020;34(2):81-93. doi:10.1016/j.tmrv.2020.02.001
134. Tomkins SE, Elford J, Nichols T, et al. Occupational transmission of hepatitis C in healthcare workers and factors associated with seroconversion: UK surveillance data. *J Viral Hepat.* 2012;19(3):199-204. doi:10.1111/j.1365-2893.2011.01543.x
135. Lim SH, Lee S, Lee YB, et al. Increased prevalence of transfusion-transmitted diseases among people with tattoos: a systematic review and meta-analysis. *PLoS One.* 2022;17(1):e0262990. doi:10.1371/journal.pone.0262990
136. Allison RD, Conry-Cantilena C, Koziol D, et al. A 25-year study of the clinical and histologic outcomes of hepatitis C virus infection and its modes of transmission in a cohort of initially asymptomatic blood donors. *J Infect Dis.* 2012;206(5):654-661. doi:10.1093/infdis/jis410
137. Parés A, Barrera JM, Caballería J, et al. Hepatitis C virus antibodies in chronic alcoholic patients: association with severity of liver injury. *Hepatology.* 1990;12(6):1295-1299. doi:10.1002/hep.1840120608
138. Salari N, Darvishi N, Hemmati M, et al. Global prevalence of hepatitis C in prisoners: a comprehensive systematic review and meta-analysis. *Arch Virol.* 2022;167(4):1025-1039. doi:10.1007/s00705-022-05382-1
139. van Beek I, Dwyer R, Dore GJ, Luo K, Kaldor JM. Infection with HIV and hepatitis C virus among injecting drug users in a prevention setting: retrospective cohort study. *BMJ.* 1998;317(7156):433-437. doi:10.1136/bmj.317.7156.433
140. Haber PS, Parsons SJ, Harper SE, White PA, Rawlinson WD, Lloyd AR. Transmission of hepatitis C within Australian prisons. *Med J Aust.* 1999;171(1):31-33. doi:10.5694/j.1326-5377.1999.tb123494.x
141. Poulin C, Courtemanche Y, Serhir B, Alary M. Tattooing in prison: a risk factor for HCV infection among inmates in the Quebec's provincial correctional system. *Ann Epidemiol.* 2018;28(4):231-235. doi:10.1016/j.annepidem.2018.02.002
142. Frank C, Mohamed MK, Strickland GT, et al. The role of parenteral antischistosomal therapy in the spread of hepatitis C virus in Egypt. *Lancet.* 2000;355(9207):887-891. doi:10.1016/s0140-6736(99)06527-7
143. Mahase E. Hepatitis C: Egypt makes "unprecedented progress" towards elimination. *BMJ.* 2023 Oct 10;383:2353. doi: 10.1136/bmj.p2353. PMID: 37816531.
144. Ruiz-Extremera Á, Muñoz-Gámez JA, Salmerón-Ruiz MA, et al. Genetic variation in interleukin 28B with respect to vertical transmission of hepatitis C virus and spontaneous clearance in HCV-infected children. *Hepatology.* 2011;53(6):1830-1838. doi:10.1002/hep.24298
145. Koziel MJ, Wong DK, Dudley D, Houghton M, Walker BD. Hepatitis C virus-specific cytolytic T lymphocyte and T helper cell responses in seronegative persons. *J Infect Dis.* 1997;176(4):859-866. doi:10.1086/516546
146. Lingala S, Ghany MG. Natural history of Hepatitis C. *Gastroenterol Clin North Am.* 2015;44(4):717-734. doi:10.1016/j.gtc.2015.07.003
147. Merican I, Sherlock S, McIntyre N, Dusheiko GM. Clinical, biochemical and histological features in 102 patients with chronic hepatitis C virus infection. *Q J Med.* 1993;86(2):119-125.
148. Fletcher NF, JA MK. Hepatitis C virus and the brain. *J Viral Hepat.* 2012;19(5):301-306. doi:10.1111/j.1365-2893.2012.01591.x
149. Stephenson J. Former addicts face barriers to treatment for HCV. *JAMA.* 2011;285(8):1003-1005. doi:10.1001/jama.285.8.1003
150. Beckman AL, Bilinski A, Puglisi L, Lockman-Fine T, Gonsalves G. *Follow California's Lead: Treat Inmates with Hepatitis C.* Accessed August 16, 2023. https://www.healthaffairs.org/do/10.1377/forefront.20180724.396136
151. Graf C, Mucke MM, Dultz G, et al. Efficacy of direct-acting antivirals for chronic hepatitis C virus infection in people who inject drugs or receive opioid substitution therapy: a systematic review and meta-analysis. *Clin Infect Dis.* 2020;70(11):2355-2365. doi:10.1093/cid/ciz696
152. Boursier J, Bertrais S, Oberti F, et al. Comparison of accuracy of fibrosis degree classifications by liver biopsy and non-invasive tests in chronic hepatitis C. *BMC Gastroenterol.* 2011;11:132. doi:10.1186/1471-230x-11-132
153. Ostapowicz G, Watson KJ, Locarnini SA, Desmond PV. Role of alcohol in the progression of liver disease caused by hepatitis C virus infection. *Hepatology.* 1998;27(6):1730-1735. doi:10.1002/hep.510270637
154. Pessione F, Degos F, Marcellin P, et al. Effect of alcohol consumption on serum hepatitis C virus RNA and histological lesions in chronic hepatitis C. *Hepatology.* 1998;27(6):1717-1722. doi:10.1002/hep.510270635
155. Anand BS, Currie S, Dieperink E, et al. Alcohol use and treatment of hepatitis C virus: results of a national multicenter study. *Gastroenterology.* 2006;130(6):1607-1616. doi:10.1053/j.gastro.2006.02.023
156. Vandenbulcke H, Moreno C, Colle I, et al. Alcohol intake increases the risk of HCC in hepatitis C virus-related compensated cirrhosis: a prospective study. *J Hepatol.* 2016;65(3):543-551. doi:10.1016/j.jhep.2016.04.031
157. Modi AA, Feld JJ, Park Y, et al. Increased caffeine consumption is associated with reduced hepatic fibrosis. *Hepatology.* 2010;51(1):201-209. doi:10.1002/hep.23279
158. AASLD/IDSA HCV Guidance Panel. Hepatitis C guidance: AASLD-IDSA recommendations for testing, managing, and treating adults infected with hepatitis C virus. *Hepatology.* 2015;62(3):932-954. doi:10.1002/hep.27950
159. Macias J, Morano LE, Tellez F, et al. Response to direct-acting antiviral therapy among ongoing drug users and people receiving opioid substitution therapy. *J Hepatol.* 2019;71(1):45-51. doi:10.1016/j.jhep.2019.02.018
160. The Lancet. Viral hepatitis elimination: a challenge, but within reach. *Lancet.* 2022;400(10348):251. doi:10.1016/S0140-6736(22)01377-0
161. Simmons B, Saleem J, Hill A, Riley RD, Cooke GS. Risk of late relapse or reinfection with hepatitis C virus after achieving a sustained virological response: a systematic review and meta-analysis. *Clin Infect Dis.* 2016;62(6):683-694. doi:10.1093/cid/civ948
162. Cepeda JA, Thomas DL, Astemborski J, et al. Impact of hepatitis C treatment uptake on cirrhosis and mortality in persons who inject drugs : a longitudinal, community-based cohort study. *Ann Intern Med.* 2022;175(8):1083-1091. doi:10.7326/M21-3846
163. Batchelder AW, Peyser D, Nahvi S, Arnsten JH, Litwin AH. "Hepatitis C treatment turned me around": psychological and behavioral transformation related to hepatitis C treatment. *Drug Alcohol Depend.* 2015;153:66-71. doi:10.1016/j.drugalcdep.2015.06.007
164. Pockros PJ. New direct-acting antivirals in the development for hepatitis C virus infection. *Therap Adv Gastroenterol.* 2010;3(3):191-202. doi:10.1177/1756283x10363055

165. Chappell CA, Scarsi KK, Kirby BJ, et al. Ledipasvir plus sofosbuvir in pregnant women with hepatitis C virus infection: a phase 1 pharmacokinetic study. *Lancet Micorbe.* 2020;1(5):e200-e208. doi:10.1016/S2666-5247(20)30062-8
166. Goldberg D, Ditah IC, Saeian K, et al. Changes in the prevalence of hepatitis C virus infection, nonalcoholic steatohepatitis, and alcoholic liver disease among patients with cirrhosis or liver failure on the waitlist for liver transplantation. *Gastroenterology.* 2017;152(5):1090-1099. e1091: doi:10.1053/j.gastro.2017.01.003
167. Arora SS, Axley P, Ahmed Z, et al. Decreasing frequency and improved outcomes of hepatitis C-related liver transplantation in the era of direct-acting antivirals—a retrospective cohort study. *Transpl Int.* 2019;32(8):854-864. doi:10.1111/tri.13424
168. Koch M, Banys P. Liver transplantation and opioid dependence. *JAMA.* 2011;285(8):1056-1058. doi:10.1001/jama.285.8.1056
169. Braun HJ, Schwab MP, Jin C, et al. Opioid use prior to liver transplant is associated with increased risk of death after transplant. *Am J Surg.* 2021;222(1):234-240. doi:10.1016/j.amjsurg.2020.11.039
170. Zhu J, Peltekian KM. Cannabis and the liver: things you wanted to know but were afraid to ask. *Can Liver J.* 2019;2(3):51-57. doi:10.3138/canlivj.2018-0023
171. Lange M, Zaret D, Kushner T. Hepatitis delta: current knowledge and future directions. *Gastroenterol Hepatol (N Y).* 2022;18(9):508-520.
172. Wedemeyer H, Schoneweis K, Bogomolov P, et al. Safety and efficacy of bulevirtide in combination with tenofovir disoproxil fumarate in patients with hepatitis B virus and hepatitis D virus coinfection (MYR202): a multicentre, randomised, parallel-group, open-label, phase 2 trial. *Lancet Infect Dis.* 2023;23(1):117-129. doi:10.1016/S1473-3099(22)00318-8
173. Riordan SM, Skouteris GG, Williams R. Metabolic activity and clinical efficacy of animal and human hepatocytes in bioartificial support systems for acute liver failure. *Int J Artif Organs.* 1998;21(6):312-318.
174. Silva MO, Roth D, Reddy KR, Fernandez JA, Albores-Saavedra J, Schiff ER. Hepatic dysfunction accompanying acute cocaine intoxication. *J Hepatol.* 1991;12(3):312-315. doi:10.1016/0168-8278(91)90832-v
175. Selim K, Kaplowitz N. Hepatotoxicity of psychotropic drugs. *Hepatology.* 1999;29(5):1347-1351. doi:10.1002/hep.510290535
176. Duysen EG, Li B, Carlson M, et al. Increased hepatotoxicity and cardiac fibrosis in cocaine-treated butyrylcholinesterase knockout mice. *Basic Clin Pharmacol Toxicol.* 2008;103(6):514-521. doi:10.1111/j.1742-7843.2008.00259.x
177. Mallat A, Dhumeaux D. Cocaine and the liver. *J Hepatol.* 1991;12(3):275-278. doi:10.1016/0168-8278(91)90826-w
178. Henry JA, Jeffreys KJ, Dawling S. Toxicity and deaths from 3,4-methylenedioxymethamphetamine ("ecstasy"). *Lancet.* 1992;340 (8816):384-387. doi:10.1016/0140-6736(92)91469-o
179. Hearn WL, Flynn DD, Hime GW, et al. Cocaethylene: a unique cocaine metabolite displays high affinity for the dopamine transporter. *J Neurochem.* 1991;56(2):698-701. doi:10.1111/j.1471-4159.1991.tb08205.x
180. Andrews P. Cocaethylene toxicity. *J Addict Dis.* 1997;16(3):75-84. doi:10.1300/J069v16n03_08
181. Tamargo JA, Sherman KE, Sekaly RP, et al. Cocaethylene, simultaneous alcohol and cocaine use, and liver fibrosis in people living with and without HIV. *Drug Alcohol Depend.* 2022;232:109273. doi:10.1016/j.drugalcdep.2022.109273
182. RJM C. MDMA-associated liver toxicity: pathophysiology, management, and current state of knowledge. *AACN Adv Crit Care.* 2019;30(3):232-248. doi:10.4037/aacnacc2019852
183. Ellis AJ, Wendon JA, Portmann B, Williams R. Acute liver damage and ecstasy ingestion. *Gut.* 1996;38(3):454-458. doi:10.1136/gut.38.3.454
184. Jones AL, Simpson KJ. Review article: mechanisms and management of hepatotoxicity in ecstasy (MDMA) and amphetamine intoxications. *Aliment Pharmacol Ther.* 1999;13(2):129-133. doi:10.1046/j.1365-2036.1999.00454.x
185. *LiverTox: Clinical and Research Information on Drug-Induced Liver Injury.* National Institute of Diabetes and Digestive and Kidney Diseases; 2012.
186. Luethi D, Liechti ME, Krähenbühl S. Mechanisms of hepatocellular toxicity associated with new psychoactive synthetic cathinones. *Toxicology.* 2017;387:57-66. doi:10.1016/j.tox.2017.06.004
187. Armen R, Kanel G, Reynolds T. Phencyclidine-induced malignant hyperthermia causing submassive liver necrosis. *Am J Med.* 1984;77(1):167-172. doi:10.1016/0002-9343(84)90455-8
188. Jenkins MG, Handslip R, Kumar M, et al. Reversible khat-induced hepatitis: two case reports and review of the literature. *Frontline Gastroenterol.* 2013;4(4):278-281. doi:10.1136/flgastro-2013-100318
189. Pantano F, Tittarelli R, Mannocchi G, et al. Hepatotoxicity Induced by "the 3Ks": Kava, Kratom and Khat. *Int J Mol Sci.* 2016;17(4):580. doi:10.3390/ijms17040580
190. SMS O, Sandven I, Berhe NB, et al. Khat chewing increases the risk for developing chronic liver disease: a hospital-based case-control study. *Hepatology.* 2018;68(1):248-257. doi:10.1002/hep.29809
191. Osborne CS, Overstreet AN, Rockey DC, Schreiner AD. Drug-induced liver injury caused by kratom use as an alternative pain treatment amid an ongoing opioid epidemic. *J Investig Med High Impact Case Rep.* 2019;7:2324709619826167. doi:10.1177/2324709619826167
192. Ishida JH, Peters MG, Jin C, et al. Influence of cannabis use on severity of hepatitis C disease. *Clin Gastroenterol Hepatol.* 2008;6(1):69-75. doi:10.1016/j.cgh.2007.10.021
193. Tam J, Liu J, Mukhopadhyay B, Cinar R, Godlewski G, Kunos G. Endocannabinoids in liver disease. *Hepatology.* 2011;53(1):346-355. doi:10.1002/hep.24077
194. Patsenker E, Stoll M, Millonig G, et al. Cannabinoid receptor type I modulates alcohol-induced liver fibrosis. *Mol Med.* 2011;17(11-12): 1285-1294. doi:10.2119/molmed.2011.00149
195. Mutlu B, Puigserver P. Controversies surrounding peripheral cannabinoid receptor 1 in fatty liver disease. *J Clin Invest.* 2021;131(22):e154147. doi:10.1172/JCI154147
196. Saxon AJ, Ling W, Hillhouse M, et al. Buprenorphine/Naloxone and methadone effects on laboratory indices of liver health: a randomized trial. *Drug Alcohol Depend.* 2013;128(1-2):71-76. doi:10.1016/j.drugalcdep.2012.08.002
197. Petrovic A, Vukadin S, Sikora R, et al. Anabolic androgenic steroid-induced liver injury: An update. *World J Gastroenterol.* 2022;28(26):3071-3080. doi:10.3748/wjg.v28.i26.3071
198. Bond P, Llewellyn W, Van Mol P. Anabolic androgenic steroid-induced hepatotoxicity. *Med Hypotheses.* 2016;93:150-153. doi:10.1016/j.mehy.2016.06.004
199. Molos MA, Litton N, Schubert TT. Talc liver. *J Clin Gastroenterol.* 1987;9(2):198-203. doi:10.1097/00004836-198704000-00018
200. Allaire GS, Goodman ZD, Ishak KG, Rabin L. Talc in liver tissue of intravenous drug abusers with chronic hepatitis. A comparative study. *Am J Clin Pathol.* 1989;92(5):583-588. doi:10.1093/ajcp/92.5.583

CHAPTER

90 Renal and Metabolic Disorders Related to Substance Use

Sarah Gilligan and Naveen Rathi

CHAPTER OUTLINE

- Introduction
- Overview of nephrology and renal clinical syndromes
- Renal and metabolic effects of alcohol
- Injection drug use–related renal disease
- Renal and metabolic effects of opioids
- Renal and metabolic effects of stimulants
- Renal and metabolic effects of inhalants
- Renal and metabolic effects of tobacco use and renal disease
- Renal and metabolic effects of cannabinoids
- Renal and metabolic effects of ketamine
- Conclusions

INTRODUCTION

Substance use can impact the kidneys in different ways, including through direct effects, the effects of contaminants and adulterants, or complications of other conditions associated with substance use, including infections acquired from injection drug use. Moreover, substance use can lead to acute or chronic metabolic or electrolyte changes. Renal complications associated with substance use encompass the spectrum of tubular, glomerular, interstitial, and vascular kidney disease, as well as many adverse pathophysiological and metabolic consequences. The causal links are apparent in some cases[1,2] such as human immunodeficiency virus (HIV)-associated nephropathy, hepatitis C–associated glomerular disease, or subcutaneous injection drug–related amyloidosis. However, with other diseases, such as accelerated hypertension or subtypes of focal and segmental glomerulosclerosis, the relationship, even if strongly suspected, has not been proven definitively.

A list of renal problems associated with commonly-used substances is found in **Table 90-1**. However, the multiplicity of behavioral risk factors and the variety of possible etiological agents sometimes make it difficult to define a clear-cut relationship between a given substance and a renal disease. Perhaps a more useful classification for the practitioner features the renal syndromes of presentation that can be related to one or more exposures connected to substance use (**Table 90-2**).

OVERVIEW OF NEPHROLOGY AND RENAL CLINICAL SYNDROMES

The main functions of the kidneys can be categorized as follows: maintenance of body fluid composition, excretion of metabolic end products and foreign substances, regulation of bone mineral metabolism, and production of important hormones like renin and erythropoietin. Later in the chapter, the pathophysiological mechanisms and consequences of derangements in kidney function as it relates to specific substances are discussed in more detail.

Acute tubular necrosis attributed to volume depletion and rhabdomyolysis remain the most common form of acute kidney injury (AKI) seen with use of alcohol and other drugs, including opioids, stimulants, and hallucinogens.[3] Injury to the kidney can also result in a multiplicity of signs and symptoms including proteinuria caused by altered permeability of capillary walls, hematuria caused by rupture of capillary walls, and azotemia (elevated serum blood urea nitrogen and creatinine) caused by impaired filtration of nitrogenous wastes. These manifestations ultimately lead to oliguria (reduced urine production <500 mL/d), edema caused by decreased renal clearance of salt and water, and hypertension caused by fluid retention and disturbed renal hormonal homeostasis. The nature and severity of disease in a given patient are dictated by the nature and severity of the underlying renal injury.

Specific renal diseases tend to produce characteristic syndromes of kidney dysfunction (**Table 90-2**). Nephrotic syndrome is defined as proteinuria greater than 3.5 g/d, hypoalbuminemia, hyperlipidemia, and edema. Nephritic syndrome is defined as glomerular hematuria, often with red blood cell casts, hypertension, and renal insufficiency/azotemia. There are also crossover syndromes with both nephritic and nephrotic features.

Measurement of Renal Function

For the clinician responsible for any patient with current or past unhealthy substance use, clinicians should consider obtaining a measurement of renal function, serum electrolytes, urinalysis, and urine protein excretion. Glomerular filtration rate (GFR) is generally accepted as the best overall index of kidney function and is one of the most important parameters to determine in the clinical evaluation of kidney function. The GFR is the rate at which blood is filtered across the glomerulus in the kidneys.

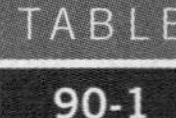

TABLE 90-1 Renal and Metabolic Complications Associated With Specific Substances or Routes of Use

Renal and Metabolic Complications Associated With Specific Substances or Routes of Use
Alcohol
Hepatorenal syndrome
Rhabdomyolysis and AKI
Increased incidence and severity of postinfectious glomerulonephritis
Electrolyte disorders
IgA nephropathy
Injection drug use
HIV nephropathy
Hepatitis C–associated glomerulopathies
Hepatitis B–associated polyarteritis nodosa
Subcutaneous injection ("skin-popping") amyloidosis
Bacterial endocarditis and acute glomerulonephritis
Opioids
Nontraumatic rhabdomyolysis (muscle compression) and AKI
Heroin nephropathy
Cocaine
Vasculitis
Rhabdomyolysis and AKI
Accelerated hypertension and renal failure
Hypertensive nephrosclerosis
Renal infarction
Thrombotic microangiopathy and renal failure
Amphetamines
Rhabdomyolysis and AKI
Accelerated hypertension and renal failure
Polyarteritis nodosa
MDMA (ecstasy)
Hyponatremia
Rhabdomyolysis and AKI
Cannabinoids
Acute tubular necrosis
Interstitial nephritis

GFR cannot be measured directly in humans, so estimation equations have been developed using serum creatinine and cystatin C. The most recent of these is the CKD EPI equation, which provides an estimate based on creatinine, cystatin C, or combined equation.[4] Both creatinine and cystatin C have advantages and disadvantages, for example creatinine is dependent on muscle mass, so using a combined equation may provide the most accurate assessment of renal function, termed eGFR.[5-8] An abrupt decline in eGFR is often due to AKI; a sustained eGFR less than 60 mL/min for 3 months or more indicates chronic kidney disease (CKD).

If proteinuria is present, quantification of total protein excretion is needed. If it is not possible to obtain a 24-hour urine collection, proteinuria can be estimated by using a spot urine protein-to-creatinine ratio. The ratio represents the approximate urinary protein excretion in a 24-hour period; for example, a ratio of 3 g/g means an approximate daily excretion of 3-g protein, though the accuracy of this estimate varies depending on hydration and muscle mass.[9]

TABLE 90-2 Renal Syndromes Commonly Associated With Substance Use

Renal Syndromes Commonly Associated With Substance Use
Nephrotic syndrome
Hepatitis B– or hepatitis C–related membranous nephropathy
HIV nephropathy (injection drug use)
Amyloidosis (subcutaneous injection drug use [IDU] ["skin popping"])
Focal and segmental glomerulosclerosis (IDU)
Nephritic-nephrotic syndrome
Hepatitis C–related membranoproliferative glomerulonephritis (IDU)
Hepatitis C–related cryoglobulinemia (IDU)
Nephritic syndrome
Bacterial endocarditis and acute glomerulonephritis (IDU)
Postinfectious glomerulonephritis (IDU)
Acute kidney injury
Rhabdomyolysis (alcohol, cocaine, MDMA [ecstasy], opioids)
Acute uric acid nephropathy ("bath salts")
Dehydration/volume depletion (MDMA [ecstasy], amphetamines, "bath salts")
Thrombotic microangiopathy (cocaine, intravenous use of PO narcotics)
Hypertension
Hepatitis B- or amphetamine-associated polyarteritis nodosa (IDU, amphetamine)
Accelerated hypertension (cocaine)

RENAL AND METABOLIC EFFECTS OF ALCOHOL

The adverse health effects of long-term heavy alcohol use and acute alcohol intoxication are well established.[10] Patients who use alcohol may present with myriad and complex fluid and electrolyte abnormalities, especially those who consume alcohol frequently and in large quantities.

Encephalopathy and loss of consciousness induced by alcohol can lead to immobilization and ischemic compression of muscle causing rhabdomyolysis and subsequent AKI.[3,11] Patients with alcohol use disorder may also present with severe anion gap acidosis following a heavy drinking episode, even if ethanol is no longer detectable in the serum. Ketoacidosis is induced by poor dietary intake and the inhibition of gluconeogenesis and acceleration of lipolysis by alcohol, though may require a serum test of beta-hydroxybutyrate for diagnosis.

Other acid-base disturbances can be seen in people with alcohol use disorder including nonanion gap acidosis secondary to diarrhea, renal tubular acidosis, and respiratory alkalosis. The latter, in part, may be secondary to impaired hepatic metabolism of progesterone, a pro-respiratory drive stimulant. As with all acid-base disturbances, measurement of serum pH is the first step in assessment.

Hypokalemia is often seen in connection with gastrointestinal losses and secondary hyperaldosteronism. Such loss may be accelerated by the use of diuretics without a potassium-sparing agent. Correction of this electrolyte abnormality is important because hypokalemia can accelerate or worsen hepatic encephalopathy, in part through the enhancement of ammoniagenesis. Hypokalemia also increases the risk for rhabdomyolysis.

One of the most frequent electrolyte abnormalities among people with alcohol use disorder is hypomagnesemia[12] due to a combination of poor nutrition and gastrointestinal losses, coupled with direct renal tubular alcohol toxicity,[13] which decreases renal magnesium reabsorption in spite of depleted body stores. Hypomagnesemia is often associated with hypocalcemia because of decreased parathyroid hormone release and bone resistance to parathyroid hormone.[14,15] In addition, if chronic pancreatitis and fat malabsorption are present, saponification (complexing) of calcium and magnesium will impair intestinal absorption of these divalent cations. Hypokalemia is worsened by concomitant hypomagnesemia, which promotes kaliuresis[16] and, like hypocalcemia, is refractory to correction unless the magnesium deficit is replaced.[17] Severe hypomagnesemia should be treated with slow intravenous (IV) infusion, whereas oral replacement can be used for milder hypomagnesemia.

Phosphate is a major intracellular anion. Hypophosphatemia is often seen in patients with alcohol use disorder and may contribute to rhabdomyolysis and encephalopathy.[18,19] Again, dietary deficiency combined with increased gastrointestinal losses and increased renal excretion of phosphorus[12,20] contributes to this deficit. Furthermore, severe and acute hypophosphatemia due to refeeding syndrome can occur in chronically malnourished patients with alcohol use disorder who begin eating again.[21]

Alcohol use may also contribute to the progression of CKD. The effect of alcohol consumption on CKD is poorly understood. In one study, light, moderate, and heavy alcohol consumption appeared to be protective against CKD in adult males[22]; however, in a another study, heavy alcohol consumption led to significantly faster progression of CKD.[23] Interestingly, the association of alcohol use with increased risk of CKD was shown in one study to be stronger in subjects with lower body mass index (BMI),[24] possibly due to poorer nutrition status.

Finally, alcohol consumption by pregnant women has been well-documented in causing fetal alcohol spectrum disorder (FASD) and spontaneous abortion.[25] However, recently there has also been a discovery of a dose-dependent effect on renal function in overweight and obese children with prenatal alcohol exposure.[26]

Hepatorenal Syndrome and Cirrhosis Associated Diseases

Chronic heavy alcohol ingestion complicated by fulminant liver failure or cirrhosis can lead to the hepatorenal syndrome (HRS). The pathogenesis and pathophysiology of this syndrome are complex and beyond the scope of this chapter and the interested reader is referred to more complete reviews.[27,28] Briefly, this syndrome is thought to reflect a state of profound renal vasoconstriction and splanchnic vasodilatation associated with severely impaired liver function, often with other systemic signs of liver failure (eg, portal hypertension, esophageal varies, and ascites). A rise in serum creatinine, oliguria, bland urine sediment, and low urinary sodium concentration—usually less than 10 mEq/L—is a characteristic presentation of HRS. Diagnosis can be complicated by falsely low creatinine in patients with cirrhosis who are often malnourished and have low muscle mass.[29]

HRS is, however, a diagnosis of exclusion. If, after cautious trials of volume replacement (salt-poor albumin or isotonic saline) and the removal of any potentially nephrotoxic agent, oliguric acute renal failure does not improve, a diagnosis of HRS is most probable. HRS is treated with albumin, vasoconstrictor sympathomimetic agents (midodrine or terlipressin), and a somatostatin analog (octreotide) to inhibit endogenous vasodilators.[30,31] These drug combinations may help to bridge the gap until liver transplantation can be performed in suitable candidates.

In postmortem studies, 50% to 100% of patients with hepatic cirrhosis due to alcohol have an associated glomerulopathy, histologically similar to immunoglobulin A (IgA) nephropathy.[32] IgA nephropathy is characterized by microhematuria and proteinuria but tends to remain clinically silent. The suspected etiology is increased levels of serum polymeric IgA and IgA immune complexes that are found in patients with alcohol-related cirrhosis and are deposited in the glomeruli.

Toxic Alcohols

The ingestion of toxic alcohols—methanol, ethylene glycol, or isopropyl alcohol (IPA)—is occasionally seen in patients who consume them as a substitute for ethanol or believing that what they are consuming is ethanol. Methanol is found in solutions used for de-icing and in some paint products, such as varnish or shellac. Ethylene glycol is found in antifreeze. The metabolic products of these alcohols (facilitated by the enzyme alcohol dehydrogenase) are severely toxic and produce organ damage and anion gap acidosis from the nonvolatile organic acids produced.

An anion gap metabolic acidosis usually is the first clue to a toxic alcohol ingestion, but the presence of an osmolar gap (ie, a difference between the calculated and measured serum osmolality >15—see below) should raise suspicion of a toxic alcohol ingestion when no other reason is apparent, such as ethanol or mannitol. In cases of ethylene glycol ingestion, the presence of calcium oxalate crystals in the urine is highly suggestive but not diagnostic. Calculated osmolality = 2 × [Na mmol/L] + [glucose mg/dL] / 18 + [BUN mg/dL] / 2.8 + [Ethanol/3.7].[33]

Ethylene Glycol

Ethylene glycol poisoning is a medical emergency. Ethylene glycol is rapidly absorbed and reaches peak serum levels 1 to 4 hours after oral ingestion. Generally, it is eliminated via exhaled carbon dioxide and through the kidneys. However, at higher doses, the kidneys become the predominant pathway for the excretion of ethylene glycol, glycolic acid, and oxalic acid. The half-life for elimination is 2.5 to 8.4 hours. Metabolic abnormalities may not be present in the early phase of presentation; therefore, diagnosis requires a high index of suspicion. Ordering an ethylene glycol level is generally not helpful because it often takes several days to result. Osmolar gap (measured minus calculated osmolality) is a characteristic, early laboratory finding that later (4-12 hours) transitions to an anion gap metabolic acidosis as ethylene glycol undergoes metabolism to its acidic derivatives. The most characteristic abnormality is the presence of large numbers of "tent-shaped" (octahedral) or needle-shaped oxalate crystals in the urine. However, its absence does not rule out ethylene glycol poisoning. Falsely elevated lactic acid on blood gas may occur due to cross-reaction of ethylene glycol metabolites glycolic acid and glyoxylic acid with L-lactate oxidase used in point-of-care blood gas analyzers.[34]

Treatment of ethylene glycol toxicity includes fomepizole, an IV medication that competitively inhibits alcohol dehydrogenase more than ethanol.[35] As long as kidney function is maintained, the alcohol will be removed by renal excretion. With severe toxicity, hemodialysis is used to remove the alcohol and the toxic products efficiently and is useful in the treatment of the concurrent metabolic acidosis. Failure to recognize and promptly treat this can lead to multiple organ system damage and failure (brain, liver, and kidney).

Isopropyl Alcohol

IPA is found in common household rubbing alcohol and other solvents. It is metabolized to acetone and excreted by the kidneys and the lung. Here, the alcohol itself rather than the products of metabolism is the toxic agent. Organic acids are not produced, so in contrast to the other toxic alcohols, the anion gap is not elevated. Patients usually appear inebriated but without the odor of ethanol on the breath. Individuals often have gastritis, ketonuria, and an osmolar gap.

Misdiagnosis of acute renal injury due to false elevation of creatinine can occur in the setting of IPA intoxication. IPA interferes with creatinine measurements when determined by colorimetric assay, but not when determined by the enzymatic Jaffe-alkaline picrate reaction assay. Measuring creatinine level by enzymatic assay in blood gas analyzer will accurately estimate serum creatinine and avoid the interference of acetone.[36]

INJECTION DRUG USE–RELATED RENAL DISEASE

Nephrotic Syndromes Associated With Injection Drug Use

HIV-Associated Nephropathy

Injection drug use is a well-known risk factor for the development of human immunodeficiency virus (HIV) infection. There are several renal diseases associated with HIV. HIVAN (HIV-associated nephropathy) typically presents as nephrotic syndrome with progressive renal failure. The development of proteinuria and impaired renal function is a harbinger of poor prognosis.[37,38] The most common histological finding is a form of focal and segmental glomerular sclerosis with collapse of the glomerular tufts, also named *collapsing focal and segmental glomerulosclerosis* (FSGS).[39] African American race, the presence of APOL1 variants (APOL1Vs) on genetic testing, low CD4 counts and positive family history of renal disease are risk factors.[40]

The pathogenesis of HIVAN is not completely understood. It is known that transgenic mice that express HIV proviral constructs in renal tissue develop disease that is identical to HIVAN in humans.[39] It has been speculated that APOL1Vs expression may render podocytes more vulnerable to different types of injury, including infections.[40]

Early on, patients with HIVAN were denied dialysis because of their short life expectancy. Today, dialysis is provided to these patients, and centers are offering stable patients the opportunity for renal transplantation.[41] This opportunity reflects the longer survival of patients with HIV on renal replacement therapy and the better outlook for those who respond and are adherent to antiretroviral treatment.[42]

Hepatitis Virus–Associated Nephrotic Syndrome

Similar to HIV, hepatitis B and C are associated with nephropathies that can be seen among people who inject drugs (PWID). All patients presenting with nephrotic syndrome of unknown etiology should be tested for hepatitis B and C virus infection.

The association between hepatitis B and membranous nephropathy is well established, with morphological studies demonstrating deposition of hepatitis B E antigen (HBeAg) in glomerular capillaries.[43] It is important to diagnose this cause of membranous nephropathy, because immunosuppressive treatment—often used in the idiopathic form of nephrotic syndrome—actually may enhance ongoing hepatitis B viral replication and is contraindicated. Moreover, antiviral therapy targeted at hepatitis B virus replication may prove beneficial.[44-46]

The most common presentation of renal disease in patients with hepatitis C is a combination of nephritic and nephrotic syndromes (ie, a urine that contains large amounts of protein, red blood cells, and red blood casts); see the following section: "Nephritic-Nephrotic Syndromes Associated With Injection Drug Use." Less often, membranous nephropathy has been described.[47,48] The detection of hepatitis C virus (HCV) protein in the glomeruli of patients with membranous nephropathy[48] strengthens this association.

Heroin-Associated Nephropathy

In the 1970s and 1980s, a heroin-associated nephropathy (HAN) was described, presenting as nephrotic syndrome among individuals who were using heroin by injection route. HAN has been considered a secondary cause of FSGS, often associated with hypertension and progression to ESRD. Occasionally, the process reversed itself with abstinence from further injection heroin use. The pathogenesis is unclear; earlier studies suggested that injection heroin, or one of its adulterants, acted as antigen leading to renal deposition of immune complexes in the kidney. More recent animal studies have shown that morphine (the active metabolite of heroin) may have a direct effect on the glomerulus, causing proliferation of fibroblasts and a decrease in degradation of renal glomerular type IV collagen.[49]

The incidence of HAN has decreased and it is now rarely encountered. This may be due to use of more purified forms of heroin and/or the removal of contaminants or adulterants that were, in fact, responsible for "heroin nephropathy," or it is possible that previous cases of HAN were actually HIVAN.[49] However, recent studies have shown a specific association between albuminuria and overuse of acidifier in dissolving heroin prior to injection.[50] Patients with FSGS, PWID, and infection with hepatitis C may present with a clinical picture similar to that of HAN.[47]

Subcutaneous Drug Use–Associated Amyloidosis

Chronic suppurative skin infections related to subcutaneous injection drug use may lead to secondary amyloidosis with renal involvement.[51-53] Secondary amyloidosis, also referred to as amyloid A (AA) amyloidosis, is a rare but serious complication of chronic inflammatory diseases and chronic infections. The kidney is the organ most frequently affected in AA amyloidosis. Clinically, these patients may be very difficult to distinguish from those with HIVAN or hepatitis-related renal disease because they present with nephrotic-range proteinuria, renal insufficiency, and normal-sized or enlarged kidneys. The presence of subcutaneous drug injection ("skin popping") or multiple skin scars or draining abscesses should alert the clinician to the possibility of this diagnosis. If alternative diagnoses are possible, a renal biopsy is indicated to confirm the presence of amyloidosis. In addition to proteinuria and renal insufficiency, tubular dysfunction, including nephrogenic diabetes insipidus and renal tubular acidosis (proximal or distal), may be present. A novel treatment agent, eprodisate, has shown promising results in the clinical management of secondary forms of systemic amyloidosis.[54]

Nephritic-Nephrotic Syndromes Associated With Injection Drug Use

Hepatitis C Virus–Related Glomerulonephritis

In addition to significant proteinuria, the presence of hematuria, hypertension, and variable degrees of renal insufficiency in the setting of past or present injection drug use should raise the suspicion of HCV-related glomerular disease. The most common pattern of injury in patients with hepatitis C infection is membranoproliferative glomerulonephritis with or without cryoglobulinemia.[55-57] Less commonly, membranous nephropathy (see foregoing) or fibrillary glomerulonephritis and immunotactoid glomerulopathy may be encountered. In the latter two instances, the clinical presentation and light microscopy findings can be indistinguishable from membranoproliferative glomerulonephritis, but organized deposits of fibrils of different sizes are detected on electron microscopy.[58]

Liver enzymes often are abnormal, but they may be minimally elevated or within normal limits, and there may be no findings in the history or physical examination that point to liver dysfunction.[59,60] In cases with associated essential mixed cryoglobulinemia, serum cryoglobulins can be detected. In addition, palpable purpura, arthralgias, peripheral neuropathy, and nonspecific systemic complaints may be present. A pattern of serum complement with decreased serum complement C4 levels and normal C3 levels is characteristic of mixed cryoglobulinemia.[61] A positive rheumatoid factor may be seen, but not consistently. Typical renal biopsy features of mixed cryoglobulinemia include intraluminal thrombi in glomerular capillaries and a substructure of curvilinear fibrils in the subendothelial space, which resemble "fingerprints" on electron microscopy.

Patients with HCV-related glomerular disease should be treated with angiotensin antagonism (with either converting enzyme inhibitors or angiotensin receptor blockers), as well as with antiviral HCV therapy. The emergence of direct-acting antivirals (DAAs) for the treatment of hepatitis C has offered the opportunity to reach sustained viral response (SVR) rates exceeding 90%. Combined antiviral therapy and immunosuppression (cyclophosphamide or rituximab with steroids) may be the treatment of choice for patients with severe renal disease (ie, cryoglobulinemia, severe nephrotic syndrome, and/or progressive renal failure).[62] Immunosuppressive therapy is still needed in these situations to stabilize the life-threatening manifestations and improve renal function.[63] While the process is clearly antigen-dependent at its onset, at least in some individuals, it may become antigen-independent and continue after viral clearance.[64] Coinfection with hepatitis C is found in up to 78% of HIV-infected PWID.[65] The course of nephropathy associated with this dual infection has been reported as aggressive, with rapid progression to ESRD.

Nephritic Syndromes Associated With Injection Drug Use

Postinfectious Glomerulonephritis

The presence of nephritic urinary sediment (proteinuria, hematuria, and often red blood cell casts), variable degrees of hypertension, and renal insufficiency in PWID should raise the suspicion of immune complex–mediated postinfectious glomerulonephritis, which can occur with bacterial sepsis, pyogenic abscesses, and acute bacterial endocarditis. The most frequent pathogen is *Staphylococcus aureus*.[66-71] Less often, *Streptococcus viridans*, gram-negative rods, or *Candida* species are isolated. Actual septic embolization of the kidneys is also encountered but is much less common. The complication of renal septic emboli is characterized by persistent fevers, gross or microscopic hematuria (occasionally accompanied by flank pain), and signs of embolization to other organs (including the brain and lungs).

Hypertension and low complement levels (C3) are present less consistently in postinfectious glomerulonephritis in PWID than in poststreptococcal glomerulonephritis, and frank nephrotic syndrome occurs only in a minority of cases.[69] Although renal failure may be irreversible in some cases, recovery of renal function usually occurs with treatment of the underlying local or systemic infection.[72]

In patients with postinfectious glomerulonephritis as a manifestation of acute endocarditis or abscesses, histological features similar to those found with poststreptococcal glomerulonephritis are seen. The pattern is one of acute proliferative glomerulonephritis with neutrophil infiltration and immune complex deposition in the mesangium and capillary walls. A higher incidence and more severe course of postinfectious glomerulonephritis in people with alcohol use disorder have been reported, but the specific reasons for this condition are unclear.[20,73,74]

When patients with bacterial endocarditis or suppurative abscesses develop renal failure days to weeks after the onset of antibiotic therapy, this should raise the suspicion of acute allergic interstitial nephritis, rather than classic postinfectious nephritis. Suggestive of this diagnosis is the finding, in the urine sediment, of renal tubular and/or white blood cells, often in cast formation. The presence or absence of urine eosinophils has been removed from the diagnostic algorithm given low sensitivity and specificity.

RENAL AND METABOLIC EFFECTS OF OPIOIDS

There is a high rate of viral, bacterial, and fungal contamination associated with injection drug use and consequently, individuals who use injection drugs are at risk of a variety of infections. As discussed above, these infections include HIV, hepatitis B and C viruses, and local pyogenic abscesses and systemic endocarditis with staphylococcal or streptococcal bacterial infections.[49] In addition to the diseases seen more broadly in association with injection drug use, opioids may have other negative consequences for the kidneys and urinary tract system.

Rhabdomyolysis

Rhabdomyolysis is a condition in which damaged skeletal muscle tissue breaks down rapidly and the breakdown products are released into the bloodstream. Some of these byproducts, such as the protein myoglobin, are harmful to the kidneys and may lead to kidney failure.

Coma from overdose or underestimated drug potency may lead to prolonged immobilization and pressure-induced muscle damage and rhabdomyolysis. Hypotension, hypoxia, acidosis, and dehydration may aggravate this potential. It has been demonstrated that rhabdomyolysis can occur in the absence of coma or evidence of muscle compression. This suggests that rhabdomyolysis could be due to a direct heroin toxic effect or an allergic response to heroin or the components in adulterated heroin admixture.[1]

Injection Use of Prescription Opioids

Thrombotic microangiopathic anemia (TMA) secondary to injection of prescription opioids is an increasingly recognized entity. Injection of oral extended-release formulations of oxymorphone and oxycodone has been associated with clinical constellation of anemia, thrombocytopenia, and evidence of hemolysis, with a negative direct Coombs test and normal ADAMTS13 activity. A case series of three patients using injected extended-release oxymorphone found thrombotic microangiopathy on renal biopsy, involving mainly the interlobular arteries, and severe endothelial cell swelling and intimal mucoid edema.[75] It is not clear whether this syndrome is attributed to the polyethylene oxide (PEO) coating on the reformulated tablets, the active medication itself, or a substance or solvent used to prepare the tablets for injection use. Few case reports were published about TMA following injection of extended-release oxymorphone.[75-78] Pathological features of TMA are described in cocaine-induced TMA section below.[79]

Urologic Effects of Opioids

Opioids can cause urinary retention, especially in older men who have underlying prostatic hyperplasia. Urinary retention is most commonly seen as an iatrogenic complication of opioid analgesia in the postoperative period.[80] Factitious nephrolithiasis has been described[81] and can be a reason for multiple visits to different healthcare settings on the part of individuals who seek prescriptions for opioid medications.

RENAL AND METABOLIC EFFECTS OF STIMULANTS

Cocaine

A wide spectrum of renal complications can occur with both acute and chronic use of cocaine. These disorders are generally renovascular (hypertension) or renal tubular (rhabdomyolysis) in origin, but there are also glomerular forms of renal injury. Many of the renal complications associated with injection cocaine use are discussed above in the section on "Injection Drug Use–Related Renal Disease"; however, there also are reports of increased prevalence of HCV infection in patients who use drugs but do not inject them. The use of shared pipes for smoking crack cocaine and transnasal transmission of HCV via contaminated drug-sniffing implements, such as straws, is the suspected potential source of viral infection as these objects come in contact with eroded intranasal blood vessels.[82]

Rhabdomyolysis

Rhabdomyolysis is a common cause of AKI associated with use of cocaine. A common presentation is of a young adult with a history of illicit drug use (especially cocaine), who is agitated, confused, combative, and hyperthermic and who has a urinalysis highly suggestive of this disease (ie, brownish-red urine positive for blood but without red blood cells on microscopy). Tonic-clonic seizures may have occurred prior to admission. In addition, blood testing usually reveals a markedly elevated serum creatine kinase (CK) level.

Muscle ischemia caused through prolonged cocaine-induced vasoconstriction of intramuscular arteries or direct myofibrillar damage is the proposed mechanism of cocaine-induced rhabdomyolysis. Cocaine may also be contaminated with arsenic or strychnine, which can also cause rhabdomyolysis.[1] Precipitating events may include volume depletion, often from fluid sequestered in damaged muscles (potentially several liters); decreased vasodilatory effect of nitric oxide, which is inactivated by myoglobin[83]; toxicity of free chelatable iron released from myoglobin[84]; and tubular obstruction by pigmented casts.[85]

Patients with total-body potassium depletion (as in malnutrition) may be predisposed to ischemic muscular injury because potassium release at the level of the microcirculation is an important mechanism for vasodilatation that sustains muscle perfusion during physical activity.[86] Total-body phosphate depletion is also a predisposing factor, but hypophosphatemia can be masked at the time of presentation because of phosphate release from injured muscle cells (even producing hyperphosphatemia). In addition to hyperactivity, compression of the muscle (crush injury) because of drug-induced stupor or coma and immobilization for prolonged periods of time can result in rhabdomyolysis (see section "Renal and Metabolic Effects of Opioids Rhabdomyolysis"). In the early phase, hypocalcemia can be secondary to deposition of calcium in necrotic muscle cells or precipitation with phosphate released from destroyed muscle cells. Hyperkalemia and hyperuricemia also may be present due to muscle cell lysis.

Treatment depends on the phase of the disease at the time of presentation. If severe renal failure is not present, aggressive intravascular volume expansion with isotonic saline is the preferred management. In the absence of hypocalcemia, the use of sodium bicarbonate to alkalinize the urine can decrease the toxicity of myoglobin. The role of mannitol in this setting is less clear.[87] Though in some early series up to 50% of patients required acute dialysis, currently most patients recover renal function without the need for long-term renal replacement therapy, perhaps reflecting more aggressive initial volume resuscitation and goal-oriented early intensive care interventions utilized today.[88]

Cocaine-Associated Vasculitis

Several case series have described vasculitis in the setting of cocaine use. This entity has recently been attributed to levamisole. At the time of a 2011 paper, approximately 70% of illicit cocaine consumed in the United States was contaminated with levamisole.[89] Though recently, it is being used much less frequently to cut cocaine. It is most commonly used as a veterinary antihelminthic agent. However, levamisole is a known immunomodulating agent.[89-91] Levamisole is added to cocaine because it potentiates its stimulant effects by inhibiting both monoamine oxidase and catechol-*O*-methyltransferase activity and consequently prolonging the action of catecholamines in the neuronal synapse and accentuating the cocaine reuptake inhibition effect.[92] Levamisole metabolites are also known to have a stimulatory effect. Moreover, levamisole adds bulk to illicit cocaine without reducing the native drug's apparent purity.[93] Both smoking and intranasal use of levamisole-contaminated cocaine have been associated with the development of vasculitis.[94]

Levamisole-induced syndrome has characteristic clinical presentation.[93,94] The skin lesions are distinctive retiform purpura, typically involving the ears, nose, cheeks, and extremities. These lesions usually resolve spontaneously within few weeks of drug discontinuation and recur with subsequent contaminated cocaine use. Renal involvement is uncommon, but when it occurs, usually presents with hematuria, proteinuria, and worsening renal function. Kidney biopsy shows necrotic crescentic lesions with or without immune complex formation. The spectrum of autoantibody findings is interesting. Perinuclear antineutrophil antibodies (p-ANCA) are almost always found in high titers (86% to 100%); cytoplasmic antineutrophil antibodies (c-ANCA) are present in about 50% of the cases.[89,93-98] Moreover, antiphospholipid antibodies and antinuclear antibodies are also often present.

The ideal treatment for levamisole-induced vasculitis is not known. Nearly all cases resolve upon the abstinence from cocaine use.[93,99-101] The role of corticosteroids is equivocal; steroids have not definitively been shown to improve or accelerate healing.[99,100,102] Use of plasmapheresis has been investigated only in few case reports.[99,100,102]

Cocaine, Hypertension, and Renal Disease

The development of acute hypertension in connection with cocaine use is well recognized and seems to be associated with the release of endothelin-1 and activation of the renin-angiotensin system,[103,104] thereby causing intense vasoconstriction. The clinical presentations of cocaine intoxication can mimic preeclampsia or scleroderma renal crisis,[105,106] and the development of accelerated hypertension and renal failure has been documented by some[107,108] but not all observers.[109] This inconsistency may reflect confounding factors, including the intensity and length of exposure, genetic predisposition, and the duration of follow-up. Immunologically, cocaine has been shown to cause mesangial proliferation by increasing the release of interleukin-6 by macrophages, which may be a cause of focal segmental glomerulosclerosis and resultant chronic renal disease and hypertension.

Cocaine-Associated Thrombotic Microangiopathy-Hemolytic Uremic Syndrome

AKI associated with thrombocytopenic microangiopathic hemolytic anemia has been described in connection with cocaine use[110-112] and possibly also with HIV infection.[113] This syndrome can have catastrophic consequences with renal cortical necrosis and permanent loss of renal function, central nervous system involvement with seizures, and the permanent sequelae of ischemic or hemorrhagic strokes.

The pathogenesis of this syndrome is not known but may involve both immunological and nonimmunological mechanisms. An autoantibody directed against the von Willebrand factor-cleaving protease has been described in some cases.[114] Direct endothelial injury, vasoconstriction, and procoagulant effects of cocaine that are thought to be involved in cases of renal infarction associated with cocaine use[115] may play a part in the development of thrombotic microangiopathic nephropathy.[116]

In patients with cocaine-associated thrombotic microangiopathy-hemolytic uremic syndrome, renal biopsy reveals fibrin thrombi in the lumen of glomerular capillaries and occluded interlobular arterioles, with swollen endothelial cells and vessel wall damage. Fibrin and red blood cells are seen in the arteriolar media in the acute phase and with "onion skin" hypertrophy of muscular arteries in the healing phase. These lesions are similar to findings associated with malignant hypertension, systemic sclerosis, and the antiphospholipid antibody syndrome. Early recognition is important because prompt treatment with plasmapheresis and infusion of fresh frozen plasma can help minimize serious bleeding complications and long-term chronic renal failure.[117]

MDMA

The amphetamine-type drug 3,4-methylenedioxymethamphetamine (MDMA) is also known as "ecstasy." MDMA is rapidly absorbed, reaching plasma peak levels in approximately 2 hours. It is metabolized by the liver and excreted by the kidney.[118] Toxicity is mostly idiosyncratic and not related to overdose. Hence, first time users tend to have more serious complications. Clinical manifestations associated with MDMA toxicity include hyponatremia, rhabdomyolysis, and hyperthermia, in addition to cardiac and neurological injury.[119,120]

MDMA induces its effect by releasing serotonin, dopamine, and norepinephrine into the CNS[121] and inhibiting their reuptake. Moreover, MDMA leads to the release of arginine vasopressin (AVP), which explains its propensity to cause hyponatremia, the most common renal complication of MDMA.[122] Hyponatremia with MDMA is at least partially dilutional given excessive water or other hypotonic beverage intake. However, the excessive release of AVP seems to be a major factor in impairing free water excretion. Cerebral edema can occur because of the acute fall in serum sodium leading to devastating complications such as mental status changes, seizures, and possibly coma and brainstem herniation, resulting in death.

MDMA-associated AKI has been described in several case reports.[123] However, it is rare and mostly associated with nontraumatic rhabdomyolysis in the setting of hyperthermia, extreme exertion, and volume depletion.[122] MDMA has also been reported to produce accelerated hypertension and AKI due to its marked sympathomimetic effects (much like cocaine).[124] Case reports of vasculitis have also been noted with use of MDMA.[125]

Therapy for acute MDMA-associated adverse events is mostly supportive care and includes aggressive cooling, IV fluids, and correction of electrolytes. Severe symptomatic hyponatremia is a medical emergency, and treatment includes 100 to 200 mL of 3% saline to be administered as soon as possible with the goal to increase the serum sodium concentration by 3 to 5 mEq/L, which should acutely lower intracranial pressure and improve symptoms.[126,127]

Amphetamines

Polyarteritis nodosa has been associated with hepatitis B and the use of some substances, especially amphetamines. Patients may present with accelerated hypertension and systemic symptoms, including malaise, arthralgia, weight loss, and asymmetric peripheral neuropathy. They may have a necrotizing vasculitis that can affect medium-sized arteries, including renal, mesenteric, coronary, and (rarely) cerebral circulation. The test result for antinuclear cytoplasmic antibodies usually is negative.[128,129] Angiography is the diagnostic procedure of choice. The finding of diffuse microaneurysms with areas of thrombosis and ischemia in multiple organs, including the kidneys, is diagnostic. Treatment usually is with steroids and cytotoxic agents. Antivirals such as lamivudine or telbivudine aimed at suppressing hepatitis B virus may prove to be effective, without the risk of enhanced viral replication with immunosuppression.

Other renal syndromes attributed to amphetamine use include AKI due to volume depletion, rhabdomyolysis, and accelerated hypertension.

Cathinones

Cathinones are stimulants that are sometimes sold as "bath salts" and include designer drugs that are derivatives of pyrrolidinopropiophenone (such as 3,4-methylenedioxopyrrovalerone) or mephedrone. There are a number of possible mechanisms for the development of AKI from bath salt intoxication. These substances may promote severe renal arteriolar vasoconstriction in a manner similar to cocaine and thereby producing renal hypoperfusion and renal ischemia, resulting in acute tubular necrosis. Rhabdomyolysis also may promote kidney injury in the setting of cathinone intoxication. Finally, hyperuricemia can be found with acute intoxication, raising the possibility of acute uric acid deposition and nephropathy contributing to the development of AKI.[130]

RENAL AND METABOLIC EFFECTS OF INHALANTS

Acute renal failure has been noted in cases of toluene intoxication from glue sniffing.[131] An unusual cause of metabolic acidosis and hypokalemia, encountered more often in teenagers, also involves toluene intoxication. The diagnosis can be difficult because patients may be reticent to report use. Patients may recover rapidly on admission to the hospital, but recurrent episodes are not uncommon.[132] Distal renal tubular acidosis has been described in this setting.[133] However, the principal mechanism producing the acidosis seems to involve increased manufacture of hippuric acid derived from toluene metabolism.[134] The hippuric acid is rapidly excreted, leading to a normal anion gap metabolic acidosis. In the distal nephron, acting as a nonreabsorbable anion, hippurate increases the excretion of sodium and potassium. If hippurate is present in sufficient amounts, severe hypokalemia may occur.

RENAL AND METABOLIC EFFECTS OF TOBACCO USE AND RENAL DISEASE

Tobacco use appears to have a deleterious effect on renal function. Cigarette smoking is related to proteinuria,[135] accelerated atherosclerotic vascular disease, and ischemic nephropathy.[136] In addition, tobacco smoking is associated with an increased risk of progression to CKD in patients with diabetes mellitus[137] and severe essential hypertension.[138] Moreover, increased risk of sustained proteinuria[135] and poorer prognosis of renal disease have been ascribed to tobacco smoking.[139] Idiopathic nodular glomerulosclerosis is a progressive vasculopathic lesion linked to hypertension and cigarette smoking. This enigmatic condition resembles nodular diabetic nephropathy, but occurs in nondiabetic patients with tobacco use and hypertension.[140]

Accelerated atherosclerotic vascular disease related to cigarette smoking can contribute to the development and progression of ischemic nephropathy. This common cause of renal failure is defined as impaired perfusion to the total renal mass and usually is associated with ischemic manifestations in other organs (cerebral vascular accidents, myocardial infarctions, and lower extremity peripheral arterial disease).[141]

RENAL AND METABOLIC EFFECTS OF CANNABINOIDS

Cannabis use may be complicated by cannabinoid hyperemesis syndrome (CHS),[142] which is characterized by abdominal pain and intractable vomiting. There have been a few case reports of AKI secondary to CHS. The unique combination of intractable vomiting and relief with hot showers seems to put CHS patients at significant risk of severe volume depletion and prerenal AKI.[143] There have also been case reports of renal infarction associated with cannabis smoking.[144]

Synthetic cannabinoids, a group of compounds with potent effects, have become more popular among young populations.[145-147] Synthetic cannabinoids (SCs), originally developed for research and drug development, produce effects similar to those of cannabis (ie, delta-9-tetrahydrocannabinol or THC). SCs are not detected by routine urine drug tests, which make them appealing to people who may undergo random urine drug testing.

Two cannabinoid receptors have been identified: cannabinoid type 1 receptor (CB1), located mostly at the CNS level, and cannabinoid type 2 (CB2) receptor, located mostly in the immune tissue.[148,149] Activation of CB1 is responsible for the neuropsychiatric effect including elation and anxiety. Activation of CB2 plays a role in signal transduction and controlling emesis and pain.[148,149] These receptors were also found to be expressed in the glomeruli and more specifically the podocytes and thought to have a beneficial role by reducing proteinuria and protecting against fibrosis.[150]

There have been reports of AKI related to the use of SC. The first case series of four patients, followed by identification of 16 cases of AKI among patients using SC, have shed light on SC as potential nephrotoxic agent.[151,152] All patients reported were young and all were men except one. Most of the patients presented with emesis, abdominal pain, or flank pain. Urine microscopy findings were variable. Ultrasound findings range from normal findings to increase echogenicity. Out of 13 kidney biopsies, 10 showed acute tubular necrosis (the most common histological finding). Interstitial nephritis was also present in three cases.[153] The pathogenesis remains elusive. Volume depletion due to nausea and vomiting causing acute tubular necrosis is possible etiology. However, most of these patients have normal blood pressure and pulse upon presentation, making volume depletion as the major cause questionable. The potential direct nephrotoxic effects of SCs or the additives has been suggested and supported by some studies.[153]

RENAL AND METABOLIC EFFECTS OF KETAMINE

Although not typically directly nephrotoxic, there is increasing evidence that ketamine use is associated with a variety of lower urinary tract symptoms.[154,155] These symptoms range from urinary frequency and urgency to sterile cystitis, bladder ulcers, and hydronephrosis. Although these symptoms are typically benign and resolve with drug discontinuation, the development of ketamine-associated hydronephrosis has been associated with decline in renal function.[155]

CONCLUSIONS

Renal disease may be seen in people who use alcohol, tobacco, and other substances. As described throughout this chapter, substance use may cause or exacerbate a wide spectrum of kidney disease. Renal and metabolic consequences of substance use are common, may be quite serious, and sometimes are difficult to diagnose and manage. Alcohol, tobacco, and other drug use must be considered in the differential diagnosis of any patient with unexplained renal pathology. Careful collaboration between nephrology, primary care, and addiction specialists can ensure safe and effective treatment of patients with substance use disorders and acute or chronic kidney disease.

REFERENCES

1. Crowe AV. Substance abuse and the kidney. *QJM.* 2000;93(3):147-152.
2. Perneger TV, Klag MJ, Whelton PK. Recreational drug use: a neglected risk factor for end-stage renal disease. *Am J Kidney Dis.* 2001;38(1):49-56.
3. Huerta-Alardin AL, Varon J, Marik PE. Bench-to-bedside review: rhabdomyolysis—an overview for clinicians. *Crit Care.* 2005;9(2):158-169.
4. Inker LA, Eneanya ND, Coresh J, et al. New creatinine- and cystatin C-based equations to estimate GFR without race. *N Engl J Med.* 2021;385:1737-1749.
5. Ye X, Liu X, Song D, et al. Estimating glomerular filtration rate by serum creatinine or/and cystatin C equations: an analysis of multi-centre Chinese subjects. *Nephrology (Carlton).* 2016;21(5):372-378.
6. Pottel H, Delanaye P, Schaeffner E, et al. Estimating glomerular filtration rate for the full age spectrum from serum creatinine and cystatin C. *Nephrol Dial Transplant.* 2017;32(3):497-507.
7. Inker LA, Schmid CH, Tighiouart H, et al. Estimating glomerular filtration rate from serum creatinine and cystatin C. *N Engl J Med.* 2012;367(1):20-29.
8. Odden MC. Cystatin C level as a marker of kidney function in human immunodeficiency virus infection: the FRAM study. *Arch Intern Med.* 2007;167(20):2213.
9. Ginsberg JM, Chang BS, Matarese RA, Garella S. Use of single voided urine samples to estimate quantitative proteinuria. *N Engl J Med.* 1983;309(25):1543-1546.
10. National Institute on Alcohol Abuse and Alcoholism Publications Catalog. *10th Special Report on the U.S. Congress on Alcohol and Health.* U.S. Dept of Health and Human Services; 2000.
11. Curry SC, Chang D, Connor D. Drug- and toxin-induced rhabdomyolysis. *Ann Emerg Med.* 1989;18(10):1068-1084.
12. Uchtenhagen A. Heroin-assisted treatment in Switzerland: a case study in policy change. *Addiction.* 2010;105(1):29-37.
13. De Marchi S, Cecchin E, Basile A, Bertotti A, Nardini R, Bartoli E. Renal tubular dysfunction in chronic alcohol abuse—effects of abstinence. *N Engl J Med.* 1993;329(26):1927-1934.
14. Laitinen K, Lamberg-Allardt C, Tunninen R, et al. Transient hypoparathyroidism during acute alcohol intoxication. *N Engl J Med.* 1991;324(11):721-727.
15. Shils ME. Magnesium, calcium, and parathyroid hormone interactions. *Ann N Y Acad Sci.* 1980;355:165-180.
16. Lin C, Wu Z, Rou K, et al. Challenges in providing services in methadone maintenance therapy clinics in China: service providers' perceptions. *Int J Drug Policy.* 2010;21(3):173-178.
17. Barbosa C, Godfrey C, Parrott S. Methodological assessment of economic evaluations of alcohol treatment: what is missing? *Alcohol Alcohol.* 2010;45(1):53-63.
18. Funabiki Y, Tatsukawa H, Ashida K, et al. Disturbance of consciousness associated with hypophosphatemia in a chronically alcoholic patient. *Intern Med.* 1998;37(11):958-961.
19. Nagata N. Hypophosphatemia and encephalopathy in alcoholics. *Intern Med.* 1998;37(11):911-912.
20. Vamvakas S, Teschner M, Bahner U, Heidland A. Alcohol abuse: potential role in electrolyte disturbances and kidney diseases. *Clin Nephrol.* 1998;49(4):205-213.
21. Marinella MA. The refeeding syndrome and hypophosphatemia. *Nutr Rev.* 2003;61(9):320-323.
22. Yuan HC, Yu QT, Bai H, Xu HZ, Gu P, Chen LY. Alcohol intake and the risk of chronic kidney disease: results from a systemic review and dose-response meta-analysis. *Eur J Clin Nutr.* 2021;75(11):1555-1567.
23. Joo YS, Koh H, Nam KH, et al. Alcohol consumption and progression of chronic kidney disease: results from the Korean cohort study for outcome in patients with chronic kidney disease. *Mayo Clin Proc.* 2021;95(2):293-305.
24. Hashimoto Y, Imaizumi T, Kato S, et al. Effect of body mass index on the association between alcohol consumption and the development of chronic kidney disease. *Sci Rep.* 2021;11(1):20440.
25. Akison LK, Moritz KM, Reid N. Adverse reproductive outcomes associated with fetal alcohol exposure: a systematic review. *Reproduction.* 2019;157(4):329-343.
26. Correia-Costa L, Schaefer F, Afonso AC, et al. Prenatal alcohol exposure affects renal function in overweight schoolchildren: birth cohort analysis. *Pediatr Nephrol.* 2020;35(4):695-702.
27. Davenport A, Ahmad J, Al-Khafaji A, Kellum JA, Genyk YS, Nadim NK. Medical management of hepatorenal syndrome. *Nephrol Dial Transplant.* 2012;27(1):34-41.
28. Wadei H. Hepatorenal syndrome: a critical update. *Semin Respir Crit Care Med.* 2012;33(01):55-69.
29. Papadakis MA, Arieff AI. Unpredictability of clinical evaluation of renal function in cirrhosis. *Am J Med.* 1987;82(5):945-952.
30. Angeli P, Volpin R, Gerunda G, et al. Reversal of type 1 hepatorenal syndrome with the administration of midodrine and octreotide. *Hepatology.* 1999;29(6):1690-1697.
31. Dobre M, Demirjian S, Sehgal AR, Navaneethan SD. Terlipressin in hepatorenal syndrome: a systematic review and meta-analysis. *Int Urol Nephrol.* 2011;43(1):175-184.
32. Newell GC. Cirrhotic glomerulonephritis: incidence, morphology, clinical features, and pathogenesis. *Am J Kidney Dis.* 1987;9(3):183-190.
33. Purssell RA, Pudek M, Brubacher J, Abu-Laban RB. Derivation and validation of a formula to calculate the contribution of ethanol to the osmolal gap. *Ann Emerg Med.* 2001;38(6):653-659.
34. Sandberg Y, Rood PP, Russcher H, Zwaans JJM, Weige JD, van Daele PLA. Falsely elevated lactate in severe ethylene glycol intoxication. *Neth J Med.* 2010;68(1):320-323.
35. Brent J, McMartin K, Phillips S, et al. Fomepizole for the treatment of ethylene glycol poisoning. *N Engl J Med.* 1999;340(11):832-838.
36. Rawan Tayseer Al Odat M, Al-Rabadi LF. American Society of Nephrology Kidney Week 2014—JASN Abstract Supplement. Accessed June 20, 2023. https://www.asn-online.org/abstracts/
37. Szczech LA, Hoover DR, Feldman JG, et al. Association between renal disease and outcomes among HIV-infected women receiving or not receiving antiretroviral therapy. *Clin Infect Dis.* 2004;39(8):1199-1206.
38. Winston JA, Klotman ME, Klotman PE. HIV-associated nephropathy is a late, not early, manifestation of HIV-1 infection. *Kidney Int.* 1999;55(3):1036-1040.
39. Izzedine H, Deray G. The nephrologist in the HAART era. *AIDS.* 2007;21(4):409-421.
40. Lan X, Rao TKS, Chander PN, Skorecki K, Singhal PC. Apolipoprotein L1 (APOL1) variants (Vs) a possible link between heroin-associated nephropathy (HAN) and HIV-associated nephropathy (HIVAN). *Front Microbiol.* 2015;6:571.
41. Gupta SK, Eustace JA, Winston JA, et al. Guidelines for the management of chronic kidney disease in HIV-infected patients: recommendations of the HIV Medicine Association of the Infectious Diseases Society of America. *Clin Infect Dis.* 2005;40(11):1559-1585.
42. Szczech LA, Eustace JA, Winston JA, et al. Protease inhibitors are associated with a slowed progression of HIV-related renal diseases. *Clin Nephrol.* 2002;57(05):336-341.
43. Lai KN, Li PK, Lui SF, et al. Membranous nephropathy related to hepatitis B virus in adults. *N Engl J Med.* 1991;324(21):1457-1463.
44. Hyman Z, Crosby F. Study of implementation of a guideline for brief alcohol intervention in primary care. *J Nurs Care Qual.* 2010;25(1):46-55.

45. Benhamou Y. Effects of lamivudine on replication of hepatitis B virus in HIV-infected men. *Ann Intern Med.* 1996;125(9):705.
46. Lai C-L, Gane E, Liaw Y-F, et al. Telbivudine versus lamivudine in patients with chronic hepatitis B. *N Engl J Med.* 2007;357(25):2576-2588.
47. Stehman-Breen C, Alpers CE, Fleet WP, Johnson RJ. Focal segmental glomerular sclerosis among patients infected with hepatitis C virus. *Nephron.* 1999;81(1):37-40.
48. Friedmann PD, Jiang L, Alexander JA. Top manager effects on buprenorphine adoption in outpatient substance abuse treatment programs. *J Behav Health Serv Res.* 2010;37(3):322-337.
49. Jaffe JA. Chronic nephropathies of cocaine and heroin abuse: a critical review. *Clin J Am Soc Nephrol.* 2006;1(4):655-667.
50. McGowan CR, Wright T, Nitsch D, et al. High prevalence of albuminuria amongst people who inject drugs: a cross-sectional study. *Sci Rep.* 2020;10(1):7059.
51. Formica R, Perazella MA. Leg pain and swelling in an HIV-infected drug abuser. *Hosp Pract.* 1998;33(10):195-197.
52. Neugarten J, Gallo GR, Buxbaum J, Katz LA, Rubenstein J, Baldwin DS. Amyloidosis in subcutaneous heroin abusers ("Skin poppers' amyloidosis"). *Am J Med.* 1986;81(4):635-640.
53. Tan AU Jr, Cohen AH, Levine BS. Renal amyloidosis in a drug abuser. *J Am Soc Nephrol.* 1995;5(9):1653-1658.
54. Dember LM, Hawkins PN, Hazenberg BPC, et al. Eprodisate for the treatment of renal disease in AA amyloidosis. *N Engl J Med.* 2007;356(23):2349-2360.
55. Agnello V, Chung RT, Kaplan LM. A role for hepatitis C virus infection in type II cryoglobulinemia. *N Engl J Med.* 1992;327(21):1490-1495.
56. Johnson RJ, Gretch DR, Yamabe H, et al. Membranoproliferative glomerulonephritis associated with hepatitis C virus infection. *N Engl J Med.* 1993;328(7):465-470.
57. Misiani R. Hepatitis C virus infection in patients with essential mixed cryoglobulinemia. *Ann Intern Med.* 1992;117(7):573.
58. Markowitz GS, Cheng JT, Colvin RB, Trebbin WM, D'Agati VD. Hepatitis C viral infection is associated with fibrillary glomerulonephritis and immunotactoid glomerulopathy. *J Am Soc Nephrol.* 1998;9:2244-2252.
59. Cheng JT, Anderson HL Jr, Markowitz GS, Appel GB, Pogue VA, D'Agati VD. Hepatitis C virus-associated glomerular disease in patients with human immunodeficiency virus coinfection. *J Am Soc Nephrol.* 1999;10(7):1566-1574.
60. Stokes MB, Cawla H, Brody RI, et al. Immune complex glomerulonephritis in patients coinfected with human immunodeficiency virus and hepatitis C virus. *Am J Kidney Dis.* 1997;29(4):514-525.
61. Haydey RP, de Rojas MP, Gigli I. A newly described control mechanism of complement activation in patients with mixed cryoglobulinemia (cryoglobulins and complement). *J Invest Dermatol.* 1980;74(5):328-332.
62. Wallack SS, Thomas CP, Martin TC, Chilingerian J, Reif S. Substance abuse treatment organizations as mediators of social policy: slowing the adoption of a congressionally approved medication. *J Behav Health Serv Res.* 2010;37(1):64-78.
63. Sise ME, Bloom AK, Wisocky J, et al. Treatment of hepatitis C virus-associated mixed cryoglobulinemia with direct-acting antiviral agents. *Hepatology.* 2016;63(2):408-417.
64. Emery JS, Kuczynski M, La D, et al. Efficacy and safety of direct acting antivirals for the treatment of mixed cryoglobulinemia. *Am J Gastroenterol.* 2017;112(8):1298-1308.
65. Quan CM, Krajden M, Grigoriew GA, Salit IE. Hepatitis C virus infection in patients infected with the human immunodeficiency virus. *Clin Infect Dis.* 1993;17(1):117-119.
66. Bakir AA, Dunea G. Drugs of abuse and renal disease. *Curr Opin Nephrol Hypertens.* 1996;5(2):122-126.
67. Hill EE, Vanderschueren S, Herijgers P, et al. Risk factors for infective endocarditis and outcome of patients with *Staphylococcus aureus* bacteremia. *Mayo Clin Proc.* 2007;82(10):1165-1169.
68. Klevens RM. Invasive methicillin-resistant *Staphylococcus aureus* infections in the United States. *JAMA.* 2007;298(15):1763.
69. Neugarten J, Baldwin DS. Glomerulonephritis in bacterial endocarditis. *Am J Med.* 1984;77(2):297-304.
70. Stachura I. Renal lesions in drug addicts. *Pathol Annu.* 1985;20(Pt 2):83-99.
71. Bernstein E, Topp D, Shaw E, et al. A preliminary report of knowledge translation: lessons from taking screening and brief intervention techniques from the research setting into regional systems of care. *Acad Emerg Med.* 2009;16(11):1225-1233.
72. Conlon PJ, Procop GW, Fowler V, Eloubeidi MA, Smith SR, Sexton DJ. Predictors of prognosis and risk of acute renal failure in patients with Rocky Mountain spotted fever. *Am J Med.* 1996;101(6):621-626.
73. Keller CK, Andrassy K, Waldherr R, Ritz E. Postinfectious glomerulonephritis—is there a link to alcoholism? *Q J Med.* 1994;87(2):97-102.
74. Bernstein E, Bernstein JA, Stein JB, Saitz R. SBIRT in emergency care settings: are we ready to take it to scale? *Acad Emerg Med.* 2009;16(11):1072-1077.
75. Ambruzs JM, Serrell PB, Rahim N, Larsen CP. Thrombotic microangiopathy and acute kidney injury associated with intravenous abuse of an oral extended-release formulation of oxymorphone hydrochloride: kidney biopsy findings and report of 3 cases. *Am J Kidney Dis.* 2014;63(6):1022-1026.
76. Amjad AI, Parikh RA. Opana-ER used the wrong way: intravenous abuse leading to microangiopathic hemolysis and a TTP-like syndrome. *Blood.* 2013;122(20):3403.
77. Kapila A, Chhabra L, Chaubey VK, Summers J. Opana ER abuse and thrombotic thrombocytopenic purpura (TTP)-like illness: a rising risk factor in illicit drug users. *BMJ Case Rep.* 2014;2014.
78. Rane M, Aggarwal A, Banas E, Sharma A. Resurgence of intravenous Opana as a cause of secondary thrombotic thrombocytopenic purpura. *Am J Emerg Med.* 2014;32(8):951.e3-951.e4.
79. Singhania G, Kallahalli SJ, Wakefield D, Kazory A. Quiz page October 2015: acute kidney injury in an intravenous drug user. *Am J Kidney Dis.* 2015;66(4):A18-A21.
80. Tammela T. Postoperative urinary retention—why the patient cannot void. *Scand J Urol Nephrol Suppl.* 1995;175:75-77.
81. Gault MH, Campbell NR, Aksu AE. Spurious stones. *Nephron.* 1988;48(4):274-279.
82. Aaron S, McMahon JM, Milano D, et al. Intranasal transmission of hepatitis C virus: virological and clinical evidence. *Clin Infect Dis.* 2008;47(7):931-934.
83. Lüscher TF, Bock HA, Yang Z, Diederich D. Endothelium-derived relaxing and contracting factors: perspectives in nephrology. *Kidney Int.* 1991;39(4):575-590.
84. Zager RA, Burkhart KM, Conrad DS, Gmur DJ. Iron, heme oxygenase, and glutathione: effects on myohemoglobinuric proximal tubular injury. *Kidney Int.* 1995;48(5):1624-1634.
85. Heyman SN, Brezis M, Rubinof CA, et al. Acute renal failure with selective medullary injury in the rat. *J Clin Invest.* 1988;82(2):401-412.
86. Knochel JP, Schlein EM. On the mechanism of rhabdomyolysis in potassium depletion. *J Clin Invest.* 1972;51(7):1750-1758.
87. Bosch X, Poch E, Grau JM. Rhabdomyolysis and acute kidney injury. *N Engl J Med.* 2009;361(1):62-72.
88. Eneas JF. The effect of infusion of mannitol-sodium bicarbonate on the clinical course of myoglobinuria. *Arch Intern Med.* 1979;139(7):801-805.
89. McGrath MM, Isakova T, Rennke HG, Mottola AM, Laliberte KA, Niles JL. Contaminated cocaine and antineutrophil cytoplasmic antibody-associated disease. *Clin J Am Soc Nephrol.* 2011;6(12):2799-2805.
90. Levamisole in rheumatoid arthritis. Final report on a randomised double-blind study comparing a single weekly dose of levamisole with placebo. Multicentre Study Group. *Ann Rheum Dis.* 1982;41(2):159-163.
91. Moertel CG, Fleming TR, Macdonald JS, et al. Levamisole and fluorouracil for adjuvant therapy of resected colon carcinoma. *N Engl J Med.* 1990;322(6):352-358.
92. Abdul-Karim R, Ryan C, Rangel C, Emmett M. Levamisole-induced vasculitis. *Proc (Bayl Univ Med Cent).* 2013;26(2):163-165.
93. Chang A, Osterloh J, Thomas J. Levamisole: a dangerous new cocaine adulterant. *Clin Pharmacol Ther.* 2010;88(3):408-411.

94. Trimarchi M, Gregorini G, Facchetti F, et al. Cocaine-induced midline destructive lesions: clinical, radiographic, histopathologic, and serologic features and their differentiation from Wegener granulomatosis. *Medicine (Baltimore)*. 2001;80(6):391-404.
95. Wiesner O, Russell KA, Lee AS, et al. Antineutrophil cytoplasmic antibodies reacting with human neutrophil elastase as a diagnostic marker for cocaine-induced midline destructive lesions but not autoimmune vasculitis. *Arthritis Rheum*. 2004;50(9):2954-2965.
96. Bhinder SK, Majithia V. Cocaine use and its rheumatic manifestations: a case report and discussion. *Clin Rheumatol*. 2007;26(7):1192-1194.
97. Buchanan JA, Oyer RJ, Patel NR, et al. A confirmed case of agranulocytosis after use of cocaine contaminated with levamisole. *J Med Toxicol*. 2010;6(2):160-164.
98. Gross RL, Brucker J, Bahce-Altunas A, et al. A novel cutaneous vasculitis syndrome induced by levamisole-contaminated cocaine. *Clin Rheumatol*. 2011;30(10):1385-1392.
99. Chung C, Tumeh PC, Birnbaum R, et al. Characteristic purpura of the ears, vasculitis, and neutropenia—a potential public health epidemic associated with levamisole-adulterated cocaine. *J Am Acad Dermatol*. 2011;65(4):722-725.
100. Walsh NM, Green PJ, Burlingame RW, Pasternak S, Hanly JG. Cocaine-related retiform purpura: evidence to incriminate the adulterant, levamisole. *J Cutan Pathol*. 2010;37(12):1212-1219.
101. Arora NP, Jain T, Bhanot R, Natesan SK. Levamisole-induced leukocytoclastic vasculitis and neutropenia in a patient with cocaine use: an extensive case with necrosis of skin, soft tissue, and cartilage. *Addict Sci Clin Pract*. 2012;7:19.
102. Pavenski K, Vandenberghe H, Jakubovic H, Adam DN, Garvey B, Streutker CJ. Plasmapheresis and steroid treatment of levamisole-induced vasculopathy and associated skin necrosis in crack/cocaine users. *J Cutan Med Surg*. 2013;17(2):123-128.
103. Nzerue CM, Hewan-Lowe K, Riley LJ. Cocaine and the kidney: a synthesis of pathophysiologic and clinical perspectives. *Am J Kidney Dis*. 2000;35(5):783-795.
104. Fine DM, Garg N, Haas M, et al. Cocaine use and hypertensive renal changes in HIV-infected individuals. *Clin J Am Soc Nephrol*. 2007;2(6):1125-1130.
105. Goodlin RC. Preeclampsia as the great impostor. *Am J Obstet Gynecol*. 1991;164(6):1577-1581.
106. Hattingh HL, Hallett J, Tait RJ. 'Making the invisible visible' through alcohol screening and brief intervention in community pharmacies: an Australian feasibility study. *BMC Public Health*. 2016;16(1):1141.
107. Norris KC, Thornhill-Joynes M, Robinson C, et al. Cocaine use, hypertension, and end-stage renal disease. *Am J Kidney Dis*. 2001;38(3):523-528.
108. Thakur V, Godley C, Weed S, Cook ME, Hoffman E. Cocaine-associated accelerated hypertension and renal failure. *Am J Med Sci*. 1996;312(6):295-298.
109. Brecklin C, Gopaniuk-Folga A, Kravetz T, et al. Prevalence of hypertension in chronic cocaine users. *Am J Hypertens*. 1998;11(11):1279-1283.
110. Kokko JP. Presidential address of the SSCI metabolic and social consequences of cocaine abuse. *Am J Med Sci*. 1990;299(6):361-365.
111. Tumlin JA, Sands JM, Someren A. Special feature: hemolytic-uremic syndrome following "Crack" cocaine inhalation. *Am J Med Sci*. 1990;299(6):366-371.
112. Volcy J, Nzerue CM, Oderinde A, Hewan-Iowe K. Cocaine-induced acute renal failure, hemolysis, and thrombocytopenia mimicking thrombotic thrombocytopenic purpura. *Am J Kidney Dis*. 2000;35(1):e3.1-e3.5.
113. Leaf AN. Thrombotic thrombocytopenic purpura associated with human immunodeficiency virus type 1 (HIV-1) infection. *Ann Intern Med*. 1988;109(3):194.
114. Furlan M, Robles R, Galbusera M, et al. von Willebrand factor-cleaving protease in thrombotic thrombocytopenic purpura and the hemolytic–uremic syndrome. *N Engl J Med*. 1998;339(22):1578-1584.
115. Sharff JA. Renal infarction associated with intravenous cocaine use. *Ann Emerg Med*. 1984;13(12):1145-1147.
116. Gu X, Herrera GA. Thrombotic microangiopathy in cocaine abuse-associated malignant hypertension: report of 2 cases with review of the literature. *Arch Pathol Lab Med*. 2007;131(12):1817-1820.
117. Kaplan BS, Meyers KE, Schulman SL. The pathogenesis and treatment of hemolytic uremic syndrome. *J Am Soc Nephrol*. 1998;9(6):1126-1133.
118. Verebey K, Alrazi J, Jaffe JH. The complications of 'ecstasy' (MDMA). *JAMA*. 1988;259(11):1649-1650.
119. Lyles J, Cadet JL. Methylenedioxymethamphetamine (MDMA, Ecstasy) neurotoxicity: cellular and molecular mechanisms. *Brain Res Brain Res Rev*. 2003;42(2):155-168.
120. Hall AP, Henry JA. Acute toxic effects of 'Ecstasy' (MDMA) and related compounds: overview of pathophysiology and clinical management. *Br J Anaesth*. 2006;96(6):678-685.
121. de la Torre R, Magi F, Roset PN, et al. Human pharmacology of MDMA: pharmacokinetics, metabolism, and disposition. *Ther Drug Monit*. 2004;26(2):137-144.
122. Campbell GA, Rosner MH. The agony of ecstasy: MDMA (3,4-methylenedioxymethamphetamine) and the kidney. *Clin J Am Soc Nephrol*. 2008;3(6):1852-1860.
123. Fahal IH, Sallomi DF, Yaqoob MM, Bell GM. Acute renal failure after ecstasy. *BMJ*. 1992;305(6844):29.
124. Bingham C, Beaman M, Nicholls AJ, Anthony PP. Necrotizing renal vasculopathy resulting in chronic renal failure after ingestion of methamphetamine and 3,4-methylenedioxymethamphetamine ('ecstasy'). *Nephrol Dial Transplant*. 1998;13(10):2654-2655.
125. Woodrow G, Turney JH. Ecstasy-induced vasculitis. *Nephrol Dial Transplant*. 1999;14:798.
126. Peate WF. Hyponatremia in marathon runners. *N Engl J Med*. 2005;353(4):427-428. author reply 427-428.
127. Maxwell DL, Polkey MI, Henry JA. Hyponatraemia and catatonic stupor after taking "ecstasy". *BMJ*. 1993;307(6916):1399.
128. Wilder CM, Brason FW IInd, Clark AK, Galanter M, Walley AY, Winstanley EL. Development and implementation of an opioid overdose prevention program within a preexisting substance use disorders treatment center. *J Addict Med*. 2014;8(3):164-169.
129. Samuels N, Shemesh O, Yinnon AM, Fisher D, Abraham AS. Polyarteritis nodosa and drug abuse: is there a connection? *Postgrad Med J*. 1996;72(853):684-685.
130. Adebamiro A, Perazella MA. Recurrent acute kidney injury following bath salts intoxication. *Am J Kidney Dis*. 2012;59(2):273-275.
131. Will AM, McLaren EH. Reversible renal damage due to glue sniffing. *Br Med J (Clin Res Ed)*. 1981;283(6290):525-526.
132. Streicher HZ, Gabow PA, Moss AH, Kono D, Kaehny WD. Syndromes of toluene sniffing in adults. *Ann Intern Med*. 1981;94(6):758-762.
133. King MD. Reversible renal damage due to glue sniffing. *Br Med J (Clin Res Ed)*. 1981;283(6296):919.
134. Carlisle EJ, Donnelly SM, Vasuvattakul S, Kamel KS, Tobe S, Halperin ML. Glue-sniffing and distal renal tubular acidosis: sticking to the facts. *J Am Soc Nephrol*. 1991;1(8):1019-1027.
135. Halimi JM, Giraudeau B, Vol S, et al. Effects of current smoking and smoking discontinuation on renal function and proteinuria in the general population. *Kidney Int*. 2000;58(3):1285-1292.
136. U.S. Department of Health and Human Services. *The Health Consequences of Smoking—50 Years of Progress: A Report of the Surgeon General*. U.S. Department of Health and Human Services, Centers for Disease Control and Prevention, National Center for Chronic Disease Prevention and Health Promotion, Office on Smoking and Health; 2014.
137. Stegmayr BG. A study of patients with diabetes mellitus (type 1) and end-stage renal failure: tobacco usage may increase risk of nephropathy and death. *J Intern Med*. 1990;228(2):121-124.
138. Regalado M, Yang S, Wesson DE. Cigarette smoking is associated with augmented progression of renal insufficiency in severe essential hypertension. *Am J Kidney Dis*. 2000;35(4):687-694.
139. Orth SR, Stöckmann A, Conradt C, et al. Smoking as a risk factor for end-stage renal failure in men with primary renal disease. *Kidney Int*. 1998;54:926-931.

140. Markowitz GS, Lin J, Valeri AM, Avila C, Nasr SH, D'Agati VD. Idiopathic nodular glomerulosclerosis is a distinct clinicopathologic entity linked to hypertension and smoking. *Hum Pathol.* 2002;33(8):826-835.
141. Greco BA, Breyer JA. The natural history of renal artery stenosis: who should be evaluated for suspected ischemic nephropathy? *Semin Nephrol.* 1996;16(1):2-11.
142. Kim HS, Anderson JD, Saghafi O, Heard KJ, Monte AA. Cyclic vomiting presentations following marijuana liberalization in Colorado. *Acad Emerg Med.* 2015;22(6):694-699.
143. Habboushe J, Sedor J. Cannabinoid hyperemesis acute renal failure: a common sequela of cannabinoid hyperemesis syndrome. *Am J Emerg Med.* 2014;32(6):690.e1-690.e2.
144. Lambrecht GL, Malbrain ML, Coremans P, Verbist L, Verhaegen H. Acute renal infarction and heavy marijuana smoking. *Nephron.* 1995;70(4):494-496.
145. EMCDDA. *Understanding the 'Spice' phenomenon*. European Monitoring Center for Drugs and Drug Addiction; 2009.
146. Castellanos D, Gralnik LM. Synthetic cannabinoids 2015: an update for pediatricians in clinical practice. *World J Clin Pediatr.* 2016;5(1):16-24.
147. U.S. Department of Justice. *Special Report: Synthetic Cannabinoids and Synthetic Cathinones Reported in NFLIS, 2009-2010*. U.S. Drug Enforcement Administration; 2011.
148. Matsuda LA, Lolait SJ, Brownstein MJ, Young AC, Bonner TI. Structure of a cannabinoid receptor and function. *Nature.* 1990;346(6284):561-564.
149. Gaoni Y, Machoulam R. Isolation, structure, and partial synthesis of an active constituent of hashish. *J Am Chem Soc.* 1646-1647;86(8):1964.
150. Nam DH, Lee MH, Kim JE, et al. Blockade of cannabinoid receptor 1 improves insulin resistance, lipid metabolism, and diabetic nephropathy in db/db mice. *Endocrinology.* 2012;153(3):1387-1396.
151. Bhanushali GK, Jain G, Fatima H, Leisch LJ, Thornley-Brown D. AKI associated with synthetic cannabinoids: a case series. *Clin J Am Soc Nephrol.* 2013;8(4):523-526.
152. Centers for Disease Control and Prevention. Acute kidney injury associated with synthetic cannabinoid use—multiple states, 2012. *MMWR Morb Mortal Wkly Rep.* 2013;62(6):93-98.
153. Pendergraft WF, Herlitz LC, Thornley-Brown D, Rosner M, Niles JL. Nephrotoxic effects of common and emerging drugs of abuse. *Clin J Am Soc Nephrol.* 2014;9(11):1996-2005.
154. Chang T, Lin CC, Lin AT, Fan Y, Chen K. Ketamine-induced uropathy: a new clinical entity causing lower urinary tract symptoms. *Low Urin Tract Symptoms.* 2012;4(1):19-24.
155. Ou SH, Wu LY, Chen HY, et al. Risk of renal function decline in patients with ketamine-associated uropathy. *Int J Environ Res Public Health.* 2020;17(19):7260.

CHAPTER

91 Gastrointestinal Disorders Related to Substance Use

Paul S. Haber and Nicholas C. Kortt

CHAPTER OUTLINE

- Introduction
- Gastrointestinal problems related to alcohol
- Gastrointestinal symptoms associated with other drugs
- Summary

INTRODUCTION

This chapter describes gastrointestinal (GI) effects of alcohol and other drugs (**Table 91-1**). Disorders of the liver are covered elsewhere (Chapter 89, "Liver Disorders Related to Substance Use").

Heavy alcohol use is associated with injury to all parts of the GI tract.[1,2] There is increasing evidence of GI injury and increased cancer risk even with moderate alcohol consumption. The gastric mucosa is a target for alcohol-related toxicity but also contributes to the oxidation of alcohol. Within the GI tract, pancreatitis is an important cause of morbidity and mortality related to heavy alcohol use. Intestinal dysfunction is common among people with alcohol use disorder causing diarrhea and malabsorption.

Tobacco use is associated with gastro-esophageal reflux, peptic ulceration, and GI malignancy but appears to protect against ulcerative colitis. Opioids have important effects on GI secretion and motility. Cannabinoids act upon the GI tract in a complex manner and can reduce GI symptoms such as nausea and vomiting in some settings but can paradoxically cause a hyperemesis syndrome. Psychostimulants such as cocaine and methamphetamine can cause GI ischemia but there is also mounting evidence that they have a detrimental impact on the gut microbiome. The body packing syndrome is rare but challenging when encountered.

GASTROINTESTINAL PROBLEMS RELATED TO ALCOHOL

The relative risk of alcohol-related GI toxicity is not well defined and appears to differ between affected tissues and between benign and neoplastic disorders. Similarly, the pattern and type of beverage has not consistently been shown to predispose to any specific GI effects. Men experience a greater burden of GI-related disease likely due to greater alcohol consumption.[3,4] This pattern may become less apparent in the future as the disparity in alcohol consumption between the sexes appears to be narrowing.[5] There is significant racial disparity in the degree to which alcohol impacts on health, which may be due to AUD treatment gaps.[6] This is the case for alcohol-related GI disease such as alcohol-related pancreatitis, which disproportionately affects African Americans,[7,8] differences that have widened during the COVID-19 pandemic.[7]

The Parotid Glands and Oral Cavity

Sialosis, a painless symmetrical enlargement of the parotid glands, is common in the context of alcohol use disorder.[9,10] It is characterized by the triad of acinar cell hypertrophy, myoepithelial degeneration and neural degeneration.[11] Salivary flow in people with heavy alcohol use has been showed to be reduced and saliva composition altered[12-14] with implications for the development of dental caries and poor oral mucosal health.

Oral mucosal epithelial atrophy, hyper-regeneration and dysplasia have been demonstrated in animal models of alcohol excess.[15-17] Human studies have identified similar effects, with necrosis involving superficial and deep tissues of the oral cavity.[18] Direct injury from ethanol is thought to induce hyper-regenerative changes[19] and enhance mucosal permeability to carcinogens.[20] Both processes may contribute to the enhanced risk of oral cancers in those who drink, and a synergistic effect is seen with concomitant tobacco consumption. Other potential mechanisms contributing to oncogenesis include the effects of alcohol on the oral microbiome, nutrition and increased generation of salivary acetaldehyde, a carcinogenic metabolite of alcohol.[21,22]

Esophagus

Both acute and chronic alcohol consumption are associated with heartburn and gastro-esophageal reflux. Acute alcohol ingestion relaxes the lower esophageal sphincter (LES).[23-25] Heartburn and other reflux symptoms are common accompaniments to alcohol intoxication and hangovers. Manometric and pH evaluation of people with alcohol use disorder have found variable effects of chronic alcohol exposure, including abnormalities of primary and secondary contractions and increased LES tone.[26-29] Consequently, cross-sectional studies have demonstrated a weak relationship between alcohol consumption and gastro-esophageal reflux symptoms[30-32] and, even then, only at higher levels of alcohol consumption.

TABLE 91-1 Gastrointestinal Disorders Related to Alcohol and Other Substances

Alcohol	Parotid enlargement Gastro-esophageal reflux Mallory-Weiss syndrome Gastropathy Peptic ulcer Pancreatic disease Small bowel dysfunction Gastrointestinal cancers
Opioids	Opioid-induced bowel dysfunction Opioid-induced gastrointestinal hyperalgesia
Laxatives	Chronic diarrhea
Anticholinergics	Constipation with anticholinergic syndrome
Tobacco	Gastro-esophageal reflux Peptic ulcer Pancreatic disease Inflammatory bowel disease Gastrointestinal cancers
Psychostimulants	Ischemic gut Alteration in microbiome
Cannabis	Antiemesis Hyperemesis syndrome
Body packing syndrome	Drug intoxication (may be life threatening)

Mallory-Weiss syndrome is linked to heavy alcohol use. It is characterized by tears in the mucosa at the cardio-esophageal junction after vomiting that can lead to significant bleeding. The syndrome accounts for almost 10% of all cases of bleeding in the upper GI tract.[33] In one series, almost half of patients with this disorder were associated with repeated retching and vomiting following heavy acute alcohol consumption.[34]

The important relationship between alcohol consumption and squamous cell esophageal carcinoma is considered later in this chapter.

Stomach

Alcohol-Related Gastritis

Alcohol-related gastritis has been variably applied to a broad range of upper GI symptoms experienced by individuals who drink heavily.[35,36]

Gastritis denotes inflammation associated with mucosal injury and alcohol has been commonly attributed as a cause of this condition.[37,38] It is often difficult to measure the role of an individual agent, such as alcohol, as the cause of gastritis due to confounding factors and difficulty measuring exposure. Despite alcohol being commonly associated with gastritis there is limited clinical evidence to support this link.

Exposure of the gastric mucosa to high concentrations of alcohol have been shown to induce apoptosis in the cells of the gastric mucosa in rats.[39] At lower concentrations of alcohol achieved during intoxication (1.0% to 4.0%) gastric endothelial cell damage has been demonstrated in an in-vitro model.[40] Active *Helicobacter pylori* (*H. pylori*) infection, a common cause of gastritis, has been associated with alcohol consumption in some settings[41] but in other settings has been identified as a potential protective factor.[42,43] Gastritis in people with alcohol use disorder is strongly associated with *H. pylori* infection and histological and clinical remission occurs with *H. pylori* eradication but not abstinence from alcohol.[44,45] *H. pylori* eradication rates with triple therapy are improved at all levels of alcohol consumption.[46] *H. pylori* expresses alcohol dehydrogenase (ADH) and exposure to alcohol generates acetaldehyde, which may be bactericidal. Furthermore, there is no link between alcohol consumption and chronic atrophic gastritis (CAG)[47]; indeed the risk of CAG is reduced with moderate alcohol consumption possibly due to reduced *H. pylori* infection.[48]

Peptic Ulcer Disease

Most studies have not shown an association between alcohol consumption and development of peptic ulcer disease (PUD) and moderate alcohol consumption may reduce the likelihood of PUD.[49,50] There is conflicting data on the risk of bleeding from peptic ulcers and alcohol. Moderate and heavy alcohol consumption has been associated with PUD bleeding in one large prospective study[51] however, this was not replicated in three further prospective studies.[52-54]

Pancreas

Alcohol-Related Pancreatitis

Pancreatic disease is an important cause of morbidity related to alcohol use. Approximately 25% of cases of acute pancreatitis in the United States (U.S.) are secondary to alcohol use and this association is more common in men.[8] Considerable variation exists in the reported proportion of cases of acute pancreatitis attributed to alcohol worldwide ranging from 5% to 70% in individual studies.[55] Alcohol has been estimated to account for 40% to 70% of all cases of chronic pancreatitis in Western countries with the incidence increasing in both the U.S. and in Europe.[56,57] There is also a significant difference in the proportion of alcohol-related pancreatitis based on ethnic background. A 2019 meta-analysis showed that alcohol has been attributed as the cause of 77% of pancreatitis in African Americans while it was attributed to 60% of cases among Aboriginal Australians.[58]

Etiology

The most common associations of acute pancreatitis in Western societies are gallstones and heavy alcohol use, which together account for approximately 75% cases. Alcohol is the most common cause of chronic pancreatitis in men (59%) but not women (28%) in whom gallstone pancreatitis occurs more often.[56,59] More than one etiology may be present in people with heavy alcohol use who have pancreatitis, including hypercalcemia and severe hypertriglyceridemia or gallstones, while around 10% of cases are idiopathic.[60]

Definitions

Acute pancreatitis refers to an acute inflammatory process of the pancreas, with variable involvement of other regional tissues or remote organ systems. The 2012 revised Atlanta classification of acute pancreatitis identified two phases of the disease: early, which can last for around a week, and late, which can persist for weeks to months. Severity is classified as mild, moderate or severe. Mild acute pancreatitis, the most common form, has no organ failure, local or systemic complications. Moderately severe acute pancreatitis is defined by the presence of transient organ failure, local complications or exacerbation of co-morbid disease. If organ failure persists for longer than 48 hours, the attack is classified as severe acute pancreatitis.[61]

Recurrent episodes of acute pancreatitis, clinical or subclinical, may lead to chronic pancreatitis. Chronic pancreatitis is characterized by chronic inflammation, glandular atrophy and fibrosis.

Susceptibility to Alcohol-Related Pancreatitis

Pancreatic disease only occurs in a minority of those who drink at risky levels. Numerous investigators have attempted to account for individual susceptibility to pancreatitis. Smoking tobacco has been linked with an increased risk,[62,63] and accelerates the progression of chronic alcohol-related pancreatitis.[64,65] Activation of pancreatic stellate cells, key players in pancreatic inflammation and fibrosis, by components of cigarette smoke has been demonstrated in vitro.[66]

Genetic factors that may contribute to increased risk of chronic pancreatitis in people with alcohol use disorder have been identified in the ADH and acetaldehyde dehydrogenase (ALDH) genes, primarily in Japanese studies.[67] A mutation of the gene coding for pancreatic secretory trypsin inhibitor PSTI (SPINK1) may account for a minority of cases.[68] Polymorphisms in the trypsin locus and Claudin-2 locus confer an increased risk of developing alcohol-induced pancreatitis.[67,69] Mutations in chymotrypsin C have been identified more frequently in alcohol-related pancreatitis compared with patients with alcohol related liver disease (2.9% and 0.7%, respectively).[70]

Despite this progress, few patients carry any individual mutation, and individual susceptibility to pancreatitis in people with heavy alcohol use remains unexplained. Studies that focused on the amount, type and pattern of alcohol consumption, diet, hypertriglyceridemia and pancreatic ischemia have not demonstrated consistent effects.[71,72]

Pathogenesis

Alcohol exposure over many years is associated with pancreatic atrophy and fibrosis that may not be clinically apparent until an acute attack of pancreatitis. A number of mechanisms have been described by which alcohol may lead to pancreatic injury.[73] Oxidative metabolism of alcohol generates reactive oxygen species (ROS) while depleting the ROS scavenger glutathione. ROS are generated by the inflammatory response triggered by autodigestion leading to cellular injury. Nonoxidative metabolism produces other toxic metabolites, fatty acid ethyl esters (FAEE), which induce organelle dysfunction. Destabilization of the organelles that contain digestive and lysosomal enzymes leads to autodigestion (**Fig. 91-1**).

Pancreatic fibrosis results from activation of pancreatic stellate cells (PSC).[66] Increased gut permeability, and hence translocation of bacterial lipopolysaccharide into the circulation, may also stimulate PSCs.[74]

Diagnosis

The diagnosis of acute pancreatitis requires two of three criteria: (1) abdominal pain consistent with pancreatitis (persistent, severe epigastric pain of acute onset over a few hours, often radiating to the back), (2) serum lipase (or amylase) levels 3 times the upper limit of normal or (3) imaging with findings characteristic of pancreatitis.[61] Gallstones should be excluded by ultrasound examination, as this is the second most common cause of pancreatitis[75] and may co-exist with unhealthy alcohol use.

The primary clinical feature of chronic pancreatitis is persisting pain and may be very severe and challenging to manage. The pain of chronic pancreatitis is typically diffusely located in the upper abdomen and may radiate to the back

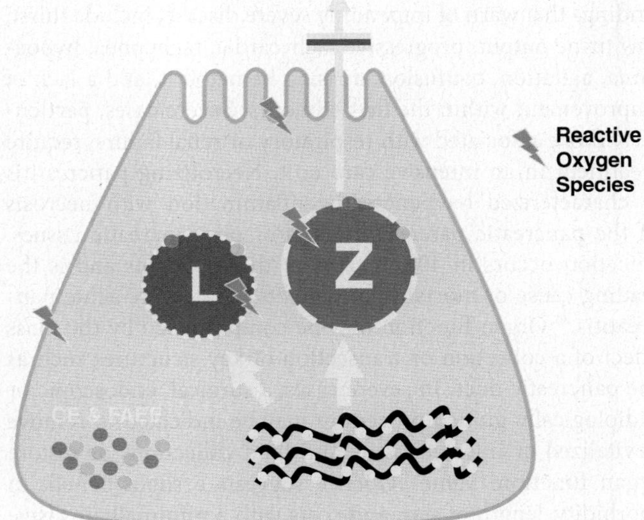

Figure 91-1. Chronic alcohol (ethanol) leads to acute pancreatitis via autodigestion through intracellular activation of digestive enzymes. CE, cholesteryl esters; FAEE, fatty acid ethyl esters; L, lysosomes; Z, zymogen granules. (Adapted from Witt H, Apte MV, Keim V, Wilson JS. Chronic pancreatitis: challenges and advances in pathogenesis, genetics, diagnosis, and therapy. *Gastroenterology*. 2007;132(4):1557-1573.)

when severe. Pain is typically associated with meals and reduces both appetite and food consumption often resulting in weight loss. A minority presents without pain. The other major manifestations are endocrine (diabetes mellitus) and exocrine insufficiency (steatorrhea). Weight loss is mild if present and vitamin deficiency is generally subclinical. Investigations may reveal malabsorption of fat-soluble vitamins and osteopenia. Other complications include pseudocyst formation, biliary or duodenal obstruction, pancreatic ascites or pleural effusion, splenic vein thrombosis, pseudoaneurysms and an increased risk of pancreatic cancer.[76]

Management of Acute Pancreatitis

Generally, pancreatitis is managed in the hospital setting. The severity is assessed clinically, biochemically and radiologically. Supportive care includes fasting, fluid resuscitation, analgesia and monitoring for complications. Intravenous opioids are typically required for analgesia, often using a patient-controlled analgesia device. No difference between opioids has been identified with regard to the risk of pancreatitis complications or serious adverse events.[77] The choice of opioid should be based on local protocol including clinician experience. For patients with mild pancreatitis, most guidelines recommend reintroduction of feeds via the oral route, returning in a stepwise fashion from a clear fluid low-fat diet to a solid diet, when abdominal pain is resolving and inflammatory markers are improving.[72] If oral intake is not likely to be restored within several days, then enteral feeding or total parenteral nutrition (TPN) is indicated.[78]

About 20% of patients with acute pancreatitis have a severe course that carries a 10% to 20% mortality rate.[79,80] Clinical findings that warn of impending severe disease, include thirst, low urine output, progressive tachycardia, tachypnea, hypoxemia, agitation, confusion, a rising hematocrit, and a lack of improvement within the first 48 hours. Severe cases, particularly those associated with respiratory or renal failure, require treatment in an intensive care unit. Necrotizing pancreatitis is characterized by pancreatic inflammation with necrosis of the pancreatic parenchyma and/or peripancreatic tissues. Infection occurs in 40% to 70% of these patients and is the leading cause of mortality in patients with severe acute pancreatitis.[80] Organ function may be compromised by the mass effect of a collection or transection of key structures such as the pancreatic duct. In severe cases, a surgical, endoscopic or radiologically-guided procedure may be indicated to remove devitalized or infected tissue and fluid collections or restore organ function. Some evidence suggests a slight benefit in morbidity, length of stay, and costs with a minimally invasive step-up approach compared with open surgical necrosectomy, but no difference in mortality has been demonstrated.[81] When required, surgery should be deferred until organization of tissues has taken place, typically after 4 weeks.[82,83] An exception is intra-abdominal catastrophe (hemorrhage, perforation, compartment syndrome), which requires immediate intervention.[84] Antibiotics are indicated for all cases of infected necrosis in acute pancreatitis. Outside of this setting, the use of antibiotics, including as prophylaxis in severe pancreatitis with necrosis, is not of proven benefit.[85]

A number of antioxidant therapies have been evaluated for both acute and chronic pancreatitis, given the role of oxidative stress in the pathogenesis of these diseases. Some promising results have been demonstrated from a meta-analysis of small randomized controlled trials for glutamine supplementation.[81,82] Most other therapies have failed to demonstrate any benefit in the treatment of acute pancreatitis.[83] Similarly, the evidence is conflicted in chronic pancreatitis (see below).

Management of Chronic Pancreatitis

Complete abstinence from alcohol is essential to minimize progression of the disease and may help to control pain. Similarly, abstinence from smoking is advisable, but this has not specifically been shown to lessen pain. Non-opioid analgesia may suffice and should be used first.[84] NSAIDs are associated with GI toxicity and persistent use should be avoided. Opioids should not be unreasonably withheld although the risk of opioid use disorder should carefully be managed according to the principles described in other chapters. Opioids are frequently ineffective and should be discontinued if ineffective. Pregabalin is more effective than placebo in providing pain relief[85] but its misuse liability is now well recognized.[86] Although data are lacking in chronic pancreatitis, antidepressants such as tricyclic antidepressants can be used for treating the component of neuropathic pain thought to be common in this condition.[84] Pancreatic enzyme supplements improve serum nutrition parameters and quality of life without significant side effects; there is limited evidence that they improve pain.[87] The use of antioxidant therapy in chronic pancreatitis has been controversial[88-90] but there is evidence that it produces significant pain relief over placebo in meta-analysis.[91,92]

Endoscopic therapy can improve pain in selected patients with outflow obstruction of the main pancreatic duct (MPD) due to strictures or intraductal stones. Endoscopic retrograde cholangio-pancreatography (ERCP) can improve drainage of the MPD by stent placement and/or by stone extraction. Complete or partial pain relief is achieved in around 60% of patients treated with this approach.[84] Celiac plexus injections are effective in around 60% of patients but pain may recur.[93] The procedure is not often performed due to limited efficacy, frequent recurrence, and significant complications[94] and generally only considered when other treatment options have failed.[84]

Exocrine insufficiency is treated by dietary modification, vitamin therapy and pancreatic enzyme replacement. Reduction of dietary fat intake reduces steatorrhea. Pancreatic enzymes are required with each meal and snack. Supplementation of fat-soluble vitamins may be required in patients with significant steatorrhea.[95]

Diabetes associated with pancreatic endocrine insufficiency is known as Type 3c (pancreatogenic) diabetes mellitus (DM). Both insulin and glucagon secretion are affected, resulting in a "brittle" diabetes. It is treated with dietary modification, treatment of malabsorption and pharmacological therapy. Insulin is typically required, though some patients respond to oral hypoglycemics with metformin being the preferred first line agent. Newer agents such as glucagon-like peptide-1 (GLP-1) agonists and dipeptidyl peptidase-4 (DPP-4) inhibitors were initially thought to increase risk of pancreatitis[96,97] and are therefore not recommended for type 3c DM. However, no increased risk of pancreatitis was identified in more recent meta-analysis.[98,99] Case reports of sodium-glucose cotransporter-2 inhibitor induced acute pancreatitis have been published[100,101] but no such risk has been identified in a meta-analysis of randomized control trials (RCT).[102] There is however insufficient evidence to support any recommendation to use these newer agents over metformin or insulin in this form of DM. Long-term surviving patients with this form of diabetes are prone to diabetic complications and should be monitored accordingly.[103]

Small Intestine

Diarrhea is common among those who drink alcohol heavily, both acutely and chronically. Multiple factors contribute to this problem including altered motility, permeability and nutritional disorders.

There are multiple mechanisms by which alcohol effects the small bowel. Alcohol promotes alteration of the normal gut flora (dysbiosis) and bacterial overgrowth, which leads to increased production of endotoxins.[104] Intestinal hyperpermeability develops from chronic alcohol exposure and small bowel mucosal injury can occur by direct contact with alcohol and may lead to loss of epithelium mainly at the villi tips.[105] These effects result in increased gut permeability resulting both in abnormal absorption of luminal content (such as endotoxin, which contributes to the pathogenesis of alcohol-associated liver and pancreatic diseases), impaired nutrient absorption and abnormal leakage of mucosal contents such as albumin.[106,107]

Many defects in absorption have been reported in people with alcohol use disorder, including water, carbohydrate, lipid, vitamins and minerals (calcium, iron, zinc and selenium).[107,108] Ethanol may exacerbate lactase deficiency, especially in African-Americans.[109] Thiamine and folate deficiency are common and clinically relevant among people with alcohol use disorder. Thiamine deficiency is due to a combination of decreased intake, decreased intestinal absorption and impaired utilization by cells.[110] Thiamine deficiency can result in Wernicke encephalopathy, which can progress to irreversible Korsakoff syndrome if left untreated. Folate deficiency occurs secondary to decreased intake, reduced intestinal absorption via inhibiting expression of the reduced folate carrier, impaired hepatic storage and decreased renal tubular reabsorption.[111] Folate deficiency can lead to macrocytic anemia and may promote the progression of alcohol-related liver disease.[112]

Colon

Portal hypertension from alcohol-related liver cirrhosis may manifest as rectal varices.[113] Hemorrhoids are not seen more commonly in patients with portal hypertension, but bleeding from these may be massive.[114] Chronic alcohol exposure has been implicated in increased mucosal hyperpermeability, dysbiosis and bacterial overgrowth of the colonic microflora. These changes are thought to promote alcohol-related liver cirrhosis secondary to increased translocation of endotoxin into the portal circulation. Alcohol use has been associated with higher risk of recurrence in patients with established inflammatory bowel disease but no association with new onset IBD has been identified.[115]

Gastrointestinal Cancer

Alcohol use is a recognized risk factor for several GI neoplasms, including tumors of the tongue, mouth, pharynx, larynx, esophagus, stomach, pancreas, colon and liver.[116,117] A comprehensive meta-analysis reported that a relatively modest average consumption of 12.5 g per day, well within the guidelines for men in many countries including the U.S., is associated with increased risk of GI cancer. For example, consumption of 12.5 g alcohol per day was associated with a relative risk (RR) of 1.13 for oropharyngeal and 1.26 for esophageal squamous cell carcinoma (SCC). Moderate levels of alcohol consumption defined as 12.5 g to 50.0 g alcohol per day were associated with a 1.17 RR for colorectal cancers and heavy consumption (>50 g per day) associated with a 2.07 RR for cancer of the liver, 1.21 for gastric cancer and 1.19 for pancreatic cancer.[118] Cancer risk rose continuously from zero alcohol consumption with no safe level, suggesting that the less alcohol consumed, the lower the risk of cancer.

There are large variations in the global burden of alcohol related cancer depending on sex and geographical location. Men in Eastern Asia and Eastern Europe have the highest rate of alcohol-related cancer and among women, Eastern Europe, Australia, New Zealand and Western Europe have the highest rates. The lowest rates are in Northern Africa and Western Asia for both sexes.[3] A multiethnic cohort study has shown an increased risk of alcohol-related colorectal cancer for Native Hawaiians, Japanese Americans, Latinos and White persons.[119] Esophageal SCC is particularly common in East Asia with studies suggesting a genetic predisposition due to a high prevalence of polymorphisms in aldehyde dehydrogenase that result in decreased activity.[120]

Alcohol use has been strongly associated with an increased incidence of esophageal (and oropharyngeal) SCC, especially in those who also smoke.[121-123] In a large landmark case-controlled study of oral and pharyngeal cancers in four areas of the U.S., Blot et al. reported a 5.8 fold increased risk among those who drink alcohol, a 7.4 fold increased risk among people who smoke tobacco cigarettes and a 38 fold increased risk among those who both drank and smoked.[124] The effect of alcohol on cancer risk appears to be dose related, rather than to the type of alcohol consumed, with a stronger association seen in men.[125] Unlike esophageal SCC, esophageal adenocarcinoma is unrelated to alcohol.[118,126]

Chronic pancreatitis is a well-known risk factor for pancreatic cancer and is commonly secondary to alcohol consumption.[127] It is difficult to determine if alcohol in the absence of pancreatitis is also a risk factor for pancreatic cancer. A large European prospective cohort study[128] attempted to control for chronic pancreatitis by sensitivity analysis. They found an association with heavy alcohol consumption (>60 g per day) and pancreatic cancer in men with hazard ratio of 1.77 indicating alcohol may play a carcinogenic role in absence of clinically evident pancreatitis.

Alcohol has long been recognized as a predisposing factor for hepatocellular carcinoma (HCC), but it is unclear whether alcohol is a direct hepatic carcinogen independent of the development of cirrhosis.[125,129] For further detail on this topic please refer to Chapter 89.

The mechanisms by which alcohol exerts its carcinogenic effect is varied and not completely understood.[130] Pure alcohol is not a carcinogen in animal studies[131] although it may aid in the penetration of other carcinogens in the digestive tract.[117] Acetaldehyde is the primary metabolite of alcohol and thought to exert direct carcinogenic effects by aberrant methylation of DNA. Chronic alcohol consumption causes increased production of ROS and oxidative stress primarily through induction of CYP2E1. Other potential mechanism that may contribute to the carcinogenic effect of alcohol include nutritional depletion such as folate deficiency, impaired immune surveillance and potential carcinogenic impurities contained in alcoholic drinks.[117,132]

GASTROINTESTINAL SYMPTOMS ASSOCIATED WITH OTHER DRUGS

Opioids

Opioids exert multiple effects on the GI tract from reducing somatic and visceral pain to inhibition of motility and secretions. Opioids act via all three receptor classes in the brain, spinal cord and enteric nervous systems. Low doses act at enteric nervous system sites and higher doses also act within the central nervous system (CNS). These effects usually are manifest as constipation, nausea, vomiting, bloating, early satiety and pain.[133] Opioid-induced bowel dysfunction (OIBD) refers to a collection of primarily GI motility disorders secondary to opioids and includes opioid-induced constipation (OIC), nausea, vomiting, bloating, early satiety and pain.[133] The primary mechanisms by which OIBD occurs is through blockade of propulsive peristalsis, inhibition of the secretion of intestinal fluids, and an increase in intestinal fluid absorption. Opioids decrease the activity of both excitatory and inhibitory neurons in the myenteric plexus. In addition, they increase smooth-muscle tone and inhibit the coordinated peristalsis required for propulsion, leading to disordered, nonpropulsive contractile activity, which contributes to nausea and vomiting as well as constipation. Longer GI transit time causes excessive water and electrolyte reabsorption from feces, and decreased biliary and pancreatic secretion further dehydrate stools.[133]

Concurrent use of other constipating drugs (eg, tricyclic antidepressants), dehydration, advancing age, immobility, metabolic abnormalities (eg, hypercalcemia), chemotherapy (particularly the vinca alkaloids) and tumor-related bowel obstruction may all contribute. Not all opioid formulations are equally constipating. Although the results of randomized trials are conflicting, a systematic review concluded that there is less constipation with transdermal fentanyl than with oral sustained-release morphine.[134] The phenomenon of nonmedical loperamide use observed with increasing frequency may produce the unintended consequence of severe constipation.[135]

Among persons receiving methadone for the treatment of opioid use disorder, constipation is common and tends to be worse early in treatment.[136,137] The high prevalence of persisting constipation suggests that tolerance to the gut effects of opioids occurs to only a limited extent. In one study, 58% of subjects in methadone maintenance experienced some degree of constipation and 10% had severe problems.[138] Constipation was equally common in people taking buprenorphine compared to methadone, but symptoms were more often described as severe in people taking methadone and also common among those using heroin.[139] Fecal impaction, and even stercoral perforation, have been described.[140] Bowel symptoms usually respond to increased fluid intake and fiber supplementation to correct for inadequate dietary intake. Laxatives are not often required but osmotic agents such as lactulose and polyethylene glycol are often used as first line agents. In the context of refractory constipation, combinations of over-the-counter laxatives, secretagogues such as lubiprostone, linaclotide and plecanatide (in countries where these are available), 5-HT4 agonists such as prucalopride and peripherally acting μ-opioid receptor agonists (PAMORAs) can be considered.[141] PAMORAs including methylnaltrexone, naloxegol and naldemedine do not cross the blood-brain barrier and have no anti-analgesic effect.[142,143] Short-term use may be considered for refractory cases in specialized settings.

An underrecognized complication of chronic opioid use is opioid-induced GI hyperalgesia (OIH; formerly "narcotic bowel syndrome"). This is a centrally-mediated disorder of GI pain and presents as a progressive and paradoxical increase in abdominal pain despite continuing or escalating doses of opioid analgesics. The diagnosis of OIH is based on the Rome IV diagnostic criteria and include: (1) chronic or frequently recurring abdominal pain that is treated with acute high-dose or chronic opioids, (2) the nature and intensity of the pain is not explained by a current or previous GI diagnosis, (3) two or more of the following: (i) the pain worsens or incompletely resolves with continued or escalating dosages of opioids, (ii) there is marked worsening of pain when the opioid dose wanes and improvement when opioids are re-instituted (soar and crash), (iii) There is a progression of the frequency, duration, and intensity of pain episodes.[144] OIH is thought to result from neuroplastic changes in the peripheral nervous system and central nervous system that lead to sensitization of pronociceptive pathways. Proposed molecular mechanisms include activation of central glutaminergic system by N-methyl-D-aspartate (NMDA) receptor activation and inhibition, increased spinal dynorphins and activation of descending spinal pathways that facilitate nociceptive processes.[145] The primary method of management is judicious opioid withdrawal.[144]

Laxatives

Surreptitious laxative use is among the more common causes for unexplained chronic diarrhea. It represents an intriguing form of substance use, in that the laxative does not directly cause euphoria and is observed in people without other substance use. These patients may present to primary care clinicians and gastroenterologists. The largest group with these issues is individuals with eating disorders such as bulimia and anorexia nervosa. The second largest group tends to be middle aged or older women who started to use laxatives for constipation and continue to overuse. In this setting, increasing doses of stimulant type laxatives reflect pharmacological tolerance. The diagnosis can be difficult and may be supported by serum hypokalemia, and stool testing where fecal electrolytes, pH and osmolality are helpful in providing evidence of laxative use. Urine laxative screening can be used to directly identify the presence of stimulant laxatives such as senna and bisacodyl.[146,147]

Anticholinergics

In high doses, anticholinergic drugs alter mood, and are occasionally used, particularly when prescribed to relieve extra-pyramidal symptoms in people receiving antipsychotic medications[148] and among those with limited access to other drugs, such as people in prison. Amitriptyline and other tricyclic antidepressant drugs may be used by people on opioid agonist treatment.[149] Clonidine and/or hyoscine prescribed for opioid withdrawal may also be used. Patients develop marked constipation and abdominal pain as well as dry mouth and blurred vision; delirium accompanies more severe cases.[150] In the authors' experience, patients have had previous substance use disorder and welcomed an explanation of their symptoms and participated in structured withdrawal of the anticholinergic medication.

Tobacco

More recently, use of electronic drug delivery devices (EDDDs) has exposed many to high doses of nicotine. Evidence of GI damage is accumulating, and inflammation of the gums, pharyngitis, nausea, vomiting, and diarrhea have been reported.[151] Alterations to the microbiome have been reported in people who use both EDDDs and tobacco.[152] The research considered below has evaluated the effects of tobacco smoking.

Gastro-Esophageal Reflux

Tobacco smoking has been linked to exacerbations of reflux symptoms. Abstinence of daily smoking was associated with an improvement in gastro-esophageal reflux symptoms from severe to minor or no symptoms with an adjusted odds ratio of 1.78 in one large prospective population-based cohort study. The association was only present among individuals with a body mass index (BMI) within normal range.[153] Nicotine has been shown to reduce LES pressure and promote gastro-esophageal reflux in response to straining during coughing and deep breathing.[154] Tobacco cigarette smoking has been associated with increased gastro-esophageal reflux that improves significantly during nonsmoking periods based on 24-hour pH monitoring.[155,156] Not all studies have yielded consistent findings. One study found that smoking did not influence basal LES pressure or esophageal motility.[157] While stopping smoking cannot be recommended as the sole treatment for reflux, it is reasonable to advise patients with gastro-esophageal reflux disease (GERD) to quit smoking based upon the association with reflux, with the expectation that GERD might improve and to prevent the myriad other adverse effects of tobacco.

Peptic Ulceration

There is considerable evidence that tobacco smoking is associated with a dose-dependent increased risk of peptic ulcer.[49] Smoking may reduce mucosal blood flow, increase gastric acid secretion, and diminish bicarbonate secretion, along with other actions that promote PUD.[158] Heavy smoking is associated with delayed ulcer healing and the risk of recurrence is increased.[159,160] Smoking increases the risk of peptic ulcer perforation.[161] Finally, the overall ulcer-related mortality is increased in those who smoke compared to those who do not.[162,163]

Pancreatic Disease

Evidence from a number of countries provides a clear link between tobacco smoking and pancreatic cancer. Several studies have consistently found a moderately increased risk of pancreatic cancer among people who smoke tobacco products, which increases significantly with increasing numbers of cigarettes smoked and smoking duration.[164,165]

Multiple studies have found positive associations between smoking and both acute and chronic pancreatitis.[166,167] A large cohort study found that the RR for smoking compared to never smoked was 3.1 for idiopathic pancreatitis and 4.9 for alcohol-related pancreatitis whereas no association was identified with gallstone pancreatitis.[167] It appears appropriate to advise patients with alcohol-related and idiopathic pancreatitis that smoking contributes to their disease and to encourage them to quit.

Inflammatory Bowel Disease

A curious relationship exists between tobacco smoking and inflammatory bowel disease. Smoking has consistently been shown to increase the risk of Crohn disease (CD) but to decrease the risk of ulcerative colitis (UC).[168]

People who smoke are more than twice as likely to develop CD as people who don't smoke.[169] Smoking may also increase the risk of recurrence of CD. Multiple studies suggest that patients who stop smoking can decrease the risk of flares and have similar risk to nonsmokers with prolonged abstinence.[170] Tobacco smoke appears to interfere with epithelial integrity and immune responses to pathogenic bacteria.[171]

Tobacco smoking is clearly associated with reduced severity of established UC, suggesting nicotine has therapeutic potential for this disease. Nicotine influences immune cellular function, increases mucin production, relaxes colonic smooth muscle, increases endogenous glucocorticoids and influences rectal blood flow and intestinal permeability.[172] The severity of UC increases after smoking abstinence, with an increase in the need for hospital admission and major medical therapy.[173] Meta-analysis of the effect of tobacco smoking on the natural history of UC have failed to show a significant benefit in preventing complications and progression of disease comparing those who smoke with those who do not and any small benefit is not thought to outweigh the other adverse effects of tobacco smoking.[174,175] Nicotine-based therapy has been explored using strategies including topical colonic administration of nicotine[176] but despite modest benefit this has not been further pursued as a commercially available therapeutic agent. A Cochrane review of transdermal nicotine patches for the treatment of mild to moderate UC has suggested that these agents can improve UC compared to placebo[177] but have significant adverse events and have not been shown to be more effective than other treatments.

Gastrointestinal Malignancy

Tobacco smoking has been linked to cancers throughout the GI tract including gastric, colorectal, biliary, hepatic and pancreatic cancer.[165,178-180] Nicotine acts on the gut acetylcholine receptors to promote cell growth factor synthesis and signal transduction. The upper GI tract is particularly exposed to the carcinogenic components of tobacco smoke. The microbiome changes also appear to play a pro-carcinogenic role.[181] Smoking is strongly associated with esophageal cancer as discussed above, and this risk is increased substantially when combined with moderate to heavy alcohol consumption.[182]

Psychostimulants

Cocaine can cause profound vasoconstriction that can lead to ischemic injury to the gut and in turn to ischemic colitis, intestinal infarction and perforation.[183] Cocaine has also been implicated as a rare cause of pancreatitis in case reports.[184] The composition of the gut microbiome may alter the behavioral response to cocaine. A novel study found that mice with reduced gut bacteria had enhanced sensitivity to cocaine reward.[185]

Similar to cocaine, methamphetamine has been reported as a rare cause of ischemic injury to the gut secondary to vasoconstriction from release of norepinephrine.[186] In some cases this can manifest with the potentially lethal complication of paralytic ileus.[187] Alterations of the GI microbiome have been identified in persons who use methamphetamine. Dopamine and norepinephrine excess stimulates alterations in the gut microbiota while bowel ischemia is associated with increased intestinal permeability. These two factors promote translocation of bacterial products into the systemic circulation, which is postulated to stimulate a systemic immune response and play a potential role in neuropsychiatric disorders.[188] Dysbiosis of the gut microbiome has been identified in men who have sex with men that use methamphetamine. This alteration resulted in an imbalanced microbiome that favored pro-inflammatory bacteria including some that have been associated with poor HIV outcomes.[189]

Cannabis

Cannabinoid receptors (CB1 and CB2) are widely expressed throughout both the upper and lower GI tract and are also expressed on hepatic stellate cells. Consequently, cannabinoids influence a range of GI functions in health and disease.[190] Evidence that cannabinoids are important in regulation of GI motility have come from various animal studies. Cannabinoids appear to decrease motility by multiple mechanisms, which include interaction with the vagal parasympathetic control of motility and modulation of cholinergic neurotransmission. The endocannabinoid system has been implicated in food intake and energy balance via bi-directional neurotransmission between the gut and brain. In a rat model, consumption of fatty food leads to endocannabinoid signaling to the brain, which is thought to reinforce hedonic eating.[191]

Nausea and vomiting are side effects of many chemotherapeutics and reduce the quality of life of patients with diabetes, cancer and acquired immune deficiency syndrome. Cannabis and other cannabinoids appear to be effective antiemetics. The synthetic cannabis-related products dronabinol and nabilone have been approved by the U.S. Food and Drug Administration for refractory chemotherapy induced nausea and vomiting.[192] Oral preparations of cannabidiol (CBD) and delta-9-tetrahydrocannabinol (THC) have benefit in reducing chemotherapy induced nausea and vomiting.[193] Most recently, a similar THC/CBD preparation provided additional benefit in patients receiving cancer chemotherapy who were also receiving guideline-consistent antiemetic prophylaxis.[194] The antiemetic effect has been demonstrated in an animal model and is related to interaction with CB1 and 5-HT3 receptors in the dorsal vagal nucleus.[192] Additional information regarding the therapeutic effectiveness of cannabis and cannabinoids and related issues are discussed in Chapter 126 of this textbook.

Despite this anti-emetic effect, cannabis has also been linked to a cannabis hyperemesis syndrome. This syndrome is characterized by cyclical nausea, vomiting and abdominal pain associated with chronic and typically heavy daily cannabis use. An almost pathognomonic characteristic of this syndrome is compulsive hot bathing for symptom relief.[195] The pathophysiology is poorly understood and multiple hypotheses have been proposed for the paradoxical emetogenic property of cannabis in chronic use. Dysregulation of the endocannabinoid system from chronic cannabis exposure leading to derangement in the body's intrinsic control of nausea and vomiting is one common hypothesis.[196] Several pharmacological approaches have been tried including benzodiazepines, haloperidol and capsaicin[197] but evidence is limited. The only treatments to be evaluated by RCT are haloperidol compared to ondansetron. Haloperidol proved superior with treatment success in 54% of patients compared to 29% for the ondansetron group.[198] Capsaicin activates the transient receptor potential vanilloid-1 receptor (TRPV-1) as does heat, suggesting a link with relief from hot showers.[199] It has been used with moderate success with a reduction in the requirement for opioids and other antiemetic agents[200] but the evidence to support this approach is currently limited. Ultimately the most effective treatment for cannabis hyperemesis syndrome is stopping cannabis use. The duration of cannabis abstinence to achieve sustained symptom relief is unknown and resumption of cannabis use is associated with recurrent symptoms.[191]

"Body Packing"

Persons smuggling illegal drugs may ingest multiple packages made from latex condoms, wax or plastic bags containing large amounts of cocaine, heroin, methamphetamine, or other drugs aiming to retrieve these after reaching their destination.[201,202] Packages may also be placed into the rectum or vagina.[202] The amount of drugs varies from small, potentially for personal use, to large scale for distribution. The incidence of this practice is unknown. The affected person may present with life-threatening symptoms of intoxication, including seizures and cardiorespiratory collapse, as well as mechanical obstruction from the ingested drug packets. Lethal drug absorption through rubber condoms may occur without rupture. Management can be challenging and involves close monitoring for complications such as drug intoxication, bowel obstruction or perforation, as well as administration of polyethylene glycol laxatives to expedite passage of packages and regular imaging with plain abdominal x-ray and/or CT until the gut is clear.[201,202]

SUMMARY

Alcohol, tobacco and other substances have a broad range of detrimental and in some cases beneficial effects on the GI tract. Heavy alcohol use is associated with injury throughout the GI tract. Males suffer the greatest alcohol-related burden of disease. There is evidence that alcohol and other substances have a negative impact on the GI microbiome with a broad range of yet to be understood implications in development of disease. Tobacco is associated with GI malignancy, GERD, peptic ulceration, and Crohn disease but is protective against ulcerative colitis. Stimulants are associated with GI ischemia that may be life-threatening. Cannabis can be an effective anti-emetic but paradoxically chronic use can contribute to the cannabis hyperemesis syndrome. Opioids commonly cause constipation and occasionally GI hyperalgesia that can limit their use.

Recognition and diagnosis of GI disturbance related to alcohol and other substances allows for better management of symptoms. Linking symptoms to substance use sets a foundation for comprehensive treatment and prevention of recurrence. Research in this area provides an opportunity to not only identify processes whereby alcohol and other substances contribute to disease but also to improve management of established GI conditions.

REFERENCES

1. Bujanda L. The effects of alcohol consumption upon the gastrointestinal tract. *Am J Gastroenterol.* 2000;95(12):3374-3382.
2. Haber PS, Kortt NC. Alcohol use disorder and the gut. *Addiction.* 2021;116(3):658-667.
3. Rumgay H, Shield K, Charvat H, et al. Global burden of cancer in 2020 attributable to alcohol consumption: a population-based study. *Lancet Oncol.* 2021;22(8):1071-1080.
4. GBD 2019 Risk Factors Collaborators. Global burden of 87 risk factors in 204 countries and territories, 1990-2019: a systematic analysis for the Global Burden of Disease Study 2019. *Lancet.* 2020;396(10258):1223-1249.
5. Keyes KM. Age, period, and cohort effects in alcohol use in the United States in the 20th and 21st centuries: implications for the coming decades. *Alcohol Res.* 2022;42(1):02.
6. Witbrodt J, Mulia N, Zemore SE, Kerr WC. Racial/ethnic disparities in alcohol-related problems: differences by gender and level of heavy drinking. *Alcohol Clin Exp Res.* 2014;38(6):1662-1670.
7. Damjanovska S, Karb DB, Cohen SM. Increasing prevalence and racial disparity of alcohol-related gastrointestinal and liver disease during the COVID-19 pandemic: a population-based national study. *J Clin Gastroenterol.* 2022;57(2):185-188.
8. Krishna SG, Kamboj AK, Hart PA, Hinton A, Conwell DL. The changing epidemiology of acute pancreatitis hospitalizations: a decade of trends and the impact of chronic pancreatitis. *Pancreas.* 2017;46(4):482-488.
9. Scully C, Bagán JV, Eveson JW, Barnard N, Turner FM. Sialosis: 35 cases of persistent parotid swelling from two countries. *Br J Oral Maxillofac Surg.* 2008;46(6):468-472.
10. Mandel L, Hamele-Bena D. Alcoholic parotid sialadenosis. *J Am Dent Assoc.* (1939). 1997;128(10):1411-1415.
11. Merlo C, Bohl L, Carda C, Gómez de Ferraris ME, Carranza M. Parotid sialosis: morphometrical analysis of the glandular parenchyme and stroma among diabetic and alcoholic patients. *J Oral Pathol Med.* 2010;39(1):10-15.
12. Dukić W, Dobrijević TT, Katunarić M, Lesić S. Caries prevalence in chronic alcoholics and the relationship to salivary flow rate and pH. *Cent Eur J Public Health.* 2013;21(1):43-47.
13. Dutta SK, Orestes M, Vengulekur S, Kwo P. Ethanol and human saliva: effect of chronic alcoholism on flow rate, composition, and epidermal growth factor. *Am J Gastroenterol.* 1992;87(3):350-354.
14. Enberg N, Alho H, Loimaranta V, Lenander-Lumikari M. Saliva flow rate, amylase activity, and protein and electrolyte concentrations in saliva after acute alcohol consumption. *Oral Surg Oral Med Oral Pathol Oral Radiol Endod.* 2001;92(3):292-298.
15. Mascrès C, Ming-Wen F, Joly JG. Morphologic changes of the esophageal mucosa in the rat after chronic alcohol ingestion. *Exp Pathol.* 1984;25(3):147-153.
16. Muller P, Hepke B, Meldau U, Raabe G. Tissue damage in the rabbit oral mucosa by acute and chronic direct toxic action of different alcohol concentrations. *Exp Pathol.* 1983;24(2-3):171-181.
17. Maier H, Weidauer H, Zoller J, et al. Effect of chronic alcohol consumption on the morphology of the oral mucosa. *Alcohol Clin Exp Res.* 1994;18(2):387-391.
18. Feng L, Wang L. Effects of alcohol on the morphological and structural changes in oral mucosa. *Pak J Med Sci.* 2013;29(4):1046-1049.

19. Simanowski UA, Stickel F, Maier H, Gartner U, Seitz HK. Effect of alcohol on gastrointestinal cell regeneration as a possible mechanism in alcohol-associated carcinogenesis. *Alcohol.* 1995;12(2):111-115.
20. Squier CA, Cox P, Hall BK. Enhanced penetration of nitrosonornicotine across oral mucosa in the presence of ethanol. *J Oral Pathol.* 1986;15(5):276-279.
21. Reidy J, McHugh E, Stassen LF. A review of the relationship between alcohol and oral cancer. *Surgeon.* 2011;9(5):278-283.
22. O'Grady I, Anderson A, O'Sullivan J. The interplay of the oral microbiome and alcohol consumption in oral squamous cell carcinomas. *Oral Oncol.* 2020;110:105011.
23. Kaufman SE, Kaye MD. Induction of gastro-oesophageal reflux by alcohol. *Gut.* 1978;19(4):336-338.
24. Mayer EM, Grabowski CJ, Fisher RS. Effects of graded doses of alcohol upon esophageal motor function. *Gastroenterology.* 1978;75(6):1133-1136.
25. Hogan WJ, Viegas de Andrade SR, Winship DH. Ethanol-induced acute esophageal motor dysfunction. *J Appl Physiol.* 1972;32(6):755-760.
26. Ferdinandis TG, Dissanayake AS, de Silva HJ. Chronic alcoholism and esophageal motor activity: a 24-h ambulatory manometry study. *J Gastroenterol Hepatol.* 2006;21(7):1157-1162.
27. Silver LS, Worner TM, Korsten MA. Esophageal function in chronic alcoholics. *Am J Gastroenterol.* 1986;81(6):423-427.
28. Grande L, Monforte R, Ros E, et al. High amplitude contractions in the middle third of the oesophagus: a manometric marker of chronic alcoholism? *Gut.* 1996;38(5):655-662.
29. Keshavarzian A, Polepalle C, Iber FL, Durkin M. Secondary esophageal contractions are abnormal in chronic alcoholics. *Dig Dis Sci.* 1992;37(4):517-522.
30. Mohammed I, Nightingale P, Trudgill NJ. Risk factors for gastro-oesophageal reflux disease symptoms: a community study. *Aliment Pharmacol Ther.* 2005;21(7):821-827.
31. Pan J, Cen L, Chen W, Yu C, Li Y, Shen Z. Alcohol consumption and the risk of gastroesophageal reflux disease: a systematic review and meta-analysis. *Alcohol Alcohol.* 2019;54(1):62-69.
32. Nocon M, Labenz J, Willich SN. Lifestyle factors and symptoms of gastro-oesophageal reflux -- a population-based study. *Aliment Pharmacol Ther.* 2006;23(1):169-174.
33. Di Fiore F, Lecleire S, Merle V, et al. Changes in characteristics and outcome of acute upper gastrointestinal haemorrhage: a comparison of epidemiology and practices between 1996 and 2000 in a multicentre French study. *Eur J Gastroenterol Hepatol.* 2005;17(6):641-647.
34. Kortas DY, Haas LS, Simpson WG, Nickel NJ III, Gates LK Jr. Mallory-Weiss tear: predisposing factors and predictors of a complicated course. *Am J Gastroenterol.* 2001;96(10):2863-2865.
35. Feinman L, Korsten MA, Lieber CS. Alcohol and the digestive tract. In: Lieber CS, ed. *Medical and Nutritional Complications of Alcoholism.* Plenum; 1992:307-340.
36. Konturek JW, Bielanski W, Konturek SJ, Domschke W. Eradication of *Helicobacter pylori* and gastrin-somatostatin link in duodenal ulcer patients. *J Physiol Pharmacol.* 1996;47(1):161-175.
37. Azer SA, Akhondi H. *Gastritis.* StatPearls Publishing; 2022. Accessed June 21, 2023. https://www.ncbi.nlm.nih.gov/books/NBK544250/
38. Dixon MF, Genta RM, Yardley JH, Correa P. Classification and grading of gastritis. The updated Sydney System. International Workshop on the Histopathology of Gastritis, Houston 1994. *Am J Surg Pathol.* 1996;20(10):1161-1181.
39. Liu ES, Cho CH. Relationship between ethanol-induced gastritis and gastric ulcer formation in rats. *Digestion.* 2000;62(4):232-239.
40. Kvietys PR, Twohig B, Danzell J, Specian RD. Ethanol-induced injury to the rat gastric mucosa. Role of neutrophils and xanthine oxidase-derived radicals. *Gastroenterology.* 1990;98(4):909-920.
41. Zhang L, Eslick GD, Xia HH, Wu C, Phung N, Talley NJ. Relationship between alcohol consumption and active *Helicobacter pylori* infection. *Alcohol Alcohol.* 2010;45(1):89-94.
42. Murray LJ, Lane AJ, Harvey IM, Donovan JL, Nair P, Harvey RF. Inverse relationship between alcohol consumption and active *Helicobacter pylori* infection: the Bristol Helicobacter project. *Am J Gastroenterol.* 2002;97(11):2750-2755.
43. Liu SY, Han XC, Sun J, Chen GX, Zhou XY, Zhang GX. Alcohol intake and *Helicobacter pylori* infection: a dose-response meta-analysis of observational studies. *Infect Dis (Lond).* 2016;48(4):303-309.
44. Uppal R, Lateef SK, Korsten MA, Paronetto F, Lieber CS. Chronic alcoholic gastritis. Roles of alcohol and *Helicobacter pylori. Arch Intern Med.* 1991;151(4):760-764.
45. Hauge T, Persson J, Kjerstadius T. *Helicobacter pylori*, active chronic antral gastritis, and gastrointestinal symptoms in alcoholics. *Alcohol ClinExp Res.* 1994;18(4):886-888.
46. Baena JM, Lopez C, Hidalgo A, et al. Relation between alcohol consumption and the success of *Helicobacter pylori* eradication therapy using omeprazole, clarithromycin and amoxicillin for 1 week. *Eur J Gastroenterol Hepatol.* 2002;14(3):291-296.
47. Adamu MA, Weck MN, Rothenbacher D, Brenner H. Incidence and risk factors for the development of chronic atrophic gastritis: five year follow-up of a population-based cohort study. *Int J Cancer.* 2011;128(7):1652-1658.
48. Gao L, Weck MN, Stegmaier C, Rothenbacher D, Brenner H. Alcohol consumption and chronic atrophic gastritis: population-based study among 9,444 older adults from Germany. *Int J Cancer.* 2009;125(12):2918-2922.
49. Rosenstock S, Jørgensen T, Bonnevie O, Andersen L. Risk factors for peptic ulcer disease: a population based prospective cohort study comprising 2416 Danish adults. *Gut.* 2003;52(2):186-193.
50. Johnsen R, Førde OH, Straume B, Burhol PG. Aetiology of peptic ulcer: a prospective population study in Norway. *J Epidemiol Community Health.* 1994;48(2):156-160.
51. Andersen IB, Jørgensen T, Bonnevie O, Grønbaek M, Sørensen TI. Smoking and alcohol intake as risk factors for bleeding and perforated peptic ulcers: a population-based cohort study. *Epidemiology.* 2000;11(4):434-439.
52. Stack WA, Atherton JC, Hawkey GM, Logan RF, Hawkey CJ. Interactions between *Helicobacter pylori* and other risk factors for peptic ulcer bleeding. *Aliment Pharmacol Ther.* 2002;16(3):497-506.
53. Imhof M, Ohmann C, Hartwig A, Thon KP, Hengels KJ, Röher HD. Which peptic ulcers bleed? Results of a case-control study. *DUSUK Study Group. Scand J Gastroenterol.* 1997;32(2):131-138.
54. Hsu PI, Lai KH, Tseng HH, et al. Risk factors for presentation with bleeding in patients with *Helicobacter pylori*-related peptic ulcer diseases. *J Clin Gastroenterol.* 2000;30(4):386-391.
55. Zilio MB, Eyff TF, Azeredo-Da-Silva ALF, Bersch VP, Osvaldt AB. A systematic review and meta-analysis of the aetiology of acute pancreatitis. *HPB (Oxford).* 2019;21(3):259-267.
56. Roberts SE, Morrison-Rees S, John A, Williams JG, Brown TH, Samuel DG. The incidence and aetiology of acute pancreatitis across Europe. *Pancreatology.* 2017;17(2):155-165.
57. Kleeff J, Whitcomb DC, Shimosegawa T, et al. Chronic pancreatitis. *Nat Rev Dis Primers.* 2017;3(1):17060.
58. Cervantes A, Waymouth EK, Petrov MS. African-Americans and Indigenous peoples have increased burden of diseases of the exocrine pancreas: a systematic review and meta-analysis. *Dig Dis Sci.* 2019;64(1):249-261.
59. Yadav D, Timmons L, Benson JT, Dierkhising RA, Chari ST. Incidence, prevalence, and survival of chronic pancreatitis: a population-based study. *Am J Gastroenterol.* 2011;106(12):2192-2199.
60. Mederos MA, Reber HA, Girgis MD. Acute pancreatitis: a review. *JAMA.* 2021;325(4):382-390.
61. Banks PA, Bollen TL, Dervenis C, et al. Classification of acute pancreatitis--2012: revision of the Atlanta classification and definitions by international consensus. *Gut.* 2013;62(1):102-111.
62. Talamini G, Bassi C, Falconi M, et al. Alcohol and smoking as risk factors in chronic pancreatitis and pancreatic cancer. *Dig Dis Sci.* 1999;44(7):1303-1311.
63. Yadav D, Lowenfels AB. The epidemiology of pancreatitis and pancreatic cancer. *Gastroenterology.* 2013;144(6):1252-1261.
64. Maisonneuve P, Lowenfels AB, Mullhaupt B, et al. Cigarette smoking accelerates progression of alcoholic chronic pancreatitis. *Gut.* 2005;54(4):510-514.

65. Kume K, Masamune A, Ariga H, Shimosegawa T. Alcohol consumption and the risk for developing pancreatitis: a case-control study in Japan. *Pancreas*. 2015;44(1):53-58.
66. Lee AT, Xu Z, Pothula SP, et al. Alcohol and cigarette smoke components activate human pancreatic stellate cells: implications for the progression of chronic pancreatitis. *Alcohol Clin Exp Res*. 2015;39(11):2123-2133.
67. Aghdassi AA, Weiss FU, Mayerle J, Lerch MM, Simon P. Genetic susceptibility factors for alcohol-induced chronic pancreatitis. *Pancreatology*. 2015;15(4 Suppl):S23-S31.
68. Witt H, Apte MV, Keim V, Wilson JS. Chronic pancreatitis: challenges and advances in pathogenesis, genetics, diagnosis, and therapy. *Gastroenterology*. 2007;132(4):1557-1573.
69. Weiss FU, Hesselbarth N, Párniczky A, et al. Common variants in the CLDN2-MORC4 and PRSS1-PRSS2 loci confer susceptibility to acute pancreatitis. *Pancreatology*. 2018;18(5):477-481.
70. Rosendahl J, Witt H, Szmola R, et al. Chymotrypsin C (CTRC) variants that diminish activity or secretion are associated with chronic pancreatitis. *Nat Genet*. 2008;40(1):78-82.
71. Apte MV, Pirola RC, Wilson JS. Individual susceptibility to alcoholic pancreatitis. *J Gastroenterol Hepatol*. 2008;23(Suppl 1):S63-S68.
72. Lankisch PG, Apte M, Banks PA. Acute pancreatitis. *Lancet*. 2015; 386(9988):85-96.
73. Apte MV, Pirola RC, Wilson JS. Mechanisms of alcoholic pancreatitis. *J Gastroenterol Hepatol*. 2010;25(12):1816-1826.
74. Vonlaufen A, Xu Z, Daniel B, et al. Bacterial endotoxin: a trigger factor for alcoholic pancreatitis? Evidence from a novel, physiologically relevant animal model. *Gastroenterology*. 2007;133(4):1293-1303.
75. Goodman AJ, Neoptolemos JP, Carr-Locke DL, Finlay DB, Fossard DP. Detection of gall stones after acute pancreatitis. *Gut*. 1985;26(2):125-132.
76. Majumder S, Chari ST. Chronic pancreatitis. *Lancet*. 2016;387(10031): 1957-1966.
77. Basurto Ona X, Rigau Comas D, Urrutia G. Opioids for acute pancreatitis pain. *Cochrane Database Syst Rev*. 2013;7:CD009179.
78. Zhao XL, Zhu SF, Xue GJ, et al. Early oral refeeding based on hunger in moderate and severe acute pancreatitis: a prospective controlled, randomized clinical trial. *Nutrition*. 2015;31(1):171-175.
79. McKay CJ, Imrie CW. The continuing challenge of early mortality in acute pancreatitis. *Br J Surg*. 2004;91(10):1243-1244.
80. Chatila AT, Bilal M, Guturu P. Evaluation and management of acute pancreatitis. *World J Clin Cases*. 2019;7(9):1006-1020.
81. Asrani V, Chang WK, Dong Z, Hardy G, Windsor JA, Petrov MS. Glutamine supplementation in acute pancreatitis: a meta-analysis of randomized controlled trials. *Pancreatology*. 2013;13(5):468-474.
82. Yong L, Lu QP, Liu SH, Fan H. Efficacy of glutamine-enriched nutrition support for patients with severe acute pancreatitis: a meta-analysis. *JPEN J Parenter Enteral Nutr*. 2016;40(1):83-94.
83. Moggia E, Koti R, Belgaumkar AP, et al. Pharmacological interventions for acute pancreatitis. *Cochrane Database Syst Rev*. 2017;4(4):CD011384.
84. Drewes AM, Bouwense SAW, Campbell CM, et al. Guidelines for the understanding and management of pain in chronic pancreatitis. *Pancreatology*. 2017;17(5):720-731.
85. Olesen SS, Bouwense SA, Wilder-Smith OH, van Goor H, Drewes AM. Pregabalin reduces pain in patients with chronic pancreatitis in a randomized, controlled trial. *Gastroenterology*. 2011;141(2):536-543.
86. Bonnet U, Scherbaum N. How addictive are gabapentin and pregabalin? A systematic review. *Eur Neuropsychopharmacol*. 2017;27(12): 1185-1215.
87. de la Iglesia-García D, Huang W, Szatmary P, et al. Efficacy of pancreatic enzyme replacement therapy in chronic pancreatitis: systematic review and meta-analysis. *Gut*. 2017;66(8):1354-1355.
88. Kirk GR, White JS, McKie L, et al. Combined antioxidant therapy reduces pain and improves quality of life in chronic pancreatitis. *J Gastrointest Surg*. 2006;10(4):499-503.
89. Bhardwaj P, Garg PK, Maulik SK, Saraya A, Tandon RK, Acharya SK. A randomized controlled trial of antioxidant supplementation for pain relief in patients with chronic pancreatitis. *Gastroenterology*. 2009;136(1):149-159.e2
90. Siriwardena AK, Mason JM, Balachandra S, et al. Randomised, double blind, placebo controlled trial of intravenous antioxidant (n-acetylcysteine, selenium, vitamin C) therapy in severe acute pancreatitis. *Gut*. 2007;56(10):1439-1444.
91. Rustagi T, Njei B. Antioxidant therapy for pain reduction in patients with chronic pancreatitis: a systematic review and meta-analysis. *Pancreas*. 2015;44(5):812-818.
92. Ahmed Ali U, Jens S, Busch OR, et al. Antioxidants for pain in chronic pancreatitis. *Cochrane Database Syst Rev*. 2014;8:CD008945.
93. Puli SR, Reddy JB, Bechtold ML, Antillon MR, Bruge WR. EUS-guided celiac plexus neurolysis for pain due to chronic pancreatitis or pancreatic cancer pain: a meta-analysis and systematic review. *Dig Dis Sci*. 2009;54(11):2330-2337.
94. Rana MV, Candido KD, Raja O, Knezevic NN. Celiac plexus block in the management of chronic abdominal pain. *Curr Pain Headache Rep*. 2014;18(2):394.
95. Struyvenberg MR, Martin CR, Freedman SD. Practical guide to exocrine pancreatic insufficiency - Breaking the myths. *BMC Medicine*. 2017;15(1):29.
96. Elashoff M, Matveyenko AV, Gier B, Elashoff R, Butler PC. Pancreatitis, pancreatic, and thyroid cancer with glucagon-like peptide-1-based therapies. *Gastroenterology*. 2011;141(1):150-156.
97. Pinto LC, Rados DV, Barkan SS, Leitão CB, Gross JL. Dipeptidyl peptidase-4 inhibitors, pancreatic cancer and acute pancreatitis: a meta-analysis with trial sequential analysis. *Sci Rep*. 2018;8(1):782.
98. Cao C, Yang S, Zhou Z. GLP-1 receptor agonists and pancreatic safety concerns in type 2 diabetic patients: data from cardiovascular outcome trials. *Endocrine*. 2020;68(3):518-525.
99. Dicembrini I, Montereggi C, Nreu B, Mannucci E, Monami M. Pancreatitis and pancreatic cancer in patientes treated with dipeptidyl peptidase-4 inhibitors: an extensive and updated meta-analysis of randomized controlled trials. *Diabetes Res Clin Pract*. 2020;159:107981.
100. Dziadkowiec KN, Stawinski PM, Proenza J. Empagliflozin-associated pancreatitis: a consideration for SGLT2 inhibitors. *ACG Case Rep J*. 2021;8(1):e00530.
101. Sujanani SM, Elfishawi MM, Zarghamravanbaksh P, Castillo FJC, Reich DM. Dapagliflozin-induced acute pancreatitis: a case report and review of literature. *Case Rep Endocrinol*. 2020;2020:6724504.
102. Tang H, Yang K, Li X, Song Y, Han J. Pancreatic safety of sodium-glucose cotransporter 2 inhibitors in patients with type 2 diabetes mellitus: a systematic review and meta-analysis. *Pharmacoepidemiol Drug Saf*. 2020;29(2):161-172.
103. Hart PA, Bellin MD, Andersen DK, et al. Type 3c (pancreatogenic) diabetes mellitus secondary to chronic pancreatitis and pancreatic cancer. *Lancet Gastroenterol Hepatol*. 2016;1(3):226-237.
104. Engen PA, Green SJ, Voigt RM, Forsyth CB, Keshavarzian A. The gastrointestinal microbiome: alcohol effects on the composition of intestinal microbiota. *Alcohol Res*. 2015;37(2):223-236.
105. Rocco A, Compare D, Angrisani D, Zamparelli MS, Nardone G. Alcoholic disease: liver and beyond. *World J Gastroenterol*. 2014;20(40):14652-14659.
106. Bishehsari F, Magno E, Swanson G, et al. Alcohol and gut-derived inflammation. *Alcohol Res*. 2017;38(2):163-171.
107. Beck IT. Small bowel injury by ethanol. In: Preedy VR, Watson RR, eds. *Alcohol and the Gastrointestinal Tract*. CRC Press; 1996:163-202.
108. Green PH. Alcohol, nutrition and malabsorption. *Clin Gastroenterol*. 1983;12(2):563-574.
109. Perlow W, Baraona E, Lieber CS. Symptomatic intestinal disaccharidase deficiency in alcoholics. *Gastroenterology*. 1977;72(4 Pt 1):680-684.
110. Martin PR, Singleton CK, Hiller-Sturmhöfel S. The role of thiamine deficiency in alcoholic brain disease. *Alcohol Res Health*. 2003;27(2): 134-142.
111. Halsted CH, Villanueva JA, Devlin AM, Chandler CJ. Metabolic interactions of alcohol and folate. *J Nutr*. 2002;132(8 Suppl):2367s-2372s.
112. Medici V, Halsted CH. Folate, alcohol, and liver disease. *Mol Nutr Food Res*. 2013;57(4):596-606.
113. Al Khalloufi K, Laiyemo AO. Management of rectal varices in portal hypertension. *World J Hepatol*. 2015;7(30):2992-2998.

114. Khalifa A, Rockey DC. Lower gastrointestinal bleeding in patients with cirrhosis-etiology and outcomes. *Am J Med Sci*. 2020;359(4):206-211.
115. White BA, Ramos GP, Kane S. The impact of alcohol in inflammatory bowel diseases. *Inflamm Bowel Dis*. 2021;28(3):466-473.
116. Connor J. Alcohol consumption as a cause of cancer. *Addiction*. 2017;112(2):222-228.
117. Boffetta P, Hashibe M. Alcohol and cancer. *Lancet Oncol*. 2006;7(2): 149-156.
118. Bagnardi V, Rota M, Botteri E, et al. Alcohol consumption and site-specific cancer risk: a comprehensive dose-response meta-analysis. *Br J Cancer*. 2015;112(3):580-593.
119. Park SY, Wilkens LR, Setiawan VW, Monroe KR, Haiman CA, Le Marchand L. Alcohol intake and colorectal cancer risk in the multiethnic cohort study. *Am J Epidemiol*. 2019;188(1):67-76.
120. Ohashi S, Miyamoto S, Kikuchi O, Goto T, Anamuma Y, Muto M. Recent advances from basic and clinical studies of esophageal squamous cell carcinoma. *Gastroenterology*. 2015;149(7):1700-1715.
121. Bagnardi V, Blangiardo M, La Vecchia C, Corrao G. A meta-analysis of alcohol drinking and cancer risk. *Br J Cancer*. 2001;85(11):1700-1705.
122. Kumagai N, Wakai T, Akazawa K, et al. Heavy alcohol intake is a risk factor for esophageal squamous cell carcinoma among middle-aged men: a case-control and simulation study. *Mol Clin Oncol*. 2013;1(5):811-816.
123. Sewram V, Sitas F, O'Connell D, Myers J. Tobacco and alcohol as risk factors for oesophageal cancer in a high incidence area in South Africa. *Cancer Epidemiol*. 2016;41:113-121.
124. Blot WJ, McLaughlin JK, Winn DM, et al. Smoking and drinking in relation to oral and pharyngeal cancer. *Cancer Res*. 1988;48(11):3282-3287.
125. Roswall N, Weiderpass E. Alcohol as a risk factor for cancer: existing evidence in a global perspective. *J Prev Med Public Health*. 2015;48(1):1-9.
126. Tramacere I, Pelucchi C, Bagnardi V, et al. A meta-analysis on alcohol drinking and esophageal and gastric cardia adenocarcinoma risk. Ann Oncol. 2012;23(2):287-297.
127. Raimondi S, Lowenfels AB, Morselli-Labate AM, Maisonneuve P, Pezilli R. Pancreatic cancer in chronic pancreatitis; aetiology, incidence, and early detection. *Best Pract Res Clin Gastroenterol*. 2010;24(3):349-358.
128. Naudin S, Li K, Jaouen T, et al. Lifetime and baseline alcohol intakes and risk of pancreatic cancer in the European Prospective Investigation into Cancer and Nutrition study. *Int J Cancer*. 2018;143(4):801-812.
129. Bassendine MF. Alcohol--a major risk factor for hepatocellular carcinoma? *J Hepatol*. 1986;2(3):513-519.
130. Rumgay H, Murphy N, Ferrari P, Soerjomataram I. Alcohol and cancer: epidemiology and biological mechanisms. *Nutrients*. 2021;13(9):31373.
131. Boyle P, Autier P, Bartelink H, et al. European Code Against Cancer and scientific justification: third version (2003). *Ann Oncol*. 2003;14(7):973-1005.
132. Haas SL, Ye W, Löhr JM. Alcohol consumption and digestive tract cancer. *Curr Opin Clin Nutr Metab Care*. 2012;15(5):457-467.
133. De Schepper HU, Cremonini F, Park MI, Camilleri M. Opioids and the gut: pharmacology and current clinical experience. *Neurogastroenterol Motil*. 2004;16(4):383-394.
134. Tassinari D, Sartori S, Tamburini E, et al. Transdermal fentanyl as a front-line approach to moderate-severe pain: a meta-analysis of randomized clinical trials. *J Palliat Care*. 2009;25(3):172-180.
135. Miller H, Panahi L, Tapia D, Tran A, Bowman JD. Loperamide misuse and abuse. *J Am Pharma Assoc*. 2017;57(2, Supplement):S45-S50.
136. Lau JY, Sung JJ, Lee KK, et al. Effect of intravenous omeprazole on recurrent bleeding after endoscopic treatment of bleeding peptic ulcers. *New Engl J Med*. 2000;343(5):310-316.
137. Yaffe GJ, Strelinger RW, Parwatikar S. Physical symptom complaints of patients on methadone maintenance. *Proc Natl Conf Methadone Treat*. 1973;1:507-514.
138. Yuan CS, Foss JF, O'Connor M, Moss J, Roizen MF. Gut motility and transit changes in patients receiving long-term methadone maintenance. *J Clin Pharmacol*. 1998;38(10):931-935.
139. Haber PS, Elsayed M, Espinoza D, Lintzeris N, Veillard AS, Hallinan R. Constipation and other common symptoms reported by women and men in methadone and buprenorphine maintenance treatment. *Drug Alcohol Depend*. 2017;181:132-139.
140. Haley TD, Long C, Mann BD. Stercoral perforation of the colon. A complication of methadone maintenance. *J Subst Abuse Treat*. 1998;15(5):443-444.
141. Farmer AD, Holt CB, Downes TJ, Ruggeri E, Del Vecchio S, De Giorgio R. Pathophysiology, diagnosis, and management of opioid-induced constipation. *Lancet Gastroenterol Hepatol*. 2018;3(3):203-212.
142. Nee J, Zakari M, Sugarman MA, et al. Efficacy of treatments for opioid-induced constipation: systematic review and meta-analysis. *Clin Gastroenterol Hepatol*. 2018;16(10):1569-1584.e2
143. Pannemans J, Vanuytsel T, Tack J. New developments in the treatment of opioid-induced gastrointestinal symptoms. *United European Gastroenterol J*. 2018;6(8):1126-1135.
144. Keefer L, Drossman DA, Guthrie E, et al. Centrally mediated disorders of gastrointestinal pain. *Gastroenterology*. 2016;S0016-5085(16):00225-0.
145. Lee M, Silverman SM, Hansen H, Patel VB, Manchikanti L. A comprehensive review of opioid-induced hyperalgesia. *Pain Physician*. 2011;14(2):145-161.
146. Roerig JL, Steffen KJ, Mitchell JE, Zunker C. Laxative abuse. *Drugs*. 2010;70(12):1487-1503.
147. Fine KD. Diarrhea. In: Feldman M, Sleisenger MH, Scharschmidt BF, eds. *Sleisenger & Fordtran's Gastrointestinal and liver disease*. 6th ed. Saunders; 1998:128-152.
148. Caplan JP, Epstein LA, Quinn DK, Stevens JR, Stern TA. Neuropsychiatric effects of prescription drug abuse. *Neuropsychol Rev*. 2007;17(3):363-380.
149. Peles E, Schreiber S, Adelson M. Tricyclic antidepressants abuse, with or without benzodiazepines abuse, in former heroin addicts currently in methadone maintenance treatment (MMT). *Eur Neuropsychopharmacol*. 2008;18(3):188-193.
150. Chiappini S, Mosca A, Miuli A, et al. Misuse of anticholinergic medications: a systematic review. *Biomedicines*. 2022;10(2):355.
151. Seiler-Ramadas R, Sandner I, Haider S, Grabovac I, Dorner TE. Health effects of electronic cigarette (e-cigarette) use on organ systems and its implications for public health. *Wien Klin Wochenschr*. 2021;133(19-20): 1020-1027.
152. Antinozzi M, Giffi M, Sini N, et al. Cigarette smoking and human gut microbiota in healthy adults: a systematic review. *Biomedicines*. 2022;10(2):510.
153. Ness-Jensen E, Lindam A, Lagergren J, Hveem K. Tobacco smoking cessation and improved gastroesophageal reflux: a prospective population-based cohort study: the HUNT study. *Am J Gastroenterol*. 2014;109(2):171-177.
154. Kahrilas PJ, Gupta RR. Mechanisms of acid reflux associated with cigarette smoking. *Gut*. 1990;31(1):4-10.
155. Kadakia SC, Kikendall JW, Maydonovitch C, Johnson LF. Effect of cigarette smoking on gastroesophageal reflux measured by 24-h ambulatory esophageal pH monitoring. *Am J Gastroenterol*. 1995;90(10):1785-1790.
156. Smit CF, Copper MP, van Leeuwen JA, Schoots IG, Stanjcic LD. Effect of cigarette smoking on gastropharyngeal and gastroesophageal reflux. *Ann Otol Rhinol Laryngol*. 2001;110(2):190-193.
157. Bhandarkar PV, Shah SK, Meshram M, Abraham P, Narayanan TS, Bhatia SJ. Effect of acute and long-term oral tobacco use on oesophageal motility. *J Gastroenterol Hepatol*. 2000;15(9):1018-1021.
158. Maity P, Biswas K, Roy S, Banerjee RK, Bandyopadhyay U. Smoking and the pathogenesis of gastroduodenal ulcer--recent mechanistic update. *Mol Cell Biochem*. 2003;253(1-2):329-338.
159. Sonnenberg A, Muller-Lissner SA, Vogel E, et al. Predictors of duodenal ulcer healing and relapse. *Gastroenterology*. 1981;81(6):1061-1067.
160. Korman MG, Hansky J, Eaves ER, Schmidt GT. Influence of cigarette smoking on healing and relapse in duodenal ulcer disease. *Gastroenterology*. 1983;85(4):871-874.
161. Svanes C, Søreide JA, Skarstein A, et al. Smoking and ulcer perforation. *Gut*. 1997;41(2):177-180.
162. Kurata JH, Elashoff JD, Nogawa AN, Haile BM. Sex and smoking differences in duodenal ulcer mortality. *Am J Public Health*. 1986;76(6):700-702.
163. Ross AH, Smith MA, Anderson JR, Small WP. Late mortality after surgery for peptic ulcer. *N Engl J Med*. 1982;307(9):519-522.

164. Lynch SM, Vrieling A, Lubin JH, et al. Cigarette smoking and pancreatic cancer: a pooled analysis from the pancreatic cancer cohort consortium. *Am J Epidemiol.* 2009;170(4):403-413.
165. Bosetti C, Lucenteforte E, Silverman DT, et al. Cigarette smoking and pancreatic cancer: an analysis from the International Pancreatic Cancer Case-Control Consortium (Panc4). *Ann Oncol.* 2012;23(7):1880-1888.
166. Tolstrup JS, Kristiansen L, Becker U, Grønbæk M. Smoking and risk of acute and chronic pancreatitis among women and men: a population-based cohort study. *Arch Internal Med.* 2009;169(6):603-609.
167. Morton C, Klatsky AL, Udaltsova N. Smoking, coffee, and pancreatitis. *Am J Gastroenterol.* 2004;99(4):731-738.
168. Mahid SS, Minor KS, Soto RE, Hornung CA, Galandiuk S. Smoking and inflammatory bowel disease: a meta-analysis. *Mayo Clin Proc.* 2006;81(11):1462-1471.
169. Silverstein MD, Lashner BA, Hanauer SB, Evans AA, Kirsner JB. Cigarette smoking in Crohn's disease. *Am J Gastroenterol.* 1989;84(1):31-33.
170. Cosnes J, Beaugerie L, Carbonnel F, Gendre JP. Smoking cessation and the course of Crohn's disease: an intervention study. *Gastroenterology.* 2001;120(5):1093-1099.
171. Verschuere S, De Smet R, Allais L, Cuvelier CA. The effect of smoking on intestinal inflammation: what can be learned from animal models? *J Crohns Colitis.* 2012;6(1):1-12.
172. Thomas GA, Rhodes J, Ingram JR. Mechanisms of disease: nicotine--a review of its actions in the context of gastrointestinal disease. *Nat Clin Pract Gastroenterol Hepatol.* 2005;2(11):536-544.
173. Beaugerie L, Massot N, Carbonnel F, Cattan S, Gendre JP, Cosnes J. Impact of cessation of smoking on the course of ulcerative colitis. *Am J Gastroenterol.* 2001;96(7):2113-2116.
174. Blackwell J, Saxena S, Alexakis C, et al. The impact of smoking and smoking cessation on disease outcomes in ulcerative colitis: a nationwide population-based study. *Aliment Pharmacol Ther.* 2019;50(5):556-567.
175. To N, Ford AC, Gracie DJ. Systematic review with meta-analysis: the effect of tobacco smoking on the natural history of ulcerative colitis. *Aliment Pharmacol Ther.* 2016;44(2):117-126.
176. Lunney PC, Leong RW. Review article: ulcerative colitis, smoking and nicotine therapy. *Aliment Pharmacol Ther.* 2012;36(11-12):997-1008.
177. McGrath J, McDonald JW, Macdonald JK. Transdermal nicotine for induction of remission in ulcerative colitis. *Cochrane Database Syst Rev.* 2004;4:CD004722.
178. Steevens J, Schouten LJ, Goldbohm RA, van den Brandt PA. Alcohol consumption, cigarette smoking and risk of subtypes of oesophageal and gastric cancer: a prospective cohort study. *Gut.* 2010;59(01):39-48.
179. Botteri E, Iodice S, Bagnardi V, Raimondi S, Lowenfels AB, Maisonneuve P. Smoking and colorectal cancer: a meta-analysis. *JAMA.* 2008;300(23):2765-2778.
180. McGee EE, Jackson SS, Petrick JL, et al. Smoking, alcohol, and biliary tract cancer risk: a pooling project of 26 prospective studies. *J Natl Cancer Inst.* 2019;111(12):1263-1278.
181. Bai X, Wei H, Liu W, et al. Cigarette smoke promotes colorectal cancer through modulation of gut microbiota and related metabolites. *Gut.* 2022;71(12):2439-2450.
182. Castellsagué X, Muñoz N, De Stefani E, et al. Independent and joint effects of tobacco smoking and alcohol drinking on the risk of esophageal cancer in men and women. *Int J Cancer.* 1999;82(5):657-664.
183. Glauser J, Queen JR. An overview of non-cardiac cocaine toxicity. *J Emerg Med.* 2007;32(2):181-186.
184. Goraya MHN, Malik A, Inayat F, et al. Acute pancreatitis secondary to cocaine use: a case-based systematic literature review. *Clin J Gastroenterol.* 2021;14(4):1269-1277.
185. Kiraly DD, Walker DM, Calipari ES, et al. Alterations of the host microbiome affect behavioral responses to cocaine. *Sci Rep.* 2016;6(1):35455.
186. Anderson JE, Brown IE, Olson KA, Iverson K, Cocanour CS, Galante JM. Nonocclusive mesenteric ischemia in patients with methamphetamine use. *J Trauma Acute Care Surg.* 2018;84(6):885-892.
187. Carlson TL, Plackett TP, Gagliano RA Jr, Smith RR. Methamphetamine-induced paralytic ileus. *Hawaii J Med Public Health.* 2012;71(2):44-45.
188. Prakash MD, Tangalakis K, Antonipillai J, Stojanovska L, Nurgali K, Apostolopoulos V. Methamphetamine: effects on the brain, gut and immune system. *Pharmacol Res.* 2017;120:60-67.
189. Cook RR, Fulcher JA, Tobin NH, et al. Alterations to the gastrointestinal microbiome associated with methamphetamine use among young men who have sex with men. *Sci Rep.* 2019;9(1):14840.
190. Pertwee RG. Cannabinoids and the gastrointestinal tract. *Gut.* 2001;48(6):859-867.
191. DiPatrizio NV. Endocannabinoids in the Gut. *Cannabis Cannabinoid Res.* 2016;1(1):67-77.
192. Taylor BN, Mueller M, Sauls RS. *Cannabinoid Antiemetic Therapy.* StatPearls Publishing; 2022. Accessed June 21, 2023. https://www.ncbi.nlm.nih.gov/books/NBK535430/
193. Duran M, Pérez E, Abanades S, et al. Preliminary efficacy and safety of an oromucosal standardized cannabis extract in chemotherapy-induced nausea and vomiting. *Br J Clin Pharmacol.* 2010;70(5):656-663.
194. Grimison P, Mersiades A, Kirby A, et al. Oral THC:CBD cannabis extract for refractory chemotherapy-induced nausea and vomiting: a randomised, placebo-controlled, phase II crossover trial. *Ann Oncol.* 2020;31(11):1553-1560.
195. Chu F, Cascella M. *Cannabinoid Hyperemesis Syndrome.* StatPearls Publishing; 2022. Accessed June 21, 2023. https://www.ncbi.nlm.nih.gov/books/NBK549915/
196. Sorensen CJ, DeSanto K, Borgelt L, Phillips KT, Monte AA. Cannabinoid hyperemesis syndrome: diagnosis, pathophysiology, and treatment—a systematic review. *J Med Toxicol.* 2017;13(1):71-87.
197. Richards JR, Gordon BK, Danielson AR, Moulin AK. Pharmacologic treatment of cannabinoid hyperemesis syndrome: a systematic review. *Pharmacotherapy.* 2017;37(6):725-734.
198. Ruberto AJ, Sivilotti MLA, Forrester S, Hall AK, Crawford FM, Day AG. Intravenous haloperidol versus ondansetron for cannabis hyperemesis syndrome (HaVOC): a randomized, controlled trial. *Ann Emerg Med.* 2021;77(6):613-619.
199. Richards JR, Lapoint JM, Burillo-Putze G. Cannabinoid hyperemesis syndrome: potential mechanisms for the benefit of capsaicin and hot water hydrotherapy in treatment. *Clin Toxicol (Phila).* 2017;1-10.
200. Wagner S, Hoppe J, Zuckerman M, Schwarz K, McLaughlin J. Efficacy and safety of topical capsaicin for cannabinoid hyperemesis syndrome in the emergency department. *Clin Toxicol (Phila).* 2020;58(6):471-475.
201. Traub SJ, Hoffman RS, Nelson LS. Body packing--the internal concealment of illicit drugs. *N Engl J Med.* 2003;349(26):2519-2526.
202. Cappelletti S, Piacentino D, Sani G, et al. Systematic review of the toxicological and radiological features of body packing. *Int J Legal Med.* 2016;130(3):693-709.

CHAPTER

92 Pulmonary Disorders Related to Substance Use

Tessa L. Steel, Corey Sadd, and Majid Afshar

CHAPTER OUTLINE

- Introduction
- Pulmonary pathophysiology and immunology of substance use
- Pulmonary effects of substance use
- Conclusion

INTRODUCTION

The respiratory tract is the body's largest surface area exposed to the external environment.[1] The airways and alveoli interact with the vascular bed of the lung and are subject to constant noxious, particulate, and antigenic challenges. As such, the respiratory system is adapted to attenuate external provocations and mediate these events at the epithelial and endothelial surfaces of the lung. Substance use may cause acute and chronic injuries to the respiratory system through various mechanisms and overwhelm the respiratory system's capacity to recover from repeated insults. As a result, substance use often leads to long-term respiratory symptoms and diseases (**Table 92-1**).

Inhalation, injection, and/or ingestion of various substances can adversely affect the airways, lung parenchyma, and pulmonary vascular bed. Respiratory failure is a common complication of unhealthy substance use. Respiratory impairment may result from central nervous system (CNS) depression (abnormal signaling in the medulla oblongata, stroke, or seizures) or respiratory muscle fatigue (respiratory compensation for metabolic acidosis or increased respiratory workload). Direct lung pathologies across airway, parenchymal, and vascular diseases include chronic obstructive pulmonary disease (COPD), aspiration events, and chronic hypoxic pulmonary vasoconstriction. Tobacco, cannabis, alcohol, opioids, cocaine, and amphetamines are the most commonly used substances resulting in pulmonary pathology. Polysubstance use is increasingly common, and clinicians should anticipate pulmonary complications due to the simultaneous use of multiple substances. This chapter provides an overview of pulmonary complications and diseases resulting from commonly used substances and common modalities of substance use (eg, inhalation, injection).

PULMONARY PATHOPHYSIOLOGY AND IMMUNOLOGY OF SUBSTANCE USE

Drugs may affect the lung through direct local inflammation, increased susceptibility to infections, airway reactivity, impairment of pulmonary vascular integrity, acute lung injury, structural injury, and derangements of gas exchange. Attributing a particular respiratory complication to a single agent can be challenging when an individual uses multiple drugs. The respiratory tract detoxifies and metabolizes proteins, drugs, and other potentially harmful substances. Unhealthy substance use can derange these critical, interrelated respiratory system functions and coexisting chronic pulmonary diseases may worsen substance use's acute and chronic physiological effects on the lungs.

Central Nervous System and Respiratory Drive

Respiration is under extensive neural control and consequently susceptible to the effects of CNS depressants and stimulants. Respiratory automaticity is regulated by the medulla oblongata within the brainstem and modulated by the reticular activating system, cerebral cortex, and peripheral sensors.[2] Respiratory depression is the inability to maintain normal ventilation. Hypoventilation from respiratory depression can lead to respiratory failure if the lungs fail to maintain normal gas exchange. Many substances discussed in this chapter inhibit respiration, causing respiratory depression or respiratory failure. Hypercapnia resulting from hypoventilation is one etiology for hypoxemia. In this setting, the hypoxemia stimulates peripheral chemoreceptors in the carotid body to trigger the CNS to increase respiratory rate and alter circulating carbon dioxide levels. However, hypoxemic drive is blunted by CNS depressants. Opioids have the most dramatic effect—binding to μ_2 receptors, blunting the CNS response to carbon dioxide, and depressing the pontine and medullary centers that regulate respiratory automaticity and cough.[2] Loss of protective gag and cough reflexes are also commonly seen in respiratory depression due to the use of CNS depressants. In contrast, stimulants (nicotine, cocaine, amphetamines) augment CNS signaling of dopamine, norepinephrine, and serotonin neurotransmitters and activate the sympathetic nervous system; this generally increases respiratory rate, dilates the airways, and does not compromise gas exchange.[3]

TABLE 92-1 Respiratory System Complications and Diseases Associated With Unhealthy Substance Use

Respiratory System	Complication	Pathogenesis	Substance/Route
Airway	Asthma/bronchospasm	Histamine release, abnormal receptor activation	Tobacco, opioids, alcohol, inhaled cocaine, cannabis, volatile inhalants
	Hemoptysis	Mucosal ulceration, mucosal burn	Freebase cocaine, any inhaled drug
	Nasal perforation	Necrosis of nasal cavity	Cocaine, opioids
Parenchymal	Chemical pneumonitis	Aspiration of low pH gastric acids	Alcohol, opioids, benzodiazepines
	Aspiration pneumonia	Infection following aspiration	Alcohol, opioids, benzodiazepines
	Cardiogenic pulmonary edema	Increased left ventricular filling pressure after adrenergic response	Cocaine, amphetamines
	Noncardiogenic pulmonary edema/ARDS	Diffuse alveolar damage, negative pressure barotrauma with pulmonary capillary leak	Tobacco, e-cigarettes (EVALI), alcohol, opioids, cocaine, amphetamines, benzodiazepines
	Pneumonia (community-acquired, atypical, and/or opportunistic)	Typical organisms: *Haemophilus* flu, *Klebsiella*, *Escherichia coli*, *Staphylococcus aureus*, atypical: tuberculosis, *Candida*	Tobacco, alcohol, opioids, cocaine, benzodiazepines, IDU
	Hypersensitivity pneumonitis	Immune response to inhaled antigen	Any inhaled drug, e-cigarettes
	Emphysema/COPD	Alveolar destruction and enlargement and small and large airway inflammation and remodeling	Tobacco, opioids, cannabis
	Lung cancer	Tumor growth via alteration of cellular and molecular genetic changes	Tobacco, opioids
	Pneumothorax	Direct needle injection of supraclavicular fossa, rupture bullous disease, cavitating septic emboli	Tobacco, cannabis, cocaine, amphetamines, IDU
	Interstitial lung disease/ bronchiolitis obliterans	Excessive accumulation of extracellular matrix and remodeling	Tobacco, e-cigarettes, cocaine, amphetamines
Indirect effects	Respiratory depression	Decreased sensitivity of chemoreceptors and activity in central respiratory centers (medulla) to pCO_2	Opioids, benzodiazepines, and other depressants
	Metabolic acidosis	Osmolar gap from alcohol	Alcohol
	Sleep-disordered breathing	Upper airway obstruction, suppress REM sleep	Alcohol, opioids, benzodiazepines
Vascular	Septic emboli	Embolization of infected material from heart valve, foreign body, or thrombus at injection site	IDU
	Needle embolization	Broken needle	IDU
	Foreign body granulomatosis and lung fibrosis	Filler agents into capillary bed with resultant macrophage and giant cell accumulation	IDU
	Hemoptysis/diffuse alveolar hemorrhage	Infarct or capillary injury	E-cigarettes, cocaine and other stimulants
	Pulmonary hypertension	Dysregulated serotonin metabolism with vascular remodeling	Cocaine, amphetamines, IV opioids

IDU, injection drug use; IV, intravenous.

Airway Pathophysiology

The airways form a connection between the external world and the respiratory units of the lung that are critical to lung function. The cough reflex and mucociliary escalator provide essential mechanical barriers to foreign matter. Ciliated cells lining the lungs' airways clear inhaled particles and act as the first line of defense against inhaled pathogens and harmful substances. Mucociliary impairment due to substance use is best described in the setting of tobacco and chronic alcohol use. Cigarette smoke causes impaired mucociliary clearance and predisposes patients to secretion retention and recurrent airway infections.[4] Cilia are exposed to ethanol via elevated circulating levels of blood alcohol in the bronchial circulation and via vaporized ethanol that is off-gassed from the bronchial circulation into the airways and exhaled—the physiologic basis for the breathalyzer test.[5] Prolonged exposure to alcohol results in dysregulation of the kinases and phosphatases that regulate cilia motility, a pathologic process called alcohol-induced ciliary dysfunction (AICD).[6]

Pulmonary Immune Function

The principal function of the respiratory system is gas exchange. An extensive network of thin-walled capillaries surrounds each alveolus. This elaborate network of airways and capillaries provides a large surface area for gas exchange and an expansive interface for the immune sampling of antigens and absorption of inhaled substances. When the upper airway fails to clear inhaled particles and pathogens, they are ingested by resident alveolar macrophages, which process, digest, and transport them to lymph nodes for antigen presentation. Alveolar macrophages also release cytokines and chemokines to recruit other immune cells to assist with pathogen clearance.[7] These mechanisms become deranged with heavy alcohol and opioid use. Alveolar macrophage production of neutrophil chemotactic cytokines is inhibited by chronic heavy alcohol use, resulting in defective neutrophil recruitment and function and poor clearance of bacteria associated with an increased risk of bacterial pulmonary infections.[8] Chronic opioid use also increases susceptibility to bacterial infections with dysregulation of the innate immune response. Opioid receptors are found within the alveolar walls of the respiratory tract and are also present within tracheal and bronchial smooth muscle tissue.[9] Opioid use causes defects in T-cell and natural killer cell function and macrophage and neutrophil phagocytosis.[10]

Tobacco smoke stimulates chemotactic cytokines leading to neutrophil and monocyte migration and cell mediators that cause alveolar epithelial injury and permeability changes.[11] Tobacco smoke causes an inflammatory response in the lower respiratory tract characterized by accumulating pigment-laden alveolar macrophages and neutrophil recruitment. These activated inflammatory cells release various mediators, including proteases, oxidants, and toxic peptides, which can damage lung structures and cause tissue destruction that leads to emphysema.[12] Electronic cigarette aerosol and vapor chemicals also disrupt the airway endothelium, create oxidative stress, and increase inflammation through neutrophil activation.[13]

Both cocaine and amphetamine-type stimulants have adverse effects on the immune system. They decrease CD4 T-helper cells, increase immunosuppressive cell signaling, switch from Th1-type cytokines to Th2-type cytokines, delay the immune response to microbial pathogens, and increase the risk for infection.[14]

There is a "gut-liver-lung axis" of oxidative stress that involves alcohol-induced gastrointestinal inflammation, translocation of gut bacteria into portal and systemic circulation, activation of hepatic resident macrophages (ie, Kupffer cells).[15] Figure 92-1 shows the interaction of alcohol use across host defense systems with upregulated proinflammatory behavior

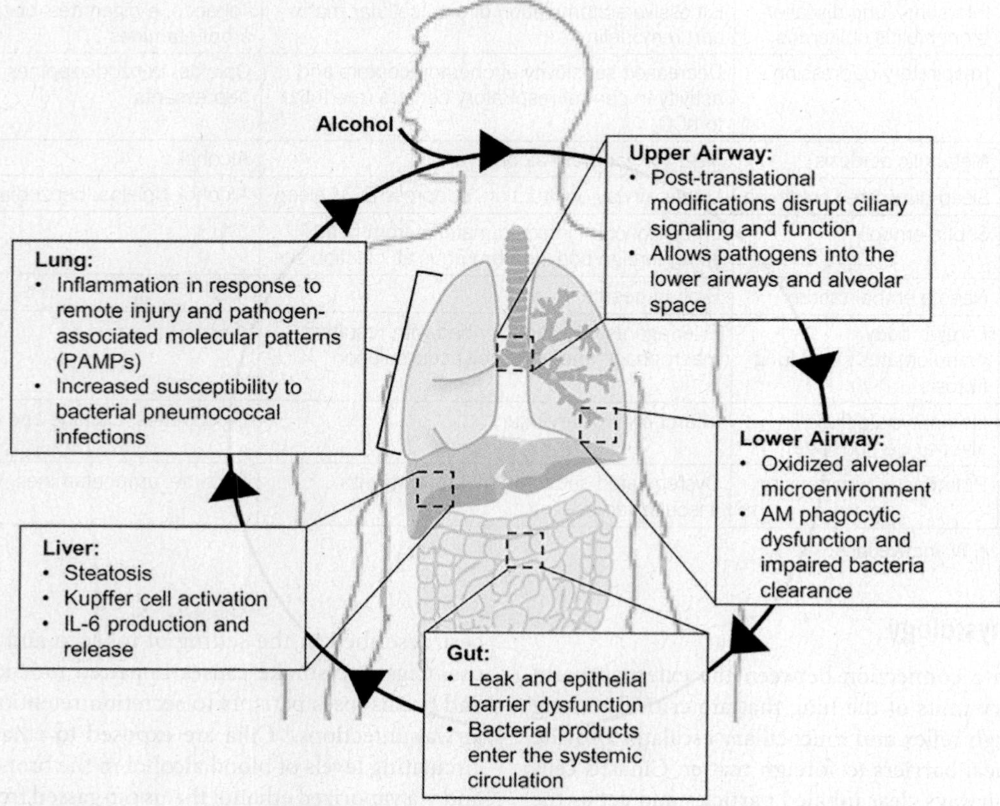

Figure 92-1. Mechanisms of lung injury and susceptibility to infection from chronic alcohol use. (From Yeligar SM, Chen MM, Kovacs EJ, Sisson JH, Burnham EL, Brown LAS. Alcohol and lung injury and immunity. *Alcohol.* 2016;55:51-59.)

and release of proinflammatory cytokines into the systemic circulation, which perpetuate abnormal alveolar macrophage function in the lungs. Depletion of glutathione (powerful antioxidant) stores, decreased intracellular zinc (affecting several zinc-dependent proteins in the lineup of antioxidant defenses), and increased production of reactive oxygen species[15] further impair bacterial clearance from the alveolar spaces and can worsen lung injury.

Pulmonary Vasculature

Large numbers of marginated leukocytes and platelets are stored within the pulmonary vasculature and are mobilized by pulmonary epithelial or endothelial cell injury, causing exudation, inflammation, and impaired gas exchange.[1] Opioids induce histamine release from mast cells that lead to pulmonary vein constriction, increased pulmonary capillary permeability and pulmonary edema, and bronchoconstriction.[16] Noncardiogenic acute pulmonary edema may occur after intravenous, freebase smoking, and nasal snorting of cocaine and amphetamine-type stimulants. Mechanisms include negative pressure pulmonary edema from high negative intrathoracic pressures during drug inhalation,[17] neurogenic pulmonary edema from sympathetic-mediated pulmonary vasoconstriction,[18] and direct toxic drug effects on alveolar epithelial and endothelial cells.[19]

The most established effects of stimulant use on respiratory function result from excessive sympathomimetic (ie, "stress-state") activation and dysregulated serotonin metabolism—both heavily implicated in cardiopulmonary vascular remodeling.[20] Amphetamines uniquely inhibit monoamine oxidase activity and have greater uptake, faster peak time, and lower clearance in the lungs compared to other organs.[21] Ecstasy/MDMA has pronounced effects on serotonin signaling,[22] binding serotonin transporters on platelets, and increasing circulating levels of serotonin two- to sevenfold.[23] Dysregulated serotonin metabolism is implicated in the pathogenesis of methamphetamine-associated pulmonary arterial hypertension.[24] Ecstasy/MDMA can bind and activate $5HT_{2B}$ serotonin receptors with similar effects as the weight loss drug fenfluramine.[25]

PULMONARY EFFECTS OF SUBSTANCE USE

Smoked (Combusted) Substance Use

Smoking produces near-instantaneous effects of various substances, including tobacco, cannabis, heroin, fentanyl, alkaloidal cocaine (freebase or "crack" cocaine), and alkaloidal methamphetamine ("ice," "crystal," or "glass"), through rapid absorption in the pulmonary circulation. The quick onset of an inhaled drug's effect with an immediate reward is the impetus for this mode of use.[26] Inhalation of drugs also introduces a variety of other substances, including pyrolysis products, contaminants, and impurities. Smoke exposure profoundly affects lung biology, altering the immunological and structural milieu. The results of smoking tobacco are best understood, but similar pathologic mechanisms apply to smoking other substances.

Smoked Tobacco

Tobacco smoke exposes the lung to over 4,500 toxins, which are associated with lung cancer, COPD, bronchitis, and airway reactivity.[27] Several factors determine the effects of tar and other pyrolysis products on the lung: (1) individual susceptibility to the various adverse effects; (2) heterozygosity for the gene that causes alpha-1-antitrypsin deficiency; (3) number of cigarettes smoked; (4) years spent smoking; and (5) behavior of smoking (eg, depth of inhalation).[28] People who smoke have a quicker decline in forced expiratory volume in 1 second (FEV1) than people who do not smoke. Reduced FEV1 is the hallmark of airflow obstruction, which leads to symptoms such as exertional dyspnea and fatigue.[29] Chronic airflow obstruction and parenchymal destruction resulting in emphysema are associated with persistent hypoxemia, which may lead to pulmonary hypertension and right heart failure (ie, cor pulmonale). [30] Reduction or abstinence from tobacco use may slow the rate of lung function decline, attenuate symptoms, lower the risk of lung cancer, and decrease the incidence of lower respiratory infections.[29]

Obstructive Airway Disease

COPD is functionally characterized by persistent airflow limitation that is often progressive over time. Spirometry is needed to diagnose airway obstruction. The diagnostic guidelines from the Global Initiative for Chronic Obstructive Lung Disease (GOLD) define fixed airway obstruction as an FEV1/forced vital capacity (FVC) less than 70% after bronchodilator administration.[31] Of note, the use of a fixed ratio to diagnose COPD does not account for expected changes in airflow limitations with age. Therefore, COPD can also be diagnosed as an FEV1/FVC below 5% of the lower limit of normal for healthy controls.

Individuals with COPD frequently have clinical manifestations of dyspnea, wheezing, chronic cough, and/or chronic (nearly daily) sputum production. Chronic bronchitis is sputum production for at least 3 months in 2 successive years without other causes of chronic cough. Airway changes in chronic bronchitis include mucus gland hypertrophy in intermediate-sized airways. Overproduction of mucus may overwhelm the mucociliary escalator, which is compromised by tobacco smoke.

Pulmonary emphysema is a common pathologic feature of COPD. Emphysema results from the destruction of alveolar walls by the deranged inflammatory response induced by tobacco smoke and irreversible enlargement of the airspaces distal to the terminal bronchiole. Associated hyperinflation and flattening of the diaphragm leads to a mechanical disadvantage for contractility of the major respiratory muscles—the diaphragm, rib cage, and abdominal muscles.[32] Lung hyperinflation and mechanical disadvantage, loss of gas-exchange surface area, and suboptimal ventilation-perfusion matching, all contribute to impaired oxygenation and carbon dioxide retention. Pneumothorax may develop from rupture of subpleural emphysematous blebs (<2 cm) or bullae (>2 cm).

Beyond spirometric evidence of obstruction (reduced FEV1/FVC), pulmonary function tests in patients with COPD often show hyperinflation (ie, increased total lung capacity), air trapping (ie, increased residual volume), and decreased diffusion capacity. The GOLD guidelines use symptoms and frequency of exacerbations to guide therapy. The mainstays of COPD management are reduction of or abstinence from tobacco use, bronchodilator therapy, inhaled or systemic steroids, antibiotics for exacerbations, supplemental oxygen therapy, and pulmonary rehabilitation.[33,34] More invasive treatments may be appropriate in select cases, including endobronchial valves or lung reduction surgery in patients with significant air trapping and upper lobe predominant emphysema. Lung transplantation is reserved for severe cases that are poorly controlled with conventional therapeutics.

Interstitial Lung Disease

Smoking is associated with an increased risk of interstitial lung disease (ILD).[35] Tobacco smoke is the primary risk factor for respiratory bronchiolitis-associated ILD (RB-ILD), desquamative interstitial pneumonia (DIP), and eosinophilic granulomatous (EG) disease, formerly known as pulmonary Langerhans cell histiocytosis. Tobacco smoking is also associated with idiopathic pulmonary fibrosis, rheumatoid arthritis-associated ILD, acute eosinophilic pneumonia, and Goodpasture syndrome.[35] Underlying pathogenesis includes bronchiolar inflammation, increased interstitial macrophages, and increased transforming growth factor-beta production, ultimately leading to pulmonary fibrosis.[36] Patients present with an insidious progression of dyspnea, dry cough, diffuse infiltrates, restrictive physiology on pulmonary function tests, and impaired diffusion capacity.[37] People who smoke are also at risk for developing a combination of pulmonary fibrosis and emphysema, which portends a worse prognosis than either condition alone.[38] Guidelines for diagnosing idiopathic pulmonary fibrosis prioritize high-resolution chest computed tomography and the involvement of a multidisciplinary diagnostic and treatment approach.[37] Bronchoscopic biopsies and bronchoalveolar lavage are helpful in the diagnosis of other types of ILD. Treatment of tobacco use disorder is a critical component of ILD management.[35] In the case of RB-ILD, DIP, and EG, abstinence from tobacco use alone may lead to stabilization of symptoms and improvement in radiographic and functional studies.

Pulmonary Hypertension and Cor Pulmonale

Chronic hypoxic vasoconstriction of the pulmonary vasculature leads to pulmonary arterial hypertension and right heart failure.[39] Pulmonary hypertension may develop among individuals with COPD and is associated with an increased rate of COPD exacerbations and mortality. Symptoms include dyspnea, fatigue, palpitations, and syncope. Patients may exhibit tachycardia, prominent neck veins, tricuspid insufficiency murmur, a prominent P2 heart sound, hepatojugular reflux, ascites, and peripheral edema. Screening for pulmonary hypertension is performed by transthoracic echocardiography and right heart catheterization confirms the diagnosis.[39]

The primary therapy for hypoxemia-related pulmonary hypertension consists of optimizing the treatment of the patient's underlying lung disease.[39] Supplemental oxygen for at least 18 hours per day prolongs survival and improves symptoms. Additional therapeutic options include anticoagulation for patients with evidence of venous thromboembolism and diuretics for patients with elevated central venous pressure. Patients with suspected pulmonary hypertension should be referred to a pulmonary hypertension specialty center for hemodynamic evaluation and consideration of advanced therapies.[39]

Pneumothorax

People who smoke have an increased risk of spontaneous pneumothorax compared to those who do not smoke.[40] Secondary spontaneous pneumothorax may occur after rupture of a subpleural bleb/bullae in patients with bullous emphysema. Cavitating infections and bronchogenic carcinomas may also cause pneumothoraces.[41]

Lung Cancer

Lung cancer is the leading cause of cancer-related death in the United States. Worldwide, tobacco smoking is linked in more than 80% of cases.[42] The risk of lung cancer is also increased in adults exposed to secondhand or indirect tobacco smoke.[43] Before lung cancer screening strategies with computed tomography, approximately 70% of lung cancers presented in advanced stages, leaving most patients with unresectable disease and a 5-year survival rate of less than 20%.[42] The United States Preventive Services Task Force guidelines recommend annual screening for lung cancer with low-dose chest computed tomography in adults aged 50 to 80 with a 20 pack-year smoking history who currently smoke or quit in the past 15 years. [44]

Patients with lung cancer may be asymptomatic with incidentally noted pulmonary nodules on imaging. Symptoms of lung cancer are weight loss, cough, chest pain, fatigue, hoarseness, superior vena cava syndrome, or hemoptysis. Diagnosis can be achieved by bronchoscopic cytological specimens, endobronchial biopsy, transbronchial biopsies, endobronchial ultrasound-guided mediastinal lymph node needle aspiration, mediastinoscopy, or surgical resection. Treatment may be definitive in the case of a completely resected, margin-free solitary pulmonary nodule, or may include radiation and/or chemotherapy, depending on the cell type and stage. Abstinence from tobacco use decreases the risk for lung cancer mortality.[45] Smoking reduction reduces the likelihood of lung cancer for patients unable to quit, albeit to a lesser extent.[46]

Acute Respiratory Distress Syndrome

Acute respiratory distress syndrome (ARDS) is clinically characterized by severe hypoxemia and bilateral pulmonary opacities on chest imaging unexplained solely by cardiac dysfunction. Pathologically, ARDS involves disruption of the pulmonary capillary-alveolar membrane and diffuse alveolar damage due to many inflammatory triggers (eg, pulmonary and nonpulmonary sepsis, trauma, and burn injuries). Both passive and active tobacco smoking confers an increased risk for ARDS in the setting of inflammatory triggers.[47,48] Active smoking increases the likelihood of ARDS in younger populations, despite lower presenting severity of illness. Regardless of risk factors, the mainstay of treatment for ARDS is lung protective ventilation and appropriate management of the underlying disease process (eg, pneumonia, trauma, etc.).

Smoked Cannabis

An accumulating body of research indicates that components of cannabis smoke have various toxic effects on the lung. High concentrations of carcinogens are present in cannabis smoke, including polycyclic aromatic hydrocarbons. Respiratory deposition of tar from cannabis smoke is four times greater than tar deposition from the same quantity of tobacco.[49] This may be partially attributable to the lack of filters in cannabis cigarettes and the deeper, longer inhalation of cannabis smoke compared to tobacco smoke.[50] While short-term cannabis use is associated with bronchodilation, chronic use through combustive mechanisms may lead to similar complications as smoking tobacco, including COPD and bullous emphysema.[51] While some uncertainty remains around the degree of harm from cannabis smoke, heavy long-term use is associated with a decline in FEV1 and an increase in COPD symptoms (cough, phlegm production, and wheezing).[52] Spontaneous pneumothorax and pneumomediastinum are also temporally associated with smoking cannabis, potentially due to Valsalva maneuvers that pressurize smoke in the lungs to enhance absorption.[53] Bronchoscopic evaluations have revealed extensive airway pathology from cannabis smoke, including epithelial damage to the central airways, replacement of ciliated bronchial epithelium with nonciliated hyperplastic mucus-secreting (goblet) cells, and squamous metaplasia of the bronchial mucosa.[54]

Smoked Opioids

Asthma, COPD, and early onset emphysema are highly prevalent in patients with unhealthy opioid use, with the strongest association in patients who smoke heroin.[55] Similar to other illicit substances (eg, cocaine, amphetamines), harmful pulmonary effects are from inhaling large amounts of particulate, smoke, and superheated gases rather than direct effects from the drug. Respiratory complications of smoking heroin include severe and fatal cases of asthma (particularly in patients with known preexisting asthma) and hypersensitivity reactions involving diffuse pulmonary infiltrates and eosinophilia on bronchoalveolar lavage.[56] However, these effects may be confounded by tobacco smoking, which is common among people who use opioids. Inhaled opioids can also precipitate severe asthma exacerbations in patients with known asthma.[57] Opioids can cause histamine release, potentially through mu receptors or IgE mediation that induce bronchospasm in histamine-sensitive asthmatics. During acute asthma exacerbations, patients with heroin use are more likely to need invasive mechanical ventilation, but this may be due to poor medication adherence among people with injection drug use.[58] Clinicians should be particularly attentive to acute asthma exacerbations triggered by heroin because patients often have poor access to health care and inconsistent maintenance therapy, associated with poorly controlled asthma and frequent exacerbations.[59]

Smoked "Crack" Cocaine and "Crystal" Methamphetamine

As with smoked tobacco and cannabis, crack cocaine exposes the lungs to various pyrolysis coproducts and contaminants, in addition to high-temperature fumes. Thermal injuries and inflammatory responses to large amounts of particulate, smoke, and superheated gases are known complications of inhaled "crack" cocaine and "ice"/"crystal" methamphetamine.[60] These lung injuries relate to the toxicities of smoking more than the direct stimulant effects. Barotrauma, pneumothorax, and pneumomediastinum are possible complications from smoking stimulants[61] through practices that expose the lungs to high pressures, such as "shotgunning" (partner-aided mouth-to-mouth administration of inhaled substances),[62] frequent and repetitive inhalation against small pipes, and Valsalva maneuvers. Individuals with crack cocaine use frequently report wheezing, cough productive of black (carbonaceous) sputum, dyspnea, and chest pain.[56] These symptoms typically resolve within days of abstinence and are related to local airway irritation from the combustible coproducts (eg, carbonaceous residue from the fuel used to ignite crack cocaine). Fatal bronchospasm may occur in individuals with preexisting asthma who smoke crack cocaine. There are fewer bronchial mucosal changes in individuals who smoke crack than in those who smoke tobacco or cannabis.[63]

Like cocaine, methamphetamine can be snorted or smoked in its alkaloidal form. Pulmonary side effects are similar to crack cocaine. Although amphetamines have bronchodilator properties and were historically used as treatment for respiratory illnesses, smoked amphetamines can produce local airway irritation, with the potential for acute bronchoconstriction and hypersensitivity reactions.[56]

"Vaping" and Electronic Cigarettes

Vaping devices heat liquid that contains a solvent (ie, propylene glycol or glycerin) that evaporates at the heating element, followed by rapid cooling to produce an aerosol. The composition of the aerosol is different from the smoke formed by combustion of tobacco. The electronic cigarette (e-cigarette) aerosol is directly inhaled ("vaped") through a mouthpiece and contains one or more flavorings with or without nicotine.[64] Independent studies show that a leading manufacturer of e-cigarettes sold cartridges/pods with nicotine levels comparable to or greater than combustive cigarettes.[65] As of 2020, there is a decline in e-cigarette use among U.S. adolescents, with 20% of high school students reporting current use of e-cigarettes compared to 28% in 2019.[66]

Commercially manufactured e-cigarettes may not expose the individual to many of the toxins in combustive tobacco smoke (eg, tars, oxidant gases, and carbon monoxide), but they do contain their own unique toxic chemical substances (flavorings, diacetyl, benzaldehyde, metals, and carcinogens like propylene glycol, glycerol).[67] Some e-cigarettes (including alleged "heat-not-burn" products) have been demonstrated to produce some degree of combustion and associated toxic products such as carbon monoxide, carcinogens, and other toxins (potentially from charring of the tobacco plug and melting of the polymer-film filter) despite claims otherwise. Given that it took 50 years to understand the risks and impacts of combusted cigarettes, with sparse long-term studies of the risks and long-term impacts of e-cigarette use (product first appeared circa 2007), our understanding of similar risks from e-cigarette use are early and incomplete. The electronic nicotine delivery system contains many components that may lead to long-term harm from not only the chemical additives but also free radicals, metal fragments, and other particulate matter that may be aerosolized and directly impact the lung and other organ systems.

Direct pulmonary toxicities of e-cigarettes have been traced to the flavoring chemicals in the liquids that are heated, aerosolized or vaporized, and inhaled.[68] There are currently over 7,500 different flavors of e-cigarettes.[69] Diacetyl is one commonly used chemical that provides a buttery or creamy flavor in e-cigarettes and is used for more ubiquitous flavors such as "tobacco," menthol, and fruit and candy flavors.[70] Occupational exposures to diacetyl and benzaldehyde have been linked to airway disease.[71] The potential risk of toxic exposure remains significant in e-cigarettes that do not contain chemical flavors. Carcinogenic carbonyls, such as formaldehyde and acetaldehyde, are degradation products of propylene glycol or glycerol, commonly used solvents with increased exposure seen in high battery output voltage devices.[72]

The direct harms to the lungs include e-cigarette or vaping product use-associated lung injury (EVALI), bronchiolitis obliterans, and acute eosinophilic pneumonia. An average inhalation from an e-cigarette includes a significant amount of e-liquid aerosols that expose the entire respiratory epithelium to potentially injurious substances.[73] A nationwide outbreak of severe lung disease associated with e-cigarettes was reported by the Center for Disease Control and Prevention (CDC).[74,75] The CDC accumulated thousands of cases where e-cigarettes were linked to EVALI with risk factors including concomitant use of tetrahydrocannabinol (THC) and contaminants like vitamin E acetate.[76] EVALI is an acute respiratory illness that can be life-threatening as a form of lung injury with diffuse alveolar damage, similar to ARDS.[77] Patients present with respiratory symptoms and bilateral opacities on chest imaging. These manifestations may also be accompanied by gastrointestinal symptoms (vomiting and diarrhea) and a smaller proportion with hemoptysis. The diagnosis is made in the absence of lung infection and the use of an e-cigarette within 90 days.

Other related conditions include acute eosinophilic pneumonia with more than 25% circulating eosinophils and, less commonly, other forms of interstitial lung disease like organizing pneumonia. Lipoid pneumonia from aspirating mineral oil and diffuse alveolar hemorrhage may also occur.[78] The treatment for EVALI is mainly supportive care with supplemental oxygen and empiric antibiotics, and some may benefit from systemic glucocorticoids. With the growing evidence around the harms of e-cigarettes and continual changes in the technology of flavorings and other chemical compounds, it is important for health providers to be mindful of pulmonary complications from e-cigarette exposure to counsel appropriately.

Acute and Chronic Unhealthy Alcohol Use

Acute Alcohol Use

Acute alcohol consumption represents a heterogeneous drinking pattern ranging between acceptable and unhealthy consumption levels, including binge consumption.[79] The respiratory effects of binge alcohol consumption, defined as greater than four or five drinks within 2 hours, rarely present with respiratory depression.[80] Only in cases of alcohol poisoning when alcohol levels above 300 mg/dL does concomitant respiratory depression occur.[81] However, this also depends on the chronicity of alcohol use because individuals with levels above 400 mg/dL have been observed to have no major consequences in their respiratory mechanics.[82] The evidence for unhealthy effects from alcohol are largely sourced among individuals with chronic alcohol consumption, but laboratory experiments have demonstrated acute derangements in inflammatory mediators and cytokines after acute consumption that may affect the host response in communicable diseases, including bacterial pneumonia.[83] More common respiratory effects from acute alcohol consumption include exacerbation of sleep disordered breathing, aspiration events with pneumonitis and pneumonia, acid-base derangements, and exacerbation of asthma.

Aspiration Syndromes

Conditions that predispose to aspiration after acute alcohol consumption include the poor response in protective airway reflexes, impaired cough and ciliary function, impaired consciousness, and disruption of normal swallowing.[84] The risk of aspirating oropharyngeal or gastric contents into the lower respiratory tract increases with impaired levels of consciousness.[85] The common aspiration syndromes include aspiration pneumonitis, aspiration pneumonia, airway obstruction, and diffuse aspiration bronchiolitis.[84] Depending on the type and quantity of material aspirated and the host's response, the clinical manifestations of aspiration can vary from transient hypoxemia, to overt pneumonia, and possibly respiratory failure with ARDS. Impaired levels of consciousness due to alcohol, drug, or hepatic failure are the most common risk factors for aspiration pneumonia.[86] Preventive care should be directed toward airway control, maintenance of at least a 30° angle for the head of the bed, avoidance of oral intake while lethargic, oral hygiene, pulmonary suctioning or "toilet," supplemental oxygen, and antibiotics as indicated. Empiric antibiotic coverage for aspiration in the absence of infiltrates and clinical and laboratory indicators of infection is not indicated.[87]

Acute Metabolic Acidosis and Respiratory Alkalosis

Alcohol may cause metabolic acidosis from alcohol-related ketoacidosis, with resultant compensatory respiratory alkalosis.[88] The most common presentation in patients with alcohol-related ketoacidosis is a history of chronic alcohol use, poor oral intake, gastrointestinal symptoms, and ketoacidosis on laboratory evaluation.[89] Patients often become tachypneic due to the acidosis, in addition to dehydration (ethanol blocks antidiuretic hormone and causes diuresis), alcohol withdrawal, and abdominal pain.[90] An elevated serum osmolal gap from ethanol may also occur in conjunction with a metabolic acidosis with concentrations exceeding 100 mosmol/kg.[91] Most often, when a patient presents to the emergency department after alcohol-related ketoacidosis, both an osmolal gap and an anion gap metabolic acidosis may coexist. However, only the osmolal gap may be found in patients who present very early after consumption, and only the anion gap metabolic acidosis may exist in patients who present very late after consumption.

Patients with alcohol intoxication and high anion gap metabolic acidosis should also be evaluated for an unexplained osmolar gap, which increases the concern for a co-ingestion and additional factors to tachypnea and respiratory alkalosis.[92] Other toxic alcohols and glycols that should be assessed are isopropanol, ethylene glycol, diethylene glycol, propylene glycol and methanol. However, co-ingestion of ethanol slows metabolism of these toxic alcohol and glycols and may reduce or even eliminate the development of the anion gap metabolic acidosis.

Asthma

Patients with asthma may experience worsening asthma symptoms after consumption of alcohol, particularly those who are histamine sensitive. Approximately a third of patients with asthma report that drinking alcohol triggered their asthma on at least two occasions.[93] Additionally, alcohol use is associated with adult-onset asthma with an increased risk for new-onset asthma in heavy daily drinkers.[94] Reactivity to low-sulfite wines may occur in a small number of individuals who report sensitivity to wines, and the sulfite additives may be the etiology for wine-induced asthmatic reactions.[95] The fractional excretion of exhaled nitric oxide is one biomarker in multiple airway diseases, including asthma. In the National Health and Examination Survey for the U.S. population, unhealthy alcohol consumption had a negative association and was an independent predictor of derangements in exhaled NO levels compared to people who never drink.[96] Furthermore, airflow obstruction increases in individuals with former heavy alcohol intake.[97] The ensuing release of histamine and other mediators of inflammation induces bronchospasm. Mutations in acetaldehyde dehydrogenase genes are associated with alcohol-induced airway reactivity.[98]

Sleep-Disordered Breathing

Acute alcohol consumption worsens the sleep architecture in individuals with sleep-disordered breathing.[99] Both duration and frequency of obstructive respiratory events are increased after acute alcohol consumption with oxyhemoglobin desaturations.[100] Snoring worsens after acute alcohol consumption and may lead to overt obstruction and obstructive sleep apnea. All patients should be advised that alcohol, among other sedating medications, may worsen obstructive sleep apnea.

Chronic Alcohol Use

Patients with chronic heavy alcohol use are at increased risk of pulmonary infections and respiratory failure with lung injury. This includes an increased risk of community-acquired pneumonia, hospital-acquired pneumonia, ARDS, and increased mortality from these conditions compared to patients without chronic heavy alcohol use.[101]

Pneumonia

Individuals with an alcohol use disorder (AUD) are disproportionately affected by bacterial pneumonia. The epidemiology in hospitalized patients with AUD shows a 2 to 3 times increased risk in the incidence of bacterial pneumonia compared to those without AUD.[102] Pneumonia in the context of AUD often progresses to systemic illness (bacteremia, sepsis, septic shock), with longer, more complicated recovery (eg, higher rates of empyema), and death from pneumonia is more common in patients with AUD compared to those without AUD.[103] Correlating with these findings, patients with AUD hospitalized with community-acquired pneumonia have an increased risk for intensive care unit admission, mechanical ventilation, pressors, and experience longer hospital stays and higher costs.[104] In addition to community-acquired pneumonia, nosocomial hospital-acquired pneumonia, including ventilator-associated pneumonia, occurs more frequently and with greater morbidity and mortality in patients with AUD.

Acute Respiratory Distress Syndrome

AUD is a major independent risk factor for ARDS.[105] As described in the pathophysiology section above, chronic alcohol use adversely affects the permeability of the pulmonary capillary-alveolar membrane.[106] Surfactant production is impaired with increases in oxidant-mediated apoptosis of alveolar epithelial cells, resulting in impaired epithelial function.[107]

Failure of the epithelial barrier leads to increased protein leak, decreased alveolar fluid clearance, and diffuse lung injury, which are the hallmark characteristics of ARDS.[108]

Respiratory Complications From Alcohol-Related Liver Disease

Cirrhosis, including alcohol-related cirrhosis, is associated with various respiratory system abnormalities. One pulmonary complication is hepatic hydrothorax in which the negative intrapleural pressure gradient causes transdiaphragmatic movement of ascites into the pleural space.[109] Ascites may also affect respiratory function through diaphragmatic restriction, reduced tidal volumes, and lower lobe atelectasis.[110] Hepatopulmonary syndrome affects 15% to 30% of patients with cirrhosis. Pulmonary microvascular vasodilation, particularly in the postcapillary pulmonary vasculature, generates a shunt with clinical findings of orthodeoxia and platypnea. Positional increases in blood flow through the lower lobes exacerbate the shunt physiology. Contrast echocardiography with agitated saline can be used to identify intrapulmonary shunting. Hepatopulmonary syndrome is reversed by liver transplant.[110]

Portopulmonary hypertension affects 2% to 5% of patients with cirrhosis. A number of vasoactive substances, genetic factors, and inflammatory processes are associated with pathologic changes in the pulmonary arterial vasculature and lead to pulmonary hypertension.[110] Portopulmonary hypertension is classified in the World Symposium on Pulmonary Hypertension as Group 1. It requires referral to a pulmonary hypertension specialty center to consider specialized disease-directed therapy (ie, pulmonary vasodilators). Transjugular intrahepatic portosystemic shunt (TIPS) procedures can acutely increase right heart preload and precipitate right heart failure in patients with portopulmonary hypertension.[111] Pulmonary arterial pressures may improve or normalize after liver transplantation, but a liver transplant is not considered a conventional treatment for the syndrome.[112]

Unhealthy Opioid Use and Injection Drug Use

Although opioids like morphine are often used to relieve dyspnea, they also exert adverse effects on the lung from both acute and chronic unhealthy use. Respiratory depression and failure, pulmonary edema, respiratory infections, COPD, septic pulmonary emboli, pulmonary hypertension, and talc-related complications are associated with chronic unhealthy use.[113] Acute use also directly affects the airways, pulmonary vasculature, and immune system, increasing the risk for pulmonary infections. Overall, pulmonary complications account for approximately 20% of opioid-related medical complications.[114]

The route of opioid administration is an important consideration. People who inject drugs with opioids may experience acute and chronic pulmonary complications, including pneumonia, septic embolization, noncardiogenic pulmonary edema, foreign body granulomatosis, emphysema, interstitial lung disease, and pulmonary vascular disease.[115] Inhalational use of opioids may induce bronchospasm, bronchitis, and hypersensitivity pneumonitis and is discussed separately in the "Smoke opioids" section.

Pneumonia

The risk for pneumonia is increased in people prescribed opioids compared to the general population.[116] People who inject drugs (PWID) have a 10-fold increased risk of pneumonia compared with the general population.[116] Community-acquired pneumonia remains the most common type of pneumonia in patients with unhealthy opioid use with the following organisms: (1) *Streptococcus pneumoniae*, (2) *Staphylococcus aureus*, (3) *Haemophilus influenzae*, (4) *Klebsiella pneumoniae*, and (5) *Escherichia coli*. Other types of respiratory infections include sinusitis, acute bronchitis, septic emboli, fungal infections, and mycobacterial infections.

The initial antibiotic regimen should target the most common bacterial pathogens in patients with typical pneumonia symptoms. Blood cultures are warranted in many patients, especially those who are toxic, ill-appearing, immunocompromised, or otherwise at high risk. Early and appropriate administration of antibiotics tailored to the suspected pathogen remains imperative to decrease mortality risk.[117] Patients with progressive disease, despite adequate bacterial coverage, should be assessed for fungal and mycobacterial agents, including *Candida* pneumonia and tuberculosis. Sputum acid-fast staining and culture may be performed if there is suspicion of mycobacterial infections and additional risk factors like HIV infection, poverty with housing insecurity, and malnutrition. In people who inject drugs, HIV infection should be assessed to consider other opportunistic pulmonary infections in addition to tuberculosis.

Pulmonary Edema

Morphine is often used as an adjunct for managing cardiogenic pulmonary edema and relieving dyspnea. However, noncardiogenic pulmonary edema is a complication of opioid overdose.[118] Dr Osler first described this phenomenon in a patient with a morphine overdose. Earlier data suggested that pulmonary edema occurs in nearly 50% of patients presenting with opioid overdose; however, recent data indicate that the incidence is lower between 1% and 10%.[119] The occurrence of pulmonary edema is not limited to intravenously administered drugs.[118] Opioid-induced pulmonary edema can occur with the first use of the drug, most commonly seen in people with less experience using the drug, but it is believed to be dose-related rather than an idiosyncratic reaction.[120]

Several mechanisms of opioid-induced noncardiogenic pulmonary edema have been proposed. One mechanism suggests that opioids directly affect the alveolar-capillary membrane, increasing permeability and allowing fluid extravasation into the alveolar spaces.[121] Alternatively, the opioid effect on the CNS may induce a neurogenic efferent response leading to alveolar-capillary permeability or pulmonary venous constriction.[18] Patients with CNS depression after an opioid overdose can develop upper airway obstruction. Breathing against the obstruction can create a strong negative pressure across the alveoli, which causes pulmonary capillary leakage. Other possibilities include a hypersensitivity reaction or acute hypoxic effect, causing increased alveolar-capillary membrane permeability.[121]

Clinically, this complication manifests as dyspnea and somnolence, usually within minutes, depending on the route of administration. Bilateral crackles may be heard on physical examination. Affected individuals become progressively hypoxemic and hypercapnic, leading to cyanosis and obtundation.[121] The chest radiograph typically reveals interstitial and/or alveolar bilateral infiltrates, often in a perihilar pattern, without cardiomegaly or pleural effusions.[118]

Treatment is supportive and may include noninvasive or invasive mechanical ventilation with supplemental oxygen and judicious use of diuretics.[118] The clinical and radiographic abnormalities generally clear within 24 hours. If there is no improvement after 48 hours, alternative diagnoses should be considered, including aspiration and superimposed pneumonia. In progressive cases of respiratory failure after an opioid overdose, ARDS should be considered as well.[122]

Septic Pulmonary Emboli

The most common reason for hospitalization in PWID is cutaneous injection-related infections, which may include thrombophlebitis at the peripheral vein sites. Emboli may originate from thrombophlebitis in the peripheral veins or from heart valves, especially the tricuspid valve. Infection may arise from drug injection under unsterile conditions with injected substance contaminated with pathogens.[123] Approximately 10% of admissions for wound infections are complicated by tricuspid valve endocarditis.[124] The organism most frequently isolated from sputum or blood cultures is *Staphylococcus aureus*.[125] Anaerobic infections may also occur from techniques used in cleaning injection equipment.

Patients typically present in an acute toxic state with fever, dyspnea, chest pain, leukocytosis, and peripheral stigmata of infective endocarditis or an audible murmur. Radiographic examination of the chest may reveal bilateral necrotizing infiltrates, or single or multiple pulmonary nodules, pulmonary gangrene, and infarctions.[126] The lesions may coalesce to form large cavities that communicate with a bronchus. Pulmonary infections from injection drug use may progress to bronchopleural fistulas, empyema, or pneumothorax.[127]

Treatment of pulmonary septic emboli requires a prolonged course of antibiotic therapy, and in some cases invasive drainage or excision. Among PWID, *Staphylococcus aureus*, aerobic gram-negative bacilli, and *Candida* species are typical organisms,[128] and individuals treated for infective endocarditis remain at risk of new bloodstream infection due to ongoing intravenous drug use.[129] Mortality associated with septic thromboemboli is greater in left-sided heart valve infection, and residual pleural scarring and fibrosis are common among survivors.[127] Inpatient addiction treatment with medication for opioid use disorder and valve surgery reduces mortality.[129]

Foreign Body Granulomatosis

Heroin is often adulterated with opioid tablets that are pulverized and frequently contain fillers. Talc, potato starch, cotton fibers, barbiturate, caffeine, magnesium stearate, silicon dioxide, and cellulose are common fillers that can enter the pulmonary capillary bed and lead to chronic inflammation and manifest as foreign body granulomatosis.[130] Occasionally, needles may break off inadvertently during injection, or entire needles may embolize if left in place after injection. This situation is more likely to occur when less accessible injection sites are used. Chest imaging may demonstrate needle fragments within chest soft tissue or lodged within the pulmonary vasculature.

Talc (magnesium silicate) is widely used as a filler in medications such as buprenorphine tablets, oxycodone, heroin, and methylphenidate. In some cases, chronic disease with talc-related fibrosis may ensue with diffuse micronodular interstitial infiltrates, particularly in the midlung zones. Dyspnea, particularly with exertion, and cough are the most common symptoms and may not manifest for years after discontinuation of IV drug use. The chest radiograph can be normal in up to half of patients with talc-related fibrosis.[131] Computed tomography will show diffuse, small centrilobular nodules or ground-glass opacities and substantial parenchymal disease that may look similar to sarcoid or asbestosis. Nodules can coalesce to opacify entire lobes as the disease progresses.[131] Pulmonary function tests reveal a low diffusion capacity.[132] Bronchoalveolar lavage may demonstrate local lymphocytosis and birefringent intracellular or free talc.[133] Lung biopsy may be required to establish the diagnosis, based on histological changes of granulomas, mononuclear inflammatory cells, lymphocytes, and fibrosis.[133]

Patients with progressive symptoms and worsening imaging and pulmonary function tests should be given a trial of systemic steroids, although the evidence is not strong around its effectiveness. In advanced stages, or if there is associated granulomatous pulmonary arterial occlusion, pulmonary hypertension and right ventricular failure can occur.[134] The retina should be examined in all patients in whom the diagnosis is being considered because talc retinopathy occurs in more than half of patients with pulmonary manifestations.[133]

Pulmonary Hypertension

PWID may develop chronic pulmonary hypertension from multiple mechanisms, including chronic hypoxemia related to ILD and vasoconstriction, pulmonary embolization of particulate matter from injected crushed tablets, and pulmonary arterial thrombosis at sites of foreign body granulomatosis.[135] Injection drug use is also a risk factor for HIV infection, which is also associated with pulmonary arterial hypertension.[136]

The most common presentation of pulmonary hypertension is dyspnea on exertion.[136] Physical examination and electrocardiogram may indicate right ventricular enlargement and failure. Treatment includes supplemental oxygen for hypoxemic patients, anticoagulation for patients at increased risk for venous thromboembolism, and diuretics for patients with right heart failure and hypervolemia. Patients with suspected pulmonary hypertension should be referred to a pulmonary hypertension center for hemodynamic evaluation and consideration of advanced therapy. Harm reduction interventions such as syringe filters may reduce pulmonary embolization of particulate matter and subsequent pulmonary hypertension.

Emphysema

Bullous emphysema may develop in people who inject drugs, associated with talc granulomatosis or idiosyncratically. The mechanism is unknown and prevalence is low, but the lung disease pattern can be different with larger, bilateral bullae in the upper lobes. Among individuals with emphysema and bullous lung disease, HIV infection and talc-containing drugs are risk factors. Opioid-related emphysematous disease manifests predominantly in the upper lobes and periphery with bullous cysts.[137]

Stimulant Use

Cocaine and amphetamine-type stimulants, including methamphetamine and amphetamine, "ecstasy" and related substances (eg, 3,4-methylenedioxymethamphetamine [MDMA]), and cathinones (eg, mephedrone, "bath salts") have a wide variety of direct and indirect toxic effects on the respiratory system. Important pulmonary pathology resulting from stimulants includes pulmonary hypertension, pulmonary edema (both cardiogenic and noncardiogenic), alveolar hemorrhage, and parenchymal processes, including eosinophilic lung disease. However, a high prevalence of polysubstance use with stimulant use (eg, concomitant tobacco use),[138] drug contamination with adulterants having toxic pulmonary effects (eg, levamisole),[139] and a lack of rigorously controlled studies make precise exposure-disease relationships elusive. Providers must ultimately be aware of various respiratory toxidromes associated with the use of stimulants to ensure timely diagnosis and effective treatment.

Consequences of Stimulant Administration

Many pulmonary complications are related to nasal insufflation, smoking, and intravenous administration of stimulants. Nasal insufflation of cocaine has well-described adverse effects on the nasal passages and upper airway. The nasal septum is particularly sensitive to the vasoconstrictive properties of cocaine as well as other amphetamine-type stimulants. Nasal septal ulceration, necrosis, and perforation may occur and are grouped as cocaine-induced midline destructive lesions (CIMDL).[140] Sinusitis, epiglottitis, and upper airway obstruction are associated with cocaine use. Immune-mediated vasculitis, due to cocaine or cocaine adulterants (ie, levamisole-induced antineutrophil cytoplasmic antibody [ANCA] positive vasculitis),[141] may be responsible for some cases of CIMDL.[140] Intravenous injection of ground tablets and contaminants of stimulants, can lead to pulmonary vascular granulomatosis, fibrosis, and pulmonary hypertension, similar to pulverized opioid tablets.[142]

Pulmonary Hypertension

The first stimulants historically implicated in the development of pulmonary arterial hypertension were prescribed as appetite suppressants for weight loss.[20] An amphetamine derivative called aminorex, used for weight loss in parts of Europe in the 1960s, was found to cause precapillary pulmonary hypertension via plexiform arteriopathy.[143] A tragic epidemic of aminorex-associated pulmonary arterial hypertension led to the first World Symposium on Pulmonary Hypertension conference in 1973.[144] Fenfluramine, another amphetamine derivative with strong serotonergic properties, was introduced in the 1970s.[143,145] Fenfluramine, commonly prescribed in combination with phentermine (aka "fen-phen"), was withdrawn from markets after several reports of cardiac valvular lesions in users, similar to those seen in carcinoid syndrome. [146] Later, the International Primary Pulmonary Hypertension Study found that using anorexic drugs like fenfluramine was associated with markedly greater odds of pulmonary hypertension.[145] Benfluorex is the most recent amphetamine derivative used in the management of overweight individuals with diabetes and is now classified as a "definite" cause of drug-induced pulmonary arterial hypertension and was withdrawn from European markets in 2009.[147]

The establishment between "idiopathic" pulmonary arterial hypertension and stimulant use arrived in the early 2000s—decades after the pulmonary arterial hypertension epidemic of amphetamine-derived appetite suppressants. Patients with idiopathic pulmonary arterial hypertension were 10 times more likely to have a history of stimulant use than patients with pulmonary arterial hypertension from other risk factors. Methamphetamine and aminorex are notably similar in chemical structure,[148] yet the first descriptions of methamphetamine-associated pulmonary arterial hypertension (meth-APAH) did not surface until 2018. The scientific reports led to methamphetamine's designation as a "definite" (as opposed to "likely") cause of pulmonary arterial hypertension at the 6th World Symposium on Pulmonary Hypertension.[149] Meth-APAH is a unique clinical phenotype of pulmonary arterial hypertension, associated with a high risk of progression and death compared to idiopathic pulmonary arterial hypertension.[150] As of 2020, patients with meth-APAH constitute 9% of the U.S.-based Pulmonary Hypertension Association Registry, but cases of meth-APAH are rising and 83% of cases in the national registry reside in the western United States.[151]

Chronic cocaine use confers a fivefold greater odds of pulmonary hypertension. An autopsy study of 20 patients who died with cocaine intoxication identified 4 patients with pulmonary artery medial hypertrophy (without foreign body embolization).[152] In the absence of more clarifying research, cocaine remains a "possible" cause of drug-induced pulmonary arterial hypertension by the World Symposium on Pulmonary Hypertension.[149] Levamisole is a common adulterant in cocaine preparations and is metabolized by the body to aminorex.[153] Overall, the science on stimulant-induced PAH raises many important hypotheses but remains in its infancy and warrants significantly more investment.

Pulmonary Edema

Cocaine and amphetamine-type stimulant use may be complicated by shortness of breath and hypoxemia due to cardiogenic pulmonary edema.[61] Perihilar, interstitial, and alveolar infiltrates on chest imaging often resolve in users after 24 to 72 hours without targeted interventions.[154] Numerous reports describing this association implicate both cardiogenic and noncardiogenic mechanisms.[61]

The sympathomimetic effects of stimulants can induce intense vasoconstriction and may acutely generate enough afterload (ie, hypertension) to overwhelm a normally functioning heart.[155] Cocaine is associated with coronary vasospasm and myocardial ischemia, which may acutely lead to systolic dysfunction and cardiogenic pulmonary edema.[156] Chronic use of stimulants is associated with systemic hypertension, left ventricular hypertrophy, and diastolic dysfunction—all of which predispose to pulmonary edema.[155] In the presence of alcohol, cocaine undergoes transesterification, forming cocaethylene.[157] Cocaethylene has a long half-life and is associated with cardiotoxicity, suggesting concurrent cocaine and alcohol use may be more potent and toxic than the use of either substance alone.[158] Amphetamine-type stimulant use is associated with dilated cardiomyopathy and systolic dysfunction, also predisposing to pulmonary edema.[159]

Diffuse Alveolar Hemorrhage

Diffuse alveolar hemorrhage may occur in several contexts related to cocaine use, though the pathobiology is not well characterized. Individuals inhaling crack cocaine without signs/symptoms of hemoptysis or spirometric abnormalities can have elevated levels of hemosiderin-positive alveolar macrophages in bronchoalveolar lavage samples.[160] Autopsy evaluations of patients who died with cocaine intoxication found acute and chronic pulmonary hemorrhage in 58% and 40% of cases, respectively.[161] Diffuse alveolar hemorrhage may be a manifestation of alveolar epithelial and endothelial injury. In symptomatic cases, diffuse alveolar hemorrhage impairs gas exchange and/or compromises the airways. Diffuse alveolar hemorrhage can also increase the risk of pulmonary infections. Alveolar macrophages in bronchoalveolar lavage samples obtained from users of crack cocaine had 5 times more iron compared to controls.[162] Iron impairs alveolar macrophage function and further disrupts the innate host immune response to infectious pathogens.[163]

Parenchymal Lung Disease

Patients who died with cocaine intoxication have histopathological evidence of interstitial pneumonitis and pulmonary fibrosis.[161] The pathogenesis of these findings is not understood, particularly the relative effects of co-smoking tobacco. "Crack lung" describes a syndrome of fever, hypoxemia, alveolar and interstitial infiltrates, pulmonary and peripheral eosinophilia, and IgE deposition associated with crack cocaine inhalation.[164] Whether reported cases of "crack lung" are a unique syndrome specific to crack use or a crack-induced hypersensitivity pneumonitis (Löffler syndrome) remains unclear.[61] It is also unclear whether crack cocaine or its contaminants are the main precipitants of this syndrome.[165] Treatment with corticosteroids has been reported to result in rapid improvement.[166] Acute eosinophilic pneumonia has separately been reported in users of amphetamine-type stimulants, but far less frequently.[167]

Lung Function

Severe bronchospasm triggered by cocaine use has been described in people with and without a history of asthma[168]; however, it is not clear that cocaine induces bronchoconstriction. Cocaine-associated bronchospasm is more likely due to local airway irritation (eg, from inhaled particles or high-temperature fumes), rather than the effects of cocaine itself.[169] Supporting this theory, crack cocaine (smoked), but not intravenous cocaine, was found to produce acute bronchoconstriction in individuals with current cocaine use who were otherwise healthy and without a history of asthma.[170] Neither acute nor chronic cocaine exposure has been found to impair diffusing capacity (DL_{CO}) in the lungs.[171] Even fewer studies have evaluated the spirometric effects of amphetamine-type stimulant use. Amphetamine-type stimulants were introduced in the United States as inhalers for asthma and nasal congestion in the early part of the last century.[172] The sympathomimetic effects of amphetamine-type stimulants are assumed to produce bronchodilation but this is not well-described.

Sedative-Hypnotics

Sedative-hypnotic drugs may exert respiratory depressant effects when hazardously used or when mixed with alcohol and opioids. Benzodiazepines, barbiturates, gamma hydroxybutyrate (GHB), and zolpidem bind gamma-aminobutyric acid (GABA) receptors normally function as targets for inhibitory neurotransmitters and promote sedation, hypnosis, anxiolysis, anterograde amnesia, and anticonvulsant activity.[173] Unhealthy use of GHB is more common in bodybuilders and those seeking its hypnotic and euphoric effects. GHB is a naturally occurring metabolite of GABA in the CNS. Unlike benzodiazepines and barbiturates that bind GABA-A receptors, GHB interacts with GABA-B receptors.

Overdose

Barbiturates were the cornerstone of sedative-hypnotic therapy until the 1970s, when benzodiazepines replaced them. Although barbiturates may be involved in a polypharmacy overdose, the most common toxic scenario with barbiturates is an accidental or intentional oral ingestion by a patient with a seizure disorder or family member with one.[174] Barbiturate overdose is more likely to result in coma or death secondary to an increased risk of respiratory depression. Clinically, sedation may progress to coma, with progressive alveolar hypoventilation and respiratory acidosis. Patients are at increased risk for aspiration and atelectasis. Hypotension, which probably is related to direct myocardial depression and vasodilatation, may ensue with cardiac arrest in barbiturate overdose.[175]

Treatment of sedative-hypnotic overdose is supportive. Decontamination with lavage and charcoal adsorption may be appropriate in patients who present within a narrow window, typically an hour, from ingestion. Supplemental oxygen, airway protection, and mechanical ventilation may be necessary. Most deaths occur due to ARDS secondary to either a chemical aspiration pneumonitis or bacterial pneumonia.

In benzodiazepine overdose, the competitive antagonist flumazenil can be administered with caution, but it is short-acting, and its ability to reverse the respiratory depressant effects is controversial. Side effects include anxiety, agitation, crying, and nausea. Seizures can be precipitated in patients with physiological dependence.[174] In barbiturate overdose, elimination can be enhanced with an alkaline diuresis. Dialysis is rarely necessary; however, hemodynamic instability refractory to fluid management is an indication for dialysis.[176] Serum drug levels often rebound after dialysis because redistribution necessitates further treatment.

GHB effects include the elevation of CNS dopamine, the elevation of CNS endorphins, and stimulating growth hormone release. Adverse respiratory effects are mainly related to respiratory depression from overdose.[177] In GHB overdose, recovery is rapid, with a full return to baseline within several hours. Generally, the prognosis is excellent with supportive care alone.

Withdrawal Syndromes

Abrupt abstinence of chronically used sedative-hypnotics may lead to withdrawal symptoms. Benzodiazepine withdrawal causes a hyperadrenergic state that increases carbon dioxide production. Tachypnea is the most common respiratory manifestation of withdrawal from benzodiazepines. Other accompanying symptoms are anxiety, tremor, headache, diaphoresis, difficulty concentrating, insomnia, hallucinations, fatigue, tachycardia, hypertension, and seizure. Increased carbon dioxide production and anxiety in patients experiencing withdrawal may lead to increased minute ventilation. It generally occurs 2 to 5 days after the last dose of the drug.[175] Management typically requires a gradual taper of a long-acting benzodiazepine or barbiturate.

Barbiturate withdrawal occurs after 2 to 7 days of abstinence. Agitation, hyperreflexia, anxiety, and tremor are most common, followed by confusion and hallucinations. Up to 75% of patients experience seizures, often refractory to phenytoin. Effective treatment requires reinstitution of a barbiturate or a cross-tolerant medication such as a benzodiazepine, administered in tapering doses. Because seizures are so common in barbiturate withdrawal, airway protection and mechanical ventilation management are the primary respiratory issues.[175]

After prolonged use of GHB, physiological dependence can occur. Initial withdrawal symptoms are similar to those in alcohol or benzodiazepine withdrawal. Later, choreatic movements and restlessness of the tongue develop. Loss of airway-protective reflexes may necessitate airway protection and mechanical ventilation. Chronic zolpidem use may be associated with rebound insomnia upon discontinuation.[178] After 3 months of nightly use, those who discontinue zopiclone or zolpidem may develop withdrawal symptoms, including anxiety, nausea, or headaches. In patients taking 20 to 30 times the recommended dose over long periods, withdrawal has been characterized as restlessness, diaphoresis, tremors, and seizures resulting in respiratory failure and aspiration.[179]

Sleep-Disordered Breathing

Benzodiazepines can worsen sleep-disordered breathing by decreasing the tone of the upper airway muscles resulting in increased obstructive events. Increased central apneas and reduced ventilatory response to carbon dioxide also lead to worse nocturnal hypoxemia.[180] Although benzodiazepines can be beneficial in treating sleep disorders by increasing total sleep time and the sense of refreshing sleep, they result in a loss of stage 3 deep sleep and less restorative sleep. Zolpidem improves sleep fragmentation and increases time in deep sleep. However, it results in increased obstructive apneic events and reduced oxygen saturation during each event. GHB does not increase obstructive events but may increase central apneas and cause increased nocturnal desaturation.

Other Substances

Use of inhalants is highly prevalent throughout the world, particularly among adolescents; 2.2% of 12- to 17-year-olds have used an inhalant in the past year with lifetime use reported between 8.6% and 13.1% among children and young adults.[181] "Fumes, gases, and vapors" remain the top substance category involved in pediatric deaths.[182] Volatile substances include aromatic and short-chain hydrocarbons, such as toluene, gasoline, butane, butyl and amyl nitrites, and organofluorines that are found in adhesives, paints, paint thinners, dry cleaning fluids, refrigerants, and propellants. Butane gas and propane gas are found in cigarette lighter refills and aerosols, alkyl nitrites (aka "poppers"), in some industrial glues, and acetone is found in nail polish remover. When sniffed or vigorously inhaled within a hermetic container ("huffed"), they are readily absorbed in the lungs. Intoxicating and dysphoric effects follow within seconds. Primary acute effects involve the CNS and include lethargy, stupor, agitation, hallucinations, dizziness, and seizures.[183]

Pulmonary complications include severe respiratory depression, barotrauma (pneumomediastinum), persistent cough, noncardiogenic pulmonary edema, and asphyxiation.[184] Nitrates and other inhalants may be directly irritating to airway mucosa, which can cause a chronic cough. Butyl and isobutyl nitrites may cause methemoglobinemia, which manifests as cyanosis with low oxygen saturation of hemoglobin but with normal partial pressure of oxygen. [185] Co-oximetry will measure methemoglobin levels and treatment is with intravenous methylene blue. Inhalant use may also result in asphyxiation from plastic bag suffocation, respiratory depression, and acute noncardiogenic pulmonary edema.[186] Metabolic acidosis may occur, with compensatory respiratory alkalosis, resulting from distal renal tubular acidosis or increased anion gap acidosis.

Nitrous oxide, also known as "laughing gas," is a widely used inhalational anesthetic-analgesic agent that also is used in a variety of commercial products (such as a propellant for whipped cream chargers) and dispensed from small metal canisters ("whippets") and inhaled from balloons.[187] It is a readily available and often used substance with euphoric effects. Pulmonary complications include pneumomediastinum, respiratory depression, and hypoxemia because of displacement of oxygen, leading to asphyxiation.[188] Treatment is supportive, including supplemental oxygen and respiratory support.

Anabolic steroids induce a prothrombotic state and may cause pulmonary embolism, strokes, and other forms of thrombosis.[189] Other respiratory complications are less common but may occur after stroke and include atelectasis, pneumonia, aspiration, neurogenic pulmonary edema, and sleep-disordered breathing.

CONCLUSION

The lung is a major organ system with constant exposure between the epithelium and the external environment, and substance use via intranasal and inhalation routes are common pathways to lung disease. Endothelial pathology may also ensue from the pulmonary blood flow via the bronchial and pulmonary circulation. Substance use via oral, subcutaneous, intramuscular, or intravenous can impact lung physiology and exacerbate existing diseases such as asthma and ARDS or initiate new diseases such pulmonary hypertension, septic emboli, and interstitial lung disease. The more common pulmonary disorders such as COPD and asthma develop or exacerbate from chronic tobacco smoke.

While smoked tobacco cigarettes remain the most frequently encountered drug leading to pulmonary disease, emerging drug markets with stimulant use and opioids are increasing the prevalence of pulmonary diseases. The growing prevalence of polysubstance use carries overlapping and synergistic effects that are harmful to the lungs. Pulmonary hypertension, ARDS, and interstitial lung disease have risk factors with substance use (ie, alcohol, opioids, methamphetamines) that are frequently underrecognized and should be considered as major risk factors. The substances may have isolated effects on the respiratory system, and many have overlapping clinical manifestations across multiple pulmonary-related diseases. When examining individuals with unhealthy substance use, health providers should consider the contributions from a wide array of substances and their interacting effects on pulmonary health.

REFERENCES

1. West JB, Luks AM. *West's Pulmonary Pathophysiology: The Essentials.* Lippincott Williams & Wilkins; 2021.
2. Hilal-Dandan R, Knollman B, Brunton L. *Goodman and Gilman's the Pharmacological Basis of Therapeutics.* 13th ed. McGraw Hill Education/Medical; 2017.
3. Kish SJ. Pharmacologic mechanisms of crystal meth. *CMAJ.* 2008; 178(13):1679-1682.
4. Ito JT, Ramos D, Lima FF, et al. Nasal mucociliary clearance in subjects with copd after smoking cessation. *Respir Care.* 2015;60(3):399-405.
5. George SC, Hlastala MP, Souders JE, Babb AL. Gas exchange in the airways. *J Aerosol Med.* 1996;9(1):25-33.
6. Price ME, Pavlik JA, Sisson JH, Wyatt TA. Inhibition of protein phosphatase 1 reverses alcohol-induced ciliary dysfunction. *Am J Physiol Lung Cell Mol Physiol.* 2015;308(6):L577-L585.
7. Aderem A, Underhill DM. Mechanisms of phagocytosis in macrophages. *Annu Rev Immunol.* 1999;17:593-623.
8. Moss M. Epidemiology of sepsis: race, sex, and chronic alcohol abuse. *Clin Infect Dis.* 2005;41(Suppl 7):S490-S497.
9. Zebraski SE, Kochenash SM, Raffa RB. Lung opioid receptors: pharmacology and possible target for nebulized morphine in dyspnea. *Life Sci.* 2000;66(23):2221-2231.
10. Peterson PK, Molitor TW, Chao CC. The opioid-cytokine connection. *J Neuroimmunol.* 1998;83(1-2):63-69.
11. Stämpfli MR, Anderson GP. How cigarette smoke skews immune responses to promote infection, lung disease and cancer. *Nat Rev Immunol.* 2009;9(5):377-384.
12. Rennard SI, Togo S, Holz O. Cigarette smoke inhibits alveolar repair: a mechanism for the development of emphysema. *Proc Am Thorac Soc.* 2006;3(8):703-708.
13. Schweitzer KS, Chen SX, Law S, et al. Endothelial disruptive proinflammatory effects of nicotine and e-cigarette vapor exposures. *Am J Physiol Lung Cell Mol Physiol.* 2015;309(2):L175-L187.
14. Pacifici R, Zuccaro P, Hernandez López C, et al. Acute effects of 3,4-methylenedioxymethamphetamine alone and in combination with ethanol on the immune system in humans. *J Pharmacol Exp Ther.* 2001;296(1):207-215.
15. Yeligar SM, Chen MM, Kovacs EJ, Sisson JH, Burnham EL, Brown LAS. Alcohol and lung injury and immunity. *Alcohol.* 2016;55:51-59.
16. Barke KE, Hough LB. Opiates, mast cells and histamine release. *Life Sci.* 1993;53(18):1391-1399.
17. Bhattacharya M, Kallet RH, Ware LB, Matthay MA. Negative-pressure pulmonary edema. *Chest.* 2016;150(4):927-933.
18. Smith WS, Matthay MA. Evidence for a hydrostatic mechanism in human neurogenic pulmonary edema. *Chest.* 1997;111(5):1326-1333.
19. Kumar K, Holden WE. Drug-induced pulmonary vascular disease—mechanisms and clinical patterns. *West J Med.* 1986;145(3):343-349.
20. Ramirez RL III, De Jesus Perez V, Zamanian RT. Stimulants and pulmonary arterial hypertension: an update. *Adv Pulm Hypertens.* 2018;17(2):49-54.
21. Volkow ND, Fowler JS, Wang G-J, et al. Distribution and pharmacokinetics of methamphetamine in the human body: clinical implications. *PLoS One.* 2010;5(12):e15269.

22. Buchanan JF, Brown CR. 'Designer drugs'. A problem in clinical toxicology. *Med Toxicol Adverse Drug Exp*. 1988;3(1):1-17.
23. Yubero-Lahoz S, Ayestas MA Jr., Blough BE, et al. Effects of MDMA and related analogs on plasma 5-HT: relevance to 5-HT transporters in blood and brain. *Eur J Pharmacol*. 2012;674(2-3):337-344.
24. Eddahibi S, Adnot S. Anorexigen-induced pulmonary hypertension and the serotonin (5-HT) hypothesis: lessons for the future in pathogenesis. *Respir Res*. 2002;3:9.
25. Setola V, Hufeisen SJ, Grande-Allen KJ, et al. 3,4-methylene-dioxymethamphetamine (MDMA, "Ecstasy") induces fenfluramine-like proliferative actions on human cardiac valvular interstitial cells in vitro. *Mol Pharmacol*. 2003;63(6):1223-1229.
26. Kral AH, Lambdin BH, Browne EN, et al. Transition from injecting opioids to smoking fentanyl in San Francisco, California. *Drug Alcohol Depend*. 2021;227:109003.
27. Smith CJ, Hansch C. The relative toxicity of compounds in mainstream cigarette smoke condensate. *Food Chem Toxicol*. 2000;38(7):637-646.
28. Sandford AJ, Chagani T, Weir TD, Connett JE, Anthonisen NR, Paré PD. Susceptibility genes for rapid decline of lung function in the lung health study. *Am J Respir Crit Care Med*. 2001;163(2):469-473.
29. Lee PN, Fry JS. Systematic review of the evidence relating FEV1 decline to giving up smoking. *BMC Med*. 2010;8:84.
30. Vassallo R, Ryu J. Tobacco smoke-related diffuse lung diseases. *Semin Resp Crit Care Med*. 2008;29(06):643-650.
31. Vogelmeier CF, Criner GJ, Martinez FJ, et al. Global Strategy for the Diagnosis, Management, and Prevention of Chronic Obstructive Lung Disease 2017 Report: GOLD Executive Summary. *Arch Bronconeumol*. 2017;53(3):128-149.
32. Polkey MI, Hamnegård C-H, Hughes PD, Rafferty GF, Green M, Moxham J. Influence of acute lung volume change on contractile properties of human diaphragm. *J Appl Physiol*. 1998;85(4):1322-1328.
33. Islam N, Rahman S. Improved treatment of nicotine addiction and emerging pulmonary drug delivery. *Drug Discov Ther*. 2012;6(3):123-132.
34. Leone FT, Zhang Y, Evers-Casey S, et al. Initiating pharmacologic treatment in tobacco-dependent adults. an official American Thoracic Society Clinical practice guideline. *Am J Respir Crit Care Med*. 2020;202(2):e5-e31.
35. Vassallo R, Ryu JH. Smoking-related interstitial lung diseases. *Clin Chest Med*. 2012;33(1):165-178.
36. Hong J-L, Lee L-Y. Cigarette smoke-induced bronchoconstriction: causative agents and role of thromboxane receptors. *J Appl Physiol*. 1996;81(5):2053-2059.
37. Raghu G, Remy-Jardin M, Richeldi L, et al. Idiopathic pulmonary fibrosis (an update) and progressive pulmonary fibrosis in adults: an official ATS/ERS/JRS/ALAT clinical practice guideline. *Am J Respir Crit Care Med*. 2022;205(9):e18-e47.
38. Lin H, Jiang S. Combined pulmonary fibrosis and emphysema (CPFE): an entity different from emphysema or pulmonary fibrosis alone. *J Thorac Dis*. 2015;7(4):767-779.
39. Nef HM, Mollmann H, Hamm C, Grimminger F, Ghofrani HA. Updated classification and management of pulmonary hypertension. *Heart*. 2010;96(7):552-559.
40. Cheng Y-L, Huang T-W, Lin C-K, et al. The impact of smoking in primary spontaneous pneumothorax. *J Thorac Cardiovasc Surg*. 2009;138(1):192-195.
41. Milroy CM, Parai JL. The histopathology of drugs of abuse. *Histopathology*. 2011;59(4):579-593.
42. Cruz CSD, Dela Cruz CS, Tanoue LT, Matthay RA. Lung cancer: epidemiology, etiology, and prevention. *Clin Chest Med*. 2011;32(4):605-644.
43. Öberg M, Jaakkola MS, Woodward A, Peruga A, Prüss-Ustün A. Worldwide burden of disease from exposure to second-hand smoke: a retrospective analysis of data from 192 countries. *Lancet*. 2011;377(9760):139-146.
44. DiGiulio S. USPSTF updates lung cancer screening guidelines. *Oncology Times*. 2021;43(9):1-11.
45. Hurt RD, Ebbert JO, Taylor Hays J, McFadden DD. Preventing lung cancer by treating tobacco dependence. *Clin Chest Med*. 2011;32(4):645-657.
46. Godtfredsen NS. Effect of smoking reduction on lung cancer risk. *JAMA*. 2005;294(12):1505.
47. Moazed F, Hendrickson C, Jauregui A, et al. Cigarette smoke exposure and acute respiratory distress syndrome in sepsis: epidemiology, clinical features, and biologic markers. *Am J Respir Crit Care Med*. 2022;205(8):927-935.
48. Calfee CS, Matthay MA, Kangelaris KN, et al. Cigarette smoke exposure and the acute respiratory distress syndrome. *Crit Care Med*. 2015;43(9):1790-1797.
49. Tashkin DP, Gliederer F, Rose J, et al. Effects of varying marijuana smoking profile on deposition of tar and absorption of CO and delta-9-THC. *Pharmacol Biochem Behav*. 1991;40(3):651-656.
50. Wu T-C, Tzu-Chin WU, Tashkin DP, Djahed B, Rose JE. Pulmonary hazards of smoking marijuana as compared with tobacco. *N Engl J Med*. 1988;318(6):347-351.
51. Tetrault JM, Crothers K, Moore BA, Mehra R, Concato J, Fiellin DA. Effects of marijuana smoking on pulmonary function and respiratory complications. *Arch Intern Med*. 2007;167(3):221-228.
52. Aldington S, Williams M, Nowitz M, et al. Effects of cannabis on pulmonary structure, function and symptoms. *Thorax*. 2007;62(12):1058-1063.
53. Miller WE, Spiekerman RE, Hepper NG. Pneumomediastinum resulting from performing Valsalva maneuvers during marihuana smoking. *Chest*. 1972;62(2):233-234.
54. Roth MD, Arora A, Barsky SH, Kleerup EC, Simmons M, Tashkin DP. Airway inflammation in young marijuana and tobacco smokers. *Am J Respir Crit Care Med*. 1998;157(3 Pt 1):928-937.
55. Alanazi AMM, Alqahtani MM, Alquaimi MM, et al. Substance use and misuse among adults with chronic obstructive pulmonary disease in the United States, 2015-2019: prevalence, association, and moderation. *Int J Environ Res Public Health*. 2021;19(1):408.
56. Tashkin DP. Airway effects of marijuana, cocaine, and other inhaled illicit agents. *Curr Opin Pulm Med*. 2001;7(2):43-61.
57. Krantz AJ, Hershow RC, Prachand N, Hayden DM, Franklin C, Hryhorczuk DO. Heroin insufflation as a trigger for patients with life-threatening asthma. *Chest*. 2003;123(2):510-517.
58. Doshi V, Shenoy S, Ganesh A, Rishi MA, Molnar J, Henkle J. Profile of acute asthma exacerbation in drug users. *Am J Ther*. 2017;24(1):e39-e43.
59. Levine M, Iliescu ME, Margellos-Anast H, Estarziau M, Ansell DA. The effects of cocaine and heroin use on intubation rates and hospital utilization in patients with acute asthma exacerbations. *Chest*. 2005;128(4):1951-1957.
60. Taylor RF, Bernard GR. Airway complications from free-basing cocaine. *Chest*. 1989;95(2):476-477.
61. Tseng W, Sutter ME, Albertson TE. Stimulants and the lung. *Clin Rev Allergy Immunol*. 2014;46(1):82-100.
62. Shesser R, Davis C, Edelstein S. Pneumomediastinum and pneumothorax after inhaling alkaloidal cocaine. *Ann Emerg Med*. 1981;10(4):213-215.
63. Auerbach O, Stout AP, Hammond EC, Garfinkel L. Changes in bronchial epithelium in relation to cigarette smoking and in relation to lung cancer. *N Engl J Med*. 1961;265:253-267.
64. Dinakar C, O'Connor GT. The health effects of electronic cigarettes. *N Engl J Med*. 2016;375(26):2608-2609.
65. Prochaska JJ, Vogel EA, Benowitz N. Nicotine delivery and cigarette equivalents from vaping a JUULpod. *Tob Control*. 2022;31(e1):e88-e93.
66. Wang TW, Neff LJ, Park-Lee E, Ren C, Cullen KA, King BA. E-cigarette use among middle and high school students—United States, 2020. *MMWR Morb Mortal Wkly Rep*. 2020;69(37):1310-1312.
67. Grana R, Benowitz N, Glantz SA. E-cigarettes: a scientific review. *Circulation*. 2014;129(19):1972-1986.
68. Farsalinos KE, Kistler KA, Gillman G, Voudris V. Evaluation of electronic cigarette liquids and aerosol for the presence of selected inhalation toxins. *Nicotine Tob Res*. 2015;17(2):168-174.
69. Zhu S-H, Sun JY, Bonnevie E, et al. Four hundred and sixty brands of e-cigarettes and counting: implications for product regulation. *Tob Control*. 2014;23(Suppl 3):iii3-iii9.
70. Allen JG, Flanigan SS, LeBlanc M, et al. Flavoring chemicals in e-cigarettes: diacetyl, 2,3-pentanedione, and acetoin in a sample of 51 products, including fruit-, candy-, and cocktail-flavored e-cigarettes. *Environ Health Perspect*. 2016;124(6):733-739.

71. Barrington-Trimis JL, Samet JM, McConnell R. Flavorings in electronic cigarettes. *JAMA*. 2014;312(23):2493.
72. Kosmider L, Sobczak A, Fik M, et al. Carbonyl compounds in electronic cigarette vapors: effects of nicotine solvent and battery output voltage. *Nicotine Tob Res*. 2014;16(10):1319-1326.
73. Chun LF, Moazed F, Calfee CS, Matthay MA, Gotts JE. Pulmonary toxicity of e-cigarettes. *Am J Physiol Lung Cell Mol Physiol*. 2017; 313(2):L193-L206.
74. Werner AK, Koumans EH, Chatham-Stephens K, et al. Hospitalizations and deaths associated with EVALI. *N Engl J Med*. 2020;382(17):1589-1598.
75. Krishnasamy VP, Hallowell BD, Ko JY, et al. Update: characteristics of a nationwide outbreak of e-cigarette, or vaping, product use-associated lung injury—United States, August 2019-January 2020. *MMWR Morb Mortal Wkly Rep*. 2020;69(3):90-94.
76. Chatham-Stephens K, Roguski K, Jang Y, et al. Characteristics of hospitalized and nonhospitalized patients in a nationwide outbreak of e-cigarette, or vaping, product use-associated lung injury—United States, November 2019. *MMWR Morb Mortal Wkly Rep*. 2019;68(46):1076-1080.
77. Butt YM, Smith ML, Tazelaar HD, et al. Pathology of vaping-associated lung injury. *N Engl J Med*. 2019;381(18):1780-1781.
78. Layden JE, Ghinai I, Pray I, et al. Pulmonary illness related to e-cigarette use in Illinois and Wisconsin—final report. *N Engl J Med*. 2020;382(10):903-916.
79. National Institute on Alcohol Abuse and Alcoholism. *Drinking Levels Defined*. Accessed May 28, 2022. https://www.niaaa.nih.gov/alcohol-health/overview-alcohol-consumption/moderate-binge-drinking
80. Johnstone RE, Witt RL. Respiratory effects of ethyl alcohol intoxication. *JAMA*. 1972;222(4):486-486.
81. Garriott JC, Aguayo EH. *Garriott's Medicolegal Aspects of Alcohol*. Lawyers & Judges Publishing Company, Inc; 2008.
82. Afshar M, Netzer G, Salisbury-Afshar E, Murthi S, Smith GS. Injured patients with very high blood alcohol concentrations. *Injury*. 2016;47(1):83.
83. Szabo G, Mandrekar P. A recent perspective on alcohol, immunity, and host defense. *Alcohol Clin Exp Res*. 2009;33(2):220-232.
84. Mandell LA, Niederman MS. Aspiration pneumonia. *N Engl J Med*. 2019;380(7):651-663.
85. Adnet F, Baud F. Relation between Glasgow Coma Scale and aspiration pneumonia. *Lancet*. 1996;348(9020):e053619.
86. Reza SM, Huang JQ, Marrie TJ. Differences in the features of aspiration pneumonia according to site of acquisition: community or continuing care facility. *J Am Geriatr Soc*. 2006;54(2):296-302.
87. Marik PE. Aspiration pneumonitis and aspiration pneumonia. *N Engl J Med*. 2001;344(9):665-671.
88. Wrenn KD, Slovis CM, Minion GE, Rutkowski R. The syndrome of alcoholic ketoacidosis. *Am J Med*. 1991;91(2):119-128.
89. Long B, Lentz S, Gottlieb M. Alcoholic Ketoacidosis: etiologies, evaluation, and management. *J Emerg Med*. 2021;61(6):658-665.
90. Jain H, Duggal M. Alcoholic ketoacidosis. In: Preedy VR, Watson RR, eds. *Comprehensive Handbook of Alcohol Related Pathology*. Elsevier; 2005:511-517.
91. Schelling JR, Howard RL, Winter SD, Linas SL. Increased osmolal gap in alcoholic ketoacidosis and lactic acidosis. *Ann Intern Med*. 1990; 113(8):580-582.
92. Kraut JA, Kurtz I. Toxic alcohol ingestions: clinical features, diagnosis, and management. *Clin J Am Soc Nephrol*. 2008;3(1):208-225.
93. Vally H, de Klerk N, Thompson PJ. Alcoholic drinks: important triggers for asthma. *J Allergy Clin Immunol*. 2000;105(3):462-467.
94. Lieberoth S, Backer V, Kyvik KO, et al. Intake of alcohol and risk of adult-onset asthma. *Respir Med*. 2012;106(2):184-188.
95. Vally H, Carr A, El-Saleh J, Thompson P. Wine-induced asthma: a placebo-controlled assessment of its pathogenesis. *J Allergy Clin Immunol*. 1999;103(1 Pt 1):41-46.
96. Afshar M, Poole JA, Cao G, et al. Exhaled nitric oxide levels among adults with excessive alcohol consumption. *Chest*. 2016; 150(1):196-209.
97. Siu S. Alcohol and lung airways function. *Perm J*. 2010;14(1):11-18.
98. Shimoda T, Kohno S, Takao A, et al. Investigation of the mechanism of alcohol-induced bronchial asthma. *J Allergy Clin Immunol*. 1996;97(1 Pt 1): 74-84.
99. Scanlan MF, Roebuck T, Little PJ, Redman JR, Naughton MT. Effect of moderate alcohol upon obstructive sleep apnoea. *Eur Respir J*. 2000;16(5):909-913.
100. Issa FG, Sullivan CE. Alcohol, snoring and sleep apnea. *J Neurol Neurosurg Psychiatry*. 1982;45(4):353-359.
101. Moss M, Burnham EL. Alcohol abuse in the critically ill patient. *Lancet*. 2006;368(9554):2231-2242.
102. Nolan JP. Alcohol as a factor in the illness of university service patients. *Am J Med Sci*. 1965;249:135-142.
103. Garcia-Vidal C, Ardanuy C, Tubau F, et al. Pneumococcal pneumonia presenting with septic shock: host- and pathogen-related factors and outcomes. *Thorax*. 2010;65(1):77-81.
104. Gupta NM, Lindenauer PK, Yu P-C, et al. Association between alcohol use disorders and outcomes of patients hospitalized with community-acquired pneumonia. *JAMA Netw Open*. 2019;2(6):e195172.
105. Moss M, Parsons PE, Steinberg KP, et al. Chronic alcohol abuse is associated with an increased incidence of acute respiratory distress syndrome and severity of multiple organ dysfunction in patients with septic shock. *Crit Care Med*. 2003;31(3):869-877.
106. Boé DM, Vandivier RW, Burnham EL, Moss M. Alcohol abuse and pulmonary disease. *J Leukoc Biol*. 2009;86(5):1097-1104.
107. Burnham EL, Moss M, Harris F, Brown LAS. Elevated plasma and lung endothelial selectin levels in patients with acute respiratory distress syndrome and a history of chronic alcohol abuse. *Crit Care Med*. 2004;32(3):675-679.
108. Moss M, Bucher B, Moore FA, Moore EE, Parsons PE. The role of chronic alcohol abuse in the development of acute respiratory distress syndrome in adults. *JAMA*. 1996;275(1):50-54.
109. Krok KL, Cárdenas A. Hepatic hydrothorax. *Semin Respir Crit Care Med*. 2012;33(1):3-10.
110. Kochar R, Nevah Rubin MI, Fallon MB. Pulmonary complications of cirrhosis. *Curr Gastroenterol Rep*. 2011;13(1):34-39.
111. Van der Linden P, Le Moine O, Ghysels M, Ortinez M, Devière J. Pulmonary hypertension after transjugular intrahepatic portosystemic shunt: effects on right ventricular function. *Hepatology*. 1996;23(5):982-987.
112. Kuo PC, Plotkin JS, Gaine S, et al. Portopulmonary hypertension and the liver transplant candidate. *Transplantation*. 1999;67(8):1087-1093.
113. Wilson KC, Saukkonen JJ. Acute respiratory failure from abused substances. *J Intensive Care Med*. 2004;19(4):183-193.
114. Rosenow EC III, Limper AH. Drug-induced pulmonary disease. *Semin Respir Infect*. 1995;10(2):86-95.
115. Han B, Gfroerer JC, Colliver JD. Associations between duration of illicit drug use and health conditions: results from the 2005-2007 national surveys on drug use and health. *Ann Epidemiol*. 2010;20(4):289-297.
116. Steffens C, Sung M, Bastian LA, Edelman EJ, Brackett A, Gunderson CG. The association between prescribed opioid receipt and community-acquired pneumonia in adults: a systematic review and meta-analysis. *J Gen Intern Med*. 2020;35(11):3315-3322.
117. Rhodes A, Evans LE, Alhazzani W, et al. Surviving sepsis campaign: international guidelines for management of sepsis and septic shock: 2016. *Intensive Care Med*. 2017;43(3):304-377.
118. Yamanaka T, Sadikot RT. Opioid effect on lungs. *Respirology*. 2013; 18(2):255-262.
119. O'Donnell AE, Pappas LS. Pulmonary complications of intravenous drug abuse. *Chest*. 1988;94(2):251-253.
120. Rosenow EC III. Drug-induced pulmonary disease. *Dis Mon*. 1994; 40(5):253-310.
121. Cooper JA Jr, White DA, Matthay RA. Drug-induced pulmonary disease. Part 2: noncytotoxic drugs. *Am Rev Respir Dis*. 1986;133(3):488-505.
122. Schiller EY, Goyal A, Mechanic OJ. Opioid overdose. *StatPearls [Internet]*. StatPearls Publishing; 2022. Accessed June 21, 2023. https://www.ncbi.nlm.nih.gov/books/NBK470415/
123. Kaushik KS, Kapila K, Praharaj AK. Shooting up: the interface of microbial infections and drug abuse. *J Med Microbiol*. 2011;60(Pt 4): 408-422.

124. Lloyd-Smith E, Wood E, Zhang R, et al. Determinants of hospitalization for a cutaneous injection-related infection among injection drug users: a cohort study. *BMC Public Health*. 2010;10:327.
125. Gordon RJ, Lowy FD. Bacterial infections in drug users. *New Engl J Med*. 2005;353(18):1945-1954.
126. Poole PS, Stark HE, Stark P. Necrotizing pneumonia, pulmonary abscess, and lung gangrene. *Contemp Diagn Radiol*. 2011;34(13):1-6.
127. Saydain G, Singh J, Dalal B, Yoo W, Levine DP. Outcome of patients with injection drug use-associated endocarditis admitted to an intensive care unit. *J Crit Care*. 2010;25(2):248-253.
128. Pericàs JM, Llopis J, Athan E, et al. Prospective cohort study of infective endocarditis in people who inject drugs. *J Am Coll Cardiol*. 2021;77(5):544-545.
129. Tan C, Shojaei E, Wiener J, Shah M, Koivu S, Silverman M. Risk of new bloodstream infections and mortality among people who inject drugs with infective endocarditis. *JAMA Netw Open*. 2020;3(8):e2012974.
130. Radke JB, Owen KP, Sutter ME, Ford JB, Albertson TE. The effects of opioids on the lung. *Clin Rev Allergy Immunol*. 2014;46(1):54-64.
131. Marchiori E, Lourenço S, Gasparetto TD, Zanetti G, Mano CM, Nobre LF. Pulmonary talcosis: imaging findings. *Lung*. 2010; 188(2):165-171.
132. Overland ES, Nolan AJ, Hopewell PC. Alteration of pulmonary function in intravenous drug abusers. Prevalence, severity, and characterization of gas exchange abnormalities. *Am J Med*. 1980;68(2):231-237.
133. Dulohery MM, Maldonado F, Limper AH. Drug-induced pulmonary disease. In: Broaddas VC, Mason RJ, Ernst JD, et al., eds. *Murray and Nadel's Textbook of Respiratory Medicine*. 6th ed. Elsevier; 2016: 1275-1294.e1217.
134. Griffith CC, Raval JS, Nichols L. Intravascular talcosis due to intravenous drug use is an underrecognized cause of pulmonary hypertension. *Pulm Med*. 2012;2012:1-6.
135. Price L, Bouillon K, John Wort S, Humbert M. Drug- and toxin-induced pulmonary arterial hypertension. *Pulmonary Vascular Disorders*. 2012;76-84.
136. Simonneau G, Montani D, Celermajer DS, et al. Haemodynamic definitions and updated clinical classification of pulmonary hypertension. *Eur Respir J*. 2019;53(1):1801913.
137. Goldstein DS, Karpel JP, Appel D, Williams MH Jr. Bullous pulmonary damage in users of intravenous drugs. *Chest*. 1986;89(2):266-269.
138. Gouzoulis-Mayfrank E, Daumann J. The confounding problem of polydrug use in recreational ecstasy/MDMA users: a brief overview. *J Psychopharmacol*. 2006;20(2):188-193.
139. Pawlik E, Mahler H, Hartung B, Plässer G, Daldrup T. Drug-related death: adulterants from cocaine preparations in lung tissue and blood. *Forensic Sci Int*. 2015;249:294-303.
140. Trimarchi M, Nicolai P, Lombardi D, et al. Sinonasal osteocartilaginous necrosis in cocaine abusers: experience in 25 patients. *Am J Rhinol*. 2003;17(1):33-43.
141. Jin Q, Kant S, Alhariri J, Geetha D. Levamisole adulterated cocaine associated ANCA vasculitis: review of literature and update on pathogenesis. *J Community Hosp Intern Med Perspect*. 2018;8(6):339-344.
142. Hind CR. Pulmonary complications of intravenous drug misuse. 1. Epidemiology and non-infective complications. *Thorax*. 1990;45(11): 891-898.
143. Rothman RB, Baumann MH. Therapeutic and adverse actions of serotonin transporter substrates. *Pharmacol Ther*. 2002;95(1):73-88.
144. Fishman AP. Primary pulmonary arterial hypertension: a look back. *J Am Coll Cardiol*. 2004;43(12 Suppl S):2S-4S.
145. Robertson CH Jr, Reynolds RC, Wilson JE III. Pulmonary hypertension and foreign body granulomas in intravenous drug abusers. Documentation by cardiac catheterization and lung biopsy. *Am J Med*. 1976;61(5):657-664.
146. Marshall EM. Valvular heart disease associated with fenfluramine-phentermine. *N Engl J Med*. 1997;337(24):1775; author reply 1775-1776.
147. Savale L, Chaumais M-C, Cottin V, et al. Pulmonary hypertension associated with benfluorex exposure. *Eur Respir J*. 2012; 40(5):1164-1172.
148. Courtney KE, Ray LA. Methamphetamine: an update on epidemiology, pharmacology, clinical phenomenology, and treatment literature. *Drug Alcohol Depend*. 2014;143:11-21.
149. Galiè N, McLaughlin VV, Rubin LJ, Simonneau G. An overview of the 6th World Symposium on Pulmonary Hypertension. *Eur Respir J*. 2019;53(1):1802148.
150. Zamanian RT, Hedlin H, Greuenwald P, et al. Features and outcomes of methamphetamine-associated pulmonary arterial hypertension. *Am J Respir Crit Care Med*. 2018;197(6):788-800.
151. Kolaitis NA, Zamanian RT, de Jesus Perez VA, et al. Clinical differences and outcomes between methamphetamine-associated and idiopathic pulmonary arterial hypertension in the Pulmonary Hypertension Association Registry. *Ann Am Thorac Soc*. 2021;18(4):613-622.
152. Murray RJ, Smialek JE, Golle M, Albin RJ. Pulmonary artery medial hypertrophy in cocaine users without foreign particle microembolization. *Chest*. 1989;96(5):1050-1053.
153. Hofmaier T, Luf A, Seddik A, et al. Aminorex, a metabolite of the cocaine adulterant levamisole, exerts amphetamine like actions at monoamine transporters. *Neurochem Int*. 2014;73:32-41.
154. Haim DY, Lippmann ML, Goldberg SK, Walkenstein MD. The pulmonary complications of crack cocaine. A comprehensive review. *Chest*. 1995;107(1):233-240.
155. Havakuk O, Rezkalla SH, Kloner RA. The cardiovascular effects of cocaine. *J Am Coll Cardiol*. 2017;70(1):101-113.
156. Talarico GP, Crosta ML, Giannico MB, Summaria F, Calò L, Patrizi R. Cocaine and coronary artery diseases: a systematic review of the literature. *J Cardiovasc Med*. 2017;18(5):291-294.
157. Laizure SC, Mandrell T, Gades NM, Parker RB. Cocaethylene metabolism and interaction with cocaine and ethanol: role of carboxylesterases. *Drug Metab Dispos*. 2003;31(1):16-20.
158. McCance-Katz EF, Kosten TR, Jatlow P. Concurrent use of cocaine and alcohol is more potent and potentially more toxic than use of either alone—a multiple-dose study. *Biol Psychiatry*. 1998;44(4):250-259.
159. Kaye S, McKetin R, Duflou J, Darke S. Methamphetamine and cardiovascular pathology: a review of the evidence. *Addiction*. 2007;102(8):1204-1211.
160. Baldwin GC, Choi R, Roth MD, et al. Evidence of chronic damage to the pulmonary microcirculation in habitual users of alkaloidal ("crack") cocaine. *Chest*. 2002;121(4):1231-1238.
161. Bailey ME, Fraire AE, Greenberg SD, Barnard J, Cagle PT. Pulmonary histopathology in cocaine abusers. *Hum Pathol*. 1994;25(2):203-207.
162. Janjua TM, Bohan AE, Wesselius LJ. Increased lower respiratory tract iron concentrations in alkaloidal ("crack") cocaine users. *Chest*. 2001;119(2):422-427.
163. O'Brien-Ladner AR, Blumer BM, Wesselius LJ. Differential regulation of human alveolar macrophage-derived interleukin-1beta and tumor necrosis factor-alpha by iron. *J Lab Clin Med*. 1998;132(6):497-506.
164. Kissner DG, Lawrence WD, Selis JE, Flint A. Crack lung: pulmonary disease caused by cocaine abuse. *Am Rev Respir Dis*. 1987;136(5):1250-1252.
165. Kon OM, Redhead JB, Gillen D, Fothergill J, Henry JA, Mitchell DM. "Crack lung" caused by an impure preparation. *Thorax*. 1996;51(9):959-960.
166. Oh PI, Balter MS. Cocaine induced eosinophilic lung disease. *Thorax*. 1992;47(6):478-479.
167. Lin S-S, Chen Y-C, Chang Y-L, Yeh DY-W, Lin C-C. Crystal amphetamine smoking-induced acute eosinophilic pneumonia and diffuse alveolar damage: a case report and literature review. *Chin J Physiol*. 2014;57(5):295-298.
168. Rebhun J. Association of asthma and freebase smoking. *Ann Allergy*. 1988;60(4):339-342.
169. Chen LC, Graefe JF, Shojaie J, Willetts J, Wood RW. Pulmonary effects of the cocaine pyrolysis product, methylecgonidine, in guinea pigs. *Life Sci*. 1995;56(1):PL7-PL12.
170. Tashkin DP, Kleerup EC, Koyal SN, Marques JA, Goldman MD. Acute effects of inhaled and IV cocaine on airway dynamics. *Chest*. 1996;110(4):904-910.

171. Kleerup EC, Koyal SN, Marques-Magallanes JA, Goldman MD, Tashkin DP. Chronic and acute effects of "crack" cocaine on diffusing capacity, membrane diffusion, and pulmonary capillary blood volume in the lung. *Chest.* 2002;122(2):629-638.
172. Benowitz NL. Clinical pharmacology and toxicology of cocaine. *Pharmacol Toxicol.* 1993;72(1):3-12.
173. Jaffe J. *Goodman and Gilman's the Pharmacological Basis of Therapeutics.* 8th ed. Pergamon Press; 1990.
174. Alkhouri I, Gibbons P, Ravindranath D, Brower K. Substance-related psychiatric emergencies. In: Riba MB, Ravindranath D, eds. *Clinical Manual of Emergency Psychiatry.* American Psychiatric Publishing; 2010:187-206.
175. Graudins AAC. *Intensive Care Medicine.* Little, Brown, Company; 1999.
176. Roberts DM, Buckley NA. Enhanced elimination in acute barbiturate poisoning—a systematic review. *Clin Toxicol.* 2011;49(1):2-12.
177. Wood DM, Brailsford AD, Dargan PI. Acute toxicity and withdrawal syndromes related to gamma-hydroxybutyrate (GHB) and its analogues gamma-butyrolactone (GBL) and 1,4-butanediol (1,4-BD). *Drug Test Anal.* 2011;3(7-8):417-425.
178. Soldatos CR, Dikeos DG, Whitehead A. Tolerance and rebound insomnia with rapidly eliminated hypnotics: a meta-analysis of sleep laboratory studies. *Int Clin Psychopharmacol.* 1999;14(5):287-303.
179. Owen RT. Extended-release zolpidem: efficacy and tolerability profile. *Drugs Today (Barc).* 2006;42(11):721.
180. Guilleminault C. Benzodiazepines, breathing, and sleep. *Am J Med.* 1990;88(3A):25S-28S.
181. Center for Behavioral Health Statistics and Quality. *Key Substance Use and Mental Health Indicators in the United States: Results From the 2015 National Survey on Drug Use and Health* (HHS Publication No. SMA 16-4984, NSDUH Series H-51). SAMHSA; 2016.
182. Mowry JB, Spyker DA, Brooks DE, Zimmerman A, Schauben JL. 2015 Annual Report of the American Association of Poison Control Centers' National Poison Data System (NPDS): 33rd Annual Report. *Clin Toxicol.* 2016;54(10):924-1109.
183. Flanagan RJ, Ives RJ. Volatile substance abuse. *Bull Narc.* 1994;46(2):49-78.
184. Anser L. Abuse of volatile substances. *Qatar Foundation Annual Research Forum.* 2013;2013(1).
185. Wright RO, Lewander WJ, Woolf AD. Methemoglobinemia: etiology, pharmacology, and clinical management. *Ann Emerg Med.* 1999;34(5):646-656.
186. Sakai K, Maruyama-Maebashi K, Takatsu A, et al. Sudden death involving inhalation of 1,1-difluoroethane (HFC-152a) with spray cleaner: three case reports. *Forensic Sci Int.* 2011;206(1-3):e58-e61.
187. Brouette T, Anton R. Clinical review of inhalants. *Am J Addict.* 2001;10(1):79-94.
188. Wagner SA, Clark MA, Wesche DL, Doedens DJ, Lloyd AW. Asphyxial deaths from the recreational use of nitrous oxide. *J Forensic Sci.* 1992;37(4):13286J.
189. Ferenchick GS, Hirokawa S, Mammen EF, Schwartz KA. Anabolic-androgenic steroid abuse in weight lifters: evidence for activation of the hemostatic system. *Am J Hematol.* 1995;49(4):282-288.

CHAPTER

93 Neurological Disorders Related to Substance Use

Emmanuelle A. D. Schindler, Mona Al Banna, Brian B. Koo, Darren C. Volpe, Hamada Hamid Altalib, and Jason J. Sico

CHAPTER OUTLINE

- Introduction
- Trauma and traumatic brain injury
- Headache
- Neurobehavioral and cognitive disorders
- Seizures
- Stroke
- Neuromuscular (nerve, muscle, and spinal cord) disorders
- Movement disorders
- Neurologic complications of substance use resulting from infections
- Other complications
- Conclusions

INTRODUCTION

This chapter addresses neurological complications of alcohol, tobacco, and other drugs (**Table 93-1**). The neurological symptoms and signs of acute toxicity and withdrawal differ widely from agent to agent, as well as the level of the neuroaxis involved. Alcohol and many other drugs can affect the brain, including cortical and subcortical areas, spinal cord, peripheral nervous system, and muscles. Frequently, more than one portion of the nervous system is affected, with acute and acute-on-chronic manifestations. For example, a patient with chronic heavy alcohol use may present acutely with delirium or an alcohol withdrawal seizure; when the acute issues improve, clinicians may find that the patient also has cognitive impairment, neuropathy, and myopathy. Potentially complicating a patient's presentation is the possibility that an individual is using more than one agent or even is intoxicated by one agent while simultaneously withdrawing from another, thereby confounding the interpretation of neurological symptoms and signs.[1,2]

This chapter is divided by types of neurological conditions (eg, stroke, seizure) and, when appropriate, is subdivided by specific substance. When subdivisions are used, the order of specific substances reflects the relative importance of that substance in a given neurological condition.

TRAUMA AND TRAUMATIC BRAIN INJURY

Trauma may be intentional (eg, assault) or unintentional (eg, falls and motor vehicle accidents). In 2019, the Centers for Disease Control and Prevention's (CDC's) National Center for Health Statistics (NHCS) reported that unintentional injuries (ie, accidents) were the third leading cause of mortality for all age groups and the leading cause of death for those aged 1 to 44.[3,4] Alcohol and other drug use plays a major role in injuries and subsequent trauma. For example, alcohol intoxication has been associated with 25% to 35% of nonfatal motor vehicle injuries and 40% to 50% of fatal motor vehicle accidents.[5]

Trauma frequently affects the central and peripheral nervous systems, resulting in both acute and chronic injuries. Trauma can acutely affect the brain, spinal cord, and peripheral nerves. Intoxication (from alcohol, alone or in combination with other substances) may be responsible, in part, for the trauma itself (eg, motor vehicle accident or unintended fall); also, coexisting intoxication at the time of injury may mask the extent of neurological injury, when present. When considering alcohol specifically, those who drink are more likely to be involved in a motor vehicle accident and that trauma is likely to be more severe than someone who was not drinking at the time of the accident.[5] Furthermore, the diagnosis of alcohol use disorder may be missed; early identification is important, given implications for acute management as well as recognizing the long-term need for continued outpatient management and rehabilitation.

When trauma affects the brain, traumatic brain injury (TBI), contusions, hemorrhage (eg, intracerebral, subarachnoid), and hematomas (eg, epidural and subdural) can result. Epidural and subdural hematomas may require surgical evacuation. Traumatic subarachnoid hemorrhages may also require neurosurgical intervention, especially if obstructive hydrocephalus develops.[6] Hemorrhage and hematomas are of special concern in people with alcohol use disorders and chronic liver disease, as they often have thrombocytopenia and abnormalities of clotting factors; moreover, alcohol acutely enhances blood-brain barrier leakage around areas of cerebral trauma.[7]

Persons sustaining head trauma may experience altered mentation, headache, nausea, vomiting, speech difficulties, and seizures. Alcohol and other drug use are the greatest risk factors for developing TBI,[8] defined as "an alteration in brain function, or other evidence of brain pathology, caused by an external force."[9] The CDC reports that in 2019 there were 223,135 TBI-related hospitalizations and in 2020, 64,362

TABLE 93-1 Important Neurologic Complications Associated With Alcohol and Other Drugs

Alcohol
Traumatic brain injury
Progressive cognitive decline (including mild cognitive impairment and dementia)
Wernicke-Korsakoff disease
Pellagra
Marchiafava-Bignami disease
Seizures
Ischemic stroke
Hemorrhagic stroke
Peripheral neuropathy
Compression neuropathy
Myopathy
Nerve and nerve root injury (including compartment syndrome)
Spinal cord injury
Movement disorders (including tremor, asterixis, and chorea)
Central nervous system infections

Other sedative-hypnotic agents (barbiturates, benzodiazepines)
Headache
Neurobehavioral (including mental clouding)
Seizures

Caffeine
Headache (from withdrawal)

Cocaine, amphetamines, and MDMA
Headache
Neurobehavioral (including shorter attention span, paranoia, impulsivity, and hallucinations)
Seizures
Ischemic stroke
Hemorrhagic stroke
Reversible cerebral vasoconstriction syndrome
Movement disorders (including "crack dancing," "boca torcida," "punding," tics, and acute dystonia)

Tobacco and nicotine
Ischemic stroke
Hemorrhagic stroke

Cannabis (marijuana) and synthetic cannabinoids
Cognitive impairment
Acute psychoses
Ischemic stroke

Heroin and opioids
Headache
Cognitive impairment (including dementia associated with "chasing the dragon")
Seizures (specifically meperidine and the combination of pentazocine and tripelennamine)
Ischemic stroke
Hemorrhagic stroke
Neuropathy
Guillain-Barré syndrome
Acute transverse myelitis
Movement disorders (including myoclonus, intractable hiccups)

Hallucinogens (LSD, psilocybin, mescaline)
Headache
Neurobehavioral (including psychosis and impaired working memory)
Seizures
Ischemic stroke

Dissociative anesthetics (ketamine, PCP)
Neurobehavioral (including schizophrenia-like symptoms)
Seizures
Ischemic stroke
Hemorrhagic stroke
Hypertensive encephalopathy

Inhalants
Dementia (toluene)
Delirium (gasoline containing tetraethyl lead)
Neuropathy (*N*-hexane)
Myelopathy (Nitrous oxide)
Seizures

Anticholinergics
Seizures

deaths attributable to TBI within the United States. These estimates do not include TBIs treated in the Emergency Department only, outpatient settings, and those not seeking evaluation.[10] The prevalence of alcohol dependence at the time of TBI is estimated to be 50% to 60%, with some 29% to 52% of those admitted with TBI having a measurable alcohol level upon arrival to an emergency department.[8] TBI can be graded as mild (synonymous with concussion), moderate, or severe, dependent on the duration of loss of consciousness, and whether alteration of consciousness, posttraumatic amnesia, and radiographic evidence of injury are present.[11] TBI can acutely cause changes in mentation, memory impairment, as well as a postconcussive syndrome, including such symptoms as vertigo, nausea, vomiting, and headaches. Longer-term TBI may cause chronic headaches, epilepsy, aberrations in sleep, and neurobehavioral (eg, increased anxiety, depression, mood swings) and neurocognitive (eg, memory and attention difficulties) changes.[12] Furthermore, the use of alcohol and other drugs is common after TBI.[8]

Spinal cord injury (from cord contusion, transection, or vascular compromise) most commonly occurs in the cervical region (C1 to C7-T1), followed in equal proportion in the thoracic (T1-T11), thoracolumbar (T11 or T12 to L1-L2), and lumbosacral (L2 to S5) regions.[13] Symptoms of spinal cord injury are referential to the level involved. Deficits on neurological examination may include weakness and sensory loss below the level of trauma, or perianal sensory loss. It is important to perform a thorough neurological (including rectal and perianal) examination in spinal cord injury patients, as prognosis for recovery is related to initial neurological deficit severity.[14]

Trauma may also cause injury to the peripheral nervous system, at the level of individual nerves, the plexus (either brachial or lumbosacral), or individual nerve roots. When evaluating patients with injury to the peripheral nervous system, it is important to (1) determine if weakness or sensory changes can be localized to a specific level of the nervous system (eg, a single nerve as seen in "Saturday night [radial] palsy" versus a plexus injury); (2) decide whether more than one injury may be present ("double-crush" injury of a single nerve and plexus or nerve root); (3) isolate the mechanism of injury (to assess if there is nerve laceration, traction, etc.); and (4) determine the time interval between onset of injury and presentation.[15] When seeing patients acutely who may have been immobilized for an extended period of time, physical examination (eg, pulselessness, poikilothermia), and laboratory assessment (eg, renal function and creatine kinase [CK] levels) for compartment syndrome are imperative, as significant morbidity and possible mortality may result with a delayed diagnosis.[15,16]

HEADACHE

Headache disorders are a group of neurological disorders driven by central and peripheral pathologies and manifesting largely with paroxysmal pain attacks in the head or face.[17,18] The term "headache" is used in this section to describe any number of possible cranial and facial pain conditions. When specific headache types are referenced (eg, migraine, cluster), they are so designated.

Associations among headache, mood, and substance use disorders have been identified, which invoke common biological mechanisms.[17,19,20] Headache and pain also have a unique relationship with substance use disorders, as they may function as the trigger or the consequence of substance use.[19,20] For instance, some patients have such debilitating headaches that they use illicit substances to relieve pain or dissociate from their symptoms. Withdrawal from such substances can then be accompanied by rebound headaches, leading to the continued use of the drug and ultimately development of a substance use disorder despite little symptom improvement.

A drug can also cause headache through both direct and indirect mechanisms. While vascular changes (eg, dilation, constriction) are often implicated, other actions in the central or peripheral nervous systems could be involved.[21] Drugs may also cause headache through indirect mechanisms, such as dehydration, anorexia, insomnia, or trauma. The associations with headache for specific substances are reviewed below.

Alcohol

Patients with headache disorders may reduce their alcohol consumption to avoid triggering attacks.[22,23] Wine is a common trigger for migraine,[24] whereas those with cluster headache commonly report beer as a trigger.[23] Nonalcohol ingredients in these beverages (eg, tyramine, sulfites) have been implicated, although the evidence to support this is variable.[24] Alcohol commonly causes a delayed headache in those with or without a prior headache history; multiple systems, including vascular, inflammatory, and endocrine, have been implicated in this *veisalgia* or "hangover" syndrome.[25] The headaches that arise in alcohol withdrawal are likely to stem from cerebrovascular dysfunction[26] and pain hypersensitivity[27] that occur in that syndrome. Furthermore, those with cirrhosis resulting from alcohol who have coagulopathy and/or platelet dysfunction are at risk for both traumatic and spontaneous intracranial hemorrhages, which can initially present as either a focal or holocephalic headache.[26] Alcohol is not considered a treatment for headache, but those with severe or frequent headaches might drink in order to escape their pain, despite the deleterious effects.[22]

Other Sedative–Hypnotic Agents (Barbiturates, Benzodiazepines)

Combination medications that include the barbiturate, butalbital, are often prescribed to patients for the treatment of headache, particularly low-pressure headache (eg, from cerebrospinal fluid leak after dural puncture). However, the American Headache Society (AHS) has released guidelines against the use of butalbital as first-line abortive therapy for recurrent headaches.[28] The frequent use of butalbital-containing medications is highly correlated with chronification of headache[29] and development of physical dependence and addiction to the medication.[30] Abrupt abstinence from any barbiturate may be associated with withdrawal seizures.[31,32] The withdrawal from benzodiazepines may also be accompanied by headaches, particularly if it is associated with paroxysmal spikes in blood pressure.[33] While benzodiazepines are not a standard treatment for headache, it has been suggested that they may offer benefit by addressing co-occurring anxiety, insomnia, somatoform symptoms, cervicogenic headaches, or neck pain, though other medications and nonpharmacological treatments may also be effective.[34]

Caffeine

A positive correlation exists between caffeine intake and headache.[35] With regular caffeine consumption, headaches can result if it is withdrawn, a phenomenon not uncommon on weekends or holidays.[35] It has been suggested that DSM-defined caffeine dependence is largely driven by withdrawal headaches and not a desire for the positive effects (eg, elevated mood, enhanced concentration)[35] or craving generated through reward circuitry. Caffeine, often used in the form of combination analgesics, also has a reasonable efficacy in treating migraine and tension-type headaches.[35] It is a standard treatment for headaches acquired after dural puncture; both intravenous (IV) and oral administrations are used.[35] Caffeine-containing energy drinks are commonly consumed by patients with cluster headache to abort attacks, though they typically confer only partial efficacy.[36] Of note, other substances in caffeine beverages may also impact headaches; coffee contains chlorogenic acid and energy drinks often contain taurine, compounds with anti-inflammatory and/or anti-headache properties.[37]

Cocaine, Amphetamines, and MDMA (Ecstasy)

Cocaine can induce headaches acutely, in delayed fashion (hours), or in times of withdrawal.[38,39] When applied to the sphenopalatine fossa, cocaine reduces the duration of nitroglycerin-induced attacks in cluster headache.[40] AHS guidelines for the management of cluster headache from the American Academy of Neurology (AAN) cite Level C evidence for the use of intranasal cocaine spray (not available in the United States; however, used clinically outside of the United States) as a "possibly effective" treatment of cluster headache.[41]

Amphetamine compounds deplete serotonin stores, posing risk for patients with migraines through a mechanism that may involve increased nitric oxide production.[42] Stimulants, including methamphetamine,[43] 3,4-methylenedioxy-*N*-methylamphetamine (MDMA)[41,44] sympathomimetic cough and cold medication,[45] prescription stimulants for attention-deficit hyperactivity disorder[46] and cocaine[47] can also cause intracranial hemorrhage or vasculopathy, which may present with headache.

Tobacco and Nicotine

Headaches are associated with both active and passive cigarette smoking.[22,48] This may be due to a number of factors, including lifestyle, carbon monoxide levels, and nicotine withdrawal.[22,48] One study identified a potential link between tobacco exposure and more severe features of cluster headache.[49] Cigarette smoke can be a trigger for those with migraine or tension-type headaches.[48] While patients with cluster headache are stereotypically people who smoke heavily, a number of studies have failed to show that smoking behaviors, including stopping smoking, influence cluster attacks, the course of cluster headaches,[23,50,51] or response to therapy.[52,53] Electronic cigarettes, which decrease many of the confounders of smoke, tar, and other nonnicotine products, can either trigger or alleviate headache.[48] There is indeed some evidence for the use of nicotine-containing products in the treatment of pain and headache.[54]

Opioids

Regular exposure to opioids sensitizes both peripheral and central arms of the trigeminal pathway and is associated with rebound or overuse headache.[55,56] Persons with opioid use disorder have a high rate of headache disorders (60%) particularly with chronic use.[39] While the use of opioids does not significantly impact preexisting headache,[39] opioid intoxication does produce a tension-like headache, whereas opioid withdrawal causes headache with migrainous features.[39] Those treated with methadone maintenance may have various headache disorders, such as cluster headache[57] and temporomandibular joint disorders.[58] Withdrawal from methadone can also lead to headaches.

The AHS has recommended against using opioids as first-line treatment of recurrent headaches given the risks for of physiological dependence (and opioid use disorder) and heightened pain sensitivity.[28,59] Despite this, opioids are frequently used in the emergency setting, with a greater than 50% increase between 2000 and 2010.[60] In community Emergency Departments, opioids are prescribed in up to 70% of migraine patients.[61] When opioids are used on an outpatient basis for headache, concerning patterns of physiological dependence and opioid use disorder emerge in almost one-fifth of patients.[56] As an exception, it is widely accepted to prescribe opioid medication to patients with cancer-related head and face pain.[39] Outside of opioid use, migraine itself is an opioid-sensitive condition; low-dose morphine induces physiological effects in opioid-naive patients with migraines, which are not seen in opioid-naive controls, including presyncope and increased respiratory rates. Furthermore, low-dose morphine is also considered a pharmacological challenge, given that it can induce migraine attacks among those living with migraine who are opioid-naive.[62]

Hallucinogens (LSD, Psilocybin, Mescaline)

Hallucinogens (also called psychedelics), such as D-lysergic acid diethylamide (LSD), psilocybin, and mescaline, can induce headaches of different types.[63] Given that hallucinogens do not have the same addiction liability properties as other substances,[64] they are unlikely to create a cycle of recurring headache. Traumatic injury during an altered state of consciousness could potentially lead to long-term headaches, though the incidence of serious injury and use of emergency services seen with hallucinogen use is dramatically lower than other substances.[64]

Hallucinogens bear chemical and pharmacological resemblance to certain medications, such as dihydroergotamine and methysergide, used in the treatment of headaches. Therefore, it comes as no surprise that there has been interest in the therapeutic use of hallucinogens for migraine and cluster headache.[64] The first double-blind, placebo-controlled clinical trial of a hallucinogen in migraine showed that a single low dose of psilocybin (10 mg/70 kg) reduced several measures of headache burden in the 2 weeks measured after administration.[65] The first randomized controlled trial of a hallucinogen (psilocybin) in cluster headache was recently completed (NCT02981173). Another with LSD is ongoing (NCT03781128).

Cannabinoids

Both endogenous and exogenous cannabinoids have been shown to modulate pain pathways.[66] For individuals with regular cannabis use, withdrawal from cannabinoid products can result in rebound headaches.[22] It has also been suggested that endocannabinoid deficiency may predispose to migraine and that cannabis may alleviate symptoms of this condition.[22] There are reports supporting the efficacy of cannabis in the treatment of migraine, though formal scientific studies are currently lacking.[22] A number of clinical trials have been initiated or are in preparation, using different cannabinoids, different doses, and in various populations, including adolescents.[67] The relaxation effect induced by the drug may account for its reported efficacy.[21] In cluster headache, cannabis is not uncommonly used, although the available data have shown equivocal efficacy,[68] or in some cases, suggest a propensity to trigger attacks.[21] Cannabis used as treatment (CUAT) is reviewed in more detail in Section 15 of this textbook.

Dissociative Anesthetics (Ketamine, PCP, and Dextromethorphan)

Ketamine's pharmacotherapeutic purview has expanded beyond its traditional use as an anesthetic agent, and may have value in the treatment of mood disorders, refractory status epilepticus, and complex regional pain syndrome.[69] Ketamine has been shown to reduce the duration and severity of migraine aura.[69,70] The AHS cites insufficient evidence and presents no formal recommendations for its use.[59] While ketamine infusion is used to manage refractory headache in certain specialty centers, more research is required to fully characterize the safety and efficacy of this treatment in specific headache disorders.[11,71]

NEUROBEHAVIORAL AND COGNITIVE DISORDERS

Substance use has effects on multiple cortical and subcortical networks subserving cognition, memory, and behavior. Functional imaging studies show changes in metabolism and cerebral blood flow in specific brain regions with the acute and chronic use of substances. During the immediate use of a substance, varying and transient levels of altered consciousness, inattention (versus hypervigilance), euphoria (versus depression), impaired memory, disinhibited behavior, and altered judgment are seen acutely. The chronic use of various substances may have long-term effects on multiple cognitive domains including executive function, memory, and attention. Abstinence can result in improvements in some neurocognitive domains, although this may be confounded by chronicity of substance use as well as genetic and other variables. A study on individuals with multiple types of substance use disorder demonstrated significant improvements in inhibitory control measures (and other cognitive domains) after 1 to 4 months of abstinence, although not in learning and memory.[72,73]

It should be noted that people with unhealthy substance use often use multiple substances and are at risk for altered mentation by indirect mechanisms, including head trauma, infection, and malnutrition. Longitudinal studies of the effects of individual substances therefore remain challenging in the setting of these confounders. Additionally, the baseline mental status of the patient before substance use is often uncertain and certain disorders or deficits may predispose one to substance use, making it difficult to draw firm conclusions. However, the accumulation of structural and functional imaging studies and the use of more sensitive neurocognitive test measures, as well as longitudinal studies, shed more light on the neurobehavioral and cognitive effects of individual substances.

In this section, the acute and chronic effects of alcohol and other substances on cognition, memory, and behavior will be discussed.

Alcohol

Acute Effects

Heavy alcohol use often leads to nutritional deficiency, notably thiamine and nicotinic acid, which may cause acute neurological symptoms. Wernicke-Korsakoff disease is caused by thiamine deficiency. Because body stores[74] are limited, this disease can occur after only a few weeks of inadequate thiamine intake.[75] In the acute syndrome, neurobehavioral symptoms evolve over days or weeks to a "global confusional state," with varying degrees of lethargy, inattentiveness, abulia, and impaired memory.[75] Abnormal eye movements are usually (but not invariably) present, characterized by nystagmus and/or limitations of abduction or horizontal gaze; progression to complete ophthalmoplegia may occur. Ataxic gait (both cerebellar and vestibular in origin) may progress to an inability to stand independently. Without treatment, there is a progression to coma and death. On pathological evaluation, there are histologically distinct abnormalities in the medial thalamus, hypothalamus and periaqueductal gray matter of the midbrain, and the periventricular areas of the pons and medulla. These regional pathological changes are often seen as hyperintense (T2-weighted) lesions on magnetic resonance imaging (MRI).[76] With early treatment (IV thiamine and multivitamins), recovery begins within hours or days and can be complete. If treatment is delayed, the mental symptoms can evolve into Korsakoff syndrome, an irreversible disorder in which the predominant abnormality is impaired memory. Specifically, patients are unable to store or retrieve recent information and have varying degrees of anterograde and retrograde amnesia. There is a prominent tendency to confabulate, especially in the acute setting, but this may persist in chronic stages. Residual nystagmus and gait ataxia also may be present.

Pellagra is caused by nicotinic acid (vitamin B3) deficiency. Affected individuals may have a skin rash, gastrointestinal symptoms (stomatitis and enteritis, with nausea, vomiting, and diarrhea), and neurobehavioral/cognitive symptoms, including dementia, delirium, irritability, insomnia, impaired memory, delusions, or hallucinations.[77] Untreated pellagra is fatal. With prompt nicotinic acid replacement, recovery can occur over hours or days.

Marchiafava-Bignami disease is specifically associated with alcohol use disorder and is characterized by demyelinating lesions in the corpus callosum and progressive neurological symptoms, often ending fatally within a few months. However, it can have a subacute or chronic course. It is rare and may sometimes exist in a more chronic dementia state. Its pathophysiology is unclear, but it is thought to be related to the nutritional deficiencies in people with alcohol use disorder.[78] Mental symptoms predominate and include depression, mania, paranoia, and dementia. Seizures are common, and hemiparesis, aphasia, dyskinesia, and ataxia are variably present. The callosal lesions do not explain the devastating neurological deterioration.

Chronic Effects

Alcohol-related dementia refers to progressive cognitive decline that is not easily attributed to another cause or a primary dementia.[79] It is gradual in onset and is manifested by more global cognitive deficits compared to the acute and specific amnesia and confabulation seen with Korsakoff syndrome. Neuropsychological testing shows cognitive impairment in 50% to 70% of people who drink heavily.[74] Enlarged cerebral ventricles and sulci are often seen on structural brain imaging, correlating with cognitive decline and improving with abstinence in some reports.[80] Neuropathological studies of individuals without evidence of nutritional deficiency describe neuronal loss in selective regions of the brain, especially the superior frontal association cortex (a pattern unlike that of Wernicke-Korsakoff disease). One study using magnetic resonance spectroscopy and *N*-acetylaspartate confirmed the vulnerability of this region.[81] Investigators have correlated frontal lobe damage with particular cognitive or behavioral abnormalities (eg, difficulty planning, problem-solving, and abstracting, as well as disinhibition and lack of insight).[82] Another prospective study examining the effects of alcohol on brain structures (characterized by MRI) over a 30-year period found that individuals consuming both high (>30 units/week) and moderate (14-21 units/week) levels of alcohol had a higher odds of hippocampal atrophy compared with those who abstained.[83]

The detrimental effects of alcohol on cognition are dose-related; a review of 19 studies found that 5 or 6 "standard U.S. drinks" daily resulted in "cognitive inefficiencies," whereas 10 or more drinks daily caused serious cognitive impairment.[84] On the other hand, epidemiological studies have suggested that low alcohol intake, compared with abstinence, is associated with a reduced risk of dementia.[85] Alcohol's effects on cognition thus follow a J-shaped curve similar to its effects on ischemic cerebrovascular disease, but these results may be explained by residual confounding. Reducing the likelihood of ischemic stroke does not fully explain the apparent cognitive benefits, which might be related to antioxidant properties of alcoholic beverages.[86]

Other Sedative-Hypnotic Agents (Barbiturates, Benzodiazepines)

Sedatives have many clinical uses, including the treatment of anxiety (usually acutely), epilepsy, alcohol withdrawal, and at times as sleep aids. Barbiturates can produce mental clouding or paradoxical hyperactivity in older adults.[87] Paradoxical effects may also be seen with benzodiazepines. Acutely, sedative-hypnotics can negatively affect cognition and memory, independent of their sedating effects.[88] Explicit memory is more affected than implicit memory.[89] As such, those under the acute influence of a sedative-hypnotic may have difficultly consciously trying to remember specific events though still able to walk or ride a bike. Meta-analyses have found cognitive dysfunction in long-term benzodiazepine treatment, with some evidence of milder residual dysfunction when they were discontinued.[90]

Cocaine, Amphetamines, and MDMA (Ecstasy)

Psychostimulant effects on cognition are thought to exist on a dose-dependent continuum, with cognitive enhancement at low doses and possible cognitive deficits with heavy or chronic use.[91] Individuals with chronic cocaine use have significant impairments in executive function, including impaired capacity to learn from errors (thus, poor decision-making and risk assessment), inability to inhibit irrelevant impulses (thus, a tendency to act impulsively), and increased perseveration.[92] Other cognitive impairments include shorter attention span, impaired working memory, and impaired visual and verbal memory.[92] Individuals with cocaine use disorder have been found to have abnormal structure and function of frontal-striatal (basal ganglia) systems as well as decreased volume of widespread regions of the cortex and cerebellum.[93] Conversely, similar to the effects of methamphetamine, cocaine has been related to the enlargement of striatal structures where it exerts most of its pharmacological effects. Widespread microvascular lesions due to cocaine use (see "Stroke" section) might contribute to cognitive dysfunction.[94]

Amphetamine, methamphetamine, and MDMA cause alterations in the transmission of monoamines acutely leading to hyperalertness, psychomotor agitation, pressured speech, elevated sense of well-being, and elation. Chronically, dextroamphetamine damages dopaminergic nerve terminals, MDMA damages serotonergic nerve terminals, and methamphetamine damages both dopaminergic and serotonergic nerve terminals.[95,96] Functional imaging studies have shown reduced neuronal integrity in the cortex and basal ganglia (proton magnetic resonance spectroscopy) and abnormal glucose metabolism in limbic and paralimbic structures (positron emission tomography).[95,96] Therefore, individuals with illicit amphetamine use have changes in brain structures involved in the regulation of mood. There is also evidence for impairments in sustained attention and vigilance in individuals with recent abstinence from methamphetamine, with structural and functional changes in the insular and anterior cingulate cortices.[38,97] Other neuropsychological effects include deficits in working memory, learning, and processing speed.

Amphetamine use, both prescription and illicit, is associated with a variety of psychiatric disorders, including anxiety disorders, mood disorders, and psychosis. The related symptoms including paranoia, hallucinations, and grandiosity may occur either with acute or chronic use. Withdrawal from amphetamines can lead to depression lasting for months. However, claims of permanent depression in individuals with stimulant use (resulting from damage to the dopaminergic mesolimbic "reward circuit") are unproven.

MDMA acutely has both amphetamine-like and hallucinogenic effects, causing euphoria, high energy, and social disinhibition. Acute adverse effects may include hyperactivity, distorted perceptions, and confusion; more serious effects may include dehydration and hyperthermia. Long-term MDMA use may cause cognitive impairment through serotonergic damage. Brain imaging studies show reductions in serotonin transporter (SERT) density and binding potential (cortex, hippocampus) and reductions in hippocampal volume.[97-99] There is also evidence for MDMA-induced programmed cell death in hippocampal neurons of rats.[100,101] Significant detrimental effects on both long-term and short-term memory and visuospatial functions have been found in neurocognitive studies of individuals who use MDMA.[101-103]

Cannabinoids

Effects of cannabis occur shortly after intake (usually smoked) and may cause a sense of well-being, mild euphoria, and relaxation. Adverse effects include dysphoria, depression, or delusions. Acutely, cannabis use leads to deficits in attention, memory, and sense of time. Chronic persistent cannabis use studied over a 20-year time frame, starting in adolescence, was correlated with broad neuropsychological impairments (including learning, memory, and executive function) that interfered with everyday cognitive functioning.[104] Specifically, impairments have been found in decision-making and risk-taking with heavy, habitual cannabis use.[105,106] Evidence from larger reviews suggests that even once weekly use of cannabis in adolescence can result in longer-term neurocognitive dysfunction and damage[107-109] and that there is a risk of impaired brain development in young people who use cannabis.[110,111] On structural imaging studies, impaired axonal connectivity was identified in the hippocampus and splenium of the corpus callosum in individuals with regular cannabis use and was more prominent when use began in early teens.[112,113] A review of neuroimaging studies in adolescents with cannabis use showed abnormal frontal-parietal network activity.[114] Moreover, cannabis use during childhood or adolescence has been associated with an increased risk for developing schizophrenia.[115-117] Synthetic cannabinoids in the form of IV delta-9-tetrahydrocannabinol, when given as a one-time dose, have been demonstrated to induce an acute psychotic reaction among individuals without a prior history of psychiatric disease.[118] The regular use of synthetic cannabinoids has also been associated with the development of psychosis.[119,120] A systematic review suggests that there are preferential impairments in executive function in synthetic and organic cannabinoid users, with more severe effects with long-term use.[73,121,122]

Opioids

The chronic effects of opioids on cognition are difficult to study in isolation because many individuals have a lifetime history of other substance use. Studies have yielded mixed results, showing variability ranging from mild to moderate levels of cognitive dysfunction.[123] A study of individuals with prescription opioid use disorder showed decreases in functional connectivity of key regions including amygdala, nucleus accumbens, and anterior insula, which[124] subserve functions including impulse control, affect, motivation, and reward/decision-making, and, therefore, may have neurobehavioral implications.[124,125] The use of opioids has been linked to significant deficits on neuropsychological tests of decision-making and strategic planning; the latter seems to demonstrate "the difficulty of [individuals with drug use] to mentally organize behavior to achieve a goal through a series of intermediate steps."[93]

Hallucinogens (LSD, Psilocybin, Mescaline)

Acutely, hallucinogens produce profound changes in perception, mood (often severe lability), and cognition, usually within 30 to 90 minutes of administration (for LSD). Acute adverse effects may include panic attacks, prolonged unpleasant experience ("bad trip"), and psychotic reactions; psychosis may rarely be prolonged or perhaps accelerated in susceptible individuals. Individuals who use hallucinogens may report depersonalization, altered sense of reality, or transcendental experiences. Additionally, some individuals may experience a recurrence of the original psychic effects days to weeks later in the absence of further drug use ("flash back"). Acutely, there are deficits in working memory and word recall; however, it is not proven that hallucinogens cause permanent cognitive alteration (except possibly MDMA, described above). Neurobiologically, the most prominent effects are upon serotonin receptors, most notably 5-HT_{2A}. The indolamines, including LSD and psilocybin, are relatively nonselective with respect to effects on serotonin receptors and also act on dopamine receptors. According to a functional imaging study on psilocybin, preferentially affected brain regions include the prefrontal cortex and posterior cingulate gyrus.[126] A review of neuroimaging studies on hallucinogens showed widespread acute effects, including inhibition of the default mode network, as well as long-term effects including thinning of the posterior cingulate cortex and thickening of the anterior cingulate cortex.[127]

Dissociative Anesthetics (Ketamine, PCP, Dextromethorphan)

Acutely, phencyclidine produces schizophrenia-like symptoms, both positive (agitation, paranoia, delusions, or hallucinations) and negative (autism, loss of ego boundaries, avolition, or catatonia). Permanent neuropsychiatric change has been claimed.[119]

Inhalants

Toluene, which is found in many solvents, paints, and glues is associated with white matter lesions and can result in dementia, often accompanied by pyramidal, cerebellar, and oculomotor signs.[120] Individuals who inhale gasoline containing tetraethyl lead may develop lead encephalopathy.[121]

SEIZURES

Every human brain, even in the absence of a structural injury, has the potential to experience a seizure if exposed to an inciting chemical milieu. Seizures can be a feature of either drug toxicity (as with psychostimulants) or withdrawal (as with alcohol or sedative-hypnotic agents).[122,123] Alcohol and other drug use is the cause of 14% of acute symptomatic seizures.[124] Medical or nonmedical use of prescription medications may also lower seizure threshold.[128] However, substance-induced seizures are often confounded by co-occurring neurological injury. In one study, among 140 patients with alcohol-related seizures, 54% had another potential seizure etiology.[129] While many substance-induced seizures will present as generalized tonic-clonic convulsions, a seizure may be focal in onset if a person has an underlying structural brain injury that becomes hyperexcitable during acute intoxication or withdrawal. For instance, if a person with a TBI and left frontal encephalomalacia experiences an alcohol-related seizure, the seizure may begin with right limb shaking with or without secondary generalization. Alternatively, a focal lesion may be a consequence of the substance use leading to a seizure.[130]

Alcohol

Alcohol is a depressant that potentiates gamma-aminobutyric acid (GABA)-ergic neurotransmission[131]; the role of acute alcohol toxicity inducing seizures is controversial. Most alcohol-related seizures are due to withdrawal or a co-occurring neurological injury, such as TBI and associated encephalomalacia, hematoma, or infection. The term "alcohol-related seizures" refers to seizures in the absence of epilepsy or other predisposing factors, such as a structural lesion.[132] Such seizures most often are a withdrawal phenomenon, occurring 6 to 48 hours after the last drink in persons with chronic heavy alcohol use or months to years of binges; however, they may occur during active drinking or more than a week after the last drink.[133] One case-control study of new-onset seizures failed to show a clear temporal relation between seizures and recent abstinence,[134] whereas another study among those with a history of epilepsy noted that 95% of alcohol-related seizures occurred within 12 hours of abstinence. The minimal duration of drinking is uncertain, but the risk is dose-related, beginning at 50 g of ethanol daily.[134]

Alcohol withdrawal seizures usually are single or occur in a brief cluster, with status epilepticus occurring in up to 10%. Alcohol withdrawal seizures are typically generalized tonic-clonic seizures. Seizures that are focal in onset suggest an underlying structural lesion. II In the absence of status epilepticus, treatment of alcohol withdrawal seizures with an anticonvulsant (other than benzodiazepines) is not advised.[133,135] In animals and humans, phenytoin fails to prevent alcohol withdrawal seizures.[136] Further, even when nonsedating anticonvulsants (eg, valproic acid and carbamazepine) have been used for alcohol withdrawal seizure management, significant side effects developed (such as nausea, vomiting, vertigo), leading to discontinuation by patients.[137] Initial management of alcohol withdrawal seizures should focus on airway, breathing, and circulation. Once these are stabilized, parenteral or oral benzodiazepines Are administered to treat and prevent further seizures and other symptoms of alcohol withdrawal.[133] Given early enough, IV lorazepam decreases the likelihood of recurrent seizures over the next several hours.[138] It should be noted that repeated episodes of alcohol withdrawal is a risk factor for developing alcohol withdrawal seizures.[130]

As suggested above, the diagnosis of alcohol-related seizures requires exclusion of other causes. Brain computed tomography or MRI is indicated if seizures are of new onset, and lumbar puncture should be performed if meningitis or subarachnoid hemorrhage is suspected. In patients with alcohol-related seizures, the electroencephalogram usually is normal.[139]

Treatment of status epilepticus during alcohol withdrawal is conventional; benzodiazepines and phenobarbital have the advantage of cross-tolerance with alcohol and, thus, efficacy in treating other withdrawal symptoms, including progression to *delirium tremens* (DTs).[135]

Other Sedative-Hypnotic Agents (Barbiturates, Benzodiazepines)

As with alcohol, seizures in people with benzodiazepine and barbiturate use disorders occur most often as a withdrawal phenomenon.[140] Benzodiazepines are sometimes associated with paradoxical toxic reactions featuring agitation, hallucinations, and, in some cases, seizures,[141] with children and the elderly being especially susceptible.[142] In a study of volunteers who had taken oral pentobarbital or secobarbital daily for several months, abrupt withdrawal produced paroxysmal electroencephalographic changes without symptoms in one-third of the subjects. Withdrawal from 600 mg/day caused minor symptoms in one-half of the subjects and a seizure in 10%. Withdrawal from 900 mg or more per day caused seizures in 75% and delirium in 65%.[143] In evaluating patients for first-time seizure within the emergency department, it is important to perform urine drug testing, as it may reveal unreported use of benzodiazepines or barbiturates.

Cocaine, Amphetamines, and MDMA (Ecstasy)

Single-site studies have reported that seizures occur in approximately 8% of patients presenting to Emergency Departments who have used cocaine. The prevalence of cocaine-associated seizures ranges from 1% to 9%.[144] Any route of administration can precipitate a seizure, but new-onset seizures most often follow IV administration of cocaine hydrochloride or smoking of alkaloidal "crack"; the reason probably is the higher dose and more rapid delivery to the brain these practices permit.

In animals, cocaine produces a "kindling" effect (repeated fixed doses of the drug progressively lower seizure threshold).[145] Seizures usually occur either immediately or within a few hours of cocaine administration. Seizures occurring many hours after use might be related to the proconvulsant properties of the cocaine metabolite, benzoylecgonine.[146] Single grand mal seizures are most common; focal seizures suggest underlying cerebral trauma, stroke, or infection. Status epilepticus tends to be refractory to treatment. Seizures have occurred in infants being breastfed by cocaine-using mothers and in infants and small children who passively inhaled cocaine smoke.[147,148] Despite the biological plausibility of an association between cocaine and seizures, a systematic review on the topic did not finding convincing evidence for a causal relationship.[140]

Stimulants such as amphetamines, methamphetamine, ephedrine, and MDMA are associated with increased risk of seizures. Theoretically, MDMA may directly lower seizure threshold by causing chronic depletion of serotonin levels. However, hyponatremia associated with excessive fluid intake and the syndrome of inappropriate antidiuretic hormone is a more common cause of seizures among individuals using MDMA.[149] In a case series of 32 patients with MDMA toxicity, 3 had seizures associated with hyponatremia (sodium ranging from 115 to 127 mEq/L); all 3 had a tonic-clonic seizure 4 to 6 hours after ingestion, presented with persistent hyperthermia, rhabdomyolysis, severe hepatotoxicity, and renal failure and were comatose for 1 to 3 days.[150] Compared with cocaine-associated seizures, which may occur without symptoms or signs of overdose, seizures associated with amphetamine-like psychostimulants, including methamphetamine, usually are accompanied by other symptoms of severe toxicity including agitation, psychosis, fever, hypertension, and cardiac arrhythmia.[151] The difference may be related to cocaine's local anesthetic properties; procaine and similar agents are epileptogenic.

Opioids

In animals, opioids are either a proconvulsant or an anticonvulsant, depending on receptor specificity and seizure model; in humans, opioids lower the seizure threshold.[152] In one study, heroin use (past and present) was found to be associated with an increased odds of first-time seizure (adjusted odds ratio [aOR] = 2.8) after adjusting for age, gender, alcohol use, and history of head trauma, hypertension, and stroke; adjustments were not made for possible concurrent drug use (eg, benzodiazepines). Heroin use within the first 24 hours of hospitalization was associated with an even higher odds of "unprovoked seizure" (aOR = 4.7).[152,153]

A number of prescription opioids are associated with seizures. Meperidine is an opioid that can cause seizures and myoclonus through the proconvulsant properties of its metabolite, normeperidine.[154] In a prospective study of the neurotoxic effects of meperidine for the treatment of postoperative pain of 67 patients, 8 had myoclonic jerks, and 2 had grand mal seizures.[155] Seizures often follow the parenteral use of the mixed agonist-antagonist opioid pentazocine when it is combined with the antihistamine tripelennamine ("Ts and Blues"); both drugs are epileptogenic.[156] Tramadol has also been associated with seizures, with an overwhelming majority of cases occurring either within 24 hours of the first dose or within 12 hours of the last dose.[157]

Cannabinoids

There is no compelling evidence that cannabis is associated with seizures. Several case reports and one small case-control study suggest that it may be protective.[152,158] In a series of informal interviews of 211 patients with epilepsy and seizures, 90% reported no relationship between cannabis use and seizures, and 7% reported decreased seizure frequency.[159] However, the study was based on patient report and may be subject to recall bias. In 2014, the AAN conducted a systematic review of the efficacy and safety of CUAT in selected neurological conditions, including seizures, reporting that there were no Class I-III studies addressing whether cannabinoids decreased seizure frequency, whereas two Class IV studies did not demonstrate significant benefit after 3 to 18 weeks of use.[160] More recent guidelines recommend, given the lack of high-quality clinical trials, that clinical application of cannabis for treatment of seizures is best suited (at this time) for medically refractory individuals with epilepsy.[161] Among children with Dravet syndrome, a rare genetic disorder associated with medically refractory epilepsy, cannabidiol therapy was associated with reduction in seizures.[158] The Epilepsy Foundation notes that some states have approved "compassionate access" to CUAT for the treatment of epilepsy and that individuals should work with their treating physicians in making decisions about pharmacological and nonpharmacological therapies for seizures.[153] The issue of cannabis to treat epilepsy is detailed further in Section 15 of this textbook.

Dissociative Anesthetics (Ketamine, PCP, Dextromethorphan)

Phencyclidine blocks *N*-methyl-D-aspartate receptors and thus would be expected to have anticonvulsant properties; however, at high doses (ie, 1 mg/kg or more), seizures and myoclonus often are encountered.[162] Such patients are likely to have other signs of overdose, including coma with extensor posturing yet open staring eyes, marked hyperthermia, myoglobinuria, respiratory depression, and hypertension progressing to hypotension.

Psychedelics (LSD, Psilocybin, Mescaline)

Seizures are not an expected toxic feature of psychedelics (eg, LSD, mescaline, or psilocin/psilocybin), but they can occur following exposure to very high doses.[163]

Inhalants

Seizures can complicate acute intoxication with inhalants (such as glues, solvents, or aerosols); in fact, toxic seizures and hallucinations are features that distinguish intoxication with inhalants from intoxication with alcohol.[164]

Other Substances

Seizures can accompany severe anticholinergic poisoning.[165] Seizures as a toxic effect are described with methaqualone, (which sometimes is combined with an antihistamine), and with glutethimide, (which has anticholinergic properties).[166] An alcohol-like withdrawal syndrome that can include seizures has been described with the sedative gamma-hydroxybutyric acid and gamma-hydroxybutyric acid precursors gamma-butyrolactone and 1,4-butanediol.[167]

STROKE

Stroke can be either ischemic (87%) or hemorrhagic (13%). Stroke-related mortality has decreased in the Western world in recent years due to improved management of cerebrovascular risk factors (eg, hypertension, hyperlipidemia, tobacco smoking) and enhanced acute stroke care.[168-170] However, the incidence continues to rise in many low- and middle-income nations as economic prosperity recapitulates the increased rate of obesity and smoking-related illnesses that occurred in higher-income countries.[171-175] Substance use can augment stroke risk factors (eg, alcohol-induced hypertension), may serve as risk factors themselves (eg, smoking), predispose to conditions that are associated with stroke (eg, endocarditis or HIV infection),[176] and complicate the secondary prevention of stroke (eg, tobacco interfering with the metabolism of antiplatelet agents). Substance use contributes to stroke pathogenesis and can cause stroke in people of all ages, even in the absence of other known vascular risk factors.[177] For this reason, it is recommended that all patients who present with ischemic or hemorrhagic stroke undergo urine drug testing, irrespective of age or comorbidities.[178] Here, we highlight some common substances implicated in stroke.

Tobacco and Nicotine

Tobacco, in the form of cigarette smoking, is a well-established, potent, and modifiable risk factor for all types of vascular disease, including coronary heart disease, peripheral vascular disease, carotid artery disease, and cerebrovascular disease. Cigarette smoking also increases the risk of every stroke type, including ischemic (eg, thrombotic, cardioembolic) and hemorrhagic stroke type (eg, intracerebral, subarachnoid). This elevated risk is more pronounced in ischemic and subarachnoid strokes compared with intracerebral hemorrhages (ICHs).[170,179] This association is especially pronounced in younger persons with cryptogenic stroke.[172]

Smoking leads to accelerated atherosclerosis, acute and chronic elevations in blood pressure, elevated fibrinogen levels, arterial wall damage, platelet dysfunction, and inhibition of prostacyclin formation.[176] Accumulation of carbon monoxide (a component of tobacco smoke) also decreases the oxygen-binding capacity of circulating red blood cells. Nicotine acutely causes effects through its sympathomimetic actions, including increases in blood pressure, pulse, and cardiac contractility. Longer-term effects of nicotine include a predisposition to developing metabolic syndrome, enhanced progression of atherosclerotic plaques, and increased incidence of hypertension.[180] Stroke risk increases with the number of cigarettes smoked daily. Men who smoked 20 or more cigarettes daily experience a twofold-increased risk of ICH and ischemic stroke and a threefold increased risk of subarachnoid hemorrhage compared to men who do not smoke.[173] Women who smoked 15 or more cigarettes daily experience a greater than twofold increased risk of ICH and fourfold increased risk of subarachnoid hemorrhage.[173] Smoking and oral contraceptive use synergistically increase the risk of cardiovascular events.[179] It is hypothesized that stroke risk is increased with exposure to passive cigarette smoking; however, a recent meta-analysis has challenged this assertion.[181] There is however recent evidence that secondhand smoking increases ischemic stroke risk and poststroke mortality rates.[168] Even smokeless tobacco has been demonstrated to increase the risk of acute ischemic stroke (particularly in the young) and the risk of cardiovascular morbidity in general.[174,175]

In addition to the direct relationship between tobacco and stroke, it is also known that tobacco smoking complicates the secondary prevention of ischemic stroke. For instance, tobacco smoking leads to an increase in blood pressure, particularly during periods of withdrawal during which there is increased sympathetic tone. In addition, active smoking decreases the efficacy of antiplatelet agents and interferes with the metabolism of oral anticoagulant agents.[182]

Recognizing the importance of tobacco use counseling and role of tobacco use as a stroke risk factor, the AHA/ASA strongly recommends:

- Counseling, alone or in conjunction with medication treatment (eg, nicotine replacement therapy [NRT], varenicline, bupropion) to aid in stopping smoking (Class I, Level of Evidence A)
- Counseling to stop smoking to lower risk of recurrent cerebrovascular event (Class I, Level of Evidence B)
- Avoidance of passive cigarette smoke (Class I, Level of Evidence B)[170,179]

NRT is one means of treatment for people who currently smoke. However, the means by which nicotine can enhance cerebrovascular risk raises concerns that NRT may also increase stroke risk. In an observational study conducted in the United Kingdom (UK) among 33,247 individuals, there was no significant increased stroke risk in the 56 days after the first prescription for NRT (incidence ratio = 1.30, 95% CI, 0.77-2.19).[183] Electronic drug delivery devices (EDDDs, including nicotine e-cigarettes), which are used as an alternative to smoking traditional cigarettes, and are increasingly being used by youth, are being studied for the purposes of promoting quitting smoking, however their short- and long-term health risks are still being explored. In one study, among people ages 18 to 44, after adjusting for sociodemographic factors, vascular risk factors, and concurrent use of traditional cigarette use, the adjusted odds ratio (aOR) of having a stroke were lower for those using EDDDs (ie, sole EDDD users) compared to those who used only traditional cigarettes (aOR = 0.69). However, people who used both EDDDs and traditional cigarettes ("dual use," a common behavior among those who use EDDDs) experienced a higher adjusted odds of having a stroke compared to those who only used traditional cigarettes (aOR = 2.91).[183] Elsewhere, and when comparing people who used EDDDs to people who have never used EDDDs, despite being younger with lower body mass indices (BMI) and lower rates of diabetes, EDDD users had a higher aOR of ischemic stroke (1.71). Thus, EDDDs are not safe. The effects of EDDDs on health, as well as their use in tobacco treatment, are reviewed in Sections 2 and 8 of this textbook.

Alcohol

In contrast to tobacco exposure, alcohol consumption is considered a "less well documented or potentially modifiable risk factor" by the American Heart Association/American Stroke Association Primary Prevention of Ischemic Stroke Guidelines.[170] The guidelines note that, "the risk of harmful alcohol consumption is not well defined," but that alcohol intake greater than 4 drinks/day (ie, >60 g/d) is associated with stroke recurrence. Heavy alcohol use is associated with an increased risk of cardiomyopathy, coronary artery disease, peripheral arterial disease, hypertension, diabetes mellitus, and hyperlipidemia.[184] Alcohol also modulates endogenous fibrinolysis and platelet aggregation as well as impairing liver synthetic function with sustained, long-term use.[184]

The association of alcohol consumption with stroke varies depending on the amount and chronicity of alcohol use. The risk of any stroke has been found to be higher for women than for men who consumed more than 3 drinks on average/day.[185] Drinking up to two drinks daily has been associated with decreased risk of ischemic stroke.[186] No differences in associations have been seen between wine, beer, and liquor. One meta-analysis concluded that heavy alcohol use increases relative risk (RR) of stroke, while light to moderate consumption may be protective against total and ischemic stroke, with a curvilinear association between ethanol consumption and risk. Consumption of less than 12 to 24 g/d of ethanol was associated with a reduced ischemic stroke risk (RR = 0.72), whereas consumption of more than 60 g/d increased the risk of both ischemic (RR = 1.69) and hemorrhagic strokes (RR = 2.18).[187] A more recent systematic review also noted a lower risk of ischemic stroke with light (ie, <1 drink/day) and moderate alcohol consumption (1-2 drinks/day) and a higher risk of ischemic stroke with high (>2-4 drinks/day) and heavy (>4 drinks/day), confirming a "J-shaped" association between alcohol consumption and ischemic stroke risk, with alcohol having a protective effect at low and moderate levels of consumption and increased risk with higher alcohol consumption. This J-shaped relationship is seen among both men and women.[170,188] In comparison, hemorrhagic stroke risk has been associated with increased alcohol consumption in a monotonic fashion.[180,189] Light and moderate alcohol consumption were neither positively nor negatively associated with hemorrhagic stroke risk (either intracerebral hemorrhage or subarachnoid hemorrhage).[189] High alcohol consumption was non-significantly associated with increased risk of both intracerebral and subarachnoid hemorrhage, whereas heavy drinking was associated with a significantly increased risk of both intracerebral (RR = 1.67) and subarachnoid (RR = 1.82) hemorrhage.[173,190-193]

Heavy alcohol use leads to many complications, including alcohol-related cardiac disease, hypertension, platelet dysfunction, synthetic liver dysfunction, accelerated atherosclerosis, acceleration of clotting cascade, decreased fibrinolysis, direct cerebral vasoconstriction, hemoconcentration, and hyperhomocysteinemia due to folate deficiency. Alcohol—even at modest doses—conveys an increased risk for atrial fibrillation and alcoholic cardiomyopathy, which confer a high risk of thromboembolism.[194] The association with reduced risk of ischemic stroke (if causal) may be related to decreased low-density lipoproteins and increased high-density lipoproteins, increased prostacyclin, decreased platelet aggregation, and decreased fibrinogen levels.[1,186]

There are a number of other indirect ways in which heavy alcohol use increases the mortality and morbidity from stroke:

1. Trauma related to alcohol intoxication can lead to epidural and subdural hematomas.
2. Alcohol use is associated with an increased risk of post-stroke seizures.[195]
3. Alcohol use increases the risk of poststroke pneumonia—a condition associated with increased length of hospital stay and increased mortality.[196]
4. Alcohol use is associated with a decreased likelihood of receiving IV thrombolytic therapy in the setting of acute stroke for unclear reasons (though it may be related to a clinician's fear of exposing a person to bleeding complications or of treating a stroke mimic in the setting of alcohol intoxication).[197]

Given the direct and indirect effects of alcohol on stroke risk, stroke prevention guidelines recommend counseling the patient to limit alcohol consumption (men should not consume more than 2 drinks per day, and nonpregnant women or those over age 65 years of age should not consume more than 1 drink per day).

Cocaine, Amphetamines, and MDMA (Ecstasy)

Cocaine significantly increases the risk of cardiovascular and cerebrovascular complications.[198] An association between stroke and cocaine was first reported in 1977.[190] Since the introduction of crack cocaine in the 1980s, a sharp rise has been seen in cases of both ischemic and hemorrhagic (both intracerebral and subarachnoid) strokes with cocaine use.[191]

Cocaine has the potential to cause a reversible vasospasm, hypertensive surges, a drug-induced arteritis and to increase platelet aggregation.[199] Chronic cocaine use modulates several functions of luminal endothelial cells predisposing to thrombus formation.[192] In addition, the use of cocaine can lead to coronary artery vasoconstriction with subsequent myocardial infarction (MI), cardiac arrhythmias, and cardiomyopathy; these may predispose one toward having an ischemic or hemorrhagic stroke. Superimposed upon all of this is the potential toxicity of chemical adulterants during the synthesis or distribution of cocaine, though the association between commonly-used adulterants and stroke is not clear.

In addition to being a local anesthetic, cocaine binds specific transport proteins, thereby blocking the presynaptic reuptake of monoamine neurotransmitters (dopamine, norepinephrine, and serotonin) at the synaptic nerve endings. These elevated monoamines, especially dopamine, mediate cerebral artery vasoconstriction and vasospasm.[193] Both cocaine and its metabolite benzoylecgonine induce vasoconstriction by blocking the reuptake of norepinephrine.[200]

Cerebral ischemia related to cocaine use has been documented as transient ischemic attacks (TIAs) and infarction of the cerebrum, thalamus, brainstem, spinal cord, and retina.[201] Hemorrhagic strokes can occur in the setting of abrupt elevation in blood pressure, mycotic aneurysm rupture (associated with endocarditis), hemorrhagic conversion of an established ischemic stroke, or venous sinus thrombosis with venous infarction. Approximately 50% of patients with cocaine-associated ICH have an underlying saccular aneurysms or vascular malformations. Injection use of cocaine increases the risk of endocarditis, which indirectly increases stroke risk.[168,175,202]

The concomitant use of cocaine and alcohol leads to production of metabolite cocaethylene, which has been associated with a 40-fold increased risk of acute cardiac events and 25-fold increase in risk of sudden death.[203] Direct cerebral vasoconstriction causes ischemia. Magnetic resonance angiography has demonstrated vasoconstriction of large arteries 20 minutes following IV cocaine use.[204] Vasculitis has been implicated based on angiographic "beading." Most autopsies fail to show evidence of vasculitis, however, with only a few cases showing trace evidence without vessel wall necrosis.[205,206] It is thought that the appearance of vasculitis may be secondary to cerebral artery vasospasm.

Treatment of cocaine-associated ischemic stroke includes acute blood pressure management. Beta-blocking agents are typically avoided, especially in the presence of concomitant cocaine-related chest pain or MI.[207] Dopamine release onto neurons that mediate cerebral artery tone is inhibited by dihydropyridine calcium channel antagonists, thereby hindering cocaine-induced vasospasm.[193] Antithrombotic agents are given to counteract vasospasm-associated thrombus formation, but are strongly avoided in cocaine-associated hemorrhages. In hemorrhagic strokes, computed tomography angiogram should be utilized to determine the presence of an underlying aneurysm or vascular malformation given that cocaine is more likely to expose an underlying lesion than to be a primary cause. Transthoracic echocardiogram and, if needed, transesophageal echocardiogram should be pursued to assess for possible endocarditis in the case of ischemic stroke in the setting of injection drug use.

Similar to cocaine, amphetamine-like medications have psychostimulant properties and cause excitability, euphoria, and heightened alertness in tandem with a significant increase in sympathetic tone, which increases blood pressure and heart rate, sometimes dramatically so. These include methylphenidate, methamphetamines, dextroamphetamines, phenylpropanolamine (PPA), ephedrine, and pseudoephedrine. Amphetamine use has been associated with hemorrhagic stroke, both with chronic use and after initial exposure.[1,208] PPA is a sympathomimetic agent found in appetite suppressants and decongestants. A significant increase in risk of hemorrhagic stroke in women who used PPA has been reported.[209] Following this, the Food and Drug Administration (FDA) ordered withdrawal of all PPA-containing products from the market. Other stimulants, such as ephedra, phentermine, and fenfluramine, have been marketed as food supplements or appetite suppressants and thus are available "over the counter." Ephedra (an herb containing varying quantities of ephedrine and pseudoephedrine), long used in Chinese medicine for respiratory illnesses, had been marketed in weight loss and energy supplements. Due to reports of hemorrhagic stroke at higher doses, as well as gastrointestinal and psychiatric side effects, the FDA banned the sale of ephedra-containing dietary supplements in 2004.[210]

Stimulants increase the effects of norepinephrine and dopamine by increasing their release and blocking presynaptic reuptake.[211] This can result in elevated heart rate and blood pressure, arrhythmia, vasospasm, and vasculitis, potentially increasing risk of stroke, MI, or sudden death. Multiple studies have failed to find a significant risk of cardiovascular events in children taking prescribed stimulants; however, lack of statistical power was a key issue for many given the low overall incidence of cerebrovascular events in children.[212] Intravenous and inadvertent carotid artery injection of crushed methylphenidate, however, can result in ischemic stroke due to foreign body emboli.[200]

Cerebral vasculitis and the reversible cerebral vasoconstriction syndrome ("RCVS") occur more commonly among those using amphetamines as opposed to cocaine; amphetamine-induced cerebral vasculitis or RCVS can cause ischemic and hemorrhagic stroke. A population-based case-control study of young women found an increased risk of hemorrhagic and ischemic stroke with amphetamine/methamphetamine use (aOR = 3.80).[213] Other studies of hospitalized people who use amphetamine have found an increased risk of hemorrhagic stroke (aOR = 4.95) but not ischemic stroke. Amphetamine use was also associated with higher mortality after hemorrhagic stroke (aOR = 2.63).[202]

Case reports have described vasculitis in children taking methylphenidate for treatment of attention deficit hyperactivity disorder.[214,215] One study reported 14 individuals with the use of more than one drug (12 of whom used IV methamphetamine) who developed a necrotizing arteritis that resembled polyarteritis nodosa.[216] Ischemic and hemorrhagic lesions were found in the cerebrum, cerebellum, and brainstem. Animal studies have confirmed evidence of cerebral vasculitis following single or repeated IV administration of methamphetamine or methylphenidate, often in vessels smaller than those typically involved in polyarteritis nodosa.[217]

MDMA has stimulant and hallucinogenic effects; both hemorrhagic and ischemic strokes have been reported in association with its use, usually in the setting of hypertensive crisis and severe hyperthermia.[218]

Opioids

Ischemic and hemorrhagic strokes have been described in the setting of heroin use.[219,220] Multiple mechanisms have been suggested. Heroin overdose can cause hypotension and respiratory depression with hypoxemia. Direct toxicity from heroin, an adulterating substance, or pharmacologically active ingredients used in heroin preparations are other possibilities,[221] and multiple strokes in the context of a hypereosinophilic syndrome due to heroin use has been described.[222] Intravenous or nasally inhaled heroin use has been associated with stroke in the absence of other risk factors.[223]

Ischemic strokes can occur secondary to endocarditis (*Staphylococcus aureus* and *Candida*) and basilar meningitis with secondary vasculitis or vasculopathy (this risk is increased if the patient in question has HIV/AIDS). Hemorrhagic strokes can also be caused by endocarditis or ruptured mycotic and saccular aneurysms or result from alterations in the clotting cascade from underlying hepatitis (with ensuing hepatic synthetic dysfunction) or nephropathy.[174,201]

Cannabinoids

Several potential precipitants of stroke have been described among individuals who use cannabis, including very large doses of cannabis being consumed, simultaneous alcohol ingestion, and sexual activity through reversible cerebral vasoconstriction.[224,225] Cannabis has been associated with arrhythmias (including atrial fibrillation), impaired cerebral autoregulation, and systemic hypotension. Additionally, a multifocal intracranial vasculopathy has been described in association with cannabis use, and in one series, this was confirmed (via formal angiography) in 21% of young people presenting with an ischemic stroke.[224,226] Young patients with stroke of unknown etiology (ie, cryptogenic stroke) should be questioned regarding their use of cannabis and other cannabinoids and have urine drug testing performed.[174,224,227]

Case reports suggest an association between synthetic cannabinoid use and the development of arterial and venous thromboses. In one report, a 25-year-old man developed a proximal right middle cerebral artery ischemic infarction the day after inhaling "Freeze," (which was found via gas chromatography to contain cannabimimetic ADB-FUBINACA).[228] In another, a 32-year-old woman developed multiple thromboembolic events during a period of smoking synthetic cannabinoids, including an ischemic stroke, a pulmonary embolism, and renal artery infarcts.[229] During periods of abstinence, she did not develop thromboembolic events.

As of 2015, 64 cases of cannabis-related stroke have been reported, with a majority being of the ischemic subtype[230]; in 81%, the stroke occurred shortly after exposure to cannabis, and 50% of had other risk factors for cerebrovascular disease.[231] In a case-control study of cannabis and stroke risk, patients 18 to 55 years old admitted with an ischemic stroke or TIA were 2.3 times more likely to have a positive urine test for cannabis.[227] However, a more recent population-based case-control study (1,090 cases, 1,152 controls) did not demonstrate an association between cannabis use (both within 24 hours and 30 days) and ischemic stroke after adjusting for sociodemographics, hypertension, diabetes, and current tobacco or alcohol use.[232]

Psychedelics (LSD, Psilocybin, Mescaline)

LSD can acutely increase blood pressure causing vasoconstriction in systemic and cerebral arteries. This can lead to narrowing and occlusion of the intracranial vasculature (seen on angiography as arterial "beading") ultimately resulting in ischemic stroke.[233] Ischemic stroke has been reported up to several days after LSD use.

Dissociative Anesthetics (Ketamine, PCP, Dextromethorphan)

PCP can cause euphoria at lower doses and psychosis at higher doses. The exact mechanism remains unclear, but it is known that PCP causes systemic hypertension lasting hours or days. Cerebral infarction, intracerebral and subarachnoid hemorrhage, and hypertensive encephalopathy have followed the use of PCP.[1]

Other Substances

Anabolic androgenic steroid ("AAS") use is common not only athletes but also casual exercise enthusiasts. AAS use has myriad physiological effects, which often go undiagnosed and unrecognized. Data thus far implicating anabolic steroids with increased risk of cardiovascular disease are limited to case reports. Stroke has been reported in the young without any concomitant cardiovascular risk factors.[234,235] Reports link anabolic steroid use with MI, cardiomyopathy, stroke, and death (including sudden death) by elevated blood pressure, increased platelet aggregation, dysrhythmias, and concentric left ventricular hypertrophy.[236,237]

NEUROMUSCULAR (NERVE, MUSCLE, AND SPINAL CORD) DISORDERS

Disorders of the muscles, peripheral nerves, and spinal cord related to substance use can have acute or chronic presentations. Manifestations of these conditions include neuropathic symptoms (loss of feeling and balance difficulties from large nerve fiber damage; tingling, burning, and increased sensitivity from small nerve fiber damage), weakness, and bowel and bladder dysfunction. Patterns of weakness and sensory symptoms are useful in determining whether the muscle, the nerve, or the spinal cord may be affected. For example, in peripheral neuropathies, sensory signs (eg, decreased vibration, "stocking and glove" distribution of pinprick loss) predominate, and weakness is predominantly distal, whereas myopathies typically present with proximal muscle weakness without sensory findings. The presence of peripheral neuropathy does not exclude the presence of a concomitant myopathy, as can be seen in heavy alcohol use. Neuromuscular damage may occur secondary to direct toxicity from the offending agent, nutritional deficiencies, a robust inflammatory response to a specific agent, or some other mechanism. A decreased level of consciousness from intoxication or withdrawal from substances can result in patients being immobilized for prolonged periods of time in unusual positions, with resultant compressive neuropathies. These can be the result of direct compression (as seen in radial nerve palsy) or associated with myoedema (as seen in compartment syndrome).

Alcohol

Neuropathy may occur with chronic heavy alcohol use. The frequency of neuropathy due to alcohol use varies from 20% to 66% based on the methods used to identify it; a 2019 systematic review estimated that peripheral neuropathy occurs among 46% of people with chronic heavy alcohol use.[238] The neuropathy can present with symptoms of motor, sensory, and/or autonomic (eg, orthostatic hypotension, bradycardia) dysfunction, leading to increased morbidity associated with falls, infections, and pain. Typical symptoms consist of numbness, paresthesias, and pain mainly in the distal legs and feet.[239] Autonomic dysfunction can occur and requires careful history to elicit symptoms. Etiology has been attributed to direct toxic effects of alcohol, as well as thiamine deficiency and other nutritional deficiencies, including folate and B_{12}.[226] The duration of direct exposure to alcohol correlates with electrophysiological changes and lends support to direct toxic effects.[240] Management consists of abstinence from alcohol as well as improved nutrition. Limited data support aggressive supplementation with B-vitamins, especially thiamine.[238] Pain should be managed symptomatically with neuropathic pain medications, including gabapentin. The long-term outcome of alcohol neuropathy is not well known, but, at a minimum, progression can be halted with abstinence. Acute compressive neuropathies most commonly involve the radial nerve ("Saturday night palsy") and the peroneal nerve causing wrist drop and foot drop, respectively; a superimposed diffuse neuropathy may leave those with alcohol use disorder more susceptible to nerve compression neuropathies.

Alcohol myopathy can present with acute and chronic manifestations. Acute myopathy may present with myalgias, weakness, and elevation of creatine kinase (CK); it may also present with acute rhabdomyolysis with myoglobinuria or asymptomatic elevation of serum CK. It may be confused with polymyositis; improvement over weeks to months without the use of corticosteroids would distinguish it from an inflammatory myopathy. Chronic heavy alcohol use is also associated with a painless, progressive proximal weakness. CK level is usually not elevated, and discontinuation of alcohol can stabilize and possibly result in improvement.[241] Continued drinking can result in progressive weakness and cardiomyopathy leading to arrhythmia and heart failure.[242] Management of this condition is symptomatic and it may be reversible in some cases.[230]

Alcohol may be associated with spinal cord trauma, as previously mentioned under "Trauma and Traumatic Brain Injury."

Opioids

The injection use of substances including opioids has been associated with nerve and muscle disorders. Neuropathies have been attributed to compression, muscle edema, and immune mechanisms. Guillain-Barré syndrome, which affects multiple nerve roots and results in an ascending pattern of weakness and sensory symptoms, has been reported in association with injection heroin use.[243] An unusual manifestation of heroin neuropathy is atraumatic brachial and lumbosacral plexopathies, most often associated with rhabdomyolysis.[244] Heroin-associated myelopathy has been reported following injection and intranasal insufflation.[245] Acute transverse myelitis has been described in the thoracic segments in individuals who use heroin. This location suggests vascular insufficiency due to the vulnerability of the spinal cord to hypotension in this region.[246]

Inhalants

N-hexane is a hydrocarbon used in glues and roofing. "Glue-sniffers' neuropathy" is a severe sensorimotor polyneuropathy that affects individuals who use products containing *N*-hexane and may progress to quadriplegia over a few weeks. Pathologically, axons are distended by masses of neurofilaments, and secondary demyelination occurs.[247] Improvement can be seen when the exposure ceases, but may not be complete.[248] Nitrous oxide use can result in a myelopathy that is similar to that caused by B_{12} deficiency. Although the effect of nitrous oxide toxicity can be ameliorated by methionine supplementation, the mechanism of myelopathy remains unknown.[249,250]

Other Substances

Cocaine, amphetamines, LSD, phencyclidine and cannabis have been associated with rhabdomyolysis in case reports. A variety of mechanisms for rhabdomyolysis have been suggested including compression, direct muscle toxicity, falls, seizure, and renal disease.[251,252] Cocaine has rarely been associated with peripheral neuropathy presenting as a mononeuritis multiplex as a result of a presumed vascular insult.[253,254]

MOVEMENT DISORDERS

The interaction between movement disorders and alcohol and other substances is complex, as there are many substances that can directly cause movement disorders, and at the same time, there are others that can be used to treat symptoms associated with these disorders. Furthermore, a movement disorder may be triggered by intoxication or withdrawal from a substance.

Movement disorders can be divided into those where there is hyperkinetic or hypokinetic movement. In general, drugs that enhance monoaminergic transmission provoke hyperkinetic movements, while drugs that stimulate inhibitory neurotransmission lessen hyperkinetic movements. Still further, chronic use, especially of the monoaminergic enhancing drugs, can result in a relatively depleted monoaminergic state and produce hypokinetic movements. Acute withdrawal, especially of the GABAergic substances, can result in worsening or emergence of hyperkinetic movements. The neurotransmitter dopamine plays an integral role in the pathophysiology of intoxication and addiction.[255] It is central to the pathogenesis of some of the best-recognized hypo- and hyperkinetic movement disorders and in fact has itself been used nonmedically by those with Parkinson disease.[256] It is not surprising, then, that a variety of movement disorders can be associated with substance use.

Alcohol

Movement disorders usually emerge in the setting of chronic alcohol use or withdrawal. As alcohol preferentially affects neurons in the cerebellum, tremor and to a lesser extent ataxia are associated with its overuse or withdrawal. Acutely, alcohol increases GABAergic transmission at cerebellar interneurons that project to Purkinje cells, resulting in a net decrease of glutamatergic transmission at these sites.[257]

Postural tremor—tremor best seen distally in the hands with outstretched arms—is the most common tremor associated with alcohol. Acute alcohol ingestion is associated with an increase in postural tremor that peaks at about 60 minutes after alcohol ingestion.[258] Alcohol withdrawal tremor occurs acutely during the first 1 to 2 days following alcohol abstinence or decreased intake. It is coarse, irregular, and seen best distally in the hands and interferes with movement. It is responsive to benzodiazepines, baclofen, and beta blockers and, in most cases, subsides after a few days of abstinence.[259] An alcohol-induced cerebellar tremor typically results gradually from long-standing heavy alcohol use. It is best seen as an intentional tremor that is worse when touching distant objects and is associated with other cerebellar signs such as a broad-based gait and difficulty performing rapid alternating movements.[260]

Other movement disorders are associated with alcohol as well. "Negative" myoclonus, seen clinically as asterixis or jerking movements resulting from transient loss of muscle tone when maintaining a posture, can be seen in patients with alcohol use disorder and liver failure.[259] Transient parkinsonian symptoms have been reported in some patients with chronic heavy alcohol use in the days to weeks following alcohol withdrawal. Transient choreiform movements and dyskinesias of the face, tongue, neck, and arms have also been associated with alcohol withdrawal, sometimes preceded by transient parkinsonism. Symptoms typically resolve without lasting sequelae; changes in dopamine receptor sensitivity are postulated to cause both of these phenomena.[261,262]

Alcohol is also often used by patients with essential tremor to decrease tremor amplitude and acutely results in amelioration of the tremor in 50% to 90% of cases.[263,264] Alcohol is typically beneficial in reducing myoclonus and to a lesser extent dystonia in the autosomal dominantly inherited myoclonus dystonia.[265] In addition, alcohol ingestion may also acutely help patient with vocal tremor, torticollis, myoclonus-dystonia,[266] and posthypoxic myoclonus, mainly by alcohol's inhibition of hyper-excitability in cerebellar and cerebellar-related networks.[267]

Cocaine, Amphetamines, and MDMA

Cocaine may result in a number of de novo hyperkinetic movement disorders, as well as exacerbation of preexisting conditions, thought to result from dopamine hyperactivity. One phenomenon is the dance-like choreoathetoid movements and dyskinesias of cocaine intoxication. Orolingual dyskinesias are also seen in persons with chronic cocaine use. Onset can be immediately after ingestion, and the movements can last several days or persist indefinitely.[260,268-270] Cocaine can also cause acute dystonic reactions, when agonist and antagonist muscles are stimulated to co-contract and posturing and muscle spasm can result.[259-261,271] Dystonic reactions are especially seen when cocaine is coadministered with neuroleptics.[271] De novo tic disorders and exacerbation of tic disorders such as Tourette syndrome have been reported with prescription central stimulants and are associated with cocaine as well.[272] The exacerbations may be sustained even after stopping cocaine use.[260] Cocaine has also been associated with a mild low-frequency resting tremor that can persist in times of abstinence.[273] With chronic and repeated cocaine use, a state of dopamine depletion can result, with decreased levels of dopamine in caudate and frontal cortex, and also decreases in vesicular monoamine transporter-2 levels.[274] The clinical pathological correlate of this dopamine-depleted state is one of the depressions and parkinsonisms.[273]

Similar to cocaine, acute amphetamine use (including methamphetamine and MDMA) can cause dyskinesias, tremor, acute dystonic reactions, and exacerbation of tics.[259,275,276] In addition, acute amphetamine intoxication has long been associated with a phenomenon termed "punding," which refers to a series of meaningless and repetitive movements or behaviors that are highly stereotyped but unique to an individual and usually related to their premorbid habits. Examples include polishing nails, picking at excoriations, sorting things, and taking apart and putting together mechanical objects. These seemingly pointless repetitive behaviors can be performed continuously for hours, sometimes to the point of self-harm.[277,278] Punding is not unique to amphetamine use and can be seen in cocaine intoxication as well.[279] Oromandibular stereotypies, including bruxism and repetitive tongue protrusion, have also been associated with amphetamine use; in fact, trauma and ulceration of the tongue and lips have been described as a sign of amphetamine use as early as 1965.[280] This behavior occurs both acutely and can persist during abstinence; in some cases, botulinum toxin therapy to the muscles of mastication may be an effective therapy.[281,282]

Opioids

Opioids, in various forms and routes of administration, have been associated with myoclonus. This is seen in both the acute intoxication and withdrawal periods. The myoclonus can be generalized, or focal as in the case of intractable hiccups. Opioid-related myoclonus is more likely to occur in patients with other co-occurring medical disorders and with coadministration of D2 agonists or other drugs (eg, nonsteroidal anti-inflammatory drugs, antidepressants) and is responsive to benzodiazepines.[260,283] Although itself not an opioid, it is worth noting that MPTP (1-methyl-4-phenyl-1,2,3,6-tetrahydropyridine) was formed as a toxic by-product for chemists to synthetically produce the opiate meperidine. In the 1980s, individuals with heroin use that injected this MPTP-laden "new heroin" developed acute levodopa-responsive parkinsonism.[284] Still to this day, MPTP is used in animal models of Parkinson disease.[260,285]

Vapors of heroin pyrolysate are often inhaled ("chasing the dragon") by people who use heroin. But when the drug is heated on an aluminum base, a cerebral and cerebellar spongiform leukoencephalopathy can develop. This state can manifest with choreoathetoid movements, tremor, or parkinsonism, as well as ataxia, dementia, blindness, quadriparesis, obtundation, and frequently death.[286] Survivors are typically left with pronounced neurological residua. The nature of the toxicity is unknown; elevated lactate in the damaged white matter suggests mitochondrial dysfunction.[287]

Tobacco and Nicotine

There is some evidence to suggest that tobacco use disorder is inversely associated with the development of Parkinson disease and that those with Parkinson disease are less prone to develop a substance use disorder. There is emerging evidence that α6β2β3 subtype nAChR expression is reduced in the striatum of patients with Parkinson disease and that this correlates to the degree of dopamine transporter loss.[288] This is interesting as data dating back more than 40 years has shown that a history of ever having smoked cigarettes is associated with a lower risk of developing Parkinson disease,[289] begging the question "Does nicotine or cigarette smoking decrease the likelihood of developing Parkinson disease?" Recent data suggests that Parkinson patients are less likely to smoke cigarettes and are more likely to perceive that stopping smoking is "easy."[290] This thought is consistent with neuropathology in Parkinson disease patients that shows up to 50% reduction in available nicotinic acetylcholine receptors in the frontal and temporal brain regions. Thus, it is possible that Parkinson disease can be used as a clinical model of a decreased potential for addiction to nicotine.

Cannabinoids

Movement abnormalities are not typically associated with cannabis use, and, in fact, there are case reports of transient amelioration of symptoms in various movement disorders, such as Huntington disease and Tourette syndrome.[159,291] As a result, there has been interest in using cannabinoids for the treatment of movement disorders, especially since the basal ganglia is rich with cannabinoid receptors.[292] The use of nabilone in a crossover study for the treatment of symptomatic Huntington disease showed no improvement.[293] Another crossover study of cannabidiol capsules for symptomatic Huntington disease found that an average daily dose of approximately 700 mg/day neither improved symptoms nor resulted in toxicities.[159] Regarding Parkinson disease, although preclinical studies have shown benefit of cannabinoids in animal models, clinical studies have been mixed. Open label and survey studies on the use of cannabis to treat PD have suggested improvement of PD tremor and bradykinesia with cannabinoids.[281,294] On the other hand, randomized controlled studies of nabilone and cannabidiol have not found that these agents benefit the motor symptoms of PD.[282,295] Cannabis used as treatment (CUAT) for neurological disorders is discussed further in Section 15 of this textbook.

Other Substances

It is important to note that in some patients, prescription medications can be used in amounts or for purposes other than intended. In addition to the nonmedical use of prescription opioids and sedatives, other medications have been noted to be used nonmedically. The dopamine dysregulation syndrome is a neurobehavioral syndrome that results most often in patients with levodopa-responsive Parkinson disease who compulsively take supratherapeutic amounts of levodopa.[285] Persons with dopamine dysregulation syndrome suffer from often violent levodopa-induced dyskinesias. Neurobehavioral symptoms can include paranoia, hypomania, hypersexuality, pathological gambling, and heightened aggression.

NEUROLOGICAL COMPLICATIONS OF SUBSTANCE USE RESULTING FROM INFECTIONS

Injection drug use is a risk factor for HIV/AIDS, which predisposes to opportunistic infections, which may involve the nervous system.[296-298] The most common neurological complications are CNS opportunistic infections (toxoplasmosis, cryptococcal meningitis/cryptococcomas, progressive multifocal leukoencephalopathy), malignancies (primary CNS lymphoma), stroke, peripheral neuropathy, and HIV-associated neurocognitive disorder (HAND).[299,300]

Individuals with injection drug use are also subject to an array of non–HIV-associated local and systemic infections, including abscesses, cellulitis, pneumonia, sepsis, endophthalmitis, osteomyelitis, and pyogenic arthritis.[301] Endocarditis (bacterial or fungal) may be complicated by meningitis, cerebral infarction, diffuse vasculitis, abscess (intraparenchymal, subdural, or epidural, including the spinal cord) or subarachnoid hemorrhage from rupture of a septic ("mycotic") aneurysm.[302,303] Infectious hepatitis can cause encephalopathy or, because of deranged clotting, hemorrhagic stroke. Vertebral osteomyelitis can cause radiculopathy or spinal cord compression.

Even before the AIDS epidemic, it was recognized that individuals with heavy alcohol use and other drug use often are immunosuppressed. Those with alcohol use disorders are prone to develop bacterial or tuberculous meningitis, which should be considered in someone who drinks excessively who presents with seizures or altered mentation, even when the clinical picture suggests intoxication, withdrawal, thiamine deficiency, hepatic encephalopathy, or hypoglycemia (any of which could coexist). Clinicians should have a low threshold for performing a lumbar puncture in someone with alcohol use disorder and altered mentation, even in the absence of fever or stiff neck. HIV-seronegative patients who are injecting drugs are also at risk for CNS infection, including fungal agents such as *Candida* or *Mucor*.[304]

Tetanus is a CNS infection that presents with muscle spasms and is rare in the developed world given widespread vaccination; however, it is a threat to all unvaccinated people especially of the developing world. Any penetrating injury, including the use of a hypodermic needle, can inoculate *Clostridium tetanus* spores into the skin, which can then readily migrate to the CNS. Generalized tetanus involves the CNS and leads to trismus (lockjaw) and dysautonomia (irritability, diaphoresis, tachycardia, blood pressure lability, fever) in the later stages of the disease. The most common physical exam findings include stiff neck, opisthotonus, risus sardonicus (sardonic smile), and periods of upper airway obstruction secondary to pharyngeal muscle contraction. Tetanus, usually severe, is associated with subcutaneous injection of heroin.[305] It is thought that the powdered form of heroin is often dissolved in mild acids followed by heating in a spoon prior to use, which creates a mildly acidic environment that kills the non–spore-forming bacteria, but allows for spore-forming bacteria such as *Clostridium tetanus* to grow.[306] The disease is rapidly progressive within a few days and most often results in death especially after entering the late stages. The treatment for tetanus includes wound management (by wound debridement to eradicate the spores and necrotic tissues) and antimicrobial therapy. Tetanus toxin is irreversibly bound to tissues, so only the unbound toxin is available for neutralization by administration of human tetanus immune globulin intramuscularly and should be the most immediate treatment if there is a suspicion of tetanus infection.[307]

Cases of botulism have been reported among people who inject drugs; this is a CNS infection that results from the introduction of *Clostridium botulinum* spores into an injection site that then secrete a toxin under anaerobic conditions. Botulism most commonly presents with bilateral symmetric cranial neuropathies such as ptosis, diplopia, blurred vision, dysphagia, dysarthria, and symmetrical descending weakness of the upper extremities. Notably, no sensory deficits occur with botulism infection. Botulism occurs at injection sites and, among those who snort cocaine, in the nasal sinuses.[308] In the U.S., an outbreak was reported in the 1990s in people using of black tar heroin, and since then, other outbreaks have been reported in Europe. Treatment of botulism is similar to that of tetanus. It consists of immediate administration of a trivalent antitoxin, antimicrobials such as IV penicillin G or metronidazole, and surgical excision of the abscess.[309,310]

Disseminated candidiasis also occurs as a result of injection drug use and can lead to CNS complication including endophthalmitis. *Candida* infection of the CNS is uncommon, but its primary risk factor is neutropenia. *Candida* endophthalmitis is a frequent and debilitating sequela of candidiasis, and all patients with candidemia should have an ophthalmological examination as it requires a longer duration of treatment. In adults, *Candida* is the second most common cause of cerebral micro-abscesses after *Staphylococcus aureus*. *Candida* infection of the CNS can present as a brain abscess sometimes with vascular involvement and basilar artery thrombosis or subarachnoid hemorrhage from a rupture of mycotic aneurysm infected with *Candida*. MRI is useful in visualizing micro-abscesses.

Injection drug use is associated with sexual behaviors that may increase the risk for acquiring sexually transmitted infections, including syphilis. In a Russian study, prevalence of syphilis was nine times higher in females who used injection drugs and was also strongly associated with being a sex worker.[311] Homosexual/bisexual men who use injection drugs were also found to have a more frequent occurrence of both HIV and syphilis coinfection, compared with heterosexual men who used injection drugs.[312] Syphilis is caused by the bacterium *Treponema pallidum*, and is called neurosyphilis when it involves the CNS. Neurosyphilis is classified into early (divided into primary and secondary stages) and late (including latent and tertiary stages) stages. The early stage occurs most commonly less than 1 year after initial infection, and symptomatology includes meningitis, cranial neuropathies, strokes (most commonly in HIV coinfected patients), and/or gummas (mass lesions). The late stage occurs years to decades after initial infection and involves the dorsal columns of the spinal cord leading to a condition called *tabes dorsalis* characterized by weakness of the extremities and loss of vibration sense and proprioception. This potentially reversible condition is diagnosed by lumbar puncture, and CSF results can reveal a lymphocytic pleocytosis and/or elevated protein. *T. pallidum* cannot be cultured, so the fluorescent treponemal antibody absorption (FTA-ABS), nontreponemal rapid plasma regain (RPR), and venereal disease research laboratory (VDRL) tests are used to diagnose the disease. The CDC recommends treatment with IV penicillin G.[313] Neurosyphilis is important to identify in a patient who has a history of distant or recent past injection drug use, whether HIV seropositive or not, because it is potentially reversible.

Human T-cell lymphotropic virus type I/II (HTLV-I/II) is a retrovirus, which like HIV can be transmitted intravenously, sexually, or perinatally (from mother to child during pregnancy). HTLV-II seroprevalence rates in North Americans with injection drug use vary between 9% and 18% with higher rates associated with female gender, non-White race, and heroin use.[296,297] HTLV-I and HTLV-II are known to cause a disease that affects the spinal cord, known as tropic spastic paraparesis (TSP) or HTLV-I-associated myelopathy (HAM), a chronic and progressive disease that is endemic to some equatorial areas of the world. Criteria for a diagnosis of TSP/HAM include hyperreflexia, often with spasticity and clonus, as well as the presence of HTLV-I or HTLV-II antibodies or antigens in serum and/or CSF. Other supportive criteria include lower extremity weakness (usually bilateral) and neurogenic bladder and/or bowel dysfunction. Most cases of TSP/HAM are caused by HTLV-I; HTLV-II-associated myelopathy also exists but is milder and more slowly progressive. In rare cases, individuals with HAM/TSP may also develop uveitis, arthritis, infectious dermatitis, and polymyositis. The most serious complication of HTLV-I infection is development of adult T-cell leukemia or lymphoma. Unfortunately, there is no known treatment of HAM/TSP.[297]

OTHER COMPLICATIONS

Impaired vision with optic atrophy is common in individuals with alcohol use disorders. The optic nerve lesions are mainly the result of nutritional deficiency, but the particular deficiency is uncertain, as are the possible toxicities of alcohol itself and of cyanide in tobacco smoke.[298,304] In one case report, a man who took large doses of a heroin mixture containing quinine developed blindness; vision improved when he resumed using heroin without quinine.[314]

Cerebellar degeneration can occur in nutritionally deficient people with alcohol use disorder in the absence of Wernicke-Korsakoff syndrome. The superior cerebellar vermis is preferentially affected, resulting in gait and sometimes leg ataxia, usually without ataxia of the arms or dysarthria.[315,316] As with other central and peripheral nerve complications of heavy alcohol use, both nutritional deficiency and alcohol toxicity are probably contributory. With abstinence and nutritional replenishment, improvement is likely, albeit usually incomplete.

Central pontine myelinolysis after over vigorous correction of hyponatremia may occur in people with alcohol use disorders. Most severely affecting the pontine base, central pontine myelinolysis can cause quadriparesis progressing to locked-in syndrome. Most extensive demyelination can impair consciousness. Extrapontine myelinolysis can cause ataxia, abnormal behavior, or movement disorders. Lesions can be identified by MRI, including diffusion-weighted imaging.[317]

CONCLUSIONS

Neurological complications of alcohol, tobacco, and other drugs occur commonly and can affect any part of the neuroaxis. Multiple portions of the nervous system can be affected simultaneously, even if a person uses only one drug. Complications can be acute or acute-on-chronic and may result from acute use, long term use, and withdrawal states. A thorough neurological examination is required to understand the extent of nervous system involvement, regardless of whether the patient is presenting to the Emergency Department, has been hospitalized, or is being seen in outpatient settings. When detected early and treated appropriately, many neurological complications associated with substance use are reversible.

REFERENCES

1. Brust J. *Neurological Aspects of Substance Abuse*. 2nd ed. Butterworth-Heinemann; 2004.
2. Goldfrank L, Flomenbaum N, Lewin N, et al. *Goldfrank's Toxicologic Emergencies*. 6th ed. Appleton & Lange; 1998.
3. Centers for Disease Control and Prevention. Accidents or Unintentional Injuries. Accessed May 24, 2022. https://www.cdc.gov/nchs/fastats/accidental-injury.htm
4. Heron M. *National Vital Statistics Reports - Deaths: Leading Causes for*; 2019. Accessed May 22, 2022. https://www.cdc.gov/nchs/data/nvsr/nvsr70/nvsr70-09-508.pdf
5. National Institute on Alcohol Abuse and Alcoholism - Alcohol Alert. Accessed September 7, 2012. http://pubs.niaaa.nih.gov/publications/aa03.htm
6. Mohr JP, Wolf PA, Grotta JC, Moskowitz MA, Mayberg MR, Kummer RV. *Stroke: Pathophysiology, Diagnosis, and Management*. 5th ed. Elsevier Saunders; 2011.
7. Halt P, Swanson R, Faden A. Alcohol exacerbates behavioral and neurochemical effects of rat spinal cord trauma. *Arch Neurol*. 1992;49:1178-1184.
8. Silver J, McAllister T, Yudofsky S. *Textbook of Traumatic Brain Injury*. American Psychiatric Publishing, Inc; 2011.
9. Menon DK, Schwab K, Wright DW, Maas AI. Position statement: definition of traumatic brain injury. *Arch Phys Med Rehabil*. 2010;91(11):1637-1640.
10. Centers for Disease Control and Prevention. *TBI Data*. Accessed February 2, 2022. https://www.cdc.gov/traumaticbraininjury/data/index.html
11. VA/DoD. *Evidence Based Practice for Management of Concussion/Mild Traumatic Brain Injury*. Accessed November 16, 2016. http://www.healthquality.va.gov/guidelines/Rehab/mtbi/
12. Tsao J, Abrams G, Alessi A, et al. Traumatic brain injury. *Continuum (Minneap Minn)*. 2010;16(6):1-218.
13. Sekhon L, Fehlings M. Epidemiology, demographics, and pathophysiology of acute spinal cord injury. *Spine*. 2001;26(24 Suppl):S2-S12.
14. Bradley W, Daroff R, Fenichel G, et al. *Neurology in Clinical Practice - The Neurological Disorders*. Vol 2. 5th ed. Elsevier Inc.; 2008.
15. Mustafa N, Hyun A, Kumar J, Yekkirala L. Gluteal compartment syndrome: a case report. *Cases J*. 2009;2:190.
16. Olson S, Glasgow R. Acute compartment syndrome in lower extremity musculoskeletal trauma. *J Am Acad Orthop Surg*. 2005;13(7):436-444.
17. Weiller C, May A, Limmroth V, et al. Brain stem activation in spontaneous human migraine attacks. *Nat Med*. Jul 1995;1(7):658-660.

18. May A, Goadsby PJ. Hypothalamic involvement and activation in cluster headache. *Curr Pain Headache Rep*. 2001;5(1):60-66. doi:10.1007/s11916-001-0011-4
19. McDermott MJ, Tull MT, Gratz KL, Houle TT, Smitherman TA. Comorbidity of migraine and psychiatric disorders among substance-dependent inpatients. *Headache*. 2014;54(2):290-302.
20. RS EI-M, Kranzler HR, Kamanitz JR. Headaches and psychoactive substance use. *Headache*. 1991;31(9):584-587. doi:10.1111/j.1526-4610.1991.hed3109584.x
21. McGeeney BE. Cannabinoids and hallucinogens for headache. *Headache*. 2013;53(3):447-458.
22. Aamodt AH, Stovner LJ, Hagen K, Bråthen G, Zwart J. Headache prevalence related to smoking and alcohol use. The Head-HUNT Study. *Eur J Neurol*. 2006;13(11):1233-1238.
23. Rozen TD, Fishman RS. Cluster headache in the United States of America: demographics, clinical characteristics, triggers, suicidality, and personal burden. *Headache*. 2012;52(1):99-113.
24. Panconesi A. Alcohol and migraine: trigger factor, consumption, mechanisms. A review. *J Headache Pain*. 2008;9(1):19-27.
25. Evans RW, Sun C, Lay C. Alcohol hangover headache. *Headache*. 2007;47(2):277-279.
26. Jochum T, Reinhard M, Boettger MK, Piater M, Bär KJ. Impaired cerebral autoregulation during acute alcohol withdrawal. *Drug Alcohol Depend*. 2010;110(3):240-246.
27. Jochum T, Boettger MK, Burkhardt C, Juckel G, Bär KJ. Increased pain sensitivity in alcohol withdrawal syndrome. *Eur J Pain*. 2010;14(7):713-718.
28. Loder E, Weizenbaum E, Frishberg B, Silberstein S. Choosing wisely in headache medicine: the American Headache Society's list of five things physicians and patients should question. *Headache*. 2013;53(10):1651-1659.
29. Bigal ME, Serrano D, Buse D, Scher A, Stewart WF, Lipton RB. Acute migraine medications and evolution from episodic to chronic migraine: a longitudinal population-based study. *Headache*. 2008;48(8):1157-1168.
30. Young WB, Siow HC. Should butalbital-containing analgesics be banned? *Yes. Curr Pain Headache Rep*. 2002;6(2):151-155.
31. Loder E, Biondi D. Oral phenobarbital loading: a safe and effective method of withdrawing patients with headache from butalbital compounds. *Headache*. 2003;43(8):904-909.
32. Mauskop A. Simplified butalbital withdrawal protocol. *Headache*. 2004;44(3):290-291.
33. Páll A, Becs G, Erdei A, et al. Pseudopheochromocytoma induced by anxiolytic withdrawal. *Eur J Med Res*. 2014;19(1):53.
34. Maizels M. Clonazepam for refractory headache: three cases illustrative of benefit and risk. *Headache*. 2010;50(4):650-656.
35. Shapiro RE. Caffeine and headaches. *Curr Pain Headache Rep*. 2008;12(4):311-315.
36. Schindler EA, Gottschalk CH, Weil MJ, Shapiro RE, Wright DA, Sewell RA. Indoleamine hallucinogens in cluster headache: results of the clusterbusters medication use survey. *J Psychoactive Drugs*. 2015;47(5):372-381.
37. Schindler EAD, Cooper V, Quine DB, et al. "You will eat shoe polish if you think it would help"-Familiar and lesser-known themes identified from mixed-methods analysis of a cluster headache survey. *Headache*. 2021;61(2):318-328.
38. Dhopesh V, Maany I, Herring C. The relationship of cocaine to headache in polysubstance abusers. *Headache*. 1991;31(1):17-19.
39. De Marinis M, Janiri L, Agnoli A. Headache in the use and withdrawal of opiates and other associated substances of abuse. *Headache*. 1991;31(3):159-163.
40. Costa A, Pucci E, Antonaci F, et al. The effect of intranasal cocaine and lidocaine on nitroglycerin-induced attacks in cluster headache. *Cephalalgia*. 2000;20(2):85-91.
41. Kahn DE, Ferraro N, Benveniste RJ. 3 cases of primary intracranial hemorrhage associated with "Molly", a purified form of 3,4-methylenedioxymethamphetamine (MDMA). *J Neurol Sci*. 2012;323(1-2):257-260.
42. Saengjaroentham C, Supornsilpchai W, Ji-Au W, Srikiatkhachorn A, Maneesri-le GS. Serotonin depletion can enhance the cerebrovascular responses induced by cortical spreading depression via the nitric oxide pathway. *Int J Neurosci*. 2015;125(2):130-139.
43. Ohta K, Mori M, Yoritaka A, Okamoto K, Kishida S. Delayed ischemic stroke associated with methamphetamine use. *J Emerg Med*. 2005;28(2):165-167.
44. Lee GY, Gong GW, Vrodos N, Brophy BP. 'Ecstasy'-induced subarachnoid haemorrhage: an under-reported neurological complication? *J Clin Neurosci*. 2003;10(6):705-707.
45. Cantu C, Arauz A, Murillo-Bonilla LM, López M, Barinagarrementeria F. Stroke associated with sympathomimetics contained in over-the-counter cough and cold drugs. *Stroke*. 2003;34(7):1667-1672.
46. Graham J, Coghill D. Adverse effects of pharmacotherapies for attention-deficit hyperactivity disorder: epidemiology, prevention and management. *CNS Drugs*. 2008;22(3):213-237.
47. Pozzi M, Roccatagliata D, Sterzi R. Drug abuse and intracranial hemorrhage. *Neurol Sci*. 2008;29(Suppl 2):S269-S270.
48. Taylor FR. Tobacco, Nicotine, and Headache. *Headache*. 2015;55(7):1028-1044.
49. Rozen TD. Cluster headache clinical phenotypes: tobacco nonexposed (never smoker and no parental secondary smoke exposure as a child) versus tobacco-exposed: results from the United States Cluster Headache Survey. *Headache*. 2018;58(5):688-699.
50. Ferrari A, Zappaterra M, Righi F, et al. Impact of continuing or quitting smoking on episodic cluster headache: a pilot survey. *J Headache Pain*. 2013;14(1):48.
51. Levi R, Edman GV, Ekbom K, Waldenlind E. Episodic cluster headache. II: high tobacco and alcohol consumption in males. *Headache*. 1992;32(4):184-187.
52. Backx AP, Haane DY, De Ceuster L, Koehler PJ. Cluster headache and oxygen: is it possible to predict which patients will be relieved? A retrospective cross-sectional correlation study. *J Neurol*. 2010;257(9):1533-1542.
53. Rozen TD, Fishman RS. Inhaled oxygen and cluster headache sufferers in the united states: use, efficacy and economics: results from the United States Cluster Headache Survey. *Headache*. 2011;51(2):191-200.
54. Gupta VK. Antimigraine action of nicotine: theoretical basis and potential clinical application. *Eur J Emerg Med*. 2007;14(4):243-244.
55. De Felice M, Porreca F. Opiate-induced persistent pronociceptive trigeminal neural adaptations: potential relevance to opiate-induced medication overuse headache. *Cephalalgia*. 2009;29(12):1277-1284.
56. Levin M. Opioids in headache. *Headache*. 2014;54(1):12-21.
57. Diot C, Eiden C, Leglise Y, Donnadieu-Rigole H, Peyrière H. Role of methadone in induction and/or exacerbation of cluster headache in patients treated for opioid addiction. *Therapie*. 2015;70(3):305-307.
58. Winocur E, Gavish A, Volfin G, Halachmi M, Gazit E. Oral motor parafunctions among heavy drug addicts and their effects on signs and symptoms of temporomandibular disorders. *J Orofac Pain*. 2001;15(1):56-63.
59. Orr SL, Friedman BW, Christie S, et al. Management of adults with acute migraine in the emergency department: The American Headache Society evidence assessment of parenteral pharmacotherapies. *Headache*. 2016;56(6):911-940.
60. Mazer-Amirshahi M, Dewey K, Mullins PM, et al. Trends in opioid analgesic use for headaches in U.S. emergency departments. *Am J Emerg Med*. 2014;32(9):1068-1073.
61. Young N, Silverman D, Bradford H, Finkelstein J. Multicenter prevalence of opioid medication use as abortive therapy in the ED treatment of migraine headaches. *Am J Emerg Med*. 2017;35(12):1845-1849.
62. Nicolodi M. Differential sensitivity to morphine challenge in migraine sufferers and headache-exempt subjects. *Cephalalgia*. 1996;16(5):297-304.
63. Johnson MW, Sewell RA, Griffiths RR. Psilocybin dose-dependently causes delayed, transient headaches in healthy volunteers. *Drug Alcohol Depend*. 2012;123(1-3):132-140.
64. van Amsterdam J, Opperhuizen A, van den Brink W. Harm potential of magic mushroom use: a review. *Regul Toxicol Pharmacol*. 2011;59(3):423-429.

65. Schindler EAD, Sewell RA, Gottschalk CH, et al. Exploratory controlled study of the migraine-suppressing effects of psilocybin. *Neurotherapeutics*. 2021;18(1):534-543.
66. Baron EP. Comprehensive review of medicinal marijuana, cannabinoids, and therapeutic implications in medicine and headache: what a long strange trip it's been .... *Headache*. 2015;55(6):885-916.
67. ClinicalTrials.gov. Accessed May 22, 2022. https://clinicaltrials.gov/ct2/results?cond=Migraine&term=cannabinoid&cntry=&state=&city=&dist=
68. Leroux E, Taifas I, Valade D, Donnet A, Chagnon M, Ducros A. Use of cannabis among 139 cluster headache sufferers. *Cephalalgia*. 2013; 33(3):208-213.
69. Lodge D, Mercier MS. Ketamine and phencyclidine: the good, the bad and the unexpected. *Br J Pharmacol*. 2015;172(17):4254-4276.
70. Kaube H, Herzog J, Käufer T, Dichgans M, Diener HC. Aura in some patients with familial hemiplegic migraine can be stopped by intranasal ketamine. *Neurology*. 2000;55(1):139-141.
71. Mojica JJ, Schwenk ES, Lauritsen C, Nahas SJ. Beyond the Raskin Protocol: ketamine, lidocaine, and other therapies for refractory chronic migraine. *Curr Pain Headache Rep*. 2021;25(12):77.
72. Schmidt TP, Pennington DL, Cardoos SL, Durazzo TC, Meyerhoff DJ. Neurocognition and inhibitory control in polysubstance use disorders: comparison with alcohol use disorders and changes with abstinence. *J Clin Exp Neuropsychol*. 2017;39(1):22-34.
73. Cohen K, Weinstein A. The effects of cannabinoids on executive functions: evidence from cannabis and synthetic cannabinoids—a systematic review. *Brain Sci*. 2018;8(3):40.
74. Martin P, Adinoff B, Weingartner H, Mukherjee A, Eckardt M. Alcoholic organic brain disease: nosology and pathophysiologic mechanisms. *Prog Neuropsychopharmacol Biol Psychiatry*. 1986;10(2):147.
75. Victor M, Adams R, Collins G. *The Wernicke-Korsakoff Syndrome*. 2nd ed. FA Davis; 1989.
76. Antunez E, Estruch R, Cardenal C, Nicolas J, Fernandez-Sola J, Urbano-Marquez A. Usefulness of CT and MR imaging in the diagnosis of acute Wernicke's encephalopathy. *AJR Am J Roentgenol*. 1998;171(4):1131.
77. Serdau M, Hausser-Hauw C, Laplane D. The clinical spectrum of alcoholic pellagra encephalopathy. *Brain*. 1988;111:829-842.
78. Ropper A, Brown R. Diseases of the nervous system caused by nutritional deficiency. In: Ropper AH, Samuels MA, eds. *Adams and Victor's Principles of Neurology*. 9th ed. McGraw Hill; 2009: ch 41.
79. Brust J. Ethanol. In: Spencer PS, Schaumberg HH, eds. *Experimental and Clinical Neurotoxicology*. 2nd ed. Oxford University Press; 2000:541-557.
80. Carlen P, Wortzman G, Holgate R, Wilkinson D, Rankin J. Reversible cerebral atrophy in recently abstinent chronic alcoholics measured by computed tomography scans. *Science*. 1978;200(4345):1076-1078.
81. Schweinsburg B, Taylor M, Alhassoon O, et al. Clinical pathology in brain white matter of recently detoxified alcoholics: a 1-H magnetic spectroscopy investigation of alcohol associated frontal lobe injury. *Alcohol Clin Exp Res*. 2001;25:924-934.
82. Brun A, Anderson J. Frontal dysfunction and frontal cortical synapse loss in alcoholism—the main cause of alcohol dementia. *Dement Geriatr Cogn Disord*. 2001;12:289-294.
83. Topiwala A, Allan CL, Valkanova V, et al. Moderate alcohol consumption as risk factor for adverse brain outcomes and cognitive decline: longitudinal cohort study. *BMJ*. 2017;357:j2353.
84. File S, Mabbutt P. Long-lasting effects on habituation and passive avoidance performance of a period of chronic ethanol administration in the rat. *Behav Brain Res*. 1990;36:171-178.
85. Mukamal K, Kuller L, Fitzpatrick A, et al. Prospective study of alcohol consumption and risk of dementia in older adults. *JAMA*. 2003;289: 1405-1413.
86. Brust J. Wine, flavanoids, and the "water of life". *Neurology*. 2002;59: 1300-1301.
87. Maytal J, Shinnar S. Barbiturates. In: Spencer PS, Schaumberg HH, eds. *Experimental and Clinical Neurotoxicology*. 2nd ed. Oxford University Press; 2000:219-225.
88. Vermeeren A, AML C. Chapter 5 - Effects of the use of hypnotics on cognition. In: HPA VD, Kerkhof GA, eds. *Progress in Brain Research*. Elsevier; 2011:89-103.
89. Curran HV. Effects of anxiolytics on memory. *Hum Psychopharmacol*. 1999;14(S1):S72-S79. doi:10.1002/(SICI)1099-1077(199908)14:1
90. Stewart S. The effects of benzodiazepines on cognition. *J Clin Psychiatry*. 2005;66(Suppl 2):9-13.
91. Wood S, Sage JR, Shuman T, Anagnostaras SG. Psychostimulants and cognition: a continuum of behavioral and cognitive activation. *Pharmacol Rev*. 2014;66(1):193-221.
92. Madoz-Gúrpide A, Blasco-Fontecilla H, Baca-García E, Ochoa-Mangado E. Executive dysfunction in chronic cocaine users: an exploratory study. *Drug Alcohol Depend*. 2011;117(1):55-58.
93. Ersche K, Barnes A, Jones P, Morein-Zamir S, Robbins T, Bullmore E. Abnormal structure of frontostriatal brain systems is associated with aspects of impulsivity and compulsivity in cocaine dependence. *Brain*. 2011;134(7):2013-2024.
94. Lim K, Choi S, Pomara N, et al. Reduced frontal white matter integrity in cocaine dependence: a controlled diffusion tensor imaging study. *Biol Psychiatry*. 2002;51:890-895.
95. Chang LAD, Ernst T, Volkow N. Structural and metabolic brain changes in the striatum associated with methamphetamine abuse. *Addiction*. 2007;102(Suppl 1):16-32.
96. London ED, Berman SM, Voytek B, et al. Cerebral metabolic dysfunction and impaired vigilance in recently abstinent methamphetamine abusers. *Biol Psychiatry*. 2005;58:770-778.
97. Reneman L, de Win MML, van den Brink W, Booij J, den Heeten GJ. Neuroimaging findings with MDMA/ecstasy: technical aspects, conceptual issues and future prospects. *J Psychopharmacol*. 2006;20: 164-175.
98. Erritzoe D, Frokjaer V, Holst K, et al. In vivo imaging of cerebral serotonintransporter and serotonin (2A) receptor binding in 3,4-methylenedioxymethamphetamine (MDMA or 'ecstasy') and hallucinogen users. *Arch Gen Psychiatry*. 2011;68:562-576.
99. Hollander BD, Schouw M, Groot P, et al. Preliminary evidence of hippocampal damage in chronic users of ecstasy. *J Neurol Neurosurg Psychiatry*. 2011;83:83-85.
100. Capela J, Araújo S, Costa V, et al. The neurotoxicity of hallucinogenic amphetamines in primary cultures of hippocampal neurons. *Neurotoxicology*. 2013;34:254-263.
101. Murphy P, Bruno R, Ryland I, et al. The effects of 'ecstasy' (MDMA) on visuospatial memory performance: findings from a systematic review with meta-analyses. *Hum Psychopharmacol*. 2012;27(2):113-138.
102. Parrott A. MDMA in humans: factors which affect the neuro-psychobiological profiles of recreational ecstasy users, the integrative role of bio-energetic stress. *J Psychopharmacol*. 2006;20:147-163.
103. Laws K, Kokkalis J. Ecstasy (MDMA) and memory function: a meta-analytic update. *Hum Psychopharmacol*. 2007;22(6):318-388.
104. Meier MH, Caspi A, Ambler A, et al. Persistent cannabis users show neuropsychological decline from childhood to midlife. *Proc Natl Acad Sci U S A*. 2012;109(40):E2657-E2664.
105. Verdejo-Garcia A, Rivas-Perez C, Lopez-Torrecillas F, Perez-Garcia M. Differential impact of severity of drug use on frontal behavioral symptoms. *Addict Behav*. 2006;31(8):1373-1382.
106. Crean RD, Crane NA, Mason BJ. An evidence based review of acute and long-term effects of cannabis use on executive cognitive functions. *J Addict Med*. 2011;5(1):1-8.
107. Lisdahl KM, Gilbart ER, Wright NE, Shollenbarger S. Dare to delay? the impacts of adolescent alcohol and marijuana use onset on cognition, brain structure, and function. *Front Psychiatry*. 2013;4:53.
108. Lisdahl KW, Wright NE, Medina-Kirchner C, Maple KE, Shollenbarger S. Considering cannabis: the effects of regular cannabis use on neurocognition in adolescents and young adults. *Curr Addict Rep*. 2014;1(2):144-156.
109. Tapert SF, Granholm E, Leedy NG, Brown SA. Substance use and withdrawal: neuropsychological functioning over 8 years in youth. *J Int Neuropsychol Soc*. 2002;8(7):873-883.
110. Volkow ND, Swanson JM, Evins AE, et al. Effects of cannabis use on human behavior, including cognition, motivation, and psychosis: a review. *JAMA Psychiatry*. 2016;73(3):292-297. doi:10.1001/jamapsychiatry.2015.3278

111. Volkow ND, Baler RD, Compton WM, Weiss SRB. Adverse health effects of marijuana use. *N Engl J Med*. 2014;370(23):2219-2227.
112. Brust J. Cognition and cannabis: from anecdote to advanced technology. *Brain*. 2012;135(7):2004-2005.
113. Zalesky A, Solowij N, Yucel M, et al. Effect of long-term cannabis on axonal fibre connectivity. *Brain*. 2012;135(7):2245-2255.
114. Lorenzetti V, Alonso-Lana S, Youssef GJ, et al. Adolescent cannabis use: what is the evidence for functional brain alteration? *Curr Pharm Des*. 2016;22(42):6353-6365.
115. Linszen D, van Amelsvoort T. Cannabis and psychosis: an update on course and biological plausible mechanisms. *Curr Opin Psychiatry*. 2007;20:116-120.
116. Bec PL, Fatseas M, Denis C, Lavie E, Auriacombe M. Cannabis and psychosis: search for a causal link through a critical and systematic review. *Encephale*. 2009;35(377-385):377.
117. Fernandez-Espejo E, Viveros MP, Núñez L, Ellenbroek BA, de Fonseca FR. Role of cannabis and endocannabinoids in the genesis of schizophrenia. *Psychopharmacology*. 2009;206:531-549.
118. Morrison PD, Zois V, McKeown DA, et al. The acute effects of synthetic intravenous Delta9-tetrahydrocannabinol on psychosis, mood and cognitive functioning. *Psychol Med*. 2009;39(10):1607-1616.
119. Fauman B, Aldinger G, Fauman M. Psychiatric sequelae of phencyclidine abuse. *Clin Toxicol*. 1976;9:529-538.
120. Filley C, Heaton R, Rosenberg N. White matter dementia in chronic toluene abuse. *Neurology*. 1990;40:532-534.
121. Valpey R, Sumi S, Copass M, et al. Acute and chronic progressive encephalopathy due to gasoline sniffing. *Neurology*. 1978;28:507-510.
122. Earnest M. Seizures. *Neurologic Clinics*. 1993;11:563-575.
123. Alldredge BK, Lowenstein DH, Simon RP. Seizures associated with recreational drug abuse. *Neurology*. 1989;39(8):1037. doi:10.1212/wnl.39.8.1037
124. Annegers J, Hauser W, Lee J, Rocca WA. Incidence of acute symptomatic seizures in Rochester, Minnesota, 1935-1984. *Epilepsia*. 1995;36: 327-333.
125. Upadhyay J, Maleki N, Potter J, et al. Alterations in brain structure and functional connectivity in prescription opioid-dependent patients. *Brain*. 2010;133(7):2098-2114.
126. Carhart-Harris R, Erritzoe D, Williams T, et al. Neural correlates of the psychedelic state as determined by fMRI studies with psilocybin. *Proc Natl Acad Sci U S A*. 2012;109(6):2138-2143.
127. Dos Santos RG, Osorio FL, Crippa JA, Hallak JE. Classical hallucinogens and neuroimaging: a systematic review of human studies: hallucinogens and neuroimaging. *Neurosci Biobehav Rev*. 2016;71:715-728. doi:10.1016/j.neubiorev.2016.10.026
128. Devinsky OHG, Patin J. Clozapine-related seizures. *Neurology*. 1991;41:369-371.
129. Rathlev N, Ulrich A, Shieh T, Callum MG, Bernstein E, D'Onofrio G. Etiology and weekly occurrence of alcohol-related seizures. *Acad Emerg Med*. 2002;9:824-828.
130. Lechtenberg R, Worner T. Seizure risk with recurrent alcohol detoxification. *Arch Neurol*. 1990;47:535-538.
131. Zhu PJ, Lovinger DM. Ethanol potentiates GABAergic synaptic transmission in a postsynaptic neuron/synaptic bouton preparation from basolateral amygdala. *J Neurophysiol*. 2006;96(1):433-441.
132. Hauser W, Ng S, Brust J. Alcohol, seizures, and epilepsy. *Epilepsia*. 1988;29(Suppl 2):S66-S78.
133. Bråthen G, Ben-Menachem E, Brodtkorb E, et al. EFNS guideline on the diagnosis and management of alcohol-related seizures: report of an EFNS task force. *Eur J Neurol*. 2005;12:575-581.
134. Ng S, Hauser W, Brust J, Susser M. Alcohol consumption and withdrawal in new-onset seizures. *N Engl J Med*. 1988;319:666-673.
135. Hughes J. Alcohol withdrawal seizures. *Epilepsy Behav*. 2009;15:92-97.
136. Alldredge B, Lowenstein D, Simon R. A placebo-controlled trial of intravenous diphenylhydantoin for the short-term treatment of alcohol withdrawal seizures. *Am J Med*. 1989;87:645-648.
137. Hillbom M, Tokola R, Kuusela V, et al. Prevention of alcohol withdrawal seizures with carbamazepine and valproic acid. *Alcohol*. 1989;6(3): 223-226.
138. D'Onofrio G, Rathlev N, Ulrich A, et al. Lorazepam for the prevention of recurrent alcohol withdrawal seizures. *Annals of Emergency Medicine*. 1994;23:513-518.
139. Fisch B, Hauser W, JCM JB, et al. The EEG response to diffuse and patterned photic stimulation during acute untreated alcohol withdrawal. *Neurology*. 1989;39:434-436.
140. Sordo L, Indave BI, Degenhardt L, et al. A systematic review of evidence on the association between cocaine use and seizures. *Drug Alcohol Depend*. 2013;133(3):795-804.
141. Fouilladieu JL, D'Engert J, Conseiller C. Benzodiazepines. *N Engl J Med*. 1984;310:464.
142. Mancuso CE, Tanzi MG, Gabay M. Paradoxical reactions to benzodiazepines: literature review and treatment options. *Pharmacotherapy*. 2004;24(9):1177-1185.
143. Fraser H, Wikler A, Essig C, Isbell H. Degree of physical dependence induced by secobarbital or pentobarbital. *JAMA*. 1958;166:126-129.
144. Majlesi N, Shih R, Fiesseler FW, Hung O, Debellonia R. Cocaine-associated seizures and incidence of status epilepticus. *West J Emerg Med*. 2010;11(2):157-160.
145. Karler R, Petty C, Calder L, Turkanis SA. Proconvulsant and anticonvulsant effects in mice of acute and chronic treatment with cocaine. *Neuropharmacology*. 1989;28:709-714.
146. Konkol R, Erickson B, Doerr J, Hoffman RG, Madden JA. Seizures induced by the cocaine metabolite benzoylecgonine in rats. *Epilepsia*. 1992;33:420-427.
147. Chaney N, Franke J, Wadington W. Cocaine convulsions in a breast-feeding baby. *J Pediatr*. 1988;112:134-135.
148. Bateman D, Heagarty M. Passive freebase cocaine ("crack") inhalation by infants and toddlers. *Am J Dis Child*. 1989;143:25-27.
149. Matthai S, Davidson D, Sills J, Alexandrou D. Cerebral oedema after ingestion of MDMA ("ecstasy") and unrestricted intake of water. *BMJ*. 1996;312:1359.
150. Brvar M, Kozelj G, Osredkar J, Mozina M, Gricar M, Bunc M. Polydipsia as another mechanism of hyponatremia after 'ecstasy' (3,4 methyldioxymethamphetamine) ingestion. *Eur J Emerg Med*. 2004;11:302-304.
151. Pascual-Leone A, Dhuna A, Altafullah I, Anderson DC. Cocaine-induced seizures. *Neurology*. 1990;40:404-407.
152. Ng SK, Brust JC, Hauser WA, Susser M. Illicit drug use and the risk of new-onset seizures. *Am J Epidemiol*. 1990;132(1):47-57.
153. Epilepsy Foundation. *Medical Marijuana*. Accessed October 6, 2017. https://www.epilepsy.com/learn/treating-seizures-and-epilepsy/other-treatment-approaches/medical-marijuana-and-epilepsy
154. Hershey L. Meperidine and central neurotoxicity. *Ann Intern Med*. 1983;98:548-549.
155. Kaiko RF, Foley KM, Grabinski PY, et al. Central nervous system excitatory effects of meperidine in cancer patients. *Ann Neurol*. 1983;13(2):180-185.
156. Caplan L, Thomas C, Banks G. Central nervous system complications of addiction to "T's and blues." *Neurology*. 1982;32:623-628.
157. Kahn LH, Alderfer RJ, Graham DJ. Seizures reported with tramadol. *JAMA*. 1997;278(20):1661.
158. Devinsky O, Cross JH, Laux L, et al. Trial of cannabidiol for drug-resistant seizures in the Dravet Syndrome. *N Engl J Med*. 2017;376(21):2011-2020.
159. Consroe P, Laguna J, Allender J, et al. Controlled clinical trial of cannabidiol in Huntington's disease. *Pharmacol Biochem Behav*. 1991;40(3):701-708.
160. Koppel BS, Brust JCM, Fife T, et al. Systematic review: efficacy and safety of medical marijuana in selected neurologic disorders. Report of the Guideline Development Subcommittee of the American Academy of Neurology. *Neurology*. 2014;82(17):1556-1563.
161. Kolikonda MK, Srinivasan K, Enja M, Sagi V, Lippmann S. Medical marijuana for epilepsy? *Innov Clin Neurosci*. 2016;13(3-4):23-26.
162. McCarron MM, Schultze BW, Thompson GA, Conder MC, Goetz WA. Acute phencyclidine intoxication: incidence of clinical findings in 1,000 cases. *Ann Emerg Med*. 1981;10:237-242.
163. Fisher D, Ungerleider J. Grand mal seizures following ingestion of LSD. *Calif Med*. 1967;106:210-211.

164. Morton H. Occurrence and treatment of solvent abuse in children and adolescents. *Pharmacol Ther.* 1987;33:449-469.
165. Mikolich J, Paulson G, Cross C. Acute anticholinergic syndrome due to jimson seed ingestion. *Ann Intern Med.* 1975;83:321-325.
166. Hoaken P. Adverse effects of methaqualone. *Can Med Assoc J.* 1975;112:685.
167. Snead III OS, Gibson KM. Gamma-hydroxybutyric acid. *N Engl J Med.* 2005;352:2721-2732.
168. Tsao CW, Aday AW, Almarzooq ZI, et al. Heart disease and stroke statistics–2022 update: a report from the American Heart Association. *Circulation.* 2022;145(8):e153-e639.
169. Burke JF, Lisabeth LD, Brown DL, Reeves MJ, Morgenstern LB. Determining stroke's rank as a cause of death using multicause mortality data. *Stroke.* 2012;43(8):2207-2211. doi:10.1161/strokeaha.112.656967
170. Kleindorfer DO, Towfighi A, Chaturvedi S, et al. 2021 Guideline for the prevention of stroke in patients with stroke and transient ischemic attack: a guideline From the American Heart Association/American Stroke Association. *Stroke.* 2021;52(7):e364-e467.
171. Feigin VL, Stark BA, Johnson CO, et al. Global, regional, and national burden of stroke and its risk factors;2019: a systematic analysis for the Global Burden of Disease Study 2019. *Lancet Neurol.* 2021;20(10): 795-820.
172. Jaffre A, Ruidavets JB, Nasr N, Guidolin B, Ferrieres J, Larrue V. Tobacco use and cryptogenic stroke in young adults. *J Stroke Cerebrovasc Dis.* 2015;24(12):2694-2700.
173. Kurth T, Kase CS, Berger K, Schaeffner ES, Buring JE, Gaziano JM. Smoking and the risk of hemorrhagic stroke in men. *Stroke.* 2003;34(5):1151-1155.
174. Asplund K. Smokeless tobacco and cardiovascular disease. *Prog Cardiovasc Dis.* 2003;45(5):383-394.
175. Vidyasagaran AL, Siddiqi K, Kanaan M. Use of smokeless tobacco and risk of cardiovascular disease: A systematic review and meta-analysis. *Eur J Prev Cardiol.* 2016;23(18):1970-1981.
176. Sico JJ, Chang C-CH, So-Armah K, et al. HIV status and the risk of ischemic stroke among men. *Neurology.* 2015;84(19):1933-1940.
177. Sultan S, Elkind MS. The growing problem of stroke among young adults. *Curr Cardiol Rep.* 2013;15(12):421. doi:10.1007/s11886-013-0421-z
178. Kalani R, Liotta EM, Prabhakaran S. Diagnostic yield of universal urine toxicology screening in an unselected cohort of stroke patients. *PLoS One.* 2015;10(12):e0144772.
179. Meschia JF, Bushnell C, Boden-Albala B, et al. Guidelines for the primary prevention of stroke. a statement for healthcare professionals from the American Heart Association/American Stroke Association. *Stroke.* 2014;45(12):3754-3832.
180. Mishra A, Chaturvedi P, Datta S, Sinukumar S, Joshi P, Garg A. Harmful effects of nicotine. *Indian J Med Paediatr Oncol.* 2015;36(1):24-31.
181. Lai MC, Chou FS, Yang YJ, Wang CC, Lee MC. Tobacco use and environmental smoke exposure among Taiwanese pregnant smokers and recent quitters: risk perception, attitude, and avoidance behavior. *Int J Environ Res Public Health.* 2013;10(9):4104-4116.
182. Gagne JJ, Bykov K, Choudhry NK, Toomey TJ, Connolly JG, Avorn J. Effect of smoking on comparative efficacy of antiplatelet agents: systematic review, meta-analysis, and indirect comparison. *BMJ.* 2013;347:f5307.
183. Parekh T, Pemmasani S, Desai R. Risk of stroke with e-cigarette and combustible cigarette use in young adults. *Am J Prev Med.* 2020;58(3):446-452.
184. Fernandez-Sola J. Cardiovascular risks and benefits of moderate and heavy alcohol consumption. *Nat Rev Cardiol.* 2015;12(10):576-587.
185. Patra J, Taylor B, Irving H, et al. Alcohol consumption and the risk of morbidity and mortality for different stroke types - a systematic review and meta-analysis. *BMC Public Health.* 2010;10(1):258.
186. Sacco RL, Elkind M, Boden-Albala B. The protective effect of moderate alcohol consumption on ischemic stroke. *JAMA.* 1999;281(1):53-60.
187. Reynolds K, Lewis B, Nolen JD, Kinney GL, Sathya B, He J. Alcohol consumption and risk of stroke: a meta-analysis. *JAMA.* 2003;289(5): 579-588.
188. Ricci C, Wood A, Muller D, et al. Alcohol intake in relation to non-fatal and fatal coronary heart disease and stroke: EPIC-CVD case-cohort study. *BMJ.* 2018;361:k934.
189. Larsson SC, Wallin A, Wolk A, Markus HS. Differing association of alcohol consumption with different stroke types: a systematic review and meta-analysis. *BMC Medicine.* 2016;14(1):178.
190. Brust JCM, Richter RW. Stroke associated with cocaine abuse? *N Y State J Med.* 1977;77:1473-1475.
191. Levine SR, Brust JC, Futrell N, et al. Cerebrovascular complications of the use of the "crack" form of alkaloidal cocaine. *N Engl J Med.* 1990;323(11):699-704.
192. Saez CG, Olivares P, Pallavicini J, et al. Increased number of circulating endothelial cells and plasma markers of endothelial damage in chronic cocaine users. *Thromb Res.* 2011;128(4):e18-e23.
193. Johnson BA, Devous MD, Ruiz P, Ait-Daoud N. Treatment advances for cocaine-induced ischemic stroke: focus on dihydropyridine-class calcium channel antagonists. *Am J Psychiatry.* 2001;158(8):1191-1198.
194. Larsson SC, Drca N, Wolk A. Alcohol consumption and risk of atrial fibrillation: a prospective study and dose-response meta-analysis. *J Am Coll Cardiol.* 2014;64(3):281-289.
195. Zhang C, Wang X, Wang Y, et al. Risk factors for post-stroke seizures: a systematic review and meta-analysis. *Epilepsy Res.* 2014;108(10): 1806-1816.
196. Matz K, Seyfang L, Dachenhausen A, et al. Post-stroke pneumonia at the stroke unit - a registry based analysis of contributing and protective factors. *BMC Neurol.* 2016;16:107.
197. Gattringer T, Enzinger C, Fischer R, et al. IV thrombolysis in patients with ischemic stroke and alcohol abuse. *Neurology.* 2015;85(18):1592-1597.
198. Sordo L, Indave BI, Barrio G, Degenhardt L, de la Fuente L, Bravo MJ. Cocaine use and risk of stroke: a systematic review. *Drug Alcohol Depend.* 2014;142:1-13.
199. Toossi S, Hess CP, Hills NK, Josephson SA. Neurovascular complications of cocaine use at a tertiary stroke center. *J Stroke Cerebrovasc Dis.* 2010;19(4):273-278.
200. Mizutani T, Lewis R, Gonatas N. Medial medullary syndrome in a drug user. *Arch Neurol.* 1980;37:425-428.
201. Brust JCM. Stroke and substance abuse. In: Caplan LR, ed. *Uncommon Causes of Stroke.* 2nd ed. Cambridge University Press; 2008:365-369.
202. Westover A, Halm E. Do prescription stimulants increase the risk of adverse cardiovascular events?: a systematic review. *BMC Cardiovasular Disorders.* 2012;12(1):41-50.
203. Keegan A. Cocaine plus alcohol, a deadly mix. *NIDA Notes.* 1991;6:18-19.
204. Kaufman MJ, Levin JM, Ross MH, et al. Cocaine-induced cerebral vasoconstriction detected in humans with magnetic resonance angiography. *JAMA.* 1998;279(5):376-380.
205. Brust JCM. Stroke and substance abuse. In: Mohr J, ed. *Stroke: Pathophysiology, Diagnosis, and Management.* 5th ed. Elsevier Saunders; 2011.
206. Krendel DA, Ditter SM, Frankel MR, Ross WK. Biopsy-proven cerebral vasculitis associated with cocaine abuse. *Neurology.* 1990;40(7): 1092-1094.
207. Egred M, Davis GK. Cocaine and the heart. *Postgrad Med J.* 2005;81(959):568-571.
208. Ohga ENT, Tomita T, et al. Increased levels of circulating I-CAM-1, VCAM-1, and L-selectin in obstructive sleep apnea syndrome. *J Appl Physiol.* 1999;87:10-14.
209. Kernan WN, Viscoli CM, Brass LM, et al. Phenylpropanolamine and the risk of hemorrhagic stroke. *N Engl J Med.* 2000;343(25):1826-1832.
210. Morgenstern LB, Viscoli CM, Kernan WN, et al. Use of ephedra-containing products and risk for hemorrhagic stroke. *Neurology.* 2003;60(1):132-135.
211. Volkow ND, Wang G-J, Fowler JS, et al. Cardiovascular effects of methylphenidate in humans areassociated with increases of dopamine in brain and of epinephrine in plasma. *Psychopharmacology (Berl).* 2003;166:264-270.
212. Westover AN, McBride S, Haley RW. Stroke in young adults who abuse amphetamines or cocaine: A population-based study of hospitalized patients. *Arch Gen Psychiatry.* 2007;64(4):495-502.

213. Petitti DB, Sidney S, Quesenberry C, Bernstein A. Stroke and cocaine or amphetamine use. *Epidemiology*. 1998;9(6):596-600.
214. Trugman J. Cerebral arteritis and oral methylphenidate. *Lancet*. 1988;1:584-585.
215. Schteinschnaider A, Plaghos LL, Garbugino S, et al. Cerebral arteritis following methylphenidate use. *J Child Neurol*. 2000;15:265-267.
216. Citron BP, Halpern M, McCarron M, et al. Necrotizing angiitis associated with drug abuse. *N Engl J Med*. 1970;283(19):1003-1011.
217. Rumbaugh C, Fang H, Higgins R, Bergeron R, Segall H, Teal J. Cerebral microvascular injury in experimental drug abuse. *Invest Radiol*. 1976;11(4):282.
218. Schifano F, Oyefeso A, Webb L, Pollard M, Corkery J, Ghodse AH. Review of deaths related to taking ecstasy, England and Wales, 1997-2000. *BMJ*. 2003;326(7380):80-81.
219. Kumar N, Bhalla MC, Frey JA, Southern A. Intraparenchymal hemorrhage after heroin use. *Am J Emerg Med*. 2015;33(8):1109.e3-4.
220. Benoilid A, Collongues N, de Seze J, Blanc F. Heroin inhalation-induced unilateral complete hippocampal stroke. *Neurocase*. 2013;19(4):313-315.
221. Caplan L, Thomas C, Banks G. Stroke and drug abuse. *Stroke*. 1982;13:869-872.
222. Bolz J, Meves SH, Kara K, Reinacher-Schick A, Gold R, Krogias C. Multiple cerebral infarctions in a young patient with heroin-induced hypereosinophilic syndrome. *J Neurol Sci*. 2015;356(1-2):193-195.
223. Brust JCM, Richter RW. Stroke associated with addiction to heroin. *J Neurol Neurosurg Psychiatry*. 1976;39:194-199.
224. Wolff V, Armspach J-P, Lauer V, et al. Cannabis-related stroke: myth or reality? *Stroke*. 2013;44(2):558-563.
225. Calabrese LH, Dodick DW, Schwedt TJ, Singhal AB. Narrative review: reversible cerebral vasoconstriction syndromes. *Ann Intern Med*. 2007;146(1):34-44. doi:10.7326/0003-4819-146-1-200701020-00007
226. Mellion M, Gilchrist JM, de la Monte S. Alcohol-related peripheral neuropathy: nutritional, toxic, or both? *Muscle Nerve*. 2011;43(3):309-316.
227. Barber PA, Pridmore HM, Krishnamurthy V, et al. Cannabis, ischemic stroke, and transient ischemic attack: a case-control study. *Stroke*. 2013;44(8):2327-2329.
228. Moeller S, Lücke C, Struffert T, et al. Ischemic stroke associated with the use of a synthetic cannabinoid (spice). *Asian J Psychiatr*. 2017;25:127-130.
229. Raheemullah A, Laurence TN. Repeated thrombosis after synthetic cannabinoid use. *J Emerg Med*. 2016;51(5):540-543.
230. Preedy VR, Ohlendieck K, Adachi J, et al. The importance of alcohol-induced muscle disease. *J Muscle Res Cell Motil*. 2003;24(1):55-63.
231. Hackam DG. Cannabis and stroke: systematic appraisal of case reports. *Stroke*. 2015;46(3):852-856.
232. Dutta T, Ryan KA, Thompson O, et al. Marijuana use and the risk of early ischemic stroke. *Stroke*. 2021;52(10):3184-3190.
233. Sobel J, Espinaso O, Friedman S. Carotid artery obstruction following LSD capsule injection. *Arch Intern Med*. 1971;5:213-215.
234. Shimada Y, Yoritaka A, Tanaka Y, et al. Cerebral infarction in a young man using high-dose anabolic steroids. *J Stroke Cerebrovasc Dis*. 2012; 21(8):906.e9-11.
235. Shamloul RM, Aborayah AF, Hashad A, Abd-Allah F. Anabolic steroids abuse-induced cardiomyopathy and ischaemic stroke in a young male patient. *BMJ Case Rep*. 2014;2014:bcr2013203033.
236. Angell P, Chester N, Green D, Somauroo J, Whyte G, George K. Anabolic steroids and cardiovascular risk. *Sports Med*. 2012;42(2):119-134. doi:10.2165/11598060-000000000-00000
237. Youssef MYZ, Alqallaf A, Abdella N. Anabolic androgenic steroid-induced cardiomyopathy, stroke and peripheral vascular disease. *BMJ Case Rep*. 2011;2011:bcr1220103650.
238. Julian T, Glascow N, Syeed R, Zis P. Alcohol-related peripheral neuropathy: a systematic review and meta-analysis. *J Neurol*. 2019;266(12):2907-2919.
239. Goforth HW, Fernandez F. Acute neurologic effects of alcohol and drugs. *Neurol Clin*. 2012;30(1):277-284. ix.
240. Ammendola A, Tata MR, Aurilio C, et al. Peripheral neuropathy in chronic alcoholism: a retrospective cross-sectional study in 76 subjects. *Alcohol Alcohol*. 2001;36(3):271-275.
241. Pascuzzi RM. Drugs and toxins associated with myopathies. *Curr Opin Rheumatol*. 1998;10(6):511-520.
242. Urbano-Marquez A, Fernandez-Sola J. Effects of alcohol on skeletal and cardiac muscle. *Muscle Nerve*. 2004;30(6):689-707.
243. Smith W, Wilson AF. Guillain-barré syndrome in heroin addiction. *JAMA*. 1975;231(13):1367-1368.
244. Dabby RDR, Gilad R, et al. Acute heroin-related neuropathy. *J Peripher Nerv Syst*. 2006;11:304-309.
245. McCreary M, Emerman C, Hanna J, Simon J. Acute myelopathy following intranasal insufflation of heroin: a case report. *Neurology*. 2000;55(2):316-317.
246. Richter RW, Pearson J, Bruun B, Challenor YB, Brust JC, Baden MM. Neurological complications of addiction to heroin. *Bull N Y Acad Med*. 1973;49(1):3-21.
247. Pastore C, Izura V, Marhuenda D, Prieto MJ, Roel J, Cardona A. Partial conduction blocks in N-hexane neuropathy. *Muscle Nerve*. 2002;26(1):132-135.
248. Misirli H, Domac FM, Somay G, Araal O, Ozer B, Adiguzel T. N-hexane induced polyneuropathy: a clinical and electrophysiological follow up. *Electromyogr Clin Neurophysiol*. 2008;48(2):103-108.
249. Shulman RM, Geraghty TJ, Tadros M. A case of unusual substance abuse causing myeloneuropathy. *Spinal Cord*. 2007;45(4):314-317.
250. Hathout L, El-Saden S. Nitrous oxide-induced B12 deficiency myelopathy: perspectives on the clinical biochemistry of vitamin B_{12}. *J Neurol Sci*. 2011;301(1-2):1-8.
251. Richards J. Rhabdomyolysis and drugs of abuse. *J Emerg Med*. 2000;19:51-56.
252. Grob D. Rhabdomyolysis and drug-related myopathies. *Curr Opin Rheumatol*. 1990;2(6):908-915.
253. Beniczky S, Tfelt-Hansen P, Fabricius M, Andersen KV. Multiple mononeuropathy following cocaine abuse. *BMJ Case Rep*. 2009;2009:bcr07.2008.0446. doi:10.1136/bcr.07.2008.0446
254. de Souza A, Desai PK, de Souza RJ. Acute multifocal neuropathy following cocaine inhalation. *J Clin Neurosci*. 2017;36:134-136.
255. Giovannoni G, O'Sullivan JD, Turner K, Manson AJ, Lees AJ. Hedonistic homeostatic dysregulation in patients with Parkinson's disease on dopamine replacement therapies. *J Neurol Neurosurg Psychiatry*. 2000;68(4):423-428.
256. Spigset O, von-Schele C. Levodopa dependence and abuse in Parkinson's disease. *Pharmacotherapy*. 1997;17(5):1027-1030.
257. Wadleigh A, Valenzuela CF. Ethanol increases GABAergic transmission and excitability in cerebellar molecular layer interneurons from GAD67-GFP knock-in mice. *Alcohol Alcohol*. 2012;47(1):1-8.
258. Jones AW, Neri A. Age-related differences in the effects of ethanol on performance and behaviour in healthy men. *Alcohol Alcohol*. 1994;29(2):171-179.
259. Brust JCM. Substance abuse and movement disorders. *Mov Disord*. 2010;25(13):2010-2020.
260. Cardoso F, Jankovic J. Movement disorders in neurologic complications of drug and alcohol abuse. *Neurol Clin*. 1993;11:625-638.
261. Cardoso FE, Jankovic J. Cocaine-related movement disorders. *Mov Disord*. 1993;8(2):175-178.
262. Shandling M, Carlen PL, Lang AE. Parkinsonism in alcohol withdrawal: a follow-up study. *Mov Disord*. 1990;5(1):36-39.
263. Koller WC, Busenbark K, Miner K. The relationship of essential tremor to other movement disorders: report on 678 patients. *Essential Tremor Study Group. Ann Neurol*. 1994;35(6):717-723.
264. Hess CW, Saunders-Pullman R. Movement disorders and alcohol misuse. *Addict Biol*. 2006;11(2):117-125.
265. Quinn NP. Essential myoclonus and myoclonic dystonia. *Mov Disord*. 1996;11(2):119-124.
266. Frucht SJ, Riboldi GM. Alcohol-responsive hyperkinetic movement disorders-a mechanistic hypothesis. *Tremor Other Hyperkinet Mov (N Y)*. 2020;10:47.
267. Wu J, Tang H, Chen S, Cao L. Mechanisms and pharmacotherapy for ethanol-responsive movement disorders. *Review. Front Neurol*. 2020;11:892.

268. Daras M, Koppel BS, Atos RE. Cocaine-induced choreoathetoid movements ('crack dancing'). *Neurology*. 1994;44(4):751-752.
269. San Luciano M. Saunders-Pullman R. Substance abuse and movement disorders. *Curr Drug Abuse Rev*. 2009;2(3):273-278.
270. Bartzokis G, Beckson M, Wirshing DA, Lu PH, Foster JA, Mintz J. Choreoathetoid movements in cocaine dependence. *Biol Psychiatry*. 1999;45(12):1630-1635.
271. Hegarty AM, Lipton RB, Merriam AE, Freeman K. Cocaine as a risk factor for acute dystonic reactions. *Neurology*. 1991;41(10):1670-1672.
272. Pascual Leone A, Dhuna A. Cocaine-associated multifocal tics. *Neurology*. 1990;40(6):999-1000.
273. Bauer LO. Resting hand tremor in abstinent cocaine-dependent, alcohol-dependent, and polydrug-dependent patients. *Alcohol Clin Exp Res*. 1996;20(7):1196-1201.
274. Büttner A. Review: The neuropathology of drug abuse. *Neuropathol Appl Neurobiol*. 2011;37(2):118-134.
275. Priori A, Bertolasi L, Berardelli A, Manfredi M. Acute dystonic reaction to ecstasy. *Mov Disord*. 1995;10(3):353-353.
276. Cosentino C. Ecstasy and acute dystonia. *Mov Disord*. 2004;19(11): 1386-1387.
277. Randrup A, Munkvad I. Stereotyped activities produced by amphetamine in several animal species and man. *Psychopharmacology*. 1967;11(4): 300-310.
278. Rylander G. Psychoses and the punding and choreiform syndromes in addiction to central stimulant drugs. *Psychiatr Neurol Neurochir*. 1972;75(3):203-212.
279. Fasano A, Barra A, Nicosia P, et al. Cocaine addiction: from habits to stereotypical-repetitive behaviors and punding. *Drug Alcohol Depend*. 2008;96(1-2):178-182.
280. Ashcroft GW, Eccleston D, Waddell JL. Recognition of amphetamine addicts. *Br Med J*. 1965;1(5426):57.
281. Sañudo-Peña MC, Patrick SL, Khen S, Patrick RL, Tsou K, Walker JM. Cannabinoid effects in basal ganglia in a rat model of Parkinson's disease. *Neurosci Lett*. 1998;248(3):171-174.
282. Venderová K, Růzicka E, Vorísek V, Visnovský P. Survey on cannabis use in Parkinson's disease: subjective improvement of motor symptoms. *Mov Disord*. 2004;19(9):1102-1106.
283. Lauterbach EC. Hiccup and apparent myoclonus after hydrocodone: review of the opiate-related hiccup and myoclonus literature. *Clin Neuropharmacol*. 1999;22(2):87-92.
284. Langston JW. Chronic Parkinsonism in humans due to a product of meperidine-analog synthesis. *Science*. 1983;219(4587):979.
285. Lopez W, Jeste DV. Movement disorders and substance abuse. *Psychiatr Serv*. 1997;48(5):634-636.
286. Buxton JA, Sebastian R, Clearsky L, et al. Chasing the dragon - characterizing cases of leukoencephalopathy associated with heroin inhalation in British Columbia. *Harm Reduct J*. 2011;8:3.
287. Kriegstein A, Shungu D, Millar W, et al. Leukoencephalopathy and raised brain lactate from heroin vapor inhalation ("chasing the dragon"). *Neurology*. 1999;53:1765-1773.
288. Bohr IJ, Ray MA, McIntosh JM, et al. Cholinergic nicotinic receptor involvement in movement disorders associated with Lewy body diseases. An autoradiography study using [(125)I]alpha-conotoxinMII in the striatum and thalamus. *Exp Neurol*. 2005;191(2): 292-300.
289. Checkoway H, Powers K, Smith-Weller T, Franklin GM, Longstreth WT Jr, Swanson PD. Parkinson's disease risks associated with cigarette smoking, alcohol consumption, and caffeine intake. *Am J Epidemiol*. 2002;155(8):732-738.
290. Ritz B, Lee P-C, Lassen CF, Arah OA. Parkinson disease and smoking revisited: Ease of quitting is an early sign of the disease. *Neurology*. 2014;83(16):1396-1402.
291. Muller-Vahl KR, Schneider U, Prevedel H, et al. Delta 9-tetrahydrocannabinol (THC) is effective in the treatment of tics in Tourette syndrome: a 6-week randomized trial. *J Clin Psychiatry*. 2003;64(4):459-465.
292. Benarroch E. Endocannabinoids in basal ganglia circuits: implications for Parkinson disease. *Neurology*. 2007;69(3):306-309.
293. Curtis A, Mitchell I, Patel S, Ives N, Rickards H. A pilot study using nabilone for symptomatic treatment in Huntington's disease. *Mov Disord*. 2009;24(15):2254-2259.
294. van Vliet SAM, Vanwersch RAP, Jongsma MJ, Olivier B, Philippens IHCHM. Therapeutic effects of Delta9-THC and modafinil in a marmoset Parkinson model. *Eur Neuropsychopharmacol*. 2008;18(5):383-389.
295. Sieradzan KA, Fox SH, Hill M, Dick JP, Crossman AR, Brotchie JM. Cannabinoids reduce levodopa-induced dyskinesia in Parkinson's disease: a pilot study. *Neurology*. 2001;57(11):2108-2111.
296. Feigal E, Murphy E, Vranizan K, et al. Human T cell lymphotropic virus types I and II in intravenous drug users in San Francisco: risk factors associated with seropositivity. *J Infect Dis*. 1991;164(1):36-42.
297. Zunt JRMS, Alarcon JO, Longstreth WT Jr, Price R, Holmes KK. Quantitative assessment of spasticity in human T-cell lymphotropic virus type I-associated myelopathy/tropical spastic paraparesis. *J Neurovirol*. 2005;11(1):70-73.
298. Chiotoroiu SM, Noaghi M, Stefaniu GI, Secureanu FA, Purcarea VL, Zemba M. Tobacco-alcohol optic neuropathy--clinical challenges in diagnosis. *J Med Life*. 2014;7(4):472-476.
299. Malouf RJG, Dobkin J, Brust JC. Neurologic disease in human immunodeficiency virus-infected drug abusers. *Arch Neurol*. 1990;47(9):1002-1007.
300. Marder K, Lu X, Stern Y, et al. Risk of human immunodeficiency virus type 1-related neurologic disease in a cohort of intravenous drug users. *Arch Neurol*. 1995;52(12):1174-1182.
301. Richter R. Infections other than AIDS. *Neurol Clin*. 1993;11:591-603.
302. Brust J, Dickinson P, Hughes J, Holtzman RN. The diagnosis and treatment of cerebral mycotic aneurysms. *Ann Neurol*. 1990;27:238-246.
303. Marantz P, Linzer M, Feiner C. Inability to predict diagnosis in febrile intravenous drug abusers. *Ann Intern Med*. 1987;106:823-828.
304. Carroll F. The etiology and treatment of tobacco-alcohol amblyopia. *Am J Ophthalmol*. 1944;27:713-725.
305. Brust JC, Richter RW. Tetanus in the inner city. *N Y State J Med*. 1974;74:1735-1742.
306. Kaushik KS, Kapila K, Praharaj AK. Shooting up: the interface of microbial infections and drug abuse. *J Med Microbiol*. 2011;60(Pt 4):408-422.
307. Afshar M, Raju M, Ansell D, Bleck TP. Narrative review: tetanus—a health threat after natural disasters in developing countries. *Ann Intern Med*. 2011;154(5):329-335.
308. Kudrow D, Henry D, Haake D, Marshall G, Mathisen GE. Botulism associated with Clostridium botulinum sinusitis after intranasal cocaine use. *Ann Intern Med*. 1988;109:984-985.
309. Merrison AFA, Chidley KE, Dunnett J, Sieradzan KA. Wound botulism associated with subcutaneous drug use. *BMJ*. 2002;325(7371):1020-1021.
310. Kalka-Moll WM, Aurbach U, Schaumann R, Schwarz R, Seifert H. Wound botulism in injection drug users. *Emerg Infect Dis*. 2007;13(6):942-943.
311. Karapetyan AF, Sokolovsky YV, Araviyskaya ER, Zvartau EE, Ostrovsky DV, Hagan H. Syphilis among intravenous drug-using population: epidemiological situation in St Petersburg, Russia. *Int J STD AIDS*. 2002;13(9):618-623.
312. Nelson KEVD, Cohn S, Odunmbaku M, Lindsay A, Antohony JC, Hook EW III Sexually transmitted diseases in population of intravenous drug users: association with seropositivity to the human immunodeficiency virus (HIV). *J Infect Dis*. 1991;164(3):457-463.
313. Marra CM. Neurosyphilis. *Continuum (Minneap Minn)*. 2015;21 (6 Neuroinfectious Disease):1714-1728.
314. Brust J, Richter R. Quinine amblyopia related to heroin addiction. *Ann Intern Med*. 1974;74:84-86.
315. Sullivan EV, Rosenbloom MJ, Deshmukh A, Desmond JE, Pfefferbaum A. Alcohol and the cerebellum: effects on balance, motor coordination, and cognition. *Alcohol Health Res World*. 1995;19(2):138-141.
316. Victor M, Adams R, Mancall E. A restricted form of cerebellar cortical degeneration occurring in alcoholic patients. *Arch Neurol*. 1959;1(6): 579-688.
317. Uchino A, Yuzuriha T, Murakami M, et al. Magnetic resonance imaging of sequelae of central pontine myelinolysis in chronic alcohol abusers. *Neuroradiology*. 2003;45:877-880.

CHAPTER

94 Human Immunodeficiency Virus, Tuberculosis, and Other Infectious Diseases Related to Substance Use

Carol A. Sulis, Ayesha Appa, and Simeon D. Kimmel

CHAPTER OUTLINE

- Introduction
- Social determinants of infectious diseases
- Host defenses
- Skin and soft tissue infections
- Gingivitis
- Endocarditis
- Noncardiac vascular infections
- Respiratory infections
- Hepatic and gastrointestinal infections
- Bone and joint infections
- Nervous system infections
- Eye infections
- Human immunodeficiency virus and acquired immunodeficiency syndrome
- Sexually transmitted diseases
- Conclusions

INTRODUCTION

Infectious diseases are common complications in patients with substance use disorders.[1,2] Skin and soft tissue infections, endocarditis, hepatitis, human immunodeficiency virus (HIV), pneumonia, and tuberculosis have been problems for people who use drugs (PWUD) for decades; COVID-19 is a relative newcomer. Infections related to substance use may occur by direct inoculation of blood-borne or environmental pathogens or risky behaviors and are often modified by dysfunctional host defenses and multiple overlapping structural vulnerabilities such as food or housing insecurity, gender discrimination, or systemic racism. While infections impact the health of PWUD, they also provide an opportunity to establish positive relationships and engage patients in substance use treatment and harm reduction services.[3,4]

This chapter focuses on common infectious complications of substance use. Standard texts and review articles should be consulted for detailed descriptions of the epidemiology, pathophysiology, clinical presentation, and management of these infectious disorders.

SOCIAL DETERMINANTS OF INFECTIOUS DISEASES

Risk for infection, addiction, and their outcomes are impacted by the social, cultural, and political environment. Poverty, homelessness, racism, and discrimination based on sexual and gender identity contribute to the risk of unhealthy substance use which in turn may increase risk of infection.[5] Co-occurring epidemics and social forces that interact with each other such as injection drug use, HIV, hepatitis C, and homelessness have been termed "syndemics."[6,7] This chapter aims to assist clinicians in the diagnosis and treatment of infections related to substance use. Clinicians and health systems must also address underlying social determinants of health to successfully treat individual patients who use substances and to combat health inequities impacting PWUD at the population level.

HOST DEFENSES

Multiple nonprescribed substances and routes of use are associated with immunocompromised states. Alcohol use can cause bone marrow suppression, malnutrition, and splenic dysfunction in patients with cirrhosis. Opioids, nicotine, cocaine, methamphetamine, and cannabis modulate the immune response in various ways. These include direct effects on innate or cellular immunity to drug-related stimulation of the hypothalamic–pituitary–adrenal axis which can alter endogenous glucocorticoid release.[8-10] The magnitude and clinical importance of these effects requires further study.

Cigarette smoking causes defective mucociliary function and predisposes to the development of sinopulmonary infections caused by encapsulated organisms such as *Streptococcus pneumoniae* or *Klebsiella pneumoniae*.[11]

Among people who inject drugs (PWID), breach of local skin and mucosal barriers by the repeated injection of nonsterile materials and colonization with resistant organisms appears to drive infection risk more than deficiencies in phagocytic function or antibody response. Repeated, nonspecific stimulation of the immune system leads to polyclonal elevation of immunoglobulin, which, in turn, can cause diagnostic confusion when caring for the patient who develops autoantibodies such as rheumatoid factor or who has a biological false-positive test for syphilis or hepatitis C.

Cell-mediated deficiencies that result from effects on T-lymphocyte function caused by infection with HIV, tuberculosis, and other intracellular pathogens are well described.[12]

SKIN AND SOFT TISSUE INFECTIONS

Skin and soft tissue infections are common among PWID and increasingly the reason for hospital admission.[13] The type of infection (cellulitis, abscess, or ulcer), its location and severity, and causative organisms are related to the duration, site, and frequency of injection, availability and adherence to harm reduction practices (hand washing, skin cleansing, use of sterile injection equipment), and local epidemiology of both infectious diseases and drug supply.[14,15] Gram-positive organisms such as *Staphylococcus aureus* and groups A, C, F, and G beta-hemolytic streptococci are most often seen.[1,16,17] Other pathogens like *Pseudomonas aeruginosa and Serratia marcescens* as well as *clostridial* and *bacillus species* (including rarely *Bacillus anthracis*) are less common.[18-21]

Methicillin-resistant *S. aureus* (MRSA) infections are common among PWID[9,22,23] and clonal lineages of MRSA can spread through injection drug networks.[24] Local antibiograms should be consulted but most isolates are sensitive to trimethoprim–sulfamethoxazole and vancomycin and many remain sensitive to doxycycline and clindamycin. Risk factors for MRSA colonization include use of alcohol, methamphetamine, injection drugs, and congregate living environments such as shelters or carceral institutions.[25] Therapy includes incision and drainage of the abscess, judicious use of appropriate antibiotics, and meticulous hygiene.[15]

PWID who mix drugs with saliva or who lick needles before injecting are particularly prone to polymicrobial infections with viridans streptococci, *Haemophilus* spp., *Eikenella corrodens*, and oral anaerobes. Infection with these organisms also occurs in bite wounds and closed-fist injuries.

Repeated injection of nonsterile, potentially vasoactive substances including opioids, stimulants, or adulterants such as xylazine can cause ischemic necrosis, rendering the damaged areas susceptible to superinfection.[26,27] Xylazine, an alpha-2 adrenergic receptor agonist approved as a veterinary sedative, is increasingly present in the drug supply and associated with skin ulcerations.[27-30] The pathophysiology and evidence for management of these ulcerations is rapidly evolving but they are at high risk for superinfection, making excellent wound care paramount.[31-33] Streptococcal infection in areas of tissue ischemia can also cause large necrotic ulcers with extensive loss of tissue. Ulcers become colonized with a mixture of environmental pathogens, so surface cultures are not useful in guiding antibiotic selection.

Most patients with cellulitis have local pain, redness, warmth, and swelling or induration of the skin. Patients who delay seeking medical care because of fear of stigma, untreated substance withdrawal, or untreated pain can develop extensive cellulitis, necrotizing fasciitis, or overwhelming sepsis.[34,35]

Patients with abscesses may describe pain or tenderness at a superficial cutaneous site and have overlying erythema, induration, or fluctuance. A deeper abscess may surround blood vessels (especially in the neck and groin) causing local bland or suppurative thrombophlebitis, or be hidden deep in muscles, mediastinum, or epidural space. Deep neck abscesses can cause internal jugular vein thrombosis, vocal cord paralysis, airway obstruction, or massive hemorrhage after eroding into the carotid artery. The presentation of deeper abscesses can be subtle and diagnosis often requires radiological imaging.

In PWID, necrotizing fasciitis, an infection of the deep fascial structures, can be caused by *Streptococcus pyogenes* (group A beta-hemolytic streptococci), MRSA, or a mixture of aerobic and anaerobic pathogens and most commonly originates at a soft tissue injection site. The most important diagnostic clue is the presence of hemodynamic instability or pain out of proportion to physical findings. Clinicians should be aware of potential bias against PWID such as attributing symptoms to "drug seeking behavior," which delay diagnosis and stigmatize PWID who present for care.[36,37] Classic findings of high fever, crepitus, and progressive edema occur late in the course. Prompt surgical and radiological evaluations are crucial for a diagnosis of fasciitis. However, imaging studies may be insufficiently sensitive to document the extent of soft tissue involvement, even when gas is present. In patients with necrotizing fasciitis, treatment with antibiotics and urgent surgical exploration with debridement are required to minimize morbidity and maximize survival.

In most other cases of skin and soft tissue infection, empiric antibiotic therapy should be directed at the most likely pathogen and then modified when results from cultures of blood or aspirated pus become available. Typically, initial empiric therapy is guided by the likely etiology, clinical presentation, and local antibiogram.[15] Early surgical evaluation and drainage of collections can minimize morbidity and continued tissue destruction. However, the clinician should carefully evaluate lesions located in the vicinity of blood vessels (especially in the groin), because a mycotic aneurysm can masquerade as an abscess and should not be blindly incised due to the potential for massive hemorrhage.

Management of skin ulcers often requires antibiotics and aggressive wound care to minimize loss of function, especially when lesions are located on the hand. However, accessing supportive environments with comprehensive, longitudinal wound care for PWID can be a challenge.

Infections in large skeletal muscles resembling tropical pyomyositis have also been recognized, especially among PWID.[38] Pyomyositis is commonly caused by *S. aureus and* characterized by the presence of a suppurative collection without myonecrosis, often without prior trauma or local drug injection at the site. Patients may have fever, pain, and swelling in the involved muscle, but often there is little evidence of local inflammation. Diagnosis is made by needle aspiration of pus, with subsequent antibiotic therapy directed by culture results.

Vibrio vulnificus is an unusual cause of cellulitis, soft tissue infection, and bacteremia in patients with cirrhosis who have been exposed to saltwater or shellfish.[39,40] Patients may develop nausea, vomiting, fever, hypotension, shock, and hemorrhagic skin bullae. Prognosis is poor, even with aggressive antibiotic and surgical management.

All patients with injection-related skin and soft tissue infections should be counseled about sterile injection technique, provided with harm reduction supplies such as clean water and sterile injection equipment, and referred to harm reduction organizations.[41,42] Screening for other injection-related infections including HIV and hepatitis C. Measuring immunity to hepatitis A and B should be routine.[43] Aggressive opioid withdrawal management and substance use treatment including buprenorphine and methadone for people with opioid use disorder should be offered.[44]

Complications related to infections with the *Clostridium* sp. that cause botulism and tetanus are discussed later, as are epidural and splenic abscess and mycotic aneurysm.

GINGIVITIS

Acute necrotizing ulcerative gingivitis (ANUG, trench mouth, Vincent angina) is characterized by severe pain, gingival necrosis, and bleeding. Patients often have fever, malaise, and fetid breath. Though associated with a variety of oral flora, the pathogenesis remains uncertain. Development of ANUG appears to be associated with smoking, stress, immunosuppression, and poor oral hygiene. Treatment may include use of antiseptic (chlorhexidine) mouthwash, systemic antibiotics such as penicillin or clindamycin, or debridement.

Oropharyngeal lesions are a common presenting symptom among people who have used cocaine adulterated with levamisole, a veterinary antihelminthic. Agranulocytosis, cutaneous vasculitis, soft tissue infections, and leukoencephalopathy have also been described.[45]

Extensive tooth decay is common among people who chronically use methamphetamine and is thought to be due to a combination of bruxism, decreased saliva production, and poor dental hygiene.[46-48] Because aggressive intervention may be required to prevent disease progression, oral health should be evaluated at each visit to facilitate recognition and expedite early referral to a dentist.

ENDOCARDITIS

(Cardiovascular complications also are addressed in Chapter 88.)

Epidemiology and Pathogenesis

Infective endocarditis (IE) is a morbid infection with a rising incidence among PWID.[49-51] Among PWID, IE usually begins during an episode of transient bacteremia related to injection. The bacteria lodge on the heart valve and form a *vegetation*, composed of layers of platelets and fibrin covering clumps of relatively sequestered microorganisms. Though most vegetations are located on heart valves, they can occur on any endothelial surface. IE in people who do not inject drugs often occurs in people with underlying cardiac lesions who experience transient bacteremia for other reasons.

In PWID, IE most often is caused by *S. aureus* (more than 50%), of which variable proportions are methicillin resistant.[52,53] Infections with streptococci (13%), enterococci (7%), and fungi, particularly nonalbicans *Candida* species (5%), are less common. In contrast, in people who do not inject drugs, IE most often is caused by viridans streptococci (30%-50%), staphylococci (40%), and enterococci (5%-10%).

Both PWID and people with alcohol use disorder have a higher proportion of IE caused by gram-negative bacilli such as *P. aeruginosa*, *Burkholderia cepacia*, and *S. marcescens*.[52-56] Underlying alcohol use disorder is identified as a risk factor in 40% of episodes of pneumococcal endocarditis, and concurrent meningitis is present in 70% of this subgroup of patients.[57]

Culture-negative endocarditis caused by *Bartonella quintana* has been described in men with alcohol use disorder experiencing homelessness.[58,59] Endocarditis caused by a vast array of additional pathogens has been described in case reports.[60-62]

The sustained bacteremia that characterizes IE occurs when microorganisms are released as the vegetation fragments, and the size of the vegetation is related to the type of pathogen. Organisms such as *S. marcescens* and *C. albicans* tend to produce large friable vegetations and bulky emboli.

Clinical Presentation

Clinical features usually include fever, accompanied by a panoply of cardiac abnormalities (murmur, conduction delay, congestive heart failure, and valvular dysfunction), complications from emboli or from metastatic seeding of other structures during the bacteremia (causing meningitis, brain abscess, osteomyelitis, or splenic abscess), and a wide spectrum of immune complex-mediated phenomena (arthritis, glomerulonephritis, aseptic meningitis, Osler nodes, Roth spots, splinter hemorrhages, and other manifestations of vasculitis).[52] Patients may report fever, night sweats, anorexia, arthralgias, myalgias (especially in the low back and upper thighs), and weight loss. However, the presence of IE cannot be predicted in febrile PWID on the basis of signs and symptoms alone.[63] Unexplained fever should prompt evaluation for endocarditis.

The most reliable clues are the presence of embolic phenomenon and visualization of vegetations on echocardiography. PWID have a high incidence of acute IE involving a previously normal tricuspid valve. These patients may have pulmonary symptoms, including cough and pleuritic chest pain from septic pulmonary emboli. Pulmonary infiltrate or effusion occurs in 75% to 85%, and evidence of septic pulmonary embolization eventually is present on 90% of chest x-rays. These emboli appear as rounded infiltrates ("cannonballs") early in the course, often in showers, and may undergo central cavitation or be complicated by empyema. In contrast, patients with left-sided endocarditis may develop congestive heart failure and stigmata of systemic embolization.

Mycotic aneurysms complicate IE in 15% of patients. Most are asymptomatic and resolve with treatment.

Diagnosis

After performing a careful history and physical examination, patients should have two or three blood cultures drawn prior to treatment with empiric antibiotics.

Definitive diagnosis requires microbiological or pathological proof of infection by histology or by culture of a sample of the vegetation or embolus obtained at surgery or autopsy.[64-66] A possible diagnosis is established by demonstrating a characteristic vegetation, valve ring abscess, or dehiscence of a prosthetic valve with echocardiography in a patient with multiple positive blood cultures obtained over an extended period.[66] However, even a negative transesophageal echocardiogram (TEE) does not exclude the diagnosis. The probability that endocarditis is present is estimated by using the Modified Duke criteria.[66]

Treatment

Effective antimicrobial therapy requires identification of the specific pathogen and assessment of its antimicrobial susceptibility. Empiric therapy should be targeted to the most likely pathogens.[52] Initial therapy with an antistaphylococcal antibiotic is appropriate for most PWID. Given high prevalence of MRSA, vancomycin should be used empirically. Addition of antibiotics directed against gram-negative pathogens should be considered based on local epidemiology, etiology of the infection, and severity of the presentation.[67]

The chosen antibiotic must achieve sufficient levels to permit passive diffusion deep into the vegetation, where microcolonies of the pathogen are located. Ultimately, antibiotic selection should be based on final culture and sensitivity results. The duration of therapy should follow standard guidelines. Most patients require a minimum of 4 to 6 weeks of intravenous antibiotics, though shorter courses can be effective in uncomplicated tricuspid valve endocarditis.[52]

Once effective antimicrobial therapy has been initiated, symptoms of fever and fatigue improve coincident with clearance of bacteremia. Blood cultures for streptococci and enterococci should become sterile after 1 to 2 days.[68,69] Blood cultures for staphylococci should become sterile after 3 to 5 days but can take 10 to 14 days to become sterile in patients treated with vancomycin.[69] As a result, short-course therapy cannot be used in regimens containing vancomycin. In some cases, additional agents with activity against MRSA such as daptomycin or ceftaroline may be substituted. Blood cultures should be obtained daily, until sterile. If initial blood cultures remain negative, the possibility of culture-negative endocarditis, an undrained focus of infection such as splenic abscess, or an alternative diagnosis should be explored. Diagnostic possibilities are best assessed with the assistance of an infectious disease specialist.

Ensuring completion of recommended courses of antibiotics is essential for curing IE. However, patients often experience acute withdrawal and untreated pain while hospitalized and are not routinely offered medication for opioid use disorder (MOUD). Hospitalizations for IE are opportunities to initiate MOUD and link patients to longitudinal outpatient treatment, which may reduce rehospitalization and death.[70,71]

PWID with IE face multiple challenges to completing their antibiotic regimen including longer hospitalizations than people with IE who do not inject drugs.[72] Historically PWID were excluded from programs delivering outpatient intravenous antibiotics through a peripherally inserted catheter (PICC) and were offered treatment only in inpatient or post-acute care settings. However, due to inequitable admission practices for PWID, access to postacute care settings is often limited.[73] In addition to withdrawal, cravings, and poorly controlled pain, PWID with IE may experience stigma, trauma, and social isolation, which contributes to high rates of patient directed discharges.[74-76]

In addition to improved integration of substance use treatment into clinical care, there are several promising developments in antibiotic treatment for IE. Providing treatment for PWID outside of the hospital with PICCs has proven safe for many patients, especially compared with high rates of premature antibiotic discontinuation among hospitalized patients.[77,78] Homelessness may make this option impractical. Emerging evidence suggests that in selected patients, a strategy of 2 weeks of intravenous antibiotics followed by oral antibiotics can be effective, although this is not currently recommended by guidelines.[79,80] Finally, though not approved for use in IE, long-acting antibiotics with activity against gram positive organisms administered every week intravenously may be another option.[81] Rigorous studies are evaluating this approach.

When developing antibiotic treatment plans for IE and all infections, special care should be taken to ensure there are no significant medication interactions with MOUD. For example, methadone's metabolism can be significantly induced by rifampin, an antibiotic that is sometimes included as part of a patient's treatment regimen.[82] Rifabutin is an alternative rifamycin medication with less significant interactions. As methadone can cause prolonged QT intervals, EKGs should be monitored when medications such as linezolid, fluoroquinolones, and antifungal agents like fluconazole that can also cause cardiac conduction delays are added.

Surgical intervention should be considered for patients who demonstrate congestive heart failure because of valvular dysfunction refractory to medical therapy, large (>10 mm) or growing vegetation, multiple clinically relevant emboli despite antibiotic therapy during first 2 weeks, infection caused by fungi or resistant organisms that may not respond to medical therapy alone (*Pseudomonas, Serratia, Enterobacter*), extension of myocardial abscess, inability to sterilize blood cultures, or infection or dehiscence of a prosthetic valve. Patients with valve ring abscess should be monitored for the development of conduction abnormalities.

These patients may require placement of a temporary pacemaker because of the risk of developing high-grade heart block.

Outcome and Prevention

A successful outcome requires adherence to antibiotic therapy and access to cardiac valve surgery when indicated. The outcome of an episode of IE is based on many factors including age of the patient, virulence of the organism, site of the infection, presence of complications (such as congestive heart failure, renal failure, rupture of a mycotic aneurysm, cardiac arrhythmia, conduction abnormalities, or cerebral embolization), and the presence of comorbid conditions. Left-sided endocarditis is associated with a worse prognosis, as is infection with gram-negative bacilli or fungi. Heart failure remains the leading cause of death. Availability of multidisciplinary endocarditis working groups, which include cardiologists, cardiac surgeons, infectious disease physicians, addiction specialists, case managers, and other specialties as needed (neurology, anesthesiology), is an emerging strategy to ensure that patients receive guideline concordant, patient-centered care.[83,84]

After cure, patients remain at a substantially increased risk of reinfection and death. As injection drug use is the most common risk factor for recurrent native valve endocarditis, ensuring access to harm reduction services and addiction treatment following discharge is essential.[70,71,84,85] Patients should be given prophylactic antibiotics when undergoing certain invasive dental procedures.[86] Administration of antibiotics solely to prevent endocarditis is no longer recommended for patients who undergo a genitourinary or gastrointestinal tract procedure. In addition, patients should be counseled about reducing the likelihood of transient bacteremia including aggressive treatment of skin infections, good dental hygiene, and treatment of the underlying substance use disorder.

NONCARDIAC VASCULAR INFECTIONS

Epidemiology and Pathogenesis

Both direct injury to blood vessels during injection drug use and substance-induced vasospasm are associated with endothelial injury and thrombus formation. Bacterial seeding of the thrombus can result in septic thrombophlebitis. Alternatively, a hematoma adjacent to the traumatized or ischemic blood vessel may serve as a nidus for superinfection. An arteriovenous fistula can occur either as a result of a direct injury or from extension of local infection.

A mycotic aneurysm results when emboli to the vasa vasorum cause a mushroom-shaped swelling, especially at arterial bifurcations. Mycotic aneurysms complicate 15% of cases of IE. They usually are silent but may become symptomatic in 3 to 5% of patients months or years after completion of appropriate therapy.

For most noncardiac endovascular lesions, the predominant pathogen is *S. aureus*; however, gram-negative bacilli (especially *P. aeruginosa*) are reported with increased frequency in PWID.

Clinical Presentation

When peripheral blood vessels are involved, clinical findings include fever with local pain, swelling, warmth, and induration. A bruit may be present. Infections of the peripheral vasculature can masquerade as cellulitis or subcutaneous abscess, and blind surgical incision should be avoided. Thrombosis of larger vessels can be associated with either pulmonary embolization or distal ischemia and may be confused with IE.

A patient with a mycotic aneurysm in the neck or groin may describe a painful, tender, enlarging, pulsatile mass with overlying bruit or thrill, accompanied by various constitutional symptoms. Ischemia of a distal extremity or signs of nerve compression may be present. Two important complications include extension of infection into surrounding soft tissue with abscess formation and massive hemorrhage from aneurysmal rupture. Mycotic aneurysms in the brain complicate 2% to 4% of cases of left-sided endocarditis. Patients may report headache, visual disturbances, or show signs of cranial nerve palsy.

Patients with endovascular infection may have sustained bacteremia and signs of clinical sepsis. Management of septic thrombophlebitis generally includes treatment with intravenous antibiotics and, in some cases, short-term anticoagulation.

Diagnosis

Successful management of a mycotic aneurysm requires early diagnosis before rupture occurs. Misdiagnosis is common, and a high index of suspicion is essential. Computed tomographic angiography with contrast enhancement and magnetic resonance angiography are most commonly used but sometimes arteriographic confirmation is required.

Treatment

Empiric antibiotics can be given after blood cultures have been obtained. Antibiotic choice should reflect local epidemiology and should include an antistaphylococcal agent with additional gram-negative coverage in geographic regions with an increased prevalence of gram-negative endovascular infection. The antibiotic regimen should be modified on the basis of culture and sensitivity results and usually is continued for 4 to 6 weeks.

Surgical excision of an enlarging mycotic aneurysm and surrounding infected tissue may be necessary to avoid rupture. Intrathoracic, intra-abdominal, and peripheral mycotic aneurysms often require surgical excision. Cerebral mycotic aneurysms usually heal with medical therapy alone but may require neurosurgical intervention if enlarging or bleeding.

RESPIRATORY INFECTIONS

(Respiratory problems are also discussed in Chapter 92.)

Epidemiology and Pathogenesis

Many factors interfere with host defenses and predispose the patient to lung infection.[11,87-94] Cigarette smoke disrupts mucociliary function and macrophage activation. Alterations in consciousness accompanied by depressed gag reflex can compromise airway protection and permit aspiration of oropharyngeal flora. In addition, alcohol use disorder is associated with oropharyngeal colonization with enteric gram-negative bacilli and abnormal phagocyte function. Smoking cannabis is associated with infections from various contaminants including *Aspergillus*. Injection drug use is associated with drug-induced bronchospasm, pulmonary edema, and the development of various types of foreign-body granuloma (cotton, starch, or talc) from contaminants in injected materials. Such nonspecific abnormalities on chest radiograph contribute to diagnostic confusion in a febrile patient with cough. An increased risk of exposure to certain pathogens related to social determinants of health (especially homelessness or incarceration) and the increased prevalence of HIV infection in this group also contribute to the increased risk of respiratory infection.

Pneumonia

Pneumonia is present in up to one-third of PWID evaluated for fever and complicates admissions for treatment of alcohol withdrawal or cocaine intoxication.[95,96] Septic pulmonary emboli associated with right-sided endocarditis or septic thrombophlebitis and tuberculosis infection are common. Most pulmonary infections are community-acquired episodes of pneumonia, caused by common respiratory pathogens such as *S. pneumoniae*, atypical bacteria (such as *Legionella* or *Chlamydia*), oral anaerobes, or viruses. PWID have an increased incidence of pneumonia caused by *Haemophilus influenzae*, *S. aureus*, and *P. aeruginosa*, especially those coinfected with HIV.

Patients with HIV are at higher risk of developing pneumonia. Though *Pneumocystis (carinii) jiroveci* is a major pulmonary pathogen in patients with AIDS, pneumonia caused by *Mycobacterium tuberculosis*, *Mycobacterium avium-intracellulare*, cytomegalovirus, and common bacterial and viral pathogens occurs with increased frequency in this group. Lung abscesses can complicate aspiration pneumonia, necrotizing bacterial pneumonia, or septic emboli. Left-sided pulmonic effusion may be a clue to an underlying splenic abscess or bacterial or tuberculous pleuritis.

Evaluation of respiratory symptoms in a febrile person who uses drugs should follow standard guidelines, with empiric management directed at likely pathogens.[97,98] Like methadone, macrolides and quinolones, common medications used for pneumonia, can cause conduction delays. When these medications are used together the QT interval should be monitored carefully.

COVID

Late in 2019 a new beta-coronavirus was identified as the cause of a cluster of pneumonia cases in China. Coronavirus disease 2019 (COVID-19) caused a severe acute coronavirus syndrome (SARS-CoV-2) that spread rapidly causing a worldwide pandemic.[99] Certain racial/ethnic communities were disproportionally effected due to social determinants of health, including structural racism.[100,101] The elderly, immunocompromised, and those with diabetes, mental health issues, obesity, pregnancy, substance use disorder, and a wide variety of chronic illnesses (cardiovascular, hepatitis, neurologic, pulmonary, and renal) were at higher risk for severe disease or death.[99] Over time, variants emerged and were often responsible for new surges of infection. Despite the rapid development of vaccines and antivirals, COVID-19 has caused hundreds of millions of cases and millions of excess deaths around the world.[102,103]

Most patients recover within 3 months. Long-term sequelae include pulmonary, neurologic, and cardiovascular changes in up to 20% of patients.[104] A syndrome of "Long Covid" characterized by fatigue, difficulty concentrating, cough, and clotting abnormalities, lasting from 3 months to over 2 years, has been reported. Studies are in progress to better define this syndrome.[99,105,106]

Treatment guidelines continue to evolve as the virus mutates. Care must be taken when using certain antiviral drugs such as nirmatrelvir/ritonavir because of its interaction with other drugs. Nirmatrelvir/ritonavir notably induces the metabolism of methadone. Patients should be made aware of this risk, monitored for evidence of withdrawal, and the methadone dose may need to be increased.

Prevention is by vaccination supplemented by social distancing, appropriate use of masks, isolation of infected patients, and quarantine of close contacts to a case.[107] Pre- and postexposure prophylaxis regimens using monoclonal antibodies are available but are not effective against all variants. Vaccination is associated with less severe illness, fewer hospitalizations, and fewer deaths. Optimal vaccine strategies are being studied. People with SUD appear to be at increased risk for COVID-19 infection and for adverse outcomes even when fully vaccinated.[108] In addition, increased unhealthy substance use during the pandemic appears to have contributed to a 25% increase in alcohol-related deaths and a 14.9% increase in opioid overdose deaths.[109,110]

Tuberculosis

Tuberculosis is a leading cause of infectious morbidity and mortality worldwide, and one-quarter of the world population has latent tuberculosis infection. In the United States, only 2% to 6% of the population has latent infection.[111] Rates of active disease fell steadily until the mid-1980s, when there was a brief resurgence coincident with immigration patterns and the spread of HIV. HIV infection has contributed to the rising case rates because of the higher likelihood of reactivation as immune function decreases and because of the risk of unusually rapid progression to active disease following new (primary) infection. In addition, patients with HIV have a higher prevalence of extrapulmonary and drug-resistant disease.[112] PWUD, especially people with alcohol use disorder and PWID, have an increased incidence of reactivation tuberculosis.[113,114] Injection drug use was implicated in a large outbreak of multidrug-resistant tuberculosis in New York City, where most transmission occurred in hospitals and jails.[115,116] Difficulties controlling this outbreak were compounded by homelessness and incomplete adherence with medical therapy.

Infection is spread by the aerosolization of acid-fast bacilli in respiratory secretions. Patients with cavitary disease are particularly infectious because of the high concentration of bacilli in their sputum. Cough-inducing procedures such as bronchoscopy, administration of aerosolized medications (including bronchodilators), and smoking (cigarettes, free base forms of cocaine, and cannabis) can increase transmission.

The classic symptoms of pulmonary tuberculosis include cough with purulent, blood-tinged sputum, increasing malaise, and the development of night sweats and weight loss as the disease progresses. High fever is seen with decreasing frequency as the level of immunosuppression increases. Diagnosis is made by culturing *M. tuberculosis* from expectorated sputum. A fully automated nucleic acid amplification test (by rapid, real-time PCR) identifies targeted nucleic acid sequences in the TB genome and provides results from unprocessed sputum samples in less than 2 hours. Tuberculin skin tests generally turn positive 4 to 6 weeks after primary infection but can be negative in up to 25% of patients at the time of diagnosis. Interpretation of the tuberculin test is stratified to reflect a combination of risk factors, including severity of underlying immunosuppression, and should follow standard algorithms.[117,118] In vitro testing using interferon gamma release assays (IGRAs) are available, but interpretation is complicated by false-positive and false-negative results. Since no diagnostic strategy has been proven superior, decisions about which test to use may be influenced by availability, cost, and convenience. IGRAs should not be used for diagnosis of active tuberculosis because of poor sensitivity and specificity. To avoid nosocomial transmission, patients with a suspicious presentation should be placed in respiratory isolation until the diagnosis is excluded.

Extrapulmonary tuberculosis occurs in one-fifth of adults and up to 60% to 80% of patients with HIV. Diagnosis is challenging because of the paucity of bacilli in extrapulmonary sites. Histopathology classically shows giant cell granulomas with central caseating necrosis. Extrapulmonary seeding commonly causes empyema, meningitis, and vertebral osteomyelitis, and diagnosis generally requires biopsy.

Because of the long delay to obtain culture and sensitivity results, treatment usually is initiated before a definitive diagnosis has been established. Treatment should follow the American Thoracic Society Guidelines.[117-119] Many patients are started on a four-drug regimen that includes isoniazid, rifampin, pyrazinamide, and ethambutol. Patients should be closely monitored for disease progression and the development of treatment-related side effects, such as hepatitis or rash. The initial regimen is adjusted once sensitivities are known. Duration of therapy is based on the severity of immunosuppression and extent of disease. PWID are at increased risk of multidrug-resistant tuberculosis (resistant to both isoniazid and rifampin). For these patients, results of sensitivity testing are crucial in planning an effective treatment regimen that should include at least two active agents.

Extra care must be taken in medication selection for patients with TB and HIV. Drugs may be poorly absorbed because of underlying enteropathy or have significant interactions with other medications. For example, rifampin should not be used with protease inhibitors or many other medications because of its effect on hepatic catabolism. Directly observed therapy is strongly encouraged when nonadherence is anticipated. Embedding directly observed therapy into opioid treatment programs is an effective treatment strategy.[120,121] People with HIV, especially those with CD4 cell counts under 200, should be monitored closely for the development of immune reconstitution inflammatory syndrome.

Most PWUD are at increased risk of tuberculosis infection and should have routine IGRAs or tuberculin skin testing. Interpretation of the skin test result and selection of a treatment regimen should follow standard guidelines.[117-119,122] For example, PWID with more than 10-mm induration on skin testing might be given a 12-week combination regimen of once-weekly isoniazid and rifapentine (3HP) by directly observed therapy after active disease is excluded. PWID with HIV may receive 3HP if there are no drug interactions, or might be given 9 months of isoniazid when there is more than a 5-mm induration on skin testing or after close contact with a case of infectious tuberculosis, regardless of skin test results. Many drug combinations and dosing schedules are available. Peripheral neuropathy can occur in patients treated with isoniazid, especially in those with preexisting nutritional deficiency, alcohol use, pregnancy, diabetes, renal failure, and HIV infection, and can be minimized by using concurrent pyridoxine. Rifampin can induce the metabolism of methadone and patients often require increasing methadone doses. PWID with underlying hepatitis or who use hepatotoxins such as alcohol have an increased risk of developing hepatitis when using isoniazid, rifampin, or pyrazinamide. These patients should be monitored for the development of anorexia, abdominal pain, nausea, vomiting, change in color of urine or stool, or jaundice.

Influenza

Most patients with underlying lung disease are at risk of increased morbidity from influenza and should be offered annual immunization.[123] The efficacy of pneumococcal vaccine to prevent invasive disease varies with the population studied. Vaccination is recommended for patients with immunocompromising conditions including HIV infection, those aged 65 or older, and those who have chronic medical conditions such as diabetes, heart, lung or liver disease, and for those who smoke cigarettes or have risky alcohol use or alcohol use disorder (CDC guidelines recommend for those with "alcoholism") due to their negative impacts on immune function and increased disease severity.[124]

HEPATIC AND GASTROINTESTINAL INFECTIONS

(Hepatic and gastrointestinal disorders are also addressed in Chapters 89 and 91, respectively.)

Viral hepatitis is common among people who use injection drugs, noninjection drugs, and alcohol and has been extensively reviewed. To achieve the goal of hepatitis C elimination and reduced transmission, it is a priority to ensure that effective and well-tolerated direct-acting antiviral medications be made available to PWID with hepatitis C in primary care, substance use treatment facilities and service organizations. Vaccination against hepatitis A and B should be encouraged.

Hepatic cirrhosis results from an irreversible chronic injury to the hepatic parenchyma that is most often caused by alcohol use, viral hepatitis, or metabolic-associated fatty liver disease. Infection is the leading cause of death in patients with cirrhosis. Gram-negative enteric bacilli such as *Escherichia coli*, *K. pneumoniae*, and encapsulated respiratory pathogens such as *S. pneumoniae* are the most frequent cause of infection in these patients; however, severe infections with many other organisms, including *V. vulnificus*, *Pasteurella multocida*, *Aeromonas hydrophila*, *Listeria monocytogenes*, and *Campylobacter* spp., and tuberculosis also have been described.

Spontaneous bacterial peritonitis (SBP) is a common and potentially fatal infectious complication in patients with cirrhosis and ascites. Pathogenesis involves translocation of bacteria from the gut to mesenteric lymph nodes and is associated with deficiencies in humoral response and phagocytic function.[125,126]

Diagnostic paracentesis should be performed in patients with ascites who have fever. Analysis of ascitic fluid should include Gram stain and culture for bacteria, mycobacteria, and fungi; measurement of albumin; absolute and differential white blood cell count; and cytopathology. Empiric antibiotic therapy is directed against suspected pathogens and should be refined once culture results become available. Because gram-negative enteric bacilli and *S. pneumoniae* are the most common cause of infection in these patients, a third-generation cephalosporin or a combination of fluoroquinolone plus clindamycin or metronidazole is a common starting regimen. Patients with SBP who develop renal failure are treated with intravenous albumin.[127] Patients who have a low ascitic fluid protein or more advanced liver disease are at increased risk of developing SBP. Some authorities recommend the use of prophylactic antibiotics to prevent SBP in this subset of patients as well as those with a prior episode of SBP.

Tuberculous peritonitis, which is uncommon, usually is diagnosed by peritoneal biopsy and culture.

BONE AND JOINT INFECTIONS

Osteomyelitis

Most microorganisms can infect the bone. Frequent pathogens include *S. aureus* (60%), *Staphylococcus epidermidis* (30%), streptococci, gram-negative bacilli, anaerobes, mycobacteria, and fungi (10%), and prevalence is related to mode of acquisition. Infection can occur by hematogenous seeding, by introduction after surgery or trauma, or by spread from a contiguous focus.[128-130] In adults, hematogenous spread of bacteria frequently involves the spine because of the vascularity of the vertebrae. Vertebral osteomyelitis in PWID usually involves the lumbosacral and cervical spine. Common pathogens include *S. aureus*, gram-negative bacilli (including *P. aeruginosa*), and fungi. Though the original source of these infections may be unknown, most are seeded hematogenously during an episode of bacterial endocarditis or locally from a contiguous soft tissue focus.

Adults may develop osteomyelitis of the hand caused by mouth flora (including *Staphylococcus* spp., *E. corrodens*, *P. multocida*, and oral anaerobes) associated with local trauma after bite wounds or closed-fist injury.

Patients with osteomyelitis report focal pain and tenderness. Fever is present in two-thirds of patients; erythema, warmth, and swelling are variably present. Lack of signs and symptoms frequently results in a delay in diagnosis.

In vertebral osteomyelitis, associated symptoms result when inflammation extends beyond the spine to cause retropharyngeal abscess, mediastinitis, subdiaphragmatic or iliopsoas abscess, meningitis, or epidural abscess with evidence of spinal cord compression. Spinal tuberculosis (Pott disease) is relatively indolent and patients may have late sequelae and extensive vertebral destruction.

Diagnosis of osteomyelitis is made by biopsy and culture of the bone. Computed tomography scan and magnetic resonance imaging are helpful in determining the extent of involvement but are not specific. Blood cultures often are negative, especially when the osteomyelitis resulted from hematogenous seeding during a remote bacteremic infection (such as endocarditis). Antibiotics alone may be sufficient therapy to cure acute osteomyelitis and should be chosen on the basis of isolated pathogens. Use of empiric therapy is suboptimal because of the wide range of potential pathogens. Surgical debridement generally is required for cure when the infection has been present for longer than 6 weeks (chronic osteomyelitis).

Establishing a regimen that is mutually acceptable to the patient and clinician is challenging because of the requirement for prolonged intravenous or oral therapy. Emerging randomized controlled trial evidence suggests that selected patients with osteomyelitis can be spared prolonged intravenous antimicrobial treatment and successfully transitioned to oral therapy.[131] As with endocarditis, it is essential to ensure both withdrawal and pain are adequately managed, that harm reduction education is provided, and that substance use treatment is offered.

Septic Arthritis

Septic arthritis occurs when bacteria seed joints previously damaged by trauma, instrumentation, osteoarthritis, or chronic inflammatory conditions. Infection with *S. aureus* is most common, though infection with many other organisms has been reported. Arthrocentesis with culture and microscopic examination of joint fluid are required for diagnosis. Differential diagnosis includes gonorrhea, crystal arthropathy, and a variety of noninfectious etiologies.

Two particular syndromes are more common among PWID than in the general population and involve fibrocartilaginous joints, which are most susceptible to hematogenous seeding. Septic arthritis of the sternoclavicular joint caused by *P. aeruginosa* has been reported primarily in PWID. Most cases occur without identification of an antecedent infection. Symptoms may be present for several months before the patient seeks evaluation for fever, tenderness and swelling over the joint, or decreased range of motion of the ipsilateral shoulder.[132] Another unusual presentation is of septic arthritis of the sacroiliac joint or symphysis pubis. Symptoms include fever and various combinations of hip, groin, thigh, or lower abdominal pain that is exacerbated by walking.[133,134] In such cases, infection may spread from the joint to contiguous soft tissues and bone. Treatment may require exploratory arthrotomy, with surgical debridement of infected material followed by prolonged antibiotic therapy directed at isolated organisms.

NERVOUS SYSTEM INFECTIONS

People who use drugs are prone to a variety of central nervous system complications that may have an infectious origin. Such manifestations are easily missed if symptoms are mistakenly attributed to intoxication or withdrawal. Delirium, acute confusional states, encephalopathy, or coma may accompany overdose, withdrawal, intoxication, infection, or a large number of noninfectious etiologies. Central nervous system mass lesions, seizures, hemorrhage, stroke syndromes, transverse myelitis, and peripheral neuropathies have a similarly broad differential. Clinical features should guide diagnostic strategies, with management based on results of lumbar puncture and neuroradiological imaging.[135]

Endocarditis can cause central nervous system symptoms in PWID and lead to meningitis (aseptic or purulent), brain abscess from septic emboli, or hemorrhage from rupture of a mycotic aneurysm.[136] Bacteremia with or without accompanying IE can cause vertebral osteomyelitis, which, in turn, can be complicated by epidural abscess, sometimes with evidence of cord compression.[137]

Brain abscess and subdural empyema in the absence of endocarditis usually are caused by a varied group of pyogenic bacteria; however, infection with many other organisms, including *Nocardia*, *Aspergillus* spp., *Cryptococcus*, mucormycosis, tuberculosis, and *Toxoplasma gondii*, has been reported, especially in immunosuppressed patients with HIV. Etiology often involves extension from a contiguous focus in the mastoid, ear, or paranasal sinuses; seeding of a preexisting subdural hematoma during an episode of transient bacteremia; or direct inoculation of the subdural space after a traumatic wound. A patient with brain abscess may have nonspecific symptoms such as headache or personality change, and an abscess can attain a large size before diagnosis. Management includes antibiotics and drainage, if indicated.

In most cases, patients with HIV who have ring-enhancing mass lesions in the brain and appropriate clinical presentation are treated empirically for toxoplasmosis. Symptoms that worsen or fail to improve after 2 weeks should prompt more aggressive evaluation, including consideration of brain biopsy.

Meningovascular syphilis has been reported in a number of patients with HIV, despite presumably effective therapy for primary syphilis infection, and should be considered in young people who present with a new stroke.[138]

Contamination of skin ulcers with spores of *Clostridium* spp. can cause neurological symptoms from elaboration of neurotoxins. Wound botulism is caused by contamination of injection sites or skin ulcers with *Clostridium botulinum* that release botulinum toxin.[139] Toxin is absorbed, disseminated, and ultimately binds to specific receptors, where it blocks acetylcholine release, resulting in a descending, symmetric, flaccid paralysis. There has been an increase in reported cases among PWID who injected black tar heroin, the dark, gummy substance derived from crude preparations of opium that may be contaminated by spore-containing adulterants such as dirt.[140] Diagnosis is established by recovering *C. botulinum* from the wound or by detecting toxin in serum, but negative findings do not exclude the diagnosis. Treatment with trivalent or type-specific antitoxin can limit disease progression. Involvement of motor neurons causes respiratory failure, and patients may require respiratory support for several months until synapses are regenerated.[139] Botulism has been reported in a patient with colonization of the paranasal sinuses after intranasal cocaine use.[141]

Tetanus is caused by the release of a potent neurotoxin by *Clostridium tetani* at the site of a wound in a person who lacks protective antibodies.[142] Wounds contaminated by dirt, feces, or saliva provide an appropriate anaerobic milieu for these vegetative bacteria. Between 2009 and 2017, there were 264 reported cases in the United States, a decline from previous years when approximately 100 cases of tetanus per year were reported.[143] Most tetanus cases have been associated with acute injury, chronic wounds, and diabetes. Fifteen to eighteen percent of the reported cases were in PWID who injected black tar heroin. Toxin travels up the axon to spinal neurons, where it blocks the release of glycine and other neurotransmitters used to inhibit afferent motor neurons. Binding results in unrestrained nerve firing with sustained muscle contractions and rigidity. Binding is irreversible, and recovery requires generation of new axon terminals. Symptoms begin 7 to 21 days after injury. Early symptoms of trismus (lockjaw) progress to dysphagia, hydrophobia, and drooling, followed by opisthotonos, with painful flexion of the arms and extension of the legs. The patient remains conscious. Very rarely, localized tetanus can cause weakness limited to a single extremity, but this weakness usually progresses to generalized tetany. Management should include antibiotics, aggressive wound debridement, tetanus immune globulin, and supportive care. Prevention requires protective antibody levels. All patients should be immunized with tetanus toxoid every 10 years after a primary series (or immediately after a high-risk wound if more than 5 years has elapsed since the last booster).

EYE INFECTIONS

PWID have an increased incidence of bacterial and fungal endophthalmitis, often as a complication of IE. Many investigators have reported *C. albicans* endophthalmitis as part of a syndrome of disseminated candidiasis in people who injected "brown heroin," presumably related to fungal contamination of the lemon juice used to dissolve the drug.[144] The most commonly reported bacterial causes include *S. aureus* and *Bacillus cereus.*

Symptoms of endophthalmitis include acute onset of blurred vision, eye pain, and decreased visual acuity.[145] Diagnosis requires a high index of suspicion; aggressive evaluation and management are required to salvage vision.[146]

Cytomegalovirus retinitis is the most common serious intraocular complication of AIDS and generally occurs after reactivation of latent infection in patients with CD4 cell counts of less than 50, especially those not receiving antiretroviral therapy (ART). Disease is characterized by retinal necrosis and edema that begins peripherally in the eye and may remain asymptomatic until there has been significant retinal destruction or detachment. Symptoms of blurring or loss of vision, floaters, or flashing lights in one or both eyes should always be evaluated with dilated ophthalmoscopy. Characteristic retinal changes include yellow-white, fluffy exudates with associated hemorrhage. Therapy with oral, intravenous, or intraocular antiviral agents can reduce the risk of vision loss. However, patients may develop significant intraocular inflammation associated with immune recovery (immune recovery uveitis) and require aggressive management to prevent permanent loss of vision.

HUMAN IMMUNODEFICIENCY VIRUS AND ACQUIRED IMMUNODEFICIENCY SYNDROME

Since the original description of HIV with *Pneumocystis carinii pneumonia* and Kaposi sarcoma in 1981 among a cluster of men who had sex with men,[147,148] enormous advances have transformed what was a universally fatal infection into a chronic disease for those able to access and continue antiretroviral treatment (ART). There are now a variety of single pill per day regimens that are effective and relatively well-tolerated as well as long-acting injectable ART formulations. Comprehensive discussions of the AIDS pandemic, including details of transmission, seroconversion, immunosuppression related to disease stage, use of ART, and prophylaxis and treatment for opportunistic infections are available.[149-152]

Epidemiology and Pathogenesis

HIV infection usually is acquired through exposure to an HIV-infected individual through sexual intercourse, exposure to blood products (injection drug use or other mechanisms), or by perinatal transmission; the relative frequency of each varies by country. In the United States, 1.19 million persons 13 years of age or older were estimated to be living with HIV as of 2019.[153] The Centers for Disease Control (CDC) estimates that 58% of HIV infections were acquired through male-to-male sexual contact, 26% through heterosexual contact, 11% through injection drug use, and 5% had overlapping risk factors for male-to-male sexual contact and injection drug use.[153,154] The estimated HIV prevalence rate in the United States by race/ethnicity demonstrates striking disparities among people of color: 1,411 Black Americans per 100,000 population and 626 Hispanic/Latinx Americans per 100,000 population are infected with HIV compared with 198 White Americans per 100,000 population. Similarly, the HIV epidemic is regionally concentrated with 46% of persons with HIV living in the South, 22% in the Northeast, 20% in the West and 12% in the Midwest as of 2019.[153]

HIV diagnoses related to injection drug use decreased 48% between 2008 and 2014, likely reflecting increased national HIV prevention and treatment efforts, including expansion of syringe service programs.[154] However between 2014 and 2018, there was an 11% increase in new diagnoses among PWID due to increasing injection drug use and an increase in syringe sharing, which has been documented in HIV outbreaks among PWID across the United States.[155-160] Driven by the syndemic of homelessness, poverty, and incarceration, PWID have lower viral suppression rates and higher mortality than people with HIV who do not inject drugs.[154] The ongoing overdose crisis may result in worsening of this disparity.

Classification

The stages of HIV infection include acute HIV infection (Stage 1) where there is an initial uncontrolled phase of high HIV viremia and, for many, an acute retroviral clinical syndrome. Chronic HIV infection (Stage 2) is followed by Acquired Immunodeficiency Syndrome (AIDS) (Stage 3) in which the CD4 lymphocytes fall below 200 cells/mm and/or opportunistic infections emerge.[150]

Primary (acute) HIV infection causes symptoms in 50% to 90% of cases and occurs 2 to 4 weeks after exposure. Symptoms of fever, adenopathy, pharyngitis, rash, and myalgias are reported by more than 50% of patients and last 1 to 4 weeks. Other nonspecific symptoms that have been reported include arthralgias, diarrhea, headache, nausea and vomiting, hepatosplenomegaly, thrush, mucocutaneous ulcers, meningoencephalitis, peripheral neuropathy, cranial nerve palsy, Guillain-Barré syndrome, radiculopathy, cognitive impairment, and psychosis.[161] High-level viremia during the acute illness permits dissemination of virus to the central nervous system and lymphatic tissue. The lymphatics are a major reservoir of HIV infection, and replication continues during the clinically latent disease stage. Plasma levels of HIV decline dramatically during the resolution of the symptomatic phase of primary HIV, presumably because of the development of humoral and cellular immune responses, and reach a nadir at 120 days.

By 6 months after transmission, 95% of patients have developed stabilization of viral load, with levels correlating with prognosis. As the disease progresses, lymph node architecture is disrupted, releasing more HIV, with an accompanying slow but progressive decline in CD4 counts in most patients. The average life expectancy in the absence of treatment is approximately 10 years, and rates of progression appear similar by gender, race, and risk category when adjusted for quality of medical care.

Diagnosis

Prior to 2006, the CDC recommended HIV screening for asymptomatic individuals based on demographic distribution of reported AIDS cases. However, 13% of people living with HIV were not aware of their diagnosis and thus were more likely to transmit the infection.[153] Late diagnosis of HIV, when the disease had progressed to Stage 3/AIDS, was common (21% in 2016).[162]

As a result, in 2006, the CDC recommended routine HIV screening for all patients aged 13 to 64 years in all health care settings.[163] Repeat screening is recommended at least once yearly for people considered at high risk for HIV acquisition, including PWID and their sex partners, people who exchange sex for money or drugs, sex partners of people with HIV, and people who have had 2 or more sex partners since their most recent HIV test. While HIV testing is voluntary, the CDC recommends opt-out screening. Opt-out HIV screening is also recommended universally for pregnant women. The CDC specifies that a positive HIV result should be personally and confidentially communicated from a clinical provider or other skilled staff to the patient, with appropriate linkage to care and treatment, even if other health problems, including substance use disorders, have not been fully treated.

Types of HIV Testing

As of 2014, the preferred HIV screening test is a laboratory-based HIV antibody/antigen test that detects both HIV-1 capsid antigen (p24) and antibodies to HIV-1 or HIV-2.[164] This combined HIV test detects 50% of cases within approximately 18 days of HIV infection and 99% of HIV cases within 45 days of infection. The CDC considers these immunoassays to have a 45-day "window period" between infection and expectation of test positivity.[165] These laboratory-based tests have relatively quick turn-around time, with results available in as little as 30 minutes. In contrast, the laboratory-based HIV antibody tests that were previously used had a "window period" of 90 days, proving to be less useful in acute or early HIV infection. There are multiple single-use, point-of-care HIV antibody tests (and at least one point-of-care HIV antigen/antibody test), which can be used in alternative clinical settings utilizing finger-stick blood collection or saliva testing with results available in as little as 40 minutes. Because all point-of-care testing modalities are associated with considerably diminished sensitivity, laboratory-based HIV antigen/antibody tests are preferred, but point-of-care "rapid" HIV tests may have an important role when follow up is unreliable, such as in the emergency department or at syringe services programs.[164,166-168]

After a positive antigen/antibody HIV immunoassay, verification of HIV infection is typically performed using an HIV antibody differentiation assay, which determines whether the patient has HIV-1 or HIV-2 infection.[168] If the differentiation assay is indeterminate or in the case of acute infection, HIV-1 nucleic acid testing to measure HIV viral load can confirm the diagnosis. Historically, antibody testing was confirmed by an HIV-1 Western blot that demonstrates at least two characteristic antigens (p24, gp41, or gp120/160), but this is no longer part of the recommended diagnostic algorithm.[168]

Acute HIV Infection

Acute HIV infection should be considered in any patient with a history of potential exposure and compatible symptoms. After performing a careful history and physical examination, the best diagnostic testing to obtain is *both* an HIV antigen/antibody test (which may or may not be positive depending on the timing of the infection) and quantitative HIV RNA testing (viral load), which should be positive 5 to 10 days following infection. If there is clinical concern that the patient is in the window period before any testing is positive, testing should be repeated within 1 week. Finally, diagnostic testing for HIV can be complicated by delayed seroconversion in people on medications for HIV preexposure prophylaxis.[169] Consultation with an HIV specialist is recommended in these clinical scenarios.

Other Testing

Once the diagnosis of HIV has been established, all patients should have quantification of their CD4 lymphocytes, evaluation of HIV resistance with genotype testing, and HIV-related health maintenance testing such as testing for viral hepatitis, syphilis, gonorrhea, chlamydia, and latent tuberculosis, serologic testing for toxoplasma, kidney and liver function tests, and Papanicolaou tests, in addition to HLA B 5701 testing for abacavir hypersensitivity, G6PD deficiency testing, and ophthalmological examination as clinically indicated.[170]

Treatment

HIV has progressed from a chronic illness with limited, relatively toxic treatments to the current era, in which there are multiple, highly effective medications that can lead to durable viral suppression.

Initiation and ART Basics

While optimal ART selection is a rapidly evolving topic, federally approved guidelines are available that describe optimal baseline evaluation, laboratory testing, and management of the patient with coinfections. Additional guidelines provide disease-specific recommendations for the prevention and treatment of common opportunistic infections, including *Pneumocystis jiroveci pneumonia*, cytomegalovirus-associated retinitis, disseminated *Mycobacterium avium–intracellulare* complex infection, and tuberculosis.[152]

Guidelines strongly support initiation of ART for all people living with HIV as soon as possible following diagnosis regardless of CD4 count, both because of demonstrated clinical benefit for the patient and for prevention of further HIV transmission. ART are classified mechanistically into the following categories: (1) entry inhibitors, (2) nucleoside reverse transcriptase inhibitors (NRTIs), (3) non-nucleoside reverse transcriptase inhibitors (NNRTIs), (4) nucleoside reverse transcriptase translocation inhibitors (NRTTI: pending FDA approval), (5) integrase strand transfer inhibitors (INSTIs), and (6) protease inhibitors (PIs). To induce and maintain viral suppression, most patients are treated with three active antiretroviral drugs, ideally in the form of a once daily, one-pill regimen; although guidelines also support two-drug therapy for certain patients. Antiretroviral regimens have been greatly simplified with the availability of a variety of single- or two-pill combinations. These are generally well tolerated and have fewer side effects and drug interactions than previous generations of antiretroviral drugs.

As of 2022, treatment is initiated with a three-drug regimen with high potency and barrier to resistance, commonly with a "backbone" of two NRTIs and an "anchor" of an INSTI, though referral to the most up-to-date guidelines is recommended.[150] Initial regimen selection and ongoing ART use should consider patient preference, comorbid medical conditions (chronic kidney disease, osteoporosis, cardiovascular disease, obesity), medication interactions, food requirements, drug resistance testing, and pretreatment HIV RNA level and CD4 count. Long-acting injectable ART or ART implants will likely become part of routine HIV treatment in coming years.[150] Consultation with an HIV specialist is recommended to determine whether certain patients (either patients with nonadherence to oral medications or stable patients who desire to transition away from oral medications) might benefit from long-acting injectable ART. Patients with HIV and OUD who receive treatment with MOUD including buprenorphine and methadone have improved ARV adherence and HIV outcomes regardless if OUD treatment is integrated into HIV treatment or ARV treatment is integrated into an opioid treatment setting.[171-176]

When initiating ART in patients with CD4 counts below 200 and high HIV RNA levels, it is important to counsel patients about the risk of immune reconstitution inflammatory syndrome (IRIS).[152,177,178] IRIS can manifest as severe or worsening symptoms of an active opportunistic infection being treated at time of ART initiation ("paradoxical IRIS") or as a new set of signs and symptoms of infection weeks following ART initiation indicating a previously undiagnosed opportunistic infection ("unmasking IRIS").

Health Maintenance for Persons With HIV and Substance Use Disorders

In addition to age-appropriate cancer screening and cardiovascular health maintenance, immunizations for hepatitis A and B, influenza, SARS-CoV-2, pneumococcus, meningococcus, varicella zoster virus, human papilloma virus, and tetanus-diphtheria-pertussis should be administered, in addition to any childhood immunizations that are not up to date.[179] Updated guidelines are published by the CDC.[180] Yearly screening for HCV with antibody or viral load testing is indicated if the patient has ongoing risk factors, along with latent tuberculosis testing based on risk factors.

Past and current behaviors and exposures that resulted in HIV infection should be reviewed and mitigation plans designed to prevent further transmission. A harm reduction approach allows for effective partnership with the patient aimed at reducing the negative consequences of the risky behavior. Continuing risky substance use should prompt provision or referral to addiction treatment services, if the patient is amenable, to improve substance use and HIV viral suppression. Developing capacity to provide integrated treatment should be a priority given evidence that co-locating HIV and OUD treatment is associated with improved HIV outcomes.[172,175,176] In addition, the patient should receive education and counseling on how to reduce the risk of exposure to opportunistic pathogens associated with food, pets, water, travel, or the environment. Indication for initiation, maintaining, and discontinuing chemoprophylaxis against opportunistic infections should be reviewed at each clinical visit.[152]

Response to HIV Treatment

Initiation and adherence to ART is central for maximal and durable suppression of viral load, restoration or preservation of immunological function, improvement in the quality of life, and reduction of HIV-related morbidity and mortality. Efficacy of therapy is evaluated by monitoring viral load, which should be undetectable (<40-50 copies per mL) 8 to 24 weeks after initiation of treatment.[151]

The proportion of patients with each of the various AIDS-defining conditions, the rate of disease progression, the rate of AIDS deaths, and the average life expectancy have changed dramatically coincident with the widespread use of ART and prophylaxis against opportunistic infections. In the past, patients with AIDS and CD4 cell count under 50 cells/mm^3 had a median survival of 12 to 18 months. However, many of these patients had received no ART or suboptimal ART by current standards. Treatment strategies now known to prolong survival include use of ART, use of primary and secondary prophylaxis for *Pneumocystis jiroveci pneumonia* and, in some cases, *Mycobacterium avium–intracellulare* complex, and care by a physician knowledgeable about both HIV and primary care.[170] This is particularly important for older individuals in whom management of other comorbidities can complicate HIV therapy.

Failure of therapy at 4 to 6 months can be ascribed to nonadherence in the context of competing priorities (such as maintaining shelter, food), nonadherence related to medication adverse effects or difficulty with dosing regimen, viral resistance, or suboptimal ART levels related to medication interactions, among other factors. It is strongly recommended that care be co-managed with an expert in HIV treatment if evaluating a patient with unknown reason for treatment failure.

Drug Interactions

Drug–drug or drug–food interactions can affect the absorption and efficacy of certain medications, though this is less common with current ART regimens. Methadone, buprenorphine, and naltrexone do not lead to low serum levels of NRTIs, INSTIs, or newer PIs. However, methadone levels can be significantly decreased when given with certain protease inhibitors (pharmacokinetic boosters like ritonavir, cobicistat that induce methadone metabolism). Interactions are more common among those using older ART regimens. Ensuring no medication interactions are present, ideally with assistance of a clinical pharmacist, is a critical step when prescribing new medications to people with HIV.

Integrase inhibitors are appealing because of their high barriers to resistance. ART regimens anchored by the protease inhibitor darunavir also provide a high barrier to resistance, but drug interactions are more numerous (CYP enzymes as a substrate, inhibitor, or inducer). For example, concurrent therapy with rifampin can decrease the concentration of a protease inhibitor by as much as 80%, so its use should be avoided to prevent development of antiretroviral resistance and treatment failure. On the other hand, use of a boosted PI (such as ritonavir- or cobicistat-boosted darunavir) along with corticosteroids or atypical antipsychotics will lead to higher-than-expected levels of the latter two drugs, which can lead to considerable morbidity. The development and severity of these adverse effects often are unpredictable; thus, assessment of toxicity should be performed frequently as part of routine follow-up care.

As the population of people living with HIV ages, long-term complications of ART are increasingly clinically relevant. Tenofovir disoproxil fumarate, one of the NRTIs, is associated with nephrotoxicity and osteoporosis, but is also associated with reductions in serum cholesterol levels. Tenofovir alafenamide, a newer NRTI, was developed to minimize serum drug levels and hence nephrotoxicity and bone toxicity, but may be associated with weight gain. Abacavir, another NRTI, has been associated in retrospective studies with increased risk of myocardial infarction. The integrase inhibitors, which are included in many initial regimens, can occasionally lead to headache and insomnia. There is some concern that INSTIs also may contribute to weight gain. Finally, PIs may lead to dyslipidemia and metabolic syndrome. Careful consideration of patient goals, comorbid conditions, and medication interactions along with close monitoring are key in designing optimal treatment regimens.

HIV Prevention

As previously noted, incidence of new HIV infections has fluctuated across demographic groups, with most new infections occurring either in young people of color who have sex with men or in clusters related to injection drug use. Among MSM, methamphetamine use is associated with higher-risk sexual activity and HIV acquisition.[181] A multi-pronged approach to HIV prevention, including optimal HIV preexposure prophylaxis (PrEP), is suggested. Patients who use substances that increase their risk of HIV acquisition either because of sexual risk or risk related to injection drug use should be offered PrEP. The importance of using a sterile syringe for every injection and the avoidance of sharing any injection-related drug paraphernalia with another person should be emphasized. Such patients should be encouraged to use a syringe service program and to safely discard syringes after one use. In areas where syringe service programs are not available, PWID should be taught to clean their injection equipment with household bleach before use. Finally, HIV PrEP is known to be underutilized with less than 20% of persons at risk for HIV in the United States prescribed PrEP and even lower rates among PWID.[182,183] Guidelines are available for prescribing and monitoring PrEP.[184] The CDC defines indications for PrEP in the sexually active adult as having an HIV-positive sexual partner, bacterial sexually transmitted infection in the prior 6 months, and/or inconsistent condom use with sexual partners in the context of anal or vaginal sex in last 6 months. Indication for PrEP among PWID include having an HIV-positive injecting partner, sharing injection equipment, or having sexual risk for acquiring HIV. The majority of PrEP studies have been done in cis-men with inclusion of trans-women related to sexual risk. Evidence for PrEP among PWID are limited to one study that found tenofovir disoproxil-fumarate was effective at reducing transmission.[185] Other options available for MSM and trans-women to prevent sexual transmission of HIV include tenofovir disoproxil-fumarate dosed on-demand, tenofovir alafenamide-emtricitabine dosed daily, and long-acting intramuscular injectable cabotegravir. Important features of PrEP prescribing include baseline HIV testing with an antigen/antibody test and consideration of HIV RNA testing, along with assessment of renal function, assessment for other STIs (syphilis, gonorrhea, and chlamydia), and hepatitis B and C. This testing should be repeated every 3 months while on PrEP. If HIV is acquired while on PrEP, it is important to convert the patient to a full ART regimen with drugs with expected activity in consultation with an HIV physician.

SEXUALLY TRANSMITTED DISEASES

The epidemiology, clinical features, diagnosis, and treatment of sexually transmitted infections other than HIV/AIDS have been reviewed extensively and treatment guidelines are available.[186] Though the prevalence is higher in people who use drugs (PWUD), the presentation, diagnosis, and management of most sexually transmitted diseases are not profoundly influenced by drug use. Methamphetamine, which can be used by PWUD (particularly MSM) to enhance the sexual experience, is associated with particularly high-risk sexual behavior (number of partners, lack of condom use) as well as acquisition of syphilis. Cases of syphilis in the United States were lowest from 2000 to 2001 but have steadily increased since that time. While MSM are disproportionately impacted, rates of primary and secondary syphilis among women also markedly increased from 2016 to 2020. Similarly, congenital syphilis cases have risen dramatically, mirroring the increase among women. Methamphetamine use, homelessness, and lack of prenatal care are commonly identified in these cases, suggesting the need for both increased screening and the need to address syndemics affecting vulnerable populations.

The clinician and patient should conduct a formal, ongoing review of STI risks.[187] Prevention messages should encourage safer sex, including the correct and consistent use of barrier protection. In selected patients, use of postexposure prophylaxis may be warranted.[184,188] There are a number of potential complications from sexually transmitted diseases and other infectious diseases that can affect the pregnant woman or her fetus. Pregnant women who use drugs should be screened according to standard protocols and aggressively treated to minimize negative maternal or fetal outcomes.

Because of the synergistic effect of cigarette smoke in the development of HPV-associated cancers, patients with diagnosed HPV should be strongly encouraged to consider smoking abstinence.

CONCLUSIONS

Identifying and treating infectious complications of substance use is important to the health of PWUD. Diagnosis, prevention, and treatment of these infections requires consideration of the patient's exposures, substance use, medical, and social issues. The social, cultural, and political determinants of health drive risks for infectious complications from substance use and structure disparities in access to and provision of clinical care for PWUD. Infectious complications are opportunities to establish a therapeutic alliance and engage PWUD in substance use treatment and other risk reduction strategies. Integrating care for infectious diseases and substance use disorder is essential to providing quality clinical care for individual PWUD and a promising approach to mitigating health inequalities at the population level.

REFERENCES

1. Brown PD, Levine DP. Infections in injection drug users. *Infect Dis Clin North Am.* 2002;16(3):xiii-xiv. doi:10.1016/S0891-5520(02)00021-1
2. Springer SA, del Rio C. Addressing the intersection of infectious disease epidemics and opioid and substance use epidemics. *Infect Dis Clin North Am.* 2020;34(3):xiii-xiv. doi:10.1016/J.IDC.2020.06.016
3. Larochelle MR, Bernstein R, Bernson D, et al. Touchpoints – opportunities to predict and prevent opioid overdose: a cohort study. *Drug Alcohol Depend.* 2019;204:107537. doi:10.1016/j.drugalcdep.2019.06.039
4. Springer SA, Korthuis PT, del Rio C. Integrating treatment at the intersection of opioid use disorder and infectious disease epidemics in medical settings: a call for action after a National Academies of Sciences, Engineering, and Medicine Workshop. *Ann Intern Med.* 2018;169(5):335-336. doi:10.7326/M18-1203
5. Dasgupta N, Beletsky L, Ciccarone D. Opioid crisis: no easy fix to its social and economic determinants. *Am J Public Health.* 2018;108(2):182-186. doi:10.2105/AJPH.2017.304187
6. Singer M, Bulled N, Ostrach B, Mendenhall E. Syndemics and the biosocial conception of health. *Lancet.* 2017;389(10072):941-950. doi:10.1016/S0140-6736(17)30003-X
7. Perlman DC, Jordan AE. The syndemic of opioid misuse, overdose, HCV, and HIV: structural-level causes and interventions. *Curr HIV/AIDS Rep.* 2018;15(2):96-112. doi:10.1007/s11904-018-0390-3
8. Alonzo NC, Bayer BM. Opioids, immunology, and host defenses of intravenous drug abusers. *Infect Dis Clin North Am.* 2002;16(3):553-569. doi:10.1016/S0891-5520(02)00018-1
9. Cohen AL, Shuler C, McAllister S, et al. Methamphetamine use and methicillin-resistant *Staphylococcus aureus* skin infections. *Emerg Infect Dis.* 2007;13(11):1707-1713. doi:10.3201/eid1311.070148
10. Friedman H, Newton C, Klein TW. Microbial infections, immunomodulation, and drugs of abuse. *Clin Microbiol Rev.* 2003;16(2):209-219. doi:10.1128/CMR.16.2.209-219.2003
11. Arcavi L, Benowitz NL. Cigarette smoking and infection. *Arch Intern Med.* 2004;164(20):2206-2216. doi:10.1001/archinte.164.20.2206
12. Moir S, MFA C. The immunology of human immunodeficiency virus infection. In: Bennett J, Dolin R, Blaser M, eds. *Mandell, Douglas, and Bennett's Principles and Practice of Infectious Diseases.* 8th ed. Saunders, Elsevier Inc; 2015:1526-1540.
13. Ciccarone D, Unick GJ, Cohen JK, Mars SG, Rosenblum D. Nationwide increase in hospitalizations for heroin-related soft tissue infections: associations with structural market conditions. *Drug Alcohol Depend.* 2016;163:126-133. doi:10.1016/j.drugalcdep.2016.04.009
14. Gordon RJ, Lowy FD. Bacterial infections in drug users. *N Engl J Med.* 2005;353(18):1945-1954. doi:10.1056/NEJMra042823
15. Stevens DL, Bisno AL, Chambers HF, et al. Executive summary: practice guidelines for the diagnosis and management of skin and soft tissue infections: 2014 update by the Infectious Diseases Society of America. *Clin Infect Dis.* 2014;59(2):147-159. doi:10.1093/cid/ciu444
16. Brook I, Frazier EH. Aerobic and anaerobic bacteriology of wounds and cutaneous abscesses. *Arch Surg.* 1990;125(11):1445-1451. doi:10.1001/archsurg.1990.01410230039007
17. Summanen PH, Talan DA, Strong C, et al. Bacteriology of skin and soft-tissue infections: comparison of infections in intravenous drug users and individuals with no history of intravenous drug use. *Clin Infect Dis.* 1995;20:S279-S282. doi:10.1093/clinids/20.Supplement_2.S279
18. Palmateer NE, Ramsay CN, Browning L, Goldberg DJ, Hutchinson SJ. Anthrax infection among heroin users in Scotland during 2009-2010: a case-control study by linkage to a national drug treatment database. *Clin Infect Dis.* 2012;55(5):706-710. doi:10.1093/cid/cis511
19. Holzmann T, Frangoulidis D, Simon M, et al. Fatal anthrax infection in a heroin user from southern Germany, June 2012. *Euro Surveill.* 2012;17(26):1-4.
20. Centers for Disease Control and Prevention (CDC). Unexplained illness and death among injecting-drug users—Glasgow, Scotland; Dublin, Ireland; and England, April-June 2000. *MMWR Morb Mortal Wkly Rep.* 2000;49(22):489-492.
21. Bangsberg DR, Rosen JL, Aragón T, Campbell A, Weir L, Perdreau-Remington F. Clostridial myonecrosis cluster among injection drug users: a molecular epidemiology investigation. *Arch Intern Med.* 2002;162(5):517-522. doi:10.1001/archinte.162.5.517
22. Allison DC, Miller T, Holtom P, Patzakis MJ, Zalavras CG. Microbiology of upper extremity soft tissue abscesses in injecting drug abusers. *Clin Orthop Relat Res.* 2007;461:9-13. doi:10.1097/BLO.0b013e31811f3526
23. Jackson KA, Bohm MK, Brooks JT, et al. Invasive methicillin-resistant *Staphylococcus aureus* infections among persons who inject drugs—six sites, 2005-2016. *MMWR Morb Mortal Wkly Rep.* 2018;67(22):625-628. doi:10.15585/mmwr.mm6722a2
24. Marks LR, Calix JJ, Wildenthal JA, et al. *Staphylococcus aureus* injection drug use-associated bloodstream infections are propagated by community outbreaks of diverse lineages. *Commun Med.* 2021;1(1):52. doi:10.1038/s43856-021-00053-9
25. Leibler JH, Liebschutz JM, Keosaian J, et al. Homelessness, personal hygiene, and MRSA nasal colonization among persons who inject drugs. *J Urban Health.* 2019;96(5):734-740. doi:10.1007/s11524-019-00379-9
26. Reyes JC, Negrón JL, Colón HM, et al. The emerging of xylazine as a new drug of abuse and its health consequences among drug users in Puerto Rico. *J Urban Health.* 2012;89(3):519-526. doi:10.1007/S11524-011-9662-6

27. Friedman J, Montero F, Bourgois P, et al. Xylazine spreads across the U.S.: a growing component of the increasingly synthetic and polysubstance overdose crisis. *Drug Alcohol Depend.* 2022;233. doi:10.1016/j.drugalcdep.2022.109380
28. Malayala SV, Papudesi BN, Bobb R, Wimbush A. Xylazine-induced skin ulcers in a person who injects drugs in Philadelphia, Pennsylvania, USA. *Cureus.* 2022;14(8). doi:10.7759/CUREUS.28160
29. Gupta R, Holtgrave DR, Ashburn MA. Xylazine—medical and public health imperatives. *N Engl J Med.* 2023;388(24):2209-2212. doi:10.1056/NEJMP2303120
30. Kovach S, Sherman SV. Xylazine-associated skin injury. *N Engl J Med.* 2023;388(24):2274-2274. doi:10.1056/NEJMICM2303601
31. NEXT Distro. *Xylazine Quick Guide for People Who Use Drugs.* Accessed June 30, 2023. https://nextdistro.org/resources-collection/xylazine-quick-guide
32. Grakyen Center for Addiction-Boston Medical Center, University of Pittsburgh. *Xylazine Wounds Handout.* Accessed June 30, 2023. https://www.addictiontraining.org/documents/resources/341_Xylazine_Wounds_Handout_-_English_Version_pocket_size.pdf
33. New York State Department of Health. *Xylazine: What Clinicians Need to Know.* Accessed June 30, 2023. https://www.health.ny.gov/publications/12044.pdf
34. Harris RE, Richardson J, Frasso R, Anderson ED. Experiences with skin and soft tissue infections among people who inject drugs in Philadelphia: a qualitative study. *Drug Alcohol Depend.* 2018;187:8-12. doi:10.1016/j.drugalcdep.2018.01.029
35. Summers PJ, Hellman JL, MacLean MR, Rees VW, Wilkes MS. Negative experiences of pain and withdrawal create barriers to abscess care for people who inject heroin. A mixed methods analysis. *Drug Alcohol Depend.* 2018;190:200-208. doi:10.1016/j.drugalcdep.2018.06.010
36. Monteiro J, Phillips KT, Herman DS, et al. Self-treatment of skin infections by people who inject drugs. *Drug Alcohol Depend.* 2020;206. doi:10.1016/j.drugalcdep.2019.107695
37. Biancarelli DL, Biello KB, Childs E, et al. Strategies used by people who inject drugs to avoid stigma in healthcare settings. *Drug Alcohol Depend.* 2019;198:80-86. doi:10.1016/j.drugalcdep.2019.01.037
38. Hsueh PR, Hsiue TR, Hsieh WC. Pyomyositis in intravenous drug abusers: report of a unique case and review of the literature. *Clin Infect Dis.* 1996;22(5):858-860. doi:10.1093/clinids/22.5.858
39. Arnold M, Woo ML, French GL. *Vibrio vulnificus* septicaemia presenting as spontaneous necrotising celluitis in a woman with hepatic cirrhosis. *Scand J Infect Dis.* 1989;21(6):727-731. doi:10.3109/00365548909021704
40. Wongpaitoon V, Sathapatayavongs B, Prachaktam R, Bunyaratvej S, Kurathong S. Spontaneous *Vibrio vulnificus* peritonitis and primary sepsis in two patients with alcoholic cirrhosis. *Am J Gastroenterol.* 1985;80(9):706-708.
41. Fernandes RM, Cary M, Duarte G, et al. Effectiveness of needle and syringe programmes in people who inject drugs—an overview of systematic reviews. *BMC Public Health.* 2017;17(1):309. doi:10.1186/s12889-017-4210-2
42. Taylor JL, Johnson S, Cruz R, Gray JR, Schiff D, Bagley SM. Integrating harm reduction into outpatient opioid use disorder treatment settings: harm reduction in outpatient addiction treatment. *J Gen Intern Med.* 2021;36(12):3810-3819. doi:10.1007/s11606-021-06904-4
43. Harvey L, Taylor JL, Assoumou SA, et al. Sexually transmitted and blood-borne infections among patients presenting to a low-barrier substance use disorder medication clinic. *J Addict Med.* 2021;15(6):461-467. doi:10.1097/ADM.0000000000000801
44. Weinstein ZM, Wakeman SE, Nolan S. Inpatient addiction consult service: expertise for hospitalized patients with complex addiction problems. *Med Clin North Am.* 2018;102(4):587-601. doi:10.1016/j.mcna.2018.03.001
45. Lee KC, Ladizinski B, Federman DG. Complications associated with use of levamisole-contaminated cocaine: an emerging public health challenge. *Mayo Clin Proc.* 2012;87(6):581-586. doi:10.1016/j.mayocp.2012.03.010
46. Saini T, Edwards PC, Kimmes NS, Carroll LR, Shaner JW, Dowd FJ. Etiology of xerostomia and dental caries among methamphetamine abusers. *Oral Health Prev Dent.* 2005;3(3):189-195.
47. Shaner JW, Kimmes N, Saini T, Edwards P. "Meth mouth": rampant caries in methamphetamine abusers. *AIDS Patient Care STDS.* 2006;20(3):146-150. doi:10.1089/apc.2006.20.146
48. Marshall BDL, Werb D. Health outcomes associated with methamphetamine use among young people: a systematic review. *Addiction.* 2010;105(6):991-1002. doi:10.1111/j.1360-0443.2010.02932.x
49. Wurcel AG, Anderson JE, KKH C, et al. Increasing infectious endocarditis admissions among young people who inject drugs. *Open Forum Infect Dis.* 2016;3(3):ofw157. doi:10.1093/ofid/ofw157
50. Schranz AJ, Fleischauer A, Chu VH, Wu LT, Rosen DL. Trends in drug use-associated infective endocarditis and heart valve surgery, 2007 to 2017: a study of statewide discharge data. *Ann Intern Med.* 2019;170(1):31-40. doi:10.7326/M18-2124
51. Deo SV, Raza S, Kalra A, et al. Admissions for infective endocarditis in intravenous drug users. *J Am Coll Cardiol.* 2018;71(14):1596-1597. doi:10.1016/j.jacc.2018.02.011
52. Baddour LM, Wilson WR, Bayer AS, et al. Infective endocarditis in adults: diagnosis, antimicrobial therapy, and management of complications: a scientific statement for healthcare professionals from the American Heart Association. *Circulation.* 2015;132(15):1435-1486. doi:10.1161/CIR.0000000000000296
53. Rodger L, Glockler-Lauf SD, Shojaei E, et al. Clinical characteristics and factors associated with mortality in first-episode infective endocarditis among persons who inject drugs. *JAMA Netw Open.* 2018;1(7):e185220. doi:10.1001/jamanetworkopen.2018.5220
54. Levine DP, Crane LR, Zervos MJ. Bacteremia in narcotic addicts at the detroit medical center. II. infectious endocarditis: a prospective comparative study. *Rev Infect Dis.* 1986;8(3):374-396. doi:10.1093/clinids/8.3.374
55. Shekar R, Rice TW, Zierdt CH, Kallick CA. Outbreak of endocarditis caused by pseudomonas aeruginosa serotype O11 among pentazocine and tripelennamine abusers in chicago. *J Infect Dis.* 1985;151(2):203-208. doi:10.1093/infdis/151.2.203
56. Mills J, Drew D. Serratia marcescens endocarditis: a regional illness associated with intravenous drug abuse. *Ann Intern Med.* 1976;84(1):29-35. doi:10.7326/0003-4819-84-1-29
57. Musher DM. Infections caused by streptococcus pneumoniae: clinical spectrum, pathogenesis, immunity, and treatment. *Clin Infect Dis.* 1992;14(4):801-807. doi:10.1093/clinids/14.4.801
58. Spach DH, Kanter AS, Daniels NA, et al. *Bartonella* (Rochalimaea) species as a cause of apparent "culture-negative" endocarditis. *Clin Infect Dis.* 1995;20(4):1044-1047. doi:10.1093/clinids/20.4.1044
59. Comer JA, Flynn C, Regnery RL, Vlahov D, Childs JE. Antibodies to *Bartonella* species in inner-city intravenous drug users in Baltimore. *Md. Arch Intern Med.* 1996;156(21):2491-2495.
60. Riancho JA, Echevarría S, Napal J, Martin Duran R, Gonzalez MJ. Endocarditis due to *Listeria* monocytogenes and human immunodeficiency virus infection. *Am J Med.* 1988;85(5):737. doi:10.1016/S0002-9343(88)80255-9
61. Bestetti RB, Figueiredo JF, Da Costa JC. *Salmonella* tricuspid endocarditis in an intravenous drug abuser with human immunodeficiency virus infection. *Int J Cardiol.* 1991;30(3):361-362. doi:10.1016/0167-5273(91)90019-L
62. Steen MK, Bruno-Murtha LA, Chaux G, Lazar H, Bernard S, Sulis C. *Bacillus cereus* endocarditis: report of a case and review. *Clin Infect Dis.* 1992;14(4):945-946. doi:10.1093/clinids/14.4.945
63. Chung-Esaki H, Rodriguez RM, Alter H, Cisse B. Validation of a prediction rule for endocarditis in febrile injection drug users. *Am J Emerg Med.* 2014;32(5):412-416. doi:10.1016/J.AJEM.2014.01.008
64. Durack DT, Lukes AS, Bright DK. Duke Endocarditis Service. New criteria for diagnosis of infective endocarditis: utilization of specific echocardiographic findings. *Am J Med.* 1994;96(3):200-209. doi:10.1016/0002-9343(94)90143-0
65. Bayer AS, Ward JI, Ginzton LE, Shapiro SM. Evaluation of new clinical criteria for the diagnosis of infective endocarditis. *Am J Med.* 1994;96(3):211-219. doi:10.1016/0002-9343(94)90144-9
66. Li JS, Sexton DJ, Mick N, et al. Proposed modifications to the Duke criteria for the diagnosis of infective endocarditis. *Clin Infect Dis.* 2000;30(4):633-638. doi:10.1086/313753

67. Wilson WR, Karchmer AW, Dajani AS, et al. Antibiotic treatment of adults with infective endocarditis due to streptococci, enterococci, staphylococci, and HACEK microorganisms. *American Heart Association. JAMA.* 1995;274(21):1706-1713.
68. Siegrist EA, Wungwattana M, Azis L, Stogsdill P, Craig WY, Rokas KE. Limited clinical utility of follow-up blood cultures in patients with streptococcal bacteremia: an opportunity for blood culture stewardship. *Open Forum Infect Dis.* 2020;7(12):1-5. doi:10.1093/OFID/OFAA541
69. Carugati M, Bayer AS, Miró JM, et al. High-dose daptomycin therapy for left-sided infective endocarditis: a prospective study from the international collaboration on endocarditis. *Antimicrob Agents Chemother.* 2013;57(12):6213. doi:10.1128/AAC.01563-13
70. Kimmel SD, Walley AY, Li Y, et al. Association of treatment with medications for opioid use disorder with mortality after hospitalization for injection drug use-associated infective endocarditis. *JAMA Netw Open.* 2020;3(10):e2016228. doi:10.1001/jamanetworkopen.2020.16228
71. Barocas JA, Morgan JR, Wang J, McLoone D, Wurcel A, Stein MD. Outcomes associated with medications for opioid use disorder among persons hospitalized for infective endocarditis. *Clin Infect Dis.* 2021;72(3):472-478. doi:10.1093/cid/ciaa062
72. Kim JH, Fine DR, Li L, et al. Disparities in United States hospitalizations for serious infections in patients with and without opioid use disorder: a nationwide observational study. *PLoS Med.* 2020;17(8):e1003247. doi:10.1371/JOURNAL.PMED.1003247
73. Kimmel SD, Rosenmoss S, Bearnot B, et al. Northeast postacute medical facilities disproportionately reject referrals for patients with opioid use disorder. *Health Aff (Millwood).* 2022;41(3):434-444. doi:10.1377/HLTHAFF.2021.01242
74. Simon R, Snow R, Wakeman S. Understanding why patients with substance use disorders leave the hospital against medical advice: a qualitative study. *Subst Abus.* 2020;41(4):519-525. doi:10.1080/08897077.2019.1671942
75. Bearnot B, Mitton JA, Hayden M, Park ER. Experiences of care among individuals with opioid use disorder-associated endocarditis and their healthcare providers: results from a qualitative study. *J Subst Abuse Treat.* 2019;102:16-22. doi:10.1016/j.jsat.2019.04.008
76. Kimmel SD, Kim JH, Kalesan B, Samet JH, Walley AY, Larochelle MR. Against medical advice discharges in injection and non-injection drug use-associated infective endocarditis: a nationwide cohort study. *Clin Infect Dis.* 2021;73(9):E2484-E2492. doi:10.1093/cid/ciaa1126
77. Suzuki J, Johnson J, Montgomery M, Hayden M, Price C. Outpatient parenteral antimicrobial therapy among people who inject drugs: a review of the literature. *Open Forum Infect Dis.* 2018;5(9). doi:10.1093/ofid/ofy194
78. Adams JW, Savinkina A, Hudspeth JC, et al. Simulated cost-effectiveness and long-term clinical outcomes of addiction care and antibiotic therapy strategies for patients with injection drug use–associated infective endocarditis. *JAMA Netw Open.* 2022;5(2):e220541-e220541. doi:10.1001/JAMANETWORKOPEN.2022.0541
79. Iversen K, Ihlemann N, Gill SU, et al. Partial oral versus intravenous antibiotic treatment of endocarditis. *N Engl J Med.* 2019;380(5):415-424. doi:10.1056/NEJMoa1808312
80. Marks LR, Liang SY, Muthulingam D, et al. Evaluation of partial oral antibiotic treatment for persons who inject drugs and are hospitalized with invasive infections. *Clin Infect Dis.* 2020;71(10):E650-E656. doi:10.1093/cid/ciaa365
81. Morrisette T, Miller MA, Montague BT, Barber GR, RB MQ, Krsak M. Long-acting lipoglycopeptides: "lineless antibiotics" for serious infections in persons who use drugs. *Open Forum Infect Dis.* 2019;6(7). doi:10.1093/ofid/ofz274
82. Kinney EM, Vijapurapu S, Covvey JR, Nemecek BD. Clinical outcomes of concomitant rifamycin and opioid therapy: a systematic review. *Pharmacother J Hum Pharmacol Drug Ther.* 2021;41(5):479-489. doi:10.1002/PHAR.2520
83. Kaura A, Byrne J, Fife A, et al. Inception of the 'endocarditis team' is associated with improved survival in patients with infective endocarditis who are managed medically: findings from a before-and-after study. *Open Hear.* 2017;4(2):e000699. doi:10.1136/openhrt-2017-000699
84. Yucel E, Bearnot B, Paras ML, et al. Diagnosis and management of infective endocarditis in people who inject drugs: JACC state-of-the-art review. *J Am Coll Cardiol.* 2022;79(20):2037-2057. doi:10.1016/J.JACC.2022.03.349
85. Islam S, Piggott DA, Moriggia A, et al. Reducing injection intensity is associated with decreased risk for invasive bacterial infection among high-frequency injection drug users. *Harm Reduct J.* 2019;16(1):38. doi:10.1186/s12954-019-0312-8
86. Wilson W, Taubert KA, Gewitz M, et al. Prevention of infective endocarditis: guidelines from the American Heart Association. *Circulation.* 2007;116(15):1736-1754. doi:10.1161/CIRCULATIONAHA.106.183095
87. Moss M, Parsons PE, Steinberg KP, et al. Chronic alcohol abuse is associated with an increased incidence of acute respiratory distress syndrome and severity of multiple organ dysfunction in patients with septic shock. *Crit Care Med.* 2003;31(3):869-877. doi:10.1097/01.CCM.0000055389.64497.11
88. O'Brien JM, Lu B, Ali NA, et al. Alcohol dependence is independently associated with sepsis, septic shock, and hospital mortality among adult intensive care unit patients. *Crit Care Med.* 2007;35(2):345-350. doi:10.1097/01.CCM.0000254340.91644.B2
89. Caiaffa WT, Vlahov D, Graham NM, et al. Drug smoking, *Pneumocystis carinii* pneumonia, and immunosuppression increase risk of bacterial pneumonia in human immunodeficiency virus-seropositive injection drug users. *Am J Respir Crit Care Med.* 1994;150(6 Pt 1):1493-1498. doi:10.1164/ajrccm.150.6.7952605
90. Wewers MD, Diaz PT, Wewers ME, Lowe MP, Nagaraja HN, Clanton TL. Cigarette smoking in HIV infection induces a suppressive inflammatory environment in the lung. *Am J Respir Crit Care Med.* 1998;158(5 Pt 1):1543-1549. doi:10.1164/ajrccm.158.5.9802035
91. Bartlett JG, Gorbach SL, Finegold SM. The bacteriology of aspiration pneumonia. *Am J Med.* 1974;56(2):202-207. doi:10.1016/0002-9343(74)90598-1
92. O'Donnell AE, Pappas LS. Pulmonary complications of intravenous drug abuse. Experience at an inner-city hospital. *Chest.* 1988;94(2):251-253. doi:10.1378/chest.94.2.251
93. Bailey ME, Fraire AE, Greenberg SD, Barnard J, Cagle PT. Pulmonary histopathology in cocaine abusers. *Hum Pathol.* 1994;25(2):203-207. doi:10.1016/0046-8177(94)90279-8
94. Edelman EJ, Gordon KS, Crothers K, et al. Association of prescribed opioids with increased risk of community-acquired pneumonia among patients with and without HIV. *JAMA Intern Med.* 2019;179(3):297-304. doi:10.1001/JAMAINTERNMED.2018.6101
95. Goss CH, Rubenfeld GD, Park DR, Sherbin VL, Goodman MS, Root RK. Cost and incidence of social comorbidities in low-risk patients with community-acquired pneumonia admitted to a public hospital. *Chest.* 2003;124(6):2148-2155. doi:10.1378/chest.124.6.2148
96. de Roux A, Cavalcanti M, Marcos MA, et al. Impact of alcohol abuse in the etiology and severity of community-acquired pneumonia. *Chest.* 2006;129(5):1219-1225. doi:10.1378/chest.129.5.1219
97. Metlay JP, Waterer GW, Long AC, et al. Diagnosis and treatment of adults with community-acquired pneumonia. *Am J Respir Crit Care Med.* 2019;200(7):E45-E67. doi:10.1164/rccm.201908-1581ST
98. O'Grady NP, Barie PS, Bartlett JG, et al. Guidelines for evaluation of new fever in critically ill adult patients: 2008 update from the American College of Critical Care Medicine and the Infectious Diseases Society of America. *Crit Care Med.* 2008;36(4):1330-1349. doi:10.1097/CCM.0b013e318169eda9
99. Centers for Disease Control. *Healthcare Workers: Information on COVID-19.* Accessed May 26, 2022. https://www.cdc.gov/coronavirus/2019-nCoV/hcp/index.html
100. Khanijahani A, Iezadi S, Gholipour K, Azami-Aghdash S, Naghibi D. A systematic review of racial/ethnic and socioeconomic disparities in COVID-19. *Int J Equity Health.* 2021;20(1):248. doi:10.1186/s12939-021-01582-4
101. Lin Q, Paykin S, Halpern D, Martinez-Cardoso A, Kolak M. Assessment of structural barriers and racial group disparities of COVID-19 mortality with spatial analysis. *JAMA Netw Open.* 2022;5(3):e220984. doi:10.1001/jamanetworkopen.2022.0984

102. COVID-19 Cumulative Infection Collaborators. Estimating global, regional, and national daily and cumulative infections with SARS-CoV-2 through Nov 14, 2021: a statistical analysis. *Lancet (London, England).* 2022;399(10344):2351-2380. doi:10.1016/S0140-6736(22)00484-6
103. World Health Organization. *Coronavirus disease (COVID-19) Weekly Epidemiological Updates and Monthly Operational Updates.* Accessed May 26, 2022. https://www.who.int/emergencies/diseases/novel-coronavirus-2019/situation-reports
104. Bull-Otterson L, Baca S, Saydah S, et al. Post-COVID conditions among adult COVID-19 survivors aged 18-64 and ≥ 65 years—United States, March 2020-November 2021. *Morb Mortal Wkly Rep.* 2022;71(21):713.
105. Huang L, Li X, Gu X, et al. Health outcomes in people 2 years after surviving hospitalisation with COVID-19: a longitudinal cohort study. *Lancet Respir Med.* 2022;1(9):863-876. doi:10.1016/S2213-2600(22)00126-6
106. Su Y, Yuan D, Chen DG, et al. Multiple early factors anticipate post-acute COVID-19 sequelae. *Cell.* 2022;185(5):881-895.e20. doi:10.1016/j.cell.2022.01.014
107. Centers for Disease Control and Prevention. *Use of COVID-19 Vaccines in the United States.* Accessed May 26, 2022. https://www.cdc.gov/vaccines/covid-19/clinical-considerations/covid-19-vaccines-us.html
108. Wang L, Wang Q, Davis PB, Volkow ND, Xu R. Increased risk for COVID-19 breakthrough infection in fully vaccinated patients with substance use disorders in the United States between December 2020 and August 2021. *World Psychiatry.* 2022;21(1):124-132. doi:10.1002/wps.20921
109. White AM, Castle IJP, Powell PA, Hingson RW, Koob GF. Alcohol-related deaths during the COVID-19 pandemic. *JAMA.* 2022;327(17):1704-1706. doi:10.1001/jama.2022.4308
110. Ahmad F, Rossen L. Sutton P. *Provisional Drug Overdose Death Counts.* Accessed June 1, 2022. https://www.cdc.gov/nchs/nvss/vsrr/drug-overdose-data.htm
111. Mancuso JD, Diffenderfer JM, Ghassemieh BJ, Horne DJ, Kao TC. The prevalence of latent tuberculosis infection in the United States. *Am J Respir Crit Care Med.* 2016;194(4):501-509. doi:10.1164/rccm.201508-1683OC
112. Dunlap NE, Bass J, Fujiwara P, et al. Diagnostic standards and classification of tuberculosis in adults and children. *Am J Respir Crit Care Med.* 2000;161(4 I):1376-1395. doi:10.1164/ajrccm.161.4.16141
113. Reichman LB, Felton CP, Edsall JR. Drug dependence, a possible new risk factor for tuberculosis disease. *Arch Intern Med.* 1979;139(3):337-339.
114. Perlman DC, Salomon N, Perkins MP, Yancovitz S, Paone D, Des Jarlais DC. Tuberculosis in drug users. *Clin Infect Dis.* 1995;21(5):1253-1264. doi:10.1093/clinids/21.5.1253
115. Frieden TR, Sterling T, Pablos-Mendez A, Kilburn JO, Cauthen GM, Dooley SW. The emergence of drug-resistant tuberculosis in New York City. *N Engl J Med.* 1993;328(8):521-526. doi:10.1056/NEJM199302253280801
116. Gordin FM, Nelson ET, Matts JP, et al. The impact of human immunodeficiency virus infection on drug-resistant tuberculosis. *Am J Respir Crit Care Med.* 1996;154(5):1478-1483. doi:10.1164/ajrccm.154.5.8912768
117. Centers for Disease Control and Prevention (CDC). *Targeted Tuberculin Testing and Treatment of Latent Tuberculosis Infection.* American Thoracic Society. MMWR Recommendations and reports. Accessed December 2, 2022. https://www.cdc.gov/mmwr/preview/mmwrhtml/rr4906a1.htm
118. Taylor Z, Nolan CM, Blumberg HM. Controlling tuberculosis in the United States. Recommendations from the American Thoracic Society, CDC, and the Infectious Diseases Society of America. Accessed December 2, 2022. https://www.cdc.gov/mmwr/preview/mmwrhtml/rr5412a1.htm
119. National Society of Tuberculosis Clinicians and National, Tuberculosis Controllers Association. *Testing and Treatment of Latent Tuberculosis Infection in the United States: Clinical Recommendations.* Accessed December 2, 2022. https://www.tbcontrollers.org/resources/tb-infection/clinical-recommendations/
120. Batki SL, Gruber VA, Bradley JM, Bradley M, Delucchi K. A controlled trial of methadone treatment combined with directly observed isoniazid for tuberculosis prevention in injection drug users. *Drug Alcohol Depend.* 2002;66(3):283-293. doi:10.1016/S0376-8716(01)00208-3
121. Gourevitch MN, Wasserman W, Panero MS, Selwyn PA. Successful adherence to observed prophylaxis and treatment of tuberculosis among drug users in a methadone program. *J Addict Dis.* 1996;15(1):93-104. doi:10.1300/J069V15N01_07
122. Getahun H, Matteelli A, Abubakar I, et al. Management of latent *Mycobacterium tuberculosis* infection: WHO guidelines for low tuberculosis burden countries. *Eur Respir J.* 2015;46(6):1563-1576. doi:10.1183/13993003.01245-2015
123. Grohskopf LA, Blanton LH, Ferdinands JM, et al. Prevention and control of seasonal influenza with vaccines: recommendations of the Advisory Committee on Immunization Practices—United States, 2022-23 influenza season. *MMWR Recomm Rep.* 2022;71(1):1-28. doi:10.15585/mmwr.rr7101a1
124. Kobayashi M, Farrar JL, Gierke R, et al. Use of 15-valent pneumococcal conjugate vaccine and 20-valent pneumococcal conjugate vaccine among U.S. adults: updated recommendations of the Advisory Committee on Immunization Practices—United States, 2022. *MMWR Morb Mortal Wkly Rep.* 2022;71(4):109-117. doi:10.15585/mmwr.mm7104a1
125. Such J, Runyon BA. Spontaneous bacterial peritonitis. *Clin Infect Dis.* 1998;27(4):669-674. doi:10.1086/514940
126. Runyon BA, Montano AA, Akriviadis EA, Antillon MR, Irving MA, McHutchison JG. The serum-ascites albumin gradient is superior to the exudate-transudate concept in the differential diagnosis of ascites. *Ann Intern Med.* 1992;117(3):215-220. doi:10.7326/0003-4819-117-3-215
127. Salerno F, Navickis RJ, Wilkes MM. Albumin infusion improves outcomes of patients with spontaneous bacterial peritonitis: a meta-analysis of randomized trials. *Clin Gastroenterol Hepatol.* 2013;11(2):123-30.e1. doi:10.1016/j.cgh.2012.11.007
128. Sapico FL, Montgomerie JZ. Vertebral osteomyelitis in intravenous drug abusers: report of three cases and review of the literature. *Rev Infect Dis.* 1980;2(2):196-206. doi:10.1093/clinids/2.2.196
129. Lew DP, Waldvogel FA. Osteomyelitis. *Lancet.* 2004;364(9431):369-379. doi:10.1016/S0140-6736(04)16727-5
130. Rao N, Ziran BH, Lipsky BA. Treating osteomyelitis: antibiotics and surgery. *Plast Reconstr Surg.* 2011;127(Suppl):177S-187S. doi:10.1097/PRS.0b013e3182001f0f
131. Li HK, Rombach I, Zambellas R, et al. Oral versus intravenous antibiotics for bone and joint infection. *N Engl J Med.* 2019;380(5):425-436. doi:10.1056/NEJMoa1710926
132. Ross JJ, Shamsuddin H. Sternoclavicular septic arthritis: review of 180 cases. *Medicine (Baltimore).* 2004;83(3):139-148. doi:10.1097/01.md.0000126761.83417.29
133. Chandrasekar PH, Narula AP. Bone and joint infections in intravenous drug abusers. *Rev Infect Dis.* 1986;8(6):904-911. doi:10.1093/clinids/8.6.904
134. Ross JJ, Hu LT. Septic arthritis of the pubic symphysis: review of 100 cases. *Medicine (Baltimore).* 2003;82(5):340-345. doi:10.1097/01.md.0000091180.93122.1c
135. Tunkel AR, Pradhan SK. Central nervous system infections in injection drug users. *Infect Dis Clin North Am.* 2002;16(3):589-605. doi:10.1016/s0891-5520(02)00015-6
136. Carneiro TS, Awtry E, Dobrilovic N, et al. Neurological complications of endocarditis: a multidisciplinary review with focus on surgical decision making. *Semin Neurol.* 2019;39(04):495-506. doi:10.1055/s-0039-1688826
137. Darouiche RO. Spinal epidural abscess. *N Engl J Med.* 2006;355(19):2012-2020. doi:10.1056/NEJMra055111
138. Centers for Disease Control and Prevention (CDC). Symptomatic early neurosyphilis among HIV-positive men who have sex with men—four cities, United States, January 2002-June 2004. *MMWR Morb Mortal Wkly Rep.* 2007;56(25):625-628.
139. Rao AK, Sobel J, Chatham-Stephens K, Luquez C. Clinical Guidelines for Diagnosis and Treatment of Botulism, 2021. *MMWR Recomm Reports.* 2021;70(2):1-36. doi:10.15585/mmwr.rr7002a1
140. Edwards LD, Gomez I, Wada S, et al. Notes from the field: wound botulism outbreak among a group of persons who inject drugs—Dallas,

Texas, 2020. *MMWR Morb Mortal Wkly Rep.* 2022;71(15):556-557. doi:10.15585/mmwr.mm7115a3

141. Kudrow DB, Henry DA, Haake DA, Marshall G, Mathisen GE. Botulism associated with *Clostridium botulinum* sinusitis after intranasal cocaine abuse. *Ann Intern Med.* 1988;109(12):984-985. doi:10.7326/0003-4819-109-12-984
142. Cherubin CE. Clinical severity of tetanus in narcotic addicts in New York City. *Arch Intern Med.* 1968;121(2):156-158.
143. Blain A, Tiwari TSP. Tetanus. In: Roush SW, Baldy LM, MAK H, eds. *Manual for the Surveillance of Vaccine-Preventable Diseases.* Centers for Disease Control and Prevention and Department of Health and Human Services; 2020. Accessed July 7, 2023. https://www.cdc.gov/vaccines/pubs/surv-manual/chpt16-tetanus.html
144. Bisbe J, Miro JM, Latorre X, et al. Disseminated candidiasis in addicts who use brown heroin: report of 83 cases and review. *Clin Infect Dis an Off Publ Infect Dis Soc Am.* 1992;15(6):910-923. doi:10.1093/clind/15.6.910
145. Usmani B, Latif A, Amarasekera S, et al. Eye-related emergency department visits and the opioid epidemic: a 10-year analysis. *Ophthalmic Epidemiol.* 2020;27(4):300-309. doi:10.1080/09286586.2020.1744165
146. Kim RW, Juzych MS, Eliott D. Ocular manifestations of injection drug use. *Infect Dis Clin North Am.* 2002;16(3):607-622. doi:10.1016/s0891-5520(02)00013-2
147. Centers for Disease Control. Pneumocystis pneumonia—Los Angeles. *MMWR Morb Mortal Wkly Rep.* 1981;30(21):250-252.
148. Centers for Disease Control. Kaposi's sarcoma and *Pneumocystis* pneumonia among homosexual men—New York City and California. *MMWR Morb Mortal Wkly Rep.* 1981;30(25):305-308.
149. Centers for Disease Control and Prevention (CDC). *HIV Surveillance Report*, 2020. Accessed July 7, 2023. https://www.cdc.gov/hiv/library/reports/hiv-surveillance.html
150. Panel on Antiretroviral Guidelines for Adults and Adolescents. *Guidelines for the Use of Antiretroviral Agents in Adults and Adolescents with HIV.* Department of Health and Human Services. Accessed July 7, 2023. https://clinicalinfo.hiv.gov/en/guidelines/hiv-clinical-guidelines-adult-and-adolescent-arv/whats-new-guidelines
151. Panel on Treatment of HIV During Pregnancy and Prevention of Perinatal Transmission. *Recommendations for the Use of Antiretroviral Drugs During Pregnancy and Interventions to Reduce Perinatal HIV Transmission in the United States.* Department of Health and Human Services; 2023. Accessed October 5, 2023. https://clinicalinfo.hiv.gov/en/guidelines/perinatal
152. Panel on Guidelines for the Prevention and Treatment of Opportunistic Infections in Adults and Adolescents with HIV. *Guidelines for the Prevention and Treatment of Opportunistic Infections in Adults and Adolescents with HIV.* National Institutes of Health, Centers for Disease Control and Prevention, the HIV Medicine Association, and the Infectious Disease Society of America; 2022. Accessed July 7, 2023. https://clinicalinfo.hiv.gov/en/guidelines/hiv-clinical-guidelines-adult-and-adolescent-opportunistic-infections/whats-new
153. Centers for Disease Control and Prevention. *Estimated HIV Incidence and Prevalence in the United States, 2015-2019.* Vol. 26; 2021. Accessed July 7, 2023. https://www.cdc.gov/hiv/pdf/library/reports/surveillance/cdc-hiv-surveillance-supplemental-report-vol-26-1.pdf
154. Mitsch AJ, Hall HI, Babu AS. Trends in HIV infection among persons who inject drugs: United States and Puerto Rico, 2008-2013. *Am J Public Health.* 2016;106(12):2194-2201. doi:10.2105/AJPH.2016.303380
155. Wejnert C, Hess KL, Hall HI, et al. Vital signs: trends in hiv diagnoses, risk behaviors, and prevention among persons who inject drugs—United States. *MMWR Morb Mortal Wkly Rep.* 2016;65(47):1336-1342. doi:10.15585/mmwr.mm6547e1
156. Peters PJ, Pontones P, Hoover KW, et al. HIV infection linked to injection use of oxymorphone in Indiana, 2014-2015. *N Engl J Med.* 2016;375(3):229-239. doi:10.1056/nejmoa1515195
157. McAuley A, Palmateer NE, Goldberg DJ, et al. Re-emergence of HIV related to injecting drug use despite a comprehensive harm reduction environment: a cross-sectional analysis. *Lancet HIV.* 2019;6(5):e315-e324. doi:10.1016/S2352-3018(19)30036-0
158. Lyss SB, Zhang T, Oster AM. Brief report: HIV diagnoses among persons who inject drugs by the urban-rural classification—United States, 2010-2018. *J Acquir Immune Defic Syndr.* 2021;88(3):238-242. doi:10.1097/QAI.0000000000002769
159. Evans ME, Labuda SM, Hogan V, et al. *Notes from the Field*: HIV infection investigation in a rural area—West Virginia, 2017. *MMWR Morb Mortal Wkly Rep.* 2018;67(8):257-258. doi:10.15585/mmwr.mm6708a6
160. Alpren C, Dawson EL, John B, et al. Opioid use fueling HIV transmission in an urban setting: an outbreak of HIV infection among people who inject drugs-Massachusetts, 2015-2018. *Am J Public Health.* 2020;110(1):37-44. doi:10.2105/AJPH.2019.305366
161. Kahn JO, Walker BD. Acute human immunodeficiency virus type 1 infection. *N Engl J Med.* 1998;339(1):33-39. doi:10.1056/NEJM199807023390107
162. Centers for Disease Control and Prevention. *Monitoring Selected National HIV Prevention and Care Objectives by Using HIV Surveillance Data.* Vol. 23. Accessed July 7, 2023. https://www.cdc.gov/hiv/pdf/library/reports/surveillance/cdc-hiv-surveillance-supplemental-report-vol-23-4.pdf
163. Branson BM, Handsfield HH, Lampe MA, et al. Revised recommendations for HIV testing of adults, adolescents, and pregnant women in health-care settings. *MMWR Recomm Rep.* 2006;55(RR-14):1-17.
164. Centers for Disease Control and Prevention and Association of Public Health Laboratories. *Laboratory Testing for the Diagnosis of HIV Infection: Updated Recommendations*; 2014. doi:10.15620/cdc.23447
165. Delaney KP, Hanson DL, Masciotra S, Ethridge SF, Wesolowski L, Owen SM. Time until emergence of HIV test reactivity following infection with HIV-1: implications for interpreting test results and retesting after exposure. *Clin Infect Dis.* 2017;64(1):53-59. doi:10.1093/CID/CIW666
166. Parker MM, Bennett SB, Sullivan TJ, et al. Performance of the Alere Determine™ HIV-1/2 Ag/Ab Combo Rapid Test with algorithm-defined acute HIV-1 infection specimens. *J Clin Virol.* 2018;104:89-91. doi:10.1016/J.JCV.2018.05.005
167. Stekler JD, Ure G, O'Neal JD, et al. Performance of Determine Combo and other point-of-care HIV tests among Seattle MSM. *J Clin Virol.* 2016;76:8-13. doi:10.1016/J.JCV.2015.12.011
168. Centers for Disease Control and Prevention. *2018 Quick Reference Guide: Recommended Laboratory HIV Testing Algorithm for Serum or Plasma Specimens.* Accessed August 8, 2022. https://stacks.cdc.gov/view/cdc/50872
169. Smith DK, Switzer WM, Peters P, et al. A strategy for PrEP clinicians to manage ambiguous HIV test results during follow-up visits. *Open Forum Infect Dis.* 2018;5(8). doi:10.1093/OFID/OFY180
170. Aberg JA, Gallant JE, Ghanem KG, Emmanuel P, Zingman BS, Horberg MA. Executive summary: primary care guidelines for the management of persons infected with HIV: 2013 update by the HIV Medicine Association of the Infectious Diseases Society of America. *Clin Infect Dis.* 2014;58(1):1-10. doi:10.1093/cid/cit757
171. Mcnamara KF, Biondi BE, Hernández-Ramírez RU, Taweh N, Grimshaw AA, Springer SA. A Systematic review and meta-analysis of studies evaluating the effect of medication treatment for opioid use disorder on infectious disease outcomes. *Open Forum Infect Dis.* 2021;8(8). doi:10.1093/OFID/OFAB289
172. Altice FL, Bruce RD, Lucas GM, et al. HIV treatment outcomes among HIV-infected, opioid-dependent patients receiving buprenorphine/naloxone treatment within HIV clinical care settings: results from a multisite study. *J Acquir Immune Defic Syndr.* 2011;56(Suppl 1). doi:10.1097/QAI.0B013E318209751E
173. Berg KM, Litwin A, Li X, Heo M, Arnsten JH. Directly observed antiretroviral therapy improves adherence and viral load in drug users attending methadone maintenance clinics: a randomized controlled trial. *Drug Alcohol Depend.* 2011;113(2-3):192-199. doi:10.1016/J.DRUGALCDEP.2010.07.025
174. Lappalainen L, Nolan S, Dobrer S, et al. Dose-response relationship between methadone dose and adherence to antiretroviral therapy among HIV-positive people who use illicit opioids. *Addiction.* 2015;110(8):1330-1339. doi:10.1111/ADD.12970
175. Lucas GM, Chaudhry A, Hsu J, et al. Clinic-based treatment of opioid-dependent HIV-infected patients versus referral to an opioid treatment

program: a randomized trial. *Ann Intern Med.* 2010;152(11):704-711. doi:10.7326/0003-4819-152-11-201006010-00003

176. Oldfield BJ, Munõz N, McGovern MP, et al. Integration of care for HIV and opioid use disorder. *AIDS.* 2019;33(5):873-884. doi:10.1097/QAD.0000000000002125
177. Schiffer JT, Sterling TR. Timing of antiretroviral therapy initiation in tuberculosis patients with AIDS: a decision analysis. *J Acquir Immune Defic Syndr.* 2007;44(2):229-234. doi:10.1097/QAI.0b013e31802e2975
178. McIlleron H, Meintjes G, Burman WJ, Maartens G. Complications of antiretroviral therapy in patients with tuberculosis: drug interactions, toxicity, and immune reconstitution inflammatory syndrome. *J Infect Dis.* 2007;196(Suppl):S63-S75. doi:10.1086/518655
179. Freedman MS, Ault K, Bernstein H. Advisory Committee on Immunization Practices recommended immunization schedule for adults aged 19 Years or older—United States, 2021. *MMWR Morb Mortal Wkly Rep.* 2021;70(6):193-196. doi:10.15585/mmwr.mm7006a2
180. Centers for Disease Control and Prevention. *Vaccination Information for Adults.* Accessed December 2, 2022. https://www.cdc.gov/vaccines/adults/rec-vac/health-conditions/hiv.html
181. Mansergh G, Purcell DW, Stall R, et al. CDC consultation on methamphetamine use and sexual risk behavior for HIV/STD infection: summary and suggestions. *Public Health Rep.* 2006;121(2):127-132. doi:10.1177/003335490612100205
182. Harris NS, Johnson AS, Huang YLA, et al. Vital signs: status of human immunodeficiency virus testing, viral suppression, and HIV preexposure prophylaxis—United States, 2013-2018. *MMWR Morb Mortal Wkly Rep.* 2019;68(48):1117-1123. doi:10.15585/mmwr.mm6848e1
183. Streed CG, Morgan JR, Gai MJ, Larochelle MR, Paasche-Orlow MK, Taylor JL. Prevalence of HIV preexposure prophylaxis prescribing among persons with commercial insurance and likely injection drug use. *JAMA Netw Open.* 2022;5(7):e2221346. doi:10.1001/JAMANETWORKOPEN.2022.21346
184. Centers for Disease Control and Prevention. U.S. Public Health Service. *Preexposure Prophylaxis for the Prevention of HIV Infection in the United States—2021 Update: A Clinical Practice Guideline.* Accessed July 7, 2023. https://www.cdc.gov/hiv/pdf/risk/prep/cdc-hiv-prep-guidelines-2021.pdf
185. Choopanya K, Martin M, Suntharasamai P, et al. Antiretroviral prophylaxis for HIV infection in injecting drug users in Bangkok, Thailand (the Bangkok Tenofovir Study): A randomized, double-blind, placebo-controlled phase 3 trial. *Lancet.* 2013;381:2083-2090.
186. Workowski KA, Bachmann LH, Chan PA, et al. Sexually transmitted infections treatment guidelines, 2021. *MMWR Recomm Rep.* 2021;70(4):1-187. Accessed August 8, 2022. www.cdc.gov/std/treatment-guidelines/STI-Guidelines-2021.pdf
187. Centers for Disease Control and Prevention (CDC). Integrated prevention services for HIV infection, viral hepatitis, sexually transmitted diseases, and tuberculosis for persons who use drugs illicitly: summary guidance from CDC and the U.S. Department of Health and Human Services. *MMWR Recomm Rep.* 2012;61(RR-5):1-40.
188. Updated Guidelines for Antiretroviral Postexposure Prophylaxis after Sexual, Injection-Drug Use, or Other Nonoccupational Exposure to HIV—United States, 2016. *MMWR Morb Mortal Wkly Rep.* 2016;65(17):458. doi:10.15585/mmwr.mm6517a5

CHAPTER

95

Sleep Disorders Related to Substance Use

Sanford Auerbach

CHAPTER OUTLINE

- Introduction
- Overview of sleep
- Disorders of sleep
- Alcohol and sleep
- Specific sleep disorders associated with alcohol use disorder
- Other drugs and sleep
- Clinical approaches to sleep disorders
- Special issues in sleep pharmacotherapy and addiction

INTRODUCTION

Sleep is a complex physiological state that is essential for normal function throughout the day. Despite its critical role, sleep appears to be quite fragile. About 35% of all adults report insomnia at some point during the preceding 6 months, and half describe it as serious.[1] Given the influence of alcohol and other drugs on sleep, sleep problems are likely to be more prevalent in persons with substance use disorder (SUD).

The coexistence of a sleep disorder with SUD is a complex problem. For example, alcohol consumption can affect "normal sleep" in people without alcohol problems, whereas the patient with alcohol use disorder (AUD) has disrupted sleep while using alcohol and withdrawing from alcohol. Alcohol also has an effect on other sleep-related disorders, particularly obstructive sleep apnea (OSA).

This chapter reviews the essential elements of clinical sleep physiology, sleep, the effects of alcohol in those with and without AUD, and alcohol withdrawal. Finally, the effects of other drugs and alcohol on other specific sleep disorders are considered.

OVERVIEW OF SLEEP

Sleep is essential for normal human function. Wakefulness (lack of sleepiness), vigilance, and performance on monotonous tasks deteriorate after a single sleepless night. Further sleep deprivation leads to more inattentiveness and performance failure. "Sleep need" is difficult to define but usually is accepted as the amount of sleep required for optimal function during wakeful periods. Sleep need varies from one individual to another in a range from 3 to 10 hours of sleep over a 24-hour period.[2] The change in sleep need with increasing age has been the subject of considerable study, but such studies often are confounded by changes in lifestyle, diet, medication use, napping patterns, and the like. These studies suggest that total sleep over a 24-hour period shows a small decrease in sleep need as an individual transitions from young adulthood into older age.[2]

The relationship of subjective to objective measures of sleep deserves further comment. In the general population, self-reports of sleep time often are subject to both overestimates and underestimates. Overestimates can be attributed, in part, to the fact that an arousal must be at least 5 to 6 minutes in duration if it is to be recalled subsequently as a sustained arousal or period of wakefulness. As a result, sleep punctuated by recurrent, yet brief, periods of arousal may be described as "sound sleep." Similarly, underestimates of sleep duration are not uncommon and are a feature of the sleep state misperception associated with paradoxical insomnia. This dissociation between subjective and objective sleep can be further compounded because healthy older adults may simply accept a decrease in sleep efficiency as a part of normal aging. However, aging also is associated with reduced ability to tolerate sleep deprivation.

Given these influences, it is clear that objective measures of sleep and sleepiness are critical to the study of sleep and the effects of alcohol on sleep. The nocturnal polysomnogram (PSG) is the standard method of determining the presence and stage of sleep by measuring electroencephalographic (EEG), electromyographic, and electrooculographic activity.[3,4] Similarly, the multiple sleep latency test is a standard and accepted measure of daytime sleepiness; it employs polysomnography while a patient is allowed to take naps on 5 separate occasions throughout a day.[5] The assessment of average sleep latency with such a standardized tool allows a quantification of "sleepiness."

Sleep Architecture

Understanding normal sleep is an essential prerequisite for understanding sleep disorders (Table 95-1). Sleep is a dynamic process, featuring fluctuations in brain wave activity, muscle tone, eye movement, and autonomic activity. It consists of two discrete states: rapid eye movement (REM) and nonrapid eye movement (NREM) sleep. Each can be defined in physiological terms by using the elements of the PSG: EEG, electrooculogram, and electromyogram. Formal criteria have been elaborated in widely accepted manuals.[3,4]

TABLE 95-1 Summary of Sleep Stages

Non-REM sleep (nonrapid eye movement sleep)
N1 (stage 1 NREM, light stage of NREM)
Low amplitude, slow-moving eye movements, some decrease in muscle tone from wake
N2 (stage 2 NREM, light stage of NREM)
Low amplitude, slight decrease in muscle tone, no eye movements
K-complexes, spindles
N3 (stages 3 and 4 NREM, slow-wave sleep [SWS], deep sleep)
High amplitude, slow-wave sleep, no eye movements, some decrease in muscle tone
Decreasing duration as percentage of total sleep with aging
REM sleep (rapid eye movement sleep, dreaming sleep, paradoxical sleep)
Low amplitude, frequency most comparable to N1, rapid eye movements
Sawtooth waves
Relative absence of muscle tone
Typical dream sleep

Nonrapid Eye Movement

NREM sleep has been subdivided into three stages (N1, N2, and N3), where N3 is often referred to as *slow-wave sleep* (SWS) or *delta sleep*. (The reader should be aware that prior to 2008, it was customary to consider NREM in four stages (1-4) with stages 3 and 4 usually consolidated and referred to as SWS.) In brief, each stage is characterized by progressively slower EEG background, lower muscle tone, and decreasing eye movements.

Rapid Eye Movement

Stage R or REM sleep does not fit into the same staging system as NREM sleep and thus sometimes is referred to as *paradoxical sleep*. Although EEG activity is relatively active, the muscle tone achieves its lowest state over a 24-hour period (relative muscle atonia). REM sleep is characterized by REMs scattered through the duration of each REM cycle. REM sleep can be further subdivided into tonic (background EEG, relative muscle atonia, hippocampal theta activity) and phasic (REMs, brief muscle twitches, "sawtooth" waves on the EEG, and ponto-geniculo-occipital spikes, as recorded in animals) components. REM sleep is associated with well-formed dreams. Individuals aroused from REM sleep will recall dreams about 80% of the time. NREM arousals may be associated with recall of isolated images or thought fragments, but not the well-formed images of REM sleep.

Nightmares are usually a reflection of the elements of REM sleep. As the individual initially awakens from a frightening dream and begins to scream, no sound emerges, because he or she still is paralyzed with the muscle atonia of REM. It is noteworthy that these components of REM sleep are not rigidly synchronized. Another example of this loose synchronization can be seen in some normal individuals with sleep paralysis as a benign condition, in which the individual is transiently "paralyzed" as he or she awakens from sleep.

Sleep Rhythms

The components of sleep do not occur randomly throughout the course of the night. In fact, a clear pattern emerges from the ultradian or short rhythms of sleep. The "light" stages of NREM are seen first. They are followed by a transition to SWS, followed by lighter stages of NREM again, and then REM sleep. Typically, there are 3 to 4 NREM-REM cycles, each lasting 90 to 120 minutes. As the night progresses, the relative amount of time spent in REM increases, and the amount of time in SWS decreases. Thus, REM usually is skewed toward the end of the sleep period and SWS toward the beginning.

More importantly, sleep-wake rhythms follow a circadian or approximately 24-hour biological pattern. Sleep-wake is considered a circadian rhythm that is tightly synchronized with circadian variations in core body temperature. The suprachiasmatic nucleus of the hypothalamus in animals, and an analogous structure in humans, with inputs from the retinohypothalamic pathways, has been identified as the endogenous pacemaker. Although individuals may have different periodicities in their clocks ("larks" and "owls"), there are many factors that maintain or influence these rhythms. Although activity levels, social cues, mealtimes, and other external scheduling factors play some role, the most powerful *zeitgeber* (light giver) has proven to be exogenous light. Presumably, light exerts its influence through the retinohypothalamic input to the suprachiasmatic nucleus.[6]

Aging results in a greater sensitivity to time zone or shift work changes. In such situations, there is a significant desynchronization between social and environmental cues and biological rhythms. The individual attempts to sleep or to stay awake at times that are not closely synchronized to biological rhythms. Older adults appear to be less tolerant of such desynchronization, as well as dealing with the clinical effects of an advancing rhythm. This implies earlier wake-up times (the lark), which persist despite later sleep-onset times. The net result is the need to nap because a sleep debt is acquired.

The "Two-Phase" Model

Normal sleep patterns are often considered as emerging from an interaction between the two major forces just discussed. These include the homeostatic drive based upon sleep need and the circadian drive. Thus, as the homeostatic component accumulates through the day, the circadian drive may not be adequate by midafternoon to sustain full wakefulness. As a consequence, one may experience the midafternoon drowsiness during the so-called siesta zone. Similarly, after falling asleep for several hours and awakening at 3 AM, the homeostatic drive has dissipated, and the individual may find it difficult to fall back to sleep for another 1 to 2 hours (**Table 95-2**).

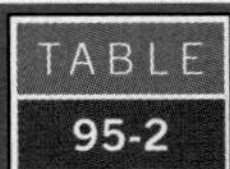

TABLE 95-2 The Two-Phase Model of Sleep

The Two-Phase Model of Sleep
Homeostatic
• Individuals usually require a certain amount of sleep over a 24-hour period.
• As sleep deprivation accumulates during the waking hours, a sleep drive starts to build.
Circadian
• Individuals have an approximately 24 hour biological clock.
• Periods of sleep-permissive and wakeful-permissive zones that occur each day in a predictable manner.
• Rhythms are influenced by scheduling to some degree, in particular to light exposure.

DISORDERS OF SLEEP

For a comprehensive listing of specific disorders and their descriptions, the reader is referred to *The International Classification of Sleep Disorders, Revised (ICSD-3)*.[7] The DSM-5 also provides a description of various disorders in the section on "Sleep-Wake Disorders." This chapter focuses first on problems related to sleep need, sleep rhythms, intrinsic sleep disorders, extrinsic factors, and medical-psychiatric factors (Table 95-3). This will then permit a brief discussion of evolving concepts of insomnia, including the concept of primary insomnia.

Specific Sleep Disorders

Although there are many intrinsic sleep disorders, the four most common disorders are restless legs syndrome (RLS), OSA, insomnia, and circadian rhythm disorders.

Restless Legs Syndrome

It has been estimated that RLS is present in 5% to 15% of the general population. It affects both sexes and has been described in both children and adults. The usual presentation is with an urge to move, usually accompanied by uncomfortable sensations. These paresthesias are usually bilateral, often more prominent in the legs than in the arms. The sensations typically are described as burning, tingling, stabbing, aching, or simple pain. Some patients complain of sensations of ants crawling or worms burrowing. Symptoms usually are subjective and vary over the course of the day. Although the paresthesias can be rather dramatic, it is actually the urge to move that is considered to be one of the essential features of RLS. They tend to be worse when the individual is inactive, especially in the evening when preparing for sleep. Another key feature is the observation that movement may relieve the symptoms for a brief period of time. Patients may have particular difficulties in enclosed areas such as airplanes, cars, or trains. Symptoms are variable and may fluctuate over time, with exacerbations and remissions.[8] Some patients develop myoclonus or sudden jerking movements.

RLS should not be confused with periodic limb movements of sleep (PLMS). PLMS occur during sleep and most commonly in N2. PLMS are repetitive limb movements occurring during sleep and may be associated with brief arousals. The clinical significance, at this point, is uncertain. RLS occurs during wakefulness and interferes with sleep at the transition between wakefulness and sleep. On the other hand, it should be noted that about 80% of cases with RLS would also exhibit PLMS.

The pathophysiology of RLS has been attributed to a disorder of iron-mediated dopamine transport within the central nervous system (CNS). Many medical problems have been found to aggravate the symptoms. Uremia, anemia, and neuropathies have been implicated in many so-called secondary cases. Although iron deficiency may be implicated

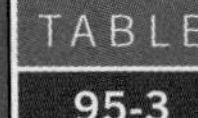

TABLE 95-3 Common Disorders of Sleep

Common Disorders of Sleep
Restless legs syndrome
Considered to be a disorder of the iron-mediated dopamine transport system
May be aggravated by certain medications, such as most antidepressants
Responsive to certain classes of medications including dopaminergic agents, alpha-2-delta ligands and opioids
Essential features:
An urge to move the limbs, usually lower extremities.
Symptoms relieved by movement or stretching.
Symptoms aggravated by inactivity.
Symptoms follow a diurnal pattern and are worse in the evening.
May be associated with subjective sensations or paresthesias.
Obstructive sleep apnea
Can be considered as an interaction between the degree of muscle relaxation of the muscles of the upper airway (in particular, the genioglossus) and the anatomy.
Common features include obesity, loud snoring, male > female, aging, and daytime sleepiness.
Commonly associated with hypertension, cardio- and cerebrovascular disorders, decreased glucose tolerance, and an increased risk for neurodegenerative disorders.
May be aggravated by certain medications—perhaps benzodiazepines.
Once recognized, OSA can be treated with positive airway pressure (PAP) therapy.
Distinct from central sleep apnea (CSA), which may be associated with congestive heart failure, CNS disorders, or opioid use.
Insomnia
Impairment of sleep onset, sleep maintenance, or early awakening with an impact on the next day function
May/may not be associated with other medical/psychiatric disorders
Has been considered as a symptom or as a comorbid disorder:
Treatment should be directed at associated medical/psychiatric disorders.
Insomnia-specific treatment:
Cognitive-Behavioral Therapy for Insomnia (CBT-I)
Specific pharmacotherapy—complicated by potential substance use disorder

in many cases, the only indication may be a serum ferritin level in the low normal range. Of particular note in addiction medicine, is the observation that RLS may be aggravated or triggered by the use of several medications, including antidepressants, lithium carbonate, neuroleptics, and caffeine.[9] In addition, caffeine, nicotine, and chocolate may aggravate RLS—critical factors in dealing with addiction medicine.[10]

Although efforts should be made to identify factors that may be aggravating symptoms, the treatment of RLS usually requires medication.[8,11] The most commonly used are the dopaminergic drugs (ropinirole, pramipexole, rotigotine, etc.) and the calcium channel alpha-2-delta ligands (gabapentin, pregabalin, gabapentin enacarbil). Success has also been demonstrated with benzodiazepines (usually clonazepam), other anticonvulsants (carbamazepine), opioids, and others such as clonidine. Opioids are of particular interest. Some patients report that they began to use opioids on a regular basis when they received them for an unrelated disorder and realized that they were able to sleep for the first time in years. Caution, however, needs to be exercised in the treatment of RLS. The dopaminergic agents may be associated with augmentation and the emergence of worsening symptoms, oftentimes during the day. Many of the other agents are of concern in patients with disorders of addiction.

Obstructive Sleep Apnea

OSA is a common syndrome. It is a treatable disorder that accounts for many of the cases of excessive somnolence and insomnia encountered in most sleep centers. Epidemiological studies have suggested that snoring occurs in 9% to 24% of middle-age men and in 4% to 14% of middle-age women,[12,13] although there is a tendency to underreport snoring.[14] The prevalence of OSA in overall population has been estimated to be 2% in women and 4% in men.[15,16] If one considers only the index of events per hour and relaxes the requirement of sleepiness, the prevalence increases to 9% in women and 24% in men with the incidence in men clearly outnumbering that in women until menopause. Common risk factors include obesity, sedative use, alcohol consumption, diabetes, stroke, and age.[16-20] Other neurological and medical conditions may also be associated with an increased risk for OSA. OSA is characterized by repetitive episodes of sleep-related upper airway obstructions that usually are associated with oxygen desaturation. OSA can be conceptualized as a disorder emerging from an interaction between anatomy and muscle relaxation especially in the upper airway dilator muscles of the oropharynx as it occurs in sleep. As muscles relax, airflow can generate vibrations in the soft tissues of the upper airway, including the soft palate.[21] Such vibration produces the noise or snoring. The role of upper airway muscle relaxation in the pathophysiology also means that certain medications, such as benzodiazepines or alcohol, may aggravate the severity of the OSA, presumably, by the enhanced degree of muscle relaxation. In some patients, snoring appears in isolation; in such cases, the term *primary snoring* is applied.

The consequences of OSA can be considered at several different levels. Firstly, there are the psychosocial implications of loud snoring that often accompanies OSA. The disrupted sleep can certainly contribute to daytime sleepiness with impairments of alertness, concentration, mood, and behavior.

There are several cardiopulmonary consequences of OSA. Feedback reflexes may be insufficient to cause arousal (arousal produces return of muscle tone on cessation of the respiratory events). Indeed, one might see significant oxygen desaturation with arrhythmia, systemic arterial hypertension, and polycythemia. These changes can become chronic, and recent epidemiological studies have suggested that OSA plays a role in the development of often-unrecognized hypertension in the general public.[22,23]

Central sleep apnea (CSA) is a disorder characterized by recurrent episodes of apnea during sleep resulting from temporary loss of ventilatory effort. CSA may be associated with desaturations and arousals, as encountered in OSA. Although CSA is much less frequently encountered when compared with OSA, it does pose a particular potential problem in addiction medicine. There are different forms of CSA, including the common form of Cheyne-Stokes respirations that may be associated with congestive heart failure or other CNS pathologies. A pattern of sleep-related irregular respirations has been referred to as ataxic breathing or Biot respirations and has been associated with chronic opioid therapy, and the risk seems to be related to the morphine dose equivalents.[24,25]

Insomnia

In brief, insomnia refers to a pattern of disrupted sleep (eg, delayed sleep onset, frequent arousals, early awakening), in an individual given sufficient opportunity to sleep, that is associated with a pattern of daytime distress and symptoms. The requirement of daytime symptoms distinguishes the person with insomnia from the individual with an insufficient sleep disorder. Insomnia may be transient or chronic, primary, or secondary. Primary insomnia is considered to be independent of other sleep disturbances or the other factors cited previously (ICSD-2). The concept of primary insomnia is interesting because most sleep specialists acknowledge that it is fairly uncommon, yet it is the target of all clinical trials of pharmacological agents seeking a U.S. Food and Drug Administration (FDA) indication for the treatment of insomnia.

In recent years, there seems to have been a paradigm shift in the approach to insomnia. In a consensus statement from a National Institutes of Health summit meeting (June 13-15, 2005), it was concluded that insomnia should be considered a comorbid disorder.[26] This represented a shift from the thinking that insomnia is a symptom and that the emphasis in management should be directed toward the underlying disorder. As an example, one might consider the relationship between pain and insomnia. Although pain may be a causative factor in the development of insomnia, it must also be considered that sleep deprivation may influence pain thresholds, and the treatment of insomnia may facilitate the management of pain. Ultimately, it may be reasonable to consider the predisposing, precipitating, and perpetuating factors involved in the individual case.[26,27]

Circadian Rhythm Disorders

For a variety of social and biological reasons, there is a tendency for the adolescent to become delayed and the older adult to become advanced. The resulting complaints typically involve insomnia and difficulty in staying awake at other times. A common experience is the transient dysfunction associated with jet lag. This is simply a situation in which the biological clock suddenly becomes desynchronized from the social environment. Because most people find it easier to "delay" their clocks, it becomes easier for most to fly from the East Coast to the West Coast, (which requires an advancement of the rhythm), than from west to east.

In addition, the circadian rhythm of the older adult appears to be more fragile and susceptible to disruption, as might be seen in shift workers or patients plagued by the nocturnal arousal of chronic pain. It is unclear how much of this change is due to biological changes in the endogenous oscillator that governs the rhythms and how much is the result of changes in exogenous factors such as light exposure, lifestyle changes, and physical activity. The rhythm can be manipulated by well-timed bright light exposure. The full range of circadian rhythm disorders, as described in the ICSD-2, includes problems related to delays, advancements, and shifting rhythms. The pathophysiology of these disorders may vary, but some can be attributed to jet travel or shift work.

Nightmare Disorder

Nightmare disorder is defined as a parasomnia or abnormal/unusual behavior during sleep. It is associated with REM sleep; hence, the characteristic features of a dream, disturbing in this case, trigger an awakening that is typically associated with a brief period of atonia or paralysis. It is of interest to those dealing with SUD because the disorder is often associated with posttraumatic stress disorder (PTSD), which is a common co-occurring problem. In fact, most of the literature on the treatment of nightmare disorder refers to PTSD-associated nightmare disorder. Furthermore, some of the medications used to treat nightmare disorder overlap with drugs with addictive potential.

A variety of behavioral psychological approaches have been suggested for the treatment of nightmare disorder, but Image Rehearsal Therapy is usually recommended. A variety of medications have been suggested, but none specifically recommended. Medications considered in the treatment of PTSD-associated nightmare disorder include several atypical antipsychotics, and several antidepressants, as well as prazosin, clonidine, gabapentin and cannabis derivatives/synthetics. The use of cannabis as treatment, including for Post Traumatic Stress Disorder, is reviewed in Chapter 126, "Therapeutic Effectiveness of Cannabis and Cannabinoids." Interestingly, it has been recommended to not use clonazepam or venlafaxine.[27]

Extrinsic Factors

Several extrinsic factors affect sleep, including exercise, the sleep environment, medications, and drug effects. Exercise has long been recognized as a factor promoting sound sleep.[28] Regular exercise, especially in the late afternoon or early evening, is conducive to sleep initiation, through either release of certain endogenous substances or subsequent cooling 5 to 6 hours later, which reinforces circadian factors.[29] Inactivity can be a factor in sleep disruption in the young as well as the old, but daytime bed rest is a greater issue in the sleep of older adults.[30,31]

Environmental stimuli, such as room temperature and light, are often factors in the initiation and maintenance of sleep. Although arousal thresholds vary from one individual to the next, aging has been associated with increased susceptibility to external arousal.[32,33]

The effect of evening meals is somewhat controversial. The conventional wisdom has been that a light bedtime snack—perhaps with a glass of milk—promotes sleep. This effect has been attributed to tryptophan or to the release of digestive hormones, which can be sedating.[34] On the other hand, there are reports that heavy bedtime snacks can be disruptive to sleep. Clinical experience suggests that these effects are variable and need to be assessed in each individual.

Medical and Psychiatric Factors

The interaction between sleep and other medical conditions can be quite complex. Certain medical conditions contribute directly to specific sleep disorders such as OSA or RLS. However, other disorders simply lead to problems with the wake-sleep transition at sleep onset or at other times through the night, including the most vulnerable time in the circadian cycle (ie, 3:00-5:00 AM). Sleep disorders have been associated with nocturia, headache, gastrointestinal illnesses, cardiopulmonary disease, menopause, and chronic pain.[35-38]

The role of psychiatric disorders always should be considered in the assessment of sleep disorders. Two specific sleep-related psychiatric disorders have been formally defined. The ICSD-2 describes an "alcohol-dependent insomnia" in people without AUD who use alcohol as a hypnotic for sleep onset for more than 30 days and who may not otherwise meet criteria for an AUD. The DSM-5 describes criteria for a "substance-induced sleep disorder," with subtypes based on the substance used.

Sleep disruption is not uncommon in any person with a comorbid psychiatric syndrome, but most of the attention has been directed toward the relationship between affective disorders and sleep. Insomnia is the prominent feature, although hypersomnia may be seen in depression, especially when the depression is a component of a bipolar disorder.[39] Similarly, during manic episodes, one may see periods of sleeplessness, with an apparent reduction in sleep need.

ALCOHOL AND SLEEP

The relationship between alcohol and sleep is complex. Alcohol consumption has been associated with an increased risk of sleep disruption,[40] with older age[41] and, possibly gender,[41] as additional contributing factors. The issue is further complicated by the use of alcohol in the self-treatment of insomnia and the relationship between insomnia and alcohol craving.[42] It may be best to first consider the impact of alcohol on sleep and sleep architecture and then, the relationship between alcohol and disorders of sleep.

Effect of Alcohol on Sleep in the Individual Without Alcohol Use Disorder

Alcohol is probably the sleep-promoting agent that is most widely used by the general public. In a population survey, 13% of survey respondents ages 18 to 45 years old reported that, in the preceding year, they had used alcohol to assist in sleep onset. Another 2% said they had used alcohol continuously for at least a month for this purpose, whereas 5% said they had used alcohol in combination with another hypnotic agent.[39] Despite this wide use, it must be remembered that alcohol can be mildly stimulating.[43] The source of the variability in its hypnotic properties is not clear, although animal studies suggest a possible role of age. In at least one study, it was demonstrated that adolescent animals developed a much more rapid tolerance to the hypnotic effects of alcohol than did older animals, although older males had a tendency to sleep longer.[44,45] Another consideration is that stimulant effects may be related to the period of absorption and low-moderate doses, whereas sedative effects are more closely linked to periods of alcohol elimination and higher doses.[46]

The effects of alcohol on the sleep architecture of the individual without AUD should be considered in terms of both direct effects and immediate withdrawal (**Table 95-4**). Because alcohol is rapidly metabolized, the direct effect of evening alcohol consumption usually is during the sleep cycle. As predicted by the hypnotic effect, sleep latency is shortened, and there is an increase in the amount of NREM sleep and SWS that occurs at the expense of REM sleep, which is suppressed during the acute phase.[47-49] As the effects of the alcohol dissipate, there is a rebound effect, in which sleep becomes lighter and more easily disrupted. REM increases, with an associated increase in dreams and nightmares. There is an increase in sympathetic arousals, with tachycardia and sweating. After adjusting for blood alcohol levels, these effects may be more prominent in women than in men.[50]

As alcohol consumption continues, the hypnotic effects may diminish, but the late sleep disruption persists.[51] Ultimately, the net effect is a feeling of fatigue during the individual's waking hours.

Alcohol's hypnotic effects were seen in a study of infants fed breast milk flavored with alcohol who fell asleep more easily, but they seemed to sleep less deeply.[52] This finding would be predicted from our knowledge of alcohol's effects in older

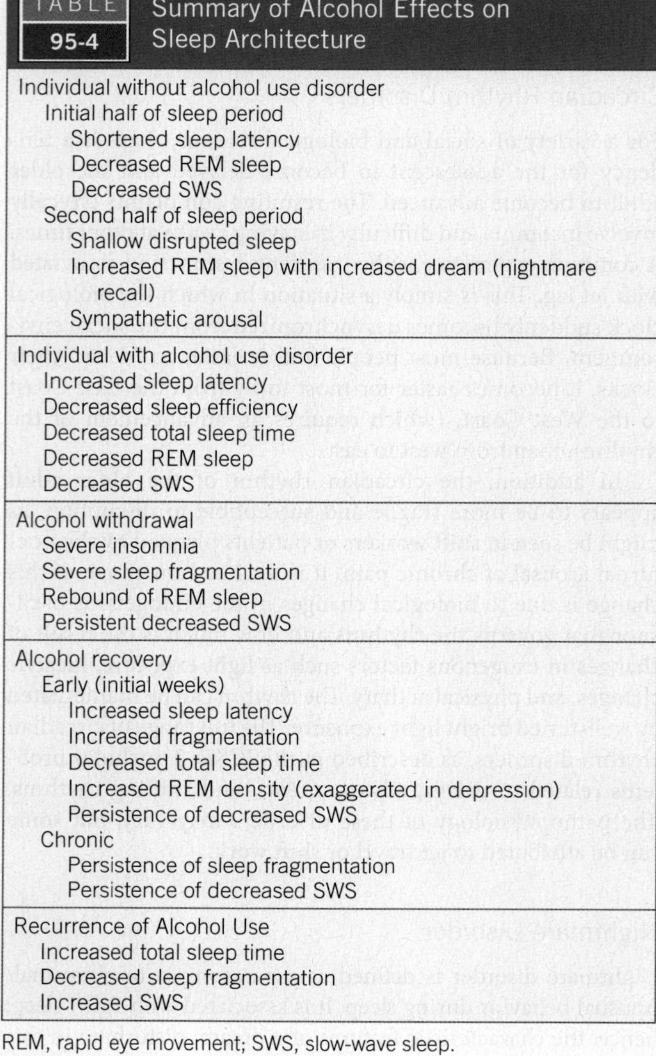

TABLE 95-4 Summary of Alcohol Effects on Sleep Architecture

Condition	Phase	Effects
Individual without alcohol use disorder	Initial half of sleep period	Shortened sleep latency
		Decreased REM sleep
		Decreased SWS
	Second half of sleep period	Shallow disrupted sleep
		Increased REM sleep with increased dream (nightmare recall)
		Sympathetic arousal
Individual with alcohol use disorder		Increased sleep latency
		Decreased sleep efficiency
		Decreased total sleep time
		Decreased REM sleep
		Decreased SWS
Alcohol withdrawal		Severe insomnia
		Severe sleep fragmentation
		Rebound of REM sleep
		Persistent decreased SWS
Alcohol recovery	Early (initial weeks)	Increased sleep latency
		Increased fragmentation
		Decreased total sleep time
		Increased REM density (exaggerated in depression)
		Persistence of decreased SWS
	Chronic	Persistence of sleep fragmentation
		Persistence of decreased SWS
Recurrence of Alcohol Use		Increased total sleep time
		Decreased sleep fragmentation
		Increased SWS

REM, rapid eye movement; SWS, slow-wave sleep.

patients. It also has been shown that a woman's daily consumption of small amounts of alcohol in the first trimester of pregnancy is associated with subsequent sleep disruption in infants, when measured by brain electrical activity.[53]

It would seem that the hypnotic effects of alcohol should be related to direct effects of alcohol on the CNS. Unfortunately, this explanation does not account for the observation that sleepiness can be observed after the alcohol is no longer detectable. Although it is customary to advise patients with sleep difficulties to avoid late-evening alcohol, there is evidence that even early-evening alcohol consumption may disrupt sleep in the last half of the night.[54] This would apply to alcohol consumed even 6 hours before sleep onset.[55] Similarly, alcohol administered early in the day has been shown to have a negative effect on multiple sleep latency tests and tests of divided attention, even when given later in the day when alcohol levels are undetectable.[55]

Finally, some data suggest that there is a synergistic interaction between alcohol exposure and prior sleepiness.

The hypnotic effects seem to be enhanced in the previously sleep-deprived individual.[56] In particular, low-dose alcohol administered after a night of reduced sleep is associated with reduced performance on a driving simulator.[51,55,57,58] The implication is that, in individuals functioning on reduced sleep, alcohol has an enhanced sedating effect even at low doses, which in turn has an effect on performance in activities such as driving.

It is important to note that many of the conclusions of the studies of the impact of alcohol on the sleep of persons without AUD have been based on studies in men. A recent study of 7 women without AUD (aged 22-25) suggested that the impact of alcohol on the sleep of women may be less intense than the impact on the sleep of men[59] (see **Table 95-4**).

Effect of Alcohol on Sleep in the Individual With Alcohol Use Disorder

It is not uncommon for persons with AUD to report some combination of insomnia, hypersomnia, circadian rhythm disorders, or parasomnias (abnormal sleep-related behaviors). Such reports usually are reflected in other, more objective measures. Various studies of patients with AUDs have demonstrated increased sleep latencies (time to fall asleep), decreased sleep efficiencies, and decreased total sleep, with reductions in both REM and SWS.[60-62] As the AUD continues, patients often report that they are no longer able to initiate sleep without a drink. After a time, the usual rhythms of sleep become quite disrupted (see **Table 95-4**).

Dream Content in Moderate to Severe Alcohol Use Disorder

Although dreams usually are correlated with REM sleep, studies of dream content in people with AUD often are conducted without the use of polysomnographic techniques. In general, these studies find that individuals with AUD suffer from nightly nightmares more often than controls.[63,64] In a more general study of patients with SUDs in a withdrawal management program, dreaming about drinking was a poor prognostic sign for recurrence of alcohol use.[65] Others have reported that among people with AUD in recovery, dreams about drinking were viewed with concern and were considered a potential trigger for recurrent use.[66]

The use of alcohol to suppress nightmares needs to be considered in the management of other disorders associated with nightmares, such as PTSD.[67] In fact, some patients may have initiated their use of alcohol or other drugs out of a desire to suppress nightmares.

Alcohol, Sleep, and Other Cardiopulmonary Functions

In addition to the effect of alcohol on OSA, it is important to be aware of the interaction between chronic obstructive pulmonary disease (COPD) and alcohol during sleep. For example, alcohol consumption before sleep by patients with COPD can worsen nocturnal hypoxemia during sleep[68] and increase ventricular ectopic activity.[69]

Sleep in Alcohol Withdrawal

The alcohol withdrawal syndrome frequently is marked by severe insomnia and sleep fragmentation. The reduction of SWS during this period has been related to a loss of restful sleep and feelings of daytime fatigue. The rebound of REM sleep has been regarded as a component of the pathophysiology of hallucinations encountered in the withdrawal syndrome. In fact, sleep during withdrawal may consist simply of fragments of REM sleep. It is of some interest that the rebound of SWS does not appear to occur.[61]

Nightmares and vivid dreams are not uncommon features of alcohol withdrawal and probably reflect the observed REM "pressure." In fact, it has been speculated that the rebound of REM encountered in acute withdrawal states such as *alcohol withdrawal delirium* may account for much of the associated clinical symptomatology.[70,71] It has been speculated that it is the early and abundant REM, with its associated dream content or hallucinations, and the accompanying sympathetic discharge that may account for much of the clinical picture of alcohol withdrawal delirium.[72] These views are consistent with attempts to record the sleep of patients with alcohol withdrawal delirium, which have found mostly stage 1 NREM and REM, with some evidence of increased muscle tone, even though these findings are clinically inconsistent.[73] The increase in muscle activity also has suggested a possible relationship with REM behavior disorder, in which patients lose the muscle atonia of sleep and actually begin to act out their dreams.[74]

Sleep During Alcohol Use Disorder Remission

In the patient with an AUD, sleep is not immediately recovered with abstinence; in fact, it may require months or even years. In the first 2 to 3 weeks of early remission, increased sleep latency may be seen, accompanied by increased sleep fragmentation and reduced total sleep time (TST). There may be a decrease in SWS and an increase in REM density[75]; such an increased density of REMs suggests an apparent rebound effect. The effects on REM may be exaggerated in patients with secondary depression, who also may exhibit a shortened REM latency (duration of onset of REM after sleep onset) and a greater percentage of sleep time spent in REM sleep.[76]

These changes may persist for months or years, with sleep time reduced and fragmented and an elevated percentage of TST spent in REM sleep.[75-77] Long-term follow-up of patients with AUD in remission has demonstrated persistent subjective and objective sleep difficulties. The most prominent feature appears to be a persistent reduction in the amount of SWS as a percentage of total sleep.[76,78,79]

Sleep disruption during recovery also has been examined from the perspective of its effect on the patient's efforts to remain sober. For example, it has been demonstrated that the presence of subjective sleep disruption increases the likelihood that the recovering individual will return to alcohol use.[80] Longitudinal studies have suggested that the persistence of objective and subjective sleep difficulties at about 1 month of sobriety predicts recurrence of use by 5 months.[78,80]

A recovering person with AUD who begins to drink again will experience an increase in SWS, with an increase in TST and reduction in fragmentation. This response, which involves a perceived immediate improvement in sleep, is thought to contribute to recurrent drinking, even though continued alcohol use inevitably leads to further sleep disruption.

Several investigators have attempted to identify the sleep measures that are the most important in predicting recurrence of drinking. Some studies suggest that the degree of SWS reduction could be correlated with a poorer prognosis for continued recovery 2 months after discharge from an inpatient treatment program.[81,82] Subsequent studies, however, suggested that measures of REM sleep were critical in predicting outcome. These studies suggested that measures of REM pressure, as defined by a shortened REM latency, increased REM density, and increased amount of time in REM sleep as a percentage of total sleep, when measured within 2 weeks of initiation of abstinence, were markers of a better prognosis for continued recovery at 3 months after discharge.[83-85] In fact, the emergence of these markers of REM pressure is among the most robust predictors of continued recovery at the 3-month mark.

It should be noted that the prognostic value of these sleep measures changes as abstinence progresses. For example, at the 5-month mark, prolonged sleep latency and poor sleep efficiency are predictors of recurrence by 1 year, but measures of REM pressure are no longer helpful.[79] Prolonged sleep latency (time to sleep onset) has an advantage over other measures because of the relative ease with which it is ascertained.

SPECIFIC SLEEP DISORDERS ASSOCIATED WITH ALCOHOL USE DISORDER

Alcohol and Sleep-Related Breathing Disorders

Patients with AUD appear to be at an increased risk of developing OSA, especially if they snore.[86-89] A large retrospective analysis suggested that these findings might, in part, be related to an association with smoking in this population and that smoking was the primary agent.[90] Nevertheless, alcohol has been found to induce obstructive apnea in healthy asymptomatic men,[91] as well as chronic snorers.[92,93] Alcohol has been shown to increase the frequency and duration of obstructive events in patients with established OSA.[94]

Two of the essential elements in the pathophysiology of OSA are the anatomy of the upper airway and the degree of relative muscle atonia associated with sleep. The decrease in muscle tone of the upper airway leads to an increase in snoring and inspiratory resistance, with an accompanying reduction in airflow.[95,96] Alcohol contributes to a reduction in muscle tone, with a selective reduction in genioglossal activity, thus aggravating any tendency to develop snoring or OSA.[95] As a consequence, there is an increase in snoring, as well as interruption in normal nocturnal respiration. The associated sleep disruption then contributes to an increase in daytime fatigue and somnolence. These changes in airflow resistance are sufficient to cause OSA in those who consume moderate to high doses of alcohol in the evening, even if they do not otherwise have OSA.[93,95]

Alcohol administration to asymptomatic men has been associated with increased episodes of desaturation, as well as an increase in frequency and duration of hypopneas and apneas.[91] Moreover, the depressant effects of alcohol can decrease the likelihood of arousal from an obstructive event, thus prolonging the duration of each respiratory event.[78,91,97] In fact, abstinence from alcohol before bedtime is considered an important step in treating OSA.[98]

Although alcohol use can induce apneas and obstructions can worsen established OSA, the relationship of alcohol to the development of OSA varies across populations. Older patients, for example, are more vulnerable to this effect.[95] Similarly, the effect is not particularly prominent in normal women.[99,100] In some studies of normal male subjects and young nonobese snorers, alcohol exerted minimal effects on the development of OSA.[94] Thus, it appears that other factors, such as age, the presence of snoring, and perhaps gender, play a role in the development of OSA.

OSA has been related to impaired performance on driving simulators and increased motor vehicle crashes even in the absence of alcohol.[55] Alcohol further decreases the performance of the patient with OSA. One small study suggested that a higher-than-expected number of sleep-related respiratory events in patient who had completed withdrawal management might contribute to impaired driving performance.[91] In patients with established severe OSA, it has been noted that consumption of two or more alcoholic drinks per day is associated with a fivefold increase in fatigue-related motor vehicle crashes when compared with those who consumed little or no alcohol.

Alcohol and Periodic Limb Movements of Sleep

In at least one survey of a large sleep clinic sample, the risk of PLMS was increased almost threefold by alcohol consumption.[101] This increase, however, was not seen in another study in which abstinent patients with DSM-IV-defined alcohol dependence were evaluated and compared with those without.[102] Nevertheless, the potential increase in fatigue and daytime somnolence associated with PLMS can play a role in the management of these patients.

OTHER DRUGS AND SLEEP

Stimulants

It is widely accepted that a primary effect of stimulants is to suppress sleep. Studies have demonstrated that stimulants such as amphetamine, methylphenidate, pemoline, or cocaine prolong sleep latency and reduce TST. Stimulants have a specific inhibitory effect on REM sleep, so that there is a prolonged REM latency with a reduction in total REM throughout the sleep period.[103] Presumably, this effect is attributable to the dopaminergic stimulation of the arousal system, although serotonergic systems also may be involved.[104] This is also true for the nonamphetamine stimulants (modafinil and armodafinil) that are thought to exert their effect through dopamine reuptake inhibition without an effect on other monoaminergic systems. When used episodically, these agents contribute to periods of sleeplessness that can last for days, but they are usually followed by a rebound hypersomnia. Tolerance to this effect can develop with continued use, even in those who take these agents for medical disorders such as narcolepsy or attention deficit hyperactivity disorder (ADHD).[105]

After a period of persistent, chronic use, withdrawal of stimulants often leads to initial insomnia, which may persist.[106] The sleep abnormalities encountered in stimulant withdrawal include a rebound effect. In particular, they include a decrease in sleep efficiency, with increased periods of nocturnal wakefulness, increased amounts of REM sleep with a shortened REM latency, and increased stage 1 NREM sleep.[107] This effect is similar to the rebound effect encountered in the second half of the night after evening alcohol consumption.

The first 2 weeks of stimulant withdrawal usually are marked by some improvement in measurements of TST, stage 1 NREM sleep, and REM density, even though changes persist.

The use of stimulants also carries a special note when one considers the management of sleep disorders. Stimulants are commonly used in the treatment of the hypersomnias. The commonly used stimulants include the amphetamine-type (methylphenidate, dextroamphetamine, etc.) and the nonamphetamine type (modafinil and armodafinil) stimulants. Obviously, care must be taken with individuals who may have difficulties with substance use.

Cocaine

Cocaine behaves like the other stimulants. Sleep difficulties are not an uncommon effect of cocaine. PSG studies also demonstrate the features commonly associated with stimulants including an increased sleep latency, reduced total sleep time, and REM suppression. During acute withdrawal, TST is also associated with reduced impaired sleep initiation and maintenance. As one might anticipate, REM latency will be shortened with an increase in the amount of REM sleep when considered as a percentage of total sleep. Similarly, SWS will also be decreased. Sleep will continue to deteriorate in a similar pattern until the patient enters the subacute phase of withdrawal. It has also been noted that the patients in withdrawal may underestimate the severity of the sleep disruption despite the fact that their performance is otherwise consistent with sleep deprivation.[108]

MDMA (Ecstasy)

Ecstasy ([±]3,4-methylenedioxymethamphetamine, MDMA) is a psychostimulant and a synthetic derivative of amphetamine. It has both stimulant and hallucinogenic properties and is structurally similar to both amphetamine and mescaline. Chronic use is associated with a significant decrease in serotonergic activity and also serves as a releaser and reuptake inhibitor of monoamines, including dopamine and norepinephrine. Acute MDMA administration disrupts sleep and REM sleep, specifically without producing daytime sleepiness such as sleep restriction does. Compared with control subjects, individuals who use MDMA showed evidence of hyperarousal and impaired REM function.[109]

Sleep is usually disrupted for 48 hours following ingestion with additional REM suppression. Chronic use has also been associated with further sleep disturbance. PSG studies done during periods of abstinence in individuals with heavy MDMA use generally show an increase in N1 and a decrease in N2 with a reduction in TST.[109-111] The REM suppression will improve over time.[8]

MDMA will disrupt nocturnal sleep but will not be associated with the daytime sleepiness that would otherwise be expected from an equivalent night of sleep deprivation.[111] Although MDMA has stimulant properties, its use will not compensate for the effects of sleep deprivation in tests of performance or driving skills.[112]

People who have used MDMA regularly, but are abstinent, appear to have long-lasting changes to their sleep architecture and quality of sleep. Although the studies have been small, when comparing those reporting prior MDMA use to healthy controls, those reported uses had reductions in total sleep and non-REM sleep, primarily reductions in stage 2 sleep.[113]

Opioids

The primary effect on sleep of acute administration of opioids to normal subjects or individuals who have achieved abstinence is to shorten sleep latency and reduce TST, sleep efficiency, REM sleep, and SWS.[114-117] Although some have attributed sedative properties of opioids to anticholinergic properties,[118] a more likely explanation may be the mu opioid receptor depression of the hypothalamic hypocretin/orexin system.[119] Chronic use, however, usually leads to tolerance to some of these effects. The REM-suppressing effects of morphine, for example, usually disappear within a week, even though sleep fragmentation may persist.[120] Even the longer-acting opioids, such as methadone, contribute to insomnia, with disruption of sleep architecture and increased arousals accompanying chronic administration.[121] This also may occur in patients undergoing opioid agonist therapy. The pathophysiology of this effect is not clear, but evidence suggests that the REM-inhibiting properties can be attributed to inhibition of acetylcholine receptors in the pontine reticular formation or to direct agonist effects at specific mu receptors.[122]

It is also important to keep in mind that opioids have been associated with three types of sleep-related breathing disorders. These include sleep-related hypoventilation, central sleep apnea (CSA) and OSA.[117] Most often the CSA follows an irregular pattern (Biot).[117]

Opioids play a role in the treatment and management of specific sleep disorders. In particular, they have been found to be quite useful in the management of RLS[123,124] and PLMS,[125] although the mechanism of this benefit is not well understood. In fact, anecdotal evidence shows that some patients with RLS or PLMS who are treated with opioids for unrelated disorders become dependent on opioids when they experience the sleep benefits. For example, a patient may suddenly realize that postoperative opioids allow for marked improvement in sleep that had been interrupted by previously undiagnosed RLS. Opioids play an obvious role in the management of sleep disorders secondary to pain syndromes.

Little has been written about the characteristics of sleep during withdrawal from opioids, but clinical experience suggests that insomnia often is cited as a troublesome feature of withdrawal and requires specific attention.

Nicotine

The effects of nicotine on sleep have not been well studied, but the available data suggest that, compared with people who don't smoke, people who smoke experience an increase in sleep latency and an increase in arousals with resulting poorer sleep maintenance and a relative increase in sleep apneas and leg movements.[126,127] The increased prevalence of sleep disruption in people who smoke has also been found to be independent of other psychiatric disturbances.[128] A possible biphasic response is that low doses promote sleep and higher doses disrupt sleep.[126,129] Unlike most of the other agents discussed in this chapter, nicotine can increase rather than decrease REM.

Withdrawal from nicotine is associated with sleep disruption and increased daytime sleepiness, marked by multiple sleep latency tests.[130] The effect of nicotine patches on sleep disruption remains unclear.[131] The variability of responses may be due to the anxiety and irritability encountered in nicotine withdrawal.

Some researchers speculate that, in addition to the direct effect of nicotine on sleep mechanisms and architecture, tobacco and the irritation it causes to the upper airway may contribute to OSA.[132] Furthermore, it has been suggested that untreated OSA may be a risk factor for smoking, suggesting that treatment of OSA may be important in the management of nicotine addiction.[133] Similarly, nicotine and smoking may also be a risk factor for OSA.[134]

Smoking and nicotine may be associated with other sleep disorders. For instance, there appears to be an association with bruxism.[134] Although nicotine has been implicated as an aggravating factor in RLS,[10] there are rare cases where it seemed to be palliative.[135,136] Care should also be taken to address drug interactions. For instance, ropinirole is commonly used to treat RLS. Ropinirole is a CYP1A2 substrate, and smoking induces cytochrome P450 isozyme CYP1A2. As a consequence, levels will be lower in people who smoke and may increase during periods of abstinence from smoking.[137]

Caffeine

As early as 1672, coffee was prescribed for disorders associated with sleepiness. The effect of coffee on sleepiness stems from caffeine. Caffeine has been consumed in some form for much of human history, but it was not officially discovered until 1819. The effects of caffeine overlap with those of other stimulants. Caffeine has a long history of use to combat fatigue and sleepiness in normal individuals[138] and to improve performance in shift workers[138] and can trigger insomnia in experimental conditions as well.[139] Unlike many other stimulants, caffeine appears to exert its effect by blocking adenosine receptors (primarily A1 and A2A) on neurons and glial cells of all brain areas. In addition, xanthines, including caffeine, will inhibit phosphodiesterases, promote calcium release from intracellular stores, and interfere with GABA-A receptors. Caffeine, through antagonism of adenosine receptors (ARs), affects brain functions such as sleep, cognition, learning, and memory.[140,141]

Sleep difficulties are not an uncommon effect of caffeine. PSG studies also demonstrate the features commonly associated with stimulants including an increased sleep latency, reduced total sleep time, and REM suppression. During acute withdrawal, TST is also associated with reduced impaired sleep initiation and maintenance. As one might anticipate, REM latency will be shortened with an increase in the amount of REM sleep when considered as a percentage of total sleep. Similarly, SWS will also be decreased. Withdrawal effects may be minimized by a small amount of morning dosed caffeine. Sleep will continue to deteriorate in a similar pattern until the patient enters the subacute phase of withdrawal. It has also been noted that the patients in withdrawal may underestimate the severity of the sleep disruption despite the fact that their performance is otherwise consistent with sleep deprivation.[110] Sleep changes related to caffeine also seem to increase with aging.[142]

Caffeine is often used in combination with alcohol, and together they can lead to even further aggravation of insomnia. Although alcohol has hypnotic properties, its half-life is much shorter than that of caffeine, and its major effects disappear within a few hours. At that point, the rebound effect of alcohol withdrawal and the persistent stimulatory effect of caffeine jointly contribute to further sleep disruption.[139]

The effect of abrupt withdrawal of caffeine should not be underestimated. Although few formal studies of caffeine withdrawal and its effects on sleep have been conducted, it has been noted that within 18 to 24 hours, some patients develop headache, fatigue, irritability, sleepiness, and flu-like symptoms.[143]

Cannabis

Cannabis is a complex of more than 400 compounds, including flavonoids, terpenoids, and cannabinoids. Cannabinoids are the active ingredients and appear to have individual interactive effects that contribute to the net effect. *Cannabis sativa* contains over 70 different cannabinoids; Δ9-tetrahydrocannabinol (Δ9-THC) and cannabidiol (CBD) are the two major constituents of this plant.[144] Although the terms cannabis and marijuana are often used interchangeably, cannabis refers to cannabis products in general and marijuana refers to cannabis products that are made from the dried flowers, leaves, stems and seeds of the cannabis plant. There has more recently been an effort to shift away from using the term marijuana, which has historical roots in playing to xenophobia and the racist war on drugs. It has long been accepted that cannabis may contribute to improved quality of sleep either by direct hypnotic activity or by an impact on pain, anxiety, and other chronic difficulties. Some of the hypnotic effect has been attributed to the ability of cannabinoids to modulate spontaneous neuronal activity and evoke inhibition of the locus coeruleus noradrenergic neurons.[133] The hypnotic properties may be of particular concern in addiction medicine. In a study of individuals with chronic cannabis use, abstinence from THC increased ratings of anxiety/depression/irritability and decreased the reported quantity and quality of sleep. It was suggested that these abstinence symptoms may contribute to continued use.[144]

The hypnotic effect of cannabis may be a bit oversimplified. Although THC has usually been implicated and its hypnotic properties described, it appears that another major constituent of cannabis, CBD, may actually induce alertness.[145] It appears that this alerting system may be modulated by CBD's impact on dopaminergic release and activation of neurons in the hypothalamus and dorsal raphe nucleus. In animal studies, perfusion of the lateral hypothalamus and the dorsal raphe nucleus has been shown to promote wakefulness and decrease REM and SWS.[146,147]

In addition, there have been a few studies that have looked specifically at the impact of cannabis on sleep architecture. Low doses of THC have been associated with a shortened sleep latency, suppression of REM with an increase in SWS and TST. Heavy doses of THC, on the other hand, have been associated with not only suppression of REM but also a decrease in SWS and an increase in sleep latency. Chronic use has been associated with persistent suppression of SWS. Abstinence seems to lead to a rebound effect with a decrease in REM latency and an increase in the relative amount of REM sleep but a decrease in SWS. In the long-term administration (more than 7 days), some tolerance probably develops to the SWS effects, but not to the REM sleep effects.[110,148-150]

There have been a few studies that have examined the value of cannabis in the treatment of specific sleep disorders. Several studies have suggested that cannabinoids may be effective in the treatment of insomnia.[151] Cannabinoids may also lead to an improvement in the frequency of obstructive sleep-related breathing effects.[152,153] Two small case series have suggested that cannabis may also be helpful in the management of RLS.[154,155] In addition, cannabinoids may play a role in the management of Nightmare Disorder, especially as related to PTSD.[27] However, a more recent review is not as encouraging (see Chapter 126 "Therapeutic Effectiveness of Cannabis and Cannabinoids" in this textbook). Unfortunately, studies examining the role of cannabinoids in the management of sleep disorders are limited and further study is required.

There have been a few studies that examined the impact of abrupt withdrawal of cannabis on sleep. Unfortunately, methodological problems limit our ability to establish any firm conclusions.[156] Nevertheless, it is likely that the increasing legalization of cannabis will lead to an increase in our knowledge of the relationship of cannabis to sleep and sleep disorders. In addition, more information may emerge about the relative effect of the different modes of consumption (oral, smoke, etc.) and different strains with varying composition of different cannabinoids.

Benzodiazepines

Benzodiazepines, first synthesized in the 1950s, are commonly used medications for help with both sleep initiation and sleep maintenance insomnia, in addition to being drugs that are used in harmful ways. Although benzodiazepines gained their height of popularity in the 1970s, the side effect profile and the potential for unhealthy or harmful use started to emerge.[157] This class of medications offers sedative/hypnotic, anxiolytic, anticonvulsant, and muscle relaxing properties with potential side effects of daytime sedation, delirium, falls, ataxia, rebound insomnia, and cognitive impairment.[157-159]

The primary effects of benzodiazepines are to shorten sleep-onset latency, reducing REM latency and decreasing nocturnal awakenings.[157,160,161] With acute and chronic use, there can be an increase in spindle activity and a decrease in the amount of SWS (slow-wave sleep). These agents bind to GABA receptors in the CNS and result in inhibition of neuronal excitation. GABA receptors are ubiquitous in the brain, including the ventral lateral preoptic area that controls sleep.[157,162] More specifically, benzodiazepines bind nonselectively to the GABA-A alpha subunits resulting in sedative, hypnotic, anticonvulsant, muscle relaxant, and anxiolytic properties and of course corresponding side effects.[163,164]

The benzodiazepines that are approved by the FDA for the short-term use of insomnia include triazolam, estazolam, temazepam, and quazepam. The duration of action and the adverse side effects of the medications are related to the elimination half-life and active metabolites. Metabolism is mostly through the liver via glucuronidation, oxidation, and nitroreduction, with little renal involvement.[163,165] As oxidative capacity is reduced with aging, all but temazepam have a prolonged half-life in the elderly, which significantly affects both the efficacy and the side effect profile. Alcohol and other CNS depressants should be avoided in conjunction with benzodiazepines.

Temazepam is the most commonly used benzodiazepine for insomnia. Short-term use of the medication is effective in improvement of TST without major CNS and behavioral adverse effects.[166,167] Unfortunately, no benzodiazepines have been studied for more than 12 weeks to assess long-term effects of chronic medication use.

Benzodiazepine use is associated with potential for physical dependence.[168,169] Typical symptoms of withdrawal, which result secondary to an abrupt discontinuation, include agitation, anxiety, dysphoria, rebound insomnia, diarrhea, tachycardia, delirium, and seizures.[170] The role of this class of medications is diminishing, and increasingly benzodiazepine use is discouraged, especially in the elderly population.

Since the 1980s, nonbenzodiazepine receptor agonist (BZRA) medications like zolpidem, zopiclone, eszopiclone, and zaleplon have steadily gained popularity and conquered the insomnia drug market.[171] These agents differ in structure from typical benzodiazepines but have a similar mechanism of effect. Similar to benzodiazepines, non BZRAs bind to the GABA-A receptor complex. Only these medications are more selective and bind to the GABA-A alpha-1 subunit, which is responsible for both sedative and hypnotic effects with less risk of negative consequences. Although originally considered as a safer, effective alternative to the classic benzodiazepines with no potential for unhealthy use, studies have emerged that highlighted unhealthy use among both men and women. Most cases are in people more likely to engage in unhealthy use of other drugs and who have psychiatric illness.[171] There is one study, published in 2007, which determined that zolpidem has a potential for unhealthy use and to be associated with SUD, and therefore should be used with caution in vulnerable populations.[172]

Gabapentin

Gabapentin, first approved in 1993 in the United States as an antiepileptic, is a commonly used medication for insomnia especially in the patient population that suffers from neuropathic pain and restless leg.[173,174]

Gabapentin was originally marketed and sold as an agent with no significant risk for unhealthy use or disorder and lacks the federal classification of a scheduled medication. It is used in the treatment of AUD and withdrawal. A number of cases have described SUD associated with gabapentin, all in patients with prior SUD, in particular co-occurring with opioid use disorder.[175] Some report euphoric effects similar but weaker to cocaine when combined with quetiapine. Some people with opioid use disorder use gabapentin to potentiate the desired opioid effects and it has been shown to increase the risk of opioid-related overdose.[175]

Withdrawal from gabapentin has also been described, which includes agitation, confusion and disorientation, diaphoresis, tremor, tachycardia, hypertension, and insomnia.[175-177]

Gabapentin is a structural analogue of GABA that does not bind to GABA but exerts a neural inhibitory role through binding to the alpha-2-delta-1 subunits of the voltage-gated calcium channels.[175,178] Gabapentin is highly lipid soluble and widely distributes through the CNS, resulting in its associated side effect of drowsiness, which is responsible for its effects on insomnia.[179,180]

Gabapentin improves WASO (wake after sleep onset) and increases TST. These results are both from objective PSG (polysomnogram) results and from subjective patient questionnaires. In addition, subjective questionnaires also indicated an improvement in overall sleep quality.[179] Adverse side effects include headaches, dizziness, and GI disturbances. Overall, it is second-line therapy for insomnia unless the patients have comorbid RLS and/or chronic neuropathic pain.

Clonidine

Clonidine is a nonselective alpha-2 adrenergic agonist that has been used to help with sleep initiation and maintenance, especially in the pediatric population. Although it is commonly used among people with SUD to help with both alcohol and opioid withdrawal, it is also a drug that is used in unhealthy ways.

Although the literature is sparse, there is some polysomnographic evidence to suggest that clonidine shortens sleep latency, overall decreases REM sleep, and improves sleep efficiency.[181,182]

Clonidine works at the level of the prefrontal cortex, mediating inattentiveness, hyperactivity, and impulsivity. At the level of the thalamus, its actions are associated with sedation. At the level of the locus coeruleus, it is associated with hypotensive and sedative effects.[182] Given the above properties, it is a commonly used medication in people with ADHD to help with inattention or hyperactivity, to potentiate the effects of stimulants, and also to help with commonly associated symptoms of both sleep initiation and sleep maintenance insomnia.[182,183]

Clonidine is also commonly used to help with sleep in children with neurodevelopmental disorders, like autism spectrum disorder (ASD). In children with ASD, it was shown to decrease sleep initiation latency and night awakenings, in addition to improving mood instability and aggressiveness.[182,184]

Clonidine has also been successful in reducing the CNS noradrenergic activity and helping in symptoms of PTSD. Open-label case series showed that clonidine reduces PTSD trauma nightmares and overall improved sleep in Cambodian refugees and improved overall PTSD symptoms in veterans.[183,184]

Clonidine has been used extensively to aid in symptoms of opioid withdrawal by reducing sympathetic overactivity like tachycardia, hypertension, seating, flashes, and restlessness.[183,185] In addition, it eases accompanying insomnia.

Of interest, according to a study that published a self-reported questionnaire of patients seeking management of withdrawal, 18% reported receiving a prescription for clonidine, 6% reported using higher than prescribed doses of clonidine, and 8% reported taking clonidine without a prescription, and the prevalence of nonprescribed use was higher among people with opioid use disorder.[186] Explanations for unhealthy clonidine use might be related to the medication's ability to potentiate opioidergic effects, including analgesia.[186] Other thoughts include clonidine's ability to reduce core withdrawal symptoms, to dampen other adverse effects of other drugs, or to self-medicate comorbid undiagnosed psychopathology.[186,187]

CLINICAL APPROACHES TO SLEEP DISORDERS

The clinical approach to patients with co-occurring sleep and SUD poses certain problems. In addition to dealing with specific sleep disorders, it is necessary to address the effect of the substance for use on sleep, the effect of withdrawal, and any comorbid psychiatric problems such as depression. In some cases, a drug may have been masking or inadvertently treating an underlying sleep disorder, as in the case of the therapeutic effects of opioids on RLS. The clinical picture may be further complicated because some of the medications used in the treatment of specific sleep disorders have a potential for unhealthy use. Therefore, a systematic approach is critical.

1. The first step is to obtain a careful history of the amount of sleep actually obtained in a 24-hour period. A diary can be used, but a careful history often elicits the necessary information.
2. The next step is to address the issue of timing and to determine the patient's probable circadian rhythm. This can be complicated by shifting work schedules and other activities. Again, the history is the most powerful tool. A sleep diary can be helpful.
3. Consider the potential for medical or psychiatric issues that can interfere with sleep. These are detected through a careful medical and psychiatric review, including an inventory of medications, exercise, nicotine, alcohol, and other drug use. Give careful attention to symptoms of anxiety, depression, nightmares, and posttraumatic stress.
4. Inquire about possible features of intrinsic sleep disorders. Is there evidence of OSA (snoring, sleep disruption, obesity, hypertension, and morning headache)? Is there a reason to suspect PLMS or RLS? Is there a history of sleep-disturbing paresthesias or a history of sleep-related movement disorder?
5. Inquire about the sleep environment. Is the sleep area conducive to the relaxation required to allow the wake-to-sleep transition? This is a relative concept; for example, a television can be hypnotic for some but stimulating for others.

Occasionally, additional diagnostic studies are required. Some of these studies are part of the medical evaluation. Expanded use of a diary can be of value. A PSG should be considered if OSA or narcolepsy is suspected. A PSG is also helpful in evaluating parasomnia (abnormal sleep-related behavior). Finally, a multiple sleep latency test can be helpful in documenting hypersomnia or the presence of early-onset REM.

After the evaluation is complete, the clinician can initiate a strategy to address the sleep problem. This approach needs to take the SUD into consideration, because problems underlying the addiction must be addressed and treated. Care must be taken in the selection of medications. Whenever possible, associated medical or psychiatric conditions should be treated. Only then can "intrinsic" sleep disorders be treated.

For example, RLS and PLMS can be treated with medications that are not subject to unhealthy use. OSA usually is treated with continuous positive airway pressure devices.

If the patient still has difficulties with sleep, an underlying cause should be sought. Often, the cause is some form of anxiety disorder that requires direct attention. At times, this may be related to a withdrawal effect. Relaxation techniques are as helpful to some patients as medications. The usual sedating or hypnotic agents can be used for transient problems. However, in working with a patient for whom addiction is an issue, it is wise to consider the sedating antidepressants or the more active agents used to treat other anxiety-related disorders, such as the selective serotonin reuptake inhibitors (SSRIs).

SPECIAL ISSUES IN SLEEP PHARMACOTHERAPY AND ADDICTION

Consideration of pharmacotherapy in patients with the potential for unhealthy use of medications may present unique challenges. For obvious reasons, the approach may not be straightforward. Later, we shall review some of these concerns.

Finally, in a particular concern for patients with SUD, one must consider the long-term impact of the substance in question. The effects of withdrawal may persist for extended periods of time. Furthermore, it is important to keep in mind that patients may also have tobacco use disorder and be dealing with nocturnal nicotine withdrawal.

Insomnia

When appropriate, nonpharmacological approaches should be considered first. Several medications can be considered in the management of insomnia. Certainly, it is important to address associated medical issues. Whether one considers the insomnia as a symptom or a comorbid disorder, it is often helpful to treat the insomnia directly. Anxiety and stress are symptoms that are often overlooked. Frequently, patients become fixated on the sleep issue and fail to recognize the contribution of anxiety to insomnia. They may become convinced that treatment of insomnia will eliminate anxiety. At this point, the standard of care is to consider Cognitive-Behavioral Therapy for Insomnia (CBT-I).

CBT-I actually consists of a several components. Although frequently used by sleep medicine behavioral specialists, many of the features can be handled by the addiction clinician. These components include: Sleep Hygiene, Stimulus Control Therapy, Sleep Restriction Therapy Cognitive Therapy and Relaxation Therapy.

1. Sleep Hygiene
   The sleep environment should be modified to allow for the relaxation required for the wake-to-sleep transition. It should be separated from work and play areas. Noise and lighting should be modified to allow for optimal relaxation.
   - The times at which caffeine, nicotine, alcohol, and other medications are used should be assessed and adjusted as necessary.
   - Regular exercise has been found to improve sleep and should be recommended.
   - Adoption of a regular sleep-wake schedule should be encouraged. Napping is permissible but will reduce the need to sleep at night.

- Finally, the patient needs to be able to separate sleep time from other stressors, allowing for a period of relaxation. The patient should be instructed to leave the bedroom whenever he or she is unable to sleep, to avoid the development of further anxiety.

2. Stimulus Control Therapy
   It is important to eliminate factors that might contribute to an inability to fall asleep. The sleep area should be free of elements that might be stimulating to the patient. For some patients who wake in the middle of the night and check the clock to see how much sleep they might lose, it will be important to remove the clock.
3. Sleep Restriction Therapy
   Restricting the time available for sleep has been shown to increase sleep efficiency. This is usually done by getting an estimate of the sleep need over a 24-hour period and restricting the time in bed to slightly less than that amount of time. Often, this includes an elimination of naps and restriction of time in bed at night.
4. Cognitive therapy
   This includes the education of the patient to sleep. It is common to experience a few awakenings. It is important to set a regular sleep timing, and so forth.
5. Relaxation Therapy
   Once other sleep disorders are addressed, a common problem is the inability to relax. The relaxation therapy should be tailored to the patient. There is no reason that any approach will be superior for all patients.

Access to a specialist in CBT-I is not always available. This should not deter the clinician from recommending some of these elements. In addition, there are programs that are available online and some are at no-cost.

The clinician may be concerned about the addition of traditional anxiolytics such as benzodiazepines—but, other nonbenzodiazepine approaches may be helpful. Frequently, SSRIs or similar agents may be helpful. Other pharmacological nonbenzodiazepine agents, which promote sleep, may be considered, such as FDA approved medications for the treatment of insomnia. Certainly, this must be considered in the context of an underlying SUD and the risks and benefits assessed, particularly for BZRAs. This group includes several of the traditional benzodiazepines and the benzodiazepine receptor agonists (zolpidem, zaleplon, and eszopiclone). Other medications approved for the treatment of insomnia include doxepin (3, 6 mg doses), ramelteon (an MT1 and MT2 agonist), and the dual-action orexin receptor antagonists or DORAs (suvorexant, lemborexant, daridorexant).

There are other medications that have been commonly used for the management of insomnia symptoms. These do not have formal FDA approval, and one needs to be mindful of side effects. The potential for unhealthy use needs to be monitored always in this population, even with medications that were not previously considered to have such potential. Gabapentin is an example of an agent with a long history of use but only recently recognized to have unhealthy use potential. Unfortunately, there is no absolute answer for the clinician. In each case, the clinician needs to weigh the potential benefits against the side effects. One also needs to consider the management of the underlying SUD. Pharmacotherapy options include:

1. Herbal agents. Several herbal ingredients have been suggested as hypnotics. Unfortunately, the use of these agents is limited by the relative lack of potency and the uncertainty of the formulation since they are not regulated as other medications.
2. Melatonin. Melatonin has been used for its sleep-promoting properties as well as for its ability to assist in the management of circadian sleep phase disorders. Although limited by the same issues cited for herbal agents, there has been a greater degree of evidence and acceptability that should make the clinician consider a trial of melatonin for the initiation of sleep.
3. Over-the-counter agents. In general, the "active ingredient" in most of the over-the-counter medications that target insomnia is an antihistamine. The most limiting factor with these medications is that the effective half-life may be a bit longer than desired.
4. Sedating antidepressants. Over the years, along with the BZRAs, this group has been most commonly prescribed as a sleep aid. The most common agents in this group are trazodone, mirtazapine, doxepin, and amitriptyline. All of these have been noted to be sedating. They all have an effective half-life that is somewhat longer than desirable for some. The implication is that the patient may experience some "hangover" effect in the morning. There may be some concern about some anticholinergic effect.
5. Sedating antipsychotics. Quetiapine is a sedating atypical antipsychotic that has also been used as a sleep aid. Again, the clinician needs to consider the potential side effects when using antipsychotics.
6. Clonidine. Clonidine is an alpha-2-adrenergic agonist with sedating properties. Care must be taken since it may have a relatively long half-life. It has been found to be helpful in a variety of anxiety-related disorders and can be helpful in sleep promotion. It may also be helpful in the management of ADHD. As noted, there is evidence to suggest that it may also be helpful in the management of RLS—a disorder that may also interfere with sleep onset. Again, the clinician must consider the use of this in the context of overall addiction management.
7. Prazosin. Prazosin is an alpha-1-adrenergic blocker that has been found to be particularly helpful in the management of nightmare disorder. Although the available evidence is primarily tagged to nightmare disorder associated with PTSD, it should be noted that most of the studies of medical management of nightmare disorder are restricted to cases associated with PTSD. Although prazosin is not specifically targeted for insomnia, there are some patients where nightmare disorder may masquerade as insomnia.
8. Calcium channel alpha-2-delta ligands. Although there is no formal indication for their use in insomnia, there has been an increase in the use of gabapentin and pregabalin

for patients with insomnia. There has also been concern about the potential for unhealthy use of these agents, so special care must be taken if these agents are to be considered in the treatment of patients with addiction.

9. BZRAs (benzodiazepine receptor agonists). This is the group of medications that include the agents with an FDA indication for the treatment of insomnia. These agents are GABA-A receptor agonists, and many feel that they should be considered as a single group. These include the traditional benzodiazepines and the receptor agonists (zolpidem, zaleplon, eszopiclone). In clinical practice, most of these agents vary according to rate of effect onset, potency, and rate of effect elimination. Again, great care must be taken if they are to be considered in the patient with addiction.
10. Ramelteon. This is an MT1/MT2 agonist that has been approved for the treatment of insomnia, particularly sleep-onset insomnia. Its role and effectiveness in this population are unclear. It appears to have little or no potential for unhealthy use; however, as described for other medications above, such problems are typically identified later—after FDA approval and widespread use, and in more generalized populations. Unfortunately, it is also considered to have low potency.
11. Dual-action orexin/hypocretin receptors antagonists (DORAs). This a relatively new class of hypnotic agents that include suvorexant and the more recently released lemborexant and daridorexant. A deficiency in the orexin/hypocretin system is considered to be the cause of many cases of narcolepsy. They can be considered for short-term and long-term treatment of insomnia. Infrequent, but notable side effects may include disruptive dreams, sleep paralysis and suicidal thoughts that appear to be dose-related.

Restless Legs Syndrome

A few words of caution arise with regard to recognition and management of RLS in this patient population. It is possible that RLS symptoms may be "unmasked" as the patient withdraws from certain drugs of addiction, especially opioids. It is also possible that symptoms may be triggered or aggravated by several of the medications cited above. In particular, antihistamines, antidepressants, and antipsychotic medications may be culprits. Similarly, caffeine and nicotine may also be aggravating factors. All of this can be complicated by the fact that RLS may "masquerade" as anxiety/insomnia (see **Table 95-3**).

REFERENCES

1. Mellinger GD, Balter MB, Uhlenhuth EH. Insomnia and its treatment: prevalence. *Arch Gen Psychiatry*. 1985;42:225-232.
2. Ohayon MM, Carskadon MA, Guilleminault C, Vitiello MV. Meta-analysis of quantitative sleep parameters from childhood to old age in healthy individuals: developing normative sleep values across the human lifespan. *Sleep*. 2004;27(7):1255-1273.
3. Rechtschaffen A, Kales A. *A Method of Standardized Terminology, Techniques and Scoring System for Sleep Stages of Human Subjects*. Brain Information Series/Brain Research Institute; 1968.
4. Berry RB, Bfooks R, Gamaldo CE, et al. *The AASM Manual for the Scoring of Sleep and Associated Events, version 2.4*. American Academy of Sleep Medicine; 2017.
5. American Sleep Disorders Association. The clinical use of the Multiple Sleep Latency Test. *Sleep*. 1992;15:265-278.
6. Czeisler C, Richardson G, Martin JB. Disorders of sleep and circadian rhythm. In: Wilson JD, Braumwald E, Fauci A, et al., eds. *Principles and Practice of Internal Medicine*. McGraw Hill; 1991.
7. The Diagnostic Classification Steering Committee. *The International Classification of Sleep Disorders Diagnostic and Coding Manual, Revised*. American Academy of Sleep Medicine; 2005.
8. Allen R, Picchietti D, Hening WA. Restless legs syndrome: diagnostic criteria, special considerations, and epidemiology. A report from the restless legs syndrome diagnosis and epidemiology workshop at the National Institutes of Health. *Sleep Med*. 2003;4:101-119.
9. Tenkerwalder C, Hening WA, Montagna P, et al. Treatment of restless legs syndrome: an evidence based review and implications for clinical practice. *Mov Disord*. 2008;23(16):2267-2302.
10. Yang C, White DP, Winkelman JW. Antidepressants and periodic leg movements of sleep. *Biol Psychiatry*. 2005;58:510-514.
11. Sforza E, Mathis J, Bassetti CL. Restless leg syndrome: pathophysiology and clinical aspects. *Schweiz Arch Neurol Psychiatr*. 2003;154:349-357.
12. Aurora RN, Kristo DA, Bista SR, et al. The treatment of restless legs syndrome and periodic limb movement disorder in adults—an update for 2012: practice parameters with an evidence-based systematic review and meta-analyses. *Sleep*. 2012;35(8):1039-1062.
13. Koskenvu M, Kapiro J, Partinen M. Snoring as a risk factor for hypertension and angina pectoris. *Lancet*. 1985;1:893-895.
14. Lugaresi E, Partinen M. Prevalence of snoring in sleep and breathing. In: Saunders N, Sullivan CE, eds. *Sleep and Breathing*. Marcel Dekker; 1994.
15. Telakivi T, Partinen M, Koskenvuo M, Salmi T, Kaprio J. Periodic breathing and hypoxia in snorers and controls: validation of snoring history and association with blood pressure and obesity. *Acta Neurol Scand*. 1987;76:69-75.
16. Young T, Palta M, Dempsey J, Skatrud J, Weber S, Badr S. The occurrence of sleep disordered breathing among middle-aged adults. *N Engl J Med*. 1993;328(17):1230-1235.
17. Lee W, Nagubsdi S, Kryger MH, Mokhlesi B. Epidemiology of obstructive sleep apnea: a population based perspective. *Expert Rev Respir Med*. 2008;2(3):349-364.
18. Schober AK, Neurath MF, Hersch IA. Prevalence of sleep apnea in diabetic patients. *Clin Respir J*. 2011;5(3):165-172.
19. Li Y, Veasey SC. Neurobiology and neuropathophysiology of obstructive sleep apnea. *Neuromolecular Med*. 2012;14(3):168-179.
20. van Dijk M, Donga E, van Dijk JG, et al. Disturbed subjective sleep characteristics in adult patients with longstanding type I diabetes mellitus. *Diabetologia*. 2011;54(8):1967-1976.
21. Guilleminault MD, Stohs R. Upper airway resistance syndrome. *Sleep Res*. 1991;20:250-257.
22. Morrill MJ, Finn L, Kim H, Peppard PE, Badr MS, Young T. Sleep fragmentation, awake blood pressure and sleep disordered breathing in a population-based study. *Am J Respir Crit Care Med*. 2000;162:2091-2096.
23. Nieto FJ, Young TB, Lind KB, et al. Association of sleep disordered breathing, sleep apnea and hypertension in a large community based study. *JAMA*. 2000;283:1829-1836.
24. Walker JM, Farney RJ, Rhondeau SM, et al. Chronic opioid use is a risk factor for the development of central sleep apnea and ataxic breathing. *J Clin Sleep Med*. 2007;3(5):455-461.
25. Walker JM, Famey RJ. Are opioids associated with sleep apnea? A review of the evidence. *Curr Pain Headache Rep*. 2009;13(2):120-126.
26. NIH State-of-the-Science Conference Statement on manifestations and management of chronic insomnia in adults. *NIH Consen State Sci Statements*. 2005;22(2):1-30.
27. Morgenthaler TI, Auerbach S, Casey KR, et al. Position paper for the treatment of nightmare disorder in adults: an American Academy of Sleep Medicine position paper. *J Clin Sleep Med*. 2018;14(6):1041-1055.
28. Shapiro CM, Warren PM, Trinder J, et al. Fitness facilitates sleep. *Eur J Appl Physiol*. 1987;53:1-4.

29. Edinger JD, Morey MC, Sullivan RJ, et al. Aerobic fitness, acute exercise and fitness in older men. *Sleep*. 1993;16(4):351-359.
30. Spielman AJ, Sakin P, Thorpy MJ. Treatment of chronic insomnia by restriction of time in bed. *Sleep*. 1987;10:145-156.
31. Rubenstein ML, Rothenberg SA, Maherwarren S, et al. Modified sleep restriction therapy in middle aged and elderly insomniacs. *Sleep Res*. 1990;19:276.
32. Zepelon H, McDonald CS, Zammit GK. Effect of age on auditory threshold. *J Gerontol*. 1984;39:284-300.
33. Harsh J, Purvis B, Badia P, Magee J. Behavioral responses in older adults. *Biol Psychol*. 1990;30:51-60.
34. Southwell PR, Evans CR, Hunt JN. The effects of a hot milk drink on movements during sleep. *Br Med J*. 1992;2:429-433.
35. Baker JC, Mitteness LS. Nocturia in the elderly. *Gerontologist*. 1989;28:99-194.
36. Cook NR, Evans DA, Funklestein H, et al. Correlates of headache in a population based cohort study of the elderly. *Arch Neurol*. 1989;46:338-344.
37. Hyppa MT, Kronholm E. Quantity of sleep and chronic illness. *J Clin Epidemiol*. 1989;42:633-638.
38. Brugge KL, Kripke DF, Ancoli-Israel S, et al. The association of menopause status and age with sleep disorders. *Sleep Res*. 1989;18:208.
39. Johnson EA, Roehrs T, Roth T, Breslau N. Epidemiology of alcohol and medications as aids to sleep in early adulthood. *Sleep*. 1988;21:178-186.
40. Hu N, Ma Y, He J, Zhu L, Cao S. Alcohol consumption and increase of sleep disorder: a systematic review and meta-analysis of cohort studies. *Drug Alcohol Depend*. 2020;217:108259.
41. Baker FC, Carskadon MA, Hasler BP. Sleep and women's health:sex- and age-specific contributors to alcohol use disorders. *J Womens Health (Larchmt)*. 2020;29(3):443-445.
42. Britton A, Fat LN, Neligan A. The association between alcohol consumption and sleep disorders among older people in the general population. *Sci Rep*. 2020;10(1):5275.
43. Papineau KL, Roehrs TA, Petricelli N, Rosenthal LD, Roth T. Electrophysiological assessment (the multiple sleep latency test) of the biphasic effects of ethanol in humans. *Alcohol Clin Exp Res*. 1988;22:231-235.
44. Silveri NM, Spear LP. Ontogeny of rapid tolerance to the hypnotic effects of ethanol. *Alcohol Clin Exp Res*. 1999;23(7):1180-1184.
45. Silveri NM, Spear LP. Decreased sensitivity to the hypnotic effects of ethanol early in ontogeny. *Alcohol Clin Exp Res*. 1998;22(3):670-676.
46. Roehrs T, Roth T. Sleep, sleepiness, sleep disorders and alcohol use and abuse. *Sleep Med Rev*. 2001;5:287-297.
47. Yules RB, Lippman ME, Freedman DX. Alcohol administration prior to sleep: the effect on EEG sleep stages. *Arch Gen Psychiatry*. 1967;16:94-97.
48. Lobo LL, Tuffik S. Effect of alcohol on sleep parameters of sleep deprived healthy volunteers. *Sleep*. 1997;20:52-59.
49. Feige B, Gann H, Brueck R, et al. Effects of alcohol on polysomnographically recorded sleep in healthy subjects. *Alcohol Clin Exp Res*. 2006;30:1527-1537.
50. Arnedt JT, Rohsenow DJ, Almeida AB, et al. Sleep following alcohol intoxication in healthy, young adults: effects of sex and family history of alcoholism. *Alcohol Clin Exp Res*. 2011;35(5):870-878.
51. Vitello MV. Sleep, alcohol and alcohol abuse. *Addict Biol*. 1997;2:151-158.
52. Mennella JA, Gerish CJ. Effects of exposure to alcohol in mothers' milk on infant sleep. *Pediatrics*. 1998;101(5):E2.
53. Scher GS, Richardson GA, Coble PA, Day NL, Stoffer DS. The effects of parental alcohol and marijuana exposure: disturbances in neonatal sleep cycling and arousal. *Pediatr Res*. 1998;24:101-105.
54. Landolt HP, Roth C, Dijk DJ. Late afternoon ethanol intake affects nocturnal sleep and the sleep EEG in middle-aged man. *J Clin Psychopharmacol*. 1996;16:428-436.
55. Roehrs T, Beare D, Zorick F. Sleepiness and ethanol effects on simulated driving. *Alcohol Clin Exp Res*. 1994;18:154-158.
56. Zwyghuizen-Doorenbos A, Roehrs T, Timms V. Individual differences in the sedating effects of alcohol. *Alcohol Clin Exp Res*. 1990;14:400-404.
57. Zwyghuizen-Doorenbos A, Roehrs T, Lamphere J. Increased daytime sleepiness enhances ethanol's sedative effects. *Neuropsychopharmacology*. 1998;1:279-286.
58. Lunley M, Roehrs T, Asker D, Zorick F, Roth T. Ethanol and caffeine effects on daytime sleepiness/alertness. *Sleep*. 1987;10:306-312.
59. Van Reen E, Jenni OG, Carskadon MA. Effects of alcohol on sleep and the sleep electroencephalogram in healthy young women. *Alcohol Clin Exp Res*. 2006;30:974-981.
60. Mello MK, Mendelson JH. Behavioral studies of sleep patterns in alcoholics during intoxication and withdrawal. *J Pharmacol Exp Ther*. 1970;175:94-112.
61. Allen RP, Wagman A, Fallace LA. Electroencephalic (EEG) sleep recovery following prolonged alcohol intoxication in alcoholics. *J Nerv Ment Dis*. 1971;153:424-433.
62. Adamson J, Berdick JA. Sleep of day alcoholics. *Arch Gen Psychiatry*. 1973;28:146-149.
63. Cernovsky Z. MMPI, nightmares in male alcoholics. *Percept Mot Skills*. 1985;61:841-842.
64. Cernovsky Z. MMPI and nightmare reports in women addicted to alcohol and other drugs. *Percept Mot Skills*. 1986;62:717-719.
65. Christo G, Franey C. Addicts' drug related dreams: their frequency and relationship to six-month outcomes. *Subst Use Misuse*. 1996;31:1-15.
66. Denizen N. Alcoholic dreams. *Alcohol Treat Q*. 1988;5:133-139.
67. Stewart SH. Alcohol abuse in individuals exposed to trauma—a critical review. *Psychol Bull*. 1996;120:83-112.
68. Easton PA, West PA, Weatherall RC, Brewster JF, Lertzman M, Kryger MH. The effect of excessive ethanol ingestion on sleep in severe chronic obstructive pulmonary disease. *Sleep*. 1987;10:224-233.
69. Dolly FR, Block AJ. Increased ventricular ectopy and sleep apnea following ethanol ingestion in COPD patients. *Chest*. 1983;83:469-472.
70. Rowland RH. Sleep onset rapid eye movement periods in neuropsychiatric disorders: implications for the pathophysiology of psychoses. *J Nerv Ment Dis*. 1997;185:730-738.
71. Johnson LC, Burdick JA, Smith J. Sleep during alcohol intake and withdrawal in the chronic alcoholic. *Arch Gen Psychiatry*. 1970;22:406-418.
72. Feinberg I. Hallucinations, dreaming and REM sleep. In: Kemp W, ed. *Origin and Mechanisms of Hallucinations*. Plenum Publishing; 1970:125-132.
73. Wolin SJ, Mello JK. The effects of alcohol on dreams and hallucinations in alcohol addicts. *Ann N Y Acad Sci*. 1973;215:266-302.
74. Mahowald MW, Shenck CH. REM sleep parasomnias. In: Kryger MH, Roth T, Dement WC, eds. *Principles and Practice of Sleep Medicine*. 3rd ed. WB Saunders; 2000.
75. Gillin JC, Smith TL, Irwin M. Short REM latency in primary alcoholics with secondary depression. *Am J Psychiatry*. 1990;147:106-109.
76. Williams HL, Rundell OH. Altered sleep physiology in chronic alcoholics: reversal with abstinence. *Alcohol Clin Exp Res*. 1981;2:318-325.
77. Ehlers CL, Phillips E, Parry BL. Electrophysiological findings during the menstrual cycle in women with and without late luteal phase dysphoric disorder: relationship to risk for alcoholism. *Biol Psychiatry*. 1996;39:720-732.
78. Brower KJ, Aldrich MS, Hall JM. Polysomnographic and subjective sleep predictors in alcoholic relapse. *Alcohol Clin Exp Res*. 1998;22:1864-1877.
79. Drummond SPA, Gillin JC, Smith TL. The sleep of abstinent pure primary alcoholic patients: natural course and relationship to relapse. *Alcohol Clin Exp Res*. 1998;22:1796-1782.
80. Brower KJ, Aldrich MS, Robinson EA, et al. Insomnia, self-medication and relapse to alcoholism. *Am J Psychiatry*. 2001;158:399-404.
81. Allen RP, Wagman AM, Funderburk FR, et al. Slow wave sleep: a predictor of individual responses to drinking. *Biol Psychiatry*. 1980;15:345-348.
82. Wagman AM, Allen RP, Funderbunk FR, Wells DT. EEG measures of functional tolerance to alcohol. *Biol Psychiatry*. 1978;13:719-728.
83. Clark CP, Gillin JC, Golshan S, et al. Increased REM density at admission predicts relapse by three months in primary alcoholics with a lifetime history of secondary depression. *Biol Psychiatry*. 1998;43:601-607.

84. Clark CP, Gillin JC, Golshan S, et al. Polysomnography and depressive symptoms in primary alcoholism with and without a lifetime history of secondary depression and inpatients with primary major depression. *J Affect Disord*. 1999;52:177-185.
85. Gillin JC, Smith TL, Irwin M. Increased pressure for rapid eye movement sleep at time of hospital admission predicts relapse in nondepressed patients with primary alcoholism at three month follow-up. *Arch Gen Psychiatry*. 1994;51:189-197.
86. Aldrich MS. Sleep disordered breathing in alcoholics: association with age. *Alcohol Clin Exp Res*. 1993;17(6):1179-1183.
87. Burgos-Sanchez C, Jones NN, Avillion M, et al. Impact of alcohol consumption on snoring and sleep apnea: a systematic review and meta-analysis. *Otolaryngol Head Neck Surg*. 2020;163(6):1078-1086.
88. Simou E, Britton J, Leonardi-Bee J. Alcohol and the risk of sleep apnea: a systematic review and meta-analysis. *Sleep Med*. 2018;42:38-46.
89. Tracy EL, Reid KJ, Baron KG. The relationship between sleep and physical activity: the moderating role of daily alcohol consumption. *Sleep*. 2021;11(10):zsab112.
90. Bloom JW, Kaltenborn WT, Quan F. Risk factors for a general population for snoring: importance of smoking and obesity. *Chest*. 1988;93:678-683.
91. Tassan V, Block A, Boysen P. Alcohol increases sleep apnea and oxygen desaturation in asymptomatic men. *Am J Med*. 1981;71:240-245.
92. Robinson R, White D, Zwilich C. Moderate alcohol ingestion increases upper airway resistance in normal subjects. *Am Rev Resp Dis*. 1985;132:1238-1241.
93. Miller M, Dawson A, Henricksen S. Bedtime alcohol increases resistance of upper airways and produces sleep apnea in asymptomatic snorers. *Alcohol Clin Exp Res*. 1988;12:801-805.
94. Scrina L, Broudy M, Nay KN, Cohn MA. Increased severity of obstructive sleep apnea after bedtime alcohol ingestion: diagnostic potential and proposed mechanism of action. *Sleep*. 1982;5:318-328.
95. Krol RC, Knuth SL, Bartlett D. Selective reduction of genioglossal muscle activity by alcohol in normal human subjects. *Am Rev Resp Dis*. 1984;129:247-250.
96. Dawson A, Bigby BG, Poceta JS, Mitler MM. Effect of bedtime alcohol on inspiratory resistance and respiratory drive in snoring and nonsnoring men. *Alcohol Clin Exp Res*. 1997;21:183-190.
97. Berry RB, Bonnet M, Light RW. Effect of ethanol on the arousal response to airway obstruction during sleep in normal subjects. *Am Rev Resp Dis*. 1992;145:445-452.
98. Issa FG, Sullivan CE. Alcohol, snoring and sleep apnea. *J Neurol Neurosurg Psychiatry*. 1982;45:353-358.
99. Block AJ, Hellard DW, Slayton PC. Minimal effect of alcohol ingestion on breathing during the sleep of postmenopausal women. *Chest*. 1985;88:181-184.
100. Block AJ, Hellard DW, Slayton PC. Effect of alcohol ingestion on breathing and oxygenation during sleep: analysis of the effects of age and sex. *Am J Med*. 1986;80:595-560.
101. Aldrich MS, Shipley JE. Alcohol use and periodic limb movements of sleep. *Alcohol Clin Exp Res*. 1993;17:192-196.
102. Le Bon O, Verbanck P. Sleep in detoxified alcoholics: impairment of most standard sleep parameters and increased risk for sleep apnea, but not for myoclonus: a controlled study. *J Stud Alcohol*. 1997;58:30-36.
103. Post RM, Gillin JC, Goodwin FK. The effect of orally administered cocaine on sleep of depressed patients. *Psychopharmacology (Berl)*. 1970;37:59-66.
104. Gillin JC, Pulverenti L, Withers N, Golshan S, Koob G. The effects of lisuride on mood and sleep during acute withdrawal in stimulant abusers: a preliminary report. *Biol Psychiatry*. 1994;35:843-849.
105. Feinberg I, Hibi S, Braun M, Caveness C, Westerman G, Small A. Sleep amphetamine effects in MBDS and normal subjects. *Arch Gen Psychiatry*. 1974;31:723-731.
106. Washington WW, Brown BS, Haertzen CA. Changes in mood, craving and sleep during short term abstinence reported by male cocaine addicts. *Arch Gen Psychiatry*. 1990;47:861-868.
107. Thompson PM, Gillin JC, Golshan S. Polygraphic sleep measures differentiate alcoholics and stimulant abusers during short-term abstinence. *Biol Psychiatry*. 1995;38:831-836.
108. Garciaa AN, Salloum IM. Polysomnographic sleep disturbances in nicotine, caffeine, alcohol, cocaine, opioid, and cannabis use: a focused review. *Am J Addict*. 2015;24:590-598.
109. Randall S, Johanson CE, Tancer M, Roehrs T. Effects of acute 3, 4-methylenedioxymethamphetamine on sleep and daytime sleepiness in MDMA users: a preliminary study. *Sleep*. 2009;32(11):1513-1519.
110. Schierenbeck T, Riemann D, Berger M, Hornyak M. Effect of illicit recreational drugs upon sleep: cocaine, ecstasy and marijuana. *Sleep Med Rev*. 2008;12(5):381-389.
111. Kirilly E, Molnar E, Balogh B, et al. Decrease in REM latency and changes in sleep quality parallel serotonergic damage and recovery after MDMA: a longitudinal study over 180 days. *Int J Neuropsychopharmacol*. 2008;11(6):795-809.
112. Bosker WM, Kuypers KP, Conen S, et al. MDMA (ecstasy) effects on actual driving performance before and after sleep deprivation, as function of dose and concentration in blood and oral fluid. *Psychopharmacology (Berl)*. 2012;222(3):367-376.
113. McCann UD, Ricaurte GA. Effects of (±) 3,4-methylenedioxymathamphetamine (MDMA) on sleep and circadian rhythms. *ScientificWorldJournal*. 2007;7:231-238.
114. Kay D, Pickworth W, Neider G. Morphine-like insomnia in nondependent human addicts. *Br J Clin Pharmacol*. 1981;11:159-169.
115. Curtis AF, Miller MB, Rathinakumar H, et al. Opioid use, pain intensity, age and sleep architecture in patients with fibromyalgia and insomnia. *Pain*. 2019;160(9):2086-2092.
116. Cutrufello NJ, Ianus VD, Rowley JA. Opioids and sleep. *Curr Opin Pulm Med*. 2020;26(6):634-641.
117. Rosen IM, Aurora RN, Kirsch DB, et al. Chronic opioid therapy and sleep. An American Academy of Sleep Medicine position paper. *J Clin Sleep Med*. 2019;15(11):1671-1673.
118. Benyamin R, Trescot AM, Datta S, et al. Opioid complications and side effects. *Pain Physician*. 2008;2(Suppl):S105-S120.
119. Li Y, van den Pol AN. Mu-opioid receptor-mediated depression of the hypothalamic hypocretin/orexin arousal system. *J Neurosci*. 2008;28(11):2814-2819.
120. Staedt J, Wassmuth F, Stoppe G, et al. Effects of chronic treatment with methadone and naltrexone on sleep in addicts. *Eur Arch Psychiatry Clin Neurosci*. 1996;246:305-309.
121. Kay D. Human sleep and EEG through a cycle of methadone dependence. *Electroencephalogr Clin Neurophysiol*. 1975;38:35-43.
122. Cronin A, Keifer JC, Baghdoyan HA. Opioid inhibition of rapid eye movement sleep by a specific mu receptor agonist. *Br J Anaesth*. 1995;74:188-192.
123. Trzepecz PT, Violette EJ, Sateia MJ. Response to opioids in three patients with restless legs syndrome. *Am J Psychiatry*. 1984;141:993-995.
124. Walters AS, Wagner ML, Henning WA. Successful treatment of the idiopathic restless legs syndrome in a randomized double-blind trial of oxycodone versus placebo. *Sleep*. 1993;16:327-332.
125. Javey N, Walters AS, Henning W, Gidro-Frank S. Opioid treatment of periodic leg movements in patients without restless legs syndrome. *Neuropeptides*. 1988;11:181-184.
126. Davila DG, Hunt RD, Offord KP, Harris CD, Shepard JW Jr. Acute effects of transdermal nicotine on sleep architecture, snoring and sleep disordered breathing in non-smokers. *Am J Respir Crit Care Med*. 1994;150:469-474.
127. Jaehne A, Unbehaun T, Feige B, Lutz UC, Batra A, Riemann D. How smoking affects sleep: a polysomnographical analysis. *Sleep Med*. 2012;10:1286-1292.
128. Cohrs S, Rodenbeck A, Riemann D, et al. Impaired sleep quality and sleep duration in smokers—results from the German Multicenter Study on Nicotine Dependence. *Addict Biol*. 2012;10:1-11.
129. Gillin JC, Landon M, Ruiz C, Golshan S, Salin-Pascual R. Dose-dependent effects of transdermal nicotine on early morning awakening

and rapid eye movement sleep time in normal nonsmoking volunteers. *J Clin Psychopharmacol*. 1994;14:264-267.

130. Salin-Pascual RJ, Drucker-Colin R. A novel effect of nicotine on mood and sleep in major depression. *Neuroreport*. 1998;9:57-60.
131. Prosise GL, Bonnet MH, Berry RB. Effect of abstinence from smoking on sleep and daytime sleepiness. *Chest*. 1994;105:1136-1141.
132. Hughes JR, Higgins ST, Bickel WK. Nicotine withdrawal versus other drug withdrawal syndromes: similarities and dissimilarities. *Addiction*. 1994;89:461-470.
133. Wetter DW, Young TB, Bidwell TR, Badr MS, Palta M. Smoking as a risk factor for sleep-disordered breathing. *Arch Intern Med*. 1994; 154:2219-2224.
134. Lin YN, Li QY, Zhang XJ. Interaction between smoking and obstructive sleep apnea: not just participants. *Chin Med J (Engl)*. 2012;125(17):3150-3156.
135. Rintakoski K, Ahlberg J, Hublin C, et al. Bruxism is associated with nicotine dependence: a Nationwide Finnish Twin Cohort Study. *Nicotine Tob Res*. 2010;12(12):1254-1260.
136. Oksenberg A. Alleviation of severe restless legs syndrome (RLS) symptoms by cigarette smoking. *J Clin Sleep Med*. 2010;6(5):489-490.
137. Lahan V, Ahmad S, Gupta R. RLS relieved by tobacco chewing: paradoxical role of nicotine. *Neurol Sci*. 2012;33:1209-1210.
138. Kelly TL, Miller NM, Bonnet MH. Sleep latency measures of caffeine effects during sleep deprivation. *Electroencephalogr Clin Neurophysiol*. 1997;102:397-400.
139. Ker K, Edwards PJ, Felix LM, Blakchall K, Roberts I. Caffeine for the prevention of injuries and errors in shift workers. *Cochrane Database Syst Rev*. 2010;5:CD008508.
140. Stradling JR. Recreational drugs and sleep. *Br Med J*. 1993;305:573-575.
141. Portas CM, Thakkar M, Rainie DG, Greene RW, McCarley RW. Role of adenosine in behavioral state modulation: a microdialysis study in the freely moving cat. *Neuroscience*. 1997;79:225-235.
142. Frozi J, de Cavalko HW, Ottoni GL, Cunha RA, Lara DR. Distinct sensitivity to caffeine-induced insomnia related to age. *J Psychopharmacol*. 2018;32(1):89-95.
143. Ribeiro JA, Sebastiao AM. Caffeine and adenosine. Role of the central ascending neurotransmitter systems in the psychostimulant effects of caffeine. *J Alzheimers Dis*. 2010;20(Suppl 1):35-49.
144. Mendelson WB. *Human Sleep: Research and Clinical Care*. Plenum Press; 1987.
145. Haney M, Gunderson EW, Rabkin J, et al. Dronabinol and marijuana in HIV-positive marijuana smokers caloric intake, mood, and sleep. *J Acquir Immune Defic Syndr*. 2007;45:545-554.
146. Paton WD, Pertwee RG. The actions of cannabis in man. In: Mechoulam R, ed. *Marijuana: Chemistry, Pharmacology, Metabolism and Clinical Effects*. Academic Press; 1973:288-334.
147. Bolla KI, Lesage SR, Gamaldo CE, et al. Polysomnogram changes in marijuana users who report sleep disturbances during prior abstinence. *Sleep Med*. 2010;11:882-889.
148. Bolla KI, Lesage SR, Gamaldo CR, et al. Sleep disturbance in heavy marijuana users. *Sleep*. 2008;31(6):901-908.
149. Murillo-Rodríguez E, Millán-Aldaco D, Palomero-Rivero M, Mechoulam R, Drucker-Colín R. Cannabidiol, a constituent of *Cannabis sativa*, modulates sleep in rats. *FEBS Lett*. 2006;580:4337-4345.
150. Teofilo L. *Medications and Their Effects on Sleep. Sleep Medicine: Essentials and Review*. Oxford University Press; 2008:35-72.
151. Kaul M, Zee PC, Sahni AS. Effects of cannabinoids on sleep and their therapeutic potential for sleep disorders. *Neurotherapeutics*. 2021;18:217-227.
152. Whiting PF, Wolff R, Deshpande S, et al. Cannabinoids for medical use: a systematic review and meta-analysis. *JAMA*. 2015;313(24):2456-2247.
153. Carley DW, Prasad B, Reid KJ, et al. Pharmacotherapy of apnea by cannabimimetic enhancement, the PACE clinical trial: effects of dronabinol in obstructive sleep apnea. *Sleep*. 2018;41(1):zsx184.
154. Megelin T, Ghorayeb I. Cannabis for restless legs syndrome: a report of six patients. *Sleep Med*. 2017;36:182-183.
155. Ghorayeb I. More evidence of cannabis efficacy in restless legs syndrome. *Sleep Breath*. 2020;24(1):277-279.
156. Gates P, Albertella L, Copeland J. Cannabis withdrawal and sleep: a systematic review of human studies. *Subst Abus*. 2016;37(1):255-269.
157. Schroeck JL, Ford J, Conway EL. Review of safety and efficacy of sleep medicines in older adults. *Clin Ther*. 2016;38:2340-2372.
158. Hutchison LC, O'Brien CE. Changes in pharmacokinetics and pharmacodynamics in the elderly patients. *J Pharm Pract*. 2007;20:4-12.
159. Greenblatt DJ, Harmatz JS, von Moltke LL, Wright CE, Shader RI. Age and gender effects of pharmacokinetics and pharmacodynamics of triazolam, a cytochrome P450 3A substrate. *Clin Pharmacol Ther*. 2004;76:467-479.
160. Albrecht S, Ihmsen H, Hering W, et al. The effect of age on the pharmacokinetics and pharmacodynamics of midazolam. *Clin Pharmacol Ther*. 1999;65:630-639.
161. Kamel NS, Gammack JK. Insomnia in the elderly: cause, approach, and treatment. *Am J Med*. 2006;119:463-469.
162. Woodward M. Hypnosedatives in the elderly. *CNS Drugs*. 1999; 11:263-279.
163. Woodward MC. Managing insomnia in older people. *J Pharmacy Pract Res*. 2007;37:236-241.
164. Ebert B, Wafford KA, Deacon S. Treating insomnia: current and investigational pharmacological approaches. *Pharmacol Ther*. 2006; 112:612-629.
165. Mohler H, Fritschy JM, Rudolph U. A new benzodiazepine pharmacology. *J Pharmacol Exp Ther*. 2002;300:2-8.
166. Bain KT. Management of chronic insomnia in the elderly person. *Am J Geriatr Pharmacother*. 2006;4:168-192.
167. Tariq SH, Pulisetty S. Pharmacotherapy for insomnia. *Clin Geriatr Med*. 2008;24:93-105.
168. Vgontzas AN, Kales A, Bixler EO, Myers DC. Temazepam 7.5mg: effects on sleep in elderly insomnia. *Eur J Clin Pharmacol*. 1994;46: 209-213.
169. Mejdi T. Benzodiazepines revisited. *Br J Med Pract*. 2012;5:a501.
170. Bogunovic OJ, Greenfield SF. Practical geriatrics: use of benzodiazepines among elderly patients. *Psychiatr Serv*. 2004;55:233-235.
171. Stranks EK, Crowe SF. The acute cognitive effects of zopiclone, zolpidem, zaleplon, and eszopiclone: a systematic review and meta-analysis. *J Cin Exp Neuropsychol*. 2014;36:691-700.
172. Voictorri-Vigneau C, Dailly E, Veyrac G, Jolliet P. Evidence of zolpidem abuse and dependence: results of the French center for evaluation and information on pharmacodependence network survey. *Br J Clin Pharmacol*. 2007;64:198-209.
173. Winkelman JW. Clinical practice. Insomnia disorder. *N Engl J Med*. 2015;373:1437-1444.
174. Lee DO, Buchfuhrer MJ, Garcia-Boreguero D. Efficacy of gabapentin enacarbil in adult patients with severe primary restless le syndrome. *Sleep Med*. 2016;19:50-56.
175. Mersfelder TL, Nocols WH. Gabapentin: abuse, dependence and withdrawal. *Ann Pharmacother*. 2016;50(3):229-233.
176. See S, Hendriks E, Hsieung L. Akathisia induced by gabapentin withdrawal. *Ann Pharmacother*. 2011;45:e31.
177. Barrueto F, Green J, Howland MA, Hoffman RS, Nelson LS. Gabapentin withdrawal presenting as status epilepticus. *J Toxicol Clin Toxicol*. 2002;40:925-928.
178. Sills GJ. The mechanism of action of gabapentin and pregabalin. *Curr Opin Pharmacol*. 2006;6:108-113.
179. Furey SA, Hull SG, Leibowitz MT, Jayawardena S, Roth T. A randomized, double-blind, placebo controlled, multicenter 28-day, PSG study of gabapentin in transient insomnia induced by sleep phase advance. *J Clin Sleep Med*. 2014;10:1101-1109.
180. Altamura AC, Moliterno D, Paletta S. Understanding the pharmacokinetics of anxiolytic drugs. *Expert Opin Drug Metab Toxicol*. 2013;9:423-440.
181. Danchin N, Genton P, Atlas P, Anconina J, Leclere J, Cherrier F. Comparative effects of atenolol and clonidine on polygraphically

recorded sleep in hypertensive men: a randomized, double-blind, crossover study. *Int J Clin Pharmacol Ther*. 1995;33(1):52-55.

182. Naguy A. Clonidine use in psychiatry: panacea or panache? *Pharmacology*. 2016;98:87-92.
183. Childress AC, Sallee RF. Revisiting clonidine: an innovative add-on option for attention-deficit/hyperactivity disorder. *Drugs Today*. 2012;48:207-217.
184. Ming X, Gordon E, Kang N, et al. Use of clonidine in children with autism spectrum disorder. *Brain Dev*. 2008;30:454-460.
185. Kleber HD, Gold MS, Riordan CE. The use of clonidine in detoxification from opiates. *Bull Narc*. 1980;32:1-10.
186. Wilens T, Zulauf C, Ryland D, Carrellas M, Catalina-Wellington I. Prescription medication misuse among opioid dependent patients seeking inpatient detoxification. *Am J Addict*. 2015;24:173-177.
187. Baird CR, Fox P, Colvin LA. Gabapentinoid abuse in order to potentiate the effect of methadone: a survey among substance misusers. *Eur Addict Res*. 2014;20:115-118.

96 Traumatic Injuries Related to Alcohol and Other Drug Use

Edouard Coupet Jr, Deepa R. Camenga, Gail D'Onofrio, and Federico E. Vaca

CHAPTER OUTLINE

- Introduction
- Epidemiology of alcohol- and other drug–related injuries
- Relationship between alcohol, other drugs, and traumatic injury
- Special considerations
- Conclusions

INTRODUCTION

Alcohol and other drug use contribute to a substantial share of injury events, including motor vehicle crashes (MVCs), falls, assaults, burns, drownings, homicides, and suicides. Injured patients with substance use disorder (SUD) suffer more frequent and severe complications than injured patients without SUD. These events are associated with significantly increased morbidity and mortality. Moreover, they also have far-reaching consequences for the individual, other individuals, their family, workplace, community, and society. This chapter discusses the role of alcohol and other drug use in traumatic injury.

To date, the majority of substance use and addiction research in the context of traumatic injury relates to alcohol. However, the body of literature related to other drugs, particularly within the emergency medicine literature continues to grow. The objective of this chapter is to provide clinicians with an overview of traumatic injury and its various forms that may occur in the context of alcohol and other drug use; the complex relationship between alcohol, other drug use, and traumatic injury; and additional special considerations that may be particularly relevant to the emergency department (ED) setting. Additional information surrounding ED-based screening and brief interventions for substance use and SUD, an important tool to identify and render treatment in this population, can be found in Section 4 of this textbook.

EPIDEMIOLOGY OF ALCOHOL- AND OTHER DRUG–RELATED INJURIES

Overall Risks

The risks of alcohol-related injury span across the entire spectrum, from drinking low-risk amounts to severe alcohol use disorder. In a study of 37 EDs across 18 countries, alcohol was estimated to be attributable to 16.4% of all injuries.[1] The proportion of injury-related ED encounters with any recent alcohol use ranges from 7.8% to as high as 81.9%.[2] Alcohol has a well-established link to nearly all categories of both unintentional and intentional injuries, particularly because of its psychomotor impairing effects.[1,3-12] Alcohol and other drug use is also a major risk factor for the 240,000 to 280,000 deaths that occur from traumatic injury annually in the United States.[13-17] In 2020, unintentional injury, suicide, and homicide were the top three leading causes of death for individuals aged 1 to 44 years, accounting for 121,477 deaths. Approximately 63% of these deaths were categorized as poisonings (including accidental poisoning and exposure to opioids, alcohol, hallucinogens, sedative-hypnotic unspecified drugs, biological substances, and other drugs/chemical agents).[17]

Unintentional Injury: Alcohol- and Motor Vehicle–Related Injuries and Fatalities

Motor vehicle crash is the leading cause of death among children and young adults in the United States.[18] According to the National Highway Traffic Safety Administration in 2020, 30% of the 38,824 MVC fatalities were alcohol related.[19] The societal cost of alcohol-related MVCs was estimated to be $49 billion in 2010 with blood alcohol concentration (BAC) levels of 0.08 g/dL or greater responsible for over 90% of this cost.[20] Previous studies show there is a strong dose-response relationship between acute alcohol consumption and the risks of MVC and MVC-related morbidity and mortality.[6,21] Drivers who drink alcohol, yet are not legally impaired, are responsible for a substantial number of fatalities as well. One study of 612,030 MVC fatalities from 2000 to 2015 found that 33,965 had a BAC less than 0.08 g/dL, corresponding to 15% of alcohol-related fatalities and 6% of all fatalities.[22] Evidence also suggests that between 70% and 90% of individuals who have received a first-time driving under the influence (DUI) offense have met the definition of alcohol use disorder in their lifetime.[23-25]

Although the rates of alcohol-related fatal MVC and DUI are greater among men compared to women, more recent evidence suggests these gender differences are narrowing.[26-29] A 2020 study of the National Drug Survey of Drug Use and Health (NSDUH) found a significant and gradual increase in alcohol-related DUI arrests among women from 1.2% in 2002, to 2.3% in 2014, to 2.5% in 2017.[28] Among all racial and ethnicity groups, Indigenous American populations have the highest rates of alcohol-related MVC fatality, while Asian populations have the lowest.[30] Alcohol-impaired young drivers, as well as their passengers, are at substantial risk for MVC mortality.[31-34]

Further, youth who ride with an alcohol-impaired driver are at increased risk of alcohol-impaired driving in the future.[35]

Unintentional Injury: Alcohol- and Non–motor Vehicle-Related Injuries and Fatalities

Alcohol is involved in 46% of pedestrian crash fatalities (32% of pedestrians with a BAC of 0.08 g/dL or higher), 49.5% of fatal drownings, 34.9% of nonfatal drownings, and up to 50% of burn injuries.[36-38] For most aquatic activities, including boating and diving, alcohol use is associated with an increased risk of injury and death. Research suggests men are at greater risk for alcohol-related drowning than women.[37] Among patients requiring hospitalization for burn injury, alcohol use was found to be associated with increased risks of inhalation-related injury and death.[39,40] A prospective study of 689 injured bicyclists presenting to a Level 1 urban trauma center found that 15.1% consumed alcohol prior to injury. Additionally, prior alcohol use was associated with decreased helmet use, greater use of hospital resources, and increased risks of severe injury and death.[15] Alcohol-related falls are also associated with more severe injury, particularly as BAC levels rise.[41]

Intentional Injury: Alcohol Use and Interpersonal Violence

In the United States, homicide is the leading cause of death for Black youth and the third leading cause for adolescents and young adults overall.[17] Alcohol consumption is closely associated with intentional injuries, such as those that result from interpersonal violence and self-harm. Alcohol is widely known to decrease inhibition and increase aggression.[42] A meta-analysis of 37 EDs across 18 countries found that 44.2% of patients reported alcohol use prior to sustaining an assault-related injury, the highest for all types of injuries. Among those with assault-related injuries, 90.7% of their injuries were attributable to alcohol use.[1] Kuhns et al. determined that 48% of homicide victims tested positive for alcohol while 33% (using the 0.08 g/dL threshold) and 35% (using the 0.10 g/dL threshold) were found to be intoxicated.[43] Black populations have the highest rates of alcohol-associated homicide deaths among all racial and ethnic groups.[30]

Alcohol use is also a risk factor for firearm-related morbidity and mortality. A systematic review encompassing 40 years of peer-reviewed studies examining the relationship between alcohol use and firearm violence in the United States determined that over one-third of firearm injury decedents had acutely consumed any amount of alcohol; over one-fourth had heavily consumed alcohol prior to death.[44] Among youth, previous evidence demonstrates that adolescents who start drinking alcohol early and more frequently are at an increased risk of perpetration and victimization of youth violence.[45] A case-control study of adolescent firearm homicide victims demonstrated that alcohol at the individual (personal history of alcohol use) and neighborhood-levels (living in a neighborhood with high densities of alcohol outlets) were both associated with increased odds of death by firearm homicide.[46]

Existing evidence also supports a connection between alcohol use and intimate partner violence. A previous study found that 30% to 40% of men and 27% to 34% of women who have perpetrated violence against their partners were consuming alcohol at the time of the event.[47] Over 40% of individuals participating in treatment for alcohol use disorder reported perpetration of intimate partner violence in the previous 12 months.[48-50] Prior research has found a small to moderate effect size for the relationship between alcohol use and male-to-female partner violence and a small effect size for female-to-male partner violence.[11] Acute alcohol consumption is also significantly associated with both intimate partner violence perpetration and victimization within same-sex couples.[51-54]

Intentional Injury: Alcohol Use and Self-harm

Suicide is among the largest contributors to premature death.[17] Approximately 22% of suicide deaths worldwide are attributable to alcohol.[55] Alcohol use is profoundly associated with psychiatric disorders, which negatively impact mental health. This association has the potential to increase the risk of suicide.[12] Alcohol was present in 36% of men and 28% of women suicide decedents.[56] As BAC levels increase, acute alcohol consumption is associated with a significantly increased odds of suicide attempt.[57] Moreover, the odds of suicidal behavior are three times higher for individuals with a diagnosis of alcohol use disorder compared to those without a diagnosis.[58] A meta-analysis of alcohol use and firearm injury found that 35% of firearm suicide decedents acutely consumed alcohol prior to their death.[44] Among men, risk factors for alcohol intoxication prior to death by suicide include younger age, Indigenous American/Alaska Native heritage, Latino heritage, being a veteran, firearm use or hanging/suffocation as a means of death, and residing in rural areas. Among women, risk factors include younger age, Indigenous American/Alaska Native heritage, and firearm use or hanging/suffocation as a means of death.[59]

Unintentional Injury: Other Drug Use and Motor Vehicle Injuries and Fatalities

Aside from alcohol, it has been widely established that many other drugs can negatively impact safe driving.[60] The most frequently identified drug, other than alcohol, in impaired drivers is cannabis. According to data from the 2018 NSDUH, 4.7% of respondents aged 16 years and older reported cannabis-impaired driving and 0.9% reported driving under the influence of illicit drugs other than cannabis in the past year.[61] From 2000 to 2018, the trend in cannabis- and cannabis- and alcohol-related MVC fatalities increased from 9.0% in 2000 to 21.5% in 2018 and 4.8% in 2000 to 10.3% in 2018, respectively.[62] As more states legalize both recreational and cannabis used as treatment, the prevalence of cannabis-impaired driving is expected to increase further. A study of annual traffic fatalities found an increase in fatality rates in Alaska, Oregon, Washington, and Colorado, all states that legalized cannabis, compared to control states that did not, postlegalization.[63]

As cannabis use increases, the risks associated with simultaneous cannabis- and alcohol-impaired driving is expected to increase as well. Literature suggests that adolescents and young adults who have used alcohol and cannabis simultaneously are at increased risks of driving impaired and riding with an impaired driver.[64-66] A study of young adults who use alcohol and cannabis simultaneously found that one-third drove after use and two-thirds rode with an impaired driver.[67] Further, the combination of alcohol and cannabis use is associated with increased risks of MVC and unsafe driving behaviors compared to using either substance separately.[68,69] Cannabis-impaired driving has also been associated with use of other drugs. A previous study found that individuals who reported cannabis-impaired driving had an increased odds of cocaine, hallucinogen, and methamphetamine use prior to driving as well.[70]

Intentional Injury: Other Drug Use and Violent Injuries

While the connection between alcohol and intentional injury is the most well studied, there is evidence to support a relationship between other drug use and interpersonal violent and self-harm injuries. A single-site retrospective study of adults with major penetrating trauma, including firearm and stab injuries, found 93% of individuals who received urine toxicology testing were positive for at least one substance. Other than alcohol, the most common drugs detected were cannabis (65.7%), benzodiazepines (30.8%), opiates (27.%), cocaine (20.4%), and amphetamines (19.7%).[71] Study samples demonstrate between 25% and 61% of individuals presenting to the ED for nonpartner violent injury reported drug use within the past year.[72-75] In ED studies, previous drug use of any type is associated with up to a sevenfold greater odds of either a previous or acute violent injury.[72,76,77] Seeking acute care for violent injury is also associated with an increased odds of previous drug use.[78,79] A systematic review of ED-based studies that screen, provide a brief intervention, and/or directly refer to treatment for drug use and drug use disorders found that cannabis was the most common drug identified among individuals injured by nonpartner violence.[72,74,76-82] This review also found that cocaine use was also associated with 2.7 to 3.1 greater odds of violent injury.[72,76,82]

Literature surrounding intimate partner violence and drug use has primarily focused on victimization for women and perpetration for men. Compared to alcohol use, drug use overall has a stronger association with intimate partner victimization.[83] Historically, there was a belief that the relationship between drug use and intimate partner violence differed by the type of drug used.[84] However, a recent meta-analysis did not find any differences between the types of drugs used, including categorization by stimulant versus nonstimulant, and intimate partner violence perpetration and victimization.[83] Among individuals who have experienced intimate partner victimization, literature suggests that 2.4% of individuals had opioid use disorder (OUD), while 46% to 50% had prescription opioid use for pain relief in the past 5 years. For perpetration, one study found that 1.5% of individuals had OUD. Among women who have experienced victimization, 32% to 75% have used opioids in the past year. Among men who have used nonprescribed opioids 58% have perpetrated intimate partner violence in their lifetimes.[85]

Intentional Injury: Other Drug Use and Self-harm

Virtually all SUDs are associated with an increased risk of suicide. Opioid use is widely understood to be a risk factor for suicide by overdose. In 2017, over 40% of overdose and suicide deaths involved opioids, a number that is likely underestimated.[86] Among SUDs other than OUD, prior literature has found that the suicide hazard ratios are 11.35 for sedative, 3.89 for cannabis, 2.83 for benzodiazepine, 2.10 for psychostimulant, and 1.35 for cocaine use disorders.[87,88]

RELATIONSHIP BETWEEN ALCOHOL, OTHER DRUGS, AND TRAUMATIC INJURY

The relationship between alcohol, other drug use, and traumatic injury is exceptionally complex. Further elucidating this relationship is challenging for a myriad of reasons including: (1) relatively few studies have been conducted examining substance use at the time of injury; (2) there is a paucity of standards for collecting and reporting data surrounding alcohol and other drug use in the context of trauma; (3) stigma surrounds alcohol, other drug use, and certain types of injuries such as those caused by interpersonal violence; (4) there are challenges with engagement given the intersection of two marginalized populations who may not seek healthcare with regularity; (5) relevant research studies have high rates of attrition (eg, unable to contact or death); and (6) there is a lack of viable and sustained community resources where patients can be referred for counseling and treatment services.[89-92] For unintentional injuries such as MVC-related injury, research shows that alcohol use has a direct, dose-dependent relationship with the risk of injury. For MVC-related injury, the odds ratio increases by 1.24 for every 10 g to 52.0 at 120 g of pure alcohol consumed.[6] Cannabis-impaired driving is associated with a 1.92 increased odds of MVC.[93] Alcohol and other drug use increase the risk of MVC-related and other unintentional injuries by impairing alertness, judgment, and both spatial and motor skills.[6,60]

The nature of the relationship between alcohol, other drug use, and intentional injury is notably more complex.[87,94] A meta-analysis found a substantial linkage between alcohol, other drug use, and both violence perpetration and victimization.[94] There are several competing theories that explain this relationship including: (1) alcohol and other drug use causing interpersonal violence through their pharmacologic effects; (2) interpersonal violence causing alcohol and other drug use (e.g., alcohol and other drug use to cope with the physical, emotional, and psychological sequelae of injury); and (3) the existence of mutually held risk factors between alcohol, other drug use, and interpersonal violence (eg, psychiatric disorders, poverty).[94,95] For self-inflicted injuries, alcohol is a known risk factor for suicide attempt and death.[87] Alcohol increases the risk of suicidal behavior directly by impairing judgement and attenuating impulse control.[12] Alcohol use is associated with a 94% increase in the risk of death by suicide.[96] This relationship is further intensified in the setting of co-occurring psychiatric disorders such as depression and bipolar disorder.[97,98]

SPECIAL CONSIDERATIONS

Electronic Cigarette Use and Injuries

Electronic cigarettes, including vapes, vape pens, mods, tanks, and e-hookahs, are nicotine delivery products that have quickly risen in popularity in the United States and worldwide. In 2019, 4.5% of all adults in the United States reported current use of these products. Electronic cigarette use was highest among adults between the ages of 18 and 24 years (9.3%), with 56.0% of these young adults reporting that they have never used cigarettes before.[99] While evolving, the literature to support the efficacy of electronic cigarette use for treating nicotine/tobacco use disorder remains inconclusive.[100-102] Yet the primary motivation for electronic cigarette use among adults is abstinence or reduction of traditional cigarette use.[103,104] Although uptake among youth has declined in recent years, electronic cigarette use is the most commonly used tobacco product among U.S. middle and high school students. Among youth who reported tobacco use in 2020, 19.6% (3.02 million) of high school and 4.7% (550,000) of middle school students reported electronic cigarette use.[105] Additional information about electronic cigarette use can be found in Chapter 22 "Electronic Drug Delivery Devices."

Individuals who use electronic cigarettes may adjust the voltage of the battery to improve the delivery of nicotine and other substances from the e-liquid, alter the thickness of the aerosol-vapor, or experience the "throat hit" during inhalation.[106-108] Certain types of manufactured electronic cigarettes have built-in timers to prevent battery overheating; however, these safety features are not present in modified devices. Consequently, the lithium ion battery can overheat, which causes an explosion and fire due to the inherent flammability of the e-liquid.[109]

This explosive capability leads to unintentional injuries such as burn and traumatic injuries. From 2015 to 2017, U.S. EDs treated 2,035 patients with electronic cigarette explosion injuries with most patients being treated and released (69%).[110] A systematic review describing 164 cases of burn injuries caused by electronic cigarette explosions found that 90% were men between the ages of 20 and 29 years old. In 65% of cases, the electronic cigarette exploded in the individual's pocket as opposed to the face or hand. The thigh, hand, genitals, and face were among the most common areas of the body that were burned. As far as severity, most burns were either second-degree (35%) or a combination of second- and third-degree (20%) burns. Case reports of other specific injuries include oral injuries such as intraoral burns and dental injuries, ocular chemical injuries, and cervical spine fractures.[111-114] In an effort to protect the public's health, in August 2016, the Food and Drug Administration gained the authority to regulate the manufacturing of electronic cigarettes.[115] However, this authority continues to be challenged in court by electronic cigarette manufacturers, resulting in eroded regulation.

COVID-19–Related Alcohol, Other Drug Use, and Injury Issues

The global coronavirus disease 2019 (COVID-19) pandemic led to extensive disruptions to public health infrastructure with requests for physical distancing to mitigate the spread of the virus. Existing literature has shown that social isolation and economic stress may have exacerbated mental health, leading to an increase in the risks of alcohol, other drug use and both unintentional and intentional injuries.[116-122] Beginning in March 2020, the United States declared COVID-19 to be a national emergency. In response to this, many states implemented stay-at-home orders. These events were associated with a 38% increase in alcohol sales.[123] Studies of alcohol and other drug screening among trauma patients found an increase in the rate of positive urine toxicology and blood alcohol tests after stay-at-home orders were implemented.[124,125] Although there were decreases in vehicle miles traveled, traffic volumes, and MVCs overall, the rates of alcohol-impaired and drug-impaired driving and MVCs increased.[122,126-129] A study of seriously and fatally injured drivers prior to and during the COVID-19 pandemic found that 64.7% of drivers tested positive for at least one drug during, compared to 50.8% prior to the pandemic. Cannabis use (32.7%) was also more prevalent than alcohol use (28.3%) among drivers during the pandemic.[130] Another study from a single Level 1 trauma center found an increase in alcohol-related MVCs during the COVID-19 pandemic compared to before, despite a decrease in the rate of MVCs overall.[122] For intentional injuries, U.S. EDs saw decreases in those that result from self-harm and interpersonal violence. This is despite a marked rise in the number of emergency calls to report intimate partner violence worldwide.[128,131] Yet, during the pandemic, studies of self-reported national data suggest that suicidal ideation and interpersonal violence were more likely to be associated with substance use.[121,132]

"Excited Delirium"

During 2020, in parallel to the COVID-19 pandemic, the United States also experienced mass protests surrounding the killings of George Floyd, Daniel Prude, and Elijah McClain, all unarmed Black men, while in law enforcement custody. The cause of these heavily publicized deaths was attributed to "excited delirium," also known as "agitated delirium" by medical examiners, lawyers, law enforcement, first responders, and expert witnesses. Wetli and Fishbain developed the diagnostic term "excited delirium" to describe "a state of extreme mental and physiological excitement, characterized by extreme agitation, hyperthermia, hostility, exceptional strength, and endurance without apparent fatigue." Originally it was used to describe six individuals who died under law enforcement custody and had nonfatal levels of cocaine in their blood with no anatomic cause of death on autopsy.[133] Since, it has been modified by multiple authors and has evolved into the most current definition, "an invariably fatal condition that is characterized by the acute onset of delirium with disturbance in consciousness and cognition, combative and violent behavior, physical restraint, and demise due to sudden cardiac death."[134] Some authors have posited that death results from a combination of stimulant drug use, particularly cocaine, and agitation prompting a cardiac calcium channel blockade. However, this phenomenon is poorly understood and there is no literature to support its existence to date.[135-137] Excited delirium is not currently listed in the *International Classification of Diseases* (ICD-9 or ICD-10), nor the *Diagnostic and Statistical Manual of Mental Disorders* (DSM-5).

In addition to its uncertain definition, excited delirium is also controversial because its features typically incite the use of force and restraints by law enforcement and first responders. A review of the role of restraint in fatal excited delirium found that death occurred in the presence of aggressive physical restraints, during which restraint-related asphyxia was considered the cause of death.[135,138] Further, the use of restraints, in combination with stimulant drug use, obesity, and the presence of other comorbid diseases, is associated with an increased risk of mortality due to the risk of asphyxiation.[139,140] For these reasons, excited delirium is seen by many as a politically charged term that may conceal the excessive use of force by law enforcement personnel, particularly toward Black men.[141] Overall, the mortality of excited delirium has been estimated to be between 8.3% and 16.5%. Independent risk factors for receiving a diagnosis of excited delirium include male sex, young age, being overweight, and Black race. Most diagnoses are made in the context of alcohol and other drug use with up to 90% of individuals having positive urine toxicology testing. The most common drug detected is cocaine.[142] Overall, clinicians should avoid use of the term "excited delirium" as there is little to no evidence to support it as a medical diagnosis.

CONCLUSIONS

Alcohol and other drugs are responsible for a broad range of injuries, from MVCs to drownings, and burns to assaults. Individuals seeking care for injury have a high prevalence of co-occurring substance use and SUD. The linkage between alcohol, other drug use, and unintentional injuries, such as those MVC-related, is well-studied. Yet its relationship with intentional injuries, such as those that result from interpersonal violence, while convincing, is more complex. The explosive capabilities of electronic cigarettes can lead to burn and other traumatic injuries. In 2020, the COVID-19 pandemic and public rallies for social justice have highlighted additional concerns at the intersection of substance use and traumatic injury.

REFERENCES

1. Cherpitel CJ, Ye Y, Bond J, et al. Alcohol attributable fraction for injury morbidity from the dose-response relationship of acute alcohol consumption: emergency department data from 18 countries. *Addiction.* 2015;110(11):1724-1732. doi:10.1111/add.13031
2. Cherpitel CJ, Ye Y, Bond J, et al. Multi-level analysis of alcohol-related injury and drinking pattern: emergency department data from 19 countries. *Addiction.* 2012;107(7):1263-1272. doi:10.1111/j.1360-0443.2012.03793.x
3. Culhane J, Silverglate B, Freeman C. Alcohol is a predictor of mortality in motor vehicle collisions. *J Safety Res.* 2019;71:201-205.
4. Cherpitel CJ. Alcohol and injuries resulting from violence: a review of emergency room studies. *Addiction.* 1994;89(2):157-165. doi:10.1111/j.1360-0443.1994.tb00874.x
5. Rehm J, Baliunas D, Borges GLG, et al. The relation between different dimensions of alcohol consumption and burden of disease: an overview. *Addiction.* 2010;105(5):817-843. doi:10.1111/j.1360-0443.2010.02899.x
6. Taylor B, Irving HM, Kanteres F, et al. The more you drink, the harder you fall: a systematic review and meta-analysis of how acute alcohol consumption and injury or collision risk increase together. *Drug Alcohol Depend.* 2010;110(1):108-116. doi:10.1016/j.drugalcdep.2010.02.011
7. Vinson DC, Borges G, Cherpitel CJ. The risk of intentional injury with acute and chronic alcohol exposures: a case-control and case-crossover study. *J Stud Alcohol.* 2003;64(3):350-357. doi:10.15288/jsa.2003.64.350
8. Shih H-C, Hu S-C, Yang C-C, Ko T-J, Wu J-K, Lee C-H. Alcohol intoxication increases morbidity in drivers involved in motor vehicle accidents. *Am J Emerg Med.* 2003;21(2):91-94. doi:10.1053/ajem.2003.50025
9. Macdonald S, Cherpitel CJ, Borges G, DeSouza A, Giesbrecht N, Stockwell T. The criteria for causation of alcohol in violent injuries based on emergency room data from six countries. *Addict Behav.* 2005;30(1):103-113. doi:10.1016/j.addbeh.2004.04.016
10. Cherpitel CJ, Ye Y, Bond J, Room R, Borges G. Attribution of alcohol to violence-related injury: self and other's drinking in the event. *J Stud Alcohol Drugs.* 2012;73(2):277-284.
11. Foran HM, O'Leary KD. Alcohol and intimate partner violence: a meta-analytic review. *Clin Psychol Rev.* 2008;28(7):1222-1234. doi:10.1016/j.cpr.2008.05.001
12. Pompili M, Serafini G, Innamorati M, et al. Suicidal behavior and alcohol abuse. *Int J Environ Res Public Health.* 2010;7(4):1392-1431. doi:10.3390/ijerph7041392
13. DiMaggio CJ, Avraham JB, Frangos SG, Keyes K. The role of alcohol and other drugs on emergency department traumatic injury mortality in the United States. *Drug Alcohol Depend.* 2021;225:108763. doi:j.drugalcdep.2021.108763
14. Afshar M, Netzer G, Murthi S, Smith GS. Alcohol exposure, injury, and death in trauma patients. *J Trauma Acute Care Surg.* 2015;79(4):643.
15. Sethi M, Heyer JH, Wall S, et al. Alcohol use by urban bicyclists is associated with more severe injury, greater hospital resource use, and higher mortality. *Alcohol.* 2016;53:1-7.
16. Brady JE, Li G. Prevalence of alcohol and other drugs in fatally injured drivers. *Addiction.* 2013;**108**(1):104-114. doi:10.1111/j.1360-0443.2012.03993.x
17. Centers for Disease Control and Prevention. *Web-Based Injury Statistics Query and Reporting System*; 2021.
18. Cunningham RM, Walton MA, Carter PM. The major causes of death in children and adolescents in the United States. *N Engl J Med.* 2018;379(25):2468-2475. doi:10.1056/NEJMsr1804754
19. Stewart T. *Overview of Motor Vehicle Crashes in 2020.* Accessed June 26, 2023. https://trid.trb.org/view/1922738
20. Blincoe L, Miller TR, Zaloshnja E, Lawrence BA. *The Economic and Societal Impact of Motor Vehicle Crashes*; 2010 (Revised). Accessed 26 June, 2023. https://crashstats.nhtsa.dot.gov/Api/Public/ViewPublication/812013
21. Van Dyke NA, Fillmore MT. Laboratory analysis of risky driving at 0.05% and 0.08% blood alcohol concentration. *Drug Alcohol Depend.* 2017;175:127-132. doi:10.1016/j.drugalcdep.2017.02.005

22. Lira MC, Sarda V, Heeren TC, Miller M, Naimi TS. Alcohol policies and motor vehicle crash deaths involving blood alcohol concentrations below 0.08%. *Am J Prev Med*. 2020;58(5):622-629.
23. LaPlante DA, Nelson SE, Odegaard SS, LaBrie RA, Shaffer HJ. Substance and psychiatric disorders among men and women repeat driving under the influence offenders who accept a treatment-sentencing option. *J Stud Alcohol Drugs*. 2008;69(2):209-217. doi:10.15288/jsad.2008.69.209
24. Keating LM, Nelson SE, Wiley RC, Shaffer HJ. Psychiatric comorbidity among first-time and repeat DUI offenders. *Addict Behav*. 2019;96:1-10. doi:10.1016/j.addbeh.2019.03.018
25. McCutcheon VV, Heath AC, Edenberg HJ, et al. Alcohol criteria endorsement and psychiatric and drug use disorders among DUI offenders: greater severity among women and multiple offenders. *Addict Behav*. 2009;34(5):432-439.
26. Vaca FE, Romano E, Fell JC. Female drivers increasingly involved in impaired driving crashes: actions to ameliorate the risk. *Acad Emerg Med*. 2014;21(12):1485-1492.
27. Tsai VW, Anderson CL, Vaca FE. Alcohol involvement among young female drivers in U.S. fatal crashes: unfavourable trends. *Inj Prev*. 2010;16(1):17. doi:10.1136/ip.2009.022301
28. Oh S, Vaughn MG, Salas-Wright CP, AbiNader MA, Sanchez M. Driving under the influence of alcohol: findings from the NSDUH, 2002-2017. *Addict Behav*. 2020;108:106439. doi:10.1016/j.addbeh.2020.106439
29. Reilly K, Woodruff SI, Hohman M, Barker M. Gender differences in driving under the influence (DUI) program client characteristics: implications for treatment delivery. *Women Health*. 2019;59(2):132-144. doi:10.1080/03630242.2018.1434589
30. Keyes KM, Liu XC, Cerda M. The role of race/ethnicity in alcohol-attributable injury in the United States. *Epidemiol Rev*. 2011;34(1):89-102. doi:10.1093/epirev/mxr018
31. Wagenaar AC, Maldonado-Molina MM, Wagenaar BH. Effects of alcohol tax increases on alcohol-related disease mortality in Alaska: time-series analyses from 1976 to 2004. *Am J Public Health*. 2009;99(8):1464-1470. doi:10.2105/AJPH.2007.131326
32. Wagenaar AC, O'Malley PM, LaFond C. Lowered legal blood alcohol limits for young drivers: effects on drinking, driving, and driving-after-drinking behaviors in 30 states. *Am J Public Health*. 2001;91(5):801.
33. Romano E, Fell J, Li K, Simons-Morton BG, Vaca FE. Alcohol-related deaths among young passengers: an analysis of national alcohol-related fatal crashes. *J Safety Res*. 2021;79:376-382.
34. National Highway Traffic Safety Administration. *Young Drivers. Traffic Safety Facts*. National Center for Statistics and Analysis; 2019.
35. Li K, Simons-Morton BG, Vaca FE, Hingson R. Association between riding with an impaired driver and driving while impaired. *Pediatrics*. 2014;133(4):620-626. doi:10.1542/peds.2013-2786
36. Davis CS, Esposito TJ, Palladino-Davis AG, et al. Implications of alcohol intoxication at the time of burn and smoke inhalation injury: an epidemiologic and clinical analysis. *J Burn Care Res*. 2013;34(1):120-126.
37. Hamilton K, Keech JJ, Peden AE, Hagger MS. Alcohol use, aquatic injury, and unintentional drowning: a systematic literature review. *Drug Alcohol Rev*. 2018;37(6):752-773.
38. National Highway Traffic Safety Administration. *Pedestrians. Traffic Safety Facts*. National Center for Statistics and Analysis; 2019.
39. Klifto KM, Shetty PN, Slavin BR, et al. Impact of nicotine/smoking, alcohol, and illicit substance use on outcomes and complications of burn patients requiring hospital admission: systematic review and meta-analysis. *Burns*. 2020;46(7):1498-1524. doi:10.1016/j.burns.2019.08.003
40. Silver GM, Albright JM, Schermer CR, et al. Adverse clinical outcomes associated with elevated blood alcohol levels at the time of burn injury. *J Burn Care Res*. 2008;29(5):784-789. doi:10.1097/BCR.0b013e31818481bc
41. Johnston JJE, McGovern SJ. Alcohol related falls: an interesting pattern of injuries. *Emerg Med J*. 2004;21(2):185. doi:10.1136/emj.2003.006130
42. World Health Organization. *Global Status Report on Alcohol and Health 2018*. World Health Organization;2019.
43. Kuhns JB, Wilson DB, Clodfelter TA, Maguire ER, Ainsworth SA. A meta-analysis of alcohol toxicology study findings among homicide victims. *Addiction*. 2011;106(1):62-72. doi:10.1111/j.1360-0443.2010.03153.x
44. Branas CC, Han S, Wiebe DJ. Alcohol use and firearm violence. *Epidemiol Rev*. 2016;38(1):32-45. doi:10.1093/epirev/mxv010
45. World Health Organization. *Preventing Youth Violence: An Overview of the Evidence*. World Health Organization; 2015.
46. Hohl BC, Wiley S, Wiebe DJ, Culyba AJ, Drake R, Branas CC. Association of drug and alcohol use with adolescent firearm homicide at individual, family, and neighborhood levels. *JAMA Intern Med*. 2017;177(3):317-324. doi:10.1001/jamainternmed.2016.8180
47. Caetano R, Schafer J, Cunradi CB. Alcohol-related intimate partner violence among white, black, and Hispanic couples in the United States. *Domestic Violence. Routledge*. 2017;153-160.
48. Taft CT, O'Farrell TJ, Doron-LaMarca S, et al. Longitudinal risk factors for intimate partner violence among men in treatment for alcohol use disorders. *J Consult Clin Psychol*. 2010;78(6):924-935.
49. Chermack ST, Fuller BE, Blow FC. Predictors of expressed partner and non-partner violence among patients in substance abuse treatment. *Drug Alcohol Depend*. 2000;58(1-2):43-54.
50. Schumacher JA, Fals-Stewart W, Leonard KE. Domestic violence treatment referrals for men seeking alcohol treatment. *J Subst Abuse Treat*. 2003;24(3):279-283.
51. Kelley ML, Milletich RJ, Lewis RJ, et al. Predictors of perpetration of men's same-sex partner violence. *Violence Vict*. 2014;29(5):784-796.
52. Lewis RJ, Mason TB, Winstead BA, Kelley ML. Empirical investigation of a model of sexual minority specific and general risk factors for intimate partner violence among lesbian women. *Psychol Violence*. 2017;7(1):110.
53. Badenes-Ribera L, Bonilla-Campos A, Frias-Navarro D, Pons-Salvador G, Monterde-I-Bort H. Intimate partner violence in self-identified lesbians: a systematic review of its prevalence and correlates. *Trauma Violence Abuse*. 2016;17(3):284-297.
54. Finneran C, Stephenson R. Antecedents of intimate partner violence among gay and bisexual men. *Violence Vict*. 2014;29(3):422-435.
55. World Health Organization. *Preventing Suicide: A Global Imperative*. World Health Organization; 2014.
56. Kaplan MS, Huguet N, McFarland BH, et al. Use of alcohol before suicide in the United States. *Ann Epidemiol*. 2014;24(8) 588-592.e2: doi:10.1016/j.annepidem.2014.05.008
57. Borges G, Bagge CL, Cherpitel CJ, Conner KR, Orozco R, Rossow I. A meta-analysis of acute use of alcohol and the risk of suicide attempt. *Psychol Med*. 2017;47(5):949-957. doi:10.1017/S0033291716002841
58. Conner KR, Bagge CL. Suicidal behavior: links between alcohol use disorder and acute use of alcohol. *Alcohol Res*. 2019;40(1):arcr.v40.1.02. doi:10.35946/arcr.v40.1.02
59. Kaplan MS, McFarland BH, Huguet N, et al. Acute alcohol intoxication and suicide: a gender-stratified analysis of the National Violent Death Reporting System. *Inj Prev*. 2013;19(1):38. doi:10.1136/injuryprev-2012-040317
60. Cafaro TW. Slipping through the cracks: why can't we stop drugged driving. *W New Eng L Rev*. 2010;32:33.
61. Azofeifa A, Rexach-Guzmán BD, Hagemeyer AN, Rudd RA, Sauber-Schatz EK. Driving under the influence of marijuana and illicit drugs among persons aged≥ 16 years—United States, 2018. *MMWR Morbid Mortal Wkly Rep*. 2019;68(50):1153.
62. Lira MC, Heeren TC, Buczek M, et al. Trends in Cannabis involvement and risk of alcohol involvement in motor vehicle crash fatalities in the United States, 2000-2018. *Am J Public Health*. 2021;111(11):1976-1985. doi:10.2105/AJPH.2021.306466
63. Kamer RS, Warshafsky S, Kamer GC. Change in traffic fatality rates in the first 4 states to legalize recreational marijuana. *JAMA Intern Med*. 2020;180(8):1119-1120. doi:10.1001/jamainternmed.2020.1769
64. Vaca FE, Li K, Hingson R, Simons-Morton BG. Transitions in riding with an alcohol/drug-impaired driver from adolescence to emerging adulthood in the United States. *J Stud Alcohol Drugs*. 2016;77(1):77-85.
65. Li K, Ochoa E, Vaca FE, Simons-Morton B. Emerging adults riding with marijuana-, alcohol-, or illicit drug-impaired peer and older drivers. *J Stud Alcohol Drugs*. 2018;79(2):277-285.
66. Cartwright J, Asbridge M. Passengers' decisions to ride with a driver under the influence of either alcohol or cannabis. *J Stud Alcohol Drugs*. 2011;72(1):86-95.

67. Patrick ME, Graupensperger S, Dworkin ER, Duckworth JC, Abdallah DA, Lee CM. Intoxicated driving and riding with impaired drivers: comparing days with alcohol, marijuana, and simultaneous use. *Drug Alcohol Depend.* 2021;225:108753. doi:10.1016/j.drugalcdep.2021.108753
68. Duckworth JC, Lee CM. Associations among simultaneous and co-occurring use of alcohol and marijuana, risky driving, and perceived risk. *Addict Behav.* 2019;96:39.
69. Subbaraman MS, Kerr WC. Simultaneous versus concurrent use of alcohol and cannabis in the National Alcohol Survey. *Alcohol Clin Exp Res.* 2015;39(5):872-879.
70. Yockey A, Vidourek R, King K. Drugged driving among U.S. adults: results from the 2016-2018 national survey on drug use and health. *J Safety Res.* 2020;75:8-13. doi:10.1016/j.jsr.2020.10.006
71. Marco CA, Sich M, Ganz E, Clark ANJ, Graham M. Penetrating trauma: relationships to recreational drug and alcohol use. *Am J Emerg Med.* 2022;52:8-12. doi:10.1016/j.ajem.2021.11.035
72. Cunningham RM, Murray R, Walton MA, et al. Prevalence of past year assault among inner-city emergency department patients. *Ann Emerg Med.* 2009;53(6):814-823.
73. Murphy DA, Shetty V, Zigler C, Resell J, Yamashita D-D. Willingness of facial injury patients to change causal substance using behaviors. *Subst Abuse.* 2010;31(1):35-42.
74. Cherpitel CJ, Borges G. Substance use among emergency room patients: an exploratory analysis by ethnicity and acculturation. *Am J Drug Alcohol Abuse.* 2002;28(2):287-305.
75. Laytin AD, Shumway M, Boccellari A, Juillard CJ, Dicker RA. Another "lethal triad"—risk factors for violent injury and long-term mortality among adult victims of violent injury. *J Emerg Med.* 2018;54(5):711-718. doi:10.1016/j.jemermed.2017.12.060
76. Grisso JA, Schwarz DF, Hirschinger N, et al. Violent injuries among women in an urban area. *N Engl J Med.* 1999;341(25):1899-1905.
77. Cunningham R, Walton M, Trowbridge M, et al. Correlates of violent behavior among adolescents presenting to an urban emergency department. *J Pediatr.* 2006;149(6):770-776.
78. Bohnert KM, Walton MA, Ranney M, et al. Understanding the service needs of assault-injured, drug-using youth presenting for care in an urban emergency department. *Addict Behav.* 2015;41:97-105.
79. Cunningham RM, Ranney M, Newton M, Woodhull W, Zimmerman M, Walton MA. Characteristics of youth seeking emergency care for assault injuries. *Pediatrics.* 2014;133(1):e96-e105.
80. Cunningham RM, Carter PM, Ranney M, et al. Violent reinjury and mortality among youth seeking emergency department care for assault-related injury: a 2-year prospective cohort study. *JAMA Pediatr.* 2015;169(1):63-70. doi:10.1001/jamapediatrics.2014.1900
81. Chermack ST, Murray R, Kraus S, et al. Characteristics and treatment interests among individuals with substance use disorders and a history of past six-month violence: findings from an emergency department study. *Addict Behav.* 2014;39(1):265-272.
82. Coupet E Jr, Dodington J, Brackett A, Vaca FE. United States emergency department screening for drug use among assault-injured individuals: a systematic review. *West J Emerg Med.* 2022;23(4):443-450.
83. Cafferky BM, Mendez M, Anderson JR, Stith SM. Substance use and intimate partner violence: a meta-analytic review. *Psychol Violence.* 2018;8(1):110.
84. Smith PH, Homish GG, Leonard KE, Cornelius JR. Intimate partner violence and specific substance use disorders: findings from the National Epidemiologic Survey on Alcohol and Related Conditions. *Psychol Addict Behav.* 2012;26(2):236-245. doi:10.1037/a0024855
85. Stone R, Rothman EF. Opioid use and intimate partner violence: a systematic review. *Curr Epidemiol Rep.* 2019;6(2):215-230. doi:10.1007/s40471-019-00197-2
86. Bohnert ASB, Ilgen MA. Understanding links among opioid use, overdose, and suicide. *N Engl J Med.* 2019;380(1):71-79.
87. Esang M, Ahmed S. A closer look at substance use and suicide. *Am J Psychiatry Res J.* 2018;13(6):6-8. doi:10.1176/appi.ajp-rj.2018.130603
88. Bohnert KM, Ilgen MA, Louzon S, McCarthy JF, Katz IR. Substance use disorders and the risk of suicide mortality among men and women in the U.S. Veterans Health Administration. *Addiction.* 2017;112(7):1193-1201.
89. Goldstein PJ. Drugs, violence, and federal funding: a research odyssey. *Subst Use Misuse.* 1998;33(9):1915-1936.
90. Roche JS, Clery MJ, Carter PM, et al. Tracking assault-injured, drug-using youth in longitudinal research: follow-up methods. *Acad Emerg Med.* 2018;25(11):1204-1215. doi:10.1111/acem.13495
91. Spagnolo PA, Montemitro C, Leggio L. New challenges in addiction medicine: COVID-19 infection in patients with alcohol and substance use disorders—the perfect storm. *Am J Psychiatry.* 2020;177(9):805-807.
92. Livingston M, Callinan S. Underreporting in alcohol surveys: whose drinking is underestimated? *J Stud Alcohol Drugs.* 2015;76(1):158-164.
93. Asbridge M, Hayden JA, Cartwright JL. Acute cannabis consumption and motor vehicle collision risk: systematic review of observational studies and meta-analysis. *BMJ.* 2012;344:e536.
94. Bogerts B. *Alcohol, Drugs and Violence. Where Does Violence Come From?* Springer; 2021:83-88.
95. Lim JY, Lui CK. Longitudinal associations between substance use and violence in adolescence through adulthood. *J Soc Work Pract Addict.* 2016;16(1-2):72-92.
96. Isaacs JY, Smith MM, Sherry SB, Seno M, Moore ML, Stewart SH. Alcohol use and death by suicide: a meta-analysis of 33 studies. *Suicide Life Threat Behav.* 2022;52(4):600-614.
97. Oquendo MA, Currier D, Liu S-M, Hasin DS, Grant BF, Blanco C. Increased risk for suicidal behavior in comorbid bipolar disorder and alcohol use disorders: results from the National Epidemiologic Survey on Alcohol and Related Conditions (NESARC). *J C Psychiatry.* 2010;71(7):902-909.
98. Holmstrand C, Bogren M, Mattisson C, Brådvik L. Long-term suicide risk in no, one or more mental disorders: the Lundby Study 1947-1997. *Acta Psychiatr Scand.* 2015;132(6):459-469.
99. Cornelius ME, Wang TW, Jamal A, Loretan CG, Neff LJ. Tobacco product use among adults—United States, 2019. *MMWR Morbid Mortal Wkly Rep.* 2020;69(46):1736-1742.
100. Hartmann-Boyce J, McRobbie H, Butler AR, et al. Electronic cigarettes for smoking cessation. *Cochrane Database Syst Rev.* 2021;9(9):CD010216.
101. Malas M, van der Tempel J, Schwartz R, et al. Electronic cigarettes for smoking cessation: a systematic review. *Nicotine Tob Res.* 2016;18(10):1926-1936.
102. Zhuang Y-L, Cummins SE, Sun JY, Zhu S-H. Long-term e-cigarette use and smoking cessation: a longitudinal study with U.S. population. *Tob Control.* 2016;25(Suppl 1):i90. doi:10.1136/tobaccocontrol-2016-053096
103. Kalkhoran S, Alvarado N, Vijayaraghavan M, Lum PJ, Yuan P, Satterfield JM. Patterns of and reasons for electronic cigarette use in primary care patients. *J Gen Intern Med.* 2017;32(10):1122-1129.
104. Patel D, Davis KC, Cox S, et al. Reasons for current e-cigarette use among U.S. adults. *Prev Med.* 2016;93:14-20.
105. Gentzke AS, Wang TW, Jamal A, et al. Tobacco product use among middle and high school students—United States, 2020. *MMWR Morbid Mortal Wkly Report.* 2020;69(50):1881-1888. doi:10.15585/mmwr.mm6950a1
106. Etter J-F. Throat hit in users of the electronic cigarette: an exploratory study. *Psychol Addict Behav.* 2016;30(1):93-100.
107. Jones CD, Ho W, Gunn E, Widdowson D, Bahia H. E-cigarette burn injuries: comprehensive review and management guidelines proposal. *Burns.* 2019;45(4):763-771. doi:10.1016/j.burns.2018.09.015
108. Talih S, Balhas Z, Eissenberg T, et al. Effects of user puff topography, device voltage, and liquid nicotine concentration on electronic cigarette nicotine yield: measurements and model predictions. *Nicotine Tob Res.* 2015;17(2):150-157.
109. Brown CJ, Cheng JM. Electronic cigarettes: product characterisation and design considerations. *Tob Control.* 2014;23(suppl 2):ii4-ii10.
110. Rossheim ME, Livingston MD, Soule EK, Zeraye HA, Thombs DL. Electronic cigarette explosion and burn injuries, U.S. Emergency Departments 2015-2017. *Tob Control.* 2019;28(4):472-474. doi:10.1136/tobaccocontrol-2018-054518
111. Norii T, Plate A. Electronic cigarette explosion resulting in a C1 and C2 fracture: a case report. *J Emerg Med.* 2017;52(1):86-88.
112. Harrison R, Hicklin D Jr. Electronic cigarette explosions involving the oral cavity. *J Am Dent Assoc.* 2016;147(11):891-896.

113. Brooks JK, Kleinman JW, Brooks JB, Reynolds MA. Electronic cigarette explosion associated with extensive intraoral injuries. *Dent Traumatol.* 2017;33(2):149-152.
114. Jamison A, Lockington D. Ocular chemical injury secondary to electronic cigarette liquid misuse. *JAMA Ophthalmol.* 2016;134(12):1443-1443.
115. Food and Drug Administration HHS. Deeming tobacco products to be subject to the Federal Food, Drug, and Cosmetic Act, as amended by the Family Smoking Prevention and Tobacco Control Act; restrictions on the sale and distribution of tobacco products and required warning statements for tobacco products. Final rule. *Federal Register.* 2016. Accessed June 26, 2023. https://www.federalregister.gov/documents/2016/05/10/2016-10685/deeming-tobacco-products-to-be-subject-to-the-federal-food-drug-and-cosmetic-act-as-amended-by-the
116. Holland KM, Jones C, Vivolo-Kantor AM, et al. Trends in U.S. emergency department visits for mental health, overdose, and violence outcomes before and during the COVID-19 pandemic. *JAMA Psychiatry.* 2021;78(4):372-379. doi:10.1001/jamapsychiatry.2020.4402
117. Horigian VE, Schmidt RD, Feaster DJ. Loneliness, mental health, and substance use among U.S. young adults during COVID-19. *J Psychoactive Drugs.* 2021;53(1):1-9.
118. Czeisler MÉ, Lane RI, Wiley JF, Czeisler CA, Howard ME, Rajaratnam SMW. Follow-up survey of U.S. adult reports of mental health, substance use, and suicidal ideation during the COVID-19 pandemic, September 2020. *JAMA Netw Open.* 2021;4(2):e2037665. doi:10.1001/jamanetworkopen.2020.37665
119. Czeisler MÉ, Lane RI, Petrosky E, et al. Mental health, substance use, and suicidal ideation during the COVID-19 pandemic—United States, June 24-30, 2020. *MMWR Morbid Mortal Wkly Report.* 2020;69(32):1049.
120. Pino EC, Gebo E, Dugan E, Jay J. Trends in violent penetrating injuries during the first year of the COVID-19 pandemic. *JAMA Netw Open.* 2022;5(2):e2145708. doi:10.1001/jamanetworkopen.2021.45708
121. Gresham AM, Peters BJ, Karantzas G, Cameron LD, Simpson JA. Examining associations between COVID-19 stressors, intimate partner violence, health, and health behaviors. *J Social Pers Relationships.* 2021;38(8):2291-2307. doi:10.1177/02654075211012098
122. Devarakonda AK, Wehrle CJ, Chibane FL, Drevets PD, Fox ED, Lawson AG. The effects of the COVID-19 pandemic on trauma presentations in a level one trauma center. *Am Surg.* 2020;87(5):686-689. doi:10.1177/0003134820973715
123. Zipursky JS, Stall NM, Silverstein WK, et al. Alcohol sales and alcohol-related emergencies during the COVID-19 pandemic. *Ann Intern Med.* 2021;174(7):1029-1032.
124. McGraw C, Salottolo K, Carrick M, et al. Patterns of alcohol and drug utilization in trauma patients during the COVID-19 pandemic at six trauma centers. *Inj Epidemiol.* 2021;8(1):1-8.
125. Young KN, Yeates EO, Grigorian A, et al. Drug and alcohol positivity of traumatically injured patients related to COVID-19 stay-at-home orders. *Am J Drug Alcohol Abuse.* 2021;47(5):605-611.
126. Kamine TH, Rembisz A, Barron RJ, Baldwin C, Kromer M. Decrease in trauma admissions with COVID-19 pandemic. *West J Emerg Med.* 2020;21(4):819-822. doi:10.5811/westjem.2020.5.47780
127. Sutherland M, McKenney M, Elkbuli A. Vehicle related injury patterns during the COVID-19 pandemic: what has changed? *Am J Emerg Med.* 2020;38(9):1710-1714. doi:10.1016/j.ajem.2020.06.006
128. Law RK, Wolkin AF, Patel N, et al. Injury-related emergency department visits during the COVID-19 pandemic. *Am J Prev Med.* 2022;63(1):43-50. doi:10.1016/j.amepre.2022.01.018
129. Woods-Fry H, Vanlaar WGM, Wicklund C, Robertson RD. *Alcohol-Impaired Driving & COVID-19 in the United States: Results From the 2020 TIRF USA Road Safety Monitor.* National Academies; 2020.
130. Thomas FD, Berning A, Darrah J, et al. *Drug and Alcohol Prevalence in Seriously and Fatally Injured Road Users Before and During the COVID-19 Public Health Emergency: United States.* National Highway Traffic Safety Administration; 2020.
131. Agüero JM. COVID-19 and the rise of intimate partner violence. *World Dev.* 2021;137:105217. doi:10.1016/j.worlddev.2020.105217
132. Tsai J, Elbogen EB, Huang M, North CS, Pietrzak RH. Psychological distress and alcohol use disorder during the COVID-19 era among middle- and low-income U.S. adults. *J Affect Disord.* 2021;288:41-49. doi:10.1016/j.jad.2021.03.085
133. Wetli CV, Fishbain DA. Cocaine-induced psychosis and sudden death in recreational cocaine users. *J Forensic Sci.* 1985;30(3):873-880.
134. DiMaio TG, DiMaio VJM. *Excited Delirium Syndrome: Cause of Death and Prevention.* CRC Press; 2005.
135. Strömmer EMF, Leith W, Zeegers MP, Freeman MD. The role of restraint in fatal excited delirium: a research synthesis and pooled analysis. *Forensic Sci Med Pathol.* 2020;16(4):680-692.
136. Vilke GM, Payne-James J, Karch SB. Excited delirium syndrome (ExDS): redefining an old diagnosis. *J Forensic Leg Med.* 2012;19(1):7-11. doi:10.1016/j.jflm.2011.10.006
137. Paquette M. Excited delirium: does it exist? *Perspect Psychiatr Care.* 2003;39(3):93-94.
138. Brody JK, Jordan A, Wakeman SE. *Excited Delirium: Valid Clinical Diagnosis or Medicalized Racism? Organized Medicine Needs to Take a Stand*; 2021. Accessed June 20, 2022. https://www.statnews.com/2021/04/06/excited-delirium-medicalized-racism-organized-medicine-take-a-stand/
139. Stratton SJ, Rogers C, Brickett K, Gruzinski G. Factors associated with sudden death of individuals requiring restraint for excited delirium. *Am J Emerg Med.* 2001;19(3):187-191.
140. Schmidt P, Madea B. Positional traumatic and restraint asphyxia. In: Madea B, ed. *Asphyxiation, Suffocation, and Neck Pressure Deaths.* CRC Press; 2020:232-239.
141. Ranson D. Excited delirium syndrome: a political diagnosis? *J Law Med.* 2012;19(4):667-672.
142. Gonin P, Beysard N, Yersin B, Carron P-N. Excited delirium: a systematic review. *Acad Emerg Med.* 2018;25(5):552-565. doi:10.1111/acem.13330

97 Endocrine and Reproductive Disorders Related to Substance Use

Priya Jaisinghani and Gwendolyne Anyanate Jack

CHAPTER OUTLINE

- Introduction
- Alcohol
- Tobacco
- Opioids
- Other drugs
- Conclusion

INTRODUCTION

The endocrine effects of alcohol and other drugs are complex. These substances can alter the secretion of hormone-releasing factors and hormones at the level of the hypothalamus and pituitary; alter the synthesis or release of hormones at the level of the thyroid, adrenal, or pancreas; alter hormone action on target organs; and alter hormone economy by affecting their metabolism or binding proteins. Multiple hormone systems can be affected, many of whose actions may conflict, leading to a lack of net clinical effect. When one adds to this inherent complexity, the effects on the endocrine system of gender, mental status, and mental illness, the heterogeneity of illegal drugs, the prevalence of polydrug use, the effects of drug withdrawal, and differences between the effects of acute and chronic substance use, it becomes clear that the study of the endocrine effects of alcohol and other drugs is multifaceted. Generalizing many of these effects to clinical practice may be even more challenging. Therefore, the most clearly recognized and clinically relevant effects are summarized in this chapter (**Table 97-1**).

ALCOHOL

Hypoglycemia

One of the most serious consequences of heavy alcohol use is hypoglycemia, which can lead to neurological damage, coma, seizures, or death. Alcohol causes hypoglycemia by producing malnutrition, reducing the body's production of glucose, and impairing the body's response to hypoglycemia. Alcohol use is a common cause of spontaneous hypoglycemia.[1,2]

Unlike other drugs, ethyl alcohol is a significant source of energy, with 7.1 kcal/g. Malnutrition can result from heavy alcohol use, as nutrients are replaced by the "empty" calories of alcohol (ie, alcohol provides energy but no other nutrients such as protein or vitamins). In addition, the normal metabolism of alcohol to acetaldehyde by alcohol dehydrogenase leads to the conversion of nicotinamide adenine dinucleotide (NAD) to its reduced form (NADH), resulting in a decrease in gluconeogenesis. NAD is a cofactor necessary for many of the reactions involved in glucose synthesis. Alcohol does not affect glucose release from glycogen stores, which in a well-fed subject can provide glucose for 12 hours or more. In a prolonged fasting state or in a state of depleted glycogen stores, as seen in people with alcohol use disorders who are malnourished, the inability to compensate for hepatic glycogen depletion can lead to hypoglycemia after acute alcohol ingestion.

Alcohol also can impair the body's hormonal responses to hypoglycemia. Several investigators have shown that alcohol impairs the release of cortisol, growth hormone, glucagon, and vasopressin in response to hypoglycemia.[3-7] Kolaczynski et al.[8] also found similar alcohol-induced reductions in cortisol, glucagon, and growth hormone levels in response to hypoglycemia but found faster glucose recovery with alcohol use, suggesting alcohol-related peripheral insulin resistance. Kerr et al.[9] found a similar suppression of growth hormone, an insignificant suppression of cortisol, and increased insulin resistance in mildly intoxicated hypoglycemic patients with type 1 diabetes. Rasmussen et al.[10] found no change, on the other hand, in glucose counter regulation during acute insulin-induced hypoglycemia in diet-treated patients with mild type 2 diabetes.

There are five classes of alcohol-induced hypoglycemia: simple alcohol-induced fasting hypoglycemia, alcohol-related ketoacidosis with hypoglycemia, alcohol-related exacerbation of insulin-induced hypoglycemia, alcohol-related exacerbation of sulfonylurea-induced hypoglycemia, and alcohol-induced reactive hypoglycemia. In simple alcohol-induced fasting hypoglycemia, patients typically present with coma and a blood glucose level of less than 40 mg/dL. Blood alcohol levels may be detectable. Because of the mechanism underlying this type of hypoglycemia, patients respond promptly to intravenous dextrose but may not respond to glucagon administration.

Alcohol-related ketoacidosis is common. Depletion of NAD resulting from alcohol metabolism leads to the increased production of beta-hydroxybutyrate, acetoacetate, and acetone. Beta-hydroxybutyrate, which is not detectable by routine urine or serum ketone testing, predominates, so the beta-hydroxybutyrate-to-acetoacetate ratio can be as high as 7:1 to 10:1, as compared to 3:1 in diabetic ketoacidosis. Insulin secretion, which ordinarily prevents the development of ketoacidosis, is suppressed by decreased serum glucose levels and

TABLE 97-1 Endocrine Syndromes Associated With Substance Use

Alcohol
- Diabetes insipidus
- Gynecomastia
- Hyperadrenalism
- Hyperglycemia
- Hypoglycemia
- Hyperlipidemia
- Hyperprolactinemia (possibly)
- Hypogonadism/infertility
- Hypertension
- Osteoporosis

Amphetamines
- Hyperadrenalism
- Hypertension
- Weight loss
- Syndrome of inappropriate antidiuretic hormone (SIADH) (MDMA)

Anabolic steroids
- Gynecomastia
- Hyperlipidemia
- Hypogonadism/infertility
- Hypertension
- Hyperthyroidism (possibly)
- Virilization

Barbiturates
- Hypoadrenalism (possibly)
- Hypothyroidism (possibly)
- Osteoporosis

Benzodiazepines
- Hypoadrenalism (possibly)
- Hypoglycemia (possibly)
- Syndrome of inappropriate antidiuretic hormone (SIADH) (possibly)

Caffeine
- Hyperglycemia
- Hyperlipidemia (possibly)
- Hypertension
- Osteoporosis (possibly)

Cocaine
- Hyperglycemia
- Hyperprolactinemia
- Hypertension
- Weight loss

Inhalants
- Hypogonadism/infertility
- Hypothyroidism (possibly)
- Osteoporosis (possibly)

Lysergic acid
- Hypertension

Cannabis
- Gynecomastia (possibly)
- Hypoadrenalism (possibly)
- Hypoglycemia (possibly)
- Hypogonadism/infertility (possibly)

Opioids
- Hyperprolactinemia
- Hypogonadism/infertility
- Osteoporosis
- Adrenal insufficiency

Phencyclidine
- None known

Tobacco
- Hyperlipidemia
- Hypogonadism/infertility
- Hypertension
- Hyperthyroidism
- Hypothyroidism (possibly)
- Osteoporosis
- Syndrome of inappropriate antidiuretic hormone

EDDDs (nicotine)
- Unknown

high catecholamine levels. The patient usually has a history of chronic heavy alcohol use and may be experiencing nausea, vomiting, abdominal pain, and metabolic acidosis. Blood alcohol levels usually are not detectable. Glucose levels may range from low to mildly elevated but typically are less than 250 mg/dL. Treatment includes dextrose and volume repletion. Marked hyperglycemia should raise the suspicion of concomitant diabetes or diabetic ketoacidosis.[11]

Patients with diabetes treated with insulin or sulfonylurea are at risk for severe hypoglycemia with alcohol use.[12-14] Though they often are the only reasonable options for achieving some measure of glucose control in patients who continue to drink heavily, insulin and sulfonylureas should be used with great caution in patients with alcohol use disorders and diabetes. Cognitive impairment and nonrecognition of hypoglycemia with alcohol use can lead to nontreatment of hypoglycemia in patients with diabetes.[15,16] Patients with diabetes must be counseled about alcohol use and its hypoglycemic consequences. In addition, sulfonylureas and insulin are metabolized in the liver and are more likely to cause severe hypoglycemia in patients with alcohol-related cirrhosis than in those without cirrhosis. Basal insulins, such as degludec and U300 glargine, are associated with lower risk for nocturnal hypoglycemia, although this has not been specifically studied in those with alcohol use disorders.[17,18] Basal insulins such as U500 insulin, which may show greater improvements in diabetes control in certain cases compared to U100 insulin, still need additional research to assess the risk of severe hypoglycemia; however, alcohol use is still cautioned with its use.[19,20]

Short-acting insulin secretagogues of the meglitinide class, such as repaglinide and nateglinide, have less hypoglycemic risk and might be considered as having a role in patients with alcohol use disorders. However, cases of severe hypoglycemia have been described with repaglinide[21] and nateglinide,[22] and Bolen et al.[23] have reported that hypoglycemia with repaglinide was comparable to that seen with sulfonylureas. Comparison of nateglinide with repaglinide has suggested a lower, albeit statistically insignificant, incidence of hypoglycemia.[24] Although antihyperglycemic medications such as metformin, rosiglitazone, and pioglitazone are not associated with hypoglycemia, caution should be exercise due to potential risk of lactic acidosis (metformin) and liver toxicity (rosiglitazone and pioglitazone).

Pharmacologic therapies including glucagonlike peptide 1 agonists(GLP-1 RAs), such as semaglutide, dulaglutide, and liraglutide, and dipeptidyl peptidase IV inhibitors(DPP4-Is), such as sitagliptin, saxagliptin, and linagliptin, and the newer combination agent glucose-dependent insulinotropic polypeptide glucagonlike peptide 1 agonist (GIP/GLP-1 RA), tirzepatide, increase incretin action, leading to glucose-dependent insulin release, reduced glucagon, and slowed gastric emptying. GLP-1 RAs and GIP/GLP-1 RAs have low hypoglycemia risk when used as monotherapy, and DPP4-Is are not associated with hypoglycemia.[25] Initial studies suggested increased risk of pancreatitis with GLP-1 RAs and DPP4-Is; however, more recent studies have not found conclusive evidence of increased risk of pancreatitis or pancreatic cancer with GLP-1 RAs and DPP4-Is.[26,27] Given the dearth of studies on the risk of pancreatitis in patients with prior history of pancreatitis, alternative antihyperglycemic therapies should be considered in patients with a prior history of pancreatitis. Patients with alcohol use disorders who are prescribed GLP-1 RAs, GIP/GLP-1 RAs, or DPP4-Is, should be counseled on signs/symptoms of pancreatitis and advised to promptly discontinue the use of GLP-1 RA or DPP4-I if pancreatitis is suspected.[28] Less commonly used therapies that have been approved for improving glycemic control in type 2 diabetes mellitus, such as colesevelam, a bile acid resin, and bromocriptine, a dopamine agonist, may be adjunctive therapies, but the former is not indicated in those with hypertriglyceridemia, and the latter may increase the risk for orthostatic hypotension and psychosis.

Alcohol abstinence is recommended to minimize the risk of hypoglycemia. The American Diabetes Association recommends limiting alcohol intake (women ≤1 drink daily and men ≤2 drinks daily) and education/awareness of the recognition and management of delayed hypoglycemia, especially if patients are using insulin or insulin secretagogues. If alcohol use persists, consumption of food with alcohol is recommended, and patients with diabetes are encouraged to monitor blood glucose frequently after drinking.[29] Diabetes care in those with alcohol-related liver disease and ongoing heavy alcohol use is difficult, and less stringent glycemic goals, as well as early consultation with a diabetologist, are reasonable.

Reactive or postprandial hypoglycemia with alcohol use can occur, depending on the carbohydrate composition of the meal consumed. O'Keefe and Marks[30] first described this phenomenon as profound hypoglycemia (mean blood glucose nadir, 48.6 mg/dL) that occurs 3 to 4 hours after the ingestion of alcohol combined with 60 g sucrose (as in gin and tonic). This phenomenon can develop in up to 10% to 20% of healthy subjects and does not appear to occur with saccharin or fructose and alcohol.[31] Work by Flanigan suggested that hypoglycemia develops because of suppression of growth hormone release.[32] A recent study also suggested increased insulin levels as a contributing mechanism while other postulated mechanisms include, hepatic insulin resistance, increased intestinal glucose absorption and altered lipid metabolism.[33]

Hyperglycemia

Alcohol-related pancreatitis can lead to pancreatic exocrine and endocrine insufficiency, with Nikkola et al. finding that 55% of those with a first episode of acute alcohol-related pancreatitis developed prediabetes or diabetes mellitus over a median of 7.5 years of follow-up. Recurrent pancreatitis episodes were strongly associated with pancreatogenic diabetes mellitus, while the severity of acute alcohol-related pancreatitis was not associated with development of diabetes mellitus.[34] However, it is important to note that there has been an evolution in the classification system for severity of acute pancreatitis. This may make it difficult to compare studies that use various scoring systems over time to draw conclusions. In addition, it is thought that alcohol and its metabolites itself lead to damage including atrophy, fibrosis, or an inflammatory response suggesting confounding variables may exist.[35] When diabetes mellitus results from pancreatic insufficiency, it is an indication that more than 90% of the pancreatic beta cells, which produce insulin, and the alpha cells, which produce glucagon, are destroyed. The secondary diabetes mellitus that results typically is an extremely labile insulin-dependent diabetes, in that those patients are absolutely insulin deficient and have normal or increased insulin sensitivity. Diabetic ketoacidosis results not simply from a lack of insulin but also from an increase in the glucagon-insulin ratio. This explains why patients with type 2 diabetes may develop ketoacidosis in the setting of severe infection and the presence of high insulin levels. In patients with pancreatitis-induced diabetes, the lack of glucagon makes the patient somewhat resistant to developing diabetic ketoacidosis but also quite prone to developing hypoglycemia.

Acute ethanol consumption has been shown to increase peripheral insulin resistance, and interested readers are directed to an extensive review from Ting and Lautt.[36] This insulin resistance is localized to skeletal muscle and may be related to ethanol-induced changes in lactate, triglyceride, norepinephrine, hepatic insulin-sensitizing substance, hepatic glutathione, and insulin binding. Despite this insulin resistance, postprandial glucose levels may be lower after preprandial consumption of 20 g of alcohol in lean, young healthy adults[37] and 15 g of alcohol after low-carbohydrate, high-fat meals in postmenopausal women.[38]

The association of alcohol use and glucose control is a complicated one, with most studies finding a U-shaped association between alcohol use and diabetes mellitus, with low consumption having the lowest risk for diabetes mellitus.[39-41] Though chronic heavy alcohol use can lead to chronic pancreatitis, pancreatic insufficiency, and subsequent diabetes mellitus, some studies have found an association between low amounts of alcohol use and improved insulin sensitivity[42-44] and a decreased risk of diabetes mellitus in men.[45] Other investigators found no effect[46,47] or lower insulin secretion with higher alcohol use.[48] Some authors have found no association, which suggests the possibility that associations in other studies are not causal[49] and there may be other contributing factors such as alcohol amount and duration effect.[50] Knott et al. indicate that there are gender-specific differences in the association between alcohol consumption and the risk of type 2 diabetes mellitus. They reported no reduction in type 2 diabetes mellitus in men regardless of alcohol consumption level, whereas in women there was decreased risk of type 2 diabetes in the setting of low amounts of alcohol consumption. The discrepancy may be linked to differences in the effects of alcohol on insulin sensitivity in men compared to women, as well as the prevalence of comorbidities and diabetes mellitus risk factors in women, or it may be due to inadequately measured confounding factors.[51] The effects of different types of alcohol on diabetes risk and control have recently been reviewed and suggest that if the effect is causal, wine may provide more protection than beer or spirits. It was proposed that resveratrol extract in wine may contribute to its glucose-lowering properties.[52]

Reproductive Consequences

The reproductive effects of alcohol use are gender specific. Alcohol use has long been known to cause sexual dysfunction and hypogonadism in men, particularly in those with alcohol-related cirrhosis.[53] Even in men without liver disease, alcohol use leads to a decrease in testosterone,[54] which may be the result of a combination of direct effects on the testicular synthesis of testosterone and hypothalamic-pituitary function[55] or on increases in sex hormone-binding globulin, which can lead to a decrease in bioavailable testosterone.[56] The incidence of gynecomastia is increased in alcohol-related cirrhosis, primarily because of increased levels of androstenedione, a precursor for estrogen synthesis.[57] Increased prolactin levels have been found in patients with alcohol-related cirrhosis,[58] though it may not be present in those with alcohol use disorders who do not have severe liver disease.[59]

In women, the effects of alcohol use depend on menopausal status and hormone therapy use. In premenopausal women, alcohol consumption was associated with increase in estradiol levels, and the effect was increased during times of gonadotropin elevation such as luteinizing hormone (LH) surge and early pregnancy. This increase in estrogen level may explain why alcohol use is associated with an increased risk of breast cancer[60] and why alcohol can be associated with a delay in menopause. Premenopausal women on hormonal contraceptives who consumed alcohol had higher levels of estradiol. In premenopausal women and postmenopausal women taking estrogen, acute alcohol consumption leads to an increase in estradiol levels through reduced metabolism of estradiol in the liver. It is thought that due to the accumulation of NADH from alcohol consumption, there is decreased conversion from estradiol to estrone, which results in estradiol excess.[61-63] In postmenopausal women not on hormonal therapy, the effects of alcohol on estrogen levels have been inconclusive.[64] Women with high or frequent alcohol intake were found to have higher rates of menstrual disorders, including amenorrhea, dysmenorrhea, and irregular menstrual periods.

Pregnant women with high alcohol intake have a higher incidence of miscarriages, placental abruption, preterm deliveries, and stillbirths than do controls.[65] An increased risk of infertility was associated with as few as one to five alcoholic drinks a week in a Danish study[66] and with as little as 12 g of alcohol a week (about 1 drink) in an American study.[67] There may be an increase in prolactin levels and a decrease in oxytocin levels in lactating women[68] and premenopausal women who are exposed to alcohol (approximately 2 drinks).[69] Despite the increase in prolactin levels, lactating women may have a slight decrease in milk production.[70]

Bone Health Consequences

Postmenopausal women who drink low amounts of alcohol may have an increased bone mineral density and a decreased risk of fractures.[65] Similar effects have been found by others,[71-73] with some finding differences in the type of alcoholic beverage, with wine or beer being associated with more benefit than spirits or liquor.[74,75] However, alcohol use disorder is associated with decreased bone mass and an increased risk of skeletal fractures.[76-79] African American men may be less susceptible to this bone loss.[80] Authors have described this phenomenon as a J-shaped association, where there is a threshold at which alcohol use transitions from conferring a protective effect on bone health to having a deleterious effect on bone density and fracture risk.[81] Alcohol consumption can increase the risk of fractures independent of bone density.[82] In addition to increased risk of falls while inebriated, other indirect factors such as lean body mass, decompensated liver disease, vitamin D deficiency, and poor nutritional status contribute to the increased risk of fractures, especially rib fractures in heavy alcohol drinkers.[83]

In addition to alterations in sex hormones and the type of fat malabsorption and vitamin D deficiency associated with liver disease, alcohol use can reversibly impair bone formation by osteoblasts.[84-86] Therefore, alcohol consumption affects bone remodeling imbalance and preferentially decreases bone formation.[87] It has been postulated that alcohol-induced oxidative stress suppresses Wnt/Dkk1 signaling pathways, thereby decreasing the formation of osteoblasts.[88] Malnutrition and low body mass and decreases in IGF-I, a bone growth factor, may play a significant role in the decreased bone mass.[89,90] Reductions in leptin with alcohol use[91,92] may also play a role in decreasing bone mass although there is some controversy about what exactly is that role.[93] In animal studies, the parathyroid hormone (PTH) may help reverse some of the bone loss although continued alcohol use impairs the response.[94]

Heavy alcohol use is associated with osteonecrosis of the bone.[95] Alcohol-associated osteonecrosis of the femoral head may be due in part to lipid or cortisol changes,[96] and, in fact, alcohol may be responsible for up to one-third of cases of femoral head osteonecrosis.[97]

Other Endocrinological Consequences

Alcohol use increases triglyceride synthesis, leading to hypertriglyceridemia and hepatic steatosis. The increased NADH/NAD ratio leads to increases in alpha-glycerophosphate, which favors hepatic triglyceride accumulation by trapping fatty acids. The excess NADH enhances fatty acid synthesis. Alcohol increases the high-density lipoprotein (HDL) fraction of cholesterol, which may be associated with reduced cardiovascular morbidity and mortality.[98]

Though glucocorticoid response to hypoglycemia can be impaired by alcohol use, patients with chronic heavy alcohol use have elevated adrenocorticotropic hormone (ACTH) and cortisol production. This response is mediated by corticotropin-releasing hormone (CRH) and the interaction with stress. This may be related to a person's genetic propensity to developing an alcohol use disorder. These effects are dose dependent.[99]

Rarely, patients with alcohol use disorder may develop the clinical stigmata of glucocorticoid excess, such as central obesity, moon facies, "buffalo hump," and biochemical evidence of nonsuppressible glucocorticoid excess that is difficult to distinguish from Cushing syndrome. This condition, which has been termed pseudo-Cushing syndrome, reverses with abstinence from alcohol for at least 1 month.[100,101] There are no clear clinical features or lab test results that distinguish pseudo-Cushing from Cushing syndrome,[101] and a period of alcohol abstinence and reversal of the syndrome may avoid the search for a nonexistent pituitary or adrenal tumor.

Alcohol may influence hormones regulating feeding behavior. Leptin levels are decreased acutely after low amounts of alcohol use[91] and in malnourished people with an alcohol use disorder.[92] Ghrelin secretion is similarly reduced, without effects on peptide YY, soon after moderate alcohol intake.[102,103] This is somewhat paradoxical given that these hormones suppress appetite and alcohol is believed to stimulate appetite.

Alcohol use has effects on plasma volume and blood pressure status. It transiently decreases vasopressin release, leading to water diuresis.[104] This condition can be problematic in patients with partial diabetes insipidus. Acute alcohol use also increases blood pressure, possibly through an increase in norepinephrine.[105] Low amounts of alcohol consumption appear to increase plasma renin activity, though such increases are believed to result from a secondary response to changes in fluid and electrolyte balance.[106] Though alcohol by itself does not affect mineralocorticoid levels, alcohol-related cirrhosis leads to elevations of aldosterone in response to decreased effective plasma volume.

Alcohol use and even periods of withdrawal or early abstinence have been associated with a lower serum thyroxine (T4) and serum triiodothyronine (T3) and blunted thyroid-stimulating hormone (TSH) in response to thyrotropin-releasing hormone (TRH).[107] As the liver is a major site for the conversion of T4 to T3, alcohol-related cirrhosis of the liver can produce decreases in T3 without producing clinical hypothyroidism in those without preexisting autoimmune thyroid disease.[108,109]

Alcohol use was reported to suppress melatonin secretion through increased norepinephrine levels, and this increase may be implicated in disturbances in sleep and performance.[110]

TOBACCO

The adverse effects of tobacco on the cardiopulmonary systems are well known. Tobacco smoke contains a myriad of chemical compounds—most notably nicotine, tar, thiocyanate, 2,3-hydroxypyridine, and carbon monoxide—which may have multiple endocrine effects. Many of these effects have been reviewed in detail.[111]

Thyroid Consequences

Passive smoke exposure may increase resting metabolic rate and thyroid hormone secretion.[112,113] Cigarette smoking increases the risk of Graves disease and Graves ophthalmopathy and can lower TSH levels.[114-120] Stopping smoking seems to be associated with reduction in the risk for Graves disease.[121] The increased risk of ophthalmopathy with cigarette smoking may be related to increased fibroblast adipogenesis associated with increased interleukin-1 levels and interleukin-6 levels and upregulation of adipocyte-related immediate early genes.[122,123] Additionally, smoking can adversely influence response to treatment modalities for Graves disease and Graves ophthalmopathy. The response to glucocorticoids or orbital radiation in patients with Graves ophthalmopathy can be dampened by smoking cigarettes.[124] Smoking also increases the risk of Graves ophthalmopathy after radioiodine therapy.[125]

Older studies have associated smoking with goiter and hypothyroidism.[126,127] This may be a consequence of the thiocyanate present in cigarette smoke, which is a goitrogen that inhibits iodide uptake and hormone synthesis and increases iodine exit from the thyroid.[128,129] Newer studies have shown that smoking may also be associated with decreased levels of serum thyroid autoantibodies,[118,130-133] with stopping smoking increasing the risk for these antibodies.[134] Some studies note that smoking may cause hypothyroidism only in those with preexisting thyroid dysfunction. Smoking appears to lower the risk of thyroid cancer.[135,136]

Insulin Resistance and Dyslipidemia

Cigarette smoking,[137] as well as nicotine gum use,[138] is associated with an increase in insulin resistance and an increased risk of developing impaired glucose tolerance and diabetes mellitus.[45,139-142] Stopping smoking does not seem to eliminate the risk of diabetes mellitus as both former smokers and current smokers have an increased risk for type 2 diabetes mellitus, affecting men more than women.[143] Secondhand smoke exposure similarly increases diabetes risk.[144] Mild decreases in HDL cholesterol and mild elevations in triglycerides, consistent with this insulin resistance, are associated with cigarette smoking,[137] though these changes may be due to components of cigarette smoke other than nicotine.[145] In adolescents, both passive smoke exposure and active smoking have been associated with the metabolic syndrome.[146] Insulin resistance and dyslipidemia may be responsible, in part, for the elevated rates of cardiovascular and atherosclerotic disease associated with cigarette use.

Reproductive Function

In women, cigarette smoking is associated with decreases in estrogen levels[147] and, in fact, can enhance estrogen degradation.[148] The decrease in estrogen levels could also impair the efficacy of oral contraceptive pills.[125,149] Smoking is also associated with early menopause[150,151] and increased ovarian age and follicular-stimulating hormone (FSH) levels.[152,153] A meta-analysis by Waylen and colleagues found that patients who smoked had poorer outcomes with assisted reproduction, with significantly lower odds of clinical pregnancy per cycle, higher odds of spontaneous miscarriage, and higher odds of ectopic pregnancy.[154] In men, cigarette smoking is associated with quantitative and qualitative decrements in sperm[155-157] and with increases in serum estrogen.[158] Unfortunately, public knowledge of the risk of smoking for these reproductive issues is low, ranging from 17% to 39%,[159] and educating patients about these unrealized dangers is paramount.

Bone Health

Cigarette smoking is associated with decreased bone mineral density and increased bone loss in postmenopausal women and elderly men[160] and is an independent risk factor for osteoporotic fracture.[161,162] This fracture risk appears, in part, due to a decrease in intestinal calcium absorption,[163,164] resulting in a negative calcium balance. Brot et al.[165] found an association between smoking and decreased serum 25-hydroxyvitamin D,

1,25-dihydroxyvitamin D, PTH, and osteocalcin levels, suggesting a more complex effect of smoking on calcium and bone metabolism. Cigarette smoking can negate the protective effect of estrogen therapy on the risk of hip fracture in postmenopausal women.[166] It also is associated with femoral head osteonecrosis,[95] possibly through impairment of vascular function or changes in blood lipids.

Other Endocrinological Effects

Cigarette smoke stimulates antidiuretic hormone release from the pituitary through an airway-mediated mechanism that does not depend on circulating nicotine.[167,168] This antidiuretic effect may cause or exacerbate hyponatremia in susceptible patients.[169,170] The nicotine found in cigarette smoke can increase the release of catecholamines from the adrenal medulla, which may precipitate a hypertensive crisis for those with pheochromocytoma. In addition, smoking is associated with hypertension and poorly controlled hypertension, apparently through stimulation of the noradrenergic nervous system[171]; such hypertension is not angiotensin II dependent.[172] Nicotine increases ACTH release and cortisol release in a dose-dependent fashion[173-175] and may have some role in nicotine/tobacco addiction. Cigarette smoking is associated with activation on the HPA axis, leading to elevated cortisol levels and loss of diurnal variation in cortisol secretion. Stopping smoking may restore the diurnal variation, thus suggesting that smoking likely has a short-term effect on cortisol levels.[176] However, moderately elevated cortisol throughout the day, as can be seen with cigarette smoking, may have clinical implications such as increased insulin resistance.[177]

Cigarettes also may increase prolactin secretion. In a study of men randomized to 0.2 or 2 mg nicotine cigarettes, in the higher dose nicotine group, prolactin levels were measured to be more than 150% above the baseline by 30 minutes and remained elevated 1 hour after smoking; however, there was no significant increase in prolactin in the low nicotine group. Whether this translates into clinical manifestations of hyperprolactinemia is unclear.[173,175] In people who smoke cigarettes chronically, there is inhibition of prolactin thought to be via activation of nictotinic receptors of the tuberoinfundibular dopamine neurons leading to release of prolactin inhibitory factor.[125]

The use of electronic drug (nicotine) delivery devices (EDDDs) such as electronic cigarettes (e-cigarettes), vape pens, hookah pens have become a popular alternative to tobacco smoking; however, the long-term health effects have not been well studied. E-cigarettes are not recommended by the FDA as an option to achieve abstinence from tobacco.[178] Due to inconsistent labeling and variability of nicotine content in the cartridges, the level of nicotine exposure remains unclear.[179] In a study on rats administered electronic cigarette refill liquid, decreased sperm density and viability, as well as testosterone levels were observed in rat testes and thought to be due to impaired oxidative balance and steroidogenesis.[180] El-Shahawy et al. found that men who used EDDDs with nicotine were more likely to report erectile dysfunction than men without reported use of EDDDs.[181] In another study using the mouse model, it was observed that EDDD exposure prior to conception, delayed implantation of the fertilized embryo by modulating receptive gene pathways that affect timely embryo attachment to the uterus, thereby reducing fertility.[182] In addition to infertility, EDDDs have been linked to development of prediabetes, where people who vaped were 22% more likely to develop prediabetes than those who have never partaken. It has been suggested that nicotine, which is in both cigarettes and EDDDs, is a significant driver of the insulin resistance that predisposes to prediabetes and elevated glucose levels. More studies are needed evaluating other endocrinological manifestations of nicotine-containing EDDDs.

OPIOIDS

The endocrine effects of acute administration of opioids occur primarily in the hypothalamus and pituitary. Gonadotropins (FSH and LH) are suppressed by inhibition of gonadotropin-releasing hormone secretion. Prolactin secretion is stimulated, while ACTH and cortisol secretion are suppressed.[183] Chronic administration of opioids can produce partial tolerance to many of the endocrine effects. Vuong et al.[184] have exhaustively reviewed the endocrine effects of opioids, and readers are directed to this review for further in depth treatment of this topic.

Male Gonadal Function

Male gonadal function in patients with opioid use disorder (OUD), and those patients with OUD who are treated with methadone, has been primarily diminished but not in all studies. In men, methadone use has been associated with a decline in serum testosterone levels in some early studies.[185-187] In contrast, Cushman and Kreek did not find changes in testosterone levels among people with opioid use disorder resulting from heroin who were treated with methadone.[188,189] Another study looking at methadone, methadone/heroin, and heroin use found normal levels of testosterone, FSH, LH, and prolactin in all but the individuals who used heroin, in whom elevated prolactin levels were found.[190] However, individuals who used only heroin, individuals who used heroin and methadone, and 45% of the individuals who took methadone in that study had diminished sperm motility. Lafisca et al.[191] looked at short-term methadone use in 30 men and found no abnormalities of estrogen, progesterone, or LH, whereas FSH showed lower values than normal, and androstenedione, dehydroepiandrosterone, and prolactin noticeably increased in many subjects. Modest variations were noted for testosterone and dihydrotestosterone. Other investigators found a decrease in basal FSH and LH levels, with a decrease in pituitary response to gonadotropin-releasing hormone, suggesting a hypothalamic cause for hypogonadism in people with opioid use disorder.[192] While Brown et al.[193] found sexual dysfunction associated with methadone dose in 14% of men attending an opioid treatment program, they did not find it associated with a decrease in testosterone level.

Daniell[194] found that men being treated with sustained-action opioids for chronic pain had decreasing testosterone levels in a dose-dependent fashion, with overtly low levels with a daily methadone dose equivalent of more than 70 mg. Many were overtly symptomatic with erectile dysfunction. Bliesener et al.[195] found that people with opioid use disorder on buprenorphine maintenance had higher testosterone levels, comparable to healthy controls, than did those treated with methadone, suggesting that hypogonadism may be mediated through mu opioid receptor since methadone is a pure mu opioid receptor agonist and buprenorphine is a partial mu opioid receptor agonist with high affinity but low intrinsic activity. Hallinan et al.[196,197] confirmed that male hypogonadism and sexual dysfunction were more common with methadone treatment than with buprenorphine.

The variability in opioid-induced male hypogonadism may be due in part to the presence of other components, as well as variable doses of opioids, in street preparations of heroin, continued use of heroin in methadone-treated individuals, and the possible effect of malnutrition on the reproductive system. A study of the endocrine effects of long-term intrathecal opioid administration for pain relief found diminished testosterone and LH levels in men but normal FSH and prolactin levels in comparison to control patients with a comparable pain syndrome but who were not treated with opioid,[198] suggesting that these are the "pure" opioid effects on the male reproductive system. A systematic review and meta-analysis by Bawor and colleagues concluded that both methadone and nonmethadone opioids are associated with a 165 ng/mL reduction in total testosterone in men.[199] There is likely some individual variation, depending on baseline testosterone and sex hormone-binding globulin levels, with regard to whether this has clinical relevance.

The male hypogonadism resulting from opioid use may increase pain sensitivity. In the Testosterone and Pain (TAP) trial, Basaria and colleagues studied 84 men on at least the equivalent of 20 mg of hydrocodone daily for 4 weeks for noncancer pain and found to have a morning serum total testosterone less than 350 ng/dL. Forty-three were randomized to 14 weeks of topical testosterone replacement and 41 to placebo. Those on testosterone replacement had greater improvements in pressure and mechanical hyperalgesia, and sexual desire, as well as decreases in body fat composition.[200]

Female Gonadal Function

In women, more than half of a group of 76 patients with opioid use disorder on methadone maintenance had menstrual irregularities.[201] Endocrinological studies on seven of the women showed alterations in hypothalamic and pituitary function leading to oligo-ovulation. A study of 21 premenopausal women who received chronic intrathecal opioids found 14 to have amenorrhea and 7 to have menstrual irregularity, with decrements in serum LH, FSH, estradiol, and progesterone concentrations.[198] In the same study, 18 postmenopausal women had serum LH and FSH levels significantly lower than did postmenopausal control subjects, further indicating impairment of gonadotropin release. Women being treated for chronic pain with sustained-action, transdermal, or oral opioids have been associated with lower sex hormones due to ovarian and adrenal suppression.[202] Opioids have been found to be competitive inhibitors of human placental aromatase, the enzyme that converts androgens to estrogens.[203,204] The clinical implications of this effect and generalizability to other tissues are unclear.

This hypogonadism may also be influenced through hyperprolactinemia. Opioids are well known to increase prolactin levels,[205] and this is likely mediated through dopaminergic mechanisms.[206] Naloxone does not affect the TRH-stimulated release of prolactin.[207]

Bone Health

Hypogonadism is a risk factor for osteoporosis. There is evidence showing a decrease in bone density with opioids[208-212] in both men and women, although two studies found it more common in men than in women and associated with a higher risk of hypogonadism.[213,214] Kim et al.[215] found a high degree of vitamin D deficiency and insufficiency among those on methadone in an opioid treatment program, which may adversely affect the bone. There is also evidence for increased fracture risk.[216,217] The effects on bone may be reversed with abstinence from the opioid.[208] If this is not possible, usual approaches to treating low bone density should be considered such as sex hormone replacement therapy, adequate calcium and vitamin D intake, weight-bearing exercise, other lifestyle changes such as moderation of alcohol use and stopping smoking, and judicious use of bisphosphonates or other osteoporosis drugs.

Other Endocrine Effects

Opioids have been associated with hypoadrenalism, whether given intrathecally,[198] orally,[218,219] or transdermally.[220] Opioids appear to inhibit the ACTH response to CRH, and their effect is blocked by naloxone.[221,222].

At high doses (ie, morphine ≥15 mg), opioids may induce growth hormone release among normal subjects but to a greater extent in those with acromegaly.[223] Naloxone may block the stimulation of growth hormone with growth hormone–releasing hormone.[224] Opioids may also stimulate TSH release,[205] an effect blocked by naloxone.[207]

Reed and Ghodse studied oral glucose tolerance testing and insulin/growth hormone/cortisol responses in 12 patients with opioid use disorder compared with age, sex, and weight-matched controls. Individuals with heroin use had evidence for insulin resistance and higher growth hormone levels, with lower cortisol levels.[225] This was confirmed by Passariello et al. who also found increased catecholamine levels in those individuals with heroin use when matched for age, sex, and weight.[226] Although a retrospective observational study found that methadone treatment, more so than buprenorphine, was associated with diabetes mellitus, there have been concerns that concomitant hepatitis C (HCV) in these patients may increase the risk for diabetes.[227] Howard et al. found an increased prevalence of diabetes mellitus in those with past and present opioid use, controlled for older age, family history of diabetes, obesity, HCV, and ethnicity. In addition, those with combined prescription opioid use together with current illicit opioid or methadone use had the highest risk for diabetes mellitus (odds ratio 2.58).[228] In a nested case-control study using the UK-based General Practice Research Database, however, Li and colleagues did not find any association between opioid use for noncancer pain and type 2 diabetes mellitus among 50,468 patients with diabetes.[229]

OTHER DRUGS

Cannabis

The major psychoactive component of cannabis is delta-9-tetrahydrocannabinol (THC), though cannabis can contain more than 400 chemicals. Factors including concomitant use of other drugs, variability in smoking technique, and variable potencies of cannabis and development of tolerance to cannabis' effects can make it difficult to generalize from study findings to clinical practice. Consistent endocrine effects of cannabis in animals have not translated to consistent findings in humans.[230]

Though some investigators have reported that heavy cannabis smoking is associated with low plasma levels of testosterone,[231] others report that chronic cannabis use has no effects on plasma testosterone or LH in men.[232] Further confusion arises from reports suggesting that smoking cannabis acutely suppresses LH in men[233] and premenopausal women in the luteal phase of their menstrual cycle but not in postmenopausal women.[234] One study of pregnant people who used cannabis found no changes in female sex hormones as compared with controls.[235] Takeda hypothesized that THC may increase estrogen receptor (ER) β expression, possibly reducing ERα signaling.[236] Brents recently reviewed the effects of cannabis and the endocannabinoid system on the female reproductive system.[237] Cannabis might affect fertility, decreasing LH, testosterone, sperm count and motility in men, and suppressing ovulation in women.

Cannabis is the most commonly used illicit drug in pregnancy, estimated at 5.2% with up to 10.7% of women during the first trimester. Cannabis has not been found to be teratogenic and has not been found to have consistent effects on pregnancy outcomes, although there have been concerns about increased potency of cannabis with an increase in THC concentration from 3.4% to 8.8% from 1993 to 2008. There are cannabinoid receptors in the uterine decidua and placenta, potentially leading to increased placental resistance and intrauterine growth restriction.[238]

There have been reports of an association between chronic cannabis use and increased risk of testicular germ cell tumors[239,240] although Lacson and colleagues found an inconsistent dose-response relationship with a clearer association of testicular germ cell tumors with individuals with former cannabis use, infrequent use, and those of shorter duration than those individuals who currently used cannabis frequently, or those with more than 10 years of use.[241]

With regard to other endocrinological effects, prolonged oral administration of 210 mg THC a day (the equivalent of smoking 6 cannabis cigarettes) for 14 days significantly suppressed the cortisol and growth hormone response to insulin-induced hypoglycemia, though the THC use did not suppress the cortisol and growth hormone response to values consistent with cortisol or growth hormone deficiency.[242] Continued cannabis use has not been found to affect the normalization of the hypothalamic-pituitary-adrenal axis in patients with opioid use disorder initiating methadone treatment.[243] Adolescents with reported early onset (9-12 years of age) of cannabis use were found to have lower salivary cortisol levels on awakening.[244] It is unclear whether the lower salivary cortisol resulted from the early cannabis use or vice versa. Heavy cannabis use may likely cause significant hypoadrenalism or impaired recovery from insulin-induced hypoglycemia only in those with preexisting adrenal disease. In animals, cannabis suppresses TSH and peripheral thyroid hormone levels,[230] and one study in humans showed a normal TSH but decreased peripheral T4 associated with an increased T3 uptake, suggesting dose-dependent decreases in thyroid-binding globulin,[245] but no clear alteration in thyroid status. Cannabis has well-recognized effects on feeding behavior ("the munchies") by its interactions with cannabinoid receptors (CB-1).[246] In a recent study in HIV-infected men, cannabis smoking increased serum leptin and ghrelin and decreased peptide YY levels, without affecting insulin levels.[247] THC may contribute to weight gain via the effects described at the cannabinoid receptor and increase in appetite secondary to hormone effects. A new study has shown that delta9-tetrahydrocannabivarin (THCV) may have appetite suppressing qualities by blocking cannabinoid receptors.[248]

Sophocleous and colleagues noted that cannabinoid receptor knockout mice were associated with increased bone mineral density but increased bone loss with aging due to effects on osteoclasts, osteoblasts, and bone marrow adiposity. They found that individuals with heavy cannabis use (>5,000 occasions) had reduced bone density Z-scores, associated with increased bone turnover markers, lower 25-hydroxyvitamin D levels, and increased risk of fractures. Most of the bone density reduction was explained by differences in body mass index, which was lower in individuals who use cannabis, and mitigated by dietary calcium intake.[249]

Cocaine

Cocaine acts primarily by blocking the reuptake of norepinephrine, dopamine, and serotonin at the synaptic junctions, resulting in increased neurotransmitter concentrations. In animal studies, cocaine can stimulate the adrenal medulla to release epinephrine and norepinephrine. By increasing catecholamines, counterregulatory hormones that antagonize insulin, stimulate glucose production and inhibit glucose clearance, hyperglycemia can result as can diabetic ketoacidosis or hyperosmolar nonketotic hyperglycemia without any other identified precipitants.[250,251] Diabetic ketoacidosis appears to occur more frequently in individuals who use cocaine, resulting from a combination of omission of insulin therapy and cocaine effects on glucose metabolism.[251]

Dopamine is an important physiological regulator of prolactin and TSH secretion. Acute cocaine use suppresses prolactin secretion with increases in dopamine levels, but with chronic use, dopamine levels become depleted, and hyperprolactinemia results.[252-254] This hyperprolactinemia persists even after cocaine withdrawal.[255] The clinical significance is unclear, but it may be a cause of hypogonadism. Though acute cocaine use produces rises in ACTH, FSH, and LH,[252,256,257] abnormalities of testosterone, cortisol, LH,[253] or thyroid function tests[258] have not been found in individuals with chronic cocaine use.

Amphetamines

Amphetamines, such as dextroamphetamine and methylamphetamine, have not been well studied with regard to the endocrinological effects of chronic use. They act primarily by stimulating the release of norepinephrine and dopamine. Well-described acute endocrine effects of amphetamine administration include increased corticosteroid release and increased growth hormone release,[259-261] each of which can be influenced by the presence of depression[262-266] or other psychoactive medications.[267] Though increased salivary cortisol response to D-amphetamine HAS been associated with personality traits of aggression and thrill-seeking,[268] the clinical implications of these findings remain unclear. The cortisol response to social stressors in chronic methamphetamine use has been variable.[269-271] In the clinical setting, amphetamine use has also been known to lead to poor bone quality and an elevated risk of osteoporosis.[272]

Preexisting hyperthyroidism may increase the risk of death due to ecstasy (3,4-methylenedioxymethamphetamine).[273] Ecstasy has also been associated with severe hyponatremia related to SIADH.[274,275]

Both cocaine and amphetamine have well-known effects on appetite suppression. In 1995, Douglass et al.[276] first described the upregulation of a peptide in response to the acute administration of cocaine and amphetamine. This peptide is now known as cocaine- and amphetamine-regulated transcript and has been shown to have a role in feeding behavior, interacting with neuropeptide Y, leptin, and cannabinoid (CB-1) receptors. Interested readers are referred to a useful review by Vicentic and Jones.[277]

Caffeine

Caffeine is one of the world's most widely used drugs. The many forms in which it is delivered and prepared, including tea, coffee, and caffeinated soft drinks, may contain other bioactive substances such as flavonoids[278] and the diterpene cafestol.[279,280] Add to this the marked range of caffeine content of a particular beverage, from a can of cola (37 mg) to a specialty coffee shop 16-oz regular coffee (330 mg),[281] and there are multiple confounds to its study.

Caffeine is a neuroendocrine stimulant with action mediated by central adenosine receptor antagonism.[282] Ingestion of 250 mg (approximately 3 cups of coffee) produces a rapid release of epinephrine from the adrenal medulla, which can increase blood pressure.[283] Immediate ingestion of 250 to 500 mg caffeine (equivalent of 3 to 6 cups of coffee) has little effect on circulating cortisol, TSH, growth hormone, prolactin, T3,[284] or norepinephrine levels. However, the ingestion of 250 mg caffeine produces an increased epinephrine and norepinephrine response to tilt-table testing[283] and increased epinephrine, norepinephrine, cortisol, and growth hormone response to hypoglycemia or low-normal glucose levels in normal healthy adults[285] and in patients with insulin-dependent diabetes.[286] Tolerance to caffeine can develop with chronic use so that these neuroendocrine changes do not become clinically relevant except after a period of abstinence. It has been suggested that caffeine can be a useful treatment for patients with diabetes without autonomic neuropathy who have hypoglycemic unawareness.[286]

Caffeine may have acute effects on glucose metabolism. Four hundred milligrams of caffeine daily for 1 week decreased insulin sensitivity in caffeine-tolerant young adults.[287] Five hundred milligrams of caffeine daily increased average glucose, and exaggerated postprandial glucose increases in caffeine-tolerant type 2 diabetics.[288] Chronic coffee consumption, however, is associated with a decreased risk of type 2 diabetes mellitus.[281,289] The effects appear to be consistent across diverse populations, with a dose-dependent response, and are also found with decaffeinated coffee and tea. For every additional cup of coffee, there is an estimated 7% reduction in the excess risk of type 2 diabetes mellitus.[289]

Caffeine is associated with increased urinary calcium excretion[290] and with decrements in serum-free estradiol[291,292] and serum insulinlike growth factor 1 levels,[293] both of which are important in maintaining bone mass. As such, it is not surprising that caffeine use in some studies has been associated with an increased risk of fracture[294,295] and an increased risk of reduced bone mass.[296,297] However, other studies do not support this increased risk.[298,299]

One report from Lu and colleagues found that a high physiological dose (approximately 5 cups of coffee), may directly suppress PTH release from parathyroid cells in vitro, which might increase bone density but impair bone formation/quality.[300] Add to this mixture the studies that show that tea can protect against hip fractures[301] and is associated with increased bone density,[278] and the overall situation becomes more confusing. If there is an effect of caffeine intake on bone health, it is not likely to be clinically significant.

The effects of caffeine intake on reproductive health and fertility have been conflicted, but the current data do not show any significant effect on fertility,[302] male sperm quality,[303] pregnancy outcomes, or outcomes of assisted reproduction.[304] Caffeine, by inducing CYP1A2 and CYP2C8, which also are implicated in metabolism of tamoxifen, may decrease the risk of early events in estrogen receptor (ER)-positive breast cancers at a dose of 2 or more cups of coffee daily and may also modulate ER status.[305]

Coffee impairs the intestinal absorption of L-thyroxine and may alter the management of hypothyroidism.[306] Thus, it is advised that levothyroxine should be taken on an empty stomach at least 30 to 60 minutes before breakfast as many foods and drinks may affect this drug.

Benzodiazepines

Benzodiazepines act by stimulating gamma-aminobutyric acidergic (GABA-ergic) neurons, which usually are inhibitory in function. Many researchers have found that benzodiazepines, such as diazepam, alprazolam, and temazepam, suppress basal serum levels of cortisol[307-310] and also suppress the body's cortisol and ACTH response to metyrapone,[311] insulin-induced hypoglycemia, CRH,[312] metabolic stress,[313] and exercise.[314] Such changes potentially could lead to a hypoadrenal crisis or prolonged hypoglycemia in persons using benzodiazepines who have preexisting adrenal disease.

Suppression of cortisol response persists despite chronic benzodiazepine use[315]; however, this finding may not apply to all benzodiazepines. Ambrosi et al.[316] found that triazolam and flurazepam did not influence cortisol release in women with insulin-induced hypoglycemia. Chronic diazepam use may lead to greater decrease in basal cortisol levels among elderly patients compared to younger patients.[317]

Benzodiazepines may variably stimulate the release of growth hormone,[318] though not all investigators have confirmed this finding.[319] This growth hormone response is blunted with long-term benzodiazepine administration[320] and hyperglycemia,[321] suggesting that significant clinical effects are unlikely. One case report described a syndrome involving inappropriate antidiuretic hormone secretion associated with the use of lorazepam.[322]

Hedrington and colleagues studied the effect of alprazolam on counterregulatory responses to hypoglycemia in healthy subjects finding a significant blunting of catecholamine release, glucagon, growth hormone, and pancreatic polypeptide but a neutral effect on cortisol release, with decreased lipolysis and glycogenolysis in response to insulin-induced hypoglycemia. In addition, there was a reduction in hypoglycemic adrenergic symptoms after alprazolam.[323] This same group found not only a similar reduction in catecholamines, glucagon, and growth hormone but also a reduction in cortisol, among healthy exercising patients[324] as well as exercising patients with type 1 diabetes mellitus.[325] As such, there may be an increased risk for severe hypoglycemia in those on hypoglycemic agents.

Barbiturates

Barbiturates are known to induce the cytochrome P450 enzyme system, leading to enhanced metabolism of many substances. Among these substances are thyroid hormone, hydrocortisone, vitamin D, and methadone. Barbiturate use or misuse can lead to increasing thyroid hormone requirements,[326] hydrocortisone requirements, osteomalacia, or opioid withdrawal. Overt hypothyroidism or hypoadrenalism is not likely in the absence of underlying thyroid or adrenal disease.

Inhalants

The inhalation of volatile solvents, such as toluene, is known to cause multiple medical complications, such as heart, liver, lung, nerve, and kidney damage.[327,328] No specific endocrine consequences have yet been described. However, these solvents can cause renal tubular dysfunction, leading to hypophosphatemia and acidosis, which can affect calcium and bone metabolism. Though recurrent nephrolithiasis was described,[329,330] no case of toluene-induced osteomalacia has been described as yet.

Cohen et al. reported a case of rapid-onset diffuse skeletal fluorosis, presenting as debilitating hip pain associated with diffuse osteosclerosis and heterotopic bone formation, from inhalant use of dust cleaner containing the refrigerant 1,1-difluoroethane.[331]

Occupational exposure to inhalants is associated with infertility, increased risk of spontaneous abortion, and multiple birth defects. In addition, case reports of children born to those who use inhalants have led to the term fetal solvent syndrome, reflecting its similarity to fetal alcohol syndrome. Interested readers are referred to the review by Jones and Balster.[332]

Anabolic Steroids

The anabolic steroids, which are testosterone derivatives, include nandrolone, oxandrolone, oxymetholone, and stanozolol. Male and female athletes often use these substances in efforts to improve athletic performance. The adverse endocrine consequences are a direct result of androgenic effects and suppression of the hypothalamic-pituitary-gonadal axis. These effects include testicular atrophy; decreases in testosterone, LH, and FSH; increases in estrone; and suppression of spermatogenesis in men,[333,334] leading to infertility.[335] Gynecomastia can result from aromatization of the androgens to estrogen in endogenous androgen suppression. In women, there can be menstrual disturbances, deepening of the voice, and development of acne and male-pattern body hair.[336] Interested readers are directed to the Endocrine Society scientific statement about the adverse health consequences of performance-enhancing drugs.[337]

Anabolic steroids can affect other hormones by decreasing hepatic synthesis of proteins, such as thyroid-binding globulin, sex hormone–binding globulin, vitamin D–binding protein, and HDL cholesterol.[334,338] There can be mild thyroidal impairment, as measured by TSH and T3 response to TRH.[339] Clinically relevant sequelae are not present without underlying hyperthyroidism. Other lipid changes include increases in low-density lipoprotein cholesterol and decreases in Lp(a).[340] There are conflicting reports regarding insulin resistance and anabolic steroid use.[341,342] Those with preexisting coronary artery disease may be at increased risk because of decreased HDL and increased low-density lipoprotein cholesterol. Hypertension, ventricular remodeling, myocardial ischemia, and sudden cardiac death each have been temporally and causally associated with anabolic steroid use.[343] Work from Basaria et al.[344] has shown an increased risk for coronary events in elderly men with heart disease treated with testosterone replacement therapy. Basaria, writing about the Testosterone's Effects on Atherosclerosis Progression in Aging Men (TEAAM) multicenter trial of testosterone replacement in men 60 years and older with low or low-normal testosterone levels, found no significant changes in carotid artery intima-media thickness or coronary artery calcium.[345] Budoff and colleagues found a significantly increased noncalcified coronary artery plaque in 65 years and older men with low testosterone levels on testosterone replacement therapy.[346] Contradicting reports, however, have suggested that androgens may have antiatherogenic and antianginal effects[347-349] in both supraphysiological and physiological doses.

No significant changes in adult bone metabolism (PTH or vitamin D metabolites) have been reported in patients treated with nandrolone.[350] Anabolic steroid use in children, however, may prematurely close epiphyseal growth plates, leading to growth stunting. Growth hormone levels can rise with anabolic steroid use; resolution of the hypothalamic-pituitary-gonadal suppression can take several months[351] and is a common cause of hypogonadotropic hypogonadism.

Other Drugs

Lysergic acid diethylamide acutely increases blood pressure, heart rate, and plasma levels of cortisol, prolactin, oxytocin, and epinephrine.[352] The clinical significance of these changes is not clear. No endocrinological consequences have been described with phencyclidine use; further research is required.

CONCLUSION

Alcohol and other drugs have complex effects on the endocrine system, with a subsequent broad range of effects on energy metabolism, electrolytes, reproduction, blood pressure control, and bone health. They can cause derangements in glucose, lipids, sodium, fertility, blood pressure, and osteoporosis. Many effects may not have clinical relevance due to development of tolerance, and these effects are reversible with abstinence from the drug. Their broad-reaching effects should be considered in the care of patients who use these drugs.

REFERENCES

1. Marks V, Teale JD. Drug-induced hypoglycemia. *Endocrinol Metab Clin North Am.* 1999;28(3):555-577.
2. Hart SP, Frier BM. Causes, management and morbidity of acute hypoglycaemia in adults requiring hospital admission. *QJM.* 1998;91(7):505-510.
3. Berman JD, Cook DM, Buchman M, Keith LD. Diminished adrenocorticotropin response to insulin-induced hypoglycemia in nondepressed, actively drinking male alcoholics. *J Clin Endocrinol Metab.* 1990;71(3):712-717.
4. Wand GS, Dobs AS. Alterations in the hypothalamic-pituitary-adrenal axis in actively drinking alcoholics. *J Clin Endocrinol Metab.* 1991;72(6):1290-1295.
5. Joffe BI, Seftel HC, Van As M. Hormonal responses in ethanol-induced hypoglycemia. *J Stud Alcohol.* 1975;36(5):550-554.
6. Chiodera P, Coiro V. Inhibitory effect of ethanol on the arginine vasopressin response to insulin-induced hypoglycemia and the role of endogenous opioids. *Neuroendocrinology.* 1990;51(5):501-504.
7. Wilson NM, Brown PM, Juul SM, Prestwich SA, Sönksen PH. Glucose turnover and metabolic and hormonal changes in ethanol-induced hypoglycaemia. *Br Med J (Clin Res Ed).* 1981;282(6267):849-853.
8. Kolaczynski JW, Ylikahri R, Harkonen M, Koivisto VA. The acute effect of ethanol on counterregulatory response and recovery from insulin-induced hypoglycemia. *J Clin Endocrinol Metab.* 1988;67(2):384-388.
9. Kerr D, Cheyne E, Thomas P, Sherwin R. Influence of acute alcohol ingestion on the hormonal responses to modest hypoglycaemia in patients with type 1 diabetes. *Diabet Med.* 2007;24(3):312-316.
10. Rasmussen BM, Orskov L, Schmitz O, Hermansen K. Alcohol and glucose counterregulation during acute insulin-induced hypoglycemia in type 2 diabetic subjects. *Metabolism.* 2001;50(4):451-457.
11. Kitabchi AE, Umpierrez GE, Murphy MB, et al. Management of hyperglycemic crises in patients with diabetes. *Diabetes Care.* 2001;24(1):131-153.
12. Arky RA, Veverbrants E, Abramson EA. Irreversible hypoglycemia. A complication of alcohol and insulin. *JAMA.* 1968;206(3):575-578.
13. Melander A, Lebovitz HE, Faber OK. Sulfonylureas. Why, which, and how? *Diabetes Care.* 1990;13(Suppl 3):18-25.
14. Richardson T, Weiss M, Thomas P, Kerr D. Day after the night before: influence of evening alcohol on risk of hypoglycemia in patients with type 1 diabetes. *Diabetes Care.* 2005;28(7):1801-1802.
15. Cheyne EH, Sherwin RS, Lunt MJ, Cavan DA, Thomas PW, Kerr D. Influence of alcohol on cognitive performance during mild hypoglycaemia; implications for type 1 diabetes. *Diabet Med.* 2004;21(3):230-237.
16. Kerr D, Macdonald IA, Heller SR, Tattersall RB. Alcohol causes hypoglycaemic unawareness in healthy volunteers and patients with type 1 (insulin-dependent) diabetes. *Diabetologia.* 1990;33(4):216-221.
17. Riddle MC, Bolli GB, Ziemen M, Muehlen-Bartmer I, Bizet F, Home PD. New insulin glargine 300 units/mL versus glargine 100 units/mL in people with type 2 diabetes using basal and mealtime insulin: glucose control and hypoglycemia in a 6-month randomized controlled trial (EDITION 1). *Diabetes Care.* 2014;37(10):2755-2762. doi:10.2337/dc14-0991
18. Zinman B, Philis-Tsimikas A, Cariou B, et al. Insulin degludec versus insulin glargine in insulin-naive patients with type 2 diabetes: a 1-year, randomized, treat-to-target trial (BEGIN Once Long). *Diabetes Care.* 2012;35(12):2464-2471.
19. Hood RC, Arakaki RF, Wysham C, Li YG, Settles JA, Jackson JA. Two treatment approaches for human regular U-500 insulin in patients with type 2 diabetes not achieving adequate glycemic control on high-dose U-100 insulin therapy with or without oral agents: a randomized, titration-to-target clinical trial. *Endocr Pract.* 2015;21(7):782-793. doi:10.4158/EP15612
20. Ramirez A, Weare-Regales N, Domingo A, et al. Clinical impact of initiation of U-500 insulin vs continuation of U-100 insulin in subjects with diabetes. *Fed Pract.* 2021;38(3):e15-e21. doi:10.12788/fp.0105
21. Flood TM. Serious hypoglycemia associated with misuse of repaglinide. *Endocr Pract.* 1999;5(3):137-138.
22. Nagai T, Imamura M, Iizuka K, Mori M. Hypoglycemia due to nateglinide administration in diabetic patient with chronic renal failure. *Diabetes Res Clin Pract.* 2003;59(3):191-194.
23. Bolen S, Feldman L, Vassy J, et al. Systematic review: comparative effectiveness and safety of oral medications for type 2 diabetes mellitus. *Ann Intern Med.* 2007;147(6):386-399.
24. Rosenstock J, Hassman DR, Madder RD, et al. Repaglinide versus nateglinide monotherapy: a randomized, multicenter study. *Diabetes Care.* 2004;27(6):1265-1270.

25. Gilbert MP, Pratley RE. GLP-1 Analogs and DPP-4 inhibitors in type 2 diabetes therapy: review of head-to-head clinical trials. *Front Endocrinol (Lausanne)*. 2020;11:178. doi:10.3389/fendo.2020.00178
26. Drab SR. Glucagon-like peptide-1 receptor agonists for type 2 diabetes: a clinical update of safety and efficacy. *Curr Diabetes Rev*. 20196;12(4):403-413. doi:10.2174/1573399812666151223093841
27. Cao C, Yang S, Zhou Z. GLP-1 receptor agonists and pancreatic safety concerns in type 2 diabetic patients: data from cardiovascular outcome trials. *Endocrine*. 2020;68(3):518-525. doi:10.1007/s12020-020-02223-6
28. Bays HE, Fitch A, Christensen S, Burridge K, Tondt J. Anti-obesity medications and investigational agents: an Obesity Medicine Association (OMA) clinical practice statement (CPS) 2022. *Obesity Pillars*. 2022;2:100018.
29. American Diabetes Association Professional Practice Committee. Facilitating Behavior Change and Well-being to Improve Health Outcomes: Standards of Medical Care in Diabetes—2022. *Diabetes Care*. 2022;45(Suppl. 1):S60-S82. doi:10.2337/dc22-S005
30. O'Keefe SJ, Marks V. Lunchtime gin and tonic a cause of reactive hypoglycaemia. *Lancet*. 1977;1(8025):1286-1288.
31. Marks V, Wright J. Alcohol-provoked reactive hypoglycemia. In: Andreani D, Lefebvre P, Marks V, eds. *Current Views on Hypoglycemia and Glucagon*. Academic Press; 1980:283.
32. Flanagan D, Wood P, Sherwin R, Debrah K, Kerr D. Gin and tonic and reactive hypoglycemia: what is important-the gin, the tonic, or both? *J Clin Endocrinol Metab*. 1998;83(3):796-800.
33. Oba-Yamamoto C, Takeuchi J, Nakamura A, et al. Combination of alcohol and glucose consumption as a risk to induce reactive hypoglycemia. *J. Diabetes Investig*. 2020;12(4):651-657. doi:10.1111/jdi.13375
34. Nikkola J, Laukkarinen J, Lahtela J, et al. The long-term prospective follow-up of pancreatic function after the first episode of acute alcoholic pancreatitis: recurrence predisposes one to pancreatic dysfunction and pancreatogenic diabetes. *J Clin Gastroenterol*. 2017;51(2):183-190.
35. A, Park WG. Acute pancreatitis and diabetes mellitus: a review. *Korean J Intern Med*. 2021;36(1):15-24. doi:10.3904/kjim.2020.505
36. Ting JW, Lautt WW. The effect of acute, chronic, and prenatal ethanol exposure on insulin sensitivity. *Pharmacol Ther*. 2006;111(2):346-373.
37. Brand-Miller JC, Fatima K, Middlemiss C, et al. Effect of alcoholic beverages on postprandial glycemia and insulinemia in lean, young, healthy adults. *Am J Clin Nutr*. 2007;85(6):1545-1551.
38. Greenfield JR, Samaras K, Hayward CS, Chisholm DJ, Campbell LV. Beneficial postprandial effect of a small amount of alcohol on diabetes and cardiovascular risk factors: modification by insulin resistance. *J Clin Endocrinol Metab*. 2005;90(2):661-672.
39. Carlsson S, Hammar N, Grill V. Alcohol consumption and type 2 diabetes meta-analysis of epidemiological studies indicates a U-shaped relationship. *Diabetologia*. 2005;48(6):1051-1054.
40. Baliunas DO, Taylor BJ, Irving H, et al. Alcohol as a risk factor for type 2 diabetes: a systematic review and meta-analysis. *Diabetes Care*. 2009;32(11):2123-2132.
41. Koppes LL, Dekker JM, Hendriks HF, Bouter LM, Heine RJ. Moderate alcohol consumption lowers the risk of type 2 diabetes: a meta-analysis of prospective observational studies. *Diabetes Care*. 2005;28(3):719-725.
42. Kiechl S, Willeit J, Poewe W, et al. Insulin sensitivity and regular alcohol consumption: large, prospective, cross sectional population study (Bruneck study). *BMJ*. 1996;313(7064):1040-1044.
43. Razay G, Heaton KW. Moderate alcohol consumption has been shown previously to improve insulin sensitivity in men. *BMJ*. 1997;314(7078):443-444.
44. Fueki Y, Miida T, Wardaningsih E, et al. Regular alcohol consumption improves insulin resistance in healthy Japanese men independent of obesity. *Clin Chim Acta*. 2007;382(1-2):71-76.
45. Rimm EB, Chan J, Stampfer MJ, Colditz GA, Willett WC. Prospective study of cigarette smoking, alcohol use, and the risk of diabetes in men. *BMJ*. 1995;310(6979):555-559.
46. Cordain L, Melby CL, Hamamoto AE, et al. Influence of moderate chronic wine consumption on insulin sensitivity and other correlates of syndrome X in moderately obese women. *Metabolism*. 2000;49(11):1473-1478.
47. Flanagan DE, Pratt E, Murphy J, et al. Alcohol consumption alters insulin secretion and cardiac autonomic activity. *Eur J Clin Invest*. 2002;32(3):187-192.
48. Crandall JP, Polsky S, Howard AA, et al. Alcohol consumption and diabetes risk in the diabetes prevention program. *Am J Clin Nutr*. 2009;90(3):595-601.
49. Saremi A, Hanson RL, Tulloch-Reid M, Williams DE, Knowler WC. Alcohol consumption predicts hypertension but not diabetes. *J Stud Alcohol*. 2004;65(2):184-190.
50. Davies MJ, Baer DJ, Judd JT, Brown ED, Campbell WS, Taylor PR. Effects of moderate alcohol intake on fasting insulin and glucose concentrations and insulin sensitivity in postmenopausal women: a randomized controlled trial. *JAMA*. 2002;287(19):2559-2562.
51. Knott C, Bell S, Britton A. Alcohol consumption and the risk of type 2 diabetes: a systematic review and dose-response meta-analysis of more than 1.9 million individuals from 38 observational studies. *Diabetes Care*. 2015;38(9):1804-1812.
52. Huang J, Wang X, Zhang Y. Specific types of alcoholic beverage consumption and risk of type 2 diabetes: a systematic review and meta-analysis. *J Diabetes Investig*. 2017;8:56-68.
53. Lloyd CW, Williams RH. Endocrine changes associated with Laennec's cirrhosis of the liver. *Am J Med*. 1948;4(3):315-330.
54. Gordon GG, Altman K, Southren AL, Rubin E, Lieber CS. Effect of alcohol (ethanol) administration on sex-hormone metabolism in normal men. *N Engl J Med*. 1976;295(15):793-797.
55. Van Thiel DH, Lester R, Vaitukaitis J. Evidence for a defect in pituitary secretion of luteinizing hormone in chronic alcoholic men. *J Clin Endocrinol Metab*. 1978;47(3):499-507.
56. Iturriaga H, Lioi X, Valladares L. Sex hormone-binding globulin in non-cirrhotic alcoholic patients during early withdrawal and after longer abstinence. *Alcohol Alcohol*. 1999;34(6):903-909.
57. Kley HK, Niederau C, Stremmel W, Lax R, Strohmeyer G, Krüskemper HL. Conversion of androgens to estrogens in idiopathic hemochromatosis: comparison with alcoholic liver cirrhosis. *J Clin Endocrinol Metab*. 1985;61(1):1-6.
58. Van Thiel DH, McClain CJ, Elson MK, McMillin MJ. Hyperprolactinemia and thyrotropin-releasing factor (TRH) responses in men with alcoholic liver disease. *Alcohol Clin Exp Res*. 1978;2(4):344-348.
59. Agner T, Hagen C, Nyboe Andersen B, Hegedüs. Pituitary-thyroid function and thyrotropin, prolactin and growth hormone responses to TRH in patients with chronic alcoholism. *Acta Med Scand*. 1986;220(1):57-62.
60. Zumoff B. The critical role of alcohol consumption in determining the risk of breast cancer with postmenopausal estrogen administration. *J Clin Endocrinol Metab*. 1997;82(6):1656-1658.
61. Mendelson JH, Mello NK, et al. Alcohol effects on naltrexone-stimulated luteinizing hormone, prolactin, and estradiol in women. *J Stud Alcohol*. 1987;48(4):287-294.
62. Mendelson JH, Lukas SE, Mello NK, Amass L, Ellingboe J, Skupny A. Acute alcohol effects on plasma estradiol levels in women. *Psychopharmacology (Berl)*. 1988;94(4):464-467.
63. Mendelson JH, Mello NK, Teoh SK, Ellingboe J. Alcohol effects on luteinizing hormone releasing hormone-stimulated anterior pituitary and gonadal hormones in women. *J Pharmacol Exp Ther*. 1989;250(3):902-909.
64. Gill J. The effects of moderate alcohol consumption on female hormone levels and reproductive function. *Alcohol Alcohol*. 2000;35(5):417-423.
65. Bradley KA, Badrinath S, Bush K, Boyd-Wickizer J, Anawalt B. Medical risks for women who drink alcohol. *J Gen Intern Med*. 1998;13(9):627-639.
66. Jensen TK, Hjollund NH, Henriksen TB, et al. Does moderate alcohol consumption affect fertility? Follow up study among couples planning first pregnancy. *BMJ*. 1998;317(7157):505-510.
67. Hakim RB, Gray RH, Zacur H. Alcohol and caffeine consumption and decreased fertility. *Fertil Steril*. 1998;70(4):632-637.
68. Mennella JA, Pepino MY, Teff KL. Acute alcohol consumption disrupts the hormonal milieu of lactating women. *J Clin Endocrinol Metab*. 2005;90(4):1979-1985.

69. Mennella JA, Pepino MY. Short-term effects of alcohol consumption on the hormonal milieu and mood states in nulliparous women. *Alcohol.* 2006;38(1):29-36.
70. Mennella JA. Short-term effects of maternal alcohol consumption on lactational performance. *Alcohol Clin Exp Res.* 1998;22(7):1389-1392.
71. Mukherjee S, Sorrell MF. Effects of alcohol consumption on bone metabolism in elderly women. *Am J Clin Nutr.* 2000;72(5):1073.
72. Rapuri PB, Gallagher JC, Balhorn KE, Ryschon KL. Alcohol intake and bone metabolism in elderly women. *Am J Clin Nutr.* 2000;72(5):1206-1213.
73. Williams FM, Cherkas LF, Spector TD, MacGregor AJ. The effect of moderate alcohol consumption on bone mineral density: a study of female twins. *Ann Rheum Dis.* 2005;64(2):309-310.
74. Tucker KL, Jugdaohsingh R, Powell JJ, et al. Effects of beer, wine, and liquor intakes on bone mineral density in older men and women. *Am J Clin Nutr.* 2009;89(4):1188-1196.
75. Yin J, Winzenberg T, Quinn S, Giles G, Jones G. Beverage-specific alcohol intake and bone loss in older men and women: a longitudinal study. *Eur J Clin Nutr.* 2011;65(4):526-532.
76. Saville PD. Changes in bone mass with age and alcoholism. *J Bone Joint Surg Am.* 1965;47:492-499.
77. de Vernejoul MC, Bielakoff J, Herve M, et al. Evidence for defective osteoblastic function. A role for alcohol and tobacco consumption in osteoporosis in middle-aged men. *Clin Orthop Relat Res.* 1983;179:107-115.
78. Bikle DD, Genant HK, Cann C, Recker RR, Halloran BP, Strewler GJ. Bone disease in alcohol abuse. *Ann Intern Med.* 1985;103(1):42-48.
79. Lalor BC, France MW, Powell D, Adams PH, Counihan TB. Bone and mineral metabolism and chronic alcohol abuse. *Q J Med.* 1986;59(229):497-511.
80. Odvina CV, Safi I, Wojtowicz CH, et al. Effect of heavy alcohol intake in the absence of liver disease on bone mass in black and white men. *J Clin Endocrinol Metab.* 1995;80(8):2499-2503.
81. Kanis JA, Johansson H, Johnell O, et al. Alcohol intake as a risk factor for fracture. *Osteoporos Int.* 2005;16(7):737-742.
82. Bang CS, Shin IS, Lee SW, et al. Osteoporosis and bone fractures in alcoholic liver disease: a meta-analysis. *World J Gastroenterol.* 2015;21(13):4038-4047.
83. González-Reimers E, Alvisa-Negrín J, Santolaria-Fernández F, et al. Vitamin D and nutritional status are related to bone fractures in alcoholics. *Alcohol Alcohol.* 2011;46(2):148-155.
84. Lindholm J, Steiniche T, Rasmussen E, et al. Bone disorder in men with chronic alcoholism: a reversible disease? *J Clin Endocrinol Metab.* 1991;73(1):118-124.
85. Pepersack T, Fuss M, Otero J, Bergmann P, Valsamis J, Corvilain J. Longitudinal study of bone metabolism after ethanol withdrawal in alcoholic patients. *J Bone Miner Res.* 1992;7(4):383-387.
86. Peris P, Pares A, Guanabens N, et al. Bone mass improves in alcoholics after 2 years of abstinence. *J Bone Miner Res.* 1994;9(10):1607-1612.
87. Maurel DB, Boisseau N, Benhamou CL, Jaffre C. Alcohol and bone: review of dose effects and mechanisms. *Osteoporos Int.* 2012;23(1):1-16.
88. Chen JR, Lazarenko OP, Shankar K, Blackburn ML, Badger TM. A role for ethanol-induced oxidative stress in controlling lineage commitment of mesenchymal stromal cells through inhibition of Wnt/β-catenin signaling. *J Bone Miner Res.* 2010;25(5):1117-1127.
89. Santolaria F, Gonzalez-Gonzalez G, Gonzalez-Reimers E, et al. Effects of alcohol and liver cirrhosis on the GH-IGF-I axis. *Alcohol Alcohol.* 1995;30(6):703-708.
90. Santolaria F, Gonzalez-Reimers E, Perez-Manzano JL, et al. Osteopenia assessed by body composition analysis is related to malnutrition in alcoholic patients. *Alcohol.* 2000;22(3):147-157.
91. Rojdmark S, Calissendorff J, Brismar K. Alcohol ingestion decreases both diurnal and nocturnal secretion of leptin in healthy individuals. *Clin Endocrinol (Oxf).* 2001;55(5):639-647.
92. Santolaria F, Perez-Cejas A, Aleman MR, et al. Low serum leptin levels and malnutrition in chronic alcohol misusers hospitalized by somatic complications. *Alcohol Alcohol.* 2003;38(1):60-66.
93. Idelevich A, Sato K, Baron R. What are the effects of leptin on bone and where are they exerted? *J Bone Miner Res.* 2013;28(1):18-21.
94. Sibonga JD, Iwaniec UT, Shogren KL, Rosen CJ, Turner RT. Effects of parathyroid hormone (1-34) on tibia in an adult rat model for chronic alcohol abuse. *Bone.* 2007;40(4):1013-1020.
95. Matsuo K, Hirohata T, Sugioka Y, Ikeda M, Fukuda A. Influence of alcohol intake, cigarette smoking, and occupational status on idiopathic osteonecrosis of the femoral head. *Clin Orthop Relat Res.* 1988;234:115-123.
96. Chang CC, Greenspan A, Gershwin ME. Osteonecrosis: current perspectives on pathogenesis and treatment. *Semin Arthritis Rheum.* 1993;23(1):47-69.
97. Antti-Poika I, Karaharju E, Vankka E, Paavilainen T. Alcohol-associated femoral head necrosis. *Ann Chir Gynaecol.* 1987;76(6):318-322.
98. Gaziano JM, Buring JE, Breslow JL, et al. Moderate alcohol intake, increased levels of high-density lipoprotein and its subfractions, and decreased risk of myocardial infarction. *N Engl J Med.* 1993;329(25):1829-1834.
99. Clarke TK, Treutlein J, Zimmermann US, et al. HPA-axis activity in alcoholism: examples for a gene-environment interaction. *Addict Biol.* 2008;13(1):1-14.
100. Kirkman S, Nelson DH. Alcohol-induced pseudo-Cushing's disease: a study of prevalence with review of the literature. *Metabolism.* 1988;37(4):390-394.
101. Besemer F, Pereira AM, Smit JW. Alcohol-induced Cushing syndrome. Hypercortisolism caused by alcohol abuse. *Neth J Med.* 2011;69(7):318-323.
102. Calissendorff J, Danielsson O, Brismar K, Röjdmark S. Inhibitory effect of alcohol on ghrelin secretion in normal man. *Eur J Endocrinol.* 2005;152(5):743-747.
103. Calissendorff J, Danielsson O, Brismar K, Röjdmark S. Alcohol ingestion does not affect serum levels of peptide YY but decreases both total and octanoylated ghrelin levels in healthy subjects. *Metabolism.* 2006;55(12):1625-1629.
104. Oiso Y, Robertson G. Effect of ethanol on vasopressin secretion and the role of endogenous opioids. In: Schrier R, ed. *Vasopressin.* Raven Press; 1985:265.
105. Howes LG, Reid JL. The effects of alcohol on local, neural and humoral cardiovascular regulation. *Clin Sci (Lond).* 1986;71(1):9-15.
106. Puddey IB, Vandongen R, Beilin LJ, Rouse IL. Alcohol stimulation of renin release in man: its relation to the hemodynamic, electrolyte, and sympatho-adrenal responses to drinking. *J Clin Endocrinol Metab.* 1985;61(1):37-42.
107. Rachdaoui N, Sarkar DK. Effects of alcohol on the endocrine system. *Endocrinol Metab Clin North Am.* 2013;42(3):593-615. doi:10.1016/j.ecl.2013.05.008
108. Chopra IJ, Solomon DH, Chopra U, Young TR, Chua Teco GN. Alterations in circulating thyroid hormones and thyrotropin in hepatic cirrhosis: evidence for euthyroidism despite subnormal serum triiodothyronine. *J Clin Endocrinol Metab.* 1974;39(3):501-511.
109. Hegedus L. Decreased thyroid gland volume in alcoholic cirrhosis of the liver. *J Clin Endocrinol Metab.* 1984;58(5):930-933.
110. Ekman AC, Leppaluoto J, Huttunen P, Aranko K, Vakkuri O. Ethanol inhibits melatonin secretion in healthy volunteers in a dose-dependent randomized double blind cross-over study. *J Clin Endocrinol Metab.* 1993;77(3):780-783.
111. Tweed JO, Hsia SH, Lutfy K, Friedman TC. The endocrine effects of nicotine and cigarette smoke. *Trends Endocrinol Metab.* 2012; 23(7):334-342.
112. Metsios GS, Flouris AD, Jamurtas AZ, et al. A brief exposure to moderate passive smoke increases metabolism and thyroid hormone secretion. *J Clin Endocrinol Metab.* 2007;92(1):208-211.
113. Soldin OP, Goughenour BE, Gilbert SZ, Landy HL, Soldin SJ. Thyroid hormone levels associated with active and passive cigarette smoking. *Thyroid.* 2009;19(8):817-823.
114. Bartalena L, Martino E, Marcocci C, et al. More on smoking habits and Graves' ophthalmopathy. *J Endocrinol Invest.* 1989;12(10):733-737.
115. Hägg E, Asplund K. Is endocrine ophthalmopathy related to smoking? *Br Med J (Clin Res Ed).* 1987;295(6599):634-635.

116. Shine B, Fells P, Edwards OM, Weetman AP. Association between Graves' ophthalmopathy and smoking. *Lancet*. 1990;335(8700):1261-1263.
117. Prummel MF, Wiersinga WM. Smoking and risk of Graves' disease. *JAMA*. 1993;269(4):479-482.
118. Belin RM, Astor BC, Powe NR, Ladenson PW. Smoke exposure is associated with a lower prevalence of serum thyroid autoantibodies and thyrotropin concentration elevation and a higher prevalence of mild thyrotropin concentration suppression in the third national health and nutrition examination survey (NHANES III). *J Clin Endocrinol Metab*. 2004;89(12):6077-6086.
119. Asvold BO, Bjøro T, Nilsen TI, Vatten LJ. Tobacco smoking and thyroid function: a population-based study. *Arch Intern Med*. 2007; 167(13):1428-1432.
120. Jorde R, Sundsfjord J. Serum TSH levels in smokers and non-smokers. The 5th Tromso study. *Exp Clin Endocrinol Diabetes*. 2006; 114(7):343-347.
121. Vestergaard P. Smoking and thyroid disorders—a meta-analysis. *Eur J Endocrinol*. 2002;146(2):153-161.
122. Cawood TJ, Moriarty P, O'Farrelly C, O'Shea D. Smoking and thyroid-associated ophthalmopathy: a novel explanation of the biological link. *J Clin Endocrinol Metab*. 2007;92(1):59-64.
123. Planck T, Shahida B, Parikh H, et al. Smoking induces overexpression of immediate early genes in active Graves' ophthalmopathy. *Thyroid*. 2014;24(10):1524-1532.
124. Xing L, Ye L, Zhu W, et al. Smoking was associated with poor response to intravenous steroids therapy in Graves' ophthalmopathy. *Br J Ophthalmol*. 2015;99(12):1686-1691.
125. Kapoor D, Jones TH. Smoking and hormones in health and endocrine disorders. *Eur J Endocrinol*. 2005;152(4):491-499.
126. Hegedüs L, Karstrup S, Veiergang D, Jacobsen B, Skovsted L, Feldt-Rasmussen U. High frequency of goitre in cigarette smokers. *Clin Endocrinol (Oxf)*. 1985;22(3):287-292.
127. Christensen SB, Ericsson UB, Janzon L, Tibblin S, Melander A. Influence of cigarette smoking on goiter formation, thyroglobulin, and thyroid hormone levels in women. *J Clin Endocrinol Metab*. 1984;58(4):615-618.
128. Fukayama H, Nasu M, Murakami S, Sugawara M. Examination of antithyroid effects of smoking products in cultured thyroid follicles: only thiocyanate is a potent antithyroid agent. *Acta Endocrinol (Copenh)*. 1992;127(6):520-525.
129. Utiger RD. Cigarette smoking and the thyroid. *N Engl J Med*. 1995;333(15):1001-1002.
130. Goh SY, Ho SC, Seah LL, Fong KS, Khoo DHC. Thyroid autoantibody profiles in ophthalmic dominant and thyroid dominant Graves' disease differ and suggest ophthalmopathy is a multiantigenic disease. *Clin Endocrinol (Oxf)*. 2004;60(5):600-607.
131. Strieder TG, Prummel MF, Tijssen JG, Endert E, Wiersinga WM. Risk factors for and prevalence of thyroid disorders in a cross-sectional study among healthy female relatives of patients with autoimmune thyroid disease. *Clin Endocrinol (Oxf)*. 2003;59(3):396-401.
132. Krassas GE, Wiersinga W. Smoking and autoimmune thyroid disease: the plot thickens. *Eur J Endocrinol*. 2006;154(6):777-780.
133. Pedersen IB, Laurberg P, Knudsen N, et al. Smoking is negatively associated with the presence of thyroglobulin autoantibody and to a lesser degree with thyroid peroxidase autoantibody in serum: a population study. *Eur J Endocrinol*. 2008;158(3):367-373.
134. Effraimidis G, Tijssen JG, Wiersinga WM. Discontinuation of smoking increases the risk for developing thyroid peroxidase antibodies and/or thyroglobulin antibodies: a prospective study. *J Clin Endocrinol Metab*. 2009;94(4):1324-1328.
135. Kabat GC, Kim MY, Wactawski-Wende J, Rohan TE. Smoking and alcohol consumption in relation to risk of thyroid cancer in postmenopausal women. *Cancer Epidemiol*. 2012;36(4):335-340.
136. Meinhold CL, Ron E, Schonfeld SJ, et al. Nonradiation risk factors for thyroid cancer in the U.S. radiologic technologists study. *Am J Epidemiol*. 2010;171(2):242-252.
137. Targher G, Alberiche M, Zenere MB, Bonadonna RC, Muggeo M, Bonora E. Cigarette smoking and insulin resistance in patients with noninsulin-dependent diabetes mellitus. *J Clin Endocrinol Metab*. 1997;82(11):3619-3624.
138. Eliasson B, Taskinen MR, Smith U. Long-term use of nicotine gum is associated with hyperinsulinemia and insulin resistance. *Circulation*. 1996;94(5):878-881.
139. Carlsson S, Midthjell K, Grill V, Nord-Trondelag study. Smoking is associated with an increased risk of type 2 diabetes but a decreased risk of autoimmune diabetes in adults: an 11-year follow-up of incidence of diabetes in the Nord-Trondelag study. *Diabetologia*. 2004;47(11):1953-1956.
140. Manson JE, Ajani UA, Liu S, Nathan DM, Hennekens CH. A prospective study of cigarette smoking and the incidence of diabetes mellitus among U.S. male physicians. *Am J Med*. 2000;109(7):538-542.
141. Foy CG, Bell RA, Farmer DF, Goff DC Jr, Wagenknecht LE. Smoking and incidence of diabetes among U.S. adults: findings from the insulin resistance atherosclerosis study. *Diabetes Care*. 2005;28(10):2501-2507.
142. Wannamethee SG, Shaper AG, Perry IJ, British Regional Heart Study. Smoking as a modifiable risk factor for type 2 diabetes in middle-aged men. *Diabetes Care*. 2001;24(9):1590-1595.
143. Spijkerman AMW, Van der ADL, Nilsson PM, et al. Smoking and long-term risk of type 2 diabetes: the EPIC-InterAct study in European populations. *Diabetes Care*. 2014;37(12):3164-3171.
144. Houston TK, Person SD, Pletcher MJ, Liu K, Iribarren C, Kiefe CA. Active and passive smoking and development of glucose intolerance among young adults in a prospective cohort: CARDIA study. *BMJ*. 2006;332(7549):1064-1069.
145. Jensen EX, Fusch C, Jaeger P, Penheim E, Horber FF. Impact of chronic cigarette smoking on body composition and fuel metabolism. *J Clin Endocrinol Metab*. 1995;80(7):2181-2185.
146. Weitzman M, Cook S, Auinger P, et al. Tobacco smoke exposure is associated with the metabolic syndrome in adolescents. *Circulation*. 2005;112(6):862-869.
147. MacMahon B, Trichopoulos D, Cole P, Brown J. Cigarette smoking and urinary estrogens. *N Engl J Med*. 1982;307(17):1062-1065.
148. Jensen J, Christiansen C, Rodbro P. Cigarette smoking, serum estrogens, and bone loss during hormone-replacement therapy early after menopause. *N Engl J Med*. 1985;313(16):973-975.
149. Rosenberg MJ, Waugh MS, Stevens CM. Smoking and cycle control among oral contraceptive users. *Am J Obstet Gynecol*. 1996;174:628-632.
150. Jick H, Porter J. Relation between smoking and age of natural menopause. report from the Boston Collaborative Drug Surveillance Program, Boston University Medical Center. *Lancet*. 1977;1(8026):1354-1355.
151. McKinlay SM, Bifano NL, McKinlay JB. Smoking and age at menopause in women. *Ann Intern Med*. 1985;103(3):350-356.
152. Windham GC, Mitchell P, Anderson M, Lasley BL. Cigarette smoking and effects on hormone function in premenopausal women. *Environ Health Perspect*. 2005;113(10):1285-1290.
153. Kinney A, Kline J, Kelly A, Reuss ML, Levin B. Smoking, alcohol and caffeine in relation to ovarian age during the reproductive years. *Hum Reprod*. 2007;22(4):1175-1185.
154. Waylen AL, Metwally M, Jones GL, Wilkinson AJ, Ledger WL. Effects of cigarette smoking upon clinical outcomes of assisted reproduction: a meta-analysis. *Hum Reprod Update*. 2009;15(1):31-44.
155. Evans HJ, Fletcher J, Torrance M, Hargreave TB. Sperm abnormalities and cigarette smoking. *Lancet*. 1981;1(8221):627-629.
156. Shaarawy M, Mahmoud KZ. Endocrine profile and semen characteristics in male smokers. *Fertil Steril*. 1982;38(2):255-257.
157. Vine MF, Margolin BH, Morrison HI, Hulka BS. Cigarette smoking and sperm density: a meta-analysis. *Fertil Steril*. 1994;61(1):35-43.
158. Barrett-Connor E, Khaw KT. Cigarette smoking and increased endogenous estrogen levels in men. *Am J Epidemiol*. 1987;126(2):187-192.
159. The Practice Committee of the American Society for Reproductive Medicine. Smoking and infertility: a committee opinion. *Fertil Steril*. 2012;98(6):1400-1406.

160. Vogel JM, Davis JW, Nomura A, Wasnich RD, Ross PD. The effects of smoking on bone mass and the rates of bone loss among elderly Japanese-American men. *J Bone Miner Res.* 1997;12(9):1495-1501.
161. National Osteoporosis Foundation. *Clinician's Guide to Prevention and Treatment of Osteoporosis.* National Osteoporosis Foundation; 2013.
162. Yoon V, Maalouf NM, Sakhaee K. The effects of smoking on bone metabolism. *Osteoporos Int.* 2012;23(8):2081-2092.
163. Krall EA, Dawson-Hughes B. Smoking and bone loss among postmenopausal women. *J Bone Miner Res.* 1991;6(4):331-338.
164. Krall EA, Dawson-Hughes B. Smoking increases bone loss and decreases intestinal calcium absorption. *J Bone Miner Res.* 1999;14(2):215-220.
165. Brot C, Jorgensen NR, Sorensen OH. The influence of smoking on vitamin D status and calcium metabolism. *Eur J Clin Nutr.* 1999;53(12):920-926.
166. Kiel DP, Baron JA, Anderson JJ, Hannan MT, Felson DT. Smoking eliminates the protective effect of oral estrogens on the risk for hip fracture among women. *Ann Intern Med.* 1992;116(9):716-721.
167. Husain MK, Frantz AG, Ciarochi F, Robinson AG. Nicotine-stimulated release of neurophysin and vasopressin in humans. *J Clin Endocrinol Metab.* 1975;41(6):1113-1117.
168. Rowe JW, Kilgore A, Robertson GL. Evidence in man that cigarette smoking induces vasopressin release via an airway-specific mechanism. *J Clin Endocrinol Metab.* 1980;51(1):170-172.
169. Allon M, Allen HM, Deck LV, Clark ML. Role of cigarette use in hyponatremia in schizophrenic patients. *Am J Psychiatry.* 1990;147(8):1075-1077.
170. Ellinas PA, Rosner F, Jaume JC. Symptomatic hyponatremia associated with psychosis, medications, and smoking. *J Natl Med Assoc.* 1993;85(2): 135-141.
171. Cryer PE, Haymond MW, Santiago JV, Shah SD. Norepinephrine and epinephrine release and adrenergic mediation of smoking-associated hemodynamic and metabolic events. *N Engl J Med.* 1976;295(11):573-577.
172. Ottesen MM, Worck R, Ibsen H. Captopril does not blunt the sympathoadrenal response to cigarette smoking in normotensive humans. *Blood Press.* 1997;6(1):29-34.
173. Wilkins JN, Carlson HE, Van Vunakis H, HillMA GE, Jarvik ME. Nicotine from cigarette smoking increases circulating levels of cortisol, growth hormone, and prolactin in male chronic smokers. *Psychopharmacology (Berl).* 1982;78(4):305-308.
174. Seyler LE Jr, Fertig J, Pomerleau O, Hunt D, Parker K. The effects of smoking on ACTH and cortisol secretion. *Life Sci.* 1984;34(1):57-65.
175. Xue Y, Morris M, Ni L, et al. Venous plasma nicotine correlates of hormonal effects of tobacco smoking. *Pharmacol Biochem Behav.* 2010;95(2):209-215.
176. Badrick E, Kirschbaum C, Kumari M. The relationship between smoking status and cortisol secretion. *J Clin Endocrinol Metab.* 2007;92(3):819-824.
177. Plat L, Leproult R, L'Hermite-Baleriaux M, et al. Metabolic effects of short-term elevations of plasma cortisol are more pronounced in the evening than in the morning. *J Clin Endocrinol Metab.* 1999;84(9):3082-3092.
178. Villanti AC, Johnson AL, Ambrose BK, et al. Use of flavored tobacco products among U.S. youth and adults; findings from the first wave of the PATH Study (2013-2014). *Am J Prev Med.* 2017;53(2):139-151.
179. Callahan-Lyon P. Electronic cigarettes: human health effects. *Tob Control.* 2014;23(Suppl 2):ii36-ii40.
180. El Golli N, Rahali D, Jrad-Lamine A, et al. Impact of electronic-cigarette refill liquid on rat testis. *Toxicol Mech Methods.* 2016;26(6):417-424.
181. El-Shahawy O, Shah T, Obisesan OH, et al. Association of e-cigarettes with erectile dysfunction: the population assessment of tobacco and health study. *Am J Prev Med.* 2022;62(1):26-38. doi:10.1016/j.amepre.2021.08.004
182. Wetendorf M, Randall LT, Lemma MT, et al. E-cigarette exposure delays implantation and causes reduced weight gain in female offspring exposed in utero. *J Endocr Soc.* 2019;3(10):1907-1916. doi:10.1210/js.2019-00216
183. Carlson H. Drugs and pituitary function. In: Melmed S, ed. *The Pituitary.* Blackwell Science; 1995:645.
184. Vuong C, Van Uum SH, O'Dell LE, Lutfy K, Friedman TC. The effects of opioids and opioid analogs on animal and human endocrine systems. *Endocr Rev.* 2010;31(1):98-132.
185. Azizi F, Vagenakis AG, Longcope C, Ingbar SH, Braverman LE. Decreased serum testosterone concentration in male heroin and methadone addicts. *Steroids.* 1973;22(4):467-472.
186. Cicero TJ, Bell RD, Wiest WG, Allison JH, Polakoski K, Robins E. Function of the male sex organs in heroin and methadone users. *N Engl J Med.* 1975;292(17):882-887.
187. Mendelson JH, Mendelson JE, Patch VD. Plasma testosterone levels in heroin addiction and during methadone maintenance. *J Pharmacol Exp Ther.* 1975;192(1):211-217.
188. Cushman P Jr. Plasma testosterone in narcotic addiction. *Am J Med.* 1973;55(3):452-458.
189. Cushman P Jr, Kreek MJ, Methadone-maintained patients. Effect of methadone on plasma testosterone, FSH, LH, and prolactin. *N Y State J Med.* 1974;74(11):1970-1973.
190. Ragni G, De Lauretis L, Bestetti O, Sghedoni D, Gambaro V. Gonadal function in male heroin and methadone addicts. *Int J Androl.* 1988;11(2):93-100.
191. Lafisca S, Bolelli G, Franceschetti F, Filicori M, Flamigni C, Marigo M. Hormone levels in methadone-treated drug addicts. *Drug Alcohol Depend.* 1981;8(3):229-234.
192. Brambilla F, Resele L, De Maio D, Nobile P. Gonadotropin response to synthetic gonadotropin hormone-releasing hormone (GnRH) in heroin addicts. *Am J Psychiatry.* 1979;136(3):314-317.
193. Brown R, Balousek S, Mundt M, Fleming M. Methadone maintenance and male sexual dysfunction. *J Addict Dis.* 2005;24(2):91-106.
194. Daniell HW. Hypogonadism in men consuming sustained-action oral opioids. *J Pain.* 2002;3(5):377-384.
195. Bliesener N, Albrecht S, Schwager A, Weckbecker K, Lichtermann D, Klingmüller D. Plasma testosterone and sexual function in men receiving buprenorphine maintenance for opioid dependence. *J Clin Endocrinol Metab.* 2005;90(1):203-206.
196. Hallinan R, Byrne A, Agho K, McMahon CG, Tynan P, Attia J. Hypogonadism in men receiving methadone and buprenorphine maintenance treatment. *Int J Androl.* 2009;32(2):131-139.
197. Hallinan R, Byrne A, Agho K, McMahon C, Tynan P, Attia J. Erectile dysfunction in men receiving methadone and buprenorphine maintenance treatment. *J Sex Med.* 2008;5(3):684-692.
198. Abs R, Verhelst J, Maeyaert J, et al. Endocrine consequences of long-term intrathecal administration of opioids. *J Clin Endocrinol Metab.* 2000;85(6):2215-2222.
199. Bawor M, Bami H, Dennis BB, et al. Testosterone suppression in opioid users: a systematic review and meta-analysis. *Drug Alcohol Depend.* 2015;149:1-9.
200. Basaria S, Travison TG, Alford D, et al. Effects of testosterone replacement in men with opioid-induced androgen deficiency: a randomized controlled trial. *Pain.* 2015;156(2):280-288.
201. Santen FJ, Sofsky J, Bilic N, Lippert R. Mechanism of action of narcotics in the production of menstrual dysfunction in women. *Fertil Steril.* 1975;26(6):538-548.
202. Daniell HW. Opioid endocrinopathy in women consuming prescribed sustained-action opioids for control of nonmalignant pain. *J Pain.* 2008;9(1):28-36.
203. Zharikova OL, Deshmukh SV, Kumar M, et al. The effect of opiates on the activity of human placental aromatase/CYP19. *Biochem Pharmacol.* 2007;73(2):279-286.
204. Zharikova OL, Deshmukh SV, Nanovskaya TN, Hankins GDV, Ahmed MS. The effect of methadone and buprenorphine on human placental aromatase. *Biochem Pharmacol.* 2006;71(8):1255-1264.
205. Devilla L, Pende A, Morgano A, Giusti M, Musso NR, Lotti G. Morphine-induced TSH release in normal and hypothyroid subjects. *Neuroendocrinology.* 1985;40(4):303-308.
206. Delitala G, Grossman A, Besser GM. The participation of hypothalamic dopamine in morphine-induced prolactin release in man. *Clin Endocrinol (Oxf).* 1983;19(4):437-444.
207. Rampinini A, Iannotta F, Rizzuto G, Colombo F, Giuliani F, Parabiaghi R. Effect of naloxone on TRH-induced PRL and TSH response in normal man. *Minerva Endocrinol.* 1989;14(2):125-128.

208. Pedrazzoni M, Vescovi PP, Maninetti L, et al. Effects of chronic heroin abuse on bone and mineral metabolism. *Acta Endocrinol (Copenh).* 1993;129(1):42-45.
209. Wilczek H, Stepan J. Bone metabolism in individuals dependent on heroin and after methadone administration. *Cas Lek Cesk.* 2003;142(10):606-608.
210. Kinjo M, Setoguchi S, Schneeweiss S, Solomon DH. Bone mineral density in subjects using central nervous system-active medications. *Am J Med.* 2005;118(12):1414.
211. Arnsten JH, Freeman R, Howard AA, Floris-Moore M, Santoro N, Schoenbaum EE. HIV infection and bone mineral density in middle-aged women. *Clin Infect Dis.* 2006;42(7):1014-1020.
212. Kim TW, Alford DP, Malabanan A, Holick MF, Samet JH. Low bone density in patients receiving methadone maintenance treatment. *Drug Alcohol Depend.* 2006;85(3):258-262.
213. Fraser LA, Morrison D, Morley-Forster P, et al. Oral opioids for chronic non-cancer pain: higher prevalence of hypogonadism in men than in women. *Exp Clin Endocrinol Diabetes.* 2009;117(1):38-43.
214. Grey A, Rix-Trott K, Horne A, Gamble G, Bolland M, Reid IR. Decreased bone density in men on methadone maintenance therapy. *Addiction.* 2011;106(2):349-354.
215. Kim TW, Alford DP, Holick MF, Malabanan AO, Samet JH. Low vitamin D status of patients in methadone maintenance treatment. *J Addict Med.* 2009;3(3):134-138.
216. Ensrud KE, Blackwell T, Mangione CM, et al. Central nervous system active medications and risk for fractures in older women. *Arch Intern Med.* 2003;163(8):949-957.
217. Vestergaard P, Rejnmark L, Mosekilde L. Fracture risk associated with the use of morphine and opiates. *J Intern Med.* 2006;260(1):76-87.
218. Pullan PT, Watson FE, Seow SS, Rappeport W. Methadone-induced hypoadrenalism. *Lancet.* 1983;1(8326 Pt 1):714.
219. Müssig K, Knaus-Dittmann D, Schmidt H, Mörike K, Häring HU. Secondary adrenal failure and secondary amenorrhoea following hydromorphone treatment. *Clin Endocrinol (Oxf).* 2007;66(4):604-605.
220. Oltmanns KM, Fehm HL, Peters A. Chronic fentanyl application induces adrenocortical insufficiency. *J Intern Med.* 2005;257(5):478-480.
221. Allolio B, Schulte HM, Deuss U, Kallabis D, Hamel E, Winkelman W. Effect of oral morphine and naloxone on pituitary-adrenal response in man induced by human corticotropin-releasing hormone. *Acta Endocrinol (Copenh).* 1987;114(4):509-514.
222. Conaglen JV, Donald RA, Espiner EA, Livesey EA, Nicholls MG. Effect of naloxone on the hormone response to CRF in normal man. *Endocr Res.* 1985;11(1-2):39-44.
223. Bhansali A, Velayutham P, Sialy R, Sethi B. Effect of opiates on growth hormone secretion in acromegaly. *Horm Metab Res.* 2005;37(7):425-427.
224. Tomasi PA, Fanciulli G, Palermo M, Pala A, Demontis MA, Delitala G. Opioid-receptor blockade blunts growth hormone (GH) secretion induced by GH-releasing hormone in the human male. *Horm Metab Res.* 1998;30(1):34-36.
225. Reed JL, Ghodse AH. Oral glucose tolerance and hormonal response in heroin-dependent males. *Br Med J.* 1973;2(5866):582-585.
226. Passariello N, Giugliano D, Quatraro A, et al. Glucose tolerance and hormonal responses in heroin addicts. A possible role for endogenous opiates in the pathogenesis of non-insulin-dependent diabetes. *Metabolism.* 1983;32(12):1163-1165.
227. Fareed A, Byrd-Sellers J, Vayalapalli S, Drexler K, Phillips L. Predictors of diabetes mellitus and abnormal blood glucose in patients receiving opioid maintenance treatment. *Am J Addict.* 2013;22(4):411-416.
228. Howard AA, Hoover DR, Anastos K, et al. The effects of opiate use and hepatitis C virus infection on risk of diabetes mellitus in the women's interagency HIV study. *J Acquir Immune Defic Syndr.* 2010;54(2):152-159.
229. Li L, Setoguchi S, Cabral H, Jick S. Opioids and risk of type 2 diabetes in adults with non-cancer pain. *Pain Physician.* 2013;16(1):77-88.
230. Brown TT, Dobs AS. Endocrine effects of marijuana. *J Clin Pharmacol.* 2002;42(11 Suppl):90S-96S.
231. Kolodny RC, Masters WH, Kolodner RM, Toro G. Depression of plasma testosterone levels after chronic intensive marihuana use. *N Engl J Med.* 1974;290(16):872-874.
232. Mendelson JH, Kuehnle J, Ellingboe J, Babor TF. Plasma testosterone levels before, during and after chronic marihuana smoking. *N Engl J Med.* 1974;291(20):1051-1055.
233. Cone EJ, Johnson RE, Moore JD, Roache JD. Acute effects of smoking marijuana on hormones, subjective effects and performance in male human subjects. *Pharmacol Biochem Behav.* 1986;24(6):1749-1754.
234. Mendelson JH, Cristofaro P, Ellingboe J, Benedikt R, Mello NK. Acute effects of marihuana on luteinizing hormone in menopausal women. *Pharmacol Biochem Behav.* 1985;23(5):765-768.
235. Braustein GD, Buster JE, Soares JR, Gross SJ. Pregnancy hormone concentrations in marijuana users. *Life Sci.* 1983;33(2):195-199.
236. Takeda S. Delta(9)-tetrahydrocannabinol targeting estrogen receptor signaling: The possible mechanism of action coupled with endocrine disruption. *Biol Pharm Bull.* 2014;37(9):1435-1438.
237. Brents LK. Marijuana, the endocannabinoid system and the female reproductive system. *Yale J Biol Med.* 2016;89(2):175-191.
238. Warner TD, Roussos-Ross D, Behnke M. It's not your mother's marijuana effects on maternal-fetal health and the developing child. *Clin Perinatol.* 2014;41(4):877-894.
239. Daling JR, Doody DR, Sun X, et al. Association of marijuana use and the incidence of testicular germ cell tumors. *Cancer.* 2009;115(6):1215-1223.
240. Trabert B, Sigurdson AJ, Sweeney AM, Strom SS, McGlynn KA. Marijuana use and testicular germ cell tumors. *Cancer.* 2011;117(4):848-853.
241. Lacson JC, Carroll JD, Tuazon E, Castelao J, Berstein L, Cortessis VK. Population-based case-control study of recreational drug use and testis cancer risk confirms an association between marijuana use and nonseminoma risk. *Cancer.* 2012;118(21):5374-5383.
242. Benowitz NL, Jones RT, Lerner CB. Depression of growth hormone and cortisol response to insulin-induced hypoglycemia after prolonged oral delta-9-tetrahydrocannabinol administration in man. *J Clin Endocrinol Metab.* 1976;42(5):938-941.
243. Nava F, Manzato E, Lucchini A. Chronic cannabis use does not affect the normalization of hypothalamic-pituitary-adrenal (HPA) axis induced by methadone in heroin addicts. *Prog Neuropsychopharmacol Biol Psychiatry.* 2007;31(5):1089-1094.
244. Huizink AC, Ferdinand RF, Ormel J, Verhulst FC. Hypothalamic-pituitary-adrenal axis activity and early onset of cannabis use. *Addiction.* 2006;101(11):1581-1588.
245. Herning RI, Better W, Cadet JL. EEG of chronic marijuana users during abstinence: relationship to years of marijuana use, cerebral blood flow and thyroid function. *Clin Neurophysiol.* 2008;119(2):321-331.
246. Kirkham TC. Cannabinoids and appetite: food craving and food pleasure. *Int Rev Psychiatry.* 2009;21(2):163-171.
247. Riggs PK, Vaida F, Rossi SS, et al. A pilot study of the effects of cannabis on appetite hormones in HIV-infected adult men. *Brain Res.* 2012;1431:46-52.
248. Abioye A, Ayodele O, Marinkovic A, Patidar R, Akinwekomi A, Sanyaolu A. Δ9-Tetrahydrocannabivarin (THCV): a commentary on potential therapeutic benefit for the management of obesity and diabetes. *J Cannabis Res.* 2020;2(1):6. doi:10.1186/s42238-020-0016-7
249. Sophocleous A, Robertson R, Ferreira NB, McKenzie J, Fraser WD, Ralston SH. Heavy cannabis use is associated with low bone mineral density and an increased risk of fractures. *Am J Med.* 2017;130(2):214-221.
250. Abraham MR, Khardori R. Hyperglycemic hyperosmolar nonketotic syndrome as initial presentation of type 2 diabetes in a young cocaine abuser. *Diabetes Care.* 1999;22(8):1380-1381.
251. Warner EA, Greene GS, Buchsbaum MS, Cooper DS, Robinson BE. Diabetic ketoacidosis associated with cocaine use. *Arch Intern Med.* 1998;158(16):1799-1802.
252. Heesch CM, Negus BH, Bost JE, Keffer JH, Snyder RW 2nd, Eichhorn EJ. Effects of cocaine on anterior pituitary and gonadal hormones. *J Pharmacol Exp Ther.* 1996;278(3):1195-1200.

253. Mendelson JH, Mello NK, Teoh SK, Ellingboe J, Cochin J. Cocaine effects on pulsatile secretion of anterior pituitary, gonadal, and adrenal hormones. *J Clin Endocrinol Metab*. 1989;69(6):1256-1260.
254. Lee MA, Bowers MM, Nash JF, Meltzer HY. Neuroendocrine measures of dopaminergic function in chronic cocaine users. *Psychiatry Res*. 1990;33(2):151-159.
255. Mendelson JH, Teoh SK, Lange U, et al. Anterior pituitary, adrenal, and gonadal hormones during cocaine withdrawal. *Am J Psychiatry*. 1988;145(9):1094-1098.
256. Mendelson JH, Teoh SK, Mello NK, Ellingboe J, Rhoades E. Acute effects of cocaine on plasma adrenocorticotropic hormone, luteinizing hormone and prolactin levels in cocaine-dependent men. *J Pharmacol Exp Ther*. 1992;263(2):505-509.
257. Teoh SK, Sarnyai Z, Mendelson JH, et al. Cocaine effects on pulsatile secretion of ACTH in men. *J Pharmacol Exp Ther*. 1994;270(3):1134-1138.
258. Dhopesh VP, Burke WM, Maany I, Ravi NV. Effect of cocaine on thyroid functions. *Am J Drug Alcohol Abuse*. 1991;17(4):423-427.
259. Besser GM, Butler PW, Landon J, Rees L. Influence of amphetamines on plasma corticosteroid and growth hormone levels in man. *Br Med J*. 1969;4(5682):528-530.
260. Rees L, Butler PW, Gosling C, Besser GM. Adrenergic blockade and the corticosteroid and growth hormone responses to methylamphetamine. *Nature*. 1970;228(5271):565-566.
261. Dommisse CS, Schulz SC, Narasimhachari N, Blackard WG, Hamer RM. The neuroendocrine and behavioral response to dextroamphetamine in normal individuals. *Biol Psychiatry*. 1984;19(9):1305-1315.
262. Langer G, Heinze G, Reim B, Matussek N. Reduced growth hormone responses to amphetamine in "endogenous" depressive patients: studies in normal, "reactive" and "endogenous" depressive, schizophrenic, and chronic alcoholic subjects. *Arch Gen Psychiatry*. 1976;33(12):1471-1475.
263. Checkley SA, Crammer JL. Hormone responses to methylamphetamine in depression: a new approach to the noradrenaline depletion hypothesis. *Br J Psychiatry*. 1977;131:582-586.
264. Checkley SA. Corticosteroid and growth hormone responses to methylamphetamine in depressive illness. *Psychol Med*. 1979;9(1):107-115.
265. Sachar EJ, Asnis G, Nathan RS, Halbriech U, Tabrizi MA, Halpern FS. Dextroamphetamine and cortisol in depression. morning plasma cortisol levels suppressed. *Arch Gen Psychiatry*. 1980;37(7):755-757.
266. Halbreich U, Sachar EJ, Asnis GM, et al. Growth hormone response to dextroamphetamine in depressed patients and normal subjects. *Arch Gen Psychiatry*. 1982;39(2):189-192.
267. Nurnberger JI Jr, Simmons-Alling S, Kessler L, et al. Separate mechanisms for behavioral, cardiovascular, and hormonal responses to dextroamphetamine in man. *Psychopharmacology (Berl)*. 1984;84(2):200-204.
268. White TL, Grover VK, de Wit H. Cortisol effects of D-amphetamine relate to traits of fearlessness and aggression but not anxiety in healthy humans. *Pharmacol Biochem Behav*. 2006;85(1):123-131.
269. Gerra G, Bassignana S, Zaimovic A, et al. Hypothalamic-pituitary-adrenal axis responses to stress in subjects with 3,4-methylenedioxy-methamphetamine ('ecstasy') use history: correlation with dopamine receptor sensitivity. *Psychiatry Res*. 2003;120(2):115-124.
270. Li SX, Yan SY, Bao YP, et al. Depression and alterations in hypothalamic-pituitary-adrenal and hypothalamic-pituitary-thyroid axis function in male abstinent methamphetamine abusers. *Hum Psychopharmacol*. 2013;28(5):477-483.
271. King G, Alicata D, Cloak C, Chang L. Psychiatric symptoms and HPA axis function in adolescent methamphetamine users. *J Neuroimmune Pharmacol*. 2010;5(4):582-591.
272. Mosti MP, Flemmen G, Hoff J, Stunes AK, Syversen U, Wang E. Impaired skeletal health and neuromuscular function among amphetamine users in clinical treatment. *Osteoporos Int*. 2016;27(3):1003-1010. doi:10.1007/s00198-015-3371-z
273. Martin TL, Chiasson DA, Kish SJ. Does hyperthyroidism increase risk of death due to the ingestion of ecstasy? *J Forensic Sci*. 2007;52(4):951-953.
274. Henry JA, Fallon JK, Kicman AT, Hutt AJ, Cowan DA, Forsling M. Low-dose MDMA ("ecstasy") induces vasopressin secretion. *Lancet*. 1998;351(9118):1784.
275. Baggott MJ, Garrison KJ, Coyle JR, et al. MDMA impairs response to water intake in healthy volunteers. *Adv Pharmacol Sci*. 2016;2016:2175896.
276. Douglass J, McKinzie AA, Couceyro P. PCR differential display identifies a rat brain mRNA that is transcriptionally regulated by cocaine and amphetamine. *J Neurosci*. 1995;15(3 Pt 2):2471-2481.
277. Vicentic A, Jones DC. The CART (cocaine- and amphetamine-regulated transcript) system in appetite and drug addiction. *J Pharmacol Exp Ther*. 2007;320(2):499-506.
278. Hegarty VM, May HM, Khaw KT. Tea drinking and bone mineral density in older women. *Am J Clin Nutr*. 2000;71(4):1003-1007.
279. Weusten-Van der Wouw MP, Katan MB, Viani R, et al. Identity of the cholesterol-raising factor from boiled coffee and its effects on liver function enzymes. *J Lipid Res*. 1994;35:721-733.
280. Mensink RP, Lebbink WJ, Lobbezoo IE, Weusten-Van der Wouw MP, Zock PL, Katan MB. Diterpene composition of oils from Arabica and Robusta coffee beans and their effects on serum lipids in man. *J Intern Med*. 1995;237(6):543-550.
281. van Dam RM. Coffee consumption and risk of type 2 diabetes, cardiovascular diseases, and cancer. *Appl Physiol Nutr Metab*. 2008;33(6):1269-1283.
282. Snyder SH, Katims JJ, Annau Z, Bruns RF, Daly JW. Adenosine receptors and behavioral actions of methylxanthines. *Proc Natl Acad Sci U S A*. 1981;78(5):3260-3264.
283. Debrah K, Haigh R, Sherwin R, Murphy J, Kerr D. Effect of acute and chronic caffeine use on the cerebrovascular, cardiovascular and hormonal responses to orthostasis in healthy volunteers. *Clin Sci (Lond)*. 1995;89(5):475-480.
284. Spindel ER, Wurtman RJ, McCall A, et al. Neuroendocrine effects of caffeine in normal subjects. *Clin Pharmacol Ther*. 1984;36(3):402-407.
285. Kerr D, Sherwin RS, Pavalkis F, et al. Effect of caffeine on the recognition of and responses to hypoglycemia in humans. *Ann Intern Med*. 1993;119(8):799-804.
286. Debrah K, Sherwin RS, Murphy J, Kerr D. Effect of caffeine on recognition of and physiological responses to hypoglycaemia in insulin-dependent diabetes. *Lancet*. 1996;347(8993):19-24.
287. MacKenzie T, Comi R, Sluss P, et al. Metabolic and hormonal effects of caffeine: randomized, double-blind, placebo-controlled crossover trial. *Metabolism*. 2007;56(12):1694-1698.
288. Lane JD, Feinglos MN, Surwit RS. Caffeine increases ambulatory glucose and postprandial responses in coffee drinkers with type 2 diabetes. *Diabetes Care*. 2008;31(2):221-222.
289. Huxley R, Lee CM, Barzi F, et al. Coffee, decaffeinated coffee, and tea consumption in relation to incident type 2 diabetes mellitus: a systematic review with meta-analysis. *Arch Intern Med*. 2009;169(22):2053-2063.
290. Bergman EA, Massey LK, Wise KJ, Sherrard DJ. Effects of dietary caffeine on renal handling of minerals in adult women. *Life Sci*. 1990;47(6):557-564.
291. London S, Willett W, Longcope C, McKinlay S. Alcohol and other dietary factors in relation to serum hormone concentrations in women at climacteric. *Am J Clin Nutr*. 1991;53(1):166-171.
292. Nagata C, Kabuto M, Shimizu H. Association of coffee, green tea, and caffeine intakes with serum concentrations of estradiol and sex hormone-binding globulin in premenopausal Japanese women. *Nutr Cancer*. 1998;30(1):21-24.
293. Landin-Wilhelmsen K, Wilhelmsen L, Lappas G, et al. Serum insulin-like growth factor I in a random population sample of men and women: relation to age, sex, smoking habits, coffee consumption and physical activity, blood pressure and concentrations of plasma lipids, fibrinogen, parathyroid hormone and osteocalcin. *Clin Endocrinol (Oxf)*. 1994;41(3):351-357.
294. Kiel DP, Felson DT, Hannan MT, et al. Caffeine and the risk of hip fracture: the Framingham Study. *Am J Epidemiol*. 1990;132(4):675-684.
295. Hernandez-Avila M, Colditz GA, Stampfer MJ, Rosner B, Speizer FE, Willett WC. Caffeine, moderate alcohol intake, and risk of fractures of the hip and forearm in middle-aged women. *Am J Clin Nutr*. 1991;54(1):157-163.

296. Hernandez-Avila M, Stampfer MJ, Ravnikar VA, et al. Caffeine and other predictors of bone density among pre- and perimenopausal women. *Epidemiology*. 1993;4(2):128-134.
297. Yano K, Heilbrun LK, Wasnich RD, Hankin JH, Vogel JM. The relationship between diet and bone mineral content of multiple skeletal sites in elderly Japanese-American men and women living in Hawaii. *Am J Clin Nutr*. 1985;42(5):877-888.
298. Tavani A, Negri E, La Vecchia C. Coffee intake and risk of hip fracture in women in northern Italy. *Prev Med*. 1995;24(4):396-400.
299. Lloyd T, Rollings N, Eggli DF, Kieselhorst K, Chinchilli VM. Dietary caffeine intake and bone status of postmenopausal women. *Am J Clin Nutr*. 1997;65(6):1826-1830.
300. Lu M, Farnebo LO, Branstrom R, Larsson C. Inhibition of parathyroid hormone secretion by caffeine in human parathyroid cells. *J Clin Endocrinol Metab*. 2013;98(8):E1345-E1351.
301. Kanis J, Johnell O, Gullberg B, et al. Risk factors for hip fracture in men from southern Europe: the MEDOS study. Mediterranean osteoporosis study. *Osteoporos Int*. 1999;9(1):45-54.
302. Peck JD, Leviton A, Cowan LD. A review of the epidemiologic evidence concerning the reproductive health effects of caffeine consumption: a 2000-2009 update. *Food Chem Toxicol*. 2010;48(10):2549-2576.
303. Karmon AE, Toth TL, Chiu YH, et al. Male caffeine and alcohol intake in relation to semen parameters and in vitro fertilization outcomes among fertility patients. *Andrology*. 2017;5(2):354-361.
304. Morgan S, Koren G, Bozzo P. Is caffeine consumption safe during pregnancy? *Can Fam Physician*. 2013;59(4):361-362.
305. Simonsson M, Soderlind V, Henningsson M, et al. Coffee prevents early events in tamoxifen-treated breast cancer patients and modulates hormone receptor status. *Cancer Causes Control*. 2013;24(5):929-940.
306. Benvenga S, Bartolone L, Pappalardo MA, et al. Altered intestinal absorption of L-thyroxine caused by coffee. *Thyroid*. 2008;18(3):293-301.
307. Schuckit MA, Hauger RL, Monteiro MG, Irwin M, Duthie LA, Mahler HI. Response of three hormones to diazepam challenge in sons of alcoholics and controls. *Alcohol Clin Exp Res*. 1991;15(3):537-542.
308. Zemishlany Z, McQueeney R, Gabriel SM, Davidson M. Neuroendocrine and monoaminergic responses to acute administration of alprazolam in normal subjects. *Neuropsychobiology*. 1990;23(3):124-128.
309. Risby ED, Hsiao JK, Golden RN, Potter WZ. Intravenous alprazolam challenge in normal subjects. Biochemical, cardiovascular, and behavioral effects. *Psychopharmacology (Berl)*. 1989;99(4):508-514.
310. Roy-Byrne PP, Cowley DS, Hommer D, Ritchie J, Greenblatt D, Nemeroff C. Neuroendocrine effects of diazepam in panic and generalized anxiety disorders. *Biol Psychiatry*. 1991;30(1):73-80.
311. Arvat E, Maccagno B, Ramunni J, et al. The inhibitory effect of alprazolam, a benzodiazepine, overrides the stimulatory effect of metyrapone-induced lack of negative cortisol feedback on corticotroph secretion in humans. *J Clin Endocrinol Metab*. 1999;84(8):2611-2615.
312. Korbonits M, Trainer PJ, Edwards R, Bresser GM, Grossman AB. Benzodiazepines attenuate the pituitary-adrenal responses to corticotrophin-releasing hormone in healthy volunteers, but not in patients with Cushing's syndrome. *Clin Endocrinol (Oxf)*. 1995;43(1):29-35.
313. Breier A, Davis O, Buchanan R, et al. Effects of alprazolam on pituitary-adrenal and catecholaminergic responses to metabolic stress in humans. *Biol Psychiatry*. 1992;32(10):880-890.
314. Deuster PA, Faraday MM, Chrousos GP, Poth MA. Effects of dehydroepiandrosterone and alprazolam on hypothalamic-pituitary responses to exercise. *J Clin Endocrinol Metab*. 2005;90(8):4777-4783.
315. Cowley DS, Roy-Byrne PP, Radant A, et al. Benzodiazepine sensitivity in panic disorder: effects of chronic alprazolam treatment. *Neuropsychopharmacology*. 1995;12(2):147-157.
316. Ambrosi F, Ricci S, Quartesan R, et al. Effects of acute benzodiazepine administration on growth hormone, prolactin and cortisol release after moderate insulin-induced hypoglycemia in normal women. *Psychopharmacology (Berl)*. 1986;88(2):187-189.
317. Pomara N, Willoughby LM, Sidtis JJ, Cooper TB, Greenblatt DJ. Cortisol response to diazepam: its relationship to age, dose, duration of treatment, and presence of generalized anxiety disorder. *Psychopharmacology (Berl)*. 2005;178(1):1-8.
318. Monteiro MG, Schuckit MA, Hauger R, Irwin M, Duthie LA. Growth hormone response to intravenous diazepam and placebo in 82 healthy men. *Biol Psychiatry*. 1990;27(7):702-710.
319. Levin ER, Sharp B, Carlson HE. Failure to confirm consistent stimulation of growth hormone by diazepam. *Horm Res*. 1984;19(2):86-90.
320. Shur E, Petursson H, Checkley S, Lader M. Long-term benzodiazepine administration blunts growth hormone response to diazepam. *Arch Gen Psychiatry*. 1983;40(10):1105-1108.
321. Ajlouni K, El-Khateeb M. Effect of glucose of growth hormone, prolactin and thyroid-stimulating hormone response to diazepam in normal subjects. *Horm Res*. 1980;13(3):160-164.
322. Engel WR, Grau A. Inappropriate secretion of antidiuretic hormone associated with lorazepam. *BMJ*. 1988;297(6652):858.
323. Hedrington MS, Farmerie S, Ertl AC, Wang Z, Tate DB, Davis SN. Effects of antecedent GABA(A) activation with alprazolam on counterregulatory responses to hypoglycemia hi healthy humans. *Diabetes*. 2010;59(4):1074-1081.
324. Hedrington MS, Tate DB, Younk LM, Davis SN. Effects of antecedent GABA A receptor activation on counterregulatory responses to exercise in healthy man. *Diabetes*. 2015;64(9):3253-3261.
325. Hedrington MS, Mikeladze M, Tate DB, Younk LM, Davis I, Davis SN. Effects of gamma-aminobutyric acid A receptor activation on counterregulatory responses to subsequent exercise in individuals with type 1 diabetes. *Diabetes*. 2016;65(9):2754-2759.
326. Hoffbrand BI. Barbiturate/thyroid-hormone interaction. *Lancet*. 1979; 2(8148):903-904.
327. Streicher HZ, Gabow PA, Moss AH, et al. Syndromes of toluene sniffing in adults. *Ann Intern Med*. 1981;94(6):758-762.
328. Meadows R, Verghese A. Medical complications of glue sniffing. *South Med J*. 1996;89(5):455-462.
329. Kaneko T, Koizumi T, Takezaki T, Sato A. Urinary calculi associated with solvent abuse. *J Urol*. 1992;147(5):1365-1366.
330. Kroeger RM, Moore RJ, Lehman TH, Giesy JD, Skeeters CE. Recurrent urinary calculi associated with toluene sniffing. *J Urol*. 1980;123(1):89-91.
331. Cohen E, Hsu R, Evangelista P, Aaron R, Rubin L. Rapid-onset diffuse skeletal fluorosis from inhalant abuse. *JBJS Case Connect*. 2014;4(4):1.
332. Jones HE, Balster RL. Inhalant abuse in pregnancy. *Obstet Gynecol Clin North Am*. 1998;25(1):153-167.
333. Bijlsma JW, Duursma SA, Thijssen JH, Huber O. Influence of nandrolondecanoate on the pituitary-gonadal axis in males. *Acta Endocrinol (Copenh)*. 1982;101(1):108-112.
334. Small M, Beastall GH, Semple CG, Cowan RA, Forbes CD. Alteration of hormone levels in normal males given the anabolic steroid stanozolol. *Clin Endocrinol (Oxf)*. 1984;21(1):49-55.
335. de Souza GL, Hallak J. Anabolic steroids and male infertility: a comprehensive review. *BJU Int*. 2011;108(11):1860-1865.
336. Strauss RH, Liggett MT, Lanese RR. Anabolic steroid use and perceived effects in ten weight-trained women athletes. *JAMA*. 1985;253(19):2871-2873.
337. Pope HG Jr, Wood RI, Rogol A, Nyberg F, Bowers L, Bhasin S. Adverse health consequences of performance-enhancing drugs: an endocrine society scientific statement. *Endocr Rev*. 2014;35(3):341-375.
338. Malarkey WB, Strauss RH, Leizman DJ, Liggett M, Demers LM. Endocrine effects in female weight lifters who self-administer testosterone and anabolic steroids. *Am J Obstet Gynecol*. 1991;165(5 Pt 1):1385-1390.
339. Deyssig R, Weissel M. Ingestion of androgenic-anabolic steroids induces mild thyroidal impairment in male body builders. *J Clin Endocrinol Metab*. 1993;76(4):1069-1071.
340. Hartgens F, Rietjens G, Keizer HA, Kuipers H, Wolffenbuttel BHR. Effects of androgenic-anabolic steroids on apolipoproteins and lipoprotein (a). *Br J Sports Med*. 2004;38(3):253-259.
341. Polderman KH, Gooren LJ, Asscheman H, Bakker A, Heine RJ. Induction of insulin resistance by androgens and estrogens. *J Clin Endocrinol Metab*. 1994;79(1):265-271.

342. Hobbs CJ, Jones RE, Plymate SR. Nandrolone, a 19-nortestosterone, enhances insulin-independent glucose uptake in normal men. *J Clin Endocrinol Metab*. 1996;81(4):1582-1585.
343. Sullivan ML, Martinez CM, Gennis P, Gallagher EJ. The cardiac toxicity of anabolic steroids. *Prog Cardiovasc Dis*. 1998;41(1):1-15.
344. Basaria S, Coviello AD, Travison TG, et al. Adverse events associated with testosterone administration. *N Engl J Med*. 2010;363(2):109-122.
345. Basaria S, Harman SM, Travison TG, et al. Effects of testosterone administration for 3 years on subclinical atherosclerosis progression in older men with low or low-normal testosterone levels: a randomized clinical trial. *JAMA*. 2015;314(6):570-581.
346. Budoff MJ, Ellenberg SS, Lewis CE, et al. Testosterone treatment and coronary artery plaque volume in older men with low testosterone. *JAMA*. 2017;317(7):708-716.
347. English KM, Mandour O, Steeds RP, Diver MJ, Jones TH, Channer KS. Men with coronary artery disease have lower levels of androgens than men with normal coronary angiograms. *Eur Heart J*. 2000;21(11):890-894.
348. Webb CM, Adamson DL, de Zeigler D, Collins P. Effect of acute testosterone on myocardial ischemia in men with coronary artery disease. *Am J Cardiol*. 1999;83(3):437-439, A9.
349. Webb CM, McNeill JG, Hayward CS, de Zeigler D, Collins P. Effects of testosterone on coronary vasomotor regulation in men with coronary heart disease. *Circulation*. 1999;100(16):1690-1696.
350. Bijlsma JW, Duursma SA, Bosch R, Huber O. Lack of influence of the anabolic steroid nandrolondecanoate on bone metabolism. *Acta Endocrinol (Copenh)*. 1982;101(1):140-143.
351. Alèn M, Rahkila P, Reinilä M, Vihko R. Androgenic-anabolic steroid effects on serum thyroid, pituitary and steroid hormones in athletes. *Am J Sports Med*. 1987;15(4):357-361.
352. Schmid Y, Enzler F, Gasser P, et al. Acute effects of lysergic acid diethylamide in healthy subjects. *Biol Psychiatry*. 2015;78(8):544-553.

CHAPTER

98 Substance Use During Pregnancy

Michael F. Weaver, Hendrée E. Jones, and Martha J. Wunsch

CHAPTER OUTLINE

- Approach to pregnant people
- Screening
- Teratogenicity
- Neonatal abstinence syndromes
- Tobacco
- Alcohol and sedatives
- Opioids
- Cannabis
- Stimulants
- Substance use disorder treatment in the pregnant and postpartum individual
- Labor and delivery
- Breastfeeding
- Legal issues
- Postpartum care
- Conclusions

APPROACH TO PREGNANT PEOPLE

While the potential consequences of substance use disorders (SUD) during pregnancy for the health and well-being of the birthing person, fetus, and neonate are concerning, SUD during pregnancy must be viewed in context and in relation to multiple other factors that can compromise healthy pregnancies. People who use substances during pregnancy (PSP) often do so in the context of intricately complex individual, social, and environmental factors, including poor nutrition, extreme stress, violence of multiple forms, poor housing conditions, exposure to environmental toxins and diseases, and depression, all of which can impact postnatal outcomes.[1,2] While people who have SUD during pregnancy often face many challenges, each patient is unique, and each patient must be viewed in the context of their own risk and protective factors to optimize treatment and outcomes for the family and child.

This chapter recognizes that not every person with the capacity for pregnancy identifies as a woman. It is important for high quality care for providers to embrace the desire to be inclusive and respect each individual's gender identity, expression, and experience, and be helpful to all who need care during the perinatal time. This chapter uses gender-inclusive language (person/people/they/them/patient) as well as woman/women in some cases. Use of such language acknowledges the long history of gender discrimination focused on women and the specialized health care documents and research that has been published on women. Further, the use of inclusive language aims to model competency and in no way aims to undermine or eliminate the primacy of women in birth. Using gender-neutral language in no way forces people to eliminate woman from their vocabulary. Rather, it sets a standard for professionals to serve a wide range of people with birthing capacity.

For the health and well-being of birthing person and child, all health care providers should be able to recognize perinatal SUD, address this medical problem, and thus reduce potential complications for the birthing person and child. The prevalence of substance use during pregnancy is substantial. Pregnant people using tobacco, alcohol, prescription medications, and illicit substances may have irregular menstrual cycles yet still can conceive. Several months may lapse before an individual realizes that they are pregnant.[3] Perinatal SUD affect individuals of all races, ethnicities, and socioeconomic levels.[4] In the 2020 National Survey on Drug Use and Health, 10.6% of pregnant people consumed alcohol, while 8.4% smoked cigarettes.[4] The prevalence of past month self-reported illicit substance use during pregnancy varies by type of psychoactive substance, with 8% reporting cannabis use, 0.4% using opioids, and 0.3% using cocaine.[4] Pregnancy motivates some, but not all, individuals to quit using substances, but others may have difficulty stopping due to the severity of their SUD or fear of withdrawal. The clinician's role is to begin to support PSP in changing their behavior to stop or substantially reduce substance use and to assist with addiction treatment referral. Whether or not an individual continues to use substances, every pregnant person should be encouraged to engage in prenatal care and have access to the services that best support their health needs.

PSP experience more prejudice and are much more stigmatized and discriminated against than nonpregnant people, so they may deny their drug use, its harmful effects, and the need to seek help.[5] Clinicians who provide health care to PSP should be sensitive to the cultural background, family context, and the patients' feelings. Systemic racism profoundly harms the mental and physical health as well as the lives of pregnant and parenting people who identify as Indigenous American/Alaska Natives, Asian, Black, Hispanic/Latinx, Pacific Islanders, and other racially and ethnically minoritized groups, often referred to as Black, Indigenous, People of Color (BIPOC).[6] To date, few studies evaluate racial or ethnic inequities among birthing people and children affected by substances including opioid use disorder (OUD). When studies report race and ethnicity data, it is often poorly described.[7] Among the studies that have carefully examined race and ethnicity related to pregnancy and SUD treatment, results show that non-Hispanic White women were more likely than non-Hispanic Black women and Hispanic women to receive medication to treat OUD during pregnancy and also use it consistently.[8] White non-Hispanic women were also more likely than non-Hispanic Black women and Hispanic women to receive buprenorphine treatment compared with methadone treatment.[9,10] Further, while 66% of women with OUD continued taking medications for OUD (MOUD) 12 months after delivery, BIPOC women had greater challenges in continuing care, likely due to issues of structural racism.[10]

Clinicians need to provide care in a supportive and nonjudgmental manner. Clinicians should be sensitive and explicitly discuss with their patients the need for and limits around confidentiality regarding SUD, because of stigma, discrimination and potential legal ramifications. In many cases, a person may have used alcohol or drugs during a previous pregnancy, experiencing the negative consequences of stigmatization and perhaps loss of custody of other children. PSP may be understandably wary of health care providers owing to previous experiences. The availability of a physician within a prenatal clinic setting able to make the determination of severity of SUD and with skills in facilitating a referral to treatment is advantageous. This process will increase access for PSP to these services. Such a strategy helps to decrease the stigma attached to specialized SUD treatment services. However, if an addiction medicine specialist physician is not available within the prenatal clinic setting, then it is well worthwhile to have other clinicians within that setting who are familiar with the principles of addiction medicine.

Encouragement and consistency in approach, expectations, and messages to PSP are important and will maximize engagement and retention in treatment.[11] Effective treatment for patients and their newborns requires collaboration among multiple providers and agencies. It is essential that there be clear and direct communication among the patient's SUD specialist, obstetricians, pediatricians, neonatologists, primary care physicians, nurses, anesthesiologists, psychiatrists, psychologists, and social workers, and this may require obtaining appropriate consent from the patient to release medical information. Clear and appropriate communication with legal agencies such as Child Protective Services is also important in order to advocate for PSP.

SCREENING

Estimates vary, but 30% to 50% of people in the general population have unintended pregnancies. For pregnant people with OUD, the rate is estimated to be 86%.[12] Prevalence estimates for pregnancies exposed to other psychoactive substances are less known, but one could expect that the overwhelming majority of PSP did not intend to become pregnant. Thus, comprehensive care for people who may become pregnant and are using substances should include reproductive health education and access to methods to provide control over their reproductive options. Drug and alcohol use during pregnancy is substantially underreported, with both amount and frequency of use being underreported by PSP who use frequently compared to those who only use occasionally.[13]

PSP may not fit the usual stereotype of a person with an SUD, making early identification difficult. Screening individuals in a prenatal clinic with specific questions about tobacco, alcohol, and drug use holds the promise of identifying, intervening, and reducing substance use during pregnancy.[14] Universal verbal screening followed when appropriate by brief intervention (SBI) and initiation of or referral to treatment for individuals with SUD is recommended in obstetric settings by the American College of Obstetrics and Gynecology (ACOG).[15] Asking directly about current substance use can identify the risk of use and of SUD to inform and educate individuals planning conception or who are currently pregnant.

Screening of pregnant people for substance use should be done at the first prenatal visit and repeated every trimester if necessary.[16] Validated screening instruments for pregnant people include the T-ACE, the TWEAK, and the AUDIT-C for alcohol, and the TAPS,[17] the 5Ps,[18] and the SURP-P,[19] which are used for multiple substances. Screening is used to determine the risk level of a pregnant individual for problems related to substance use during pregnancy. Those at low risk can simply receive brief advice, and those at high risk should be further evaluated for a diagnosis of SUD and treatment initiation. Individuals at moderate risk benefit most from a brief intervention delivered by the clinician. Pregnant people at moderate risk are those who have a history of SUD with high quantities, who have recent SUD treatment, who stopped using during pregnancy, and who continue sporadic low-level use during pregnancy. The purpose of screening is to allow for treatment of the SUD, not to punish or prosecute the pregnant patient. To normalize this process, it may be useful to standardize the approach to screening and set expectations with the patient at the outset of the visit.

Information from a thorough history (including medical problems and social stressors) and a physical examination can provide clues to the use of specific substances during pregnancy. Pregnant people are often introduced to and supplied with drugs by a partner; therefore, substance use by a current significant other should increase the index of concern.[20] Given that approximately 90% of drug treatment-enrolled pregnant people smoke cigarettes, the use of nicotine and/or cannabis may be an important indicator of other SUD.[21] If any of these risk factors are present, there is increased likelihood of perinatal use and/or SUD, and the expectant parent should be asked about the spectrum of substance use.

Although limitations in assessing the extent of physical abuse and differing definitions of what constitute physical abuse create difficulties in precisely estimating the extent of physical abuse in pregnant individuals, estimates suggest a prevalence rate of around 6% in the general population of pregnant people.[22]

In contrast, it is estimated that 34% of PSP report physical abuse, usually intimate partner violence.[23] This rate is similar to rates of victimization among nonpregnant women with SUD, so pregnancy is not a protective factor against domestic violence.[24] Physical, sexual, and verbal abuse by a partner is also common among women with alcohol use disorder, so eliciting a thorough social history adds information about consequences of addiction. These high rates of domestic violence among PSP should prompt clinicians to ask all pregnant people about the possibility of physical or sexual abuse, violence, or injury, especially when substance use is also identified in the individual or their partner. There is no single recommended way to address this issue. Clinicians are encouraged to implement screening with whatever method is comfortable and opportune (written form in waiting room, asking as part of other screening questions on a list, or working into a general interview at an appropriate time based on clinician judgment). There are three screening tools available—Women Abuse Screen Tool (WAST), Abuse Assessment Screen (AAS), and Humiliation, Afraid, Rape, and Kick (HARK)—that are identified as having strong psychometrics and validation for women and could be useful for identifying pregnant people at risk for intimate partner violence.[25]

Cognizance and discussion of risks and/or indications of use or SUD with pregnant individuals can help enhance honest communication about substance use throughout pregnancy. Once identified, options for treatment of acute withdrawal syndromes or other pharmacotherapy and behavioral treatments can be offered to PSP, if applicable.

Routine office visits for prenatal care provide an opportunity to screen for depression and other mental health issues, as co-occurring psychiatric disorders are common in this population. Appropriate obstetric care also includes evaluation for sexually transmitted infections with treatment of the individual and ideally treatment of the partner. Office visits allow ongoing evaluation of the psychosocial support system and may include referral to appropriate community services, if not available in the prenatal clinic setting.

Prenatal education about labor, delivery, and care of the newborn may prevent misunderstandings. Discussions with the PSP should include details of the birth plan, including the treatment of pain during labor and postpartum, education about the potential need for treatment of neonatal withdrawal due to maternal medications, and appropriate contraceptive methods postpartum. When possible, involvement of the patient's significant other and support system, with their consent, is helpful. Supporting patients in touring birthing hospitals and identifying providers that are compassionate and knowledgeable about SUD and neonatal withdrawal is helpful.

Laboratory Testing

The decision to implement any tool for health care, including drug testing, should be grounded in the aim to improve patient care and outcomes. The ethical principle of autonomy indicates that a patient's informed consent is needed before a urine drug test can be performed on either the birthing person or the infant. This is important given the potential legal and social consequences of the testing results.[26] Infant urine, as well as urine from the birthing parent, are biological matrices that have been tested to identify use of legal and illegal drugs. As with any medical diagnostic evaluation, laboratory evaluation of biological matrices must have a confirmation test (eg, liquid chromatography-mass spectrometry) and be accompanied by a review of the pregnant person's records, medical and psychiatric history, and for those PSP identified at the time of the birth, a complete evaluation for substance use during pregnancy. Such action is important given that patients have lost custody of their infants based on false positive tests that lacked later confirmation of drug use.[27] In addition to helping in a diagnostic evaluation of the newly identified PSP, negative results may be helpful in validating a birthing person's history of engagement in treatment, recovery, and abstinence. However, it is important to remember that a positive biological test does *not* (1) diagnose a current SUD, (2) provide a result of parenting ability, or indicate, by itself, child harm,[28] or (3) indicate amount, frequency, or route of substance use.

The decision to perform drug testing on a pregnant person is often influenced by unconscious bias, ethnic stereotypes, and racial discrimination held by the physician.[29] This bias has harmed patients. For example, non-Hispanic Black patients are significantly more likely than their White counterparts to receive urine drug testing.[30] Then, once referred to Child Welfare, Black patients are more likely to be separated from their children, for longer durations and are less likely to be reunited with their children compared to their White counterparts.[31] Individuals of reproductive age are very supportive of laws mandating universal verbal screening and urine drug testing of pregnant people and newborns, and that pregnant individuals should not be able to decline such screening.[32] However, the same population was not supportive of targeting low-income individuals for testing, underscoring the experience of lived discrimination and reminder that substance use problems occur in every socioeconomic level.

The advantage of testing urine is ease of collection; however, results only reflect use and fetal exposure shortly before delivery due to the short window of detection for most substances in urine. Any positive toxicology test result should be discussed with the patient, and results of a definitive test should be utilized if the patient's self-report is not consistent with the presumptive test.[33]

ASAM recommends against meconium or cord tissue testing for many reasons including: (1) the detection window is long and not reflective of behavioral changes during pregnancy, (2) results may reflect iatrogenic exposure to medications administered to the neonate and, (3) such test results are a measure of "social risk" rather than an indication for clinical care. The ASAM policy stated that, "Infant meconium, umbilical cord, and cord blood testing often takes 5 to 7 days to result, lack clinical utility in guiding the management of hospitalized infants, and are not recommended."[33]

Any toxicology testing during the perinatal period should be standardized in hospital policies and include the birthing parent and/or child care response to such test results that goes beyond surveillance and reporting. Such testing results should be used only when clinical indications suggest it is necessary, obtained with informed, written consent, except in emergency situations.[34] True informed consent ensures risks and benefits have been reviewed given the unique legal and social consequences of testing for pregnant and postpartum people. The goal of testing needs to be clear to the patient and clinician as well as who will have access to the results, the protections of such data and the possible ramifications of a positive test. Refusing a toxicology test should be seen as neither indication of use nor detract from clinical care of the patient (ASAM policy cited above).

Alcohol use often accompanies illicit substance use and/or nonmedical use of prescription medications in pregnancy; the biomarkers ethyl glucuronide (EtG), ethyl sulfate (EtS), and fatty acid ethyl esters (FAEE) in urine have been validated in outpatient settings.[34] Biomarker positive evidence of alcohol use may be present from 72 hours to 7 weeks after use. Variations in results depend upon chosen lower limits for reporting positive results. EtG and FAEE are correlated in pregnancy.[35] Among pregnant nurses using alcohol-containing mouthwash and hand cleansers during hospital shifts, there were no false-positive results for EtG and EtS.[36] Clinician judgment in interpretation is necessary, as results indicate exposure to alcohol throughout pregnancy, which is an indicator of risk, but not an assessment of parenting ability.

Confirmed or suspected history of SUD in the birthing parent should lead to screening for hepatitis B and C, human immunodeficiency virus (HIV), and other sexually transmitted infections. Infants born to PSP are at higher risk for these infections because of the association of drug use with high-risk sexual behaviors, and intranasal and parenteral routes of administration. Screening facilitates early treatment and may help prevent further transmission or other complications of infection.

TERATOGENICITY

It is not necessary for a pregnant person to meet diagnostic criteria for a SUD for disruption of fetal growth and development to occur. Exposure in the first trimester can result in significant problems, including pregnancy loss. Most of the development and organogenesis occurs in the first 12 weeks of pregnancy; however, exposure during any trimester can result in poor health outcomes.[37]

A teratogen is a substance that may produce an alteration in the offspring's physical structures and/or behavior when used during gestation. The time of exposure and amount of chemical will affect whether congenital malformations or neurobehavioral problems that persist into later lifetime will occur. In many cases, a "subthreshold exposure" will not lead to malformations, whereas in others, a small dose during critical embryogenesis can lead to significant teratogenicity. It is difficult to attribute causation to exposure when there are confounding variables such as malnutrition, severe stress, and concurrent use of other substances. Alcohol and tobacco, alone and in combination with other substances, are known to have the most potential to cause teratogenicity in the human, but any psychoactive substance use in pregnancy, whether illicit or medicinal, always involves some degree of risk of some form of teratogenicity to the developing embryo.[38]

Since the late 1990s, use of illicit and licit opioids has increased, including during pregnancy. This has been associated with increased rates of neonatal abstinence syndrome (NAS).[39] From 2010 to 2017, the overall incidence of NAS increased from 4.0 to 7.3 per 1,000 birth hospitalizations. This is an increase of 3.3 cases per 1,000 birth hospitalization and a relative increase of 82%. Regarding demographics and source of payment, infants with NAS were more likely to be non-Hispanic White (77.5% versus 52.2%), cases that were Medicaid-billed (84.0% versus 46.3%), and pregnant people were more likely to reside in zip codes in the lowest quartile of median income (38.1% versus 28.1%). Although rates of NAS vary by state, significantly more cases occur in nonmetropolitan counties (22.1% versus 13.4%), a trend that has been maintained since 2004.

Use of more than one substance, sometimes referred to as multi-substance use, is the norm rather than the exception in many substance-exposed pregnancies; thus, it is often difficult to determine specific effects of exposure to individual psychoactive substances.[40] Reports of congenital malformations due to in utero opioid exposure come from individuals prescribed opioids for treatment of pain and those prescribed methadone or buprenorphine for OUD, two different populations. In utero opioid exposures may be associated with cardiac malformations (ventricular septal defect, secundum atrial septal defect/patent foramen ovale), neural tube defect, clubfoot, and oral clefts.[41] In two population-based cohort studies, the absolute risk of congenital anomalies was low from first trimester exposures among pregnant people with chronic pain. A small increased risk of some organ system anomalies was identified in one group; among the other cohort there were no cardiac defects, however, there was a small increase in the risk of oral clefts.[42,43] Among pregnant people with OUD, confounds of socioeconomic stresses including adverse childhood events and exposure to other substances (specifically tobacco and alcohol) and the postpartum environment affect neurodevelopmental outcomes. Reports of congenital and developmental adverse outcomes among methadone or buprenorphine in utero exposed infants and children are rare and must be weighed against the results of ongoing active opioid use of opioids, illicit and licit, among pregnant people.[44,45]

NEONATAL ABSTINENCE SYNDROMES

Use of psychoactive substances during pregnancy can require assessment and treatment of the newborn for intoxication or withdrawal in the absence of diagnosis of SUD. When a pregnant person reports use of prescribed or illicit substances, there is a documented history of use during pregnancy, or a urine drug test is confirmed positive, the newborn should have regular assessment for withdrawal or intoxication beginning at birth or as soon as possible. Asking about the use of tobacco, including electronic nicotine delivery devices, or "vaping," is important as this may not seem significant to the pregnant or postpartum person and is not included in a UDS. An infant born to a person currently prescribed medications for treatment of SUD, specifically MOUD, should be assessed for withdrawal and intoxication, remembering that other substances may be present.

The terminology used to describe in utero exposure to psychoactive substances can be confusing. While neonatal opioid withdrawal (NOW) refers specifically to the effects of in utero exposure to opioids, NAS is a broader term encompassing exposures to any illicit or licit substance with potential for harmful use. Describing an infant with NAS or NOW as "substance exposed" or "in utero exposed," instead of "addicted newborns," is an important distinction that increases linguistic accuracy and decreases stigma. Efforts are currently being made to implement a standardized definition of opioid withdrawal in the neonate. This new bedside definition includes both a known history of in utero opioid exposure (not necessarily by toxicology testing) with or without the presence of other psychotropic substances, and the presence of at least two of the most common clinical signs characteristic of withdrawal (excessive crying, fragmented sleep, tremors, increased muscle tone, gastrointestinal dysfunction).[46]

In the newborn, signs of intoxication and/or withdrawal from psychoactive substances are generally characterized by autonomic instability, central nervous system (CNS) irritability, sleep/wake cycle disturbance, and feeding difficulties.[37] The duration and severity of intoxication and the onset of withdrawal syndrome will depend upon the time of the last substance exposure, the combination of substances, and the metabolism and excretion of the drug.[47] Intoxication can be mistaken for withdrawal given the primitive nature of the newborn CNS. For example, an infant exposed in the few days before birth to a stimulant such as cocaine may display stimulant intoxication for the first 48 to 72 hours after birth. This infant will be irritable, have sleep/wake cycle disruption, and feed poorly; stimulant intoxication could be confused with opioid withdrawal. If the same infant has also been alcohol exposed shortly before birth, symptoms may be more severe, as alcohol and cocaine form coca ethylene, a potent long-lasting stimulant.[48] Obtaining the history of substance use from the pregnant person, evaluating urine drug testing during pregnancy and at birth, and knowing the history of use during pregnancy are important in diagnosing intoxication versus withdrawal.

Timing of substance withdrawal is consistent with the characteristics and pharmacology of the substance. In the case of the infant exposed to opioids, withdrawal signs will generally emerge in the first 24 hours of life for the newborn if the primary substance exposure was to a short acting substance such as fentanyl or heroin. In contrast, if methadone is prescribed, signs of withdrawal usually present later, 24 to 72 hours postbirth, while signs of withdrawal from buprenorphine usually present later than with methadone, 48 to 96 hours postbirth.[49] Similarly, withdrawal from a sedative will be consistent with characteristics of the substance. Withdrawal from alprazolam will emerge earlier than that from diazepam. Clinical signs and symptoms in the substance exposed newborn should not be attributed solely to drug withdrawal or intoxication without appropriate assessment and diagnostic tests to rule out other causes. Consultation with a neonatologist is important in cases where presentation is not straightforward, the course is difficult, or the infant is not responding to supportive care and pharmacotherapy.

It is optimal to observe substance exposed newborns in the hospital for at least 72 to 96 hours after birth to monitor for signs of a neonatal intoxication or a withdrawal syndrome. If an infant is discharged prior to this time, the postpartum individual and the support network should be well informed about signs of NAS and have clear access to medical care regarding NAS.

It is important for providers to implement a standardized hospital protocol for NAS assessment and treatment as it improves infant outcomes (eg, reduces length of hospital stay).[50] The Finnegan Neonatal Abstinence Scoring System (FNASS) is most widely used measure to assess and treat infants with NAS. However, the Eat, Sleep, Console (ESC) method decreased both the use of medication to treat NAS and length of hospital stay compared to FNASS.[51] The assessment and treatment of neonatal opioid withdrawal in the neonate is discussed in more detail the section entitled *Neonatal Opioid Withdrawal/Neonatal Abstinence Syndrome.*

TOBACCO

Fifty percent of individuals who smoke and become pregnant quit during pregnancy.[52] In the United States, 4.9% to 15% of pregnant people use electronic cigarettes.[53] All pregnant individuals should be asked directly about tobacco (all forms) including via electronic drug delivery devices (EDDDs)/ electronic cigarettes, and any quit attempts. ACOG recommends clinicians strongly advise all pregnant people who use tobacco/nicotine to quit.[54] Nicotine replacement therapy (NRT) does not appear to have negative health impacts on the pregnant person or baby,[55] so should be considered for pregnant people for whom behavioral interventions alone have not been successful. In fact, higher doses of NRT may be necessary due to higher nicotine metabolism during pregnancy to control withdrawal and achieve abstinence.[56] Varenicline and bupropion are alternative pharmacotherapies for stopping smoking. A meta-analysis found no evidence of harmful effects associated with use of bupropion or varenicline during pregnancy.[57] However, both medications can be found in breast milk. Thus, it is suggested that health care providers focus on brief office-based interventions coupled with referral to tobacco/nicotine treatment programs specifically developed for pregnant people.

Finally, PSP should be reminded that quitting at any time during their pregnancy is advantageous to themselves, their fetus, and their other children.[58]

Cigarette use exposes the fetus to carbon monoxide, nicotine, and tar, which contains multiple chemicals including cyanide and lead. Nicotine is quickly absorbed, crosses the placenta, and is active in the developing CNS, causing developmental neurological problems.[59] An inverse relationship exists between birth weight and the number of cigarettes smoked per day. Neonates born to pregnant people who smoked during pregnancy weigh an average of 200 g (range, 100-400 g) less and have lower birth lengths than neonates born to those who did not smoke during pregnancy.[60] Fortunately, a period of accelerated growth occurs during the first year of life, and generally, no differences in body weight or length are observed among infants at 1 year of age. Smoking during pregnancy increases the risk of obstetric complications, including spontaneous abortions, placental abruption, premature labor, and preterm birth.[60] Infants have higher risk for morbidity from smoking when born to pregnant people with slower nicotine metabolism, which includes disproportionate representation of Black individuals.[61] Smokeless tobacco use during pregnancy results in increased rates of fetal morbidity and mortality.[62]

Because nicotine is a stimulant, infants born to pregnant individuals who smoke or otherwise use tobacco/nicotine may also be irritable and difficult to calm. Infants exposed to tobacco were more excitable and hypertonic with indications of disturbance in the CNS, gastrointestinal system, and visual response.[63]

Neurobehavioral abnormalities have been identified in the newborn period in infants exposed to tobacco in utero.[63] Multiple studies have examined the causal link between sudden infant death syndrome (SIDS) and smoking. Given the confounding effect of postnatal exposure to cigarette smoking, an analysis of more than 60 studies concluded that nearly one-third of SIDS deaths may be prevented with abstinence from smoking in pregnancy.[64,65]

ALCOHOL AND SEDATIVES

Public health messaging emphasizes there is no safe amount of alcohol consumption during pregnancy. Exposure of as little as one standard drink/day during pregnancy can impact neurodevelopment, particularly during gastrulation.[66,67] Effects of alcohol exposure in utero include stillbirth, miscarriage, preterm delivery, SIDS, and in the most severe cases, fetal alcohol spectrum disorder.[68] Nonetheless, use of alcohol continues to increase among people who can become pregnant ages 18 to 49, and rates of alcohol consumption during pregnancy in the United States increased between 2011 and 2018.[69] Between 2018 and 2020, 13.5% of pregnant individuals reported current drinking and 5.2% reported binge drinking, an increase from 2015 to 2017. During pregnancy, alcohol use and binge drinking were more likely among persons with frequent mental distress, and lack of a regular health care provider was associated with higher amounts of current drinking.

Sedative Use in Pregnant People

Use of multiple substances is common among pregnant people. Individuals with a sedative use disorder using alcohol may also use benzodiazepines, barbiturates, and other sedatives such as gamma-hydroxybutyrate and the benzodiazepine subtype agonist class of medications to treat insomnia.

Progression to severe withdrawal from alcohol or sedatives carries a significant mortality risk, so early recognition and treatments are essential. However, the normal physiological changes that accompany pregnancy can make it difficult to recognize early withdrawal. Treatment for acute withdrawal from sedatives (including alcohol) in PSP should be accomplished in an inpatient setting that allows for medical supervision in collaboration with an obstetrician. Uncontrolled withdrawal symptoms may be life-threatening to both the pregnant parent and fetus. Benzodiazepines and barbiturates can adversely affect the fetus when given during pregnancy, so this should be considered when beginning treatment for acute withdrawal symptoms. However, the risk to both the pregnant individual and fetus from untreated sedative withdrawal is usually greater than the potential risk to the fetus from exposure to these medications in a controlled setting.

Prenatal Alcohol Exposure

In the pregnant person, when alcohol is consumed, it is absorbed into the maternal bloodstream, quickly crosses the placenta, and enters fetal circulation.[66] Alcohol is found in significant levels in the amniotic fluid even after a single moderate dose. As fetal hepatic circulation does not metabolize alcohol as efficiently as in the adult, alcohol is not eliminated from the amniotic fluid as rapidly as it is from maternal circulation.

The effects of consuming alcohol during pregnancy vary depending upon the amount used, timing of exposure during gestation, concurrent use of other psychoactive substances, and maternal factors such as stress, nutrition, and life circumstances. For example, there are known negative effects of binge drinking during pregnancy on child cognition, however, effects of low to "moderate" average weekly alcohol consumption on child neuropsychological behavior up to 5 years are less clear.[70] Fetal alcohol syndrome (FAS) was initially described by Lemoine in the 1960s in France and Jones in United States in 1973.[71] In some affected individuals the results of prenatal alcohol exposure (PAE) may be microscopic. Alternatively, the neurodevelopmental and behavioral consequences of PAE may be present, and the history of use in pregnancy may not be available. The umbrella term fetal alcohol spectrum disorder (FASD) was introduced to describe those infants and children lacking the cardinal diagnostic criteria of FAS (prenatal and postnatal growth retardation, small head circumference [microcephaly], and facial and nonfacial dysmorphology), but still with effects of alcohol exposure in utero.[72] While FASD adequately describes the varying effects of in utero alcohol exposure, this categorization is an umbrella term and not a recognized diagnostic term. See **Table 98-1**.

TABLE 98-1 Diagnostic Criteria for Four Conditions Within the FASD Spectrum According to CoFASP

Diagnostic criterion	FAS		Partial FAS		ARND	ARBD
Confirmed prenatal alcohol exposure[a]	Yes	No	Yes	No	Yes	Yes
Facial dysmorphology[b]	Required	Required	Required	Required	Not required	N/A
Growth deficiency[c]	Required	Required	Not required	Required if brain abnormality is not present	Not required	N/A
Brain abnormality[d]	Required	Required	Not required	Required if growth deficiency is not present	Not required	N/A
Cognitive or behavioral impairment[e]	Required	Required	Required	Required	Required[f]	N/A
Other systemic malformation	Not required	Not required	Not required	Not required	Not required	Required

[a]Defined as 6 or more drinks/week for 2 weeks or 3 or more drinks on 2 or more occasions; documentation of maternal intoxication in records; positive biomarker for alcohol; or evidence of risky maternal drinking on a validated screening tool.

[b]Defined as 2 or more of the following: short palpebral fissures, thin vermilion border, and smooth philtrum.

[c]Defined as height and/or weight equal to or less than the 10th centile based on racially/ethnically normed charts.

[d]Defined as head circumference equal to or less than the 10th centile, structural brain anomaly, or recurrent nonfebrile seizures.

[e]Cognitive impairment is defined as global cognitive impairment, verbal or spatial IQ, or individual neurocognitive domain greater than or equal to 1.5 SD below mean. Behavioral impairment is defined as impairment of self-regulation greater than or equal to 1.5 SD below mean. For children under age 3, developmental delay is required.

[f]ARND requires two behavioral or cognitive deficits if IQ is not greater than or equal to 1.5 SD below the mean.

Note: ARBD, alcohol-related birth defects; ARND, alcohol-related neurodevelopmental disorder; FAS, fetal alcohol syndrome; N/A, not applicable.

Many diagnostic criteria and schemata have described the spectrum of structural anomalies and neurocognitive disabilities associated with PAE. A new diagnostic classification is described in the DSM-5, Neurobehavioral Disorder with Prenatal Alcohol Exposure (ND-PAE). This categorization addresses the spectrum of neurodevelopmental and mental health problems and symptoms experienced by affected adults and children. The diagnosis of ND-PAE includes impairments and deficits in neurocognitive, self-regulatory, and adaptive functioning.[73]

Evaluation of elementary age children in predominantly White and middle-class areas in the Midwest and Rocky Mountain region described the prevalence of alcohol-exposed pregnancies in these communities. These studies predate the DSM-5 introduction of ND-PAE and use FAS, partial FAS, and FASD terminology. In the Midwestern city, FAS was reported in 6 to 9 per 1,000 children (midpoint, 7.5), PFAS from 11 to 17 per 1,000 children (midpoint, 14), or an estimation of the rate of FASD of 24 to 48 per 1,000 children or 2.4% to 4.8% of the population (midpoint, 3.6%). Prevalence rates of FASD were similar for children in the Rocky Mountain City (FAS is 2.9 to 7.5 per 1,000, PFAS is 7.9 to 17.7 per 1,000, and combined prevalence is 10.9 to 25.2 per 1,000 or 1.1%).[74]

The NIAAA-funded Collaboration on FASD Prevalence (CoFASP) is the first major, multi-sample, multi-site effort to report a population prevalence of the full continuum of FASD and maternal risk factors for PAE in the United States.[67] **Table 98-1** lists the diagnostic criteria developed by CoFASP for diagnoses represented within FASD: FAS, partial FAS, alcohol-related neurodevelopmental disorder (ARND) and alcohol-related birth defects (ARBD). In one midwestern city, there was no significant difference of FASD prevalence among differing self-identified ethnic/racial identities.[75] There were no socio-economic factors linked to exposure other than unmarried status. Risk factors for a PAE were personally reported use of alcohol during the pregnancy, use of tobacco and cocaine, less prenatal care initiated at a later gestational date, delayed recognition of pregnancy, lower body mass index (BMI), and smaller head circumference.

Pregnant people may have exposure to other sedatives besides alcohol. Benzodiazepines and benzodiazepine subtype agonists have been reported to decrease birth weight and increase odds of preterm birth.[76] Studies of sole exposure to this class of drugs were of patients taking prescribed medications for sleep and anxiety.[77] The National Birth Defect Prevention Study (1997-2011) reported some esophageal, cardiac, and congenital malformations with benzodiazepine exposures.[78] However, a cohort in Norway studied over a similar time frame showed an absence of an association of exposure to benzodiazepines or benzodiazepine subtype agonists with birth weight relative to gestational age and sex.[76] As with other in utero substance exposures, study results have been mixed and more long-term data is needed.

Addiction treatment is an opportunity to intervene with the current pregnancy and prevent further alcohol affected pregnancies. The addiction specialist may be the first professional with whom a birth parent shares concern about other children's development. Addiction medicine specialists providing primary care will find the NIAAA publication "Recognizing Alcohol-Related Neurodevelopmental Disorder (ARND) in Primary Healthcare of Children" helpful in identifying PAE children for further evaluation.[79] Formal diagnosis of ND-PAE is made through evaluation by a multidisciplinary team including geneticists, psychologists, physicians, and allied health professionals. Families and patients can find information about ND-PAE and support through the Fetal Alcohol Spectrum Disorders United (www.FASDUnited.org).

OPIOIDS

The use of heroin or nonmedical use of prescription opioid medications may continue into pregnancy because attempts to quit lead to obvious withdrawal symptoms, but PSP may be reluctant to disclose information about their opioid use.

Pharmacotherapy in Pregnancy

Opioid withdrawal syndrome during pregnancy can lead to fetal distress and premature labor owing to increased oxygen consumption by both the PSP and fetus. Even minimal symptoms in the pregnant individual may indicate fetal distress, as the fetus may be more susceptible to withdrawal symptoms than the birthing person. Methadone is frequently used to treat acute withdrawal symptoms from illicit opioids. Methadone may be used by a clinician for temporary maintenance when a patient with an OUD is admitted to a hospital for an illness other than OUD that may be complicated by opioid withdrawal. This includes admission for evaluation for preterm labor, which may be induced by acute opioid withdrawal. Naloxone should not be given to a pregnant person maintained on an opioid agonist medication or using opioid agonists illicitly, except as a last resort in life-threatening opioid overdose, as withdrawal precipitated by an opioid antagonist can result in spontaneous abortion, premature labor, or stillbirth.

Medically assisted withdrawal of the pregnant individual with an OUD is not recommended because of high rates of return to opioid use and increased risk to the fetus of intrauterine death. MOUD with methadone has served as the longtime standard of treatment.[80] Buprenorphine is now a first-line medication alongside methadone. Being on an adequate and stable dose of MOUD decreases fluctuations in the pregnant individual's opioid blood concentration, which is thought to reduce stress on the fetus related to rapid cycles of intoxication and withdrawal. Fluctuations between opioid intoxication and withdrawal result in adverse fetal effects, such as premature labor and spontaneous abortion. Illicitly bought heroin/fentanyl is likely adulterated with other compounds that may be harmful to the fetus, and access to illicit prescription opioids may be unpredictable, so elimination of any opioid use with adequate doses of MOUD prevents harm to the fetus from exposure to these other compounds. Engagement in MOUD improves maternal health and nutrition, reduces obstetric complications, and improves the health of the infant at delivery. Other advantages of opioid agonist pharmacotherapy over illicit opioid use are reduction of acquisitive crime and the risk of incarceration and decreased disruption of the birthing person-child dyad.[81] MOUD enhances the ability of PSP to participate in prenatal care and SUD treatment, thus giving the PSP and the family the opportunity to adequately prepare for the arrival of the infant.

Pregnant people with OUD should be initiated without barrier on MOUD either through their OB if they feel comfortable offering buprenorphine or by being referred to a local addiction treatment program, if available. Most programs assign high priority to pregnant individuals, so the patient may be able to enter treatment sooner than if they were not pregnant. Pregnant people maintained on methadone or buprenorphine should have their dose monitored regularly throughout the pregnancy and the postpartum period and their dose adjusted as necessary.

Certain factors need to be considered when treating PSP with methadone. The dose given during pregnancy does not correlate with neonatal abstinence symptoms, so the benefits of prescribing methadone are not offset by harm to the newborn.[82] Effective daily methadone doses in pregnant individuals with OUD may vary.[83] It is reasonable to expect the methadone dose requirement to increase during the third trimester of pregnancy due to larger plasma volume, decreased plasma protein binding, increased tissue binding, increased methadone metabolism, and increased methadone clearance. As a result, the half-life of methadone is shortened as pregnancy progresses, and the pregnant individual may experience mild withdrawal symptoms unless adjustments are made to the methadone dose. Dividing the total daily requirement into 2 or more doses, given throughout the day, is preferred, if possible. This split-dose procedure provides a more even blood concentration throughout each day.[84]

Sublingual buprenorphine, a partial μ agonist and κ antagonist prescribed for the treatment of OUD, has been used successfully in pregnant people and should not be considered "off-label" use. It is available in an office setting or opioid treatment program. Induction onto buprenorphine is not more complex than methadone, the initial dose may need to be divided into 2 or 3 doses, and it may take a few days for dose stability to occur. This medication has been well tolerated by pregnant people. Newborns of individuals prescribed buprenorphine have a lower incidence of NAS compared to methadone. Buprenorphine exposed newborns require less morphine to stabilize NAS and a shorter duration of treatment than neonates exposed in utero to methadone.[82] The onset of treatment for NAS due to exposure to buprenorphine may be longer when compared to methadone exposure, however still occurs still within 4 days of hospital observation.[82] MOUD as part of comprehensive care for pregnant women who use heroin/fentanyl and/or illicit prescription opioids improves maternal psychosocial function and birth outcomes.[85]

Although medically assisted withdrawal of the pregnant individual with OUD is not recommended, there is some research on naltrexone as MOUD in pregnant patients. Over 25 published prenatal naltrexone implant exposure cases are published and all showed normal birth outcomes.[86-89] While potential confounding factors were not controlled, the results suggest no evidence of an increased risk for poor neonatal outcomes with prenatal naltrexone exposure.[90] However, maternal return to illicit opioid use may occur in a short time period if naltrexone is discontinued and there is an increased risk of fatal overdose following naltrexone discontinuation.

Neonatal Opioid Withdrawal/Neonatal Abstinence Syndrome

Identification and Treatment of the In Utero Opioid-Exposed Newborn

No matter what specific identification schemata and/or pharmacologic and nonpharmacologic interventions are used, the overall goal of identification and treatment of the substance exposed newborn should include the family, particularly the birthing parent-infant dyad, to empower families and decrease the stigma associated with the pregnancy and substance use.[91] Reviews of the treatment of neonatal abstinence syndrome (NAS) and neonatal opioid withdrawal (NOW) reveal that standard, evidence-based approaches for managing NOW are not present nationwide. Until recently, there was little consistency across nurseries in the assessment, medication, and nonpharmacologic treatments of NAS. A comprehensive review of 53 studies (2007-2017) with 11,907 unique birthing parent-infant dyads, revealed a paucity of evidence to support specific diagnostic or treatment approaches for NAS.[92]

Beginning in the 1970s, one assessment to identify the newborn at risk for withdrawal and initiate treatment for NAS was the Finnegan Neonatal Abstinence Scoring System (FNASS). The limitations of the FNASS led to development of other assessment tools and treatment approaches.[93] A refinement of the FNASS was developed as part of The Maternal Opioid Treatment: Human Experimental Research (MOTHER) project. The MOTHER NAS scale shortened the number of signs measured and clearly specified and defined item-by-item infant signs and symptoms with weighted scores. This modified scale included considerations of comorbid exposure to tobacco or other stimulants, a noisy environment and overstimulation, or whether the infant is hungry or not.[82]

Another approach to assessment and treatment of NAS is Eat, Sleep, Console (ESC, see **Table 98-2**).[91,94] ESC implements specific environmental strategies prior to initiation of medication.[95] In a comparison of ESC to a modified FNASS (M-FNASS) in a nursery implementing ESC while still using M-FNASS scores, there was significant correlation between the two scoring schemata.[96] However, outcomes differed as infants managed with ESC had shorter overall lengths of stay

TABLE 98-2 Eat, Sleep, Console: Parameters for Infant Assessment

EAT	The newborn should eat an appropriate amount based on days of age. For the 1- to 2-day-old, this may be less than an ounce per feeding. For 3 days old or greater, this should be 1 or more ounce(s) per feed. Breastfeeding quality should be "good" as defined by the mother and nursing staff assessment. Baby coordinates feeding within 10 minutes of showing hunger AND/OR is able to sustain feeding for 10 minutes at breast or with 10 cc of finger- or bottle-feeding.
SLEEP	The newborn should be able to sleep undisturbed for a minimum of 1 hour. Holding the newborn to support an undisturbed sleep period is often necessary.
CONSOLE	Determine whether the newborn can be consoled within 10 minutes. If not, nonpharmacological interventions should be increased including a second caregiver making attempts to console the newborn. If the newborn remains inconsolable, this would be an indication that the newborn may need pharmacological treatment and the medical team should be notified.

and less frequently required pharmacologic treatment. For infants who required pharmacologic treatment, the duration of treatment and length of stay were shorter. An advantage of the ESC approach is that it allows newborns and parent(s) to room together on inpatient units and, in most instances, infants are treated exclusively with nonpharmacologic interventions. In a qualitative study of the experience of parents of infants with NAS treated with ESC, four themes emerged. Parents may experience gaps in communication about what to expect in the hospital immediately after delivery and during their infant's hospital stay. They may also experience feelings of guilt, fear, and stress when the infant requires treatment and need increased support. Parents were supportive of fewer interventions and normalizing of newborn care in the ESC approach and felt encouraged to lead their infant's NAS care. The engagement of parents may have contributed to the success of the ESC approach.[97]

Pharmacologic Treatment of Neonatal Abstinence Syndrome

When nonpharmacologic measures are inadequate to calm an infant, opioids are prescribed as first line therapy in most cases. The most common opioid prescribed for NOW was morphine (82%) followed by methadone (22%), buprenorphine (4%) and clonidine (2%).[98] Phenobarbital and clonidine are most prescribed as second line agents, most commonly when infants do not respond to single treatment with an opioid.[99] Methadone, thought to be efficacious given the long half-life, was compared to morphine and found to be efficacious and

TABLE 98-3 Pharmacotherapy for Neonatal Opioid Withdrawal Syndrome

	Dosing		
Medication	**Initial dose**	**Increment**	**Maximum dose**
Oral morphine	0.04 mg/kg every 3-4 h	0.04 mg/kg per dose	0.2 mg/kg per dose
Oral methadone	0.05-0.1 mg/kg q6h	0.05 mg/kg per dose	To effect
Oral clonidine	0.5 µg/kg every 3-6 h	Not studied	1 µg/kg every 3 h
Sublingual buprenorphine	5.3 µg/kg q8 hours	Up-titration rate 25% Maximum number of up-titrations 6	20 µg/kg q8 hours

Adapted from Desmond MM, Wilson GS. Neonatal abstinence syndrome: recognition and diagnosis. *Addict Dis Int J.* 1975;2:113-121.

Oral morphine sulfate directions based on Berghella et al.[81]

Sublingual buprenorphine based on Kraft et al.[178]

Note that a secondary medication of phenobarbital was added if the maximum buprenorphine dose did not control withdrawal signs. Kraft also noted, "The weaning phase makes up the majority of time of treatment, so optimization of dosing in this period has the larger potential impact for reducing duration of treatment. Given the half-life and excellent safety profile, changing the dosing interval after stabilization from q8 to q12 or even q24 could facilitate transition to an outpatient setting."[178]

safe.[100] See **Table 98-3**. In the MOTHER trial, methadone was compared to buprenorphine for NOW among pregnant people treated for OUD with methadone and buprenorphine themselves. Both medications were found to be effective, with buprenorphine requiring fewer days of treatment.[82] Buprenorphine is being prescribed for NOW in many centers as evaluations are ongoing.[47]

CANNABIS

Cannabis is the most common drug used during pregnancy, with 7% of pregnant people reporting use,[101] and up to 14.6% of pregnant adolescents.[102] Most people who use cannabis will quit when they discover they are pregnant, but 30% will continue to use.[103] The legalization of recreational cannabis and cannabis used as treatment (CUAT) at the state level is increasing, which has also led to an increase in other forms of use of cannabis such as via electronic cigarettes, edibles, lollipops, and lotions. Unfortunately, many pregnant people believe that cannabis is relatively safe to use in pregnancy, with increasing rates of cannabis use due to reductions in perceived risk and stigma.[104] The amount of delta-9-tetrahydrocannabinol (THC), the active ingredient in various cannabis products, varies significantly depending on the extraction process from the cannabis plant. Individuals who may become pregnant are using greater quantities of cannabis or cannabis products with higher THC concentrations, especially after legalization, so that neonates had substantially more exposure to cannabis in the postlegalization period.[105] Pregnant patients who report cannabis use are more likely to be young, single, primigravida, and Black.[106] Factors that help predict cannabis use during pregnancy include employment status, use of tobacco cigarettes, and pre-pregnancy cannabis use.[107]

THC easily crosses the placenta, and the fetus is exposed to the active chemical as well as carbon monoxide. Numerous studies have documented neurodevelopmental deficits in children prenatally exposed to cannabis.[108] The concurrent use of alcohol and tobacco in pregnancy confounds understanding of the teratogenicity of cannabis, but there does not appear to be any teratogenic pattern unique to cannabis. There is an association between cannabis use and preterm birth, low birthweight, and higher chance for neonatal intensive care.[109] Neonatal effects take the form of impaired regulatory control, including irritability, tremors and sleep disturbances.[110,111] Preteen children who were exposed in utero have demonstrated behavioral problems and reduced attention span.[112] During adolescence, studies have shown that children exposed to cannabis in utero had lower scores on tests of visual problem solving, visual-motor coordination, and visual analysis compared to unexposed children.[113,114]

Cannabis is neither regulated nor evaluated by the U.S. Food and Drug Administration, so there are no approved indications and no standardized formulations, dosages, or delivery systems. There is no known safe level of cannabis use during preconception, pregnancy, or lactation, so ACOG and the American Academy of Pediatrics recommend that pregnant people abstain from cannabis during pregnancy and breastfeeding.[115]

STIMULANTS

Stimulants include cocaine, methamphetamine, methylenedioxy-methamphetamine (MDMA, or ecstasy), and synthetic cathinones ("bath salts").

The withdrawal syndrome from stimulants is subtle and complex and consists primarily of depression and craving. As abrupt discontinuation of stimulants does not cause gross physiological sequelae, they are not tapered off or replaced with a cross-tolerant drug during medically supervised withdrawal treatment.[116] Pregnant people withdrawing from stimulants should not receive medication except in cases of extreme agitation. Low doses of a benzodiazepine may be used if necessary.

An abstinence syndrome for intrauterine cocaine exposure has not been clearly defined, although effects of cocaine intoxication on neurobehavioral status have been identified. Intoxicated newborns may be irritable, difficult to quiet, and have feeding difficulties.[117] Infants with prenatal exposure to methamphetamine may develop jitteriness, drowsiness, and respiratory distress, although very few require pharmacologic intervention.[118]

When cocaine is used, the active drug and its metabolites readily cross the placenta. As fetal pH normally is lower than maternal pH and the fetal liver does not metabolize cocaine efficiently, cocaine is more highly concentrated in amniotic fluid. Cocaine use during pregnancy is associated with higher odds of preterm birth, shorter gestational age at delivery, and small for gestational age neonates.[119] The effects of cocaine are thought to be through direct neurotoxicity by disrupting monoaminergic pathways and causing vascular damage.[120] Multiple studies have identified neurological, developmental, and behavioral deficiencies in the infant, toddler, and young child exposed prenatally to cocaine.[121] Cognitive differences, motor delays, language delays, and fine-motor problems have been identified, and there may be a dose-response effect of cocaine on newborn head circumference.[122] However, many confounders of these effects have been identified, not the least of which is the use of alcohol with cocaine.[123] For example, Frank et al. completed a systematic review that excluded studies that lacked control groups, used unblinded examiners, did not prospectively enroll participants, or suffered from other serious methodological limitations.[124] On the basis of these studies, the authors concluded that: "there is no convincing evidence that prenatal cocaine exposure is associated with developmental toxic effects that are different in severity, scope or kind from the sequelae of multiple other risk factors." This review helped to debunk the "crack baby" myth as findings once thought to be specific effects of gestational cocaine exposure were shown to be correlated with other factors, including prenatal exposure to alcohol, cannabis, tobacco, and the quality of the child's environment. Studies published after this systematic review that controlled for a number of medical and social risk factors, reported differences between in utero exposed and nonexposed children on measures of attention, language and perceptual reasoning. Yet, results of such studies are mixed, the effect sizes are often small and findings are only single rather than multiple components of attention and language. The extent to which such findings are meaningful for predicting later learning disorders and associated problems in school is not clear.[125]

There is some concern about neurobehavioral alterations occurring with prenatal exposure to therapeutic and nontherapeutic use of amphetamines.[126] Newborns exposed to methamphetamines in utero may be small for gestational age, have lower birth weight, smaller head circumference, and are at risk for neurodevelopmental abnormalities,[127] including poorer cognitive function by age 7 years.[128] Exposure to MDMA is associated with fine and gross motor delays and lower milestone attainment.[129] There are no studies currently available on the maternal, fetal, or childhood effects of synthetic cathinones.[130]

SUBSTANCE USE DISORDER TREATMENT IN THE PREGNANT AND POSTPARTUM INDIVIDUAL

Simple supportive statements to stop using are sometimes helpful if substance use is identified early, but in most cases of SUD that is moderate to severe such education does not change behavior. SUD treatment is more likely to be effective when begun during pregnancy than afterward. **Table 98-4** provides a set of key components of compassionate care to complete with the pregnant and postpartum patient using substances. In certain cases, therapy for PSP who are actively using illicit substances begins with management of withdrawal, but this is merely a first step in overall treatment. Patients are likely to benefit from different types of treatment programs, depending on the primary drug used and severity of SUD, as well as the patient's life context, including their past experience in treatment or recovery. The ability of PSP to follow through with treatment may be compromised by guilt, lack of supportive significant others (including family), and uncertainty about the success of treatment. However, the possibility of being reunited with children that may have been placed with another family member or in temporary foster care is often an incentive for a pregnant or postpartum person to enter treatment. Providing dyadic care treatment, where both the birthing parent and child are together in treatment, reduces the burden on the foster care system by increasing the safety of the family in a therapeutic environment.

Unique factors and problems must be considered when providing treatment to pregnant people. Access to treatment for PSP may be limited by lack of treatment program openings, transportation problems, lack of childcare, or poverty.[131] SUD treatment programs must provide childcare to be effective, but few do so.[132,133] Twelve-step mutual-help group attendance and/or formal treatment programs, whether inpatient, residential, or outpatient, must address these unique challenges to be optimally effective. Specialty residential treatment programs for PSP, specifically those that provide care for their infants, are economically justified because comprehensive treatment programs for this population are successful.[134] **Figure 98-1** shows the domains of treatment that comprise dyadic care.

Pharmacotherapy may be an option for some PSP, though some medications are contraindicated in pregnancy. Individuals prescribed medication for an alcohol use disorder should inform their health care provider if they are planning to become pregnant. Some forms of long-term SUD pharmacotherapy are not appropriate in pregnancy. Disulfiram is contraindicated during pregnancy because of the association with specific birth defects.[135] Acamprosate and naltrexone do not appear to be associated with substantial risk of congenital

TABLE 98-4 Care Considerations for Birthing Person and Child

	Compassionate care of the birthing person and child		
	Prenatal	**Labor and delivery**	**Postpartum**
Emphasize	Patient engagement in prenatal care • Regardless of substance use • With respect for treatment choices	Honor the birth plan • Communicate with parent about newborn care	Continued engagement and care with health providers after birth • Postpartum visits every 2 weeks to support and care for the birthing parent and neonate
Screen	• Substance use, HIV, hepatitis, STIs. • Co-occurring disorders: ADHD, major depressive disorder, anxiety disorders, eating disorders	(*If not already done*) • Substance use, HIV, hepatitis, STIs. • Co-occurring disorders: ADHD, major depressive disorder, anxiety disorders, eating disorders	• Postpartum depression or other co-occurring disorders • Need for more support in housing, relationships, transportation, parenting, and medical, social service issues
Assess	• Housing and employment • Relationships and support system • Needs specific to each individual	• Pain in birthing parent • Newborn for NAS if parent has OUD • Newborn for effects of other medications prescribed or substances used	• Adequate pain management • Establishment of feeding/comfort with breast/chest feeding
Treat	• Is the dose of maintenance medication for OUD adequate for stabilization? • Is the timing of dosing appropriate: BID, QID or more often doses may be needed? • Is split dosing of medications for OUD needed?	Medications prescribed for the treatment of opioid use disorder (buprenorphine, methadone) do NOT provide adequate analgesia in labor, delivery and postpartum. • Continue maintenance medications through labor and delivery Patients with SUDs should have adequate pain management, even if actively using • Spinal anesthesia should be considered • Short-acting full opioid agonists may be required	
		Treat pain with nonpharmacological and medication interventions Note: Possible higher tolerance to opioids Avoid • Dilaudid due to euphorigenic properties • Partial agonists/antagonists pain medications for OUD patients	• Substance use disorder • Co-occurring psychiatric disease • Other medical diseases • According to recovery needs, medication for addiction treatment, Medications for Prevention of return to use. • Postpartum pain
Assist and support	• Develop birth plan • Choose support person during birth • What to pack in birthing bag • Tour hospital • Identify/interview pediatrician	• Support of birthing parent's choice of infant feeding (breast, chest, bottle) • Recognize that sexual trauma may play a role in breast/chest feeding decisions • Support the birthing parent and neonate in bonding, skin to skin, eye gazing and learning each other's cues	• Discuss and support choice in reproductive life planning • Social support and/or mutual self-help • Parenting support • Support of birthing parent and child if state agency for child welfare • Sleep hygiene • Nutrition while breastfeeding • Postpartum visits every 2 weeks that address care for the birthing parent and neonate • Pediatric care including immunizations

Educate	• Nutrition and prenatal vitamins
	• Naloxone for OD
	• Plan for treatment of pain after birth
	• Neonatal medication exposure and need for treatment of withdrawal
		• Care of the newborn
		• The signs and symptoms of neonatal withdrawal
		• How to help nursing staff care for the infant
		• Treatment of infant withdrawal
		  • Eat, Sleep, Console Protocols
		  • Other treatment approaches
			• Support parent in recognizing developmental milestones of child and seeking and receiving support with any questions about the child's health and well-being

Coordinate	Team Care plans including Medical, Nursing, Social Service providers throughout the prenatal, labor and delivery, and postpartum course		

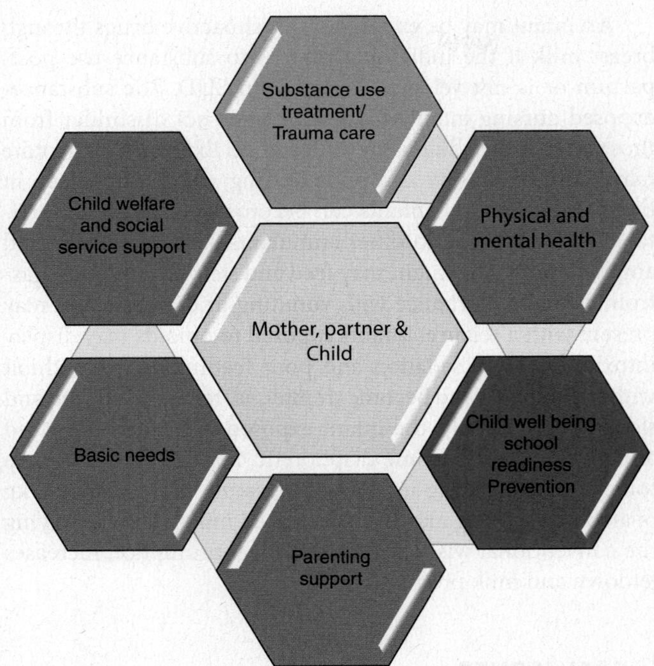

Figure 98-1. Aspects of care to address for the birthing person and child note: The items in *green* represent aspects of care that include the birthing person and the child, items in *purple* are specific to the child and items in *blue* are specific to the birthing person. (Adapted from: Rutman, D, Hubberstey C, Van Bibber M, Poole N, Schmidt RA. *Stories and Outcomes of Wraparound Programs Reaching Pregnant and Parenting Women at Risk*. Nota Bene Consulting Group; 2021.)

malformation or other serious consequences, so should be considered for treatment of pregnant people with AUD based on current evidence, although more research is warranted.[136] Clinicians should discuss options regarding whether to start or continue acamprosate or naltrexone and the preferences of the pregnant person. Buprenorphine or methadone treatment is first-line therapy for pregnant women using opioids and requires dose monitoring throughout pregnancy. Maintenance until after delivery is recommended as opposed to tapering off during pregnancy.

LABOR AND DELIVERY

One of the most common complications of substance use during pregnancy is preterm labor with occurrence varying according to the substance. Rates from opioid use may be as high as 29% to 41%.[11] Rates for other illicit drugs are generally lower, with around 6% attributable to cocaine.[137]

Pregnant individuals may return to substance use as they near the end of pregnancy. They may confuse early signs of labor with signs of acute withdrawal, so may use illicit prescription opioids and/or heroin during the early hours of labor and arrive at the hospital in labor with high concentrations of substances from recent use. This increases the chances of fetal stress and distress. Some PSP may use opioids immediately before presenting for delivery in anticipation of the pain and stress of labor. Reassuring the individual that they will have access to adequate analgesia may help to allay some fears. The delivery method should be selected based solely on obstetric considerations. The staff on a labor and delivery unit should be aware that pregnant people who use stimulants may display bizarre and potentially abusive behavior.[11]

Delivery is a clinical situation with nearly universal acute pain and a reasonably defined onset and resolution.[138] Patients who use illicit drugs are subject to pain in the same manner as any other patient, so can benefit from appropriate treatment for pain (if the drug used is an opioid, they may have tolerance and thus require higher doses of opioids for pain relief). PSP should be assessed for appropriate analgesia, and anesthesia options and adequate pain management should be provided at the time of delivery. ACOG recommends including strategies to avoid or minimize opioid analgesics, highlighting alternative therapies such as nonpharmacologic (exercise, physical therapy, behavioral approaches) and nonopioid pharmacologic treatment.[15] Regional anesthesia may be the procedure of choice during delivery and for postpartum pain. Placement of an epidural catheter with infusion of a local anesthetic such as bupivacaine can reduce or eliminate the need for opioid analgesics. Pain medication should not be withheld based on the presence of current or past SUD. There is no reason to withhold or alter the dose or timing of MOUD in labor and delivery or postpartum. Adjust the pain medication dose based on the patient's reported pain level using a pain scale. Splitting the daily dose of buprenorphine in four (ie, administering every 6 hours) may take advantage of the analgesic properties of the medication.[139] One study found that pregnant people stable in treatment with methadone or buprenorphine experienced adequate pain control postpartum with the use of other opioids in combination with acetaminophen and a nonsteroidal anti-inflammatory drug.[140] These results suggest that routine pain management protocols are effective in reducing pain in buprenorphine- or methadone-maintained patients following a vaginal delivery. A second study showed that individuals prescribed methadone during pregnancy had similar analgesic requirements and response during labor, but required more opioid analgesic after cesarean delivery when compared to individuals not prescribed methadone.[138] Pregnant people using heroin/fentanyl or prescribed chronic opioids (including MOUD) should not receive opioid agonist/antagonist pain medications (such as pentazocine or butorphanol) for acute pain because these medications may cause an acute opioid withdrawal syndrome.[141]

After delivery, opioid analgesics may be necessary, especially after cesarean section, vaginal laceration, or episiotomy repair. Guidelines from the Centers for Disease Control and Prevention recommend prescribing the lowest effective dose of immediate-release opioid.[142] For nonsurgical pain, a prescription for an opioid for 3 days or fewer is usually sufficient, and for postoperative pain, 7 to 10 days, along with nonopioid pain medications as indicated.

BREASTFEEDING

Individuals actively engaged in recovery, including those in SUD treatment, should be encouraged to breastfeed as long as UDS are negative and the person is negative for HIV.[143] Those infected with either hepatitis B or C may also breastfeed as long as the nipple and surrounding areola are not cracked and/or bleeding to avoid direct contact with the birthing parent's blood.[144] In such cases, individuals should be encouraged to pump and discard breast milk and to resume nursing after the skin has healed. Breastfeeding builds a strong parent-infant bond while providing optimal nutrition and passive immunization for the child. Individuals with SUD may struggle with the responsibilities and role of parenthood, sometimes having lost custody of infants and children or having been exposed to SUD in their own families as children. Therefore, successful establishment of breastfeeding by a recovering person is particularly empowering.

After birth, the pregnant person can breastfeed while on MOUD.[143] The American Academy of Pediatrics lists methadone as a medication compatible with breastfeeding.[144] Nonetheless, individuals in methadone programs are sometimes discouraged from breastfeeding or are told that their "dose is too high." Such a position is contrary to the evidence that negligible amounts of methadone are excreted in human milk across the dose range; thus, there is no contraindication to nursing while prescribed methadone.[145] Although little methadone is transferred in breast milk, small amounts may ease neonatal withdrawal from opioids. Buprenorphine is likewise appropriate to be continued for an individual who becomes pregnant while on MOUD. Small amounts of buprenorphine are excreted in breast milk, so breastfeeding should also be encouraged in individuals prescribed buprenorphine.[146] A recent meta-analysis showed that breastfeeding is associated with reduced initiation and duration of pharmacological treatment and length of stay for NAS.[147] Insufficient information about the extent to which naloxone passes into breast milk is available to provide guidance with regard to breastfeeding. Clinicians should discuss options regarding whether to continue buprenorphine without or with naloxone and the preferences of the birthing parent.

Breastfeeding when individuals are using benzodiazepines should be discouraged. Diazepam and its active metabolite, *N*-desmethyldiazepam, have been found in both breast milk and infant blood. However, the relative concentrations in breast milk and infant blood plasma are not currently known. Breastfeeding should likewise be discouraged during any period of cocaine use.[148] Cocaine is present in breast milk, which the newborn easily absorbs. Moreover, metabolism of cocaine in infants is quite slow, and it may be several days before cocaine does not appear in urine assay of the newborn. Breastfeeding during any period of cannabis use should also be discouraged. Cannabinoids have been shown to pass through breast milk.[149] THC is found in breast milk at levels elevated to maternal blood plasma levels. ACOG discourages clinicians from prescribing or suggesting the use of cannabis for treatment purposes during preconception, pregnancy, and lactation.[150]

An infant may be exposed to psychoactive drugs through breast milk if the individual returns to substance use postpartum or is not yet in recovery from SUD. The substance-exposed nursing infant will display signs not dissimilar from those seen in the adult using a substance. Exposure to nicotine may cause irritability and poor feeding and disrupt sleep in the infant. Similarly, infants can become intoxicated and irritable with exposure to other stimulants such as cocaine and amphetamine. The infant may feed and sleep poorly, have gastrointestinal disturbance with vomiting or diarrhea, and may present with a seizure. Infants exposed to opioids may display intoxication with sedation and poor feeding or may exhibit withdrawal signs and become tremulous, restless, and feed and sleep poorly. Finally, the infant exposed to alcohol may feed and grow poorly, become diaphoretic, and have poor muscle tone. A breastfeeding individual ingesting more than 1 g/kg of alcohol each day may have decreased milk letdown, belying the conventional wisdom that alcohol consumption increases letdown and milk production.[151]

LEGAL ISSUES

Patient history or physician examination may lead a physician to request laboratory screening for substances in a pregnant person and/or newborn child, in the interest of the health of both. Testing should not be done without the patient's (pregnant person's) knowledge. A request for bodily fluid testing must be accompanied by informed consent, because testing without this violates the constitutional rights of the parent and child and the patient's autonomy.[152] Newborn testing to avoid parental consent is unethical and should not be done in practice.[153] Some states have laws that present terrible dilemmas to clinicians because they equate positive drug testing with child abuse or criminal offenses, which can interfere with successful treatment of SUD.[154] However, in many cases across the nation, legislators and the courts have ruled that SUD in pregnancy is not a criminal matter and there is no evidence that punitive approaches work.[152,155]

The intersectionality of systemic racism, pregnancy, and substance use often leads to faulty logic that substance use without any other contextual factors should be reported to Child Protective Services (CPS). Such biases also lead to hospitals enforcing the practice of "test and report" with an overreliance on urine drug testing as a proxy for parental "fitness." ACOG cautions that such a practice is both unethical and ineffective in reducing drug use among pregnant people.[156]

The proportion of children reported to CPS with parental "drug abuse" increased from 18% to 31% from 2010 to 2019.[157] Foster care data indicates that child removals due to parental drug use increased 60% between 2007 and 2017.[158] Historically, Black and Indigenous American/Alaska Native children have been overrepresented in the foster care system and data shows that despite comparable rates of detection of substance use in Black and White mothers, Black newborns are more likely to be reported to CPS in spite of universal urine drug testing.[159] For example, 12% of Black children and 15% of Indigenous American/Alaska Native children enter the foster care system before they turn 18, compared to 6% of all U.S. children.[160] Recently, the largest increase of child removals due to substance use was observed for White children ages 0-4 (49.9% increase), followed by ages 5+ White children with substance removals (39.7 % increase). The number of BIPOC children with substance removals also increased over time for both ages 0-4 (22.7%) and ages 5+ (6.1%; an increase of 731 children), although to a smaller degree than White children.[158] Although more White children were removed because of parental substance use, findings suggest they are more likely than BIPOC children to be reunified. The parent receiving medication to treat OUD significantly increased these odds of reunification.[158]

The federal Child Abuse Prevention and Treatment Act requires states to have policies and procedures to notify CPS of substance-exposed newborns.[161] Specifically, notifications are required when the birthing person or neonate has a toxicology test that is positive for substances and/or the neonate exhibits physical, neurological, or behavioral symptoms consistent with prenatal substance exposure, withdrawal symptoms from prenatal substance exposure, or FASD. The mandate to report varies significantly, and thus clinicians should be familiar with legislation in their state and community. Upon receiving a notification of a neonate with prenatal substance exposure, CPS makes an initial assessment to determine whether the neonate meets the State's definition of child abuse or neglect. If the neonate does not meet criteria for abuse or neglect, the family should be referred to a community agency for a needs assessment. If the neonate meets the state's criteria for abuse or neglect, the neonate and family will be referred to CPS for a family assessment or investigation. If the neonate and family are screened in for services, CPS conducts a safety assessment to determine the extent to which the child will be safe in the home. The criteria for safety determination include: the parents' ability to perform essential parental responsibilities, the birthing person's behavior and interaction/bonding with the newborn, the family's support system, and home environment including a crib, clothing, and formula (if not breast/chest feeding). Assessment of all other adults and children living in the home is also included.[161]

Substance use during pregnancy is not, in and of itself, abuse or neglect. However, many states require hospitals to report pregnant people suspected of heavy alcohol or other drug use to local public health authorities or the criminal justice system when they present for delivery, whether or not treatment was sought for SUD. The threshold for amount of alcohol or other substances such as cannabis that triggers reporting to authorities may not be specified by state legislation and left up to the judgment of the clinician. This reporting may rightfully cause PSP to be even more wary of acknowledging that they have a problem. For this reason, it is very important for a physician who recognizes perinatal SUD to address this issue with the patient in a compassionate, nonjudgmental manner, thus advocating for both parent and child. Mandatory reporting of positive UDS during pregnancy or aggressive prosecution of PSP may cause individuals to avoid disclosure of SUD during pregnancy. Some PSP avoid prenatal care and hospital delivery, particularly if they have other children in the custody of CPS or living with relatives, because they fear the loss of their children. Punitive state policies do not reduce rates of NAS.[162] However, mandatory reporting legislation may provide an incentive for PSP to enter treatment prior to delivery in order to avoid potential prosecution. Continued custody of the child may be contingent upon adherence to a treatment plan determined by CPS. Every effort should be made to coordinate appropriate placement of the infant (with the birthing parent, another family member, or in foster care) when an individual is in need of SUD treatment. With such support, the pregnant or postpartum person can continue to build a bond with the infant, and it provides positive motivation for them to attend treatment and enter recovery. Laws vary greatly across the United States and are often unclear regarding charges of child abuse for PSP.[155] Education and support of PSP about applicable state legislation can help enhance motivation to enter SUD treatment prior to delivery.

POSTPARTUM CARE

Substance-use-related death, those deaths from poisoning caused by substances (legal, illegal, or prescribed medications), is a leading cause of death among reproductive age individuals. The maternal mortality rate in 2019 (20.1 deaths per 100,000 live births) was significantly higher than the rate in 2018 (17.4 deaths per 100,000 live births). In 2019, the maternal mortality rate for non-Hispanic Black women was 44.0 deaths per 100,000 live births, 2.5 times the rate for non-Hispanic White women (17.9) and 3.5 times the rate for Hispanic women (12.6). Rates for non-Hispanic Black women were significantly higher than rates for non-Hispanic White and Hispanic women. The increase in the maternal mortality rate from 2018 (14.9) to 2019 for non-Hispanic White women was statistically significant.

Substance-use-related pregnancy-associated deaths are occurring primarily in the postpartum period, often after birthing people have stopped seeing their obstetrical provider. In Wisconsin, Utah, Massachusetts, and Colorado, most substance-use-related pregnancy-associated deaths occurred in the postpartum year.[163-165] Contact with the health care system is not uncommon before maternal death as nearly two-thirds of individuals had at least 1 emergency department visit or inpatient hospital admission before their death, suggesting that the health care system can intervene and potentially prevent their deaths.[166]

For those with OUD, postpartum medication is a noted risk factor for overdose.[163,167] Several studies found an association between loss of custody and discontinuation of treatment postpartum.[168,169] Multiple stresses such as high rates of postpartum depression, CPS involvement, and other forms of patient-centered chaos are recognized as risk factors for treatment disengagement.[170,171] An important barrier in the continuity of OUD treatment is loss of medical insurance in the postpartum period.[165]

Solutions to the mortality problem in the year after delivery include treating OUD as a lifelong condition requiring chronic care, not simply acute or episodic care: reimburse frequent follow-up of postpartum patients that include postpartum support, education about the signs of postpartum depression and anxiety, plan for sleep and medication management, creating a plan of safe care, and discussing the role of CPS. Furthermore, health care systems need to extend the range of concerns beyond the strictly medical issues. States with Medicaid expansion had a 6% decrease in opioid overdose deaths compared with states without expansion.[172] Expansion of Medicaid coverage to a year postpartum to ensure uninterrupted mental health and substance use care is quite literally life-saving.[173]

SUD is not sufficient to determine at-risk parenting; however, it is within a cumulative risk framework. Identifying children who were exposed in utero to substances can be a launching point to help optimize the health and well-being of the birthing parent and child.[174] Further, the link between parental SUD and child maltreatment has been affirmed in the Adverse Childhood Experiences Study.[175] Effectively treating a parent is the most important intervention for the child exposed to substances, both prenatally and during childhood.[176] Particularly in the case of PSP, the additional stresses of meeting the developmental needs of a newborn, possibly together with rearing older children, lack of family and social support, depression and other psychiatric problems, inadequate housing or homelessness, exposure to violence, and financial difficulties, may pose as much risk to successful child rearing as SUD.[175] Comprehensive ongoing SUD treatment, tailored to help the parent address other stressors besides SUD, reduces the chance of an adverse outcome for both. Otherwise, these factors can hamper the recovering patient's effectiveness as a parent, thus contributing to the risk of return to SUD.[177]

If a parent is successful in treatment, they may be able to retain custody of children. For the parent whose children have been removed from the home, a goal of treatment and recovery should be reunification of the family. Prolonged hospitalization of newborns or foster care for children born to PSP is highly disruptive to bonding and family cohesion as well as an economic burden on society. Effective treatment and intervention is cost-effective in the short and long term and becomes the first and most effective prevention intervention for children. For PSP without an SUD, the goal of brief counseling is to prevent a return to hazardous substance use, particularly during a subsequent pregnancy.

Following birth, parental treatment plans should be expanded to address newborn medical problems such as infection and developmental problems due to substance exposure. Bonding with the infant may be more difficult, so the parent may need to be taught specific skills to calm and feed the infant. Older children may need to be evaluated for developmental problems if the parent is concerned or gives a history of substance use in earlier pregnancies. Communication links developed during the pregnancy should be expanded to include physicians, social workers, and allied health professionals caring for the infant and older children. Such interventions can have a positive impact on development of every child in the family and prevent another substance-exposed pregnancy.[175]

CONCLUSIONS

At every visit and with every patient interaction, providers have an opportunity to help improve outcomes of patients with substance use problems during pregnancy and the postpartum times. Compassionate, nonjudgmental care can be the catalyst for patients to seek and obtain the help they need. Screening with one of several validated screening tools for substance use should be performed for all pregnant people at the initial prenatal visit and repeated if necessary. Screening for co-occurring disorders and domestic violence is also valuable. Clinicians must be aware of mandated reporting requirements in their jurisdiction during pregnancy or after delivery, and testing should never occur without consent of the pregnant/birthing person. Once identified, PSP should be offered low barrier access to pharmacotherapy for OUD, as well as for withdrawal syndromes, notably for alcohol or sedatives. Pregnant people should also be offered appropriate options for pain management at and after delivery and education about breastfeeding as well as postpartum care and support. Unfortunately, there is still work to be done regarding racial and ethnic disparities in access to MOUD and other addiction treatment, but clinicians can address structural racism by providing supportive and nonjudgmental care to all PSP. Clinicians can also play a role in advocating for PSP at the public policy and legislative level by working to change problematic regulations requiring mandatory reporting to CPS for substance exposure.

REFERENCES

1. Effects of in utero exposure to street drugs. *Am J Public Health.* 1993;83(Suppl):1-32. doi:10.2105/ajph.83.suppl.1
2. Jones HE. Treating opioid use disorders during pregnancy: historical, current, and future directions. *Substance Abuse.* 2013;34(2):89-91. doi:10.1080/08897077.2012.752779
3. Engs RC. *Women: Alcohol and Other Drugs.* Kendall/Hunt Publishing Company; 1990.
4. Substance Abuse and Mental Health Services Administration. *2020 National Survey on Drug Use and Health: Women.* Accessed January 3, 2023. https://www.samhsa.gov/data/release/2020-national-survey-drug-use-and-health-nsduh-releases
5. Bolnick JM, Rayburn WF. Substance use disorders in women: special considerations during pregnancy. *Obstet Gynecol Clin North Am.* 2003;30(3):545-558. doi:10.1016/S0889-8545(03)00068-8
6. Paradies Y, Ben J, Denson N, et al. Racism as a determinant of health: a systematic review and meta-analysis. *PLoS ONE.* 2015;10(9):e0138511. doi:10.1371/journal.pone.0138511
7. Schiff DM, Work EC, Foley B, et al. Perinatal opioid use disorder research, race, and racism: a scoping review. *Pediatrics.* 2022;149(3):e2021052368. doi:10.1542/peds.2021-052368

8. Peeler M, Gupta M, Melvin P, et al. Racial and ethnic disparities in maternal and infant outcomes among opioid-exposed mother-infant dyads in Massachusetts (2017-2019). *Am J Public Health.* 2020;110(12):1828-1836. doi:10.2105/AJPH.2020.305888
9. Schiff DM, Nielsen TC, Hoeppner BB, et al. Methadone and buprenorphine discontinuation among postpartum women with opioid use disorder. *Am J Obstet Gynecol.* 2021;225(4):424.e1-424.e12. doi:10.1016/j.ajog.2021.04.210
10. Schiff DM, Nielsen T, Hoeppner BB, et al. Assessment of racial and ethnic disparities in the use of medication to treat opioid use disorder among pregnant women in Massachusetts. *JAMA Netw Open.* 2020;3(5):e205734. doi:10.1001/jamanetworkopen.2020.5734
11. Wright A, Walker J. Management of women who use drugs during pregnancy. *Semin Fetal Neonatal Med.* 2007;12(2):114-118.
12. Heil SH, Jones HE, Arria A, et al. Unintended pregnancy in opioid-abusing women. *J Subst Abuse Treat.* 2011;40(2):199-202.
13. Garg M, Garrison L, Leeman L, et al. Validity of self-reported drug use information among pregnant women. *Matern Child Health J.* 2016;20(1):41-47.
14. Chang G, Wilkins-Haug L, Berman S, Goetz MA. Brief intervention for alcohol use in pregnancy: a randomized trial. *Addiction.* 1999; 94(10):1499-1508.
15. American College of Obstetricians and Gynecologists (ACOG). Opioid use and opioid use disorder in pregnancy. Committee Opinion No. 711. *Obstet Gynecol.* 2017;130:e81-94.
16. Wright TE, Terplan M, Ondersma SJ, et al. The role of screening, brief intervention, and referral to treatment in the perinatal period. *Am J Obstet Gynecol.* 2016;215(5):539-547.
17. McNeely J, Wu L, Subramaniam G, et al. Performance of the tobacco, alcohol, prescription medication, and other substance use (TAPS) tool for substance use screening in primary care patients. *Ann Intern Med.* 2016;165:690-699.
18. Kennedy C, Finkelstein N, Hutchins E, Mahoney J. Improving screening for alcohol use during pregnancy: the Massachusetts ASAP program. *Matern Child Health J.* 2004;8(3):137-147.
19. Yonkers KA, Gotman N, Kershaw T, Forray A, Howell HB, Rounsaville BJ. Screening for prenatal substance use: development of the Substance Use Risk Profile-Pregnancy scale. *Obstet Gynecol.* 2010;116(4):827-833.
20. Tuten M, Jones HE. A partner's drug-using status impacts women's drug treatment outcome. *Drug Alcohol Depend.* 2003;70(3):327-330.
21. Jones H, Heil S, O'Grady K, et al. Smoking in pregnant women screened for an opioid agonist medication study compared to related pregnant and non-pregnant patient samples. *Am J Drug Alcohol Abuse.* 2009;35(5):375-380.
22. Martin SL, Mackie L, Kupper LL, Buescher PA, Moracco KE. Physical abuse of women before, during, and after pregnancy. *JAMA.* 2001;285(12):1581-1584.
23. Haller DL, Miles DR. Victimization and perpetration among perinatal substance abusers. *J Interpers Violence.* 2003;18(7):760-780.
24. Martin SL, Kilgallen B, Dee DL, Dawson S, Campbell J. Women in a prenatal care/substance abuse treatment program: links between domestic violence and mental health. *Matern Child Health J.* 1998; 2(2):85-94.
25. Arkins B, Begley C, Higgins A. Measures for screening for intimate partner violence: a systematic review. *Psychiatr Ment Health Nurs.* 2016;23(3-4):217-235.
26. Zizzo N, Di Pietro N, Green C, Reynolds J, Bell E, Racine E. Comments and reflections on ethics in screening for biomarkers of prenatal alcohol exposure. *Alcohol Clin Exp Res.* 2013;37(9):1451-1455.
27. Hickey K. *Woman Who Lost Custody After False-positive Drug Test Wins Settlement.* November 14, 2017. Hickey & Hull Law Partners. Accessed June 27, 2023. https://www.hickeyandhull.com/legal-blog/woman-who-lost-custody-after-false-positive-drug-test-wins-settlement
28. The White House Executive Office of the President Office of National Drug Control Policy. *Substance use Disorder in Pregnancy: Improving Outcomes for Families.* Accessed 27 June, 2023. https://www.whitehouse.gov/wp-content/uploads/2021/10/ONDCP_Report-Substance-Use-Disorder-and-Pregnancy.pdf
29. Kerker BD, Horwitz SM, Leventhal JM. Patients' characteristics and providers' attitudes: predictors of screening pregnant women for illicit substance use. *Child Abuse Negl.* 2004;28(2):209-223.
30. Winchester ML, Shahiri P, Boevers-Solverson E, et al. Racial and ethnic differences in urine drug screening on labor and delivery. *Matern Child Health J.* 2022;26(1):124-130. doi:10.1007/s10995-021-03258-5
31. Harp KLH, Bunting AM. The racialized nature of child welfare policies and the social control of black bodies. *Soc Polit.* 2020;27(2):258-281. doi:10.1093/sp/jxz039
32. Tucker Edmonds B, McKenzie F, Austgen MB, Carroll AE, Meslin EM. Women's opinions of legal requirements for drug testing in prenatal care. *J Matern Fetal Neonatal Med.* 2017;30(14):1693-1698.
33. American Society of Addiction Medicine. *Substance use and substance use disorder among pregnant and postpartum people.* Accessed June 27, 2023. https://www.asam.org/advocacy/public-policy-statements/details/public-policy-statements/2022/10/12/substance-use-and-substance-use-disorder-among-pregnant-and-postpartum-people
34. Dahl H, Voltaire Carlsson A, Hillgren K, Helander A. Urinary ethyl glucuronide and ethyl sulfate testing for detection of recent drinking in an outpatient treatment program for alcohol and drug dependence. *Alcohol.* 2011;46(3):278-282.
35. Cabarcos P, Tabernero MJ, Otero JL, et al. Quantification of fatty acid ethyl esters (FAEE) and ethyl glucuronide (EtG) in meconium for detection of alcohol abuse during pregnancy: correlation study between both biomarkers. *J Pharm Biomed Anal.* 2014;100:74-78.
36. Ondersma SJ, Beatty JR, Rosano TG, Strickler RC, Graham AE, Sokol RJ. Commercial ethyl glucuronide (EtG) and ethyl sulfate (EtS) testing is not vulnerable to incidental alcohol exposure in pregnant women. *Subst Use Misuse.* 2016;51(1):126-130.
37. Etemadi-Aleagha A, Akhgari M. Psychotropic drug abuse in pregnancy and its impact on child neurodevelopment: a review. *World J Clin Pediatr.* 2022;11(1):1-13. doi:10.5409/wjcp.v11.i1.1
38. Thompson BL, Levitt P, Stanwood GD. Prenatal exposure to drugs: effects on brain development and implications for policy and education. *Nat Rev Neurosci.* 2009;10(4):303. doi:10.1038/NRN2598
39. Hirai AH, Ko JY, Owens PL, Stocks C, Patrick SW. Neonatal abstinence syndrome and maternal opioid-related diagnoses in the U.S., 2010-2017. *JAMA.* 2021;325(2):146-155. doi:10.1001/jama.2020.24991
40. Jarlenski MP, Paul NC, Krans EE. Polysubstance use among pregnant women with opioid use disorder in the united states, 2007-2016. *Obstet Gynecol.* 2020;136(3):556. doi:10.1097/AOG.0000000000003907
41. Lind JN, Interrante JD, Ailes EC, et al. Maternal use of opioids during pregnancy and congenital malformations: a systematic review. *Pediatrics.* 2017;139(6): doi:10.1542/PEDS.2016-4131
42. Bowie AC, Werler MM, Velez MP, et al. Prescribed opioid analgesics in early pregnancy and the risk of congenital anomalies: a population-based cohort study. *CMAJ.* 2022;194(5):E152-E162. doi:10.1503/cmaj.211215
43. Bateman BT, Hernandez-Diaz S, Straub L, et al. Association of first trimester prescription opioid use with congenital malformations in the offspring: population based cohort study. *BMJ.* 2021;372:n102. doi:10.1136/bmj.n102
44. Lee SJ, Bora S, Austin NC, Westerman A, Henderson JMT. Neurodevelopmental outcomes of children born to opioid-dependent mothers: a systematic review and meta-analysis. *Acad Pediatr.* 2020;20(3):308-318. doi:10.1016/j.acap.2019.11.005
45. Nelson LF, Yocum VK, Patel KD, Qeadan F, Hsi A, Weitzen S. Cognitive outcomes of young children after prenatal exposure to medications for opioid use disorder: a systematic review and meta-analysis. *JAMA Netw Open.* 2020;3(3):e201195. doi:10.1001/jamanetworkopen.2020.1195
46. Jilani SM, Jones HE, Grossman M, et al. Standardizing the clinical definition of opioid withdrawal in the neonate. *J Pediatr.* 2022;243: 33-39.e1.
47. Devlin LA, Young LW, Kraft WK, et al. Neonatal opioid withdrawal syndrome: a review of the science and a look toward the use of

buprenorphine for affected infants. *J Perinatol.* 2022;42(3):300-306. doi:10.1038/S41372-021-01206-3

48. Chiriboga CA, Kuhn L, Wasserman GA. Prenatal cocaine exposures and dose-related cocaine effects on infant tone and behavior. *Neurotoxicol Teratol.* 2007;29(3):323. doi:10.1016/J.NTT.2006.12.002
49. Gaalema DE, Heil SH, Badger GJ, Metayer JS, Johnston AM. Time to initiation of treatment for neonatal abstinence syndrome in neonates exposed in utero to buprenorphine or methadone. *Drug Alcohol Depend.* 2013;133(1):266-269. doi:10.1016/j.drugalcdep.2013.06.004
50. Patrick SW, Schumacher RE, Horbar JD, et al. Improving care for neonatal abstinence syndrome. *Pediatrics.* 2016;137(5):e20153835. doi:10.1542/peds.2015-3835
51. Nicholson S, Waskosky A. The eat, sleep, console method: a literature review. *Neonatal Netw.* 2022;41(6):333-340. doi:10.1891/NN-2021-0003
52. Cooper S, Orton S, Leonardi-Bee J, et al. Smoking and quit attempts during pregnancy and postpartum: a longitudinal UK cohort. *BMJ Open.* 2017;7(11):e018746.
53. Gould GS, Havard A, Lim LL, The PSANZ Smoking in Pregnancy Expert Group, Kumar R. Exposure to tobacco, environmental tobacco smoke and nicotine in pregnancy: a pragmatic overview of reviews of maternal and child outcomes, effectiveness of interventions and barriers and facilitators to quitting. *Int J Environ Res Public Health.* 2020;17(6):2034.
54. American College of Obstetrics and Gynecology. Committee opinion no. 471: smoking cessation during pregnancy. *Obstet Gynecol.* 2010;116(5):1241-1244.
55. Bar-Zeev Y, Lim LL, Bonevski B, Gruppetta M, Gould GS. Nicotine replacement therapy for smoking cessation during pregnancy. *Med J Aust.* 2018;208(1):46-51.
56. Bowker K, Lewis S, Coleman T, Cooper S. Changes in the rate of nicotine metabolism across pregnancy: a longitudinal study. *Addiction.* 2015;110(11):1827-1832.
57. Turner E, Jones M, Vaz LR, Coleman T. Systematic review and meta-analysis to assess the safety of bupropion and varenicline in pregnancy. *Nicotine Tob Res.* 2019;21(8):1001-1010.
58. England LJ, Kendrick JS, Wilson HG, Merritt RK, Gargiullo PM, Zahniser SC. Effects of smoking reduction during pregnancy on the birth weight of term infants. *Am J Epidemiol.* 2001;154(8):694-701.
59. Andres RL, Day MC. Perinatal complications associated with maternal tobacco use. *Semin Neonatol.* 2000;5(3):231-241.
60. Rogers JM. Tobacco and pregnancy. *Reprod Toxicol.* 2009;28:152-160.
61. Stroud LR, Papandonatos GD, Jao NC, Niaura R, Buka S, Benowitz NL. Maternal nicotine metabolism moderates the impact of maternal cigarette smoking on infant birth weight: a Collaborative Perinatal Project investigation. *Drug Alcohol Depend.* 2022;233:109358.
62. Zhou S, Rosenthal DG, Sherman S, Zelikoff J, Gordon T, Weitzman M. Physical, behavioral, and cognitive effects of prenatal tobacco and postnatal secondhand smoke exposure. *Curr Probl Pediatr Adolesc Health Care.* 2014;44(8):219-241.
63. Law KL, Stroud LR, LaGasse LL, Niaura R, Liu J, Lester BM. Smoking during pregnancy and newborn neurobehavior. *Pediatrics.* 2003;111 (6 Pt 1):1318-1323.
64. Mitchell EA, Milerad J. Smoking and the sudden infant death syndrome. *Rev Environ Health.* 2006;21(2):81-103.
65. Zhang K, Wang X. Maternal smoking and increased risk of sudden infant death syndrome: a meta-analysis. *Leg Med (Tokyo).* 2013;15(3):115-121.
66. Centers for Disease Control and Prevention. *Fetal Alcohol Spectrum Disorders (FASDs).* Accessed March 18, 2022. https://www.cdc.gov/ncbddd/fasd/index.html
67. NIAAA 50th Anniversary Festschrift. *Alcohol Research: Current Reviews.* Accessed March 18, 2022. https://arcr.niaaa.nih.gov/topic-series/niaaa-50th-anniversary-festschrift
68. Bailey BA, Sokol RJ. Prenatal alcohol exposure and miscarriage, stillbirth, preterm delivery, and sudden infant death syndrome. *Alcohol Res Health.* 2011;34(1):86.
69. Denny CH, Acero CS, Terplan M, Kim SY. Trends in alcohol use among pregnant women in the U.S., 2011-2018. *Am J Prev Med.* 2020;59(5):768-769. doi:10.1016/j.amepre.2020.05.017
70. Flak AL, Su S, Bertrand J, Denny CH, Kesmodel US, Cogswell ME. The association of mild, moderate, and binge prenatal alcohol exposure and child neuropsychological outcomes: a meta-analysis. *Alcohol Clin Exp Res.* 2014;38(1):214-226. doi:10.1111/acer.12214
71. Jones KL, Smith DW. Recognition of the fetal alcohol syndrome in early infancy. *Lancet.* 1973;302(7836):999-1001. doi:10.1016/S0140-6736(73)91092-1
72. Sokol RJ, Delaney-Black V, Nordstrom B. Fetal alcohol spectrum disorder. *JAMA.* 2003;290(22):2996-2999. doi:10.1001/jama.290.22.2996
73. Hagan JF, Balachova T, Bertrand J, et al. Neurobehavioral disorder associated with prenatal alcohol exposure. *Pediatrics.* 2016;138(4):e20151553.
74. May PA, Baete A, Russo J, et al. Prevalence and characteristics of fetal alcohol spectrum disorders. *Pediatrics.* 2014;134(5):855-866. doi:10.1542/peds.2013-3319
75. May PA, Hasken JM, Baete A, et al. Fetal alcohol spectrum disorders in a midwestern city: child characteristics, maternal risk traits, and prevalence. *Alcohol Clin Exp Res.* 2020;44(4):919-938. doi:10.1111/acer.14314
76. Huitfeldt A, Sundbakk LM, Skurtveit S, Handal M, Nordeng H. Associations of maternal use of benzodiazepines or benzodiazepine-like hypnotics during pregnancy with immediate pregnancy outcomes in Norway. *JAMA Network Open.* 2020;3(6):e205860. doi:10.1001/jamanetworkopen.2020.5860
77. Lupattelli A, Chambers CD, Bandoli G, et al. association of maternal use of benzodiazepines and Z-hypnotics during pregnancy with motor and communication skills and attention-deficit/hyperactivity disorder symptoms in preschoolers. *JAMA Netw Open.* 2019;2(4):e191435. doi:10.1001/jamanetworkopen.2019.1435
78. Tinker SC, Reefhuis J, Bitsko RH, et al. Use of benzodiazepine medications during pregnancy and potential risk for birth defects, National Birth Defects Prevention Study, 1997-2011. *Birth Defects Res.* 2019;111(10):613-620. doi:10.1002/BDR2.1497
79. National Institute on Alcohol Abuse and Alcoholism (NIAAA). *Recognizing Alcohol-Related Neurodevelopmental Disorder (ARND) in Primary Health Care of Children.* Accessed March 19, 2022. https://www.niaaa.nih.gov/about-niaaa/our-work/ICCFASD/proceedings/2011
80. World Health Organization. *Guidelines for the Identification and Management of Substance Use and Substance Use Disorders in Pregnancy*; 2014.
81. Berghella V, Lim PJ, Hill MK, Cherpes J, Chennat J, Kaltenbach K. Maternal methadone dose and neonatal withdrawal. *Am J Obstet Gynecol.* 2003;189(2):312-317. doi:10.1067/S0002-9378(03)00520-9
82. Jones HE, Kaltenbach K, Heil SH, et al. Neonatal abstinence syndrome after methadone or buprenorphine exposure. *New Engl J Med.* 2010; 363(24):2320-2331. doi:10.1056/nejmoa1005359
83. Wittmann BK, Segal S. A comparison of the effects of single- and Split-dose methadone administration on the fetus: ultrasound evaluation. *Subst Use Misuse.* 1991;26(2):213-218. doi:10.3109/10826089109053183
84. Jones HE, Deppen K, Hudak ML, et al. Clinical care for opioid-using pregnant and postpartum women: the role of obstetric providers. *Am J Obstet Gynecol.* 2014;210(4):302-310. doi:10.1016/j.ajog.2013.10.010
85. Ebner N, Rohrmeister K, Winklbaur B, et al. Management of neonatal abstinence syndrome in neonates born to opioid maintained women. *Drug Alcohol Depend.* 2007;87(2-3):131-138. doi:10.1016/j.drugalcdep.2006.08.024
86. Hulse G, O'Neil G. Using naltrexone implants in the management of the pregnant heroin user. *Aust NZ J Obstet Gynaecol.* 2002;42:569-573.
87. Hulse GK, Arnold-Reed DE, O'Neil G, Hansson RC. Naltrexone implant and blood naltrexone levels over pregnancy. *Aust NZ J Obstet Gynaecol.* 2003;43:386-388.
88. Hulse GK, O'Neill G. A possible role for implantable naltrexone in the management of the high-risk pregnant heroin user. *Aust NZ J Obstet Gynaecol.* 2002;42:93-94.
89. Hulse GK, O'Neil G, Arnold-Reed DE. Methadone maintenance versus implantable naltrexone treatment in the pregnant heroin user. *Int J Gynaecol Obstet.* 2004;85:170-171.

90. Jones HE, Chisolm MS, Jansson LM, Terplan M. Naltrexone in the treatment of opioid-dependent pregnant women: the case for a considered and measured approach to research. *Addiction*. 2013;108(2):233-247.
91. Grisham LM, Stephen MM, Coykendall MR, Kane MF, Maurer JA, Bader MY. Eat, sleep, console approach: a family-centered model for the treatment of neonatal abstinence syndrome. *Adv Neonatal Care*. 2019;19(2):138-144. doi:10.1097/ANC.0000000000000581
92. Wachman EM, Schiff DM, Silverstein M. Neonatal abstinence syndrome: advances in diagnosis and treatment. *JAMA*. 2018;319(13):1362-1374. doi:10.1001/jama.2018.2640
93. Schiff DM, Grossman MR. Beyond the finnegan scoring system: novel assessment and diagnostic techniques for the opioid-exposed infant. *Semin Fetal Neonatal Med*. 2019;24(2):115. doi:10.1016/j.siny.2019.01.003
94. Grossman MR, Lipshaw MJ, Osborn RR, Berkwitt AK. A novel approach to assessing infants with neonatal abstinence syndrome. *Hosp Pediatr*. 2018;8(1):1-6. doi:10.1542/hpeds.2017-0128
95. Velez M, Jansson LM. The Opioid dependent mother and newborn dyad: non-pharmacologic care. *J Addict Med*. 2008;2(3):113-120. doi:10.1097/ADM.0B013E31817E6105
96. Ryan K, Moyer A, Glait M, et al. Correlating scores but contrasting outcomes for eat sleep console versus modified finnegan. *Hosp Pediatr*. 2021;11(4):350-357. doi:10.1542/hpeds.2020-003665
97. McRae K, Sebastian T, Grossman M, Loyal J. Parent perspectives on the eat, sleep, console approach for the care of opioid-exposed infants. *Hosp Pediatr*. 2021;11(4):358-365. doi:10.1542/hpeds.2020-002139
98. Snowden JN, Akshatha A, Annett RD, et al. The ACT NOW clinical practice survey: gaps in the care of infants with neonatal opioid withdrawal syndrome. *Hosp Pediatr*. 2019;9(8):585-592. doi:10.1542/hpeds.2019-0089
99. Merhar SL, Ounpraseuth S, Devlin LA, et al. Phenobarbital and clonidine as secondary medications for neonatal opioid withdrawal syndrome. *Pediatrics*. 2021;147(3):e2020017830. doi:10.1542/peds.2020-017830
100. Davis JM, Shenberger J, Terrin N, et al. Comparison of safety and efficacy of methadone vs morphine for treatment of neonatal abstinence syndrome a randomized clinical trial. *JAMA Pediatrics*. 2018;172(8):741-748. doi:10.1001/jamapediatrics.2018.1307
101. Volkow ND, Han B, Compton WM, McCance-Katz EF. Self-reported medical and nonmedical cannabis use among pregnant women in the United States. *JAMA*. 2019;322(2):167-169. doi:10.1001/jama.2019.7982
102. Salas-Wright CP, Vaughn MG, Ugalde J, Todic J. Substance use and teen pregnancy in the United States: evidence from the NSDUH 2002-2012. *Addict Behav*. 2015;45:218-225. doi:10.1016/j.addbeh.2015.01.039
103. Mark K, Gryczynski J, Axenfeld E, Schwartz RP, Terplan M. Pregnant women's current and intended cannabis use in relation to their views toward legalization and knowledge of potential harm. *J Addict Med*. 2017;11(3):211-216.
104. Wilkinson ST, Yarnell S, Radhakrishnan R, Ball SA, D'Souza DC. Marijuana legalization: impact on physicians and public health. *Annu Rev Med*. 2016;67:453-466. doi:10.1146/annurev-med-050214-013454
105. Jones JT, Baldwin A, Shu I. A comparison of meconium screening outcomes as an indicator of the impact of state-level relaxation of marijuana policy. *Drug Alcohol Depend*. 2015;156:e104-e105. doi:10.1016/j.drugalcdep.2015.07.290
106. Chabarria KC, Racusin DA, Antony KM, et al. Marijuana use and its effects in pregnancy. *Am J Obstet Gynecol*. 2016;215(4):506e1-506e7. doi:10.1016/j.ajog.2016.05.044
107. Pike CK, Sofis MJ, Budney AJ. Correlates of continued cannabis use during pregnancy. *Drug Alcohol Depend*. 2021;227:108939. doi:10.1016/j.drugalcdep.2021.108939
108. Chasnoff IJ. Medical marijuana laws and pregnancy: implications for public health policy. *Am J Obstet Gynecol*. 2017;216(1):27-30.
109. Corsi DJ, Walsh L, Weiss D, et al. association between self-reported prenatal cannabis use and maternal, perinatal, and neonatal outcomes. *JAMA*. 2019;322(2):145-152. doi:10.1001/jama.2019.8734
110. Fried PA, Makin JE. Neonatal behavioural correlates of prenatal exposure to marihuana, cigarettes and alcohol in a low risk population. *Neurotoxicol Teratol*. 1987;9(1):1-7. doi:10.1016/0892-0362(87)90062-6
111. Scher MS, Richardson GA, Coble PA, Day NL, Stoffer DS. The effects of prenatal alcohol and marijuana exposure: Disturbances in neonatal sleep cycling and arousal. *Pediatr Res*. 1988;24(1):101-105. doi:10.1203/00006450-198807000-00023
112. Goldschmidt L, Day NL, Richardson GA. Effects of prenatal marijuana exposure on child behavior problems at age 10. *Neurotoxicol Teratol*. 2000;22(3):325-336. doi:10.1016/S0892-0362(00)00066-0
113. Willford JA, Chandler LS, Goldschmidt L, Day NL. Effects of prenatal tobacco, alcohol and marijuana exposure on processing speed, visual-motor coordination, and interhemispheric transfer. *Neurotoxicol Teratol*. 2010;32(6):580-588. doi:10.1016/j.ntt.2010.06.004
114. Fried PA, Watkinson B, Gray R. Differential effects on cognitive functioning in 13- to 16-year-olds prenatally exposed to cigarettes and marihuana. *Neurotoxicol Teratol*. 2003;25(4):427-436. doi:10.1016/S0892-0362(03)00029-1
115. American College of Obstetrics and Gynecology. Marijuana use during pregnancy and lactation. *Obstet Gynecol*. 2017;130(4):e205-e209. doi:10.1097/AOG.0000000000002354
116. Weaver M, Schnoll S. Stimulants—amphetamines, cocaine. In: McCrady BS, Epstein EE, eds. *Addictions: A Comprehensive Guidebook*. Oxford University Press; 1999:105-120.
117. Karmel BZ, Gardner JM. Prenatal cocaine exposure effects on arousal-modulated attention during the neonatal period. *Dev Psychobiol*. 1996;29(5):463-480.
118. Smith L, Yonekura ML, Wallace T, Berman N, Kuo J, Berkowitz C. Effects of prenatal methamphetamine exposure on fetal growth and drug withdrawal symptoms in infants born at term. *J Dev Behav Pediatr*. 2003;24(1):17-23.
119. Gouin K, Murphy K, Shah PS. Effects of cocaine use during pregnancy on low birthweight and preterm birth: systematic review and metaanalyses. *Am J Obstet Gynecol*. 2011;204(4):340.e1-340.e12. doi:10.1016/j.ajog.2010.11.013
120. Lester BM, Tronick EZ, LaGasse L, et al. The maternal lifestyle study: effects of substance exposure during pregnancy on neurodevelopmental outcome in 1-month-old infants. *Pediatrics*. 2002;110(6 I):1182-1192. doi:10.1542/peds.110.6.1182
121. Scanlon JW. The neuroteratology of cocaine: background, theory, and clinical implications. *Reprod Toxicol*. 1991;5(2):89-98. doi:10.1016/0890-6238(91)90037-G
122. Bateman DA, Chiriboga CA. Dose-response effect of cocaine on newborn head circumference. *Pediatrics*. 2000;106(3):E33.
123. Lumeng JC, Cabral HJ, Gannon K, Heeren T, Frank DA. Pre-natal exposures to cocaine and alcohol and physical growth patterns to age 8 years. *Neurotoxicol Teratol*. 2007;29(4):446-457.
124. Frank DA, Augustyn M, Knight WG, Pell T, Zuckerman B. Growth, development, and behavior in early childhood following prenatal cocaine exposure. *JAMA*. 2001;285(12):1613-1625.
125. Hurt H, Betancourt LM, Malmud EK. Children with and without gestational cocaine exposure: a neurocognitive systems analysis. *Neurotoxicol Teratol*. 2009;31(6):334-341.
126. Golub M, Costa L, Crofton K, et al. NTP-CERHR expert panel report on the reproductive and developmental toxicity of amphetamine and methamphetamine. *Birth Defects Res B Dev Reprod Toxicol*. 2005;74(6):471-584. doi:10.1002/bdrb.20048
127. Kalaitzopoulos DR, Chatzistergiou K, Amylidi AL, Kokkinidis DG, Goulis DG. Effect of methamphetamine hydrochloride on pregnancy outcome: a systematic review and meta-analysis. *J Addict Med*. 2018;12(3):220-226. doi:10.1097/ADM.0000000000000391
128. Diaz SD, Smith LM, Lagasse LL, et al. Effects of prenatal methamphetamine exposure on behavioral and cognitive findings at 7.5 years of age. *J Pediatr*. 2014;164(6):1333-1338. doi:10.1016/j.jpeds.2014.01.053
129. Singer LT, Moore DG, Min MO, et al. Motor delays in MDMA (ecstasy) exposed infants persist to 2 years. *Neurotoxicol Teratol*. 2016;54:22-28. doi:10.1016/j.ntt.2016.01.003

130. Smid MC, Metz TD, Gordon AJ. Stimulant use in pregnancy: an under-recognized epidemic among pregnant women. *Clin Obstet Gynecol.* 2019;62(1):168-184. doi:10.1097/GRF.0000000000000418
131. Roberts LW, Dunn LB. Ethical considerations in caring for women with substance use disorders. *Obstet Gynecol Clin North Am.* 2003;30(3):559-582. doi:10.1016/S0889-8545(03)00071-8
132. Smith IE, Dent DZ, Coles CD, Falek A. A comparison study of treated and untreated pregnant and postpartum cocaine-abusing women. *J Subst Abuse Treat.* 1992;9(4):343-348. doi:10.1016/0740-5472(92)90029-N
133. Howell EM, Heiser N, Harrington M. A review of recent findings on substance abuse treatment for pregnant women. *J Subst Abuse Treat.* 1999;16(3):195-219. doi:10.1016/S0740-5472(98)00032-4
134. McCollister KE, French MT, Cacciola J, Durell J, Stephens RL. Benefit-cost analysis of addiction treatment in Arkansas: specialty and standard residential programs for pregnant and parenting women. *Subst Abuse.* 2002;23(1):31-51. doi:10.1080/08897070209511473
135. Jessup M, Green JR. Treatment of the pregnant alcohol-dependent woman. *J Psychoactive Drugs.* 1987;19(2):193-203. doi:10.1080/02791072.1987.10472403
136. Kelty E, Terplan M, Greenland M, Preen D. Pharmacotherapies for the treatment of alcohol use disorders during pregnancy: time to reconsider? *Drugs.* 2021;81(7):739-748. doi:10.1007/s40265-021-01509-x
137. Nace EP, Birkmayer F, Sullivan MA, et al. Socially sanctioned coercion mechanisms for addiction treatment. *Am J Addict.* 2007;16(1):15-23. doi:10.1080/10550490601077783
138. Meyer M, Wagner K, Benvenuto A, Plante D, Howard D. Intrapartum and postpartum analgesia for women maintained on methadone during pregnancy. *Obstetr Gynecol.* 2007;110(2 I):261-266. doi:10.1097/01.AOG.0000275288.47258.e0
139. Alford DP, Compton P, Samet JH. Acute pain management for patients receiving maintenance methadone or buprenorphine therapy. *Ann Intern Med.* 2006;144(2):127-134. doi:10.7326/0003-4819-144-2-200601170-00010
140. Jones HE, O'Grady K, Dahne J, et al. Management of acute postpartum pain in patients maintained on methadone or buprenorphine during pregnancy. *Am J Drug Alcohol Abuse.* 2009;35(3):151-156. doi:10.1080/00952990902825413
141. Strain EC, Preston KL, Liebson IA, Bigelow GE. Precipitated withdrawal by pentazocine in methadone-maintained volunteers. *J Pharmacol Exp Ther.* 1993;267(2):624-634.
142. Dowell D, Haegerich TM, Chou R. CDC guideline for prescribing opioids for chronic pain-United States, 2016. *JAMA.* 2016;315(15):1624-1645. doi:10.1001/jama.2016.1464
143. McCarthy JJ, Posey BL. Methadone levels in human milk. *J Hum Lact.* 2000;16(2):115-120. doi:10.1177/089033440001600206
144. Eidelman AI, Schanler RJ. Breastfeeding and the use of human milk. *Pediatrics.* 2012;129(3): doi:10.1542/peds.2011-3552
145. Jansson LM, Velez M, Harrow C. Methadone maintenance and lactation: a review of the literature and current management guidelines. *J Hum Lact.* 2004;20(1):62-71. doi:10.1177/0890334403261027
146. Marquet P, Chevrel J, Lavignasse P, Merle L, Lachâtre G. Buprenorphine withdrawal syndrome in a newborn. *Clin Pharmacol Ther.* 1997;62(5):569-571. doi:10.1016/S0009-9236(97)90053-9
147. Chu L, McGrath JM, Qiao J, et al. A meta-analysis of breastfeeding effects for infants with neonatal abstinence syndrome. *Nurs Res.* 2022;71(1):54-65. doi:10.1097/NNR.0000000000000555
148. Wong S, Ordean A, Kahan M, et al. Substance use in pregnancy. *J Obstet Gynaecol Can.* 2011;33(4):367-384. doi:10.1016/S1701-2163(16)34855-1
149. Perez-Reyes M, Wall ME. Presence of delta9-tetrahydrocannabinol in human milk. *N Engl J Med.* 1982;307(13):819-820.
150. American College of Obstetrics and Gynecology. Committee opinion No. 637: marijuana use during pregnancy and lactation. *Obstet Gynecol.* 2015;126(1):234-238.
151. National Library of Medicine. Drugs and Lactation Database (LactMed). *Alcohol.* Accessed 27 June, 2023. https://www.ncbi.nlm.nih.gov/books/NBK501469/
152. Harris LH, Paltrow L. The status of pregnant women and fetuses in U.S. criminal law. *JAMA.* 2003;289(13):1697-1699.
153. Polak K, Kelpin S, Terplan M. Screening for substance use in pregnancy and the newborn. *Semin Fetal Neonatal Med.* 2019;24(2):90-94.
154. Kimbel AS. Pregnant drug abusers are treated like criminals or not treated at all: a third option proposed. *J Contemp Health Law Policy.* 2004;21(1):36-66.
155. Abel EL, Kruger M. Physician attitudes concerning legal coercion of pregnant alcohol and drug abusers. *Am J Obstet Gynecol.* 2002;186(4):768-772.
156. American College of Obstetricians and Gynecologists. *Opposition to Criminalization of Individuals During Pregnancy and the Postpartum Period. Position Statement.* Accessed August 9, 2022. https://www.acog.org/clinical-information/policy-and-position-statements/statements-of-policy/2020/opposition-criminalization-of-individuals-pregnancy-and-postpartum-period
157. Children's Bureau/ACYF/ACF/HHS. *Child Maltreatment 2018.* The Administration for Children and Families. Accessed August 9, 2022. https://www.acf.hhs.gov/cb/report/child-maltreatment-2018
158. Lloyd Sieger MH. Reunification for young children of color with substance removals: an intersectional analysis of longitudinal national data. *Child Abuse Negl.* 2020;108. doi:10.1016/j.chiabu.2020.104664
159. Hill RB. Institutional racism in child welfare. *Race Soc.* 2004;7(1):17-33. doi:10.1016/j.racsoc.2004.11.004
160. Wildeman C, Edwards FR, Wakefield S. The cumulative prevalence of termination of parental rights for U.S. children, 2000-2016. *Child Maltreat.* 2020;25(1):32-42. doi:10.1177/1077559519848499
161. Child Welfare Information Gateway. *Parental Drug Use as Child Abuse.* U.S. Department of Health and Human Services, Children's Bureau; 2016.
162. Atkins DN, Durrance CP. State policies that treat prenatal substance use as child abuse or neglect fail to achieve their intended goals. *Health Aff (Millwood).* 2020;39(5):756-763. doi:10.1377/hlthaff.2019.00785
163. Schiff DM, Nielsen T, Terplan M, et al. Fatal and nonfatal overdose among pregnant and postpartum women in Massachusetts. *Obstet Gynecol.* 2018;132(2):466-474. doi:10.1097/AOG.0000000000002734
164. Metz TD, Rovner P, Hoffman MC, Allshouse AA, Beckwith KM, Binswanger IA. Maternal deaths from suicide and overdose in Colorado, 2004-2012. *Obstet Gynecol.* 2016;128(6):1233-1240. doi:10.1097/AOG.0000000000001695
165. Smid MC, Stone NM, Baksh L, et al. Pregnancy-associated death in utah: contribution of drug-induced deaths. *Obstet Gynecol.* 2019;133(6):1131-1140. doi:10.1097/AOG.0000000000003279
166. Goldman-Mellor S, Margerison CE. Maternal drug-related death and suicide are leading causes of postpartum death in California. *Am J Obstet Gynecol.* 2019;221(5):489.e1-489.e9. doi:10.1016/j.ajog.2019.05.045
167. Wilder C, Lewis D, Winhusen T. Medication assisted treatment discontinuation in pregnant and postpartum women with opioid use disorder. *Drug Alcohol Depend.* 2015;149:225-231. doi:10.1016/j.drugalcdep.2015.02.012
168. Clark HW. Residential substance abuse treatment for pregnant and postpartum women and their children: treatment and policy implications. *Child Welfare.* 2001;80(2):179-198.
169. Schauberger CW, Borgert AJ, Bearwald B. Continuation in treatment and maintenance of custody of newborns after delivery in women with opioid use disorder. *J Addict Med.* 2020;14(2):119-125. doi:10.1097/ADM.0000000000000534
170. Mattocks KM, Clark R, Weinreb L. Initiation and engagement with methadone treatment among pregnant and postpartum women. *Womens Health Issues.* 2017;27(6):646-651. doi:10.1016/j.whi.2017.05.002
171. Kelly PJ, Blacksin B, Mason E. Factors affecting substance abuse treatment completion for women. *Issues Ment Health Nurs.* 2001;22(3):287-304. doi:10.1080/01612840152053110
172. Faherty LJ, Kranz AM, Russell-Fritch J, et al. Association of punitive and reporting state policies related to substance use in pregnancy with rates of neonatal abstinence syndrome. *JAMA Netw Open.* 2019;2(11):e1914078. doi:10.1001/jamanetworkopen.2019.14078

173. Normile B, Hanlon C, Eichner H. *State Options for Promoting Recovery among Pregnant and Parenting Women with Opioid or Substance Use Disorder*. National Academy for State Health Policy; 2018.

174. Doris JL, Meguid V, Thomas M, Blatt S, Eckenrode J. Prenatal cocaine exposure and child welfare outcomes. *Child Maltreat*. 2006;11(4):326-337.

175. Nair P, Schuler ME, Black MM, Kettinger L, Harrington D. Cumulative environmental risk in substance abusing women: early intervention, parenting stress, child abuse potential and child development. *Child Abuse Negl*. 2003;27(9):997-1017.

176. Johnson JL, Leff M. Children of substance abusers: overview of research findings. *Pediatrics*. 1999;103(5 Pt 2):1085-1099.

177. Ingersoll KS, Lu IL, Haller DL. Predictors of in-treatment relapse in perinatal substance abusers and impact on treatment retention: a prospective study. *J Psychoactive Drugs*. 1995;27(4):375-387.

178. Kraft WK, Adeniyi-Jones SC, Chervoneva I, et al. Buprenorphine for the treatment of the neonatal abstinence syndrome. *N Engl J Med*. 2017;376(24):2341-2348.

Perioperative Management of Patients With Substance Use

Zoe M. Weinstein, Megan E. Buresh, and Daniel P. Alford

CHAPTER OUTLINE

- Introduction
- Perioperative care of the patient with unhealthy alcohol use
- Perioperative care of the patient with an opioid use disorder
- Perioperative care of the patient with benzodiazepine use disorder
- Perioperative care of the patient with nicotine use
- Perioperative care of the patient with cannabis use
- Perioperative care of the patient with stimulant use disorder
- High-risk surgeries in patients with substance use disorders
- Conclusions

INTRODUCTION

Surgery may be required for complications of alcohol and other drug use such as the management of traumatic injuries, infections of the skin, soft tissue, bones, and joints, infective endocarditis, and certain cancers. It is estimated that in the perioperative setting, one in five patients has an alcohol use disorder, one in three has a nicotine use disorder and one in ten patients has a another substance use disorder (SUD).[1]

Substance use and its associated chronic medical conditions can increase the risk of postoperative complications. Careful preoperative evaluation may detect clinical signs of chronic diseases secondary to alcohol or other drug use that increase surgical risk, such as diseases affecting the heart, lungs, kidney, liver, nervous system, and pancreas. In an older retrospective study of patients presenting with traumatic mandibular fractures in which two-thirds reported current or past alcohol or other drug use disorders, postoperative complications including wound infections and poor healing were up to five times more likely in groups with substance use compared to individuals who did not use substances.[2] Orthopedic surgery in patients with an active opioid use disorder was associated with an increased inpatient mortality and morbidity including respiratory failure, surgical site infection, pneumonia, myocardial infarction, and postoperative ileus.[3,4]

Hospitalization for surgery may be the first time that a patient with a SUD does not have access to alcohol or other drugs, putting them at risk for withdrawal. Acute withdrawal syndromes may complicate surgery and the postoperative course presenting as tachycardia, hypertension, anxiety, delirium, pain, and seizures. Therefore, providers of perioperative care must identify SUDs and be comfortable with the management of substance withdrawal syndromes.

The care of patients with SUDs is also complicated by a potential mutual distrust that exists between patients and their medical team, with physician fear of being deceived and patient fear of being mistreated and stigmatized.[5] In addition, patients may use substances to manage their pain and have their own beliefs about the safety of the use of substances or analgesics in the perioperative period, and thus this is a critical time for patient education.[6] Treating physicians should not expect to cure the patient's SUD during the perioperative hospitalization but should focus on getting the patient through the surgery safely and then offering the patient referral to long-term addiction treatment. This chapter focuses on relevant perioperative issues in the patient with alcohol or other substance use.

PERIOPERATIVE CARE OF THE PATIENT WITH UNHEALTHY ALCOHOL USE

Unhealthy alcohol use is common especially in patients seeking medical and surgical care.[7] The prevalence of alcohol use disorders is as high as 40% in emergency room and various surgical inpatient settings and up to 50% in patients with trauma.[8] Many chronic medical conditions that can complicate or necessitate surgery, including dilated cardiomyopathy, cirrhosis, pancreatitis, and oral and esophageal cancers, are attributable to alcohol. The incidence of symptomatic alcohol withdrawal in hospitalized patients is as high as 8% and is two to five times higher in hospitalized trauma and surgical patients.[9-11] Chronic alcohol use can increase the risk of postoperative mortality[12] and morbidity through immune suppression, reduced cardiac function, and dysregulated homeostasis including alterations in platelet production, aggregation, and changes in fibrinogen levels.[13,14] Preoperative alcohol use is an independent predictor of pneumonia, sepsis, superficial surgical site infection, wound complications, and longer hospital stays.[15] Postoperative complications appear to show a dose-response relationship with alcohol consumption, that is the more alcohol consumed, the higher risk for postoperative complications.[16] Therefore, universal preoperative screening for unhealthy alcohol use and withdrawal risk is important.

Preoperative Evaluation

In addition to a complete history and focused examination, the preoperative evaluation should assess for the risk of acute alcohol withdrawal and the presence of diseases associated with heavy alcohol use. Historically, physicians failed to identify alcohol use disorders. In one study, only 16% of people with alcohol use disorder were identified in the perioperative setting.[17] The amount of alcohol consumed is a risk factor for postoperative complications.[18] When screening for alcohol use disorders, it is important to remember that patients with unhealthy alcohol use are often asymptomatic and may minimize consumption. Quantity and frequency questions are essential but are generally not sensitive or specific for diagnosing an alcohol use disorder, except for specific items that have been validated for this purpose. Laboratory tests such as blood alcohol levels and liver function tests are not sensitive or specific.

Adults undergoing preoperative evaluation should be screened using validated questionnaires such as the single item screening question (SISQ), Alcohol Use Disorder Identification Test (AUDIT), or the AUDIT-C. The 3-item AUDIT-C can identify patients at risk for postoperative complications but also for increased postoperative health care utilization (ie, hospital length of stay, more ICU days).[19,20]

In the surgical setting, screening for risk of withdrawal and medical comorbidities are the priorities. Consider including one or more of the following questions regarding alcohol withdrawal in the preoperative evaluation:

- Have you ever gone through alcohol withdrawal, such as having tremor or the shakes?
- Have you ever had problems or gotten sick when you stopped drinking?
- Have you ever had a seizure, hallucinations, alcohol withdrawal delirium, or been confused after cutting down or stopping drinking?

The spectrum of withdrawal ranges from anxiety, mild tremor, hallucinosis, to seizures and delirium. In the postoperative period, withdrawal can mimic many postoperative complications including acute pain and sepsis. Risk factors associated with severe and prolonged alcohol withdrawal include amount and duration of alcohol use, multiple recurrent withdrawal episodes, older age, and co-occurring diseases.[21] It is also important to note that sedatives and analgesics given during surgery and the postoperative period may delay, partially treat, or obscure some symptoms of alcohol withdrawal. Use of other substances, (eg, benzodiazepines, stimulants) is common and should also be screened for.

Physical examination should evaluate for evidence of liver, pancreatic, nervous system, and cardiac disease. The spectrum of alcohol-associated liver disease ranges from fatty liver with normal or mild elevations in aminotransaminases to acute hepatitis and cirrhosis. Clinicians should look for evidence of cirrhosis including jaundice, palmar erythema, gynecomastia, spider telangiectasia, as well as findings consistent with portal vein hypertension, namely splenomegaly, ascites, hemorrhoids, and caput medusa (dilation of the periumbilical veins on the abdominal wall). Pancreatitis can present as acute and chronic abdominal pain as well as exocrine (ie, malabsorption) and endocrine dysfunction (ie, glucose intolerance). Alcohol-associated dementia, Korsakoff syndrome, hepatic and Wernicke encephalopathy, myelopathies, and polyneuropathies are nervous system disorders associated with long-term regular heavy alcohol use. These neurological conditions can worsen during the perioperative period and may be confused with other postoperative neurological complications. Therefore, preoperative baseline mental status and cognition should be assessed and well documented. Preoperative evaluation for congestive heart failure should be considered because up to one-third of patients with long-standing heavy alcohol use have a decreased cardiac ejection fraction.[22] Because of the association between heavy alcohol use/alcohol use disorders and nicotine use disorder, patients should also be evaluated for smoking-related comorbidities such as coronary heart disease and chronic obstructive pulmonary disease (COPD).

Preoperative laboratory studies should include electrolytes, liver function tests, coagulation studies, and a complete blood count. Anemia is common in patients with alcohol use disorders as well as decreased platelet count from alcohol-associated bone marrow suppression and splenic sequestration. Patients are at increased risk of perioperative bleeding secondary to coagulopathies and thrombocytopenia. It is also important to identify patients who are in remission from alcohol or other drug use preoperatively because they may have concerns and questions about perioperative exposure to sedative-hypnotics and opioid analgesics.

Management of Alcohol Withdrawal

One of the most common complications of hospitalized patients with alcohol use disorder is withdrawal. The spectrum of alcohol withdrawal ranges from minor symptoms of autonomic hyperactivity including diaphoresis, tachycardia, systolic hypertension to tremor, insomnia, hallucinations, nausea, vomiting, psychomotor agitation, anxiety, and grand mal seizures to life-threatening alcohol withdrawal delirium. Withdrawal symptoms may appear within hours of decreased intake; however, during the perioperative period, the administration of anesthetics, sedatives, and analgesics may delay the onset of withdrawal. Recognizing withdrawal risk and treating early withdrawal can prevent the complications of severe withdrawal. Because alcohol withdrawal is especially dangerous during the postoperative period, asymptomatic but at-risk patients should receive prophylactic treatment to prevent withdrawal. Although many medications have been used to treat alcohol withdrawal, benzodiazepines are the medications of choice for both the prevention and management of alcohol withdrawal.[23,24] For most patients, benzodiazepines with a long half-life such as diazepam or chlordiazepoxide should be chosen. However, patients with severe liver disease should receive shorter-acting agents that are not metabolized by hepatic oxidation (often impaired in severe liver disease), such as lorazepam, to avoid excessive and prolonged sedation.

Treatment of withdrawal should be based on the severity of symptoms and signs. The Clinical Institute Withdrawal Assessment Scale for Alcohol, revised, is a validated tool that can be used to rate the severity for alcohol withdrawal[25] however it may be difficult to use in the postoperative period in patients unable to verbally communicate and may be less reliable in patients with acute medical or surgical illnesses. Alternatively, for patients who are in severe withdrawal and unable to respond to questions, the Minnesota Detoxification Scale (MINDS) protocol could be used.[26] Goals for management of alcohol withdrawal include treatment of withdrawal symptoms, prevention of initial and recurrent seizures, and prevention and treatment of alcohol withdrawal delirium. Alcohol withdrawal is covered in more detail in Chapter 56, "Management of Alcohol Intoxication and Withdrawal."

Alcohol Use and Surgical Risk

In addition to alcohol withdrawal, observational studies have demonstrated that heavy alcohol use, even in the absence of clinical liver disease or alcohol use disorder per se, is an independent risk factor for postoperative complications. Higher rates of postoperative complications were seen after spinal surgery, transurethral prostatectomy, colonic surgery, and hysterectomy.[27-30] There is a dose-response effect, with increased alcohol consumption being associated with both increased postoperative complications and prolonged hospital stay. The most dramatic differences were in groups who drank more than 60 g of alcohol (>4 drinks) per day.[31] The postoperative complications reported were an increased rate of infection, bleeding, and delayed wound healing. Patients with alcohol use disorders also have longer intensive care unit stays, more postoperative septicemia, and pneumonia requiring mechanical ventilation as well as increased overall mortality.[32]

Five possible pathological mechanisms have been identified to account for the increased rate of postoperative complications including immune incompetence, subclinical cardiac insufficiency, hemostatic imbalances, abnormal stress response, and wound healing dysfunction.[9] Heavy alcohol use suppresses T-cell–dependent activity and decreases macrophage, monocyte, and neutrophil mobilization, and phagocytosis. The decreased cardiac function associated with heavy alcohol use is thought to be secondary to direct alteration in the electromechanical coupling and contractility of cardiac myocytes. This alcohol-associated cardiac dysfunction may be reversible, with 50% of patients showing improvement after 6 months of abstinence.[33] The hemostatic dysfunction in people with an alcohol use disorder is due to a modification in coagulation and fibrinolysis pathways as well as a decrease in the number and function of platelets. Wound healing problems seem related to poor accumulation of collagen.

Abstinence before surgery decreases postoperative morbidity. A meta-analysis of two small randomized clinical trials evaluating the effect of intensive preoperative alcohol abstinence interventions including pharmacological strategies showed a decrease of overall postoperative complications but no significant reduction of in-hospital and 30-day mortality rates.[34] It suggests that when possible, treatment of alcohol use disorder should occur preoperatively, with treatments proven to decrease alcohol use or achieve abstinence (eg, pharmacotherapies and proven psychosocial approaches).

Alcohol-Associated Liver Disease

The spectrum of liver disease associated with the spectrum of unhealthy alcohol use includes asymptomatic fatty liver, to acute hepatitis, and finally chronic cirrhosis. Each form of liver disease carries some degree of surgical risk and requires special preoperative considerations.

Fatty Liver

Alcohol-associated fatty liver (hepatic steatosis) occurs in 90% of heavy drinkers and is often asymptomatic and reversible. Signs and symptoms, when present, include nausea, vomiting, and right upper quadrant pain and tenderness. Laboratory tests often demonstrate a mild elevation in liver transaminases but with preserved liver synthetic function with normal bilirubin, albumin, and coagulation studies. These signs and symptoms usually resolve within 2 weeks of abstinence.[35] Patients with fatty liver seem to tolerate surgery well; however, there are no known studies evaluating perioperative risk in these patients. It is prudent to delay elective surgery until resolution of clinical signs and symptoms, and if possible, abstinence is achieved.

Hepatitis

Alcohol-associated hepatitis is a serious inflammatory disease of the liver, which occurs in up to 40% of people who drink heavily. The pathological mechanisms include hepatocyte swelling, liver infiltration with polymorphonuclear cells, and hepatocyte necrosis. Patients often present extremely ill with nausea, vomiting, anorexia, abdominal pain, fever, and jaundice. Elevated transaminases and prolonged coagulation studies are common. Surgical risk is very high in this group, with 100% mortality rates reported in older series.[36] Therefore, hepatitis should be considered a contraindication to elective surgery. It is recommended that elective surgery be delayed until clinical and laboratory parameters normalize, sometimes taking up to 12 weeks.

Cirrhosis

Cirrhosis occurs in 15% to 20% of individuals with heavy alcohol use and refers to the irreversible necrosis, nodular regeneration, and fibrosis of the liver. Cirrhosis is associated with abnormal hepatic circulation, resulting in portal vein hypertension. Clinically, patients may present with ascites, peripheral edema, poor nutritional status, muscle wasting, coagulopathies, gastrointestinal bleeding from esophageal varices, encephalopathy, and renal insufficiency as well as hypoxia secondary to hepatopulmonary syndrome and pulmonary hypertension. The need for surgery is common in patients with cirrhosis, with up to 10% requiring a surgical procedure during the last 2 years of life.[37]

Depending on the severity of cirrhosis, surgery can be extremely risky. The most common causes of perioperative mortality in patients with cirrhosis are sepsis, hemorrhage, and hepatorenal syndrome.[37] Although currently used anesthetic agents are not hepatotoxic, surgical stress, in itself, causes hemodynamic changes in the liver resulting in postoperative elevations in liver function tests in patients with no underlying liver disease.[38] Patients with underlying liver dysfunction are at increased risk for hepatic decompensation during surgical stress because anesthetic agents decrease hepatic blood flow by as much as 50% and therefore decrease hepatic oxygen uptake.[39] Intraoperative traction on abdominal viscera may also decrease hepatic blood flow.

Effect of Cirrhosis on Surgical Risk

Surgery in patients with cirrhosis is high risk. A study of patients undergoing total knee arthroplasty found that both local and systemic complications were as high as 44% in patients with cirrhosis versus 6% in a control group.[40] The preoperative factors associated with increased surgical morbidity and mortality include emergent surgery, upper abdominal surgery, poor hepatic synthetic function, anemia, ascites, malnutrition, and encephalopathy.[38] These patients are at increased risk for uncontrolled bleeding, infections, and delirium. Coagulopathies and thrombocytopenia result in difficult perioperative hemostasis. Ascites increases the risk of intra-abdominal infections, abdominal wound dehiscence, and abdominal wall herniation. Nutritional deficiencies result in poor wound healing and an increased risk of skin breakdown, and encephalopathy decreases the patient's ability to effectively participate in postoperative rehabilitation. The action of anesthetic agents may be prolonged and increases the risk of delirium.

Cholecystectomy is a particularly risky surgery in patients with cirrhosis and portal hypertension because of intra-abdominal collateral circulation. This collateral circulation increases the vascularity of the gallbladder bed and places the patient at greater risk for severe perioperative hemorrhage. In a group of patients with cirrhosis undergoing cholecystectomy, those considered decompensated preoperatively by the presence of ascites and prolonged coagulation studies had an 83% morality rate compared with 10% in compensated patients.[41]

In trying to risk stratify patients preoperatively, it is important to look for clinical signs of cirrhosis and portal hypertension. There are two scoring systems in use to predict whether patients with advanced liver disease will survive surgery.[42] In 1964, the Child and Turcotte Classification stratified patients with cirrhosis into three classes based on "hepatic reserve" and therefore surgical risk before portacaval shunt surgery.[43] Class A was the most compensated, whereas class C was the most decompensated group. Variables included laboratory values of bilirubin and albumin as well as clinical ascites, encephalopathy, and nutritional status. Garrison found good correlation between Child and Turcotte Classification and abdominal surgical mortality with class A, B, and C mortality rates of 10%, 31%, and 76%, respectively.[44] Some of the limitations of the Child and Turcotte Classification scheme included the subjective nature and interobserver variation in the assessment of nutritional status, encephalopathy, and ascites. In an attempt to decrease the subjective nature of the classification scheme, Pugh et al. modified the Child and Turcotte Classification[45] (**Table 99-1**). The Pugh modification separates hepatic encephalopathy into five grades depending on various signs and symptoms (**Table 99-2**). The subjective evaluation of nutritional status is changed to objective measured prolongation in prothrombin time and the assignment of class based on a total point score. Using pooled surgical data, the Pugh Classification scheme has proven to be a good preoperative risk stratifier (**Table 99-3**).

A second scoring system is the Model for End-Stage Liver Disease (MELD), which was designed to predict survival after transjugular intrahepatic portosystemic shunt treatment of bleeding esophageal varices.[46] The MELD score is used to prioritize patients for liver transplantation and, more recently, as a predictor of survival after nontransplant surgery.[47] The MELD score is calculated using the patient's international normalized ratio (INR) and serum creatinine and bilirubin. Because the MELD formula is complex, scores can be calculated using an online score calculator at http://www.unos.org/resources/meldpeldcalculator.asp.

TABLE 99-1 Pugh Classification (Modified Child and Turcotte Classification)

	Points		
	1	2	3
Encephalopathy (grade)	None	I-II	III-IV
Ascites	Absent	Slight	Moderate
Bilirubin (mg/dL)	1-2	2-3	>3
Albumin (g/dL)	>3.5	2.8-3.5	<2.8
Prothrombin time (seconds prolonged) or international normalized ratio	1-3 <1.7	4-6 1.7-2.3	>6 >2.3

Class A 5-6 points; Class B 7-9 points; Class C 10-15 points.

Adapted from Pugh RN, Murray-Lyon IM, Dawson JL, et al. Transection of the oesophagus for bleeding oesophageal varices. *Br J Surg.* 1973;60:646-649.

TABLE 99-2 Encephalopathy Grade

Encephalopathy Grade
Grade 0: normal
Grade I: consists of personality changes with altered sleep patterns (eg, sleep day-night reversal) and inappropriate behavior, constructional apraxia
Grade II: consists of mental confusion, disorientation to time and place, drowsiness, asterixis, and fetor hepaticus
Grade III: consists of severe mental confusion, stuporous but arousable, incoherent, asterixis, fetor hepaticus, rigidity, and hyperreflexia
Grade IV: consists of deep coma, unresponsive to stimuli, not arousable, decerebrate and decorticate posturing, fetor hepaticus, decreased muscle tone, and decreased reflexes

Adapted from Trey C, Burns DG, Saunders SJ. Treatment of hepatic coma by exchange blood transfusion. *N Engl J Med.* 1966;274:473-481.

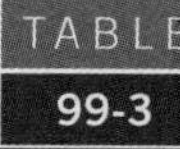

TABLE 99-3 Child Class, Operative Risk, and Operability

Child Class, Operative Risk, and Operability
Child A 2%-10% mortality risk • No limitation • Normal response to all operations • Normal ability of liver to regenerate
Child B 6%-31% mortality risk • Some limitation in liver function • Altered response to all operations but good tolerance with preparation
Child C 20%-76% mortality risk • Severe limitation of liver function • Poor response to all operations regardless of preparation

Adapted from Stone HH. Preoperative and postoperative care. *Surg Clin North Am.* 1977;57(2):409-419. Copyright 1977, with permission from Elsevier.

Preoperative Considerations in Patients With Cirrhosis

Preoperative abstinence should be the goal before all elective procedures. Since coagulopathies may develop as a result of vitamin K deficiency due to malnutrition or intestinal bile salt deficiency, attempts at correction should start with the administration of vitamin K. If there is no effect in 12 hours, it is most likely secondary to decreased hepatic production of coagulation factors, and perioperative use of fresh frozen plasma should be considered. Thrombocytopenia secondary to bone marrow suppression, hypersplenism, and splenic sequestration should be considered for preoperative prophylactic platelet transfusions when counts fall below 50,000/mm^3.[48] In addition, units of packed red blood cells should be on hold in the blood bank.

Ascites secondary to portal hypertension and hypoalbuminemia can impede abdominal wall healing, increase the risk of abdominal wall dehiscence and herniation, and restrict effective mechanical ventilation. Therefore, ascites should be optimally managed preoperatively with sodium restriction and appropriate diuretic therapy. In patients with peripheral edema, a more aggressive approach including large-volume paracentesis (≥5 L) should be considered. Electrolytes should be monitored closely. Perioperative hemodynamic monitoring is often needed because these patients may have large fluid shifts, especially during abdominal surgeries.

Preoperative antibiotic prophylaxis against secondary and spontaneous bacterial peritonitis may be appropriate. Perioperative changes in volume status and hemodynamics may adversely affect renal function, which should be monitored closely. These patients are at risk for renal insufficiency secondary to prerenal azotemia as well as developing hepatorenal syndrome. Any potential nephrotoxic agent should be used with extreme caution. Many perioperative conditions can exacerbate hepatic encephalopathy such as gastrointestinal bleeding, constipation, azotemia, hypoxia, and the use of sedatives. Aggressive preoperative treatment of hepatic encephalopathy using lactulose and dietary protein restriction is recommended. Patients with known gastroesophageal varices should be monitored closely for gastrointestinal bleeding and should be considered for beta-blocker prophylaxis preoperatively.

The nutritional status of patients with cirrhosis is usually poor, and they are often deficient in thiamine, folate, vitamin C, and B vitamins. Nutritional status should be optimized with multivitamins, thiamine, folate, and nutritional supplementation preoperatively. From a pulmonary standpoint, patients with decompensated cirrhosis may desaturate because of the development of pulmonary shunts in hepatopulmonary syndrome; therefore, continuous monitoring oxygen saturation should be part of the postoperative care. There is increasing evidence that laparoscopic procedures in patients with cirrhosis may be safer than open procedures regardless of Child Classification.[44] Patients with cirrhosis undergoing surgery may benefit from a multidisciplinary approach including a hepatologist (and nephrologist if the patient has renal insufficiency).

Bariatric Surgery and the Risk of Alcohol-Related Problems

There is now strong empirical evidence showing that individuals who undergo bariatric surgery are at an elevated risk of developing alcohol-related problems, ranging from increased alcohol use to alcohol use disorder (AUD) and alcohol-related liver disease. The prevalence of AUD at 1-year postbariatric surgery is similar to the rate in the general population, but exceeds the general population over time with over 16% meeting criteria for AUD 7 years following surgery.[49] The increased risk for AUD is likely multifactorial including alterations in alcohol absorption.[50] Another controversial hypothesis is related to an addiction transfer from food to alcohol and that patients may have previously used food as a coping strategy and increase alcohol use as an alternative to consuming food.[51]

Preoperative risk factors for postoperative problematic alcohol use include younger adults, higher preoperative alcohol use, depression and maladaptive eating patterns, including emotional eating and purging.[50]

Management of Patients on Naltrexone (Opioid Antagonist) Pharmacotherapy

Patients with AUD treated with naltrexone (oral daily or depot monthly) pharmacotherapy are becoming more common. Because naltrexone is an opioid antagonist and will block the effects of co-administered opioid agonists, patients requiring opioid analgesics during the perioperative period will need to discontinue naltrexone.[52] The half-life of a single dose of oral naltrexone is 14 hours. The recommendation that oral naltrexone be discontinued at least 72 hours before surgery is based on experimental studies showing that 50% of the oral naltrexone blockade effect was gone after 72 hours.[53] Because a degree of opioid resistance will remain, patients should be observed closely for respiratory depression and sedation. After intramuscular depot injection of naltrexone, peak plasma levels occur within 2 to 3 days with a decline in plasma concentrations beginning approximately 14 days after dosing. For patients on depot naltrexone, elective surgery should be postponed, if possible, for a month after the last naltrexone injection. Patients requiring opioids for pain management after emergent surgery should have naltrexone discontinued and opioids analgesics administered under close observation. Animal studies have shown that naltrexone blockade can be overcome resulting in analgesia and no significant respiratory depression or sedation with either hydrocodone or fentanyl at 10 to 20 times the usual doses.[54] An anesthesiologist should be consulted to assist with perioperative pain management including the use of nonopioid alternatives and regional analgesia.

Naltrexone can be restarted when the patient no longer requires opioid analgesics. In order to avoid precipitating opioid withdrawal, patients must be opioid free for a minimum of 7 to 10 days before restarting naltrexone if they are physically dependent on opioids. This opioid-free time period may be longer if patients are taking extended-release/long-acting opioids. However, if patients have only been briefly on opioids in the postoperative period and are not physically dependent, providers may consider resuming naltrexone treatment within 24 to 48 hours after the last short-acting analgesic opioid medication. If there is concern for precipitated withdrawal, a naloxone challenge can be performed using naloxone before naltrexone administration.[55]

PERIOPERATIVE CARE OF THE PATIENT WITH AN OPIOID USE DISORDER

The goal during the perioperative period is to get the patient with an opioid use disorder (OUD) safely through the surgical period and presents an opportunity to engage patients in treatment. Persons with OUD are at high risk for complications that require surgical intervention. Most of these complications are a consequence of both active and past high-risk practices such as lack of access to sterile injection equipment among people who inject drugs, and the direct toxic effects of the drug and additives being injected. Infections of the skin, soft tissue, bones, and joints are common and often require surgical drainage and debridement. Infectious endocarditis may require emergent or urgent heart valve replacement. Functional bowel obstruction has also been described in patients with chronic opioid use and may require surgical management. Acute hepatitis B and chronic hepatitis C infections are common in patients with injection drug use and are among leading causes of liver disease requiring transplantation.[56] Chronic diseases associated with risky opioid use, such as pulmonary hypertension secondary to talc granulomatosis, renal insufficiency secondary to heroin-associated nephropathy, HIV, chronic hepatitis B and C, and congestive heart failure from valvular heart disease secondary to endocarditis, can all increase surgical risk. Acute opioid withdrawal can also complicate the perioperative period.

Preoperative Evaluation

Patients with current or past injection drug use should be evaluated for past endocarditis and the need for antibiotic prophylaxis. They should also be evaluated for HIV and active hepatitis B and C. Hospitalized patients with OUD are at risk for acute opioid withdrawal. The onset and severity of withdrawal will depend on which opioid is being used and on the degree of physical dependence, which is related to the duration and amount used. Daily use for at least 2 to 3 weeks is generally required before significant physical dependence (and thus clinically significant withdrawal) occurs. Withdrawal from heroin and short-acting prescription opioids typically begins within 4 to 6 hours of the time of last use. Withdrawal from extended-release, long-acting opioids such as methadone and sustained-release oxycodone and morphine may not occur for up to 24 to 36 hours. Fentanyl withdrawal is more unpredictable due to its high lipophilicity and slow distribution from tissues into the plasma. Active opioid use can be verified using urine drug tests. Heroin and other semisynthetic opioids will be detected as morphine or codeine in the urine for up to 72 hours. Synthetic opioids (such as methadone and fentanyl) are not always included in standard urine drug tests, so if synthetic opioid use is suspected, the laboratory should be asked to test for the specific synthetic opioid of concern. Depending on the opioid used, acute withdrawal usually peaks at 2 to 3 days and can last for up to 14 days. The Clinical Opiate Withdrawal Scale (54)[57] and the Short Opiate Withdrawal Scale (55)[58] are useful clinical opioid withdrawal assessment instruments.

Management of Opioid Withdrawal

Opioid withdrawal can be effectively treated using a long-acting opioid agonist such as methadone or buprenorphine.[59]

Adjunctive medications such as clonidine, antiemetics and antimotility agents can be used to treat physiological manifestations of opioid withdrawal while buprenorphine or methadone is taking effect. A starting dose of 10 to 30 mg of methadone orally or 2 to 4 mg of buprenorphine sublingually lessens the signs and symptoms of withdrawal in most patients. The patient should be reassessed for continued withdrawal in 2 to 3 hours; if withdrawal persists, additional doses of 5 to 10 mg of methadone or 2 to 4 mg of buprenorphine may be given; total dose during the first 24 hours should typically not exceed 40 mg of methadone or 16 mg of buprenorphine, unless an addiction specialist familiar with these medications is consulted. Patients using illicitly-manufactured fentanyl and its analogs may be at higher risk of precipitated withdrawal from buprenorphine up to 24 to 48 hours after last fentanyl use and may be better treated using methadone or a low-dose buprenorphine initiation strategy.[60] Opioid withdrawal is covered in more detail in Chapter 58.

After a stable dose of opioid agonist has been achieved, it should be given daily to prevent the reemergence of withdrawal. It is important to openly discuss this treatment plan with the patient and nursing staff to avoid unnecessary anxiety and conflict between the patient and health care team. If the patient on methadone is unable to take oral medications during the perioperative period, methadone can be administered parenterally (IV, SQ, or IM) at 50% of the total daily oral dose administered in a divided dose every 12 hour (eg, 40 mg by mouth every day = 10 mg IV every 12 hours).[61-63]

After acute withdrawal is controlled, discuss with the patient continued daily dosing (recommended) versus daily dose taper until the day of discharge. For patients desiring continuation of medication, further up-titration of buprenorphine and methadone can continue during the perioperative period. All patients should be offered continuation of medication postoperatively with active linkage to ongoing treatment posthospitalization.

Low-Dose Buprenorphine Initiation

Traditionally, starting buprenorphine requires abstinence from all full-agonist opioids and waiting until patients experience opioid withdrawal prior to giving first buprenorphine dose to avoid precipitated withdrawal. However, in the perioperative setting, many patients require ongoing opioids for pain. Low-dose buprenorphine initiation[64] involves administering small and gradually increasing doses of buprenorphine while continuing a full-agonist opioid.[64,65] Thus, patients can start buprenorphine without experiencing opioid withdrawal. Low-dose initiation can be considered for patients with recent fentanyl or methadone use and those receiving ongoing opioids for pain. To date, evidence for low-dose initiation is based on case series and retrospective reviews. There are published inpatient protocols using a variety of buprenorphine formulations with initial doses equivalent to 0.2 to 0.5 mg SL with gradually increasing doses over 3 to 7 days.[66-68] When available, low-dose initiation is best done with the assistance of an addiction specialist.

Management of Patients on Medications for Opioid Use Disorders

Patients may be maintained on opioid *agonist* therapy (OAT) with methadone or buprenorphine or on opioid *antagonist* therapy with naltrexone. Patients on OAT should be maintained on their usual maintenance dose equivalent during the perioperative period and treated with additional full agonist opioids as needed for perioperative analgesia. The correct maintenance dose should be determined by calling the patient's methadone program or buprenorphine prescriber. Buprenorphine dose may also be verified through prescription drug monitoring programs (PDMP). Patients treated with naltrexone maintenance will need to discontinue naltrexone preoperatively to achieve benefit from postoperative opioid analgesics. The patient's addiction treatment program or physician prescriber should be notified at time the patient is discharged from the hospital to assure continuity of addiction care. Some methadone-maintained patients who have impaired mobility postoperatively may be eligible for additional take-home doses of methadone from their addiction treatment provider. Due to varying clinic policies, this should be arranged directly with opioid treatment program clinic staff.

Management of Acute Pain in Patients on Opioid Agonist Therapy

Management of acute postoperative pain in patients maintained on long-acting OAT can be challenging; however, recommendations have been published[69-72] (**Tables 99-4** and **99-5**). The daily methadone or buprenorphine dose a patient receives will not provide analgesia for acute pain. Patients on

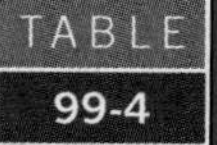
TABLE 99-4 General Principles for Pain Management in Patients With Opioid Use Disorder

- Reassure the patient that addiction history will not prevent adequate pain management.
- Use conventional analgesics, including opioids, to aggressively treat the painful condition.
- Utilize multimodal pain management with nonopioid medications (NSAID, acetaminophen, epidural/spinal analgesia, nerve blocks) as indicated.
- Continue the usual dose (or equivalent) of opioid agonist.
- Opioid cross-tolerance and patient's increased pain sensitivity will necessitate higher opioid analgesic doses at shorter intervals.
- Write for continuous scheduled dosing rather than as needed orders.
- At maximum, patient should be on one long-acting opioid (eg, methadone, buprenorphine, morphine sulfate) and one short-acting opioid for breakthrough pain (eg, hydromorphone, oxycodone).
- Avoid using mixed agonist/antagonist opioids as they will precipitate an acute withdrawal syndrome.
- All patients who can take PO should be preferentially given oral opioids instead of IV.
- Outpatient treatment providers should be notified of medications received in hospital that may impact follow-up drug test results.

TABLE 99-5 Specific Recommendations for Management of Pain and Opioid Use Disorder Pharmacotherapy

Home medication	Management of OUD	Pain management: Mild pain (pain score 4 or less)	Pain management: Moderate to severe pain (pain score 5 or greater)	Discharge planning
Buprenorphine	Continue buprenorphine at home dose	1) Start with nonopioid analgesics 2) Split buprenorphine dose into Q6-8h dosing; can increase total daily dose up to 32 mg	**Add ONE short-acting full agonist opioid (eg, oxycodone, hydromorphone) for breakthrough pain** (if buprenorphine is given first, giving additional opioids will NOT precipitate withdrawal) Higher doses of opioids will be needed compared to opioid-naive patients (eg, oxycodone 15-20 mg PO instead of 5-10 mg) Pain control should be re-assessed after every dose	Patient's outpatient buprenorphine prescriber should be contacted prior to discharge with the following goals: (1) to notify of opioids received while in hospital; (2) arrange for follow-up appointment; and (3) inform of any dose changes and if patient will be discharged on additional opioids for pain An X-waivered buprenorphine prescriber will need to write a discharge prescription to bridge to their next outpatient appointment
Methadone	Confirm methadone dose with outpatient methadone program and continue at home dose	Start with nonopioid analgesia Consider splitting total daily methadone dose into two or three times daily dosing Patient's methadone program should be contacted prior to any methadone dose changes		Prior to discharge, patient's methadone clinic should be contacted to resume dosing and to ensure that there will not be any gaps in receiving methadone. Methadone prescriptions for opioid use disorder cannot be written on discharge. Methadone may only be dispensed for up to 72 hours if provider has specific DEA exception[a]
Naltrexone	STOP naltrexone	No opioids should be given for pain until oral naltrexone has been stopped for 3 days	Higher than usual doses of opioids may be attempted to overcome naltrexone's opioid antagonist effects. This must be done with continuous pulse oximetry with close observation for respiratory depression	Prior to discharge, patient's outpatient naltrexone prescriber should be notified of opioids prescribed and planned duration in order to plan re-initiation of naltrexone
Not on medication for opioid use disorder as outpatient	**Offer patient methadone or buprenorphine to manage opioid deficit** (reminder—buprenorphine must be given prior to full agonist opioids for pain and patient must be in withdrawal from any street opioids used prior to first dose of buprenorphine to avoid precipitating withdrawal)	1) Start with nonopioid analgesics 2) Split buprenorphine dose into Q6-8h dosing; can increase total daily dose up to 32 mg	**Choose ONE short-acting full agonist opioid (eg, oxycodone, hydromorphone) for breakthrough pain** (if buprenorphine is given first, giving additional opioids will NOT precipitate withdrawal)	If patient desires to continue buprenorphine maintenance on discharge or to be linked to methadone, outpatient follow-up should be arranged, and plan made for interim prescription Patient should be discharged with no more than 1- to 2-week supply of opioids for pain and will need close outpatient follow-up

From Drug Enforcement Agency. *DEA's Commitment to Expanding Access to Medication-Assisted Treatment*. Accessed May 13, 2022. https://www.dea.gov/press-releases/2022/03/23/deas-commitment-expanding-access-medication-assisted-treatment; Drug Enforcement Agency. *Instructions to Request Exception to 21CFR1306.07*. Published online March 23, 2022. https://www.deadiversion.usdoj.gov/drugreg/Instructions-to-request-exception-to-21CFR1306.07(b)-3-day-rule-(EO-DEA248)-Clean.pdf

OAT have high tolerance to other opioids and often require higher and more frequent doses of opioid analgesics to adequately treat acute pain. Both methadone and buprenorphine have long plasma half-lives (15-40 hours), with different durations of action for analgesia (4-8 hours) and for suppression of opioid withdrawal (24-36 hours). The appropriate treatment of acute pain in these patients includes uninterrupted OAT to address the patient's baseline opioid requirement for addiction treatment and providing additional medication for aggressive pain management. Continuing the usual dose of OAT avoids worsening pain symptoms because of the increased pain sensitivity associated with opioid withdrawal. While it has been accepted practice to continue methadone perioperatively, there has been debate about whether to continue or discontinue buprenorphine preoperatively.[69] Preclinical and clinical studies now suggest that concurrent use of opioid analgesics in patients maintained on buprenorphine is effective[73-76] and is associated with decreased perioperative pain scores,[77,78] and decreased need for opioid prescription on discharge.[77] Despite this, there continue to be high rates of perioperative buprenorphine dose holds.[79]

To decrease anxiety, patients should be reassured that their OUD treatment will continue and their pain will be aggressively treated. As with all patients suffering acute pain, multimodal pain management and nonopioid analgesics should be aggressively implemented first line. However, patients with moderate to severe acute pain will often require opioid analgesics. Because of cross-tolerance with OAT, adequate pain control will generally necessitate higher opioid doses at shorter intervals. Analgesic dosing should be continuous or scheduled rather than as needed. Allowing pain to reemerge before administering the next analgesic dose causes unnecessaryf suffering and anxiety and increases tension between patient and treatment team. In these cases, one short-acting opioid should be chosen (eg, oxycodone or hydromorphone), with consideration that higher doses will be needed compared to opioid-naive patients (eg, oxycodone 10-20 mg every 4 hours or hydromorphone 4-6 mg every 4 hours for patients tolerating oral medications, or equivalent IV dose if not able to take oral medications) with reassessment of pain control after every dose until adequate analgesia is achieved. Clinical experience supports consideration of PCA use in patients on OAT with increased patient control over analgesia minimizing patient anxiety over pain management. In a retrospective cohort study of patients with OUD on buprenorphine or methadone maintenance, there was no significant correlation between first 24-hour PCA usage and preoperative buprenorphine or methadone dose.[74] Patients who did not receive baseline buprenorphine or methadone dose on day after surgery required longer duration of PCA.

Mixed agonist/antagonist opioid analgesics such as pentazocine and butorphanol must be avoided because they may displace the methadone or buprenorphine from the mu receptor, thus precipitating acute opioid withdrawal in these patients. Racial disparities for treatment of acute pain is well-documented, with particularly poor pain treatment for Black patients.[80] In order to decrease these disparities, providers should examine their own racial bias and strive to standardize pain treatment for all patients.

Management of Acute Pain in Patients on Opioid Antagonist Therapy

Patients with OUD treated with naltrexone (oral daily and depot monthly) maintenance therapy are becoming more common. See section above entitled "Management of Patients on Naltrexone (Opioid Antagonist) Pharmacotherapy" for guidance on acute pain management of patients maintained on naltrexone.

PERIOPERATIVE CARE OF THE PATIENT WITH BENZODIAZEPINE USE DISORDER

Benzodiazepines, which are commonly prescribed to treat panic attacks, anxiety, and insomnia, have a high potential for risky use. Patients who use benzodiazepines in a risky manner often use other substances.[81] Benzodiazepine use has been associated with increased risk for postoperative adverse events,[82] including higher rates of postoperative mechanical ventilation and intensive care requirements among trauma surgery patients.[83] Chronic benzodiazepine use can result in physical dependence, with an acute withdrawal syndrome that can be life threatening. The withdrawal syndrome ranges from severe anxiety, insomnia, and autonomic hyperactivity (including tachycardia and hypertension) to seizures and delirium.

Patients with physical dependence to prescribed benzodiazepines should be maintained on their usual dose during the perioperative period to prevent acute withdrawal and subsequent postoperative complications. Patients physically dependent on illicit benzodiazepines should be maintained on an equivalent dose of long-acting benzodiazepine (eg, diazepam, chlordiazepoxide) during the perioperative period with psychiatric and addiction specialist consultation for guidance on a safe benzodiazepine taper during the postoperative period, noting that patients physically dependent on long-acting benzodiazepines may not exhibit withdrawal symptoms for 5 to 7 days after the last dose.

PERIOPERATIVE CARE OF THE PATIENT WITH NICOTINE USE

People who currently smoke tobacco have a 1.38 times higher likelihood of 30-day postoperative mortality compared to people who have never smoked. People who currently smoke also have greater odds of postoperative cardiovascular events (ie, cardiac arrest, myocardial infarction, stroke), infections (ie, pneumonia, incision infections, sepsis), and unplanned intubation.[84] Risk for pulmonary infections is increased due to abnormalities in their respiratory epithelium leading to retained secretions and abnormal lung immune responses.[85]

Healing is impaired because of decreased tissue oxygenation and inhibition of normal immune responses. A 20-pack-year history and smoking more than 20 cigarettes a day seem to be the threshold of this increased risk. In observational studies of patients undergoing cardiothoracic surgery, the increased risk decreases only after 8 weeks after stopping smoking and was unrelated to pulmonary function test results.[86] Preoperative evaluation should include assessment of physical dependence on nicotine and risk of withdrawal. In addition, preoperative evaluation should include assessment for evidence of cardiovascular disease and COPD. Patients with COPD have increased risk of postoperative pulmonary complications, including pneumonia, respiratory failure with prolonged mechanical ventilation, and COPD exacerbations.[87]

Preoperative interventions for nicotine/tobacco use have been shown to reduce the incidence of postoperative complications.[88] Pharmacotherapy, including nicotine replacement, bupropion, and varenicline, consistently increases abstinence rates and should be considered preoperatively.[89] Nicotine replacement therapy also should be offered postoperatively to patients at risk for nicotine withdrawal.

PERIOPERATIVE CARE OF THE PATIENT WITH CANNABIS USE

Compared with tobacco, the airway effects of smoking cannabis are mild, but with acute use, upper airway edema can occur and a chronic cough and mild airflow obstruction can develop with long-term use.[90] However, cannabis use has not to date been associated with negative surgical outcomes, and a small cohort study of trauma patients showed that those who had cannabis positive toxicology were less likely to need vasopressors intraoperatively.[91] Patients with occasional cannabis use may have lower pain preoperatively,[92] and occasional use of cannabis has not be shown to impact long-term postoperative outcomes.[93] However, patients with a cannabis use disorder may experience dysphoria or other withdrawal symptoms with prolonged hospitalization and may have worse pain and increased risk of infection in the postoperative period.[94,95] Thus, not only screening for use, but for physiological dependence and a use disorder may be beneficial for perioperative counseling.

PERIOPERATIVE CARE OF THE PATIENT WITH STIMULANT USE DISORDER

Cocaine and methamphetamine may be ingested, snorted, smoked, injected, or taken rectally. Injection stimulant use may result in all the complications attributable to injection drug use such as endocarditis, pulmonary hypertension, hepatitis, and HIV. Stimulants negatively impact the immune system via multiple mechanisms, including inducing oxidative stress, increasing inflammatory cytokines and causing break down of the body's physical and chemical barriers allowing for microbial translocation.[96,97] Acute stimulant intoxication can be a life-threatening condition because of excessive adrenergic stimulation and vasospasm resulting in acute psychosis, hypertensive crisis, hyperthermia, arrhythmias, seizures, bowel ischemia, myocardial infarction, and cerebrovascular accident. Patients who use stimulants may require surgical interventions due to the acute and chronic effects of these drugs. Methamphetamine use may lead to traumatic injuries, severe periodontal disease, chemical burns, and skin abscesses from compulsive skin picking. Smoked stimulants can increase surgical risk by causing pulmonary edema.

Long-term stimulant use can result in medical conditions that increase surgical risk such as cardiac dysfunction from myocardial infarction or dilated cardiomyopathy. Up to 7% of asymptomatic people who chronically use cocaine have left ventricular systolic dysfunction,[98] while young people who use methamphetamine were found to have a 3.7-fold increased odds of cardiomyopathy.[99] Left ventricular hypertrophy is a known risk factor for ventricular arrhythmias.[100,101] Therefore, it is critically important to identify stimulant use during preoperative assessment and to evaluate carefully for clinical evidence of cardiac disease.

Concurrent use of cocaine and alcohol is common, because alcohol prolongs the effects of cocaine through the metabolite cocaethylene. Cocaethylene increases the rate of cardiac complications. Therefore, all patients who use cocaine should be screened for concurrent alcohol use. The period of cocaine intoxication is generally brief (~60 minutes) and should not increase the risk of most surgery. However, methamphetamine's longer half-life of 12 hours could adversely affect emergent surgical procedures. Intoxicated patients should be placed in a calm and quiet environment and managed with sedatives such as benzodiazepines. Depression and hypersomnolence are common in stimulant withdrawal and may mimic or be confused with other postoperative neurological complications.

HIGH-RISK SURGERIES IN PATIENTS WITH SUBSTANCE USE DISORDERS

Organ Transplant

Hepatitis B and C infections from injection drug use and alcohol-associated liver disease are the most common causes of end-stage liver disease requiring liver transplantation in the United States. In the past, patients with a history of substance use disorder have been kept off transplantation lists because of fears of posttransplant nonadherence, with subsequent loss of graft but also because of moralistic arguments that the patients had "self-inflicted" diseases. Some studies have demonstrated posttransplant recurrence of use rates as high as 49%, with lower overall survival rates in patients who failed to complete addiction treatment.[102] This has resulted in the widely used "6-month abstinence" rule despite a lack of evidence validating its use in predicting recurrence of use.[103] Other studies found no difference in 1-year survival rate between patients with alcohol use disorders who maintained sobriety and patients who had no history of an alcohol use disorder.[104] Among people with alcohol use disorders selected for liver transplant, most (71%) abstained or nearly completely abstained.[105] A study identified preoperative risk factors that were predictive of recurrence of use after transplantation that included shorter length of abstinence before transplantation, greater than one episode of alcohol withdrawal before transplantation, younger age at time of transplantation, and an alcohol use disorder in first-degree relatives.[106] Patients with a current or past SUDs need to be offered treatment for their SUD, assessed for risk of recurrence of use and social support systems before transplantation. Addiction specialists should be part of the transplant team. A history of SUD or active treatment, including treatment with methadone or buprenorphine, should not be a reason to decline a patient from transplant listing; indeed doing so is a violation of the American with Disabilities Act. Additionally, transplant teams should be vigilant about how provider bias and systemic racism impact patient care. Black patients are more likely to be denied a liver transplant compared to White patients due to cited concerns about substance use,[107] even though on a population level Black people are less likely to have a SUD.[108]

Valve Surgery for Endocarditis

The diagnosis of endocarditis is associated with a 20% short-term and 37% long-term mortality[109] and growing rates of hospitalization, especially related to injection drug use.[110] Early surgical intervention has been shown to reduce morbidity and mortality[111]; however, surgery may be delayed or withheld due to concerns about postoperative substance use.[112(p201),113] There is no evidence to support withholding life-saving surgery due to history of or active substance use, and "treatment contracts" or other punitive mechanisms should be actively discouraged.[114,115] Multidisciplinary endocarditis teams can increase the proportion of patients to receive guideline-concordant care (including surgery), significantly reducing mortality and addressing stigma toward people who inject drugs.[116,117] The use of multidisciplinary teams is now explicitly recommended in multiple endocarditis treatment guidelines.[118,119] In addition, initiation of treatment for SUDs is critical, but often neglected.[120] Being on medication for opioid use disorder substantially improved mortality among patients with endocarditis and opioid use disorder.[121]

CONCLUSIONS

Patients with substance use disorders have high rates of hospitalization and surgery. The underlying history of addiction may not be apparent initially, but thorough history-taking and the use of effective screening tools can elicit information about past or current drug and alcohol use disorders. Careful evaluation also can detect clinical signs of chronic diseases of the heart, lungs, and liver related to drug and alcohol use. The importance of identifying addiction preoperatively cannot be overstated. Perioperative morbidity associated with acute withdrawal syndromes can be prevented with proper preoperative treatment. If possible, elective surgery should be postponed allowing for completion of substance withdrawal. Sedative-hypnotics and opioid analgesics should be used as indicated perioperatively; however, these drugs have a risk of harmful use in patients with addiction, so they should be prescribed with caution. Management of patients with addiction going for surgery often requires consultation with addiction and pain specialists. All patients with current addiction should be offered and encouraged to engage in addiction treatment perioperatively. Providers should advocate that all patients receive medically necessary care and be vigilant for stigma impacting a patient's ability to get necessary surgery.

REFERENCES

1. Kork F, Neumann T, Spies C. Perioperative management of patients with alcohol, tobacco and drug dependency. *Curr Opin Anesthesiol.* 2010;23(3):384-390. doi:10.1097/ACO.0b013e3283391f79
2. Passeri LA, Ellis E, Sinn DP. Relationship of substance abuse to complications with mandibular fractures. *J Oral Maxillofac Surg.* 1993;51(1):22-25. doi:10.1016/s0278-2391(10)80383-0
3. Menendez ME, Ring D, Bateman BT. Preoperative opioid misuse is associated with increased morbidity and mortality after elective orthopaedic surgery. *Clin Orthop.* 2015;473(7):2402-2412. doi:10.1007/s11999-015-4173-5
4. Sodhi N, Anis HK, Acuña AJ, et al. Opioid use disorder is associated with an increased risk of infection after total joint arthroplasty: a large database study. *Clin Orthop Relat Res.* 2020;478(8):1752-1759. doi:10.1097/CORR.0000000000001390
5. Merrill JO, Rhodes LA, Deyo RA, Marlatt GA, Bradley KA. Mutual mistrust in the medical care of drug users. *J Gen Intern Med.* 2002;17(5):327-333. doi:10.1046/j.1525-1497.2002.10625.x
6. Fernandez AC, Lin LA, Bazzi AR, Boissoneault J, Borsari B, Blow F. Beliefs about perioperative opioid and alcohol use among elective surgical patients who report unhealthy drinking: a qualitative study. *Pain Med.* 2021;22(10):2384-2392. doi:10.1093/pm/pnab104
7. Saitz R. Unhealthy alcohol use. *N Engl J Med.* 2005;352(6):596-607. doi:10.1056/NEJMcp042262
8. D'Onofrio G, Bernstein E, Bernstein J, et al. Patients with alcohol problems in the emergency department, Part 1: improving detection. *Acad Emerg Med.* 1998;5(12):1200-1209. doi:10.1111/j.1553-2712.1998.tb02696.x
9. Spies C, Tønnesen H, Andreasson S, Helander A, Conigrave K. Perioperative morbidity and mortality in chronic alcoholic patients. *Alcohol Clin Exp Res.* 2001;25(5 Suppl ISBRA):164S-170S. doi:10.1097/00000374-200105051-00028
10. Foy A, Kay J. The incidence of alcohol-related problems and the risk of alcohol withdrawal in a general hospital population. *Drug Alcohol Rev.* 1995;14(1):49-54. doi:10.1080/09595239500185051
11. Gordon AJ, Olstein J, Conigliaro J. Identification and treatment of alcohol use disorders in the perioperative period. *Postgrad Med.* 2006;119(2):46-55. doi:10.3810/pgm.2006.07.1743
12. Masoomi H, Kang CY, Chen A, et al. Predictive factors of in-hospital mortality in colon and rectal surgery. *J Am Coll Surg.* 2012;215(2):255-261. doi:10.1016/j.jamcollsurg.2012.04.019
13. Tønnesen H. Influence of alcohol on several physiological functions and its reversibility: a surgical view. *Acta Psychiatr Scand Suppl.* 1992;369:67-71.

14. Zhang P, Bagby GJ, Happel KI, Raasch CE, Nelson S. Alcohol abuse, immunosuppression, and pulmonary infection. *Curr Drug Abuse Rev.* 2008;1(1):56-67. doi:10.2174/1874473710801010056
15. Nath B, Li Y, Carroll JE, Szabo G, Tseng JF, Shah SA. Alcohol exposure as a risk factor for adverse outcomes in elective surgery. *J Gastrointest Surg.* 2010;14(11):1732-1741. doi:10.1007/s11605-010-1350-4
16. Tønnesen H, Nielsen PR, Lauritzen JB, Møller AM. Smoking and alcohol intervention before surgery: evidence for best practice. *Br J Anaesth.* 2009;102(3):297-306. doi:10.1093/bja/aen401
17. Mehta AJ. Alcoholism and critical illness: a review. *World J Crit Care Med.* 2016;5(1):27-35. doi:10.5492/wjccm.v5.i1.27
18. Tønnesen H, Petersen KR, Højgaard L, et al. Postoperative morbidity among symptom-free alcohol misusers. *Lancet.* 1992;340(8815):334-337. doi:10.1016/0140-6736(92)91405-w
19. Rubinsky AD, Sun H, Blough DK, et al. AUDIT-C alcohol screening results and postoperative inpatient health care use. *J Am Coll Surg.* 2012;214(3):296-305.e1. doi:10.1016/j.jamcollsurg.2011.11.007
20. Bradley KA, Rubinsky AD, Sun H, et al. Alcohol screening and risk of postoperative complications in male va patients undergoing major non-cardiac surgery. *J Gen Intern Med.* 2011;26(2):162-169. doi:10.1007/s11606-010-1475-x
21. Saitz R. Recognition and management of occult alcohol withdrawal. *Hosp Pract 1995.* 1995;30(6):49-54, 56-58. doi:10.1080/21548331.1995.11443214
22. Regan TJ. Alcohol and the cardiovascular system. *JAMA.* 1990; 264(3):377-381. doi:10.1001/jama.1990.03450030101041
23. Pace CA, Samet JH. Substance use disorders. *Ann Intern Med.* 2016;164(7):ITC49. doi:10.7326/AITC201604050
24. Mayo-Smith MF, Beecher LH, Fischer TL, et al. Management of alcohol withdrawal delirium: an evidence-based practice guideline. *Arch Intern Med.* 2004;164(13):1405-1412. doi:10.1001/archinte.164.13.1405
25. Sullivan JT, Sykora K, Schneiderman J, Naranjo CA, Sellers EM. Assessment of alcohol withdrawal: the revised clinical institute withdrawal assessment for alcohol scale (CIWA-Ar). *Br J Addict.* 1989;84(11):1353-1357.
26. DeCarolis DD, Rice KL, Ho L, Willenbring ML, Cassaro S. Symptom-driven lorazepam protocol for treatment of severe alcohol withdrawal delirium in the intensive care unit. *Pharmacotherapy.* 2007;27(4):510-518. doi:10.1592/phco.27.4.510
27. Tønnesen H, Schütten BT, Tollund L, Hasselqvist P, Klintorp S. Influence of alcoholism on morbidity after transurethral prostatectomy. *Scand J Urol Nephrol.* 1988;22(3):175-177. doi:10.1080/00365599.1988.11690408
28. Felding C, Jensen LM, Tønnesen H. Influence of alcohol intake on postoperative morbidity after hysterectomy. *Am J Obstet Gynecol.* 1992;166(2):667-670. doi:10.1016/0002-9378(92)91695-7
29. Blood AG, Sandoval MF, Burger E, Halverson-Carpenter K. Risk and protective factors associated with surgical infections among spine patients. *Surg Infect.* 2017;18(3):234-249. doi:10.1089/sur.2016.183
30. Amri R, Dinaux AM, Kunitake H, Bordeianou LG, Berger DL. Risk stratification for surgical site infections in colon cancer. *JAMA Surg.* 2017;152(7):686-690. doi:10.1001/jamasurg.2017.0505
31. Tonnesen H, Kehlet H. Preoperative alcoholism and postoperative morbidity. *Br J Surg.* 1999;86(7):869-874. doi:10.1046/j.1365-2168.1999.01181.x
32. Jensen NH, Dragsted L, Christensen JK, Jørgensen JC, Qvist J. Severity of illness and outcome of treatment in alcoholic patients in the intensive care unit. *Intensive Care Med.* 1988;15(1):19-22. doi:10.1007/BF00255630
33. Vecchia LL, Bedogni F, Bozzola L, Bevilacqua P, Ometto R, Vincenzi M. Prediction of recovery after abstinence in alcoholic cardiomyopathy: role of hemodynamic and morphometric parameters. *Clin Cardiol.* 1996;19(1):45-50. doi:10.1002/clc.4960190109
34. Oppedal K, Møller AM, Pedersen B, Tønnesen H. Preoperative alcohol cessation prior to elective surgery. *Cochrane Database Syst Rev.* 2012;7):CD008343: doi:10.1002/14651858.CD008343.pub2
35. Rizvon MK, Chou CL. Surgery in the patient with liver disease. *Med Clin North Am.* 2003;87(1):211-227. doi:10.1016/s0025-7125(02)00153-0
36. Greenwood SM, Leffler CT, Minkowitz S. The increased mortality rate of open liver biopsy in alcoholic hepatitis. *Surg Gynecol Obstet.* 1972;134(4):600-604.
37. Patel T. Surgery in the patient with liver disease. *Mayo Clin Proc.* 1999;74(6):593-599. doi:10.4065/74.6.593
38. Friedman LS. Surgery in the patient with liver disease. *Trans Am Clin Climatol Assoc.* 2010;121:192-205.
39. Cowan RE, Jackson BT, Grainger SL, Thompson RPH. Effects of anesthetic agents and abdominal surgery on liver blood flow. *Hepatology.* 1991;14(6):1161-1166. doi:10.1002/hep.1840140634
40. Shih LY, Cheng CY, Chang CH, Hsu KY, Hsu RWW, Shih HN. Total knee arthroplasty in patients with liver cirrhosis. *J Bone Joint Surg Am.* 2004;86(2):335-341. doi:10.2106/00004623-200402000-00017
41. Aranha GV, Sontag SJ, Greenlee HB. Cholecystectomy in cirrhotic patients: a formidable operation. *Am J Surg.* 1982;143(1):55-60. doi:10.1016/0002-9610(82)90129-5
42. Suman A, Carey WD. Assessing the risk of surgery in patients with liver disease. *Cleve Clin J Med.* 2006;73(4):398-404.
43. Child CG, Turcotte JG. Surgery and portal hypertension. *Major Probl Clin Surg.* 1964;1:1-85.
44. Garrison RN, Cryer HM, Howard DA, Polk HC. Clarification of risk factors for abdominal operations in patients with hepatic cirrhosis. *Ann Surg.* 1984;199(6):648-655. doi:10.1097/00000658-198406000-00003
45. Pugh RN, Murray-Lyon IM, Dawson JL, Pietroni MC, Williams R. Transection of the oesophagus for bleeding oesophageal varices. *Br J Surg.* 1973;60(8):646-649. doi:10.1002/bjs.1800600817
46. Malinchoc M, Kamath PS, Gordon FD, Peine CJ, Rank J, ter Borg PCJ. A model to predict poor survival in patients undergoing transjugular intrahepatic portosystemic shunts. *Hepatology.* 2000;31(4):864-871. doi:10.1053/he.2000.5852
47. Suman A, Barnes DS, Zein NN, Levinthal GN, Connor JT, Carey WD. Predicting outcome after cardiac surgery in patients with cirrhosis: a comparison of Child-Pugh and MELD scores. *Clin Gastroenterol Hepatol.* 2004;2(8):719-723. doi:10.1016/S1542-3565(04)00296-4
48. Kaufman RM, Djulbegovic B, Gernsheimer T, et al. Platelet Transfusion: a clinical practice guideline from the AABB. *Ann Intern Med.* 2015;162(3):205-213. doi:10.7326/M14-1589
49. Miller-Matero LR, Hamann A, LaLonde L, et al. Predictors of alcohol use after bariatric surgery. *J Clin Psychol Med Settings.* 2021;28(3):596-602. doi:10.1007/s10880-020-09751-3
50. Ivezaj V, Benoit S, Davis J, et al. Changes in alcohol use after metabolic and bariatric surgery: predictors and mechanisms. *Curr Psychiatry Rep.* 2019;21(9):85. doi:10.1007/s11920-019-1070-8
51. Steffen KJ, Engel SG, Wonderlich JA, Pollert GA, Sondag C. Alcohol and other addictive disorders following bariatric surgery: prevalence, risk factors and possible etiologies. *Eur Eat Disord Rev.* 2015;23(6):442-450. doi:10.1002/erv.2399
52. Vickers AP, Jolly A. Naltrexone and problems in pain management. *BMJ.* 2006;332(7534):132-133. doi:10.1136/bmj.332.7534.132
53. Verebey K. The clinical pharmacology of naltrexone: pharmacology and pharmacodynamics. *NIDA Res Monogr.* 1981;28:147-158.
54. Dean RL, Todtenkopf MS, Deaver DR, et al. Overriding the blockade of antinociceptive actions of opioids in rats treated with extended-release naltrexone. *Pharmacol Biochem Behav.* 2008;89(4):515-522. doi:10.1016/j.pbb.2008.02.006
55. Sullivan MA, Garawi F, Bisaga A, et al. Management of relapse in naltrexone maintenance for heroin dependence. *Drug Alcohol Depend.* 2007;91(2-3):289-292. doi:10.1016/j.drugalcdep.2007.06.013
56. Aranda-Michel J, Dickson RC, Bonatti H, Crossfield JR, Keaveny AP, Vasquez AR. Patient selection for liver transplant: 1-year experience with 555 patients at a single center. *Mayo Clin Proc.* 2008;83(2):165-168. doi:10.4065/83.2.165
57. Wesson DR, Ling W. The clinical opiate withdrawal scale (COWS). *J Psychoactive Drugs.* 2003;35(2):253-259. doi:10.1080/02791072.2003.10400007
58. Gossop M. The development of a short opiate withdrawal scale (SOWS). *Addict Behav.* 1990;15(5):487-490. doi:10.1016/0306-4603(90)90036-W

59. Donroe JH, Holt SR, Tetrault JM. Caring for patients with opioid use disorder in the hospital. *CMAJ*. 2016;188(17-18):1232-1239. doi:10.1503/cmaj.160290
60. Varshneya NB, Thakrar AP, Hobelmann JG, Dunn KE, Huhn AS. Evidence of buprenorphine-precipitated withdrawal in persons who use fentanyl. *J Addict Med*. 2022;16(4):e265-e268. doi:10.1097/ADM.0000000000000922
61. Shaiova L, Berger A, Blinderman CD, et al. Consensus guideline on parenteral methadone use in pain and palliative care. *Palliat Support Care*. 2008;6(2):165-176. doi:10.1017/S1478951508000254
62. McPherson MLM. *Demystifying Opioid Conversion Calculations: A Guide for Effective Dosing*. American Society of Health-System Pharmacists; 2010.
63. Kornick CA, Kilborn MJ, Santiago-Palma J, et al. QTc interval prolongation associated with intravenous methadone. *Pain*. 2003;105(3):499-506.
64. Hämmig R, Kemter A, Strasser J, et al. Use of microdoses for induction of buprenorphine treatment with overlapping full opioid agonist use: the Bernese method. *Subst Abuse Rehabil*. 2016;7:99-105. doi:10.2147/SAR.S109919
65. De Aquino JP, Parida S, Sofuoglu M. The pharmacology of buprenorphine microinduction for opioid use disorder. *Clin Drug Investig*. 2021;41(5):425-436. doi:10.1007/s40261-021-01032-7
66. Cohen SM, Weimer MB, Levander XA, Peckham AM, Tetrault JM, Morford KL. Low dose initiation of buprenorphine: a narrative review and practical approach. *J Addict Med*. 2022;16(4):399-406. doi:10.1097/ADM.0000000000000945
67. Button D, Hartley J, Robbins J, Levander XA, Smith NJ, Englander H. Low-dose buprenorphine initiation in hospitalized adults with opioid use disorder: a retrospective cohort analysis. *J Addict Med*. 2022;16(2):e105-e111. doi:10.1097/ADM.0000000000000864
68. Bhatraju EP, Klein JW, Hall AN, et al. Low dose buprenorphine induction with full agonist overlap in hospitalized patients with opioid use disorder: a retrospective cohort study. *J Addict Med*. 2022;16(4):461-465. doi:10.1097/ADM.0000000000000947
69. Alford DP, Compton P, Samet JH. Acute pain management for patients receiving maintenance methadone or buprenorphine therapy. *Ann Intern Med*. 2006;144(2):127-134.
70. Hickey T, Abelleira A, Acampora G, et al. Perioperative buprenorphine management: a multidisciplinary approach. *Med Clin North Am*. 2022;106(1):169-185. doi:10.1016/j.mcna.2021.09.001
71. Veazie S, Mackey K, Peterson K, Bourne D. Managing acute pain in patients taking medication for opioid use disorder: a rapid review. *J Gen Intern Med*. 2020;35(Suppl 3):945-953. doi:10.1007/s11606-020-06256-5
72. Alford DP. Chapter 12: Acute and chronic pain. In: Renner JA, Levounis P, LaRose AT, eds. *Office-Based Buprenorphine Treatment of Opioid Use Disorder*. 2nd ed. American Psychiatric Association Publishing, Inc; 2018.
73. Vilkins AL, Bagley SM, Hahn KA, et al. Comparison of post-cesarean section opioid analgesic requirements in women with opioid use disorder treated with methadone or buprenorphine. *J Addict Med*. 2017;11(5):397-401. doi:10.1097/ADM.0000000000000339
74. Macintyre PE, Russell RA, Usher KAN Gaughwin M, Huxtable CA. Pain relief and opioid requirements in the first 24 hours after surgery in patients taking buprenorphine and methadone opioid substitution therapy. *Anaesth Intensive Care*. 2013;41(2):222-230.
75. Jones HE, O'Grady K, Dahne J, et al. Management of acute postpartum pain in patients maintained on methadone or buprenorphine during pregnancy. *Am J Drug Alcohol Abuse*. 2009;35(3):151-156. doi:10.1080/00952990902825413
76. Niel JCG van, Schneider J, Tzschentke TM. Efficacy of full μ-opioid receptor agonists is not impaired by concomitant buprenorphine or mixed opioid agonists/antagonists—preclinical and clinical evidence. *Drug Res*. 2016;66(11):562-570. doi:10.1055/s-0042-109393
77. Quaye A, Potter K, Roth S, Acampora G, Mao J, Zhang Y. Perioperative continuation of buprenorphine at low–moderate doses was associated with lower postoperative pain scores and decreased outpatient opioid dispensing compared with buprenorphine discontinuation. *Pain Med*. 2020;21(9):1955-1960. doi:10.1093/pm/pnaa020
78. Komatsu R, Nash M, Peperzak KA, Wu J, Dinges EM, Bollag LA. Postoperative pain and opioid dose requirements in patients on sublingual buprenorphine: a retrospective cohort study for comparison between postoperative continuation and discontinuation of buprenorphine. *Clin J Pain*. 2022;38(2):108-113. doi:10.1097/AJP.0000000000000996
79. Wyse JJ, Herreid-O'Neill A, Dougherty J, et al. Perioperative management of buprenorphine/naloxone in a large, national health care system: a retrospective cohort study. *J Gen Intern Med*. 2022;37(12):2998-3004. doi:10.1007/s11606-021-07118-4
80. Meghani SH, Byun E, Gallagher RM. Time to Take Stock: a meta-analysis and systematic review of analgesic treatment disparities for pain in the United States. *Pain Med*. 2012;13(2):150-174. doi:10.1111/j.1526-4637.2011.01310.x
81. Moro RN, Geller AI, Weidle NJ, et al. Emergency department visits attributed to adverse events involving benzodiazepines, 2016-2017. *Am J Prev Med*. 2020;58(4):526-535. doi:10.1016/j.amepre.2019.11.017
82. Gaulton TG, Wunsch H, Gaskins LJ, et al. Preoperative sedative–hypnotic medication use and adverse postoperative outcomes. *Ann Surg*. 2021;274(2):e108. doi:10.1097/SLA.0000000000003556
83. Cheng V, Inaba K, Johnson M, et al. The impact of pre-injury controlled substance use on clinical outcomes after trauma. *J Trauma Acute Care Surg*. 2016;81(5):913-920. doi:10.1097/TA.0000000000001229
84. Turan A, Mascha EJ, Roberman D, et al. Smoking and perioperative outcomes. *Anesthesiology*. 2011;114(4):837-846. doi:10.1097/ALN.0b013e318210f560
85. Chalon J, Tayyab MA, Ramanathan S. Cytology of respiratory epithelium as a predictor of respiratory complications after operation. *Chest*. 1975;67(1):32-35. doi:10.1378/chest.67.1.32
86. Warner MA, Offord KP, Warner ME, Lennon RL, Conover MA, Jansson-schumacher U. Role of preoperative cessation of smoking and other factors in postoperative pulmonary complications: a blinded prospective study of coronary artery bypass patients. *Mayo Clin Proc*. 1989;64(6):609-616. doi:10.1016/S0025-6196(12)65337-3
87. Hong CM, Galvagno SM. Patients with chronic pulmonary disease. *Med Clin North Am*. 2013;97(6):1095-1107. doi:10.1016/j.mcna.2013.06.001
88. Thomsen T, Villebro N, Møller AM. Interventions for preoperative smoking cessation. *Cochrane Database Syst Rev*. 2014;2014(3):CD002294. doi:10.1002/14651858.CD002294.pub4
89. Webb AR, Coward L, Meanger D, Leong S, White SL, Borland R. Offering mailed nicotine replacement therapy and Quitline support before elective surgery: a randomised controlled trial. *Med J Aust*. 2022;216(7):357-363. doi:10.5694/mja2.51453
90. Moran S, Thorndike AN, Armstrong K, Rigotti NA. Physicians' missed opportunities to address tobacco use during prenatal care. *Nicotine Tob Res*. 2003;5(3):363-368. doi:10.1080/1462220031000094150
91. Yeung BG, Ma MW, Scolaro JA, Nelson AM. Cannabis exposure decreases need for blood pressure support during general anesthesia in orthopedic trauma surgery. *Cannabis Cannabinoid Res*. 2022;7(3):328-335. doi:10.1089/can.2021.0009
92. Medina SH, Nadarajah V, Jauregui JJ, et al. Orthopaedic surgery patients who use recreational marijuana have less pre-operative pain. *Int Orthop*. 2019;43(2):283-292. doi:10.1007/s00264-018-4101-x
93. Albelo FD, Baker M, Zhang T, et al. Impact of pre-operative recreational marijuana use on outcomes two years after orthopaedic surgery. *Int Orthop*. 2021;45(10):2483-2490. doi:10.1007/s00264-021-05069-3
94. Wiseman LK, Mahu IT, Mukhida K. The effect of preoperative cannabis use on postoperative pain following gynaecologic oncology surgery. *J Obstet Gynaecol Can*. 2022;44(7):750-756. doi:10.1016/j.jogc.2022.01.018
95. Weisberg MD, Ng MK, Magruder ML, Vakharia RM, Roche MW, Erez O. The association of cannabis use disorder and perioperative complications after primary total knee arthroplasty. *J Am Acad Orthop Surg*. 2022;30(7):313-320. doi:10.5435/JAAOS-D-21-00703
96. Salamanca SA, Sorrentino EE, Nosanchuk JD, Martinez LR. Impact of methamphetamine on infection and immunity. *Front Neurosci*. 2015;8:445. doi:10.3389/fnins.2014.00445

97. Volpe GE, Ward H, Mwamburi M, et al. Associations of cocaine use and HIV infection with the intestinal microbiota, microbial translocation, and inflammation. *J Stud Alcohol Drugs*. 2014;75(2):347-357.
98. Bertolet BD, Freund G, Perchalski DL, Pepine CJ, Martin CA, Williams CM. Unrecognized left ventricular dysfunction in an apparently healthy cocaine abuse population. *Clin Cardiol*. 1990;13(5):323-328. doi:10.1002/clc.4960130505
99. Yeo KK, Wijetunga M, Ito H, et al. The association of methamphetamine use and cardiomyopathy in young patients. *Am J Med*. 2007;120(2):165-171. doi:10.1016/j.amjmed.2006.01.024
100. Lange RA, Hillis LD. Cardiovascular complications of cocaine use. *N Engl J Med*. 2001;345(5):351-358. doi:10.1056/NEJM200108023450507
101. Afonso L, Mohammad T, Thatai D. Crack whips the heart: a review of the cardiovascular toxicity of cocaine. *Am J Cardiol*. 2007;100(6):1040-1043. doi:10.1016/j.amjcard.2007.04.049
102. Stowe J, Kotz M. Addiction medicine in organ tansplantation. *Prog Transplant Aliso Viejo Calif*. 2001;11(1):50-57. doi:10.7182/prtr.11.1.n86031643h5n248p
103. Shawcross DL, O'Grady JG. The 6-month abstinence rule in liver transplantation. *The Lancet*. 2010;376(9737):216-217. doi:10.1016/S0140-6736(10)60487-4
104. Starzl TE, Van Thiel D, Tzakis AG, et al. Orthotopic liver transplantation for alcoholic cirrhosis. *JAMA J Am Med Assoc*. 1988;260(17):2542-2544.
105. DiMartini A. Natural history of alcohol use disorders in liver transplant patients. *Liver Transpl*. 2007;13(S2):S76-S78. doi:10.1002/lt.21342
106. Perney P, Bismuth M, Sigaud H, et al. Are preoperative patterns of alcohol consumption predictive of relapse after liver transplantation for alcoholic liver disease? *Transpl Int*. 2005;18(11):1292-1297. doi:10.1111/j.1432-2277.2005.00208.x
107. DeBlasio RN, Myaskovsky L, DiMartini AF, et al. The combined roles of race/ethnicity and substance use in predicting likelihood of kidney transplantation. *Transplantation*. 2022;106(4):e219-e233. doi:10.1097/TP.0000000000004054
108. Center for Behavioral Health Statistics and Quality. *Racial/Ethnic Differences in Substance Use, Substance Use Disorders, and Substance Use Treatment Utilization Among People Aged 12 or Older (2015-2019)*. SAMHSA; 2021. Accessed June 27, 2023. https://www.samhsa.gov/data/sites/default/files/reports/rpt35326/2021NSDUHSUChartbook102221B.pdf
109. Abegaz TM, Bahagavathula AS, Gebreyohannes EA, Mekonnen AB, Abebe TB. Short- and long-term outcomes in infective endocarditis patients: a systematic review and meta-analysis. *BMC Cardiovasc Disord*. 2017;17:291. doi:10.1186/s12872-017-0729-5
110. Wurcel AG, Anderson JE, Chui KKH, et al. Increasing infectious endocarditis admissions among young people who inject drugs. *Open Forum Infect Dis*. 2016;3(3):ofw157. doi:10.1093/ofid/ofw157
111. Kang DH, Kim YJ, Kim SH, et al. Early surgery versus conventional treatment for infective endocarditis. *N Engl J Med*. 2012;366(26):2466-2473. doi:10.1056/NEJMoa1112843
112. Hull SC, Jadbabaie F. When is enough enough? The dilemma of valve replacement in a recidivist intravenous drug user. *Ann Thorac Surg*. 2014;97(5):1486-1487. doi:10.1016/j.athoracsur.2014.02.010
113. Hayden M, Moore A. Attitudes and approaches towards repeat valve surgery in recurrent injection drug use-associated infective endocarditis: a qualitative study. *J Addict Med*. 2020;14(3):217-223. doi:10.1097/ADM.0000000000000558
114. Wurcel AG, Yu S, Pacheco M, Warner K. Contracts with people who inject drugs following valve surgery: unrealistic and misguided expectations. *J Thorac Cardiovasc Surg*. 2017;154(6):2002. doi:10.1016/j.jtcvs.2017.07.020
115. DiMaio JM, Salerno TA, Bernstein R, Araujo K, Ricci M, Sade RM. Ethical obligation of surgeons to noncompliant patients: can a surgeon refuse to operate on an intravenous drug-abusing patient with recurrent aortic valve prosthesis infection? *Ann Thorac Surg*. 2009;88(1):1-8. doi:10.1016/j.athoracsur.2009.03.088
116. Carrasco-Chinchilla F, Sánchez-Espín G, Ruiz-Morales J, et al. Influence of a multidisciplinary alert strategy on mortality due to left-sided infective endocarditis. *Rev Espanola Cardiol Engl Ed*. 2014;67(5):380-386. doi:10.1016/j.rec.2013.09.010
117. El-Dalati S, Cronin D, Riddell J, et al. The clinical impact of implementation of a multidisciplinary endocarditis team. *Ann Thorac Surg*. 2022;113(1):118-124. doi:10.1016/j.athoracsur.2021.02.027
118. Habib G, Lancellotti P, Antunes MJ, et al. 2015 ESC guidelines for the management of infective endocarditis: The Task Force for the Management of Infective Endocarditis of the European Society of Cardiology (ESC) Endorsed by: European Association for Cardio-Thoracic Surgery (EACTS), the European Association of Nuclear Medicine (EANM). *Eur Heart J*. 2015;36(44):3075-3128. doi:10.1093/eurheartj/ehv319
119. Pettersson GB, Coselli JS, Pettersson GB, et al. 2016 The American Association for Thoracic Surgery (AATS) consensus guidelines: surgical treatment of infective endocarditis: executive summary. *J Thorac Cardiovasc Surg*. 2017;153(6):1241-1258.e29. doi:10.1016/j.jtcvs.2016.09.093
120. Rosenthal ES, Karchmer AW, Theisen-Toupal J, Castillo RA, Rowley CF. Suboptimal addiction interventions for patients hospitalized with injection drug use-associated infective endocarditis. *Am J Med*. 2016;129(5):481-485. doi:10.1016/j.amjmed.2015.09.024
121. Kimmel SD, Walley AY, Li Y, et al. Association of treatment with medications for opioid use disorder with mortality after hospitalization for injection drug use-associated infective endocarditis. *JAMA Netw Open*. 2020;3(10):e2016228. doi:10.1001/jamanetworkopen.2020.16228

SECTION

12

Co-occurring Addiction and Other Psychiatric Disorders

Associate Editor: Richard N. Rosenthal
Lead Section Editor: Edward V. Nunes
Section Editor: R. Jeffrey Goldsmith

CHAPTER

100 Substance-Induced Mental Disorders

Mark H. Duncan, R. Jeffrey Goldsmith, Matthew Iles-Shih, and Richard K. Ries

CHAPTER OUTLINE

- Introduction
- Diagnosis of substance-induced mental disorders
- Prevalence and course of substance-induced mental disorders
- Specific substances: substance-induced symptoms
- Diagnosing substance-induced mental disorders
- Treatment of substance-induced mental disorders
- Conclusions

INTRODUCTION

The focus of this chapter is to help clinicians understand, differentially diagnose, and treat a person with substance-induced psychiatric syndromes that mimic traditional psychiatric disorders such as depression, anxiety, and psychotic disorders. Because there is often overlap between the pharmacodynamics of potentially addictive substances as well as many psychiatric disorders, it should not be surprising that many patients with substance use disorders (SUDs) (including withdrawal) may appear to have a free-standing psychiatric disorder or at least appear to have significant psychiatric symptoms.

The revised chapter of "Substance-Related and Addictive Disorders" in the fifth edition of the *Diagnostic and Statistical Manual of Mental Disorders* (DSM-5) of the American Psychiatric Association[1] includes changes to grouping of the disorders so that substance-induced disorders are discussed in general terms in the chapter "Substance-Related and Addictive Disorders," while the specific substance-induced psychiatric disorder is discussed in the chapter discussing that specific disorder (ie, substance-induced depressive disorder (SIDD) is found in the chapter on Depressive Disorders). In addition, there are two additional substance-induced psychiatric disorders in DSM-5: Substance-Induced Bipolar and Related Disorder (SIBD) and Substance-Induced Obsessive-Compulsive and Related Disorder (SIOCD).

This chapter in the DSM-5 describes the diagnostic criteria in the DSM-5, reviews the epidemiological data, and discusses the clinical strategies needed to manage these disorders. Eleven substance-induced mental disorders (SIMDs) are outlined:

- Substance/Medication-Induced Delirium
- Substance/Medication-Induced Major or Mild Neurocognitive Disorder
  - □ Nonamnestic-Confabulatory Type
  - □ Amnestic-Confabulatory Type
- Substance/Medication-Induced Persisting Amnestic Disorder
- Substance/Medication-Induced Psychotic Disorder
- Substance/Medication-Induced Depressive Disorder
- Substance/Medication-Induced Bipolar and Related Disorder
- Substance/Medication-Induced Anxiety Disorder
- Substance/Medication-Induced Obsessive-Compulsive and Related Disorder
- Hallucinogen Persisting Perception Disorder
- Substance/Medication-Induced Sexual Dysfunction
- Substance/Medication-Induced Sleep Disorder

Here, we will focus on those that are most confounding in terms of differential *psychiatric* presentation (substance-induced depression, anxiety, psychotic, bipolar, OCD, and neurocognitive disorders). These will be referred to as substance-induced mental disorders (SIMD). We will also highlight substance-induced suicidal behavior, due to the risk and frequency of suicidal behavioral in the context of substance use. However, substance-induced suicidal behavior is not a separate diagnosis in the DSM-5. Substance-induced disorders that are not the focus of this chapter include Substance/Medication-Induced Delirium, Substance-Induced Sexual Dysfunction, and Substance-Induced Sleep Disorder.

DIAGNOSIS OF SUBSTANCE-INDUCED MENTAL DISORDERS

According to DSM-5, there are several classes of chemicals that may induce mental disorders as well as a variety of toxins and medications. The addictive substances that can induce mental disorders are alcohol, cannabis, phencyclidine (PCP) and other hallucinogens/dissociatives, inhalants, opioids, sedative-hypnotic/anxiolytic drugs, stimulants, caffeine, and tobacco (nicotine). In the DSM-5,[1] there are five (A-E) criteria for diagnosis of all substance/medication-induced mental disorders:

A. The disorder represents a clinically significant symptomatic presentation of a relative mental disorder.
B. There is evidence from history, physical examination, or laboratory findings of both of the following:
   1. The disorder developed during or within 1 month of a substance intoxication or withdrawal or taking a medication.

2. The involved substance/medication is capable of producing the mental disorder.

C. The disorder is not better explained by an independent mental disorder. Such evidence of an independent mental disorder could include the following:
1. The disorder preceded the onset of severe intoxication or withdrawal or exposure to a medication.
2. The full mental disorder persisted for a substantial period of time (eg, at least 1 month) after the cessation of acute withdrawal or severe intoxication or taking the medication. This criterion does not apply to substance-induced neurocognitive disorders or Hallucinogen Persisting Perception Disorder, which persist beyond the cessation of acute intoxication or withdrawal.

D. The disorder does not occur exclusively during the course of a delirium.

E. The disorder causes clinically significant distress or impairment in social, occupational, or other important areas of functioning.

The International Classification of Diseases (ICD) constitutes another widely used diagnostic classification system published by the World Health Organization (WHO). The ICD is now in its eleventh revision (ICD-11), approved by the World Health Assembly in 2019. It includes a series of "substance-induced mental disorders," each explicitly defined in relation to the specific substance producing the syndrome.

PREVALENCE AND COURSE OF SUBSTANCE-INDUCED MENTAL DISORDERS

Substance-Induced Depressive Disorder

Alcohol and Substance-Induced Depressive Disorder

People with an alcohol use disorder are 2.3 times as likely to have a major depressive disorder in the past year than those without an alcohol use disorder.[2] Depressive disorders appear commonly in treatment-seeking adults. In a study looking at nearly 3,000 treatment-seeking patients with alcohol dependence per the DSM-III R, 15.2% were found to have a primary Major Depressive Disorder, and 26% were found to have a substance-induced disorder.[3] In comparison, a general national survey of over 40,000 respondents from 2004, where 9% were reported to have any substance use disorder, and less than 1% were found to have a substance-induced depressive disorder.[2]

The course of symptoms between a substance induced depressive disorder and a primary depressive disorder is notably different. In a study of treatment-seeking men with an average of 9 days of abstinence leading into the study, 42% endorsed moderate to severe depressive symptoms at the beginning of treatment.[4] By the 2nd week, only 12% of subjects were still depressed and by the 4th week only 6% remained depressed, demonstrating that most substance-induced depressive symptoms will resolve fairly quickly with abstinence. In contrast, Ramsey et al. studied AUD patients with SIDD and found that over a course of a year, 26.4% of those diagnosed with SIDD were reclassified as having an independent MDD because of meeting full criteria for the diagnosis of MDD after 1 month of sobriety.[5] In this study, those with a history of past independent MDD were five times more likely to be reclassified from SIDD to independent MDD. Patients who had lower severity of DSM-IV alcohol dependence were also more likely to be reclassified as having independent MDD.

Stimulants and Substance-Induced Depressive Disorder

The prevalence of cocaine-induced depressive disorder is not clear, but studies of treatment-seeking patients with a cocaine use disorder have classified 30% to 60% with a lifetime cocaine-induced depressive disorder.[6,7] In a study of 160 patients in a treatment facility that used the Psychiatric Research Interview for Substance and Mental Diseases for evaluation, 38.7% of the sample who had a co-occurring lifetime depressive episode met criteria for a primary major depressive disorder, and 61.3% who had a co-occurring lifetime depressive episode met criteria for a cocaine-induced major depressive episode.[7] In an older study of 298 patients in treatment-seeking adults at an addiction clinic, around 30% of the sample were reported to have depressive disorders that remitted within 10 days of cocaine abstinence.[6]

People with methamphetamine use disorders are also reported to have high rates of depressive symptoms and suicidal behavior during active use as well as during withdrawal and early abstinence. Among a large study of psychiatric symptoms among 1,016 methamphetamine users presenting for treatment, 57% reported some depressive symptoms that ranged from mild to severe, and 27% had attempted suicide in the past.[8] In a 3-year follow-up study of 526 participants of the original cohort, 15.2% were eventually diagnosed with a major depressive disorder.[9] Those found to have a major depressive disorder were found to have worse outcomes in employment, substance use, and other psychiatric symptoms. Another study looking at 400 treatment-seeking participants with methamphetamine use disorder diagnosed 40% with a major depressive disorder on entry and an additional 44% with a substance-induced depressive disorder.[10] Participants in this study used other substances, with 87% using both alcohol and cannabis. One potentially unique feature of methamphetamine-induced depression is its relationship to a co-occurring methamphetamine-induced psychosis. In a study of 164 participants who did not have a primary psychotic disorder and who were followed monthly for 12 months, the three core cluster of psychiatric symptoms exacerbated by methamphetamine use included psychotic symptoms, affective symptoms (depression, suicidality, hostility, and self-neglect), and psychomotor agitation.[11] Methamphetamine-induced depressive symptoms significantly and rapidly declined in the absence of methamphetamine use. This was seen in the context of a cohort of 21 participants in an inpatient setting for methamphetamine dependence, where depression symptoms reduced over 3 weeks to minimal or mild symptoms in 65% of the group.[12]

Opioids and Substance-Induced Depressive Disorders

Depressive disorders are the most common psychiatric comorbidity among people with OUD. Estimated prevalence rates range between 16% and 32%.[13] In a study of 500 patients with opioid use disorder seeking treatment, 54.8% were found to have a substance-induced depressive disorder and 7.4% were found to have a major depressive disorder.[14] When in treatment with medications for opioid use disorder, depressive symptoms often resolve. In a 24-week trial of 570 patients with OUD and taking either buprenorphine-naloxone or extended-release naltrexone, two-thirds of the 232 patients with mild to severe depression symptoms had a 50% reduction in symptoms from baseline or had a complete remission of symptoms from baseline at 4 weeks. There was no difference in symptom reduction between either medication. Those with moderate to severe symptoms at baseline, using the Hamilton Depression Rating Scale, were less likely to remit and likely represent a primary depressive disorder.[15]

Substance-Induced Anxiety Disorder (SIAD)

The disproportionate co-occurrence of SUDs and many anxiety disorders (eg, GAD, SAD, panic disorder), and PTSD are well established and associated with greater severity and longer duration of both sets of mental health disorders.[16-19] The relationship between anxiety disorders/PTSD and SUDs is often complicated, etiologically, by overlapping genetic, physiologic, and psychosocial risk factors.[20,21] Even so, the epidemiology of SIADs remains poorly described and may vary significantly between populations based on substance of use as well as demographic factors. For example, preliminary evidence suggests that whereas Social Anxiety Disorder is a predisposing risk factor for development of AUD (and not the reverse), daily cannabis use appears to predispose individuals to developing SAD.[22-24] As with depressive symptoms, anxiety symptoms show similar changes over the early sobriety phase. Several studies have reported high rates of anxiety symptoms among patients with AUD in withdrawal, with 80% of such male subjects experiencing repeated panic attacks during alcohol withdrawal.[25] In the same study, 50% to 67% of the AUD subjects had high scores on the state anxiety measures, which resembled generalized anxiety and social phobia. Brown et al. reported that 40% of recently detoxified men with AUD scored above the 75th percentile on the state anxiety subscale of the State Trait Anxiety Inventory. At discharge after 4 weeks, 12% scored that high, whereas at 3-month follow-up, only 5% remained above the 75th percentile. This finding suggests that 35% had SIAD.

Substance-Induced Psychotic Disorders

Psychosis during intoxication is common among those using psychotomimetic substances, which include cannabis, cocaine, amphetamines and related stimulants, hallucinogens, novel psychoactive substances, and dissociative drugs such as PCP, ketamine, and dextromethorphan. Regarding the prevalence of substance-induced psychotic disorders (SIPD), Brady et al.[26] evaluated individuals admitted for treatment of cannabis use disorder and found that 53% reported transient cocaine-induced psychosis. Caton et al.[27] evaluated individuals with psychosis and SUDs presenting to a psychiatric emergency department in New York using PRISM-IV and reported a prevalence of 44% for SIPD, while the other 56% had primary psychotic disorder (PPD) with concurrent substance use. In a later study by Fraser et al.,[28] the PRISM-IV differentially diagnosed 56% of first-episode psychosis patients with SIPD and 44% with PPD. An Australian study using PRISM-IV was done by Hides et al.[29] to investigate the rates of PPDs and SIPD compared to no psychotic disorder among people who used methamphetamine accessing needle and syringe programs. More than half of the study subjects met DSM-IV criteria for a lifetime psychotic disorder including 80% with SIPD and 20% with PPD.

Most cases of SIPD are short-lived and resolve within a few days to 2 weeks with the exception of methamphetamine and synthetic cannabinoid-induced psychosis since persistent psychotic symptoms after heavy and/or long-term use has been well documented in several studies.[29-31] Those with SIPD had higher rates of substance use and SUD, had higher levels of insight, were more likely to have a forensic and trauma history, and had more severe hostility and anxiety symptoms compared to those with non–drug-induced psychosis.[28] Although SIPD is thought to have a better prognosis than PPD, a recent study documents that SIPD transitions to a permanent schizophrenia spectrum disorder in about 10.9% to 24.3% of cases followed in Taiwan.[30] In a Finnish register-based study of over 18,000 inpatients with SIPD, the 8-year cumulative risk of SIPD converting to a diagnosis of schizophrenia spectrum disorder was 46% for those diagnosed with cannabis-induced psychosis and 30% for those with amphetamine-induced psychosis.[31]

Substance-Induced Bipolar and Related Disorder

According to DSM-5, this disorder is defined as a prominent and persistent disturbance in mood characterized by elevated, expansive, or irritable mood with or without depressed mood or markedly diminished interest or pleasure in almost all activities. The prevalence of substance-induced bipolar disorder (SIBD) is unknown as there are no epidemiological studies. In clinical practice, methamphetamine is typically associated with a SIBD and in studies dating back to the 1950s highlight the prevalence of a methamphetamine-induced bipolar disorder ranging from 5% to 24%.[32] More recent case reports suggest that a methamphetamine-induced bipolar disorder is often characterized by abrupt and frequent mood changes than is typically seen in a primary bipolar disorder.[32] Often, substances such as cannabis and alcohol can increase the risk for recurrence of manic symptoms and worsen one's overall bipolar course, but do not appear to result in a substance-induced manic disorder.[33,34]

Substance/Medication-Induced Obsessive-Compulsive and Related Disorders

Obsessions, compulsions, skin picking, hair pulling, and other body-focused repetitive behaviors can occur during substance intoxication or withdrawal, use of a medication, or exposure to heavy metals or toxins. Stimulants such as methamphetamine, amphetamine, cocaine, and substituted cathinones are associated with this diagnosis (ie, methamphetamine-induced excoriation [skin-picking] disorder). The prevalence of SIOCD is considered rare; however, one study of amphetamine-induced obsessive-compulsive disorder (AIOCD) in Iran showed the prevalence of AIOCD to be 6.9% in patients with amphetamine use disorder presenting for treatment.[21]

Substance-Induced Neurocognitive Disorders

Neurocognitive deficits are highly correlated with substance use and widespread among individuals who regularly use substances.[35] Both DSM-5[1] and ICD-11[36] recognize mild and major substance/medication-induced neurocognitive disorders (SINCD) that persist beyond periods of intoxication and withdrawal and are not attributable to another medical condition or better explained by another psychiatric disorder. In the DSM-5, these diagnoses require that, first, the individual meet criteria for a major or mild neurocognitive disorder (NCD) and then that the purported causal relationship between symptoms and substance use be biologically plausible.

Risk factors for SINCD include substance use of longer duration, early onset, greater intensity, older age, persistence of use past the 4th decade, and the use of specific substances or substance combinations.[37] Still, discerning a SINCD can be a challenge given numerous confounders and effect modifiers, including co-occurring psychiatric disorders, enhanced TBI risk, nutritional status, and SUD-associated major organ system disease with neurocognitive sequelae (including cirrhosis, cerebrovascular disease, and renal failure). For example, in ADHD, dysfunction in dopaminergic pathways appear to overlap with some of the neurophysiologic circuit abnormalities related to reward that are seen in individuals with SUDs.[38] Thus, not only does ADHD predispose individuals to developing SUDs, symptoms of executive dysfunction may exist subclinically at baseline in people with SUDs and overlap with acute and subacute intoxication and withdrawal states of multiple substances. Discerning etiology, therefore, requires careful history-taking (including collateral regarding childhood symptomatology or enforced abstinence, when possible) and possibly serial observation during future periods of abstinence.[39] Stimulant-associated SINCDs may also involve deficits in memory, learning, and executive function due to either or both direct neurotoxic effects of these substances or stimulant-related cerebrovascular injury. Although comparatively rare on a population level, inhalant-induced mild and major NCD exhibits, disproportionately, cognitive slowing and impaired executive function.[40] Among those experiencing OUD, research has identified a pattern of milder generalized cognitive dysfunction with more pronounced deficits in complex psychomotor activities.[41]

Substance-Associated Suicidal Behavior

Substance-associated suicidal behavior (SASB) includes thoughts, planning, attempts, and completed suicides. SASB is a common finding in people who use intoxicating substances. It can also be seen in both states of intoxication and chronic use and is as dangerous as most psychiatric disorders in terms of the risk of suicide. In a recent review of addiction and suicide, Youdelis-Flores concluded that persons with alcohol use disorders had rates of suicide 5 to 15 times that of the general public, with higher rates related to severity of the AUD; and those with opioid use disorders 10 to 14 times the rate.[42] Henriksson et al.[43] reported that nearly half (43%) of a group of suicide victims in Finland had the diagnosis of AUD and that 48% of those with AUDs had co-occurring depression, 42% had a personality disorder, and 36% had a significant Axis III medical disorder. Salloum et al.[44] studied patients who had been hospitalized psychiatrically and found that more than half of the subjects in all three groups studied (with alcohol use disorder, cannabis use disorder, or AUD plus CUD combined) had a history of suicide attempts. Zweben et al.[8] also found a high prevalence of prior suicide attempts (27%) in patients with methamphetamine use disorders presenting for treatment. Elliott et al.[45] found that hospitalized patients who made medically severe suicide attempts had a statistically higher rate of substance use related attempts than did patients who made less severe suicide attempts. Moreover, many of the patients with substance-induced mood disorder did not meet the criteria for chronicity of substance dependence. This finding is consistent with the findings of Asnis et al.[46] and Murphy and Wetzel,[47] who argued that alcohol intoxication dysregulates mood independent of use patterns, suggesting that some individuals are at risk of suicide regardless of the chronicity of their alcohol use. Conner et al.[48] analyzed suicidal behavior in 3,729 individuals with AUD and concluded that both independent and substance-induced depression are associated with suicidal ideation and planning, whereas alcohol-related aggression predicts suicide attempts. Aharonovich et al.[49] studied depressed people with a substance use disorder who had attempted suicide and found that patients with SIDD were as likely as those with independent MDD to have attempted suicide. Ries et al.[50] studied acutely suicidal psychiatric inpatients with SIDD and found that this subgroup had higher severity of suicidal ideation but improved more quickly than other patients and tended to have shorter lengths of stay. Opioid overdoses are now one of the leading causes of death in the United States with more recent increases associated with the use of fentanyl.[51] Research has shown a great deal of overlap in characteristics between those who die by overdose and those who die by suicide, with 1 in 5 of those who were receiving inpatient treatment for OUD reporting an intention to die prior to their most recent opioid overdose.[52] Since previous overdoses or suicide attempts are among the strongest predictors of future overdoses or suicide attempts and there is marked overlap, clinicians should always ask about both these past actions and current risks. Assessment of suicidal ideations should be done at the beginning and throughout treatment. Developing a clinic-wide strategy for assessing suicide risk with an accompanying safety plan as needed. Further information on addressing suicidal thoughts and behaviors in substance use treatment can be found here: Substance Abuse and Mental Health Services Administration (SAMHSA)—Addressing Suicidal Thoughts and Behaviors in Substance Abuse Treatment—and The Colombia Lighthouse Project: https://cssrs.columbia.edu.

Tools to Screen for Suicide

- The Columbia-Suicide Severity Rating Scale (C-SSRS)[53] is the recommended tool to assess suicide risk. This 6-question tool has been widely studied and validated in multiple countries and languages. It is the only tool that assesses for intensity, frequency, and changes of suicidal ideation over time. Although frequently used, it has not been validated in patients with substance use disorders.
- Relying on the 9th question of the PHQ-9 to screen for suicide risk is insufficient as it results in too many false positives and does not assess current suicidal plans or intent.[54] If the PHQ-9 is to be used for preliminary assessment of suicide risk, a follow-up questionnaire, like the C-SSRS, should be used for a more complete assessment.

SPECIFIC SUBSTANCES: SUBSTANCE-INDUCED SYMPTOMS

The occurrence of psychiatric symptoms as a result of legal and illegal drug use has been well documented. It is common medical knowledge that hallucinogens and dissociative agents cause hallucinations, stimulants cause euphoria, and chronic sedative use can result in depression. It is common medical knowledge that in acute withdrawal, alcohol, and sedative-hypnotics cause anxiety. It is less obvious that a distinct set of symptoms appear when psychoactive substances are used over a long period. Symptoms reported for each of the major psychoactive substances are reviewed below to establish a basis on which to understand the syndromes that can arise.

Caffeine, at average consumption levels, has no significant impairing psychiatric symptoms, with the exception of those with some genetic predisposition to the negative effects of caffeine that will result in anxiety symptoms.[55,56] However, energy drinks can contain anywhere from 80 to 500 mg of caffeine whereas an 8-oz cup of coffee is around 80 to 100 mg.[57] Symptoms concerning for a substance-induced disorder are typically seen only at high doses over 500 to 600 mg of caffeine in a day and can include anxiety, restlessness, insomnia, gastrointestinal upset, tremors, tachycardia, and psychomotor agitation.[57]

Nicotine is the deadliest psychoactive drug in the form of tobacco products, and while still under early study may also have harmful effects as delivered by electronic drug delivery devices (EDDDs, such as e-cigarettes or "vaping"). Nicotine use is frequently co-occurring with psychiatric disorders.[58] The self-medication hypothesis explaining this relationship has given way over time to research suggesting that smoking may cause anxiety, depression, ADHD and schizophrenia.[59-62] Further strengthening this relationship is the observation that stopping smoking is significantly associated with decreased anxiety, depression, and improvements in mood and quality of life.[63] That said, this relationship is not typically described as a substance-induced disorder as the relationship between nicotine and psychiatric symptoms and disorders are quite complex.[62] Currently, it is thought that nicotine may increase the vulnerability to psychiatric disorders, and smoking may help alleviate those symptoms initially, but then worsen them over time. In contrast, depression and anxiety symptoms can clearly be a function of nicotine withdrawal independent of an underlying anxiety or depressive disorder.[64] Nicotine withdrawal peaks within 2 to 3 days and can last 3 to 4 weeks or longer.[65]

Alcohol use is common among American adolescents and young adults. Although light consumption of alcohol is associated with a slight euphoria or "buzz," moderate to heavy consumption may be associated with depression, suicidal feelings, or psychotic symptoms in some individuals.[66] Anxiety symptoms are also common in alcohol use disorders and are most pronounced within a state of withdrawal. In those who are physiologically dependent, one usually sees a hyperadrenergic state during withdrawal that is characterized by agitation, anxiety, tremor, malaise, hyperreflexia, mild tachycardia, increasing blood pressure, sweating, insomnia, nausea or vomiting, and perceptual distortions. After acute withdrawal from alcohol, some persons suffer from continued mood instability, with moderate lows, fatiguability, insomnia, reduced sexual interest, and hostility. In addition to alcohol-related hallucinosis secondary to alcohol withdrawal, a unique alcohol-induced psychotic disorder has also been described that includes auditory hallucinations and delusions of persecutions, jealousy, or grandeur.[66] This can be seen in the context of heavy drinking and resolved within 18 to 35 days with antipsychotic treatment.

With *sedative-hypnotics and anxiolytics*, particularly the benzodiazepines, acute use can produce a "high" similar to that seen with alcohol. The drug effects are perceived as relaxing, producing a social ease, but sedatives also can induce depression, anxiety, and even withdrawal-induced psychosis with prolonged use. Withdrawal symptoms include mood instability with anxiety or depression, sleep disturbance, autonomic hyperactivity, tremor, nausea or vomiting, transient hallucinations or illusions, and grand mal seizures. A protracted withdrawal syndrome has been reported to include anxiety, depression, paresthesia, perceptual distortions, muscle pain and twitching, tinnitus, dizziness, headache, derealization and depersonalization, and impaired concentration. These symptoms can last for weeks, and some (such as anxiety, depression, tinnitus, and paresthesia) have been reported for a year or more after withdrawal.[67]

Stimulants: *cocaine*, *amphetamine/methamphetamine*, and other stimulant use often is associated with an intense euphoria or "rush," with hyperactive behavior and speech, racing thoughts, hypersexuality, anorexia, insomnia, inattention, anxiety, and manic/labile mood swings. The route of administration and the dose alter the intensity of the experience. Depressive symptoms and cognitive problems as well as hypersomnia, decreased energy, and increased appetite commonly occur during a stimulant withdrawal phase. After a methamphetamine binge of several days, individuals will often be hostile and agitated, which is referred to as "tweaking" as they stop their use, or they may use other drugs such as benzodiazepines or alcohol to moderate the agitation. Up to 40% of people who use methamphetamine become paranoid and delusional after prolonged heavy use.[68] Once abstinence is maintained for several weeks to months, the psychotic symptoms usually attenuate and resolve but many of those with SIPD go on to develop a persistent psychotic disorder.[31] Persons with stimulant use disorders report a prolonged withdrawal state that is dysphoric and prominently marked by anhedonia and/or anxiety, but which does not meet the symptom severity criteria to qualify as a DSM-5 disorder. This anhedonic state can persist for weeks to months. Individuals with stimulant use disorder frequently report hallucinatory symptoms that are visual ("coke snow") and tactile ("meth mites" or formication). Sleep disturbances are prominent in the intoxicated and withdrawn states, as is sexual dysfunction. Methylenedioxymethamphetamine (MDMA), more commonly known as "ecstasy," intoxication produces stimulant effects similar to cocaine and amphetamine as well as empathogenic effects such as empathy, a sense of well-being, and sociability due to serotonergic activity.[69] Withdrawal states are characterized by depression, hypersomnia, poor concentration, and fatigue. People who use MDMA chronically may develop more severe longer-term problems such as dysphoric states and cognitive impairments in memory, concentration, and executive functioning, which are thought to be due to serotonergic neurotoxicity.[69]

Opioids: Opioid effects are dose- and tolerance-dependent and can include analgesia, anxiolysis, euphoria, sedation, respiratory depression, miosis, nausea, decreased GI motility. In contrast to stimulants, when used to produce an altered state (a "high" or "rush") opioid intoxication is usually associated with a mellow, intensely pleasurable, calmly euphoric state and sense of well-being. Intensity of effect can be enhanced through dose and route of administration, with rapid onset achieved through injection or inhalation. However, if opioids are used for an extended period, paradoxical effects such as moderate to severe depression and hyperalgesia are common. Signs and symptoms of opioid withdrawal include irritability, restlessness, agitation, craving, anxiety, dysphoria, insomnia, anorexia, generalized joint aches and muscle cramping, diaphoresis, chills, piloerection, tremor, lacrimation and rhinorrhea, yawning, mydriasis, tachycardia, and gastrointestinal symptoms (nausea, cramping, and diarrhea). In the setting of physiologic dependence and abstinence of short-acting opioids (eg, heroin, morphine, IR oxycodone), onset of symptoms can occur within hours. Alternatively, withdrawal can be delayed and prolonged with abstinence from longer-acting opioids and opioidlike substances (including methadone, buprenorphine, kratom/*Mitragyna speciosa*) and fentanyl (which sequesters in adipose with repeated use, then gradually redistributes following abstinence). Anxiety, depression, sleep disturbance, and cravings often persist, in a milder form, for weeks to months as a protracted withdrawal syndrome that gradually subsides. In overdose, opioids produce respiratory depression, decreased tidal volume, depressed mental status, miotic pupils, and decreased bowel sounds with potential for respiratory arrest and death.

Classical hallucinogens such as lysergic acid diethylamide (LSD), mescaline, psilocybin, and dimethyltryptamine (DMT) produce visual distortions and frank hallucinations. All hallucinogens are associated with drug-induced panic reactions that feature panic, paranoia, and even delusional states in addition to the hallucinations. However, they are not associated with a withdrawal syndrome. Some people who use hallucinogens experience chronic reactions, involving (1) prolonged psychotic reactions; (2) suicidality; (3) and flashbacks.[70] A flashback is the re-experiencing of hallucinogen-induced perceptual distortions, despite no recent hallucinogen use. The DSM-5 refers to these flashbacks as "Hallucinogen Persisting Perception Disorder" and requires that they be distressing or impairing to the patient.

Cannabis and hashish or hash oil contain *tetrahydrocannabinol* (THC). Intoxication with THC augments appetite and causes sedation with euphoria. Some people who use it experience a marked sense of time distortion and feelings of depersonalization. A cannabis withdrawal syndrome can emerge that is generally mild and consists of anxiety, irritability, physical tension, depressed mood, decreased appetite, restlessness, and craving. Recent literature has emerged that early use of cannabis is a risk factor for the later development of psychotic disorders[71] and the cumulative 8-year risk of cannabis-induced psychosis converting to permanent psychosis is 46%.[31]

PCP, an arylcyclohexylamine, and *ketamine* are N-methyl-D-aspartate (NMDA) antagonists and dissociative drugs that cause hallucinations and dissociative states. Dextromethorphan is a codeinelike drug that when metabolized is converted to dextrorphan, which is also an NMDA antagonist. All three are known for their dissociative and delusional properties. PCP is also associated with violent behavior and amnesia of the intoxication. Whereas ketamine is known for its anesthesia and impaired verbal learning and spatial memory. Chronic use of ketamine has been thought to produce schizophrenia-like positive and negative symptoms.[72] Dextromethorphan at high doses can lead to delusions, hallucinations, and paranoia that have been reported to persist after several days of abstinence requiring treatment with an antipsychotic.[73]

Novel psychoactive substances also known as designer drugs and other emerging substances often found on the internet and advertised as "legal highs" have been appearing with increasing frequency over the past decades. The United Nations Office on Drugs and Crime tracks emerging new psychoactive substances around the world and continues to document the growth of substances like synthetic cathinones and synthetic cannabinoids. *Synthetic cathinones* popularly known as "bath salts" are all synthetic analogs of cathinone derived from leaves of the khat plant (*Catha edulis*), a stimulant chewed for centuries in Yemen, Somalia, Eritrea, and Ethiopia.[74] The cathinone derivatives found in bath salts are primarily *3,4-methylenedioxypyrovalerone (MDPV)*, *mephedrone*, and *methylone*, which are structurally similar to methamphetamine and MDMA, and produce similar stimulant effects as well as psychotic effects in susceptible individuals. Other new psychoactive substances of which we have little medical knowledge include *methoxetamine*, a "legal" ketamine analog that is an NMDA receptor antagonist that causes hallucinations, and the *piperazine derivatives* that have central serotonergic and amphetamine-like effects.[74]

Salvia divinorum, a herb in the mint family that has become more popular of late, is native to Southern Mexico and is used for its mind-altering effects. The plant can be chewed, smoked, or vaporized and is not controlled under the United States Controlled Substances Act. *Salvia divinorum* is, however, controlled by a large number of states and had been widely available via the internet or local "head shops." Psychotropic properties are due to the chemical *salvinorin A*, a kappa opioid receptor agonist. Effects include hallucinations, visual distortions, perceptual disturbances, anxiety, confusion, and dysphoria.[75] Some people who use it describe synesthesia (where one sensory perception takes on the appearance of another, ie, hearing colors or smelling sounds), while others endorse a dissociative or "out of body experience." Effects can last as long as 24 hours.[75]

Synthetic cannabinoids such as "spice" and "K2" consist of inert plant material sprayed with chemical compounds originally designed by pharmaceutical companies as research drugs with cannabinoid receptor agonist activity.[75] Psychotropic effects that occur when "spice" is smoked include alterations in mood, perception, as well as anxiety, agitation, nausea, vomiting, tachycardia, elevated blood pressure, tremor, seizures, hallucinations, paranoid behavior, and unresponsiveness to external stimulation.[74]

DIAGNOSING SUBSTANCE-INDUCED MENTAL DISORDERS

Diagnosing substance-induced mental disorders can be challenging and requires a working knowledge of what psychiatric symptoms substances can induce, as well as, the potential course of those symptoms over time, as outlined above. That will allow providers to characterize the role of substances in substance-induced mental disorders, including identifying a potential SUD, as the first step in making this diagnosis. The substance-induced symptoms must be differentiated from the symptoms of independent psychiatric disorders in the second step.

Tips to help providers in sorting out substance-induced versus primary psychiatric disorders:

- Make sure you ask about patient history of psychiatric symptoms over a lifetime. People with primary psychiatric disorders often have psychiatric symptoms before the onset of their substance use. The timeline of psychiatric symptomatology, especially around persistence of symptoms during periods of prolonged abstinence, can be helpful in highlighting a primary psychiatric diagnosis.
- Do they have a substance use disorder? People with SUDs have a higher risk of developing a substance-induced mental disorder.
- How severe are the psychiatric symptoms? More severe psychiatric symptoms in someone with a SUD suggest the presence of a primary psychiatric disorder.
- Effective past psychiatric treatment.
- Toxicology screens help because people may be reticent to disclose their substance use, or unaware of all different substances that might be mixed with each other. Be clear that you have consent to get a drug screen. New psychoactive substances, synthetic cannabinoids, Kratom, PCP, MDMA, hallucinogens, and others may not show up on a substance test and special orders may be needed for the lab to look for these substances. See Chapter 32, "Laboratory Diagnosis," for further details.
- Past substance use–related ED visits or inpatient/residential SUD treatment.
- Collateral information (family, friends, and PDMP).
- Use screening and measurement-based tools, such as the Patient Health Questionnaire-9 (PHQ-9), the Generalized Anxiety Disorder-7 (GAD-7), the PTSD Checklist for DSM-5 (PCL-5, the Adult Symptom Rating Scale v1.1 (ASRS v1.1) for ADHD, the Patient Mania Questionnaire (PMQ-9) to help identify independent psychiatric disorders.
- Continue to monitor psychiatric symptoms during and after substance use treatment in case the presumed substance-induced symptoms transition into a primary mental health disorder. The use of symptom tracking tools, as listed above can help monitor symptoms over time.

TREATMENT OF SUBSTANCE-INDUCED MENTAL DISORDERS

Once psychiatric symptoms have been identified, it is important to take them into consideration when determining the appropriate level of care for a patient. As per the ASAM criteria (see Chapter 47, "The ASAM Criteria and Matching Patients to Treatment"), psychiatric complications will help determine whether a patient needs inpatient management or a less restrictive option. If a patient is acutely suicidal or psychotic and unable to care for themselves, inpatient placement will be needed. In some cases, this will necessitate admission to an involuntary psychiatric unit in place of an addiction inpatient facility, to stabilize a patient's mental health crisis before addressing their substance use problems. Withdrawal management is typically provided in inpatient psychiatric settings, but ongoing substance treatment post discharge can fall through the cracks and should be discussed before discharge.

The need to treat psychiatric symptoms before diagnostic certainty will vary from patient to patient. In the case of acute psychotic or manic symptoms, the use of antipsychotics are typically needed and used in both inpatient and outpatient settings. For depression, anxiety, inattention, and other symptoms, a more conservative approach can be taken, with close monitoring of these symptoms over time. That said, waiting until a patient is "completely sober" to begin treatment of a co-occurring psychiatric disorder may lead to a delay in psychiatric treatment and the patient dropping out of SUD treatment. As it can be challenging to clarify a primary psychiatric disorder, treating psychiatric symptoms with both medications and therapy as indicated, within 4 weeks of abstinence or identification of symptoms, can be worthwhile to help keep people engaged and prevent a delay in treatment. However, ongoing evaluation for treatment response and diagnostic clarification is needed. Further details on treating co-occurring psychiatric disorders can be found in the Chapters 101 to 107.

Case 1: Diagnostic Considerations

At this point, the clinician has enough information to diagnose AUD. His mood disturbance is prominent and is more severe than that experienced by people who drink alcohol and most persons with an AUD. His depressive symptoms seem sufficiently severe to suggest major depression; however, there is no evidence of depression at the times that Mr B is not drinking heavily, suggesting an alcohol-induced depressive disorder. The AUD seems to be primary since it began before the depressive symptoms. This sequence of symptoms suggests SIDD. It is possible that Mr B has two independent disorders: AUD and MDD; however, there is no evidence of that at present.

Treatment Considerations

A trial of abstinence is indicated in a safe and supportive environment to help address his risk of suicide, sort out his diagnoses, and start treatment. The *ASAM Criteria* (see Chapter 47, "The ASAM Criteria and Matching Patients to Treatment"), can help provide a guideline for multidimensional assessment and criteria for treatment of addictive, substance-related, and co-occurring conditions, and how to decide the appropriate level of care. In the absence of that resource, providers should consider the following:

(1) Identify the patient's goals around drinking and specifically his desire for abstinence.
(2) If the patient wants to stop drinking, the provider will need to consider the potential for complicated withdrawal and the appropriate setting for withdrawal management (see Chapter 56, "Management of Alcohol Intoxication and Withdrawal"). If the patient does not want to stop drinking, harm reduction approaches should be taken, and close follow-up of his drinking and depressive symptoms are needed.
(3) The severity of his psychiatric symptoms and elevated risk for suicide indicate the need for a suicide safety plan.

Case 1

Mr B is a 46-year-old divorced White man who works as a house painter. He came to his PCP because of persistent suicidal ideas without plan or intent, which frightened him. He had become increasingly depressed over the preceding month and was afraid that he was "going crazy." He has experienced 1 to 2 day long depressive periods over the preceding 7 years (since his divorce), but nothing like this. He has never been diagnosed or treated psychiatrically for depression. On further evaluation for additional etiologies, the PCP finds out that Mr B has increased his drinking to about a case of beer a day for the past month. He reports that the alcohol use is the only way he can cope with his depression. Mr B also endorses being hospitalized once, 4 years ago, for alcohol withdrawal management, but received no further treatment. He denies any loss of control of his drinking but is experiencing difficulty in getting to work on time since becoming depressed and is in trouble with his supervisor. He denies morning tremors and says that he never has experienced seizures, delirium tremens, or hallucinations when withdrawing. Mr B admits that his ex-wife complained about his drinking. He has had only one period of abstinence for more than a year, while on probation for his second DUI. He does not think his alcohol use is contributing to his depressive symptoms. He denies hallucinations and obsessions. He denies any manic episodes. A point of care toxicology test is negative for benzodiazepines, opioids, barbiturates, and cocaine, but positive for alcohol. His PHQ9 is a 21 out of 27 (severe symptoms) and his GAD7 is a 12 out of 21 (severe symptoms).

Special attention will need to be directed at reducing access to his gun during this acute time. Family and friends can be very helpful in managing this risk.

(4) Decides to treat or monitor his depressive symptoms.

Whether or not the patient starts treatment for his alcohol use disorder, it is reasonable to monitor the symptoms of his depression with a validated measuring tool, like the PHQ9, for 2 to 4 months. If his symptoms persist or worsen, starting treatment for his depressive symptoms with therapy or an antidepressant would be reasonable due to the severity of his symptoms regardless of alcohol use treatment status. Finally, if the patient does stop drinking and enters treatment for his AUD ongoing recovery support through an addiction treatment program, and support by friends and family should be pursued. FDA-approved medications for AUD such as naltrexone, acamprosate, disulfiram, and injectable naltrexone, are most helpful when the patient is open to the idea of abstinence from alcohol, and willing to engage in psychosocial treatment. Various off-label medications may also have effectiveness for AUD (such as topiramate, gabapentin, etc.). Patients with a strong connection to Alcoholics Anonymous do better with both their addiction and depression symptoms and should be offered as a treatment option to all patients seeking abstinence.

Case 2: Diagnostic Considerations

Based on the information provided, we can diagnosis severe AUD and co-occurring PTSD as two primary disorders. His timeline provides evidence that they interact, through a bidirectional positive reinforcement. His disordered sleep appears likely of mixed etiology with components of PTSD as well as direct and indirect effects of alcohol. Finally, he is experiencing an acute alcohol withdrawal syndrome and has a distant history of severe withdrawal.

Treatment Considerations

In considering their shared approach to treatment, Mr M and his care provider(s) will need to work collaboratively to identify treatment priorities based on clinical acuity and patient values. First, Mr M and his PCP were able to agree that acute withdrawal management was the most pressing concern. In light of his history of complex withdrawal and more recent levels of use, accompanying withdrawal symptomatology, and limited access to monitoring and support outside in the community, they agreed that treatment in an acute care setting was warranted.

Having the patient engage with the full treatment team including addiction specialists (counselors, physicians, and peer

Case 2

Mr M is a 64-year-old housed, divorced, and unemployed Black Army Veteran. He is seen infrequently in the health care system but presented to his PCP today with a chief complaint of insomnia, which has worsened over the past 4 to 6 months. During his appointment, he reports that he has been struggling with intermittent awakenings and disturbing dreams at night and recurrent unpleasant thoughts and memories during the day. He notes that these symptoms were prominent "years ago, but it died down for a long while" until resurfacing about a year ago. In this context, he started drinking alcohol—both during the day to address anxiety/distress and, at night, to fall asleep. He thought this was helpful at first but, over the past 6 months, he finds that he has become increasingly anxious, jumpy and irritable, and that his sleep is now more disrupted then before. He finds that he is further isolating himself from his friends and drinking more. He notes hand tremors and some sweating in the mornings, which resolve with a few shots of whiskey. He does not "keep tabs" but estimates that he has been drinking at least a fifth of whiskey daily for a few months, and likely even more over the past few weeks. Expressing genuine concern, the PCP uses a structured but patient-centered approach to obtain additional history relating to mental health, substance use, and other pertinent medical and psychosocial factors. Mr M notes that his father struggled with alcohol use, but he is not aware of other addiction or psychiatric family history. He quit smoking in his 40s and, aside from alcohol, denies other substance use history. He describes being diagnosed with combat-related PTSD several decades ago and he was reluctant to engage in formal PTSD treatment. He notes a period of eight years beginning in his early-40s when "I was a full-on alcoholic," experiencing physiologic dependence and tolerance and a loss of control with an inability to limit use despite experiencing a range of significant interpersonal, social, legal, and medical consequences. After being treated for severe alcohol withdrawal he found support through AA and his religious community. During the subsequent decade-plus of sobriety, his anxiety and PTSD symptoms significantly improved. However, about a year ago he was a witness to and nearly the victim of a shooting in his neighborhood. Afterwards, he experienced a re-emergence of nightmares, flashbacks, intrusive thoughts, panic attacks, hypervigilance and avoidance. It was in this context he began to drink again, "at first just a little, just to try to sleep, but it's like it woke something in me and I feel like I'm back where I was years ago." He notes, "now my withdrawals are bad, I can't stop drinking for very long before I get shaky and sick." He indicates that he last drank 4 to 5 hours ago and his CIWA is scored at 9. He has been trying to taper himself over the past week but has not been successful. He is motivated to stop drinking.

Case 3

Mr S, a 20-year-old gay man, was brought by the police to the local emergency department after threatening his partner with a knife. He presented with acute agitation, hostility, paranoia, and delusions of reference. He expressed fear that his partner was a "necrophiliac" and a serial murderer. Over the past month, Mr S had begun to arm himself with a knife to protect himself and others from possible attack. Other symptoms included frequent anger episodes, increased libido, insomnia, tachycardia, weight loss, and anxiety. On physical exam, he was found to have scattered scarring and sores on his face, arms, and legs. The patient reported having used methamphetamine on many occasions over the past year, smoked, and later injected over weekends to "party with friends." During his partying experiences, he related repeated unsafe sexual practices including receptive anal intercourse and he requested an HIV test. He described frequent withdrawal effects after a weekend of partying that included hypersomnia, increased appetite, poor concentration, and dysphoria that would last several days and culminate in craving until his next methamphetamine binge. In addition to methamphetamine use, the patient also reported frequent alcohol and cannabis use but denied a history to support a SUD including withdrawal from those substances. He denied all other drug use including tobacco.

specialists), psychiatry, and members of the spiritual care service, is recommended. In this case to help Mr M feel respected and develop a greater understanding of how his AUD and PTSD interact and the importance of addressing both concurrently. Prior to hospital discharge for alcohol withdrawal management, starting pharmacotherapy for co-occurring conditions should be considered such as a combination of naltrexone and gabapentin for AUD as well as a serotonin specific reuptake inhibitor for PTSD. A decision around the use of prazosin can be deferred to outpatient follow-up. Assigning a peer navigator to help patients follow-up with a complicated and diverse treatment plan that can include multiple clinical settings, providers, and meetings can be very useful.

Case 3: Diagnostic Considerations

This case appears to be methamphetamine-induced psychotic disorder. However, given his young age, the possibility of a PPD cannot be ruled out. A drug toxicology screen should be obtained to rule out other drugs despite his denial of use since street drugs are often contaminated with other compounds. He appears delusional and dangerous with very poor insight as he has armed himself with a knife over the last month and believes his partner may be trying to kill him. Hostility is a frequent symptom of methamphetamine psychosis[50] but is also common in untreated paranoid psychosis. He does not appear to have negative symptoms of schizophrenia, but there may have been a prodromal period of increasing delusional and paranoid thoughts, which is common for people who become psychotic from frequent use of methamphetamine. He also appears to have maniclike agitation, mood lability, and excessive sexual behavior accompanying his insomnia alternating with depressive periods and hypersomnia. This is characteristic of people who use stimulants chronically, and experience repeated binge and withdrawal episodes. His weight loss, tachycardia, and mild hypertension are probably effects of the stimulant, but a thyroid disorder should be ruled out. His skin lesions are likely due to "meth mites" or formication and the chronic skin picking frequently seen in those who use methamphetamine. In DSM-5, this is diagnosed as stimulant-induced excoriation disorder and is considered a stimulant-induced obsessive-compulsive-related disorder. However, the lesions may also represent a parasitic infestation such as lice, scabies, or bed bugs or a sexually transmitted disease (STD) such as a rash or chancre associated with syphilis since he has had indiscriminate and unsafe sexual behavior that is frequently associated with recreational methamphetamine use. An HIV test, as well as other STD tests, should be done.

Treatment Issues

This patient is frightened but also hostile and delusional with poor insight and threatening behavior. He also has intense craving associated with his withdrawal periods, which likely will prompt him to leave against medical advice. If he declines admission for stabilization, then involuntary psychiatric hospitalization is required as well as acute treatment of the agitation and psychosis with benzodiazepines and atypical antipsychotics. Mr S will need extensive education about the origin of his psychosis followed by inpatient and then outpatient addiction treatment for prevention of return to use. His partner should be warned if homicidal ideation is present and advised to seek a protective order. He will also need close follow-up after hospitalization to ensure that his paranoia attenuates with abstinence and antipsychotic treatment.

Treatment Considerations

Prognosis will depend primarily on his motivation and success in addiction treatment, and it is essential that he understand the role methamphetamine has played in his decompensation and the likelihood of worsening and prolonged psychosis should he return to substance use. If psychosis persists despite a month of abstinence, a PPD must be considered. Subspecialized culturally appropriate addiction treatment for sexual minorities with methamphetamine use disorder is available in most large urban areas and can include education about unsafe

Case 4

Ms A is a 35-year-old woman who was brought to the emergency department (ED) after overdosing on heroin and clonazepam. She was revived by bystanders using naloxone. When evaluated in the ED, she reported severe anxiety, panic attacks, and feeling very despondent over the past few weeks with suicidal ideation. She reported her overdose was an attempt to "escape the pain" but not necessarily to end her life, rather, end her suffering. She endorsed chronic pain due to past trauma from domestic violence and had been on prescription opioids for several years. Over the past year, she began to use heroin after her physician retired, and the new provider did not want to continue prescribing opioids. She related that she has had untreated depression and anxiety in the past, but her symptoms began to worsen when she started injecting heroin and using clonazepam to supplement her "highs." Ms A reported that she would use 1 to 3 mg daily of clonazepam that she bought on the streets to "help" with withdrawal and symptoms of anxiety and panic, but she took 5 mg on the day of her overdose.

sexual practices and harm reduction. Twelve-step groups such as "Crystal Meth Anonymous" and "Strength Over Speed" are very helpful if available, and are "gay friendly." AA and NA groups will also suffice. As yet, there is no FDA-approved pharmacological treatment for methamphetamine use disorder.

Case 4: Diagnostic Considerations

Ms A's overdose and suicidal ideation brought her to the emergency department. She also endorsed prominent anxiety and depression, which is consistent with opioid and benzodiazepine use disorders and withdrawal symptoms. Her past psychiatric history is not clear as to whether she has a primary mood or anxiety disorder, but it is important to further evaluate this after withdrawal symptoms have been managed and consider other diagnoses such as PTSD or a personality disorder. It is possible that she has both an independent psychiatric disorder as well as SIMD. Some may be tempted to take this overdose less seriously due to her clear opioid and benzodiazepine use disorders and unclear psychiatric disorder. However, a desire to die has been found to be common in people with nonfatal opioid overdoses.[52] Also women with multiple SUDs are more likely than men to have underlying co-occurring disorders, and risk for suicide attempts and completed suicide is high.[42] Her suicide attempt was very dangerous, and continuing her use of both heroin and benzodiazepines (both now often laced with fentanyl) will likely result in further overdoses and eventual death—either accidental or deliberate. Investigating unsafe sexual practices and needle sharing and screening for HIV disease and viral hepatitis is necessary for anyone using intravenous drugs, and it would be wise to obtain a comprehensive toxicology screen to rule out other unreported substance use. Further assessing for domestic violence and PTSD is also very important.

Treatment Considerations

Patient safety related to overdose and suicidality, are primary issues here. The clinician must assess the severity of the suicidal impulse and the social supports available before deciding whether Ms A should be referred for inpatient psychiatric treatment, residential addiction treatment, or if outpatient treatment is appropriate. In addition, the clinician should assess what type of suicidal thoughts she is having, whether she has a plan to carry out the idea, whether she has the means to complete the plan, whether she has made prior attempts and, if so, how serious were the attempts. It is important to explore reasons to continue living and whether there are other alternatives to committing suicide. Inducting her on buprenorphine in the Emergency Department should be considered as it may be lifesaving and provide another mechanism for engagement.[76] Evaluating for any past addiction treatments, what type of treatment received and the outcomes are important to formulate the next steps. Ongoing treatment will need to assess anxiety, depression, and PTSD. People with multiple SUDs and serious intravenous drug use are often demoralized because of treatment failures and severe psychosocial stressors, which contribute to a sense of hopelessness and shame. It is essential to engage Ms A in a motivational manner and assure her that her pain and addiction, as well as depression and anxiety can be managed through a combination of pharmacotherapy and psychotherapy, such as buprenorphine or methadone, talk therapy, and adjunctive nonaddictive medications for residual psychiatric disorders. A trauma-informed substance treatment program for women would be ideal for Ms A.

Safety from benzodiazepine withdrawal is also an important issue that must be considered. She may be minimizing her benzodiazepine use and thus will need ongoing monitoring for withdrawal symptoms. Serious benzodiazepine withdrawal is best handled in an inpatient setting and can be assessed and treated along with her opioid use disorder, psychiatric symptoms, and suicidality.

Assessing a patient's motivation to follow through may be difficult if the patient is previously unknown to the clinician. As referenced above, buprenorphine may be key for engagement, and will likely decrease future craving and prevent overdoses. Engagement in an addiction treatment program will depend on availability, insurance, and the patient's denial, motivation, and awareness of the centrality of drugs and alcohol in her life. How well addiction treatment will fit in the context of her other social relationships such as children, significant others, and family members, and employment needs will also need to be considered. Attention to these psychosocial issues may be the key to engagement. Using motivational strategies by highlighting how a women's AA or NA groups will be able to address issues she is dealing with, is indicated. Successful integration of these factors in an intervention remains part of the art of medicine.

CONCLUSIONS

The SIMDs are common illnesses that often are associated with (but are not limited to) SUDs. Although they frequently are short-lived, these disorders are by no means clinically insignificant. Serious self-injury is reported with SIDD, and safety is an important clinical issue. This situation can present a clinical dilemma in determining the proper level of care. Services that treat co-occurring addiction and other psychiatric disorders in parallel rather than in series often provide improved clinical and cost-effective outcomes. Confusion about the diagnosis can delay interventions; therefore, achieving clarification through a comprehensive evaluation is the first order of business after safety is addressed. However, in cases of severe psychiatric distress with an unclear diagnosis, symptomatic treatment may be necessary. Although abstinence is a critical factor in recovery from SIMD, it is not always the only factor. Ongoing engagement around a person's substance use disorder and psychiatric disorder at the same time is often needed. When the patient's behavior is unsafe or unmanageable, a psychiatric unit may be necessary until the patient's behavior is less risky. Such patient-treatment matching should be done on an individual basis, depending on the patient's needs, the resources available, and the skills and preferences of the clinicians involved.

REFERENCES

1. American Psychiatric Association. *Diagnostic and Statistical Manual of Mental Disorders*. 5th ed. APA; 2013.
2. Grant BF, Stinson FS, Dawson DA, et al. Prevalence and co-occurrence of substance use disorders and independent mood and anxiety disorders: results from the National Epidemiologic Survey on Alcohol and Related Conditions. *Arch Gen Psychiatry*. 2004;61(8):807-816. doi:10.1001/archpsyc.61.8.807
3. Schuckit MA, Tipp JE, Bergman M, Reich W, Hesselbrock VM, Smith TL. Comparison of induced and independent major depressive disorders in 2,945 alcoholics. *Am J Psychiatry*. 1997;154(7):948-957. doi:10.1176/ajp.154.7.948
4. Brown SA, Schuckit MA. Changes in depression among abstinent alcoholics. *J Stud Alcohol*. 1988;49(5):412-417. doi:10.15288/jsa.1988.49.412
5. Ramsey SE, Kahler CW, Read JP, Stuart GL, Brown RA. Discriminating between substance-induced and independent depressive episodes in alcohol dependent patients. *J Stud Alcohol*. 2004;65(5):672-676. doi:10.15288/jsa.2004.65.672
6. Rounsaville BJ, Anton SF, Carroll K, Budde D, Prusoff BA, Gawin F. Psychiatric diagnoses of treatment-seeking cocaine abusers. *Arch Gen Psychiatry*.1991;48(1):43-51.doi:10.1001/archpsyc.1991.01810250045005
7. Alías-Ferri M, García-Marchena N, Mestre-Pintó JI, et al. Cocaine and depressive disorders: when standard clinical diagnosis is insufficient. *Adicciones*. 2021;33(3):193-200. Trastorno por uso de cocaína y depresión: cuando el diagnóstico clínico no es suficiente. doi:10.20882/adicciones.1321
8. Zweben JE, Cohen JB, Christian D, et al. Psychiatric symptoms in methamphetamine users. *Am J Addict*. 2004;13(2):181-190. doi:10.1080/10550490490436055
9. Glasner-Edwards S, Marinelli-Casey P, Hillhouse M, Ang A, Mooney LJ, Rawson R. Depression among methamphetamine users: association with outcomes from the Methamphetamine Treatment Project at 3-year follow-up. *J Nerv Ment Dis*. 2009;197(4):225-231. doi:10.1097/NMD.0b013e31819db6fe
10. McKetin R, Lubman DI, Lee NM, Ross JE, Slade TN. Major depression among methamphetamine users entering drug treatment programs. *Med J Aust*. 2011;195(S3):S51-S55. doi:10.5694/j.1326-5377.2011.tb03266.x
11. McKetin R, Dawe S, Burns RA, et al. The profile of psychiatric symptoms exacerbated by methamphetamine use. *Drug Alcohol Depend*. 2016;161:104-109. doi:10.1016/j.drugalcdep.2016.01.018
12. McGregor C, Srisurapanont M, Jittiwutikarn J, Laobhripatr S, Wongtan T, White JM. The nature, time course and severity of methamphetamine withdrawal. *Addiction*. 2005;100(9):1320-1329. doi:10.1111/j.1360-0443.2005.01160.x
13. Bastien G, Del Grande C, Dyachenko A, et al. Preferences for research design and treatment of comorbid depression among patients with an opioid use disorder: a cross-sectional discrete choice experiment. *Drug Alcohol Depend*. 2021;226:108857. doi:10.1016/j.drugalcdep.2021.108857
14. Ahmadi J, Majdi B, Mahdavi S, Mohagheghzadeh M. Mood disorders in opioid-dependent patients. *J Affect Disord*. 2004;82(1):139-142. doi:10.1016/j.jad.2003.09.015
15. Na PJ, Scodes J, Fishman M, Rotrosen J, Nunes EV. Co-occurring depression and suicidal ideation in opioid use disorder: prevalence and response during treatment with buprenorphine-naloxone and injection naltrexone. *J Clin Psychiatry*. 2022;83(3):21m14140. doi:10.4088/JCP.21m14140
16. Kessler RC, Chiu WT, Demler O, Merikangas KR, Walters EE. Prevalence, severity, and comorbidity of 12-month DSM-IV disorders in the National Comorbidity Survey Replication. *Arch General Psychiatry*. 2005;62(6):617-627. doi:10.1001/archpsyc.62.6.617
17. Sartor CE, Lynskey MT, Heath AC, Jacob T, True W. The role of childhood risk factors in initiation of alcohol use and progression to alcohol dependence. *Addiction*. 2007;102(2):216-225. doi:10.1111/j.1360-0443.2006.01661.x
18. Norman SB, Haller M, Hamblen JL, Southwick SM, Pietrzak RH. The burden of co-occurring alcohol use disorder and PTSD in U.S. Military veterans: comorbidities, functioning, and suicidality. *Psychol Addict Behav*. 2018;32(2):224-229. doi:10.1037/adb0000348
19. Boschloo L, Vogelzangs N, van den Brink W, et al. Alcohol use disorders and the course of depressive and anxiety disorders. *Br J Psychiatry*. 2012;200(6):476-484. doi:10.1192/bjp.bp.111.097550
20. Koob GF, Volkow ND. Neurobiology of addiction: a neurocircuitry analysis. *Lancet Psychiatry*. 2016;3(8):760-773. doi:10.1016/s2215-0366(16)00104-8
21. Vorspan F, Mehtelli W, Dupuy G, Bloch V, Lépine JP. Anxiety and substance use disorders: co-occurrence and clinical issues. *Curr Psychiatry Rep*. 2015;17(2):4. doi:10.1007/s11920-014-0544-y
22. Torvik FA, Rosenström TH, Gustavson K, et al. Explaining the association between anxiety disorders and alcohol use disorder: a twin study. *Depress Anxiety*. 2019;36(6):522-532. doi:10.1002/da.22886
23. Lowe DJE, Sasiadek JD, Coles AS, George TP. Cannabis and mental illness: a review. *Eur Arch Psychiatry Clin Neurosci*. 2019;269(1):107-120. doi:10.1007/s00406-018-0970-7
24. Cougle JR, Hakes JK, Macatee RJ, Chavarria J, Zvolensky MJ. Quality of life and risk of psychiatric disorders among regular users of alcohol, nicotine, and cannabis: an analysis of the National Epidemiological Survey on Alcohol and Related Conditions (NESARC). *J Psychiatric Res*. 2015;66-67:135-141. doi:10.1016/j.jpsychires.2015.05.004

25. Brown SA, Irwin M, Schuckit MA. Changes in anxiety among abstinent male alcoholics. *J Stud Alcohol*. 1991;52(1):55-61. doi:10.15288/jsa.1991.52.55
26. Brady KT, Lydiard RB, Malcolm R, Ballenger JC. Cocaine-induced psychosis. *J Clin Psychiatry*. 1991;52(12):509-512.
27. Caton CL, Drake RE, Hasin DS, et al. Differences between early-phase primary psychotic disorders with concurrent substance use and substance-induced psychoses. *Arch Gen Psychiatry*. 2005;62(2):137-145. doi:10.1001/archpsyc.62.2.137
28. Fraser S, Hides L, Philips L, Proctor D, Lubman DI. Differentiating first episode substance induced and primary psychotic disorders with concurrent substance use in young people. *Schizophr Res*. 2012;136(1-3):110-115. doi:10.1016/j.schres.2012.01.022
29. Hides L, Dawe S, McKetin R, et al. Primary and substance-induced psychotic disorders in methamphetamine users. *Psychiatry Res*. 2015;226(1):91-96. doi:10.1016/j.psychres.2014.11.077
30. Chen WL, Hsieh CH, Chang HT, Hung CC, Chan CH. The epidemiology and progression time from transient to permanent psychiatric disorders of substance-induced psychosis in Taiwan. *Addict Behav*. 2015;47:1-4. doi:10.1016/j.addbeh.2015.02.013
31. Niemi-Pynttäri JA, Sund R, Putkonen H, Vorma H, Wahlbeck K, Pirkola SP. Substance-induced psychoses converting into schizophrenia: a register-based study of 18,478 Finnish inpatient cases. *J Clin Psychiatry*. 2013;74(1):e94-e99. doi:10.4088/JCP.12m07822
32. Ikawa H, Kanata S, Akahane A, Tochigi M, Hayashi N, Ikebuchi E. A case of methamphetamine use disorder presenting a condition of ultra-rapid cycler bipolar disorder. *SAGE Open Med Case Rep*. 2019;7:2050313x19827739. doi:10.1177/2050313x19827739
33. Sideli L, Quigley H, La Cascia C, Murray RM. Cannabis use and the risk for psychosis and affective disorders. *J Dual Diagn*. 2020;16(1):22-42. doi:10.1080/15504263.2019.1674991
34. Preuss UW, Hesselbrock MN, Hesselbrock VM. A prospective comparison of bipolar i and ii subjects with and without comorbid alcohol dependence from the COGA dataset. *Front Psychiatry*. 2020;11:522228. doi:10.3389/fpsyt.2020.522228
35. Aharonovich E, Garawi F, Bisaga A, et al. Concurrent cannabis use during treatment for comorbid ADHD and cocaine dependence: effects on outcome. *Am J Drug Alcohol Abuse*. 2006;32(4):629-635. doi:10.1080/00952990600919005
36. International Classification of Diseases, Eleventh Revision (ICD-11). World Health Organization. Accessed June 28, 2023. https://icd.who.int/browse11
37. Stavro K, Pelletier J, Potvin S. Widespread and sustained cognitive deficits in alcoholism: a meta-analysis. *Addict Biol*. 2013;18(2):203-213. doi:10.1111/j.1369-1600.2011.00418.x
38. Lee SS, Humphreys KL, Flory K, Liu R, Glass K. Prospective association of childhood attention-deficit/hyperactivity disorder (ADHD) and substance use and abuse/dependence: a meta-analytic review. *Clin Psychol Rev*. 2011;31(3):328-341. doi:10.1016/j.cpr.2011.01.006
39. Iqbal MN, Levin CJ, Levin FR. Treatment for substance use disorder with co-occurring mental illness. *Focus (Am Psychiatr Publ)*. 2019;17(2):88-97. doi:10.1176/appi.focus.20180042
40. Marín-Navarrete R, Toledo-Fernández A, Villalobos-Gallegos L, Pérez-López A, Medina-Mora ME. Neuropsychiatric characterization of individuals with inhalant use disorder and polysubstance use according to latent profiles of executive functioning. *Drug Alcohol Depend*. 2018;190:104-111. doi:10.1016/j.drugalcdep.2018.06.005
41. Wollman SC, Hauson AO, Hall MG, et al. Neuropsychological functioning in opioid use disorder: a research synthesis and meta-analysis. *Am J Drug Alcohol Abuse*. 2019;45(1):11-25. doi:10.1080/00952990.2018.1517262
42. Yuodelis-Flores C, Ries RK. Addiction and suicide: a review. *Am J Addict*. 2015;24(2):98-104. doi:10.1111/ajad.12185
43. Henriksson MM, Aro HM, Marttunen MJ, et al. Mental disorders and comorbidity in suicide. *Am J Psychiatry*. 1993;150(6):935-940. doi:10.1176/ajp.150.6.935
44. Salloum IM, Daley DC, Cornelius JR, Kirisci L, Thase ME. Disproportionate lethality in psychiatric patients with concurrent alcohol and cocaine abuse. *Am J Psychiatry*. 1996;153(7):953-955. doi:10.1176/ajp.153.7.953
45. Elliott AJ, Pages KP, Russo J, Wilson LG, Roy-Byrne PP. A profile of medically serious suicide attempts. *J Clin Psychiatry*. 1996;57(12):567-571. doi:10.4088/jcp.v57n1202
46. Asnis GM, Friedman TA, Sanderson WC, Kaplan ML, van Praag HM, Harkavy-Friedman JM. Suicidal behaviors in adult psychiatric outpatients, I: description and prevalence. *Am J Psychiatry*. 1993;150(1):108-112. doi:10.1176/ajp.150.1.108
47. Murphy GE, Wetzel RD. The lifetime risk of suicide in alcoholism. *Arch Gen Psychiatry*. 1990;47(4):383-392. doi:10.1001/archpsyc.1990.01810160083012
48. Conner KR, Hesselbrock VM, Meldrum SC, et al. Transitions to, and correlates of, suicidal ideation, plans, and unplanned and planned suicide attempts among 3,729 men and women with alcohol dependence. *J Stud Alcohol Drugs*. 2007;68(5):654-662. doi:10.15288/jsad.2007.68.654
49. Aharonovich E, Liu X, Nunes E, Hasin DS. Suicide attempts in substance abusers: effects of major depression in relation to substance use disorders. *Am J Psychiatry*. 2002;159(9):1600-1602. doi:10.1176/appi.ajp.159.9.1600
50. Ries RK, Yuodelis-Flores C, Comtois KA, Roy-Byrne PP, Russo JE. Substance-induced suicidal admissions to an acute psychiatric service: characteristics and outcomes. *J Subst Abuse Treat*. 2008;34(1):72-79. doi:10.1016/j.jsat.2006.12.033
51. Ahmad FB CJ, Rossen LM, Sutton P. *Provisional Drug Overdose Death Counts*. Accessed June 28, 2023. https://www.cdc.gov/nchs/nvss/vsrr/drug-overdose-data.htm#citation
52. Connery HS, Weiss RD, Griffin ML, et al. Suicidal motivations among opioid overdose survivors: replication and extension. *Drug Alcohol Depend*. 2022;235:109437. doi:10.1016/j.drugalcdep.2022.109437
53. Project TCL. *About the Protocol*. Accessed June 21, 2022. https://cssrs.columbia.edu/the-columbia-scale-c-ssrs/about-the-scale/
54. Na PJ, Yaramala SR, Kim JA, et al. The PHQ-9 Item 9 based screening for suicide risk: a validation study of the Patient Health Questionnaire (PHQ)-9 Item 9 with the Columbia Suicide Severity Rating Scale (C-SSRS). *J Affect Disord*. 2018;232:34-40. doi:10.1016/j.jad.2018.02.045
55. Yang A, Palmer AA, de Wit H. Genetics of caffeine consumption and responses to caffeine. *Psychopharmacology*. 2010;211(3):245-257. doi:10.1007/s00213-010-1900-1
56. Persad LA. Energy drinks and the neurophysiological impact of caffeine. *Front Neurosci*. 2011;5:116. doi:10.3389/fnins.2011.00116
57. Cappelletti S, Piacentino D, Sani G, Aromatario M. Caffeine: cognitive and physical performance enhancer or psychoactive drug? *Curr Neuropharmacol*. 2015;13(1):71-88. doi:10.2174/1570159x13666141210215655
58. Prochaska JJ, Das S, Young-Wolff KC. Smoking, mental illness, and public health. *Annu Rev Public Health*. 2017;38:165-185. doi:10.1146/annurev-publhealth-031816-044618
59. Breslau N, Novak SP, Kessler RC. Daily smoking and the subsequent onset of psychiatric disorders. *Psychol Med*. 2004;34(2):323-333. doi:10.1017/s0033291703008869
60. Steuber TL, Danner F. Adolescent smoking and depression: which comes first? *Addict Behav*. 2006;31(1):133-136. doi:10.1016/j.addbeh.2005.04.010
61. Weiser M, Reichenberg A, Grotto I, et al. Higher rates of cigarette smoking in male adolescents before the onset of schizophrenia: a historical-prospective cohort study. *Am J Psychiatry*. 2004;161(7):1219-1223. doi:10.1176/appi.ajp.161.7.1219
62. Kutlu MG, Parikh V, Gould TJ. Nicotine addiction and psychiatric disorders. *Int Rev Neurobiol*. 2015;124:171-208. doi:10.1016/bs.irn.2015.08.004
63. Taylor G, McNeill A, Girling A, Farley A, Lindson-Hawley N, Aveyard P. Change in mental health after smoking cessation: systematic review and meta-analysis. *BMJ*. 2014;348:g1151. doi:10.1136/bmj.g1151

64. Edwards AC, Kendler KS. Nicotine withdrawal-induced negative affect is a function of nicotine dependence and not liability to depression or anxiety. *Nicotine Tob Res.* 2011;13(8):677-685. doi:10.1093/ntr/ntr058
65. Hughes JR, Higgins ST, Bickel WK. Nicotine withdrawal versus other drug withdrawal syndromes: similarities and dissimilarities. *Addiction.* 1994;89(11):1461-1470. doi:10.1111/j.1360-0443.1994.tb03744.x
66. Masood B, Lepping P, Romanov D, Poole R. Treatment of alcohol-induced psychotic disorder (alcoholic hallucinosis)-a systematic review. *Alcohol Alcohol.* 2018;53(3):259-267. doi:10.1093/alcalc/agx090
67. Ashton H. Protracted withdrawal syndromes from benzodiazepines. *J Subst Abuse Treat.* 1991;8(1-2):19-28. doi:10.1016/0740-5472(91)90023-4
68. Glasner-Edwards S, Mooney LJ. Methamphetamine psychosis: epidemiology and management. *CNS Drugs.* 2014;28(12):1115-1126. doi:10.1007/s40263-014-0209-8
69. Thomasius R, Petersen KU, Zapletalova P, Wartberg L, Zeichner D, Schmoldt A. Mental disorders in current and former heavy ecstasy (MDMA) users. *Addiction.* 2005;100(9):1310-1319. doi:10.1111/j.1360-0443.2005.01180.x
70. Schlag AK, Aday J, Salam I, Neill JC, Nutt DJ. Adverse effects of psychedelics: From anecdotes and misinformation to systematic science. *J Psychopharmacol.* 2022;36(3):258-272. doi:10.1177/02698811211069100
71. Livne O, Shmulewitz D, Sarvet AL, Wall MM, Hasin DS. Association of cannabis use-related predictor variables and self-reported psychotic disorders: U.S. adults, 2001-2002 and 2012-2013. *Am J Psychiatry.* 2022;179(1):36-45. doi:10.1176/appi.ajp.2021.21010073
72. Liu Y, Lin D, Wu B, Zhou W. Ketamine abuse potential and use disorder. *Brain Res Bull.* 2016;126(Pt 1):68-73. doi:10.1016/j.brainresbull.2016.05.016
73. Martinak B, Bolis RA, Black JR, Fargason RE, Birur B. Dextromethorphan in cough syrup: the poor man's psychosis. *Psychopharmacol Bull.* 2017;47(4):59-63.
74. Luethi D, Liechti ME. Designer drugs: mechanism of action and adverse effects. *Arch Toxicol.* 2020;94(4):1085-1133. doi:10.1007/s00204-020-02693-7
75. Rosenbaum CD, Carreiro SP, Babu KM. Here today, gone tomorrow… and back again? A review of herbal marijuana alternatives (K2, Spice), synthetic cathinones (bath salts), kratom, Salvia divinorum, methoxetamine, and piperazines. *J Med Toxicol.* 2012;8(1):15-32. doi:10.1007/s13181-011-0202-2
76. D'Onofrio G, O'Connor PG, Pantalon MV, et al. Emergency department-initiated buprenorphine/naloxone treatment for opioid dependence: a randomized clinical trial. *JAMA.* 2015;313(16):1636-1644. doi:10.1001/jama.2015.3474

CHAPTER

101 Co-occurring Mood Disorders and Substance Use Disorders

Edward V. Nunes and Jungjin Kim

CHAPTER OUTLINE

- Overview and diagnostic criteria
- Prevalence and prognostic effects of co-occurring mood and substance use disorders
- Differential diagnosis
- Management of co-occurring mood and substance use disorders
- Summary and future directions

OVERVIEW AND DIAGNOSTIC CRITERIA

Significance

Depressive disorders, major depression and persistent depressive disorder (dysthymia), are among the most common psychiatric disorders in the general population. Estimates from community surveys show that over 10% of the general population has experienced a depressive disorder at some point in their lifetime, and the prevalence of substance use disorders (SUDs) is increased by a factor of two or more among individuals with major depression.[1] Major depression is the most common co-occurring psychiatric disorder encountered among patients presenting for treatment for SUDs, with lifetime prevalence rates ranging from 15% to 50% across samples studied from various treatment settings.[2] Among patients with SUDs, major depression has been associated with worse outcome, including worse substance use outcome, worse psychiatric symptoms, and increased suicide risk. Clinical trials suggest that treatment of depression among patients with co-occurring SUDs with medication or behavioral therapy can improve outcome. Thus, it is very important for clinicians working with such patients to be able to recognize and treat depression or make appropriate referrals for treatment.

Bipolar disorder is more rare in the general population, with estimates of the lifetime prevalence of bipolar I disorder ranging from 1% to 3%, another 1% for bipolar II disorder, and 2% or more having subthreshold disorders in the bipolar spectrum, each of which is associated with moderate to severe functional impairment.[3,4] Bipolar disorder is correspondingly less common than major depression among samples of patients seeking treatment for SUDs in routine outpatient settings. However, the strength of association between bipolar disorders and SUDs is larger than for depressive disorders, with the presence of a bipolar disorder increasing the likelihood of an SUD by a factor of four or more. Hence, among patients with bipolar disorder, the prevalence of SUDs is 40% or more,[5] and patients with both substance and bipolar disorders are especially likely to be encountered on inpatient settings or other clinical programs serving psychiatric or so-called dual diagnosis populations. As with unipolar depression, co-occurring bipolar and SUD is associated with worse prognosis, and clinical trials suggest that proper treatment of bipolar disorder improves substance use outcome. Further, many patients with bipolar disorder (particularly those who have had bipolar disorder for a long time) will present with a depressive syndrome, but the treatment recommendations for bipolar depression are different from unipolar depression. For bipolar disorder, mood stabilizer medications (eg, lithium, valproate, carbamazepine, lamotrigine) are the mainstay of pharmacotherapy, rather than antidepressant medications, and second generation neuroleptics (eg, quetiapine, olanzapine, risperidone, aripiprazole) are often effective as well. Thus, it is very important for clinicians working with patients with SUDs to be able to recognize bipolar disorder, distinguish unipolar depression from bipolar disorder, and either treat or make appropriate referrals for treatment.

Substance-induced mood disorder (depressive or bipolar) is a persistent mood disturbance (eg, depressed mood or pervasive loss of interest in the case of depressive disorder) that impairs functioning and warrants clinical attention, but which has occurred only in the context of active substance use. This category was introduced in DSM-IV to recognize that there exist mood syndromes that are more than just the usual intoxication or withdrawal effects of substances on the one hand but cannot be clearly diagnosed as independent depressive or bipolar disorders on the other. Research suggests that substance-induced depression has prognostic significance and may convert to independent depression over a subsequent follow-up period with the depression persisting or emerging during abstinence from substances.[6]

Disruptive mood dysregulation disorder (DMDD) is a new diagnosis, added in DSM-5[7] under the category of depressive disorders, consisting of severe recurrent temper outbursts, accompanied by a persistent irritable or angry mood most of the time. Onset is in childhood, before the age of 10. This diagnosis was introduced in DSM-5 in part because of the recognition of a subgroup of children with severe irritability and temper outbursts, who were being over-diagnosed as childhood bipolar disorder despite an absence of sustained episodes of hypomania or mania and major depression required for the bipolar diagnosis. The diagnosis is only recognized in childhood and adolescence. As children with DMDD pass into adulthood, bipolar disorder rarely emerges, but rather depressive or anxiety disorders may emerge. The early onset, prior to the age of risk for substance use disorders, makes DMDD an important syndrome to probe in the developmental history, as its presence indicates a mood disorder independent of substance use.

DSM-5 Criteria for Mood Disorders

An overview of DSM-5 depressive disorders and bipolar disorders[7] is provided in **Tables 101-1** and **101-2**. Much of the epidemiologic and clinical trials evidence on co-occurrence of mood and substance use disorders is based on earlier criteria sets, mainly DSM-IV[8] and DSM-III. However, the criteria for depressive and bipolar disorders have remained relatively consistent across DSM versions, other than the addition of substance-induced disorders (first appeared in DSM-IV) and DMDD in DSM-5. Readers who are less familiar with how to take a history to detect these disorders are encouraged to obtain experience with one of the semi-structured psychiatric diagnostic interviews such as the Structured Clinical Interview for DSM-5 (SCID),[9] the Psychiatric Research Interview for Substance and Mental Disorders (PRISM),[10] or the Mini-International Neuropsychiatric Interview (MINI).[11] These interviews guide the clinician in how to ask about each of the symptoms and apply the DSM criteria.

Depressive Disorders

DSM-5 defines a major depressive episode (see **Table 101-1**) as a period of persistent depressed mood or pervasive loss of pleasure or interest in usual activities, with associated depressive symptoms (disturbances in weight, appetite, or sleep, low energy, agitation or motor slowing, diminished concentration, feelings of worthlessness or guilt, thoughts of death or suicide), lasting at least two weeks, and that interferes with functioning. Persistent depressive disorder (dysthymia) is a period of milder but chronic depression lasting at least 2 years. Major depressive disorder is diagnosed when there have been one or more major depressive episodes. Major depression may occur as a single isolated episode, may run a chronic episodic course with multiple recurrences, or may be chronic and unremitting. Major depressive episodes may also be superimposed on a chronic dysthymic pattern. At its most severe, there can be psychosis, often involving delusions of paranoia or guilt or medical illness (eg, the patient begins to believe he or she has committed a terrible crime and will be punished, or has a serious illness despite negative medical workup). Risk factors for depressive disorders include a genetic component, as well as stress (eg, setbacks or losses) and trauma. Thus, in taking a history, it is important to ask about family history and about stressors and traumatic experiences. DSM-5 also requires that a depressive disorder is not caused by substance use (alcohol, drugs, or a medication) or a medical condition (eg, hypothyroidism or other systemic illnesses). Thus, a medical history and workup can be an important component of the diagnostic evaluation. Finally, when evaluating a patient presenting with a major depressive episode or a syndrome of dysthymia, it is important to review the history for past episodes of mania, hypomania, or mixed mood episodes (episodes containing both depressive and manic features simultaneously). The presence of one of these indicates that the patient has a bipolar disorder.

Bipolar Disorders

Bipolar disorders consist of episodes of major depression or dysthymia, alternating with episodes of mania or hypomania, at some time during the lifetime course. Bipolar I disorder is diagnosed when there are one or more episodes of mania over the lifetime, although most such patients also have depressive episodes. Mania is a severe disturbance consisting of euphoric, expansive, or irritable mood, high energy, less need for sleep (eg, only a few hours per night), grandiose thinking (eg, believing one has special powers, religious revelations), and increased speech and activity level. Functioning is severely impaired with disorganized, inappropriate behavior, and patients often become psychotic with hallucinations and delusions that may be grandiose ("I am the messiah") or paranoid ("the CIA is after me"). Mixed states also occur, in which the patient meets displays symptoms of both mania and major depression during the same episode. Bipolar II disorder describes patients with a history of hypomania and of major depressive episodes. Hypomania is a milder form of mania, without psychosis and with less functional impairment. In some cases, functioning may temporarily improve during hypomania, with high levels of productivity and creativity. In most cases of bipolar disorder, depressive episodes are predominant (particularly later in the course of the disorder), with less frequent mania or hypomania. Thus, patients with bipolar disorder often present with major depression, or dysthymia, and a careful lifetime history is needed to determine whether there have been past episodes of mania or hypomania. It is useful to interview family members who may provide more objective observations about a patient's hypomania or mania, since patients themselves often have little insight during mania or hypomania and may not experience these states as abnormal. As with depressive disorders, genetics, stress, and trauma are risk factors, so that family history and history of stress and trauma exposure are important. Drug intoxications (particularly stimulants), medications, or medical illnesses that might mimic bipolar disorder symptoms (eg, hyperthyroidism) need to be ruled out.

Disruptive Mood Dysregulation Disorder

DMDD is a syndrome with onset in children between ages 6 and 10, consisting of severe recurrent temper outbursts, which may involve physical aggression as well as verbal aggression, accompanied by a persistent irritable or angry mood most of the time. Severe Mood Dysregulation (SMD) was a similar

TABLE 101-1 Synopsis of Diagnostic Criteria for DSM-5 Depressive Disorders and Important Issues to Consider in Diagnosing Depressive Disorders in Patients Who Are Using Drugs or Alcohol

Overview of DSM-5 criteria for depressive disorders[6]	Notes on making the diagnosis in patients using drugs or alcohol
Major depressive disorder	
Consists of one or more episodes of major depression over the course of the lifetime. May occur as single episode or recurrent episodes or may run a chronic course. Other subtypes include anxious, melancholic, atypical, postpartum, psychotic, catatonic, and seasonal. The mixed subtype includes hypomanic or manic symptoms in addition to depression symptoms and suggests likely underlying bipolar disorder.	• Take a careful history of the course of depressive episodes over the lifetime (eg, age of first onset, age at subsequent episodes, duration and quality of episodes). • Relate lifetime course of depression to the lifetime course of substance use and substance use disorders.
Major depressive episode	
• At least 2 weeks of persistent core mood disturbance: 1. Depressed mood 2. Loss of interest or pleasure in most activities Plus associated symptoms: 3. Weight loss or gain 4. Insomnia or hypersomnia 5. Psychomotor agitation or retardation 6. Fatigue or loss of energy 7. Feelings of worthlessness or excessive guilt 8. Poor concentration or indecisiveness 9. Thoughts of death or suicide or suicidal behavior • A total of at least five symptoms are needed, including either (1) or (2). • Symptoms must be persistent: "most of the day, every day." • Not due to drug or alcohol use or another physiological cause such as a medical illness.	• Most depressive symptoms occur as part of intoxication or withdrawal syndromes of one or more substances (see also **Table 101-3**), so care is needed in attributing a symptom to a depressive disorder, as opposed to effects of a substance. • Look for persistence of depressive symptoms ("most of the day, every day") through increases or decreases in substance use or abstinent periods; symptoms that emerge and then resolve in step with substance use are more consistent with intoxication or withdrawal effects (eg, insomnia that occurs only on nights after episodes of cocaine use).
Persistent depressive disorder (dysthymia)	
A low-grade but chronic depression—at least 2-yr duration, feeling depressed "most of the day, more days than not," plus at least two associated symptoms (appetite disturbance, sleep disturbance, low energy, low self-esteem, poor concentration or indecisiveness, hopelessness); not due to drug or alcohol use or another physiological cause such as medical illness.	• Fewer and milder symptoms may be more difficult to distinguish from substance intoxication or withdrawal effects, but chronicity may be more indicative of a disorder that is independent of substance effects. • Look for the chronicity and persistence ("most of the day, more days than not") of symptoms, despite ups and downs in levels of substance use or periods of abstinence.
Premenstrual dysphoric disorder	
Depressive symptoms occur in the week before menstruation and resolve after menses. Not merely a worsening of another disorder like major depression.	• For women, ask about variation in symptoms over the menstrual cycle.
Other specified depressive disorders Unspecified depressive disorder	
Residual categories for depressive syndromes that fall short of diagnostic criteria for major depression or dysthymia (eg, not enough symptoms or not sufficient duration or persistence) but appear clinically significant.	• Little research on this residual category. • Given fewer and milder symptoms, more concern about distinguishing from intoxication or withdrawal effects. • But depressive disorders lie on a continuum, and milder forms may still be clinically significant.
Depressive disorder due to another medical condition	
Depressive symptoms or syndrome that can be caused by a medical condition.	• Chronic infections or metabolic conditions are common among patients with chronic substance problems (eg, HIV, HCV, liver failure, thyroid disease). Medical history, review of systems, physical exam, and other appropriate medical workup should be considered.
Substance-induced depression	
Depressive syndrome that cannot be established to be independent of drug or alcohol use (eg, by history, it seems to occur only during periods of substance use), but depressive symptoms are "sufficiently severe to warrant independent clinical attention" and are most severe or long lasting than typical symptoms of intoxication or withdrawal.	• See **Table 101-6** related text for more discussion. • Bear in mind that this is not simply intoxication or withdrawal effects (a common misconception, encouraged by the term "substance induced") but rather mood symptoms in excess of substance effects.

Mood disorders, grouped into depressive disorders and bipolar disorders, consist of combinations of mood episodes (major depressive episode, manic episode, hypomanic episode, mixed episode). For detailed criteria, see the full DSM-5 criteria and accompanying discussion.[7]

TABLE 101-2 Synopsis of Diagnostic Criteria for DSM-5 Bipolar Disorders and Important Issues to Consider in Diagnosing Bipolar Disorders in Patients Who Are Using Drugs or Alcohol

Synopsis of DSM-5 criteria for bipolar disorders[6]	Notes on making the diagnosis in patients using drugs or alcohol
• **Bipolar I Disorder:** at least one episode of mania. Often a series of episodes of mania, hypomania, and major depression. Subtypes include anxious, with mixed features (episodes with combinations of symptoms of depression and mania), rapidly cycling, melancholic, psychotic, peripartum, or seasonal. • **Bipolar II Disorder:** episodes of major depression plus episodes of hypomania. Depression often predominates the history. • A rapid-cycling pattern is diagnosed when there are at least four episodes in a year (eg, switches between mania or hypomania and depression).	• Take a careful history of the course of depressive episodes over the lifetime (eg, age of first onset, age at subsequent episodes, duration and quality of episodes). • Relate lifetime course of depression to the lifetime course of substance use and substance use disorders. • Rapid cycling has been associated with substance use disorder, though care must be taken not to mistake shifts in mood from euphoric to depressed caused by alternating periods of intoxication and withdrawal.
Manic episode	
• At least 1 week of persistently elevated, expansive, or irritable mood, and markedly increased goal-directed activity or energy, lasting at least a week, and accompanied by at least three of the following: 1. Grandiosity, inflated self-esteem (eg, patient believes they have special powers or insights [eg, on a mission from God]) 2. Decreased need for sleep (sleeps less, yet feels well rested) 3. More talkative, pressured speech, hard to interrupt 4. Flight of ideas—patient may report feeling of racing thoughts, or clinician may observe rapid expression of ideas 5. Distractibility—attention easily drawn to outside stimuli 6. Increase in activity level—may be goal directed (such as increased activity at school or work, socially, or sexually) or may present as agitation 7. Excessive involvement in activities with high potential for bad consequences (displaying seemingly poor judgment) (eg, buying sprees [buying large quantities of things the patient may have had little interest in previously], sexual adventures, foolish business ventures) • Marked impairment in functioning, or needing hospitalization, or psychotic • Not due to drug or alcohol use or other physiological causes	• Mania resembles stimulant intoxication (cocaine, amphetamines), including development of psychosis; other intoxication syndromes, including alcohol, PCP, or hallucinogens, might also resemble features of mania. • Manic-like symptoms that are part of intoxication should resolve quickly as intoxication wears off. • Duration (persistence) and severity of symptoms of mania usually make it easy to distinguish mania from intoxication effects.
Hypomanic episode	
Essentially same criteria as manic episode but may be of shorter duration (4 d) and not severe enough to meet criteria for mania (no psychosis, no hospitalization, no marked impairment in functioning); there must be a change in functioning, which may cause impairment but may sometimes enhance functioning (eg, patient becomes more productive or creative at work).	• Milder symptoms may be more difficult to distinguish from substance intoxication, but intoxication symptoms should resolve quickly as intoxication wears off. • Look for persistence of symptoms, despite ups and downs in levels of substance use or periods of abstinence.
Cyclothymic disorder	
Chronic course (at least 2 y) with periods of hypomanic symptoms and periods of depressive symptoms (not reaching criteria for major depression).	• Fewer and milder symptoms more difficult to distinguish from binge–crash pattern of cocaine/stimulant intoxication and withdrawal. • Look for persistence of symptoms, despite ups and downs in levels of substance use or periods of abstinence.
Other specified or unspecified bipolar disorders	
Residual categories for syndromes that fall short of criteria for bipolar I and II, or cyclothymia	• Same caveats in regard to fewer/mild symptoms as for cyclothymic disorder
Substance-induced mood disorder	
Bipolar syndrome that cannot be established to be independent of drug or alcohol use (seems to occur only during periods of substance use), and the substance involved is capable of producing the symptoms (eg, alcohol, stimulants, PCP, hallucinogens).	• Not simply intoxication or withdrawal effects (eg, cocaine intoxication symptoms that resolve rapidly after a binge) but rather mood symptoms "in excess" of expected substance effects. • There has been little research on substance-induced bipolar disorder per se. • Often possible to recognize independent bipolar disorder through a careful history, without needing to invoke the substance-induced category.

Bipolar disorders consist of combinations of mood episodes (major depressive episode, manic episode, hypomanic episode, mixed episode). For detailed criteria, see the full DSM criteria and accompanying discussion.[7]

syndrome of chronic irritability in childhood developed and studied prior to the formulation of DMDD into DSM-5. The diagnosis of DMDD should not be made if the syndrome is better explained by another disorder, such as a depressive or anxiety disorder, PTSD or ADHD, though it may co-occur with these disorders. The diagnosis should not be made in the presence of bipolar disorder or oppositional defiant disorder. Children and adolescents with DMDD have elevated levels of psychosocial impairment and co-occurring psychiatric disorders.[12] In adolescence and adulthood the symptoms of DMDD may persist, or evolve into depressive or anxiety disorders, while emergence of bipolar disorder is less common. Treatment research is limited, though a range of options have been suggested, including antidepressants, anticonvulsant/mood stabilizers, stimulants, neuroleptics, and alpha-2 agonists and behavioral therapies.[13]

In adolescence, co-occurrence of a syndrome of irritability, similar to DMDD, with heavy cannabis use has been described, responding to the anticonvulsant valproate.[14] DMDD was associated with an increased risk of substance use disorders among 13- to 18-year-olds in the National Comorbidity Survey—Adolescent Supplement.[15] The differential diagnosis of irritability among adolescents or adults with SUDs includes that irritability and aggression can be features of a number of intoxication or withdrawal syndromes and are also common in antisocial personality, which has high comorbidity with SUDs. It is important to examine the past history and developmental history for evidence of chronic problems with irritability or aggression that began in childhood and appear independent of substance use during adolescence and adulthood. A useful opening question is to ask whether the patient frequently got into fights during childhood. If a DMDD diagnosis appears to have been present in childhood, this suggests a disorder independent of substance use and would strengthen the case for diagnosing mood or anxiety syndromes in adolescence or adulthood as independent of substance use, and prompt consideration of corresponding pharmacotherapy or behavioral therapy.

Distinguishing Substance-Related Mood Symptoms From Mood Disorders

The problem of distinguishing mood symptoms caused by substance intoxication or withdrawal or chronic exposure to substances from independent mood disorders is a common challenge for clinicians working with substance-using patients. Mood symptoms (eg, sadness, apathy, irritability, pessimism, hopelessness, suicidal ideation, fatigue, appetite changes, anxiety, insomnia or hypersomnia, euphoria, hyperactivity) are very common among patients with drug or alcohol use problems. Often, such symptoms are components of substance intoxication or withdrawal and will resolve with abstinence; in that case, the indicated treatment is aggressive treatment of the substance problem. At other times, the mood symptoms are components of an independent mood disorder that needs to be treated in addition to treating the substance problems. In between are the substance-induced mood disorders, where the mood symptoms exceed what would be expected from intoxication or withdrawal but cannot be established as independent of substance use by history. For more on substance induced disorders, please see Chapter 100, "Substance Induced Mental Disorders."

Table 101-3 provides a summary of the overlap between symptoms of substance intoxication and withdrawal as listed in DSM-5 and symptoms of depressive and bipolar disorders. It is a worthwhile exercise to review the descriptions in DSM-5 (and the criteria) of the various substance intoxication and withdrawal syndromes. It is also important to consider the time courses of the intoxication and withdrawal syndromes. Intoxication syndromes typically resolve within hours of last substance exposure. Withdrawal syndromes typically resolve with a few days of last substance exposure, although there is greater variation across substances. Cannabis withdrawal, for example, may not begin until several days after abstinence from cannabis and may last for 1 to 2 weeks.

Abstinence or Initiation of Substance Treatment Improves Depression

This point cannot be overemphasized. Studies among pre–DSM-5 defined alcohol-,[16-18] opioid-,[19] and cocaine-dependent patients[20,21] have documented elevated scores on depression symptom scales that improve substantially after initiation of abstinence upon treatment entry, such as hospitalization for withdrawal management or initiation of maintenance treatment with methadone,[22] buprenorphine or extended-release naltrexone.[23] Thus, initiation of treatment for the substance use problem and efforts to achieve abstinence should always be a first step in the treatment of a patient with co-occurring mood and SUDs.

Some Cases of Depression Will Persist Despite Abstinence or Substance Treatment

This point deserves equal emphasis. Despite abstinence, or reductions in substance use, some cases of depression will persist. Evidence suggests that a careful clinical history can distinguish mood disorders that are independent of substance use and will persist in abstinence from those that will resolve with abstinence. For example, in a now classic series of studies, Brown and Schuckit[17,24] divided patients with DSM-defined alcohol dependence entering a 4-week inpatient stay into those with no history of mood disorder, those with a "secondary" mood disorder (onset after the onset of alcohol use disorder), and those with a "primary" mood disorder (mood disorder onset prior to the onset of alcohol use disorder). All three groups had substantially elevated Hamilton Depression Scale (HDS) scores at the outset. After 1 to 2 weeks of abstinence, the groups with no mood disorder or a secondary mood disorder experienced reductions of over 50% in their HDS scores, with

TABLE 101-3 Similarities and Differences Between DSM-5 Intoxication or Withdrawal Symptoms and Symptoms of DSM-5 Mood Disorders

	Intoxication or withdrawal symptoms that resemble major depression or dysthymia	Intoxication or withdrawal symptoms that resemble mania or hypomania	Intoxication or withdrawal symptoms that are distinct from symptoms of mood disorders
Alcohol or sedatives	**Intoxication:** mood lability **Withdrawal:** anxiety, insomnia	**Intoxication:** inappropriate sexual or aggressive behavior, mood lability, impaired judgment **Withdrawal:** insomnia, agitation, auditory hallucinations	**Intoxication:** slurred speech, incoordination, unsteady gait, nystagmus, impaired memory, stupor, coma **Withdrawal:** autonomic hyperactivity (eg, sweating, increased pulse, blood pressure, temperature), tremor, nausea/vomiting, visual or tactile hallucinations, seizures, delirium
Cocaine or other stimulants as amphetamines	**Intoxication:** anxiety, anger, psychomotor agitation or retardation, weight loss **Withdrawal:** dysphoria, fatigue, insomnia or hypersomnia, increased appetite, psychomotor agitation or retardation	**Intoxication:** euphoria, increased sociability, hypervigilance, anger, impaired judgment, impaired functioning, agitation, paranoia **Withdrawal:** insomnia, agitation	**Intoxication:** stereotyped behaviors, vital sign abnormalities, pupillary dilation, sweating or chills, nausea or vomiting, respiratory depression, cardiac symptoms (chest pain, arrhythmias), confusion, coma, dyskinesia, dystonia, seizures **Withdrawal:** vivid unpleasant dreams
Cannabis	**Intoxication:** social withdrawal, anxiety, increased appetite **Withdrawal:** depressed mood, irritability, anxiety, insomnia, decreased appetite, restlessness	**Intoxication:** euphoria, impaired judgment **Withdrawal:** irritability, anger, increased aggression, insomnia	**Intoxication:** impaired coordination, conjunctival injection, tachycardia, dry mouth, sense of time slowing down **Withdrawal:** strange dreams, headache, shakiness, sweating, stomach upset, nausea, sweating
Opioids	**Intoxication:** apathy, dysphoria, psychomotor retardation **Withdrawal:** dysphoria (irritability, anxiety), insomnia, fatigue	**Intoxication:** euphoria, agitation, impaired judgment or social functioning **Withdrawal:** irritability, insomnia	**Intoxication:** pupillary constriction, slurred speech, drowsiness, respiratory depression, stupor, coma (pupillary dilation and other signs of anoxia) **Withdrawal:** nausea, vomiting, muscle aches, lacrimation, rhinorrhea, pupillary dilation, piloerection, sweating, diarrhea, yawning, fever
Hallucinogens	**Intoxication:** anxiety, depression, paranoia	**Intoxication:** euphoria, paranoia, impaired judgment or functioning	**Intoxication:** ideas of reference, fear of losing one's mind, perceptual changes (depersonalization, derealization, hallucinations, synesthesia), pupillary dilation, tachycardia, sweating, palpitations, tremors, blurred vision, incoordination
PCP	**Intoxication:**	**Intoxication:** belligerence, impulsiveness, agitation, impaired judgment or functioning	**Intoxication:** nystagmus, tachycardia, hypertension, decreased responsiveness to pain, unsteady gait, slurred speech, muscular rigidity, seizures, coma, hyperacusis
Nicotine	**Withdrawal:** dysphoria, insomnia, irritability, anxiety, difficulty concentrating, restlessness, increased appetite, weight gain	**Withdrawal:** irritability, impaired concentration, restlessness, insomnia	**Withdrawal:** bradycardia

Note: The table lists DSM-5 symptoms for intoxication or withdrawal from each of the main substance classes and shows where there is overlap with similar symptoms of DSM-5 depressive syndromes (major depression, dysthymia) in column 2 or bipolar syndromes (mania, hypomania) in column 3; column 4 lists intoxication and withdrawal symptoms that are not consistent with mood disorder symptoms and would be helpful to distinguish substance effects from mood disorders.

scores dropping into the normal or mildly depressed range, so no specific treatment for depression is needed. However, in the group with primary mood disorder, there was no change in the depression scores over three weeks of abstinence, and two-thirds of those patients had HDS scores greater than 20 after 3 weeks of abstinence, consistent with severe depression. For these patients, aggressive treatment of the alcohol use disorder did not take care of the depression, and most clinicians and researchers would now agree that these patients with primary depression, identified with a careful lifetime psychiatric history, need to receive treatment for their depressive disorder, in addition to continued treatment for the alcohol use disorder.

PREVALENCE AND PROGNOSTIC EFFECTS OF CO-OCCURRING MOOD AND SUBSTANCE USE DISORDERS

Mood Disorders Among Patients Seeking Treatment for Substance Use Disorders

Numerous studies have been published examining the prevalence of mood disorders among patients admitted to alcohol or drug treatment programs, mainly inpatient withdrawal management or rehabilitation units, outpatient programs, or opioid maintenance programs. Reviews of this literature[2] show lifetime prevalence rates of major depression ranging from 20% to 50%, with rates of current major depression in the 10% to 20% range, substantially exceeding rates found in the general population. These high rates of comorbidity may occur in part because depression may be a factor that motivates patients with SUDs to seek treatment. Bipolar disorder is less common in these samples, consistent with its low prevalence rate in the general population. Thus, clinicians seeing patients in these typical addiction treatment settings should expect to see high rates on co-occurring depression but should also remain alert for cases of bipolar disorder, mindful that bipolar disorder often presents as depression, and review of the past history is needed to identify past episodes of mania or hypomania.

Comorbidity of Mood and Substance Use Disorders in the General Population

Table 101-4 summarizes the odds ratios of association between SUDs and mood and other psychiatric disorders, derived from three major community surveys—the Epidemiologic Catchment Area (ECA) Study,[25] the National Comorbidity Survey (NCS),[26,27] and the National Epidemiologic Survey on Alcohol and Related Conditions (NESARC).[1,3] As can be seen in **Table 101-4**, odds ratios are at least 2.0 for most combinations of disorders, showing that the presence of an SUD at least doubles the odds of a mood disorder, or other disorders, being present. It is notable that the odds ratios for major depression and dysthymia (persistent depressive disorder in

TABLE 101-4 Odds Ratios[a] Reflecting the Strength of Association or Co-occurrence Between Alcohol or Drug Dependence Disorders and Affective and Other Selected Disorders From Three Community Surveys

	ECA		NCS				NESARC	
			Alcohol dependence		Other drug dependence			
	Alcohol dependence	Other drug dependence	Men	Women	Men	Women	Alcohol dependence	Other drug dependence
Mood disorders								
Major depressive disorder	1.6	3.7	3.0	4.1	2.0[b]	2.0[b]	3.7	9.0
Dysthymia	2.3	3.6	3.8	3.6	1.3[b]	1.3[b]	2.8	11.3
Bipolar disorder	4.6	8.3	12.0[c]	5.3[c]			5.7[c]	13.9[c]
Other disorders								
Panic disorder	3.3	4.4	2.3	3.0			3.6[d]	10.5[d]
Social phobia	1.6	2.2	2.4	2.6	2.6[b]	2.6[b]	2.5	5.4
Posttraumatic stress disorder	—	—	3.2	3.6	3.0	4.5	—	—
Attention deficit hyperactivity disorder (ADHD)	—	—	2.8[b]	2.8[b]	7.9[b]	7.9[b]	—	—
Antisocial personality	14.7	15.6	8.3	17.0			7.1	18.5

Note: Data taken from three community surveys: the Epidemiologic Catchment Area (ECA) Study, the National Comorbidity Survey (NCS), and the National Epidemiologic Survey on Alcohol and Related Conditions (NESARC); odds ratio can be interpreted roughly as the multiple by which the prevalence of a disorder across the rows (major depression, dysthymia, etc.) is increased when alcohol or drug dependence is present, compared to individuals without alcohol or drug dependence.

[a]ECA and NCS report odds ratios on lifetime prevalences of co-occurring disorders; NESARC reports odds ratios on 12-month prevalences of co-occurring disorders.

[b]For these co-occurring disorders in NCS, odds ratios are reported for men and women combined.

[c]For NCS and NESARC, odds ratios are for bipolar I disorder with a history of full mania.

[d]For NESARC, odds ratios shown are for panic disorder with agoraphobia; odds ratios for panic disorder without agoraphobia were similar.

DSM-5) are similar. Thus, while dysthymia is often thought of as a mild version of depression, it should not be discounted in the clinical evaluation. The hallmark of dysthymia is its chronicity, and the presence of chronic depressive symptoms across the course of an SUD, even if the depressive symptoms are milder, should be taken seriously.

For bipolar disorder, the odds ratios are substantially larger than for major depression or dysthymia. When depressive symptoms are present, it is important to search the history carefully for past episodes of mania or hypomania, since bipolar illness has a particularly strong association with SUDs, and it has specific treatment implications that differ from those for unipolar depression.

Depression May Signal the Presence of ADHD, PTSD, or Other Disorders

As can be seen in **Table 101-4**, other common disorders, including attention deficit hyperactivity disorder (ADHD), posttraumatic stress disorder (PTSD), and other anxiety disorders, have odds ratios of association with SUDs that are as large as or larger than the associations for depressive disorders. These disorders are covered in detail in other chapters in this text. The point here is that these disorders often co-occur with depression, may be more easily distinguished from toxic and withdrawal effects of substances, and have distinct treatment implications. Thus, in patients with SUDs who present with depressive symptoms, it is important to look in the history for these other disorders.

For common anxiety disorders (social phobia, panic disorder with or without agoraphobia, and PTSDs), which often co-occur with depression, the cardinal symptoms (fear of social interactions, spontaneous panic attacks and fear of public places, and re-experiencing symptoms triggered by reminders of traumatic events) are distinctive and not attributable to substance intoxication or withdrawal. Thus, the presence of one of these anxiety syndromes in a depressed person with an SUD strongly suggests the presence of an independent disorder, warranting specific treatment. Like depression, the anxiety disorders often respond to treatment with antidepressant medications, although they have distinct behavioral therapeutic indications.

ADHD has strong associations with SUDs, with odds ratios of 2.8 and 7.9, respectively,[28] as well as strong associations with major depression (odds ratio = 2.7), dysthymia (odds ratio = 7.5), and bipolar disorder (odds ratio = 7.4).[28] The symptoms of inattention and hyperactivity begin in early childhood and can often be recognized in the developmental history as problems with school performance in elementary school, well before the onset of drug or alcohol use. The symptoms, particularly poor attention and poor organization skills, often persist into adulthood and are responsible for substantial functional impairment and poor role performance during adulthood (eg, poor job performance, high divorce rate). This in turn lends itself to the development of depression. ADHD has distinct treatment implications, responding to stimulant medications, or guanfacine, atomoxetine, or noradrenergic antidepressants. For more on ADHD, see Chapter 104, "Co-Occurring Addictive Disorder and Attention Deficit Hyperactivity Disorder."

Antisocial personality is included in **Table 101-4** to illustrate its strong association with SUDs. Patients with SUDs will often have antisocial features, but it is important to bear in mind that the presence of antisocial features, or disorder, does not rule out the presence of a mood or anxiety disorder, and they often co-occur. In addition, antisocial features may develop secondary to an SUD, that may resolve with recovery.

Prognostic Effects

A review of studies of longitudinal follow up of people with co-occurring mood and substance use disorders[2] shows that studies examining a lifetime diagnosis of major depression (ie, major depression at any point during the lifetime) found little prognostic effect on outcome of substance use or use disorder. In contrast, a current diagnosis of major depression has been consistently associated with worse outcome of substance use problems over follow-up periods ranging from 6 months to 5 years. This adverse prognostic effect holds for major depression diagnosed at an initial evaluation[29-32] and for major depression diagnosed during the follow-up period,[33,34] among those with alcohol use disorder,[31-35] methadone-maintained patients with opioid use disorders,[29,30] and patients with cocaine use disorders.[36]

Another important pattern in the results from longitudinal studies is that depressive symptoms at the time of entry into treatment, as measured by an elevated score on a standard scale such as the Beck Depression Inventory (BDI) or HDS, have inconsistent prognostic effects.[2] For example, in a study of inpatients with pre-DSM-5–defined alcohol dependence, Greenfield et al.[31] showed that an elevated HDS score at baseline was not associated with outcome across a 1-year follow-up, whereas a diagnosis of major depression at baseline did predict relapse to heavy drinking during follow-up. Dysthymia (ie, low-grade chronic depression) has received little study in terms of its prognostic effects on substance use outcome. However, there is some evidence that depressive symptoms have adverse prognostic effects when they persist during or after treatment of an SUD.[34,37,38] This suggests that persistent depressive symptoms, even if not meeting criteria for major depression, should be taken seriously among patients with SUDs. Depressive symptoms among patients with co-occurring bipolar and alcohol use disorder have been associated with subsequent increased heavy drinking.[39]

Taken together, these data have clinical implications. Depression symptom scales such as the Beck Depression Scale or Hamilton Depression Scale or PHQ-9 can be useful as screening tools, but these need to be followed up with a careful clinical history, establishing the presence or absence of depressive disorder. A past history of a depressive disorder is an important component of a complete history, but it is current major depression that is most clearly associated with worse outcome among patients with SUDs and should be attended to in the treatment plan. Chronic low-grade depression (dysthymia) and depression that persists after initiation of treatment for the substance problem also warrant clinical attention.

Primary Care and Psychiatric Populations

The majority of individuals with SUDs, depression, and other common mental disorders present, not at specialty mental health or addiction treatment settings, but at the offices of primary care physicians or other medical settings,[40] where SUDs and depression are more likely to go undetected and may be associated with over- or underutilization of services and poor outcome.[41] Patients may be unaware of these problems or may avoid discussing them with health care providers because of the stigma attached to the idea of having a "psychiatric" problem. This presents a challenge to addiction specialists to reach out to these other settings with programs of screening and brief intervention.[42]

Among outpatients seeking treatment for depression in one large study (STAR*D), the prevalence of concurrent AUDs was 13% and drug use disorders 8%.[43] Such rates are modest but exceed what would be expected in the general population. Among psychiatric inpatients, a more severely ill group, SUDs are common among both patients with major depression and bipolar disorder.[44] Rates of current SUDs of 30% or higher have been observed among patients in treatment for bipolar disorder.[5,44] The co-occurrence of mood and SUDs may be especially common among patients with serious co-occurring medical disorders such as HIV.[45,46]

DIFFERENTIAL DIAGNOSIS

Etiological Relationships Between Mood and Substance Use Disorders

When approaching the diagnostic evaluation, it is important to consider the multiple potential etiological relationships between mood symptoms or syndromes and SUDs. A summary of these is presented in Table 101-5, along with possible underlying mechanisms and implications for diagnostic assessment and treatment.

There are two important clinical implications here. The first is to appreciate the complexity and to avoid viewing patients in simplistic terms during diagnostic evaluation. All mood symptoms are not caused by toxic and withdrawal effects of substances, nor is all substance use a result of underlying psychopathology (as in "self-medication"). The second point is to be cautious in formulating causal mechanisms between co-occurring disorders. For example, when depression resolves with treatment of an SUD and establishment of abstinence, this is consistent with the inference that depression was a toxic effect of substance use. However, it is also possible that there was an independent mood disorder that responded to supportive elements of the behavioral therapy used to treat the SUD, with the potential to re-emerge at some future point.

DSM-5 Primary Versus Substance-Induced Mood Disorders Versus Expected Effects of Substances (Intoxication and Withdrawal)

Prior to DSM-IV, co-occurring disorders were often classified as "primary" versus "secondary," referring to the order of first onset—a major depressive disorder would be considered primary if its age at onset preceded the age at onset of an SUD or secondary if the SUD came first. "Primary" was also used in a more conceptual sense to convey causality—the primary disorder is the main disorder, which drives any secondary disorders. In DSM-III, an "organic mood disorder" could be used to categorize a mood disorder caused by substance use. DSM-IV and DSM-5 advanced the field by synthesizing pre–DSM-IV approaches to define primary (or independent) mood disorders and creating the new category of substance-induced mood disorder, which is in turn distinct from and exceeds in severity and duration the usual intoxication and withdrawal effects of substances. The DSM-5 criteria, and our interpretation of them, are summarized in Table 101-6. Because the DSM-5 criteria, as stated, leave some details vague, a suggested operationalization is also included in Table 101-6, based on data from the diagnostic approach taken by the PRISM interview and its demonstrated prognostic significance.[10,34]

Primary (Independent) Mood Disorder

DSM-5 defines a primary or independent mood disorder as one that precedes the onset of substance use or persists during significant periods of abstinence (one month or more is suggested as a rule of thumb). We have found that the historical data needed to establish these criteria (ages at onset, presence of periods of abstinence, and mood syndromes occurring during abstinent periods) can be determined with good reliability from a clinical history[47] and have established good reliability for the categorical diagnosis with both a modified SCID[47] and the PRISM diagnostic interviews.[10]

Substance-Induced Mood Disorder

The category of substance-induced mood disorder was established to recognize the phenomenon of co-occurring mood syndromes that cannot be established as chronologically independent of substance use (hence, not meeting the definition of primary), yet the mood symptoms seem to exceed what would be expected from the usual intoxication or withdrawal effects of the substance(s) a patient is taking. A typical example would be a patient with a long-standing, chronic history of heavy substance use, who also has a syndrome consistent with major depression that has occurred only during substance use, yet the syndrome seems substantial enough to warrant clinical attention and perhaps specific antidepressant treatment.

TABLE 101-5 Summary of Possible Etiological Relationships Between Co-occurring Affective Symptoms/Syndromes and Substance Use Disorders

Relationship	Mechanism	Clinical presentation and implications
Substance use causes affective symptoms.	Substance intoxication, withdrawal, or biological effects of chronic substance use—DSM-5 substance-induced disorder.	Substance use disorder is chronologically primary; mood symptoms resolve with abstinence or reduced substance use; treatment focuses on substance use disorder.
Substance use causes affective syndrome, which then takes on a life of its own.	Stress and loss (eg, relationships, jobs) engendered by substance use disorder promote depression; biological effects of chronic substance exposure trigger a vulnerability to mood disorder.	Affective syndrome is chronologically secondary but persists after abstinence (DSM-5 primary or independent mood disorder); treat both affective and substance use disorders.
Affective syndrome causes substance use disorder.	Self-medication (taking substances to relieve symptoms of affective disorder—eg, low mood, low energy, poor sleep in depression, lack of sleep, excessive energy in mania or hypomania).	Affective syndrome is chronologically primary or emerges during abstinence, preceding relapse; pure self-medication—in which self-medication is the only mechanism operating and treatment can focus exclusively on the affective disorder—is relatively rare.
Substance use is part of a pattern of increased activity and impulsivity in mania or hypomania.	Impulsivity, seeking out new experiences.	Substance use is chronologically secondary, beginning during episodes of mania or hypomania, and resolves with return to euthymia or depression; treatment can focus on bipolar disorder, but as with pure self-medication, this may be relatively rare.
Affective syndrome causes substance use disorder, which then takes on a life of its own.	Exposure to substances during an episode of affective disorder triggers a vulnerability to substance use disorder.	Substance use disorder is chronologically secondary but persists after mood disorder is treated; treat both disorders.
Independent disorders.	Both affective and substance use disorders are common in the general population and will co-occur by chance.	Any chronological pattern; each disorder persists during remissions of the other; treat both disorders.
Affective and substance use disorders stem from common underlying risk factors.	Common genetic factors, stress, trauma.	Any chronological pattern; both disorders need to be treated; reduction of stress may help both.
Affective symptoms and substance use become related over time.	Moods become a conditioned cue triggering substance use.	Substance use disorder may be chronologically primary, but moods (eg, sadness, anger) trigger episodes of substance use or cravings; management of unpleasant moods becomes an important part of therapy.
Co-occurrence worsens prognosis.	Presence of multiple disorders interferes with coping or treatment seeking.	Any chronological pattern; each disorder needs specific treatment.
Affective symptoms/syndrome may prompt treatment seeking for substance problems.	Affective symptoms (sad mood, trouble sleeping, functional impairment) engender motivation.	Any chronological pattern; focus on treatment of substance use, but affective disorder may need to be treated if it persists.

Distinguishing Substance-Induced Mood Disorder From Expected Effects of Substances

Expected intoxication or withdrawal effects of substances, and their overlap with symptoms of mood disorders, are summarized in **Table 101-3**. DSM-5 clearly specifies that the symptoms of either a primary (independent) or a substance-induced mood disorder must exceed the expected effects of intoxication or withdrawal from the substances the patient is taking (see **Tables 101-1** to **101-3**). The term "substance induced" is somewhat confusing in that it implies cause and effect (substances causing mood symptoms). Thus, clinicians sometimes use "substance induced" to describe intoxication or withdrawal effects, when DSM-5 in fact excludes these from a diagnosis of substance-induced mood disorder. For this reason, we have recommended a more neutral term, such as "substance-associated," that might be considered to replace "substance-induced."[48]

A substance-induced mood disorder should, according to the criteria, resolve if abstinence is achieved. However, it has been shown that if rigorous criteria are set for making the diagnosis (see Diagnostic Methods, below), a substantial proportion of such cases diagnosed as substance-induced major depression at an index evaluation will persist during future

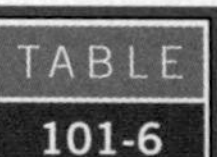

TABLE 101-6 Summary of DSM-5 Scheme for Classifying Co-Occurring Mood and Substance Use Disorders[a] and Suggestions for Operationalization of Criteria Based on SCID-SAC or PRISM Interviews[b]

DSM-5 criteria	Suggested operationalization based on the PRISM or SCID-SAC interviews
Independent (primary) mood disorder • Mood symptoms precede the onset of substance use. • Mood symptoms persist for a substantial period of time after the cessation of acute withdrawal or severe intoxication. DSM-5 suggests 1 month, but 1 or 2 weeks may be considered, given most withdrawal syndromes clear up within that timeframe. • Mood symptoms substantially in excess of what would be expected given the type or amount of the substance used or the duration of use. • Other evidence of an independent mood disorder (eg, a past history of recurrent episodes of major depression, clear family history of mood disorder).	Full criteria for DSM-5 mood disorder are met and include at least one of the following: 1. Age at onset of mood disorder precedes the onset of regular substance use. 2. Past episodes of mood disorder occurred during past periods of abstinence (SCID-SAC asks for past abstinence periods of 6 months or more; although this may be unnecessarily long). 3. Mood disorder persists after induction of abstinence in the current episode (DSM-5 recommends persistence of mood disorder during at least one month of abstinence; arguments can be made for shorter or longer durations, although we lean toward shorter duration—eg, 1-2 weeks). 4. Mood disorder is chronic (symptoms substantially in excess of usual effects of substances). This criterion seems difficult to operationalize, since it is a gradation based mainly on clinical judgment; long duration of mood disorder [eg, 3–6 mo or more] is more objective.
Substance-induced mood disorder • "Prominent and persistent disturbance in mood" (depressed mood or loss of interest/pleasure or elevated/expansive or irritable). • Mood symptoms develop during substance intoxication or withdrawal. • "Mood symptoms sufficiently severe to warrant independent clinical attention." • Mood symptoms exceed what would usually be associated with the intoxication or withdrawal syndrome. • Not better accounted for by an independent mood disorder. • "Substance induced" terminology may be a point of confusion, since it implies that substance causes the symptoms, prompting clinicians to think of intoxication or withdrawal when assigning this diagnosis; however, DSM-5 distinguishes substance-induced mood disorder as distinct from usual substance effects, warranting "independent clinical attention."	• Full criteria for a DSM-5 mood disorder are met (eg, "Substance-Induced Major Depression" or "Substance-Induced Dysthymia") (DSM-5 only specifies that the core mood symptoms be present). • PRISM asks the interviewer to judge that each symptom contributing to the diagnosis exceeds the usual effects of intoxication or withdrawal of the substances concurrently being taken (eg, insomnia not better explained by nightly cocaine use) and refers interviewer to DSM-IV criteria lists for alcohol and drug intoxication and withdrawal syndromes. • Mood disorder is chronic (symptoms exceeding the usual effects of substances seem difficult to operationalize as a criterion, since it is a gradation based mainly on clinical judgment; long duration of mood disorder [eg, 3-6 months or more] is more objective and may be a proxy).
Usual effects of substances DSM-5 suggests a diagnosis of substance intoxication or withdrawal should be made unless the mood symptoms are sufficiently severe or exceed what would be expected from intoxication or withdrawal effects.	PRISM asks the interviewer to judge that each symptom contributing to the diagnosis exceeds the usual effects of intoxication or withdrawal of the substances concurrently being taken and refers the interviewer to DSM-*5* criteria lists for alcohol and drug intoxication and withdrawal syndromes.

[a]For a complete statement of the criteria, see DSM-5 section on substance-induced depressive disorder.[7]

[b]Structured Clinical Interview for DSM-5, Substance Abuse Comorbidity Version (SCID-SAC)[47]; Psychiatric Research Interview for Substance and Mental Disorders (PRISM).[10]

abstinent periods, thus in effect converting to primary major depression.[6,49] Thus, substance-induced depression may be viewed as a sort of in-between category, where a mood disorder syndrome is present, but whether it is temporally independent of substance use (and hence primary or independent) is uncertain at the time of evaluation. This highlights the importance of identifying and following substance-induced depression, as it may convert to primary (independent) depression over time and as efforts are made to reduce or eliminate substance use.

Diagnostic Methods and Predictive Validity

One of the problems with the DSM-IV/5 approach is that the criteria are left vague in certain respects. For example, the criteria for substance-induced depression require only a persistent depressed mood or loss of interest, without any mention of associated depressive symptoms (eg, appetite, sleep, energy, etc.) nor how many symptoms need to be present. **Table 101-6** summarizes the DSM-5 criteria in the first column and suggests further operationalized criteria in the second column, based on the PRISM interview.[10,34] To make a diagnosis of substance-induced mood disorder, PRISM requires full criteria for a mood disorder (eg, major depression or dysthymia) to be met and that each symptom contributing to the diagnosis (eg, insomnia, loss of appetite, low energy) exceeds the expected effects of the substances that the patients are taking; the interviewer is referred to the DSM-5 criteria sets for intoxication and withdrawal syndromes for the various substances (see **Tables 101-1** and **101-2** for symptoms likely to overlap between mood and substance intoxication/withdrawal). The PRISM interview has been computerized and may be used as a clinical diagnostic instrument and a way for clinicians to gain experience with the history taking needed to evaluate DSM-IV/5 mood disorders among patients with SUDs (for more information on PRISM see https://www.columbiapsychiatry.org/profile/deborah-hasin-phd).

Evidence for the predictive validity of the operationalization of the diagnostic criteria reflected in the PRISM comes from a longitudinal study of patients with SUDs (alcohol, cocaine, or opioids) interviewed with the PRISM at an index hospitalization on a co-occurring disorder inpatient unit and then followed for one year.[6,34] About half of this sample had current major depression syndromes. About half of these major depression syndromes were diagnosed as independent (or primary) and half as substance induced. A PRISM diagnosis of substance-induced major depression was associated with failure of the SUD to remit, while a diagnosis of independent (or primary) major depression during a period of abstinence over the follow-up period was associated with a greater risk of return to SUD.[34] Both disorders were associated with suicidal behavior or ideation.[50] Further, of those cases diagnosed with a current substance-induced major depression, more than half converted into an independent major depression over the 1-year follow-up by being shown to persist during at least a 1-month period of abstinence.[6] Another study, using similar diagnostic methods, found a similar high rate of conversion to independent depression over a longitudinal follow-up.[49] When predictors of the likelihood of depression occurring over the course of the 1-year follow-up were examined, a past history of independent major depression and the presence of concurrent anxiety disorders were both associated with increased likelihood of depression.[6] This highlights the importance of a thorough clinical history on the lifetime course of depression, as well as inquiring about anxiety and other common co-occurring disorders.

Ries et al.[51] tested a simplified method of operationalizing the DSM-IV approach to co-occurring mood disorders. Specifically, they created a Likert-type scale that asks the evaluating clinician, after completing the clinical history, to rate the degree to which a mood disorder is independent or substance induced. This is reminiscent of the approach taken by the Structured Clinical Interview for DSM-5 (SCID),[9] which includes a module for substance-induced depression that simply asks the interviewer to make judgment based on the criteria. Mood disorders rated toward the substance-induced end of the spectrum on Ries' Likert scale were more likely to remit but were also associated with suicidal ideation and risk.[52] This work suggests that the judgment of experienced clinicians may be relied upon to make valid distinctions between substance-induced and independent mood disorders. However, experience with psychiatric diagnosis supports erecting criteria that are as objective as possible in order to maximize reliability and validity.

Diagnosing Bipolar Disorder in the Setting of Substance Use Disorder

Intoxication with cocaine or other stimulants may resemble hypomanic or even sometimes manic symptoms such as irritability, grandiosity, hyperactivity, talkativeness, impulsivity, insomnia, and paranoia. The impulsivity of alcohol or sedative intoxication may occasionally also resemble that of mania (see **Table 101-3**). However, full-blown mania (see **Table 101-2**) must last for at least a week, during which the symptoms should be persistent, whereas symptoms of intoxication are usually intermittent. For example, in mania, high energy and other symptoms can go on for days despite little or no sleep. In contrast, in cocaine intoxication, these symptoms usually last a matter of hours after cocaine use and are followed by a crash with increased sleep and low energy. Further, the marked impairment or psychosis required for mania is usually well in excess of what would be produced by intoxication. For example, cocaine intoxication may produce paranoia that lasts for a few hours and resolves during the crash period, whereas the psychosis characteristic of mania, often either paranoid or grandiose, is persistent over days and weeks. The nature of paranoid symptoms due to cocaine intoxication as opposed to mania is often distinct as well. For example, cocaine-induced paranoia symptoms are often focused on drug-related issues ("someone is coming to steal my drugs; the police are after me"), whereas manic symptoms may focus on special powers or more bizarre paranoid ideas (eg, ideas of reference). Hence, in establishing a diagnosis of mania, nature of symptoms, persistence of symptoms over time, and severity of impairment are key markers, as well as occurrence of the symptoms during clear periods of abstinence. Frank mania is distinctive, despite ongoing substance use.

Hypomania, which involves the same core symptoms as mania but may be briefer (at least 4 days) and with less impairment in functioning, may be more difficult to distinguish from substance intoxication or withdrawal effects. The same is true with cyclothymia, which may be difficult to distinguish from alternating periods of intoxication and withdrawal, mimicking hypomanic and depressive symptoms, respectively (see **Table 101-2**). Thus, it is particularly important to try to establish episodes of the mood disturbances during periods of abstinence or predating onset of significant substance use, to distinguish an independent mood disorder.

Rapid-cycling bipolar disorder is diagnosed when there have been at least four mood episodes over the past 12 months, punctuated either by periods of remission or by switches in polarity (from mania to depression, or vice versa). On the order of 20% of cases of bipolar disorder are rapid cycling, and the pattern is associated with greater impairment and poorer response to treatment.[53,54] Some evidence suggests that the rapid-cycling subtype is associated with increased prevalence of SUDs.[55] Thus, it is important to look for this pattern in the history. However, as for hypomania or cyclothymia, a pattern or multiple switches in mood states become more difficult to distinguish from the ups and downs of substance intoxication and withdrawal. It is important to establish in the history that hypomanic or manic syndromes have persisted over days or weeks before switching to depression, as well as seeking to establish occurrence of the symptoms during periods of abstinence.

Substance intoxication is likely to exacerbate the disinhibition and poor judgment associated with mania and is associated with poor medication adherence,[56] which promotes relapse. Thus, patients who present to emergency departments or other acute psychiatric settings with worsening mania are likely to also have SUD in the clinical picture.

For most patients with bipolar disorder, particularly those who have had the disorder for an extended period of time, the clinical course predominantly consists of depression, with occasional episodes of mania or hypomania. Thus, in a depressed patient with an SUD, it is important to carefully review the past history for episodes of mania or hypomania. In patients with chronic SUDs, clear-cut episodes of mania or hypomania, because they are distinctive from the usual effects of substances, are valuable in establishing that a primary (independent) mood disorder is indeed present and in need of treatment.

Summary of Recommendations for Diagnosis of Co-occurring Mood Disorders

The accumulated evidence suggests steps that the clinician can take during the clinical history to make this differential diagnosis between primary (independent) mood disorders, substance-induced mood disorders, and usual intoxication or withdrawal effects of substances (**Table 101-7**). These include:

- Establishing the presence of a full DSM-5 syndrome (eg, major depression, dysthymia, hypomania).[10]
- Establishing that each of the component criteria that make up the diagnosis exceeds the symptomatology that might be expected from the substances the patient is taking (eg, insomnia in a stimulant user).[10]
- Establishing the relative ages of onset and offset of mood disorder episodes in relation to periods of active substance

TABLE 101-7 Summary of Diagnostic and Historical Features Useful in Making the Differential Diagnosis of DSM-5 Independent Mood Disorder (as Opposed to Substance-Induced Mood Disorder)

Diagnostic/historical feature	Rationale and comment
Essential diagnostic features	
(1) Presence of a full DSM-5 syndrome (eg, major depression, dysthymia, hypomania)	Essential diagnostic feature.
(2) Each component criterion that makes up the diagnosis exceeds what symptomatology might be expected from concurrent substances the patient is taking	Implied in DSM-5, this feature applies if patient is currently using substances and may also be applied to DSM-5 substance-induced mood disorder, as in the PRISM interview.[10]
(3) Pattern of relative ages of onset and offset of mood disorder episodes in relation to periods of active substance use, such that the mood syndrome (including past episodes) precedes the onset of significant substance use or has persisted during abstinent periods	Essential DSM-5 diagnostic feature.
Associated historical features	
(4) History of serious suicide attempts	Serious suicide attempts are associated with depressive and bipolar disorders; suicidality by itself is not a toxic or withdrawal effect of any substance.
(5) History of co-occurring anxiety disorders	Anxiety disorders have symptoms that are distinctive from toxic or withdrawal effects (eg, spontaneous panic attacks, agoraphobia, social phobia, re-experiencing symptoms of PTSD) and high co-occurrence with mood disorders.
(6) Developmental history for early-onset mood disorder, anxiety disorders, or attention deficit hyperactivity disorder	Elementary school (if not junior high school) generally precedes onset of substance use, and mood or anxiety disorders sometimes have such early onset; ADHD has early onset and high co-occurrence with both depressive and bipolar disorder among adults.
(7) Family history for mood, anxiety, or other nonsubstance axis I disorders	Mood disorders are heritable, and a positive family history of mood disorder suggests proband may carry similar vulnerability.
(8) History of response to prior treatments for substance use disorders and depression	This can be a useful source of information for treatment planning; treatment approaches (behavioral therapies or medications) that have been successful in the past should be considered to be reinstituted; if treatment approaches have clearly failed despite adequate trials, these might best be avoided.

use, to determine whether the mood syndrome (including past episodes) precedes the onset of substance use or has persisted during abstinent periods.[12]

- Probing for a history of serious suicide attempts.[57]
- Probing for a history of trauma, PTSD and other co-occurring anxiety disorders.[58]
- Probing the developmental history for early-onset anxiety disorders, ADHD, or irritability and aggression consistent with DMDD.
- Probing the family history for mood, anxiety disorders, or other nonsubstance disorders.[57-59]
- Documenting response to past treatment efforts, including psychosocial/behavioral or medication treatments for substance use and for depression, as these data may guide treatment planning going forward.

MANAGEMENT OF CO-OCCURRING MOOD AND SUBSTANCE USE DISORDERS

Depressive Disorders

Antidepressant Medication

Effect of Antidepressant Medication on Outcome of Co-occurring Depression

Antidepressant medication has been the most thoroughly studied treatment modality for co-occurring mood and SUDs with numerous placebo-controlled trials in the literature. Two meta-analyses[60,61] reached similar conclusions that antidepressant medication is more effective than placebo in improving outcome among patients with co-occurring alcohol use disorder and depressive disorder, with the evidence less clear among patients with cocaine or opioid use disorder (the latter may be due to fewer high-quality studies, as some studies found positive results and others have not). Nunes and Levin[60] identified 14 placebo-controlled trials that selected patients with depressive disorders (major depression or dysthymia) co-occurring with alcohol, cocaine, or opioid use disorders and conducted an in-depth analysis of depression outcome, substance use outcome, and moderators of medication effects. The effect size (Cohen's d: standardized difference between means of Hamilton Depression Scale [HDS] score at outcome between medication and placebo groups) for the effect of medication on depression outcome was 0.38 (95% confidence interval 0.18 to 0.58), a small- to medium-sized effect that is in the same range and that observed in clinical trials of medications for treatment of routine outpatient depression.[62] The magnitude of the effect size was strongly related to placebo response—the greater the placebo response, the smaller the effect of medication.

Effects of Antidepressant Medication on Substance Use Outcome

In the Nunes and Levin meta-analysis,[60] among studies that showed medium to large effect sizes of antidepressant medication in improving depression outcome (Cohen's d > 0.5 standard deviations),[63-68] an effect size in the medium range was also observed on outcome measures of self-reported quantity of substance use,[60] whereas among studies with smaller effects on depression outcome the effect size for self-reported substance use outcome was near zero.[68-75] Categorical outcome measures reflecting criteria for remission or substantial improvement in substance use showed significant but smaller superiority of medication over placebo and overall modest rates of remission. This suggests the conclusion that treatment of a co-occurring depression with antidepressant medication may be helpful in reducing substance use when the depression improves.

Torrens et al.[61] cast a wider net in their meta-analysis and analyzed placebo-controlled trials of antidepressant medications for SUDs, dividing studies into those that did or did not require co-occurring depression and focusing on substance use outcomes. They found a significant favorable effect of antidepressant medication on drinking outcome among patients with co-occurring alcohol use disorder and depressive disorders, with equivocal findings for patients with co-occurring cocaine or opioid use disorder and depression, although they conclude that further research in each of these populations is needed.

Results of Recent Trials

Placebo-controlled trials of antidepressants published since these meta-analyses have produced a similar pattern of results, as have more recent meta-analyses.[76,77] Several negative trials have been published that had high placebo mood response,[78-82] while several studies with low to moderate placebo response showed some evidence of beneficial effects, at least on depression outcome.[83-85]

Association Between Mood Outcome and Substance Use Outcome

In addition to the finding that beneficial effects of medication on substance use outcome were observed in trials that demonstrated larger effects of medication on mood outcome,[56] some trials also reported the correlation between mood improvement and substance use improvement within the trial data set. In these analyses, the relationship between improvement in mood and improvement in substance use outcome is consistently strong and positive.[67,69,75,82,84] One study was able to show clearly that mood improvement mediates the effect of medication on substance use outcome,[67] but most of such trials lack this type of mediational analysis. These data suggest that depression and substance use outcomes are, at least in part, causally related and support the idea of concurrently treating both disorders.

Moderators of Antidepressant Medication Effect

Nunes and Levin[60] in their meta-analysis also studied moderators of medication effect—that is, features of the trials that predicted greater or lesser effect of medication compared to placebo on the outcome of depression. These bear detailed discussion, because they are useful in developing guidelines for management of patients with co-occurring depression and SUDs (see Table 101-8).

Placebo Response

Low placebo response rate was the strongest moderator of medication effect, accounting for approximately 70% of the variance in effect sizes across studies.[60] Placebo response was quantified as the percent improvement in the Hamilton Depression Scale (HDS) score between baseline and end of study in the placebo group of each respective trial. Studies with low placebo response rates (in the 20%-30% range) showed large medication versus placebo differences. In contrast, about half the studies had high placebo response rates in the 40% to 60% range; for this group of studies, the effect sizes hovered around zero, meaning no benefit of medication over placebo. High placebo response in these studies may represent improvement due to the background treatment that

TABLE 101-8 Factors (Moderators) Associated With Efficacy of Antidepressant Medications in Clinical Trials Among Patients With Co-occurring Depression and Substance Use Disorders and Implications for Clinical Practice

Moderator	Evidence	Implications for clinical practice
Placebo response	• Low placebo response associated with greater effect of antidepressant medication in a meta-analysis.[60] • High placebo response associated with lack of effect of antidepressant medication.	• Always treat the substance use disorder; in clinical trials, placebo response represents a response to the background treatment of substance use disorder, which may improve mood without resort to specific antidepressant treatment.
Establishment of abstinence before diagnosing depression	• Studies that required abstinence or enforced abstinence on an inpatient unit prior to diagnosis and treatment of mood disorder yielded larger medication effects.[60]	• Treat the substance use disorder and try to establish abstinence or reduction in substance use prior to diagnosis and treatment of depression. • Careful clinical history to establish evidence of independent depressive disorder as suggested in DSM-5 (see **Tables 101-6** and **101-7** for guidelines on diagnosis).
Class of antidepressant medication	• More consistent evidence for efficacy of TCAs and other noradrenergic or mixed-mechanism antidepressants.[60,61] • Less consistent evidence for efficacy of SSRIs, although some studies show robust efficacy of SSRIs when depression is diagnosed during abstinence,[66,68] and many negative studies have high placebo response.[60] • SSRIs associated with worse drinking outcome among early-onset type of alcohol use disorder (not selected for depression but characterized by early substance onset, antisocial personality features, and moderately elevated depression symptoms).[88,89]	• Consider SSRIs as first-line medication treatment due to good tolerability and safety characteristics in setting of ongoing substance use. • Switch to non-SRI antidepressant if SRI trial fails; TCAs may be considered but need to weigh risks, including sedation, overdose, and seizures; consider other newer antidepressant medications with noradrenergic or mixed mechanisms of action (eg, venlafaxine, duloxetine, mirtazapine, nefazodone). • Proceed with caution with SSRIs in patients with early-onset alcohol or drug use disorders and antisocial personality features.
Concurrent manual-guided psychosocial intervention	• Most of the clinical trials of antidepressant medication that were negative implemented a manual-guided psychosocial intervention as the background treatment received by all participating patients.[60]	• Initiate treatment of substance use disorder with an evidence-based treatment as elements of that treatment or resultant improvement in substance use may improve mood without resort to specific antidepressant treatment.
Diagnosis of depressive disorder (vs depressive symptoms)	• Meta-analysis[61] found little evidence for efficacy of antidepressants among alcohol- or drug-dependent patients without depressive disorders	• Careful clinical history to establish evidence of independent depressive disorder as suggested in DSM-5 (see **Tables 101-6** and **101-7** for guidelines on diagnosis). • More research needed on treatment response to antidepressant medications among patients with DSM-5 substance-induced depression. • Bear in mind that antidepressant medications may have beneficial effects for alcohol or drug use disorders that are separate from their antidepressant effects (eg, effect of nortriptyline for nicotine use disorder is related not to past history of major depression but rather to reduction of postquit dysphoria.[90])

all patients receive, which in these trials involved some form of psychosocial treatment for the SUD. This is part of what underlies our recommendation that treatment of the SUD is a first priority in the management of patients with co-occurring depression and substance problems. Treatment of the SUD may, in many cases, result in improvement in both substance use and depression.

Antidepressant Response in Patients With Alcohol Versus Drug Use Disorders

Consistent with the findings of Torrens et al.,[61] Nunes and Levin[60] found greater evidence for efficacy of antidepressant medications among depressed patients with alcohol use disorders than among those with drug use disorders. Across studies of patients with drug use disorders (cocaine or opioid use disorders), there is more heterogeneity, meaning some studies demonstrating benefits of antidepressants and others do not. The studies of patients with drug use disorders tended to have high placebo response, whereas more of the studies of patients with alcohol use disorders had methodological features associated with low placebo response and larger medication effects, namely, diagnosis of depression during a period of abstinence, treatment with a tricyclic or other noradrenergic medications (as opposed to a selective serotonin reuptake inhibitor [SSRI]), and absence of a manual-guided psychosocial intervention.

Notably, a recent trial of venlafaxine among patients with major depression and cannabis use disorder showed high placebo response and no difference between medication and placebo on mood outcome over and above placebo. Counter to expectations, outcome of cannabis use was worse on venlafaxine compared to placebo.[81]

Another recent trial recruited from people who used intravenous opioids and were not engaged in any treatment and tested a combination of cognitive-behavioral therapy (CBT) plus the SSRI antidepressant citalopram.[85] The combined treatment was superior to an assessment-only control condition in terms of proportion achieving remission from depression, and remission was associated with treatment adherence. Most people engaged in unhealthy opioid use are not engaged in any treatment, and this trial[85] is of particular interest because it suggests the potential of targeting depression as a way of engaging more such patients in treatment. It also suggests the utility of a combined pharmacological-behavioral treatment approach, which may have the potential to benefit more patients than either treatment alone.

Diagnosis of Depression During a Period of Initial Abstinence

Four placebo-controlled trials were conducted among patients with alcohol use disorder, who were diagnosed after at least 1 week of abstinence from alcohol.[63,65,66,86] These studies yielded medium to large effects of antidepressant medication on both depression and drinking outcomes. Three of those studies[63,66,86] worked with hospitalized patients with alcohol use disorder with relatively severe depressive disorders that were shown to persist after withdrawal management and enforced abstinence on the inpatient unit. This finding suggests that, when possible, an effort should be made to help patients initiate abstinence and observe the response of the depression during early abstinence, prior to initiating antidepressant medication. Depression that persists during an initial period of abstinence would be consistent with what DSM-5 would call a primary or independent depression. Greater severity of depression is also known to be associated with stronger effects of antidepressant medication in clinical trials.

With the advent of managed care and cost containment, hospitalization, particularly of several weeks' duration, is less of an option than it was when these antidepressant trials were conducted. Further, many patients will resist hospitalization or be unable to set aside work or family responsibilities to go into a hospital. Many of the studies in which patients were diagnosed on an outpatient basis implemented efforts to obtain a systematic clinical history to establish that depression was independent of substance use on a lifetime basis. Some of these studies observed significant benefits of medication,[64,65,67,83,84] although others that applied similarly careful historical criteria and methods failed to observe benefits of medication.[70,71] A recent large clinical trial among outpatient DSM-IV–defined alcohol dependence required both a brief period (1 week) of initial abstinence and a DSM-IV diagnosis of independent major depression using the PRISM interview (see **Table 101-6**), yet a substantial placebo response rate and no clear advantage of medication are still observed.[79] One possible explanation is that even independent major depression among such patients may often respond to the milieu and background psychosocial treatment offered as part of medication trials, resulting in high placebo response and less of a role for medication.

Class of Antidepressant Medication

Each of the meta-analyses that examined class of medication as a factor,[60,61,77] reached a similar conclusion that the evidence of efficacy for SSRIs is less robust than the evidence for efficacy of tricyclics, mainly desipramine or imipramine, and other medications with mixed modes of action. Many of the negative studies with SSRIs also had high placebo response rates, which do not suggest an inherent lack of efficacy of the medication. Further, several of the largest effects of medication (versus placebo) were observed with SSRIs, fluoxetine[66] or sertraline,[86] among hospitalized patients with co-occurring alcohol use disorder and severe depression.

Among placebo-controlled trials with patients with alcohol use disorder not selected specifically for depression, there is evidence that SSRIs may produce worse drinking outcome compared to placebo among patients with type B alcohol use disorder (high-risk/high-severity subtype). Type B is characterized by severe alcohol problems, high levels of externalizing psychopathology, and early onset of alcohol problems. In contrast, patients with less severe/late-onset alcohol use disorder (type A) may benefit from SSRIs.[87-89] An analogous finding was obtained among patients with PTSD; sertraline produced worse drinking outcome among patients with severe alcohol problems and later-onset PTSD, while sertraline was superior to placebo among patients with early-onset PTSD and less severe alcohol problems.[90] Another trial among veterans with PTSD and alcohol use disorder found desipramine superior to the SSRI paroxetine on drinking outcomes.[91] Similarly, venlafaxine, an SSRI with some noradrenergic reuptake inhibition (SNRI), made cannabis use worse compared to placebo among patients with cannabis use and major depression,[81] and cannabis use disorder typically has adolescent onset. Thus, it may be that SSRIs are less effective, perhaps even counterproductive in depressed patients with SUDs who have externalizing symptoms and/or early onset of SUD.

In terms of clinical recommendations, SSRIs have the advantage of being generally well tolerated, with less potential for sedation or other adverse effects. In contrast, tricyclic antidepressants (TCAs) generate a number of concerns including risks of sedation, overdose, QT prolongation, and seizures. Thus, we would continue to recommend SSRIs as the first-line treatment and move to a non-SSRI antidepressant, such as venlafaxine, duloxetine, mirtazapine,[92] or bupropion, or a TCA if the SSRI trial fails. The exception might be a patient with early-onset substance use and prominent externalizing symptoms or antisocial personality features, for whom the data suggest caution in the use of SSRIs.

Concurrent Psychosocial Intervention

One of the more intriguing findings to emerge from the meta-analysis[60] was that placebo-controlled trials that offered a manual-guided psychosocial intervention as the background treatment (ie, received by all participating patients) tended to have high placebo response rates and lesser medication effects.[72-74] These were interventions for SUD, including various cognitive-behavioral interventions or 12-step facilitation. Such interventions generally have components that focus on managing mood symptoms and thus may have inherent antidepressant effects. Also, these interventions may help reduce substance use, which in turn improves mood. A recent multisite sertraline trial, also a negative study with a high placebo response rate, offered all patients a medical management type of intervention, which was manual guided and emphasized abstinence and treatment adherence.[79] In terms of clinical recommendations, these findings reinforce the importance of initiating treatment for the SUD as the first step with any patient with co-occurring SUD and depression. Treatment of the SUD may be enough to produce improvement in depression.

Behavioral Treatments for Co-occurring Depression and Substance Use Disorders

A number of controlled studies have been conducted on psychosocial treatments for depression among patients with SUDs. These studies support the effectiveness of behavioral therapies for treatment of co-occurring depression and SUDs. A recent systematic review of studies of cognitive-behavioral treatments for concurrent depression and substance problems concluded this approach has promise, but more research is needed.[93] A recent meta-analysis of controlled trials of combined CBT and motivational interviewing for patients with alcohol use disorder and major depression found small but significant effect sizes for improvement of both mood and alcohol outcome.[94] Some of these are technology-based interventions, delivered over the internet, not requiring an expert therapist, and thus have potential for widespread dissemination.[95]

The community reinforcement approach (CRA) combined with voucher incentives is arguably the most effective behavioral treatment for SUDs. It is of interest for treatment of depression because it emphasizes increasing a patient's experience of reward and increasing pleasant activities (eg, family, friends, work, recreation). This has much in common with the behavioral activation component of CBT for depression.[96] Several trials suggest the promise of CRA with voucher incentives for treatment of co-occurring SUDs and depression.[97-99] Behavioral activation itself has been tested in a small controlled trial among patients with co-occurring drug use disorders and depressive symptoms and found superior to a treatment as usual control on outcome of mood symptoms.[100]

Referral to self-help groups such as Alcoholics Anonymous is a standard practice in treatment of SUDs. A 12-step facilitation was among the background treatments associated with high placebo response in the antidepressant trials reviewed above.[60] One observational study suggests that participation in Alcoholics Anonymous may reduce suicide risk.[101] On the face of it, 12-step groups contain elements including social support that would seem likely to benefit both depression and substance problems among individuals who become engaged in the groups.

Medication Treatments for Substance Use Disorders

Effective medications, such as disulfiram, naltrexone,[102,103] buprenorphine, or methadone, should also be considered in the treatment of patients with co-occurring depression and SUDs. The importance of initiating effective treatment for the SUD among patients with co-occurring depression has already been emphasized, and these medications are highly effective in reducing substance use. For example, depressive symptoms decrease substantially during the first 1 to 2 weeks of methadone maintenance treatment for opioid use disorder,[19] and about half of major depressive syndromes in patients presenting for methadone maintenance can be expected to resolve during those initial weeks of treatment.[67] Depression has also been shown to improve substantially among patients with opioid use disorder treated with sublingual buprenorphine or extended-release injection naltrexone.[23] Naltrexone and disulfiram were both shown to be safe and effective among patients with co-occurring alcohol use disorder and psychiatric disorders, including major depression.[102,103]

Combining Medications for Depression and Substance Use Disorder

A recent controlled trial among patients with co-occurring DSM-IV-TR–defined alcohol dependence and major depression found the combination of the antidepressant sertraline plus naltrexone superior to either medication alone or placebo on drinking outcomes.[104] A small pilot trial found the addition of disulfiram to imipramine useful in patients with co-occurring depression and alcohol use disorder whose drinking did not respond to imipramine alone.[105] These findings suggest the potential utility of combining medications for depression with medications for SUDs.

Adolescents and Treatment of Co-occurring Depression and Substance Use Disorder

SUDs often have their onset in adolescence, as do mood disorders, and the combination is associated with expected risk factors such as physical or sexual abuse[106] and with worse clinical outcome.[107] Effective intervention early in the course of these disorders has the potential to improve functioning during adolescence and prevents progression to chronic mood and substance use problems during adulthood. Treatment research on mood and SUDs in adolescents is limited. Controlled trials of antidepressant medication treatments among depressed adolescents (not selected for SUDs) have produced mixed results, often with high placebo response rates. An NIH-sponsored, multisite, randomized two by two trial of fluoxetine and CBT found fluoxetine superior to placebo on depression outcome, with the best outcome overall for the group receiving both fluoxetine and CBT.[108,109]

Several open-label trials support the effectiveness of fluoxetine for adolescents with combined depression and SUDs.[107,110] In a placebo-controlled trial of fluoxetine among adolescents with depression and an alcohol use disorder,[80] no difference in outcome between medication and placebo was observed. However, all patients in this trial received intensive CBT and motivational enhancement therapy (MET), and significant improvement from baseline in both depression and drinking was observed in the placebo group, as well as the group that received fluoxetine. In the other trial, adolescents with SUDs, major depression, and conduct disorder (CD) were randomized to fluoxetine or placebo while all received CBT; fluoxetine was superior to placebo on one of the two main depression outcome measures. The placebo response rate was high, with substantial overall improvements in depressive symptoms, conduct disorder symptoms, and self-reported substance use in both fluoxetine and placebo groups; fluoxetine was not superior to placebo on any of the substance use outcome measures, and in fact, urine toxicology outcome was slightly better on placebo than on fluoxetine.[111] These two studies support the effectiveness of combined fluoxetine and CBT for treating adolescents with combined depression and SUDs. However, the high placebo response rates observed in both these trials echo the finding among trials in adults that included a manual-guided intervention as the platform treatment[60] and suggest manual-guided psychosocial treatments like CBT alone may be effective for many depressed, substance-using adolescents. The lack of a favorable fluoxetine effect on substance use outcome, observed here, is also reminiscent of concerns, deriving from trials in adults, about poor substance use outcome with SSRIs among those with type B alcohol use disorder (see discussion in section "Class of Antidepressant Medication"). Type B is characterized by early onset of alcohol problems and externalizing psychopathology; these adolescent samples had early onset (by definition) and in one trial also carried diagnoses of conduct disorder. The results are also consistent with the observation from the meta-analysis[60] that the effect of medication on depression may be more robust than the effect on substance use outcome.

Late Life and Treatment of Co-occurring Depression and Substance Use Disorders

Although often thought of as a disease of the youth, SUDs occur in the elderly and may be an underrecognized problem in this population. The pattern of substances used may differ, with more alcohol and prescription drug problems among the elderly, often undiagnosed and untreated.[112,113] In addition to depression among the elderly, problems with sleep and painful medical conditions, prompting prescriptions of tranquilizers or narcotic analgesics, may contribute. Sleep problems and pain need to be treated, but clinicians working with the elderly should take a careful history for risk factors (eg, past history and family history of substance use problems), proceed cautiously, warn patients of the risks and warning signs of addiction, and monitor patients for the development of warning signs, such as development of tolerance, escalating dose, and substance-related impairment. As patients with SUDs who are under treatment grow older, for example, among methadone-maintained patients, the diseases of aging, such as cardiac and pulmonary disease and arthritis, become more prevalent along with depression and other psychiatric disorders, complicating clinical management.[114] Importantly, identification and effective treatment of depression (either with pharmacotherapy or behavioral therapy) may improve sleep, pain tolerance, and general functioning and in that instance could be expected to reduce the need for other prescription medications.

Research on treatment of SUDs and co-occurring substance use and depression among the elderly is limited, but results to date are encouraging in suggesting that treatment methods developed for young and middle-aged adults can be cautiously extrapolated to the elderly. Findings include that alcohol intake at treatment outset does not interfere with the treatment of depression[110] and that depression and drinking outcome tend to be correlated.[115,116] Since elderly patients with co-occurring disorders are most likely to present in primary medical or psychiatric care settings, a major challenge is to improve screening and intervention. One large trial showed that an integrated model of care (care for depression and SUDs within primary care) was superior to a referral-based model in promoting engagement in treatment of depression and alcohol problems.[117]

Suicidal Behavior and Co-occurring Depression/ Substance Use

Depression and substance use are both important risk factors for suicide, and thus, the potential for suicide needs to be carefully assessed in any patient presenting with this combination of disorders. Recent evidence suggests that both DSM-IV independent and substance-induced depression are associated with increase of suicidal thinking and behavior among patients with SUDs.[50,52,57] Other common risk factors for suicide such as family history of suicide, history of trauma, history of irritability or violence, current support systems, and physical illness should also be evaluated.[118,119]

In recent years, considerable concern has been aroused by reports of antidepressants being associated with increased risk of suicide, particularly among adolescents and young adults, resulting in the addition of explicit warnings being added to the prescribing information of these medications. Certainly, suicide risk (thinking, intent, and behavior) needs to be followed carefully in any depressed patient with a SUD during a course of treatment, whether or not it was present at baseline. A general consensus, based on recent data,[120,121] is that the benefits of antidepressant treatment (in terms of improved symptoms) outweigh the risks, although exacerbations of suicidal thinking or behavior may occur, and patients should be informed and closely monitored. Among patients with co-occurring depression and alcohol use disorder admitted to an inpatient unit, most of whom had substantial suicidal thinking at admission, treatment with fluoxetine improved depression and drinking outcome, and there were no suicide attempts.[66]

Interventions at the Level of Service Delivery and Primary Care

Most patients with depression, substance use problems, or both depression and substance use problems present to primary care physicians or to treatment providers in settings such as emergency rooms or primary care clinics (rather than to specialty practitioners or treatment providers in specialty clinics). Given evidence from randomized controlled trials supporting the effectiveness of treating depression among patients with SUDs, an important challenge is how to translate this finding into a program of care that is effective and can be implemented in primary health care settings. Watkins et al.[122] conducted a group-level randomized trial in which over 20,000 patients participating in managed care organizations were screened, and those screening positive for depression were randomly assigned to usual care or to one of two quality improvement programs, one focusing on implementation of antidepressant medications and one focusing on implementing psychotherapy for depression. The primary care clinics at which these patients were treated were randomized to usual care or to implement one of the two quality improvement programs. For patients with both depression and substance use problems, both quality improvement programs were associated with increased likelihood of prescription of antidepressant medications and improved depression outcome compared to usual care. In the STAR*D study, where over 2,000 depressed patients in primary care psychiatric or medical settings were treated openly with citalopram, the rate of depression response was just as good among those patients with SUDs compared to patients without SUDs, although there was a somewhat lower rate of remission of depression.[123] These studies suggest that efforts to increase treatment of combined depression and unhealthy substance use in primary care settings would have favorable effects and should encourage more efforts to develop programs of screening and intervention in primary care settings.

Another important question is whether patients with combinations of psychiatric and SUDs benefit when services for both problems are integrated into one treatment program, as opposed to a model in which psychiatric and substance problems are treated at separate programs. One large randomized trial found integrated services for patients with depression or problematic alcohol use resulted in superior outcome compared to a model in which patients were referred out to separate clinics for each problem.[117] Whether services are best delivered with an integrated model or through referral out to specialty clinics depends on the availability of integrated services and the severity and complexity of each component problem. Referrals can also be effective, especially when efforts are made to enhance communication between treatment teams and different programs.[124]

Depression and the Treatment of Nicotine/Tobacco Use Disorder

The prevalence of nicotine use disorder (mainly smoking) is increased among patients with mood disorders and is very high among patients with SUDs. Yet, nicotine use disorder is often overlooked during the evaluation and treatment of both mood disorders and SUDs—perhaps because it does not cause immediate impairment in the same way as mood or drug and alcohol problems, or perhaps staff are fearful of increased patient behavioral problems, including against medical advice discharges, should smoking be prohibited during treatment. Nonetheless, nicotine use disorder should be a focus of treatment planning, due to its substantial adverse long-term effects on health. Evidence on the co-occurrence of nicotine use disorder and depression also serves to illustrate the potential complexity of co-occurring psychiatric and SUDs.

Interest in this comorbidity began, in part, with observations that a history of major depression was common among patients seeking treatment to quit cigarette smoking and that a history of depression was an adverse prognostic factor, predicting lower likelihood of successfully quitting smoking.[125] Case histories, and a subsequent series, documented the emergence of severe depression after quitting smoking, which resolved only when smoking was resumed, suggesting that nicotine may function like an antidepressant medication for some patients.[126] Studies suggest that treatment for nicotine use disorder is effective among patients with depression.[127] However, few studies have evaluated the treatment of current depression among patients with nicotine use disorder, and in fact, current major depression has been an exclusion criterion from most clinical trials of treatments for nicotine use disorder.

Clinical trials of treatments for nicotine use disorder have often examined the history of major depression as a moderator, also with surprising findings. These include the finding that noradrenergic antidepressant medications bupropion and the tricyclic nortriptyline are effective agents for treating nicotine use disorder, but their effect does not appear to depend upon a history of depression.[128,129] For example, in a two by two trial, patients with nicotine use disorder were randomly assigned to nortriptyline or placebo and to either a cognitive-behavioral treatment or a control psychotherapy, and the patients were stratified into those with and without a history of major depression; a history of major depression was not associated with greater effectiveness of nortriptyline, although it was associated with a greater effectiveness of the cognitive therapy; analysis of mediators suggested that nortriptyline was having its beneficial effect by reducing the initial dysphoria experienced by patients after they quit smoking.[128] Thus, this would appear to be an example of an antidepressant medication having a beneficial effect on substance-induced mood symptoms. Several other studies have suggested addition of CBT for depression to nicotine use disorder treatment improved smoking outcome among patients with histories of major depression or greater severity of depression symptoms.[130,131]

Reminiscent of the questions raised above about the effectiveness of SSRI antidepressants among patients with SUDs, a meta-analysis suggests SSRIs are ineffective for nicotine use disorder.[132] For example, fluoxetine has been found to be ineffective as treatment for nicotine use disorder[133] or perhaps even counterproductive.[134] An exception is that one trial did find evidence of a beneficial effect of fluoxetine among smokers with more severe depressive symptoms at the outset of treatment.[135]

Summary of Treatment Recommendations for Co-occurring Depression

- *Treat the substance use disorder*. For any patient presenting with drug or alcohol problems, an important priority is to address the SUD. This can be easy to overlook when a clinician is called to consult about depression or when the patient is most bothered by the depressive symptoms. Substantial evidence, across substances, shows that treatment of SUDs, especially if abstinence is achieved, is associated with improvement of depressive symptoms. The full range of treatment options should be considered, including different levels of care, evidence-based behavioral interventions, as well as medications (eg, disulfiram, naltrexone, buprenorphine).
- *Evaluate the mood symptoms and look for other commonly co-occurring disorders (eg, PTSD, ADHD)*. Screening for depression can be accomplished during a review of systems in the initial clinical interview or with an instrument such as the Beck Depression Inventory (BDI) or the Patient Health Questionnaire (PHQ-9).[136] Patients who screen positive should be followed with a more in-depth psychiatric history, according to the DSM-5 (see **Tables 101-6** and **101-7**), to arrive at a diagnostic assessment of independent depressive disorder, substance-induced depressive disorder, or depressive symptoms as usual effects of substances. The history should be probed for evidence of bipolar disorder (history of mania or hypomania), since the treatment approach for bipolar disorder differs from that of depressive disorders, as well as severity of depression and suicide risk, as these will influence the urgency with which treatment of depression is initiated. Other disorders that frequently co-occur with depression, including PTSD, other anxiety disorders, and ADHD, should also be explored in the history, as these also have distinct treatment implications.
- *Treat the depression and other co-occurring disorders*. As the evidence reviewed above shows, primary or independent (as defined by DSM-5) major depression or dysthymia (persistent depressive disorder) among patients with SUDs should be treated. A guideline such as the Texas Medication Algorithm Project (TMAP)[137,138] can be applied to select antidepressant medications. Evidence-based behavioral therapies such as CBT or related approaches, as reviewed above (eg, behavioral activation, the community reinforcement approach), have also shown promise. Behavioral therapies avoid the potential for medication-substance interactions. Thus, it is worth considering as a first-line treatment for depression if personnel trained in the delivery of effective methods are available. To the extent that the depression is more severe with greater symptom levels, impairment, or suicide risk, medication should be preferred as the first-line treatment, perhaps in conjunction with behavioral treatment. The TMAP algorithm[137,138] recommends SSRI antidepressants as the first line of treatment due to their good tolerability and evidence of efficacy, unless the patient has a history of failure to respond to past adequate trials. However, as reviewed above, some evidence suggests SSRIs may be ineffective or even counterproductive for some patients with co-occurring substance and depressive disorders, namely those with early age of onset of substance problems. TCAs have the most consistent evidence of efficacy from the clinical trials reviewed, although their side effect profile makes them less than ideal for patients with SUDs, including risk for overdose in the setting of opioid use disorders.

Other medications with noradrenergic or mixed modes of action, such as venlafaxine, duloxetine, mirtazapine, or nefazodone, should be considered, mindful that fewer clinical trials have tested these agents for treatment of combined substance and depressive disorders. If other co-occurring disorders are present, such as bipolar disorder, anxiety disorders, or ADHD, these need to be considered in the treatment plan.

Bipolar Disorder

Pharmacological Treatments

Overview of Medication Treatment for Bipolar Illness

Pharmacological treatment is the mainstay of the treatment for bipolar disorder. More comprehensive reviews of pharmacotherapy for bipolar disorder can be found elsewhere,[139,140] and the TMAP is a useful guideline.[141] Briefly, treatment can be divided into the management of acute mania or hypomania, the management of bipolar depression, and maintenance medication to prevent recurrent mood episodes once an acute episode has resolved or improved.

Acute mania is typically treated with both a mood stabilizer (lithium, or an anticonvulsant) and an antipsychotic medication. Mood stabilizers that are FDA approved for the treatment of mania include lithium and the anticonvulsants valproate and carbamazepine. The combination is often preferable because mood stabilizers take longer time to work, while the antipsychotic medications work rapidly and are particularly useful in exerting rapid control over acute manic symptoms such as racing thoughts, agitation, and insomnia, and psychosis. Both first-generation (eg, chlorpromazine, haloperidol, perphenazine) and second-generation (eg, risperidone, olanzapine, quetiapine) antipsychotic medications are effective. Frank mania is a medical/psychiatric emergency due to the potential for psychosis and/or severely impaired judgment, either of which can lead to dangerous and self-destructive behavior. Patients with mania often have little or no insight into their condition and may be uncooperative. Thus, these patients should be brought to an emergency room for acute pharmacological management and considered for inpatient psychiatric admission to achieve full symptom control. Disordered substance use often accompanies acute mania or hypomania, and brief hospitalization can begin to bring this under control as well by establishing initial abstinence and allowing time for evaluation of the relationship between manic symptoms and substance use.

During the maintenance phase, the patient has already achieved relative euthymia, or stable mood. Here, the treatment goal is prevention of future mood episodes. To do this, the patient may continue the same medication that treated the acute mood episode or switch to a different medication that may be better-tolerated long-term. Valproate has been favored in recent years, perhaps because lithium has a narrow therapeutic window with serious toxicity and death if the levels become too high, thus requiring careful monitoring and a reliable patient with a low risk of overdose. However, lithium is often uniquely effective and reduces the risk of suicide; it should thus be considered in cooperative patients or in those with a significant other who can be involved to help monitor medication administration. Antipsychotics are less desirable as maintenance treatments because of significant side effects that can develop with chronic use, including tardive dyskinesia, weight gain, and metabolic syndrome. However, an antipsychotic often proves necessary, in conjunction with mood stabilizers, to maintain stable mood. Also, antipsychotics, taken at bedtime, provide a nonaddictive alternative to benzodiazepines for sleep. This is helpful because insomnia is a common symptom of bipolar disorder. During long-term antipsychotic treatment, clinicians should monitor abnormal movements and metabolic parameters, such as body mass index and serum glucose and triglycerides. Another benefit of antipsychotic medication is the availability of long-acting depot injections. Six antipsychotics are available as long-acting depot injections: haloperidol, fluphenazine, aripiprazole, paliperidone , olanzapine and risperidone. The long-acting injectable antipsychotics are especially useful, in combination with mood stabilizers, for patients who struggle with medication adherence or in whom relapse is regularly preceded by discontinuing medication. The long-acting injection guarantees that at least some mood stabilizing medication is on board, even if the patient stops the other medications, and this can attenuate the severity of the recurrent mood episode and facilitate intervention.

Substance use disorder is more likely to occur in manic or hypomanic episodes than in depressive phases of bipolar illness,[142] although it can certainly occur in conjunction with depression or during periods of euthymia as well. Hence, clinicians need to be prepared to medically manage acute intoxication or withdrawal when treating any phase of bipolar disorder. Of note, if the patient is undergoing acute alcohol withdrawal, lithium should be avoided due to potential toxicity from volume depletion. Anticonvulsants like valproic acid, on the other hand, may mitigate alcohol withdrawal symptoms.[143]

Management of Bipolar Depression. In most cases of bipolar disorder, depression is the predominant mood disturbance, with mania or hypomania occurring much less frequently.[144] Also, bipolar disorder patients are more likely to present for treatment of depression because depression is painful, whereas mania or hypomania can sometimes (but not always) be experienced as pleasurable, or the patient lacks insight into the adverse consequences of mania. Thus, as noted previously, it is very important to review the longitudinal mood history of a depressed patient for evidence of past episodes of mania or hypomania or family history of bipolar illness. The management of bipolar depression differs significantly from the management of unipolar depression. Antidepressant medication, either given alone or in combination with antipsychotics or mood stabilizers, is often ineffective and may even be harmful, as it can induce mania, mixed mood states, or rapid cycling of mood. Patients with bipolar depression often respond best to a mood stabilizer (lithium or anticonvulsant) or combination of a mood stabilizer with a low to moderate dose of a second-generation antipsychotic. Only five agents—olanzapine-fluoxetine combination, quetiapine, lurasidone, cariprazine and lumateperone—have regulatory approval for acute bipolar depression. Lamotrigine is not approved for acute bipolar depression but is commonly used due to evidence of its efficacy.[145] Lamotrigine may cause life-threatening skin reaction (Stevens-Johnson syndrome), and thus, the medication should be started at low dose (25 mg) and titrated slowly to the target dose range of 100 to 300 mg/d, with careful monitoring for dermatological reactions. However, once a maintenance dose is established without skin problems, lamotrigine is generally well tolerated and often quite effective in treating bipolar depression and preventing relapse.

Medication Treatments for Co-occurring Bipolar and Substance Use Disorders

Medications for Bipolar Disorder

Compared to bipolar disorder alone, there has been less research focused specifically on pharmacotherapy for co-occurring bipolar disorder and SUD. Therefore, clinicians should select medications based on the usual considerations given to each illness. The usual considerations include clinical evidence of effectiveness, adverse effect profile, family history of response, and the likelihood of adherence. Only a handful of double-blind, placebo-controlled trials have been conducted on patients with bipolar and SUDs. Salloum et al.[146] showed in a double-blind trial among individuals with co-occurring bipolar and SUDs that valproate combined with lithium was superior to lithium plus placebo in reducing the number of heavy drinking days. In another well-designed, placebo-controlled trial among hospitalized adolescents with bipolar and SUDs, lithium improved both mood and substance use outcome.[147] A third placebo-controlled trial examined carbamazepine among patients with cocaine use disorder with or without co-occurring mood disorders[148]; the mood disorder group included both major depressive disorder and bipolar disorder, many of those being bipolar II; among the subgroup with mood disorders, carbamazepine improved depression outcome with a trend toward reduced cocaine use as well, while the medication had no significant effects in the subgroup without mood disorders. Other open-label trials of anticonvulsant mood stabilizers among patients with SUDs and bipolar disorder have also shown evidence of good tolerability and efficacy, including lamotrigine,[149,150] valproate,[151,152] and gabapentin.[153]

Anticonvulsants have been studied as treatments for SUDs, based on hypotheses of beneficial effects on the pathophysiology of addiction (eg, augmentation of GABAergic inputs to the brain reward system). For example, substantial clinical trials suggest the efficacy of topiramate[154] and gabapentin[155] for alcohol use disorder, and a small trial suggests promise for topiramate[156] for cocaine use disorder. Topiramate and gabapentin have limited evidence as monotherapy for bipolar disorder, but may be useful as an adjunctive mood stabilizer.[157]

Second-generation neuroleptic medications have also shown promise among patients with co-occurring substance use and bipolar disorders, including small open-label, uncontrolled trials on quetiapine[158] and aripiprazole.[159] Quetiapine has been the subject of three randomized clinical trials. A double-blind, placebo-controlled trial of quetiapine (up to 600 mg/d), added to other mood stabilizers in patients with bipolar disorder (mainly depressed) and SUDs (mainly alcohol), showed quetiapine superior to placebo on depression outcome; there was no main effect of quetiapine treatment on substance use outcome, but improvement in drinking outcome measures did correlate with improvement in depression scores.[160] A second study[161] of quetiapine as an adjunct to either lithium or divalproex therapy for this population showed no benefit over placebo in drinking outcomes. Finally, a more recent study[162] compared quetiapine versus placebo in 90 patients with bipolar disorder and alcohol use disorder who were already taking a mood stabilizer. Quetiapine offered no advantage over placebo either in alcohol-related or mood outcomes. Taken together, the results of these trials resemble the larger literature on antidepressant medications among unipolar depressed patients[60] in suggesting that appropriate pharmacological treatment of a carefully diagnosed co-occurring DSM-IV/5 independent mood disorder improves mood symptoms, and in some studies, substance use improves as well. In each of the controlled trials, steps were taken in the diagnostic workup to establish the presence of an independent bipolar disorder (according to DSM-IV criteria), either through establishing persistence of mood symptoms during abstinence on an inpatient unit[147] or through a careful history.[146,148] The same caveat applies that medication treatment of the mood disorder is generally not likely to adequately or fully treat the SUD, so that specific attention in the treatment plan to behavioral or medication treatment for SUD also needs to be considered.

Medications for Substance Use Disorders

There is little evidence regarding the use of medications for targeted treatment of SUDs among patients with bipolar illness. Medications for SUD can be chosen as one would choose in SUD patients without bipolar disorder. Patients with bipolar disorder and alcohol use disorder, for instance, may first consider naltrexone, acamprosate, or disulfiram. Patients with bipolar disorder and opioid use disorder may opt for extended-release naltrexone, buprenorphine, or methadone. When prescribing multiple medications, drug-drug interactions should always be kept in mind. For example, carbamazepine chosen for bipolar disorder may cause opioid withdrawal when administered to patients maintained on buprenorphine or methadone, because carbamazepine accelerates hepatic breakdown of these medications.

As a general principle, if a medication for SUD is indicated (eg, methadone or buprenorphine for opioid use disorder or naltrexone for alcohol use disorder), it should be initiated with careful monitoring. For example, disulfiram, a potent deterrent against alcohol use disorder has been associated with rare cases of psychosis, thought to be due to its inhibitory effect on dopamine beta-hydroxylase, which in turn increases brain dopamine levels.[163] However, disulfiram and naltrexone have both been used safely and effectively in patients with co-occurring alcohol use disorder and other severe mental illnesses (including bipolar disorder).[102]

An open-label trial suggested that naltrexone, an effective treatment for alcohol use disorder, was safe and associated with both improved mood and improved alcohol use among patients with co-occurring bipolar and alcohol use disorder[164]; the majority of patients in that trial were depressed at the outset. A follow-up to this trial, a double-blind placebo-controlled trial with 50 patients, demonstrated a statistically nonsignificant trend favoring naltrexone on the outcome of drinking days.[164] A cautionary note, however, has been sounded by a report of two cases in which treatment with naltrexone in patients with mania and concurrent alcohol use disorder was poorly tolerated, producing marked nausea.[165] Similarly, in the open trial of naltrexone,[166] more of the patients who dropped out had mania or hypomania. New-onset hypomania has been observed in a patient with opioid dependence after withdrawal management and induction onto naltrexone.[167] This suggests that clinicians should carefully monitor patients with co-occurring bipolar and alcohol use disorders for side effects or clinical worsening when using naltrexone.

Finally, one study has been conducted using acamprosate for 33 patients with co-occurring bipolar disorder and alcohol use disorder; this trial showed no benefit of acamprosate over placebo regarding drinking outcomes.[168]

Other Medication Approaches

An intriguing and potentially promising medication for the treatment of patients with bipolar disorder and co-occurring SUDs is citicoline (cytidine-5′-diphosphate choline [CDP-choline]), a mononucleotide consisting of choline, cytosine, pyrophosphate, and ribose. Citicoline increases incorporation of phospholipids into membranes, enhances synthesis of structural phospholipids, and has been studied as a treatment for ischemic stroke, Parkinson disease, traumatic brain injury, and glaucoma. Citicoline may increase production in cholinergic brain neurons of acetylcholine, a substance thought to be important in learning and memory. Similarly, in elderly patients with mild cognitive impairment, citicoline treatment produced greater improvements in verbal memory. Citicoline has been examined in three separate studies of patients with bipolar disorder and stimulant use disorders. A small, proof-of-concept study ($N = 44$) of those with bipolar disorder and cocaine use disorder found that patients receiving citicoline were significantly less likely than those receiving placebo to have a cocaine-positive urine test at the end of a 12-week study.[169] In a larger subsequent study ($N = 130$), those receiving citicoline had better cocaine use outcomes, particularly early in treatment.[170] A study of citicoline in depressed patients (including those with bipolar depression) with DSM-IV-TR methamphetamine dependence ($N = 60$) showed a beneficial effect of citicoline on depressive symptoms but not on methamphetamine use.[171]

Behavioral Treatments

While medications are essential for treating most cases of bipolar disorder, behavioral treatments are also important to improve clinical outcome. The goals of behavioral and psychosocial treatment for bipolar disorder include (1) maintaining a treatment alliance and continuity of care, (2) securing adherence to medication treatment, and (3) coping with symptoms and addressing stressors or other circumstances that may lead to symptomatic exacerbations.[172,173] An SUD may undermine each of these goals, and thus, an important related goal is to identify and address substance use problems. Bipolar disorder generally runs a chronic, often waxing and waning, course, and maintaining continuity of care is an essential challenge. Patients may become impulsive or lose insight into their illness, particularly during manic or hypomanic phases, or lose sight of the need for ongoing treatment during periods of remission or relative quiescence of symptoms. Poor adherence to medications is a frequent cause of relapse and poor outcome in bipolar disorder. Patients may be bothered by side effects of medications. Patients may miss certain aspects of their mood fluctuations that are blunted by mood stabilizing medications. While this is particularly true of manic or hypomanic phases that are often experienced as pleasurable, some patients with bipolar disorder ironically resist the blunting of depressed mood as well, viewing their depression as a reflection of their "true" feelings. Finally, stressful life events, such as family conflict, and irregularity of daily routines and the sleep-wake cycle may contribute at a physiological level to the mood instability of bipolar disorder.[172,173] These types of issues—medication adherence, insight into illness, and management of stress—should be addressed in the behavioral/psychosocial management of patients with bipolar and SUDs.

Several specific behavioral/psychosocial treatments for bipolar disorder have been developed and have shown evidence of efficacy, including psychoeducation,[174-176] CBT,[177] Interpersonal Social Rhythm Therapy,[178-180] and Family-Focused Therapy.[181] Each to varying degrees addresses the common issues outlined above, including alliance, understanding the illness and its signs and symptoms, the importance of treatment adherence in general and medication adherence in particular, and the role of stressors and daily routines. Psychoeducation follows a medical model and emphasizes medication adherence, early recognition of symptoms, and social and occupational functioning. In addition to those basic goals, CBT seeks to understand and address connections between maladaptive thoughts or behaviors and mood disturbances. Interpersonal Social Rhythm Therapy, derived from interpersonal therapy for depression,[178] addresses the impact of relationships on mood fluctuations and also emphasizes the importance of normalizing routines and the sleep-wake cycle and targets disturbances in these areas, particularly disturbances in sleep, as warning signs. Reduced sleep or insomnia are frequently harbingers of mania, and hypersomnia often signals impending depression. Family-Focused Therapy is based on evidence that a stressful family environment has been associated with worse outcome; this treatment approach seeks to reduce tension and improve family functioning and coping strategies. Readers working with patients with bipolar and SUDs are encouraged to become familiar with these approaches. Patients and their families and significant others need to understand bipolar disorder, recognize signs of relapse, and have strategies on how to intervene; each of these approaches affords a range of useful strategies.

Behavioral Approaches to Co-occurring Bipolar and Substance Use Disorders

Integrated Group Therapy (IGT)[182,183] is the first group-based behavioral approach developed specifically for patients with both bipolar disorder and SUDs and has been shown to be effective in reducing substance use in two randomized controlled trials.[184,185] IGT is a manual-guided group treatment designed to serve as an adjunct to pharmacotherapy for bipolar disorder. It is assumed that the medications are managed during separate individual sessions with each patient's physician. Founded on cognitive-behavioral principles and focused on relapse prevention, IGT incorporates aspects of the above reviewed behavioral treatments for bipolar disorder while addressing the unique interrelationships between bipolar and SUDs. The superior substance-related outcomes of IGT across the two RCTs suggest that contextualizing SUD treatment in light of co-occurring mood symptoms is an important treatment element.

The core principles of IGT include the idea that similar patterns of thought and behavior promote relapse to both mood episodes and substance use and patients are encouraged to approach their problems as a single disorder—"bipolar substance use disorder"—rather than as a pair of distinct disorders. This counteracts the tendency of patients to view one of the disorders as predominant and minimize the other. Each session is focused on a topic, such as "dealing with depression without misusing substances" and "recovery versus relapse thinking." Each session begins with a "check-in" in which group members all report on their week in terms of substance use, mood symptoms, medication adherence, high-risk situations, and coping strategies employed. This is followed by a review of the topic of the previous week, followed by a presentation of the current topic and related coping skills to be learned; patients are given handouts and homework assignments to practice recovery skills during the coming week. The emphasis throughout is on similarities in the relapse and recovery process between the two disorders and the interrelationships between relapse to substance use and to mood episodes. There is also a strong emphasis on medication adherence, combating pessimism, and on maintaining daily routines and a regular sleep cycle. Since IGT is designed as an adjunctive treatment, it can be incorporated into a range of practice settings including either treatment programs for SUDs or psychiatric clinics serving bipolar patients or office-based practice.

An individual cognitive-behavioral approach has also been developed for patients with combined substance and mood disorders.[186] This approach includes medication monitoring plus 16 individual cognitive-behavioral sessions focused on an integrated approach to mood and substance use problems. In a randomized controlled trial among patients with bipolar disorder and SUDs, where the control group was medication monitoring alone, patients receiving this CBT had better medication adherence and fewer depressive symptoms compared to controls, but no difference in substance use outcome. Interestingly, the opposite pattern was observed in the initial trial of IGT, in which patients assigned to IGT had superior substance use outcome, but mood symptoms were actually somewhat worse on IGT compared to the Group Drug Counseling control; the latter mood symptoms were in the mild range and could reflect greater awareness and hence greater reporting of mood symptoms on IGT. In the second trial of IGT, however, the number of patients who had a "good clinical outcome," defined as being abstinent and having no mood episodes during the previous month, was more than twice as high for IGT patients than for patients receiving Group Drug Counseling.[185] Taken together, the results of these trials suggest there may be a role for individual CBT approaches to patients with combined bipolar and SUDs.

In addition to the integrated psychotherapeutic approaches described above, the entire treatment programs can offer an integrated approach, as developed by Farren et al.[187-189] This program, which consists of a combination of psychoeducation, individualized interpersonal therapy, relapse prevention group therapy, medications, and self-help groups, combines patients with bipolar and unipolar depression as well as SUDs.

An important line of research has examined the effectiveness of integrated approaches to treatment of patients with severe mental illness and substance use problems, as opposed to the traditional approach of referring patients to different agencies for psychiatric and substance treatment, respectively. In addition to patients with schizophrenia, the severely mentally ill population includes patients with severe cases of bipolar disorder, major depression, or schizoaffective disorder. For example, Assertive Community Treatment (ACT) is carried out by treatment teams that seek to deliver all needed services (eg, treatment for psychiatric disorder, treatment for SUD, and social services) to patients without resort to outside referrals. ACT and other integrated treatment models have a strong empirical evidence base,[190,191] including evidence of efficacy specifically among patients with bipolar and SUDs.[192] As an alternative to integrated models, efforts to enhance cooperation between separate agencies focusing on diverse combinations of psychiatric and substance problems can also be successful.

Summary of Treatment Recommendations for Co-occurring Bipolar Disorder

Initiation of effective treatment for the SUD is an important priority. However, the evidence on behavioral or psychosocial interventions suggests the importance of approaching the treatment of combined bipolar and SUDs simultaneously in an integrated fashion. If the diagnostic assessment establishes a clear-cut diagnosis of bipolar I or II disorder, this is almost certainly independent of SUD, and medication treatment for bipolar disorder is generally indicated. Bipolar disorder often runs a severe and disabling course, and medications are usually essential to achieving a good outcome. Several specific behavioral approaches have also been developed, which are useful as adjuncts to medication treatment of bipolar disorder. These behavioral treatments emphasize medication adherence; establishing a healthy, well-regulated lifestyle and sleep cycle; and addressing distorted cognitions that may exacerbate mood swings or substance use. An acute episode of mania, hypomania, mixed mood episode, or severe bipolar depression often rises to the level of medical emergency, requiring emergency room management and hospitalization. Suicide is a significant risk with bipolar disorder, and patients should be monitored for warning signs and risk factors. The available evidence on the use of mood stabilizers and antipsychotic medications among patients with combined bipolar and SUDs suggests these medications are effective in improving both bipolar symptoms and substance use outcome. Guidelines for pharmacotherapy of bipolar disorder can be followed, bearing in mind that a satisfactory outcome may depend upon combinations of medications with consideration for drug-drug interactions, patient preference and goals, and likelihood of adherence.

When the diagnostic assessment suggests a bipolar spectrum disorder (eg, cyclothymia or subthreshold bipolar disorder), the differential diagnosis between an independent bipolar disorder and a substance-induced mood disorder may be less clear. This differential is more difficult if the mood swings are less severe, of shorter duration, and consonant with intoxication or withdrawal symptoms of the substances the patient is using. In this instance, aggressive treatment of the SUD, combined with careful monitoring of the mood symptoms, may be warranted. Resolution of the mood symptoms with abstinence or improvement in the substance problems would add more credence to the substance-induced diagnosis, although mood swings may occur considerably later. Conversely, persistence of the mood symptoms despite improvement in substance use would suggest the presence of co-occurring bipolar disorder.

Available evidence suggests that the behavioral management of patients with combined bipolar and SUDs is important and should involve approaching both disorders in an integrated fashion, emphasizing common behavior patterns promoting recovery and relapse in both disorders and the importance of medication adherence and fostering a lifestyle conducive to recovery from both disorders. Manual-guided interventions[182,184] are available as well as integrated approaches at the programmatic level for patients with SUDs and mood disorders[184,186,187] or those who are severely ill and disabled.[189,190]

SUMMARY AND FUTURE DIRECTIONS

This chapter has attempted to serve as a primer on the diagnosis and treatment of mood disorders and presents the evidence on diagnosis and treatment of mood disorders among patients with SUDs. Several common themes emerge from the literature on depressive disorders and bipolar disorders co-occurring with SUDs. Initiation and maintenance of treatment for the SUD are always a priority that should not be overlooked. Careful diagnostic assessment and a lifetime clinical history are important for distinguishing between independent mood disorders, requiring specific treatment, versus substance-induced mood disorders that may resolve with abstinence or reduction in substance use. It is ideal to be able to observe the course of mood symptoms after reduction in substance use or abstinence, although abstinence will not always be achieved among outpatients and treatment will often need to be initiated without this information. To the extent that they have been tested in clinical trials, independent depressive or bipolar disorders seem to respond to the same medication or behavioral treatments that are effective for mood disorders in the absence of SUDs. Behavioral approaches may be effective as an alternative to antidepressant medication among substance-dependent patients with depression, while among bipolar patients, behavioral techniques have emphasized adherence to mood stabilizing medications and an integrated approach to substance and bipolar problems.

Despite substantial evidence on the diagnosis and treatment of mood disorders, SUDs, and their co-occurrence, many questions remain unanswered and indicate further research. Work is needed on the DSM diagnostic criteria and associated clinical features, to improve the important differential diagnosis between independent and substance-induced mood disorders. More research is needed on medication and behavioral treatments. There is, to date, only limited research on the prognostic and treatment indications of substance-induced mood disorders. Finally, the co-occurrence of mood and SUDs invites a range of studies seeking to understand the connection between these domains of disorders at a fundamental biological level. Examples may include studies on the effect of chronic exposure to specific substances (eg, cannabis, nicotine) on the development of mood disorders and vice versa, using genetics, brain imaging, and other biological markers. Such research promises to yield insights into the biology of each disorder as well as their combination and should help to place psychiatric diagnosis and treatment on a more sound pathophysiological footing, as is the ultimate goal beyond DSM-IV and DSM-5.

REFERENCES

1. Hasin DS, Goodwin RD, Stinson FS, Grant BF. Epidemiology of major depressive disorder: results from the National Epidemiologic Survey on Alcoholism and Related Conditions. *Arch Gen Psychiatry.* 2005;62(10):1097-1106.
2. Hasin D, Nunes E, Meydan J. Comorbidity of alcohol, drug and psychiatric disorders: epidemiology. In: Kranzler HR, Tinsley JA, eds. *Dual Diagnosis and Treatment: Substance Abuse and Comorbid Disorders*. 2nd ed. Marcel Dekker; 2004:1-34.
3. Grant BF, Stinson FS, Hasin DS, et al. Prevalence, correlates, and comorbidity of bipolar I disorder and axis I and II disorders: results from the National Epidemiologic Survey on Alcohol and Related Conditions. *J Clin Psychiatry.* 2005;66(10):1205-1215.
4. Merikangas KR, Akiskal HS, Angst J, et al. Lifetime and 12-month prevalence of bipolar spectrum disorder in the National Comorbidity Survey replication. *Arch Gen Psychiatry.* 2007;64(5):543-552.
5. Cerullo MA, Strakowski SM. The prevalence and significance of substance use disorders in bipolar type I and II disorder. *Subst Abuse Treat Prev Policy.* 2007;2:29.
6. Nunes EV, Liu X, Samet S, Matseoane K, Hasin D. Independent versus substance-induced major depressive disorder in substance-dependent patients: observational study of course during follow-up. *J Clin Psychiatry.* 2006;67(10):1561-1567.
7. American Psychiatric Association. *Diagnostic and Statistical Manual of Mental Disorders*. 5th ed. (DSM-5). American Psychiatric Association Publishing; 2013.
8. American Psychiatric Association. *Diagnostic and Statistical Manual of Mental Disorders*. 4th ed. American Psychiatric Association Publishing; 1994.
9. First MB, Williams JBW, Karg RS, Spitzer RL. *Structured Clinical Interview for DSM-5 Disorders, Clinician Version (SCID-5-CV)*. American Psychiatric Association Publishing; 2016.
10. Hasin D, Samet S, Nunes E, Meydan J, Matseoane K, Waxman R. Diagnosis of comorbid psychiatric disorders in substance users assessed with the Psychiatric Research Interview for Substance and Mental Disorders for DSM-IV. *Am J Psychiatry.* 2006;163:689-696.
11. Sheehan DV, Lecrubier Y, Sheehan KH, et al. The Mini-International Neuropsychiatric Interview (M.I.N.I.): the development and validation of a structured diagnostic psychiatric interview for DSM-IV and ICD-10. *J Clin Psychiatry.* 1998;59(Suppl 20):22-33.
12. Bruno A, Celebre L, Torre G, et al. Focus on disruptive mood dysregulation disorder: a review of the literature. *Psychiatry Res.* 2019;279:323-330.
13. Tourian L, LeBoeuf A, Breton JJ, et al. Treatment options for the cardinal symptoms of disruptive mood dysregulation disorder. *J Can Acad Child Adolesc Psychiatry.* 2015;24(1):41-54.
14. Donovan SJ, Nunes EV. Treatment of comorbid affective and substance use disorders. Therapeutic potential of anticonvulsants. *Am J Addict.* 1998;7(3):210-220.
15. Althoff RR, Crehan ET, He JP, Burstein M, Hudziak JJ, Merikangas KR. Disruptive mood dysregulation disorder at ages 13-18: results from the National Comorbidity Survey-Adolescent Supplement. *J Child Adolesc Psychopharmacol.* 2016;26(2):107-113.
16. Schuckit MA. Genetic and clinical implications of alcoholics and affective disorder. *Am J Psychiatry.* 1986;143:140-147.
17. Brown SA, Schuckit MA. Changes in depression among abstinent alcoholics. *J Stud Alcohol.* 1988;49:412-417.
18. Liappas J, Paparrigopoulos E, Tzavellas G, Christodoulou G. Impact of alcohol detoxification on anxiety and depressive symptoms. *Drug Alcohol Depend.* 2002;68:215-220.
19. Strain EC, Stitzer ML, Bigelow GE. Early treatment time course of depressive symptoms in opiate addicts. *J Nerv Ment Dis.* 1991;179(4):215-221.
20. Weddington WW, Brown BS, Haertzen CA, et al. Changes in mood, craving, and sleep during short-term abstinence reported by male cocaine addicts. *Arch Gen Psychiatry.* 1990;47:861-868.
21. Satel SL, Price LH, Palumbo JM, et al. Clinical phenomenology and neurobiology of cocaine abstinence: a prospective inpatient study. *Am J Psychiatry.* 1991;148:1712-1716.
22. Nunes EV, Sullivan MA, Levin FR. Treatment of depression in patients with opiate dependence. *Biol Psychiatry.* 2004;56(10):793-802.
23. Na PJ, Scodes J, Fishman M, Rotrosen J, Nunes EV. Co-occurring depression and suicidal ideation in opioid use disorder: prevalence and response during treatment with buprenorphine-naloxone and injection naltrexone. *J Clin Psychiatry.* 2022;83(3):21m14140.
24. Brown SA, Inaba RK, Gillin JC, Schuckit MA, Stewart MA, Irwin MR. Alcoholism and affective disorder: clinical course of depressive symptoms. *Am J Psychiatry.* 1995;152(1):45-52.
25. Regier DA, Farmer ME, Rae DS, et al. Comorbidity of mental disorders with alcohol and other drug abuse—results from the Epidemiological Catchment Area (ECA) Study. *JAMA.* 1990;263:2511-2518.
26. Kessler R, McGonagle K, Zhao S, et al. Lifetime and 12-month prevalence of DSM-III-R psychiatric disorders in the United States. Results from the National Comorbidity Survey. *Arch Gen Psychiatry.* 1994;51:8-19.
27. Kessler RC. Epidemiology of psychiatric comorbidity. In: Tsuang MT, Tohen M, GEP Z, eds. *Textbook in Psychiatric Epidemiology*. Wiley-Liss; 1995:179-197.
28. Kessler RC, Adler L, Barkley R, et al. The prevalence and correlates of adult ADHD in the United States: results from the National Comorbidity Survey Replication. *Am J Psychiatry.* 2006;163(4):716-723.
29. Rounsaville BJ, Weissman MM, Crits-Christoph K, Wilber C, Kleber H. Diagnosis and symptoms of depression in opiate addicts; course and relationship to treatment outcome. *Arch Gen Psychiatry.* 1982;39:151-156.
30. Rounsaville BJ, Kosten TR, Weissman MM, Kleber HD. Prognostic significance of psychopathology in treated opiate addicts; a 2.5 year follow-up study. *Arch Gen Psychiatry.* 1986;43:739-745.
31. Greenfield SF, Weiss RD, Muenz LR, et al. The effect of depression on return to drinking: a prospective study. *Arch Gen Psychiatry.* 1998;55(3):259-265.
32. Dixit AR, Crum RM. Prospective study of depression and the risk of heavy alcohol use in women. *Am J Psychiatry.* 2000;157(5):751-758.
33. Hasin D, Tsai W, Endicott J, Mueller T, Corvell W, Keller M. The effects of major depression on alcoholism: five year course. *Am J Addict.* 1996;5:144-155.
34. Hasin D, Liu X, Nunes E, McCloud S, Samet S, Endicott J. Effects of major depression on remission and relapse of substance dependence. *Arch Gen Psychiatry.* 2002;59(4):375-380.
35. Rounsaville BJ, Dolinsky ZS, Babor TF, Meyer RE. Psychopathology as a predictor of treatment outcome in alcoholics. *Arch Gen Psychiatry.* 1987;44:505-513.
36. Carroll KM, Power ME, Bryant K, Rounsaville BJ. One-year follow-up status of treatment-seeking cocaine abusers. Psychopathology and dependence severity as predictors of outcome. *J Nerv Ment Dis.* 1993;181:71-79.
37. Brown RA, Monti PM, Myers MG, et al. Depression among cocaine abusers in treatment: relation to cocaine and alcohol use and treatment outcome. *Am J Psychiatry.* 1998;155(2):220-225.
38. Curran GM, Flynn HA, Kirchner J, Booth BM. Depression after alcohol treatment as a risk factor for relapse among male veterans. *J Subst Abuse Treat.* 2000;19(3):259-265.
39. Prisciandaro JJ, DeSantis SM, Chiuzan C, Brown DG, Brady KT, Tolliver BK. Impact of depressive symptoms on future alcohol use in patients with co-occurring bipolar disorder and alcohol dependence: a prospective analysis in an 8-week randomized controlled trial of acamprosate. *Alcohol Clin Exp Res.* 2012;36(3):490-496.
40. Nordström A, Bodlund O. Every third patient in primary care suffers from depression, anxiety or alcohol problems. *Nord J Psychiatry.* 2008;62(3):250-255.
41. Ford JD, Trestman RL, Tennen H, Allen S. Relationship of anxiety, depression and alcohol use disorders to persistent high utilization and potentially problematic under-utilization of primary medical care. *Soc Sci Med.* 2005;61(7):1618-1625.

42. Babor TF, McRee BG, Kassebaum PA, Grimaldi PL, Ahmed K, Bray J. Screening, Brief Intervention, and Referral to Treatment (SBIRT): toward a public health approach to the management of substance abuse. *Subst Abuse.* 2007;28(3):7-30.
43. Davis LL, Frazier EC, Gaynes BN, et al. Are depressed outpatients with and without a family history of substance use disorder different? A baseline analysis of the STAR*D cohort. *J Clin Psychiatry.* 2007;68(12):1931-1938.
44. Brady K, Casto S, Lydiard RB, Malcolm R, Arana G. Substance abuse in an inpatient psychiatric sample. *Am J Drug Alcohol Abuse.* 1991;17(4):389-397.
45. Haller DL, Miles DR. Suicidal ideation among psychiatric patients with HIV: psychiatric morbidity and quality of life. *AIDS Behav.* 2003;7(2):101-108.
46. Berger-Greenstein JA, Cuevas CA, Brady SM, Trezza G, Richardson MA, Keane TM. Major depression in patients with HIV/AIDS and substance abuse. *AIDS Patient Care STDS.* 2007;21(12):942-955.
47. Nunes EV, Goehl L, Seracini A, et al. A modification of the structured clinical interview for DSM-III-R to evaluate methadone patients: test-retest reliability. *Am J Addict.* 1996;5(3):241-248.
48. Nunes EV, Rounsaville BJ. Comorbidity of substance use with depression and other mental disorders: from Diagnostic and Statistical Manual of Mental Disorders, fourth edition (DSM-IV) to DSM-V. *Addiction.* 2006;101(Suppl 1):89-96.
49. Ramsey SE, Kahler CW, Read JP, Stuart GL, Brown RA. Discriminating between substance-induced and independent depressive episodes in alcohol dependent patients. *J Stud Alcohol.* 2004;65(5):672-676.
50. Aharonovich E, Liu X, Nunes E, Hasin DS. Suicide attempts in substance abusers: effects of major depression in relation to substance use disorders. *Am J Psychiatry.* 2002;159(9):1600-1602.
51. Ries RK, Demirsoy A, Russo JE, Barrett J, Roy-Byrne PP. Reliability and clinical utility of DSM-IV substance-induced psychiatric disorders in acute psychiatric inpatients. *Am J Addict.* 2001;10(4):308-318.
52. Ries RK, Yuodelis-Flores C, Comtois KA, Roy-Byrne PP, Russo JE. Substance-induced suicidal admissions to an acute psychiatric service: characteristics and outcomes. *J Subst Abuse Treat.* 2008;34(1):72-79.
53. Bauer M, Beaulieu S, Dunner DL, Lafer B, Kupka R. Rapid cycling bipolar disorder—diagnostic concepts. *Bipolar Disord.* 2008;10(1 Pt 2): 153-162.
54. Schneck CD, Miklowitz DJ, Calabrese JR, et al. Phenomenology of rapid-cycling bipolar disorder: data from the first 500 participants in the Systematic Treatment Enhancement Program. *Am J Psychiatry.* 2004;161(10):1902-1908.
55. Kupka RW, Luckenbaugh DA, Post RM, et al. Comparison of rapid-cycling and non-rapid-cycling bipolar disorder based on prospective mood ratings in 539 outpatients. *Am J Psychiatry.* 2005;162(7):1273-1280.
56. Manwani SG, Szilagyi KA, Zablotsky B, et al. Adherence to pharmacotherapy in bipolar disorder patients with and without co-occurring substance use disorders. *J Clin Psychiatry.* 2007;68(8):1172-1176.
57. Schuckit MA, Tipp JE, Bergman M, Reich W, Hesselbrock VM, Smith TL. Comparison of induced and independent major depressive disorders in 2,945 alcoholics. *Am J Psychiatry.* 1997;154(7):948-957.
58. Preuss UW, Schuckit MA, Smith TL, et al. A comparison of alcohol-induced and independent depression in alcoholics with histories of suicide attempts. *J Stud Alcohol.* 2002;63(4):498-502.
59. Schuckit MA, Smith TL, Danko GP, et al. A comparison of factors associated with substance-induced versus independent depressions. *J Stud Alcohol Drugs.* 2007;68(6):805-812.
60. Nunes EV, Levin FR. Treatment of depression in patients with alcohol or other drug dependence: a meta-analysis. *JAMA.* 2004;291(15):1887-1896.
61. Torrens M, Fonseca F, Mateu G, Farré M. Efficacy of antidepressants in substance use disorders with and without comorbid depression. A systematic review and meta-analysis. *Drug Alcohol Depend.* 2005;78(1):1-22.
62. Walsh BT, Seidman SN, Sysko R, Gould M. Placebo response in studies of major depression; variable, substantial, and growing. *JAMA.* 2002;287:1840-1847.
63. Altamura AC, Mauri MC, Girardi T, Panetta B. Alcoholism and depression: a placebo-controlled study with viloxazine. *Int J Clin Pharmacol Res.* 1990;10(5):293-298.
64. Nunes EV, McGrath PJ, Quitkin FM, et al. Imipramine treatment of cocaine abuse; possible boundaries of efficacy. *Drug Alcohol Depend.* 1995;39:185-195.
65. Mason BJ, Kocsis JH, Ritvo EC, Cutler RB. A double-blind, placebo-controlled trial of desipramine for primary alcohol dependence stratified on the presence or absence of major depression. *JAMA.* 1996;275:761-767.
66. Cornelius JR, Salloum IM, Ehler JG, et al. Fluoxetine in depressed alcoholics. A double-blind, placebo-controlled trial. *Arch Gen Psychiatry.* 1997;54:700-705.
67. Nunes EV, Quitkin FM, Donovan SJ, et al. Imipramine treatment of opiate-dependent patients with depressive disorders. A placebo-controlled trial. *Arch Gen Psychiatry.* 1998;55:153-160.
68. Kleber HD, Weissman MM, Rounsaville BJ, Wilber CH, Prusoff BA, Riordan CE. Imipramine as treatment for depression in addicts. *Arch Gen Psychiatry.* 1983;40:649-653.
69. McGrath PJ, Nunes EV, Stewart JW, et al. Imipramine treatment of alcoholics with primary depression: a placebo-controlled clinical trial. *Arch Gen Psychiatry.* 1996;53:232-240.
70. Petrakis I, Carroll KM, Nich C, Gordon L, Kosten T, Rounsaville B. Fluoxetine treatment of depressive disorders in methadone-maintained opiate addicts. *Drug Alcohol Depend.* 1998;50:221-226.
71. Roy-Byrne PP, Pages KP, Russo JE, et al. Nefazodone treatment of major depression in alcohol-dependent patients: a double-blind, placebo-controlled trial. *J Clin Psychopharmacol.* 2000;20:129-136.
72. Schmitz JM, Averill P, Stotts AL, Moeller FG, Rhoades HM, Grabowski J. Fluoxetine treatment of cocaine-dependent patients with major depressive disorder. *Drug Alcohol Depend.* 2001;63:207-214.
73. Pettinati HM, Volpicelli JR, Luck G, Kranzler HR, Rukstalis MR, Cnaan A. Double-blind clinical trial of sertraline treatment for alcohol dependence. *J Clin Psychopharmacol.* 2001;21:143-153.
74. Moak DH, Anton RF, Latham PK, Voronin KE, Waid RL, Durazo-Arvizu R. Sertraline and cognitive behavioral therapy for depressed alcoholics: results of a placebo-controlled trial. *J Clin Psychopharmacol.* 2003;23:553-562.
75. Carpenter KM, Brooks AC, Vosburg SK, Nunes EV. The effect of sertraline and environmental context on treating depression and illicit substance use among methadone maintained opiate dependent patients: a controlled clinical trial. *Drug Alcohol Depend.* 2004;74(2):123-134.
76. Hobbs JD, Kushner MG, Lee SS, Reardon SM, Maurer EW. Meta-analysis of supplemental treatment for depressive and anxiety disorders in patients being treated for alcohol dependence. *Am J Addict.* 2011;20(4):319-329.
77. Iovieno N, Tedeschini E, Bentley KH, Evins AE, Papakostas GI. Antidepressants for major depressive disorder and dysthymic disorder in patients with comorbid alcohol use disorders: a meta-analysis of placebo-controlled randomized trials. *J Clin Psychiatry.* 2011;72(8):1144-1151.
78. Gual A, Balcells M, Torres M, Madrigal M, Diez T, Serrano L. Sertraline for the prevention of relapse in detoxicated alcohol dependent patients with a comorbid depressive disorder: a randomized controlled trial. *Alcohol Alcohol.* 2003;38(6):619-625.
79. Kranzler HR, Mueller T, Cornelius J, et al. Sertraline treatment of co-occurring alcohol dependence and major depression. *J Clin Psychopharmacol.* 2006;26(1):13-20.
80. Cornelius JR, Bukstein OG, Wood DS, Kirisci L, Douaihy A, Clark DB. Double-blind placebo-controlled trial of fluoxetine in adolescents with comorbid major depression and an alcohol use disorder. *Addict Behav.* 2009;34(10):905-909.
81. Levin FR, Mariani J, Brooks DJ, et al. A randomized double-blind, placebo-controlled trial of venlafaxine-extended release for co-occurring cannabis dependence and depressive disorders. *Addiction.* 2013;108(6):1084-1094.
82. Raby WN, Rubin EA, Garawi F, et al. A randomized, double-blind, placebo-controlled trial of venlafaxine for the treatment of depressed cocaine-dependent patients. *Am J Addict.* 2014;23(1):68-75.

83. Hernandez-Avila CA, Modesto-Lowe V, Feinn R, Kranzler HR. Nefazodone treatment of comorbid alcohol dependence and major depression. *Alcohol Clin Exp Res.* 2004;28(3):433-440.
84. McDowell D, Nunes EV, Seracini AM, et al. Desipramine treatment of cocaine-dependent patients with depression: a placebo-controlled trial. *Drug Alcohol Depend.* 2005;80(2):209-221.
85. Stein MD, Solomon DA, Herman DS, et al. Pharmacotherapy plus psychotherapy for treatment of depression in active injection drug users. *Arch Gen Psychiatry.* 2004;61(2):152-159.
86. Roy A. Placebo-controlled study of sertraline in depressed recently abstinent alcoholics. *Biol Psychiatry.* 1998;44:633-637.
87. Kranzler HR, Burleson JA, Brown J, Babor TF. Fluoxetine treatment seems to reduce the beneficial effects of cognitive-behavioral therapy in type B alcoholics. *Alcohol Clin Exp Res.* 1996;20(9):1534-1541.
88. Pettinati HM, Volpicelli JR, Kranzler HR, Luck G, Rukstalis MR, Cnaan A. Sertraline treatment for alcohol dependence: interactive effects of medication and alcoholic subtype. *Alcohol Clin Exp Res.* 2000;24(7):1041-1049.
89. Kranzler HR, Feinn R, Armeli S, Tennen H. Comparison of alcoholism subtypes as moderators of the response to sertraline treatment. *Alcohol Clin Exp Res.* 2012;36(3):509-516.
90. Brady KT, Sonne S, Anton RF, Randall CL, Back SE, Simpson K. Sertraline in the treatment of co-occurring alcohol dependence and posttraumatic stress disorder. *Alcohol Clin Exp Res.* 2005;29(3):395-401.
91. Petrakis IL, Ralevski E, Desai N, et al. Noradrenergic vs serotonergic antidepressant with or without naltrexone for veterans with PTSD and comorbid alcohol dependence. *Neuropsychopharmacology.* 2012;37(4):996-1004.
92. Cornelius JR, Chung TA, Douaihy AB, et al. A review of the literature of mirtazapine in co-occurring depression and an alcohol use disorder. *J Addict Behav Ther Rehabil.* 2016;5(4):159.
93. Hides L, Samet S, Lubman DI. Cognitive behaviour therapy (CBT) for the treatment of co-occurring depression and substance use: current evidence and directions for future research. *Drug Alcohol Rev.* 2010;29(5):508-517.
94. Riper H, Andersson G, Hunter SB, de Wit J, Berking M, Cuijpers P. Treatment of comorbid alcohol use disorders and depression with cognitive–behavioural therapy and motivational interviewing: a meta-analysis. *Addiction.* 2014;109(3):394-406.
95. Kay-Lambkin FJ, Baker AL, Kelly B, Lewin TJ. Clinician-assisted computerised versus therapist-delivered treatment for depressive and addictive disorders: a randomised controlled trial. *Med J Aust.* 2011;195(3):S44-S50.
96. Hopko DR, Lejuez CW, Ruggiero KJ, Eifert GH. Contemporary behavioral activation treatments for depression: procedures, principles, and progress. *Clin Psychol Rev.* 2003;23(5):699-717.
97. Carpenter KM, Aharonovich E, Smith JL, Iguchi MY, Nunes EV. Behavior therapy for depression in drug dependence (BTDD): results of a stage Ia therapy development pilot. *Am J Drug Alcohol Abuse.* 2006;32(4):541-548.
98. Carpenter KM, Smith JL, Aharonovich E, Nunes EV. Developing therapies for depression in drug dependence: results of a stage 1 therapy study. *Am J Drug Alcohol Abuse.* 2008;34(5):642-652.
99. Higgins ST, Sigmon SC, Wong CJ, et al. Community reinforcement therapy for cocaine-dependent outpatients. *Arch Gen Psychiatry.* 2003;60(10):1043-1052.
100. Daughters SB, Braun AR, Sargeant MN, et al. Effectiveness of a brief behavioral treatment for inner-city illicit drug users with elevated depressive symptoms: the life enhancement treatment for substance use (LETS Act!). *J Clin Psychiatry.* 2008;69(1):122-129.
101. Mann RE, Zalcman RF, Smart RG, Rush BR, Suurvali H. Alcohol consumption, alcoholics anonymous membership, and suicide mortality rates, Ontario, 1968-1991. *J Stud Alcohol.* 2006;67(3):445-453.
102. Petrakis IL, Poling J, Levinson C, et al. Naltrexone and disulfiram in patients with alcohol dependence and comorbid psychiatric disorders. *Biol Psychiatry.* 2005;57(10):1128-1137.
103. Petrakis I, Ralevski E, Nich C, et al. Naltrexone and disulfiram in patients with alcohol dependence and current depression. *J Clin Psychopharmacol.* 2007;27(2):160-165.
104. Pettinati HM, Oslin DW, Kampman KM, et al. A double-blind, placebo-controlled trial combining sertraline and naltrexone for treating co-occurring depression and alcohol dependence. *Am J Psychiatry.* 2010;167(6):668-675.
105. Nunes EV, McGrath PJ, Quitkin FM, et al. Imipramine treatment of alcoholism with comorbid depression. *Am J Psychiatry.* 1993;150(6):963-965.
106. Clark DB, De Bellis MD, Lynch KG, Cornelius JR, Martin CS. Physical and sexual abuse, depression and alcohol use disorders in adolescents: onsets and outcomes. *Drug Alcohol Depend.* 2003;69(1):51-60.
107. Cornelius JR, Clark DB, Bukstein OG, Birmaher B, Salloum IM, Brown SA. Acute phase and five-year follow-up study of fluoxetine in adolescents with major depression and a comorbid substance use disorder: a review. *Addict Behav.* 2005;30(9):1824-1833.
108. March J, Silva S, Petrycki S, et al. Fluoxetine, cognitive-behavioral therapy, and their combination for adolescents with depression: Treatment for Adolescents With Depression Study (TADS) randomized controlled trial. *JAMA.* 2004;292(7):807-820.
109. March JS, Silva S, Petrycki S, et al. The Treatment for Adolescents With Depression Study (TADS): long-term effectiveness and safety outcomes. *Arch Gen Psychiatry.* 2007;64(10):1132-1143.
110. Riggs PD, Mikulich SK, Coffman LM, Crowley TJ. Fluoxetine in drug-dependent delinquents with major depression: an open trial. *J Child Adolesc Psychopharmacol.* 1997;7(2):87-95.
111. Riggs PD, Mikulich-Gilbertson SK, Davies RD, Lohman M, Klein C, Stover SK. A randomized controlled trial of fluoxetine and cognitive behavioral therapy in adolescents with major depression, behavior problems, and substance use disorders. *Arch Pediatr Adolesc Med.* 2007;161(11):1026-1034.
112. Weintraub E, Weintraub D, Dixon L, et al. Geriatric patients on a substance abuse consultation service. *Am J Geriatr Psychiatry.* 2002;10(3):337-342.
113. Holroyd S, Duryee JJ. Substance use disorders in a geriatric psychiatry outpatient clinic: prevalence and epidemiologic characteristics. *J Nerv Ment Dis.* 1997;185(10):627-632.
114. Lima JE, Reid MS, Smith JL, et al. Medical and mental health status among drug dependent patients participating in a smoking cessation treatment study. *J Drug Issues.* 2009;39(2):293-312.
115. Oslin DW, Katz IR, Edell WS, Ten Have TR. Effects of alcohol consumption on the treatment of depression among elderly patients. *Am J Geriatr Psychiatry.* 2000;8(3):215-220.
116. Oslin DW. Treatment of late-life depression complicated by alcohol dependence. *Am J Geriatr Psychiatry.* 2005;13(6):491-500.
117. Bartels SJ, Coakley EH, Zubritsky C, et al. Improving access to geriatric mental health services: a randomized trial comparing treatment engagement with integrated versus enhanced referral care for depression, anxiety, and at-risk alcohol use. *Am J Psychiatry.* 2004;161(8):1455-1462.
118. Roy A. Characteristics of cocaine-dependent patients who attempt suicide. *Am J Psychiatry.* 2001;158(8):1215-1219.
119. Phillips J, Carpenter KM, Nunes EV. Suicide risk in depressed methadone-maintained patients: associations with clinical and demographic characteristics. *Am J Addict.* 2004;13(4):327-332.
120. Kutcher S, Gardner DM. Use of selective serotonin reuptake inhibitors and youth suicide: making sense from a confusing story. *Curr Opin Psychiatry.* 2008;21(1):65-69.
121. Bridge JA, Iyengar S, Salary CB, et al. Clinical response and risk for reported suicidal ideation and suicide attempts in pediatric antidepressant treatment: a meta-analysis of randomized controlled trials. *JAMA.* 2007;297(15):1683-1696.
122. Watkins KE, Paddock SM, Zhang L, Wells KB. Improving care for depression in patients with comorbid substance misuse. *Am J Psychiatry.* 2006;163(1):125-132.
123. Davis LL, Wisniewski SR, Howland RH, et al. Does comorbid substance use disorder impair recovery from major depression with SSRI

treatment? An analysis of the STAR*D level one treatment outcomes. *Drug Alcohol Depend.* 2010;107(2-3):161-170.
124. Rosenheck RA, Resnick SG, Morrissey JP. Closing service system gaps for homeless clients with a dual diagnosis: integrated teams and interagency cooperation. *J Ment Health Policy Econ.* 2003;6(2):77-87.
125. Glassman AH. Cigarette smoking: implications for psychiatric illness. *Am J Psychiatry.* 1993;150(4):546-553.
126. Glassman AH, Covey LS, Stetner F, Rivelli S. Smoking cessation and the course of major depression: a follow-up study. *Lancet.* 2001;357(9272):1929-1932.
127. Barnett PG, Wong W, Hall S. The cost-effectiveness of a smoking cessation program for out-patients in treatment for depression. *Addiction.* 2008;103(5):834-840.
128. Hall SM, Reus VI, Muñoz RF, et al. Nortriptyline and cognitive-behavioral therapy in the treatment of cigarette smoking. *Arch Gen Psychiatry.* 1998;55(8):683-690.
129. Brown RA, Niaura R, Lloyd-Richardson EE, et al. Bupropion and cognitive-behavioral treatment for depression in smoking cessation. *Nicotine Tob Res.* 2007;9(7):721-730.
130. Brown RA, Kahler CW, Niaura R, et al. Cognitive-behavioral treatment for depression in smoking cessation. *J Consult Clin Psychol.* 2001;69(3):471-480.
131. Patten CA, Martin JE, Myers MG, Calfas KJ, Williams CD. Effectiveness of cognitive-behavioral therapy for smokers with histories of alcohol dependence and depression. *J Stud Alcohol.* 1998;59(3):327-335.
132. Hughes JR, Stead LF, Lancaster T. Antidepressants for smoking cessation. *Cochrane Database Syst Rev.* 2007;1:CD000031.
133. Saules KK, Schuh LM, Arfken CL, Reed K, Kilbet MM, Schuster CR. Double-blind placebo-controlled trial of fluoxetine in smoking cessation treatment including nicotine patch and cognitive-behavioral group therapy. *Am J Addict.* 2004;13(5):438-446.
134. Spring B, Doran N, Pagoto S, et al. Fluoxetine, smoking, and history of major depression: a randomized controlled trial. *J Consult Clin Psychol.* 2007;75(1):85-94.
135. Blondal T, Gudmundsson LJ, Tomasson K, et al. The effects of fluoxetine combined with nicotine inhalers in smoking cessation—a randomized trial. *Addiction.* 1999;94(7):1007-1015.
136. Kroenke K, Spitzer RL, Williams JB. The PHQ-9: validity of a brief depression severity measure. *J Gen Intern Med.* 2001;16(9):606-613.
137. Crismon ML, Trivedi M, Pigott TA, et al. The Texas Medication Algorithm Project: report of the Texas Consensus Conference Panel on medication treatment of major depressive disorder. *J Clin Psychiatry.* 1999;60(3):142-156.
138. Trivedi MH, Rush AJ, Crismon ML, et al. Clinical results for patients with major depressive disorder in the Texas Medication Algorithm Project. *Arch Gen Psychiatry.* 2004;61(7):669-680.
139. Thase ME. STEP-BD and bipolar depression: what have we learned? *Curr Psychiatry Rep.* 2007;9(6):497-503.
140. Goodwin GM, Haddad PM, Ferrier IN, et al. Evidence-based guidelines for treating bipolar disorder: revised third edition recommendations from the British Association for Psychopharmacology. *J Psychopharmacol.* 2016;30(6):495-553.
141. Suppes T, Dennehy EB, Hirschfeld RM, et al. The Texas implementation of medication algorithms: update to the algorithms for treatment of bipolar I disorder. *J Clin Psychiatry.* 2005;66(7):870-886.
142. Weiss RD, Mirin SM, Griffin ML, Michael JL. Psychopathology in cocaine abusers: changing trends. *J Nerv Ment Dis.* 1988;176:719-725.
143. Hammond CJ, Niciu MJ, Drew S, Arias AJ. Anticonvulsants for the treatment of alcohol withdrawal syndrome and alcohol use disorders. *CNS Drugs.* 2015;29(4):293-311.
144. Judd LL, Schettler PJ, Akiskal HS, et al. Long-term symptomatic status of bipolar I vs. bipolar II disorders. *Int J Neuropsychopharmacol.* 2003;6(2):127-137.
145. Calabrese JR, Bowden CL, Sachs GS, Ascher JA, Monaghan E, Rudd GD. A double-blind placebo-controlled study of lamotrigine monotherapy in outpatients with bipolar I depression. Lamictal 602 Study Group. *J Clin Psychiatry.* 1999;60:79-88.
146. Salloum IM, Cornelius JR, Daley DC, Kirisci L, Himmelhoch JM, Thase ME. Efficacy of valproate maintenance in patients with bipolar disorder and alcoholism: a double-blind placebo-controlled study. *Arch Gen Psychiatry.* 2005;62:37-45.
147. Geller B, Cooper TB, Sun K, et al. Double-blind and placebo-controlled study of lithium for adolescent bipolar disorders with secondary substance dependency. *J Am Acad Child Adolesc Psychiatry.* 1998;37:171-178.
148. Brady KT, Sonne SC, Malcolm RJ, et al. Carbamazepine in the treatment of cocaine dependence: subtyping by affective disorder. *Exp Clin Psychopharmacol.* 2002;10(3):276-285.
149. Brown ES, Perantie DC, Dhanani N, Beard L, Orsulak P, Rush AJ. Lamotrigine for bipolar disorder and comorbid cocaine dependence: a replication and extension study. *J Affect Disord.* 2006;93(1-3):219-222.
150. Rubio G, Lopez-Munoz F, Alamo C. Effects of lamotrigine in patients with bipolar disorder and alcohol dependence. *Bipolar Disord.* 2006;8(3):289-293.
151. Brady KT, Sonne SC, Anton R, Ballenger JC. Valproate in the treatment of acute bipolar affective episodes complicated by substance abuse: a pilot study. *J Clin Psychiatry.* 1995;56(3):118-121.
152. Salloum IM, Douaihy A, Cornelius JR, Kirisci L, Kelly TM, Hayes J. Divalproex utility in bipolar disorder with co-occurring cocaine dependence: a pilot study. *Addict Behav.* 2007;32(2):410-415.
153. Perugi G, Toni C, Frare F, et al. Effectiveness of adjunctive gabapentin in resistant bipolar disorder: is it due to anxious-alcohol abuse comorbidity? *J Clin Psychopharmacol.* 2002;22(6):584-591.
154. Johnson BA, Rosenthal N, Capece JA, et al. Topiramate for treating alcohol dependence: a randomized controlled trial. *JAMA.* 2007;298(14):1641-1651.
155. Mason BJ, Quello S, Goodell V, Shadan F, Kyle M, Begovic A. Gabapentin treatment for alcohol dependence: a randomized clinical trial. *JAMA Intern Med.* 2014;174(1):70-77.
156. Kampman KM, Pettinati H, Lynch KG, et al. A pilot trial of topiramate for the treatment of cocaine dependence. *Drug Alcohol Depend.* 2004;75(3):233-240.
157. Roy Chengappa KN, Schwarzman LK, Hulihan JF, et al. Adjunctive topiramate therapy in patients receiving a mood stabilizer for bipolar I disorder: a randomized, placebo-controlled trial. *J Clin Psychiatry.* 2006;67(11):1698-1706.
158. Brown ES, Nejtek VA, Perantie DC, Bobadilla L. Quetiapine in bipolar disorder and cocaine dependence. *Bipolar Disord.* 2002;4(6):406-411.
159. Brown ES, Jeffress J, Liggin JD, Garza M, Beard L. Switching outpatients with bipolar or schizoaffective disorders and substance abuse from their current antipsychotic to aripiprazole. *J Clin Psychiatry.* 2005;66(6):756-760.
160. Brown ES, Garza M, Carmody TJ. A randomized, double-blind, placebo-controlled add-on trial of quetiapine in outpatients with bipolar disorder and alcohol use disorders. *J Clin Psychiatry.* 2008;69(5):701-705.
161. Stedman M, Pettinati HM, Brown ES, Kotz M, Calabrese JR, Raines S. A double-blind, placebo-controlled study with quetiapine as adjunct therapy with lithium or divalproex in bipolar I patients with coexisting alcohol dependence. *Alcohol Clin Exp Res.* 2010;34(10):1822-1831.
162. Brown ES, Davila D, Nakamura A, et al. A randomized, double-blind, placebo-controlled trial of quetiapine in patients with bipolar disorder, mixed or depressed phase, and alcohol dependence. *Alcohol Clin Exp Res.* 2014;38(7):2113-2118.
163. Nunes E, Quitkin F. Disulfiram and bipolar affective disorder. *J Clin Psychopharmacol.* 1987;7(4):284.
164. Brown ES, Carmody TJ, Schmitz JM, et al. A randomized, double-blind, placebo-controlled pilot study of naltrexone in outpatients with bipolar disorder and alcohol dependence. *Alcohol Clin Exp Res.* 2009;33(11):1863-1869.
165. Sonne SC, Brady KT. Naltrexone for individuals with comorbid bipolar disorder and alcohol dependence. *J Clin Psychopharmacol.* 2000;20(1):114-115.
166. Brown ES, Beard L, Dobbs L, Rush AJ. Naltrexone in patients with bipolar disorder and alcohol dependence. *Depress Anxiety.* 2006;23(8):492-495.

167. Sullivan MA, Nunes EV. New-onset mania and psychosis following heroin detoxification and naltrexone maintenance. *Am J Addict.* 2005;14(5):486-487.
168. Tolliver BK, Desantis SM, Brown DG, Prisciandaro J, Brady KT. A randomized, double-blind, placebo-controlled clinical trial of acamprosate in alcohol-dependent individuals with bipolar disorder: a preliminary report. *Bipolar Disord.* 2012;14(1):54-63.
169. Brown ES, Gorman AR, Hynan LS. A randomized, placebo-controlled trial of citicoline add-on therapy in outpatients with bipolar disorder and cocaine dependence. *J Clin Psychopharmacol.* 2007;27(5):498-502.
170. Brown ES, Todd JP, Hu LT, et al. A randomized, double-blind, placebo-controlled trial of citicoline for cocaine dependence in bipolar I disorder. *Am J Psychiatry.* 2015;172(10):1014-1021.
171. Brown ES, Gabrielson B. A randomized, double-blind, placebo-controlled trial of citicoline for bipolar and unipolar depression and methamphetamine dependence. *J Affect Disord.* 2012;143(1-3):257-260.
172. Craighead WE, Miklowitz DJ. Psychosocial interventions for bipolar disorder. *J Clin Psychiatry.* 2000;61(Suppl 13):58-64.
173. Scott J, Gutierrez MJ. The current status of psychological treatments in bipolar disorders: a systematic review of relapse prevention. *Bipolar Disord.* 2004;6:498-503.
174. Colom F, Vieta E. A perspective on the use of psychoeducation, cognitive-behavioral therapy and interpersonal therapy for bipolar patients. *Bipolar Disord.* 2004;6:480-486.
175. Colom F, Vieta E, Martinez-Aran A, et al. A randomized trial on the efficacy of group psychoeducation in the prophylaxis of recurrences in bipolar patients whose disease is in remission. *Arch Gen Psychiatry.* 2003;60:402-407.
176. Colom F, Vieta E, Sánchez-Moreno J, et al. Group psychoeducation for stabilised bipolar disorders: 5-year outcome of a randomised clinical trial. *Br J Psychiatry.* 2009;194(3):260-265.
177. Lam DH, Watkins ER, Hayward P, et al. A randomized controlled study of cognitive therapy for relapse prevention for bipolar affective disorder: outcome of the first year. *Arch Gen Psychiatry.* 2003;60:145-152.
178. Frank E, Kupfer DJ, Ehlers LC, et al. Interpersonal and social rhythm therapy for bipolar disorder: integrating interpersonal and behavioral approaches. *Behav Ther.* 1994;17:143-149.
179. Frank E, Swartz HA, Kupfer DJ. Interpersonal and social rhythm therapy: managing the chaos of bipolar disorder. *Biol Psychiatry.* 2000;48:593-604.
180. Frank E, Kupfer DJ, Thase ME, et al. Two-year outcomes for interpersonal and social rhythm therapy in individuals with bipolar I disorder. *Arch Gen Psychiatry.* 2005;62:996-1004.
181. Miklowitz DJ, George EL, Richards JA, Simoneau TL, Suddath RL. A randomized study of family-focused psychoeducation and pharmacotherapy in the outpatient management of bipolar disorder. *Arch Gen Psychiatry.* 2003;60(9):904-912.
182. Weiss RD. Treating patients with bipolar disorder and substance dependence: lessons learned. *J Subst Abuse Treat.* 2004;27:307-312.
183. Weiss RD, Griffin ML, Kolodziej ME, et al. A randomized trial of integrated group therapy versus group drug counseling for patients with bipolar disorder and substance dependence. *Am J Psychiatry.* 2007;164(1):100-107.
184. Weiss RD, Connery HS. *Integrated Group Therapy for Bipolar Disorder and Substance Abuse.* Guilford Press; 2011.
185. Weiss RD, Griffin ML, Jaffee WB, et al. A "community-friendly" version of integrated group therapy for patients with bipolar disorder and substance dependence: a randomized controlled trial. *Drug Alcohol Depend.* 2009;104(3):212-219.
186. Schmitz J, Averill P, Sayre S, et al. Cognitive-behavioral treatment of bipolar disorder and substance abuse: a preliminary randomized study. *Addict Disord Treat.* 2002;1:17-24.
187. Farren CK, McElroy S. Treatment response of bipolar and unipolar alcoholics to an inpatient dual diagnosis program. *J Affect Disord.* 2008;106(3):265-272.
188. Farren CK, McElroy S. Predictive factors for relapse after an integrated inpatient treatment programme for unipolar depressed and bipolar alcoholics. *Alcohol Alcohol.* 2010;45(6):527-533.
189. Farren CK, Snee L, McElroy S. Gender differences in outcome at 2-year follow-up of treated bipolar and depressed alcoholics. *J Stud Alcohol Drugs.* 2011;72(5):872-880.
190. Grella CE, Stein JA. Impact of program services on treatment outcomes of patients with comorbid mental and substance use disorders. *Psychiatr Serv.* 2006;57(7):1007-1015.
191. Drake RE, Mueser KT, Brunette MF. Management of persons with co-occurring severe mental illness and substance use disorder: program implications. *World Psychiatry.* 2007;6(3):131-136.
192. Drake R, Xie H, McHugo G, Shumway M. Three-year outcome of long-term patients with co-occurring bipolar and substance use disorders. *Biol Psychiatry.* 2004;56:749-756.

102 Co-occurring Substance Use, Anxiety Disorders, and Obsessive-Compulsive Disorders

Alyssa Braxton, Eric T. Dobson, and Karen J. Hartwell

CHAPTER OUTLINE

- Introduction
- Prevalence
- Screening and differential diagnosis
- General treatment considerations
- Alcohol and anxiety
- Tobacco products and anxiety disorders
- Opioids and anxiety disorders
- Cannabis and anxiety disorders
- Obsessive-compulsive disorder
- Stimulants and anxiety disorders
- Conclusions

INTRODUCTION

Numerous studies suggest that anxiety disorders, symptoms of anxiety, and substance use disorders (SUDs) commonly co-occur. The interaction between these disorders and symptoms is bidirectional and variable. Anxiety disorders may be a risk factor for the development of SUDs. Anxiety disorders modify the presentation and outcome of treatment for SUDs, just as substance use and SUDs modify the presentation and outcome of treatment for anxiety disorders. Anxiety symptoms commonly emerge during the course of chronic intoxication and withdrawal. Individuals who are defined as having co-occurring anxiety and SUDs should meet criteria for the anxiety disorder independent of periods of acute intoxication and withdrawal. **Table 102-1** provides brief descriptions of the major anxiety disorders. Obsessive-compulsive disorder (OCD) has historically been classified as an anxiety disorder and will be included in this chapter, although DSM-5 has now moved OCD and related disorders into their own category. In this chapter, the area of co-occurring SUDs and anxiety and OCDs are reviewed. Prevalence, diagnostic, and treatment issues are addressed.

PREVALENCE

General Population

A meta-analysis of 22 epidemiological studies from 1990 to 2014 including the National Epidemiologic Survey on Alcohol and Related Conditions (NESARC) with a sample size of 504,319 adults found significant association (OR 2.91) between illicit drug use and any anxiety disorder. Likewise, the association of alcohol use disorders (AUDs) co-occurring with anxiety disorders was significant with OR of 2.11. The OR for DSM-IV–defined dependence was higher than abuse irrespective of diagnosis.[1] A large study examining the relationship between anxiety and DSM-IV substance dependence in young adults found that the onset of one or more anxiety disorders without other co-occurring psychiatric disorders such as depression preceded the onset of alcohol and/or other substance dependence 80% of the time.[2] In a clinical sample of individuals diagnosed with OCD, 27% met criteria for a lifetime SUDs and 70% of individuals with a co-occurring SUD reported that the OCD preceded the onset of the SUD by at least 1 year.[3]

Note that in this chapter we will refer for the most part to "Substance Use Disorders," reflecting the current DSM-5 diagnostic criteria and terminology for substance-related disorders. We may still refer to the earlier DSM-IV entities "Substance Dependence" and "Substance Abuse" when needed if the data being cited specifically identifies them, as in the studies discussed above. DSM-5 adopted the single entity "Substance Use Disorder," both for scientific reasons (the criteria items for the former "Abuse" and "Dependence" were found to fall on a continuum consistent with a single disorder, varying in severity), and because the older terms were felt to be stigmatizing.

Primary Care Populations

Anxiety disorders are common within primary care settings and associated with functional impairment, distress, and high utilization of medical care services.[4] In a large random sample of consecutive primary clinic patients, approximately 20% had at least one anxiety disorder with generalized anxiety disorder (GAD) most common (8%), followed by panic disorder (PD) (7%) and social anxiety disorder (SAD) (6%).[5] Within primary care, the identification of problems with anxiety is poor with only 23% of patients with anxiety disorders recognized compared to 56% of depressive disorders.[6] Substance use is also common among primary care populations with estimates of 26% past-year use of illicit substances and 62% past-year alcohol use and 44% past-year tobacco use. Among other substances, cannabis is the commonly used illicit substance (21%) followed by cocaine (7%) and prescription medications

TABLE 102-1 Brief Descriptions of Major Anxiety Disorders

Disorder	Description
Panic disorder (PD)	Panic attacks are described as episodes of intense fear or discomfort in the absence of real danger associated with both physical and cognitive symptoms such as rapid heartbeat, shortness of breath, shaking, chest pain, nausea, fear of dying or going crazy, derealization, or depersonalization. They can occur in the context of any anxiety disorder, mood disorders, substance-induced disorders, and from some general medical problems. PD is characterized by recurrent unexpected panic attacks frequently followed by persistent worry and concern about additional attacks
Agoraphobia (AG)	AG is described as anxiety about being in places or situations from which escape may be difficult or help is unavailable, leading to avoidant behavior and distress. Often associated with panic attacks and concern about having a panic attack in such places or situations
Social anxiety disorder (SAD)	SAD or social phobia is characterized by a persistent and marked fear or anxiety about scrutiny in social or performance situations leading to embarrassment or humiliation. Feared situations are usually avoided or endured with great distress or anxiety
Generalized anxiety disorder (GAD)	GAD is characterized by excessive worry and anxiety for 6 months or longer, causing significant impairment in functioning or distress, present for more days than not
Obsessive-compulsive disorder (OCD)	OCD is characterized by recurrent obsessions (unwanted, repetitive, often disturbing intrusive thoughts) and compulsions (repetitive behaviors, such as checking or counting, and efforts to suppress engender anxiety) that either are time consuming or cause significant impairment or distress. The DSM-5 categorizes obsessive-compulsive and related disorders separately from anxiety disorders
Substance/medication-induced anxiety disorder (SIAD)	SIAD is described as the development of anxiety or panic attacks during substance intoxication or withdrawal or exposure to medication known to cause anxiety. Exceeds usual intoxication or withdrawal effects. Resolves with abstinence from substances (DSM-5 suggests resolution within a month of abstinence)

From American Psychiatric Association. *Diagnostic and Statistical Manual of Mental Disorders*. 5th ed. American Psychiatric Association; 2013.

including opioids, sedatives, and stimulants (7%).[7] In a recent survey of about 13,000 primary care patients across multiple European countries, approximately 9% met criteria for DSM-IV alcohol dependence, of whom only 22% had received treatment.[8]

SCREENING AND DIFFERENTIAL DIAGNOSIS

Based on prevalence data, individuals seeking treatment for anxiety should be assessed for the presence of a SUD, and conversely, individuals seeking SUD treatment should be assessed for co-occurring psychiatric disorders, including anxiety disorders. However, differentiating co-occurring anxiety disorders and SUDs is a diagnostic conundrum. Substance use and withdrawal can mimic nearly every psychiatric disorder (see Chapter 100, "Substance-Induced Mental Disorders"). Substance intoxication and withdrawal syndromes are defined in DSM-5 with characteristic symptom clusters that may include anxiety or related symptoms that resolve during the time frame consistent with the action of the substance. Substance-induced disorders exceed the usual expected effects of intoxication or withdrawal. The various substances have profound effects on neurotransmitter systems involved in the pathophysiology of anxiety disorders, and chronic substance use may unmask a vulnerability to anxiety or cause neurobiological changes that may manifest as an anxiety disorder. The best way to differentiate substance-induced, transient symptoms of anxiety from an independent anxiety disorder that warrant treatment is through observation during a period of abstinence. Transient substance-related states will typically improve with time. The duration of abstinence necessary to distinguish independent from substance-induced disorders is not precisely defined by DSM-5 and remains controversial. DSM-5 suggests 1 month of abstinence as a general rule. However, this is likely to be based on both the diagnosis being assessed and the substance used. For example, long half-life drugs (eg, some benzodiazepines, methadone) may require longer for a substance-induced disorders to subside, while shorter-acting substances (eg, alcohol, cocaine, short half-life benzodiazepines) require shorter periods of abstinence to make accurate diagnoses. It is also possible that substance use may engender a syndrome consistent with an anxiety disorder that is more long-lasting, although at some point, this would become more consistent in DSM-5 with an independent disorder. A family history of anxiety disorders, the onset of anxiety symptoms before the onset of SUD, and sustained anxiety symptoms during lengthy periods of abstinence all suggest an independent anxiety disorder.

Because of the high rate of co-occurrence of anxiety and SUDs, screening patients at primary care, substance use, or mental health treatment settings is critical. This is especially important considering that early diagnosis and treatment can improve treatment outcomes and avoid unnecessary use of medications that can lead to a SUD. A number of screening tools are available and easily integrated into everyday practice. For example, the Mini-International Neuropsychiatric Interview has a brief form that contains screening questions for PD, agoraphobia (AG), SAD, and OCD, among others.[9] The screener contains one "yes or no" question for each anxiety disorder, and all are based on the DSM-5 criteria (**Table 102-2**). Numerous self-report questionnaires have been developed to screen for anxiety disorders in the primary care settings. For example, the Four-Dimensional Symptom Questionnaire (4DSQ) is a

TABLE 102-2 Screening Questions for Anxiety Disorders Adapted From the Mini-International Neuropsychiatric Interview

Diagnosis	Screening question
Panic disorder	Have you, more than once, had episodes or attacks of sudden anxiety, fear, or uneasiness in situations where most people would not feel that way? Did the episodes peak within 10 minutes of starting?
Social anxiety disorder	In the past *month*, did you have persistent fear and anxiety when being watched or being the focus of attention? Fearful of being embarrassed, rejected, or humiliated? This includes things like being in social settings, speaking in public, eating in public, or writing while someone watches.
Generalized anxiety disorder	Have you worried *excessively* or been anxious about several routine things over the past 6 months?
Obsessions	In the past *month*, have you been bothered by recurrent thoughts, impulses, or images that were undesired, distasteful, inappropriate, intrusive, or distressing (eg, thoughts you were dirty, contaminated, *or* had germs; *or* fear of contaminating others; *or* fear of harming someone even though it is distressing or fearing you would act on some impulse; *or* fear or superstitions that you would be responsible for things going wrong; obsessions with sexual thoughts, images, or impulses; *or* hoarding, collecting, *or* religious obsessions)?
Compulsions	In the past *month*, did you do something repeatedly without being able to resist doing it, like washing or cleaning excessively; counting or checking things over and over; repeating, collecting, or arranging things; or other superstitious rituals?

From Sheehan DV. *MINI International Neuropsychiatric Interview* English Version 7.0.2 for DSM-5. 2016. http://harmresearch.org

50-item self-rating questionnaire developed to distinguish depression, anxiety, and somatization from general distress.[10] The Hospital Anxiety and Depression Scale (HADS) is a 14-item self-rating questionnaire that measures both depression and anxiety.[11] In a multisite trial, the 4DSQ and the HADS were administered to 295 patients on sick leave due to psychological problems excluding patients with known depressive or anxiety disorders.[12] The 4DSQ demonstrated superiority compared to the HADS in detecting PD, agoraphobia, and social anxiety requiring treatment. The Obsessive-Compulsive-Inventory-4 is a brief 4-item version of the OCD-Revised, and it shows promise as a practical screening tool.[13] These self-rating questionnaires and other screening tools can be administered by support staff in the office setting and can help to identify high-risk individuals. However, because of symptom overlap and diagnostic difficulties, a detailed interview is needed to fully differentiate substance-induced symptoms from primary mood/anxiety disorders.

GENERAL TREATMENT CONSIDERATIONS

For patients presenting with anxiety and SUDs, a first principle is to initiate treatment for the substance use disorder, since reduction of or abstinence from substance use is likely to lead to improvement in anxiety, particularly for substance-induced anxiety. Consider psychosocial treatments or medication treatments or both. In one example, Petrakis and colleagues studied 254 outpatients with DSM-IV alcohol dependence and a variety of co-occurring psychiatric disorders,[14] investigating the efficacy of disulfiram and naltrexone or their combination in a 12-week randomized trial. Participants treated with naltrexone or disulfiram, as compared with placebo, had significantly more consecutive weeks of abstinence and fewer drinking days per week. In comparison to naltrexone-treated participants, disulfiram-treated participants reported less craving from pre- to posttreatment. The effects of the medications by specific co-occurring psychiatric disorder were not discussed, but active medication was associated with greater symptom improvement (eg, less anxiety).

The integration of services and effective treatments from both psychiatric and SUD fields is essential to the optimal treatment of individuals with co-occurring disorders. It is important to maximize the use of nonpharmacological treatments. Some research suggests that some traditional therapies, including group therapies and Alcoholics or Narcotics Anonymous, may be more challenging for individuals with anxiety disorders. A study of individuals entering community-based intensive outpatient substance treatment found that clinically significant social anxiety interfered with recovery-related activities such as attending 12-step recovery meetings, finding a sponsor, and speaking up in groups.[15] Learning strategies to self-regulate anxiety can disrupt the cycle of substance use to combat intolerable subjective states and help individuals to acquire alternative coping strategies. Among psychosocial treatments, cognitive-behavioral therapies (CBTs) are among the most effective for both anxiety disorders and SUDs with techniques such as muscle relaxation, behavioral activation, coping skills, and sleep hygiene being utilized. The effectiveness of CBT for all of the anxiety disorders is well established in both clinical trials and naturalistic settings,[16] and CBT has been utilized extensively in the treatment of SUDs.[17]

Individuals in recovery often have complex, conflicting feelings and attitudes about medications and may see the need for pharmacotherapy as a sign of defectiveness or failure. For some patients, there is a struggle surrounding the use of medication and the belief that total abstinence from all psychoactive substances (including medications to treat addiction) is necessary for recovery.[18] It is important to address the individual's concerns about taking medication and to address the need for adherence in a proactive manner.

In cases where the relationship of psychiatric symptoms and substance use is unclear, a careful assessment of the risks and benefits of using medications must be considered. Pharmacotherapies for anxiety disorders are well established and reviewed in detail in the literature.[19-22] Pharmacotherapy decisions should generally follow routine clinical practice for treatment of the anxiety disorder with some exceptions. It is important to pay attention to potential toxic interactions between the prescription medications and illicit drugs and alcohol in case of recurrence of substance use. It is also important to use the medication with the least addictive potential. A recent review of pharmacotherapies for the treatment of anxiety disorders indicated that selective serotonin retake inhibitors (SSRIs) as a class are generally considered as first-line medications due to overall effectiveness, tolerability, and safety.[19] Serotonin-norepinephrine reuptake inhibitors (SNRIs) are typically seen as alternate first-line medications and utilized after failure or inadequate response to an SSRI. Venlafaxine and duloxetine are efficacious in the treatment of GAD, and venlafaxine is also indicated for the treatment of GAD and SAD.[19,20] Mirtazapine has shown promise in several open trials in PD and GAD with mixed results in SAD.[23] Other antidepressants, such as the tricyclic antidepressants and monoamine oxidase inhibitors, are generally used as second- or third-line medications primarily due to problems with tolerability and lethality in overdose. Because of its limited effectiveness, buspirone is generally only utilized for the treatment of uncomplicated GAD.[20] Anticonvulsants may also have a role. For the treatment of GAD, pregabalin has the greatest amount of support from multiple double-blind placebo-controlled randomized clinical trials (RCTs) and is approved for treatment of GAD by the European Medicines Agency.[20] Gabapentin demonstrated promise in a double-blind RCT for SAD, in a subset of patients with more severe PD with agoraphobia, anxiety in breast cancer survivors, and in several studies of surgery-related anxiety.[24] Hydroxyzine used as needed is also indicated for anxiety and likely attenuates anxiety by inhibiting the histamine H_1 and serotonin 2a receptors.[25] The serotonergic properties of the atypical antipsychotics are thought to augment the action of antidepressants in the treatment of depression, and as a result, these medications are also being investigated in the treatment of anxiety disorders. However, double-blind placebo-controlled RCTs of the atypical antipsychotics are still quite limited, and these agents should be reserved for use after failure of other interventions.[20]

Benzodiazepines have demonstrated efficacy in the treatment of PD, GAD, and SAD.[19,20] However, benzodiazepine adverse side effects include aberrant use and addiction potential, problematic sedation, cognitive impairment, risk of falls, and with prolonged use, tolerance and withdrawal. In patients without risk of substance use disorders, their use should generally be limited to patients who have not responded to at least three previous treatments such as an SSRI, an SNRI, and a psychotherapeutic intervention. As a rule, benzodiazepines should be avoided in patients with a current SUD or at risk for a substance use disorder (eg, past history of a SUD). Hydroxyzine is an alternative to benzodiazepines that can be used as needed to provide relief of anxiety symptoms with less risk of nonmedical or addiction.

ALCOHOL AND ANXIETY

Though the relationship between alcohol and anxiety disorders varies to some degree across specific disorders, drinking to self-medicate anxiety may make both occurrence and persistence of AUDs more likely.[26-28] The relationship between anxiety and alcohol use may predispose young people to develop an AUD, with early-onset anxiety disorders associated with an earlier age of first alcohol use.[29] The short-term relief of anxiety from alcohol use, in combination with longer-term anxiety induction from chronic drinking and withdrawal, may also initiate a feed-forward cycle of increasing anxiety symptoms and alcohol consumption.[30]

A 2015 Cochrane systematic review concluded that the evidence base of pharmacotherapy for co-occurring alcohol and anxiety disorders was both of very poor quality and inconclusive.[31] Guidelines recommend treating co-occurring anxiety disorders with antidepressant medications while limiting the use of benzodiazepines to acute withdrawal management.[32] Previous research has indicated that alcohol use appears to attenuate the efficacy of anxiety disorder treatment.[33,34] There is some evidence from a meta-analysis that treatment of anxiety disorders can be integrated in to the treatment of alcohol use disorder with improvements in outcomes for both alcohol and anxiety disorders.[35]

Generalized Anxiety Disorder

Community surveys including the National Comorbidity Study, NESARC-II, and the National Survey of Mental Health & Well-being reported strong odds of association (odds ratio [OR] of 3.0-4.6) between AUD and GAD, reflecting increased prevalence of GAD among those with AUD, and vice versa.[36] Subsequently, the NESARC-III survey, conducted 2012-2013 study, using DSM-5 criteria for diagnoses, found weaker odds of association between AUD and lifetime GAD, when controlling for other co-occurring disorders (eg, depression, bipolar disorder, etc.) (OR 1.05-1.39).[36,37] Clinically, this suggests that the presence of GAD in a patient with AUD should prompt a search for additional co-occurring disorders.

Differential Diagnosis

GAD symptoms overlap with alcohol withdrawal symptoms. A DSM-5 diagnosis of GAD requires that symptomatology is not attributable to the physiological effects of a substance. Therefore, distinguishing substance-induced anxiety symptoms from GAD is important. As patients engage in recovery, ongoing clinical assessment of anxiety symptoms and syndromes is important, as a substance-induced anxiety syndrome should improve as substance use diminishes, while persistence of an anxiety syndrome despite reduction of or abstinence from substance use suggests an independent anxiety disorder.

Treatment

The most current guidelines for the pharmacological treatment of GAD are from the National Collaborating Centre for Mental Health.[21] First-line medications are SSRIs, followed by an alternative SSRI or SNRI in the case of lack of efficacy. There are a number of alternatives, or adjunctive medications to consider if SSRIs or SNRIs are not effective. Buspirone or other types of antidepressants (eg, mirtazapine, tricyclic antidepressants) can be considered. Pregabalin can be considered in the case of SSRI and SNRI intolerance. Benzodiazepines should only be used short-term during crises, while antipsychotics should only be considered for refractory cases. Although effective for some individuals, controlled trials do not support the use of beta-blockers. Because GAD has a remitting-recurring chronic course, and favorable evidence that antidepressants prevent recurrence, long-term treatment of GAD is often indicated.[36]

There is little evidence-based research to direct treatment decisions for individuals with GAD and co-occurring AUDs. Although SSRIs have not been well studied in individuals with co-occurring GAD and SUDs, they are efficacious in the treatment of uncomplicated GAD and relatively safe to use in individuals with SUDs.[38] Pregabalin has demonstrated efficacy for GAD and mild-moderate alcohol withdrawal syndrome but has not been evaluated in co-occurring AUD and GAD.[39] Buspirone, a serotonin 5HT1A receptor partial agonist, should be considered as it has few side effects, no potential for nonmedical use, and is effective for treatment of GAD. A 12-week, placebo-controlled trial in patients with alcohol use disorder who had elevated anxiety that persisted after withdrawal from alcohol, found buspirone reduced anxiety, reduced drinking, and improved retention in treatment.[40]

Social Anxiety Disorder

Community surveys have shown increased odds of AUD in the presence of SAD, or vice versa (ORs of 1.5-3.0).[41] Similar to the findings with GAD, in the NESARC-III study, this association was weakened after controlling for other co-occurring disorders.[37] Again, this suggests that clinically detection of SAD should prompt a search in the patient's history for other disorders such as depression.

Self-medication has been suggested as a mechanism for the association between SAD and AUDs, given evidence that SAD symptoms often precede onset of SUDs.[41] This is consistent with patients' anecdotal reports that alcohol reduces anxiety acutely making it more tolerable to go into social situations. This suggests the importance of a careful developmental history to detect early onset SAD, and other disorders or risk factors such as early trauma or adverse childhood experiences (ACEs).

Differential Diagnosis

The key symptom of SAD, fear of performance or social situations, is specific to SAD and not generally associated with substance use or withdrawal, making diagnosis easier than for other co-occurring anxiety disorders. SAD is often first evident in childhood, and a careful developmental history should be taken, looking for anxiety in school and social situations, as well as other disorder and childhood risk factors such as ACEs. One possible clinical presentation is that of an adolescent who was anxious in school since childhood, and meets criteria for SAD, who discovers alcohol reduces anxiety in social gatherings with peers and begins to drink alcohol. This can then lead to maladaptive behaviors or heavy alcohol use and development of an alcohol use disorder. Conversely, a pattern of binge drinking in adolescence should prompt exploration of the history for SAD and other co-occurring disorders.

Treatment

Current treatment guidelines for SAD emphasize psychotherapy with CBT being preferred, with psychodynamic psychotherapy being second line. Initial pharmacological treatment recommendations for SAD include SSRIs, with preference for sertraline or escitalopram. For those with inadequate treatment response, second-line therapy includes alternative SSRIs with preference for fluvoxamine or paroxetine, or an SNRI (venlafaxine), with MAOIs being third-line (phenelzine).[22] Two small placebo-controlled studies of paroxetine in co-occurring AUD and SAD have demonstrated significant improvement in social anxiety with paroxetine treatment but no significant group differences in alcohol use in either study.[42,43] A subsequent controlled trial integrating a brief alcohol intervention into treatment failed to demonstrate decreased alcohol use or drinking behavior in people with SAD who were consuming alcohol in at-risk patterns.[44] Finally, a recent RCT allocated participants with AUD and SAD ($N = 117$) to integrated CBT and motivational enhancement or to a control (alcohol-focused) intervention. Integrated treatment improved SAD and quality of life but not AUD-related outcomes.[45]

In a longitudinal study of outcome after hospitalization in patients with AUD with and without SAD, no difference was found between groups in treatment adherence, including attendance at Alcoholics Anonymous and other outcomes. However, individuals with SAD chaired Alcoholics Anonymous meetings less often, were more ashamed of attendance, felt less integrated into the group, and were less likely to feel better after a meeting.[46] This suggests individual therapy may be better suited for patients whose social anxiety makes it difficult for them to tolerate groups.

Obsessive-Compulsive Disorder

The association of OCD and AUDs is less robust than for other anxiety disorders. In the National Comorbidity Survey Replication study, OCD was negatively correlated with AUD.[47]

Differential Diagnosis

Craving in SUDs can be intrusive and recurrent, comparable to the intrusive recurrent thoughts that drive behavior in OCD.[48] DSM-5 diagnostic criteria specify that a diagnosis of OCD should not be made when symptoms are better explained by a substance-related disorder or SUD. The thoughts and compulsions in individuals with AUDs are generally restricted to alcohol use and easily distinguished from OCD.

Treatment

Current guidelines recommend CBT (exposure and response prevention), pharmacotherapy, or combined treatment as first line for OCD. First-line medications for OCD are SSRIs, followed by switching to a different SSRI, clomipramine or mirtazapine, or augmenting with an antipsychotic.[49,50] There are no controlled studies of pharmacological treatment of co-occurring OCD and SUDs. One recent study of intensive OCD-oriented residential treatment found lower past-year alcohol use predicted better treatment response.[51]

Panic Disorder With or Without Agoraphobia

In the NESARC-III study, lifetime history of an AUD was associated with increased odds of PD (OR 1.12-1.44).[37] In one review of the literature, the risk of PD in the presence of AUDs was 2 to 4 times higher than in the absence of AUD.[52]

Differential Diagnosis

Individuals with panic attacks may use alcohol to decrease panic symptoms, precipitating an AUD.[52] Because alcohol withdrawal may increase anxiety to the point of panic-like severity, a diagnosis of PD should only be made following several weeks of abstinence if temporal onset of PD prior to AUD is not clear. Panic attacks may also be difficult to distinguish from surges of anxiety as part of intoxication from stimulants or cannabis, or withdrawal from opioids or sedatives. Panic Disorder is often accompanied by agoraphobia. Characteristic fear of specific types of public places, (bridges, trains, etc.), is distinct from substance-induced anxiety, and may clarify the diagnosis of an independent anxiety disorder, even if the patient cannot be assessed after achieving abstinence.

Treatment

Current guidelines for pharmacological treatment of PD recommend against benzodiazepine, antihistamine and antipsychotic prescribing, in favor of SSRIs followed by imipramine or clomipramine in poor responders.[22] Without treatment, the risk of return to alcohol use is increased.[53] A few studies support CBT in the treatment of PD co-occurring with AUD. One study compared hybrid CBT targeting both alcohol and panic versus treatment as usual in a 28-day SUD program, demonstrating that CBT improved both drinking and PD outcomes.[54]

TOBACCO PRODUCTS AND ANXIETY DISORDERS

Between 2004 and 2011, smoking rates have declined significantly ($p < 0.001$) among individuals without mental illness (from 20% to 16%); however, comparable declines ($p = 0.50$) were not seen in individuals with mental illness (from 29% to 27%), including anxiety disorders.[55] Indeed, higher baseline anxiety is associated with decreased likelihood of abstinence from tobacco. Menthol brands are associated with greater odds of depression and anxiety, and from 2003 to 2019 became more popular among certain populations of people who were currently smoking (28%-34%), as well as those who were non-Hispanic Black (73%-77%), young adults (32%-38%), and females (32%-40%).[56] The use of chewing tobacco is also increased among individuals with anxiety including PD (OR 1.5).[57] As of 2019, the use of e-cigarettes in adults has increased (4.5%) particularly among adults ages 18 to 24 (9.3%) with over half (56.0%) of young e-cigarette users reporting they have never smoked cigarettes.[58] Nicotine withdrawal remains problematic in electronic drug delivery devices (EDDDs) that deliver nicotine, especially as this rate of nicotine delivery increasingly mimics traditional cigarettes; and anxiety is a symptom of nicotine withdrawal, which often drives recurrent dosing throughout the day (negative reinforcement). Thus, use of rapid delivery nicotine products can generate anxiety, which then can drive recurrent use, resulting in nicotine/tobacco use disorder.

Despite strong associations between nicotine use and anxiety disorders, there has been little investigation of causal connections or treatment. Previous research has suggested that nicotine can alleviate anxiety, but other studies indicate that nicotine use and withdrawal can cause anxiety.[59] The Netherlands Study of Depression and Anxiety, a longitudinal naturalistic cohort study, found that the onset of anxiety disorders was 5 years earlier for early-onset as compared to late-onset smoking, and this relationship remained after controlling for gender, education, and childhood trauma.[60] Additionally, a recent Cochrane review found quitting smoking does not worsen mental health and, in fact, may be associated with small-to-moderate improvements in mental health, including anxiety.[61]

Differential Diagnosis

The anxiety and arousal associated with nicotine withdrawal can be distinguished from independent anxiety disorders by time course. Prospective research suggests nicotine withdrawal symptoms typically return to baseline within 10 days[62] and anxiety related to nicotine typically decreases within 4 weeks of quitting smoking.[63] Anxiety persisting beyond the withdrawal period warrants further investigation. It is important to note that when individuals enter inpatient or residential treatment, their cigarette smoking is generally significantly curtailed. Anxiety related to nicotine withdrawal should be taken into consideration in any assessment of anxiety in individuals hospitalized for the treatment of either SUDs or psychiatric disorders. Administration of nicotine replacement therapy may be helpful in removing anxiety due to nicotine withdrawal.

Panic Disorder

The relationship between PD and smoking tobacco is the best studied of all the anxiety disorders, with studies supporting a strong relationship between PD and smoking. In NESARC-III, PD was associated with DSM-5 nicotine use disorder (OR 2.72).[64] In a clinical sample of individuals with anxiety disorders, the PD group had the highest proportion of people who smoked, 40.4%, and these were more likely to smoke heavily compared to the SAD group, 20%.[65] A history of panic attacks has been associated with daily, heavy smoking (20 or more cigarettes/day), DSM-IV nicotine dependence, and a history of failed quit attempts.[66]

Early smoking increases the risk for the development of PD,[67] and initiation may precede the onset of PD by many years (median, 12 years).[68] Breslau found that current but not past smoking was associated with the subsequent onset of PD and agoraphobia, and the risk decreased with increasing time since quitting.[69] Potential neurobiologic explanations include a shared vulnerability to both disorders, the release of norepinephrine by nicotine producing panic-like symptoms, self-medication, and the result of respiratory abnormalities from smoking.[70]

Social Anxiety Disorder

NESARC-III found a significant association between SAD and nicotine use disorder (OR 1.8).[64] Although some studies have failed to demonstrate a relationship,[71] one prospective longitudinal study of adolescents and young adults found that both social fears and SAD were significantly associated with higher rates of DSM-IV nicotine dependence.[72] Approximately 50% reported the onset of SAD before smoking. SAD often has early onset and can be detected on developmental history. Among individuals with SAD, cigarette smoking may be used to attenuate social anxiety in anticipation of and during social situations. In a clinical laboratory study, young adults who smoked tobacco and who had elevated social anxiety who smoked a cigarette had significantly reduced negative affect during a social stress task compared to those with average social anxiety scores.[73]

Generalized Anxiety Disorder

In NESARC-III, GAD was significantly associated with nicotine use disorder (OR 2.1).[64] In one prospective longitudinal study of adolescents and young adults, heavy smoking (≥20 cigarettes per day) was associated with an increased risk of GAD (21%, OR 5.5) during young adulthood.[71] GAD is about twice as common in women than in men, and men are more likely to have nicotine addiction, use alcohol and nonprescribed medications to relieve symptoms, and less likely to seek treatment.[74]

Obsessive-Compulsive Disorder

The prevalence of smoking tobacco is significantly lower among adults with OCD and parents of youth with OCD, suggesting that the low prevalence of smoking may be familial and stimulating effect of nicotine may exacerbate OCD symptoms.[75] OCD is a heterogeneous disorder, however, and smoking status differs based on distinct subcategories of OCD. In a clinical sample, the rate of smoking was highest among individuals with symmetry-counting-repeating-ordering symptoms compared to those with washing symptoms and taboo.[76]

Tobacco/Nicotine Treatment

Current guidelines for treating tobacco/nicotine use disorder recommend a combination of counseling and medication. Pharmacotherapy is recommended in all individuals attempting to quit unless contraindicated. Medications that reliably increase long-term smoking abstinence include bupropion sustained release (SR), all forms of nicotine replacement therapy (nicotine gum, nicotine inhaler, nicotine nasal spray, nicotine lozenge, and nicotine patch), and varenicline.[77] In clinical trials, participants with a history of an anxiety disorder were less likely to be abstinent at 8 weeks or 6 months post quit.[78] They were also twice as likely to report stress and nearly 4 times as likely to endorse negative affect as a reason for return to use.[79]

A recent secondary analysis of a large ($N = 4{,}092$) placebo and active (NRT) controlled RCT of varenicline and bupropion for quitting smoking revealed comparative efficacy of interventions in subjects with mood, anxiety, or psychotic disorders.[80] All treatments were superior to placebo in subjects with co-occurring anxiety disorders with varenicline being significantly superior to bupropion.

Bupropion can cause anxiety and agitation in some individuals, so it should be used with caution in anxious patients. Buspirone (up to 60 mg/d) had a beneficial effect on abstinence in people who smoked tobacco and were also highly anxious in one RCT. However, buspirone decreased abstinence in the low-anxiety group.[81]

A recent study of Web-based tobacco/nicotine use disorder (TUD) interventions in subjects with various co-occurring psychiatric disorders found that participants with PD, GAD and SAD all rated online treatment as more acceptable than those without co-occurring mood or anxiety issues; however they had lower utilization of Web-based TUD tools and lower quit rates than those without anxiety disorders.[82] Morissette[59] suggested that interoceptive exposure therapy may be helpful in reducing distress and anxiety during withdrawal by teaching individuals to tolerate internal cues such as negative affect, craving, and withdrawal symptoms.

OPIOIDS AND ANXIETY DISORDERS

In 2020, approximately 9.5 million people aged 12 or older used opioids nonmedically, accounting for 3.4% of the population.[83] Lifetime anxiety disorder were identified in approximately 60.9% with DSM-IV opioid dependence and 28.6% with DSM-IV opioid abuse in the NESARC study. Particularly strong associations were found for panic disorder with agoraphobia and co-occurring opioid use with an odds ratio of 13.8.

Of note, associations between panic disorder and any opioid use disorder were higher for women when compared to men.[84]

Diagnosis

The release of endogenous opioids in response to stress has a modulating effect on anxiety, and conversely blocking the opioid system with an antagonist produces anxiety symptoms in human volunteers.[85] Opioid withdrawal, which causes noradrenergic overactivity and higher anxiety, can make distinguishing an underlying anxiety disorder difficult.[86] Panic attacks, restlessness and increased anxiety are common during opioid withdrawal and can contribute to risk of return to use on opioids. Stabilization in treatment including pharmacotherapy for opioid withdrawal and psychosocial treatments can significantly reduce opioid withdrawal-related symptoms quickly allowing for better diagnostic clarity of underlying anxiety disorders.

Treatment

While no clinical trials of treatments for co-occurring anxiety disorders have been conducted, general treatment principles apply. Patients presenting for treatment of opioid use disorders should be screened for anxiety, and the temporal relationship of anxiety symptoms to opioid use and addiction should be assessed. A comprehensive treatment plan is necessary to address the opioid use, anxiety, other comorbid SUDs, and chronic pain if present. Initial components should include medical withdrawal management and initiation of one of the effective medications, for example, buprenorphine or methadone. If anxiety persists after withdrawal management and stabilization, then specific treatments for anxiety should be considered. Clinicians should choose anxiety medications with efficacy for the specific anxiety disorder being treated, offer CBT if available, and provide attention to special considerations described in this chapter. If chronic pain is an issue, consultation with a pain specialist may be helpful.

CANNABIS AND ANXIETY DISORDERS

Cannabis contains over 100 cannabinoids with most research focused on the most potent psychoactive compounds, Δ-9-tetrahydrocannabinol (THC) and cannabidiol (CBD). THC is responsible for the intoxicating euphoric effects and undesirable experiences such as anxiety and paranoia. CBD is not euphorigenic, attenuates the action of THC and has anticonvulsant properties. For both, the claims of benefit (analgesia, anxiolysis) are not well characterized. Cannabis products, available either at legal dispensaries or on black market, vary widely in potency, with trend being increased THC concentrations, and increasing risk of adverse psychoactive effects. For further information on cannabis used as treatment (CUAT), please read the two chapters on this subject in Section 15 of this textbook.

Diagnosis

The relationship between cannabis and anxiety varies across individuals, and likely with the dosage and type of cannabis. Some report use of cannabis helps with sleep or anxiety. On the other hand, cannabis use can result in acute anxiety during intoxication[87] and withdrawal.[88] There is significant evidence for an association between the development and persistence of psychotic disorders and cannabis, however the relationship with anxiety disorders remains unclear when controlling for confounding factors.[89] For example, a 2014 meta-analysis of 31 studies found a small positive association between cannabis use and cannabis use disorder and anxiety.[90] In contrast, analysis from NESARC wave 1 and wave 2 found that, after adjusting for confounders, cannabis use or CUD was not associated with an increased incidence of most anxiety disorders and inversely the majority of anxiety disorders were not associated with cannabis use or CUD.[91] Meta-analysis, longitudinal, and epidemiologic evidence of an association between anxiety disorders and cannabis use disorders demonstrates that the onset of anxiety seems to occur prior to cannabis use disorder onset for the majority of adults with co-occurring disorders.[92,93]

Treatment

Treatment for cannabis use disorder may be affected by co-occurring anxiety, though this is understudied. One study suggests anxious people who use cannabis and use cannabis to manage negative emotions experience more severe withdrawal, reduced self-efficacy to refrain from use in emotionally distressing situations, and coping-motivated use.[94] In a large multisite trial investigating the effectiveness of two psychosocial treatments for cannabis use disorder, higher anxiety prior to treatment was associated with increased depression at baseline and increased cannabis-related problems at baseline and both follow-up time points.[95] Of note, the results also suggested patients with cannabis use disorder may benefit from treatment focused on the development of skills to manage anxiety, as anxiety reduction was associated with improved cannabis outcomes. A study comparing people with cannabis use disorder who were successful versus unsuccessful in ending their cannabis use found that those who were successful were more likely to employ coping strategies such as alternative ways to relax and deal with unpleasant emotions than those who were unsuccessful.[96] In sum, the relationship between cannabis and anxiety disorders is complex. Most research to date has found an association between anxiety and cannabis use and disorders, though causality and degree of mediation by confounders is not entirely determined.

OBSESSIVE-COMPULSIVE DISORDER

The limited research on cannabinoids and OCD is limited and consists of case reports, small observational studies, and a few laboratory investigations with mixed results. Emerging research suggests that the endocannabinoid system may play a role in symptoms of OCD and is a potential target for novel medication development.[97] A preliminary Internet survey of cannabis using adults with OCD found 90% were using high-potency cannabis products, 42% met criteria for a CUD, 29% used to manage OCD, with most reporting (self-reported) symptom improvement in the absence of evidence-based care.[98] One small, randomized placebo-controlled human laboratory study found smoked cannabis, whether primarily THC or CBD, had little acute impact on self-reported OCD symptoms with smaller reductions in anxiety compared to placebo.[99]

STIMULANTS AND ANXIETY DISORDERS

There is limited research on co-occurring anxiety disorders and cocaine, methamphetamine, and amphetamine use. These agents stimulate noradrenergic systems, and acute intoxication may be associated with anxiety. Because of these anxiogenic effects, it has been postulated that individuals who are vulnerable to anxiety may be less likely to use this class of drugs nonmedically or develop substance use disorders with them.[100] On the other hand, the stimulant high may transiently override anxiety. When anxiety symptoms are reported in individuals with stimulant use disorders, it is useful to ascertain whether anxiety precedes stimulant use, or emerges after stimulant use, appearing to be a substance-induced effect.

Prevalence

Thirty-nine percent of individuals with amphetamine use disorders and 31% of those with cocaine use disorders reported lifetime anxiety disorders. Of individuals with anxiety disorders, 4.8% reported lifetime amphetamine use disorder and 5.4% reported lifetime cocaine use disorder.[84] Studies of treatment-seeking individuals indicate that anxiety disorders are less common in cocaine-using treatment-seeking patients as compared with patients with alcohol and other SUDs.[101] One study[102] found lifetime prevalence of SAD in a population with DSM-IV cocaine dependence to be 13.9%, with SAD preceding the onset of cocaine dependence in nearly all cases. In the Methamphetamine Treatment Project, participants completed self-report measures of anxiety.[103] Women reported higher levels of anxiety than did men. The frequency of methamphetamine use was positively associated with severity of general anxiety and phobic anxiety. At 3-year follow-up, 26.2% of participants met criteria for current or past anxiety disorder, with GAD being most common. Among those with anxiety disorders, treatment adherence was worse, and self-reported methamphetamine use was significantly higher during the follow-up period.[104] In a review of two community surveys, lifetime stimulant use was associated with lifetime diagnoses of nearly every anxiety disorder.[105]

Diagnosis

The repetitive, stereotyped behavior that can occur during acute intoxication of cocaine has commonalities with that of OCD. These symptoms generally occur only during acute intoxication and withdrawal and do not meet diagnostic criteria for OCD. According to DSM-5, a diagnosis of excoriation disorder should not be made when skin-picking behavior is attributable to substance use. DSM-5 does suggest a diagnosis of substance-induced obsessive-compulsive and related disorder should be considered when symptoms of OCD occur in the setting of substance use.[106] Cocaine has been reported to precipitate panic attacks in patients without previous PD.[107] Methamphetamine and cocaine withdrawal symptoms include low levels of anxiety in the early days of abstinence.[108,109] Therefore, a period of abstinence is warranted before diagnosing an anxiety disorder in individuals with stimulant use disorders.

Treatment

There are a number of psychosocial treatments with demonstrated efficacy in the treatment of DSM-defined stimulant use disorder including contingency management and CBT.[110] Individuals with co-occurring anxiety/anxiety disorders should be engaged in evidence-based psychosocial treatment for their stimulant use, as reduction of or abstinence from stimulant use may help the anxiety.

There is a paucity of research focused on treatments targeting co-occurring stimulant use and anxiety disorders. In one case series, patients with cocaine-induced PD had substantial symptom improvement after treatment with either carbamazepine or clonazepam.[111] Anticonvulsant agents, such as valproate and carbamazepine, have demonstrated efficacy in the treatment of PD. PD in patients with co-occurring stimulant use may be linked to a sensitization mechanism and may respond to anticonvulsant medications. This hypothesis warrants further investigation. When an independent anxiety disorder is diagnosed in the setting of a stimulant use disorder, treatment of the anxiety disorder, with medication or behavioral therapy or both, are viable options.

CONCLUSIONS

Because of the high co-occurrence of anxiety disorders and SUDs and the high prevalence of both sets of disorders in the population, primary care and mental health providers will encounter these conditions frequently in the course of their work. It is essential that providers address anxiety in patients with substance use disorders as a routine part of treatment. This requires careful differential diagnosis that requires at least a brief period of sustained abstinence. Behavioral treatments, such as various forms of CBT, are a mainstay of treatment for both anxiety disorders and SUDs and are a good way to initiate treatment. Providers should also consider appropriate medication treatments for anxiety disorders (eg, SSRI antidepressants) and substance use disorders (eg, naltrexone for alcohol or opioid use disorder, buprenorphine for opioid use disorder, or nicotine replacement or bupropion for nicotine use disorder). Medications with low risk for nonmedical use are preferable.

REFERENCES

1. Lai HMX, Cleary M, Sitharthan T, Hunt GE. Prevalence of comorbid substance use, anxiety and mood disorders in epidemiological surveys 1990-2014: a systematic review and meta-analysis. *Drug Alcohol Depend.* 2015;154:1-13.
2. Lopez B, Turner RJ, Saavedra LM. Anxiety and risk for substance dependence among late adolescents/young adults. *J Anxiety Disord.* 2005;19:275-294.
3. Mancebo MC, Grant JE, Pinto A, Eisen JL, Rasmussen SA. Substance use disorders in an obsessive-compulsive disorder clinical sample. *J Anxiety Disord.* 2009;23:429-435.
4. Gurmankin Levy A, Maselko J, Bauer M, Richman L, Kubzansky L. Why do people with an anxiety disorder utilize more nonmental health care than those without? *Health Psychol.* 2007;26:545-553.
5. Kroenke K, Spitzer RL, Williams JB, Monahan PO, Löwe B. Anxiety disorders in primary care: prevalence, impairment, comorbidity, and detection. *Ann Intern Med.* 2007;146:317-325.
6. Bakken K, Landheim AS, Vaglum P. Axis I and II disorders as long-term predictors of mental distress: a six-year prospective follow-up of substance-dependent patients. *BMC Psychiatry.* 2007;7:29.
7. McNeely J, Wu LT, Subramaniam G, et al. Performance of the tobacco, alcohol, prescription medication, and other substance use (TAPS) tool for substance use screening in primary care patients. *Ann Intern Med.* 2016;165:690-699.
8. Rehm J, Allamani A, Elekes Z, et al. Alcohol dependence and treatment utilization in Europe—a representative cross-sectional study in primary care. *BMC Fam Pract.* 2015;16:90.
9. Sheehan DV. *MINI International Neuropsychiatric Interview.* English Version 7.0.2 for DSM-5. Accessed June 28, 2023. http://harmresearch.org
10. Terluin B, van Marwijk HW, Ader HJ, et al. The Four-Dimensional Symptom Questionnaire (4DSQ): a validation study of a multidimensional self-report questionnaire to assess distress, depression, anxiety and somatization. *BMC Psychiatry.* 2006;6:34.
11. Zigmond AS, Snaith RP. The hospital anxiety and depression scale. *Acta Psychiatr Scand.* 1983;67:361-370.
12. Terluin B, Brouwers EP, van Marwijk HW, Veerhak PFM, van der Horst HE. Detecting depressive and anxiety disorders in distressed patients in primary care; comparative diagnostic accuracy of the Four-Dimensional Symptom Questionnaire (4DSQ) and the Hospital Anxiety and Depression Scale (HADS). *BMC Fam Pract.* 2009;10:58.
13. Abramovitch A, Abramowitz JS, McKay D. The OCI-4: an ultra-brief screening scale for obsessive-compulsive disorder. *J Anxiety Disord.* 2021;78:102354.
14. Petrakis IL, Poling J, Levinson C, et al. Naltrexone and disulfiram in patients with alcohol dependence and comorbid psychiatric disorders. *Biol Psychiatry.* 2005;57:1128-1137.
15. Book SW, Thomas SE, Dempsey JP, Randall PK, Randall CL. Social anxiety impacts willingness to participate in addiction treatment. *Addict Behav.* 2009;34:474-476.
16. Kaczkurkin AN, Foa EB. Cognitive–behavioral therapy for anxiety disorders: an update on the empirical evidence. *Dialogues Clin Neurosci.* 2015;17:337-346.
17. McHugh RK, Hearon BA, Otto MW. Cognitive behavioral therapy for substance use disorders. *Psychiatr Clin North Am.* 2010;33:511-525.
18. Ronel N, Gueta K, Abramsohn Y, Caspi N, Adelson M. Can a 12-step program work in methadone maintenance treatment? *Int J Offender Ther Comp Criminol.* 2011;55:1135-1153.
19. Bystritsky A, Khalsa SS, Cameron ME, Schiffman J. Current diagnosis and treatment of anxiety disorders. *P T.* 2013;38:30-57.
20. Baldwin DS, Anderson IM, Nutt DJ, et al. Evidence-based pharmacological treatment of anxiety disorders, post-traumatic stress disorder and obsessive-compulsive disorder: a revision of the 2005 guidelines from the British Association for Psychopharmacology. *J Psychopharmacol.* 2014;28:403-439.
21. *National Collaborating Centre for Mental Health (UK). Generalized Anxiety in Adults: Management in Primary, Secondary, and Community Care.* British Psychological Society; 2011.
22. National Collaborating Centre for Mental Health. *National Institute for Health and Care Excellence: Clinical Guidelines Social Anxiety Disorder: recognition, Assessment and Treatment.* British Psychological Society and The Royal College of Psychiatrists; 2013.
23. Alam A, Voronovich Z, Carley JA. A review of therapeutic uses of mirtazapine in psychiatric and medical conditions. *Prim Care Companion CNS Disord.* 2013;15:PCC.13r01525.
24. Berlin RK, Butler PM, Perloff MD. Gabapentin therapy in psychiatric disorders: a systematic review. *Prim Care Companion CNS Disord.* 2015;17(5):10.4088/PCC.15r01821. doi:10.4088/PCC.15r01821
25. Guaiana G, Barbui C, Cipriani A. Hydroxyzine for generalized anxiety disorder. *Cochrane Database Syst Rev.* 2010;12:CD006815.
26. Pacek LR, Storr CL, Mojtabai R, et al. Comorbid alcohol dependence and anxiety disorders: a national survey. *J Dual Diagn.* 2013;9. doi:10.1080/15504263.2013.835164
27. Menary KR, Kushner MG, Maurer E, Thuras P. The prevalence and clinical implications of self-medication among individuals with anxiety disorders. *J Anxiety Disord.* 2011;25:335-339.
28. Crum RM, Mojtabai R, Lazareck S, et al. A prospective assessment of reports of drinking to self-medicate mood symptoms with the incidence and persistence of alcohol dependence. *JAMA Psychiat.* 2013;70:718-726.
29. Birrell L, Newton NC, Teesson M, Tonks Z, Slade T. Anxiety disorders and first alcohol use in the general population. Findings from a nationally representative sample. *J Anxiety Disord.* 2015;31:108-113.
30. Kushner MG, Abrams K, Borchardt C. The relationship between anxiety disorders and alcohol use disorders: a review of major perspectives and findings. *Clin Psychol Rev.* 2000;20:149-171.
31. Ipser JC, Wilson D, Akindipe TO, Sager C, Stein DJ. Pharmacotherapy for anxiety and comorbid alcohol use disorders. *Cochrane Database Syst Rev.* 2015;1:CD007505.
32. Reus VI, Fochtmann LJ, Bukstein O, et al. The American Psychiatric Association Practice Guideline for the Pharmacological Treatment of Patients with Alcohol Use Disorder. *Am J Psychiatry.* 2018;175:86-90.
33. Gajecki M, Berman AH, Sinadinovic K, et al. Effects of baseline problematic alcohol and drug use on Internet-based cognitive behavioral therapy outcomes for depression, panic disorder and social anxiety disorder. *PLoS One.* 2014;9:e104615.
34. Hesse M. Integrated psychological treatment for substance use and co-morbid anxiety or depression vs. treatment for substance use alone. A systematic review of the published literature. *BMC Psychiatry.* 2009;9:6.
35. Hobbs JD, Kushner MG, Lee SS, Reardon SM, Maurer EW. Meta-analysis of supplemental treatment for depressive and anxiety disorders in patients being treated for alcohol dependence. *Am J Addict.* 2011;20:319-329.
36. Smith JP, Randall CL. Anxiety and alcohol use disorders: comorbidity and treatment considerations. *Alcohol Res.* 2012;34(4):414-431.
37. Grant BF, Goldstein RB, Saha TD, et al. Epidemiology of DSM-5 alcohol use disorder: results from the National Epidemiologic Survey on Alcohol and Related Conditions III. *JAMA Psychiatry.* 2015;72:757-766.
38. Donovan MR, Glue P, Kolluri S, Emir B. Comparative efficacy of antidepressants in preventing relapse in anxiety disorders—a meta-analysis. *J Affect Disord.* 2010;123:9-16.
39. Oulis P, Konstantakopoulos G. Pregabalin in the treatment of alcohol and benzodiazepines dependence. *CNS Neurosci Ther.* 2010;16:45-50.
40. Kranzler HR, Burleson JA, Del Boca FK, et al. Buspirone treatment of anxious alcoholics. A placebo-controlled trial. *Arch Gen Psychiatry.* 1994;51(9):720-731.

41. Goodwin RD, Stein DJ. Anxiety disorders and drug dependence: evidence on sequence and specificity among adults. *Psychiatry Clin Neurosci*. 2013;67:167-173.
42. Randall CL, Johnson MR, Thevos AK, et al. Paroxetine for social anxiety and alcohol use in dual-diagnosed patients. *Depress Anxiety*. 2001;14:255-262.
43. Book SW, Thomas SE, Randall PK, Randall CL. Paroxetine reduces social anxiety in individuals with a co-occurring alcohol use disorder. *J Anxiety Disord*. 2008;22:310-318.
44. Book SW, Thomas SE, Smith JP, et al. Treating individuals with social anxiety disorder and at-risk drinking: phasing in a brief alcohol intervention following paroxetine. *J Anxiety Disord*. 2013;27:252-258.
45. Stapinski LA, Sannibale C, Subotic M, et al. Randomised controlled trial of integrated cognitive behavioural treatment and motivational enhancement for comorbid social anxiety and alcohol use disorders. *Aust N Z J Psychiatry*. 2021;55:207-220.
46. Terra MB, Barros HM, Stein AT, et al. Does co-occurring social phobia interfere with alcoholism treatment adherence and relapse? *J Subst Abuse Treat*. 2006;31:403-409.
47. Kessler RC, Chiu WT, Demler O, Merikangas KR, Walters EE. Prevalence, severity, and comorbidity of 12-month DSM-IV disorders in the National Comorbidity Survey Replication. *Arch Gen Psychiatry*. 2005;62:617-627.
48. Modell JG, Glaser FB, Cyr L, Mountz JM. Obsessive and compulsive characteristics of craving for alcohol in alcohol abuse and dependence. *Alcohol Clin Exp Res*. 1992;16:272-274.
49. Koran LM, Hanna GL, Hollander E, Nestadt G, Simpson HB. Practice guideline for the treatment of patients with obsessive-compulsive disorder. *Am J Psychiatry*. 2007;164(7 Suppl):5-53.
50. Katzman MA, Bleau P, Blier P, et al. Canadian clinical practice guidelines for the management of anxiety, posttraumatic stress and obsessive-compulsive disorders. *BMC Psychiatry*. 2014;14(Suppl 1):S1.
51. Brennan BP, Lee C, Elias JA, et al. Intensive residential treatment for severe obsessive-compulsive disorder: characterizing treatment course and predictors of response. *J Psychiatr Res*. 2014;56:98-105.
52. Cosci F, Schruers KR, Abrams K, Griez EJL. Alcohol use disorders and panic disorder: a review of the evidence of a direct relationship. *J Clin Psychiatry*. 2007;68:874-880.
53. Kushner MG, Abrams K, Thuras P, Hanson KL, Brekke M, Sletten S. Follow-up study of anxiety disorder and alcohol dependence in comorbid alcoholism treatment patients. *Alcohol Clin Exp Res*. 2005;29:1432-1443.
54. Kushner MG, Sletten S, Donahue C, et al. Cognitive-behavioral therapy for panic disorder in patients being treated for alcohol dependence: moderating effects of alcohol outcome expectancies. *Addict Behav*. 2009;34:554-560.
55. Cook BL, Wayne GF, Kafali EN, Liu Z, Shu C, Flores M. Trends in smoking among adults with mental illness and association between mental health treatment and smoking cessation. *JAMA*. 2014;311:172-182.
56. Seaman EL, Corcy N, Chang JT, et al. Menthol cigarette smoking trends among united states adults, 2003-2019. *Cancer Epidemiol Biomarkers Prev*. 2022;31:1959-1965.
57. Fu Q, Vaughn MG, Wu LT, Heath AC. Psychiatric correlates of snuff and chewing tobacco use. *PLoS One*. 2014;9:e113196.
58. Cornelius ME, Wang TW, Jamal A, Loretan CG, Neff LJ. Tobacco product use among adults—United States, 2019. *MMWR Morb Mortal Wkly Rep*. 2020;69:1736-1742.
59. Morissette SB, Tull MT, Gulliver SB, Kamholz BW, Zimering RT. Anxiety, anxiety disorders, tobacco use, and nicotine: a critical review of interrelationships. *Psychol Bull*. 2007;133:245-272.
60. Jamal M, Does AJ, Penninx BW, Cuijpers P. Age at smoking onset and the onset of depression and anxiety disorders. *Nicotine Tob Res*. 2011;13:809-819.
61. Taylor GM, Lindson N, Farley A, et al. Smoking cessation for improving mental health. *Cochrane Database Syst Rev*. 2021;3:CD013522.
62. Shiffman S, Patten C, Gwaltney C, et al. Natural history of nicotine withdrawal. *Addiction*. 2006;101:1822-1832.
63. West R, Hajek P. What happens to anxiety levels on giving up smoking? *Am J Psychiatry*. 1997;154:1589-1592.
64. Chou SP, Goldstein RB, Smith SM, et al. The epidemiology of DSM-5 nicotine use disorder: results from the National Epidemiologic Survey on Alcohol and Related Conditions-III. *J Clin Psychiatry*. 2016;77:1404-1412.
65. McCabe RE, Chudzik SM, Antony MM, Young L, Swinson RP, Zolvensky MJ. Smoking behaviors across anxiety disorders. *J Anxiety Disord*. 2004;18:7-18.
66. Cougle JR, Zvolensky MJ, Fitch KE, Sachs-Ericsson N. The role of comorbidity in explaining the associations between anxiety disorders and smoking. *Nicotine Tob Res*. 2010;12:355-364.
67. Bernstein A, Zvolensky MJ, Schmidt NB, Sachs-Ericsson N. Developmental course(s) of lifetime cigarette use and panic attack comorbidity: an equifinal phenomenon? *Behav Modif*. 2007;31:117-135.
68. Amering M, Bankier B, Berger P, Griengl H, Windhaber J, Katschnig H. Panic disorder and cigarette smoking behavior. *Compr Psychiatry*. 1999;40:35-38.
69. Breslau N, Novak SP, Kessler RC. Daily smoking and the subsequent onset of psychiatric disorders. *Psychol Med*. 2004;34:323-333.
70. Cosci F, Knuts IJ, Abrams K, Griez EJL, Schruers KRJ. Cigarette smoking and panic: a critical review of the literature. *J Clin Psychiatry*. 2010;71:606-615.
71. Johnson JG, Cohen P, Pine DS, Klein DF, Kasen F, Brook JS. Association between cigarette smoking and anxiety disorders during adolescence and early adulthood. *JAMA*. 2000;284:2348-2351.
72. Sonntag H, Wittchen HU, Höfler M, Kessler RC, Stein MB. Are social fears and DSM-IV social anxiety disorder associated with smoking and nicotine dependence in adolescents and young adults? *Eur Psychiatry*. 2000;15:67-74.
73. Dahne J, Hise L, Brenner M, Lejuez CW, MacPherson L. An experimental investigation of the functional relationship between social phobia and cigarette smoking. *Addict Behav*. 2015;43:66-71.
74. Vesga-Lopez O, Schneier FR, Wang S, et al. Gender differences in generalized anxiety disorder: results from the National Epidemiologic Survey on Alcohol and Related Conditions (NESARC). *J Clin Psychiatry*. 2008;69:1606-1616.
75. Abramovitch A, Pizzagalli DA, Geller DA, Reuman L, Wilhelm S. Cigarette smoking in obsessive-compulsive disorder and unaffected parents of OCD patients. *Eur Psychiatry*. 2015;30:137-144.
76. Tan O, Tas C. Symptom dimensions, smoking and impulsiveness in obsessive-compulsive disorder. *Psychiatr Danub*. 2015;27:397-405.
77. Fiore MCB, Bailey WC, Cohen SJ, et al. *Treating Tobacco Use and Dependence: 2008 Update-Clinical Practice Guideline*. Agency for Healthcare Research and Quality: P.H.S. U.S. Department of Health and Human Services; 2008.
78. Piper ME, Cook JW, Schlam TR, Jorenby DE, Baker TB. Anxiety diagnoses in smokers seeking cessation treatment: relations with tobacco dependence, withdrawal, outcome and response to treatment. *Addiction*. 2011;106:418-427.
79. Tulloch HE, Pipe AL, Clyde MJ, Reid RD, Els C. The quit experience and concerns of smokers with psychiatric illness. *Am J Prev Med*. 2016;50:709-718.
80. Evins AE, Benowitz NL, West R, et al. Neuropsychiatric safety and efficacy of varenicline, bupropion, and nicotine patch in smokers with psychotic, anxiety, and mood disorders in the EAGLES trial. *J Clin Psychopharmacol*. 2019;39:108-116.
81. Cinciripini PM, Lapitsky L, Seay S, Wallfisch A, Meyer WJ 3rd, van Vunakis H. A placebo-controlled evaluation of the effects of buspirone on smoking cessation: differences between high- and low-anxiety smokers. *J Clin Psychopharmacol*. 1995;15:182-191.
82. Watson NL, Heffner JL, Mull KE, McClure JB, Bricker JB. Comparing treatment acceptability and 12-month cessation rates in response to Web-based smoking interventions among smokers who do and do not screen positive for affective disorders: secondary analysis. *J Med Internet Res*. 2019;21:e13500.
83. Substance Abuse and Mental Health Services Administration. *Key substance use and mental health indicators in the United States: Results from the 2020 National Survey on Drug Use and Health* (HHS Publication

No. PEP21-07-01-003, NSDUH Series H-56). Center for Behavioral Health Statistics and Quality, SAMHSA; 2021.

84. Conway KP, Compton W, Stinson FS, Grant BF. Lifetime comorbidity of DSM-IV mood and anxiety disorders and specific drug use disorders: results from the National Epidemiologic Survey on Alcohol and Related Conditions. *J Clin Psychiatry*. 2006;67:247-257.
85. Colasanti A, Rabiner EA, Lingford-Hughes A, Nutt DJ. Opioids and anxiety. *J Psychopharmacol*. 2011;25:1415-1433.
86. Harris AC, Gewirtz JC. Elevated startle during withdrawal from acute morphine: a model of opiate withdrawal and anxiety. *Psychopharmacology (Berl)*. 2004;171:140-147.
87. Green B, Kavanagh D, Young R. Being stoned: a review of self-reported cannabis effects. *Drug Alcohol Rev*. 2003;22:453-460.
88. Raphael B, Wooding S, Stevens G, Connor J. Comorbidity: cannabis and complexity. *J Psychiatr Pract*. 2005;11:161-176.
89. Hanna RC, Perez JM, Ghose S. Cannabis and development of dual diagnoses: a literature review. *Am J Drug Alcohol Abuse*. 2017;43:442-455.
90. Kedzior KK, Laeber LT. A positive association between anxiety disorders and cannabis use or cannabis use disorders in the general population—a meta-analysis of 31 studies. *BMC Psychiatry*. 2014;14:136.
91. Feingold D, Weiser M, Rehm J, Lev-Ran S. The association between cannabis use and anxiety disorders: results from a population-based representative sample. *Eur Neuropsychopharmacol*. 2016;26:493-505.
92. Wittchen HU, Frohlich C, Behrendt S, et al. Cannabis use and cannabis use disorders and their relationship to mental disorders: a 10-year prospective-longitudinal community study in adolescents. *Drug Alcohol Depend*. 2007;88:S60-S70.
93. Buckner JD, Heimberg RG, Schneier FR, Liu SM, Wang S, Blanco C. The relationship between cannabis use disorders and social anxiety disorder in the National Epidemiological Study of Alcohol and Related Conditions (NESARC). *Drug Alcohol Depend*. 2012;124:128-134.
94. Buckner JD, Walukevich KA, Zvolensky MJ, Gallagher MW. Emotion regulation and coping motives serially affect cannabis cessation problems among dually diagnosed outpatients. *Psychol Addict Behav*. 2017;31:839-845.
95. Buckner JD, Carroll KM. Effect of anxiety on treatment presentation and outcome: results from the Marijuana Treatment Project. *Psychiatry Res*. 2010;178:493-500.
96. Rooke SE, Norberg MM, Copeland J. Successful and unsuccessful cannabis quitters: comparing group characteristics and quitting strategies. *Subst Abuse Treat Prev Policy*. 2011;6:30.
97. Kayser RR, Snorrason I, Haney M, Lee FS, Simpson HB. The endocannabinoid system: a new treatment target for obsessive compulsive disorder? *Cannabis Cannabinoid Res*. 2019;4:77-87.
98. Kayser RR, Senter MS, Tobet R, Raskin M, Patel S, Simpson HB. Patterns of cannabis use among individuals with obsessive-compulsive disorder: results from an Internet survey. *J Obsessive Compuls Relat Disord*. 2021;30:100664.
99. Kayser RR, Haney M, Raskin M, Arout C, Simpson HB. Acute effects of cannabinoids on symptoms of obsessive-compulsive disorder: a human laboratory study. *Depress Anxiety*. 2020;37:801-811.
100. De Wit H, Uhlenhuth EH, Johanson CE. Individual differences in the reinforcing and subjective effects of amphetamine and diazepam. *Drug Alcohol Depend*. 1986;16:341-360.
101. Rounsaville BJ, Anton SF, Carroll K, Budde D, Prusoff BA, Gawin F. Psychiatric diagnoses of treatment-seeking cocaine abusers. *Arch Gen Psychiatry*. 1991;48:43-51.
102. Myrick H, Brady KT. Social phobia in cocaine-dependent individuals. *Am J Addict*. 1997;6:99-104.
103. Zweben JE, Cohen JB, Christian D, et al. Psychiatric symptoms in methamphetamine users. *Am J Addict*. 2004;13:181-190.
104. Glasner-Edwards S, Mooney LJ, Marinelli-Casey P, et al. Anxiety disorders among methamphetamine dependent adults: association with post-treatment functioning. *Am J Addict*. 2010;19:385-390.
105. Sareen J, Chartier M, Paulus MP, Stein MB. Illicit drug use and anxiety disorders: findings from two community surveys. *Psychiatry Res*. 2006;142:11-17.
106. American Psychiatric Association. *Diagnostic and Statistical Manual of Mental Disorders*. 5th ed. American Psychiatric Association; 2013.
107. Aronson TA, Craig TJ. Cocaine precipitation of panic disorder. *Am J Psychiatry*. 1986;143:643-645.
108. McGregor C, Srisurapanont M, Jittiwutikarn J, Laobhripatr S, Wongtan T, White JM. The nature, time course and severity of methamphetamine withdrawal. *Addiction*. 2005;100:1320-1329.
109. Erb S. Evaluation of the relationship between anxiety during withdrawal and stress-induced reinstatement of cocaine seeking. *Prog Neuropsychopharmacol Biol Psychiatry*. 2010;34:798-807.
110. Roll JM. Contingency management: an evidence-based component of methamphetamine use disorder treatments. *Addiction*. 2007;102(Suppl 1): 114-120.
111. Louie AK, Lannon RA, Ketter TA. Treatment of cocaine-induced panic disorder. *Am J Psychiatry*. 1989;146:40-44.

CHAPTER

103 Co-occurring Psychosis and Substance Use Disorders

Douglas Ziedonis, Xiaoduo Fan, Snehal Bhatt, and Stephen A. Wyatt

CHAPTER OUTLINE

- Introduction
- Definition of psychotic disorders
- Prevalence of co-occurring substance use disorder and psychosis
- Diagnostic assessment
- Differential diagnosis
- Clinical presentation of substance-induced psychosis
- Management of co-occurring substance use disorder and psychosis
- Other outpatient treatment approaches
- Longer-term management
- Conclusion

INTRODUCTION

The occurrence of psychotic symptoms by an individual using substances poses special diagnostic and treatment challenges for clinicians in all treatment settings, such as mental health, addiction, emergency room, and primary care. This chapter focuses on the tasks of assessment, diagnosis, and acute and long-term treatment considerations of co-occurring substance use and psychosis. The acute management of substance-induced psychosis is discussed in addition to the acute and long-term management of co-occurring substance use or use disorder and psychosis. There is a need for a comprehensive assessment and integrated treatment that addresses the complex differential diagnosis and treatment challenges in this patient population. However, most addiction treatment programs tend not to include individuals with more severe and persistent schizophrenia or other psychotic syndromes in longer-term rehabilitation treatment programs. The American Society of Addiction Medicine (ASAM) created organizational criteria characterizing addiction treatment programs as either "capable" or "enhanced" in regards to their capabilities in treating people with co-occurring mental illness and addiction (see Chapter 47, "ASAM Criteria and Matching Patients to Treatment"). Programs labeled "capable" are able to assess and manage relatively stable patients with a co-occurring psychotic illness, while the enhanced programs are more fully integrated and have enhanced treatment services and staff to treat less stable or new onset co-occurring patients with psychosis. Historically, traditional mental health settings have had to adapt and in many locales could not refuse to treat individuals with schizophrenia just because they had a co-occurring substance use disorder (SUD), although it is clear that prior to focused efforts by SAMHSA starting in the mid-1980s to increase the attention to co-occurring mental disorder and SUD, patients with active SUD were routinely excluded from treatment in many mental health treatment programs due to the lack of adequate training of mental health professionals about SUD diagnosis and treatment. Similarly, many addiction treatment programs at that time routinely excluded patients with active psychotic and other mental disorders, given that clinical staff were not trained to treat severe mental illness. Given that most individuals with a psychotic disorder are treated in traditional mental health treatment settings, these settings need to enhance their capabilities to screen, assess, coordinate, and provide treatment or integrated care through referral.

DEFINITION OF PSYCHOTIC DISORDERS

Psychosis is defined as a gross impairment in reality testing that is characterized by distortions of perception (as manifested by hallucinations or illusions) or thought (as manifested by delusions). According to the current edition of the *Diagnostic and Statistical Manual of Mental Disorders* (DSM-5),[1] key features that define the psychotic disorders include delusions, hallucinations, disorganized thinking, grossly disorganized or abnormal motor behavior (including catatonia), and negative symptoms (**Table 103-1**). Hallucinations (eg, auditory, visual, tactile, olfactory) and delusions (paranoid, persecutory, grandiose, etc.) are labeled "positive" symptoms. "Negative" symptoms greatly impact interpersonal communication and include diminished emotional expression, lack of motivation, anhedonia, decreased speech, and social withdrawal. Psychotic disorders include schizophrenia, schizoaffective disorder, delusional disorder, substance- or medication-induced psychotic disorder, psychotic disorder due to another medical condition, and others.

PREVALENCE OF CO-OCCURRING SUBSTANCE USE DISORDER AND PSYCHOSIS

Substance-Induced Psychosis

Varying degrees of transient substance-induced psychotic symptoms are not uncommon among those who present while intoxicated or during withdrawal. Psychotic symptoms can be

TABLE 103-1 Key Features That Define the Psychotic Disorders

- *Delusion* is a firmly held false belief based on incorrect inference about reality.
- *Hallucination* is a false sensory perception that has the compelling sense of reality and occurs without stimulation of the relevant sensory organ.
- *Disorganized thinking (speech)* often presents as looseness of association (where there is a lack of continuity in thought between sentences or subjects) or, in the extreme, can be completely incoherent (lack of continuity in thought within a sentence or phrase).
- *Grossly disorganized or abnormal motor behavior (including catatonia) may manifest as* difficulty in performing activities of daily living, poor hygiene, appearing markedly disheveled, unusual dress, inappropriate sexual behavior, or unpredictable agitation.
- *Catatonia* is a marked and bizarre motor abnormality that is characterized by immobility. It may involve certain types of excessive activity, mutism, resistance to being moved, assumption of unusual body positions, and echoing the sound last heard or action last seen.
- *Negative symptoms* are characterized by diminished emotional expression, avolition (reduced ability to initiate and complete goals), alogia (poverty of speech), anhedonia (inability to experience pleasure), and asociality (lack of interest in social interactions).

induced by a variety of substances, such as alcohol, cocaine, cannabis (including synthetic cannabinoids), amphetamines, dissociatives, and hallucinogens, often in combination. Opioid use is less commonly associated with inducing psychosis; however, given the fentanyl crisis, this substance is often mixed in other substances such as methamphetamine and cannabis. Fentanyl and other opioids can result in psychosis symptoms during use or withdrawal. The combination of fentanyl with stimulants and cannabis can make management more complex.

Further delineation can be made in the examination of the persistence of substance-induced psychosis during abstinence. Psychotic symptoms may persist after substance abstinence. A recent meta-analysis reported that the pooled proportion of transition from substance-induced psychosis to schizophrenia was 25%.[2] In general, psychotic symptoms need to persist for at least a month after abstinence from substance use prior to establishing the diagnosis of a primary psychotic disorder comorbid with substance use.[3,4] The rates of transition from substance-induced psychosis to schizophrenia vary across different types of substance with highest rates associated with cannabis, hallucinogens, and amphetamines.[2]

Primary Psychotic Disorder With Co-Occurring Substance Use Disorder

Several studies have examined rates of co-occurring substance use and schizophrenia and found that up to half of individuals with schizophrenia have a lifetime prevalence of at least one SUD, excluding tobacco/nicotine use disorder, which is even more common.[5,6] In the classic Epidemiologic Catchment Area community-based study, 34% of those with schizophrenia had an alcohol use disorder (AUD) and 28% had nonalcohol SUDs, including 16% who used cocaine.[5] More recently, the National Epidemiologic Survey on Alcohol and Related Conditions (NESARC) suggested that schizophrenia is associated with increased transition from abstinence to use, particularly for cannabis.[7] The odds of those with schizophrenia also carrying a SUD diagnosis are 4.6-fold higher than those of the general population.[4,8] Mental health treatment settings report rates of current nonnicotine SUDs in the population of individuals with schizophrenia in the range from 25% to 75%. However, these epidemiologic data represent a "best guess" of the true rates, given the challenges of diagnosing an SUD in the presence of schizophrenia and the problems of diagnosing schizophrenia in the context of an SUD. Even an objective measure, such as routine urine drug screening in hospitals, may fail to detect or underestimate substance use.[9] Of note, studies suggest that 70% to 90% of patients with schizophrenia have tobacco/nicotine use disorder, and nicotine is not routinely included in reported rates of SUDs, making the actual rates even higher.

A Canadian study of 203 patients with first episode psychosis identified more than half (52%) presented with a comorbid SUD, most often alcohol or cannabis.[10] A British survey of 123 patients with first episode psychosis found that the frequency of substance use is twice that of the general population and more common in men than women; cannabis was the most commonly used drug (51%), followed by alcohol (43%).[11] The NIH funded Clinical Antipsychotic Trial of Intervention Effectiveness (CATIE) study was conducted across 57 U.S. clinical sites and included 1,460 individuals with DSM-IV schizophrenia. At baseline, 60% individuals of the study sample were found to use at least one substance (alcohol or other drugs), including 37% with evidence of an SUD.[12] When compared with people who did not use substances, those who used alcohol and/or other drugs (with or without a diagnosed SUD) were more likely to be male, African American, less educated, and recently homeless. Furthermore, they were more likely to report childhood conduct problems, a history of major depression, and to have suffered a recent exacerbation of schizophrenia. Interestingly, substance use was generally associated with higher or equivalent overall psychosocial functioning at baseline compared to abstinence from substance use.[13] From the same study, a report examined the relationship between severity of illicit substance use at the time of study entry and 18-month longitudinal outcomes. It was found that those with moderate to heavy use of substances had significantly poorer outcomes in the domains of psychosis, depression, and quality of life compared with both those with mild use and abstaining.[14]

Some data suggest that the use of alcohol or other drugs can lead to the earlier onset of schizophrenia in an already vulnerable individual.[15] Cannabis is linked to an earlier onset of schizophrenia and more severe positive symptoms among individuals with schizophrenia.[10,16,17] Substance use is also associated with nonadherence with treatment.[18,19] In patients with first-episode psychosis, substance use is also associated with poorer functional outcome, more frequent return to use, and a greater symptom burden.[20] In patients with schizophrenia, the use of even relatively small amounts of substance over a short period can result in exacerbation of psychiatric problems, increased risks of return to substance use and hospitalization, increased use of emergency department services, increased risks of HIV or hepatitis B or C infections, suicidal behavior, loss of housing, increased vulnerability to exploitation (sexual, physical, or other),[16] and poorer prognosis of medical conditions, such as diabetes.[21] In addition, medication nonadherence and substance use were found to negatively impact hospital readmission in a study of Australian patients with psychosis.[17]

As noted, nicotine/tobacco use disorder is very common amongst people with psychotic disorders as well as SUD (70%-90%) and is a major contributor to the increased morbidity and mortality in these populations.[22] A meta-analysis suggested that daily tobacco use is associated with an increased risk of psychosis and an earlier age of onset of psychotic illness; however, whether or not there is a causal link between tobacco use and psychosis remains unknown and merits further examination.[23] Reduction in tobacco use and potential abstinence should be an important consideration in the treatment plan.[24,25] Effective strategies to address tobacco use in mental health and addiction treatment settings require broader system-level changes, supportive of and consistent with program missions and patient recovery goals.[26,27] Treatment of co-occurring nicotine/tobacco use disorder among individuals with schizophrenia often requires a combination of medication, psychosocial treatment, and community-based approaches, including continuity of care between primary care providers and community tobacco treatment resources.[22] Organizational change strategies have been effective in decreasing tobacco use in addiction and mental health settings and addressing barriers to integrated care.[26,27] With adequate training, mental health clinicians can effectively help people with co-occurring nicotine/tobacco use disorder and schizophrenia improve their motivation and achieve tobacco abstinence.[28] The Learning About Healthy Living (LAHL) treatment manual is available online and has been demonstrated to help individuals with lower motivation to learn more about the risks of ongoing tobacco use, increase motivation to change, increase orientation to wellness, and attempt to quit tobacco use.[29]

DIAGNOSTIC ASSESSMENT

At the time of the patient's initial presentation for evaluation and treatment, the clinician should have four primary goals: patient safety, staff safety, elicitation of the patient's history, and formulation of initial impressions. Following the assessment, a set of treatment recommendations can be established in an effort to appropriately manage agitation, psychotic symptoms, and possible withdrawal symptoms.[4] Often, as a result of the acuity of the presenting episode, the emergency department is the setting most adequately prepared for the evaluation of an acutely psychotic patient. Some, mostly urban, communities have a psychiatric triage setting where a well-prepared staff can conduct a safe and appropriate evaluation. Staff members in these settings should be trained to treat such patients in an effective, safe, and nonjudgmental manner. If available, a psychiatric specialist may be asked to participate in the patient evaluation.

Patient safety should be addressed by providing a setting in which external stimuli are minimized and a modicum of dignity is established, while maintaining the physical safety of the patient and staff. Whenever possible, patients should be placed in a quiet, low stimulus room with staff trained in de-escalation in an attempt to reduce a patient's level of anxiety and agitation. Physical restraints are used less frequently in mental health settings but may be necessary and require ongoing observation and documentation throughout the period of restraint. Sedating medications, for example, benzodiazepines and antipsychotic medications, may be warranted in an attempt to prevent harm to self or others. These medications should be given, if possible, after the primary assessment has taken place and a well-documented attempt has been made at relieving agitation by establishing a low stimulus environment and counseling. The sedative effect of medications may disguise the presenting clinical symptoms and the effects of these medications may interact negatively with substances the patient used prior to admission. Of note, there is variability globally on the acceptance and use of chemical restraints, including considering a wider range of nonpharmacological interventions.

The patient's mental status should be assessed, with particular attention given to cognitive impairments and fluctuations of mental status. Initial assessment of vital signs should be obtained. Variations in pulse, blood pressure, and respiratory function are not uncommon in the presentation of many toxic states and should be monitored until stable. Structured instruments are available to help in assessing severity of withdrawal symptoms, such as Clinical Institute Withdrawal Assessment Alcohol Scale Revised (CIWA-AR), Clinical Opiate Withdrawal Scale (COWS) (see Section 7, Management of Intoxication and Withdrawal). Consideration should be given to the need for protection of the airway and possible establishment of intravenous access.

Multiple substance use of a range of combinations (alcohol, cannabis, tobacco, stimulants, opioids) does make assessments more complicated, including the dosing for treating withdrawal. Electronic drug delivery device (EDDD, or e-cigarettes) technology has expanded, and open system EDDDs allow any combination or substance to be delivered via the lungs.

Included in the primary assessment is the gathering of history from anyone with information about the patient before his or her arrival at the hospital. Collateral history obtained from family, friends, or others is often very helpful in establishing the patient's social, physical, and mental health history. Emergency personnel or police should be questioned for details of the scene at which they first encountered the patient and their observations of the patient during transport. This information can provide significant insights into the prehospital mental status of the patient and possible involvement of substances (as indicated, eg, by a pattern of confusion or a waxing and waning of signs and symptoms).

Initial laboratory information should include a complete blood count, electrolytes, liver enzymes, glucose, blood urea nitrogen, calcium, thyroid screen, blood alcohol, and urine analysis with a comprehensive drug screen. The five most common drugs in a standard urine toxicology screen include cocaine, amphetamines, cannabis, phencyclidine (PCP), and some opioids; however, there are many other types of substances that might be considered such as an expanded panel for more/most opioids including fentanyls, synthetic cannabinoid products, MDMA (ecstasy), bath salts (cathinones), methylphenidate, ketamine, dextromethorphan, etc. Clinicians can check with the toxicology laboratories they use to assess if these other substances can be evaluated in situations where the patients reports that the psychosis or other unusual symptoms are new symptoms from their usual substance (these substances might be unknown additives) or when patients or others note that there is an increase in a particular substance in the community. State toxicology laboratories can be excellent sources of information in learning about substances in the community, including additive mixes.[30]

If the patient lapses into coma, the administration of parenteral thiamine, glucose, magnesium, and naloxone may be appropriate, even before the laboratory results are available. Computed tomography (CT) scan of the brain is of little help in differentiating between schizophrenia and drug-induced psychosis.[31] However, head CT of an acutely psychotic patient should be considered if the blood and urine drug screens are negative, and the patient presents first-episode psychosis. One should note, however, that head CT scans are most helpful in cases of skull fractures, subdural or intracranial hematomas, and contusions but will only be positive in 20% to 50% of cases of diffuse axonal injury.[32] If the blood and urine evaluation is not diagnostic and the CT scan is negative, lumbar puncture may be warranted, especially for patients without a history of psychiatric disorders and with an acute change of mental status.

TABLE 103-2 Psychosis Secondary to Medical Conditions

- *Neurologic conditions*: neoplasms, stroke, epilepsy, auditory nerve injury, deafness, migraine, central nervous system infection, etc.
- *Endocrine conditions*: hyperthyroid or hypothyroid, parathyroid, or hypoadrenocorticism
- *Metabolic conditions*: hypoxia, hypercarbia, hypoglycemia
- *Fluid or electrolyte imbalances*
- *Hepatic or renal failure*
- *Autoimmune disorders* with central nervous system involvement (systemic lupus erythematosus)
- *Delirium*
- *Dementia*: Alzheimer disease, vascular, HIV related, Parkinson disease, Huntington disease, head trauma, and the like
- *Neoplasm*: lung

TABLE 103-3 Substances That Cause Psychotic Symptoms

During intoxication associated with excessive use

- Sedatives (alcohol, benzodiazepines, barbiturates)
- Stimulants (amphetamine, cocaine)
- Designer drugs (MDMA; substituted cathinones)
- Cannabis/THC/synthetic cannabinoids
- Hallucinogens (LSD, dimethyltryptamine, psilocin, psilocybin, etc.)
- Opioids
- Dissociatives (phencyclidines, ketamine, dextromethorphan)
- Steroids

During withdrawal after abrupt discontinuation

- Sedatives (alcohol, benzodiazepines, barbiturates)
- Anesthetics and analgesics
- Anticholinergic agents
- Anticonvulsants
- Antihistamines
- Antihypertensives
- Antimicrobial medications
- Antiparkinson medications
- Cardiovascular medications
- Chemotherapeutic agents
- Corticosteroids
- Gastrointestinal medications
- Muscle relaxants
- Nonsteroidal anti-inflammatory drugs
- Various over-the-counter medications
- Toxins (anticholinesterase, organophosphate insecticides, nerve gases, carbon monoxide, and volatile substances such as fuel or paint)

DIFFERENTIAL DIAGNOSIS

A new patient presenting with both psychotic symptoms and active substance use can be a diagnostic dilemma, and the differential diagnosis must be broad. In addition to a primary psychotic disorder, clinicians must consider the possibility that these symptoms are caused by a general medical condition (**Table 103-2**) or substance intoxication or withdrawal (**Table 103-3**). Psychotic symptoms can occur as the presenting symptoms or may be part of a more complex syndrome of cognitive disorders, such as delirium or dementia. Psychotic symptoms can occur in the context of other categories of mental disorders, particularly affective disorders. For example, delusions or hallucinations may be symptoms of major depression or the manic phase of bipolar disorder. Co-occurring substance use is common in patients with major depression or bipolar disorder.

The type and duration of psychotic symptoms are important in making a differential diagnosis. The following are general considerations; the DSM-5-TR should be consulted for more specific, definitive guidance. Psychotic symptoms that have a sudden onset and that last more than 1 day but less than 1 month suggest a brief psychotic disorder. If the symptoms have been present for more than 1 month, but less than 6 months, a diagnosis of schizophreniform disorder may be considered. If the symptoms last longer than 6 months and include prominent delusions or hallucinations, a diagnosis of schizophrenia or schizoaffective disorder should be considered. In making a diagnosis of a psychotic disorder, the clinician needs to rule out mood disorder, substance-induced disorder, and other medical causes.

In clinical practice, patients are often seen with a mix of symptoms that may not fit neatly into a diagnostic category such as schizophrenia or bipolar disorder. Schizoaffective disorder is diagnosed when symptoms of a psychotic disorder and a mood disorder (depression, mania, or mixed states) co-occur typically during the same time period in the course of the illness. In contrast to major depression with psychotic features, schizoaffective disorder features a period of psychotic symptoms in the absence of mood disorder symptoms. A delusional disorder is considered when nonbizarre delusions are present, and little other pathology is seen with no marked impairment in functioning.

Several common scenarios can be challenging for clinicians in differentiating the diagnosis of schizophrenia or an SUD induced psychosis. One common and challenging scenario is when the clinician is evaluating a new patient who presents with both psychotic symptoms and ongoing substance use. This is particularly true when no patient history of serious mental illness is available. It is often difficult to establish the exact chronology of the onset of the psychotic symptoms and that of substance use. Therefore a definitive diagnosis of a psychotic disorder cannot be established, resulting in the need to treat the coexisting psychosis and SUD simultaneously. In one longitudinal diagnostic study of 165 patients with chronic psychosis and cocaine use, a definitive diagnosis could not be established in 93% of the cases.[33] To establish a definitive diagnosis of schizophrenia in this study, the researchers required that a patient meet diagnostic criteria (DSM-III-R) for schizophrenia only after 6 weeks of abstinence. Using these strict guidelines, the primary reasons a diagnosis could not be established were insufficient abstinence (78%), poor memory (24%), or inconsistent reporting (20%) on the part of the patient. A review of hospital records and collateral information addressed the problems of poor memory and inconsistent reporting, leaving insufficient abstinence as the primary barrier to establish a diagnosis. The finding that most patients continued to use substances reflects the difficulty of treating this population and underscores the need to make clinical decisions in the context of diagnostic uncertainty.

A second common and challenging scenario occurs when the clinician is re-evaluating a known psychiatric patient with schizophrenia, who presents with new symptoms and an undiagnosed SUD. The patient may contribute to a misdiagnosis by downplaying or denying his or her substance-related problems or by pointing to other causes of such problems. One study of patients with schizophrenia who presented at hospital emergency departments found that 33% had recently used cocaine, but half of those persons reported no recent use.[33] Thus, urine toxicology[9] and alcohol breathalyzer tests are strongly advised as adjuncts to self-report. The clinician should be careful not to dwell exclusively on the amount of substance used, because the diagnosis of an SUD generally does not rely on quantity or frequency measures.

Schanzer et al. reported that clinicians in psychiatric emergency rooms tend to attribute psychotic symptoms to a primary psychotic disorder rather than to co-occurring substance use.[34] This may result in difficulties for the patient, in that an incorrect diagnosis may have long-term negative implications including the associated stigma, unnecessary inpatient hospitalization, and inappropriate treatment with antipsychotic medications. Clinicians might consider referring these patients to an integrated treatment program that can treat the psychosis and provide enhanced care and monitoring of the ongoing substance use and further determine if there is a SUD that needs treating.

There should be arrangements for continued observation and follow-up due to the fact that the diagnosis of these patients may change over time from substance-induced psychotic disorder to a primary psychotic disorder, especially in individuals with significant family history of psychotic disorder, poor premorbid adjustment, lack of awareness, and under-reporting of psychotic symptoms.[4,35,36] A recent large-scale registry study in Finland[37] found that the 8-year cumulative risk to receive a schizophrenia spectrum diagnosis was 46% for those with a diagnosis of cannabis-induced psychosis and 30% for those with an amphetamine-induced psychosis. The conversion to schizophrenia spectrum diagnosis was particularly rapid for cannabis-induced psychosis. Importantly, patients who use substances nonmedically are associated with poor adherence to treatment plans including medication management. Consequently, a presenting with a recurrence of psychosis may be the result of both nonadherence of antipsychotic medication treatment and continued use of alcohol or other substances.

CLINICAL PRESENTATION OF SUBSTANCE-INDUCED PSYCHOSIS

The following discussion focuses on the unique relationship of certain psychoactive substances to the development of psychotic symptoms.

Alcohol Use Disorders and Psychosis

Psychotic symptoms in the context of alcohol use disorders (AUD) can occur during either intoxication or withdrawal. Though emergence of psychotic symptoms associated with alcohol generally occurs in the context of recent discontinuation of alcohol use, usually within 3 to 5 days.[38,39] Delirium tremens, which may include visual, auditory, or tactile hallucinations, is considered a medical emergency and confers a high risk of death if left untreated (See Chapter 56, "Management of Alcohol Intoxication and Withdrawal").

By contrast, alcohol-induced psychotic disorder (AIPD)—traditionally referred to as *alcoholic hallucinosis*—is a clinical condition that is distinct from alcohol-withdrawal delirium, Wernicke-Korsakoff syndrome, and alcohol-induced dementia.[40] The prevalence of AIPD has been estimated to be around 4% in individuals with AUD,[41] and symptoms are based in the still-undefined interplay of chronic AUD with the gamma-aminobutyric acid type A, *N*-methyl-D-aspartic acid (NMDA), and dopamine receptors.[41] DSM-5 requires that symptoms begin during or soon after alcohol intoxication or withdrawal, do not precede alcohol use and do not exclusively occur during a delirium.[40] According to the ICD-10, the symptoms of AIPD begin within 2 weeks of alcohol use and must persist for more than 48 hours. Symptoms should not be a part of alcohol intoxication or withdrawal and clouding of consciousness should be no more than minor.[42] Patients who develop AIPD also commonly have co-occurring psychiatric illnesses, along with psychosocial stressors, such as low income, unemployment, and lack of social supports.[43] Clinical experience suggests that AIPD may develop sometimes when a person with physiologic dependence cuts back to a lower daily alcohol volume, for example, from a quart to a pint, but does not stop alcohol intake.

Hallucinations in AIPD most often are of the auditory type, and may be threatening, or command-type. Hallucinations may also be accompanied by delusions, often of persecutory nature, along with anxiety, in the presence of a clear consciousness.[44] Individuals can be in an extremely agitated and paranoid state because of the hallucinations and physical discomfort. Psychotic symptoms, particularly paranoia, may persist for hours to weeks. Some evidence suggests that individuals with symptoms that are prolonged for weeks or months may have a predisposition to a psychotic illness.[45] There can be great similarity between this psychotic appearance and schizophrenia, although patients with AIPD may be less likely to display negative symptoms.[44] Historically, research suggests that 10% to 20% of patients with alcohol-related psychosis may develop a chronic psychotic disorder similar to schizophrenia.[46] By contrast, a more recent study[47] showed that the cumulative risk of progression to schizophrenia for patients with AIPD was just under 5%. Importantly, this study demonstrated that individuals with alcohol and drug induced psychosis who progress to develop schizophrenia have the same genetic vulnerability to develop schizophrenia as do other patients with schizophrenia—a vulnerability not shared by individuals with alcohol and drug induced psychosis that do not go on to develop schizophrenia. Importantly, AIPD has been associated with considerable mortality,[43] highlighting the value of continuing to better understand and manage this condition.

Recent literature has begun to highlight the factors that may influence this relationship between AUD and psychosis. Kendler[47] demonstrated that schizophrenia that follows alcohol or drug induced psychotic disorder may appropriately be viewed as a substance precipitated disorder in vulnerable individuals. Supporting this conclusion is a recent study[48] showing that AUD and schizophrenia share significant genetic correlations. Yet another recent study[44] shed light into the possible role of the perisylvian language network. The perisylvian language network includes Broca's and Wernicke's areas responsible for language. Altered connectivity or lesions of this network are associated with auditory hallucinations in schizophrenia, as well as with impaired immediate verbal memory that is seen in patients with AIPD.

Cannabis and Psychosis

Data from the NESARC and NESARC-III show that both cannabis use and cannabis dependence, based on the DSM-IV criteria, have increased in the last decade.[49] This includes a rise in adolescent and young adult use of cannabis.[50] Alarmingly, the most recent Monitoring the Future Study demonstrated that use of cannabis among young adults has increased significantly reaching a historic high in 2021.[51]

The past decade has seen changes in cannabis laws and patterns of recreational use. More potent strains and forms of cannabis, corresponding to higher delta-9-tetrahydrocannabinol (THC) percentage, have become more prevalent. Additionally, more people are using oral cannabis products ("edibles"), vaporizers, and cannabis concentrates ("wax," "shatter," "dabs"), which can have substantially higher concentrations of THC.[52] Edible products are particularly associated with impairing intoxication symptoms in inexperienced consumers due to prolonged absorption and manufacturing inconsistencies.[53]

Typically, psychosis associated with cannabis is acute and of short duration. Intoxication symptoms vary depending on individual variation, dosage, route of administration methods, chronicity, and environment. The most frequent effects of cannabis at levels of moderate intoxication are euphoria, an awareness of alteration in thought processes, suspiciousness and paranoid ideation, alteration in the perception of time, a sensation of heightened visual perception, impaired psychomotor performance and, at higher doses, auditory and visual hallucinations.[54] These effects have been reproduced in the laboratory and appear to be partially dose dependent. A recent study showed that patients presenting with first episode psychosis with a history of daily use of high potency cannabis—defined in this study as having concentration of THC of more than 10%—display more positive and fewer negative symptoms compared to patients with no or low-potency cannabis use.[55] First-time use, large amounts, and route of ingestion (oral more so than smoked) may be factors in the higher incidence of cannabis-related psychosis.[56,57] With recent legalization in certain U.S. states and rising potency, hospital visits due to cannabis intoxication have increased.[58] Individuals with chronic cannabis use may continue to screen positive for cannabis use after weeks or even months of abstinence due to the accumulation and slow release of tetrahydrocannabinol from adipose tissue. There is evidence to suggest that some individuals seek the more psychotomimetic effects achieved through chronic use of large amounts of cannabis[59] or by use of high-potency cannabis.[60]

There is now mounting evidence that chronic use of cannabis is related to the onset of a primary psychotic disorder.[61,62] Of all substance-induced psychotic disorders, cannabis-induced psychotic disorder is the most likely to progress to schizophrenia, and this can happen in up to 34% of cases.[2,63] Cannabis use and cannabis use disorder (CUD) are highly prevalent in patients admitted for First Episode Psychosis, and the onset of cannabis use generally precedes the onset of symptoms.[64] Indeed, cannabis is considered "one of the few potentially modifiable risk factors in schizophrenia,"[36] especially in those with subclinical psychotic symptoms, family history of schizophrenia, or recent functional decline. There is also growing evidence that rising prevalence of cannabis use, coupled with the use of high potency cannabis, may be contributing to rising rates of psychotic disorders. Livne[65] reported a nearly 2.5 times increase in self-reported psychosis when comparing data from NESARC conducted in 2001 to 2002 with data from NESARC III conducted in 2012 to 2013. In both sets of data, individuals with CUD and individuals with any cannabis use were more likely to report psychosis compared to individuals with no cannabis use, and, pertinently, people who used cannabis were more likely to self-report psychosis in NESARC III compared to NESARC. Focusing on population-level data, Hjorthoj[66] reported that in Denmark, the proportion of cases of schizophrenia that can be attributable to cannabis increased nearly four-fold in the past two decades—from 2% in 1995, to 8% in 2010.

Recent research has identified several risk factors that may increase the risk of cannabis-induced psychotic disorders. A number of genetic polymorphisms have been identified in genes that directly (*COMT, DRD2, DAT*) or indirectly (*AKT1*) modulate dopamine pathways and may contribute to this risk. Of note, evidence points toward the importance of interplay between genetic and environmental factors, including cannabis use and childhood trauma.[67] Potency of cannabis also appears to increase the risk of psychosis in multiple studies.[55,66,68,69] The age of initiation,[70] and weekly or more frequent pattern of use,[55,71,72] may also be associated with the risk of psychosis in individuals using cannabis. Kline[68] showed that earlier age at first exposure was associated with a younger age at onset of prodromal psychosis, a younger age at onset of psychotic symptoms, and worse premorbid functioning in individuals being admitted for first episode psychosis. DiForti et al.[69] showed that daily use of what the authors defined as "high potency" (>10% THC, which is lower than a majority of strains currently found in the market in the United States) cannabis was associated with a nearly 5-fold increased risk of developing a psychotic disorder. The authors concluded that if high-potency cannabis was no longer available, up to 12.2% of cases of first episode psychosis may not occur. Of note, across the 11 European study sites there were higher associations, rising to 30.3% in London and 50.3% in Amsterdam, where the highest potency cannabis is generally found. These findings highlight the importance of public health education on potential harms of the daily use of cannabis products that contain high levels of THC and the association with psychosis.

The question of whether a patient is experiencing chronic psychosis due to cannabis is a difficult one to answer for a variety of reasons: Is the patient remaining abstinent? What other substances might the patient have used? Is there predisposing psychopathology? Did the individual with a prodromal psychotic illness find refuge in the use of cannabis? And did cannabis, in turn, open a "genetic window" in an already predisposed patient at an earlier age?[73] Often, collateral information is needed to obtain this information. These are important diagnostic questions to consider given the link between cannabis use and psychosis. There is a near 2-fold increase in the odds of developing a psychotic illness in the cannabis-using population.[74,75] There is also evidence that patients with recent onset of a psychotic illness have more severe psychotic and disorganized symptoms if consistently using cannabis,[76] as well as increased potential for recurrence of symptoms and treatment nonadherence.[77] When observed over a 10-year period, there is evidence that cannabis use is associated with more severe psychotic symptoms.[78] This study further indicated that the severity of schizophrenia symptoms and cannabis use were bidirectional predictors of each other with severe schizophrenia being correlated with higher risk of cannabis use.[78] Based upon this knowledge, treatment should target psychosis and cannabis use in a parallel, integrated manner. There is evidence that using nonpharmacological approaches, such as contingency management (CM), or cognitive-based interventions, may improve outcome.[79]

Cocaine and Psychosis

Transient paranoia is a common feature of chronic cocaine intoxication,[80,81] appearing in 33% to 50% of patients. A recent meta-analysis[82] reported a 54.7% prevalence of lifetime cocaine-induced psychosis, and a 16% prevalence of lifetime cocaine-induced psychotic disorder. Psychotic symptoms associated with cocaine use are almost exclusively seen in the intoxication phase and rarely extend beyond the "crash" phase in the patient who does not have a primary psychotic illness.[39] There are multiple indicators that high-dose use of cocaine over time is strongly associated with the onset of psychotic symptoms, especially in younger people.[36,81,83] There also is strong evidence that sensitization occurs with chronic administration of cocaine and amphetamines.[36,84] Sensitization results in psychotic symptoms occurring following repeated use even at lower doses of the stimulant. Onset of psychotic symptoms is associated with reduction in individual doses, use, and the desire for treatment.[83] The most frequently reported psychotic symptoms related to cocaine use are persecutory delusions and hallucinations. Auditory hallucinations are the most common and often are associated with persecutory delusions. Visual hallucinations are the next most common, followed by tactile hallucinations.[83] Visual hallucinations have been associated with chronic mydriatic pupils and the appearance of geometric shapes. Nearly all the hallucinations are associated with antecedent drug use. Evidence suggests that the character of the psychotic symptoms experienced is associated with the setting in which drugs are ingested.[85] Stereotypic behavior also can be associated with psychosis. Such repeated, purposeless, gross motor movements occasionally continue after the intoxication subsides.

Amphetamines and Psychosis

Amphetamine-induced psychosis can develop over prolonged exposure in association with large amounts of the drug, which is delivered by any route of administration. The strongest correlation has been seen in those individuals who use large amounts by intravenous injection. Indeed, a recent review by Arunogiri[86] showed that the frequency of use, amount of use, along with the severity of methamphetamine dependence, are most consistently associated with psychosis. Other factors that increase the risk of psychosis may include concurrent use of other substances, particularly alcohol and cannabis, major depressive disorder, antisocial personality disorder, as well as a family history of psychotic disorders.[87] A recent review[88] reported that the most commonly reported symptoms in methamphetamine associated psychosis are persecutory delusions and auditory and visual hallucinations, followed by hostility, disorganization, and depression. Negative symptoms are relatively uncommon in this population. Typically, this altered mental state lasts only during the period of intoxication, although there are reports of it persisting for days to weeks. Amphetamine psychosis can progress through three stages of severity. Initially, symptoms can include increased curiosity and repetitive examining, searching, and sorting behaviors. In the second stage, these behaviors are followed by increased suspiciousness. In the final stage, symptoms may include ideas of reference, persecutory delusions, and auditory or visual hallucinations, which are marked by a fearful, panic-stricken, agitated, overactive state.[84]

Clinical experience suggests that amphetamine psychosis can last for 3 to 6 months in extreme cases of high-dose use. There is little evidence to suggest that these drugs directly cause schizophrenia, but the interaction of amphetamine use and preexisting vulnerability may account for increased rates of schizophrenia onset among those with more extensive use.[89] Indeed, a nationwide Finnish registry study[37] reported that the 8-year cumulative risk of a schizophrenia spectrum diagnosis was 30% for those admitted with an amphetamine-induced psychosis. There is also potential for long-term affective instability, a moderate to severe anxiety state, and underlying suspiciousness.

Hallucinogens and Psychosis

Hallucinogens, also termed classic psychedelics, are a group of compounds, including lysergic acid diethylamide (LSD), psilocybin, mescaline, and *N,N*-dimethyltryptamine (DMT), which share a common mechanism of action, mainly through agonism at the serotonin 5-HT2A receptors.

Results from the 2020 National Survey on Drug Use and Health[90] indicated an estimated lifetime use and past year use of hallucinogens at 15.9% and 2.6% respectively among those individuals aged 12 years or older. Notably, nearly 40% of those that used these substances in the last year represented the highly vulnerable ages between 12 and 25 years old.

The primary model for psychedelics is lysergic acid diethylamide (LSD), an indole-type drug with structural similarities to serotonin. LSD crosses the blood-brain barrier readily and has a potent affinity for the 5-HT2A receptor. Its half-life is approximately 100 minutes. The onset of LSD effects in humans begins 30 to 90 minutes after administration, with subjective and physiological effects generally lasting five to ten hours after drug administration. The acute subjective and psychological effects of classic psychedelics can vary widely from individual to individual, and even within the same individual. Effects are highly dependent on the *"set"*—an individual's own expectations, hopes, fears, intentions, preparation, and mental state—and the *"setting"*—the substance, the dose, as well as the environment in which experience takes place. The initial, and most common, level of the experience is sensory, which can include alterations in perception of objects, vivid imagery with eyes closed, illusions, and more rarely, pseudo hallucinations during which reality testing may remain intact. Synesthesia may be experienced, and time may slow down or even stop. Individuals commonly have a very affect-laden experience, and a whole range of emotions may be experienced. These may change rapidly or even occur simultaneously during a single session. Derealization, depersonalization, and paranoia may be experienced. Biographical material and memories may be experienced in an emotionally connected manner, and existential, spiritual, and symbolic themes may emerge. Mystical experiences tend to occur frequently at higher doses. A study by Carhart-Harris et al.[91] administered LSD 75 µg IV to 20 healthy participants. Acutely, there were increases in an index of psychosis-like symptoms. However, 2 weeks post-LSD, there were no changes in delusional thinking. Additionally, 2 weeks postadministration, increased optimism and trait openness were observed after LSD, but not after placebo. Also notably, there was a positive correlation between impaired/disorganized thinking acutely, and trait openness 2 weeks post-LSD.

No clear evidence exists that LSD directly causes a prolonged psychotic-like illness. Niemi-Pynttäri et al.'s[37] Finnish registry study reported a 24% conversion to schizophrenia spectrum disorder in the 8 years following admission with hallucinogen-induced psychosis. Such longitudinal studies, however, cannot control for all preexisting psychopathology or the high rate of adulterants in the formulation of the drugs. Nichols et al. concluded that although acute psychotic reactions may occur with LSD use, the incidence of prolonged reactions is extremely rare—particularly when LSD is administered in a research context—and may be attributed to premorbid vulnerability.[92] Intriguingly, in a retrospective stratified analysis of over 21,000 subjects, lifetime psychedelic use was significantly associated with a lower rate of seven core psychotic symptoms.[93] The psychiatric diagnosis most commonly associated with post-LSD psychosis is a form of schizoaffective disorder. The appearance of some affective instability-involving a feeling of an altered state of consciousness and recurrent perceptual disorder, primarily visual, are the most common symptoms seen in patients with associated chronic psychosis. Hallucinogen persisting perception disorder (HPPD) differs from classic psychosis in that the experience is purely perceptual, and reality testing is intact. Unfortunately, there are no evidence-based treatments for HPPD. At the same time, more recent clinical and population-based studies have not supported the idea of "flashbacks" or HPPD associated with classic psychedelics.[93] An individual with schizophrenia who uses LSD has been shown to have an earlier age of onset and better premorbid social functioning than the non–drug-using individual with schizophrenia.[94,95]

Dissociatives and Psychosis

The cyclohexylamine anesthetics phencyclidine (PCP) and ketamine hydrochloride as well as dextromethorphan, (which is converted to dextrorphan). each result in psychotic-like experiences during intoxication. Evidence suggests that, with PCP, the psychotic-like state can last for prolonged periods beyond intoxication.

Ketamine, at a potency 10 to 50 times lower than PCP, has been shown to produce far fewer of these psychotic-like episodes and was originally developed for use as an anesthetic without the psychotogenic effects of PCP. While ketamine—due to its NMDA, glutamate receptor, blocking effects—has been used in investigations of animal models of schizophrenia, it has not led to prolonged psychotic reactions at therapeutic doses in humans. In healthy research participants, as well as in individuals with schizophrenia, dissociative and psychotic symptoms induced by ketamine generally resolve within 2 to 3 hours of administration. There are a growing number of reports showing the benefits of ketamine in treatment of individuals with treatment resistant depression with psychosis, though more rigorous research is clearly needed to demonstrate safety and efficacy.[96] Interestingly, children do not appear to develop the associated psychotic-like symptoms with ketamine.

Early observations of patients treated with PCP noted the similarities between dissociative and schizophrenia spectrum disorders.[97,98] The clinical appearance is that of altered sensory perception, bizarre and impoverished thought and speech, impaired attention, disrupted memory, and disrupted thought processes in healthy individuals. There also may be protracted psychosis.[99] There is considerable symptom variation, depending on dose. At lower doses of PCP (20-30 ng/mL), one is likely to observe sedation, mood elevation, irritability, impaired attention and memory, mutism, hyperactivity, and stereotypy. As serum levels rise to 30 to 100 ng/mL, mood changes, psychosis, analgesia, paresthesia, and ataxia can occur. These levels are associated with profound paranoia, aggression, and violent behavior. Higher levels (>100 ng/mL) can cause stupor, hyperreflexia, hypertension, seizure, coma, and/or death.

There is widespread nonmedical use of over-the-counter cough and cold medicines that contain dextromethorphan, a nonopioid synthetic analog of codeine. These formulations often also contain antihistamines, acetaminophen, or pseudoephedrine, which can complicate treatment for dextromethorphan poisoning. The major active metabolite of dextromethorphan is dextrorphan. This compound, like phencyclidine and ketamine, is a noncompetitive antagonist of the NMDA receptor, which is conducive to nonmedical use, and potential toxicity, and psychosis.[100] There is initially a mild stimulatory effect followed by hallucinations and delusions. A bottle of OTC cough syrup may contain over 350 mg of dextromethorphan. At low doses of 1.5 to 2.5 mg/kg, or approximately 100 to 200 mg of dextromethorphan in a 70 kg individual, restless and anxiety may be noted. Consuming one, 350 mg, bottle of OTC cough syrup can generate altered perceptions and closed-eye hallucinations, which are seen at doses of 2.5 to 7.5 mg/kg. Partial dissociation, along with mania, panic, and altered consciousness are noted at doses of 7.5 to 15 mg/kg, or two bottles of OTC cough syrup. This can progress to complete dissociation at doses over 15 mg/kg, or three bottles of OTC cough syrup or a total of 1,050 mg of dextromethorphan.[101-104] Excessive doses have resulted in respiratory depression, tachycardia, and hypertension.[105] These doses may also result in false-positive urine immunoassay for phencyclidine.[106]

MDMA ("Ecstasy") and Psychosis

3,4-Methylenedioxymethamphetamine (MDMA or "ecstasy") is a derivative of methamphetamine, which has a mixed spectrum of effects, including stimulant, empathogenic, and hallucinogenic. MDMA increases the release and inhibits the reuptake of serotonin, dopamine, and norepinephrine from presynaptic neurons, as well as decreasing their degradation by inhibiting monoamine oxidase.[107] MDMA has received breakthrough drug status from the FDA for the treatment of PTSD based upon a series of phase 2 and one phase 3 clinical trial.[108,109]

Those who use MDMA report enhanced empathy, feelings of closeness to others, euphoria, mood elevation, greater tendency to socialize, increased self-esteem, and altered visual perceptions.[36] Hallucinations associated with use generally are mild but can be intense and severe. There is little data on psychosis associated with MDMA use, but case reports exist. Deaths have occurred in cases that presented as a syndrome featuring severe hyperthermia, altered mental status, autonomic dysfunction, and dystonia.[110] The mechanism is unclear, but, as with a serotonin syndrome, MDMA can have a direct effect on the thermoregulatory mechanisms that potentiate the context of the drug use. For example, MDMA is often used in the setting of dance parties where there is sustained physical activity, high temperatures, and inadequate fluid intake resulting in dehydration and an electrolyte imbalance.

There is also concern about the long-term neurotoxicity of MDMA. Long-term use can result in serotonin neural injury associated with psychiatric presentation of psychosis, panic attacks, anxiety, depression, flashbacks, and memory disturbances.[111] In general, neurodegenerative effects of MDMA have been demonstrated in experimental animals through a variety of mechanisms including accumulation of toxic metabolites, hyperthermia, increased oxidative stress, glial cell activation, excitotoxicity, and even mitochondrial dysfunction. On the other hand, the evidence of lasting serotonergic or dopaminergic neurotoxicity in humans is growing but as yet is inconclusive.[112] Use of MDMA must be ruled out with new onset of psychosis.

New Psychoactive Substances and Psychosis

New Psychoactive Substances (NPS) are defined as "substances…that are not controlled under the Single Convention on Narcotic Drugs of 1961, or the Convention on Psychotropic Substances of 1971, but that may pose a threat to public health."[113] Some of these substances may be analogues of existing controlled substances; some may be newly synthesized to mimic the effects of controlled substances; some may have been around for a long time with a recent increase in use. NPS are a very large group of diverse substances. Between 2009 to 2021, 134 countries reported over 1,127 such substances to the United Nations Office on Drugs and Crime (UNODC). These substances are also fluid—entering and leaving the market as a result of popularity and control policies—and in 2021, over 500 of these substances were available globally. The use of any given NPS tends to be lower than controlled substances, with past year prevalence of less than 1% reported in 21 countries. The use of NPS tends to be higher in high school students, with a median of 2.2% across 44 countries. Encouragingly, UNODC has reported a gradual decline in the use of NPS globally.[113] While the overall public health burden of NPS is lower compared to internationally controlled substances, they can still have major adverse effects on an individual's health. This section will focus on NPS associated with psychosis. Of note, this section will not cover certain NPS associated with psychosis due to having been covered elsewhere, (eg, MDMA, ketamine), or due to effects being very similar to what has been covered elsewhere, (eg, plant-based psychedelics, or psychedelic tryptamines).

Synthetic cannabinoids represent the most prevalent category of NPS globally and in the United States. Over the past decade, the use of synthetic cannabinoid receptor agonists such as JWH-018, JWH-073, and CP 47,497, which are marketed as "K2" and "Spice," has been a major public health concern. In a small, 2014, survey of adults who used cannabis regularly,[114] half reported smoking synthetic cannabinoids and one-quarter reported use in the previous month. Since then, the use of these substances has declined. According to the UNODC, the annual prevalence of synthetic cannabinoids among 12th grade students in the United States declined from just under 12% in 2010 to under 4% in 2019. The use also remains far below that of cannabis—with 28% of 10th graders reporting past year use of "marijuana" versus 2.5% reporting past year use of "synthetic marijuana."[113] At the same time, over 20 novel synthetic cannabinoids have been reported between 2017 and 2021. These newer synthetic cannabinoids display an increased affinity and activity at the CB-1 receptor, leading to greater potential for adverse effects, including psychotic symptoms.[115] Studies of the association between synthetic cannabinoids and psychosis are scarce but some small studies support the occurrence of psychotic symptoms as a consequence to high doses of synthetic cannabinoids.[116-118] Bassir-Nia et al.[119] reported that compared to cannabis induced psychosis, synthetic cannabinoid induced psychosis required higher doses of antipsychotic medications and longer hospital stays. In their comprehensive review, Schifano et al.[120] also report recurrence or worsening of preexisting psychotic disorder, as well as emergence of persisting psychotic disorder following heavy synthetic cannabinoid use.

Between 2016 and 2020, novel stimulants were the most common category of NPS by effect.[113] Synthetic cathinones, colloquially known as "bath salts," are one category of stimulant-type NPS. Synthetic cathinones are derived from *Catha edulis*, also known as *khat*, a shrub native to east Africa, whose leaves and stems are chewed for a mild stimulant effect. Cathinone, the active compound in *Catha edulis*, has several derivatives, termed synthetic cathinones, which have been used globally. The exact effects of synthetic cathinones vary upon their pharmacological properties, but in general are similar to methamphetamine. Piperazines, often sold as "legal ecstasy," or "benzo fury," represent another major category of stimulant type NPS. The major compound in piperazines, *N*-benzylpiperazine, is structurally similar to amphetamine. Another major category of NPS is phenethylamines, a large and fascinating category of NPS. Several synthetic phenethylamines are used in the United States and globally, including 2C-B-FLY, 2C-E, DOI, DOC, bromo-dragonfly, MBDB, and PMMA.[113] Phenethylamines act on serotonergic receptors, leading to psychedelic effects, but also may inhibit NE/DA reuptake. Depending upon dose and chemical structure, the effects of phenethylamines can vary greatly, from psychedelic to stimulant-like to entactogenic, that is, promoting empathy, emotional openness, and relatedness. MDMA—a phenethylamine—has been covered earlier.[120]

Ketamine, covered earlier, is considered an NPS by UNDOC. There are also related dissociatives that are available but less commonly used, including 4-MeO-PCP and methoxetamine. Sold on the Internet as a "legal high" under a variety of names such as "mexxy," or "special M," these agents act as noncompetitive NMDA receptor antagonists but may also exert effects on opioid and monoamine receptors. Effects can include perceptual disturbances, hallucinations, derealization, and depersonalization in a dose-dependent fashion.[121]

Finally, one plant-based NPS associated with psychotic symptoms and not considered a classic psychedelic is *Salvia divinorum*, known as "diviner's sage," "magic mint," "Sally D," or "Maria Pastora." The active compound within this plant is salvinorin A, which acts as a kappa opioid antagonist. Potent and unique hallucinogenic effects have been reported within seconds of inhalation, with a duration of effects of 20 to 30 minutes. In addition to hallucinations and perceptual disturbances, users report synesthesia, dissociative and "out of body" experiences, as well as a sense of fractured reality.[122] Extreme dysphoria and anxiety may be associated with use. There is little literature on acute management, which is largely supportive. Benzodiazepines may be used to address anxiety and distress. Rates of *Salvia divinorum* use have been declining steadily after peaking over a decade ago. The annual prevalence among U.S. 12th graders was 5.5% in 2010 and had declined to under 1% in 2019.[113]

Multiple Substance Use and Psychosis

Multiple substance use of a range of combinations (alcohol, stimulants, cannabis, opioids, tobacco) and associated psychosis continue to be a major clinical challenge. Opioid use is less likely to result in psychosis symptoms; however, psychosis symptoms can occur in some people. Also, fentanyl is now ubiquitous in the drug selling culture and this substance is often mixed in illegal drugs, including stimulants, cannabis, etc. Fentanyl and other opioids by themselves can result in psychotic symptoms during use or withdrawal. The combination of fentanyl with stimulants and cannabis can make assessment and treatment more complex. Additional research is needed on how fentanyl combination impacts psychotic symptoms as well as the development of new intervention strategies.

MANAGEMENT OF CO-OCCURRING SUBSTANCE USE DISORDER AND PSYCHOSIS

Management of Psychosis

Pharmacological Treatment

Antipsychotic medications are often an important component of the treatment of co-occurring substance use and psychosis. Medications should be complemented by psychosocial interventions that facilitate patient engagement and help patients develop skills in interpersonal communication, crisis management, and recovery.

The potential interactions between the substances used and the possible medication choices should be taken into consideration. For example, clinicians should avoid prescribing medications that cause sedation when treating patients who use sedating substances nonmedically. In addition, clinicians generally should avoid prescribing medications with addictive potential.

Patients who present with active substance use (with or without a confirmed SUD), co-occurring psychotic symptoms, and medication nonadherence can be difficult to manage as outpatients. Improving medication adherence can be enhanced by reducing the patient's psychotic symptoms and providing psychotherapy and medication education. Patient follow-up should include continued use of motivational enhancement techniques, establishing between-visit telephone contact, and strong consideration of the use of long-acting injectable antipsychotic medication if patients are unable or refuse to take oral medications. Patients may require more intense monitoring and services via admission to a level of care higher than outpatient service, such as partial hospitalization or intensive outpatient service levels. The ASAM Criteria has six dimensions that can be used to help decide what is the right level of care (acute intoxication and/or withdrawal; biomedical conditions and complications; emotional, behavioral, or cognitive conditions and complications; readiness to change; return to use, continued use, or continued problem potential; and recovery/living environment). The severity level on these six dimensions is associated with the different levels of care: outpatient treatment, intensive outpatient and partial hospitalization, residential/inpatient treatment, medically managed intensive, and inpatient treatment.[123]

Over the past decades, atypical antipsychotic medications have been approved by the U.S. Food and Drug Administration (FDA) for the treatment of schizophrenia. Some of these medications also have been studied for the treatment of SUDs (with and without coexisting schizophrenia).[8,16,124] This class of medication has the benefit of decreasing extrapyramidal side effects, when compared with conventional antipsychotics. In addition to acting on the dopamine system, atypical antipsychotics also bind to the serotonin receptors, which is thought to play an important role in substance craving and addiction. An accumulating body of literature has suggested that some atypical antipsychotics might be beneficial in reducing craving and substance use.[125]

Clinical judgment based on the individual patient's situation should guide the choice of antipsychotic medications. Some studies have found no difference between conventional and atypical antipsychotics used to treat patients with co-occurring substance use and psychosis,[126] while others have found that atypical antipsychotics may have some advantages.[8,16,127-130] For example, clozapine appears to be more effective than risperidone[8,16,124,131] and olanzapine[130] in reducing alcohol and/or cannabis use and/or craving among patients with schizophrenia or schizoaffective disorder. A study by Brunette et al.[132] indicates that clozapine may also prevent recurrence of use in patients with schizophrenia using alcohol, cannabis, or cocaine. Furthermore, risperidone and clozapine appear to reduce the likelihood of return to use for patients with opioid use disorder.[133] In a 14-week trial comparing olanzapine and risperidone in the treatment of patients with co-occurring schizophrenia and cocaine/cannabis use, Akerele and Levin showed some potential benefit of olanzapine for the treatment of cocaine dependence in individuals with schizophrenia.[134] In another study, risperidone and ziprasidone increased patients' retention in co-occurring treatment compared with olanzapine or conventional antipsychotics.[135] More recently, a systematic review and meta-analysis reported that clozapine was superior to other antipsychotics for reduction of substance use and risperidone to olanzapine for craving in SUD individuals.[136] Craving was evaluated in these studies using different questionnaires, and in the most recent DSM version, craving is now a diagnostic criterion for SUDs.[136]

Interactions Between Substances and Antipsychotic Medications

Substances can interact with antipsychotic medications and, therefore, affect their efficacy and side effects in schizophrenia treatment. For example, in the CATIE study, illegal substance use and alcohol (with or without SUD) was shown to attenuate the apparent superiority of olanzapine over the other antipsychotics based on the primary outcome measure of time to all-cause treatment discontinuation.[137] The interactions are both pharmacokinetic and pharmacodynamic.

By-products of tobacco smoking, particularly the polycyclic aromatic hydrocarbons, are metabolic inducers of the cytochrome P-450 1A2 isoenzyme (CYP1A2). Smoking is known to decrease blood levels of haloperidol, fluphenazine and thiothixene, olanzapine, and clozapine.[130,138-140] Abstinence from smoking increases blood levels of antipsychotic medications. People who smoke usually are prescribed approximately double the dose of conventional antipsychotic medications that is given to those that do not smoke.[141] There is a report of clozapine toxicity and seizure in the context of a quit attempt, presumably related to a sudden increase in serum levels of the drug.[142] The effect on metabolism is important in making treatment decisions regarding inpatients whose smoking is restricted as well as the patient who is attempting to quit smoking.

Caffeine is more than 90% dependent on CYP1A2 for its metabolism. Near 90% of the adult U.S. population consume caffeine.[143] Patients with schizophrenia consume significant more caffeine than the general population.[144] Caffeine increases the levels of clozapine and olanzapine through competitive inhibition on CYP1A2.[145]

One meta-analysis suggests that patients with co-occurring schizophrenia and SUD (especially cocaine related) are more likely to experience extrapyramidal adverse effects with antipsychotic medication.[146] Substance use has been associated with earlier and more severe cases of tardive dyskinesia.[147-149] However, other studies suggested that substance use had no effect on movement disorders when important covariates were considered.[141,150,151]

Additional Medication Decisions

After clinicians have chosen a primary medication treatment option that stabilizes the psychotic symptoms, they can consider the use of additional medication, as necessary, to manage comorbid depression, or other psychiatric conditions. Further, medications are used to manage substance-induced intoxication or withdrawal symptoms as needed.

Psychosocial Interventions

Individuals with co-occurring substance use and psychosis will benefit from both comprehensive psychosocial interventions and pharmacological treatments.[152] This section will, however, focus on those individuals with a primary psychotic disorder and SUDs, as opposed to individuals with substance-induced psychosis (see Chapter 100, "Substance-Induced Mental Disorders"). Research has demonstrated the importance of therapist empathy[153] and developing a positive therapeutic alliance as a cornerstone of psychosocial treatment.[154,155]

Beyond the therapeutic alliance, there are several core treatment strategies that can improve the lives of such patients. Carey[156] has suggested a five-step "collaborative, motivational, harm reduction" approach: establish and develop a working alliance,[157] help the patient evaluate the cost-benefit ratio of continued substance use (decisional balance in motivational enhancement therapy [MET]),[10] help the patient develop individual goals,[158] help build a supportive environment[159] and a lifestyle that is conducive to abstinence, and helping learn to anticipate and cope with crises.[17,156]

Some individuals with schizophrenia report that using substances helps them cope with symptoms of their schizophrenia.[24,160] While clinicians are likely to hear "self-medication" explanations from their patients, the skilled clinician will listen thoughtfully but understand that the research data supporting the concept are mixed[161]; however, the patient's explanation helps understand at least part of their motivation to use substances. For example, psychotic symptoms in individuals diagnosed with schizophrenia can improve temporarily after nicotine use; however, chronic tobacco use disorder has led to great health disparities in this population, including shorter life span and common morbidities from tobacco use. On the other hand, quitting smoking leads to significant improvements in anxiety, depression, and stress in both psychiatric and nonpsychiatric populations.[162] Clinicians need to understand these motivations of "self-medication" in order to help individuals develop alternative ways to manage the symptoms they are self-treating with substances. Additionally, counseling can introduce other possible explanations for the individual's ongoing use attributed to self-medicating, such as they are treating withdrawal symptoms (not necessarily non–SUD-related stress and anxiety).

Nonetheless, working with these patients requires that the clinician be direct in addressing inconsistencies. For example, if a patient has recent positive cocaine urine samples, yet denies any use during the preceding month, the clinician should be understanding of the initial stage of recovery but point out the discrepancy. Abstinence may be a goal; however, the poorly motivated individuals may benefit from motivational interviewing to increase motivation to stop using substances, address their ambivalence, and to in the future move to a higher motivational level when they are able to engage in treatment.

Keeping patients engaged requires efforts to treat their schizophrenia and to provide encouragement and other "rewards" for small steps toward reducing substance use. It is important to evaluate outcomes other than total abstinence; for example, the clinician might assess the patient for reduced quantity or frequency of substance use, participation in treatment or other activities, adherence to medications and keeping appointments, progress toward short-term goals, and involvement of family or significant others in treatment. These commonsense process outcomes, which align with the ASAM Criteria dimensions 4, 5, 6 but are different, are all important steps toward abstinence and recovery.

Management of Substance Use Disorder With Co-Occurring Psychosis

Pharmacological Treatment

For the treatment of AUD, the U.S. FDA has approved the use of three adjunctive medications: disulfiram, acamprosate, and naltrexone. Disulfiram, a medication used to promote alcohol abstinence, shows some benefits in patients with schizophrenia and AUD.[4,8,16,131] The clinical trial results of disulfiram are mixed, and a meta-analysis showed no difference between treatment and control groups in blinded studies.[163] However, positive findings were reported in open-label studies. The possibility of an alcohol-disulfiram reaction requires that it be given only to patients who comprehend the consequences of alcohol consumption when taking disulfiram. According to some clinicians, administration of disulfiram at high doses (1,000 mg) has produced psychotic symptoms in patients not diagnosed with psychotic disorders. Roncero et al.[125] caution against the use of disulfiram in patients with a history of affective disorders, suicidality, cognitive deterioration, or poor impulse control. Liver function should be monitored when patients receive disulfiram treatment.[8,16] Individuals with poor impulse control may not be good candidates for this medication option. Overdose of disulfiram is not common, but possible, and might include symptoms of ataxia, dizziness, low blood pressure, seizures, vomiting, and coma. Purposeful excessive alcohol use while on the medication may be a possible suicide attempt option.

Clinical studies of naltrexone, an opioid antagonist, are supportive of its use in patients with co-occurring SUD and psychosis.[164] Naltrexone is a relatively safe medication that can be used with patients who are at risk of return to use of alcohol; no alcohol and naltrexone interaction has been reported. Even though there are no systematic studies of the use of naltrexone and acamprosate in patients with co-occurring schizophrenia and AUD, they may be used in combination with psychotropic medications, and there are no known drug-drug interactions. Naltrexone can precipitate opioid withdrawal, so clinicians should carefully assess patients' use of prescription or nonmedical opioid prior to the administration of this medication. Naltrexone's most common side effects include headache and nausea. Liver function should be monitored when using naltrexone.

Patients with agitation and transient psychotic symptoms (with or without schizophrenia) in the setting of alcohol withdrawal often are treated with benzodiazepines in the same way one would treat uncomplicated withdrawal. However, in the severely agitated patient with persistent psychotic symptoms, antipsychotics may be warranted. Alcohol withdrawal has been associated with the development of extrapyramidal symptoms, including dystonia, akathisia, choreoathetosis, and parkinsonism[165]; therefore, particular attention should be given to the possible development of extrapyramidal symptoms in a patient treated with antipsychotics during acute alcohol withdrawal. Other medical issues that influence the choice of medication in heavy drinkers in alcohol withdrawal are the risk for withdrawal seizures and the possibility of impaired hepatic function that may increase the risk of serious adverse effects. Pertinently, phenothiazine and butyrophenone antipsychotics, such as haloperidol, can further reduce the seizure threshold. Due to these reasons, antipsychotics should only be used if significant psychotic symptoms remain present even after providing definitive treatment for alcohol withdrawal. Patients should also be closely monitored for suicidality. The prognosis of treating the positive symptoms of AIPD with antipsychotic medication and abstinence is fair. Treatment of the negative symptoms of AIPD—more associated with alcohol encephalopathy—remains less clear and has proven to be more challenging, although there is a suggestion in the literature that abstinence may be beneficial.[166]

For cocaine addiction, there are no FDA-approved medications. For individuals with schizophrenia and cocaine addiction, there are numerous small studies that suggest some promise for a range of medications (desipramine, selegiline, mazindol, and amantadine); however, there is no strong evidence that any are effective. The best option is often to provide integrated psychosocial treatment and adjust the antipsychotic medication as needed.[140,155,159]

A randomized controlled trial[167] including 45 patients compared risperidone and aripiprazole for amphetamine-induced psychosis over a 6-week period and found that risperidone had a greater effect on positive symptoms, while aripiprazole was more effective for negative symptoms. Treatment of amphetamine intoxication should be initiated by providing a safe, secure, and quiet place for the patient. The potential for agitation and violence is significant in acutely intoxicated patients. Physical restraints should be avoided or used in a time-limited fashion so as not to complicate the presentation with worsening hyperthermia, dehydration, rhabdomyolysis, and possible renal failure. One should keep in mind the potential of amphetamines for lowering seizure threshold, inducing hyperpyrexia, and stimulating cardiovascular compromise, particularly in the patient who is using large amounts of methamphetamine in a chronic pattern. In such patients, antipsychotics with greater potential for lowering the seizure threshold, for example, olanzapine or haloperidol, should be avoided.[168] Risperidone and aripiprazole are associated with a lower incidence of potential seizures and are more commonly recommended. Benzodiazepines may help treat hypertension and tachycardia associated with stimulant intoxication and may also help protect against seizures.

For classic psychedelics, the typical emergency visit secondary to use of the drug occurs as a result of anxiety, a concurrent accident, or suicidal behavior. "Talking down" the patient through providing a calm, reassuring environment and supportive therapy, is the most common way to ease his or her anxiety around the psychotic symptoms of LSD and related drugs. The persistently agitated patient may be treated pharmacologically with a quick-acting benzodiazepine, such as lorazepam. Antipsychotic use is rarely indicated. If supportive therapy and benzodiazepines do not alleviate psychotic symptoms, or if the psychotic symptoms continue to worsen and present a risk of harm to self or others, haloperidol (1-5 mg), or an equivalent dose of high-potency antipsychotic medication, may be appropriate. Monitoring for neuroleptic side effects such as rigidity, akathisia, and tremor is important.

Treatment of the acutely disturbing effects of PCP-like drugs can be achieved with benzodiazepines in doses equivalent to diazepam 10 mg and greater, titrated until the patient is satisfactorily sedated. Intravenous administration is preferable to intramuscular injection. The patient's respiratory status should be continually monitored. There may be a dramatic reduction in aggressive behavior and a significant improvement in the psychotic symptoms with benzodiazepines, and this can minimize the need for the use of antipsychotic medications. Neuroleptics also can be considered for treatment of psychotic symptoms in rare cases if benzodiazepines do not help improve symptoms. Phenothiazine and butyrophenone antipsychotics, such as haloperidol, should generally be avoided, as they can reduce the seizure threshold and interfere with heat dissipation. Previously, urine acidification with ammonium chloride to facilitate urinary excretion of PCP was recommended. However, doing so can lead to metabolic acidosis, which in turn can result in other problems, including worsening of rhabdomyolysis and renal damage. Urine acidification has not been studied in cases of ketamine toxicity. As a result, urine acidification is not recommended in cases of ketamine or PCP toxicity. Management of acute dextromethorphan toxicity includes gastrointestinal decontamination with activated charcoal and reversal of respiratory compromise with naloxone,[169] though observation and symptomatic treatment are often sufficient.

Treatment of acute toxicity of synthetic cathinones is similar to that of other substances with sympathomimetic properties. Spiller et al.[170] described a retrospective case series of 236 patients who were reported to poison centers after consuming synthetic cathinones, in which over one-third of these acute cases experienced hallucinations and paranoia, respectively. Of note, agitation was seen in over 80%, and combative behavior in 56%. Benzodiazepines are considered the first line treatment for managing agitation and psychosis, but antipsychotic medications may be used cautiously in case of lack of response. Acute toxicity, and clinical management, of piperazines are similar to that described above for synthetic cathinones.[121]

Pharmacological treatment for tobacco addiction includes FDA-approved medications such as nicotine replacements (transdermal patch, gum, lozenge, spray, or inhaler), bupropion, or varenicline. These medications combined with specialized tobacco treatment programs appear to benefit patients with tobacco addiction and psychosis.[139,157,159] Moreover, a recent large trial[171] compared varenicline and bupropion to nicotine patch or placebo in individuals with psychiatric disorders including psychosis and found no significant increase in subsequent risk of a diverse range of adverse effects. Despite modest evidence of an increased risk of psychosis due to bupropion,[172] as an adjunct to antipsychotic medication, bupropion can help patients with co-occurring disorders who want to stop smoking,[16,131] without adversely affecting their mental state.[173] However, its potential to reduce the seizure threshold limits its use in the presence of an antipsychotic with similar effect, such as clozapine.[125] There is some evidence that patients also prescribed atypical antipsychotics will have higher rates of abstinence, lower rates of attrition, and lower levels of expired carbon monoxide compared to those on typical antipsychotics.[157] An important finding was that psychiatric symptoms were not exacerbated with abstinence.[157,174] Please also see Section 7 of this textbook for a discussion of intoxication and withdrawal syndromes and their management.

Psychosocial Interventions

Psychosocial interventions are considered an integral part of managing co-occurring SUD and psychosis.[175] Various psychosocial interventions appear to be helpful, and there was not any relative advantage of any specific psychosocial intervention for those with SUD and serious mental illness.[175-179] Three specific approaches that are commonly used and fundamental to the treatment program for co-occurring disorders are MET,[180] Relapse Prevention,[181] and 12-step facilitation.[182] However, for each approach, modifications from their original form are required due to the biological, cognitive, affective, and interpersonal issues often present among individuals with schizophrenia. These modifications of conventional addiction treatments should consider the common features among individuals with schizophrenia, including low motivation and self-efficacy, cognitive deficits, and lack of interpersonal skills. These unique features highlight both the need and sometimes difficulty to develop a strong treatment alliance.[147] The 12-step approach has been modified for people with co-occurring disorders, who often have reported some difficulty in engaging in 12-step groups in several ways. There are dedicated 12-step groups that focus on co-occurring disorders,[183] and there are 12-step brochures that provide guidance to patients and providers on the appropriate use of medications when indicated.[184] There have been few studies of 12-step facilitation alone for individuals with schizophrenia; however, this approach has been used routinely with other psychosocial treatments in integrated treatment programs.

Several treatment approaches with similar behavioral therapy models for co-occurring disorders have been suggested. The Motivation-Based Dual Diagnosis Treatment model employs a stage-matching approach that combines mental health and addiction treatments, based on the patient's motivational level, severity of illness, and dual diagnosis subtype. The Motivation-Based Dual Diagnosis Treatment approach acknowledges the distinctive features of the schizophrenia-addiction subtype.[185] This approach has been used in the different levels of care described in the ASAM Criteria and best relates to help improve the 4, 5, and 6 dimensions (Readiness to Change; Return to Use, Continued Use or Continued Problem Potential; and Recovery and Living Environment)—particularly the readiness to change. The model uses stages of change in assessing the patient and matches treatment strategies and goals (such as abstinence or harm reduction, medication compliance, session attendance) to the individual's stage of readiness to change. MET is a primary psychosocial approach for patients with poor motivation. However, when the traditional MET approach is used with co-occurring disorders, clinicians should recognize the need for adjustments, which include the following:

- The clinician should play a more active role in offering practical, useful solutions to the patient's concerns about everyday survival. The clinician should not assume that such patients are able to solve problems effectively on their own while actively engaged in addiction-related behaviors.
- MET should be formulated as a continuing component of treatment rather than being limited to the four sessions that have been envisioned for those with a diagnosis of SUD without schizophrenia. Motivational interviewing was the first psychosocial treatment approach in this area; however, MET was developed in the PROJECT MATCH study as a shortened four-session version of motivational interviewing, and added specific items of personalized feedback, decisional balance, and consideration of the Prochaska motivational levels of change.
- The decision balance intervention (pros/cons), a cornerstone of MET, might be employed in other aspects of treatment beyond SUD matters to include other related topics such as the pros/cons of taking antipsychotic medication.
- The clinician should acknowledge that individuals with co-occurring disorders may not consistently accept the diagnosis of schizophrenia, may vary in their willingness to maintain medication for schizophrenia, and may fluctuate in their motivational stages between denial, ambivalence, and ready for making change in their substance use.

Attending to the role of motivational stage is important to the success of the treatment plan. Clinicians must work to help the patient strengthen their motivation to reduce or quit their substance use and address the challenges related to their schizophrenia treatment including the importance of medications in managing both SUD and psychosis. In addition to internal motivators for change, external motivators can also be helpful, such as support from family and friends, employment, healthy relationships, reducing legal consequences, and others. The community reinforcement and contingency management approaches have been used in substance use treatment[186]; however, there are few studies in patients with psychosis and SUD. These approaches could be a way to increase external motivators and explore a range of possible motivators—disability income, probation, family, etc.[187]

Dual Recovery Therapy (DRT) integrates substance use Relapse Prevention, social skills training, MET, and the "recovery language" of 12-step programs in linked group and individual treatment sessions.[185] DRT best relates to help improve the 4, 5, and 6 dimensions of the ASAM criteria (Readiness to Change; Return to Use, Continued Use or Continued Problem Potential; and Recovery and Living Environment). MET and recovery language are added to address patients' often low levels of motivation for change and to take advantage of the common lexicon of the 12-step programs, with which many patients already are familiar. The resulting treatment is designed to enhance intrinsic motivation for change, bolster the patients' sense of self-efficacy, improve their social skills, and give them tools for coping with high-risk situations. Training is grounded in cognitive-behavioral theory and targets the cognitive difficulties in patients with schizophrenia. The ability to communicate and solve problems is developed through role-plays that can be introduced in both group and individual therapy, whereas the understanding and management of their substance use problems are improved through an emphasis on coping strategies (eg, how to organize one's time). The clinician gives ongoing consideration to both substance use and co-occurring psychiatric conditions, monitors their interaction, and adjusts the treatment emphasis accordingly. A patient's motivation to address the symptoms of schizophrenia may not be the same as his or her motivation to address substance use, and treatment is best tailored to the individual's motivation for each problem area.

The first month of DRT involves twice-weekly individual sessions. Motivation is assessed and enhanced in these early individual sessions, while the clinician works on building a strong therapeutic alliance. A plan for change is discussed, and basic skills that will be necessary for later group sessions are introduced. Subsequent individual sessions focus on reinforcing material discussed in group therapy.

Ongoing DRT includes individual and group-based treatments. The group and individual sessions are linked, in that individual sessions are used to reinforce the material discussed during the group sessions. Group sessions follow a standard format, which begins with a relaxation exercise, followed by an update report from each client. Group structure is provided by focusing on a specific topic each week (eg, Relapse Prevention, mood management, symptom management, increasing pleasurable activities, communication skills, asking for help, and medication compliance). Because skill building plays a central role in dual recovery therapy, behavioral rehearsal and role-playing are used regularly. DRT has been used in all levels of care described by ASAM Criteria; however, it is most common in outpatient treatment, including partial hospitalization and intensive outpatient treatment settings.

OTHER OUTPATIENT TREATMENT APPROACHES

In addition to the standard evidence-based treatments for addiction, new innovative approaches have been developed in recent years. For example, virtual-reality (VR)-based therapy has been observed to reduce craving and increase coping mechanisms for a variety of SUDs.[87,188,189] It is thought that VR-based therapy works on a number of cognitive processes related to substance use by allowing patients to experience highly controlled and highly interactive three-dimensional environments where they can work through personalized real-life addiction related situations, thereby offering a novel solution to many of the problems presented by traditional exposure-based therapies.[190] A growing number of studies have been conducted using VR-based therapy for psychosis. A review of 50 studies suggests that VR-based therapy appears safe and well-tolerated, and has demonstrated benefit for auditory hallucinations, paranoia, depression, anxiety, and social and cognitive functioning in psychotic patients.[191] VR-based therapy holds great promise in helping individuals with co-occurring addiction and psychosis and could be used in all levels of care described by The ASAM Criteria. however, it is most common in outpatient treatment, including partial hospitalization and intensive outpatient treatment settings.

Mindfulness-based relapse prevention (MBRP) represents another novel therapeutic technique with potential use for co-occurring disorders. MBRP embodies a combination of CBT and mindfulness techniques and aims to help improve coping mechanisms and decrease risk of relapse in SUDs.[192] MBRP is based on the mindfulness-based stress reduction approach that includes education and skill development of mindfulness meditation practice (formal practice) as well as everyday awareness of small moments exercise. These exercises increase focus on a particular behavior (taking a shower, drinking a cup of coffee, etc.), and noticing senses at that time. This ability to focus and notice when distracted is very relevant to craving, especially cue reactive craving to a known craving stimulus. MBRP has been shown to decrease substance craving and depressive symptoms for patients with SUD and comorbid depression.[193] MBRP is helpful in increasing awareness of cravings and what else might be going on at that time, including setting, people around, and moods. A meta-analysis of mindfulness- and acceptance-based interventions for psychosis revealed that such interventions significantly reduced positive and negative symptoms of psychosis.[194] A recent narrative review suggests that mindfulness-based interventions can reduce psychotic symptoms, improve emotional regulation, reduce substance use, and decrease re-hospitalization rates in patients with schizophrenia.[195] As such, MBRP appears to be an emerging novel treatment approach for co-occurring SUD and psychosis. MBRP could be used in all levels of care described by The ASAM Criteria; however, it is most common in outpatient treatment, including partial hospitalization and intensive outpatient treatment settings.

LONGER-TERM MANAGEMENT

Ongoing treatment of co-occurring psychosis and SUD requires integrated treatment that attempts to reduce the likelihood of recurrence of substance use and earlier management of psychotic symptoms and promotes recovery and wellness. Some patients will continue to display psychotic symptoms and actively use substances. If the diagnosis is uncertain and the patient is able to achieve prolonged abstinence, the clinician then can consider a medication-free period. Psychotic symptoms that continue despite abstinence will require formal treatment. The optimal long-term management for schizophrenia is a combination of antipsychotic treatment, psychosocial intervention for both the SUD and the psychosis, and case management as needed. Long-term psychotherapy should address both substance use and psychosis.

For individuals with schizophrenia and SUD, the prognosis for long-term improvement and recovery depends on a treatment strategy that addresses both substance use and schizophrenia, that responds to the unique biological and psychosocial vulnerabilities of the individual, and that takes an empathic and collaborative approach that includes shared decision making and has a recovery-oriented approach to empowerment, connecting with others, and hope for the future.

Training programs should be designed to develop basic co-occurring disorders assessment and treatment competencies for health care providers. Clinicians should have skills and knowledge in integrating mental health and addiction treatment approaches, with special emphasis on MET, relapse prevention, and 12-step facilitation for addiction, as well as social skills training and behavioral therapies for psychiatric disorders. Other helpful strategies include DRT, behavioral contracting, community reinforcement approaches, money management, peer support/counseling, vocational/educational counseling, and family therapies.[196,197]

Recovery

People with lived experience of SUD and psychosis may attend 12-step meetings or have other types of peer support as part of their treatment. In these settings and now in routine treatment, the importance of an orientation toward personal recovery has been identified. A recovery orientation emphasizes living a satisfying, hopeful, and contributing life even within the limitations caused by illness, has been increasingly recognized in substance use and mental health treatment. The Substance Abuse and Mental Health Services Administration (SAMHSA) defines recovery as "a process of change through which individuals improve their health and wellness, live a self-directed life, and strive to reach their full potential."[198] Within this broad definition, SAMHSA identified four major domains that support recovery: health, home, purpose, and community. In practical terms, mental health recovery focuses on minimizing the effect of illness on quality of life, rather than just simple symptom reduction, and on fostering patient-centered, autonomy-supporting care.[199,200]

Recovery is a journey of healing and transformation enabling a person with mental disorders and/or SUD to live a meaningful life in the community of his or her choice while striving to achieve his or her full potential.[201] It is often not a linear process and requires the patient and the health care provider to have patience and respect for the process. In fact, the journey often involves exacerbations and remissions that are all part of the process. Recovery is a personal journey; however, it can benefit from support by the providers, family or friends, a recovery network (such as 12-Step Groups or Dual Diagnosis Groups). Recovery from SUD also considers the importance of connecting with others in recovery, attending to a personal plan for enhancing their lives, and a goal of abstinence from substances. However, stopping substance use is just part of a long and complex recovery process that extends beyond abstinence alone. The 12-step model outlines steps for increased awareness, learning from past behaviors, connecting with others, being able to acknowledge problems, having spiritual or other supports such as meditation, and helping others on a similar journey. Addiction often causes serious negative consequences in an individual's life. Therefore, treatment should address needs on physical health, social, occupational, family, and legal aspects to be successful.

CONCLUSION

The co-occurrence of substance use and psychosis represents a unique challenge to patients, health care providers, and policymakers. There are various evidence-based treatment approaches available to address these complex needs. Such approaches represent an opportunity for significant improvement in clinical outcomes, morbidity, mortality, and quality of life among individuals with both conditions.

ACKNOWLEDGMENTS

The authors would like to acknowledge Dr Marc Steinberg, Makenzie Tonelli, Aurelia Bizamcer, David Smelson, Celine Larkin, and Adrienne Vaiana for their contributions in previous editions of this chapter.

REFERENCES

1. American Psychiatric Association. *Diagnostic and Statistical Manual of Mental Disorders (DSM-5).* American Psychiatric Association; 2013.
2. Murrie B, Lappin J, Large M, Sara G. Transition of substance-induced, brief, and atypical psychoses to schizophrenia: a systematic review and meta-analysis. *Schizophr Bull.* 2020;46(3):505-516.
3. Mathias S, Lubman DI, Hides L. Substance-induced psychosis: a diagnostic conundrum. *J Clin Psychiatry.* 2008;69(3):358-367.
4. Tsuang J, Fong TW. Treatment of patients with schizophrenia and substance abuse disorders. *Curr Pharm Des.* 2004;10:2249-2261.
5. Regier DA, Farmer ME, Rae DS, et al. Comorbidity of mental disorders with alcohol and other drug abuse: results from the Epidemiologic Catchment Area (ECA) study. *JAMA.* 1990;264(19):2511-2518.
6. Swofford CD, Scheller-Gilkey G, Miller AH, Woolwine B, Mance R. Double jeopardy: schizophrenia and substance use. *Am J Drug Alcohol Abuse.* 2000;26(3):343-353.
7. Martins SS, Gorelick DA. Conditional substance abuse and dependence by diagnosis of mood or anxiety disorder or schizophrenia in the U.S. population. *Drug Alcohol Depend.* 2011;119(1-2):28-36.
8. Wobrock T, Soyka M. Pharmacotherapy of patients with schizophrenia and substance abuse. *Expert Opin Pharmacother.* 2009;10(3):353-367.
9. Reidy LJ, Junquera P, Van Dijck K, Steele BW, Nemeroff CB. Underestimation of substance abuse in psychiatric patients by conventional hospital screening. *J Psychiatr Res.* 2014;59:206-212.
10. Addington J, Addington D. Patterns, predictors and impact of substance use in early psychosis: a longitudinal study. *Acta Psychiatr Scand.* 2007;115(4):304.
11. Barnett JH, Werners U, Secher SM, et al. Substance use in a population-based clinic sample of people with first-episode psychosis. *Br J Psychiatry.* 2007;190(6):515-520.
12. Swartz MS, Wagner HR, Swanson JW, et al. Substance use in persons with schizophrenia: baseline prevalence and correlates from the NIMH CATIE study. *J Nerv Ment Dis.* 2006;194(3):164-172.
13. Swartz MS, Wagner HR, Swanson JW, et al. Substance use and psychosocial functioning in schizophrenia among new enrollees in the NIMH CATIE study. *Psychiatr Serv.* 2006;57(8):1110-1116.
14. Kerfoot KE, Rosenheck RA, Petrakis IL, et al. Substance use and schizophrenia: adverse correlates in the CATIE study sample. *Schizophr Res.* 2011;132(2):177-182.
15. Mueser K, Bellack A, Blanchard J. Comorbidity of schizophrenia and substance abuse: implications for treatment. *J Consult Clin Psychol.* 1992;60(6):845-856.
16. Green AI, Noordsy DL, Brunette MF, O'Keefe C. Substance abuse and schizophrenia: pharmacotherapeutic intervention. *J Subst Abuse Treat.* 2008;34(1):61-71.
17. Hunt G, Bergen J, Bashir M. Medication compliance and comorbid substance abuse in schizophrenia: impact on community survival 4 years after a relapse. *Schizophr Res.* 2002;54(3):253.
18. Coldham E, Addington J, Addington D. Medication adherence of individuals with a first episode of psychosis. *Acta Psychiatr Scand.* 2002;106(4):286-290.
19. Colizzi M, Carra E, Fraietta S, et al. Substance use, medication adherence and outcome one year following a first episode of psychosis. *Schizophr Res.* 2016;170(2-3):311-317. doi:10.1016/j.schres.2015.11.016
20. Turkington A, Mulholland CC, Rushe TM, et al. Impact of persistent substance misuse on 1-year outcome in first-episode psychosis. *Br J Psychiatry.* 2009;195(3):242-248.
21. Jackson C, Covell N, Drake R, Essock S. Relationship between diabetes and mortality among persons with co-occurring psychotic and substance use disorders. *Psychiatr Serv.* 2007;58(2):270-272.
22. Ziedonis D, Hitsman B, Beckham JC, et al. Tobacco use and cessation in psychiatric disorders: National Institute of Mental Health report. *Nicotine Tob Res.* 2008;10(12):1691-1715.
23. Gurillo P, Jauhar S, Murray RM, MacCabe JH. Does tobacco use cause psychosis? Systematic review and meta-analysis. *Lancet Psychiatry.* 2015;2(8):718-725.
24. American Psychiatric Association. Practice guideline for the treatment of patients with nicotine dependence. *Am J Psychiatry.* 1996;153(10 Suppl):1-31.
25. Fiore M, Bailey W, Cohen S, et al. *Treating Tobacco Use and Dependence: Quick Reference Guide for Clinicians.* U.S. Department of Health and Human Services: The Public Health Service; 2000.
26. George T, Ziedonis D. Addressing tobacco dependence in psychiatric practice: promises and pitfalls. *Can J Psychiatry.* 2009;54(6):353-355.
27. Ziedonis D, Parks J, Zimmermann MH, McCabe P. Program and system level interventions to address tobacco amongst individuals with schizophrenia. *J Dual Diagn.* 2007;3(3-4):151-175.
28. Williams JM, Steinberg ML, Zimmermann MH, et al. Comparison of two intensities of tobacco dependence counseling in schizophrenia and schizoaffective disorder. *J Subst Abuse Treat.* 2010;38(4):384-393.
29. Williams JM, Ziedonis DM, Vreeland B, et al. A wellness approach to addressing tobacco in mental health settings: learning about healthy living. *Am J Psychiatr Rehabil.* 2009;12(4):352-369.
30. Mukherji P, Azhar Y, Sharma S. *Toxicology Screening.* StatPearls Publishing; 2021. Accessed June 28, 2023. https://www.ncbi.nlm.nih.gov/books/NBK499901/
31. Wiesbeck GA, Taeschner K-L. A cerebral computed tomography study of patients with drug-induced psychoses. *Eur Arch Psychiatry Clin Neurosci.* 1991;241(2):88-90.
32. Gallagher CN, Hutchinson PJ, Pickard JD. Neuroimaging in trauma. *Curr Opin Neurol.* 2007;20(4):403-409.

33. Shaner A, Roberts L, Eckman T, et al. Sources of diagnostic uncertainty for chronically psychotic cocaine abusers. *Psychiatr Serv.* 1998;49(5):684-690.
34. Schanzer BM, First MB, Dominguez B, Hasin DS, Caton CL. Diagnosing psychotic disorders in the emergency department in the context of substance use. *Psychiatr Serv.* 2006;57(10):1468-1473.
35. Caton CL, Hasin DS. Shrout PE, et al. Stability of early-phase primary psychotic disorders with concurrent substance use and substance-induced psychosis. *Br J Psychiatry.* 2007;190(2):105-111.
36. Wearne TA, Cornish JL. A comparison of methamphetamine-induced psychosis and schizophrenia: a review of positive, negative,and cognitive symptomatology. *Front Psychiatry.* 2018;9:491.
37. Niemi-Pynttäri JA, Sund R, Putkonen H, Vorma H, Wahlbeck K, Pirkola SP. Substance-induced psychoses converting into schizophrenia: a register-based study of 18,478 Finnish inpatient cases. *J Clin Psychiatry.* 2013;74(1):e94-e99.
38. Isbell H, Fraser H, Wikler A, Belleville R, Eisenman AJ. An experimental study of the etiology of "rum fits" and delirium tremens. *Q J Stud Alcohol.* 1955;16(1):1-33.
39. Mendelson JH, Ladou J. Experimentally induced chronic intoxication and withdrawal in alcoholics. 2. Psychophysiological findings. *Q J Stud Alcohol.* 1964;25:14-39.
40. Jordaan GP, Emsley R. Alcohol-induced psychotic disorder: a review. *Metab Brain Dis.* 2014;29(2):231-243.
41. Tabakoff B, Hoffman PL. Alcohol addiction: an enigma among us. *Neuron.* 1996;16(5):909-912.
42. Masood B, Lepping P, Romanov D, Poole R. Treatment of alcohol-induced psychotic disorder (alcoholic hallucinosis)—a systematic review. *Alcohol Alcohol.* 2018;53(3):259-267.
43. Perälä J, Kuoppasalmi K, Pirkola S, et al. Alcohol-induced psychotic disorder and delirium in the general population. *Br J Psychiatry.* 2010;197(3):200-206.
44. Hendricks ML, Emsley RA, Nel DG, Thornton HB, Jordaan GP. Cognitive changes in alcohol-induced psychotic disorder. *BMC Res Notes.* 2017;10(1):1-8.
45. Victor M, Hope J. The phenomenon of auditory hallucinations in chronic alcoholism; a critical evaluation of the status of alcoholic hallucinosis. *J Nerv Ment Dis.* 1958;126(5):451-481.
46. Soyka M. Pharmacological treatment of alcohol hallucinosis. *Alcohol Alcohol.* 2008;43(6):719-720.
47. Kendler KS, Ohlsson H, Sundquist J, Sundquist K. Prediction of onset of substance-induced psychotic disorder and its progression to schizophrenia in a Swedish national sample. *Am J Psychiatry.* 2019;176(9):711-719.
48. Johnson EC, Kapoor M, Hatoum AS, et al. Investigation of convergent and divergent genetic influences underlying schizophrenia and alcohol use disorder. *Psychol Med.* 2023;53(4):1196-1204.
49. Hasin DS, Saha TD, Kerridge BT, et al. Prevalence of marijuana use disorders in the United States between 2001-2002 and 2012-2013. *JAMA Psychiatry.* 2015;72(12):1235-1242.
50. Ganesh S, D'Souza DC. Cannabis and psychosis: recent epidemiological findings continuing the "Causality Debate". *Am J Psychiatry.* 2022;179(1):8-10.
51. Patrick ME, Schulenberg JE, Miech RA, Johnston LD, O'Malley PM, Bachman JG. *Monitoring the Future Panel Study Annual Report: National Data on Substance Use Among Adults Ages 19 to 60, 1976-2021.* Monitoring the Future Monograph Series. University of Michigan Institute for Social Research; 2022. doi:10.7826/ISR- UM.06.585140.002.07.0001.2022
52. Spindle TR, Bonn-Miller MO, Vandrey R. Changing landscape of cannabis: novel products, formulations, and methods of administration. *Curr Opin Psychol.* 2019;30:98-102.
53. Monte AA, Zane RD, Heard KJ. The implications of marijuana legalization in Colorado. *JAMA.* 2015;313(3):241-242.
54. Ashton CH. Pharmacology and effects of cannabis: a brief review. *Br J Psychiatry.* 2001;178(2):101-106.
55. Quattrone D, Ferraro L, Tripoli G, et al. Daily use of high-potency cannabis is associated with more positive symptoms in first-episode psychosis patients: the EU-GEI case–control study. *Psychol Med.* 2021;51(8):1329-1337.
56. Chaudry H, Moss H, Bashir A, Suliman T. Cannabis psychosis following bhang ingestion. *Br J Addict.* 1991;86(9):1075-1081.
57. Tennant FS, Groesbeck CJ. Psychiatric effects of hashish. *Arch Gen Psychiatry.* 1972;27(1):133-136.
58. Wang GS, Buttorff C, Wilks A, Schwam D, Tung G, Pacula RL. Impact of cannabis legalization on healthcare utilization for psychosis and schizophrenia in Colorado. *Int J Drug Policy.* 2022;104:103685.
59. Ghodse AH. Cannabis psychosis. *Br J Addict.* 1986;81(4):473-478.
60. Caton CL. The need for close monitoring of early psychosis and co-occurring substance misuse. *Psychiatr Bull.* 2011;35(7):241-243.
61. Kuepper R, van Os J, Lieb R, Wittchen HU, Hofler M, Henquet C. Continued cannabis use and risk of incidence and persistence of psychotic symptoms: 10 year follow-up cohort study. *BMJ.* 2011;342:d738.
62. Moore TH, Zammit S, Lingford-Hughes A, et al. Cannabis use and risk of psychotic or affective mental health outcomes: a systematic review. *Lancet.* 2007;370(9584):319-328.
63. Tandon R, Shariff SM. Substance-induced psychotic disorders and schizophrenia: pathophysiological insights and clinical implications. *Am J Psychiatry.* 2019;176(9):683-684.
64. Kline ER, Ferrara M, Li F, D'Souza DC, Keshavan M, Srihari VH. Timing of cannabis exposure relative to prodrome and psychosis onset in a community-based first episode psychosis sample. *J Psychiatr Res.* 2022;147:248-253.
65. Livne O, Shmulewitz D, Sarvet AL, Wall MM, Hasin DS. Association of cannabis use-related predictor variables and self-reported psychotic disorders: U.S. adults, 2001-2002 and 2012-2013. *Am J Psychiatry.* 2022;179(1):36-45.
66. Hjorthøj C, Posselt CM, Nordentoft M. Development over time of the population-attributable risk fraction for cannabis use disorder in schizophrenia in Denmark. *JAMA Psychiatry.* 2021;78(9):1013-1019.
67. Carvalho C, Vieira-Coelho MA. Cannabis induced psychosis: a systematic review on the role of genetic polymorphisms. *Pharmacol Res.* 2022;181:106258.
68. Petrilli K, Ofori S, Hines L, Taylor G, Adams S, Freeman TP. Association of cannabis potency with mental ill health and addiction: a systematic review. *Lancet Psychiatry.* 2022;9(9):736-750.
69. Di Forti M, Quattrone D, Freeman TP, et al. The contribution of cannabis use to variation in the incidence of psychotic disorder across Europe (EU-GEI): a multicentre case-control study. *Lancet Psychiatry.* 2019;6(5):427-436.
70. Lawn W, Mokrysz C, Lees R, et al. The CannTeen Study: cannabis use disorder, depression, anxiety, and psychotic-like symptoms in adolescent and adult cannabis users and age-matched controls. *J Psychopharmacol.* 2022;36(12):1350-1361.
71. Robinson T, Ali MU, Easterbrook B, Hall W, Jutras-Aswad D, Fischer B. Risk-thresholds for the association between frequency of cannabis use and the development of psychosis: a systematic review and meta-analysis. *Psychol Med.* 2023;53(9):3858-3868
72. Kiburi SK, Molebatsi K, Ntlantsana V, Lynskey MT. Cannabis use in adolescence and risk of psychosis: are there factors that moderate this relationship? A systematic review and meta-analysis. *Subst Abuse.* 2021;42(4):527-542.
73. Hambrecht M, Häfner H. Cannabis, vulnerability, and the onset of schizophrenia: an epidemiological perspective. *Aust N Z J Psychiatry.* 2000;34(3):468-475.
74. Arseneault L, Cannon M, Witton J, Murray RM. Causal association between cannabis and psychosis: examination of the evidence. *Br J Psychiatry.* 2004;184(2):110-117.
75. Smit F, Bolier L, Cuijpers P. Cannabis use and the risk of later schizophrenia: a review. *Addiction.* 2004;99(4):425-430.
76. Grech A, Van Os J, Jones PB, Lewis SW, Murray RM. Cannabis use and outcome of recent onset psychosis. *Eur Psychiatry.* 2005;20(4):349-353.
77. Zammit S, Moore TH, Lingford-Hughes A, et al. Effects of cannabis use on outcomes of psychotic disorders: systematic review. *Br J Psychiatry.* 2008;193(5):357-363.

78. Foti DJ, Kotov R, Guey LT, Bromet EJ. Cannabis use and the course of schizophrenia: 10-year follow-up after first hospitalization. *Am J Psychiatry*. 2010;167(8):987-993.
79. Hamilton I, Sumnall H. Are we any closer to identifying a causal relationship between cannabis and psychosis? *Curr Opin Psychol.* 2021;38:56-60.
80. Manschreck T, Laughery J, Weisstein C, et al. Characteristics of freebase cocaine psychosis. *Yale J Biol Med.* 1988;61(2):115-122.
81. Satel SL, Southwick SM, Gawin FH. Clinical features of cocaine-induced paranoia. *Am J Psychiatry*. 1991;148(4):495-498.
82. Sabe M, Zhao N, Kaiser S. A systematic review and meta-analysis of the prevalence of cocaine-induced psychosis in cocaine users. *Prog Neuropsychopharmacol Biol Psychiatry*. 2021;109:110263.
83. Brady K, Lydiard R, Malcolm R, Ballenger J. Cocaine-induced psychosis. *J Clin Psychiatry*. 1991;52(12):509-512.
84. Ellinwood E Jr, Sudilovsky A, Nelson L. Evolving behavior in the clinical and experimental amphetamine (model) psychosis. *Am J Psychiatry*. 1973;130(10):1088-1093.
85. Sherer MA. Intravenous cocaine: psychiatric effects, biological mechanisms. *Biol Psychiatry*. 1988;24(8):865-885.
86. Arunogiri S, Foulds JA, McKetin R, Lubman DI. A systematic review of risk factors for methamphetamine-associated psychosis. *Aus N Z J Psychiatry*. 2018;52(6):514-529.
87. Chiang M, Lombardi D, Du J, et al. Methamphetamine-associated psychosis: clinical presentation, biological basis, and treatment options. *Hum Psychopharmacol.* 2019;34(5):e2710.
88. Voce A, Calabria B, Burns R, Castle D, McKetin R. A systematic review of the symptom profile and course of methamphetamine-associated psychosis: substance use and misuse. *Subst Use Misuse*. 2019;54(4):549-559.
89. Bramness JG, Gundersen OH, Guterstam J, et al. Amphetamine-induced psychosis—a separate diagnostic entity or primary psychosis triggered in the vulnerable? *BMC Psychiatry*. 2012;12:221.
90. NIDA. Hallucinogens. 2011. Accessed November 14, 2016. https://www.samhsa.gov/data/release/2020-national-survey-drug-use-and-health-nsduh-releases. 2011 [cited 2016 November 14].
91. Carhart-Harris RL, Kaelen M, Bolstridge M, et al. The paradoxical psychological effects of lysergic acid diethylamide (LSD). *Psychol Med.* 2016;46(7):1379-1390.
92. Nichols DE. Hallucinogens. *Pharmacol Ther*. 2004;101(2):131-181.
93. Krebs T, Johansen P. Psychedelics and mental health: a population study. *PLoS One*. 2012;8(8):e63972.
94. Breakey WR, Goodell H, Lorenz PC, McHugh PR. Hallucinogenic drugs as precipitants of schizophrenia. *Psychol Med*. 1974;4(03):255-261.
95. Bowers MB. Acute psychosis induced by psychotomimetic drug abuse: I. Clinical findings. *Arch Gen Psychiatry*. 1972;27(4):437-440.
96. Le TT, Di Vincenzo JD, Teopiz KM, et al. Ketamine for psychotic depression: an overview of the glutamatergic system and ketamine's mechanisms associated with antidepressant and psychotomimetic effects. *Psychiatry Res*. 2021;306:114231.
97. Cohen BD, Rosenbaum G, Luby ED, Gottlieb JS. Comparison of phencyclidine hydrochloride (Sernyl) with other drugs: simulation of schizophrenic performance with phencyclidine hydrochloride (Sernyl), lysergic acid diethylamide (LSD-25), and amobarbital (Amytal) sodium; II. Symbolic and sequential thinking. *Arch Gen Psychiatry*. 1962;6(5):395-401.
98. Davies BM, Beech H. The effect of 1-arylcyclohexylamine (Sernyl) on twelve normal volunteers. *Br J Psychiatry*. 1960;106(444):912-924.
99. Fauman B, Aldinger G, Fauman M, Rosen P. Psychiatric sequelae of phencyclidine abuse. *Clin Toxicol*. 1976;9(4):529-538.
100. Rammer L, Holmgren P, Sandler H. Fatal intoxication by dextromethorphan: a report on two cases. *Forensic Sci Int*. 1988;37(4):233-236.
101. Boyer EW. Dextromethorphan abuse. *Pediatr Emerg Care*. 2004;20(12):858-863.
102. Cranston J, Yoast R. Abuse of dextromethorphan. *Arch Fam Med*. 1998;8(2):99-100.
103. Silvasti M, Karttunen P, Tukiainen H, Kokkonen P, Hänninen U, Nykänen S. Pharmacokinetics of dextromethorphan and dextrorphan: a single dose comparison of three preparations in human volunteers. *Int J Clin Pharmacol Ther Toxicol*. 1987;25(9):493-497.
104. Antoniou T, Juurlink DN. Dextromethorphan abuse. *CMAJ*. 2014;186(16):E631.
105. Bem J, Peck R. Dextromethorphan. An overview of safety issues. *Drug Saf.* 1991;7(3):190-199.
106. Schier J. Avoid unfavorable consequences: dextromethorpan can bring about a false-positive phencyclidine urine drug screen. *J Emerg Med*. 2000;18(3):379-381.
107. Battaglia G, De Souza EB. Pharmacologic profile of amphetamine derivatives at various brain recognition sites: selective effects on serotonergic systems. *NIDA Res Monogr*. 1989;94:240-258.
108. Mithoefer MC, Feduccia AA, Jerome L, et al. MDMA-assisted psychotherapy for treatment of PTSD: study design and rationale for phase 3 trials based on pooled analysis of six phase 2 randomized controlled trials. *Psychopharmacology (Berl)*. 2019;236(9):2735-2745.
109. Mitchell JM, Bogenschutz M, Lilienstein A, et al. MDMA-assisted therapy for severe PTSD: a randomized, double-blind, placebo-controlled phase 3 study. *Nat Med*. 2021;27(6):1025-1033.
110. Mueller PD, Korey WS. Death by "ecstasy": the serotonin syndrome? *Ann Emerg Med*. 1998;32(3):377-380.
111. Graeme KA. New drugs of abuse. *Emerg Med Clin North Am*. 2000;18(4):625-636.
112. Costa G, Gołembiowska K. Neurotoxicity of MDMA: main effects and mechanisms. *Exp Neurol*. 2022;347:113894.
113. United Nations Office on Drugs and Crime. *World Drug ReportBooklet 4—Drug Market Trends: Cocaine*. New Psychoactive Substances. Accessed August 9, 2022: Amphetamine-Type Stimulants; *2022* doi:https://www.unodc.org/unodc/en/data-and-analysis/world-drug-report-2022.html
114. Gunderson EW, Haughey HM, Ait-Daoud N, Joshi AS, Hart CL. A survey of synthetic cannabinoid consumption by current cannabis users. *Subst Abus*. 2014;35(2):184-189.
115. Malaca S, Busardò FP, Nittari G, Sirignano A, Ricci G. Fourth generation of synthetic cannabinoid receptor agonists: a review on the latest insights. *Curr Pharm Des*. 2022;28(32):2603-2617.
116. Every-Palmer S. Synthetic cannabinoid JWH-018 and psychosis: an explorative study. *Drug Alcohol Depend*. 2011;117(2-3):152-157.
117. Hermanns-Clausen M, Kneisel S, Szabo B, Auwarter V. Acute toxicity due to the confirmed consumption of synthetic cannabinoids: clinical and laboratory findings. *Addiction*. 2013;108(3):534-544.
118. Hoyte CO, Jacob J, Monte AA, Al-Jumaan M, Bronstein AC, Heard KJ. A characterization of synthetic cannabinoid exposures reported to the National Poison Data System in 2010. *Ann Emerg Med*. 2012;60(4):435-438.
119. Bassir Nia A, Medrano B, Perkel C, Galynker I, Hurd YL. Psychiatric comorbidity associated with synthetic cannabinoid use compared to cannabis. *J Psychopharmacol*. 2016;30(12):1321-1330.
120. Schifano F, Napoletano F, Chiappini S, et al. New/emerging psychoactive substances and associated psychopathological consequences. *Psychol Med*. 2021;51(1):30-42.
121. Wallach J, Kang H, Colestock T, et al. Pharmacological investigations of the dissociative 'legal highs' diphenidine, methoxphenidine and analogues. *PLoS One*. 2016;11(6):e0157021.
122. Ventura L, Carvalho F, Dinis-Oliveira RJ. Opioids in the frame of new psychoactive substances network: a complex pharmacological and toxicological issue. *Curr Mol Pharmacol*. 2018;11(2):97-108.
123. Chuang E, Wells R, Alexander JA, Friedmann PD, Lee IH. Factors associated with use of ASAM criteria and service provision in a national sample of outpatient substance abuse treatment units. *J Addict Med*. 2009;3(3):139-150. doi:10.1097/ADM.0b013e31818ebb6f
124. Smelson DA, Dixon L, Craig T, et al. Pharmacological treatment of schizophrenia and co-occurring substance use disorders. *CNS Drugs*. 2008;22(11):903-916.

125. Roncero C, Barral C, Grau-Lopez L, et al. Protocols of dual diagnosis intervention in schizophrenia. *Addict Disord Their Treat.* 2011;10(3):131-154.
126. Post R. Cocaine psychoses: a continuum model. *Am J Psychiatry.* 1975;132(3):225-231.
127. Drake RE, Xie H, McHugo GJ, Green AI. The effects of clozapine on alcohol and drug use disorders among patients with schizophrenia. *Schizophr Bull.* 2000;26(2):441-449.
128. Smelson D, Losonczy M, Castles-Fonseca K, Stewart P, Kaune M, Ziedonis D. Preliminary outcomes from a booster case management program for individuals with a co-occurring substance abuse and a persistent psychiatric disorder. *J Dual Diagn.* 2005;3(1):47-59.
129. Smelson DA, Roy A, Roy M. Risperidone diminishes cue-elicited craving in withdrawn cocaine-dependent patients. *Can J Psychiatry.* 1997;42(9):984.
130. Zhornitsky S, Rizkallah É, Pampoulova T, et al. Antipsychotic agents for the treatment of substance use disorders in patients with and without comorbid psychosis. *J Clin Psychopharmacol.* 2010;30(4):417-424.
131. Green A, Drake R, Brunette M, Noordsy D. Schizophrenia and co-occurring substance use disorder. *Am J Psychiatry.* 2007;164(3):402-408.
132. Brunette MF, Drake RE, Xie H, McHugo GJ, Green AI. Clozapine use and relapses of substance use disorder among patients with co-occurring schizophrenia and substance use disorders. *Schizophr Bull.* 2006;32(4):637-643.
133. Ho AP, Tsuang JW, Liberman RP, et al. Achieving effective treatment of patients with chronic psychotic illness and comorbid substance dependence. *Am J Psychiatry.* 1999;156(11):1765-1770.
134. Akerele E, Levin FR. Comparison of olanzapine to risperidone in substance-abusing individuals with schizophrenia. *Am J Addict.* 2007;16(4):260-268.
135. Stuyt EB, Sajbel TA, Allen MH. Differing effects of antipsychotic medications on substance abuse treatment patients with co-occurring psychotic and substance abuse disorders. *Am J Addict.* 2006;15(2):166-173.
136. Krause M, Huhn M, Schneider-Thoma J, Bighelli I, Gutsmiedl K, Leucht S. Efficacy, acceptability and tolerability of antipsychotics in patients with schizophrenia and comorbid substance use. a systematic review and meta-analysis. *Eur Neuropsychopharmacol.* 2019;29(1):32-45.
137. Swartz MS, Wagner HR, Swanson JW, et al. The effectiveness of antipsychotic medications in patients who use or avoid illicit substances: results from the CATIE study. *Schizophr Res.* 2008;100(1-3):39-52.
138. Ereshefsky L, Saklad SR, Watanabe MD, Davis CM, Jann MW. Thiothixene pharmacokinetic interactions: a study of hepatic enzyme inducers, clearance inhibitors, and demographic variables. *J Clin Psychopharmacol.* 1991;11(5):296-301.
139. George T, Sernyak M, Ziedonis D, Woods S. Effects of clozapine on smoking in chronic schizophrenic outpatients. *J Clin Psychiatry.* 1995;56(8):344-346.
140. McEvoy J, Freudenreich O, McGee M, VanderZwaag C, Levin E, Rose J. Clozapine decreases smoking in patients with chronic schizophrenia. *Biol Psychiatry.* 1995;37(8):550-552.
141. Ziedonis D, Kosten T, Glazer W. The impact of drug abuse on psychopathology and movement disorders in chronic psychotic outpatients. In: Harris L, ed. *Problems of Drug Dependence 1994.* NIDA Research Monograph 153. National Institute on Drug Abuse; 1994.
142. Skogh E, Bengtsson F, Nordin C. Could discontinuing smoking be hazardous for patients administered clozapine medication? A case report. *Ther Drug Monit.* 1999;21(5):580-582.
143. de Leon J. Atypical antipsychotic dosing: the effect of smoking and caffeine. *Psychiatr Serv.* 2004;55(5):491-493.
144. Potvin S, Blanchet P, Stip E. Substance abuse is associated with increased extrapyramidal symptoms in schizophrenia: a meta-analysis. *Schizophr Res.* 2009;113(2-3):181-188.
145. Binder RL, Kazamatsuri H, Nishimura T, McNiel DE. Smoking and tardive dyskinesia. *Biol Psychiatry.* 1987;22(10):1280-1282.
146. Fulgoni VL, III, Debra R Keast, Harris R Lieberman. Trends in intake and sources of caffeine in the diets of U.S. adults: 2001-2010. *Am J Clin Nutr.* 2015;101(5):1081-1087. doi:10.3945/ajcn.113.080077
147. Larson CA, Carey KB. Caffeine: brewing trouble in mental health settings? *Prof Psychol Res Pr.* 1998;29(4):373-376. doi:10.1037/0735-7028.29.4.373
148. Olivera AA, Kiefer MW, Manley NK. Tardive dyskinesia in psychiatric patients with substance use disorders. *Am J Drug Alcohol Abuse.* 1990;16(1-2):57-66.
149. Zaretsky A, Rector NA, Seeman MV, Fornazzari X. Current cannabis use and tardive dyskinesia. *Schizophr Res.* 1993;11(1):3-8.
150. Goff DC, Henderson DC, Amico E. Cigarette smoking in schizophrenia: relationship to psychopathology and medication side effects. *Am J Psychiatry.* 1992;149(9):1189-1194.
151. Hughes JR, Hatsukami DK, Mitchell JE, Dahlgren LA. Prevalence of smoking among psychiatric outpatients. *Am J Psychiatry.* 1986;143(8):993-997.
152. Murthy P, Chand P. Treatment of dual diagnosis disorders. *Curr Opin Psychiatry.* 2012;25(3):194-200.
153. Moyers TB, Houck J, Rice SL, Longabaugh R, Miller WR. Therapist empathy, combined behavioral intervention, and alcohol outcomes in the COMBINE research project. *J Consult Clin Psychol.* 2016;84(3):221-229. doi:10.1037/ccp0000074
154. Clarke N, Mun EY, Kelly S, White HR, Lynch K. Treatment outcomes of a combined cognitive behavior therapy and pharmacotherapy for a sample of women with and without substance abuse histories on an acute psychiatric unit: do therapeutic alliance and motivation matter? *Am J Addict.* 2013;22(6):566-573. doi:10.1111/j.1521-0391.2013.12013.x
155. Bourke E, Barker C, Fornells-Ambrojo M. Systematic review and meta-analysis of therapeutic alliance, engagement, and outcome in psychological therapies for psychosis. *Psychol Psychother.* 2021;94(3):822-853. doi:10.1111/papt.12330
156. Carey KB. Substance use reduction in the context of outpatient psychiatric treatment: a collaborative, motivational, harm reduction approach. *Community Ment Health J.* 1996;32(3):291-306; discussion 307-310.
157. Addington J, el-Guebaly N, Campbell W, Hodgins DC, Addington D. Smoking cessation treatment for patients with schizophrenia. *Am J Psychiatry.* 1998;155(7):974-976.
158. Adler LE, Hoffer LD, Wiser A, Freedman R. Normalization of auditory physiology by cigarette smoking in schizophrenic patients. *Am J Psychiatry.* 1993;150(12):1856-1861.
159. Ziedonis D, Fisher W. Motivation-based assessment and treatment of substance abuse in patients with schizophrenia. *Hatherleigh Guide to Treating Substance Abuse.* Part 2. Hatherleigh Press; 1996:270-287.
160. Kelly C, McCreadie RG. Smoking habits, current symptoms, and premorbid characteristics of schizophrenic patients in Nithsdale. *Scotland. Am J Psychiatry.* 1999;156(11):1751-1757.
161. Brunette MF, Mueser KT, Xie H, Drake RE. Relationships between symptoms of schizophrenia and substance abuse. *J Nerv Ment Dis.* 1997;185(1):13-20.
162. Taylor G, McNeill A, Girling A, Farley A, Lindson-Hawley N, Aveyard P. Change in mental health after smoking cessation: systematic review and meta-analysis. *BMJ.* 2014;348:g1151.
163. Skinner MD, Lahmek P, Pham H, Aubin HJ. Disulfiram efficacy in the treatment of alcohol dependence: a meta-analysis. *PLoS One.* 2014;9(2):e87366.
164. Ziedonis DM, Smelson D, Rosenthal RN, et al. Improving the care of individuals with schizophrenia and substance use disorders: consensus recommendations. *J Psychiatr Pract.* 2005;11(5):315-339.
165. Shen W. Extrapyramidal symptoms associated with alcohol withdrawal. *Biol Psychiatry.* 1984;19(7):1037-1043.
166. Jordaan GP, Warwick JM, Nel DG, Hewlett R, Emsley R. Alcohol-induced psychotic disorder: brain perfusion and psychopathology—before and after anti-psychotic treatment. *Metab Brain Dis.* 2012;27(1):67-77.
167. Farnia V, Shakeri J, Tatari F, et al. Randomized controlled trial of aripiprazole versus risperidone for the treatment of amphetamine-induced psychosis. *Am J Drug Alcohol Abuse.* 2014;40(1):10-15.
168. Khoury R, Ghossoub E. Antipsychotics and seizures: what are the risks. *Curr Psychiatry.* 2019;18:21-33.

169. Schneider SM, Michelson EA, Boucek CD, Ilkhanipour K. Dextromethorphan poisoning reversed by naloxone. *Am J Emerg Med.* 1991;9(3):237-238.
170. Spiller HA, Ryan ML, Weston RG, Jansen J. Clinical experience with and analytical confirmation of "bath salts" and "legal highs" (synthetic cathinones) in the United States. *Clin Toxicol.* 2011;49(6):499-505.
171. Anthenelli RM, Benowitz NL, West R, et al. Neuropsychiatric safety and efficacy of varenicline, bupropion, and nicotine patch in smokers with and without psychiatric disorders (EAGLES): a double-blind, randomised, placebo-controlled clinical trial. *Lancet.* 2016;387(10037):2507-2520.
172. Kumar S, Kodela S, Detweiler JG, Kim KY, Detweiler MB. Bupropion-induced psychosis: folklore or a fact? A systematic review of the literature. *Gen Hosp Psychiatry.* 2011;33(6):612-617.
173. Tsoi DT, Porwal M, Webster AC. Efficacy and safety of bupropion for smoking cessation and reduction in schizophrenia: systematic review and meta-analysis. *Br J Psychiatry.* 2010;196(5):346-353.
174. Dalack GW, Becks L, Hill E, Pomerleau OF, Meador-Woodruff JH. Nicotine withdrawal and psychiatric symptoms in cigarette smokers with schizophrenia. *Neuropsychopharmacology.* 1999;21(2):195-202.
175. Hunt GE, Siegfried N, Morley K, Sitharthan T, Cleary M. Psychosocial interventions for people with both severe mental illness and substance misuse. *Cochrane Database Syst Rev.* 2013;(10):CD001088.
176. Docherty J. The individual psychotherapies: efficacy, syndrome-based treatments, and the therapeutic alliance. In: Lazare A, ed. *Outpatient Psychiatry: Diagnosis and Treatment.* Williams & Wilkins; 1980.
177. Drake RE, Noordsy DL. Case management for people with coexisting severe mental disorder and substance use disorder. *Psychiatr Ann.* 1994;24(8):427-431.
178. U.S. Department of Health and Human Services. *Reducing Tobacco Use.* A Report of the Surgeon General. U.S. Department of Health and Human Services, Centers for Disease Control and Prevention, National Center for Chronic Disease Prevention and Health Promotion, Office on Smoking and Health; 2000.
179. Wilkins JN. Pharmacotherapy of schizophrenia patients with comorbid substance abuse. *Schizophr Bull.* 1997;23(2):215-228.
180. Minkoff K. An integrated treatment model for dual diagnosis of psychosis and addiction. *Hosp Community Psychiatry.* 1989;40(10):1031-1036.
181. Marlatt G, Gordon J. *Relapse Prevention: Maintenance Strategies in the Treatment of Addictive Behaviors.* Guilford Press; 1985.
182. Dixon L, Rebori T. Psychosocial treatment of substance abuse in schizophrenic patients. In: Shriqui CL, Nasrallah HA, eds. *Contemporary Issues in the Treatment of Schizophrenia.* American Psychiatric Press; 1995.
183. Bogenschutz MP, Rice SL, Tonigan JS, et al. 12-step facilitation for the dually diagnosed: a randomized clinical trial. *J Subst Abuse Treat.* 2014;46(4):403-411. doi:10.1016/j.jsat.2013.12.009
184. Alcoholics Anonymous. *The A.A. Member—Medications & Other Drugs.* Accessed July 7, 2023. doi:https://www.aa.org/aa-member-medications-and-other-drugs
185. Ziedonis DM, D'Avanzo K. Schizophrenia and substance abuse. In: Kranzler HR, Rounsaville BJ, eds. *Dual Diagnosis and Treatment: Substance Abuse and Comorbid Medical and Psychiatric Disorders.* Marcel Dekker; 1998:427-465.
186. Hilton T. Pharmacological issues in the management of people with mental illness and problems with alcohol and illicit drug misuse. *Crim Behav Ment Health.* 2007;17(4):215-224.
187. Desrosiers JJ, Tchiloemba B, Boyadjieva R, Jutras-Aswad D. Implementation of a contingency approach for people with co-occurring substance use and psychiatric disorders: acceptability and feasibility pilot study. *Addict Behav Rep.* 2019;10:100223. doi:10.1016/j.abrep.2019.100223
188. Chen XJ, Wang DM, Zhou LD, et al. Mindfulness-based relapse prevention combined with virtual reality cue exposure for methamphetamine use disorder: study protocol for a randomized controlled trial. *Contemp Clin Trials.* 2018;70:99-105.
189. Culbertson C, Nicolas S, Zaharovits I, et al. Methamphetamine craving induced in an online virtual reality environment. *Pharmacol Biochem Behav.* 2010;96(4):454-460.
190. Pot-Kolder RM, Geraets CN, Veling W, et al. Virtual-reality-based cognitive behavioural therapy versus waiting list control for paranoid ideation and social avoidance in patients with psychotic disorders: a single-blind randomised controlled trial. *Lancet Psychiatry.* 2018;5(3):217-226.
191. Rus-Calafell M, Garety P, Sason E, Craig TJ, Valmaggia LR. Virtual reality in the assessment and treatment of psychosis: a systematic review of its utility, acceptability and effectiveness. *Psychol Med.* 2018;48(3):362-391.
192. Bowen S, Witkiewitz K, Clifasefi SL, et al. Relative efficacy of mindfulness-based relapse prevention, standard relapse prevention, and treatment as usual for substance use disorders: a randomized clinical trial. *JAMA Psychiatry.* 2014;71(5):547-556.
193. Zemestani M, Ottaviani C. Effectiveness of mindfulness-based relapse prevention for co-occurring substance use and depression disorders. *Mindfulness.* 2016;7(6):1347-1355.
194. Louise S, Fitzpatrick M, Strauss C, Rossell SL, Thomas N. Mindfulness- and acceptance-based interventions for psychosis: our current understanding and a meta-analysis. *Schizophr Res.* 2018;192:57-63.
195. Fattahi C, Hamada K, Chiang M, et al. A narrative review of mindfulness-based therapy for schizophrenia, co-occurring substance use and comorbid cardiometabolic problems. *Psychiatry Res.* 2021;296:113707.
196. Mueser KT, Gingerich S. Treatment of co-occurring psychotic and substance use disorders. *Soc Work Public Health.* 2013;28(3-4):424-439. doi:10.1080/19371918.2013.774676
197. Cather C, Brunette MF, Mueser KT, et al. Impact of comprehensive treatment for first episode psychosis on substance use outcomes: a randomized controlled trial. *Psychiatry Res.* 2018;268:303-311. doi:10.1016/j.psychres.2018.06.055
198. SAMHSA. *SAMHSA Announces a Working Definition of "Recovery" from Mental Disorders and Substance Use Disorders.* Substance Abuse and Mental Health Services Administration. 2011. Accessed November 14, 2016. https://store.samhsa.gov/product/SAMHSA-s-Working-Definition-of-Recovery/PEP12-RECDEF
199. Davidson L, Roe D. Recovery from versus recovery in serious mental illness: one strategy for lessening confusion plaguing recovery. *J Ment Health.* 2007;16(4):459-470.
200. Deegan PE. Recovery: the lived experience of rehabilitation. *Psychiatr Rehabil J.* 1988;11(4):11-19.
201. SAMHSA. *Substance Abuse and Mental Health Services Administration. National Consensus Statement on Mental Health Recovery.* U.S. Department of Health and Human Services; 2006.

CHAPTER

104 Co-occurring Attention Deficit Hyperactivity Disorder and Substance Use Disorders

David Saunders and Frances Rudnick Levin

CHAPTER OUTLINE

- Introduction
- Diagnosis of ADHD
- Epidemiology of ADHD and substance use disorders
- Possible reasons for linkage of ADHD and substance use disorders
- Genetic and neural underpinnings of ADHD, and implications for substance use disorder vulnerability
- The impact of having ADHD alone and with substance use disorders
- Treatment of co-occurring ADHD and substance use disorder
- Child and adolescent treatment considerations
- Summary

INTRODUCTION

This chapter examines two common psychiatric problems: attention deficit hyperactivity disorder (ADHD) and substance use disorders (SUDs). Over the past three decades, it has become increasingly clear that most individuals diagnosed with childhood ADHD continue to have impairing symptoms into adulthood. Indeed, one recent study found that 90% of children diagnosed with ADHD will continue to have at least residual symptoms in young adulthood, often exacerbated during times of stress, and frequently with only temporary periods of remission.[1,2] The coexistence of a SUD makes it more difficult to treat the ADHD symptoms in adulthood.[3] Similarly, untreated ADHD may make it less likely that standard treatments for SUD will be as effective.[4-7] The overrepresentation of ADHD in persons with SUDs, the reasons for this association, the diagnostic issues related to making the diagnosis of ADHD in adults with an SUD, child and adolescent treatment considerations, and the implications for treatment are discussed.

DIAGNOSIS OF ADHD

ADHD is a neurodevelopmental disorder characterized by inattention, impulsivity, and hyperactivity. To meet DSM-5 criteria for ADHD, individuals should have either (1) six symptoms of inattention in childhood or five symptoms at age 17 years or older (inattentive presentation) or (2) six symptoms of impulsivity and hyperactivity in childhood or five symptoms at age 17 years of older (impulsive/hyperactive presentation) or (3) both (combined presentation). Individuals who met full criteria in childhood but currently in adulthood have fewer than six symptoms of inattention or hyperactivity/impulsivity are described as having ADHD, in partial remission. Some ADHD symptoms need to occur prior to the age of 12. This represents a change from DSM-IV where the age criterion required impairing symptoms prior to the age of 7; it is expected that this change will raise the prevalence rates in general and treatment populations. Further, some impairments from these symptoms need to be present in two or more settings, and the symptoms must produce clear evidence of significant impairment. Moreover, the symptoms cannot be better accounted for by another mental disorder.[8]

The ADHD criteria emphasize both the developmental aspect of the disorder and the fact that childhood behavior problems often are context dependent. The more settings in which aberrant behavior occurs, the more likely the behavior interferes with the child's functioning and therefore warrants a diagnosis. The multi-setting requirement for the diagnosis of ADHD underscores the importance of obtaining collateral not only from parents, but also from school (or work in older adolescents/adults). For example, a child who appears distracted and inattentive in only one setting (such as at school) but can listen well and pay attention in other settings, may have a learning disability rather than ADHD[9] or may have a co-occurring learning disability.[10] Or alternatively, a unique stressor in a single context (eg, bullying at school) could be the source of symptoms that present like ADHD. In this setting, addressing the underlying cause could eliminate the presenting symptoms and thus argue against a diagnosis of ADHD.

Utility of ADHD Screening Instruments in Substance-Using Populations

Although ADHD is common among those with nicotine, alcohol, and other SUDs, it is often not assessed.[11] While it is not unreasonable to intensively evaluate all persons with a SUD for ADHD, a quick and more cost-effective approach, particularly in clinical settings, is to administer a reliable screening instrument followed by a standardized diagnostic interview for likely cases.[12] Three commonly used instruments include the Wender Utah Rating Scale (WURS, 25 items),[12] which screens for childhood ADHD, the Conners' Adult ADHD Rating Scale (CAARS, 18 items),[13] and Adult ADHD Self-Report Scale Version 1.1 (ASRS-vI.I, 6 items).[14] Each of these screens has been used in the general and treatment populations with good results.[12,13,15-19]

The utility of these instruments in persons with an active SUD has also been studied in individuals with SUD. For example, in a small Spanish sample of individuals with substance use problems ASRS-v1.1, was found to have good sensitivity (87.5%).[20] Another ADHD screening instrument, the Attention-Deficit Scales for Adults (ADSA), has also been evaluated in persons with an active SUD. This questionnaire, somewhat longer than the other instrument (54 items), was found to have reasonable sensitivity (0.79) and specificity (0.64).[21]

Recently, a study was conducted to assess the clinical utility of three of the short, commonly administered instruments (eg, the WURS, the CAARS [18-item], and the ASRS-v1.1) in a population of individuals currently seeking treatment for cocaine use disorder.[22] The validity of the instruments was tested by comparing the screening results to the Conners' Adult ADHD Diagnostic Interview for the DSM-IV (CAADID).[23] All three instruments demonstrated adequate sensitivity, specificity, and positive/negative predictive values, with the CAARS outperforming the rest on predictive parameters and the WURS having the greatest sensitivity. While these findings suggest that standard ADHD screening instruments may be reasonably applied in persons with an active SUD, the study was relatively small and conducted with people who primarily used cocaine. In a subsequent study, the validity of the ASRS-v1.1 was assessed in a large sample ($N > 1{,}000$) of treatment seekers coming for treatment for various SUDs. The sensitivity was good (at 0.84). Although the positive predictive validity was relatively low (0.26), the negative predictive validity was high (0.97), suggesting that few cases of ADHD were missed.[24] The ASRS-v1.1 may be uniquely practical in that it is much shorter (only six items) and has reasonable sensitivity and specificity. Thus, the implementation of these instruments with populations with ongoing SUDs is reasonable but should not replace a careful diagnostic evaluation.

Use of Neuropsychological Testing to Confirm ADHD Diagnosis

ADHD is a clinical diagnosis that is best made by carrying out a comprehensive assessment that includes developmental history, learning history, evaluation of other psychiatric comorbidities, and medical evaluation. Although various neuropsychological tests, electrophysiologic data, and neuroimaging tests have found differences among adults with and without ADHD,[25-27] no test has adequate specificity to "diagnose" an individual with ADHD.[28,29] However, continuous performance tests are the most evidence based of currently available psychological tests, demonstrating reasonable sensitivity and specificity and promising positive predictive power.[28]

Computer testing shows areas of dysfunction that may or may not be consistent with ADHD. However, testing may be useful for treatment or educational planning[11,28,30] since learning disabilities and academic underachievement are common in individuals with ADHD.[31,32] While the utility of these tests in active substance-using populations has not been established,[11] observing how individuals behave while taking neurocognitive tests can provide useful clinical information. An individual who demonstrates short latency responses, uncritical and careless performance with frequent false starts, off-task behaviors, and concentration problems might indicate the presence of ADHD.[33]

Difficulties in Diagnosing Adult ADHD in Substance-Using Populations

Although the DSM-5 provides clear-cut criteria for making the diagnosis of adult ADHD, diagnostic ambiguity often arises when one attempts to apply these criteria to individuals who have hazardous use of alcohol and other drugs. Specifically, common ADHD symptoms can be difficult to identify and disentangle when an individual is actively using or withdrawing from substances. Two approaches for clarifying whether ADHD is present are particularly effective. First, when possible, it is best to assess individuals when they have been abstinent for 2 to 4 weeks to ensure the acute effects of alcohol or drugs or withdrawal from alcohol and/or drugs are not confounding the diagnosis. Second, obtaining a developmental history is critical. For example, if a patient displayed symptoms of ADHD prior to using substances, they are naturally more likely to have ADHD. Because patients cannot always recall their developmental history, obtaining collateral history can be especially important when the diagnosis is unclear. However, if one cannot wait 2 to 4 weeks or obtain a developmental history, this should not preclude making a diagnosis, especially if ADHD is likely present and the patient is unable to maintain abstinence.

Potential Reasons for Underdiagnosis

Recalling symptoms that began at an early age can be problematic. While this is somewhat mitigated by the raising of the age of onset from less than 7 to less than 12 years with DSM-5, many adults have difficulty remembering symptoms occurring while in elementary or middle school. Individuals with a SUD may have memory deficits due to drug use, making both current and past ADHD symptom recall even more difficult. In assessing a child for ADHD symptoms, child psychiatrists or pediatricians often seek information from a teacher or parent; however, these sources of information often are not available during assessment of the adult patient, particularly a substance-using patient. The patient may be estranged from his/her family. Even when an older family member or parent is available, the reliability of the information may be questionable. The older family member may have had an alcohol/drug problem or other dysfunction to a degree that his or her ability to recall the patient's childhood behavior may be limited. Another good way to obtain historical data is to ask the patient to provide elementary school report cards. These can afford an accurate "snapshot" of the patient as a child. Although many parents may not have kept such school records, it is worthwhile to inquire.

If the patient or family cannot recall symptoms prior to age 12 but does remember substantial impairment related to ADHD symptoms in high school, it is reasonable to make the unspecified ADHD diagnosis. Additionally, recent longitudinal studies suggest that some individuals may not meet full symptom criteria until late adolescence or early adulthood.[34-36] Researchers have hypothesized two potential explanations for these findings. Some have argued that these data support a variant of ADHD that is not developmentally driven. Others have argued that parental structure, higher IQ, or milder childhood symptomatology may obfuscate the full manifestation of symptoms until supportive "environmental scaffolding" is removed, often when an individual is out of their childhood environment or in college.[37] In other words, a more intelligent and/or motivated child, or a child with extensive parental support, may not receive a diagnosis because the symptoms do not sufficiently impair them. The upshot for clinicians is that if a patient cannot recall symptoms prior to the age of 12 this should not rule out the diagnosis of ADHD.

In addition to the lack of good historical information, several other reasons for underdiagnosis of ADHD may be identified. First, many persons with both SUDs and adult ADHD were not diagnosed as children and attribute their impatience, restlessness, or procrastination to character traits of being "hotheaded," "easily bored," or "lazy." Second, many of the consequences of ADHD (such as work failure and poor educational attainment) also are associated with SUD. Persons with undiagnosed ADHD may assume that it is their alcohol or drug use that prevents them from attaining their full potential. Third, patients often develop ways to partially compensate for their ADHD symptoms, so that the symptoms of the disorder may not be obvious to the evaluating clinician. For example, adults who feel restless may learn to get up from the table and serve others as a socially appropriate way to handle their need for increased activity. Fourth, because questions regarding childhood behaviors—particularly behaviors associated with ADHD—are not always part of the "standard" intake interview, it can be an easy diagnosis to overlook. Unlike depression or psychosis, which causes episodic changes in functioning that may be incapacitating or require hospitalization, the symptoms of ADHD are more chronic and usually do not have such dramatic consequences. The latter are thus less likely to be noticed and attributed to a psychiatric disorder.

Potential Reasons for Overdiagnosis

Screening instruments can be useful in identifying individuals with child and adult ADHD, but overreliance on such instruments can lead to overdiagnosis. However, the growing literature suggests that these instruments have clinical utility and reasonable psychometric properties[22,24,38] such that they might be reasonable to administer in SUD treatment settings as a first step followed by a clinical interview for those who screen positive.

Overdiagnosis of adult ADHD also can occur if one ignores the functional impairment criterion. For example, it is common for individuals to procrastinate when faced with difficult projects. The difference is that adults with ADHD have had significant occupational, interpersonal, or psychological impairment owing to their impaired ability to start and complete tasks. It is incumbent on the clinician to ensure that a patient's current symptoms of ADHD are not limited to one setting. An individual who is completing difficult projects at home but is unable to finish assigned projects at work may be experiencing job dissatisfaction rather than ADHD. Moreover, the ADHD symptoms need to be impairing, not merely bothersome.

Another way in which the clinician may over diagnose ADHD is by failing to confirm that a patient shows a continuity of symptoms from childhood to adulthood. Levin et al.[39] have observed that some individuals with cocaine use disorder have impairing ADHD-like symptoms that occur only after a period of regular drug use, but they cannot recall having experienced ADHD symptoms in childhood. Other clinicians have also noted that intoxication of certain substances or withdrawal symptoms overlap with ADHD symptoms.[40] Therefore, taking a good longitudinal history is critical. Further, a good medical evaluation is important since anemia and thyroid problems may mimic some of the symptoms associated with ADHD.[29] However, sudden development of "ADHD symptoms" due to medical causes should not be confused with ADHD if a good longitudinal history is obtained.

Finally, some individuals may feign symptoms of ADHD to get special consideration with test taking, or to obtain stimulant medication for recreational use, diversion, or performance enhancement in high school/college or athletics.[41,42]

Co-occurring Psychiatric Disorders

Another issue that complicates assessment and often leads to diagnostic confusion is that of additional co-occurring psychiatric disorders. Generally, because ADHD symptoms are present in elementary school and precede the SUD, ADHD can be more readily identified as an independent, longstanding disorder—verified by collateral from childhood or adolescence, when appropriate, and evidence-based scales—compared with disorders that usually are episodic in nature and may first manifest later in life, including after the initiation of heavy substance use, (which would be termed a "substance-induced" syndrome).

The last criterion listed in the DSM-5 for ADHD emphasizes that ADHD should not be diagnosed if the observed symptoms are better accounted for by another mental disorder. Unfortunately, some clinicians may interpret this to mean that if depression or bipolar illness is present, ADHD should not be diagnosed. In reality, these disorders may coexist. For example, common or associated symptoms found in either a depressive disorder or ADHD include inattention, concentration difficulties, psychomotor agitation, and sleep difficulties. In an active substance use, these symptoms can be exacerbated. Similarly, ADHD and hypomania and mania share many symptoms such as distractibility, talkativeness, impulsivity, mood swings/anger outburst, and increased psychomotor activity.

Kessler et al.[15] found that 12-month prevalence rates of major depression, bipolar illness, and anxiety disorders are substantially higher among those with ADHD compared to non-ADHD adults. The prevalence rate of depression was 18.6% in the ADHD group and 7.8% in the non-ADHD group. Similarly, the prevalence rate of bipolar illness was 19.4% in the ADHD group and 3.1% in the non-ADHD group. The presence of certain symptoms provides helpful clues in discerning whether one or both disorders are present. Individuals with major depression may experience symptoms of inattention but are less likely to have hyperactivity and talkativeness associated with ADHD. Further, if there is a diminished interest in activities, depressed mood, or suicidality, this is unlikely to be from ADHD alone. Further, symptoms of decreased concentration as part of a depressive syndrome should resolve when the depression improves, either concurrently or by history.

Although bipolar illness and ADHD share certain symptoms, certain features common to bipolar illness are relatively uncommon in those with ADHD (eg, elevated mood, grandiosity, flight of ideas). Further, individuals with bipolar illness are more likely to describe discrete periods of increased restlessness, talkativeness, hyperactivity, and the like, whereas those with adult ADHD will be more likely to describe a lifelong constellation of these symptoms to a lesser degree. Importantly, individuals with ADHD typically do not exhibit psychotic symptoms. If these are present, they indicate the likelihood of an additional mood disturbance and/or a substance-induced psychotic disorder. That said, it is important to keep in mind the high comorbidity of ADHD and mood disorders and that a patient may have both disorders.

Often, adults with ADHD have first-degree relatives with ADHD; their presence may suggest that the individual in question has ADHD. However, depression and bipolar illness also are overrepresented in families of individuals diagnosed with ADHD,[43,44] complicating the diagnostic picture. Determining whether an individual has ADHD alone, has multiple psychiatric disorders, or has a psychiatric disorder other than ADHD rests on clinical judgment. Initial treatment is usually focused on the more severe illness present. However, this should not preclude attention to the other disorder when improvement in symptoms of the more severe illness occurs.[45] Again, a comprehensive diagnostic assessment that addresses psychiatric comorbidity and pertinent family history is needed prior to initiating any pharmacotherapy.

EPIDEMIOLOGY OF ADHD AND SUBSTANCE USE DISORDERS

ADHD is the most common behavioral disorder of childhood, affecting 8% to 18% of children and adolescents worldwide.[46] In terms of young adulthood, recent studies suggest that there are variable patterns of remission from ADHD, and that the symptom course typically fluctuates between childhood and young adulthood. One recent follow-up study of the Multimodal Study of ADHD (MTA), a seminal study of ADHD symptom course and treatment, indicates that the majority of children with ADHD will experience a waxing and waning of symptoms across development. Specifically, while 30% of children with ADHD will experience a period or periods of full remission at some point between childhood and young adulthood, 60% of those children will experience recurrence of ADHD thereafter. Relatively few children have either full remission (9.1% of this sample) or stable persistence of ADHD (10.8%).[2] These findings may explain the variable rates of adult ADHD observed in the literature. The findings also appear to support what many clinicians observe, namely, that young adult patients may not meet full criteria for ADHD at a given time point, but do continue to have significant impairment because of persistent though fluctuating ADHD symptoms.

Several studies have demonstrated that the onset of substance use occurs earlier among adolescents with ADHD, and particularly those with hyperactive-impulsive symptoms.[47,48] Further, SUD is overrepresented among those with both ADHD symptoms and the full ADHD diagnosis.[49,50] In the National Comorbidity Survey Replication study, 15.2% of those with ADHD, compared to 5.6% of those without ADHD, had an SUD,[15] demonstrating that SUDs are overrepresented in the general population of ADHD adults. In a subsequent study using the National Comorbidity Adolescent sample, Kessler et al.[51] found that the onset of adolescent substance use was earlier for those with ADHD compared to those without ADHD, but those with conduct disorder had an even earlier onset of substance use. Using another large sample of adolescents (the National Health and Nutrition Examination Survey), Brinkman et al.[52] found that ADHD and conduct disorder were associated with earlier onset of tobacco and alcohol use than having neither disorder. ADHD alone was associated with increased tobacco but not alcohol use.

In a recent analysis of the National Epidemiology Survey on Alcohol and Related Disorders (NESARC), over 33,000 respondents were queried about ADHD symptoms, substance use, and SUDs.[53] Even after adjusting for conduct disorders, both substance use and SUDs were associated with having ADHD symptoms (not the full diagnosis of ADHD at 17 years or younger), ADHD-combined, ADHD-hyperactive/impulsive, and ADHD-inattentive subtypes. Notably, regardless of ADHD diagnostic subtype, the lifetime prevalence rates for alcohol, nicotine, or cannabis use disorders were 20% or greater, with the highest rates consistently in the combined group. Similar to work of others,[47,54] having ADHD-hyperactive/impulsive symptoms was more reliably associated with substance use or SUD compared to having inattentive ADHD symptoms.[53] Taken together, these studies suggest that ADHD and substance use disorders are not independent disorders and that their association is not the result of ascertainment bias.

Individuals with ADHD also have a greater likelihood of nicotine use disorder, as evidenced by multiple studies. Adults with ADHD have higher rates of nicotine use disorder than the general population (40% versus 26%). The odds of current smoking in adolescents with clinically significant inattentive ADHD symptoms were 2.8 times greater than for those without inattentive ADHD symptoms.[55,56] Analysis of the Longitudinal Study of Adolescent Health, a large perspective epidemiologic survey of adolescents, found that for each self-reported inattentive and hyperactive symptom, the risk of lifetime tobacco smoking increased. Further, for those reporting ever smoking, increase in symptoms was associated with earlier age of smoking and number of cigarettes smoked.[57] In meta-analyses conducted by Charach et al.[58] and Lee et al.,[49] ADHD was associated with nicotine use and nicotine use disorders, along with other SUD.

In a prospective study, Lambert and Hartsough[59] noted that individuals with ADHD had early onset of regular smoking and adults with ADHD were more likely to smoke daily than were controls. Additionally, adults with ADHD who smoke cigarettes have been found to experience more severe withdrawal when they cease smoking compared to those without ADHD.

Similar and perhaps more striking than community samples is the overrepresentation of ADHD in treatment populations. Following up on smaller prevalence studies,[60,61] a recent large multisite sample prevalence study conducted in 10 countries found that the mean rates of ADHD in adults seeking treatment for their SUDs were 14% using DSM-IV criteria and 17% using DSM-5 criteria. Moreover, a meta-analysis of 29 studies evaluating for ADHD in adolescents and adults with various SUDs obtained an overall rate of 23%, with a confidence interval of 19% to 27%.[62] Taken together, ADHD is commonly found among those seeking treatment for their SUD and yet surprisingly goes unrecognized in psychiatric as well as substance use treatment populations.[63]

POSSIBLE REASONS FOR LINKAGE OF ADHD AND SUBSTANCE USE DISORDERS

Myriad pathways lead from ADHD to the development of an SUD. In a comprehensive review, Molina and Pelham[64] put forth some of the underlying variables associated with ADHD (eg, biologic vulnerabilities, impulsive anger, neurocognitive deficits) as well as intervening variables (eg, social difficulties, academic difficulties, conduct problems) that may lead to substance use and SUD. Because it is beyond the scope of this chapter, we will only focus on a few of these important variables: conduct disorder and impulsivity.

There is considerable evidence that individuals diagnosed with childhood ADHD who also have conduct disorder as children are more likely to develop problems related to substance use.[65-68] Further, in some clinical samples, the presence of ADHD is associated with more severe conduct disorder symptoms and greater number of DSM-IV-defined substance dependence for multiple substances.[67] Of note, in a 2-year follow-up study of adolescents with co-occurring DSM-IV substance dependence and conduct disorder, severity of initial conduct disorder and age of onset, but not severity of ADHD or treatment duration, predicted worse substance dependence outcomes.[69]

While some prospective studies suggest that the increased risk for substance use among ADHD children is mediated by conduct disorder[70-72] other studies suggest that ADHD confers a risk for substance use, even in the absence of conduct disorder.[73,74] Further, several investigators have found that a substantial proportion of individuals with adult ADHD have an ongoing SUD in the absence of Anti-Social Personality Disorder (ASPD),[47,75,76] a diagnosis that requires a diagnosis of conduct disorder before age 15. In one review of 10 longitudinal studies, Lee et al. concluded that the risk of developing an SUD may be partially or fully accounted for by disruptive behavior disorders such as oppositional defiant disorder or conduct disorder (CD).[49] A subsequent meta-analysis by Serra-Pinheiro[77] of 16 studies found that when conduct disorder was controlled for, ADHD no longer conferred a risk for either illegal substance use or SUDs, though they acknowledged that they were unable to look at different ADHD subtypes because of power limitations. Moreover, the authors note that it may be the ADHD that results in school failure, deviant peer groups, and the likelihood of both conduct disorder and substance use. Indeed, Molina and Pelham[64] conclude that trying to control for CD when trying to determine the risk for SUD may "miss the potential for the cascading pattern of vulnerability that starts with temperament, childhood escalation of disruptive behaviors such as rule breaking and defiance and culminates with expanded behaviors that include early/heavier/escalating problematic substance use." Regardless of how critical it is to focus on ADHD with CD or ADHD alone, it remains an open question whether ADHD alone confers a risk for illegal substance use and SUD in adolescents. Perhaps more important is whether the ADHD symptoms persist into late adolescence and adulthood. Once regular substance use is established, the presence of ADHD symptoms may increase the likelihood of heavy and impairing use, even in the absence of a disruptive behavior disorder.

Impulsivity is another factor that may facilitate the initiation and persistence of drug use among individuals with ADHD. A growing preclinical and clinical literature suggests that impulsivity is associated with increased likelihood of developing or having a substance use problem.[78-80] Impulsivity, a common feature of ADHD, is defined as the inability to inhibit responses. Increased impulsivity may facilitate risk-taking behavior, involvement with drug-using peers, and poor cognitive skills to weigh the negative consequences of drug experimentation and continued substance use.[55,56] Consistently, some investigators have found that ADHD individuals with hyperactivity/impulsivity, but not inattentive symptoms, are more likely to have early-onset substance use or eventual substance use problems than those without any ADHD symptoms, even in the absence of conduct disorder behaviors.[47,48] While impulsivity may lead to substance use problems, individuals with ADHD may choose to use and eventually use various substances to mitigate ADHD symptoms or associated dysphoria.[81,82]

Some researchers (and popular news outlets) have suggested that treatment of ADHD with stimulants puts one at higher risk for SUDs.[83] This theoretical risk is proposed to occur by (1) the process of behavioral sensitization or (2) patients' belief that, because a stimulant medication has been prescribed, they can use cocaine or other drugs without difficulty. However, multiple recent studies have debunked this theory with respect to childhood onset ADHD. For example, a recent meta-analysis, Humphreys et al.[84] found that stimulant treatment does not increase the risk of nonmedical substance use or use disorder. A longitudinal study found that stimulant treatment of ADHD in childhood, particularly when administered from an early age, was actually associated with a lower risk for a SUD.[85] Further, another recent meta-analysis that looked at longitudinal studies that target cigarette smoking found that stimulant treatment reduced the likelihood of cigarette smoking while controlling for conduct disorder.[86] A recent analysis of 10 cohorts of high school seniors from the Monitoring the Future study found that among ADHD adolescents those administered ADHD medication from an earlier age or for longer duration were less likely to be currently smoking or have past year use of illegal drugs.[87] Consistent with this, a large Swedish registration study, which assessed individuals between 1960 and 1968, found that longer duration and earlier initiation of ADHD stimulant medication were associated with significant reduction in having an SUD at follow-up in 2009.[54] Taken together, these new data support that treatment of ADHD as a child or adolescent, including with stimulants, was associated with lower risk of SUDs, not higher. Indeed, from a clinical perspective, an untreated child is more likely to function poorly in school, seek out other marginalized peers, and become involved with alcohol or drugs. Moreover, one might postulate that sustained improvement in ADHD symptoms would be more likely to enhance psychosocial functioning and reduce the likelihood of SUD.

Whenever prescribing a medication with potential for nonmedical use or diversion, particularly among patients with substance use disorders, those risks need to be considered and weighed against possible benefits. Untreated ADHD is associated with significant functional impairment, morbidity, and mortality. Treatment of ADHD with stimulant medications is effective and associated with substantial improvements in functioning. Extended-release formulations of stimulants have been shown in short-term clinical trials to be safe and effective for treatment of patients with stimulant use disorders (such as cocaine or methamphetamine), improving ADHD symptoms, and promoting abstinence, with little evidence of nonmedical use in those trials.[88] Extended-release formulations are preferred, because the pharmacokinetic profile of slow absorption and elimination is less likely to produce the rewarding effects that might promote nonmedical use.[88] However, there is always the risk that exposure to stimulant medications can lead to nonmedical use, diversion, or a use disorder. The group at highest risk would be late adolescents and adults whose medications are not being monitored by their parents. Clinicians prescribing stimulant medications for ADHD to any patient, and especially to those with substance use disorders, need to remain mindful of this risk, monitoring patients regularly for appropriate use of the medication, telltale signs of nonmedical use, or for worsening of substance problems.

GENETIC AND NEURAL UNDERPINNINGS OF ADHD, AND IMPLICATIONS FOR SUBSTANCE USE DISORDER VULNERABILITY

The systematic study of the shared genetic, neural, and environmental underpinnings of ADHD and SUD is difficult. First, both disorders are complex and heterogeneous. As such, the subtleties and nuances of the relationship between ADHD and SUD etiology are only beginning to be understood. Secondly, comparatively few genetic and neural studies have focused specifically on individuals with both ADHD and SUDs. While a few such studies exist (ie, Soler Artigas[89]), in general, the study of the relationship between SUD and ADHD consists of comparing the individual literatures on ADHD and SUD.[89]

Genetics

Evidence supporting the genetic basis of ADHD derives from family, twin, and adoption studies, as well as molecular genetics. Twin studies have yielded a heritability estimate of 80% for ADHD, suggesting that the genetic contribution is strong.[90-92] Indeed, genetic contribution to risk is higher for ADHD than any other psychiatric condition according to heritability estimates based on a large national sibling study.[92] By comparison, other psychiatric conditions had significantly lower heritability estimates, including autism spectrum disorder (≈62%), schizophrenia (≈58%) bipolar disorder (≈52%), and obsessive compulsive disorder (≈38%), to name a few.

Early molecular genetic studies employed candidate-gene strategies to identify risk loci based on proposed pathophysiology, which point to multiple neurotransmitters, including dopamine, noradrenaline, and serotonin.[93,94] Such molecular genetics studies support the notion that ADHD is a heterogeneous disorder, dependent on several interacting genes, and there is a shared genetic risk profile with substance use disorders. Prominent among these are the genes for the dopamine transporter (DAT) and the D4 dopamine receptor (DRD4).[90,91,94-97] Notably, 9-repeat allele carriers of the DAT have been associated with enhanced neural responsivity to nicotine cues and may have a role in alcohol use disorder, whereas 10-repeat homozygosity of DAT1 may contribute to susceptibility to ADHD,[98-100] suggesting that certain genetic aberrations of the DAT genotype are associated with higher risk for ADHD and SUDs. In individuals with ADHD, the 10-repeat DAT1 allele is associated with decreased cortical thickness of the right prefrontal cortex (PFC).[101] Altered DRD4 expression results in reduced receptor effectiveness and increased gamma-aminobutyric acid transmission, thereby decreasing pyramidal cell firing.[45] Various polymorphisms of the DRD4 alleles have been shown to be associated with heroin addiction, alcohol use disorder, and ADHD.[102-105] Further, medications that inhibit the DAT, such as methylphenidate, increase synaptic dopamine levels and ameliorate the symptoms of ADHD. Other candidate genes of interest that have been associated with ADHD include (1) SNAP-25, which is associated with neuronal release of DA[90,106]; (2) serotonin 1B receptor (HTR1B) (9)[107]; (3) tryptophan hydroxylase 2 (TPH2), which catalyzes tryptophan to produce a precursor to serotonin[106,107]; and (4) alpha-1A adrenergic receptors (ADRA1A).[107,108]

However, the individual mutations identified by candidate gene studies account for only a small percentage of heritability in ADHD. Thus, more recently, researchers have employed genome-wide association studies (GWAS), which can look for 100,000s of single nucleotide polymorphisms to better characterize risk for ADHD. This strategy recently identified 12 risk loci, none of which were implicated in the aforementioned candidate-gene studies, but rather pointed to genes known to be critical for brain development (ie, FOXP2).[109] Interestingly, these loci were also implicated in other psychiatric disorders, including major depressive disorder and autism spectrum disorder, indicating that there is a shared genetic risk profile across disorders,[110] consistent with the high comorbidity among these disorders. In terms of shared genetic underpinnings with substance use disorders, a recent meta-analysis suggests that ADHD and cannabis use disorder share a background of common genetic variants, including on the aforementioned FOXP2 site.[89] This study estimates that individuals with ADHD are 7.9 times more likely to consume cannabis than individuals without ADHD. Still, 12 aforementioned loci only accounted for 22% of the heritability of ADHD (let alone the shared heritability with SUDs), suggesting that almost 50% of the heritability of the disorder is unexplained.[94] In summary, as with other psychiatric disorders, genetic risk for ADHD is likely conveyed by dozens of genes, each exerting small effects. Further research is thus needed to elucidate the genetic underpinnings of ADHD, including its association with substance use disorders.

Finally, recent research has focused on the role of epigenetic modifications, which have suggested that DNA methylation of genes relevant to ADHD pathophysiology and neurodevelopment play a role in the development of ADHD.[111] One upshot of epigenetics is that it has the potential to further characterize complex gene-environment interactions involving environmental factors, such as in utero exposure to substances and/or postnatal exposure to social stressors. Further characterization of these risk pathways will be critical in the coming years to understand the inheritance patterns of ADHD and SUDs.

Neuroimaging

Neuroimaging studies of ADHD include multiple modalities, including structural magnetic resonance imaging (MRI), resting state functional connectivity MRI, task-based functional MRI (fMRI) and Positron Emission Tomography (PET). Structurally, several consistent findings have been identified in the literature, with varying effect sizes.[112,113] Individuals with ADHD have been shown to have reduced volume of the PFC.[114] This finding is sensible given current proposed pathophysiological mechanisms of ADHD in that the PFC is densely populated with DA receptors (especially D1) and NE receptors, and balanced DA tone in the PFC is essential for normal working memory function and attention regulation.[45,115] Studies have also identified smaller volumes in individuals with ADHD in specific regions, including, the dorsolateral PFC, cerebellum, and subcortical structures[116,117] and Castellanos et al.[118] found a that ADHD was associated with smaller total cerebral brain volumes from childhood through adolescence. Bernanke and colleagues[119] note, however, that studies that identified the greatest differences between ADHD and control subjects were underpowered. Further, resting state fMRI connectivity analyses of patients with ADHD have consistently shown altered activity involving networks with a diverse array of functions. For example, altered activity has been observed within the Default Mode Network—a network of brain regions that demonstrate highly correlated activity at rest and are associated with task-irrelevant mental processes, encompassing the precuneus/posterior cingulate cortex, the medial prefrontal cortex, and the lateral and inferior parietal cortex.[120] Further, individuals with ADHD have also been shown to have altered functional connectivity *between* the DMN and the cognitive control network, a region implicated in attention regulation and executive function that includes the dorsal anterior cingulate cortex/supplementary motor area, the posterior parietal cortex, the anterior insular cortex, the dorsolateral prefrontal cortex, and inferior frontal junction.[120] But studies have also shown that patients with ADHD demonstrate aberrations in connectivity within the dopaminergic mesolimbic system, which includes the nucleus accumbens, the amygdala and the ventral tegmental area,[94] which is associated with learning, motivation and anticipation of outcomes. For a thorough review of these findings, see Posner et al.[94,120]

Finally, task-based fMRI studies in individuals with ADHD have demonstrated dysfunction in two circuits involving attention and inhibition. Specifically, a recent meta-analysis of 607 subjects with ADHD identified reduced activation during inhibitory control tasks in the right inferior frontal cortex, the supplementary motor area, and the anterior cingulate cortex.[121] They also observed reduced activation in attention-based tasks in the right dorsolateral prefrontal cortex, thalamic and parietal regions, and the posterior basal ganglia.[121]

How do these structural MRI, functional MRI, and connectivity findings in individuals with ADHD relate to SUD? A recent systematic review on the neural correlates of increased risk of SUD in adolescent ADHD proposed three different potential mechanisms that might differentiate individuals with ADHD and SUD (or at risk for SUD) from those with ADHD alone (or at low risk for SUD).[122] The first theory proposes exaggerated abnormalities in the inhibitory control and reward processing networks; the second proposes abnormalities in just reward processing; and the third proposes exaggerated abnormalities in just inhibitory control. Indeed, multiple structural MRI, functional MRI, and diffusion tensor imaging (DTI) studies support the first two hypotheses.[123-125] While there is no evidence in the literature to support the third theory, it is theoretically plausible that impaired inhibitory control alone distinguishes those with ADHD and SUD from those with ADHD alone.[122] Regardless of which theory holds true, the evidence is clear that (1) the networks implicated in ADHD are also relevant to SUD; and (2) there may be differences in these networks that distinguish those with ADHD alone relative to those with ADHD and SUD or high-risk for SUD.

Finally, in a comprehensive review Kalivas and Volkow[126] note that most all substances with nonmedical use liability produce their euphorigenic effects through their direct or indirect release of dopamine in the "reward" system of the brain consisting of the ventral tegmental area and the nucleus accumbens (with some possible exceptions, ie, hallucinogens). With chronic drug use, derangements in the dopaminergic system produce a relative hypodopaminergic state. Supporting this, Nutt et al.[127] reviewed numerous studies that used PET imaging and 11C-raclopride PET binding to assess stimulant–dopamine release in persons with a chronic alcohol and substance use disorder and found that regardless of the substance used, synaptic ventral striatal dopamine levels were lower in the persons with an SUD compared to those without a SUD. Interestingly, one study found that high-risk young adults who had not yet developed an SUD were more likely to have diminished dopamine signaling compared to controls—not unlike the hypodopaminergic functioning observed in prefrontal regions of the brain among individuals with ADHD.[128-130] This finding would seem to suggest that there may be impaired dopamine transmission *prior* to the onset of an SUD in individuals with ADHD.

THE IMPACT OF HAVING ADHD ALONE AND WITH SUBSTANCE USE DISORDERS

ADHD has substantial morbidity in and of itself. In an individual with ADHD, occupational and social deficits attributed to substance use may be due in small or large part to persistent ADHD symptoms. Mannuzza and Klein[32] noted that children with ADHD who were followed into adulthood were more likely to have completed less schooling, to hold occupations with less professional or social status, to suffer from poor self-esteem, to have social skill deficits, and to have antisocial personality disorder (ASP). Murphy and Barkley[13] found that, as adults, individuals who were diagnosed with ADHD in childhood were more likely to have had their driver's licenses suspended, to have incurred speeding violations, to have quit or been fired from a job, and to have been married multiple times. ADHD symptoms appear to place these individuals at great risk for ASPD, mood and anxiety disorders, and SUDs.[32,47,131-133] Women with ADHD may be particularly vulnerable to eating disorders, such as bulimia.[134] In a longitudinal study, women with ADHD had fewer romantic relationships and poorer self-esteem than those without ADHD.[135] Moreover, persistent symptoms seem to place individuals at greatest risk for early substance use.[48,136] Individuals with ADHD have higher rates of incarcerations, criminal recidivism, and violent criminal behavior.[131,137,138]

When ADHD symptoms are co-occurring with those of an SUD, the severity of impairment of each disorder is likely to increase. Moreover, the individual's response to addiction treatment is adversely affected by co-occurring ADHD. Biederman et al. found that following a period of SUD, adults with ADHD were more likely to transition from an alcohol use disorder to a drug use disorder and to continue to use substances than were similar patients without ADHD.[139] Likewise, among individuals with a lifetime history of an SUD, those who also had ADHD evinced a longer duration of having an SUD and a slower remission rate.[65]

Carroll and Rounsaville compared the clinical course of cocaine use among individuals with and without childhood histories of ADHD.[7] Those with childhood ADHD had an earlier onset of regular cocaine use, more frequent and intense cocaine use, and greater lifetime treatment exposure. Similarly, Levin et al. found that among individuals with DSM-IV cocaine dependence entering a therapeutic community, those with ADHD were less likely to graduate from the program compared to those with depression (and no ADHD) or those without ADHD or depression.[16] Graduation is an important milestone associated with better long-term outcome.

Based on these findings, it is increasingly evident that ADHD may exert a negative effect on the course of a SUD and that treatment needs to be targeted at both the psychiatric and substance use disorders. Functioning in modern society, be it in school, a job, relationships (co-workers, friends, spouse), requires a great deal of organization, attention to detail, and reliable adherence to schedules, commitments, and performance of repetitive, tedious tasks, all of which are more difficult with ADHD. SUDs likewise disrupt social and emotional functioning. Engaging in treatment for a SUD alone, without ADHD, requires adhering to a schedule, engagement with clinicians, and concerted effort, let alone the changes needed to achieve recovery, including controlling impulses to use substances and rebuilding social and occupational functioning. Thus, it is easy to imagine how ADHD and SUD would compound each other, how ADHD would interfere with treatment for SUD, and why concurrent treatment of ADHD along with the SUD would be important.

TREATMENT OF CO-OCCURRING ADHD AND SUBSTANCE USE DISORDER

Patients with co-occurring ADHD and SUD present a formidable challenge for any clinician treating such individuals. First, as previously described, it is often difficult to accurately diagnose ADHD in patients seeking treatment for SUD, since the symptoms of substance use or withdrawal can mimic ADHD. Furthermore, ADHD symptoms are chronic in nature and do not necessarily attract clinical attention upon initial presentation for SUD treatment. Finally, because stimulants remain the primary treatment modality for adult ADHD without co-occurring anxiety or depressive disorders, many clinicians are reluctant to prescribe such medications to patients presenting with SUD. ADHD and SUD *with* co-occurring anxiety or depression is distinct, and stimulants or SSRIs alone might be insufficient.[140] Indeed, patients with co-occurring ADHD may not have an adequate therapeutic response to antidepressants if the ADHD is not treated, motivating the Canadian ADHD Resource Alliance (for example) to recommend the use of a long-acting stimulant in addition to an antidepressant, or bupropion, which improves depressive and ADHD symptoms in some patients.[140] In any case, the identification and treatment of co-occurring ADHD in patients with SUD (with or without co-occurring anxiety or depression) is an increasing clinical priority, and the judicious use of stimulants when patients are diagnosed with ADHD using evidence-based scales, ought to be considered.[141]

Critically, compared to other patients with SUDs, individuals with ADHD may have greater difficulties in processing information and in sitting through group meetings—a common format for addiction treatment. Because individuals with ADHD tend to act impulsively, they also may be more likely than those without ADHD to drop out of treatment. Counselors and other patients may find individuals with untreated ADHD to be "frustrating." By recognizing and treating the ADHD, patients' attentional and behavioral problems may be alleviated, and as a result, their treatment outcomes may be improved.

In this section, we will provide an overview of the pharmacologic and nonpharmacologic therapies available, offer some general guidelines in choosing the most appropriate therapeutic option, and discuss optimal treatment strategies for the treatment of ADHD in a patient with SUD.

Pharmacotherapeutic Options for Treatment of ADHD

Amphetamine analogs and methylphenidate have been the most widely studied pharmacotherapies for adult ADHD without co-occurring SUD, although nonstimulant medications, including atomoxetine, tricyclic antidepressants, bupropion, monoamine oxidase inhibitors (MAOIs), alpha-2 agonists, and venlafaxine, have been studied as well. Modafinil, a novel stimulant medication with seemingly lower potential for nonmedical use than traditional stimulant medications, has also been studied for the treatment of ADHD. While there is substantial evidence for the efficacy of these agents in adults with ADHD, there are only a limited number of studies of patients with co-occurring ADHD and SUD. In a meta-analysis reviewing stimulant and nonstimulant treatments for adult ADHD (typically without co-occurring SUD), Torgersen et al. found that methylphenidate, amphetamines, and nonstimulants (desipramine, bupropion, atomoxetine) were superior to placebo.[142] Notably, in a subsequent meta-analysis, Faraone and Glatt found that stimulant medications are more effective than nonstimulants in treating ADHD. In another meta-analysis focused on methylphenidate trials,[143] Koesters et al. found that methylphenidate was superior to placebo,[144] but the effect size was substantially lower than an earlier meta-analysis by Faraone and Glatt (0.42 versus 0.73).[143] This is partially explained in that the Koesters analysis included studies of adults with a SUD with ADHD, a group that has been shown to be less responsive to medication.

Stimulant Medications

Amphetamine analogs and methylphenidate are the stimulant medications most used to treat ADHD in children and adults in the United States. Methylphenidate is a piperidine derivative that primarily acts extracellularly. Specifically, it partially blocks the dopamine transporter (DAT), whose function it is to remove dopamine from the presynaptic cell.[145] Thus by inhibiting DAT-mediated reuptake, methylphenidate increases the amount of dopamine available in the synapse for neurotransmission. Amphetamine analogs also prevent reuptake of dopamine via blockade of DAT. Critically, however, amphetamine also enters the presynaptic neuron and stimulates release of dopamine. In this way, amphetamine increases the availability of dopamine via both reuptake inhibition from the synapse and release from the presynaptic neuron via multiple mechanisms.[146]

The release of dopamine stimulated by both methylphenidate and amphetamine have a downstream effect on several relevant neural systems, including the reticular activating system, frontal circuits involved in cognitive control, and reward circuits. In each case, the overall clinical effect is to improve alertness and focus, reduce impulsivity, and render tedious tasks more rewarding.

Methylphenidate has been one of the first-line treatments for ADHD in children for decades and has been demonstrated to be safe and effective for the treatment of ADHD in adults.[147] It is available in multiple immediate- and sustained-release preparations for delayed absorption. Amphetamine analogs, also first-line treatments for ADHD in adults and children 6 years of age and older, have also been shown to be effective for the treatment of ADHD in both children and adults.[148] However, most of the studies discussed herein did not assess populations with ADHD and co-occurring SUDs. Commercially available amphetamine analogs include methamphetamine, dextroamphetamine, mixed amphetamine salts (MAS), and lisdexamfetamine. Methamphetamine is only available in an immediate-release preparation and is rarely prescribed due to concerns of nonmedical use and diversion. Dextroamphetamine is available in immediate- and sustained-release preparations. MAS is a fixed-combination amphetamine composed of equal amounts of dextroamphetamine saccharate, dextroamphetamine sulfate, racemic amphetamine aspartate monohydrate, and racemic amphetamine sulfate. MAS is available in immediate- and sustained-release preparations. Lisdexamfetamine is FDA approved for childhood and adult ADHD. Because it is a prodrug, it is a therapeutically inactive molecule until it is cleaved to L-lysine and active D-amphetamine, and it is associated with a longer duration of effect and reduced nonmedical use potential.[149] Side effects most associated with amphetamine and methylphenidate administration include insomnia, emotional lability, nausea/vomiting, nervousness, palpitations, elevated blood pressure, and rapid heart rate. Rare but serious adverse effects include severe hypertension, seizures, psychosis, and myocardial infarction. Clinical trials, which have mostly studied extended-release formulations of stimulants, suggest that nonmedical use of prescribed stimulants is uncommon among patients with SUDs who are interested in addressing their substance use and are *carefully diagnosed with co-occurring ADHD using evidence-based scales and, if possible, collateral history*, but patients should be carefully monitored for evidence of nonmedical use.

Modafinil, a novel wake-promoting agent that is FDA approved for narcolepsy and shift work sleep, has been shown to improve ADHD symptoms in children and adolescents, albeit less so than traditional stimulant medication.[133,142,150-152] Although modafinil has some stimulant-like properties (eg, promoting wakefulness), it has minimal reported nonmedical use potential. While there are some data supporting its efficacy in reducing cocaine use among those without alcohol use disorders,[153,154] it has not been evaluated for its efficacy in reducing ADHD symptoms among those with cocaine or other SUDs. At present, it would be considered a second-line agent for the treatment of ADHD.

Nonmedical Use Potential of Psychostimulants

While methylphenidate and amphetamine analogs are widely used in the treatment of ADHD, concern exists with respect to their nonmedical use potential, particularly in patients with SUD. Wilens et al.[42] define nonmedical use (described in the 2008 paper as "misuse," a value-attributing term we no longer support) of ADHD medications as "taking ADHD prescriptions not prescribed to the individual or taking medication differently than they were prescribed (eg, more than prescribed, taking alcohol or other drugs)". Diversion of stimulants was defined as the transfer of ADHD prescription medications from one individual who does have a prescription to another individual who does not have a prescription. This transfer includes the "selling, trading, or giving away prescription medication." Such aberrant behaviors should be distinguished from prescription stimulant use disorder.

According to the 2020 National Survey on Drug Use and Health, 0.5% of Americans aged 12 years or older reported current (last 30 days) nonmedical use of prescription stimulant medications, and 1.8% in the past year.[155] While these rates are lower than current nonmedical use of pain relievers (0.9% and 3.3% in the past month and year, respectively), the risks of prescribing stimulant medications in a population vulnerable to nonmedical use must be considered carefully (ie, college students engaging in unhealthy use of alcohol or other drugs).

In terms of populations that are especially susceptible to nonmedical stimulant use, the rates of past-year nonmedical use ranges from 1% to 10% among high school students, and between 3% and 10% in young adults.[155-158] Further, among young adults who used any prescription stimulants in the past year, more than 45% used them nonmedically[155] and more than two-third were approached to divert their medications.[156] Importantly, nonmedical use was associated with impulsivity and other substance use, and the primary reason endorsed for nonmedical use was performance enhancement, for example to cram for exams or complete required papers.[158] Interestingly, the method of procurement of the stimulant may predict whether one goes on to develop a stimulant disorder. Indeed one study suggested that those who obtained prescription drugs via theft, fake prescriptions, purchases, or multiple sources, were more likely to report past year SUDs, and also had the most severe risk profiles.[158]

Finally, the increased risk of diversion or nonmedical use as compared to medical use with stimulants is higher than with other medications.[156,158] Individuals who receive medication for ADHD are three times as likely to be asked to divert their medication as those receiving pain medication, and more than twice as likely as those receiving medications for sleep or anxiety.[156] Further, a study conducted at the University of Maryland found that students are more likely to receive a medication to treat pain than stimulants to treat ADHD, but the percentage of diverted prescribed medication is substantially higher for stimulants compared to pain relievers, 62% versus 35%.[159] Sharing of stimulant medications among high school or college students is commonly reported, often to help prepare for exams or other challenging academic assignments, and while this may be relatively harmless for some individuals, for those vulnerable to stimulant use disorder—such as those with co-occurring SUD—it may kindle the addiction, a significant risk.

Nonmedical Use Liability of Short Versus Long-Acting Formulations of Prescription Stimulants

The studies described above often do not make a distinction between immediate-release preparations and long-acting (aka extended-release) formulations, and there may be substantive differences in the subjective effects and nonmedical use liability of different stimulant preparations. Long-acting preparations of stimulant medications were initially developed to reduce the frequency of dosing and provide consistent therapeutic blood levels throughout the day. However, evidence is accumulating that long-acting preparations may have lower nonmedical use potential and may have particular utility for patients with co-occurring SUD.[160-162] Since the reinforcing effects of stimulants are associated with rapid changes in serum concentrations,[163] sustained-release preparations of methylphenidate or amphetamine, which slow the rate of onset of the drug's effect, are likely to be associated with less positive subjective drug effects. In a large internet survey of over 10,000 participants, long-acting stimulants, and in particular lisdexamfetamine and OROS methylphenidate, were much less likely to be used nonmedically than immediate-release preparations.[164]

Consistent with this, in a neuroimaging study conducted by Spencer et al., non–substance-using adults without ADHD were administered immediate-release methylphenidate or

OROS methylphenidate (Concerta) with similar maximum methylphenidate concentration.[165] Not surprisingly, the time to reach maximum concentration and dopamine receptor occupancy was longer in the OROS methylphenidate group, and this was associated with significantly lower ratings of "feeling an effect" or "liking the effect." These data suggest that long-acting stimulants may be less likely to be used nonmedically, for their euphorigenic effects. An additional advantage of delayed-release preparations is greater difficulty in using via a nonoral route (eg, injected or intranasally), which should also reduce the potential for nonmedical use and diversion.

In a 10-year longitudinal study in which 98 subjects were receiving psychotropic medication, Wilens et al. found that most ADHD individuals, predominately those with conduct disorders, used their medications appropriately.[166] However, those with conduct disorder or SUDs reported more nonmedical use and diversion, and there appeared to be more nonmedical use and diversion of immediate-release compared to extended-release stimulants.[42,166] For people with DSM-IV cocaine dependence, Collins et al. found that those with ADHD experienced similar subjective effects to cocaine as those without ADHD.[167] However, the subjective effects of cocaine were lessened when people with co-occurring cocaine dependence and ADHD were maintained on higher doses of sustained-released methylphenidate compared to a lower dose of sustained-release methylphenidate or placebo.

Even though nonmedical use and diversion of prescription stimulants, particularly long-acting preparations, may be of less concern for many patients with ADHD and SUD, there is reason for concern, especially in populations that are actively using and not seeking treatment. Notably, the rates of nonmedical use and diversion are substantially higher in adolescence and young adults. In most cases, there is a lack of physician oversight for such individuals, and therefore, there is no cardiovascular screening or warnings about possible interactions with other stimulants or over the counter nonstimulant preparations. It is crucial that patients who are prescribed stimulants for their ADHD, regardless of whether they are individuals with a current or past SUD, or have no history of nonmedical use, be warned about the risks associated with prescription stimulant use (including unhealthy use and addiction), understand why it is important not to "share" their medication with others, and be given strategies of how to safeguard their medication so that it is not diverted.

Nonstimulant Medications

A diverse group of nonstimulant medications has been identified as having some efficacy for the treatment of ADHD, although none have been shown to be therapeutically equivalent to stimulant medications. Except for atomoxetine and guanfacine extended release (which are FDA approved for use in both pediatric and adult ADHD), all other nonstimulant medications are "off- label" for ADHD and are generally considered second- or third-line treatments. There are certain instances where nonstimulant medications might be considered first line, such as if a motor tic disorder is present, cardiovascular disease, or co-occurring anxiety or depression.

Atomoxetine is a centrally acting noradrenergic reuptake inhibitor.[168,169] Onset of the therapeutic effects of atomoxetine is more gradual than that experienced with stimulant medications and may take several weeks to manifest, much akin to antidepressant treatment for depression. Common side effects of atomoxetine include sedation, appetite suppression, nausea, vomiting, and headache. Rare but serious side effects reported in children and adolescents include increased suicidal ideation and hepatotoxicity. Atomoxetine has no known nonmedical use potential, so it is an attractive candidate medication for study in the treatment of ADHD in patients with SUDs, although published data are limited.

Guanfacine extended release, a noradrenergic alpha-2 agonist, has been shown to be nearly as effective as stimulants in youth,[170] and although it has not been as extensively studied in adults, there is evidence that it is effective in treating adult ADHD symptoms as well.[143] It has also been shown to further reduce ADHD symptoms among those that have had a partial response to stimulants.[171] Common side effects of guanfacine include somnolence, headaches, sedation, and hypotension.[172] ADHD improvements have been observed after 1 week of medication administration.[173]

Finally, several antidepressant agents, typically those with stimulating properties, have been studied for the treatment of ADHD. Tricyclic antidepressants, which block the reuptake of norepinephrine, have some efficacy in reducing ADHD symptoms but are considered to be less effective than the stimulant medications.[174] The antidepressant bupropion is mainly a norepinephrine reuptake inhibitor, but also has some dopaminergic effect, and has been reported to be effective in the treatment of ADHD,[175] although when studied in patients with SUD, it offered no benefit over placebo.[11,176,177] Venlafaxine, a norepinephrine-serotonin reuptake inhibitor antidepressant medication, has limited evidence of efficacy in ADHD in uncontrolled and small placebo-controlled clinical trials.[178,179] Monoamine oxidase inhibitors (MAOIs) have demonstrated efficacy for ADHD, but the potential for hypertensive crises associated with tyramine-containing foods and medications (both illicit and prescribed) limits their utility, thus MAOIs should be considered relatively contraindicated in patients with SUD.

Pharmacotherapy Selection for ADHD and Co-occurring SUD

At present, there are no clear-cut guidelines regarding the appropriate use of traditional stimulant medications—methylphenidate and amphetamine analogs—in the treatment of adult ADHD and SUD. To our knowledge, there have been fourteen double-blind treatment studies conducted in individuals with an active co-occurring SUD with ADHD in which only three evaluated a nonstimulant medication (**Table 104-1**). None of the nonstimulant trials found the medication (bupropion or atomoxetine) to be superior to placebo in reducing substance use on the primary outcome measures. However,

TABLE 104-1 Psychopharmacologic Treatment of ADHD and SUD: 14 Double-Blind Trials

	N	Drug	Medication	Results
Stimulant trials				
Schubiner et al.[180]	48	Cocaine	MPH	ADHD: mixed SUD: negative
Riggs et al.[181]	69	Various	Pemoline*	ADHD: mixed SUD: negative
Carpentier et al.[182]	25	Various	MPH	ADHD: negative
Levin et al.[183]	98	Methadone/cocaine	MPH + bupropion	ADHD: negative SUD: negative
Levin et al.[177]	106	Cocaine	MPH	ADHD: mixed SUD: mixed
Winhusen et al.[184]	255	Nicotine	MPH	ADHD: positive SUD: mixed
Konstenius et al.[185]	24	Methamphetamine	MPH	ADHD: negative SUD: negative
Riggs et al.[186]	303	Most cannabis	MPH	ADHD: mixed SUD: mixed
Konstenius et al.[187]	54	Amphetamine	MPH	ADHD: positive SUD: positive
Kollins et al.[188]	32	Nicotine	Lisdexamfetamine	ADHD: positive SUD: negative
Levin et al.[189]	126	Cocaine	Mixed amphetamine salt XR	ADHD: positive SUD: negative
Nonstimulant trials				
Wilens et al.[42]	147	Alcohol	Atomox	ADHD: positive SUD: mixed
McRae-Clark et al.[190]	38	Cannabis	Atomox	ADHD: mixed SUD: negative
Thurstone et al.[191]	70	Various	Atomox	ADHD: negative SUD: negative

***Pemoline is a rarely used stimulant**

	Sample size	Drug	RX use results
Schubiner et al.[180]	48	Cocaine	MPH/mixed for ADHD, cocaine: negative
Riggs et al.[181]	69	Various	Pemoline/mixed ADHD, SUD: negative
Carpentier et al.[182]	25	Various	MPH/inpatient study ADHD: negative
Levin et al.[183]	98	Methadone/cocaine	MPH/bupropion/ADHD and cocaine: both negative
Levin et al.[177]	106	Cocaine	MPH/mixed for ADHD and cocaine
Wilens et al.[42]	147	Alcohol	Atomox/ADHD: positive: mixed alcohol
Winhusen et al.[184]	255	Nicotine	MPH/ADH: positive; mixed smoking
Konstenius et al.[185]	24	Methamphetamine	MPH/ADHD and methamphetamine: negative
McRae-Clark et al.[190]	38	Cannabis	Atomox/ADHD: mixed; THC: negative
Thurstone et al.[191]	70	Various	Atomox/ADHD neg; SUD neg
Riggs et al.[186]	303	Most cannabis	MPH/mixed ADHD and SUD
Konstenius et al.[187]	54	Amphetamine	MPH/ADHD positive; SUD: positive
Kollins et al.[188]	32	Nicotine	Lisdexamfetamine/ADHD positive; nicotine negative
Levin et al.[189]	126	Cocaine	Mixed amphetamine salt XR/ADHD and cocaine: both positive

atomoxetine was found to be superior to placebo in treating ADHD in individuals with DSM-IV alcohol dependence and outperformed the placebo group on some secondary alcohol outcome measures.[42] The therapeutic use of stimulant medications has been studied in patients with co-occurring adult ADHD and SUD, with mixed reports of efficacy.

In a recent meta-analysis, Cunill et al. found that ADHD pharmacotherapies modestly reduced ADHD symptoms but were not more effective than placebo in reducing substance use or promoting abstinence in ADHD individuals with SUDs.[192] However, the meta-analysis incorporated studies that varied considerably in terms of ADHD pharmacotherapies tested. Further, the Cunill et al. study did not include two studies that found that stimulant medication was superior on ADHD and substance use primary outcomes.[192]

Most of the studies have shown some "signal" in terms of reducing ADHD symptoms on either the primary or secondary outcome, and a minority of studies have shown some benefit of pharmacotherapy in reducing substance use, particularly if there is a large ADHD response.[177,193]

Some possible reasons for the modest response to medications for persons with an SUD with ADHD include (1) inadequate dosing; (2) less responsiveness if actively using substances; (3) lack of abstinence to clarify the ADHD diagnosis; (4) use of older, poorly absorbed sustained-release stimulant formulations; (5) additional comorbidities; and (6) poor medication adherence.

Despite these issues, there is no need for therapeutic nihilism. Two large clinical trials were conducted as part of the NIDA Clinical Trials Network (CTN) and two more recent studies in which robust dosing of stimulant medication suggests that pharmacotherapies may be useful for treating both ADHD and the SUD. The two large CTN studies compared osmotic release oral system (OROS) methylphenidate (72 mg/d) to placebo. In one study with substance-using adolescents, the active medication group was superior to placebo on some ADHD outcome measures (those that were parent-rated), although not the primary one (those that were self-rated by the adolescents). Similarly, the substance use primary outcome (self-reported drug use) was not superior in the medication arm, but the secondary outcome (urine screens) was superior in the active treatment arm compared to the placebo arm. In a secondary analysis of these data, Tamm et al. found that those who had co-occurring conduct disorder were more likely to show reductions in their substance use if they received OROS MPH compared to placebo.[194]

In the second trial with adults who had co-occurring DSM-IV nicotine dependence and ADHD, OROS MPH in combination with a nicotine patch was superior to the patch alone in reducing ADHD symptoms but not in stopping smoking.[195] However, secondary analyses have shown that certain subgroups may be more responsive to an active medication intervention. Nunes et al. found that those with greater baseline severity of ADHD symptoms or greater improvement in ADHD symptoms were more likely to become nicotine abstinent compared to placebo.[193] However, those with low ADHD severity or reduction in ADHD symptoms did not show higher abstinence rates if they received OROS-MPH compared to placebo.

Two additional published trials led to the same conclusion, namely, that robust doses of prescribed stimulant medication may be needed to effectively treat both ADHD and stimulant use disorders. Whereas a standard dose of OROS MPH (72 mg/d) was not superior to placebo in reducing ADHD symptoms or amphetamine use in ADHD adults with amphetamine use disorders,[185] a much higher dose (up to 180 mg/d) was superior in both outcome measures in a sample of recently released people with criminal offense histories, including reduction in ADHD symptoms as measured by the CAARS:SV (95% CI −14.18 to −3.28, $p = 0.002$).[187] A larger study conducted in ADHD adults with cocaine use disorder compared two robust doses of extended-release MASs (60 and 80 mg/d) to placebo and found that active medication was also more effective than placebo in reducing ADHD symptoms and promoting abstinence[189] (60 mg/d OR = 2.82, 95% CI 1.15-7.42, while 80 mg/d OR = 5.46, 95% CI, 2.25-13.27). While both studies suggest that higher than standard FDA-approved doses may be necessary to achieve a clinically meaningful effect, this work needs to be replicated among those with stimulant use disorders. Moreover, it remains an open question whether high doses are needed in other SUDs (eg, those with alcohol use disorders or cannabis use disorders). At present, there are no additional studies confirming these results.

What these studies suggest is that under closely monitored conditions and carefully selected populations, stimulant medication can be given safely to persons with an active SUD. There are two specific reasons for enhanced monitoring when prescribing stimulant medications to persons with an SUD: adverse medical and psychiatric effects, and nonmedical use and/or diversion. With respect to the former, all patients on stimulant medications should be closely monitored for adverse effects, and the same is true for those with co-existing SUDs. Prescribers should monitor for changes in blood pressure, reductions in appetite, changes in sleep, increased irritability, and signs of psychosis or mania. Caution is warranted if a patient has hypertension, or a patient is suspected of actively using other legal and illegal stimulants given the risk for compounding the risk for these side effects. Notably, one should not prescribe stimulants if a patient is taking monoamine oxidase inhibitors. Fortunately, given the short half-lives of stimulants, many of these side effects are reversible with discontinuation of the medication. Additionally, the most severe adverse effects—including mania, psychosis, extreme changes in blood pressure—are far less common than reductions in appetite, irritability, or changes in sleep. In any case, careful monitoring is always warranted.

Second, concerns arise about prescribing controlled substances to patients with ADHD. Notably, however, none of the studies evaluating a stimulant formulation reported substantial nonmedical use of medications provided. Supporting this, Winhusen et al. explored drug liking and nonmedical use of medication provided in two large CTN studies that compared OROS MPH to placebo.[195] One trial was conducted in ADHD adolescents with SUDs[186] and the other was conducted in ADHD adults with DSM-IV nicotine dependence.[184] Winhusen et al. found that adolescents with SUDs were not more likely than adults with tobacco use disorder to describe feeling euphoric with OROS MPH.[195] While the adolescents were more likely to lose pills and need replacement pills than the adults, there was no difference between those taking MPH and placebo. Nevertheless, careful monitoring for signs of nonmedical use and diversion are warranted given the potential risk.

In choosing between stimulant and nonstimulant agents for co-occurring ADHD and SUD, the risk of untreated ADHD symptoms versus the risk of stimulant nonmedical use and diversion should be balanced. In developing a treatment plan for co-occurring ADHD and SUD, these risks must be considered in light of the individual characteristics of the patient in question. The appropriateness of the medication choice should be regularly reassessed based on the patient's clinical response and overall clinical status. General recommendations for pharmacotherapy management of ADHD and co-occurring SUD follow.

To help organize treatment planning and decision-making, we propose classifying patients with co-occurring ADHD and SUD into three risk groups: lower, moderate, and severe (**Table 104-2**). The most important clinical variable in considering the use of stimulant medication is whether the SUD is active or in remission. Patients with a remote history of an SUD and a long period of abstinence from substance use likely represent a lower-risk group for prescribing stimulant medications. Patients should be counseled that their history of SUD may put them at increased risk, and general prescribing precautions should be employed (eg, use of delayed-release preparations, monitoring prescription renewal times, random pill counts, drug testing to verify medication-taking while also providing one form of surveillance for evidence of other substance use).

Patients with ongoing substance use, but not those with a diagnosis of an SUD, likely represent an increased risk of nonmedical use and diversion of prescription stimulants. For patients who are at elevated risk, additional controls need to be in place to use prescription stimulants safely. More frequent office visits, urine toxicology testing, and monitoring the pattern of substance use are prudent measures. Involvement of a responsible significant other to help monitor the medication may be considered. Alternatively, nonstimulants may be appropriate, although there may be a less robust response.

Patients with an active SUD represent a high-risk group for prescription stimulant treatment of ADHD. For these patients, given the elevated risk of nonmedical use or diversion, nonstimulant medications are likely to be a first-line choice. However, in cases where response to nonstimulant medications is suboptimal, stimulant medications may be considered in certain circumstances. For example, stimulant

TABLE 104-2 Suggested Treatment Stratification for Co-occurring ADHD/SUD

Lower-risk group (eg, 20 years abstinent from alcohol, no current illicit drug use) • Brief office intervention • Advise of the risk of combining prescription stimulants with other substances • Warn about diversion • Ongoing monitoring • ADHD response • Use vs nonmedical use pattern • Use delayed absorption formulation when prescribing stimulants
Moderate-risk group (eg, some substance use but not current use disorder; nonmedical use of stimulants in past) • Include strategies for the low-risk group • More frequent office visits • Very close attention to patterns of alcohol/drug use • Urine toxicology testing • Use delayed absorption formulation when prescribing stimulants
High-risk group (eg, active SUD) • Include strategies for the moderate-risk group • May try nonstimulants first • If poor response to nonstimulant, switch to long-acting stimulant • Require counseling, involvement with the self-help group, or referral to appropriate SUD treatment • If severe, SUD may refer for intensive intervention prior to starting medication • May need to avoid stimulants if they have history or current use disorder due to prescription stimulants or high risk of diversion of medication (ie, sold medication in the past)

treatment of a patient with an active SUD may be indicated in an intensive structured and monitored outpatient treatment program. Certain precautions are warranted when using stimulants in patients engaging in nonmedical substance use. Keeping careful records of prescriptions written and the number of pills given is crucial. By seeing the patient on a frequent basis, the number of pills per prescription can be reduced, the patient's treatment response can be closely monitored, and any potential interactions between the stimulant and other nonmedically used substances can be identified. It should be made clear to patients that urine toxicology screens will be conducted routinely and that if the patient does not show a clinically significant reduction in alcohol or drug use, other treatment strategies will be implemented. Patients should ingest their medication on a regular schedule, rather than on an as-needed basis, to avoid inadequate and intermittent relief of symptoms. Our recommendation would be to use long-acting preparations for ADHD in patients with SUD to reduce the potential for nonmedical use. Novel delivery systems such as the crush-resistant shell of Concerta,[186] the FDA-approved methylphenidate skin patch Daytrana, or the prodrug, lisdexamfetamine, are more resistant to nonmedical use and may be desirable alternatives in patients with co-occurring ADHD and SUD.

Finally, persons with co-occurring ADHD and SUD who are treated with stimulants may use them nonmedically or divert their medication. Thus, these possibilities should be discussed with the patient before a stimulant is prescribed. Like other areas of clinical uncertainty, good clinical judgment becomes crucial when deciding who will benefit from a pharmacologic treatment intervention and which medication(s) should be used. With careful ongoing monitoring and surveillance, emergent problems can be identified early, and the treatment plan modified. Possible signs and symptoms of nonmedical use of prescription stimulant medications include frequent lost prescriptions or discordant pill counts, demands for immediate-release preparations, continuously escalating doses, psychosis, agitation, and physiologic toxicity (hypertension, tachycardia, or chest pain).

Psychotherapeutic Interventions for ADHD and Substance Use Disorder

Compared to the pharmacologic treatment literature, there are fewer clinical data to suggest which nonpharmacologic approaches work best for persons with ADHD and SUDs. As in the treatment of individuals with SUDs with other psychiatric disorders, concurrently treating the symptoms of both the SUD and the ADHD is more likely to produce a positive treatment outcome than treating one disorder alone. While there has been a growing literature of psychotherapeutic approaches used to treat adult ADHD, most of these studies have combined pharmacotherapies with psychotherapy. The types of interventions studied include cognitive-behavioral therapy (CBT), which provides an assortment of cognitive and behavioral tools to address ADHD-related impairment, including assistance with organization and planning, psychoeducation about the impact of ADHD, as well as strategies to enhance problem solving and adaptive thinking, and reduce distractibility. Mindfulness-based interventions, metacognitive training, and psychoeducation alone have also been studied, though to a lesser extent. Overall, these studies suggest that combination therapy (medication and mostly cognitive therapy) is more effective than medication alone or medication plus psychoeducation.[196-198]

To our knowledge, there has not been a controlled treatment trial directly comparing psychotherapy or medication alone as a treatment for ADHD and SUD. Adults, in contrast to children, may have a greater potential to understand the effects of ADHD symptoms on their lives and thus may be better able to utilize cognitive-behavioral approaches without medication, particularly if their ADHD symptoms are not too severe. Notably, such approaches may need to be modified for persons with ADHD and SUD. For example, less emphasis should be placed on homework and more emphasis on in-session work, which might include attention and memory strategies like writing down essential information, breaking down tasks into small steps, establishing clear expectations in advance about what is to be learned, and repeating instructions to make certain a message is understood, among others. Weinstein has suggested that such strategies may have specific clinical utility for individuals with ADHD in addiction treatment settings.[199]

Using a manualized relapse prevention approach that targeted ADHD symptoms and substance use, Aviram et al.[200] found that the challenge for therapists is to identify the links among the cognitive, behavioral, and physiologic symptoms associated with ADHD and those associated with drug use. Limitations stemming from ADHD, as well as feelings of negative self-worth, may lead to substance use, which is self-reinforcing and further limits the patient's coping abilities. The limitations must be countered in treatment by providing tangible coping skills and techniques, many of which are incorporated into the relapse prevention model. To this end, one recent clinical trial of 119 adults with co-occurring ADHD SUDs compared an integrated CBT approach that targeted both ADHD symptoms and substance use to a CBT intervention that targeted substance use alone.[201] The researchers found that integrated CBT was more effective than CBT for SUD for reducing ADHD symptoms immediately posttreatment. However, ADHD symptoms did not differ between the two groups at 2-month follow-up, nor were there difference in SUD outcomes.

One experimental approach that also might be useful for persons with ADHD and SUD is node-link mapping, or NLM. Node-link mapping consists of drawing spatial-verbal displays to represent interrelationships among ideas, feelings, facts, and experiences.[200,202] Although Dansereau et al. did not specifically assess subjects for adult ADHD, they compared the efficacy of NLM to standard counseling in reducing SUD among methadone-maintained patients.[203] Individuals who received standard therapy and/or had poor attention did less well in methadone treatment. However, NLM-enhanced counseling reduced the negative effects of poor attention. Unfortunately, this promising preliminary work has not been studied more extensively.

Given that CBT is a standard empirically-based psychotherapeutic approach in treating SUDs, it is not surprising that most of the clinical trials conducted in adolescents and adults with ADHD and SUDs have used CBT as a behavioral platform. Interestingly, several studies that compared active medication and CBT to placebo and CBT found that both groups did equally well in terms of reduction in ADHD symptoms and substance use, suggesting that for some individuals CBT may be effective as a singular treatment.[177,186,190] Notably, in a secondary analysis conducted by Nunes et al., adults with co-occurring ADHD and nicotine use disorder and low severity of ADHD symptoms had greater rates of abstinence if they received CBT and placebo rather than CBT and OROS MPH; the reverse (OROS MPH superior to placebo) was true if their ADHD symptomatology was high.[193] This suggests that certain patients might benefit from CBT alone, whereas others might do better with combined treatment. However, this remains an empirical question and needs to be tested in other SUD adolescent and adult populations with ADHD.

CHILD AND ADOLESCENT TREATMENT CONSIDERATIONS

As discussed above, the evidence is clear that ADHD in children and adolescents is longitudinally associated with SUD outcomes in adolescence and young adulthood, including increased risk of SUDs. Specifically, one meta-analysis found that childhood ADHD increases the risk for alcohol use disorder during young adulthood (OR = 1.35, 95% CI = 1.11-1.64, $p < 0.01$), cannabis use disorder in young adulthood (OR = 1.51, 95% CI = 1.02-2.24, $p = 0.04$), DSM-IV psychoactive SUDs in young adulthood (ie, any alcohol or drug use; OR = 1.59, 95% CI = 1.12-2.25, $p < 0.01$), and nicotine use in middle adolescence (OR = 2.36, 95% CI 1.71-3.27, $p < 0.01$).[58] Given such adverse outcomes, early diagnosis and treatment of ADHD is critical in children and adolescents.

However, many parents are hesitant to start their children on medication for ADHD, especially stimulants, even though it is the gold standard treatment.[204,205] There are at least three reasons that parents are hesitant to treat their child's ADHD with medication. First, many worry that taking stimulants increases the risk of SUD. Second, many worry that starting their child on a medication at such a young age means they will have to be on medications their entire lives. Third, many are concerned about long-term side effects of ADHD medications, specifically stimulants. It is important for clinicians to be aware of and address these concerns head on.

Regarding the first of these, parents need to be informed that treatment of ADHD in childhood reduces the risk of future SUD, despite fears that treatment with stimulants increases the risk of SUDs—fears that are sometimes stoked in the popular press.[83,206] Owing to this concern, some parents will categorically refuse to start medication, or wait until the child is so clinically impaired that they have no choice. However, many can and will be persuaded by evidence from the scientific literature, so clinicians working with children and adolescents should be prepared to share such data.

The question of when medication for ADHD should be discontinued is still an open question. However, one recent study reported that discontinuation of treatment after 2 years of continuous treatment resulted in 40.4% of participants worsening, particularly in younger children.[207] These data suggest that continuation beyond 2 years is indicated for a sizeable portion of patients with ADHD. On the other hand, almost 60% of participants "did not worsen" after discontinuation, leading the authors to conclude that patients with ADHD should be assessed for discontinuation at least annually. Because many of these patients will worsen, however, medication should restarted at the first sign of relapse.

In terms of long-term side effects, a recent meta-analysis found that treatment with stimulants was associated with statistically significant reductions in height and weight. However, the effect size was small, and the clinical significance was minimal, as a 10-year-old boy treated with stimulants for 2 years could expect to slow height gain by 1.39 cm (0.54 inches), and slow weight gain by 1.96 kg (less than 1 lb). Notably, age, baseline physical characteristics, and dose did not moderate any of these associations.[208]

In summary, some parents may be hesitant to start their children on stimulants. However, discussing the considerable benefits of treating ADHD for future SUD and limited costs may convince them to reconsider.

SUMMARY

ADHD is a widely prevalent disorder in children, adolescents, and adults. It is overrepresented in substance-using populations and persons with an SUD have higher than expected rates of ADHD. There are several proposed mechanisms underlying the association between ADHD and SUDs, with support from genetic and neuroimaging studies. Several ADHD instruments may have utility for screening individuals with an SUD with ADHD, though a comprehensive diagnostic history is required to accurately diagnose adolescents and adults with an SUD with ADHD. Recent trials have suggested that treatment of ADHD by stimulants may lead to reduction in both ADHD symptoms and drug use across the lifespan. Fewer data exist to support the use of nonstimulants or nonpharmacologic treatment alone for adults with ADHD and an SUD. In summary, given the high co-occurrence, patients with SUDs should be evaluated for ADHD, and when ADHD is present it should be considered in formulating treatment plans.

REFERENCES

1. Barkley R. *Attention-Deficit Hyperactivity Disorder*. Guilford Press; 2006.
2. Sibley MH, Arnold LE, Swanson JM, et al. Variable patterns of remission from ADHD in the multimodal treatment study of ADHD. *Am J Psychiatry*. 2022;179:142-151.
3. Mariani JJ, Mariani JJ, Levin FR. Treatment strategies for co-occurring ADHD and substance use disorders. *Am J Addict*. 2007;16:45-56.
4. Stratton J, Gailfus D. A new approach to substance abuse treatment. Adolescents and adults with ADHD. *J Subst Abus Treat*. 1998;15:89-94.
5. Levin FR, Evans SM, Vosburg SK, Horton T, Brooks D, Ng J. Impact of attention-deficit hyperactivity disorder and other psychopathology on treatment retention among cocaine abusers in a therapeutic community. *Addict Behav*. 2004;29:1875-1882.
6. Sullivan MA, Levin FR. Attention deficit/hyperactivity disorder and substance abuse: diagnostic and therapeutic considerations. *Adult Attention Deficit Disorder: Brain Mechanisms and Life Outcomes*. Annals of the New York Academy of Sciences; 2001.
7. Carroll KM, Rounsaville BJ. History and significance of childhood attention deficit disorder in treatment-seeking cocaine abusers. *Compr Psychiatry*. 1993;34:75-82.
8. American Psychiatric Association. *Diagnostic and Statistical Manual of Mental Disorders*. American Psychiatric Association; 2000.
9. Adler LA, Faraone SV, Spencer TJ, et al. The reliability and validity of self- and investigator ratings of ADHD in adults. *J Atten Disord*. 2008;11:711-719.
10. Knivsberg AM, Andreassen AB. Behaviour, attention and cognition in severe dyslexia. *Nord J Psychiatry*. 2008;62:59-65.
11. Levin FR. Diagnosing ADHD in adults with substance use disorder: DSM-IV criteria and differential diagnosis. *J Clin Psychiatry*. 2007;68:e18.
12. Ward MF, Wender PH, Reimherr FW. The Wender Utah Rating Scale: an aid in the retrospective diagnosis of childhood attention deficit hyperactivity disorder. *Am J Psychiatry*. 1993;150:885-890.

13. Murphy K, Barkley RA. Prevalence of DSM-IV symptoms of ADHD in adult licensed drivers: implications of clinical diagnosis. *J Atten Disord.* 1996;1:147-161.
14. Kessler RC, Berglund P, Demler O, Jin R, Merikangas KR, Walters EE. Lifetime prevalence and age-of-onset distributions of DSM-IV disorders in the National Comorbidity Survey Replication. *Arch Gen Psychiatry.* 2005;62:593-602.
15. Kessler RC, Adler L, Barkely R, et al. The prevalence and correlates of adult ADHD in the United States: results from the National Comorbidity Survey Replication. *Am J Psychiatry.* 2006;163:716-723.
16. Levin FR, Evans SM, McDowell DM, Brooks DJ, Nunes E. Bupropion treatment for cocaine abuse and adult attention-deficit/hyperactivity disorder. *J Addict Dis.* 2002;21:1-16.
17. Stein MA, Sandoval R, Szumowski E, et al. Psychometric characteristics of the Wender Utah Rating Scale (WURS): reliability and factor structure for men and women. *Psychopharmacol Bull.* 1995;31:425-433.
18. Kessler RC, Adler LA, Gruber MJ, Sarawate CA, Spencer S, Van Brunt DL. Validity of the World Health Organization Adult ADHD Self-Report Scale (ASRS) Screener in a representative sample of health plan members. *Int J Methods Psychiatr Res.* 2007;16:52-65.
19. Adler L, Cohen J. Diagnosis and evaluation of adults with attention-deficit/hyperactivity disorder. *Psychiatr Clin North Am.* 2004;27:187-201.
20. Özgen H, Spijkerman R, Noack M, et al. International consensus statement for the screening, diagnosis, and treatment of adolescents with concurrent attention-deficit/hyperactivity disorder and substance use disorder. *Eur Addict Res.* 2020;26:223-232.
21. McCann BS, Roy-Byrne P. Screening and diagnostic utility of self-report attention deficit hyperactivity disorder scales in adults. *Compr Psychiatry.* 2004;45:175-183.
22. Dakwar E, Mahony A, Pavlicova M, et al. The utility of attention-deficit/hyperactivity disorder screening instruments in individuals seeking treatment for substance use disorders. *J Clin Psychiatry.* 2021;73:22036.
23. Connors C, Epstein J, Johnson D. *Conners' Adult ADHD Diagnostic Interview for DSM-IV.* Multi-Health Systems Inc; 2001.
24. van de Glind G, van den Brink W, Koeter MWJ, et al. Validity of the Adult ADHD Self-Report Scale (ASRS) as a screener for adult ADHD in treatment seeking substance use disorder patients. *Drug Alcohol Depend.* 2013;132:587-596.
25. Mayes SD, Calhoun SL, Crowell EW. Learning disabilities and ADHD. *J Learn Disabil.* 2000;33:417-424.
26. Johnson DE, Waid LR, Anton RF. Childhood hyperactivity, gender, and Cloninger's personality dimensions in alcoholics. *Addict Behav.* 1997;22:649-653.
27. Johnson DE, Epstein JN, Waid LR, Latham PK, Voronin KE, Anton RF. Neuropsychological performance deficits in adults with attention deficit/hyperactivity disorder. *Arch Clin Neuropsychol.* 2001;16:587-604.
28. Gordon M, Barkley RA, Lovett BJ. Tests and observational measures. *Attention-Deficit Hyperactivity Disorder: Handbook for Diagnosis and Treatment.* 3rd ed. Guilford Press; 2006:369-289.
29. Murphy Gordon M. Assessment of adults with ADHD. *Attention-Deficit Hyperactivity Disorder: Handbook for Diagnosis and Treatment.* 3rd ed. Guilford Press; 2006:425-450.
30. Barkley RA, Fischer M, Smallish L, Fletcher K. Young adult outcome of hyperactive children: adaptive functioning in major life activities. *J Am Acad Child Adolesc Psychiatry.* 2006;45:192-202.
31. Biederman J, Faraone SV, Spencer T, et al. Patterns of psychiatric comorbidity, cognition, and psychosocial functioning in adults with attention deficit hyperactivity disorder. *Am J Psychiatry.* 1993;150:1792-1798.
32. Mannuzza S, Klein RG. Long-term prognosis in attention-deficit/hyperactivity disorder. *Child Adolesc Psychiatr Clin N Am.* 2000;9:711-726.
33. Gascon GG, Johnson R, Burd L. Central auditory processing and attention deficit disorders. *J Child Neurol.* 1986;1:27-33.
34. Moffitt TE, Houts R, Asherson P, et al. Is adult ADHD a childhood-onset neurodevelopmental disorder? evidence from a four-decade longitudinal cohort study. *Am J Psychiatry.* 2015;172:967-977.
35. Caye A, Rocha TBM, Anselmi L, et al. Attention-deficit/hyperactivity disorder trajectories from childhood to young adulthood: evidence from a birth cohort supporting a late-onset syndrome. *JAMA Psychiatry.* 2016;73:705-712.
36. Agnew-Blais JC, Polanczyk GV, Danese A, Wertz J, Moffitt TE, Arseneault L. Evaluation of the persistence, remission, and emergence of Attention-deficit/hyperactivity disorder in young adulthood. *JAMA Psychiatry.* 2016;73:713-720.
37. Faraone SV, Biederman J. Can attention-deficit/hyperactivity disorder onset occur in adulthood? *JAMA Psychiatry.* 2016;73:655-656.
38. Daigre Blanco C, Ramos-Quiroga JA, Valero S, Bosch R, Roncero C, Gonzalvo B. Adult ADHD Self-Report Scale (ASRS-v1.1) symptom checklist in patients with substance use disorders. *Actas Esp Psiquiatr.* 2009;37:299-305.
39. Levin FR, Evans SM, McDowell DM, Kleber HD. Methylphenidate treatment for cocaine abusers with adult attention-deficit/hyperactivity disorder: a pilot study. *J Clin Psychiatry.* 1998;59:300-305.
40. Vergara-Moragues E, González-Saiz F, Rojas OL, et al. Diagnosing adult attention deficit/hyperactivity disorder in patients with cocaine dependence: discriminant validity of Barkley executive dysfunction symptoms. *Eur Addict Res.* 2011;17:279-284.
41. Avois L, Robinson N, Saudan C, Baume N, Mangin P, Saugy M. Central nervous system stimulants and sport practice. *Br J Sports Med.* 2006;40(Suppl 1):i16-i20.
42. Wilens TE, Adler LA, Adams J, et al. Misuse and diversion of stimulants prescribed for ADHD: a systematic review of the literature. *J Am Acad Child Adolesc Psychiatry.* 2008;47:21-31.
43. Biederman J, Faraone SV, Keenan K, Knee D, Tsuang MT. Family-genetic and psychosocial risk factors in DSM-III attention deficit disorder. *J Am Acad Child Adolesc Psychiatry.* 1990;29:526-533.
44. Biederman J, Faraone SV, Keenan K, et al. Further evidence for family-genetic risk factors in attention deficit hyperactivity disorder. Patterns of comorbidity in probands and relatives psychiatrically and pediatrically referred samples. *Arch Gen Psychiatry.* 1992;49:728-738.
45. Staller JA, Faraone SV. Targeting the dopamine system in the treatment of attention-deficit/hyperactivity disorder. *Expert Rev Neurother.* 2007;7:351-362.
46. Xu G, Strathearn L, Liu B, Yang B, Bao W. Twenty-year trends in diagnosed attention-deficit/hyperactivity disorder among US children and adolescents, 1997-2016. *JAMA Netw Open.* 2018;1:e181471.
47. Elkins IJ, McGue M, Iacono WG. Prospective effects of attention-deficit/hyperactivity disorder, conduct disorder, and sex on adolescent substance use and abuse. *Arch Gen Psychiatry.* 2007;64:1145-1152.
48. Chang Z, Lichtenstein P, Larsson H. The effects of childhood ADHD symptoms on early-onset substance use: a Swedish twin study. *J Abnorm Child Psychol.* 2012;40:425-435.
49. Lee SS, Humphreys KL, Flory K, Liu R, Glass K. Prospective association of childhood attention-deficit/hyperactivity disorder (ADHD) and substance use and abuse/dependence: a meta-analytic review. *Clin Psychol Rev.* 2011;31:328-341.
50. Bernardi S, Faraone SV, Cortese S, et al. The lifetime impact of attention deficit hyperactivity disorder: results from the National Epidemiologic Survey on Alcohol and Related Conditions (NESARC). *Psychol Med.* 2012;42:875-887.
51. Kessler RC, Avenevoli S, McLaughlin KA, et al. Lifetime co-morbidity of DSM-IV disorders in the US National Comorbidity Survey Replication Adolescent Supplement (NCS-A). *Psychol Med.* 2012;42:1997-2010.
52. Brinkman WB, Epstein JN, Auinger P, Tamm L, Froehlich TE. Association of attention-deficit/hyperactivity disorder and conduct disorder with early tobacco and alcohol use. *Drug Alcohol Depend.* 2015;147:183-189.
53. De Alwis D, Lynskey MT, Reiersen AM, Agrawal A. Attention-deficit/hyperactivity disorder subtypes and substance use and use disorders in NESARC. *Addict Behav.* 2014;39:1278-1285.
54. Chang Z, Lichtenstein P, Halldner L, et al. Stimulant ADHD medication and risk for substance abuse. *J Child Psychol Psychiatry.* 2014;55:878-885.

55. Pomerleau OF, Downey KK, Stelson FW, Pomerleau CS. Cigarette smoking in adult patients diagnosed with attention deficit hyperactivity disorder. *J Subst Abus.* 1995;7:373-378.
56. Tercyak KP, Lerman C, Audrain J. Association of attention-deficit/hyperactivity disorder symptoms with levels of cigarette smoking in a community sample of adolescents. *J Am Acad Child Adolesc Psychiatry.* 2002;41:799-805.
57. Kollins SH, McClernon JF, Fuemmeler BF. Association between smoking and attention-deficit/hyperactivity disorder symptoms in a population-based sample of young adults. *Arch Gen Psychiatry.* 2005;62:1142-1147.
58. Charach A, Yeung E, Climans T, Lillie E. Childhood attention-deficit/hyperactivity disorder and future substance use disorders: comparative meta-analyses. *J Am Acad Child Adolesc Psychiatry.* 2011;50:9-21.
59. Lambert NM, Hartsough CS. Prospective study of tobacco smoking and substance dependencies among samples of ADHD and non-ADHD participants. *J Learn Disabil.* 1998;31:533-544.
60. Levin FR, Evans SM, Kleber HD. Prevalence of adult attention-deficit hyperactivity disorder among cocaine abusers seeking treatment. *Drug Alcohol Depend.* 1998;52:15-25.
61. King VL, Brooner RK, Kidorf MS, Stoller KB, Mirsky AF. Attention deficit hyperactivity disorder and treatment outcome in opioid abusers entering treatment. *J Nerv Ment Dis.* 1999;187:487-495.
62. van Emmerik-van Oortmerssen K, van der Glind G, Koeter MWJ, et al. Psychiatric comorbidity in treatment-seeking substance use disorder patients with and without attention deficit hyperactivity disorder: results of the IASP study. *Addiction.* 2014;109:262-272.
63. Ginsberg Y, Quintero J, Anand E, Casillas M, Upadhyaya HP. Underdiagnosis of attention-deficit/hyperactivity disorder in adult patients: a review of the literature. *Prim Care Companion CNS Disord.* 2014;16:PCC.13r01600.
64. BSG M, Pelham WE. Attention-deficit/hyperactivity disorder and risk of substance use disorder: developmental considerations, potential pathways, and opportunities for research. *Annu Rev Clin Psychol.* 2014;10:607-639.
65. Wilens TE, Biederman J, Mick E. Does ADHD affect the course of substance abuse? Findings from a sample of adults with and without ADHD. *Am J Addict.* 1998;7:156-163.
66. Gittelman R, Mannuzza S, Shenker R, Bonagura N. Hyperactive boys almost grown up. I. Psychiatric status. *Arch Gen Psychiatry.* 1985;42:937-947.
67. Thompson LL, Riggs PD, Mikulich SK, Crowley TJ. Contribution of ADHD symptoms to substance problems and delinquency in conduct-disordered adolescents. *J Abnorm Child Psychol.* 1996;24:325-347.
68. Milberger S, Biederman J, Faraone SV, Wilens T, Chu MP. Associations between ADHD and psychoactive substance use disorders. Findings from a longitudinal study of high-risk siblings of ADHD children. *Am J Addict.* 1997;6:318-329.
69. Crowley TJ, Mikulich SK, MacDonald M, Young SE, Zerbe GO. Substance-dependent, conduct-disordered adolescent males: severity of diagnosis predicts 2-year outcome. *Drug Alcohol Depend.* 1998;49: 225-237.
70. Brook DW, Brook JS, Zhang C, Koppel J. Association between attention-deficit/hyperactivity disorder in adolescence and substance use disorders in adulthood. *Arch Pediatr Adolesc Med.* 2010;164:930-934.
71. Pardini D, White HR, Stouthamer-Loeber M. Early adolescent psychopathology as a predictor of alcohol use disorders by young adulthood. *Drug Alcohol Depend.* 2007;88(Suppl 1):S38-S49.
72. Flory K, Milich R, Lynam DR, Leukefeld C, Clayton R. Relation between childhood disruptive behavior disorders and substance use and dependence symptoms in young adulthood: individuals with symptoms of attention-deficit/hyperactivity disorder and conduct disorder are uniquely at risk. *Psychol Addict Behav.* 2003;17:151-158.
73. Mannuzza S, Klein RG, Addalli KA. Young adult mental status of hyperactive boys and their brothers: a prospective follow-up study. *J Am Acad Child Adolesc Psychiatry.* 1991;30:743-751.
74. Wilens TE, Martelon M, Joshi G, et al. Does ADHD predict substance-use disorders? A 10-year follow-up study of young adults with ADHD. *J Am Acad Child Adolesc Psychiatry.* 2011;50:543-553.
75. Biederman J, Wilens T, Mick E, Milberger S, Spencer TJ, Faraone SV. Psychoactive substance use disorders in adults with attention deficit hyperactivity disorder (ADHD): effects of ADHD and psychiatric comorbidity. *Am J Psychiatry.* 1995;152:1652-1658.
76. Mannuzza S, Klein RG, Bessler A, Malloy P, LaPadula M. Adult outcome of hyperactive boys. Educational achievement, occupational rank, and psychiatric status. *Arch Gen Psychiatry.* 1993;50:565-576.
77. Serra-Pinheiro MA, Coutinho ESF, Souza IS, et al. Is ADHD a risk factor independent of conduct disorder for illicit substance use? A meta-analysis and metaregression investigation. *J Atten Disord.* 2013;17:459-469.
78. Dalley JW, Fryer TD, Brichard L, et al. Nucleus accumbens D2/3 receptors predict trait impulsivity and cocaine reinforcement. *Science.* 2007;315:1267-1270.
79. Hoffman WF, Moore M, Templin R, McFarland B, Hitzemann RJ, Mitchell SH. Neuropsychological function and delay discounting in methamphetamine-dependent individuals. *Psychopharmacol.* 2006; 188:162-170.
80. Kelly TH, Robbins G, Martin CA, et al. Individual differences in drug abuse vulnerability: d-amphetamine and sensation-seeking status. *Psychopharmacology.* 2006;189:17-25.
81. Khantzian EJ. An extreme case of cocaine dependence and marked improvement with methylphenidate treatment. *Am J Psychiatry.* 1983;140:784-785.
82. Khantzian EJ. The self-medication hypothesis of addictive disorders: focus on heroin and cocaine dependence. *Am J Psychiatry.* 1985;142:1259-1264.
83. Schwarz A. Concerns About ADHD Practices and Amphetamine Addiction. *New York Times.* Accessed July 7, 2023. https://www.nytimes.com/2013/02/03/us/concerns-about-adhd-practices-and-amphetamine-addiction.html
84. Humphreys KL, Eng T, Lee SS. Stimulant medication and substance use outcomes: a meta-analysis. *JAMA Psychiatry.* 2013;70:740-749.
85. Groenman AP, Oosterlaan J, Rommelse N, et al. Substance use disorders in adolescents with attention deficit hyperactivity disorder: a 4-year follow-up study. *Addiction.* 2013;108:1503-1511.
86. Schoenfelder EN, Faraone SV, Kollins SH. Stimulant treatment of ADHD and cigarette smoking: a meta-analysis. *Pediatrics.* 2014;133:1070-1080.
87. McCabe SE, Dickinson K, West BT, Wilens TE. Age of onset, duration, and type of medication therapy for attention-deficit/hyperactivity disorder and substance use during adolescence: a multi-cohort national study. *J Am Acad Child Adolesc Psychiatry.* 2016;55:479-486.
88. Heikkinen M, Taipale H, Tanskanen A, Mittendorfer-Rutz E, Lähteenvuo M, Tiihonen J. Association of pharmacological treatments and hospitalization and death in individuals with amphetamine use disorders in a Swedish nationwide cohort of 13,965 patients. *JAMA Psychiatry.* 2023;80(1):31-39. doi:10.1001/jamapsychiatry.2022.3788
89. Soler Artigas M, Sánchez-Mora, Rovira P, et al. Attention-deficit/hyperactivity disorder and lifetime cannabis use: genetic overlap and causality. *Mol Psychiatry.* 2020;25:2493-2503.
90. Faraone SV, Perlis RH, Doyle AE, et al. Molecular genetics of attention-deficit/hyperactivity disorder. *Biol Psychiatry.* 2005;57:1313-1323.
91. Sharp SI, McQuillin A, HMD G. Genetics of attention-deficit hyperactivity disorder (ADHD). *Neuropharmacology.* 2009;57:590-600.
92. Pettersson E, Lichtenstein P, Larsson H, et al. Genetic influences on eight psychiatric disorders based on family data of 4 408 646 full and half-siblings, and genetic data of 333,748 cases and controls. *Psychol Med.* 2019;49:1166-1173.
93. Faraone SV, Biederman J, Spencer T, et al. Diagnosing adult attention deficit hyperactivity disorder: are late onset and subthreshold diagnoses valid? *Am J Psychiatry.* 2006;163:1720-1729.
94. Posner J, Polanczyk GV, Sonuga-Barke E. Attention-deficit hyperactivity disorder. *Lancet.* 2020;395:450-462.
95. Faraone SV, Biederman J. Neurobiology of attention-deficit hyperactivity disorder. *Biol Psychiatry.* 1998;44:951-958.

96. Thapar A, O'Donovan M, Owen MJ. The genetics of attention deficit hyperactivity disorder. *Hum Mol Genet.* 2005;14 Spec No. 2: R275-R282.
97. Dadds MR, Schollar-Root O, Lenroot R, Moul C, Hawes DJ. Epigenetic regulation of the DRD4 gene and dimensions of attention-deficit/hyperactivity disorder in children. *Eur Child Adolesc Psychiatry.* 2016;25:1081-1089.
98. Shook D, Brady C, Lee PS, et al. Effect of dopamine transporter genotype on caudate volume in childhood ADHD and controls. *Am J Med Genet B Neuropsychiatr Genet.* 2011;156B:28-35.
99. Franklin TR, Wang Z, Li Y, et al. Dopamine transporter genotype modulation of neural responses to smoking cues: confirmation in a new cohort. *Addict Biol.* 2011;16:308-322.
100. Grzywacz A, Samochowiec J. Case-control, family based and screening for DNA sequence variation in the dopamine transporter gene polymorphism DAT 1 in alcohol dependence. *Psychiatr Pol.* 2008;42: 443-452.
101. Fernández-Jaén A, López-Martín S, Albert J, et al. Cortical thickness differences in the prefrontal cortex in children and adolescents with ADHD in relation to dopamine transporter (DAT1) genotype. *Psychiatry Res.* 2015;233:409-417.
102. Lai JH, Zhu YS, Huo ZH, et al. Association study of polymorphisms in the promoter region of DRD4 with schizophrenia, depression, and heroin addiction. *Brain Res.* 2010;1359:227-232.
103. Muglia P, Jain U, Macciardi F, Kennedy JL. Adult attention deficit hyperactivity disorder and the dopamine D4 receptor gene. *Am J Med Genet.* 2000;96:273-277.
104. George SR, Cheng R, Nguyen T, Israel Y, O'Dowd BF. Polymorphisms of the D4 dopamine receptor alleles in chronic alcoholism. *Biochem Biophys Res Commun.* 1993;196:107-114.
105. Comings DE, Gonzalez N, Wu S, et al. Studies of the 48 bp repeat polymorphism of the DRD4 gene in impulsive, compulsive, addictive behaviors: tourette syndrome, ADHD, pathological gambling, and substance abuse. *Am J Med Genet.* 1999;88:358-368.
106. Lasky-Su J, Anney RJL, Neale BM, et al. Genome-wide association scan of the time to onset of attention deficit hyperactivity disorder. *Am J Med Genet B Neuropsychiatr Genet.* 2008;147B:1355-1358.
107. Gizer IR, Ficks C, Waldman ID. Candidate gene studies of ADHD: a meta-analytic review. *Hum Genet.* 2009;126:51-90.
108. Elia J, Capasso M, Zaheer Z, et al. Candidate gene analysis in an on-going genome-wide association study of attention-deficit hyperactivity disorder: suggestive association signals in ADRA1A. *Psychiatr Genet.* 2009;19:134-141.
109. Demontis D, Walters RK, Martin J, et al. Discovery of the first genome-wide significant risk loci for attention deficit/hyperactivity disorder. *Nat Genet.* 2019;51:63-75.
110. Stergiakouli E, Martin J, Hamshere ML, et al. Association between polygenic risk scores for attention-deficit hyperactivity disorder and educational and cognitive outcomes in the general population. *Int J Epidemiol.* 2017;46:421-428.
111. Walton E, Pingault JB, Cecil CAM, et al. Epigenetic profiling of ADHD symptoms trajectories: a prospective, methylome-wide study. *Mol Psychiatry.* 2017;22:250-256.
112. Hoogman M, Muetzel R, Guimaraes JP, et al. Brain imaging of the cortex in ADHD: a coordinated analysis of large-scale clinical and population-based samples. *Am J Psychiatry.* 2019;176:531-542. doi:10.1176/appi.ajp.2019.18091033
113. Hoogman M, Bralten J, Hibar DP, et al. Subcortical brain volume differences in participants with attention deficit hyperactivity disorder in children and adults: a cross-sectional mega-analysis. *Lancet Psychiatry.* 2017;4:310-319.
114. Sowell ER, Thompson PM, Welcome SE, Henkenius AL, Toga AW, Peterson BS. Cortical abnormalities in children and adolescents with attention-deficit hyperactivity disorder. *Lancet.* 2003;362:1699-1707.
115. Arnsten AFT. Fundamentals of attention-deficit/hyperactivity disorder: circuits and pathways. *J Clin Psychiatry.* 2006;67:7-12.
116. Spencer TJ, Biederman J, Mick E. Attention-deficit/hyperactivity disorder: diagnosis, lifespan, comorbidities, and neurobiology. *Ambul Pediatr.* 2007;7:73-81.
117. Seidman LJ, Valera EM, Makris N. Structural brain imaging of attention-deficit/hyperactivity disorder. *Biol Psychiatry.* 2005;57:1263-1272.
118. Castellanos FX, Lee PP, Sharp W, et al. Developmental trajectories of brain volume abnormalities in children and adolescents with attention-deficit/hyperactivity disorder. *JAMA.* 2002;288:1740-1748.
119. Bernanke J, Luna A, Chang L, Bruno E, Dworkin J, Posner J. Structural brain measures among children with and without ADHD in the Adolescent Brain and Cognitive Development Study cohort: a cross-sectional US population-based study. *Lancet Psychiatry.* 2022;9:222-231.
120. Posner J, Park C, Wang Z. Connecting the dots: a review of resting connectivity MRI studies in attention-deficit/hyperactivity disorder. *Neuropsychol Rev.* 2014;24:3-15.
121. Hart H, Radua J, Nakao T, Mataix-Cols D, Rubia K. Meta-analysis of functional magnetic resonance imaging studies of inhibition and attention in attention-deficit/hyperactivity disorder. *JAMA Psychiatry.* 2013;70:185.
122. Adisetiyo V, Gray KM. Neuroimaging the neural correlates of increased risk for substance use disorders in attention-deficit/hyperactivity disorder—a systematic review. *Am J Addict.* 2017;26:99-111.
123. Castellanos-Ryan N, Struve M, Whelan R, et al. Neural and cognitive correlates of the common and specific variance across externalizing problems in young adolescence. *Am J Psychiatry.* 2014;171:1310-1019.
124. Hulvershorn LA, Finn P, Hummer TA, et al. Cortical activation deficits during facial emotion processing in youth at high risk for the development of substance use disorders. *Drug Alcohol Depend.* 2013;131:230-237.
125. van Ewijk H, Groenman AP, Zwiers MP, et al. Smoking and the developing brain: altered white matter microstructure in attention-deficit/hyperactivity disorder and healthy controls. *Hum Brain Mapp.* 2015;36:1180-1189.
126. Kalivas PW, Volkow ND. The neural basis of addiction: a pathology of motivation and choice. *Am J Psychiatry.* 2005;162:1403-1413.
127. Nutt DJ, Lingford-Hughes A, Erritzoe D, PRA S. The dopamine theory of addiction: 40 years of highs and lows. *Nat Rev Neurosci.* 2015;16:305-312.
128. Casey KF, Benkelfat C, Cherkasova MV, Baker GB, Dagher A, Leyton M. Reduced dopamine response to amphetamine in subjects at ultra-high risk for addiction. *Biol Psychiatry.* 2014;76:23-30.
129. Prince J. Catecholamine dysfunction in attention-deficit/hyperactivity disorder: an update. *J Clin Psychopharmacol.* 2008;28:S39-S45.
130. Valera EM, Faraone SV, Murray KE, Seidman LJ. Meta-analysis of structural imaging findings in attention-deficit/hyperactivity disorder. *Biol Psychiatry.* 2007;61:1361-1369.
131. Klein RG, Mannuzza S, Ramos Olazagasti MA, et al. Clinical and functional outcome of childhood attention-deficit/hyperactivity disorder 33 years later. *Arch Gen Psychiatry.* 2012;69:1295-1303.
132. Greenfield B, Hechtman L, Weiss G. Two subgroups of hyperactives as adults: correlations of outcome. *Can J Psychiatry.* 1988;33:505-508.
133. Biederman J, Mick E, Surman C, et al. A randomized, placebo-controlled trial of OROS methylphenidate in adults with attention-deficit/hyperactivity disorder. *Biol Psychiatry.* 2006;59:829-835.
134. Biederman J, Petty CR, Monuteaux MC, et al. Adult psychiatric outcomes of girls with attention deficit hyperactivity disorder: 11-year follow-up in a longitudinal case-control study. *Am J Psychiatry.* 2010;167:409-417.
135. Babinski DE, Pelham WE Jr, Molina BSG, et al. Women with childhood ADHD: comparisons by diagnostic group and gender. *J Psychopathol Behav Assess.* 2011;33:420-429.
136. Molina BSG, Pelham WE, Pelham WE Jr. Childhood predictors of adolescent substance use in a longitudinal study of children with ADHD. *J Abnorm Psychol.* 2003;112:497-507.
137. Young S, Wells J, Gudjonsson GH. Predictors of offending among prisoners: the role of attention-deficit hyperactivity disorder and substance use. *J Psychopharmacol.* 2011;25:1524-1532.

138. González RA, Gudjonsson GH, Wells J, Young S. The role of emotional distress and ADHD on institutional behavioral disturbance and recidivism among offenders. *J Atten Disord.* 2016;20:368-378.
139. Biederman J, Wilens TE, Mick E, Faraone SV, Spencer T. Does attention-deficit hyperactivity disorder impact the developmental course of drug and alcohol abuse and dependence? *Biol Psychiatry.* 1998;44:269-273.
140. Katzman MA, Bilkey TS, Chokka PR, Fallu A, Klassen LJ. Adult ADHD and comorbid disorders: clinical implications of a dimensional approach. *BMC Psychiatry.* 2017;17(1):302. doi:10.1186/s12888-017-1463-3
141. Kast KA, Rao V, Wilens TE. Pharmacotherapy for attention-deficit/hyperactivity disorder and retention in outpatient substance use disorder treatment: a Retrospective Cohort Study. *J Clin Psychiatry.* 2021;82(2):20m13598. doi:10.4088/JCP.20m13598
142. Torgersen T, Gjervan B, Rasmussen K. Treatment of adult ADHD: is current knowledge useful to clinicians? *Neuropsychiatr Dis Treat.* 2008;4:177-186.
143. Faraone SV, Glatt SJ. A comparison of the efficacy of medications for adult attention-deficit/hyperactivity disorder using meta-analysis of effect sizes. *J Clin Psychiatry.* 2010;71:754-763.
144. Koesters M, Becker T, Kilian R, Fegert JM, Weinmann S. Limits of meta-analysis: methylphenidate in the treatment of adult attention-deficit hyperactivity disorder. *J Psychopharmacol.* 2009;23:733-744.
145. Iversen L. Neurotransmitter transporters and their impact on the development of psychopharmacology. *Br J Pharmacol.* 2006;147:S82-S88.
146. Heal DJ, Smith SL, Gosden J, Nutt DJ. Amphetamine, past and present—a pharmacological and clinical perspective. *J Psychopharmacol.* 2013;27:479-496.
147. Faraone SV, Spencer T, Aleardi M, Pagano C, Biederman J. Meta-analysis of the efficacy of methylphenidate for treating adult attention-deficit/hyperactivity disorder. *J Clin Psychopharmacol.* 2004;24:24-29.
148. Spencer T, Biederman J, Wilens T, et al. Efficacy of a mixed amphetamine salts compound in adults with attention-deficit/hyperactivity disorder. *Arch Gen Psychiatry.* 2001;58:775-782.
149. Jasinski DR, Krishnan S. Abuse liability and safety of oral lisdexamfetamine dimesylate in individuals with a history of stimulant abuse. *J Psychopharmacol.* 2009;23:419-427.
150. Connor DF, Fletcher KE, Swanson JM. A meta-analysis of clonidine for symptoms of attention-deficit hyperactivity disorder. *J Am Acad Child Adolesc Psychiatry.* 1999;38:1551-1559.
151. Greenhill LL, Biederman J, Boellner SW, et al. A randomized, double-blind, placebo-controlled study of modafinil film-coated tablets in children and adolescents with attention-deficit/hyperactivity disorder. *J Am Acad Child Adolesc Psychiatry.* 2006;45:503-511.
152. Swanson JM, Greenhill LL, Lopez FA, et al. Modafinil film-coated tablets in children and adolescents with attention-deficit/hyperactivity disorder: results of a randomized, double-blind, placebo-controlled, fixed-dose study followed by abrupt discontinuation. *J Clin Psychiatry.* 2006;67:137-147.
153. Dackis CA, Kampman KM, Lynch KG, Pettinati HM, O'Brien CP. A double-blind, placebo-controlled trial of modafinil for cocaine dependence. *Neuropsychopharmacology.* 2005;30:205-211.
154. Dackis CA, Kampman KM, Lynch KG, et al. A double-blind, placebo-controlled trial of modafinil for cocaine dependence. *J Subst Abuse Treat.* 2012;43:303-312.
155. SAMHSA. *Key Substance Use and Mental Health Indicators in the United States: Results from the 2020 National Survey on Drug Use and Health.* HHS Publication No. PEP21-07-01-003, NSDUH Series H-56. Accessed July 7, 2023. https://ia802303.us.archive.org/28/items/2020-nsduh/2020%20nsduh.pdf
156. SE MC, West BT, Teter CJ, Boyd CJ. Trends in medical use, diversion, and nonmedical use of prescription medications among college students from 2003 to 2013: connecting the dots. *Addict Behav.* 2014;39:1176-1182.
157. Goodhines PA, Taylor LE, Zaso MJ, Antshel KM, Park A. Prescription stimulant misuse and risk correlates among racially-diverse urban adolescents. *Subst Use Misuse.* 2020;55:2258-2267.
158. SE MC, Teter CJ, Boyd CJ, Wilens TE, Schepis TS. Sources of prescription medication misuse among young adults in the United States. *J Clin Psychiatry.* 2018;79:33-40.
159. Garnier LM, Arria AM, Caldeira KM, Vincent KB, O'Grady KE, Wish ED. Sharing and selling of prescription medications in a college student sample. *J Clin Psychiatry.* 2010;71:262-269.
160. Findling RL. Evolution of the treatment of attention-deficit/hyperactivity disorder in children: a review. *Clin Ther.* 2008;30:942-957.
161. Mao AR, Babcock T, Brams M. ADHD in adults: current treatment trends with consideration of abuse potential of medications. *J Psychiatr Pract.* 2011;17:241-250.
162. Mariani JJ, Levin FR. Psychostimulant treatment of cocaine dependence. *Psychiatr Clin North Am.* 2012;35:425-439.
163. Volkow ND, Swanson JM. Variables that affect the clinical use and abuse of methylphenidate in the treatment of ADHD. *Am J Psychiatry.* 2003;160:1909-1918.
164. Cassidy TA, Varughese S, Russo L, Budman SH, Eaton TA, Butler SF. Nonmedical use and diversion of ADHD stimulants among U.S. adults ages 18-49: a National Internet Survey. *J Atten Disord.* 2015;19:630-640.
165. Spencer TJ, Biederman J, Ciccone PE, et al. PET study examining pharmacokinetics, detection and likeability, and dopamine transporter receptor occupancy of short- and long-acting oral methylphenidate. *Am J Psychiatry.* 2006;163:387-395.
166. Wilens TE, Gignac M, Swezey A, Monuteaux MC, Biederman J. Characteristics of adolescents and young adults with ADHD who divert or misuse their prescribed medications. *J Am Acad Child Adolesc Psychiatry.* 2006;45:408-414.
167. Collins SL, Levin FR, Foltin RW, Kleber HD, Evans SM. Response to cocaine, alone and in combination with methylphenidate, in cocaine abusers with ADHD. *Drug Alcohol Depend.* 2006;82:158-167.
168. Adler LA, Spencer TJ, Milton DR, Moore RJ, Michelson D. Long-term, open-label study of the safety and efficacy of atomoxetine in adults with attention-deficit/hyperactivity disorder: an interim analysis. *J Clin Psychiatry.* 2005;66:294-299.
169. Michelson D, Adler L, Spencer T, et al. Atomoxetine in adults with ADHD: two randomized, placebo-controlled studies. *Biol Psychiatry.* 2003;53:112-120.
170. Faraone SV, Buitelaar J. Comparing the efficacy of stimulants for ADHD in children and adolescents using meta-analysis. *Eur Child Adolesc Psychiatry.* 2010;19:353-364.
171. Spencer TJ, Greenbaum M, Ginsberg LD, Murphy WR. Safety and effectiveness of coadministration of guanfacine extended release and psychostimulants in children and adolescents with attention-deficit/hyperactivity disorder. *J Child Adolesc Psychopharmacol.* 2009;19:501-510.
172. Connor DF, Findling RL, Kollins SH, et al. Effects of guanfacine extended release on oppositional symptoms in children aged 6-12 years with attention-deficit hyperactivity disorder and oppositional symptoms: a randomized, double-blind, placebo-controlled trial. *CNS Drugs.* 2010;24:755-768.
173. Sallee FR, Lyne A, Wigal T, JJ MG. Long-term safety and efficacy of guanfacine extended release in children and adolescents with attention-deficit/hyperactivity disorder. *J Child Adolesc Psychopharmacol.* 2009; 19:215-226.
174. Wolraich ML, Wibbelsman CJ, Brown TE, et al. Attention-deficit/hyperactivity disorder among adolescents: a review of the diagnosis, treatment, and clinical implications. *Pediatrics.* 2005;115:1734-1746.
175. Conners CK, Casat CD, Gualtieri CT, et al. Bupropion hydrochloride in attention deficit disorder with hyperactivity. *J Am Acad Child Adolesc Psychiatry.* 1996;35:1314-1321.
176. Levin FR, Bisaga A, Raby W, et al. Effects of major depressive disorder and attention-deficit/hyperactivity disorder on the outcome of treatment for cocaine dependence. *J Subst Abus Treat.* 2008;34:80-89.
177. Levin FR, Evans SM, Brooks DJ, Garawi F. Treatment of cocaine dependent treatment seekers with adult ADHD: double-blind comparison of methylphenidate and placebo. *Drug Alcohol Depend.* 2007;87(1):20-29.
178. Olvera RL, Pliszka SR, Luh J, Tatum R. An open trial of venlafaxine in the treatment of attention-deficit/hyperactivity disorder in children and adolescents. *J Child Adolesc Psychopharmacol.* 1996;6:241-250.

179. Amiri S, Farhang S, Ghoreishizadeh MA, Malek A, Mohammadzadeh S. Double-blind controlled trial of venlafaxine for treatment of adults with attention deficit/hyperactivity disorder. *Hum Psychopharmacol.* 2012;27:76-81.
180. Schubiner H, Saules KK, Arfken CL, et al. Double-blind placebocontrolled trial of methylphenidate in the treatment of adult ADHD patients with comorbid cocaine dependence. *Exp Clin Psychopharmacol.* 2002;10(3):286-294.
181. Riggs PD, Hall SK, Mikulich-Gilbertson SK, Lohman M, Kayser A. A randomized controlled trial of pemoline for attention-deficit/hyperactivity disorder in substance-abusing adolescents. *J Am Acad Child Adolesc Psychiatry.* 2004;43(4):420-429.
182. Carpentier PJ, de Jong CA, Dijkstra BA, Verbrugge CA, Krabbe PF. A controlled trial of methylphenidate in adults with attention deficit/hyperactivity disorder and substance use disorders. *Addiction.* 2005;100(12):1868-1874.
183. Levin FR, Evans SM, Brooks DJ, Kalbag AS, Garawi F, Nunes EV. Treatment of methadone-maintained patients with adult ADHD: double-blind comparison of methylphenidate, bupropion and placebo. *Drug Alcohol Depend.* 2006;81(2):137-148.
184. Winhusen TM, Somoza EC, Brigham GS, et al. Impact of attention-deficit/hyperactivity disorder (ADHD) treatment on smoking cessation intervention in ADHD smokers: a randomized, double-blind, placebo-controlled trial. *J Clin Psychiatry.* 2010;71:1680-1688.
185. Konstenius M, Jayaram-Lindström N, Beck O, Franck J. Sustained release methylphenidate for the treatment of ADHD in amphetamine abusers: a pilot study. *Drug Alcohol Depend.* 2010;108:130-133.
186. Riggs PD, Winhusen T, Davies RD, et al. Randomized controlled trial of osmotic-release methylphenidate with cognitive-behavioral therapy in adolescents with attention-deficit/hyperactivity disorder and substance use disorders. *J Am Acad Child Adolesc Psychiatry.* 2011;50:903-914.
187. Konstenius M, Jayaram-Lindström N, Guterstam J, Beck O, Philips B, Franck J. Methylphenidate for attention deficit hyperactivity disorder and drug relapse in criminal offenders with substance dependence: a 24-week randomized placebo-controlled trial. *Addiction.* 2014;109:440-449.
188. Kollins SH, English JS, Itchon-Ramos N, et al. A pilot study of lis-dexamfetamine dimesylate (LDX/SPD489) to facilitate smoking cessation in nicotine-dependent adults with ADHD. *J Atten Disord.* 2014;18(2):158-168. doi:10.1177/1087054712440320
189. Levin FR, Mariani JJ, Specker S, et al. Extended-release mixed amphetamine salts vs placebo for comorbid adult attention-deficit/hyperactivity disorder and cocaine use disorder: a randomized clinical trial. *JAMA Psychiatry.* 2015;72:593-602.
190. McRae-Clark AL, Carter RE, Killeen TK, Carpenter MJ, White KG, Brady KT. A placebo-controlled trial of atomoxetine in marijuana-dependent individuals with attention deficit hyperactivity disorder. *Am J Addict.* 2010;19:481-489.
191. Thurstone C, Riggs PD, Salomonsen-Sautel S, Mikulich-Gilbertson SK. Randomized, controlled trial of atomoxetine for attention-deficit/hyperactivity disorder in adolescents with substance use disorder. *J Am Acad Child Adolesc Psychiatry.* 2010;49(6):573-582. doi:10.1016/j.jaac.2010.02.013
192. Cunill R, Castells X, Tobias A, Capellà D. Atomoxetine for attention deficit hyperactivity disorder in the adulthood: a meta-analysis and meta-regression. *Pharmacoepidemiol Drug Saf.* 2013;22:961-969.
193. Nunes EV, Covey LS, Brigham G, et al. Treating nicotine dependence by targeting attention-deficit/hyperactivity disorder (ADHD) with OROS methylphenidate: the role of baseline ADHD severity and treatment response. *J Clin Psychiatry.* 2013;74:983-990.
194. Tamm L, Trello-Rishel K, Riggs P, et al. Predictors of treatment response in adolescents with comorbid substance use disorder and attention-deficit/hyperactivity disorder. *J Subst Abuse Treat.* 2013;44:224-230.
195. Winhusen TM, Lewis DF, Riggs PD, et al. Subjective effects, misuse, and adverse effects of osmotic-release methylphenidate treatment in adolescent substance abusers with attention-deficit/hyperactivity disorder. *J Child Adolesc Psychopharmacol.* 2011;21:455463.
196. March JS, Swanson JM, Arnold LE, et al. Anxiety as a predictor and outcome variable in the multimodal treatment study of children with ADHD (MTA). *J Abnorm Child Psychol.* 2000;28:527-541.
197. Safren SA, Sprich S, Mimiaga MJ, et al. Cognitive behavioral therapy vs relaxation with educational support for medication-treated adults with ADHD and persistent symptoms: a randomized controlled trial. *JAMA.* 2010;304:875-880.
198. Philipsen A. Psychotherapy in adult attention deficit hyperactivity disorder: implications for treatment and research. *Expert Rev Neurother.* 2012;12:1217-1225.
199. Weinstein CS. Cognitive remediation strategies: an adjunct to the psychotherapy of adults with attention-deficit hyperactivity disorder. *J Psychother Pract Res.* 1994;3:44-57.
200. Aviram RB, Rhum M, Levin FR. Psychotherapy of adults with comorbid attention-deficit/hyperactivity disorder and psychoactive substance use disorder. *J Psychother Pr Res.* 2001;10:179-186.
201. van Emmerik-van Oortmerssen K, Vedel E, Kramer FJ, et al. Integrated cognitive behavioral therapy for ADHD in adult substance use disorder patients: results of a randomized clinical trial. *Drug Alcohol Depend.* 2019;197:28-36.
202. Dees SM, Dansereau DF, Simpson DD. A visual representation system for drug abuse counselors. *J Subst Abus Treat.* 1994;11:517-523.
203. Dansereau DF, Joe GW, Simpson DD. Attentional difficulties and the effectiveness of a visual representation strategy for counseling drug-addicted clients. *Int J Addict.* 1995;30:371-386.
204. Vitulano LA, Mitchell JT, Vitulano ML, et al. Parental perspectives on attention-deficit/hyperactivity disorder treatments for children. *Clin Child Psychol Psychiatry.* 2022;27(4):1019-1032. doi:10.1177/13591045221108836
205. Pliszka S. Practice parameter for the assessment and treatment of children and adolescents with attention-deficit/hyperactivity disorder. *J Am Acad Child Adolesc Psychiatry.* 2007;46:894-921.
206. Wedge M. Are ADHD drugs safe in the long term? *Psychology Today.* Accessed July 7, 2023. https://www.psychologytoday.com/us/blog/suffer-the-children/201405/are-adhd-drugs-safe-in-the-long-term
207. Matthijssen AFM, Dietrich A, Bierens M, et al. Continued benefits of methylphenidate in ADHD after 2 years in clinical practice: a randomized placebo-controlled discontinuation study. *Am J Psychiatry.* 2019;176:754-762.
208. Carucci S, Balia C, Gagliano A, et al. Long term methylphenidate exposure and growth in children and adolescents with ADHD. A systematic review and meta-analysis. *Neurosci Biobehav Rev.* 2021;120:509-525.

CHAPTER

105 Co-occurring Personality Disorders and Substance Use Disorders

Stephen Ross, Adam Demner, Daniel Roberts, Petros Petridis, and Michael Torres

CHAPTER OUTLINE

- Introduction
- Definitions/classification
- Epidemiology
- Diagnosis: Theoretical issues
- Diagnosis: Practical issues
- Treatment
- Conclusions

INTRODUCTION

Personality disorders (PDs) are defined by DSM-5 as enduring patterns of inner experience and behavior that deviate markedly from the expectations of the individual's culture that are deep-seated, pervasive, and produce psychopathological symptoms affecting cognition, emotion, interpersonal functioning, and impulse regulation.[1] The patterns cause repeated conflicts with one's social and occupational environment and lead to emotional distress.

DEFINITIONS/CLASSIFICATION

The DSM-5 employs a categorical classification system placing the PDs into three *clusters* based on symptom similarities (A, B, C) that produce 10 distinct disorders.

- Cluster A (paranoid, schizoid, schizotypal): These disorders are characterized by odd or eccentric cognition and behavior related to the schizophrenia spectrum.[2]
- Cluster B (antisocial, borderline, histrionic, narcissistic): These disorders are marked by emotional, dramatic, or erratic behavior and are related to trait impulsivity and/or affect dysregulation and are on the spectrum with impulse disorders.[3]
- Cluster C (avoidant, dependent, obsessive-compulsive): These disorders are marked by anxious symptoms, are related to trait anxiety or compulsivity, and are on the spectrum with anxiety disorders.[4]

The onset of PDs is in late adolescence or early adulthood when personality trait patterns become stable.[1] Although PDs tend to have a chronic course of illness, longitudinal studies have generally supported the notion that PDs tend to improve over time from the perspective of decreases in clinical symptomatology, although the evidence is more mixed for clusters A and C disorders.[5-9]

PDs and substance use disorders (SUDs) are highly associated with each other, especially in mental health and SUD treatment settings where they represent the norm in terms of comorbidity.[10,11] Screening and the use of standardized assessment instruments are vital components of diagnostic formulation to determine the presence of a PD, which is distinguishable from or co-occurring with an SUD. Given the epidemiological data where the majority of patients with a PD have a co-occurring SUD and vice versa,[10] an *a priori* diagnostic assumption should be that there are two separate problems until proven otherwise. Patients with co-occurring SUDs and PDs can benefit from treatment as much as those without PDs, but the presence of a PD does negatively affect the course of treatment of the SUD and is associated with worse outcomes.[12] This chapter will review the following regarding PDs and co-occurring SUDs: epidemiology; diagnostic assessment (theoretical and practical); and treatment (outcomes, psychosocial, pharmacological).

EPIDEMIOLOGY

PDs and SUDs are both prevalent in the general population. In looking at 5 well-designed (ie, use of DSM-IV, or ICD-10 diagnostic criteria and structured or semistructured interviews) community surveys of PDs published since 2000 with sample sizes ranging from 214 (NCS-R) to 43,093 (NESARC), the estimated prevalence of any PD in the general population ranged from 4.4% to 13.4% with a median of 9.6% and with cluster C disorders (obsessive-compulsive personality disorder [OCPD] and avoidant PD) being the most commonly diagnosed.[13] In comparison, SUDs affect 40.2 million (14.5% of the population) individuals 12 years of age or older, including both alcohol or illicit drugs usage.[14] This does not include nicotine/tobacco use disorders, which affect 13% of the population.[15]

In addition to both being prevalent conditions by themselves in the general population, PDs and SUDs are intimately related in community samples. For instance, in a nonpatient sample of 790 individuals who were relatives of both controls and psychiatric patients, of those who had any PD, 43% and 53%, respectively, met criteria for a lifetime alcohol use disorder (AUD) or drug use disorder (DUD).[16] Using revised diagnostic criteria from the NESARC community sample, Trull and colleagues found that each PD was strongly associated with lifetime DSM-IV-TR substance dependence syndromes with the highest rates of co-occurrence as follows: alcohol dependence co-occurring with anti-social personality disorder (ASPD) (51%), histrionic PD (50%), and borderline personality disorder (BPD) (47%); drug dependence co-occurring with histrionic PD (30%), dependent PD (27%), and ASPD (25%); and nicotine dependence co-occurring with ASPD (57%), BPD (54%), and dependent PD (54%).[11]

The rates of PDs in psychiatric or addiction treatment settings are also significantly increased.[10,16] In selecting well-designed studies (ie, random selection, sample size ≥100, use of standardized diagnostic instruments), Verheul reported on the prevalence rates of PDs: 45% to 80% (median 60%) in psychiatric patients and 35% to 73% (median 57%) in patients treated for SUDs.[10] Even though cluster C diagnoses (OCPD, avoidant PD) are the most common PD diagnoses in the general population, cluster B disorders (ASPD and BPD) are the most commonly associated with SUDs in either community or treatment (SUD or traditional psychiatric) samples. In one study examining PDs in first-admission patients with SUDs, 46% of the patients with an SUD had at least one PD with ASPD being most prevalent (16%) followed closely by BPD (13%) and then paranoid, avoidant, and obsessive-compulsive PDs (all at 8%). In a review of comorbidity data between BPD and SUD, Trull et al. reported that among those seeking addiction treatments, rates of BPD ranged from 10% to 72.7% and conversely among those receiving treatment for BPD, the prevalence of current SUDs is between 28.5% and 72.7%.[17] From the ECA study, ASPD (among men) was more frequently diagnosed with an SUD than any other Axis I or II disorder with 83% of individuals with ASPD also meeting criteria for an SUD and with ASPD being diagnosed in 18% of those with a DUD and 14% with an AUD.[18]

In summary, there is substantial co-morbidity of PDs and SUDs in community and treatment samples with ASPD and BPD being most commonly associated with SUDs. In treatment settings, clinicians should be aware of this epidemiologic data to optimize diagnostic assessment and treatment planning.

DIAGNOSIS: THEORETICAL ISSUES

Before discussing the practical aspects of clinical diagnostic assessments for patients with co-occurring PDs and SUDs, a brief discussion of the etiological theories of these disorders is in order as well as any evidence that supports a particular model. Given the markedly high co-occurrence of SUDs and PDs (especially ASPD and BPD), a correlation between the two has long been assumed, theorized, and studied with the evidence for an association derived from genetic, epidemiological, retrospective, and longitudinal studies.[19] In addition to a discussion about the etiology of PDs, two main classification systems to model PDs comorbid with SUDs will be discussed: *etiological and co-occurring.*

Etiology of PDs

PDs are thought to arise from an interaction between biological (genes, temperament), psychological, familial, and sociocultural risk factors over time, with the risk increasing with the number of risk factors involved. *Temperament* is an individual's biologically determined innate disposition or pattern of thinking, feeling, and behaving, and accounts for the majority of variance in *personality traits.*[20] The biological basis of temperament is supported by animal and human studies with parallels seen in temperament structure (ie, defensive reactions to fear and anger; approach reactions of activity and pleasure to high-intensity stimulation; attention and orienting).[21,22] There is no simple relationship between single genes and temperament and it is likely that temperament is polygenetically determined.[23] *Personality traits* are defined as individual variation in behavior, cognition, and affect that are stable over time and represent a combination of temperament and longitudinal experience.[24] In dimensional models of personality psychopathology, PDs represent an amplification and psychopathological expression of normative personality traits leading to functional impairment.[5] Both personality traits[25-27] and PDs have a genetic, heritable component with twin studies demonstrating heritability of PDs ranging from 40% (for cluster A disorders) to 60% (for cluster B and C disorders).[28] Longitudinal studies have demonstrated a considerable link between temperament, adult personality, and personality psychopathology.[29]

Co-Occurring Models

In co-occurring models, there is the presence of two distinct disorders, one psychiatric other than an SUD and one substance related. One possibility relating the two disorders is that both have unique and independent etiological determinants and that both disorders *co-occur randomly*. Alternatively, in the *common factor* model, the co-occurrence of both a PD and an SUD is caused by shared vulnerabilities or risk factors, ranging from genetic to sociocultural. This model would be most applicable to the interaction between SUD and certain PDs (ASPD and BPD) because of the considerable comorbidity as mentioned above. This model is best evaluated by twin, family and adoption studies. If shared genetic risk factors to both a PD and SUD were to account for the increased comorbidity, an elevated incidence of the one disorder (ie, SUD) would be expected in relatives of individuals with the other disorder (ie, PD). However, there is little evidence to support this model other than some data suggesting common genetic influences on symptom clusters that account for a significant genetic etiology for both alcohol dependence and conduct disorder/ASPD.[30-33]

Etiological Models

Etiological diagnoses come in two varieties: *secondary SUD* and *secondary psychopathological* models. In the *secondary SUD models*, the presence of a PD or pathological personality traits are risk factors contributing to the development of an SUD. Since the traits within a PD usually have some early manifestations in childhood and adolescence, it is possible to prospectively examine the relationship between maladaptive traits, seen prior to exposure to addictive substances, and the subsequent development of SUD. A number of traits have been identified that appear commonly in both SUDs and PDs (such as sensation seeking, novelty seeking, impulsivity, negative emotionality), and prospective studies have assessed the link between these traits identified in children or adolescents with later onset of SUDs.

Several pathways have been proposed that might explain how certain personality traits or symptoms of a PD might lead to an SUD.[30]

a. *Behavioral disinhibition pathway*: In this pathway, traits such as impulsivity, behavioral undercontrol, aggression, and diminished conscientiousness predict substance initiation and use syndromes presumably mediated through affiliation with deviant peer groups and poor socialization,[32-34] consistent with ASPD and possibly BPD. Evidence for this comes from epidemiological studies that demonstrate a strong link between SUDs and other psychiatric disorders along the impulsive spectrum and longitudinal studies that demonstrate a link between the aforementioned antisocial traits that predate and predict the development of an SUD in adolescents and young adults.[35-39] and is associated with earlier initiation of substance use, earlier onset of SUDs, and a more severe form of the illness.[40]
b. *Stress reduction pathway*: In this pathway, individuals with high neuroticism traits (ie, stress sensitivity, negative emotionality, mood instability) can be predicted to develop an SUD in an attempt to self-treat unpleasant affective and cognitive states. Khantzian "self-medication hypothesis" (SMH) is an example of a stress reduction pathway and views preexisting difficulties in self-esteem regulation, modulation of dysphoric affect, and self-care as establishing a vulnerability to development of an SUD.[41,42] The data supporting the SMH in general are mixed. Despite some studies from treatment samples suggesting specificity between a particular substance being used for a particular mental illness,[43-46] the majority of the data across a broad spectrum of mental illnesses do not reveal a strong relationship between type of mental illness and type of substance.[47] However, there is evidence that patients may use substances to medicate unpleasant emotional states, across a variety of diagnoses, to alleviate the dysphoria.[48] Several longitudinal studies have shown that high neuroticism traits in children are predictive of SUDs in adolescence and young adulthood[34,35,49,50] and might explain the comorbidity of SUDs seen in avoidant and BPD.[19]
c. *Reward sensitivity pathway*: This pathway suggests that individuals who show traits of novelty seeking, reward responsivity, and extraversion are at increased risk for developing an SUD. The mechanism hypothesizes that these individuals experience an exaggerated reward response with addictive substances, which leads to a sensitization process, further reinforcing the addictive behavior. Some evidence from longitudinal studies supports this model,[34,37,49,51] and it might account for the co-occurrence of SUDs seen in narcissistic, histrionic, and antisocial PDs.[19]

In the *secondary psychopathology model*, substance use precedes and causes personality disorders. Though this model has a paucity of empirical support relative to the secondary SUD models, it remains pertinent from a conceptual perspective to the overall understanding of co-occurring PDs and SUDs; furthermore, this model may be a key element to avoid misdiagnosis of PDs. It is a frequent clinical observation that active addiction generates significant characterological symptoms that can be indistinguishable from the symptoms of a PD (See *Substance Use Masquerading as PDs* in assessment section below). An example of this would be "secondary sociopathy," symptoms consistent with antisocial PD occasioned by drug use.[52] Certain drugs (ie, IV heroin; crack cocaine), especially those that are illegal and perceived as very harmful, are associated with antisocial behaviors. These apparent symptoms of personality psychopathology should remit with sobriety without a preexisting PD.

In all of these models, substance initiation and continued use secondary to personality psychopathology eventually translates into an independent SUD; over a long enough period of time, the neurobiology of the normative reward system can be sufficiently hijacked and corrupted leading to chronic neuroadapative changes associated with the transition from at-risk substance use to increasingly severe SUD.[31,53] Once physical dependence or other SUD-related criteria reach a collective threshold, the SUD is now established and can continue independent of its original relationship to the mental disorder causing it, even if the original offending psychiatric condition (ie, PD) is treated with remission of illness. However, there will remain negative bidirectional effects now that there are two distinct problems.

DIAGNOSIS: PRACTICAL ISSUES

Screening is a crucial step prior to diagnostic formulation. Since patients with PDs tend to have more severe pathology and more frequent treatment contact, they are more likely to present in the situations with the least time for assessment, such as emergency rooms or incarcerated settings.[54,55] However, most screening questionnaires focus on specific PDs or require too much time to be used in routine clinical practice. The use of standardized assessment instruments is important in diagnosing PDs because traditional unstructured clinical diagnostic interviews are poorly reliable and are associated with missed and incorrect diagnoses.[56-58] There are a number of formal assessment tools used in evaluating personality pathology, although they were not specifically designed for an SUD population. The ones mentioned in this section demonstrate good reliability and validity from research. These tools range from self-report questionnaires to semistructured and structured diagnostic interviews. Self-report questionnaires that offer a comprehensive assessment of PDs from the DSM perspective include the Millon Clinical Multiaxial Inventory-III (MCMI-III),[59] (perhaps the most widely used in research and clinical practice), the Personality Diagnostic Questionnaire-4,[60] the Minnesota Multiphasic Personality Inventory (MMPI) Personality Disorder Scales,[61] and the Coolidge Axis II Inventory (CATI),[62] although the MMPI and the CATI are not specifically coordinated with DSM. Other self-administered questionnaires are more specific for particular PDs, such as the Psychopathic Personality Inventory,[63] the Narcissistic Personality Inventory,[64] and the Schizotypal Personality Questionnaire.[65] Although self-report questionnaires assessing PDs have the advantage of being highly sensitive and therefore useful as screening tools, they have the disadvantage of a significant false-positive rate leading to overdiagnoses of PDs.[66] This effect may be pronounced for an SUD population, since the questionnaires do not differentiate the effects of substance use from personality traits. Clinical interviews are important here to determine if a particular behavior is substance related or more global. The Structured Interview of Personality Organization (STIPO) is a semistructured interview designed to assess a psychodynamically oriented model of personality health and disorder, which is designed for the dimensional assessment of identity, primitive defenses, and reality testing.[67] These three primary domains are central to the model of personality pathology, notably borderline personality organization, elaborated by Kernberg and do not correlate to the totality of DSM diagnostic criteria.[68] Examples of clinician-administered diagnostic interviews include the Structured Clinical Interview for DSM-5 Personality Disorders (SCID-5-PD),[69] which is the updated version of the SCID-II[70] developed for the DSM-IV, the Diagnostic Interview for DSM-IV Personality Disorders,[71] and the Structured Interview for DSM-IV Personality Disorders.[72] Though such assessments are useful to formally establish DSM diagnoses, they can be labor intensive and time-consuming to administer, diminishing their feasibility and utility in routine clinical settings.

Diagnostic Challenges

The ultimate goal of assessment is to determine the presence of a PD, which is distinguishable from or co-occurring with an SUD. Several factors can help in this process (see **Table 105-1**). Given the epidemiological data where the majority of patients with a PD (especially BPD and ASPD) have a co-occurring SUD and vice versa, a diagnostic a priori assumption should be that there are two separate problems until proven otherwise by a process of exclusion (ie, that it is a case of an etiological diagnosis). As a general clinical rule, symptoms that persist beyond 1 month of abstinence are more likely to be primary.

Any assessment tool must be considered along with other information sources, such as unstructured patient interviews, collateral information, and longitudinal assessment. Collateral contacts can be essential in elucidating long-standing behavior patterns, can provide information that the patient is not able or willing to provide, and can increase the convergent validity of diagnoses.[73] Risk assessment for suicidality, nonsuicidal self-injury, and violence deserve special attention, particularly in patients with BPD and ASPD.[74] Given the high-risk nature of these patients, a team-based approach and access to referral services is ideal for optimal management.

In addition to a careful substance history and risk assessment, important areas of focus include a history of trauma (physical, sexual, and emotional abuse, neglect, conflict in the household), familial history of personality dysfunction, and quality/quantity of current and past interpersonal relationships (ie, object relations). Inflexible or maladaptive coping skills are the hallmark of a PD. Close attention to interpersonal style and transference/countertransference can yield important diagnostic information. For example, patients with BPD tend to develop transference quickly and intensely, and to have extreme and rapid oscillations; the clinician is experienced as all good and ideal, and then suddenly all bad and malicious after a seemingly small disappointment. Schizoid or avoidant patients may be especially deferential or reserved in a clinical encounter.

Psychiatric Illness Masquerading as PDs

It is also important to rule out other co-occurring psychiatric disorders whose symptom presentation may mimic symptoms of various PDs. For example, bipolar disorders should be excluded before diagnosing BPD, and social anxiety disorder should be ruled out before diagnosing avoidant personality disorder. A detailed temporal history and longitudinal assessment is key to differentiate acute *state* phenomenon usually associated with nonpersonality psychopathological disorders (ie, acute mood instability associated with mania or substance use) versus longer-term *traits* associated with PDs.

Substance Use Masquerading as PDs

Substances can mimic a wide variety of personality phenomenology and pathology along a temporal spectrum from acute to chronic. From a diagnostic perspective, it is important to know these effects to take into account when considering etiological (ie, secondary psychopathology) versus co-occurring diagnostic models. Below are salient examples, as categorized by DSM-5 personality disorder clusters A, B, and C:

Cluster A

Consider psychotogenic substances. These include NMDA antagonists (eg, PCP, ketamine, dextromethorphan), 5HT2a agonists (eg, LSD, DMT), kappa opioid agonists (eg, *Salvia divinorum*), stimulants (eg, cocaine, methamphetamines, substituted cathinones [ie, mephedrone, "bath salts," "flakka"]), CB1 agonists (eg, cannabis, synthetic cannabinoids), inhalants (eg, nitrous oxide, toluene), and chronic heavy alcohol use. Heavy methamphetamine or PCP use can occasion psychotic states that last for weeks to months even in the absence of underlying psychotic spectrum illnesses, including affective psychoses,[75,76]

TABLE 105-1 Diagnostic Formulation

1. Family history (FH): for both PDs and SUDs. Since both have approximately a 50% genetic involvement, a strong family history would be suggestive of an independent diagnostic entity (ie, strong family history of ASPD would suggest the presence of ASPD in a particular patient where secondary sociopathy was a possibility).
2. Age of onset
   a. Age of onset: Onset of PDs typically occurs in the late adolescent/early adulthood period.
3. Premorbid symptom pattern
   a. Example: Conduct disorder diagnosis and symptoms would be highly suggestive of the presence of ASPD in an adult.
   b. Example: Premorbid paranoid or schizotypal personality traits and changes are associated with the prodrome of schizophrenia so caution would be advised in diagnosing cluster A disorders in those who are experiencing a prodrome of schizophrenia.
4. Temporal history to determine order of onset of SUD vs PD vs medical disorders and to assess the relationship between the three variables
   a. Example: Conduct disorder typically precedes the development of an SUD.
5. Periods of abstinence: The continued presence of PD symptoms during significant periods of abstinence suggests dual or multiple diagnoses, and conversely, their absence suggests the presence of an SUD without a co-occurring PD.
   a. Example: The remission of PD symptoms during sustained abstinence would suggest pseudo-PDs, or continued presence would suggest comorbidity.
6. Collateral history: family, friends, case managers, treatment providers.
7. Toxicology monitoring: urine testing as the most common method.
8. Use structured or semistructured measures such as the SCID-PD to enhance the reliability and validity of diagnoses.
9. Use serial, longitudinal assessments to increase reliability and validity of diagnoses as opposed to relying on single assessments, especially those done in acute settings (ie, a patient admitted to an inpatient dual diagnosis unit actively in withdrawal, psychotic, and suicidal).
10. Use multiple sources to gather data such as clinician-administered structured or semistructured interviews, self-report, collateral information, physical examination, and laboratory tests.
11. Beware of making PD diagnoses during periods of active intoxication and withdrawal.
12. Rule out non-PD psychiatric disorders whose symptoms may mimic those of a particular PD and better account for a given clinical scenario.
    a. Example: Symptoms of bipolar disorder can mimic symptoms of BPD.
13. Rule out substances that can mimic PD symptoms depending on the particular cluster (See *Substance Use Masquerading as PDs* in assessment section below).
14. Rule out medical conditions that can acutely or chronically cause symptoms consistent with PDs (See *Substance Use Masquerading as PDs* in assessment section below).

From Widiger TA. The DSM-III-R categorical personality disorder diagnoses: a critique and an alternative. *Psychol Inquiry.* 1993;4(2):75-90; American Psychiatric Association. *Diagnostic and Statistical Manual of Mental Disorders: DSM-5*. Vol. 5. American Psychiatric Association; 2013; Ross S. The mentally ill substance abuser. In: Galanter M, Kleber M, eds. *Textbook of Substance Abuse Treatment.* 4th ed. The American Psychiatric Publishing; 2008:537-554; Jang KL, Livesley WJ, Vernon PA, et al. Heritability of personality disorder traits: a twin study. *Acta Psychiatr Scand.* 1996;94:438-444.

and could be incorrectly diagnosed as schizotypal or paranoid personality disorder. Of all substances, alcohol is the most psychotogenic and can cause chronic psychotic disorders (ie, alcohol-induced psychotic disorder, with hallucinations, Korsakoff syndrome, Marchiafava-Bignami syndrome). This chronic psychotic state could appear like the new onset of cluster A symptoms especially if the psychotic symptoms were attenuated.[76]

Cluster B

The affective instability of BPD can be mimicked by the intoxication and/or withdrawal states of many substances. Interpersonal difficulties, impulsivity, transient paranoia, and identity disturbance are all features that can be seen in patients with active addiction. One should be especially cautious of diagnosing ASPD during states of active drug use, since patients can be manipulative or resort to criminal activity to maintain their addiction. If there is no history of conduct disorder or criminal activity prior to the onset of SUD, "secondary sociopathy" is the more likely diagnosis.

Cluster C

Consider anxiogenic substances, such as stimulants, CB1 agonists, and the serotonergic hallucinogens (ie, LSD), especially when used in uncontrolled settings. While alcohol and opioids are both acute-acting anxiolytics, chronic use can lead to marked anxiety during periods of withdrawal, and protracted withdrawal can last for months.[77]

Medical Illness Masquerading as PDs

In addition to harmful use of drugs, there are other general medical conditions that can sufficiently alter physiological brain processes to produce changes in personality, either acutely or over a longer period of time. Examples of conditions that can cause *acute changes* in personality include infections (ie, herpes encephalitis, meningitis, sepsis), hematomas (ie, epidural, subdural), and metabolic syndromes (ie, hyperglycemia, hyperthyroidism, hypoxia, hypercarbia, delirium). Examples of medical conditions that can occasion *longer-term changes* in personality include frontal lobe traumatic brain injury (ie, Phineas Gage), dementing syndromes (ie, Pick, Alzheimer, Huntington, Wilson), infectious illness (ie, Creutzfeldt-Jakob disease), CNS tumors (ie, frontal lobe, pituitary), strokes, porphyrias, and chronic temporal lobe epilepsy. Traumatic brain injury predominantly damages frontal and temporal brain regions irrespective of etiology such as hemorrhages, contusions, or diffuse axonal injury.[78] One of the most common effects of frontal lobe damage can be dramatic changes in personality and behavior. At least three major syndromes have been identified depending on the specific frontal cortical area damaged: *medial frontal regions* (including anterior cingulate and superior medial frontal regions) resulting in "pseudodepression" marked by avolition, lethargy, anhedonia, and delays in cognitive processing speed; *orbitofrontal cortex* leading to "pseudopsychopathy" marked by aggression, disinhibition, impulsivity, lack of empathy, and childish behavior; *ventro and dorsolateral frontal* areas leading to "pseudodementia" or "dysexecutive syndrome" marked by impairments in organization, reasoning, planning, motivation, and self-monitoring.[79]

TREATMENT

Treatment Outcomes

When examining co-occurring PDs and SUDs, the data are mixed as to whether co-occurring PDs in individuals with SUDs predict a worse response to treatment. A growing number of studies have consistently demonstrated that personality psychopathology, although associated with pre- and posttreatment problem severity, is not a strong predictor of clinical improvement in this population.[80-86] Alternatively, a number of studies have shown that PDs can predict a shorter time to return to use, worse SUD outcomes in general, increased treatment discontinuation rates, or lack of aftercare compliance after discharge in patients with SUDs.[87-90] One systematic review looking at 122 studies with nearly 200,000 participants revealed an increased vulnerability for dropping out of treatment associated with younger patients, those with cognitive dysfunction, and individuals having a diagnosis of ASPD and histrionic PD.[91] Studies focusing on "normal" personality traits in individuals with SUDs have delineated low persistence, high novelty seeking, high neuroticism, and low conscientiousness as strong predictors of a shorter time to recurrence of use.[92]

Factors that have been identified as positively affecting treatment outcomes in individuals with co-occurring PDs and SUDs include higher level of motivation for change, longer length of time in treatment, and increased therapist alliance.[84,88,93] Regarding the comorbidity of PDs and other psychiatric disorders, it has been demonstrated that PDs are associated with worse outcomes for patients with a broad range of psychiatric disorders and SUDs.[94] Prospective longitudinal outcome studies of SUD patients with both PDs and other psychiatric disorders suggest that having a combination of both disorders predicted worse outcomes such as increased likelihood of return to use[95] or worse psychosocial outcomes.[95,96] Co-occurring non-SUD psychiatric pathology in individuals with PDs and SUDs ("triply diagnosed") has also been associated with worse treatment outcomes in terms of aftercare compliance.[90]

General Treatment Strategies

Below is a list of evidence-based psychosocial and pharmacological treatments for personality disorders, including treatments designed for co-occurring PDs and SUDs. See **Table 105-2** for general principles for treating patients with co-occurring PDs and SUDs.

Psychosocial Treatments

Cluster A Disorders

The recommendation of psychosocial treatments for this cluster of PDs is mostly derived from several case reports or uncontrolled studies, although there have been a few RCTs focused on schizotypal PD.[97] The treatment guidelines have suggested utilizing certain psychosocial techniques, such as CBT, social skills training, psychodynamic approaches, supportive, group, or mixed approaches.[98-102] An additional treatment consideration is that a more structured setting (ie, an inpatient or day program) with a greater dosed intensity of psychosocial treatment may be better than nonintensive outpatient treatment.[103]

Consistent with social and cognitive impairment being hallmarks of schizotypal PD,[104] data from the few RCTs in this area suggest that interventions focused on social skills training and cognitive remediation (ie, cognitive skills training in the areas most impaired in psychotic spectrum disorders, such as attention and concentration, psychomotor speed, learning and memory, and executive functions) may be useful psychosocial interventions for patients with schizotypal PD. In an RCT comparing 79 patients with schizotypal PD who received integrated treatment (consisting of a community treatment model focused on young first-episode psychotic patients with social skills training and psychoeducation) versus treatment as usual, at 2-year follow-up, those randomized to integrated treatment were significantly less likely to be diagnosed with a psychotic disorder (25.0% compared to 48.3% in the standard group).[105] In another RCT, McClure et al. enrolled 28 participants with schizotypal PD in an 8-week, randomized, double-blind, placebo-controlled trial to receive cognitive remediation and social skills training plus either guanfacine or placebo, and those participants in the experimental arm showed statistically significant improvements in reasoning, problem solving, and functional capacity.[106]

Cluster B Disorders

The cluster B disorders have by far received the most attention in the psychotherapy literature compared to either the cluster A or C disorders, with the majority of psychotherapy RCTs being conducted for these disorders.[107]

TABLE 105-2 General Treatment Principles

1. Employ evidence-based psychosocial treatments for PDs, SUDs, or those that have been demonstrated to be beneficial for both disorders (ie, DBT-S).
2. Combine symptom-targeted pharmacotherapy with psychotherapy for the PD and use evidence-based pharmacotherapies for the SUD (ie, FDA-approved medications for alcohol, opioid, nicotine/tobacco use disorders).
3. Focus on therapeutic alliance, as it is associated with positive treatment outcomes.[97]
4. Use longer-term treatments as they have been associated with positive outcomes for PDs,[98-101] SUDs,[102] and co-occurring PDs and SUDs.[7]
5. Risk assessment is a crucial aspect of initial and ongoing evaluation especially for those PDs (ie, BPD, ASPD) associated with self-harm or violence toward others.
6. Treatment should be integrated to focus on both the PD and the SUD from the beginning and care should be delivered in an integrated system of care model rather than sequential or parallel ones.[99,100,103,104]
7. Often, the ideal treatment environment is highly structured, such as a day hospital or a federally regulated methadone clinic especially with greater severity of PD illness.[105,106]
8. Patients with co-occurring PDs and SUDs can exhaust the resources of individual clinicians and systems alike, so staff working with these patients should have additional training in PD and SUD, and should take advantage of opportunities for supervision and consultation.[7]
9. Participation in an aftercare program is highly recommended.
10. Utilize intensive case management services for certain individuals such as those with greater severity of illness, homelessness, and a history of noncompliance.
11. Focus on addressing maladaptive traits or impairments in personality functioning (such as cognitive distortions, affect dysregulation, motivational impairment, perceptual problems, and interpersonal dysfunction) especially as it relates to recurrence of SUD symptoms.
12. Aggressively treat co-occurring non-SUD psychiatric disorders.

From Widiger TA. The DSM-III-R categorical personality disorder diagnoses: a critique and an alternative. *Psychol Inquiry.* 1993;4(2):75-90; American Psychiatric Association. *Diagnostic and Statistical Manual of Mental Disorders: DSM-5.* Vol. 5. American Psychiatric Association; 2013; Ross S. The mentally ill substance abuser. In: Galanter M, Kleber M, eds. *Textbook of Substance Abuse Treatment.* 4th ed. The American Psychiatric Publishing; 2008:537-554; Jang KL, Livesley WJ, Vernon PA, et al. Heritability of personality disorder traits: a twin study. *Acta Psychiatr Scand.* 1996;94:438-444.

Borderline PD

Several psychotherapeutic interventions for BPD have been developed and evaluated in RCTs: specialized treatments such as dialectical behavioral therapy (DBT),[108,109] mentalization-based therapy (MBT),[110,111] transference-focused psychotherapy (TFP),[112,113] schema-focused therapy (SFT),[114-116] and generalist approaches such as general psychiatric management (GPM)[117,118] and structured clinical management (SCM).[110,119,120]

DBT was the first psychotherapy specifically designed to treat BPD and has received the most empirical attention in research settings. DBT combines cognitive-behavioral techniques for reality testing and emotional regulation with interventions focused on distress tolerance, acceptance, and mindfulness, to specifically address skill deficits, maladaptive cognitions, and self-injurious behavior in patients with BPD.[108] Mindfulness is one of the core components of DBT and is considered central to the other skills taught in DBT, in being able to help individuals with BPD accept and tolerate difficult and overwhelming emotions. Derived from traditional contemplative meditative traditions and practices, mindfulness can be described as "moment-to-moment, non-judgmental awareness, cultivated by paying attention in a specific way, that is, in the present moment, and as non-reactively, as non-judgmentally, and as openheartedly as possible."[121] As applied to DBT, mindfulness is the capacity to pay attention and live fully in the present moment, experience the full range of emotions and physical sensations, and to accept difficult situations (ie, radical acceptance) without judgment.[108]

The modified version adapted for patients with SUD is DBT Substance Abuse (DBT-S), which includes the standard components of DBT plus a focus on abstinence issues, improving motivation for change, additional modified skills, and strategies to strengthen the therapeutic alliance by enhancing the therapist's skills and motivation to engage difficult, "easily lost" patients.[122] Several RCTs in both inpatient and outpatient settings have demonstrated the efficacy of DBT compared to a control group (usually treatment as usual [TAU]), and the most recent Cochrane Database review of psychotherapies for BPD (including 75 RCTs) supports the primary role of psychotherapy in BPD treatment, with a sufficient number and strength of the included studies for the authors to conclude that DBT is efficacious for BPD.[123-125] A 2022 follow-up analysis by Stoffers-Winterling et al. further supports the primary role of psychotherapies in BPD treatment, and found statistically significant effect estimates (supported by at least low-certainty quality evidence) only for DBT and MBT.[126]

MBT is derived from both classical psychoanalytic concepts and newer developments from attachment theory and social cognition research, which theorizes that impairments in mentalization (defined as the capacity to understand thoughts, emotions, and behaviors and how they are associated with specific mental states in ourselves and others) lead to core pathologies associated with BPD, specifically difficulties in differentiating mental states of self and others.[127] Like DBT, MBT can be delivered in individual and group formats. It focuses on improving the patient's ability to "mentalize" (ie, differentiate and separate out their own thoughts, feelings, and behaviors from others in the context of relationships).[111] Several RCTs of MBT have demonstrated efficaciousness of MBT in terms of improvements in core BPD symptoms, fewer self-harm and suicidal behaviors, and improved psychosocial functioning.[110,125,126,128-130]

TFP is a psychoanalytically-oriented treatment built upon the theoretical conceptualization that primitive psychological defense mechanisms (eg, splitting) are a core source of pathology in BPD leading to identify diffusion, affect dysregulation, and interpersonal dysfunction.[131,132] The treatment, which involves twice-weekly individual psychotherapy sessions, focuses on the utilization and analysis of the relationship between patient and therapist to allow the patient to more accurately perceive and optimally respond to intrapsychic and interpersonal dynamics.[98,119] TFP has been evaluated in a small number of RCTs.[125,133,134] In one RCT with 104 participants randomized to outpatient TFP versus treatment by experienced community clinicians, the TFP group demonstrated statistically significant improvements in core BPD symptoms, improved psychosocial functioning, fewer suicide attempts, less inpatient admissions, and approximately a 50% lower treatment discontinuation rate.[135] In another RCT of 90 participants randomized to year-long outpatient treatment of TFP versus DBT versus supportive dynamic psychotherapy, all three modalities demonstrated significant reductions in depression and anxiety as well as improvements in global functioning. In this study, DBT and TFP were significantly associated with reductions in suicidal behavior, but only TFP was significantly predictive of reductions in irritability, impulsivity, and aggressive behavior toward others.[136]

SFT is a cognitive-behavioral intervention based on identifying maladaptive cognitive schemas that developed as a result of adverse childhood events and lead to cognitive distortions associated with BPD.[119] A small number of RCTs have demonstrated the efficacy of SFT for BPD in outpatient settings.[115,125,137] In a comparative effectiveness RCT of 88 participants randomized to SFT versus TFP, at 3-year follow-up, both groups demonstrated significant improvements in all core BPD symptoms and improved quality of life, though SFT was noted to be more effective on all measures.[115] A recent RCT by Arntz et al., which included 495 participants with BPD in five countries, strengthened the established evidence that SFT is an efficacious treatment for BPD, with the additional finding that the combination of individual and group SFT is more effective than individual SFT alone.[114]

A limitation of these treatment modalities is that they require significant specialized training and clinical resources, so there has been a move to develop less intensive evidence-based treatments, such as GPM and SCM.[117,119] GPM is based upon a case management model, which conceptualizes interpersonal hypersensitivity as a core feature of BPD psychopathology, and combines supportive, cognitive-behavioral, and psychodynamic principles and strategies to promote functioning in endeavors outside of treatment.[117,119] In a RCT of GPM versus DBT, GPM was shown to match DBT in significant improvements on all measured outcomes (eg, suicidal and nonsuicidal self-injury and BPD symptoms), which continued out to 1- and 2-year posttreatment follow up.[118,119] SCM was developed in the United Kingdom, and similar to GPM, involves a structured framework for treating BPD that is meant to be utilized by mental health clinicians with minimal additional training.[119] In a RCT of SCM versus MBT, patients receiving MBT improved somewhat more quickly and showed improved outcomes compared to SCM at 18 months follow up, but those in the SCM group were noted to be as clinically improved as those in the MBT group, with a faster reduction in self harm behavior, at the 6-month timepoint.[110,119]

Antisocial PD

ASPD, especially the psychopathic variant, has long been considered the one PD that will not respond to psychotherapy.[99,138,139] According to the National Collaborating Centre for Mental Health 2010 and the most recent Cochrane Database review, there is not enough good quality evidence to assess the value of psychosocial interventions in persons with ASPD.[139-141] However, it is important to note that most of the studies included in such systematic reviews involved participants with diagnoses other than ASPD.[139] In the one psychotherapy RCT that evaluated ASPD, 52 adult men with ASPD with acts of aggression in the 6 months prior to study entry were randomized to 6 months of CBT plus TAU versus TAU alone, which revealed a trend toward improvement of the CBT-augmented group with respect to problematic drinking, social functioning, and beliefs about others.[142]

While awaiting larger and longer-term studies to evaluate the efficacy and effectiveness of psychosocial treatments for ASPD, research over the past few decades has explored the efficacy of family-based interventions for antisocial youths (ie, those with conduct disorder, a precursor to ASPD).[98] Several controlled trials have suggested the efficacy of multisystemic family therapy (MSFT) in juvenile offenders in terms of lower rates of recidivism, reductions in deviant peer affiliation, and improved familial communication.[143-145]

In terms of comorbidity, a RCT of 175 persons with ASPD (seeking or currently in SUD treatment) comparing a short-term psychoeducational program designed to address impulsive and self-destructive behaviors versus TAU found that the psychoeducation program improved adherence to SUD treatment[146]; and a post-hoc secondary analysis found that the program increased subjects' sense of having received help for their ASPD, which in turn was associated with more days abstinent, fewer treatment drop outs, and increased treatment satisfaction.[147]

Narcissistic PD and Histrionic PD

Although psychotherapy is commonly recommended to treat narcissistic personality disorder (NPD) and histrionic personality disorder (HPD), the evidence base from RCTs is lacking.[99,100,148] Regarding NPD (a disorder characterized by grandiosity, sense of superiority, wish for admiration, entitlement, arrogance, envy, lack of empathy, exploitation of others), psychotherapeutic treatments have been developed from the psychoanalytic/psychodynamic and CBT models. The most prominent psychodynamically oriented psychotherapies adapted for the treatment of NPD, derived from BPD treatment, are TFP and MBT. TFP in NPD focuses on exploration of the patient's envy, grandiosity, aggression, and defensiveness.[149] Diana Diamond and colleagues have adapted TFP to develop a specialized treatment platform for pathological narcissism and NPD (TFP-N) although the intervention has not yet been systematically studied.[150,151] Regarding MBT in the treatment of NPD, there are a few case reports in the literature suggesting the utility of using MBT to treat NPD[152] or narcisisstic traits.[153,154]

CBT treatments adapted to treat NPD have included schema-focused therapy (a form of CBT designed to treat PDs that incorporates elements from object relationships, psychodynamic and gestalt therapies and focuses on early maladaptive schemas regarding relationships to self or others)[155] and DBT.[149] Cognitive techniques, such as reframing and problem-solving, combined with behavioral modification such as reducing grandiosity and impulse control, have been suggested as ways to strengthen the therapeutic alliance and increase treatment adherence in NPD.[156] Open-label and RCTs are needed to assess the efficacy of CBT interventions to treat NPD.

Cluster C Disorders

A variety of psychosocial interventions have been studied to treat cluster C disorders including CBT, social skills training, and psychodynamic psychotherapy.[98] Of the therapies studied, psychodynamic psychotherapy appears to have the strongest evidence base. Three controlled trials conducted in a cohort of patients with a variety of cluster C disorders provided preliminary evidence for the efficacy of short term dynamic psychotherapy to treat core symptoms of Cluster C disorder.[157-160]

Integrated PD and SUD Psychosocial Treatments

There have been two major attempts to develop integrated psychosocial treatments for PDs co-occurring with SUDs: dual-focus schema therapy (DFST) and DBT for substance abusers (DBT-S).

DFST is a manualized cognitive-behavioral therapy developed as an integrated approach across the spectrum of PDs that co-occur with SUDs.[161] It is delivered in an individual psychotherapy format focusing on maladaptive cognitive schemas associated with various PDs, and acquiring new coping skills for symptom-focused relapse prevention. Three RCTs have evaluated the efficacy of DFST with mixed results and it has not been implemented as a standard of care intervention.[162-164]

In contrast to DFST, the evidence base for DBT-S as an integrated PD-SUD psychotherapy, to treat co-occurring BPD and an SUD, is more robust. There have been two RCTs of DBT-S conducted in outpatients with comorbid BPD and an SUD. The first study compared DBT-S to a community-based TAU, and the second study compared DBT-S to comprehensive validation therapy plus a 12-step approach (CVT + 12S). In the first RCT, the DBT-S group had significantly greater reductions in substance use throughout the treatment period including final follow-up at 16 months; this group also had significantly superior improvements in global and social functioning relatively to the TAU group.[165] In the second RCT, the DBT-S group maintained reductions in opioid use throughout the entire 12 months of treatment while the CVT + 12S group significantly increased opioid use during the final 4 months of treatment; both groups demonstrated significant reductions in psychopathology from baseline to the 16-month follow-up point.[166] Given the substantial evidence base in support of DBT for BPD and the data from the two above-mentioned RCTs of DBT-S in those with BPD and co-occurring SUDs, one could include DBT or DBT-S as a standard treatment for those with co-occurring BPD and SUDs.

Although not specifically designed as an integrated psychosocial treatment for co-occurring PDs and SUDs, *therapeutic communities* (TCs), developed in the 1960s, include components that address both SUDs and co-occurring antisocial traits. The core principles underlying TCs include provision of a highly structured daily routine; "community as method" approach where the peer-led community provides the active treatment ingredient through a combination of positive reinforcement, negative reinforcement, and coercion; promoting personal responsibility and self-reliance by developing vocational and independent living skills; and promoting prosocial values within a hierarchical social network that sustains abstinence and recovery (see Chapter 76).[167,168] Community-based residential TCs have demonstrated efficacy in reducing substance use and criminality and increasing employment in prospective, longitudinal trials.[169-171] RCTs have demonstrated the efficacy of prison-based TCs in reducing substance use and recidivism relative to the control condition,[172,173] and a meta-analysis of 15 trials evaluating TCs in correctional settings concluded that TCs were associated with significant positive reductions in recidivism.[174] Despite the promising evidence base for TCs in this patient population, there are only a handful of programs available in the United States.

Pharmacological Treatments

Beginning in the early 90s, the PD field underwent a paradigm shift in conceptualizing personality pathologies as purely psychological to also neurobiological in origin.[175] Siever and Davis[2] provided one of the first neurobiological models of PDs and categorized PD symptoms along several dimensions common with other psychiatric disorders: (1) *affective instability* (ie, labile mood, rejection sensitivity) continuous with mood disorders; (2) *cognitive-perceptual organization* (ie, paranoid ideation, derealization) continuous with psychotic spectrum disorders; (3) *impulsivity* (ie, aggression, self-injury) continuous with impulse control disorders; and (4) *inhibition* (ie, anxiety) continuous with anxiety spectrum disorders. With this neurobiological framework, psychopharmacological treatments were theorized to modulate neurotransmitter systems at brain regions common across both personality and nonpersonality disorders.[176] This led to an increase in pharmacology research in PDs, which had previously been treated using only psychotherapeutic interventions.

Of the domains listed above, the first three (affective, cognitive, and impulsive) have garnered the most attention as they tend to produce more problematic and urgent symptoms such as violence and suicidal behaviors.[176] BPD has been by far the most studied PD in terms of psychopharmacological research followed by schizotypal PD (SPD) and then ASPD. The other PDs have essentially not been empirically studied from a pharmacological intervention standpoint. Although there has never been an FDA-approved pharmacotherapy to treat any PD, pharmacotherapies can be used adjunctively to treat symptom clusters of some PDs and may augment first-line psychosocial treatments.

Borderline PD

BPD consists of several symptom domains of dysfunction: affective instability, intense and unstable relationships, identity disturbance, fear of abandonment, transient paranoid ideation, impulsivity, inappropriate anger, chronic feelings of emptiness, and recurrent self-harm.[177] Although the data do not suggest that pharmacotherapies lead to disease remission in BPD, there is an evidence base supporting efficacy in treating a spectrum of symptom clusters in BPD.[178]

Several meta-analyses and systemic reviews of RCTs have revealed that mood stabilizers and second-generation antipsychotics ameliorate a number of core BPD symptoms.[179-184] Valproic acid has been shown to improve impulsivity, anger, hostility, self-harm, and affective instability.[185-187] Similarly, the anticonvulsants topiramate[45,188,189] and lamotrigine[190,191] have been shown to decrease impulsivity, anger, and affective instability. It is worth noting that the benefits of using an anticonvulsant must be weighed against their risks, which can include drowsiness, fatigue, tremor, Stevens-Johnson Syndrome, cognitive impairments, and birth defects.[178]

Among the second-generation antipsychotics, both aripiprazole[192,193] and olanzapine[194-196] have been shown to treat cognitive-perceptual symptoms (ie, paranoid ideation), irritability, anger, affective instability, and impulsivity in BPD patients. As with all medications, BPD patients treated with antipsychotics should be monitored for side effects, which include metabolic derangements, development of movement disorders, and more.[178] Antidepressant medications including selective serotonin reuptake inhibitors, tricyclic antidepressants, and monoamine oxidase inhibitors have been largely ineffective at treating core BPD symptoms.[179-181,184,197]

Schizotypal PD

Cognitive-perceptual abnormalities and interpersonal dysfunction are the hallmarks of schizotypal personality disorder (SPD), a disorder falling on a spectrum with schizophrenia.[177] Several meta-analyses and systematic reviews of RCTs have revealed that both first and second-generation antipsychotics have demonstrated efficacy in reducing cognitive-perceptual symptoms and improving mood in patients with SPD.[97,183,198] Besides SPD, there is little evidence to suggest the utility of using antipsychotics in schizoid or paranoid PDs.[199]

Antisocial PD

A meta-analysis of RCTs investigating pharmacotherapy to treat ASPD has been conducted on phenytoin, desipramine, nortriptyline, bromocriptine, and amantadine and currently there is no evidence base to suggest the use of any pharmacotherapy in ASPD.[200]

CONCLUSIONS

- PDs commonly occur in both traditional psychiatric and SUD treatment settings and there is considerable co-occurrence between these disorders and SUDs, especially with ASPD and BPD.
- Screening, standardized diagnostic assessments, family history, age of symptom onset, premorbid symptom patterns, temporal history of PD symptoms relative to substance initiation and use, periods of abstinence, collateral history, serial and longitudinal assessments, and ruling out harmful substance use or medical conditions that can masquerade as PD symptoms are key to establishing the diagnosis of a PD independent from an SUD.
- Patients with co-occurring PDs and SUDs can benefit from treatment as much as those without PDs, but the presence of a PD does negatively affect the treatment course of the SUD and is associated with treatment noncompliance and return to use.
- It is important to provide comprehensive care, optimally within a structured environment (ie, Coexisting Disorder Day Program, MMTP, TC) with a dual focus (ie, PD and SUD), in an integrated system utilizing symptom-targeted pharmacotherapy when indicated as an adjunct to psychosocial interventions.
- Although there are no FDA-approved pharmacotherapies to treat any PD, pharmacotherapies can be used adjunctively to treat symptom clusters of some PDs (ie, BPD, SPD) and may augment first-line psychosocial treatments.

REFERENCES

1. American Psychiatric Association. *Diagnostic and Statistical Manual of Mental Disorders: DSM-5*. American Psychiatric Association; 2013.
2. Siever LJ, Davis KL. A psychobiological perspective on the personality disorders. *Am J Psychiatry.* 1991;148(12):1647-1658. doi:10.1176/ajp.148.12.1647
3. Zanarini MC. Borderline personality disorder as an impulse spectrum disorder. *Borderline Personality Disorder: Etiology and Treatment.* 1993:67-86.
4. Livesley WJ, Jang KL. Toward an empirically based classification of personality disorder. *J Pers Disord.* 2000;14(2):137-151. doi:10.1521/pedi.2000.14.2.137

5. Grilo CM, Sanislow CA, Gunderson JG, et al. Two-year stability and change of schizotypal, borderline, avoidant, and obsessive-compulsive personality disorders. *J Consult Clin Psychol.* 2004;72(5):767-775. doi:10.1037/0022-006x.72.5.767
6. Johnson JG, Cohen P, Kasen S, Skodol AE, Hamagami F, Brook JS. Age-related change in personality disorder trait levels between early adolescence and adulthood: a community-based longitudinal investigation. *Acta Psychiatr Scand.* 2000;102(4):265-275. doi:10.1034/j.1600-0447.2000.102004265.x
7. Lenzenweger MF. Stability and change in personality disorder features: the Longitudinal Study of Personality Disorders. *Arch Gen Psychiatry.* 1999;56(11):1009-1015. doi:10.1001/archpsyc.56.11.1009
8. Shea MT, Stout R, Gunderson J, et al. Short-term diagnostic stability of schizotypal, borderline, avoidant, and obsessive-compulsive personality disorders. *Am J Psychiatry.* 2002;159(12):2036-2041. doi:10.1176/appi.ajp.159.12.2036
9. Seivewright H, Tyrer P, Johnson T. Change in personality status in neurotic disorders. *Lancet.* 2002;359(9325):2253-2254. doi:10.1016/s0140-6736(02)09266-8
10. Verheul R. Co-morbidity of personality disorders in individuals with substance use disorders. *Eur Psychiatry.* 2001;16(5):274-282. doi:10.1016/s0924-9338(01)00578-8
11. Trull TJ, Jahng S, Tomko RL, Wood PK, Sher KJ. Revised NESARC personality disorder diagnoses: gender, prevalence, and comorbidity with substance dependence disorders. *J Pers Disord.* 2010;24(4):412-426. doi:10.1521/pedi.2010.24.4.412
12. Verheul R, Andrea H, Berghout CC, et al. Severity Indices of Personality Problems (SIPP-118): development, factor structure, reliability, and validity. *Psychol Assess.* 2008;20(1):23-34. doi:10.1037/1040-3590.20.1.23
13. Samuels J. Personality disorders: epidemiology and public health issues. *Int Rev Psychiatry.* 2011;23(3):223-233. doi:10.3109/09540261.2011.588200
14. SAMHSA. *Results from the 2020 National Survey on Drug Use and Health: National Findings.* Office of Applied Studies. DHHS Publication; 2020.
15. Cornelius ME, Wang TW, Jamal A, Loretan CG, Neff LJ. Tobacco product use among adults—United States, 2019. *MMWR Morb Mortal Wkly Rep.* 2020;69(46):1736-1742. doi:10.15585/mmwr.mm6946a4
16. Zimmerman M, Coryell W. DSM-III personality disorder diagnoses in a nonpatient sample. Demographic correlates and comorbidity. *Arch Gen Psychiatry.* 1989;46(8):682-689. doi:10.1001/archpsyc.1989.01810080012002
17. Trull TJ, Freeman LK, Vebares TJ, Choate AM, Helle AC, Wycoff AM. Borderline personality disorder and substance use disorders: an updated review. *Borderline Personal Disord Emot Dysregul.* 2018;5:15. doi:10.1186/s40479-018-0093-9
18. Regier DA, Farmer ME, Rae DS, et al. Comorbidity of mental disorders with alcohol and other drug abuse. Results from the Epidemiologic Catchment Area (ECA) Study. *JAMA.* 1990;264(19):2511-2518.
19. Verheul R, van den Bosch LM, Ball SA. Substance abuse. In: Oldham J, Skodol AE, Bender DS, eds. *Textbook of Personality Disorders.* The American Psychiatric Publishing; 2005.
20. Plomin R, DeFries JC, GE MC. *Behavioral Genetics.* Macmillan; 2008.
21. Andersen AM, Bienvenu OJ. Personality and psychopathology. *Int Rev Psychiatry.* 2011;23(3):234-247. doi:10.3109/09540261.2011.588692
22. Rothbart MK. Temperament, development, and personality. *Curr Direct Psychol Sci.* 2007;16(4):207-212.
23. Rutter M, Plomin R. Opportunities for psychiatry from genetic findings. *Br J Psychiatry.* 1997;171(3):209-219.
24. Paris J. A current integrative perspective on personality disorders. In: Oldham J, Skodol AE, Bender DS, eds. *Textbook of Personality Disorders.* The American Psychiatric Publishing; 2005.
25. Livesley WJ, Jang KL, Jackson DN, Vernon PA. Genetic and environmental contributions to dimensions of personality disorder. *Am J Psychiatry.* 1993;150(12):1826-1831. doi:10.1176/ajp.150.12.1826
26. Livesley WJ, Jang KL, Vernon PA. Phenotypic and genetic structure of traits delineating personality disorder. *Arch Gen Psychiatry.* 1998;55(10):941-948. doi:10.1001/archpsyc.55.10.941
27. Gillespie NA, Cloninger CR, Heath AC, Martin NG. The genetic and environmental relationship between Cloninger's dimensions of temperament and character. *Pers Individ Dif.* 2003;35(8):1931-1946. doi:10.1016/s0191-8869(03)00042-4
28. Jang KL, Livesley WJ, Vernon PA, Jackson DN. Heritability of personality disorder traits: a twin study. *Acta Psychiatr Scand.* 1996;94(6):438-444. doi:10.1111/j.1600-0447.1996.tb09887.x
29. Caspi A, Harrington H, Milne B, Amell JW, Theodore RF, Moffitt TE. Children's behavioral styles at age 3 are linked to their adult personality traits at age 26. *J Pers.* 2003;71(4):495-513. doi:10.1111/1467-6494.7104001
30. Verheul R, Van den Brink W. Causal pathways between substance use disorders and personality pathology. *Aus Psychologist.* 2005;40(2):127-136.
31. Ross S, Peselow E. The neurobiology of addictive disorders. *Clin Neuropharmacol.* 2009;32(5):269-276.
32. Sher KJ, Trull TJ. Personality and disinhibitory psychopathology: alcoholism and antisocial personality disorder. *J Abnorm Psychol.* 1994;103(1):92.
33. Krueger RF, Hicks BM, Patrick CJ, Carlson SR, Iacono WG, McGue M. Etiologic connections among substance dependence, antisocial behavior, and personality: modeling the externalizing spectrum. *J Abnorm Psychol.* 2002;111(3):411-424.
34. Wills TA, Windle M, Cleary SD. Temperament and novelty seeking in adolescent substance use: convergence of dimensions of temperament with constructs from Cloninger's theory. *J Pers Soc Psychol.* 1998;74(2):387.
35. Caspi A, Begg D, Dickson N, et al. Personality differences predict health-risk behaviors in young adulthood: evidence from a longitudinal study. *J Pers Soc Psychol.* 1997;73(5):1052-1063. doi:10.1037//0022-3514.73.5.1052
36. Krueger RF, Caspi A, Moffitt TE, Silva PA, McGee R. Personality traits are differentially linked to mental disorders: a multitrait-multidiagnosis study of an adolescent birth cohort. *J Abnorm Psychol.* 1996;105(3):299.
37. Masse LC, Tremblay RE. Behavior of boys in kindergarten and the onset of substance use during adolescence. *Arch Gen Psychiatry.* 1997;54(1):62-68.
38. Sher KJ, Bartholow BD, Wood MD. Personality and substance use disorders: a prospective study. *J Consult Clin Psychol.* 2000;68(5):818.
39. Bahlmann M, Preuss UW, Soyka M. Chronological relationship between antisocial personality disorder and alcohol dependence. *Eur Addict Res.* 2002;8(4):195-200.
40. Verheul R, Hartgers C, Van den Brink W, Koeter M. The effect of sampling, diagnostic criteria and assessment procedures on the observed prevalence of DSM-III-R personality disorders among treated alcoholics. *J Stud Alcohol.* 1998;59(2):227-236.
41. Khantzian EJ. The self-medication hypothesis of addictive disorders: focus on heroin and cocaine dependence. In: Allen D, ed. *The Cocaine Crisis.* Springer; 1987:65-74.
42. Khantzian EJ. The self-medication hypothesis of substance use disorders: a reconsideration and recent applications. *Harv Rev Psychiatry.* 1997;4(5):231-244.
43. Tournier M, Sorbara F, Gindre C, Swendsen JD, Verdoux H. Cannabis use and anxiety in daily life: a naturalistic investigation in a non-clinical population. *Psychiatry Res.* 2003;118(1):1-8.
44. Carrigan MH, Randall CL. Self-medication in social phobia: a review of the alcohol literature. *Addict Behav.* 2003;28(2):269-284.
45. Nickel MK, Nickel C, Mitterlehner FO, et al. Topiramate treatment of aggression in female borderline personality disorder patients: a double-blind, placebo-controlled study. *J Clin Psychiatry.* 2004;65(11):1515-1519. doi:10.4088/jcp.v65n1112
46. Ogborne AC, Smart RG, Weber T, Birchmore-Timney C. Who is using cannabis as a medicine and why: an exploratory study. *J Psychoactive Drugs.* 2000;32(4):435-443.
47. Kessler RC. The epidemiology of dual diagnosis. *Biol Psychiatry.* 2004;56(10):730-737.

48. Mueser KT, Drake RE, Wallach MA. Dual diagnosis: a review of etiological theories. *Addict Behav.* 1998;23(6):717-734.
49. Cloninger CR, Sigvardsson S, Bohman M. Childhood personality predicts alcohol abuse in young adults. *Alcohol Clin Exp Res.* 1988;12(4):494-505.
50. Conrod PJ, Pihl RO, Vassileva J. Differential sensitivity to alcohol reinforcement in groups of men at risk for distinct alcoholism subtypes. *Alcohol Clin Exp Res.* 1998;22(3):585-597.
51. Schuckit MA, Klein J, Twitchell G, Smith TL. Personality test scores as predictors of alcoholism almost a decade later. *Am J Psychiatry.* 1994;151(7):1038-1042.
52. Mariani JJ, Horey J, Bisaga A, et al. Antisocial behavioral syndromes in cocaine and cannabis dependence. *Am J Drug Alcohol Abuse.* 2008;34(4):405-414.
53. Slutske WS, Cronk NJ, Sher KJ, Madden PA, Bucholz KK, Heath AC. Genes, environment and individual differences in alcohol expectancies among female adolescents and young adults. *Psychol Addict Behav.* 2002;16(4):308.
54. Nace EP, Davis CW, Gaspari JP. Axis II comorbidity in substance abusers. *Am J Psychiatry.* 1991;148(1):118-120.
55. Bender DS, Dolan RT, Skodol AE, et al. Treatment utilization by patients with personality disorders. *Am J Psychiatry.* 2001;158(2):295-302.
56. Rogers R. Standardizing DSM-IV diagnoses: the clinical applications of structured interviews. *J Pers Assess.* 2003;81(3):220-225.
57. Zimmerman M, Mattia JI. Differences between clinical and research practices in diagnosing borderline personality disorder. *Am J Psychiatry.* 1999;156(10):1570-1574.
58. Zimmerman M, Mattia JI. Psychiatric diagnosis in clinical practice: is comorbidity being missed? *Compr Psychiatry.* 1999;40(3):182-191.
59. Millon T. *Millon Clinical Multiaxial Inventory-III [Manual Second Edition].* Pearson Assessments; 1997.
60. Hyler SE. *Personality Diagnostic Questionnaire-4.* New York State Psychiatric Institute; 1994.
61. Morey LC, Waugh MH, Blashfield RK. MMPI scales for DSM-III personality disorders: their derivation and correlates. *J Pers Assess.* 1985;49(3):245-251.
62. Coolidge FL, Merwin MM. Reliability and validity of the Coolidge Axis II Inventory: a new inventory for the assessment of personality disorders. *J Pers Assess.* 1992;59(2):223-238.
63. Lilienfeld SO, Andrews BP. Development and preliminary validation of a self-report measure of psychopathic personality traits in noncriminal population. *J Pers Assess.* 1996;66(3):488-524.
64. Raskin R, Terry H. A principal-components analysis of the Narcissistic Personality Inventory and further evidence of its construct validity. *J Pers Soc Psychol.* 1988;54(5):890.
65. Raine A. The SPQ: a scale for the assessment of schizotypal personality based on DSM-III-R criteria. *Schizophr Bull.* 1991;17(4):555-564.
66. McDermut W. Assessment instruments and standardized evaluation. In: Oldham J, Skodol AE, Bender DS, eds. *Textbook of Personality Disorders.* American Psychiatric Publishing, Inc; 2005.
67. Stern BL, Caligor E, Clarkin JF, et al. Structured Interview of Personality Organization (STIPO): preliminary psychometrics in a clinical sample. *J Pers Assess.* 2010;92(1):35-44.
68. Kernberg OF. *Severe Personality Disorders: Psychotherapeutic Strategies.* Yale University Press; 1993.
69. First M, Williams J, Benjamin L, Spitzer R. *User's Guide for the SCID-5-PD (Structured Clinical Interview for DSM-5 Personality Disorder).* American Psychiatric Association; 2015.
70. First M, Gibbon R, Spitzer R, et al. *Structured Clinical Interview for DSM-IV Axis II Personality Disorders (SCID-II).* American Psychiatric Press; 1997.
71. Zanarini MC, Frankenburg FR, Sickel AE. *Diagnostic Interview for DSM-IV Personality Disorders.* Laboratory for the Study of Adult Development, McLean Hospital and the Department of Psychiatry, Harvard University; 1996.
72. Pfohl B, Blum N, Zimmerman M. *Structured Interview for DSM-IV Personality.* American Psychiatric Press; 1997.
73. Widiger TA. The DSM-III-R categorical personality disorder diagnoses: a critique and an alternative. *Psychol Inquiry.* 1993;4(2):75-90.
74. Preuss UW, Koller G, Barnow S, Eikmeier M, Soyka M. Suicidal behavior in alcohol-dependent subjects: the role of personality disorders. *Alcohol Clin Exp Res.* 2006;30(5):866-877.
75. Grelotti DJ, Kanayama G, Pope HG Jr. Remission of persistent methamphetamine-induced psychosis after electroconvulsive therapy: presentation of a case and review of the literature. *Am J Psychiatry.* 2010;167(1):17-23.
76. Ross S, Peselow E. Co-occurring psychotic and addictive disorders: neurobiology and diagnosis. *Clin Neuropharmacol.* 2012;35(5):235-243.
77. Weiss F, Ciccocioppo R, Parsons LH, et al. Compulsive drug-seeking behavior and relapse: neuroadaptation, stress, and conditioning factors. *Ann N Y Acad Sci.* 2001;937(1):1-26.
78. Stuss DT. Traumatic brain injury: relation to executive dysfunction and the frontal lobes. *Curr Opin Neurol.* 2011;24(6):584-589.
79. Zappala G, de Schotten MT, Eslinger PJ. Traumatic brain injury and the frontal lobes: what can we gain with diffusion tensor imaging? *Cortex.* 2012;48(2):156-165.
80. Alterman AI, Rutherford MJ, Cacciola JS, McKay JR, Boardman CR. Prediction of 7 months methadone maintenance treatment response by four measures of antisociality. *Drug Alcohol Depend.* 1998;49(3):217-223. doi:10.1016/s0376-8716(98)00015-5
81. Cacciola JS, Alterman AI, Rutherford MJ, Snider EC. Treatment response of antisocial substance abusers. *J Nerv Ment Dis.* 1995;183(3):166-171. doi:10.1097/00005053-199503000-00007
82. Cacciola JS, Rutherford MJ, Alterman AI, McKay JR, Snider EC. Personality disorders and treatment outcome in methadone maintenance patients. *J Nerv Ment Dis.* 1996;184(4):234-239. doi:10.1097/00005053-199604000-00006
83. Cecero JJ, Ball SA, Tennen H, Kranzler HR, Rounsaville BJ. Concurrent and predictive validity of antisocial personality disorder subtyping among substance abusers. *J Nerv Ment Dis.* 1999;187(8):478-486. doi:10.1097/00005053-199908000-00004
84. Crits-Christoph P, Siqueland L, Blaine J, et al. Psychosocial treatments for cocaine dependence: National Institute on Drug Abuse Collaborative Cocaine Treatment Study. *Arch Gen Psychiatry.* 1999;56(6):493-502. doi:10.1001/archpsyc.56.6.493
85. Powell BJ, Penick EC, Nickel EJ, et al. Outcomes of co-morbid alcoholic men: a 1-year follow-up. *Alcohol Clin Exp Res.* 1992;16(1):131-138. doi:10.1111/j.1530-0277.1992.tb00649.x
86. Verheul R, van den Brink W, Koeter MW, Hartgers C. Antisocial alcoholic patients show as much improvement at 14-month follow-up as non-antisocial alcoholic patients. *Am J Addict.* 1999;8(1):24-33. doi:10.1080/105504999306054
87. Thomas VH, Melchert TP, Banken JA. Substance dependence and personality disorders: comorbidity and treatment outcome in an inpatient treatment population. *J Stud Alcohol.* 1999;60(2):271-277. doi:10.15288/jsa.1999.60.271
88. Verheul R, van den Brink W, Hartgers C. Personality disorders predict relapse in alcoholic patients. *Addict Behav.* 1998;23(6):869-882. doi:10.1016/s0306-4603(98)00065-3
89. Kosten TA, Kosten TR, Rounsaville BJ. Personality disorders in opiate addicts show prognostic specificity. *J Subst Abuse Treat.* 1989;6(3):163-168. doi:10.1016/0740-5472(89)90003-2
90. Ross S, Dermatis H, Levounis P, Galanter M. A comparison between dually diagnosed inpatients with and without Axis II comorbidity and the relationship to treatment outcome. *Am J Drug Alcohol Abuse.* 2003;29(2):263-279. doi:10.1081/ada-120020511
91. Brorson HH, Ajo Arnevik E, Rand-Hendriksen K, Duckert F. Drop-out from addiction treatment: a systematic review of risk factors. *Clin Psychol Rev.* 2013;33(8):1010-1024. doi:10.1016/j.cpr.2013.07.007
92. van den Bosch LM VR, Ball SA. Substance abuse. In: Oldham JM, Skodol A, Bender DS, eds. *Textbook of Personality Disorders.* American Psychiatric Association; 2005:463-475.
93. Gerstley L, McLellan AT, Alterman AI, Woody GE, Luborsky L, Prout M. Ability to form an alliance with the therapist: a possible marker of prognosis for patients with antisocial personality disorder. *Am J Psychiatry.* 1989;146(4):508-512. doi:10.1176/ajp.146.4.508

94. Pettinati HM, Pierce JD Jr, Belden PP, Meyers K. The relationship of Axis II personality disorders to other known predictors of addiction treatment outcome. *Am J Addict.* 1999;8(2):136-147. doi:10.1080/105504999305947
95. Cacciola JS, Alterman AI, Rutherford MJ, McKay JR, Mulvaney FD. The relationship of psychiatric comorbidity to treatment outcomes in methadone maintained patients. *Drug Alcohol Depend.* 2001;61(3):271-280. doi:10.1016/s0376-8716(00)00148-4
96. Westermeyer J, Thuras P. Association of antisocial personality disorder and substance disorder morbidity in a clinical sample. *Am J Drug Alcohol Abuse.* 2005;31(1):93-110.
97. Kirchner SK, Roeh A, Nolden J, Hasan A. Diagnosis and treatment of schizotypal personality disorder: evidence from a systematic review. *NPJ Schizophr.* 2018;4(1):20. doi:10.1038/s41537-018-0062-8
98. Dixon-Gordon KL, Turner BJ, Chapman AL. Psychotherapy for personality disorders. *Int Rev Psychiatry.* 2011;23(3):282-302. doi:10.3109/09540261.2011.586992
99. Gabbard GO. *Psychodynamic Psychiatry in Clinical Practice.* 5th ed. American Psychiatric Publishing, Inc; 2014.
100. Leichsenring F, Leibing E. The effectiveness of psychodynamic therapy and cognitive behavior therapy in the treatment of personality disorders: a meta-analysis. *Am J Psychiatry.* 2003;160(7):1223-1232.
101. Leichsenring F, Rabung S. Long-term psychodynamic psychotherapy in complex mental disorders: update of a meta-analysis. *Br J Psychiatry.* 2011;199(1):15-22.
102. Stone MH. *Paranoid, Schizotypal, and Schizoid Personality Disorders. Gabbard's Treatments of Psychiatric Disorders.* 5th ed. American Psychiatric Publishing, Inc; 2014:999-1014.
103. Bartak A, Andrea H, Spreeuwenberg MD, et al. Patients with cluster a personality disorders in psychotherapy: an effectiveness study. *Psychother Psychosom.* 2011;80(2):88-99.
104. McClure MM, Harvey PD, Bowie CR, Iacoviello B, Siever LJ. Functional outcomes, functional capacity, and cognitive impairment in schizotypal personality disorder. *Schizophr Res.* 2013;144(1-3):146-150. doi:10.1016/j.schres.2012.12.012
105. Nordentoft M, Thorup A, Petersen L, et al. Transition rates from schizotypal disorder to psychotic disorder for first-contact patients included in the OPUS trial. A randomized clinical trial of integrated treatment and standard treatment. *Schizophr Res.* 2006;83(1):29-40.
106. McClure MM, Graff F, Triebwasser J, et al. Guanfacine augmentation of a combined intervention of computerized cognitive remediation therapy and social skills training for schizotypal personality disorder. *Am J Psychiatry.* 2019;176(4):307-314.
107. Duggan C, Huband N, Smailagic N, Ferriter M, Adams C. The use of psychological treatments for people with personality disorder: a systematic review of randomized controlled trials. *Personal Ment Health.* 2007;1(2):95-125.
108. Linehan MM. *Cognitive–Behavioral Treatment of Borderline Personality Disorder.* Guilford Press; 2018.
109. Linehan MM, Comtois KA, Murray AM, et al. Two-year randomized controlled trial and follow-up of dialectical behavior therapy vs therapy by experts for suicidal behaviors and borderline personality disorder. *Arch Gen Psychiatry.* 2006;63(7):757-766.
110. Bateman A, Fonagy P. Randomized controlled trial of outpatient mentalization-based treatment versus structured clinical management for borderline personality disorder. *Am J Psychiatry.* 2009;166(12):1355-1364. doi:10.1176/appi.ajp.2009.09040539
111. Fonagy P, Luyten P. A developmental, mentalization-based approach to the understanding and treatment of borderline personality disorder. *Dev Psychopathol.* 2009;21(4):1355-1381. doi:10.1017/S0954579409990198
112. Kernberg OF, Yeomans FE, Clarkin JF, Levy KN. Transference focused psychotherapy: overview and update. *Int J Psychoanal.* 2008;89(3):601-620. doi:10.1111/j.1745-8315.2008.00046.x
113. Levy KN, Draijer N, Kivity Y, Yeomans FE, Rosenstein LK. Transference-focused psychotherapy (TFP). *Curr Treat Options Psychiatry.* 2019;6(4):312-324.
114. Arntz A, Jacob GA, Lee CW, et al. Effectiveness of predominantly group schema therapy and combined individual and group schema therapy for borderline personality disorder: a randomized clinical trial. *JAMA Psychiatry.* 2022;79(4):287-299. doi:10.1001/jamapsychiatry.2022.0010
115. Giesen-Bloo J, van Dyck R, Spinhoven P, et al. Outpatient psychotherapy for borderline personality disorder: randomized trial of schema-focused therapy vs transference-focused psychotherapy. *Arch Gen Psychiatry.* 2006;63(6):649-658. doi:10.1001/archpsyc.63.6.649
116. Young JE. *Cognitive Therapy for Personality Disorders: A Schema-Focused Approach.* Professional Resource Press/Professional Resource Exchange; 1999.
117. Gunderson J, Masland S, Choi-Kain L. Good psychiatric management: a review. *Curr Opin Psychol.* 2018;21:127-131. doi:10.1016/j.copsyc.2017.12.006
118. McMain SF, Links PS, Gnam WH, et al. A randomized trial of dialectical behavior therapy versus general psychiatric management for borderline personality disorder. *Am J Psychiatry.* 2009;166(12):1365-1374.
119. Choi-Kain LW, Finch EF, Masland SR, Jenkins JA, Unruh BT. What works in the treatment of borderline personality disorder. *Curr Behav Neurosci Rep.* 2017;4(1):21-30.
120. Bateman AW, Krawitz R. *Borderline Personality Disorder: An Evidence-Based Guide for Generalist Mental Health Professionals.* Oxford University Press; 2013.
121. Kabat-Zinn J. Mindfulness. *Mindfulness.* 2015;6(6):1481-1483. doi:10.1007/s12671-015-0456-x
122. Dimeff LA, Linehan MM. Dialectical behavior therapy for substance abusers. *Addict Sci Clinical Pract.* 2008;4(2):39.
123. Clarkin JF, Levy KN, Lenzenweger MF, Kernberg OF. Evaluating three treatments for borderline personality disorder: a multiwave study. *Am J Psychiatry.* 2007;164(6):922-928. doi:10.1176/ajp.2007.164.6.922
124. Kliem S, Kröger C, Kosfelder J. Dialectical behavior therapy for borderline personality disorder: a meta-analysis using mixed-effects modeling. *J Consult Clin Psychol.* 2010;78(6):936.
125. Storebø OJ, Stoffers-Winterling JM, Völlm BA, et al. Psychological therapies for people with borderline personality disorder. *Cochrane Database Syst Rev.* 2020;5:CD012955.
126. Stoffers-Winterling JM, Storebø OJ, Kongerslev MT, et al. Psychotherapies for borderline personality disorder: a focused systematic review and meta-analysis. *Br J Psychiatry.* 2022;221(3):538-552.
127. Choi-Kain LW, Unruh BT. Mentalization-based treatment: a common-sense approach to borderline personality disorder. *Psychiatric Times.* 2016;33(3).
128. Bateman A, Fonagy P. Treatment of borderline personality disorder with psychoanalytically oriented partial hospitalization: an 18-month follow-up. *Am J Psychiatry.* 2001;158(1):36-42. doi:10.1176/appi.ajp.158.1.36
129. Bateman A, Fonagy P. 8-year follow-up of patients treated for borderline personality disorder: mentalization-based treatment versus treatment as usual. *Am J Psychiatry.* 2008;165(5):631-638. doi:10.1176/appi.ajp.2007.07040636
130. Bateman AW, Fonagy P. Effectiveness of psychotherapeutic treatment of personality disorder. *Br J Psychiatry.* 2000;177(2):138-143.
131. Kernberg O, Caligor E. A psychoanalytic theory of personality disorders. In: Lenzenweger MF, Clarkin JF, eds. *Major Theories of Personality Disorder.* Guilford Press; 2005:114-145.
132. Yeomans FE, Clarkin JF, Levy KL. Psychodynamic psychotherapies and psychoanalysis. In: Oldham JM, Skodol AE, Bender DS, eds. *The American Psychiatric Association Publishing Textbook of Personality Disorders*; 2014.
133. Kernberg OF. New developments in transference focused psychotherapy. *Int J Psychoanal.* 2016;97(2):385-407.
134. Buchheim A, Hörz-Sagstetter S, Doering S, et al. Change of unresolved attachment in borderline personality disorder: RCT study of transference-focused psychotherapy. *Psychother Psychosom.* 2017;86(5):314-316. doi:10.1159/000460257
135. Doering S, Horz S, Rentrop M, et al. Transference-focused psychotherapy v. treatment by community psychotherapists for borderline personality disorder: randomised controlled trial. *Br J Psychiatry.* 2010;196(5):389-395. doi:10.1192/bjp.bp.109.070177

136. Levy KN, Meehan KB, Kelly KM, et al. Change in attachment patterns and reflective function in a randomized control trial of transference-focused psychotherapy for borderline personality disorder. *J Consult Clin Psychol.* 2006;74(6):1027.
137. Farrell JM, Shaw IA, Webber MA. A schema-focused approach to group psychotherapy for outpatients with borderline personality disorder: a randomized controlled trial. *J Behav Ther Exp Psychiatry.* 2009;40(2):317-328.
138. Salekin RT. Psychopathy and therapeutic pessimism. Clinical lore or clinical reality? *Clin Psychol Rev.* 2002;22(1):79-112. doi:10.1016/s0272-7358(01)00083-6
139. Black DW, Blum NS. Antisocial personality disorder and other antisocial behavior. *The American Psychiatric Publishing Textbook of Personality Disorders.* The American Psychiatric Publishing; 2014:429.
140. Gibbon S, Khalifa NR, Cheung N-Y, Völlm BA, McCarthy L. Psychological interventions for antisocial personality disorder. *Cochrane Database Syst Rev.* 2020;9:CD007668. doi:10.1002/14651858.CD007668.pub3
141. National Collaborating Centre for Mental Health (UK). *Antisocial Personality Disorder: Treatment, Management and Prevention.* British Psychological Society; 2010.
142. Davidson K, Tyrer P, Tata P, et al. Cognitive behaviour therapy for violent men with antisocial personality disorder in the community: an exploratory randomized controlled trial. *Psychol Med.* 2009;39(4): 569-577.
143. Borduin CM, Schaeffer CM, Heiblum N. A randomized clinical trial of multisystemic therapy with juvenile sexual offenders: effects on youth social ecology and criminal activity. *J Consult Clin Psychol.* 2009;77(1):26.
144. Henggeler SW, Melton GB, Smith LA. Family preservation using multisystemic therapy: an effective alternative to incarcerating serious juvenile offenders. *J Consult Clin Psychol.* 1992;60(6):953.
145. Henggeler SW, Melton GB, Smith LA, Schoenwald SK, Hanley JH. Family preservation using multisystemic treatment: long-term follow-up to a clinical trial with serious juvenile offenders. *J Child Fam Stud.* 1993;2(4):283-293.
146. Thylstrup B, Hesse M. Impulsive lifestyle counseling to prevent dropout from treatment for substance use disorders in people with antisocial personality disorder: a randomized study. *Addict Behav.* 2016;57:48-54.
147. Thylstrup B, Schrøder S, Fridell M, Hesse M. Did you get any help? A post-hoc secondary analysis of a randomized controlled trial of psychoeducation for patients with antisocial personality disorder in outpatient substance abuse treatment programs. *BMC Psychiatry.* 2017;17(1):1-10.
148. Perry JC, Banon E, Ianni F. Effectiveness of psychotherapy for personality disorders. *Am J Psychiatry.* 1999;156(9):1312-1321.
149. Yakeley J. Current understanding of narcissism and narcissistic personality disorder. *BJPsych Adv.* 2018;24(5):305-315.
150. Diamond D, Yeomans F, Keefe JR. Transference-Focused Psychotherapy for Pathological Narcissism and Narcissistic Personality Disorder (TFP-N). *Psychodyn Psychiatry.* 2021;49(2):244-272.
151. Diamond D, Yeomans FE, Stern BL, Kernberg OF. *Treating Pathological Narcissism with Transference-Focused Psychotherapy.* Guilford Press; 2021.
152. Cherrier J-F. Reflections on mentalization-based treatment and its adaptation for men presenting a narcissistic personality disorder and a not otherwise specified personality disorder. *Sante Ment Que.* 2013;38(1):243-258.
153. Seligman S. Mentalization and metaphor, acknowledgment and grief: Forms of transformation in the reflective space. *Psychoanal Dialogues.* 2007;17(3):321-344.
154. Rossouw TI. The use of mentalization-based treatment for adolescents (MBT-A) with a young woman with mixed personality disorder and tendencies to self-harm. *J Clin Psychol.* 2015;71(2):178-187.
155. Young JE. Schema-focused therapy for personality disorders. *Cognitive Behaviour Therapy.* Routledge; 2014:215-236.
156. Cukrowicz KC, Poindexter EK, Joiner TE Jr. Cognitive behavioral approaches to the treatment of narcissistic personality disorder. In: Campbell WK, Miller JD, eds. *The Handbook of Narcissism and Narcissistic Personality Disorder*; 2011:457-465.
157. Winston A, Laikin M, Pollack J, Wallner Samstag L, McCullough L, Muran JC. Short-term psychotherapy of personality disorders. *Am J Psychiatry.* 1994;151(2):190-194.
158. Hellerstein DJ, Rosenthal RN, Pinsker H, Samstag LW, Muran JC, Winston A. A randomized prospective study comparing supportive and dynamic therapies: outcome and alliance. *J Psychother Pract Res.* 1998;7(4):261-271.
159. Svartberg M, Stiles TC, Seltzer MH. Randomized, controlled trial of the effectiveness of short-term dynamic psychotherapy and cognitive therapy for cluster C personality disorders. *Am J Psychiatry.* 2004;161(5):810-817.
160. Keefe JR, McMain SF, McCarthy KS, et al. A meta-analysis of psychodynamic treatments for borderline and cluster C personality disorders. *Personal Disord.* 2020;11(3):157-169. doi:10.1037/per0000382
161. Ball SA, Cecero JJ. Addicted patients with personality disorders: traits, schemas, and presenting problems. *J Pers Disord.* 2001;15(1):72-83.
162. Ball SA. Comparing individual therapies for personality disordered opioid dependent patients. *J Pers Disord.* 2007;21(3):305-321.
163. Ball SA, Cobb-Richardson P, Connolly AJ, Bujosa CT, O'neall TW. Substance abuse and personality disorders in homeless drop-in center clients: symptom severity and psychotherapy retention in a randomized clinical trial. *Compr Psychiatry.* 2005;46(5):371-379.
164. Ball SA, Maccarelli LM, LaPaglia DM, Ostrowski MJ. Randomized trial of dual-focused versus single-focused individual therapy for personality disorders and substance dependence. *J Nerv Mental Dis.* 2011;199(5):319-328.
165. Linehan MM, Schmidt H, Dimeff LA, Craft JC, Kanter J, Comtois KA. Dialectical behavior therapy for patients with borderline personality disorder and drug-dependence. *Am J Addict.* 1999;8(4):279-292.
166. Linehan MM, Dimeff LA, Reynolds SK, et al. Dialectical behavior therapy versus comprehensive validation therapy plus 12-step for the treatment of opioid dependent women meeting criteria for borderline personality disorder. *Drug Alcohol Depend.* 2002;67(1):13-26.
167. De Leon G. Therapeutic communities. In: Galanter M, Kleber HD, eds. *The American Psychiatric Publishing Textbook of Substance Abuse Treatment.* American Psychiatric Publishing, Inc; 2008:459-475.
168. Sacks S, Chaple M, Sacks JY, McKendrick K, Cleland CM. Randomized trial of a reentry modified therapeutic community for offenders with co-occurring disorders: crime outcomes. *J Subst Abuse Treat.* 2012;42(3): 247-259.
169. De Leon G. *The Therapeutic Community: Study of Effectiveness.* US Department of Health and Human Services, Public Health Service, Alcohol, Drug Abuse, and Mental Health Administration, National Institute on Drug Abuse; 1984.
170. Hubbard RL, Rachal JV, Craddock SG, Cavanaugh ER. Treatment Outcome Prospective Study (TOPS): client characteristics and behaviors before, during, and after treatment. *NIDA Res Monogr.* 1984;51:42-68.
171. Simpson DD, Sells SB. Effectiveness of treatment for drug abuse: an overview of the DARP research program. *Adv Alcohol Subst Abuse.* 1982;2(1):7-29.
172. Hser Y-I, Anglin MD, Powers K. A 24-year follow-up of California narcotics addicts. *Arch Gen Psychiatry.* 1993;50(7):577-584.
173. Wexler HK, Falkin GP, Lipton DS. Outcome evaluation of a prison therapeutic community for substance abuse treatment. *Crim Just Behav.* 1990;17(1):71-92.
174. Lipton DS, Pearson FS, Cleland CM, Yee D. The effects of therapeutic communities and milieu therapy on recidivism. In: McGuire J, ed. *Offender Rehabilitation and Treatment: Effective Programmes and Policies to Reduce Re-offending*; 2002:39-77.
175. American Psychiatric Association. *Textbook of Personality Disorders.* 3rd ed. American Psychiatric Association Publishing; 2021.
176. Soloff P. Somatic treatments. In: Oldham J, Skodol A, Bender D, eds. *Textbook of Personality Disorders.* American Psychiatric Publishing; 2005:387-403.

177. American Psychiatric Association. *Diagnostic and Statistical Manual of Mental Disorders 5-TR ed.* American Psychiatric Association; 2022.
178. Nelson K, Tsheringla S. Pharmacological management. In: Skodol A, Oldham J, eds. *Textbook of Personality Disorders*. 3rd ed. American Psychiatric Association; 2021:465-492.
179. Stoffers J, Vollm BA, Rucker G, Timmer A, Huband N, Lieb K. Pharmacological interventions for borderline personality disorder. *Cochrane Database Syst Rev.* 2010;6:CD005653. doi:10.1002/14651858.CD005653.pub2
180. Lieb K, Vollm B, Rucker G, Timmer A, Stoffers JM. Pharmacotherapy for borderline personality disorder: cochrane systematic review of randomised trials. *Br J Psychiatry.* 2010;196(1):4-12. doi:10.1192/bjp.bp.108.062984
181. Vita A, De Peri L, Sacchetti E. Antipsychotics, antidepressants, anticonvulsants, and placebo on the symptom dimensions of borderline personality disorder: a meta-analysis of randomized controlled and open-label trials. *J Clin Psychopharmacol.* 2011;31(5):613-624. doi:10.1097/JCP.0b013e31822c1636
182. Bellino S, Rinaldi C, Bozzatello P, Bogetto F. Pharmacotherapy of borderline personality disorder: a systematic review for publication purpose. *Curr Med Chem.* 2011;18(22):3322-3329. doi:10.2174/092986711796504682
183. Ingenhoven T, Lafay P, Rinne T, Passchier J, Duivenvoorden H. Effectiveness of pharmacotherapy for severe personality disorders: meta-analyses of randomized controlled trials. *J Clin Psychiatry.* 2010;71(1):14-25. doi:10.4088/jcp.08r04526gre
184. Gartlehner G, Crotty K, Kennedy S, et al. Pharmacological treatments for borderline personality disorder: a systematic review and meta-analysis. *CNS Drugs.* 2021;35(10):1053-1067. doi:10.1007/s40263-021-00855-4
185. Hollander E, Allen A, Lopez RP, et al. A preliminary double-blind, placebo-controlled trial of divalproex sodium in borderline personality disorder. *J Clin Psychiatry.* 2001;62(3):199-203. doi:10.4088/jcp.v62n0311
186. Frankenburg FR, Zanarini MC. Divalproex sodium treatment of women with borderline personality disorder and bipolar II disorder: a double-blind placebo-controlled pilot study. *J Clin Psychiatry.* 2002;63(5):442-446. doi:10.4088/jcp.v63n0511
187. Bellino S, Bozzatello P, Rocca G, Bogetto F. Efficacy of omega-3 fatty acids in the treatment of borderline personality disorder: a study of the association with valproic acid. *J Psychopharmacol.* 2014;28(2):125-132. doi:10.1177/0269881113510072
188. Loew TH, Nickel MK, Muehlbacher M, et al. Topiramate treatment for women with borderline personality disorder: a double-blind, placebo-controlled study. *J Clin Psychopharmacol.* 2006;26(1):61-66. doi:10.1097/01.jcp.0000195113.61291.48
189. Nickel MK, Nickel C, Kaplan P, et al. Treatment of aggression with topiramate in male borderline patients: a double-blind, placebo-controlled study. *Biol Psychiatry.* 2005;57(5):495-499. doi:10.1016/j.biopsych.2004.11.044
190. Tritt K, Nickel C, Lahmann C, et al. Lamotrigine treatment of aggression in female borderline-patients: a randomized, double-blind, placebo-controlled study. *J Psychopharmacol.* 2005;19(3):287-291. doi:10.1177/0269881105051540
191. Reich DB, Zanarini MC, Bieri KA. A preliminary study of lamotrigine in the treatment of affective instability in borderline personality disorder. *Int Clin Psychopharmacol.* 2009;24(5):270-275. doi:10.1097/YIC.0b013e32832d6c2f
192. Nickel MK, Muehlbacher M, Nickel C, et al. Aripiprazole in the treatment of patients with borderline personality disorder: a double-blind, placebo-controlled study. *Am J Psychiatry.* 2006;163(5):833-838. doi:10.1176/ajp.2006.163.5.833
193. Nickel MK, Loew TH, Pedrosa GF. Aripiprazole in treatment of borderline patients, part II: an 18-month follow-up. *Psychopharmacology (Berl).* 2007;191(4):1023-1026. doi:10.1007/s00213-007-0740-0
194. Bogenschutz MP, George NH. Olanzapine versus placebo in the treatment of borderline personality disorder. *J Clin Psychiatry.* 2004;65(1):104-109. doi:10.4088/jcp.v65n0118
195. Soler J, Pascual JC, Campins J, et al. Double-blind, placebo-controlled study of dialectical behavior therapy plus olanzapine for borderline personality disorder. *Am J Psychiatry.* 2005;162(6):1221-1224. doi:10.1176/appi.ajp.162.6.1221
196. Schulz SC, Zanarini MC, Bateman A, et al. Olanzapine for the treatment of borderline personality disorder: variable dose 12-week randomised double-blind placebo-controlled study. *Br J Psychiatry.* 2008;193(6):485-492. doi:10.1192/bjp.bp.107.037903
197. Stoffers-Winterling J, Storebo OJ, Lieb K. Pharmacotherapy for borderline personality disorder: an update of published, unpublished and ongoing studies. *Curr Psychiatry Rep.* 2020;22(8):37. doi:10.1007/s11920-020-01164-1
198. Jakobsen KD, Skyum E, Hashemi N, Schjerning O, Fink-Jensen A, Nielsen J. Antipsychotic treatment of schizotypy and schizotypal personality disorder: a systematic review. *J Psychopharmacol.* 2017;31(4):397-405. doi:10.1177/0269881117695879
199. Stoffers-Winterling J, Vollm B, Lieb K. Is pharmacotherapy useful for treating personality disorders? *Expert Opin Pharmacother.* 2021;22(4):393-395. doi:10.1080/14656566.2021.1873277
200. Khalifa NR, Gibbon S, Vollm BA, Cheung NH, McCarthy L. Pharmacological interventions for antisocial personality disorder. *Cochrane Database Syst Rev.* 2020;9:CD007667. doi:10.1002/14651858.CD007667.pub3

106 Co-occurring Posttraumatic Stress Disorder and Substance Use Disorders

Tanya C. Saraiya, Sudie E. Back, Michael E. Saladin, Therese K. Killeen, and Kathleen T. Brady

CHAPTER OUTLINE

- Introduction
- Phenomenology
- Epidemiology
- Etiological relationship between PTSD and SUDs
- Neurobiological factors in co-occurring PTSD and SUDs
- Assessment of PTSD in SUDs
- Treatment of PTSD and co-occurring PTSD-SUD
- Concluding comments

INTRODUCTION

For centuries in the Western hemisphere, symptoms of posttraumatic stress disorder (PTSD) have been recognized first in combat veterans, then in survivors of rape, and referred to by various names, including soldier's heart, shell shock, and combat neurosis, among others.[1] In 1980, the diagnosis of PTSD was first included in the *Diagnostic and Statistical Manual of Mental Disorders*, Third Edition (DSM-III), which resulted in a growing body of translational research investigating the etiology, neurobiology, comorbidity, and treatment of PTSD.[2] Over the past four decades, epidemiologic studies have investigated PTSD and its co-occurring disorders, finding substance use disorders (SUD) to be particularly common among individuals with a diagnosis of PTSD. Across civilians and veterans in the United States with PTSD, the prevalence of lifetime SUD is estimated to be between 30% to 76% compared to 10% to 34.9% among individuals without PTSD.[3-7] One study found that in almost half a million veterans, 63% with an alcohol use disorder also showed a diagnosis of PTSD and 76% with any SUD also showed a diagnosis of PTSD.[7] These data point to the highly co-occurring nature of PTSD and SUD and indicates that persons presenting to treatment for either PTSD or SUD should be screened for both disorders to ensure accurate assessment and the provision of appropriate treatment.

Regarding treatment, studies demonstrate a more complicated clinical course and worse treatment outcomes among individuals with co-occurring PTSD and SUD. In general, individuals with co-occurring PTSD and SUD have poorer treatment outcomes than those with SUD alone, a poorer quality of life, and more social and legal problems, suicide attempts, co-occurring mood and anxiety disorders, and violence.[8,9] They tend to have a longer duration of substance use, a greater number of SUD symptoms, undergo more episodes of SUD treatment, demonstrate less improvement during treatment than their counterparts with SUD alone, and simultaneously show more severe PTSD presentations. In a study of veterans with co-occurring PTSD and SUD ($N = 81$), high rates of suicide attempts (27.2%) and suicidal ideation (42.0%) were reported.[10] Another study examining the health and well-being of civilian men ($N = 65$) and women ($N = 68$) with SUD found that the presence of co-occurring PTSD was associated with significantly more chronic physical, cardiovascular, and neurological symptoms, as well as poorer mental health functional status.[11] These studies are part of a much larger body of literature examining the impact of co-occurring PTSD and SUD on various parameters of functioning and demonstrate the necessity of a thorough assessment of individuals with co-occurring PTSD-SUD. In this chapter, we address the phenomenology, epidemiology, assessment, and treatment of patients with co-occurring PTSD and SUD to assist clinicians in providing informed and effective care.

PHENOMENOLOGY

In the DSM-5-TR, PTSD is no longer classified as an anxiety disorder but was moved to the category of "Trauma and Stressor-Related Disorders."[12] The DSM-5 outlines the following criteria recommended to diagnose PTSD for adults, adolescents, and children over the age of 6 years old:

- The occurrence of a traumatic event (criterion A).
- Greater than 1 month of symptoms (criterion F) within the four symptom criteria of intrusion (criterion B), avoidance (criterion C), negative alterations in cognitions and mood (criterion D), and arousal and reactivity (criterion E), all of which cannot be due to the effects of a substance or medical condition (criterion H).
- Impaired functioning or significant distress (criterion G).
- If the onset of symptoms is 6 months or more after the traumatic event, the disorder is considered to have a delayed expression or onset.[12]

The definition of a qualifying traumatic event has also changed in DSM-5. An individual must have directly experienced or witnessed a traumatic event or learned about an event happening to a close family member or friend. The traumatic event must involve "actual or threatened death" or "serious injury to self or others." If an individual reports learning that the traumatic event happened to a close family member or friend, the event must be accidental or involve violence. Sexual violence replaced "threat to physical integrity," and repeated and extreme exposure to aversive details of the traumatic event have been included. The latter is meant to include first responders, such as police officers and emergency medical personnel, and is clarified in DSM-5-TR to not include exposure to electronic media unless such exposure is work related. The "intense fear, helplessness, or horror" response at the time of the trauma has been eliminated in DSM-5.[12]

There are many ways in which patients with PTSD re-experience (criterion B) traumatic events. They may report unpleasant dreams related to the trauma, intrusive involuntary memories of the event, or behave as if an event were currently happening (ie, dissociative flashbacks). Re-experiencing may also occur through cues that elicit memories of the trauma(s) and then trigger intense or prolonged psychological distress or physiological reactivity, thus leading to avoidance behaviors (criterion C). Patients may avoid distressing memories, thoughts, and feelings (C1), and/or, activities, places, conversations, or people (C2) associated with the trauma. Individuals must meet at least one of the two avoidance symptoms to meet diagnostic criteria for PTSD.[12]

The new symptom cluster, negative alterations in cognition and mood (criterion D), consists of: (1) three numbing symptoms from the DSM-IV avoidance cluster (amnesia of dissociative nature [D1], diminished interest [D5], detachment or estrangement [D6]); (2) two new symptoms involving distorted cognitions leading to blame of self and others (D3) and negative emotional states, such as fear, shame, anger, or guilt (D4); and (3) two symptoms that have been altered from DSM-IV: exaggerated negative beliefs about self, others or the world (D2) and a persistent inability to experience positive emotions (D7).[12,13]

The symptoms of alterations in arousal and reactivity (criterion E) include irritable behavior and/or angry outbursts involving verbal or physical aggression toward people or objects (E1), hypervigilance (E3), exaggerated startle response (E4), problems with concentration (E5), and sleep disturbance (E6). One additional symptom, reckless or destructive behavior, has been added to this criterion (E2). The addition of two symptoms related to depersonalization and derealization recognizes a dissociative subtype of PTSD.[12,13]

The DSM-5-TR recognizes that although the criterion A index trauma is used as the basis of symptom endorsement, many patients with multiple closely related events have symptoms that exist prior to the index event. Thus, for symptoms in criterion D and E, individuals with multiple closely related events can experience either onset or exacerbation of symptoms following the index event. However, the avoidance and re-experiencing symptoms must have an onset following the index trauma.[13]

Of note, after experiencing a traumatic event, many patients present with some symptoms of PTSD, but do not meet the threshold for a formal diagnosis of PTSD. This clinical presentation is termed subthreshold PTSD and can be diagnosed as "Unspecified Trauma/Stressor-Related Disorder." Various definitions have been proposed for subthreshold PTSD in the research literature,[14,15] where the greatest consensus suggests that subthreshold PTSD is meeting two to three of criterion B thru E. There is some evidence that subthreshold PTSD is more common among individuals witnessing traumatic events happening to loved ones,[15] but additional work should continue to examine formal definitions of subthreshold of PTSD to capture the breadth of responses to traumatic events.

It has been estimated that between 39% and 90% of the population has been exposed to a traumatic event,[16] and of those who experience a traumatic event, 10% to 20% will develop PTSD[17] where a greater percentage will report subthreshold PTSD symptoms.[14,15] However, specific subsets of the population, namely individuals holding a diverse identity, show higher prevalence rates. Specifically, greater trauma exposure and PTSD diagnosis is evidenced among racial and ethnic minority communities,[18-22]sexual minorities,[23] and women.[24] Higher risk to trauma exposure and PTSD diagnosis among these communities with structural and systemic inequities increases the risk of oppression, discrimination, and thus, trauma exposure and PTSD.[25] This risk for greater trauma exposure along with other health concerns based on individual identity is considered among the social determinants of health. Such social determinants of health also increase the risk of other traumas and stressors which may be closely related or fall outside the scope of criterion A. These traumas include racial trauma, discrimination, incarceration, adverse childhood experiences, historical trauma, and intergenerational trauma, and are under investigation for their association with PTSD development and severity.[26-30]

Although DSM-5-TR yielded lower prevalence rates than DSM-IV (lifetime 8.3% versus 9.8%, respectively), there is still a high degree of concordance.[31] The differences are largely attributed to the more restrictive criterion A and needing at least one of the two avoidance symptoms (criterion C) to meet PTSD diagnosis. The revisions made to DSM-5 add more objectivity and clarity when assessing qualifying trauma events and PTSD symptoms.[13]

EPIDEMIOLOGY

Several epidemiological studies have examined the rates of co-occurring PTSD and SUD. The National Comorbidity Survey (NCS), a large-scale epidemiologic survey ($N = 5,877$) conducted in the early 1990s, examined psychiatric disorders in the U.S. general population. Using DSM-III-Revised criteria, the NCS found the overall lifetime prevalence rate for PTSD at 7.8%, and those with PTSD were 2 to 4 times more likely than their counterparts without PTSD to meet criteria for a SUD.[17] The National Comorbidity Survey Replication (NSC-R), which took place approximately one decade after the NCS, found a similar overall lifetime PTSD prevalence rate (6.8%) using DSM-IV criteria.[32] The National Epidemiologic Survey on Alcohol and Related Conditions (NESARC) was conducted in two waves and Wave 2 assessed for PTSD using DSM-IV-TR from 2004 to 2005 ($N = 34,653$). It was estimated in the NESARC Wave 2 that 1.6% of the U.S. population meets criteria for co-occurring alcohol dependence and PTSD.[3] The NESARC-III was conducted between 2012 and 2013 and included 36,309 civilians. Using modified DSM-5 criteria (modified to require three or more symptoms in D and E), it was found that the odds ratios for a co-occurring SUD was 1.3 among those with PTSD in the past 12 months and 1.5 among those with PTSD in their lifetime.[33] Finally, the National Survey on Drug Use and Health Mental Health Surveillance Survey (NSDUH-MHSS) assessed PTSD among a sample from 2008 and 2012 using DSM-IV-TR definitions of PTSD ($N = 5,653$) and found that adults with exposure to potentially traumatic events (ie, termed "potentially" since data was collected via survey rather than clinical interview) were more likely to use substances than those who had no history of such exposure.[34] Therefore, large epidemiological studies of the U.S. population support the strong co-occurrence between PTSD and SUD.

The prevalence of co-occurring PTSD and SUDs has been examined in various populations, with U.S. veterans being one of the most extensively investigated groups. Among a nationally representative sample of 1,484 veterans in 2013, lifetime DSM-5 PTSD probability was estimated to be 8.1% and PTSD was associated with increased odds of SUD (OR = 3.9-4.5).[35] Co-occurring PTSD and SUD has been associated with serious health consequences. A recent study examining 272,509 veterans with PTSD receiving services within the Veterans Health Administration between 2005 and 2007 found that SUD was associated with increased mortality, and SUD was a stronger predictor among veterans under the age of 45 for non-injury-related mortality, and for older age groups SUD was a stronger predictor for injury-related mortality.[36]

Similarly, minority groups in the U.S. have also evidenced higher prevalence rates of PTSD and SUD singularly[20,37-40] suggesting higher prevalence rates of co-occurring PTSD and SUD. However, limited work has investigated such disparities,[41] calling for a much-needed area of future investigation. Nevertheless, collectively, present data indicate a high prevalence of this co-occurrence in a variety of clinical populations, suggesting a unique and potent interconnectedness between PTSD and SUD, and raising questions about the relationship between these two disorders.

ETIOLOGICAL RELATIONSHIP BETWEEN PTSD AND SUDs

Various theories have been proposed to characterize the development of co-occurring PTSD and SUD. As one of the most prominent, the self-medication hypothesis,[42-49] postulates that substance use serves to alleviate PTSD symptoms and this alleviation of symptoms is negatively reinforcing. That is, in the case of primary PTSD (ie, person first develops PTSD and subsequently develops SUD), the substance use may be driven largely by the need to relieve negative mood states and distress associated with PTSD symptoms. In the case of secondary PTSD (ie, person first develops SUD and is later exposed to trauma and develops PTSD), the alcohol/drug use may be driven largely by the need for relief from a state of deficit caused by neuroadaptations that occur due to chronic substance use (ie, withdrawal, chronic heavy use), which is also negatively reinforcing and a form of self-medication. An additional mechanism for secondary PTSD is that substance use can increase the risk of trauma exposure, and chronic substance use can in turn increase the likelihood that such trauma exposure develops into PTSD.[49] The causes of substance use in patients with SUD and PTSD are multifaceted and likely not mutually exclusive.[49] However, in short, whether PTSD is primary or secondary, dually afflicted individuals may use substances to relieve negative mood/anxiety associated with PTSD, relieve aversive withdrawal states associated with chronic substance use, or both.

As mentioned above, sometimes the onset of the SUD precedes the development of PTSD. This is called the high-risk model wherein the probability of developing PTSD is increased via three potential causal pathways. The first potential pathway may be through the cognitive impairments caused by using substances. Use of many substances, including alcohol, impairs decision-making and can attenuate fear responses. Combined, this can put an individual at risk of experiencing a potentially traumatic event while intoxicated.[50,51] Second, the lifestyle of a person who uses substances, which is typically considered to be high-risk with dangerous environments and behaviors associated with obtaining or using alcohol or drugs, may increase the likelihood of experiencing a traumatic event and subsequently developing PTSD. Finally, the increased anxiety and arousal that accompanies chronic substance use may increase the biologic vulnerability to develop PTSD after trauma exposure.[52]

Lastly, there is some evidence that other factors may play a role in the development of co-occurring PTSD and SUD. Plausible factors that have been investigated include brain structure and connectivity abnormalities, hypothalamic-pituitary-adrenal axis, genetics, and psychosocial factors, all of which appear to be influenced by social determinants of health.[53,54] The direction of the causal relationship between co-occurring PTSD and SUD is likely to vary from one individual to another and may not be unidirectional. Therefore, it is important to assess the temporal course of onset of PTSD and SUD among each patient, as well as their reasons for current alcohol/drug use in order to help develop the most effective treatment plan for that particular patient.[49]

NEUROBIOLOGICAL FACTORS IN CO-OCCURRING PTSD AND SUDs

Research has delineated common neurobiological factors and dysregulation associated with PTSD and SUDs.[55] In relation to brain structure and connectivity, PTSD and SUD are associated with changes in corticolimbic structures, in particular the amygdala (AMY) and prefrontal cortex (PFC).[56] Individuals with PTSD exhibit hypoactive executive functioning (PFC) and hyperactive fear circuitry (AMY) activity.[57] Additionally, disconnection between the PFC and AMY has been found in those with PTSD,[58] which may explain failure to extinguish fear responses.[59,60] Alcohol and/or drug cues stimulate AMY and PFC activity[61,62] and individuals with DSM-IV defined alcohol dependence have lower AMY volume, which is associated with increased craving and alcohol consumption.[63] Research shows that chronic use of alcohol produces long-term plasticity in the medial PFC and impairs the extinction of fear, suggesting that alcohol may facilitate the development and/or maintenance of PTSD.[64] Dysregulation in corticolimbic structures common to both PTSD and SUD is also likely to reduce ability to regulate intrusive trauma-related memories and craving-related thoughts. As such, corticolimbic impairment may be an important target for intervention for individuals with PTSD and SUD. For instance, transcranial magnetic stimulation (TMS) noninvasively stimulates brain tissue and has shown preliminary, albeit small and sometimes conflicting, improvements in PTSD samples by targeting the corticolimbic system requiring further investigation.[65,66] In addition, deep brain stimulation (DBS) is a more surgically invasive method where electrodes stimulate the brain. Case studies have suggested promise with DBS for reductions in PTSD symptoms, but additional work is needed, and the surgical risks of this intervention remain high.[65]

The hypothalamic-pituitary-adrenal (HPA) axis and the autonomic nervous system are also key components in the development and maintenance of PTSD and SUD.[67,68] These neurobiological systems regulate the human physiological response to stress. As illustrated in **Figure 106-1** the HPA axis response involves the release of corticotropin releasing factor (CRF) from the hypothalamus, which stimulates adrenocorticotrophin hormone (ACTH) release from the anterior pituitary and, in turn, stimulates the release of cortisol from the adrenal glands. On the other hand, the autonomic nervous system response to stress is activated through the release of epinephrine (EPI) and norepinephrine (NE). Both CRF and autonomic nervous system dysfunction has been implicated in PTSD and SUD. Individuals with PTSD have higher levels of CRF and corticotropin-releasing hormone (CRH) compared to controls.[69,70] In laboratory animal models stress has been shown to reinstate previously extinguished drug seeking behavior, and CRF and noradrenergic pathways appear involved.[71] In animal models administration of CRH leads to reinstatement of drug taking following extinction.[71] Further, among people with DSM-IV defined cocaine dependence, CRH administration increased drug craving and subjective stress.[72] Thus in individuals with PTSD, high CRH, EPI and NE levels may further increase anxiety, craving, and lead to exacerbated withdrawal symptoms upon cessation of substances.[52]

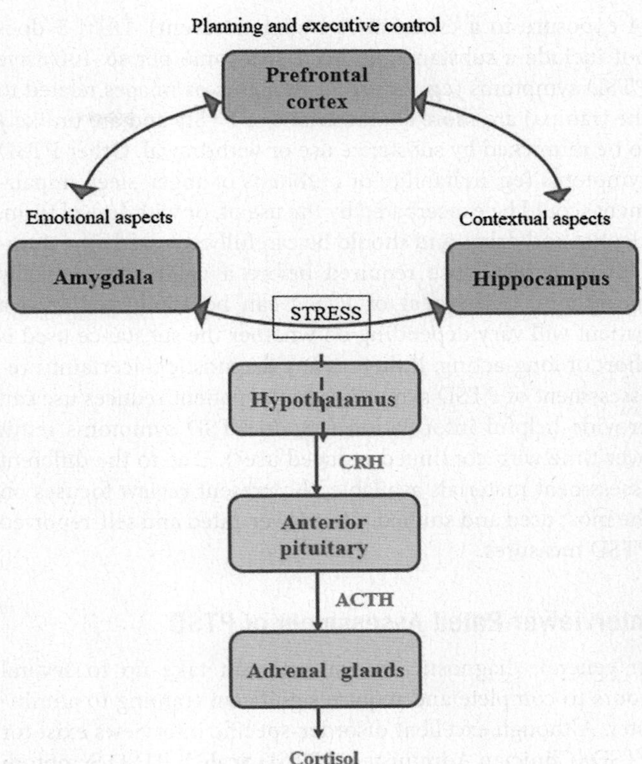

Figure 106-1. Corticolimbic structures and the hypothalamic-pituitary-adrenal axis. (Adapted from Groeneweg FL, et al. Rapid non-genomic effects of corticosteroids and their role in the central stress response. *J Endocrinol.* 2011;209(2):153-167.)

ASSESSMENT OF PTSD IN SUDs

Given the high rates of trauma and PTSD among individuals with SUD, it is important to screen all SUD patients. Numerous interviewer-rated and self-report assessments for PTSD are available.[73,74] Reviews of the literature have found that brief PTSD measures (ie, 30 items or less) appear to be as good as longer, more complicated measures.[75,76] Accordingly, the assessment of PTSD in persons with SUD can be completed more quickly and efficiently from a clinical resource management perspective (eg, staff/clinician time). In fact, the gains to be achieved in terms of quality of care far exceed any resource expenditures. In this section, we highlight some of the most commonly used and psychometrically sound interview and self-report instruments for assessing PTSD,[75,76] with revised recommendations made given the changes in the diagnostic criteria of PTSD in the DSM-5[77] and noted measurement invariance across specific populations with PTSD and SUD.[78,79]

PTSD assessment should be conducted after a patient has emerged from acute alcohol or drug intoxication and withdrawal.[80] In contrast to other anxiety disorders (eg, generalized anxiety disorder), less abstinence may be required to establish a diagnosis of PTSD among SUD patients because of the unique nature of the diagnostic criteria (ie, requirement of exposure to a criterion A traumatic event). DSM-5 does not include a substance-induced syndrome per se. Intrusive PTSD symptoms (eg, recurrent thoughts or images related to the trauma) are more characteristic of PTSD and are unlikely to be mimicked by substance use or withdrawal. Other PTSD symptoms (eg, irritability or outbursts of anger, sleep impairment) could be exacerbated by the use of, or withdrawal from, alcohol and drugs and should be carefully assessed. The duration of reduced use required before a valid and clinically meaningful assessment of PTSD can be conducted with a patient will vary depending on whether the substance used is short or long-acting. If there is any diagnostic uncertainty, reassessment of PTSD symptoms as the patient reduces use can provide helpful information (eg, do PTSD symptoms remit over time with continued reduced use?). Due to the different assessment materials available, the present review focuses on the most used and studied interviewer-rated and self-reported PTSD measures.

Interviewer-Rated Assessment of PTSD

In general, diagnostic assessments can take up to several hours to complete and require significant training to administer. Although excellent disorder-specific interviews exist for PTSD (Clinician Administered PTSD Scale,[81] PTSD Symptom Scale—Interview Version[82]), interviews designed to assess the full spectrum of psychiatric disorders may be better suited for treatment planning, especially in samples with high rates of co-occurring psychiatric disorders (eg, SUD, major depressive disorder). One of the best examples of this is the Structured Clinical Interview of DSM-5 Disorders (SCID[83]). Additional structured clinical interviews include the Mini International Neuropsychiatric Interview,[84] which also provides the DSM diagnoses but takes approximately half the time to administer relative to the SCID. Of note, novel research utilizing advanced statistical methods has assessed the validity of PTSD assessments among diverse populations. Morgan-López et al. found that some PTSD measurements are less accurate and show risk of bias and poorer accuracy among some populations (ie, measurement invariance whereby certain items/symptoms are weighted more heavily to represent PTSD).[79] Morgan-López et al. found that the Clinician Administered PTSD Scale for DSM-5 (CAPS-5[81]; see below) showed bias among incarcerated women and African Americans by rating them to have lower severity of PTSD than their true symptom presentations.[79] These findings suggest that while these assessments are critical to clinical practice, assessors should be aware of possible bias in scores among some individuals. Future work in this area is needed to increase the validity of PTSD assessments.

Clinician-Administered PTSD Scale for DSM-5 (CAPS-5)

The most widely used interviewer-rated PTSD assessment is the *Clinician Administered PTSD Scale for DSM-5* (CAPS-5).[81] This is a 30-item structured interview that was developed at the National Center for PTSD and is designed for use by clinicians and trained paraprofessionals. A Life Event Checklist of potentially traumatic events is included at the beginning of the interview to assess lifetime trauma exposure. Twenty items assess the frequency and intensity of diagnostic PTSD symptoms (eg, re-experiencing, avoidance, numbing, hyperarousal). In addition, items assess onset and duration of symptoms, subjective distress, social and occupational functioning, symptom change for repeated administration, overall response validity, overall PTSD severity, and specifications for the dissociative subtype. The CAPS-5 can be used to make current diagnosis of PTSD (past month), lifetime diagnosis of PTSD, and assess PTSD symptom severity. In addition, the past week CAPS-5 can assess for symptom change from the past week. The full CAPS-5 interview takes 45 to 60 minutes to administer.

PTSD Symptom Scale—Interview for DSM-5

The PTSD Symptom Scale—Interview for DSM-5 (PSSI-5)[82] is a 24-item clinician-rater, semi-structured interview for PTSD. The measure begins with an assessment of trauma exposure, and continues to assess the 20 symptoms of PTSD as defined in the DSM-5: intrusions, avoidance, changes in mood and cognition, and arousal and hyperactivity. Frequency and severity scores are rated for each symptom. The remaining items assess distress, interference, and duration of the symptoms. Studies comparing the PSSI-5 and CAPS-5 have demonstrated similar reliability for each measure.[82] The PSSI-5 takes approximately 30 minutes to complete.

Structured Clinical Interview for DSM-5 Disorders

The Structured Clinical Interview for DSM-5 Disorders (SCID)[83] is a semi-structured interview designed to diagnose most DSM-5 disorders (eg, depressive, psychotic, anxiety, substance use, and eating disorders). The DSM-III-R SCID[85] was the first comprehensive semi-structured interview for the diagnosis of PTSD. The SCID has been revised to reflect modifications for each version of the DSM.[83,85,86] The SCID contains a section that briefly reviews lifetime exposure to traumatic events and the age of occurrence, followed by diagnostic questions to assess PTSD symptoms. If multiple traumas exist, the diagnostic questions are asked in relation to the trauma that has most affected the patient.

MINI International Neuropsychiatric Interview PTSD Module

The MINI[84] is a brief structured clinical interview that, like the SCID, assesses most major psychiatric disorders, including PTSD. The MINI PTSD module assesses diagnostic PTSD symptoms during the past month. Relative to the SCID and CAPS-5, this instrument has the advantage of significantly shorter administration time, but with similar reliability findings.[84]

Composite International Diagnostic Interview

The Composite International Diagnostic Interview (CIDI)[87,88] is a standardized interview and it assesses most major mental disorders. Unlike the other interviewer-rated measures mentioned in this chapter, the CIDI provides diagnosis according to the *International Classification of Diseases*, 10th Edition (ICD-10), which is slightly different from the DSM with regard to PTSD diagnostic criteria, and demonstrates similar reliability findings to that of the SCID.[89] The CIDI is suitable for lay interviewers. Versions are available to assess past 12 months and lifetime symptoms. In addition, a computerized version of the CIDI is available.

In general, clinical interviewing of trauma can pose some challenges for clinicians as patients may be reluctant to talk about trauma, struggle to identify trauma in their lifetime (ie, patients may believe their traumas are "natural" or "a normal part of living") or have experienced so many traumas that the interview can become longer than anticipated. While it is important to assess for trauma exposure since it informs symptomatic presentations, interviewers are advised to hold a balance of compassion and efficiency to complete trauma interviews within the time allotted. This presents as having a welcoming, trusting, and safe presence to encourage disclosures of trauma while acknowledging time limitations. Statements such as, "I know we have a lot to cover today. Could you briefly tell me about any difficult experiences you have lived through where you feared for your life or the life of others? For instance, this could be physical assault, sexual assault, losing someone suddenly, combat, or something else." If an interview begins to become too long, interviews can be respectfully shortened by saying statements such as, "I'm so sorry you went through this experience. Unfortunately, we have limited time today, but I am making note of these experiences to ensure we give you the proper time and care to attend to what you've lived through in your future treatment planning." Most patients are receptive to gentle directing in clinical interviewing given that asking about trauma and providing space for it to be discussed can be healing in and of itself. Allow patients the opportunity to give only as much information about their trauma as they feel comfortable.

Self-Report Assessment of PTSD

Once a PTSD diagnosis has been established, symptom frequency and severity are the next essential components to treatment planning and monitoring. Several measures have been developed for monitoring PTSD symptoms. These measures are generally brief, self-report assessments of the 20 symptoms associated with PTSD. Some of the most widely used include the PTSD Checklist for DSM-5 (PCL-5)[90,91] and the Posttraumatic Diagnostic Scale for DSM-5 (PDS-5).[92] These measures provide quick feedback regarding symptom severity and include cutoff scores to inform a provisional diagnostic status, which can be verified with a validated clinical interview. Self-report measures are an excellent tool to assess changes in symptom severity particularly when a PTSD diagnosis has already been established or when requiring a briefer assessment. Separate trauma-specific versions of symptom severity measures also have been developed (eg, military versus civilian[73,93]). In addition, briefer versions have been proposed to further reduce the time demands, although less accuracy of symptom severity compared to questionnaires such as the PTSD Checklist for DSM-5.[94]

PTSD Checklist for DSM-5

The PCL-5[90] is a 20-item self-report measure that assesses PTSD symptoms according to the DSM-5 criteria experienced in the last month. Items assess symptoms across the four symptom clusters of PTSD (re-experiencing, numbing, avoidance, and hyperarousal) on a 0 to 4 Likert scale. Total scores range from 0 to 80, with a score of 31 to 33 indicating probable PTSD.[91] PCL-5 scores of 31 to 33 have shown high sensitivity (0.88) and specificity (0.69) when compared to the CAPS-5 among two samples of veterans.[91] These values suggest that the PCL-5 is good at assessing PTSD symptoms among those with PTSD but can have slightly more false positives than the gold standard CAPS-5 clinical interview. Versions of the PCL have been studied for the DSM-IV and DSM-5, as well as different trauma foci, each of which have received support for their reliability and validity in the literature.[73]

Posttraumatic Diagnostic Scale for DSM-5

The PDS-5[92] is a 24-item self-report measure of DSM-5 PTSD criteria and symptom severity for all four symptom clusters. The PDS-5 begins with two screen questions to assess trauma exposure, and then focuses the symptom questions on a single traumatic event. The next items assess the 20 symptoms of PTSD as defined in the DSM-5-TR: intrusions (items 1-5), avoidance (items 6-7), changes in mood and cognition (items 8-14), and arousal and hyperactivity (items 15-20). The remaining items assess overall distress and interference, and onset and duration of the symptoms. This self-report measure mirrors the interviewer-rated assessment developed by the same authors (PSSI-5).[82]

TREATMENT OF PTSD AND CO-OCCURRING PTSD-SUD

A broad range of traditional and specialized therapies have been promoted for the treatment of PTSD, several of which have received considerable empirical scrutiny. More recently, there has been a growth of studies of therapies specifically designed to address PTSD and SUD concurrently. Whether one considers the treatment of PTSD alone or PTSD-SUD comorbidity, treatments tend to fall into two general classes: psychotherapy and pharmacotherapy (or their combination). This section will briefly describe, discuss, and evaluate these two general classes of interventions with respect to the treatment of PTSD and co-occurring PTSD-SUD.

An exhaustive review of the treatment literature is not possible given space limitations, so consequently we have adopted the following focus. First, three types of cognitive-behavioral therapies (CBTs) for PTSD will be discussed; namely, (1) exposure-based therapy, (2) cognitive-focused therapy, and (3) anxiety/stress management therapy. CBTs for PTSD are emphasized here because they are widely accepted as the most empirically valid treatments for PTSD.[95] Additionally, results from some studies suggest that the treatment of one disorder in people with more than one psychiatric disorder often yields clinical benefits for the untreated co-occurring disorder.[96] This being the case, treatment of PTSD in people with co-occurring PTSD-SUD is important because it can be expected to have a positive impact on substance use. Second, we will outline and discuss integrative CBTs for the concurrent treatment of PTSD and SUD. These are relatively recent and comprehensive treatments that make an explicit attempt to concurrently address PTSD and SUD symptomatology. Each treatment will be described in some detail to elucidate both unique features and specific commonalities, and important research findings will be briefly outlined. Third, we will examine pharmacotherapies for PTSD and, fourth, we will describe developments in pharmacotherapy for co-occurring PTSD-SUD. These latter two sections will be relatively brief, as this type of treatment has not yielded efficacy findings on par with CBT.

Although this chapter will focus on treatments for PTSD, it is important to note that some investigators have explored the use of psychotherapeutic techniques soon after trauma exposure to prevent the development of PTSD. A psychosocial intervention delivered directly after the trauma, called single-session critical incident stress debriefing, has not been shown to be effective in preventing the development of PTSD, and may also be harmful.[97] However, delivering CBT to individuals with Acute Stress Disorder (ASD; which is diagnosed at least two days after the trauma) has been shown to mitigate or prevent the development of chronic PTSD.[98,99] Since CBT techniques used for ASD treatment are the same as those used for PTSD treatment (eg, exposure and cognitive therapy strategies), this section will focus primarily on CBTs designed to treat PTSD.

CBT for PTSD

Exposure-Based Therapy

There are several forms of exposure-based therapy,[100-103] and as a group, they represent the longest-standing empirically validated psychotherapies for PTSD. Exposure therapies are based on conditioning[104-106] and information processing[107] theories of fear acquisition and attenuation. Conditioning models assert that fear abatement results from behavioral extinction,[108] which is simply a procedure of repeated exposure to fear-eliciting situations or stimuli (eg, physical location where a motor vehicle accident occurred) in the absence of the feared outcome (eg, motor vehicle accident) until the fear response subsides. This is a form of inhibitory learning where the expression of the fear response is opposed and thereby provides memory for new learning (eg, absence of a motor vehicle accident in the physical location where the motor vehicle accident occurred). Contemporary neuropsychological models suggest that fear reduction occurs via the formation of a new memory during behavioral extinction that inhibits fear responding.[108-110] Similarly, information processing models highlight that fear attenuation occurs when an individual processes new information that contrasts with, and modifies, the pathological elements of a traumatic memory.

Procedurally, individuals are either exposed to in vivo or imaginal fear-eliciting cues. In the former case, exposure is performed via confronting situations in real life that one associates with the traumatic experience, whereas in the latter case, exposure is performed via confronting the memory of the traumatic experience (eg, revisiting the trauma memory aloud during session). One of the major advantages of imaginal exposure over in vivo exposure methods is that trauma cues that would otherwise be difficult and/or unethical (ie, physical conditions present in a combat situation, distant locations where an assault occurred) to use in exposure therapy can be easily integrated into an imagery-based procedure. Both in vivo and imaginal procedures reduce avoidance behavior and promote self-mastery.

One of the most extensively studied exposure treatments for PTSD is Prolonged Exposure therapy or PE.[111] Briefly, the treatment consists of several primary components including: (1) psychoeducation about common reactions to traumatic events, (2) relaxation via breathing retraining, (3) prolonged imaginal exposure to the trauma via detailed, therapist guided, revisiting of the event(s), and (4) in vivo exposure to trauma-related situations that are safe but avoided because they elicit fear. Although the duration of PE therapy can vary, a typical course is completed in 8 to 12 sessions, with each session lasting about 60 to 90 minutes.[112] However, some patients may experience marked improvements in symptoms with as few as 3 to 5 sessions. One study, for example, found that 35% of their participants achieved significant and sudden gains between sessions 3 and 5 of PE.[113] In addition, PE has been modified for primary care settings as a brief, 4 to 6 session, 30 minute treatment to attend to patients in the primary care setting with sub-threshold PTSD and has shown positive outcomes.[114] In general, it is standard practice to monitor PTSD symptoms throughout treatment and tailor treatment length as needed. Furthermore, PE has also been modified to attend to racial trauma among Black/African Americans,[115] although larger randomized clinical trials are needed to assess the efficacy of these modifications.

There is another form of exposure-based therapy that requires brief consideration. Shapiro[116-118] forwarded an extension of Wolpe's[106] systematic desensitization therapy that was initially named eye movement desensitization (EMD therapy). Shapiro later added the term 'reprocessing' (hence, EMDR therapy) to denote a conceptual shift towards an information processing interpretation of the therapy's mechanism of action. In line with emotional and information processing theories, EMDR is presumed to exert its effects by assisting patients in reprocessing the trauma memory and modifying any problematic/unhelpful associations or components of the memory. Although EMDR is not typically categorized as an exposure-based therapy in the literature more broadly, certain aspects of this therapy overlap with imaginal exposure. Specifically, one of its central elements involves the therapist eliciting vivid trauma-related imagery while having the patient rehearse alternative interpretations of the imagined traumatic event(s). This aspect of EMDR is similar to exposure with cognitive therapy features.

EMDR differs from standard exposure-based and cognitive therapies in several important ways. First, therapists encourage patients to engage in free associations that emerge after recalling the trauma memory. Thus, a wide array of memories and associations may be discussed during a given EMDR session. The second difference, and perhaps the most unique feature of EMDR, is that therapists conduct the imaginal exposure while the patient simultaneously engages in bilateral stimulation eye movements. Bilateral stimulation originally included visually tracking the back-and-forth movement of a therapist-manipulated object (eg, the therapist's finger), although other forms of bilateral stimulation have been used in EMDR, such as audio stimulation or tactile sensations like hand tapping. Some experimental research in healthy controls suggests that bilateral stimulation may reduce vividness and emotional associations for autobiographical memories.[119] Accordingly, Shapiro and colleagues have proposed that bilateral stimulation may facilitate distress reduction, reducing avoidance of the trauma memory, and increasing the ability to process the trauma memory and develop more adaptive trauma-related thoughts and associations.[116]

Finally, a recently developed form of exposure therapy is Written Exposure Therapy.[120] Written Exposure Therapy consists of five individual, 60-minute sessions which focus on (1) psychoeducation about common reactions to trauma and PTSD, (2) imaginal exposure with the therapist where the patient writes the trauma narrative in each session for 30 minutes, and (3) cognitive and emotional processing of the patient's experience writing the trauma narrative. Unlike PE, Written Exposure Therapy does not have between-session homework or in vivo exposures and is significantly shorter in treatment length, all of which has been shown to enhance treatment retention.[121,122] The evidence base of Written Exposure Therapy is continuing to grow and demonstrate its advantages as a brief exposure-based treatment for PTSD.

Cognitive-Focused Therapy

There are essentially two therapies that comprise this class, cognitive therapy (CT) and cognitive processing therapy (CPT). Cognitive therapy refers to a broad class of therapy that was originally developed as a treatment for depression[123,124] and subsequently extended to address anxiety[125,126] as well as SUD.[127] As applied to PTSD, the therapy is built conceptually around the notion that it is the *meaning* that individuals assign to traumatic events, rather than the traumatic events, which determines the duration and intensity of emotion/mood states that ensue. Accordingly, interpretations or meanings that are negatively biased or irrational give rise to negative mood states such as fear and anxiety. The goal of CT then is to aid individuals in implementing corrective cognitive procedures to identify and challenge inaccurate, irrational thoughts and beliefs and to replace them with ones that are more evidence-based, rational, and beneficial. For example, patterns of thinking challenged in CT for PTSD could include unhelpful beliefs about the trauma (eg, self-blame or guilt), about oneself (eg, perception of one's own control or capacity to cope), or about the world and others (eg, perceptions of safety and trustworthiness).

The other therapy in this class, CPT, is like CT but has a decidedly more emotional focus. CPT is a PTSD-specific treatment protocol developed by Resick and Schnicke[128,129] that combines a cognitive focus with elements of exposure therapy. Although originally developed to address PTSD resulting from sexual assault, it has been extended to victims of other types of traumas.[130,131] This therapy has several important elements that are presumed to have therapeutic potency. There is a psychoeducation component in which an information-processing model of PTSD is presented. The exposure element consists of a writing-reading task where the individual develops a detailed narrative of their traumatic experience(s). The goal of this component is for the individual to maximize emotional processing of the trauma and to identify areas of incomplete processing or unhelpful thought/belief patterns related to the trauma. The primary feature of this treatment is the cognitive therapy component that involves identification and challenging of key cognitive distortions. Specific areas of belief that are targeted for challenge relate to themes of safety, trust, power, esteem, and intimacy. The therapy generally concludes with an analysis of beliefs, including changes to dysfunctional thinking, and discussion of future goals. Completion of CPT can be achieved in approximately twelve 60-to-90-minute therapy sessions. Akin to work on PE, the need for greater personalization of treatments to diverse individuals has led to the cultural modification of CPT to specific communities, such as Indigenous Americans[132,133] and low- and middle-income countries, such as the Democratic Republic of the Congo.[134] This work has shown that evidence-based treatments for PTSD are modifiable to the unique needs of diverse populations.

Anxiety Management Therapy

While there are several therapies that could be considered members of this category (eg, biofeedback and relaxation training[135]), one of the most widely known and studied is Stress Inoculation Training[136-138] or SIT. This treatment is based on Lazarus and Folkman's[139] model that stress occurs when the demands of a situation are viewed as outweighing one's ability to cope. As applied to PTSD,[140,141] the main goal of this therapy is to provide individuals with a sense of mastery over their PTSD symptoms by teaching them a variety of coping skills and then permitting them to practice the skills both inside and outside of treatment sessions. SIT can be used in both individual and group formats and has broad application to a variety of anxiety disorders (eg, panic disorder). Common elements of SIT are relaxation training, breathing training, thought-stopping, self-instruction training, assertiveness training, cognitive restructuring, anger management, and problem-solving training. After learning new coping skills, patients practice them in increasingly anxiety-provoking situations such as graduated exposures, as a method of "inoculation" against relapse and preparation for coping with future difficulties. These skills can be taught and practiced over 8 to 12 sessions, and the therapy can be adapted to briefer psycho-educational formats.

Effectiveness of CBT for PTSD

A detailed review of the efficacy literature is not possible given space limitations, and readers are referred to several recent reviews and meta-analyses of CBT for PTSD.[95,142-153] An important caveat to consider is that the findings from these reviews may have limited generalizability to co-occurring PTSD-SUD; one review[148] noted that 62% of PTSD therapy studies reviewed excluded individuals with a co-occurring SUD. With this caveat in mind, there are some general and a few specific conclusions that can be drawn from the extant literature.

First and foremost, all CBTs produce clinically significant reductions in PTSD symptomatology relative to wait-list or treatment as usual (TAU) comparisons. The treatments also tend to produce appreciable benefits on collateral symptoms of depression and generalized anxiety. The treatments appear to benefit a range of populations including those with civilian and combat-related PTSD. A recent meta-analysis showed that treatment discontinuation rates from evidence-based treatments for PTSD are on average, 14% to 18%[154] although many studies have reported higher rates closer to 20% to 40%.[155,156]

While differences among the treatments are difficult to discern from this vast and complex literature of clinical trials, the reviews suggest several qualified generalizations. One such generalization is that imaginal exposure procedures lead to substantial symptom reduction beyond what can be achieved with anxiety management procedures such as SIT or CT. This has been evidenced through the advent of Written Exposure Therapy.[121,122,157] A second conclusion is that the combination of in vivo and imaginal exposure produces substantial and persistent symptom reduction. There is some evidence suggesting that exposure therapy benefits are maximized with the combination of in vivo and imaginal exposure and that the addition of other cognitive and anxiety management therapy elements does not appreciably enhance exposure-based therapy outcomes. It also appears that CPT, a cognitive therapy with exposure elements, is as effective as PE in the treatment of PTSD, and that CPT might be more beneficial in addressing trauma-related guilt.[158]

An additional novel therapy, Trauma-Informed Guilt Reduction Therapy (TriGR), is a 6-session, 90-minute, individual therapy which has demonstrated superior efficacy in reducing PTSD, depression, and anxiety symptoms than in comparison to supportive therapy.[159,160] TriGR attends the emotional focus of guilt, shame, and moral injury in PTSD, rather than fear and anxiety as in exposure-based therapies by combining elements of psychoeducation and cognitive restructuring of guilt cognitions in accordance with one's values. The authors reported a 50% PTSD recovery rate which they tentatively attributed to the therapy's ability to address the predominantly guilt emotional focus of the PTSD.[160] Thus, it appears that certain strategic integrations of cognitive and exposure therapy elements may offer unique benefits, at least with some subgroups of individuals with PTSD.

Lastly, EMDR has been the focus of much controversy[161-165] and research, primarily because of the unusual assumption that the bilateral stimulation eye movements are essential to its efficacy, and because EMDR was touted as an effective treatment for a variety of disorders including PTSD. Over a decade of research has now shown that the eye movement feature does not appear relevant to treatment outcome[166-172] and that EMDR is no more effective than any other more theoretically grounded exposure therapy.[169,171-175] Thus, EMDR is an efficacious treatment for PTSD, but its efficacy is likely attributable to its exposure and cognitive therapy elements.

In sum, the bulk of clinical studies point to the combination of exposure therapy, emotional processing, and cognitive restructuring as the dominant therapeutic approaches for resolving PTSD. While this assertion may be questionable under some conditions and/or with some subgroups of persons with PTSD, it is consistent with the fact that the National Academy of Medicine, Department of Veterans Affairs, Department of Defense, and the International Society for Traumatic Stress Studies have selected PE, CPT, and EMDR as evidence-based, first line treatments for PTSD.[176-179]

Integrated CBT for Co-occurring PTSD-SUD

In general, psychotherapy is an important part of treatment for PTSD and SUD. However, most patients with PTSD and co-occurring SUD receive treatment for the SUD only.[180,181] It is important to note that historically, political and public health systems have responded punitively to substance use (eg, the crack/cocaine epidemic) with stigmatization, criminalization, and court-mandated treatment.[182] This societal response alongside ongoing sociodemographic and neighborhood inequities has led to health disparities in the perception, receipt, and access to care for SUD treatment. Less resourced communities and individuals, typically holding a minoritized identity (ie, race, gender, sexuality, ethnicity, etc.) are more likely to be denied treatment, perceived negatively, incarcerated, or die due to their substance use.[183-185] One study showed that among Black Americans in the United States, opioid overdose deaths have increased at a higher rate than non-Hispanic, White Americans.[183] These disparities continue to persist in SUD treatment and have worsened due to the COVID-19 pandemic.[186] Accordingly, the field must take an active approach in changing beliefs around SUD and increasing equitable access to care. Many community programs have responded astutely to these health disparities by adopting trauma-informed care for patients with PTSD and SUD, such as screening for trauma/PTSD, evidence-based treatments, harm reduction models, and medications for opioid use disorder.

Many clinicians still argue the SUD should be treated first or that abstinence is necessary before diagnosis and a management plan can be made.[187] Subsequent to the successful completion of SUD treatment, patients are often, but not always, referred to PTSD treatment.[188] It is unknown how many referred patients seek out and complete PTSD treatment. Proponents of this treatment model, known as "sequential" treatment, in which the SUD is first treated and then the PTSD is treated, posit that continued substance use during therapy impedes therapeutic efforts to address PTSD, and that addressing the trauma increases the risk of return to use.[189,190] Importantly, there is little empirical data over the past two decades to support these concerns and there is a growing body of literature to support the alternative.

Clinicians often perceive individuals with co-occurring PTSD and SUD as being more difficult to treat than individuals with either PTSD or SUD alone.[191] This is likely due to more difficult treatment engagement, higher rates of attrition, lower treatment adherence, and poorer treatment outcomes.[192] "Integrated" treatment models, in which both the SUD and PTSD are simultaneously addressed in therapy, have been developed over the past decade. Findings from studies of integrated treatments show that alcohol and drug use typically decrease significantly and do not increase with the addition of trauma-focused interventions.[192-196] Proponents of integrated treatments assert that PTSD symptoms may, at least in part, drive substance use and that untreated PTSD symptoms place patients at risk of return to use. In so far as substance use represents self-medication of PTSD symptoms,[42] addressing traumas early in treatment may improve long-term recovery from SUD.[197-199] Furthermore, a substantial proportion of patients with co-occurring PTSD-SUD express a preference for integrated treatment.[180,200,201]

To date, most published research on integrated treatment models has fallen into two broad categories: (1) exposure-based trauma therapies delivered concurrently with established evidence-based SUD interventions[188,194,202,203] and (2) non-exposure based therapies that focus on CBT or coping skills. Seeking Safety (SS) is the most widely known and empirically studied integrated CBT to date.[204,205] SS is a 25-session, present-focused, manualized treatment that provides psychoeducation, teaches coping skills, and helps patients gain more control over their lives. SS was first developed for adult women in a group modality, but has since been expanded to men, adolescents, and individual therapy. The findings from most studies suggest that SS leads to improvement in substance use, PTSD symptoms, depressive symptoms, and interpersonal functioning.[206-208] In a randomized controlled trial, Hien and colleagues[209] compared SS to the "gold standard" SUD treatment, relapse prevention (RP), and to treatment-as-usual (TAU) among 107 women. At the end of treatment, patients who received TAU failed to demonstrate significant improvement, or in the case of PTSD symptoms, worsened over time. In contrast, patients who received either SS or RP demonstrated significant improvements in substance use, PTSD, and psychiatric symptom severity. SS and RP, however, did not differ from one another on treatment outcomes. Hien and colleagues[210] extended this research by comparing group-based SS to a group-based women's health education group + TAU. Notably, clinically significant reductions in trauma symptoms were found for both the experimental and control conditions but no significant between group differences were observed. Seeking Safety has also demonstrated successful outcomes in challenging populations, such as prisoners,[211] adolescents,[208] and veterans.[207] See www.seekingsafety.org for more detailed information on SS.

Other integrated CBTs that use exposure-based techniques, the gold standard psychosocial treatment for PTSD, have also been developed. Triffleman and colleagues[212] pioneered the systematic examination of interventions that integrates exposure-based techniques for PTSD with empirically validated treatments for SUD by developing Substance Dependence Posttraumatic Stress Disorder Therapy (SDPT).[212,213] SDPT is a 20-week manualized outpatient treatment that utilizes RP, coping skills, psychoeducation, and in vivo exposure (but not imaginal exposure) for individuals with PTSD. In a small, controlled pilot trial (N = 19) using methadone maintained subjects who also engaged in cocaine use, SDPT was compared to Twelve-Step Facilitation Therapy. Patients in both groups showed improvements in PTSD and drug use, but no statistically significant differences between treatment conditions were observed. This may have been due to the small sample size and the short-follow up period of one month.

Back, Brady, and colleagues[202,214] developed a manualized treatment that combined PE and cognitive-behavioral RP for individuals with PTSD and cocaine dependence. The treatment protocol, initially called Concurrent Treatment of PTSD and Cocaine Dependence (CTPCD) included 16 individual sessions. Results from an uncontrolled study (N = 39) showed that patients demonstrated significant pre- to posttreatment reductions in all three clusters of PTSD symptoms, as measured by clinician-rated and self-report measures.[214] Significant reductions in cocaine use were also observed. Approximately 10% of urine drug screen (UDS) tests were positive each week and this rate did not increase during treatment as PTSD was more directly addressed with exposure techniques. The treatment was later modified to a 12-session version that addresses PTSD and all types of co-occurring SUD (eg, alcohol, cocaine, cannabis) and is named "COPE" which stands for Concurrent Treatment of PTSD and Substance Use Disorders using Prolonged Exposure."[215] Several RCTs of COPE among national and international populations has shown that COPE yields significant reductions in PTSD symptom severity and significant or equivalent reductions in SUD severity in comparison to TAU. Importantly, the use of PE in COPE did not increase substance use or return to use rates highlighting the feasibility of integrated, trauma-focused, treatment for PTSD and SUD.[10,216-218] In Back et al., significantly more veterans in COPE (83%), as compared to RP (36%), no longer met diagnostic criteria for PTSD at the end of the 12-session treatment.[10]

Coffey and Colleagues[219] explored a modified version of the original CTPCD among inner-city patients at a community mental health center (CMHC). They used both individual and group therapy format and a team-based treatment approach including an individual therapist, group therapist, case managers, and psychiatrist. They also included a dialectical behavior therapy (DBT) psychosocial skills training group. The findings suggest that the treatment leads to reductions in trauma-related symptoms, improvements in SUD outcomes, and is well tolerated.[219]

Additionally, Sannibale and colleagues[220] compared Integrated CBT for PTSD and alcohol use disorder (AUD) against CBT for AUD and supportive counseling. Participants in both conditions received alcohol treatment based on the Project MATCH CBT manual and Combined Behavioral Intervention Manual (COMBINE). The AUD and supportive counseling treatment solely targeted AUD symptoms rather than PTSD symptoms, while the CBT for PTSD and AUD integrated CBT for AUD with exposure-based elements from PE and cognitive restructuring elements similar to CPT. Both groups demonstrated significant reductions in PTSD symptoms. Interestingly, participants who had received at least one session of exposure therapy were twice as likely to show significant changes in CAPS severity than those who did not receive any exposure therapy. Those in the CBT for AUD plus supportive counseling group demonstrated greater reductions in alcohol use, dependence severity, and AUD-related problems than those in the CBT for PTSD and AUD condition. However, those in the CBT for AUD condition were significantly more likely to seek treatment services outside of the study during follow-up, likely confounding findings.

The findings from these and other investigations[192,194] provide evidence that integrated treatments are beneficial to many patients with trauma/PTSD and co-occurring SUD. They also show that imaginal and in vivo exposure techniques for PTSD can be used safely and effectively with SUD patients. Concerns that exposure therapy for PTSD would exacerbate substance use among SUD patients have not been borne out. Findings show that addressing trauma via present or past-oriented treatments does not worsen patients' symptoms, but rather it significantly improves PTSD, substance use and general psychiatric distress. More randomized controlled trials are needed, however, to determine whether and for whom integrated PTSD-SUD treatments are superior to SUD-only treatments. To attend to this question, Hien, Morgan-López, and colleagues are conducting the first ever individual patient data meta-analysis where patient data across more than 30 randomized controlled trials is being psychometrically harmonized to compare the efficacy of integrated, non-integrated, trauma-focused, and pharmacotherapy treatments for PTSD and SUD as well as putative mechanisms of action underlying treatment efficacy.[79,203] This investigation is, to our knowledge, the first of its kind and will allow head-to-head comparisons of diverse treatments for PTSD and SUD which have as of yet not been possible. Preliminary results have developed a nomenclature for integrated trauma-focused treatments and found PTSD assessments vary in precision and accuracy across populations (ie, measurement nonequivalence), which point to field-wide changes to consider in the diagnosis and treatment of PTSD.[78,79,203,221] Furthermore, their primary outcome results which are under review show that for the treatment of PTSD and SUD, the combination of trauma-focused psychotherapy with pharmacotherapy for alcohol use disorder showed the highest efficacy in treatment outcomes.[222]

There has been a significant growth of research on integrated treatments to investigate the combination of CBT and pharmacotherapy approaches.[223-229] For instance, one study[230] reported that sertraline treatment of PTSD was significantly augmented by the addition of PE (although the augmentation effect was restricted to persons who were partial responders to sertraline). Other studies have examined the combination of 3,4-methylenedioxymethamphetamine or MDMA[231] and methylthioninium chloride or methylene blue[232] with psychotherapy for PTSD. Across these studies, the combination of pharmacotherapies with PTSD treatment has increased reductions in PTSD symptoms.

Pharmacotherapy of PTSD

The primary goals of the pharmacologic treatment of PTSD include decreasing PTSD symptoms, improving overall functioning, improving resilience to future stressors, decreasing symptoms of co-occurring psychiatric conditions (eg, depression, SUDs), and reducing risk of PTSD recurrence.[233] Long term pharmacologic treatment (eg, 1 year) is recommended based on evidence that PTSD is likely to return following discontinuation of shorter treatment.[97]

A recent meta-analysis comparing psychotherapy and pharmacotherapy treatments for PTSD evidenced that trauma-focused psychotherapy treatments are superior in long-term PTSD reductions than pharmacotherapies for PTSD.[227] However, pharmacotherapies can assist in managing PTSD symptoms, and two medications, both selective serotonin reuptake inhibitors (SSRIs), are currently FDA-approved for the treatment of PTSD: sertraline and paroxetine. These are considered the first line pharmacotherapeutic treatment options for PTSD based on their demonstrated efficacy in treating PTSD and other co-occurring conditions, and their relative safety in overdose.[97,227,233-238] SSRIs have been shown to improve all four symptom clusters of PTSD and overall quality of life, particularly among civilian PTSD patients.[237] In addition, serotonin and norepinephrine reuptake inhibitor (SNRIs) can be used, such as venlafaxine (ie, Effexor, an FDA-approved antidepressant which has been shown to reduce PTSD symptoms in placebo-controlled investigations.[227,239,240] Other pharmacologic agents have been investigated for the treatment of PTSD and some have shown promise, but none are FDA-approved. On example is nefazodone, which decreased PTSD symptoms in the short term but was taken off market due to risk of hepatoxicity. Thus, at present, pharmacotherapies are a second line treatment for PTSD.[227]

Generally, clinical guidelines suggest that trauma-focused psychotherapy is the first-line treatment for PTSD followed by, or alongside, SSRIs. SSRIs alone are a second line of treatment. However, there are some exceptions to this general clinical guidance. First, if a patient prefers pharmacotherapy treatments to trauma-focused treatments, medications can be started first. Secondly, if there are symptoms that would interfere with the initiation and engagement in psychotherapy—particularly in the areas of mood, sleep, and hyperarousal—pharmacotherapy treatment can be started first to provide stabilization. Among pharmacotherapy treatments, SSRIs or SNRIs are first prescribed and following 8 to 10 weeks of use if there is a poor response, it is recommended to try a second SSRI or SNRI. Antipsychotics can be used as an adjunct to SSRIs or SSNRIs if there is poor response to either of the antidepressants or if there are psychotic features alongside PTSD.[241,242]

Historically, while some tricyclic antidepressants (TCAs) and monoamine oxidase inhibitors (MAOIs) have been shown to be effective in improving PTSD and associated symptoms, they are no longer commonly used due to cardiovascular and anticholinergic side effects, risk of seizures with TCAs, and strict dietary restrictions and risk of hypertensive crisis with MAOIs.[233,243] Findings from other studies examining the use of mood stabilizers and anticonvulsants fail to show benefit in the management of PTSD.[233] Encouraging evidence exists that antipsychotic medications, in particular risperidone, may be beneficial as an augmentation medication to partial responders of SSRIs.[233,243] The risk of side effects with the use of antipsychotics, however, needs to be considered when choosing a medication.[237] Benzodiazepines, which help alleviate anxiety and sleep impairment, are contraindicated as a monotherapy or preventative strategy based on preliminarily findings that their use was associated with increased risk of PTSD symptom recurrence relative to placebo.[97,237] Benzodiazepines are also contraindicated for exposure-based therapies because they suppress the fear response.[244] Finally, medications that reduce central nervous system activity (eg, clonidine, prazosin) may be helpful in decreasing nightmares and hyperarousal symptoms, which do not respond particularly well to SSRIs.[243] Additional randomized controlled trials are needed to better assess their spectrum of efficacy, and the evaluation of treatments across multiple psychotherapies and pharmacotherapies as in the individual patient data meta-analysis will provide such evidence.[79,203]

Research on the pharmacologic prevention of PTSD is limited and methodologically problematic. Consequently there are no medications that effectively prevent/curtail the development of PTSD.[233] Translational research has led to mixed findings that would support cautious optimism. Numerous preclinical studies have implicated the noradrenergic system, likely via action in the basolateral amygdala, in both the formation and maintenance of fear-related memories.[245-250] Several studies using fear-conditioning paradigms in animals have suggested a role for the β-adrenoreceptor in memory recall that is prompted by the presentation of cues associated with aversive outcomes.[246,251,252] These promising animal studies led to research with human participants suggesting that β-adrenergic antagonists (eg, propranolol) may selectively interfere with emotional memory.[253-255] In one of these studies,[255] participants with PTSD and non-PTSD controls treated with propranolol (a β-blocking agent) versus placebo evidenced reduced recall of the emotionally arousing content of a story told to them one week earlier. However, additional studies failed to replicate these results and showed mixed findings. A recent systematic review and meta-analysis found that across studies, there is no benefit from using propranolol to reduce the development of PTSD.[256] Collectively, these findings suggest that the there is a lack of evidence to support the strategic use of β-blocking agents (eg, propranolol) to prevent PTSD development.

Pharmacotherapy of Co-occurring PTSD-SUD

There is limited research on pharmacotherapy for co-occurring PTSD and SUD.[257-260] Most studies, however, show promise and suggest that patients with PTSD and co-occurring AUD respond as well to standard PTSD pharmacotherapies as compared to patients without co-occurring SUD. There is a paucity of research on pharmacotherapies for PTSD and other SUD beyond AUD.

Several studies have examined the use of SSRIs, the pharmacologic treatment of choice for PTSD, among patients with co-occurring SUDs. All these studies have evaluated sertraline. The first was a small ($N = 9$) open-label trial among outpatients with DSM-IV defined alcohol dependence and PTSD.[261] Decreases in alcohol use severity (eg, number of drinking days, number of drinks per day) were shown and approximately half (4/9) of the patients were abstinent during the 12-week follow-up period. In addition, significant reductions in all three PTSD symptom clusters were reported.

A second investigation extended the Brady et al. study and examined the efficacy of 12 weeks of sertraline versus placebo among 94 outpatients with alcohol dependence and PTSD.[261,262] Both groups showed improvement in alcohol use severity, but no significant between group differences were revealed. A more recent study by Hien et al., compared the combination of Seeking Safety, a trauma-focused cognitive behavioral treatment, with sertraline with Seeking Safety and placebo over 12 weeks.[223] Among 69 participants that were primarily female and identified as Black/African American, the combination of Seeking Safety with sertraline group showed greater reductions in PTSD symptoms than the Seeking Safety plus placebo control group. Both groups improved in alcohol use disorder severity, but there was no difference between groups in alcohol use outcomes.[223]

Recent placebo-controlled trials have evaluated the effects of prazosin (with target dose of 16 mg per day) on co-occurring PTSD and alcohol use disorder (AUD). Though an initial 6-week pilot trial ($N = 30$) indicated reduced drinking in the prazosin group relative to the placebo group and similar PTSD symptom reductions between the medication and placebo groups,[263] a subsequent larger 13-week trial in veterans (N = 96) revealed no between-group differences in alcohol use or PTSD outcomes.[264] Another recent pilot study trial evaluated the effect of topiramate (300 mg/d) among 30 veterans with PTSD and AUD. In comparison to placebo, veterans with PTSD and AUD who received topiramate showed significant reductions in alcohol use, alcohol craving, and PTSD symptom severity, with a particular decrease in hyperarousal symptoms.[265] However, topiramate has also been shown to cause cognitive disturbances, warranting caution.[266]

Among larger trials, a 12-week trial of the FDA approved alcohol use disorder medications disulfiram, naltrexone, and their combination (N = 254) was conducted among individuals with co-occurring psychiatric disorders and alcohol use disorder included 93 individuals with PTSD.[267] Among the PTSD subgroup, active medication, relative to placebo, yielded better alcohol outcomes, and disulfiram appeared particularly associated with reductions in PTSD symptoms. More recently, Foa and colleagues[268] examined the efficacy of PE with and without naltrexone in a sample of people with alcohol dependence (N = 165) and co-occurring PTSD. Participants were randomly assigned to receive: PE plus naltrexone (100 mg/d), PE plus placebo medication, supportive counseling plus naltrexone (100 mg/d), or supportive counseling plus placebo medication. Significant reductions in PTSD symptoms and percentage of days drinking were observed in all four groups. Those who received naltrexone had significantly lower numbers of drinking days than those who did not receive the medication regardless of receiving PE versus supportive counseling. Importantly, at 6-month follow-up, all groups had increases in the percentage of drinking days, but those in the PE plus naltrexone group had the smallest increase.

As aforementioned, developing research also indicates a potential for D-cycloserine to enhance exposure-based treatment outcomes with anxiety-disordered individuals (eg, PTSD) and may have potential as an innovative treatment for co-occurring PTSD-SUD. The medication, D-cycloserine (DCS), is a partial NMDA agonist and an FDA approved antibiotic treatment for tuberculosis. As already noted, exposure-based therapy is founded on the principles of conditioned fear extinction and has demonstrated efficacy in the treatment of several anxiety disorders including PTSD.[269] Building upon the animal studies demonstrating DCS-facilitated extinction of conditioned fear responses,[270-275] a number of recent clinical trials have examined the potential facilitative effects of DCS on extinction of fear-based responses and symptoms associated with anxiety disorders. To date, a recent meta-analysis identified 13 studies on DCS where it was shown that DCS can facilitate extinction of anxiety/fear symptomatology in PTSD, obsessive-compulsive disorder, panic disorder, social anxiety disorder, acrophobia, and snake phobia at a moderate effect, d = -0.34.[269] The existing clinical data strongly suggests that DCS might enhance exposure-based treatment outcome for severe anxiety disorders, including PTSD. Animal based studies have thus begun to examine how DCS may augment reductions in PTSD and SUD.[276,277]

In addition to its potential for advancing exposure therapy for PTSD, the ability of DCS to facilitate extinction might be fruitfully explored with respect to exposure-based treatment of SUD,[278-280] known as cue exposure therapy (CE). Briefly, CE involves exposing individuals with SUD to stimuli that have acquired the ability, via Pavlovian conditioning, to elicit craving and other reactions (eg, increase in heart rate) because of a history of contiguous pairings with drug or alcohol administration. These craving and other cue-elicited reactions are assumed to have an important role in the maintenance of, and recurrence of, substance use.[281-284] The goal of CE is to attenuate or eliminate craving and reactivity via extinction, thereby reducing risk of further substance use (ie, maintaining abstinence). To date, CE therapy has been associated with modest efficacy[277,285] but medication developments such as DCS hold promise for bolstering the effects of CE. Furthermore, future clinical studies involving people with co-occurring PTSD-SUD could investigate the possibility of DCS-enhanced outcomes of an integrated exposure-based therapy consisting of PE and CE.[280]

Additional emerging research has examined at over-the-counter adjunctive treatments to enhance evidence-based PTSD and SUD treatment. Briefly, N-acetylcysteine (NAC), is an antioxidant that targets glutamate modulation in the nucleus accumbens. Translational studies have shown that NAC significantly reduces nicotine and cocaine administration.[286,287] Novel randomized clinical trials among PTSD and SUD samples have shown a similar pattern: NAC shows high tolerability and feasibility among human participants and significantly reduces PTSD symptoms, craving, and alcohol use.[224,225] Although additional work is needed, the accessibility of NAC shows promise for feasible adjunctive PTSD and SUD treatments.

CONCLUDING COMMENTS

It is well-established that SUD frequently co-occurs with PTSD and that this co-occurrence is profoundly detrimental to physical and psychological well-being. Theory and research about the nature of the causal relationship between the two disorders suggests that even though no single model has received unequivocal empirical support, it appears that PTSD most often precedes the development of SUD, thereby highlighting the key role of PTSD in the subsequent development of SUD. While the contribution of neurobiological factors to the etiology and maintenance of PTSD-SUD co-occurrence are not completely understood, there is considerable evidence of shared causal processes. Chief among these processes is dysregulation of both the HPA axis and noradrenergic systems. In addition, both PTSD and SUD are associated with deficits in neural circuitry related to executive functioning and limbic system regulation. It is likely that these shared mechanisms contribute to the co-occurrence of PTSD-SUD and may provide important treatment targets to help reduce severity of both disorders. Moreover, social determinants of health increase the disproportionate risk to be exposed to trauma and develop co-occurring PTSD and SUD. It will be important to harness prevention and treatment efforts to reduce disparities in the development of these co-occurring disorders as well as attend to existing health inequities (from the systemic to individual level) in the receipt of evidence-based PTSD and SUD treatments.

The effective management of co-occurring PTSD-SUD begins with a comprehensive assessment. Numerous interview and self-report measures are available that allow clinicians to efficiently assess history of trauma exposure, PTSD symptoms, history of substance use, and SUD symptoms. As always, the integrity of assessment findings will be enhanced by ensuring that a sufficient period of reduced use has occurred prior to conducting the assessment.

Some of the best treatments for people with co-occurring PTSD-SUD are those that concurrently address both disorders. Several highly efficacious cognitive behavioral therapies for the treatment of PTSD can be readily employed with individuals with SUD, as evidenced by positive findings of integrated PTSD-SUD behavioral treatments.[193,203,288,289] Exposure-based interventions (eg, PE) are considered the gold standard of CBTs; other cognitive-focused and anxiety-focused therapies have been employed with considerable success. In addition, investigations are underway to identify pharmacotherapies that may[265] help reduce symptoms of both disorders among individuals with co-occurring PTSD-SUD.[224,259,264,268,290,291] Since treatment of any form can often prove challenging to the recipient, clinicians should employ strategies to enhance retention, such as telephone contact between sessions and continue outpatient care for at least 3 months after treatment completion.[292,293]

REFERENCES

1. Sadock B, Sadock VA. *Kaplan & Sadock's Synopsis of Psychiatry*. Lippincott Williams & Wilkins; 2003.
2. American Psychological Association. *Diagnostic and Statistical Manual of Mental Disorders*. American Psychiatric Press, Inc; 1980.
3. Blanco C, Xu Y, Brady K, Pérez-Fuentes G, Okuda M, Wang S. Comorbidity of posttraumatic stress disorder with alcohol dependence among US adults: results from National Epidemiological Survey on Alcohol and Related Conditions. *Drug Alcohol Depend*. 2013;132(3):630-638.
4. Petrakis IL, Rosenheck R, Desai R. Substance use comorbidity among veterans with posttraumatic stress disorder and other psychiatric illness. *Am J Addict*. 2011;20(3):185-189.
5. Smith SM, Goldstein RB, Grant BF. The association between posttraumatic stress disorder and lifetime DSM-5 psychiatric disorders among veterans: data from the National Epidemiologic Survey on Alcohol and Related Conditions-III (NESARC-III). *J Psychiatr Res*. 2016;82:16-22.
6. Pietrzak RH, Goldstein RB, Southwick SM, Grant BF. Prevalence and Axis I comorbidity of full and partial posttraumatic stress disorder in the United States: results from Wave 2 of the National Epidemiologic Survey on Alcohol and Related Conditions. *J Anxiety Disord*. 2011;25(3):456-465.
7. Seal KH, Cohen G, Waldrop A, Cohen BE, Maguen S, Ren L. Substance use disorders in Iraq and Afghanistan veterans in VA healthcare, 2001-2010: implications for screening, diagnosis and treatment. *Drug Alcohol Depend*. 2011;116(1-3):93-101.
8. Norman SB, Haller M, Hamblen JL, Southwick SM, Pietrzak RH. The burden of co-occurring alcohol use disorder and PTSD in U.S. Military veterans: comorbidities, functioning, and suicidality. *Psychol Addict Behav*. 2018;32(2):224-229.
9. Vujanovic AA, Back SE. *Posttraumatic Stress and Substance Use Disorders: A Comprehensive Clinical Handbook*. Routledge; 2019.
10. Back SE, Killeen T, Badour CL, et al. Concurrent treatment of substance use disorders and PTSD using prolonged exposure: A randomized clinical trial in military veterans. *Addict Behav*. 2019;90:369-377.
11. Ouimette P, Goodwin E, Brown PJ. Health and well being of substance use disorder patients with and without posttraumatic stress disorder. *Addict Behav*. 2006;31(8):1415-1423.
12. American Psychiatric Association. *Diagnostic and Statistical Manual of Mental Disorders. Text Revision*. 5th ed. American Psychiatric Association; 2022.
13. Weathers FW, Marx BP, Friedman MJ, Schnurr PP. Posttraumatic stress disorder in DSM-5: new criteria, new measures, and implications for assessment. *Psychol Injury Law*. 2014;7(2):93-107.
14. Franklin CL, Raines AM, Chambliss JL, Walton JL, Maieritsch KP. Examining various subthreshold definitions of PTSD using the Clinician Administered PTSD Scale for DSM-5. *J Affect Disord*. 2018;234:256-260.
15. McLaughlin KA, Koenen KC, Friedman MJ, et al. Subthreshold posttraumatic stress disorder in the world health organization world mental health surveys. *Biol Psychiatry*. 2015;77(4):375-384.
16. Brunello N, Davidson JR, Deahl M, Kessler RC, et al. Posttraumatic stress disorder: diagnosis and epidemiology, comorbidity and social consequences, biology and treatment. *Neuropsychobiology*. 2001;43(3):150-162.
17. Kessler RC, Sonnega A, Bromet E, Hughes M, Nelson CB. Posttraumatic stress disorder in the National Comorbidity Survey. *Arch Gen Psychiatry*. 1995;52(12):1048-1060.
18. Spoont MR, McClendon J. Racial and ethnic disparities in PTSD. *PTSD Res Q*. 2020;31(4).
19. Alegría M, Fortuna LR, Lin JY, et al. Prevalence, risk, and correlates of posttraumatic stress disorder across ethnic and racial minority groups in the United States. *Med Care*. 2013;51(12):1114-1123.
20. Roberts AL, Gilman SE, Breslau J, et al. Race/ethnic differences in exposure to traumatic events, development of post-traumatic stress disorder, and treatment-seeking for post-traumatic stress disorder in the United States. *Psychol Med*. 2011;41(1):71-83.
21. Bassett D, Buchwald D, Manson S. Posttraumatic stress disorder and symptoms among American Indians and Alaska Natives: a review of the literature. *Soc Psychiatry Psychiatr Epidemiol*. 2014;49(3):417-433.
22. Gillespie CF, Bradley B, Mercer K, et al. Trauma exposure and stress-related disorders in inner city primary care patients. *Gen Hosp Psychiatry*. 2009;31(6):505-514.
23. Roberts AL, Austin SB, Corliss HL, Vandermorris AK, Koenen KC. Pervasive trauma exposure among US sexual orientation minority adults and risk of posttraumatic stress disorder. *Am J Public Health*. 2010;100(12):2433-2441.
24. López-Castro T, Saraiya T, Hien DA. *Women, Trauma, and PTSD, in Women's Mental Health Across the Lifespan: Challenges, Vulnerabilities, and Strengths*. Routledge. 2017;175-193.
25. Williams MT, Haeny AM, Holmes SC. Posttraumatic stress disorder and racial trauma. *PTSD Res Q*. 2021;32(1).
26. Bernard DL, Calhoun CD, Banks DE, Halliday CA, Hughes-Halbert C, Danielson CK. Making the "C-ACE" for a culturally-informed adverse childhood experiences framework to understand the pervasive mental health impact of racism on Black youth. *J Child Adolesc Trauma*. 2021;14(2):233-247.
27. Williams MT, Osman M, Gran-Ruaz S, Lopez J. Intersection of racism and PTSD: assessment and treatment of racial stress and trauma. *Curr Treat Options Psychiatry*. 2021;8(4):167-185.
28. Holmes SC, Facemire VC, DaFonseca AM. Expanding criterion A for posttraumatic stress disorder: considering the deleterious impact of oppression. *Traumatology*. 2016;22(4):314-321.

29. Sibrava NJ, Bjornsson AS, Pérez Benítez ACI, Moitra E, Weisberg RB, Keller MB. Posttraumatic stress disorder in African American and Latinx adults: clinical course and the role of racial and ethnic discrimination. *Am Psychol*. 2019;74(1):101-116.
30. Williams MT, Holmes S, Zare M, Haeny A, Faber S. An evidence-based approach for treating stress and trauma due to racism. *Cogn Behav Pract*. 2022.
31. Kilpatrick D, Resnick HS, Milanak ME, Miller MW, Keyes KM. National estimates of exposure to traumatic events and PTSD prevalence using DSM-IV and DSM-5 criteria. *J Trauma Stress*. 2013;26(5):537-547.
32. Kessler RC, Berglund P, Demler O, Jin R, Merikangas KR, Walters EE. Lifetime prevalence and age-of-onset distributions of DSM-IV disorders in the National Comorbidity Survey Replication. *Arch Gen Psychiatry*. 2005;62(6):593-602. Erratum appears in *Arch Gen Psychiatry*. 2005;62(7):768.
33. Goldstein RB, Smith SM, Chou SP, et al. The epidemiology of DSM-5 posttraumatic stress disorder in the United States: results from the National Epidemiologic Survey on Alcohol and Related Conditions-III. *Soc Psychiatry Psychiatr Epidemiol*. 2016;51(8):1137-1.
34. Forman-Hoffman VL, Bose J, Batts KR, et al. *Correlates of Lifetime Exposure to One of More Potentially Traumatic Events and Subsequent Posttraumatic Stress Among Adults in the United States: Results from the Mental Health Surveillance Study, 2008-2012.* Center for Behavioral Health Statistics and Quality Data Review. Accessed July 1, 2022. https://www.samhsa.gov/data/report/correlates-lifetime-exposure-one-or-more-potentially-traumatic-events-and-subsequent.
35. Wisco BE, Marx BP, Miller MW, et al. Probable posttraumatic stress disorder in the US veteran population according to DSM-5: results from the National Health and Resilience in Veterans Study. *J Clinical Psychiatry*. 2016;77(11):1503-1510.
36. Bohnert KM, Ilgen MA, Rosen CS, Desai RA, Austin K, Blow FC. The association between substance use disorders and mortality among a cohort of Veterans with posttraumatic stress disorder: variation by age cohort and mortality type. *Drug Alcohol Depend*. 2013;128(1):98-103.
37. Smith SM, Stinson FS, Dawson DA, Goldstein R, Huang B, Grant BF. Race/ethnic differences in the prevalence and co-occurrence of substance use disorders and independent mood and anxiety disorders: results from the National Epidemiologic Survey on Alcohol and Related Conditions. *Psychol Med*. 2006;36(7):987-998.
38. Lee RD, Chen J. Adverse childhood experiences, mental health, and excessive alcohol use: examination of race/ethnicity and sex differences. *Child Abuse Negl*. 2017;69:40-48.
39. Meshberg-Cohen S, Presseau C, Thacker LR, Hefner K, Svikis D. Posttraumatic stress disorder, health problems, and depression among African American women in residential substance use treatment. *J Womens Health (Larchmt)*. 2016;25(7):729-737.
40. Vasilenko SA, Evans-Polce RJ, Lanza ST. Age trends in rates of substance use disorders across ages 18-90: differences by gender and race/ethnicity. *Drug Alcohol Depend*. 2017;180:260-264.
41. Torchalla I, Strehlau V, Li K, Linden IA, Noel F, Krausz M. Posttraumatic stress disorder and substance use disorder comorbidity in homeless adults: prevalence, correlates, and sex differences. *Psychol Addict Behav*. 2014;28(2):443-452.
42. Khantzian EJ. The self-medication hypothesis of addictive disorders: focus on heroin and cocaine dependence. *Am J Psychiatry*. 1985;142(11):1259-1264.
43. Khantzian EJ. Self-regulation and self-medication factors in alcoholism and the addictions. Similarities and differences. *Recent Dev Alcohol*. 1990;8:255-271.
44. Khantzian EJ. The self-medication hypothesis of substance use disorders: a reconsideration and recent applications. *Harv Rev Psychiatry*. 1997;4(5):231-244.
45. Reed PL, Anthony JC, Breslau N. Incidence of drug problems in young adults exposed to trauma and posttraumatic stress disorder: do early life experiences and predispositions matter? *Arch Gen Psychiatry*. 2007;64(12):1435-1442.
46. Dvorak RD, Pearson MR, Day AM. Ecological momentary assessment of acute alcohol use disorder symptoms: associations with mood, motives, and use on planned drinking days. *Exp Clin Psychopharmacol*. 2014;22(4):285.
47. Kaysen D, Stappenbeck C, Rhew I, Simpson T. Proximal relationships between PTSD and drinking behavior. *Eur J Psychotraumatol*. 2014;5:26518.
48. Simpson TL, Stappenback CA, Luterek JA, Lehavot K, Kaysen DL. Drinking motives moderate daily relationships between PTSD symptoms and alcohol use. *J Abnorm Psychol*. 2014;123(1):237.
49. Maria-Rios CE, Morrow JD. Mechanisms of shared vulnerability to post-traumatic stress disorder and substance use disorders. *Front Behav Neurosci*. 2020;14:6.
50. Steele CM, Josephs RA. Alcohol myopia: its prized and dangerous effects. *Am Psychol*. 1990;45(8):921.
51. Testa M, Livingston JA. Alcohol consumption and women's vulnerability to sexual victimization: can reducing women's drinking prevent rape? *Subst Use Misuse*. 2009;44(9-10):1349-1376.
52. Jacobsen LK, Southwick SM, Kosten TR. Substance use disorders in patients with posttraumatic stress disorder: a review of the literature. *Am J Psychiatry*. 2001;158(8):1184-1190.
53. Fani N, Carter SE, Harnett NG, Ressler KJ, Bradley B. Association of racial discrimination with neural response to threat in Black women in the U.S. exposed to trauma. *JAMA Psychiatry*. 2021;78(9):1005-1012.
54. Fani N, Harnett NG, Bradley B, et al. Racial discrimination and white matter microstructure in trauma-exposed Black women. *Biol Psychiatry*. 2022;91(3):254-261.
55. Gilpin NW, Weiner JL. Neurobiology of comorbid posttraumatic stress disorder and alcohol-use disorder. *Genes Brain Behav*. 2017;16(1):15-43.
56. Morey RA, Haswell CC, Hooper SR, De Bellis MD. Amygdala, hippocampus, and ventral medial prefrontal cortex volumes differ in maltreated youth with and without chronic posttraumatic stress disorder. *Neuropsychopharmacology*. 2016;41(3):791-801.
57. Huang M-X, Yurgil KA, Robb A, et al. Voxel-wise resting-state MEG source magnitude imaging study reveals neurocircuitry abnormality in active-duty service members and veterans with PTSD. *NeuroImage Clin*. 2014;5:408-419.
58. Jin C, Qi R, Yin Y, et al. Abnormalities in whole-brain functional connectivity observed in treatment-naive post-traumatic stress disorder patients following an earthquake. *Psychol Med*. 2014;44(9):1927-1936.
59. Milad MR, Pitman RK, Ellis CB, et al. Neurobiological basis of failure to recall extinction memory in posttraumatic stress disorder. *Biol Psychiatry*. 2009;66(12):1075-1082.
60. Marek R, Strobel C, Bredy TW, Sah P. The amygdala and medial prefrontal cortex: partners in the fear circuit. *J Physiol*. 2013;591(10):2381-2391.
61. Beck A, Wüstenberg T, Genauck A, et al. Effect of brain structure, brain function, and brain connectivity on relapse in alcohol-dependent patients. *Arch Gen Psychiatry*. 2012;69(8):842-852.
62. Sinha R, Li CSR. Imaging stress- and cue-induced drug and alcohol craving: Association with relapse and clinical implications. *Drug Alcohol Rev*. 2007;26(1):25-31.
63. Wrase J, Makris N, Braus DF, et al. Amygdala volume associated with alcohol abuse relapse and craving. *Am J Psychiatry*. 2008;165(9):1179-1184.
64. Holmes A, Fitzgerald PJ, MacPherson KP, et al. Chronic alcohol remodels prefrontal neurons and disrupts NMDAR-mediated fear extinction encoding. *Nat Neurosci*. 2012;15(10):1359-1361.
65. Larkin MB, McGinnis JP, Snyder RI, et al. Neurostimulation for treatment-resistant posttraumatic stress disorder: an update on neurocircuitry and therapeutic targets. *J Neurosurg*. 2021;134(6):1711-1713.
66. Edinoff AN, Hegerfeld TL, Petersen M, et al. Transcranial magnetic stimulation for post-traumatic stress disorder. *Front Psychiatry*. 2022;13:701348.
67. Rivier C. Role of hypothalamic corticotropin-releasing factor in mediating alcohol-induced activation of the rat hypothalamic–pituitary–adrenal axis. *Front Neuroendocrinol*. 2014;35(2):221-233.

68. Daskalakis NP, Lehrner A, Yehuda R. Endocrine aspects of post-traumatic stress disorder and implications for diagnosis and treatment. *Endocrinol Metab Clin North Am*. 2013;42(3):503-513.
69. Baker DG, West SA, Nicholson WE, et al. Serial CSF corticotropin-releasing hormone levels and adrenocortical activity in combat veterans with posttraumatic stress disorder. *Am J Psychiatry*. 1999;156(4):585-588.
70. Bremner JD, Randall P, Vermetten E, et al. Magnetic resonance imaging-based measurement of hippocampal volume in posttraumatic stress disorder related to childhood physical and sexual abuse—a preliminary report. *Biol Psychiatry*. 1997;41(1):23-32.
71. Shaham Y, Funk D, Erb S, Brown TJ, Walker CD, Stewart J. Corticotropin-releasing factor, but not corticosterone, is involved in stress-induced relapse to heroin-seeking in rats. *J Neurosci*. 1997;17(7):2605-2614.
72. Brady KT, McRae AL, Moran-Santa Maria MM, et al. Response to corticotropin-releasing hormone infusion in cocaine-dependent individuals. *Arch Gen Psychiatry*. 2009;66(4):422-430.
73. Orsillo SM. Measures for acute stress disorder and posttraumatic stress disorder. In: Antony MM, Orsillo SM, Roemer L, eds. *Practitioner's Guide to Empirically Based Measures of Anxiety*. Springer; 2002:255-307.
74. Wilson JP, Keane TM, eds. *Assessing Psychological Trauma and PTSD*. Guildford Press; 1997.
75. Brewin CR. Systematic review of screening instruments for adults at risk of PTSD. *J Trauma Stress*. 2005;18(1):53-62.
76. Keane TM, Brief DJ, Pratt EM, Miller MW. Assessment of PTSD and its comorbidities in adults. In: Friedman MJ, Schnurr PP, Keane TM, eds. *Handbook of PTSD: Science and Practice*. Guilford Press; 2007:279-305.
77. American Psychiatric Association. *Diagnostic and Statistical Manual of Mental Disorders (DSM-5®)*. American Psychiatric Publishing; 2013.
78. Saavedra LM, Morgan-López AA, Back SE, et al. Measurement error-corrected estimation of clinically significant change trajectories for interventions targeting comorbid PTSD and substance use disorders in OEF/OIF veterans. *Behav Ther*. 2022;53(5):1009-1023.
79. Morgan-López AA, Hien DA, Saraiya TC, et al. Estimating posttraumatic stress disorder severity in the presence of differential item functioning across populations, comorbidities, and interview measures: introduction to Project Harmony. *J Trauma Stress*. 2022;35(3):926-940.
80. Read JP, Bollinger AR, Sharkansky E. Assessment of comorbid substance use disorder and posttraumatic stress disorder. In: Ouimette P, Brown PJ, eds. *Trauma and Substance Abuse: Causes, Consequences, and Treatment of Comorbid Disorders*. American Psychological Association; 2003:111-125.
81. Weathers F, Bovin MJ, Lee DJ, et al. *The Clinician-Administered PTSD Scale for DSM-5 (CAPS-5). National Center for PTSD*. Accessed July 11, 2023. https://www.ptsd.va.gov/professional/assessment/adult-int/caps.asp
82. Foa EB, McLean CP, Zang Y, et al. Psychometric properties of the posttraumatic stress disorder symptom scale interview for DSM–5 (PSSI–5). *Psychol Assess*. 2016;28(10):1159-1165.
83. First MB, Williams JBW, Karg RS, Spitzer Robert L. *Structured Clinical Interview for DSM-5 Disorders—Clinician Version (SCID-5-CV)*. American Psychiatric Association; 2015.
84. Sheehan DV, Lecrubier Y, Sheehan KH, et al. The Mini-International Neuropsychiatric Interview (M.I.N.I.): the development and validation of a structured diagnostic psychiatric interview for DSM-IV and ICD-10. *J Clin Psychiatry*. 1998;59(Suppl 20):22-33. quiz 34-57
85. Spitzer RL, Williams JB, Gibbon M, First MB. The structured clinical interview for DSM-III-R (SCID) I: history, rationale, and description. *Arch Gen Psychiatry*. 199249(8):624-629.
86. First MB, Spitzer RL, Gibbon M, et al. *Structured Clinical Interview for DSM-IV-TR Axis I Disorders, Research Version, Patient Edition (SCID-I/P)*. Biometrics Research, New York State Psychiatric Institute; 1995.
87. Wittchen HU. Reliability and validity studies of the WHO-Composite International Diagnostic Interview (CIDI): a critical review. *J Psychiatric Res*. 1994;28(1):57-84.
88. World Health Organization. *Composite International Diagnostic Interview (CIDI)*. WHO; 1990.
89. Kessler RC, Calabrese JR, Farley PA, et al. Composite International Diagnostic Interview screening scales for DSM-IV anxiety and mood disorders. *Psychol Med*. 2013;43(8):1625-1637.
90. Weathers FW, Litz BT, Keane TM, Palmieri PA, Marx BP, Schnurr PP. *The PTSD Checklist for DSM-5 (PCL-5)*. 2013. http://www.ptsd.va.gov
91. Bovin MJ, Marx BP, Weathers FW, et al. Psychometric properties of the PTSD Checklist for Diagnostic and Statistical Manual of Mental Disorders-Fifth Edition (PCL-5) in veterans. *Psychol Assess*. 2016;28(11):1379-1391.
92. Foa EB, McLean CP, Zang Y, et al. Psychometric Properties of the Posttraumatic Diagnostic Scale for DSM–5 (PDS–5). *Psychol Assess*. 2016;28(10):1166-1171.
93. Steenkamp MM, Litz BT, Gray MJ, et al. A brief exposure-based intervention for service members with PTSD. *Cogn Behav Pract*. 2011;18(1):98-107.
94. Price M, Szafranski DD, van Stolk-Cooke K, Gros DF. Investigation of abbreviated 4 and 8 item versions of the PTSD Checklist 5. *Psychiatry Res*. 2016;239:124-130.
95. Nemeroff CB, Bremner JD, Foa EB, Mayberg HS, North CS, Stein MB. Posttraumatic stress disorder: a state-of-the-science review. *J Psychiatr Res*. 2006;40(1):1-21.
96. Foa EB, Hembree EA, Cahill SP, et al. Randomized trial of prolonged exposure for posttraumatic stress disorder with and without cognitive restructuring: outcome at academic and community clinics. *J Consult Clin Psychol*. 2005;73(5):953-964.
97. Ballenger JC, Davidson JRT, Lecrubier Y, et al. Consensus statement update on posttraumatic stress disorder from the international consensus group on depression and anxiety. *J Clin Psychiatry*. 2004;65 (Suppl 1):55-62.
98. Bryant RA, Moulds ML, Nixon RV. Cognitive behaviour therapy of acute stress disorder: a four-year follow-up. *Behav Res Ther*. 2003;41(4):489-494.
99. Bryant RA, Moulds ML, Nixon RDV, Mastrodomenico J, Felmingham K, Hopwood S. Hypnotherapy and cognitive behaviour therapy of acute stress disorder: a 3-year follow-up. *Behav Res Ther*. 2006;44(9):1331-1335.
100. Brom D, Kleber RJ, Defares PB. Brief psychotherapy for posttraumatic stress disorders. *J Consult Clin Psychol*. 1989;57(5):607-612.
101. Foa EB, Dancu CV, Hembree EA, Jaycox LH, Meadows EA, Street GP. A comparison of exposure therapy, stress inoculation training, and their combination for reducing posttraumatic stress disorder in female assault victims. *J Consult Clin Psychol*. 1999;67(2):194-200.
102. Hyer L, Woods MG, Bruno R, Boudewyns P. Treatment outcomes of Vietnam veterans with PTSD and the consistency of the MCMI. *J Clin Psychol*. 1989;45(4):547-552.
103. Tarrier N, Pilgrim H, Sommerfield C. A randomized trial of cognitive therapy and imaginal exposure in the treatment of chronic posttraumatic stress disorder. *J Consult Clin Psychol*. 1999;67(1):13-18.
104. Mowrer OA. *Learning Theory and Behavior*. Wiley; 1960.
105. Stampfl TG, Levis DJ. Essentials of implosive therapy: a learning-theory-based psychodynamic behavioral therapy. *J Abnorm Psychol*. 1967;72(6):496-503.
106. Wolpe J. *Psychotherapy by Reciprocal Inhibition*. Stanford University Press; 1958.
107. Foa EB, Huppert JD, Cahill SP. Emotional processing theory: an update. In: Rothbaum BO, ed. *Pathological Anxiety: Emotional Processing in Etiology and Treatment*. Guilford Press; 2006:3-24.
108. Pavlov IP. *Conditioned Reflexes*. Dover Publications; 1927.
109. Konorski J. *Conditioned Reflexes and Neuronal Organization*. Cambridge University Press; 1948.
110. Rescorla RA. Spontaneous recovery. *Learn Mem*. 2004;11(5):501-509.
111. Foa EB, Hembree EA, Rothbaum BO, Rauch SAM. *Prolonged Exposure Therapy for PTSD: Emotional Processing of Traumatic Experiences—Therapist Guide*. 2nd ed. Oxford University; 2019.
112. Foa EB, Bredemeier K, Acierno R, et al. The efficacy of 90-min versus 60-min sessions of prolonged exposure for PTSD: a randomized controlled trial in active-duty military personnel. *J Consult Clin Psychol*. 2022;90(6):503-512.
113. Doane LS, Feeny NC, Zoellner LA. A preliminary investigation of sudden gains in exposure therapy for PTSD. *Behav Res Ther*. 2010;48(6):555-560.
114. SAM R, Cigrang J, Austern D, Evans A; STRONG STAR Consortium. Expanding the reach of effective PTSD treatment into primary care: prolonged exposure for primary care. *Focus (Am Psychiatr Publ)*. 2017;15(4):406-410.

115. Williams MT, Malcoun E, Sawyer BA, Davis DM, Nouri LB, Bruce SL. Cultural adaptations of prolonged exposure therapy for treatment and prevention of posttraumatic stress disorder in African Americans. *Behav Sci (Basel)*. 2014;4(2):102-124.
116. Shapiro F, Maxfield L. Eye movement desensitization and reprocessing (EMDR): information processing in the treatment of trauma. *J Clin Psychol*. 2002;58(8):933-946.
117. Shapiro F. *Eye Movement Desensitization and Reprocessing: Basic Principles, Protocols, and Procedures*. 2nd ed. Guilford Press; 2001: xxiv, 472.
118. Shapiro F. Efficacy of the Eye movement desensitization procedure in the treatment of traumatic memories. *J Trauma Stress*. 1989;2(2):199-223.
119. van den Hout M, Muris P, Salemink E, Kindt M. Autobiographical memories become less vivid and emotional after eye movements. *Br J Clin Psychol*. 2001;40(2):121-130.
120. Sloan DM, Marx BP. *Written Exposure Therapy for PTSD: A Brief Treatment Approach for Mental Health Professionals*. *American Psychological Association*. 2019;xiii:115.
121. LoSavio ST, Worley CB, Aajmain ST, Rosen CS, Stirman SW, Sloan DM. Effectiveness of written exposure therapy for posttraumatic stress disorder in the Department of Veterans Affairs Healthcare System. *Psychol Trauma*. 2023;15(5):748-756.
122. Sloan DM, Marx BP, Acierno R, Messina M, Cole TA. Comparing written exposure therapy to prolonged exposure for the treatment of PTSD in a veteran sample: a non-inferiority randomized design. *Contemp Clin Trials Commun*. 2021;22:100764.
123. Beck AT. *Cognitive Therapy and the Emotional Disorders*. International Universities Press; 1976.
124. Beck AT. *Cognitive Therapy of Depression*. Guilford Press; 1979.
125. Beck AT, Emery G, Greenberg RL. *Anxiety Disorders and Phobias: A Cognitive Perspective*. 15th anniversary ed. Basic Books; 2005.
126. Clark DM. A cognitive approach to panic. *Behav Res Ther*. 1986; 24(4):461-470.
127. Beck AT, Wright FD, Newman CF, Liese BS. *Cognitive Therapy of Substance Abuse*. Guilford Press; 1993.
128. Resick PA, Schnicke MK. Cognitive processing therapy for sexual assault victims. *J Consult Clin Psychol*. 1992;60(5):748-756.
129. Resick PA, Schnicke MK. *Cognitive Processing Therapy for Rape Victims: A Treatment Manual*. Sage Publishing; 1993.
130. Monson CM, Schnurr PP, Resick PA, Friedman MJ, Young-Xu Y, Stevens SP. Cognitive processing therapy for veterans with military-related posttraumatic stress disorder. *J Consult Clin Psychol*. 2006;74(5):898-907.
131. Ahrens J, Rexford L. Cognitive processing therapy for incarcerated adolescents with PTSD. *J Aggress Maltreat Trauma*. 2002;6(1):201-216.
132. Pearson CR, Kaysen D, Huh D, Bedard-Gilligan M. Randomized control trial of culturally adapted cognitive processing therapy for PTSD substance misuse and HIV sexual risk behavior for Native American women. *AIDS Behav*. 2019;23(3):695-706.
133. Pearson CR, Smartlowit-Briggs L, Belcourt A, Bedard-Gilligan M, Kaysen D. Building a tribal-academic partnership to address PTSD, substance misuse, and HIV among American Indian women. *Health Promot Pract*. 2019;20(1):48-56.
134. Kaysen D, Stappenbeck CA, Carroll H, et al. Impact of setting insecurity on Cognitive Processing Therapy implementation and outcomes in eastern Democratic Republic of the Congo. *Eur J Psychotraumatol*. 2020;11(1):1735162.
135. Silver SM, Brooks A, Obenchain J. Treatment of Vietnam War veterans with PTSD: a comparison of eye movement desensitization and reprocessing, biofeedback, and relaxation training. *J Trauma Stress*. 1995;8(2):337-342.
136. Meichenbaum D. Stress inoculation training. *Psychology Practitioner Guidebooks*. Pergamon Press; 1985.
137. Meichenbaum D. *Clinical Handbook/Therapist Manual for Assessing and Treating Adults with PTSD*. Institute Press; 1994.
138. Meichenbaum D. Self-instructional training. In: Kanfer FH, Goldstein AP, eds. *Helping People Change*. Pergamon Press; 1975:357-391.
139. Lazarus RS, Folkman S. *Stress, Appraisal and Coping*. Springer; 1984.
140. Veronen LJ, Kilpatrick DG. Stress management for rape victims. In: Meichenbaum D, Jaremko ME, eds. *Stress Reduction and Prevention*. Plenum Press; 1983:341-374.
141. Foa EB, Rothbaum BO, Riggs DS, Murdock TB. Treatment of posttraumatic stress disorder in rape victims: a comparison between cognitive-behavioral procedures and counseling. *J Consult Clin Psychol*. 1991;59(5):715-723.
142. Yadin E, Foa E. Cognitive behavioral treatments for posttraumatic stress disorder. In: Kirmayer LJ, Lemelson R, Barad M, eds. *Understanding Trauma: Integrating Biological, Clinical, and Cultural Perspectives*. Cambridge University Press; 2007:178-193.
143. Foa EB, Cahill SP. Psychological treatments for PTSD: an overview. In: Neira Y, Gross R, Marshall RD, eds. *9/11: Public Health in the Wake of Terrorist Attacks*. Cambridge University Press; 2006:457-474.
144. Foa EB. Psychosocial therapy for posttraumatic stress disorder. *J Clin Psychiatry*. 2006;67(Suppl 2):40-45.
145. Bisson JI, Ehlers A, Matthews R, Pilling S, Richards D, Turner S. Psychological treatments for chronic post-traumatic stress disorder. Systematic review and meta-analysis. *Br J Psychiatry*. 2007;190:97-104.
146. Keane TM, Marshall AD, Taft CT. Posttraumatic stress disorder: etiology, epidemiology, and treatment outcome. *Annu Rev Clin Psychol*. 2006;2:161-197.
147. Bisson J, Andrew M. Psychological treatment of post-traumatic stress disorder (PTSD). *Cochrane Database of Syst Rev*. 2007;18(3):CD003388.
148. Bradley R, Greene J, Dutra S, Westen D. A multidimensional meta-analysis of psychotherapy for PTSD. *Am J Psychiatry*. 2005;162(2):214-227.
149. Foa E, Rothbaum BO, Furr JM. Augmenting exposure therapy with other BT procedures. *Psychiatric Ann*. 2003;33(1):47-53.
150. Watts BV, Schnurr PP, Mayo L, Young-Xu Y, Weeks WB. Meta-analysis of the efficacy of treatments for posttraumatic stress disorder. *J Clin Psychiatry*. 2013;74(6):e541-e550.
151. Carpenter JK, Andrews LA, Witcraft SM, Powers MB, Smits JAJ, Hofmann SG. Cognitive behavioral therapy for anxiety and related disorders: a meta-analysis of randomized placebo-controlled trials. *Depress Anxiety*. 2018;35(6):502-514.
152. Powers MB, Halpern JM, Ferenschak MP, Gillihan SJ, Foa EB. A meta-analytic review of prolonged exposure for posttraumatic stress disorder. *Clin Psychol Rev*. 2010;30(6):635-641.
153. Suomi A, Evans L, Rodgers B, Taplin S, Cowlishaw S. Couple and family therapies for post-traumatic stress disorder (PTSD). *Cochrane Database Syst Rev*. 2019;12(12):CD011257.
154. Lewis C, Roberts NP, Gibson S, Bisson JI. Dropout from psychological therapies for post-traumatic stress disorder (PTSD) in adults: systematic review and meta-analysis. *Eur J Psychotraumatol*. 2020;11(1):1709709.
155. Kehle-Forbes SM, Meis LA, Spoont MR, Polusny MA. Treatment initiation and dropout from prolonged exposure and cognitive processing therapy in a VA outpatient clinic. *Psychol Trauma*. 2016;8(1):107-114.
156. Niles BL, Polizzi CP, Voelkel E, Weinstein ES, Smidt K. Initiation, dropout, and outcome from evidence-based psychotherapies in a VA PTSD outpatient clinic. *Psychol Serv*. 2018;15(4):496-502.
157. Thompson-Hollands J, Marx BP, Lee DJ, Resick PA, Sloan DM. Long-term treatment gains of a brief exposure-based treatment for PTSD. *Depress Anxiety*. 2018;35(10):985-991.
158. Grunert BK, Weis JM, Smucker MR, Christianson HF. Imagery rescripting and reprocessing therapy after failed prolonged exposure for posttraumatic stress disorder following industrial injury. *J Behav Ther Exp Psychiatry*. 2007;38(4):317-328.
159. Norman S. Trauma-informed guilt reduction therapy: overview of the treatment and research. *Curr Treat Options Psychiatry*. 2022;9(3):115-125.
160. Norman SB, Capone C, Panza KE, et al. A clinical trial comparing trauma-informed guilt reduction therapy (TrIGR), a brief intervention for trauma-related guilt, to supportive care therapy. *Depress Anxiety*. 2022;39(4):262-273.
161. Acierno R et al. Review of the validation and dissemination of eye-movement desensitization and reprocessing: a scientific and ethical dilemma. *Clin Psychol Rev*. 1994;14(4):287-299.

162. McNally RJ. EMDR and mesmerism: a comparative historical analysis. *J Anxiety Disord*. 1999;13(1-2):225-236.
163. Herbert JD, Lilenfeld SO, Lohr JM, et al. Science and pseudoscience in the development of eye movement desensitization and reprocessing: implications for clinical psychology. *Clin Psychol Rev*. 2000;20(8):945-971.
164. Rosen GM, McNally RJ, Lohr JM, Devilly GJ, Herbert JD, Lilenfeld SO. A realistic appraisal of EMDR. *Calif Psychologist*. 1998;31:25-27.
165. McNally R. Research on eye movement desensitization and reprocessing (EMDR) as a treatment for PTSD. In: Friedman MJ, ed. *PTSD Research Quarterly*. VA Medical and Regional Office Center; 1999:1-8.
166. Lohr JM, Lilenfeld SO, Tolin DF, Herbert JD. Eye movement desensitization and reprocessing: an analysis of specific versus nonspecific treatment factors. *J Anxiety Disord*. 1999;13(1-2):185-207.
167. Lohr JM, Kleinknecht RA, Tolin DF, Barrett RH. The empirical status of the clinical application of eye movement desensitization and reprocessing. *J Behav Ther Exp Psychiatry*. 1995;26(4):285-302.
168. Lohr JM, Kleinknecht RA, Conley AT, Dal Cerro S, Schmidt J, Sonntag ME. A methodological critique of the current status of eye movement desensitization (EMD). *J Behav Ther Exp Psychiatry*. 1992;23(3):159-167.
169. Pitman RK, Orr SP, Altman B, Longpre RE, Poiré RE, Macklin ML. Emotional processing during eye movement desensitization and reprocessing therapy of Vietnam veterans with chronic posttraumatic stress disorder. *Compr Psychiatry*. 1996;37(6):419-429.
170. Lohr JM, Tolin DF, Lilienfeld SO. Efficacy of eye movement desensitization and reprocessing: implications for behavior therapy. *Behav Ther*. 1998;29(1):123-156.
171. Cahill SP, Carrigan MH, Frueh BC. Does EMDR work? And if so, why?: a critical review of controlled outcome and dismantling research. *J Anxiety Disord*. 1999;13(1-2):5-33.
172. Davidson PR, Parker KC. Eye movement desensitization and reprocessing (EMDR): a meta-analysis. *J Consult Clin Psychol*. 2001;69(2):305-316.
173. Rothbaum BO, Astin MC, Marsteller F. Prolonged exposure versus eye movement desensitization and reprocessing (EMDR) for PTSD rape victims. *J Trauma Stress*. 2005;18(6):607-616.
174. Macklin ML, Metzger LJ, Lasko NB, Berry NJ, Orr SP, Pitman RK. Five-year follow-up study of eye movement desensitization and reprocessing therapy for combat-related posttraumatic stress disorder. *Compr Psychiatry*. 2000;41(1):24-27.
175. Renfrey G, Spates CR. Eye movement desensitization: a partial dismantling study. *J Behav Ther Exp Psychiatry*. 1994;25(3):231-239.
176. Committee on Treatment of Posttraumatic Stress Disorder Board on Population Health and Public Health Practice. *Treatment of PTSD: An Assessment of the Evidence*. National Academies Press; 2007.
177. Cusack K, Jonas DE, Forneris CA, et al. Psychological treatments for adults with posttraumatic stress disorder: a systematic review and meta-analysis. *Clin Psychol Rev*. 2016;43:128-141.
178. McSweeney LB, Rauch SAM, Norman SB, Hamblen JL. *Prolonged Exposure for PTSD Treatment*. 2020.
179. Forbes D, Bisson JI, Monson CM, Berliner L. (Eds.). *Effective treatments for PTSD: Practice guidelines from the International Society for Traumatic Stress Studies* (3rd ed.). The Guilford Press; 2020. https://psycnet.apa.org/record/2020-23029-000
180. Najavits LM, Sullivan TP, Schmitz M, Weiss RD, Lee CSN. Treatment utilization by women with PTSD and substance dependence. *Am J Addict*. 2004;13(3):215-224.
181. Young HE, Rosen CS, Finney JW. A survey of PTSD screening and referral practices in VA addiction treatment programs. *J Subst Abuse Treat*. 2005;28(4):313-319.
182. Volkow ND. Addiction should be treated, not penalized. *Neuropsychopharmacology*. 2021;46(12):2048-2050.
183. Furr-Holden D, Milam AJ, Wang L, Sadler R. African Americans now outpace whites in opioid-involved overdose deaths: a comparison of temporal trends from 1999 to 2018. *Addiction*. 2021;116(3):677-683.
184. Trangenstein PJ, Greene N, Eck RH, Milam AJ, Furr-Holden CD. Alcohol advertising and violence. *Am J Prev Med*. 2020;58(3):343-351.
185. Xu Y, Okuda M, Hser Y-I, et al. Twelve-month prevalence of psychiatric disorders and treatment-seeking among Asian Americans/Pacific Islanders in the United States: results from the National Epidemiological Survey on Alcohol and Related Conditions. *J Psychiatr Res*. 2011;45(7):910-918.
186. Hien DN, Bauer AG, Franklin L, Lalwani T, Pean K. Conceptualizing the COVID-19, opioid use, and racism syndemic and its associations with traumatic stress. *Psychiatr Serv*. 2022;73(3):353-356.
187. Busuttil W. Complex post-traumatic stress disorder: a useful diagnostic framework? *Psychiatry*. 2009;8(8):310-314.
188. Flanagan JC, Korte KJ, Killeen TK, Back SE. Concurrent treatment of substance use and PTSD. *Curr Psychiatry Rep*. 2016;18(8):70.
189. Nace EP. Posttraumatic stress disorder and substance abuse. *Clinical issues. Recent Dev Alcohol*. 1988;6:9-26.
190. Pitman RK, Altman B, Greenwald E, et al. Psychiatric complications during flooding therapy for posttraumatic stress disorder. *J Clin Psychiatry*. 1991;52(1):17-20.
191. Schäfer I, Najavits LM. Clinical challenges in the treatment of patients with posttraumatic stress disorder and substance abuse. *Curr Opin Psychiatry*. 2007;20(6):614-618.
192. Roberts NP, Roberts PA, Jones N, Bisson JI. Psychological interventions for post-traumatic stress disorder and comorbid substance use disorder: a systematic review and meta-analysis. *Clin Psychol Rev*. 2015;38:25-38.
193. Torchalla I, Nosen L, Rostam H, Allen P. Integrated treatment programs for individuals with concurrent substance use disorders and trauma experiences: a systematic review and meta-analysis. *J Subst Abuse Treat*. 2012;42(1):65-77.
194. van Dam D, Ehring T, Vedel E, Emmelkamp PMG. Trauma-focused treatment for posttraumatic stress disorder combined with CBT for severe substance use disorder: a randomized controlled trial. *BMC Psychiatry*. 2013;13(1):172.
195. Simpson TL, Lehavot K, Petrakis IL. No wrong doors: findings from a critical review of behavioral randomized clinical trials for individuals with co-occurring alcohol/drug problems and posttraumatic stress disorder. *Alcohol Clin Exp Res*. 2017;41(4):681-702.
196. Meshberg-Cohen S, MacLean RR, Schnakenberg Martin AM, Sofuoglu M, Petrakis IL. Treatment outcomes in individuals diagnosed with comorbid opioid use disorder and posttraumatic stress disorder: a review. *Addict Behav*. 2021;122:107026.
197. Back SE, Brady KT, Sonne SC, Verduin ML. Symptom improvement in co-occurring PTSD and alcohol dependence. *J Nerv Ment Dis*. 2006;194(9):690-696.
198. Ouimette P, Courtney A, Moos RH, Finney JW. Posttraumatic stress disorder in substance abuse patients: relationships to 1 year posttreatment outcomes. *Psychol Addict Behav*. 1997;1(1):34-47.
199. Hien DA, Litt LC, Cohen LR, Miele GM, Campbell A. *Trauma Services for Women in Substance Abuse Treatment: An Integrated Approach*. American Psychological Association; 2009.
200. Back SE, Brady KT, Jaanimägi U, Jackson JL. Cocaine dependence and PTSD: a pilot study of symptom interplay and treatment preferences. *Addict Behav*. 2006;31(2):351-354.
201. Brown PJ, Stout RL, Gannon-Rowley J. Substance use disorder-PTSD comorbidity: patients' perceptions of symptom interplay and treatment issues. *J Subst Abuse Treat*. 1998;15(5):445-448.
202. Back SE, Dansky BS, Carroll KM, Foa EB, Brady KT. Exposure therapy in the treatment of PTSD among cocaine-dependent individuals: description of procedures. *J Subst Abuse Treat*. 2001;21(1):35-45.
203. Hien DA, Fitzpatrick S, Saavedra LM, et al. What's in a name? A data-driven method to identify optimal psychotherapy classifications to advance treatment research on co-occurring PTSD and substance use disorders. *Eur J Psychotraumatol*. 2022;13(1):2001191.
204. Najavits LM. *Seeking Safety: A Treatment Manual for PTSD and Substance Abuse*. Guilford Press; 2002.
205. Najavits LM, Weiss RD, Shaw SR, Muenz LR. "Seeking safety": outcome of a new cognitive-behavioral psychotherapy for women with posttraumatic stress disorder and substance dependence. *J Trauma Stress*. 1998;11(3):437-456.
206. Zlotnick C, Najavits LM, Rohsenow DJ, Johnson DM. A cognitive-behavioral treatment for incarcerated women with substance abuse

disorder and posttraumatic stress disorder: findings from a pilot study. *J Subst Abuse Treat*. 2003;25(2):99-105.

207. Boden MT, Kimerling R, Jacons-Lentz J, et al. Seeking safety treatment for male veterans with a substance use disorder and post-traumatic stress disorder symptomatology. *Addiction*. 2012;107(3):578-586.
208. Najavits LM, Gallop RJ, Weiss RD. Seeking safety therapy for adolescent girls with PTSD and substance use disorder: a randomized controlled trial. *J Behav Health Serv Res*. 2006;33(4):453-463.
209. Hien DA, Cohen LR, Miele GM, Litt LC, Capstick C. Promising treatments for women with comorbid PTSD and substance use disorders. *Am J Psychiatry*. 2004;161(8):1426-1432.
210. Hien DA, Wells EA, Jiang H, et al. Multisite randomized trial of behavioral interventions for women with co-occurring PTSD and substance use disorders. *J Consult Clin Psychol*. 2009;77(4):607-619.
211. Zlotnick C, Johnson J, Najavits LM. Randomized controlled pilot study of cognitive-behavioral therapy in a sample of incarcerated women with substance use disorder and PTSD. *Behav Ther*. 2009;40(4):325-336.
212. Triffleman E, Carroll K, Kellogg S. Substance dependence posttraumatic stress disorder therapy. An integrated cognitive-behavioral approach. *J Subst Abuse Treat*. 1999;17(1-2):3-14.
213. Triffleman E. Gender differences in a controlled pilot study of psychosocial treatments in substance dependent patients with post-traumatic stress disorder: design considerations and outcomes. *Alcohol Treat Q*. 2000;18(3):113-126.
214. Brady KT, Dansky BS, Back SE, Foa EB, Carroll KM. Exposure therapy in the treatment of PTSD among cocaine-dependent individuals: preliminary findings. *J Subst Abuse Treat*. 2001;21(1):47-54.
215. Back SE, Foa EB, Killeen TK, et al. *Concurrent Treatment of PTSD and Substance Use Disorders Using Prolonged Exposure (COPE): Therapist Guide*. Oxford University Press; 2015.
216. Ruglass LM, Lopez-Castro T, Papini S, Killeen T, Back SE, Hien DA. Concurrent treatment with prolonged exposure for co-occurring full or subthreshold posttraumatic stress disorder and substance use disorders: a randomized clinical trial. *Psychother Psychosom*. 2017;86(3):150-161.
217. Norman SB, Trim R, Haller M, et al. Efficacy of integrated exposure therapy vs integrated coping skills therapy for comorbid posttraumatic stress disorder and alcohol use disorder: a randomized clinical trial. *JAMA Psychiatry*. 2019;76(8):791-799.
218. Mills KL, Teesson M, Back SE, et al. Integrated exposure-based therapy for co-occurring posttraumatic stress disorder and substance dependence: a randomized controlled trial. *JAMA*. 2012;308(7):690-699.
219. Coffey SF, Stasiewicz PR, Hughes PM, Brimo ML. Trauma-focused imaginal exposure for individuals with comorbid posttraumatic stress disorder and alcohol dependence: revealing mechanisms of alcohol craving in a cue reactivity paradigm. *Psychol Addict Behav*. 2006;20(4):425-435.
220. Sannibale C, Teesson M, Creamer M, et al. Randomized controlled trial of cognitive behaviour therapy for comorbid post-traumatic stress disorder and alcohol use disorders. *Addiction*. 2013;108(8):1397-1410.
221. Ruglass LM, Morgan-López AA, Saavedra LM, et al. Measurement nonequivalence of the Clinician-Administered PTSD Scale by race/ethnicity: implications for quantifying posttraumatic stress disorder severity. *Psychol Assess*. 2020;32(11):1015-1027.
222. Hien DA, Morgan-López AA, Saavedra LM, et al. Project Harmony: a meta-analysis with individual patient data of behavioral and pharmacologic trials for comorbid posttraumatic stress, alcohol and other drug use disorders. *Am J Psychiatry*. 2023;180(2):155-166.
223. Hien DA, Levin FR, Ruglass LM, et al. Combining seeking safety with sertraline for PTSD and alcohol use disorders: a randomized controlled trial. *J Consult Clin Psychol*. 2015;83(2):359-369.
224. Back S, McCauley JL, Korte KJ, et al. A double-blind, randomized, controlled pilot trial of N-Acetylcysteine in veterans with posttraumatic stress disorder and substance use disorders. *J Clin Psychiatry*. 2016;77(11):e1439-e1446.
225. Back SE, Gray K, Santa Ana E, et al. N-acetylcysteine for the treatment of comorbid alcohol use disorder and posttraumatic stress disorder: design and methodology of a randomized clinical trial. *Contemp Clin Trials*. 2020;91:105961.
226. McRae-Clark AL, Baker NL, Moran-Santa Maria M, Brady KT. Effect of oxytocin on craving and stress response in marijuana-dependent individuals: a pilot study. *Psychopharmacology (Berl)*. 2013;228(4):623-631.
227. Lee DJ, Schnitzlein CW, Wolf JP, Vythilingham M, Rasmusson AM, Hoge CW. Psychotherapy versus pharmacotherapy for posttraumatic stress disorder: systemic review and meta-analyses to determine first-line treatments. *Depress Anxiety*. 2016;33(9):792-806.
228. Gray KM, Carpenter MJ, Baker NL, et al. A double-blind randomized controlled trial of N-acetylcysteine in cannabis-dependent adolescents. *Am J Psychiatry*. 2012;169(8):805-812.
229. Ray LA, Meredith LR, Kiluk BD, Walthers J, Carroll KM, Magill M. Combined pharmacotherapy and cognitive behavioral therapy for adults with alcohol or substance use disorders: a systematic review and meta-analysis. *JAMA Netw Open*. 2020;3(6):e208279.
230. Rothbaum BO, Cahill SP, Foa EB, et al. Augmentation of sertraline with prolonged exposure in the treatment of posttraumatic stress disorder. *J Trauma Stress*. 2006;19(5):625-638.
231. Mitchell JM, Bogenschutz M, Lilienstein A, et al. MDMA-assisted therapy for severe PTSD: a randomized, double-blind, placebo-controlled phase 3 study. *Nat Med*. 2021;27(6):1025-1033.
232. Zoellner LA, Telch M, Foa EB, et al. Enhancing extinction learning in posttraumatic stress disorder with brief daily imaginal exposure and methylene blue: a randomized controlled trial. *J Clin Psychiatry*. 2017;78(7):e782-e789.
233. Zhang W, Davidson JR. Post-traumatic stress disorder: an evaluation of existing pharmacotherapies and new strategies. *Expert Opin Pharmacother*. 2007;8(12):1861-1870.
234. Brady K, Pearlstein T, Asnis GM, et al. Efficacy and safety of sertraline treatment of posttraumatic stress disorder: a randomized controlled trial. *JAMA*. 2000;283(14):1837-1844.
235. Davidson J, Pearlstein T, Londborg P, et al. Efficacy of sertraline in preventing relapse of posttraumatic stress disorder: results of a 28-week double-blind, placebo-controlled study. *Am J Psychiatry*. 2001;158(12):1974-1981.
236. Ipser J, Seedat S, Stein DJ. Pharmacotherapy for post-traumatic stress disorder—a systematic review and meta-analysis. *S Afr Med J*. 2006;96(10):1088-1096.
237. Davidson JR. Pharmacologic treatment of acute and chronic stress following trauma: 2006. *J Clin Psychiatry*. 2006;67(Suppl 2):34-39.
238. Marshall RD, Beebe KL, Oldham M, Zaninelli R. Efficacy and safety of paroxetine treatment for chronic PTSD: a fixed-dose, placebo-controlled study. *Am J Psychiatry*. 2001;158(12):1982-1988.
239. Davidson J, Baldwin D, Stein DJ, et al. Treatment of posttraumatic stress disorder with venlafaxine extended release: a 6-month randomized controlled trial. *Arch Gen Psychiatry*. 2006;63(10):1158-1165.
240. Davidson J, Rothbaum BO, Tucker P, Asnis G, Benattia I, Musgnung JJ. Venlafaxine extended release in posttraumatic stress disorder: a sertraline- and placebo-controlled study. *J Clin Psychopharmacol*. 2006;26(3):259-267.
241. Ursano RJ, Bell C, Eth S, et al. Practice guideline for the treatment of patients with acute stress disorder and posttraumatic stress disorder. *Am J Psychiatry*. 2004;161(11 Suppl):3-31.
242. Stein MB. Management of posttraumatic stress disorder in adults. In: Roy-Byrne PP, ed. *UpToDate*. 2023.
243. Schoenfeld FB, Marmar CR, Neylan TC. Current concepts in pharmacotherapy for posttraumatic stress disorder. *Psychiatr Serv*. 2004;55(5):519-531.
244. Spiegel DA, Bruce TJ. Benzodiazepines and exposure-based cognitive behavior therapies for panic disorder: conclusions from combined treatment trials. *Am J Psychiatry*. 1997;154(6):773-781.
245. Berlau DJ, McGaugh JL. Enhancement of extinction memory consolidation: the role of the noradrenergic and GABAergic systems within the basolateral amygdala. *Neurobiol Learn Mem*. 2006;86(2):123-132.
246. Debiec J, Ledoux JE. Disruption of reconsolidation but not consolidation of auditory fear conditioning by noradrenergic blockade in the amygdala. *Neuroscience*. 2004;129(2):267-272.

247. Lee JL, Di Ciano P, Thomas KL, Everitt BJ. Disrupting reconsolidation of drug memories reduces cocaine-seeking behavior. *Neuron*. 2005;47(6):795-801.
248. McGaugh JL. Memory—a century of consolidation. *Science*. 2000;287(5451):248-251.
249. Nader K. Memory traces unbound. *Trends Neurosci*. 2003;26(2):65-72.
250. Sara SJ. Retrieval and reconsolidation: toward a neurobiology of remembering. *Learn Mem*. 2000;7(2):73-84.
251. Cahill L, Pham CA, Setlow B. Impaired memory consolidation in rats produced with beta-adrenergic blockade. *Neurobiol Learn Mem*. 2000;74(3):259-266.
252. Morris RW, Westbrook RF, Killcross AS. Reinstatement of extinguished fear by beta-adrenergic arousal elicited by a conditioned context. *Behav Neurosci*. 2005;119(6):1662-1671.
253. Cahill L, Prins B, Weber M, McGaugh JL. Beta-adrenergic activation and memory for emotional events. *Nature*. 1994;371(6499):702-704.
254. O'Carroll RE, Drysdale E, Cahill L, Shajahan P, Ebmeier KP. Stimulation of the noradrenergic system enhances and blockade reduces memory for emotional material in man. *Psychol Med*. 1999;29(5):1083-1088.
255. Reist C, Duffy JG, Fujimoto K, Cahill L. beta-Adrenergic blockade and emotional memory in PTSD. *Int J Neuropsychopharmacol*. 2001;4(4):377-383.
256. Raut SB, Canales JJ, Ravindran M, et al. Effects of propranolol on the modification of trauma memory reconsolidation in PTSD patients: a systematic review and meta-analysis. *J Psychiatr Res*. 2022;150:246-256.
257. Brady KT, Verduin ML. Pharmacotherapy of comorbid mood, anxiety, and substance use disorders. *Subst Use Misuse*. 2005;40(13-14):2021-2041, 2043-2048.
258. Lingford-Hughes AR, Welch S, Nutt DJ. Evidence-based guidelines for the pharmacological management of substance misuse, addiction and comorbidity: recommendations from the British Association for Psychopharmacology. *J Psychopharmacol*. 2004;18(3):293-335.
259. Shorter D, Hsieh J, Kosten TR. Pharmacologic management of comorbid post-traumatic stress disorder and addictions. *Am J Addict*. 2015;24(8):705-712.
260. Petrakis IL, Simpson TL. Posttraumatic stress disorder and alcohol use disorder: a critical review of pharmacologic treatments. *Alcohol Clin Exp Res*. 2017;41(2):226-237.
261. Brady KT, Sonne SC, Roberts JM. Sertraline treatment of comorbid posttraumatic stress disorder and alcohol dependence. *J Clin Psychiatry*. 1995;56(11):502-505.
262. Brady KT, Sonne S, Anton RF, Randall CL, Back SE, Simpson K. Sertraline in the treatment of co-occurring alcohol dependence and posttraumatic stress disorder. *Alcohol Clin Exp Res*. 2005;29(3):395-401.
263. Simpson TL, Malte CA, Dietel B, et al. A pilot trial of prazosin, an alpha-1 adrenergic antagonist, for comorbid alcohol dependence and posttraumatic stress disorder. *Alcohol Clin Exp Res*. 2015;39(5):808-817.
264. Petrakis IL, Desai N, Gueorguieva R, et al. Prazosin for veterans with posttraumatic stress disorder and comorbid alcohol dependence: a clinical trial. *Alcohol Clin Exp Res*. 2016;40(1):178-186.
265. Batki SL, Pennington DL, Lasher B, et al. Topiramate treatment of alcohol use disorder in veterans with posttraumatic stress disorder: a randomized controlled pilot trial. *Alcohol Clin Exp Res*. 2014;38(8):2169-2177.
266. Mula M. Topiramate and cognitive impairment: evidence and clinical implications. *Ther Adv Drug Saf*. 2012;3(6):279-289.
267. Petrakis IL, Poling J, Levinson C, et al. Naltrexone and disulfiram in patients with alcohol dependence and comorbid post-traumatic stress disorder. *Biol Psychiatry*. 2006;60(7):777-783.
268. Foa EB, Yusko DA, McLean CP, et al. Concurrent naltrexone and prolonged exposure therapy for patients with comorbid alcohol dependence and PTSD: a randomized clinical trial. *JAMA*. 2013;310(5):488-495.
269. Rodrigues H, Figueira I, Loipes A, et al. Does d-cycloserine enhance exposure therapy for anxiety disorders in humans? A meta-analysis. *PLoS One*. 2014;9(7):e93519.
270. Ledgerwood L. *Effects of D-Cycloserine on the extinction of conditioned freezing in rats*. Dissertation Abstracts International: B, Sciences and Engineering; 2004.
271. Ledgerwood L, Richardson R, Cranney J. Effects of d-cycloserine on extinction of conditioned freezing. *Behav Neurosci*. 2003;117(2):341-349.
272. Ledgerwood L, Richardson R, Cranney J. d-Cycloserine and the facilitation of extinction of conditioned fear: consequences for reinstatement. *Behav Neurosci*. 2004;118(3):505-513.
273. Ledgerwood L, Richardson R, Cranney J. d-Cycloserine facilitates extinction of learned fear: effects on reacquisition and generalized extinction. *Biol Psychiatry*. 2005;57(8):841-847.
274. Walker DL, Ressler KJ, Lu K-T, Davis M. Facilitation of conditioned fear extinction by systemic administration or intra-amygdala infusions of D-cycloserine as assessed with fear-potentiated startle in rats. *J Neurosci*. 2002;22(6):2343-2351.
275. Yang YL, Lu KT. Facilitation of conditioned fear extinction by d-cycloserine is mediated by mitogen-activated protein kinase and phosphatidylinositol 3-kinase cascades and requires de novo protein synthesis in basolateral nucleus of amygdala. *Neuroscience*. 2005;134(1):247-260.
276. Thanos PK, Bermeo C, Wang G-J, Volkow ND. d-Cycloserine accelerates the extinction of cocaine-induced conditioned place preference in C57bL/c mice. *Behav Brain Res*. 2009;199(2):345-349.
277. Santa Ana EJ, Rounsaville BJ, Frankforter TL, et al. d-Cycloserine attenuates reactivity to smoking cues in nicotine dependent smokers: a pilot investigation. *Drug Alcohol Depend*. 2009;104(3):220-227.
278. Drummond DC, Tiffany ST, Glautier S, Remington B, eds. *Addictive Behavior: Cue Exposure Theory and Practice*. Wiley; 1995.
279. Drobes DJ, Saladin ME, Tiffany ST. Classical conditioning mechanisms in alcohol dependence. In: Heather N, Peters TJ, Stockwell T, eds. *International Handbook of Alcohol Dependence and Problems*. Wiley; 2001:281-297.
280. Byrne SP, Haber P, Baillie A, Giannopolous V, Morley K. Cue exposure therapy for alcohol use disorders: what can be learned from exposure therapy for anxiety disorders? *Subst Use Misuse*. 2019;54(12):2053-2063.
281. Childress AR, Ehrman R, McLellan AT, O'Brien C. Conditioned craving and arousal in cocaine addiction: a preliminary report. *NIDA Res Monogr*. 1988;81:74-80.
282. O'Brien CP, Childress AR, Ehrman R, Robbins SJ. Conditioning factors in drug abuse: can they explain compulsion? *J Psychopharmacol*. 1998;12(1):15-22.
283. Sinha R, Fuse T, Aubin LR, O'Malley SS. Psychological stress, drug-related cues and cocaine craving. *Psychopharmacology (Berl)*. 2000;152(2):140-148.
284. Wise RA. The neurobiology of craving: implications for the understanding and treatment of addiction. *J Abnorm Psychol*. 1988;97:118-132.
285. Conklin CA, Tiffany ST. Applying extinction research and theory to cue-exposure addiction treatments. *Addiction*. 2002;97:155-167.
286. Knackstedt LA, LaRowe S, Mardikian P, et al. The role of cystine-glutamate exchange in nicotine dependence in rats and humans. *Biol Psychiatry*. 2009;65(10):841-845.
287. LaRowe SD, Kalivas PW, Nicholas JS, Randall PK, Mardikian P, Malcolm RJ. A double-blind placebo-controlled trial of N-acetylcysteine in the treatment of cocaine dependence. *Am J Addict*. 2013;22(5):443-452.
288. Roberts NP, Roberts PA, Jones N, Bisson JL. Psychological therapies for post-traumatic stress disorder and comorbid substance use disorder. *Cochrane Database Syst Rev*. 2016;4(4):CD010204.
289. Back SE, Killeen T, Foa EB, Santa Ana EJ, Gros DF, Brady KT. Use of an integrated therapy with prolonged exposure to treat PTSD and comorbid alcohol dependence in an Iraq veteran. *Am J Psychiatry*. 2012;169(7):688-691.
290. Ralevski E, Olivera-Figueroa LA, Petrakis I. PTSD and comorbid AUD: a review of pharmacological and alternative treatment options. *Subst Abuse Rehabil*. 2014;5:25-36.
291. Schiff M, Nacasch N, Levit S, Katz N, Foa EB. Prolonged exposure for treating PTSD among female methadone patients who were survivors of sexual abuse in Israel. *Soc Work Health Care*. 2015;54(8):687-707.
292. Ouimette P, Brown PJ, eds. *Trauma and Substance Abuse: Causes, Consequences, and Treatment of Comorbid Disorders*. American Psychological Association; 2003.
293. Riggs DS, Rukstalis M, Volpicelli JR, Kalmanson D, Foa EB. Demographic and social adjustment characteristics of patients with comorbid posttraumatic stress disorder and alcohol dependence: potential pitfalls to PTSD treatment. *Addict Behav*. 2003;28(9):1717-1730.

CHAPTER

107 Co-occurring Eating Disorders and Substance Use Disorders

Lisa J. Merlo, Nicole Avena, Ashley N. Gearhardt, and Mark S. Gold

CHAPTER OUTLINE

- Introduction
- Definitions
- Prevalence of eating disorders
- Differential diagnosis
- Screening instruments
- Treatment
- Biological management
- Psychological management
- Recovery issues
- Areas for further study
- Summary

INTRODUCTION

This chapter describes commonalities between, and co-occurrence of, substance use disorders (SUDs) and disturbances in eating. Anorexia nervosa (AN), bulimia nervosa (BN), binge eating disorder (BED), and obesity are serious clinical conditions with significant medical and psychological consequences. BN, BED, and obesity share many similarities with SUDs and frequently co-occur, complicating the assessment, diagnosis, treatment, and long-term recovery processes for both conditions.

DEFINITIONS

Eating Disorders

Eating disorders constitute a category of psychiatric illnesses characterized by disturbed eating patterns and dysfunctional attitudes related to food, eating, and body shape.[1] Available data suggest that AN, BN, and BED are closely associated with SUDs.[2] Indeed, eating disorders and SUDs frequently co-occur, and twin studies reveal shared genetic variance between these conditions.[3] Whereas SUDs can be understood as an individual's biological sensitivity and pathological attachment to drugs or alcohol, the eating disorders can be similarly described as a pathological relationship with food.[4]

Anorexia Nervosa

Readers are referred to the current *Diagnostic and Statistical Manual of Mental Disorders* (DSM)[1] for a full listing of diagnostic criteria for AN. There are two types of AN: (1) the restricting type, where extreme calorie limitation is the means of weight loss, and (2) the binge/purge subtype, where periods of food intake are compensated for through behaviors like excessive exercise, vomiting, and laxative use.[1] Individuals with AN are characterized by significantly low body weight, though they are often adamant in their denial of the disorder[5] and may go to great lengths to mask their impairment or hide their symptoms (eg, by avoiding eating around other people, wearing baggy clothing to hide their emaciated frame, creating/eating elaborate meals when there are witnesses). Associated physical symptoms, which may initially provide the impetus for seeking treatment, include constipation, cold intolerance, lethargy, and in some cases lanugo (fine body hair that develops along the midsection and appendages). AN can result in significant medical complications, including hypothalamic-pituitary-adrenal axis dysfunction, pubertal delay or interruption, growth retardation, bone mass reduction, and osteopenia/osteoporosis. Other possible symptoms include bradycardia, hypotension, cardiac arrhythmias, mitral valve prolapse, metabolic alkalosis or acidosis, hypokalemia, hypoglycemia, leukopenia, anemia, carotenemia, acrocyanosis, thrombocytopenia, peripheral neuropathy, hypothermia, dehydration, hair loss, and dry skin.[6-8] The mortality rate for individuals with AN is extremely high, ranging from 7% to 10% in studies spanning 8 years.[9,10] Rates of completed suicide in this population range from 0.9% to 6.3%.[11]

Bulimia Nervosa

The diagnostic criteria for BN are outlined in the current DSM.[1] BN differs from AN in that markedly low body weight is not a symptom, but the presence of binge eating and compensation for bingeing is necessary for the diagnosis. If low body weight is present, the binge/purge subtype of AN may be the better diagnostic fit. Compensatory actions involve purging by self-induced vomiting in approximately 90% of BN cases, but may also include use of laxatives, diuretics, and/or enemas; excessive exercise; periods of fasting; or severe caloric restriction. Because of the frequency of vomiting, it is common for dental enamel to show significant erosion.[12] Other significant medical complications associated with BN include fluid and electrolyte abnormalities (eg, hypokalemia, metabolic alkalosis or acidosis), cardiac arrhythmias, parotid enlargement, submandibular adenopathy, menstrual irregularity, constipation, and reproductive problems.[8,13]

Binge Eating Disorder

The key distinction from BN is that individuals with BED do not engage in compensatory behavior for their overeating. Binge eating episodes often involve eating rapidly, eating more than intended (eg, eating until uncomfortably full or bingeing when not hungry), eating alone (often owing to embarrassment or shame regarding the excessive food intake), and feeling disgusted, guilty, or depressed after binge eating.[1] Some report feelings of dissociation during episodes of binge eating, and most with BED view their binge eating as unwanted and distressing. Approximately 20% of individuals with BED are overweight, and approximately 70% are obese.[14] Additionally, 30% of individuals who are obese are diagnosed with BED.[15] The most common medical complications associated with BED result from consequences of morbid obesity, including hypertension, type II diabetes, cardiovascular disease and stroke, osteoarthritis, increased risk for cancer, chronic muscular pain, joint pain, gastrointestinal problems including irritable bowel syndrome, and early menarche.[16-18]

Obesity

Obesity is another serious condition related, in part, to disturbance in eating. The diagnosis of obesity is made based on an individual's body mass index (BMI) score. BMI is calculated by dividing weight in kilograms by height in meters squared. Standard cut points are used to determine the weight range: underweight (BMI < 18.5), normal weight (BMI 18.5-24.9), overweight (BMI 25-29.9), and obese (BMI ≥ 30). BMI from 30 to 34.9 is considered stage 1 obesity, from 35 to 39.9 is stage 2 obesity, and 40 or higher is stage 3 obesity (also called morbid obesity).

"Food Addiction"

Though not a clinical diagnosis, the construct of "food addiction" (FA)[19] was originally conceptualized by applying the DSM-IV-TR[20] criteria for substance dependence to highly processed food as an addictive substance. Updated criteria based on DSM-5 are listed in **Table 107-1**. Although it was ultimately decided that sufficient evidence did not yet exist to include FA in the DSM-5 or ICD-10, additional clinical and research findings have demonstrated that pathological attachment to food (particularly highly processed foods high in refined carbohydrates and fat) is similar to SUD in virtually all spheres, including neurobiological.[21-24] Results of functional magnetic resonance imaging (fMRI) studies comparing scores on a measure of FA with brain activity suggested that neural activation patterns are similar for individuals who demonstrate addictive behavior toward either food or drugs.[25,26] Further, neural alterations in the ventral and dorsal striatum are associated with food craving and weight gain, consistent with patterns seen in other addictive behaviors.[27] Interestingly, signs of FA are sometimes endorsed in AN, particularly the binge/purge subtype. This may reflect subjective (rather than objective) feelings of being "addicted" to food.[28] In addition, studies demonstrate that 40.5% to 56.8% of individuals with BED can be classified with FA,[29,30] and 72.2% of obese individuals with FA can be diagnosed with BED.[31]

TABLE 107-1 Proposed Criteria for Food Addiction Based on DSM-5 Substance Use Disorder Criteria

A problematic pattern of food consumption causing clinically significant impairment or distress, as evidenced by at least two of the following within any year (mild 2-3 symptoms, moderate 4-5 symptoms, severe 6 or more symptoms:
The need for increased food consumption to achieve the same level of satisfaction; or decreased satisfaction over time when consuming a consistent amount of food (tolerance)
The development of physiological or cognitive symptoms when consumption of food (or certain types of food, such as carbohydrates) is decreased abruptly; or continued consumption to prevent such symptoms (withdrawal)
Consuming larger amounts of food or eating for longer periods of time than intended
Continuing desire to control eating or repeated unsuccessful attempts to cut down or control eating (ie, dieting)
Spending significant periods of time obtaining, preparing, or consuming food or recovering from overeating
Reduction or impairment in important activities as a result of food consumption or its effects
Persistent overeating despite medical or psychological consequences
Intense cravings/urges to consume the food
Consuming the food in physically hazardous situations
Continuing food intake in the same manner despite interpersonal problems
Pattern of food intake causes failure to fulfill daily role obligations

PREVALENCE OF EATING DISORDERS

General Population

Lifetime prevalence rates for the primary eating disorders are listed in **Table 107-2**.[32-35] Symptom onset rarely occurs past the age of 40 years,[1] and point prevalence rates are much higher during adolescence and early adulthood. For example, the prevalence of subclinical AN among girls ages 16 to

TABLE 107-2 Lifetime Prevalence Rates for Eating Disorders

	Lifetime Prevalence Female	Lifetime Prevalence Male
Anorexia nervosa (AN)	0.9%-1.9%	0.29%-0.3%
Bulimia nervosa (BN)	1.5%-2.9%	~0.5%
Binge eating disorder (BED)	1.9%-3.5%	0.3%-2.0%

25 is estimated to be about 10%.[36] The onset of BN occurs most commonly between the ages of 14 and 22.[32] BED onset typically occurs later than AN or BN, most frequently in the early to mid-20s, though many patients do not present for treatment until their 40s.[37] The percentage of the population afflicted with disordered eating rises dramatically when obesity is included. As of 2014, 36.5% of American adults aged 20 or older were obese (ie, BMI ≥ 30), as well as 17% of youth.[38] In addition, recent meta-analyses estimated that 20% of adults and 15% of adolescents and children met the proposed criteria for FA.[39,40] As with SUDs, heritability appears to be an important factor in the development of eating disorders.[41] An international investigation, the Eating Disorders Genetics Initiative, is actively investigating the role of genes and environment in AN, BN, and BED,[42] and genome-wide association studies have suggested that future AN studies focus on genes related to metabolism and the gastrointestinal tract.[43]

Patients With Substance Use Disorders

Among individuals receiving SUD treatment, approximately 0.02% to 3.4% also currently suffer from an eating disorder.[44,45] Treating one condition may exacerbate the other, but ignoring one may cause a new life-threatening disease to emerge. Thus, careful consideration to co-occurring eating disorders must be part of the comprehensive care of SUDs and vice versa. Results of the National Comorbidity Survey Replication study suggested that lifetime co-occurrence of alcohol use disorders and eating disorders ranges from 24% to 25%, whereas lifetime co-occurrence between drug use disorders and eating disorders is 18% to 26%.[32] Among adolescents being treated for eating disorders, approximately 35% display "regular or risky substance use" (as compared to those with "no or occasional use," as defined by the study authors), with rates of SUDs estimated at 1.1% for alcohol, 3.2% for cannabis, 1.1% for other drugs, and 14.7% for tobacco.[46]

Binge eating is frequently associated with excessive alcohol consumption,[47,48] with up to 57% of men and 28% of women with BED meeting criteria for a SUD.[49] Rates of BN are also significantly higher among women who use alcohol in an unhealthy manner than those in the general population, with greater than two-thirds identifying themselves as "binge eaters" with or without purging.[50] Individuals with a history of overeating may develop SUDs after improving their eating habits (eg, following bariatric surgery).[51] In addition, animal research has demonstrated that abstaining from alcohol may promote bingeing on sugary foods, whereas restricting sugary food intake may promote excessive alcohol consumption.[52] Human studies have demonstrated that drug withdrawal may promote overeating[53] and that treatment and recovery from SUDs are frequently associated with weight gain.[54,55] However, in the absence of BED, obesity may actually serve a protective function against substance use. Research has demonstrated that, as BMI increases, the percentage of women who have consumed alcohol or smoked cannabis in the previous year decreases significantly.[56,57]

Conversely, dieting and purging are frequently associated with the use of cocaine and other stimulants.[48,58,59] Although individuals with food-restricting habits are less likely to use stimulants than individuals who binge or purge, they still display increased use of stimulants compared to the general population.[48] Patients with AN also frequently use prescription and over-the-counter medication in unhealthy ways (eg, they may use psychostimulants for weight management).[60] Unhealthy use of caffeine and laxatives is common among both individuals with restricting behaviors and those with purging behaviors.[61] Many people who chronically use tobacco cite fear of weight gain as a deterrent to their cessation efforts,[62] and the presence of an eating disorder may impede treatment. However, female adolescents with restricting habits are actually less likely to use tobacco, alcohol, and cannabis than are individuals in the general population.[61]

Patients With Psychiatric Disorders

The most common co-occurring psychiatric disorders among individuals with AN are mood disorders, with approximately 94% of AN patients meeting criteria for a depressive disorder.[58] Between 56% and 66% of those with an eating disorder experience one or more anxiety disorders.[58,63] Obsessive-compulsive disorder is common, with a prevalence rate between 29.5% and 41% among individuals with AN or BN.[64-66] Social phobia has a 20% rate of co-occurrence,[64] and about 68% of patients meet diagnostic criteria for one or more personality disorders, based on DSM-IV criteria,[66] though rates vary between 21% and 97%.[67] Patients with AN most commonly display cluster C (anxious/avoidant) personality disorders, whereas those with BN are more likely to display cluster B (dramatic/erratic) personality disorders.[67] Finally, individuals with BED are three times more likely to suffer from major depressive disorder than are individuals from the general population,[68] and co-occurring personality disorders are frequently associated with the severity of binge eating.[49] Obesity is also associated with increased psychiatric conditions, including major depressive disorder and generalized anxiety disorder.[69]

Primary Care or Other Health Care Populations

Within a family practice setting, the prevalence of AN is estimated to be between 4.2% and 6.3%, and the prevalence of BN is estimated to be between 6.3% and 12.2%.[70,71] Up to one-third of female adolescents with type I diabetes exhibit disordered eating behaviors.[72] With regard to BED, the prevalence is approximately 5% to 30% among obese individuals.[73,74] In fact, there is almost a fivefold increase in risk for BED among individuals whose BMI is at least 40 compared to those whose BMI is within the normal range, and the risk for displaying subclinical binge eating behavior shows the same trend.[75] Heredity may play a role in the development of BED, as 20.2% of individuals who are related to an overweight or obese person with BED also develop BED, compared to only 9.6% of individuals who are related to an overweight or obese person without BED. Relatives of the BED group are also more likely to have higher current BMI and elevated rates of obesity.[75] In addition, among female athletes, rates of subclinical eating disorders range from 15% to 32%,[76] and these symptoms also commonly occur among male athletes. Participation in aesthetic sports (eg, ballet, gymnastics, figure skating) or sports in which "making weight" is required (eg, wrestling, horse racing) results in increased risk for disordered eating.[77]

DIFFERENTIAL DIAGNOSIS

Identifying Eating Disorders

Patients with eating disorders often resist acknowledging their symptoms and are often in extreme denial of their illness, even when referred for treatment by a parent or friend. Individuals with AN may surreptitiously increase their weight for weigh-ins using weights, heavy clothing, or water loading.[78] When self-referred, they may neglect to mention their disordered eating, instead presenting with nonspecific symptoms such as fatigue, lack of energy, or dizziness[63] or associated complaints such as intolerance to cold, throat or abdominal pain, digestive problems, heart palpitations, or changes in drinking or urination.[79] Several medical disorders share symptoms with eating disorders, complicating the diagnostic process. For example, hyperthyroidism, diabetes, tumors, gastrointestinal disorders (eg, inflammatory bowel disease), nutrient malabsorption, immunodeficiency, chronic infections, and Addison disease may all result in weight changes and associated symptoms.[79]

Eating Disorders in Patients With Substance Use Disorders

Detection of eating disorders may be particularly difficult among patients who have SUDs that appear to "explain" the symptoms. For example, alcohol-related disorders can result in vomiting (as seen in AN and BN) and lethargy (as seen in AN, BN, BED, and obesity). Cannabis use may result in binge eating (as in BN, BED, and obesity). Use of amphetamines, methamphetamine, cocaine, MDMA (3,4-methylenedioxy-methamphetamine), and opioids can result in decreased eating and significant weight loss (as in AN), and some individuals even report using low doses of MDMA specifically for weight management.[80] Thus, regardless of whether an eating disorder is initially suspected, addiction clinicians should specifically inquire about eating disturbances, as well as weight-related drug use (eg, use of "diet pills," laxatives, stimulants). Individuals with eating disorders are unlikely to offer this information spontaneously, but the presence of a co-occurring eating disorder may affect SUD treatment decisions.

All patients with SUD would also benefit from analysis of diet, exercise, eating behaviors,[74] and BMI. In particular, patients undergoing treatment for alcohol use disorder should always be evaluated for binge eating symptoms; those in treatment for a stimulant use disorder should always be assessed for purging behaviors and excessive dieting; and patients with unhealthy use of caffeine or laxatives should always undergo a general eating disorder screening. The addiction clinician should also routinely include an assessment of current and past eating habits when recording the medical history, in order to obtain a comprehensive understanding of the patient and be alert to signs of an underlying or co-occurring eating disorder. As treatment for the SUD progresses, the patient's weight and BMI should be monitored to track significant gain or loss. Many instruments are available to assist with eating disorder screening and assessment, which can take place during the initial SUD evaluation and intermittently throughout treatment.

SCREENING INSTRUMENTS

Eating Disorders Inventory, Third Edition

The *Eating Disorders Inventory*, Third Edition (EDI-3),[81] can be used to assist in the diagnosis of an eating disorder. The EDI-3 contains 12 subscales (91 items) assessing specific eating disorder symptoms (eg, drive for thinness, body dissatisfaction, bulimia) and related psychological constructs (eg, ineffectiveness, perfectionism). It is appropriate for individuals 12 years and older and can be completed in about 20 minutes.

Eating Disorder Diagnostic Scale

The Eating Disorder Diagnostic Scale (EDDS)[82] is a 19-item self-report questionnaire that assesses eating disorder symptoms over the previous 3 months. It is useful in differential diagnosis for AN, BN, and BED and requires about five minutes to complete. Most items are scored using a 7-point Likert-type scale. The authors have developed algorithms to determine whether diagnostic criteria are met for AN, BN, and/or BED.

Eating Disorder Examination Questionnaire

The Eating Disorder Examination Questionnaire (EDE-Q)[83] assesses disordered eating behaviors and attitudes over the previous 4 weeks, in order to assist with diagnosis of AN and BN. The EDE-Q contains 36 items that are scored using a 7-point forced-choice scale. It takes about 10 minutes to complete.

Bulimia Test—Revised

The Bulimia Test—Revised (BULIT—R)[84] is a 36-item self-report measure of BN symptoms (eg, binge eating, compensatory behaviors, and body shape disturbance). It can be used specifically to assist with the diagnosis of BN and can be completed in 5 to 10 minutes. Items are scored using a 5-point Likert-type scale. The BULIT—R is recommended for individuals 16 years and older.

Binge Eating Scale

The Binge Eating Scale (BES)[85] is a 16-item measure used to assess binge eating symptoms and assist with diagnosis of

BED. For each item, respondents choose from four statements to determine which statement describes them best. The BES has published cutoffs to determine whether an individual displays clinically significant binge eating symptoms. It can be completed in less than 5 minutes.

Night Eating Symptom Scale

The Night Eating Symptom Scale (NESS)[86] is a self-report instrument that contains 12 items specifically assessing symptoms of night-eating syndrome (ie, overeating during the nighttime hours), such as percentage of food consumed after supper and frequency of nighttime snacking. It takes less than 5 minutes to complete.

Yale Food Addiction Scale, Version 2.0

The Yale Food Addiction Scale Version 2.0 (YFAS 2.0)[87] is used to screen for "food addiction" (FA) and includes 35 items assessing symptomatic behaviors. Respondents use a 7-point scale ranging from "never" to "every day" to rate the frequency of each behavior. The scale provides a measure of FA symptoms and a "diagnosis" of food addiction based on DSM-5 SUD criteria. It takes less than five minutes to complete.

TREATMENT

The treatment of eating disorders can be a long and arduous process marked by alternating periods of recurrence and recovery. Continued diligence is needed, as there is an increased risk of suicide attempts and completions among individuals who have an eating disorder diagnosis and their relatives.[88]

Acute Treatment

For serious cases, and particularly for adolescent patients, treatment may commence on a coerced or even involuntary basis through enrollment in an inpatient or residential program. A focus on refeeding takes precedence in order to medically stabilize the patient and restore cognitive functioning so that he or she is able to participate in the treatment process.

Subacute Treatment

The patient is more likely to be successful if he or she agrees to treatment and is motivated to change his or her behavior. As a result, motivational interviewing interventions may be useful in helping the patient to recognize the need for treatment and to increase his or her willingness to enter and participate in a treatment program.[89,90]

Long-Term Treatment

Management of an eating disorder typically involves a multidisciplinary team and includes psychosocial, behavioral, and pharmacological interventions. Psychotherapy is an important component of treatment and may include both individual and family sessions.[91] Depending on the severity of symptoms and presence of co-occurring disorders, treatment may be administered in outpatient, partial hospitalization, inpatient, or residential settings. No matter the treatment milieu or modality, development of a treatment contract specifying goals and expectations related to each disorder may be beneficial.

BIOLOGICAL MANAGEMENT

Acute Biological Management of AN

Generally, patients who are medically or psychiatrically unstable are referred for inpatient care.[92] Individuals with co-occurring SUDs may also be referred for more intensive treatment owing to the increased psychological strain associated with attempting to simultaneously abstain from two maladaptive coping mechanisms (ie, substance use and disordered eating or purging) and the increased medical risks associated with these conditions. Whether the patient has a co-occurring SUD or not, the medical management of AN begins with a comprehensive medical and neurological evaluation and treatment of co-occurring medical conditions. Rehydrating and refeeding safely are the keys to medical intervention. While the establishment of weight gain is a goal, it is important to be certain that an electrolyte, cardiac, or other disease does not kill the patient or compromise the patient's ability to be treated or recover.

Subacute Biological Management of AN

In cases of co-occurring AN and SUDs, integrative treatment targeting both disorders is recommended. If this is not available, it is generally recommended that SUD treatment take priority unless the patient is at immediate medical risk due to malnutrition. Once the patient achieves stable sobriety, the treatment for AN may begin. Individuals with AN are generally terrified of gaining weight, so weight gain should be implemented gradually (eg, 0.5-1.0 lb/wk). The American Dietetic Association recommends nutrition intervention and nutritional counseling by a registered dietician as an integral part of treatment for AN.[93] Thus, every addiction clinician should establish contact with a credible referral source to assist with this component of treatment. Referral to a mental health professional is typically helpful, especially one with experience treating eating disorders. Among adolescents, weight gain may best be achieved using a family intervention referred to as the *Maudsley Method*. This approach involves encouraging parents to take an active role in promoting their child's weight regain.[94] However, neither this method nor other forms of family therapy are generally efficacious for adult patients with AN.[95,96] Nutritional rehabilitation and weight restoration treatment for adult patients and some adolescents generally consist of utilizing behavioral reinforcement to reward eating. It has been suggested that parenteral nutrition and nasogastric feeding be avoided, if possible, due to concerns that the patient may relapse or develop other symptoms (eg, purging) to compensate for her or his weight gain.[97] However, there is some evidence that nocturnal nasogastric feeding may increase weight gain.[98]

Long-Term Biological Management of AN

The process of gaining weight is often very stressful for patients with AN, and the addiction clinician may wish to monitor the patient more closely during the weight restoration period to assess for signs of recurrent substance use. Thus far, no pharmacological treatments have proven effective in treatment of the primary symptoms of AN.[95,99] However, selective serotonin reuptake inhibitors (SSRIs) may help to decrease associated symptoms such as depression, obsessive-compulsive symptoms, and lack of interoceptive awareness.[100,101] Like parenteral feeding, it is recommended that medications to promote weight gain be used judiciously in order to avoid overwhelming the patient. However, use of calcium supplements and a multivitamin is recommended.[102] Oral contraceptives or hormone replacement therapy may be prescribed to help regulate the menstrual cycle, mitigate effects of hypoestrogenemia, and minimize bone loss.[103] Though benzodiazepines are sometimes prescribed to patients with AN with the goal of helping them remain calm at meal time, benzodiazepines are *not* indicated for the treatment of any eating disorder and should be tapered and discontinued during the course of SUD treatment.

Acute Biological Management of BN

Management of medical complications associated with BN may be necessary. For example, estrogen replacement may be indicated to combat hypothalamic hypogonadism. Physicians should monitor patients with BN to assess for fluid and electrolyte abnormalities, cardiac arrhythmias, gastrointestinal symptoms, and reproductive problems. Patients with BN plus co-occurring SUDs are more likely to have medical complications; a general medical workup may be indicated for these patients.

Subacute Biological Management of BN

Integrative treatment is recommended for patients with co-occurring BN and SUD. If not available, patients should be treated first for their SUD due to higher mortality risk in SUDs compared to BN. Once in stable sobriety, biological management of BN generally involves medication with an SSRI. Specifically, fluoxetine has demonstrated efficacy in reducing the core symptoms of BN and has been shown to lower treatment discontinuation rates.[104] It is the only medication approved by the Food and Drug Administration (FDA) for the treatment of BN, with suggested dosage of approximately 60 mg/d. Sertraline, escitalopram, and fluvoxamine are also used off-label in patients who do not tolerate fluoxetine, or have insufficient treatment response. Other medications with demonstrated off-label efficacy include desipramine, up to 300 mg/d[105]; imipramine, up to 300 mg/d[106]; and topiramate, titrated from 25 mg/d up to 250 mg/d or 400 mg/d.[107,108] However, the potential risks of these medications should be carefully considered, particularly for individuals with history of malnutrition, electrolyte imbalance, or cardiac concerns.

Long-Term Biological Management of BN

It is recommended that any pharmacotherapy be combined with cognitive-behavioral therapy (CBT), as described later.[108-111] Individuals with a co-occurring SUD who prefer not to take prescription medication should be referred directly for CBT. Among those who are willing to take medications, pharmacotherapy for co-occurring psychiatric conditions should also be considered. Given the detrimental effects of digestive juices on tooth enamel and oral health, a dental exam is recommended for patients with BN who engage in purging through vomiting,[110] as well as those with the binge-purge subtype of AN.

Biological Management of BED

Lisdexamfetamine dimesylate became the first medication to be approved by the FDA for the treatment of BED in adults[112]; however, the medication has significant addiction potential and is therefore not recommended as a first-line treatment for individuals with history of SUD. Psychostimulant medications, in general, may be most useful for treatment of BED with co-occurring attention deficit/hyperactivity disorder (ADHD) among individuals with no history of SUD. However, even among this group, there are risks and benefits of psychostimulant medications to consider, including diversion, nonmedical use and stimulant use disorder/addiction, cardiovascular side effects, and unintended weight loss.[113] Several SSRIs (eg, sertraline, 50-200 mg/d; fluvoxamine, 50-300 mg/d; fluoxetine, 20-80 mg/d; and citalopram, 20-60 mg/d) have also demonstrated efficacy in the treatment of BED.[114-116] In addition, topiramate (50-600 mg/d) has utility in decreasing the number of binge eating episodes per week, decreasing BMI, and shortening the time to recovery.[117] Sibutramine 15 mg/d has shown promise in reducing binge episodes and promoting weight loss.[118] Pharmacological treatment of co-occurring psychiatric conditions in BED patients may also be warranted. Further, given that overweight and obesity may be consequences of BED, additional medical management may be necessary to prevent or treat associated conditions (eg, hypertension, type II diabetes, hypercholesterolemia, hyperlipidemia). Recent proof-of-concept studies demonstrated positive preliminary results for transcranial direct current stimulation (tDCS) as a potential nonpharmacological biological treatment for BED[119] and AN.[120] More research will be needed to assess safety and efficacy of this treatment option.

Acute Biological Management of Obesity

Treating obesity is both difficult and complex because of the short and long feedback loops and the importance of eating to survive.[121] Biological management of obesity is generally considered a three-tiered approach that begins with changes in diet and increased exercise. If additional assistance is needed, medications can be added, or devices/surgery can be considered. When patients display morbid obesity, particularly with additional risk factors such as hypertension and type II diabetes, Roux-en-Y gastric bypass surgery or lap-band surgery may be performed. These surgeries result in sustained weight loss with decreased prevalence of health conditions (eg, type II diabetes) related to obesity.[122-124] Unfortunately, though these surgeries can be lifesaving for many patients, they are associated with risk of rehospitalization (eg, due to ventral hernia repair and gastric revision)[125] and early mortality, particularly in elderly patients.[126] Bariatric surgery should not be considered without a full psychiatric evaluation, including an SUD assessment, as co-occurring psychiatric and substance use disorders are common among bariatric surgery candidates[127] and can affect the success of surgery. Clinical evidence suggests that individuals who undergo bariatric surgery may be at increased risk of developing a SUD postoperatively, and patients with a history of SUDs may be particularly at risk, as alcohol absorption and metabolism change considerably.[128,129] Medical devices approved by the FDA include the Maestro Rechargeable electrical stimulation system,[130] and the ReShape Integrated Dual Balloon System and ORBERA Intragastric Balloon System, which are considered short-term treatments that should be removed after 6 months.[131] Finally, the AspireAssist device helps to control calorie absorption through surgical placement of a drainage tube designed to decrease stomach contents after feedings.[132] Due to side effects and known risks of the surgical placement procedure, this device is recommended only for obese patients who have failed to manage their weight with nonsurgical methods.

Subacute Biological Management of Obesity

If surgery is not yet indicated, antiobesity medication may be utilized. Glucose lowering medications, particularly glucagon-like peptide 1 (GLP-1) receptor agonists (GLP-1RAs), have provided new hope and options for treatment of obesity with or without diabetes. In 2014, liraglutide was the first GLP-1 agonist to be FDA-approved for weight management in obese patients without diabetes. However, it comes with a warning regarding risk of thyroid cancer and requires close monitoring by a physician.[133] In 2021, the GLP-1 agonist semaglutide was also approved for this indication, based on consistent favorable clinical outcomes.[134-137] It is indicated in patients with a body mass index (BMI) equal to or more than 30 kg/m^2, or a BMI equal to or more than 27 kg/m^2 with comorbidities. Prior to these new treatments, weight loss medication effects were inconsistent or short-lived. Two of the FDA-approved obesity medications (phentermine and diethylpropion) are appetite suppressants for short-term (ie, less than a year) use only. A third medication is orlistat, a fat absorption inhibitor.

Other approved medications or medication combinations appear to support the "food addiction" hypothesis,[23] and also suggest an important role for addiction theory in treatment of obesity. One combines the FDA-approved medications bupropion SR and naltrexone SR.[138] Another medication combining the drugs phentermine (an appetite suppressant) and topiramate XR (an anticonvulsant with weight loss side effects) has demonstrated efficacy in promoting weight loss,[139] but the FDA recommends monitoring patients for cardiovascular risk, with an indication against use by pregnant women.[140]

Long-Term Biological Management of Obesity

Lifestyle changes, including improved diet and increased exercise, are recommended for long-term management of obesity, including for patients who take anti-obesity medication or undergo bariatric surgery.

PSYCHOLOGICAL MANAGEMENT

Acute Psychological Management

Many of the same issues arise during therapy for both SUDs and eating disorders. Thus, participation in SUD treatment may provide a strong foundation from which to work toward management of disordered eating symptoms. For example, learning better ways to communicate with family and handle conflict may reduce the need for maladaptive coping through both substance use and disordered eating. Practicing these strategies during SUD treatment may give the patient confidence to implement similar strategies in order to manage eating disorder symptoms. For example, establishing a daily routine, self-monitoring using a food journal, developing structured meal times, ensuring the availability of nutritious and "safe" foods, and limiting exposure to triggers for bingeing or purging can be effective ways to promote recovery from an eating disorder.

For patients with AN, both family therapy and individual therapy have demonstrated efficacy, though family therapy may be particularly beneficial for younger patients.[141] Cognitive-behavioral therapy (CBT) has consistently been shown to reduce the risk for recurrence of disease and improve outcome for patients with AN.[94,142,143] Again, many of the skills developed during CBT for SUD can be easily transferred to eating disorder treatment (eg, challenging dysfunctional cognitions, behavioral experiments). Management of BN is generally enhanced by combining pharmacotherapy with CBT, though CBT is currently recommended as the first-line treatment for BN, given its demonstrated efficacy in multiple trials.[144] CBT can be administered either individually or in a group setting and is generally included as part of both residential and outpatient treatment programs. Among patients with BED without co-occurring SUDs, psychotherapy appears to be most successful when administered as either individual or group CBT,[95] though interpersonal psychotherapy has also demonstrated efficacy.[145] With regard to obesity symptoms, behavioral weight loss strategies have demonstrated positive outcomes in the short term, particularly for weight loss[146]; however, CBT appears to be a superior treatment for the symptoms of BED over time.[147] Again, when the eating disorder patient has a co-occurring SUD, it is important to continue monitoring the patient closely in order to be vigilant for signs of recurrence of substance use or SUD. Therapy should focus on developing new adaptive coping skills to replace the SUD and eating disorder symptoms.

Subacute Psychological Management

Social support can be beneficial to individuals as they undergo treatment and recovery. As in SUD treatment, group therapy may be an appropriate and useful component of treatment in which patients learn they are not alone in their struggles with disordered eating, share their challenges and successes, and learn from one another's experiences. However, for individuals admitted to treatment involuntarily (and particularly those with AN), group therapy may be contraindicated. In some cases, this may lead to competition among the patients to be the "thinnest" in the group or sharing of maladaptive strategies to continue losing weight.

Eating disorders occur frequently within close-knit groups (eg, "cliques" of friends, sports teams, sororities), particularly among adolescent females and young adults.[148] Socially valued behaviors (eg, food restriction) often increase with social proximity, whereas nonvalued behaviors (eg, binge eating, purging) decrease.[149] However, levels of binge eating appear to grow more similar among females as their friendship grows closer.[150] As a result, large-scale prevention and intervention programs are important and can be effective in managing the incidence and prevalence of AN, BN, and BED.[151,152]

Long-Term Psychological Management

Among motivated individuals, and particularly those who have participated successfully in Alcoholics Anonymous (AA) or Narcotics Anonymous (NA), referral to a 12-step program for eating disorders may be beneficial. Eating Disorders Anonymous (EDA) follows many of the tenets of AA (eg, 12 steps and 12 traditions), but—given that food is necessary for survival—it focuses on "balance" rather than "abstinence" as the goal. Eating disorder symptoms (eg, restricting, bingeing, purging) are viewed as ways of coping with stress, so the program focuses more on developing alternate adaptive coping strategies rather than focusing on eating habits per se. EDA participants are encouraged to work with a sponsor or "buddy" on their path to recovery. Similarly, Overeaters Anonymous (OA) is a 12-step fellowship program following in the tradition of AA. OA meetings focus primarily on the needs of individuals with compulsive eating or binge eating symptoms. It may be particularly useful for individuals who appear to suffer from "food addiction." OA participants view overeating as similar to a SUD and work toward the goal of abstaining from overeating.

RECOVERY ISSUES

Co-Occurring Substance Use Disorders

Co-occurring SUDs and eating disorders may negatively affect SUD treatment prognosis,[153] and many publicly-funded SUD treatment programs are not able to admit/treat patients with co-occurring eating disorders.[154] In fact, eating disorder symptoms may serve as a coping mechanism for some patients with SUDs. When a SUD is co-occurring with AN, it is generally suggested that treatment occur in a residential treatment facility where both issues can be addressed.[155] Recovery rates for AN with co-occurring SUDs, especially involving alcohol, are generally poor. This combination is a strong predictor of fatal outcome.[156] Patients with BN plus a co-occurring SUD have treatment outcomes similar to those without a history of SUD,[10] though SUD patients with bingeing symptoms may have a worse outcome than those without bingeing.[157] Individuals who suffer from BED with a co-occurring SUD generally show outcomes similar to those without a SUD.[49]

General Recovery Rates

Research has demonstrated recovery rates for eating disorders to be between about 40% and 94%, with better recovery rates and outcome for BN than for AN.[158,159] BN generally is not fatal, whereas the mortality rate for those with AN is about 10%.[1] Among BED patients, there is some evidence that the disorder will spontaneously remit over time,[160] though other research has suggested a more chronic nature, particularly among patients who are older, more obese, and meet full diagnostic criteria.[161] As is seen among individuals recovering from SUDs, the vacillation between dieting (ie, "abstinence") and overeating (ie, "active use") is common among individuals struggling with obesity or BED.[162]

Disordered Eating After Substance Use Disorder Treatment

After SUD treatment, some individuals who are abstaining from drug or alcohol use may compensate for this lack of chemical reinforcement by overeating. Preliminary research has demonstrated significant weight gain among a group of adolescents who completed treatment and maintained abstinence from addictive substances.[54] In addition, one study has documented the significant rates of past SUDs among extremely obese individuals considering bariatric surgery. Kalarchian et al.[163] reported that one-third of these individuals were in recovery from a SUD, whereas fewer than 2% had a current diagnosis. Though information was not available regarding their weight at the time of active SUD, clinical experience suggests that many of these individuals became obese after treatment for their SUDs. In addition, the presence of an eating disorder is associated with increased risk for return to substance use. Individuals who are attempting to manage their disordered eating symptoms may turn to drugs or alcohol as an alternate coping strategy. As a result, the addiction clinician should be vigilant to symptoms of overeating or disordered eating among SUD patients and should provide all patients with preventative counseling and referral to a registered dietitian.

AREAS FOR FURTHER STUDY

As research data accumulate demonstrating similarities among the various eating disorders and SUDs, the addiction clinician will likely need to gain further experience with the identification and treatment of these serious diseases. Regardless of which condition precedes the other, SUDs contribute to the high mortality rates observed in patients with eating disorders.[164] More research is needed to further explore and evaluate the subtypes of disordered eating and to determine whether "food addiction" is an independent diagnostic entity that is predictive of treatment outcome.[165] Future work might focus on the development of brief screening devices (eg, a "CAGE"-type questionnaire for eating disorders) as well as alternate treatment strategies built on the principles developed within the field of addiction medicine. For example, eating disorder treatments may increasingly capitalize on methods such as contingency management, pharmacotherapies, and long-term residential care for eating disorders and obesity. Addiction clinicians and eating disorder specialists would likely benefit from opportunities to network and share methods and ideas in order to maximize care for these commonly co-occurring disorders.

SUMMARY

Eating disorders (especially AN, BN, and BED) are serious conditions that necessitate timely detection and intervention. These disorders have both psychological and medical consequences that can be life threatening. Co-occurring SUDs are common, and it is recommended that all individuals undergoing treatment for a SUD be screened for disordered eating behaviors and vice versa. When present, serious disordered eating symptoms may complicate treatment for SUDs. Individuals with eating disorders should be medically stabilized before beginning SUD treatment, though treatments for both disorders are frequently complementary.

REFERENCES

1. American Psychiatric Association. *Diagnostic and Statistical Manual of Mental Disorders*. 5th ed. American Psychiatric Association; 2013.
2. Devoe DJ, Dimitropoulos G, Anderson A, et al. The prevalence of substance use disorders and substance use in anorexia nervosa: a systematic review and meta-analysis. *J Eat Disord*. 2021;9(1):161.
3. Munn-Chernoff MA, Johnson EC, Chou YL, et al. Shared genetic risk between eating disorder- and substance-use-related phenotypes: evidence from genome-wide association studies. *Addict Biol*. 2021;26(1):e12880.
4. Ayton A, Ibrahim A, Dugan J, Galvin E, Wright OW. Ultra-processed foods and binge eating: a retrospective observational study. *Nutrition*. 2021;84:111023.
5. Couturier J, Lock J. Denial and minimization in adolescents with anorexia nervosa. *Int J Eat Disord*. 2006;39:212-216.
6. Katzman DK. Medical complications in adolescents with anorexia nervosa: a review of the literature. *Int J Eat Disord*. 2005;37 (Suppl):S52-S59.
7. Miller KK, Grinspoon SK, Ciampa J, Hier J, Herzog D, Klibanski A. Medical findings in outpatients with anorexia nervosa. *Arch Intern Med*. 2005;165:561-566.
8. Cartwright MM. Eating disorder emergencies: understanding the medical complexities of the hospitalized eating disordered patient. *Crit Care Nurs Clin North Am*. 2004;16:515-530.
9. Eddy KT, Keek PK, Dorer DJ, Delinsky SS, Franko DL, Herzog DB. Longitudinal comparison of anorexia nervosa subtypes. *Int J Eat Disord*. 2002;31:191-201.
10. Franko DL, Dorer DJ, Keel PK, Jackson S, Manzo MP, Herzog DB. How do eating disorders and alcohol use disorder influence each other? *Int J Eat Disord*. 2005;38:200-207.
11. Franko DL, Keel PK. Suicidality in eating disorders: occurrence, correlates, and clinical implications. *Clin Psychol Rev*. 2006;26:769-782.
12. Rytomaa I, Jarvinen V, Kanerva R, Heinonen OP. Bulimia and tooth erosion. *Acta Odontol Scand*. 1998;56:36-40.
13. Mehler PS, Crews C, Weiner K. Bulimia: medical complications. *J Womens Health*. 2004;13:668-675.
14. Gruzca RA, Przybeck TR, Cloninger CR. Prevalence and correlates of binge eating disorder in a community sample. *Compr Psychiatry*. 2007;48:124-131.
15. Pagoto S, Bodenlos JS, Kantor L, Gitkind M, Curtin C, Ma Y. Association of major depression and binge eating disorder with weight loss in a clinical setting. *Obesity*. 2007;15:2557-2559.
16. Bulik CM, Reichborn-Kjennerud T. Medical morbidity in binge eating disorder. *Int J Eat Disord*. 2003;34:S39-S46.
17. Raman RP. Obesity and health risks. *J Am Coll Nutr*. 2002;21:S134-S139.
18. Pi-Sunyer FX. The medical risks of obesity. *Obes Surg*. 2002;12:S6-S11.
19. Gearhardt AN, Corbin WR, Brownell KD. Food addiction: an examination of the diagnostic criteria for dependence. *J Addict Med*. 2009;3:1-7.
20. American Psychiatric Association. *Diagnostic and Statistical Manual of Mental Disorders*. 4th ed. American Psychiatric Association; 2000.
21. Avena NM, Gold JA, Kroll C, Gold MS. Further developments in the neurobiology of food and addiction: update on the state of the science. *Nutrition*. 2012;28:341-343.
22. Brown RM, Kupchik YM, Spencer S, et al. Addiction-like synaptic impairments in diet-induced obesity. *Biol Psychiatry*. 2017;81:797-806.
23. Blumenthal DM, Gold MS. Neurobiology of food addiction. *Curr Opin Clin Nutri Metab Care*. 2010;13:359-365.
24. Gearhardt AN, Schulte EM. Is food addictive? A review of the science. *Ann Rev Nutrition*. 2021;41:387-410.
25. Gearhardt AN, Yokum S, Orr PT, Stice E, Corbin WR, Brownell KD. Neural correlates of food addiction. *Arch Gen Psychiatry*. 2011;68:808-816.
26. Ravichandran S, Bhatt RR, Pandit B, et al. Alterations in reward network functional connectivity are associated with increased food addiction in obese individuals. *Sci Rep*. 2021;11:3386.
27. Contreras-Rodríguez O, Martín-Pérez C, Vilar-López R, Verdejo-Garcia A. Ventral and dorsal striatum networks in obesity: link to food craving and weight gain. *Biol Psychiatry*. 2017;81:789-796.
28. Tran H, Poinsot P, Guillaume S, et al. Food addiction as a proxy for anorexia nervosa severity: new data based on the Yale Food Addiction Scale 2.0. *Psychiatry Res*. 2020;293:113472.
29. Cassin SE, von Ranson KM. Is binge eating experienced as an addiction? *Appetite*. 2007;49:687-690.
30. Gearhardt AN, White MA, Masheb RM, Morgan PT, Crosby RD, Grilo CM. An examination of the food addiction construct in obese patients with binge eating disorder. *Int J Eat Disord*. 2012;45:657-663.
31. Davis C, Curtis C, Levitan RD, Carter JC, Kaplan AS, Kennedy JL. Evidence that "food addiction" is a valid phenotype of obesity. *Appetite*. 2011;57:711-717.

32. Hudson JI, Hiripi E, Pope HG Jr, Kessler RC. The prevalence and correlates of eating disorders in the National Comorbidity Survey Replication. *Biol Psychiatry.* 2007;61:348-358.
33. Bulik CM, Sullivan PF, Tozzi F, Furberg H, Lichtenstein P, Pedersen NL. Prevalence, heritability, and prospective risk factors for anorexia nervosa. *Arch Gen Psychiatry.* 2006;63:305-312.
34. Wade TD, Bergin JL, Tiggemann M, Bulik CM, Fairburn CG. Prevalence and long-term course of lifetime eating disorders in an adult Australian twin cohort. *Aust N Z J Psychiatry.* 2006;40:121-128.
35. Ackard DM, Fulkerson JA, Neumark-Sztanier D. Prevalence and utility of DSM-IV eating disorder diagnostic criteria among youth. *Int J Eat Disord.* 2007;40:409-417.
36. Walsh JM, Wheat ME, Freund K. Detection, evaluation, and treatment of eating disorders: the role of the primary care physician. *J Gen Intern Med.* 2000;15:577-590.
37. Spurrell EB, Wilfley DE, Tanofsky MB, Brownell KD. Age of onset for binge eating: are there different pathways to binge eating? *Int J Eat Disord.* 1997;21:55-65.
38. Ogden CL, Carroll MD, Fryar CD, et al. *Prevalence of Obesity Among Adults and Youth: United States 2011–2014.* NCHS Data Brief, No. 219. National Center for Health Statistics; 2015.
39. Yekaninejad MS, Badrooj N, Vosoughi F, Lin C-Y, Potenza MN, Pakpour AH. Prevalence of food addiction in children and adolescents: a systematic review and meta-analysis. *Obes Reviews.* 2021;22(6):e13183.
40. Praxedes DR, Silva-Júnior AE, Macena ML, et al. Prevalence of food addiction determined by the Yale Food Addiction Scale and associated factors: a systematic review with meta-analysis. *Eur Eat Dis Rev* 2022;30(2):85-95.
41. Hübel C, Abdulkadir M, Herle M, et al. One size does not fit all. Genomics differentiates among anorexia nervosa, bulimia nervosa, and binge-eating disorder. *Int J Eat Disord.* 2021;54(5):785-793.
42. Bulik CM, Thornton LM, Parker R, et al. The Eating Disorders Genetics Initiative (EDGI): study protocol. *BMC Psychiatry.* 2021;21(1):234. doi:10.1186/s12888-021-03212-3
43. Bulik CM, Carroll IM, Mehler P. Reframing anorexia nervosa as a metabo-psychiatric disorder. *Trends Endocrinol Metab.* 2021;32(10): 752-761. doi:10.1016/j.tem.2021.07.010
44. Hasin D, Sarnet S, Nunes E, Meydan J, Matseoane K, Waxman R. Diagnosis of comorbid psychiatric disorders in substance users assessed with the psychiatric research interview for substance and mental disorders for DSM-IV. *Am J Psychiatry.* 2006;163:689-696.
45. Castel S, Rush B, Urbanoski K, Toneatto T. Overlap of clusters of psychiatric symptoms among clients of a comprehensive addiction treatment service. *Psychol Addict Behav.* 2006;20:28-35.
46. Castro-Fornieles J, Díaz R, Goti J, et al. Prevalence and factors related to substance use among adolescents with eating disorders. *Eur Addict Res.* 2010;16(2):61-68.
47. Piran N, Robinson SR. Associations between disordered eating behaviors and licit and illicit substance use and abuse in a university sample. *Addict Behav.* 2006;31:1761-1775.
48. Conason AH, Sher L. Alcohol use in adolescents with eating disorders. *Int J Adolesc Med Health.* 2006;18:31-36.
49. Wilfley DE, Friedman MA, Dounchis JZ, Stein RI, Welch RR, Ball SA. Comorbid psychopathology in binge eating disorder: relation to eating disorder severity at baseline and following treatment. *J Consult Clin Psychol.* 2000;68:641-649.
50. Stewart S, Brown CG, Devoulyte K, Theakston J, Larsen SE. Why do women with alcohol problems binge eat? Exploring connections between binge eating and heavy drinking in women receiving treatment for alcohol problems. *J Health Psychol.* 2006;11:409-425.
51. Steffen KJ, Engel SG, Wonderlich JA, Pollert GA, Sondag C. Alcohol and other addictive disorders following bariatric surgery: prevalence, risk factors and possible etiologies. *Eur Eat Disord Rev.* 2015;23(6):442-450.
52. Avena NM, Carrillo CA, Needham L, Leibowitz SF, Hoebel BG. Sugar-dependent rats show enhanced intake of unsweetened ethanol. *Alcohol.* 2004;34:203-209.
53. Edge PJ, Gold MS. Drug withdrawal and hyperphagia: lessons from tobacco and other drugs. *Curr Pharm Des.* 2011;17:1173-1179.
54. Hodgkins CC, Jacobs WS, Gold MS. Weight gain after adolescent drug addiction treatment and supervised abstinence. *Psychiatr Ann.* 2003;33:112-116.
55. Neale J, Nettleton S, Pickering L, Fischer J. Eating patterns among heroin users: a qualitative study with implications for nutritional interventions. *Addiction.* 2012;107:635-641.
56. Kleiner KD, Gold MS, Frost-Pineda K, Lenz-Brunsman B, Perri MG, Jacobs WS. Body mass index and alcohol use. *J Addict Dis.* 2004;23:105-118.
57. Warren M, Frost-Pineda K, Gold MS. Body mass index and marijuana use. *J Addict Dis.* 2005;24:95-100.
58. Blinder BJ, Cumella EJ, Sanathara VA. Psychiatric comorbidities of female inpatients with eating disorders. *Psychosom Med.* 2006;68:454-462.
59. Piran N, Robinson S. The association between disordered eating and substance use and abuse in women: a community-based investigation. *Women Health.* 2006;44:1-20.
60. Teter CJ, McCabe SE, LaGrange K, Cranford JA, Boyd CJ. Illicit use of specific prescription stimulants among college students: prevalence, motives, and routes of administration. *Pharmacotherapy.* 2006;26:1501-1510.
61. Stock SL, Goldberg E, Corbett S, Katzman DK. Substance use in female adolescents with eating disorders. *J Adolesc Health.* 2002; 31:176-182.
62. Pomerleau CS, Zucker AN, Stewart AJ. Characterizing concerns about postcessation weight gain: results from a national survey of women smokers. *Nicotine Tob Res.* 2001;3:51-60.
63. Mehler PS. Diagnosis and care of patients with anorexia nervosa in primary care settings. *Ann Intern Med.* 2001;134:1048-1059.
64. Kaye WH, Bulik CM, Thornton L, Barbarich N, Masters K. Comorbidity of anxiety disorders with anorexia nervosa and bulimia nervosa. *Am J Psychiatry.* 2004;161:2215-2221.
65. Milos G, Spindler A, Ruggiero G, Klaghofer R, Schnyder U. Comorbidity of obsessive-compulsive disorders and duration of eating disorders. *Int J Eat Disord.* 2002;31:284-289.
66. Milos G, Spindler A, Schnyder U. Psychiatric comorbidity and Eating Disorder Inventory (EDI) profiles in eating disorder patients. *Can J Psychiatry.* 2004;49:179-184.
67. Westen D, Harnden-Fischer J. Personality profiles in eating disorders: rethinking the distinction between axis I and axis II. *Am J Psychiatry.* 2001;158:547-562.
68. Telch CF, Stice E. Psychiatric comorbidity in women with binge eating disorder prevalence rates from a non-treatment seeking sample. *J Consult Clin Psychol.* 1998;66:768-776.
69. Kasen S, Cohen P, Chen H, Must A. Obesity and psychopathology in women: a three decade prospective study. *Int J Obes (Lond).* 2007;32:558-566.
70. Currin L, Schmidt U, Treasure J, Jick H. Time trends in eating disorder incidence. *Br J Psychiatry.* 2005;186:132-135.
71. Turnbull S, Ward A, Treasure J, Hick J, Derby L. The demand for eating disorder care: an epidemiological study using the general practice research database. *Br J Psychiatry.* 1996;169:705-712.
72. Rodin G, Craven J, Littlefield C, Murray M, Daneman D. Eating disorders and intentional insulin undertreatment in adolescent females with diabetes. *Psychosomatics.* 1991;32:171-176.
73. Bruce B, Agras WS. Binge eating in females: a population-based investigation. *Int J Eat Disord.* 1992;12:365-373.
74. Bruce B, Wilfley DE. Binge eating among the overweight population: a serious and prevalent problem. *J Am Diet Assoc.* 1996;96:58-61.
75. Hudson J, Lalonde JK, Berry JM, et al. Binge-eating disorder as a distinct familial phenotype in obese individuals. *Arch Gen Psychiatry.* 2006;63:313-319.
76. Beals KA, Manore MM. Disorders of the female athlete triad among collegiate athletes. *Int J Sport Nutr Exerc Metab.* 2002;12:281-293.
77. Reinking MF, Alexander LE. Prevalence of disordered-eating behaviors in undergraduate female collegiate athletes and nonathletes. *J Athl Train.* 2005;40:47-51.

78. Kreipe RE, Birndorf SA. Eating disorders in adolescents and young adults. *Med Clin North Am.* 2000;84:1027-1049.
79. Pritts SD, Susman J. Diagnosis of eating disorders in primary care. *Am Fam Physician.* 2003;67:297-304.
80. Strote J, Lee JE, Wechsler H. Increasing MDMA use among college students: results of a national survey. *J Adolesc Health.* 2002;30:64-72.
81. Garner DM. Eating disorder inventory-3. Professional Manual. Lutz, FL: Psychological Assessment Resources. *Int J Eat Dis.* 2004;35(4):478-479.
82. Stice E, Telch CF, Rizvi SL. Development and validation of the Eating Disorder Diagnostic Scale: a brief self-report measure of anorexia, bulimia, and binge eating disorder. *Psychol Assess.* 2000;12:123-131.
83. Fairburn CG, Beglin SJ. Assessment of eating disorders: interview or self-report questionnaire? *Int J Eat Disord.* 1994;16:363-370.
84. Thelen MH, Farmer J, Wonderlich S, et al. A revision of the Bulimia Test: the BULIT-R. *Psychol Assess.* 1991;3:119-124.
85. Gormally J, Black S, Daston S, Rardin D. The assessment of binge eating severity among obese persons. *Addict Behav.* 1982;7:47-55.
86. O'Reardon JP, Stunkard AJ, Allison KC. Clinical trial of sertraline in the treatment of night eating syndrome. *Int J Eat Disord.* 2004;35:16-26.
87. Gearhardt AN, Corbin WR, Brownell KD. Development of the Yale Food Addiction Scale Version 2.0. *Psychol Addict Behav.* 2016; 30(1):113-121.
88. Yao S, Kuja-Halkola R, Thornton LM, et al. Familial liability for eating disorders and suicide attempts: evidence from a population registry in Sweden. *JAMA Psychiatry.* 2016;73(3):284-291.
89. Dunn EC, Neighbors C, Larimer ME. Motivational enhancement therapy and self-help treatment for binge eaters. *Psychol Addict Behav.* 2006;20:44-52.
90. Macdonald P, Hibbs R, Corfield F, Treasure J. The use of motivational interviewing in eating disorders: a systematic review. *Psychiatry Res.* 2012;200(1):1-11.
91. Costa MB, Melnik T. Effectiveness of psychosocial interventions in eating disorders: an overview of Cochrane systematic reviews. *Einstein (Sao Paulo).* 2016;14(2):235-277.
92. American Psychiatric Association. Practice guidelines for the treatment of patients with eating disorders revisions. *Am J Psychiatry.* 2000;157:1-39.
93. American Dietetic Association. Position of the American Dietetic Association: nutrition intervention in the treatment of anorexia nervosa, bulimia nervosa, and other eating disorders. *J Am Diet Assoc.* 2006;106:2073-2082.
94. LeGrange D. The Maudsley family-based treatment for adolescent anorexia nervosa. *World Psychiatry.* 2005;4:142-146.
95. Bulik CM, Berkman ND, Brownley KA, Sedway JA, Lohr KN. Anorexia nervosa treatment: a systematic review of randomized controlled trials. *Int J Eat Disord.* 2007;40:310-320.
96. Wilson GT. Psychological treatment of eating disorders. *Annu Rev Clin Psychol.* 2005;1:439-465.
97. Tiller J, Schmidt U, Treasure J. Compulsory treatment for anorexia nervosa: compassion or coercion? *Br J Psychiatry.* 1993;162:649-680.
98. Robb AS, Silber TJ, Orrell-Valente JK, et al. Supplemental nocturnal nasogastric refeeding for better short-term outcome in hospitalized adolescent girls with anorexia nervosa. *Am J Psychiatry.* 2002;159:1347-1353.
99. Becker AE. Outpatient management of eating disorders in adults. *Curr Womens Health Rep.* 2003;3:221-229.
100. Santonastaso P, Friederici S, Favaro A. Sertraline in the treatment of restricting anorexia nervosa: an open controlled trial. *J Child Adolesc Psychopharmacol.* 2001;11:143-150.
101. Fassino S, Leombruni P, Daga G, et al. Efficacy of citalopram in anorexia nervosa: a pilot study. *Eur Neuropsychopharmacol.* 2002;12:453-459.
102. Berger MM, Shenkin A. Vitamins and trace elements: practical aspects of supplementation. *Nutrition.* 2006;22:952-955.
103. Klibanski A, Biller BMK, Schoenfield DA, Herzog DB, Saxe VC. The effects of estrogen administration on trabecular bone loss in young women with anorexia nervosa. *J Clin Endocrinol Metab.* 1995;80:898-904.
104. Berkman ND, Bulik CM, Brownley KA, et al. Management of eating disorders. *Evid Rep Technol Assess (Full Rep).* 2006;135:1-166.
105. Walsh BT, Wilson GT, Loeb KL, et al. Medication and psychotherapy in the treatment of bulimia nervosa. *Am J Psychiatry.* 1997;154: 523-531.
106. Agras WS, Rossiter EM, Arnow B, et al. Pharmacologic and cognitive behavioral treatment for bulimia nervosa: a controlled comparison. *Am J Psychiatry.* 1992;149:82-87.
107. Nickel C, Tritt K, Muehlbacher M, et al. Topiramate treatment in bulimia nervosa patients: a randomized, double-blind, placebo-controlled trial. *Int J Eat Disord.* 2005;38:295-300.
108. Hoopes SP, Reimherr FW, Hedges DW, et al. Treatment of bulimia nervosa with topiramate in a randomized, double-blind, placebo-controlled trial, part 1: improvement in binge and purge measures. *J Clin Psychiatry.* 2003;64:1335-1341.
109. Hay PJ, Backaltchuk J. Extracts from "clinical evidence": bulimia nervosa. *BMJ.* 2001;323:33-37.
110. Hay PJ. Understanding bulimia. *Aust Fam Physician.* 2007;36:708-712.
111. Ramoz N, Versini A, Gorwood P. Eating disorders: an overview of treatment responses and the potential impact of vulnerability genes and endophenotypes. *Expert Opin Pharmacother.* 2007;8:2049-2044.
112. U.S. Food and Drug Administration. *FDA Expands Uses of Vyvanse to Treat Binge-Eating Disorder.* January 30, 2015. Accessed December 1, 2016. http://www.fda.gov/NewsEvents/Newsroom/PressAnnouncements/ucm432543.htm
113. Keshen A, Bartel S, Frank GKW, et al. The potential role of stimulants in treating eating disorders. *Int J Eat Disord.* 2021;55(3):318-331. doi:10.1002/eat.23650
114. McElroy SL, Hudson JI, Malhotra S, Welge JA, Nelson EB, Keck PE Jr. Citalopram in the treatment of binge-eating disorder: a placebo-controlled trial. *J Clin Psychiatry.* 2003;64:807-813.
115. Arnold LM, McElroy SL, Hudson JI, Welge JA, Bennett AJ, Keck PE. A placebo-controlled, randomized trial of fluoxetine in the treatment of binge-eating disorder. *J Clin Psychiatry.* 2002;63:1028-1033.
116. McElroy SL, Casuto LS, Nelson EB, et al. Placebo-controlled trial of sertraline in the treatment of binge eating disorder. *Am J Psychiatry.* 2000;157:1004-1006.
117. McElroy SL, Hudson JI, Capece KB, et al. Topiramate for the treatment of binge-eating disorder associated with obesity: a placebo-controlled study. *Biol Psychiatry.* 2007;61:1039-1048.
118. Wilfley DE, Crow SJ, Hudson JI, et al. Efficacy of sibutramine for the treatment of binge eating disorder: a randomized multicenter placebo-controlled double-blind study. *Am J Psychiatry.* 2008;165:51-58.
119. Burgess EE, Sylvester MA, Morse KE, et al. Effects of transcranial direct current stimulation (tDCS) on binge-eating disorder. *Int J Eat Disord.* 2016;49(10):930-936.
120. Woodside DB, Dunlop K, Sathi C, Lam E, McDonald B, Downar J. A pilot trial of repetitive transcranial magnetic stimulation of the dorsomedial prefrontal cortex in anorexia nervosa: resting fMRI correlates of response. *J Eat Disord.* 2021;9(1):52. doi:10.1186/s40337-021-00411-x
121. Valentino MA, Lin JE, Waldman SA. Central and peripheral molecular targets for antiobesity pharmacotherapy. *Clin Pharmacol Ther.* 2010;87:652-662.
122. Ben-David K, Rossidis G. Bariatric Surgery: indications, safety and efficacy. *Curr Pharm Des.* 2011;17:1209-1217.
123. Mingrone G, Panunzi S, De Gaetano A, et al. Bariatric surgery versus conventional medical therapy for type 2 diabetes. *N Engl J Med.* 2012;366:1577-1585.
124. Schauer PR, Kashyap SR, Wolski K, et al. Bariatric surgery versus intensive medical therapy in obese patients with diabetes. *N Engl J Med.* 2012;366:1567-1576.
125. Birkmeyer NJ, Dimick JB, Share D, et al. Hospital complication rates with bariatric surgery in Michigan. *JAMA.* 2010;304:435-442.
126. Maciejewski ML, Livingston EH, Smith VA, et al. Survival among high-risk patients after bariatric surgery. *JAMA.* 2011;305:2419-2426.
127. Rosenberger PH, Henderson KE, Grilo CM. Psychiatric disorder comorbidity and association with eating disorders in bariatric surgery patients: a cross-sectional study using structured interview-based diagnosis. *J Clin Psychiatry.* 2006;67:1080-1085.

128. Maluenda F, Csendes A, De Aretxabala X, et al. Alcohol absorption modification after a laparoscopic sleeve gastrectomy due to obesity. *Obes Surg.* 2010;20:744-748.
129. Woodard GA, Downey J, Hernandez-Boussard T, Morton JM. Impaired alcohol metabolism after gastric bypass surgery: a case-crossover trial. *J Am Coll Surg.* 2011;212:209-214.
130. Hwang SS, Takata MC, Fujioka K. Update on bariatric surgical procedures and an introduction to the implantable weight loss device: the Maestro Rechargeable System. *Med Devices (Auckl).* 2016;9:291-299.
131. Gleysteen JJ. A history of intragastric balloons. *Surg Obes Relat Dis.* 2016;12(2):430-435.
132. U.S. Food and Drug Administration. *FDA Approves AspireAssist Obesity Device.* June 14, 2016. Accessed December 1, 2016. http://www.fda.gov/NewsEvents/Newsroom/PressAnnouncements/ucm506625.htm
133. U.S. Food and Drug Administration. *FDA Approves Weight Management Drug Saxenda.* December 23, 2014. Accessed December 6, 2016. http://www.fda.gov/NewsEvents/Newsroom/PressAnnouncements/ucm427913.htm
134. Wilding JPH, Batterham RL, Calanna S, et al. Once-weekly semaglutide in adults with overweight or obesity. *N Engl J Med.* 2021;384(11):989.
135. Wadden TA, Bailey TS, Billings LK, et al. Effect of subcutaneous semaglutide vs placebo as an adjunct to intensive behavioral therapy on body weight in adults with overweight or obesity: the STEP 3 randomized clinical trial. *JAMA.* 2021;325(14):1403-1413.
136. Rubino D, Abrahamsson N, Davies M, et al. Effect of continued weekly subcutaneous semaglutide vs placebo on weight loss maintenance in adults with overweight or obesity: the STEP 4 randomized clinical trial. *JAMA.* 2021;325(14):1414-1425.
137. Kushner RF, Calanna S, Davies M, et al. Semaglutide 2.4 mg for the treatment of obesity: key elements of the STEP Trials 1 to 5. *Obesity.* 2020;28:1050-1061.
138. Plodkowski RA, Nguyen Q, Sundaram U, Nguyen L, Chau DL, St JS. Bupropion and naltrexone: a review of their use individually and in combination for the treatment of obesity. *Expert Opin Pharmacother.* 2009;10:1069-1081.
139. Gadde KM, Allison DB, Ryan DH, et al. Effects of low-dose, controlled-release, phentermine plus topiramate combination on weight and associated comorbidities in overweight and obese adults (CONQUER): a randomised, placebo-controlled, phase 3 trial. *Lancet.* 2011;377:1341-1352.
140. Salazar S. Assessment and management of the obese adult female: a clinical update for providers. *J Midwifery Womens Health.* 2006;51:202-207.
141. Eisler I, Dare C, Russell GF, Szmukler G, le Grange D, Dodge E. Family and individual therapy in anorexia nervosa: a 5-year follow-up. *Arch Gen Psychiatry.* 1997;54:1025-1030.
142. McIntosh VV, Jordan J, Carter FA, et al. Three psychotherapies for anorexia nervosa: a randomized, controlled trial. *Am J Psychiatry.* 2005;162:741-747.
143. Pike KM, Walsh BT, Vitousek K, Wilson GT, Bauer J. Cognitive behavior therapy in the posthospitalization treatment of anorexia nervosa. *Am J Psychiatry.* 2003;160:2046-2049.
144. Lewandowski LM, Gebing TA, Anthony JL, O'Brien WH. Meta-analysis of cognitive behavioral treatment studies for bulimia. *Clin Psychol Rev.* 1997;17:703-718.
145. Wilfley DE, Welch RR, Stein RI, et al. A randomized comparison of group cognitive behavioral therapy and group interpersonal psychotherapy for the treatment of overweight individuals with binge eating disorder. *Arch Gen Psychiatry.* 2002;59:713-721.
146. Nauta H, Hospers H, Kok G, Jansen A. A comparison between a cognitive and a behavioral treatment for obese binge eaters and obese non-binge eaters. *Behav Ther.* 2000;31:441-461.
147. Nauta H, Hospers H, Jansen A. One-year follow-up effects of two obesity treatments on psychological well-being and weight. *Br J Health Psychol.* 2001;6:271-284.
148. Paxton SJ, Schutz HK, Wertheim EH, Muir SL. Friendship clique and peer influences on body image concerns, dietary restraint, extreme weight-loss behaviors, and binge eating in adolescent girls. *J Abnorm Psychol.* 1999;108:255-266.
149. Meyer C, Waller G. Social convergence of disturbed eating attitudes in young adult women. *J Nerv Ment Dis.* 2001;189:114-119.
150. Crandall CS. Social contagion of binge eating. *J Pers Soc Psychol.* 1988;55:588-598.
151. Becker CB, Smith LM, Ciao AC. Peer-facilitated eating disorder prevention: a randomized effectiveness trial of cognitive dissonance and media advocacy. *J Couns Psychol.* 2006;53:550-555.
152. Becker CB, Smith LM, Ciao AC. Reducing eating disorder risk factors in sorority members: a randomized trial. *Behav Ther.* 2005;36:245-253.
153. Bonfà F, Cabrini S, Avanzi M, Bettinardi O, Spotti R, Uber E. Treatment dropout in drug-addicted women: are eating disorders implicated? *Eat Weight Disord.* 2008;13:81-86.
154. Gordon SM, Johnson JA, Greenfield SF, Cohen L, Killeen T, Roman PM. Assessment and treatment of co-occurring eating disorders in publicly funded addiction treatment programs. *Psychiatr Serv.* 2008;59:1056-1059.
155. Woodside BD, Staab R. Management of psychiatric comorbidity in anorexia nervosa and bulimia nervosa. *CNS Drugs.* 2006;20:655-663.
156. Herzog DB, Greenwood DN, Dorer DJ, et al. Mortality in eating disorders: a descriptive study. *Int J Eat Disord.* 2000;28:20-26.
157. Cohen LR, Greenfield SF, Gordon S, et al. Survey of eating disorder symptoms among women in treatment for substance abuse. *Am J Addict.* 2010;19:245-251.
158. Couturier J, Lock J. What is recovery in adolescent anorexia nervosa? *Int J Eat Disord.* 2006;39:550-555.
159. Fichter MM, Quadflieg N. Twelve-year course and outcome of bulimia nervosa. *Psychol Med.* 2004;34:1395-1406.
160. Fairburn CG, Cooper Z, Doll HA, Norman P, O'Connor M. The natural course of bulimia nervosa and binge eating disorder in young women. *Arch Gen Psychiatry.* 2000;57:659-665.
161. Pope HG, Lalonde JK, Pindyck LJ, et al. Binge eating disorder: a stable syndrome. *Am J Psychiatry.* 2006;163:2181-2183.
162. Jeffery RW, Drewnowski A, Epstein LH, et al. Long-term maintenance of weight loss: current status. *Health Psychol.* 2000;19:5-16.
163. Kalarchian MA, Marcus MD, Levine MD, et al. Psychiatric disorders among bariatric surgery candidates: relationship to obesity and functional health status. *Am J Psychiatry.* 2007;164:328-334.
164. Mellentin AI, Mejldal A, Guala MM, et al. The impact of alcohol and other substance use disorders on mortality in patients with eating disorders: a nationwide register-based retrospective cohort study. *Am J Psychiatry.* 2022;179(1):46-57. doi:10.1176/appi.ajp.21030274
165. National Center on Addiction and Substance Abuse. *Understanding and Addressing Food Addiction: A Science-based Approach to Policy, Practice and Research.* National Center on Addiction and Substance Abuse; 2016. Accessed May 16, 2018. https://ce-classes.com/exam_format/5b57f674ca03e7e842461973da964fa3.pdf

SECTION

13

Pain and Addiction

Associate Editor: Shannon C. Miller
Lead Section Editor: Martin D. Cheatle
Section Editor: William C. Becker

CHAPTER

108 The Pathophysiology of Chronic Pain and Clinical Interfaces With Substance Use Disorder

Laura Morgan Frankart and Michael F. Weaver

CHAPTER OUTLINE

- Introduction
- Chronic pain
- Clinical interface between pain and substance use disorders
- Conclusions

INTRODUCTION

Chronic pain, our society's most common and most costly chronic illness[1] and globally the most burdensome illness[2] has the potential to change a person's life trajectory, sometimes catastrophically, when treated inadequately or unwisely. Patients with unrelieved pain, vulnerable to the promise of cure or relief and desperate to restore their lives but without access to evidence-based treatments or clinical teams with the appropriate expertise, may try unproven medical and nonmedical treatments. Opioid analgesics pose a particular dilemma. While they can provide important benefit particularly in acute and end-of-life pain, they can also strongly impact the reward systems in the brain that play a key role in the activation and perpetuation of substance use disorder (SUD). Thus, the two together—chronic pain and SUD—present a "perfect storm" of complexity and a challenge to clinicians, healthcare systems, and society at large. Patients, their families, their employers, their communities, and their healthcare providers share the burden of chronic pain and SUD. All of these groups have a role to play in improving the outcomes of chronic pain and the outcomes of SUD, particularly when they complicate each other.

For purposes of this chapter, we will not be considering cancer pain caused by malignant cells that damage tissues and the nervous system; rather, we will be referring to the cluster of noncancer conditions and diseases associated with persistent pain (eg, musculoskeletal conditions, neurological damage) that share common neuropathophysiological mechanisms, using the term chronic noncancer pain (CNCP). Similarly, we will not be focusing on occasional risky use of addictive substances, but rather drug using behaviors in patterns consistent with the diagnosis of SUD. Unraveling the biopsychosocial factors that perpetuate both of these chronic diseases and addressing these factors in an organized, prioritized, goal-oriented management plan challenge our understanding of behavioral neuroscience and our core competencies in the use of available medical and team-based therapies, our capacity for empathy, and our patience and perseverance.[3] This challenge extends to the optimization of our healthcare system so that it models a chronic disease approach to treatment and incentivizes outcomes instead of profit. The pathophysiology of CNCP and SUD do not alone account for their variable symptomatic and behavioral expression and psychosocial complexity. Neural and glial networks regulating pain perception and behavior interact with emotional regulation and reward systems influencing SUDs. Physiological responses in both are worthy of examination with the expectation that the coexistence of CNCP and SUD will lead to complex interactions, that is, SUD altered by pain and pain altered by SUD.

This chapter reviews the pathophysiology of CNCP and the theoretical and clinical phenomenology of its overlap with SUD. The mechanisms of pain perception and modulation in CNCP are reviewed, with discussion of those aspects likely to be impacted by the presence of SUD. In this regard, the role of central sensitization and kindling and affective responses including depression and anxiety in CNCP is discussed, particularly since these processes and comorbidities also play a role in the phenomenology and treatment of SUD. Finally, ideas about potential interactions between CNCP and SUD are suggested, focusing on how the general state of SUD, inherited characteristics of the individual, and neuroadaptations specific to opioid use patterns might affect the co-expression of these phenomena.

CHRONIC PAIN

In contrast to our ability to prevent, minimize, and manage acute pain, the management of CNCP often presents a daunting challenge. First, the physiology of pain after initial onset becomes much more complex almost immediately—the longer the pain, the more complex the process. The concept of "chronification" increasingly supplants the older, less useful, dimensional division between acute and chronic pain.[4] Pain is now more accurately described as a continuum of experience from the moment of its onset until its cessation, and that experience informs the next experience of pain, through the glial cellular and neuronal network memory systems.

Chronic **nociceptive** pain, such as from arthritis, involves processes that include *transduction/activation, transmission, modulation/augmentation*, and *perception*, whereas chronic **neuropathic** pain, caused by damage to neural tissue, is often independent of *transduction* and involves persistent *activation, transmission, modulation/augmentation,* and *perception.* These processes will be discussed below in more detail. In both types of persistent pain, a number of biopsychosocial factors can potentially influence neuroplastic changes in the central nervous system (CNS) that will, in turn, determine the salience of the pain for a person, the impact of pain on their life, and pain's resistance to treatments that focus on the nociceptive stimulus.[4,5] These factors include, but are not limited to, environmental context, meaning of pain, attention, mood and affect, anxiety, catastrophizing, and social and cognitive attention/reinforcement.

Although experiments using laboratory-induced nociception in animals can control for much genetic and experiential variability, this is not possible in humans suffering chronic or episodic pain. Every new episode or change in pain intensity, character, or localization activates neural and inflammatory mechanisms informed by prior nociceptive experience and cognitive-emotional processes influenced by current context and meaning conditioned by past experience. These processes involve inflammatory glial activating systems in the CNS interacting with neural networks subserved by a myriad of chemical messengers that communicate among sensory systems and various cognitive-emotional processing and behavioral systems.[6,7]

Pain is always an intensely personal and unique experience. However, pain experiences do cluster in specific, predictable patterns that can be diagnostically informative, for example, the pattern of pain can be nearly diagnostic in such conditions as lumbar radiculitis in S1 dermatome distribution (secondary to lumbar nerve root irritation or mechanical compression of the S1 nerve root), migraine, fibromyalgia, diabetic neuropathy, and postherpetic neuralgia. Clinicians caring for patients with CNCP face the challenge of formulating the plan of care for each patient, to the degree possible in any particular clinical setting, a plan of care that addresses the interaction of biopsychosocial factors and neurobehavioral processes that activate and perpetuate chronic pain. Then they must devise a feasible treatment plan that has the best chance of remediating the most salient factors to improve the longitudinal outcome.

Pain Anatomy and Physiology

Wall and Melzack's[8] postulation of the gate theory of pain provided the first pathophysiological model to coherently explain the phenomenology of pain perception and modulation observed clinically. Gate theory proposed that the final experience of pain was not fully shaped by nociceptive or tissue transduction processes, but that pain transmission (and ultimately perception) could be "gated" or modulated by other neurophysiological inputs. Factors such as psychological state and its physiological effects somehow affected the transmission of pain sensation and its experiential severity. Examples abound of the phenomenon of environmental conditions and psychological state altering pain experience following normally very painful nociceptive injury—such as injured athletes not experiencing pain during competition or wounded soldiers not experiencing pain during battle.

There are multiple targets for pain treatments. Some aim to reduce the stimulus itself—for example, weight loss to reduce weight-bearing stress on injured or diseased joints in the lower limbs or lower spine or postural and ergonomics training in musculoskeletal diseases leading to less "transduction" (activation of nociceptors). Others aim to block the stimulus from reaching the spinal cord (transmission), for example, peripheral nerve blocks, or aim to deactivate the transmission of the pain signal in the spinal cord rostrally to the brain (transmission), for example, neuromodulation. And others target CNS responses and pathological neuroplasticity—for example, neural reprogramming using cognitive–behavioral and psychomotor trainings to improve coping and reverse pathological neuroplastic changes.[9,10] In the hopes of positively affecting all of these processes, clinicians commonly combine treatments, each targeting different mechanisms.[3-5,11]

This additive, integrated approach improves pain control and outcomes as demonstrated by meta-analytic studies of comprehensive rehabilitation center populations.[12] Although scientific comparisons of a single proven treatment with combinations of two or more proven treatments are prohibitively expensive, multimodality treatment to improve functional outcomes, not just pain control, is relatively well established as the most effective and longest-lasting treatment for CNCP.

The neurobiological basis for Wall and Melzack's functional gating system, now better understood, provides a conceptual framework for understanding the clinical presentation of pain and helps explain the often complementary effects of different treatments for pain. **Figure 108-1** simplistically depicts the anatomy of the systems for pain perception and transmission. For convenience, the very complex phenomenology of pain can be characterized as three major "stages" involving different mechanisms depending on the nature and time course of the originating stimulus.[13] The stages are (1) nociception, the consequences of a brief noxious stimulus; (2) persistent and/or repeated nociception, the consequences of a prolonged or repetitive noxious stimulus leading to tissue damage and peripheral inflammation; and (3) the consequences of neurological damage, including peripheral neuropathies and peripheral and central sensitization. These stages are not mutually exclusive and overlap temporally and physiologically through the complex interaction among various brain regions and ascending and descending messages between the CNS and the body. Their end result is chronic pain perpetuated by one or more of several mechanisms: chronic inflammation or recurrent injury peripherally; ectopic excitability of peripheral pain neurons; excitation and priming of spinal microglial cells; structural reorganization (eg, neuroplasticity) of neural networks in the periphery and CNS so that touch, movement, temperature, and emotional changes cause and/or increase the

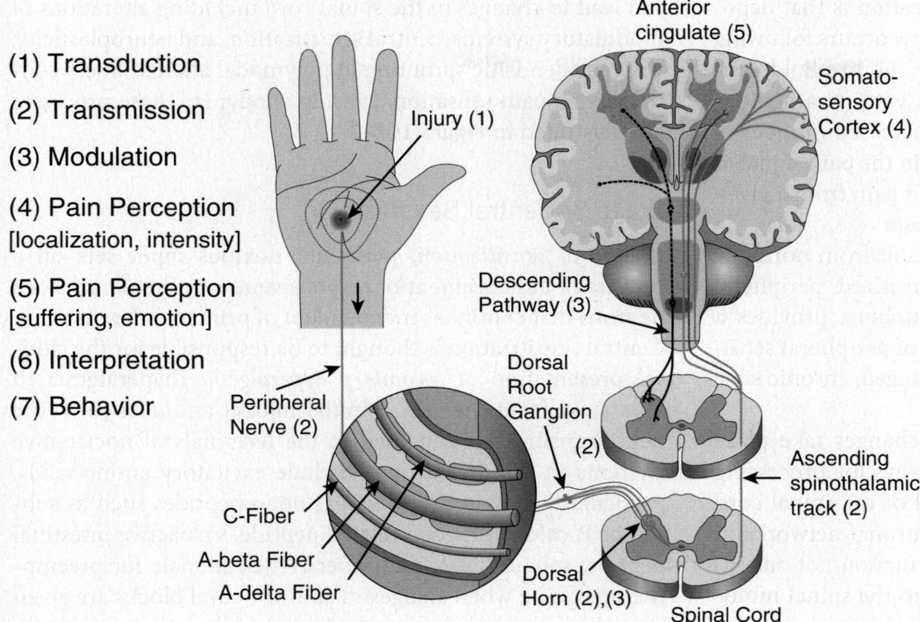

Figure 108-1. Anatomy of pain perception.

sensation of pain (discussed later—see **Table 108-1**); and loss of descending inhibitory controls. At any given time, one or a combination of these pathophysiological mechanisms may be contributing to the experience of CNCP.

Stage 1: Nociception

A sufficiently strong noxious stimulus (mechanical, thermal, or chemical) activates nociceptors leading to depolarization of pain afferents (A delta and C fibers) that transmit the pain message from the peripheral tissue to the dorsal horn of the spinal cord. If the signal is strong enough (many nociceptive neurons firing) and/or repetitive enough, second-order neurons depolarize, sending the message rostrally to the lateral and medial thalamus. There, projections to the somatosensory cortex convey localization and intensity information resulting in the conscious perception of pain. Projections from the medial thalamus to the limbic system, specifically the anterior cingulate cortex and insular cortex, activate suffering and the emotional aspect of pain, as in **Figure 108-1**. Once this entire system is activated, repetitive nociceptor stimulation in the periphery can trigger a hyper-response of the second-order neuron, increasing pain despite no increase in nociceptor input.

TABLE 108-1 Simple Bedside Examination Techniques, Findings and their Meaning

Exam Technique	Finding	Meaning
Palpation	Tenderness, soreness, guarding	Sensitization, inflammation
	Pain intensity increased relative to stimulus	Hyperalgesia or hyperpathia
Straight leg raise	Patient's pain complaint is reproduced	Nerve root disease; radiculopathy, esp. in lower back pain
Deep tendon reflexes	Diminished or absent	Neuropathic involvement

From Rathmell JP, Fields HL. Pain: pathophysiology and management. In: Loscalzo J, Fauci A, Kasper D, Hauser S, Longo D, Jameson J, eds. *Harrison's Principles of Internal Medicine.* 21st ed. McGraw Hill; 2022; Engstrom JW. Back and neck pain. In: Loscalzo J, Fauci A, Kasper D, Hauser S, Longo D, Jameson J, eds. *Harrison's Principles of Internal Medicine.* 21st ed. McGraw Hill; 2022.

Stage 2: Peripheral Sensitization

The situation changes in stage 2 pain when a noxious stimulus is very intense or prolonged leading to tissue damage and inflammation. Many nociceptors are inactive and unresponsive under normal circumstances; however, cell damage and death from injury or disease and accompanying inflammation can cause an "awakening" of nociceptors, which may spontaneously discharge and become more sensitive to peripheral stimulation.[13,14] This is one type of *peripheral sensitization.* The sensitization of nociceptors occurs when such inflammatory mediators as bradykinin, prostaglandins, serotonin, and histamine[15] are released in damaged tissue. They bind to specific receptors on nociceptive afferents, which elicits the activation of second messenger systems. Ultimately, this leads to phosphorylation of receptors, influx of Ca^{2+} ions, (which further sensitizes the cell), and release of such chemicals as substance P, which promote continued release of inflammatory mediators. Several types of pharmacological receptors, including opioid, γ-aminobutyric acid (GABA), bradykinin, histamine, serotonin, and, more recently, capsaicin,[16] have also been identified on the surface membrane of sensory axons.

The consequence of peripheral sensitization is that depolarization of primary afferent pain fibers now occurs following a stimulus that previously would have been subthreshold; sensitized fibers may even fire spontaneously, without a noxious stimulus being present. The firing of an increased number of nociceptive afferents codes for an increase in the pain signal to the spinal cord and brain, causing increased pain from a given noxious stimulus—this is termed *hyperalgesia*.

Also in this circumstance, pain can result from normally innocuous light touch that activates sensitized peripheral neurons[17]—this is termed *allodynia*. A sunburn provides a good clinical example of a temporary state of peripheral sensitization, whereas arthritis would be a prolonged, chronic state (as in **Table 108-1**).

Along with nociceptor sensitization, changes take place in the central pathways. The central pathways for processing nociceptive information begin at the level of the spinal cord (and medullary) dorsal horn. The interneuronal networks in the dorsal horn transmit nociceptive information not only to neurons that project to the brain but also to the spinal motor neurons, which may lead to enhanced reflex actions, including muscle spasm, in response to a noxious stimuli. Other sensory inputs (eg, counterstimulation with an acupuncture needle or icing) can result in inhibition of projection neurons. The balance of these excitatory and inhibitory processes provides an explanatory basis for gate theory of pain transmission.[18]

Following damage to peripheral nerves, whether by neurological disease, amputations, surgery, radiation, or chemotherapy, pain fibers can fire spontaneously, can be triggered by trivial stimuli, and can fire in response to adrenergic outflow (such as occurs with psychological stress). Continual firing can lead to changes in the spinal cord including alterations of modulatory systems, central sensitization, and neuroplasticity, whereby dendritic sprouting in polymodal afferent fibers contributes to pain sensation, causing allodynia. These processes are illustrated in **Figure 108-2**.

Stage 3: Central Sensitization

In *central sensitization*, persistent noxious input sets off a process of enhancement of responsiveness in the dorsal horn neurons that continues independent of primary afferent drive. Central sensitization is thought to be responsible for the clinical presentation of *secondary hyperalgesia* (hyperalgesia in sites away from the site of initial injury) and *allodynia*. The neurotransmitters contained in the terminals of nociceptive afferents in the dorsal horn include excitatory amino acids, particularly glutamate, as well as neuropeptides such as substance P, calcitonin gene-related peptide, vasoactive intestinal peptide, somatostatin, and others. The rationale for preemptive analgesia, when analgesics and/or neural blocks are given prior to a surgical procedure, is that such interventions are thought to prevent central sensitization.[19] Inhibition of nociceptive circuits, mediated by a number of neurotransmitters, including amino acids such as 5-hydroxytryptamine, GABA, and glycine as well as neuropeptides such as enkephalins, forms the basis of many pharmacological interventions.

These chronic pain states are generally the consequence of chronic inflammation secondary to structure injury (eg, arthritis), damage to peripheral nerves (eg, neuropathy), damage to the CNS (eg, thalamic stroke, multiple sclerosis), or changes in the CNS itself, for example, neuroplasticity,

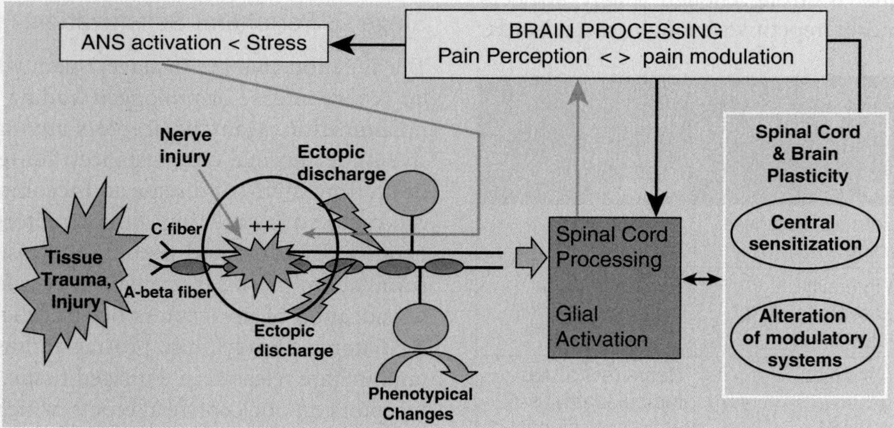

Figure 108-2. Key: After injury to first-order nociceptive fibers, they spontaneously and repetitively discharge, activating the biochemical cascade, leading to central sensitization and neuroplasticity. Pain activates the stress response, including the sympathetic system, which can also be activated by emotional states such as anxiety or frustration not directly related to pain. Sympathetic terminals on injured nerves and/or nociceptors release norepinephrine, respectively, increasing ectopic discharge of injured nerves and/or lowering nociceptor firing threshold in injured tissue. This pathophysiological process increases pain such that commonly patients with CNCP are known to isolate socially, avoiding interpersonal contact and other situations that might aggravate them and worsen their pain. (Adapted from Woolf CJ, Mannion RJ. Neuropathic pain: aetiology, symptoms, mechanisms, and management. *Lancet*. 1999;353(9168):1959-1964; Attal N, Bouhassira D. Mechanisms of pain in peripheral neuropathy. *Acta Neurol Scand Suppl*. 1999;173:12-24; discussion 48-52.)

central sensitization, and alteration in modulatory systems like descending inhibitory systems (eg, complex regional pain syndrome, as in **Fig. 108-2**). CNCP is often characterized by a lack of correlation between the intensity of a peripheral stimulus and the intensity of pain (manifest by exaggerated responses to noxious stimuli) and also by pain that is spontaneous or triggered by innocuous physical or psychological stimuli.[20]

Descending control from supraspinal centers inhibits ascending nociceptive transmission; this control is proportional to the afferent nociceptive input by C fibers. It has been suggested that loss of a proportion of the normal input after peripheral nerve damage produces a lifting of descending inhibition, which could be responsible for enhanced pain perception, particularly for the phenomenon of *hyperalgesia*, in which there is an exaggerated pain response to a noxious stimulus.[13] However, the development of stage 3 pain may also involve genetic, cognitive, and emotional factors that remain to be clarified.[18]

Recent brain imaging studies suggest that more rostral changes in the CNS also mediate sensitization. This finding supports a widely held clinical belief that stimulating, goal-directed activity and exercise suppress pain, enable improvements in functional ability, and even reduce the manifestations of central sensitization (eg, allodynia and hyperpathia). This phenomenon is thought to be one reason for the effectiveness of comprehensive rehabilitation programs in treating chronic pain. Regions in the cingulate gyrus have now been identified that are responsible for modulating behavioral responses to pain, attention to pain, pain induced fear, and learning and pain.[21]

Adult hippocampal neurogenesis (AHN) is implicated in learning, emotional functions, and is disrupted in negative mood disorders.[22] Recent evidence indicates that AHN is decreased in persistent pain consistent with the idea that chronic pain is a major stressor, associated with negative moods and abnormal memories. Various manipulations blocking AHN decreased postinjury neuropathic or inflammatory pain behaviors. Negative mood could be dissociated from persistent pain. These results suggest that AHN mediated hippocampal neurogenesis-related learning mechanisms are involved in emergence of persistent pain.[22]

Figure 108-3 illustrates the sequence of biopsychosocial processes involved in the transition from acute injury to CNCP and its related comorbidities and disability. Treatment involves a comprehensive approach that identifies the patient's biopsychosocial profile in this phenomenological pathway and addresses specific pathophysiological factors perpetuating pain and pain-related and disease-related impairments and comorbidities (see **Fig. 108-3**).

Pain and Emotions

Emotional states that activate sympathetic arousal, such as anxiety or anger, can increase acute pain and reactivate or worsen chronic pain. When depression and anxiety disorders, or other related disorders such as posttraumatic stress disorder (PTSD), and CNCP are comorbid, they complicate each other's treatment, such that treating one condition without treating the other effectively increases the likelihood of treatment failure. Functional MRI studies have been inconclusive in finding an association between anxiety or depressive symptoms and alterations in gray matter morphology.[23] Certain personal traits, such as external locus of control[24,25] and a tendency to catastrophize[26] predict worse outcomes. Pain catastrophizing has been associated with alterations in gray matter in brain areas involved in somatosensory, motor, and pain processing. Catastrophizing is related to pain processing including reduced engagement of the descending pain inhibitory system, and activation of areas related to attention

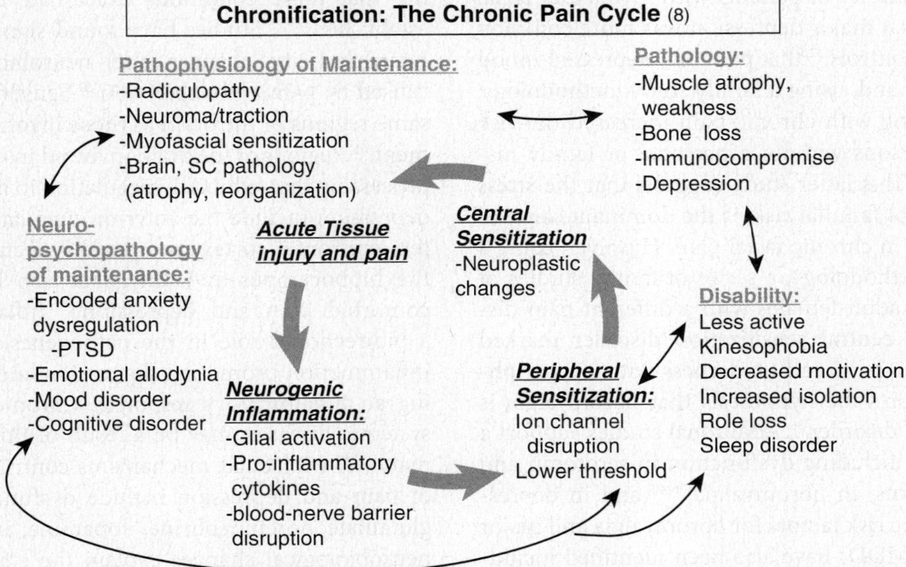

Figure 108-3. Acute to chronic pain cycle. (From Gallagher RM. Pharmacological approaches to pain management. In: Ebert M, Kerns R, eds. *Behavioral and Psychopharmacological Pain Management*. Cambridge University Press; 2010:129-141.)

to pain, emotion, and motor activity.[23] These observations underlie the demonstrated value of empowering patients with CNCP in self-management to strengthen internal controls and in cognitive reframing to reduce catastrophizing. Finally, comorbid substance use may complicate the use of opioid analgesics for pain control. Due to the high rate of opioid overdoses and questions about long-term benefit, the use of opioids for acute and chronic pain was re-examined first in 2016 and again in 2022 by the Centers for Disease Control and Prevention (CDC)[27,28] which suggested limiting long-term exposure to opioids as it might not improve function and might activate SUD mechanisms in patients at risk. Substance use, by interfering with the sustained, goal-oriented behavior needed for functional restoration, leads to poor outcomes of pain treatment generally. The mechanisms for this effect will be discussed in more detail below. Thus, identifying and managing these comorbidities are critical to effectively treating pain.

Evolving Understanding of Psychosomatic Concepts

A review of rigorous epidemiological studies over several decades demonstrates a strong association between depressive and anxiety disorders and chronic pain.[29] Although chronic pain generally affects psychological health and functional status consistently across cultures,[30] the relationship is more complex when considering specific painful diseases. For example, a mechanism for the high association between depression, anxiety disorders, and arthritis is suggested by recent studies linking the presence of depression to an impaired capacity to regulate the inflammatory cascade during stress.[31]

The causal direction of the relationships among chronic pain disorders and psychiatric comorbidities and the relative influence of environmental factors and genetic/familial factors, "nature versus nurture," are also being studied. For example, a series of studies of patients with myofascial facial pain demonstrated that major depression was more common than in community controls,[32] that pain and depressed mood seasonally covaried,[33] and, using a family study methodology, that the stress of living with chronic pain increased the risk for depression in persons without a personal or family history of depression.[34] This latter study suggests that the stress of living with pain, not familial risk, is the dominant cause of comorbid depression in chronic facial pain. However, using a similarly rigorous methodology, a series of family studies of community-dwelling adult females with a different pain disease, fibromyalgia, a central sensitization disorder marked by generalized muscle pain and tenderness with no peripheral pathology, supports the hypothesis that fibromyalgia is an affective spectrum disorder.[35] Additional studies support a shared pathogenesis, including dysfunction in serotonin and norepinephrine systems, in fibromyalgia,[36-40] and in depression.[41,42] Shared genetic risk factors for fibromyalgia and major depressive disorder (MDD) have also been identified including genetic polymorphisms in serotonin-related genes in fibromyalgia.[43-48] Thus, the increase in rates of major depression in families of persons with fibromyalgia, with or without depression, may reflect vulnerability in these neurotransmitter systems that influence both disorders.

The effects of some environmental factors on the pathogenesis of pain disorders and depressive disorders and SUD may be shared. Stress and trauma, implicated in both facial pain[34] and depression[49-52] and SUD, may alter the course of pain in subjects with existing pain. In a prospective study of a community sample of fibromyalgia and major life trauma (the 9/11 World Trade Center attack), exposure to stress was not associated with an increase in rates of fibromyalgia in controls (community subjects without fibromyalgia) but was associated with increases in pain in community subjects with fibromyalgia already confirmed by research diagnostic criteria.[53]

One interpretation of these aforementioned studies is that central states such as fibromyalgia and MDD share a genetic or other biologically mediated vulnerability to respond to stressful or traumatic events with psychological and pain-related symptoms. This interpretation is consistent with two recent studies, one showing that persons with fibromyalgia symptoms are more likely than community controls to develop PTSD in response to a fixed level of exposure to traumatic events[53] and another demonstrating that during experimental interpersonal stress, women with fibromyalgia who were primed to experience negative mood prior to stress showed greater subsequent pain elevations than similarly primed women with osteoarthritis.[54] Genetic studies suggest that a functional polymorphism in the promoter region of the serotonin transporter gene affects the influence of stressful life events on depression,[55] a region that has also been implicated in some investigations of fibromyalgia.[44,45]

Pain and Depression

The coexistence of pain and depression and the understanding that these conditions exacerbate one another is well-established.[56-59] Studies have found significant overlap in the neuroplasticity changes and neurobiological mechanisms caused by pain and depression.[60] Sensory pathways share the same regions of the brain as those involved in mood management.[61] Regions of the brain involved in emotional and reward processing that exhibit dysregulation in both chronic pain and depression include the anterior cingulate cortex, insular cortex, prefrontal cortex, and nucleus accumbens. Additionally, the hippocampus and amygdala also likely play a role in comorbid pain and depression.[62] Inflammation may have a bidirectional role in the pathogenesis of depression with inflammation promoting depression and depression facilitating an inflammatory response. Chronic pain, among other systemic diseases, may be a result of this heightened inflammation.[63] Molecular mechanisms contributing to coexistence of pain and depression include dysfunction in signaling of glutamate, norepinephrine, dopamine, and serotonin.[62] These neurobiological changes explain the effectiveness of current therapeutic approaches such as serotonin norepinephrine reuptake inhibitors and tricyclic antidepressants.

Pain and Anxiety

The experimental and epidemiological evidence points to a strong association between anxiety and pain[29,30] mediated in part by the amygdala, which appears to play a key role in the regulation of the emotional response to pain. The "nociceptive amygdala" can be influenced by a wide range of environmental and internal stimuli to modulate the subjective experience of pain. The hippocampus, a structure with robust connections to the amygdala, is a center for memory formation, storage, and retrieval. It provides information from detailed memories processed by the amygdala and given a particular emotional value, which may influence the development of "pain memory" after central sensitization. The emotional value the amygdala places on a particular memory is then fed back to the hippocampus, which integrates this information and either strengthens or weakens the memory. This is why it is believed that events associated with high emotional content, and often painful injury, such as a car accident or being wounded in battle, tend to be remembered in greater detail, as observed in PTSD, than those experiences with little emotional significance (eg, back pain on your drive to work every morning or working in the garden on the weekend). Exposure to novel, "interesting" environments can reverse hippocampal sensitization in pain experiments. Studies of disorders such as complex regional pain syndrome (formerly called reflex sympathetic dystrophy) show that specific sequences of mental activities[64] and biofeedback using brain imaging[9] reduce pain. These studies support the usefulness of rehabilitative approaches emphasizing patient involvement in goal-oriented, motivating, engrossing activities.[10]

PTSD, which is often comorbid with chronic pain associated with physical injury, is associated with changes in the amygdala, hippocampus, and other areas of the limbic system (the neural circuits of complex emotional experience). Neuroimaging studies have found consistent reductions in either total hippocampal volume or blood flow in men and women with PTSD.[65-67]

Other research on structures within this fear circuit has expanded our understanding of how cortical structures influence the amygdala. Human imaging studies have found that the fusiform gyrus, prefrontal gyrus, and anterior cingulate gyrus are preferentially activated in response to fearful stimuli.[68,69] The orbitofrontal cortex (OFC), which is involved in the evaluation of risk and reward and social norms, may also have a direct role in regulation of anxiety via its connection to the amygdala.[70] The cortex plays an essential role in the categorization, appraisal, and attenuation of our reactions to fearful stimuli, such as pain. The higher cortical connections to the more primitive fight, flight, and reward circuitry provide a degree of conscious recognition and control over these processes. These connections and their conditioning suggest the biological basis for the effects of behavioral treatments used widely in chronic pain, such as relaxation and biofeedback. They also suggest specific targets for neuromodulation.

Gamma-aminobutyric acid (GABA) appears to be a potential marker of pain severity in chronic nociceptive pain states independent of negative affect.[71] The pain–γ-aminobutyric acid interrelation remained strong when controlling for depression. Combined levels of glutamine and glutamate were unrelated to psychometric or to pain thresholds. The findings suggest that GABAergic disinhibition of the salience network may underlie sensitization to averse stimuli as a mechanism contributing to pain chronification.

More recent functional brain chemistry research has provided neuroanatomical evidence for the overlap between the processing and perception of pain and anxiety. In an experiment comparing patients with chronic low back pain to normal controls, significant differences were found in two regions of the association cortex (OFC and dorsolateral prefrontal cortex [DLPFC]), the cingulate gyrus (part of the limbic system), and the thalamus.[72] The study showed that persons with chronic low back pain have differences in regional brain chemistry in the OFC and DLPFC when compared with those without pain. Additionally, persons with chronic low back pain and anxiety had changes in chemistry suggesting increased interaction among all four brain regions, whereas anxious controls only had changes observed in the OFC. Anxiety and pain, therefore, share common neurochemical pathways and can interact in a way that leads to the reorganization of perceptual pathways in the brain. Living with chronic pain is stressful and is thought to be associated with physiological and psychological changes, yet there is a knowledge gap regarding brain elements involved in such conditions. Studies with fMRI suggest that the subjective spontaneous pain of chronic back pain involves specific spatiotemporal neuronal mechanisms, distinct from those observed for acute experimental pain, implicating a salient role for the emotional brain concerning the self.[73]

CLINICAL INTERFACE BETWEEN PAIN AND SUBSTANCE USE DISORDERS

Multiple points of interface exist between pain and SUD, and these become significant at the clinical level. Patients with SUD can express their stress level or anxiety by utilizing the word "pain" or reporting a high pain level. Pain and drug reward share common neuroanatomical and neurochemical substrates, and the physiological sequela of SUD (ie, tolerance, physiological dependence, and altered stress response) have clear effects on pain management. Reinforcing drugs often have analgesic properties, yet the disease of SUD brings with it malaise, mood states, behaviors, and social losses that serve to worsen the pain experience. The clinical interaction of pain and SUD is particularly complex in the case of opioid use disorder, as these drugs appear to be imbued with both analgesic and hyperalgesic properties. And finally, common comorbid or experiential disorders including anxiety, depression, and trauma may predispose to both conditions.

Neurobiological Interface of Pain and Substance Use Disorder

A patient with CNCP may be tolerant to or physiologically dependent on the effects of an opioid without being addicted to it. SUD is identified by a cluster of aberrant patterns of behavior that, while partially motivated by these physiological changes, is evident in much broader domains.

In considering the interplay between the neurobiological systems that underlie pain and SUD, several points of overlap can be identified. First, many reinforcing drugs have inherent analgesic properties and thereby recruit ascending and descending pain pathways to diminish the perception of pain. In addition, the disorder of SUD brings with it physical and psychological consequences that serve to worsen or facilitate the pain experience. Of these, the negative affective states that characterize chronic pain and SUD share allostatic changes in reward systems resulting in the chronification and treatment-resistant nature of both. Finally, it appears that opioid use may bring specific hyperalgesic changes to pain systems, which can further complicate the experience and management of chronic pain.

Analgesic Effects of Reinforcing Drugs

As points of interface between the physiology of pain and SUD are considered, it is important to recognize that many classes of reinforcing drugs have analgesic properties. The opioids are defined by their direct analgesic effects, and at high doses, alcohol is a potent anesthetic and analgesic. The sedative hypnotics, particularly benzodiazepines, are used to treat the pain sustained by muscle spasticity secondary to upper motor neuron damage[74] and are a standard anxiolytic adjunct for procedural sedation and analgesia.[75,76] CNS stimulants, such as cocaine and caffeine, produce and potentiate analgesia, presumably by increasing neurotransmitter activity in descending inhibitory pain pathways.

Of current interest are the effects of cannabinoids on pain perception. In 1992, Devane et al.[77] developed a high-affinity synthetic cannabinoid ligand, confirming the presence of endogenous cannabinoid G protein-coupled receptors in the human body,[78] with central subtype receptors widely distributed in the cortex, basal ganglia, cerebellum, and hippocampus.[79] Of the two receptor subtypes identified as integral to the endocannabinoid system, cannabinoid receptor 1 is thought to have the most direct influence on neuronal pain processing pathways. Two mechanisms of pain modulation by cannabinoids have been proposed: (1) inhibition at the dorsal root ganglia resulting in inhibition of ascending nociceptive pain signals and (2) modulation at the brain stem suppressing descending nociceptive signals.[80] While preclinical data has suggested cannabinoid modulation occurs in the peripheral nervous system,[81-83] human studies have not replicated these results.[80]

While clinical trials of cannabinoids in multiple sclerosis have suggested a benefit for neuropathic pain,[84,85] human studies of cannabinoid-mediated analgesia have been limited by study size, heterogeneous patient populations, subjective outcome measures, and variable drug pharmacokinetics.[86] Recent meta-analyses have found no evidence that cannabinoids effectively treat acute,[87] fibromyalgia[88] or rheumatic pain.[89] There are reports of moderate efficacy to treat cancer pain[90,91] although there is insufficient evidence for its use as an adjunct in this context.[92] It is identified as a fourth-line analgesic for the management of neuropathic pain, behind the more effective antiepileptics, tricyclic antidepressants, serotonin and norepinephrine reuptake inhibitors, and opioids.[93,94] However, all reviews note that the paucity of well-controlled clinical trials on cannabinoids as analgesics limits comprehensive evaluation of efficacy. Further information on the use of cannabis as treatment can be found in Section 15 of this textbook.

General Effects of Substance Use Disorders on Pain

Careful examination of the extant literature provides evidence that physiological states consistent with SUD can affect nociceptive input, processing, and/or modulation in several different ways. SUD facilitates the experience of pain in multiple ways, including its associated sympathetic arousal and negative mood states. These changes are related to both the discrete effects of certain classes of drugs and the effects of all reinforcing drugs on reward-relevant systems.

For example, important psychological sequelae, including sleep disorders and psychiatric illness, are characteristic of SUD and, as previously noted, can contribute to the experience of chronic pain and decrease the efficacy of analgesic interventions. SUDs commonly co-occur with mood disorders,[95] which—if not corrected—can increase the perception of pain. Depression has been demonstrated to increase the discomfort associated with pain and to impair function in studies of chronic pain patients. Symptoms frequently improve with effective antidepressant treatment.[96] Drug use in those with SUD is characterized by frequent and rapid fluctuations in blood levels of the drug. Reinforcing substances tend to be ingested in short-acting formulations and via routes with rapid onset (ie, inhalation, intravenous) to boost psychoactive effect. These use patterns result in rapidly alternating states of intoxication and subtle (or sometimes full-blown) withdrawal.

Strong and persistent negative affective states accompany withdrawal from many such drugs. Individuals with SUDs experiencing withdrawal suffer from negative symptoms such as anhedonia, prolonged dysphoria, and irritability,[97] which have been attributed to dopamine (DA) depletion in the reward pathways (reward deficiency). A second component of the negative emotional states common to all reinforcing drugs is the activation of brain stress systems such as corticotropin-releasing factor, norepinephrine, and dynorphin. Clearly, the negative feeling states associated with drug withdrawal can augment the subjective discomfort associated with pain.

Finally, and not insignificantly, the interpersonal conflicts, role adjustments, and social support losses that characterize the social context of SUD can worsen the experience of pain, making the individual less able to manage or cope with discomfort. The chaotic and drug-oriented lifestyle of the person with a SUD makes it difficult to comply with prescribed pain management regimes and engage in pain reduction activities (exercise, mindful meditation). Empirical support for a worsened pain experience in individuals with active SUD has been demonstrated in the case of experimental pain, as compared to those in drug-free recovery. Persons with active SUD are significantly less tolerant of cold pressor pain than drug-free people with SUD in remission, whether the drug was a CNS stimulant (cocaine) or opioid.[98]

Potential Neurobiological Basis for Overlap of the Allostatic States of Substance Use Disorders and Pain

Allostatic states secondary to ongoing drug use in the brain systems underlying learning and memory can drive aberrant drug-seeking behaviors, especially under conditions of withdrawal or, in the absence of withdrawal, with recurrent craving.[99]

The development of aversive or negative emotional states that constitute negative reinforcers in SUD has been linked to the two distinct neurobiological processes noted above: loss of function in the reward systems or reward deficiency (within-system neuroadaptations) and recruitment of brain stress or antireward systems (between-system neuroadaptations).[100] Reward deficiency is identified by decreased sensitivity to natural reinforcers and by decreased activity of dopaminergic pathways[101] in the motivational circuits of the ventral striatum-extended amygdala. Overall, reward function is diminished, and persistent negative affective states reflected in depression and anhedonia predominate. Conversely, antireward processes include the release of corticotropin-releasing factors, norepinephrine, epinephrine, and dynorphin, which serve to further reinforce negative affect (including fear and anxiety)[102] and motivate rigid directed behaviors to provide relief.[97] Pain generates a negative emotional state that can exacerbate the negative emotional state associated with SUD and vice versa. Building upon historical models of pain and reward as existing on a continuum, pain can also be conceptualized as a disorder of reward function. Reward deficiency and antireward mechanisms result in the "chronification" of both pain and SUD.[103] In this model, the preoccupation and compulsive seeking of comfort are homologous in the patient with both CNCP and SUD. For those with CNCP, the reward associated with pain relief would be less salient in the context of reward deficiency and concurrent antireward stress responses.[104] In the case of the patient with SUD, ongoing reward deficiency amplifies the reinforcement of drug use, which also alleviates the distress associated with antireward.[105] Interestingly, the combination of reward deficiency and antireward processes in midbrain and cortical systems is hypothesized to explain the high rates of suicidality in both patients with chronic pain and those with SUD.[106]

Unique Effects of Opioid Use Disorder on Pain

The effects of opioid use disorder (OUD) on pain become especially pertinent in the case of individuals with opioid use disorder because the class of drug with disordered use is also the primary pharmacological tool for the treatment of moderate to severe clinical pain. OUD and opioid analgesia are dependent upon opioid agonist activity at the mu opioid receptor; the reinforcing and analgesic effects of morphine, for example, can be blocked by the administration of mu receptor antagonists and are absent in mu opioid receptor gene knockout mice. In that the same receptor is central to both OUD and pain systems, it is reasonable to expect that perturbations in the latter might be evident in individuals chronically exposed to opioids (agonists or antagonists) in the context of the former. Although drug reward and analgesia are distinct processes, opioids activate their shared anatomical substrate, the mu opioid receptor, inducing the interrelated CNS changes of tolerance and physiological dependence. In addition to the ventromedial medulla, mu receptors are located in the cortex, thalamus, periaqueductal gray, spinal cord, and peripheral sensory neurons. Individuals with OUD may seek psychoactive effects yet are not immune to the effects of these drugs on central and peripheral opioid-relevant pain systems.

Genetics of Pain and Opioid Use Disorder

Individual differences in pain tolerance and opioid response have long been appreciated at the clinical level, and the genetic factors, which underlie these differences, are increasingly elucidated. For example, heritable differences in hepatic P450 isoenzyme activity affect both the amount of reward and analgesia received from opioids metabolized by this system. Individuals who are extensive "metabolizers" of opioids (ie, those with high P450 activity) receive less analgesia and reward from a given opioid dose[107] theoretically putting them at decreased risk for opioid use disorder but increased risk for unrelieved pain.[108]

With the advent of molecular genetics, investigators in both the pain and SUD fields have been focusing on polymorphisms in the mu opioid receptor gene (*OPRM1*) as candidates underlying phenotypes for pain sensitivity,[109] opioid analgesic response,[110] and OUD.[111] Probably best characterized is the single nucleotide polymorphism *A118G* of *OPRM1*, such that normal human subjects with the variant allele have been shown to require almost twice as high a plasma level of morphine to achieve the analgesic response as those with the nonmutated allele.[112] Other genes linked to pain and opioid responses include those that code for the delta opioid receptor, the capsaicin-sensing vanilloid receptor,[113] the neurotransmitter enzyme catechol-*O*-methyltransferase,[114] and the melanocortin-1 receptor gene.[115]

Epigenetic mechanisms (nongenetic influences on gene expression) underlying the development of SUD and chronic pain are receiving increased attention. In the case of alcohol use disorder, epigenetic modifications in the amygdala have been demonstrated to contribute to the negative affective states characteristic of the allostatic changes associated with SUD,[116] whereas cocaine intake appears to alter gene expression in reward-relevant pathways in the nucleus accumbens.[117] Such epigenetic regulation may be especially significant during windows of neurodevelopmental vulnerability (prenatal, adolescence)[118] and explain the link between early substance use and SUD later in life. In the case of chronic pain, there is evidence that inflammation and tissue or neural injury can induce epigenetic modifications in the CNS resulting in pain hypersensitivity,[119] including allodynia and hyperalgesia. Portending overlap between epigenetic mechanisms that mediate both chronic pain and SUD, Descalzi and colleagues describe chronic pain-induced modifications in brain reward systems, analogous to those induced by exposure to reinforcing drugs.[120] Epigenetically mediated histone methyltransferase G9a regulation appears to be a common adaptive response of neurons to compensate for the negative effects of chronic drug use on the brain, and this might also be true for the negative effects of pain.[121]

Opioid-Induced Hyperalgesia

Broadly conceptualized as an opponent process, the hyperalgesia induced by opioids is theorized to counter the analgesia these drugs provide. Opioid-induced hyperalgesia (OIH) is defined as increased sensitivity to pain resulting from opioid administration and characterized by increase in pain sensation to external stimuli over time and spreading of pain to locations beyond the initial pain site. It has been best demonstrated in animal models, wherein pain-free rodents have significantly decreased nociceptive thresholds from baseline following single or repeated administration of opioids. These preclinical studies have shown that OIH generalizes across nociceptive stimuli (thermal, chemical, electrical), opioid agent (heroin, fentanyl, morphine), and route of administration (IV, SC, IT, IP, oral). The hyperalgesia is dose dependent (cumulative dose/cumulative exposure) and appears to resolve in a time course similar to its development, with increased magnitude of response correlated to its duration. It intensifies with antagonist precipitated withdrawal and worsens with repeated withdrawal episodes.[122] Evident in increased incisional (wound) hyperalgesia, OIH appears to share mechanisms underlying the development of neuropathic pain.

Withdrawal Hyperalgesia

The phenomenon of hyperalgesia has long been recognized as a fundamental symptom of the opioid withdrawal syndrome in animal models of OUD and although not extensively studied, hyperalgesia and spontaneous muscle and bone pain have long been considered cardinal symptoms of opioid withdrawal in humans. The time course, opioid dose-response relationship, and opioid pretreatment parameters of withdrawal hyperalgesia have been carefully characterized in preclinical models for over 30 years, such that it occurs following single or long-term opioid exposure and is variable in duration and intensity depending on opioid, opioid dose, route of administration, and duration of use.[123]

Heightened pain perception has been long observed in people with OUD during abstinence.[124] Individuals with OUD maintained on either methadone or the partial agonist buprenorphine showed increased sensitivity to cold pressor pain.[125] Indeed, Ren et al.[126] found that a hyperalgesic state can persist for up to 5 months in abstinent subjects with OUD and that those with more pain sensitivity also displayed greater cue-induced craving at this time point. Thus, individuals with OUD and poor pain tolerance may suffer a more severe form of OUD, have difficulty tolerating the discomfort (pain) inherent in withdrawal management and early abstinence, and be more likely to return to use.

OIH and Tolerance

The presence of hyperalgesia with ongoing opioid use provides an alternate conceptualization of analgesic tolerance. As eloquently hypothesized by Colpaert[127] and Célèrier,[128] that which appears to be opioid analgesic tolerance, and therefore increased opioid need, may in fact be an organismic response to an opioid-induced hypersensitivity to pain or "apparent tolerance." Essentially, opioids lose their analgesic effectiveness in the face of decreased tolerance for pain. That OIH might contribute to the variable and incompletely understood phenomenon of analgesic tolerance in the clinical setting is a paradigm-shifting idea; analgesic tolerance may reflect underlying neuroadaptive changes that reflect the possibility of OIH. Clinically, tolerance provides a certain amount of protection for the user, such as with the respiratory depressant effects of opioids or the anesthetic effects of ethanol. However, tolerance does not develop to all physiological drug effects; for example, in the case of opioids, tolerance to the opioid-induced bowel dysfunction, and more specifically opioid-induced constipation, does not diminish over time.[129]

Through their preclinical work exploring the molecular mechanisms of hyperalgesia, Mao et al.[130] demonstrated the similarities between opioid analgesic tolerance and OIH. In an important series of studies, these investigators provide credible evidence that the development of opioid analgesic tolerance via intermittent morphine dosing induces hyperalgesia, while animals made hyperalgesic via neuropathic injury concomitantly exhibit opioid analgesic tolerance (results replicated with heroin by Célèrier et al.[128]).

Mechanisms of OIH

Various physiological explanations for the development of OIH have been offered and have focused on both spinal and supraspinal systems as the site of action.[131-142] A common pathway for the development of morphine tolerance/hyperalgesia is activation of ionotropic NMDA receptors on dorsal horn spinal cord neurons, with subsequent intracellular increases in protein kinase C and nitric oxide. Here, OIH is conceptualized as a variant of central sensitization and, like the hyperalgesia of neuropathic origin,[136] can be prevented by *N*-methyl-D-aspartate (NMDA) receptor antagonism and calcium channel blockers.[138-140] The latter finding has spurred interest in the potential utility of NMDA receptor antagonists as a means to enhance the effectiveness of opioid analgesia[141,142] and complements the ongoing work of OUD scientists on the utility of these agents to reverse opioid tolerance and physiological dependence.[143-147]

There is preclinical evidence[137] that OIH may in fact be the result of the activation of descending pain facilitation systems arising from mu opiate receptor activation[138] in the rostral ventromedial medulla (RVM).[134,137,147] Specifically implicated are opioid-induced increased levels of the pronociceptive peptide cholecystokinin (CCK) in the RVM. Increases in CCK appear to play a role in the development of opiate analgesic tolerance as well.[148] It is suggested that CCK activity in the medulla drives descending pain facilitatory mechanisms, resulting in spinal hyperalgesic responses to nociceptive input.[136,137]

Various spinal neuropeptides, distinct from excitatory amino acid systems, have also been implicated in the development of OIH. Interestingly, the hyperalgesic effects of opioids have been reversed by the administration of an antagonist to the neurokinin-1 receptor, which is the receptor mediating the nociceptive neuropeptide substance P. Particularly active in pain of inflammatory origin, substance P involvement suggests a neuroinflammatory component to the development of OIH.[149]

Emerging evidence suggests a key role for neuroimmune processes in the development of OIH.[150,151] In this model, exogenously administered opioids are theorized to bind to mu receptors located on the astrocytes of the blood–brain barrier, activating these and resulting in the subsequent expression and release of proinflammatory chemokines and cytokines. Specifically, peripheral immune cells activated in response to opioid administration are hypothesized to bind to glial cells and induce specific classes of central proinflammatory (and therefore pronociceptive) cytokines, thus resulting in a state of heightened pain sensitivity.[150,152-157] Reviewing the literature, Ossipov[149] commented that, "opioid-induced abnormal pain may share a molecular signature with pain of inflammatory origin" (p. 320).

Finally, more than 30 years ago, Seigel et al. demonstrated a conditioned component to OIH. A robust hyperalgesia was observed in animals receiving saline in an environment previously paired with morphine administration.[158,159] This work showed that rats receiving acute morphine doses (3-9 doses separated by 48 hours) in a specific environment demonstrate significant hyperalgesia in the same setting as compared to rats receiving morphine unpaired with setting or saline control rats. Because conditioned responses to medications typically are opposite in direction to unconditioned drug effects, the learned responses were ascribed a causal role in the development of drug tolerance.

Clinical Evidence of OIH

Evidence for OIH in humans has primarily been demonstrated in three populations: patients taking medications for OUD (methadone, buprenorphine), patients administered opioids during the surgical period, and healthy volunteers administered opioids acutely and then evaluated with experimental pain assays. Less common, but of increased interest in the era of the prescription opioid epidemic, are data to support the presence of OIH in patients with chronic pain on opioid therapy; the degree to which prescribed opioids worsen outcomes in patients with chronic pain is an important area of investigation (see **Table 108-2** for proposed differential diagnosis of increased pain in patients on opioid therapy).

Opioid Agonist Treatment with Methadone

As early as 1965, Martin and Inglis[131] described significantly lower tolerance for cold pressor-induced pain in a sample of incarcerated, known opioid-using women, in comparison to matched controls without OUD. Ho and Dole[160] found that both methadone-maintained (MM) and non-MM individuals with OUD had significantly lower thresholds for cold pressor pain than did matched nonaddicted sibling controls. Subsequent work supports that, at methadone trough conditions, cold pressor pain *threshold* does not differ between MM and non-MM patients with OUD but is significantly lower for MM patients in comparison to matched normal controls.[161] Under the same conditions, MM patients' cold pressor pain *tolerance* is less than that in both matched non-MM patients with OUD[98] and matched controls.[161] A similar nonsignificant trend for decreased pain tolerance in MM patients was noted for electrical pain stimulation, although a significant analgesic effect for methadone on cold pressor, electrical, and pressure pain 2 to 4 hours post dose was reported.[161] With respect to perceived pain severity, Schall et al.[162] found no difference

TABLE 108-2 Proposed Differential Diagnosis for Increased Complaints of Pain in Patient on Opioid Therapy

Differential dx	Nature of pain	Onset	Response to opioid administration
Increased pain pathology	Localized to pain site	Variable	Pain improves
Opioid tolerance	Localized to pain site	Gradual	Pain improves
Opioid withdrawal	Diffuse, hyperalgesia	Abrupt	Pain improves
Opioid-induced hyperalgesia	Diffuse, hyperalgesia	Abrupt or gradual	Pain worsens
Pseudo-addiction	Localized to pain site	Ongoing	Pain improves
Addiction	Diffuse, hyperalgesia	Ongoing	Pain worsens

between MM and control subjects in their perception of pressure pain (measured on a scale of 1-10) immediately prior to methadone dosing.

Across nociceptive stimuli, MM patients reliably demonstrate poor tolerance for experimental pain and are, on average, between 42% and 76% less tolerant of cold pressor pain than are normal controls matched on age, gender, and ethnicity.[125,161,163,164] Pilot data suggest that degree of hyperalgesia may vary with the intrinsic activity of the opioid maintenance agent, such that patients maintained on the partial agonist buprenorphine are less hyperalgesic than those maintained on methadone, a full agonist.[163] These data are correlational in nature, resulting in controversy as to whether or not the diminished tolerance in pain noted in persons on opioid agonist therapy for opioid use disorder is in fact "opioid induced." It is possible that patients prone to OUD are pain intolerant by nature and therefore patients on medication for opioid use disorder (MOUD) are more likely to display reduced cold pressor pain tolerance due to that intrinsic characteristic as opposed to being an effect of opioids.

Surgical Patients

Data suggest the presence of OIH in postoperative patients who received opioids intraoperatively and perhaps in a dose-dependent manner.[165,166] Data show that in patients undergoing various abdominal surgeries, postoperative reports of pain severity at rest and/or opioid consumption were significantly higher in those patients receiving intrathecal or intravenous short-acting opioids (fentanyl and remifentanil) during surgery in comparison to those receiving placebo[166] or low-dose opioids.[165,167-169] The hyperalgesia is most pronounced early in the postoperative period (24 hours) and with high-dose remifentanil administration; patients receiving high-dose intraoperative opioids utilized approximately 18 mg more of morphine sulfate during the postoperative period and had larger margins of wound hyperalgesia than those in patients with lower intraoperative opioid exposure. The hyperalgesia was minimized if the cumulative intraoperative opioid dose was kept below 40 μg/kg; if co-administered with ketamine,[170-172] magnesium,[173] dexmedetomidine,[174] pregabalin,[175] propofol,[176] nitrous oxide, and clonidine; or if tapered slowly. In that it is elicited with the abrupt offset of intraoperative remifentanil infusion suggests that rather than OIH, withdrawal hyperalgesia may be the source of increased sensitivity to pain.

Healthy Controls

Similarly, in healthy controls, remifentanil or fentanyl administered by bolus or slow (90-100 minutes) infusion has been shown to increase the perceived severity of heat pain and cold pressor pain two hours following administration, and wound, electric burn, or topical capsaicin hyperalgesia from 30 minutes to seven hours following administration. Again, in these instances, hyperalgesia was evaluated following offset of acute opioid effect; thus, it is unclear if withdrawal hyperalgesia accounted for the findings. In fact, healthy controls receiving a single dose of parenteral morphine or hydromorphone evidenced significant hyperalgesia following an acute naloxone challenge.[124]

Patients With Chronic Pain

Across a number of case studies, the emergence of hyperalgesia and allodynia has been reported in patients with cancer on large or rapidly escalating doses of morphine or fentanyl,[177-180] in at least one case resolving with discontinuation and switching to a weaker opioid.[181] A similar pattern of OIH induced with intrathecal sufentanil and clearing with opioid discontinuation has been described in a single case report of a woman with chronic noncancer low back pain (failed back syndrome),[182] suggesting that regardless of the etiology of chronic pain (cancer versus noncancer), OIH becomes evident in certain individuals in the context of high-dose opioid therapy. OIH in these patients often presents with a constellation of neuroexcitatory signs, including agitation, myoclonus, and delirium.

In the case of chronic pain, few prospective studies exist. In this work, comparators typically include patients receiving low-dose opioids or placebo. As opioid dose increases (>100 mg MED), hyperalgesia worsens, and "high-grade" tolerance is more likely to co-occur with OIH; there appears to be a negative correlation between OIH and opioid-derived analgesia,[183] and OIH is more robust in the presence of neuropathic, as opposed to nociceptive pain. Unknown is the degree to which the presence of chronic pain accounts for baseline hyperalgesia, which is reflected in OIH responses. Interestingly, those patients with chronic pain screened at higher risk for OUD were also more likely to report increased pain sensitivity to punctuate mechanical stimuli, regardless of whether they were receiving no opioids, low-dose opioids, or high-dose opioids, suggesting that hyperalgesia may be less related to opioid prescription and more related to propensity for OUD.[184]

A single study by Chu et al.[122] demonstrated the development of OIH in a small sample of patients with chronic non-cancer low back pain following 1 month of oral sustained-release morphine treatment (median dose 75 mg/d). In these six individuals, 30 days of morphine at therapeutic doses not only resulted in analgesic tolerance to challenge doses of remifentanil but also diminished tolerance to cold pressor pain by almost 25% from baseline. Similarly, Suzan and colleagues found that tolerance to heat pain diminished significantly following 4 weeks of oral hydromorphone therapy in patients with chronic pain, a finding that was not duplicated in matched healthy controls.[185] In a sample of cancer patients with pain undergoing a standardized lidocaine injection, self-reported ratings of pain and unpleasantness, as well as pain behaviors associated with the procedure increased by daily MED opioid dose.[186] When evaluating patients with chronic pain on methadone for the treatment of OUD, Hay and colleagues report diminished pain tolerance on the cold pressor assay in those both with and without chronic pain.[187]

Despite appreciating analgesia, the experimental and clinical pain responses of these patients suggest the presence of opioid-induced hyperalgesic changes.

Genetics and Opioid-Induced Hyperalgesia

Ongoing work provides evidence that OIH may arise from the epigenetic modifications associated with opioid tolerance. For example, He and Wang suggest that microRNA activity regulates the expression of mu opioid receptors, thereby interfering with both opioid analgesic and reward activity.[188] Further, to the degree that histone modification underlies the development of neuropathic pain, these mechanisms are likewise implicated in the initiation and maintenance of opioid tolerance and OIH.[119] Human studies of patients taking opioids for the treatment of OUD or chronic pain suggest that opioid-induced DNA methylation is related to increased chronic pain severity, which at the level of the patient is expressed as OIH.[120,189]

CONCLUSIONS

Pain is the most modulated of the sensory modalities. How a given, quantifiable stimulus is processed by the nervous system can be modified at the level of the nociceptor, the peripheral nerve, the spinal cord neurons and tracts, the spinal cord microglia, and the thalamus and its interactions with the cortex and various activating centers such as the amygdala. Modulation typically occurs as a dynamic interaction of processes among these sites. The unique susceptibility of pain to neuromodulation and allostasis portends a significant role for SUD in altering the pain experience. SUD physiology underlies the pathophysiological processing of the motivational system encoding reward and stress/antireward; stimuli that are by nature stressful and unrewarding, such as pain, are likely to be preferentially affected by the presence of SUDs.

Hypotheses about how the neurophysiological overlap between chronic pain and SUD might clinically manifest must take into account how holistic human responses to their combined presence may alter or mask predicted physiological responses.

Several points of overlap exist between the physiological bases of pain and SUD. Specific avenues by which the chronic use of reinforcing drugs might alter the processing of noxious stimuli include mediation of reward and stress response, withdrawal phenomena affecting emotional processes, and opioid tolerance. Further, genetic and epigenetic influences on phenotype expression of interrelated pain and reward systems play a role in the ultimate pain experience. Across this literature, a trend toward decreased pain tolerance in SUD can be discerned; thus, the presence of SUD appears to augment the experience of pain.

With respect to OUD specifically, the development or presence of OIH has the potential to complicate pain management. Less well studied but intriguing is evidence that individuals vary in their propensity to both OUD and pain responses; the link between the two may arise from inborn differences in endogenous opioid system tone or opioid-induced epigenetic changes, which underlie homeostatic and allostatic processes.

Consideration of the physiological bases of pain and SUD, and how they overlap, provides direction for the management of pain in this population. The human phenomena of pain and SUD are not separate but interrelated; knowledgeable management of the former must reflect the extent to which, even at the physiological level, its expression and response are affected by the latter.

ACKNOWLEDGMENT

The authors wish to recognize the contributions of the authors of previous versions of this chapter: Rollin Gallagher, Peggy Compton, and Adrian Popescu.

REFERENCES

1. Institute of Medicine. Relieving Pain in America: A Blueprint for Transforming Prevention, Care, Education, and Research. Accessed July 19, 2023. https://www.ncbi.nlm.nih.gov/books/NBK91497/
2. Global Burden of Disease Study 2013 Collaborators. Global, regional, and national incidence, prevalence, and years lived with disability for 301 acute and chronic diseases and injuries in 188 countries, 1990–2013: a systematic analysis for the Global Burden of Disease Study 2013. *Lancet*. 2015;386:743-800.
3. Fishman SM, Young HM, Arwood EL. Core competencies for pain management: results of an interprofessional consensus summit. *Pain Med*. 2013;14:971-981.
4. Hashmi JA, Baliki MN, Huang L, et al. Shape shifting pain: chronification of back pain shifts brain representation from nociceptive to emotional circuits. *Brain*. 2013;136:2751-2768.
5. Vachon-Presseau E, Roy M, Martel MO, et al. The stress model of chronic pain: evidence from basal cortisol and hippocampal structure and function in humans. *Brain*. 2013;136(Pt 3):815-827.
6. Milligan ED, Watkins LR. Pathological and protective roles of glia in chronic pain. *Nat Rev Neurosci*. 2009;10(1):23-36.
7. Loram LC, Taylor FR, Strand KA, et al. Prior exposure to glucocorticoids potentiates lipopolysaccharide induced mechanical allodynia and spinal neuroinflammation. *Brain Behav Immun*. 2011;25(7):1408-1415.
8. Melzack R, Wall PD. Pain mechanisms: a new theory. *Science*. 1965;150(3699):971-979.
9. deCharms RC, Maeda F, Glover GH, et al. Control over brain activation and pain learned by using real-time functional MRI. *Proc Natl Acad Sci U S A*. 2005;102(51):18626-18631.
10. Gallagher RM. Rational integration of pharmacologic, behavioral, and rehabilitation strategies in the treatment of chronic pain. *Am J Phys Med Rehabil*. 2005;84(3 Suppl):S64-S76.
11. Baron R, Maier C, Attal N, et al. Peripheral neuropathic pain: a mechanism-related organizing principle based on sensory profiles. *Pain*. 2017;158:261-272.
12. Guzmán J, Esmail R, Karjalainen K, Malmivaara A, Irvin E, Bombardier C. Multidisciplinary bio-psycho-social rehabilitation for chronic low back pain. *Cochrane Database Syst Rev*. 2002;1:CD000963.
13. Cervero F, Laird JM. Mechanisms of touch-evoked pain (allodynia): a new model. *Pain*. 1996;68(1):13-23.
14. Mendell JR, Sahenk Z. Clinical practice. Painful sensory neuropathy. *N Engl J Med*. 2003;348(13):1243-1255.
15. Schaible HG, Schmidt RF. Activation of groups III and IV sensory units in medial articular nerve by local mechanical stimulation of knee joint. *J Neurophysiol*. 1983;49(1):35-44.

16. Tal M, Bennett GJ. Extra-territorial pain in rats with a peripheral mononeuropathy: mechano-hyperalgesia and mechano-allodynia in the territory of an uninjured nerve. *Pain*. 1994;57(3):375-382.
17. Sandkuler J. Models and mechanisms of hyperalgesia and allodynia. *Physiol Rev*. 2009;89(2):707-758.
18. Willis WD, Westlund KN. Neuroanatomy of the pain system and of the pathways that modulate pain. *J Clin Neurophysiol*. 1997;14(1):2-31.
19. Woolf CJ, Mannion RJ. Neuropathic pain: aetiology, symptoms, mechanisms, and management. *Lancet*. 1999;353(9168):1959-1964.
20. Rome HP Jr, Rome JD. Limbically augmented pain syndrome (LAPS): kindling, corticolimbic sensitization, and the convergence of affective and sensory symptoms in chronic pain disorders. *Pain Med*. 2000; 1(1):7-23.
21. Vogt BA. Pain and emotion interactions in subregions of the cingulate gyrus. *Nat Rev Neurosci*. 2005;6(7):533-544.
22. Apkarian AV, Mutso AA, Centeno MV, et al. Role of adult hippocampal neurogenesis in persistent pain. *Pain*. 2016;157(2):418-428.
23. Malfliet A, Coppieters I, Van Wilgen P, et al. Brain changes associated with cognitive and emotional factors in chronic pain: a systematic review. *Eur J Pain*. 2017;21(5):769-786.
24. Iles RA, Davidson M, Taylor NF. Psychosocial predictors of failure to return to work in non-chronic non-specific low back pain: a systematic review. *Occup Environ Med*. 2008;65(8):507-517.
25. Gallagher RM, Rauh V, Haugh LD, et al. Determinants of return-to-work among low back pain patients. *Pain*. 1989;39(1):55-67.
26. Vowles KE, McCracken LM, Eccleston C. Patient functioning and catastrophizing in chronic pain: the mediating effects of acceptance. *Health Psychol*. 2008;27(2 Suppl):S136-S143.
27. Dowell D, Haegerich TM, Chou R. CDC guideline for prescribing opioids for chronic pain—United States, 2016. *JAMA*. 2016;315(15):1624-1645. doi:10.1001/jama.2016.1464
28. Dowell D, Ragan KR, Jones CM, Baldwin GT, Chou R. CDC clinical practice guideline for prescribing opioids for pain—United States, 2022. *MMWR Recomm Rep*. 2022;71(3):1-95.
29. Gallagher RM, Verma S. Mood and anxiety disorders in chronic pain. In: Dworkin R, Brieghtbart W, eds. *Psychosocial and Psychiatric Aspects of Pain: A Handbook for Health Care Providers. Progress in Pain Research and Management*. Vol. 27. IASP Press; 2004.
30. Gureje O, Von Korff M, Simon GE, Gater R. Persistent pain and well-being: a World Health Organization study in primary care. *JAMA*. 1998;280(2):147-151.
31. Miller GE, Rohleder N, Stetler C, Kirschbaum C. Clinical depression and regulation of the inflammatory response during acute stress. *Psychosom Med*. 2005;67(5):679-687.
32. Gallagher RM, Marbach JJ, Raphael KG, Dohrenwend BP, Cloitre M. Is major depression comorbid with temporomandibular pain and dysfunction syndrome? A pilot study. *Clin J Pain*. 1991;7(3):219-225.
33. Gallagher RM, Marbach J, Raphael K, et al. Myofascial face pain: seasonal variability in pain intensity and demoralization. *Pain*. 1995;61(1):113-120.
34. Dohrenwend BP, Raphael KG, Marbach JJ, Gallagher RM. Why is depression comorbid with chronic myofascial face pain? A family study test of alternative hypotheses. *Pain*. 1999;83(2):183-192.
35. Raphael KG, Janal MN, Nayak S, Schwartz JE, Gallagher RM. Familial aggregation of depression in fibromyalgia: a community-based test of alternate hypotheses. *Pain*. 2004;110(1–2):449-460.
36. Arnold LM, Hudson JI, Hess EV, et al. Family study of fibromyalgia. *Arthritis Rheum*. 2004;50(3):944-952.
37. Russell IJ, Michalek JE, Vipraio GA, Fletcher EM, Javors MA, Bowden CA. Platelet 3H-imipramine uptake receptor density and serum serotonin levels in patients with fibromyalgia/fibrositis syndrome. *J Rheumatol*. 1992;19(1):104-109.
38. Russell IJ, Vaeroy H, Javors M, Nyberg F. Cerebrospinal fluid biogenic amine metabolites in fibromyalgia/fibrositis syndrome and rheumatoid arthritis. *Arthritis Rheum*. 1992;35(5):550-556.
39. Yunus MB, Dailey JW, Aldag JC, Masi AT, Jobe PC. Plasma and urinary catecholamines in primary fibromyalgia: a controlled study. *J Rheumatol*. 1992;19(1):95-97.
40. Schwarz MJ, Spath M, Müller-Bardorff H, Pongratz DE, Bondy B, Ackenheil M. Relationship of substance P, 5-hydroxyindole acetic acid and tryptophan in serum of fibromyalgia patients. *Neurosci Lett*. 1999;259(3):196-198.
41. Charney DS. Monoamine dysfunction and the pathophysiology and treatment of depression. *J Clin Psychiatry*. 1998;59(Suppl 14):11-14.
42. Hirschfeld RM. History and evolution of the monoamine hypothesis of depression. *J Clin Psychiatry*. 2000;61(Suppl 6):4-6.
43. Bondy B, Spaeth M, Offenbaecher M, et al. The T102C polymorphism of the 5-HT2A-receptor gene in fibromyalgia. *Neurobiol Dis*. 1999; 6(5):433-439.
44. Cohen H, Buskila D, Neumann L, Ebstein RP. Confirmation of an association between fibromyalgia and serotonin transporter promoter region (5-HTTLPR) polymorphism, and relationship to anxiety-related personality traits. *Arthritis Rheum*. 2002;46(3):845-847.
45. Gursoy S. Absence of association of the serotonin transporter gene polymorphism with the mentally healthy subset of fibromyalgia patients. *Clin Rheumatol*. 2002;21(3):194-197.
46. Offenbaecher M, Bondy B, de Jonge S, et al. Possible association of fibromyalgia with a polymorphism in the serotonin transporter gene regulatory region. *Arthritis Rheum*. 1999;42(11):2482-2488.
47. Arnold LM, Fan J, Russell IJ, et al. The fibromyalgia family study: a genome-wide linkage scan study. *Arthritis Rheum*. 2013;65(4):1122-1128.
48. D'Agnelli S, Arendt-Nielsen L, Gerra MC, et al. Fibroymalgia: genetics and epigenetics insights may provide the basis for the development of diagnostic biomarkers. *Molecular Pain*. 2019;15(1):1-12.
49. Kendler KS, Kessler RC, Neale MC, Heath AC, Eaves LJ. The prediction of major depression in women: toward an integrated etiologic model. *Am J Psychiatry*. 1993;150(8):1139-1148.
50. Riso LP, Miyatake RK, Thase ME. The search for determinants of chronic depression: a review of six factors. *J Affect Disord*. 2002;70(2):103-115.
51. Shrout PE, Link BG, Dohrenwend BP, Skodol AE, Stueve A, Mirotznik J. Characterizing life events as risk factors for depression: the role of fateful loss events. *J Abnorm Psychol*. 1989;98(4):460-467.
52. Tennant C. Life events, stress and depression: a review of recent findings. *Aust N Z J Psychiatry*. 2002;36(2):173-182.
53. Raphael KG, Natelson BH, Janal MN, Nayak S. A community-based survey of fibromyalgia-like pain complaints following the World Trade Center terrorist attacks. *Pain*. 2002;100(1-2):131-139.
54. Davis MC, Zautra AJ, Reich JW. Vulnerability to stress among women in chronic pain from fibromyalgia and osteoarthritis. *Ann Behav Med*. 2001;23(3):215-226.
55. Caspi A, Sugden K, Moffitt TE, et al. Influence of life stress on depression: moderation by a polymorphism in the 5-HTT gene. *Science*. 2003;301(5631):386-389.
56. von Knorring L, Perris C, Eisemann M, Eriksson U, Perris H. Pain as a symptom in depressive disorders. II. Relationship to personality traits as assessed by means of KSP. *Pain*. 1983;17(4):377-384.
57. Aguera-Ortiz L, Failde I, Mico JA, Cervilla J, Lopez-Ibor JJ. Pain as a symptom of depression: prevalence and clinical correlates in patients attending psychiatric clinics. *J Affect Disord*. 2011;130(1):106-112.
58. Bair MJ, Robinson RL, Katon W, Kroenke K. Depression and pain comorbidity: a literature review. *Arch Int Med*. 2003;163(20):2433-2445.
59. Williams LS, Jones WJ, Shen J, Robinson RL, Weinberger M, Kroenke K. Prevalence and impact of depression and pain in neurology outpatients. *J Neurol Neurosurg Psychiatry*. 2003;74(11):1587-1589.
60. Sheng J, Liu S, Wang Y, Cui R, Zhang X. The link between depression and chronic pain: neural mechanisms in the brain. *Neural Plast*. 2017;2017:9724371.
61. Meerwijk EL, Ford JM, Weiss SJ. Brain regions associated with psychological pain: implications for a neural network and its relationship to physical pain. *Brain Imaging Behav*. 2013;7:1-14.
62. Doan L, Manders T, Wang J. Neuroplasticity underlying the comorbidity of pain and depression. *Neural Plast*. 2015;2015:504691.
63. Kiecolt-Glase JK, Derry HM, Fagundes CP. Inflammation: depression fans the flames and feasts on the heat. *Am J Psychiatry*. 2015; 172(11):1075-1091.

64. Moseley GL. Is successful rehabilitation of complex regional pain syndrome due to sustained attention to the affected limb? A randomised clinical trial. *Pain*. 2005;114(1-2):54-61.
65. Bremner JD, Vythilingam M, Vermetten E, et al. MRI and PET study of deficits in hippocampal structure and function in women with childhood sexual abuse and posttraumatic stress disorder. *Am J Psychiatry*. 2003;160(5):924-932.
66. Lindauer RJ, Vlieger EJ, Jalink M, et al. Smaller hippocampal volume in Dutch police officers with posttraumatic stress disorder. *Biol Psychiatry*. 2004;56(5):356-363.
67. Hedges DW, Farrer TJ, Brown BL. Association between C-reactive protein and cognitive deficits in elderly men and women: a meta-analysis. *Int Psychogeriatr*. 2012;24(9):1387-1392.
68. Hadjikhani N, de Gelder B. Seeing fearful body expressions activates the fusiform cortex and amygdala. *Curr Biol*. 2003;13(24):2201-2205.
69. Hariri AR, Mattay VS, Tessitore A, Fera F, Weinberger DR. Neocortical modulation of the amygdala response to fearful stimuli. *Biol Psychiatry*. 2003;53(6):494-501.
70. Morris JS, Dolan RJ. Dissociable amygdala and orbitofrontal responses during reversal fear conditioning. *Neuroimage*. 2004; 22(1):372-380.
71. Peek AL, Leaver AM, Foster S, et al. Increased GABA+ in people with migraine, headache, and pain conditions- a potential marker of pain. *J Pain*. 2021;22(12):1631-1645.
72. Grachev ID, Fredrickson BE, Apkarian AV. Brain chemistry reflects dual states of pain and anxiety in chronic low back pain. *J Neural Transm*. 2002;109(10):1309-1334.
73. Baliki MN, Apkarian AV. Nociception, pain, negative moods, and behavior selection. *Neuron*. 2015;87(3):474-491.
74. Taricco M, Pagliacci MC, Telaro E, Adone R. Pharmacological interventions for spasticity following spinal cord injury: results of a Cochrane systematic review. *Eura Medicophys*. 2006;42(1):5-15.
75. Bahn EL, Holt KR. Procedural sedation and analgesia: a review and new concepts. *Emerg Med Clin North Am*. 2005;23(2):503-517.
76. Mazurek MS. Sedation and analgesia for procedures outside the operating room. *Semin Pediatr Surg*. 2004;13(3):166-173.
77. Devane WA, Hanus L, Breuer A, et al. Isolation and structure of a brain constituent that binds to the cannabinoid receptor. *Science*. 1992;258(5090):1946-1949.
78. Herkenham M. In: Pertwee RG, ed. *Cannabinoid Receptors*. Academic Press; 1995:145-166.
79. Matsuda LA, Lolait SJ, Brownstein MJ, Young AC, Bonner TI. Structure of a cannabinoid receptor and functional expression of the cloned cDNA. *Nature*. 1990;346(6284):561-564.
80. Milligan AL, Szabo-Pardi TA, Burton MD. Cannabinoid receptor type 1 and its role as an analgesic: an opioid alternative? *J Dual Diagn*. 2020;16(1):106-119.
81. Mao J, Price DD, Lu J, Keniston L, Mayer DJ. Two distinctive antinociceptive systems in rats with pathological pain. *Neurosci Lett*. 2000;280(1):13-16.
82. Palazzo E, Marabese I, de Novellis V, et al. Metabotropic and NMDA glutamate receptors participate in the cannabinoid-induced antinociception. *Neuropharmacology*. 2001;40(3):319-326.
83. Palazzo E, de Novellis V, Marabese I, Rossi F, Maione S. Metabotropic glutamate and cannabinoid receptor crosstalk in periaqueductal grey pain processing. *Curr Neuropharmacol*. 2006;4(3):225-231.
84. Rog DJ, Nurmikko TJ, Young CA. Oromucosal delta9-tetrahydrocannabinol/cannabidiol for neuropathic pain associated with multiple sclerosis: an uncontrolled, open-label, 2-year extension trial. *Clin Ther*. 2007;29(9):2068-2079.
85. Wade DT, Makela P, Robson P, House H, Bateman C. Do cannabis-based medicinal extracts have general or specific effects on symptoms in multiple sclerosis? A double-blind, randomized, placebo-controlled study on 160 patients. *Mult Scler*. 2004;10(4):434-441.
86. Hosking RD, Zajicek JP. Therapeutic potential of cannabis in pain medicine. *Br J Anaesth*. 2008;101(1):59-68.
87. Stevens AJ, Higgins MD. A systematic review of the analgesic efficacy of cannabinoid medications in the management of acute pain. *Acta Anaesthesiol Scand*. 2017;61(3):268-280. doi:10.1111/aas.12851
88. Walitt B, Klose P, Fitzcharles MA, Phillips T, Häuser W. Cannabinoids for fibromyalgia. *Cochrane Database Syst Rev*. 2016;7:CD011694. doi:10.1002/14651858.CD011694.pub2
89. Fitzcharles MA, Häuser W. Cannabinoids in the management of musculoskeletal or rheumatic diseases. *Curr Rheumatol Rep*. 2016;18(12):76.
90. Tateo S. State of the evidence: cannabinoids and cancer pain-a systematic review. *J Am Assoc Nurse Pract*. 2017;29(2):94-103. doi:10.1002/2327-6924.12422
91. Tsang CC, Giudice MG. Nabilone for the management of pain. *Pharmacotherapy*. 2016;36(3):273-286. doi:10.1002/phar.1709
92. van den Beuken-van Everdingen MH, de Graeff A, et al. Pharmacological treatment of pain in cancer patients: the role of adjuvant analgesics, a systematic review. *Pain Pract*. 2017;17:409-419. doi:10.1111/papr.12459
93. Deng Y, Luo L, Hu Y, Fang K, Liu J. Clinical practice guidelines for the management of neuropathic pain: a systematic review. *BMC Anesthesiol*. 2016;16:12. doi:10.1186/s12871-015-0150-5
94. Beaulieu P, Boulanger A, Desroches J, Clark AJ. Medical cannabis: considerations for the anesthesiologist and pain physician. *Can J Anaesth*. 2016;63(5):608-624. doi:10.1007/s12630-016-0598-x
95. Schuckit MA. Comorbidity between substance use disorders and psychiatric conditions. *Addiction*. 2006;101(Suppl 1):76-88.
96. Krebs EE, Gaynes BN, Gartlehner G, et al. Treating the physical symptoms of depression with second-generation antidepressants: a systematic review and metaanalysis. *Psychosomatics*. 2008;49(3):191-198.
97. Koob GF. A role for brain stress systems in addiction. *Neuron*. 2008;59(1):11-34.
98. Compton MA. Cold-pressor pain tolerance in opiate and cocaine abusers: correlates of drug type and use status. *J Pain Symptom Manage*. 1994;9(7):462-473.
99. Nestler EJ. Neurobiology. Total recall-the memory of addiction. *Science*. 2001;292(5525):2266-2267.
100. Koob GF, Volkow ND. Neurocircuitry of addiction. *Neuropsychopharmacology*. 2010;35:217-238.
101. Martikainen IK, Nuechterlein EB, Peciña M, et al. Chronic back pain is associated with alterations in dopamine neurotransmission in the ventral striatum. *J Neurosci*. 2015;35(27):9957-9965. doi:10.1523/JNEUROSCI.4605-14.2015
102. LeBlanc DM, McGinn MA, Itoga CA, Edwards S. The affective dimension of pain as a risk factor for drug and alcohol addiction. *Alcohol*. 2015;49(8):803-809. doi:10.1016/j.alcohol.2015.04.005
103. Borsook D, Linnman C, Faria V, Strassman AM, Becerra L, Elman I. Reward deficiency and anti-reward in pain chronification. *Neurosci Biobehav Rev*. 2016;68:282-297. doi:10.1016/j.neubiorev.2016.05.033
104. Becker S, Ghandi W, Schweinhardt P. Cerebral interactions of pain and reward and their relevance for chronic pain. *Neurosci Lett*. 2012;520:182-187.
105. Rosen LG, Sun N, Rushlow W, Laviolette SR. Molecular and neuronal plasticity mechanisms in the amygdala-prefrontal cortical circuit: implications for opiate addiction memory formation. *Front Neurosci*. 2015;9:399. doi:10.3389/fnins.2015.00399
106. Elman I, Boorsock D, Volkow ND. Pain and suicidality: insights from reward and addiction neuroscience. *Prog Neurobiol*. 2013;109:1-27.
107. Otton SV, Schadel M, Cheung SW, Kaplan HL, Busto UE, Sellers EM. CYP2D6 phenotype determines the metabolic conversion of hydrocodone to hydromorphone. *Clin Pharmacol Ther*. 1993; 54(5):463-472.
108. Oertel B, Lotsch J. Genetic mutations that prevent pain: implications for future pain medication. *Pharmacogenomics*. 2008;9(2):179-194.
109. Stamer UM, Stuber F. Genetic factors in pain and its treatment. *Curr Opin Anaesthesiol*. 2007;20(5):478-484.
110. Flores CM, Mogil JS. The pharmacogenetics of analgesia: toward a genetically-based approach to pain management. *Pharmacogenomics*. 2001;2(3):177-194.

111. Mayer P, Hollt V. Pharmacogenetics of opioid receptors and addiction. *Pharmacogenet Genomics*. 2006;16(1):1-7.
112. Lotsch J, Geisslinger G. Relevance of frequent mu-opioid receptor polymorphisms for opioid activity in healthy volunteers. *Pharmacogenomics J*. 2006;6(3):200-210.
113. Caterina MJ, Leffler A, Malmberg AB, et al. Impaired nociception and pain sensation in mice lacking the capsaicin receptor. *Science*. 2000;288(5464):306-313.
114. McKemy DD, Neuhausser WM, Julius D. Identification of a cold receptor reveals a general role for TRP channels in thermosensation. *Nature*. 2002;416(6876):52-58.
115. Mogil JS, Ritchie J, Smith SB, et al. Melanocortin-1 receptor gene variants affect pain and mu-opioid analgesia in mice and humans. *J Med Genet*. 2005;42(7):583-587.
116. Pandey SC, Kyzar E, Zhang H. Epigenetic basis of the dark side of alcohol addiction. *Neuropharmacology*. 2017;122:74-84. doi:10.1016/j.neuropharm.2017.02.002
117. Cadet JL, McCoy MT, Jayanthi S. Epigenetics and addiction. *Clin Pharmacol Ther*. 2016;99(5):502-511. doi:10.1002/cpt.345
118. Cecil CA, Walton E, Viding E. Epigenetics of addiction: current knowledge, challenges, and future directions. *J Stud Alcohol Drugs*. 2016;77(5):688-691.
119. Liang L, Lutz BM, Bekker A, Tao YX. Epigenetic regulation of chronic pain. *Epigenomics*. 2015;7(2):235-245. doi:10.2217/epi.14.75
120. Descalzi G, Ikegami D, Ushijima T, Nestler EJ, Zachariou V, Narita M. Epigenetic mechanisms of chronic pain. *Trends Neurosci*. 2015;38(4):237-246. doi:10.1016/j.tins.2015.02.001
121. Gerra MC, Dallabona C, Arendt-Nielsen L. Epigenetic alterations in prescription opioid misuse: new strategies for precision pain management. *Genes (Basel)*. 2021;12(8):1226.
122. Chu LF, Angst MS, Clark D. Opioid-induced hyperalgesia in humans: molecular mechanisms and clinical considerations. *Clin J Pain*. 2008;24(6):479-496.
123. Kim DH, Fields HL, Barbaro NM. Morphine analgesia and acute physical dependence: rapid onset of two opposing, dose-related processes. *Brain Res*. 1990;516(1):37-40.
124. Compton P, Athanasos P, Elashoff D. Withdrawal hyperalgesia after acute opioid physical dependence in nonaddicted humans: a preliminary study. *J Pain*. 2003;4:511-519.
125. Compton P, Charuvastra VC, Ling W. Pain intolerance in opioid-maintained former opiate addicts: effect of long-acting maintenance agent. *Drug Alcohol Depend*. 2001;63(2):139-146.
126. Ren Z-Y, Shi J, Epstein DH, et al. Abnormal pain response in pain sensitive opiate addicts after prolonged abstinence predicts increased drug craving. *Psychopharmacology (Berl)*. 2009;204:423-429.
127. Colpaert FC. Mechanisms of opioid-induced pain and antinociceptive tolerance: signal transduction. *Pain*. 2002;95(3):287-288.
128. Célèrier E, Laulin JP, Corcuff JB, Le Moal M, Simonnet G. Progressive enhancement of delayed hyperalgesia induced by repeated heroin administration: a sensitization process. *J Neurosci*. 2001;21(11):4074-4080.
129. Müller-Lissner S, Bassotti G, Coffin B, et al. Opioid-induced constipation and bowel dysfunction: a clinical guideline. *Pain Med*. 2017;18:1837-1863. doi:10.1093/pm/pnw255
130. Mao J, Price DD, Mayer DJ. Mechanisms of hyperalgesia and morphine tolerance: a current view of their possible interactions. *Pain*. 1995;62(3):259-274.
131. Martin JE, Inglis J. Pain tolerance and narcotic addiction. *Br J Soc Clin Psychol*. 1965;4(3):224-229.
132. Dogrul A, Bilsky EJ, Ossipov MH, Lai J, Porreca F. Spinal L-type calcium channel blockade abolishes opioid-induced sensory hypersensitivity and antinociceptive tolerance. *Anesth Analg*. 2005;101(6):1730-1735.
133. Gardell LR, Wang R, Burgess SE, et al. Sustained morphine exposure induces a spinal dynorphin-dependent enhancement of excitatory transmitter release from primary afferent fibers. *J Neurosci*. 2002;22(15):6747-6755.
134. King T, Gardell LR, Wang R, et al. Role of NK-1 neurotransmission in opioid-induced hyperalgesia. *Pain*. 2005;116(3):276-288.
135. Lim G, Wang S, Zeng Q, Sung B, Mao J. Evidence for a long-term influence on morphine tolerance after previous morphine exposure: role of neuronal glucocorticoid receptors. *Pain*. 2005;114(1-2):81-92.
136. Vanderah TW, Gardell LR, Burgess SE, et al. Dynorphin promotes abnormal pain and spinal opioid antinociceptive tolerance. *J Neurosci*. 2000;20(18):7074-7079.
137. Vanderah TW, Suenaga NM, Ossipov MH, Malan TP Jr, Lai J, Porreca F. Tonic descending facilitation from the rostral ventromedial medulla mediates opioid-induced abnormal pain and antinociceptive tolerance. *J Neurosci*. 2001;21(1):279-286.
138. Gardell LR, King T, Ossipov MH, et al. Opioid receptor-mediated hyperalgesia and antinociceptive tolerance induced by sustained opiate delivery. *Neurosci Lett*. 2006;396(1):44-49.
139. Larcher A, Laulin JP, Celerier E, Le Moal M, Simonnet G. Acute tolerance associated with a single opiate administration: involvement of *N*-methyl-d-aspartate-dependent pain facilitatory systems. *Neuroscience*. 1998;84(2):583-589.
140. Richebe P, Rivat C, Creton C, et al. Nitrous oxide revisited: evidence for potent antihyperalgesic properties. *Anesthesiology*. 2005;103(4):845-854.
141. Price DD, Mayer DJ, Mao J, Caruso FS. NMDA-receptor antagonists and opioid receptor interactions as related to analgesia and tolerance. *J Pain Symptom Manage*. 2000;19(1 Suppl):S7-S11.
142. Weinbroum AA, Rudick V, Paret G, Ben-Abraham R. The role of dextromethorphan in pain control. *Can J Anaesth*. 2000;47(6):585-596.
143. Bisaga A, Popik P. In search of a new pharmacological treatment for drug and alcohol addiction: *N*-methyl-d-aspartate (NMDA) antagonists. *Drug Alcohol Depend*. 2000;59(1):1-15.
144. Elliott K, Hynansky A, Inturrisi CE. Dextromethorphan attenuates and reverses analgesic tolerance to morphine. *Pain*. 1994;59(3):361-368.
145. Pasternak GW, Kolesnikov YA, Babey AM. Perspectives on the *N*-methyl-D-aspartate/nitric oxide cascade and opioid tolerance. *Neuropsychopharmacology*. 1995;13(4):309-313.
146. Trujillo KA. Effects of noncompetitive *N*-methyl-d-aspartate receptor antagonists on opiate tolerance and physical dependence. *Neuropsychopharmacology*. 1995;13(4):301-307.
147. Compton PA, Ling W, Torrington MA. Lack of effect of chronic dextromethorphan on experimental pain tolerance in methadone-maintained patients. *Addict Biol*. 2008;13(3-4):393-402.
148. Xie JY, Herman DS, Stiller CO, et al. Cholecystokinin in the rostral ventromedial medulla mediates opioid-induced hyperalgesia and antinociceptive tolerance. *J Neurosci*. 2005;25(2):409-416.
149. Ossipov MH, Lai J, King T, et al. Antinociceptive and nociceptive actions of opioids. *J Neurobiol*. 2004;61(1):126-148.
150. DeLeo JA, Tanga FY, Tawfik VL. Neuroimmune activation and neuroinflammation in chronic pain and opioid tolerance/hyperalgesia. *Neuroscientist*. 2004;10(1):40-52.
151. Watkins LR, Maier SF. The pain of being sick: implications of immune-to-brain communication for understanding pain. *Annu Rev Psychol*. 2000;51:29-57.
152. Wieseler-Frank J, Maier SF, Watkins LR. Immune-to-brain communication dynamically modulates pain: physiological and pathological consequences. *Brain Behav Immun*. 2005;19(2):104-111.
153. Song P, Zhao ZQ. The involvement of glial cells in the development of morphine tolerance. *Neurosci Res*. 2001;39(3):281-286.
154. Johnston IN, Westbrook RF. Inhibition of morphine analgesia by LPS: role of opioid and NMDA receptors and spinal glia. *Behav Brain Res*. 2005;156(1):75-83.
155. Johnston IN, Milligan ED, Wieseler-Frank J, et al. A role for proinflammatory cytokines and fractalkine in analgesia, tolerance, and subsequent pain facilitation induced by chronic intrathecal morphine. *J Neurosci*. 2004;24(33):7353-7365.
156. Hendrie CA. Naloxone-sensitive hyperalgesia follows analgesia induced by morphine and environmental stimulation. *Pharmacol Biochem Behav*. 1989;32(4):961-966.
157. McNally GP. Pain facilitatory circuits in the mammalian central nervous system: their behavioral significance and role in morphine analgesic tolerance. *Neurosci Biobehav Rev*. 1999;23(8):1059-1078.

158. Krank MD, Hinson RE, Siegel S. Conditional hyperalgesia is elicited by environmental signals of morphine. *Behav Neural Biol.* 1981;32(2):148-157.
159. Siegel S, Hinson RE, Krank MD. The role of predrug signals in morphine analgesic tolerance: support for a Pavlovian conditioning model of tolerance. *J Exp Psychol Anim Behav Process.* 1978;4(2):188-196.
160. Ho A, Dole VP. Pain perception in drug-free and in methadone-maintained human ex-addicts. *Proc Soc Exp Biol Med.* 1979;162(3): 392-395.
161. Doverty M, White JM, Somogyi AA, Bochner F, Ali R, Ling W. Hyperalgesic responses in methadone maintenance patients. *Pain.* 2001;90(1–2):91-96.
162. Schall U, Katta T, Pries E, Klöppel A, Gastpar M. Pain perception of intravenous heroin users on maintenance therapy with levomethadone. *Pharmacopsychiatry.* 1996;29(5):176-179.
163. Athanasos P, Smith CS, White JM, Somogyi AA, Bochner F, Ling W. Methadone maintenance patients are cross-tolerant to the antinociceptive effects of very high plasma morphine concentrations. *Pain.* 2006;120(3):267-275.
164. Pud D, Cohen D, Lawental E, Eisenberg E. Opioids and abnormal pain perception: new evidence from a study of chronic opioid addicts and healthy subjects. *Drug Alcohol Depend.* 2006;82(3):218-223.
165. Carcoba LM, Contreras AE, Cepeda-Benito A, Meagher MW. Negative affect heightens opiate withdrawal-induced hyperalgesia in heroin dependent individuals. *J Addict Dis.* 2011;30(3):258-270.
166. Liebmann PM, Lehofer M, Moser M, et al. Persistent analgesia in former opiate addicts is resistant to blockade of endogenous opioids. *Biol Psychiatry.* 1997;42(10):962-964.
167. Prosser JM, Steinfeld M, Cohen LJ, et al. Abnormal heat and pain perception in remitted heroin dependence months after detoxification from methadone-maintenance. *Drug Alcohol Depend.* 2008;95(3):237-244.
168. Treister R, Eisenberg E, Lawental E, Pud D. Is opioid-induced hyperalgesia reversible? A study on active and former opioid addicts and drug naïve controls. *J Opioid Manag.* 2012;8(6):343-349. doi:10.5055/jom.2012.0134
169. Chia YY, Liu K, Wang JJ, Kuo MC, Ho ST. Intraoperative high dose fentanyl induces postoperative fentanyl tolerance. *Can J Anaesth.* 1999;46(9):872-877.
170. Fletcher D, Martinez V. How can we prevent opioid induced hyperalgesia in surgical patients? *Br J Anaesth.* 2016;116(4):447-449. doi:10.1093/bja/aew050
171. Fletcher D, Martinez V. Opioid-induced hyperalgesia in patients after surgery: a systematic review and a meta-analysis. *Br J Anaesth.* 2014;112(6):991-1004. doi:10.1093/bja/aeu137
172. Angst MS. Intraoperative use of remifentanil for TIVA: postoperative pain, acute tolerance, and opioid-induced hyperalgesia. *J Cardiothorac Vasc Anesth.* 2015;29(Suppl 1):S16-S22. doi:10.1053/j.jvca.2015.01.026
173. Lyons PJ, Rivosecchi RM, Nery JP, Kane-Gill SL. Fentanyl-induced hyperalgesia in acute pain management. *J Pain Palliat Care Pharmacother.* 2015;29(2):153-160. doi:10.3109/15360288.2015.1035835
174. Richebé P, Pouquet O, Jelacic S, et al. Target-controlled dosing of remifentanil during cardiac surgery reduces postoperative hyperalgesia. *J Cardiothorac Vasc Anesth.* 2011;25(6):917-925. doi:10.1053/j.jvca.2011.03.185
175. Leal PC, Salomão R, Brunialti MK, Sakata RK. Evaluation of the effect of ketamine on remifentanil-induced hyperalgesia: a double-blind, randomized study. *J Clin Anesth.* 2015;27(4):331-337. doi:10.1016/j.jclinane.2015.02.002
176. Loftus RW, Yeager MP, Clark JA. Intraoperative ketamine reduces perioperative opiate consumption in opiate-dependent patients with chronic back pain undergoing back surgery. *Anesthesiology.* 2010;113(3):639-646. doi:10.1097/ALN.0b013e3181e90914
177. Tverskoy M, Oz Y, Isakson A, Finger J, Bradley EL Jr, Kissin I. Preemptive effect of fentanyl and ketamine on postoperative pain and wound hyperalgesia. *Anesth Analg.* 1994;78(2):205-209.
178. Song JW, Lee YW, Yoon KB, Park SJ, Shim YH. Magnesium sulfate prevents remifentanil-induced postoperative hyperalgesia in patients undergoing thyroidectomy. *Anesth Analg.* 2011;113(2):390-397. doi:10.1213/ANE.0b013e31821d72bc
179. Lee C, Kim YD, Kim JN. Antihyperalgesic effects of dexmedetomidine on high-dose remifentanil-induced hyperalgesia. *Korean J Anesthesiol.* 2013;64(4):301-307. doi:10.4097/kjae.2013.64.4.301
180. Lee C, Lee HW, Kim JN. Effect of oral pregabalin on opioid-induced hyperalgesia in patients undergoing laparo-endoscopic single-site urologic surgery. *Korean J Anesthesiol.* 2013;64(1):19-24. doi:10.4097/kjae.2013.64.1.19
181. Kaye AD, Chung KS, Vadivelu N, Cantemir C, Urman RD, Manchikanti L. Opioid induced hyperalgesia altered with propofol infusion. *Pain Physician.* 2014;17(2):E225-E228.
182. Ali NM. Hyperalgesic response in a patient receiving high concentrations of spinal morphine. *Anesthesiology.* 1986;65(4):449.
183. Mercadante S, Ferrera P, Villari P, Arcuri E. Hyperalgesia: an emerging iatrogenic syndrome. *J Pain Symptom Manage.* 2003;26(2):769-775.
184. Mercadante S, Arcuri E. Hyperalgesia and opioid switching. *Am J Hosp Palliat Care.* 2005;22(4):291-294.
185. Sjøgren P, Jonsson T, Jensen NH, Drenck NE, Jensen TS. Hyperalgesia and myoclonus in terminal cancer patients treated with continuous intravenous morphine. *Pain.* 1993;55(1):93-97.
186. Okon TR, George ML. Fentanyl-induced neurotoxicity and paradoxic pain. *J Pain Symptom Manage.* 2008;35(3):327-333.
187. Devulder J. Hyperalgesia induced by high-dose intrathecal sufentanil in neuropathic pain. *J Neurosurg Anesthesiol.* 1997;9(2):146-148.
188. Kest B, Hopkins E, Palmese CA, Adler M, Mogil JS. Genetic variation in morphine analgesic tolerance: a survey of 11 inbred mouse strains. *Pharmacol Biochem Behav.* 2002;73(4):821-828.
189. Kest B, Palmese CA, Hopkins E, Adler M, Juni A, Mogil JS. Naloxone-precipitated withdrawal jumping in 11 inbred mouse strains: evidence for common genetic mechanisms in acute and chronic morphine physical dependence. *Neuroscience.* 2002;115(2):463-469.

CHAPTER

109 Psychological Issues in the Management of Pain

Martin D. Cheatle

CHAPTER OUTLINE

- Introduction
- Mind-body connection
- Psychological modulation of pain
- Pain and common co-occurring psychological issues
- Psychological processes of pain
- Classification of pain syndromes
- The role of the environment
- Developmental issues
- Assessing co-occurring psychological and substance use disorders
- Biopsychosocial approach to the treatment of pain
- Conclusions

INTRODUCTION

Chronic pain remains a significant health care problem. Population-based estimates of the prevalence of chronic pain in U.S. adults ranges from 11% to 40%[1] with variation in subgroups. A more granular assessment of chronic pain revealed that 20.4 % (50 million) of the U.S. adult population prevalence endorse having experienced chronic pain and 8% (19.6 million) noted high-impact chronic pain defined as pain causing major limitations in life domains (work, avocations, social, self-care).[2] Later estimates revealed that 4.3% of U.S. adults experience high-impact chronic pain, associated with more severe pain, more severe mental health and cognitive impairment than those with chronic pain without disability, and have a have greater likelihood of disability than those with stroke or kidney failure.[3] Individuals most affected by both chronic pain and high-impact chronic pain are women, older adults, unemployed adults, adults living in poverty, adults with public health insurance, and adults living in rural areas.[2] Chronic pain not only causes individual suffering and disability but also affects the patient's family and society. The National Academy of Medicine (NAM, formerly the Institute of Medicine) 2011 report "Relieving pain in America: A blueprint for transforming prevention, care, education and research"[4] estimated the annual cost of chronic pain in the United States to be between $560 and $600 billion dollars, including health care costs ($261-$300 billion) and lost productivity ($297-$336 billion). Medications for chronic pain management alone has been estimated to cost 17.8 billion dollars annually.[5]

The NAM report emphasized that the chronic pain experience is complicated and multifaceted, stating, "We believe pain arises in the nervous system but represents a complex and evolving interplay of biological, behavioral, environmental, and societal factors." Commonly, patients with chronic pain have multiple medical and psychiatric co-occurring conditions. It has been estimated that 40 to 60% of patients with chronic pain experience major depression[6,7]; 35% any anxiety disorder[8]; 9% to 10% posttraumatic stress disorder[9]; greater than 50% experience sleep disturbance[10] and 8 to 10% develop opioid use disorder.[11] In this chapter psychological factors in the development and maintenance of the pain experience will be discussed as well as assessment and treatment strategies. While this chapter addresses primarily chronic noncancer pain (CNCP), many of the principles discussed may be applicable in acute, subacute, and cancer related pain as well.

MIND-BODY CONNECTION

Cartesian dualism, mostly associated with the philosophy of Rene Descartes, suggested that the mind (mental function) and the body are distinct, separate entities, and therefore, one can exist without the other. Although there is a robust literature on the effect of the mind-body connection in maintaining health or contributing to the development of illnesses, in many ways, the current medical methodology including pain management still practices this dualistic approach. There are many examples of the strong influence of an individual's emotional state, social milieu, and attitudes on physical symptoms and disability. The tendency to separate the mind from the body, the psychological from the so-called organic, does not allow the clinician to fully understand the person's pain experience and also leads to biases in diagnosing and treating the whole person leading to poorer outcomes. In spite of the incredible advances in diagnostic imaging, pharmacotherapy, pharmacogenetics, and refinement in surgical interventions, the number of individuals suffering and becoming disabled from chronic pain grows each year. This is the result in part from our failure to adequately address the psychological aspects of CNCP and the focus of our health care system on the organic pathology rather than the person. This is in the face of compelling evidence that psychosocial variables predict onset, chronicity, and outcomes in back pain (one of the most prevalent pain conditions) more than do somatic variables. These influences frequently supersede existing tissue damage in determining the experience of the person who has pain. As noted, pain is complex and influenced by biological, psychological, motivational, cultural and social factors that cannot be assessed or managed by a traditional biomedical approach.

For example, in a 4-year prospective study of 3,020 aircraft workers, job dissatisfaction and poor performance appraisals strongly predicted reports of acute back pain at work.[12] Subjects who "hardly ever" enjoyed their jobs were more than twice as likely to report a back injury as were those who "almost always" enjoyed their work. Another prospective study of 1,412 pain-free employees confirmed that those dissatisfied with their work were twice as likely to seek care for low back pain (LBP) during a 12-month period as those who were satisfied, while those who felt underpaid were nearly four times as likely, and those in the lowest socioeconomic stratum were almost five times as likely to seek care for LBP.[13] A systematic review evaluated the role of psychological factors in the transition to chronic low back pain and found that emotional distress, depressive mood, and somatization were predictors of developing chronic low back pain.[14] One of the most common and preventable forms of chronic pain is chronic postsurgical pain (CPSP). The International Association for the Study of Pain defines CPSP as pain that develops or increases in intensity after a surgical procedure, persists beyond the tissue healing process (>3 months), and is localized to the surgical field or innervation territory of nerve located in surgical field. Certain surgeries put patients at higher risk for developing CPSP, such as thoracotomy, mastectomy, abdominal and orthopedic surgeries, such as total joint arthroplasties. Preoperative risk factors include symptoms of psychological distress in particular depression, anxiety, or pain catastrophizing, which can be conceptualized as magnified, exaggerated negative focus on pain.[15-17]

These studies underscore that the traditional biomedical approach to pain care is inadequate in assessing important psychosocial and neurobehavioral mechanisms such as anxiety, depression, kinesiophobia (defined as an irrational fear that movement or activity will lead to reinjury or heightened pain), and catastrophizing that are common in patients with pain and can modify the manifestation and maintenance of pain.

This chapter will discuss key psychological factors that can significantly affect the individual's pain experience and pain-related functional impairment and outline evidenced-based treatments demonstrated to be efficacious in improving functionality and mood.

PSYCHOLOGICAL MODULATION OF PAIN

Relationship Between Emotions and Pain

Patients with CNCP often are not provided a plausible explanatory medical diagnosis. This can foster a sense of being discounted and vilified leaving the patient feeling that their pain experience is purely psychological or "the pain is only in my head." This not only erodes the clinician-patient therapeutic relationship but also can facilitate poor adherence to possibly beneficial prescribed therapies. Historically, clinicians have been trained in the biomedical, linear approach to health care: eliciting symptoms, assigning a diagnosis, and prescribing a treatment. This linear approach can erroneously lead clinicians either to doubt the reality of the symptoms or to assume that they were caused psychologically if there is no identified organic pathology or specific biomarker. While it has been well documented that beliefs, fears, expectations, and affect can both exacerbate and reduce the pain experience, this should not be taken as evidence that psychological processes are the root cause of the pain.[18]

Pain is primarily a function of the nervous system and, especially in the case of protracted and/or neuropathic pain, may bear little relation to the intensity of peripheral stimulation. The classical single pathway theory of pain as a signal transmitted from the receptor to the cortex is an oversimplification, since it does not incorporate processes such as sensitization, descending inhibition and facilitation of pain, and neuroplastic changes, which fully account for several previously classified idiopathic conditions.[19-21]

A primary example of this misinterpretation is the condition of fibromyalgia. Patients with fibromyalgia present with reports of widespread musculoskeletal pain with diffuse hyperalgesia and/or allodynia with no apparent evidence of initiating trauma or tissue damage and experiencing concomitant other central nervous system (CNS)-mediated symptoms such as sleep disturbance, fatigue, memory problems, and mood disturbance. Fibromyalgia was initially considered a psychiatric or somatic disorder due to the paucity of identifiable organic pathology and the diffuse nature of the pain complaints and related symptoms. Findings from functional neuroimaging studies have supported the theory that fibromyalgia is related to a problem with augmented pain or sensory processing in the CNS and imbalances in levels of neurotransmitters that affect pain and sensory transmission.[22] There is also evidence that individuals with fibromyalgia may have elevated endogenous opioid activity at baseline (ie, already working at full levels and thus cannot increase with new pain stimuli), thus causing high baseline occupancy of opioid receptors, even among opioid naive patients. Cerebrospinal fluid (CSF) of patients with fibromyalgia show higher enkephalins compared to controls. Unlike the opioid system, the serotonergic/noradrenergic system is hypofunctional in these patients with decreased norepinephrine and serotonin metabolites in CSF.[23] This explains the efficacy of medications that raise serotonin and norepinephrine in relieving pain (duloxetine, venlafaxine). There is also evidence of increased levels of substance P and glutamate in CSF of patients with fibromyalgia versus controls,[24,25] which explains why exercise is effective for fibromyalgia as it alters endogenous neurotransmission by increasing antinociceptive neurotransmitters and reducing glutamate.

There has been growing interest in genomics and pain. For example, animal studies have demonstrated genetic vulnerability to developing neuropathic pain,[26] and human studies have identified genetic variations that modify pain perception or opioid responsivity.[27]

This emerging literature on the variability of pain perception and predisposition to developing painful conditions having a strong genetic component should obviate the tendency of clinicians to attribute unexplained pain solely to psychological processes. Unfortunately, core competencies in pain science and practice are lacking in most medical school curriculums. In a study by Fishman et al.,[28] 1,506 random questions from the United States Medical Licensing Examination (USMLE) were reviewed by a panel of pain experts. Results revealed that only 15.4% of the 1,506 USMLE questions reviewed were assessed as being fully or partially related to pain, rather than just mentioning pain but not testing knowledge of its mechanisms and their implications for treatment. The large majority of questions related to pain (88%) focused on assessment rather than safe and effective pain management, or the context of pain.[28] This paucity of basic training in pain medicine to clinicians can perpetuate myths regarding the psychological etiology of poorly defined pain conditions causing additional unneeded suffering.

Emotional Distress

It is very common for patients with CNCP to experience concomitant mood and anxiety symptoms that often do not meet criteria for a psychiatric diagnosis but can nonetheless exacerbate pain and contribute to the individual's suffering. Emotional states can influence pain perception acutely, predict its persistence, and impact treatment response. For example, Berna et al.[29] found that experimentally induced negative (sad) mood states in healthy volunteers led to increased unpleasantness of experimental pain. Imaging with functional MRI demonstrated that this was associated with increased activity in the prefrontal cortex, anterior cingulate, and hippocampus. Those with the largest increase in pain unpleasantness showed the greatest activation of the inferior frontal gyrus and amygdala. Previous studies demonstrated that experimental pain perception was modified by induction of happy or sad moods by short stories, hypnotic induction, and other methods.[30,31] Notably, these changes are not contingent on the person's meeting criteria for a psychiatric diagnosis of depression or anxiety but only on the presence of the mood state.

PAIN AND COMMON CO-OCCURRING PSYCHOLOGICAL ISSUES

In clinical populations, mood and anxiety disorders are common in patients with chronic nonmalignant pain (CNMP). McWilliams et al.[8] employed data from the National Comorbidity Survey to evaluate the associations between CNCP and common mood and anxiety disorders in a sample representative of the general U.S. civilian population. Participants completed the Composite International Diagnostic Interview to establish psychiatric diagnoses. Participants with chronic pain (arthritis) as compared to the general population had a higher prevalence of depression (20.2% versus 9.3%), any anxiety disorder (35.1% versus 18.1%), and PTSD (10.7% versus 3.3%). In another study, a telephone survey of a community sample was conducted and revealed that the prevalence of pain in this cohort was 21.9% and that 35% of these patients with pain reported experiencing concomitant depression.[32]

Bair et al.[6] performed a Medline literature review of mood and anxiety disorders and pain. They found that the prevalence of pain in patients with depression ranged from 15% to 100% with a mean prevalence of 65%. The wide prevalence range could be attributable to modest sample sizes and variable assessments of both pain condition including intensity, location, and also depression. In reviewing the prevalence of major depression in patients identified as having pain, the authors discovered that the prevalence varied based on clinic setting and ranged from 85% in dental clinics specializing in chronic facial pain to 52% in pain clinics, 27% in primary care clinics, and 18% in population-based settings. In a subsequent investigation by Bair et al.,[33] 500 patients with chronic musculoskeletal pain were evaluated for mood and anxiety disorders. Results indicated that 20% of this population had co-occurring depressive disorders, 3% co-occurring anxiety disorders, and 23% had both. Variations in rates often reflect differences in settings, methodology, and criteria, as well as diagnostic ambiguity resulting from the overlap of affective symptoms with those of pain and pain-related sequelae. For example, sleep disturbance due to effects of medications and pain itself, lower energy (anergia) due to insomnia and deconditioning, and lower libido due to medication effects (eg, opioid-induced androgen deficiency) can mimic symptoms of mood disorder leading to misdiagnosis.

Though it is well documented that there is a high prevalence of depression in individuals with CNCP, the underlying mechanism of this relationship is not well understood. There is growing interest in exploring the common biological substrates of depression and pain. Maletic and Raison reviewed evidence supporting a biological relationship between depression, fibromyalgia, and neuropathic pain. These conditions may share genetic vulnerabilities and overlapping neurochemistry and can be triggered or modulated by environmental stressors.[34] Kim et al. found that the brain indoleamine 2,3-dioxygenase 1 (IDO1), a rate-limiting enzyme in tryptophan metabolism, plays a key role. Rats in which chronic pain was produced by inflammatory arthritis developed both depressive behavior and IDO1 upregulation in the hippocampus. In humans, they found elevated plasma IDO1 activity in patients with both pain and depression, and in rats, this was found after induction of "anhedonia" by chronic social stress. *IDO1* gene knockout or pharmacological inhibition of hippocampal IDO1 attenuated both nociceptive and depressive behavior.[35] Rome and Rome[36] coined the term "limbically augmented pain syndrome" to describe a model of pain and affect based on neuroplastic processes in corticolimbic structures linking sensory and affective domains of pain. In this model, exposure to a noxious stimulus can lead to a sensitized corticolimbic state with kindling properties of amplification, neuroanatomic spreading, and cross-sensitization. The advent of more advanced neuroimaging (fMRI, PET) technology will promote more needed research in this area of the biological substrates of the relationship between emotional states and the pain experience.

It has been highly debated which comes first, pain leading to depression or pain being a symptom of depression. There is evidence that each condition can predict the future development of the other[37] and each condition can compromise successful treatment of the other.[38-40] A recent cross-sectional study assessed depression, pain intensity, physical function, and demographics in 102 patients with upper extremity musculoskeletal pain. Results indicated that pain intensity and depression were partial mediators of their respective and independent effects on physical functioning. The authors concluded that there was a bidirectional mediation of pain intensity and depression on their respective effects on physical function.[41]

While depression has been a primary focus of research in pain and co-occurring psychiatric disorders, anxiety is very common in patients with CNCP and is the most prevalent type of psychiatric disorders. For example, McWilliams et al.[32] evaluated survey data from a representative sample of 3,032 U.S. adults. Both medical and psychiatric information was collected in particular diagnoses of depression, panic attacks, and generalized anxiety disorder (GAD) and pain conditions including arthritis, migraine, and back pain. Logistic regression analyses showed statistically significant positive associations between each pain condition and psychiatric disorders (odds ratio [OR] ranged from 1.48 to 3.86). The survey respondents with pain were more likely to have depression (OR 1.48-2.84) but even more so to have an anxiety disorder (OR 2.09-3.86). The authors concluded that while there has been an emphasis on depression and pain, anxiety appears to be more common and deserving of further evaluation.

Anxiety and depression not only can add to the suffering of patients with pain but also can influence treatment outcomes and chronification of pain (the transformation of acute to chronic pain). In one study, baseline anxiety, as well as depression, predicted functional and symptomatic outcome in patients with sciatica.[42] Research into the factors that predict "chronification" has also implicated depression and anxiety. Shaw et al.[43] studied 140 men with first-onset LBP of approximately 8 weeks' duration. Chronification was predicted by lifetime history of depression (OR 4.99), lifetime GAD (OR 2.45), PTSD (OR 3.23), and pre-DSM-5–defined nicotine dependence (OR 2.49). In a prospective, observational, longitudinal study, neuropathic pain symptoms, severity, interference, and baseline characteristics were assessed at the time of hospital admission and 4 months after a traumatic musculoskeletal injury ($N = 205$). Approximately a third of the patients developed chronic moderate to severe pain by 4 months after the initial injury. Statistically significant predictors of the development and maintenance of pain included high general anxiety while in the hospital immediately after the injury and posttraumatic stress symptoms at 4 months following the injury.[44]

Another common psychiatric disorder in patients with pain is PTSD. PTSD in the DSM-IV was classified under anxiety disorders, but in the DSM-5 it is included in a new category: Trauma- and Stressor-Related Disorders. The diagnostic criteria for PTSD in the DSM-5 identify the trigger to PTSD as exposure to actual or threatened death, serious injury, or sexual violation. PTSD is highly prevalent in patients with CNCP. In a group of veterans seeking treatment for PTSD, Shipherd et al. found that 66% had chronic pain as well.[45] Defrin et al. found that, compared to healthy controls and those with anxiety disorders, patients with PTSD had higher rates of chronic pain, more intense pain, and pain in more body regions. Thresholds to experimental pain were higher than the control groups; however, when the thresholds were exceeded, patients experienced the pain as much more intense.[46] In a meta-analysis of the prevalence of PTSD in persons with chronic pain, PTSD varied from 0% to 57%. Analysis of subgroups revealed that PTSD prevalence was 20.5% (95% CI, 9.5-39.0) among patients with widespread pain, 11.2% (95% CI, 5.7-22.8) in patients with headache, and 0.3% (95% CI, 0.0-2.4) in patients with back pain.[47] Another study evaluated the relationship between PTSD and CNCP and possible mediators. Patients seeking treatment for CNCP with a diagnosis of PTSD had higher pain intensity, pain-related interference, depression, and lower levels of pain-related acceptance and committed action. The authors concluded that psychological flexibility (acceptance, cognitive fusion, committed action, self as context) mediated the relationship between PTSD and CNCP.[48]

PSYCHOLOGICAL PROCESSES OF PAIN

Anxiety Sensitivity

Anxiety sensitivity (AS) has garnered renewed interest as a key factor in understanding the subjective pain experience. AS refers to an abnormal fear of the normal sensations associated with anxiety or fear of anxiety-related symptoms. AS has been established as a risk factor for both panic episodes and anxiety disorders. Relative to pain, AS has been postulated as an important factor in the development and maintenance of chronic pain by intensifying the tendency to develop fear of pain. According to this theory, this fear of pain leads to pain-related avoidance promoting deconditioning and increased pain, and thus a vicious cycle of fear-avoidance-deconditioning-pain-fear.[49] This model was subsequently modified to include the cognitive variables of appraisals and expectations of pain contributing to pain catastrophizing, which leads to pain-related fear and avoidance behavior.[50] AS is associated with muscular, abdominal, and head pain, as well as with impaired coping.[51,52] AS has also been associated with acute pain, with recent work using an experimental pain model (cold pressure test [CPT]) demonstrating that high AS subjects reporting more anticipatory fear prior to CPT experienced heightened subjective pain, which appeared to be related to autonomic nervous system reactivity.[53]

Anger, Forgiveness, Empathy

Other emotional states and attitudes, while not considered disorders, can influence physical and emotional suffering and functionality. For example, anger, which is not uncommon in patients with CNCP, has been shown to cause added suffering and reduce function and moderate response to treatment,[54-57] whereas forgiveness[58] and gratitude can have a positive therapeutic effect and promote psychological resilience.[59-62] Likewise, it has been demonstrated that empathetic feedback from an observer can have a positive effect on pain appraisal and physiological arousal.[63]

To summarize, the relationship between emotions and pain is complex. It appears that mood and anxiety can elicit or exacerbate pain and pain can elicit or exacerbate a mood or anxiety disorder. Either state can lead to the other being treatment resistant. Mood and anxiety can predict the chronification of acute pain; and there is emerging evidence that pain and emotions have shared biological substrates.

Attention and Pain Perception

A number of experimental and clinical studies have revealed compelling evidence that attention can significantly alter pain perception. When an individual with either acute experimental pain or chronic pain is distracted from their pain by engaging in a competing cognitive task, pain is perceived as less intense. A growing number of neuroimaging studies have begun to provide insight into the underlying neurobiological mechanisms of these effects.[64-69] CNS areas involved in the effect of attention on pain modulation include the spinal cord dorsal horn. This results from the influence of descending inhibitory and facilitatory pathways regulated by the nucleus raphe magnus,[65] which is, in turn, under the influence of descending fibers from the amygdala[68] Bushnell et al.[67] found that distraction from a painful stimulus diminished both pain report and activation of the primary somatosensory cortex. Sprenger et al.[68] used high-resolution fMRI to show that a distracting memory task inhibited afferent signals of thermal pain at the level of the dorsal horn. Petrovic et al.[69] demonstrated that a maze task reduced the experience of pain and activity in the somatosensory association areas and periaqueductal gray/midbrain in subjects given the cold pressor test.

Individuals with pain often isolate themselves either due to concomitant mood disorders or due to pain-related limitations, which engenders an environment lacking competing or challenging stimuli to distract themselves from their pain. The pain can become all-consuming and the focus of their existence, leading to more pain and suffering.

Expectations and Goal Setting

Patient expectations and treatment goals are often not assessed but can be important in influencing treatment outcomes and pain perception. Several studies have suggested that patient expectations of recovery predicted return to work and pain-related disability.[70,71] Likewise, patient expectations can influence response to specific interventions. Kalauokalani et al.[72] in a cohort of patients receiving massage and acupuncture for LBP found that patient expectations correlated with response to each treatment and with which treatment produced better results. Results of these studies were correlational and did not determine causality, so it is difficult to distinguish if patients are able to accurately predict their own outcomes or if low patient expectations encumber recovery and response to treatments. Related but less studied is patient goal-setting determining treatment outcomes. Tan et al.[73] prospectively assessed the association between a number of personal attributes, vocational factors, and return to work outcome in a cohort of patients admitted to a university pain treatment program. Age, marital status, educational level, and length of unemployment were all predictive of eventual return to work. Overall, listing return to work as a baseline treatment goal was the most significant best predictor of return to employment outcome. Results from experimental pain studies also suggest that expectations can change perception. For example, Koyama and colleagues[74] showed that altering expectations of experimental pain produced not only influenced a subject's pain report but also resulted in concordant activation of select brain regions including the thalamus, insula, prefrontal cortex, and anterior cingulate cortex. Sawamoto et al.[75] created the expectation of pain with a series of painful thermal stimulations and then administered a comfortably warm stimulation. When a painful stimulus was expected, there was activation of the nucleus accumbens and posterior insula in response to the neutral stimulus, as reflected in fMRI. There was also an increase in the perceived unpleasantness of the stimulation.

This line of research suggests that providers should be cognizant of patient's expectations and their goals for treatment outcomes as they can have a strong influence on pain perception and treatment response.

Kinesiophobia and Fear-Avoidance Model of Pain

A subgroup of patients will heal from an initial trauma but go on to develop chronic pain and related disabilities in part due to certain psychological processes. One that is common in patients with CNCP is kinesiophobia. The fear-avoidance model of chronic pain postulated by Vlaeyen and Linton[76,77] focuses on patient's adaptive and maladaptive interpretation of pain. If a patient interprets their pain as nonthreatening (in other words temporary), they tend to resume usual and therapeutic physical activities after the initial recovery from an injury. On the other hand, if a patient misinterprets their pain as a sign of a serious injury or pathological state that they have little control over, this leads to catastrophic fear of pain or further injury and can generalize to fear of any physical activity. This fear-avoidance creates a vicious cycle of inactivity causing physical deconditioning leading to more pain, psychological distress and disability. Pain-related fear was found to be more predictive of subsequent functional impairment than pain severity alone.[78,79] At times, inordinate fear may be iatrogenic[80] and fostered by physician comments such as "you will eventually need surgery; it is inevitable" or "this is the worst case of spinal stenosis I have seen; it is amazing you can still walk" or "you have a slipped disc."

In chronic pain, information can be therapeutic or counterproductive. Clinicians should be cautious in explaining the etiology of pain, prognosis, and expectations regarding potential outcome from prescribed therapies and attempt to balance optimism with reality. Cheatle suggests that the initial encounter with a patient should follow the principle of VEET: *Validate* that the patients' pain is real and not psychological; *Educate* the patient on the neurobiology of chronic pain, setting the stage for a biopsychosocial approach; *Evaluate*—conduct a thorough biobehavioral examination; and finally, *Treat*—based on the comprehensive evaluation, develop a personalized treatment plan keeping in mind the patients' goals and expectations.[81]

Cognitions and Coping

The role of cognition in supporting healthy moods and attitudes and contributing to psychiatric conditions has been recognized for over three decades[82] and has been extended to the area of chronic pain.[83,84] The underlying premise of cognitive theories is that individuals react to their interpretation and understanding of events, rather than to the events themselves. In the depressed patient, their view of the world is clouded by irrational, maladaptive thoughts that perpetuate and deepen the depression. Maladaptive cognitions have the quality of being automatic and habitual, so that they rarely are examined for validity. The patient accepts these distorted thoughts as real, even when they are clearly illogical to others. These theories on cognition form the basis for the well-validated treatment approach of cognitive-behavioral therapy (CBT) and acceptance and commitment therapy, which will be discussed later in the chapter.

Catastrophizing

Cognitive factors affect pain in a number of ways.[85,86] The aversive quality of pain and therefore suffering is modified by its interpretation,[87,88] so that it is more distressing if thought to be a warning of potential bodily harm. Catastrophizing is a well-studied cognitive factor that is associated with poor pain tolerance and coping,[89] sleep disturbance,[90] and suicidal ideation[91] in patients with CNCP. Catastrophizing can be conceptualized as a negative cognitive-affective response to pain. For example, appraisals such as "this pain will kill me" and "I may become paralyzed" can increase dysfunction, worsen pain, and hinder coping.[92,93] Negative thoughts that reduce pain tolerance include those emphasizing the aversiveness of the situation, the inadequacy of the person to bear it, or the physical harm that could occur.[86] Catastrophizing can also be a risk factor for a patient developing opioid use disorder.[94]

Providers can reduce catastrophic thinking by (1) validating the patient's complaint as real but manageable, (2) supporting the patient's self-efficacy in controlling the pain and maintaining function, and (3) providing clear guidance as to which activities the patient can safely perform—even if they are painful. Cognitive-behavioral therapy is designed to target both catastrophizing and kinesiophobia to support the patient being proactive rather than reactive in managing their pain.

Helplessness Versus Self-Efficacy

Cognitive influences include not only beliefs regarding pain but also those regarding the person experiencing it and their beliefs about their ability to control the pain. Seligman's[95] model of learned helplessness in depression suggests that those who feel unable to control events in their lives will respond passively to them, become depressed, and experience increased disability and pain. Conversely, belief in self-efficacy is a major determinant of successful coping[96,97] and predicts better functioning in fibromyalgia and arthritis.[98,99] These beliefs are favorably associated not only with pain and function but also with treatment outcomes. For example, Costa et al.[100] assessed the association of self-efficacy with pain and function in chronic back pain and fear of movement. They followed patients for a year and found that self-efficacy predicted improvements in pain and function much better than did fear of movement.

In summary, while working with patients with CNCP, it is important to encourage and support a rational view of their pain, self-efficacy, and self-responsibility.

CLASSIFICATION OF PAIN SYNDROMES

How pain syndromes have been described and classified has evolved from the pejorative, less useful classifications to more evidence-based, clinically practical ones.

DSM-IV and DSM-5

The diagnosis of somatoform disorders in the DSM-IV was predicated primarily on the presence of medically unexplained symptoms. This was quite problematic, since a number of pains conditions that were previously "medically unexplained" and therefore thought to be "nonphysiologic or functional" have now been explained by such processes as central sensitization, neuroplasticity, and glial activation. The category of "somatoform disorders" has now been eliminated, and the DSM-5 category of "somatic symptom disorders" will apply to many patients previously diagnosed with somatoform disorders.[101,102] Whether the symptoms are medically explained is no longer a criterion for the diagnosis; instead, the emphasis is on distress, dysfunction, and disproportionate thoughts, feelings, and behaviors.

The DSM-IV condition "pain disorder" was characterized by significant pain (causing distress or impairment) "that is judged to be psychologically caused, exacerbated, or perpetuated." The criteria for making this judgment were not provided.[103] This diagnosis has been eliminated, as has "somatization disorder," which required a multitude of medically unexplained symptoms (four of them are pain related). These have been replaced with "somatic symptom disorder," which offers a specifier for "with predominant pain," if applicable. These newer diagnoses may be easier to apply clinically. Somatic symptom disorder involves one or more somatic symptoms that are distressing or result in significant disruption of daily life. Excessive feelings, thoughts, or behaviors related to the somatic symptoms or associated health concerns are manifested by at least one of the following: disproportionate and persistent thoughts about the seriousness of one's symptoms, persistently high level of anxiety about health symptoms, or excessive time and energy devoted to these symptoms or health concerns. Although any one somatic symptom may not be continuously present, the state of being symptomatic is persistent (typically more than 6 months).[104]

Chronic Pain Syndrome

Chronic pain syndrome (CPS) is a somewhat archaic and pejorative term that is still often heard, perhaps because it is a useful concept. It must be distinguished from CNCP. The term was used to describe patients with inordinate impairment and behavioral abnormalities[105] and was defined as intractable pain of 6 months' or more duration, accompanied by marked alterations of behavior, with depression or anxiety, marked restriction in daily activities, excessive use of medication and frequent use of medical services, no clear relationship to organic pathology, and typically a history of multiple, nonproductive tests, treatments, and surgeries. Thus, CPS is predominantly a behavioral syndrome that affects a minority of patients with chronic pain. The term properly directs therapy toward the reversal of regression and away from an exclusive focus on nociception but does not substitute for a careful diagnosis of the underlying physiological, psychological, and conditioning components of the syndrome. Some of the controversy regarding long-term opioid therapy may actually be an argument between those who have found opioids useful in treating chronic *pain* and those who have found them harmful in chronic pain *syndrome*. Patients with pain who have an active SUD are probably at increased risk for chronic pain *syndrome*, since they may be predisposed to inordinate disability, symptom exaggeration, and high levels of health care utilization.

Malingering

Factitious disorder is driven by the aim to assume the role of being ill, impaired, or injured but without any obvious *external* rewards for such behavior.[104] This aim has been understood to be driven by the *internal* reward received by obtaining sympathy, nurturance, or attention by assuming the sick role. It is distinguished from malingering, which involves the intentional reporting of symptoms for personal gain/reward (such as disability payments or avoidance of an unpleasant situation). The distinction is not always clear. While both result in the conscious/intentional feigning or physical production of symptoms, the motivation or decision-making process to produce these symptoms is fully conscious in the malingering person (who thus can be held accountable for their actions); on the contrary, the motivation or decision-making is instead unconscious and not intentional in the factitious patient—and thus is due to psychiatric disease. Malingering is not a somatoform disorder, not a form of psychogenic pain, and not a diagnosable disorder. It is simply a form of fraud that uses faux illness to obtain benefit. It is included in this section because it may be confused with or conflated with somatic symptom and related disorders such as factitious disorder, and because when symptoms seem inexplicable; malingering, somatization, and factitious processes are in the differential diagnosis. It is generally considered to be rare in patients reporting CNCP, but this belief may be based less on objective data than on the clinician's need to believe patients in order to function well as a caregiver and advocate.

The burden of proof must be on the clinician to demonstrate the presence of conscious, willful motivation and deception prior to labeling a patient as malingering, and for most conditions, that can only be accomplished through covert or overt observation. It is difficult to make this distinction, since it relies primarily on patient intent and consciousness of the situation, which are not readily observable. Surveillance may be the only way to diagnose some cases accurately, though grossly discordant findings (eg, a person with prolonged inability to tolerate hand touch due to allodynia who has calluses and grease under the nails) suggest malingering.

Malingering is not rare in people seeking external gain, and many of us have been chagrined to receive a surveillance video from a worker's compensation case manager showing the "disabled" patient we have been caring for easily pushing a lawn mower.

Mailis-Gagnon et al.[106] reported that 4 out of 15 women referred for presumed complex regional pain syndrome had self-inflicted illness, characterized by limb ligation, ulcers, and "bizarre migrating wounds" that abated with casting. Other studies have shown a not-negligible prevalence of malingering in patients reporting pain,[107] diarrhea,[108] deafness,[109] and cognitive dysfunction.[110] Gervais et al.[111] found that patients with fibromyalgia who were receiving or seeking disability income were likely to demonstrate faking on tests of memory complaints, in contrast to patients with rheumatoid arthritis or fibromyalgia who were not seeking or receiving disability income.

It is important when characterizing patients with CNCP to avoid terms that are vilifying and having no clinical utility in developing a meaningful and efficacious treatment plan or developing a therapeutic alliance promoting adherence.

THE ROLE OF THE ENVIRONMENT

There are two primary environmental factors having impact on the pain experience and pain behaviors: (1) stressors can affect the amount of pain experienced in a given situation, and

(2) incentives (reinforcements) can influence the pain experienced and the behaviors associated with it.

Stress

Preclinical studies have convincingly demonstrated that stressful environments and experiences not only appear to magnify pain (hyperalgesia) but may generate it de novo. Rivat et al.[112] found that repeated social defeat induced hyperalgesia in rats that was associated with expression of proinflammatory genes (iNOS and COX-2) in the spinal cord. The effect was reversed by an antagonist of cholecystokinin, a transmitter in the descending pain facilitatory system. Le Roy et al.[113] demonstrated that nonnociceptive stress in rat models, especially if repeated, predisposed to development of hyperalgesia in response to pressure and inflammation. Green et al.[114] found that rats exposed to unpredictable sound stress developed an enhanced and prolonged response to cytokine-induced mechanical hyperalgesia, cutaneous and masseter hyperalgesia, as well as visceromotor hyperactivity and anxiety, thought to be reminiscent of fibromyalgia.

Human studies tend to focus on more extreme stress, such as that associated with combat. Chronic diffuse pain is one constellation of symptoms commonly reported in Gulf War veterans and is closely associated with psychiatric symptoms.[115] Stress, of course, not only amplifies pain but also has the potential to create incentives for pain behaviors such as when such behavior provides escape from stress.

Behavioral Contingencies

Operant conditioning is a behavioral model of learning for voluntary and automatic animal and human responses. In this learning model, all overt behaviors are strongly influenced by their consequences and the context in which the behaviors occur. Fundamentally, behaviors that are reinforced increase in frequency and those not reinforced or the reinforcement is removed "extinguish." A positive reinforcement is when a behavior is followed by a pleasant consequence and a negative reinforcement is when an aversive stimulus is removed due to a specific behavior. Key points regarding operant conditioning include the observations that (1) it often occurs without the knowledge of the trainer or trainee; (2) in most cases, repetition is required for conditioning to occur, so that the concepts are more important in chronic conditions than acute ones; and (3) the timing of reinforcement is critical. An immediate small reinforcer may outweigh a delayed large one, as reflected in the human penchant for behaviors that produce immediate small rewards despite substantial delayed adverse consequences. Addiction-related behavior may be driven at least in part by this phenomenon.

Because of conditioning, "illness behaviors" may become contingent on incentives and may increase or decrease regardless of nociception.

Wilbert Fordyce pioneered applying the model of operant conditioning to pain management and developed the first U.S. pain program based on operant conditioning principles. In this approach, pain behaviors such as pain-focused conversation, limping, and rubbing body parts are maintained by external reinforcers (solicitous response by family, caregivers), and these maladaptive behaviors can be extinguished by not responding to them and, instead, reinforcing competing adaptive behaviors, such as exercise. Results were impressive, as individuals who had been disabled for years began to exercise, relinquish assistive devices, and engage in conversations about non–pain-related topics.[116,117] The operant conditioning-based program developed by Fordyce was soon emulated by hundreds of programs in several countries. The response of severely dysfunctional individuals to environmental contingencies in these programs lent support to the belief that much unnecessary functional impairment is maintained by environmental rewards. A Cochrane review of 30 randomized clinical trials of behavioral therapies for chronic LBP found moderate quality evidence that operant conditioning was effective in improving function.[118]

More recently, there has been a focus on informal social support and pain behavior. Based on the operant conditioning model, most studies in this area have focused on one specific form of social support: solicitousness. Solicitousness involves attentiveness to patients' pain behaviors, offering assistance and taking over his/her duties, and is often associated with higher pain severity and disability and lower physical and psychological functioning.[119] For example, Pence et al.[120] reviewed studies of the impact of spousal behaviors (typically characterized as solicitous, punishing, or distracting) on patients' activity level, pain, and mood. Additionally, they studied 64 patients with headache by means of a self-report questionnaire. Patients reporting that their spouses responded negatively to well behaviors had more pain and pain behavior. Spousal responses judged to facilitate well behavior had no observable effect. Solicitous responses were associated with more pain, pain behavior, depression, and pain interference with life activities. In another study of data recorded from home accelerometer monitoring of new patients in a chronic pain clinic, Alschuler et al.[121] examined pain sensitivity, fear avoidance, and solicitous spousal responses. They found that the operant conditioning model accounted for the preponderance of variance in physical activity. Patients were more active when spouses were less solicitous, less punishing, and more distracting. When evaluating potential reinforcers of maladaptive pain-related behaviors, it is important to observe the interaction of the patient and close family members and it is recommended having close family members attend office visits.

Secondary and Tertiary Gains and Disability

While primary gains (solicitous spouse) can reinforce maladaptive behaviors and increase pain, so can secondary gains (external gains that accrue due to illness or symptoms).[122] In a comparison of 3,802 pain patients and 3,849 controls,

Rohling et al.[123] found that financial compensation was associated with greater pain and reduced medical and surgical treatment efficacy. However, when the incentives for wellness are powerful, function may be preserved despite serious illness. In a study of injured workers, return to work correlated strongly with preinjury wages, both in those who underwent spine surgery and those who did not.[124]

Tertiary gains refer to incentives for illness that may also modify the family's behavior. For example, the wife of an unskilled worker in a floundering industry may sense that the family's security is contingent on his disabled status. She therefore may defend his disability and support his helplessness. A particularly insidious form of tertiary gain is seen in the not uncommon situation in which a patient with chronic pain receives many hours of care per week from a "home health aide," who happens to be a family member. The family member has income only so long as the patient remains unable to function.

This discussion of the various "gains" that can result from being disabled due to a pain condition should not be mistaken as implying that these individuals are not suffering. While disability income may provide a modicum of typically meager financial security, the vast majority of pain sufferers incur numerous losses (work and family roles, isolation, sense of being a burden on one's family and society), which often lead to depression and despair.

DEVELOPMENTAL ISSUES

When a patient presents with ill-defined pain complaints with no identified organic cause and a history of childhood trauma, increasingly referred to as adverse childhood experiences (ACEs), often they are categorized as having psychogenic pain or a somatization disorder. Sources of trauma have included abandonment, neglect, insufficient nurture, and physical or sexual abuse.[125-130]

Studies in this area have typically compared patients with CNCP that have an identified medical cause to patients with poorly defined or unknown etiology, such as fibromyalgia or patients diagnosed as having a somatoform pain disorder. For example, Imbierowicz et al.[131] compared the childhood experiences of controls (medically explained chronic pain) with patients with fibromyalgia and with somatoform pain. They found that the latter two groups had more ACEs, including sexual and physical maltreatment, poor emotional relationships with parents, lack of physical affection, parental quarreling, unhealthy substance use in the mother, separation, and financial stress, prior to the age of seven. In another study, Brown et al.[132] used a structured interview to compare 22 patients with a diagnosis of "somatization disorder" to 19 medical comparison subjects. Somatization disorder patients reported significantly more childhood emotional abuse, family conflict, and more severe forms of physical abuse and less family cohesion. Chronic emotional abuse was the best predictor of unexplained physical symptoms. Sexual abuse, separation/loss, and witnessing violence were equally common in the two groups. The somatization disorder group reported significantly more family conflict and less family cohesion. Sachs-Ericsson et al.[133] examined data from 5,877 subjects who received Part II of the National Comorbidity Survey in the 1990s. Participants with current (12 months) health problems were queried about their current pain. Those with abuse histories reported more pain, and the difference was not explained by depression.

Results from human[134] and animal experimental studies[135,136] further support the relationship between early trauma and subsequent "exaggerated" or unexplained pain.

Suggested mechanisms of the association between early developmental deprivation, neglect, and abandonment possibly leading to physical symptoms include insecure attachment[137] and increased vigilance and anxiety.[138]

Emerging evidence strongly supports the concept that psychological trauma, especially when the nervous system is developing in early life, can cause significant neurological changes. Landa et al.[139] reviewed evidence that childhood neglect and trauma are associated with later life somatization. They cite a convergence of information from genetics, developmental neurobiology, and other fields, suggesting that there may be a shared neural system underlying physical and social pain and that this system can be disrupted by deficiencies in the early infant/caregiver relationship. Rome and Rome[36] speculated that psychological trauma, in a process akin to kindling, can evoke a hypersensitivity not unlike that seen in neurogenic sensitization and that this hypersensitivity involves cross-sensitization, so that the individuals are hypersensitive to psychic (loss, humiliation) and physical (injury) trauma, both of which elicit both physical and affective symptoms.

The advent of advanced neuroimaging has demonstrated an underlying biological substrate of many pain conditions often thought of as purely psychological. Thus, the use of terms such as "somatization" and "psychogenic" becomes pejorative and potentially harmful to patients with CNCP who already feel stigmatized. Many of these "psychogenic" conditions such as fibromyalgia, irritable bowel syndrome, vulvodynia, and interstitial cystitis have been classified as functional pain syndromes (FPS). FPS have been characterized as central sensitivity syndromes, an overlapping group of conditions that share a common pathophysiological mechanism of pain and/or sensory amplification. Individuals with FPS tend to exhibit diffuse pain sensitivity (hyperalgesia) and diminished pain thresholds (allodynia) without an initiating painful stimulus.[21] Using this explanatory model of pain in patients with FPS reduces resistance to psychological interventions and promotes a more collaborative clinician-patient relationship.

ASSESSING CO-OCCURRING PSYCHOLOGICAL AND SUBSTANCE USE DISORDERS

Given the high prevalence of mood and anxiety disorders in patients with CNCP and the effect of these psychological processes on the pain experience, it is important that every patient seen for chronic pain undergo at least a brief screening for the presence of anxiety and depression. There are a variety of validated and reliable mental health screening tools. An expert consensus group on measuring emotional functioning in chronic pain[140] recommended the Beck Depression Inventory (BDI)[141] and the Profile of Mood States (POMS).[142] The BDI is a 21-question self-report measure of depression severity over the past week. The POMS has a full-length version (65 items) and a short-length version (35 questions) both consisting of seven scales. Three of these scales are very pertinent to the pain population (anger/hostility, depression/rejection, and tension/anxiety). In busy practices, the brief screener PHQ-4[143] can be used. The PHQ-4 is a four-item screening tool for depression and anxiety. Mood and anxiety symptoms are dynamic and not static and these conditions should be routinely assessed.

Assessing for SUDs in patients with CNCP can be challenging especially if they are legitimately prescribed medications that can have euphoric or anxiolytic effects. Every patient with CNCP should be initially screened for unhealthy opioid use or the presence of a SUD; and if prescribed opioids long-term, periodically monitored for the development of aberrant medication-taking behaviors (AMTB). A note of caution, AMTB are not necessarily surrogates for a patient developing a SUD. The only validated tool for assessing risk of OUD in patients with CNCP receiving opioids is the Opioid Risk Tool-OUD.[144] Examples of opioid screening tools and general substance use screening assessments are outlined in **Table 109-1**.

TABLE 109-1 Examples of Unhealthy Opioid Use Risk and Substance Use Disorder Screening Tools

Patients considered for long-term opioid therapy	Items	Administered
ORT (Opioid Risk Tool)	5	By patient
SOAPP (Screener and Opioid Assessment for Patients with Pain)	24, 14, and 5	By patient
DIRE (Diagnosis, Intractability, Risk, and Efficacy Score)	7	By clinician
Characterize misuse once opioid treatments begin		
PMQ (Pain Medication Questionnaire)	26	By patient
COMM (Current Opioid Misuse Measure)	17	By patient
PDUQ (Prescription Drug Use Questionnaire)	40	By clinician
Risk of developing an OUD in patients with CNCP		
ORT-OUD (Opioid Risk Tool-Opioid Use Disorder)	13	By patient
Not specific to pain populations		
CAGE-AID (Cut Down, Annoyed, Guilty, Eye-Opener Tool, Adjusted to Include Drugs)	4	By clinician
RAFFT (Relax, Alone, Friends, Family, Trouble)	5	By patient
DAST (Drug Abuse Screening Test)	28	By patient
SBIRT (Screening, Brief Intervention, and Referral to Treatment)	Varies	By clinician
AUDIT-C (Alcohol Use Disorders Identification Test for Consumption)	3	By patient

BIOPSYCHOSOCIAL APPROACH TO THE TREATMENT OF PAIN

The traditional biomedical, linear approach to pain assessment, and treatment is inadequate in addressing the various psychosocial and neurobehavioral mechanisms that can lead to and maintain pain. There is persuasive evidence that a biopsychosocial approach to pain management improves pain, function, mood, and general quality of life.[145-148] A biopsychosocial program typically includes a graded exercise program, CBT and Acceptance Commitment Therapy (ACT), and rational pharmacotherapy.[81]

Exercise

Exercises and physical therapy have been shown to improve pain and function in those with CNCP.[149,150] Exercise not only can enhance the release of endogenous opioids (endorphins) thus potentially reducing the use of prescription opioids, but can also reduce the mortality and morbidity related to major health conditions. Recent data from randomized studies suggest that aerobic exercise also significantly improves function and quality of life in patients with chronic LBP. Exercise has proven to be a potent anxiolytic as it both blunts the body's response to cortisol and increases brain serotonin levels; epidemiological studies have shown that exercise both prevents anxiety disorders and effectively treats them.[151,152] Patients with CNCP usually have had a number of trials of physical therapy. Often their experience with physical therapy is not positive as they either are exposed to a "no pain, no gain" approach, which typically leads to pain flares and reinforcing their fear-avoidance to exercise, or a passive approach (massage, electrical stimulation, heat, etc.), which supports passive dependency. An effective physical therapy program for patients with CNCP pain should involve (1) acquiring first aid techniques for pain relief at home for patients to self-manage pain flares, such as the use of transcutaneous electrical nerve stimulation (TENS), rest, ice, compression, elevation (RICE), heat, and use of over-the-counter medications such as responsible dosing of non-steroidal anti-inflammatories), etc. This can engender a sense of empowerment over their pain and independence and (2) establish a well-balanced, independent exercise program in a very graded fashion as these patients typically have had poor experiences with traditional physical therapy and tend to catastrophize. Weekly achievable and agreed upon goals should be established that will not lead to an increase in pain.

Cognitive-Behavioral Therapy for CNCP

Patients with CNCP often present with concomitant mood and anxiety disorders and maladaptive behaviors and thought processes that contribute to suffering. There are a number of psychological interventions that have been shown to be effective in improving function and mood in patients with CNCP. These include relaxation therapy, assertiveness training, motivational interviewing, acceptance and commitment therapy, and mindfulness meditation. CBT includes a number of these strategies.

Cognitive Therapy

Patients with CNCP tend to engage in maladaptive thinking (catastrophizing) and maladaptive behavior (kinesiophobia), both of which contribute to depression, low self-efficacy, and disability. The process of CBT typically includes specific skill acquisition such as mindfulness-based stress reduction and cognitive restructuring, followed by skill consolidation, rehearsal, and relapse training.[153] The process of cognitive restructuring consists of identifying and modifying negative/irrational thought patterns and substituting more rational/functional cognitions to aid the patient to reframe and reconceptualize his/her own personal view of pain, thus promoting the patient to being more proactive, rather than passive, and encouraging a sense of competence and self-efficacy.[154]

CBT has been found to be cost-effective and clinically effective in improving mood and function in a variety of chronic pain disorders including arthritis,[155] chronic LBP,[156,157] lupus,[158] fibromyalgia,[159] and sickle cell disease.[160] A Cochrane review by Bernardy et al.[161] assessed the effectiveness of CBT for fibromyalgia. The authors evaluated 23 studies that met the inclusion criteria with a total of 2,231 patients. Results indicated that CBT was superior to groups receiving a control condition in terms of reducing negative mood, decreasing disability, and reducing pain, both at treatment completion and 6-month posttreatment completion.

Another application of CBT relevant to improving pain is in improving sleep disorders. Sleep disturbance is highly prevalent in patients with CNCP.[162,163] The association between persistent pain and sleep disturbance is bidirectional in nature. Pain may lead to poor sleep quality and decreased total sleep time, therefore exacerbating pain and further impairing mood and contributing to decreased function and increased disability.[164,165] A CBT insomnia (CBT-I) program typically includes six components: *psychoeducation* regarding insomnia, *stimulus control* techniques to promote a strong association between the bed and rapid-onset sleep (eg, removing the TV from the bedroom, restricting the use of bed for only sleep and sex, maintaining a regular wake/sleep cycle), *sleep restriction* (limiting the time spent in bed to only actual time of asleep), *sleep hygiene* (targets behaviors and environmental conditions that can promote or interfere with sleep such as timing of exercise, certain foods, bright lights, reading, or watching material that is emotionally charged), *relaxation therapy* (facilitates reducing physical and mental tension via mediation, guided imagery, etc.), and *cognitive therapy* (addresses how beliefs and attitudes toward sleep can affect sleep and identifies and replaces maladaptive thoughts with rational, adaptive ones). Wiles et al. performed a meta-analytic review of 14 randomized controlled trials (RCTs) comparing CBT-I to a number of control groups. They found that CBT-I had a medium to large effect size in improving insomnia, and these effects were durable after the completion of treatment.[166] A systematic review by Mitchell et al. compared CBT-I to prescription and over-the-counter medications for sleep. Results revealed that CBT-I was more effective than benzodiazepine and nonbenzodiazepine drugs in improving sleep.[167] CBT-I has also been applied to patients with sleep disturbance and CNCP demonstrating improved sleep and significantly greater reductions in depression, fatigue, and pain-related interference as compared to control groups.[168,169]

Mindfulness Meditation

CBT has evolved over the years and increasingly focuses on such concepts as mindfulness and "acceptance and commitment therapy" (ACT). In part, these concepts and their associated therapies embody a recognition that the quest for a cure of illness and elimination of symptoms can become self-defeating and ultimately constitute a part of the problem. The newer work holds that there can be value in surrender and that symptom control strategies can be harmful if they fail, dominate the person's life, or lead to loss of valued activities and goals.[170] In 105 patients with chronic pain, McCracken et al.[171] found that baseline mindfulness, as reflected in the Mindfulness Attention Awareness Scale, was associated with reduced depression, pain-related anxiety, and both physical and psychological functional impairment. There is early evidence that mindfulness and acceptance correlated with improved function and reduced opioid use in patients with chronic LBP.[172]

Zeidan et al.[173] extensively reviewed the literature related to pain and mindfulness, which they characterized as including (1) regulated, sustained attention to the moment-to-moment quality and character of sensory, emotional, and cognitive events; (2) the recognition of such events as momentary, fleeting, and changeable (past and future representations of those events being considered cognitive abstractions); and (3) a consequent lack of emotional or cognitive appraisal and reactions to these events. Mindfulness is taught by one of several forms of meditation training. Although it originated in the Buddhist tradition, contemporary training is usually fully secular. Zeidan's group found compelling support for the ability of both "focused attention" and "open monitoring" forms of meditation to reduce both the perception of pain and its associated unpleasantness. Further, they reviewed imaging studies demonstrating differences in regional brain activation in meditators versus nonmeditators on exposure to noxious stimuli. The amount of training required to produce meaningful differences in pain perception was as small as four 20-minute sessions. A recent review of mindfulness meditation for fibromyalgia found convincing evidence that mindfulness-based interventions were effective in decreasing fibromyalgia-related pain and psychological symptoms, especially when combined with other treatments such as exercise and CBT.[174]

Acceptance and Commitment Therapy

Acceptance and commitment therapy (ACT) is a form of CBT that is a directive and experiential type of therapy based on rational frame theory. The goal of ACT is to experience life mindfully and reinforce psychological flexibility. The core processes of ACT include (1) contact with the present moment, (2) self as context, (3) defusion (disentangling ourselves from our maladaptive thoughts and emotions), (4) acceptance, (5) values, and (6) committed action. A number of RCTs of ACT for CNCP have demonstrated ACT to be effective in improving mood and function. In a meta-analysis of 22 acceptance-based studies, including mindfulness and ACT, Veehof et al. found evidence of efficacy for pain (effect size 0.37) and depression (effect size 0.32). Benefit was also found for anxiety, physical well-being, and quality of life. The authors concluded that, although results were not as strong as those supporting CBT, the acceptance-based treatments were a viable alternative to them.[175] Vowles et al. followed a group of 171 subjects with chronic musculoskeletal pain who had completed a course of ACT. At a 3-year follow-up, 68% of the cohort continued to note improvement in key outcomes including pain-related anxiety, physical and psychosocial disability, and depression.[176]

ACT is a promising new intervention for patients with CNCP that requires additional research on the underlying mechanisms of action and the characteristics of the patients who would best respond to this type of treatment. Clinically, patients who are able to accept that their pain as a chronic disease that needs to be managed and not seek a cure (repeated surgeries, etc.) tend to have less psychological stress and find ways to have a fulfilling life in spite of the pain.

CBT/ACT for Pain and Co-occurring Substance Use Disorders

There is persuasive, evolving evidence of the potential efficacy of CBT/ACT in improving outcomes in patients with CNCP and co-occurring nicotine use disorder[177]; alcohol use disorder[178]; patients with chronic pain, substance use disorder and hepatitis C virus[179]; patients with CNCP and opioid use disorder[180] and compelling evidence of neurophysiological mechanisms in ACT among patients with co-occurring OUD and chronic pain.[181]

Assertiveness Training

There is scant research specifically on the efficacy of assertiveness training in patients with CNCP, but assertiveness training is one cornerstone of a comprehensive biopsychosocial program. Over time, many patients with CNCP tend to become either passive or aggressive in their communication styles. Poor skills in communicating one's needs, difficulties resisting the demands of others, and tendencies to feel victimized in interpersonal encounters can create strong incentives for the "sick role." Pain can become an excuse for saying no when people lack the skills and confidence for refusing gracefully. Cultural proscriptions of unkindness to the sick may buffer nonassertive against others' insensitivity. Assertiveness training provides alternative strategies that facilitate relinquishing the sick role and promoting improvement in the clinician-patient relationship and within the family.

Family Therapy

Pain clearly can greatly affect the patient but also the patient's family members who can have a major influence on the patient's functional impairment and mood.[182] The influences are bidirectional—living with a person who has chronic pain can stress the family emotionally and financially and often leads to family-wide reductions in recreation and socialization. The family is likely to feel obligated to take on the role of caretaker. Role reversal is common, and patients frequently express remorse for the fact that their small children have begun to parent them or their spouse has had to return to work.

McCracken[183] studied 228 consecutive patients referred to an inpatient rehabilitation program and confirmed that both solicitous and punishing responses from significant others were negatively associated with acceptance of pain.

Alschuler et al.[121] equipped patients with LBP with inertial activity monitors and investigated the relative influence of pain, fear/avoidant issues, and operant factors (family behaviors that were solicitous, punishing, or distracting) in predicting function. Family operant factors were the best predictors of physical activity. The authors suggested that training family members in operant principles could be a critical step in pain rehabilitation.

Based on this literature and that on contingency management, it is imperative that family members be included in the assessment and the therapeutic process. It is crucial to evaluate potential family dynamics that may discourage the patient from engaging in adaptive behaviors or reinforcing the sick role. Therapeutically, including the family in treatment can encourage effective, healthy interactions and support the patient in achieving independence and restoring confidence.

Messages for Families

1. Support, validation, and positive regard are important.
2. Rewarding "pain behavior" promotes its increase; thus, positive statements and attention should be contingent on behaviors that are not intrinsic to pain or the sick role (eg, comments about emotions or current life events should receive more response than comments about pain, medications, and treatments).

3. Overprotection promotes invalidism. Movements in the direction of normal behavior should elicit enthusiastic encouragement, not dissuasion and cautions. Offers to accompany the patient on an outing are a better gesture of affection than suggestions for rest in the recliner.
4. Criticizing "pain behavior" is likely to promote its increase while helping to engender depression.
5. It may be helpful to think in terms of reversing the role change to that of caregiver and replacing it with that of companion, friend, lover, or playmate.

A critical issue is that advice to ignore pain behaviors not be misinterpreted as advice to ignore the person.

The distress of family members often warrants specific management. They may find their lives controlled by a loved one's illness. They feel duty bound to give yet receive little. Self-blame and guilt coexist with resentment. They may feel helpless and depressed, and their own lives often become unmanageable. Family discord often becomes a major source of stress for the patient with pain. Individual counseling, group therapy involving family members of pain patients, and conventional family therapy have all been used with success. Restoration of good quality of life to the nonpain sufferers is also a valid treatment goal.

Interdisciplinary Pain Programs

Patients with CNCP are complex often presenting with multiple psychiatric and medical comorbidities and behavioral and family issues that require a holistic and multifaceted approach such as is offered in Interdisciplinary Pain Programs (IPP). The first IPPs were modeled on the original behavioral program designed by Fordyce; however, various combinations of interventions have been employed in subsequent pain treatment centers. Typical services in IPPs include education, activating physical therapy, rational pharmacotherapy, operant conditioning, psychotherapy (personal and family), medication weaning, addiction treatment, and treatment of co-occurring psychiatric disorders. Interventions such as TENS, spinal cord stimulation, and nerve blocks may be included. IPPs have been found to be clinically efficacious in improving the quality of life and functional abilities of disabled patients with CNCP and effective economically in reducing health care costs and promoting return to work. In an early meta-analysis of 65 studies of IPP, Flor et al.[184] found improvements in pain, mood, and interference with life activities, including work. Health care utilization declined, and benefits were stable over time. Turk reviewed outcome studies of IPPs and found pain reductions of 14% to 60%, opioid reductions of up to 73%, and dramatic increases in levels of activity.[185] Forty-three percent more patients were working after treatment than before. One of his reviewed studies[186] found a 90% reduction in physician visits following treatment. There were 50% to 65% fewer surgeries in treated than in untreated patients and 65% fewer hospitalizations. Thirty-five percent fewer patients were on disability income supplementation. Turk estimated that IPPs led to 27 fewer surgeries per 100 patients, for an average (in 1995 dollars) of $4,050 saved per patient (at $15,000 per surgery). He estimated overall medical costs at more than $13,000 per year pretreatment and $5,600 in the year after treatment. This suggests a saving of $7,700 per year per patient following treatment. Disability savings approximated $400,000 per person removed from permanent disability. Subsequently, Gatchel and Okifuji reviewed studies of IPP effectiveness and concluded that such treatment is the most efficacious and cost-effective, evidence-based treatment extant for CNMP.[187]

In 2007, Turk and Swanson reviewed studies of the effectiveness and costs of a number of treatments for chronic pain and cited studies showing the mean pain reduction from IPPs to be 37%, which occurred along with 63% reduction in pain medication use.[188] In contrast to many treatments (eg, stimulators, pumps, pharmaceuticals) that require substantial continuing health care utilization, IPP treatment was typically associated with a reduction in health care and associated expenditures. IPPs were two to four times more cost-effective than spinal cord stimulator or intrathecal analgesia for increasing physical function. IPPs were shown to be 12 times more cost-effective than conventional medical care, 17.5 times more cost-effective than spinal cord stimulator, and 30 times more cost-effective than surgery for the goal of return to work.

Unfortunately, in spite of this persuasive body of literature supporting efficacy of IPPs, in the United States, interdisciplinary pain clinics are now the exception rather than the rule.[189] Pain care has become procedure driven, and reimbursement for IPPs has progressively been reduced leaving few IPPs in operation.

Barriers to Receiving Psychological Care

While psychological therapies have been proven to be effective in improving pain, mood, and function in patients with CNCP, there are a number of barriers to receiving these necessary services. Ehde et al.[190] outlined some of these barriers, which included:

- Financial (lack of insurance coverage for mental health care)
- Environmental (lack of transportation or lack of clinicians in the geographic region)
- Patient attitude related (stigma associated with receiving psychological care)
- Health care system barriers (no existing referral system to psychologists)

Potential solutions to these barriers include employing non-psychologists who otherwise routinely interact with patients to deliver CBT/operant therapy to their patients with pain. This might include dental hygienists for temporomandibular joint pain, physical and occupational therapists, and certified nursing assistants, among others. This may be successful with minimal training for less complex cases, but a well-trained mental health provider is needed for patients who have more complicated co-occurring mood and anxiety disorders.

Another avenue for providing psychological care to this patient population is through e-health such as computer-assisted CBT, telemedicine, and smartphone apps. Initial work in this area is promising. Rini et al.[191] conducted an RCT comparing an automated, internet-based, 8-week pain coping skills training program to a control group of patients with osteoarthritis pain. The experimental group had a high session completion adherence (91%) and overall reported significantly less pain as compared to the control group. Dear et al.[192] tested an enhanced clinician-guided internet-based CBT (iCBT) program for pain that included five iCBT sessions, homework assignments, weekly emails, or telephone contact with a clinical psychologist compared to a waitlist control group. Results demonstrated that the treatment group had significantly greater improvements in anxiety, depression, average pain intensity, and disability as compared to the control group. The psychologists' mean total time calling the subjects was 81.54 minutes. Use of smartphone apps has been less well studied for pain,[193] and use of telemedicine has been highly effective in treating very refractory conditions such as PTSD[194] but has not been fully explored in delivering pain care.

CONCLUSIONS

Compelling evidence demonstrates that separating the mind from the body and treating them separately is not only ineffective in managing complex pain conditions but does not allow for advancing our understanding of this complex interaction and developing novel interventions. Psychological traumas can produce lasting alterations in CNS function and even structure. At the same time, studies have shown that numerous painful symptoms thought to be "psychogenic" or "somatization" have their explanation in central sensitization and neuroplasticity.

At the societal level, chronic pain is a significant health care problem affecting more than 30% of the U.S. adult population with this number increasing yearly. The 2011 NAM report on pain describes pain as "a national challenge" requiring a "cultural transformation to better prevent, assess, treat and understand pain of all types."[2] In spite of this valiant effort of the NAM to encourage reform in how we care for patients in CNCP, the current model of care tends to be unimodal such as interventional pain medicine or at best multimodal (interventions and pharmacotherapy). A biopsychosocial-based, interdisciplinary care that includes rational pharmacotherapy, restorative, activating physical therapy, and psychological interventions (eg, CBT, ACT, family therapy) have been demonstrated to significantly improve functional status, psychological well-being, reduce pain severity and opioid use, and decrease health care utilization. Unfortunately, there are few of these programs available in the United States, and we need further health care economics research to support improved access to interdisciplinary pain care, behavioral health, and SUD treatment. Other future directions include developing and testing novel delivery systems for psychological interventions for pain and additional research on the biological substrates of the mind-body interaction in pain.

ACKNOWLEDGMENTS

We would like to acknowledge the significant contribution of Edward C. Covington, MD, and Margaret M. Katz, DO, to this chapter from their previous version.

REFERENCES

1. Interagency Pain Research Coordinating Committee. *National Pain Strategy: A Comprehensive Population Health-Level Strategy for Pain.* U.S. Department of Health and Human Services, National Institutes of Health; 2016.
2. Dahlhamer J, Lucas J, Zelaya C, et al. Prevalence of chronic pain and high-impact chronic pain among adults - United States, 2016. *MMWR Morb Mortal Wkly Rep.* 2018;67(36):1001-1006.
3. Pitcher MH, Von Korff M, Bushnell MC, Porter L. Prevalence and profile of high-impact chronic pain in the United States. *J Pain.* 2019;20(2):146-160.
4. Institute of Medicine (IOM). *Relieving Pain in America: A Blueprint for Transforming Prevention, Care, Education, and Research: A Call for Public Action.* The National Academies Press; 2011.
5. Rasu RS, Vouthy K, Crowl AN, et al. Cost of pain medication to treat adult patients with nonmalignant chronic pain in the United States. *J Manag Care Spec Pharm.* 2014;20(9):921-928.
6. Bair MJ, Robinson RL, Katon W, Kroenke K. Depression and pain comorbidity: a literature review. *Arch Intern Med.* 2003; 163(20):2433-2445.
7. Miller LR, Cano A. Comorbid chronic pain and depression: who is at risk? *J Pain.* 2009;10(6):619-627.
8. McWilliams LA, Cox BJ, Enns MW. Mood and anxiety disorders associated with chronic pain: an examination in a nationally representative sample. *Pain.* 2003;106(1-2):127-133.
9. Fishbain DA, Pulikal A, Lewis JE, Gao J. Chronic pain types differ in their reported prevalence of post-traumatic stress disorder (PTSD) and there is consistent evidence that chronic pain is associated with PTSD: an evidence-based structured systematic review. *Pain Med.* 2017;18:711-735.
10. Cheatle MD, Foster S, Pinkett A, Lesneski M, Qu D, Dhingra L. Assessing and managing sleep disturbance in patients with chronic pain. *Sleep Med Clin.* 2016;11(4):531-541.
11. Vowles KE, McEntee ML, Julnes PS, Frohe T, Ney JP, van der Goes DN. Rates of opioid misuse, abuse, and addiction in chronic pain: a systematic review and data synthesis. *Pain.* 2015;156(4):569-576.
12. Bigos SJ, Battie MC, Spengler DM, et al. A prospective study of work perceptions and psychosocial factors affecting the report of back injury. *Spine.* 1991;16(1):1-6.
13. Papageorgiou AC, Macfarlane GJ, Thomas E, Croft PR, Jayson MI, Silman AJ. Psychosocial factors in the workplace—do they predict new episodes of low back pain? Evidence from the South Manchester Back Pain Study. *Spine.* 1997;22(10):1137-1142.
14. Pincus T, Burton AK, Vogel S, Field AP. A systematic review of psychological factors as predictors of chronicity/disability in prospective cohorts of low back pain. *Spine.* 2002;27(5):E109-E120.
15. Lavand'homme P. Transition from acute to chronic pain after surgery. *Pain.* 2017;158(4):S50-S54.
16. Katz J, Seltzer Z. Transition from acute to chronic postsurgical pain: risk factors and protective factors. *Expert Rev Neurother.* 2009;9(5):723-744.
17. Althaus A, Hinrichs-Rocker A, Chapman R, et al. Development of a risk index for the prediction of chronic post-surgical pain. *Eur J Pain.* 2012;16(6):901-910.
18. Covington EC. Psychogenic pain: what it means, why it doesn't exist, and how to diagnose it. *Pain Med.* 2000;1(4):287-294.

19. Xu Q, Yaksh TL. A brief comparison of the pathophysiology of inflammatory versus neuropathic pain. *Curr Opin Anaesthesiol.* 2011;24(4):400-407.
20. Latremoliere A, Woolf CJ. Central sensitization: a generator of pain hypersensitivity by central neural plasticity. *J Pain.* 2009;10(9):895-926.
21. Woolf CJ. Central sensitization: implications for the diagnosis and treatment of pain. *Pain.* 2011;152:S2-S15.
22. Sluka KA, Clauw DJ. Neurobiology of fibromyalgia and chronic widespread pain. *Neuroscience.* 2016;338:114-129.
23. Mease PJ. Further strategies for treating fibromyalgia: the role of serotonin and norepinephrine reuptake inhibitors. *Am J Med.* 2009;122(12 Suppl):S44-S55.
24. Tsilioni I, Russell IJ, Stewart JM, Gleason RM, Theoharides TC. Neuropeptides CRH, SP, HK-1, and inflammatory cytokines IL-6 and TNF are increased in serum of patients with fibromyalgia syndrome, implicating mast cells. *J Pharmacol Exp Ther.* 2016;356(3):664-672.
25. Pyke TL, Osmotherly PG, Baines S. Measuring glutamate levels in the brains of fibromyalgia patients and a potential role for glutamate in the pathophysiology of fibromyalgia symptoms: a systematic review. *Clin J Pain.* 2017;33(10):944-954.
26. Ziv-Sefer S, Raber P, Barbash S, Devor M. Unity vs. diversity of neuropathic pain mechanisms: allodynia and hyperalgesia in rats selected for heritable predisposition to spontaneous pain. *Pain.* 2009;146(1-2):148-157.
27. Lötsch J, Geisslinger G. Current evidence for a modulation of nociception by human genetic polymorphisms. *Pain.* 2007;132(1-2):18-22.
28. Fishman SM, Carr DB, Hogans B, et al. Scope and nature of pain- and analgesia-related content of the United States Medical Licensing Examination (USMLE). *Pain Med.* 2018;19(3):449-459.
29. Berna C, Leknes S, Holmes EA, Edwards RR, Goodwin GM, Tracey I. Induction of depressed mood disrupts emotion regulation neurocircuitry and enhances pain unpleasantness. *Biol Psychiatry.* 2010;67(11):1083-1090.
30. Zelman DC, Howland EW, Nichols SN, Cleeland CS. The effects of induced mood on laboratory pain. *Pain.* 1991;46:105-111.
31. Rainville P, Bao QVH, Chrétien P. Pain-related emotions modulate experimental pain perception and autonomic responses. *Pain.* 2005;118(3):306-318.
32. McWilliams LA, Goodwin RD, Cox BJ. Depression and anxiety associated with three pain conditions: results from a nationally representative sample. *Pain.* 2004;111(1-2):77-83.
33. Bair MJ, Wu J, Damush TM, Sutherland JM, Kroenke K. Association of depression and anxiety alone and in combination with chronic musculoskeletal pain in primary care patients. *Psychosom Med.* 2008;70(8):890-897.
34. Maletic V, Raison CL. Neurobiology of depression, fibromyalgia and neuropathic pain. *Front Biosci.* 2009;14:5291-5338.
35. Kim H, Chen L, Lim G, et al. Brain indoleamine 2,3-dioxygenase contributes to the comorbidity of pain and depression. *J Clin Invest.* 2012;122(8):2940-2954.
36. Rome HP Jr, Rome JD. Limbically augmented pain syndrome (LAPS): kindling, corticolimbic sensitization, and the convergence of affective and sensory symptoms in chronic pain disorders. *Pain Med.* 2000;1(1):7-23.
37. Vranceanu AM, Bachoura A, Weening A, Vrahas M, Smith RM, Ring D. Psychological factors predict disability and pain intensity after skeletal trauma. *J Bone Joint Surg Am.* 2014;96(3):e20.
38. Gureje O, Simon GE, Von Kor M. A cross-national study of the course of persistent pain in primary care. *Pain.* 2001;92:195-200.
39. Williams LS, Jones WJ, Shen J, Robinson RL, Kroenke K. Outcomes of newly referred neurology outpatients with depression and pain. *Neurology.* 2004;63(4):674-677.
40. Kroenke K, Shen J, Oxman TE, Williams JW Jr, Dietrich AJ. Impact of pain on the outcomes of depression treatment: results from the RESPECT trial. *Pain.* 2008;134(1-2):209-215.
41. Talaei-Khoei M, Fischerauer SF, Jha R, Ring D, Chen N, Vranceanu AM. Bidirectional mediation of depression and pain intensity on their associations with upper extremity physical function. *J Behav Med.* 2018;41(3):309-317. doi:10.1007/s10865-017-9891-6
42. Edwards RR, Klick B, Buenaver L, et al. Symptoms of distress as prospective predictors of pain-related sciatica treatment outcomes. *Pain.* 2007;130(1-2):47-55.
43. Shaw WS, Means-Christensen AJ, Slater MA, et al. Psychiatric disorders and risk of transition to chronicity in men with first onset low back pain. *Pain Med.* 2010;11(9):1391-1400.
44. Rosenbloom BN, Katz J, Chin KY, et al. Predicting pain outcomes after traumatic musculoskeletal injury. *Pain.* 2016;157(8):1733-1743.
45. Shipherd JC, Keyes M, Jovanovic T, et al. Veterans seeking treatment for posttraumatic stress disorder: what about comorbid chronic pain? *J Rehabil Res Dev.* 2007;44(2):153-166.
46. Defrin R, Ginzburg K, Solomon Z, et al. Quantitative testing of pain perception in subjects with PTSD—implications for the mechanism of the coexistence between PTSD and chronic pain. *Pain.* 2008;138(2):450-459.
47. Siqveland J, Hussain A, Lindstrøm JC, Ruud T, Hauff E. Prevalence of posttraumatic stress disorder in persons with chronic pain: a meta-analysis. *Front Psychiatry.* 2017;8:164.
48. Åkerblom S, Perrin S, Rivano Fischer M, McCracken LM. The relationship between posttraumatic stress disorder and chronic pain in people seeking treatment for chronic pain: the mediating role of psychological flexibility. *Clin J Pain.* 2018;34(6):487-496.
49. Asmundson GJ, Norton PJ, Norton GR. Beyond pain: the role of fear and avoidance in chronicity. *Clin Psychol Rev.* 1999;19(1):97-119.
50. Norton PJ, Asmundson GJ. Anxiety sensitivity, fear, and avoidance behavior in headache pain. *Pain.* 2004;111(1-2):218-223.
51. Stewart SH, Asmundson GJ. Anxiety sensitivity and its impact on pain experiences and conditions: a state of the art. *Cogn Behav Ther.* 2006;35(4):185-188.
52. Thompson T, Keogh E, French CC, et al. Anxiety sensitivity and pain: generalisability across noxious stimuli. *Pain.* 2008;134(1-2):187-196.
53. Dodo N, Hashimoto R. The effect of anxiety sensitivity on psychological and biological variables during the cold pressor test. *Auton Neurosci.* 2017;205:72-76.
54. Fishbain DA, Lewis JE, Bruns D, Disorbio JM, Gao J, Meyer LJ. Exploration of anger constructs in acute and chronic pain patients vs. community patients. *Pain Pract.* 2011;11(3):240-251.
55. Trost Z, Vangronsveld K, Linton SJ, Quartana PJ, Sullivan MJL. Cognitive dimensions of anger in chronic pain. *Pain.* 2012;153(3):515-517.
56. Fernandez E, Turk DC. The scope and significance of anger in the experience of chronic pain. *Pain.* 1995;61(2):165-175.
57. Kerns RD, Rosenberg R, Jacob MC. Anger expression and chronic pain. *J Behav Med.* 1994;17(1):57-67.
58. Carson JW, Keefe FJ, Goli V, et al. Forgiveness and chronic low back pain: a preliminary study examining the relationship of forgiveness to pain, anger, and psychological distress. *J Pain.* 2005;6(2):84-91.
59. Wood AM, Froh JJ, Geraghty AW. Gratitude and well-being: a review and theoretical integration. *Clin Psychol Rev.* 2010;30(7):890-905.
60. Fernando GA. Bloodied but unbowed: resilience examined in a South Asian community. *Am J Orthopsychiatry.* 2012;82(3):367-375.
61. Froh JJ, Yurkewicz C, Kashdan TB. Gratitude and subjective well-being in early adolescence: examining gender differences. *J Adolesc.* 2009;32(3):633-650.
62. Ng MY, Wong WS. The differential effects of gratitude and sleep on psychological distress in patients with chronic pain. *J Health Psychol.* 2013;18(2):263-271.
63. Fauchon C, Faillenot I, Perrin AM, et al. Does an observer's empathy influence my pain? Effect of perceived empathetic or unempathetic support on a pain test. *Eur J Neurosci.* 2017;46(10):2629-2637. doi:10.1111/ejn.13701
64. Legrain V, Damme SV, Eccleston C. A neurocognitive model of attention to pain: behavioral and neuroimaging evidence. *Pain.* 2009;144(3):230-232.
65. Fields HL, Malick A, Burstein R. Dorsal horn projection targets of ON and OFF cells in the rostral ventromedial medulla. *J Neurophysiol.* 1995;74(4):1742-1759.

66. Neugebauer V, Li W, Bird GC, Han JS. The amygdala and persistent pain. *Neuroscientist.* 2004;10(3):221-234.
67. Bushnell MC, Duncan GH, Hofbauer RK, Ha B, Chen JI, Carrier B. Pain perception: is there a role for primary somatosensory cortex? *Proc Natl Acad Sci U S A.* 1999;96(14):7705-7709.
68. Sprenger C, Eippert F, Finsterbusch J, Bingel U, Rose M, Büchel C. Attention modulates spinal cord responses to pain. *Curr Biol.* 2012;22(11):1019-1022.
69. Petrovic P, Petersson KM, Ghatan PH, Stone-Elander S, Ingvar M. Pain-related cerebral activation is altered by a distracting cognitive task. *Pain.* 2000;85:19-30.
70. Iles RA, Davidson M, Taylor NF, O'Halloran P. Systematic review of the ability of recovery expectations to predict outcomes in non-chronic non-specific low back pain. *J Occup Rehabil.* 2009;19(1):25-40.
71. Clay FJ, Newstead SV, Watson WL, Ozanne-Smith J, Guy J, McClure RJ. Bio-psychosocial determinants of persistent pain 6 months after non-life-threatening acute orthopaedic trauma. *J Pain.* 2010;11(5):420-430.
72. Kalauokalani D, Cherkin DC, Sherman KJ, Koepsell TD, Deyo RA. Lessons from a trial of acupuncture and massage for low back pain: patient expectations and treatment effects. *Spine.* 2001;26(13):1418-1424.
73. Tan V, Cheatle MD, Macklin S, Moberg PJ, Esterhai JL. Goal setting as a predictor of return to work in a population of chronic musculoskeletal pain patients. *Int J Neurosci.* 1997;92(3-4):161-170.
74. Koyama T, McHaffie JG, Laurientit PJ, Coghill RC. The subjective experience of pain: where expectations become reality. *Proc Natl Acad Sci U S A.* 2005;102(36):12950-12955.
75. Sawamoto N, Honda M, Okada T, et al. Expectation of pain enhances responses to nonpainful somatosensory stimulation in the anterior cingulate cortex and parietal operculum/posterior insula: an event-related functional magnetic resonance imaging study. *J Neurosci.* 2000;20(19):7438-7445.
76. Vlaeyen JWS, Linton SJ. Fear-avoidance and its consequences in chronic musculoskeletal pain: a state of the art. *Pain.* 2000;85:317-332.
77. Vlaeyen JW, Linton SJ. Fear-avoidance model of chronic musculoskeletal pain: 12 years on. *Pain.* 2012;153(6):1144-1147.
78. McCracken LM, Spertus IL, Janeck AS, Sinclair D, Wetzel FT. Behavioral dimensions of adjustment in persons with chronic pain: pain-related anxiety and acceptance. *Pain.* 1999;80:283-289.
79. Crombex G, Vlaeyen JW, Heuts PH, Lysens R. Pain-related fear is more disabling than pain itself: evidence on the role of pain-related fear in chronic back pain disability. *Pain.* 1999;80:329-339.
80. Vlaeyen JW, Linton SJ. Are we "fear-avoidant"? *Pain.* 2006;124(3):240-241.
81. Cheatle MD. Biopsychosocial approach to assessing and managing patients with chronic pain. *Med Clin North Am.* 2016;100(1):43-53.
82. Beck AT, Rush AJ, Shaw BF, Emery G. *Cognitive Therapy of Depression.* Guilford Press; 1979.
83. Turk DC, Meichenbaum D, Genest M. *Pain and Behavioral Medicine: A Cognitive-Behavioral Perspective.* Guilford Press; 1983.
84. Turk DC, Rudy TE. Assessment of cognitive factors in chronic pain: a worthwhile enterprise? *J Consult Clin Psychol.* 1986;54(6):760-768.
85. Jensen MP, Turner JA, Romano JM, Karoly P. Coping with chronic pain: a critical review of the literature. *Pain.* 1991;47:249-283.
86. Affleck G, Urrows S, Tennen H, Higgins P. Daily coping with pain from rheumatoid arthritis: patterns and correlates. *Pain.* 1992;51:221-229.
87. Melzack R. Neurophysiology of pain. In: Sternbach RA, ed. *The Psychology of Pain.* 2nd ed. Raven Press; 1986.
88. Ahles TA, Blanchard EB, Ruckdeschel JC. The multidimensional nature of cancer-related pain. *Pain.* 1983;17:277-288.
89. Weissman-Fogel I, Sprecher E, Pud D. Effects of catastrophizing on pain perception and pain modulation. *Exp Brain Res.* 2008;186(1):79-85.
90. Byers HD, Lichstein KL, Thorn BE. Cognitive processes in comorbid poor sleep and chronic pain. *J Behav Med.* 2016;39(2):233-240.
91. Sansone RA, Watts DA, Wiederman MW. Pain, pain catastrophizing, and history of intentional overdoses and attempted suicide. *Pain Pract.* 2014;14(2):E29-E32.
92. Turk DC, Rudy TE. Cognitive factors and persistent pain: a glimpse into Pandora's box. *Cognit Ther Res.* 1992;16(2):99-122.
93. Keefe FJ, Brown GK, Wallston KA, Caldwell DS. Coping with rheumatoid arthritis pain: catastrophizing as a maladaptive strategy. *Pain.* 1989;37:51-56.
94. Compton P. Chronic pain and addiction: worry about the worrier. *Am J Drug Alcohol Abuse.* 2019;45(5):430-431.
95. Seligman ME. Learned helplessness. *Annu Rev Med.* 1972;23:407-412.
96. Bandura A. Self-efficacy: toward a unifying theory of behavioral change. *Psychol Rev.* 1977;84:191-215.
97. Jensen MP, Turner JA, Romano JM. Self-efficacy and outcome expectancies: relationship to chronic pain coping strategies and adjustment. *Pain.* 1991;44:263-269.
98. Maly MR, Costigan PA, Olney SJ. Self-efficacy mediates walking performance in older adults with knee osteoarthritis. *J Gerontol A Biol Sci Med Sci.* 2007;62(10):1142-1146.
99. Buckelew SP, Huyser B, Hewett J, et al. Self-efficacy predicting outcome among fibromyalgia subjects. *Arthritis Care Res.* 1996;9(2):97-104.
100. Menezes Costa LDC, Maher CG, McAuley JH, Hancock MJ, Smeets RJEM. Self-efficacy is more important than fear of movement in mediating the relationship between pain and disability in chronic low back pain. *Eur J Pain.* 2011;15(2):213-219.
101. Hamilton JC, Eger M, Razzak S, Feldman MD, Hallmark N, Cheek S. Somatoform, factitious, and related diagnoses in the national hospital discharge survey: addressing the proposed DSM-5 revision. *Psychosomatics.* 2013;54(2):142.
102. Dimsdale J, Creed F; DSM-5 Workgroup on Somatic Symptom Disorders. The proposed diagnosis of somatic symptom disorders in DSM-5 to replace somatoform disorders in DSM-IV—a preliminary report. *J Psychosom Res.* 2009;66(6):473-476.
103. American Psychiatric Association. *Diagnostic and Statistical Manual of Mental Disorders.* 4th Text Revision ed. American Psychiatric Association; 2000.
104. American Psychiatric Association. *Diagnostic and Statistical Manual of Mental Disorders.* 5th ed. American Psychiatric Association; 2013.
105. U.S. Commission on the Evaluation of Pain. *Report of the Commission on the Evaluation of Pain, Appendix C: Summary of the National Study of Chronic Pain Syndrome.* Social Security Administration, Office of Disability; 1987.
106. Mailis-Gagnon A, Nicholson K, Blumberger D, Zurowski M. Characteristics and period prevalence of self-induced disorder in patients referred to a pain clinic with the diagnosis of complex regional pain syndrome. *Clin J Pain.* 2008;24(2):176-185.
107. Fishbain DA, Cutler R, Rosomoff HL, Rosomoff RS. Chronic pain disability exaggeration/malingering and submaximal effort research. *Clin J Pain.* 1999;15(4):244-274.
108. Bytzer P, Stokholm M, Andersen I, Klitgaard NA, Schaffalitsky de Muckadell OB. Prevalence of surreptitious laxative abuse in patients with diarrhea of uncertain origin: a cost benefit analysis of a screening procedure. *Gut.* 1989;30(10):1379-1384.
109. Rickards FW, De Vidi S. Exaggerated hearing loss in noise induced hearing loss compensation claims in Victoria. *Med J Aust.* 1995; 163(7):360-363.
110. Schmand B, Lindeboom J, Schagen S, Heijt R, Koene T, Hamburger HL. Cognitive complaints in patients after whiplash injury: the impact of malingering. *J Neurol Neurosurg Psychiatry.* 1998;64(3):339-343.
111. Gervais RO, Russell AS, Green P, Allen LM III, Ferrari R, Pieschl SD. Effort testing in patients with fibromyalgia and disability incentives. *J Rheumatol.* 2001;28(8):1892-1899.
112. Rivat C, Becker C, Blugeot A, et al. Chronic stress induces transient spinal neuroinflammation, triggering sensory hypersensitivity and long-lasting anxiety-induced hyperalgesia. *Pain.* 2010;150(2):358-368.
113. Le Roy C, Laboureyras E, Gavello-Baudy S, Chateauraynaud J, Laulin JP, Simonnet G. Endogenous opioids released during non-nociceptive environmental stress induce latent pain sensitization via a NMDA-dependent process. *J Pain.* 2011;12(10):1069-1079.
114. Green PG, Alvarez P, Gear RW, Mendoza D, Levine JD. Further validation of a model of fibromyalgia syndrome in the rat. *J Pain.* 2011;12(7):811-818.

115. Kuzma J, Black D. Chronic widespread pain and psychiatric disorders in veterans of the first Gulf War. *Curr Pain Headache Rep.* 2006;10(2):85-89.
116. Fordyce WE, Fowler RS, Lehman F, Delateur BJ, Sand PL, Trieschmann RB. Operant conditioning in the treatment of chronic pain. *Arch Phys Med Rehabil.* 1973;54(9):399-408.
117. Fordyce WE. *Behavioral Methods for Chronic Pain and Illness.* C.V. Mosby; 1976.
118. Henschke N, Ostelo RW, van Tulder MW, et al. Behavioural treatment for chronic low-back pain. *Cochrane Database Syst Rev.* 2010;7:CD002014.
119. Bernardes SF, Forgeron P, Fournier K, Reszel J. Beyond solicitousness: a comprehensive review on informal pain-related social support. *Pain.* 2017;158(11):2066-2076.
120. Pence LB, Thorn BE, Jensen MP, Romano JM. Examination of perceived spouse responses to patient well and pain behavior in patients with headache. *Clin J Pain.* 2008;24(8):654-661.
121. Alschuler KN, Hoodin F, Murphy SL, Rice J, Geisser ME. Factors contributing to physical activity in a chronic low back pain clinical sample: a comprehensive analysis using continuous ambulatory monitoring. *Pain.* 2011;152(11):2521-2527.
122. Fishbain DA, Rosomoff HL, Cutler RB, Rosomoff RS. Secondary gain concept: a review of the scientific evidence. *Clin J Pain.* 1995;11:6-21.
123. Rohling ML, Binder LM, Langhinrichsen-Rohling J. Money matters: a meta-analytic review of the association between financial compensation and the experience and treatment of chronic pain. *Health Psychol.* 1995;14(6):537-547.
124. Nguyen TH, Randolph DC, Talmage J, Succop P, Travis R. Long-term outcomes of lumbar fusion among workers' compensation subjects: a historical cohort study. *Spine.* 2011;36(4):320-331.
125. Hagekull B, Bohlin G. Predictors of middle childhood psychosomatic problems: an emotion regulation approach. *Infant Child Dev.* 2004; 13:389-405.
126. Payne B, Norfleet MA. Chronic pain and the family: a review. *Pain.* 1986;26:1-22.
127. Roy R. Marital and family issues in patients with chronic pain: a review. *Psychother Psychosom.* 1982;37:1-12.
128. Roy R. Pain-prone patient: a revisit. *Psychother Psychosom.* 1982; 37:202-213.
129. Bendixen M, Muus KM, Schei B. The impact of child sexual abuse—a study of a random sample of Norwegian students. *Child Abuse Negl.* 1994;18(10):837-847.
130. Walsh CA, Jamieson E, Macmillan H, Boyle M. Child abuse and chronic pain in a community survey of women. *J Interpers Violence.* 2007;22(12):1536-1554.
131. Imbierowicz K, Egle UT. Childhood adversities in patients with fibromyalgia and somatoform pain disorder. *Eur J Pain.* 2003;7(2): 113-119.
132. Brown RJ, Schrag A, Trimble MR. Dissociation, childhood interpersonal trauma, and family functioning in patients with somatization disorder. *Am J Psychiatry.* 2005;162:899-905.
133. Sachs-Ericsson N, Kendall-Tackett K, Hernandez A. Childhood abuse, chronic pain, and depression in the National Comorbidity Survey. *Child Abuse Negl.* 2007;31(5):531-547.
134. Ringel Y, Drossman DA, Leserman JL, et al. Effect of abuse history on pain reports and brain responses to aversive visceral stimulation: an FMRI study. *Gastroenterology.* 2008;134(2):396-404.
135. Coutinho SV, Plotsky PM, Sablad M, et al. Neonatal maternal separation alters stress-induced responses to viscerosomatic nociceptive stimuli in rat. *Am J Physiol Gastrointest Liver Physiol.* 2002;282(2):G307-G316.
136. Green PG, Chena X, Alvareza P, Ferrari LF, Levine JD. Early-life stress produces muscle hyperalgesia and nociceptor sensitization in the adult rat. *Pain.* 2011;152:2549-2556.
137. Porter LS, Davis D, Keefe FJ. Attachment and pain: recent findings and future directions. *Pain.* 2007;128(3):195-198.
138. McWilliams LA, Asmundson GJG. The relationship of adult attachment dimensions to pain-related fear, hypervigilance, and catastrophizing. *Pain.* 2007;127(1-2):27-34.
139. Landa A, Peterson BS, Fallon BA. Somatoform pain: a developmental theory and translational research review. *Psychosom Med.* 2012; 74(7):717-727.
140. Dworkin R, Turk DC, Farrar JT, et al. Core outcome measures for chronic pain trials: IMMPACT recommendations. *Pain.* 2005;113(1-2):9-19.
141. Beck A, Ward C, Mendelson M, Mock J, Erbaugh J. An inventory for measuring depression. *Arch Gen Psychiatry.* 1961;4:561-571.
142. McNair D, Lorr M, Droppleman L. *Profile of Mood States.* Educational and Industrial Testing Service; 1971.
143. Kroenke K, Spitzer RL, Williams JB, Lowe B. An ultrabrief screening scale for anxiety and depression: the PHQ-4. *Psychosomatics.* 2009;50(6):613-621.
144. Cheatle MD, Compton PA, Dhingra L, Wasser TE, O'Brien CP. Development of the revised opioid risk tool to predict opioid use disorder in patients with chronic nonmalignant pain. *J Pain.* 2019;20(7):842-851.
145. Turk DC, Swanson K. Efficacy and cost-effectiveness treatment of chronic pain: an analysis and evidence-based synthesis. In: Schatman ME, Campbell A, eds. *Chronic Pain Management: Guidelines for Multidisciplinary Program Development.* Informa Healthcare; 2007:15-38.
146. Oslund S, Robinson RC, Clark TC, et al. Long-term effectiveness of a comprehensive pain management program: strengthening the case for interdisciplinary care. *Proc (Bayl Univ Med Cent).* 2009;22(3):211-214.
147. Cheatle MD, Gallagher RM. Chronic pain and comorbid mood and substance use disorders: a biopsychosocial treatment approach. *Curr Psychiatry Rep.* 2006;8(5):371-376.
148. McCracken LM, Turk TC. Behavioral and cognitive-behavioral treatment for chronic pain: outcome, predictors of outcome, and treatment process. *Spine.* 2002;27(22):2564.
149. Sullivan AB, Scheman J, Venesy D, Davin S. The role of exercise and types of exercise in the rehabilitation of chronic pain: specific or nonspecific benefits. *Curr Pain Headache Rep.* 2012;16(2):153-161.
150. Murtezani A, Hundozi H, Orovcanec N, Sllamniku S, Osmani T. A comparison of high intensity aerobic exercise and passive modalities for the treatment of workers with chronic low back pain: a randomized, controlled trial. *Eur J Phys Rehabil Med.* 2011;47(3):359-366.
151. Heldt SA, Stanek L, Chhatwal JP, Ressler KJ. Hippocampus-specific deletion of BDNF in adult mice impairs spatial memory and extinction of aversive memories. *Mol Psychiatry.* 2007;12(7):656-670.
152. Wipfli BM, Rethorst CD, Landers DM. The anxiolytic effects of exercise: a meta-analysis of randomized trials and dose-response analysis. *J Sport Exerc Psychol.* 2008;30(4):392-410.
153. Turk DC, Flor H. Etiological theories and treatments for chronic back pain. II. Psychological models and interventions. *Pain.* 1984; 19(3):209-233.
154. Ashar YK, Gordon A, Schubiner H, et al. Effect of pain reprocessing therapy vs placebo and usual care for patients with chronic back pain: a randomized clinical trial. *JAMA Psychiatry.* 2022;79(1):13-23.
155. Keefe FJ, Caldwell DS. Cognitive behavioral control of arthritis pain. *Med Clin North Am.* 1997;81:277-290.
156. Linton SJ. A 5-year follow-up evaluation of the health and economic consequences of an early cognitive behavioral intervention for back pain: a randomized, controlled trial. *Spine.* 2006;31(8):853-858.
157. Lamb SE, Hansen Z, Lall R, Castelnuovo E, Withers EJ, Nichols V. Group cognitive behavioral treatment for low-back pain in primary care: a randomized controlled trial and cost-effectiveness analysis. *Lancet.* 2010;375:916-923.
158. Greco CM, Rudy TE, Manzi S. Effects of a stress-reduction program on psychological function, pain, and physical function of systemic lupus erythematosus patients: a randomized controlled trial. *Arthritis Rheum.* 2004;51(4):625-634.
159. Thieme K, Flor H, Turk D. Psychological pain treatment in fibromyalgia syndrome: efficacy of operant behavioral and cognitive behavioral treatments. *Arthritis Res Ther.* 2006;8(4):R121.
160. Chen E, Cole SW, Kato PM. A review of empirically supported psychosocial interventions for pain and adherence outcomes in sickle cell disease. *J Pediatr Psychol.* 2004;29:1997-2009.

161. Bernardy K, Klose P, Busch AJ, Choy EH, Häuser W. Cognitive behavioural therapies for fibromyalgia. *Cochrane Database Syst Rev.* 2013;9:CD009796. doi:10.1002/14651858.CD009796.pub2
162. Tang NK, Wright KJ, Salkovskis PM. Prevalence and correlates of clinical insomnia co-occurring with chronic back pain. *J Sleep Res.* 2007;16(1):85-95.
163. McCracken LM, Williams JL, Tang NK. Psychological flexibility may reduce insomnia in persons with chronic pain: a preliminary retrospective study. *Pain Med.* 2011;12(6):904-912.
164. Haythornthwaite JA, Hegel MT, Kerns RD. Development of a sleep diary for chronic pain patients. *J Pain Symptom Manage.* 1991;6(2):65-72.
165. Chiu YH, Silman AJ, Macfarlane GJ, et al. Poor sleep and depression are independently associated with a reduced pain threshold. Results of a population based study. *Pain.* 2005;115(3):316-321.
166. Wiles NJ, Thomas L, Turner N, et al. Long-term effectiveness and cost-effectiveness of cognitive behavioural therapy as an adjunct to pharmacotherapy for treatment-resistant depression in primary care: follow-up of the CoBalT randomised controlled trial. *Lancet.* 2016;3(2):137-144.
167. Mitchell MD, Gehrman P, Perlis M, Umscheid CA. Comparative effectiveness of cognitive behavioral therapy for insomnia: a systematic review. *BMC Fam Pract.* 2012;13:40.
168. Jungquist CR, Tra Y, Smith MT, et al. The durability of cognitive behavioral therapy for insomnia in patients with chronic pain. *Sleep Disord.* 2012;2012:679648.
169. Tang NK, Goodchild CE, Salkovskis PM. Hybrid cognitive-behavior therapy for individuals with insomnia and chronic pain: a pilot randomized controlled trial. *Behav Res Ther.* 2012;50(12):814-821.
170. McCracken LM, Carson JW, Eccleston C, Keefe FJ. Acceptance and change in the context of chronic pain. *Pain.* 2004;109(1-2):4-7.
171. McCracken LM, Gauntlett-Gilbert J, Vowles KE. The role of mindfulness in a contextual cognitive-behavioral analysis of chronic pain-related suffering and disability. *Pain.* 2007;131(1-2):63-69.
172. Potter JS. *NIH Pain Consortium 7th Annual NIH Symposium on Advances in Research*. Washington, DC; 2012.
173. Zeidan F, Grant JA, Brown CA, McHaffie JG, Coghill RC. Mindfulness meditation-related pain relief: evidence for unique brain mechanisms in the regulation of pain. *Neurosci Lett.* 2012;520(2):165-173.
174. Adler-Neal AL, Zeidan F. Mindfulness meditation for fibromyalgia: mechanistic and clinical considerations. *Curr Rheumatol Rep.* 2017; 19(9):59.
175. Veehof MM, Oskam MJ, Schreurs KM, Bohlmeijer ET. Acceptance-based interventions for the treatment of chronic pain: a systematic review and meta-analysis. *Pain.* 2011;152:533-542.
176. Vowles KE, McCracken LM, O'Brien JZ. Acceptance and values-based action in chronic pain: a three-year follow-up analysis of treatment effectiveness and process. *Behav Res Ther.* 2011;49(11):748-755.
177. McDougal JC, Ock S, Demers LB, Sokolove RL. Cognitive behavioral therapy and pharmacotherapy for the treatment of tobacco use disorder in primary care for resident physicians. *MedEdPORTAL.* 2019;15:10812.
178. Byrne SP, Haber P, Baillie A, Costa DSJ, Fogliati V, Morley K. Systematic reviews of mindfulness and acceptance and commitment therapy for alcohol use disorder: should we be using third wave therapies? *Alcohol.* 2019;54(2):159-166.
179. Morasco BJ, Greaves DW, Lovejoy TI, Turk DC, Dobscha SK, Hauser P. Development and preliminary evaluation of an integrated cognitive-behavior treatment for chronic pain and substance use disorder in patients with the hepatitis C virus. *Pain Med.* 201617(12):2280-2290.
180. Vowles KE, Witkiewitz K, Cusack KJ, et al. Integrated behavioral treatment for veterans with co-morbid chronic pain and hazardous opioid use: a randomized controlled pilot trial. *Pain.* 202021(7-8): 798-807.
181. Smallwood RF, Potter JS, Robin DA. Neurophysiological mechanisms in acceptance and commitment therapy in opioid-addicted patients with chronic pain. *Psychiatry Res Neuroimaging.* 2016;250:12-14.
182. Lewandowski W, Morris R, Draucker CB, Risko J. Chronic pain and the family: theory-driven treatment approaches. *Issues Ment Health Nurs.* 2007;28(9):1019-1044.
183. McCracken LM. Social context and acceptance of chronic pain: the role of solicitous and punishing responses. *Pain.* 2005;113:155-159.
184. Flor H, Fydrich T, Turk DC. Efficacy of multidisciplinary pain treatment centers: a meta-analytic review. *Pain.* 1992;49:221-230.
185. Turk DC. Efficacy of multidisciplinary pain centers in the treatment of chronic pain. In: MJM C, Campbell NJ, eds. *Pain Treatment Centers at a Crossroads: A Practical and Conceptual Reappraisal. Progress in Pain Research and Management*. Vol. 7 IASP Press; 1996:257-273.
186. Tollison CD, Kriegel ML, Downie GR. Chronic low back pain: results of treatment at the Pain Therapy Center. *South Med J.* 1985;78(11):1291-1295.
187. Gatchel RJ, Okifuji A. Evidence-based scientific data documenting the treatment and cost-effectiveness of comprehensive pain programs for chronic nonmalignant pain. *J Pain.* 2006;7(11):779-793.
188. Turk DC, Swanson K. Efficacy and cost-effectiveness treatment for chronic pain: an analysis and evidence-based synthesis. In: Schatman ME, Campbell A, eds. *Chronic Pain Management: A Guidebook for Multidisciplinary Program Development.* Informa Healthcare; 2007:15-38.
189. Schatman ME. Interdisciplinary chronic pain management: international perspectives. *ISAP Pain Clin Updates.* 2012;20(7):1-5.
190. Ehde DM, Dillworth TM, Turner JA. Cognitive-behavioral therapy for individuals with chronic pain: efficacy, innovations, and directions for research. *Am Psychol.* 2014;69(2):153-166.
191. Rini C, Porter LS, Somers TJ, et al. Automated Internet-based pain coping skills training to manage osteoarthritis pain: a randomized controlled trial. *Pain.* 2015;156(5):837-848.
192. Dear BF, Titov N, Perry KN, et al. The pain course: a randomized controlled trial of a clinician-guided Internet-delivered cognitive behavior therapy program for managing chronic pain and emotional well-being. *Pain.* 2013;154(6):942-950.
193. Lalloo C, Jibb LA, Rivera J, Agarwal A, Stinson JN. "There's a Pain App for That": review of patient-targeted smartphone applications for pain management. *Clin J Pain.* 2015;31(6):557-563.
194. Tuerk PW, Yoder M, Ruggiero K, Gros DF, Acierno R. A pilot study of prolonged exposure therapy for posttraumatic stress disorder delivered via telehealth technology. *J Trauma Stress.* 2010;23:116-123.

CHAPTER

110 Assessing and Mitigating Risk of Suicide in Patients With Pain and Substance Use Disorders

Martin D. Cheatle

CHAPTER OUTLINE

- Introduction
- Chronic pain and suicide
- Suicide and substance use disorders
- Pain, substance use disorders and suicide: Risk factors
- Assessing risk for suicide
- Mitigation strategies
- Pharmacologic and nonpharmacologic interventions
- Summary

INTRODUCTION

Suicide has become a global epidemic. The Word Health Organization published an executive summary, "Preventing Suicide, A Global Imperative."[1] In this summary, there were some distressing facts: every 40 seconds someone in the world dies of suicide; an estimated 804,000 suicide deaths occurred worldwide in 2012; the annual global suicide rate was 11.4/100,000 population (15.0 male and 8.0 female); and in the age group of 15 to 29 it is the second leading cause of death. Suicide constitutes 54% of the 1.5 million violent deaths per year globally. Over 75% of suicides occur in low and middle-income families, and these numbers continue to burgeon annually. In 2020 suicide was the 12th leading cause of death in the United States.[2] Suicide is the second leading cause of death in people aged 10 to 34 and the fifth leading cause in people aged 35 to 54.[2] There are certain populations that are at high risk for suicide including individuals who suffer from chronic pain and those with substance use disorders (SUDs).

CHRONIC PAIN AND SUICIDE

The prevalence of suicidal ideation in patients with pain is not inconsequential, ranging anywhere from 18% to 50%.[3-18] For example, Tang and Crane[15] completed a systematic review of the literature on pain and risk of suicide, which revealed that the risk of successful suicide was doubled in patients with chronic pain as compared to nonpain controls. Hitchcock et al.[3] found that 50% of patients with chronic pain endorsed experiencing suicidal ideation directly related to pain intensity. In another study Ilgen et al.[16] evaluated a large cohort obtained from the Veterans Affairs' database ($N = 260{,}254$) and discovered that veterans experiencing severe pain were more likely to end their life by suicide than veterans with no, mild, or moderate pain (HR: 1.33; 95% CI: 1.15-1.54). Cheatle et al.[13] evaluated suicide risk and potential predictors of suicidal ideation in a sample of 466 patients with chronic noncancer pain (CNCP) enrolled in a behaviorally based pain program. Results revealed a high rate of suicidal ideation (26%) and logistic regression of suicidal ideation revealed that history of sexual abuse (beta = 0.825; $p < 0.020$; OR = 2.657 [95% CI = 1.447-4877]), family history of suicidal ideation (beta = 0.471; $p < 0.006$; OR = 1.85 [95% CI = 1.234-3.070]) and being socially withdrawn (beta = 0.482; $p < 0.001$; OR = 2.226 [95% CI = 1.413-3.505]) were predictive of suicidal ideation. Campbell et al.[17] examined data from the 2007 Australian National Survey of Mental Health and Wellbeing. This nationally representative household survey of 8,841 individuals revealed that the odds ratio of lifetime and past 12-month suicidal ideation and suicidal behavior was two to three times greater in individuals with CNCP than those without CNCP. In a subsequent study by Campbell et al.[18] the prevalence and correlates of suicidal ideation and suicidal behavior were evaluated in a sample of 1,514 community-based subjects with CNCP receiving opioid therapy. Past 12-month suicidal ideation was acknowledged by 36.5% of the sample and 16.4% reported a lifetime suicide attempt after the onset of their pain.

SUICIDE AND SUBSTANCE USE DISORDERS

Individuals with SUDs, like those suffering from chronic pain can experience depression, suicidal ideation, alienation, loss of relationships, financial problems and a sense of hopelessness which are risk factors for suicidal ideation. Approximately 40% of patients seeking treatment for SUDs report a history of suicide attempts.[19-21] Compared to the general population, individuals with an alcohol use disorder are almost 10 times more likely to die by suicide and those who inject drugs are approximately 14 times more likely to commit suicide as compared to the general public.[22]

Patients with co-occurring pain and SUD are at high risk for attempting and ending their lives by suicide.

PAIN, SUBSTANCE USE DISORDERS AND SUICIDE: RISK FACTORS

General risk factors for suicide include gender (female); age (>45 years old); having co-occurring mental disorders (especially depression, suicidal ideation and SUD); acute losses and stressors (relationships, job, finances); enduring chronic medical illnesses; experiencing conflict, disaster, discrimination; past psychiatric hospitalizations; frequency of suicidal ideation; severity of psychiatric disorder; poor social support and the strongest predictor of suicide is a previous suicide attempt.[1,23] While patients with pain and those with SUDs commonly share some of not to these general risk factors such as personal and vocational losses, isolation, mood, and anxiety disorders; there are risk factors that are more specific to pain and SUD.

Substance Use Disorders and Suicide: Risk Factors

A number of mental health, personality traits, social and developmental risk factors for suicidality in patients with SUDs have been identified. Yuodelis-Flores and Ries[24] evaluated characteristics of suicidal ideation and suicide attempts in patients with SUDs. Results indicated that a history of attempted suicide was a strong predictor of future suicide. Several personality traits such as impulsiveness, aggression, pessimism, and hopelessness, along with acute stressors such as loss of relationships or income and a history of childhood sexual abuse all were key factors contributing to the risk of suicide in patients with SUD. Certain mental disorders also strongly predicted the risk of suicide attempts in patients with SUD, in particular, major depressive disorder, bipolar disorder, PTSD, and borderline personality disorder. In another study by Archambault and colleagues suicidal ideation and past suicide attempts were evaluated in a cohort of 202 patients with opioid use disorder (OUD) entering a residential treatment center. They found that patients with a diagnosed mood disorder were 2.48 times more likely to endorse suicidal ideation and 2.64 times more likely to report a history of a suicide attempt. Patients with an anxiety diagnosis were 2.41 times more likely to report suicidal ideation and patients experiencing co-occurring chronic pain were 2.59 times more likely to report suicidal ideation. Lastly, the probability of reporting suicidal ideation was 5.09 times higher in patients with suspected or diagnosed personality disorders.[25]

Chronic Pain and Suicide: Risk Factors

Pain specific risk factors for suicide include pain type, sleep disturbance, pain intensity, pain coping, and opioid dosing.

Pain Type

A meta-analysis of the impact on pain on current and lifetime suicidal ideation and suicidal behavior revealed that any type of physical pain (headache, spine, chest, musculoskeletal, pelvic, fibromyalgia, abdominal, or unexplained pain) was a consistent risk factor for suicidality.[26] Patients with certain pain conditions are particularly vulnerable to suicide including fibromyalgia, migraine, and complex regional pain syndromes. Jimenez-Rodriguez et al.[27] assessed the risk of suicidal ideation and suicidal behavior in patients with fibromyalgia (FM) compared to nonpain controls and patients suffering from low back pain (LBP). The percent of population expressing suicidal ideation in the control group was 4%, LBP 18.8% (OR = 4.583; 95% CI = 0.826-25.432; p value 0.082). and patients with FM was 41% (OR = 26.889; 95% CI = 5.72-126.42; $p < 0.0001$). Novic et al.[28] conducted a systematic review of the literature on the relationship between migraine and suicidal ideation. Seventeen papers met inclusion criteria of having empirical analyses. Results indicated that there was a strong association between migraine and suicidal ideation and suicidal behavior especially in the subtype of migraine with aura.

Patients with migraine and concomitant FM have a particularly high risk of suicide. Risk of suicidal ideation and suicidal behavior in a cohort of 1,318 patients with migraine with 10.1% of this sample having comorbid FM were examined. Patients with both migraine and FM had a higher rate of headache frequency and headache-related disability, poorer sleep and were more depressed and anxious as compared to patients that only experienced migraine. Patients with both headache and FM had a statistically higher rate of suicidal ideation (58.3% versus 24%) and attempt (17.6% versus 5.7%).[29] In a study by Do-Hyeong Lee et al. patients with complex regional pain syndrome (CRPS) type 1 and type 2 were evaluated and revealed that 74.9% of patients with CRPS were at high risk as compared to 25.6% that were at low risk for suicidal ideation. Risk factors associated with suicidal ideation in this cohort included depression, pain severity, and low functionality.[30]

Sleep Disturbance

Sleep disturbance is highly prevalent in patients with chronic pain ranging from 50% to 80%[12,31-37] and has been postulated as a potential risk factor of suicidal ideation in this patient population. Smith et al.[36] assessed 51 outpatients with CNCP and 24% endorsed current suicidal ideation. A discriminant analysis revealed that sleep onset insomnia and pain intensity accounted for greater than 84% of these cases of suicidal ideation which was independent of depression severity. Racine et al.[12] examined 88 patients with CNCP who completed a self-administered questionnaires at intake to three pain clinics in Canada. Like the findings of Smith et al.,[36] 24% of these patients endorsed experiencing suicidal ideation. Poor sleep quality was the only significant variable predictor of suicidal ideation. Although sleep disturbance is common in patients with pain it is often not evaluated or effectively treated.[37]

Pain Intensity

Pain intensity has been postulated as predictive of suicidal ideation and suicidal behavior in patients with chronic pain. Ilgen et al.[16] analyzed a large cohort of Veterans Affairs' medical records and the National Death Index (N = 260,254) evaluating the association between self-assessed pain severity and suicidal behavior in veterans. They discovered after controlling for demographic and psychiatric factors that veterans with severe pain were more likely to die by suicide than ones with mild or moderate pain (HR: 1.33; 95% CI: 1.15-1.54).

Pain Coping

Patients with chronic pain can engage in maladaptive thinking-pain catastrophizing, which can be conceptualized as magnified, exaggerated negative focus on pain that can contribute to depression and disability and in turn exacerbate an individual's experience of pain and suffering.[38] In a large cohort of 1,515 patients with CNCP the association between suicidal ideation and individual differences in the use of pain-related coping strategies and pain catastrophizing was evaluated. Results revealed that 32% of the subjects reported recent suicidal ideation and that depression and pain catastrophizing best predicted the occurrence and suicidal ideation. Demographic variables, pain intensity and pain duration were not highly significant predictors of suicidal ideation.[14] Patients suffering from headaches are a high-risk group for suicidal ideation. The extent of headache disability, pain-related catastrophizing and suicidality was examined in a cohort of 200 patients with headache. The degree of headache disability and pain catastrophizing was strongly associated with suicidal ideation and actual suicide attempts. Brown et al. analyzed the longitudinal association between two styles of pain coping, catastrophizing, and hoping/praying, as predictors of subsequent suicidal ideation in patients with CNCP receiving long-term opioid therapy. Catastrophizing was a statistically significant predictor of increased subsequent suicidal ideation, whereas hoping/praying did not protect against future suicidal ideation or behavior. The relationship between catastrophizing and future suicidal ideation was mediated by depression, but not social support or pain interference.[39]

Opioid Dosing

Another identified risk factor or suicidal ideation in patients with CNCP is opioid dosing. Ilgen et al.[40] evaluated the risk of suicide stratified by different opioid doses in a retrospective analysis of veterans with CNCP. After controlling for demographic and other relevant clinical factors (depression, PTSD etc.) the results indicated that higher opioid doses were associated with increased risk of suicide mortality. Compared with individuals that received 20 mg or less morphine equivalent daily dose (MEDD), those prescribed 20 to 50 MEDD had a hazard ratio (HR) of 1.48 (95% CI: 1.25-1.75); 50 to 100 MEDD HR of 1.69 (95% CI: 1.33-2.14); and 100+ a HR of 2.15 (95% CI: 1.64-2.81).

In managing patients with CNCP, clinicians should be cognizant of these risk factors and screen patients routinely for SUDs, mood disorders, pain catastrophizing, sleep disturbance, pain intensity, opioid dosing and have a plan of action if patients are identified as high risk for suicide.

ASSESSING RISK FOR SUICIDE

Assessing risk for suicide in patients with CNCP should include routinely evaluating mood, sleep disturbance, presence of SUDs and specific tools for suicidal ideation and suicidal behavior.

Mental Health Screening

There are several validated depression and anxiety assessment tools. The Initiative on Methods, Measurements and Pain Assessment in Clinical Trials (IMMPACT) consensus group[41] recommended the Beck Depression Inventory (BDI)[42] and the Profile of Mood States (POMS)[43] for measuring emotional function in chronic pain. The BDI is a 21-item self-report measure of the severity of depressive symptoms over the past week, whereas the POMS assesses distinct mood states including depression, anxiety, and anger, thought to be the most relevant factors in the pain population. Another commonly used depression screening tool developed for use in primary care is the Patient Health Questionnaire (PHQ-9),[44] which is a self-rating instrument that includes nine symptoms of depression based on the DSM-IV TR criteria for major depression. Two measures of anxiety that are highly valid and reliable are the Beck Anxiety Inventory (BAI)[45] and the State-Trait Anxiety Inventory.[46] A brief screener for both anxiety and depression is the PHQ-4.[47]

Sleep Disturbance

Assessing sleep disturbance can include polysomnography (typically used if sleep apnea is suspected, especially if a patient is on opioid therapy), actigraphy (eg, Fitbit, Apple watch, etc.) and patient self-report measures. Self-report measures assess different characteristics of sleep disturbance. For example, Wolff's Morning Questions[48] and Kryger's Subjective Measurements[49] are types of postsleep evaluations assessing sleep onset, sleep latency and morning restfulness. There are also tools that assess sleep quality such as the Pittsburgh Sleep Quality Index.[50] Another tool often used is the PROMIS Sleep Disturbance Measure–Short Form, a brief eight-item self-report measure that assesses sleep quality and disturbances over the last week.[51]

Substance Use Disorders

Since patients with pain and concomitant SUDs are at particular risk for suicide it is important to assess for presence of unhealthy substance use and for risk of developing an opioid use disorder if patients are being considered for opioid therapy or receiving long term opioid therapy. Examples of assessment tools for general SUDs include the CAGE-AID (Cut down, Annoyed, Guilty, Eye-opener Tool),[52] which assesses for both unhealthy alcohol and drug use and consists of four questions and is administered by the clinician, the RAFFT (Relax, Along, Friends, Family, Trouble),[53] a five-item patient self-report questionnaire; the DAST (Drug Abuse Screening Test), which has 28, 20 and 10-question versions and is a patient self-report measure[54,55] and the SBIRT (Screening, Brief Intervention and Referral to Treatment), which varies on number of items and is administered by the clinician.[56]

Risk assessment tools for potential prescription opioid misuse and unhealthy use when considering long term opioid therapy include the Opioid Risk Tool (ORT),[57] the Screener and Opioids Assessment for Patients with Pain (SOAPP),[58] and the Diagnosis, Intractable Risk and Efficacy Score (DIRE).[59] These three instruments are examples of assessing risk for potential aberrant drug-related behavior (ADRB) but are not validated to assess risk of developing an opioid use disorder. The Opioid Risk Tool-Opioid Use Disorder is a valid assessment tool for assessing risk of developing an opioid use disorder in patients with CNCP.[60] Examples of assessment tools to monitor opioid misuse in patients on long term opioid therapy initiated include the Pain Medication Questionnaire (PMQ),[61] Current Opioid Misuse Measure (COMM),[62] and the Prescription Drug Use Questionnaire (PDUQ).[63]

Screening Tools for Suicide

Many depression screening tools have a question on suicide risk for example question 9 on the PHQ-9,[55] which asks, "Thoughts that you are better off dead or of hurting yourself in some way." More specific assessment tools for suicidal ideation and suicidal intentionality include the P-4 Brief Assessment, which assess **P**ast suicide attempts, a **P**lan for suicide, **P**robability of completing suicide and **P**reventive factors.[64] The Columbia Suicide Severity Rating Scale (C-SSRS) has been frequently used for clinical trials on new medications and in clinical practice. The C-SSRS assesses several domains of suicide including ideation, intention, behaviors, severity of self-injury and potential lethality of suicide attempts.[65] Another commonly employed assessment tool is the Beck Scale for Suicide Ideation. It consists of 19 items and was developed to detect current intensity of a patient's attitudes, plans and behaviors towards suicide. It also contains two additional items that assess the number of previous attempts and the intensity of the strength of the intent to die during the last attempt.[67]

The Suicide Assessment Five-Step Evaluation and Triage (SAFE-T) assessment tool was developed in collaboration with Substance Abuse and Mental Health Services Administration (SAMHSA). The SAFE-T assesses risk factors such as suicidal behavior, current and past psychiatric disorders, key symptoms, family history, change in treatment and access to fire arms; protective factors, both internal, such as the ability to cope with stress, spiritual or religious beliefs and frustration tolerance, and external, such as responsibility to children or others, and having a positive therapeutic relationship and good social supports; suicidal inquiry, which asks specific questions about thoughts, plans, behaviors, intents, risk level and intervention; assesses the risk level based on the clinical judgment after completing the first three steps. Patients are stratified into low, moderate, and high risk, with specific interventions indicated for each risk level. And unlike other suicide assessment tools the SAFE-T documents the risk level and rationale for the treatment plan to address or reduce the risk.[66]

MITIGATION STRATEGIES

Risk Stratification and Treatment Options

Patients who screen as having moderate to severe depression with or without endorsing suicidal ideation or specific plans should be ideally co-managed with a mental health provider until the depression improves and stabilizes. Patients who acknowledge active suicidal plans may require intensive outpatient or inpatient psychiatric care depending on certain factors such as: the severity of depression and the suicidal ideation, if the patient has vague or specific plans for suicide including having access to means (potentially lethal medications such as opioids and benzodiazepines or owns a gun), history of past suicide attempts or evidence of impulsivity. Mitigating factors include the patient having a strong social support system, someone the patient would feel safe in confiding in; have demonstrated good impulse control; and lastly, they have an open and collaborative relationship with their health care provider. These patients may be considered for outpatient management of their suicidal ideation. If the patient is in the acute phase, they may require more intense treatment consisting of possibly pharmacotherapy and/or possibly frequent psychotherapy sessions. Patients who are high risk for suicidality or have chronic suicidal ideation, should be considered for more intensive mental health care.[67] For an extended list of potential risk factors and protective factors (see **Table 110-1**).

TABLE 110-1 List of Potential Risk Factors and Protective Factors for Suicide

Risk Factors	Protective Factors
Males under age 25 and over 65	No personal or family history of severe psychiatric disorders
Past history of self-harm (not just suicide)	Sense of belonging and purpose
Family history of suicidal behavior	Personal beliefs that discourage suicide
Active unhealthy substance use	Active engagement in mental health and community services
History of impulsivity	History of good impulse control, coping with life stressors
Changes in mood	Financial, housing, health stability
Sense of feeling hopeless/ worthless	Good support system
Poor social support system	Good support system
Access to lethal means (medications, gun, etc.)	Open and positive relationship with healthcare providers
Major life stressor (loss of relationship, acute medical condition, loss of job, income, housing	A sense of optimism, hope and being future oriented

PHARMACOLOGIC AND NONPHARMACOLOGIC INTERVENTIONS

Pharmacologic Interventions

In managing patients with co-occurring pain and SUDs who may be at increased risk for suicide, a pharmacologic strategy should include managing depressive symptomatology, improving sleep disturbance, and reducing pain. If opioid or benzodiazepine use is medically necessary, these medications should be prescribed cautiously, in small amounts and should be held and administered by a family member. Further, the patient should be monitored closely with frequent urine drug screening and checking the state prescription drug monitoring program.[67]

Certain antidepressants have been found efficacious for co-occurring depression and pain such as venlafaxine, duloxetine, milnacipran (not FDA-approved for the treatment of depression), and desvenlafaxine. Antiepileptic medications such as gabapentin and pregabalin can target certain types of pain conditions such as fibromyalgia, neuropathic pain conditions (diabetic neuralgia, complex regional pain syndrome) and in some cases provide mood stabilization and improve sleep. However, this medication has some concern for risk for aberrant medication taking behaviors and SUD. There has been some concern regarding the association between suicide and antidepressant and antiepileptic medication[68] such that the clinician should closely monitor a patient for increased risk of suicide when initiating antidepressant and antiepileptic therapy.

For patients with co-occurring CNCP and opioid use disorder who are expressing suicidal ideation, there is growing evidence of the efficacy of buprenorphine for pain relief, treating their opioid use disorder, and in reducing suicidal ideation.[69] Lastly there is evidence potentially supporting the use of within-clinic administration of ketamine for pain reduction, mood improvement and in reducing suicidal ideation, but this needs further investigation.[70]

Nonpharmacologic Interventions

Patients with CNCP, and CNCP and SUD, commonly experience co-occurring depression, anxiety, and sleep disturbance, which can increase the risk for suicide. Pharmacotherapy by itself has limited efficacy in managing these co-occurring conditions and the most effective approach is combining rational pharmacotherapy and nonpharmacologic interventions such as cognitive-behavioral therapy (CBT) and Acceptance Commitment Therapy (ACT).

Cognitive-Behavioral Therapy

There is a robust literature supporting the efficacy of CBT in improving mood and anxiety disorders, PTSD and other conditions including pain, sleep, and SUDs.

a. CBT-Pain

Patients experiencing chronic pain tend to engage in maladaptive thinking patterns most commonly catastrophizing (which is an irrational thought pattern that a current or future situation is worse than it is) and maladaptive behaviors (eg, kinesiophobia/fear of movement), which can result in further deconditioning, increased pain and social isolation—thus exacerbating depression and risk for suicide. As noted previously, catastrophizing has been identified as a significant risk factor for suicidal ideation in patients with chronic pain.[13] CBT typically includes specific evidenced-based techniques to assist and support the patient in identifying maladaptive behaviors and/or dysfunctional thought patterns that may diminish the patient's ability to adjust to and cope with their chronic pain thus contributing to their related depression and anxiety. CBT techniques can include mindfulness-based stress reduction, progressive muscle relaxation training, pacing, effective communication, cognitive restructuring, followed by skill consolidation, rehearsal, and relapse training.[71] Cognitive restructuring is a technique to address catastrophizing and involves the patient being cognizant of recurrent negative, dysfunctional/irrational thoughts and challenging these cognitions to promote the patient to reframe and reconceptualize their subjective view of pain and support the patient to be more proactive, rather than reactive, thereby reinforcing a sense of competence and self-efficacy.

There is persuasive literature supporting the clinical efficacy and cost-effectiveness of CBT in improving mood, anxiety, and functionality in several chronic pain disorders, including chronic low back pain, arthritis, lupus, fibromyalgia, and sickle cell disease.[72-78]

b. CBT-Insomnia

CBT-insomnia (CBT-I) has been effective in improving sleep disturbance, sleep efficiency and sleep quality and is equal to or superior to sleep medications.[79] Sleep disturbance is highly prevalent in patients with CNCP, pain and sleep are bidirectional and sleep disturbance is a known risk factor for suicide in patients with CNCP.

CBT-I typically includes psychoeducation about sleep and insomnia; stimulus control; sleep restriction; sleep hygiene; relaxation training; and cognitive restructuring. CBT-I can be delivered in an individual, group and computer-assisted format with generally equal effectiveness. There has been some effort to combine CBT-P and CBT-I into a hybrid program to target both pain and insomnia with promising results in improving sleep, mood, and function.[80]

c. CBT, Pain and SUD

There has been national attention to the opioid crisis with increasing rates of unhealthy prescription opioid use and opioid-related fatalities, although current opioid-related overdoses and deaths are increasingly related to fentanyl contamination or use. While the rate of true of opioid use disorders in patients with CNCP exposed to opioids is relatively low, opioid use not meeting DSM5 criteria for opioid use disorder is more common. There is compelling evidence that CBT can potentially reduce the risk of unhealthy prescription opioid use in high-risk patients by providing nonopioid therapy targeted to improve mood, anxiety, sleep, and pain coping skills and in improving outcomes in patients with pain who have a history of a SUD. Morasco et al.[81] evaluated the efficacy of CBT in patients with hepatitis C who also experienced chronic pain and had a history of SUD that were enrolled in an 8-sessions integrated group CBT program for chronic pain and SUD. Results revealed improvement in key outcomes including pain-related interference, reduction in cravings for alcohol and other substances, and a decrease in past-month alcohol and substance use.

Acceptance and Commitment Therapy

ACT is a form of therapy based on rational frame theory that is directive and experiential. ACT emphasizing experiencing one's life mindfully. The core processes of ACT include: Contact with the present moment; Self-as-context; Diffusion; Acceptance; Values; and Committed action. The goal of ACT is for the patient to strive for psychological flexibility to cope with pain more effectively. Several randomized clinical trials have demonstrated treatment efficacy and long-term durability of ACT in patients with CNCP. For example, Vowles et al.[82] demonstrated improvement in physical and emotional well-being in a cohort of patients with CNCP that completed a course of ACT for pain and these improvements were maintained three years after treatment by 64.8% of these patients. ACT has also been employed in treating SUDs and shown reduced rates of relapse and improved quality of life as compared to treatment as usual care.[83]

SUMMARY

Managing patients with CNCP is challenging and more so in individuals suffering from both CNCP and SUD. These patients often present with significant medical, social, and psychiatric co-occurring disorders. Suicidal ideation is highly prevalent in this vulnerable population. Risk factors for suicide that are both general and unique to patients with pain and SUD have been identified and there is emerging literature on effective pharmacologic and nonpharmacologic interventions to mitigate the risk of suicide in these patients. Clinicians who are involved in the treatment of CNCP and SUD should be cognizant of the silent epidemic of suicide, assess for risk of suicide on an ongoing basis and have a plan of action if a patient is identified as being at risk for suicide.

REFERENCES

1. *Preventing Suicide: A Global Imperative.* World Health Organization; 2014. Accessed May 20, 2022. http://apps.who.int/iris/bitstream/10665/131056/1/9789241564779_eng.pdf?ua=1&ua=1
2. National Center for Health Statistics. *About Multiple Cause of Death, 1999–2020.* CDC WONDER online database. Accessed July 19, 2023. https://wonder.cdc.gov/mcd-icd10.html
3. Hitchcock L, Ferrell B, McCaffery M. The experience of chronic nonmalignant pain. *J Pain Symptom Manage.* 1994;9:312-318.
4. Stenager EN, Stenager E, Jensen K. Attempted suicide, depression and physical diseases: a 1-year follow-up study. *Psychother Psychosom.* 1994;61:65-73.
5. Fishbain DA, Goldberg M, Rosomoff RS, Rosomoff H. Completed suicide in chronic pain. *Clin J Pain.* 1991;7:29-36.
6. Fishbain DA. The association of chronic pain and suicide. *Semin Clin Neuropsychiatry.* 1999;4:221-227.
7. Smith MT, Edwards RR, Robinson RC, Dworkin RH. Suicidal ideation, plans and attempts in chronic pain patients: factors associated with increased risk. *Pain.* 2004;111:201-208.
8. Braden JB, Sullivan MD. Suicidal thoughts and behavior among adults with self-reported pain conditions in the national comorbidity survey replication. *J Pain.* 2008;9:1106-1115.
9. Ilgen MA, Zivin K, McCammon RJ, Valenstein M. Pain and suicidal thoughts, plans and attempts in the United States. *Gen Hosp Psychiatry.* 2008;30:521-527.
10. Ratcliffe GE, Enns MW, Belik SL, Sareen J. Chronic pain conditions and suicidal ideation and suicide attempts: an epidemiologic perspective. *Clin J Pain.* 2008;24:204-210.
11. Substance Abuse and Mental Health Services Administration. *Drug Abuse Warning Network, 2007: Estimates of Drug-Related Emergency Department Visits.* SAMHSA; 2010. https://www.samhsa.gov/data/sites/default/files/DAWN2k10ED/DAWN2k10ED/DAWN2k10ED.htm.
12. Racine M, Choinière M, Nielson WR. Predictors of suicidal ideation in chronic pain patients: an exploratory study. *Clin J Pain.* 2014;30(5):371-378.
13. Cheatle M, Wasser T, Foster C, Olugbodi A, Bryan J. Prevalence of suicidal ideation in patients with chronic noncancer pain referred to a behaviorally based pain program. *Pain Phys.* 2014;17(3):E359-E367.
14. Edwards RR, Smith MT, Kudel I, Haythornthwaite J. Pain-related catastrophizing as a risk factor for suicidal ideation in chronic pain. *Pain.* 2006;126:272-279.
15. Tang NK, Crane C. Suicidality in chronic pain: a review of the prevalence, risk factors and psychological links. *Psychol Med.* 2006;36:575-586.
16. Ilgen MA, Zivin K, Austin KL, et al. Severe pain predicts greater likelihood of subsequent suicide. *Suicide Life Threat Behav.* 2010;40(6):597-608.
17. Campbell G, Darke S, Bruno R, Degenhardt L. The prevalence and correlates of chronic pain and suicidality in a nationally representative sample. *Aust N Z J Psychiatry.* 2015;49(9):803-811.
18. Campbell G, Bruno R, Darke S, et al. Prevalence and correlates of suicidal thoughts and suicide attempts in people prescribed pharmaceutical opioids for chronic pain. *Clin J Pain.* 2016;32(4):292-301.
19. Roy A, Janal MN. Risk factors for suicide among alcohol-dependent patients. *Arch Suicide Res.* 2007;11:211-217.
20. Roy A. Characteristics of cocaine dependent patients who attempt suicide. *Arch Suicide Res.* 2009;13:46-51.
21. Roy A. Risk factors for attempting suicide in heroin addicts. *Suicide Life Threat Behav.* 2010;40:416-420.
22. Wilcox HC, Conner KR, Caine ED. Association of alcohol and drug use disorders and completed suicide: an empirical review of cohort studies. *Drug Alcohol Depend.* 2004;76:S11-S19.
23. Centers for Disease Control and Prevention (CDC). National Center for Injury Prevention and Control; 2010. Accessed May 10, 2022. https://www.cdc.gov/suicide/
24. Yuodelis-Flores C, Ries RK. Addiction and suicide: a review. *Am J Addict.* 2015;24(2):98-104.
25. Archambault L, Jutras-Aswad D, Touré EH, et al. Profiles of patients with opioid use disorders presenting a history of suicidal ideations and attempts. *Psychiatr Q.* 2022;93(2):637-650.
26. Calati R, Laglaoui Bakhiyi C, Artero S, Ilgen M, Courtet P. The impact of physical pain on suicidal thoughts and behaviors: meta-analyses. *J Psychiatr Res.* 2015;71:16-32.
27. Jimenez-Rodríguez I, Garcia-Leiva JM, Jimenez-Rodriguez BM, Condés-Moreno E, Rico-Villademoros F, Calandre EP. Suicidal ideation and the risk of suicide in patients with fibromyalgia: a comparison with non-pain controls and patients suffering from low-back pain. *Neuropsychiatr Dis Treat.* 2014;10:625-630.

28. Nović A, Kõlves K, O'Dwyer S, De Leo D. Migraine and suicidal behaviors: a systematic literature review. *Clin J Pain.* 2016;32(4):351-364.
29. Liu HY, Fuh JL, Lin YY, Chen WT, Wang SJ. Suicide risk in patients with migraine and comorbid fibromyalgia. *Neurology.* 2015;85(12):1017-1023.
30. Lee D-H, Noh EC, Kim YC, et al. Risk factors for suicidal ideation among patients with complex regional pain syndrome. *Psychiatry Investig.* 2014;11(1):32-38.
31. Tang NK, Wright KJ, Salkovskis PM. Prevalence and correlates of clinical insomnia co-occurring with chronic back pain. *J Sleep Res.* 2007;16(1):85-95.
32. McCracken LM, Williams JL, Tang NK. Psychological flexibility may reduce insomnia in persons with chronic pain: a preliminary retrospective study. *Pain Med.* 2011;12(6):904-912.
33. Allen KD, Renner JB, DeVellis B, Helmick C, Jordan JM. Osteoarthritis and sleep: the Johnston County Osteoarthritis Project. *J Rheumatol.* 2008;35:1102-1107.
34. Artner J, Cakir B, Spiekermann JA, et al. Prevalence of sleep deprivation in patients with chronic neck and back pain: a retrospective evaluation of 1016 patients. *J Pain Res.* 2013;6:1-6.
35. Alsaadi SM, McAuley JH, Hush JM, Maher CG. Prevalence of sleep disturbance in patients with low back pain. *Eur Spine J.* 2011;20(5):737-743.
36. Smith MT, Perlis ML, Haythornthwaite JA. Suicidal ideation in outpatients with chronic musculoskeletal pain: an exploratory study of the role of sleep onset insomnia and pain intensity. *Clin J Pain.* 2004;20(2):111-118.
37. Cheatle MD, Foster S, Pinkett A, Lesneski M, Qu D, Dhingra L. Assessing and managing sleep disturbance in patients with chronic pain. *Anesthesiol Clin.* 2016;34(2):379-393.
38. Turner JA, Aaron LA. Pain-related catastrophizing: what is it? *Clin J Pain.* 2001;17(1):65-71.
39. Brown LA, Lynch KG, Cheatle M. Pain catastrophizing as a predictor of suicidal ideation in chronic pain patients with an opiate prescription. *Psychiatry Res.* 2020;286:112893.
40. Ilgen MA, Bohnert AS, Ganoczy D, Bair MJ, McCarthy JF, Blow FC. Opioid dose and risk of suicide. *Pain.* 2016;157(5):1079-1084.
41. Dworkin R, Turk DC, Farrar JT, et al. Core outcome measures for chronic pain trials: IMMPACT recommendations. *Pain.* 2005;113(1-2):9-19.
42. Beck A, Ward C, Mendelson M, Mock J, Erbaugh J. An inventory for measuring depression. *Arch Gen Psychiatry.* 1961;4:561-571.
43. McNair D, Lorr M, Droppleman L. *Profile of Mood States.* Educational and Industrial Testing Service; 1971.
44. Kroenke K, Spitzer RL, Williams JB. The PHQ-9: validity of a brief depression severity measure. *J Gen Intern Med.* 2001;16(9):606-613.
45. Beck AT, Epstein N, Brown G, Steer RA. An inventory for measuring clinical anxiety: psychometric properties. *J Consult Clin Psychol.* 1988;56(6):893-897.
46. Spielberg C, Gorsuch R, Lushene R. *Manual for the State-Trait Anxiety Inventory.* Consulting Psychologists; 1970.
47. Kroenke K, Spitzer RL, Williams JBW, Löwe B. An ultra-brief screening scale for anxiety and depression: the PHQ–4. *Psychosomatics.* 2009;50(6):613-621.
48. Wolff BB. Evaluation of hypnotics in outpatients with insomnia using a questionnaire and a self-rating technique. *Clin Pharmacol Ther.* 1974;15(2):130-140.
49. Kryger MH, Steljes D, Pouliot Z, Neufeld H, Odynski T. Subjective versus objective evaluation of hypnotic efficacy: experience with zolpidem. *Sleep.* 1991;14(5):399-407.
50. Buysse DJ, Reynolds CF III, Monk TH, Berman SR, Kupfer DJ. The Pittsburgh Sleep Quality Index: a new instrument for psychiatric practice and research. *Psychiatry Res.* 1989;28(2):193-213.
51. Yu L, Buysse DJ, Germain A, et al. Development of short forms from the PROMIS™ sleep disturbance and Sleep-Related Impairment item banks. *Behav Sleep Med.* 2011;10(1):6-24.
52. Brown RL, Rounds LA. Conjoint screening questionnaires for alcohol and other drug abuse: criterion validity in a primary care practice. *Wis Med J.* 1995;94(3):135-140.
53. Bastiaens L, Riccardi K, Sakhrani D. The RAFFT as a screening tool for adult substance use disorders. *Am J Drug Alcohol Abuse.* 2002;28(4):681-691.
54. Skinner HA. The drug abuse screening test. *Addict Behav.* 1982;7(4):363-371.
55. Cocco KM, Carey KB. Psychometric properties of the Drug Abuse Screening Test in psychiatric outpatients. *Psych Assess.* 1998;10(4):681-691.
56. Screening, Brief Intervention, and Referral to Treatment (SBIRT). Accessed December 18, 2016. https://www.samhsa.gov/sbirt
57. Webster LR, Webster RM. Predicting aberrant behaviors in opioid-treated patients: preliminary validation of the Opioid Risk Tool. *Pain Med.* 2005;6:432-442.
58. Butler SF, Fernandez K, Benoit C, Budman SH, Jamison RN. Validation of the revised screener and opioid assessment for patients with pain. *J Pain.* 2008;9:360-372.
59. Belgrade MJ, Schamber CD, Lindgren BR. The DIRE score: predicting outcomes of opioid prescribing for chronic pain. *J Pain.* 2006;7:671-681.
60. Cheatle MD, Compton PA, Dhingra L, Wasser TE, O'Brien CP. Development of the revised opioid risk tool to predict opioid use disorder in patients with chronic nonmalignant pain. *J Pain.* 2019;20(7):842-851.
61. Adams LL, Gatchel RJ, Robinson RC, et al. Development of a self-report screening instrument for assessing potential opioid medication misuse in chronic pain patients. *J Pain Symptom Manage.* 2004;27:440-459.
62. Butler SF, Budman SH, Fernandez KC, et al. Development and validation of the Current Opioid Misuse Measure. *Pain.* 2007;130:144-156.
63. Compton PA, Wu SM, Schieffer B, Pham Q, Naliboff BD. Introduction of a self-report version of the Prescription Drug Use Questionnaire and relationship to medication agreement noncompliance. *J Pain Symptom Manage.* 2008;36:383-395.
64. Posner K, Brown GK, Stanley B, et al. The Columbia-Suicide Severity Rating Scale: initial validity and internal consistency findings from three multisite studies with adolescents and adults. *Am J Psychiatry.* 2011;168(12):1266-1277.
65. Beck AT, Steer RA, Ranieri WF. Scale for suicide ideation: psychometric properties of a self-report version. *J Clin Psychol.* 1988;44(4):499-505.
66. SAMSHA. Suicide Assessment Five-Step Evaluation and Triage (SAFE-T). Accessed May 5, 2022. http://store.samhsa.gov/shin/content//SMA09-4432/SMA09-4432.pdf
67. Cheatle MD. Depression, chronic pain, and suicide by overdose: on the edge. *Pain Med.* 2011;12(Suppl 2):S43-S48.
68. Bailly F, Belaid H. Suicidal ideation and suicide attempt associated with antidepressant and antiepileptic drugs: implications for treatment of chronic pain. *Joint Bone Spine.* 2021;88(1):105005. doi:10.1016/j.jbspin.2020.04.016
69. Cameron CM, Nieto S, Bosler L, et al. Mechanisms underlying the anti-suicidal treatment potential of buprenorphine. *Adv Drug Alcohol Res.* 2021;1:10009. doi:10.3389/adar.2021.10009
70. Tran K, McCormack S. *Ketamine for Chronic Non-Cancer Pain: A Review of Clinical Effectiveness, Cost-Effectiveness, and Guidelines.* Canadian Agency for Drugs and Technologies in Health; 2020.
71. Turk DC, Flor H. Etiological theories and treatments for chronic back pain. II. Psychological models and interventions. *Pain.* 1984;19(3):209-233.
72. Lamb SE, Hansen Z, Lall R, Castelnuovo E, Withers EJ, Nichols V. Group cognitive behavioral treatment for low-back pain in primary care: a randomized controlled trial and cost-effectiveness analysis. *Lancet.* 2010;375:916-923.
73. Linton SJ. A 5-year follow-up evaluation of the health and economic consequences of an early cognitive behavioral intervention for back pain: a randomized, controlled trial. *Spine.* 2006;31(8):853-858.
74. Keefe FJ, Caldwell DS. Cognitive behavioral control of arthritis pain. *Med Clin North Am.* 1997;81:277-290.
75. Greco CM, Rudy TE, Manzi S. Effects of a stress-reduction program on psychological function, pain, and physical function of systemic lupus erythematosus patients: a randomized controlled trial. *Arthritis Rheum.* 2004;51(4):625-634.
76. Thieme K, Flor H, Turk D. Psychological pain treatment in fibromyalgia syndrome: efficacy of operant behavioral and cognitive behavioral treatments. *Arthritis Res Ther.* 2006;8(4):R121.

77. Chen E, Cole SW, Kato PM. A review of empirically supported psychosocial interventions for pain and adherence outcomes in sickle cell disease. *J Pediatr Psychol.* 2004;29:1997-2009.
78. Bernardy K, Klose P, Busch AJ, Choy EH, Häuser W. Cognitive behavioral therapies for fibromyalgia. *Cochrane Database Syst Rev.* 2013;(9):CD009796. doi:10.1002/14651858.CD009796.pub2
79. Svertsen B, Omvik S, Pallesen S, et al. Cognitive behavioral therapy vs zopiclone for treatment of chronic primary insomnia in older adults: a randomized controlled trial. *JAMA.* 2006;295(24):2851-2858.
80. Tang NK, Goodchild CE, Salkovskis PM. Hybrid cognitive-behavior therapy for individuals with insomnia and chronic pain: a pilot randomized controlled trial. *Behav Res Ther.* 2012;50(12):814-821.
81. Morasco BJ, Greaves DW, Lovejoy TI, Turk DC, Dobscha SK, Hauser P. Development and preliminary evaluation of an integrated cognitive-behavior treatment for chronic pain and substance use disorder in patients with the hepatitis C virus. *Pain Med.* 2016;17(12):2280-2290.
82. Vowles KE, McCracken LM, O'Brien JZ. Acceptance and values-based action in chronic pain: a three-year follow-up analysis of treatment effectiveness and process. *Behav Res Ther.* 2011;49(11):748-755.
83. Lee EB, An W, Levin ME, Twohig MP. An initial meta-analysis of Acceptance and Commitment Therapy for treating substance use disorders. *Drug Alcohol Depend.* 2015;155:1-7.

CHAPTER

111 Rehabilitation Approaches to Pain Management

Steven Stanos and Randy L. Calisoff

CHAPTER OUTLINE

- Introduction
- Active physical therapy
- Occupational therapy
- Psychological interventions as part of a pain rehabilitation plan
- Therapeutic methods used in acute and chronic pain conditions
- Conclusion

INTRODUCTION

Chronic pain and substance use disorder (SUD) are highly prevalent and represent conditions with potentially negative synergy between them. An estimated 50 million Americans report chronic pain—pain on most days or every day—in the past 6 months. Additionally, 20 million Americans report high impact chronic pain, pain that limits life or work on most days during the same timeframe, many of which may be at risk for substance use problems and greater psychosocial distress.[1] Although causative and developmental factors of SUDs and chronic pain may negatively impact each other, successful rehabilitation efforts for both conditions should focus on active interventions (eg, physical therapy [PT], exercises) and behavioral health interventions. Rehabilitation may be described as a "return to ability ... the return to the fullest physical, mental, social, vocational, and economic usefulness that is possible for the individual." The focus is placed more on one's abilities rather than his or her disabilities.[2] The patient with SUD may be faced with an additional challenge of comorbid chronic pain. A recent systematic review found that people who use prescription opioids nonmedically had two to three times higher prevalence rates of mental health conditions and pain than did the general population.[3] Incorporating a rehabilitation-based approach to treating chronic pain can serve as a valuable tool for managing patients with chronic pain with and without co-occurring SUD.[4,5]

A number of chronic and acute pain conditions can benefit from a wide range of nonpharmacological interventions. A rehabilitation-based approach focuses on a staged approach to addressing the range of acute to chronic pain conditions. A focused history and physical exam can help to identify areas of impairment and guide subsequent treatment interventions and the development of a comprehensive rehabilitation plan. More chronic presentations may need psychological and vocational interventions as well. In carefully selected patients, some interventional procedures (eg, epidural injections for acute radicular pain or trigger point injections for myofascial pain) may provide additional tools for the pain clinician but will not be the focus of this chapter. The chapter overviews active and passive therapies for acute and chronic pain conditions, including "restorative therapies" such as active physical and occupational therapy (OT), and team approaches to comprehensive care. In response to the growing overdose epidemic and increasing prevalence of chronic pain, a multidisciplinary Health and Human Services task force defined the range of pain management interventions that should be considered when developing a patient-centered pain management plan including medications, restorative therapies, interventional procedures, behavioral health approaches, and complementary and integrative health therapies[6] (**Fig. 111-1**). Therapeutic methods including specific physical agents, sometime referred to as "modalities" are also considered restorative interventions, and commonly include the usage of hot/cold packs, ultrasound, phonophoresis, and iontophoresis, the subject of which will be discussed further in the chapter.

The World Health Organization (WHO) and federal agencies have embraced the concept of a "biopsychosocial model" for assessing and treating patients with chronic pain, including those with co-occurring SUD or other psychiatric disorders.[6,7] A rehabilitation approach for assessing and treating pain is based on a conceptualization of the experience of pain as only one part of the dynamic interplay between physical changes in the nervous system and psychological factors. Nociceptive pathways can be affected by tissue-related changes as well as psychosocial factors including stress, anxiety, depression, external factors such as the environment, and past experiences. The resulting pain experienced by the patient will be manifested by overt pain behaviors and suffering.[8] From a rehabilitation perspective, all of these biopsychosocial factors should be considered when developing and delivering a pain management treatment program.

In assessing complaints, one should focus on the patient's individual "impairments" (ie, physical or psychological abnormality), the effects of these impairments on function or "disability" where there is a restriction or lack of ability to perform a specific job related to physical or psychological impairments, and how that affects his or her place in society.[9] The WHO has broadened the concept of "chronic pain" to include the unique relationship among an individual patient's pain and related

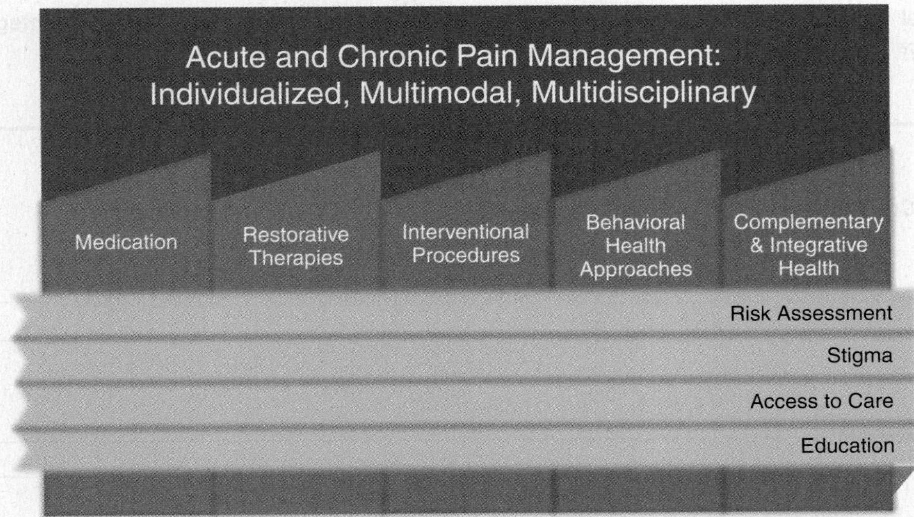

Figure 111-1. Acute and chronic pain management interventions. (From United States Department of Health and Human Services. *Pain Management Best Practices. Inter-agency Task Force Report: Updates, Gaps, Inconsistencies, and Recommendations.* US Department of Health and Human Services; 2019. pmtf-final-report-2019-05-23.pdf (hhs.gov))

activities, function, and participation in society, including the influence of related environmental and personal factors[10] (see **Fig. 111-2**).

A conceptual model based on disease management approaches similar to those for diabetes, heart disease, and asthma can be applied to the treatment of many chronic pain conditions[11] (see **Fig. 111-3**). In this model, moving from left (parallel practice) to right (integrative management) includes moving from a biomedical, disease-focused approach to a collaborative, integrative, team-based treatment model. Moving across the continuum, the philosophy emphasizes the whole person and flexible roles among clinicians with little reliance on hierarchy. Acute pain conditions typically respond to a biomedical approach focused on acute management, decreasing local soft tissue swelling and immobilization. Similarly, parallel practice, for example, could involve an emergency team working efficiently on a patient presenting with cardiac pain. Individual roles are specifically defined, and extensive

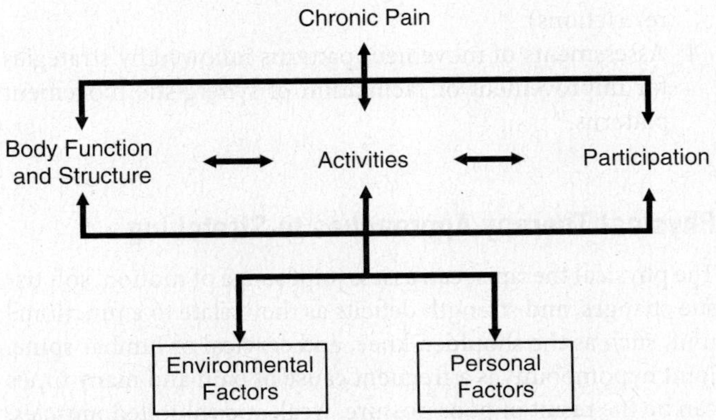

Chronic Pain

Body Function and Structure

Activities

Participation

Environmental Factors

Personal Factors

Figure 111-2. The WHO model of factors interacting with chronic pain and activity.

communication is often not necessary. Collaborative models may involve a physician referring a patient to a different specialist for consultation. Coordinated models may include the additional use of a case manager to help coordinate delivery and communication of care. A "multidisciplinary" approach includes the use of one or a number of allied health disciplines, such as a physical therapist or occupational therapist directed by a senior provider. In a multidisciplinary care, clinicians need not be in the same facility, and communication may vary, as may the transfer of records and reports. As the presenting complaint becomes more chronic, a more collaborative approach involving the coordination of multiple caregivers defines an "interdisciplinary approach."[12]

In an interdisciplinary model, care is usually provided at one facility, where patients participate in a number of therapies, working with multiple disciplines and health care providers. Treatments may include restorative therapies such as physical and occupational therapy, behavioral health therapies (eg, cognitive-behavioral therapy, mindfulness training) and relaxation training, aerobic conditioning, education, vocational rehabilitation, medical management, and pain education. Pain rehabilitation programs include individual and group sessions, and can vary in intensity from 4 hours per day, 1 to 2 days per week to more comprehensive 6 to 8 hours per day, 4 to 5 days per week, for 15 to 20 days. Such programs are usually provided in an outpatient setting.[13,14] Outcomes from interdisciplinary treatment programs have demonstrated not only improvement in pain and psychophysical functioning but significant success for tapering or elimination of opioids.[15,16] A recent DoD/VA review examined outcomes across multiple programs with similar interdisciplinary models demonstrating medium to large effect sizes regardless of preprogram opioid use status, a diagnosis of OUD, or daily morphine equivalent dose.[17]

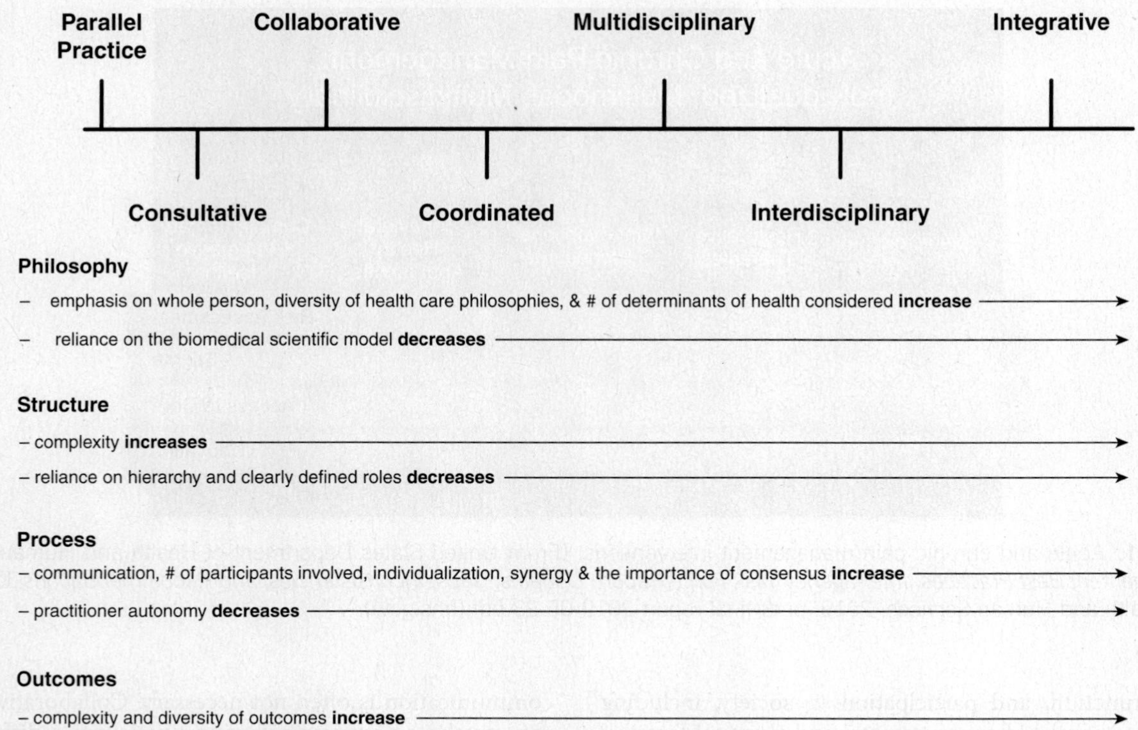

Figure 111-3. Models of medical care. (From Boon H, Verhoef M, O'Hara D, Findlay B. From parallel practice to integrative health care: a conceptual framework. *BMC Health Serv Res.* 2004;4:15.)

Treatments focus on helping the patient acquire pain management skills, decrease pain, improve psychosocial functioning, and return to leisure and vocational function. We will describe allied health disciplines that can be used in a unimodal manner or as part of a comprehensive rehabilitation-based treatment plan.

ACTIVE PHYSICAL THERAPY

Physical therapy promotes the human body's complex movement system and includes, among other interventions, the application of therapeutic methods, therapeutic exercise, functional training in home and work activities, and manual therapy (https://www.apta.org/siteassets/pdfs/policies/guiding-principles-to-achieve-the-vision.pdf).

Physical therapy treatment primarily includes 1-hour sessions, which can include patient education, instruction in exercises and stretches, core strengthening, gait training, manual therapy, and pool or aquatic therapy, with progression of activities over several therapy visits. Patients are given short- and long-term therapy goals and instruction in exercises and stretches. The physical therapist may also dispense equipment, braces, and supports.

The addiction medicine clinician can refer patients for evaluation and treatment to a physical therapist. Follow-up should include monitoring for compliance. Often, reviewing a patient's exercise program and stretches will help reinforce with the patient the importance of the patient's active role in the rehabilitation process.

The goal of any referral to a physical therapist is to establish a patient in a therapeutic exercise program that they continue to pursue on their own at home, often written as a prescription. The basic principles of a therapeutic exercise prescription include the following:

1. Functional evaluation and assessment of dysfunction and impairments.
2. Evaluation and management of motor control (eg, strength and balance).
3. Identification and management of bony and joint kinematic limitations (eg, joint contracture, soft tissue restrictions).
4. Assessments of movement patterns followed by strategies for improvement or facilitation of synergistic movement patterns.[18]

Physical Therapy Approaches to Stretching

The physical therapist can assess joint range of motion, soft tissue changes, and strength deficits as they relate to a functional unit, such as the shoulder, knee, and cervical or lumbar spine. Joint hypomobility is a frequent cause of pain and many times can be the result of poor posture, weak and inhibited muscles, and tight soft tissue. Muscles surrounding the affected area may also develop compensatory activation patterns and neural dysfunction. Various stretching techniques can be used and guided by the therapist and over time performed individually by the patient. Basic types of stretching include ballistic, passive, static, and neuromuscular facilitation. Ballistic stretching uses repetitive rapid application of force in a jerking or bouncing manner in which momentum helps to carry the body part through a range of motion until muscles are stretched to their physiological maximums. More commonly used stretching for chronic pain includes static stretching and proprioceptive neuromuscular facilitation (PNF).

Static stretching techniques involve stretching an antagonist muscle passively by putting the segment in a maximal position of stretch and holding for 10 to 60 seconds. This stretching is repeated four to six times and often incorporates the patient's own body weight, the assistance of a therapist, or stretching equipment.[19] PNF techniques can be also useful for improving flexibility. Different types of PNF exercises include contract-relax, useful when range of motion is limited by muscle or soft tissue tightness, and hold-relax, which includes additional light pressure from the therapist, producing maximal stretch of the involved antagonist muscle groups. Myofascial release is a physical or occupational therapy technique that requires specific training and can accomplish stretching of deeper fascia and connective tissue. In some states, therapists may also be licensed in such interventional approaches for myofascial pain as dry needle insertion and trigger point injections.[20,21]

A growing area of therapy includes stretching the perineural tissues or "neurodynamic therapy," commonly used in cervical and lumbar radicular pain or peripheral nerve compression disorders (eg, ulnar neuropathy of the elbow, median neuropathy at the wrist).[22] Here, neural tissue may become constrained in tight muscle or soft tissue causing increased nerve excitability and such symptoms as paresthesias and dysesthesias in the distribution of specific nerves. Butler and others have eloquently described stretching techniques that can be taught to a patient as part of a therapy program.[23]

Aquatic Therapy

Numerous studies have found aquatic therapy to be beneficial in a variety of acute and chronic pain conditions, including fibromyalgia, spinal cord injury, osteoarthritis, and various orthopedic injuries.[24] Therapy is usually supervised by a physical therapist, occupational therapist, or trainer. Treatment is usually in a group setting with the goal of instructing patients in the performance of exercises that can be performed in the water and continued independently. The beneficial effects of aquatic therapy include decreases in joint compression forces, the counteraction of gravitational obstacles by buoyancy, decreased pain, and reduced protective muscle spasm.[25]

The physical properties of water that are useful include "weightlessness" and resistive forces against which patients can apply force.

Common indications for therapy include peripheral edema, decreased range of motion and strength, impaired balance, weight-bearing restrictions due to injury or surgery, gait abnormalities, and cardiovascular deconditioning.[26,27] In chronic neck and low back pain, aquatic therapy may be provided initially, until improved conditioning permits successful application of land-based therapy. Aquatic therapy may help to eliminate fear-related avoidance of movement, to improve range of motion, and to initiate stretching and strengthening.

A significant percentage of chronic pain conditions involve disorders of the neck and lumbar spine, which accounts for a large proportion of those in need of treatment. Besides passive treatments used for acute pain management (see below), PT-directed exercises may help patients improve function and decrease pain. Patients with acute and chronic low back pain may benefit from referral to a physical therapist for instruction in one of a number of programs, such as lumbar stabilization or core strengthening, or for specialized directional preference treatments such as McKenzie-based therapy. Additional specialty PT care also includes integrating nervous system pain education, which helps patients understand how biological, psychological, and neurological changes can cause pain and also be targets of retraining pain processing, described as pain neuroscience education interventions.[28] A summary of common PT approached for neck- and lumbar-related pain conditions is included in **Table 111-1**.[28,29]

Lumbar and Cervical Stabilization

Stabilization exercises focus on strengthening weak and inhibited muscles and strengthening or "stabilizing" muscles that surround the spine, thereby improving muscular support.[30] Assessing and improving the "core" is the cornerstone of any stabilization program for the lumbar spine, and similar principles can be applied to cervical- and joint-related pain conditions.[31] The *core* is defined as the lumbopelvic-hip complex, thought to include over 29 muscles attaching in this region of the body. Key lumbopelvic-hip muscles include those attaching to the lumbar spine (transversospinalis group, erector spinae, quadratus lumborum, and latissimus dorsi), abdominal muscles (rectus abdominis, external and internal obliques, and transversus abdominis), and key hip muscles (gluteus maximus, gluteus medius, and psoas).[32] Cervical stabilization focuses on improving spine mechanics (cervical flexion, extension, side bending, and rotation), improving maladaptive postures, increasing cervical extensor and posterior scapular muscle strength, and usually stretching restricted anterior pectoralis and shoulder muscles.

The goals of core training include improving dynamic postural control, establishing optimal muscular balance and joint movement around the affected region, maximizing functional strength and endurance, and increasing postural control.[33] Core stabilization also provides proximal stability in the spine for more efficient movement in the lower extremities.

Common muscle impairment patterns seen in many patients with acute and chronic low back pain include weak buttock muscles (eg, gluteus medius), weak abdominals (rectus and transverse abdominis), overactive synergist muscles

TABLE 111-1 Common Physical Therapy Interventions for Low Back Pain

Treatment intervention	Description
1. Manual therapy	Thrust and nonthrust mobilization and manipulation directed by physical therapist. May include soft tissue, muscle release, and joint mobilization
2. Trunk coordination, strengthening, and endurance exercises	Lumbar coordination, strength, and exercises focus on motor control and strengthening of deep and superficial abdominal and trunk muscles. Endurance training (ie, walking, treadmill walking, aquatic exercises) can be coordinated into the treatment plan
3. Centralization and directional preference exercises and procedures	Repeated movements, exercises, or procedures that promote centralization to decrease leg symptoms. Direction of exercises is determined by the physical therapist and consider moderate to high-intensity exercise for patients with chronic low back pain without generalized pain and progressive, low-intensity, submaximal fitness and endurance exercises for patients with chronic low back pain with generalized pain
4. Flexion exercises	Flexion exercises of the spine (seated, supine, standing) may be appropriate with a subset of patients including those with spinal stenosis to help improve cross-sectional area of the spinal canal potentially decreasing compression of nerve roots and improve spinal flexibility
5. Nerve mobilization procedures and traction	Identify tissue restrictions (ie, muscle, tendon, joint) contributing to radicular or lower limb neuropathic pain and direct therapist applied or self-directed nerve mobilization stretches
6. Traditional patient education and counseling	Education and advice related to cause of pain, identifying and problem solving around functional tasks (lifting, bending, carrying), and may include basic education on breathing and relaxation techniques to be incorporated in daily activities Counsel patients to remain active, avoid bed rest, and educate on the natural history of low back pain
7. Pain Neuroscience Education (PNE)	Education and training based on a neuroscience understanding of pain and sensitization of the nervous system and a deemphasis on pathoanatomic causes of pain focusing on patients understanding concepts like the purpose of pain, pain's influence on thoughts, emotions, and actions, as well as the impact of pain on peripheral nerves such as signal transmission and pain neurotransmitters, and central nervous system and the brain's role in producing pain, and the influence of one's beliefs, and attention on a persons' pain experience

Adapted from Delitto A, George S, Van Dillen L, et al. Low back pain: clinical practice guidelines lined to the International Classification of Functioning, Instability, and Health from the Orthopaedic Section of the American Physical Therapy Association. *J Orthop Sports Phys Ther.* 2011;42(4):A1-A57; Louw A, Diener I, Butler D, Puentedura E. The effect of neuroscience education on pain, disability, anxiety, and stress in chronic musculoskeletal pain. *Arch Phys Med Rehab.* 2011;92(12):2041-2056.

such as piriformis and hamstring, and shortened antagonist muscles (thigh adductors and iliopsoas).[34] In the cervical spine, many patients with neck pain present with weak trapezius and scapular muscles, overactive levator scapulae, and shortened antagonists, such as the pectoralis. They often show maladaptive postures and positions of the cervical spine. All of these impairments may contribute to pain and disability and may be specific areas of assessment and treatment by the properly trained therapist. A therapy program could include strengthening exercises on an exercise ball or without specific equipment.

Mechanical Diagnosis and Therapy (McKenzie Therapy)

Mechanical diagnosis and therapy, commonly referred to as McKenzie therapy, is a common, specialized approach in which specially trained therapists instruct patients through a number of active positions of motion in the lumbar spine and determine whether patients are able to decrease or change the pain referral pattern from the extremities to more "centralized" low back or neck pain. This is based on the theory that an intact nucleus pulposus (cervical or lumbar), responsible for generating referred pain to a limb, will produce different symptoms in certain positions with repeated standardized end range test movements (eg, lumbar extension [seated or standing], lumbar flexion, side bending). The most common movement is lumbar extension, although a small percentage of patients may "centralize" their symptoms with repeated flexion or trunk side bending. Those patients who respond to repeated positioning (such as lumbar extension, flexion, or side bending) are given those same exercises to do on a daily basis to help decrease symptoms.[35,36]

Pain Neuroscience Education

Pain neuroscience education (PNE) consists of educational sessions guided by a trained physical or occupational therapist focused on a neuroscience-based understanding of pain and related sensitization of the nervous system. Education and training deemphasizes pathoanatomic causes of pain shifting toward the patient's own understanding of strategies to increase pain thresholds with exercises, decrease fear, and decrease brain activity in areas of pain with the use of metaphors and stories. Educational instruction includes, for example, the purpose of pain; pain's influence on one's thoughts, emotions, and actions; the impact of pain on peripheral nerves such as signal transmission and pain neurotransmitters; and the central nervous system and brain's role in producing pain. It also emphasizes the influence of one's beliefs and attention on a person's pain experience. Therapists undergo additional training and certification to provide this type of treatment that is integrated with a standard active physical therapy program.[23,37,38]

OCCUPATIONAL THERAPY

OT consists of assessment and training of patients in areas related to functional activities. Areas addressed may include specific activities of daily living (ADLs), posture, ergonomics, and body mechanics. Work site analyses may be conducted. Patients may be fitted for braces and splints. In the United States, OT may be provided in postoperative orthopedic care, such as after carpal tunnel release or upper limb fracture. An occupational therapist assesses range of motion, strength, and strength with an emphasis on improving functional, vocational, avocational (leisure), or sports-specific activities.

Posture and Body Mechanics

Many chronic musculoskeletal pain conditions of the cervical and lumbar spine, large joints (shoulder, hip), small joints (hand, wrist, ankle), and soft tissue structures (eg, tendons, muscles, and ligaments) may be aggravated by poor posture. Basic assessment of sitting and standing posture and retraining may be a focus of individual OT sessions and can be applied at home and work. Proper standing and sitting posture will help reduce stress and strain over bony and soft tissue structures.

Body mechanics assessment and retraining can be an important clinical focus of OT in many chronic pain conditions. Proper lifting and reaching mechanics, similar to posture training, can help to improve function, decrease pain, increase tolerance for an activity, and limit injury. Simple instructions to patients to improve posture and decrease pain are included below:

Standing:

Feet shoulder width apart, shoulders even over hips.
Even weight distributed over both feet.
Knees straight and unlocked.
Pelvis level.
Stomach muscles slightly engaged.
Ears lined up over shoulders.

Sitting:

Pelvis level, and weight is even over ischial tuberosities.
Hips and knees at 90° or greater.
Knees and feet shoulder/hip width apart.
Feet flat on floor or stable surface.
Knees over ankles.
Stomach muscles slightly engaged.
Shoulders evenly aligned over hips.[39]

Ergonomics is the science of designing equipment with the aim of increasing productivity and reducing fatigue and discomfort. This is an additional area in which OT can be of value to a patient with chronic pain. With the increased use of computers, keypads, handheld devices, and prolonged sedentary work mostly on a computer, there has been an increase in chronic neck, shoulder, upper limb musculoskeletal conditions, as well as low back pain. An ergonomic evaluation helps the OT to optimize positioning of equipment, keyboards, and other work site tools to help improve function and tolerance, decrease pain, and prevent injury. Physical rehabilitation programs that include ergonomic interventions for upper limb and neck pain have been found to be effective in decreasing pain and improving function in a number of studies.[40,41]

Occupational Work Rehabilitation

OT can assist in addressing patient-specific work goals. Occupational therapists, by reviewing job descriptions and performing job site analyses, can thereby help to determine whether job site or specific job modifications are needed to enable a worker or patient to perform a job safely. Occupational therapists can perform functional baseline testing to clarify an individual's specific physical abilities and tolerances or can provide more structured and extensive testing via a functional capacity evaluation (FCE).[42] FCEs are done by specially trained physical or occupational therapists and usually take place over a 3- to 4-hour period. They help determine physical tolerance for lifting, pulling, grasping, and pushing capabilities, which are typically integrated with validity testing.[43] The FCE can help to determine whether a patient can meet specific job demands as defined by the U.S. Department of Labor.[44] Work or physical demand levels include *sedentary*, *light*, *medium*, and *heavy* and clarify both the amount of time an activity is done (infrequent, occasional, frequent, and constant) as a percentage of the work day and the frequency of repetitions (see **Table 111-2**).

A general familiarity with physical demand levels is helpful to the clinician when asked to determine work restrictions for patients and safety for return to work. Formal FCE testing coupled with visual observation of the patient during the examination may also provide objective measures (eg, heart rate, blood pressure) for documenting inconsistencies of effort, validity of effort, and responses to work.[45]

PSYCHOLOGICAL INTERVENTIONS AS PART OF A PAIN REHABILITATION PLAN

In addition to physical and occupational therapy, pain rehabilitation relies heavily on psychological interventions.[46] The reader is referred to the chapter within this section of the textbook on psychological therapies for pain (see Chapter 109,

TABLE 111-2 Dictionary of Occupational Titles System for Classifying the Strength Demands of Work

Physical demand level	Occasional (0%-33% of workday)	Frequent (34%-66% of workday)	Constant (67%-100% of workday)
Sedentary	10 lb	Negligible	Negligible
Light	20 lb	10 lb and/or walk/stand/ push/pull or arm/leg controls	Negligible and/or push/pull of arm/leg controls while seated
Medium	20-50 lb	10-25 lb	10 lb
Heavy	50-100 lb	25-50 lb	10-20 lb
Very heavy	Over 100 lb	Over 50 lb	Over 20 lb

"Psychological Issues in the Management of Pain"). The table below summarizes the range of psychological interventions that may be incorporated into a focused treatment plan or more comprehensive multi- or interdisciplinary treatment program[47] (see **Table 111-3**).

THERAPEUTIC METHODS USED IN ACUTE AND CHRONIC PAIN CONDITIONS

Passive PT

The final section will overview passive therapeutic methods commonly used for acute musculoskeletal and soft tissue injuries and in carefully selected chronic pain cases. It includes heat and cold therapies; ultrasound; electrical stimulation, including transcutaneous electrical nerve stimulation (TENS) as well as iontophoresis and soft tissue massage. These passive therapeutic methods should be used judiciously to augment an active self-management program (see **Tables 111-4** and **111-5**).[48]

Heat Therapy

For millennia, thermal therapeutic methods have often been used for soft tissue dysfunction and to assist with pain management. Physiologically, heat applied to soft tissues produces an elevated temperature and an increase in blood flow to the affected region. With increased blood flow, hydrostatic pressure and increased capillary permeability lead to an increase in inflammatory mediators in the region, serving an important role in early healing. It is important for the practitioner to note that heat to affected regions is contraindicated in edematous regions, as heat can exacerbate edema.[49,50]

Pain relief from heat therapy is due to vasodilation in the affected region. This reduces muscle spasms, allowing for a greater tolerance in connective tissue stretching.[51] The transfer of heat can be accomplished through conduction (hot packs, paraffin baths), convection (fluidotherapy, hydrotherapy), and conversion (radiant heat). There are two types of heat treatments commonly used: hot packs and ultrasound therapy.

Hot Packs

Hot packs, also known as hydrocollator packs, contain silica gel. This silica gel is heated to a temperature of about 170°F in a hot water tank. The hot packs are subsequently wrapped in four to six layers of towels and applied to the affected region on the patient's skin for 20 to 30 minutes. It is necessary to check the patient every 5 minutes during this procedure to avoid risk of burns.[52] Indications for hot pack application include painful muscle spasms, abdominal muscle cramping, menstrual cramps, and superficial thrombophlebitis. Contraindications of hydrocollator therapy include peripheral vascular disease, superficial skin eruptions at the site of application, desensitized skin, altered sensation in the affected region, or

TABLE 111-3 Psychological Interventions for Pain Rehabilitation Management

Self-regulatory approaches	Behavioral approaches	Cognitive-behavioral therapy (CBT)	Acceptance and commitment therapy
• Utilize interaction between biologic and psychological factors to increase the individual's sense of control over pain • Include biofeedback, relaxation training, hypnosis, and mindfulness	• Target pain behaviors • Include operant behavioral therapy and treatment of fear avoidance	• Addresses pain maladaptive emotions/behaviors/cognitions through a goal-oriented systematic procedure • Main components are understanding the treatment rationale, learning coping skills/training, and applying/maintaining coping skills	• Acceptance- and mindfulness-based intervention • Emphasizes recognition and acceptance of emotions and cognitions, rather than recognition and change (ie, CBT)

From Kerns R, Sellinger J, Goodin B. Psychological treatment of chronic pain. *Annu Rev Clin Psychol.* 2011;7:411-434.

TABLE 111-4 Superficial and Deep Heat Modalities

	Composition	Effect	Contraindications
Superficial heat			
Hydrocollator packs and hot packs	• Bags of silica gel heated in stainless steel containers in water to a temperature of about 170°F • Applied to affected region over towels	Increases temperature of tissues by 38°F	Peripheral vascular disease, skin compromise, desensitized skin, new skin
Paraffin baths	Paraffin wax and mineral oil in 7:1 ratio heated to 130°F Body part dipped in paraffin bath, repeated 7-12 times, and then wrapped in plastic wax paper and covered by towel	Increases temperature of tissues by 42°F	Same as above
Deep heat			
Ultrasound	Electrical current applied to quartz crystal	• Produces acoustic vibration above the audible range • 1 MHz Ultrasound heats tissues at a rate of 0.36°F per minutes per Watt/cm^2	Pregnancy, laminectomy sites, ischemic regions, eyes, sites of arthroplasty, near reproductive organs, and tumors
Phonophoresis	Topical anti-inflammatory medications driven into tissues via ultrasound		Same as above

From Stanos S, McLean J, Rader L. Physical medicine rehabilitation approaches to pain. *Anesthesiol Clin.* 2007;25:721-759.

new skin.[53] In one study, application of a hydrocollator pack in patients with myofascial pain of the upper trapezius for 30 minutes three times per day for a period of 2 weeks resulted in improved pain and anxiety levels.[54]

Ultrasound

Ultrasound provides the deepest heat of all of the heat therapies used.[55] Therapeutic ultrasonography uses a frequency range of 0.8 to 1.0 MHz. This is achieved by applying electrical energy to a crystal, which vibrates at a high frequency, thus producing ultrasonic waves. These waves can be delivered in a pulsed or continuous fashion, thereby providing a high heating intensity to the affected area. The ultrasonic waves vibrate tissues deep inside the affected region, creating heat that increases blood flow into the tissues, assisting with the healing process.[56] Continuous ultrasound produces analgesia through temperature elevation, increasing capillary permeability, increasing protein synthesis, and activating immune response near the tissue injury site, which may stimulate regeneration of damaged tissues.[57]

Ultrasound is used to treat joint and muscle sprains, bursitis, and tendonitis. In addition to causing increases in tissue relaxation, local blood flow, and scar tissue breakdown, ultrasound can also be used to help reduce local swelling and chronic inflammation.[58] Ultrasound can also be used in phonophoresis, in which ultrasound is used to drive a topical agent, such as diclofenac, into the tissues.[59] The agent can be mixed with the ultrasound gel and applied under the ultrasound head, where the ultrasonic sound waves drive the medication into the tissues, potentially reducing inflammation and related pain.[60] A randomized, single-blind, placebo-controlled

TABLE 111-5 Transcutaneous Electrical Nerve Stimulation (TENS)

TENS type	Amplitude/frequency	Indication	Duration	Setting changes
Conventional (low intensity, high frequency)	1-2 mA/50-100 Hz	Acute and chronic pain states	• 1-20 min for rapid relief • 30 min to 2 h for short duration of analgesia • Repeat as needed	Increase amplitude or pulse width to avoid adaptation and maintain analgesia
Iontophoresis	Current of 2-4 mA used by practitioner to drive medications into affected tissues through the use of TENS unit	Reduction in pain and inflammation	TENS unit pads are applied for about 10 min during treatment session	Works as a fixed percutaneous drug delivery system to drive topical agents bypassing first-pass metabolism

From Stanos S, McLean J, Rader L. Physical medicine rehabilitation approaches to pain. *Anesthesiol Clin.* 2007;25:721-759.

trial showed that phonophoresis with capsaicin and exercises in the treatment of chronic neck pain were superior in reducing pain and disability compared to capsaicin and exercises alone.[61]

Typical ultrasound treatments last from 3 to 5 minutes, depending on the size of the affected area. The dosage of the treatment is determined by the intensity and duration of stimulus. The intensity of sound energy available from the ultrasound head is typically expressed as watts per square centimeter. In acute conditions, low-intensity treatment is required. Chronic conditions may require a higher intensity. Indications for ultrasound include joint contractures, joint adhesions, calcific bursitis, neuromas, fibrosis, phantom limb pain, and myofascial pain.[62] Contraindications for ultrasound include pregnancy, laminectomy sites, and ischemic regions. Application of ultrasound over surgically implanted hardware remains an area of controversy and should be performed with caution.[63] Paraffin baths are another form of heat therapy utilizing conduction and are useful in contractures due to rheumatoid arthritis, burns, and scleroderma. Paraffin can be applied to the patient's extremities. Since the specific heat of paraffin is one-half that of water, a higher temperature (55 °C) is tolerable without risk of tissue burns when using paraffin compared to water (42-45 °C). Solid paraffin forms a protective and insulating coat over the skin, and the paraffin bath is maintained at the melting point of 51.7 °C to 54.4 °C in an insulated, thermostatically controlled container.[64] Methods of paraffin bath application involve dipping, immersion, brush application, pouring, and casting/wrapping.[65]

Cold Therapy

Superficial treatments with cold and pressure have long been used in treating painful conditions.[66] Cryotherapy, or the use of cold, is used by therapists using superficial agents that are inexpensive and easy to use. These include ice, cold water, vaporizing liquids, refrigerated units, and chemical packs, often requiring little preparation on the part of the practitioner.[67] Historically, cold therapy has been used more than heat in the acute phase of tissue injury. Application of cold to an affected body part in the acute phase can have several effects that may help modify pain. First, by cooling the surface of the affected region and underlying tissues, cold therapy results in blood vessel narrowing, or vasoconstriction, thus leading to a decrease in the amount of blood being delivered to the site of injury and decreasing the amount of soft tissue swelling. Second, the effects of cold slow down pain signal transmission, leading to decrease hyperexcitability as well as nerve transmission in pain fibers. Lastly, cold therapy helps to release endorphins at the site of tissue injury leading to a reduction in neurogenic inflammation and raising the pain threshold.[68,69] After several minutes, the blood vessels then dilate allowing blood to return to the region. Muscular spasm often occurs in response to pain, and ice has been shown to reduce this. Cold temperature environment caused by ice reduces the conduction velocity of sensory and motor nerves, thereby ultimately reducing motor activity.[70] In addition, the risk of cell death due to increased oxygen demands during tissue injury is reduced by cold therapy, which reduces the oxygen requirements of cells in the affected region.[71] Continuous cryotherapy devices demonstrated the best outcome for patients after knee arthroscopy procedures, showing a significant reduction in pain, swelling, and analgesic consumption and increase in range of motion.[72]

Ice pack treatment begins with placement of a dry terry cloth towel over the region to prevent direct contact of the ice with the skin. The ice pack is then applied to the affected region for no more than 20 minutes. Studies have shown that application of an ice pack containing at least 0.6 kg of ice leads to more cooling than does a 0.3-kg ice pack. When applied for 20 minutes to the painful region, the 0.6-kg ice pack produced a mean skin temperature of 6.0 °C, compared to 9.6 °C with the 0.3-kg ice pack. Thus, clinicians should consider using ice packs weighing at least 0.6 kg for cold treatment.[73]

Another method of cold therapy is ice baths, which are fashioned by filling a tub half way with cold water and ice and submerging the injured body part into the tub. The disadvantage of ice baths is that no compression is involved, though it is thought that rest, ice, compression, and elevation (the RICE principle) are most effective in combination.[74]

Ice massage is another cold therapy in which water is placed into a foam cup and frozen. The top of the cup is then peeled back, and ice is massaged into the painful region using a constant circular motion. It is important to avoid holding the ice in one area for more than 3 minutes in order to prevent frostbite. This method can be repeated two to three times daily.

Gel packs can be an effective method of cold therapy because they are reusable and portable. They are useful in the clinic setting because they are a clean means of providing cold therapy. Gel packs are applied to the affected region through a towel or cloth to prevent frostbite.

Another cold treatment known as vapocoolant sprays effectively removes heat from the skin by evaporating quickly when in contact with the affected body part. This method of cold therapy only provides a very superficial cooling effect but is often used before a contracted muscle is stretched (commonly referred to as the "spray and stretch technique").[75]

General indications for cold therapy include acute musculoskeletal trauma, pain, muscular spasm, and spasticity. Precautions and contraindications for cold therapy include ischemia, cold intolerance, Raynaud phenomenon, cold allergy, and skin insensitivity.[76]

Electrical Stimulation Therapy

Electrical stimulation is a nonpharmacological physical modality that has been shown to strengthen muscles, promote healing, increase circulation to affected tissues, and ultimately reduce pain.[60] This modality has demonstrated efficacy in a variety of pain conditions, including chronic low back pain, hemiplegic shoulder pain, and arthritic pain.[77] With transcutaneous electrical nerve stimulation (TENS) therapy, described in more detail below, a current generator delivers electrical current through electrodes applied to the body causing a tingling sensation and/or muscle contractions. This electrical signal disrupts the pain signals being from the affected area.[78]

Transcutaneous Electrical Nerve Stimulation

This type of electrotherapy applies a low-voltage electrical pulse to the nervous system using surface electrodes placed onto the skin in the affected area. TENS has been used in both acute and chronic pain states with the goal of pain reduction. The analgesia produced by TENS is likely explained by the gate control theory of pain, developed by Melzack and Wall in 1965.[78] This theory posits that stimulating large, highly myelinated afferent A-beta fibers blocks or gates the transmission of pain signals through small nociceptive fibers (myelinated A-δ and unmyelinated C fibers) at the level of the spinal cord, resulting in decreased pain; TENS is thought to create this effect.[78]

The electrodes used in TENS are typically placed over the regions where pain perceived, most commonly in the upper or lower back region. While different types of stimulation devices are available, the most common type of stimulation has been high-frequency (40-150 Hz) and low-intensity (10-30 mA) stimulation, with the amplitude adjusted to result in minimal discomfort to the patient. This type of stimulation is known as conventional mode TENS (in contrast to low-frequency/high-intensity stimulation). Patients are instructed to place the electrodes over the affected regions and set the TENS unit at a comfortable amplitude for 30-minute intervals, two to three times daily.

While the use of TENS is common, studies of efficacy have shown conflicting results. One study by Oosterhof et al.[79] found a statistically significant difference between conventional and sham TENS, in which the conventional TENS group had higher rates of patient satisfaction; however, no statistically significant differences in pain intensity were found between the two groups. In another study focusing on the use of TENS in diabetic neuropathic pain, no statistically significant differences in pain relief were found when TENS was compared to placebo.[80] In a systematic literature search, the Therapeutics and Technology Assessment Subcommittee of the American Academy of Neurology found two class II studies showing benefit of TENS versus sham treatment in chronic low back pain but two class I studies and another class II study not showing benefit. The committee concluded that TENS is ineffective for chronic low back pain but probably is effective for painful diabetic neuropathy (two class II studies).[81] One systematic review and meta-analysis of 381 randomized controlled trials looking at the effect of TENS on both acute and chronic pain (the meta-TENS study) found that there was moderate-certainty evidence that pain intensity is lower during or immediately after TENS compared with placebo and without serious adverse events.[82] The only common adverse effects are intolerance of the sensation of stimulation and skin irritation, which is likely if the intensity of the unit is too high. This can be rectified by frequently shifting electrode positions as well as using a different conducting gel.[83]

Precautions and Contraindications of TENS Therapy

Electrical stimulation therapy should be avoided over regions such as the heart and anterior cervical region or in patients with malignancies. Electrodes should never be placed on or near the eyes, in the mouth, transcerebrally, or on the front of the neck. Electrical stimulation should not be used during pregnancy or at any time around infected tissue. In addition, this type of therapy should not be used by individuals with pacemakers, defibrillators, or other implanted electrical devices due to potential for interference and failure of the pacemaker itself as well as the potential of defibrillator/electrical device discharge.[84] Caution should be utilized when employing electrical stimulation over insensate skin, as this can cause superficial or more serious burns.

TENS and Interferential Current Therapy

Interferential current therapy (IFC) therapy involves the production of low frequency current (usually uncomfortable when delivered in isolation) in body tissue by the simultaneous application of two different medium frequency currents with a low frequency current produced by interference of two different medium frequency currents thus described as "interferential current." The medium frequency adjusted with amplitude-modulated frequency (AMF) at low frequency (1-250 Hz), produces higher penetration of the electrical stimulation in the tissue by reducing tissue impedance.[85] Analgesia, in this case, is explained similarly to when TENS is used, achieved by the same physiological mechanisms.[86] In a randomized, placebo-controlled trial examining TENS and IFC for chronic low back pain, both TENS and IFC presented an immediate analgesic effect in chronic low back pain, especially using the interferential current of 4 kHz modulated at 100 Hz.[87]

Iontophoresis

Iontophoresis uses TENS therapy to drive topical medications, such as dexamethasone, into the affected tissues.[88,89] This is followed by attaching a TENS unit to the region, with a current of 2 to 4 mA applied for about 10 minutes. Once this process has been completed, the electrical pads are removed, and the area is cleaned. By working as a percutaneous drug delivery system, iontophoresis allows drug delivery directly to the target region. In addition, iontophoresis avoids the risks and inconveniences of parenteral therapy, prevents the variation in the absorption and metabolism seen with oral medication administration, and effectively bypasses hepatic "first-pass" elimination commonly seen with oral medication administration.[90] Typical medications used with iontophoresis include topical steroids and other nonsteroidal anti-inflammatory medications.[91] Clinical applications of iontophoresis include conditions such as bursitis and plantar fasciitis.

Massage Therapy

Massage therapy involves pressure and stretching provided for 5- to 15-minute duration in a rhythmic fashion to affected regions. The physiological effects include reflex vasodilation with improvement in circulation, assistance in venous blood return from the periphery to the central nervous system, increased lymphatic drainage, decreased muscular tightness, and softening of adhesions/scars.[92] There are several types of therapeutic massage, including effleurage, petrissage (kneading), tapotement (percussion), friction massage, soft tissue mobilization (forceful massage of the fascia-muscle system), myofascial release, and acupressure. Please refer to **Table 111-6** for a description of each type of massage.[93-96]

Work from the Ottawa Panel investigated multiple pain conditions (ie, low back pain, neck pain, and osteoarthritis) and treatments including massage. The Ottawa Panel was able to demonstrate that massage therapy showed beneficial results for mechanical low back pain when compared to acupuncture, self-care/education, relaxation therapies, conventional physiotherapy, and placebo. In addition, the Ottawa Panel recommended the use of massage therapy in the management of subacute and chronic low back pain in view of immediate posttreatment improvement in pain and disability and short-term relief when combined with therapeutic exercise and education.[97]

Massage should not be performed over areas containing malignancies or over infected areas or regions containing nerve entrapments. Additional contraindications include the presence of deep venous thromboses, severe varicosities, severe clotting or bleeding disorders, and therapeutic anticoagulation.

TABLE 111-6 Massage Therapy Techniques

Massage type	Description
Effleurage	Gliding movement of skin without deep muscle involvement
Petrissage (kneading)	Used for muscle relaxation
Tapotement (percussion)	Helps with desensitization
Friction massage	Prevents adhesions in acute muscle injuries
Soft tissue mobilization	A forceful massage of the fascia-muscle system, which is used for reduction of contractures
Myofascial release	Prolonged light pressure applied in specific directions to stretch focal regions of muscle Often used in myofascial pain states
Acupressure	Finger pressure applied over acupuncture points in order to decrease pain

CONCLUSION

The patient with a prior or current SUD and co-occurring chronic pain can benefit from a wide array of active therapeutic interventions including physical and occupational therapies, pain education training, and a range of passive treatments for acute and chronic pain conditions. The focus of care, as in SUD-related treatment, should encompass a biopsychosocial multimodal approach. Psychological interventions, including behavioral, cognitive-behavioral therapy, mindfulness training, and acceptance- and commitment-based therapies, may be integrated into rehabilitation-based programs. Additionally, participation in more comprehensive multi- and interdisciplinary treatment programs may also be helpful to decrease pain and learn skills to improve psychosocial functioning.

In some patients, the use of passive treatments may be used as an additional tool for treating acute musculoskeletal and soft tissue disorders or for ongoing maintenance management of chronic pain. The active and passive treatments and more formal multi- and interdisciplinary treatment interventions reviewed in this chapter can be integrated easily into an ongoing treatment program of patients with substance use and addiction disorders. In more challenging cases, the addiction specialist can refer patients to their colleagues in physical medicine and rehabilitation, occupational medicine, and pain medicine. Patient referral to physical and occupational therapy should include follow-up and monitoring for compliance, assessing the ability for the patient to incorporate skills learned in treatment into their daily lives and during flare-ups. Better self-management of pain may help to reduce pain, improve psychosocial functioning, and, in many instances, help to reduce the incidence of recurrence of addiction-related behaviors and relapse.

REFERENCES

1. Dahlhamer J, Lucas J, Zelaya C, et al. Prevalence of chronic pain and high-impact chronic pain among adults—United States, 2016. *MMWR Morb Mortal Wkly Rep.* 2018;67:1001-1006. doi:10.15585/mmwr.mm6736a2
2. Hopkins HL, Smith HD, Tiffany EG. Rehabilitation. In: Hopkins HL, Smith HD, eds. *Willard and Spackman's Occupational Therapy.* 6th ed. JB Lippincott; 1983.
3. Fisher B, Lusted A, Roerecke M, Taylor B, Rehm J. The prevalence of mental health and pain symptoms in a population samples reporting nonmedical use of prescription opioids: a systematic review and meta-analysis. *J Pain.* 2012;13:1029-1044.
4. Turk DC. Efficacy of multidisciplinary pain centers in the treatment of chronic pain. *Prog Pain Res Manag.* 1996;7:57-74.
5. Kessler R. Impact of substance abuse in the diagnosis, course, and treatment of mood disorders: the epidemiology of dual diagnosis. *Biol Psychiatry.* 2004;56:730-737.
6. United States Department of Health and Human Services. *Pain Management Best Practices. Inter-agency Task Force Report: Updates, Gaps, Inconsistencies, and Recommendations.* U.S. Department of Health and Human Services; 2019.
7. World Health Organization. *International Classification of Functioning, Disability and Health.* WHO; 2001. https://www.who.int/standards/classifications/international-classification-of-functioning-disability-and-health

8. Kidd BL, Urban LA. Mechanisms of inflammatory pain. *Br J Anaesth.* 2001;87:3-11.
9. American Physical Therapy Association. The guide to physical therapist practice. Second Edition. *Phys Ther.* 2001;81(1):9-738.
10. Weigl M, Cieza C, Cantista P, Stucki G. Physical disability due to musculoskeletal conditions. *Best Pract Res Clin Rheumatol.* 2007;21:167-190.
11. Boon H, Verhoef M, O'Hara D, Findlay B. From parallel practice to integrative health care: a conceptual framework. *BMC Health Serv Res.* 2004;4:15.
12. Stanos S, Houle TT. Multidisciplinary and interdisciplinary management of chronic pain. *Phys Med Rehabil Clin N Am.* 2006;17(2):435-450.
13. Stanos SP. Developing an interdisciplinary multidisciplinary chronic pain management program: nuts and bolts. In: Schatman M, Campbell A, eds. *Chronic Pain Management: Guidelines for Multidisciplinary Program Development*. Informa Healthcare; 2007.
14. Stanos S. Interdisciplinary pain management. In: Benzon H, ed. *Practical Management of Pain*. 6th ed. Elsevier; 2023.
15. Hooten W, Townsend C, Sletten C, Bruce B, Rome J. Treatment outcomes after multidisciplinary pain rehabilitation with analgesic medication withdrawal for patients with fibromyalgia. *Pain Med.* 2007;8(1):8-16.
16. Huffman K, Sweis G, Gase A, Scheman J, Covington E. Opioid use 12 months following interdisciplinary pain rehabilitation and weaning. *Pain Med.* 2013;14:1908-1917.
17. Murphy J, Palyo S, Schmidt Z, et al. The resurrection of interdisciplinary pain rehabilitation: outcomes across a Veterans Affairs collaborative. *Pain Med.* 2021;22:430-443.
18. Cook G. *The Four Ps (Exercise Prescription). Functional Exercise Training Course Manual.* North American Sports Medicine Institute, ACE; 1997.
19. Humphrey LD. Flexibility. *J Phys Educ Recreat Dance.* 1981;52:41.
20. Keirns M. *Myofascial Release in Sports Medicine*. Human Kinetics; 2000.
21. Travell JG, Simons DG. *Myofascial Pain and Dysfunction: The Trigger Point Manual.* Vol. 2. Lippincott Williams & Wilkins; 1992.
22. Butler DS. *The Sensitive Nervous System*. 2nd ed. Noigroup Publications; 2006.
23. Butler DS, Moseley L. *Explain Pain*. Noigroup Publications; 2013.
24. Hurley R, Turner C. Neurology and aquatic therapy. *Clin Manage.* 1991;1(1):26-27.
25. Thein JM, Thein BL. Aquatic-based rehabilitation and training for the elite athlete. *J Orthop Sports Phys Ther.* 1998;27(1):32-41.
26. Irion JM. Aquatic therapy. In: Brandy WD, Sanders B, eds. *Therapeutic Exercise: Techniques for Intervention*. Lippincott Williams & Wilkins; 2011.
27. Sova R. *Aquatic Activities Handbook*. Jones & Bartlett; 1993.
28. Louw A, Diener I, Butler D, Puentedura E. The effect of neuroscience education on pain, disability, anxiety, and stress in chronic musculoskeletal pain. *Arch Phys Med Rehab.* 2011;92(12):2041-2056.
29. Delitto A, George S, Van Dillen L, et al. Low back pain: clinical practice guidelines lined to the International Classification of Functioning, Instability, and Health from the Orthopaedic Section of the American Physical Therapy Association. *J Orthop Sports Phys Ther.* 2011;42(4):A1-A57.
30. Richardson C, Jull G, Hodges P, Hides J. *Therapeutic Exercise for Spinal Stabilization and Low Back Pain*. Churchill Livingstone; 1999.
31. King M. Core stability: creating a foundation for functional rehabilitation. *Athl Ther Today.* 2000;5(2):6-13.
32. Porterfield J, DeRosa C. *Mechanical Low Back Pain: Perspectives in Functional Anatomy*. Saunders; 1991.
33. Gracovetsky S, Farfan H. The optimum spine. *Spine.* 1986;11:543-573.
34. Geraci M. Rehabilitation of the hip and pelvis. In: Kibler WB, ed. *Functional Rehabilitation of Sports and Musculoskeletal Injuries*. Aspen Publishers; 1998.
35. McKenzie RA, May S. *Mechanical Diagnosis and Therapy: The Lumbar Spine*. Spinal Publication Ltd; 2002.
36. Donelson R, Grant W, Kamps C, Medcalf R. Pain response to sagittal end range spinal motion: a multi-centered, prospective, randomized trial. *Spine.* 1991;16:S206-S212.
37. Louw A, Zimmney K, Puentedura E, Diener I. The efficacy of pain neuroscience education on musculoskeletal pain: a systematic review of the literature. *Physiother Theory Pract.* 2016;32:332-355.
38. Rufa A, Beissner K, Dolphin M. The use of pain neuroscience education in older adults with chronic back and/or lower extremity pain. *Physiother Theory Pract.* 2019;35(7):603-613.
39. Rehabilitation Institute of Chicago, Center for Pain Management. *Pain Program Workbook*. Rehabilitation Institute of Chicago; 2013.
40. Povlsen B. Physical rehabilitation with ergonomic intervention of currently working keyboard operators with nonspecific Type II work-related upper limb disorder: a prospective study. *Arch Phys Med Rehabil.* 2012;93:78-81.
41. Fabrizio P. Ergonomic intervention in the treatment of a patient with upper extremity and neck pain. *Phys Ther.* 2009;89:351-360.
42. Matheson LN, Mooney V, Grant JE, Leggett S, Kenny K. Standardized evaluation of work capacity. *J Back Musculoskelet Rehabil.* 1996;6:249-264.
43. Matheson L. Functional capacity evaluation. In: Andersson G, Demeter S, Smith G, eds. *Disability Evaluation*. Mosby Yearbook; 1996.
44. U.S. Department of Labor. *Dictionary of Occupational Titles*. U.S. Government Printing Office; 1986.
45. Reneman MF, Fokkens AS, Dijkstra PU, Geertzen JH, Groothoff JW. Testing lifting capacity: validity of determining effort level by means of observation. *Spine.* 2005;30(2):E40-E46.
46. Turk D, Okifuji A. Psychological factors in chronic pain: evolution and revolution. *J Consult Clin Psychol.* 2002;70(3):678-690.
47. Kerns R, Sellinger J, Goodin B. Psychological treatment of chronic pain. *Annu Rev Clin Psychol.* 2011;7:411-434.
48. Stanos S, McLean J, Rader L. Physical medicine rehabilitation approaches to pain. *Anesthesiol Clin.* 2007;25:721-759. doi:10.1016/j.anclin.2007.07.008
49. Reyes T. *Introduction to Physical Therapy and Patient Care. Hydrotherapy, Traction and Massage*. 2nd ed. UST Press; 1985:121.
50. Dontigny RL, Sheldon KW. Simultaneous use of heat and cold in treatment of muscle spasm. *Arch Phys Med Rehabil.* 1962;43:235-237.
51. Greenberg RS. The effects of hot packs and exercise on local blood flow. *Phys Ther.* 1972;52(3):273-278.
52. Yeshurun L, Azhari H. Non-invasive measurement of thermal diffusivity using high-intensity focused ultrasound and through-transmission ultrasonic imaging. *Ultrasound Med Biol.* 2016;42(1):243-256.
53. Lehmann JF. *Therapeutic Heat and Cold*. 4th ed. FA Davis; 1990:417-581.
54. Im SH, Han EY. Improvement in anxiety and pain after whole body whirlpool hydrotherapy among patients with myofascial pain syndrome. *Ann Rehabil Med.* 2013;37(4):534-540. doi:10.5535/arm.2013.37.4.534
55. Robertson VJ, Baker KG. A review of therapeutic ultrasound: effectiveness studies. *Phys Ther.* 2001;81(7):1339-1350.
56. Wong RA, Schumann B, Townsend R, Phelps CA. A survey of therapeutic ultrasound use by physical therapists who are orthopaedic certified specialists. *Phys Ther.* 2007;87(8):986-994.
57. Dantas LO, Osani MC, Bannuru RR. Therapeutic ultrasound for knee osteoarthritis: a systematic review and meta-analysis with grade quality assessment. *Braz J Phys Ther.* 2021;25(6):688-697.
58. Rosim GC, Barbieri CH, Lanças FM, Mazzer N. Diclofenac phonophoresis in human volunteers. *Ultrasound Med Biol.* 2005;31(3):337-343.
59. Shestack R. *Handbook of Physical Therapy*. 3rd ed. Springer Publishing; 1977:47.
60. Gladwell PW, Badlan K, Cramp F, Palmer S. Direct and indirect benefits reported by users of transcutaneous electrical nerve stimulation for chronic musculoskeletal pain: qualitative exploration using patient interviews. *Phys Ther.* 2015;95(11):1518-1528.
61. Durmus D, Alayli G, Tufekci T, Kuru O. A randomized placebo-controlled clinical trial of phonophoresis for the treatment of chronic neck pain. *Rheumatol Int.* 2014;34(5):605-611.
62. Miller DL, Smith NB, Bailey MR, et al. Overview of therapeutic ultrasound applications and safety considerations. *J Ultrasound Med.* 2012;31(4):623-634.
63. Abramson DI, Tuck S Jr, Chu LS, Agustin C. Effect of paraffin bath and hot fomentations on local tissue temperatures. *Arch Phys Med Rehabil.* 1964;45:87-94.

64. Stimson CW, Rose GB, Nelson PA. Paraffin bath as thermotherapy: an evaluation. *Arch Phys Med Rehabil.* 1958;39(4):219-227.
65. Helfand AE, Bruno J. Therapeutic modalities and procedures. Part I: cold and heat. *Clin Podiatry.* 1984;1(2):301-313.
66. Britton NF, Skevington SM. A mathematical model of the gate control theory of pain. *J Theor Biol.* 1989;137(1):91-105.
67. Basford JR. Physical agents and biofeedback. In: DeLisa JA, Gans BM, Bockenek WL, eds. *Rehabilitation Medicine: Principles and Practice.* JB Lippincott; 1988:257-271.
68. Chung MK, Wang S. Cold suppresses agonist-induced activation of TRPV1. *J Dent Res.* 2011;90(9):1098-1102.
69. Abramson DI, Chu LS, Tuck S Jr, Lee SW, Richardson G, Levin M. Effect of tissue temperatures and blood flow on motor nerve conduction velocity. *JAMA.* 1966;198:1082-1088.
70. Koç M, Tez M, Yoldaş O, Dizen H, Göçmen E. Cooling for the reduction of postoperative pain: prospective randomized study. *Hernia.* 2006;10(2):184-186.
71. Janwantanakul P. The effect of quantity of ice and size of contact area on ice pack/skin interface temperature. *Physiotherapy.* 2009;95(2): 120-125.
72. Kunkle B, Kothandaraman V, Goodlow J, et al. Orthopaedic application of cryotherapy: a comprehensive review of the history, basic science, methods, and clinical effectiveness. *JBJS Rev.* 2021;9(1):e20.00016.
73. Järvinen TA, Kääriäinen M, Järvinen M, Kalimo H. Muscle strain injuries. *Curr Opin Rheumatol.* 2000;12(2):155-161.
74. Kostopoulos D, Rizopoulos K. Effect of topical aerosol skin refrigerant (spray and stretch technique) on passive and active stretching. *J Bodyw Mov Ther.* 2008;12(2):96-104.
75. Swenson C, Sward L, Karlsson J. Cryotherapy in sports medicine. *Scand J Med Sci Sports.* 1996;6(4):193-200.
76. Poitras S, Brosseau L. Evidence-informed management of chronic low back pain with transcutaneous electrical nerve stimulation, interferential current, electrical muscle stimulation, ultrasound and thermotherapy. *Spine J.* 2008;8:226-233.
77. Buchmuller A, Navez M, Milletre-Bernardin M, et al. Value of TENS for relief of chronic low back pain with or without radicular pain. *Eur J Pain.* 2012;16(5):656-665.
78. Melzack R, Wall PD. Pain mechanisms: a new theory. *Science.* 1965;150:971-979.
79. Oosterhof J, Samwel HJA, de Boo TM, Wilder-Smith OHG, Oostendorp AB, Crul BJP. Predicting outcome of TENS in chronic pain: a prospective, randomized, placebo controlled trial. *Pain.* 2008;136(1-2):11-20.
80. Gossrau G, Wähner M, Kuschke M, et al. Microcurrent transcutaneous electric nerve stimulation in painful diabetic neuropathy: a randomized placebo-controlled study. *Pain Med.* 2011;12(6):953-960.
81. Dubinsky RM, Miyasaki J. Assessment: efficacy of transcutaneous electric nerve stimulation in the treatment of pain in neurologic disorders (an evidence-based review): report of the Therapeutics and Technology Assessment Subcommittee of the American Academy of Neurology. *Neurology.* 2010;74(2):173-176.
82. Johnson M, Paley C, Jones G, Mulvey MR, Wittkopf PG. Efficacy and safety of transcutaneous electrical nerve stimulation (TENS) for acute and chronic pain in adults: a systematic review and meta-analysis of 381 studies (the meta-TENS study). *BMJ Open.* 2022;12(2):e051073.
83. Fary RE, Briffa NK. Monophasic electrical stimulation produces high rates of adverse skin reactions in healthy subjects. *Physiother Theory Pract.* 2011;27(3):246-251.
84. Holmgren C, Carlsson T, Mannheimer C, Edvardsson N. Risk of interference from transcutaneous electrical nerve stimulation on the sensing function of implantable defibrillators. *Pacing Clin Electrophysiol.* 2008;31(2):151-158.
85. Fuentes JP, Armijo Olivo S, Magee DJ, Gross DP. Effectiveness of interferential current therapy in the management of musculoskeletal pain: a systematic review and meta-analysis. *Phys Ther.* 2010;90:1219-1238.
86. Dohnert MB, Bauer JP, Pavao TS. Study of the effectiveness of interferential current as compared to transcutaneous electrical nerve stimulation in reducing chronic low back pain. *Braz J Pain.* 2015;16:27-33.
87. Dias L, Cordeiro M, Schmidt de Sales R, et al. Immediate analgesic effect of transcutaneous electrical nerve stimulation (TENS) and interferential current (IFC) on chronic low back pain: randomised placebo-controlled trial. *J Bodyw Mov Ther.* 2021;27:181-190.
88. Gurney AB, Wascher DC. Absorption of dexamethasone sodium phosphate in human connective tissue during iontophoresis. *Am J Sports Med.* 2008;36:753-759.
89. McLaughlin GW, Arastu H, Harris J, et al. Biphasic transdermal iontophoretic drug delivery platform. *Ann Int Conf IEEE Eng Med Biol Soc.* 2011;1225-1228.
90. Costello T, Jeske A. Iontophoresis: applications in transdermal medication delivery. *Phys Ther.* 1995;75:554-563.
91. Weerapong P, Hume PA, Kolt GS. The mechanisms of massage and effects on performance, muscle recovery and injury prevention. *Sports Med.* 2005;35(3):235-256.
92. Braddom RL. *Physical Medicine and Rehabilitation.* 4th ed. Elsevier Health Sciences; 2010.
93. Ernst E. The safety of massage therapy. *Rheumatology.* 2003;42(9):1101-1106.
94. Atkins D, Eichler D. The effects of self-massage on osteoarthritis of the knee: a randomized controlled trial. *Int J Ther Massage Bodywork.* 2013;6(1):4-14.
95. Little P, Lewish G, Webley F, et al. Alexander technique lessons, exercise and massage (ATEAM) for S19 Self-Care Therapies for Chronic Pain chronic or recurrent back pain. *Evid Based Med.* 2008;42(12):965-968.
96. Crawford C, Lee C, May T; Active Self-Care Therapies for Pain (PACT) Working Group. Physically-oriented therapies for the self-management of chronic pain symptoms. *Pain Med.* 2014;15(Suppl 1):S54-S65.
97. Brosseau L, Wells GA, Poitras S, et al. Ottawa panel evidence-based clinical practice guidelines on therapeutic massage for low back pain. *J Bodyw Mov Ther.* 2012;16(4):424-455.

CHAPTER

112 Nonopioid Pharmacotherapy of Pain

Emily R. Casey and Tanya J. Uritsky

CHAPTER OUTLINE

- Introduction
- Nonopioid pharmacological agents
- Opioid alternative analgesics
- Summary
- Acknowledgments

INTRODUCTION

Pharmacotherapy is a balancing act of the benefits versus the risks of a medication with the patients' ability to tolerate side effects and to adhere to dosing schedules. Managing patients with pain and selecting the appropriate analgesic requires correctly diagnosing and classifying pain as somatic or neuropathic. Nonopioid pharmacotherapy is part of a multimodal approach to pain management and has a growing role in the treatment of pain, in particular in patients with pain and co-occurring substance use disorders. Acetaminophen, nonsteroidal anti-inflammatory drugs (NSAIDs) and opioids are the principal medications for somatic pain. Opioid alternative analgesics such as antidepressants, antiepileptic drugs (AEDs), anesthetics, and adrenergic agents are not primary analgesics but have analgesic efficacy in certain conditions and are more commonly used for neuropathic pain. The appropriate use of both types of medications can greatly improve analgesia as well as overall pain management. After the appropriate class of nonopioid medication has been selected, the choice of a specific drug is determined by its side effects, route of administration, and individual patient characteristics such as risks and co-occurring conditions. When opioid alternative analgesics (eg, gabapentin, amitriptyline) fail to treat moderate to severe neuropathic pain effectively, evidence suggests opioids may still yield a good response in well selected and monitored patients as was demonstrated in clinical trials with tramadol, low-dose methadone, or morphine.[1-4] In patients at increased risk for harms with the use of opioids, carefully consider using and selecting agents with improved safety profiles, such as buprenorphine, which is discussed in Chapter 113, "Opioid Therapy of Pain." Other alternative treatment methods include interventional techniques, physical modalities, and behavioral and integrative medicine approaches. In the management of chronic pain, these alternative treatment methods serve as adjuncts to primary therapy and may not be effective substitutes for pharmacotherapy. This chapter provides an overview of nonopioid and opioid alternative analgesic pharmacotherapy mechanisms of action and indications. (Integrative medicine and behavioral approaches, which are integral to a multidisciplinary approach to pain management, are reviewed in Chapters 109 and 111. The use of opioid medications is discussed in Chapter 113.)

NONOPIOID PHARMACOLOGICAL AGENTS

Acetaminophen

Acetaminophen is an analgesic and antipyretic agent often utilized first line to treat mild to moderate pain. Acetaminophen is converted to a metabolite, p-aminophenol which crosses the blood-brain barrier and is then converted into AM404. AM404 then acts on both TRPV1 and CB1 receptors to produce analgesia.[5] It is also possible that acetaminophen inhibits COX pathways in the central nervous system producing analgesia without producing anti-inflammatory effects.[5] In a Cochrane review including 51 studies evaluating pain control after surgery, 50% of participants who received a single oral dose of acetaminophen after a surgical procedure reported pain relief compared to only 20% of patients who received placebo. In this same review it was found that the analgesic effect of acetaminophen 1,000 mg in the postoperative period was comparable to low dose NSAIDs including ibuprofen 100 mg, celecoxib 200 mg, and naproxen 200 to 220 mg.[6] Acetaminophen should be provided on a scheduled basis to maximize its analgesic potential and to permit stronger analgesics with greater risk of toxicity, like NSAIDs or opioids, to be used more sparingly.

While adverse reactions due to acetaminophen are rare, there is the potential for the development of hematological, metabolic, and electrolyte abnormalities. Acetaminophen also has a potential for causing hepatotoxicity and has been implicated in the development of liver failure, resulting in the need for a liver transplant, or in some severe cases, death. Acetaminophen-associated hepatotoxicity is typically due to ingestion of doses that are higher than the maximum daily recommended dose. Acetaminophen is an ingredient in many over the counter products marketed for the treatment of pain, allergies, cold, and flu and the risk of accidental ingestion of high doses of acetaminophen is a serious concern. In adult patients without evidence of hepatic impairment, the maximum recommended daily dose of acetaminophen is 4,000 mg.[7] In patients with hepatic dysfunction, such as chronic liver disease or cirrhosis the maximum recommended daily dose of acetaminophen ranges from 2,000 to 3,000 mg.

The use of acetaminophen in pregnant persons is considered appropriate for the treatment of pain and fever. There have been multiple observational studies and case reports that have reported on adverse events in children who had acetaminophen exposure in utero, such as asthma or ADHD, though none have proven a causal relationship.[8-10]

Nonsteroidal Anti-Inflammatory Drugs

Nonsteroidal anti-inflammatory drugs (NSAIDs), the most widely used analgesics, are indicated for somatic pain of mild to moderate intensity. They are most useful in bone and joint pain but can be used in conjunction with opioids for all types of pain. The primary mechanism of action of the NSAID class includes inhibition of cyclooxygenase-1 (COX-1) and cyclooxygenase-2 (COX-2) activity, which in turn inhibits prostaglandin, thromboxane, and prostacyclin production.[11,12] Prostaglandin inhibition is primarily responsible for the analgesic activity of NSAIDs as prostaglandins sensitize peripheral nerve endings to noxious stimuli and are key to the inflammatory cascade.[11] Prostaglandins also influence many other body functions, acting as potent vasodilators in the peripheral vasculature and influencing the degree of sodium, water, and potassium secretion. Therefore, the inhibition of prostaglandin production not only produces beneficial analgesic effects, but can also result in adverse effects such as vasoconstriction and increased sodium, water, and potassium retention. This class of analgesics also requires both hepatic and renal clearance.[13] When one of these systems is impaired, drug accumulation can occur and dose adjustment is required.

The toxicity of NSAIDs is well recognized. Renal damage is a major toxic effect, particularly for those with compromised renal function.[14] Primarily, renal injury from NSAIDs is due to the lack of prostaglandin activity leading to vasoconstriction of the renal tubules and subsequently causing a decrease in renal blood flow that can lead to medullary ischemia.[15] Renal tubule vasoconstriction can lead to an acute kidney injury (AKI) or worsening chronic kidney disease. A useful rule of thumb is to avoid the use of NSAIDs in any patient with proteinuria and decreased glomerular filtration rate (eGFR < 30 mL/min/1.73^2). Use of NSAIDs in patients with hepatic dysfunction is also a concern due to lower serum albumin concentrations leading to a higher concentration of unbound NSAID in the serum, lending itself to a greater toxicity potential. NSAIDs increase the risk of gastrointestinal (GI) and variceal hemorrhage, development of ascites, and renal dysfunction in patients with hepatic dysfunction.[16] In patients with cirrhosis, NSAIDs should be avoided due to risk of hepatorenal syndrome.

GI toxicity is a concern with NSAID use. Several studies suggest that the rate of significant GI problems, such as ulceration and bleeding, is about 10%. More mild adverse effects such as abdominal discomfort, nausea, and vomiting are commonly reported with NSAID use.[17] These effects can be attributed to prostaglandin inhibition, which results in the loss of the protective GI mucosa, and topical irritation where the drug itself disrupts the mucosal barrier and erodes epithelial cells. GI effects can be mitigated through correct use of NSAIDs. Specific modifications such as taking the medication with food or directly after eating can decrease the incidence of GI upset. Additionally, proton pump inhibitors (PPIs) are clinically accepted and suggested by both the American College of Rheumatology and the American Gastroenterological Association for patients with GI risk factors when alternatives such as acetaminophen or COX-1 alternatives cannot be employed.[18] If utilizing PPI prophylaxis therapy in this patient population, providers should ensure that the PPI is de-prescribed when NSAID use is no longer indicated. It should also be noted that prophylaxis therapy with H_2 receptor antagonists is not recommended. While H_2 receptor antagonists may be an effective therapy to treat duodenal ulcers, they are less effective than PPI therapy for the treatment of NSAID-associated gastric ulcers.[19] Prophylaxis with misoprostol can also be useful,[20] but it is expensive and its long-term effects are unknown. Consequently, it should be reserved for patients who have a known sensitivity to NSAIDs and for after PPI failure.

Beyond renal, hepatic, and GI toxicities, hematological and cardiovascular toxicities are additional concerns with NSAID use. Most NSAIDs inhibit platelet aggregation through thromboxane inhibition.[21] This effect may pose a concern for elderly persons or those taking concomitant antiplatelet or anticoagulant agents as there is a risk for prolonged bleeding time. In adult patients who do not have risk factors for increased or prolonged bleeding, the clinical relevance of this effect is limited. In a study of 11 healthy adults who underwent a seven-day course of ibuprofen 600 mg orally every eight hours, platelet dysfunction occurred in 63% of participants, though it normalized within 24 hours of completion of the NSAID regimen in all participants.[22] Through this same mechanism, NSAIDs compete with aspirin (ASA) for platelet binding sites. Because of this, NSAIDs have the potential to reverse the protective effect of ASA on strokes and myocardial infarction. For this reason, the Food and Drug Administration (FDA) has recommended that, if patients are taking both NSAIDs and immediate-release ASA for anticoagulation, NSAIDs should be taken 8 hours before or 30 minutes after ASA.[23] In patients with cardiovascular risk factors who may be taking ASA for prevention of cardiovascular events, NSAID use should be carefully considered. The NSAID class is also known to cause a transient increase in blood pressure and exacerbate congestive heart failure (CHF) through mechanisms mentioned previously, vasoconstriction, sodium, and water retention.[24] In 2015, the FDA also strengthened its warning that NSAIDs can increase the risk of a heart attack or stroke.[25]

In an attempt to decrease the toxicity of traditional NSAIDs, COX-2 selective inhibitors were developed. The COX-2 enzyme is thought to have less impact on gastric mucosa production and platelet aggregation when compared to COX-1. This is because COX-1 enzymes are ubiquitous while COX-2 enzymes are found only in certain tissues such as renal, tracheal epithelial, and gut—to a lesser extent when compared to COX-1.[26] The use of COX-2 selective inhibitors has diminished in recent years as clinical trials and retrospective meta-analysis demonstrated increased myocardial infarctions and strokes in recipients of COX-2 inhibitors compared to traditional NSAIDs.[27,28] The NSAIDs as a class display a spectrum of COX inhibition. This class's activity ranges from ketorolac, which displays near complete COX-1 activity, to naproxen and ibuprofen, which are considered nonselective agents yet display slightly more COX-1 than COX-2 inhibition, to meloxicam, which displays slightly more COX-2 than COX-1 activity yet is typically also regarded as nonselective, to rofecoxib, which has been removed from the market due to risks associated with its near complete COX-2 inhibition. The only currently available NSAID that is considered a COX-2 selective inhibitor is celecoxib, which carries a black box warning for cardiovascular risk, but displays more balanced COX-1 and 2 activity compared to the other COX-2 selective agents and is considered safe for continued use.

An alternative strategy to mitigate the adverse effects of NSAIDs includes using topical formulations. NSAIDs come in a variety of topical formulations such as gel, or patches. While the side effects of topical NSAIDs are generally noted to be the same as oral NSAIDs, adverse effects of topical formulations occur at a markedly lower incidence when compared to systemic formulations. Patients that may benefit from topical NSAIDs such as diclofenac gel or patch include those with osteo- or rheumatoid arthritis.[29]

The use of NSAIDs among pregnant persons is controversial in the literature. A study by Daniel et al. in 2014 showed that with the exception of indomethacin, there was no increased risk of spontaneous abortion following exposure to a specific NSAID, including both COX-2 selective or nonselective inhibitors.[30] Most of the participants in this study, however, were exposed solely to nonselective inhibitors and therefore the study was limited by a small sample size of participants exposed to COX-2 selective inhibitors, with an unadjusted increased risk of spontaneous abortion following exposure to COX-2 selective inhibitors. In 2020, the FDA recommended that pregnant persons avoid the use of NSAIDs at 20 weeks or later due to concern of low amniotic fluid and the potential of injury to neonate kidneys. This recommendation was based on 35 cases of low amniotic fluid levels or neonate renal dysfunction that were reported to the FDA, all of which were serious.[30] The FDA did report that in most cases the condition was reversible if NSAID use was ceased.

Significant interactions between NSAIDs and other medications are common. The most important of these involve the potentiation of renal and hematologic toxicity of co-administered drugs and variation in drug levels like lithium and methotrexate. NSAIDs should be used cautiously in patients taking medications that act on the renin-angiotensin-aldosterone system (RAAS) such as angiotensin-converting enzyme inhibitors (ACE-i) and angiotensin-II receptor blockers (ARB).[31] The co-administration of these classes of medications with NSAIDs puts patients at an increased risk for AKI and hyperkalemia.[31] These effects are mitigated through increased renal reabsorption of potassium and an overall decrease in renal blood flow. Dramatic and dangerous increases in serum levels of lithium, widely used in psychiatric therapy, can result from concomitant NSAID use resulting from decreased renal clearance.[32] As previously mentioned, NSAIDs should be used cautiously in patients taking concomitant anticoagulant or antiplatelet agents due to the potential increased risk of bleeding. For the same reason, selective serotonin re-uptake inhibitors (SSRIs), should be used cautiously when co-administered with NSAIDs as serotonin binds platelets resulting in decreased platelet aggregation.

Adverse drug effects are dose and duration-related and there is a ceiling level to the analgesic effect of NSAIDs, beyond which increasing the dose does not improve analgesia and increases the incidence of adverse drug events. This ceiling varies from patient to patient, requiring individualized titration of dose. Patients who do not respond sufficiently to one class may have excellent results with a different class. Patients with advanced disease and pain sufficiently severe to interfere with their activities of daily living may require additional therapy.

OPIOID ALTERNATIVE ANALGESICS

Medications that have a primary indication other than analgesia, but which have analgesic properties in certain conditions, are referred to as opioid alternative analgesics. Most of these medications enhance the body's own pain-modulating mechanisms or the effectiveness of other analgesics. Several different classes of medications are used as opioid alternative analgesics, including antidepressants, anti-epileptic drugs (AEDs), local anesthetics, adrenergic agonists, capsaicin, botulinum toxin, and muscle relaxants.

Antidepressants

Tricyclic antidepressants (TCAs) have been used for many years for the management of neuropathic pain. Their analgesic effect appears to be independent of their antidepressant activity. There is evidence to suggest that TCAs work to enhance the body's own pain-modulating pathways through inhibition of serotonin and norepinephrine reuptake, which propagates inhibition of synaptic transmission.[33,34] TCAs exhibit further analgesic action via blockade of voltage gated sodium and calcium channels.[34] TCAs are effective therapeutic options for neuropathic pain, including peripheral nerve injuries, postherpetic neuralgia (PHN) and diabetic peripheral neuropathy (DPN), but appear to have poor efficacy in HIV neuropathy.[35,36] The greatest evidence for analgesic efficacy is with the older, tertiary amine antidepressants, such as amitriptyline, imipramine, and doxepin. Secondary amine tricyclics, such as desipramine and nortriptyline, are also effective and have less sedation and anticholinergic side effects.[37] The half-life of the TCA class is generally about 24 hours and onset of action is slow, requiring several weeks for the full drug effect to be achieved. TCAs display a significant number of side effects, the most common of which is sedation. In certain cases where pain overnight leads to sleep disturbance, these medications may not only treat the pain but also help promote sleep. TCA use may result in anticholinergic effects such as constipation, urinary retention, dry mouth, cardiac arrhythmias, blurry vision, and confusion. Hypotension can also occur and is more directly attributed to alpha blockade effects. TCAs are contraindicated in patients with glaucoma and prolonged QT syndrome and should be used with caution in patients with urinary outlet obstruction or those taking concomitant medications that may prolong the QT interval such as methadone.[38,39] Due to these adverse effects, TCAs also appear on the Beer's Criteria Medication List, which is a guideline for healthcare professionals that lists medications which may be inappropriate for use in older adults. The risk of experiencing side effects can be mitigated through utilizing strategies such as choosing a secondary amine tricyclic, starting at a low dose and escalating at weekly intervals, and instructing the patient to take the medication 10 to 12 hours before rising, rather than at bedtime. The usual starting dose for amitriptyline for pain is between 10 and 25 mg, and most patients find benefit at ranges between 50 and 150 mg.[39,40] It should be noted that the risk of suicidality increases with the initiation of TCA therapy. This risk should be weighed against the potential analgesic benefit of TCA therapy and close psychiatric assessment may be warranted.

Some patients are not able to tolerate TCAs and may benefit from some of the newer antidepressants. In general, serotonin-norepinephrine reuptake inhibitors (SNRIs) are superior for pain reduction when compared to selective serotonin reuptake inhibitors (SSRIs), and typically, the more selective the antidepressant is for serotonin, the less it is associated with analgesic efficacy. Venlafaxine, duloxetine, and milnacipran are SNRIs that have shown efficacy in pain of neuropathic origin and other painful conditions.[41] In a well-designed crossover study, venlafaxine (225 mg/d) and imipramine (150 mg/d) similarly improved symptoms of painful polyneuropathy where patients rated pain paroxysms, constant pain, and pressure-evoked pain.[42] Venlafaxine has also been shown to be effective in postmastectomy pain syndrome, fibromyalgia, migraine and tension headache, and painful DPN.[43,44] Typical dosing for venlafaxine ranges from 37.5 mg daily to 225 mg daily with a target dose of more than 150 mg when utilized for pain as there is some evidence that venlafaxine may be more effective for the treatment of pain at higher doses due to greater norepinephrine activity.[44] Duloxetine has also been shown to be useful in neuropathic pain. Multiple clinical trials with duloxetine have demonstrated efficacy in restoring functional status and decreasing pain scores in DPN when given in doses of 60 mg daily or twice daily.[45,46] In practice duloxetine is often dosed at a maximum of 60 mg once daily as twice daily dosing resulted in more significant adverse drug events and offered no additional analgesic benefit.[47] A randomized blinded trial of DPN demonstrated that duloxetine is comparable to amitriptyline in efficacy, but overall, participants preferred duloxetine.[48] Duloxetine has also improved global pain scores in fibromyalgia, for which it has an FDA indication (with and without co-occurring depression). Milnacipran is also indicated for the treatment of fibromyalgia and when dosed at 50 mg twice daily was found provide a similar reduction in pain scores and rate of adverse effects as duloxetine. In this same review, duloxetine displayed a significant difference in improved mood compared to milnacipran.[49] Duloxetine and venlafaxine may be the preferred drugs for the treatment of depression with co-occurring pain syndromes, regardless of whether these pain syndromes have classic etiologies (eg, DPN, radicular pain) or are nonspecific pain associated with depression. SNRIs are associated with adverse effects such as nausea and vomiting, dizziness, and fatigue. Venlafaxine specifically may result in hypertension, which can be a dose limiting adverse effect. Reports suggest SNRIs should be used with caution in patients on anticoagulants or with bleeding diathesis, as SNRIs reduce platelet serotonin content and therefore influence hemostasis and prolong bleeding duration.[50] Advantages of SNRIs over classic TCAs include fewer anticholinergic effects, less alpha blockade, absence of QT prolongation and general improved tolerability.

Antiepileptic Drugs

Carbamazepine, gabapentin, and several other AEDs have efficacy in neuropathic pain.[51] Modes of action vary but generally relate to sodium channel blockade, GABA-ergic action, or modulation of calcium channels. AEDs may reduce pain by reducing neuronal excitability and local neuronal discharges. They appear to be helpful in pain syndromes that are characterized by paroxysmal or lancinating pain, as well as burning pain and allodynia.[52,53] Phenytoin was the first AED used for pain and was found to be effective in trigeminal neuralgia in 1942; however, it is no longer in common use as newer drugs are less toxic, have fewer interactions, and have more approved indications. For example, carbamazepine remains first-line therapy for trigeminal neuralgia and has been well studied and used successfully in a variety of neuropathic pain states such as fibromyalgia.[54] Carbamazepine exerts its mechanism of action primarily through modulation of sodium and calcium voltage gated ion channels, rendering them inactive and thereby inhibiting generation and firing of action potentials. Important side effects include dizziness, somnolence, and significant leukopenia, as well as Stevens-Johnson Syndrome (SJS). Hyponatremia also can occur as an idiosyncratic reaction. When utilized for pain syndromes, carbamazepine is typically initiated at a dose of 200 mg daily. Carbamazepine is metabolized via the cytochrome P450 3A4 (CYP 3A4) enzyme and has significant autoinduction of metabolism and is associated with many drug interactions. Escalating doses may be required to achieve the same plasma levels and clinical effect over time and medications such as protease inhibitors, azole antifungals, and macrolides may increase plasma carbamazepine levels, while medications such as phenobarbital, phenytoin, and rifampin may decrease serum carbamazepine levels. Carbamazepine may also affect plasma concentrations of other medications resulting in increased levels of medications such as protease inhibitors, some antipsychotics, and warfarin. Like carbamazepine, oxcarbazepine also works to inhibit of neuronal firing through binding to sodium channels and there is some evidence that oxcarbazepine may be useful in pain of spinal cord injury (SCI), radiculopathy, and DPN, as well as carbamazepine nonresponsive trigeminal neuralgia.[55] Adverse effects of oxcarbazepine include dizziness, sedation, and fatigue. Hyponatremia is a frequent problem, particularly when combined with a number of psychotropic drugs. When utilized for neuropathic pain oxcarbazepine dosing is initiated at 300 mg daily and may be titrated to a maximum of 1,800 mg daily. Oxcarbazepine is associated with fewer drug interactions when compared to carbamazepine although it has been noted to increase serum concentration levels of phenobarbital and phenytoin when used concomitantly.

Valproic acid (VPA) is another AED that has been used for the management of lancinating pain, with mixed results, and for pain of DPN. VPA has multiple mechanisms of action such as NMDA antagonism, blockade of voltage gated sodium and calcium channels, and inhibition of glutamate resulting in upregulation of GABA. There are no large studies demonstrating long-term effectiveness for VPA use in the management of pain syndromes, and a recent Cochrane Review found support to be poor for its use in neuropathic pain.[56] There is, however, extensive evidence of its usefulness for migraine, both as an abortive and as a prophylactic agent and the recommended dose for migraine prophylaxis is typically 500 mg daily.[57,58] The most common side effects associated with VPA include dizziness, appetite changes, and insomnia. VPA is also associated with more serious, yet less common, adverse effects such as SJS, pancreatitis, hyperammonemia, and significant hepatic dysfunction. VPA is associated with a large number of drug interactions. Carbapenem antibiotics and rifampin can lower serum VPA levels, while aspirin and felbamate can increase serum VPA levels. VPA may also affect the serum concentration of concomitantly used medications such as increasing levels of phenobarbital, phenytoin, and warfarin.

Several newer AEDs have been found to be useful in treating neuropathic pain. Gabapentin, a calcium channel modulating agent via the alpha-2-delta subunit, has demonstrated efficacy in both lancinating and continuous dysesthetic pain.[59-61] Gabapentin is generally well-tolerated with few drug interactions and a favorable side effect profile. Gabapentin has a 5- to 7-hour half-life with nonlinear absorption, necessitating a three times a day dosage. Treatment is typically started at 300 mg daily and then escalated in increments of 100 to 300 mg every 3 to 5 days, up to a maximum of 3,600 mg daily in divided doses. Due to saturable kinetics, doses higher than 3,600 mg are not well absorbed, so doses above this are of questionable utility.[62] Gabapentin has recently been made available in two other formulations: a gastro-retentive, extended release formulation (gabapentin ER) and a twice-daily dosed actively transported prodrug (gabapentin enacarbil) designed for dose-proportional exposure. A 2014 Cochrane Review of gabapentin and its newer formulations showed that evidence was too limited to determine an optimal dose-response relationship for PHN, painful DPN, and mixed neuropathic pain.[63] For treatment of mixed neuropathic pain, a recent clinical trial comparing gabapentin with nortriptyline found that combination of these two medications resulted in a significantly greater pain reduction (52.8%) than did gabapentin alone (31.1%) or nortriptyline alone (38.8%).[64] The most commonly reported side effect is somnolence, which generally diminishes after the first 2 weeks of therapy. Accordingly, preoperative gabapentin (typically 900-1,200 mg/d) reduces the amount of opioid required to achieve adequate postoperative pain control and associated classic opioid side effects, but is associated with increased acute sedation.[64] Gabapentin is excreted renally and dose adjustments are required when utilized in those with renal impairment.

Pregabalin has the same mechanism of action and a similar adverse effect profile to gabapentin. In multiple large-scale trials, 150 to 600 mg/d of pregabalin had good efficacy in controlling neuropathic pain in both PHN and DPN.[65,66] Similar to trials with gabapentin, typically, more than 50% benefit was quantified with the McGill pain questionnaire, average daily pain scores, patient and clinical global impression of change, sensory/affective pain scores, and other efficacy measures. Additionally, sleep interference scores improved across multiple studies. Despite efficacy in PHN and DPN, recent studies suggest that pregabalin is not effective in treatment of HIV neuropathy.[67] Pregabalin is typically initiated at 50 mg three times per day and increased to 100 mg three times per day over a week. Best pain control usually occurs after 1 week of dosing. Dosing of 450 mg/d is recommended in fibromyalgia, and various neuropathic pain syndromes may require up to 600 mg/d to achieve efficacy.[68-70] The efficacy of pregabalin in the setting of fibromyalgia has been demonstrated through a handful of RCTs that demonstrated significant improvement in sleep quality, as well as change in scores on the Fibromyalgia Impact Questionnaire, and the Patient's Global Impression of Change Scale compared to placebo.[71] Most common side effects reported were dizziness and somnolence, which generally resolved with drug habituation. Weight gain is also common. Absolute platelet number can be decreased with pregabalin; thus, it should be used with caution in patients prone to thrombocytopenia. As with gabapentin, dose adjustments are required when utilized in those with renal impairment. Pregabalin is a controlled substance and carries a risk of unhealthy use including addiction, which is also a concern with gabapentin.[72]

Other less commonly utilized AEDs demonstrate less comparative efficacy and are associated with significant tolerability issues. Lamotrigine binds to voltage gated sodium channels and has been shown to have modest efficacy in treatment of DPN and HIV neuropathy at doses of 200 to 400 mg daily.[73,74] Lamotrigine is associated with side effects such as dizziness, nausea, and fatigue as well as more serious reactions such as drug reaction with eosinophilia and systemic symptoms (DRESS) and blood dyscrasias. Due to the potential for SJS and other dermatological side effects, lamotrigine initiation requires slow titration. There are also many drug interactions associated with lamotrigine. VPA increases lamotrigine levels significantly while carbamazepine, phenytoin, phenobarbital, rifampin, and protease inhibitors significantly decrease lamotrigine levels. Topiramate, which also works to inhibit voltage gated sodium channels, has little to no efficacy comparable to established agents in the various pain syndromes. It does have well-established efficacy in migraine prophylaxis and dosing is initiated at 25 mg daily then increased by 25 mg weekly until the recommended dose of 50 mg twice daily.[75] Side effects include cognitive issues such as difficulty with memory or concentration, dizziness, and weight loss. When administered with phenytoin, carbamazepine, VPA, or lamotrigine a reduction in the plasma concentration of topiramate is observed.

Clonazepam is a benzodiazepine with anticonvulsant properties that has been used for lancinating pain. The evidence for its use in this subset of pain is not lacking and derives mostly from case reports and anecdotal experience. Clonazepam also has utility in the treatment of muscle spasms as well as myoclonus.[76,77] The usual starting dose is 0.5 mg in the evening, escalating up to 2 mg three times per day if needed. Clonazepam is best used in patients with co-occurring anxiety and due to the propensity to produce significant dysphoria, it should be used cautiously when depression is present. As with all benzodiazepines, it is recommended to avoid use when possible in those with previous or co-occurring substance use disorders. Use with opioids also significantly increases the risk for respiratory depression. In a case cohort study evaluating the relationship between benzodiazepine prescribing and the risk of overdose in U.S. veterans receiving opioids, about half of the deaths observed occurred when benzodiazepines and opioids were concomitantly prescribed. The hazards ratio for risk of death from overdose for veterans with a current prescription for benzodiazepines compared to those without a prescription was 3.86.[78] The concomitant use of opioids and any other medication that results in central nervous system depression, such as benzodiazepines, gabapentinoids, or muscle relaxants, results in increased sedation and can result in increased risk for respiratory depression and associated mortality.[79,80]

Anesthetics

Neuropathic pain has been found to respond transiently to high doses of intravenous (IV) anesthetics, such as lidocaine.[81-83] IV lidocaine is traditionally utilized as a treatment for ventricular arrhythmias as well as a local anesthetic. Lidocaine exerts its analgesic mechanism of action through modulation of voltage gated sodium channels resulting in alteration of neuron conduction and is thought to have anti-inflammatory effects via reduction of inflammatory cytokines.[84] The onset of action of IV lidocaine ranges from 45 to 90 seconds and the drug has a half-life of about 2 hours. When dosed for analgesia, a 1 to 2 mg/kg bolus is administered followed by a continuous infusion ranging from 0.5 mg/kg/hr to a maximum of 3 mg/kg/hr.[85] Adverse effects of lidocaine include bradycardia, hypotension, QRS prolongation, as well as other dysrhythmias. Toxicity from lidocaine typically presents as lightheadedness, tongue numbness, or metallic taste and can progress to more serious effects such as confusion, paresthesias, tremor, or seizure.[86] Toxicity can occur with serum levels greater than 5 mcg/mL. If any of the signs or symptoms of lidocaine toxicity are recognized, it is recommended to check a serum lidocaine level. IV lidocaine should be avoided or used cautiously in patients with CHF, hepatic, or renal dysfunction as accumulation can occur and may result in fatal toxic effects. IV lidocaine has proven to be effective in acute pain scenarios such as limb trauma and perioperative pain.[87-89] A systematic review that included 26 articles evaluating IV lidocaine for neuropathic pain found that IV lidocaine was effective in treating neuropathic pain, though the analgesic effect wore off quickly after lidocaine infusions were stopped.[90,91]

Lidocaine is also available in a variety of topical formulations such as cream, gel, ointment, solution, or patch. Dosing for topical lidocaine varies based on the formulation utilized. All formulations of topical lidocaine should be applied to intact skin and over the site of the pain. Adverse effects of topical lidocaine formulations are typically limited to skin reactions such as itching, redness, or rash.[92] While systemic adverse effects of topical lidocaine are rare, certain interventions such as applying heat directly to the area where topical lidocaine was applied can increase the rate of absorption and therefore result in systemic adverse effects and should be avoided. Topical lidocaine formulations such as creams or ointments can be used on irritated areas of the skin for some analgesia and are typically applied two to three times daily. Formulations such as gel or solution can be used for pain or irritation in the mouth. Patches have proven to be effective for PHN and anecdotally, are used in a variety of both acute and chronic pain conditions such as acute musculoskeletal pain, or pain associated with placement of things like percutaneous endoscopic gastrostomy (PEG) tubes.[93,94] Eutectic mixture of local anesthetics (EMLA) is a 1:1 mixture of prilocaine and lidocaine, which can penetrate the skin and produce local anesthesia. It has been helpful in patients with peripheral nerve lesions and in reducing pain associated with venipuncture. EMLA has been particularly helpful in PHN.[95]

Mexiletine is an oral local anesthetic that is structurally similar to lidocaine, works via modulation of voltage gated sodium channels, and may be useful for neuropathic pain. The onset of action for analgesia is about one hour and the half-life is about 10 hours, which may be increased in renal dysfunction. Mexiletine is primarily eliminated via hepatic metabolism though cytochrome P450 2D6 (CYP2D6). Concomitant use of mexiletine with CYP2D6 inhibitor such as fluoxetine or bupropion will result in increased serum concentration of mexiletine. Evidence of analgesic efficacy of mexiletine is contradictory, but it seems that higher doses may show benefit.[96,97] The starting dose is 150 mg/d and may be increased in 150-mg increments every 3 to 5 days, up to a dose of 300 mg three times per day or until side effects occur. The most common side effects are dose related and include nausea, dizziness, and tremors. In a small randomized controlled trial, mexiletine, at doses of 150 mg twice daily, was found to reduce the number of cramps and severity of cramps significantly in patients with amyotrophic lateral sclerosis (ALS).[98]

Ketamine, an *N*-methyl-D-aspartate (NMDA) receptor antagonist, has a role in both acute and chronic pain management.[99,100] Ketamine is administered in a variety of formulations including intravenous, intramuscular, intranasal, oral and topical. The onset of action typically ranges from about one minute when IV ketamine is used to about 30 minutes when taken orally. The major active hepatic metabolite of ketamine is norketamine, which retains both psychoactive and anaesthetic effects. As ketamine utilizes CYP enzymes for metabolism, there are a number of interactions associated with this medication. The plasma concentration of ketamine will be reduced if used concomitantly with inducers like rifampin, and can be increased by 2.5 times when given with inhibitors like clarithromycin. Adverse effects of ketamine include hypertension, tachycardia, dizziness, as well as other CNS effects such as confusion or delirium. Ketamine use should be avoided in patients with a history of psychiatric illness such as psychosis or delirium due to the potential for emergence reactions. If emergence reactions occur, they should be treated with administration of a benzodiazepine. Ketamine also has risk for unhealthy use including addiction. Ketamine is generally used as an adjunctive agent in patients that have a poor or inadequate response to opioid and adjunctive analgesic therapy. A variety of ketamine dosing regimens can be found in the literature with IV infusion rates ranging from 0.05 to 1 mg/kg/h for the treatment of acute pain.[101] There is less literature surrounding the use of ketamine for chronic pain.[102] A meta-analysis evaluating the use of IV ketamine in patients with chronic pain disorders found that the median dose of ketamine infusion was 0.35 mg/kg, though a wide range of infusion regimens were found. This meta-analysis also found that most patients reported a reduction in pain scores somewhere between 48 hours and 2 weeks after infusion, with the analgesic effect waning somewhere between 4 and 8 weeks after infusion.[103] Oral ketamine is typically initiated at doses of 10 mg every 6 hours and may be increased by 10 mg every 24 hours. Effective doses of oral ketamine range from 1.5 to 3 mg daily.[104] There is limited evidence on intranasal ketamine, although small sample-size data supports its use in the treatment of breakthrough pain in patients with chronic pain at doses up to 50 mg resulting in rapid-onset pain relief that lasted up to 50 minutes.[105] There are conflicting data about the efficacy of topical ketamine at different potencies, with promising data in the treatment of chemotherapy-induced peripheral neuropathy and complex regional pain syndrome, although doses and formulations vary between studies and more studies are needed.[106,107]

Cannabis Used as Treatment

Many patients have refractory chronic pain for which cannabis may play a role. The active molecules in cannabis are delta-9-tetrahydrocannabinol (THC) and cannabidiol (CBD). These molecules act on cannabinoid receptors (CB_1, CB_2) which are present throughout the body. CB_1 receptors appear primarily in the CNS while CB_2 receptors appear more abundantly in immune-related cells. The effect of cannabis on pain is multifactorial and includes activation of both CB_1 and CB_2 receptors to inhibit the release of glutamate, modulate inhibitory pain pathways, and decrease inflammation.[108]

Cannabis is available in a variety of formulations for use in treatment. Cannabis may be inhaled, used topically, taken sublingually, or ingested in the form of an edible product or a liquid tincture. Based on the formulation administered, differences in onset of action are observed, with inhaled cannabis typically taking effect within 10 minutes while the onset of alternative formulations varies from 30 minutes to over one hour. An analysis of survey data from adults in the U.S. and Canada who utilize cannabis for treatment of chronic pain found that 45% of respondents utilized both inhalation and noninhalation routes and this group reported more significant improvements in health when compared to using either formulation alone ($p < 0.001$).[109]

While evidence suggests there may be benefit for cannabis in the treatment of chronic pain, studies are limited by heterogeneous data and small sample sizes. A retrospective review analyzing the efficacy of cannabis used as treatment (CUAT) in 38 patients with fibromyalgia found that patients utilizing cannabis via the inhalation route reported significantly lower pain scores at 1, 3, and 12 months of treatment ($p < 0.001$). The most common adverse effects reported included somnolence, confusion, and dizziness.[110] Similarly, a 2015 meta-analysis conducted by Whiting et al. found moderate-quality evidence supporting the benefit of smoked THC and nabiximols for treatment of chronic neuropathic or cancer pain.[111] Meanwhile, a 2015 meta-analysis by Deshpande et al. showed that there is evidence for the use of low-dose nonsynthetic cannabis in refractory neuropathic pain in conjunction with traditional analgesics, although the evidence was limited by dosing and THC strength variations and short trial durations.[112]

The data surrounding use of cannabidiol (CBD) alone is similarly heterogeneous. A randomized controlled trial evaluated the efficacy of cannibidiol compared to placebo when utilized as an add-on analgesic therapy in 136 patients experiencing pain due to hand osteoarthritis or psoriatic arthritis. The primary outcome was pain intensity at 12 weeks, in which there was no difference found between the CBD and placebo treated groups ($p = 0.96$). The group treated with CBD did experience a significant decrease from baseline in the Health Assessment Questionnaire ($p < 0.01$).[113] A number of small studies recently published demonstrate some benefit to utilizing CBD in treating peripheral neuropathy and pain associated with temporomandibular disorders.[108,114] A fuller and longer-term understanding of which cannabinoids are most useful for which symptoms and in which doses awaits further research.

Cannabis use, especially smoked cannabis, does raise safety concerns, as current evidence on long-term effects is limited and there is a lack of standardization of potency and routes of administration. Potential concerns include exacerbation of psychiatric illness, development of a substance use disorder, and effects on cognition including deficits in memory and ability to focus.[115] Recently published evidence from participants of the Dunedin Longitudinal study show that long term cannabis use may be associated with cognitive deficits. Long term cannabis users (reported cannabis use weekly or more during more than one questionnaire over multiple years) displayed a decline in IQ from childhood and self-reported memory and attention problems more commonly when compared to peer cohorts of long term tobacco, long term alcohol, and midlife recreational cannabis users.[115] There is no FDA approval for the use of cannabis or cannabis extracts for any condition, and the Institute of Medicine and the American Society of Addiction Medicine (ASAM) recommend that additional research be conducted before cannabis is recommended by a physician for an unapproved clinical indication. Please also see chapters relating to CUAT in Section 15 of this textbook.[116]

Alpha-Agonists

The α2-adrenergic agonists, most commonly clonidine, have been studied in a variety of pain syndromes including chronic neuropathic pain, myofascial pain, and complex regional pain syndrome. The mechanisms of action are presumed to be an enhancement of endogenous pain-modulating systems and, in the case of sympathetically maintained pain, sympatholytic effects. Administration can be epidural, intrathecal, oral, or transdermal.[117,118] Major limiting factors of use are hypotension and sedation. Although these are not pronounced in otherwise healthy patients, in the presence of neuropathy, blood pressure fluctuations can be increased.

While a randomized, double-blind, placebo-controlled, parallel-group, multicenter trial of 182 participants showed that 0.1% clonidine gel formulation, used at total daily dose of 3.9 mg/d, improved pain in patients suffering from painful diabetic neuropathy,[119] the Phase III trial ultimately failed to show a statistically significant difference. A two-phase double-blind crossover placebo-controlled study showed that a clonidine patch, started at 0.1 mg/d and titrated up to either to the maximum dose of 0.3 mg/d, did show a statistically significant decrease in the pain intensity associated with painful diabetic neuropathy. Post hoc analysis suggested that patients with intermittent, sharp, and shooting pain sensations may receive the greatest benefit. Clonidine patches are administered weekly at doses of 0.1, 0.2, and 0.3 mg/d.[120]

Capsaicin

Topical agents, like capsaicin, are useful for several types of continuous pain. Their action is local rather than systemic, and therefore, they are most effective in pain states that have a predominantly peripheral etiology. These include painful neuropathies, herpetic and PHN, and, occasionally, painful arthropathies. Topical agents alone are usually insufficient to produce total pain relief, but they can be helpful in patients who experience adverse effects from other drugs. Capsaicin, a naturally occurring pepper extract, has been found to be useful in reducing pain from DPN.[121] The capsaicin preparation is applied to the area of greatest discomfort several times a day with a delay in pain relief of several days. On initial application, many patients complain of markedly worsened pain and burning. This resolves after several applications and may be due to the local release of substance P. Unfortunately, the burning can be severe, and may lead to premature discontinuation of the drug. Multiple studies have demonstrated weak to moderate efficacy of capsaicin for neuropathic and musculoskeletal pain.[122] It should be reserved for combination therapy or when typical analgesics have failed. In a study of 200 patients with chronic neuropathic pain, pain was significantly reduced by the combination of topical 3.3% doxepin and 0.025% capsaicin. Absolute pain reduction was similar to either agent alone, but with a more rapid onset with the combination.[123,124] The capsaicin 8% dermal patch, has demonstrated efficacy in PHN, HIV-associated neuropathy, and chronic neuropathic pain.[125,126]

Botulinum Toxin

Botulinum toxin is a neurotoxin that produces muscle relaxation through blockade of acetylcholine release at neuromuscular junctions. Botulinum toxin is a widely accepted intervention for preventative treatment of migraines. When compared to topiramate in a RCT, botulinum toxin was shown to have superior tolerability in patients with chronic migraine. Botulinum toxin has yet to be compared to newer migraine agents, CGRPs, in head-to-head trials. The American Academy of Neurology states that botulinum toxin should be offered as a treatment option to patients with chronic migraine to increase the number of headache free days.[127] There have been several small studies showing the efficacy of intradermal and submucosal injections as well as topical botulinum toxin for various types of neuropathic pain. A meta-analysis including 21 RCTs evaluating the use of botulinum toxin in treatment of neuropathic pain found that botulinum toxin provides greater benefit in reducing pain intensity when compared to placebo in patients with trigeminal neuralgia, PHN, and diabetic neuropathy. The use of botulinum toxin in each of these disease states is promising, though larger RCTs are needed to decipher dosing regimens.[128,129]

Muscle Relaxants

The muscle relaxant class includes a group of diverse medications such as cyclobenzaprine, carisoprodol, methocarbamol, and chlorzoxazone. Cyclobenzaprine is a tricyclic agent that has been marketed as a muscle relaxant. Its major site of action appears to be in the brainstem, although the exact mechanism of action is unclear. It is indicated for short-term use only. Initial recommended cyclobenzaprine dosing begins at 5 mg three times a day. While cyclobenzaprine may be titrated to 10 mg three times a day, this increased dose has not been shown to have greater efficacy than 5 mg three times a day and is associated with a greater incidence of sedation.[130] It is quite sedating and should be used cautiously with other serotonergic medications. Methocarbamol, carisoprodol, and chlorzoxazone are agents whose exact mode of action remains unclear although largely thought to be due to CNS depressant effects. For each of these medications, the appropriateness of therapy should be continuously evaluated, treatment should not be extended beyond a couple of weeks and due to their potential for unhealthy use including addiction, these medications should be avoided when possible. It should also be noted that there is a risk of additive sedation when any of these medications are used with other medications that result in CNS depression, such as opioids or gabapentin, and concomitant use should be avoided whenever possible.[131]

Anti-Spasmodic Agents

There are various anti-spasmodic medications. This class includes medications such as baclofen and tizanidine. These medications are useful for conditions that produce flexor and extensor spasms because of neural injury, as well as chronic muscle spasm. Baclofen is a GABA-ergic drug with affinity for the presynaptic $GABA_B$ receptors. It suppresses excitatory transmitter release and action at the spinal cord level. There is some evidence that it also blocks transmitter release at cutaneous nociceptive nerve endings.[132] Patients with spasticity related to cerebral palsy, multiple sclerosis or upper motor neuron lesions or spastic hemiplegia from trauma, cerebrovascular disease or accident, or degenerative disease might benefit from baclofen. There is also some anecdotal literature suggesting that it may be useful for facial pain. Initial recommended dosing for oral baclofen is 5 to 10 mg up to three times daily as needed. Baclofen may also be delivered intrathecally via a surgically inserted pump in cases of severe spasticity. When used intrathecally, baclofen is administered as either a continuous infusion or periodic bolus. In both cases, intrathecal baclofen is titrated to effect.[133] The major side effects of baclofen are sedation and the occurrence of seizures with abrupt discontinuation. Patients may require additional antispasmodic medications for treatment of these disease states. Tizanidine, an $alpha_2$-adrenergic agonist, may be as effective as baclofen in decreasing spasticity but produces less muscle weakness. Initial dosing recommendations range from 2 to 4 mg every 8 to 12 hours as needed, with a maximum recommended dose of 24 mg daily.[134] Similar to the muscle relaxants, each of these medications increases the risk for additive sedation if used concomitantly with other medications that result in CNS depression.[131]

SUMMARY

There are multiple classes of nonopioid and opioid alternative analgesic medications that produce varying degrees of pain reduction associated with several different mechanisms of action. Choosing an appropriate analgesic requires careful attention to adverse drug reactions as well as drug-drug and drug-disease interactions. A summary of nonopioid medication and opioid alternative medication classes, mechanisms of actions, indications, and interactions is provided in **Table 112-1**. Nonopioid medications are often used in combinations, although studies supporting this practice are few. Their effect on chronic pain is to mitigate it and only rarely to eliminate it. The overarching goal of therapy should be to improve function as part of a multi-faceted approach to pain management.

TABLE 112-1 Summary of Nonopioid Pharmacotherapy by Drug Class

Medication Class	Mechanism(s)	Indication(s)	Interactions/Cautions	Place in Practice
Acetaminophen	• Agonist at TPRV1 and CB1 receptors	• Somatic pain of mild to moderate intensity	• Risk for hepatic toxicity when used at doses greater than maximum daily recommended dose	• First line agent for mild to moderate acute pain
Traditional nonsteroidal anti-inflammatory drugs (NSAIDs)	• Anti-inflammatory • Variable selectivity for inhibition of cyclooxygenase (COX)-1 and COX-2 activity leading to inhibition of prostaglandin production	• Somatic pain of mild to moderate intensity	• Enhanced side effects in older adults and patients with renal, hepatic, or hematological disease • Increased risk of GI bleed • Controversial use in pregnancy • Increased risk of myocardial infarction and stroke	• May be used safely in patients without hepatic or renal dysfunction who are not taking concomitant • Risk of adverse effects is dose and duration-related • Topical NSAIDs should be considered for patients who have increased risk and who have pain that is superficial and localized

(Continued)

TABLE 112-1 Summary of Nonopioid Pharmacotherapy by Drug Class *(Continued)*

Medication Class	Mechanism(s)	Indication(s)	Interactions/Cautions	Place in Practice
COX-2 selective NSAIDs (celecoxib)	• Anti-inflammatory • Inhibition of COX-2 activity >> inhibition of COX1 activity	• Somatic pain of mild to moderate intensity	• Enhanced side effects in older adults and patients with renal, hepatic, or hematological disease • Increased risk of myocardial infarction and stroke	• May be useful in certain pain states such as osteoarthritis in patients without cardiovascular risk
Tricyclic antidepressants (TCAs) (imipramine, amitriptyline, desipramine, nortriptyline, doxepin)	• Inhibition of serotonin and norepinephrine reuptake (analgesia) • Antagonist of alpha-1, alpha-2, muscarinic, and histaminergic receptors (adverse effects)	• Continuous, burning, or dysesthetic pain	• Contraindicated in patients with glaucoma, cardiac arrhythmias, and prolonged QT syndrome • Avoid use in older patients and in those with urinary outlet obstruction	• Second or third line agents for neuropathic pain • Cause anticholinergic effects that increase sedation, constipation, risk of falls and lead to difficulty with tolerability
Serotonin-norepinephrine uptake inhibitors (SNRIs) (venlafaxine, desvenlafaxine, duloxetine, milnacipran, levomilnacipran)	• Serotonin and norepinephrine reuptake inhibition	• Neuropathic pain syndromes • Fibromyalgia • Migraine • Tension headache • Osteoarthritis of the knee	• Use with caution in patients on anticoagulation or with increased risk of GI bleed	• First line for neuropathic pain • Generally improved tolerability over TCAs
Antiepileptic drugs (AEDs) (phenytoin, carbamazepine, oxcarbazepine, valproic acid, gabapentin, pregabalin, lamotrigine, topiramate, clonazepam)	• Variable • Generally involve sodium channel blockade, GABA-ergic action, or modulation of calcium channels	• Neuropathic pain syndromes characterized by paroxysmal or lancinating pain, as well as burning pain and allodynia	• Many drug interactions • Use caution in patients with hyponatremia, leukopenia, thrombocytopenia, depression, or hepatic or renal dysfunction • Several agents require monitoring for dermatological side effects including Stevens-Johnson syndrome	• Gabapentin and pregabalin are first line agents for most indications; other AEDs are considered third line due to risk of interactions and adverse effects • Carbamazepine is typically regarded as first line for trigeminal neuralgia • Topiramate is utilized to treat pain due to migraine
Systemic anesthetics (lidocaine, mexiletine, ketamine)	• Modes of action vary • Lidocaine and mexiletine block voltage-gated sodium channels. • Ketamine is an NMDA receptor antagonist	• Neuropathic pain and continuous dysesthetic pain	• Use with caution in patients with blood dyscrasias or with history of substance use disorder • In higher doses, monitor for cognitive effects and psychosis	• Typically utilized for the treatment of refractory pain syndromes • Ketamine and lidocaine have a role in patients with significant opioid tolerance as multimodal analgesia • If emergence reaction occur, treat with a benzodiazepine
Cannabis	• Modulation of cannabinoid receptors	• Chronic pain • Pain secondary to multiple sclerosis • Cancer pain	• Use with caution in patients with history of substance use disorder • Limited evidence about long-term side effects	• Laws for use vary by state • Need more data in the treatment of chronic pain
α2-Adrenergic agonists (clonidine)	• Enhancement of endogenous pain-modulating systems and sympatholysis	• Chronic neuropathic pain • Myofascial pain • Complex regional pain syndrome	• Use with caution in patients with labile blood pressure or heart rate	• May be used as adjunctive agent in the setting of spasmodic pain

TABLE 112-1 Summary of Nonopioid Pharmacotherapy by Drug Class *(Continued)*

Medication Class	Mechanism(s)	Indication(s)	Interactions/Cautions	Place in Practice
Capsaicin	• Local activity on Substance P	• Pain of peripheral etiology including chronic neuropathies, herpetic and postherpetic neuralgia	• Monitor for adverse dermatological reactions • Local burning with application	• Adjunctive agent for the treatment of neuropathic pain • Must be applied four times daily for effect • Topical patch beneficial for patients with post-herpetic neuralgia
Muscle relaxants (cyclobenzaprine, carisoprodol, methocarbamol, and chlorzoxazone)	• GABA-ergic blockade of neurotransmitter release at cutaneous nociceptive nerve endings • Central nervous system depression	• Spasticity	• Use with caution in patients with history of substance use disorder • Co-prescription of CNS depressants with opioid analgesics increases risk for respiratory depression and death	• Should be used for a maximum of up to 14 days at a time to treat acute painful muscle spasms
Anti-spasmodic agents (baclofen, tizanidine)	• Baclofen works via GABA-ergic activity • Tizanidine is an alpha$_2$-adrenergic agonist	• Spasticity	• Abrupt discontinuation of baclofen can cause seizures and death • Tizanidine can cause decreases in blood pressure and heart rate	• Useful in the setting muscle spasm due to neural injury or chronic muscle spasm

ACKNOWLEDGMENTS

We would like to recognize Simy K. Parikh, Michael Perloff, and James A.D. Otis for their work on the original version of this chapter.

REFERENCES

1. Raja SN, Haythornthwaite JA, Pappagallo M, et al. Opioids versus antidepressants in postherpetic neuralgia: a randomized, placebo-controlled trial. *Neurology.* 2002;59:1015-1021.
2. Hollingshead J, Duhmke RM, Cornblath DR. Tramadol for neuropathic pain. *Cochrane Database Syst Rev.* 2006;3:CD003726.
3. Morley JS, Bridson J, Nash TP, Miles JB, White S, Makin MK. Low-dose methadone has an analgesic effect in neuropathic pain: a double-blind randomized controlled crossover trial. *Palliat Med.* 2003;17:576-587.
4. Norrbrink C, Lundeberg T. Tramadol in neuropathic pain after spinal cord injury: a randomized, double-blind, placebo-controlled trial. *Clin J Pain.* 2009;25:177-184.
5. Ohashi N, Kohno T. Analgesic effect of acetaminophen: a review of known and novel mechanisms of action. *Front Pharmacol.* 2020;11:580289.
6. Toms L, McQuay HJ, Derry S, Moore RA. Single dose oral paracetamol (acetaminophen) for postoperative pain in adults. *Cochrane Database Syst Rev.* 2008;2008(4):CD004602.
7. Bunchorntavakul C, Reddy KR. Acetaminophen-related hepatotoxicity. *Clin Liver Dis.* 2013;17(4):587-607, viii.
8. Cheelo M, Lodge CJ, Dharmage SC, et al. Paracetamol exposure in pregnancy and early childhood and development of childhood asthma: a systematic review and meta-analysis. *Arch Dis Child.* 2015;100(1):81-89.
9. Lourido-Cebreiro T, Salgado FJ, Valdes L, Gonzalez-Barcala FJ. The association between paracetamol and asthma is still under debate. *J Asthma.* 2017;54(1):32-38.
10. Scialli AR, Ang R, Breitmeyer J, Royal MA. A review of the literature on the effects of acetaminophen on pregnancy outcome. *Reprod Toxicol.* 2010;30(4):495-507.
11. Vane J. Inhibition of prostaglandin synthesis as a mechanism of action for aspirin-like drugs. *Nature.* 1971;234:231-238.
12. Phillips WJ, Currier BL. Analgesic pharmacology: II. Specific analgesics. *J Am Acad Orthop Surg.* 2004;12(4):221-233.
13. Verbeeck RK, Blackburn JL, Loewen GR. Clinical pharmacokinetics of non-steroidal anti-inflammatory drugs. *Clin Pharmacokinet.* 1983;8(4):297-331.
14. Kincaid-Smith P. Effects of non-narcotic analgesics on the kidney. *Drugs.* 1986;32(Suppl 4):109-128.
15. Lucas GNC, Leitão ACC, Alencar RL, Xavier RMF, Daher EF, Silva Junior GBD. Pathophysiological aspects of nephropathy caused by non-steroidal anti-inflammatory drugs. *J Bras Nefrol.* 2019;41(1):124-130.
16. Chandok N, Watt KD. Pain management in the cirrhotic patient: the clinical challenge. *Mayo Clin Proc.* 2010;85(5):451-458.
17. Loeb DS, Ahlquist DA, Talley NJ. Management of gastroduodenopathy associated with use of nonsteroidal anti-inflammatory drugs. *Mayo Clin Proc.* 1992;67:354-364.
18. Gwee KA, Goh V, Lima G, Setia S. Coprescribing proton-pump inhibitors with nonsteroidal anti-inflammatory drugs: risks versus benefits. *J Pain Res.* 2018;11:361-374.
19. Targownik LE, Metge CJ, Leung S, et al. The relative efficacies of gastroprotective strategies in chronic users of nonsteroidal anti-inflammatory drugs. *Gastroenterology.* 2008;134:937-944.
20. Driver B, Marks DC, van der Wal DE. Not all (N)SAID and done: effects of nonsteroidal anti-inflammatory drugs and paracetamol intake on platelets. *Res Pract Thromb Haemost.* 2019;4(1):36-45.
21. Goldenberg NA, Jacobson L, Manco-Johnson MJ. Brief communication: duration of platelet dysfunction after a 7-day course of ibuprofen. *Ann Intern Med.* 2005;142:506-509.
22. U.S. Food and Drug Administration. *Information for Healthcare Professionals: Concomitant Use of Ibuprofen and Aspirin.* Accessed December 20, 2016. https://www.fda.gov/media/76636/download
23. Varga Z, Sabzwari SRA, Vargova V. Cardiovascular risk of nonsteroidal anti-inflammatory drugs: an under-recognized public health issue. *Cureus.* 2017;9(4):e1144.
24. U.S. Food and Drug Administration. *FDA Drug Safety Communication: FDA strengthens warning that non-aspirin nonsteroidal anti-inflammatory*

drugs (NSAIDs) can cause heart attacks or strokes. Accessed December 19, 2016. http://www.fda.gov/Drugs/DrugSafety/ucm451800.htm.

25. Brooks P, Emery P, Evans JF, et al. Interpreting the clinical significance of the differential inhibition of cyclooxygenase-2 and cyclooxygenase-2. *Rheumatology*. 1999;38:779-788.
26. Bavry AA, Khaliq A, Gong Y, Handberg EM, Cooper-Dehoff RM, Pepine CJ. Harmful effects of NSAIDs among patients with hypertension and coronary artery disease. *Am J Med*. 2011;124:614-620.
27. Gudbjornsson B, Thorsteinsson SB, Sigvaldason H, et al. Rofecoxib, but not celecoxib, increases the risk of thromboembolic cardiovascular events in young adults—a nationwide registry-based study. *Eur J Clin Pharmacol*. 2010;66:619-625.
28. Derry S, Conaghan P, Da Silva JA, Wiffen PJ, Moore RA. Topical NSAIDs for chronic musculoskeletal pain in adults. *Cochrane Database Syst Rev*. 2016;4(4):CD007400.
29. Sharon D, Koren G, Lunefeld E, Bilenko N, Ratzon R, Levy A. Fetal exposure to nonsteroidal anti-inflammatory drugs and spontaneous abortions. *CMAJ*. 2014;186(5):E177-E182.
30. U.S. Food and Drug Administration. *FDA Recommends Avoiding Use Of NSAIDs In Pregnancy At 20 Weeks Or Later Because They Can Result In Low Amniotic Fluid*. Accessed July 20, 2023. https://www.fda.gov/drugs/drug-safety-and-availability/fda-recommends-avoiding-use-nsaids-pregnancy-20-weeks-or-later-because-they-can-result-low-amniotic
31. Moore N, Pollack C, Butkerait P. Adverse drug reactions and drug–drug interactions with over-the-counter NSAIDs. *Ther Clin Risk Manag*. 2015;11:1061-1075.
32. Monji A, Maekawa T, Miura T, et al. Interactions between lithium and non-steroidal antiinflammatory drugs. *Clin Neuropharmacol*. 2002;25:241-242.
33. Maroon JC, Bost JW, Maroon A. Natural anti-inflammatory agents for pain relief. *Surg Neurol Int*. 2010;1:80. doi:s10.4103/2152-7806.73804
34. Casas R, Sacanella E, Urpi-Sarda M, et al. The effects of the Mediterranean diet on biomarkers of vascular wall inflammation and plaque vulnerability in subjects with high risk for cardiovascular disease. A randomized trial. *PloS One*. 2014;9(6):e100084.
35. Feinmann C. Pain relief by antidepressants: possible modes of action. *Pain*. 1985;23:1-8.
36. Sindrup SH, Otto M, Finnerup NB, Jensen TS. Antidepressants in the treatment of neuropathic pain. *Basic Clin Pharmacol Toxicol*. 2005;96:399-409.
37. Kieburtz K, Simpson D, Yiannoutsos C, et al. A randomized trial of amitriptyline and mexiletine for painful neuropathy in HIV infection. AIDS Clinical Trial Group 242 Protocol Team. *Neurology*. 1998;51:1682-1688.
38. Shlay JC, Chaloner K, Max MB, et al. Acupuncture and amitriptyline for pain due to HIV-related peripheral neuropathy: a randomized controlled trial. Terry Beirn Community Programs for Clinical Research on AIDS. *JAMA*. 1998;280:1590-1595.
39. Godfrey RG. A guide to the understanding and use of tricyclic antidepressants in the overall management of fibromyalgia and other chronic pain syndromes. *Arch Intern Med*. 1996;156:1047-1052.
40. Gillman PK. Tricyclic antidepressant pharmacology and therapeutic drug interactions updated. *Br J Pharmacol*. 2007;151(6):737-748.
41. Sindrup SH, Bach FW, Madsen C, Gram LF, Jensen TS. Venlafaxine versus imipramine in painful polyneuropathy: a randomized, controlled trial. *Neurology*. 2003;60:1284-1289.
42. Reuben SS, Makari-Judson G, Lurie SD. Evaluation of efficacy of the perioperative administration of venlafaxine XR in the prevention of postmastectomy pain syndrome. *J Pain Symptom Manage*. 2004;27:133-139.
43. Amr YM, Yousef AA. Evaluation of efficacy of the perioperative administration of venlafaxine or gabapentin on acute and chronic postmastectomy pain. *Clin J Pain*. 2010;26:381-385.
44. Aiyer R, Barkin RL, Bhatia A. Treatment of neuropathic pain with venlafaxine: a systematic review. *Pain Med*. 2017;18(10):1999-2012.
45. Armstrong DG, Chappell AS, Le TK, et al. Duloxetine for the management of diabetic peripheral neuropathic pain: evaluation of functional outcomes. *Pain Med*. 2007;8:410-418.
46. Arnold LM, Pritchett YL, D'Souza DN, Kajdasz DK, Iyengar S, Wernicke JF. Duloxetine for the treatment of fibromyalgia in women: pooled results from two randomized, placebo-controlled clinical trials. *J Womens Health (Larchmt)*. 2007;16:1145-1156.
47. Murakami M, Osada K, Ichibayashi H, et al. An open-label, long-term, phase III extension trial of duloxetine in Japanese patients with fibromyalgia. *Mod Rheumatol*. 2017;27(4):688-695.
48. Kaur H, Hota D, Bhansali A, Dutta P, Bansal D, Chakrabarti A. A comparative evaluation of amitriptyline and duloxetine in painful diabetic neuropathy: a randomized, double-blind, cross-over clinical trial. *Diabetes Care*. 2011;34:818-822.
49. Hauser W, Petzke F, Sommer C. Comparative efficacy and harms of duloxetine, milnacipran, and pregabalin in fibromyalgia syndrome. *J Pain*. 2010;11(6):505-521.
50. Lopponen P, Tetri S, Juvela S, et al. Association between warfarin combined with serotonin-modulating antidepressants and increased case fatality in primary intracerebral hemorrhage: a population based study. *J Neurosurg*. 2014;120(6):1358-1363.
51. Johannessen LC. Antiepileptic drugs in non-epilepsy disorders: relations between mechanisms of action and clinical efficacy. *CNS Drugs*. 2008;22:27-47.
52. Galer BS. Neuropathic pain of peripheral origin: advances in pharmacologic treatment. *Neurology*. 1995;45:S17-S25; discussion S35-S36.
53. McQuay H, Carroll D, Jadad AR, Wiffen P, Moore A. Anticonvulsant drugs for management of pain: a systematic review. *BMJ*. 1995;311:1047-1052.
54. Moosa RS, McFadyen ML, Miller R, Rubin J. Carbamazepine and its metabolites in neuralgias: concentration-effect relations. *Eur J Clin Pharmacol*. 1993;45:297-301.
55. Gomez-Arguelles JM, Dorado R, Sepulveda JM, et al. Oxcarbazepine monotherapy in carbamazepine-unresponsive trigeminal neuralgia. *J Clin Neurosci*. 2008;15:516-519.
56. Gill D, Derry S, Wiffen PJ, Moore RA. Valproic acid and sodium valproate for neuropathic pain and fibromyalgia in adults. *Cochrane Database Syst Rev*. 2011;(10):CD009183.
57. Bakhshayesh B, Seyed Saadat SM, Rezania K, Hatamian H, Hossieninezhad M. A randomized open-label study of sodium valproate vs sumatriptan and metoclopramide for prolonged migraine headache. *Am J Emerg Med*. 2013;31(3):540-544.
58. Silberstein SD, Holland S, Freitag F, et al. Quality Standards Subcommittee of the American Academy of Neurology and the American Headache Society. Evidence-based guideline update: pharmacologic treatment for episodic migraine prevention in adults: report of the Quality Standards Subcommittee of the American Academy of Neurology and the American Headache Society. *Neurology*. 2012;78(17):1337-1345.
59. Segal AZ, Rordorf G. Gabapentin as a novel treatment for postherpetic neuralgia. *Neurology*. 1996;46:1175-1176.
60. Rowbotham M, Harden N, Stacey B, Bernstein P, Magnus-Miller L. Gabapentin for the treatment of postherpetic neuralgia: a randomized controlled trial. *JAMA*. 1998;280:1837-1842.
61. Moore RA, Wiffen PJ, Derry S, McQuay HJ. Gabapentin for chronic neuropathic pain and fibromyalgia in adults. *Cochrane Database Syst Rev*. 2014;27(4):CD007938.
62. Gilron I, Bailey JM, Tu D, Holden RR, Jackson AC, Houlden RL. Nortriptyline and gabapentin, alone and in combination for neuropathic pain: a double-blind, randomised controlled crossover trial. *Lancet*. 2009;374:1252-1261.
63. Elwes RD, Binnie CD. Clinical pharmacokinetics of newer antiepileptic drugs. Lamotrigine, vigabatrin, gabapentin and oxcarbazepine. *Clin Pharmacokinet*. 1996;30:403-415.
64. Ho KY, Gan TJ, Habib AS. Gabapentin and postoperative pain—a systematic review of randomized controlled trials. *Pain*. 2006;126:91-101.
65. Richter RW, Portenoy R, Sharma U, Lamoreaux L, Bockbrader H, Knapp LE. Relief of painful diabetic peripheral neuropathy with pregabalin: a randomized, placebo-controlled trial. *J Pain*. 2005;6:253-260.

66. Dworkin RH, Corbin AE, Young JP Jr, et al. Pregabalin for the treatment of postherpetic neuralgia: a randomized, placebo-controlled trial. *Neurology.* 2003;60:1274-1283.
67. Simpson DM, Schifitto G, Clifford DB, et al. Pregabalin for painful HIV neuropathy: a randomized, double-blind, placebo-controlled trial. *Neurology.* 2010;74:413-420.
68. Rosenstock J, Tuchman M, LaMoreaux L, Sharma U. Pregabalin for the treatment of painful diabetic peripheral neuropathy: a double-blind, placebo-controlled trial. *Pain.* 2004;110:628-638.
69. Lesser H, Sharma U, LaMoreaux L, Poole RM. Pregabalin relieves symptoms of painful diabetic neuropathy: a randomized controlled trial. *Neurology.* 2004;63:2104-2110.
70. Raouf M, Atkinson TJ, Crumb MW, Fudin J. Rational dosing of gabapentin and pregabalin in chronic kidney disease. *J Pain Res.* 2017;10:275-278.
71. Sabatowski R, Galvez R, Cherry DA, et al. Pregabalin reduces pain and improves sleep and mood disturbances in patients with post-herpetic neuralgia: results of a randomised, placebo-controlled clinical trial. *Pain.* 2004;109:26-35.
72. Buscaglia M, Brandes H, Cleary J. Special report: the abuse potential of gabapentin & pregabalin. *Pract Pain Manag.* 2019;19(4).
73. Eisenberg E, Lurie Y, Braker C, Daoud D, Ishay A. Lamotrigine reduces painful diabetic neuropathy: a randomized, controlled study. *Neurology.* 2001;57:505-509.
74. Simpson DM, Olney R, McArthur JC, Khan A, Godbold J, Ebel-Frommer K. A placebo-controlled trial of lamotrigine for painful HIV-associated neuropathy. *Neurology.* 2000;54:2115-2119.
75. Huntington J, Yuan CL. Topiramate for migraine prevention. *Am Fam Physician.* 2005;72(8):1563-1564.
76. Bartusch SL, Sanders BJ, D'Alessio JG, Jernigan JR. Clonazepam for the treatment of lancinating phantom limb pain. *Clin J Pain.* 1996;12:59-62.
77. Eisele JH Jr, Grigsby EJ, Dea G. Clonazepam treatment of myoclonic contractions associated with high-dose opioids: case report. *Pain.* 1992;49:231-232.
78. Park TW, Saitz R, Ganoczy D, Ilgen MA, Bohnert AS. Benzodiazepine prescribing patterns and deaths from drug overdose among US veterans receiving opioid analgesics: case-cohort study. *NMJ.* 2015;350:h2698.
79. National Institute of Heath. *Benzodiazepines and Opioids.* Accessed June 27, 2022. https://nida.nih.gov/research-topics/opioids/benzodiazepines-opioids
80. Liu S, O'Donnell J, Gladden RM, McGlone L, Chowdhury F. Trends in nonfatal and fatal overdoses involving benzodiazepines—38 States and the District of Columbia, 2019-2020. *MMWR Morb Mortal Wkly Rep.* 2021;70(34):1136-1141.
81. Glazer S, Portenoy RK. Systemic local anesthetics in pain control. *J Pain Symptom Manage.* 1991;6:30-39.
82. Rowbotham M, Reisner L, Fields HL. Both IV lidocaine and morphine reduce the pain of post-herpetic neuralgia. *Neurology.* 1991;41:1024-1028.
83. Tremont-Lukats IW, Challapalli V, McNicol ED, Lau J, Carr DB. Systemic administration of local anesthetics to relieve neuropathic pain: a systematic review and meta-analysis. *Anesth Analg.* 2005;101:1738-1749.
84. Masic D, Liang E, Ling C, Sterk EJ, Barbas B, Rech MA. Intravenous lidocaine for acute pain: a systematic review. *Pharmacotherapy.* 2018;38(12):1250-1259.
85. Eipe N, Gupta S, Penning J. Intravenous lidocaine for acute pain: an evidence-based clinical update. *BJA Education.* 2016;16(9):292-298.
86. Marra DE, Yip D, Fincher EF, Moy RL. Systemic toxicity from topically applied lidocaine in conjunction with fractional photothermolysis. *Arch Dermatol.* 2006;142(8):1024-1026.
87. Farahmand S, Hamrah H, Arbab M, Sedaghat M, Ghafouri HB, Bagheri-Hariri S. Pain management of acute limb trauma patients with intravenous lidocaine in emergency department. *Am J Emerg Med.* 2018;36(7):1231-1235.
88. Tauzin-Fin P, Bernard O, Sesay M, et al. Benefits of intravenous lidocaine on post-operative pain and acute rehabilitation after laparoscopic nephrectomy. *J Anaesthesiol Clin Pharmacol.* 2014;30(3):366-372.
89. Yue H, Zhou M, Lu Y, Chen L, Cui W. Effect of intravenous lidocaine on postoperative pain in patients undergoing intraspinal tumor resection: study protocol for a prospective randomized controlled trial. *J Pain Res.* 2020;13:1401-1410.
90. Zhu B, Zhou X, Zhou Q, Wang H, Wang S, Luo K. Intra-venous lidocaine to relieve neuropathic pain: a systematic review and meta-analysis. *Front Neurol.* 2019;10:954.
91. Kandil E, Melikman E, Adinoff B. Lidocaine infusion: a promising therapeutic approach for chronic pain. *J Anesth Clin Res.* 2017;8(1):697.
92. Rowbotham MC, Davies PS, Verkempinck C, Galer BS. Lidocaine patch: double-blind controlled study of a new treatment method for post-herpetic neuralgia. *Pain.* 1996;65(1):39-44.
93. Bai Y, Millet T, Tan M, Law LSC, Gan TJ. Lidocaine patch for acute pain management: a meta analysis of prospective controlled trials. *Curr Med Res Opin.* 2015;3:1-7.
94. Voute M, Morel V, Pickering G. Topical lidocaine for chronic pain treatment. *Drug Des Devel Ther.* 2021;15:4091-4103.
95. Stow PJ, Glynn CJ, Minor B. EMLA cream in the treatment of post-herpetic neuralgia. *Efficacy and pharmacokinetic profile. Pain.* 1989;39:301-305.
96. Carroll IR, Kaplan KM, Mackey SC. Mexiletine therapy for chronic pain: survival analysis identifies factors predicting clinical success. *J Pain Symptom Manage.* 2008;35(3):321-326.
97. Chabal C, Jacobson L, Mariano A, Chaney E, Britell CW. The use of oral mexiletine for the treatment of pain after peripheral nerve injury. *Anesthesiology.* 1992;76:513-517.
98. Oskarsson B, Moore D, Mozaffar T, et al. Mexiletine for muscle cramps in amyotrophic lateral sclerosis: a randomized, double-blind crossover trial. *Muscle Nerve.* 2018; doi:10.1002/mus.26117
99. Bell RF, Kalso EA. Ketamine for pain management. *Pain Rep.* 2018;3(5):e674.
100. Schwenk ES, Viscusi ER, Buvanendran A, et al. Consensus guidelines on the use of intravenous ketamine infusions for acute pain management from the American Society of Regional Anesthesia and Pain Medicine, the American Academy of Pain Medicine, and the American Society of Anesthesiologists. *Reg Anesth Pain Med.* 2018;43(5):456-466.
101. Orhurhu V, Orhurhu MS, Bhatia A, Cohen S. Ketamine infusions for chronic pain: a systemic review and meta-analysis of randomized controlled trials. *Anesth Analg.* 2019;129(1):241-254.
102. Culp C, Kim HK, Abdi S. Ketamine use for cancer and chronic pain management. *Front Pharmacol.* 2021;11:599721. doi:10.3389/fphar.2020.599721
103. Buvanendran A, Kroin JS, Rajagopal A, Robison SJ, Moric M, Tuman KJ. Oral ketamine for acute pain management after amputation surgery. *Pain Med.* 2018;19(6):1265-1270.
104. Carr DB, Goudas LC, Denman WT, et al. Safety and efficacy of intranasal ketamine for the treatment of breakthrough pain in patients with chronic pain: a randomized, double-blind, placebo-controlled, crossover study. *Pain.* 2004;108(1-2):17-27.
105. Mahoney JM, Vardaxis V, Moore JL, Hall AM, Haffner KE, Peterson MC. Topical ketamine cream in the treatment of painful diabetic neuropathy: a randomized, placebo-controlled, double-blind initial study. *J Am Podiatr Med Assoc.* 2012;102(3):178-183.
106. Barton DL, Wos EJ, Qin R, et al. A double-blind, placebo-controlled trial of a topical treatment for chemotherapy-induced peripheral neuropathy: NCCTG trial N06CA. *Support Care Cancer.* 2011;19(6):833-841.
107. Finch PM, Knudsen L, Drummond PD. Reduction of allodynia in patients with complex regional pain syndrome: a double-blind placebo-controlled trial of topical ketamine. *Pain.* 2009;145(3):18-25.
108. Vučković S, Srebro D, Vujović KS, Vučetić Č, Prostran M. Cannabinoids and pain: new insights from old molecules. *Front Pharmacol.* 2018;9:1259.
109. Boehnke KF, Yakas L, Scott JR, et al. A mixed analysis of cannabis use routines for chronic pain management. *J Cannabis Res.* 2022;4(1):7.
110. Mazza M. Medical cannabis for the treatment of fibromyalgia syndrome: a retrospective, open-label case series. *J Cannabis Res.* 2021;3(1):4.

111. Whiting PF, Wolff RF, Despande S, et al. Cannabinoids for medical use: a systematic review and meta-analysis. *JAMA*. 2015;313(24):2456-2473.
112. Deshpande A, Mailis-Gagnon A, Zoheiry N, Lakha SF. Efficacy and adverse effects of medical marijuana for chronic noncancer pain: systematic review of randomized controlled trials. *Can Fam Physician*. 2015;61(8):e372-e381.
113. Vela J, Dreyer L, Petersen KK, Nielsen LA, Duch KS, Kristensen S. Cannabidiol treatment in hand osteoarthritis and psoriatic arthritis. *Pain*. 2022;163:1206-1214.
114. Nitecka-Buchta A, Nowak-Wachol A, Wachol K, et al. Myorelaxant effect of transdermal cannabidiol application in patients with TMD: a randomized, double-blind trial. *J Clin Med*. 2019;8(11):1886.
115. Meier MH, Caspi A, Knodt AR, et al. Long term cannabis use and cognitive reserves and hippocampal volume in midlife. *Am J Psychiatry*. 2022;179(5):362-374.
116. National Academies of Sciences, Engineering and Medicine, Health and Medicine Division. Board on Population Health and Public Health Practice, Committee on the Health Effects of Marijuana: An Evidence Review and Research Agenda. *The Health Effects of Cannabis and Cannabinoids: The Current State of Evidence and Recommendations for Research*. National Academies Press; 2017.
117. Zeigler D, Lynch SA, Muir J, Benjamin J, Max MB. Transdermal clonidine versus placebo in painful diabetic neuropathy. *Pain*. 1992;48:403-408.
118. Uhle EI, Becker R, Gatscher S, Bertalanffy H. Continuous intrathecal clonidine administration for the treatment of neuropathic pain. *Stereotact Funct Neurosurg*. 2000;75:167-175.
119. Campbell CM, Kipnes MS, Stouch BC, et al. Randomized control trial of topical clonidine for treatment of painful diabetic neuropathy. *Pain*. 2012;153(9):1815-1823.
120. Byas-Smith MG, Max MB, Muir J, Kingman A. Transdermal clonidine compared to placebo in painful diabetic neuropathy using a two-stage 'enriched enrollment' design. *Pain*. 1995;60(3):267-274.
121. The Capsaicin Study Group. Treatment of painful diabetic neuropathy with topical capsaicin. A multicenter, double-blind, vehicle-controlled study. *Arch Intern Med*. 1991;151:2225-2229.
122. Mason L, Moore RA, Derry S, Edwards JE, McQuay HJ. Systematic review of topical capsaicin for the treatment of chronic pain. *BMJ*. 2004;328:991.
123. McCleane G. Topical application of doxepin hydrochloride, capsaicin and a combination of both produces analgesia in chronic human neuropathic pain: a randomized, double-blind, placebo-controlled study. *Br J Clin Pharmacol*. 2000;49:574-579.
124. Irving G, Backonja M, Rauck R, Webster LR, Tobias JK, Vanhove GF. NGX-4010, a capsaicin 8% dermal patch, administered alone or in combination with systemic neuropathic pain medications, reduces pain in patients with postherpetic neuralgia. *Clin J Pain*. 2012;28:101-107.
125. Derry S, Lloyd R, Moore RA, McQuay HJ. Topical capsaicin for chronic neuropathic pain in adults. *Cochrane Database Syst Rev*. 2009; CD007393.
126. Simpson DM, Brown S, Tobias J. Controlled trial of high-concentration capsaicin patch for treatment of painful HIV neuropathy. *Neurology*. 2008;70:2305-2313.
127. Becker WJ. Botulinum toxin in the treatment of headache. *Toxins (Basel)*. 2020;12(12):803.
128. Egeo G, Fofi L, Barbanti P. Botulinum neurotoxin for the treatment of neuropathic pain. *Front Neurol*. 2020;11(716).
129. Oh HM, Chung ME. Botulinum toxin for neuropathic pain: a review of the literature. *Toxins*. 2015;7(8):3127-3154.
130. Borenstein DG, Korn S. Efficacy of a low dose regimen of cyclobenzaprine hydrochloride in acute skeletal muscle spasm: results of two placebo-controlled trials. *Clin Ther*. 2003;25(4):1056-1073.
131. Watanabe JH, Yang J. Hospitalization and combined use of opioids, benzodiazepines, and muscle relaxants in the United States. *Hosp Pharm*. 2020;55(5):286-291.
132. Hwang AS, Wilcox GL. Baclofen, gamma-aminobutyric acid B receptors and substance P in the mouse spinal cord. *J Pharmacol Exp Ther*. 1989;248:1026-1033.
133. Vats A, Amit A, Cossar M, Bhatt P, Cozens A. Intrathecal baclofen trial using a temporary indwelling intrathecal catheter – a single institution experience. *J Clin Neurosci*. 2019;68:33-38.
134. Malanga G, Reiter R, Garay E. Update on tizanidine for muscle spasticity and emerging indications. *Expert Opin Pharmacother*. 2008;9(12):2209-2215.

CHAPTER

113 Opioid Therapy of Pain

Peggy Compton and Friedhelm Sandbrink

CHAPTER OUTLINE

- Introduction
- Historical perspectives on opioids
- Prevalence of pain
- Opioids in the treatment of pain
- Special issues in the use of opioids
- Clinical variables in the use of opioids
- Responsible opioid prescribing to mitigate risks
- Summary
- Acknowledgment

INTRODUCTION

Opioids are the most potent analgesic agents clinically available. They have wide efficacy and utility in the treatment of acute and cancer-related pain. While opioids may be helpful as one component within a multimodal pain management plan for chronic non–cancer-related pain in some patients, the risks of long-term opioid therapy are considerable and for many patients may outweigh the potential benefit. Opioid pain medication use can present serious risks, including respiratory depression and sedation, and patients with mental health disorders and a history of substance use disorder (SUD) are particularly vulnerable. This chapter addresses key conceptual, pharmacologic, and clinical issues related to opioids as a basis for weighing the potential benefits and risks of their use in the treatment of pain, and presents clinical strategies to optimize safety and effectiveness, including for persons with, or at risk for, SUDs. To provide context, we begin with brief discussion of the historical use of opioids, the prevalence of pain in our society, and contemporary views on the use of opioids in the treatment of pain.

HISTORICAL PERSPECTIVES ON OPIOIDS

Opioids have been used for medicinal purposes for millennia. One of the first records of the use of opioids comes in the Sumerian ideogram of *hul gil*, the "plant of joy," inscribed more than 5,000 years ago.[1] Theophrastus, the Greek philosopher and popularizer of science, provides the first written account of the use of opium to relieve pain in 300 BCE.[2] During this time, the Greek physicians Hippocrates and Galen used opium to treat headaches, coughing, asthma, and melancholy. In 1805, morphine was purified from opium, but use did not become widespread until the development of the hypodermic syringe by Alexander Wood in 1853, which allowed morphine to be introduced directly into the circulatory system[3]; it is reported that the first recorded case of an opioid overdose was that of Mrs. Alexander Wood via the delivery of morphine by this route. This led to the widespread use of morphine for the injuries and secondary pain syndromes such as causalgia suffered by hundreds of soldiers in the U.S. Civil War.[4] Heroin was introduced as an over-the-counter drug by the Bayer Company in 1895 and widely marketed as a panacea for numerous medical conditions.[5]

By the early 1900s, both appropriate therapeutic use and unhealthy use of opioids were widespread in the United States. The Institute of Medicine estimates that approximately 300,000 Americans were "opioid addicted" at that time: with a total population of a little over 75,000,000 in 1900, this would be about 1 in every 250 people.[6] The medical community came to recognize the problem of opium addiction, and in a 1900 article in the *Journal of the American Medical Association*, Dr. John Witherspoon, referring to opioids, exhorted physicians to "save our people from the clutches of this hydra-headed monster which stalks the civilized world, wrecking lives and happy homes, filling our jails and lunatic asylums…"[7]

Opioids were subsequently subjected to regulation and taxation through the Harrison Narcotics Tax Act in 1914, with legal use restricted to "legitimate medical purposes." In 1919, a federal ruling held that treatment of opioid addiction, now termed opioid use disorder (OUD), was "outside the realm of legitimate medical interest,"[8] creating a conundrum that allowed physicians to treat pain but not OUD that sometimes occurred in the context of medical use. Prescribing of opioids decreased and remained relatively low into the 1960s. An article on managing cancer pain in the *Journal of the American Medical Association* in 1941 reflects the low esteem in which opioids were held, "The use of narcotics in the terminal cancer patient is to be condemned … due to undesirable side effects … dominant in the list of these … is addiction."[9]

The hospice and palliative care movement blossomed in England in the mid-1960s under the leadership of Dame Cicely Saunders at St Christopher's hospice. With demonstration that opioid use could be safe, effective, and provide comfort at the end of life, the movement spread rapidly to the United States.[10] With observation of favorable outcomes in hospice patients, aggressive management of acute pain emerged. The 1970 Federal Controlled Substances Act classified controlled substances into risk categories and required registration of providers; this provided a structure that both supported and allowed control of use of opioids and other controlled substances. Cancer pain specialists noted favorable long-term results from opioid therapy of pain in cancer survivors without the inevitable evolution of tolerance or OUD. A one-paragraph letter by Porter and Jick to the editor of the *New England Journal of Medicine* in 1980 reported on low incidence of OUD in patients who received opioid pain medication during hospitalization, although no follow-up following discharge was attempted.[11] Portenoy and Foley published a case series in 1986 with favorable outcome in 24 of 38 carefully selected patients with chronic noncancer pain, opening a debate about use of opioids for wider variety of pain.[12] The publication of Melzack's classic paper, *The Tragedy of Needless Pain*, in 1990 signaled the beginning of two decades of more liberal opioid prescribing for pain in the U.S.[13]

The introduction of extended-release oxycodone in 1996 was associated with aggressive marketing for use in noncancer pain, with the argument that extended-release formulations would improve pain management by providing more stable blood levels and thus more consistent relief. Professional organizations and national initiatives began to promote more aggressive pain management including the use of opioid medications. In 1996, the president of the American Pain Society promoted the concept of pain as a vital sign in order to elevate awareness of pain treatment among healthcare professionals. The same year the American Academy of Pain Medicine and American Pain Society issued a consensus statement supporting long-term opioid therapy as an option for chronic noncancer pain, stating that the risk for de novo OUD was low, respiratory depression induced by opioids was short-lived and was antagonized by pain, and tolerance was not a prevalent limitation to long-term opioid use.[14] In 2000, the U.S. Veterans Health Administration (VHA) declared pain the "fifth vital sign,"[15] and in 2001, the Joint Commission on Accreditation of Hospital Organizations implemented assessment and management of pain as a quality measure[16]; subsequently, state rules pertaining to opioid prescribing were relaxed. Indicative of this growing consensus was a 2001 Joint Statement from 21 Health Organizations and the Drug Enforcement Administration (DEA). Among the 21 health organizations joining the DEA in the statement were such respected and mainstream organizations as the American Medical Association (AMA), American Cancer Association, and American Academy of Family Physicians. The consensus statement began by asserting the "fact" that "Undertreatment of pain is a serious problem in the United States, including pain among patients with chronic conditions" and that "pain should be aggressively treated."[17] This era of aggressive pain management resulted in increased utilization of opioid medications for patients with chronic non–cancer-related pain in combination with pressure on providers to document lowering of pain scores, while at the same time health insurance reimbursements for interdisciplinary pain management teams dwindled.

Prescribing of opioid medication increased steadily from the 1980s until 2012. In the early 2000s, the first reports of increases in prescription opioid overdoses emerged, and in 2005, Franklin and colleagues published data from the Washington State workers' compensation system on opioid overdose deaths of injured workers, noting an association with escalating dosages of high potency opioids including long-acting formulations.[18] By 2007, deaths from overdoses of prescription opioids exceeded the deaths from heroin and cocaine combined,[15] and by 2008, drug overdoses, mostly from prescribed opioids, surpassed auto fatalities as leading cause of accidental death in the United States.[19] The *New England Journal of Medicine* highlighted the epidemic of at-risk drug use and overdose deaths involving prescription opioid pain relievers in the 2010 article titled "A Flood of Opioids, a Rising Tide of Deaths."[20] After approval of a risk evaluation and mitigation strategies (REMS) program by the FDA for transmucosal immediate-release fentanyl products in 2011, the FDA implemented the extended-release/long-acting (ER/LA) opioids REMS program with voluntary training for prescribers in 2012,[21] and even consumer groups published warnings about the dangers of opioid use for pain.[22]

In 2016, the Centers for Disease Control and Prevention (CDC) published the highly influential *Guideline for Prescribing Opioids for Chronic Pain*,[23] which had a chilling effect on opioid prescribing, driving limits on the dose and duration of opioid prescriptions.[24] As a consequence, many clinicians implemented opioid tapers—sometimes even abrupt discontinuations—in patients with chronic pain, including many without evidence of harm or use disorder. Concerns that haphazard and/or guideline discordant opioid tapering in patients with chronic pain brings harm (including increasing suicidality),[25-27] were subsequently voiced by pain advocates and clinicians alike[28-31] resulting in the CDC issuing a revised statement in 2019 encouraging clinicians and policy makers to not "misapply" the 2016 guideline.[32] At that time, the FDA issued a drug safety communication warning against sudden discontinuation of opioid pain medicines and requiring label changes to guide prescribers on gradual, individualized tapering.[33] Subsequently published studies indeed documented risks related to discontinuation or tapering of long-term opioid therapy, including increased risk of illicit opioid use,[34] high incidence of emergency department visits and opioid-related hospitalizations,[35] increased incidence of mental health crises and overdose events,[26] and increased risk of death from suicide or overdose.[36]

In June 2020, the AMA recommended that the CDC make additional revisions to the 2016 guideline in order to attempt to ensure that patients with pain would not be denied appropriate opioid prescriptions.[37] In November 2022, the CDC published an update to their 2016 opioid guideline recommending that "clinicians should carefully weigh benefits and risks and exercise care when reducing or continuing opioid dosage" for patients already receiving higher opioid dosages, while noting, "Unless there are indications of a life-threatening issue, such as warning signs of impending overdose, eg, confusion, sedation, or slurred speech, opioid therapy should not be discontinued abruptly, and clinicians should not abruptly or rapidly reduce opioid dosages from higher dosages."[38]

Despite these successful efforts to decrease the use of prescription opioids, opioid-related deaths continue to escalate in the U.S., including dramatic increases in overdoses from heroin since 2010 and fentanyl and its derivatives since 2013.[39] These trends have only escalated during the COVID-19 pandemic. Provisional data from CDC's National Center for Health Statistics indicate an estimated 100,306 drug overdose deaths during 12-month period ending in April 2021, an increase of 28.5% from the 78,056 deaths during the same period the year before. The new data documents that the estimated overdose deaths from opioids specifically increased to 75,673 in the 12-month period ending in April 2021, up from 56,064 the year before.[40]

PREVALENCE OF PAIN

Pain is one of the most common ailments for which patients seek medical care. Acute pain following trauma or injury, including surgical intervention, is nearly ubiquitous and integral to the healing process. A large systematic review of pain following traumatic musculoskeletal injury found that a large proportion (28% to 93%) of patients experiencing traumatic musculoskeletal injury will develop persistent pain for a period of up to 84 months, although the severity of pain generally decreases over time.[41] Similarly, a significant number of patients develop chronic postsurgical pain (CPSP), which is often rated as severe, and includes treatment-resistant neuropathic components.[42,43] For example, rates of persistent pain are alarmingly high following total knee arthroplasty, with Petersen and colleagues reporting that between 44% to 53% patients develop CPSP, including 15% to 19% who rate their pain as severe.[44,45]

Chronic noncancer pain impacts the daily lives of fully one-quarter of Americans between the ages of 45 and 64, and 30.8% of persons 65 years of age and older, with the prevalence of high impact chronic pain being 7.4% in all adults in the U.S. Non-Hispanic White adults (23.6%) were more likely to have chronic pain compared with non-Hispanic Black (19.3%), Hispanic (13.0%), and non-Hispanic Asian (6.8%) adults.[46] According to a 2011 report of the Institute of Medicine, the costs of chronic pain is approximately 600 billion dollars a year when lost productivity and medical costs are combined, dwarfing the costs of other chronic illnesses. These numbers are expected to grow as the baby boom generation ages, obesity rates rise, and persons increasingly survive traumatic injuries and cancer.[47]

Pain also continues to be a common symptom in patients with cancer. A recent systematic review and meta-analysis of 117 studies including over 63,500 patients found pain prevalence rates to be 39.3% after curative treatment, 55.0% during cancer treatment, and 66.4% in advanced, metastatic, or terminal disease. Pain of moderate to severe severity was reported by 38.0% of all patients.[48] As increasing numbers of patients survive a cancer diagnosis, chronic pain among cancer survivors is an increasingly appreciated clinical problem.[49] A recent analysis of the 2016 to 2017 National Health Interview Survey suggested that 34.6% of cancer survivors reported having chronic pain and 16.1% reported having high intensity chronic pain, defined as chronic pain limiting life or work activities on most days or every day in the past 6 months.[50] Among patients with a cancer diagnosis, chronic pain was associated with greater odds of feeling depressed, feeling worried/nervous/anxious, being unable to work, and needing assistance with activities of daily living.[51]

The prevalence of chronic pain among persons with SUDs may be significantly higher than that of the general population, with studies suggesting chronic pain occurs in up to 50% to 60% of patients taking medications for OUD (methadone, buprenorphine), in which 25% to 35% of cases, the pain is rated as severe.[52,53] More severe chronic pain in patients with SUD is associated with more chronic illness, poorer psychosocial, physical and social functioning, and higher rates of mental illness (primarily major depression).[54-60] The presence of chronic pain portends poorer OUD treatment outcomes, such that patients with pain are more likely to engage in continued polydrug use, require higher doses of methadone, experience higher ratings of opioid craving, and are more likely to return to opioid use.[61-63] Persons with alcohol and other SUDs are vulnerable to traumatic injury,[64] which may contribute to a relatively higher prevalence of chronic pain in persons with SUDs.[65]

OPIOIDS IN THE TREATMENT OF PAIN

Opioids are the most potent analgesic agents available. For severe acute post-surgical or trauma-induced pain, opioid therapy is usually included in the pain treatment plan, which also includes nonopioid analgesics and non-pharmacological interventions as appropriate. Opioids are not recommended as first-line therapy in patients with mild-to-moderate acute pain, and the recommendation is always to keep the dosage as low as possible and the duration as short as possible and as needed for the severity of the pain condition.[23,66,67] Increasingly, multimodal analgesia, including regional analgesia, acetaminophen, nonsteroidal anti-inflammatory agents, gabapentinoids, tramadol, lidocaine, and/or the *N*-methyl-D-aspartate class of glutamate receptor antagonists have been shown to be effective adjuncts to opioid analgesia post-operatively, resulting in less opioid need and acceptable pain outcomes.[68-71]

Opioids remain standard in the treatment of advanced or progressive cancer-related pain, occupying steps two and three of the widely accepted "therapeutic ladder" developed by the World Health Organization,[72] although recent metanalyses suggest that their efficacy may be overstated[73] and multimodal pain treatment is being implemented more widely.[74,75] To ensure that patients with cancer have adequate access to opioids as needed while minimizing risks, opioid stewardship programs have been developed and put in place in many medical institutions including hospitals and specialized cancer care settings.[76-80] As cancer treatment has improved and cancer for many people has become a chronic illness with long-term survival, there is ongoing reevaluation of the role of opioids in treatment of long-term non-progressive cancer-related pain.[54]

It is estimated that between 5 and 8 million Americans use opioids daily for chronic pain management.[81] Recent guidelines suggest that the role of opioids in the treatment of chronic noncancer pain or pain not associated with a terminal illness is limited at best.[23,66] Based on systematic assessments that there is a lack of high-quality evidence to suggest long-term benefit in pain and function for patients with chronic noncancer pain treated with opioid therapy when compared to no opioids, and epidemiological evidence of possible harms associated with long-term opioid therapy (including overdose and motor vehicle injury), the 2022 CDC Clinical Practice Guideline for Prescribing Opioids for Pain[38]) express notable caution against long-term opioid therapy and recommended frequent reassessment of harm and benefit among those already prescribed. Similarly, the 2022 VA/DoD Clinical Practice Guideline for Opioid Therapy of Chronic Pain recommended against initiation of opioid therapy in patients with noncancer pain altogether and notes the particularly high risks of poor outcomes in younger patients, those with concurrent SUD, and in the presence of benzodiazepine co-prescribing.[66] As noted, concern has been expressed by both patient advocates and professional organizations that these guidelines have gone too far and risk compelling providers to withhold opioids from patients who would benefit from their use[32]; however, they have undoubtedly resulted in more thoughtful and informed opioid prescribing practices.

Essentially, the role of opioids in the treatment of chronic noncancer pain is limited less by the nature of the medications and more by the nature of the pain.[82] Chronic noncancer pain typically has multiple etiologic components that include pathophysiologic, psychosocial, and behavioral factors, and it impacts diverse biopsychosocial domains of experience. Over time, the originating pathophysiologic source of pain, which might have responded to opioid analgesia initially, contributes less to the pain experience, whereas affective and cognitive components predominate. Because of this, the most effective treatments of chronic pain demand a multimodal interdisciplinary biopsychosocial treatment approach that addresses maladaptive feelings and thoughts the patient holds about the pain.[83] Such approaches include cognitive-behavioral therapy, mindfulness-based therapy, and acceptance and commitment therapy,[84-86] which enable patients to achieve maximal levels of functionality despite the presence of ongoing pain.

SPECIAL ISSUES IN THE USE OF OPIOIDS

As do all medications, opioids have the potential for both benefit and harm. In addition to a range of physical side effects, opioids have specific pharmacologic effects, including physical dependence, tolerance, and hyperalgesia, which may complicate their use for pain treatment and require special care in management. Further, like other controlled substances, opioids deserve special consideration for their capacity to provide reward and to result in unhealthy use, diversion, and associated harms, including use disorder and overdose in certain at-risk individuals.

These issues may be of less significance in the treatment of acute and cancer pain than in the management of chronic non–cancer-related pain, given the often time-limited duration of use in these situations, but a thorough understanding of these issues improves decision-making in all three contexts. Each issue is considered separately below, whereas other side effects of opioids, including the critical issue of respiratory depression, are reviewed with clinical variables in the use of opioids.

Physical Dependence

Physical dependence may be defined as a physiologic adaptation to the continuous presence of a drug that produces symptoms of withdrawal when the drug effect significantly diminishes or stops.[87] Physical dependence occurs not only to drugs with reward potential, such as opioids and benzodiazepines, but also to those with little or no reward potential, such as alpha-2 adrenergic agonists (eg, clonidine) and tricyclic antidepressants. It results in a drug class-specific withdrawal syndrome that can be produced by abrupt cessation, rapid dose reduction, decreasing blood level of the drug, and/or administration of an antagonist. Such physical dependence is an expected occurrence in all patients after 2 to 10 days of regular administration of an opioid, and therefore is not diagnostic of an OUD. The character and intensity of the withdrawal syndrome vary, depending on the dose, half-life and duration of opioid administration and a variety of host factors, including previous experience with withdrawal, prior long-term administration of opioids, and the patient's expectations regarding withdrawal.[88]

Common symptoms of opioid withdrawal include autonomic signs and symptoms, such as diarrhea, piloerection, sweating, mydriasis, and mild increases in blood pressure and pulse, as well as signs of central nervous system (CNS) arousal such as irritability, anxiety, and sleeplessness. These negative emotional states and stress-like responses in withdrawal have been ascribed to diminished function of the dopamine reward system as well as activation of certain brain stress neurotransmitters, such as corticotropin-releasing factor and dynorphin.[89] Craving for the medication is expected in the course of withdrawal, and pain—most often experienced as abdominal cramping, deep bone pain, or diffuse muscle aching—is common.[90] Providing evidence for opioid withdrawal hyperalgesia, patients with chronic pain may experience an intensified level of their usual pain syndrome during opioid withdrawal.[91-93] In patients who are physically dependent on opioids, the use of short-acting opioids may result in intermittent withdrawal between doses, which may result in an increase in perceived pain.[94] Sympathetic arousal and muscular tension associated with withdrawal may also play a role in increased pain. Such rebound phenomena can theoretically be avoided by carefully scheduling doses to maintain constant blood levels, but stable blood levels are easier to achieve with longer-acting medications; however, there are concerns that around-the-clock administration of opioids contributes to the development of physical dependence and tolerance and thus may lead to dosage escalation over time and increased risk.

Exhibiting withdrawal symptoms is one of the diagnostic criteria for OUD, but, according to the DSM-5,[95] should not be considered for individuals taking opioids solely under appropriate medical supervision. Conflating OUD with physical dependence is both inaccurate and problematic as it raises misperceptions about both persons with OUD who are physically dependent on medications to treat OUD (methadone, buprenorphine) despite continuing in a state of recovery, and individuals without OUD who become physically dependent on opioid analgesic medications (given under medical supervision) without developing the defining characteristics of OUD.[96] Physical dependence, however, manifests itself with withdrawal symptoms of hyperalgesia (increased pain sensation) and anhedonia (inability to feel pleasure), which are powerful drivers of opioid-seeking, and opioid medication tapering may thus result in opioid craving, a symptom of OUD, thus the distinction between physical dependence and OUD clinically can be difficult to discern.[97]

Tolerance

Tolerance is indicated by the need for increasing doses of a medication to achieve the initial effects of the drug,[87,98] or less of an effect from the same dose over time. Tolerance may occur differentially—in terms of timing and extent—to a drug's analgesic effects and to such side effects as respiratory depression, sedation, or nausea. Tolerance can be innate due to inherent genetic characteristics of the individual (in response the particular opioid), or it can be acquired in response to ongoing exposure to the opioid. Acquired tolerance may be due to both pharmacokinetic factors, such as changes in drug absorption and metabolism that reduce blood concentration, and to pharmacodynamic factors such as receptor desensitization or other density changes at the level of opioid receptors.[99,100] Changes in central immune signaling and in *N*-methyl-D-aspartate (NMDA) receptor activity are involved in the evolution of opioid tolerance.[101,102] Behavioral opioid tolerance evident in mood and affect has been attributed to opponent adaptive processes in the **mesocorticolimbic reward circuitry**.[103] The patterns of occurrence of tolerance in clinical settings have not been well described, and animal studies suggest that tolerance to the analgesic effects of medications can occur in some contexts but not in others.[99] Human studies of the management of acute pain document the development of progressive tolerance to the analgesic effects of opioids when they are administered on a continuous basis over a period of several days.[104] Over a period of weeks to months, however, some studies suggest that the continuing development of progressive tolerance to the analgesic effects of opioids may not regularly occur,[98] though other studies suggest progressive gradual tolerance does occur in chronic pain in many, if not most patients.[105]

While absolute tolerance to the analgesic effects of opioids does not appear to be a critical limiting factor to the treatment of acute pain or cancer-related pain in most patients, in the context of chronic pain not associated with life-threatening illness, there is increasing evidence of diminishing benefit and potential harm associated with high-dose opioid use, and thus progressive tolerance may be a prohibitive factor in long-term use of opioids in this context. It is conceivable that around-the-clock dosing of short-acting (immediate release) or long-acting opioids used regularly may increase the likelihood or degree of tolerance, as such prescribing results in greater dosage increases over time. As with physical dependence, tolerance may occur in any individual who uses an opioid over time and is not alone diagnostic of OUD. Exhibiting tolerance is one of the diagnostic criteria for OUD, according to the DSM-5, but should not be considered for individuals taking opioids solely under appropriate medical supervision.[95]

Hyperalgesia

Hyperalgesia is a physiologic state in which there is sensitization to nociceptive stimuli resulting in lowered pain threshold and/or decreased tolerance to pain. We understand now that there are many factors that may result in hyperalgesia and sensitization, including the long-term presence of pain itself, and physiological and psychological stressors such as sleep deprivation,[106] possibly mediated by aberrant glial activation.[107] Certain pain disorders are understood as central sensitization syndromes with hyperalgesia as a typical feature of these conditions (eg, fibromyalgia),[108] and opioid therapy is generally not recommended in their management.[109]

Opioid use may worsen pain in some contexts, a phenomenon termed opioid-induced hyperalgesia (OIH). Observational studies have long indicated that some individuals with chronic pain who use opioids on a long-term basis experience improvement in pain after tapering or simple withdrawal of opioids, without the institution of other major pain interventions.[110-114] These studies include observations of patients with pain and OUD in both pain treatment and addiction treatment settings. Though higher levels of pain on opioids in some of these studies may have been mediated by intermittent withdrawal-induced hyperalgesia associated with short-acting opioids, it is increasingly appreciated that opioids may result in hyperalgesia as well.

OIH has been demonstrated in both animals and human models.[115-120] The mechanisms of hyperalgesia are not fully defined but appear to involve both glutamate-mediated activation of NMDA receptors and induction of inflammatory cytokines in the CNS.[121-123] Similar systems appear to be involved in the development of OIH and opioid tolerance, however, the clinical and neurophysiologic relationships between opioid tolerance and OIH continue to be elucidated.[124-127] The extent to which hyperalgesia occurs in clinical settings and its relevance for patients who use opioids on a long-term basis is not known and may vary between individuals. There is evidence that opioids administered in the intraoperative period induce post-operative hyperalgesia, apparent in significantly higher pain scores at rest and more postoperative opioid use and being most pronounced early in the first 24 hours following surgery.[128-131] Upon pain testing, patients with high intraoperative opioid use (most commonly fentanyl or remifentanil) demonstrate significantly decreased pain thresholds and larger margins of wound hyperalgesia. These findings have spurred current interest in evaluating opioid-sparing peri- and intraoperative procedures, such as preoperative administration of gabapentinoids, co-administration of nonopioid analgesics including NSAIDs and acetaminophen, ketamine, magnesium, propofol, nitrous oxide, and clonidine to minimize post-operative OIH.[132,133]

While hyperalgesia does not present a clinical issue in many patients with chronic pain maintained on opioids for months to years, two small prospective studies show increased sensitivity to thermal pain following one month of opioid therapy.[134,135] In another sample of patients with chronic pain, Kim and colleagues showed that pain sensitivity to a standardized lidocaine injection increased with daily dose of opioid.[136] Acknowledging that hyperalgesia commonly accompanies chronic pain, it is unclear the degree to which pain-generated hyperalgesia contributes to OIH noted in this population; however, Hay and colleagues found similar degrees of hyperalgesia in opioid-maintained samples with and without pain.[137] Several structured evidence-based reviews conclude that there is insufficient evidence to determine whether clinically significant OIH occurs in the context of long-term opioid use in clinical settings.[138,139] A 2017 systematic review of patient outcomes in voluntary dose reduction or discontinuation of long-term opioid therapy suggests that pain, function, and quality of life may improve with opioid dose reduction.[140]

The Reward Cycle

Commonly used opioid analgesics act primarily on mu opioid receptors. Mu opioid agonists produce pleasant feelings ranging from contentedness to euphoria in many, though not all, individuals.[142] Some persons, in fact, experience dysphoria or no mood changes in association with opioid use. These pleasant feelings are said to be "rewarding" in that they motivate persons to repeat opioid administration to reproduce these pleasant sensations aka the reward cycle. Kappa opioid agonists (such as butorphanol, pentazocine, or nalbuphine) can also produce euphoria, though do so less commonly than mu opioid agonists, and are more often associated with dysphoria.[143] The potential for opioids to further activate and potentiate the reward system when used for pain is a critical factor to consider in all patients, and especially when treating persons at risk for unhealthy substance use or with co-occurring SUDs. A clear understanding of the potential issues that modulate the reward experiences when opioids are used for analgesia are helpful to optimize clinical management strategies, particularly in persons at risk for unhealthy use or use disorders.

Mechanisms of Reward

Human brain reward systems are complex and discussed in more detail in Chapter 1, "Drug Addiction: The Neurobiology of Motivation Gone Awry" of this textbook. One critical step through which opioids produce reward is by binding to GABAergic interneurons that inhibit dopamine production in the limbic reward system, resulting in increased dopaminergic activity and a cascade of secondary effects producing feelings of reward or euphoria. In some contexts, particularly terminal illness, euphoria may in fact be a valued side effect. However, when euphoria becomes the primary motivation for the use of opioids, it may undermine pain treatment and become problematic,[144] particularly if it leads to compulsive use despite harm, a hallmark of OUD. Understanding the factors that affect the rewarding properties of opioids provide guidance in clinical pain treatment settings.

Factors Affecting Reward

Rate of Increase (T_{max})

Both animal drug self-administration studies and human drug-liking studies have demonstrated that reward is greater when the rate of rise in drug blood levels increases: the faster the onset, the more intense the high.[145,146] The intravenous (IV) route of administration causes a more rapid rise in blood levels and therefore provides more euphoria than the oral route for a given drug at a given dose, with intramuscular and subcutaneous administration providing intermediate effects (**Fig. 113-1**). Among opioids given orally, those with an inherently slower time to peak effect (such as methadone or levorphanol) are expected to produce weaker reward effects than opioids with relatively rapid onset, such as immediate-release oxycodone, hydrocodone, or hydromorphone. Similarly, rapid-onset transmucosal formulations of fentanyl are expected to have higher reward than fentanyl administered

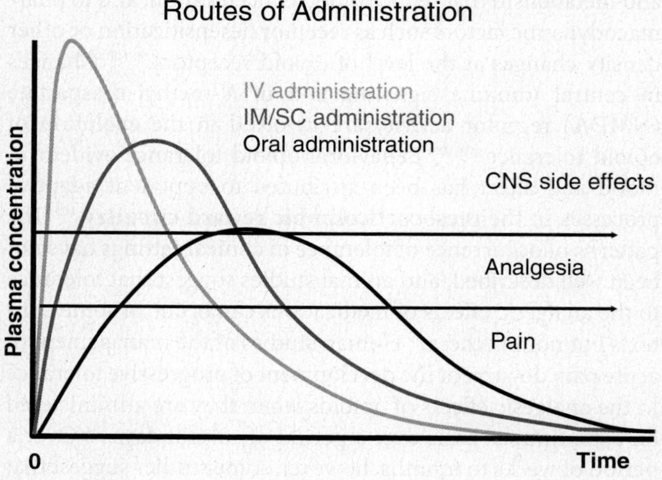

Figure 113-1. Routes of administration. IV, intravenous; IM/SC, intramuscular/subcutaneous; CNS, central nervous system.

transdermally, and the transmucosal immediate release fentanyl risk evaluation and mitigation strategy[147] is an FDA-required program when prescribing the transmucosal formulations. Based on the increased reward associated with rapid onset of opioids, it is not surprising that many persons who use opioids for euphoric effects alter the delivery system by crushing tablets and snorting or injecting the contents to increase reward.

Peak Blood Levels Attained (C_{max})

The higher the opioid blood level relative to the individual's tolerance for the drug, the greater the reward, thus reward is dose dependent. An opioid-naive individual with little or no tolerance may experience euphoria with a drug blood level that would cause no significant reward effect in a more tolerant individual. As described above, a dose of an opioid given intravenously achieves a higher peak blood level than the same dose administered by the oral route, with subcutaneous and intramuscular again providing intermediate reward (see **Fig. 113-1**).

Changes in Blood Levels

As the rise in blood levels of a drug is associated with onset of euphoria, stable levels generally produce less euphoria than intermittently rising and falling levels. This key principle underlies the effectiveness of methadone maintenance therapy for OUD. Extrapolating to pain treatment, continuous IV infusion of an opioid is expected to trigger less reward than intermittent boluses and controlled-release opioids (used by the intended route at the intended time interval), or intrinsically long-acting opioids (such as methadone or levorphanol) would be less rewarding than frequently dosed short-acting medications (**Fig. 113-2**). Of note, patient-controlled analgesia (PCA) is not expected to provide significant reward because the incremental doses are very small and spaced at intervals that do not permit a rapid, high rise in blood levels.

Interference of Reward with Pain

Early research in both human and animal models suggested that opioids were less rewarding in the presence of pain,[148-150] although pain relief itself is inherently rewarding, both in its amelioration of suffering as well as its potential to enable rewarding activities in life to resume. This hypothesis is supported by reports from patients who say that opioids relieve their pain without providing psychoactive effects, and also report appreciation of their ability to function when they receive pain relief from effective treatment of all kinds, including nonopioids. As well, many patients experience dysphoria or other uncomfortable symptoms (eg, sedation, constipation, nausea) rather than euphoria, when given opioids for their pain and often stop them for this reason alone[151-153] or in combination with an improvement in their pain condition.

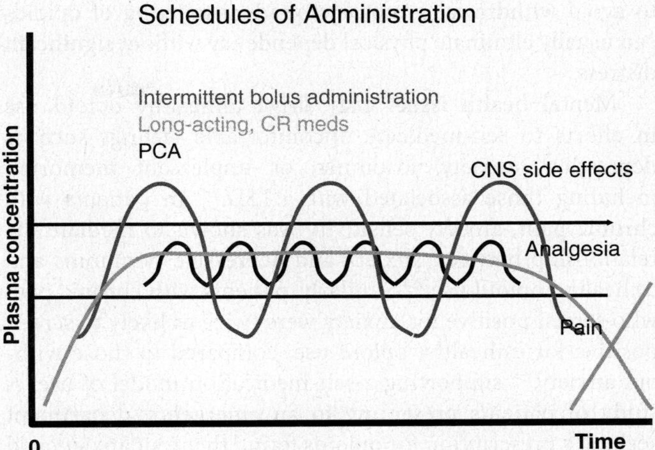

Figure 113-2. Schedules of administration. CR, controlled release; PCA, patient-controlled analgesia; CNS, central nervous system.

Nevertheless, based on our current understanding that up to 10% of patients treated with long-term opioids meet diagnostic criteria for OUD, the presence of pain cannot be considered a sufficiently protective factor against reward to occur, particularly in those at risk.[23,154,155]

Unhealthy Opioid Use

In the context of pain management, unhealthy opioid use is defined as any use that increases the risk or likelihood for health consequences (hazardous use) or has already led to health consequences (harmful use).[156] Patients use opioids for a variety of unhealthy reasons with a wide range of implications (**Table 113-1**). It is important to distinguish clinically between different causes of unhealthy opioid use in order to address each case appropriately.

A common cause of unhealthy use is simply misunderstanding how opioids are supposed to be used; clear written instructions, with engagement of support systems for those with cognitive challenges, can reduce this type of use. Patients who have become physically dependent on opioids may continue to use the drugs after the pain has resolved in order

TABLE 113-1 Differential Diagnosis of Unhealthy Use of Analgesic Opioids

- Misunderstanding of dosing instructions
- Self-medication of:
  - Mood/stress
  - Insomnia
  - Disturbing memories
  - Anxiety
  - Undertreated pain
- Compulsive use due to the presence of an opioid use disorder
- Diversion for profit

to avoid withdrawal symptoms; gradual tapering of opioids can usually eliminate physical dependency without significant distress.

Mental health issues may drive unhealthy opioid use in efforts to self-medicate uncomfortable feelings such as depression, anxiety, insomnia, or unpleasant memories, including those associated with PTSD.[157] In patients with chronic pain, anxiety sensitivity was shown to mediate the relationship between anxiety and depressive symptoms and unhealthy opioid use.[158] Similarly, patients with chronic pain who screen positive for anxiety were twice as likely to screen positive for unhealthy opioid use, compared to those without anxiety,[159] supporting a self-medication model of use. A study of patients presenting to an emergency department seeking a prescription for opioids found that trait anxiety and panic disorder correlated with a positive screen for risk of unhealthy opioid use.[160] These patients usually benefit from more directed treatment of co-occurring psychiatric or other problems.

It has been posited that some patients exhibit distress, use opioid medication more frequently than prescribed and/or engage in behaviors aimed at obtaining more medication because they are experiencing unrelieved pain. The term *pseudoaddiction* has been used to indicate that undertreatment of pain is the main reason for drug-seeking behavior in these patients, rather than the presence of an OUD.[161] It has been suggested that pseudoaddictive behavior could be distinguished from addiction by the fact that, when adequate analgesia is achieved such as by increasing the dosage or frequency of opioid treatment, the patient's drug seeking behavior would resolve. Empirical evidence, however, to support pseudoaddiction as a clinical diagnosis distinct from a use disorder is lacking; the clinical construct is now considered questionable and may have contributed to dosage escalations in patients vulnerable to or with OUD and thus is considered to have contributed to the opioid crisis in the U.S.[162,163]

A previous history of SUD is clearly a major risk factor for unhealthy use of prescription opioids. Longitudinal administrative data on 15,160 veterans showed that a history of SUD was a strong predictor of unhealthy opioid use, and co-occurring mental health disorder was a moderately strong predictor of recognized DSM-IV–defined prescription opioid abuse and dependence.[164] A more controlled study of 127 veterans prescribed opioids in a primary care setting found that patients with a history of an SUD were three to six times more likely to use opioid medications in an unhealthy manner than patients without a history of an SUD.[165] In a large pain clinic, younger age, history of unhealthy alcohol use or current cannabis or cocaine use, and history of legal problems with alcohol or drugs increased the risk of unhealthy prescribed opioid use,[166] while in another primary care VHA sample, individuals with evidence of cocaine use were much less likely to resolve unhealthy opioid use in a structured prescribing program than other patients.[167] Medication craving,[168,169] and current tobacco use have been identified as predictors of unhealthy prescribed opioid use,[170] suggesting that underlying vulnerability in the limbic reward system may drive this use.

Several screening tools exist to predict the risk of a patient with pain engaging in unhealthy medication use behaviors, sometimes referred to as aberrant use behaviors, however recent meta-analyses found insufficient evidence for their effectiveness in reducing unhealthy medication use or the development of SUD.[171,172] For example, the Opioid Risk Tool (ORT), a five-question screen that is based on the patient's personal and family history, has shown reasonable ability to discriminate between patients at high and low risk of aberrant opioid use behaviors,[173] and the Screener and Opioid Assessment for Patients in Pain—Revised (SOAPP-R), a 24-item self-report screen reports good predictive ability.[174] Validity data have also been reported for a more recent screener, the Brief Risk Interview (BRI), which is composed of 12 items and designed to be administered by a clinician.[175] However, studies comparing the predictive accuracy for unhealthy medication use of the ORT, the SOAPP-R, and the BRI found highly variable and inconsistent rates of sensitivity and specificity; similarly, likelihood ratios for both the ORT and SOAPP-R were evaluated as essentially noninformative.[176,177] The VHA has mandated risk assessment by providers when initiating new opioid therapy and data-based risk reviews for patients exposed to opioid therapy and considered very high risk by a predictive analytic tool, the Stratification Tool for Opioid Risk Mitigation (STORM) that provides estimates for death from opioid overdose or suicide.[178]

It is important to be aware that none of these tools have been specifically validated for use in populations with identified SUDs. Though not a screen for risk of unhealthy use per se, the Addiction Behaviors Checklist (ABC)[179] and the Prescription Drug Use Questionnaire (PDUQ)[180] can be used to track behaviors of concern between clinic visits. Another promising tool to detect unhealthy opioid use is the Current Opioid Misuse Measure, which has demonstrated 77% specificity and 77% sensitivity in identifying current prescription unhealthy opioid use in a primary care setting.[181] Due to the limitations associated with the predictive and concurrent validity associated with these screeners, composite indices have also been described combining scores from tools with urine toxicology results. For example, Wasan and colleagues created the Aberrant Drug Behavior Index and the Drug Misuse Index which combine PDUQ or ABC scores with urine toxicology to predict relative risk of unhealthy opioid use.[182] Common across these tools is the presence of a family history of a SUD, the presence of a personal history of a SUD, and the presence of co-occurring psychiatric disorder as putting the patient at risk for unhealthy medication use behaviors.

Substance and Opioid Use Disorders

In the context of pain treatment with opioids, SUD must be diagnosed through the observation of a constellation of maladaptive behaviors rather than by the neurophysiologic phenomena of physical dependence and tolerance. SUD in the context of opioid therapy for pain has been characterized by the presence of a combination of observations suggesting *adverse consequences* due to use of the drugs, *loss of control* over drug use, and *preoccupation* with obtaining opioids despite the presence of adequate analgesia. As noted, physical dependence on opioids and the development of tolerance to their effects do not, of themselves, constitute a use disorder.[96] Physical dependence, however, manifests itself with withdrawal symptoms of hyperalgesia (increased sensitivity to pain) and anhedonia (inability to feel pleasure) that are powerful drivers of opioid seeking, thus opioid medication taper or withdrawal may result in opioid craving which appears symptomatic of OUD.[97]

Adverse consequences that are suggestive of a use disorder include persistent sedation or euphoria, deteriorating function despite relief of pain, or increase in distresses such as anxiety, sleep disturbance, or depressive symptoms. *Loss of control* over use might be reflected in exhausting prescriptions before the expected renewal date, obtaining prescriptions from multiple sources, or obtaining opioids from illicit sources. *Preoccupation* with opioid use may be reflected in noncompliance with nonopioid components of the pain treatment plan, inability to recognize non-nociceptive components of pain, and the perception that no interventions other than opioids have any effect on pain. It is important to recognize that such behaviors may occur on an occasional basis for a variety of reasons in the context of successful opioid therapy for pain. By contrast, a pattern of persistent occurrences and decline in function should prompt concern and further assessment (**Table 113-2**). The adverse consequences, loss of control and preoccupation characteristic of SUD are captured in the diagnostic criteria for SUD in the DSM-5.[183]

As reviewed, early twentieth century studies led to a perception that the iatrogenic creation of SUDs through medical use of opioids was a very frequent occurrence.[184,185] In contrast, a number of retrospective surveys in the 1980s of never-addicted medical patients suggested that the risk of development of the same in the course of long-term opioid therapy for pain was very low,[12,186] leading to an underappreciation of the risks. Recent guidelines regarding long-term opioid therapy for chronic pain are based on the understanding that any exposure to opioid medication for pain in at-risk individuals can result in the development of OUD.[96,187]

Studies of the incidence of addiction in the context of pain treatment have generally examined a wide variety of unhealthy use or aberrant behaviors rather than specifically assessing for use disorders, and have been variable in methodology, operative definitions, and quality. In addition, many studies that assess opioid use in pain populations excluded high-risk groups (eg, those with a prior history of SUD). Current best estimates for carefully diagnosed OUD in patients taking opioids for chronic pain range from 8% to 12%,[155] which is only somewhat higher than the prevalence of SUDs in the U.S. population in general (6.6%),[188] suggesting that those same factors that put an individual at risk for developing SUD (family history, co-occurring psychiatric disorders, early onset of use) are also involved in the development of the same in persons with chronic pain and on opioid therapy.[172,189,190]

When SUD is identified in the course of opioid therapy for pain, it is important to address it swiftly and comprehensively, so that the pain is effectively controlled and to prevent the debilitating sequelae of SUDs. With an active, untreated OUD, patients will, by definition, be unable to control their opioid use and achieve the desired functional outcomes of effective pain management. Institution of appropriate addiction treatment services, tightening the structure of opioid treatment to maintain safety, and involving the patient's social support system in supporting treatment and recovery are important first steps. As such patients cannot be expected to control their opioid use and adhere to prescribed limits, continuation of opioid therapy for pain is associated with high risks including overdose, and they should be treated according to guidelines for OUD care including transition to evidence-based medication therapy for OUD that may include a low or very low dose protocol for buprenorphine or overlap approach to allow gradual transition from the opioid therapy for pain to buprenorphine therapy for OUD.[191] Some patients may be tapered off the opioid therapy for pain successfully, especially if OUD is mild by diagnostic criteria, but the extent to which this is possible is unpredictable for a given patient. Patients with moderate to

TABLE 113-2 Definition and Indicators of Substance Use Disorder in Pain Patients

Substance use disorder
American Society of Addiction Medicine (ASAM), American Pain Society (APS), American Academy of Pain Medicine (AAPM)
A primary, chronic, neurobiologic disease with genetic, psychosocial, and environmental factors influencing its development and manifestations characterized by behaviors that include one or more of the following:

ASAM-APS-AAPM behavioral criteria	Examples of specific behaviors in opioid therapy for pain
Impaired control over use, compulsive use	Frequent loss/theft reported, calls for early renewals, withdrawal noted at appointments
Continued use despite harm due to use	Declining function, intoxication, persistent over sedation
Preoccupation with use, craving	Nonopioid interventions ignored, opioids only intervention considered, recurrent requests for opioid increase/complaints increasing pain in absence of disease progression despite titration[a]

[a]May reflect tolerance or hyperalgesia.

severe OUD to prescription opioid therapy should be treated similar to patients with OUD to other opioids, but with modifications such as dosing buprenorphine at least 3 to 4 times per day to provide better analgesia.

CLINICAL VARIABLES IN THE USE OF OPIOIDS

Opioids are often the mainstay of treatment of moderate to severe acute pain and pain associated with progressive or terminal illnesses. As noted, when used in the treatment of chronic, noncancer pain, they should only be used as one component of multimodal and multidisciplinary pain, and at the lowest dosage and for the shortest duration to achieve the pain treatment goals.[23,66] Goals of pain treatment generally include reduction in pain, enhanced level of function, and improved quality of life. There is increasing evidence that long-term opioid therapy is likely more harmful than beneficial to achieve these goals and the VA/DoD Clinical Practice Guideline for Opioid Therapy of Chronic Pain recommends against initiation of long-term opioid therapy.[66]

A number of variables must be considered when considering opioid therapy for pain. In addition to consideration of the special issues addressed above, important variables include drug selection, dose titration and scheduling, and potential side effects. It also is critically important to understand how to appropriately change opioid formulations or withdraw opioids when indicated. Finally, there are clinical practices that are consistent with responsible prescribing of these medications; in that opioids that have inherent risks associated with their use, and the prescriber is responsible to engage in directed clinical practices to mitigate these risks.

Drug Selection

Opioids produce their analgesia and side effects primarily through activation of mu, kappa, and delta opioid receptors.[192] Most of the commonly used opioid analgesics have predominantly mu receptor agonist activity, however, some analgesic opioids have agonist-antagonist or partial mu agonist activity. Each of these opioid classes is considered here.

Mu opioid agonists are the most commonly prescribed class of opioid analgesics and include morphine, oxycodone, hydromorphone, oxymorphone, methadone, hydrocodone, and fentanyl (**Table 113-3**). Full mu agonists usually have no ceiling analgesic effect and may be titrated as needed to achieve analgesia, limited only by side and adverse effects. Higher dosages are associated with increased risk for overdose and development of OUD, with guidelines recommending against dosage increases to high dosage therapy. Tolerance to some side effects (eg, respiratory depression) generally occurs more rapidly than tolerance to analgesia but is usually incomplete and in particular monitoring for respiratory depression and sedation is always important, and especially in opioid-naive individuals, as doses are increased, or as specific opioids formulations are changed.

Though most mu agonists are interchangeable if attention is paid to relative potencies and onset and duration of action, individuals may respond differently to different opioids in terms of both analgesia and side effects. This may in part be due to variability in mu opioid receptor expression in different individuals as well as to variable opioid receptor specificity of the different drugs.[193] Some mu receptor polymorphisms may require higher agonist dosing to achieve maximal analgesic efficacy.[194] Additionally, known individual differences have been demonstrated in opioid metabolic pathways due to variations in cytochrome 450 enzyme expressions.[195] Recognition of variability in both opioid receptor expression and opioid metabolism can explain observed differences in patient responses to different opioids and holds promise for the use of pharmacogenetic testing in matching individuals with opioids that may be most effective for them with fewest side effects.[196-198]

Methadone differs from other mu agonists in several ways, and while it may have potentially advantageous properties compared to other opioids used for pain management, it is also associated with increased risk of overdose and mortality, in part due to its cardiac side effects, the complex pharmacokinetic and pharmacodynamic properties including its variable half-life and multiple drug interactions, which together make it more difficult to use safely than other opioids.[199,200] Thus, methadone should only be initially prescribed or increased in dosage by providers experienced with its use.[66] Methadone has a long and unpredictable elimination half-life (usually 15-60 hours, rarely as high as 120 hours) that necessitates prescribing at low dosage and especially careful titration in steps sufficiently long (>5-7 days) to allow for steady state to be achieved. The analgesic duration of methadone is much shorter than its long serum half-life, and thus for pain treatment, methadone is usually prescribed at least BID to TID.[200] Its dextro-isomer has NMDA receptor antagonist activity, and it has been suggested that this may result in greater efficacy in treating neuropathic pain, though this has not been demonstrated clearly in clinical trials.[201] Methadone is metabolized by the cytochrome 450 system, and its blood levels may be critically affected by other drugs that induce or inhibit this system.[202] Further, the potency ratio of methadone to morphine is strongly dose dependent and ranges from 2:1 for low dose methadone therapy to 16 to even 20:1 in higher dose ranges.[200] The incomplete cross-tolerance between methadone and other mu opioid agonists requires the use of a much lower than calculated equianalgesic dose of methadone in the patient who is transitioning from other mu agonists. Current guidelines recommend a starting dosage of 2.5 BID to TID for opioid naive patients with chronic non-cancer pain,[66,200] and up to 5 mg BID to TID when faster titration is desired.[66] Conversely, patients who are changed from methadone to other opioids may experience poor analgesia for reasons that are not fully understood.[203] Methadone is known to cause significant QTc prolongation in some patients and has been associated with *torsades de pointes* syndrome. EKG testing prior to starting methadone and during the course of titration is recommended for all patients,

TABLE 113-3 Opioids Commonly Prescribed for Pain With Key Characteristics

Opioid	Example brands/preparations	Special pain issues	Special issues associated with unhealthy use
Mu agonists			
Morphine	Morphine IR, MS Contin (12-hour controlled release [CR]), Kadian, Avinza (24-hour CR), Oramorph (intermediate release [IR])	CR mechanism provides relatively stable blood levels	Abuse-deterrent CR formulation available
Oxycodone	Percocet (IR and acetaminophen), Percodan (IR and aspirin), OxyContin (12 CR) generic CRs	CR mechanism provides relatively stable blood levels	Abuse-deterrent CR formulations available
Oxymorphone	Opana IR and CR, Numorphan	CR mechanism provides relatively stable blood levels	Abuse-deterrent CR formulations available
Hydrocodone	Vicodin (IR and acetaminophen), Lortab (IR and acetaminophen)	Most commonly prescribed opioid	Most common opioid used in an unhealthy manner
Hydromorphone	Dilaudid (IR), Exalgo (CR)		Quick onset, relatively high reward value Abuse-deterrent CR formulation available
Fentanyl	Duragesic (72-hour CR patch), Transmuscosal immediate release fentanyl (TIRF): Abstral sublingual tablet, Actiq (fentanyl citrate) oral transmucosal lozenge, Fentora (fentanyl citrate) buccal tablet, Lazanda (fentanyl) nasal spray, and Onsolis (fentanyl) buccal soluble film	Patch provides very stable blood levels when used as prescribed Transmucosal immediate release fentanyl (TIRF) products are subject to FDA-mandated REMS program	Unhealthy use less common with patch but dangerous when used in an unhealthy manner due to concentrated dosing
Methadone	Methadose, Dolophine	Second analgesic mechanism: *N*-methyl-D-aspartate (NMDA) receptor antagonist. Possibly less tolerance and greater efficacy in neuropathic pain indications	Pharmacologic properties make unhealthy use particularly risky; used to treat opioid addiction
Tapentadol	Nucynta	Second analgesic mechanism: reduces reuptake of norepinephrine. Possible greater efficacy in neuropathic pain	Abuse-deterrent CR formulation available
Codeine	Tylenol #3 (IR with acetaminophen)	Prodrug with ceiling effect	
Partial mu agonists			
Tramadol	Ultram (IR), Ultracet (IR with acetaminophen)	Second analgesic mechanism (increase serotonin/norepinephrine); limited dose due to seizures	Relatively low rates of unhealthy use and reward documented, though does occur in some persons
Buprenorphine	Approved for pain: Butrans (transdermal system) 7-day patch Belbuca (buccal film) Approved for opioid use disorder: Subutex (sublingual tab)Suboxone (plus naloxone, sublingual film) Zubsolv (plus naloxone, sublingual tab) Bunavail (plus naloxone, buccal film) Sublocade (extended-release injection) Probuphine (implant)	Partial agonist; ceiling effect; may cause precipitated withdrawal in patients already on opioids Formulations approved for pain are relatively lower doses, may be used at lowest dosage in opioid-naive patients Formulations for treatment of opioid use disorder may be used off-label for pain Dosing is usually 3-4 times per day for buccal/sublingual forms when used for pain	Considered safer than high potency full mu agonists regarding respiratory depression and overdose deaths; some unhealthy use reported; may be used illicitly for prevention of withdrawal Useful agents in patients with pain and co-occurring opioid use disorder
Kappa opioids		**Mu antagonist actions**	
Butorphanol	Stadol (intravenous [IV] or intranasal)	Rapid onset of intranasal, ceiling analgesic effects	Less reward in some but intranasal route is quick onset
Nalbuphine	Nubain (IV only)	Ceiling analgesic effects	Less reward in some than mu agonist medications
Pentazocine	Talwin, Talwin NX (with naltrexone; oral only)	Ceiling analgesic effects	Less reward in some but formulated with naltrexone due to unhealthy intravenous use in 1960s

Adapted from Savage SR, Passik S, Kirsch K. Challenges in using opioids to treat pain in persons with substance use disorders. *Addict Sci Clin Pract.* 2008;4(2):4-25.

with follow up EKG within 2 to 4 weeks after initiation in for patients with risk factors for dysrhythmias. Methadone should not be started with QTc above 450 ms, and, for those already on treatment, discontinuation should be considered at QTc between 450 and 500 ms, and strongly recommended above 500 ms.[200] EKG monitoring becomes particularly important when methadone is combined with other drugs that prolong QT intervals.

Agonist-antagonist—or kappa agonist—opioids, including pentazocine, nalbuphine, and butorphanol, have predominantly kappa agonist effects while antagonizing the mu receptor. These drugs have been widely regarded as having less potential for unhealthy use than the pure full mu agonists, though the development of use disorders to these medications have been observed. The actions of kappa agonists are complex and may include analgesia as well as antagonism of the effects of rewarding drugs, which has made their study a focus for addiction treatment and analgesic drug development.[204-206] Their clinical usefulness as analgesics is limited by a number of factors. They exhibit a ceiling effect in terms of analgesia and cannot be titrated for severe pain. Their use sometimes is associated with dysphoric reactions. Because of their mu antagonist activity, they may reverse analgesia and precipitate withdrawal in individuals who are physically dependent on mu agonists. Consequently, no clear advantages of agonist–antagonist drugs have been demonstrated in the treatment of pain, though they may be a reasonable choice in some patients. There is some evidence that kappa agonists may have greater analgesic efficacy in women.[207]

Partial mu agonists, including buprenorphine, provide analgesia via mu opioid receptors but have lower intrinsic activity than full mu agonists. Buprenorphine is a partial agonist of the mu opioid receptor with complex pharmacology that also includes action on the delta and kappa receptors.[208] It is available in parenteral, sublingual, buccal and transdermal preparations, and more recently a depot formulation. It has a long half-life and high receptor affinity and is effective in treatment of OUD.[209] In the United States, sublingual or transmucosal buprenorphine is FDA-approved for treatment of OUD by physicians, physician assistants, and nurse practitioners with waivers from the Substance Abuse and Mental Health Services Administration (SAMHSA) to provide this treatment.[210] Buprenorphine is also available in the U.S. in transdermal and buccal forms with indications for the treatment of moderate-to-severe pain.[211,212] In addition, a transmucosal/buccal form (Belbuca®) has been approved by the FDA for severe pain. This is lower dosed, however, than the transmucosal/sublingual forms approved for OUD. The latter may also be used off label for moderate-to-severe pain, usually at 6- to 8-hour intervals.[213] Buprenorphine has traditionally been thought to have a ceiling effect as an analgesic and, therefore, not able to provide continuously increasing analgesia beyond a certain dose titration; however, this belief has been challenged.[211] The 2022 VA DoD Clinical Practice Guideline for Opioid Therapy suggests the use of buprenorphine instead of full agonist opioids for patients receiving daily opioids for the treatment of chronic pain due to lower risk of overdose and unhealthy use, with overall similar efficacy for analgesia.[66] While buprenorphine's unhealthy use potential has been thought to be relatively low, it appears to have diversion potential as a means to prevent withdrawal in persons who are physically dependent on illicit opioids.[214-216]

Tramadol and tapentadol are dual-mechanism opioids that combine action on the mu opioid receptor with a second analgesic mechanism mediated by their inhibitory action on serotonin and norepinephrine reuptake. Tramadol, which generally is used in oral form, is a partial mu agonist and has a second mechanism of analgesia through its function as serotonin and norepinephrine reuptake inhibitor (SNRI). Doses are limited by a significant potential for seizures at levels above 400 mg per day, which thus is its effective analgesic ceiling. It appears to have less unhealthy use potential than pure mu opioid analgesics, although as with buprenorphine, there have been reports of such unhealthy use.[217] Tapentadol combines mu opioid receptor agonist action with norepinephrine reuptake inhibition. It also inhibits serotonin reuptake, but serotonergic activity is much lower than noradrenergic activity. Tapentadol may be used to treat musculoskeletal and neuropathic pain conditions,[218,219] has a favorable profile for avoiding non-serious adverse events or discontinuation of treatment due to adverse events compared to other opioids; however, the clinical implications of these findings are unclear. No opioid should be taken concomitantly with alcohol due to potentiating risk including sedation and overdose, and in addition, alcohol can increase the serum concentration of tapentadol.

Routes of Administration

Opioids may be administered orally, rectally, transmucosally, intranasally, intravenously, subcutaneously, transdermally, and intraspinally. The oral, enteral, or transdermal routes generally are preferred when feasible because they are not invasive and usually provide satisfactory analgesia, even when high doses are required. However, when these routes are not feasible (as when patients are unable to take medications orally) or in the case of acute pain crisis when rapid onset is critical (eg, myocardial infarction), parenteral routes are preferred. Note that parenteral routes increase both speed of onset and peak blood levels obtained, which may be favorable in terms of analgesia but also may increase reward, a consideration in persons at risk for SUDs, as well as increase sedation and other side effects.

IV access may be difficult in individuals with a history of injection drug use; for such patients, surgical venous access may be necessary, or continuous subcutaneous infusions may be used. Intramuscular injections are effective but discouraged because of the pain involved in repeated injections and the variable blood levels obtained. If side effects of systemic use are not acceptable, intraspinal opioids may be indicated. Epidural administration is commonly used postoperatively when a catheter may already be in place. For longer-term use, intrathecal analgesia is more commonly provided. Rectal preparations may be useful for patients who are vomiting or who are unable to take oral medications. Sublingual or transmucosal administration of some preparations is clinically effective as well; these have a rapidity of onset and peak levels generally intermediate to oral and IV use.

Dose Titration and Scheduling

Measuring Efficacy

The efficacy of opioids is most commonly established by measuring the amount of pain (or pain relief) experienced. The serial use of a pain severity rating scale, such as a numerical 0 to 10 rating scale or a visual analogue faces scale, is helpful in assessing response to pain treatment. In treating chronic pain, it is often helpful to obtain a numerical score for the worst pain, least pain, and average (or typical) pain experienced in a particular period of time, such as the past week. In patients who cannot use a numerical rating scale, verbal descriptors such as none, mild, moderate, severe, and excruciating may be preferred. In the context of chronic pain treatment, assessment of pain interference, quality of life, and functioning (physical, psychological and social) may have equal or greater importance than measurement of pain severity. A simple measurement tool recommended for monitoring of response to pain management including opioid therapy is the PEG tool that measure *p*ain severity, pain interference with *e*njoyment of life, and pain interference with *g*eneral activity (each on a 0-10 numeric rating scale).[23] Pain ratings may be affected by myriad co-occurring issues and experiences, so rather than relying on target numbers as indication of satisfactory treatment, providers should involve the patient in setting individualized specific treatment goals, such as by using SMART goals that are specific, measurable, action-oriented, realistic, and time-bound,[66,220] as discussed in Chapter 111, "Rehabilitation Approaches to Pain Treatment."

Dose Requirements

Several factors must be considered in determining the dose and interval of administration that will provide effective analgesia in a given patient for a given amount of pain, however it is recommended to use the lowest dose of opioids as indicated by patient-specific risks and benefits, with short-acting formulations and using lower doses is always recommended (see Responsible Opioid Prescribing to Mitigate Risk below). The CDC Clinical Practice Guideline for Prescribing Opioids for Pain[23] recommends prescribing the lowest effective dosage and the VA/DoD Clinical Practice Guideline for Opioid Therapy recommend using the lowest dose of opioid and the shortest duration as indicated by patient specific risk and benefits.[66] The pharmacokinetics and potencies of the drugs must be taken into consideration, along with idiosyncratic or individual patient responses to different opioids as reviewed above. Finally, the tolerance of individuals who have been exposed to opioids on a prolonged basis (whether therapeutically or due to OUD) must be accommodated. Individuals currently using opioids or have used them persistently in the past are likely to be relatively tolerant or may develop rapid tolerance to the analgesic effects of opioids and, therefore, may require relatively high doses at relatively short intervals to achieve analgesia. If the patient has used opioids on a daily basis prior to the onset of acute pain, then his or her usual dose of opioids cannot be expected to provide analgesia for acute pain, and additional treatment should be provided.

Long-Acting Versus Short-Acting Medications

Long-acting medications include those that are intrinsically long acting, such as methadone, levorphanol, and buprenorphine, and medications that are long acting by virtue of being formulated for slow release, such as controlled-release and transdermal preparations. Most other opioids are shorter acting and immediate release.

When patients have persistent pain on an around-the-clock basis, longer-acting medications at least theoretically offer the advantage of providing relatively stable drug blood levels and, therefore, more consistent analgesia than frequent doses of short-acting medications. Fewer peaks and valleys may result in fewer side effects, including less reward. When longer-acting medications are taken on a scheduled basis, it is believed that patients are less driven to focus on pain and medication use because there is usually less opportunity for pain or mild withdrawal symptoms to recur and less need to watch the clock to note when medication is due.

Despite these theoretical advantages of long-acting or sustained-release opioids, recent literature reviews found no evidence that continuous, time-scheduled use of extended-release/long-acting (ER/LA) opioids is more effective or safer than intermittent use of immediate-release opioids or that time-scheduled use of ER/LA opioids reduces risks for unhealthy opioid use or OUD.[23,66] In addition, it is unclear whether around-the-clock or intermittent dosing is more likely to drive tolerance, hyperalgesia and/or physical dependence. ER/LA opioids are now considered more risky than short-acting/immediate release opioids due to the relatively large amount of opioid they contain, and any theoretical advantages of long-acting opioids, therefore, must be weighed against other clinical issues.

It is important to be aware that most controlled-release opioids can be altered to become immediate-release drugs through chewing, crushing, snorting, or extracting and injecting. Currently, a number of abuse-deterrent formulations are available, and the FDA has released guidance to industry on the development of future abuse-deterrent medications,[221] though it is unlikely that any system will be entirely abuse-proof as taking more doses of a medication—the most common form of unhealthy use—is still possible.[222] Strategies employed to reduce potential for at-risk use include embedding the opioid with the antagonist naltrexone (eg, Embeda®) that is released with tampering or, as with the reformulation of OxyContin® in 2010, creating a chemical matrix from which the opioid cannot easily be released with chewing, crushing, or chemical extraction.[223-226]

Scheduled Versus As-Needed (Rescue) Opioids (PRN)

Shorter acting opioid medications may be considered for intermittent pain, for acute pain conditions and acute exacerbation of chronic pain, or for evoked increases of chronic pain, when not sufficiently controlled by nonopioid pharmacological and nonpharmacological modalities. There are several issues to consider in scheduling opioids, particularly in individuals with, or at risk for, unhealthy substance use or SUD. First, pairing the perception of pain with the administration of a rewarding, and therefore potentially reinforcing, drug can theoretically reinforce the perception of pain and lead to increased use of the drug and increasing distress.[227,228] Such potential reinforcement of pain may be modified by making opioid use time-contingent or activity-contingent rather than contingent on the experience of pain. In time-contingent dosing, a patient who routinely develops pain in the afternoon and evening, for example, might receive a routine dose of short-acting opioid at noon and 5 PM only. In activity-contingent dosing, someone with unmanageable pain in association with certain valued activities (such as gardening or periodically being required to perform an activity at work that activates disabling pain), might be instructed to take medication 30 minutes before the activity. In addition to reducing reinforcement of pain and medication taking, such strategies may improve pain control by preempting it.

Scheduling opioid doses in supervised care settings, such as hospitals or nursing homes, also eliminates the need for patients to request medications, which can result in delayed treatment and create a perception that the patient is "constantly seeking opioids." When opioids are scheduled, the patient may decline doses if pain is well-controlled.

For constant pain at a moderate level of intensity, when an opioid is indicated, a relatively low dose of a long-acting pure mu agonist (such as methadone or a controlled-release preparation of morphine, oxycodone, or other opioid) or a combination product containing an opioid and acetaminophen or an NSAID may be appropriate. For severe pain, a pure mu agonist is usually indicated unless a neural blocking procedure or other intervention controls the pain. The selected opioid should be without a ceiling effect, rather than a mixed agonist-antagonist or product containing acetaminophen or salicylate (which can be toxic with titration) and should not have toxic metabolites.

If pain is continuous, patient-controlled analgesia (PCA), a continuous parenteral infusion, can be used for temporary pain control, or a long-acting oral or transdermal medications, depending on the context, is appropriate. As per the CDC opioid guideline,[23] however, it is strongly recommended to avoid using an extended-release formulation at initiation of opioid therapy. In acute or cancer pain, rescue doses of PRN medications are usually provided for breakthrough pain or exacerbations of baseline pain. The frequency and doses of rescue doses must be determined according to the context.[229,230] When multiple doses are required each day, this generally indicates a need for a higher baseline dose of long-acting medications.

In the chronic noncancer pain setting, when long-acting opioids are used for continuous baseline pain, it is preferable that patients manage the daily "ups and downs" of pain with activity pacing and use of nonopioid interventions (heat, ice, stretching, relaxation, etc.) to prevent or address mild exacerbations, rather than using frequent doses of PRN medications. Some clinicians provide a few PRN doses per month or per week for more major exacerbations of pain to deter unnecessary frequent ER or clinic visits. However, some patients with chronic pain have predictable activity-related pain that may require regular short-acting doses in association with the activity, such as keeping a job when there are no work adjustments available such as eliminating pain-causing work activities or shifting to lighter work that does not exacerbate the pain-causing condition. Care must be taken to assure that the cognitive effects of PRN dosing does not impair safe work and function.

Patient-Controlled Analgesia

As noted above, PCA can be used successfully for the management of acute pain and may be a preferred method of providing postoperative and posttraumatic pain control, including and in particular in individuals with SUD.[231] It often is used in the setting of advanced cancer pain as well. PCA allows the patient to self-administer small incremental doses of opioids intravenously or subcutaneously and thus provides stable analgesic blood levels. It usually produces more uniform pain relief at a lower total dose of medications than bolus dosing or continuous infusions. It avoids peaks (which may cause sedation or intoxication) and valleys (which may result in pain, anxiety, and drug craving). As with scheduled dosing, the use of PCA eliminates the need for the patient to request opioids and thus avoids potential conflicts between patients and staff, which can unfortunately arise when persons with SUD request opioids.[228] For persons with significant opioid tolerance and severe pain, a basal infusion may be used with PCA, under close monitoring to detect respiratory depression. Basal rate should not be initially used in opioid-naive patients.

Opioid Side Effects and Management

Opioid side effects can be categorized as those associated with acute and long-term opioid use.

Acute Use Side Effects

Common acute physical side effects of opioid use include respiratory depression, constipation, nausea and vomiting, urinary retention, and pruritus. Respiratory depression deserves special consideration because it can be life threatening.

Respiratory Depression

Respiratory depression is a potentially fatal side effect of opioid administration and demands awareness throughout treatment, particularly when opioids are first introduced or when doses are increased, or specific opioids changed.[232] Opioid-induced respiratory depression results from depression of brainstem respiratory responses to carbon dioxide (CO_2) in a dose dependent manner.[233] Respiratory depression may be significant, in particular, when higher-dose opioids are used for acute pain in opioid-naive patients, or in elderly or debilitated patients. Patients with sleep disordered breathing from obstructive or central sleep apnea who rely on CO_2 response to awaken them during sleep if hypoventilation occurs are at particularly high risk for respiratory depression. In patients with sleep apnea, opioid therapy should be generally avoided.[66] If opioid therapy is truly required due to severity of the pain condition and failure to respond to other treatment options in those with sleep apnea, the dosage should be kept as low as possible, in particular for the sleeping hours, and with use of continuous positive airway pressure (CPAP) during sleep. At particularly high risk for respiratory depression are patients who are also using other drugs with respiratory depressive action, in particular sedative-hypnotics including benzodiazepines.[23,66] In a retrospective cohort study, the risk for opioid overdose was highest for individuals on long-term opioid therapy for chronic pain who also received concurrent long-term benzodiazepine therapy.[234] The same study also showed increased risk for overdose in patients receiving zolpidem in combination with opioids, albeit lower than for benzodiazepines.

Sedation may in part be due to hypoventilation and accumulation of CO_2 (ie, the result of early respiratory depression) and thus signals the urgent need to hold opioid medication until sedation has resolved and decrease future dosing. Respiratory depression is rarely a problem in long-term opioid administration in individuals without specific risk factors, if doses are increased gradually in response to analgesic tolerance, because tolerance to respiratory depression tends to occur more rapidly than to analgesia. All patients should be closely followed, however, with each dosage change, and in particular, when doses are abruptly increased or when patients are rotated from one opioid to another.[235] Special care also should be exercised in titrating opioids with long half-lives, such as methadone or levorphanol, because delayed respiratory depression may occur several days after dosage increase. Withholding of opioids and respiratory support are the first-line treatments for this side effect. An opioid antagonist such as naloxone should be used in emergency situations with awareness that it may precipitate acute withdrawal in persons with physical dependence; co-prescription of naloxone to all patients prescribed long-term opioid therapy is increasingly considered a cornerstone of responsible opioid prescribing.[236,237] Whether it is sufficiently safe to resume opioid therapy after the recovery from the overdose event at a lower dosage needs to be carefully reviewed.

The issuance of naloxone to patients with opioid therapy or with history of OUD is now a generally accepted risk mitigation strategy to reverse respiratory depression in overdose situations. The 2022 CDC opioid guideline recommends, "Before starting and periodically during continuation of opioid therapy, clinicians should evaluate risk for opioid related harms and discuss risk with patients. Clinicians should work with patients to incorporate into the management plan strategies to mitigate risk, including offering naloxone… ."[23] The VHA recommends issuing naloxone to all patients with diagnosis of OUD and to patients undergoing or having recently completed opioid tapering or discontinuation.[66]

Pain acts as a stimulant for wakefulness and ventilation, so care should be taken when a patient using opioids for pain control undergoes a definitive procedure that alleviates pain, such as a nerve block or spinal cord ablation; in the sudden absence of pain, pre-procedure doses of opioids may result in sudden sedation or hypoventilation. Doses should be reduced as indicated in response to reduced pain.

Other Acute Side Effects and Management

Side effects sometimes are specific to a particular opioid in a particular individual, and it is often appropriate to simply substitute a different opioid to avoid a side effect such as nausea or pruritus. With the exception of constipation, side effects may improve with continued use of opioids at a stable dose. While persistent side effects can often be alleviated through treatments such as stool softeners, antiemetics, or antihistamines, often the best approach is to discuss with the patient reduction of opioid dosage and possibly discontinuation of opioid therapy. Some side effects correlate with blood levels and may be minimized by limiting peak levels through scheduled doses of ER/LA opioids when oral preparations are used. Continuous infusions or PCA achieves the same goal when parenteral administration is required.

Constipation is a persistent side effect that usually does not resolve without treatment. It is attributed to direct action on opioid receptors in the intestinal wall. This causes a decrease in intestinal motility and results in dehydration of stool. It generally is advisable, therefore, to give both a stool softener and a bowel stimulant to effectively manage constipation. When long-term and/or high-dose use of opioids is anticipated, introduction of such treatment on a preemptive basis is recommended.[238] For many patients, the best strategy to treat constipation is lowering the opioid dosage, but stool softeners and stimulants may still be needed. Transdermal administration instead of oral administration of the opioid lessens the gastrointestinal side effects including constipation.[239]

Hepatic, renal, and other organ toxicity generally are not reported with opioids as they are with many nonopioid analgesics, such as acetaminophen and NSAIDs. However, close observation and dose adjustments may be appropriate in persons who have impaired hepatic or renal function, which may result in reduced drug clearance.

CNS side effects of opioids may include sedation, cognitive dysfunction, and affective changes. Sedation and mild cognitive changes are common when opioids are introduced or when the dose is increased and may resolve once a stable therapeutic dose of opioid is achieved and sustained for a period of time.[240] Sedation may be considered a warning sign for respiratory depression and is a risk for injury due to falls or accidents, and thus should usually result in holding the medication and/or reducing the dosage. CNS effects may persist, particularly when long-acting medications are used in elderly or frail patients, and patients on methadone may be of particular high risk.[241] Like many other side effects, sedation and cognitive dysfunction are usually managed or avoided by reducing the opioids dosage. Administration of a treatment medication (stimulant) to counteract the sedating effect of opioids in chronic noncancer pain is controversial. When significant persistent opioid-induced sedation occurs in cancer pain patients or patients with other severe intractable pain, stimulants such as methylphenidate and dextroamphetamine may be helpful.[242] The use of stimulants, which may be used in an unhealthy manner by some individuals, requires the same caution in patients with SUD as that required in the use of opioids.

Long-Term Use Side Effects

Side effects of long-term opioid use may include hyperalgesia, respiratory depression, and constipation (all previously discussed), as well as additional effects on the endocrine and immune systems.

Endocrine Effects

Opioids affect the hypothalamic-pituitary-adrenal and the hypothalamic-pituitary-gonadal axes. Effects in human and animal models include alterations in activity of growth hormone, prolactin, luteinizing hormone, testosterone, estradiol, oxytocin, thyroid-stimulating hormone, vasopressin, and adrenocorticotropic hormone.[243] Interactions between opioids and endocrine systems are complex and vary with the type and duration of opioid used as well as the gender and medical comorbidities of users. However, clinically significant effects with prolonged use may include androgen deficiency and bone loss.[244]

Androgen deficiency, including low testosterone levels in men, can manifest in depressive symptoms, fatigue, low libido, and erectile dysfunction.[245] Many experts recommend routine testing of all men receiving long-term opioid therapy, and there is clear evidence of symptom improvement when symptomatic low testosterone levels are identified and treated.[246,247] In women, gonadotropin dysfunction has been shown to include lowered levels of follicle-stimulating hormone, luteinizing hormone, estradiol, dehydroepiandrosterone, and testosterone with common clinical manifestations of oligomenorrhea or amenorrhea. Estrogen replacement therapy in consultation with an endocrinologist is sometimes indicated.[248]

Increased rates of osteopenia and osteoporosis have been observed in people who use opioids long-term and may be related to opioid-induced changes in bone metabolism and endocrine function.[249,250] However, studies to date have been confounded by numerous variables including medications, activity levels, nutrition, smoking, and others, so the mechanisms are not clear; it is also unclear whether bone density screening may be indicated for all persons receiving long-term opioids.[251] The concern is of special significance, however, in older persons who may be at risk for falls and fractures related to the use of opioids.[252]

Immune Effects

Effects of opioids on the immune system have been demonstrated, with numerous early studies both in animals and humans suggesting immunosuppressive effects, particularly on cell-mediated immunity.[253] Specifically, opioids have repeatedly been demonstrated to have broad immunosuppressant effects[254,255] attributed to decreases in macrophage activity, and interfering with production and release of cytokines necessary to mount an effective inflammatory response.[256,257] More recently, diminished NF-kappa B activation in stimulated immune cells in response to opioids (morphine and fentanyl) has been reported in several in vitro examinations.[258,259] Although the clinical relevance of this opioid-induced immunosuppression is disputed, the association between opioid use and postoperative infection continues to be a concern.[258-266]

Conversely, there are reports of acute opioid administration increasing circulating levels of several proinflammatory cytokines, including NF-kappa B.[267] For example, within hours of heroin or morphine administration, mice demonstrate increased serum levels of IL-6,[268] and splenocyte production of IL-1β, IFN-γ, IL-12, and TNFα,[269] effects antagonized by naltrexone.[270] Proinflammatory consequences are suggested by parallel evidence for decreased expression of the anti-inflammatory cytokines, IL-10 and IL-4, following acute opioid exposure.[271,272] Further, via toll-like receptors, opioids induce proinflammatory effects on spinal glial cells, which is thought to lead to increases in cytokines in the plasma.[273-275]

The potential for immunosuppressive effects and carcinogenesis associated with the use of opioids may provide additional rationale for limiting the use of opioids in acute and chronic pain treatment settings.[276] However, no clear clinically significant effects of opioids on immune function have been demonstrated to date, and the clinical relevance of these findings is therefore uncertain. In addition, pain itself has been demonstrated to have both immunosuppressive[277] and proinflammatory effects, making the relative balance of these effects difficult to determine[278-280] when opioids are administered in the context of pain.

Opioid Rotation

Because side effects can vary from one opioid to another in different patients, rotation from one opioid to another may be helpful in resolving side effects that do not resolve over time or that do not respond to pharmacologic treatment. Transition from one opioid or form of opioid to another may be indicated in a number of circumstances, such as when tolerance occurs to a specific opioid with loss of analgesic efficacy, when a patient on long-term oral opioids becomes unable to swallow oral medication, or when significant side effects occur and persist. Opioid rotation may result in improved analgesia when tolerance is present, and sometimes on significantly lower equivalent doses of the new opioid. Rotation back to the original opioid—or an alternative—can occur if tolerance develops to the new opioid.[281] Opioid rotation has been found to be clinically useful in both cancer-related pain and chronic non–cancer-related pain.[282,283]

Traditionally, opioid analgesic equivalency charts have been used to calculate equianalgesic doses, and the new opioid has been given at 50% to 75% of the calculated equianalgesic dose to account for incomplete cross-tolerance (except when methadone is the new medication, in which case the dose reduction is much lower—to 10% to 25% of the calculated dose or less). However, this practice has been called into question as potentially unsafe for several reasons: equianalgesic studies are based on single-dose studies rather than long-term administration; equianalgesic charts vary significantly in dose equivalents listed; and charts cannot take into account inter-patient variability in opioid responsiveness and tolerance.[284] In addition, it has been observed that there is a risk of overdose when new opioids are started, suggesting the need for a new paradigm of rotation.[285] It should be noted that some methadone conversion tables in use are clearly incorrect and suggest a 2:1 methadone to morphine potency ratio with oral morphine, which is only true at very low doses of methadone. At higher doses, the ratio is closer to 16:1 or even 20:1.[200] This, plus the extreme inter-patient variability in methadone half-life, renders the use of any conversion ratio hazardous when rotating to methadone from other opioids. Each patient must be individually titrated, starting with quite low doses of methadone.

As an alternative, it is suggested that equianalgesic charts be used to guide starting doses and intervals of administration of the new opioid, and the new opioid should be given within its usual range of effective starting doses and titrated gradually with careful observation.[285] If the patient is reliable in managing their opioid medication, PRN doses of short-acting opioid can be provided and used if analgesia is inadequate and there is no sedation present. It is critical to be aware of the potential of delayed respiratory depression, particularly with drugs with long half-lives such as methadone and to monitor carefully and instruct a patient to hold medication for sedation (which most often precedes respiratory depression).

Sometimes, the transition from one opioid to another is better tolerated if the patient is gradually cross-tapered from one medication to another. In this process, the old medication is gradually tapered while the new medication is increased incrementally over a few days or weeks. This permits observation of the patient's response to the new drug and adjustment of the dose to avoid side effects and maintain analgesia.

Opioid Tapering

In the acute pain setting, most patients taper their medications without incident as pain gradually improves. However, tapering sometimes is impeded by fear, withdrawal, or craving. The goal of tapering is to provide fairly stable but decreasing blood levels of opioid so as to prevent precipitous troughs. Though stable blood levels usually are only approximated with the use of short-acting medications, most patients do not experience significant withdrawal while gently tapering in the acute pain context. If the patient has been using an intermittently administered medication such as bolus parenteral morphine or oral oxycodone, the interval of administration can be decreased somewhat as the dose is decreased in order to avoid low blood levels between doses. Some patients may benefit from having their medications dispensed daily or dose-by-dose while tapering in order to assist in controlling use as the dose is decreasing.

In the context of chronic noncancer pain, continuation of opioid therapy may be appropriate in some patients if it is helping pain and function and if there are no significant adverse consequences associated with use, after careful education of the patient about risks and alternatives and in agreement with patient preference. There is no clear evidence, however, that opioid medication provides long-term benefit for chronic noncancer pain.[23,66,286] If opioid therapy does not continue to achieve its goals of improved pain and function, or if therapy cannot be structured to maintain safety owing to unhealthy use, or if the patient would like to reduce or stop the use of opioid medication, or if pain improves or resolves, it may be appropriate to gradual reduce and discontinue opioid treatment. Opioids should be tapered to avoid withdrawal and a rebound increase in pain. In case of evidence of medication diversion, however, opioid prescribing is usually terminated immediately and further opioid dispensing should generally be avoided. Alternative treatments should be provided for pain and any withdrawal symptoms that occur. If an OUD is identified, treatment for it should be initiated or intensified. If pain cannot be satisfactorily managed without opioids and the patient exhibits unhealthy opioid use, referral for medication for OUD should be considered.

The goal of opioid tapering is to improve the balance of risks and clinically meaningful benefits for patients on long-term opioid therapy. For patients on higher-dose opioid therapy who are not experiencing improvement in function or quality of life, opioid taper has been recommended to improve chronic pain outcomes, citing self-reports of decreased pain and medication use following dose reduction.[92,110,115,287-290] According to a systematic review of patient outcomes after dose reduction or discontinuation of long-term opioid therapy, improvement was reported in pain severity (8 of 8 fair-quality studies), function (5 of 5 fair-quality studies), and quality of life (3 of 3 fair-quality studies).[140] In a small sample of veterans, opioid tapers to an average of 54% of baseline dose resulted in either no change in pain or less pain when compared to baseline pain severity in 70% of subjects.[290] A study of patients with chronic pain assigned to an opioid taper treatment had significant improvements at 22 weeks in ratings on pain interference, pain self-efficacy and perceived opioid problems, even though absolute daily MME did not significantly decrease.[291]

A cognitive-behavioral intervention that decreased opioid use in patients with chronic pain concomitantly led to significant improvements in pain severity, function and increased use of pain coping strategies.[292] A 2020 review of 49 studies suggested improvements in pain scores among patients tapering opioids while participating in intensive multimodal pain interventions, and mostly unchanged pain in patients tapering opioid therapy with less intensive or nonspecific cointerventions.[141]

With respect to effective opioid taper protocols, no clear evidence-based regimen is recommended, but it is generally understood that slower dosage reductions are better tolerated than faster tapers. In their 2016 guideline, the CDC recommended reducing weekly dosage by 10% to 50% of the original dosage, and rapid taper over 2 to 3 weeks in the case of a severe adverse event such as overdose, and notes that slower tapers such as 10% per month might be appropriate and better tolerated than more rapid tapers, particularly when patients have been taking opioids for longer durations (eg, for years).[23] The updated 2022 CDC guideline uses even more cautious language by stating that opioid tapers "can be completed over several months to years depending on the opioid dosage and should be individualized based on patient goals and concerns. Longer durations of previous opioid therapy might require longer tapers. Tapers of 10% per month or slower are likely to be better tolerated than more rapid tapers, particularly when patients have been taking opioids for longer durations (eg, for a year or longer).[38]" Once patients reach low dosages, it is common to slow the tapering speed, and when the smallest available dose is reached, the interval between doses can be extended or a lower potency drug may be used instead. As noted by the CDC, patient agreement and interest in tapering is likely to be a key component of successful tapers. The VA/DoD recommends a collaborative, patient-centered and individualized approach to tapering.[66] Factors that would suggest a more gradual taper include higher opioid dose and longer duration of opioid therapy, whereas more rapid taper are indicated by non-adherence to the treatment plan and escalating high-risk medication-related behaviors. Both guidelines suggest that in patients with longstanding high dosage opioid therapy, such tapering may require months or even years.[23,66] For some patients, pauses in the taper for weeks or months may be helpful to allow for physiological and psychological adaptation during the tapering process. The rate of opioid dosage reduction may need to be adjusted during the course of opioid tapering and should be reevaluated after each dose change.

When opioids are reduced or discontinued, clinicians must remain vigilant about any symptoms and signs of opioid withdrawal, and adverse consequences should be minimized or avoided as much as possible. As noted above, risks related to discontinuation or tapering of long-term opioid therapy include higher risk of illicit opioid use,[34] high incidence of emergency department visits and opioid-related hospitalizations,[35] increased incidence of mental health crises and overdose events,[26] and increased risk of death from suicide or overdose.[36] For patients with high risk on opioid medication unable or unwilling to taper, the conversion to buprenorphine therapy provides another option to lessen risk while maintaining pain control, and gradual switching over using a low or very low dose of protocol of buprenorphine initiation avoids patients having to stop their full mu agonist opioid medication prior to the transition.

The clinical team's key management strategies leading to successful tapers include[29,140,141,287,291,293-295]:

- Closely monitoring for the emergence of psychiatric symptoms, including suicidality, and for risk of craving and the potential of illicit drug use, and managing appropriately.
- Providing social support and empathetic and encouraging communication between the patient and clinician.
- Creating a trusted provider-patient relationship to motivate and implement the opioid tapering process with the patient successfully.
- Working with the patient to obtain patient agreement and motivation to reduce dosage, following principles of shared decision making.
- Advising that after opioid taper to lower dosage or discontinuation has been accomplished, most patients have stable or improved physical and cognitive function, anxiety, and mood, and that patients' pain levels are commonly stable or even decreased.
- Educating the patient and family about acute and protracted opioid withdrawal symptoms and management. Nevertheless, provide reassurance that opioid reductions are generally implemented slowly to avoid severe withdrawal symptoms.
- Educating the patient that symptoms such as insomnia or increased pain may occur temporarily,[29,84,287,296-298] and usually improve or resolve over time. Providing reassurance that you will be supporting them during the transition
- Making a concerted effort to ensure that the patient does not feel abandoned during the opioid tapering process, particularly maintaining frequent contact with the patient. This includes scheduling follow-up contacts even after opioid therapy has stopped due to higher risk in the subsequent weeks to months.
- If patients are receiving both long-acting and short-acting opioids, the decision regarding which formulation to be tapered first needs to be individualized based on safety, medical history, mental health diagnoses, and patient preference. Reducing the long-acting medication initially first to lower dosage level may be easier tolerated by the patient, and sometimes the long-acting and short-acting medication may be reduced simultaneously.
- Once the lowest dose of medication is reached, dosing frequency can be decreased and eventually stopped once taken less than once a day.
- In particular, patients must be made aware that it takes as little as a week to lose tolerance to their prior opioid dose and that they are at high risk of overdose if they resume their prior dose.[23,66]
- Issuance of naloxone to patients undergoing opioid tapering or with recently stopped opioid medication.

Management of Opioid Withdrawal

While abrupt discontinuation of opioids should generally be avoided, it may be justified when a patient exhibits dangerous behaviors (eg, threatening behaviors, persistent and serious disruptive behavior, suicidal ideation or behaviors) but should be coupled with mental health support and medical care for the management of opioid withdrawal. When there is evidence for diversion, the clinician should discontinue opioid therapy.

If abrupt cessation of opioids is necessary, an acute withdrawal syndrome may be attenuated through the prescription of medications for symptom control.[299] An alpha-2-adrenergic drug such as clonidine or lofexidine may be helpful in attenuating autonomic signs and symptoms of withdrawal.[300,301] The alpha-2 agonist tizanidine showed benefit in patients tapering from long-term, high-dose opioids for chronic pain.[298] NSAIDs, acetaminophen or topical menthol/methylsalicylate can relieve muscular aching. A gastrointestinal antispasmodic such as dicyclomine may relieve gastric cramping distress, and loperamide or bismuth subsalicylate are used for diarrhea. Prochlorperazine, promethazine and ondansetron may relieve nausea. While benzodiazepine or other sedative–hypnotic used on a short-term basis may reduce irritability, anxiety, and sleeplessness, these medications are typically avoided in this setting due to risks including but not limited to unhealthy use and overdose. Alternatively, sedating medications such as trazodone, doxepin, or gabapentin have been demonstrated to have similar effects in reducing withdrawal symptoms including sleep disturbance.

It is important to note that withdrawal of opioids used for pain can be legally supervised by any physician with a DEA license, however, withdrawal management as a component of OUD treatment with buprenorphine can only be done by a waivered buprenorphine provider or with methadone by a federally licensed methadone maintenance treatment center.

RESPONSIBLE OPIOID PRESCRIBING TO MITIGATE RISKS

Due to the unique risks associated with opioids, especially when prescribed for ongoing or long-term use, it is incumbent upon the provider to put in place certain controls to ensure that the medications are used safely and consistent with the principles of effective pain care. While not strictly evidence-based,[96,302] the 2016 *CDC Guideline for Prescribing Opioids for Chronic Pain*[23] and the 2022 update to this guideline[38] provide a guiding framework for the responsible prescribing of opioid analgesics in a manner that minimizes risk. These and similar guidelines[66,303,304] address the primary risks of concern, which include overdose, unhealthy use and use disorders, not only for the patients for whom the opioids are prescribed, but also for family members or others who may have access to the medications.

Firstly, opioids should only be considered first-line therapies for moderate to severe acute pain and active cancer, palliative, and end of life care. Nonpharmacologic therapy and nonopioid pharmacologic therapy are preferred for chronic pain, and if used, opioids should be combined with nonpharmacologic therapy and nonopioid pharmacologic therapy; opioid therapy should only be considered if the benefits for both pain and function are anticipated to outweigh risks to the patient. Before starting opioid therapy for chronic pain, the clinician should establish treatment goals with the patients, including realistic goals for pain and function, and establish that opioid therapy will be discontinued if benefits are not appreciated.

In this conversation with the patient with chronic pain, the clinician should emphasize that improvement in function is the primary goal, even if there are no absolute changes in pain severity. The patient must be *advised about the serious adverse effects of opioids* including possible fatal respiratory depression as well as unhealthy use including OUD, and the common adverse effects of opioids such as constipation, nausea, vomiting, pruritus and physical dependence. In addition, the potential adverse effects that opioids may have on the ability to safely operate a vehicle should be discussed. This conversation is commonly documented in an *opioid treatment agreement* signed by both the patient and provider (see **Fig. 113-3**), which typically stipulates the understanding that the patient will obtain opioids from a single provider only; take opioid in doses, frequency and for symptoms only as prescribed; follow the refill policy; fully engage in all nonopioid and nonpharmacological pain management treatment interventions; submit random urine samples for toxicology for analysis; refrain from the use of other psychoactive drugs or substances (including alcohol); and store the medication securely so that no other family members or visitors can gain access to it.[305-307] Such opioid agreements are not legally binding contracts, and patients may be hesitant to sign. Instead, a written informed consent with the emphasis on educating the patient about risks and benefits of opioid therapy, alternatives to opioid medication, and providing guidance on opioid tapering and discontinuation can support the patient-provider relationship and allows for documentation of appropriate patient education including safety concerns and risk mitigation expectations in a patient-centered format. Written informed consents are mandated for patients on long-term opioid therapy in the VA, with few exceptions such as for cancer pain.[308] The corresponding patient education guide is freely available.[309]

Previously reviewed were *screening tools* that can be used to predict risk for or identify unhealthy opioid use behaviors; these do not predict the development of a use disorder. Recently published is the Opioid Risk Tool for OUD (ORT-OUD) (see **Table 113-4**) which has demonstrated high sensitivity and specificity for identifying patients with chronic pain and prescribed opioid who will develop OUD.[310] Opioids should be used cautiously, if at all, in patients who score at high risk; because the risk factors for OUD generalize across substances, SUD assessment and intervention should be instituted, as an active SUD will interfere with improvements in pain outcomes.

Informed Consent / Agreement for the Use of Opioid Medication in Chronic Pain

"Opioid" is the medical name for a type of strong painkillers. Like all medications, opioids have potential to help people and cause harm. The purpose of this document is to outline the overall benefits and harms so that together with your practitioner you can determine whether an opioid trial is suitable for you at this time. Using opioid medication is always a trial and if the goals of using the opioid are not met, the opioid should always be gradually stopped. Not everyone will benefit from an opioid. In those who do, pain relief is generally modest. For example, your pain may only decrease by about 10% to 30%. The possible side effects are the same for all the opioids but different people react to each opioid individually. What might work well for you with few side effects may be terrible for the next person. Most side effects are worst when the medication is first started and can be effectively managed. Some side effects are more problematic with higher doses and longer term use.

The potential harms of using these medications are:

Some Possible Side Effects

Side Effects

- Constipation (common & persistent)
- Nausea and vomiting (usually only in first few days)
- Reduced production of testosterone (may cause reduced sex drive and fertility in men)
- Reduced production of estrogen & progesterone (may cause periods to stop, reduced sex drive & fertility in women)
- Excessive sweating
- Weight gain
- Swollen ankles/legs
- Sedation, drowsiness, clouded thinking
- Sleep apnea
- Hyperalgesia (opioid makes pain worse rather than better)

Addiction is a disease that occurs in some individuals. Like becoming overweight does not necessarily mean you will become diabetic, taking opioids does not necessarily cause addiction, however, if you have risk factors for addiction (such as a strong family history of drug or alcohol abuse) or have had problems with drugs or alcohol in the past you must notify your practitioner since using opioids will put you at greater risk. The extent of this risk is not certain.

- I have notified my practitioner of any personal or family history of drug or alcohol abuse. ________ (INITIALS)

Physical dependence means that if the opioid medication is abruptly stopped or not taken as directed, a withdrawal symptom can occur. This is a normal response to some medications and also occurs, for instance, with antidepressants. Stopping opioids is uncomfortable but not usually dangerous if done with a controlled, gradual approach. Having withdrawal after stopping or reducing prescribed opioids in no way implies that you are addicted. (It does if the drug is alcohol though). The withdrawal syndrome could include sweating, nervousness, stomach cramps, diarrhea, goose bumps, feeling worried, irritable or moody. Those who have been on higher doses for longer periods of time will experience greater withdrawal symptoms. Sometimes a temporary withdrawal pain may occur and this usually resolves within 4 weeks.

Tolerance means that over time the body becomes "used to" the medication and it feels less effective. The dose of the opioid may have to be adjusted to a dose that produces benefit and a *realistic* decrease of your pain yet does not have intolerable side effects. Sometimes this is not possible and the opioid will have to be stopped and/or alternate therapy explored.

- I am aware that drowsiness or clouded thinking may make it dangerous for me to drive or operate heavy machinery. Alcohol or other medications that also cause drowsiness may worsen this effect. I agree not to drive or operate heavy machinery or sign legal documents while my practitioner is starting me on these new medications, significantly increasing my dose, or if I feel in any way impaired from this therapy at other times.

  ________ (INITIALS)

- I understand the use of alcohol and opioids together is potentially dangerous. I have been advised not do this.

  ________ (INITIALS)

Figure 113-3. Sample opioid treatment agreement. (Used with permission from RxFiles Academic Detailing [http://www.rxfiles.ca].)

Urine drug testing (UDT) includes urine drug screening (UDS) and confirmatory testing for further characterization, if clinically indicated such as for unexpected or irregular results on UDS. UDT should be performed prior to initiating opioid therapy and as part of long-term opioid treatment in order to document use of the prescribed medication and to exclude the use of illicit or nonprescribed substances.[311,312] UDS panels differ in the drugs that are detected and false positive or negative results may occur. In general, UDS fairly reliably detects opiates, naturally occurring opioids such as morphine or codeine, if present in significant concentration. UDS tests generally have lower sensitivity for semi-synthetic opioids (eg, oxycodone) and usually do not detect synthetic opioids such as fentanyl or buprenorphine.[313] Therefore, it is recommended to be sure the screening assay includes oxycodone, which may require a separate order. Buprenorphine and fentanyl

Safeguards for Best Practice to Protect Patient and Society
Opioids are controlled substances and there are numerous laws and regulations regarding the prescribing of them that your practitioner has to adhere to. The following requests are considered standard best practice and help this healthcare practice and you comply with these laws and regulations.

The patient agrees:

1. To fill prescriptions only at one pharmacy located at ______________________________.*

   ***physician will send a copy of this agreement to the above pharmacy*
2. That all prescriptions for pain medications will, except in an emergency, only come from my practitioner or the clinic. **This includes over-the-counter codeine products, e.g. Tylenol #1.**
3. To reliably attend appointments with the practitioner.
4. To not use any illegal substances, such as cocaine, etc. while taking an opioid.
5. To take the opioid as prescribed by the practitioner.
6. To not request earlier prescription refills or decide to use more without the knowledge and consent of the practitioner if a specific quantity of medication is prescribed to last until the next scheduled appointment.
7. To explore and participate in other pain consultations/management strategies as recommended.
8. To safely store the medication. (This is REALLY important as most of the prescription opioids now on the street were stolen from a regular user). Use a locked box and do not keep them where others might see or have access to them.
9. To contact the appropriate travel authority (usually the consulate website of the country you are going to) and obtain a note from my practitioner before travel, as traveling out of country with opioids may pose problems.
10. That lost/stolen/spilt medications will not be replaced. (With apologies but we must be like the bank and money in this regard).
11. To periodic urine drug tests as required by the practitioner (including coming in for random screens).
12. To a planned process to reduce and/or discontinue the opioid if goals/benefits are not realized or harms outweigh benefits.
13. To periodic pill counts as requested by the pharmacist (including coming in for random counts).

Single Provider
Use of Other Psychoactive Substances
Refill Policy
Take as Prescribed
Treatment Engagement
Safe Storage
Urine Testing

The practitioner agrees:

1. To be able to see you within a reasonable time for follow up
2. To discuss the results of urine drug testing with you before making any decisions
3. To explore treatment for your pain with other non-opioid therapies (drug and/or non-drug) as may be indicated

Signature Lines

______________________ Practitioner signature ______________ Date

______________________ Patient signature ______________ Date

______________________ Patient name (print)

Forms available at:
Word (modifiable): http://www.rxfiles.ca/rxfiles/uploads/documents/Opiod-Informed-Consent-And-Agreement.docx
Pdf: http://www.rxfiles.ca/rxfiles/uploads/documents/Opiod-Informed-Consent-And-Agreement.pdf

Figure 113-3. Continued

screening assays are also available and should be included if (1) a patient is prescribed either of these medications or (2) illicit use of them is a concern. Unexpected findings on a screening test should prompt confirmation usually by liquid or gas chromatography coupled with mass spectroscopy.[311,314]

UDT should be approached in a patient-centered way. Unexpected findings should trigger a discussion with the patient and lead to enhanced treatment of the individual depending on the reason for the finding.[38,315] Care may need to be revised or changed, but UDT results should be understood

TABLE 113-4 Opioid Risk Tool for Opioid Use Disorder

Mark each box that applies	YES	NO
Family history of substance abuse		
Alcohol	1	0
Illegal drugs	1	0
Rx drugs	1	0
Personal history of substance abuse		
Alcohol	1	0
Illegal drugs	1	0
Rx drugs	1	0
Age between 16-45 years	1	0
Psychological disease		
ADD, OCD, bipolar, schizophrenia	1	0
Depression	1	0
Scoring totals		

This tool should be administered to patients upon an initial visit prior to beginning or continuing opioid therapy for pain management. A score of 2 or lower indicates low risk for future opioid use disorder; a score of 3 or more indicates high risk for opioid use disorder.

From Cheatle MD, Compton PA, Dhingra L, Wasser TE, O'Brien CP. Development of the revised opioid risk tool to predict opioid use disorder in patients with chronic nonmalignant pain. *J Pain.* 2019;20(7):842-851.

as a single point of information among many in the rich array of information the clinician has regarding the patient. In persons with no appreciated risk for unhealthy medication use, UDT is done randomly at a minimum of annual basis by many experts, though a recent expert consensus panel funded by a urine toxicology testing company recommended more frequent routine screening.[316] In veterans, close monitoring including greater use of UDT was associated with reduced risk of suicide attempts,[317] and for persons at higher risk, testing should be done more often, such as monthly or even weekly, especially during periods of high stress.

As previously noted, opioids should always be prescribed at the *lowest effective dose* and in *immediate-release, short-acting formulations* as possible. Extant data provide good evidence that opioid-related overdose risk is dose-dependent. In comparison to patients with chronic pain on low-dose opioids (defined as < 20 morphine mg equivalents [MME]/day), the odds of overdose increased between 1.3 and 1.9 for dosages of 20 to less than 50 MME/day, between 1.9 and 4.6 for dosages of 50 to less than 100 MME/day, and between 2.0 and 8.9 for dosages of 100 or more MME/day.[318-320] Similarly, fatal overdose risk increased with MME daily dose; compared to low dose, risk increased by 0.15% for 50 up to 99 MME/day, and 0.25% for 100 or more MME/day.[56] These findings were supported in a more recent study showing that opioid overdose fatalities in chronic pain patients were prescribed higher average daily opioid dosages (98 MME/day versus 48 MME/day).[321] Based upon these data, recent guidelines suggest that clinicians should implement additional precautions, including increased frequency of follow up, for patients on opioid dosages above 50 mg MME/day, and generally should avoid increasing dosage to greater 90 MME/day without careful justification based on diagnosis and on individualized assessment of benefits and risks.[23,66]

In addition to overdose, higher dose opioids appear to be related to a lower quality of life. A study of 801 primary care patients with chronic pain on opioid therapy found that quality of life, measured as physical functioning, was lowest in patients on high dose opioids (>105 MME/day), whereas those taking 5 to 40 mg MME/day had better quality of life scores than those at high dosage or not on opioid therapy at all, though this could be due to multiple factors including the underlying pain condition.[322] However, most of the studies on opioid dosage and function suffer from being cross-sectional[323-326] and the phenomenon of selection bias: since generally patients are not started on opioids unless they have failed other common medications such as acetaminophen or NSAIDs, it is not possible to determine whether opioids lead to worse clinical status or whether the correlation reflects the fact that sicker patients with more co-morbidities are more likely to start on opioids and escalate to high doses of medication.

Importantly, epidemiologic studies suggest that concurrent use of benzodiazepines with opioids prescribed for chronic pain increases risk for fatal overdose,[327,328] thus *co-prescription of CNS depressants should be avoided.*[23,66] Clinicians should review the patient's history of controlled substance prescriptions using *state prescription drug monitoring program* (PDMP) data to determine whether patients are receiving additional opioids, benzodiazepines or other sedative-hypnotics that increase risk of overdose. If concurrent benzodiazepine use is detected, these should be tapered gradually, as abrupt withdrawal can be associated with rebound anxiety, hallucinations, seizures, delirium, tremors and, in rare cases, death. Alternative approaches for treating anxiety, such as cognitive–behavioral therapy or certain antidepressants, should be considered. In that persons with sleep-disordered breathing are also at high risk for opioid-induced respiratory depression, opioids should be cautiously prescribed for these patients. In all patients provided an ongoing opioid prescription, *naloxone should be co-prescribed*, and a family member trained on the signs of opioid toxicity and naloxone administration.

SUMMARY

Opioids have an important role in relieving human suffering. At the same time, it is important to respect their potential to cause harm in vulnerable individuals and their limitations in management of chronic pain. In order to use opioids effectively and safely when they are indicated, clinicians must understand pharmacologic and clinical issues related to opioids and carefully structure treatment with respect to the particular benefits and risks for individual patients. It is to be hoped that, over time, science and clinical experience will provide a fuller understanding of ways to harness the full potential of opioids to relieve suffering while eliminating the harmful consequences of their use. In the meantime, the art of pain care should be combined with the science of pain care to give patients the best quality of life possible, given the reality of their clinical diagnoses.

ACKNOWLEDGMENT

An earlier version of this chapter was written by Seddon Savage, which provided the basis of the current chapter.

REFERENCES

1. Krikorian AD. Were the opium poppy and opium known in the ancient Near East? *J Hist Biol.* 1975;8:95-114.
2. Kritikos PG, Papadaki SP. *The history of the poppy and of opium and their expansion in antiquity in the eastern Mediterranean area.* United Nations Office on Drugs and Crime. *Bulletin on Narcotics.* 1967;3. Accessed July 20, 2023. https://www.unodc.org/unodc/en/data-and-analysis/bulletin/bulletin_1967-01-01_3_page004.html
3. Ellis H. Alexander Wood: inventor of the hypodermic syringe and needle. *Br J Hosp Med (Lond).* 2017;78(11):647.
4. Wier MS. *Injuries of Nerves and Their Consequences.* Lippincott Williams & Wilkins; 1872.
5. Booth M. *Opium: A History.* St Martins Press; 1996.
6. Institute of Medicine. A century of American narcotic policy. In: Courtwright D, ed. *Treating Drug Problems*, Vol. 2. IOM; 1992:1-62.
7. Witherspoon JA. A protest against some of the evils in the profession of medicine. *JAMA.* 1900;34:1589-1592.
8. Webb v. United States, *249 U.S.* 1919;96: Accessed August 15, 2022. https://tile.loc.gov/storage-services/service/ll/usrep/usrep249/usrep249096/usrep249096.pdf
9. Lee LE Jr. Medication in the control of pain in terminal cancer. *JAMA.* 1941;116:216-219.
10. Rhymes J. Hospice care in America. *JAMA.* 1990;242(3):369-372.
11. Porter J, Jick H. Addiction rare in patients treated with narcotics. *N Engl J Med.* 1980;302:123.
12. Portenoy RK, Foley KM. Chronic use of opioid analgesics in non-malignant pain: report of 36 cases. *Pain.* 1986;25(2):171-186.
13. Melzack R. The tragedy of needless pain. *Sci Am.* 1990;262(2):27-33.
14. [no author listed]. The use of opioids for the treatment of chronic pain. A consensus statement from the American Academy of Pain Medicine and the American Pain Society. *J Pain.* 1997;13(1):6-8.
15. US Veterans Health Administration. *Pain as the Fifth Vital Sign Toolkit.* US Veterans Health Administration; 2000.
16. Frasco PD, Sprung J, Trentman TL. The impact of the Joint Commission for accreditation of healthcare organization pain initiative on perioperative opiate consumption and recovery room length of stay. *Anesth Analg.* 2005;100:162-168.
17. Drug Enforcement Administration. A joint statement from 21 health organizations and the Drug Enforcement Administration. Promoting pain relief and preventing abuse of pain medications: a critical balancing act. *J Pain Symptom Manage.* 2002;24(2):147.
18. Franklin GM, Mai J, Wickizer T, Turner JA, Fulton-Kehoe D, Grant L. Opioid dosing trends and mortality in Washington State workers' compensation, 1996-2002. *Am J Ind Med.* 2005;48(2):91-99.
19. Paulozzi LJ, Jones C, Mack K, Rudd R. Vital signs: overdoses of prescription opioid pain relievers—United States, 1999-2008. *MMWR Morb Mortal Wkly Rep.* 2011;60:1487-1492.
20. Okie S. A flood of opioids, a rising tide of deaths. *N Engl J Med.* 2010;363(21):1981-1985.
21. Food and Drug Administration (FDA). *Questions and Answers: FDA approves a Risk Evaluation and Mitigation Strategy (REMS) for Extended-Release and Long-Acting (ER/LA) Opioid Analgesics.* Accessed October 17, 2023. https://www.fda.gov/drugs/information-drug-class/questions-and-answers-fda-approves-risk-evaluation-and-mitigation-strategy-rems-extended-release-and
22. Consumer Report. *Should you take opioids to treat pain?* Accessed on October 30, 2017. https://www.consumerreports.org/cro/2012/07/should-you-take-opioids-to-treat-pain/index.htm
23. Dowell D, Haegerich TM, Chou R. CDC Guideline for prescribing opioids for chronic pain — United States, 2016. *MMWR Recomm Rep.* 2016;65(1):1-49.
24. Bohnert ASB, Guy GP Jr, Losby JL. Opioid prescribing in the United States before and after the Centers for Disease Control and Prevention's 2016 opioid guideline. *Ann Intern Med.* 2018;169(6):367-375.
25. Demidenko MI, Dobscha SK, Morasco BJ, Meath THA, Ilgen MA, Lovejoy TI. Suicidal ideation and suicidal self-directed violence following clinician-initiated prescription opioid discontinuation among long-term opioid users. *Gen Hosp Psychiatry.* 2017;47:29-35.
26. Agnoli A, Xing G, Tancredi DJ, Magnan E, Jerant A, Fenton JJ. Association of dose tapering with overdose or mental health crisis among patients prescribed long-term opioids. *JAMA.* 2021;326(5):411-419. doi:10.1001/jama.2021.11013
27. Hallvik SE, El Ibrahimi S, Johnston K, et al. Patient outcomes after opioid dose reduction among patients with chronic opioid therapy. *Pain.* 2022;163(1):83-90. doi:10.1097/j.pain.0000000000002298
28. Mackey K, Anderson J, Bourne D, Chen E, Peterson K. *Evidence Brief: Benefits and Harms of Long-term Opioid Dose Reduction or Discontinuation in Patients with Chronic Pain.* Evidence Synthesis Program, Health Services Research and Development Service, Office of Research and Development, Department of Veterans Affairs. VA ESP Project #09-199; 2019. Accessed July 20, 2023. https://www.hsrd.research.va.gov/publications/esp/tapering-opioid.cfm
29. Kroenke K, Alford DP, Argoff C, et al. Challenges with implementing the Centers For Disease Control and Prevention opioid guideline: a consensus panel report. *Pain Med.* 2019;20(4):724-735.
30. Schatman ME, Ziegler SJ. Pain management, prescription opioid mortality, and the CDC: is the devil in the data? *J Pain Res.* 2017;10:2489-2495.
31. Dowell D, Haegerich T, Chou R. No shortcuts to safer opioid prescribing. *N Engl J Med.* 2019;380(24):2285-2287.
32. Centers for Disease Control and Prevention. *CDC Advises Against Misapplication of the Guideline for Prescribing Opioids for Chronic Pain.* Accessed August 12, 2022. https://www.cdc.gov/media/releases/2019/s0424-advises-misapplication-guideline-prescribing-opioids.html
33. Food and Drug Administration. *FDA identifies harm reported from sudden discontinuation of opioid pain medicines and requires label changes to guide prescribers on gradual, individualized tapering.* Accessed August 6, 2022. https://www.fda.gov/drugs/drug-safety-and-availability/fda-identifies-harm-reported-sudden-discontinuation-opioid-pain-medicines-and-requires-label-changes?
34. Coffin PO, Rowe C, Oman N, et al. Illicit opioid use following changes in opioids prescribed for chronic non-cancer pain. *PLoS One.* 2020;15(5):e0232538-e0232538.
35. Mark TL, Parish W. Opioid medication discontinuation and risk of adverse opioid-related health care events. *J Subst Abuse Treat.* 2019;103:58-63.
36. Oliva EM, Bowe T, Manhapra A, et al. Associations between stopping prescriptions for opioids, length of opioid treatment, and overdose or suicide deaths in US veterans: observational evaluation. *BMJ.* 2020;368:m283.
37. American Medical Association. *AMA recommendation to CDC, June 16, 2020 urging the CDC Guideline to start recognizing the need for individualized care for patients with pain.* Accessed August 15, 2022. https://searchlf.ama-assn.org/letter/documentDownload?uri=%2Funstructured%2Fbinary%2Fletter%2FLETTERS%2F2020-6-16-Letter-to-Dowell-re-Opioid-Rx-Guideline.pdf

38. Centers for Disease Control and Prevention. *Federal Register Notice: CDC's updated Clinical Practice Guideline for Prescribing Opioids is now open for public comment*. Accessed August 9, 2022. https://www.cdc.gov/media/releases/2022/s0210-prescribing-opioids.html
39. Center for Disease Control and Prevention. *Prescription Opioid Data*. Accessed August 15, 2022. https://www.cdc.gov/drugoverdose/deaths/prescription/
40. Centers for Disease Control and Prevention. *Drug Overdose Deaths in the U.S. Top 100,000 Annually*. Accessed August 15, 2022. https://www.cdc.gov/nchs/pressroom/nchs_press_releases/2021/20211117.htm
41. Rosenbloom BN, Khan S, McCartney C, Katz J. Systematic review of persistent pain and psychological outcomes following traumatic musculoskeletal injury. *J Pain Res.* 2013;6:39-51.
42. Lavand'homme P. Transition from acute to chronic pain after surgery. *Pain.* 2017;158(4):S50-S54.
43. Richebe P, Capdevila X, Rivat C. Persistent postsurgical pain: pathophysiology and preventive pharmacologic considerations. *Anesthesiology.* 2018;129:590-607.
44. Petersen KK, Simonsen O, Laursen MB, Nielsen TA, Rasmussen S, Arendt-Nielsen L. Chronic postoperative pain after primary and revision total knee arthroplasty. *Clin J Pain.* 2015;31(1):1-6. doi:10.1097/AJP.0000000000000146
45. Petersen KK, Graven-Nielsen T, Simonsen O, Laursen MB, Arendt-Nielsen L. Postoperative pain mechanisms assessed by cuff algometry are associated with chronic postoperative pain relief after total knee replacement. *Pain.* 2016;157(7):1400-1406.
46. Zelaya CE, Dahlhamer JM, Lucas JW, Connor EM. Chronic pain and high-impact chronic pain among U.S. adults, 2019. *NCHS Data Brief.* 2020;(390):1-8.
47. Institute of Medicine of National Institutes of Health. *Relieving Pain in America: a Blueprint for Transforming Prevention, Care, Education and Research.* National Academies Press; 2011.
48. van den Beuken-van Everdingen MH, Hochstenbach LM, Joosten EA, Tjan-Heijnen VC, Janssen DJ. Update on prevalence of pain in patients with cancer: systematic review and meta-analysis. *J Pain Symptom Manage.* 2016;51(6):1070-1090.e9. doi:10.1016/j.jpainsymman.2015.12.340
49. Paice JA, Portenoy R, Lacchetti C, et al. Management of chronic pain in survivors of adult cancers: American Society of Clinical Oncology clinical practice guideline. *J Clin Oncol.* 2016;34(27):3325-3345. doi:10.1200/JCO.2016.68.5206
50. Jiang C, Wang H, Wang Q, Luo Y, Sidlow R, Han X. Prevalence of chronic pain and high-impact chronic pain in cancer survivors in the United States. *JAMA Oncol.* 2019;5(8):1224-1226. doi:10.1001/jamaoncol.2019.1439
51. Sanford NN, Sher DJ, Butler SS, et al. Prevalence of chronic pain among cancer survivors in the United States, 2010-2017. *Cancer.* 2019;125(23):4310-4318. doi:10.1002/cncr.32450
52. Cicero TJ, Lynskey M, Todorov A, Inciardi JA, Surratt HL. Co-morbid pain and psychopathology in males and females admitted to treatment for opioid analgesic abuse. *Pain.* 2008;139(1):127-135.
53. Voon P, Hayashi K, Milloy MJ, et al. Pain among high-risk patients on methadone maintenance treatment. *J Pain.* 2015;16(9):887-894.
54. Barry DT, Cutter CJ, Beitel M, Kerns RD, Liong C, Scottenfeld RS. Psychiatric disorders among patients seeking treatment for co-occurring chronic pain and opioid use disorder. *J Clin Psychiatry.* 2016;77(10):1413-1419.
55. Potter JS, Shiffman SJ, Weiss RD. Chronic pain severity in opioid-dependent patients. *Am J Drug Alcohol Abuse.* 2008;34(1):101-107.
56. Rosenblum A, Joseph H, Fong C, Kipnis S, Cleland C, Portenoy RK. Prevalence and characteristics of chronic pain among chemically dependent patients in methadone maintenance and residential treatment facilities. *JAMA.* 2003;289(18):2370-2378.
57. Jamison RN, Kauffman J, Katz NP. Characteristics of methadone maintenance patients with chronic pain. *J Pain Symptom Manage.* 2000;19(1):53-62.
58. Peles E, Schreiber S, Gordon J, Adelson M. Significantly higher methadone dose for methadone maintenance treatment (MMT) patients with chronic pain. *Pain.* 2005;113(3):340-346.
59. Karasz A, Zallman L, Berg K, Gourevitch M, Selwyn P, Arnsten JH. The experience of chronic severe pain in patients undergoing methadone maintenance treatment. *J Pain Symptom Manage.* 2004;28(5):517-525.
60. Ilgen MA, Trafton JA, Humphreys K. Response to methadone maintenance treatment of opiate dependent patients with and without significant pain. *Drug Alcohol Depend.* 2006;82(3):187-193.
61. Novak SP, Herman-Stahl M, Flannery B, Zimmerman M. Physical pain, common psychiatric and substance use disorders, and the non-medical use of prescription analgesics in the United States. *Drug Alcohol Depend.* 2009;100(1-2):63-70.
62. Tsui JI, Lira MC, Cheng DM, et al. Chronic pain, craving, and illicit opioid use among patients receiving opioid agonist therapy. *Drug Alcohol Depend.* 2016;166:26-31.
63. Griffin ML, McDermott KA, McHugh RK, Fitzmaurice GM, Jamison RN, Weiss RD. Longitudinal association between pain severity and subsequent opioid use in prescription opioid dependent patients with chronic pain. *Drug Alcohol Depend.* 2016;163:216-221.
64. West SL. Substance use among persons with traumatic brain injury: a review. *NeuroRehabilitation.* 2011;29(1):1-8.
65. MacLeod JB, Hungerford DW. Alcohol-related injury visits: do we know the true prevalence in U.S. trauma centres. *Injury.* 2011;42(9):922-926.
66. Department of Defense, Department of Veterans Affairs. *VA/DoD Clinical Practice Guideline: Management of Opioid Therapy for Chronic Pain.* 2022. Accessed on August 8, 2022. https://www.healthquality.va.gov/guidelines/Pain/cot/
67. Department of Defense, Department of Veterans Affairs. *VA/DoD Clinical Practice Guideline: Diagnosis and Treatment of Low Back Pain (LBP).* 2022. Accessed August 15, 2022. https://www.healthquality.va.gov/guidelines/Pain/lbp/
68. Wick EC, Grant MC, Wu CL. Postoperative multimodal analgesia pain management with nonopioid analgesics and techniques: a review. *JAMA Surg.* 2017;152(7):691-697. doi:10.1001/jamasurg.2017.0898
69. McEvoy MD, Raymond BL, Krige A. Opioid-sparing perioperative analgesia within enhanced recovery programs. *Anesthesiol Clin.* 2022;40(1):35-58. doi:10.1016/j.anclin.2021.11.001
70. Cheung CK, Adeola JO, Beutler SS, Urman RD. Postoperative pain management in enhanced recovery pathways. *J Pain Res.* 2022;15:123-135. doi:10.2147/JPR.S231774
71. Tan M, Law LS, Gan TJ. Optimizing pain management to facilitate Enhanced Recovery After Surgery pathways. *Can J Anaesth.* 2015;62(2):203-218. doi:10.1007/s12630-014-0275-x
72. World Health Organization. *Cancer Pain Relief: With a Guide to Opioid Availability.* 2nd ed. World Health Organization; 1996.
73. Wiffen PJ, Wee B, Derry S, Bell RF, Moore RA. Opioids for cancer pain – an overview of Cochrane reviews. *Cochrane Database Syst Rev.* 2017;7:CD012592.
74. Zajączkowska R, Kocot-Kępska M, Leppert W, Wordliczek J. Bone pain in cancer patients: mechanisms and current treatment. *Int J Mol Sci.* 2019;20(23):6047. doi:10.3390/ijms20236047
75. Yoon SY, Oh J. Neuropathic cancer pain: prevalence, pathophysiology, and management. *Korean J Intern Med.* 2018;33(6):1058-1069. doi:10.3904/kjim.2018.162
76. Rodrigue D, Winkelmann J, Price M, Kalandranis E, Klempner L, Kapoor-Hintzen N. Opioid misuse: an organizational response while managing cancer-related pain. *Clin J Oncol Nurs.* 2020;24(2):170-176. doi:10.1188/20.CJON.170-176
77. Reddy A, de la Cruz M. Safe opioid use, storage, and disposal strategies in cancer pain management. *Oncologist.* 2019;24(11):1410-1415. doi:10.1634/theoncologist.2019-0242
78. Gaertner J, Boehlke C, Simone CB II, Hui D. Early palliative care and the opioid crisis: ten pragmatic steps towards a more rational use of opioids. *Ann Palliat Med.* 2019;8(4):490-497. doi:10.21037/apm.2019.08.01
79. American Hospital Association. *Stem the Tide: Opioid Stewardship Measurement and Implementation Guide.* 2020. Accessed August 15, 2022. https://www.aha.org/system/files/media/file/2020/07/HIIN-opioid-guide-0520.pdf

80. Weiner SG, Price CN, Atalay AJ, et al. A health system-wide initiative to decrease opioid-related morbidity and mortality. *Jt Comm J Qual Patient Saf.* 2019;45(1):3-13. doi:10.1016/j.jcjq.2018.07.003
81. Reuben DB, Alvanzo AA, Ashikaga T, et al. National Institutes of Health Pathways to Prevention Workshop: the role of opioids in the treatment of chronic pain. *Ann Intern Med.* 2015;162(4):295-300.
82. Clauw DJ, Essex MN, Pitman V, Jones KD. Reframing chronic pain as a disease, not a symptom: rationale and implications for pain management. *Postgrad Med.* 2019;131(3):185-198. doi:10.1080/00325481.2019.1574403
83. Rusu AC, Gajsar H, Schlüter MC, Bremer YI. Cognitive biases toward pain: implications for a neurocognitive processing perspective in chronic pain and its interaction with depression. *Clin J Pain.* 2019;35(3): 252-260. doi:10.1097/AJP.0000000000000674
84. U.S. Department of Health and Human Services. *Pain Management Best Practices Inter-Agency Task Force Report: Updates, Gaps, Inconsistencies, and Recommendations.* Accessed October 17, 2023. https://www.hhs.gov/sites/default/files/pain-mgmt-best-practices-draft-final-report-05062019.pdf
85. McCracken LM, Vowles KE. Acceptance and commitment therapy and mindfulness for chronic pain: model, process, and progress. *Am Psychol.* 2014;69(2):178-187. doi:10.1037/a0035623
86. Bernard P, Romain AJ, Caudroit J, et al. Cognitive behavior therapy combined with exercise for adults with chronic diseases: systematic review and meta-analysis. *Health Psychol.* 2018;37(5):433-450. doi:10.1037/hea0000578
87. Savage SR, Joranson DE, Covington EC, Schnoll SH, Heit HA, Gilson AM. Definitions related to the medical use of opioids: evolution towards universal agreement. *J Pain Symptom Manage.* 2003;26(1):655-667.
88. Evans CJ, Cahill CM. Neurobiology of opioid dependence in creating addiction vulnerability. *F1000Res.* 2016;5:F1000 Faculty Rev-1748. doi:10.12688/f1000research.8369.1
89. Koob GF, Volkow ND. Neurobiology of addiction: a neurocircuitry analysis. *Lancet Psychiatry.* 2016;3(8):760-773.
90. Jaffe J. Opiates: clinical aspects. In: Lowinson J, Ruiz P, Millman R, eds. *Substance Abuse: A Comprehensive Textbook.* Williams & Wilkins; 1992:186-194.
91. Younger J, Barelka P, Carroll I, et al. Reduced cold pain tolerance in chronic pain patients following opioid detoxification. *Pain Med.* 2008;9:1158-1163.
92. Hooten WM, Mantilla CB, Sandroni P, Townsend CO. Associations between heat pain perception and opioid dose among patients with chronic pain undergoing opioid tapering. *Pain Med.* 2010;11(11):1587-1598.
93. Wang H, Akbar M, Weinsheimer N, Gantz S, Schiltenwolf M. Longitudinal observation of changes in pain sensitivity during opioid tapering in patients with chronic low-back pain. *Pain Med.* 2011;12:1720-1726.
94. Brodner RA, Taub A. Chronic pain exacerbated by long-term narcotic use in patients with non-malignant disease: clinical syndrome and treatment. *Mt Sinai J Med.* 1978;45:233-237.
95. American Psychiatric Association. *About DSM-5-TR.* Accessed August 15, 2022. https://www.psychiatry.org/psychiatrists/practice/dsm/about-dsm.
96. Volkow ND, McLellan AT. Opioid abuse in chronic pain--misconceptions and mitigation strategies. *N Engl J Med.* 2016;374(13):1253-1263.
97. Ballantyne JC, Sullivan MD, Kolodny A. Opioid dependence vs addiction: a distinction without a difference? *Arch Intern Med.* 2012;172(17):1342-1343.
98. Foley K. Clinical tolerance to opioids. In: Basbaum A, Besson J, eds. *Towards a New Pharmacotherapy of Pain.* John Wiley & Sons; 1991:181-203.
99. Taylor DA, Fleming WW. Unifying perspectives of the mechanisms underlying the development of tolerance and physical dependence to opioids. *J Pharmacol Exp Ther.* 2001;297:11-18.
100. Williams JT, Ingram SL, Henderson G, et al. Regulation of mu-opioid receptors: desensitization, phosphorylation, internalization, and tolerance. *Pharmacol Rev.* 2013;65:223-254.
101. Collins E, Cesselin F. Neurobiological mechanisms of opioid tolerance and dependence. *Clin Neuropharmacol.* 1991;14:465-488.
102. Sánchez-Blázquez P, Rodríguez-Muñoz M, Berrocoso E, Garzón J. The plasticity of the association between mu-opioid receptor and glutamate ionotropic receptor N in opioid analgesic tolerance and neuropathic pain. *Eur J Pharmacol.* 2013;716(1-3):94-105.
103. Cahill CM, Walwyn W, Taylor AM, Pradhan AA, Evans CJ. Allostatic mechanisms of opioid tolerance beyond desensitization and downregulation. *Trends Pharmacol Sci.* 2016;37(11):963-976.
104. Hutchinson MR, Shavit Y, Grace PM, Rice KC, Maier SF, Watkins LR. Exploring the neuroimmunopharmacology of opioids: an integrative review of mechanisms of central immune signaling and their implications for opioid analgesia. *Pharmacol Rev.* 2011;63(3):772-810.
105. Roth SH, Fleischmann RM, Burch FX, et al. Around-the-clock, controlled-release oxycodone therapy for osteoarthritis-related pain: placebo-controlled trial and long-term evaluation. *Arch Intern Med.* 2000;27(160):853-860.
106. Schuh-Hofer S, Wodarski R, Pfau DB, et al. One night of total sleep deprivation promotes a state of generalized hyperalgesia: a surrogate pain model to study the relationship of insomnia and pain. *Pain.* 2013;154(9):1613-1621.
107. Nijs J, Loggia ML, Polli A, et al. Sleep disturbances and severe stress as glial activators: key targets for treating central sensitization in chronic pain patients? *Expert Opin Ther Targets.* 2017;21(8):817-826.
108. Sluka KA, Clauw DJ. Neurobiology of fibromyalgia and chronic widespread pain. *Neuroscience.* 2016;338:114-129.
109. Goldenberg DL, Clauw DJ, Palmer RE, Clair AG. Opioid use in fibromyalgia: a cautionary tale. *Mayo Clin Proc.* 2016;91(5):640-648.
110. Baron MJ, McDonald PW. Significant pain reduction in chronic pain patients after detoxification from high dose opioids. *J Opioid Manag.* 2006;2(5):277-282.
111. Krumova EK, Bennemann P, Kindler D, Schwarzer A, Zenz M, Maier C. Low pain intensity after opioid withdrawal as a first step of a comprehensive pain rehabilitation program predicts long-term nonuse of opioids in chronic noncancer pain. *Clin J Pain.* 2013;29:760-769.
112. Darchuk KM, Townsend CO, Rome JD, Bruce BK, Hooten WM. Longitudinal treatment outcomes for geriatric patients with chronic non-cancer pain at an interdisciplinary pain rehabilitation program. *Pain Med.* 2010;11:1352-1364.
113. Hayhurst CJ, Durieux ME. Differential opioid tolerance and opioid-induced hyperalgesia: a clinical reality. *Anesthesiology.* 2016;124(2):483-488.
114. Compton P, Halabicky OM, Aryal S, Badiola I. Opioid taper is associated with improved experimental pain tolerance in patients with chronic pain: an observational study. *Pain Ther.* 2022;11(1):303-313. doi:10.1007/s40122-021-00348-8
115. Miller NS, Swiney T, Barkin RL. Effects of opioid prescription medication dependence and detoxification on pain perceptions and self-reports. *Am J Ther.* 2006;13(5):436-444.
116. Yi P, Pryzbylkowski P. Opioid induced hyperalgesia. *Pain Med.* 2015;16(Suppl 1):S32-S36.
117. Brush DE. Complications of long-term opioid therapy for management of chronic pain: the paradox of opioid-induced hyperalgesia. *J Med Toxicol.* 2012;8(4):387-392.
118. Lee M, Silverman SM, Hansen H, Patel VB, Manchikanti L. A comprehensive review of opioid-induced hyperalgesia. *Pain Physician.* 2011;14(2):145-161.
119. Célèrier E, Rivat C, Jun Y, et al. Long-lasting hyperalgesia induced by fentanyl in rats: preventive effect of ketamine. *Anesthesiology.* 2000;92:465-472.
120. Liang DY, Liao G, Wang J, et al. A genetic analysis of opioid-induced hyperalgesia in mice. *Anesthesiology.* 2006;104:1054-1062.
121. Angst MS, Clark JD. Opioid-induced hyperalgesia: a qualitative systematic review. *Anesthesiology.* 2006;104:570-587.
122. Chang G, Chen L, Mao J. Opioid tolerance and hyperalgesia. *Med Clin North Am.* 2007;91(2):199-211. doi:10.1016/j.mcna.2006.10.003
123. Roeckel LA, Le Coz GM, Gavériaux-Ruff C, Simonin F. Opioid-induced hyperalgesia: cellular and molecular mechanisms. *Neuroscience.* 2016;338:160-182.
124. Jin H, Sun YT, Guo GQ, et al. Spinal TRPC6 channels contributes to morphine-induced antinociceptive tolerance and hyperalgesia in rats. *Neurosci Lett.* 2017;639:138-145.
125. Donaldson R, Sun Y, Liang DY, et al. The multiple PDZ domain protein Mpdz/MUPP1 regulates opioid tolerance and opioid-induced hyperalgesia. *BMC Genomics.* 2016;17:313.

126. Kim SH, Stoicea N, Soghomonyan S, Bergese SD. Remifentanil-acute opioid tolerance and opioid-induced hyperalgesia: a systematic review. *Am J Ther.* 2015;22(3):e62-e74.
127. Liang DY, Li X, Clark JD. Epigenetic regulation of opioid-induced hyperalgesia, dependence, and tolerance in mice. *J Pain.* 2013;14(1):36-47.
128. Fletcher D, Martinez V. Opioid-induced hyperalgesia in patients after surgery: a systematic review and a meta-analysis. *Br J Anaesth.* 2014;112(6):991-1004.
129. Malik OS, Kaye AD, Urman RD. Perioperative hyperalgesia and associated clinical factors. *Curr Pain Headache Rep.* 2017;21(1):4.
130. Yu EH, Tran DH, Lam SW, Irwin MG. Remifentanil tolerance and hyperalgesia: short-term gain, long-term pain? *Anaesthesia.* 2016;71(11):1347-1362.
131. Angst MS. Intraoperative use of remifentanil for tiva: postoperative pain, acute tolerance, and opioid-induced hyperalgesia. *J Cardiothorac Vasc Anesth.* 2015;29(Suppl 1):S16-S22.
132. Fletcher D, Martinez V. How can we prevent opioid induced hyperalgesia in surgical patients? *Br J Anaesth.* 2016;116(4):447-449.
133. Weinbroum AA. Postoperative hyperalgesia–A clinically applicable narrative review. *Pharmacol Res.* 2017;120:188-205.
134. Chu LF, Clark D. Opioid-induced hyperalgesia in humans: molecular mechanisms and clinical considerations. *Clin J Pain.* 2008;24(6):479-496.
135. Suzan E, Eisenberg E, Treister R, Haddad M, Pud D. A negative correlation between hyperalgesia and analgesia in patients with chronic radicular pain: is hydromorphone therapy a double-edged sword? *Pain Physician.* 2013;16(1):65-76.
136. Kim SH, Yoon DM, Choi KW, Yoon KB. High-dose daily opioid administration and poor functional status intensify local anesthetic injection pain in cancer patients. *Pain Physician.* 2013;16(3):E247-E256.
137. Hay JL, White JM, Bochner F, Somoygi AA, Semple TJ, Rounsefell B. Hyperalgesia in opioid-managed chronic pain and opioid-dependent patients. *J Pain.* 2009;10(3):316-322.
138. Chu LF, Clark DJ, Angst MS. Opioid tolerance and hyperalgesia in chronic pain patients after one month of oral morphine therapy: a preliminary prospective study. *J Pain.* 2006;7:43-48.
139. Fishbain DA, Cole B, Lewis JE, Gao J, Rosomoff RS. Do opioids induce hyperalgesia in humans? An evidence-based structured review. *Pain Med.* 2009;10(5):829-839.
140. Frank JW, Lovejoy TI, Becker WC, et al. Patient outcomes in dose reduction or discontinuation of long-term opioid therapy. *Ann Intern Med.* 2017;167:181-191.
141. Mackey K, Anderson J, Bourne D, Chen E, Peterson K. Benefits and harms of long-term opioid dose reduction or discontinuation in patients with chronic pain: a rapid review. *J Gen Intern Med.* 2020;35(Suppl 3):935-944. doi:10.1007/s11606-020-06253-8
142. Le Merrer J, Becker JA, Befort K, Kieffer BL. Reward processing by the opioid system in the brain. *Physiol Rev.* 2009;89(4):1379-1412.
143. Wang YH, Sun JF, Tao YM, Chi ZQ, Liu JG. The role of kappa-opioid receptor activation in mediating antinociception and addiction. *Acta Pharmacol Sin.* 2010;31(9):1065-1070.
144. Hurd YL. Perspectives on current directions in the neurobiology of addiction disorders relevant to genetic risk factors. *CNS Spectr.* 2006;11(11):855-862.
145. Bieber CM, Fernandez K, Borsook D, et al. Retrospective accounts of initial subjective effects of opioids in patients treated for pain who do or do not develop opioid addiction: a pilot case–control study. *Exp Clin Psychopharmacol.* 2008;16(5):429-434.
146. Marsch LA, Bickel WK, Badger GJ, et al. Effects of infusion rate of intravenously administered morphine on physiological, psychomotor, and self-reported measures in humans. *J Pharmacol Exp Ther.* 2001;299(3):1056-1065.
147. Food and Drug Administration. *Transmucosal Immediate-Release Fentanyl (TIRF) Medicines.* Accessed August 15, 2022. https://www.fda.gov/drugs/information-drug-class/transmucosal-immediate-release-fentanyl-tirf-medicines
148. Pasternak GW. Opioid and their receptors: are we there yet? *Neuropharmacology.* 2013;1(13):135-144.
149. Zacny JP, Klafta JM, Coalson DW, et al. The effects of cold water emersion on the reinforcing and subjective effects of fentanyl in health volunteers. *Drug Alcohol Depend.* 1996;42(3):197-200.
150. Martin TJ, Ewan E. Chronic pain alters drug self-administration: implications for addiction and pain mechanisms. *Exp Clin Psychopharmacol.* 2008;16(5):357-366.
151. Moore RA, McQuay HJ. Prevalence of opioid adverse events in chronic non-malignant pain: systematic review of randomised trials of oral opioids. *Arthritis Res Ther.* 2005;7(5):R1046-R1051.
152. Furlan AD, Sandoval JA, Mailis-Gagnon A, Tunks E. Opioids for chronic noncancer pain: a meta-analysis of effectiveness and side effects. *CMAJ.* 2006;174(11):1589-1594.
153. Eisenberg E, McNicol E, Carr DB. Opioids for neuropathic pain. *Cochrane Database Syst Rev.* 2006;(3):CD006146.
154. Vowles KE, McEntee ML, Julnes PS, Frohe T, Ney JP, van der Goes DN. Rates of opioid misuse, abuse, and addiction in chronic pain: a systematic review and data synthesis. *Pain.* 2015;156(4):569-576. doi:10.1097/01.j.pain.0000460357.01998.f1
155. Boscarino JA, Hoffman SN, Han JJ. Opioid-use disorder among patients on long-term opioid therapy: impact of final DSM-5 diagnostic criteria on prevalence and correlates. *Subst Abuse Rehabil.* 2015;6:83-91.
156. Saitz R, Miller SC, Fiellin DA, Rosenthal RN. Recommended use of terminology in addiction medicine. *J Addict Med.* 2021;15(1):3-7. doi:10.1097/ADM.0000000000000673
157. Rogers AH, Zvolensky MJ, Ditre JW, Buckner JD, Asmundson GJG. Association of opioid misuse with anxiety and depression: a systematic review of the literature. *Clin Psychol Rev.* 2021;84:101978. doi:10.1016/j.cpr.2021.101978
158. Rogers AH, Garey L, Bakhshaie J, Viana AG, Ditre JW, Zvolensky MJ. Anxiety, depression, and opioid misuse among adults with chronic pain: the role of anxiety sensitivity. *Clin J Pain.* 2020;36(11):862-867. doi:10.1097/AJP.0000000000000870
159. Feingold D, Brill S, Goor-Aryeh I, Delayahu Y, Lev-Ran S. Misuse of prescription opioids among chronic pain patients suffering from anxiety: a cross-sectional analysis. *Gen Hosp Psychiatry.* 2017;47:36-42. doi:10.1016/j.genhosppsych.2017.04.006
160. Wilsey B, Fishman S, Tsodikov A, Ogden C, Symreng I, Ernst A. Psychological co-morbidities predicting prescription opioid abuse among patient in chronic pain presenting to the emergency department. *Pain Med.* 2008;9:1107-1117.
161. Weissman DE, Haddox JD. Opioid pseudoaddiction: an iatrogenic syndrome. *Pain.* 1989;36:363-366.
162. Greene MS, Chambers RA. Pseudoaddiction: fact or fiction? An investigation of the medical literature. *Curr Addict Rep.* 2015;2(4):310-317.
163. Kaczmarek E. Promoting diseases to promote drugs: the role of the pharmaceutical industry in fostering good and bad medicalization. *Br J Clin Pharmacol.* 2022;88(1):34-39. doi:10.1111/bcp.14835
164. Edlund MJ, Steffick D, Hudson T, Harris KM, Sullivan M. Risk factors for clinically recognized opioid abuse and dependence among veterans using opioid for chronic non-cancer pain. *Pain.* 2007;129:355-362.
165. Morasco B, Dobscha S. Prescription medication misuse and substance use disorder in VA primary care patients with chronic pain. *Gen Hosp Psychiatry.* 2008;30:93-99.
166. Ives TJ, Chelminski PR, Hammett-Stabler CA, et al. Predictors of opioid misuse in patients with chronic pain: a prospective cohort study. *BMC Health Serv Res.* 2006;6:46. doi:10.1186/1472-6963-6-46
167. Meghani SH, Wiedemer NL, Becker WC, Gracely EJ, Gallagher RM. Predictors of resolution of aberrant drug behavior in chronic pain patients treated in a structured opioid risk management program. *Pain Med.* 2009;10(5):858-865.
168. Wasan AD, Butler SF, Budman SH, et al. Does report of craving opioid medication predict aberrant drug behavior among chronic pain patients? *Clin J Pain.* 2009;25:193-198.
169. Martel MO, Dolman AJ, Edwards RR, Jamison RN, Wasan AD. The association between negative affect and prescription opioid misuse in patients with chronic pain: the mediating role of opioid craving. *J Pain.* 2014;15(1):90-100.

170. Cheatle MD, Obrien CP, Mathai K, Hansen M, Grasso M, Yi P. Aberrant behaviors in a primary care-based cohort of patients with chronic pain identified as misusing prescription opioids. *J Opioid Manag.* 2013;9(5):315-324.
171. Keall R, Keall P, Kiani C, Luckett T, McNeill R, Lovell M. A systematic review of assessment approaches to predict opioid misuse in people with cancer. *Support Care Cancer.* 2022;30(7):5645-5658. doi:10.1007/s00520-022-06895-w
172. Chou R, Fanciullo GJ, Fine PG, Miaskowski C, Passik SD, Portenoy RK. Opioids for chronic noncancer pain: prediction and identification of aberrant drug-related behaviors: a review of the evidence for an American Pain Society and American Academy of Pain Medicine clinical practice guideline. *J Pain.* 2009;10(2):131-146. doi:10.1016/j.jpain.2008.10.009
173. Webster LR, Webster RM. Predicting aberrant behaviors in opioid-treated patients: preliminary validation of the Opioid Risk Tool. *Pain Med.* 2005;6(6):432-442.
174. Butler SF, Budman SH, Fernandez KC, Fanciullo GJ, Jamison RN. Cross validation of a screener to predict opioid misuse in chronic pain patients (SOAPP-R). *J Addict Med.* 2009;3(2):66-73.
175. Jones T, Lookatch S, Grant P, McIntyre J, Moore T. Further validation of an opioid risk assessment tool: the Brief Risk Interview. *J Opioid Manag.* 2014;10:353-364.
176. Jones T, Moore T, Levy JL, et al. A comparison of various risk screening methods in predicting discharge from opioid treatment. *Clin J Pain.* 2012;28:93-100.
177. Moore TM, Jones T, Browder JH, Daffron S, Passik SD. A comparison of common screening methods for predicting aberrant drug-related behavior among patients receiving opioids for chronic pain management. *Pain Med.* 2009;10:1426-1433.
178. Oliva EM, Bowe T, Tavakoli S, et al. Development and applications of the Veterans Health Administration's Stratification Tool for Opioid Risk Mitigation (STORM) to improve opioid safety and prevent overdose and suicide. *Psychol Serv.* 2017;14(1):34-49. doi:10.1037/ser0000099
179. Wu SM, Compton P, Bolus R, et al. The addiction behaviors checklist: validation of a new clinician-based measure of inappropriate opioid use in chronic pain. *J Pain Symptom Manage.* 2006;32(4):342-351.
180. Compton P, Wu SM, Schieffer B, Pham Q, Naliboff BD. Introduction of self-report version of the prescription drug use questionnaire and relationship to medication agreement non-compliance. *J Pain Symptom Manage.* 2008;36(4):383-395.
181. Meltzer EC, Rybin D, Saitz R, et al. Identifying prescription opioid use disorder in primary care: diagnostic characteristics of the current opioid misuse measure (COMM). *Pain.* 2011;152(2):397-402.
182. Jamison RN, Ross EL, Michna E, Chen LQ, Holcomb C, Wasan AD. Substance misuse treatment for high-risk chronic pain patients on opioid therapy: a randomized trial. *Pain.* 2010;150(3):390-400.
183. American Psychiatric Association. *Diagnostic and Statistical Manual of Mental Disorders, Fifth Edition.* Text Revision (DSM-5-TR). American Psychiatric Association Publishing; 2022.
184. Kolb L. Types and characteristics of drug addicts. *Ment Hyg.* 1925;9:300.
185. Rayport M. Experience in the management of patients medically addicted to narcotics. *JAMA.* 1954;165:684-691.
186. Perry S, Heindrich G. Management of pain during debridement: a survey of U.S. burn units. *Pain.* 1982;13:12-14.
187. Volkow ND, Koob GF, McLellan AT. Neurobiologic advances from the brain disease model of addiction. *N Engl J Med.* 2016;374(4):363-371. doi:10.1056/NEJMra1511480
188. Substance Abuse and Mental Health Services Administration. *Key substance use and mental health indicators in the United States: Results from the 2020 National Survey on Drug Use and Health (HHS Publication No. PEP21-07-01-003, NSDUH Series H-56).* Center for Behavioral Health Statistics and Quality, Substance Abuse and Mental Health Services Administration; 2021.
189. Turk D, Swanson K, Gatchel R. Predicting opioid misuse by chronic pain patients: a systematic review and literature synthesis. *Clin J Pain.* 2008;24:497-508.
190. Seghal N, Manchikanti L, Smith H. Prescription opioid abuse in chronic pain: a review of opioid abuse predictors and strategies to curb opioid abuse. *Pain Physician.* 2012;15:ES67-ES92.
191. Ahmed S, Bhivandkar S, Lonergan BB, Suzuki J. Microinduction of buprenorphine/naloxone: a review of the literature. *Am J Addict.* 2021;30(4):305-315. doi:10.1111/ajad.13135
192. Pasternak GW. Preclinical pharmacology and opioid combinations. *Pain Med.* 2012;13(Suppl 1):4-11.
193. Somogyi AA, Barratt DT, Collier JK. Pharmacogenetics of opioids. *Clin Pharmacol Ther.* 2007;81(3):429-444.
194. Lötsch J, Geisslinger G. Are mu-opioid receptor polymorphisms important for clinical opioid therapy? *Trends Mol Med.* 2005;11(2):82-89.
195. Stamer UM, Zhang L, Stuber F. Personalized therapy in pain management: where do we stand? *Pharmacogenetics.* 2010;11(6):843-864.
196. Branford R, Droney J, Ross JR. Opioid genetics: the key to personalized pain control? *Clin Genet.* 2012;82(4):301-310.
197. Gray K, Adhikary SD, Janicki P. Pharmacogenomics of analgesics in anesthesia practice: a current update of literature. *J Anaesthesiol Clin Pharmacol.* 2018;34(2):155-160. doi:10.4103/joacp.JOACP_319_17
198. Peiró AM. Pharmacogenetics in pain treatment. *Adv Pharmacol.* 2018;83:247-273. doi:10.1016/bs.apha.2018.04.004
199. Chou R, Weimer MB, Dana T. Methadone overdose and cardiac arrhythmia potential: findings from a review of the evidence for an American Pain Society and College on Problems of Drug Dependence clinical practice guideline. *J Pain.* 2014;15(4):338-365.
200. Chou R, Cruciani RA, Fiellin DA, et al. Methadone safety: a clinical practice guideline from the American Pain Society and College on Problems of Drug Dependence, in collaboration with the Heart Rhythm Society. *J Pain.* 2014;15(4):321-337.
201. McNicol ED, Ferguson MC, Schumann R. Methadone for neuropathic pain in adults. *Cochrane Database Syst Rev.* 2017;5:CD012499.
202. Kharash ED, Stubbert K. The role of cytochrome p4502B6 in methadone metabolism and clearance. *J Clin Pharmacol.* 2013;53(3):305-313.
203. Moryl N, Santiago-Palma J, Kornick C, et al. Pitfalls of opioid rotation: substituting another opioid for methadone in patients with cancer pain. *Pain.* 2002;96:325-328.
204. Wee S, Koob GF. The role of the dynorphin-kappa opioid system in the reinforcing effects of drugs of abuse. *Psychopharmacology (Berl).* 2010;210(2):121-135.
205. Kaski SW, White AN, Gross JD, Siderovski DP. Potential for kappa-opioid receptor agonists to engineer nonaddictive analgesics: a narrative review. *Anesth Analg.* 2021;132(2):406-419. doi:10.1213/ANE.0000000000005309
206. Paton KF, Atigari DV, Kaska S, Prisinzano T, Kivell BM. Strategies for developing κ opioid receptor agonists for the treatment of pain with fewer side effects. *J Pharmacol Exp Ther.* 2020;375(2):332-348. doi:10.1124/jpet.120.000134
207. Fillingim RB, Gear RW. Sex differences in opioid analgesia: clinical and experimental findings. *Eur J Pain.* 2004;8(5):413-425.
208. Lutfy K, Cowan A. Buprenorphine: a unique drug with complex pharmacology. *Curr Neuropharmacol.* 2004;2(4):395-402.
209. Wakhlu S. Buprenorphine: a review. *J Opioid Manag.* 2009;5(1):59-64.
210. Substance Abuse and Mental Health Services Administration. *Waiver Elimination (MAT Act).* Accessed October 17, 2023. https://www.samhsa.gov/medications-substance-use-disorders/waiver-elimination-mat-act#:~:text=What%20does%20this%20mean%20for,on%20opioid%20use%20disorder%20prescriptions
211. Vadivelu N, Hines RL. Management of chronic pain in the elderly: focus on transdermal buprenorphine. *Clin Interv Aging.* 2008;3(3):421-430.
212. Plosker GL. Buprenorphine 5, 10 and 20 μg/h transdermal patch: a review of its use in the management of chronic non-malignant pain. *Drugs.* 2011;71(18):2491-2509.
213. Heit HA, Gourlay DL. Buprenorphine: new tricks with an old molecule for pain management. *Clin J Pain.* 2008;24(2):93-97.
214. Yokell MA, Zaller ND, Green TC, Rich JD. Buprenorphine and buprenorphine/naloxone diversion, misuse, and illicit use: an international review. *Curr Drug Abuse Rev.* 2011;4(1):28-41.

215. Allen B, Harocopos A. Non-prescribed buprenorphine in New York city: motivations for use, practices of diversion, and experiences of stigma. *J Subst Abuse Treat.* 2016;70:81-86. doi:10.1016/j.jsat.2016.08.002
216. Chilcoat HD, Amick HR, Sherwood MR, Dunn KE. Buprenorphine in the United States: motives for abuse, misuse, and diversion. *J Subst Abuse Treat.* 2019;104:148-157. doi:10.1016/j.jsat.2019.07.005
217. Cicero TJ, Inciardi JA, Adams EH, et al. Rates of abuse of tramadol remain unchanged with the introduction of new branded and generic products: results of an abuse monitoring system, 1994-2004. *Pharmacoepidemiol Drug Saf.* 2005;14(12):851-859.
218. Santos J, Alarcao J, Fareleira F, Vaz-Carneiro A, Costa J. Tapentadol for chronic musculoskeletal pain in adults. *Cochrane Database Syst Rev.* 2015;5:CD009923.
219. Schwartz S, Etropolski M, Shapiro DY, et al. Safety and efficacy of tapentadol ER in patients with painful diabetic peripheral neuropathy: results of a randomized-withdrawal, placebo-controlled trial. *Curr Med Res Opin.* 2011;27(1):151-162.
220. Doran GT. There's a S.M.A.R.T. way to write management's goals and objectives. *Management Review.* 1981;70(11):35-36.
221. Food and Drug Administration. *Abuse Deterrent Opioids- Evaluation and Labeling.* Accessed August 15, 2022. http://www.fda.gov/downloads/Drugs/GuidanceComplianceRegulatoryInformation/Guidances/UCM334743.pdf
222. Bannwarth B. Will abuse-deterrent formulations of opioid analgesics be successful in achieving their purpose? *Drugs.* 2012;72(13):1713-1723. doi:10.2165/11635860-000000000-00000
223. Stanos SP, Bruckenthal P, Barkin RL. Strategies to reduce the tampering and subsequent abuse of long-acting opioids: potential risks and benefits of formulations with physical or pharmacologic deterrents to tampering. *Mayo Clin Proc.* 2012;87(7):683-694.
224. Lourenço LM, Matthews M, Jamison RN. Abuse-deterrent and tamper-resistant opioids: how valuable are novel formulations in thwarting non-medical use? *Expert Opin Drug Deliv.* 2013;10(2):229-240.
225. Rana D, Salave S, Benival D. Emerging trends in abuse-deterrent formulations: technological insights and regulatory considerations. *Curr Drug Deliv.* 2022;19(8):846-859. doi:10.2174/1567201818666211208101035
226. Pergolizzi JV Jr, Raffa RB, Taylor R Jr, Vacalis S. Abuse-deterrent opioids: an update on current approaches and considerations. *Curr Med Res Opin.* 2018;34(4):711-723. doi:10.1080/03007995.2017.1419171
227. Fordyce W. Opioids, pain and behavioral outcomes. *Am Pain Soc J.* 1992;1(4):282-284.
228. Højsted J, Sjøgren P. Addiction to opioids in chronic pain patients: a literature review. *Eur J Pain.* 2007;11(5):490-518.
229. Smith H. A comprehensive review of rapid onset opioids for breakthrough pain. *CNS Drugs.* 2012;26(6):509-535.
230. Zeppetella G, Davies AN. Opioids for the management of breakthrough pain in cancer patients. *Cochrane Database Syst Rev.* 2013;(10):CD004311.
231. Mehta V, Langford RM. Acute pain management for opioid dependent patients. *Anaesthesia.* 2006;61(3):269-276.
232. MacIntyre PE, Loadsman JA, Scott DA. Opioids, ventilation and acute pain management. *Anaesth Intensive Care.* 2011;39(4):545-558.
233. Zutler M, Holty JE. Opioid, sleep and sleep-disordered breathing. *Curr Pharm Des.* 2011;17(15):1443-1449.
234. Turner BJ, Liang Y. Drug overdose in a retrospective cohort with non-cancer pain treated with opioids, antidepressants, and/or sedative-hypnotics: interactions with mental health disorders. *J Gen Intern Med.* 2015;30(8):1081-1096.
235. Dahan A, Overdyk F, Smith T, Aarts L, Niesters M. Pharmacovigilance: a review of opioid-induced respiratory depression in chronic pain patients. *Pain Physician.* 2013;16(2):E85-E94.
236. Jones CM, Compton W, Vythilingam M, Giroir B. Naloxone co-prescribing to patients receiving prescription opioids in the Medicare Part D Program, United States, 2016-2017. *JAMA.* 2019;322(5):462-464. doi:10.1001/jama.2019.7988
237. Watson A, Guay K, Ribis D. Assessing the impact of clinical pharmacists on naloxone co-prescribing in the primary care setting. *Am J Health Syst Pharm.* 2020;77(7):568-573. doi:10.1093/ajhp/zxaa007
238. Brock C, Olesen SS, Olesen AE, Frøkjaer JB, Andresen T, Drewes AM. Opioid-induced bowel dysfunction: pathophysiology and management. *Drugs.* 2012;72(14):1847-1865.
239. Wolff RF, Aune D, Truyers C, et al. Systematic review of efficacy and safety of buprenorphine versus fentanyl or morphine in patients with chronic moderate to severe pain. *Curr Med Res Opin.* 2012;28(5):833-845.
240. Zacny J. A review of the effects of opioids on psychomotor and cognitive functioning in humans. *Exp Clin Psychopharmacol.* 1995;3:432-466.
241. Van Ojik AL, Jansen PAF, Brouwers JRBJ, van Roon EN. Treatment of chronic pain in older people: evidence-based choice of strong-acting opioids. *Drugs Aging.* 2012;29(8):615-625.
242. Prommer E. Methylphenidate: established and expanding roles in symptom management. *Am J Hosp Palliat Care.* 2012;29(6):483-490.
243. Vuong C, Van Uum SH, O'Dell LE, Lutfy K, Friedman TC. The effects of opioids and opioid analogs on animal and human endocrine systems. *Endocr Rev.* 2010;31(1):98-132.
244. Brennan M. The effect of opioid therapy on endocrine function. *Am J Med.* 2013;126(3):S12-S18.
245. Smith HS, Elliott JA. Opioid-induced androgen deficiency (OPIAD). *Pain Physician.* 2012;15(3 Suppl):ES145-ES156.
246. De Maddalena C, Bellini M, Berra M, Meriggola MC, Aloisi AM. Opioid-induced hypogonadism: why and how to treat it. *Pain Physician.* 2012;15(Suppl 3):ES111-ES118.
247. Blick G, Khera M, Bhattacharya RK, Nguyen D, Kushner H, Miner MM. Testosterone replacement therapy outcomes among opioid users: the Testim Registry in the United States (TRiUS). *Pain Med.* 2012;13(5):688-698.
248. Daniell HW. Opioid endocrinopathy in women consuming prescribed sustained-action opioids for control of nonmalignant pain. *J Pain.* 2008;9(1):28-36.
249. Nelson RE, Nebeker JR, Sauer BC, LaFleur J. Factors associated with screening or treatment initiation among male United States veterans at risk for osteoporosis fracture. *Bone.* 2012;50(4):983-988.
250. Kim TW, Alford DP, Malabanan A, Holick MF, Samet JH. Low bone density in patients receiving methadone maintenance treatment. *Drug Alcohol Depend.* 2006;85(3):258-262.
251. Fortin JD, Bailey GM, Vilensky JA. Does opioid use for pain management warrant routine bone mass density screening in men? *Pain Physician.* 2008;11(4):539-541.
252. Miller M, Stürmer T, Azrael D, Levin R, Solomon DH. Opioid analgesics and the risk of fractures in older adults with arthritis. *J Am Geriatr Soc.* 2011;59(3):430-438.
253. Sacerdote P. Opioids and the immune system. *Palliat Med.* 2006;20(Suppl 1):9-15.
254. Beilin B, Shavit Y, Hart J, et al. Effects of anesthesia based on large vs. small doses of fentanyl on natural killer cell cytotoxicity in the perioperative period. *Anesth Analg.* 1996;82(3):492-497.
255. McCarthy L, Wetzel M, Sliker JK, Eisenstein TK, Rogers TJ. Opioids, opioid receptors, and the immune response. *Drug Alcohol Depend.* 2001;62(2):111-123.
256. Bussiere JL, Adler MW, Rogers TJ, Eisenstein TK. Cytokine reversal of morphine-induced suppression of the antibody response. *J Pharmacol Exp Ther.* 1993;264(2):591-597.
257. Eisenstein EM, Jaffe JS, Strober W. Reduced interleukin-2 (IL-2) production in common variable immunodeficiency is due to a primary abnormality of CD4+ T cell differentiation. *J Clin Immunol.* 1993;13(4):247-258.
258. Bastami S, Norling C, Trinks C, et al. Inhibitory effect of opiates on LPS mediated release of TNF and IL-8. *Acta Oncol.* 2013;52(5):1022-1033.
259. Mizota T, Tsujikawa H, Shoda T, Fukuda K. Dual modulation of the T-cell receptor-activated signal transduction pathway by morphine in human T lymphocytes. *J Anesth.* 2013;27(1):80-87.
260. Brack A, Rittner HL, Stein C. Immunosuppressive effects of opioids—clinical relevance. *J Neuroimmune Pharmacol.* 2011;6(4):490-502.
261. Garcia JB, Cardoso MG, Dos-Santos MC. Opioid and the immune system: clinical relevance. *Rev Bras Anestesiol.* 2012;62(5):709-718.

262. Al-Hashimi M, Scott SW, Thompson JP, Lambert DG. Opioids and immune modulation: more questions than answers. *Br J Anaesth.* 2013;111(1): 80-88.
263. Ninkovic J, Roy S. Role of the mu-opioid receptor in opioid modulation of immune function. *Amino Acids.* 2013;45(1):9-24.
264. Chen L, Wang Q, Li D, Chen C, Li Q, Kang P. Meta-analysis of retrospective studies suggests that the pre-operative opioid use is associated with an increased risk of adverse outcomes in total hip and or knee arthroplasty. *Int Orthop.* 2021;45(8):1923-1932. doi:10.1007/s00264-021-04968-9
265. Abdel Shaheed C, Beardsley J, Day RO, McLachlan AJ. Immunomodulatory effects of pharmaceutical opioids and antipyretic analgesics: mechanisms and relevance to infection. *Br J Clin Pharmacol.* 2022;88(7): 3114-3131. doi:10.1111/bcp.15281
266. Chung BC, Bouz GJ, Mayfield CK, et al. Dose-dependent early postoperative opioid use is associated with periprosthetic joint infection and other complications in primary TJA. *J Bone Joint Surg Am.* 2021;103(16):1531-1542. doi:10.2106/JBJS.21.00045
267. Roy S, Cain KJ, Chapin RB, Charboneau RG, Barke RA. Morphine modulates NF kappa B activation in macrophages. *Biochem Biophys Res Commun.* 1998;245(17):392-396.
268. Houghtling RA, Mellon RD, Tan RJ, Bayer BM. Acute effects of morphine on blood lymphocyte proliferation and IL-6 levels. *Ann N Y Acad Sci.* 2000;917:771-777.
269. Pacifici R, di Carlo S, Bacosi A, Pichini S, Zuccaro P. Pharmacokinetics and cytokine production in heroin and morphine-treated mice. *Int J Immunopharmacol.* 2000;22(8):603-614.
270. Holan V, Zajicova A, Krulova M, Blahoutová V, Wilczek H. Augmented production of proinflammatory cytokines and accelerated allotransplantation reactions in heroin-treated mice. *Clin Exp Immunol.* 2003;132(1):40-45.
271. Sacerdote P. Effects of in vitro and in vivo opioids on the production of IL-12 and IL-10 by murine macrophages. *Ann N Y Acad Sci.* 2003;992:129-140.
272. Kelschenbach J, Barke RA, Roy S. Morphine withdrawal contributes to TH cell differentiation by biasing cells toward the TH2 lineage. *J Immunol.* 2005;175:587-595.
273. Hutchinson MR, Bland ST, Johnson KW, Rice KC, Maier SF, Watkins LR. Opioid-induced glial activation: mechanisms of activation, dependence, and reward. *Sci World J.* 2007;7:98-111.
274. Watkins LR, Hutchinson MR, Johnston IN, Maier SF. Glia: novel counter-regulators of opioid analgesia. *Trends Neurosci.* 2005;28(12):661-669.
275. Hutchinson MR, Coats BD, Lewis SS, et al. Proinflammatory cytokines oppose opioid-induced acute and chronic analgesia. *Brain Behav Immun.* 2008;22(8):1178-1189.
276. Kosciuczuk U, Knapp P, Lotowska-Cwiklewska AM. Opioid-induced immunosuppression and carcinogenesis promotion theories create the newest trend in acute and chronic pain pharmacotherapy. *Clinics (Sao Paulo).* 2020;75:e1554. doi:10.6061/clinics/2020/e1554
277. Page GG. The immune-suppressive effects of pain. *Adv Exp Med Biol.* 2003;521:117-125.
278. Greisen J, Juhl C, Grøfte T, Vilstrup H, Jensen TS, Schmitz O. Acute pain induces insulin resistance in humans. *Anesthesiology.* 2001;95(3):578-584.
279. Edwards RR, Kronfli T, Haythornwaite JA, Smith MT, McGuire L, Page GG. Association of catastrophizing with interleukin-6 responses to acute pain. *Pain.* 2008;140(10):135-144.
280. Griffis CA, Crabb Breen E, Compton P, et al. Acute painful stress and inflammatory mediator production. *Neuroimmunomodulation.* 2013;20(3):127-133.
281. Quigley C. Opioid switching to improve pain relief and drug tolerability. *Cochrane Database Syst Rev.* 2004;3:CD004847.
282. Vadalouca A, Moka E, Argyra E, Sikioti P, Siafaka I. Opioid rotation in patients with cancer: a review of the current literature. *J Opioid Manag.* 2008;4(4):213-250.
283. Vissers KC, Besse K, Hans G, Devulder J, Morlion B. Opioid rotation in the management of chronic pain: where is the evidence? *Pain Pract.* 2010;10(2):85-93.
284. Knotkova H, Fine PG, Portenoy RK. Opioid rotation: the science and the limitations of the equianalgesic dose table. *J Pain Symptom Manage.* 2009;38(3):426-439.
285. Webster LR, Fine PG. Review and critique of opioid rotation practices and associated risks of toxicity. *Pain Med.* 2012;13(4):562-570.
286. Krebs EE, Gravely A, Nugent S, et al. Effect of opioid vs nonopioid medications on pain-related function in patients with chronic back pain or hip or knee osteoarthritis pain: the SPACE randomized clinical trial. *JAMA.* 2018;319(9):872-882. doi:10.1001/jama.2018.0899
287. Berna C, Kulich RJ, Rathmell JP. Tapering long-term opioid therapy in chronic noncancer pain: evidence and recommendations for everyday practice. *Mayo Clin Proc.* 2015;90(6):828-842.
288. Franklin GM; American Academy of Neurology. Opioids for chronic noncancer pain: a position paper of the American Academy of Neurology. *Neurology.* 2014;83(14):1277-1284.
289. Taylor CB, Zlutnick SI, Corley MJ, Flora J. The effects of detoxification, relaxation, and brief supportive therapy on chronic pain. *Pain.* 1980;8(3):319-329.
290. Harden P, Ahmed S, Ang K, Wiedemer N. Clinical implications of tapering chronic opioids in a veteran population. *Pain Med.* 2015;16(10):1975-1981.
291. Sullivan MD, Turner JA, DiLodovico C, D'Appollonio A, Stephens K, Chan YF. Prescription opioid taper support for outpatients with chronic pain: a randomized controlled trial. *J Pain.* 2017;18(3):308-318.
292. Naylor MR, Naud S, Keefe FJ, Helzer JE. Therapeutic Interactive Voice Response (TIVR) to reduce analgesic medication use for chronic pain management. *J Pain.* 2010;11(12):1410-1419.
293. Matthias MS, Johnson NL, Shields CG, et al. "I'm not gonna pull the rug out from under you": patient-provider communication about opioid tapering. *J Pain.* 2017;18(11):1365-1373. doi:10.1016/j.jpain.2017.06.008
294. Frank JW, Levy C, Matlock DD, et al. Patients' perspectives on tapering of chronic opioid therapy: a qualitative study. *Pain Med.* 2016;17(10):1838-1847.
295. Darnall BD, Ziadni MS, Stieg RL, Mackey IG, Kao MC, Flood P. Patient-centered prescription opioid tapering in community outpatients with chronic pain. *JAMA Intern Med.* 2018;178(5):707-708. doi:10.1001/jamainternmed.2017.8709
296. Goesling J, Moser SE, Zaidi B, et al. Trends and predictors of opioid use after total knee and total hip arthroplasty. *Pain.* 2016 Jun;157(6):1259-1265. doi:10.1097/j.pain.0000000000000516
297. Manhapra A, Arias AJ, Ballantyne JC. The conundrum of opioid tapering in long-term opioid therapy for chronic pain: a commentary. *Subst Abus.* 2018;39(2):152-161. doi:10.1080/08897077.2017.1381663
298. Sturgeon JA, Sullivan MD, Parker-Shames S, Tauben D, Coelho P. Outcomes in long-term opioid tapering and buprenorphine transition: a retrospective clinical data analysis. *Pain Med.* 2020;21(12):3635-3644. doi:10.1093/pm/pnaa029
299. Rahimi-Movaghar A, Gholami J, Amato L, Hoseinie L, Yousefi-Nooraie R, Amin-Esmaeili M. Pharmacological therapies for management of opium withdrawal. *Cochrane Database Syst Rev.* 2018;6(6):CD007522. doi:10.1002/14651858.CD007522.pub2
300. Jasinski D, Johnson R, Kocher T. Clonidine in morphine withdrawal: differential effects on sign and symptoms. *Arch Gen Psychiatry.* 1985;42:1063-1065.
301. Gowing L, Farrell M, Ali R, White JM. Alpha$_2$-adrenergic agonists for the management of opioid withdrawal. *Cochrane Database Syst Rev.* 2016;2016(5):CD002024. doi:10.1002/14651858.CD002024.pub5
302. Chou R, Turner JA, Devine EB, et al. The effectiveness and risks of long-term opioid therapy for chronic pain: a systematic review for a National Institutes of Health Pathways to Prevention Workshop. *Ann Intern Med.* 2015;162(4):276-286. doi:10.7326/M14-2559
303. McCarberg BH. Pain management in primary care: strategies to mitigate opioid misuse, abuse, and diversion. *Postgrad Med.* 2011;123(2):119-130.
304. Turner HN, Oliver J, Compton P, et al. Pain management and risks associated with substance use: practice recommendations. *Pain Manag Nurs.* 2022;23(2):91-108. doi:10.1016/j.pmn.2021.11.002

305. Penko J, Mattson J, Miaskowski C, Kushel M. Do patients know they are on pain medication agreements? Results from a sample of high-risk patients on chronic opioid therapy. *Pain Med.* 2012;13(9):1174-1180.
306. Argoff CE, Kahan M, Sellers EM. Preventing and managing aberrant drug-related behavior in primary care: systematic review of outcomes evidence. *J Opioid Manag.* 2014;10(2):119-134.
307. Cheatle MD, Savage SR. Informed consent in opioid therapy: a potential obligation and opportunity. *J Pain Symptom Manage.* 2012;44(1):105-116.
308. Sandbrink F, Oliva EM, McMullen TL, et al. Opioid prescribing and opioid risk mitigation strategies in the Veterans Health Administration. *J Gen Intern Med.* 2020;35(Suppl 3):927-934. doi:10.1007/s11606-020-06258-3
309. U.S. Department of Veterans Affairs. *Safe and Responsible Use of Opioids for Chronic Pain. A Patient Information Guide.* Accessed August 10, 2022. https://www.ethics.va.gov/docs/policy/Safe_and_Responsible_Use_of_Opioids.pdf
310. Cheatle MD, Compton P, Dhingra L, Wasser T, O'Brien C. Development of the revised opioid risk tool to predict opioid use disorder in patients with chronic non-malignant pain. *J Pain.* 2019;20(7):842-851. doi:10.1016/j.jpain.2019.01.011
311. Christo PJ, Manchikanti L, Ruan X, et al. Urine drug testing in chronic pain. *Pain Physician.* 2011;14(2):123-143.
312. Compton P. Trust but verify. *Pain Med.* 2014;15(12):1999-2000.
313. Reisfield GM, Goldberger BA, Bertholf RL. Choosing the right laboratory: a review of clinical and forensic toxicology services for urine drug testing in pain management. *J Opioid Manag.* 2015;11(1):37-44.
314. Pesce A, West C, Egan City K, Strickland J. Interpretation of urine drug testing in pain patients. *Pain Med.* 2012;13(7):868-885.
315. Heit HA, Gourlay DL. Using urine drug testing to support healthy boundaries in clinical care. *J Opioid Manag.* 2015;11(1):7-12.
316. Peppin JF, Passik SD, Couto JE, et al. Recommendations for urine drug monitoring as a component of opioid therapy in the treatment of chronic pain. *Pain Med.* 2012;13(7):886-896.
317. Im JJ, Shachter RD, Oliva EM, et al. Association of care practices with suicide attempts in US veterans prescribed opioid medications for chronic pain management. *J Gen Intern Med.* 2015;30(7):979-991.
318. Bohnert AS, Valenstein M, Bair MJ, et al. Association between opioid prescribing patterns and opioid overdose-related deaths. *JAMA.* 2011;305(13):1315-1321.
319. Gomes T, Mamdani MM, Dhalla IA, Paterson JM, Juurlink DN. Opioid dose and drug-related mortality in patients with nonmalignant pain. *Arch Intern Med.* 2011;171(7):686-691.
320. Dunn KM, Saunders KW, Rutter CM, et al. Opioid prescriptions for chronic pain and overdose: a cohort study. *Ann Intern Med.* 2010;152(2):85-92.
321. Bohnert AS, Logan JE, Ganoczy D, Dowell D. A detailed exploration into the association of prescribed opioid dosage and overdose deaths among patients with chronic pain. *Med Care.* 2016;54(5):435-441.
322. Dillie KS, Fleming MF, Mundt MP, French MT. Quality of life associated with daily opioid therapy in a primary care chronic pain sample. *J Am Board Fam Med.* 2008;21(2):108-117.
323. Dersh J, Mayer TG, Gatchel RJ, Polatin PB, Theodore BR, Mayer EA. Prescription opioid dependence is associated with poorer outcomes in disabling spinal disorders. *Spine (Phila Pa 1976).* 2008;33(20):2219-2227.
324. Kidner CL, Gatchel RJ, Mayer TG. MMPI disability profile is associated with degree of opioid use in chronic work-related musculoskeletal disorders. *Clin J Pain.* 2010;26(1):9-15.
325. Kidner CL, Mayer TG, Gatchel RJ. Higher opioid doses predict poorer functional outcome in patients with chronic disabling occupational musculoskeletal disorders. *J Bone Joint Surg Am.* 2009;91(4):919-927.
326. Quinlan J. The use of a subanesthetic infusion of intravenous ketamine to allow withdrawal of medically prescribed opioids in people with chronic pain, opioid tolerance and hyperalgesia: outcome at 6 months. *Pain Med.* 2012;13(11):1524-1525.
327. Dasgupta N, Funk MJ, Proescholdbell S, Hirsch A, Ribisl KM, Marshall S. Cohort study of the impact of high-dose opioid analgesics on overdose mortality. *Pain Med.* 2015;17(1):85-98.
328. Jones CM, McAninch JK. Emergency department visits and overdose deaths from combined use of opioids and benzodiazepines. *Am J Prev Med.* 2015;49:493-501.

CHAPTER

114 Co-occurring Pain and Substance Use Disorders

William C. Becker and Declan T. Barry

CHAPTER OUTLINE

- Introduction
- Problems of co-occurring issues
- Evolving guidance on the use of opioids in the treatment of chronic pain
- Gourlay and Heit
- Treating pain in the presence of an SUD
- Treating addiction in the presence of pain
- Conclusion

INTRODUCTION

In the late 1980s and early 1990s, experts bemoaned clinicians' inability to distinguish between patients with pain and patients with "addiction" (substance use disorders [SUDs]). To the present day, insistence on forcing this false dichotomy clouds assessment and treatment of both conditions. Unfortunately, the conditions are far from mutually exclusive; in fact, each can increase vulnerability to the other, often obscures the diagnosis of the other, and sometimes impedes treatment of the other. A significant percentage of the patients seeking treatment for SUDs suffer from co-occurring chronic pain. Rosenblum et al., for example, surveyed 390 patients from opiate treatment programs (OTPs) and 531 from short-term inpatient SUD treatment programs in New York State. They found that 37% of patients receiving methadone reported severe chronic pain, as did 24% of the inpatients.[1] Patients with other SUDs also appear to have a relatively high prevalence of pain; in a population of patients in outpatient SUD treatment, 29% reported *severe* chronic pain.[2]

Historically, estimates of the prevalence of SUDs in those with chronic pain have varied widely, in large part due to variable methodology, including differences in substance types, SUD assessments, and SUD definitions, which, when accounting for prevalence of OUD among patients with chronic pain on long-term opioid therapy (LTOT), may confuse patients not taking medications as prescribed and true OUD. A 2021 systematic review estimated the prevalence of "problematic opioid use," defined by the authors as "any type of problematic behavior related to opioid intake; namely, abuse, misuse, addiction, dependence, and aberrant behavior/use" among patients with chronic pain to be 36.3% (95% confidence interval: 27.4% to 45.2%; I2 = 99.64%).[3] In contrast to studies examining aberrant medication taking behaviors, others have used formal diagnostic OUD criteria. For example, in a large cohort study of patients with chronic pain receiving LTOT, Boscarino and colleagues[4] found that 35% of them met DSM-5 criteria for lifetime (including pre-existing to starting the LTOT) OUD (22% for moderate OUD and 13% for severe OUD). In the most rigorous systematic review to date, Vowles et al. estimated that the prevalence of OUD in patients with chronic pain ranged from 8% to 12%.[5]

PROBLEMS OF CO-OCCURRING ISSUES

Reciprocal Vulnerability

As implied by the epidemiological data above, persons with SUDs are at higher than average risk of developing a chronic pain condition. This is not unexpected, given that individuals with SUDs are more susceptible to incurring traumas and of developing painful illnesses such as pancreatitis, cirrhosis, stroke, HIV infection, and peripheral arterial disease. The converse situation, in which having pain increases the vulnerability to SUD, is also the case, mainly via the mechanism of increased likelihood of exposure to controlled substances. However, in studies examining the incidence of unhealthy substance use and SUD among patients with pain prescribed opioids, several concluded that unhealthy substance use problems preceded therapeutic opioid exposure. As far back as 1993, Polatin et al.[6] showed that when chronic low back pain and DSM-IIIR defined substance abuse coexisted, the substance abuse had preceded the pain in 94% of cases. Similarly, Potter et al.[7] found that of 48 patients hospitalized for extended-release (ER) oxycodone OUD, 77% had a nonopioid substance use problem prior to taking oxycodone ER. In a highly selected group of patients undergoing pain rehabilitation, Covington et al. found that 33% of those with OUD began with medical exposure, 64% was with recreational use, and 3% was undetermined.[8] Importantly, chronic pain and SUDs share several risk factors, including childhood trauma/neglect, adult trauma, and posttraumatic stress disorder.[9] A paucity of research has examined order of condition onset among patients seeking treatment for co-occurring chronic pain and OUD. In a study of patients entering clinical trials of treatments for co-occurring chronic pain and OUD ($N = 170$), 52% reported chronic pain preceded OUD (ie, pain first), 35% reported the reverse (ie, OUD first), and the remainder (13%) reported that both conditions emerged during the same time period.[10] Differences in co-occurring psychiatric disorders associated with order of condition onset (eg, the OUD first group had higher rates of nonopioid SUDs and personality disorders than the pain first group) suggest that varying pathways may exist for the emergence of OUD and chronic pain.

Diagnostic Confounds

SUD may complicate the diagnosis of pain, since it provides an incentive, which may or may not be consciously appreciated by the patient, to minimize reports of benefit from nonopioid therapies. Given that most chronic pain is due less to peripheral nociception than to central sensitization, the clinician is placed into a challenging situation in which the primary diagnostic finding guiding decision making is patient report. Although self-report is the gold-standard assessment of pain, some clinicians who treat patients with suspected or documented OUD question its validity.[11,12] Thus, the risk of undertreating actual pain coexists with the risk of inappropriately supporting OUD (not that these are mutually exclusive), and there are few objective guides as to optimal choices.

Pain also complicates the diagnosis of SUD insofar as pain probably makes it harder for patients—and clinicians—to recognize that a SUD has developed. This may be especially the case for individuals with no prior history of SUDs who were prescribed opioids for analgesic purposes and proceeded to develop an addiction (ie, iatrogenic addiction). Loss of control may be subtle, or even not clear, as patients with pain may increase use citing pain flares. Furthermore, harms putatively due to opioid use, particularly high-dose therapy, for example, declining function, opioid induced hyperalgesia, may be in part due to worsening of the pain condition. Thus, adjudicating the DSM-5 criterion "Use is continued despite knowledge of persistent or recurrent physical or psychological problems likely to have been caused or exacerbated by the opioid" can be challenging. Efforts are ongoing to explore if there should be a separate diagnostic entity for patients on LTOT for pain for whom harms outweigh benefits—thus for whom tapering is indicated—but who struggle to taper.[13] Creating a new diagnostic classification may serve two purposes: helping clinicians reduce the tendency to inappropriately diagnose OUD in cases where patients only have physiologic dependence and establishing better treatment pathways for patients feeling stuck on ineffective LTOT. Counselors in opioid treatment programs (OTPs) report that patients with co-occurring OUD and chronic pain sometimes view themselves as "pain patients" and different from those with OUD alone.[12] Many factors may confirm to patients with pain that they are "not like those people" with "addiction" or SUD.

Treatment Impediments

Treating chronic pain can be challenging in the presence of SUD. Patients with OUD may not respond readily to nonopioid pain treatments such as other medications, injections, physical therapy, or cognitive-behavioral interventions. A patient-centered approach, being as transparent as possible with concerns about the low likelihood for long-term benefit of opioid therapy and relatively greater likelihood of long-term harm, can be effective. Patients may ultimately be dissatisfied with nonopioid treatment recommendations, but they may be markedly more dissatisfied if they receive those recommendations accompanied by a perception that they were not listened to, or their pain was not taken seriously.

The therapeutic relationship can be complicated by the presence of SUD. For example, in patients receiving LTOT, those who engage in nonmedical opioid use may believe that they are doing so to relieve pain, while their prescriber may suspect that the pain complaints reflect "drug seeking" wherein the patient's requests for prescribed opioids are not to relieve pain but rather to pursue opioid-related high (or relief of withdrawal). An impasse may develop, with escalating mutual mistrust and hostility. Similarly, treatment of SUD is complicated by chronic pain. Clinicians in office-based and OTP settings report a lack of expertise in addressing co-occurring chronic pain and OUD or unhealthy opioid use and may feel overwhelmed by the psychiatric and medical complexity of patients with these conditions.[11,12]

EVOLVING GUIDANCE ON THE USE OF OPIOIDS IN THE TREATMENT OF CHRONIC PAIN

March 2016 saw the release of the Centers for Disease Control and Prevention's (CDC) Guideline for Prescribing Opioids for Chronic Pain,[14] a landmark effort that received widespread publicity and raised some controversies. It stands in marked contrast to the last major guideline (2009's APS/AAPM Clinical Guidelines for the Use of Chronic Opioid Therapy in Chronic Noncancer Pain)[15] as decidedly "opioid avoidant" insofar as it promotes nonopioid and nonpharmacological treatment options as preferred in the treatment of chronic pain; identifies recommended limits in dosages prescribed; and advocates for heightened vigilance in surveilling for indications to taper down or discontinue opioids among patients already on LTOT (ie, when benefit no longer outweighs harm). The CDC Guideline also placed much greater emphasis on the lack of evidence demonstrating long-term efficacy of LTOT (as is the case for the other treatments for chronic pain)[16] and the persuasive evidence of potential harm, especially at higher doses.

The 2016 CDC Guideline was decried by critics over their perception of its excessive emphasis on arbitrary LTOT dose thresholds and that many recommendations were based on low-quality evidence. While it clearly does not advocate forced tapers, it seems to have been invoked by various stakeholders as rationale to implement them. Thus, a revised Guideline was released in late 2022 that, among other changes, emphasized the need to tailor treatment recommendations to each patient's needs. Taken together, these guidelines mark a growing appreciation that high-quality pain care means a blend of nonpharmacological and pharmacological options; that treatments where patients take an active role (eg, yoga) are particularly valuable; that self-management skill building is low-cost and effective and promotes nonreliance on the health care system. However, the lack of availability of some of these approaches (especially outside of integrated health systems) and their inconsistent reimbursement are barriers to their dissemination. There is also increased recognition that it may be in patients' best interests in the near, intermediate, and especially long term to reduce or avoid taking opioids. This latter realization has less to do with the worry that patients may develop an OUD but more to do with the observational data and emerging RCT data that patients may experience accelerated decline in wellbeing and accrue a variety of bothersome and sometimes serious harms on long-term, and especially high-dose, opioids. However, for people already on LTOT for whom benefit *is* outweighing harm, LTOT (and ongoing close monitoring of it) should be continued. Involuntary tapering of patients not experiencing harm is not evidence-based, not guideline concordant, and may have its own set of serious risks.[17]

Monitoring for Unhealthy Use and Opioid Use Disorder

Like its predecessor, the 2022 CDC Guideline did not proscribe initiation of LTOT and also advocated tapering or tapering and discontinuation of extant LTOT only when benefit does not outweigh harm. Thus, like previous guidelines, the 2022 CDC Guideline recommends ongoing monitoring of patients prescribed opioid analgesics for, among other things, aberrant medication-taking behaviors, as well as incident OUD. The CDC Guideline recommends specific risk reduction strategies including seeing the patient receiving LTOT in follow up every 3 months or more frequently if the patient is at high risk, routinely querying the state prescription drug monitoring program and performing urine drug testing. More detailed, non–consensus-based guidance on monitoring was published by Gourlay and Heit[18] using the term Universal Precautions, meant to invoke the Infectious Disease concept that all are at risk of harm and a standard, nonjudgmental, patient centered approach may mitigate that risk (**Table 114-1**).

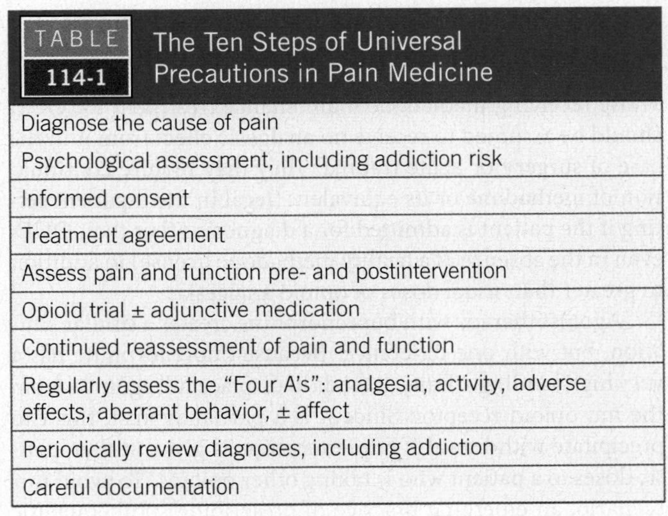

TABLE 114-1 The Ten Steps of Universal Precautions in Pain Medicine

Diagnose the cause of pain
Psychological assessment, including addiction risk
Informed consent
Treatment agreement
Assess pain and function pre- and postintervention
Opioid trial ± adjunctive medication
Continued reassessment of pain and function
Regularly assess the "Four A's": analgesia, activity, adverse effects, aberrant behavior, ± affect
Periodically review diagnoses, including addiction
Careful documentation

GOURLAY AND HEIT

Diagnosis of Opioid Use Disorder in Chronic Pain

The criteria for a diagnosis of OUD in the patient with chronic pain are similar to those in patients without pain; however, they may be more difficult to discern because many of the OUD criteria may arise in part due to impairments in social role functioning caused by pain. To help resolve this conundrum, we rely on clear communication with the patient of what constitutes unsafe use. However, as noted above, the issue of diagnosis of OUD in the setting of LTOT remains a murky one but emerging paradigms may provide clarity.[19]

The DSM-5 defines OUD as a maladaptive pattern of opioid use leading to significant impairment or distress, as manifested by at least two of the following, occurring within a 12-month period (abbreviated)[20]:

1. The opioid is often taken in larger amounts or over a longer period than intended.
2. There is a persistent desire or unsuccessful efforts to cut down or control use.
3. A great deal of time is spent in activities necessary to obtain, use, or recover from opioid effects.
4. Recurrent use results in failure to fulfill major role obligations.
5. There is continued use despite persistent or recurrent social or interpersonal problems caused or exacerbated by the substance.
6. Important social, occupational, or recreational activities are reduced because of use.
7. There is recurrent use in situations in which it is physically hazardous.
8. Use is continued despite knowledge of persistent or recurrent physical or psychological problems likely to have been caused or exacerbated by the opioid.
9. Tolerance (*not counted for those taking opioid analgesics under medical supervision*).
10. Withdrawal (*not counted for those taking opioid analgesics under medical supervision*).
11. Craving or a strong desire or urge to use the opioid.

The indicators of iatrogenic OUD (ie, occurring in the course of medically supervised opioid analgesic therapy) are often subtler than in the case of recreational OUD. Loss of control may be manifested by an inability to ration medication (eg, consistent early opioid medication refills). Use despite adverse consequences may be less likely to be shown by legal entanglements (patients who have a prescription may be less likely to steal medications, and those who do not drive due to pain do not receive citations for driving under the influence) than by family reports that the person loses the thread of a conversation, falls asleep at the dinner table, or takes medications to go on a family excursion only to fall asleep. Having or seeking multiple prescribers may occur in the person who has developed prescription OUD and often may only be identified by reviewing the online state prescription drug monitoring program records. Families may be much less clear in confirming that their loved one has iatrogenic OUD than they would be in the case of cocaine or alcohol and may see the adverse consequences of opioids as simply the price that must be paid for some measure of pain relief. Guidelines to date tend to be mute on specific steps prescribers should take when concerning medication-taking behaviors become evident, but emerging consensus guidance may help fill this void.[21]

TREATING PAIN IN THE PRESENCE OF AN SUD

SUD poses challenges for the safe and successful treatment of both acute and chronic pain and, perhaps the most challenging of all, the so-called acute-on-chronic pain. The optimal strategies vary, depending on whether the patient is actively using substances, in abstinence-based recovery, or enrolled in active treatment (with or without pharmacotherapy), as well as on whether the target is acute or chronic pain.

Acute Pain

Substance use increases the likelihood of developing acute pain through a number of mechanisms, especially those related to trauma.[22] Substance use also increases the likelihood that the resulting pain will not be optimally managed.[23] Patients actively using licit or illicit opioids may not receive indicated opioid therapy (eg, IV morphine in the setting of myocardial infarction), as providers fail to account for the presence of tolerance or fear being duped into "feeding the addiction."[24] Poor postoperative analgesia may result from provision of "standard" doses of opioids that not only fail to relieve pain but may not even be sufficient to prevent the compounding of surgical pain by opioid withdrawal. The patient with OUD is especially likely to benefit from multimodal analgesia, in which a variety of regional and systemic interventions are combined, thereby reducing the need to rely solely on opioids.[25]

Acute-on-Chronic Pain

This term is used to describe the presence of acute pain in a patient who has preexisting chronic pain. Those who have taken long-term high-dose opioids for pain, whether with co-occurring OUD or not, and who then undergo surgery are especially vulnerable to poor perioperative pain control.[26] This may result in part due to a failure of providers to either accurately document preoperative opioid use and/or to act on this information on the part of those providing postoperative care. These patients require not only their typical maintenance dose as a baseline that provides little or no analgesia but also additional analgesic doses that will likely be greater than those required by a nontolerant person.

Even when appropriate attention is paid to this issue, it is much more difficult to achieve satisfactory analgesia in the highly tolerant patient and aggressive treatment is more

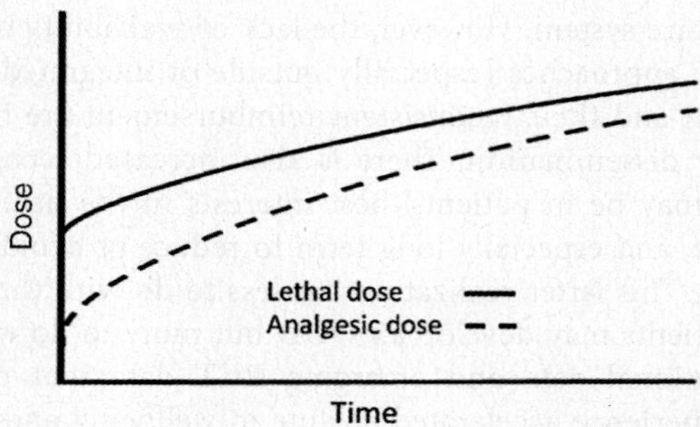

Figure 114-1. Hypothetical graph of narrowed therapeutic window with increasing opioid tolerance in patients taking chronic high-dose opioids.

hazardous. Despite greater doses of opioids, tolerant patients have both more postoperative pain and more opioid-induced sedation.[26] Tolerance develops to opioid effects at different rates; for example, tolerance to sedation and respiratory depression occurs more rapidly than to miosis and constipation. Although data are difficult to locate, it also appears that tolerance to opioid toxicity and opioid analgesia develops at different rates, such that the therapeutic window that exists in initiates becomes narrower over time as the effective dose approaches the lethal dose (**Fig. 114-1**). A not uncommon scenario is a patient with chronic back pain who has taken the equivalent of high-dose oral morphine daily for several years and then undergoes lumbar intervertebral fusion because of persistent pain. The opioid dose that failed to control preoperative chronic pain will have little effect on the first postoperative days, when the chronic pain is compounded by surgical pain. In such cases, regional analgesia and nonopioid systemic analgesia are often required, in addition to nonpharmacological interventions. (It is likely that opioid-induced hyperalgesia [OIH][27] plays a role in the phenomena described here; that is, OIH rather than or in addition to analgesic tolerance may cause the failure of postoperative analgesia, in which case the strategy of maximizing nonopioid interventions is even more appropriate.)

Acute or Acute-on-Chronic Pain Among Patients Receiving Opioid Agonist Therapy for OUD

Those receiving methadone maintenance treatment for OUD should be assumed to receive no analgesic effect from it in the case of surgery or acute trauma. They may require continuation of methadone or its equivalent (legal in the inpatient setting if the patient is admitted for a diagnosis other than OUD, even in the absence of a facility methadone license) in addition to greater than usual doses of opioid analgesia.

Agonist therapy with buprenorphine creates a similar situation, but with one difference. Because buprenorphine has a very high binding affinity, it tends to displace full agonists from the mu opioid receptor. Since it is a partial agonist, this can precipitate withdrawal if buprenorphine is given at therapeutic doses to a patient who is taking other opioids. To avoid this scenario, an emerging practice of prescribing subtherapeutic doses of buprenorphine and increasing to therapeutic dose over several days—while continuing full agonist use—appears to be a promising alternative approach to requiring patients abruptly stop full agonist opioid use, await withdrawal symptoms and then initiate buprenorphine.[28,29] Conversely, full mu agonists can be given to treat pain in a patient taking buprenorphine, though aggressive dose titration may be required due to buprenorphine's avid binding and the need for the new opioid to displace it at the receptor. Some clinicians prefer to wean buprenorphine and replace it with a full mu agonist in preparation for surgery; however, emerging practices in need of randomized trial evidence suggest that (1) buprenorphine itself may be adequate for peri-operative opioid therapy and if the patient is on a relatively low dose of buprenorphine, it can be titrated for postoperative analgesia, given either sublingually or parenterally as needed and (2) maintaining some buprenorphine throughout the perioperative period and using full agonists briefly "on top of" buprenorphine may lead to better pain control.[30]

Although patients in treatment with oral or depot naltrexone, a competitive opioid antagonist, experience markedly attenuated effects from opioid administration, the blockade can be overcome with high-dose therapy. This creates a risk of overdose, since the dose of opioid necessary to overcome the naltrexone block may become toxic as naltrexone is metabolized. Such patients therefore require close monitoring for as long as both the opioid and the naltrexone are in the bloodstream.

Frequent Emergency Department Visits

While the U.S. National Center for Health Statistics reported in 2006 that 39% of all ambulatory encounters in which opioids were prescribed, administered, or continued occurred in emergency departments (EDs),[31] more recent studies indicate that the rates of opioid prescribing in EDs are declining. Data from the 2006-2017 National Hospital Ambulatory Medical Care Survey found that the rates of ED visits by adults with opioids prescribed at discharge increased from 2006 to 2007 (19.0%) through 2010 to 2011 (21.5%) and then decreased from 2010 to 2011 through 2016 to 2017 (14.6%).[32] Similarly, in a retrospective cohort study from July 1, 2012 to June 30, 2018 of patients presenting to two EDs with a pain-related problem, the rates of opioid analgesic receipt at discharge decreased from 37.8% to 13.3% over the 6-year period.[33] Emergency facilities encounter patients with OUD who present with complaints of severe pain and request opioids, without objective evidence of acute illness. Since ignoring suffering and rewarding aberrant medication-taking behaviors are both problematic, states and hospitals have developed guidelines designed to ensure that patients receive appropriate care while minimizing the contribution to opioids in circulation and avoiding the promotion of drug-seeking behavior. The guidelines typically emphasize avoiding provisions of opioid medications for chronic pain in the emergency setting, avoiding prescriptions for long-acting opioids, not refilling lost or stolen prescriptions for opioids given for pain or OUD, avoiding parenteral opioids, using nonopioids whenever possible, and creating a care plan for frequent patients that provides for continuity of care with a nonemergency clinician.[34,35] When opioids are provided, it is recommended prescribing only small quantities. We note that while a recent systematic review of 63 studies found that most interventions aimed at reducing opioid prescribing at ED discharge lowered the opioid prescription rate, the opioid quantity prescribed was largely unaffected.[36]

Chronic Pain

Nonpharmacological treatments for chronic pain include physical therapy/exercises/fitness/yoga and similar activities that reduce pain or lumbago, migraine, fibromyalgia, and other conditions. Psychological treatments are reviewed elsewhere in this text (see Chapter 109, "Psychological Issues in the Management of Pain"). They can reduce pain and increase patients' ability to cope with residual pain, while improving quality of life. Treatments such as transcutaneous electrical neurostimulation, massage, and osteopathic manipulative therapies may provide pain reduction without compromising the abstinence of a person in recovery.

Of all studied treatments for disabling chronic pain, interdisciplinary pain rehabilitation programs have the best outcomes and have demonstrated lasting benefit following treatment. These programs typically eschew both opioids and invasive therapies, relying instead on such interventions as behavioral treatments, cognitive therapies, physical reconditioning, and adjuvant analgesics. A large number of studies have demonstrated that these interdisciplinary pain programs improve pain, physical function, psychological distress, and inordinate health care utilization.[37] Studies are limited by the impossibility of blinding and the lack of randomization, although one military study did randomize patients and showed similar outcomes.[38] Unfortunately, such programs are unavailable for most patients who are disabled with chronic pain. Schatman[39] reviewed estimates that the number of programs has declined by 85%, so that now there is one program for every 670,000 patients with chronic pain, leaving the bulk of chronic pain care to primary care providers, who may lack comfort and/or competence to manage it.

Techniques involving regional anesthesia may provide relief of sufficient duration to favorably impact the life of the patient with chronic pain. A more detailed review of these techniques is beyond the scope of this chapter; however, a few examples may be given[40]: botulinum toxin is approved for chronic migraine in addition to its role in conditions involving muscle spasm.[41] Celiac plexus blockade can produce months of relief of pain from the upper abdominal viscera. Trigger point injections and injections of superficial bursae may reduce pain and thereby facilitate rehabilitation.

Neuromodulation, involving the electrical stimulation of neural structures, is useful for several chronic pain syndromes.[40] Spinal cord stimulation reduces chronic radicular pain, complex regional pain syndrome (CRPS), and some cases of axial spine pain.[42] Peripheral nerve stimulation often reduces pain from peripheral mononeuropathies.[43] Deep brain stimulation has been used in intractable cases of post stroke pain,[44] and motor cortex stimulation has relieved CRPS.[45] Magnetic stimulation has also been studied.[46]

Numerous nonopioid pharmacological treatments for chronic pain have been shown to be effective[47,48] (see also Chapter 112, "Nonopioid Pharmacotherapy of Pain"). Gabapentinoids are useful for neuropathic pain, migraine prophylaxis, and treatment of fibromyalgia but emerging data on their liability for unhealthy use, and additive risk of overdose when combined with opioids means caution must be exercised. Other antiepileptics have shown benefit for a variety of neuropathic pains, including tic douloureux and multiple sclerosis. The "SNRIs" (serotonin and norepinephrine reuptake inhibitors) and tricyclic antidepressants, which also inhibit uptake of serotonin and norepinephrine, may be useful for neuropathic pain, migraine, and fibromyalgia pain. They have shown benefit in chronic low back pain, irritable bowel syndrome, temporomandibular joint syndrome, vulvodynia, and other hyperalgesic states. Topical analgesics, such as capsaicin, diclofenac gel and patches, and transdermal lidocaine, are effective for selected pains and lack psychoactive effects. Acetaminophen should not be forgotten as an analgesic that relieves minor pains and can reduce other analgesic requirements in more serious ones. The anti-inflammatory drugs are most effective for nociceptive pains, especially those of inflammatory or bony origin, and have clear opioid-sparing effects when used after surgery or trauma.[49] However, long-term use of acetaminophen and NSAIDs carries a risk of serious adverse effects of hepatotoxicity, gastric bleeding, increased risk of myocardial infarction, stroke, etc. Cannabis for chronic pain conditions is an active area of research; to date, systematic reviews suggest there may be some short-term benefit but longer term studies are needed to explore both long-term benefit and potential harms. The topic of cannabis used as treatment is covered in section 15 of this textbook.

There is very little data concerning the use of LTOT in those with a history of SUD. The safest treatments for people with co-occurring SUD and chronic pain are those that avoid controlled substances; however, there are some causes of severe nociceptive pain where opioids may need to be considered because of the absence of good alternatives. Chronic pancreatitis pain and ischemic pain from peripheral arterial disease are examples, although the former has been managed with pancreatectomy/islet cell autotransplant.[50] Given the evidence that LTOT provides less than 50% pain reduction to less than 50% of those entering treatment and the paucity of evidence of improved quality of life in most pain conditions, it should not be considered essential to effective management.[51-53]

Sublingual buprenorphine, although only approved for treatment of OUD, is also an excellent analgesic and can therefore offer the side benefit of pain efficacy for patients receiving it for OUD who also have pain.[54,55] It is less likely than full mu agonists to produce respiratory depression, may cause less immune suppression, and may elicit less analgesic tolerance.[56] The fact that the approved form (for long-term use) in the United States is combined with naloxone makes it less subject to diversion and to altered routes of administration. For the person who requires both opioid agonist treatment for OUD and long-term opioid analgesia, buprenorphine has unique advantages. It should be noted that the relative safety of buprenorphine is attenuated if combined with benzodiazepines.[57]

Chronic Pain Among Patients on Opioid Agonist Therapy for OUD

Chronic pain is highly prevalent in patients receiving opioid agonist therapy for OUD with buprenorphine or methadone,[1,58] and the majority of patients with OUD entering treatment with chronic pain would benefit from integrated SUD/pain management services.[59,60] Often, OTPs target OUD and ignore chronic pain.[61] Proposed strategies for managing chronic pain in patients receiving opioid agonist therapy for OUD often focus on pharmacotherapy, including opioid medications (see below). Three pilot studies[62-64] and three randomized clinical trials[65-67] support the efficacy of cognitive-behavioral therapy in managing coexisting chronic pain and substance-related disorders. One pilot demonstrated preliminary efficacy for an integrated treatment using Acceptance and Commitment Therapy for chronic pain and Mindfulness Based Relapse Prevention for opioid misuse. Group treatments that promote relaxation training, exercise, and psychoeducation have demonstrated feasibility in OTPs and warrant further examination.[68] Studies have found that whereas addiction counselors in OTPs report a lack of expertise in managing chronic pain,[12] they can be trained to proficiently provide brief and targeted group interventions to address pain as well as individual CBT psychoeducation sessions with exercise goal setting.[69]

LTOT is incompatible with naltrexone treatment, since it would be neither reasonable nor safe to prescribe naltrexone and then attempt to chronically overcome it with opioids. When patients taking methadone or buprenorphine are thought to need higher doses of opioids for chronic analgesia, there is little data to guide providers. Essentially, all studies of LTOT have been conducted with doses well below those provided by agonist treatment of OUD, and there is evidence that opioid overdose deaths are proportional to dose prescribed.[70] Therefore, consistent with CDC guidance, nonopioid-based therapies should be preferred when a patient receiving opioid agonist therapy for OUD needs more aggressive, multimodal pain treatment on an ongoing basis.

Additional Rewarding Medications

Since patients with CNCP and SUDs often have co-occurring psychiatric conditions, most commonly anxiety and/or depression,[71] they may be prescribed anxiolytics and sedative-hypnotics. Anxiolytics, sedative-hypnotics and gabapentinoids may be used nonmedically and, when combined with opioids, lead to increased overdose risk.[72] These risks should be considered when contemplating the potential benefits of prescribing anxiolytics or sedative-hypnotics in patients with chronic pain who are receiving LTOT or in patients with co-occurring OUD and chronic pain who are receiving opioid agonist treatment; alternative treatments for anxiety, muscle spasm, and insomnia should be considered. Most antidepressants have anxiolytic properties, are typically first-line therapy for anxiety disorders, and are not subject to unhealthy use.[73-77] Chronic pain is also strongly associated with sleep disorders,[78,79] which tend to amplify pain. These should be addressed; however, prolonged use of the potentially addictive substances is best avoided in those with SUD, and they tend to be of only transient benefit in any case.[80,81] Most so-called muscle relaxants have sedative effects and are indicated only for short-term use.

TREATING ADDICTION IN THE PRESENCE OF PAIN

Chronic pain complicates SUD treatment. Patients receiving opioid agonist treatment report using a variety of licit (eg, nicotine) and illicit substances (eg, heroin) to manage pain. Some patients may attribute poor functioning to pain and not substance use. It may weaken the family's support of abstinence, as they may be unsure whether rewarding drugs are an asset or liability to the patient, or perhaps both. Since clinicians in SUD and office-based settings have difficulty securing referrals for the management of chronic pain accompanied by confirmed or suspected OUD, onsite interventions for these co-occurring conditions is an important area for future research.[12,69]

Agonist or Abstinence?

Abstinence-based treatment of OUD has a high rate of return to nonmedical opioid use, such that pharmacotherapy is recommended for most.[82] Moore et al.[83] studied 200 primary care patients treated with buprenorphine/naloxone and found better treatment retention and a higher percent of opioid negative urine samples in patients with prescription OUD than those with heroin use disorder. A study that examined order of condition onset among patients seeking treatment for co-occurring OUD and chronic pain found that compared to those whose pain preceded OUD, patients whose OUD preceded pain were more likely to have co-occurring nonopioid SUDs.[11] While these findings are preliminary they suggest different clinical needs may be present in subgroups of individuals with chronic pain and OUD or unhealthy opioid use.

CONCLUSION

The concurrence of CNCP and SUD is challenging for patients and has been a particularly challenging overlap for health care clinicians with regard to both assessment and treatment. That historically unprecedented levels of opioid prescribing in the United States led to increased incidence of OUD adds a layer of complexity to management. Clinicians would do well to first appreciate that chronic pain often co-occurs with OUD and to rely on the fundamentals of assessment to establish if and when either or both are present. The CDC's new guideline stands to bring increasing clarity to the fore: if there are preferred options to LTOT for all patients with chronic pain, health care systems can focus on making those treatments available and accessible to all, rather than expending energy on ascertaining who is and is not appropriate for LTOT. Evidence-based treatments are emerging for the overlap of chronic pain and SUDs.

REFERENCES

1. Rosenblum A, Joseph H, Fong C, Kipnis S, Cleland C, Portenoy RK. Prevalence and characteristics of chronic pain among chemically dependent patients in methadone maintenance and residential treatment facilities. *JAMA*. 2003;289(18):2370-2378.
2. Sheu R, Lussier D, Rosenblum A, et al. Prevalence and characteristics of chronic pain in patients admitted to an outpatient drug and alcohol treatment program. *Pain Med.* 2008;9(7):911-917.
3. Jantarada C, Silva C, Guimarães-Pereira L. Prevalence of problematic use of opioids in patients with chronic noncancer pain: a systematic review with meta-analysis. *Pain Pract.* 2021;21(6):715-729.
4. Boscarino JA, Rukstalis MR, Hoffman SN, et al. Prevalence of prescription opioid-use disorder among chronic pain patients: comparison of the DSM-5 vs. DSM-4 diagnostic criteria. *J Addict Dis.* 2011;30:185-194.
5. Vowles KE, McEntee ML, Julnes PS, Frohe T, Ney JP, van der Goes DN. Rates of opioid misuse, abuse, and addiction in chronic pain: a systematic review and data synthesis. *Pain.* 2015;156(4):569-576.
6. Polatin P, Kinney R, Gatchel R, Lillo E, Mayer TG. Psychiatric illness and chronic low-back pain; the mind and the spine-which goes first? *Spine.* 1993;18:66-71.
7. Potter JS, Hennessy G, Borrow JA, Greenfield SF, Weiss RD. Substance use histories in patients seeking treatment for controlled-release oxycodone dependence. *Drug Alcohol Depend.* 2004;76(2):213-215.
8. Covington EC, Kotz MM. *Pain Reduction With Opioid Elimination.* American Academy of Pain Medicine Annual meeting. American Academy of Pain Medicine; 2002.
9. National Center on Addiction and Substance Abuse at Columbia University. *Addiction Medicine: Closing the Gap Between Science and Practice.* Accessed May 2023. https://cdn-01.drugfree.org/web/prod/wp-content/uploads/2012/06/19202800/Addiction-medicine-closing-the-gap-between-science-and-practice_1.pdf?_gl=1
10. Barry D, Beitel M, Cutter CJ, et al. Psychiatric comorbidity and order of condition onset among patients seeking treatment for chronic pain and opioid use disorder. *Drug Alcohol Depend.* 2021;221:108608. doi:10.1016/j.drugalcdep.2021.108608
11. Barry DT, Irwin KS, Jones ES, et al. Opioids, chronic pain, and addiction in primary care. *J Pain.* 2010;11(12):1442-1450.
12. Beitel M, Oberleitner L, Kahn M, et al. Drug counselor responses to patients' pain reports: a qualitative investigation of barriers and facilitators to treating patients with chronic pain in methadone maintenance treatment. *Pain Med.* 2017;18:2152-2161.
13. Edmond SN, Snow JL, Pomeranz J, Van Cleve R, Becker WC. Arguments for and against a new diagnostic entity for patients with chronic pain on long-term opioid therapy for whom harms outweigh benefits. *J Pain.* 2022;23(6):958-966.
14. Dowell D, Haegerich T, Chou R. CDC Guideline for prescribing opioids for chronic pain—United States. 2016. *MMWR Recomm Rep.* 2016;65(1):1-49.

15. Chou R, Fanciullo GJ, Fine PG, et al. Clinical guidelines for the use of chronic opioid therapy in chronic noncancer pain. *J Pain.* 2009;10(2):113-130.
16. Tayeb BO, Barreiro AE, Bradshaw YS, Chui KK, Carr DB. Durations of opioid, nonopioid drug, and behavioral clinical trials for chronic pain: adequate or inadequate? *Pain Med.* 2016;17(11):2036-2046.
17. Kertesz SG. Turning the tide or riptide? The changing opioid epidemic. *Subst Abus.* 2017;38(1):3-8.
18. Gourlay DL, Heit HA, Almahrezi A. Universal precautions in pain medicine: a rational approach to the treatment of chronic pain. *Pain Med.* 2005;6(2):107-112.
19. Manhapra A, Arias AA, Ballantyne JC. The conundrum of opioid tapering in long-term opioid therapy for chronic pain: a commentary. *Subst Abus.* 2018;39(2):152-161.
20. American Psychiatric Association. DSM-5 Development web site. Accessed September 4, 2012. http://www.dsm5.org/ProposedRevisions/Pages/proposedrevision.aspx?rid=460
21. Merlin JS, Young SR, Azari S, et al. Management of problematic behaviours among individuals on long-term opioid therapy: protocol for a Delphi study. *BMJ Open.* 2016;6(5):e011619.
22. MacLeod JB, Hungerford DW. Alcohol-related injury visits: do we know the true prevalence in U.S. trauma centres? *Injury.* 2011;42(9):922-926.
23. Bourne N. Acute pain management in the opioid-tolerant patient. *Nurs Stand.* 2010;25(12):35-39.
24. Rapp SE, Ready LB, Nessly ML. Acute pain management in patients with prior opioid consumption: a case-controlled retrospective review. *Pain.* 1995;61(2):195-201.
25. Richebé P, Beaulieu P. Perioperative pain management in the patient treated with opioids: continuing professional development. *Can J Anaesth.* 2009;56(12):969-981.
26. Chapman CR, Davis J, Donaldson GW, Naylor J, Winchester D. Postoperative pain trajectories in chronic pain patients undergoing surgery: the effects of chronic opioid pharmacotherapy on acute pain. *J Pain.* 2011;12(12):1240-1246.
27. Angst MS, Clark JD. Opioid-induced hyperalgesia: a qualitative systematic review. *Anesthesiology.* 2006;104(3):570-587.
28. Becker WC, Frank JW, Edens EL. Switching from high-dose, long-term opioids to buprenorphine: a case series. *Ann Intern Med.* 2020;173(1):70-71.
29. Cohen SM, Weimer MB, Levander XA, Peckham AM, Tetrault JM, Morford KL. Low dose initiation of buprenorphine: a narrative review and practical approach. *J Addict Med.* 2022;16(4):399-406.
30. Hickey T, Abelleira A, Acampora G, et al. Perioperative buprenorphine management: a multidisciplinary approach. *Med Clin North Am.* 2022;106(1):169-185.
31. Raofi S, Schappert SM. Medication therapy in ambulatory medical care: United States, 2003-04. *Vital Health Stat 13.* 2006;(163):1-40.
32. Rui P, Santo L, Ashman JJ. *Trends in Opioids Prescribed at Discharge From Emergency Departments Among Adults: United States, 2006-2017.* National Health Statistics Reports; no. 135. National Center for Health Statistics; 2020.
33. Gleber R, Vilke GM, Castillo EM, Brennan J, Oyama L, Coyne CJ. Trends in emergency physician opioid prescribing practices during the United States opioid crisis. *Am J Emerg Med.* 2020;38(4):735-740. doi:10.1016/j.ajem.2019.06.011
34. American College of Emergency Physicians. *Opioid Prescribing in the ED.* Accessed March 2023. https://www.acep.org/by-medical-focus/mental-health-and-substanc-use-disorders/opioids/Opioid-Prescribing-in-the-ED
35. Daoust R, Paquet J, Marquis M, et al. Evaluation of interventions to reduce opioid prescribing for patients discharged from the emergency department: a systematic review and meta-analysis. *JAMA Netw Open.* 2022;5(1):e2143425. doi:10.1001/jamanetworkopen.2021.43425
36. Turk DC, Swanson K. Efficacy and cost-effectiveness treatment for chronic pain: an analysis and evidence-based synthesis. In: Schatman ME, Campbell A, eds. *Chronic Pain Management: A Guidebook for Multidisciplinary Program Development.* Informa Healthcare; 2007: 15-38.
37. Gatchel RJ, McGeary DD, Peterson A, et al. Preliminary findings of a randomized controlled trial of an interdisciplinary military pain program. *Mil Med.* 2009;174(3):270-277.
38. Schatman ME. Interdisciplinary chronic pain management: international perspectives. *Pain.* 2012;20(7):1-5.
39. American Society of Anesthesiologists Task Force on Chronic Pain Management; American Society of Regional Anesthesia and Pain Medicine. Practice guidelines for chronic pain management: an updated report by the American Society of Anesthesiologists Task Force on Chronic Pain Management and the American Society of Regional Anesthesia and Pain Medicine. *Anesthesiology.* 2010;112(4):810-833.
40. Allergan Inc. Package insert. Accessed July 23, 2023. http://www.allergan.com/assets/pdf/botox_pi.pdf.
41. Oakley JC. Spinal cord stimulation: patient selection, technique, and outcomes. *Neurosurg Clin N Am.* 2003;14(3):365-380.
42. de Leon-Casasola OA. Spinal cord and peripheral nerve stimulation techniques for neuropathic pain. *J Pain Symptom Manage.* 2009;38(2 Suppl):S28-S38.
43. Levy RM. Deep brain stimulation for the treatment of intractable pain. *Neurosurg Clin N Am.* 2003;14(3):389-399.
44. Plow EB, Pascual-Leone A, Machado A. Brain stimulation in the treatment of chronic neuropathic and non-cancerous pain. *J Pain.* 2012;13(5):411-424.
45. Nizard J, Lefaucheur JP, Helbert M, de Chauvigny E, Nguyen JP. Non-invasive stimulation therapies for the treatment of refractory pain. *Discov Med.* 2012;14(74):21-31.
46. Substance Abuse and Mental Health Services Administration. *Managing Chronic Pain in Adults With or in Recovery From Substance Use Disorders.* Treatment Improvement Protocol (TIP) Series 54. HHS Publication No. (SMA) 12-4671. Substance Abuse and Mental Health Services Administration; 2011.
47. Bair MJ, Sanderson TR. Coanalgesics for chronic pain therapy: a narrative review. *Postgrad Med.* 2011;123(6):140-150.
48. McQuay HJ, Moore A. NSAIDs and coxibs: clinical use. In: McMahon S, Koltzenburg M, eds. *Wall and Melzack's Textbook of Pain.* 5th ed. Churchill Livingstone; 2005:474-480.
49. Bellin MD, Sutherland DE, Robertson RP. Pancreatectomy and autologous islet transplantation for painful chronic pancreatitis: indications and outcomes. *Hosp Pract (1995).* 2012;40(3):80-87.
50. Noble M, Treadwell JR, Tregear SJ, et al. Long-term opioid management for chronic noncancer pain. *Cochrane Database Syst Rev.* 2010;(1):CD006605.
51. Ballantyne JC. "Safe and effective when used as directed": the case of chronic use of opioid analgesics. *J Med Toxicol.* 2012;8(4):417-423.
52. Kalso E, Edwards JE, Moore RA, McQuay HJ. Opioids in chronic non-cancer pain: systematic review of efficacy and safety. *Pain.* 2004;112(3):372-380.
53. Daitch J, Frey ME, Silver D, Mitnick C, Daitch D, Pergolizzi J Jr. Conversion of chronic pain patients from full-opioid agonists to sublingual buprenorphine. *Pain Physician.* 2012;15(3 Suppl):ES59-ES66.
54. Davis MP. Twelve reasons for considering buprenorphine as a frontline analgesic in the management of pain. *J Support Oncol.* 2012;10(6):209-219.
55. Likar R. Transdermal buprenorphine in the management of persistent pain—safety aspects. *Ther Clin Risk Manag.* 2006;2(1):115-125.
56. Poisnel G, Dhilly M, Le Boisselier R, Barre L, Debruyne D. Comparison of five benzodiazepine-receptor agonists on buprenorphine-induced mu-opioid receptor regulation. *J Pharmacol Sci.* 2009;110(1):36-46.
57. Barry DT, Savant JD, Beitel M, et al. Pain and associated substance use among opioid dependent individuals seeking office-based treatment with buprenorphine–naloxone: a needs assessment study. *Am J Addict.* 2013;22(3):212-217.
58. Barry DT, Beitel M, Cutter CJ, Joshi D, Falcioni J, Schottenfeld RS. Conventional and non-conventional pain treatment utilization among opioid dependent individuals with pain seeking methadone maintenance treatment: a needs assessment study. *J Addict Med.* 2010;4(2):81-87.
59. Barry DT, Savant JD, Beitel M, et al. Use of conventional, complementary, and alternative treatments for pain among individuals seeking

primary care treatment with buprenorphine-naloxone. *J Addict Med.* 2012;6(4):274-279.

60. Scimeca MM, Savage SR, Portenoy R, Lowinson J. Treatment of pain in methadone-maintained patients. *Mt Sinai J Med.* 2000;67(5-6):412-422.
61. Morasco BJ, Greaves DW, Lovejoy TI, Turk DC, Dobscha SK, Hauser P. Development and preliminary evaluation of an integrated cognitive-behavior treatment for chronic pain and substance use disorder in patients with the hepatitis c virus. *Pain Med.* 2016;17(12):2280-2290.
62. Ilgen MA, Haas E, Czyz E, Webster L, Sorrell JT, Chermack S. Treating chronic pain in veterans presenting to an addictions treatment program. *Cogn Behav Pract.* 2011;18(1):149-160.
63. Currie SR, Hodgins DC, Crabtree A, Jacobi J, Armstrong S. Outcome from integrated pain management treatment for recovering substance abusers. *J Pain.* 2003;4(2):91-100.
64. Ilgen MA, Bohnert AS, Chermak S, et al. A randomized trial of a pain management intervention for adults receiving substance use disorder treatment. *Addiction.* 2016;111(8):1385-1393.
65. Ilgen MA, Coughlin LN, Bohnert AS, et al. Efficacy of a psychosocial pain management intervention for men and women with substance use disorders and chronic pain: a randomized clinical trial. *JAMA Psychiatry.* 2020;77(12):1225-1234. doi:10.1001/jamapsychiatry.2020.2369
66. Barry DT, Beitel M, Cutter CJ, et al. An evaluation of the feasibility, acceptability, and preliminary efficacy of cognitive-behavioral therapy for opioid use disorder and chronic pain. *Drug Alcohol Depend.* 2019;194:460-467.
67. DiMeola KA, Haynes J, Barone M, et al. A pilot investigation of nonpharmacological pain management intervention groups in methadone maintenance treatment. *J Addict Med.* 2022;16(2):229-234. doi:10.1097/ADM.0000000000000877
68. Butner JL, Bone C, Ponce Martinez CC, et al. Training drug counselors to deliver a brief psychosocial intervention for chronic pain among patients in opioid agonist treatment: a pilot investigation. *Subst Abus.* 2018;39:199-205.
69. Dunn KM, Saunders KW, Rutter CM, et al. Opioid prescriptions for chronic pain and overdose: a cohort study. *Ann Intern Med.* 2010;152(2):85-92.
70. Barry DT, Cutter CJ, Beitel M, Kerns RD, Liong C, Schottenfeld RS. Psychiatric disorders among patients seeking treatment for co-occurring chronic pain and opioid use disorder. *J Clin Psychiatry.* 2016;77(10):1413-1419.
71. Park TW, Saitz R, Ganoczy D, Ilgen MA, Bohnert AS. Benzodiazepine prescribing patterns and deaths from drug overdose among US veterans receiving opioid analgesics: case-cohort study. *BMJ.* 2015;350:h2698.
72. Gomes T, Juurlink DN, Antoniou T, Mamdani MM, Paterson JM, van den Brink W. Gabapentin, opioids, and the risk of opioid-related death: a population-based nested case–control study. *PLoS Med.* 2017;14(10):e1002396.
73. D'Elia G, von Knorring L, Marcusson J, Mattsson B, Perris C, Persson G. A double blind comparison between doxepin and diazepam in the treatment of states of anxiety. *Acta Psychiatr Scand Suppl.* 1974;255:35-46.
74. Bianchi GN, Phillips J. A comparative trial of doxepin and diazepam in anxiety states. *Psychopharmacologia.* 1972;25(1):86-95.
75. Rickels K, Downing R, Schweizer E, Hassman H. Diazepam vs trazodone vs imipramine for generalized anxiety disorder. Antidepressants for the treatment of generalized anxiety disorder. A placebo-controlled comparison of imipramine, trazodone, and diazepam. *Arch Gen Psychiatry.* 1993;50(11):884-895.
76. Kapczinski F, Lima MS, Souza JS, Schmitt R. Antidepressants for generalized anxiety disorder. *Cochrane Database Syst Rev.* 2003;(2):CD003592.
77. Saletu-Zyhlarz GM, Abu-Bakr MH, Anderer P, et al. Insomnia related to dysthymia: polysomnographic and psychometric comparison with normal controls and acute therapeutic trials with trazodone. *Neuropsychobiology.* 2001;44(3):139-149.
78. Smith MT, Huang MI, Manber R. Cognitive behavior therapy for chronic insomnia occurring within the context of medical and psychiatric disorders. *Clin Psychol Rev.* 2005;25:559-592.
79. Stiefel F, Stagno D. Management of insomnia in patients with chronic pain conditions. *CNS Drugs.* 2004;18:285-296.
80. Morin CM, Vallières A, Guay B, et al. Cognitive behavioral therapy, singly and combined with medication, for persistent insomnia: a randomized controlled trial. *JAMA.* 2009;301(19):2005-2015.
81. Smith MT, Perlis ML, Park A, et al. Comparative meta-analysis of pharmacotherapy and behavior therapy for persistent insomnia. *Am J Psychiatry.* 2002;159(1):5-11.
82. Center for Substance Abuse Treatment. *Medication-Assisted Treatment for Opioid Addiction in Opioid Treatment Programs.* Treatment Improvement Protocol (TIP) Series 43. DHHS Publication No. (SMA) 05-4048. Substance Abuse and Mental Health Services Administration; 2005. Accessed July 24, 2023. http://www.ncbi.nlm.nih.gov/books/NBK64164/pdf/TOC.pdf
83. Moore BA, Fiellin DA, Barry DT, et al. Primary care office-based buprenorphine treatment: comparison of heroin and prescription opioid dependent patients. *J Gen Intern Med.* 2007;22(4):527-530.

CHAPTER

115 Legal and Regulatory Considerations in Opioid Prescribing

David J. Copenhaver, Rohit Nalamasu, Wesley R. Prickett, Julia Megan Webb, and Scott M. Fishman

CHAPTER OUTLINE

- Introduction
- Federal opioid regulations
- State-controlled substance regulations
- Opioid prescribing when federal and state law conflict
- Roles and recommendations from federal agencies and organizations
- Prescribing guidelines
- Prescription drug monitoring programs
- Opioids and the supreme court
- Summary

DISCLAIMER: The authors do not offer legal advice. Readers seeking legal or risk management advice in any of the areas discussed in this chapter should seek expert guidance from risk management and/or legal professionals.

INTRODUCTION

The National Academy of Medicine (previously the Institute of Medicine), in a landmark report entitled "Relieving Pain in America," detailed the epidemic of chronic pain in the United States. This 2011 report estimated that chronic pain affects nearly 100 million American adults.[1] The use of opioids to treat chronic nonmalignant pain went from uncommon to too common over several recent decades. In some instances, prescribers became complacent in using opioids to treat a variety of chronic pain complaints of varying severity with minimal assessment of functional benefit achieved, implementation of safety measures, or consideration of nonopioid pain management. National attention to responsible opioid prescribing has only grown in light of reports from the Centers for Disease Control and Prevention (CDC) underscoring unintended overdose from prescription opioids as a leading cause of accidental death in adults aged 25 to 64.[2,3] In 2019, 70,630 drug overdose deaths occurred in the United States, with an increase of 4% from 2018 to 2019. Approximately 50,000 of these deaths (or 70%) were due to opioids. This trend was initially noted in the year 2000 at which time it appeared that these unintended overdose deaths were largely driven by excessive opioid prescribing. In a second phase, these overdose deaths appeared to be driven by increasing rates of heroin use, and later by nonprescription synthetic opioid use (**Fig. 115-1**). Prescriptions for opioids in the U.S. appear to have peaked in 2012 and currently have decreased by half that amount (**Table 115-1**). Currently, the main driver of opioid-involved overdose deaths is thought to be related to synthetic opioids,[4] as suggested by the current findings of unintended overdose deaths that are increasing despite substantially reduced rates of opioid prescribing. This evolving predicament challenges clinicians, regulators, and lawmakers to establish a framework of guidelines to better guide prescribers on how to achieve a tenable balance between the goals of alleviating suffering and minimizing harm to the patient and society.

Rapidly expanding evidence describing the wide range of serious risks associated with chronic opioid therapy requires that any prescriber of opioids have, at minimum, a foundational understanding of evolving federal and state regulations governing the use of all controlled substances, not just opioids. The following chapter will highlight some of these regulations and provide a brief overview.

FEDERAL OPIOID REGULATIONS

Federal regulations governing controlled substances are intended to balance the need for the therapeutic use of these substances with the mandate to protect consumers. Historically, controlled substance regulations have been driven by two major concepts: transparency or truth in labeling, the domain of the Food and Drug Administration (FDA), and the appropriate distribution and use of controlled substances, the domain of the Drug Enforcement Administration (DEA). Truth in labeling protects consumers from an educational standpoint, and the appropriate use of controlled substances, in theory, limits access to these substances, thereby protecting the public at large from diversion and unhealthy use of prescribed controlled drugs. Federal regulation of medications, including controlled substances, began in the United States over 100 years ago with the Pure Food and Drug Act of 1906. This statute was enacted to ensure that medications had proper labeling and were unadulterated before reaching the consumer.[5] Established in 1914, the Harrison Narcotics Tax Act was developed to impede diversion and unhealthy use of opioids and was followed by the Marijuana Tax Act of 1937.[5] Amphetamines, barbiturates, and hallucinogens were brought under regulation in 1965 under the Federal Food, Drug, and Cosmetic Act.[5]

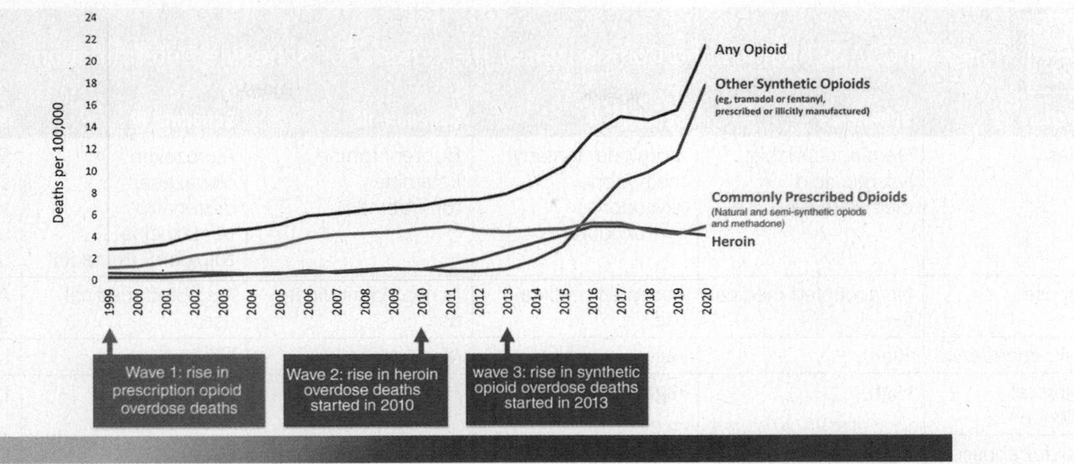

Figure 115-1. Three waves of opioid overdose deaths. (From Centers for Disease Control and Prevention. *Understanding the Opioid Overdose Epidemic*. National Vital Statistics System Morality File. https://www.cdc.gov/opioids/basics/epidemic.html)

The U.S. Congress sought to consolidate the various federal regulatory statutes governing drugs of potential unhealthy use or substance use disorders (SUD), and in 1970, the Comprehensive Drug Abuse Prevention and Control Act was created. Title II of this policy is the Controlled Substances Act (CSA), which is the primary set of federal regulations that govern the medical use of controlled substances in the United States. Under the CSA, controlled substances are divided into five schedules based on the following characteristics: potential for abuse [sic], pharmacological effects, scientific properties, pattern of abuse, public health risk, psychological or physiological dependence, liability, and whether the substance is an immediate precursor of a substance already classified under a CSA schedule.[6] As reflected in **Table 115-2**, Schedule II-IV drugs all have accepted medical use and primarily differ based on varying degrees of physical/psychological dependence and unhealthy use potential. Each drug schedule also carries differing criminal penalties for unlawful use outside of accepted standard medical practice. The implementation and enforcement of the CSA are currently assigned to the DEA in the Department of Justice. The classification of drugs within these schedules is subject to review and may be adjusted if evidence is sufficient as was the case in 2014 when hydrocodone was rescheduled from a Schedule III to a Schedule II drug and tramadol became a Schedule IV drug.[7]

TABLE 115-1 Total Number and Rate of Opioid Prescriptions Dispensed, United States, 2006-2020

Year	Total Number of Prescriptions	Opioid Dispensing Rate Per 100 Persons
2006	215,917,663	72.4
2007	228,543,773	75.9
2008	237,860,213	78.2
2009	243,738,090	79.5
2010	251,088,904	81.2
2011	252,167,963	80.9
2012	255,207,954	81.3
2013	247,090,443	78.1
2014	240,993,021	75.6
2015	226,819,924	70.6
2016	214,881,662	66.5
2017	191,909,384	59.0
2018	168,158,611	51.4
2019	153,260,450	46.7
2020	142,816,781	43.3

From Centers for Disease Control and Prevention. *U.S. Opioid Dispensing Rate Maps*. https://www.cdc.gov/drugoverdose/rxrate-maps/index.html

Federal regulations allow opioids to be prescribed for legitimate medical purposes, including both for acute pain and chronic pain.[8] Methadone and buprenorphine are used to treat pain as well as medication for opioid use disorder (MOUD) in the setting of withdrawal management and opioid use disorder (OUD). Although no special DEA registration is required to prescribe buprenorphine or methadone for pain, when methadone and buprenorphine are prescribed as MOUD, additional regulations and requirements for prescribers are required as additional precautions must be taken.[9-11] The specific licensing requirements to prescribe buprenorphine and methadone as MOUD are beyond the scope of this chapter and are covered elsewhere in this textbook. Clinicians should be aware of specific exceptions to these rules to provide patients with OUD appropriate care in an acute setting. The DATA 2000 amendment to the CSA allows physicians to administer, not prescribe, buprenorphine or methadone for agonist treatment or withdrawal management in patients with opioid dependence or OUD who are admitted for a primary

TABLE 115-2 The Five CSA Schedules and Comparison of the Criteria for Schedule Determination

CSA schedule	Schedule I	Schedule II	Schedule III	Schedule IV	Schedule V
Examples	Heroin, cannabis, lysergic acid diethylamide	Morphine, fentanyl, methadone, oxycodone, hydrocodone	Buprenorphine, ketamine (dronabinol)	Alprazolam, clonazepam, diazepam, pentazocine, zolpidem, tramadol	Pregabalin, substances with small amounts of codeine or diphenoxylate
Medical use	No accepted medical use	Accepted medical use	Accepted medical use	Accepted medical use	Accepted medical use
Physical dependence	High	High	Moderate to low	Limited	Limited
Psychological dependence	High	High	High	Limited	Limited
Potential for abuse	High	High	Moderate (less than CSA Schedule I-II)	Low	Low

From Drug Enforcement Agency. *Drug Scheduling.* Accessed November 28, 2016. https://www.dea.gov/druginfo/ds.shtml

Fishman S. Regulating opioid prescribing through prescription monitoring programs: balancing drug diversion and treatment of pain. *Pain Med.* 2004;5(3):309-324.

problem other than opioid dependence. This allows physicians to manage these patients for whom opioid withdrawal would complicate treatment of the presenting medical or surgical condition, such as myocardial infarction, without obtaining an official waiver.[12] The "three-day rule" allows clinicians who are not registered to treat OUD to administer, but not prescribe, opioids for a maximum of 72 hours to relieve acute withdrawal symptoms in a patient with pre-DSM-IV defined opioid dependence, while a referral is arranged for treatment.[12]

STATE-CONTROLLED SUBSTANCE REGULATIONS

In addition to federal laws, states may adopt state regulations that can be more or less restrictive or proscriptive than federal laws. State medical policy can vary widely from state to state, and for this reason, prescribers must be fully aware of the legal statutes in their state. Some specific state variations of interest include possible limits on the amount of opioids that can be dispensed, listing opioids as a treatment of last resort, requiring that opioids result in documented functional improvement, requirement for evaluation by a pain specialist, or provider continuing medical education (CME) requirements in opioid prescribing or pain management. Some states may require consultation with an addiction medicine specialist if chronic opioid therapy is to be used in a patient in whom the provider suspects SUD or unhealthy drug use.[13]

OPIOID PRESCRIBING WHEN FEDERAL AND STATE LAW CONFLICT

Physicians are expected to comply with both state and federal prescribing regulations. The Supremacy Clause of Constitution Article VI, as well as the doctrine known as pre-emption, suggests that when in conflict, federal law prevails over state law.[14] In general, where state and federal regulations are in conflict, clinicians are advised to adhere to the most conservative or restrictive standards. As such, the exact course of action for adherence to the law may not be straightforward, and clinicians must refer to official legal counsel for specific advice.[14]

As an example, federal law classifies cannabis as a Schedule I substance: one with no accepted medical use and a high unhealthy use potential. In recent years, a growing number of states have adopted new laws addressing cannabis/marijuana (18 states plus the District of Columbia as of April 2022),[15] ranging from decriminalizing possession to legalizing the use of cannabis as treatment or for recreational use. As the continued prescribing of a controlled substance to individuals known to be using a Schedule I drug is typically inappropriate or illegal,[16] physicians who prescribe opioids in states where cannabis use is legal to varying degrees may find themselves in conflict between federal and state law.

Another example of variability of state laws and possible conflict with federal requirements involves breach of doctor-patient relationships and responses to illegal behavior of patients with respect to controlled substance prescriptions. If a prescriber knows that an opioid prescription has been forged, but the crime did not take place on the prescriber's premises, there is some controversy over whether reporting such a crime to law enforcement might constitute a violation of the prescriber's requirement to confidentiality of protected health information as set forth by the Health Insurance Portability and Accountability Act (HIPAA).[17] Tennessee specifically requires a health care provider with knowledge that a person has secured or has attempted to secure a controlled substance through deceit to report the offense to law enforcement.[18] It appears that such specific state law would offer an exemption to the HIPAA privacy requirement. A few other states appear to have provisions within their state laws that may authorize health care professionals to inform law enforcement when they reasonably believe that a patient may have obtained or sought to obtain a fraudulent prescription for controlled substances.[19-21]

ROLES AND RECOMMENDATIONS FROM FEDERAL AGENCIES AND ORGANIZATIONS

The Drug Enforcement Administration

State medical boards are charged with upholding standards of professional practice and assuring compliance of practitioners with both state and federal regulations. However, with respect to prescribing controlled substances for pain, their role may overlap with that of the Drug Enforcement Administration (DEA). As part of the U.S. Department of Justice, the DEA does not directly regulate medical practice, but it may investigate practitioners who do not comply with the laws regarding distribution of controlled substances.[22] These investigations can lead to revocation of the provider's DEA registration or to criminal prosecution.

According to the DEA, common behaviors that result in investigation include issuing prescriptions for controlled substances without a physician-patient relationship, issuing prescriptions in exchange for sex, charging fees commensurate with "drug dealing" rather than providing medical services, issuing prescriptions using fraudulent names, and self-prescribing or misuse by practitioners.[22] The DEA reported in 2006 that, in any given year, less than 0.01% of physicians in the United States lose their controlled substance registrations based on a DEA investigation, and most investigations of physicians that result in loss of DEA registration are initiated by the state medical board.[22] The number of cases of disciplined physicians has risen over the past decade from previous historically low levels. In 2012, it was reported that 0.5% of all licensed physicians in the United States were disciplined by state medical boards.[23]

Health care providers who wish to prescribe controlled substances must be registered and obtain a provider number through the DEA. Federal DEA registrations are valid for 3 years, and the DEA certificate of registration must be kept at the registered location and be readily retrievable for inspection purposes.[24] Currently, requirements to obtain a DEA number are associated with the provider meeting criteria for licensing, but there are no initial requirements for demonstration of knowledge or competence related to controlled substance prescribing and no requirements for continuing medical education credits.

In 2006, the DEA released an updated Practitioner's Manual that summarizes the federal regulations regarding controlled substances and the CSA. The complete manual can be found at www.deadiversion.usdoj.gov under resources: significant guidance documents and an updated version has not been released as of mid-2022.[25] Also in 2006, the DEA released a statement entitled "Dispensing Controlled Substances for the Treatment of Pain."[22] Health care providers are encouraged to familiarize themselves with these two documents as they provide important information regarding federal regulations on prescribing controlled substances. These documents emphasize the need for appropriate documentation, security of medications both on the part of the patient and the dispenser, and the need for careful monitoring of medication use and amount.[22]

In 2007, the DEA limited the amount of Schedule II controlled substances that can be prescribed within a single prescription to no more than a 90-day supply with a new prescription being required if continued use is deemed medically necessary beyond this period.[26] Prescribers also must follow their state law that may have limits that are less than the federal 90-day period and/or dose unit requirements. Although refills on Schedule II drugs are never allowed, practitioners may provide patients with multiple prescriptions, to be filled sequentially, for the same Schedule II controlled substance.[26] In states where this practice is legal, issuing multiple, sequential prescriptions allows practitioners to provide up to a 90-day supply of a Schedule II medication without interval office visits. In some cases, this practice may be used to tightly control prescribing, for example, providing four prescriptions for 1 week each, thus limiting the amount available to a week's supply at a time but not requiring an office visit until a month later. When using such sequential prescriptions, the prescriber indicates that the prescription should not be filled until a later date that is clearly written on the prescription. However, postdating these prescriptions is not allowed, and each prescription must be dated on the day it was written. Thus, multiple prescriptions might each have the same date (indicating the date they were written) but different fill dates for when a pharmacist can fill the prescriptions. Issuing multiple prescriptions in this way is not permitted in every state, and providers must ensure compliance with the more stringent regulation. In 2010, the DEA determined that practitioners who are registered with the DEA can prescribe scheduled substances electronically through special procedures,[27] though state laws vary with respect to electronic prescribing.

The Food and Drug Administration and Risk Evaluation and Mitigation Strategies

The Food and Drug Administration (FDA) has the authority to require pharmaceutical manufacturers to develop Risk Evaluation and Mitigation Strategies (REMS) under the Food and Drug Administration Amendments Act (FDAAA) of 2007.[28] The REMS requirement ensures that the benefits of the substance outweigh potential risks and provide drug class-specific education to prescribers.[28] Historically, the FDA has used various risk management strategies for other drugs before the REMS requirement was applied to opioids.[29]

The FDA initially released a REMS for transmucosal immediate-release fentanyl (TIRF) in December of 2011 and modified it in 2020, essentially to ensure that patients receiving a TIRF medication were opioid tolerant at the time of receiving the TIRF prescription.[30] Going beyond the issue of TIRF medications, the FDA sought to address the much larger and growing problem of opioid related overdose and inappropriate use related to opioid medications that were prescribed for chronic pain. In 2011, the FDA, in collaboration with the White House Office of the National Drug Control Policy, issued a directive requiring stakeholders to develop comprehensive REMS for long-acting opioids (LAOs) and requested that certain manufacturers of LAOs develop REMS for their products.[31,32] The manufacturers of LAOs are required to provide financial support for the development and implementation of this voluntary continuing medical education (CME) related to their products. The FDA released the final REMS requirements for extended-release/long-acting opioids (LAOs) in July of 2012.[27] These include extended-release products of morphine, oxycodone, and transdermal fentanyl, as well as intrinsically long-acting medications such as methadone. These REMS have drawn criticism because providers participate in the CME education on a voluntary basis. Some have suggested that voluntary CME education is unlikely to make a substantial difference in the epidemic of prescription related OUD and that ineffective REMS education may necessitate mandatory education for prescribers of these medications. In fact, some states have already adopted mandatory CME on opioid-related topics. The FDA is continually evaluating substances, and the updated list of REMS can be found at https://www.accessdata.fda.gov/scripts/cder/rems/index.cfm.[33]

The FDA has issued several consumer warnings on the disposal of controlled substances. The transdermal fentanyl patch has been highlighted by the FDA for its potential serious risk to children or others who may find and use discarded patches. One can extrapolate similar concerns for any controlled substance product that leaves residual drug to be discarded following proper use such as transdermal buprenorphine patches and possibly transmucosal fentanyl products as well as others. These warnings have highlighted the growing necessity for prescribers to educate their patients and the patient's family or caregivers about the safe use, storage, and disposal of controlled substances. The Secure and Responsible Drug Disposal Act of 2010, an amendment to the CSA, authorized the DEA to advance rules allowing the transfer of legally obtained prescribed controlled substances to authorized collectors for safe disposal.[34] The DEA sponsors the National Prescription Drug Take-Back Days and provides and authorizes "Take-Back" collection sites. When a Take-Back program is not available, the FDA and DEA recommend flushing used or unwanted opioid medications, including transdermal formulations, immediately down the toilet.[35] Alternatively, patients may prefer to dispose of their opioids at a local pharmacy, however not all pharmacies will participate. There has been recent research on the utility of mail home disposal kits provided at the time of discharge.[36,37]

Responsible opioid prescribing necessitates that patient education is featured prominently in the provider-patient treatment agreement.[38] Patient education resources can be found in many locations, including two websites from the National Institutes of Health (NIH)–NIDA https://www.drugabuse.gov/drugs-abuse/opioids and the CDC at https://www.cdc.gov/opioids/patients/materials.html.[39]

PRESCRIBING GUIDELINES

Centers for Disease Control and Prevention and the 2016 Opioid Prescribing Guidelines

The Centers for Disease Control and Prevention (CDC) is part of the U.S. Department of Health and Human Services and "serves as the national focus for developing and applying disease prevention and control, environmental health, and health promotion and health education activities designed to improve the health of the people of the United States."[40] To this end, the CDC provides advice and recommendations to the federal government through federal advisory committees and communicates with the public via weekly publications of the *Morbidity and Mortality Weekly Report* (MMWR).

The *CDC Guideline for Prescribing Opioids for Chronic Pain* was published in March 2016.[41] The guideline is intended to provide "recommendations to primary care physicians who are prescribing opioids for chronic pain outside of active cancer treatment, palliative care, and end-of-life care." It addresses three domains of concern including when to initiate or continue opioids for chronic pain; opioid selection, dose, duration, follow-up, and discontinuation; and assessment of risk and mitigation of harm. Five key clinical questions (KQ) are addressed: (1) effectiveness of long-term opioid therapy; (2) risks of opioids including misuse, addiction, and overdose; (3) effectiveness of opioid dosing strategies; (4) accuracy of risk prediction and effectiveness of risk mitigation strategies; and (5) effects on long-term opioid use due to prescribing of opioids for acute pain.[42] Among the more specific recommendations contained in the guideline are that the clinician should carefully assess individual risks and benefits of opioid therapy within 1 to 4 weeks of initiating or increasing opioids and that these risks and benefits be re-evaluated at least every three months during therapy and when increasing opioids to 50 or more morphine milligram equivalents (MME)/d. The guideline suggests extra caution when escalating to or maintaining doses at 90 or more MME/d. Other recommendations include offering naloxone to patients at increased risk for opioid overdose and obtaining a urine drug test and consultation with a Prescription Drug Monitoring Program (PDMP) prior to and at least every 3 months during long-term opioid therapy. The guideline recognizes that long-term opioid use often begins with prescribing opioids for acute pain, including postsurgical pain. The guideline recommends clinicians to prescribe only the amount of immediate-release opioids required to treat "pain severe enough to require opioids." The guideline also suggests that "3 days or less will often be sufficient" for treating most forms of acute pain and "more than 7 days will rarely be needed." A full discussion and description of the recommendations is beyond the scope of this chapter.

TABLE 115-3 CDC Recommendations for Prescribing Opioids for Chronic Pain Outside of Active Cancer, Palliative, and End-of-Life Care[a]

Determining when to initiate or continue opioids for chronic pain
1. Nonpharmacological therapy and nonopioid pharmacological therapy are preferred for chronic pain. Clinicians should consider opioid therapy only if expected benefits for both pain and function are anticipated to outweigh risks to the patient. If opioids are used, they should be combined with nonpharmacological therapy and nonopioid pharmacological therapy, as appropriate. 2. Before starting opioid therapy for chronic pain, clinicians should establish treatment goals with all patients, including realistic goals for pain and function, and should consider how therapy will be discontinued if benefits do not outweigh risks. Clinicians should continue opioid therapy only if there is clinically meaningful improvement in pain and function that outweighs risks to patient safety. 3. Before starting and periodically during opioid therapy, clinicians should discuss with patients the known risks and realistic benefits of opioid therapy and patient and clinician responsibilities for managing therapy.
Opioid selection, dosage, duration, follow-up, and discontinuation
1. When starting opioid therapy for chronic pain, clinicians should prescribe immediate-release opioids instead of extended-release/long-acting (ER/LA) opioids. 2. When opioids are started, clinicians should prescribe the lowest effective dosage. Clinicians should use caution when prescribing opioids at any dosage, should carefully reassess evidence of individual benefits and risks when increasing dosage to ≥50 morphine milligram equi valents (MME)/d, and should avoid increasing dosage to ≥90 MME/d or carefully justify a decision to titrate dosage to ≥90 MME/d. 3. Long-term opioid use often begins with treatment of acute pain. When opioids are used for acute pain, clinicians should prescribe the lowest effective dose of immediate-release opioids and should prescribe no greater quantity than needed for the expected duration of pain severe enough to require opioids. Three days or less will often be sufficient; more than seven days will rarely be needed. 4. Clinicians should evaluate benefits and harms with patients within 1-4 weeks of starting opioid therapy for chronic pain or of dose escalation. Clinicians should evaluate benefits and harms of continued therapy with patients every 3 months or more frequently. If benefits do not outweigh harms of continued opioid therapy, clinicians should optimize other therapies and work with patients to taper opioids to lower dosages or to taper and discontinue opioids.
Assessing risk and addressing harms of opioid use
1. Before starting and periodically during continuation of opioid therapy, clinicians should evaluate risk factors for opioid-related harms. Clinicians should incorporate into the management plan strategies to mitigate risk, including considering offering naloxone when factors that increase risk for opioid overdose, such as history of overdose, history of substance use disorder, higher opioid dosages (≥50 MME/d), or concurrent benzodiazepine use, are present. 2. Clinicians should review the patient's history of controlled substance prescriptions using state Prescription Drug Monitoring Program (PDMP) data to determine whether the patient is receiving opioid dosages or dangerous combinations that put him or her at high risk for overdose. Clinicians should review PDMP data when starting opioid therapy for chronic pain and periodically during opioid therapy for chronic pain, ranging from every prescription to every 3 months. 3. When prescribing opioids for chronic pain, clinicians should use urine drug testing before starting opioid therapy and consider urine drug testing at least annually to assess for prescribed medications as well as other controlled prescription drugs and illicit drugs. 4. Clinicians should avoid prescribing opioid pain medication and benzodiazepines concurrently whenever possible. 5. Clinicians should offer or arrange evidence-based treatment (usually medication-assisted treatment with buprenorphine or methadone in combination with behavioral therapies) for patients with opioid use disorder.

[a]All recommendations are category A (apply to all patients outside of active cancer treatment, palliative care, and end-of-life care) except recommendation 10 (designated category B, with individual decision-making required); see full guideline for evidence ratings.

Reproduced from Box 1 of the CDC guideline for prescribing opioids for chronic pain—United States, 2016. https://www.cdc.gov/mmwr/volumes/65/rr/rr6501e1.htm

The 2016 recommendations are summarized in **Table 115-3**, and the full report is available at https://www.cdc.gov/mmwr/volumes/65/rr/rr6501e1.htm.

Although the CDC guideline is not a federal statute, the recommendations are intended to shape opioid prescribing practices, and the specificity of the recommendations are likely to influence what is considered the standard of care. Some states have adopted elements of the guideline as state-specific opioid prescribing rules.

Misapplication of CDC Guidelines

Since the 2016 CDC opioid guidelines were introduced, there have been unintended applications of these guidelines. These issues include confusion with opioid tapering, misapplication of guideline for MOUD, misunderstanding regarding opioid dosage recommendations resulting in hard limits or abrupt discontinuation, and misapplication to other unintended patient populations other than chronic pain patients. Moreover, concerns have been raised about overdose, mental health crises, and even suicide associated with involuntary or aggressive tapering as well as abstinence from long-standing opioid dosing.[42] The authors of the original guidelines have asserted these misconceptions were never intended and that misapplication of the guidelines could result in unintended patient health and safety consequences.[43] The 2016 CDC guidelines were intended for primary care physicians to help aid decision making when treating patients with chronic pain. The CDC and the original authors of the guideline have recently come forward to emphasize that the CDC guideline was never meant to provide absolute rules of practice. The CDC continues to admonish clinicians "to continue to use their clinical judgment, base treatment on what they know about their patients, maximize use of safe and effective non-opioid treatments, and consider the use of opioids only if their benefits are likely to outweigh their risks."[44] The advice from the CDC in avoiding misapplication of their opioid guideline involve these key points: (1) the guideline was intended for PCP's treating chronic pain for greater than 3 months, and not for patients with cancer, acute sickle cell crises, or postoperative pain; they did not intend to set "Hard Dosing Limits" or advise abrupt tapering, "cutting off" opioids or sudden discontinuation of opioids, and that the guidelines were intended to address opioids for chronic pain and not medication assisted therapy for OUD.[44] As a result of this, the American Medical Association has called for a major revision of the CDC guideline.

Federation of State Medical Board Guidelines

State medical boards are responsible for physician licensing. The regulations and requirements regarding licensing can vary significantly from state to state. Should concerns arise in the practice of a prescribing physician, these state boards are also responsible for determining whether these clinicians are practicing within or below the standards of medical practice in their state. Medical boards usually look to experts and particularly to professional groups to help determine the standard of care.[45]

The Federation of State Medical Boards (FSMB), a national nonprofit organization representing 70 medical and osteopathic boards, published one of the earliest policies regarding the use and prescribing of controlled substances. Many states have turned to these recommendations for guidance when drafting local state legislation and medical policy. Originally adopted in 1998 and revised in 2013, the FSMB released its "Model Policy on the Use of Opioid Analgesics in the Treatment of Chronic Pain."[46] This policy was developed to assist medical and osteopathic medical boards when evaluating cases involving the prescribing of opioid analgesics.

The former FSMB "Model Policy on the Use of Opioid Analgesics in the Treatment of Chronic Pain"[46] was replaced in 2017 with the FSMB "Guidelines for the Chronic Use of Opioid Analgesics" in April of 2017.[47] In updating the existing policy, the FSMB intended this new policy to provide direction for overall safe and evidence based opioid prescribing without creating a specific standard of care.

Other Guidelines and Guideline Challenges START

The evidence to guide decisions about the efficacy of opioid use in chronic noncancer pain (CNCP) remains weak to inadequate. The American Pain Society (APS) and the American Academy of Pain Medicine (AAPM) produced "Clinical Guidelines for the Use of Chronic Opioid Therapy (COT) in Chronic Non-Cancer Pain (CNCP)" in 2009.[48] In 2010, the Cochrane collaboration released its "Long-term Opioid Management for CNCP," which represented an interpretation of the data available.[49] The summary statement from the Cochrane review states "The findings of this systematic review suggest that proper management of a type of strong painkiller (opioids) in well-selected patients with no history of substance addiction or abuse can lead to long-term pain relief for some patients with a very small (though not zero) risk of developing addiction, abuse, or other serious side effects. However, the evidence supporting these conclusions is weak, and longer-term studies are needed to identify the patients who are most likely to benefit from treatment." In 2012, the American Society of Interventional Pain Physicians released its "Guidelines for Responsible Opioid Prescribing in Chronic Non-Cancer Pain." Among the many provisions, this evidence-based guideline stressed many expectations associated with responsible opioid prescribing, which are listed in **Table 115-4**.[50] The result of the National Summit for Opioid Safety, which convened in the Fall of 2012, was a document entitled "Principles for more selective and cautious opioid prescribing," which is summarized in **Table 115-5**.[51] Most recently, the Agency for Healthcare Research and Quality (AHRQ) released a report titled "The Effectiveness and Risks of Long-Term Opioid Treatment of Chronic Pain" in October 2014, which reported that the evidence for long-term opioid therapy for chronic pain is very limited and that the increased risk of serious harms appears to be dose dependent.[52] The CDC guideline details and incorporates many of these documents and concerns.

PRESCRIPTION DRUG MONITORING PROGRAMS

In an attempt to help prescribers or law enforcement professionals prevent unhealthy use including addiction to controlled substances, many states have created PDMPs or Prescription Monitoring Programs (PMPs). PDMPs vary by state, but all are intended to track prescribing and dispensing of controlled substance prescriptions.[53] PDMPs have been present in several states since the 1940s, but after the creation of the Harold Rogers PDMP by the Department of Justice in 2002 and the National All Schedules Prescription Electronic Reporting Act (NASPER), passed by Congress in 2005, there has been a substantial increase in the number of states using PDMPs.[54,55] There has also been an increase in the number of states employing electronic PDMP systems intended to assist clinicians at the point of care. These point-of-care PDMP systems are designed to help clinicians detect when patients are receiving prescriptions for controlled substances from multiple physicians and/or multiple pharmacies. These secure electronic PDMPs are usually directly accessible by health care providers and/or law enforcement personnel. Updated PDMP information can be found at the National Alliance for Model State Drug Laws using the following internet link: https://namsdl.org/wp-content/uploads/Prescription-Drug-Monitoring-Programs-Evidence-Based-Practices-to-Optimize-Prescriber-Use.pdf.[56]

TABLE 115-4 Major Provisions of the 2012 American Society of the Interventional Pain Physicians Guidelines for Responsible Opioid Prescribing in Chronic Noncancer Pain

- Comprehensive assessment and documentation.
- Screening for opioid use to identify and reduce aberrant medication taking behaviors and opioid use disorder.
- Implement prescription drug monitoring programs.
- Urine drug testing implemented from initiation along with subsequent adherence monitoring.
- Establish diagnosis (physical and psychological) prior to prescribing.
- Risk stratification (low, medium, or high risk).
- Obtain pain management consultation for nonpain physicians.
- Establish medical necessity prior to initiation or maintenance of chronic opioid therapy (COT).
- Establish treatment goals of opioid therapy with regard to pain relief and improvement in function.
- Limit high-dose LAO to specific circumstances with severe intractable pain not amenable to short-acting or moderate doses of LAOs.
- Use a robust treatment agreement.
- Initiate opioids at low doses and short-acting drugs with appropriate monitoring.
- Use methadone for late stages after failure of other opioid therapies and only by clinicians with specific training in the risks and uses:
  - Monitor electrocardiogram prior to initiation, 30 days, and yearly thereafter.
- Evaluate relative and absolute contraindications to opioid use in chronic noncancer pain:
  - Including respiratory instability, acute psychiatric instability, uncontrolled suicide risk, active or history of alcohol or other substance use disorders, confirmed allergy to opioid agents, coadministration of drugs capable of inducing life-limiting drug interaction, concomitant use of benzodiazepines, active diversion of controlled substances, and concomitant use of heavy doses of central nervous system depressants.
- Dose stratification (oral morphine mg equivalents).
  - Low dose, ≤40 mg
  - Moderate dose, 41-90 mg
  - High dose, >91 mg
- COT may be continued, with continuous adherence monitoring, in well-selected populations, in conjunction with or after failure of other modalities of treatments with improvement in physical and functional status and minimal adverse effects.

Federal grant funding, under the Harold Rogers Prescription Drug Monitoring Program, has been available to support state PDMPs, but the responsibility for the upkeep and regulation of each PDMP is predominantly at the state level. The information recorded by each PDMP is variable. For instance, some states monitor all scheduled medications, whereas other states only track certain drug schedules. The state agency responsible for the maintenance of the PDMP also varies from state to state but includes state health departments, boards of pharmacy, law enforcement agencies, and professional licensing boards.[55]

TABLE 115-5 National Summit for Opioid Safety—Principles for More Selective and Cautious Opioid Prescribing

Principles for all chronic noncancer pain patients

1. Self-care is the foundation for effective chronic noncancer pain care.
2. Your relationship with the patient supports effective self-care.
3. Guide care by progress toward resuming activities.
4. Prioritize long-term pain and function effectiveness over short-term pain relief.

Principles when considering long-term use of opioids

1. Put patient safety first.
2. Think twice before prescribing long-term opioids for axial low back pain, headache, and fibromyalgia.
3. Systematically evaluate risks.
4. Consider intermittent opioid use.
5. Do not sustain opioid use long term without decisive benefits.
6. Keep opioid doses as low as possible.

Principles for patients using opioids long term

1. Clearly communicate standardized expectations to reduce risks.
2. Adhere to recommended precautions.
3. Avoid prescribing opioids and sedatives concurrently.
4. Revisit discontinuing opioids or lowering dose.
5. Identify and treat prescription opioid misuse/disorders.

Electronic interstate data sharing began in 2010, and currently communication between states with PDMPs is becoming more common. As of January 2021, all state PDMPs, with the exception of California, Guam, and the Northern Mariana Islands, participate in PDMP electronic data sharing. This is increasingly more common over border states, with 38 of PDMP programs communicating with border partners. Recommended best practice remains that PDMPs should have the ability to communicate with other states, but at a minimum communicate with border states.[57] A lack of communication can be especially problematic for health care providers who service a population area composed of multiple states or when patients initiate care in a new state. Also, the effectiveness of the PDMP for diminishing controlled substance unhealthy use including addiction is difficult to determine due to their high variability, but in many states, PDMPs are a critical component of risk management evaluation in the prescribing of controlled substances. The White House has clearly stated that PDMPs are a pillar in the fight against the epidemic of prescription related OUD and overdose. As such, the need for the exchange of information between state-based PDMPs will likely spur state systems that can communicate across state lines or perhaps even a unified federal PDMP system. Moreover, where available, the use of the PDMP is expected on the part of prescribers and/or dispensers.

OPIOIDS AND THE SUPREME COURT

On June 27, 2022, the U.S. Supreme Court unanimously ruled in favor of two physicians who individually, in different cases, had previously been found guilty of improper prescribing of opioids.[58] In each of the two distinct cases, the court found that the jury had not been adequately informed of the knowledge basis for "wrongdoing" that would be required to support a criminal conviction. The court stated that the government had an obligation to demonstrate that an otherwise authorized physician "knowingly or intentionally" prescribed the drug for other than a "legitimate medical purpose" and outside the "usual course of professional practice." A minority opinion suggested that prescribers could still be prosecuted under the Controlled Substance Act for prescribing that is "foreign to medicine, such as facilitating addiction or recreational drug abuse." In this landmark case, convictions for the prescribing physicians, including their substantial sentences (21 and 25 years respectively), were remanded back to lower courts for new trials. Thus, the court did not justify the practice for these physicians, but instead made a clear statement that physician prosecutions for inappropriate prescribing must address physician intent and context. This ruling suggests potential benefits for prescribing clinicians through documenting prescriber intent through cogent medical decision-making supported by transparent analysis of risk and benefits.

SUMMARY

This chapter has outlined regulatory and legal considerations surrounding opioid prescribing. The debate about appropriate pain management and particularly about the appropriate use of controlled substances is important and ongoing. Over the past decade, we have witnessed substantial swings in extreme positions on both sides of the debate, and more recently have seemed to come to greater consensus on balancing the risks and benefits of these drugs. The risks of prescription opioids have become increasingly apparent over the past several decades, especially considering alarming data on unintended overdose deaths. Emerging evidence suggests that most patients with chronic, nonmalignant pain can be managed well on nonopioid therapies. Other evidence suggests some groups may be harmed with long-term opioid therapy and in highly selected patients, the benefits of opioids may outweigh the risk. Moreover, we have most recently become aware of the harms that can come with sudden abstinence or involuntary tapering of opioids in some patients on long-standing or high dosages. There is a paucity of evidence to determine exactly which subgroups of patients may benefit and which may be harmed by opioid therapy. Therefore, great care and monitoring are essential when opioids are started, managed, or discontinued. As the opioids epidemic has now evolved, there has been a corresponding paradigm shift toward significant risk management in the use of opioids. Nonetheless, the need for clinicians to apply thoughtful consideration to each individual patient to address the many facets of the pain experience has not changed. The recent ruling of the Supreme Court, that endorsed the important role of prescriber intent in criminal determination of improper prescribing, should encourage prescribers to demonstrate intent through documented and transparent analysis of risks and benefits, which forms the cornerstone of all medical decisions.

The legal considerations involved in opioid prescribing are complex but have evolved to promote safe use. Health care providers are strongly encouraged to work with legal experts in this area for legal advice when confronted with challenging situations, to familiarize themselves with their local and national laws and regulations, and to stay abreast of the changing political landscape regarding opioid prescribing.

REFERENCES

1. Institute of Medicine. *Relieving Pain in America: A Blueprint for Transforming Prevention, Care, Education, and Research.* National Academies Press; 2011.
2. Rudd RA, Aleshire N, Zibble JE, Gladden MR. Increases in drug and opioid overdose deaths—United States, 2000-2014. *MMWR Morb Mortal Wkly Rep.* 2016;64(50-51):1378-1382. Accessed August 21, 2022. http://www.cdc.gov/mmwr/preview/mmwrhtml/mm6450a3.htm
3. CDC: National Center for Injury Prevention and Control. *Ten Leading Causes of Death and Injury.* Accessed August 21, 2022. http://www.cdc.gov/injury/images/lc-charts/leading_causes_of_injury_deaths_unintentional_injury_2014_1040w740h.gif
4. Centers for Disease Control and Prevention. *Death Rate Maps and Graphs.* Accessed August 21, 2022. www.cdc.gov/drugoverdose/deaths/index.html
5. U.S. Food and Drug Administration. *Milestones in U.S. Food and Drug Law.* Accessed August 21, 2022. https://www.fda.gov/about-fda/fda-history/milestones-us-food-and-drug-law
6. United States House of Representatives. *Comprehensive Drug Abuse Prevention and Control Act of 1970.* HRRep No. 91-1444. 1970.
7. Drug Enforcement Agency. *Scheduling Actions, Chronological Order.* Accessed August 21, 2022. https://www.deadiversion.usdoj.gov/schedules/orangebook/b_sched_chron.pdf
8. Drug Enforcement Administration. *Pharmacist's Manual: An Informational Outline of the Controlled Substance Act, Revised 2010.* Accessed July 25, 2023. https://deadiversion.usdoj.gov/GDP/(DEA-DC-046R1)(EO-DEA154R1)_Pharmacist's_Manual_DEA.pdf
9. 21 U.S.C. § 823.
10. Substance Abuse and Mental Health Service Administration (SAMHSA). *Buprenorphine*; 2016:10. Accessed August 21, 2023. http://www.samhsa.gov/medication-assisted-treatment/treatment/buprenorphine
11. 42 CFR-PART 8. *Medication Assisted Treatment for Opioid Use Disorders.* Accessed July 25, 2023. https://www.ecfr.gov/current/title-42/chapter-I/subchapter-A/part-8
12. 21 Code of Federal Regulations §1306.07. *Administering or Dispensing of Narcotic Drugs.* Accessed July 25, 2023. https://www.ecfr.gov/cgi-bin/text-idx?SID=dd3324c93ad659b4a55e8cca8156a65c&node=se21.9.1306_107&rgn=div8
13. Ohio Administrative Code, chapter 4731-21-02 section 4(c). *Utilizing Prescription Drugs for the Treatment of Chronic Pain.*
14. Martineau RJ. In state-federal conflicts, the supremacy clause wins. *Chicago Herald Tribune.* 2010;28.
15. Mayorquin O. In what states is weed legal? Here is the list. *USA Today,* Gannett Satellite Information Network. Accessed August 21, 2022. https://www.usatoday.com/story/news/nation/2022/04/20/states-with-legal-weed-recreational/7371071001/
16. Pain & Policy Studies Group, University of Wisconsin School of Medicine and Public Health, Paul P. Carbone Cancer Center. *Achieving Balance in State Pain Policy: A Guide to Evaluation.* 2014. Accessed July 25, 2023.

https://www.fightcancer.org/sites/default/files/National%20Documents/Achieving%20Balance%20in%20State%20Pain%20Policy.pdf

17. Singh N, Fishman S, Rich B, Orlowski A. Prescription opioid forgery: reporting to law enforcement and protection of medical information. *Pain Med.* 2013;14(6):792-798.
18. Tenn. Code Ann. § 53-11-309.
19. Virginia Va. Code Ann. § 32.1-127.1:03.
20. Louisiana La. Rev. Stat. Ann. § 40:971.
21. Maine Me. Rev. Stat. Ann. Tit. 17-A, § 1108.
22. Department of Justice, Drug Enforcement Administration. *Dispensing Controlled Substances for the Treatment of Pain, Part V*. 2006. Accessed August 21, 2022. https://www.deadiversion.usdoj.gov/fed_regs/notices/2006/fr09062.htm
23. Dineen KK, DuBois. Between a rock and a hard place: can physicians prescribe opioids to treat pain adequately while avoiding legal sanction? *Am J Law Med.* 2016;42(1):7-52. doi:10.1177/0098858816644712
24. Drug Enforcement Administration. *Certificate of Registration Information*. Accessed August 21, 2022. https://deadiversion.usdoj.gov/drugreg/index.html
25. U.S. Department of Justice. *Practitioner's Manual: An Informational Outline of the Controlled Substances Act*. 2006 edition. Accessed August 21, 2022. https://www.in.gov/pla/files/DEA_Practitioner_Manual.pdf
26. U.S. Department of Justice. *Questions & Answers*. 2007. Accessed August 21, 2022. https://www.deadiversion.usdoj.gov/faq/index.html
27. U.S. Department of Justice. *Electronic Prescriptions for Controlled Substances (EPCS)*. Accessed August 21, 2022. http://www.deadiversion.usdoj.gov/ecomm/e_rx
28. House of Representatives, 110th Congress. H.R. Report No. 3580 Food and Drug Administration Amendments Act of 2007.
29. Leiderman D. Risk management of drug products and the U.S. food and drug administration: evolution and context. *Drug Alcohol Depend.* 2009;105(Suppl 1):S9-S13.
30. Center for Drug Evaluation and Research. U.S. Food and Drug Administration. *Questions and Answers: FDA Approves a Class Risk Evaluation and Mitigation Strategy (REMS) for Transmucosal Immediate-Release Fentanyl (TIRF) Medicines*. Accessed August 21, 2022. https://www.fda.gov/drugs/information-drug-class/questions-and-answers-fda-approves-class-risk-evaluation-and-mitigation-strategy-rems-transmucosal
31. Food and Drug Administration. *New Safety Measures Announced for Extended-Release and Long-Acting Opioids*. Accessed August 21, 2022. https://www.fda.gov/drugs/information-drug-class/new-safety-measures-announced-extended-release-and-long-acting-opioids
32. Opioid REMS meeting invitation template. Accessed August 21, 2022. https://www.fda.gov/advisory-committees/advisory-committee-calendar/may-3-4-2016-joint-meeting-drug-safety-and-risk-management-advisory-committee-and-anesthetic-and-analgesic-drug-products-advisory-committee
33. U.S. Food and Drug Administration. *Approved Risk Evaluation and Mitigation Strategies (REMS)*. Accessed August 21, 2022. https://www.accessdata.fda.gov/scripts/cder/rems/index.cfm
34. Drug Enforcement Agency. *Drug Disposal Information*. Accessed August 21, 2022. https://www.deadiversion.usdoj.gov/drug_disposal/
35. Food and Drug Administration. *Drug Disposal: FDA's Flush List for Certain Medicines*. Accessed August 21, 2022. https://www.fda.gov/drugs/disposal-unused-medicines-what-you-should-know/drug-disposal-fdas-flush-list-certain-medicines
36. Talebi R, Miller C, Abboudi J, et al. How patients dispose of unused prescription opioids: a survey of over 300 postoperative patients. *Cureus.* 2022;14(8):e28111. doi:10.7759/cureus.28111
37. Agarwal AK, Lee D, Ali Z, et al. Effect of mailing an at-home disposal kit on unused opioid disposal after surgery: a randomized clinical trial. *JAMA Netw Open.* 2022;5(5):e2210724. doi:10.1001/jamanetworkopen.2022.10724
38. Fishman S. *Responsible Opioid Prescribing. A Clinician's Guide*. 2nd ed. Federation of State Medical Boards/Waterford Life Sciences; 2011.
39. Centers for Disease Control. *Helpful Materials for Patients*. Accessed August 21, 2022. https://www.cdc.gov/opioids/patients/materials.html
40. Centers for Disease Control. Accessed August 21, 2022. http://www.cdc.gov/maso/pdf/cdcmiss.pdf
41. Dowell D, Haegerich T. *Chou R. CDC Guideline for Prescribing Opioids for Chronic Pain-United States*; 2016. Accessed August 21, 2022. http://www.cdc.gov/mmwr/volumes/65/rr/rr6501e1.htm
42. Agnoli A, Xing G, Tancredi TJ, Magnan E, Jerant A, Fenton JJ. Association of dose tapering with overdose or mental health crisis among patients prescribed long-term opioids. *JAMA.* 2021;326(5):411-419.
43. Dowell D, Haegerich T, Chou R. No shortcuts to safer opioid prescribing. *N Engl J Med.* 2019;380(24):2285-2287.
44. Centers for Disease Control and Prevention. *CDC Advises Against Misapplication of the Guideline for Prescribing Opioids for Chronic Pain*. Accessed August 21, 2022. https://www.cdc.gov/media/releases/2019/s0424-advises-misapplication-guideline-prescribing-opioids.html
45. National Alliance for Model State Drug Laws. *Prescription Drug Monitoring Program (PDMP/PMP) Basics*. Accessed August 21, 2022. https://namsdl.org/wp-content/uploads/Prescription-Drug-Monitoring-Program-PDMP-PMP-Basics.pdf
46. The Federation of State Medical Boards. *Model Policy on the Use of Opioid Analgesics in the Treatment of Chronic Pain*. 2013. Accessed August 21, 2022. http://www.fsmb.org/Media/Default/PDF/FSMB/Advocacy/pain_policy_july2013.pdf
47. Federation of State Medical Boards. *Guidelines for the Chronic Use of Opioid Analgesics*. Accessed August 21, 2022. https://www.fsmb.org/siteassets/advocacy/policies/opioid_guidelines_as_adopted_april-2017_final.pdf
48. American Pain Society (APS) and the American Academy of Pain Medicine (AAPM). Clinical guidelines for the use of chronic opioid therapy (COT) in chronic noncancer pain (CNCP). *J Pain.* 2009;10:113-130.
49. Nobel M. Long-term opioid management for chronic noncancer pain. *Cochrane Database Syst Rev.* 2010;(1):CD006605.
50. Manchikanti L. Guidelines for responsible opioid prescribing in chronic non-cancer pain: part 1 and part 2. *Pain Physician.* 2012;15:S1-S116.
51. Group Health. *National Summit on Opioid Safety*. Accessed August 21, 2022. https://www.slideshare.net/grouphealth/national-summit-on-opioid-safety
52. Pacific Northwest Evidenced-based Practice Center. *The Effectiveness and Risks of Long-term Opioid Treatment of Chronic Pain*. Agency for Healthcare Research and Quality; 2014:216.
53. Legislative Summary Memo. A.10623. Internet System for Tracking Over-prescribing (iSTOP). 2012, chapter 447 of the L. New York.
54. Department of Justice. *Harold Rogers Prescription Drug Monitoring Program*. Accessed August 21, 2022. https://bja.ojp.gov/funding/opportunities/o-bja-2022-171290
55. HR Rep No. 1132, 109th Congress. National All Schedules Prescription Electronic Reporting Act of 2005.
56. The PEW Charitable Trusts. *Prescription Drug Monitoring Programs*. Accessed April 24, 2022. https://namsdl.org/wp-content/uploads/Prescription-Drug-Monitoring-Programs-Evidence-Based-Practices-to-Optimize-Prescriber-Use.pdf
57. Fishman S. Regulating opioid prescribing through prescription monitoring programs: balancing drug diversion and treatment of pain. *Pain Med.* 2004;5(3):309-324.
58. Supreme Court of the United States. Xiulu Ruan v. United States. Accessed August 21, 2022. https://www.supremecourt.gov/opinions/21pdf/20-1410_1an2.pdf

SECTION

14

Children and Adolescents

Associate Editor: Sharon Levy
Lead Section Editor: J. Wesley Boyd
Section Editors: Sarah M. Bagley and Sion Kim Harris

CHAPTER

116 Screening and Brief Intervention for Adolescents

Jessica B. Calihan and Lydia A. Shrier

CHAPTER OUTLINE

- Introduction
- Setting the stage
- Incorporating screening into the visit
- Screening
- Response to screening and assessment
- Referral to treatment
- Involving the family
- Follow-up
- Resources
- Summary

INTRODUCTION

Substance use (SU) in adolescence increases risk of future substance use disorder (SUD) and has important adverse developmental, cognitive, psychiatric, and medical outcomes.[1,2] SUD is a chronic disorder characterized by persistent SU despite negative consequences.[3] Screening, brief intervention, and referral to treatment (SBIRT) is a comprehensive approach to addressing SU that can be universally incorporated into routine adolescent care to prevent and intervene on adolescent SUD and its sequelae. This chapter will describe screening and brief intervention practices that can be implemented in primary care to efficiently and effectively evaluate alcohol and drug-related risk, provide brief intervention, and plan appropriate follow-up.

Adolescence is a period of developmental vulnerability during which the brain is particularly susceptible to the adverse effects of psychoactive substances. SUD is a neurologically-based chronic disorder whereby repeated exposure to substances disrupts brain circuitry, particularly in the reward center.[4,5] Much of adolescent neurodevelopment occurs in regions of the brain associated with reward, as well as with impulsivity and motivation. Developmental perturbations in these areas with substance exposure, as well as an imbalance between the underdeveloped cognitive control system and developed emotion and reward system, help to explain why adolescent SU is a risk factor for progression to SUD.[2,6-9] Approximately 75% of adults with SUD report initiation of SU under the age of 18.[10] Younger age of substance initiation and use is also associated with elevated risk of depression, anxiety, and psychosis related to SU,[11-13] as well as adverse neurodevelopmental effects on cognition, memory, and learning.[2,14-16] In the short term, SU can result in cognitive problems such as poor concentration and memory, changes in mood and behavior, declines in school performance, and risk-taking behaviors, as well as various physical problems depending on the type of substance. Most concerningly, the last few years have seen a greater increase in overdose deaths for adolescents, relative to the overall population, with a 94% increase from 2019 to 2020 and 20% increase from 2020 to 2021.[17]

One way to prevent and intervene on adolescent SU is to incorporate SBIRT into routine adolescent care to determine whether an adolescent is using substances, provide positive feedback for youth who have not used substances, assess risk for developing a SUD for youth who have used substances, advise at-risk youth about the potential consequences of SU, and refer adolescents at high risk to additional assessment and treatment.[18] SBIRT has been effectively implemented in primary care practices, community mental health organizations, emergency rooms, and schools. In these settings, SBIRT is cost-effective, well-received by youth and providers, and associated with improved adolescent access to appropriate brief interventions, increased engagement in follow-up treatment, reduced SU, and increased intention to avoid initiation.[19-28]

Primary care providers (PCPs) have a unique opportunity to provide preventive guidance, identify SU early, and intervene before substance-related consequences occur. Most adolescents see a physician for a yearly visit incorporating preventive screening as recommended by the Maternal and Child Health Bureau, American Academy of Pediatrics (AAP), American Medical Association, and American Academy of Family Physicians.[29,30] Access has expanded since implementation of the Affordable Care Act, with increases in primary care utilization by publicly insured, low-income, Black, and Hispanic adolescents.[29] Pediatricians have often built trusting, long-term relationships with patients, and most report screening for SU annually.[31] However, providers also cite barriers to effective SBIRT, including limited time, concerns about confidentiality, and insufficient knowledge and/or resources to address positive screens.[31]

SETTING THE STAGE

Adolescents may be reluctant to discuss SU with their provider, particularly if they perceive the provider may be critical or if they are not yet comfortable sharing personal details. SU is highly stigmatized, which may further limit adolescents' willingness to discuss concerns. To effectively engage youth in these conversations, providers can use a nonjudgmental and empathetic interviewing style, avoid making any assumptions, and employ motivational interviewing (MI) strategies. Such strategies include asking open-ended questions to assess substance-related risks and using reflective statements to explore ambivalence, link an individual's goals with their behaviors, and elicit motivation to change.[32-34] It is also important to assure conditional confidentiality, normalize screening, build rapport prior to screening, and review SU within a broader psychosocial assessment. Please see Sidebar 118 SB1 on "Confidentiality in Caring for Adolescents" in Section 14 of this textbook for additional discussion of this topic.

Providers can begin asking adolescents about SU as soon as the adolescent is old enough to be interviewed without a parent ("parent" is used to broadly refer to guardians and involved family members) present, typically between 11 and 13 years. The National Institute on Alcohol Abuse and Alcoholism (NIAAA) recommends screening for alcohol use in patients as young as nine years when appropriate,[35] while the AAP recommends starting at age 11 years.[36]

INCORPORATING SCREENING INTO THE VISIT

Screening is incorporated into annual visits as part of the psychosocial assessment. It is also important to screen youth who present with health concerns potentially related to SU (eg, accidents and injuries, recurrent gastrointestinal problems), new mental health symptoms or diagnoses, frequent school absences, behavior changes such as increased oppositional or impulsive behavior, dramatic mood changes, loss of interest in activities, and/or disengagement with school and/or extracurriculars.[35] Providers should review confidentiality with the adolescent and their family before speaking with an adolescent alone, ideally at the start of any visit that may incorporate SBIRT. Confidentiality is a crucial aspect of comprehensive care for adolescents (see Sidebar 118 SB1), and reassurance regarding confidentiality often influences whether patients will engage around sensitive topics and answer questions honestly.[18,37,38] Once the adolescent is alone, providers can build rapport by asking general questions about the youth's experiences, strengths, and goals. It is helpful to normalize the conversation by reminding adolescents that screening is a routine part of health care for all youth.

SU screening is typically integrated into preexisting frameworks for evaluating adolescent psychosocial behaviors and risk factors. The Home, Education, Activities, Drugs, Sex, Suicidality (HEADSS) psychosocial interview starts with assessment of adolescents' home and school environment before transitioning to more personal questions, including about SU.[39] The Strengths, School, Home, Activities, Drugs and SU, Emotions, Sexuality, and Safety (SSHADESS) assessment is similar, but begins by highlighting a youth's strengths to increase comfort and promote confidence to change.[40]

SCREENING

Starting the Screening Conversation

SBIRT begins with screening, which aims to identify adolescents at risk of substance-related consequences and/or SUD. To screen, providers should use a validated brief screening tool (see below), particularly as clinical impressions tend to underestimate the severity of adolescent SU.[41] In younger adolescents, it is helpful to evaluate what they know about substances and to ask about any SU among peers, as this begins the conversation in a less-threatening way, provides information about the environment in which the youth is making decisions about substances, and helps providers identify patients at early stages of substance involvement who may benefit from advice around risks of peer use.[35,42]

Screening Methods

Screening may be accomplished using in-person, paper, or electronic questionnaires, the latter of which can be completed in the office waiting room or at home prior to the visit.[43] Although national surveys and screening instrument research trials consistently find higher rates of adolescent SU than clinical samples, suggesting paper or electronic screens may be more accurate, there are no differences in sensitivity and specificity between electronic and verbal screens.[42,44-48] Electronic or paper questionnaires are preferred by adolescents, acceptable to providers, and feasible to implement, although care should be taken to maintain confidentiality for adolescents who lack space at home or in clinic to complete the questionnaire alone.[43,49,50] Computerized screens are also time-efficient, allowing providers to use limited clinic time for behavioral counseling.[46,51] Furthermore, computerized versions that incorporate immediate personalized feedback for adolescents and/or offer providers recommended talking points may facilitate effective brief interventions.[25,50,52]

Validated Screen Options

Presumptive and specific questions that identify frequency, such as "In the past year, on how many days have you used alcohol?" from the Brief Screening Instrument for Adolescent Tobacco, Alcohol, and Drug Use (BSTAD), have high sensitivity and specificity for use, and may help reduce ambiguity and concerns about stigma.[53-55] There are several other validated screens that can be used in pediatric primary care, including the S2BI (Screening to Brief Intervention), NIAAA (National Institute on Alcoholism and Alcohol Abuse) Youth Alcohol Screening Tool, CRAFFT (Car, Relax, Alone, Family, Forget, Trouble), and ASSIST (Alcohol, Smoking and Substance Involvement Screening Test).[35,42,55-57] See **Table 116-1** for details of each tool. Screens validated only in adults, such as the CAGE questionnaire, are not appropriate for use with adolescents.

The S2BI and BSTAD, which are recommended by the National Institute on Drug Abuse (NIDA), are time-efficient

TABLE 116-1 Screening Tools for Adolescent Substance Use

Screen	S2BI (Screening to Brief Intervention)[58] https://www.drugabuse.gov/adolescent-substance-use-screening-tools	BSTAD (Brief Screener for Tobacco, Alcohol, and other Drugs)[2] https://www.drugabuse.gov/adolescent-substance-use-screening-tools	NIAAA Youth Alcohol Screening Tool[3,4] https://pubs.niaaa.nih.gov/publications/Practitioner/YouthGuide/YouthGuide.pdf	CRAFFT version 2.1[5-7] www.crafft.org	ASSIST (Alcohol, Smoking and Substance Involvement Screening Test)[8] https://www.who.int/publications/[10]
Ages	12-17 years	12-17 years	9-18 years	12-18 years	12-17 years
Items	*In the **past year**, how many times have you used…?* (never, 1-2 times, monthly, weekly or more) Three questions on tobacco, alcohol, and cannabis. Response other than "never," question about frequency for four other substance categories	*In the **past year**, on how many days have you…?* Three questions on tobacco, alcohol, and cannabis. If response other than "0," question about any use for nine other substance categories	Age 9-11 *Do you have any friends who drank….in the **past year**?* *How about you—have you **ever** had …?"* Age 11-14 *Do you have any friends who drank….in the **past year**?* *How about you—in the **past year,** on how many days have you had…?* Age 14-18 *In the **past year,** on how many days have you had…?* *If your friends drink, how many drinks…on an occasion?*	*During the **past 12 months**, on how many days did you…?* Three questions on alcohol, marijuana, & other drugs. If any use, query problems related to use: Car, Relax, Alone, Forget, Family/ Friends, Trouble. If no use, Car question only (riding with driver under the influence).	Q1: *In your **life**, which of the following substances have you ever used (nonmedical use only)?* 9 substance categories If "none," end interview. If "yes," ask for each substance: Q2 *In the past three months, how often …?* If any use in past three months, three additional questions about problematic use. If any SU on Q1, three additional questions about high-risk use.
Positive screen	Never → No use Once or twice → Lower risk Monthly or more → Higher risk	0 days → No use 1 day → Lower risk 2+ days → Higher risk	Age 9-11: Use → Problem use Age 12-15: 1-5 → Problem use; 6+ → AUD Age 16: 6-11 → Problem use; 12+ → AUD Age 17: 6-23 → Problem use; 24+ → AUD Age 18: 12-51 → Problem use; 52+ → AUD	2+ yes responses on CRAFFT questions → Problem use	Alcohol: 0-10 → Low risk 11-26 → Moderate risk 27+ → High risk Other Substances: 0-3 → Low risk 3-26 → Moderate risk 27+ → High risk **Calculate score by adding Q2-Q7 for each substance*
Sensitivity & specificity	Alcohol use disorder Sensitivity 53% Specificity 94% Cannabis use disorder Sensitivity 81% Specificity 92%	Alcohol use disorder Sensitivity 96% Specificity 85% Cannabis use disorder Sensitivity 80% Specificity 93%	Depends on age and sex. Problem use Sensitivity 93%-100% Specificity 66%-95% Severe disorder Sensitivity 81%-100% Specificity 71%-99%	Any substance use Sensitivity 96% Specificity 81% Problem SU/SUD Sensitivity 79% Specificity 97% SUD Sensitivity 91% Specificity 93%	Tobacco problem use Sensitivity 97% Specificity 95% Tobacco use disorder Sensitivity 95% Specificity 93% Alcohol problem use Sensitivity 90% Specificity 82% Alcohol use disorder Sensitivity 100% Specificity 79% Cannabis problem use Sensitivity 98% Specificity 91% Cannabis use disorder Sensitivity 98% Specificity 87%

(Continued)

TABLE 116-1 Screening Tools for Adolescent Substance Use (*Continued*)

Screen	S2BI (Screening to Brief Intervention)[58] https://www.drugabuse.gov/adolescent-substance-use-screening-tools	BSTAD (Brief Screener for Tobacco, Alcohol, and other Drugs)[2] https://www.drugabuse.gov/adolescent-substance-use-screening-tools	NIAAA Youth Alcohol Screening Tool[3,4] https://pubs.niaaa.nih.gov/publications/Practitioner/YouthGuide/YouthGuide.pdf	CRAFFT version 2.1[5-7] www.crafft.org	ASSIST (Alcohol, Smoking and Substance Involvement Screening Test)[8] https://www.who.int/publications/[10]
Comments	Includes tobacco. Places responses (including no use) into actionable categories that align with AAP recommendations.[9]	Includes tobacco.	Only for alcohol. Tailors questions and cutpoints for risk to adolescent age/stage. Queries friends' drinking (predicts patient's future drinking). Validated for use in primary care,[10] emergency departments,[11] and subspecialty care.[12]	Version 2.1 added three consumption frequency questions to the original 6-item CRAFFT; 2.1+N includes vaping/tobacco use and Hooked on Nicotine Checklist.[13,14] All adolescents questioned about driving after use or riding with driver under the influence	Developed for adults. Questions provide information on consequences of use to inform brief intervention. Score corresponds with actionable intervention response.

Adapted from Burke P, Shrier LA. "Adolescent Substance Use: Screening and Intervention Strategies for the Primary Care Office", AAP 2019 Session I3089. Courtesy of the National Library of Medicine.

and provide substance-specific risk based on frequency of use. Both tools are available online at https://nida.nih.gov/. The NIAAA Youth Alcohol Screening Tool is very brief (two items), queries peer alcohol use, and has been validated in multiple settings, but does not include other substances.[42,54,59,60] The ASSIST and CRAFFT are slightly longer instruments that can be used to evaluate consequences of SU and to inform subsequent intervention conversations.[56,57] The CRAFFT is a commonly used screen that incorporates frequency questions with a 6-item screen for SU-related problems and is recommended by the AAP. The CRAFFT problem questions may be administered after the CRAFFT frequency questions or after another brief frequency screen (eg, S2BI).[61] It has been translated into, and validated in, many languages, and is available online at https://crafft.org/.[62-66] In adults, the ASSIST provides substance-specific risk scores for nine categories of substances; however, in adolescent-focused research, ASSIST has only been validated to establish problem use of alcohol, nicotine, and cannabis, and is not validated to determine SUD severity.[56]

Additional Assessment

Following a positive screen, additional information is used to determine next intervention steps. In general, providers can use open-ended questions to evaluate the pattern of SU over time, perceived benefits and consequences of ongoing use, whether the adolescent has attempted to reduce SU in the past, reasons for those attempts, and why those attempts were or were not successful. In addition, providers may ask about tension with family or friends, changes in school or extracurricular performance, suspensions or expulsions, physical or verbal fights, medical problems (eg, overdose or getting sick), motor vehicle collisions, unintentional injury, unwanted sexual contact, or legal concerns. These questions provide valuable information for subsequent personalized brief interventions to enhance motivation for change.

When an adolescent endorses SU, it is also important to assess related medical, psychiatric, and cognitive consequences (**Table 116-2**). Signs and symptoms of SU are often nonspecific and may include sleep disturbance, gastrointestinal reflux, appetite or weight changes, changes in mood or behavior, cognitive problems such as poor memory and concentration, injection or skin-popping marks, ulcers or irritation around the nose or mouth suggestive of inhalant use, recurrent injuries suggestive of alcohol use, and/or chronic cough, decreased exercise tolerance or dyspnea on exertion suggestive of e-cigarette/vaping associated lung injury (EVALI). Questions about experienced or witnessed overdose are recommended. Of note, injection drug use, polysubstance use, psychiatric comorbidity, witnessing an overdose, being unstably housed, and sedative (opioid, tranquilizer, alcohol, benzodiazepine) use are all associated with overdose in adolescents and young adults.[67] PCPs may also consider screening for co-occurring mental health disorders, which are common and may require further assessment by a behavioral health clinician.[58]

Laboratory testing is often included in the comprehensive evaluation of adolescents with SUD. There are many biological options for testing, including urine, blood, breath, saliva, sweat, and hair.[68] Urine testing is the most frequently used

TABLE 116-2 Signs of Acute Substance Use, Withdrawal, and Chronic Use in Adolescents

Substance	Acute use	Withdrawal	Chronic use
Nicotine/tobacco	Alertness, reduced appetite, palpitations, elevated blood pressure and heart rate, smell of tobacco/smoke/electronic cigarette flavorings	Anxiety, irritability, difficulty concentrating, restlessness, hunger, tremor, sweating, dizziness, headaches	E-cigarette or vaping associated lung injury (EVALI), heart disease, lung cancer, throat and mouth cancer, chronic obstructive pulmonary disease
Alcohol	Fruity smelling breath, disinhibited or silly, clumsy, vomiting, poor decision-making	Headache, nausea, vomiting, dry mouth, tremor, anxiety, seizures, delirium tremens (rare in adolescents)	Enlarged liver, acute or chronic liver disease, hypertension
Cannabis	Erythematous conjunctivae, tachycardia, dry mouth, increased talking, euphoria, smell of burned cannabis, paranoia, hallucinations	Anxiety, nervousness, decreased appetite	Chronic cough, wheezing, EVALI, cannabis hyperemesis syndrome
Cocaine	Hyperalert state, increased talking, hyperthermia, nausea, dry mouth, dilated pupils, sweating, cardiac arrhythmias	Depression, anhedonia, insomnia, lethargy, mental slowing	Erosion of dental enamel, gingival ulceration, chronic rhinitis, epistaxis, perforated nasal septum, midline granuloma, cardiac arrhythmias, hypertension, paranoia, psychosis
Amphetamines	Similar to cocaine		Choreoathetoid movement disorders, skin picking and ulcerations
Opioids	Constricted pupils, drowsiness, slowed respirations, bradycardia, slurred speech, slowed comprehension, constipation, needle injection marks, skin/soft tissue infections, phlebitis, abscesses	Flulike symptoms, muscle and joint aches, dilated pupils, coryza, lacrimation, sweating, abdominal cramps, nausea, vomiting, diarrhea, hot and cold flashes, piloerection, yawning, tremors, anxiety, irritability	Abscesses, cellulitis, phlebitis and scarring (from injection use), endocarditis, chronic constipation, malnutrition
Benzodiazepines	Drowsiness, slowed respirations, slurred speech, slowed comprehension	Tremors, anxiety, irritability, restlessness, seizures	Sleep difficulties, anxiety, personality changes
Hallucinogens	Toxic psychosis, paranoia, anxiety, tachycardia, hypertension, dry mouth, nausea, vomiting	—	Psychosis, depression, personality changes
Inhalants	Euphoria, slurred speech, ataxia, diplopia, lacrimation, rhinorrhea, salivation, irritation of the mucus membranes, nausea, vomiting, arrhythmias, metallic paint residues around facial area or fingers	Headaches, sleepiness, depression	Irritation of mucus membranes, changes in neurologic exam
Ecstasy	Euphoria, decreased interpersonal boundaries, tachycardia, hypertension, hyperthermia, sweating, muscle spasms, bruxism, blurred vision, chills, nystagmus	Depression, anxiety, paranoia, dehydration	Cognitive deficits

because it has a long period of detection for multiple substances and is well studied and standardized. However, samples may be tampered with, and collection requires an invasion of privacy. Blood tests are useful for detecting acute use, but are invasive, costly, and have a short period of detection for many substances. Breath testing, which can be used to detect nicotine or alcohol use, gives information about acute use but does not correspond with impairment.[68] Testing modalities are discussed in further detail in Section 4 of this textbook. Testing comes in multiple forms and can be used, with an adolescent's consent, to complement their self-report and inform safety concerns. Of note, the AAP cautions against involuntary drug testing in adolescents, even at parental request, due to concerns about limited efficacy in reducing SU, issues of interpretability, and potential unintended consequences, such as negative effects on the parent-child relationship or school breach of confidentiality.[68] Interpretability may be limited by inability to detect certain synthetic or "designer" substances, interfering medications or foods causing false positives, and variations in substance detection time due to chronicity of use, test characteristics, and individual metabolism.[68] When used, providers and families should understand that laboratory testing is only one piece of information that needs to be interpreted in the broader context of the patient's history.

RESPONSE TO SCREENING AND ASSESSMENT

General Approach

The second step of SBIRT, Brief Intervention (BI), is a MI-based conversation focused on eliciting and strengthening adolescents' motivation to make healthy choices that prevent, reduce, or stop SU-associated risks. See **Table 116-3** and the descriptions below for recommended BI strategies based on screening results. Providers start by giving feedback on screening and assessment results, transition to provide education about the potential cognitive, psychiatric, and physical harms of SU, and end by giving clear advice regarding abstinence or cessation.[18] For effective BI, providers use the information they gained during screening and assessment to provide tailored feedback, help youth recognize a link between SU and related consequences, and guide adolescents to make personalized and relevant goals to reduce or cease use. Although these conversations require time, even succinct guidance can be impactful, and studies have suggested that many adolescent-serving providers can provide counseling and brief advice in less than 5 minutes.[25,69]

Providers can perform BI immediately after verbal screening. When electronic or paper screens are utilized previsit, providers may want to incorporate BI into the psychosocial assessment, when the adolescent is alone, and confidentiality has already been established. If available, behavioral health clinicians embedded in primary care practices can help implement BI.[26,70] However, PCP provision of BI ensures greater availability for adolescents given that the need for referral and transfer of care may serve as a barrier to receipt of behavioral health clinician intervention.[71,72]

In general, BI is most effective when providers use MI strategies to elicit an adolescent's own motivation for changing behavior. In MI, providers work to engage the patient through careful listening and reflection, focus on shared purpose, evoke desire and resources for change while recognizing ambivalence, and, if the individual is ready, partner to plan salient goals.[34] Core MI skills include emphasizing autonomy, providing information, reflecting to affirm and summarize, and questioning to explore an individuals' perspectives and ideas.[34] Ideally, providers avoid the urge to tell a patient their behavior is problematic and outline steps to fix it. Instead, providers respect an individual's autonomy and perspective without judgment, listen closely to patient's goals and barriers, and compassionately prioritize individual's well-being with the overall goal of strengthening patients' intrinsic motivation to change. Providers may use affirming and/or reflective statements to rephrase and emphasize what a patient said, provide additional information about health risks with permission, and summarize the conversation to empower behavior change and help patients accomplish their goals.

TABLE 116-3 Brief Interventions Tailored to Screening Result

Screening result	Recommended approach
No use	Positive reinforcement *Goal:* Encourage choice to remain abstinent
Low risk of SUD	Brief advice *Goal:* Prevent additional use and risk behaviors
Moderate risk SUD/ problem use	Motivational intervention *Goal:* Reduce use and associated risk behaviors
High risk SUD	Motivational intervention *Goals:* Reduce use and associated risk behaviors, refer to treatment

SUD, substance use disorder.

No Use: Positive Reinforcement

Sarah is a 15-year-old girl who presents for her annual physical visit. When the provider uses the S2BI to screen for substance use, Sarah denies using tobacco/nicotine, alcohol, or cannabis in the past year. Adolescents who have not tried substances can receive positive feedback that frames abstinence as a choice. Providers may encourage delayed SU initiation until the brain is more mature, which may be viewed as protective against the developmental neurocognitive effects of early substance initiation.[18] Affirming statements such as "*You have made the healthy choice to avoid alcohol and drugs. This is the best choice for your health. If this ever changes, I hope you will feel comfortable talking to me about it*," provide positive feedback for abstinence and open opportunities for future discussion. "Normative correction" statements, such as "*most people your age choose not to use*" help clarify that use is not developmentally appropriate, common, or expected at this age.[18]

Substance Use without SUD: BI

Nikhil is a 14-year-old boy who comes to clinic with his mother, who is concerned about his friend's recent suspension for vaping in school. When screened alone, Nikhil shares that a few of his friends vape cannabis regularly, and he says that he has vaped cannabis only once. Further screening with CRAFFT reveals he once was driven home by an older friend who had been vaping cannabis. This patient is at low risk for SUD and would benefit from BI incorporating education on substance-related risks, including riding with an impaired driver (see below), and advice to abstain. Ideally this conversation would recognize and emphasize personal strengths and values, such as school or extracurricular achievement, and incorporate knowledge of any health concerns, such as the risk of alcohol use for individuals with diabetes. For example, a provider may tell Nikhil: "*You are an amazing soccer player, so you may find it helpful to know that vaping cannabis can affect your endurance and reaction time. My recommendation is that you avoid cannabis as well as alcohol and other drugs because they can harm your health.*" In this statement, the provider personalizes advice and provides a clear recommendation to not use substances based on the potential negative health effects that may be salient to the specific patient.

Riding/Driving Risk Counseling

Providers can give all families of adolescents the "Contract for Life (https://crafft.org/contract/)," a document developed by Students Against Destructive Decisions (SADD) that asks adolescents to commit to avoiding destructive decisions that jeopardize health, safety, and overall well-being, including driving under the influence or riding with an impaired drive. Parents also sign to commit to communicating with youth about these decisions and to providing transportation home without questions when necessary.[73] An analysis of brief primary care counseling incorporating the contract found significant short-term reductions in risk of riding with an impaired driver, although additional research is needed to determine best practices for addressing adolescent impaired driving.[74] Families should be reassured that the purpose of using the contract is to ensure safe transportation, not to avoid conversations. Instead, parents may be encouraged to discuss the event later, when parents and adolescent are neither intoxicated nor angry, and to explore how the situation may be avoided in the future. Given that 1 in 12 adolescents have driven with an intoxicated parent or adult family member, it may be beneficial to give the contract directly to parents if they are present.[75] Risk reduction counseling is recommended for all adolescents who have ridden with or been an impaired driver, with attention to challenges to safe driving or riding and plans to use alternative transportation strategies if needed. This intervention may be particularly important as substance-influenced risking/driving behaviors have been associated with future increased SU and related consequences.[76]

Mild to Moderate SUD: BI Utilizing MI

Elijah is a 16-year-old boy with a history of anxiety who, when screened during his annual visit, endorses monthly cannabis use. He occasionally uses alone, and his parents grounded him after finding vapes in his room. This patient may have mild-moderate SUD based on monthly use reported on S2BI screen and positive CRAFFT (ie, score of 2 or more, indicating problematic use). As discussed above, additional assessment using the Elicit-Provide-Elicit framework is warranted to evaluate additional consequences of Elijah's use and inform MI-based BI. The provider starts by eliciting what Elijah knows about the effects of cannabis on mental health, school and extracurriculars, and family dynamics. Reflective statements, such as "*you use cannabis to help you to manage your anxiety, and, at the same time, your parents are upset about your use and you're worried about how it affects your concentration in school*" acknowledges both the benefits and the risks of the cannabis use, demonstrating that the provider is listening in a nonjudgmental way. By ending with the risks, the provider can then move the conversation to enhancing the patient's motivation to change by offering information about substance-related risks specific to the patient. The provider asks permission, "*If it's okay with you, may I share some information about how cannabis can affect concentration and anxiety?*" and, if permission is granted, then provides the information. Given that legalization of medical and recreational cannabis use has been associated with decreased perception of cannabis-associated risks among adolescents,[44,77] providers may want to note that readily available products with higher tetrahydrocannabinol (THC) concentrations have been temporally correlated with increased hospitalizations for cannabis hyperemesis syndrome, injury and fatal car crashes, and risk of psychiatric disorders such as anxiety, major depression, suicidality, psychosis, and schizophrenia.[11,12,78-80]

Next, the provider elicits the client's reaction: what do they think of the information given, have they tried to decrease use before, and are they are motivated to address use. Providers may query where patients are on the readiness ruler, a 0-10 continuum indicating desire to change, and then ask "*Why not a (lower number)?*" to reinforce reasons for change, and "*Why not a (higher number)?*" to assess barriers to change.[81,82] If the patient is ready to change, providers can help the patient set salient goals, identify concrete strategies to achieve those goals, and brainstorm solutions to any barriers. Lastly, providers should summarize the conversation, highlighting the patient's reasons for change, change plan, and solutions to any barriers, and ensure close follow-up to assess goal progression and need for additional treatment.

Severe SUD: BI and Referral to Treatment

Christine is a 16-year-old girl whose parents are concerned about her depressed mood, frequent school absences, and recent decision to quit theater, which she previously enjoyed. When screened alone, she endorses daily alcohol use and monthly opioid use. She describes using alone, frequent cravings for alcohol, and loss of friendships due to her use. Although she is worried about the risks of opioid use, she does not feel her alcohol use is problematic. This high-risk patient has frequent SU and multiple symptoms consistent with severe SUD. Next steps to care for patients with severe SUD include a safety assessment, evaluation of co-occurring mental health disorders, comprehensive evaluation of SU-associated risks, and referral to addiction specialists for comprehensive evaluation and treatment. Adolescents who are high risk of overdose (see **Table 116-4**) may benefit from expedited referral regardless of SU severity. Referral may be limited by availability of specialty care, as only 1% of addiction medicine board-certified providers are

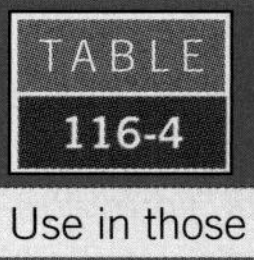

TABLE 116-4 High-Risk Substance Use Features

High-Risk Substance Use Features
Use in those aged 14 years or younger
Use of opioids, methamphetamines, cocaine, or combinations of sedatives (ie, alcohol and benzodiazepines)
History of overdose
History of severe intoxication requiring urgent evaluation
Co-occurring substance use and mental health disorders
Escalating behavioral or functional impairment
Significant mental health concerns

pediatricians, and only a quarter of U.S. addiction treatment facilities serve adolescents.[83] Providers can utilize the Substance Abuse and Mental Health Services Administration (SAMHSA) treatment services locator (https://www.samhsa.gov/find-help) to find resources in their area.

For adolescents engaging in high-risk SU, the goal of the PCP is to support engagement in specialty SU care. The PCP may use an MI approach to assess perceived consequences of use, substance-related goals, and ambivalence about change. Providers may also counsel about addiction as a neurologic disorder that can be effectively treated and encourage and empower adolescents' intrinsic motivation for change. Family involvement (see below) is also often beneficial and may include an assessment of family's prior efforts to address their youth's use, individual or community resources, facilitators and barriers to accessing treatment, and experience with relatives' SU and treatment.[84]

REFERRAL TO TREATMENT

Adolescents with severe SUD or high-risk features benefit from treatment by an addiction specialist. The American Society of Addiction Medicine (ASAM) defines multiple levels of care for adolescents that correspond to addiction severity, related concerns, and potential for recovery. Options range from outpatient treatment by addiction specialists (Level 1) to intensive inpatient services with medical management (Level 4).[85] Please see Chapter 47, "The ASAM Criteria and Matching Patients to Treatment," as well as Chapter 118, "Placement Criteria and Strategies for Adolescent Treatment Matching" for further details. Adolescents are best treated in the least-restrictive environment possible and, ideally, voluntarily engage in their care. As of 2021, 35 states and the District of Columbia allow the involuntary commitment and treatment of individuals with SUD if their SU either affects their ability to care for themselves or is at high risk of causing imminent physical harm to themselves or others.[86] While these policies may provide an option for concerned families of youth who are unable to otherwise engage in care, compulsory treatment is not associated with improved outcomes, does not necessarily include evidence-based treatment such as pharmacotherapy, and, in adults, has been associated with increased risk of overdose following discharge.[87,88]

There are many barriers to specialty addiction treatment, including stigma surrounding SUD, insufficient provider referrals to care, severely limited addiction services for adolescents, and family denial about the seriousness of the disease and associated consequences.[71,83] In practice, less than 8% of adolescents, and 4% of young adults, with past-year SUD receive SU treatment.[47] As mentioned previously, the low proportion of adolescents requiring SUD treatment who receive it is in part due to insufficient resources.[83] Furthermore, there is a significant need for more evidence-based strategies to engage adolescents in available treatment.[18] Research suggests that most youth with problematic SU are not referred to specialty care,[71] and one study found that fewer than one-half of adolescents who receive referrals successfully engage in addiction treatment.[27]

INVOLVING THE FAMILY

One way to support adolescent engagement in care is to involve family members when possible. Parents may be the first to bring concerns about their child's SU to a provider's attention, and in those cases, it can be helpful to query parents' observations and concerns. In situations where adolescents disclose SU first, providers can work with them to decide when and how best to involve their families. It is often helpful to speak with parents, who may provide additional history or share concerning changes they have noticed in their child or home environment, such as missing prescriptions or changes in school performance, that warrant additional evaluation. Parents may also provide important details on family history of SUD and treatment, as well as family substance-related practices in the home, which have been associated with increased risk of adolescent SU.[89]

Family engagement in SU prevention and treatment is also crucial for improving health outcomes for all family members, preventing adolescent SU initiation, and improving treatment outcomes.[90] Providers may use MI strategies to help parents recognize consequences of their child's SU, increase desire to support behavior change and engagement in treatment, and set behavioral expectations for their child. Family therapy may also be a particularly efficacious intervention to reduce SU.[91] Although there remains a need for additional evidence-based strategies, there are multiple ways providers can help families support their child's care, access information about addiction and treatment, and address the impact of their child's use on their health and well-being.[84]

FOLLOW-UP

Care of youth with problematic SU does not end with BI and referral to treatment. Through close follow-up, providers can continue to support an individual's or family's efforts to decrease use and engage with treatment. Clear documentation of screening results and BI goals in the chart may help facilitate treatment and follow-up, particularly when youth are followed by multiple providers. For youth with mild or moderate SUD, close follow-up provides an opportunity to assess and encourage adolescents' success in implementing strategies to decrease use. Clinicians can give youth who have reduced their use positive feedback, the opportunity to discuss how they overcame barriers, support in recognizing ongoing and future barriers, and an assessment of motivation that will continue to support abstinence. Youth who have continued or increased use may benefit from reassessment of goals and/or referral to specialized treatment. Patients with severe SUD may benefit from additional MI and assessment of SU-related risks while awaiting specialized addiction treatment. For all patients, situations such as overdose, emergency room or hospital evaluation for intoxication, injection drug use, self-injurious behaviors, driving while intoxicated, and/or other high-risk behaviors warrant urgent referral to a higher level of care. If the adolescent consents, providers can help facilitate transition to addiction care by providing a "warm hand-off" to specialists detailing the adolescent's medical and psychiatric history, SU-related concerns, and need for further treatment.

RESOURCES

There are multiple online resources available for providers caring for adolescents with SU. The SAMHSA (https://www.samhsa.gov/sbirt) and the NIDA (https://www.drugabuse.gov/nidamed-medical-health-professionals/science-to-medicine/screening-substance-use/in-pediatric-adolescent-medicine-setting) provide helpful information and resources for both providers and families. Education on evidence-based prevention and treatment of opioid use disorder is available from the Opioid Response Network (https://opioidresponsenetwork.org) and the Providers Clinical Support System (PCSS; https://pcssnow.org).

SUMMARY

Adolescent SU is a prevalent behavior that may have numerous short- and long-term adverse consequences for youth. SBIRT can be feasibly and effectively implemented in pediatric primary care to identify adolescents at risk of having a SUD. Universal screening with validated tools can identify adolescents at risk for SUD and guide BIs to prevent or reduce substance-related harms. BI based in MI principles can be utilized to counsel and support youth with all levels of risk. Youth at low risk can be effectively counseled in primary care about the health risks of SU. Youth at risk for mild to moderate SUD can receive additional assessment of substance-related risks and consequences, BI aimed at establishing motivation for change, and close follow-up in primary care. Youth at risk for severe SUD or who have high-risk behaviors need to be referred to an appropriate level of specialty care.

REFERENCES

1. Kirsch DE, Lippard ETC. Early life stress and substance use disorders: the critical role of adolescent substance use. *Pharmacol Biochem Behav.* 2022;215:173360. doi:10.1016/j.pbb.2022.173360
2. Gray KM, Squeglia LM. Research review: what have we learned about adolescent substance use? *J Child Psychol Psychiatry.* 2018;59(6):618-627. doi:10.1111/jcpp.12783
3. American Psychiatric Association. *Diagnostic and Statistical Manual of Mental Disorders.* 5th ed. American Psychiatric Association; 2013.
4. Kim S, Kwok S, Mayes LC, Potenza MN, Rutherford HJV, Strathearn L. Early adverse experience and substance addiction: dopamine, oxytocin, and glucocorticoid pathways. *Ann N Y Acad Sci.* 2017;1394(1):74-91. doi:10.1111/nyas.13140
5. Volkow ND, Li TK. Drug addiction: the neurobiology of behaviour gone awry. *Nat Rev Neurosci.* 2004;5(12):963-970. doi:10.1038/nrn1539
6. Chambers RA, Taylor JR, Potenza MN. Developmental neurocircuitry of motivation in adolescence: a critical period of addiction vulnerability. *Am J Psychiatry.* 2003;160(6):1041-1052.
7. Nixon K, McClain JA. Adolescence as a critical window for developing an alcohol use disorder: current findings in neuroscience. *Curr Opin Psychiatry.* 2010;23(3):227-232. doi:10.1097/YCO.0b013e32833864fe
8. Richmond-Rakerd LS, Slutske WS, Wood PK. Age of initiation and substance use progression: a multivariate latent growth analysis. *Psychol Addict Behav.* 2017;31(6):664-675. doi:10.1037/adb0000304
9. Irons DE, Iacono WG, McGue M. Tests of the effects of adolescent early alcohol exposures on adult outcomes. *Addiction.* 2015;110(2):269-278. doi:10.1111/add.12747
10. Substance Abuse and Mental Health Services Administration. *Age of Substance Use Initiation among Treatment Admissions Aged 18 to 30.* Substance Abuse and Mental Health Services Administration; 2014. Accessed July 25, 2023. https://www.samhsa.gov/data/sites/default/files/WebFiles_TEDS_SR142_AgeatInit_07-10-14/TEDS-SR142-AgeatInit-2014.htm
11. French L, Gray C, Leonard G, et al. Early cannabis use, polygenic risk score for schizophrenia and brain maturation in adolescence. *JAMA Psychiatry.* 2015;72(10):1002-1011. doi:10.1001/jamapsychiatry.2015.1131
12. Hines LA, Freeman TP, Gage SH, et al. Association of high-potency cannabis use with mental health and substance use in adolescence. *JAMA Psychiatry.* 2020;77(10):1044-1051. doi:10.1001/jamapsychiatry.2020.1035
13. Moore THM, Zammit S, Lingford-Hughes A, et al. Cannabis use and risk of psychotic or affective mental health outcomes: a systematic review. *Lancet.* 2007;370(9584):319-328.
14. Frolli A, Ricci MC, Cavallaro A, et al. Cognitive development and cannabis use in adolescents. *Behav Sci (Basel).* 2021;11(3):37. doi:10.3390/bs11030037
15. Castellanos-Ryan N, Pingault JB, Parent S, Vitaro F, Tremblay RE, Séguin JR. Adolescent cannabis use, change in neurocognitive function, and high-school graduation: a longitudinal study from early adolescence to young adulthood. *Dev Psychopathol.* 2017;29(4):1253-1266. doi:10.1017/S0954579416001280
16. Crean RD, Crane NA, Mason BJ. An evidence based review of acute and long-term effects of cannabis use on executive cognitive functions. *J Addict Med.* 2011;5(1):1-8. doi:10.1097/ADM.0b013e31820c23fa
17. Friedman J, Godvin M, Shover CL, Gone JP, Hansen H, Schriger DL. Trends in drug overdose deaths among U.S. adolescents, January 2010 to June 2021. *JAMA.* 2022;327(14):1398-1400. doi:10.1001/jama.2022.2847
18. Levy SJL, Williams JF, Committee on Substance Use and Prevention, et al. Substance use screening, brief intervention, and referral to treatment. *Pediatrics.* 2016;138(1):e20161211. doi:10.1542/peds.2016-1211
19. Neighbors CJ, Colby SM, Monti PM. Cost-effectiveness of a motivational intervention for alcohol-involved youth in a hospital emergency department. *J Stud Alcohol Drugs.* 2010;71(3):384-394. doi:10.15288/jsad.2010.71.384
20. Mitchell SG, Gryczynski J, Gonzales A, et al. Screening, brief intervention, and referral to treatment (SBIRT) for substance use in a school-based program: services and outcomes. *Am J Addict.* 2012;21:S5-S13. doi:10.1111/j.1521-0391.2012.00299.x

21. Chadi N, Levy S, Wisk LE, Weitzman ER. Student experience of school screening, brief intervention, and referral to treatment. *J Sch Health.* 2020;90(6):431-438. doi:10.1111/josh.12890
22. Lunstead J, Weitzman ER, Kaye D, Levy S. Screening and brief intervention in high schools: school nurses' practices and attitudes in Massachusetts. *Subst Abuse.* 2017;38(3):257-260. doi:10.1080/08897077.2016.1275926
23. Maslowsky J, Whelan Capell J, Moberg DP, Brown RL. Universal school-based implementation of screening brief intervention and referral to treatment to reduce and prevent alcohol, marijuana, tobacco, and other drug use: process and feasibility. *Subst Abuse Res Treat.* 2017;11:117822181774666. doi:10.1177/1178221817746668
24. Parthasarathy S, Kline-Simon AH, Jones A, et al. Three-year outcomes after brief treatment of substance use and mood symptoms. *Pediatrics.* 2021;147(1):e2020009191. doi:10.1542/peds.2020-009191
25. Harris SK, Csémy L, Sherritt L, et al. Computer-facilitated substance use screening and brief advice for teens in primary care: an international trial. *Pediatrics.* 2012;129(6):1072-1082. doi:10.1542/peds.2011-1624
26. Sterling S, Kline-Simon AH, Jones A, et al. Health care use over 3 years after adolescent SBIRT. *Pediatrics.* 2019;143(5):e20182803. doi:10.1542/peds.2018-2803
27. Stanhope V, Manuel JI, Jessell L, Halliday TM. Implementing SBIRT for adolescents within community mental health organizations: a mixed methods study. *J Subst Abuse Treat.* 2018;90:38-46. doi:10.1016/j.jsat.2018.04.009
28. Levy S, Wisk LE, Minegishi M, et al. Association of screening and brief intervention with substance use in Massachusetts middle and high schools. *JAMA Netw Open.* 2022;5(8):e2226886. doi:10.1001/jamanetworkopen.2022.26886
29. Adams SH, Park MJ, Irwin CE. Adolescent and young adult preventive care: comparing national survey rates. *Am J Prev Med.* 2015;49(2):238-247. doi:10.1016/j.amepre.2015.02.022
30. Adams SH, Park MJ, Twietmeyer L, Brindis CD, Irwin CE. Increasing delivery of preventive services to adolescents and young adults: does the preventive visit help? *J Adolesc Health.* 2018;63(2):166-171. doi:10.1016/j.jadohealth.2018.03.013
31. Hammond CJ, Parhami I, Young AS, et al. Provider and practice characteristics and perceived barriers associated with different levels of adolescent SBIRT implementation among a national sample of US pediatricians. *Clin Pediatr (Phila).* 2021;60(9-10):418-426.
32. Barnett E, Sussman S, Smith C, Rohrbach LA, Spruijt-Metz D. Motivational interviewing for adolescent substance use: a review of the literature. *Addict Behav.* 2012;37(12):1325-1334. doi:10.1016/j.addbeh.2012.07.001
33. Steele DW, Becker SJ, Danko KJ, et al. Brief behavioral interventions for substance use in adolescents: a meta-analysis. *Pediatrics.* 2020;146(4):e20200351. doi:10.1542/peds.2020-0351
34. Naar S, Suarez M. *Motivational Interviewing with Adolescents and Young Adults.* 2nd ed. Guilford Press; 2021.
35. National Institute on Alcohol Abuse and Alcoholism. *Alcohol Screening and Brief Intervention for Youth: A Practitioner's Guide.* National Institute on Alcohol Abuse and Alcoholism; 2021.
36. Hagan JF, Shaw JS, Duncan PM. *Bright Futures: Guidelines for Health Supervision of Infants, Children and Adolescents.* 4th ed. American Academy of Pediatrics; 2017.
37. Ford CA. Influence of physician confidentiality assurances on adolescents' willingness to disclose information and seek future health care. A randomized controlled trial. *JAMA.* 1997;278(12):1029-1034. doi:10.1001/jama.278.12.1029
38. Gilbert AL, Rickert VI, Aalsma MC. Clinical conversations about health: the impact of confidentiality in preventive adolescent care. *J Adolesc Health.* 2014;55(5):672-677. doi:10.1016/j.jadohealth.2014.05.016
39. Neinstein LS, Katzman DK, Callahan ST, Gordon CM, Joffe A, Rickert VI. *Neinstein's Adolescent and Young Adult Health Care: A Practical Guide.* 6th ed. Wolters Kluwer; 2016.
40. Ginsburg KR. Viewing our adolescent patients through a positive lens. *Contemporary Pediatrics.* Accessed May 5, 2022. https://www.contemporarypediatrics.com/view/viewing-our-adolescent-patients-through-positive-lens
41. Wilson CR, Sherritt L, Gates E, Knight JR. Are clinical impressions of adolescent substance use accurate? *Pediatrics.* 2004;114(5):e536-e540. doi:10.1542/peds.2004-0098
42. Kelly SM, Gryczynski J, Mitchell SG, Kirk A, O'Grady KE, Schwartz RP. Validity of brief screening instrument for adolescent tobacco, alcohol, and drug use. *Pediatrics.* 2014;133(5):819-826. doi:10.1542/peds.2013-2346
43. Jasik CB, Berna M, Martin M, Ozer EM. Teen preferences for clinic-based behavior screens: who, where, when, and how? *J Adolesc Health.* 2016;59(6):722-724. doi:10.1016/j.jadohealth.2016.08.009
44. Johnston LD, Miech RA, O'Malley PM, Bachman JG, Schulenberg JE, Patrick ME. *Monitoring the Future National Survey Results on Drug Use: 2020 Overview Key Findings on Adolescent Drug Use*; 2021.
45. Gryczynski J, Mitchell SG, Schwartz RP, et al. Disclosure of adolescent substance use in primary care: comparison of routine clinical screening and anonymous research interviews. *J Adolesc Health.* 2019;64(4):541-543. doi:10.1016/j.jadohealth.2018.10.009
46. Harris SK, Knight JR Jr, Van Hook S, et al. Adolescent substance use screening in primary care: validity of computer self-administered versus clinician-administered screening. *Subst Abuse.* 2016;37(1):197-203. doi:10.1080/08897077.2015.1014615
47. Center for Behavioral Health Statistics and Quality, Substance Abuse and Mental Health Services Administration. *Key Substance Use and Mental Health Indicators in the United States: Results from the 2020 National Survey on Drug Use and Health*; 2021.
48. Soberay A, Pietruszewski P, DeSorrento L, Levy S. Rates and predictors of substance use in pediatric primary care clinics. *Subst Abuse.* 2022;43(1):1094-1099.
49. Knight JR, Harris SK, Sherritt L, et al. Adolescents' preferences for substance abuse screening in primary care practice. *Subst Abuse.* 2007;28(4):107-117. doi:10.1300/J465v28n04_03
50. Gibson EB, Knight JR, Levinson JA, Sherritt L, Harris SK. Pediatric primary care provider perspectives on a computer-facilitated screening and brief intervention system for adolescent substance use. *J Adolesc Health.* 2021;69(1):157-161. doi:10.1016/j.jadohealth.2020.09.037
51. Gadomski AM, Fothergill KE, Larson S, et al. Integrating mental health into adolescent annual visits: impact of pre-visit comprehensive screening on within-visit processes. *J Adolesc Health.* 2015;56(3):267-273. doi:10.1016/j.jadohealth.2014.11.011
52. Richardson L, Parker EO, Zhou C, Kientz J, Ozer E, McCarty C. Electronic health risk behavior screening with integrated feedback among adolescents in primary care: randomized controlled trial. *J Med Internet Res.* 2021;23(3):e24135. doi:10.2196/24135
53. Chung T, Smith GT, Donovan JE, et al. Drinking frequency as a brief screen for adolescent alcohol problems. *Pediatrics.* 2012;129(2):205-212. doi:10.1542/peds.2011-1828
54. Spirito A, Bromberg JR, Casper TC, et al. Reliability and validity of a two-question alcohol screen in the pediatric emergency department. *Pediatrics.* 2016;138(6):e20160691. doi:10.1542/peds.2016-0691
55. Levy S, Weitzman ER, Marin AC, Magane KM, Wisk LE, Shrier LA. Sensitivity and specificity of S2BI for identifying alcohol and cannabis use disorders among adolescents presenting for primary care. *Subst Abuse.* 2021;42(3):388-395. doi:10.1080/08897077.2020.1803180
56. Gryczynski J, Kelly SM, Mitchell SG, Kirk A, O'Grady KE, Schwartz RP. Validation and performance of the Alcohol, Smoking and Substance Involvement Screening Test (ASSIST) among adolescent primary care patients: WHO ASSIST for adolescents. *Addiction.* 2015;110(2):240-247. doi:10.1111/add.12767
57. Knight JR, Sherritt L, Shrier LA, Harris SK, Chang G. Validity of the CRAFFT substance abuse screening test among adolescent clinic patients. *Arch Pediatr Adolesc Med.* 2002;156(6):607. doi:10.1001/archpedi.156.6.607
58. Essau CA. Comorbidity of substance use disorders among community-based and high-risk adolescents. *Psychiatry Res.* 2011;185(1-2):176-184. doi:10.1016/j.psychres.2010.04.033
59. Levy S, Dedeoglu F, Gaffin JM, et al. A screening tool for assessing alcohol use risk among medically vulnerable youth. *PLoS One.* 2016;11(5):e0156240. doi:10.1371/journal.pone.0156240
60. D'Amico EJ, Parast L, Meredith LS, Ewing BA, Shadel WG, Stein BD. Screening in primary care: what is the best way to identify at-risk youth

for substance use? *Pediatrics.* 2016;138(6):e20161717. doi:10.1542/peds.2016-1717

61. Committee on Substance Use and Prevention. Substance use screening, brief intervention, and referral to treatment. *Pediatrics.* 2016;138(1):e20161210. doi:10.1542/peds.2016-1210
62. Boston Children's Hospital. Get the CRAFFT. Accessed July 25, 2023. https://crafft.org/get-the-crafft
63. Rial A, Kim-Harris S, Knight JR, et al. Empirical validation of the CRAFFT Abuse Screening Test in a Spanish sample. *Adicciones.* 2019;31(2):160-169.
64. Källmén H, Berman AH, Jayaram-Lindström N, Hammarberg A, Elgan TH. Psychometric properties of the AUDIT, AUDIT-C, CRAFFT and ASSIST-Y among Swedish adolescents. *Eur Addict Res.* 2019;25(2):68-77. doi:10.1159/000496741
65. Song Y, Kim H, Park SY. An item response theory analysis of the Korean version of the CRAFFT scale for alcohol use among adolescents in Korea. *Asian Nurs Res.* 2019;13(4):249-256. doi:10.1016/j.anr.2019.09.003
66. Bernard M, Bolognini M, Plancherel B, et al. French validity of two substance-use screening tests among adolescents: a comparison of the CRAFFT and DEP-ADO. *J Subst Use.* 2005;10(6):385-395. doi:10.1080/14659890412331333050
67. Lyons RM, Yule AM, Schiff D, Bagley SM, Wilens TE. Risk factors for drug overdose in young people: a systematic review of the literature. *J Child Adolesc Psychopharmacol.* 2019;29(7):487-497. doi:10.1089/cap.2019.0013
68. Levy S, Siqueira LM; Committee on Substance Abuse. Testing for drugs of abuse in children and adolescents. *Pediatrics.* 2014;133(6):e1798-e1807. doi:10.1542/peds.2014-0865
69. Levy S, Wiseblatt A, Straus JH, Strother H, Fluet C, Harris SK. Adolescent SBIRT practices among pediatricians in Massachusetts. *J Addict Med.* 2020;14(2):145-149. doi:10.1097/ADM.0000000000000551
70. Sterling S, Kline-Simon AH, Satre DD, et al. Implementation of screening, brief intervention, and referral to treatment for adolescents in pediatric primary care: a cluster randomized trial. *JAMA Pediatr.* 2015;169(11):e153145. doi:10.1001/jamapediatrics.2015.3145
71. Mitchell SG, Gryczynski J, Schwartz RP, et al. Adolescent SBIRT implementation: generalist vs. specialist models of service delivery in primary care. *J Subst Abuse Treat.* 2020;111:67-72. doi:10.1016/j.jsat.2020.01.007
72. Barbosa C, Wedehase B, Dušek K, et al. Costs and implementation effectiveness of generalist versus specialist models for adolescent screening and brief intervention in primary care. *J Stud Alcohol Drugs.* 2022;83(2):231-238.
73. SADD: Students Against Destructive Decisions. *SADD Nation.* Accessed June 1, 2022. https://www.sadd.org/resources
74. Knight JR, Csemy L, Sherritt L, et al. Screening and brief advice to reduce adolescents' risk of riding with substance-using drivers. *J Stud Alcohol Drugs.* 2018;79(4):611-616. doi:10.15288/jsad.2018.79.611
75. Harris SK, Johnson JK, Sherritt L, Copelas S, Rappo MA, Wilson CR. Putting adolescents at risk: riding with drinking drivers who are adults in the home. *J Stud Alcohol Drugs.* 2017;78(1):146-151. doi:10.15288/jsad.2017.78.146
76. Osilla KC, Seelam R, Parast L, D'Amico EJ. Associations between driving under the influence or riding with an impaired driver and future substance use among adolescents. *Traffic Inj Prev.* 2019;20(6):563. doi:10.1080/15389588.2019.1615620
77. Carliner H, Brown QL, Sarvet AL, Hasin DS. Cannabis use, attitudes, and legal status in the U.S: a review. *Prev Med.* 2017;104:13-23. doi:10.1016/j.ypmed.2017.07.008
78. Farmer CM, Monfort SS, Woods AN. Changes in traffic crash rates after legalization of marijuana: results by crash severity. *J Stud Alcohol Drugs.* 2022;83(4):494-501. doi:10.15288/jsad.2022.83.494
79. Levine A, Clemenza K, Rynn M, Lieberman J. Evidence for the risks and consequences of adolescent cannabis exposure. *J Am Acad Child Adolesc Psychiatry.* 2017;56(3):214-225. doi:10.1016/j.jaac.2016.12.014
80. Nemer L, Lara LF, Hinton A, Conwell DL, Krishna SG, Balasubramanian G. Impact of recreational cannabis legalization on hospitalizations for hyperemesis. *Am J Gastroenterol.* 2021;116(3):609-612. doi:10.14309/ajg.0000000000001182
81. Maisto SA, Krenek M, Chung TA, Martin CS, Clark D, Cornelius JR. A comparison of the concurrent and predictive validity of three measures of readiness to change alcohol use in a clinical sample of adolescents. *Psychol Assess.* 2011;23(4):983-994. doi:10.1037/a0024136
82. Maisto SA, Krenek M, Chung T, Martin CS, Clark D, Cornelius J. Comparison of the concurrent and predictive validity of three measures of readiness to change marijuana use in a clinical sample of adolescents. *J Stud Alcohol Drugs.* 2011;72(4):592-601.
83. Alinsky RH, Hadland SE, Matson PA, Cerda M, Saloner B. Adolescent-serving addiction treatment facilities in the United States and the availability of medications for opioid use disorder. *J Adolesc Health.* 2020;67(4):542-549. doi:10.1016/j.jadohealth.2020.03.005
84. Bagley SM, Ventura AS, Lasser KE, Muench F. Engaging the family in the care of young adults with substance use disorders. *Pediatrics.* 2021;147(Supplement 2):S215-S219. doi:10.1542/peds.2020-023523C
85. American Society of Addiction Medicine. *The ASAM Criteria: Treatment Criteria for Addictive, Substance-Related, and Co-Occurring Conditions.* 3rd ed. American Society of Addiction Medicine; 2013. Accessed January 31, 2022. https://www.asam.org/asam-criteria
86. Prescription Drug Abuse Policy System. *Involuntary Commitment for Substance Use.* Accessed November 1, 2023. https://pdaps.org/datasets/civil-commitment-for-substance-users-1562936854
87. Werb D, Kamarulzaman A, Meacham MC, et al. The effectiveness of compulsory drug treatment: a systematic review. *Int J Drug Policy.* 2016;28:1-9. doi:10.1016/j.drugpo.2015.12.005
88. Rafful C, Orozco R, Rangel G, et al. Increased non-fatal overdose risk associated with involuntary drug treatment in a longitudinal study with people who inject drugs. *Addict Abingdon Engl.* 2018;113(6):1056-1063. doi:10.1111/add.14159
89. Trucco EM. A review of psychosocial factors linked to adolescent substance use. *Pharmacol Biochem Behav.* 2020;196:172969. doi:10.1016/j.pbb.2020.172969
90. Ventura AS, Bagley SM. To improve substance use disorder prevention, treatment and recovery: engage the family. *J Addict Med.* 2017;11(5):339-341.
91. Tanner-Smith EE, Wilson SJ, Lipsey MW. The comparative effectiveness of outpatient treatment for adolescent substance abuse: a meta-analysis. *J Subst Abuse Treat.* 2013;44(2):145-158. doi:10.1016/j.jsat.2012.05.006

Sidebar 1

Neurobiological Determinants of Addiction in Children and Adolescents

Marisa M. Silveri, Andie Stallman, and Jennifer T. Sneider

INTRODUCTION

The societal impacts of addiction are numerous and widespread, with some estimates indicating that the lives of seven people are affected for each individual with addiction and the associated biopsychosocial consequences.[1,2] The age of onset of first use is one of the strongest predictors of later substance use disorders (SUDs),[3,4] given associations with elevated risk for psychosocial problems (eg, family problems, depression, anxiety, unhealthy substance use, sexual abuse, and violence). Such factors can describe individuals relative to the social environment and how these affect physical and mental health.[3,4] Indeed, initiation of use, rapid escalation in quantity and frequency of intake, and increasing prevalence of SUDs often occur during the critical period of adolescent brain development.

Adolescence is characterized by substantial biological, psychological, and social changes across many domains: structural, functional, and neurochemical brain changes, sleep physiology, hormones and puberty, cognition, motivation, reward sensitivity, stress, adversity, mental health, social function, and impacts of cultural, familial, and intergenerational influences.[5-8] The biopsychosocial model considers biological (genetics, neurobiology, physiology), psychological (mental and emotional wellness, behavior, cognition), and social factors (life traumas, stressors, early life experiences, familial and intergenerational, cultural, and community relationships) and their complex interactions in development, mental health, and addiction.[9,10] The examination of the interplay of biopsychosocial factors has considerable potential to identify causes, characterize manifestation, and implement early prevention, screening, and timely interventions among people who begin substance use at an early age.

Biopsychosocial Model of Addiction

Biological risks for addiction can include a family history of substance use problems, physiological responses to substances, and brain changes that can be antecedents to and consequences of use. Psychological risk factors include the appetitive effects of substances, mental health conditions (eg, depression, anxiety, etc.), impulsivity, and emotional regulation. Social risk factors include peer pressure, social support networks, past traumatic events, adjustment difficulties, and societal acceptance of substance use. Applying a biopsychosocial model to addiction permits a holistic, multifaceted conceptualization of the disorder instead of identifying a singular cause.[11] Considering only biological makeup has significant drawbacks, given research documenting that addiction is a complex phenomenon and the fact that there is no "addiction gene" or genetic sequence that accounts for the notable variance in the expression of addiction. On the contrary, it has become well-accepted that a constellation of factors contributes to a person being more or less at risk for addiction. Grisel[12] noted, "the bottom line is that there are likely as many pathways to becoming a (person with an addiction disorder) as there are (people with addiction disorders)."[12]

Medical Model of Addiction

The medical model categorizes SUD as a disease. As defined by the American Society of Addiction Medicine: "Addiction is a primary, chronic disease of brain reward, motivation, memory, and related circuitry." To date, there is mounting evidence of neurobiological correlates of substance-related loss of control, compulsive substance use, inflexible behavior, and dysregulated emotional states. Substances such as alcohol can impair learning and memory, disrupt planning, increase impulsivity, decrease behavioral inhibition, increase poor decision-making, and alter emotion regulation and reward.[13,14] Some cognitive abilities are particularly vulnerable to being impaired by chronic, heavy use, for example, executive functions, including working memory and response inhibition, controlled/effortful processing of novel information, selective/divided attention, and spatial, episodic, and autobiographical memory. Other areas of cognition are spared, such as general intelligence, over-learned knowledge, and automatic information processes.[15] A sizeable proportion of persons (estimated 35%-70%) diagnosed with a SUD display some neurocognitive deficits relative to those without a SUD, while many have subtle or transient cognitive disruptions.[13,16-19] Unhealthy substance use is linked to structural and functional brain abnormalities[20] and altered neurochemistry.[21] With repeated, chronic substance exposure, altered receptor function adapts to new homeostatic states in the presence of substances. Indeed, homeostatic conditions are disrupted during abstinence and can be detected and persist before a return (recovery) to nonaffected levels. In support of neurobiological evidence of harmful substance use, molecular targets and vulnerable brain circuitries that undergo maladaptive alterations in response to repeated substance exposure can be minimized or eliminated by medications developed to treat SUDs.[22]

It is vital to appreciate the limitations of the disease model, which assumes that the origins of addiction exist solely within the individual, therefore failing to consider important influences related to psychosocial factors, including social learning and culture, and social determinants of health such as poverty and discrimination (biopsychosocial perspective). The psychodynamic approach to understanding addiction examines how past events, thoughts and circumstances shape substance use and other harmful behaviors. Through a psychodynamic lens, substance use reflects a need to escape internal struggles of malaise and seek self-containment, referred to as the self-medication hypothesis.[23] The self-medication hypothesis includes factors that include, but are not limited to, self-deceptive attempts at adaptation and affect regulation associated with insecure attachment, inability to prioritize self-care or delay gratification, novelty seeking and impulsivity, and adverse childhood experiences.[23,24] On the one hand, psychological factors are often interpreted as reflecting a choice to use substances and, as such, a character flaw that led to unhealthy substance use. The medical model of addiction, however, points to a disease that is not a choice, decreasing the notion that addiction is the fault of the individual. Ultimately, a combination of these models offers the best approach to understanding risks and treating addiction. A goal of determining characteristics of risk, from behavior to mental health to neurobiology, is to help develop prevention efforts and create early intervention strategies to reduce the incidence of use and risky behaviors associated with harmful patterns of use and the development of addiction.[1,25]

Reaching Neurobiological Adulthood

Given the growing evidence of alterations associated with adolescent alcohol, cannabis, and other drug use (**Table 116-5**),[26] there has been a sizeable shift in focus to prospectively characterizing brain development prior to the onset of use to identify neurobiological signatures of risk for addiction and, increasingly, establishing relationships between biopsychosocial factors and addiction.[6,27]

Over the past two decades, magnetic resonance imaging (MRI) techniques have dramatically improved our understanding of the developmental profile of adolescent brain development due in part to the rapid evolution and availability of higher field-strength scanners, hardware and software innovations, and advanced imaging sequences. As a result, neuroimaging studies have significantly advanced the understanding of neuromaturational changes from childhood through adolescence[28,29] and into late adolescence/emerging adulthood.[30]

Brain imaging studies show that as one ages there is a general linear increase in white matter (WM), thought to

TABLE 116-5 2021 Monitoring the Future Survey Results: Adolescent Lifetime Use of Alcohol and Other Substances

Substance		8th Graders	10th Graders	12th Graders
Alcohol	Any use	21.7%	34.7%	54.1%
	Been drunk	8.3%	17.8%	38.9%
Cannabis		10.2%	22.0%	38.6%
Nicotine	Cigarettes	7.0%	10.0%	17.8%
	Smokeless	4.6%	4.9%	8.6%
Vaping	Nicotine	17.5%	29.7%	40.5%
	Cannabis	6.5%	16.5%	25.7%
	Flavoring only	12.0%	19.6%	25.2%
	JUUL	10.3%	19.8%	28.5%
Amphetamines		5.8%	5.2%	4.9%
Methamphetamine		0.3%	0.4%	0.6%
Ecstasy (MDMA)		1.0%	1.4%	2.8%
Inhalants		11.3%	7.2%	5.0%
LSD		1.2%	2.5%	4.9%
Hallucinogens (not LSD)		1.3%	2.5%	5.3%
Any illicit drug		15.9%	25.0%	41.3%
Any illicit drug (not cannabis)		8.8%	9.1%	12.8%

Percent prevalence for each substance is taken directly from Table 5 of Johnston LD, O'Malley PM, Miech RA, et al. *Monitoring the Future National Survey Results on Drug Use 1975-2021: Overview, Key Findings on Adolescent Drug Use*. Institute for Social Research. University of Michigan; 2022.

reflect myelination of axons and improved brain connectivity, and a nonlinear decrease in gray matter (GM), attributed to proliferation followed by pruning of synaptic connections that reduces neuronal redundancy and improves neuronal efficiency.[8,28] The last region of the brain to mature is the frontal lobe, with improved WM connectivity observed among widely distributed brain networks, for example, reward and limbic (emotion regulation) circuitries,[31,32] and frontally-based regions and functionally connected subcortical structures. Neuromaturation also is observed at the level of neurochemistry, with age-related increases in brain gamma aminobutyric acid (GABA),[33] the major inhibitory neurotransmitter in the mammalian brain.[34] Not surprisingly, adolescent brain reorganization, refinements, and functional improvements map onto enhanced cognitive abilities. Accordingly, functional magnetic resonance imaging (fMRI) studies document significant increases in the magnitude of frontal lobe activity during the performance of frontally mediated executive tasks, highlighting the importance of maturation of this region in contributing to age-related improvements in cognitive control. Furthermore, the medial prefrontal cortex (mPFC) and anterior cingulate cortex (ACC), areas of the frontal lobe heavily involved in self-regulation, together form a major node of the default mode network (DMN). The DMN is a collection of prefrontal, posterior cingulate/precuneus, and parietal regions that function together in an organized manner when an individual is at rest. The activity of the DMN is suspended or suppressed during goal-directed behaviors.[35] The functioning of DMN not only matures during healthy brain development,[36] but is compromised in addiction.[37] As frontally mediated networks mediate self-regulation, the vulnerability of these networks also contributes to risky behaviors and harmful use of substances in adolescents. Indeed, parallel to brain development is an increased propensity to seek novel stimulation and engage in risk-taking behaviors.

Characterizing the neurobiology underlying immature cognitive and behavioral responses, which result in suboptimal self-regulatory control, has been an area of extensive investigation. While neurobiological refinement is associated with improvements in higher-order cognitive domains,[38,39] for example, dramatic improvements in executive function and emotion regulation, remodeling also extends to regions implicated in learning and memory. Recent work highlights the essential role of integrating the prefrontal cortex (PFC) and hippocampal circuitries during adolescence in incorporating past experience into current decision-making and thus promoting adaptive behaviors necessary for successful developmental transitions.[40]

Child and Adolescent Brain Vulnerabilities

It has been well established that many substances with addiction liability are toxic to the brain, particularly to developing regions that overlap with those most vulnerable to alcohol and other potentially addictive substances. Studies confirm that the most common region neurobiologically impacted by substance use in youth is the frontal lobe (~63%).[41] Observed effects could also reflect biopsychosocial contributions associated with antecedents of use, for example, age of initiation of substance use; family history of addiction; childhood maltreatment; and other types of childhood adversity (environmental); and co-occurring psychiatric conditions.

Substance use is associated with deficits across several domains of cognition, with executive functioning and memory domains most vulnerable to disruptions by alcohol.[42,43] MRI and fMRI, employed to characterize neurobiological factors underlying alcohol-related cognitive deficits, have revealed alterations in brain structure and brain activation during the performance of cognitive tasks. Adolescents who initiated heavy drinking exhibited reduced fMRI responses at baseline during a visual working memory task, but then had increased frontal and parietal activation at a follow-up visit, relative to those adolescents who did not initiate drinking.[44] Similarly, adolescents with limited substance use at baseline who then transitioned to heavy alcohol use exhibited less neural activation in frontal, parietal, and left cingulate regions during inhibitory processing at follow-up.[45] These longitudinal results suggest evidence for unique patterns of brain activation in adolescents prior to initiating substance use, perhaps reflecting a neurobiological predictor of risk for increased future substance use problems.[46] Because of high rates of alcohol and cannabis, nicotine, and other substance co-use, substance-specific alterations are difficult to disentangle. Some work suggests greater impairments related to alcohol consumption, while other studies have identified more associations with cannabis use and minimal influence of alcohol use. Paradoxically, individuals who use both cannabis and alcohol have more similar patterns of brain activation to controls than users of either substance alone. While cannabis may have properties that attenuate alcohol-related neurotoxicity, this notion is not supported by the literature, which offers substantial evidence of alterations in people who use cannabis and who also drink. Methodological differences and a lack of consideration of biopsychosocial factors may contribute to contradictory results. Differences may be confounded by age, sex and gender, racial/ethnic and cultural factors, socioeconomic status, childhood adversity, timing and frequency of use, length of intervals between measurements, and thorough characterization of psychiatric and substance use histories. In addition, it is plausible that one imaging methodology alone may be insufficient for fully delineating the complex nature of substances and independent and interactive influences on biopsychosocial factors. Conversely, it is noteworthy that alcohol, cannabis, nicotine, and other drug effects are evident among even people who use at more moderate levels with no SUD, such as those meeting subdiagnostic criteria for binge drinking or people who smoke nicotine.

Utility of Prospective Studies—Predicting Risk

Federally funded initiatives are now underway to more thoroughly examine risk factors for and the longitudinal impacts of substance use in extensive, multisite studies of adolescents: the National Consortium on Alcohol and NeuroDevelopment in Adolescence (N-CANDA)[47,48] (cross-sequential design, ages 12-21) and the Adolescent Brain Cognitive Development Study (ABCD Study, https://abcdstudy.org) (longitudinal, ages 9-10, examined yearly for 10 years).[49-53] The ABCD Study is an open-science, multisite, prospective, longitudinal study following over 11,800 9- and 10-year-old youths for 10 years into early adulthood. This national effort is uniquely positioned to address pressing public health concerns from a biopsychosocial perspective. The ABCD study uses sophisticated technologies to conduct a study of sufficient size and statistical power to identify benchmarks for healthy neurodevelopment and to track the onset and course of mental health conditions, including substance use. To date, few studies have investigated sex effects on the impacts of alcohol and other substance use.[54-56] Per the mandate from the National Institutes of Health (NIH), the ABCD study includes comparable proportions of sexes and genders to begin to parse sex and gender effects on mental health and addiction outcomes. Youths and their families provide rich details about their environmental experiences and undergo extensive phenotypic, cognitive, genetic, emotional, health, and neuroimaging assessments to advance understanding of how multiple aspects of youth experiences (eg, culture and environment, etc.) relate to developmental outcomes, including the age of onset of substance use and patterns of use that follow. It remains to be determined to what degree neurobiological consequences may resolve with extended abstinence or continue to decline with increasing use. To that end, long-term prospective multimodal studies are helping to elucidate the impacts of various use trajectories during the developmental period, especially during adolescence, that endure later in life.

SUMMARY

Adolescents have an increased propensity to seek novel stimulation and engage in risk-taking behaviors as well as heightened neurobiological vulnerability, particularly to alcohol and other substances. To understand brain development in the context of healthy brain maturation and substance use onset, regular and escalating use, and addiction, many investigations have identified substance-related alterations associated with adolescent alcohol, cannabis, and other drug use. Over the past two decades, better characterization of neurodevelopmental changes and milestones have been captured noninvasively using MRI. Moreover, incorporating complementary multimodal measures of brain function and neuroplasticity offers valuable insight into the dynamic processes of brain maturation. Establishing maturational profiles of central target sites of action of alcohol and other substances may reveal underpinnings of risk for initiation of use, while identifying neural signatures associated with the onset and escalation of adolescent substance use. Together with data from animal models demonstrating adolescence to be a period of unique sensitivity to addictive substances, there are increasing translational opportunities that will ultimately further our understanding of the consequences of alcohol and other substance use on the adolescent brain.

Future studies must continue to elucidate how adolescent brain development unfolds, what brain regions and networks are affected by alcohol and substances when early exposure occurs, and what biopsychosocial factors influence risk and consequences of SUDs in children and adolescents. Regardless of antecedent or consequence, there is a vital need for initiatives that bridge gaps in the elucidation of the biopsychosocial factors that increase addiction risk in adolescents.[9,10,57,58] Such information is crucial for primary care physicians[59-62] who can offer preventive advice and brief interventions to individuals and their families and for mental health practitioners who provide clinical care and treatment for adolescents at risk for alcohol and other substance use disorders.[1,63-65]

REFERENCES

1. Potenza MN. Biological contributions to addictions in adolescents and adults: prevention, treatment, and policy implications. *J Adolesc Health.* 2013;52(2 Suppl 2):S22-S32. doi:10.1016/j.jadohealth.2012.05.007
2. Volkow ND, Baler RD, Goldstein RZ. Addiction: pulling at the neural threads of social behaviors. *Neuron.* 2011;69(4):599-602. doi:10.1016/j.neuron.2011.01.027
3. Grant BF, Dawson DA. Age of onset of drug use and its association with DSM-IV drug abuse and dependence: results from the National Longitudinal Alcohol Epidemiologic Survey. *J Subst Abuse.* 1998;10(2):163-173. doi:S0899-3289(99)80131-X [pii]
4. Poudel A, Gautam S. Age of onset of substance use and psychosocial problems among individuals with substance use disorders. *BMC Psychiatry.* 2017;17(1):10. doi:10.1186/s12888-016-1191-0
5. Bjork JM, Straub LK, Provost RG, Neale MC. The ABCD study of neurodevelopment: identifying neurocircuit targets for prevention and treatment of adolescent substance abuse. *Curr Treat Options Psychiatry.* 2017;4(2):196-209. doi:10.1007/s40501-017-0108-y
6. Dick AS, Lopez DA, Watts AL, et al. Meaningful associations in the adolescent brain cognitive development study. *Neuroimage.* 2021;239:118262. doi:10.1016/j.neuroimage.2021.118262
7. Spear LP. The adolescent brain and age-related behavioral manifestations. *Neurosci Biobehav Rev.* 2000;24(4):417-463. doi:10.1016/s0149-7634(00)00014-2
8. Spear LP. Adolescent neurodevelopment. *J Adolesc Health.* 2013;52 (2 Suppl 2):S7-S13. doi:10.1016/j.jadohealth.2012.05.006
9. Skewes MC, Gonzalez VM. The biopsychosocial model of addiction. In: Miller PM, ed. *Principles of Addiction: Comprehensive Addictive Behaviors and Disorders.* Vol. 1. 2013:61-70.
10. Haslam SA, Haslam C, Jetten J, Cruwys T, Bentley SV. Rethinking the nature of the person at the heart of the biopsychosocial model: exploring social changeways not just personal pathways. *Soc Sci Med.* 2021;272:113566. doi:10.1016/j.socscimed.2020.113566
11. Marlatt GA, Baer JS, Donovan DM, Kivlahan DR. Addictive behaviors: etiology and treatment. *Annu Rev Psychol.* 1988;39:223-252. doi:10.1146/annurev.ps.39.020188.001255
12. Grisel J. *Never Enough: Neuroscience and Experience of Addiction.* Scribe; 2019.
13. Oscar-Berman M, Valmas MM, Sawyer KS, Ruiz SM, Luhar RB, Gravitz ZR. Profiles of impaired, spared, and recovered neuropsychologic processes in alcoholism. *Handb Clin Neurol.* 2014;125:183-210. doi:10.1016/B978-0-444-62619-6.00012-4
14. Sullivan EV, Pfefferbaum A. Neurocircuitry in alcoholism: a substrate of disruption and repair. *Psychopharmacology (Berl).* 2005;180(4):583-594. doi:10.1007/s00213-005-2267-6 [doi]

15. Bates ME, Buckman JF, Nguyen TT. A role for cognitive rehabilitation in increasing the effectiveness of treatment for alcohol use disorders. *Neuropsychol Rev.* 2013;23(1):27-47. doi:10.1007/s11065-013-9228-3
16. Stavro K, Pelletier J, Potvin S. Widespread and sustained cognitive deficits in alcoholism: a meta-analysis. *Addict Biol.* 2013;18(2):203-213. doi:10.1111/j.1369-1600.2011.00418.x
17. Fernández-Serrano MJ, Pérez-García M, Perales JC, Verdejo-García A. Prevalence of executive dysfunction in cocaine, heroin and alcohol users enrolled in therapeutic communities. *Eur J Pharmacol.* 2010;626(1):104-112. doi:10.1016/j.ejphar.2009.10.019
18. Gould TJ. Addiction and cognition. *Addict Sci Clin Pract.* 2010;5(2):4-14.
19. Cutuli D, Ladrón de Guevara-Miranda D, Castilla-Ortega E, Santín LJ, Sampedro-Piquero P. Highlighting the role of cognitive and brain reserve in the substance use disorder field. *Curr Neuropharmacol.* 2019;17(11):1056-1070. doi:10.2174/1570159x17666190617100707
20. Buhler M, Mann K. Alcohol and the human brain: a systematic review of different neuroimaging methods. *Alcohol Clin Exp Res.* 2011;35(10):1771-1793. doi:10.1111/j.1530-0277.2011.01540.x
21. Meyerhoff DJ, Durazzo TC, Ende G. Chronic alcohol consumption, abstinence and relapse: brain proton magnetic resonance spectroscopy studies in animals and humans. *Curr Top Behav Neurosci.* 2013;13:511-540. doi:10.1007/7854_2011_131
22. Koob GF, Volkow ND. Neurocircuitry of addiction. *Neuropsychopharmacology.* 2009;35(1):217-238. doi:10.1038/npp2009110
23. Alfonso CA. An overview of the psychodynamics of addiction. *Psychodyn Psychiatry.* 2021;49(3):363-369. doi:10.1521/pdps.2021.49.3.363
24. Schindler A. Attachment and substance use disorders-theoretical models, empirical evidence, and implications for treatment. *Front Psychiatry.* 2019;10:727. doi:10.3389/fpsyt.2019.00727
25. Singh S, Windle SB, Filion KB, et al. E-cigarettes and youth: patterns of use, potential harms, and recommendations. *Prev Med.* 2020;133:106009. doi:10.1016/j.ypmed.2020.106009
26. Johnston LD, O'Malley PM, Miech RA, et al. *Monitoring the Future National Survey Results on Drug Use 1975-2021: Overview, Key Findings on Adolescent Drug Use*. Institute for Social Research, University of Michigan; 2022.
27. Lisdahl KM, Tapert S, Sher KJ, et al. Substance use patterns in 9-10 year olds: baseline findings from the adolescent brain cognitive development (ABCD) study. *Drug Alcohol Depend.* 2021;227:108946. doi:10.1016/j.drugalcdep.2021.108946
28. Casey BJ, Getz S, Galvan A. The adolescent brain. *Dev Rev.* 2008;28(1):62-77. doi:10.1016/j.dr.2007.08.003
29. Gogtay N, Giedd JN, Lusk L, et al. Dynamic mapping of human cortical development during childhood through early adulthood. *Proc Natl Acad Sci U S A.* 2004;101(21):8174-8179.
30. Sullivan EV, Pfefferbaum A, Rohlfing T, Baker FC, Padilla ML, Colrain IM. Developmental change in regional brain structure over 7 months in early adolescence: comparison of approaches for longitudinal atlas-based parcellation. *Neuroimage.* 2011;57(1):214-224. doi:10.1016/j.neuroimage.2011.04.003
31. Casey BJ, Giedd JN, Thomas KM. Structural and functional brain development and its relation to cognitive development. *Biol Psychol.* 2000;54(1-3):241-257.
32. Pfefferbaum A, Mathalon DH, Sullivan EV, Rawles JM, Zipursky RB, Lim KO. A quantitative magnetic resonance imaging study of changes in brain morphology from infancy to late adulthood. *Arch Neurol.* 1994;51(9):874-887.
33. Silveri MM, Sneider JT, Crowley DJ, et al. Frontal lobe gamma-aminobutyric acid levels during adolescence: associations with impulsivity and response inhibition. *Biol Psychiatry.* 2013;74(4):296-304. doi:10.1016/j.biopsych.2013.01.033
34. Coyle JT, Enna SJ. Neurochemical aspects of the ontogenesis of GABAnergic neurons in the rat brain. *Brain Res.* 1976;111(1):119-133. doi:10.1016/0006-8993(76)91053-2
35. Raichle ME, MacLeod AM, Snyder AZ, Powers WJ, Gusnard DA, Shulman GL. A default mode of brain function. *Proc Natl Acad Sci U S A.* 2001;98(2):676-682. doi:10.1073/pnas.98.2.676
36. Stevens MC, Pearlson GD, Calhoun VD. Changes in the interaction of resting-state neural networks from adolescence to adulthood. *Hum Brain Mapp.* 2009;30(8):2356-2366. doi:10.1002/hbm.20673
37. Sutherland MT, McHugh MJ, Pariyadath V, Stein EA. Resting state functional connectivity in addiction: lessons learned and a road ahead. *Neuroimage.* 2012;62(4):2281-2295. doi:10.1016/j.neuroimage.2012.01.117
38. Casey BJ, Galvan A, Hare TA. Changes in cerebral functional organization during cognitive development. *Curr Opin Neurobiol.* 2005;15(2):239-244.
39. Paus T. Mapping brain maturation and cognitive development during adolescence. *Trends Cogn Sci.* 2005;9(2):60-68. doi:10.1016/j.tics.2004.12.008
40. Murty VP, Calabro F, Luna B. The role of experience in adolescent cognitive development: integration of executive, memory, and mesolimbic systems. *Neurosci Biobehav Rev.* 2016;70:46-58. doi:10.1016/j.neubiorev.2016.07.034
41. Silveri MM, Dager AD, Cohen-Gilbert JE, Sneider JT. Neurobiological signatures associated with alcohol and drug use in the human adolescent brain. *Neurosci Biobehav Rev.* 2016;70:244-259. doi:10.1016/j.neubiorev.2016.06.042
42. Oscar-Berman M. Neuropsychological vulnerabilities in chronic alcoholism. In: Noronha A, Eckardt M, Warren K, eds. *Review of NIAAA's Neuroscience and Behavioral Research Portfolio*. National Institutes of Health; 2000:437-472.
43. Oscar-Berman M, Marinkovic K. Alcoholism and the brain: an overview. *Alcohol Res Health.* 2003;27(2):125-133.
44. Squeglia LM, Pulido C, Wetherill RR, Jacobus J, Brown GG, Tapert SF. Brain response to working memory over three years of adolescence: influence of initiating heavy drinking. *J Stud Alcohol Drugs.* 2012;73(5):749-760.
45. Wetherill R, Tapert SF. Adolescent brain development, substance use, and psychotherapeutic change. *Psychol Addict Behav.* 2013;27(2):393-402. doi:10.1037/a0029111
46. Norman AL, Pulido C, Squeglia LM, Spadoni AD, Paulus MP, Tapert SF. Neural activation during inhibition predicts initiation of substance use in adolescence. *Drug Alcohol Depend.* 2011;119(3):216-223. doi:10.1016/j.drugalcdep.2011.06.019
47. Brown SA, Brumback T, Tomlinson K, et al. The National Consortium on Alcohol and NeuroDevelopment in Adolescence (NCANDA): a multisite study of adolescent development and substance use. *J Stud Alcohol Drugs.* 2015;76(6):895-908. doi:10.15288/jsad.2015.76.895
48. Sullivan EV, Brumback T, Tapert SF, et al. Cognitive, emotion control, and motor performance of adolescents in the NCANDA study: contributions from alcohol consumption, age, sex, ethnicity, and family history of addiction. *Neuropsychology.* 2016;30(4):449-473. doi:10.1037/neu0000259
49. Feldstein Ewing SW, Bjork JM, Luciana M. Implications of the ABCD study for developmental neuroscience. *Dev Cogn Neurosci.* 2018;32:161-164. doi:10.1016/j.dcn.2018.05.003
50. Jernigan TL, Brown SA; ABCD Consortium Coordinators. Introduction. *Dev Cogn Neurosci.* 2018;32:1-3. doi:10.1016/j.dcn.2018.02.002
51. Lisdahl KM, Sher KJ, Conway KP, et al. Adolescent brain cognitive development (ABCD) study: overview of substance use assessment methods. *Dev Cogn Neurosci.* 2018;32:80-96. doi:10.1016/j.dcn.2018.02.007
52. Luciana M, Bjork JM, Nagel BJ, et al. Adolescent neurocognitive development and impacts of substance use: overview of the adolescent brain cognitive development (ABCD) baseline neurocognition battery. *Dev Cogn Neurosci.* 2018;32:67-79. doi:10.1016/j.dcn.2018.02.006
53. Volkow ND, Koob GF, Croyle RT, et al. The conception of the ABCD study: from substance use to a broad NIH collaboration. *Dev Cogn Neurosci.* 2018;32:4-7. doi:10.1016/j.dcn.2017.10.002
54. Hammerslag LR, Gulley JM. Sex differences in behavior and neural development and their role in adolescent vulnerability to substance use. *Behav Brain Res.* 2016;298(Pt A):15-26. doi:10.1016/j.bbr.2015.04.008
55. Hardee JE, Cope LM, Munier EC, Welsh RC, Zucker RA, Heitzeg MM. Sex differences in the development of emotion circuitry in adolescents at risk for substance abuse: a longitudinal fMRI study. *Soc Cogn Affect Neurosci.* 2017;12(6):965-975. doi:10.1093/scan/nsx021

56. Heitzeg MM, Hardee JE, Beltz AM. Sex differences in the developmental neuroscience of adolescent substance use risk. *Curr Opin Behav Sci.* 2018;23:21-26. doi:10.1016/j.cobeha.2018.01.020
57. Hickie IB, Scott EM, Cross SP, et al. Right care, first time: a highly personalised and measurement-based care model to manage youth mental health. *Med J Aust.* 2019;211(Suppl 9):S3-S46. doi:10.5694/mja2.50383
58. Lehman BJ, David DM, Gruber JA. Rethinking the biopsychosocial model of health: understanding health as a dynamic system. *Soc Personal Psychol Compass.* 2017;11(8):e12328. https://doi.org/10.1111/spc3.12328
59. Byregowda H, Flynn AL, Knight JR, Harris SK. Perceived risk of harm mediates the effects of primary care alcohol use screening and brief advice in adolescents. *J Adolesc Health.* 2022;70(3):442-449. doi:10.1016/j.jadohealth.2021.09.029
60. Harris SK, Csémy L, Sherritt L, et al. Computer-facilitated substance use screening and brief advice for teens in primary care: an international trial. *Pediatrics.* 2012;129(6):1072-1082. doi:10.1542/peds.2011-1624
61. Knight JR, Kuzubova K, Csemy L, Sherritt L, Copelas S, Harris SK. Computer-facilitated screening and brief advice to reduce adolescents' heavy episodic drinking: a study in two countries. *J Adolesc Health.* 2018;62(1):118-120. doi:10.1016/j.jadohealth.2017.08.013
62. Knight JR, Sherritt L, Gibson EB, et al. Effect of computer-based substance use screening and brief behavioral counseling vs usual care for youths in pediatric primary care: a pilot randomized clinical trial. *JAMA Netw Open.* 2019;2(6):e196258. doi:10.1001/jamanetworkopen.2019.6258
63. Chambers RA, Taylor JR, Potenza MN. Developmental neurocircuitry of motivation in adolescence: a critical period of addiction vulnerability. *Am J Psychiatry.* 2003;160(6):1041-1052.
64. Rutherford HJ, Mayes LC, Potenza MN. Neurobiology of adolescent substance use disorders: implications for prevention and treatment. *Child Adolesc Psychiatr Clin N Am.* 2010;19(3):479-492. doi:10.1016/j.chc.2010.03.003
65. Feldstein Ewing SW, Tapert SF, Molina BS. Uniting adolescent neuroimaging and treatment research: recommendations in pursuit of improved integration. *Neurosci Biobehav Rev.* 2015;62:109-114. doi:10.1016/j.neubiorev.2015.12.011

Sidebar 2

Governmental Policy on Cannabis Legalization and Use: Impact on Youth

Ziming Xuan, Lynsie Ranker, and Sion Kim Harris

The past few decades have seen the general liberalization of cannabis laws both within the United States (U.S.) and abroad. While in the U.S. cannabis remains illegal at the federal level (considered a Schedule 1 substance), states have moved toward decriminalization as well as legalization either for "medical" or recreational use (for individuals 21 or older). As of mid-2023, 38 states, plus the District of Columbia (DC), as well as several U.S. territories have passed medical cannabis (hereafter more accurately termed cannabis used as treatment) laws (CUATL).[1] A growing number of states have enacted recreational cannabis laws (RCL), moving from eight states in 2016 to 23 states (plus DC and Guam) as of mid-2023.[1] This is in addition to other regulatory transitions including decriminalization (laws providing protection against arrest or conviction for personal use and/or possession) of cannabis. Nearly all states have implemented some more liberal form of cannabis legislation; a few states legalized only the use/sale of high cannabidiol/low delta-9-tetrahydrocannabinol (THC) products.[1] Globally, other countries have similarly moved toward legalization and/or decriminalization. Uruguay and Canada were the first two countries to nationally legalize the sale and consumption of recreational cannabis. Along with policy shifts have come increased public support for legalization.[2]

The general trend toward legalization has continued the debate surrounding the safety and health effects of cannabis use. There is some evidence of medicinal benefits of cannabinoids, including neuropathic pain relief, sleep, and management of chronic spasticity.[3] However, effects have overall been deemed as modest, particularly when weighed against the risks associated with acute or chronic use such as motor vehicle-related injury/death, adverse mental health outcomes, poor respiratory function, cardiovascular disease, and cannabis use disorder/addiction.[4] Further information on risks and therapeutic potential of cannabis, as well as legal and ethical issues relevant to the clinician considering recommending cannabis to a patient are each covered in section 15 of this textbook. Health-related consequences may be particularly relevant among adolescents, a vulnerable population still undergoing physical, mental, and social development.

Early initiation of cannabis use in adolescents is linked with increased use frequency and cannabis use disorder (CUD).[5] Among youth who use cannabis, 17% may go on to develop CUD. Initiating use of cannabis by age 16 has been associated with a nearly threefold increase in risk of CUD.[6] Moderate evidence links cannabis use with uptake of other substances,[7] although studies have also suggested cannabis may be a substitute rather than a compliment to other substance use.[5] Cannabis use has also been associated with increased risk of adverse mental health outcomes including psychosis, depression, anxiety, and suicidality.[5,8,9] A meta-analysis of 11 studies found cannabis use in adolescence was associated with depression and suicidal ideation and attempts in young adulthood.[9] However, assessing causality is challenging due to temporality concern where individuals with pre-existing subclinical mental health issues may self-medicate with cannabis. In addition, the mental and behavioral health effects (ie, psychosis, substance use disorder) may depend on the potency and amount consumed, information not always collected in studies.

An additional concern regarding youth is the effect of cannabis use on brain development and cognition during a sensitive neurodevelopmental period.[10] Studies suggest that even low levels of cannabis use in early adolescence may affect brain structure and function (compared to those with no use),[11] which could impact reasoning, attention, concentration, decision-making, working memory, and anxiety/stress.[9,11] Effects on executive functioning, learning, and memory are exacerbated by frequency of use and age of initiation.[12,13] In addition, there is strong evidence that cannabis use in adolescence negatively impacts academic success and educational attainment.[14,15]

Based on a social ecological framework,[16] it is important to consider how macrosystem-level factors such as cannabis policies shape social changes that may influence cannabis use among youth. As the U.S. and other countries are moving toward legalization, cannabis use may become more socially acceptable and accessible to youth. Understanding the impacts of cannabis policies on youth is therefore a public health priority. Below we outline the current state of evidence on cannabis policies and adolescent health.

EVIDENCE OF LEGALIZATION IMPACTS ON YOUTH

Cannabis is one of the most popular drugs among youth. In 2019, 22% of U.S. high school students reported using cannabis in the past 30 days, an increase from 20% in 2017.[17] This is in contrast to consistent declines in youth alcohol use.[18] One 2019 survey of online panels of Canadian, U.S., and English youth, found that past-year, past 30-day and daily cannabis use were higher in the U.S. and Canada (both countries with more liberalized cannabis laws).[19] Roughly 4% of adolescents in the U.S. and Canada report daily use.[19] Some studies have also documented increased frequency of cannabis use among adolescents[20] and shifts in patterns of use toward higher potency products.[19,21] A longitudinal analysis among high school youth in Canada found no significant changes on cannabis use following the Cannabis Act legalizing recreational cannabis use for adults effective in October 2018, although repeated cross-sectional analysis on a larger youth sample in the same study found a small increase in use after legalization.[22] Data from 20 European countries based on the European School Survey Project on Alcohol and Other Drugs (ESPAD) showed restrictive policies reduced the prevalence of cannabis use, and more liberal policy changes were associated with increases in the proportion of students initiating cannabis use, although no evidence was found with frequent use.[23]

Because there have been rapid changes in U.S. cannabis policies in the past two decades, resulting in considerable heterogeneity across states, there has been a growing body of research aimed at understanding the impacts on youth health attributable to cannabis policy changes. Both CUATL and RCL may influence perceived harms of cannabis use by youth and impact youth access (cost, avenues for obtaining) as well as use patterns among youth. Evidence to date from studies of CUATL and RCL on adolescents show mixed findings. Difference-in-differences analysis of 2009 to 2019 Youth Risk Behavior Surveillance System (YRBS) survey data found RML was associated with higher lifetime and current use among adolescents in Alaska, which enacted RML, as compared to Hawaii, which did not enact RML.[24] However, analysis of weighted national and all available state YRBS data from 1993 to 2019 found no significant association between enactment of RCLs or CUATLs and cannabis use.[25] Sarvet et al.[26] conducted a meta-analysis on 11 studies on CUATL and found no significant change in past-month adolescent cannabis use,[26] and another review found consistent negative or insignificant associations among those under 21 years old across early CUATL studies.[27]

On the other hand, a recent study of 7th, 9th, and 11th grade students in California found RCL implementation was associated with increased likelihood of lifetime and past-30-day cannabis use, with the degree of association varying by age, gender, and race/ethnicity.[28] Another study found that RCL in Washington state led to decreases in perceived harm and increased use in adolescents, but found no effects for Colorado legalization.[29] A 2016 study using the Monitoring the Future Survey (a national survey of U.S. youth), found 8th graders attending schools less than five miles from a CUAT dispensary were more likely to report recent cannabis use.[30] A retrospective cohort study of adolescent (11-17 years) hospitalizations at children's hospitals between 2008 and 2019 found increased cannabis-related hospitalization in CUATL states and RCL states.[31] Melchior et al.[32] conducted a systematic review and meta-analysis and found no significant change of youth cannabis use related to CUATL and decriminalization, but detected small increases in youth cannabis consumption related to RCL.[32] Increases in youth past-month cannabis use in response to RCL, especially for young women and for people who binge drank, were also summarized in a narrative review of 32 studies.[33] Thus far, RCL evaluations in the U.S. have focused on early adopting states (Oregon, Colorado, and Washington) with fairly robust CUAT dispensary systems prior to recreational legalization.[27]

While effects of legalization are equivocal for adolescents, studies show a clear pattern of increased use among adults, including among young adults aged 19 to 22.[34] For adults, CUATL enactment led to increased prevalence of use, with the stringency of provisions potentially affecting uptake.[27] Specifically, studies that examined specific CUATL provisions found use may be higher when CUATLs are less stringent (eg, retail dispensaries, broader definitions of pain to quality).[35-37] There is some evidence that states with CUATL have higher CUD prevalence among adults[35,37]; however, the results are mixed and evidence on how CUATLs are connected to CUD and CUD-related treatment and hospitalizations remains limited.

HIGH POTENCY CANNABIS USE

Although U.S. studies to date may show little effect of cannabis legalization on overall use prevalence among adolescents, studies show recent changes in their use patterns (types and content), including increases in frequency of use[20,38] and use preference shifts toward use of higher potency cannabis products through vaping and edibles.[19,39] Legalization status has been associated with proliferation of types and methods of consumption.[27] Specifically, adolescents in more liberalized states (versus other states) are more likely to report lifetime vaping and edible cannabis use, and use of cannabis concentrates, particularly in areas with higher dispensary density.[40-42] Also, studies have found increases in THC levels in cannabis products within states upon CUAT and recreational legalization.[21] Increased use of high THC potency cannabis products is concerning. Studies suggest that THC sensitivity may vary by age, with adolescents experiencing more acute behavioral and cognitive effects, such as psychotic symptoms, anxiety, depression and suicidality, compared to adults.[43,44] Concentrates may have THC concentrations of 70% or higher.[45]

OTHER SUBSTANCE USE AND HARMS

Associations between cannabis legalization and alcohol use, alcohol-related outcomes, and the co-use of cannabis and alcohol are thus far inconclusive, with studies finding decreases in alcohol use associated with cannabis policy liberalization yet showing no policy impact on cannabis use itself.[46] Similarly mixed results and debates continue related to opioid use.[27] An earlier study found that, from 1999 to 2010, states with CUATL experienced slower increase in opioid overdose mortality.[47] A more recent study using the same approach extending through 2017 found no support of reduced mortality over the longer period, either with CUATL or RCL states.[48] For tobacco, there is some evidence that legalization decreases tobacco use or has limited impacts on tobacco use.[49,50] However, the majority of studies have focused specifically on combustible cigarettes,[27] failing to address the rise in popularity of e-cigarettes and other electronic nicotine devices among adolescents during these time periods.[51] Analyses of the first four waves (2013-2018) of the Population Assessment of Tobacco and Health Study found that among adolescents who were cannabis naive at baseline, past-30-day e-cigarette use at baseline was associated with past-30-day cannabis use at 12-month follow-up, and this association is stronger among those living in states that legalized adult recreational cannabis use.[52]

Analysis of claims data from 2003 to 2017 found that the rate of self-harm injury for young males under 21 years old were associated with recreational cannabis states, and RCLs permitting dispensaries and lacking dose-related restrictions were associated with significant increases in assault for males and females younger than 21 years.[53] Recreational legalization has also been associated with increases in the proportion of drivers involved in fatal crashes testing positive for THC (19.1% compared to 9.3% prior to implantation) and that THC concentrations recorded also increased.[54]

LIMITATIONS OF CURRENT EVIDENCE

Changes in cannabis-related perceptions and behaviors among youth have coincided with cannabis regulatory shifts. Yet, the limitations of current CUATL/RCL evaluations must be considered. As Smart and Pacula note, the majority of evidence of effects on adolescents come from only three different datasets (Monitoring the Future, Youth Risk Behavior Survey, National Survey of Drug Use and Health) across similar time frames.[27] Moreover, the causal connection between policy change and adolescent use is challenging to tease out. Often states that adopt CUATL or RCL have higher prevalence of use and lower risk perceptions among youth prior to policy adoption (an example of reverse causation).[55] For example, outlet density can affect consumption, yet it is also possible that demand at the local level can influence supply and affect dispensary location, density, and related retail activities, which are all subject to cannabis policies.

In addition to the limitation due to potential reverse causation, most cannabis policy studies, for example, those conducted in the U.S., have thus far focused on the impact of single and broader classification of states based on legalization status (eg, decriminalized, CUATL or RCL) without attention to heterogeneity of discrete policies within the single legalization category. Current cannabis policy taxonomy, taking recreational cannabis policies as an example, covers an extensive collection of policies including taxation, pricing restriction, retail restriction, underage prohibition, advertising restrictions, home delivery, impaired driving, product types, cultivation restriction, and so on.[56] A convenient indicator-based approach based on legalization status masks important nuance of how a given state regulates cannabis production, distribution, sales, and consumption. Because states derive revenue and sustain harm from legalizing cannabis use, this simple approach also fails to assess the role of the overall state policy control environment on youth use and related outcomes at both individual and population levels.

Other limitations of the current cannabis policy literature include reliance on repeated cross-sectional analyses on only a few different datasets, lack of in-depth outcome measures of cannabis use patterns and longitudinal outcomes and related use trajectories, and short postlegalization period that may not allow outcomes to develop and manifest. These limitations, as a whole, could contribute to these mixed findings.

FUTURE RESEARCH DIRECTIONS

As the wave of cannabis liberalization continues and cannabis policies evolve across states, it is critical to comprehensively characterize the cannabis policy control environment and assess the impact of the aggregate policy environment on cannabis use and related health outcomes among youth. Research on youth alcohol use shares similar characteristics and challenges and may serve as a helpful example of future research priorities. Alcohol is one of the most commonly used drugs among youth, and alcohol policies are mostly implemented at the state level. Prior work has demonstrated that a more stringent state alcohol policy environment (as assessed via a combined measures of multiple alcohol policies) was associated with lower youth alcohol use and binge drinking, and that adult consumption mediated policy–youth consumption association.[57] In addition to studying the overall control environment, it is important to evaluate key policy changes influencing youth consumption—especially those that affect economic affordability (eg, taxation and pricing strategies), physical availability (eg, dispensary density, retail restrictions on days and hours of sale, state monopoly, types of products sold), and perceived acceptability (eg, advertising and marketing). More systematic policy panel data collection and methodologies for characterizing cannabis policy environment are needed to enhance research rigor. In addition, rigorous quasi-experimental study designs (eg, interrupted time series design, regression discontinuity design) can be used to evaluate policy change in local contexts to assess the impact of policy change on youth health outcomes.

Nationally representative longitudinal cohort data on youth with detailed outcome data on patterns of use, product types, concurrent use with other substances, mental health, and other risky behaviors (including harms to others) should be collected to understand how policies shape the developmental and behavioral trajectories related to the use of cannabis. It is also important to build nationwide and state-specific surveillance systems to monitor product types, potency levels, and dispensary locations, and for these systems to integrate geographical, socioeconomic, and school-district indicators. Because substance co-use or poly-use is common among youth, researchers must exert effort to study the interactions of substance-specific policies on youth concurrent use of multiple substances. This is particularly relevant given the decline of alcohol and tobacco use among youth and uptrends of e-cigarette use among adolescents and cannabis use among young adults.

As improved tools are developed to facilitate the measurement of THC level, it is critical to evaluate the role of per se limits or zero tolerance policies in reducing cannabis-related driving injuries and death involving youth. Policy evaluations can learn from the alcohol literature where a myriad of strategies have been evaluated including population-wide policies (eg, higher price, minimum legal drinking age), context-specific enforcement (eg, sobriety check point, ignition interlock), restricted transportation (eg, graduated driver license), and administrative and financial incentive (eg, raising minimum legal drinking age as a condition of receiving highway funds[58]).

Because cannabis remains a Schedule 1 substance, direct advertising for cannabis on most major social media venues is banned. However, cannabis businesses in RCL states may establish social media profiles to represent their brands and attract followers to promote user engagement. Online surveys of adolescents age 15 to 19 years from four RCL states found exposure to cannabis advertising and marketing through social media was associated with past-year cannabis use.[59] This adds to earlier literature examining trajectories of past-three-months exposure to CUAT ads within a longitudinal youth cohort in California, which found increased intentions and use over 7 years.[60] Given nearly all teens use some form of social media, and exposure to cannabis advertising and promotion on social media is conducive to engagement, research is urgently needed to evaluate potential strategies of regulating cannabis advertising and marketing on social media.

Experiences of structural racism, poverty, criminalization, discrimination, and stigma as well as other forms of social inequality are related to heightened levels of psychological distress in certain vulnerable subpopulations. The responses to cope with these psychosocial stressors through substance use may contribute to substantial variation in cannabis use patterns and related harms. Disparities also exist in how groups based on these vulnerability characteristics respond to various socio-ecological factors including social media platforms, availability of cannabis product types, and state cannabis policies. Because states gain revenue from legalizing cannabis, it is imperative for state policymakers to ensure that youth subpopulations, especially marginalized minority groups, are not harmed disproportionately as cannabis is becoming more accessible by youth. Future research must incorporate issues of equity into the policy literature.

As legalization and new policies around cannabis continue to evolve, it will be critical for researchers to continue to ascertain the effect of these changes on youth health and development. Public health practitioners will need to seek new data sources, methods, and critically evaluate current literature to inform policy and intervention responses in this rapidly changing cannabis landscape.

REFERENCES

1. Hartman M. *Cannabis Overview.* National Conference of State Legislators. Accessed November 3, 2023. https://www.ncsl.org/research/civil-and-criminal-justice/marijuana-overview.aspx#1
2. Schaeffer K. *7 Facts About Americans and Marijuana.* Pew Research Center. Accessed August 5, 2022. https://www.pewresearch.org/fact-tank/2021/04/26/facts-about-marijuana/
3. Whiting PF, Wolff RF, Deshpande S, et al. Cannabinoids for medical use: a systematic review and meta-analysis. *JAMA.* 2015;313(24):2456-2473. doi:10.1001/jama.2015.6358
4. Hall W, Degenhardt L. Adverse health effects of non-medical cannabis use. *Lancet.* 2009;374(9698):1383-1391. doi:10.1016/S0140-6736(09)61037-0
5. National Academies of Sciences Engineering and Medicine. *The Health Effects of Cannabis and Cannabinoids.* Vol. 15(2). The National Academies Press; 2017:88-92. doi:10.17226/24625

6. Swift W, Coffey C, Carlin JB, Degenhardt L, Patton GC. Adolescent cannabis users at 24 years: trajectories to regular weekly use and dependence in young adulthood. *Addiction.* 2008;103(8):1361-1370. doi:10.1111/J.1360-0443.2008.02246.X
7. Osibogun O, Erinoso O, Gautam P, Bursac Z, Osibogun A. Marijuana use modifies the association between heavy alcohol consumption and tobacco use patterns among U.S. adults: findings from Behavioral Risk Factor Surveillance System, 2020. *Addict Behav.* 2022;135:107435. doi:10.1016/j.addbeh.2022.107435
8. Agrawal A, Nelson EC, Bucholz KK, et al. Major depressive disorder, suicidal thoughts and behaviours, and cannabis involvement in discordant twins: a retrospective cohort study. *Lancet Psychiatry.* 2017;4(9):706-714. doi:10.1016/S2215-0366(17)30280-8
9. Gobbi G, Atkin T, Zytynski T, et al. Association of cannabis use in adolescence and risk of depression, anxiety, and suicidality in young adulthood: a systematic review and meta-analysis. *JAMA Psychiatry.* 2019;76(4):426-434. doi:10.1001/jamapsychiatry.2018.4500
10. Ladegard K, Thurstone C, Rylander M. Marijuana legalization and youth. *Pediatrics.* 2020;145(Suppl 2):S165-S174. doi:10.1542/PEDS.2019-2056D
11. Orr C, Spechler P, Cao Z, et al. Grey matter volume differences associated with extremely low levels of cannabis use in adolescence. *J Neurosci.* 2019;39(10):1817-1827. doi:10.1523/JNEUROSCI.3375-17.2018
12. Castellanos-Ryan N, Pingault JB, Parent S, Vitaro F, Tremblay RE, Séguin JR. Adolescent cannabis use, change in neurocognitive function, and high-school graduation: a longitudinal study from early adolescence to young adulthood. *Dev Psychopathol.* 2017;29(4):1253-1266. doi:10.1017/S0954579416001280
13. Scott JC, Slomiak ST, Jones JD, Rosen AFG, Moore TM, Gur RC. Association of cannabis with cognitive functioning in adolescents and young adults: a systematic review and meta-analysis. *JAMA Psychiatry.* 2018;75(6):585-595. doi:10.1001/jamapsychiatry.2018.0335
14. Silins E, Fergusson DM, Patton GC, et al. Adolescent substance use and educational attainment: an integrative data analysis comparing cannabis and alcohol from three Australasian cohorts. *Drug Alcohol Depend.* 2015;156:90-96. doi:10.1016/j.drugalcdep.2015.08.034
15. D'Amico EJ, Tucker JS, Miles JNV, Ewing BA, Shih RA, Pedersen ER. Alcohol and marijuana use trajectories in a diverse longitudinal sample of adolescents: examining use patterns from age 11 to 17 years. *Addiction.* 2016;111(10):1825-1835. doi:10.1111/ADD.13442
16. Bronfenbrenner U. *The Ecology of Human Development: Experiments by Nature and Design.* Harvard University Press; 1979.
17. Jones CM, Clayton HB, Deputy NP, et al. Prescription opioid misuse and use of alcohol and other substances among high school students—Youth Risk Behavior Survey, United States, 2019. *MMWR Suppl.* 2020;69(1):38-46. doi:10.15585/MMWR.SU6901A5
18. Slade T, Chapman C, Swift W, Keyes K, Tonks Z, Teesson M. Birth cohort trends in the global epidemiology of alcohol use and alcohol-related harms in men and women: systematic review and metaregression. *BMJ Open.* 2016;6(10):e011827. doi:10.1136/BMJOPEN-2016-011827
19. Hammond D, Wadsworth E, Reid JL, Burkhalter R. Prevalence and modes of cannabis use among youth in Canada, England, and the U.S., 2017 to 2019. *Drug Alcohol Depend.* 2021(219):108505. doi:10.1016/j.drugalcdep.2020.108505
20. Keyes KM, Kreski NT, Ankrum H, et al. Frequency of adolescent cannabis smoking and vaping in the United States: trends, disparities and concurrent substance use, 2017-19. *Addiction.* 2022;117(8):2316-2324. doi:10.1111/add.15912
21. Sevigny EL, Pacula RL, Heaton P. The effects of medical marijuana laws on potency. *The Int J Drug Policy.* 2014;25(2):308-319. doi:10.1016/J.drugpo.2014.01.003
22. Zuckermann AME, Battista KV, Bélanger RE, et al. Trends in youth cannabis use across cannabis legalization: data from the COMPASS prospective cohort study. *Prev Med Rep.* 2021;22:101351. doi:10.1016/j.pmedr.2021.101351
23. Benedetti E, Resce G, Brunori P, Molinaro S. Cannabis policy changes and adolescent cannabis use: evidence from Europe. *Int J Environ Res Public Health.* 2021;18(10). doi:10.3390/ijerph18105174
24. Lee MH, Kim-Godwin YS, Hur H. Adolescents' marijuana use following recreational marijuana legalization in Alaska and Hawaii. *Asia Pac J Public Health.* 2022;34(1):65-71. doi:10.1177/10105395211044917
25. Anderson DM, Rees DI, Sabia JJ, Safford S. Association of marijuana legalization with marijuana use among U.S. high school students, 1993-2019. *JAMA Netw Open.* 2021;4(9):e2124638. doi:10.1001/jamanetworkopen.2021.24638
26. Sarvet AL, Wall MM, Fink DS, et al. Medical marijuana laws and adolescent marijuana use in the United States: a systematic review and meta-analysis. *Addiction.* 2018;113(6):1003-1016. doi:10.1111/ADD.14136
27. Smart R, Pacula RL. Early evidence of the impact of cannabis legalization on cannabis use, cannabis use disorder, and the use of other substances: findings from state policy evaluations. *Am J Drug Alcohol Abuse.* 2019;45(6):644-663. doi:10.1080/00952990.2019.1669626
28. Paschall MJ, García-Ramírez G, Grube JW. Recreational marijuana legalization and use among California adolescents: findings from a statewide survey. *J Stud Alcohol Drugs.* 2021;82(1):103-111. doi:10.15288/jsad.2021.82.103
29. Cerdá M, Wall M, Feng T, et al. Association of state recreational marijuana laws with adolescent marijuana use. *JAMA Pediatr.* 2017;171(2):142-149. doi:10.1001/jamapediatrics.2016.3624
30. Shi Y. The availability of medical marijuana dispensary and adolescent marijuana use. *Prev Med.* 2016;91:1-7. doi:10.1016/j.ypmed.2016.07.015
31. Masonbrink AR, Richardson T, Hall M, Catley D, Wilson K. Trends in adolescent cannabis-related hospitalizations by state legalization laws, 2008-2019. *J Adolesc Health.* 2021;69(6):999-1005. doi:10.1016/j.jadohealth.2021.07.028
32. Melchior M, Nakamura A, Bolze C, et al. Does liberalisation of cannabis policy influence levels of use in adolescents and young adults? A systematic review and meta-analysis. *BMJ Open.* 2019;9(7):e025880. doi:10.1136/bmjopen-2018-025880
33. Lachance A, Bélanger RE, Riva M, Ross NA. A systematic review and narrative synthesis of the evolution of adolescent and young adult cannabis consumption before and after legalization. *J Adolesc Health.* 2022;70(6):848-863. doi:10.1016/j.jadohealth.2021.11.034
34. Patrick ME, Schulenberg JE, Miech RA, Johnston LD, O'Malley PM, Bachman JG. *Monitoring the Future Panel Study Annual Report: National Data on Substance Use Among Adults Ages 19 to 60, 1976-2021.* Monitoring the Future Monograph Series. University of Michigan Institute for Social Research. doi:10.7826/ISR-UM.06.585140.002.07.0001.2022
35. Williams AR, Santaella-Tenorio J, Mauro CM, Levin FR, Martins SS. Loose regulation of medical marijuana programs associated with higher rates of adult marijuana use but not cannabis use disorder. *Addiction.* 2017;112(11):1985-1991. doi:10.1111/add.13904
36. Wen H, Hockenberry JM, Cummings JR. The effect of medical marijuana laws on adolescent and adult use of marijuana, alcohol, and other substances. *J Health Econ.* 2015;42:64-80. doi:10.1016/j.jhealeco.2015.03.007
37. Hasin DS, Sarvet AL, Cerdá M, et al. US adult illicit cannabis use, cannabis use disorder, and medical marijuana laws: 1991-1992 to 2012-2013. *JAMA Psychiatry.* 2017;74(6):579-588. doi:10.1001/jamapsychiatry.2017.0724
38. Palamar JJ, Le A, Han BH. Quarterly trends in past-month cannabis use in the United States, 2015-2019. *Drug Alcohol Depend.* 2021;219:108494. doi:10.1016/j.drugalcdep.2020.108494
39. Lim CCW, Sun T, Leung J, et al. Prevalence of adolescent cannabis vaping: a systematic review and meta-analysis of US and Canadian studies. *JAMA Pediatr.* 2022;176(1):42-51. doi:10.1001/jamapediatrics.2021.4102
40. Borodovsky JT, Crosier BS, Lee DC, Sargent JD, Budney AJ. Smoking, vaping, eating: is legalization impacting the way people use cannabis? *Int J Drug Policy.* 2016;36:141-147. doi:10.1016/j.drugpo.2016.02.022
41. Borodovsky JT, Lee DC, Crosier BS, Gabrielli JL, Sargent JD, Budney AJ. U.S. cannabis legalization and use of vaping and edible products among youth. *Drug Alcohol Depend.* 2017;177:299-306. doi:10.1016/j.drugalcdep.2017.02.017
42. Daniulaityte R, Zatreh MY, Lamy FR, et al. A Twitter-based survey on marijuana concentrate use. *Drug Alcohol Depend.* 2018;187:155-159. doi:10.1016/j.drugalcdep.2018.02.033

43. Murray CH, Huang Z, Lee R, de Wit H. Adolescents are more sensitive than adults to acute behavioral and cognitive effects of THC. *Neuropsychopharmacology.* 2022;47(7):1331-1338. doi:10.1038/s41386-022-01281-w
44. Vargas G, Shrier LA, Chadi N, Harris SK. High potency cannabis use in adolescence. *J Pediatr.* 2023;252:191-197. doi:10.1016/j.jpeds.2022.07.034
45. Stuyt E. The problem with the current high potency THC marijuana from the perspective of an addiction psychiatrist. *Mo Med.* 2018;115(6): 482-486.
46. Pacula RL, Smart R, Lira MC, Pessar SC, Blanchette JG, Naimi TS. Relationships of cannabis policy liberalization with alcohol use and co-use with cannabis: a narrative review. *Alcohol Res.* 2022;42(1):06. doi:10.35946/arcr.V42.1.06
47. Bachhuber MA, Saloner B, Cunningham CO, Barry CL. Medical cannabis laws and opioid analgesic overdose mortality in the United States, 1999-2010. *JAMA Intern Med.* 2014;174(10):1668-1673. doi:10.1001/jamainternmed.2014.4005
48. Shover CL, Davis CS, Gordon SC, Humphreys K. Association between medical cannabis laws and opioid overdose mortality has reversed over time. *Proc Natl Acad Sci U S A.* 2019;116(26):12624-12626. doi:10.1073/pnas.1903434116
49. Kerr DCR, Bae H, Phibbs S, Kern AC. Changes in undergraduates' marijuana, heavy alcohol and cigarette use following legalization of recreational marijuana use in Oregon. *Addiction.* 2017;112(11):1992-2001. doi:10.1111/add.13906
50. Choi A, Dave D, Sabia JJ. Smoke gets in your eyes: medical marijuana laws and tobacco cigarette use. *Am J Health Econ.* 2019;5(3):303-333. doi:10.1162/AJHE_A_00121
51. Miech R, Leventhal A, Johnston L, O'Malley PM, Patrick ME, Barrington-Trimis J. Trends in use and perceptions of nicotine vaping among US youth from 2017 to 2020. *JAMA Pediatr.* 2021;175(2):185-190. doi:10.1001/jamapediatrics.2020.5667
52. Duan Z, Wang Y, Weaver SR, et al. Effect modification of legalizing recreational cannabis use on the association between e-cigarette use and future cannabis use among US adolescents. *Drug Alcohol Depend.* 2022;233:109260. doi:10.1016/j.drugalcdep.2021.109260
53. Matthay EC, Kiang MV, Elser H, Schmidt L, Humphreys K. Evaluation of state cannabis laws and rates of self-harm and assault. *JAMA Network Open.* 2021;4(3):e211955. doi:10.1001/jamanetworkopen.2021.1955
54. Tefft BC, Arnold LS. Estimating cannabis involvement in fatal crashes in Washington state before and after the legalization of recreational cannabis consumption using multiple imputation of missing values. *Am J Epidemiol.* 2021;190(12):2582-2591. doi:10.1093/AJE/KWAB184
55. Wall MM, Poh E, Cerdá M, Keyes KM, Galea S, Hasin DS. Adolescent marijuana use from 2002 to 2008: higher in states with medical marijuana laws, cause still unclear. *Ann Epidemiol.* 2011;21(9):714-716. doi:10.1016/j.annepidem.2011.06.001
56. Klitzner MD, Thomas S, Schuler J, Hilton M, Mosher J. The new cannabis policy taxonomy on APIS: making sense of the cannabis policy universe. *J Prim Prev.* 2017;38(3):295-314. doi:10.1007/S10935-017-0475-6
57. Xuan Z, Blanchette JG, Nelson TF, et al. Youth drinking in the United States: relationships with alcohol policies and adult drinking. *Pediatrics.* 2015;136(1):18-27. doi:10.1542/peds.2015-0537
58. King R. The politics of denial: the use of funding penalties as an implementation device for social policy. *Policy Sci.* 1987;20(4):307-337. doi:10.1007/BF00135869
59. Whitehill JM, Trangenstein PJ, Jenkins MC, Jernigan DH, Moreno MA. Exposure to cannabis marketing in social and traditional media and past-year use among adolescents in states with legal retail cannabis. *J Adolesc Health.* 2020;66(2):247-254. doi:10.1016/j.jadohealth.2019.08.024
60. D'Amico EJ, Rodriguez A, Tucker JS, Pedersen ER, Shih RA. Planting the seed for marijuana use: changes in exposure to medical marijuana advertising and subsequent adolescent marijuana use, cognitions, and consequences over seven years. *Drug Alcohol Depend.* 2018;188:385-391. doi:10.1016/j.drugalcdep.2018.03.031

CHAPTER

117 Assessing Adolescent Substance Use

Ken C. Winters, Randy Stinchfield, and Shelby Franklin

CHAPTER OUTLINE

- Introduction
- Principles of assessment
- Developmental considerations
- Validity of self-report
- Course of substance use disorders
- Instrumentation
- Key points

INTRODUCTION

Adolescent onset of alcohol and other drug use (heretofore, referred to as "substance use") greatly increases the estimated risk for developing a substance use disorder (SUD) and can lead to a variety of other negative consequences, including school failure, risky sexual behavior, delinquency, incarceration, suicidality, motor vehicle injuries/fatalities, possible damage to the brain's memory region, and significant medical healthcare costs.[1] Precise assessment of adolescent substance use is essential to gain an accurate understanding of the nature and extent of substance use by adolescents and to inform possible treatment needs.

PRINCIPLES OF ASSESSMENT

Screening is the first step in identifying whether a youth may be involved in substance use. Screening results inform the clinician response, including prevention messages for youth who have not yet started substance use and determining the need for a more comprehensive assessment for those reporting use. The comprehensive assessment is used to explore the extent and nature of substance involvement and consequential problems, and to guide treatment decisions. Despite a lack of national standards from licensing and accreditation organizations, it is recommended that adolescent substance treatment facilities routinely use at least one adolescent-specific and psychometrically sound assessment instrument as part of intake and treatment planning.[2,3]

Comprehensive Assessment

If an adolescent's presenting problem, history or collateral history suggests a serious substance use problem, comprehensive assessment is indicated. This process seeks to determine the details regarding substance use history (eg, age of onset; recent and history of the type, frequency, and variety of substances used), consequences, psychosocial risk and protective factors (eg, peer affiliation, home life), situations and contexts in which substance use is common (eg, "Do you use when you are down in the dumps?"), whether criteria is met for a SUD, problem recognition and readiness for treatment, and symptoms of other behavioral and mental co-occurring problems. Ideally, assessment should combine self-administered questionnaires that have been validated for use with adolescents with an interview.

DEVELOPMENTAL CONSIDERATIONS

Identifying Clinical Significance

Most often, adolescent substance use involves alcohol, tobacco/nicotine, cannabis, or a combination of these. The majority of youth who use substances will not develop a substance use disorder, though early initiation during the teenage years is associated with a significantly elevated risk of developing a SUD later in life.[1] Also, the likelihood of having a SUD during adulthood is significantly elevated if adolescent use is associated with the presence of several SUD symptoms.[4] The brain, particularly the prefrontal cortex region, undergoes significant development during adolescence and is not fully mature until early adulthood.[5] The developing adolescent brain is more vulnerable to harms from substance use, including addiction, cognitive impairment and mental health disorders, compared to a fully mature brain.[4,6]

Substance Use Disorder Criteria

In the *Diagnostic and Statistical Manual* 5th edition (DSM-5) substance use disorders[7] are modified by three severity levels (mild [2-3 symptoms], moderate [4-5 symptoms], severe [6 or more symptoms]), indicating that the disorder exists as a spectrum. Certain criteria are difficult to interpret in adolescents. For example, the two physiological symptoms, tolerance and withdrawal, may not be as prevalent in young people who are (1) going through physical and neurodevelopmental changes, (2) and not yet chronic users of substances. At the same time, some criteria such as craving and withdrawal may not be clearly understood by adolescents who are relatively inexperienced with the effects of substances, and may lead to higher rates of false-positive endorsements.[8] Despite these limitations, the DSM-5 is used to diagnose SUD in adolescents similarly to adults.

VALIDITY OF SELF-REPORT

Self-report is a hallmark of clinical assessment, given its convenience, comprehensiveness, low cost, and because the individual is the most knowledgeable reporter. Self-report formats include self-administered questionnaire (often via an electronic format) (SAQ), interview, timeline follow-back (TLFB), and computer-assisted interview (CAI). SAQs and interviews are the primary approaches used by clinicians. Research on the concordance of SAQ, interview, TLFB, and CAI formats suggests that, for the most part, the various formats yield similar levels of disclosure.[2]

Though commonly used, the overall validity and reliability of the self-report method for assessing adolescent substance use and related problems are still debated. Under-reporting of the quantity and type of substance use on self-report measures by adolescents can occur. Youth may also see the self-report assessment as an opportunity to "cry for help" or exaggerate their responses. Laboratory testing (discussed below) can be used to corroborate adolescent self-report of substance use in some instances. Despite possible limitations, the validity of self-report for adolescent substance use in clinical situations has been supported by several lines of evidence. For example, only a small percentage of youth endorse improbable questions; adolescent self-reports often agree with corroborating sources of information, such as archival records and, for the most part, bioassay techniques; and the prevalence rate of elevations on "faking-good" and "faking-bad" scales and other statistical techniques to detect invalid self-report, is relatively low.[9] Regardless, an important condition for detailed and valid self-disclosure is good rapport and assurances of allowable confidentiality between the patient and clinician (see sidebar in Chapter 118 on confidentiality).

Alternatives to Self-Report

Collateral Reports

Whereas parents are usually willing to provide a report about their adolescent, it is not likely that they can provide detailed reports about the types, frequency, and quantity of substance use by their child.[10] Information from peers is usually not available.

Clinical Observation

A 14-item checklist of observable signs that may indicate a substance problem is contained in the Simple Screening Instrument for Alcohol and Other Drug Abuse.[11]

Laboratory Testing

Urinalysis, hair analysis, saliva testing, blood, breath and sweat testing are all used to detect exposure to substances. Newer biomarkers for alcohol, such as ethyl glucuronide (urine or hair) phosphatidylethanol (blood), and serum carbohydrate deficient transferrin (CDT) are approaches to detect alcohol for longer periods (days) compared to standard procedures and with greater accuracy. Methods for accurately detecting recent use of cannabis are still being developed. All bioassays are susceptible to both false negatives and false positives. Additional considerations are cost, access, tampering vulnerability, invasiveness, and reliability. More detail on laboratory testing can be found in section 4 of this textbook.

COURSE OF SUBSTANCE USE DISORDERS

Understanding SUD risk factors provides a vital perspective in our understanding of the onset of substance use problems and the progression to a SUD. Among adolescents that have initiated substance use, three major domains increase the risk of developing a SUD: (1) early onset, (2) psychosocial risk factors, and (3) a pre-existing behavioral or mental disorder(s), such as attention–deficit/hyperactivity disorder (ADHD), conduct disorder, or PTSD.[12]

Psychosocial Factors

Psychosocial dimensions provide valuable assessment information.[13] Variables include interpersonal relationships, school and employment, legal involvement and delinquency, recreational activities, and sexual behavior and orientation.

Peer Factors

Peer variables are one of the most prominent factors contributing to the onset and maintenance of substance use. Adolescents who associate with substance-using peers are far more likely to use compared to adolescents who do not associate with substance-using peers.[14]

Family Factors

Family influences encompass genetic risk and parenting practices. Children whose parents have a current or prior substance use problem are at increased risk for developing an SUD.[15] The importance of parenting factors cannot be understated; lack of effective limit setting, supervision and discipline, places adolescents at higher risk of an SUD. Antisocial parent behavior and lack closeness or affection also increase SUD liability in children.[14]

Psychological Benefits

Some adolescents turn to substance use to address unsatisfied psychological needs. These include, mood enhancement, stress reduction, and relief from boredom among others.

Co-occurring Mental or Behavioral Disorders

Most adolescents with substance use problems or disorders have co-occurring behavioral and/or mental disorders, and their presence can negatively impact recovery.[2]

Childhood aggression, rebelliousness, theft, and destructiveness, along with related externalizing disorders such as conduct disorder and oppositional defiant disorder, are common among youth with a SUD.[16] Delinquent behaviors and Attention Deficit Hyperactivity Disorder (ADHD) during childhood are also predictive of adolescent-onset substance use. The symptoms of these externalizing disorders impact one another; for example, treating ADHD in childhood lowers the risk of developing an SUD in adolescence.

Internalizing disorders such as anxiety disorders, posttraumatic stress disorder (PTSD), and mood disorders also are associated with increased risk of SUD.[17] Difficult or negative emotions may contribute to seeking psychological relief. However, in some instances, substance use may further aggravate these negative states, prolonging or worsening the disorder.

Impact on Treatment Outcome

The variables discussed above predict the course of SUD among adolescents receiving treatment.[2] Pretreatment characteristics that are associated with more favorable substance use outcomes include a lower substance use severity level at intake, greater readiness to change, and fewer conduct problems or other co-occurring psychopathologies. Factors influencing better outcomes during treatment include a longer length of treatment and family involvement. Posttreatment predictors of better outcome include participation in aftercare, low levels of peer substance use, ability to use coping skills, and continued commitment to abstain.

INSTRUMENTATION

Several summaries of adolescent screening and comprehensive assessments are available as book chapters,[2,18] and assessment tool databases are provided by the PhenX Toolkit (https://www.phenxtoolkit.org) and the University of Washington (http://lib.adai.washington.edu/instruments).

Screening Tools

Substance Use Screens

Self-reported substance use screening is a brief and efficient procedure generally used in primary care to identify adolescents who are at risk of a substance use disorder and direct the appropriate level of intervention. Screening tools are discussed in detail in (see Chapter 116, "Screening and Brief Intervention for Adolescents").

Comprehensive Screens

The 40-item *Personal Experience Screening Questionnaire* (PESQ) consists of a problem severity scale, substance use history, select psychosocial problems, and response distortion tendencies ("faking good" and "faking bad").[19,20]

The *Global Appraisal of Individual Needs—Short Screener* (GAIN-SS) consists of 20 items that screen for substance use and related problems.[21,22]

The 81-item adolescent version of the *Substance Abuse Subtle Screening Inventory*, now in its 4th edition, yields scores for several scales, including face-valid alcohol, face-valid other substances, obvious attributes, subtle attributes, and defensiveness.[23,24]

Screens for Nonalcohol Substances

The *Drug Abuse Screening Test for Adolescents* was adapted from Skinner's adult tool.[25,26] This 27-item questionnaire is also associated with favorable reliability data and was found to be highly predictive of DSM-IV substance use-related disorder when tested among adolescent psychiatric inpatients. There is a 10-item DAST, the DAST-10,[2] yet its psychometric adequacy with youth has not been established.

Multi-Problem Screens

The 139-item *Problem Oriented Screening Instrument for Teenagers* is part of the Adolescent Assessment and Referral System developed by the National Institute on Drug Abuse. It tests for 10 functional adolescent problem areas.[27,28]

The *Substance Use Screening Inventory-Revised* is a 159-item instrument that describes substance use problem severity and related problems. It produces scores on 10 subscales and a lie scale.[29,30]

Comparisons of Screens

A comparison of four screening tools—NIAAA's two-item screen, *Alcohol Use Disorders Identification Test*, CRAFFT, and PESQ was conducted by D'Amico and colleagues.[31] The CRAFFT and PESQ performed equally as the best among these four in predicting a SUD. Another study compared the CRAFFT, GAIN-SS, and PESQ; all three were equivalent in terms of reliability and the PESQ was slightly better on the validity indices.[20]

Comprehensive Assessment Instruments

If an initial screening indicates the need for further assessment, clinicians and researchers can employ various diagnostic interviews, problem-focused interviews, and multiscale questionnaires.

Diagnostic Interviews

Diagnostic interviews address numerous DSM-based psychiatric disorders, including SUDs. The *Diagnostic Interview for Children and Adolescents* (DICA) is a structured interview used widely among researchers and clinicians.[32] Another useful instrument that has undergone several adaptations is the *Diagnostic Interview Schedule for Children* (DISC).[33] Both the DICA and the DISC have parent and youth versions.

Problem-Focused Interviews

These instruments measure several problem areas associated with adolescent substance involvement, but generally do not focus on assessing a broad range of mental disorders at the diagnostic level. A very well-established example is the *Global Appraisal of Individual Needs*; as a semi-structured interview it covers recent and lifetime functioning in several areas, including substance use, legal and school functioning, and psychiatric symptoms.[34] Other examples include the *Adolescent Diagnostic Interview, Substance Use Screening Inventory,* and the *Comprehensive Addiction Severity Index for Adolescents*.[2]

Multiscale Questionnaires

This group of self-administered, multiscale questionnaires, such as the *Adolescent Self-Assessment Profile*[35] and the *Personal Experience Inventory*,[36] measures both substance use problem severity and related psychosocial risk factors, and some provide scales to detect response distortion tendencies (eg, faking bad, faking good).

KEY POINTS

1. Assessment of adolescent substance involvement and SUDs is a critical first step when addressing the intervention or treatment needs for the teenager. Early initiation of alcohol and other substance use significantly elevates the risk to develop a SUD.
2. Brain development is ongoing during adolescence, particularly in the prefrontal cortex brain region which governs judgment. Immaturity and socio-cultural factors unique to adolescents require use of assessments that are tailored to youth.
3. Many factors influence the course of adolescent substance use and resulting consequences. Therefore, comprehensive evaluation and treatment is recommended for all adolescents with substance use disorders.

ACKNOWLEDGMENTS

The authors wish to extend gratitude to Tamara Fahnhorst, Andria Botzet, and Ali Nicholson for their contributions to an earlier version of this chapter.

REFERENCES

1. Volkow ND, Wargo EM. Association of severity of adolescent substance use disorders and long-term outcomes. *JAMA Netw Open.* 2022;5:e225656.
2. Winters KC, Botzet AM, Lee S. Assessing adolescent substance use problems and other areas of functioning: state of the art. In: Monti P, Colby S, O'Leary T, eds. *Adolescents, Alcohol and Substance Use: Reaching Teens Through Brief Intervention.* 2nd ed. Guilford Press; 2018:83-107.
3. Levy S, Williams JF. Committee on Substance Use and Prevention. Substance use screening, brief intervention, and referral to treatment. *Pediatrics.* 2016;138(1):e20161211. doi:10.1542/peds.2016-1211
4. McCabe SE, Schulenberg JE, Schepis TS, McCabe VV, Veliz PT. Longitudinal analysis of substance use disorder symptom severity at age 18 years and substance use disorder in adulthood. *JAMA Netw Open.* 2022;5:e225324.
5. Giedd JN. Structural magnetic resonance imaging of the adolescent brain. *Ann N Y Acad Sci.* 2004;1021(1):77-85.
6. Volkow ND, Baler RD, Compton WM, Weiss SR. Adverse health effects of marijuana use. *N Engl J Med.* 2014;370(23):2219-2227.
7. American Psychiatric Association. *Diagnostic and Statistical Manual of Mental Disorders (DSM-5).* American Psychiatric Association; 2013.
8. Winters KC, Martin CS, Chung T. Substance use disorders in DSM-5 when applied to adolescents. *Addiction.* 2011;106(5):882-884.
9. Williams RJ, Nowatzki N. Validity of adolescent self-report of substance use. *Subst Use Misuse.* 2005;40(3):299-311.
10. Piehler TF, Lee S, Nicholson A, Winters KC. The correspondence of parent-reported measures of adolescent alcohol and cannabis use with adolescent-reported measures: a systematic review. *Subst Abuse.* 2019;41:437-450.
11. Winters KC, Zenilman JM. *Simple Screening Instruments for Outreach for Alcohol and Other Drug Abuse and Infectious Diseases: Treatment Improvement Protocol (TIP) Series.* US Department of Health and Human Services. Public Health Service, Substance Abuse and Mental Health Services Administration, Center Substance Abuse Treatment; 1994.
12. Montano G, Chung T. Diagnosis, epidemiology, and course of youth substance use and Substance Use Disorders. In: Kaminer Y, Winters KC, eds. *Clinical Manual of Adolescent Addictive Disorders.* American Psychiatric Association Publishing; 2018:3-24.
13. Clark D, Winters KC. Measuring risks and outcomes in substance use disorders prevention research. *J Consult Clin Psychol.* 2002;70:1207-1223.
14. Windle M. Parental, sibling, and peer influences on adolescent substance use and alcohol problems. *Appl Dev Sci.* 2000;4(2):98-110.
15. McGue M. Behavioral genetics models of alcoholism and drinking. In: Leonard KE, Blane HT, eds. *Psychological Theories of Drinking and Alcoholism.* 2nd ed. Guilford Press; 1999:372-421.
16. Clark DB, Moss H, Kirisci L, Mezzich AC, Miles R, Ott P. Psychopathology in preadolescent sons of substance abusers. *J Am Acad Child Adolesc Psychiatry.* 1997;36:495-502.
17. O'Neil KA, Conner BT, Kendall PC. Internalizing disorders and substance use disorders in youth: comorbidity, risk, temporal order, and implications for intervention. *Clin Psychol Rev.* 2011;31(1):104-112.
18. Welsh JW, Knight JR. Screening and assessment of substance use. In: Maruish ME, ed. *Handbook of Pediatric Psychological Screening and Assessment in Primary Care.* Routledge; 2018:343-357.
19. Winters KC. Development of an adolescent alcohol and other drug abuse screening scale: personal experience screening questionnaire. *Addict Behav.* 1992;17(5):479-490.
20. Carney T, Myers B, Louw J; Reliability of the GAIN-SS. CRAFTT and PESQ screening instruments for substance use among South African adolescents. *S Afr J Psychiatr.* 2016;22:10.4102/sajpsychiatry.v22i1.932.
21. Dennis ML, Chan YF, Funk RR. Development and validation of the GAIN Short Screener (GSS) for internalizing, externalizing and substance use disorders and crime/violence problems among adolescents and adults. *Am J Addict.* 2006;15(Suppl 1):80-91.
22. Stucky BD, Edelen MO, Ramchand R. A psychometric assessment of the GAIN Individual Severity Scale (GAIN-GISS) and Short Screeners (GAIN-SS) among adolescents in outpatient treatment programs. *J Subst Abuse Treat.* 2014;46:165-173.
23. Miller G. *The Substance Abuse Subtle Screening Inventory—Adolescent Version.* SASSI Institute; 1985.
24. Erford BT, Atalay Z, Bardhoshi G. Systematic review of psychometric characteristics of the SASSI–3. *Meas Eval Couns Dev.* 2020;53:62-74.
25. Martino S, Grilo CM, Fehon DC. The development of the drug abuse screening test for adolescents (DAST-A). *Addict Behav.* 2000;25:57-70.

26. Yudko E, Lozhkina O, Fouts A. A comprehensive review of the psychometric properties of the Drug Abuse Screening Test. *J Subst Abuse Treat.* 2007;32:189-198.
27. Rahdert E, ed. The adolescent assessment/referral system manual. *DHHS Pub No.(ADM).* U.S. Department of Health and Human Services, ADAMHA, National Institute on Drug Abuse; 1991:91-1735.
28. Kelly SM, O'Grady KE, Gryczynski J, Mitchell SG, Kirk A, Scwartz RP. The concurrent validity of the Problem Oriented Screening Instrument for Teenagers (POSIT) substance use/abuse subscale in adolescent patients in an urban federally qualified health center. *Subst Abuse.* 2017;38:382-388.
29. Tarter RE, Laird SB, Bukstein O, et al. Validation of the adolescent drug use screening inventory: preliminary findings. *Psychol Addict Behav.* 1992;6:233-236.
30. Kirisci L, Tarter R, Mezzich A, Reynolds M. Screening current and future diagnosis of psychiatric disorders using the revised drug use screening inventory. *Am J Drug Alcohol Abuse.* 2008;34:653-665.
31. D'Amico EJ, Parast L, Meredith LS, Ewing BA, Shadel WG, Stein BD. Screening in primary care: what is the best way to identify at-risk youth for substance use? *Pediatrics.* 2016;138(6):e20161717.
32. Reich W, Shayla JJ, Taibelson C. *The Diagnostic Interview for Children and Adolescents-Revised (DICA-R).* Washington University; 1992.
33. Shaffer D, Fisher P, Dulcan M. The NIMH Diagnostic Interview Schedule for Children (DISC 2.3): description, acceptability, prevalence, and performance in the MECA study. *J Am Acad Child Adolesc Psychiatry.* 1996;35:865-877.
34. Dennis ML. *Global Appraisal of Individual Needs (GAIN): Administration Guide for the GAIN and Related Measures.* Lighthouse Publications; 1999.
35. Wanberg K. *Adolescent Self-Assessment Profile (ASAP).* Center for Addictions Research and Evaluation; 1992.
36. Winters KC, Henly GA. *Personal Experience Inventory and Manual.* Western Psychological Services; 1989.

SUGGESTED READINGS

Angold A, Erkanli A, Copeland W, Goodman R, Fisher PW, Costello EJ. Psychiatric diagnostic interviews for children and adolescents: a comparative study. *J Am Acad Child Adolesc Psychiatry.* 2012;51:506-517.

Knight DK, Becan JE, Landrum B, Joe GW, Flynn PM. Screening and assessment tools for measuring adolescent client needs and functioning in substance abuse treatment. *Subst Use Misuse.* 2014;49:902-918.

Welsh JW, Knight JR. Screening and assessment of substance use. In: Maruish ME, ed. *Handbook of Pediatric Psychological Screening and Assessment in Primary Care.* Routledge; 2018:343-357.

Winters KC, Botzet AM, Lee S. Assessing adolescent substance use problems and other areas of functioning: state of the art. In: Monti P, Colby S, O'Leary T, eds. *Adolescents, Alcohol and Substance Use: Reaching Teens Through Brief Intervention.* 2nd ed. Guilford Press; 2018:83-107.

CHAPTER

118 Placement Criteria and Strategies for Adolescent Treatment Matching

Marc Fishman

CHAPTER OUTLINE

- Introduction
- Developmental considerations in adolescent placement
- The ASAM criteria
- Conclusions

INTRODUCTION

Although the fields of adolescent substance use disorder treatment and outcomes research in particular are still in their early stages compared to work in adults, recent progress has been considerable. Advances have been made in assessment, adolescent-specific treatment needs, modalities and techniques. Over the past 30 years, much has been learned about the effectiveness and limitations of current adolescent treatment methods and programs.

Treatment for adolescent substance use disorders (SUDs) has clearly and repeatedly been shown to be effective. Reviews of the published literature have shown favorable outcomes out to one year following treatment and beyond, across various modalities and levels of care. These results are further enhanced by favorable comparisons of treatment groups to waiting-list controls, substance-specific treatments to nonspecific treatment controls, treatment completers compared to those who did not engage or left treatment early, and carefully organized research-based treatment to loosely organized "treatment as usual."[1-7]

It is well established that favorable outcomes in treatment of adolescent SUDs, (including both abstinence and reductions in substance use short of abstinence), are associated with substantial reductions in adolescent morbidity and improvements in psychosocial function. Such improvements in function extend to school, family, criminal behaviors, psychological adjustment, and other psychosocial domains.[5,8]

While the research to date on adolescent SUD treatment has been very encouraging, there has been very little comparative examination of the broad range of current treatment modalities, levels of care, and program models.[5,9] Little is known about the differential effectiveness of various treatment strategies, intensities, and treatment program components.[10] Perhaps most important, little empirical work has been done to explore hypotheses of adolescent treatment matching and placement. Nevertheless, questions of which patient should receive what treatment have been the subject of extensive expert consideration, with progressive agreement on fundamental principles and approaches. For example, work with adults consistently shows that assessment-based stratification of severity can predict treatment response.[11,12] Using insights such as this, consensus-based "best practices" in the area of adolescent treatment matching and placement are steadily improving. This chapter provides an introduction to the developing area of adolescent treatment matching and placement, with special attention to one particular placement tool, the adolescent patient placement criteria, contained in the ASAM criteria developed by the American Society of Addiction Medicine (ASAM).

DEVELOPMENTAL CONSIDERATIONS IN ADOLESCENT PLACEMENT

One of the most important advances in the field of adolescent treatment is the articulation of approaches that are developmentally specific. This is in response to increased recognition that adolescents respond differently from adults because of differences in their levels of emotional, cognitive, physical, social, and moral development.

Examples of developmental issues that are fundamental to adolescent assessment and treatment include the extremely potent influence of peers and family. It is critical that adolescent assessments include collateral informants, to augment and clarify (and, often, correct) the history as presented by the adolescent patient. Such key informants may include family, peers, adult friends or surrogate parent figures, school and court officials, court-appointed special advocates, social service workers, and previous treatment providers.

Adolescents' use of substances frequently impairs their emotional and intellectual growth. Substance use can prevent a young person from completing the maturational tasks of adolescence, which involve formation of personal relationships, acquisition of social skills, psychological development, identity formation, individuation, education, employment, and family role responsibilities. It is one of the special challenges and unique opportunities of adolescent treatment to modify risk factors that are still actively evolving. Adolescent treatment thus often requires habilitative rather than rehabilitative approaches, emphasizing the acquisition of new capacities, rather than the restoration of lost ones.

In general, adolescents are immature in executive functioning, and are therefore less able to formulate strategies to achieve longer-term goals and to delay gratification compared to adults. Younger adolescents have a very narrow view of the world, with little capacity to think about implications of their actions. As such, appeals to change behavior in order to avoid long-term health effects of substance use are usually ineffective. Though some adolescents may adopt a pseudo-mature ("streetwise") posture, this can be misleading since immaturity usually remains prominent despite appearances.

Most adolescents have not yet acquired the skills for independent living and, even without the impairments associated with substance use, must rely heavily on the guidance of adults. As a result, adolescents typically require greater amounts of external assistance and support than adult patients, both to protect them from the sequelae of substance use and to engage them in the recovery process. In general, for a given degree of severity or functional impairment, adolescents require greater intensity of treatment than adults. This is reflected in clinical practice by a greater tendency to place adolescents in more intensive levels of care.

Transitional Age Youth

The definition of adolescence is better understood as a matter of a dimensional developmental stage, rather than a categorical cutoff of chronological age. Some youth transition out of adolescence into more adult-like functioning earlier than average, some later. On the other hand, it is useful to have an approximate age range for practical purposes, and age range definitions may be written into local regulatory language. In general, most regulatory definitions encompass the age ranges of 13 to 18 or 13 to 21, with some local variation. From a clinical perspective, these ranges should be viewed flexibly. Although payers or regulators may choose to apply a rigid age cutoff, in many cases adolescent criteria would be more appropriate than adult criteria for older adolescents or young adults.

Young adults or transitional age youth generally between ages 17 to 26 who have a foot in both worlds: adolescence and adulthood. This group is typically both emerging into independence and still relying a great deal on the support of parents or other caregiving adults.

The mixed features of both adolescence and adulthood for transition age youth require a special approach. Some providers have begun to develop specialized programming for this group and its unique clinical needs. Eventually, the separation of a third category (adolescent, adult, and transition age youth) of developmental programming may become standard. The tensions inherent in their transition often require a balancing act between emerging independence and persistent dependence. For example, tricky issues of confidentiality versus open sharing of information with parents/caregivers are common. Other common issues include financial support, shared living environments with parents, and extension of standard insurance coverage under parental policies until age 26 with the Affordable Care Act.

As an example of the vulnerability of this group, young adults have been disproportionately affected by the current opioid crisis with the highest rates of opioid use among all age groups.[13] Additionally, young adults have poorer outcomes for medication treatment of opioid use disorder than older adults. Given these realities, it is clear that developmentally-specific approaches are needed to address such discrepancies.

THE ASAM CRITERIA

The ASAM's *The ASAM Criteria: Treatment Criteria for Addictive, Substance-Related, and Co-Occurring Conditions*, 3rd ed.[14] is a clinical guide that has been widely adopted to assist in matching patients to appropriate treatment settings. It contains separate sets of criteria for adolescents and adults, and highlights adolescent-specific issues in call-out boxes throughout the narrative material explaining the criteria decision rules. The criteria, which have undergone evolutionary change and improvement since publication of the first edition in 1991, use multidimensional assessments for placement decisions. Six dimensions are specified; placements are recommended according to gradations of problem severity within each dimension.

Assessment-Based Treatment Matching and Clinical Appropriateness

The ASAM criteria use decision rules to guide placement across a continuum of levels of care. They attempt to standardize program specifications for each level of care, including guidelines for minimum staffing levels and general program components. They do not, however, specify these in detail, nor do they attempt to prescribe program models, specific treatment modalities, or techniques.

The principal goal of the ASAM criteria is to facilitate the process of matching patients in need of treatment for SUDs with appropriate treatment services and settings in order to maximize the accessibility, effectiveness, and efficiency of the treatment experience. The criteria are based on "clinical appropriateness," which emphasizes quality and efficiency over cost. This is in contrast with "medical necessity," which has been interpreted as avoiding imminent danger from acute medical or psychiatric concerns (dimensions 1, 2, and 3), and has become associated with restrictions on utilization. In contrast, "clinical appropriateness" conveys the notion that patients should be treated in the most suitable placements, defined by the extent of their problems and priorities in all six of the ASAM assessment dimensions.

Because the elements of assessment in the ASAM criteria are not concretely operationalized (as they would be, for example, in standardized assessment instruments), they allow for and require considerable clinical judgment. They are best used as illustrations of underlying principles of matching, rather than as exact prescriptions or rigid rules. The criteria avoid assumptions regarding the length of service. Rather, they provide guidelines in the form of general decision rules for continued service versus discharge/transfer, which are applied to the original admission problems in the six assessment dimensions. Under these decision rules, a patient should remain at a given level of care as long as the problems that created the need for admission persist (or new problems requiring that level of care emerge).

The criteria reflect a tension between an attempt to promote a broader treatment continuum while reflecting the real world of treatment service delivery. As a result, the criteria do not articulate some of the innovative sublevels of intensity and treatment settings that should (and in some places do) exist. The reality of limited availability of services is a substantial problem, particularly in the treatment of adolescents. One or more of the levels of care may not exist or be accessible in a given community. Logistical issues such as long waiting lists and limited insurance or other funding coverage can render a treatment setting practically unavailable. Variations in programming within a level of care might result in specific services being unavailable even if a program meets the criteria more generally. When the criteria designate a treatment placement that is not available, a patient may access recommended services through a combination of placements, erring on the side of safety and effectiveness. This may require increasing the intensity of services, usually through placement at a more intensive level of care.

The ASAM criteria outline a full range of treatment services appropriate to the needs of all adolescents with substance use disorders, whether they are privately insured, publicly insured, underinsured, or uninsured. Adolescents from underserved families and communities may need an even broader continuum of services than those with greater resources. In general, adolescents with fewer supports, less resiliency, and lower levels of baseline functioning need a higher intensity of services and longer lengths of service at all levels of care than do those with the benefits conferred by economic advantage and better social supports. All too frequently, the continuum of services described are not available to underserved populations.

One goal of the ASAM criteria has been to encompass more explicitly the circumstances of adolescents in the public sector. For example, there are specific references to adolescents involved in the juvenile legal system, where many adolescents may have had extended periods of enforced abstinence, but usually have not had active treatment. In this context, the assessment of severity and treatment needs should be made by a full multidimensional assessment that emphasizes the adolescent's acquisition of recovery skills and capacity for reintegration into the community rather than a narrow standard based on recency of use. Hopefully, active treatment, including the full continuum of care reflected in the ASAM criteria, will increasingly become the rule rather than the exception for this group.

Treatment at every level of care requires coordination of a broad array of interrelated treatment services to respond to the needs of the individual patient. This is sometimes accomplished by direct provision of multiple treatment services, and sometimes by linkages with other service providers, usually through referral. Examples include psychiatric assessment and treatment, medical assessment and treatment, engagement with a primary care provider, psychological and/or educational testing for learning disorders, special or alternative education services, family therapies, juvenile legal system probation and supervision, foster care support services, public benefit coordination or other social service agency interventions, vocational and prevocational training, child care, and transportation. In general, the greater the severity of an adolescent's problems, the greater the need for such broad and diverse adjunctive services. To deliver this array of services, treatment programs at all levels of care should develop active affiliations with programs and agencies that offer other services or levels of care and should help patients access treatment fluidly across the continuum. Barriers to treatment integration remain a fundamental and profound problem for the field, which are beginning to be addressed,[15] at least partially in response to adoption of the ASAM criteria by state agencies, third-party payers, and treatment providers.

Placement and Treatment Considerations by Assessment Dimension

The ASAM criteria organize the assessment of the substance-using adolescent into six dimensions, specifying appropriate placements according to gradations of problem severity within each dimension (**Table 118-1**).

Dimension 1: Intoxication and Withdrawal

The ASAM criteria include Dimension 1 assessment elements by specific drug classes. This highlights the range of intoxication and withdrawal symptoms, which all too often are overlooked in adolescents, and emphasizes the importance of their treatment. Common examples include memory impairment caused by cannabis intoxication, which can persist for many weeks following abstinence (substance-induced persisting amnestic disorder); sensory disturbance or "flashbacks" caused by hallucinogens, which can persist for weeks to months following abstinence (hallucinogen persisting perception disorder); and delirium and other states of cognitive disorganization caused by inhalants, which can persist for weeks or more following abstinence. Another very common example is insomnia as a symptom of extended subacute withdrawal from various substances (including cannabis, opioids, and alcohol), which can be a powerful trigger for relapse.

For most substances, most adolescents do not develop pronounced physiological withdrawal symptoms. Opioids are a notable exception in which withdrawal symptoms are common. However, adolescents are more susceptible than adults to developing tolerance, and DSM-IV symptoms of

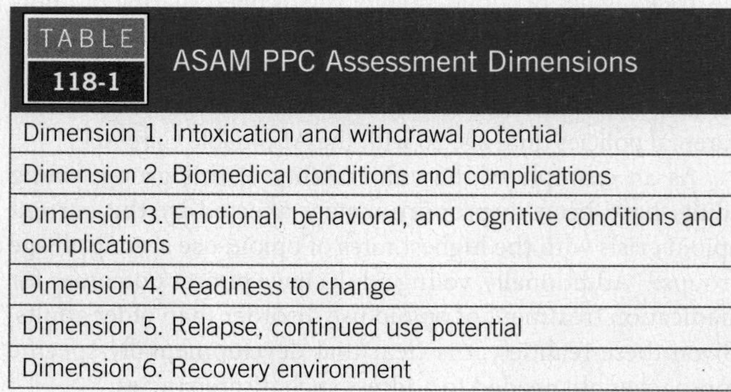

TABLE 118-1 ASAM PPC Assessment Dimensions
Dimension 1. Intoxication and withdrawal potential
Dimension 2. Biomedical conditions and complications
Dimension 3. Emotional, behavioral, and cognitive conditions and complications
Dimension 4. Readiness to change
Dimension 5. Relapse, continued use potential
Dimension 6. Recovery environment

substance dependence later in life if exposed to alcohol, cannabis, or nicotine during the teenage years.[16] The progression from casual use to a use disorder and from one substance to others is accelerated in adolescents compared to adults.[17]

Withdrawal management includes the attenuation of physiological and psychological features of intoxication and withdrawal syndromes and the process of interrupting habitual, compulsive use in adolescents. This phase of treatment frequently requires a greater initial intensity in order to establish treatment engagement and patient role induction, and is critical because it is so difficult for patients to participate in treatment while cycling between frequent intoxication and recovery.

Managing withdrawal symptoms in a setting separate from other treatment services is clinically undesirable because of the developmental issues involved in the care of adolescents. Withdrawal management ("detoxification") alone without more comprehensive attention to the broad range of problems and vulnerabilities in other domains typical of adolescents, is never sufficient. Withdrawal management should always be closely linked to next steps in ongoing treatment and continuing care. Moreover, there is no evidence that ambulatory withdrawal treatments that have become increasingly common for severe withdrawal in adults are effective with adolescents.

Dimension 2: Biomedical Conditions and Complications

Medical sequelae of addiction are less common and generally less severe in adolescents than adults, though when present, play a role in placement decisions. Some of the common medical complications of substance use in this age group include traumatic injuries (either accidental or due to victimization), respiratory depression caused by opioid or other sedative overdose, sudden inhalant death syndrome (from cardiac arrhythmia and hypoxia), and seizures caused by stimulant or inhalant intoxication. Acute alcohol poisoning is a severe medical complication that is more typical of adolescents than adults. The sequelae of injection drug use are well known, including cellulitis, HIV, endocarditis, hepatitis B, and especially hepatitis C.

Some of the less severe but more common and often underrecognized medical sequelae of substance use include gastritis caused by alcohol use, pulmonary injury from inhalational drug use, dental disease caused by poor self-care, and weight loss and malnourishment caused by self-neglect and/or the appetite-suppression that is typical with stimulants. Another notable area of medical complication in adolescents is the exacerbation of chronic illness such as diabetes, asthma, or sickle cell disease that results from impaired self-care and poor adherence to indicated medical treatments.

Sexually transmitted diseases are common among adolescents and young adults and include chlamydial and gonococcal infections, syphilis, pelvic inflammatory disease, HIV, and hepatitis B (HBV). Both urethritis in boys and cervicitis in girls are common but frequently overlooked because they are often asymptomatic. The special needs and medical vulnerabilities of pregnant substance-using teenagers require particular care in selecting treatment services. Overall, the need for contraception and other medical prevention and treatment services related to sexual behaviors in drug-involved adolescents cannot be overemphasized.

Dimension 3: Emotional, Behavioral, and Cognitive Conditions and Complications

The treatment of co-occurring psychiatric disorders and sequelae is vital in youth with SUDs.[18] Drug-involved adolescents typically demonstrate a very high degree of co-occurring psychopathology, which frequently does not remit with abstinence. The rates of co-occurring mental health disorders are higher in adolescents than in adults,[19] and the need for co-occurring enhanced or combined behavioral health programming is great. There is mounting evidence that identifying and treating depression in substance-involved youth improve substance use outcomes and vice versa.[20] There is a growing awareness of the association between of cannabis use in youth and psychotic disorders[21] and anxiety disorders[22]; these problems are worse with synthetic cannabinoids ("K2," "spice," etc.)[22] and with higher THC doses.

Even adolescents who have not been diagnosed with a psychiatric disorder often have problems in Dimension 3 that impact treatment decisions. Examples include hyperactivity or distractibility that may occur without a diagnosis of attention deficit hyperactivity disorder (ADHD), mood lability and explosive temper without a diagnosis of bipolar disorder, or dysphoric mood and loss of interests without a diagnosis of depression. Various nonspecific symptoms—such as problems with anger management or impulse control, suspiciousness, and social withdrawal—may be substance induced or substance exacerbated. Nonspecific features of immature and/or impaired executive functioning are very common in drug-involved adolescents, including impulsiveness, explosiveness, poor affective self-regulation, poor strategic planning and disinhibition.

The inclusion of cognitive conditions in Dimension 3 emphasizes the importance of cognitive abilities, as well as global or focal cognitive impairments, in an adolescent's functional capacity. Whether cognitive problems are due to preexisting conditions such as borderline intellectual functioning, fetal alcohol effects, assorted attentional deficits, or learning disorders[23,24] or are complications of substance use (such as cannabis-induced amnestic disorder), they often contribute to the severity of SUDs and interfere significantly with treatment and recovery.

To be most effective, treatment adaptations are needed to respond to adolescents' cognitive vulnerabilities and to capitalize on strengths. Cognitive function should be considered in a developmental perspective because cognition evolves dynamically over time.

One of the keys to treating adolescents is to use methods that account for issues of normal adolescent development and delayed development that often accompanies substance use and co-occurring mental health disorders. Most therapies are best delivered in time-limited components, with frequent breaks to account for limited attention spans. Adolescent engagement and learning are promoted by the use of experiential recovery activities that involve active participation rather than passive reception of information and that are somewhat energetic, noisy, and fun while at the same time delivering serious therapeutic content. Engagement is enhanced by the acknowledgement and even partial endorsement of adolescent culture, including its typical stance of nonconformity with adult and mainstream norms.

Managing adolescent behavior, even when developmentally appropriate, is another feature of treatment in Dimension 3. The expectation of mature behavior is developmentally unrealistic in adolescent settings. The acquisition of self-regulation skills is a developmental milestone for all adolescents and an essential treatment goal for people with substance use disorders at all ages. Recognizing that adolescents are still emerging from childhood, treatment programs must constantly seek a balance between limit setting and tolerance of small transgressions. Rule-breaking is not always an indicator of antisocial traits. On the other hand, careful assessment of the broad range of adolescent misbehavior forms the basis of very powerful treatment interventions that target improvements in family monitoring, supervision, and behavioral management.

In the ASAM criteria, Dimension 3 has been expanded and divided into subdomains for greater emphasis on psychiatric comorbidity. These subdomains are intended to enrich the detail and guide the assessment of risk and treatment needs for emotional, behavioral, and cognitive problems. The organization of the Dimension 3 severity specifications by subdomains emphasizes that placement decisions emerge out of the assessment of symptomatic functional impairment rather than any specific categorical diagnosis (**Table 118-2**).

For example, the subdomain titled "Dangerousness/Lethality" refers to the extent of risk of imminent harm to self or others. Assessment considerations may include suicidality, homicidality or threat to assault another, risk of victimization, and exposure to the elements. Treatment decisions in this subdomain focus on safety and protection from dangerous consequences and may include such interventions as residential containment or high-intensity family monitoring between outpatient sessions.

The subdomain titled "Interference with Addiction Recovery Efforts" refers to the extent to which psychological and behavioral symptoms are a distraction from treatment participation or engagement. Examples include difficulty attending to treatment sessions because of problems with concentration, difficulty in completing recovery assignments or absorbing treatment materials because of problems with memory or comprehension, inability to attend treatment consistently because of running away, inability to participate in treatment because of disruptive behavior, and distraction caused by preoccupying worries.

The subdomain titled "Social Functioning" refers to the extent to which emotional, behavioral, and cognitive problems cause impairments in meeting responsibilities in major social arenas such as family, school, work, and personal relationships. Examples of assessment considerations in this subdomain include peer or family conflict, legal and conduct problems, truancy or school failure, ungovernability at home, and narrowing of social repertoire and isolation.

The subdomain titled "Ability for Self-Care" refers to the extent to which the adolescent has problems in managing activities of daily living and personal care. Assessment considerations include behaviors associated with patterns of victimization, high-risk or indiscriminate sexual behaviors, disorganization that interferes with emerging independent living skills, poor self-regulation or poor cooperation with external regulation of daily routine, and problems with hygiene or nutrition.

The subdomain titled "Course of Illness" refers to an interpretation of the adolescent's present situation and symptoms in the context of his or her history and response to treatment, with a goal of predicting future course and relative stability. For example, the adolescent's history may suggest that a mood disorder may decompensate rapidly with medication noncompliance, suggesting a higher severity and indicating the need for more urgent and/or more intensive treatment than if the course deteriorates more slowly. Other examples include an adolescent who has tended to run away soon after an episode of family conflict or an adolescent who return to substance use following recurrence of depressive symptoms.

TABLE 118-2 Dimension 3 Subdomains

Dimension 3 Subdomains
Dangerousness/lethality
Interference with addiction recovery efforts
Social functioning
Ability for self-care
Course of illness

Dimension 4: Readiness to Change

Assessment of treatment readiness is an essential component of treatment matching for adolescents. In the ASAM criteria, Dimension 4 "Readiness to Change" highlights the active, dynamic concept of treatment engagement. Placement decisions based on Dimension 4 include consideration of stage of change for both the adolescent and family. Different interventions will be effective at different stages of change. Adolescents tend to present at earlier stages of readiness to change than adults because external pressures commonly push them into treatment, even more so than adults.[25] Low perceptions of harm are strongly correlated with use of substances, and the wide popularity of the attitude that cannabis is "no problem" is increasingly prominent in the current environment of decreased stigma and increased access to cannabis with legalization and cannabis used as treatment.

Engagement and role induction are critical components of treatment. Significant advances have been made in expanding treatment engagement from simply attempting to overcome the adolescent's resistance to appreciating the adolescent's own set of motivations and goals and incorporating them into a treatment agenda. Motivational interviewing and other motivational enhancement techniques have formed the basis of a variety of intervention models at various levels of care, including early intervention[26] and outpatient treatment.[27] Strategies that take advantage of touchpoints upstream from specialty care where adolescents can be engaged in their natural environments can be very productive, literally "meeting them where they are." School-based intervention is an important example and strongly emphasizes motivational approaches.[28]

Assessments of readiness to change take into account a variety of change processes, including the processes used by adolescents,[29] families,[30] and external systems, such as the coercive influence of the juvenile legal system. Readiness for change is conceived of as a balance of internal experiential contingency motivations (such as social frustrations; symptoms of intoxication or withdrawal; loss of achievements, interests, and enjoyment; unpleasant or frightening experiences, including violence, victimization, high-risk motor vehicle use, or unwelcome sexual experiences) and external contingency motivations (such as parental mandates, legal threats, drug testing, peer group affiliations and influences, and loss of status). The question is how these factors combine and how and in what setting to make best use of them in enhancing the adolescent's motivation for treatment and change. Additional factors in treatment engagement include problem identification, help-seeking orientation, self-efficacy, and hopefulness. Cultural factors also are important components in assessing readiness to change, as they influence likelihood of seeking and receiving treatment, likelihood of perceiving treatment as helpful, and consideration of cultural context in devising treatment engagement strategies.

Dimension 5: Relapse, Continued Use, or Continued Problem Potential

Dimension 5 entails an estimation of the likelihood of resumption or continuation of substance use. The assessment of reuse potential (or, reciprocally, remission potential) includes a number of key factors. Although not incorporated directly into the criteria, a schema for incorporating four subdomains for more detailed ASAM criteria Dimension 5 assessments has been proposed.[11,p.345] These subdomains are as follows: (1) historical pattern of use (including amount, frequency, chronicity, and treatment response), (2) pharmacological response to the effects from particular substances (including positive reinforcement such as pleasure with use and cravings and negative reinforcement such as relief from withdrawal or other negative experiences), (3) response to external stimuli (including reactivity to environmental triggers and acute or chronic stress), and (4) cognitive and behavioral vulnerability and resiliency factors (including traits of impulsivity, passivity, locus of control, and overall coping capacities).

The "historical pattern of use" concept is similar to the "course of illness" subdomain in Dimension 3. That is, history and treatment response are likely to predict the future course of illness, including potential return to use. For example, some adolescents are more likely to have a rapid course of full reinstatement of a SUD with severe impairment following a single lapse episode, while others are likely to have a more indolent course, with only gradual escalation of use. This suggests the need for individualized treatment- and placement-matching decisions. Response to past treatment also may be a way of using individualized treatment effectiveness as a guide to placement. If a particular dose of treatment or modality or level of care led to a significant period of improvement for an adolescent in the past, repeating that treatment following return to use may be logical. On the other hand, if a particular dose or placement was not effective in the past, a more intensive intervention may be warranted.

Dimension 6: Recovery/Living Environment

Dimension 6 aims to assess the ability of the adolescent's home environment to support or impede treatment and recovery. For adolescents, the most important features of the recovery environment generally involve family and peers. The need for inclusion of families or other caretakers in assessment and treatment is paramount. In many cases, it is unreasonable to expect that the adolescent will be the initial or most important locus of change. Rather, it often is more effective to help the family improve its approach to monitoring, supervision, and home intervention, with the expectation that the family as the primary locus of change will in turn change the adolescent.

Families, and their needs and involvement, can be broadly considered, including extended families, surrogate families, and other caretakers. It also is important to address cultural context and to use cultural competence as a critical tool for engaging families in treatment.

Problems in Dimension 6 that typically affect placement include chaotic home environments in which substance use, illegal behaviors, abuse, neglect, and lack of supervision are prominent, or a broader community in which substance use and crime are endemic. Many adolescents have a social network composed primarily or even exclusively of family members or peers who are involved in substance use or criminal behaviors. This social context may portray deviance as normative. There may not be readily apparent role models for the rewards of abstinence. Some adolescents may have had *no* experience of living in an environment that fosters healthy prosocial development and functioning.

There is an chronic shortage of programs that provide environments that support youth recovery. These structured, protective living environments are frequently vital to support ongoing treatment that might be integrated into the living environment itself or more commonly coordinated with programming off-site. Frequently, they serve the function of a supervised context where adolescents can sustain and rehearse therapeutic gains initiated at a more intensive level of care. This need for step-down, lower-intensity residential support is perhaps even more vital in the continuum of care for youth than for adults because of their lack of independence and reliance on the support or partial support of caregiving adults. For younger adolescents, these programs would typically be level 3.1 (see below), often group homes or similar programs. For young adults, these programs could also be level 3.1, though there is also a need for less intensive Recovery Housing programs, with more supervision than typical adult-style self-organized sober housing (eg, Oxford Houses), or adult-style Recovery House boarding houses that have minimal supervision, but perhaps with less intensity than the typical 3.1 or halfway house.

Placement and Treatment Considerations by Levels of Care

The adolescent levels of care in the ASAM criteria are similar to the levels of care described and endorsed in other expert consensus documents[31] (Table 118-3).

Level 0.5: Early Intervention

Early intervention services are designed to explore and address the adolescent's problems or risk factors that appear to be related to early stages of substance use. Their goal is to help the adolescent recognize the potentially harmful consequences of substance use, before such use escalates into a SUD. Level 0.5 services may be delivered in a variety of settings, including primary care medical clinics, schools (often through organized student assistance programs), social service and juvenile justice agencies, and driving-under-the-influence intervention programs.

Early intervention services are intended to combine prevention and treatment services for youth who are at risk because of their exposure to or use of substances. Populations that warrant special attention at level 0.5 are the children of parents with SUDs, siblings of people who use substances, and adolescents with other emotional or behavioral problems.

Early intervention is not appropriate for adolescents who meet criteria for a diagnosis of a SUD. If an adolescent's pattern of substance use is causing a persistent pattern of impairment treatment services are best provided at a more intensive level of care.

TABLE 118-3 ASAM PPC-2R Adolescent Levels of Care

Level 0.5: Early intervention
Level 1: Outpatient treatment
Level 2: Intensive outpatient treatment 2.1 Intensive outpatient 2.5 Partial hospitalization
Level 3: Residential treatment 3.1 Clinically managed low-intensity residential 3.5 Clinically managed medium-intensity residential 3.7 Medically monitored high-intensity residential/inpatient
Level 4: Medically managed intensive inpatient (hospital) treatment

Level 1: Outpatient Treatment

Outpatient treatment is by far the most frequently utilized level of care. It may be the initial level of care for an adolescent whose lesser severity of illness warrants this intensity of treatment. Level 1 also may be employed as a "step-down" program for the adolescent who has made progress at a more intensive level of care.

Outpatient treatment is indicated when safety and progress toward recovery goals can be expected without either the immersion intensity of level 2 services or the residential support and protection of level 3 services.

One of the advantages of outpatient treatment is the possibility of achieving therapeutic goals in the context of the patient's own home environment, where new behaviors can be practiced and solidified in real-life circumstances.

Outpatient services may be useful for the adolescent patient who is in the early stages of readiness to change and who has not yet committed to recovery. While an adolescent at this stage may require a more intensive level of care (sometimes including coerced treatment) to address dangerousness or high degrees of resistance and denial, such an increase in intensity can be counterproductive in certain situations. An alternative approach is to use a less intensive level of care to engage the resistant adolescent in treatment by enhancing his or her motivation and/or by modifying the response(s) of the various systems that affect the adolescent. In such situations, "discovery" may be a more appropriate outpatient treatment goal than "recovery." Such an approach may prepare the adolescent for more intensive treatment services or even forestall the need for a more intensive level of care.

Outpatient treatment often includes a prolonged continuing care maintenance phase, sometimes referred to as "aftercare." In this phase, strategies such as relapse prevention and strengthening protective factors are critical components of treatment. This phase focuses on anticipation of difficulties and the guidance of adolescents through the periodic recurrence of stressors without return to or exacerbation of substance use. Ongoing monitoring such as supporting parental supervision, scrutinizing school performance and peer relationships, and reviewing warning signs and triggers is a goal of outpatient treatment. The term "recovery checkups" has sometimes been used to refer to such a monitoring phase in which the intensity/frequency may be low but nevertheless explicitly organized and scheduled rather than triggered only on an ad hoc or "as-needed" basis.

Level 2: Intensive Outpatient Treatment, Partial Hospitalization

Intensive outpatient programs (IOPs) generally offer at least 6 hours of structured programming per week. However, the precise number of hours of service delivered is adjusted to meet each patient's needs. Six hours a week will be too few for many adolescents; for example, those who are early in their treatment or who are stepping down from a more intensive level of care may need 9, 12, or even 15 hours a week of IOP services.

Partial hospitalization programs (PHP, also sometimes known as "day programs") generally offer 20 or more hours of clinically intensive programming per week. They feature daily or near-daily contact and thus provide more intensive monitoring and supervision than IOP or level 1 outpatient treatment.

Intensive outpatient (level 2.1) programs typically differ from partial hospitalization (level 2.5) programs in the severity of patient disorders that they can manage. IOPs may have less capacity to effectively treat adolescents who have substantial or unstable emotional or behavioral problems; such patients are better placed in PHPs. PHPs often have direct access to, or close referral relationships with, psychiatric and medical services. They are thus better able than level 2.1 programs to meet needs identified in Dimensions 1, 2, and 3, which may warrant daily monitoring or management, but which can be appropriately addressed in a structured outpatient setting. Some PHPs can provide an intensity of treatment services approaching that of residential care if the patient's home environment can support safety, stability, and treatment progress between PHP sessions.

With both IOPs and PHPs, there are varying approaches to the program schedule and structure. Some programs employ a single fixed schedule of service hours. Others modify their service hours throughout the stages of treatment, tapering the number of hours according to a prescribed schedule. Yet another approach is to match intensity and hours of service flexibly with the severity of the patient's problems.

Adolescent IOPs generally meet after school or work hours or on weekends. Partial hospitalization may occur during school hours, and many programs, especially if they are longer term, have access to educational services for adolescent patients. PHP programs that do not provide educational services may coordinate with a school system in order to assess and meet their adolescent patients' educational needs.

Level 3: Residential Treatment

The ASAM criteria divides level 3 residential treatment into three particular subtypes:

- Level 3.1: Clinically Managed Low-Intensity Residential Treatment.
- Level 3.5: Clinically Managed Medium-Intensity Residential Treatment.
- Level 3.7: Medically Monitored High-Intensity Residential/Inpatient Treatment.

Level 3.1 (Clinically Managed Low-Intensity Residential Treatment) programs typically are provided in programs that emphasize longer-term community reintegration (sometimes referred to as "halfway houses" or "extended-care") and group homes. Such programs offer several hours a week of low-intensity treatment sessions in addition to their most important feature: a stable living environment, staffed 24 hours a day, that provides sufficient structure and supervision to prevent or minimize reuse or continued use and continued problem potential (Dimension 5). Additional treatment services and intensity may be provided through concurrent involvement in outpatient treatment at level 1 or 2.

Treatment is directed toward applying recovery skills, preventing relapse, improving social functioning by practicing interpersonal and group living skills, improving ability for self-care by organizing the activities of daily living, promoting personal responsibility through successful concurrent involvement in regular productive activities (such as school or work), developing a social network supportive of recovery, and reintegrating the adolescent into the community and (if appropriate) the family.

Treatment at level 3.1 is most often warranted as a substitute for or supplement to deficits in the adolescent's recovery environment (Dimension 6). Problems in Dimension 6 that might warrant placement in a residential program include home environments that are abusive, chaotic, or expose the adolescent to ongoing substance use such that extended separation and residential treatment support are required to overcome their toxic influences. Some adolescents require the structure of a level 3.1 program to achieve engagement in treatment (Dimension 4). Those who are in the early stages of readiness to change may benefit from being removed from an unsupportive living environment.

The length of stay in a clinically managed level 3.1 program tends to be longer than more intensive residential levels of care. In some cases, an extended period in level 3.1 treatment is needed to sustain and consolidate therapeutic gains made at more intensive levels of care because of the adolescent's functional deficits (including developmental immaturity, greater than average susceptibility to peer influence, or lack of impulse control). In some situations, there is no effective substitute for extended residential containment as reliable protection from the toxic influences of substance exposure, problematic or substance-infested environments, or the cultures of substance-involved and antisocial behaviors. Level 3.1 programs may require relatively long stays to allow certain adolescents to acquire basic living skills and mastery of coping and recovery skills. Such patients require the intensity and duration of treatment found in a level 3.5 program to accomplish some of the tasks of habilitation in a temporary "home" that can imprint the features of a successful recovery environment (Dimension 6).

Level 3.5 (Clinically Managed Medium-Intensity Residential Treatment) programs include medium-intensity settings such as therapeutic group homes, therapeutic community programs, psychosocial model residential treatment centers, or extended residential rehabilitation programs. As a group, these sometimes are referred to simply as "residential programs."

Level 3.5 programs are designed to provide relatively extended subacute treatments, with the goal of achieving fundamental personal change for the adolescent who has significant social and psychological problems. The goals and modalities of treatment focus not only on the adolescent's substance use but also on a holistic view of the adolescent that takes into account his or her behavior, emotions, attitudes, values, learning, family, culture, lifestyle, and overall health. Such programs are characterized by their reliance on the treatment community or milieu as a therapeutic agent of change. In addition to the stable recovery environment found at level 3.1, these programs utilize intensive active programming and containment to create a community or milieu that promotes both recovery skills and basic life skills. Critical treatment interventions that require intensity and persistence over extended periods of time, such as modeling prosocial patterns of behavior and adaptive patterns of emotional responsiveness, have sometimes been likened to "surrogate" or "remedial parenting." Just as important can be the induction into a healthy peer group, with the formation of a group identity that emphasizes recovery and overcoming adversity.

The adolescent who is appropriately placed in a level 3.5 program may have a variety of psychological or psychiatric problems (Dimension 3). Particularly suitable for level 3.5 treatments are the entrenched patterns of maladaptive behavior, extremes of temperament, and developmental or cognitive abnormalities related to mental health symptoms or disorders. Co-occurring disorders that often require extended treatment at level 3.5 include conduct disorder and oppositional defiant disorder, as well as the persistent patterns of disruptive behavior that may be associated with other disorders, even after they have responded to acute treatment.

Level 3.5 programs frequently work with aspects of adolescent temperament—including the impulsive, extroverted, dramatic, antisocial, thrill-seeking, or other personality traits—that may otherwise have the potential to solidify as components of emerging personality disorders. Goals of treatment include overcoming oppositionality through a combination of motivational enhancement, supportive limit setting, and judicious confrontation; teaching anger management and acquisition of conflict resolution skills; values clarification and moral habilitation; character molding and education; development of effective behavioral contingency strategies; establishment of a reliable response to external structure; and the internalization of structure through self-regulation skills.

Level 3.5 also is appropriate for the adolescent whose problems include severe delinquency and juvenile justice involvement. This level of care often is warranted for adolescents who have severe conduct problems, a progressive history of illegal behaviors, a pattern of emerging criminality, or an incipient antisocial value system. One of the key purposes of level 3.5 treatment for this set of problems is assessment and monitoring of safety, with particular attention to issues of potential safety outside of the contained setting. In this context, treatment must proceed in a contained, safe, and structured environment to allow teaching, practicing of prosocial behaviors, and facilitation of healthy reintegration into the community.

Treatment in a level 3.5 program may be used to address problems in treatment engagement and readiness to change (Dimension 4). Many adolescents do not respond to outpatient treatment due to lack of engagement, either because of a lack of personal connection to treatment, because the systems surrounding the adolescent (family, school, juvenile legal system, and the like) have not coordinated sufficiently to motivate the adolescent, or both. The immersion experience of a level 3.5 program may be needed to promote treatment role induction and introduce the adolescent into a peer group that is struggling to form a group identity that emphasizes recovery and the need for treatment. An additional goal of treatment at level 3.5 should be to promote coordination of the multiple systems surrounding the adolescent and to help devise and implement motivational strategies for ongoing engagement in treatment.

Like level 3.1, level 3.5 programs may require relatively longer stays to allow certain adolescents to acquire and consolidate basic living skills and coping skills. Such patients require longer exposure to monitoring, supervision, and the intensity of treatment interventions found in a level 3.5 program to practice and master the application of recovery skills.

Level 3.7 (Medically Monitored High-Intensity Residential/Inpatient Treatment) programs are appropriate for adolescents whose problems are so severe that they require medically monitored residential treatment, but who do not need the full resources of an acute care hospital or medically managed inpatient treatment program (level 4). Medically monitored services are provided under the supervision of physicians who are specialists in addiction medicine, and the programs tend to operate under the so-called medical model.

The adolescent who is appropriately placed in a medically monitored program may have problems in Dimensions 1, 2, or 3 that require direct medical or nursing services. Services typically provided in a level 3.7 program include medical withdrawal management, titration of a psychopharmacological regimen, and high-intensity behavior modification. Alternatively, the adolescent may have problems that do not so much require direct medical or nursing services as the overall high intensity of a program and treatment milieu that draws on the staffing pattern and availability of an interdisciplinary professional team.

An adolescent may be admitted directly to a level 3.7 program or transferred from a less intensive level of care if he or she has been refractory to treatment or as bursts of more intensive services become necessary. An adolescent also may be transferred to a level 3.7 program for continuing care from a level 4 program when he or she no longer requires the intensity of services or staffing pattern of a hospital. A common scenario is that of an adolescent who is admitted to a level 4 hospital program on an emergency basis because of a medical or psychiatric crisis situation and then is transferred to a level 3.7 program for further assessment and treatment in a substance-free state to help sort out difficult diagnostic questions regarding subacute intoxication, withdrawal, and co-occurring psychiatric disorders.

Problems in Dimension 3 are probably the most common reason for admission to level 3.7 programs. Such problems include co-occurring psychiatric disorders (such as depressive disorders, bipolar disorders, and ADHD) or symptoms (such as hypomania, severe disorganization or impulsiveness, and aggressive behaviors).

Treatment at level 3.7 often is necessary simply to orient an adolescent with addiction to the structure of daily life using organizing principles other than "getting high" and "being high." Initial forced abstinence through confinement in a level 3.7 program provides many adolescents with a much-needed reintroduction to their own patterns of emotional and cognitive experience without intoxication.

Problems in Dimension 1 that require level 3.7 services include moderate to severe withdrawal or risk of withdrawal, for example, withdrawal management from heroin or illicit prescription opioids requiring pharmacological management. Adolescents also may need medically monitored treatment because of acute or subacute intoxication. Lingering drug-induced impairments of cognitive and/or executive function (eg, by inhalants) or with psychosis (eg, by cannabis, synthetic cannabinoids, or methamphetamine) may lead to disorganization, poor judgment, aggressiveness, and/or increased impulsivity. These may require periods of close assessment and high-intensity management. Medical interventions in Dimension 5 such as initiation and stabilization on relapse prevention medications (eg, buprenorphine or extended-release naltrexone) are often most effectively accomplished in level 3.7 based on the need for intensive medical monitoring.

Level 4: Medically Managed Intensive Inpatient (Hospital) Treatment

Level 4 medically managed intensive inpatient treatment is delivered in an acute care inpatient setting in which the full resources of a general and/or psychiatric hospital are available. It is appropriate for adolescents whose acute problems are so severe that they require primary medical and nursing care on a daily basis. Although treatment is specific to SUDs, the skills of the interdisciplinary team and the availability of support services allow the conjoint treatment of any withdrawal, medical conditions, or psychiatric disorders that need to be addressed. Admissions to level 4 are most commonly provoked by urgent concerns regarding safety and/or imminent danger. Level 4 treatment tends to be brief, generally consisting of emergency or crisis interventions aimed at stabilization in preparation for transfer to a less intensive level of care for ongoing treatment.

Treatment Dose and Utilization Management

The ASAM criteria conceptualize treatment as a dynamic, longitudinal process, rather than a discrete episode of care or particular program enrollment. However, current treatment delivery systems do not generally support the necessary continuum of care. For example, a longitudinal view of treatment might call for the services of a designated care provider to coordinate (or even provide) treatment across discrete placements, but use of such a provider is unusual in most communities and systems of care.

Many difficulties arise over utilization management issues. For example, there are currently no data to guide the optimal dose of treatment for adolescents at any level of care. While the field seems to be moving away from a fixed, length of stay-based, program-driven treatment to a more flexible, assessment-based, clinically driven treatment, much of the development of adolescent programs has focused on standardized protocols with prescribed content and length of service. There has been little examination of the dose-response relationship for adolescent treatment, and further research into this issue is needed. It may turn out that certain minimum threshold lengths of service are associated with specific therapeutic gains. In particular, the needs of juvenile legal system-involved adolescents in public sector programs that use coercive treatment engagement methods (such as a court order or probationary mandate) may be best served by more predictable, though not rigid, lengths of service. Physicians and the courts must collaborate closely to assure that the interests of each adolescent patient are assessed and met. When a treatment plan does not result in sufficient progress, it calls for reassessment, which may indicate the need for more treatment, or the need to adopt a different treatment plan with a change in strategy, modality, or scope of treatment. Failure to reach treatment goals often implies a need for an increase in intensity but also can suggest a change in approach rather than in level of care. The criteria should be applied within the context of local resources and realistically designed follow-up plans.

While utilization criteria can be used as an impetus to overcoming treatment barriers through creative systems approaches, they have also been misused as a cynical justification for giving up or limiting payment for care as "fruitless." The ASAM criteria are *not* intended to imply that ongoing problems, even severe treatment-refractory problems (including continued use, return to use, lack of attendance, lack of participation), suggest inability to solve treatment problems. Changes in level of care or treatment approach should be a part of the therapeutic strategy of a longitudinal treatment plan that anticipates ongoing and future progress.

Given that SUDs often have a chronic, remitting/relapsing course, it is reasonable to expect a treatment plan to be long term. An older, presumably outdated, approach views discrete time-limited episodes of program enrollment as constituting "treatment" with any further continuing care regarded as "aftercare" rather than ongoing care, as if the active part of treatment were finished. The more appropriate view of chronic care for a chronic disorder supports therapeutic optimism for the treatment-refractory patient and reinforces the need for ongoing attention, even in the improved patient. This view is compatible with the common experience that a subset of adolescents, especially those with broader supports and higher levels of premorbid functioning, may respond to more time-limited interventions or seem to "grow out of" their difficulties with developmental maturation.

A critical feature of successful adolescent treatment across a continuum is ease of transfer across the levels of care. It is generally difficult for patients to move back and forth between levels of care due to structural issues. One reason for prolonged lengths of stay at higher levels of care is the barriers to stepping down to appropriate lower levels. Acute episodes of treatment at higher levels of care often are needed to overcome hurdles at lower levels. Repeated acute episodes of high-intensity care should be an expected modality of treatment for exacerbations, as they would be with any chronic relapsing disorder.

Ongoing treatment at less intensive levels of care to consolidate gains initiated at more intensive levels of care is also a critical feature of successful treatment. Since enduring treatment effectiveness may be tempered by the attenuation of treatment effect over time, the need for "booster" doses should be anticipated. Moreover, ongoing active treatment often is required to consolidate and sustain therapeutic gains. Finally, the long-term (sometimes indefinite) maintenance phase of treatment too often is overlooked. Treatment successes, such as a period of abstinence or improvement in functioning are sometimes misinterpreted as completion of treatment. In fact, long-term maintenance and monitoring of short-term successes are essential goals of active outpatient treatment.

Linkages Between Levels of Care

Issues regarding continuity of care, continuing care, and longitudinal follow-up are critical, especially for adolescents because they are so dynamic in their developmental changes and needs. Long-term relationships with youth and families, with the expectation of accommodating dropping in and dropping out, with changing needs over time, should be standard. The notion that patients are cured after a discrete episode of care is both common and incorrect. The need for continuity between linked treatment episodes at different levels of care based on need is vital—role induction, coordination, communication, warm hand-offs, assertive outreach, and overlapping levels of care.

Validation of Placement Criteria

The ASAM criteria were developed as a consensus-based guide to "best practices" by committees of experts and diverse stakeholders. As such, their application is not concretely operationalized or based on standardized assessment instruments, and their use relies on sound clinical judgment. The ongoing process of further operationalizing the adult ASAM criteria through its computer version named Continuum shows one possible future direction for increased reliability.

Encouraging work has been done with the adult ASAM placement criteria to support its validity. Research versions of the criteria, operationalized through standardized assessment instruments to increase reliability, have been shown to have utility and stability as multidimensional severity ratings. Additionally, limited experimental testing of treatment outcomes using earlier versions of the adult criteria has been promising. One study[11] followed posttreatment outcomes in adults randomized to placements following ASAM Patient Placement Criteria (PPC)-prescribed matching versus deliberate mismatching. Outcomes were worse when patients received mismatches to the lower-intensity level of care (LOC) instead of the appropriately matched LOC prescribed by the ASAM PPC.

There has been very little research on either the reliability or validity of the adolescent criteria. However, preliminary work suggests that clinicians who use the criteria in "real-world" settings are able to discriminate levels of clinical severity. A retrospective analysis of adolescents assigned to placements using the ASAM criteria within a single private provider's system of care found that adolescents referred to inpatient treatment had greater severity than those referred to outpatient treatment.[32] While the two groups were not different demographically, the adolescents placed in inpatient care had significantly greater severity in a variety of substance use indicators, including frequency of use, number of previous treatment episodes, number of diagnoses of DSM-defined substance dependence as opposed to substance abuse, and prevalence of physiological dependence (as primarily indicated by the symptom of tolerance). Because unhealthy substance use by adolescents is so clearly associated with problems in a wide range of related psychosocial domains, any attempt to stratify severity and treatment needs also must take these into account and not consider substance use alone. This work also demonstrated that patients referred to inpatient treatment based on the ASAM criteria had greater severity on measures of health problems, a variety of mental health symptoms, and conduct problems.

Finally, Dennis et al. developed a profile approximating the ASAM assessment dimensions, using calculated subscales from a highly reliable standardized assessment instrument (the Global Appraisal of Individual Needs—[GAIN]). In a retrospective comparison, this standardized research ASAM profile also supported the discrimination of severity and the placement decisions made by clinicians who used their own non-standardized intake assessments and the ASAM criteria.[33]

To date, there is no clear empirical evidence of the effectiveness of adolescent placement- or treatment-matching criteria based on treatment outcome data. However, there are encouraging preliminary indications that case-mix adjustments based on the ASAM criteria can help explain a considerable amount of the variance in treatment outcomes for different levels of care.[34] These indications suggest that the ASAM criteria, when refined and better operationalized, might in fact lead to predictors of treatment response. There also is work underway to use models of adherence to the ASAM criteria to determine retrospectively whether "appropriate" level of care placements leads to better outcomes.

Dennis' group has refined and expanded its ASAM criteria assessment profile based on the GAIN[35] into a computer-generated clinical tool that has proven useful in practice for approximating and highlighting treatment-matching needs. Consensus development of computerized algorithmic decision rules based on the GAIN is currently being implemented as an expansion of that tool[36] and will be the subject of future testing and research. The profile of level of care treatment matching is also highlighted by work showing differential patterns of treatment outcomes at different levels of care in community settings.[37] Along with a general endorsement of the effectiveness of community treatment, this profile begins to show the effectiveness of level of care sorting with higher-severity adolescents appropriately sorted into residential treatment, and their outcomes at 12 months show improvements with severity measures reduced and stabilized at the levels of outpatients. The computerized version of the ASAM criteria Continuum does not yet have an adolescent version.

CONCLUSIONS

At present, the adolescent population is significantly underserved, with fewer than 10% of adolescents who exhibit symptoms of problem drug use in the preceding year ever having received formal treatment.[13] It is hoped that the use of organized assessment tools, such as the ASAM Criteria, that employ gradations of severity and risk to guide treatment-matching and placement decisions will help to encourage the creation of adequate treatment resources.

The field is in need of valid assessment instruments, further operationalization of gradations of severity and risk and research to support the effectiveness of treatment matching. At the same time, it is important to resist the illusion of technique and to avoid the error of assuming that the reliability and precision of standardized instruments guarantee validity.

Treatment-matching hypotheses and practices must be refined beyond level of care to include specific interventions, services, modalities, and doses. It will be important to discern relevant subtypes that might be expected to be associated with differential treatment response within the heterogeneous population of adolescents with substance use disorders, and the validity of treatment matching will need to be demonstrated empirically.

The ASAM adolescent placement criteria continue to evolve in response to ongoing progress in the field of adolescent addiction medicine. Currently, the criteria are based predominantly on consensus best practices. As the results of additional adolescent treatment outcome research become available, future revisions of the criteria will be based increasingly on empirically verified principles of treatment matching, placement, and effectiveness. At the same time, the ASAM criteria and other clinical treatment-matching guidelines will drive research hypotheses that will lead to improved treatment and treatment access for all adolescents in need.

REFERENCES

1. Williams RJ, Chang SY; Addiction Centre Adolescent Research Group. A comprehensive and comparative review of adolescent substance abuse treatment outcome. *Clin Psychol Sci Pract.* 2000;7:138-166.
2. Hser Y, Grella CE, Hubbard RL, et al. An evaluation of drug treatment for adolescents in four U.S. cities. *Arch Gen Psychiatry.* 2001;58:689-695.
3. Winters K. Treating adolescents with substance use disorders: an overview of practice issues and treatment outcomes. *Subst Abus.* 1999;20:203-223.
4. Morral A, McCaffrey D, Ridgeway G. Effectiveness of community based treatment for substance abusing adolescents: 12-month outcomes of youths entering phoenix academy or alternative probation dispositions. *Psychol Addict Behav.* 2004;18:257-268.
5. Dennis M, Godley S, et al. The Cannabis Youth Treatment (CYT) Study: main findings from two randomized trials. *J Subst Abuse Treat.* 2004;27:197-213.
6. Muck R, Zempolich K, Titus J, Fishman M, Godley MD, Schwebel R. An overview of the effectiveness of adolescent substance abuse treatment models. *Youth Soc.* 2001;33(2):143-168.
7. Clemmey P, Payne L, Fishman M. Clinical characteristics and treatment outcomes of adolescent heroin users. *J Psychoactive Drugs.* 2004;36(1):85-94.
8. Brown SA, Myers MG, Vik PW. Correlates of success following treatment for adolescent substance abuse. *Appl Prevent Psychol.* 1994;3:61-73.
9. Tanner-Smith EE, Wilson SJ, Lipsey MW. The comparative effectiveness of outpatient treatment for adolescent substance abuse: a meta-analysis. *J Subst Abuse Treat.* 2013;44(2):145-158. doi:10.1016/j.jsat.2012.05.006
10. Dennis M, Dowud-Noursi S, Muck R, et al. The need for developing and evaluating adolescent treatment models. In: Stevens S, Morral A, eds. *Adolescent Substance Abuse Treatment in the United States: Exemplary Models from a National Evaluation Study.* Haworth Press; 2002.
11. Gastfriend DR, McLellan AT. Placement matching: theoretic basis and practical implications. *Med Clin North Am.* 1997;81:945-966.
12. Gastfriend D, ed. *Addiction Treatment Matching: Research Foundations of the American Society of Addiction Medicine (ASAM) Patient Placement Criteria.* Haworth Press; 2003.
13. Fishman M, Wenzel K, Scodes J, et al. Young adults have worse outcomes than older adults: secondary analysis of a medication trial for opioid use disorder. *J Adolesc Health.* 2020;67:778-785.
14. MeeLee D, Shulman GD, Fishman M, Gastfriend D, Miller M, eds. *The ASAM Criteria: Treatment Criteria for Addictive, Substance-Related, and Co-Occurring Conditions.* 3rd ed. The Change Companies; 2014.
15. Hunter BD, Godley MD, Godley SH. Feasibility of implementing the Adolescent Community Reinforcement Approach in school settings for adolescents with substance use disorders. *Adv School Mental Health Promot.* 2014;7:105-122.
16. Dennis M, McGeary K. Adolescent alcohol and marijuana treatment: kids need it now. *TIE Communique.* Substance Abuse and Mental Health Services Administration, Center for Substance Abuse Treatment; 1999.
17. Clark DB, Kirisci Tarter RE. Adolescent versus adult onset and the development of substance use disorders in males. *Drug Alcohol Depend.* 1998;49(2):115-121.
18. Fishman M. The relationship between substance use disorders and psychiatric comorbidity: implications for integrated health services. In: Kaminer Y, Buckstein O, eds. *Youth Substance Abuse and Co-Occurring Disorders.* APPI; 2015.
19. Kandel DB, Johnson JG, Bird HR, et al. Psychiatric disorders associated with substance use among children and adolescents: findings from the Methods for Epidemiology of Child and Adolescent Mental Disorders (MECA) study. *J Abnorm Child Psychol.* 1997;25:121-132.
20. Riggs PD, Mikulich-Gilbertson SK, Davies RD, Lohman M, Klein C, Stover SK. A randomized controlled trial of fluoxetine and cognitive behavioral therapy in adolescents with major depression, behavior problems, and substance use disorders. *Arch Pediatr Adolesc Med.* 2007;161(11):1026-1034. doi:10.1001/archpedi.161.11.1026
21. Gage SH, Munafò MR, MacLeod J, Hickman M, Smith GD. Cannabis and psychosis. *Lancet Psychiatry.* 2015;2(5):380. doi:10.1016/S2215-0366(15)00108-X

22. Kedzior KK, Laeber LT. A positive association between anxiety disorders and cannabis use or cannabis use disorders in the general population—a meta-analysis of 31 studies. *BMC Psychiatry.* 2014;14:136. doi:10.1186/1471-244X-14-136
23. Hops HA, Davis B, Lewin LM. The development of alcohol and other substance use: a gender study of family and peer context. *J Stud Alcohol Suppl.* 1999;13:22-31.
24. Tapert SF, Baratta BS, Abrantes BA, Brown SA. Attention dysfunction predicts substance involvement in community youth. *J Am Acad Child Adolesc Psychiatry.* 2002;41(6):690-686.
25. Deas D, Riggs P, Langenbucher J, Goldman M, Brown S. Adolescents are not adults: developmental considerations in alcohol users. *Alcohol Clin Exp Res.* 2000;24:232-237.
26. Colby SM, Monti PM, Barnett NP, et al. Brief motivational interviewing in a hospital setting for adolescent smoking: a preliminary study. *J Consult Clin Psychol.* 1998;66:574-578.
27. Sampl S, Kadden R. Motivational enhancement therapy and cognitive behavioral therapy for adolescent cannabis users: 5 sessions. *Cannabis Youth Treatment (CYT) Series.* Vol. 1. Center for Substance Abuse Treatment, Substance Abuse and Mental Health Services Administration; 2001.
28. Onrust SA, Otten R, Lammers J, Smit F. School-based programmes to reduce and prevent substance use in different age groups: what works for whom? Systematic review and meta-regression analysis. *Clin Psychol Rev.* 2016;44:45-59. doi:10.1016/j.cpr.2015.11.002
29. Brown S. Facilitating change for adolescent alcohol problems; a multiple options approach. In: Wagner E, Waldron H, eds. *Innovations in Adolescent Substance Abuse Interventions.* Pergamon; 2001:169-188.
30. Liddle HA, Hogue A. Multidimensional family therapy for adolescent substance abuse. In: Wagner E, Waldron H, eds. *Innovations in Adolescent Substance Abuse Interventions.* Pergamon; 2001:229-261.
31. Center for Substance Abuse Treatment. Treatment of adolescents with substance use disorders. *Treatment Improvement Protocol (TIP) Series 32.* SAMHSA; 1999.
32. Godley SH, Godley MD, Dennis ML. Assertive aftercare protocol for adolescent substance abusers. In: Wagner E, Waldron H, eds. *Innovations in Adolescent Substance Abuse Interventions.* Pergamon; 2001:313-331.
33. Dennis M, Funk R, McDermeit M, et al. Towards better placement and case mix adjustments in adolescent and adult substance abuse treatment systems. *Presented at the 8th International Conference on Treatment of Addictive Behavior.* Santa Fe, NM; January 1988.
34. Dennis M, Scott C, Godley M, et al. Predicting outcomes in adult and adolescent treatment with case mix vs. level of care: findings from the drug outcome monitoring study. *Presentation at the College on Problems of Drug Dependence.* San Juan, PR; June 2000.
35. Dennis M, White M, Titus J, Unsicker J. *Global Appraisal of Individual Needs: Administration Guide for the GAIN and Related Measures.* Sec 6. https://chestnut.app.box.com/v/GAIN-I-Materials/file/63671257181
36. Stevens L, Dennis M, Fishman M. Using the new GAIN patient placement summary to support individual treatment planning, placement and program evaluation. *Workshop at the Joint Meeting on Adolescent Treatment Effectiveness.* Baltimore, MD; March 28, 2006.
37. Dasinger L, Shane P, Martinovich Z. Assessing the effectiveness of community-based substance abuse treatment for adolescents. *J Psychoactive Drugs.* 2004;36(1):85-94.

Sidebar 1

Confidentiality in Caring for Adolescents

Connor J. Buchholz and Scott E. Hadland

Confidentiality is an essential component of health care for adolescents. Without some promise of confidentiality at the beginning of an office visit, the adolescent patient is less likely to disclose information about his or her behaviors, particularly concerning sensitive topics such as sexual activity or substance use. On the other hand, the clinician who promises unconditional confidentiality ("everything you tell me will be kept private") may find himself or herself party to information that he or she has promised not to reveal but that, if allowed to continue without disclosure, could jeopardize the health of the adolescent. For example, a teen who regularly drinks and drives is at risk of harming themselves or others, and disclosure to a parent or caregiver could be critical to addressing this risk. Health care professionals must understand the key principles underlying confidentiality and its limits.

Protection of confidentiality is a commitment to respect the dignity of patients. The promise of confidential care increases the likelihood that patients will seek care and offer frank disclosures of health concerns. Both are especially important in the care of adolescents, who are seeking autonomy and learning to make appropriate decisions about a variety of issues, including healthy behaviors and seeking health care. Research has suggested that most adolescents (age 14-18) demonstrate moral–psychological development similar enough to adults to be consistent with adequate capacity for decision-making.[1]

By providing a confidential setting in which adolescents can discuss their concerns, particularly ones they view as sensitive and/or embarrassing or wish to keep private from parents, clinicians help support this critical developmental process. However, more recent work on the neurodevelopment and neurophysiology of adolescence emphasizes that adolescent decision-making is not the same as adult decision-making. Adolescents may have less capacity to incorporate long-term outcomes into decisions, incompletely developed impulse control, which has potential to improve with age, and heightened reactivity to stress.[2-4]

Confidential care for adolescents, then, requires the provider to evaluate individual capacity for specific decisions.

RESEARCH INTO CONFIDENTIALITY ISSUES

Much of the research related to confidentiality and adolescents focuses on the importance of confidentiality as a necessary condition for optimizing adolescents' access to effective care. More than two decades of research demonstrates how much value adolescents place on confidentiality. Carroll et al.[5] reported via a systematic review of adolescents' views on school health services that disclosure and confidentiality are key themes in willingness to use available services. Cheng et al.[6] surveyed high school students and found that more than half had health concerns they wished to keep private from their parents, and that more than half would not access a familiar medical provider for issues they wished to keep private. Britto et al.[7] identified the complexity with which adolescents view privacy in clinical care. In addition to informational privacy or traditional confidentiality, adolescents reported concern about psychological privacy and a reluctance to discuss personal behaviors if a provider appeared judgmental.

Ford,[8] in a classic study, used simulated office visits to explore adolescents' views about confidentiality. Adolescents were randomized to listen to one of three standardized audiotape depictions of an office visit. On one tape, the physician promised unconditional confidentiality; on another, he or she promised conditional confidentiality; and on the third, confidentiality was not discussed. Assurances of confidentiality significantly increased the percentage of teenagers who were willing to disclose information about their sexual behaviors, drug use, and mental health concerns, and increased the percentage who were willing to seek future health care; this was true whether the confidentiality assured was conditional or unconditional. These studies affirm the importance of confidentiality for adolescents: many adolescents will not seek health care for sensitive issues unless their complex expectations of privacy are granted, though absolute confidentiality is not necessary. Furthermore, another study showed that adolescents with the greatest numbers of risk factors—hence, the ones perhaps most in need of support—are most likely to cite confidentiality concerns as a reason for forgoing health care.[9] In this study, both boys and girls who cited confidentiality as a concern were more likely to report poor parental communication, endorse higher levels of depressive symptoms, endorse suicidal ideation and attempts, and girls were also more likely to report unprotected sex, or use alcohol. Failing to ensure confidentiality increases the risk of adolescents' delaying seeking or not receiving care until serious consequences arise, while offering nuanced conditional confidentiality may signal respect for agency.

POLICIES ON CONFIDENTIALITY

Physicians' professional organizations long have supported the concept of confidential care for adolescents. In 1967, the American Medical Association adopted a position that the epidemic of sexually transmitted diseases among young people required that minors be able to receive treatment for those infections without parental notification.[10] The American Academy of Pediatrics, the Society for Adolescent Health and Medicine, the National Medical Association, the American College of Obstetricians and Gynecologists, and the American Academy of Family Physicians have jointly endorsed recommendations on confidentiality, concluding that "ultimately, the health risks to adolescents are so impelling that legal barriers and deference to parental involvement should not stand in the way of needed care."[11]

The Health Insurance Portability and Accountability Act and its accompanying Privacy Rule (2001) protect adolescents as much as adults. Adolescents who are legally able to consent to care are generally treated by the Privacy Rule as protected in their own right. The Privacy Rule defers to "state or other applicable law" in terms of parents having access to their children's health information.[12] As most states grant adolescents the right to seek confidential care, the Health Insurance Portability and Accountability Act broadly supports confidentiality. The American Academy of Pediatrics recent policy statement "Achieving Quality Healthcare for Adolescents"[13] "*offers specific health recommendations for health information and the medical home to promote confidentiality, continuity of care, patient-care transitions, and overall quality of care. These include criteria for electronic health records that encompass flexibility and specific technological capabilities and are compatible with state-specific laws as well as billing systems.*" However, the specifics of confidentiality protection vary from state to state; hence, clinicians must be knowledgeable about their own state's regulations.[14]

DECIDING WHEN DISCLOSURE IS NECESSARY

How then to handle a situation in which an adolescent discloses information that the clinician believes poses a serious threat to the health of the adolescent? Is it permissible to break confidentiality under these circumstances? Is the clinician required to do so?

Most experts do not recommend a blanket or unconditional assurance of confidentiality, and indeed, disclosure is mandated by law in certain circumstances. These typically include but may not be limited to reports of sexual or physical abuse perpetrated either on the adolescent minor or by the adolescent to another minor, or immediate risk of suicide or homicide against a readily identifiable individual. In such circumstances, clinicians must work to balance the competing duties to respect the (developing) autonomy of an adolescent patient and to avoid harm. In some cases, obeying legal duties to report threats of violence carry considerable weight as well.

In anticipation of situations such as these, most experts in adolescent health recommend a preventive ethics approach and suggest statements that offer *conditional* confidentiality. Using this approach, the adolescent is assured that most information revealed to the physician will be kept private, but he or she is cautioned that there are some limits to these assurances. One sample statement, developed by the American Medical Association's Department of Adolescent Health, is as follows: "I want to assure you that the information we discuss today is between you and me. It's confidential. In other words, I am not going to tell anyone without your permission, unless there is a situation which I believe might threaten your life or another's life or seriously endanger your health."[15] However, research suggests that adolescents prefer more specific descriptions of what kinds of discussions will be held confidential.[16] Additionally, documentation by a clinician in the medical record may be read by others; adolescents may not be aware that this information is available to other health care providers and should be informed of this.

Regardless of the exact assurance that the clinician offers, it ultimately rests with his or her judgment as to whether and when a given adolescent's behavior poses a level of risk that warrants a breach of confidentiality. In such cases, the clinician must perform a sufficiently comprehensive assessment to understand how the behavior poses a threat to the adolescent's health. An assessment of the adolescent's capacity for decision-making specific to the question at hand is also advised.

It is important to note that the clinician's belief that a given behavior is wrong in the context of the clinician's own personal, moral, or religious code is not sufficient justification for breaking confidentiality. For example, a personal belief that premarital sex is wrong would not justify disclosing to a parent that an adolescent is sexually active. On the other hand, if an adolescent discloses smoking cannabis but is doing well in school, maintains good relations with his or her parents, and never drives or attends school while "high," then that behavior does not warrant disclosure even if a health care provider believes that cannabis use is unhealthy.

Even if the clinician concludes that an adolescent's behavior is sufficiently risky to warrant parental involvement, immediate disclosure is not necessarily indicated. The clinician might first discuss his or her concerns with the adolescent and develop a plan whereby the adolescent can demonstrate a change in the risky behavior. An example would be asking an adolescent who is using cannabis and leaving the house late at night (a potential, though perhaps not immediate, safety concern) to refrain from smoking for several weeks. In advance, the adolescent would be told that if they continue to use, the clinician will disclose their concerns to a parent or caregiver after this period of time.

After a clinician concludes that a breach of confidentiality is warranted, the adolescent should be told in advance and given options about how the disclosure will occur. These might include the adolescent revealing the information to his or her parents in the presence of the clinician, the adolescent telling the parents alone, or the clinician disclosing the information to the parents. In some cases, an adolescent may request that one but not both parents be involved. If the adolescent agrees to informing parents without the clinician present, clinician follow up with a parent to ensure that safety information has been transmitted clearly and accurately is recommended.

SPECIAL CIRCUMSTANCES

The foregoing discussion pertains to typical clinical encounters. In some special circumstances, different rules of confidentiality may apply. For example, the interaction between the adolescent and clinician may be ordered by a court or required as a condition of return to school. Federal and state regulations also may stipulate conditions of confidentiality for adolescents in drug treatment programs. Under these circumstances, the adolescent, the parents, and the clinician should be clear about the nature of the physician-patient relationship, including the boundaries of confidentiality and who will have access to the adolescent's medical record, including any test results.

FAMILY INVOLVEMENT

While allowing adolescents privacy and confidentiality in medical settings is crucial, working with adolescents to bring in parents (or other legal caregivers) for support when possible is also important. Family therapies are among the most effective for mental and behavioral health problems, including substance use disorders. Furthermore, parents can help their children navigate complex treatment systems by helping with scheduling, transportation, filling prescriptions, and navigating insurance. If an adolescent initially asks to exclude their parent from treatment, exploring reasons why can help guide their care plan. For example, an adolescent who seeks treatment for a substance use disorder may not want their parents to know because they fear disclosure may result in physical violence, or because they worry that parents will be disappointed in them. The recommended clinical approach in each of these situations would be very different. The first case requires further exploration of the household dynamics and possibly mandated reporting. In the second circumstance, offering to assist the adolescent to invite a parent into a supportive role may be very helpful and can be considered a treatment goal that can be attained in partnership with the adolescent rather than a breach of confidentiality.

ACKNOWLEDGEMENT

This chapter represents an update and revision of previous chapters in this series, most recently by Dr Margaret Moon from the last edition. We are indebted to Dr Moon for her work and retain much of her prose in this current edition.

REFERENCES

1. Raymundo MM, Goldim JR. Moral-psychological development related to the capacity of adolescents and elderly patients to consent. *J Med Ethics*. 2008;34(8):602-605.
2. Uy JP, Galván A. Acute stress increases risky decisions and dampens prefrontal activation among adolescent boys. *NeuroImage*. 2017;146:679-689.
3. Lorenz C, Kray J. Are mid-adolescents prone to risky decisions? The influence of task setting and individual differences in temperament. *Front Psychol*. 2019;10:1497.

4. Salter EK. Conflating capacity & authority: why we're asking the wrong question in the adolescent decision-making debate. *Hastings Cent Rep.* 2017;47(1):32-41.
5. Carroll C, Lloyd-Jones M, Cooke J, Owen J. Reasons for the use and non-use of school sexual health services: a systematic review of young people's views. *J Public Health.* 2012;34(3):403-410.
6. Cheng TL. Confidentiality in health care. A survey of knowledge, perceptions, and attitudes among high school students. *JAMA.* 1993;269(11):1404-1407.
7. Britto MT, Tivorsak TL, Slap GB. Adolescents' needs for health care privacy. *Pediatrics.* 2010;126(6):e1469-e1476.
8. Ford CA, Millstein SG, Halpern-Felsher BL, Irwin CE. Influence of physician confidentiality assurances on adolescents' willingness to disclose information and seek future health care. A randomized controlled trial. JAMA. 1997;278(12):1029-1034.
9. Lehrer JA, Pantell R, Tebb K, Shafer MA. Forgone health care among U.S. adolescents: associations between risk characteristics and confidentiality concern. *J Adolesc Health.* 2007;40(3):218-226.
10. Coble YD. Confidential health services for adolescents. *JAMA.* 1993;269(11):1420.
11. Confidentiality in Adolescent Health Care: ACOG Committee Opinion, Number 803. *Obstet Gynecol.* 2020;135(4):e171-e177.
12. *Summary of the HIPAA Privacy Rule.* Accessed July 27, 2023. http://www.hhs.gov/sites/default/files/privacysummary.pdf
13. Adolescence CO, Adelman W, Braverman PK, et al. Achieving quality health services for adolescents. *Pediatrics.* 2016;138(2):e20161347.
14. Tebb KP, Sedlander E, Pica G, Diaz A, Peake K, Brindis CD. *Protecting Adolescent Confidentiality Under Health Care Reform: The Special Case Regarding Explanation of Benefits (EOBs).* Philip R. Lee Institute for Healthy Policy Studies and Division of Adolescent and Young Adult Medicine, Department of Pediatrics, University of California, San Francisco. Accessed July 27, 2023. https://www.hivlawandpolicy.org/sites/default/files/EOB%20Policy%20Brief-%20Protecting%20Adolescent%20Confidentiality%20Under%20Health%20Care%20Reform.pdf
15. Levenberg PB, Elster AB. *Guidelines for Adolescent Preventive Services (GAPS): Clinical Evaluation and Management Handbook.* American Medical Association, Dept. of Adolescent Health; 1995.
16. Ford CA, Thomsen SL, Compton B. Adolescents' interpretations of conditional confidentiality assurances. *J Adolesc Health.* 2001;29(3): 156159.

Sidebar 2

Drug Testing Adolescents in School

J. Wesley Boyd and John R. Knight

BACKGROUND

Efforts to intervene with adolescents who are using substances are an important part of health care given that substance use is associated with increased mortality and numerous adverse health and behavioral outcomes.[1] Several intervention efforts have focused on schools. During the George W. Bush presidential administration, the White House encouraged public schools to drug test students and exclude those who tested positive from participating in varsity sports and other high school activities.[2] This recommendation engendered significant debate among medical, legal and ethical communities. The American Academy of Pediatrics multiple policy statements on school drug testing have all concluded that mandatory drug testing in schools is both ineffective and ethically perilous, given that it could cause more harm than good.[3-5] Here, we review mandatory school drug testing with respect to the four basic bioethical principles: beneficence, nonmaleficence, autonomy, and justice.[6]

Beneficence

Beneficence refers to actions that promote the well-being of others. If mandatory school drug testing decreases student drug use, then it would promote beneficence for reasons of general health and school performance. Several experimental studies have examined the impact of mandatory drug testing policies on student drug use. While results have been mixed, there is no evidence that school-based drug testing has long-term positive effects on student drug use. A large study that used nationally representative survey data from schools (Youth, Education, and Society) and students (Monitoring the Future) found that drug testing was not associated with students' reported substance use.[7]

Nonmaleficence

The principle of nonmaleficence refers to the obligation not to harm others and/or to prevent harm from being done. The AAP has detailed potential harms associated with school drug testing. First, students might see the school environment as hostile and punitive, potentially leading to higher rates of drop out. Second, all laboratory testing, and drug testing in particular,[8] has the potential for false positive and false negative results. False positive drug tests could result in inappropriate consequences while false negative results could inappropriately reassure adults and inadvertently facilitate ongoing drug use. Finally, some adolescents who are subject to drug testing may risk harm by using dangerous substances that are not included on testing panels, or ingest toxic substances in an effort to adulterate a urine sample. Harms associated with student drug testing have not been rigorously studied, though the extent of potential harms calls for extreme caution.

Autonomy

Honoring the principle of autonomy is a moving target when it comes to adolescents, given that the amount of autonomy a youth ought to be granted varies depending on the individual's mental capacity and age. The principle of autonomy suggests that individuals should be able to choose for themselves whether they use drugs or not, and some might argue that, especially as they approached adulthood, adolescents ought to be free to choose to use intoxicating substances to some degree without harsh repercussions. Of course, given the downstream negative impact of even modest drug use on psychological functioning, advocating for autonomy in this way seems naive—to put it mildly—and needs to be balanced with promoting nonmaleficence.

The principle of autonomy comes into play in other ways as well. For example, a compelling argument can be made that even if adolescents choose to use drugs, they should not be prohibited from autonomously choosing to participate in sports or to attend school. Given that adolescents make many decisions that are not in their best interests, why should drug use in particular be the sole factor that prohibits these individuals from participating in sports or being able to attend school more generally? Why not, for example, exclude youth who smoke tobacco or overeat instead of those who use illicit substances? We do not believe that a compelling argument can be made for why substance use ought to be singled out for harsh consequences among youths.

Justice

Justice refers to fair and equitable treatment. Some schools have instituted "zero tolerance policies" that ban students who test positive for substances from extracurricular activities or suspend them from school. Instead of banning such students from extracurricular activities, justice would be better served by considering substance use as a health problem, and referring students who are identified as using substances for assessment and therapeutic intervention. This is particularly true for minority youth because educators are less likely to tolerate substance use related misconduct from minority youth and more likely to respond in ways that jeopardize a youth's future,[9] as evidenced by the dramatic over representation of Black youth referred to U.S. juvenile courts.[10] Thus, any policy that institutes punishments for drug use must be scrutinized through the lens of justice.

CONCLUSION

While school drug testing may be a well-intentioned effort to address a serious behavioral health problem, it is ethically perilous because of the potential for harms. Punishing students who use substances by excluding them from school or extracurricular activities—or reporting them to legal authorities—is not in the best interest of the student or the school community. Finding alternative methods of preventing substance use and identifying students with substance use problems is vitally needed.

REFERENCES

1. National Institutes of Health. *Percentage of adolescents reporting drug use decreased significantly in 2021 as the COVID-19 pandemic endured.* Accessed August 31, 2023. https://www.nih.gov/news-events/news-releases/percentage-adolescents-reporting-drug-use-decreased-significantly-2021-covid-19-pandemic-endured
2. Office of National Drug Control Policy. *What You Need to Know About Drug Testing in Schools.* U.S. Government Printing Office; 2002.
3. Knight JR, Mears CJ; Committee on Substance Abuse, Council on School Health, American Academy of Pediatrics. Testing for drugs of abuse in children and adolescents: addendum—testing in schools and at home. *Pediatrics.* 2007;119(3):627-630.
4. Mears CJ, Knight JR; Council on School Health, Committee on Substance Abuse, American Academy of Pediatrics. The role of schools in combating illicit substance abuse. *Pediatrics.* 2007;120(6):1379-1384.
5. Levy S, Schizer M, Ammerman SD; Committee on Substance Abuse, American Academy of Pediatrics. Adolescent drug testing policies in schools. *Pediatrics.* 2015;135(4):e1107-e1112.
6. Beauchamp TL, Childress JF. *Principles of Biomedical Ethics.* 6th ed. Oxford University Press; 2008.
7. Yamaguchi R, Johnston LD, O'Malley PM. Relationship between student illicit drug use and school drug-testing policies. *J School Health.* 2003;73:159-164. doi:10.1111/j.1746-1561.2003.tb03596.x
8. Moeller KE, Kissack JC, Atayee RS, Lee KC. Clinical interpretation of urine drug tests: what clinicians need to know about urine drug screens. *Mayo Clin Proc.* 2017;92(5):774-796.
9. Simon KM. Them and me — the care and treatment of black boys in America. *N Engl J Med.* 2020;383(20):1904-1905.
10. Office of Juvenile Justice and Delinquency Prevention. *Juvenile Court Statistics, 2018.* Accessed January 23, 2022. https://ojjdp.ojp.gov/library/publications/juvenile-court-statistics-2018

CHAPTER

119 Treating Substance Use Disorders in Carceral-Involved Youth

Kevin M. Simon

CHAPTER OUTLINE

- The "criminal justice" system
- Introduction
- Shared risk factors for substance use and carceral involvement
- Outcomes of youth with substance use and carceral system involvement
- Screening and assessment within juvenile carceral system
- Substance use disorder screening tools for carceral-involved youth
- Interventions for carceral-involved youth with substance use disorders
- Challenges providing substance use disorder interventions to carceral-involved youth
- An overlooked crowd: transitional age youth
- Summary

THE "CRIMINAL JUSTICE" SYSTEM

The criminal justice system is not *just*. It is, in fact, demonstrably unjust as to whom it criminalizes. This reality has prompted a shift in actively referring to it as the *carceral system*, which is the nomenclature used throughout this chapter. While much of the information presented in other chapters of this text also applies to carceral-involved youth (CIY), health care professionals who focus on youth should be aware of the distinctive characteristics and needs of CIY. This chapter discusses shared risk factors for substance use disorders (SUD) among youth involved in the carceral system, outcomes for these high-risk youth, the importance of universal substance use screening, the assessment process, and possible interventions for CIY; unique intervention challenges, and the often-overlooked population of transitional age youth within juvenile carceral systems. Understanding the experiences of CIY, specifically those within the system, can help clinicians better meet the needs of these youth when they are back in the community and with their families. Understanding carceral system health care can also enhance practitioners' ability to advocate for public policies that advance youth rehabilitation during and following juvenile carceral system involvement.

INTRODUCTION

The intersection of substance use disorders and carceral involvement among youth presents a complex and multifaceted challenge for healthcare providers. Despite a substantial decline in arrests of persons under 18, with an estimated 424,300 arrests made in 2020 compared to 2011, a considerable number of youth remain involved in the carceral system.[1-3] Approximately two thirds of CIY are children of color and are disproportionately represented in the carceral system.[4] CIY are likelier than noninvolved youth to have co-occurring disorders (ie, a mental health condition and co-occurring substance use/disorder).[5,6] Among adjudicated youth, approximately two-thirds report a history of substance use, and over one-third meet DSM criteria for a SUD.[7,8] Conversely, one study found that 58% of youth receiving substance use treatment were involved in the carceral system.[9]

The circumstances in which youth live, or the social and political determinants of health, including food, housing, income security, and access to education and health, strongly contribute to their health status.[10] In addition to high rates of substance use, CIY have are more likely to face other challenges that differentiate them from non-CIY. For instance, CIY are more likely than peers to have learning disabilities and school failure. As a group, CIY tend to have academic deficits in math, reading, and language due to either learning disabilities or other educational risk factors (eg, negative attitudes toward school, frequent school transitions, low academic aspirations, suspensions, and expulsions).[11] In a study of CIY ages 10 to 20, nearly 20% had a specific learning disability, and youth with mental health symptoms were even more likely to have learning problems.[12] CIY also have high rates of involvement with the child welfare system. More than half of youth considered "serious offenders" (viewed as one who has at least one recorded offense that inflicted substantial harm or one who has an official record containing offenses that cumulatively involve the infliction of substantial harm) in juvenile detention have a history of child welfare involvement due to child maltreatment.[13,14] Youth with a substantiated history of maltreatment have about 50% more contact with the juvenile carceral system compared to youth with such a history, and approximately 16% of youth placed in foster care engage with the juvenile carceral system.[15,16]

SHARED RISK FACTORS FOR SUBSTANCE USE AND CARCERAL INVOLVEMENT

Risk factors are those predictors associated with an increased likelihood of problematic substance use or other behavioral disorders. Risk factors for SUDs among CIY encompass individual-level measures (eg, genetics), social environment including family (eg, conflict), school (eg, school failure), friends (eg, negative peer pressure), and their community (eg, neighborhood distress and availability of substances). Many risk factors for problematic substance use are etiological risk factors for other problems, including carceral involvement. Because they predict future issues, malleable risk factors are potential targets for prevention.

The link between adolescent substance use and juvenile delinquency is complex. Given the high rates of reported substance use among CIY, it is unsurprising that for many, shared risk factors interact and increase adverse outcomes. These risk factors exist throughout a youth's development. At an individual level, mental health conditions like externalizing disorders (eg, oppositional defiant disorder), learning disabilities, and ADHD are associated with both substance use and juvenile carceral involvement.[17,18] Youth who initiate substance use early are more likely to develop SUDs and more likely to have carceral involvement.[19] Another shared risk factor for substance use and SUD and carceral involvement is childhood trauma. CIY experience violent victimization and trauma at higher rates than any other youth population.[20,21] One study of detained youth found that the majority (93%) reported at least one traumatic experience, most reported more than one (84%), and youth with trauma-related mental health disorders were more likely to have a SUD.[6,21,22]

At the family level, low parental attachment, low income, high family conflict, and use corporal punishment are associated with substance use and carceral involvement.[21,23,24] Involvement in the foster care system and child welfare services are known risk factors for both.[13,14] Siblings and peers who are substance involved or use substances increases a youth's risk of developing a SUD and contact with the carceral system. At the community level, poor quality schools, neighborhood poverty, substance availability, exposure to community violence, and racial prejudice show a link to both outcomes.[25,26]

Evidence shows that observable treatment barriers and biases in identification exist for substance use problems in the carceral system. Specifically, the rates of referral to and receipt of substance use services among CIY depend on specific youth characteristics rather than solely on service needs. For instance, minority youth are less likely to be referred to substance use treatment.[27,28] These disparities likely worsen other racial disparities, such as higher rates of minority youth in the carceral system and lower mental health and substance use treatment access for them, regardless of their involvement in the carceral system.[29]

Given the significant evidence linking social determinants to mental health outcomes, it is essential to implement multilevel interventions that address systemic social inequalities in areas such as access to education and employment opportunities, healthy food, secure housing, and safe neighborhoods.

OUTCOMES OF YOUTH WITH SUBSTANCE USE AND CARCERAL SYSTEM INVOLVEMENT

Youth with substance use problems and SUDs who are not in treatment are more likely to engage in crimes and violence and consequently come into contact with the carceral system more than their nonsubstance-engaged peers.[13,30] These youth also have more severe delinquent behavior and recidivate (reengaging criminal activity) more frequently, both as youth and during adulthood, compared with CIY without substance use problems.[31] CIY who use substances fair worse across educational, occupational, and health outcomes and are at a heightened risk of contracting HIV and other sexually transmitted infections.[32,33] Many of these youth are diagnosed with multiple mental and behavioral health disorders, in addition to SUDs.[5,27,34]

SCREENING AND ASSESSMENT WITHIN JUVENILE CARCERAL SYSTEM

Over the past decade, substance use and SUD assessment have gained traction, and most states have implemented screening and assessment procedures within juvenile carceral programs.[35]

The carceral system prioritizes public safety, so assessments typically focus on identifying risk factors that professionals can address through treatment or programming to reduce the likelihood of recurrence of substance use. Screening and evaluations can occur at any stage during involvement in the carceral system, and the results serve various purposes, such as determining the suitability for diversion programming, deciding placement during sentencing, or defining the frequency of community supervision. It is crucial to distinguish between "screening" and "assessment," which, although often used interchangeably, refer to two different processes. Assessment collects more extensive information when a screen positively identifies a potential problem or risk. Earlier chapters provide detail on screening and assessment tools for substance use problems. Below, we highlight tools developed explicitly for CIY.

SUBSTANCE USE DISORDER SCREENING TOOLS FOR CARCERAL-INVOLVED YOUTH

Massachusetts Youth Screening Instrument

The Massachusetts Youth Screening Instrument—Second Version (MAYSI-2), is a 52-item (5-10 minutes) screening tool designed especially for juvenile carceral system programs and facilities.[35-37] The MAYSI-2 aims to identify alcohol, drug use, mental health needs, and emotional disturbances in youths 12 through 17 years. Administering and using the MAYSI-2 requires does not require professional training provided the user follows proper administration guidance in the MAYSI-2 manual. The questions ask the youth to answer YES or NO to having experienced various thoughts, feelings, or behaviors in the past few months. The measure provides cut-offs for "Caution" (indicating "possible clinical significance") and "Warning" (indicating, "the youth has scored exceptionally high in comparison to other youths in the juvenile carceral system"). The caution/warning cut-off scores are 4/7 (alcohol/drug use), 5/8 (angry/irritable), 3/6 (depressed/anxious), 3/6 (somatic complaints), 2/3 (suicidal ideation), and 1/2 (thought disturbance). The MAYSI-2 comes with computer software that can read questions aloud to youth. The MAYSI-2 is the most widely used screening tool for behavioral health needs in detention centers when the state requires mental health screening.[38]

Youth Level of Service/Case Management Inventory

The Youth Level of Service/Case Management Inventory 2.0™ (YLS/CMI 2.0/CMI 2.0™) is a risk/needs assessment and a case management tool combined into one convenient system.[39] The YLS is a valid and reliable risk instrument that assesses the risk for recidivism (re-engaging in criminal activity) by measuring 42 risk/need factors over the following eight domains: prior and current offenses, family circumstances/parenting, education/employment, peer relations, substance use, leisure/recreation, personality/behavior, and attitudes/orientation.

Youth Assessment and Screening Instrument

The Youth Assessment and Screening Instrument (YASI) includes a 33-item prescreen and 88-item full assessment of risk, needs, and strengths among CIY.[40,41] The prescreen classifies risk and protective factors as low, moderate, or high. A positive screen of moderate or high risk warrants a thorough professional assessment. The assessment evaluates ten domains: (1) legal history, (2) family history, (3) education, (4) community and peers, (5) alcohol and substances, (6) mental health, (7) aggression and violence, (8) attitude, (9) skills, and (10) employment and use of free time. The YASI includes a review of the official criminal record, a semistructured interview with the youth, and information gathering from key informants (eg, parents/guardians, police, and school officials). The YASI recommends specific treatment options based on each youth's needs and guides case management planning.

Structured Assessment and Screening Instrument

The Structured Assessment and Screening Instrument (SAVRY) is composed of 24 items (10-15 minutes) in three risk domains (historical risk factors, social/contextual risk factors, and individual/clinical factors), drawn from existing research and the professional literature on adolescent development as well as on violence and aggression in youth 12 to 18 years,[42-44] and six protective factors rated as either present or absent. Each risk item has a three-level rating structure with specific rating guidelines (low, moderate, and high). Items are "critical" if deemed by the assessor to be strongly related to the youths' offending and needing immediate intervention. The SAVRY uses a structured professional judgment approach. The assessor provides the final Summary Risk Rating (low, moderate, or high) informed by the assessment items and based on professional judgment.

Juvenile probation settings typically complete risk assessments for re-offending, while screening and assessment for behavioral health problems are more common in detention and correctional facilities.[35,45] However, screening and evaluation of CIY have yielded mixed results in efforts to reduce recidivism rates. One study found that implementing a risk/needs assessment reduced formal supervision rates and recidivism, whereas substance use treatment lowered recidivism in youth with substance use problems.[46] Nevertheless, youth received similar levels of mental health services regardless of their assessed risk, and receiving mental health services did not lower the recidivism rate.[46]

INTERVENTIONS FOR CARCERAL-INVOLVED YOUTH WITH SUBSTANCE USE DISORDERS

The juvenile carceral system is the largest referral source for treating youth substance use.[47] Therefore, it is recommended that clinicians who treat adolescents who use substances or have SUDs become familiar with issues specific to CIY. Treatment has been incorporated throughout the juvenile carceral continuum in the past several decades, including detention centers, community-based supervision, juvenile drug court, and community reentry programs.[48,49] Many substance use treatment approaches discussed in previous chapters apply to CIY, while other interventions have been designed specifically for this population.

Some interventions developed for delinquent adolescents can be ineffective or even harmful. Unfortunately, some widely used programs fall into this category, such as scared straight or prison visitation programs, guided group interaction, positive peer culture, military-style programs, and wilderness challenges.[50] Programs that do not provide evidence-based treatments are more likely to have adverse effects. One reason for adverse effects is the group format, which can lead to deviant peer contagion or deviancy training. Youth exit these programs and engage in more externalizing behaviors, delinquency, and substance use.[50] Processing in the juvenile court system alone can increase the chances of future offending, partly due to exposure to other youth with access to drugs, weapons, and gang affiliations. Therefore, it is essential to consider the type of intervention and the format. While some studies suggest that substance use treatment in group formats can be effective for delinquent adolescents, it is essential to take certain precautions.[51] On the other hand, certain conditions, such as the tension between youth who committed the same crime, mandatory long prison terms, group counseling by probation officers, and younger youth being brought into contact with older delinquent youth, may increase the risk of adverse effects.[50]

Since CIY have high rates of SUD,[52] many substance use interventions discussed in previous chapters have been studied specifically with youth in the carceral system. Comprehensive reviews of substance use treatment of adolescents have yielded mixed results for CIY.[53-55] There has been mixed evidence regarding motivational interviewing (MI) and motivational enhancement therapy (MET) as stand-alone approaches for effecting long-term reductions in adolescent substance use, although they are currently best described as *probably efficacious* in treating adolescent SUD.[53,54] However, the adolescent community reinforcement approach reduced substance use more than treatment as usual among adolescents under community supervision, although this study excluded youth with violent offenses.[53]

Evidence suggests that several interventions explicitly developed for carceral populations can reduce re-offending, externalizing behaviors, and substance use. These interventions include multi-systemic therapy (MST) and functional family therapy (FFT), which are intensive family-based treatments that target risk factors at multiple levels of the youth's environment, including the individual, family, peer, and school levels.[56] Both interventions have positive findings from studies with a range of youth offenders (eg, chronic and violent juvenile offenders), outcomes (ie, substance use and delinquent behaviors), and durability of effects (ie, short-term and long-term outcomes).

Interventions developed for CIY and nonoffending youth with substance use problems often overlap. For example, juvenile drug courts were introduced in the mid-90s to divert incarceration by offering court supervision, mental health and substance use treatment, and regular monitoring. A review of juvenile drug courts failed to find overall evidence for their effectiveness, likely due to the lack of evidence-based principles employed in their management. However, studies have shown that when juvenile drug courts use evidence-based interventions such as MST and contingency management (CM), they can effectively reduce adolescent substance use and recidivism.[53]

Recently, within the juvenile drug court system, treatments such as CM, ecological family-based treatments (eg, multidimensional family therapy, FFT), and group cognitive-behavioral therapy have been evaluated separately or in combination. Overall, these treatments have been found in individual studies to reduce substance use among carceral involved use. However, a combination of ecological family-based treatments and CM, known as risk reduction therapy, was not found to improve substance use beyond the effects of juvenile drug courts and usual services.[53]

CHALLENGES PROVIDING SUBSTANCE USE DISORDER INTERVENTIONS TO CARCERAL-INVOLVED YOUTH

Despite the high rates of substance use problems among CIY, the availability of substance use treatment, particularly evidence-based treatment, is woefully limited, likely due to a variety of factors. The carceral system's top priority is public safety rather than the rehabilitation. Thus, assessment and treatment of substance use and other behavioral health needs are secondary concerns (to the carceral system) despite the evidence that successfully addressing these problems reduces recidivism and thus positively impacts public safety.[57]

Youth in the carceral system face varying degrees of access to substance use treatment and barriers to care depending on their placement. Most youths are under community supervision rather than in locked settings. Among youth processed and adjudicated by the carceral system in 2014, 26% were placed in residential settings, 63% were placed on probation, and 11% received other sanctions.[58] Despite the majority being in the community, a small percent (8.0%-16.4%) of youth receive treatment.[27] An additional issue among youth engaged in SUD treatment is a lack of familial support. Family involvement is a positive factor for treatment completion among youth.[59] Another concern is that the group format of many treatments in correctional facilities can have unintended negative consequences.[60] Finally, the lack of continuity of care for youth transitioning from treatment providers in correctional facilities to community-based providers remains an ongoing issue.

The accessibility of health care coverage for carceral-involved youth presents significant challenges, resulting in limited access to necessary services in their communities. These challenges are rooted in various factors, including inadequate health care coverage, navigating complex health care systems, and limited service providers in local communities. Due to the rarity of private health insurance among carceral-involved youth, funding for substance use treatment services often relies on alternative sources, such as federal block grants and public insurance mechanisms. While these sources offer coverage for a substantial portion of carceral-involved youth, interruption of coverage during incarceration is common. Reinstatement of coverage following release can be difficult, resulting in coverage gaps. Even when youth have adequate health coverage and the resources to navigate the health care system, some communities do not have sufficient substance use treatment providers to meet youth needs.[61,62] This shortage of providers is particularly true in rural areas. CIY from rural communities are less likely to access substance use treatment.

Age is also a significant predictor of treatment access, with younger adolescents more likely to be referred for treatment independent of treatment needs.[34] Thus, although the need for substance use treatment should be the determining factor in referral to receipt of services, other factors have been shown to influence access among CIY.

CIY with problematic substance use or SUDs often remain untreated, and even when treatments are available, they are unlikely to be evidence-based. This lack of evidence-informed treatment is primarily due to the multiple treatment needs of this population, which frequently include co-occurring mental health disorders. However, providing effective and comprehensive substance use treatment for this high-risk population can lead to positive outcomes and reduce the likelihood of recidivism.

AN OVERLOOKED CROWD: TRANSITIONAL AGE YOUTH

The term transitional age youth (TAY) or emerging adult refers to individuals ages 16 to 25.[62] Compared with youth from all other age groups, TAY report the highest initiation rates and use of illicit substances. Additionally, although TAY make up less than 10% of the U.S. population, they account for 28% of arrests, 26% of probation, and 28% of the jail population.[63] The rise in criminal activity is compounded by the transition to adulthood because the carceral system no longer reviews such behavior with a juvenile lens, and the young person may face criminal rather than juvenile delinquency charges.

TAY with substance use problems are at risk for poor outcomes. They have a fourfold greater probability of incarceration between ages 18 and 24 compared with those without substance use problems and are more likely to recidivate and continue offending into adulthood.[19,57] Despite these individuals' great need for substance use services, only 2% of TAY with recognized substance use treatment needs report receiving any treatment services.[64] Service utilization declined sharply during the transition age because of the multiple barriers to services, including loss of health care coverage and the transition from child to adult service systems. TAY have the highest dropout rates from substance use treatment and evidence of the worst treatment outcomes, though these may vary based on the type of substance use treatment received.[61,65,66]

Youth who struggle during the transition to adulthood often experience multiple problems, and multiple transitions during this period is a compounding factor. This period involves several expected social role transitions, such as leaving home, achieving financial and decision-making independence, committing to a romantic relationship, starting a career, becoming a parent, and engaging with the community and the broader social world. Success in these domains results from a complex interaction between adolescents, their families and communities, and available opportunities. Even the most well-adjusted youth encounter challenges during this transitional phase as they assume new responsibilities.

TAY in the carceral system have multiple barriers to a successful transition into adulthood compared with non-CIY peers, many revolving around risk factors previously discussed. For example, making a successful transition from adolescence to adulthood depends more and more on financial and other material support from family, even beyond adolescence, as well as on advantages that many youths who have been in trouble with the law do not have. CIY have high rates of learning disabilities and school failure, making successful vocational and or higher education transitions difficult.[12] High involvement rates with the child welfare system, substantial history of maltreatment, and increased likelihood of being placed in group home settings leave carceral-involved TAY with significantly compromised natural supports for transitioning to adulthood.[67]

The carceral system struggles to balance punishing delinquent acts and providing rehabilitative services in the youth's best interest. Clinicians working with TAY need to know about the aforementioned challenges and be prepared to assist them in navigating the various systems and developmental milestones that interact during this critical life stage. Unfortunately, despite a great need, there are no evidence-based practices targeting carceral-related behaviors for this age group. Further, there are no established treatments for substance use problems in general for TAY.[53] Therefore, much more support and research are needed to close the gap on the unmet needs of this vulnerable and often overlooked population.

SUMMARY

Substance use and delinquent behavior share overlapping risk factors, and substance use often predicts worse outcomes for youth involved in the carceral system, such as high recidivism rates. Interventions that include family members and target family-level risk factors for substance use are essential for youth in the carceral system. Group treatments for these youth are best provided by experienced clinicians. Providing services across multiple providers, accessing providers trained to work with carceral-involved youth, and engaging families are unique intervention challenges for this population. Transitional-age youth in the carceral system face additional difficulties navigating the youth and adult systems. Therefore, special attention is required to address their unique developmental needs and challenges. Providing evidence-based SUDs care for CIY promotes positive outcomes and reduces recidivism.

REFERENCES

1. Hockenberry S. *National Report Series Access OJJDP Publications Online at ojjdp.ojp.gov A Message From OJJDP*; 2016.
2. Initiative PP, Sawyer W. *Youth Confinement: The Whole Pie 2019*. Accessed March 19, 2023. https://www.prisonpolicy.org/reports/youth2019.html
3. Ryan L, La Vigne N. Trends in youth arrests for violent crimes. *Juvenile Justice Statistics: National Report Series Fact Sheet*. 2022. https://ojjdp.ojp.gov/publications/trends-in-youth-arrests.pdf
4. Children's defense fund. *The State of America's Children 2023: Youth Justice*. Accessed November 13, 2023. https://www.childrensdefense.org/the-state-of-americas-children/soac-2023-youth-justice/
5. Wasserman GA, McReynolds LS, Schwalbe CS, Keating JM, Jones SA. Psychiatric disorder, comorbidity, and suicidal behavior in juvenile justice youth. *Crim Justice Behav.* 2010;37(12):1361-1376. doi:10.1177/0093854810382751
6. Abram KM, Zwecker NA, Welty LJ, Hershfield JA, Dulcan MK, Teplin LA. Comorbidity and continuity of psychiatric disorders in youth after detention: a prospective longitudinal study. *JAMA Psychiatry.* 2015;72(1):84-93. doi:10.1001/jamapsychiatry.2014.1375
7. Dennis ML, Smith CN, Belenko S, et al. Operationalizing a behavioral health services cascade of care model: lessons learned from a 33-site implementation in juvenile justice community supervision. *Feb Probat.* 2019;83:52-64.
8. Sales JM, Wasserman G, Elkington KS, et al. Perceived importance of substance use prevention in juvenile justice: a multi-level analysis. *Health Justice.* 2018;6(1):12. doi:10.1186/s40352-018-0070-9
9. Hser YI, Grella CE, Hubbard RL, et al. An evaluation of drug treatments for adolescents in 4 U.S. cities. *Arch Gen Psychiatry.* 2001;58(7):689-695. doi:10.1001/ARCHPSYC.58.7.689

10. Dawes DE. The future of health equity in America: addressing the legal and political determinants of health. *J Law Med Ethics.* 2018;46(4):838-840. doi:10.1177/1073110518821976
11. Foley RM. Academic characteristics of incarcerated youth and correctional educational programs: a literature review. *J Emot Behav Disord.* 2001;9(4):248-259. doi:10.1177/106342660100900405
12. Cruise KR, Evans LJ, Pickens IB. Integrating mental health and special education needs into comprehensive service planning for juvenile offenders in long-term custody settings. *Learn Individ Differ.* 2011;21(1):30-40. doi:10.1016/J.LINDIF.2010.11.004
13. Langrehr KJ. Racial distinctions in the psychosocial histories of incarcerated youth. *Psychol Serv.* 2011;8(1):23-35. doi:10.1037/A0021795
14. Goodkind S, Shook J, Kolivoski K, Pohlig R, Little A, Kim K. From child welfare to jail: mediating effects of juvenile justice placement and other system involvement. *Child Maltreat.* 2020;25(4):410-421. doi:10.1177/1077559520904144
15. Ryan JP, Testa MF, Zhai F. African American males in foster care and the risk of delinquency: the value of social bonds and permanence. *Child Welfare.* 2008;87(1):115-150.
16. Zajac K, Sheidow AJ, Davis M. Juvenile justice, mental health, and the transition to adulthood: a review of service system involvement and unmet needs in the U.S. *Child Youth Serv Rev.* 2015;56:139. doi:10.1016/j.childyouth.2015.07.014
17. Molina BSG, Pelham WE. Attention-deficit/hyperactivity disorder and risk of substance use disorder: developmental considerations, potential pathways, and opportunities for research. *Annu Rev Clin Psychol.* 2014;10:607-639. doi:10.1146/annurev-clinpsy-032813-153722
18. Morin JFG, Afzali MH, Bourque J, et al. A population-based analysis of the relationship between substance use and adolescent cognitive development. *Am J Psychiatry.* 2019;176(2):98-106. doi:10.1176/appi.ajp.2018.18020202
19. Hoeve M, McReynolds LS, Wasserman GA, McMillan C. The influence of mental health disorders on severity of reoffending in juveniles. *Crim Justice Behav.* 2013;40(3):289-301. doi:10.1177/0093854812459639
20. Dube SR, Felitti VJ, Dong M, Chapman DP, Giles WH, Anda RF. Childhood abuse, neglect, and household dysfunction and the risk of illicit drug use: the adverse childhood experiences study. *Pediatrics.* 2003;111(3):564-572. doi:10.1542/peds.111.3.564
21. Mandavia A, GG NR, Bradley B, Ressler KJ, Powers A. Exposure to childhood abuse and later substance use: indirect effects of emotion dysregulation and exposure to trauma. *J Trauma.* 2016;29:422-429. doi:10.1002/jts.22131
22. Whitlock J, Muehlenkamp J, Eckenrode J, et al. Nonsuicidal self-injury as a gateway to suicide in young adults. *J Adolesc Health.* 2013;52(4):486-492. doi:10.1016/j.jadohealth.2012.09.010
23. Shakya HB, Christakis NA, Fowler JH. Parental influence on substance use in adolescent social networks. *Arch Pediatr Adolesc Med.* 2012;166(12):1132-1139. doi:10.1001/archpediatrics.2012.1372
24. Rusby JC, Light JM, Crowley R, Westling E. Influence of parent-youth relationship, parental monitoring, and parent substance use on adolescent substance use onset. *J Fam Psychol.* 2018;32(3):310-320. doi:10.1037/FAM0000350
25. Whittle HJ, Sheira LA, Frongillo EA, et al. Longitudinal associations between food insecurity and substance use in a cohort of women with or at risk for HIV in the United States. *Addiction.* 2019;114(1):127-136. doi:10.1111/add.14418
26. Morris AS, Squeglia LM, Jacobus J, Silk JS. Adolescent brain development: implications for understanding risk and resilience processes through neuroimaging research. *J Res Adolesc.* 2018;28(1):4. doi:10.1111/jora.12379
27. Yonek JC, Dauria EF, Kemp K, Koinis-Mitchell D, Marshall BDL, Tolou-Shams M. Factors associated with use of mental health and substance use treatment services by justice-involved youths. *Psychiatr Serv.* 2019;70(7):586-595. doi:10.1176/appi.ps.201800322
28. Marotta PL, Tolou-Shams M, Cunningham-Williams RM, Washington DM, Voisin D. Racial and ethnic disparities, referral source and attrition from outpatient substance use disorder treatment among adolescents in the United States. *Youth Soc.* 2022;54(1):148-173. doi:10.1177/0044118X20960635
29. Vinson SY, Coffey TT, Jackson N, McMickens CL, McGregor B, Leifman S. Two systems, one population: mental health care, criminal justice, and marginalized populations living with mental illness. *Psychiatr Clin North Am.* 2020;43(3). doi:10.1016/j.psc.2020.05.006
30. Maynard BR, Salas-Wright CP, Vaughn MG. High school dropouts in emerging adulthood: substance use, mental health problems, and crime. *Community Ment Health J.* 2015;51(3):289-299. doi:10.1007/s10597-014-9760-5
31. Young DW, Dembo R, Henderson CE. A national survey of substance abuse treatment for juvenile offenders. *J Subst Abuse Treat.* 2007;32(3):255-266. doi:10.1016/j.jsat.2006.12.018
32. Office of Justice Programs. *Drug Use and Delinquent Behavior: A Growth Model of Parallel Processes Among High-Risk Youths.* Accessed August 15, 2022. https://www.ojp.gov/ncjrs/virtual-library/abstracts/drug-use-and-delinquent-behavior-growth-model-parallel-processes
33. Chassin L, Knight G, Vargas-Chanes D, Losoya SH, Naranjo D. Substance use treatment outcomes in a sample of male serious juvenile offenders. *J Subst Abuse Treat.* 2009;36(2):183-194. doi:10.1016/J.JSAT.2008.06.001
34. McClelland GM, Elkington KS, Teplin LA, Abram KM. Multiple substance use disorders in juvenile detainees. *J Am Acad Child Adolesc Psychiatry.* 2004;43(10):1215-1224. doi:10.1097/01.chi.0000134489.58054.9C
35. Christian DD. Mandatory mental health screening for justice-involved youth: a national priority. *Youth Justice.* 2021;23(1):49-57. doi:10.1177/14732254211052334
36. Wasserman GA, McReynolds LS, Ko SJ, et al. Screening for emergent risk and service needs among incarcerated youth: comparing MAYSI-2 and Voice DISC-IV. *J Am Acad Child Adolesc Psychiatry.* 2004;43(5):629-639. doi:10.1097/00004583-200405000-00017
37. Gilbert AL, Grande TL, Hallman J, Underwood LA. Screening incarcerated juveniles using the MAYSI-2. *J Correct Health Care.* 2015;21(1):35-44. doi:10.1177/1078345814557788
38. Hay C, Widdowson AO, Bates M, Baglivio MT, Jackowski K, Greenwald MA. Predicting recidivism among released juvenile offenders in Florida: an evaluation of the residential positive achievement change tool. *Youth Violence Juv Justice.* 2016;16(1):97-116. doi:10.1177/1541204016660161
39. Pusch N, Holtfreter K. Gender and risk assessment in juvenile offenders: a meta-analysis. *Crim Justice Behav.* 2017;45(1):56-81. doi:10.1177/0093854817721720
40. Skeem JL, Kennealy PJ, Tatar JR, Hernandez IR, Keith FA. How well do juvenile risk assessments measure factors to target in treatment? Examining construct validity. *Psychol Assess.* 2017;29(6):679-691. doi:10.1037/PAS0000409
41. Bowser D, Henry BF, Wasserman GA, et al. Comparison of the overlap between juvenile justice processing and behavioral health screening, assessment and referral. *J Appl Juv Justice Serv.* 2018;2018:97.
42. Borum R. Assessing violence risk among youth. *J Clin Psychol.* 2000;56(10):1263-1288. doi:10.1002/1097-4679(200010)56:10<1263::aid-jclp3>3.0.co;2-d
43. Lodewijks HPB, Doreleijers TAH, de Ruiter C, Borum R. Predictive validity of the Structured Assessment of Violence Risk in Youth (SAVRY) during residential treatment. *Int J Law Psychiatry.* 2008;31(3):263-271. doi:10.1016/J.IJLP.2008.04.009
44. McGowan MR, Horn RA, Mellott RN. The predictive validity of the structured assessment of violence risk in youth in secondary educational settings. *Psychol Assess.* 2011;23(2):478-486. doi:10.1037/a0022304
45. Funk R, Knudsen HK, McReynolds LS, et al. Substance use prevention services in juvenile justice and behavioral health: results from a national survey. *Health Justice.* 2020;8(1):1-8. doi:10.1186/S40352-020-00114-6/TABLES/2
46. Vincent GM, Perrault R, Director P. *Risk Assessment And Behavioral Health Screening (RABS) Project Final Technical Report.* The Office of Juvenile Justice and Delinquency Prevention; 2018.
47. Ives, Chan Y-F, Modisette KC, Dennis ML. Characteristics, needs, services, and outcomes of youths in juvenile treatment drug courts as compared to adolescent outpatient treatment. *Drug Court Rev.* 2010;7(1):10-56.

48. National Institute on Drug Abuse. *Principles*. Accessed August 30, 2022. https://archives.nida.nih.gov/publications/principles-drug-abuse-treatment-criminal-justice-populations-research-based-guide
49. Perker SS, Chester LEH. The justice system and young adults with substance use disorders. *Pediatrics*. 2021;147(Suppl 2):S249-S258. doi:10.1542/PEDS.2020-023523H
50. Dodge KA, Dishion TJ, Lansford JE. Deviant peer influences in programs for youth: problems and solutions. *Guilford Press*. 2006;462.
51. Burleson JA, Kaminer Y, Dennis ML. Absence of iatrogenic or contagion effects in adolescent group therapy: findings from the Cannabis Youth Treatment (CYT) study. *Am J Addict*. 2006;15(SUPPL 1):s4-s15. doi:10.1080/10550490601003656
52. Hockenberry S, Puzzanchera C. *Juvenile Court Statistics*; 2015. Accessed November 11, 2020. https://calio.dspacedirect.org/handle/11212/3859
53. Hogue A, Henderson CE, Becker SJ, Knight DK. Evidence base on outpatient behavioral treatments for adolescent substance use, 2014-2017: outcomes, treatment delivery, and promising horizons. *J Clin Child Adolesc Psychol*. 2018;47(4):499-526. doi:10.1080/15374416.2018.1466307
54. Fadus MC, Squeglia LM, Valadez EA, Tomko RL, Bryant BE, Gray KM. Adolescent substance use disorder treatment: an update on evidence-based strategies. *Curr Psychiatry Rep*. 2019;21(10). doi:10.1007/S11920-019-1086-0
55. Simon KM, Levy SJ, Bukstein OG. Adolescent substance use disorders. *NEJM Evid*. 2022;1(6). doi:10.1056/EVIDRA2200051
56. Agency for Healthcare Research and Quality. *Interventions for Substance Use Disorders in Adolescents: A Systematic Review*. Accessed January 26, 2022. https://effectivehealthcare.ahrq.gov/products/substance-use-disorders-adolescents/protocol
57. Hoeve M, McReynolds LS, Wasserman GA. Service referral for juvenile justice youths: Associations with psychiatric disorder and recidivism. *Adm Policy Ment Health*. 2014;41(3):379-389. doi:10.1007/s10488-013-0472-x
58. Office of Justice Programs. *Delinquency Cases in Juvenile Court, 2014*. Accessed August 31, 2022. https://www.ojp.gov/ncjrs/virtual-library/abstracts/delinquency-cases-juvenile-court-2014
59. Wakefield SM, McPherson P, Brennan SL. Factors associated with successful completion of juvenile mental health court. *J Am Acad Psychiatry Law Online*. 2023;51(1):72-81. doi:10.29158/JAAPL.220035-21
60. Hogue A, Becker SJ, Wenzel K, et al. Family involvement in treatment and recovery for substance use disorders among transition-age youth: research bedrocks and opportunities. *J Subst Abuse Treat*. 2021;129:108402. doi:10.1016/j.jsat.2021.108402
61. Hadland SE, Bagley SM, Rodean J, et al. Receipt of timely addiction treatment and association of early medication treatment with retention in care among youths with opioid use disorder. *JAMA Pediatr*. 2018;172(11):1029-1037. doi:10.1001/jamapediatrics.2018.2143
62. Silverstein M, Hadland SE, Hallett E, Botticelli M. Principles of care for young adults with substance use disorders. *Pediatrics*. 2021;147(2):S195-S203. doi:10.1542/PEDS.2020-023523B
63. Justice Policy Institute. *Defining Violence: Reducing Incarceration by Rethinking America's Approach to Violence*. Accessed September 2, 2022. https://justicepolicy.org/research/reports-2016-defining-violence-reducing-incarceration-by-rethinking-americas-approach-to-violence
64. Substance Abuse and Mental Health Services Administration. *2020 National Survey of Drug Use and Health (NSDUH) Releases*. Accessed January 17, 2022. https://www.samhsa.gov/data/release/2020-national-survey-drug-use-and-health-nsduh-releases
65. Alinsky RH, Hadland SE, Matson PA, Cerda M, Saloner B. Adolescent-serving addiction treatment facilities in the United States and the availability of medications for opioid use disorder. *J Adolesc Health*. 2020;67(4):542-549. doi:10.1016/j.jadohealth.2020.03.005
66. Simons I, Mulder E, Breuk R, Rigter H, van Domburgh L, Vermeiren R. Determinants of parental participation in family-centered care in juvenile justice institutions. *Child Fam Soc Work*. 2019;24(1):59-68. doi:10.1111/cfs.12581
67. Vidal S, Prince D, Connell CM, Caron CM, Kaufman JS, Tebes JK. Maltreatment, family environment, and social risk factors: determinants of the child welfare to juvenile justice transition among maltreated children and adolescents. *Child Abuse Negl*. 2017;63:7-18. doi:10.1016/J.CHIABU.2016.11.013

CHAPTER

120 Treatment of Addiction-Related Disorders in Adolescents

Steven L. Jaffe, Justine Welsh, and Peter R. Cohen

CHAPTER OUTLINE

- Introduction
- Treatment modalities
- Individual behavioral treatments
- Family therapies
- Twelve-step approaches
- Treatment of opioid use disorder
- Using multiple therapies
- Return to use and continuing care
- Gender-responsive approaches to substance use
- Race and cultural factors

INTRODUCTION

The treatment of substance use disorder (SUD) in adolescents often requires unique considerations distinct from adults with SUD. An adolescent's biopsychosocial and developmental levels are important considerations in decision making. For example, it is normative for younger adolescents (age 12-14 years) to be egocentric, experience mood shifts, and have fluctuating capacity for introspection. Effective behavioral interventions reflect an application of skills in conjunction with developmental age, differing between younger and older adolescents. Since adolescents develop within a family system, including family members or caregivers can improve the effectiveness of treatment and help ensure safety. Education and parent management strategies are crucial in implementing change and increasing external motivation for abstinence or harm reduction. Adolescents differ from adults in their patterns of substance use. For example, inhalant use peaks in early adolescence, while daily cannabis, club and designer drugs, benzodiazepines, and opioid use are more common in middle and late adolescence. Adolescents have also been impacted by the opioid overdose epidemic, with a 94% increase in the overdose death rates from 2019 to 2020.[1] Although the prevalence of substance use is not more common, the introduction of synthetic opioids into the drug supply has made use riskier.[1] Use of high dose cannabis products especially by vaping has become a significant recent problem. In addition, certain studies have demonstrated that co-occurring psychiatric disorders are more common among adolescents than adults. Integrated treatment of co-occurring conditions and high-risk behaviors is recommended as the standard of care for adolescents.[2] Individualized determinations as to the appropriate setting for assessment, diagnosis and treatment of an adolescent presenting with substance use concerns is imperative. The American Society of Addiction of Medicine has developed placement criteria for adolescent treatment that include the dimensions of treatment readiness, reuse potential, and recovery environment (see Chapter 118, "Placement Criteria and Strategies for Adolescent Treatment Matching").[3]

TREATMENT MODALITIES

The National Institute on Drug Abuse, the National Institute on Alcohol Abuse and Alcoholism, and the Center for Substance Abuse Treatment have increased their support and direction for controlled studies of adolescent treatment, as well as for the development of clinical researchers to study such treatment. Improved standardized screening instruments and adolescent-specific outcome measures have been developed including tools such as the CRAFFT interview,[4] and the Screening to Brief Intervention (S2BI).[5]

Several treatment approaches have been used alone or in various combinations for the treatment of adolescent SUDs that include both behavioral and pharmacological options. Pharmacotherapy for treatment of adolescent SUD are discussed in greater detail in Chapter 117, "Assessing Adolescent Substance Use." A recent systematic review of the literature on evidence-based psychosocial treatments for adolescent SUDs found that longer duration of treatment, increased readiness to change, and family involvement were associated with better outcomes.[6] This review concluded that three treatment approaches—multidimensional family therapy (MDFT), functional family therapy (FFT), and group cognitive-behavioral therapy (CBT)—emerge as well-established models for treatment of this population. The researchers also concluded that none of the treatment approaches appeared clearly superior and that other therapeutic modalities were efficacious as well.[6] These and other important modalities are reviewed below.

INDIVIDUAL BEHAVIORAL TREATMENTS

Cognitive-Behavioral Therapy

Cognitive-behavioral therapy combines the learning principles of classical and operant conditioning with approaches to correct cognitive distortions and underlying negative belief systems. Treatment involves teaching the adolescent specific techniques to avoid substance use and engage in healthier, prosocial behaviors. Specific skills to refuse alcohol and drugs are taught and practiced in role-playing exercises. For example, the adolescent may be taught to immediately say "no" in a firm manner, making direct eye contact with the person who offers alcohol or drugs. They then practice suggesting an alternative activity or, if that is not successful, to simply tell the person to stop asking. Cognitive-behavioral coping skills to deal with urges, manage thoughts of substance use, and handle emergencies and reuse are taught and practiced. Because deficits in coping skills for negative feelings and life stresses contribute to continued substance use, more general coping strategies (such as communication skills, problem-solving strategies, anger and mood management, and relaxation training) also are taught and practiced. CBT interventions that improve self-efficacy, or confidence in the ability to refrain from substance use, have been associated with better outcomes.[7]

Findings from the Cannabis Youth Treatment (CYT) study provide support for both group and individual CBT interventions for adolescents with SUDs. In this large clinical trial, 600 adolescents who used cannabis participated in two multisite randomized clinical trials consisting of five interventions: 5 sessions of motivational enhancement therapy (MET, see below) plus CBT (MET/CBT5), 12 sessions of MET and CBT (MET/ CBTl2), Family Support Network, Adolescent Community Reinforcement Approach (A-CRA), and MDFT. All CYT interventions across both trials and all four sites produced significant reductions of cannabis use and negative consequences of use from pretreatment to 3-month follow-up that were sustained through 12 months. The most cost-effective interventions were MET/CBT5 and MET/CBT12 and ACRA. While all interventions were effective, only 35% to 40% of participants were identified as in recovery at 1 year, and 40% were lost to follow up,[8] indicating a need for new approaches to enhance treatment retention.

Two randomized clinical trials also have found CBT to be promising. In a direct comparison of CBT group therapy with interactional group therapy (IT) among adolescents with co-occurring substance use and psychiatric disorders, CBT reduced substance use and was equivalent to IT at 15 month follow up.[9] A small randomized clinical trial compared 8 weeks of CBT versus process-experiential therapy (PET) outpatient group psychotherapy for adolescents.[10] Participants in both groups reported declines in substance use from baseline to 3 and 9 months, and older youth and male participants in the CBT condition had a significantly lower rate of positive urinalysis compared to PET participants.[10]

Motivational Treatment

Prochaska and DiClemente[11] have described a series of stages that mark the progress of an individual toward abstinence from alcohol or drug use. These stages are designated as precontemplation, in which the person is not even thinking about stopping and does not recognize any problem with alcohol or drug use; contemplation, which is marked by ambivalence in which the person goes back and forth between reasons to change and reasons not to change; preparation, in which the person increases the commitment to change; action, in which the person stops using substances; and maintenance, in which the person develops a lifestyle to avoid returning to use.[11] These stages are considered progressive; therapeutic intervention involves helping the patient in an empathetic, nonconfrontational manner to move through the stages. Miller and Rollnick developed motivational interviewing (MI), which uses the strategies of expressing empathy, developing discrepancy, avoiding argumentation, rolling with resistance, and supporting self-efficacy to enhance changes along the stages. MET applies the principles of MI to specific exercises. MET was manualized for adolescents in the CYT study which demonstrated that greater motivation to change is associated with lower rates of substance use, and supported the efficacy of this modality.[12]

Two randomized trials also support the efficacy of MET with adolescents and young adults. A single 45-minute motivational intervention conducted in an emergency department with adolescents whose injuries were related to alcohol use found that the adolescents who received the intervention had fewer subsequent alcohol-related problems compared to those who received standard care.[13] A randomized trial of college freshmen who reported drinking heavily in high school found that participants who received an individual intervention had significantly greater reductions in negative consequences during a 4-year follow-up period compared to high risk controls.[13]

Adolescent Community Reinforcement Approach

The A-CRA uses prosocial activities so that abstinence is more rewarding than drinking or substance use. This modality, originally developed for adults, was adapted for adolescents and manualized and evaluated as part of the CYT Study, which demonstrated efficacy and cost-effectiveness.[8] Adolescents and caregivers/parents participate in both individual and joint sessions. A-CRA is largely based on CBT and uses reinforcers to support positive behavior change. Skills-based procedures are used to enhance communication skills, problem solving and drug refusal. Functional analyses of baseline and recent episodes of use identify internal/external triggers and highlight potential short-term positive consequences and long-term negative consequences specific to the patient. A-CRA also includes reuse prevention, sobriety sampling and healthy social and recreational activities. Clinical effectiveness has been shown in independent replications.[14] A-CRA has been studied in adolescents and young adults with opioid use disorder, demonstrating preliminary effectiveness in treatment retention and clinical improvement.[15,16]

Contingency Management

Contingency management (CM) is a behavioral treatment based on operant conditioning. CM uses concrete positive rewards (often monetary) to enhance attendance, participation, and abstinence. Numerous studies have demonstrated CM's efficacy in treatment of SUD in adult populations although it has been slow to implement due to lack of reimbursement.[17] There is a growing body of evidence that CM works for adolescents who use nicotine and cannabis in home, clinical, and justice settings.[16,18-20]

Mindfulness-Based Approaches

Mindfulness-based approaches have been successfully applied to the treatment of SUDs.[21] They include mindfulness-based cognitive therapy,[22] acceptance and commitment therapy (ACT),[23] dialectical behavioral therapy (DBT),[24] mindfulness-based relapse prevention (MBRP),[25] and mindfulness-based therapeutic community (MBTC) treatment.[26] The basis for mindfulness-based approaches is the cultivation of a nonjudgmental awareness, curiosity, openness, and acceptance of internal and external experiences, with the intended goal of eliciting greater reflection and acceptance, especially in regard to negative affect.[27] Mindfulness seeks to diminish the escalation of negative emotional reactivity (secondary negative affect in reaction to transient negative emotion) during stressful periods.[27] During mindfulness training, individuals learn to become more aware of habit-linked affective states and cravings, thus "de-automating" this largely habitual process.[28,29]

Improving distress tolerance is an important target of mindfulness-based SUD treatment.[30] In behavioral terms, mindfulness-based approaches for SUDs are described as a process of desensitization to negative affect through exposure, which helps to extinguish automatic avoidance of negative emotions and consequential substance use.[31]

Another benefit of mindfulness training in treatment is that it may concurrently target co-occurring disorders.[32] This may be of particular importance for adolescents with suicidal behavior and co-occurring affective and anxiety disorders. A controlled pilot study of young adults who used cannabis found a significant decrease of days of use when a two-session MI and mindfulness intervention were compared to a control group.[33]

Dialectical behavior therapy (DBT) is an empirically validated therapy developed by Linehan[24] that is effective in decreasing self-harming and self-defeating behaviors. This psychotherapy is now being used for adolescents with SUDs.[34] DBT combines the CBT techniques for emotional regulation with the skills of mindfulness, distress tolerance, and interpersonal effectiveness. These skills are taught in individual or group sessions and include self-reflective diary cards, individual adolescent sessions, homework assignments, parent training sessions, family therapy sessions, and phone contact for emergencies. In several studies, DBT has been shown to be efficacious in reducing suicidal behavior among adults. Linehan and colleagues have described a modification of DBT that has demonstrated preliminary efficacy in reducing substance use among adults.[35] Modifications of DBT for use with adolescents, which include family involvement, have also been described.

Unfortunately, to date, there are no published well-designed controlled studies demonstrating the effectiveness of interventions for adolescents with SUDs experiencing suicidality. This may in part be due to the risk involved and complexity of problems often found in this population. Indeed, research studies focused on interventions for substance use problems often exclude youths experiencing suicidality, just as some treatment studies for suicidal ideation exclude youths with the most serious substance use problems.

FAMILY THERAPIES

Several types of family therapy have been developed and manualized. Classic family therapy is based on the hypothesis that there is a connection between family relationships and the development or maintenance of substance use and targets interpersonal family processes. Structural–strategic family therapy emphasizes establishing a family hierarchy, with appropriate rules and authority. MDFT combines substance use treatment with multiple system assessments and interventions within the family and the surrounding psychosocial environment. Multisystemic Therapy (MST) integrates family therapy with interventions across multiple interacting systems involving the individual, school, peer group, and community.[36] FFT integrates behavioral and cognitive interventions with ecological-family relationship strategies.[37] Behavioral Family Therapy (BFT) combines family therapy with behavior therapy such that parents reinforce drug incompatible activities, supervise home assignments related to cravings, and supervise and employ written behavioral contracts with contingent reinforcers.[38,39] Brief Strategic Family Therapy (BSFT) uses a structural family systems framework to focus on correcting familial relationships that may lead to distressing experiences in youths aged 6 to 18.[40,41] A meta-analysis of family treatment of adolescents with substance use examined the efficacy of BSFT, FFT, MDFT, and MST. All four had modest but statistically significant effects compared to treatment as usual or alternate therapies.[42]

Multidimensional Family Therapy

Liddle's MDFT has the most empirical support.[6,43,44] MDFT usually involves therapy sessions one to three times per week over 3 to 6 months both in the home and at the clinic in an effort to create an empowering, nonpunitive atmosphere with a strong therapeutic alliance. Treatment domains include adolescent, parents, family, and extrafamilial interactions. A therapy assistant may help with school, economic assistance, or substance use treatment for other family members. MDFT was one of the interventions in the CYT study that demonstrated efficacy.[8] A randomized clinical trial found that adolescents who received MDFT had greater reductions in substance use and significantly improved academic achievement and family functioning at 12 months compared to those who received a multifamily educational intervention or group therapy.[43,45]

Multisystemic Therapy

Henggeler's MST promotes responsible behavior among all family members and attempts to develop each individual's capacity to manage his or her own problems. Therapists work intensively with each adolescent and family in the home, school, and even neighborhood peer group. MST has demonstrated excellent retention rates and favorable outcomes.[36] A randomized clinical trial of adolescents with legal involvement and a diagnosis of SUD compared MST to community service provided through the local office of the state substance use commission and found significantly reduced substance use at posttreatment for the MST group. While these differences disappeared by 6 months,[46] the total days of out-of-home placement for participants in the MST condition were reduced by 50% at 6-month follow-up compared to patients in the community treatment condition.[46] At 4-year follow-up, aggressive behavior was significantly reduced in participants from the MST group.[47]

A recent review of therapies for adolescents with co-occurring SUD and conduct disorder found that family therapy had the best outcomes with MST showing the most compelling evidence.[48] Another study found that integrating MST into juvenile drug court improved substance use outcomes.[49]

TWELVE-STEP APPROACHES

Twelve-step approaches are an adjunct to SUD treatment among adults that help to maintain and enhance motivation for abstinence (see Chapter 84, "Twelve-Step and Other Programs in Addiction Recovery").[50] The effectiveness of this approach with adolescents has been the subject of relatively recent investigation. There is a growing evidence base demonstrating improved outcomes including enhanced recovery capital with more frequent 12-step attendance.[51,52] Twelve-step programs provide the opportunity to attend free Alcoholics Anonymous (AA) or Narcotics Anonymous (NA) meetings, which are conducted several times a day in almost every city and town in the United States and most other countries. Thus, they are available during high stress times like weekends and holidays when recurrence of use often occurs. In the past several years, there has been an exponential growth of recovery groups and programs. In addition to the thousands of mutual help groups including Alcoholics Anonymous, Narcotics Anonymous, Cocaine Anonymous and Smart Recovery, the recovery movement has extended to the development of sober high schools and sober college programs. These programs can offer relationships with peers in recovery and mentoring relationships in the form of sponsors, who are older members with at least a year of abstinence who can provide support and guidance on how to achieve abstinence.

The 12 steps guide changes in actions, thoughts, feelings, and beliefs that an individual slowly undergoes in order to establish a state of recovery and abstinence. A summary of first five steps modified to be developmentally appropriate for adolescents can be found in **Table 120-1**.[53]

TABLE 120-1 Modifying the 12 Steps for Youth

Step	Classic 12-Step model	Adaptations for youth
1	We admitted we were powerless over alcohol (or other drugs)— that our lives had become unmanageable.	Adolescents examine the negative consequences of their alcohol and drug use. The concept of powerlessness or surrender often does not resonate with adolescents so the focus is on enhancing their power by stopping alcohol and drug use.
2	Came to believe that a Power greater than ourselves could restore us to sanity.	Adolescents are asked to recognize that the void left by stopping their use be filled by a positive higher power or spiritual feeling. This does not have to a religious belief but a spiritual one. Often, this may be the positive feelings of love within their nurturing relationships.
3	Made a decision to turn our will and our lives over to the care of God as we understood Him.	Adolescents are asked to commit themselves to working the steps and having a positive spiritual power. Learning a reflective practice, such as meditation, is an important part of this step.
4	Made a searching and fearless moral inventory of ourselves.	In this step, adolescents answer numerous detailed questions covering all aspects of their childhood and present life, which for many includes past trauma and abuse.
5	Admitted to God, to ourselves, and to another human being the exact nature of our wrongs.	In this step, the adolescent verbalizes an inventory to a counselor or a sponsor.

Studies of 12-step adolescent programs have been limited due to lack of random assignment and focus on inpatient programs.[54] However, reviews of programs that explicitly mention AA/NA as part of treatment obtain results comparable to other treatment modalities.[55] It also appears that teens that reported feeling connected to others, engaged in a higher frequency of meditation and prayer, and endorsed a more spiritual orientation to life were those who expressed a greater preference for spirituality and the 12-step approaches.[55]

Observational studies have found that among adolescents who participate in 12-step groups, abstinence rates averaged 30% to 40% across studies and time points.[55] A Comprehensive Assessment and Treatment Outcome Research (CATOR) residential treatment follow-up study found that adolescents who attended two or more meetings per week were almost six times more likely to report abstinence at 1 year than those who never attended.[56] Another study found that adolescents who completed 12-step–based treatment were approximately twice as likely to be abstinent or have minimal use compared with adolescents who needed treatment but did not receive it.[57] The favorable effect persisted at 5-year follow-up for the treatment group, especially those attending aftercare NA or AA meetings.[58] A study of adolescents following inpatient treatment found that 12-step attendance was associated with improved outcomes, with one third of participants completely abstinent during first and second 3-month intervals and the entire sample abstinent on 82% of all days at 6 months.[50] A study of youth 8 years after inpatient treatment found that attending one meeting per week was associated with significant benefit, and attending 2 to 3 meetings was associated with abstinence.[59] A study of outpatients in a combined CBT, MET, and 12-step model program found that only a minority of patients attended community 12-step meetings, though more frequent attendance was associated with greater abstinence, and both contact verbal participation and contact with a sponsor appeared to be important.[60]

TREATMENT OF OPIOID USE DISORDER

Given the rising rates of opioid-related overdose, greater attention is required to the treatment of opioid use disorder in this age group. Although there may be some promising behavioral therapies, medication is the recommended of treatment in youth and has been found to reduce opioid use enhance treatment retention, and improve mortality (see Chapter 121, "Pharmacotherapy for Adolescents with Substance Use Disorders").[61,62] Studies evaluating medication efficacy in youth with OUD often include different behavioral therapies.

Given the significant mortality benefit of pharmacological treatment, there have been few studies evaluating the primary use of behavioral therapies. A recent review identified three studies that evaluated the efficacy of behavioral intervention in this population, although none were randomized controlled trials.[63] Two of the studies reviewed the use of A-CRA, CBT and MI.[15,64] In a national sample of adolescents ages 12 to 17, those with primary opioid use who received A-CRA had similar rates of treatment engagement, retention and degree of substance use reduction as those who presented primarily for problems related to alcohol or cannabis use.[15] A separate comparison of individuals 12 to 29 who received A-CRA had shorter latency to opioid use than the other modalities compared to treatment as usual (such as supportive counseling or 12-step facilitation), CBT, or MET/CBT.[64] The study did not evaluate outcomes such as OUD symptoms or days of use. An observational study of group therapy for patients ages 16 to 22 focusing on psychosocial skills, reuse-prevention and drug refusal and separate engagement of parents/guardians found that about half of the participants reported abstinence during the 13-week group program and the majority also endorsed improvement in knowledge around relapse prevention and drug refusal skills; the majority of these patients also received medication for opioid treatment.[65]

USING MULTIPLE THERAPIES

No single behavioral treatment modality has been demonstrated to be clearly superior. All therapies have demonstrated mixed results in different patient populations and on different outcome measures, resulting in the need for a tailored treatment approach based on the individual and family system. Multiple approaches are being integrated in an attempt to improve outcomes. For example, family therapies are combined with MET, CBT, CM, DBT, and 12-step treatments to increase success.

RETURN TO USE AND CONTINUING CARE

One of the most pressing concern in adolescent SUD treatment is the lack of adolescent treatment providers. For adolescents who do enter treatment, noncompletion (which range from 30% to 50% in clinical settings) and the extremely high recurrence rate (40%-60% regardless of the treatment used) are significant issues. Ongoing care is recommended upon completion of a higher level of care, and for those who continue to use substances, a different treatment modality or more intensive setting is indicated. Assessing reasons for continued use is important to better understand an adolescent's motivations and match their goals with appropriate treatment. From a qualitative study of adolescents who had returned to use, four risk pathways have been described, including peers who use substances, presence of co-occurring psychiatric disorders, denial, and access to substances.[66] A recent qualitative study with adolescents and young adults enrolled in SUD treatment programs found that 90% involved emotional triggers that involved coping with negative feelings, 85% involved life stresses that including parental criticism and school failure, 65% involved socialization processes that including peer pressure, 75% involved cognitive factors that included decreases in motivation and cravings, and 55% involved environmental issues including availability and triggers.[67]

A commonly used treatment modality in adult studies is cognitive-behavioral reuse prevention (RP). High-risk situations are identified, and cognitive and behavioral skills are taught. In mindfulness-based reuse prevention (MBRP), the patient is taught awareness of environmental cues as well as cognitive and emotional states that have triggered relapse. This includes learning to tolerate negative affect that is often a precipitant of reuse. An adult trial of 8 weeks of RP, MBRP, or group 12-step–based treatment as usual found that RP and MBRP groups did better than TAU at 6 months and the MBRP group did better than all of the others at 1 year.[68] The positive findings suggest that this modality should be studied in adolescents, and that mindfulness practices may be added to other modalities to help adolescents cope with cravings and anhedonia.

When counseling an adolescent during return to use, the clinician can minimize guilt and shame by offering validation that the youth continues to stay engaged. Additionally, clinicians can facilitate conversations with the adolescent and their families regarding safety planning, including securing access to harm reduction strategies such as naloxone, the opioid-overdose reversal agent. Reducing stigma around medications such as naloxone and buprenorphine can be crucial to its use in pediatric populations. Assertive Continuing Care (ACC) is one approach where continued contact is the responsibility of the therapist. Monitoring by telephone and/or home visits involves education, support, and reintervention. A study of adolescents following residential treatment found that nearly half in the ACC group were abstinent for cannabis at 3 months compared to about one third in the usual continuing care group.[69] A study of aftercare for adolescents discharged from an alcohol program compared 50-minute individual MET/CBT, 15-minute MET/CBT therapeutic phone contacts, and a no intervention control group and found positive results for both active care groups[70] that were maintained over 12 months.[71] Mobile phone-based psychosocial interventions are currently in development to take advantage of adolescents heavy involvement with technology.[72]

GENDER-RESPONSIVE APPROACHES TO SUBSTANCE USE

Due to a combination of societal, neurobiological, psychosocial and psychiatric risk factors for adolescent substance use, gender-responsive approaches have been suggested in the literature. Adolescent boys are more likely to enter treatment for substance use and are more likely to be referred through the legal system,[73,74] while adolescent girls have more severe mental health symptoms, a greater likelihood of sexual abuse and family-related stress.[75] Potential developmental and gender-related treatment targets in treatment include coping skills and stress management in girls, and impulse control and sensation seeking in boys,[76] though there has been limited attention to gender issues in adolescent populations. Developmentally appropriate adaptations of gender specific substance use programming from older adults to younger patient populations may provide a platform to better fit some of the unique treatment needs of these populations.[77] The use of technology-based applications for gender-responsive substance use intervention may also have promise in younger populations.[78]

There is a growing need for screening, prevention and treatment strategies tailored towards sexual and gender minority youth. Sexual minority youth such as those who identify as members of the LGBTQIA+ community have an earlier age of initiation of substance use and higher rates of SUDs as compared to cis-gendered and heterosexual peers.[79,80] Gender minority youth (including those who are transgender and nonbinary) are also at elevated risk of unhealthy substance use when compared to cisgender youth.[79] Unique stressors such as discrimination faced by these patient populations as well as interpersonal and cultural factors driven by social context and norms are largely thought to influence substance use patterns in these subgroups.[79] To date, there has been limited research on LGBTQIA+ specific interventions. One recent review identified only two studies focused on reducing substance use in these populations, including a three session online intervention and the impact of a systems of care framework of community-based services.[81-83]

RACE AND CULTURAL FACTORS

The recent doubling of overdose deaths among U.S. teens during 2020 and 2021 was especially prevalent in minority adolescents with increased rates in Indigenous American/Alaska Native, Latinx, and Black youth.[1] Discrimination and racism have resulted in disparities of care for minority youth with decreased availability of substance use treatment. A 2014 editorial in the *Journal of Adolescent Health* summarizes the research, which then demonstrated critical racial and ethnic gaps in substance use treatment of minority youth, They cite the following documented factors for minority youth: (1) a scarcity of nearby Medicaid-funded programs; (2) a lower likelihood of having health insurance; (3) a lower proportion identified and referred for SUD; (4) a higher mistrust of providers; (5) more competing life stresses; (6) higher unexplained rates of treatment noncompletion; (7) inadequate treatment program cultural competence and/or insufficient language services; and (8) a shortage of specialty trained providers in adolescent addiction treatment who offer culturally competent care.[84] As in adult populations, there remains an urgent need to address and identify barriers to care for minoritized youth.

CASE STUDY

Jim is a 16-year-old male who was admitted to an intensive outpatient program after being arrested for selling cocaine. His substance use history included daily cannabis use for the past year, alcohol use on the weekends, occasional inhalation of his stimulant medication, and weekly cocaine for the past month. The counselors of the IOP program established a milieu of enthusiastic sobriety where the emphasis was on having fun without substances. During the first 2 weeks of the intensive outpatient program, Jim was passively adherent to attending groups, lectures, and activities. The staff used a motivational interviewing approach, but Jim was resistant to acknowledging any negative effects of his substance use except for legal issues. In family therapy, the parents worked through some of their anger and resentment at each other that had resulted from their divorce and learned to become more unified in setting appropriate limits with Jim. Using contingency management techniques, they began to reward positive behavior and removed his computer and cell phone when he attempted to contact friends with whom he used substances. By the 3rd week, he reported thinking more clearly, and the staff emphasized that the acute effects of cannabis had resolved. He now could make meaningful connections between actions and consequences. He was able to realize how substances had interfered with several areas of his life, including putting others in danger because of driving while impaired, worsening depression, falling grades, and breaking the law. This 3rd week of treatment became a turning point in his program. At a young people AA meeting, the staff connected him to a young man with 2 years of recovery who became his sponsor. They formed a very positive relationship such that they would talk on the phone three times a week and together attend AA or NA meetings. He became more active in the CBT skills training groups and learned substance refusal skills and techniques to manage urges. Because of his chronic depression and his history of ADHD, he started the antidepressant bupropion. Weekly urine drug screens became negative. In the 3rd, 4th, and 5th week of treatment, he wrote his first three steps. He learned that he had turned over his life to the negative power of substances, and now he was following a positive life direction. After discharge, he continued individual, group, and family therapy medication management and AA/NA meetings with his sponsor and other recovering peers.

ACKNOWLEDGMENT

The authors would like to acknowledge Siara Sitar, MS for assistance with formatting and referencing.

REFERENCES

1. Friedman J, Godvin M, Shover CL, Gone JP, Hansen H, Schriger DL. Trends in drug overdose deaths among US adolescents, January 2010 to June 2021. *JAMA*. 2022;327(14):1398-1400. doi:10.1001/jama.2022.2847
2. Welsh JW, Mataczynski M, Sarvey DB, Zoltani JE. Management of complex co-occurring psychiatric disorders and high-risk behaviors in adolescence. *Focus (Am Psychiatr Publ)*. 2020;18(2):139-149. doi:10.1176/appi.focus.20190038
3. Mee-Lee D, Shulman GD, Fishman M, Gastfriend DR, Griffith JH. *ASAM Patient Placement Criteria for the Treatment of Substance-Related Disorders: Revised (ASAM PPC-ZR)*. Second Edition-Revised. American Society of Addiction Medicine; 2001.
4. Knight JR, Shrier LA, Bravender TD, Farrell M, Bilt JV, Shaffer HJ. A New brief screen for adolescent substance abuse. *Arch Pediatr Adolesc Med.* 1999;153(6):591-596. doi:10.1001/archpedi.153.6.591
5. Levy S, Weiss R, Sherritt L, et al. An electronic screen for triaging adolescent substance use by risk levels. *JAMA Pediatr.* 2014;168(9):822-828. doi:10.1001/jamapediatrics.2014.774
6. Waldron HB, Turner CW. Evidence-based psychosocial treatments for adolescent substance abuse. *J Clin Child Adolesc Psychol.* 2008;37(1):238-261. doi:10.1080/15374410701820133
7. Burleson JA, Kaminer Y. Self-efficacy as a predictor of treatment outcome in adolescent substance use disorders. *Addict Behav.* 2005;30(9):1751-1764. doi:10.1016/j.addbeh.2005.07.006
8. Dennis M, Godley SH, Diamond G, et al. The Cannabis Youth Treatment (CYT) Study: main findings from two randomized trials. *J Subst Abuse Treat.* 2004;27(3):197-213. doi:10.1016/j.jsat.2003.09.005
9. Kaminer Y, Burleson JA. Psychotherapies for adolescent substance abusers: 15-month follow-up of a pilot study. *Am J Addict.* 1999;8(2):114-119. doi:10.1080/105504999305910
10. Kaminer Y, Burleson JA, Goldberger R. Cognitive-behavioral coping skills and psychoeducation therapies for adolescent substance abuse. *J Nerv Ment Dis.* 2002;190(11):737-745. doi:10.1097/00005053-200211000-00003
11. Prochaska JO, DiClemente CC. Transtheoretical therapy: toward a more integrative model of change. *Psychother Theory Res Pract.* 1982;19(3):276-288. https://doi.org/10.1037/h0088437
12. Miller W, Rollnick S. *Motivational Interviewing: Preparing People for Change*. 2nd ed. Guilford Press; 2002.
13. Baer JS, Kivlahan DR, Blume AW, McKnight P, Marlatt GA. Brief intervention for heavy-drinking college students: 4-year follow-up and natural history. *Am J Public Health.* 2001;91(8):1310-1316. Accessed May 25, 2018. https://www.ncbi.nlm.nih.gov/pmc/articles/PMC1446766/
14. Henderson CE, Wevodau AL, Henderson SE, et al. An independent replication of the adolescent-community reinforcement approach with justice-involved youth. *Am J Addict.* 2016;25(3):233-240. doi:10.1111/ajad.12366
15. Godley MD, Passetti LL, Subramaniam GA, Funk RR, Smith JE, Meyers RJ. Adolescent Community Reinforcement Approach implementation and treatment outcomes for youth with opioid problem use. *Drug Alcohol Depend.* 2017;174:9-16. doi:10.1016/j.drugalcdep.2016.12.029
16. Stanger C, Budney AJ. Contingency management: using incentives to improve outcomes for adolescent substance use disorders. *Pediatr Clin North Am.* 2019;66(6):1183-1192. doi:10.1016/j.pcl.2019.08.007
17. Oluwoye O, Kriegel L, Alcover KC, McPherson S, McDonell MG, Roll JM. The dissemination and implementation of contingency management for substance use disorders: a systematic review. *Psychol Addict Behav.* 2020;34(1):99-110. doi:10.1037/adb0000487
18. Rudes DS, Viglione J, Sheidow AJ, McCart MR, Chapman JE, Taxman FS. Juvenile probation officers' perceptions on youth substance use varies from task-shifting to family-based contingency management. *J Subst Abuse Treat.* 2021;120:108144. doi:10.1016/j.jsat.2020.108144
19. Godley MD, Godley SH, Dennis ML, Funk RR, Passetti LL, Petry NM. A randomized trial of assertive continuing care and contingency management for adolescents with substance use disorders. *J Consult Clin Psychol.* 2014;82(1):40-51. doi:10.1037/a0035264
20. Stanger C, Lansing AH, Budney AJ. Advances in research on contingency management for adolescent substance use. *Child Adolesc Psychiatr Clin N Am.* 2016;25(4):645-659. doi:10.1016/j.chc.2016.05.002
21. Zgierska A, Rabago D, Chawla N, Kushner K, Koehler R, Marlatt A. Mindfulness meditation for substance use disorders: a systematic review. *Subst Abuse.* 2009;30(4):266-294. doi:10.1080/08897070903250019
22. Segal ZV, Williams JMG, Teasdale JD. *Mindfulness-Based Cognitive Therapy for Depression: A New Approach to Preventing Relapse. Guilford Press.* 2002;xiv, 351.
23. Hayes SC, Strosahl KD, Wilson KG. *Acceptance and Commitment Therapy: An Experiential Approach to Behavior Change. Guilford Press.* 1999;xvi, 304.
24. Linehan M. *Cognitive Behavior Therapy of Borderline Personality Disorder*. Guilford Press; 2003.
25. Witkiewitz K, Bowen S. Depression, craving, and substance use following a randomized trial of mindfulness-based relapse prevention. *J Consult Clin Psychol.* 2010;78(3):362-374. doi:10.1037/a0019172
26. Zgierska A, Marcus MT. Mindfulness-based therapies for substance use disorders: part 2. *Subst Abuse.* 2010;31(2):77-78. doi:10.1080/08897071003641248
27. Praissman S. Mindfulness-based stress reduction: a literature review and clinician's guide. *J Am Acad Nurse Pract.* 2008;20(4):212-216. doi:10.1111/j.1745-7599.2008.00306.x
28. Brewer JA, Bowen S, Smith JT, Marlatt GA, Potenza MN. Mindfulness-based treatments for co-occurring depression and substance use disorders: what can we learn from the brain? *Addiction.* 2010;105(10):1698-1706. doi:10.1111/j.1360-0443.2009.02890.x
29. Teasdale JD, Segal Z, Williams JM. How does cognitive therapy prevent depressive relapse and why should attentional control (mindfulness) training help? *Behav Res Ther.* 1995;33(1):25-39. doi:10.1016/0005-7967(94)e0011-7

30. Sinha R. The role of stress in addiction relapse. *Curr Psychiatry Rep.* 2007;9(5):388-395. doi:10.1007/s11920-007-0050-6
31. Grabovac AD, Lau MA, Willett BR. Mechanisms of mindfulness: a buddhist psychological model. *Mindfulness.* 2011;2(3):154-166. doi:10.1007/s12671-011-0054-5
32. Dimeff LA, Linehan MM. Dialectical behavior therapy for substance abusers. *Addict Sci Clin Pract.* 2008;4(2):39-47. doi:10.1151/ascp084239
33. de Dios MA, Herman DS, Britton WB, Hagerty CE, Anderson BJ, Stein MD. Motivational and mindfulness intervention for young adult female marijuana users. *J Subst Abuse Treat.* 2012;42(1):56-64. doi:10.1016/j.jsat.2011.08.001
34. Linehan MM, Comtois KA, Murray AM, et al. Two-year randomized controlled trial and follow-up of dialectical behavior therapy vs therapy by experts for suicidal behaviors and borderline personality disorder. *Arch Gen Psychiatry.* 2006;63(7):757-766. doi:10.1001/archpsyc.63.7.757
35. Rathus JH, Miller AL. Dialectical behavior therapy adapted for suicidal adolescents. *Suicide Life Threat Behav.* 2002;32(2):146-157. doi:10.1521/suli.32.2.146.24399
36. Henggeler SW, Pickrel SG, Brondino MJ, Crouch JL. Eliminating (almost) treatment dropout of substance abusing or dependent delinquents through home-based multisystemic therapy. *Am J Psychiatry.* 1996;153(3):427-428. doi:10.1176/ajp.153.3.427
37. Waldron HB, Slesnick N, Brody JL, Turner CW, Peterson TR. Treatment outcomes for adolescent substance abuse at 4- and 7-month assessments. *J Consult Clin Psychol.* 2001;69(5):802-813.
38. Azrin NH, Donohue B, Besalel VA, Kogan ES, Acierno R. Youth drug abuse treatment: a controlled outcome study. *J Child Adolesc Subst Abuse.* 1994;3(3):1-16. doi:10.1300/J029v03n03_01
39. Azrin NH, Donohue B, Teichner GA, Crum T, Howell J, DeCato LA. A controlled evaluation and description of individual-cognitive problem solving and family-behavior therapies in dually-diagnosed conduct-disordered and substance-dependent youth. *J Child Adolesc Subst Abuse.* 2001;11(1):1-43. doi:10.1300/J029v11n01_01
40. Robbins MS, Szapocznik J. *Brief Strategic Family Therapy.* Accessed August 16, 2022. https://www.ojp.gov/pdffiles1/ojjdp/179285.pdf
41. Szapocznik J, Williams RA. Brief Strategic Family Therapy: twenty-five years of interplay among theory, research and practice in adolescent behavior problems and drug abuse. *Clin Child Fam Psychol Rev.* 2000;3(2):117-134. doi:10.1023/a:1009512719808
42. Baldwin SA, Christian S, Berkeljon A, Shadish WR. The effects of family therapies for adolescent delinquency and substance abuse: a meta-analysis. *J Marital Fam Ther.* 2012;38(1):281-304. doi:10.1111/j.1752-0606.2011.00248.x
43. Liddle HA, Dakof GA, Parker K, Diamond GS, Barrett K, Tejeda M. Multidimensional family therapy for adolescent drug abuse: results of a randomized clinical trial. *Am J Drug Alcohol Abuse.* 2001;27(4):651-688. doi:10.1081/ada-100107661
44. Hogue A, Henderson CE, Becker SJ, Knight DK. Evidence base on outpatient behavioral treatments for adolescent substance use, 2014–2017: outcomes, treatment delivery, and promising horizons. *J Clin Child Adolesc Psychol.* 2018;47(4):499-526. doi:10.1080/15374416.2018.1466307
45. Liddle HA. Family-based therapies for adolescent alcohol and drug use: research contributions and future research needs. *Addiction.* 2004;99(Suppl 2):76-92. doi:10.1111/j.1360-0443.2004.00856.x
46. Henggeler SW, Pickrel SG, Brondino MJ. Multisystemic treatment of substance-abusing and dependent delinquents: outcomes, treatment fidelity, and transportability. *Ment Health Serv Res.* 1999;1(3):171-184. doi:10.1023/a:1022373813261
47. Henggeler SW, Clingempeel WG, Brondino MJ, Pickrel SG. Four-year follow-up of multisystemic therapy with substance-abusing and substance-dependent juvenile offenders. *J Am Acad Child Adolesc Psychiatry.* 2002;41(7):868-874. doi:10.1097/00004583-200207000-00021
48. Spas J, Ramsey S, Paiva AL, Stein LAR. All might have won, but not all have the prize: optimal treatment for substance abuse among adolescents with conduct problems. *Subst Abuse Res Treat.* 2012;6:141-155. doi:10.4137/SART.S10389
49. Saldana L, Scott W. Henggeler. Improving outcomes and transporting evidence-based treatments for youth and families with serious clinical problems. *J Child Adolesc Subst Abuse.* 2008;17:1-10. doi:10.1080/15470650802071564
50. Kelly JF, Myers MG, Brown SA. A multivariate process model of adolescent 12-step attendance and substance use outcome following inpatient treatment. *Psychol Addict Behav.* 2000;14(4):376-389.
51. Kelly JF, Stout RL, Greene MC, Slaymaker V. Young adults, social networks, and addiction recovery: post treatment changes in social ties and their role as a mediator of 12-step participation. *PLoS One.* 2014;9(6):e100121. doi:10.1371/journal.pone.0100121
52. Hennessy EA, Finch AJ. Adolescent recovery capital and recovery high school attendance: an exploratory data mining approach. *Psychol Addict Behav.* 2019;33(8):669-676. doi:10.1037/adb0000528
53. Jaffe SL. *Workbook for Adolescent Chemical Dependency Recovery: A Guide to the First Five Steps.* American Psychiatric Press Inc; 1990.
54. Kelly JF, Myers MG. Adolescents' participation in Alcoholics Anonymous and Narcotics Anonymous: review, implications and future directions. *J Psychoactive Drugs.* 2007;39(3):259-269. doi:10.1080/02791072.2007.10400612
55. Sussman S. A review of Alcoholics Anonymous/ Narcotics Anonymous programs for teens. *Eval Health Prof.* 2010;33(1):26-55. doi:10.1177/0163278709356186
56. Harrison P, Hoffman N. *Cator Report: Adolescent Treatment Completion One Year Later.* Ramsey Clinic; 1989.
57. Winters KC, Stinchfield RD, Opland E, Weller C, Latimer WW. The effectiveness of the Minnesota Model approach in the treatment of adolescent drug abusers. *Addiction.* 2000;95(4):601-612. doi:10.1046/j.1360-0443.2000.95460111.x
58. Winters KC, Stinchfield R, Latimer WW, Lee S. Long-term outcome of substance-dependent youth following 12-step treatment. *J Subst Abuse Treat.* 2007;33(1):61-69. doi:10.1016/j.jsat.2006.12.003
59. Kelly JF, Brown SA, Abrantes A, Kahler CW, Myers M. Social recovery model: an 8-year investigation of adolescent 12-step group involvement following inpatient treatment. *Alcohol Clin Exp Res.* 2008;32(8):1468-1478. doi:10.1111/j.1530-0277.2008.00712.x
60. Kelly JF, Urbanoski K. Youth recovery contexts: the incremental effects of 12-step attendance and involvement on adolescent outpatient outcomes. *Alcohol Clin Exp Res.* 2012;36(7):1219-1229. doi:10.1111/j.1530-0277.2011.01727.x
61. Wakeman SE, Larochelle MR, Ameli O, et al. Comparative effectiveness of different treatment pathways for opioid use disorder. *JAMA Netw Open.* 2020;3(2):e1920622. doi:10.1001/jamanetworkopen.2019.20622
62. Mintz CM, Presnall NJ, Sahrmann JM, et al. Age disparities in six-month treatment retention for opioid use disorder. *Drug Alcohol Depend.* 2020;213:108130. doi:10.1016/j.drugalcdep.2020.108130
63. Welsh JW, Mataczynski MJ, Nguyen MD, McHugh RK. A review of behavioral therapies in adolescents with opioid use disorder. *Harv Rev Psychiatry.* 2020;28(5):305-315. doi:10.1097/HRP.0000000000000272
64. Davis JP, Prindle JJ, Eddie D, Pedersen ER, Dumas TM, Christie NC. Addressing the opioid epidemic with behavioral interventions for adolescents and young adults: a quasi-experimental design. *J Consult Clin Psychol.* 2019;87(10):941-951. doi:10.1037/ccp0000406
65. Pugatch M, Knight JR, McGuiness P, Sherritt L, Levy S. A group therapy program for opioid-dependent adolescents and their parents. *Subst Abuse.* 2014;35(4):435-441. doi:10.1080/08897077.2014.958208
66. Jaffe S. Pathways to relapse in chemically dependent adolescents. *J Child Adolesc Couns.* 1994;55:42-44.
67. Gonzales R, Anglin MD, Beattie R, Ong CA, Glik DC. Understanding recovery barriers: youth perceptions about substance use relapse. *Am J Health Behav.* 2012;36(5):602-614. doi:10.5993/AJHB.36.5.3
68. Bowen S, Witkiewitz K, Clifasefi SL, et al. Relative efficacy of mindfulness-based relapse prevention, standard relapse prevention, and treatment as usual for substance use disorders: a randomized clinical trial. *JAMA Psychiatry.* 2014;71(5):547-556. doi:10.1001/jamapsychiatry.2013.4546

69. Godley MD, Godley SH, Dennis ML, Funk R, Passetti LL. Preliminary outcomes from the assertive continuing care experiment for adolescents discharged from residential treatment. *J Subst Abuse Treat.* 2002;23(1):21-32. doi:10.1016/S0740-5472(02)00230-1
70. Kaminer Y, Burleson JA, Burke RH. Efficacy of outpatient aftercare for adolescents with alcohol use disorders: a randomized controlled study. *J Am Acad Child Adolesc Psychiatry.* 2008;47(12):1405-1412. doi:10.1097/CHI.0b013e318189147c
71. Burleson J, Kaminer Y. *Outcomes at Nine Month Follow up of Aftercare for Adolescents with Alcohol use Disorders*. Presentation presented at the Annual Meeting of the Research Society on Alcoholism, San Diego, CA; 2009.
72. Marsch L, Borodovsky JT. Technology based interventions for preventing and treating substance use among youth. *Child Adolesc Psychiat Clin N Am.* 2016;25(4):755-768.
73. Stevens SJ, Estrada B, Murphy BS, Mcknight KM, Tims F. Gender differences in substance use, mental health, and criminal justice involvement of adolescents at treatment entry and at three, six, twelve and thirty month follow-up. *J Psychoactive Drugs.* 2004;36(1):13-25.
74. Haughwout SP, Harford TC, Castle IJP, Grant BF. Treatment utilization among adolescent substance users: findings from the 2002 to 2013 National Survey on Drug Use and Health. *Alcohol Clin Exp Res.* 2016;40(8):1717-1727. doi:10.1111/acer.13137
75. Anderberg M, Dahlberg M. Gender differences among adolescents with substance abuse problems at Maria clinics in Sweden. *Nord Stud Alcohol Drugs.* 2018;35(1):24-38. doi:10.1177/1455072517751263
76. Dir AL, Bell RL, Adams ZW, Hulvershorn LA. Gender differences in risk factors for adolescent binge drinking and implications for intervention and prevention. *Front Psychiatry.* 2017;8:289-289. doi:10.3389/fpsyt.2017.00289
77. Welsh JW, Hunnicutt-Ferguson K, Cattie JE, et al. Adaptation and pilot testing of the Women's Recovery Group for Young Adults (WRG-YA). *Alcohol Treat Q.* 2021;39(2):225-237. doi:10.1080/07347324.2020.1837044
78. Sugarman DE, Meyer LE, Reilly ME, Rauch SL, Greenfield SF. Exploring technology-based enhancements to inpatient and residential treatment for young adult women with co-occurring substance use. *J Dual Diagn.* 2021;17(3):236-247. doi:10.1080/15504263.2021.1940412
79. Mereish EH. Substance use and misuse among sexual and gender minority youth. *Curr Opin Psychol.* 2019;30:123-127. doi:10.1016/j.copsyc.2019.05.002
80. Fish JN, Bishop MD, Russell ST. Developmental differences in sexual orientation and gender identity–related substance use disparities: findings from population-based data. *J Adolesc Health.* 2021;68(6):1162-1169. doi:10.1016/j.jadohealth.2020.10.023
81. Coulter RWS, Egan JE, Kinsky S, et al. Mental health, drug, and violence interventions for sexual/gender minorities: a systematic review. *Pediatrics.* 2019;144(3):e20183367. doi:10.1542/peds.2018-3367
82. Schwinn TM, Thom B, Schinke SP, Hopkins J. Preventing drug use among sexual-minority youths: findings from a tailored, web-based intervention. *J Adolesc Health.* 2015;56(5):571-573. doi:10.1016/j.jadohealth.2014.12.015
83. Painter KR, Scannapieco M, Blau G, Andre A, Kohn K. Improving the mental health outcomes of LGBTQ youth and young adults: a longitudinal study. *J Soc Serv Res.* 2018;44(2):223-235. doi:10.1080/01488376.2018.1441097
84. Hadland SE, Baer TE. The racial and ethnic gap in substance use treatment: implications for U.S. healthcare reform. *J Adolesc Health.* 2014;54(6):627-628. doi:10.1016/j.jadohealth.2014.03.015

CHAPTER 121

Pharmacotherapy for Adolescents With Substance Use Disorders

Jacqueline Deanna Wilson and Paula Goldman

CHAPTER OUTLINE

- Introduction
- Empirical support for pharmacotherapies in the treatment of adolescent SUDs
- Clinical considerations

INTRODUCTION

Exposure to tobacco, alcohol, and other substances during adolescence increases the risk of long-term use and the development of substance use disorder (SUD).[1,2] Evidence suggests both the rewarding and damaging effects from substances to the adolescent brain may be greater during the period of rapid myelination and maturation.[2] At the same time, adolescents have incompletely developed prefrontal cortices, leading to suboptimal conceptualization of future risks and consequences and reduced ability to regulate substance use behaviors. Additionally, individual and developmental differences in risk taking and impulsivity may explain vulnerabilities in certain youth developing SUD.[3] Thus, SUD may be conceptualized as a developmental disorder.[1,2]

Despite risks and negative sequelae, adolescents continue to use substances at high levels in the United States. Among those aged 12 to 17, 6.3% or 1.7 million, reported meeting criteria for SUD in 2020, and fewer than 10% receive treatment.[4] Even among those who do access SUD treatment, youth are significantly less likely than adults to be offered evidence-based pharmacotherapy.[5]

These patterns underscore the need for effective treatment for adolescents with SUDs. To date, several psychosocial/behavioral treatment approaches have been shown to be effective in the treatment of youth with SUD, mostly with small to moderate effect sizes.[6,7] These are discussed in Chapter 120, "Treatment of Addiction-Related Disorders in Adolescents." There is growing evidence to support the use of pharmacotherapy for treating youth with SUD, though the research remains limited. Compared to adults, youth may have differential responses to both therapeutic and side effects of pharmacotherapies necessitating well-designed and adequately powered clinical trials in pediatric populations.

In this chapter, we review the state of scientific research evaluating various pharmacotherapies for the treatment of adolescent SUDs. As there is often a lack of youth-specific research in the management of acute ingestion, overdose, and withdrawal management, and treatment tends to be similar to that of adults, we provide only a brief overview based on available evidence. We focus on the commonly used pharmacotherapies in the treatment of youth SUD's and review relevant youth studies and implications from pertinent adult trials. We also discuss the complementary and crucial role of psychosocial treatment, especially in combination with medications for adolescent SUDs. The chapter also includes a review of harm reduction tools to mitigate substance use-related consequences in youth, and reviews the importance of engaging families to support youth recovery goals.

EMPIRICAL SUPPORT FOR PHARMACOTHERAPIES IN THE TREATMENT OF ADOLESCENT SUDs

Below, we provide a summary of the research evaluating pharmacotherapies in the treatment of a variety of SUDs, including nicotine, alcohol, cannabis, opioids, stimulants, and other substances relevant to youth.

Tobacco/Nicotine

The majority of adults who smoke began using tobacco as adolescents. Some evidence suggests that smoking behavior among teens may differ from that of their adult counterparts, with adolescents smoking fewer cigarettes and less frequently than adults who smoke. However, nicotine addiction develops rapidly in youth, with approximately 25% of adolescents who smoke exhibiting signs of addiction within a month of smoking initiation.[8] Nicotine impacts the maturing adolescent brain differently than adults, for example, leading to diminished attention span and enhanced impulsivity among those who initiate nicotine exposure during adolescence but not afterwards. There are persistent changes in neuronal signaling sensitizing the adolescent brain and priming youth to use other substances.[9] In addition to the long-term harms,[10] smoking during adolescence is associated with immediate health effects, including poorer fitness, and is associated with other SUDs, mental health disorders, and conduct disorder.[11]

Nicotine use among teens remains a significant problem, however patterns of use and route of consumption have changed over time. Cigarette use among high school students has been declining since 1997. Vaping (although commonly used, "vaping" is an inaccurate term, as this involves the inhalation of a nicotine-containing aerosol from electronic drug delivery devices/EDDDs) has become a major avenue for nicotine consumption; in 2021 the lifetime prevalence of nicotine vaping was considerably higher than lifetime prevalence of cigarette use across grades.[12] There is growing evidence that vaping during adolescence predicts future cigarette use.[13] Additional health effects of vaping among adolescents are emerging as well, including associations with increased depression, increased suicidal ideation and suicide attempts,[14] lower academic performance,[15] and increased high risk sexual behaviors.[16] e-Cigarette or Vaping Use-Associated Lung Injury (EVALI), is a potentially life-threatening pulmonary complication of vaping[17]; milder forms of pulmonary impairment have also been associated with vaping, including in youth.[18]

Adolescents who smoke often report attempting to quit on their own. However, quit rates among teens who try to quit on their own are extremely low, estimated at about 4% to 6% annually. The literature on effective strategies for nicotine abstinence among adolescents is less robust than adults, and the portion of this literature reporting on the efficacy of pharmacotherapy for adolescents is limited. Several medications have been approved by the U.S. Food and Drug Administration (FDA) for the treatment of tobacco (nicotine) use disorder among adults. These include nicotine replacement medications (eg, nicotine gum, inhaler, lozenges, nasal spray, and patch), bupropion (a nicotine receptor antagonist and norepinephrine and dopamine reuptake inhibitor) and varenicline (a nicotinic receptor partial agonist). None of these medications have been approved for individuals under the age of 18 years. A 2018 meta-analysis of nine randomized controlled trials, which included 1,188 adolescents who smoked ages 12 to 20, conducted a pooled analysis of various pharmacotherapies prescribed for a total of 6 weeks to 90 days, and found increased abstinence rates at 4 weeks; however this difference was not maintained at longer follow-up intervals of 8 to 52 weeks. Only bupropion was associated with an increased abstinence rate at longer follow-up periods.[19] However, these studies were plagued by high rates of drop out and nonadherence.

The United States Preventative Task Force asserts that there is insufficient evidence to assess the benefits and harms of interventions for the abstinence from tobacco use in children and adolescents.[20] The U.S. Department of Health and Human Services[21] recommends counseling as a first line treatment for TUD in youth, with medications being offered on a case by case basis due to the limited evidence. The American Academy of Pediatrics advocates for the "Ask-Counsel-Treat" model, which entails first screening, then counseling regarding tobacco cessation, then offering treatment including behavioral treatment and pharmacotherapy when indicated.[20,22,23]

Nicotine Replacement Therapy

Nicotine replacement therapy (NRT) medications exert their effects as agonists or partial agonists and promote reduction in craving and withdrawal symptoms. Five published, randomized controlled trials have evaluated the efficacy of NRT with adolescents who smoke, showing some evidence of efficacy for the nicotine patch. Hanson et al.[24] randomly assigned adolescents who smoked to receive either the nicotine patch (with doses and titration schedules based on the level of smoking) or placebo; all participants also received behavioral treatment. The nicotine patch did not increase abstinence rates but resulted in reduced craving and withdrawal symptoms compared to placebo. No youth dropped out as a result of adverse events.

A second randomized trial evaluated nicotine patches ($N = 49$) versus placebo ($N = 49$) with adolescents who smoked regularly.[25] Overall, adherence rates and abstinence rates were low, and the authors concluded that nicotine patches did not appear to have clinical utility for this population of youth. A third trial, conducted by Moolchan et al.[26] compared nicotine gum ($N = 46$) versus nicotine patch ($N = 34$) versus placebo ($N = 40$) in adolescents who smoked greater than one half a pack per day of cigarettes for at least 6 months and scored greater than 5 on the Fagerstrom Test for Nicotine Dependence. Overall, adherence rates were greatest for those who received the patch, with 21% abstinence at the end of treatment, compared with 9% in the gum group and 5% in the placebo group. A small study[27] compared weekly group based counseling alone ($N = 17$) versus weekly group-based counseling plus nicotine nasal spray ($N = 23$). Compliance with the use of the nasal spray was low and abstinence outcomes did not differ across groups. In a study conducted in the Netherlands by Scherphof et al.[28] 257 adolescents were randomized to nicotine patch or placebo for 6 or 9 weeks, depending on the number of cigarettes smoked at baseline. Those assigned to nicotine patch reported significantly higher abstinence at two weeks but not end of treatment or at 6- or 12-month follow-up. However, end-of-treatment abstinence rates were significantly higher among those who were medication (patch) adherent.[29] A 2017 Cochrane Review combined three small studies of NRT in adolescents and concluded there was no clear evidence for the effectiveness of NRT in increasing abstinence from smoking at 6 months, although confidence intervals were wide (RR 1.11, 95% CI 0.48-2.58).[30]

Bupropion

Bupropion exerts its effect as a nicotine receptor antagonist and norepinephrine and dopamine reuptake inhibitor. The FDA previously issued a black box warning for bupropion to highlight the risk of mental health changes when taking this medication (eg, depressed mood, thoughts of suicide) and instructing clinicians to monitor changes in mood and behavior after prescribing this medication. However, this black box warning has since been removed (http://www.fda.gov/Drugs/DrugSafety/ucm532221.htm).

In one open-label pilot study, sustained-release bupropion (150 mg twice daily) appeared to be safe and clinically useful in reducing number of cigarettes smoked in a small sample of adolescents.[31] A double-blind, controlled trial[32] compared 150 mg/day of bupropion versus placebo and found higher rates of self-reported smoking abstinence among youth who received bupropion. A larger controlled trial[33] evaluated the efficacy of bupropion in augmenting behavioral therapy for adolescents. Among 312 adolescents receiving bupropion 150 mg/day or 300 mg/day, those receiving 300 mg/day achieved higher rates of abstinence compared to placebo at the end of 6 weeks of treatment.

Gray et al.[34] examined the combined efficacy of bupropion sustained release (SR) along with a contingency management (CM) behavioral intervention. The combination of medication plus CM produced greater smoking abstinence rates compared to the no-intervention condition. The combined behavioral-pharmacological treatment also produced better outcomes compared to either active intervention alone at various time points during treatment. More than half of participants across groups experienced at least one adverse event such as headache, insomnia, irritability, or dream disturbances, though there was no significant difference in adverse events between groups. The relative effectiveness of nicotine patch plus bupropion versus nicotine patch alone in adolescents who smoked was evaluated in an RCT.[35] Both groups demonstrated modest reductions in number of cigarettes smoked, with no significant difference.

Varenicline

Varenicline exerts its effects as a partial nicotinic acetylcholine receptor agonist and, like bupropion, was previously subject to a black box warning to monitor changes in mental health after starting patients on varenicline (http://www.fda.gov/Drugs/DrugSafety/ucm532221.htm), though the warning was dropped in 2016 (https://www.jwatch.org/fw112367/2016/12/19/fda-removes-black-box-warning-vareniclines-label). One study, which evaluated the pharmacokinetics, safety, and tolerability of various doses of varenicline based on body weight in teens who smoked, suggested it was generally well-tolerated.[36] Adverse events, were experienced by more than half of participants in each group; most were considered mild (dizziness, nausea, vomiting, and headache) though some participants reported psychiatric adverse events (eg, abnormal dreams). No participant discontinued varenicline due to adverse events.

Studies supporting the efficacy of varenicline in youth are mixed. A small pilot study by Gray et al. compared varenicline ($N = 15$) to bupropion XL ($N = 14$) among youth aged 15 to 20 in a double-blind, randomized trial. Both medications were associated with marked reductions in cigarettes smoked per day.[37] A larger trial that included 157 youth ages 14 to 21 enrolled from a single clinical site randomized participants to 12 weeks of varenicline versus placebo; participants in both groups received developmentally-appropriate counseling. Varenicline was well tolerated but did not improve end-of-treatment abstinence compared to placebo.[38] A trial that randomized an international sample of 312 treatment-seeking adolescents ages 12-19 to 12 weeks of high versus low dose varenicline versus placebo and developmentally-appropriate counseling found that abstinence rates did not differ between the groups.[39]

In summary, evidence supporting use of pharmacotherapy for youth in the treatment of tobacco use disorder (TUD) is limited and modest. NRT patches appear to improve craving, withdrawal symptoms, and short-term abstinence rates, though the utility of NRT in increasing long term abstinence is unclear. Bupropion appears to be safe for teens and associated with increases in long term abstinence, while studies of varenicline in youth have so far reported mixed results. To date, studies have primarily enrolled adolescents who smoke; there is less evidence regarding the efficacy of pharmacotherapy for adolescents who vape nicotine and pending, but no completed trials, for youth who exclusively vape nicotine.

Alcohol

Use of alcohol is common during adolescence, with more than half of teens having tried alcohol before completing high school and nearly 40% having experienced intoxication.[12] The severity and chronicity of adolescent alcohol use disorders are predictive of alcohol use disorders during adulthood, underscoring the importance of interventions targeting adolescent alcohol use disorders.[40]

Acute Ingestion and Withdrawal

Treatment for alcohol intoxication in youth is primarily supportive, including monitoring and managing for respiratory depression, treating electrolyte and metabolic disturbances, and managing hypovolemia and hypothermia.[41]

Symptomatic alcohol or sedative withdrawal, while rare in youth,[42] can be potentially fatal and may require the use of benzodiazepines[40] and cardiovascular monitoring delivered in withdrawal management settings or emergency departments. Although there is little literature about the management of benzodiazepines for alcohol withdrawal specific to adolescents, acute management is similar to adult patients presenting with acute alcohol or sedative withdrawal. The purpose of benzodiazepine therapy is to prevent seizures and mitigate delirium tremens. The expected time course of alcohol withdrawal is onset of mild symptoms in 6 to 24 hours from last drink, peak of symptoms in 24 to 48 hours, and resolution by about 96 hours. The preferred approach to benzodiazepine administration is symptom-triggered dosing based on Clinical Institute Withdrawal Assessment (CIWA) scores. Fixed-schedule regimens are also an option when frequent CIWA scoring is not feasible, however compared to symptom-triggered treatment these regimens are associated with increased total doses of benzodiazepines, increased risk of overmedication, and increased health care costs.[43,44] There is growing evidence supporting the use of phenobarbital in the management of acute alcohol withdrawal with a retrospective study showing patients receiving phenobarbital have similar outcomes to those treated with benzodiazepines with respect to seizures, delirium tremens, alcoholic hallucinosis, length of hospital stay, ICU admission, and medication-related adverse events.[45] There was also no difference in subsequent benzodiazepine use or return to alcohol use.[46]

However, phenobarbital has not yet been studied for alcohol withdrawal management in adolescent populations. Similarly, there is growing evidence among adults supporting the use of fixed-dose gabapentin to ameliorate acute alcohol withdrawal symptoms and promote abstinence, although the effect is predominantly on reducing a return to drinking (defined as percentage of days with heavy drinking) compared to placebo. The effect was greatest among those with more alcohol withdrawal symptoms historically.[47] As the study excluded those at elevated risk for moderate to severe withdrawal (for example, excluding those who could not maintain abstinence for three days before study start, those who were medically unstable, those with a 3-fold higher elevation in liver enzymes at baseline, or those with a history of alcohol withdrawal seizure or a CIWA-AR score of 10 or more during the initial assessment), it is unclear if gabapentin works as well as benzodiazepines in preventing alcohol withdrawal related seizures. Although it needs additional study in teens and among those with moderate to severe withdrawal risk, gabapentin may be a safer and still effective option for the outpatient management of youth at-risk for acute alcohol withdrawal.

Pharmacotherapy for Alcohol Use Disorder

Naltrexone

Naltrexone is an FDA-approved medication for the treatment of alcohol use disorders for those ages 18 and older, which exerts its effects as an opioid antagonist and by decreasing craving. There is emerging evidence supporting the safety and efficacy of naltrexone in adolescents. A small ($N = 5$), 6-week, open-label trial of 25 to 50 mg of oral naltrexone conducted by Deas and colleagues found that youth who received naltrexone showed significant reductions in number of drinks per day, in alcohol craving, and alcohol-related compulsions.[48] In a small ($N = 28$ youth 15-19 years of age) crossover trial by Miranda and colleagues, that randomized participants to receive 8 to 10 days of oral naltrexone (50 mg/daily) or placebo followed by a washout period and then switch to the opposite study condition found that naltrexone reduced heavy drinking, blunted craving and altered subjective responses to alcohol consumption, providing preliminary evidence of efficacy for the management of alcohol use disorder in youth.[49] Further studies are needed to evaluate the use of injectable, extended-release naltrexone in youth, as this is the preferred formulation in adults with alcohol use disorder and may have added benefit with respect to adherence and tolerability.

Disulfiram

Disulfiram is a medication that impairs the breakdown of alcohol and causes an unpleasant reaction to alcohol consumption. A small, double-blinded, placebo-controlled study[50] conducted with 26 adolescents, aged 16 to 19, randomized youth to receive placebo or disulfiram found that youth who received disulfiram had a lower rate of returning to use. A similar beneficial effect was observed in a study comparing disulfiram versus naltrexone in adolescents with alcohol use disorders ($N = 58$). Although disulfiram has shown preliminary efficacy, it is recommended for use only with individuals who are committed to abstinence, and treatment with this medication requires careful medical supervision due to risks of hepatotoxicity associated with disulfiram and potentially lethal risks of combining disulfiram and alcohol.[40]

Other Medications

Only one, small, open-label study has been conducted evaluating the 5-HT_3 receptor antagonist ondansetron (intended to reduce alcohol craving) in adolescents with alcohol dependence.[51,52] In this 8-week study, youth receiving ondansetron (4 mcg/kg twice daily) showed significant reductions in drinks per day and increases in number of days abstinent.[52]

Additional medications have shown promise in reducing alcohol use among adults with alcohol use disorder (AUD), including acamprosate, which is FDA approved to treat AUD in populations ages 18 years and older. However, acamprosate and other medications such as topiramate, and baclofen, have not been systematically studied in adolescent populations, and thus, their clinical utility with teens is not yet known.

In summary, pharmacotherapy in the treatment of youth with AUDs is limited but promising; additional studies are needed to identify the best formulations and further evaluate emerging treatments. The greatest data supports the use of naltrexone as an effective agent to blunt cravings and reduce the likelihood of returning to alcohol use. While the majority of studies test oral naltrexone, the added efficacy of injectable, extended-release naltrexone in studies of patients ages 18 years of age and older suggests there may also be an added benefit for adherence and tolerability in this age group. Small studies show a benefit for disulfiram in reducing the use of alcohol in a sample of youth highly highlight committed to abstinence, although its effect profile limit its applicability to youth broadly.

Cannabis

Cannabis remains the most commonly used illicit substance worldwide[53] and is the most commonly used substance other than alcohol and nicotine among youth.[12] Cannabis use among adolescents is associated with greater likelihood and persistence of use in adulthood, and use of cannabis before the age of 17 is associated with a markedly increased risk for developing substance use disorders in adulthood.[54] As with many other substances, cannabis use among teens is associated with lower academic performance, lower levels of educational and occupational achievement, and comorbid psychopathology. Additionally, cannabis use among adolescents has been associated with poorer cognitive functioning.[55]

Acute Ingestion and Withdrawal

Management of acute cannabis intoxication is focused on managing associated dysphoria, anxiety, or paranoia with reassurance, environmental measures such as decreased stimulation, and at times, short-acting benzodiazepines to mitigate acute anxiety. Synthetic cannabinoids are often much more potent than naturally occurring ones; anxiety, psychosis, seizures, and cardiotoxicity associated with synthetic cannabinoid use have been reported.[56-58] According to American Association of Poison Control Centers,[59,60] calls for human exposure to synthetic cannabinoids rose to a peak in 2015 before decreasing in 2016 with the majority of these involving people 25 years and younger. These cases have been managed in ED settings, requiring a spectrum of care, ranging from the use of benzodiazepines, antipsychotics, and/or IV fluids to intubation in intensive care units.[57]

Although often under-recognized, cannabis can result in a withdrawal syndrome.[61] A recent systematic review and meta-analysis of adult populations identified nearly half (47%) of individuals experienced cannabis withdrawal syndrome with a greater prevalence in those with concurrent tobacco and other substance use disorders as well as daily use. Treatment is supportive and focused on treating associated symptoms (eg, sleep hygiene, medication to address sleep disruption, and anxiety).[61]

Treatment

To date, no medications have been FDA approved for the treatment of cannabis use disorder in adults or children.[62] The primary treatments are psychosocial; cognitive-behavioral therapy is considered first-line treatment in adults and older youths.[63] Young adults may be more likely to identify a harm reduction versus abstinence goal. Evidence supports focusing on a reduction in frequency rather than quantity of cannabis use as a reduction in days is more consistently associated with improved functioning and improved quality of life.[64,65]

N-Acetyl Cysteine

A double-blind, randomized, controlled trial evaluated the efficacy of *N*-acetyl cysteine (NAC), a glutamate-modulating agent with activity at the nucleus accumbens. The study enrolled 116 youths ages 15 to 21 years with cannabis dependence for an 8-week period.[66] Youth participants received either 1,200 mg NAC or placebo twice daily along with twice weekly contingency management and weekly brief abstinence counseling. Results indicated that NAC was well-tolerated. Findings showed promise in reducing cannabis use (as evidenced by more than twofold reduction in positive urine samples compared to placebo).[66] A larger trial of older participants (18-50 years of age), found no differences in cannabis use between the NAC and placebo groups at 12 weeks.[67]

Topiramate

A randomized trial comparing topiramate plus motivational enhancement therapy (MET) to placebo plus MET enrolled 66 youths (ages 15-24) with heavy cannabis use.[68,69] While there was no reduction in abstinence, days with cannabis use, or urine tests, individuals in the topiramate group reduced the reported number of grams of cannabis smoked per day. High drop out in the topiramate treatment group because of adverse effects may have biased findings.

Emerging Therapies

There are small trials among adult populations suggesting potential treatments for cannabis use disorder: for example, gabapentin reduced cannabis use and withdrawal symptoms[70]; nabiximols, a cannabis whole-plant extract containing 1:1; ratio of THC and cannabidiol showed early promising but ultimately mixed effects on use[68,69]; and a phase 2a, double-blind, placebo-controlled, randomized, adaptive Bayesian trial that included participants 16 years of age and older showed cannabidiol at daily doses of 400 and 800 mg over 4 weeks were safe and more efficacious than placebo in reducing cannabis use.[71] A 6-week pilot trial of varenicline, a selective nicotinic acetylcholine receptor agonist, showed a greater reduction in percentage of days of cannabis use and greater rate of self-reported weekly cannabis abstinence, although it was not designed to detect statistically significant between-group differences.[72] Additional rigorous trials are needed to determine the ultimate efficacy of these types of therapies in reducing cannabis use, particularly among young people.

In summary, no FDA-approved medications for the treatment of cannabis use disorder exist for youth (or adults). Small trials found evidence for 1,200 mg of NAC twice daily in reducing cannabis use disorder in youth. Topiramate may have reduced the amount of cannabis used but was not well-tolerated by youth. Early data suggests that varenicline may reduce days of cannabis use and increase cannabis abstinence, although robust evaluation in clinical trials is needed.

Opioids

Youth have not been spared from the opioid-related overdose crisis impacting the United States.[73] Starting in 2020, youth experienced a greater relative increase in overdose deaths compared to adults.[74] The rising rates of deaths were driven by synthetic opioids, such as fentanyl, which increased as a cause of death 2925% between 1999 and 2016. The high morbidity and mortality from the widespread use of potent synthetic opioids highlights the need for urgent interventions to increase access to evidence-based opioid used disorder (OUD) treatment for youth.

Several pharmacotherapies have been evaluated in the treatment of OUD among adolescents, including the partial μ-opioid agonist buprenorphine, the antagonist naltrexone, and the μ-opioid agonist methadone. There is growing evidence that these medications are safe and effective for adolescents and strong evidence these medications reduce mortality in adults.[75] However, adolescents are significantly less likely than adults to receive pharmacotherapy for OUD: a retrospective review found that of youth accessing specialty treatment for OUD, only 2.4% and 4% of those using heroin and prescription opioids respectively received pharmacotherapy compared to 26.3% and 12% of adults using the same substances.[76] Chatterjee et al. demonstrated that fewer than 5% of youth with OUD received pharmacotherapy in the 12 months leading up to an overdose event.[5] Even after an overdose, only 8% of adolescents received pharmacotherapy for OUD, compared to 29% of adults. The high morbidity and mortality from the widespread use of potent synthetic opioids highlights the need for urgent interventions to increase access to evidence-based OUD treatment for youth.

Acute Ingestion and Withdrawal Management

While many adolescents nonmedically use opioids in a sporadic, experimental manner, those with physiologic dependence will often experience withdrawal upon abstinence. The expected time course of withdrawal from short-acting opioids is onset of mild symptoms in 6 to 12 hours from last use, peak of symptoms in 24 to 48 hours, and resolution by about 120 hours. While opioid withdrawal is not typically life-threatening in otherwise healthy individuals, it can cause significant distress and puts individuals at risk for return to use. Thus, it is important to offer evidence-based pharmacotherapy to mitigate withdrawal symptoms.

While clonidine (an alpha-2 adrenergic agonist) has historically been widely used to treat opioid withdrawal in youth, evidence supports the use of buprenorphine as first line treatment for adolescents. One double-blind, randomized controlled trial demonstrated that sublingual buprenorphine produced markedly better opioid abstinence and treatment retention rates compared to clonidine, although both medications appeared safe and well-tolerated in this youth sample.[77] A multisite randomized controlled trial ($N = 152$) in youth with opioid dependence found that a longer period of stabilization on sublingual buprenorphine, defined as 12 weeks as compared to up to 2 weeks, resulted in better opioid and injection use outcomes[78] and was more cost-effective.[79] Similarly, a study ($N = 53$) in which youth were assigned to either an 8- or 4-week buprenorphine taper found that those receiving a longer taper had significantly better opioid use and treatment retention outcomes.[80] A Cochrane review demonstrated that adolescents receiving buprenorphine for withdrawal management were more likely to successfully transition to maintenance therapy.[81]

Buprenorphine

Buprenorphine is a μ-opioid receptor partial agonist that reduces opioid cravings and withdrawal symptoms. It has been studied in three rigorous experimental trials in youth with OUD and has shown considerable promise as a pharmacotherapy for adolescents. It is FDA-approved for youth ages 16 and older with OUD and is a first-line agent in the treatment for youth with OUD. Buprenorphine improves psychosocial functioning[82] and is safe and effective for treating youth with OUD involving either heroin or prescription opioids.[83] Two double-blind, placebo controlled, multicenter randomized controlled trials have demonstrated benefits in adolescents, including reduction in opioid-positive urine samples, reduction in self-reported injection use and overall use, and increased treatment retention.[78,80] A retrospective cohort study of youth ages 13 to 22 receiving Medicaid found that those receiving buprenorphine were 42% less likely to drop out of treatment during the follow-up period compared to those who received behavioral treatment alone.[84] Youth factors that increase the likelihood of treatment success include receipt of ancillary treatments, success in the first 2 weeks and completion of 12 weeks of treatment.[85] Unlike methadone, which requires treatment in a specialty addiction treatment program, buprenorphine treatment can be accessed in a wide array of health care settings, including primary care. A growing number of injectable and implantable formulations of buprenorphine that may improve adherence are now FDA-approved, but there are no published studies comparing the efficacy of different formulations in adolescents nor is their adolescent-specific data highlighting best practices or strategies for inducting youth on buprenorphine during the fentanyl era.

Naltrexone

Naltrexone, an opioid antagonist, has shown promise in preventing return to opioid use among youth who have achieved abstinence from opioids.[77] The role and timing of naltrexone administration for OUD is distinct from buprenorphine because naltrexone can precipitate withdrawal symptoms if initiated earlier than 7 to 10 days after abstinence. Several observational and pilot trials suggest that naltrexone is feasible and effective in youth though no large clinical trials with this age group have been published. Monthly intramuscular injections of extended-release naltrexone may be the most promising formulation. This approach increases adherence and is more effective than oral naltrexone in the adult population. A case series of adolescents showed that monthly intramuscular injections of extended-release naltrexone appear to be well-tolerated, feasible to administer, and clinically useful for the treatment of OUD in this age group.[86] In 2021, Mitchell et al. conducted a small randomized controlled trial of 288 youth ages 15 to 21 at a residential SUD treatment program who were randomized to either extended-release naltrexone or treatment-as-usual. Intention to treat analysis did not reach significance, which may have been impacted by high rates of nonadherence. However, there was a significant reduction in opioid use for those who actually received naltrexone.[87] Further studies are needed to better understand the acceptability and efficacy of naltrexone treatment among youth with OUD.

Methadone

To our knowledge, no experimental, controlled research studies have been conducted evaluating the safety and effectiveness of methadone with adolescents; however, several reports have suggested clinical utility in youth with OUD.[88] Methadone's mechanism of action is both as a full opioid agonist and NMDA receptor antagonist, resulting in reducing craving and withdrawal symptoms. An evaluation conducted more than 40 years ago compared outcomes among teens with opioid dependence who received either methadone maintenance, therapeutic community-based treatment, outpatient "drug-free treatment" or withdrawal management. All treatment approaches were associated with reduced opioid use among youth, but treatment retention among youth who used opioids daily was greatest with methadone maintenance. More recent retrospective and observational studies have similarly demonstrated that methadone is effective for retaining adolescents with OUD in treatment. A retrospective cohort study conducted by Kellogg et al. among 147 youth ages 15 to 23 in a methadone treatment program in the United States found a 12-month retention rate of 48%,[89] and that youth retained in treatment had a higher likelihood of opioid-negative urine. Another observational study of 120 youth age 18 years found a 43% retention rate at 1 year.[90] Retrospective cohort data from adolescents and young adults receiving Medicaid found that youth receiving methadone were 68% less likely to drop out of treatment compared to those receiving behavioral treatment alone.[84] When compared to buprenorphine, a small retrospective chart review of 60 adolescents found that youth receiving methadone were retained in treatment longer than those treated with buprenorphine.[91]

Despite evidence suggesting efficacy, there are many barriers to adolescents accessing methadone therapy in the United States. Methadone is typically offered in the context of a specialized opioid treatment program (OTP) with daily observed dosing. Most OTPs do not enroll youth under age 18 years and for those who are eligible, they must often meet stringent guidelines and often require consent from a parent or legal guardian.

In summary, pharmacotherapy is recommended for youth with moderate and severe OUD at the time of their diagnosis and should be considered in those with mild OUD. Buprenorphine is the first line agent with the most robust data supporting its efficacy in youths. Oral and injectable formulations of naltrexone have less robust evidence in youth and studies are impacted by high rates of nonadherence. Naltrexone appears well-tolerated, and acceptable, with evidence for efficacy among those who are adherent. Evidence supporting methadone use for youth with OUD is limited and its use is complicated by regulatory hurdles. Equitable access to these medications remain a challenge with a cohort study of Medicaid-enrolled youths showing only 1 in 54 youths received treatment with evidence-based medications following an opioid-related overdose, and rates among Black or Latinx youth were less than 1%.[92] More work is needed to support equitable implementation of these medications, particularly with rising racial disparities in overdose rates.[93]

Cocaine, Methamphetamines, and Other Stimulants

While cocaine and methamphetamine use remain uncommon among youths (with 0.7% of youth ages 12-17 endorsing past year use of cocaine and 0.3% of methamphetamine in the United States), more than one in every six adolescents in the United States reports having ever used prescription stimulants medically or nonmedically.[94,95] Prescription stimulants remain first-line treatment for attention deficit hyperactivity disorder with 2.8 million youth prescribed these medications annually,[96] and they are one of the most frequently diverted medications among youth[97-101] with rates of 3% to 9% of middle and high school students and 3% to 25% among college students depending on the population.[102-105] There is a paucity of literature reporting on the treatment of stimulant use disorders in adolescents with the bulk supporting behavioral interventions, such as contingency management.[106] For prescription stimulants, short interventions, such as training providers to ask patients about diversion have shown modest reductions in diversion of prescribed stimulants.[107,108] Studies of adults with stimulant use disorders often generate modest treatment effects and/or inconsistent efficacy.

Acute Ingestion and Withdrawal Management

Acute and chronic use of stimulants may lead to a host of stimulant-related psychoactive effects from agitation and confusion to anxiety, panic attacks, and paranoia and physical effects including hyperthermia and hypertension. Acute management may require aggressive treatment of agitation with intravenous benzodiazepines, or first-generation antipsychotics for adjunctive therapy. Even otherwise healthy young patients are at risk for cardiac arrhythmias and other cardiotoxic effects.[109]

Synthetic cathinones are amphetamine analogs. These are marketed as "bath salts" and have a similar mechanism of action to methamphetamine. They block reuptake of dopamine, norepinephrine and serotonin and stimulate release of dopamine. Research to better understand the actions, toxicology, and unhealthy use potential of these agents remain limited, but overdose on synthetic cathinones, similar to MDMA or amphetamine, may require emergency management of cardiovascular and agitation/psychotic symptoms (with benzodiazepines and/or antipsychotics) and in rare cases may result in death.[110,111]

The number of fatal overdoses involving polysubstance use, often driven often by co-ingestion (intentionally or otherwise) of stimulants and synthetic opioids, such as fentanyl, is increasing.[112] Offering youth both anticipatory guidance on the risks of unwitting opioid exposure from a contaminated stimulant supply is now crucial along with also offering evidence-based risk reduction strategies such as naloxone and fentanyl test strips.

Treatment

To date, no pharmacotherapies have been FDA approved for the treatment of cocaine use disorder in the United States.

Although some antidepressants have shown promise in the treatment of cocaine use disorder among adults, the literature to date does not support their effectiveness.[113] Two case reports have examined the tricyclic antidepressant, desipramine, for cocaine dependence among teens and results were inconclusive.[114,115]

Psychostimulants have shown promise in adults with cocaine dependence, but remain controversial as an approach to treatment.[116,117] Long-acting amphetamine and methamphetamine have been tested in small trials of patients with stimulant disorders in adult populations with mixed results. Modafinil showed promise in small trials of adult populations, but larger trials found mixed effects.[118-120] Please refer to Chapter 64, "Pharmacological Treatment of Stimulant Use Disorder" for more information about treatment of stimulant disorder.

Although not tested in adolescents, the TA-CD vaccine stimulates production of cocaine-specific antibodies preventing them from crossing the blood-brain barrier and reducing the euphoric and reinforcing effects of cocaine. Although initial studies were promising, efficacy was mixed in subsequent studies.[121,122]

Bupropion and Extended-Release Naltrexone

Although studied in adult populations, there is emerging data suggesting a modest effect of combination bupropion and extended-release naltrexone on methamphetamine use. A double-blind, two-stage, placebo-controlled trial of 403 participants with methamphetamine use disorder received either injectable extended-release naltrexone with oral extended-release bupropion or placebo. Participants had a modest reduction in methamphetamine negative urines among the treatment group although the response rate was low overall (13.6% in the treatment group versus 2.5% in the placebo group).[123] Studies examining the efficacy of bupropion alone showed poor efficacy in reducing methamphetamine use.[124]

Mirtazapine

Mirtazapine is a mixed monoamine agonist-antagonist, which increases levels of serotonin, norepinephrine, and dopamine release and is hypothesized to reduce methamphetamine craving and withdrawal symptoms.[125] A double-blind randomized controlled trial of mirtazapine (30 mg orally) versus placebo in patients with methamphetamine use disorder found a reduction in methamphetamine-positive urine test results at 36 weeks in the treatment group compared to placebo. While adolescents were not included, the study warrants additional investigation, particularly in youth populations.

In summary, there are no FDA approved medications to treat stimulant use disorder in youth. While studies in adult populations support the modest effects of mirtazapine and combination bupropion and extended-release naltrexone in the treatment of methamphetamine use disorder, these have not been studied in adolescent and young adult populations.

CLINICAL CONSIDERATIONS

Evidence for the use of most medications to treat adolescent SUD is preliminary and emerging, with the exception of OUD. While treatment with medications, particularly buprenorphine is now the gold standard approach for youth with OUD, first line treatment for youth with other SUDs is typically a combination of psychosocial and behavioral treatments. When clinically appropriate, we recommend that clinicians engage in patient-centered discussions with youth (and their families if available) about medication options. We recommend that providers familiarize themselves with their state's rules and regulations on the need for parental consent for the treatment of adolescents with SUD, including psychotropic medications and medications for SUD, before writing a prescription. In addition to obtaining assent from minor patients and informed consent from parents, we recommend engaging the parent or caregiver to monitor medication usage to enhance adherence and support safety monitoring and reporting of adverse events and to provide an additional source of feedback regarding its efficacy. Polysubstance use is common and increases the complexity of treatment planning. In the case of youth who meet SUD criteria for multiple substances, in the absence of empirical evidence, the practitioner may consider a hierarchical treatment plan, focusing first on the substance most likely to result in medical or safety complication and utilizing a systematic and strategic combination of medications and/or psychosocial treatments to address concomitant substances and co-occurring conditions.

Another aspect of using pharmacotherapies for youth is determining an appropriate duration of treatment. As most published studies have tested the efficacy of study medications *only* for relatively short periods, we recommend that clinicians carefully discuss the limitations of currently available science at the beginning of treatment. Treatment duration in youth can be guided by treatment adherence, side effects and adverse events, clinical efficacy in reducing substance use, and global improvements in level of functioning.

Psychosocial Treatments

Although this chapter is intended to provide a review of the state of the science evaluating various pharmacotherapies for the treatment of adolescent SUDs, optimal treatment outcomes among youth are achieved when pharmacotherapy is provided along with psychosocial treatment. It is well documented that substance use among youth is highly comorbid with mental health problems. Psychosocial treatments offer the opportunity to address the full array of adolescent problems, including mental health disorders, family conflict, behavioral concerns, academic/school problems, anger management, communication, goal setting/tracking, and other important life skills training. Clinicians may consider combining pharmacotherapies for adolescents with SUDs with one or more evidence-based behavioral treatments.

Future Directions

There are numerous and wide gaps in medication treatment research among youth that urgently need to be addressed. Adequately powered replication studies to test the safety and efficacy in youth of existing FDA-approved medications for adults are obvious targets of such research. Research examining the efficacy of medications targeting the neurobehavioral and frontal lobe function deficits seen in youth with SUD such as impaired executive function, impulsivity, delay discounting, and low stress tolerance, may show promise in arresting the development of SUDs. Large scale studies that not only build and create the evidence base for SUD pharmacotherapy for youth are needed, and also hybrid trials and implementation studies showing how best to implement and integrate evidence-based practices into clinical care.

REFERENCES

1. Chen CY, Storr CL, Anthony JC. Early-onset drug use and risk for drug dependence problems. *Addict Behav.* 2009;34(3):319-322. doi:10.1016/j.addbeh.2008.10.021
2. Steinfeld MR, Torregrossa MM. Consequences of adolescent drug use. *Transl Psychiatry.* 2023;13:313. https://doi.org/10.1038/s41398-023-02590-4
3. Casey BJ, Jones RM. Neurobiology of the adolescent brain and behavior: implications for substance use disorders. *J Am Acad Child Adolesc Psychiatry.* 2010;49(12):1189-1201; quiz 1285. doi:10.1016/j.jaac.2010.08.017
4. Mericle A, Arria AM, Meyers K, Cacciola J, Winters KC, Kirby K. National Trends in Adolescent Substance Use Disorders and Treatment Availability: 2003–2010. *J Child Adolesc Subst Abuse.* 2015;24(5):255-263.
5. Chatterjee A, Larochelle MR, Xuan Z, et al. Non-fatal opioid related overdoses among adolescents in Massachusetts 2012-2014. *Drug Alcohol Depend.* 2019;194:28-31.
6. Tanner-Smith EE, Wilson SJ, Lipsey MW. The comparative effectiveness of outpatient treatment for adolescent substance abuse: a meta-analysis. *J Subst Abuse Treat.* 2013;44(2):145-158. doi:10.1016/j.jsat.2012.05.006
7. Waldron HB, Turner CW. Evidence-based psychosocial treatments for adolescent substance abuse. *J Clin Child Adolesc Psychol.* 2008;37(1):238-261. doi:10.1080/15374410701820133
8. Karpinski JP, Timpe EM, Lubsch L. Smoking cessation treatment for adolescents. *J Pediatr Pharmacol Ther.* 2010;15(4):249-263.
9. Yuan M, Cross SJ, Loughlin SE, Leslie FM. Nicotine and the adolescent brain. *J Physiol.* 2015;593(16):3397-3412. doi:10.1113/JP270492
10. Mathers M, Toumbourou JW, Catalano RF, Williams J, Patton GC. Consequences of youth tobacco use: a review of prospective behavioural studies. *Addiction.* 2006;101(7):948-958. doi:10.1111/j.1360-0443.2006.01438.x
11. Alvarado GF, Breslau N. Smoking and young people's mental health. *Curr Opin Psychiatry.* 2005;18(4):397-400. doi:10.1097/01.yco.0000172058.48154.14
12. Johnston LD, Miech RA, O'Malley PM, Bachman JG, Schulenberg JE, Patrick ME. *Monitoring the Future National Survey Results on Drug Use, 1975-2021: Overview, Key Findings on Adolescent Drug Use.* Institute for Social Research: University of Michigan; 2022.
13. Soneji S, Barrington-Trimis JL, Wills TA, et al. Association between initial use of e-cigarettes and subsequent cigarette smoking among adolescents and young adults: a systematic review and meta-analysis. *JAMA Pediatr.* 2017;171(8):788-797. doi:10.1001/jamapediatrics.2017.1488
14. Javed S, Usmani S, Sarfraz Z, et al. A scoping review of vaping, e-cigarettes and mental health impact: depression and suicidality. *J Community Hosp Intern Med Perspect.* 2022;12(3):33-39. doi:10.55729/2000-9666.1053
15. Dearfield CT, Chen-Sankey JC, McNeel TS, Bernat DH, Choi K. E-cigarette initiation predicts subsequent academic performance among youth: results from the PATH Study. *Prev Med.* 2021;153:106781. doi:10.1016/j.ypmed.2021.106781
16. Rigsby DC, Keim SA, Milanaik R, Adesman A. Electronic vapor product use and sexual risk behaviors in US adolescents. Pediatrics. 2021;147(6):8.
17. Jonas A. Impact of vaping on respiratory health. *BMJ.* 2022;378:e065997. doi:10.1136/bmj-2021-065997
18. Hamberger ES, Halpern-Felsher B. Vaping in adolescents: epidemiology and respiratory harm. *Curr Opin Pediatr.* 2020;32(3):378-383. doi:10.1097/MOP.0000000000000896
19. Myung SK, Park JY. Efficacy of pharmacotherapy for smoking cessation in adolescent smokers: a meta-analysis of randomized controlled trials. *Nicotine Tob Res.* 2019;21(11):1473-1479. doi:10.1093/ntr/nty180
20. Sargent JD, Unger JB, Leventhal AM. Recommendations from the USPSTF for prevention and cessation of tobacco use in children and adolescents. *JAMA.* 2020;323(16):1563-1564. doi:10.1001/jama.2019.22312
21. Fiore M, Jaen C, Baker T, Benowitz L, Curry S. Treating tobacco use and dependence: 2008 update. *Clinical Practice Guidelines.* US Department of Health and Human Services Public Health Service. Accessed July 27, 2023. https://www.ncbi.nlm.nih.gov/books/NBK63952/
22. Sims TH; the Committee on Substance Abuse. Tobacco as a substance of abuse. *Pediatrics.* 2009;124(5):e1045-e1053. doi:10.1542/peds.2009-2121
23. American Academy of Pediatrics. *Tobacco Use: Considerations for Clinicians.* Accessed September 8, 2022. https://www.aap.org/en/patient-care/tobacco-control-and-prevention/youth-tobacco-cessation/tobacco-use-considerations-for-clinicians/
24. Hanson K, Allen S, Jensen S, Hatsukami D. Treatment of adolescent smokers with the nicotine patch. *Nicotine Tob Res.* 2003;5(4):515-526. doi:10.1080/1462220031000118559
25. Roddy E, Romilly N, Challenger A, Lewis S, Britton J. Use of nicotine replacement therapy in socioeconomically deprived young smokers: a community-based pilot randomised controlled trial. *Tob Control.* 2006;15(5):373-376. doi:10.1136/tc.2005.014514
26. Moolchan ET, Robinson ML, Ernst M, et al. Safety and efficacy of the nicotine patch and gum for the treatment of adolescent tobacco addiction. *Pediatrics.* 2005;115(4):e407-e414. doi:10.1542/peds.2004-1894
27. Rubinstein ML, Benowitz NL, Auerback GM, Moscicki AB. A randomized trial of nicotine nasal spray in adolescent smokers. *Pediatrics.* 2008;122(3):e595-e600. doi:10.1542/peds.2008-0501
28. Scherphof CS, van den Eijnden RJJM, Engels RCME, Vollebergh WAM. Short-term efficacy of nicotine replacement therapy for smoking cessation in adolescents: a randomized controlled trial. *J Subst Abuse Treat.* 2014;46(2):120-127. doi:10.1016/j.jsat.2013.08.008
29. Scherphof CS, Eijnden RJJM, Engels RCME, Vollebergh WAM. Long-term efficacy of nicotine replacement therapy for smoking cessation in adolescents: a randomized controlled trial. *Drug Alcohol Depend.* 2014;140:217-220. doi:10.1016/j.drugalcdep.2014.04.007
30. Fanshawe TR, Halliwell W, Lindson N, Aveyard P, Livingstone-Banks J, Hartmann-Boyce J. Tobacco cessation interventions for young people. *Cochrane Database Syst Rev.* 2017;11:CD003289. doi:10.1002/14651858.CD003289.pub6
31. Upadhyaya HP, Brady KT, Wang W. Bupropion SR in adolescents with comorbid ADHD and nicotine dependence: a pilot study. *J Am Acad Child Adolesc Psychiatry.* 2004;43(2):199-205. doi:10.1097/00004583-200402000-00016
32. Niederhofer H, Huber M. Bupropion may support psychosocial treatment of nicotine-dependent adolescents: preliminary results. *Pharmacotherapy.* 2004;24(11):1524-1528. doi:10.1592/phco.24.16.1524.50953
33. Muramoto ML, Leischow SJ, Sherrill D, Matthews E, Strayer LJ. Randomized, double-blind, placebo-controlled trial of 2 dosages of sustained-release bupropion for adolescent smoking cessation. *Arch Pediatr Adolesc Med.* 2007;161(11):1068-1074. doi:10.1001/archpedi.161.11.1068

34. Gray KM, Carpenter MJ, Baker NL, et al. Bupropion SR and contingency management for adolescent smoking cessation. *J Subst Abuse Treat.* 2011;40(1):77-86. doi:10.1016/j.jsat.2010.08.010
35. Killen JD, Robinson TN, Ammerman S, et al. Randomized clinical trial of the efficacy of bupropion combined with nicotine patch in the treatment of adolescent smokers. *J Consult Clin Psychol.* 2004;72(4):729-735. doi:10.1037/0022-006X.72.4.729
36. Faessel H, Ravva P, Williams K. Pharmacokinetics, safety, and tolerability of varenicline in healthy adolescent smokers: a multicenter, randomized, double-blind, placebo-controlled, parallel-group study. *Clin Ther.* 2009;31(1):177-189. doi:10.1016/j.clinthera.2009.01.003
37. Gray KM, Carpenter MJ, Lewis AL, Klintworth EM, Upadhyaya HP. Varenicline versus bupropion XL for smoking cessation in older adolescents: a randomized, double-blind pilot trial. *Nicotine Tob Res.* 2012;14(2):234-239. doi:10.1093/ntr/ntr130
38. Gray KM, Baker NL, McClure EA, et al. Efficacy and safety of varenicline for adolescent smoking cessation: a randomized clinical trial. *JAMA Pediatr.* 2019;173(12):1146-1153. doi:10.1001/jamapediatrics.2019.3553
39. Gray KM, Rubinstein ML, Prochaska JJ, et al. High-dose and low-dose varenicline for smoking cessation in adolescents: a randomised, placebo-controlled trial. *Lancet Child Adolesc Health.* 2020;4(11):837-845. doi:10.1016/S2352-4642(20)30243-1
40. Clark DB. Pharmacotherapy for adolescent alcohol use disorder. *CNS Drugs.* 2012;26(7):559-569. doi:10.2165/11634330-000000000-00000
41. Piccioni A, Tarli C, Cardone S, et al. Role of first aid in the management of acute alcohol intoxication: a narrative review. *Eur Rev Med Pharmacol Sci.* 2020;24(17):9121-9128. doi:10.26355/eurrev_202009_22859
42. Chung T, Martin CS, Armstrong TD, Labouvie EW. Prevalence of DSM-IV alcohol diagnoses and symptoms in adolescent community and clinical samples. *J Am Acad Child Adolesc Psychiatry.* 2002;41:546-554. doi:10.1097/00004583-200205000-00012
43. Sachdeva A, Chandra M, Deshpande SN. A comparative study of fixed tapering dose regimen versus symptom-triggered regimen of lorazepam for alcohol detoxification. *Alcohol Alcohol.* 2014;49(3):287-291. doi:10.1093/alcalc/agt181
44. Soravia LM, Wopfner A, Pfiffner L, Bétrisey S, Moggi F. Symptom-triggered detoxification using the alcohol-withdrawal-scale reduces risks and healthcare costs. *Alcohol Alcohol.* 2018;53(1):71-77. doi:10.1093/alcalc/agx080
45. Nisavic M, Nejad SH, Isenberg BM, et al. Use of phenobarbital in alcohol withdrawal management—a retrospective comparison study of phenobarbital and benzodiazepines for acute alcohol withdrawal management in general medical patients. *Psychosomatics.* 2019;60(5):458-467. doi:10.1016/j.psym.2019.02.002
46. Askgaard G, Hallas J, Fink-Jensen A, Molander AC, Madsen KG, Pottegård A. Phenobarbital compared to benzodiazepines in alcohol withdrawal treatment: a register-based cohort study of subsequent benzodiazepine use, alcohol recidivism and mortality. *Drug Alcohol Depend.* 2016;161:258-264. doi:10.1016/j.drugalcdep.2016.02.016
47. Anton RF, Latham P, Voronin K, et al. Efficacy of gabapentin for the treatment of alcohol use disorder in patients with alcohol withdrawal symptoms: a randomized clinical trial. *JAMA Intern Med.* 2020;180(5):728-736. doi:10.1001/jamainternmed.2020.0249
48. Deas D, May MPHK, Randall C, Johnson N, Anton R. Naltrexone treatment of adolescent alcoholics: an open-label pilot study. *J Child Adolesc Psychopharmacol.* 2005;15(5):723-728. doi:10.1089/cap.2005.15.723
49. Miranda R, Ray L, Blanchard A, et al. Effects of naltrexone on adolescent alcohol cue reactivity and sensitivity: an initial randomized trial. *Addict Biol.* 2014;19(5):941-954. doi:10.1111/adb.12050
50. Niederhofer H, Staffen W. Comparison of disulfiram and placebo in treatment of alcohol dependence of adolescents. *Drug Alcohol Rev.* 2003;22(3):295-297. doi:10.1080/0959523031000154436
51. Dawes MA, Johnson BA, Ma JZ, Ait-Daoud N, Thomas SE, Cornelius JR. Reductions in and relations between "craving" and drinking in a prospective, open-label trial of ondansetron in adolescents with alcohol dependence. *Addict Behav.* 2005;30(9):1630-1637. doi:10.1016/j.addbeh.2005.07.004
52. Dawes MA, Johnson BA, Ait-Daoud N, Ma JZ, Cornelius JR. A prospective, open-label trial of ondansetron in adolescents with alcohol dependence. *Addict Behav.* 2005;30(6):1077-1085. doi:10.1016/j.addbeh.2004.10.011
53. United Nations Office on Drugs and Crime. *World Drug Report 2021.* Accessed September 8, 2022. https://www.unodc.org/unodc/en/data-and-analysis/wdr2021.html
54. Lynskey MT, Heath AC, Bucholz KK, et al. Escalation of drug use in early-onset cannabis users vs co-twin controls. *JAMA.* 2003;289(4):427. doi:10.1001/jama.289.4.427
55. Squeglia LM, Jacobus J, Tapert SF. The influence of substance use on adolescent brain development. *Clin EEG Neurosci.* 2009;40(1):31-38.
56. Young AC, Schwarz E, Medina G, et al. Cardiotoxicity associated with the synthetic cannabinoid, K9, with laboratory confirmation. *Am J Emerg Med.* 2012;30(7):1320.e5-e7. doi:10.1016/j.ajem.2011.05.013
57. Gunderson EW, Haughey HM, Ait-Daoud N, Joshi AS, Hart CL. "Spice" and "K2" herbal highs: a case series and systematic review of the clinical effects and biopsychosocial implications of synthetic cannabinoid use in humans. *Am J Addict.* 2012;21(4):320-326. doi:10.1111/j.1521-0391.2012.00240.x
58. Simmons J, Cookman L, Kang C, Skinner C. Three cases of "spice" exposure. *Clin Toxicol (Phila).* 2011;49(5):431-433. doi:10.3109/15563650.2011.584316
59. Bronstein AC, Spyker DA, Cantilena LR, Green JL, Rumack BH, Dart RC. 2010 Annual Report of the American Association of Poison Control Centers' National Poison Data System (NPDS): 28th Annual Report. *Clin Toxicol (Phila).* 2011;49(10):910-941. doi:10.3109/15563650.2011.635149
60. American Association of Poison Control Centers. Accessed September 8, 2022. https://aapcc.org/
61. Bahji A, Stephenson C, Tyo R, Hawken ER, Seitz DP. Prevalence of cannabis withdrawal symptoms among people with regular or dependent use of cannabinoids. *JAMA Netw Open.* 2020;3(4):e202370. doi:10.1001/jamanetworkopen.2020.2370
62. Danovitch I, Gorelick DA. State of the art treatments for cannabis dependence. *Psychiatr Clin North Am.* 2012;35(2):309-326. doi:10.1016/j.psc.2012.03.003
63. Gates PJ, Sabioni P, Copeland J, Le Foll B, Gowing L. Psychosocial interventions for cannabis use disorder. *Cochrane Database Syst Rev.* 2016;(5):CD005336. doi:10.1002/14651858.CD005336.pub4
64. Tomko RL, Gray KM, Huestis MA, Squeglia LM, Baker NL, McClure EA. Measuring within-individual cannabis reduction in clinical trials: a review of the methodological challenges. *Curr Addict Rep.* 2019;6(4):429-436.
65. Brezing CA, Choi CJ, Pavlicova M, et al. Abstinence and reduced frequency of use are associated with improvements in quality of life among treatment-seekers with cannabis use disorder. *Am J Addict.* 2018;27(2):101-107. doi:10.1111/ajad.12660
66. Gray KM, Carpenter MJ, Baker NL, et al. A double-blind randomized controlled trial of N-acetylcysteine in cannabis-dependent adolescents. *Am J Psychiatry.* 2012;169(8):805-812. doi:10.1176/appi.ajp.2012.12010055
67. Gray KM, Sonne SC, McClure EA, et al. A randomized placebo-controlled trial of N-acetylcysteine for cannabis use disorder in adults. *Drug Alcohol Depend.* 2017;177:249-257. doi:10.1016/j.drugalcdep.2017.04.020
68. Lintzeris N, Bhardwaj A, Mills L, et al. Nabiximols for the treatment of cannabis dependence: a randomized clinical trial. *JAMA Intern Med.* 2019;179(9):1242-1253. doi:10.1001/jamainternmed.2019.1993
69. Trigo JM, Soliman A, Quilty LC, et al. Nabiximols combined with motivational enhancement/cognitive behavioral therapy for the treatment of cannabis dependence: a pilot randomized clinical trial. *PLoS One.* 2018;13(1):e0190768. doi:10.1371/journal.pone.0190768
70. Mason BJ, Crean R, Goodell V, et al. A proof-of-concept randomized controlled study of gabapentin: effects on cannabis use, withdrawal and executive function deficits in cannabis-dependent adults. *Neuropsychopharmacology.* 2012;37(7):1689-1698. doi:10.1038/npp.2012.14

71. Freeman TP, Hindocha C, Baio G, et al. Cannabidiol for the treatment of cannabis use disorder: a phase 2a, double-blind, placebo-controlled, randomised, adaptive Bayesian trial. *Lancet Psychiatry.* 2020;7(10):865-874. doi:10.1016/S2215-0366(20)30290-X
72. McRae-Clark AL, Gray KM, Baker NL, et al. Varenicline as a treatment for cannabis use disorder: a placebo-controlled pilot trial. *Drug Alcohol Depend.* 2021;229(Pt B):109111. doi:10.1016/j.drugalcdep.2021.109111
73. Substance Abuse and Mental Health Services Administration, Office of the Surgeon General. *Facing Addiction in America: The Surgeon General's Report on Alcohol, Drugs, and Health.* US Department of Health and Human Services; 2016. Accessed September 8, 2022. http://www.ncbi.nlm.nih.gov/books/NBK424857/
74. Friedman J, Godvin M, Shover CL, Gone JP, Hansen H, Schriger DL. Trends in drug overdose deaths among US adolescents, January 2010 to June 2021. *JAMA.* 2022;327(14):1398-1400. doi:10.1001/jama.2022.2847
75. Larochelle MR, Bernson D, Land T, et al. Medication for opioid use disorder after nonfatal opioid overdose and association with mortality: a cohort study. *Ann Intern Med.* 2018;169(3):137-145. doi:10.7326/M17-3107
76. Feder KA, Krawczyk N, Saloner B. Medication-assisted treatment for adolescents in specialty treatment for opioid use disorder. *J Adolesc Health.* 2017;60(6):747-750. doi:10.1016/j.jadohealth.2016.12.023
77. Marsch LA, Bickel WK, Badger GJ, et al. Comparison of pharmacological treatments for opioid-dependent adolescents: a randomized controlled trial. *Arch Gen Psychiatry.* 2005;62(10):1157-1164. doi:10.1001/archpsyc.62.10.1157
78. Woody GE, Poole SA, Subramaniam G, et al. Extended vs short-term buprenorphine-naloxone for treatment of opioid-addicted youth: a randomized trial. *JAMA.* 2008;300(17):2003-2011. doi:10.1001/jama.2008.574
79. Polsky D, Glick HA, Yang J, Subramaniam GA, Poole SA, Woody GE. Cost-effectiveness of extended buprenorphine-naloxone treatment for opioid-dependent youth: data from a randomized trial. *Addiction.* 2010;105(9):1616-1624. doi:10.1111/j.1360-0443.2010.03001.x
80. Marsch LA, Moore SK, Borodovsky JT, et al. A randomized controlled trial of buprenorphine taper duration among opioid-dependent adolescents and young adults. *Addiction.* 2016;111(8):1406-1415. doi:10.1111/add.13363
81. Minozzi S, Amato L, Bellisario C, Davoli M. Detoxification treatments for opiate dependent adolescents. *Cochrane Database Syst Rev.* 2014;(4):CD006749. doi:10.1002/14651858.CD006749.pub3
82. Moore SK, Marsch LA, Badger GJ, Solhkhah R, Hofstein Y. Improvement in psychopathology among opioid-dependent adolescents during behavioral-pharmacological treatment. *J Addict Med.* 2011;5(4):264-271. doi:10.1097/ADM.0b013e3182191099
83. Motamed M, Marsch LA, Solhkhah R, Bickel WK, Badger GJ. Differences in treatment outcomes between prescription opioid-dependent and heroin-dependent adolescents. *J Addict Med.* 2008;2(3):158-164. doi:10.1097/ADM.0b013e31816b2f84
84. Hadland SE, Bagley SM, Rodean J, et al. Receipt of timely addiction treatment and association of early medication treatment with retention in care among youths with opioid use disorder. *JAMA Pediatr.* 2018;172(11):1029-1037. doi:10.1001/jamapediatrics.2018.2143
85. Subramaniam GA, Warden D, Minhajuddin A, et al. Predictors of abstinence: NIDA multi-site buprenorphine/naloxone treatment trial in opioid dependent youth. *J Am Acad Child Adolesc Psychiatry.* 2011;50(11):1120-1128. doi:10.1016/j.jaac.2011.07.010
86. Fishman MJ, Winstanley EL, Curran E, Garrett S, Subramaniam G. Treatment of opioid dependence in adolescents and young adults with extended release naltrexone: preliminary case-series and feasibility. *Addiction.* 2010;105(9):1669-1676. doi:10.1111/j.1360-0443.2010.03015.x
87. Mitchell S, Monico L, Gryczynski J, Fishman M, O'Grady KE, Schwartz R. Extended-release naltrexone for youth with opioid use disorder. *J Subst Abuse Treat.* 2021;130.
88. Hopfer CJ, Khuri E, Crowley TJ, Hooks S. Adolescent heroin use: a review of the descriptive and treatment literature. *J Subst Abuse Treat.* 2002;23(3):231-237. doi:10.1016/s0740-5472(02)00250-7
89. Kellogg S, Melia D, Khuri E, Lin A, Ho A, Kreek MJ. Adolescent and young adult heroin patients: drug use and success in methadone maintenance treatment. *J Addict Dis.* 2006;25(3):15-25. doi:10.1300/J069v25n03_03
90. Smyth BP, Elmusharaf K, Cullen W. Opioid substitution treatment and heroin dependent adolescents: reductions in heroin use and treatment retention over twelve months. *BMC Pediatrics.* 2018;18(1):151. doi:10.1186/s12887-018-1137-4
91. Bell J, Mutch C. Treatment retention in adolescent patients treated with methadone or buprenorphine for opioid dependence: a file review. *Drug Alcohol Rev.* 2006;25(2):167-171. doi:10.1080/09595230500537670
92. Alinsky RH, Zima BT, Rodean J, et al. Receipt of addiction treatment after opioid overdose among medicaid-enrolled adolescents and young adults. *JAMA Pediatr.* 2020;174(3):e195183. doi:10.1001/jamapediatrics.2019.5183
93. Khatri UG, Pizzicato LN, Viner K, et al. Racial/ethnic disparities in unintentional fatal and nonfatal emergency medical services–attended opioid overdoses during the COVID-19 pandemic in Philadelphia. *JAMA Netw Open.* 2021;4(1):e2034878. doi:10.1001/jamanetworkopen.2020.34878
94. McCabe SE, West BT. Medical and nonmedical use of prescription stimulants: results from a national multicohort study. *J Am Acad Child Adolesc Psychiatry.* 2013;52(12):1272-1280. doi:10.1016/j.jaac.2013.09.005
95. McCabe SE, Veliz P, Wilens TE, Schulenberg JE. Adolescents' prescription stimulant use and adult functional outcomes: a national prospective study. *J Am Acad Child Adolesc Psychiatry.* 2017;56(3):226-233.e4. doi:10.1016/j.jaac.2016.12.008
96. Danielson ML, Bitsko RH, Ghandour RM, Holbrook JR, Kogan MD, Blumberg SJ. Prevalence of parent-reported ADHD diagnosis and associated treatment among U.S. children and adolescents, 2016. *J Clin Child Adolesc Psychol.* 2018;47(2):199-212. doi:10.1080/15374416.2017.1417860
97. Harstad E, Levy S; Committee on Substance Abuse. Attention-deficit/hyperactivity disorder and substance abuse. *Pediatrics.* 2014;134(1):e293-e301. doi:10.1542/peds.2014-0992
98. Looby A, De Young KP, Earleywine M. Challenging expectancies to prevent nonmedical prescription stimulant use: a randomized, controlled trial. *Drug Alcohol Depend.* 2013;132(1-2):362-368. doi:10.1016/j.drugalcdep.2013.03.003
99. Molina BSG, Kipp HL, Joseph HM, et al. Stimulant diversion risk among college students treated for ADHD: primary care provider prevention training. *Acad Pediatr.* 2020;20(1):119-127. doi:10.1016/j.acap.2019.06.002
100. Stock ML, Litt DM, Arlt V, Peterson LM, Sommerville J. The prototype/willingness model, academic versus health-risk information, and risk cognitions associated with nonmedical prescription stimulant use among college students. *Br J Health Psychol.* 2013;18:490-507. doi:10.1111/j.2044-8287.2012.02087.x
101. Faraone SV, Rostain AL, Montano CB, Mason O, Antshel KM, Newcorn JH. Systematic review: nonmedical use of prescription stimulants: risk factors, outcomes, and risk reduction strategies. *J Am Acad Child Adolesc Psychiatry.* 2020;59(1):100-112. doi:10.1016/j.jaac.2019.06.012
102. Teter CJ, McCabe SE, Boyd CJ, Guthrie SK. Illicit methylphenidate use in an undergraduate student sample: prevalence and risk factors. *Pharmacotherapy.* 2003;23(5):609-617. doi:10.1592/phco.23.5.609.34187
103. Wilens TE, Adler LA, Adams J, et al. Misuse and diversion of stimulants prescribed for ADHD: a systematic review of the literature. *J Am Acad Child Adolesc Psychiatry.* 2008;47(1):21-31. doi:10.1097/chi.0b013e31815a56f1
104. Viana AG, Trent L, Tull MT, et al. Non-medical use of prescription drugs among Mississippi youth: constitutional, psychological, and family factors. *Addict Behav.* 2012;37(12):1382-1388. doi:10.1016/j.addbeh.2012.06.017
105. Compton WM, Han B, Blanco C, Johnson K, Jones CM. Prevalence and correlates of prescription stimulant use, misuse, use disorders, and motivations for misuse among adults in the U.S. *Am J Psychiatry.* 2018;175(8):741-755. doi:10.1176/appi.ajp.2018.17091048

106. Stanger C, Budney AJ. Contingency management approaches for adolescent substance use disorders. *Child Adolesc Psychiatr Clin N Am.* 2010;19(3):547-562. doi:10.1016/j.chc.2010.03.007
107. Verdi G, Weyandt LL, Zavras BM. Non-medical prescription stimulant use in graduate students: relationship with academic self-efficacy and psychological variables. *J Atten Disord.* 2016;20(9):741-753. doi:10.1177/1087054714529816
108. Teter CJ, McCabe SE, LaGrange K, Cranford JA, Boyd CJ. Illicit use of specific prescription stimulants among college students: prevalence, motives, and routes of administration. *Pharmacotherapy.* 2006;26(10):1501-1510. doi:10.1592/phco.26.10.1501
109. Ruha A, Yarema M. Pharmacologic treatment of acute methamphetamine toxicity. *Pediatric Emergency Care.* 2006;22(12):782.
110. Prosser JM, Nelson LS. The toxicology of bath salts: a review of synthetic cathinones. *J Med Toxicol.* 2012;8(1):33-42. doi:10.1007/s13181-011-0193-z
111. Spiller HA, Ryan ML, Weston RG, Jansen J. Clinical experience with and analytical confirmation of "bath salts" and "legal highs" (synthetic cathinones) in the United States. *Clin Toxicol (Phila).* 2011;49(6):499-505. doi:10.3109/15563650.2011.590812
112. Lim JK, Earlywine JJ, Bagley SM, Marshall BDL, Hadland SE. Polysubstance involvement in opioid overdose deaths in adolescents and young adults, 1999-2018. *JAMA Pediatr.* 2021;175(2):194-196. doi:10.1001/jamapediatrics.2020.5035
113. Pani PP, Trogu E, Vecchi S, Amato L. Antidepressants for cocaine dependence and problematic cocaine use. *Cochrane Database Syst Rev.* 2011;(12):CD002950. doi:10.1002/14651858.CD002950.pub3
114. Kaminer Y. Desipramine facilitation of cocaine abstinence in an adolescent. *J Am Acad Child Adolesc Psychiatry.* 1992;31(2):312-317. doi:10.1097/00004583-199203000-00020
115. Kaminer Y. Cocaine craving. *J Am Acad Child Adolesc Psychiatry.* 1994;33(4):592. doi:10.1097/00004583-199405000-00022
116. Mariani JJ, Levin FR. Psychostimulant treatment of cocaine dependence. *Psychiatr Clin North Am.* 2012;35(2):425-439. doi:10.1016/j.psc.2012.03.012
117. Rush CR, Stoops WW. Agonist replacement therapy for cocaine dependence: a translational review. *Future Med Chem.* 2012;4(2):245-265. doi:10.4155/fmc.11.184
118. Anderson AL, Reid MS, Li SH, et al. Modafinil for the treatment of cocaine dependence. *Drug Alcohol Depend.* 2009;104(1-2):133-139. doi:10.1016/j.drugalcdep.2009.04.015
119. Dackis CA, Kampman KM, Lynch KG, Pettinati HM, O'Brien CP. A double-blind, placebo-controlled trial of modafinil for cocaine dependence. *Neuropsychopharmacology.* 2005;30(1):205-211. doi:10.1038/sj.npp.1300600
120. Dackis CA, Kampman KM, Lynch KG, et al. A double-blind, placebo-controlled trial of modafinil for cocaine dependence. *J Subst Abuse Treat.* 2012;43(3):303-312. doi:10.1016/j.jsat.2011.12.014
121. Martell BA, Orson FM, Poling J, et al. Cocaine vaccine for the treatment of cocaine dependence in methadone-maintained patients: a randomized, double-blind, placebo-controlled efficacy trial. *Arch Gen Psychiatry.* 2009;66(10):1116-1123. doi:10.1001/archgenpsychiatry.2009.128
122. Kosten TR, Domingo CB, Shorter D, et al. Vaccine for cocaine dependence: a randomized double-blind placebo-controlled efficacy trial. *Drug Alcohol Depend.* 2014;140:42-47. doi:10.1016/j.drugalcdep.2014.04.003
123. Trivedi MH, Walker R, Ling W, et al. Bupropion and naltrexone in methamphetamine use disorder. *N Engl J Med.* 2021;384(2):140-153. doi:10.1056/NEJMoa2020214
124. Anderson A, Li S, Markova D, et al. Bupropion for the treatment of methamphetamine dependence in non-daily users: a randomized, double-blind, placebo-controlled trial. *Drug Alcohol Depend.* 2015;150:170-174.
125. Coffin PO, Santos G, Hern J. Effects of mirtazapine for methamphetamine use disorder among cisgender men and transgender women who have sex with men: a placebo-controlled randomized clinical trial. *JAMA Psychiatry.* 2020;77(3):246-255.

CHAPTER

122 Co-occurring Psychiatric Disorders in Adolescents With Addiction-Related Issues

Martha J. Ignaszewski and Oscar Bukstein

CHAPTER OUTLINE

- Introduction
- Prevalence of substance use disorders and co-occurring disorders
- Diagnosis and management
- Pharmacotherapy
- Psychosocial interventions
- Depressive disorders
- Bipolar disorder
- Anxiety disorders
- Posttraumatic stress disorder
- Developmental disabilities
- Schizophrenia
- ADHD, oppositional defiant disorder, and conduct disorder
- Eating disorders
- Conclusions

INTRODUCTION

Despite studies showing that levels of adolescent alcohol and illicit substance use have decreased over time, adolescent substance use and its impact remains a major concern.[1,2] Adolescents who use substances and those who meet criteria for substance use disorders (SUDs) exhibit a high prevalence of psychiatric disorders compared to the general population along with many far reaching negative effects.[3,4] Studies of treatment-seeking adolescents with SUDs have documented that 50% to 90% also have co-occurring psychiatric disorders.[5,6] Specific psychiatric disorders and other psychosocial problems such as suicide, violence and pregnancy are all associated with an increased risk of substance use. This chapter reviews substance use disorders in adolescents and considers diagnosis and management.

In this chapter, SUDs as psychiatric diagnoses are defined by the *Diagnostic and Statistical Manual of Mental Disorders*, 5th edition (DSM 5-TR) of the American Psychiatric Association.[1] Adolescents who initially seek treatment for an SUD may be different from those who seek care for a psychiatric disorder.[7,8] The terms *concurrent* and *co-occurring disorders* are used interchangeably to refer to patients who meet the criteria for both substance-related and addictive disorders and for another psychiatric diagnosis.

Many of the treatment issues posed by SUDs and common co-occurring psychiatric disorders are identical for adults and adolescents. In both populations, the course and treatment of the same two disorders may vary depending on which one is the primary—in other words, which disorder preceded the other[4]—and their relative severity. Not all patients with co-occurring disorders have the same problems and require the same treatment.[9,10] The prevalence of co-occurring disorders among adolescent inpatients with SUDs is high[4] though there is inconsistent evidence regarding the relationship, timing, and onset of psychiatric symptoms secondary to the SUDs and how many have a primary or co-occurring psychiatric diagnosis.[4]

PREVALENCE OF SUBSTANCE USE DISORDERS AND CO-OCCURRING DISORDERS

Much of the data regarding SUD prevalence comes from the National Survey on Drug Use and Health (NSDUH), which assessed SUD diagnoses using DSM-5 criteria for the first time in 2020. This impacts the ability to generate comparisons from previous years.[11] Some research shows disproportionate increases in past year prevalence estimates for alcohol and opioid use disorders (AUD, OUD) compared to DSM-IV prevalence,[12-14] while other research suggests high rates of concordance between DSM-IV and 5.[15] This is an even more complex question in youth.

DSM-5 diagnostic criteria for SUDs have not been validated in adolescent populations, and the applicability of the criteria has been questioned due to differences in substance use patterns.[16] Using DSM-5 criteria for youth may be associated with diagnostic net widening due to capturing of adolescents who were considered diagnostic orphans under DSM-IV criteria,[17] with higher likelihood of meeting diagnostic criteria. Chung et al. found the rates of tobacco (nicotine) use disorders are twice as high using DSM-5 criteria compared to DSM-IV.[18] Kelly et al.[17] reproduced these findings in a pediatric population showing more prevalent DSM-5 criteria diagnoses compared to DSM-IV for tobacco (4.0% versus 2.7%), alcohol (4.6% versus 3.8%), and cannabis (10.7% versus 8.2%).[17] Diagnostic criteria remain unchanged for SUDs in the updated DSM-5TR.[1]

In 2020, 1.6 million adolescents aged 12 to 17 (6.4% of the population) needed treatment for a substance use problem though only 7.6% of adolescents with diagnosed SUDs received any substance use treatment in the past year[5] and only 0.9% received both substance use treatment at a specialty facility and mental health treatment. The low rates of treatment participation are troubling particularly because prevalence estimates show high rates of co-occurring disorders. The COVID-19 pandemic affected the availability and mode of mental health and substance use treatment service delivery shifting it towards virtual care, which has been shown to be effective.[5]

There is a bidirectional relationship between mental health and substance use. Ninety percent of adults who develop SUDs initiated their substance use in adolescence.[4] Adolescents with prior lifetime mental disorders had high rates of both alcohol (10.3%) and illicit DSM-IV–defined substance (14.9%) abuse, with or without dependence. Alcohol and drug use were highest among adolescents with prior anxiety disorders (17.3% and 20%, respectively) and behavior disorders (15.6% and 24%, respectively). Any prior disorder significantly increased the risk of transition from nonuse to first use and from use to problematic use of either alcohol or illicit drugs.

Evidence suggests a complex, multifactorial interplay between risk factors for vulnerability for mental health disorders, substance use and SUDs and several etiologic factors. There are likely heritable links between mental illness and SUDs with common genetic, environment, family, personal, and traumatic risk factors. There are also parallel and common neurobiological processes in SUDs and mental illness with disturbances in neurotransmitter function affecting the motivation and reward system, and affecting regulation and behavioral inhibition. The self-medication hypothesis puts forward the notion that childhood trauma may contribute to the development of psychopathology, as could coping with untreated traumas, psychological pressures as they relate to maturation and underlying psychiatric conditions that may lead to substance use and risky related behaviors. Psychiatric co-occurring disorders, especially depression, anxiety, attention deficit hyperactivity disorder (ADHD) and posttraumatic stress disorder (PTSD), have been found to be mediating factors for concurrence of SUDs. In some individuals, consequences of substance use can cause secondary development of mental health problems either directly due to pharmacogenic features of substance use or indirectly relating to financial difficulties, dysfunctional relationships and other stressors and dysfunction secondary to substance use.[19,20]

Estimates vary between clinical, community, and specialty settings; however, 64% to 88% of adolescents with SUD meet criteria for co-occurring psychiatric diagnoses.[3,7,8] In specialty SUD treatment settings, more than half of adolescents have three or more co-occurring psychiatric disorders. Youth with psychiatric diagnoses have earlier initiation of substance use, more rapid progression of use with telescoping to meet SUD criteria with greater severity, and a more treatment refractory course with poorer treatment outcomes and higher recurrence rates[6,7,8] in part secondary to noncompletion of treatment and more rapid attrition.[21] Adolescents with SUD and co-occurring mental health disorders were significantly more psychologically distressed, compared to adolescents with SUD only.

The most common co-occurring psychiatric disorders among youth in addiction treatment include externalizing disorders such as conduct disorder (CD) and ADHD; however, internalizing disorders such as mood disorders (eg, depression) and trauma-related symptoms are also common.[22,23] The risk of co-occurring disorders increases with age during adolescence.

Among patients with an SUD, children aged 12 and under (95%) and females (75%-100%) have high rates of co-occurring disorders; Black people are more likely than White people to be diagnosed with CD, impulse-control, and psychotic diagnoses, while White people are more likely to be diagnosed with anxiety disorders (AD), ADHD, mood disorders (MD), personality disorders (PD), relational, and eating diagnoses. Patients with an SUD used more inpatient treatment than patients without a SUD (43% versus 21%); children, females, and Black people had elevated odds of inpatient psychiatric treatment.[24] Adolescents with onset of any psychiatric disorder, including SUD, prior to age 14 are six times as likely to have one, and 12 times as likely to have two, additional disorders by 18 years of age than those with later onset of psychiatric disorders.[25] This finding suggests that the clinician's index of suspicion for co-occurring disorders must be particularly high for younger patients with SUDs.

DIAGNOSIS AND MANAGEMENT

Psychiatric assessment of substance using youth is complex and requires careful evaluation. Youths with substance use, frequent intoxication, and withdrawal states demonstrate various behavioral changes that can overlap with other types of psychopathology. For instance, changes in mood, cognition, disinhibition, hyperactivity and agitation, and perceptual changes can all occur secondary to intoxication. Further, the manifestations of substance use and intoxication vary with the substance and amount used, as well as experience.

Health care professionals need to be equipped to appropriately evaluate and treat the patients they encounter, many of whom will have co-occurring psychiatric diagnoses. Universal screening for substance use in clinical settings where high risk individuals are treated is recommended. If a screen is positive, the recommended steps include (1) conducting a comprehensive evaluation including diagnostic assessment and psychiatric review of systems, mental status examination; (2) obtaining information from multiple sources; (3) having a high index of suspicion for co-occurring disorders in treatment seeking adolescents, especially in those whose conditions do not respond to treatment or who present challenges in treatment; (4) individualizing treatment to accommodate both the substance use and psychiatric diagnoses; (5) obtaining a comprehensive history of alcohol, tobacco/nicotine, and other substance use; and (6) knowing when to consult an addiction specialist or mental health professional. Psychopathology is a risk factor for substance use in adolescents and adults and associated with the etiology of SUDs.[26]

In some patients, the use of substances—particularly alcohol, methamphetamine, cannabis, cocaine, ecstasy, hallucinogens, and inhalants—is associated with acute and residual cognitive damage.[27] The possibility of a substance-induced neurocognitive disorder should be considered in adolescents who have difficulty coping with the cognitive and organizational demands of a structured and supportive program. Some adolescents will be able to use the program if instructions are simplified. Improvement in cognitive functioning may be rapid, but continues to improve for as long as a year or more after cessation of the chemical assault to the brain. Some may be left with residual impairments. Adolescents and their families should be informed of the cognitive consequences of their substance use in a way that does not engender despair but clearly warns against further alcohol or drug use. The presence of cognitive deficits, if they persist, should be considered in rehabilitation, educational, and vocational planning. Such patients need neuropsychological evaluation and follow-up.

PHARMACOTHERAPY

As a general guide, integrated mental health and substance use treatment is recommended and pharmacotherapy can be used safely and effectively in youth with SUDs. However, the presence of SUDs may necessitate the use of non–first-line pharmacologic agents for select diagnoses where medications may have inherent potential for unhealthy use (ie, considering the use of bupropion or serotonin-noradrenergic reuptake inhibitors over a stimulant for the management of ADHD in youth with SUDs, and preferential use of medications with lower potential for unhealthy use in anxiety management). Targeting psychiatric diagnoses with pharmacological treatment may result in improvement in mental health but is unlikely to have any specific effect on substance use or SUD without specific and concurrent psychotherapy.[26]

The reader is referred to Chapter 121, "Pharmacotherapy for Adolescents with Substance Use Disorders."

PSYCHOSOCIAL INTERVENTIONS

Psychosocial treatment, including family-based therapy, cognitive behavioral therapy (CBT), motivational interviewing, and contingency management represents the cornerstone of management of youth SUDs.[28] Recent evidence suggests that psychosocial treatments such as family-based therapy, CBT, and multicomponent approaches remain the most effective methods of treatment; however, innovative ways of improving these treatment strategies may include digital and culturally based interventions. New advances in adjunctive treatments such as pharmacotherapy, exercise, mindfulness, and recovery-oriented educational centers may have clinical utility.[29] Hogue et al.[28] provide a comprehensive overview of individual, group and family therapies for adolescent SUD.

Clinically, there exists a need for a coordinated intervention[30] as piecemeal treatments targeting isolated diagnoses have a higher risk of failure than those that simultaneously target both disorders.[31] Barriers to integrating treatment for co-occurring disorders include: (1) the historical separation of substance use and mental health services; (2) a limited number of clinicians and researchers who focus on youth with co-occurring disorders; and (3) the tendency to exclude youth with SUDs from clinical pharmacotherapy trials for psychiatric disorders.

DEPRESSIVE DISORDERS

Much has been written about the interplay between depression and substance use.[3,4,25,26] Adolescents, compared to adults, are more likely to have depressive symptoms that are characterized by irritability instead of sadness and may have more symptoms of hypersomnia and anxiety. Depression interferes with treatment through lack of concentration, motivation, hope, perseveration, and a tendency toward isolation.[1]

Rao et al.[31] found depressed adolescents developed earlier SUD, and adolescents with co-occurring SUD and depression had significantly more psychosocial distress than those with depression alone. Adolescents with past year major depressive episode are more likely to report past year and past month substance use compared to peers. Annual past year rates of illicit drug use, cannabis use, binge drinking (defined as four or more drinks on the same occasion in one day for men and four or more for women), and tobacco/nicotine use are also higher among youth with major depressive episode (28.6% versus 10.7%, 22% versus 7.9% 6.2% versus 3.8%, 12.9 versus 5.1%, respectively).[5] Adolescents who use cannabis are 37% more likely to develop depression in young adulthood than those who do not use cannabis[32] raising public health concerns regarding the high prevalence of adolescent cannabis use.

Treatment of adolescent depression has the potential to impact substance use trajectories. This outcome was explored using data from two large multi-site randomized controlled trials of treatments for adolescent depression: the Treatment of Adolescent Depression Study (TADS)[33] and Treatment of Selective Serotonin Reuptake Inhibitor (SSRI)-Resistant Depression in Adolescents Study (TORDIA).[34] In TADS, adolescents who responded positively to depression treatment had a lower likelihood of developing SUDs compared to youth with limited benefit. Similarly, in TORDIA, there was significant improvement in substance-related impairment among adolescents who responded to depression treatment. The strongest benefits were seen in youth with low substance-related impairment at the end of the 12-week acute treatment period, regardless of their baseline levels of substance-related impairment. In TADS, baseline levels of substance use were associated with poorer response to depression treatment. Other research shows the converse to be true as well, namely that interventions for

SUDs may be helpful to reduce depressive symptoms in adolescents. Four hundred eighty adolescents aged 12 to 17 who received treatment for DSM-IV defined substance abuse as part of the Brief Strategic Family Therapy (BSFT) effectiveness trial[35] had significant reductions in depressive symptoms with effect sizes in the small to medium range.

Adolescents with combined depression and SUD have higher rates of perceived service needs and receive more treatment services as compared with SUD alone.[33] Unlike adults, the secondary depression in adolescents did not remit with abstinence. This finding, if replicated, would argue for more vigorous treatment of depressive syndromes in adolescents.

Trends in suicide attempts and deaths by suicide have been increasing among adolescents. Among adolescents aged 12 to 17 in 2020, 12.0% (or 3.0 million people) had serious thoughts of suicide, 5.3% (or 1.3 million people) made a suicide plan, and 2.5% (or 629,000 people) attempted suicide in the past year.[5] The "gender paradox" refers to rates of suicide attempts in females being 3 to 9 times more common than in males; however, that the completion rates are 2 to 4 times higher in males.[36] These gender differences in suicidal behavior may relate to high rates of externalizing disorders in males, high rates of internalizing disorders in females, and associated differences in emotional and behavior problems.[37] SUDs are a risk factor for suicidal behaviors in adolescents, including ideation, attempts, and completed suicide. In one study, adolescents who reported cannabis use were 50% more likely to have suicidal ideation and 3.46 times more likely to make a suicide attempt.[32]

Evidence-based psychosocial therapies for depression in youth include cognitive-behavioral, interpersonal, cognitive, and to a lesser extent, family-based interventions.[38] As summarized by Volkow, treatment of adolescents with co-occurring disorders should include interventions for both disorders because lack of adequate treatment of one of the disorders might interfere with recovery.[30]

Due to insufficient resources, antidepressants are used more frequently than psychological interventions for management of pediatric depression and anxiety.[39] Serotonin and noradrenergic-specific agents have a relatively safe profile for side effects.[26,39] If there are doubts about the diagnosis of depression or about how to treat, consultation with a psychiatrist experienced in treating adolescents with SUDs is indicated; immediate consultation is recommended for concerns regarding suicidal behavior.[26] Medication adherence rates in adolescents are poor, and few remain on antidepressants for the recommended 6-month period.[40] It is likely that there is an interaction between antidepressants and use of psychoactive substances such as alcohol or cannabis,[41] and the current literature suggests that antidepressants are less effective for adolescents with depression/anxiety who frequently use cannabis.[42]

There are extensive disparities in access to treatment for SUD and depressive disorders.[43] A study that surveyed adolescents aged 12 to 17 years found persistent treatment gaps for co-occurring major depression and SUDs with unmet treatment needs that were significantly higher among Hispanic, Asian, Native Hawaiian, or Pacific Islander adolescents. Males were also substantially less likely to receive treatment for both conditions, as were older and uninsured adolescents. Culturally unique barriers and systemic racism prevent racial and ethnic minority adolescents from seeking and accessing mental health treatment. Some identified barriers include language barriers, cultural mistrust of health care practitioners, lack of social support and limited provision of community services.

BIPOLAR DISORDER

Bipolar disorder may be among the most difficult diagnosis to make in children and adolescents[44] and is even more difficult in teens who use substances. Issues such as changes in sleeping patterns or mood swings can be symptoms of bipolar disorder, substance use, or even normal adolescence. Careful assessment including a temporal relationship between substance use and psychiatric symptomatology and collateral information is required to appropriately evaluate for bipolar disorder. This diagnosis should be considered in substance-using youth, particularly those with a binge pattern.

Bipolar disorder often begins during late adolescence.[1,4,44] Childhood onset of bipolar disorder is more common in the United States than other countries around the world, with one quarter occurring before age 13 and two-thirds before age 19.[45] Generally, childhood onset bipolar disorder has a more difficult course and poorer outcomes than adult onset illness. Some authors have even suggested that pediatric bipolar disorder is a distinct subtype and that early onset and substance use are genetically related.[46] Childhood onset comes with significant risk of later substance use with 32% of youth developing new onset SUD within 2.7 years of diagnosis,[47] and a lifetime prevalence of 60% for the development of a SUD.[48] Wilens et al.[49] reported that youth with adolescent-onset bipolar disorder had an 8.8 times greater risk of SUD.

Children who were diagnosed with bipolar disorder and treated appropriately at a younger age had a lower subsequent risk for substance use.[47] Because bipolar disorder onset most commonly precedes SUD among youth, there is a window of opportunity for prevention. Strategies include screening for substance use among youth with bipolar disorder beginning at age 10 irrespective of other risk factors, providing family education and intervention, and implementing preventive interventions that have been successful in other populations.

Some patients may use substances, particularly alcohol, to calm themselves during a manic phase and intoxication can present with overlapping symptomatology. If a patient exhibits symptoms after a period of abstinence, the diagnosis of bipolar disorder should be considered. Valproic acid, carbamazepine, and other anticonvulsants and atypical antipsychotics, such as olanzapine and risperidone, are used as mood stabilizers.[46] Naturalistic studies suggest that youth treated with lithium have superior long-term outcomes including more euthymic days, fewer days of depression, and less suicidality compared to treatment with other mood stabilizers or other treatments.[50,51]

In a study of lithium for adolescents with SUDs and bipolar disorder,[50] symptoms of mania and use of alcohol also decreased. The advantages of lithium treatment must be balanced with the narrow therapeutic window and potential side effects, which require regular blood tests and medication adherence.

ANXIETY DISORDERS

Anxiety disorders are the most common psychiatric diagnoses, with a lifetime prevalence of over 30%, and are among the psychiatric conditions most often co-occurring in adolescents and adults with SUDs.[1] Anxiety disorders may be difficult to identify unless symptoms are overt and severe and therefore are frequently untreated, especially when present in combination with depression or SUDs.[1,4] A careful interview for anxiety symptoms and family history of anxiety disorders may be quite revealing.

A 2018 systematic review in adolescents and young adults in North America assessed use of the three most commonly used psychoactive substances in youth with depression and anxiety.[4] They identified significant associations with anxiety symptomatology and the use of alcohol (OR 1.54), cannabis (OR 1.36), and tobacco (2.21). Another systematic review found significant positive association between cannabis use at baseline and anxiety at follow-up.[52]

Lemyre et al.[53] explored the associations between anxiety and alcohol and other substance use in adolescents and whether general anxiety or symptoms of social phobia are associated with frequent alcohol use, frequent drunkenness, and cannabis use. Results found that anxiety preceded substance use and that anxiety symptoms increased the incidence of substance use and frequent alcohol use. Overall, generalized anxiety disorder places adolescents at risk for co-occurring and subsequent substance use. Previously, shyness and social anxiety had been shown to be associated with lower rates of tobacco, alcohol, cannabis and other drug use, and thus protective due to social withdrawal, concern about negative consequences of substance use and worries about cognitive or behavioral impairment.[54] Physiological symptoms of anxiety may be associated with substance use, whereas cognitive worrying is not. Social anxiety disorder is increasingly recognized as a prevalent, unremitting, and highly symptomatic disorder, associated with more use of tobacco, cannabis and drugs.[55] Adolescents with internalizing symptoms may need help coping with the symptoms even if the symptoms do not fulfill the criteria of mood or anxiety disorder.

Some adolescents (and adults) believe that drugs and alcohol may contribute to reduction of anxiety and stress, and this belief may lead them to initiate or continue use. Sometimes, a closer examination of patients who resist attending self-help meetings may reveal a social phobia or agoraphobia. Excessive use of legal substances such as caffeine, energy drinks and nicotine, illicit stimulants, or various withdrawal states including benzodiazepines and opioids may confound the clinical picture.

Behavioral treatment, including CBT, exposure, and/or relaxation training, often is helpful for anxiety disorders.[3,8,21] Interventions that address anxiety as well as the roots of substance use and negative consequences associated with use are recommended as treating only one disorder is usually less effective. However, patients may report a reduction in some anxiety symptoms during detoxification or early recovery.[55]

Pharmacotherapy may reduce symptoms of anxiety, although treatment selection must be judicious. Most clinicians consider the use of benzodiazepines as contraindicated in anyone with a history of a SUD due to the risk of addiction and unhealthy use. SSRIs are first line management for severe anxiety disorders in youth, but should not be taken with alcohol and may be less effective with concurrent cannabis use.[41] Buspirone hydrochloride and SSRIs are recommended as nonaddictive antianxiety agents. If abstinence has been established, adequate trials of behavioral or cognitive therapy[21] and alternative medications have failed, and the patient adheres to the treatment and medication regimen, the judicious use of a long-acting benzodiazepine, such as clonazepam, may be justified in a time limited fashion while longer term medications such as SSRIs or serotonin-norepinephrine reuptake inhibitors (SNRIs) are being titrated to reach clinical effect and/or skills are being developed in psychotherapy. Therapeutic skills to focus on may include distress tolerance, self-regulation and adaptive coping skills in cognitive-behavioral therapy, dialectical behavior therapy and group therapy. Shy and socially anxious youth may experience anxiety in group focused therapy that is delivered in many SUD treatment programs.

POSTTRAUMATIC STRESS DISORDER

There is a strong association between adverse childhood experiences (ACEs), trauma and PTSD diagnoses, adolescent substance use and lifetime SUDs.[2,4,9,56,57] ACEs can include stressful or traumatic events such as abuse and neglect though may also include household dysfunction such as experience of interpersonal violence in the childhood home and growing up with family members with active substance use.

The incidence of severe trauma and symptoms of PTSD is high among adolescents. Overall, 28% of youth have experienced physical abuse, 21% have experienced sexual abuse and more than 40% have experienced two or more ACEs. Adolescents exposed to multiple forms of trauma may be at high risk for psychiatric and behavioral problems.[57] Presence of additional ACES increases the rate of smoking 2.2 times, AUD 7.4 times, and intravenous illicit substance use 11.3 times. The converse relationship is also true. Lifetime prevalence of PTSD is thought to range between 26% and 52% in people with SUDs.[58] Prevalence of an SUD is associated with a 1.5 to 1.6 increased odds of having PTSD.[59,60]

Trauma and ACEs are also associated with high-risk behaviors such as risky sexual behavior with multiple partners in a dose-response relationship. This association has been referred to as a "trauma organized lifestyle," which predisposes individuals to a wide range of mental and physical illnesses and is associated with chronicity of conditions and increased morbidity and mortality with limited access to appropriate health care.[61-63] Co-occurring PTSD and SUDs are highly complex and associated with worse treatment outcomes, such as lower rates of remission and faster relapse, poorer treatment response, more cognitive difficulties, worse social functioning, greater risk of suicide attempt, and heightened mortality.[55,64] Compared to individuals with isolated diagnoses of PTSD or AUD, presence of both disorders is associated with more co-occurring psychiatric disorders, an increased risk of suicide, more severe symptoms, and greater disability.[65]

Screening for trauma and associated symptoms is recommended as part of an SUD evaluation, and, if present, symptoms can be acknowledged without arousing anxiety or risking re-traumatization. There has historically been debate about treatment of SUDs and PTSD—whether this should occur concurrently or sequentially due to concerns about use of substances as a method to cope with managing distressing trauma symptoms such as hyperarousal, negative mood, or intrusive reexperiencing. Effective treatment suggests that integrated PTSD- and SUD-focused cognitive-behavioral and family treatment for adolescents with co-occurring abuse-related PTSD and SUD may optimize outcomes for this population.[66] In addition to strong empiric support, integrated treatment appears to be preferable to youth and their families and are increasingly considered the standard of care.[64,66,67] Despite ample evidence that concurrent treatment can be effective, these historical anxieties have contributed to infrequent treatment—individuals with PTSD and SUD are frequently only treated for SUD and many individuals in SUD treatment settings are not even assessed for PTSD.[58] Whereas treatment for SUDs alone rarely leads to improvement in PTSD symptoms, reducing PTSD symptoms can significantly reduce heavy substance.[68]

Seeking Safety was the first psychotherapy developed for concurrent treatment for PTSD and SUDs. In outpatient treatment of adolescent girls, effect sizes were moderate to high for substance use and associated problems, some trauma-related symptoms, cognitions related to SUD and PTSD, and several areas of pathology not targeted in the treatment (eg, anorexia, somatization) and were sustained at follow-up.[69]

Risk Reduction through Family Therapy, which is an integrative and exposure-based risk-reduction and treatment approach for adolescents who have had traumatic experiences, is associated with fewer substance using days and reduction in PTSD symptoms.[70,71] These results suggest that this exposure-based treatment is safe, feasibly delivered by community-based clinicians, and offers an effective approach to inform clinical practice, though other research is ongoing.[72]

DEVELOPMENTAL DISABILITIES

Emerging evidence and increased attention has revealed that individuals with neurodevelopmental conditions such as autism spectrum disorder (ASD) and intellectual disability may be at increased risk for developing SUDs and experience more severe consequences of substance use despite lower or similar rates of substance use compared to the general adolescent population.[73,74] This increased risk may be due to lower tolerance for recreational substance use and heightened risk for adverse consequences due to differential intellectual, social and communicative levels of functioning. Furthermore, academic and social behavior between the ages of 7 and 9 can predict substance use at age 14 or 15 in this group.[75] Therefore, early detection of developmental disabilities including learning disorders is essential to reduce the risk of developing a SUD.

A review found that screening for SUD among individuals with ASD or mild to borderline intellectual disability (MBID) often does not occur as part of routine clinical assessments and the frequency of SUD among individuals with ASD or MBID is currently unknown.[76] Another systematic review explored the frequency across 11 studies and found wide ranging rates of SUD in patients with ASD from 0.7% to 36%, leading the authors to conclude that ASD and MBID may be associated with lower rates of SUD. The existing data are difficult to compare due to differences in the studied population including varying levels of intellectual disability, treatment settings, co-occurring psychiatric diagnoses, and methodological and measurement issues. Individuals with MBID appear to be overrepresented in addiction treatment settings, accounting for up to 30% to 40% of patients.[73]

Individuals with MBID and ASD may experience barriers to SUD treatment and accessibility of treatment offered with lower rates of initiation, engagement and higher rates of attrition. Motivational interviewing and cognitive techniques are accepted as effective in SUD treatment to build skills to resist substances and manage cravings, replace substance use with constructive and rewarding activities, improve problem solving skills and facilitate better interpersonal relationships.[74] Minor adaptations in communication may be necessary to increase substance-related knowledge for adolescents with MBID and ASD. Parents and caretakers can be integrated into treatment to support modeling of healthy behaviors and prosocial activities.

SCHIZOPHRENIA

It can be extremely difficult to distinguish between substance induced psychotic-like experiences and re-exacerbation or initial onset of a psychotic disorder. Further, the variety of substances able to provoke an episode of acute psychosis has increased dramatically over the last decades, including synthesis of new drugs such as cannabinoids and cathinones.[77] The propensity to develop psychosis and persistent symptoms appears to be associated with the severity and frequency of use of particular substances.[78] Characteristics that suggest primary psychotic disorders include earlier age of onset of psychosis compared to drug-induced psychosis, more "unusual thought content" at baseline, more positive and fewer negative symptoms, less insight and a weaker family history of psychotic disorders.[79] Substance use is reported in 30% to 70% of first episode psychosis.[80] Cannabis specifically is associated with an increased, dose-dependent risk: heavy users had a fourfold increased risk of development of psychosis compared to twofold for moderate users.[81]

Individuals who develop psychotic symptoms after substance use are more likely to develop a primary psychotic illness such as schizophrenia or a schizophrenia-spectrum disorder.[82,83] Starzer[84] investigated rates of conversion from substance induced psychosis to schizophrenia and bipolar disorder and found that about one-third of patients with substance-induced psychosis were later diagnosed with either bipolar or schizophrenia-spectrum disorders. Schizophrenia and bipolar disorder were most common in individuals with cannabis-induced psychosis with nearly half ultimately going on to diagnosis. Half of the cases of conversion to schizophrenia occurred within 3.1 years after a substance-induced psychosis, and half the cases of conversion to bipolar disorder occurred within 4.4 years. Younger age at the onset of substance use was a significant risk factor. Patients who simultaneously meet the criteria for schizophrenia and a SUD are less likely to receive treatment in an addiction treatment program than in a psychiatric unit.[77]

Increasingly, younger patients with schizophrenia use substances,[4] some in an attempt to manage or reduce their symptoms. However, few studies have supported the self-medication hypothesis of substance use in patients with schizophrenia to lessen or decrease symptoms or antipsychotic treatment side effects. Substance use interferes with treatment for psychotic disorders and is associated with clinical exacerbations of psychosis, nonadherence with treatment recommendations, poor global functioning, violence, suicide, and increased rates of reuse and rehospitalization.[85] Such patients are best managed in special "dual diagnosis" programs for psychotic patients, where the psychosis and the substance use are addressed in parallel.[77,85]

Several theories have been proposed to explain the connection between SUD and schizophrenia. There may be a reward deficiency dysfunction in schizophrenia that underlies the use of substances to compensate[85,86] and clozapine and other atypical antipsychotics may be effective in the treatment of co-occurring schizophrenia and SUD.[87] Green et al.[87] suggested that clozapine may be effective because of its weak blockade of D-2 receptors, its potent blockade of norepinephrine alpha-2 receptors, and its ability to release norepinephrine in the brain, which may allow amelioration of the brain reward circuit deficit in schizophrenic patients that underlie their substance use. Long-acting injectable second generation antipsychotics show efficacy and good tolerability for people with schizophrenia and are associated with enhanced adherence and reduced relapse rates.[88] They deserve special consideration in youth with co-occurring schizophrenia-SUDs.

Psychosocial approaches that have been studied for treatment of co-occurring schizophrenia and SUDs include Motivational Interviewing and Motivational Enhancement Therapy, relapse prevention training, and CBT. These interventions have been shown to have moderate efficacy in this population, particularly for improvements in SUD related outcomes such as abstinence or use reductions.[89] However, psychosocial treatments are recommended in conjunction with pharmacotherapy as a multi-faceted approach rather than stand alone treatment.

ADHD, OPPOSITIONAL DEFIANT DISORDER, AND CONDUCT DISORDER

ADHD, Oppositional Defiant Disorder (ODD), and Conduct Disorder (CD) are the most common co-occurring psychiatric disorders in youth with SUDs.[26,90] Rates of ADHD are higher in substance using youth and treatment seeking SUD patients compared to the general public with prevalence of 28%[3] and 44%,[90] respectively. ADHD is associated with a twofold increased risk for AUD, 2.5 times higher risk for tobacco/nicotine use disorder, and 1.5 to 2.5 times increased risk for developing of any SUD.[91] All youth with ADHD are at risk of experiencing higher rates of personal and familial dysfunction, academic and occupational challenges, and involvement with the legal system, with worse functional outcomes with persistence of symptoms and absence of treatment.[91]

Studies suggest that co-occurring ADHD and SUD may be secondary to common vulnerability factors in the inhibitory and reward system of the brain affecting genetic predispositions. Hechtman et al.[91] proposed the following causal pathways: poor executive functioning associated with poor decision-making around substance use in adolescence, impulsivity and poor response inhibition directly increases SUD risk, limited coping skills, and self-medication of symptoms. These pathways may also inform the relationship between ADHD, CD, substance use and SUDs.[22]

Nicotine use requires a special consideration in this group, as some youth may use nicotine to mitigate symptoms of ADHD. Nicotine may increase attention, reduce hyperactivity and impulsivity, and help with behavioral regulation in individuals with ADHD. Prevalence of smoking is twice as high in individuals diagnosed with ADHD compared to the general population and quit rates are 15% lower.[92] Cigarette smoking increases the risk for subsequent drug and alcohol use disorders among individuals with ADHD, and is a risk factor for other unhealthy substance use with 4 to 5 times increased likelihood of progressing to heavy cigarette and cannabis use. Pharmacotherapy for ADHD offers promise to lower the risk of smoking during adolescence.[93]

Given the high rates of concurrence of ADHD and other disruptive behavior disorders and their significance as risk factors for the development of substance use and SUDs, screening and evaluation for ADHD is recommended for all adolescents in treatment for SUD.

Treatment for co-occurring ADHD and SUDs covers the spectrum from psychosocial and behavioral interventions targeting family therapy, development of problem solving and emotional and self-regulation skills, to pharmacologic targets. Pharmacotherapy for adolescents has been controversial due to concerns about risk associated with the use of psychostimulants in substance using patient populations, though evidence suggests that appropriate treatment does not increase, and may decrease, the risk of SUD. Ozgen et al. in 2021[94] published a systematic review of controlled studies assessing the effectiveness of pharmacologic, psychosocial, and complementary treatments of ADHD in adolescents with and without co-occurring SUD and concluded that appropriate pharmacologic management of ADHD in childhood may be protective against the development of SUD in adolescence or young adulthood, high dose stimulant treatment may be an effective treatment in co-occurring disorder management, and that CBT may be particularly beneficial but that more research is needed to draw strong clinical recommendations and definitive conclusions. Their second conclusion was based on synthesis of findings from a first meta-analysis of six longitudinal studies showing a 90% greater risk of later SUD in children with ADHD who had not received stimulant treatment. They also reviewed four prospective cohort studies with findings showing no harmful effect for developing SUD with low or high stimulant exposure in childhood, that stimulant treatment was associated with a lower risk of SUD (but not nicotine dependence), that youth with later stimulant treatment initiation had a higher risk of developing SUD in adulthood, and lastly that adequate psychostimulant treatment (early, high dose, and long duration) was associated with reduced risk of SUD in adolescence.

To date, there have only been four randomized clinical trials and one systematic meta-analysis pertaining to the efficacy and safety of pharmacologic treatment of patients with co-occurring ADHD and SUD[94] and results are conflicting. Compared with placebo, methylphenidate (OR = 2.02) and atomoxetine (OR = 1.71) significantly reduced ADHD symptoms, but pemoline, bupropion, and lisdexamfetamine did not. None of the medications were effective in increasing abstinence from substances (OR = 1.09); however, the meta-analysis did not distinguish between adolescents and adults. A single study reviewing atomoxetine in youth with ADHD and SUD showed no group differences in ADHD or substance use based on self-report and urinalysis.[95] Several authors have suggested that higher stimulant doses may be required in ADHD patients with co-occurring SUD.

Most guidelines on management of ADHD have a limited focus on youth with co-occurring SUD. Existing guidelines provide general recommendations to screen adolescents with ADHD for symptoms of unhealthy substance use and SUD, to use medications with limited potential for unhealthy use, and to be alert for signs of unhealthy use or diversion of ADHD medication in this group.[96–99] Though practical treatment of co-occurring ADHD and SUD may include psychostimulant treatment, use of atomoxetine, alpha agonists, and other medications such as bupropion and venlafaxine should be considered in youth with ongoing active substance use, stimulant use disorder, and limited response to first line medications. Prior to starting stimulants, the following questions are recommended:

1. Have nonstimulant medications been tried or are there specific reasons why stimulants make sense as a first-line treatment?
2. Does the patient use substances currently?
3. If so, has the family been warned about potential risks of using stimulants?
4. Is the patient reliable and can parents be trusted to help manage the safe distribution of the medication and in the treatment plan?
5. If the patient currently uses substances, is he/she motivated and actively involved in treatment?
6. Has the patient had an established period of abstinence?
7. Is there a history of nonmedical use of amphetamine or other stimulants?
8. If the individual used stimulants nonmedically, was the intent instrumental (ie, to improve focus) or recreational?[68]

Though convention suggests pairing pharmacotherapy for ADHD with psychosocial interventions, there are no randomized trials or meta-analyses conducted in youth with co-occurring ADHD and SUD exploring the effect of these treatments. There is a small beneficial effect in trials of adolescents with ADHD without co-occurring SUDs for CBT, behavioral therapeutic approaches, motivational interviewing, psychoeducation, parent training, and training to improve planning, organizational skills, social skills, and academic/homework skills.[100] These interventions can be aimed at adolescents themselves or others in their social environment (eg, parents) and effects are often evaluated across different targets, settings, and outcome measures, including ADHD symptoms, social, planning and organizational skills, academic performance, etc.

Half of youth with combined type ADHD and a quarter of youth with inattentive type ADHD also meet criteria for oppositional defiant disorder. Conduct disorder is the most frequently co-occurring diagnosis in youth with ADHD and SUD with a prevalence rate of up to 69%.

Conduct disorder and antisocial personality disorder are the diagnoses that most often co-occur with SUDs, particularly in males.[1,91,101] Conduct problems, substance use, and risky sexual behavior have been shown to coexist among adolescents, which may lead to significant health problems.[93] Across all substances (tobacco/nicotine, binge drinking, and cannabis use), higher levels of childhood conduct problems during kindergarten predicted a greater probability of classification into more problematic adolescent trajectory classes and over time. Results highlight the importance of studying the conjoint relations among conduct problems, substance use, and risky sexual behavior in a unified model.

EATING DISORDERS

The incidence of eating disorders (EDs) and substance use in the adolescent population has increased[1,4] and the health care field is progressively identifying food addiction as a process addiction akin to SUDs. One-fourth of all patients who have an eating disorder either have a history of SUD or currently are using substances,[102] and women with EDs are more likely to use substances compared to those without EDs.

Substance use problems occur frequently in adolescents with EDs, and adolescents with EDs use substances at 20% to 40% higher rates than the general population.[103] Historically, bulimic patients were found to have a greater risk for substance use than those with restrictive ED, followed by those with binge-eating disorder though recent studies have documented that co-occurring anorexia nervosa AN and SUDs may be more prevalent than previously recognized, particularly for those with AN with bulimic features.[102] The most common occurrence is between bulimia nervosa and alcohol use disorder. Binge-purge behavior in AN and bulimia nervosa (BN) is associated with high risk of tobacco/nicotine, AUD and other substance use. In adolescents, two-thirds of those with BN have used alcohol, one-third had used cigarettes at least once, one-third have used illegal drugs at least once. Cannabis is the most frequently used illicit drug followed by cocaine then amphetamines.

Research has identified a direct association between the amount of alcohol consumed in one occasion and risk of having or developing EDs. Adolescents with binge eating are more likely to drink more than intended at each occasion and drink more than peers those who do not binge eat. Alcohol consumption likely serves as trigger for binge eating, and efforts to restrict alcohol use are followed by binge drinking. Dietary restriction can contribute to binge drinking in patients with BN. Persons with an eating disorder may use substances nonmedically to lose weight. For example, caffeine, tobacco, and amphetamines may be used as appetite suppressants or as a method to distract from thinking about food.[104]

Screening for substance use and especially AUD in patients with EDs is recommended. Co-occurring disorders can be treated using common therapeutic interventions, such as psychoeduation regarding associated risks and deleterious effects of ED behaviors and substance use, dietary education and planning, cognitive challenging of eating disordered thoughts and beliefs, building alternative skills and coping mechanisms and identifying and developing strategies to prevent relapse. Both CBT and DBT have been frequently used in the treatment of co-occurring EDs and SUDs; however, there are no randomized controlled trials.

CONCLUSIONS

In summary, psychiatric disorders and SUDs often occur together, complicating assessment and treatment. An awareness of the prevalence and manifestations of psychiatric diagnoses is essential to high-quality treatment of adolescents. Keeping current on psychopharmacological interventions and an ongoing relationship with a psychiatrist and addiction specialist who can be available for consultation as needed are helpful.[27,105] Often, the use of psychiatric medications such as antidepressants, mood stabilizers, and others is beneficial. However, care must be taken to avoid potential interactions between the illicit drugs and the prescribed medications.[26] Self-help groups such as Al-Ateen, Alcoholics Anonymous, Narcotics Anonymous, or "Double-Trouble" groups for patients with co-occurring psychiatric and SUDs can be a useful adjunct to treatment.[26] Careful observation, history taking, and appropriate consultation result in better detection and treatment of comorbid disorders and, ultimately, of the initial substance use problem.

REFERENCES

1. American Psychiatric Association. *Diagnostic and Statistical Manual of Mental Disorders*. 5th ed., text rev. APA; 2022.
2. Johnston LD, Miech RA, O'Malley PM, Bachman JG, Schulenberg JE, Patrick ME. *Monitoring the Future National Survey Results on Drug Use 1975-2021: Overview, Key Findings on Adolescent Drug Use.* Institute for Social Research, University of Michigan; 2022.
3. Brewer S, Godley MD, Hulvershorn LA. Treating mental health and substance use disorders in adolescents: what is on the menu? *Curr Psychiatry Rep.* 2017;19(1):5. doi:10.1007/s11920-017-0755-0
4. Esmaeelzadeh S, Moraros J, Thorpe L, Bird Y. Examining the association and directionality between mental health disorders and substance use among adolescents and young adults in the U.S. and Canada—a systematic review and meta-analysis. *J Clin Med.* 2018;7(12):543. doi:10.3390/jcm7120543
5. Substance Abuse and Mental Health Services Administration. *Key Substance Use and Mental Health Indicators in the United States: Results From the 2020 National Survey on Drug Use and Health.* HHS Publication No. PEP21-07-01-003, NSDUH Series H-56. Center for Behavioral Health Statistics and Quality, Substance Abuse and Mental Health Services Administration; 2021. Accessed July 27, 2023. https://www.samhsa.gov/data/sites/default/files/reports/rpt35325/NSDUHFFRPDFWHTMLFiles2020/2020NSDUHFFR1PDFW102121.pdf
6. Armstrong TD, Costello EJ. Community studies on adolescent substance use, abuse, or dependence and psychiatric comorbidity. *J Consult Clin Psychol.* 2002;70(6):1224-1239. doi:10.1037//0022-006x.70.6.1224
7. Deas D. Adolescent substance abuse and psychiatric comorbidities. *J Clin Psychiatry.* 2006;67(Suppl 7):18-23.
8. Hawkins EH. A tale of two systems: co-occurring mental health and substance abuse disorders treatment for adolescents. *Annu Rev Psychol.* 2009;60:197-227. doi:10.1146/annurev.psych.60.110707.163456
9. Hasin D, Kilcoyne B. Comorbidity of psychiatric and substance use disorders in the United States: current issues and findings from the NESARC. *Curr Opin Psychiatry.* 2012;25(3):165-171. doi:10.1097/YCO.0b013e3283523dcc
10. Grant BF, Goldstein RB, Saha TD, et al. Epidemiology of DSM-5 alcohol use disorder: results from the National Epidemiologic Survey on Alcohol and Related Conditions III. *JAMA Psychiatry.* 2015;72(8):757-766. doi:10.1001/jamapsychiatry.2015.0584
11. Substance Abuse and Mental Health Services Administration. *Impact of the DSM-IV to DSM-5 Changes on the National Survey on Drug Use and Health.* Substance Abuse and Mental Health Services Administration; 2016.
12. Agrawal A, Heath AC, Lynskey MT. DSM-IV to DSM-5: the impact of proposed revisions on diagnosis of alcohol use disorders. *Addiction.* 2011;106(11):1935-1943. doi:10.1111/j.1360-0443.2011.03517.x
13. Peer K, Rennert L, Lynch KG, Farrer L, Gelernter J, Kranzler HR. Prevalence of DSM-IV and DSM-5 alcohol, cocaine, opioid, and cannabis

use disorders in a largely substance dependent sample. *Drug Alcohol Depend.* 2013;127(1-3):215-219. doi:10.1016/j.drugalcdep.2012.07.009

14. Goldstein RB, Chou SP, Smith SM, et al. Nosologic comparisons of DSM-IV and DSM-5 alcohol and drug use disorders: results from the National Epidemiologic Survey on Alcohol and Related Conditions-III. *J Stud Alcohol Drugs.* 2015;76(3):378-388. doi:10.15288/jsad.2015.76.378
15. Chung T, Cornelius J, Clark D, Martin C. Greater prevalence of proposed ICD-11 alcohol and cannabis dependence compared to ICD-10, DSM-IV, and DSM-5 in treated adolescents. *Alcohol Clin Exp Res.* 2017;41(9):1584-1592. doi:10.1111/acer.13441
16. Kaminer Y, Winters KC. DSM-5 Criteria for youth substance use disorders: lost in translation? *J Am Acad Child Adolesc Psychiatry.* 2015;54(5):350-351. doi:10.1016/j.jaac.2015.01.016
17. Kelly SM, Gryczynski J, Mitchell SG, Kirk A, O'Grady KE, Schwartz RP. Concordance between DSM-5 and DSM-IV nicotine, alcohol, and cannabis use disorder diagnoses among pediatric patients. *Drug Alcohol Depend.* 2014;140:213-216. doi:10.1016/j.drugalcdep.2014.03.034 Published correction appears in *Drug Alcohol Depend.* 2016;168:203.
18. Chung T, Martin CS, Maisto SA, Cornelius JR, Clark DB. Greater prevalence of proposed DSM-5 nicotine use disorder compared to DSM-IV nicotine dependence in treated adolescents and young adults. *Addiction.* 2012;107(4):810-818. doi:10.1111/j.1360-0443.2011.03722.x
19. Sadock BJ, Sadock VA, Ruiz P. *Kaplan and Sadock's Concise Textbook of Clinical Psychiatry*. 4th ed. Wolters Kluwer; 2016.
20. Khantzian EJ. The self-medication hypothesis of substance use disorders: a reconsideration and recent applications. *Harv Rev Psychiatry.* 1997;4(5):231-244. doi:10.3109/10673229709030550
21. Krawczyk N, Feder KA, Saloner B, Crum RM, Kealhofer M, Mojtabai R. The association of psychiatric comorbidity with treatment completion among clients admitted to substance use treatment programs in a U.S. national sample. *Drug Alcohol Depend.* 2017;175:157-163.
22. Ignaszewski MJ, Mirza KAH, Bukstein OG. Assessment and treatment of co-occurring externalizing disorders: attention deficit—disruptive behavior disorders and substance use disorders in adolescents. In: Kaminer Y, Winters KC, eds. *Clinical Manual of Youth Addictive Disorders*. 3rd ed. American Psychiatric Association; 2020.
23. O'Neil KA, Conner BT, Kendall PC. Internalizing disorders and substance use disorders in youth: comorbidity, risk, temporal order, and implications for intervention. *Clin Psychol Rev.* 2011;31(1):104-112. doi:10.1016/j.cpr.2010.08.002
24. Wu P, Goodwin RD, Fuller C, et al. The relationship between anxiety disorders and substance use among adolescents in the community: specificity and gender differences. *J Youth Adolesc.* 2010;39(2):177-188. doi:10.1007/s10964-008-9385-5
25. Giaconia RM, Reinherz HZ, Silverman AB, Pakiz B, Frost AK, Cohen E. Ages of onset of psychiatric disorders in a community population of older adolescents. *J Am Acad Child Adolesc Psychiatry.* 1994;33(5):706-717. doi:10.1097/00004583-199406000-00012
26. Bukstein OG, Bernet W, Arnold V, et al. Practice parameter for the assessment and treatment of children and adolescents with substance use disorders. *J Am Acad Child Adolesc Psychiatry.* 2005;44(6):609-621. doi:10.1097/01.chi.0000159135.33706.37
27. Verdejo-Garcia A, Garcia-Fernandez G, Dom G. Cognition and addiction. *Dialogues Clin Neurosci.* 2019;21(3):281-290. doi:10.31887/DCNS.2019.21.3/gdom
28. Hogue A, Henderson CE, Becker SJ, Knight DK. Evidence base on outpatient behavioral treatments for adolescent substance use, 2014-2017: outcomes, treatment delivery, and promising horizons. *J Clin Child Adolesc Psychol.* 2018;47(4):499-526. doi:10.1080/15374416.2018.1466307
29. Tomko RL, Jones JL, Gilmore AK, Brady KT, Back SE, Gray KM. N-acetylcysteine: a potential treatment for substance use disorders. *Curr Psychiatr.* 2018;17(6):30-55.
30. Volkow ND. The reality of comorbidity: depression and drug abuse. *Biol Psychiatry.* 2004;56(10):714-717. doi:10.1016/j.biopsych.2004.07.007
31. Rao U, Ryan ND, Dahl RE, et al. Factors associated with the development of substance use disorder in depressed adolescents. *J Am Acad Child Adolesc Psychiatry.* 1999;38:1109-1117.
32. Gobbi G, Atkin T, Zytynski T, et al. Association of cannabis use in adolescence and risk of depression, anxiety, and suicidality in young adulthood: a systematic review and meta-analysis. *JAMA Psychiatry.* 2019;76(4):426-434. doi:10.1001/jamapsychiatry.2018.4500. Published correction appears in *JAMA Psychiatry*. 2019;76(4):447.
33. March J, Silva S, Petrycki S, et al. Fluoxetine, cognitive-behavioral therapy, and their combination for adolescents with depression: Treatment for Adolescents With Depression Study (TADS) randomized controlled trial. *JAMA.* 2004;292(7):807-820. doi:10.1001/jama.292.7.807
34. Brent D, Emslie G, Clarke G, et al. Switching to another SSRI or to venlafaxine with or without cognitive behavioral therapy for adolescents with SSRI-resistant depression: the TORDIA randomized controlled trial. *JAMA.* 2008;299(8):901-913. doi:10.1001/jama.299.8.901. Published correction appears in *JAMA*. 2019;322(17):1718.
35. Horigian VE, Weems CF, Robbins MS, et al. Reductions in anxiety and depression symptoms in youth receiving substance use treatment. *Am J Addict.* 2013;22(4):329-337. doi:10.1111/j.1521-0391.2013.12031.x
36. Miranda-Mendizabal A, Castellví P, Parés-Badell O, et al. Gender differences in suicidal behavior in adolescents and young adults: systematic review and meta-analysis of longitudinal studies. *Int J Public Health.* 2019;64(2):265-283. doi:10.1007/s00038-018-1196-1
37. Mergl R, Koburger N, Heinrichs K, et al. What are reasons for the large gender differences in the lethality of suicidal acts? An epidemiological analysis in four European countries. *PLoS One.* 2015;10(7):e0129062. doi:10.1371/journal.pone.0129062
38. Goldston DB, Curry JF, Wells KC, et al. Feasibility of an integrated treatment approach for youth with depression, suicide attempts, and substance use problems. *Evid Based Pract Child Adolesc Ment Health.* 2021;6(2):155-172. doi:10.1080/23794925.2021.1888664
39. Cipriani A, Furukawa TA, Salanti G, et al. Comparative efficacy and acceptability of 21 antidepressant drugs for the acute treatment of adults with major depressive disorder: a systematic review and network meta-analysis. *Focus (Am Psychiatr Publ).* 2018;16(4):420-429.
40. Hamrin V, Iennaco JD. Evaluation of motivational interviewing to improve psychotropic medication adherence in adolescents. *J Child Adolesc Psychopharmacol.* 2017;27(2):148-159. doi:10.1089/cap.2015.0187
41. Vaughn SE, Strawn JR, Poweleit EA, Sarangdhar M, Ramsey LB. The impact of marijuana on antidepressant treatment in adolescents: clinical and pharmacologic considerations. *J Pers Med.* 2021;11(7):615. doi:10.3390/jpm11070615
42. Hen-Shoval D, Weller A, Weizman A, Shoval G. Examining the use of antidepressants for adolescents with depression/anxiety who regularly use cannabis: a narrative review. *Int J Environ Res Public Health.* 2022;19(1):523. doi:10.3390/ijerph19010523
43. Lu W, Muñoz-Laboy M, Sohler N, Goodwin RD. Trends and disparities in treatment for co-occurring major depression and substance use disorders among US adolescents from 2011 to 2019. *JAMA Netw Open.* 2021;4(10):e2130280. doi:10.1001/jamanetworkopen.2021.30280
44. Post RM, Grunze H. The challenges of children with bipolar disorder. *Medicina (Kaunas).* 2021;57(6):601. doi:10.3390/medicina57060601
45. Post RM, Altshuler LL, Kupka R, et al. More childhood onset bipolar disorder in the United States than Canada or Europe: implications for treatment and prevention. *Neurosci Biobehav Rev.* 2017;74(Pt A):204-213. doi:10.1016/j.neubiorev.2017.01.022
46. Lin PI, McInnis MG, Potash JB, et al. Clinical correlates and familial aggregation of age at onset in bipolar disorder. *Am J Psychiatry.* 2006;163(2):240-246. doi:10.1176/appi.ajp.163.2.240
47. Goldstein BI, Strober M, Axelson D, et al. Predictors of first-onset substance use disorders during the prospective course of bipolar spectrum disorders in adolescents. *J Am Acad Child Adolesc Psychiatry.* 2013;52(10):1026-1037. doi:10.1016/j.jaac.2013.07.009
48. Tolliver BK. Bipolar disorder and substance abuse: overcome the challenges of 'dual diagnosis' patients. *Current Psychiatry.* 2010;9:33-38.
49. Wilens TE, Biederman J, Millstein RB, Wozniak J, Hahesy AL, Spencer TJ. Risk for substance use disorders in youths with child- and adolescent-onset bipolar disorder. *J Am Acad Child Adolesc Psychiatry.* 1999;38(6):680-685. doi:10.1097/00004583-199906000-00014

50. Geller B, Tillman R, Bolhofner K, Zimerman B. Pharmacological and non-drug treatment of child bipolar I disorder during prospective eight-year follow-up. *Bipolar Disord.* 2010;12(2):164-171. doi:10.1111/j.1399-5618.2010.00791.x
51. Hafeman DM, Rooks B, Merranko J, et al. Lithium versus other mood-stabilizing medications in a longitudinal study of youth diagnosed with bipolar disorder. *J Am Acad Child Adolesc Psychiatry.* 2020;59(10):1146-1155. doi:10.1016/j.jaac.2019.06.013
52. Kedzior KK, Laeber LT. A positive association between anxiety disorders and cannabis use or cannabis use disorders in the general population—a meta-analysis of 31 studies. *BMC Psychiatry.* 2014;14:136. doi:10.1186/1471-244X-14-136
53. Lemyre A, Gauthier-Légaré A, Bélanger RE. Shyness, social anxiety, social anxiety disorder, and substance use among normative adolescent populations: a systematic review. *Am J Drug Alcohol Abuse.* 2019;45(3):230-247. doi:10.1080/00952990.2018.1536882
54. Dyer ML, Easey KE, Heron J, Hickman M, Munafò MR. Associations of child and adolescent anxiety with later alcohol use and disorders: a systematic review and meta-analysis of prospective cohort studies. *Addiction.* 2019;114(6):968-982. doi:10.1111/add.14575
55. McHugh RK. Treatment of co-occurring anxiety disorders and substance use disorders. *Harv Rev Psychiatry.* 2015;23(2):99-111. doi:10.1097/HRP.0000000000000058
56. Clark DB, Lesnick L, Hegedus AM. Traumas and other adverse life events in adolescents with alcohol abuse and dependence. *J Am Acad Child Adolesc Psychiatry.* 1997;36(12):1744-1751. doi:10.1097/00004583-199712000-00023
57. Oral R, Ramirez M, Coohey C, et al. Adverse childhood experiences and trauma informed care: the future of health care. *Pediatr Res.* 2016;79(1-2):227-233. doi:10.1038/pr.2015.197
58. Vujanovic AA, Bonn-Miller MO, Petry NM. Co-occurring posttraumatic stress and substance use: emerging research on correlates, mechanisms, and treatments—introduction to the special issue. *Psychol Addict Behav.* 2016;30(7):713-719. doi:10.1037/adb0000222
59. Grant BF, Saha TD, Ruan WJ, et al. Epidemiology of DSM-5 drug use disorder: results from the National Epidemiologic Survey on Alcohol and Related Conditions-III. *JAMA Psychiatry.* 2016;73(1):39-47. doi:10.1001/jamapsychiatry.2015.2132
60. Goldstein RB, Smith SM, Chou SP, et al. The epidemiology of DSM-5 posttraumatic stress disorder in the United States: results from the National Epidemiologic Survey on Alcohol and Related Conditions-III. *Soc Psychiatry Psychiatr Epidemiol.* 2016;51(8):1137-1148. doi:10.1007/s00127-016-1208-5
61. Felitti VJ, Anda RF, Nordenberg D, et al. REPRINT OF: Relationship of childhood abuse and household dysfunction to many of the leading causes of death in adults: the adverse childhood experiences (ACE) Study. *Am J Prev Med.* 2019;56(6):774-786. doi:10.1016/j.amepre.2019.04.001
62. Kessler RC, McLaughlin KA, Green JG, et al. Childhood adversities and adult psychopathology in the WHO World Mental Health Surveys. *Br J Psychiatry.* 2010;197(5):378-385. doi:10.1192/bjp.bp.110.080499
63. Brown DW, Anda RF, Tiemeier H, et al. Adverse childhood experiences and the risk of premature mortality. *Am J Prev Med.* 2009;37(5):389-396. doi:10.1016/j.amepre.2009.06.021
64. Schumm JA, Gore WL. Simultaneous treatment of co-occurring posttraumatic stress disorder and substance use disorder. *Curr Treat Options Psych.* 2016;3:28-36. https://doi.org/10.1007/s40501-016-0071-z
65. Blanco C, Xu Y, Brady K, Pérez-Fuentes G, Okuda M, Wang S. Comorbidity of posttraumatic stress disorder with alcohol dependence among US adults: results from National Epidemiological Survey on Alcohol and Related Conditions. *Drug Alcohol Depend.* 2013;132(3):630-638.
66. Simpson TL, Lehavot K, Petrakis IL. No wrong doors: findings from a critical review of behavioral randomized clinical trials for individuals with co-occurring alcohol/drug problems and posttraumatic stress disorder. *Alcohol Clin Exp Res.* 2017;41(4):681-702. doi:10.1111/acer.13325
67. Flanagan JC, Korte KJ, Killeen TK, Back SE. Concurrent treatment of substance use and PTSD. *Curr Psychiatry Rep.* 2016;18(8):70. doi:10.1007/s11920-016-0709-y
68. Hien DA, Jiang H, Campbell AN, et al. Do treatment improvements in PTSD severity affect substance use outcomes? A secondary analysis from a randomized clinical trial in NIDA's Clinical Trials Network. *Am J Psychiatry.* 2010;167(1):95-101. doi:10.1176/appi.ajp.2009.09091261
69. Najavits LM, Gallop RJ, Weiss RD. Seeking safety therapy for adolescent girls with PTSD and substance use disorder: a randomized controlled trial. *J Behav Health Serv Res.* 2006;33(4):453-463. doi:10.1007/s11414-006-9034-2
70. Danielson CK, McCart MR, Walsh K, de Arellano MA, White D, Resnick HS. Reducing substance use risk and mental health problems among sexually assaulted adolescents: a pilot randomized controlled trial. *J Fam Psychol.* 2012;26(4):628-635. doi:10.1037/a0028862
71. Danielson CK, Adams Z, McCart MR, et al. Safety and efficacy of exposure-based risk reduction through family therapy for co-occurring substance use problems and posttraumatic stress disorder symptoms among adolescents: a randomized clinical trial. *JAMA Psychiatry.* 2020;77(6):574-586. doi:10.1001/jamapsychiatry.2019.4803
72. Hahn AM, Adams ZW, Chapman J, et al. Risk reduction through family therapy (RRFT): protocol of a randomized controlled efficacy trial of an integrative treatment for co-occurring substance use problems and posttraumatic stress disorder symptoms in adolescents who have experienced interpersonal violence and other traumatic events. *Contemp Clin Trials.* 2020;93:106012. doi:10.1016/j.cct.2020.106012
73. van Duijvenbode N, VanDerNagel JEL. A systematic review of substance use (disorder) in individuals with mild to borderline intellectual disability. *Eur Addict Res.* 2019;25(6):263-282. doi:10.1159/000501679
74. Arnevik EA, Helverschou SB. Autism spectrum disorder and co-occurring substance use disorder—a systematic review. *Subst Abuse.* 2016;10:69-75. doi:10.4137/SART.S39921
75. Hops H, Davis B, Lewin LM. The development of alcohol and other substance use: a gender study of family and peer context. *J Stud Alcohol Suppl.* 1999;13:22-31. doi:10.15288/jsas.1999.s13.22
76. Hetland J, Braatveit KJ, Hagen E, Lundervold AJ, Erga AH. Prevalence and characteristics of borderline intellectual functioning in a cohort of patients with polysubstance use disorder. *Front Psychiatry.* 2021;12:651028. doi:10.3389/fpsyt.2021.651028
77. Fiorentini A, Cantù F, Crisanti C, Cereda G, Oldani L, Brambilla P. Substance-induced psychoses: an updated literature review. *Front Psychiatry.* 2021;12:694863. doi:10.3389/fpsyt.2021.694863
78. Fiorentini A, Volonteri LS, Dragogna F, et al. Substance-induced psychoses: a critical review of the literature. *Curr Drug Abuse Rev.* 2011;4(4):228-240. doi:10.2174/1874473711104040228
79. Wilson L, Szigeti A, Kearney A, Clarke M. Clinical characteristics of primary psychotic disorders with concurrent substance abuse and substance-induced psychotic disorders: a systematic review. *Schizophr Res.* 2018;197:78-86. doi:10.1016/j.schres.2017.11.001
80. Abdel-Baki A, Ouellet-Plamondon C, Salvat É, Grar K, Potvin S. Symptomatic and functional outcomes of substance use disorder persistence 2 years after admission to a first-episode psychosis program. *Psychiatry Res.* 2017;247:113-119. doi:10.1016/j.psychres.2016.11.007
81. Marconi A, Di Forti M, Lewis CM, Murray RM, Vassos E. Meta-analysis of the association between the level of cannabis use and risk of psychosis. *Schizophr Bull.* 2016;42(5):1262-1269. doi:10.1093/schbul/sbw003
82. Ghose S. Substance-induced psychosis: an indicator of development of primary psychosis? *Am J Psychiatry.* 2018;175(4):303-304. doi:10.1176/appi.ajp.2018.17121395
83. Caton CL, Hasin DS, Shrout PE, et al. Stability of early-phase primary psychotic disorders with concurrent substance use and substance-induced psychosis. *Br J Psychiatry.* 2007;190:105-111. doi:10.1192/bjp.bp.105.015784
84. Starzer MSK, Nordentoft M, Hjorthøj C. Rates and predictors of conversion to schizophrenia or bipolar disorder following substance-induced psychosis. *Am J Psychiatry.* 2018;175(4):343-350. Published correction appears in *Am J Psychiatry.* 2019;176(4):324.
85. Khokhar JY, Dwiel LL, Henricks AM, Doucette WT, Green AI. The link between schizophrenia and substance use disorder: a unifying hypothesis. *Schizophr Res.* 2018;194:78-85. doi:10.1016/j.schres.2017.04.016

86. Jones HJ, Stergiakouli E, Tansey KE, et al. Phenotypic manifestation of genetic risk for schizophrenia during adolescence in the general population. *JAMA Psychiatry.* 2016;73(3):221-228. doi:10.1001/jamapsychiatry.2015.3058
87. Green AI, Zimmet SV, Strous RD, Schildkraut JJ. Clozapine for comorbid substance use disorder and schizophrenia: do patients with schizophrenia have a reward-deficiency syndrome that can be ameliorated by clozapine? *Harv Rev Psychiatry.* 1999;6(6):287-296. doi:10.3109/10673229909017206
88. Coles AS, Knezevic D, George TP, Correll CU, Kane JM, Castle D. Long-acting injectable antipsychotic treatment in schizophrenia and co-occurring substance use disorders: a systematic review. *Front Psychiatry.* 2021;12:808002. doi:10.3389/fpsyt.2021.808002
89. Bennett ME, Bradshaw KR, Catalano LT. Treatment of substance use disorders in schizophrenia. *Am J Drug Alcohol Abuse.* 2017;43(4):377-390. doi:10.1080/00952990.2016.1200592
90. Zulauf CA, Sprich SE, Safren SA, Wilens TE. The complicated relationship between attention deficit/hyperactivity disorder and substance use disorders. *Curr Psychiatry Rep.* 2014;16(3):436. doi:10.1007/s11920-013-0436-6
91. Hechtman L, Swanson JM, Sibley MH, et al. Functional adult outcomes 16 years after childhood diagnosis of attention-deficit/hyperactivity disorder: MTA results. *J Am Acad Child Adolesc Psychiatry.* 2016;55(11):945-952.e2. doi:10.1016/j.jaac.2016.07.774. Published correction appears in *J Am Acad Child Adolesc Psychiatry.* 2017;56(7):628; published correction appears in *J Am Acad Child Adolesc Psychiatry.* 2018;57(3):225.
92. van Amsterdam J, van der Velde B, Schulte M, van den Brink W. Causal factors of increased smoking in ADHD: a systematic review. *Subst Use Misuse.* 2018;53(3):432-445. doi:10.1080/10826084.2017.1334066
93. Miranda A, Colomer C, Berenguer C, Roselló R, Roselló B. Substance use in young adults with ADHD: comorbidity and symptoms of inattention and hyperactivity/impulsivity. *Int J Clin Health Psychol.* 2016;16(2):157-165. doi:10.1016/j.ijchp.2015.09.001
94. Özgen H, Spijkerman R, Noack M, et al. Treatment of adolescents with concurrent substance use disorder and attention-deficit/hyperactivity disorder: a systematic review. *J Clin Med.* 2021;10(17):3908. doi:10.3390/jcm10173908
95. Thurstone C, Riggs PD, Salomonsen-Sautel S, Mikulich-Gilbertson SK. Randomized, controlled trial of atomoxetine for attention-deficit/hyperactivity disorder in adolescents with substance use disorder. *J Am Acad Child Adolesc Psychiatry.* 2010;49(6):573-582. doi:10.1016/j.jaac.2010.02.013
96. ADHD Guideline Development Group. *Australian evidence-based clinical practice guideline for attention deficit hyperactivity.* Australian ADHD Professionals Association; 2022. https://adhdguideline.aadpa.com.au
97. Kooij JJS, Bijlenga D, Salerno L, et al. Updated European Consensus Statement on diagnosis and treatment of adult ADHD. *Eur Psychiatry.* 2019;56:14-34. doi:10.1016/j.eurpsy.2018.11.001
98. Canadian ADHD Resource Alliance (CADDRA). *Canadian ADHD Practice Guidelines.* 4th ed. CADDRA; 2018.
99. National Institute for Health and Care Excellence. *Attention Deficit Hyperactivity Disorder: Diagnosis and Management.* NICE Guideline [NG87]. NICE; 2019.
100. Subcommittee on Attention-Deficit/Hyperactivity Disorder; Steering Committee on Quality Improvement and Management; Wolraich M, et al. ADHD: clinical practice guideline for the diagnosis, evaluation, and treatment of attention-deficit/hyperactivity disorder in children and adolescents. *Pediatrics.* 2011;128(5):1007-1022. doi:10.1542/peds.2011-2654
101. Wolraich ML, Hagan JF, Allan C, et al.; Subcommittee on Children and Adolescents with Attention-Deficit/Hyperactive Disorder. Clinical practice guideline for the diagnosis, evaluation, and treatment of attention-deficit/hyperactivity disorder in children and adolescents. *Pediatrics.* 2019;144(4):e20192528.
102. Gregorowski C, Seedat S, Jordaan GP. A clinical approach to the assessment and management of co-morbid eating disorders and substance use disorders. *BMC Psychiatry.* 2013;13:289. doi:10.1186/1471-244X-13-289
103. Denoth F, Siciliano V, Iozzo P, Fortunato L, Molinaro S. The association between overweight and illegal drug consumption in adolescents: is there an underlying influence of the sociocultural environment? *PLoS One.* 2011;6(11):e27358. doi:10.1371/journal.pone.0027358
104. Conason AH, Sher L. Alcohol use in adolescents with eating disorders. *Int J Adolesc Med Health.* 2006;18(1):31-36. doi:10.1515/ijamh.2006.18.1.31
105. Scott K, Becker SJ, Helseth SA, et al. Pharmacotherapy interventions for adolescent co-occurring substance use and mental health disorders: a systematic review. *Fam Pract.* 2022;39(2):301-310. doi:10.1093/fampra/cmab096

SECTION

15

Ethical, Legal, and Liability Issues in Addiction Practice

Associate Editor: Andrew J. Saxon

Lead Section Editor: Timothy K. Brennan

Section Editors: Robert L. DuPont and Corrine L. Shea

CHAPTER

123 Ethical Issues in Addiction Practice

Timothy K. Brennan and H. Westley Clark

CHAPTER OUTLINE

- Introduction
- Core ethical principles
- Dealing with denial
- Establishing an ethical stance
- Future developments

INTRODUCTION

Ethics amount to a set of moral principles that govern an individual's behavior, regardless of whether that person is a clinician or a patient. In fact, the ethical principles that apply to both addiction research and practice are similar to the ethical principles that apply to general medical care. The long tradition of Western medicine that evolved from Hippocrates more than 2,000 years ago has matured through the activities of various professional organizations such as the American Medical Association (AMA), the American Hospital Association, the American Nurses Association, the American Psychiatric Association (APA), the American Psychological Association, and the National Association of Social Workers, to name just a few. These organizations have promulgated codes of conduct and behavior predicated on the imperative that clinicians must behave in an ethical manner in their interactions with patients and in the conduct of health-related matters.

In this regard, it is important to recognize that what is deemed to be *ethical* may sometimes conflict with what is deemed to be *legal*. What is *legal* is governed by laws or regulations that are codified and published and ever-changing, whereas what is *ethical* is governed by a unique situation that is specific to a particular clinician and patient. However, ethical principles are commonly encoded as standards by organized medicine and other professional organizations related to law, divinity, education, finance, etc.

Many people enter the practice of medicine guided by a spirit of altruism—that is, acting with regard to the well-being of others. This is a near-universal trait among healthcare providers and one that is easy to embody, as sick people generate empathy in others quite easily. However, within addiction medicine, where there may be preconceived notions of certain moral implications of the disease of addiction, an ethical framework becomes much more essential and worthy of continued inquiry.

Addiction medicine professionals routinely encounter clinical situations that raise ethical questions and concerns. For many years, a guiding document for practitioners has been the work of Beauchamp and Childress,[1] who promulgated the concepts of *autonomy*, *beneficence*, *nonmaleficence*, and *justice* Of course these four principles are not exclusive to the practice of medicine, where they are joined by the principle of *fidelity*, which has at least two sub-components: *confidentiality* and *veracity*. Medicine has been immersed in ethical concepts from the time of Hippocrates to the modern Belmont Report of 1979. Operationalizing and incorporating these ethical concepts into clinical practice are an obligation of all practitioners.[2]

The attitudes of individual practitioners and society as a whole can be influenced by the acts of individuals affected by substance use disorder (SUD). Unlike many medical conditions—such as cancer, neurodegenerative conditions or genetic disease—many people still argue that an individual could have avoided the SUD in the first place if they had not consumed the particular substance in excess. Sadly, even some healthcare providers may still view an SUD as a self-inflicted moral failing that should respond to the proper exercise of free will. Others view the condition as a true biologic disorder that can respond to treatment if the affected individual desires such treatment.[3] Because the sequelae of SUDs are personal, familial, and societal, nearly everyone has an opinion about the disease. Practitioners are inevitably drawn into the tension inherent in these varying opinions and need to professionally navigate the resulting ethical issues.[4]

For guidance in this process, physicians can turn to groups such as the AMA, the APA, the American Society of Addiction Medicine (ASAM), and state boards of medical licensure for information about ethical practices, as well as behaviors that are considered unethical.

CORE ETHICAL PRINCIPLES

As previously noted, five general principles provide a basis from which to explore the ethical questions and concerns that arise in the treatment of SUDs: autonomy, beneficence, nonmaleficence, justice, and fidelity.[1,5,6]

Autonomy

A primary principle in modern medicine is that clinicians should respect the right of individuals to determine what course of action is appropriate for themselves. In other words, a person acts in their own self-interest as a rational actor. Thus, the clinician is obligated to treat the patient as autonomous and avoid actions that would diminish the patient's ability to exercise personal liberty.[2,5]

Customarily, the patient's capacity to decide is presumed.[5] However, the underlying assumption of competent self-determination may be questioned when a patient is suffering from a SUD[6] because psychoactive substances interfere with cognitive processes and decision-making ability. Compromised competence is an important consideration for clinicians because it can influence how the clinician should respond to the exercise of autonomy by a patient. Further, an individual who is competent to exercise decision-making under the principle of autonomy also must accept responsibility for the consequences of such decisions, as well as the limits of the clinician's authority under that circumstance.

Thus, a clinician should have some means to assess the ongoing competence of a patient being treated for a SUD. Conditions that cause competence to wax and wane may be especially vexing for both patient and clinician. Conditions that have a progressively deteriorating effect on competence also can create dilemmas, as it becomes critical to assess the course and rate of the deterioration to determine the degree to which the clinician should respect the patient's autonomy and right to self-determination.

It is essential that the patient is able to understand the nature and consequences of the healthcare issues at stake, the risks and benefits associated with any proposed intervention, and any alternative options for care. The decisions and choices made by the patient should not be distorted by others, including the clinician, or by a medical or psychiatric condition that compromises the patient's ability to make a free choice.

SUDs can occur across the lifespan. While there is a peak in prevalence among young adults, no age group is spared the effects. Hence, neurocognitive assessments can be very important in determining the complexity of instructions for care and the nature of recovery-oriented strategies presented to the patient.

It is in the arena of diminished capacity or impairment that the ethical concept of paternalism has currency.[5] In this situation, the clinician or some other authority makes key decisions for the patient. Nevertheless, despite the clinician's belief that a patient has diminished ability to make appropriate decisions about their care, an effort should be made to explain every aspect of care to the patient, from the results of an assessment to any medications deemed appropriate.

As the so-called "Baby Boomer" generation ages, more individuals with SUDs and possible cognitive impairment may present for screening, brief intervention, and/or treatment. As this occurs, the tension between professional paternalism and patient autonomy may become more pronounced. However, Baby Boomers also may lead the way in maintaining durable powers of attorney for purposes of health care and otherwise. Such legal instruments can delegate to friends or family the autonomy that the patient otherwise would exercise. Should a patient's condition deteriorate dramatically in the absence of a legal instrument that memorializes the patient's intentions, a court may have to be petitioned to assign a legal guardian for decision-making purposes.

Tension between the values of the clinician and those of the patient also may surface in situations where the patient is under the jurisdiction of the legal system or has obligations to the child welfare system or to an employer. For example, in a case where the patient is obligated to report progress to an external agency (such as a court or child welfare agency) and that report, if accurate, could contain damaging information—such as multiple missed appointments or toxicology screens that are positive for drugs—a patient may ask the clinician to either omit or misrepresent the damaging information. In such a situation, especially in the absence of diminished competency, the clinician could be seen as disrespecting the autonomy of the patient by agreeing to the patient's request because autonomy requires the exercise of responsibility.[2]

In many cases, it may be extremely difficult not to "push" the patient toward a decision by emphasizing certain information. If nothing else, such biases should be acknowledged to the patient, who then will be able to listen to the information with an awareness of the bias. An added benefit is that the patient may be more open to therapies the physician is advocating at another stage of treatment because they were not "pushed" early on.[6]

Voluntariness Versus Coercion

A growing number of patients in addiction treatment have been forced or compelled into such treatment by their families, employers, or the legal system. For example, a spouse may give their partner an ultimatum: "get help or else." An employer may require treatment as a condition of retaining a job. A legal agency may require a defendant to enter treatment as a condition of probation, parole, or suspension of charges.

Critics of coerced treatment contend that it is unethical because it violates the principle of autonomy.[7] Some critics are particularly concerned when the legal system mandates treatment or offers inducements such as the possibility that a criminal defendant will avoid incarceration, because they view the power imbalance in such circumstances as especially annihilative to the principle of autonomy.[8]

Proponents of coerced treatment counter that while such coercion unquestionably impinges on a patient's autonomy, it does not violate it altogether, even in the context of the legal system.[8] The patient may not wish to enter treatment but always has a choice about whether to do so and retains the right to refuse. The patient may not like the consequences of refusal (losing a spouse, losing a job, or being incarcerated on criminal charges) but still retains the autonomy to make the decision in question. Proponents also point out that patients who stay in treatment for at least 90 days have better outcomes than do those who leave earlier. To the extent that coercion raises retention rates, they argue, it works to improve the chances that the patient will eventually have a positive outcome.

Much of the discussion presented here dovetails with the concept of *informed consent*. As a critical component of autonomy, informed consent is the process of communication between a patient and a clinician that allows the clinician to provide specific medical treatments to the patient. As the AMA has pointed out, the communication process associated with informed consent is both a legal requirement and an ethical obligation.[9]

Beneficence

The principle of beneficence assumes that an individual wishes to help others and implies a moral obligation to act for the benefit of the patient. Inherent in the physician-patient relationship is an obligation on the part of the physician to aid the patient and avoid harming them. However, there are limits to this obligation, and the practitioner should guard against becoming overly involved with the patient's personal affairs.

Defining the boundaries of what is "good for the patient" also is tied to the notion that a licensed practitioner is, in part, an agent of the state and, as such, an agent of social good. If the "good" in addiction medicine is recovery, then the boundaries of that "good" could become limitless, with the life of the clinician intertwined with the life of the patient. Such an outcome would invoke paternalism and a diminution of patient autonomy. Consequently, beneficence must have natural, ethical limits. While there may not be a natural boundary to the legitimate practice of addiction medicine, involving the patient in shared decision-making about their care can lead to consensus between the clinician and patient as to the way forward.

Consulting with colleagues in a legally permissible manner broadens the clinician's insight, so that boundary violations are avoided and the risk of the clinician over-identifying with the patient's struggles is minimized.[1,4]

Nonmaleficence

This ethical principle means "to do no harm." In treating patients with SUDs, the clinician must not knowingly provide ineffective treatments or act with malice toward a patient. This principle is *not* about avoiding exposing a patient to the known or unknown risks of a particular therapeutic intervention; in fact, there are risks associated with many effective treatments. Rather, the principle suggests that a clinician's bias for or against a particular type of treatment should be informed by best practices, scientific research, and/or objective clinical experience.[1,4,5]

An example of nonmaleficence is seen in the actions of a primary care physician who prescribes opioid analgesics for the treatment of pain. Because there is an inherent risk of physical dependence and/or addiction associated with the long-term use of opioids, the failure to explain that risk to a patient would be "doing harm." Further, the physician could be seen as causing harm because they lack the knowledge needed to monitor the patient's progress and adjust the analgesic as indicated. In another example, if a physician who treats SUD has no DEA waiver or federal registration to prescribe buprenorphine for the treatment of opioid use disorder, that could be seen as violating the obligation to do no harm by erecting a roadblock to patients' access to an important potential therapy. It is clear, then, that the intersection of doing good (the principle of beneficence) and causing no harm (nonmaleficence) can produce a conundrum of sorts for the addiction medicine specialist. However, patients should be aware of all treatment options available to them, regardless of the personal beliefs of the clinician who is treating them.

An example of the intersection between doing good and not causing harm can be found in the Housing First paradigm,[10] which promotes access to housing for persons who are chronically homeless, some of whom also have SUDs or disabling psychiatric conditions. A clinician working within this paradigm may be confronted with the belief that a patient should be offered housing without a corresponding requirement to participate in mental health or SUD treatment. In such situations, the clinician must find a way to respect the autonomy of the patient while promoting abstinence from unhealthy substance use. In such situations, the "stages of change" model advocated by Prochaska and DiClemente[11] offers the clinician a moral framework within which to operate.

Nonmaleficence also applies to the selection of therapies, including medications that have little empirical evidence to support their effectiveness. With the off-label use of medications, the clinician may be relying on studies involving small sample sizes or the idiosyncratic experience of a single program. Where there is limited empirical support for a medication or other therapy, there is insufficient information to educate the patient about the effectiveness of the approach in question; hence, the principle of autonomy is undermined, and that therapy should be avoided, or ideally used with very careful consideration, informed consent, documentation into the medical record, and reasonable monitoring.

The use of some psychoactive substances is a source of controversy. As of 2022, a majority of states have legalized the sale of so-called "medical" cannabis (more accurately referred to as "cannabis used as treatment"), and 18 states and Washington, DC have legalized adult use of cannabis, also known as "recreational" cannabis.[12] In those states, clinicians are faced with a dilemma in working with patients who use cannabis, which may be legal under state law but remains a violation of federal law. What is the moral position of the clinician in such a situation, especially since authority to practice comes from state governments while the authority to schedule controlled substances comes from both states and the federal government? Can the ethical principle of nonmaleficence guide the clinician?

Another example of conflicting interpretations of the principle of nonmaleficence is found in the debate over abstinence versus harm reduction approaches to the treatment of SUDs. For example, advocates of abstinence argue that a harm reduction approach is dangerous because it allows a patient to continue using substances and communicates a mixed message about the dangers of their continued use. In contrast, advocates of harm reduction argue that the abstinence-based model does not allow for compassion or for meeting the basic healthcare needs of individuals who are in the throes of addiction.[4] If people are going to inject heroin, it is reasonable that they be given the opportunity inject themselves with clean needles.

Some advocates for harm reduction also assert that the abstinence-based model may prevent recovery because it does not permit the patient to progress through the stages of change envisioned by theorists such as Prochaska and DiClemente but instead imposes a rigid clinical philosophy on the patient. Given that there are many pathways to recovery, each of these arguments creates an ethical dilemma for the clinician at both a personal and professional level.

A final issue related to the principle of nonmaleficence can be found in the context of the so-called "difficult patient." Such a patient may miss appointments or violate the treatment agreement or otherwise fail to cooperate with the clinician. Some clinicians might be inclined to discharge such a patient or to transfer them to another clinician. While the patient has a personal responsibility under the ethical principle of autonomy to honor the therapeutic agreement, the clinician has a professional obligation to do no harm. In tort law, there is a corollary to this situation, in that a clinician must not abandon a patient in the patient's hour of need. While neither nonmaleficence nor the tort concept of nonabandonment bind the clinician to the patient in perpetuity, both concepts recognize that the clinician has a duty to work with the patient to achieve the best outcome. Importantly, there are mechanisms in place that allow physicians to terminate a relationship with a patient provided that the physician gives reasonable notice, assists in providing the patient with a reasonable opportunity to find new care and assists in the transfer of medical records. The licensee's state medical board policy on this topic should be consulted. Patients are of course free to terminate a relationship with the physician at any time that they wish.

To avoid violating the principle of nonmaleficence, clinicians should establish clear guidelines with every patient at the beginning of treatment, renew the understanding of those guidelines periodically, and address the clinical issues associated with noncompliance during the course of treatment. There should be a clear understanding of what is treatment, so that a patient can decide whether the provider in question is the provider for them.

Finally, because patients suffering from SUDs are vulnerable, they are at risk for exploitation. State boards of medicine, psychology, social work, and counseling have regulations that address (and provide penalties for) sexual or financial exploitation of patients and other unacceptable behaviors on the part of practitioners. In addition, sexual or financial exploitation of patients and other unacceptable behaviors may give rise to either civil or criminal liability for the provider, resulting in financial settlements or incarceration.

Justice

This ethical principle requires that, at a macrolevel, society distributes goods and services—including medical goods and services—fairly. At the microlevel, it means that clinicians will treat patients with equal conditions equally. In a normative sense, the principle of justice would require that medical needs are determined according to (1) the benefit that would accrue to a patient from the services offered, (2) the acuity of the patient's need, (3) the potential enhancement of the patient's quality of life, and (4) the duration of the benefit.[5]

In an ideal world, nonmedical criteria would not limit the services that a patient would receive. The AMA's Code of Ethics affirms that "Non-medical criteria, such as ability to pay, age, social worth, perceived obstacles to treatment, patient contribution to illness, or past use of resources should not be considered."[5] Despite these views, there are wide disparities in the ability of patients to pay for services, just as there is a wide difference in the cost of services offered by addiction treatment providers. While a wide spectrum of treatment facilities and services are available, from volunteer non–profit-run organizations to government-financed programs to privately operated facilities, some patients are unable to afford SUD treatment, especially in non-Medicaid expansion states. Furthermore, cash-based treatment creates equity issues for those without the discretionary finances to afford such care.

A larger issue may be the absence of demand for services. Data collected by the Substance Abuse and Mental Health Services Administration (SAMHSA) show that more than 90% of those who meet the clinical criteria for SUD do not seek or receive such treatment, with over 96% not perceiving the need for treatment.[13] Moreover, although there was a hope that enactment of the Affordable Care Act and the Mental Health Parity and Addiction Equity Act would allow millions more people to access mental health and addiction services,[14] there is a difference between having financial access to services and perceiving a need for such services. While the number of individuals accessing buprenorphine treatment has increased, the number of individuals accessing SUD treatment in general has not.

It has been argued that healthcare practitioners have a responsibility to advocate for their patients and to be involved in establishing humane policies of resource allocation at both the institutional and societal levels.[15] Thus, to give meaning to the principle of justice in the context of addiction, practitioners should make efforts to educate their colleagues and patients and to promote societal awareness of the need for SUD treatment.

The promise of broader insurance coverage for addiction services also carries with it other derivative themes as part of the principle of justice. For example, nonaddiction specialist healthcare practitioners may find that their comfort level is being challenged as increasing numbers of persons with SUDs seek care (and thus constitute a larger portion of their caseloads). While it is normal to have biases, it is important to recognize when and how such biases affect one's ability to practice within the principle of justice, so that no patient is discriminated against or denied access to treatment that other patients receive. Staff training is an important component of efforts to give currency to the principle of justice because such training can help prevent discrimination against patients with

SUDs. This helps to ensure a general level of fairness regardless of an individual clinician's personal feelings about SUDs and can help promote an atmosphere of impartiality and equality in the treatment setting.[6]

Fidelity

The principle of fidelity focuses on the quality of being faithful or loyal to the duties and obligations of a caregiver to a patient. It encompasses telling the truth and keeping actual and implicit promises to the patient, that is, veracity. It also involves not representing fiction as truth. In establishing a relationship with a patient, the clinician creates a set of expectations. These include honoring the treatment agreement, adhering to professional codes of ethics, maintaining an acceptable level of competence through training and continuing education, and following the policies and procedures of the treatment organization and all applicable laws. It also means that the information provided to the clinician will remain confidential to the extent permitted by law.[4]

Among other things, fidelity invokes the Hippocratic Oath: "What I may see or hear in the course of the treatment or even outside of treatment of the patient in regard to the life of men, which on no account one must spread abroad, I will keep to myself, holding such things to be shameful to be spoken about.[16]"

Although 42 CFR Part 2[17] provides a legal framework for confidentiality that governs federally funded treatment programs, it is not the law alone upon which a patient relies in their relationship with a clinician. Confidentiality is both an implicit and explicit promise by the clinician not to divulge a patient's personal information without that patient's permission.

If a physician is going to maintain fidelity by keeping promises, it is essential to be clear in advance about which promises may have to be broken and the circumstances under which that might occur. Federal regulations offer a limited list of exceptions to confidentiality in the context of addiction treatment. For example, if a patient appears to be suicidal or homicidal, confidentiality may need to be breached. Additionally, some states may require that pregnant people who use substances be reported to child protection agencies. Also, if a patient violates certain aspects of the treatment agreement, the relationship between the clinician and patient may be terminated. It is important that the clinician be very clear about the limits to fidelity, so there are no surprises later.[4]

Fidelity and its two subcomponents, veracity and confidentiality, create a level of trust in the therapeutic relationship that is necessary for the patient to make progress in treatment. Such trust can be tested in situations involving group therapy or family therapy. While the patient is always the principal focus of the clinician, information must be shared in the group or with family members if they are to be useful resources. Thus, the patient should have a clear understanding of the limits of confidentiality in the situation of group and family therapy. Ideally, written information would be provided to the patient, describing the boundaries of confidentiality in those situations, so that the patient can make an informed judgment as to whether to participate.

As noted earlier, the principle of fidelity requires that the clinician be as knowledgeable as possible about SUD treatment so that the patient can rely on the clinician to recommend specific treatment modalities or programs. There should be no financial, clinical, or philosophical conflict of interest on the part of the physician in terms of the recommended course of treatment. For example, a patient who has opioid use disorder might benefit from evidence-based medication treatment, but if the clinician recommends only nonpharmacologic therapies, that may be a violation of the principle of fidelity. Such a situation also represents a breach of the principle of autonomy because the patient is not being provided with critical information needed to decide which course of treatment is the most likely to be beneficial.

Fidelity and veracity apply not only to the relationship between the clinician and the patient but also to the relationship between the clinician and society as a whole. For instance, a patient might ask a clinician to withhold critical information in a report to a judge, child welfare agency, or employer. While the patient can opt to ask the clinician not to file a report, they should not ask the clinician to misrepresent or withhold information that would appear in such a report.

Fidelity and veracity also militate against dual relationships, as in situations where the patient and clinician have either a past social relationship or contemplate a future social relationship. It is difficult for the clinician to act in the best interests of a patient if either the clinician's or the patient's emotional or mental processes are distorted by the dynamics of such a social relationship.[4]

In terms of health insurance coverage, neither the patient nor the clinician should misrepresent the patient's eligibility for certain benefits or utilization of those benefits. In situations in which a patient may be eligible for disability benefits, neither patient nor clinician should misrepresent findings relevant to a determination of eligibility.

DEALING WITH DENIAL

Historically, practitioners in primary care settings did not inquire about a patient's substance use unless it was directly related to the presenting complaint, and annual physical examinations rarely included questions about alcohol or drug use. The U.S. Preventive Services Task Force (USPSTF) recommends screening by asking questions about unhealthy drug use in adults aged 18 or older. Nevertheless, when a clinician suspects that a patient may be engaging in unhealthy alcohol or other drug use, they must take the initiative to raise the issue, even if the patient has not previously disclosed it. Similarly, if a clinician suspects that a patient may have an abdominal mass, they are obligated to share that finding with the patient and make a referral for an appropriate clinical workup. SUDs are no different. The clinician has an ethical duty to act if there is reason to believe that the patient's use of alcohol or drugs is negatively affecting that patient's health.

In such situations, a difficulty commonly encountered by clinicians is that raising the issue may not be enough. Denial is an integral part of SUDs. Individuals in denial fail to recognize or are reluctant to acknowledge their problem or find ways to deny or minimize the extent of their substance use because they are ambivalent about changing that use. In such situations, what is the proper balance between respect for the principle of autonomy and the physician's responsibility for the patient's health? Should the physician raise the issue and then drop it if the patient is resistant?

As previously discussed, fidelity and veracity must be bidirectional in order to give substance to autonomy. Nevertheless, denial may be about shame, stigma, guilt, and substance-induced distortion of memories. While shame, stigma, and guilt can be attenuated through good clinical care and solid therapeutic relationships, distortion of memory is another matter.

Talking to the Patient

To fulfill the ethical responsibility to the patient, the clinician must do more than simply raise an issue. They should provide relevant information, engage the patient in discussion, and, if the patient shows resistance, follow up during future visits in a compassionate and nonconfrontational manner. Unless a firm foundation of trust and understanding has been established, persistent questions or a forceful confrontation can backfire and ultimately reinforce the patient's reluctance to engage in treatment. It also may become clear that the patient does not have an accurate memory of the substance use, in which case a "surrogate historian" such as a friend or family member may be helpful, but only with the consent of the patient.[4]

Ordering Laboratory Tests

Must, or should, a patient's consent be obtained before a drug screen is ordered? It is likely that the law does not require the patient's consent. Ordinarily, a clinician does not ask a patient to sign a consent form before sending blood or urine specimen for other types of testing. However, ordering laboratory tests to screen patients for SUDs has different implications, and failing to consult the patient can damage the physician-patient relationship and undermine efforts to induce the patient to acknowledge the presence of a problem.

Further, screening urine or blood for drugs is not a routine practice in primary care settings. Patients expect to be screened for blood sugar and cholesterol, but they do not expect to be screened for drug use. Patients confronted with the results of tests they did not know were being conducted and for which they did not give specific consent may feel that their trust in the clinician has been betrayed. Such a patient is likely to be angry that the physician did not show respect for the patient's autonomy.[4,18] As a result, the patient may refuse to participate in further discussions about substance use. Therefore, the better practice is to obtain the patient's permission for blood or urine tests for alcohol or other drug use.[18]

A second reason that physicians should obtain a patient's permission before ordering laboratory drug screens has to do with the patient's right to privacy. If the physician orders a test, the patient's insurance company or other third-party payer will know about the test and perhaps even its result, so even the decision to order a drug screen discloses a good deal, regardless of whether the test result is positive or negative. Therefore, it is the patient, not the physician, who should decide whether it is necessary and appropriate for the health insurer to have that information.

A third reason to seek the patient's permission is financial. The patient's benefits plan may not cover drug screens. In such a case, the patient should have the opportunity to decide whether they are willing to pay for the test out of pocket, which is a decision that should be made before a test is ordered.

Unfortunately, if the physician consults the patient, there is a good chance that the patient will refuse permission to perform a drug test. However, this leaves the door open to further discussion with the patient about possible substance use. The patient likely will appreciate the clinician's concern for their autonomy and privacy and thus may be more open to future discussions about substance use. The clinician might begin such a discussion by asking, in a neutral way, why the patient does not wish to have a drug screen performed.

Older Patients

The clinician who suspects that an older adult is engaging in unhealthy substance use should proceed with caution. As we age, we become more sensitive to perceived threats to our autonomy.[19] Because of the stigma surrounding SUDs, a patient whose clinician suggests that they may be engaging in unhealthy substance use (legal or illegal) may conclude that the physician is suggesting that whatever brought the patient to the physician's office for a medical visit has an emotional basis or that the patient's functioning or capacity is diminished. If an older adult thinks that their autonomy is being threatened, the patient may point to the "normal" infirmities of old age as the source of the difficulty, rather than acknowledging a problem with a substance.[20]

Most older adults are unaware that the way their bodies metabolize substances (including prescription medications) changes as they age and that the amount of alcohol or drugs they consumed without obvious adverse consequences when they were younger can harm their health and even incapacitate them as they grow older.[20] Moreover, many older adult patients take multiple prescription medications to control their cholesterol, blood pressure, and other age-related disorders. They may not be aware that their prescription medications can interact with each other and with any alcohol or over-the-counter or other drugs that they consume, thus interfering with the therapeutic effects of the medications. An approach that emphasizes these issues provides an opportunity to engage an older adult in a discussion about SUDs without posing a threat to their autonomy.

ESTABLISHING AN ETHICAL STANCE

Clinicians can avoid or minimize potential ethical dilemmas if they remain aware of the sources of potential conflicts of interest, keep the purposes of the ethical principles in mind, discuss potential conflicts with patients at the beginning of treatment, and take steps to reduce the potential for conflicts.[18]

Resources for Resolving Ethical Dilemmas

Resources for obtaining professional guidance on ethical issues can be found through consultation with colleagues, accessing professional standards or codes of ethics, and obtaining legal consultation. Each has strengths and drawbacks, and each is more relevant to some types of ethical dilemmas than are others.[4,18]

Consultation

Consultation can involve peers, senior staff, or other providers within the community. Confidentiality needs to be assured in seeking consultation. If there is a chance that information cannot be shared without accidentally divulging confidential information, the provider should find a consultant in another geographic locale. Identifying information must not be shared without the patient's consent.

Professional Standards or Codes of Ethics

Many medical organizations have adopted professional standards and codes of ethics, as have organizations in social work, nursing, and psychology. While such standards do not provide answers to every ethical dilemma, they do provide useful parameters for acceptable and unacceptable professional behavior. They also may help the professional frame questions that clarify the underlying issues and thus move the situation toward a decision.

Legal Consultation

For many providers, obtaining legal advice may seem unrealistic given limited resources, but there are low-cost strategies for obtaining advice in certain situations. Most bar associations have a pro bono legal component that may provide consultation at no charge or at a reduced rate. Legal service agencies that operate as a social service to the community may have expertise regarding certain ethical dilemmas. In addition, state regulatory agencies may have resources available with legal issues related to treatment.

Although ethical issues are complex and every case requires an individual evaluation, hospitals, addiction treatment programs, and other organizations should formally articulate practices that establish a process for approaching ethical issues. Given the ambiguous nature of ethical dilemmas, it is helpful to clarify the process for resolving them, even if the actual resolution may differ from case to case.[18]

Summary: A Step-by-Step Model for Making Ethical Decisions

By following the steps outlined below, health care professionals can move toward a more rational level of decision-making about ethical issues.[4,6,18]

Identify the Ethical Issue

What is the clinician's reaction to the situation? Ethical issues often are revealed when the practitioner has a "gut instinct" that something is not right. Confusion, anxiety, and uncertainty also are indicators that an ethical issue may be involved. If basic principles seem to be compromised, the clinician should stop and evaluate further. A significant step is to examine one's own feelings about the situation.

Review the Principles at Stake

What is the true dilemma? So much can be occurring with a patient that it is difficult to see the real issue, as well as to assess how significant that issue may be.

Consider Possible Solutions

At this point, the next step—or at least several options—may be clear. If there are multiple choices, it is useful to list the options and carefully examine each one. A further step is to list the pros and cons of each option.

Take Action

Having arrived at this point, the clinician should be ready to make a decision. Sometimes, the decision may not be one that everyone is comfortable with, but it may be the least objectionable plan. The patient should be helped to understand the rationale for the decision that has been made and thoroughly involved in the decision-making process.

Follow Up and Evaluate the Outcome

The outcomes of ethical decisions should be evaluated and their impact on patients carefully monitored, both as a form of resolution of the current situation and as a reference point for addressing similar dilemmas in the future.

FUTURE DEVELOPMENTS

The coming decades promise exciting breakthroughs in the treatment of SUDs. Yet, if the past is any guide to the future, each new discovery will bring with it new challenges to the core ethical obligations of honoring informed consent, protecting confidentiality, and respecting justice while also protecting the public from harm and ensuring good care of individual patients.[6]

As pointed out by Ashcroft et al.[19] in their review of ethical issues raised by progress in addiction research, "There is significant potential for great social and individual benefit from developments in this area, but these need to be evaluated alongside some potentially significant risks of harm or limitations on individual freedom that might undermine the value or acceptability of these developments." The authors point out that concerns about the ethical implications of scientific developments are given greater urgency by the stigma and discrimination still attached to addiction and to the persons who suffer from this medical disorder.

For example, with the growth of managed care, the physician and patient no longer have an exclusive relationship. Third-party payers have intruded into the relationship in multiple ways, as by shifting some financial risk to the physician or awarding bonuses to physicians whose patients do not use expensive (or extensive) services. Under other plans, contracts limit the services for which a physician will be reimbursed. (Note that such contracts do not limit the services the physician can provide—only those for which they will be paid.) In this way, many managed care plans create incentives that can impinge on sound medical judgment.

If a clinician allows financial incentives or disincentives to influence their treatment recommendations, or lead the clinician to discharge a patient who has exhausted benefits under a health insurance contract, that clinician has placed financial interests before their obligation to the patient, which is a clear ethical violation.

Because health insurers and other third-party payers place (often hidden) limits on certain forms of treatment, ethicists have begun to suggest that clinicians should inform their patients about any economic issues that could influence either the clinician's recommendation or the patient's decision. Providing an opportunity for the patient to give "economic informed consent" ensures that the patient knows about such limitations before making a decision about the proposed course of care.

If clinicians can adapt to the "new normal," these unprecedented paradigm shifts can influence health care decision-making in a reasoned and balanced fashion, and there is real hope that the cultural stigma and disenfranchisement underlying health disparities in addiction treatment may move in the direction of compassionate and competent care for all those who suffer from addiction.[4,18,19]

REFERENCES

1. Page K. The four principles: can they be measured and do they predict ethical decision making? *BMC Med Ethics.* 2012;13:10. Accessed January 13, 2010. https://bmcmedethics.biomedcentral.com/articles/10.1186/1472-6939-13-10
2. Fisher CB. Addiction research ethics and the Belmont principles: do drug users have a different moral voice? *Subst Use Misuse.* 2011;46(6):728-741.
3. Schaler JA. *Addiction is a Choice.* Open Court Publishers; 2000.
4. Substance Abuse and Mental Health Services Administration. *Substance Abuse Treatment for Persons with HIV/AIDS. Treatment Improvement Protocol (TIP) 37.* SAMHSA, Center for Substance Abuse Treatment; 2000.
5. American Medical Association. *Code of Medical Ethics.* The Association. Accessed June 22, 2013. https://code-medical-ethics.ama-assn.org/
6. White WL, Popovits RM. *Critical Incidents: Ethical Issues in the Prevention and Treatment of Addiction.* Chestnut Health Systems; 2001.
7. Ridgely M, Iguchi M, Chiesa J; National Research Council and the Institute of Medicine. The use of immunotherapies and sustained-release formulations in the treatment of drug addiction: will current law support coercion? *New Treatments for Addiction: Behavioral, Ethical, Legal, and Social Questions.* National Academics Press; 2004:173-187.
8. Wild TC, Roberts AB, Cooper EL. Compulsory substance abuse treatment: an overview of recent findings and issues. *Eur Addict Res.* 2002;8:84-93.
9. American Medical Association. *Resource Center: Informed Consent.* The Association. Accessed July 31, 2023. https://code-medical-ethics.ama-assn.org/ethics-opinions/informed-consent
10. Kertesz SG, Crouch K, Milby JB, Cusimano RE, Schumacher JE. Housing first for homeless persons with active addiction: are we overreaching? *Milbank Q.* 2009;87(2):495-534.
11. Prochaska JO, DiClemente CC. *The Transtheoretical Approach: Towards a Systematic Eclectic Framework.* Dow Jones Irwin; 1984.
12. National Conference of State Legislatures. *State Medical Marijuana Laws.* NCSL. Accessed November 27, 2016. http://www.ncsl.org/research/health/state-medical-marijuana-laws.aspx
13. Substance Abuse and Mental Health Services Administration. Results from the 2011 National Survey on Drug Use and Health: Summary of National Findings. *NSDUH Series H-44, HHS Publication No. (SMA).* SAMHSA; 2012:12-4713.
14. Beronio K, Po R, Skopec L, Wagner SG. Affordable Care Act will expand mental health and substance use disorder benefits and parity protections for 62 million Americans. *ASPE Research Brief.* USDHHS; 2013.
15. Junkerman J, Derse A, Schiedermayer D. *Practical Ethics for Students, Interns, and Residents.* 3rd ed. University Publishing Group; 2008.
16. Lasagna L. *Hippocratic Oath (Modern Version).* Sheridan Libraries, Johns Hopkins University School of Medicine; 1964. Accessed 13 December, 2023. https://www.nlm.nih.gov/hmd/greek/greek_oath.html
17. Code of Federal Regulations. *42 U.S. Code of Federal Regulations, Part 2.* Federal Register. Accessed July 31, 2023. http://www.archives.gov/federal-register/cfr/subject-title-42.html
18. Geppert CM, Bogenschutz MP. Ethics in substance use disorder treatment. *Psychiatr Clin North Am.* 2009;32(2):283-297.
19. Ashcroft R, Campbell AV, Capps B. Ethical aspects of developments in neuroscience and drug addiction. *Foresight Brain Science, Addiction and Drugs Project. British Ministry of* Health; 2007.
20. Substance Abuse and Mental Health Services Administration. Screening and assessment for older adults. *Treatment Improvement Protocol (TIP) 26.* Center for Substance Abuse Treatment, SAMHSA; 2008.

CHAPTER

124 Consent and Confidentiality Issues in Addiction Practice

Louis E. Baxter Sr and Nan Gallagher

CHAPTER OUTLINE

- Informed consent
- Agreement to treatment
- Confidentiality protections
- Special issues in treating health care professionals

The principle of autonomy is enshrined in the Constitution, and U.S. courts have repeatedly confirmed Americans' right to make decisions for themselves, including decisions about which information about their health care may be disclosed and to whom. Whenever a physician asks a patient to sign an "informed consent" agreement or to consent to disclosure of certain information, they are affirming that the patient has the right to make decisions about their medical care and the sanctity of their confidential medical records.

INFORMED CONSENT

Informed consent has two components: information and voluntariness. First, the patient's decision to undergo a course of treatment must be based on knowledge and competency. The physician must give the patient the kind and amount of information the patient needs to make an intelligent ("informed") choice, and the patient must be capable of understanding the information and making a decision. Second, the patient's decision must be voluntary—that is, a product of their free will.[1]

Informed Consent = Knowledge Plus Competency

While physicians do not ask patients to sign informed consent forms each time medical decisions are made, such forms generally are used to indicate consenting to treatment whenever the patient will undergo an invasive procedure that poses a risk of adverse physical consequences, when the patient chooses a treatment that the physician has warned may be ineffective, or when the law requires the physician to obtain informed consent because the test can result in serious adverse *legal* or *psychological* consequences. In such cases, asking the patient to sign the form impresses on them the importance of the decision to be made (eg, in some states, a patient must sign an informed consent form when an HIV test is performed).

Information

The physician is obligated to give the patient all the information they need to make a decision.[2] This information should include the physician's opinion of the patient's diagnosis, an outline of the available treatment alternatives, a description of what each alternative involves (including its benefits and risks), an explanation of the consequences should the patient decline treatment altogether, and responses to the patient's questions. Often, the physician also helps the patient evaluate the treatment alternatives in accordance with the patient's values, hopes, and fears.

Competency (Decisional Capacity)

The concept of informed consent is based on the assumption that the patient has the capacity to make rational decisions (referred to as "decisional capacity"). Decisional capacity is defined as a state in which a patient is able to understand the physician's explanation of the diagnosis, prognosis, treatment alternatives, and likely outcome if treatment is refused, and is able to go through the complex process of assessing that information in accordance with their personal system of values. Most patients have decisional capacity. However, the physician may encounter questions about decisional capacity in dealing with two groups: adolescents and older adults.

Special Issues in Dealing With Adolescents

The situation is somewhat different for adolescents because they do not have the legal status of full-fledged adults.[3] There are certain decisions that society will not allow them to make: for example, below a certain age—which varies by state and by issue—adolescents must attend school, may not marry without parental consent, may not drive, and cannot sign binding contracts.[4] (See Section 14 in this textbook for a more detailed discussion of how this affects adolescents' right to consent to treatment.) Nevertheless, in common law, there is no minimum age at which individuals are able to consent to medical treatment and no age below which they are unable to consent. Adolescents' right to self-determination is based on their ability to understand and appreciate the information relevant to the medical decision and on their ability to consent voluntarily and freely. There is a consensus in the literature that, around age 14 years, adolescents have the cognitive ability to understand information necessary for consent.[5] However, there are limited empirical data regarding adolescents' ability to appreciate the information and to make a voluntary decision.

In more than half the states in the United States, adolescents have the right to consent to screening, assessment, or treatment for substance use disorders (SUDs). In other states, a parent must be notified of and/or consent to such care.[6] In states that do not require parental consent, the physician has no ethical dilemma; they can provide whatever treatment is appropriate and to which the adolescent patient consents. In such states, the physician should involve adolescents in the consent process to the extent possible, assessing their capacity to consent to treatment on an individual basis, recognizing that such capacity may evolve as the adolescent's cognitive capacities and values mature.[5]

It is in those states that require parental consent or notification that the physician sometimes encounters a complex ethical quandary. The difficulty arises when an adolescent who seeks assessment or treatment refuses to permit communication with a parent. Presumably, a parent whose child seeks treatment would consent. A parent or guardian who refuses to consent to treatment that a physician believes is necessary to an adolescent's well-being could face charges of child neglect.

If the physician believes that the adolescent does need treatment, they have three choices.

Option 1: Treat the Adolescent Without Consulting a Parent

The physician who treats an adolescent without parental consent or notification is acting in accordance with the ethical principles of putting the patient's health first and respecting the patient's autonomy (and privacy) but may be violating the law. Although violation of the parental consent/notification law most likely is not a criminal offense, it could put the physician's professional license at risk or expose them to a lawsuit by the adolescent's parents. It is unlikely, however, that a physician treating an adolescent would be faced with either eventuality if the treatment provided is not controversial or intrusive, does not put the adolescent at risk, and is carried out in a responsible, non-negligent manner. In such circumstances, it would be difficult for a parent (or licensing authority) to show that any harm was done. This is particularly true if the physician made a reasoned decision and acted in good faith and out of concern for the adolescent. Contrary to popular belief, most lawyers do not chase after cases that are complex, time-consuming, expensive, and difficult to win. Convincing an attorney to take on such a case would not be easy.

The physician who is considering whether to offer treatment without parental consent or notification in a state that requires it should consider the following factors.

- *The adolescent's age.* Society accords adolescents more autonomy as they get older. A physician who might decline to treat a 14-year-old patient without parental consent in a state that requires it might have fewer qualms about treating a 17-year-old patient in similar circumstances.
- *The adolescent's maturity.* Chronologic age clearly is not the only measure. There are 14-year-olds who have maturity beyond their years and emotionally immature 17-year-olds with poor social skills and reasoning ability.
- *The adolescent's family situation.* Adolescents in need of addiction disorder treatment may be estranged from their families. Those who refuse to permit parental notification may have good reason to do so. Forcing them to involve parents who have failed them is neither ethical nor good clinical practice. Reconciliation with the family may be vital to an adolescent's recovery, but circumstances may dictate that it be abandoned or postponed to a later stage of treatment.
- *The severity of the adolescent's addiction disorder* and the danger it poses to their life or health.
- *The kind of treatment to be provided.* The more intrusive and intensive the proposed treatment, the more risk the physician assumes in treating an adolescent without parental consent. For example, a physician offering an outpatient course of treatment is on firmer ground than one proposing intensive inpatient or residential treatment.
- *The physician's possible liability for refusing to treat the patient.* State law may impose a duty to treat patients in need and impose sanctions for "abandoning" patients.
- *The financial consequences.* If the physician treats an adolescent without parental consent, they may not be paid.

Option 2: Try to Obtain Consent to Treatment From the Adolescent's Parent

Calling the parent and treating the adolescent complies with the letter of state law and is in accordance with the ethical principle that puts the patient's health first. However, it clearly violates the adolescent's right to privacy. Moreover, the federal confidentiality rules complicate this choice.

Federal confidentiality regulations prohibit physicians and others who provide alcohol and drug screening, assessment, and treatment from communicating with anyone, including a parent, unless the adolescent consents. The sole exception allows the director of an addiction treatment program to communicate "facts relevant to reducing a threat to the life or physical well-being of the [adolescent seeking services] or any other individual to the minor's parent, guardian, or other person authorized under state law to act in the minor's behalf, when the program director believes that the adolescent, because of extreme youth or mental or physical condition, lacks the capacity to decide rationally whether to consent to the notification of a parent or guardian," or because "The program director believes the disclosure to a parent or guardian is necessary to cope with a substantial threat to the life or physical well-being of the adolescent or someone else" (42 CFR §§2.14(c) and (d)).

Option 3: Refuse to Treat the Adolescent

Refusing to treat the adolescent adheres to the letter of state laws that consider adolescents incompetent to make medical decisions, and it shows respect for the patient's privacy, but it may violate the ethical principle that requires the physician to put the patient's interests first. In some states, it also violates a law requiring physicians to treat patients in medical need.

Special Issues in Treating Older Adults

Most older adults are fully capable of understanding medical information, weighing treatment alternatives, and making and articulating decisions.[7] However, a small percentage of older patients clearly are incapable of participating in a decision-making process. In such cases, the older adult may have signed a health care proxy or may have a court-appointed guardian who is authorized to make such decisions.[8]

The difficulty arises when a physician is screening or assessing an older adult whose mental capacity lies between those two points on the continuum. The patient may have fluctuating capacity, with "good days" and "bad days," or periods of greater or lesser alertness depending on the time of day. The patient's condition may be transient or deteriorating. Diminished capacity may affect some parts of their ability to comprehend information and make complex decisions, but not others.

In caring for an older adult patient whose decisional capacity is less than optimal, how can the physician help the patient to understand the information presented, appreciate the implications of each alternative treatment, and make a "rational" decision, based on the patient's best interests? And what can the physician do if the patient appears not to be competent to make their own health care decisions? Although there are no easy answers to these questions, there are several possible approaches.

Present Information Carefully

The physician can help the patient who appears to have diminished capacity through a gradual information-gathering and decision-making process. Information should be presented in a way that allows the patient to absorb it gradually, clarify and restate information as necessary, and summarize the issues at regular intervals. Each alternative approach to care and its consequences should be laid out and examined separately. Finally, the physician can help the patient identify their values and link those values to the alternatives. By helping the patient narrow their focus and then proceeding step by step, the physician may be assured that the patient has understood the choices and acted in their own best interests.

Enlist the Help of a Mental Health Professional or Other Specialist

If helping the patient through a process of gradual information-gathering and decision-making is not working, the physician can suggest that physician and patient jointly consult a mental health professional or other physician who is familiar with the patient's history and who thus may have a better understanding of the obstacles to decision-making. Or the physician could suggest a specialist (such as a geriatrician) who can help determine why the patient is having difficulty and whether they have the capacity to give informed consent.

Enlist the Help of Family or Close Friends

Another approach is for the physician to suggest that the patient call in a family member or close friend who can help organize the information and sort through the alternatives. Asking the patient who would be helpful could gain endorsement of this approach.

Consult a Family Member or Friend

If the patient cannot grasp the information or come to a decision, the physician might ask the patient to allow the physician to consult a family member or close friend. If the patient consents, the physician should lay out the concerns to the family member or friend. It may be that the patient already has planned for the possibility of incapacity and has signed a durable power of attorney or health care proxy.

Guardianship

A guardian is a person appointed by a court to manage some or all aspects of another person's life. Anyone seeking appointment of a guardian must show the court that the individual is disabled in some way by disease, illness, or a neurocognitive disorder and that the disability prevents that individual from performing the tasks necessary to manage one or more areas of their life.

Each U.S. state handles guardianship proceedings differently, but some principles apply across the board: guardianship is not an all-or-nothing state. Courts generally require that the person seeking appointment of a guardian prove the individual's incapacity in a variety of tasks or areas. Courts can apply different standards to different life tasks—managing money, managing a household, making health care decisions, entering contracts. A person can be found incompetent to make contracts and manage money but competent to make their own health care decisions (or vice versa) and the guardianship limited accordingly.

Guardianship limits the older adult's autonomy and is an expensive process. It should be considered only as a last resort.

AGREEMENT TO TREATMENT

As part of the informed consent process, the physician should discuss the risks and benefits of treatment with the patient and, with appropriate consent of the patient, with family members, significant other(s), or a guardian. This type of discussion is best accompanied by a written agreement between the physician and patient addressing issues such as (1) alternative treatment options, (2) agreement to regular toxicological testing for drug use and therapeutic drug levels (if available and indicated), and (3) the reasons for which treatment may be altered or discontinued.[8]

The written treatment plan should describe the objectives that will be used to determine treatment success, such as freedom from intoxication, improved physical function, psychosocial function, and compliance and should indicate whether any further diagnostic evaluations are planned, as well as counseling, psychiatric management, or other ancillary services.

The plan should be reviewed periodically. After treatment begins, the physician should adjust therapy to the individual medical needs of each patient. Treatment goals, other treatment modalities, or a rehabilitation program should be evaluated and discussed with the patient. If possible, every attempt should be made to involve significant others or immediate family members in the treatment process, with the patient's consent.[9]

The treatment plan also should specify contingencies, such as intensification of treatment or referral to a higher level of care for poor adherence to the treatment plan (such as failure to attend appointments, ongoing use of nonprescribed substances, or evidence that prescribed medications are not being taken).

CONFIDENTIALITY PROTECTIONS

Ensuring confidentiality is perhaps the strongest element in the foundation of a therapeutic relationship,[6,10] in that patients must have reasonable assurance that what they say to a treatment professional is protected information. Moreover, medicine historically attaches a high value to patients' privacy because it is critical that patients give their physicians accurate information. By affording privacy protections to medical information, society assures patients that they can discuss sensitive subjects with their physicians without worrying about what use others might make of such information.

Nevertheless, the right to privacy is not without limits, and understanding the purpose and implications of those limits frequently poses problems for physicians and other health care professionals.[6] The nature of managed care requires more extensive justification for treatment, and the number of individuals who demand information about a patient's care is growing. Additionally, the growing use of electronic health records and other computerized data can further jeopardize the concept of protected information.

It is the ethical responsibility of health care professionals to be honest with patients as to what data need to be reported to insurance companies and what information needs to be shared with other agencies or individuals. It is the legal responsibility of the provider to obtain consent for any information shared outside of the physician-patient relationship.[10]

Basis of Confidentiality

Confidentiality is especially important when a patient has an addiction disorder because of the widespread perception that such persons are weak and/or morally impaired.[6] A patient considering treatment might be concerned that, if an insurer or HMO learns that their traumatic injuries were related to alcohol use disorder, it will be difficult or impossible to obtain coverage for hospitalization costs or that their insurance will be canceled. Similarly, a patient may fear that their relationships with a spouse, parents, children, an employer, or friends would suffer if they learned about their problems with alcohol or drugs. If a patient has marital problems, information about an addiction disorder could have an effect on divorce or custody proceedings. A patient whose problem becomes known to his employer could lose an expected promotion or their job. Adverse consequences such as these can deter patients from admitting to problems with alcohol or drugs and from obtaining treatment for those problems.

As with consent, laws governing adolescent confidentiality vary from state to state, but there are federal guidelines and common law concepts that are applicable throughout the United States. HIPAA also provides guidelines for confidential care to minors.[11]

Physicians and other medical care providers also need to manage confidentiality issues in drug testing, billing of services, and medical records and to collaborate with clinical administrative staff to clarify and implement policies to maintain confidentiality.[12]

Federal Laws Governing Confidentiality

In the early 1970s, Congress passed legislation to protect information about patients in addiction disorder treatment and directed the Department of Health and Human Services (DHHS) to issue regulations protecting patients' confidentiality. The law is codified at 42 U.S.C. §290dd-2. The implementing federal regulations, titled "Confidentiality of Alcohol and Drug Abuse Patient Records," are contained in 42 CFR Part 2 (Volume 42 of the Code of Federal Regulations, Part 2). The federal rules permit disclosures in only nine limited circumstances:

1. When a patient signs a consent form that complies with the regulations' requirements.
2. When a disclosure does not identify the patient as an individual with a substance use disorder.
3. When treatment staff consult among themselves.
4. When the disclosure is to a "qualified service organization" that provides services to the patient.
5. When there is a medical emergency.
6. When the law requires reporting of child abuse or neglect.
7. When a patient commits a crime at the treatment program or against its staff members.
8. When the information is for research, audit, or evaluation purposes.
9. When a court issues a special order authorizing disclosure.

Federal confidentiality rules apply to almost all specialized programs that treat SUDs in the United States. They prohibit staff and treatment personnel from disclosing any information (written or oral) about any applicant, patient, or former patient unless (1) the patient has consented in writing (on the form required by the regulations) or (2) another very limited exception specified in the regulations applies. The rules apply regardless of whether the individual seeking the information already has the information, has other ways of obtaining it, has official status, is authorized by state law, or has a subpoena or search warrant. In many instances, federal law and regulations restrict communications more tightly than do either the physician-patient or the attorney-client privilege. Violations of the regulations are punishable by fines of up to $500 for a first offense and up to $5,000 for each subsequent offense (42 CFR §2.4).

Physicians who practice primary care probably are not subject to the provisions of 42 CFR Part 2. However, when a general care practice includes someone whose primary function is to provide treatment for SUDs, and the practice benefits from "federal assistance," it must comply with the federal rules for handling information about patients who have SUDs. Although most primary care physicians are not subject to the federal rules, they are well advised to manage information about patients' SUDs with great care. The best practice for those who are not required to follow the rules is voluntary compliance. In 1996, the Congress passed another law, the Health Insurance Portability and Accountability Act, Public Law 104-191 (HIPAA), which mandated the establishment of standards for the privacy of "individually identifiable health information." To carry out this mandate, the Department of Health and Human Services in 2000 issued a set of regulations governing patients' privacy that applies to a wide range of "health care providers." The HIPAA regulations appear in Volume 45 of the Code of Federal Regulations, Parts 160 and 164. HIPAA regulations are not as restrictive as the requirements of 42 CFR Part 2. Practitioners who are subject to both sets of rules must follow the more restrictive federal standard.

State Laws Governing Confidentiality

State laws also afford some protection to medical information. Most physicians and patients think of these laws as the "physician-patient privilege." Strictly speaking, the physician–patient privilege is a rule of evidence that governs whether a physician can be compelled to testify in court about a patient. However, in many states the laws offer wider protection, and some states have special confidentiality laws that explicitly prohibit practitioners from divulging information about a patient without that patient's consent. States often include such prohibitions in their professional licensing laws, which generally prohibit licensed professionals from divulging information about patients. Many also make unauthorized disclosures grounds for disciplinary action, including license revocation.

Each state has its own set of rules, which means that the scope of protection offered by state law varies widely. Whether a communication (or laboratory test result) is "privileged" or "protected" depends on a number of factors:

- *The type of professional holding the information* and whether they are licensed or certified by the state. Most state laws do cover licensed physicians.
- *The context in which the information was communicated.* Some states limit protection to information a patient communicates to a physician in private, in the course of a medical consultation, but do not protect information disclosed to a physician in the presence of a third party such as a spouse. Other states protect information the patient tells the physician when others are present as well as information the physician gains during private consultations or examination.
- *The circumstances in which "confidential" information will be or was disclosed.* Some states protect medical information only when that information is sought in a court proceeding. If a physician divulges information about a patient in any other setting, the law does not recognize that there has been a violation of the patient's right to privacy. Other states protect medical information in many different contexts.
- *How the right to privacy is enforced.* Legal protection of medical information is useful only when it is backed by enforcement of the law.

Although enforcement actions remain relatively rare, states have the authority to discipline health professionals who violate patients' privacy. This is often done through states' agencies such as licensing boards and offices of civil rights. State also can allow patients to sue physicians for damages over violations of patient privacy.

Exceptions to Confidentiality Requirements

Exceptions to any general rule protecting the confidentiality of medical information generally include:

- *Consent*: All states permit physicians to disclose information if the patient consents, although states have different requirements regarding consent (eg, in some states, it must be written, while in others, it can be oral). Some states require different consent forms for disclosures about different medical disorders. Of course, the patient can revoke their consent at any time.
- *Reporting infectious diseases*: All states require physicians to report certain infectious diseases to public health authorities, although states' definitions of reportable diseases vary.
- *Reporting child abuse and neglect*: All states require physicians to report child abuse and neglect to child protective services, but again, states' definitions of child abuse vary.
- *Duty to warn*: Most states also require physicians to report a patient's credible threat to harm others.

When Confidentiality Conflicts With Other Principles

Laws differ in defining whether a physician's obligation is to the patient or another individual or class of individuals.

Employer Versus Employee

To whom does a physician owe loyalty when treating a patient who has been referred by an employer as a condition of retaining a job? Is it to the employer, who is relying on the physician to help the employee recover and remain (or return) to work? Or is it to the patient (the employee)? The employer likely will require reports from the physician on the patient's progress in treatment. What should the physician do if the employee is not attending or adhering to the treatment plan? This question appears most starkly when the employee is in a safety-sensitive position, and the physician is concerned that their behavior poses an immediate risk to other employees or to the public. To which ethical principle should the physician adhere: the obligation to safeguard the patient's privacy or the obligation to protect those who might be harmed by the patient's actions?

The best way to avoid having to grapple with this problem in an emergency (always a difficult and unpleasant experience) is to create agreed-upon ground rules before treatment begins. If an employer requires reports, the physician must have the patient sign a consent form authorizing communications with the employer and defining the kinds of information that will be reported (this agreement should be made part of the consent form). Of course, the employer also must be willing to accept whatever limitations the agreement places on the kinds of information to be provided.

Reports to employers usually include information about participation and progress in treatment. In most cases, it would be inappropriate for the physician to include detailed clinical information in such reports. However, employers can require more information when safety-sensitive employees are in treatment. For example, the employers may want to know about positive results from a urine drug test, and the physician may want to be able to report continued drug use by an employee in a safety-sensitive position. The physician can discharge their duty to the public at large (and to the employer) without violating the patient's right to privacy if the patient signs a consent form that documents their understanding that certain types of behavior will be reported to the employer.

Society Versus Patient

Most physicians know that society already has determined that their duty to warn supersedes their duty to protect a patients' privacy. The law requires a warning to the potential victim or someone in a position to protect the potential victim. The duty to warn, however, does not completely nullify the patient's right to privacy. The physician can warn others of potential danger without disclosing extraneous information about the patient, including information about their use of drugs and alcohol. Physicians who are subject to the terms of 42 CFR Part 2 are required to issue the warning in a way that minimizes harm to the patient's privacy.

SPECIAL ISSUES IN TREATING HEALTH CARE PROFESSIONALS

Special concerns regarding consent and confidentiality arise when treating and monitoring health care professionals for SUDs. Such professionals are at least as likely to experience SUDs as anyone in the general population. On the other hand, physicians and other health care professionals who access treatment through specialized professional assistance programs and subsequent monitoring have been found to have remarkable recovery rates.[13]

Dealing with an impaired colleague is a difficult, emotionally charged job for physician leaders and hospital administrators, who often have had little training in how to manage such a situation. State professional assistance programs have expertise in managing these problems, including the special issues around confidentiality and consent that arise in this population.[13]

Special Issues With Health Care Professionals

As with other patients, the assurance of confidentiality is important in engaging the patient in treatment and ongoing monitoring. However, the treatment of health care professionals presents additional responsibilities and considerations because breach of confidentiality can have a devastating effect on health care professionals' careers, while failure to disclose certain information raises patient safety concerns.

There also are issues regarding "patients' right to know" that must be evaluated and addressed.

This right to know about the capability of caregivers can conflict with the confidentiality rights of health care professionals who seek or have sought treatment for a substance use or related disorder. Thus, the balance between confidentiality and potential risks to patient safety must be carefully weighed.

As an example of the special issues that arise in treating health care professionals, their patient records are subject to interpretations of 42 CFR Part 2 and HIPAA, and also are affected by requirements of the National Practitioners Data Bank (NPDB), health insurance panels, and professional liability insurance carriers.

Engagement and Enrollment in Treatment

Many referrals to professional assistance programs come from hospitals, residency programs, medical groups, and family members. However, some patients are self-referred. At the time of entry into most professional assistance programs, the health care professional's enrollment and participation are immediately covered by 42 CFR Part 2. However, there are important exceptions. For example, some professional assistance programs operate an "anonymous" treatment track, which is approved by the state medical licensing board. Patients enrolled in such tracks are assigned a code number, are followed by the board only under that number. Patients in the anonymous track are monitored by the program for an established period of time, with quarterly reports of progress and compliance submitted to the board. Patients retain their anonymity unless they fail to comply with the program requirements.

Patients who are referred by hospitals, residency programs, or group practices also are afforded confidentiality under 42

CFR Part 2, with reports going only to persons authorized to receive them.

Treatment Records

Treatment records are privileged under the terms of 42 CFR Part 2. As such, they not released without a signed consent from the patient or a court order. Such records sometimes are requested as part of various litigation, professional liability, hospital privileging, and health insurance applications. In situations such as these (and assuming the patient's permission has been obtained), a case summary letter is preferable to release of actual medical records. Such a summary letter might contain a general acknowledgement of successful treatment for an impairing condition, ongoing stability, and assurance that ongoing monitoring is in place, along with an agreement to notify the requesting agency if the patient's status changes. In other cases, licensees waive their confidentiality rights to licensing boards in order to comply with mandates imposed as a condition of reinstatement.

Quarterly and Monthly Reports

In many situations, employers, medical staffs, and others require quarterly or monthly status reports, which serve to assure that program participants are adhering to their treatment program and doing well. In such cases, it is prudent to adhere to the reporting guidelines outlined above.

Duty to Report

In most states, there is a "duty to report" licensees who become impaired by virtue of alcohol and drug use or other causes. Some states allow such reports to be made to the approved professional assistance program. while other states require that reports be made directly to the licensing board.

Protections for Patient Records

As discussed earlier, the confidentiality rights of patients who are being treated for SUDs are protected by three federal laws[6]:

- *The Americans with Disability Act* (ADA), which prohibits discrimination against individuals who are in recovery from an impairing medical condition. The ADA has been used very effectively to protect the interests of patients in recovery who have employment issues.
- *The Rehabilitation Act of 1973,* which forbids any government agency that receives federal funding from engaging in discrimination of any kind. This law has been very helpful to health care professionals because many of their positions are associated with hospitals, most of which receive federal funding.
- *The terms of 42 CFR Part 2,* which protect the privacy of treatment records and can be accessed only with written permission of the patient to disclose specific information. Significantly, it does not allow re-disclosure of the protected information.

As important as any of these rights is the patient's right to recover. Patients who are engaged in treatment for a SUD are entitled to the same protections and considerations that would be extended to patients being treated for any other medical condition.

REFERENCES

1. Forman RF, Nagy PD. *Substance Abuse: Administrative Issues in Outpatient Treatment.* Treatment Improvement Protocol [TIP] 46. Center for Substance Abuse Treatment, SAMHSA; 2006.
2. Federation of State Medical Boards. *Model Policy for Opioid Addiction Treatment in the Medical Office.* Accessed July 31, 2023. https://meridian.allenpress.com/jmr/article/89/1/35/470720/Model-Policy-Guidelines-for-Opioid-Addiction
3. Winters KC. *Treatment of Adolescent Substance Use.* Treatment Improvement Protocol [TIP] 32. Center for Substance Abuse Treatment, SAMHSA; 1999.
4. Winters KC. *Screening and Assessment for Adolescent Substance Use.* Treatment Improvement Protocol [TIP] 31. Center for Substance Abuse Treatment, SAMHSA; 1999.
5. Schachter D, Kleinman I, Harvey W. Informed consent and adolescents. *Can J Psychiatry.* 2005;50(9):534-540.
6. Substance Abuse and Mental Health Services Administration. *Confidentiality of Patient Records for Alcohol and Other Drug Treatment.* Technical Assistance Publication [TAP] 13. Center for Substance Abuse Treatment, SAMHSA; 1994.
7. Blow FC. *Screening and Assessment for Older Adults.* Treatment Improvement Protocol [TIP] 26. Center for Substance Abuse Treatment, SAMHSA; no date.
8. McNicholas LF. *Clinical Guidelines for the Use of Buprenorphine in the Treatment of Opioid Addiction.* Treatment Improvement Protocol [TIP] 40. Center for Substance Abuse Treatment, SAMHSA; 2004.
9. Legal Action Center. *Confidentiality and Communication: A Guide to the Federal Alcohol & Drug Confidentiality Law and HIPAA, Revised.* LAC; 2006.
10. Batki SL, Selwyn PA. *Substance Abuse Treatment for Persons with HIV/AIDS.* Treatment Improvement Protocol [TIP] 37. Center for Substance Abuse Treatment, SAMHSA; 2000.
11. Berlan ED, Bravender T. Confidentiality, consent, and caring for the adolescent patient. *Curr Opin Pediatr.* 2009;21(4):450-456.
12. Weddle M, Kokotailo P. Adolescent substance abuse: Confidentiality and consent. *Pediatr Clin North Am.* 2002;49(2):301-315.
13. Seppala MD, Berge KH. The addicted physician. A rational response to an irrational disease. *Minn Med.* 2010;93(2):46-49.

CHAPTER

125 Clinical, Ethical, and Legal Considerations in Prescribing Medications With Potential for Nonmedical Use and Addiction

James W. Finch, Theodore V. Parran Jr, and Steven Prakken

CHAPTER OUTLINE

- Introduction and clinical background
- Factors contributing to inappropriate medication prescribing and use
- Universal precautions in prescribing controlled medications
- Ethical considerations when prescribing medications with potential for unhealthy use and addiction
- Regulatory and legal requirements regarding controlled medications
- Conclusions

INTRODUCTION AND CLINICAL BACKGROUND

Many medications in common use have a clearly documented potential for nonmedical use, overuse and addiction. These include medications such as opioid analgesics, stimulants, sedative-hypnotics, and for some states, cannabinoids. Although varying widely in terms of primary effects, all can have neurocognitive actions that produce euphoria or other brain rewarding effects, giving them their potential for nonmedical use, unhealthy use, and addiction.

The Drug Enforcement Administration (DEA) attempts to address this by placing certain drugs and their various formulations (often referred to as "controlled medications") into schedules that rank them in relation to presumed risk, ranging from one (highest) to five (lowest). Schedule I drugs, deemed to have no therapeutic use, are not available by prescription, while Schedule II through V medications are available, and their DEA assigned risk category determined by a number of variables.[1,2] It is important to recognize that these schedules provide only a rough estimate of the medication's potential for unhealthy use and that regardless of schedule, all controlled medications have some level of risk. Differing levels of risk are based primarily on a medication's rewarding neurocognitive effects but also on the predispositions and reactions of different individuals to those effects. As a result, these medications have risk for all individuals but are of particular risk in those with increased susceptibility such as those with a history of a substance use disorder (SUD) or mental health disorders.[3-5] Even for those with no clear vulnerability, they still have the risk of acute impairment and injury as well as the risk of physical dependence with chronic use. This highlights the importance of universal application of individual risk assessment prior to prescribing any of these medications, dictating whether they are safe to use and what level of monitoring is needed for safe use.[6,7]

However, it is important to emphasize that these medications, despite their potential risks, can be valuable therapeutic tools in the treatment of pain, anxiety, insomnia, attention deficit disorder, and other medical and psychiatric conditions. It is this challenging interplay that requires that *every* decision to prescribe such medication should be made judiciously with due consideration of the risks as well as the potential benefits of the medication and its alternatives. This also requires active engagement with the patient to provide an adequate understanding of these risks, allowing for genuine informed consent, and mandates that prescribing must be followed by monitoring appropriate to the identified level of risk.

As stated, individuals who have a history of SUD pose special challenges related to prescribing controlled medications. Such patients are at the highest risk of unhealthy medication use, induced cravings, as well as return to use of prior substances, even with short-term use. On the other hand, individuals with SUDs also are at elevated risk of physical and emotional trauma, chronic pain, debilitating mood disorders, attention deficit disorder, and undertreatment of these conditions also has risks of profound suffering and the triggering of substance use.[8]

Fortunately, for most of the conditions for which these controlled medications are prescribed, there are also clinically effective alternatives to controlled medications (with similar benefit and lower risks for SUD patient populations), although their use varies based on availability and prescriber choice. The choice of treatment requires thoughtful attention by the prescriber. It also requires that the choices stay within the prescriber's "comfort zone": comfort in using these medications as well as working with the pain, mental health or SUDs that frequently coexist.[9]

FACTORS CONTRIBUTING TO INAPPROPRIATE MEDICATION PRESCRIBING AND USE

Factors contributing to inappropriate prescribing of these medications vary widely in relation to patient characteristics and clinical settings. Multiple factors relate to clinician behaviors and concerns,[10-12] pointing to areas needing clarification:

1. What are the current guidelines or recommendations for controlled medications, and how can they be used to provide a reasonable and ethical standard of care?
2. What is the clinical utility and potential risk of the commonly prescribed controlled medications: opioids, sedatives, and stimulants?
3. How do SUDs related to controlled medications develop and present and how can they be distinguished from other high-risk or addictive drug use?
4. What are functional, nonavoidant, therapeutic responses by clinicians to problematic, high-risk medication related behaviors or SUDs when identified in patients?
5. What are current regulatory expectations regarding controlled medications, and what is a realistic perspective on clinician concerns related to potential scrutiny?

This chapter will address the potential benefits and risks of commonly prescribed controlled medications, standards of care in relation to evaluation, prescribing, monitoring, adapting treatment, and responding to problematic behaviors, including intervening when there is evidence of SUDs. In addition, ethical dilemmas in this area are explored, and challenges to identifying SUDs related to controlled medications are described.

Benefits and Potential Risks for Common Controlled Medications

Benzodiazepines

Like alcohol and barbiturates, all benzodiazepines work on GABA neurons in the brain and can trigger an acute surge of dopamine from the midbrain to the forebrain and thus a sense of euphoria. In addition, benzodiazepines and other sedative-hypnotics tend to worsen depressive and some anxiety state symptoms over time. Two primary clinical effects are relaxation or decreased anxiety, and sleepiness. The anxiety relieving effects of benzodiazepines were maintained over time with little development of tolerance and were not associated with dose escalation in one large cohort when followed for 2 years of continuous use.[13] However, the sleep promoting effects are short lived with rapid development of tolerance. As a result, benzodiazepines should only be used intermittently for the management of insomnia. While benzodiazepines may maintain efficacy as a part of the management of some anxiety disorders over time, they are not indicated in the management of PTSD, and long term use for any diagnosis requires careful consideration of risk and adequate monitoring.[14,15]

Most recommendations for the use of benzodiazepines focus on short term use and discourage long term prescribing for anxiety disorders, strongly emphasizing non–sedative-hypnotic and nonpharmacological modalities, and using benzodiazepines only if treatment with nonbenzodiazepines is inadequate.[16] However, contrary to these recommendations, a substantial amount of benzodiazepine prescribing involves long-term often daily dosing, which results in additional risk and can be very challenging to discontinue when that is needed. This risk is especially increased in older adults, in those being prescribed concomitant opioids or those with co-occurring SUDs. Any use of benzodiazepines, particularly ongoing use, should be part of a treatment plan that includes behavioral and pharmacological interventions, monitoring (including state pharmacy data monitoring programs, urine drug screening, etc.) and periodic reassessment. Patients needing escalating doses over time require re-evaluation for a worsening underlying disease, diversion, missed diagnosis, or the emergence of a SUD.

As noted, a high-risk group with respect to prescribing of benzodiazepines is those with current or past SUD, particularly alcohol or other sedatives, and for these patients benzodiazepines are generally contraindicated. However, this history is not necessarily an absolute contraindication, particularly for short term prescribing. The relative risk for a particular individual can vary considerably dependent upon whether the SUD is active or in remission, how severe it was and what drugs were involved, the complexity of co-occurring psychiatric conditions, and is there active engagement in recovery support or psychotherapy.[17,18] In addition, there are reliable reports of use of these medications over time without the development of a sedative-hypnotic use disorder or recurrence of substance use in relation to a prior SUD.[19,20] Regardless, if considered, it should be after other nonbenzodiazepine options are tried and with additional attention to close monitoring and ongoing periodic reassessment.[19,21]

Stimulants

All psychostimulants elevate norepinephrine systemically and also elicit an acute surge of dopamine from the midbrain to the forebrain and thus a sense of euphoria that varies dramatically across classes. Stimulant effects include varying degrees of decreased fatigue, longer sleep latency, insomnia, anxiety, increased ability to focus, increased energy and decreased appetite. The euphoriant effect is similar to other psychostimulants like cocaine or methamphetamine, when used inappropriately but can be mitigated by the use of slower onset, sustained release formulations.[22] Importantly, the attention increasing effects of stimulants appear to be maintained over time with little development of tolerance while tolerance to the euphoria producing effect develops quickly. The use of psychostimulants is optimal when they are part of an overall patient management approach that includes counseling, behavior modification, pharmacological interventions, monitoring and periodic careful reassessment.

A diagnosis of attention deficit hyperactivity disorder is largely clinical, should be well-documented as meeting diagnostic criteria (such as the DSM-5), and should be ideally supported by third party historians (such as parent ratings of symptoms, or those by a spouse or other person who knows the patient well). A key diagnostic item is that symptoms should not be limited to just work or school time and should persist throughout other settings and have an onset prior to the age of 12.[23] Since symptoms associated with ADHD and SUD often overlap, emphasis should be given to drug-free periods of the person's life and confounding factors such as alcohol use, disordered or inadequate sleep, mood disorders, overwork and other stressors which all affect attention and can lead to misdiagnosis. Most recommendations for the use of stimulants in the treatment of attention deficit hyperactivity disorder are for their longitudinal use, especially during school or work, and these medications generally do not result in the development of a related SUD in that setting.[24] However, they are generally not recommended as first line agents in patients with a history of SUD or co-occurring mood or anxiety disorders. In those cases, atomoxetine, a nonstimulant, which is FDA approved for ADHD, can be tried. Serotonin-norepinephrine reuptake inhibitors may be helpful when there is co-occurring depression and anxiety, and bupropion may also enable effective treatment of the attention deficit hyperactive disorder and co-occurring depression, although it may worsen associated anxiety. Again, there is little evidence of the need to increase doses of stimulants over time since evidence of tolerance to their clinical indication is generally lacking. Patients needing escalating doses of stimulants require re-evaluation for worsening situational factors, other underlying diseases, a missed diagnosis, emergence of SUD or diversion. Requests for escalating doses could also indicate the emergence of a stimulant use disorder and thus prompt a switch to noneuphorigenic alternatives.

As stated above, a special high-risk group for prescribing psychostimulants is those with current or past SUD. Psychostimulants, like all controlled drugs, can be highly reinforcing, especially in those predisposed to SUDs, and prescribing them for patients with this history should generally be avoided. Some subgroups with SUDS are at additional risk, such as adolescents, young adults and those with a history of stimulant use disorder, but any SUD history should be considered high risk.[25] By no means does this mean that the ADHD should not be treated along with the SUD, since it has been shown that untreated ADHD can worsen overall outcomes.[26] However, in all cases, the first-line treatments are focused psychotherapies and nonstimulant medications, such as bupropion or atomoxetine. Since these medications may take longer to demonstrate a positive effect, it is critical to reinforce the need for adequate time for effective trials. If ADHD symptoms continue to impair function and are considered to threaten ongoing SUD recovery, a trial of stimulant medication can be carefully considered with a clear understanding by clinician and patient that close monitoring will be required. In that situation, formulations that are considered less reinforcing, such as long-acting methylphenidate or extended release formulations like OROS-MPH or lisdexamfetamine should be used.[22,26] However, although considered less reinforcing, these medications are still psychostimulants, so their use does not mitigate the need for ongoing monitoring for as long as they are prescribed.[24]

Opioids

The use of opioids in the treatment of chronic pain continues to stimulate debate and concern, and this class of medication is given added attention in the sidebar, "Guidance on the Use of Opioids to Treat Chronic Pain," as well as in Section 13, "Pain and Addiction" in this textbook.

Risk of SUDs Related to Controlled Medications

All medications have risks, but with controlled medications, many clinicians have concerns beyond those with noncontrolled medications[27]: Concerns arise about being "scammed" or manipulated, or inadvertently contributing to or not recognizing the development of addiction. Although these are genuine risks, they should be kept in proper perspective and are lessened by a better understanding of SUDs and a thoughtful risk-mitigating approach to prescribing.

Many studies and reviews have demonstrated that serious nonmedical use or addictive use of controlled medications is relatively uncommon in general medical practice,[28,29] even in settings where it might be expected such as emergency departments or pain clinics.[30-32] Patients who develop problems with their use of controlled prescription medications are most often those with current or past histories of SUD or diversion, or those with currently unstable mental health issues. Although problems infrequently develop in the rest of the patient population, all patients should be monitored according to relative risk as described below in the Universal Precaution sections. Fraud and diversion (getting "scammed") certainly do occur but are infrequent, and use of real-time prescription drug monitoring programs (PDMPs) is designed to decrease the likelihood of "doctor shopping" (seeking controlled medications from multiple providers). In addition, electronic prescribing makes forgery more difficult. The routine use of urine toxicology makes it easier to verify whether the patient is actually taking the prescribed medication and to identify patients not being forthcoming about other drug or alcohol use.[33]

Prescription Medication SUDs Compared to SUDs Involving Nonprescribed Substances

When patients develop a SUD involving controlled prescription medications, there are several special considerations and management challenges. First is that the medication was initially introduced by a prescription to treat a medical illness or symptom complex, not to induce euphoria. This fact influences patient behavior and can worsen resistance to a SUD diagnosis. Many clinicians have heard the phrases "it was prescribed," or "I am only taking it for 'XYZ,'" or "it was recommended by my provider so it must be safe."[12]

Second, it can be difficult to establish when the prescribed medication use transitions from treating a condition to contributing to a SUD. Third, it also can be difficult to withdraw the controlled medication prescription since withdrawal from most controlled drugs produces an increase in the very same symptoms for which the medication was initially prescribed. Even if these withdrawal issues are addressed, it should be expected that the original symptom complex will re-emerge with the removal of the controlled medication and must be addressed. Managing the now combined original condition and the superimposed controlled medication SUD can be very challenging.[4]

With the advent of Prescription Monitoring Programs (PMPs), it is often possible to identify other clinicians who are contributing to a patient's controlled drug SUD. This necessitates decisions about when and how to contact the other prescribers and what information can be shared. On rare occasions information emerges from one or a series of PMP checks that bring into question the quality and competence of other prescribers and potential obligations to report such patterns to employers, group practices, licensure boards or even law enforcement.

Finally, once the prescription medication SUD has emerged, there is the challenge of changing the treatment plan away from the problematic controlled medications, possibly to other less problematic controlled medications like methadone or buprenorphine that the patient may not prefer. This can produce a major clinical relationship challenge. The effective alternatives to controlled medications often take time to work. SSRIs and cognitive-behavioral therapy for example have substantial efficacy in the treatment of some anxiety disorders but can take weeks to work well. Reconditioning, stretching and pain psychology have substantial efficacy in many chronic pain syndromes but are similarly slow to take effect. Controlled medications on the other hand tend to have a quick almost immediate effect on symptoms, so they are very reinforcing to patients with SUD by both their euphoria producing and rapid symptom relieving effects. This can prompt even stronger patient resistance, and comments like "I have tried everything else" and "it is the only thing that works." It can be very difficult to maintain boundaries in these situations, even when the risk is clear and serious.[34,35]

In summary, when the SUD involves a prescription medication, rationalizing that "it's safe," "it's prescribed," "it's the only thing that works," can provide powerful rationalization for continued use, even in the face of mounting problems. Regardless, when a pathologic pattern has developed, the DSM criteria for SUDs still apply, whether the drug is a prescribed medication or an illegal drug.

Challenges in Diagnosing Prescription Medication SUDs

Sometimes when problems are clear or high-risk, like illegality or injecting, diagnosing a SUD can be obvious. However, as with all SUDs, the development of a controlled medication associated SUD is often slow and difficult to identify. Family systems and medical practice systems can adapt to the existence of the slowly evolving SUD and associated behaviors over time.[36] SUD screening tools, even though strongly recommended in all controlled medication prescribing guidelines, are often not used in clinical practice.[37] Patient behaviors that can indicate the emergence of a prescription associated SUD are often not reflected in the medical record until the controlled medication has been prescribed for many months to years.[38]

The DSM diagnostic criteria require careful application in identifying SUDs involving prescribed medications. When a controlled medication is prescribed, particularly for a long-term condition such as a chronic pain or an anxiety disorder, applying the DSM criteria can be more difficult and can lead to over or under diagnosing.[39] Most importantly, as stated in the DSM criteria, with prescribed medication, tolerance, and withdrawal these may be assessed as present, but they are not to be counted toward the number of criteria needed to confirm a diagnosis of SUD if the controlled medication is being taken under medical supervision. Taking these medications on a regular basis, particularly daily, may lead to tolerance and/or physical dependence and withdrawal as expected physiological findings. This is not indicative of a SUD in and of itself, but patients, family and some clinicians may misinterpret this as "addiction," prompting unnecessary stigma.

Clinical judgment is needed in applying other DSM criteria as well. Craving or "strong desire or urge to use the substance," making it "difficult to think of anything else" is one criterion. But behaviors such as insistence on a particular medication or anxiety around refills (behaviors sometimes labeled as "drug seeking"), and "stockpiling" the medication, might be interpreted by some as craving and therefore suggestive of a SUD. But for someone requiring these medications to manage pain, control anxiety or maintain day to day function, these behaviors are understandable and even reasonable. Accidents, or decreased function when adapting to a change in dose or new medication might not imply a SUD but rather a possible problem with the change. Even temporary impairment from overuse might imply poor judgment rather than loss of control, unless it becomes a pattern of impulsive overuse despite adjustment in treatment. Problems that respond to therapeutic interventions will lead to decreased clinical concerns, whereas problematic behaviors that progress over time will show themselves to be more consistent with a SUD. It may become clear to the clinician, and at times to the patient, that they not only have a problem with pain, or anxiety, or attention or insomnia but also a serious problem with their medication and realize that problem will only improve when the medication is discontinued. This confusing and conflicting mix of behaviors, needs and goals, can be extremely challenging and can contribute to high risk prescribing practices.[34,35,40,41] It underscores the importance of clearly understood goals, mutually established early in treatment, the importance of ongoing monitoring and the maintenance of clear professional boundaries.

Paramount to the discussion above is the need to document these behaviors or concerns regarding patients, document any aberrant medication-taking behaviors, clearly document your discussions with patients as well as other pertinent and more objective data (results from pill counts, drug testing, state prescribing database checks, third party historians after consent is obtained, etc.) in the medical record at the time that they occur.[36] Also consider getting a second opinion any time your clinical judgment feels insecure. When in doubt, prescribe conservatively and use the universal precautions outlined below.

UNIVERSAL PRECAUTIONS IN PRESCRIBING CONTROLLED MEDICATIONS

Prescribing medications with the potential for unhealthy use and addiction requires thoughtful application of standard elements of good medical care. One model applied specifically to controlled medication prescribing is referred to as Universal Precautions, akin to the infectious disease model that emphasizes using the same approach for all patients, regardless of presumed level of risk.[42] Key elements include:

1. Conduct a patient assessment adequate to formulate a diagnosis and to assess the risk of potentially prescribing a controlled medication. These risks include misuse, diversion, SUD as well as other adverse events (ie, benzodiazepines worsening depression, stimulants worsening anxiety or insomnia, or benzodiazepines or opioids complicating obstructive sleep apnea or COPD). That is, establish an indication for prescribing and rule out contraindications.
2. Propose a treatment plan and discuss it with the patient. For adequate informed consent, discuss risks associated with use and if long term use, discuss risk for a SUD and the likelihood of physiologic dependence and withdrawal upon abrupt abstinence.
3. Before prescribing a controlled medication, especially if it is anticipated to be long term, always use a written informed consent ("treatment agreement") that sets forth the expectations and obligations of both the patient and the prescriber.
4. Initiate an appropriate "trial" of medication therapy to support specific identified goals.
5. Monitor response to therapy, including adverse events or aberrant behavior and continue, revise, or terminate medication therapy as needed.
6. Keep records of the initial evaluation and each follow-up visit, adequate to justify decisions.

By acknowledging that all controlled medication use involves some level of risk above and beyond the prescribing of noncontrolled drugs, universal precautions encourage a consistent and respectful approach to all patients, thus minimizing stigma while reducing overall risk. Universal precautions are incorporated in one form or another in most of the most recent guidelines.[6,7,43-45]

Conduct Initial Evaluation Adequate to Establish Diagnoses and Stratify Risk

The initial assessment is to determine if there is a clear indication for a particular medication, in this case a controlled medication, based on its effectiveness for an identified diagnosis. This is an obvious question that must be answered clearly: A complaint of "pain" is not sufficient to indicate the need for an opioid analgesic, just as "anxiety" or "nerves" does not alone indicate the need for a benzodiazepine, and "feeling scattered" does not indicate the need for a stimulant. These are presenting complaints that should initiate an evaluation adequate to identify the related diagnoses and thereby gauge the potential effectiveness of known treatments. If a controlled medication is being considered, there is also the need for an equally important assessment of potential risk. Along with the necessary mental health and SUD history described below, the current standard for risk evaluation prior to prescribing controlled medications includes routine toxicology testing and a review of the patient's PDMP report.

As noted, current or past SUDs or a history of diversion are among the strongest risk factors to assess when considering controlled medication use. The next most serious risk factors include past or active mental health conditions, a history of trauma or abuse, and a history of substantial nonadherence.[3-5] Risk assessment should also include current nicotine/tobacco use and gambling, given their association with SUDs and mental health disorders. This assessment should be completed before the decision to prescribe[6,7] and is facilitated by screening tools such as the AUDIT, CAGE-AID, PHQ-9, Patient Stress Questionnaire or Life Events Questionnaire (see **Table 125-1**: SAMHSA links: screening tools). Initial assumed level of risk is an estimate, to be modified over time as additional information is obtained through monitoring. If the PDMP review reveals prescribed controlled medications, the requirement for release of information to communicate with other prescribers should be done for coordination of care and to assure safe medication use.[6,7] Unprescribed controlled medications (or prescribed controlled medications that were not verbalized to the clinician as part of the routine assessment above) or illegal drugs identified on toxicology should clearly be discussed and considered very serious risks. Obtaining a release to gather functional information (including the family-CAGE) from one or more family members or significant others can be extremely valuable. This is discussed further in the Ethical Considerations section of this chapter.

Risk stratification is often less clear than deciding if a medication is indicated. It involves integrating information from multiple domains, each of which may present along a continuum from low to high risk. For example, a distant SUD history may be considered a moderate risk if it was followed by long-term recovery, while recognizing that a controlled medication prescriptions in a patient with extended abstinence can certainly trigger a return to substance use in some patients. The relative risk is thought to be lower if the prescription is short term (eg, several days duration, with no refills) and particularly if the controlled medication prescribed was not in the same class as the prior SUD. More recent SUD would be a higher risk, higher still if involving a similar drug class, higher still if the prescribing is long term, and even higher still without current active identified SUD treatment.[4,8,46] Active SUD would generally be a strong often absolute contraindication to long term controlled medication prescribing.[12,38,47] Likewise,

TABLE 125-1 State Guidelines, Regulations and Other Resources for Controlled Medication Prescribing

State by state guidelines and regulations related to controlled medication prescribing	
Pain management policies	www.fsmb.org/siteassets/advocacy/key-issues/pain-management-by-state.pdf
Pain management legislative summary	https://track.govhawk.com/reports3/KgjqQO9mkwxa
State prescription drug monitoring programs (PDMP) policy sites	www.fsmb.org/siteassets/advocacy/key-issues/prescription-drug-monitoring-programs-by-state.pdf
CME requirements related to opioid/controlled medication/pain management	www.fsmb.org/siteassets/advocacy/opioids/pdfs/opioid-and-pain-management-cme-Requirements.pdf
Medical Cannabis (Marijuana) policies	www.fsmb.org/siteassets/advocacy/key-issues/medical-marijuana-requirements-by-state.pdf
Treatment of opioid addiction in medical office	www.fsmb.org/siteassets/advocacy/policies/model-policy-on-data-2000-and-treatment-of-opioid-addiction-in-the-medical-office.pdf
Drug Enforcement Administration (DEA) links	
Registration	www.deadiversion.usdoj.gov/drugreg/
Practitioner's Manual	https://www.deadiversion.usdoj.gov/pubs/manuals/index.html
Centers for Disease Control and Prevention (CDC) links	
2022 practice guidelines for prescribing opioids	https://www.cdc.gov/drugoverdose/index.html
Prescription opioid and benzodiazepine medications: occupational safety and health	www.cdc.gov/niosh/docs/2021-116/default.html
Clinical tools for primary care providers (eg, MMEs, UDS, tapering, alternatives)	www.cdc.gov/opioids/providers/prescribing/clinical-tools.html
U.S. Health and Human Services (HHS) links	
Opioid tapering guidelines	www.hhs.gov/guidance/sites/default/files/hhs-guidance-documents/Opioid-Tapering-DSC-Final2019.pdf
Managing the benefits and risks of medications	www.fda.gov/drugs/information-consumers-and-patients-drugs/think-it-through-managing-benefits-and-risks-medicines
Substance Abuse and Mental Health Services Administration (SAMHSA) links	
SUD treatment for people with co-occurring disorders: Screening tools	https://store.samhsa.gov/sites/default/files/SAMHSA_Digital_Download/PEP20-02-01-004_Final_508.pdf
Training video links (while targeting pain management, these apply equally well to clinical issues related to all controlled medications)	
• Responding to patient questions when implementing current pain management guidelines • Understanding the pain patient • Treating complex/difficult pain patients • Discontinuing opioids: giving news patients do not want to hear	https://opioid.governorsinstitute.org/training-videos/

Note: Most state policies related to controlled medications focus primarily on the use of opioids, even those that are labeled "Controlled Medication" policies. The links above in the state-by-state guidelines provide access to medical board policies and legislative statutes related to pain (acute, chronic, intractable, end of life) and associated policies such as naloxone access, e-prescribing, PDMP use, CME requirements, and office-based treatment of OUD. See Regulatory section for further background related to their application.

a history of mood or other psychiatric disorders as well as histories of trauma or abuse add significantly to risk, but also present along a continuum in terms of severity, time course and response to treatment. All of these summate into the clinician's perception of risk, either informally or through the use of instruments such as the DIRE,[48,49] validated for opioid prescribing but applicable more broadly. Finally, as noted, perception of the relative risk level will likely evolve, based on new information or the patient's behavior, including treatment consistency, results of monitoring, and demonstrated emotional stability and functionality, any of which might lower or raise the perceived risk level over time.[36]

Discuss the Proposed Treatment Plan and Obtain Informed Consent

Adequate informed consent includes not only information related to the known effectiveness of the treatment but also its risks. This is imperative in the patient's decision to use a controlled medication. With opioids and sedatives, this would include acute side effects such as cognitive and psychomotor impairment, additive effect with alcohol or other sedatives and the risk of falls and overdose. Stimulants have an acute risk of increasing anxiety or insomnia, agitation or worsening some psychiatric symptoms. With longer term use of any controlled medication, the risks of tolerance, withdrawal, addiction and overdose should be discussed.

The treatment plan and goals should provide clear-cut, individualized, mutually agreed upon goals to guide the choice of therapies both pharmacologic and nonpharmacologic.[6,7,10] One possible patient misperception that must be addressed is the belief that complete elimination of symptoms is an attainable goal. Rather, the goals of treatment with controlled medications involve, in descending levels of importance, (1) patient safety; (2) maintenance or improvement of function; (3) reasonably attainable improvement in symptoms and quality of life; (4) improvement in associated symptoms such as sleep disturbance, depression, and anxiety; and (5) avoidance of unnecessary or excessive use of medications.[46]

Specific objectives that will be used to evaluate treatment progress should not only include subjective symptom relief but concrete and observable activities and functional improvements, preferably corroborated by significant others observation.[7] In pain management as well as mental health and SUD treatment, multimodal and multidisciplinary approaches are generally given priority. Other ancillary treatments, further diagnostic evaluations or treatment referrals should be discussed and defined as needed.[6]

Every decision to prescribe these medications must be tempered by the prescriber's knowledge and comfort level for the specific diagnosis as well as any identified co-occurring SUD or other mental health issues. When working in areas of less clinical experience there is great benefit to consulting with other clinicians with expertise or complementary experience with SUDs, mental health conditions or pain. Identifying the need for consultation prior to prescribing has the advantage of being discussed with the patient up front and making them part of the initial treatment plan rather than later after problems have developed. It will also reinforce the utility of a multi-modal approach to treatment and de-emphasize reliance on the medication alone.[6,7]

Document Decisions in a Written Informed Consent Form or Treatment Agreement

Treatment agreements are often used to outline and document the joint responsibilities of the patient and the prescriber.[50,51] Typically, they address the following:

- Goals of treatment in terms of symptom management, restoration of function, and safety.
- Patient's responsibility for safe medication use: using as prescribed, no unilateral change in use.
- Storing the medications in a secure location, safely disposing of unused medication.
- Abstaining from illegal drug use, adhering to expectations regarding alcohol, cannabis, or other controlled medications.
- Obtaining this medication only from current prescriber or practice.
- Permission to contact other clinicians for evaluation and monitoring: may vary according to risk level and may include significant others. Individuals and information being gathered are listed.
- Patient's agreement to periodic drug testing. May include random call backs and pill counts if needed for risk level.
- Prescriber's responsibility to be available or have a covering prescriber available to maintain access to refills.

The above is a basic list but items may vary in frequency or intensity depending on risk level or clinical situation. For example, it may include expectations of referral and additional treatment, such as counseling or physical therapy.

Initiate Therapeutic Trial: Goals and Medication Selection and Dosing

Once discussed and agreed upon, controlled medications should be presented to the patient as a "therapeutic trial" for a defined length of time (typically a few weeks to months), with specified evaluation points, to be monitored for both benefit and harm. If benefit is shown in terms of the patient's therapeutic goals, it will be continued. If it is not helpful, it will be modified, tapered or discontinued. If adverse events or demonstrated risks to safety are not resolved, it will be discontinued.[6,7]

Choices related to dose, schedule and formulations are important considerations,[43] with some particular issues in the setting of controlled medications. It was thought that rapid onset and short duration of action made some medications riskier than others and that slower onset, longer-acting preparations are generally of less risk for unhealthy use or addiction/SUD but are not risk-free and increase the likelihood of physical dependence. Recent evidence from the prescription opioid epidemic has brought this into question.[47] Prior experience with a particular medication or class of medications may steer selection away from or toward certain choices. Presence of rewarding effects such as euphoric mood or enhanced energy, beyond the clinical need, should be avoided and should be monitored during the therapeutic trial and is why the minimum effective dose and duration when prescribing is so important. Finally, so-called abuse-deterrent formulations can be an important lower risk option if available. However, lower risk formulations do not necessarily make controlled drugs safe in high risk patient populations.

Consideration should also include the possible functional impact from commonly expected side effects. Side effects such as weight gain or loss, sedation, or stimulation are not always possible to avoid and can at times be judiciously used to optimize function while treating the targeted disease process. Sedation as a side effect could be useful in improving sleep or a stimulation effect could help with depression, but clinicians should be on the watch for interactions with noncontrolled medication, such as added sedation from medications like gabapentin or topiramate. Clinicians generally choose to prescribe controlled medications for their anticipated analgesic, anxiolytic or other psychotropic effects, but how an individual responds to a particular medication cannot be assumed. It can only be assessed from direct, nonjudgmental questioning. For example, a prescribed opioid may provide analgesia as intended but may also have a calming effect, which the patient finds helpful for anxiety or sedation that helps them with insomnia. However, for some patients, opioids may have a paradoxical energizing effect that they may find helps with fatigue or depression.[52] Likewise, patients with ADHD often describe feeling calmer with prescribed stimulants rather than excitable, but on close questioning some may report an energizing effect above what is desired therapeutically. Exploring these individualized responses is not only needed for monitoring therapeutic effectiveness but may also identify behaviors that could become problematic, such as using the medications for conditions other than intended or escalating doses as tolerance to some of these side effects develops.[32]

Finally, the prescriber should convey that any medication, no matter how helpful, is only part of a multimodal treatment plan. Emphasizing this perspective from the beginning of treatment and as part of the trial of medication can help alleviate or counter a patient who focuses on continued dose increases as the solution to continuing distress.[6] Persistently requesting dose increases, while de-emphasizing or ignoring alternative strategies can be a worrying sign and requires careful re-evaluation of diagnosis, co-occurring disorders, and the appropriateness of the controlled medication. Long term controlled medications can inhibit help-seeking behaviors including participation in physical therapy and re-conditioning or mental health counseling.[53]

Special Precautions with Controlled Medications

At the time of prescribing, patients should be educated that it is illegal to sell, give away, or share a controlled medication with others, including family members. A corollary is the necessity to have a safe locked storage for the medication. Leaving medications where they can be stolen or ingested by children is an important source of diversion in the former instance and can contribute to accidental toxicity or overdose in both situations.[54]

One concern for clinicians is the new patient who presents or transfers already on controlled medications through another prescriber, sometimes on high doses. When the patient presents requesting refills and in danger of withdrawal or acute decompensation, the clinician, having confirmed the patient's medication history through the PDMP, having checked for the presence of the medications in the point-of-care drug screen, and having gotten a release and contacted the immediate past prescriber, can consider prescribing enough of a medication/s to meet the patient's needs for a limited time and with no additional prescriptions until an adequate evaluation is done. When the doses or combinations of medications are of significant concern, the clinician must decide what doses are needed to avoid withdrawal or decompensation while staying within the prescriber's scope of practice and expertise. To that end, when a new patient visit is initially scheduled, staff should ask if a controlled medication prescription is involved. If so, the patient should give consent to obtain prior records and the patient's PDMP report. Having all of this available at the time of the first prescriber visit can be exceedingly helpful. Once transferred to the new clinician's practice, that clinician should not feel obligated to continue a controlled medication from the previous prescriber if they feel the risks outweigh the benefits, or if safety is an issue. The patient has now become the new clinician's responsibility, as do the prescribing decisions.

Monitor Response to Medications and Presence of High-Risk Behaviors

Monitoring effectiveness has always been needed to continue medication treatment. Documenting effectiveness can be recorded as a clinical impression but can benefit from the use of measurement tools to reassess the patient's level of symptoms, function, and quality of life (see CDC link in **Table 125-1**: Clinical Tools). The Pain, Enjoyment of Life and General Activity (PEG) scale is a brief, time efficient instrument for monitoring response to pain treatment, including opioid analgesics, that can be self-administered or elicited by interview and has been validated in general medical settings.[55] Similar tools are available in the areas of anxiety, attention deficit hyperactivity disorder, and depression (see **Table 125-1**: SAMHSA link: Screening Tools). Corroborating effectiveness of treatment can also be done by asking one or more significant others about function/quality of life before and after treatment.

Recent guidelines have given increased emphasis on monitoring for high-risk behaviors.[6,7,43-45] As outlined in the Treatment Agreement, monitoring is individualized but should be some combination of noting the date when the prescription was started, the expected period of time on the medication, the use of periodic toxicology (including intermittent metabolite) testing and PDMP reports, the importance of tracking refills, and evaluating adherence with other aspects of care such as scheduled visits, consults, referrals, therapy, and other prescriptions. Frequency of monitoring varies with risk level but also with time in treatment, and stability. If needed, additional elements can be added such as random call-backs, pill counts, serum levels or contact with family members.

It is important that requirements regarding monitoring be explained to each patient at the initiation of treatment, presented in a non-pejorative yet non-negotiable way, as a "routine standard" of providing safe access to these medications (see **Table 125-1**: Training Videos: Responding to Patient Questions). The patient should be encouraged to play an active role in this monitoring by keeping track of symptoms, side effects, and other problems.

Therapeutic drug testing has become an expected part of both initial evaluation and ongoing monitoring, analogous to following glycosylated hemoglobin levels when managing diabetes. However, clinicians need to be aware of the limitations of various point of care screening tests, such as cross reactivities that result in false positive results, lack of sensitivity for some opioids and limited sensitivity to some benzodiazepines, that may cause erroneous interpretations.[56] It is advisable to verify significant or unexpected results through more sensitive and specific confirmatory laboratory studies. Consultation with the testing laboratory's toxicologist should be available when needed. Toxicology results that suggest possible nonmedical use of the medication or other drugs should be discussed with the patient in a nonaccusatory manner. Toxicology tests, like all lab tests, have the potential for error and misinterpretation. They are useful but are also just one piece of information that should be interpreted in the overall context of treatment: is the result an outlier in an otherwise stable and functional patient, or is it part of a worrisome pattern? Discussing with the patient in a mode of clinical curiosity is generally most productive. It is less likely to elicit defensiveness and therefore more likely to gather information that is useful in assisting treatment. Is there confusion regarding instructions, or complicating conditions that need to be addressed, such as untreated insomnia, mood disorder, pain, or unrecognized SUD issues.[31] This approach can strengthen the physician-patient relationship, supporting healthy behaviors as well as encouraging needed behavioral changes that are documented in the medical record.[6,8]

Patients share with prescribers the responsibility for safe access to needed medications, including providing the clinician with complete and accurate information. Some patients, intentionally or unintentionally, are less than forthcoming or give inconsistent or inaccurate reports. Clinical curiosity may reveal misunderstandings, unidentified problems or nonrecreational sharing of medications, a behavior common across age groups, with over 50% of respondents in one study reporting borrowing someone's medication and 22% reporting lending a medication to someone else.[54] But there are also those who are using their prescribed medication recreationally, or diverting for financial gain or for maintaining an undiagnosed SUD, who mislead in order to obtain medications to sustain dangerous or illegal behavior or to avoid withdrawal. Although these are the patients that most clinicians worry about, fortunately they are a small minority of those that the average clinician will encounter.[28,31] These issues are discussed further in the Ethical Considerations section of this chapter.

Whenever the clinician is uncertain about a patient's worrisome behavior or lack of clinical progress, it is advisable to seek help from an expert in the area of clinical concern, such as a pain, mental health or SUD consultant, preferably sooner rather than later. Clinicians place themselves and their patients at risk if they continue to prescribe controlled medications in the presence of concerning behaviors, and consultation can be helpful in protecting both parties from medicolegal consequences.

Based on Response: Continue, Revise, or Terminate Medication

The prescriber and patient should regularly weigh the potential benefits and risks of continued treatment. A satisfactory response would be indicated by reduced severity of symptoms, increased level of function and quality of life in the absence of concerning behaviors.

When monitoring outcome, focusing on role function and quality of life, and whether they are improving or worsening with the use of the medication can be a pivotal aspect of monitoring both effectiveness and harm. Unlike the subjectivity of reported symptom relief, functional status is observable, both by the clinician and others in the patient's life. But one caveat should be kept in mind: function has to be assessed with an eye towards "before and after" the medication, not on an absolute or ideal function. For example, back pain or severe anxiety, not treated or inadequately treated, will likely have impaired someone's function prior to starting the current medication: "Is the person's function better or worse with use of the medication?" This question is important in monitoring the effectiveness of the medication trial and the need for adjustments. It is also at the heart of sorting untoward effects from an evolving SUD.

If a decision is made to continue medication therapy, the treatment plan may need to be adjusted to support further clinical improvement or to support safe and appropriate medication use. In some cases of taking the medication incorrectly or overuse, steps such as simplifying the drug regimen and patient education can improve adherence, as can follow up phone calls, home visits by nursing personnel, or using tools such as weekly medication holders.[7] Some medication holders now have locking bins and reminder alarms to enhance compliance. More frequent visits or smaller numbers of doses per prescription can give additional structure. Having family or responsible others supervise the patient's medication use is an option but should be thought through carefully. Asking other responsible adults to dispense doses or manage supplies for impulsive or distracted patients might be appropriate. However, asking them to do this with patients who are exhibiting out-of-control or active SUD behaviors may be dangerous to the family the patient, and even the prescriber.

Reasons to Taper or Stop Prescribing a Controlled Medication

Reasons for tapering or discontinuing medication therapy include resolution of the condition being treated, emergence of intolerable side effects, inadequate medication effect, failure to improve the patient's quality of life despite adequate dosing, evidence of deteriorating function, or significant aberrant medication-taking behaviors.[8,12] Obviously, the urgency, timing and strategies needed for these different scenarios can differ dramatically, particularly when they involve dangerous or illegal activities which, though infrequent, do occur.

In most circumstances, including ineffective medication response or difficulty dealing with aberrant behaviors such as unhealthy prescription use or illegal drug use, the essential steps are (1) inform and discuss with the patient what your observations and concerns are, emphasize safety and other paramount treatment goals, and ideally seek consensus in planning the next steps for taper or discontinuation (see **Table 125-1**: Training video: Giving News Patients Don't Want to Hear), (2) educate and plan treatment in relation to clinical need, including likelihood of withdrawal, (3) assure the patient that they will continue to receive care from you with this new plan in place, (4) optimize the support system, and then (5) stop or taper the medication. This may include engaging the family or partner, referral to SUD treatment or psychotherapy, or suggesting involvement in peer support.[6,46,57] For stimulants, transferring to another formulation, such as a nonstimulant like bupropion, or from an immediate onset stimulant to a sustained release or slower onset formulation may result in better management without complete discontinuation.[22] However, evidence of drug diversion, prescription forgery, obvious impairment, use of illegal stimulants in addition to the prescribed stimulant and abusive or assaultive behaviors require stronger responses, typically including discontinuing the controlled substance prescribing.[34] For opioid use disorders that emerge in patients with pain and opioid prescriptions, referral to methadone treatment at an opioid treatment program (OTP) or initiation of buprenorphine in an OTP or office based setting can be a safe way to still provide opioids yet limit risk.

Discontinuing Medication Therapy

When a decision is made to discontinue medication therapy, any patient who has become physically dependent should be provided with a structured treatment plan that addresses not only the management of tapering to prevent or minimize substance withdrawal but also provides treatment for the possible rebound of underlying pain or mood disorders. The decision to discontinue the medication has typically been made either because the controlled medication was not helpful or because of serious safety concerns related to its use. But if worsening of the underlying conditions are not attended to, the risk to the patient is only partly alleviated. Untreated pain, anxiety, or attention deficit or hyperactivity have their own risks ranging from deteriorating function at home and at work to death from suicide or overdose.[58] One dramatic example is that the risk of suicide has been shown to be five to seven times greater in patients with pain syndromes while they are being tapered.[59]

The prescriber must first decide if such discontinuation constitutes a clinical emergency requiring referral for inpatient or outpatient withdrawal management, an urgent situation dictating an outpatient structured taper over several weeks, or a nonurgent situation that could be appropriate for a gradual taper over several months. Nonurgent and some urgent tapers can be managed on an outpatient basis by the prescribing clinician or may need referral to a SUD specialist. When tapering, it is important to be realistic regarding the patient's ability to comply and tailoring the plan accordingly. For example, providing limited prescriptions for relatively brief time periods, and if safety allows smaller incremental drops at the initiation of the taper to alleviate anticipatory anxiety. Tapering may also be easier if another agent is used in place of the discontinued medication, such as longer half-life buprenorphine for oxycodone or long-acting diazepam or chlordiazepoxide or clonazepam for short acting alprazolam or lorazepam. Along with withdrawal or rebound, anticipated challenges may arise, like insomnia or anxiety when tapering sedatives or an energy slump when discontinuing stimulants, and should be addressed preferably with means other than delaying the taper. More specific information about substance withdrawal syndromes and their management is in Section 7 of this textbook.

More frequent check-ins and drug screens and greater involvement of family or other caregivers may be required. As noted, emotional and functional status should be monitored as well as physical withdrawal and may require supportive assistance. If, over time, it becomes clear that the patient is not able to comply with the tapering plan, alternatives should be considered, such as referral for inpatient or more intensive outpatient withdrawal management. As mentioned above, for opioid withdrawal in the setting of an opioid use disorder, referral for agonist therapy with methadone or office initiation of buprenorphine can be an effective and less emotionally disruptive alternative.[60] Unfortunately, similar lower-risk medication options are not available for sedative substitution. In all cases, patients should be given the benefit of the clinician's concern and attention, remembering that these patients may have very real medical or psychiatric problems that require attention. With a few exceptions noted below, termination of prescribing the controlled medication should not mark the end of treatment, which should continue with other modalities, as available. However, not having the controlled medication available may challenge the clinician's expertise in pain or mental health disorders and require referral to a specialist for transfer or collaborative care. Health professionals, who from frustration or fear, abruptly terminate the clinician patient relationship when they stop prescribing controlled medications run the risk of breaching not only their own code of medical ethics but also the accepted standard of care and the rules of their State Medical Board. Some clinicians have a very difficult time stopping controlled medication prescribing once they have started even in high risk situations like overdosing.[34] If this exists, then consultation or second opinion should be sought and documented, and clear clinic protocols and referral sources for SUD and psychiatry should be made available for the patient as well.

Behaviors that are dangerous, illegal or abusive require a more urgent and decisive response.[34,46] In the setting of overdose due to suicidal ideation or unstable psychiatric conditions with risk of further deterioration and/or suicide, immediate admission to an inpatient setting should be considered, which at times may require involuntary commitment.

For abusive or assaultive behaviors, such as may occur when early refills or other requests are denied, the individual can be provided with other options for urgent care and promptly discharged from the practice as long as Medical Board rules are followed regarding termination of a therapeutic relationship. Acts or threats of violence may also indicate a need to contact local police to ensure safety. If available, discussing the patient's needs in a disruptive behavior hospital committee or other similar venue may mitigate risk and optimize care. With illegal behaviors, such as clear evidence of diversion, the medication can be discontinued with no need for further prescribing and possibly no further follow up with the above stated Medical Board requirement caveat. One exception is that if it is found that the fraudulent behavior was to support the patient's previously unrecognized SUD. If seeking the medication is found to be related to a SUD with evidence of physical dependence, then it does not suggest discharge but the need for a withdrawal strategy off the controlled substance and transition to a safer medication alternative, with initiation of SUD treatment.

ETHICAL CONSIDERATIONS WHEN PRESCRIBING MEDICATIONS WITH POTENTIAL FOR UNHEALTHY USE AND ADDICTION

Much of medical care involves treatments that are intended to help but through side effects or other unintended consequences have the potential for harm as well. The traditional approach to ethical decision making is to consider available treatment options in terms of potential benefit (beneficence), potential for harm (nonmaleficence or "do no harm") and respect for patient autonomy through the process of adequate informed consent.[61] Although other ethical considerations have been proposed, these three provide a practical framework to consider decisions related to prescribing controlled medications and provide guidance in discussing ethical dilemmas that might arise. That said, it is important to acknowledge that ethical decision making, that is, deciding the "right" thing to do, involves not just knowledge regarding clinical options, but also engages emotions and value laden concepts like professionalism, therapeutic relationship, confidentiality and justice. Since legal and regulatory expectations exist to promote ethical behavior among medical professionals, consideration of these perspectives not only promotes good care but may help to avoid regulatory sanctions as well.

Professionalism, Collaboration, Bias

To provide good care a clinician should be knowledgeable and apply care based on evidence and research, a seemingly values-free process. But that knowledge must be up to date, and that requires a commitment to the value of professionalism that requires ongoing self-assessment and training. The clinician must value veracity, presenting information that is fair and balanced, and not biased by outside interests or personal gain. In promoting and providing access to care that is nondiscriminatory, the clinician demonstrates a commitment to justice and social cohesion. It is also important to recognize that concepts such as "benefit" and "harm" involve the values and perceptions of both the patient and clinician, colored by their individual experiences, attitudes, and needs. Avoiding misjudgments therefore relies on open communication, and a willingness to listen, a style of professionalism that values collaborative decision making rather than paternalistic care, and which actively supports the third ethical imperative, adequate informed consent. True informed consent rests on both patient and clinician having a shared understanding of the potential benefits and harms as they apply to the patient's goals or needs, not to the clinician's preferences.

Even with good intent by the clinician, unconscious, unrecognized attitudes can short-circuit this ethically grounded approach. Prior negative experiences with substance use or mental illness, involving themselves, close relations, or prior clinical encounters may lead to stigmatizing assumptions, such as doubting the patient's sincerity or minimizing their distress. This can lead to self-fulfilling negative expectations. Unfortunately, evidence has shown that many physicians' negative expectations related to SUD treatment outcome are actually worsened during training.[27] Personality traits of clinicians may also complicate effective ethical behavior. Some made uneasy by the risks associated with these medications or with SUDs may tend toward more paternalistic or even autocratic styles to feel more in control, falling back on arbitrary rules or even punitive responses to behaviors. Others may choose to avoid this clinical cohort entirely or, on the contrary, avoid "hassles" by being the "good guy" and avoiding needed forthright discussions while loosely prescribing controlled medications, potentially putting their patient at risk. Finally, lack of knowledge or unrecognized attitudes related to race, gender or ethnicity may interfere with even conscientious care.

Thinking Through Ethical Aspects of Common Clinical Scenarios

The following segments discuss ethical perspectives and dilemmas related to a number of clinical situations that commonly occur when prescribing controlled medications.

Disagreements Over Medication-Related Treatment Choice

Regardless of best intent, clinicians and their patients are not always going to agree on choices related to prescribing, such as when the patient requests a particular medication, and the clinician does not think that the benefits outweigh the risks. Ethicists often give patient autonomy preeminence among the core ethical principles with respect to agreeing to a given treatment plan or initiation of a medications.[58] However, how does that precept apply when the clinician believes that the patient's choice is unlikely to be clinically effective or that it may be high-risk or unsafe? The response that still gives value to patient autonomy, while also respecting the clinician's commitment to effectiveness and safety, would ideally be clinical curiosity along with a willingness to openly listen to each other's responses. Motivational theory frames this as exploring the patient's "ambivalence" rather than reacting to it as "resistance."[62] If the clinician responds in a paternalistic or dogmatic mode, both are likely to become more reactive and entrenched, leading to more pushback from the patient, frustration for the clinician and ultimately worse outcomes.[63] But if ambivalence is seen as an expected and normal response to change and choice, there is an opening for exploration and possible resolution. Some issues may be nonconflictual and relatively easy to explore and resolve: Is there an adequate understanding of benefits and risks by the patient? Has the patient's concern been identified or addressed? Are clinical goals clear? Of course, not all disagreements will be resolved, but this approach is more likely to be effective and less aggravating for both parties. Ultimately, the conclusion should revolve around "safety first" but some situations may allow for a monitored "therapeutic trial," which may proceed well or will provide further direct evidence of the need for a different option.

In disagreements with an escalation in emotionality, the clinician should be sensitive to possible contributing factors: Is there a clash of personality styles, paternalistic or dogmatic by the clinician, avoidant or combative by the patient? Is this exacerbated by unrecognized transference or countertransference (eg, the clinician's style evokes memories of an abusive parent, or the patient evokes memories of a child or spouse who wouldn't accept help). Could some of the conflict be secondary to "cultural" differences or could there be unrecognized bias related to race, class or gender leading to discounting of one or the other's perspective. Does the clinician have a balanced perspective or stigmatize all patients as "drug seeking?"

Treatment Agreements

Required behaviors when using controlled medications are often listed in signed "Treatment Agreements," often including agreement to monitoring (eg, drug screens), waiver of confidentiality (eg, access to records, feedback from family), mandating certain treatments (eg, counseling) and excluding certain others (eg, no use of prescribed anxiolytics). In using these mandated agreements, ethical questions should be considered regarding harm/benefit/autonomy: Are the mandated elements known to improve outcome? Does that apply to this patient (eg, Is counseling needed?) Are the risks for this patient recognized (eg, involving an abusive, controlling spouse)? Is there risk of interrupting treatment? And are the benefits strong enough to justify overriding autonomy?[64] Language using the term "contract" should be avoided in clinical practice, and the use of the term "agreement" or "informed consent form" should be substituted.

None of these considerations exclude the use of such agreements. In fact, to not use one would go against many guidelines. However, clinicians should not use them or their requirements indiscriminately. Which items would likely be beneficial and not harmful to a particular patient? Also, consider how these "agreements" are presented. Are they presented as requirements ("my way or the highway") and is questioning them seen as hiding something or "lack of motivation?" Or, more productively, are they discussed as recommendations based on the individuals' risks and their own chosen identified goals? That is, presented as supportive of the patient's personal treatment goals and therefore supportive extensions of those chosen goals.

Asking a patient to agree to allow the clinician communication with spouses, parents, or others so as to monitor for safe medication use, if presented as "required" or "non-negotiable" could be considered coercive and not respectful of patient autonomy. But if expectations respect the patient's desire for confidentiality, such as only requesting feedback and not divulging clinical information unless agreed upon, and concerns are addressed rather than dismissed, it is thereby presented as in the interest of the patient's safety and to provide ongoing access to potentially helpful medicines that would not be available otherwise. It frames the choice in terms of maximizing benefit while minimizing harm in the interest of the patient's identified goals, rather than simply a required expectation of the prescriber. If the patient refuses to agree to aspects of the Treatment Agreement, then the clinician will not deny care as a whole, instead the clinician will simply not include a specific kind of care (the controlled medication) that is no longer considered safe.

Notifying Others of Aberrant Medication-Taking Behaviors

Are there situations related to controlled medication prescribing that allow breaching confidentiality, which is generally considered a core ethical precept of medical practice? It is an accepted standard within general medical practice that confidentiality can be breached when there is knowledge of an immediate and foreseeable threat to the safety of the individual, or others around them. It is worth noting that substance use or even addictive behavior in and of itself is not generally considered to meet the criteria of immediate risk, even considering the potential for injury, neglect or accidental overdose. For example, knowing that a patient is overusing their sedative medication and that they are responsible for a child at home would justify tapering or even discontinuing the medication, based on a change in relative benefit versus harm considerations but would not be considered adequate justification for notifying another family member or child protective services without signed release of information (and one that specifically includes substance use disorder or psychiatric information to be shared, along with typical medical information). On the other hand, when the patient expresses what is perceived by the clinician as a credible threat to a specific individual, even if while intoxicated or otherwise impaired, there may be a "duty to warn" without the need for consent. Likewise, the clinician's assessment of suicidality or homicidality may indicate the need for involuntary commitment in spite of the patient's withholding of voluntary consent. These are generally the standards that apply in these situations but can vary state to state, and clinicians should seek counsel before acting.

Cognitive Impairment and Disordered Impulse Control in Relation to Informed Consent and Patient Autonomy

As noted, a core aspect of autonomy is the patient's right to make informed, reasonable choices regarding their treatment. How is this applied when the ability to make reasonable choices is compromised by chronic pain, mood disorders, cognitive impairment, attention deficit, poor impulse control, or SUD. If there is acute patient impairment such as when under the influence or when cognition or focus is compromised by severe pain or depression, decisions that are not emergent should be delayed, or more time may be needed to assure attention or understanding. Emergent decisions may require temporary management, or rely on decisions by appropriate surrogates; decisions which should be revisited when the patient has improved cognition. Even without impairment, impulsivity or behaviors interpreted as consistent with SUD, raise concerns about the patient's decision-making processes and should be brought up and discussed openly as a source of risk: "I know you have severe pain (anxiety) but you also haven't been able to safely manage opioids (or benzodiazepines) in the past. Let's look at some safer alternatives to achieve your treatment goals." Regardless, in these cases, concerns regarding potential harm can be ethically considered to supersede the patient's desire for their chosen or preferred treatment option.

Discontinuing Prescribing or "Firing" From Practice

Is it unethical for a clinician to discontinue prescribing a controlled medication against a patient's wishes or even discharge them from care for problematic behaviors? Some, emphasizing patient autonomy, might consider this to be unethical,[65] but the overriding issue here is safety: Do the problematic behaviors put the patient or others at significant foreseeable risk, and has the patient demonstrated an inability to moderate their high-risk behavior? If so, the appropriate clinical and ethical response is to inform the patient that for reasons of safety, you will no longer continue to prescribe that medication. This is not discharging the patient from practice and is not abandonment. Care can continue but without the use of the problematic medication. If tapering or withdrawal management is needed, that can be provided, or a referral can be made.

In situations where the clinician is responding to behavior that was violent or threatening to the clinician or staff, then the safety of others is considered to override the ethical need to continue care, and the patient can be notified that care is discontinued. The patient may be told not to return to the clinical site, and contact will be by phone or other electronic option. The clinician may decide on further contact after a cooling off period depending on perceived level of risk and prior patterns of behavior. Importantly, it is necessary even in these circumstances to adhere to State Medical Board rules regarding the termination of the therapeutic relationship. These rules vary between states but typically include offering a month of emergency advice (but not necessarily controlled medication prescriptions), and offering assistance in identifying another provider and in transfer of medical records. One important caveat: if the clinician believes the behavior was related to a SUD, it is appropriate, indeed encouraged, to change the treatment plan to treatment or referral for the addiction. If that treatment is refused, and the patient is physically dependent, they should be advised of alternatives for withdrawal management.

Illegal Medication-Related Behavior

What is an appropriate way to respond to forgery or fraudulent illegal behavior, such as misrepresentation of information to obtain prescriptions or diversion of prescribed medications? Is it ethically justifiable to discontinue treatment and to report the patient to authorities? This clinical decision regarding continuing treatment would depend on ethical considerations regarding the relative risks to the patient and others and how this behavior applies to the therapeutic relationship. Whether or not to report the illegal behavior to others, including law enforcement is a complex interplay between the ethical expectations for confidentiality and federal and state mandates related to societal safety.

Individuals who have sought medications for diversion and resale have obtained the medications for financial gain in the absence of clinical need, so in terms of the ethical mandate to balance therapeutic benefit while minimizing the risk of harm, there is no ethical mandate because there is no legitimate therapeutic need and no medical risk of stopping, while there is a broader risk to others in the community if it is continued. Having fraudulently obtained the medications through misinformation and deceit, it is reasonable to conclude that no legitimate medical purpose exists that would justify continued prescribing. In these cases, summarily discontinuing the prescriptions is justifiable or even necessary, and decisions regarding continuing to provide medical care without controlled medication prescribing should be guided by the above outlined consideration relating to ending a therapeutic relationship.

Does that also void the individual's right to confidentiality and justify reporting this behavior to others, including law enforcement? Medical ethics would generally give preeminence to the mandate for confidentiality inherent in the clinician-patient relationship although questions about the legitimacy of a therapeutic relationship based on fraud make this less emphatic.[66] Many in law enforcement consider it justified to report felonious behavior to authorities on the basis of societal safety, and this is indeed mandated in the laws of some states. A review of these sometimes conflicting mandates would suggest that unless state law specifically requires reporting to law enforcement, confidentiality should take precedence. Discussing these concerns with other prescribers identified through the prescription monitoring program could be considered a legitimate therapeutic communication under HIPAA.[66] Needless to say, given the complexity of this decision, advice through the medical board counsel should be sought before action is taken.

One other mitigating factor is important in these difficult situations: when an individual has misrepresented information to obtain medication for self-medication, although legally considered fraud, many would conclude that this does not require discharging from care or reporting but does require a clinical response, particularly if the behavior was related to physical dependency and the need to avoid withdrawal. In these cases, clarity with the patient that their behavior was illegal with serious legal consequences could be a "therapeutic opportunity" to prompt the individual to seek or accept treatment.

REGULATORY AND LEGAL REQUIREMENTS REGARDING CONTROLLED MEDICATIONS

The surge in opioid overdose deaths, initially related to opioid analgesics, has resulted in a large number of recommendations for their use, including medical board guidelines and even legislative mandates in many states. Confusion and over-reaction to these recommendations have been noted to influence clinicians' willingness to prescribe these medications, leading to potential undertreatment of debilitating pain conditions.[67]

It should be noted that the actual risk of investigation related to controlled medication prescribing is extremely low[68]; the overwhelming majority of physicians prescribe in a manner that does not warrant or receive scrutiny by federal or state regulatory agencies. Fewer than one in 10,000 physicians are reported to have lost a DEA registration to prescribe controlled substances on the basis of a DEA investigation, so fear of regulatory actions need not deter the use of these medications if prescribers are thoughtful in their diagnostic assessment, treatment, and record-keeping.[69]

The two basic requirements that allow clinicians to legally prescribe, dispense, or administer a controlled medication are that they must be actively licensed by the state in which they practice and must be currently registered and licensed with the U.S. Drug Enforcement Administration (DEA). Details of these requirements are referenced in the Practitioner's Manual of the U.S. Drug Enforcement Administration, which is available on the DEA website.[1,2]

In addition, they must be in compliance with all applicable federal and state laws and regulations. But as various organizations have responded to the increase in opioid overdose deaths related to prescribing practices, the specifics of these expectations have become somewhat confusing and a source of concern for many clinicians. One untoward consequence appears to have been that these guidelines have affected clinicians' willingness to prescribe these medications leading to potential undertreatment of debilitating pain conditions.[67] Guidelines have been published by specialty organizations and state and federal agencies, most notably the CDC. In addition, most state medical boards have revised their own guidelines, often based on guidelines from the Federation of State Medical Boards or referencing those of the CDC. To add to the complexity, many state legislatures have passed laws mandating certain expectations of clinicians and pharmacies. Although there is much overlap among these various documents they do vary as applied by individual states. Most posted guidelines relate to prescribing opioids for acute or chronic pain, while some are identified as "controlled medication" guidelines, and some relate to narrow, specific actions, such as CME requirements, regular use of PDMPs, naloxone access, electronic prescribing or even dosing limits. Finally, the advent of state laws related to cannabis used as treatment (CUAT), including the role of licensed medical clinicians vary dramatically from state to state. So prescribers are strongly recommended to refer to their own state regulations as referenced in **Table 125-1**.

A significant percentage of controlled medication prescribing is done by Physician Assistants (PA) and Nurse Practitioners (NP). As for physician prescribers, these clinicians must be duly licensed to practice within a given state or states and must possess up to date DEA certification. PA prescribing falls within the purview of the state medical boards, NP prescribing usually falls within the purview of the state nursing boards.

Table 125-1 includes links, available through the Federation of State Medical Boards and other organizations, to documents related to each individual state. Keep in mind when reviewing these posted materials, that they fall into different categories, ranging from recommendations or guidelines to legal mandates and therefore, relate differently in terms of regulatory expectations: guidelines are just that, "guidelines." They are recommendations, sometimes evidence based, often combined with expert opinion, intended to update clinicians and promote an appropriate standard of practice. When these guidelines are endorsed by state medical or licensing boards, they carry an additional weight but still do not qualify as "regulations" (rules or laws).

When a state board is responding to a complaint or concern regarding a prescriber's behavior, these guidelines will be referenced by the board or its reviewers in terms of what is expected to meet the "minimum standard" of care in this area of practice, even though optional. The individual prescriber still has clinical discretion as to how these recommendations are applied in the specific clinical situations, particularly in regard to recommendations. However, deviation from regulations or laws would require a strong clinical rationale that justified the deviation. Obviously, in both cases the supportive thought process should be well documented. Clearly, legislative statutes are in the category of "law" and therefore mandated and may even carry sanctions such as fines if the clinician is noncompliant. Medical boards are often given the responsibility of implementing or monitoring compliance of these laws, often incorporating them into their rules and regulations.[6]

In conclusion, most of the laws and regulations related to prescribing controlled medications are state specific. There are federal regulations as well, such as those related to ordering and dispensing methadone in an opioid treatment program or prescribing buprenorphine for opioid use disorder, but they are further reinforced by state statute. It is strongly encouraged that prescribers familiarize themselves with these state expectations, not only in the interest of providing good care but also to allay concerns about regulatory oversight by being knowledgeable about what is expected by the states within which they practice.

The Prescription Order

The federal Controlled Substances Act defines a "lawful prescription" as one that is issued for a legitimate medical purpose by a practitioner acting in the usual course of professional practice.[1] Prescriptions can be delivered by verbal order, written paper prescription or electronic transmission. Regardless of method of delivery, careful execution of the prescription order can minimize errors in dispensing by the pharmacist and misinterpretation by patients. Additional care with written prescriptions can also minimize opportunities for manipulation by the patient who is intent on fraud. Taking time to spell out numbers, such as dose, number dispensed and number of refills, can help avoid manipulation.

Specific DEA regulations related to prescribing controlled medications are detailed in the above referenced Practitioner's Manual. For example, federal law requires that written prescription orders for controlled substances must be signed and dated on the day they are written, not allowing them to be prewritten and does not allow phone orders or refills on Schedule II controlled medications. However, it does allow the prescriber to write up to three Schedule II prescriptions to be filled at later dates, allowing them an option to limit the amounts per prescription when there are concerns about safe management. In this case the DEA requires that each prescription state the date after which it can be filled, but all three prescriptions are dated for the day they were written.

Many states now require controlled substances to be prescribed electronically. Though transition to this mandate has been very difficult for some small or rural practices, it has clearly reduced the risk of manipulated or stolen written prescriptions. However, the requirements for electronic prescribing vary from state to state, and prescribers should be aware of those in their particular state. Finally, patients who are seeking controlled substances for nonmedical use are still on the lookout for blank prescription forms, so they should be stored in a safe place, preferably locked, as opposed to being left in exam rooms The capacity for electronic prescribing has diminished the risks of theft and forgery of controlled substance prescriptions just as the wide availability of PDMPs has lessened the risk of "doctor shopping." However, a prescriber should immediately report the theft or loss of blank prescription forms to the nearest field office of the DEA and to the State Board of Medicine or Pharmacy.

Maintaining Adequate Medical Records

Adequate medical records are crucial to providing good clinical care, particularly longitudinal care, and in the event of a legal or regulatory challenge, detailed medical records are the foundations of the clinician's defense. State laws and medical board rules may differ substantially from one state to another but at a minimum, records should contain the following[7]:

1. *Patient history and physical examination*: Providing adequate detail to indicate that an evaluation similar to that which is outlined under Universal Precautions was given attention, including adequate risk assessment.
2. *Treatment plan*: Should document the working diagnoses as well as the assessment of risk underlying treatment choices. Medication trials and individualized treatment goals should be documented.
3. *Informed consent or treatment agreement*: Necessary discussions should be documented. Signed written treatment agreement, easily accessible in response to adverse behaviors.
4. *Prescription orders*: All prescription orders, written, electronic or telephoned should be documented, including off hours or by other practice prescribers and should be easily accessible for monitoring.
5. *Consultation reports*: The need for and results of all consultations and effects on treatment.
6. *Monitoring*: Activities should be recorded in visit notes or as separate activities (toxicology screenings, PDMPs, pill counts, contact with others).
7. *Treatment progress/outcomes*: Document in terms of identified goals. Give rationale for adjustments, including response to high-risk behaviors.

CONCLUSIONS

Like all clinical tools, use of controlled medications must be considered in terms of potential risks and benefits. These medications can be effective in managing a number of challenging clinical syndromes but also can be the source of serious morbidity and mortality. It is the premise of this chapter that judicious use of these medications, with attention to proper assessment, collaborative informed consent, adequate monitoring, and intervention as needed can improve clinical outcome and minimize the likelihood of nonmedical use and its risks.

On the other hand, avoiding all use of controlled medications, out of lack of knowledge, frustration, or fear, runs the risk of denying a useful treatment modality to those seeking therapeutic relief. The Universal Precautions approach to prescribing these medications is an excellent way to systematically ensure that prescribing is for a legitimate medical purpose, is within the currently expected standard of care, and keeps patient safety paramount, thereby avoiding the twin risks of over or under prescribing.

REFERENCES

1. Drug Enforcement Agency. *Drug Scheduling and Controlled Substances Act (CSA)*. Accessed November 2022. https://www.dea.gov/drug-information/csa.
2. Drug Enforcement Administration, Office of Diversion Control. Physician's Manual: An Informational Outline of the Controlled Substances Act of 1970. DEA, U.S. Department of Justice; 1990.
3. White AG, Birnbaum HG, Schiller M, Tang J, Katz NP. Analytic models to identify patients at risk for prescription opioid abuse. *Am J Manag Care*. 2009;15(12):897-906.
4. Isaacson JH, Hopper JA, Alford DP, Parran T. Prescription drug use and abuse: risk factors, red flags, and prevention strategies. *Postgrad Med.* 2005;118:19-26.
5. Webster LR. Risk factors for opioid-use disorder and overdose. *Anesth Analg.* 2017;125(5):1741-1748.
6. Federation of State Medical Boards. *Guidelines for the Chronic Use of Opioid Analgesics*. The Federation; 2017.
7. Fishman S. *Responsible Opioid Prescribing: A Clinician's Guide*. 2nd ed. FSMB Foundation. Waterford Life Sciences; 2014.
8. Finch J. Prescription Drug Abuse. *Prim Care.* 1993;20(1):231-239.
9. Agency for Healthcare Research and Quality. *Nonopioid Pharmacologic Treatments for Chronic Pain*. AHRQ; 2020. Accessed July 31, 2023. https://effectivehealthcare.ahrq.gov/products/nonopioid-chronic-pain/research
10. Wilford BW, Finch J, Czechowicz J, Warren D. An overview of prescription drug abuse: misuse and defining the problem and seeking solutions. *J Law Med Ethics.* 1994;22(3):197-203.
11. Yang YT, Larochelle MR, Haffajee RL. Managing increasing liability risks related to opioid prescribing. *Am J Med.* 2017;130(3):249-250.
12. Parran T. Prescription drug abuse: a question of balance. *Med Clin North Am.* 1997;81(4):967-978.
13. Soumerai SB, Simoni-Wastila L, Singer C, et al. Lack of relationship between long-term use of benzodiazepines and escalation to high doses. *Psychiatric Serv.* 2003;54(7):1006-1011.
14. Ballenger JC, Davidson JRT, Lecrubier Y, et al. Consensus statement update on posttraumatic stress disorder from the international consensus group on depression and anxiety. *J Clin Psychiatry.* 2004;65(Suppl 1):55-62.
15. Davidson JR. Pharmacologic treatment of acute and chronic stress following trauma: 2006. *J Clin Psychiatry.* 2006;67(Suppl 2):34-39.
16. Davidson JR. First-line pharmacotherapy approaches for generalized anxiety disorder. *J Clin Psychiatry*. 2009;70(Suppl 2):25-31.
17. Marel C, Sunderland M, Mills K, Slade T, Teesson M, Chapman C. Conditional probabilities of SUD and associated risk factors: progression from first use to use disorder on alcohol, cannabis, stimulants, sedatives and opioids. *Drug Alcohol Depend.* 2019;194:136-142.
18. McHugh R. Treatment of co-occurring anxiety disorders and substance use disorders. *Harv Rev Psychiatry.* 2015;23(2):99-111.
19. Mueller T, Pagano M, Rodriquez B, Bruce S, Stout R, Keller M. Long term use of benzodiazepines in participants with comorbid anxiety and alcohol use disorders. *Alcohol Clin Exp Res.* 2005;29(8):1411-1418.
20. Brunette M, Noordsy D, Xie H, Drake R. Benzodiazepine use and abuse among patients with severe mental illness and co-occurring substance use disorders. *Psychiatr Serv.* 2003;54(10):1395-1401.
21. Clark R. Benzodiazepine prescription practices and substance abuse in persons with severe mental illness. *J Clin Psychiary.* 2004;65(2):151-155.
22. Volkow ND. Stimulant medications: how to minimize their reinforcing effects. *Am J Psychiatry.* 2006;163(3):359-361.
23. National Library of Medicine. *DSM-5 Changes: Implications for Child Serious Emotional Disturbance*. Accessed July 31, 2023. https://www.ncbi.nlm.nih.gov/books/NBK519712/table/ch3.t3/
24. Biederman J, Monuteaux M, Spencer T, Wilens T, MacPherson H, Faraone S. Stimulant therapy and risk for subsequent substance use disorders in male adults with ADHD: a naturalistic controlled 10-year follow-up study. *Am J Psychiatry.* 2008;165:597-603.
25. Parran TV, Jasinski DR. IV ritalin abuse: prototype for prescription drug abuse. *Arch Intern Med.* 1991;151:781-783.
26. Crunelle C, van den Brink W, Moggi F, et al. International consensus statement on screening and diagnosis and treatment of substance use disorders with co-morbid ADHD. *Eur Addict Res.* 2018;24:43-51.
27. Avery J, Han BH, Zerbo E, et al. Changes in psychiatry residents' attitudes towards individuals with substance use disorders over the course of residency training. *Am J Addict.* 2017;26(1):75-79.
28. Huang B, Dawson D, Stinson F, et al. Prevalence, correlates, and comorbidity of nonmedical prescription drug use and drug use disorders in the United States: results of the National Epidemiologic Survey on Alcohol and Related Conditions. *J Clin Psychiatry.* 2006;67(7):1062-1073.
29. Fleming MF, Balousek SL, Klessig CL, Mundt MP, Brown DD. Substance use disorders in a primary care sample receiving daily opioid therapy. *J Pain.* 2007;8:573-582.
30. Nadeau S, Wu JK, Lawhern R. Opioids and chronic pain: an analytic review of the clinical evidence. *Front Pain Res.* 2021;2:721357.
31. Substance Abuse and Mental Health Services Administration. *Key Substance Use and Mental Health Indicators in the United States: Results from the 2020 National Survey on Drug Use and Health.* SAMHSA; 2021. Accessed July 31, 2023. www.samhsa.gov/data/sites/default/files/reports/rpt35325/NSDUHFFRPDFWHTMLFiles2020/2020NSDUHFFR1PDFW102121.pdf
32. Vowles K. Rates of opioid misuse, abuse, and addiction in chronic pain: a systematic review and data synthesis. *J Pain.* 2015;156(4):569-576.
33. Moride Y, Lemieux-Uresandi D, Castillon G, et al. A systematic review of interventions and programs targeting appropriate prescribing of opioids. *Pain Physician.* 2019;22(3):229-240.
34. Larochelle MR, Liebschutz JM, Zhang F, Ross-Degnan D, Wharam JF. Opioid prescribing after nonfatal overdose and association with repeated overdose: a cohort study. *Ann Intern Med.* 2016;164(1):1-9.
35. Lembke A. Why doctors prescribe opioids to known opioid abusers. *N Engl J Med.* 2012;367:1580-1581.
36. Carrington Reid M, Engles-Horton LL, Weber MB, et al. Use of opioid medications for chronic noncancer pain syndromes in primary care. *J Gen Intern Med.* 2002;17(3):173-179. doi:10.1046/j.1525-1497.2002.10435.x
37. Starrels JL, Becker WC, Weiner MG, Li X, Heo M, Turner BJ. Low use of opioid risk reduction strategies in primary care even for high risk patients with chronic pain. *J Gen Intern Med.* 2011;26(9):958-964. doi:10.1007/s11606-011-1648-2
38. Dowell D, Kunins HV, Farley TA. Opioid analgesics—risky drugs, not risky patients. *JAMA.* 2013;309(21):2219-2220. doi:10.1001/jama.2013.5794
39. Meltzer E, Rybin D, Meshesha LZ, et al. Aberrant drug-related behaviors: unsystematic documentation does not identify prescription drug use disorder. *Pain Med.* 2012;13(11):1436-1443.
40. Manhapra A, Sullivan MD, Ballantyne JC, MacLean RR, Becker WC. Complex persistent opioid dependence with long-term opioids: a gray area that needs definition, better understanding, treatment guidance, and policy changes. *J Gen Intern Med.* 202035(Suppl 3):964-971.
41. Ballantyne JC, Sullivan MD, Kolodny A. Opioid dependence vs addiction: a distinction without a difference? *Arch Intern Med.* 2012;172(17):1342-1343.
42. Gourlay DL, Heit HA. Universal precautions in pain medicine: a rational approach to the treatment of chronic pain. *Pain Med.* 2005;6:107-112.
43. Dowell D, Ragan KR, Jones CM, Baldwin GT, Chou R. CDC clinical practice guideline for prescribing opioids for pain—United States, 2022. *Recs and Reports.* 2022;71(3):1-95.
44. Chou R, Fanciullo GJ, Fine PG, et al. Clinical guidelines for the use of chronic opioid therapy in chronic noncancer pain. *J Pain.* 2009;10(2):113-130.
45. Washington State Department of Health, Agency Medical Directors' Group (AMDG). *Interagency Guideline on Prescribing Opioids for Pain*. 3rd ed. AMDG; 2015. Accessed July 31, 2023. www.doh.wa.gov/Portals/1/Documents/2300/2017/AMDG-Guidelines.pdf

46. Parran T. Pain management considerations. In: Norton M, ed. *The Pharmacist's Guide to Opioid Use Disorders*. American Society of Health-System Pharmacists; 2018.
47. Volkow ND, McLellan AT. Opioid abuse in chronic pain—misconceptions and mitigation strategies. *N Engl J Med*. 2016;374:1253-1263. doi:10.1056/NEJMra1507771
48. Belgrade MJ, Schamber CD, Lindgren BR. The DIRE score: predicting outcomes of opioid prescribing for chronic pain. *J Pain*. 2006;7:671-681.
49. Ducharme J, Moore S. Opioid use disorder assessment tools and drug screening. *Mo Med*. 2019;116(4):318-324.
50. Starrels JL, Becker WC, Alford DP, Kapoor A, Williams AR, Turner BT. Systematic review: treatment agreements and urine drug testing to reduce opioid misuse in patients with chronic pain. *Ann Intern Med*. 2010;152(11):712-720.
51. Arnold RM, Han PK, Seltzer D. Opioid contracts in chronic nonmalignant pain management. Objectives and uncertainties. *Am J Med*. 2006;1119:292.
52. Barbour A, Asbury ML, Riordan PA, Webb JA, Prakken SD. Opioid-induced somatic activation: prevalence in a population of patients with chronic pain. *Cureus*. 2020;12(5):e7911. doi:10.7759/cureus.7911
53. Large RG, Schug SA. Opioids for chronic pain of non-malignant origin—caring or crippling? *Health Care Anal*. 1995;3(1):5-11.
54. Beyene K, Sherican J, Aspden T. Prescription sharing: a systematic review of the literature. *Am J Pub Health*. 201410(4):e15-e26.
55. Krebs EE, Lorenz KA, Bair MJ, et al. Development and initial validation of the PEG, a three item scale assessing pain intensity and interference. *J Gen Intern Med*. 2009;24(6):733-738.
56. Gourlay D, Heit HA, Caplan Y. *Urine Drug Testing in Clinical Practice*. PharmaCom Group, Inc. For the American Academy of Family Physicians; 2010.
57. Frank J. Patient outcomes in dose reduction or discontinuation of long-term opioid therapy: a systematic review. *Ann Intern Med*. 2017;167(3):181-191.
58. Gillon R. Ethics needs principles—four can encompass the rest—and respect for autonomy should be first among equals. *J Med Ethics*. 2003;29(5):307.
59. Oliva E, Bowe T, Manhapra A, et al. Associations between stopping prescriptions for opioids, length of opioid treatment, and overdose or suicide deaths in U.S. veterans: observational evaluation. *BMJ*. 2020;368:m283.
60. Powell VD, Rosenberg JM, Yaganti A, et al. Evaluation of buprenorphine rotation in patients receiving long-term opioids for chronic pain: a systematic review. *JAMA Netw Open*. 2021;4(9):e2124152.
61. Beauchamp TL, Childress JF. *Principles of Biomedical Ethics*. 5th ed. Oxford University Press; 2001.
62. Miller WR, Rollnick S. *Motivational Interviewing: Helping People Change*. 3rd ed. Guilford Press; 2013.
63. Rubak S, Sandbaek A, Lauritsen T, Christensen B. Motivational interviewing: a systematic review and meta-analysis. *Br J Gen Pract*. 2005;55(513):305-312.
64. Arnold RM, PKH H, Seltzer D. Opioid contracts in chronic nonmalignant pain management: objectives and uncertainties. *Am J Med*. 2006;119(4):292-296.
65. Kertesz SG, Manhapra A, Gordon AJ. Nonconsensual dose reduction mandates are not justified clinically or ethically: an analysis. *J Law Med Ethics*. 2020;48(2):259-267.
66. Singh N, Fishman S, Rich B, Orlowski A. Prescription opioid forgery: reporting to law enforcement and protection of medical information. *Pain Med*. 2013;14(6):792-798.
67. Dowell D, Haegerich T, Chou R. No shortcuts to safer opioid prescribing. *N Engl J Med*. 2019;380:2285-2287.
68. Goldenbaum D, Christopher M, Gallagher RM, et al. Physicians charged with opioid analgesic-prescribing offenses. *Pain Med*. 2008;9(6):737-747.
69. Crane M. Treating pain without fear. *Med Econ*. 2008;85(13):62-67.

Sidebar 1

Drug Control Policy: History and Future Directions

John J. Coleman and Robert L. DuPont

Modern global drug control traces its origin to 19th century Asia and efforts to halt the British opium trade between India and China. By mid-century, two opium wars had been waged between China and Great Britain over the drug trade. China lost both of these wars, and was forced to permit the continued importation of British opium. The societal harm from opium smoking in China was staggering. By century's end, *The Times of London* reported that an estimated 70% of adult males in China regularly used the drug for its euphoric effect.[1]

The United States had relatively little interest in the Asian opium trade until 1898, following the Spanish-American War, when the United States suddenly became a colonial power in Asia through the acquisition of the Philippines and Guam. While under Spanish rule, the Philippines maintained a government-run monopoly that distributed opium to the nation's large Chinese immigrant population.[2] U.S. Governor-General of the Philippines William Howard Taft was in favor of keeping the opium monopoly in place and using the profits for an educational program but President Theodore Roosevelt disagreed and in 1905 Congress followed suit and mandated an absolute prohibition on the use of opium for any purpose other than medicinal.[3]

In 1909, the United States proposed an international conference to regulate the opium trade and, as the drug's greatest victim, China agreed to host it. Called the Shanghai Opium Commission, thirteen members, mostly representing European nations with colonial interests in Asia, met to discuss regulating the opium trade. There were disputes over basic concepts such as the definitions of medicinal and nonmedicinal uses of opium. The differences not only affected drug control policies in overseas colonies but also had repercussions at home. Gootenberg notes that in the 1920s, most European states had welfare policies that "legitimized the medicalized, national, and social approaches to problems of drug addiction."[4]

The Shanghai meeting accomplished little other than a nonbinding agreement that measures should be taken by nations within their own territories and possessions to control the manufacture, sale and distribution of opium.[5] In retrospect, despite the diversity of views expressed by the attendees, the Shanghai Opium Commission probably was the birthplace of the supply reduction paradigm, the strategy that would govern global drug control policy for another century.

A second, more substantive meeting was proposed by the United States and hosted by the Netherlands in 1912. This meeting was designated a *convention* to signal participants that binding proposals to control the commerce in opium would be on the agenda. As in the case of the Shanghai meeting, the United States was elected by the member states to chair the convention that met at The Hague several times over the next 2 years.[6]

The Hague Opium Convention attendees considered several novel proposals, including licensing producers and manufacturers of medicinal products made from opium, publishing uniform production and sales records, and moving member states to enact domestic regulatory laws to control opium and medicinal products made from it. Members agreed, at least in principle, to regulate the production of opium, to ensure its availability for medical and scientific purposes, and to prohibit other uses of it.[7]

Within days of the drafting of a treaty and the final meeting of delegates in 1914, Archduke Franz Ferdinand of Austria was assassinated, an event that precipitated the start of World War I and put a halt to further meetings of the Opium Convention. By war's end, the Convention's treaty had been ratified by only seven nations, including the United States.[7]

The United States successfully negotiated to include the Convention's opium treaty in the Treaty of Versailles that, among other things, called for establishing a *League of Nations*. British and American leaders advanced the belief that the League should promulgate a *world-wide rule of international law* to prevent future wars.[8] With this in mind, the allied powers agreed to include international drug control as an appropriate peacetime endeavor of the League.[7]

Although the U.S. senate failed to ratify the Treaty of Versailles, it did ratify the Opium Convention's treaty and Congress complied with its provisions by enacting the Harrison Narcotics Tax Act of 1914.[3] The Act provided for the "registration of, with collectors of internal revenue, and to impose a special tax on all persons who produce, import, manufacture, compound, deal in, dispense, sell, distribute, or give away opium or coca leaves, their salts, derivatives, or preparations… ."[9]

While Germany, Hungary, and Turkey opposed the Convention's opium treaty before the war, as defeated powers, they were forced as a condition of surrender to accept its provisions.[6,8,9] At the very first meeting of the League, a Special Advisory Committee on Traffic in Opium and Other Dangerous Drugs also known as the Opium Advisory Committee ("OAC") was established to operate the League's international drug control program.[10]

Over the next two decades, until the beginning of World War II, the OAC met frequently to consider global drug control policies and worked closely with the League's Health Committee (a predecessor to the World Health Organization).[7] Although the United States never joined the League, deference sometimes was afforded by League members to positions expressed by U.S. observers, often in hopes of winning public support at home and in Congress for U.S. membership.[7]

From the start, the League's approach to the global drug problem continued to focus on what today would be considered a *supply control* strategy. This approach favored economic calculations, regulatory statutes, and other rule enforcement measures intended to control the global commerce in opium and other dangerous drugs.[4]

In what may have been the first formal contact with the League on the drug issue, the Warren G. Harding administration sent former Surgeon-General Rupert Blue to the January 1923 meeting of the OAC.[7] Blue emphasized strong control measures, elimination of excess production of opium and a refining of the definitions of medical and nonmedical drug use. Blue's views differed with those of the OAC's colonial powers that considered the *quasi-medical* use of opium to be purely a domestic concern.[7] The initial description of "medicalized addiction" was the routine prescribing and dispensing of heroin to keep an addicted person hooked and prevent withdrawal. There was no "pharmacotherapy" intention whatsoever either on the part of the prescriber/dispenser or the recipient of the drug. In 1919, the Supreme Court in *Webb vs USA* decided that medicalized addiction was unlawful and to be controlled under the Harrison Narcotic Tax Act. The Court's reasoning was that giving an addicted person heroin or any drug simply to maintain the addiction was not considered "legitimate medical treatment."

U.S. policy continued to focus on supply reduction by regulating the production and distribution of drugs. Perhaps reflecting upon domestic alcohol controls ("Prohibition") at home, U.S. observers at OAC meetings typically pressed for similarly tight controls on the international drug trade.[11]

The Geneva International Opium Convention, convened from 1924 to 1925, was the first attempt by member states of the League to institute production controls on drugs with addiction potential. A setback occurred when the U.S. observer delegation "walked out" over the failure of the League to set manufacturing limits that, among other things, would end colonial era opium monopolies. Despite deep divisions among the members, the convention managed to accomplish several worthwhile goals, for example, the creation of the Permanent Central Opium Board, a system for keeping import and export records to prevent diversion, adoption of provisions to enhance domestic controls, adding restrictions on the trade of coca leaves and cannabis (referred to then as "marihuana"), placing controls on processed drugs, and adopting procedures for adding new drugs to the list of controlled substances.[7]

The treaty that resulted from the Geneva meetings may have looked good on paper, but it was weak in its execution. Signatories were not bound by its provisions and could opt out of them simply by recording their objections. The American delegation's walkout polarized key issues and intensified differences among the member states. Despite these difficulties, there was unanimity among the members for the reporting of *legitimate* drug imports and exports, for addressing the issues of coca and cannabis, and for establishing the Permanent Central Opium Board, a nongovernmental expert committee that would outlive the League itself and persist until the 1960s.[4,7]

Despite disagreements among attendees to the 1924 to 1925 sessions of the OAC, by the next round of talks in 1931, supply control advocates were firmly back in charge of the League's focus.[7] Use of drugs for nonmedical purposes, to the extent that it was discussed at all, was considered a minor aspect of supply control. Attendees sought to limit drug production to legitimate needs, to ensure affordable and adequate supplies of medicine, and to eliminate as much as possible illicit diversion and trafficking of drugs.[7]

At the 1931 meeting, the League proposed the Limiting the Manufacture and Regulating the Distribution of Narcotic Drugs Treaty that defined clear boundaries between the illicit and licit drug trade.[7] The treaty provided for the establishment of paper trails for transactions and required signatories to disclose production levels of manufactured drugs, their import and export volumes, and each member's estimated annual requirements of regulated drugs for medical and scientific use. Controlled substances were divided into two groups ("tiers") based on their relative addictive propensity. The United States ratified this treaty in April 1932, and it became law in July 1933.[12]

Among the reservations recorded by the U.S. delegation that signed the 1931 treaty was the right to impose "measures stricter than the provisions of the Convention."[12] This, according to a State Department historian, likely reflected America's frustration that despite the work of the League to enforce the provisions of the 1912 treaty, virtually no measurable progress had been made since then in reducing the global production of opium and cocaine.[7]

Historian Quincy Wright, writing about the 1931 Convention, noted that efforts to reduce opium and coca production had been stymied by the hesitancy of members to sacrifice their sovereignty for the general good. He questioned whether Americans after the "rise and fall" of alcohol prohibition might be skeptical about being able to control the use of drugs. Even so, Wright reasoned that public opinion in the United States was far more united on the policy of confining narcotic drugs to medical and scientific uses than it ever was on confining alcohol to such uses.[10]

Despite progress on the diplomatic front, the United States continued to experience problems at home with the nonmedical use of drugs. The Harrison Act had ended so-called "medicalized" addiction by prohibiting the prescribing and dispensing of narcotics for maintenance purposes.[10,13] According to some contemporary critics of American drug policy, the strict enforcement of this policy may have increased the underground commerce in banned drugs by creating a market for them.[14,15]

Historian and drug policy expert David Musto, however, offers a different opinion. Musto compared the street cost of 25 cents for 100 mg of cocaine in New York City before the Harrison Act to the cost of $10 dollars for the same amount of the drug purchased in the mid-1980s.[16] Comparing the average hourly wage and the drug's street cost for the two periods, Musto, concluded that the profit margins from cocaine sales before and after the Harrison Act were about the same.[16]

In 1930, with the Bureau of Prohibition about to be phased out with the repeal of prohibition approaching, President Herbert Hoover established the Federal Bureau of Narcotics ("FBN") to enforce the Harrison Act and to crack down on the burgeoning illicit drug trade.[17] Harry J. Anslinger, a former assistant commissioner in the Bureau of Prohibition, was appointed to head FBN and would do so for the next 32 years.[17] As FBN Commissioner, Anslinger was part of the official U.S. observer delegation to the League's Opium Commission.[7] Anslinger was known at home and abroad for his advocacy of strict drug control.[4,17]

Throughout the 1930s, Anslinger lobbied hard for a federal statute to ban cannabis. His efforts helped to enact the Marihuana Tax Act of 1937 that prohibited commerce in cannabis except for medicinal purposes when prescribed by a physician registered by the government pursuant to the Act.[3]

World War II brought about many changes in the world, including the dissolution of the League whose primary mission, ironically, was to prevent war. At the end of the war, representatives of 50 nations met in San Francisco to draw up what would become the charter for the successor to the League of Nations.[18] Called the *United Nations* ("UN"), this world body would be headquartered in New York City and given responsibility for many of the functions previously overseen by the League, including those dealing with international drug control.[18,19]

In 1961, after more than a decade of work, the UN proposed a Single Convention on Narcotics Drugs ("Single Convention"), a comprehensive drug treaty that prohibited production and supply of controlled substances except for medical and scientific purposes. The Single Convention increased from two to four the number of drug tiers or "schedules" and updated the list of drugs regulated under the 1931 treaty. The Single Convention came into force in 1964 after being ratified by 40 nations, including the United States.[20]

As in the case of previous drug treaties, the Single Convention called for participating states to enact domestic legislation, as needed, to comply with the treaty's provisions. The U.S. completed this task in 1970 with the enactment of the Controlled Substances Act ("CSA").[21] The CSA consolidated existing drug laws and included additional provisions to comply with the treaty. The CSA adopted the Convention's scheduling matrix for drugs and added an additional schedule ("Schedule I") to designate drugs and other substances *not* approved for medical use in the United States.[21,22]

A notable feature of the CSA was its treatment of medicinal controlled substances. Since passage of the Pure Food and Drug Act of 1906, responsibility for regulating medicinal substances rested with medical officers employed initially by the Department of Agriculture, and since 1930, the Food and Drug Administration ("FDA").[23] To continue this important work under the CSA, Congress divided responsibility for approving and scheduling medicinal controlled substances between the Secretary of the Department of Health, Education, and Welfare ("HEW")[24] and the Attorney General.[25]

The Department of Justice drafted a uniform statute fashioned after the federal CSA for use as model legislation for states to adopt. Some 46 states initially adopted what was called the Uniform Controlled Substances Act ("UCSA") that mirrored most provisions of the federal act but left penalty provisions up to the individual states.[26]

The CSA prohibited states from establishing laws in positive conflict with it.[27] This is particularly relevant today, given the widespread legalization by states of cannabis used as treatment and/or recreational use, a practice that technically violates the CSA cannabis provisions. Since 2013, however, the Department of Justice has *deferred* "its right to challenge [state cannabis] legalization laws… ."[28] As of January 2022, according to an industry source, cannabis used as treatment-only is *legal* in 35 states and is *legal* for both this and recreational use in 18 states and the District of Columbia.[29]

Enforcement responsibility for the CSA was given to the Attorney General who delegated it initially to the Director of the Bureau of Narcotics and Dangerous Drugs (1970-1973), and later (1973-present) to the Administrator of the Drug Enforcement Administration ("DEA").[30] To carry out the CSA provisions as they pertain to medicinal controlled substances, about 500 specially trained Diversion Investigators were hired by DEA to regulate the import/export, manufacture, prescribing, and dispensing of medicinal controlled substances. Besides performing field inspections and audits, DEA's Diversion Control Division manages the registration of approximately 1.8 million registrants consisting mainly of pharmaceutical companies, drug distributors, hospitals, pharmacies, and individual practitioners registered and authorized by the agency to handle medicinal controlled substances.[31-33]

Until the late 1990s, DEA's Diversion Control Division worked mostly behind the scenes conducting cyclic inspections and an occasional criminal case with state and local regulatory officials or DEA Special Agents.[34] With the introduction of OxyContin® (Purdue Pharma LP) in 1996 and the subsequent widespread diversion and nonmedical use of this long-acting form of oxycodone, DEA's Diversion Control Division was pressed into duty.[35] DEA was not alone; in 2007, Congress enacted the Food and Drug Administration Amendments Act that included for the first time a provision requiring the FDA to consider nonmedical drug use and overdose, whether accidental or intentional, as adverse events to be weighed against the benefits of drugs being considered for marketing approval.[19]

While the DEA focused on errant registrants, including wholesale distributors, pharmacies, and practitioners charged with civil and/or criminal law violations, the FDA focused on tightening controls on medicines with recreational and addiction potential. In 2009, the FDA issued industry guidance in the form of a draft report titled, "Format and Content of Proposed Risk Evaluation and Mitigation Strategies" ("REMS").[36] An FDA-approved REMS was required by sponsors of drugs with risk factors for recreational use and addiction.[36] The purpose of the REMS was to ensure that actions taken by the sponsors to mitigate the risks of recreational use and addiction would cause the benefits of a drug to outweigh those risks.[36] Depending upon the FDA's risk evaluation, a low-risk drug might require simply a sponsor's warning to prescriber and patient or, as in the case of high-risk fentanyl drugs, a restricted distribution program implemented by the prescriber and/or dispenser.[37]

Despite including a number of medicinal controlled substances in the FDA's REMS program, including all long-acting opioids and transmucosal immediate-release fentanyl drugs, the effect, if any, was minimal—likely because individuals who recreationally use these substances tend to use diverted drugs. A 2013 report from the Department of Health and Human Services' Office of Inspector General faulted the FDA for the program's lack of effectiveness.[38]

Faced with a rapidly increasing unhealthy use of prescription drugs in the mid-2010s, several states enacted regulations to curtail drug diversion. State medical boards, through their rule-making and licensing authority, are empowered to regulate the healthcare industry. Boards may promulgate standards of care, set rules for the dispensing of controlled substances by physicians and pharmacists, establish licensing standards for healthcare practitioners, and enforce rules governing the ownership and operation of hospitals and pain clinics.[39,40]

States also have the authority to adopt prescription drug monitoring programs (PDMPs) and require that practitioners use them. Currently, all 50 states, the District of Columbia, and at least one U.S. territory have established PDMPs to track the prescribing and dispensing of controlled substances. PDMP information is sent electronically from dispensing pharmacies to a state-managed database from which it may be accessed, in most jurisdictions, by practitioners (for their patient care only) and state officials. Several states require practitioners, under certain circumstances, to query the state's PDMP *before* prescribing a Schedule II or Schedule III controlled substance for chronic nonmalignant pain.[41]

Perhaps the most effective drug control action by a state was taken by Florida in July 2011 when the state legislature declared a health emergency and enacted special legislation that, in effect, closed half of the state's 1,000 "pill mills" (operating as pain clinics) immediately and curtailed the operation of the other half.[42] Lax controls on Florida's pill mills caused this criminal enterprise to flood the East Coast and Mid-West with tens of millions of dosage units of drugs with addiction potential.[43] At the peak of the pill mill trade, the DEA reported that 90 of the top 100 oxycodone purchasing physicians were registered in Florida.[44] With Florida under control by 2012, volumes of prescribed opioids began to subside throughout the United States.[44]

To be sure, some state actions to control drug diversion were not universally embraced by practitioners or their patients. Some claim that they impeded access to needed medications for legitimate medical purposes.[24] In addition, some in the medical community objected to what they viewed as arbitrary standards of care imposed by medical boards and state legislatures that appeared more interested in curbing nonmedical drug use than caring for patients with legitimate pain. In Washington State, for example, objections were raised over a law requiring general practitioners to refer noncancer patients to a pain specialist for consultation *before* prescribing more than the equivalent of 120 mg of morphine per day.[45]

According to the CDC, between 1999 and 2021, more than a million people died in the United States from drug overdoses, with more than 100,000 such deaths occurring in 2021, alone.[46,47] While the early years of the epidemic involved overdose deaths resulting mostly from pharmaceutical opioids, this, according to the CDC, changed dramatically in 2013 with the introduction and widespread use of illicitly manufactured fentanyl and fentanyl analogs used alone or combined with heroin or cocaine.[48] Tragically, the CDC reports that in 2020, young people ages 15 to 24 saw the biggest year-to-year increase in fatal overdoses with deaths up 49%.[49]

Most illicit fentanyl sold in the United States is produced in Chinese factories that in some cases manufacture both legitimate and illicit counterfeit versions of the same drug.[50,51] The counterfeit products, including fentanyl and fentanyl precursors, are sold openly online or via the dark web to customers all over the world.[51] Drug cartels in Mexico import fentanyl or precursors to make fentanyl, and then smuggle the product into the United States.[51]

Counterfeit pills made to look like branded and generic opioids and benzodiazepines often contain fentanyl and can be deadly. A recent safety alert issued by the DEA advised that in the first nine months of 2021, more than 9.5 million counterfeit pills containing fentanyl or methamphetamine were seized in the United States.[52] Most of the counterfeit pills seized in the United States are made in Mexico, with China supplying the chemicals for the manufacturing of fentanyl in Mexico.[52] In 2019, China acceded to a U.S. demand to place fentanyl precursors on its list of controlled substances.[53] Since then, according to a 2020 intelligence report by the DEA, some Chinese fentanyl sources have moved their operations to India where conditions are reportedly more conducive for conducting this illicit commerce.[54]

The control mechanisms developed and promulgated by the League of Nations and the UN in the last century appear no longer effective in reducing illicit drug supply or demand. Future solutions may come from unexpected places. For example, the time may be right to revisit the concept of "abuse-deterrent" formulations ("ADF").[55,56] Initially introduced in the early 2000s, ADF delivery systems were found to increase production costs and some drugs developed safety problems and were recalled or discontinued.[57,58] Perhaps more sophisticated delivery systems may avoid the fate of the first generation ADF models. The FDA continues to support the development of abuse-deterrent technologies and has issued guidance for industry explaining how ADF products may qualify for special labeling claims.[59,60]

While the misuse of prescription opioids has abated since the peak years of 2011 and 2012, most of the gains have been offset by huge increases in the use of illicit opioids like heroin, fentanyl, and novel synthetic drugs known as New Psychoactive Substances ("NPS"). This is an unusual category of dangerous drugs that after being available intermittently for several years, emerged prominently in mid-2000s and spread quickly around the globe via the internet.[61] Many NPS products contain cathinones and synthetic cannabinoids in herbal smoking mixtures promoted as *legal alternatives* to controlled substances.[61] Many have colorful names and labels identifying them as bath salts or herbal incense, and their packaging often includes statements that the products are not to be used for human consumption.[61] Four general classes of NPS products have been identified: synthetic stimulants; synthetic cannabinoids; synthetic hallucinogens; and synthetic depressants (including synthetic opioids and benzodiazepines).[62]

In 2018, a total of 892 individual NPS products, reported by 119 countries, were monitored by the UN's Office of Drug Control.[62] Control of NPS products is made difficult by their number and the identification of their ingredients. In the United States, as of 2019, a DEA report stated that law enforcement authorities had identified 300 unique NPS substances, with some being placed under emergency scheduling because of their prevalence of recreational use and toxicity.[63] Of greater concern than the NPS products themselves is the unfounded but widespread belief that these so-called legal alternatives to controlled substances are safe to use.[62]

Presently, fentanyl and fentanyl analogs dominate the NPS opioid category but a report from Sweden in 2020 identified two novel NPS opioids (AH-7921 and MT-45).[64] The latter, identified as "a former analgesic drug candidate," according to the report from Sweden, "induced not only typical opioid toxicity but also unexpected severe skin and hearing problems and even blindness requiring surgery."[64] The sudden popularity of NPS products and their largely unregulated sales online and in specialty shops threaten to render obsolete most of our existing drug control models, especially those based on 20th century control paradigms.

For 21st century drug control to be effective, authorities may need to focus more on the patient or person using substances and less attention on the drugs themselves. Looking back at past control strategies, what appears to have been missing, or at least under-emphasized, was a focus on the pathophysiology of addiction, the disordered mental and physical processes associated with substance use disorders. It has been said that "Every problem contains within itself the seeds of its solution." Solving the mystery of why some individuals use drugs while others do not, and why some go on to have substance use disorders while others do not, may provide some of the elusive answers we have been searching for since 1909.

REFERENCES

1. Hanes WT III, Sanello F. *The Opium Wars: The Addiction of One Empire and the Corruption of Another*. Sourcebooks, Inc; 2002.
2. Jonnes J. *Hep-Cats, Narcs, and Pipe Dreams: A History of America's Romance with Illegal Drugs*. Scribner; 1996.
3. Musto DF, ed. *Drugs in America*. New York University Press; 2002.
4. Gootenberg P. *Building the global drug regime: origins and impact, 1909-1990s*. In: Idler A, Vergara JCG, eds. *Transforming the War on Drugs*. Oxford University Press; 2021.

5. Booth M. *Opium: A History.* St. Martin's Griffin; 1996.
6. Musto DF. The history of legislative control over opium, cocaine, and their derivatives. In: Hamowy R, ed. *Dealing with Drugs: Consequences of Government Control.* D.C. Heath and Company; 1987.
7. McAllister WB. *Drug Diplomacy in the Twentieth Century: An International History.* Routledge; 2000.
8. Berdahl CA. The United States and the League of Nations. *Michigan Law Review.* 1929;XXVII(6):607-636.
9. United States Congress. *Harrison Narcotic Tax Act.* 1914. Accessed March 16, 2022. http://www.druglibrary.org/schaffer/history/e1910/harrisonact.htm
10. Wright Q. The Narcotics Convention of 1931. *Am J Int Law.* 1934;28(3):475-486.
11. Musto DF. *The American Disease.* 3rd ed. Oxford University Press; 1999.
12. League of Nations, Office of the Secretariat, Geneva, Switzerland. *Limiting Manufacture and Regulating Distribution of Narcotic Drugs. U.S. Treaty Series 863, 48 Stat. 1543 (Ratified April 8, 1932 by U.S.).* 1931. Accessed March 16, 2022. https://www.loc.gov/law/help/us-treaties/bevans/m-ust000003-0001.pdf
13. U.S. Congress. *Harrison Narcotic Tax Act (P.L. 63-223, 38 Stat. 785).* 1914. Accessed March 10, 2022. http://www.druglibrary.org/schaffer/history/e1910/harrisonact.htm
14. Quinn TM, McLaughlin GT. *The Evolution of Federal Drug Control Legislation. Cath U L Rev*; 1973.
15. Brown LS Jr. Substance abuse and America: historical perspective on the federal response to a social phenomenon. *J Natl Med Assoc.* 1981;73(6):497-506.
16. Rierden A. Connecticut Q&A: Dr. David F. Musto; drug laws and attitudes in closer harmony. *The New York Times.* May 10, 1992.
17. McWilliams JC. *The Protectors: Harry J. Anslinger and the Federal Bureau of Narcotics, 1930-1962.* Associated University Presses; 1990.
18. United Nations. *The San Francisco Conference.* 1999 [March 16, 2022]; Available from https://www.un.org/en/about-us/history-of-the-un/san-francisco-conference
19. United Nations. *Secretariat: New York.* 1999. Accessed March 16, 2022. https://www.un.org/en/about-us/secretariat
20. United Nations, Office on Drugs and Crime. *Single Convention on Narcotic Drugs, 1961.* Accessed March 16, 2022. https://www.unodc.org/unodc/en/treaties/single-convention.html
21. Comprehensive Drug Abuse Prevention and Control Act, Title II: Controlled Substances Act. *Pub. L. No. 91-513, 84 Stat. 1236, Title 21, United States Code, Sect 811(d)(1) International treaties, conventions, and protocols requiring control, etc.* Accessed March 16, 2022. http://uscode.house.gov/
22. Comprehensive Drug Abuse Prevention and Control Act, Title II: Controlled Substances Act. *Pub. L. No. 91-513, 84 Stat. 1236, Title 21, United States Code, Sect 812(b)(1) Schedule I.* 1970 Accessed March 16, 2022. http://uscode.house.gov/
23. Food and Drug Administration. *Milestones in U.S. Food and Drug Law.* Accessed March 16, 2022. https://www.fda.gov/about-fda/fda-history/milestones-us-food-and-drug-law
24. Department of Health and Human Health Services. *HHS Historical Highlights.* Accessed March 16, 2022. https://www.hhs.gov/about/historical-highlights/index.html
25. Spillane JF. Debating the controlled substances act. *J Drug Alcohol Depend.* 2004;76(1):17-29.
26. National Criminal Justice Association. *A Guide to State Controlled Substances Acts (Prepared in cooperation with the U.S. Department of Justice, Bureau of Justice Assistance).* Accessed March 16, 2022. https://www.ncjrs.gov/pdffiles1/Digitization/184295NCJRS.pdf
27. Controlled Substances Act. *Title 21, United States Code, Sect. 903; Application of State Law.* Accessed March 16, 2022. http://uscode.house.gov/search/criteria.shtml
28. Department of Justice, Office of Public Affairs. *Justice Department Announces Update to Marijuana Enforcement Policy.* Accessed October 13, 2014. http://www.justice.gov/opa/pr/2013/August/13-opa-974.html
29. Weednews. *Map of Marijuana Legalization by States in 2022 (Medical & Recreational).* Accessed March 14, 2022. https://www.weednews.co/marijuana-legality-states-map/
30. Code of Federal Regulations. *Subpart R - Drug Enforcement Administration: General functions: delegated authority to another Department of Justice official by Attorney General (28 CRF Sect. 0.100).* Accessed March 16, 2022. https://www.govinfo.gov/content/pkg/CFR-2021-title28-vol1/xml/CFR-2021-title28-vol1.xml#seqnum0.100
31. Office of the Inspector General, U.S. Department of Justice. *Review of the Drug Enforcement Administration's Regulatory and Enforcement Efforts to Control the Diversion of Opioids.* Accessed June 12, 2021. https://oig.justice.gov/reports/2019/e1905.pdf
32. Department of Justice, Office of Inspector General, Evaluation and Inspections Division. *The Drug Enforcement Administration's Adjudication of Registrant Actions.* Accessed August 22, 2014. http://www.justice.gov/oig/reports/2014/e1403.pdf
33. Drug Enforcement Administration. *Drug Enforcement Administration: A Tradition of Excellence, 1973-2008.* DEA; 2008.
34. Department of Justice, Office of Inspector General. *Review Of The Drug Enforcement Administration's (DEA): Control Of The Diversion Of Controlled Pharmaceuticals (Report # I-2002-010).* Accessed March 16, 2022. https://oig.justice.gov/reports/DEA/e0210/background.htm
35. Drug Enforcement Administration. *DEA Congressional Testimony: Written Statement of Joseph T. Rannazzisi, Deputy Assistant Administrator, Office of Diversion Control, Drug Enforcement Administration, in testimony given May 16th before U.S. Senate Judiciary Committee.* Accessed May 2, 2016. https://www.dea.gov/sites/default/files/pr/speechestestimony/2015t/050515t.pdf
36. Federal Register. *Draft Guidance for Industry on Format and Content of Proposed Risk Evaluation and Mitigation Strategies (REMS) [74 FR 50801].* Accessed March 10, 2022. https://www.govinfo.gov/content/pkg/FR-2009-10-01/pdf/E9-23616.pdf
37. Food and Drug Administration. *Transmucosal Immediate Release Fentanyl (TIRF): Risk Evaluation and Mitigation Strategy (REMS).* Accessed December 11, 2023. https://www.fda.gov/drugs/information-drug-class/transmucosal-immediate-release-fentanyl-tirf-medicines
38. Department of Health and Human Services, Office of Inspector General. *FDA Lacks Comprehensive Data to Determine Whether Risk Evaluation and Mitigation Strategies Improve Drug Safety.* Accessed October 1, 2016. https://oig.hhs.gov/oei/reports/oei-04-11-00510.pdf
39. Federation of State Medical Boards. *FSMB Overview.* Accessed August 29, 2016. https://www.fsmb.org/about-fsmb/fsmb-overview
40. Drew C, Thompson JN. The role of state medical boards. *Virtual Mentor.* 2005;7(4): virtualmentor.2005.7.4.pfor1-0504.
41. National Alliance for Model State Drug Laws. *Prescription Drug Monitoring Programs.* Accessed March 16, 2022. https://namsdl.org/wp-content/uploads/Prescription-Drug-Monitoring-Programs-Evidence-Based-Practices-to-Optimize-Prescriber-Use.pdf
42. Kennedy-Hendricks A, Richey M, McGinty EE, Stuart EA, Barry CL, Webster DW. Opioid overdose deaths and florida's crackdown on pill mills. *Am J Public Health.* 2016;106(2):291-297.
43. Surratt HL, O'Grady C, Kurtz SP, et al. Reductions in prescription opioid diversion following recent legislative interventions in Florida. *Pharmacoepidemiol Drug Saf.* 2014;23(3):314-320.
44. Drug Enforcement Administration. *Florida Doctors No Longer Among The Top Oxycodone Purchasers In The United States.* Accessed March 10, 2022. https://www.dea.gov/press-releases/2013/04/05/florida-doctors-no-longer-among-top-oxycodone-purchasers-united-states
45. Washington State Department of Health. *Pain Management; Morphine Equivalent Dosage (Med) Frequently Asked Questions.* Accessed March 16, 2022. http://www.doh.wa.gov/ForPublicHealthandHealthcareProviders/HealthcareProfessionsandFacilities/PainManagement/FrequentlyAskedQuestionsforPractitioners/MorphineEquivalentDosageMed
46. National Public Radio. *More than a million Americans have died from overdoses during the opioid epidemic (broadcast 12/30/21).* Accessed March 10, 2022. https://www.npr.org/2021/12/30/1069062738/more-than-a-million-americans-have-died-from-overdoses-during-the-opioid-epidemi#:~:text=A%20study%20released%20Thursday%20

by%20the%20National%20Center,shows%20another%20100%2C000%20drug%20deaths%20expected%20in%202021

47. Centers for Disease Control and Prevention. *Drug Overdose Deaths in the U.S. Top 100,000 Annually*. Accessed March 10, 2022. https://www.cdc.gov/nchs/pressroom/nchs_press_releases/2021/20211117.htm
48. Centers for Disease Control and Prevention. *Health Advisory: Increase in Fatal Drug Overdoses Across the United States Driven by Synthetic Opioids Before and During the COVID-19 Pandemic*. Accessed March 10, 2022. https://emergency.cdc.gov/han/2020/han00438.asp
49. Centers for Disease Control and Prevention. *Drug Overdose Deaths in the United States, 1999-2020*. Accessed March 10, 2022. https://www.cdc.gov/nchs/products/databriefs/db428.htm
50. Eban K. *Bottle of Lies: The Inside Story of the Generic Drug Boom*. Harper Collins; 2019.
51. Westhoff B. *Fentanyl Inc: How rogue chemists are creating the deadliest wave of the opioid epidemic*. Atlantic Monthly Press; 2019.
52. Drug Enforcement Administration. *DEA Issues Public Safety Alert on Sharp Increase in Fake Prescription Pills Containing Fentanyl and Meth*. Accessed March 14, 2022. https://www.dea.gov/press-releases/2021/09/27/dea-issues-public-safety-alert
53. Martina M. U.S. welcomes China's expanded clampdown on fentanyl. *Reuters News*. 2019.
54. Drug Enforcement Administration. *Intelligence Report: Fentanyl Flow to the United States (Report #DEA-DCT-DIR-008-20)*. DEA; 2020.
55. Coleman JJ, Schuster CR, DuPont RL. Reducing the abuse potential of controlled substances. *Pharma Med*. 2010;24(1):21-36.
56. Simon K, Worthy SL, Barnes MC, Tarbell B. Abuse-deterrent formulations: transitioning the pharmaceutical market to improve public health and safety. *Ther Adv Drug Saf*. 2015;6(2):67-79.
57. Food and Drug Administration. *FDA requests removal of Opana ER for risks related to abuse*. Accessed March 12, 2022. https://www.fda.gov/news-events/press-announcements/fda-requests-removal-opana-er-risks-related-abuse
58. Food and Drug Administration. *Current and Resolved Drug Shortages and Discontinuations Reported to FDA: Morphine Sulfate and Naltrexone Hydrochloride (EMBEDA®) Extended-Release Capsules Status: Discontinuation*. Accessed March 12, 2022. https://www.accessdata.fda.gov/scripts/drugshortages/dsp_ActiveIngredientDetails.cfm?AI=Morphine%20Sulfate%20and%20Naltrexone%20Hydrochloride%20(EMBEDA%C2%AE)%20Extended-Release%20Capsules%20&st=d
59. Food and Drug Administration. *Abuse-Deterrent Opioids — Evaluation and Labeling; Guidance for Industry*. Accessed March 17, 2022. https://www.fda.gov/media/84819/download
60. Food and Drug Administration. *Abuse-Deterrent Opioid Analgesics*. Accessed March 17, 2022. https://www.fda.gov/drugs/postmarket-drug-safety-information-patients-and-providers/abuse-deterrent-opioid-analgesics
61. Peacock A, Bruno R, Gisev N, et al. New psychoactive substances: challenges for drug surveillance, control, and public health responses. *Lancet*. 2019;394(10209):1668-1684.
62. Shafi A, Berry AJ, Sumnall H, Wood DM, Tracey DK. New psychoactive substances: a review and updates. *Ther Adv Psychopharmacol*. 2020;10:2045125320967197.
63. Drug Enforcement Administration. *About Synthetic Drugs*. Accessed March 17, 2022. https://www.deadiversion.usdoj.gov/synthetic_drugs/about_sd.html#:~:text=Law%20enforcement%20has%20encountered%20over%20300%20NPS%2C%20the,dangerous%20substances%20may%20result%20in%20a%20prosecutable%20offense
64. Helander A, Bäckberg M, Beck O. Drug trends and harm related to new psychoactive substances (NPS) in Sweden from 2010 to 2016: Experiences from the STRIDA project. *PloS One*. 2020;15(4):e0232038-e0232038.

Sidebar 2

Guidance on the Use of Opioids to Treat Chronic Pain

Steven Prakken and James W. Finch

The use of opioids in the treatment of chronic noncancer pain (CNCP) continues to stimulate debate, with valid concerns expressed by those wishing to avoid using opioids and those seeing a clear role for their continued use. In the face of the ever-increasing opioid overdose rate, does the limited evidence for long-term benefit of opioids and the risk of opioid use disorder (OUD) outweigh the real, and commonly unmet need of the 20% of U.S. adults who comprise the country's chronic pain population?[1] Are the risks of using opioids on par with the risks inherent in chronic pain with its disabling impact on soma and psyche?[2] It is important to parse out the essential factual aspects of this debate to find solutions to this growing and critically important public health dilemma.[3,4]

Though we know a great deal about the physiology and psychology of pain and have guidelines (or mandates) related to using opioids in CNCP, does that adequately equip the practicing pain clinician?[5-7] When faced with a patient with their specific and complex constellation of pain symptoms, how does one sort out the most ethical and clinically appropriate course for that individual? As uncertainty and fear regarding the use of opioids naturally arises in the clinician's mind, what is important to consider?

Guidance for using opioids in CNCP is more complex than a simple binary yes or no. One useful approach places chronic pain-related scenarios into three primary case types: treatment naive or partially treated patients; patients with inadequate response to first-line, nonopioid treatment modalities; and "legacy" patients, that is, patients with a history of long-term opioid treatment and sometimes with relatively high opioid morphine milligram equivalents (MMEs).

TREATMENT NAIVE OR PARTIALLY TREATED

There is little debate that opioids should be the last choice option for treatment naive individuals. If physical therapy, behavioral therapy, adjunctive medication, or interventional treatments have been successful in reaching functional goals, then opioids are not needed. In those not meeting their functional goals, it is important to remember that partial treatment may result from sensitization (nociplastic pain), essentially creating a secondary pain condition. Trials of serotonin norepinephrine reuptake inhibitors (SNRIs) or other medication helpful for neuropathic pain may be helpful, though close observation for sedation and cognitive impairment is required. In particular, gabapentinoids, which have gained increasing usage in recent years, have significant risk of functional impairment and may provide minimal benefit, even with neuropathic pain but particularly when used injudiciously for non-neuropathic pain.

INADEQUATE TREATMENT RESPONSE

In patients who seem nonresponsive to nonopioid modalities, consider maximizing dosages, augmentation strategies, and retrials of prior medications. But chronic pain is notoriously difficult to treat, and patient dissatisfaction is common, complicating determining what qualifies as "nonresponsive." Clear, realistic, and mutually agreed upon functional goals are crucial, and if functional goals have not been met and high impact pain persists (eg, poor mobility and substantial social or emotional disability), then considering a trial of opioids is appropriate to consider.

It is true that data do not support opioid use in CNCP for long-term pain control or improved function, but additional facts also apply: opioids are commonly used to treat cancer pain with supporting data no more robust than that for CNCP, and the commonly favored nonopioid treatments, although considered first-line, have no better documented efficacy than opioids while the side effects from these medications can reduce function well beyond any pain relief benefit.[8] Finally, the lack of data showing benefit of opioids also reflects the limitations of the available data, an example of "absence of evidence is not evidence of absence." Research tends to show the effects on groups, not individuals, and some data do indicate benefit in select individuals over the long-term.[9]

The risk of developing an OUD is an important consideration but should be kept in perspective. The belief that OUD commonly starts after the use of legitimately prescribed pain medication is no longer accurate, particularly as the availability of nonprescribed illicit opioids has escalated. Studies on OUD associated with analgesics showed that the opioids were rarely prescribed to the person, but were medications diverted from someone else. Recent studies further clarify the relative risk of OUD within pain management while prescribing opioids. Of CNCP patients on prescribed opioids, only 0.7% to 7% are estimated to go on to develop OUD,[10] and the overall OUD rate in all treated CNCP patients, with or without prescribed opioids, is 7% to 12%.[11] While this risk is relatively small, it is a very real concern and should be managed carefully. But there are also dramatic risks associated with undertreatment of pain. While the risk of death from overdose is a recognized risk from OUD, it is less frequently noted that the risks of suicide in the setting of CNCP, often attributed to inadequately managed pain, is seven times the risk of death from overdose.[12]

If a trial of opioids is initiated, the following protocol can mitigate the inherent risks. Ensure the use of universal precautions and well-defined functional goals. Aggressively treat co-occurring psychiatric disease (eg, depression, anxiety, ADHD), which can benefit function as well as response to pain management. When initiating opioid treatment, start with safer choices than classic full agonist opioids, such as tramadol, tapentadol, or buprenorphine.

LEGACY PATIENTS

Most practitioners have encountered CNCP patients who have been taking opioids for an extended period, even for decades. The most challenging are those with MME well over 100. But regardless of MME, there are several essential issues to consider. Trials of opioid taper can be appropriate, but tapers done rapidly or against the patient's will have shown suboptimal and at times dangerous results. Data initially appeared to show a benefit to tapering, but these were mostly studies of volunteers in settings with numerous treatment alternatives and high levels of support not available to most CNCP patients.[13] In addition, a recent VA study indicated that the longer patients were on opioids, the more likely they were to have suicidal ideation and overdose with tapering.[14] At this time, there is little evidence that tapering or abstinence from opioids is safer or improves outcomes in the absence of aberrant medication use, contraindication, OUD, etc.[13]

The emphasis on a specific upper limit for MME when treating CNCP resulted from the 2016 CDC guidelines, which attempted to reduce opioid use. Although the guidelines clearly state that any reduction is to be collaborative and not unilateral, some practitioners and institutions were overly aggressive in their application.[5] Plus, the data supporting the dosing limits of 50 and 90 MME now appear derived from poor evidence.[5] The large majority of overdoses are with patients taking less than 90 MME,[15] and there is no change in the shape of the risk curve above 90 MME.[16] Establishing the correct MME clinically for a particular patient has been recently revisited by the DHHS Pain Management Best Practices,[9] the AMA,[17] and the new CDC draft guidelines.[18]

The treatment of legacy patients should target function, not MME. Tapering the patient's dose should be mutually agreed upon, done slowly (5%-10% per month at most), and reversed if function is reduced.

Across categories, a central tenet in CNCP treatment is the application of "universal precautions" detailed in the chapter, but one element rates added emphasis: using treatment goals defined by functional outcomes rather than simply reported pain relief. Function is the determining element assigning success or failure to all clinical decisions when managing pain and thus needs to be clear, realistic, well-documented, and above all, collaborative. Functional status (psychological and physical) needs to remain stable or improved following all clinical interventions. Relatively brief periods of worsening or instability can be tolerated if improvement is forthcoming. But if longer-term deterioration occurs, the clinical decision likely needs to be revised or reversed.

SPECIAL TREATMENT SITUATIONS RELATED TO CNCP

Use of Opioids Other Than as Medically Intended

Concerns should be well-documented including specific behavior, isolated or recurrent, and patient's stated reason, with corroboration from the PDMP, urine drug screens and collateral information. If there are dangerous levels of impulsivity and misuse, even that do not meet criteria for OUD, then reducing the dispensed amount from monthly to weekly, random pill-counts, or other medication controls can be instituted. Studies document that 80% of misuse is related to patients' attempts to manage pain, tension, sleep, or mood. Addressing these issues directly and more aggressively may resolve many cases of use.[19] In some cases, transitioning to buprenorphine can reduce risk of harm in those who are using.

Atypical Medication Reactions

Opioids are well-known for side effects such as sedation, cognitive impairment, and respiratory depression. Atypical reactions are also common but less well-known, including stimulation. Close questioning may reveal that a patient is using this side-effect to help with unrecognized co-occurring conditions such as depression, ADHD or fatigue, which can then be addressed more therapeutically.[20] Since opioids prescribed for CNCP may improve these comorbid conditions it is important when tapering opioids to consider whether shifting symptoms, such as deterioration of mood, cognition, fatigue, or sleep problems can be attributed to lower opioid dosage.

Opioids and Benzodiazepines

The concomitant use of opioids and sedative-hypnotics, in particular benzodiazepines, is a challenge and should be avoided where possible due to the potential risk for severe sedation or other impairment or the risk of respiratory depression. First line treatments for anxiety disorders include psychotherapy or nonbenzodiazepine medications such as buspirone and antidepressants. However, there are some patients with pain and co-morbid anxiety for whom this combination may be considered, such as transiently during initiation of other therapy or when treating an anxiety disorder that is not responsive to other medications or therapy and is seriously interfering with function;. This treatment is discussed in "Pain Management Best Practices" and the new draft CDC guidelines.[5,9]

Opioid Use Disorder (OUD) and Pain Management

The use of buprenorphine as an analgesic is common and effective and useful for those with CNCP or those with co-occurring OUD and CNCP. Someone taking buprenorphine in acute pain, such as from an injury or following surgery, can be dealt with safely, including the brief use of short acting full agonist opioids, which has shown success in this setting.

NATIONAL AND STATE GUIDELINES

Of the multiple guidelines published in recent years, two merit particular attention: The 2016 guidelines published by the Centers for Disease Control and Prevention (CDC)[5] which were revised and republished in 2022[18] and those developed in 2017 by the Federation of State Medical Boards (FSMB).[7] Most boards subsequently revised their own guidelines, often based on those from the FSMB or referencing those of the CDC. Many states have also added specific expectations by legislative statute. Practitioners should familiarize themselves with the regulations specific to their states. Table 125-1 includes links to each state's specific guidelines, regulations, and statutes. Recognize that these categories represent different levels of regulatory expectations, which is addressed in more detail in the chapter's Regulatory section.

REFERENCES

1. Institute of Medicine, Board on Health Sciences Policy, Committee on Advancing Pain Research, Care, and Education. *Relieving Pain in America: A Blueprint for Transforming Prevention, Care, Education, and Research (Consensus Study Report).* National Academies Press; 2011.
2. Agency for Healthcare Research and Quality. *The Effectiveness and Risks of Long-Term Opioid Treatment of Chronic Pain.* U.S. DHHS; 2014.
3. Finch JW. Challenges of chronic pain management: public health consequences and considered responses. *NC Med J.* 2013;74(3):243-248.
4. Ballantyne JC. Opioids for the treatment of chronic pain: mistakes made, lessons learned, and future directions. *Anesth Anal.* 2017; 125(5):1769-1778.
5. Centers for Disease Control and Prevention. *Guideline for Prescribing Opioids for Chronic Pain.* CDC, U.S. Department of Health and Human Services; 2017.
6. Washington State Department of Health, Agency Medical Directors' Group (AMDG). *Interagency Guideline on Prescribing Opioids for*

Pain. 3rd ed. Accessed August 7, 2023. www.doh.wa.gov/Portals/1/Documents/2300/2017/AMDG-Guidelines.pdf

7. Federation of State Medical Boards. *Guidelines for the Chronic Use of Opioid Analgesics.* The Federation; Accessed 7 August, 2023. https://www.fsmb.org/siteassets/advocacy/policies/opioid_guidelines_as_adopted_april-2017_final.pdf
8. Nonopioid Pharmacologic Treatments for Chronic Pain: Agency for Healthcare Research and Quality (AHRQ). 2020. U.S. DHHS. Accessed August 7, 2023. https://effectivehealthcare.ahrq.gov/products/nonopioid-chronic-pain/research
9. Pain Management Best Practices Inter-Agency Task Force Report DHHS2019. Accessed August 7, 2023. www.hhs.gov/sites/default/files/pain-mgmt-best-practices-draft-final-report-05062019.pdf
10. Volkow N. Opioid abuse in chronic pain -misconceptions and mitigation strategies. *N Engl J Med.* 2016;374:1253-1263.
11. Vowles K. Rates of opioid misuse, abuse, and addiction in chronic pain: a systematic review and data synthesis. *J Pain.* 2015;156(4):569-576.
12. Oquendo MA. Suicide: a silent contributor to opioid-overdose deaths. *N Engl J Med.* 2018;378:1567-1569.
13. Frank J. Patient outcomes in dose reduction or discontinuation of long-term opioid therapy: a systematic review. *Ann Intern Med.* 2017;167(3):181-191.
14. Oliva E. Associations between stopping prescriptions for opioids, length of opioid treatment, and overdose or suicide deaths in U.S. veterans: observational eval. *BMJ.* 2020;368:m283.
15. Bohnert A. A detailed exploration into the association of prescribed opioid dosage and overdose deaths among patients with chronic pain. *Med Care.* 2016;54(5):435-441.
16. Dasgupta N. Cohort study of the impact of high-dose opioid analgesics on overdose mortality. *Pain Med.* 2016;17:85-98.
17. AMA. AMA backs update to CDC opioid prescribing guidelines. Accessed August 7, 2023. www.ama-assn.org/press-center/press-releases/ama-backs-update-cdc-opioid-prescribing-guidelines
18. Dowell D, Ragan KR, Jones CM, Baldwin GT, Chou R. *CDC Clinical Practice Guideline for Prescribing Opioids for Pain-United States, 2022. Recomm Rep.* 2022;71(3):1-95.
19. Substance Abuse and Mental Health Services Administration. *Key Substance Use and Mental Health Indicators in the United States: Results from the 2020 National Survey on Drug Use and Health.* Accessed August 7, 2023. www.samhsa.gov/data/sites/default/files/reports/rpt35325/NSDUHFFRPDFWHTMLFiles2020/2020NSDUHFFR1PDFW102121.pdf
20. Barbour A, Asbury ML, Riordan PA, Webb JA, Prakken SD. Opioid-induced somatic activation: prevalence in a population of patients with chronic pain. *Cureus.* 2020;12(5):e7911. doi:10.7759/cureus.7911

CHAPTER

126 Therapeutic Effectiveness of Cannabis and Cannabinoids

Jag H. Khalsa, Gregory C. Bunt, Marc Galanter, Mahmoud A. El-Sohly, and Shyam Kottilil

CHAPTER OUTLINE

- Facts about cannabis and cannabinoids
- Cannabis or cannabinoids used as treatment
- The physician's role in prescribing cannabis or cannabinoids used as treatment
- Conclusion
- Summary
- Key points

Plants and plant-derived chemical constituents have been used by humans as medicine for thousands of years. Cannabis is the designation of the plant, *Cannabis sativa* L., where the *Cannabis* genus belongs comprises species of the Cannabinaceae family, first classified by Carl Linnaeus in 1793.[1] Of the many varieties of cannabis cultivated in various parts of the world, three most used are *Cannabis sativa* L., *C. indica* L., and *C. ruderalis* Janisch, corresponding to useful, Indian, and wild cannabis plants, respectively. According to the 1961 United Nations Single Convention on Narcotic Drugs,[2] cannabis is defined as the flowering tops of the cannabis plant from which resin has not been extracted. Cannabis resin is the separated resin from the cannabis plant. Marijuana, the name often used in the United States and elsewhere, refers to the desiccated leaves, flowers, stems, and seeds from the hemp plant, *Cannabis sativa*. Generally, authors in the European literature tend to use the term cannabis and medicinal or medical cannabis, while those in the American literature, tend to use the term, marijuana and "medical," or rarely "medicinal marijuana." But the American literature is rapidly moving to using the term "cannabis" in part because "marijuana" has historical roots that can be stigmatizing to certain populations. As well, "used as treatment" is favored over "medical" because of concerns that the model used currently does not adhere to typical medical constraints and an evidence base in ways that are typical in the practice of medicine, and because "cannabis used as treatment" (CUAT) is a more accurate description of its use, is a less politically charged term, and is less stigmatizing to patients than the term "medical marijuana"—please see Chapter 1, "Recommended Use of Terminology in Addiction Medicine" for the origins of the term "cannabis used as treatment." In this chapter, we will present clinical research on the therapeutic potential of cannabis and its chemical constituents, known as cannabinoids.

FACTS ABOUT CANNABIS AND CANNABINOIDS

Epidemiology

Cannabis continues to be the most frequently used illegal drug in the world today. According to the 2021 World Drug Report, there were an estimated 200 million people who used cannabis in 2019 representing 4% of the global population.[3] In the United States, 48.2 million people, or about 18% of Americans, used it at least once in 2019.[4] Recent research estimates that approximately three in ten people who use cannabis have cannabis use disorder (CUD).[5] For people who begin using cannabis before age 18, the risk of developing CUD is even greater.[6] An estimated 3.9% of recent-onset users develop a DSM-defined cannabis dependence syndrome during the interval since first use (median interval duration approximately 12 months).[7] In 2021, an estimated 7.1%, 17.3%, and 30.5% of 8th, 10th, and 12th grade students, respectively, smoked cannabis in the past month.[8] Cannabis use by young people has increased or decreased at various times during the last decade, possibly due either to its potency, which has been on the rise, from about 4% concentration of delta-9-tetrahyrocannabinol (THC), cannabis's active chemical constituent, in 1995 to about 17% to 28% in 2019[9,10] and possibly due to changes in the perceptions of youth about dangers of cannabis use. Cannabis use usually peaks in the late teens to early twenties, and then declines in the later years.[11] Among adults in the U.S. during 2002 to 2017, past-year prevalence of DSM-5 CUD remained stable at 1.5% to 1.4%, but past year cannabis use increased from 10.4% (or 21.9 million) in 2002 to 15.3% (or 37.8 million) in 2017, a 72.6% increase in the number of U.S. adults who used cannabis, and daily/near daily use increased from 1.9% to 4.2%, and mild DSM-5 CUD increased from 1.4% to 1.9%. Among adults who used cannabis, past-year prevalence of DSM-5 CUD decreased from 14.8% to 9.3%, daily/near daily use increased from 18.0% to 27.2%, and DSM-5 moderate (4-5 criteria) and severe (6+ criteria) CUD decreased from 4.3% to 3.1% and from 2.4% to 1.3%, respectively.[12,13]

The Chemistry of Cannabis and Cannabinoids

The cannabis plant, like any other plant, has hundreds of chemical constituents of which only a few are known to be pharmacologically active. Of the 567 identified and characterized chemicals in cannabis, 125 are classified as cannabinoids, while the remaining belong to several classes of chemicals such as terpenes and flavonoids.[14] Of the 125 cannabinoids, only two, THC and cannabidiol (CBD), have been extensively studied for their potential therapeutic applications. Some of the active cannabinoids in cannabis are: (1) THC, the most active psychoactive component; (2) CBD, known for its anticonvulsant activity and now approved by the FDA for the treatment of intractable epilepsy; (3) THCV (tetrahydrocannabivarin), found primarily in strains of African and Asian cannabis, increases the speed and intensity of THC effects, but also causes the subjective experience to end depending on the dose; (4) CBC (cannabichromene), probably not psychoactive in its pure form but is thought to interact with THC to enhance the subjective experience and exhibits anti-inflammatory properties; (5) CBL (cannabicyclol), in the presence of light, is converted from CBC; (6) delta-8-THC, although it exists in negligible amounts in the plant, has psychoactive properties about 80% that of delta-9-THC.[15]

There are endocannabinoids that are neurotransmitters in the brain or in the periphery and act on cannabinoid receptors in the brain (CB1), or receptors in the periphery (CB2).[16] According to Wei and Piomelli,[17] "CB_1 receptor expression is high in the regions of the human brain that are implicated in the psychological and physiological effects of marijuana. For example, substantial numbers of receptors are found in the structures involved in cognitive functions and reward processing as well as in the areas that control movement and activity of the autonomic nervous system. CB_1 is also present in many cell types outside the brain, including pain-sensing neurons, innate-immune cells (eg, macrophages), adipocytes, hepatocytes, and skeletal myocytes. This broad distribution reflects the importance of endogenous cannabinoid (endocannabinoid) messengers in the peripheral control of energy balance, pain, and inflammation, among other functions. In addition to CB_1, the brain contains a relatively small number of CB_2 receptors. However, this subtype is expressed at much higher levels in cells of the immune system (eg, B lymphocytes, macrophages, and microglia) as well as in osteoclasts and osteoblasts." Further, according to Wei and Piomelli,[17] the contributions of CB_2 to endocannabinoid signaling in the brain appear to be important but are still the subject of unsettled debate. In addition, there are synthetic cannabinoids that are structurally unrelated to either phytocannabinoids or endocannabinoids but are made to interact with the cannabinoid receptors (CB_1 and CB_2), and therefore have cannabimimetic properties. CBD has been postulated to have many pharmacologic mechanisms of action ranging from immunosuppressive, anti-inflammatory, analgesic, neuroprotective, antiepileptic to antipsychotic effects.[18,19] But data from case reports or randomized clinical trials have been limited to a few of these uses where CBD alone was truly tested for efficacy; instead, versions used include either smoked cannabis, cannabis extract, or its two cannabinoids, THC and CBD. In the case of other cannabinoids such as THCV, CBC, and cannabigerol (CBG), although these have potential for developing as therapeutic agents, currently limited clinical data are available to support their use in medicine.

CANNABIS OR CANNABINOIDS USED AS TREATMENT

Since the first description of cannabis used as treatment (CUAT) by the Chinese Emperor Shen-Nung in 2737 BCE,[20] many preparations of cannabis have been used for recreational and treatment purposes.[21-23] The biological plausibility of CUAT is because the endocannabinoid system is involved in a broad range of bodily functions, including analgesia, gastrointestinal function, immune system regulation, appetite, cognitive processes and motor control, and the cannabinoids such as THC, CBD and others act by interacting with CB_1 and CB_2 receptors in the body. The CB_1 receptor is the most common G-protein-couple receptor in the brain. It is widely distributed with high levels in the hippocampus, cerebellum, basal ganglia, and neocortex in addition to peripheral nerve terminals. The CB_1 receptor has been reported to have analgesic, antispasmodic, antitremor, anti-inflammatory, appetite stimulant and antiemetic properties. CB_2 receptors are found largely within the periphery, including cells of the immune system, and have also been reported to have anti-inflammatory, analgesic, anticonvulsant, antipsychotic, antioxidant, and neuroprotective activities.[23] Thus, both THC and CBD have been tested for their therapeutic potential.[18] Currently, the approved cannabinoids are: dronabinol, a synthetic THC, approved for the treatment of anorexia associated with weight loss in AIDS patients and chemotherapy-induced nausea and vomiting; nabilone, also a synthetic cannabinoid similar to THC, approved for treatment of nausea and vomiting in patients undergoing cancer treatment; and nabiximols, a mouth spray containing two cannabis derived cannabinoids: THC and CBD in 1:1 ratio, approved in 28 countries but not the U.S., for moderate to severe spasticity due to multiple sclerosis (MS) for patients who have not responded adequately to other treatments. In addition, based on data from several clinical studies and trials (further discussed below), cannabis-derived CBD has been approved by the FDA for the treatment of a rare form of epilepsy known as Lennox-Gastaut and Dravet syndromes in children two years and older, and seizures from a rare brain tumor known as tuberous sclerosis (https://www.fda.gov/news-events/press-announcements/fda).

In the case of cannabidiol, the half-life of CBD is between 1.4 and 10.9 hours after oromucosal spray, 2 to 5 days after chronic oral administration, 24 hours after IV and 31 hours after smoking. Bioavailability following smoking is 31%, however no other studies attempted to report the absolute bioavailability of CBD following other routes in humans, despite intravenous formulations being available. The plasma concentration of CBD increased dose-dependently and the maximum concentration is reached quicker following smoking/inhalation compared to oral/oromucosal routes.[24,25] Regarding the action of CBD and THC on brain function, Batalla et al.[26] report that in healthy volunteers, as compared to placebo and THC, acute CBD enhanced fronto-striatal resting state connectivity and modulated brain activity. CBD had opposite effects when compared to THC following task-specific patterns during various cognitive paradigms, such as emotional processing (fronto-temporal), verbal memory (fronto-striatal), response inhibition (fronto-limbic-striatal), and auditory/visual processing (temporo-occipital). In individuals at clinical high risk for psychosis and patients with established psychosis, acute CBD showed intermediate brain activity compared to placebo and healthy controls during cognitive task performance. CBD modulated resting limbic activity in subjects with anxiety and metabolite levels in patients with autism spectrum disorders. But a recent review of the published research on CBD/THC[27] shows that the quality of evidence (quality and study design), as judged by using the Oxford Centre for Evidence-Based Medicine, ranges between strong to weakest, which in turn may lead to various levels of recommendations—such as grade A (strong) to grade B (moderate), grade C (weak), and grade D (weakest). Data show a moderate level of recommendation for CBD and CBD-containing compounds such as nabiximols in alleviating symptoms of cannabis-related disorders, schizophrenia, social anxiety disorder, and co-occurring autism spectrum disorder (ASD) and attention-deficit/hyperactivity disorder (ADHD). However, there is weaker evidence for insomnia, anxiety, bipolar disorder, posttraumatic stress disorder (PTSD), and Tourette syndrome. The evidence for the use of CBD and CBD-containing compounds for psychiatric disorders needs to be explored in future studies, especially large-scale and well-designed randomized clinical trials. During the last couple of decades numerous clinical studies and trials have been conducted with a few to hundreds of patients treated with a single cannabinoid like THC, CBD, or a combination of the two (THC+CBD in 1:1 ratio; nabiximols), cannabis plant extract or smoked cannabis for one or the other clinical conditions. These clinical conditions have ranged from chemotherapy-induced nausea and vomiting to loss of appetite, pain, epilepsy, autism, multiple sclerosis, spinal cord injuries, Tourette syndrome, epilepsy, glaucoma, Parkinson disease, dystonia, and PTSD.[28-30] A few recent studies also show that CBD may be effective in treating tobacco, opioid, and CUDs, and infections that co-occur in people with substance use disorders, but almost every author has suggested that additional randomized clinical trials are needed to confirm the efficacy of cannabinoid(s), cannabis plant extract or smoked cannabis. The clinical data on various medical conditions for which either smoked cannabis, whole cannabis extract, or isolated cannabinoids have been tested are discussed below in the order of strength of available evidence for a specific condition.

Antiemetic Effects

Clinical evidence from at least 15 clinical trials involving a total of 600 patients confirmed the antiemetic effects of synthetic THC. Nabilone, a synthetic cannabinoid, was approved by the U.S. Food and Drug Administration (FDA) in 2006 for treating chemotherapy-induced nausea and vomiting.[31] Similarly, data from 14 clinical trials involving 681 patients showed that synthetic THC, dronabinol was also effective for treating nausea and vomiting. It was approved by the FDA in 1985 for treating nausea, and for appetite stimulation in 1992. Health Canada also approved it in 1995 for treating nausea and vomiting undergoing cancer therapy. Nabilone was also effective in the treatment of chemotherapy induced nausea and vomiting.[32] Both nabilone and dronabinol were found to be equipotent or superior to currently available traditional nonherbal medications such as chlorpromazine, haloperidol, and others. However, because of their undesirable side effects such as drowsiness, euphoria, sedation, their use has declined. Levonantradol, another synthetic cannabinoid, was found to be slightly superior to chlorpromazine in about 50% of patients with severe nausea and vomiting refractory to conventional antiemetic therapy tested in an open phase II study but has not been widely used due to its unpleasant adverse profile of drowsiness and thought disturbance.[33]

In the case of *smoked cannabis,* the evidence for treating emesis has not been impressive. In one randomized double-blind placebo-controlled trial with 15 patients with osteogenic sarcoma, Chang and colleagues[34] observed significant antiemetic effect of smoked cannabis cigarette containing 1.9% THC, but 80% of patients experienced sedation. In a later randomized double-blind cross-over study of eight patients with various tumors, smoked cannabis showed no antiemetic effect.[35] Levitt and colleagues[36] also compared smoked cannabis with oral THC for antiemetic effect in a randomized double-blind cross over placebo-controlled study. Of the twenty patients, 20% showed efficacy and preferred smoked cannabis, 35% showed improvement but preferred oral THC, while the remaining patients did not show any preference. Interestingly, these cannabinoids have not been compared with newer antiemetic drugs such as 5HT3 antagonists or neurokinin-1-receptor antagonists.[37] Although CBD showed some antiemetic effects in animals, there are no data available from studies in humans. Similarly, there are no clinical data available on antiemetic effects of other cannabinoids. But there is no doubt that CBD and other cannabigerolic-(CBG)-derived cannabinoids, that act as agonists and antagonists at multiple targets including CB_1 and CB_2 receptors, transient receptor potential (TRP) channels, peroxisome proliferator-activated receptors (PPARs), serotonin 5-HT_{1a} receptors and others, have a potential to treat many clinical conditions including nausea and vomiting.[38,39]

Appetite Stimulant Effect

Patients on cancer therapy or infected with human immunodeficiency virus (HIV) often develop cachexia (extreme loss of body weight). In two randomized clinical trials oral THC stimulated appetite and helped retard weight loss and thereby significantly improved weight gain. In one study, among patients with HIV/AIDS (acquired immune deficiency syndrome) on dronabinol, 22% gained two or more kilograms compared with 10.3% of patients on placebo[40] and was found to be safe[41]; in another study, 75% of patients gained weight better when treated with megestrol than dronabinol.[42] Smoked cannabis (one to three cigarettes with THC content of 3.9%

daily) also significantly increased body weight gain without increasing the viral load in patients with HIV/AIDS.[43] Health Canada has approved the oral THC as an appetite stimulant for treating AIDS-associated anorexia and weight loss. On the other hand, CBD appears to decrease the appetite.[44]

Analgesic Effect

Several cannabis products including oral cannabis plant extract,[45] sublingual spray,[46] intravenous THC,[47] single cannabinoids such as THC or CBD or a combination of both, have been tested for analgesic activity in a total of 353 patients in 14 small clinical studies or trials.[48-57] For example, a sublingual single spray containing THC and CBD in 1:1 ratio (nabiximols; 2.5 mg each) for 4 weeks was effective as an analgesic in 34 patients with chronic pain.[46] The adverse reactions reported were dry mouth, drowsiness, euphoria/dysphoria, and dizziness. THC at oral doses of 15 mg and 20 mg was effective against pain in 10 patients, but most patients developed frequent drowsiness and confusion, while the lower dose of 10 mg THC was not effective.[48,49] Similarly, 10 mg and 20 mg doses of oral THC were comparable to 60 mg and 120 mg of codeine in 36 patients with cancer pain, respectively; but the higher dose of THC produced drowsiness, dizziness, sedation, mental clouding, disorientation, and impaired memory in patients. But in a study of 40 women with postoperative pain, 5 mg of oral THC was ineffective as an analgesic.[54] CBD was also ineffective at 45 mg/day for one week in patients with chronic neuropathic pain.[28] In a more recent study of 21 patients, a single inhalation dose of 25 mg of cannabis with 9.4% THC content three times daily for 5 days reduced the intensity of pain, improved sleep and was well tolerated by patients with neuropathic pain, while the lower doses of THC at 2.5% and 6.0% were ineffective.[57] An intravenous dose of THC was ineffective as an analgesic in a group of 10 healthy volunteers undergoing tooth extraction.[47] Gedin et al.[58] conducted a meta-analysis of 20 placebo-controlled trials involving almost 1500 subjects (62% female, aged between 33 and 62). They showed that cannabis or cannabis products (cannabis, THC, CBD, or nabilone; administered via pill, spray, oil or smoked) are no better at relieving variety of different pain conditions including neuropathic than a placebo. The analysis further showed that pain was rated as being significantly less intense after treatment with a placebo, with a moderate to large effect depending on each person. There was no significant difference between cannabis and a placebo for reducing pain.

One review of the published research[59] suggested that CBD could treat cancer pain with mild to moderate side effects such as drowsiness, nausea, vomiting, and dry mouth, while the other review[60] concluded that the potential benefits of cannabis-based treatment (herbal cannabis, plant-derived or synthetic THC, and THC+CBD oromucosal spray) in chronic neuropathic pain might be outweighed by their potential harms. Häuser et al.[61] also concluded that there is limited evidence for a benefit of THC+CBD spray in the treatment of neuropathic pain, and there is inadequate evidence for any benefit of cannabinoids (dronabinol, nabilone, medical cannabis, or THC+CBD spray) to treat cancer pain, pain of rheumatic or GI origin, anorexia in cancer or AIDS. Nevertheless, CBD/THC combination (nabiximols) is approved for MS-related spasticity and pain in several countries but not the United States. It is important to note that treatment with cannabis-based medicines is associated with CNS and psychiatric side effects and that the public perception of the efficacy, tolerability, and safety of cannabis-based medicines in pain management and palliative medicine conflicts with the findings of systematic reviews and prospective observational studies conducted according to the standards of evidence-based medicine.

There is limited evidence to support CBD for treating pain. Although CBD alone did reduce sensory pain and pain aversiveness in rats,[62] CBD at a dose of 45 mg/day for 1 week was found to be ineffective in 10 patients with chronic neuropathic pain.[28] However, it has been postulated that the combination of CBD and THC would decrease the addictive potential of THC while preserving its therapeutic effects. But without sufficient evidence that CBD reduces the addictive potential of THC, medical insurance payments for the use of nabiximols to treat neuropathic pain should be evaluated with great caution as the potentially addictive, intoxicating, and adverse effects of the use of high dose THC for prolonged periods could be facilitated by commercial interests and careless public policy that has been historical with addictive substances exploited by certain entities. Although other cannabinoids such as tetrahydrocannabivarin (THCV), cannabidivarin (CBDV), CBG, and CBC have shown anti-inflammatory activity, currently there are no data from clinical studies to support the use of these cannabinoids in treating any type of pain in humans.

Epilepsy

Based on the fact that CBD possesses affinity for multiple targets across a range of target classes, namely transient receptor potential vanilloid-1 (TRPV1), the orphan G-protein-coupled receptor-55 (GPR55) and the equilibrative nucleoside transporter 1 (ENT-1), resulting in functional modulation of neuronal excitability, relevant to the pathophysiology of many disease types, including epilepsy,[63] anecdotal scores, clinical studies, and trials have been conducted to determine if cannabis and/or cannabinoids could treat epilepsy in humans.[30,64] In a prospective cohort study in 59 children with drug-resistant epileptic encephalopathies (DEEs), long-term (20 months) treatment of CBD-enriched medical cannabis as an adjuvant therapy to antiseizure therapy was safe, well tolerated, and effective in reducing seizure frequency and improved the quality of daily living.[65] In a study by Tzadok and colleagues,[66] children with intractable epilepsy were treated with CBD-enriched cannabis. The selected formula contained CBD and tetrahydrocannabinol at a ratio of 20:1 dissolved in olive oil. The CBD dose ranged from 1 to 20 mg/kg/d. Seizure frequency was assessed by parental report during clinical visits. Results showed a significant positive effect on seizure load. Most of the children (66/74, 89%) reported reduction in seizure frequency: 13 (18%) reported 75% to 100% reduction, 25 (34%) reported 50% to 75% reduction, 9 (12%) reported 25% to 50% reduction, and 19 (26%) reported less than 25% reduction. Five (7%) patients reported aggravation of seizures, and adverse reactions including somnolence, fatigue, GI disturbances and irritability, which led to withdrawal of CBD patients. Among the treated patients, there was improvement in behavior, alertness, language, communication, motor skills and sleep. In a randomized, double-blind, parallel group study of 15 patients, one group of eight patients, in addition to their conventional medications, received oral CBD at 200 to 300 mg/day for 8 to 18 weeks, while the second group of seven control patients received placebo.[67] Of the eight patients on CBD, four remained seizure-free for the duration, and three showed clinical improvement. Six of the seven patients on placebo remained unchanged. Drowsiness was seen in four of the treated patients. In an open clinical trial, Devinsky and colleagues[68] also reported efficacy of CBD in treating intractable epilepsy. In an open-label interventional clinical trial, CBD, 2 to 5 mg/kg/d was tested in patients (1-30-year-old) with severe intractable, childhood-onset, treatment-resistant epilepsy, who were receiving stable doses of antiepileptic drugs before study entry in 11 epilepsy centers across the United States. The primary objective was to establish the safety and tolerability of CBD, and the primary efficacy endpoint was median percentage change in the mean monthly frequency of motor seizures at 12 weeks. Of the 214 enrolled patients, 137 (64%) were included in the efficacy analysis. In the safety and tolerability group, 33 (20%) patients had Dravet syndrome (characterized by frequent, prolonged seizures often triggered by hyperthermia, developmental delay, speech impairment, ataxia, hypotonia, sleep disturbances, and other health problems), and 31 (19%) patients had Lennox-Gastaut syndrome (characterized by muscle weakness in the head, abdomen, arms, or legs, often resulting in a gradual slump, subtle jerking [myoclonic] movements, and loss of awareness). The remaining patients had intractable epilepsies of different causes and types, thereby suggesting variable response to treatment with CBD. Adverse events were reported in 128 (79%) of the 162 patients within the safety group. Adverse events were reported in 10% (41) of patients that included somnolence (25%), decreased appetite (19%), diarrhea (19%), fatigue (13%), and convulsions (11%). Five patients discontinued treatment. Serious adverse events were reported in 48 (30%) patients, including one death—a sudden unexpected death in epilepsy but regarded as unrelated to study drug; 12% of patients had severe adverse events possibly related to cannabidiol use, the most common of which was status epilepticus ($N = 9$ [6%]). The median monthly frequency of motor seizures was 30.0 (IQR 11.0-96.0) at baseline and 15.8 (5.6-57.6) over the 12-week treatment period. The median reduction in monthly motor seizures was 36.5% (IQR 0-64.7). The authors concluded that CBD might reduce seizure frequency and might have an adequate safety profile in children and young adults with highly treatment-resistant epilepsy but recommended that randomized controlled trials are warranted to characterize the safety profile and true efficacy of CBD. Data from a phase II open-label prospective study of 35 subjects of 2 to 16 years of age also demonstrated that CBD at doses of 5 mg/kg/d raised to a maximum of 25 mg/kg/d was safe and significantly reduced seizure frequency by 61%, and improved quality of life (QOL), behavior deficits, sleep disruption, improved irritability, hyperactivity, and general health in children with drug-resistant epilepsy.[69] Thus, based on evidence from several clinical studies and trials, CBD is approved for the treatment of two rare forms of epilepsy, Lennox-Gastaut and Dravet syndromes in children 2 years and older. More recently, CBD was also approved for treating a rare genetic condition known as tuberous sclerosis, where people suffer from seizures from benign tumors in the brain.

Besides CBD, other cannabinoids like CBG, CBDV, and THCV have shown potential to treat epilepsy. Several mechanisms seem to be involved in the antiepileptic activity of CBDV. CBDV may act via CB1 and CB2 receptors and modulate neuronal excitability and neuroinflammation, may act via transient *receptor* potential cation channel subfamily V member 1 (TRPV1), CB_1-independent mechanisms[70-72] including voltage gated potassium and sodium channels, g-protein coupled receptor (GPR55123), desensitization of TPRV1148, GABAergic system[73] or through the expression of epilepsy-related genes (*Fos, Casp3, Ccl3, Cc14, Npy, Arc, Penk, Cam2a, Bdnf,* and *Egr1*) in the hippocampus, neocortex, and prefrontal cortex.[74] These results provide the first molecular confirmation of behaviorally observed effects of CBDV upon chemically induced seizures and serve to underscore its suitability for clinical development. In the case of THCV, preclinical data show that it suppressed in vitro epileptiform and in vivo seizure activity in rats.[75,76] Currently, there are no data from clinical studies to support the use of THCV for treating epilepsy.

Multiple Sclerosis

Clinical evidence from numerous small and large studies show that cannabis products may have a positive effect on multiple sclerosis (MS). Several formulations of cannabis including smoked cannabis, hashish, oral THC in capsule, oral extracts of *C. sativa* in oral and sublingual spray forms containing THC, cannabidiol, or a combination of the two and oral nabilone were tested in 13 controlled studies involving 939 patients to determine if any could treat multiple sclerosis. For example, in a double-blind randomized placebo-controlled trial of 630 patients, Zajicek and colleagues[77,78] evaluated oral THC in capsule (206 patients), and oral cannabis extract 2.5 mg THC+1.25 mg CBD, plus less than 5% other cannabinoids in a capsule (211 patients) and 213 subjects on placebo for 15 weeks. There were no objective effects on spasticity, but subjective improvement in spasticity was observed; there was objective improvement in mobility and decreased hospitalizations with oral THC. Adverse drug reactions (ADRs) were mild and tolerable. Overall, at one year follow-up there were positive effects on spasticity. In another study of 160 patients, investigators[79] evaluated oral nabiximols (THC 2.5 mg plus 2.5 mg CBD) at doses of 2.5 to 120 mg/daily for 6 weeks. There was a significant reduction in spasticity, better sleep quality and mobility in patients treated with nabiximols compared to placebo. Adverse events were mild and were well-tolerated. In another small randomized, double-blind, parallel groups, placebo-controlled study of 32 subjects in each group, Rog and colleagues[80] reported beneficial effects of nabiximols (THC+CBD, 1:1 ratio) for 4 weeks on pain and sleep disturbance. Adverse effects were dizziness, dry mouth, and somnolence; cognitive effects were limited to long-term memory storage. The oromucosal spray formulation of nabiximols was also effective in MS patients with resistant spasticity.[81-84] Overall, these studies showed positive effects of nabiximols on MS associated spasticity with mild and tolerable side effects. For its anti-inflammatory and neuroprotective effects, CBD alone could also be used to improve mobility in patients with MS.[85] In the case of other cannabinoids, Granja and colleagues[86] suggested that for its antineuroinflammatory effects, CBG could be developed to treat patients with MS. Currently, there is no evidence from clinical studies or trials to show that any other cannabinoid can be used to treat MS.

Autism

Autism spectrum disorder (ASD) is a neurodevelopmental disorder characterized by core deficits in social communication and restricted, repetitive patterns of behavior. Currently, there are no approved medications for the core symptoms of ASD, and only two medications, risperidone, and aripiprazole, have been approved by the FDA for autism associated irritability. Prescribed medications for ASD symptoms show a range of levels of efficacy, safety, and tolerability among the heterogeneous ASD population. There are also several side effects associated with medications such as aggression, anxiety, irritability, and a negative effect on cognition, leading many patients to discontinue use as the side effects outweigh benefits.[87] Neuropeptides like oxytocin and vasopressin as well as SSRIs have been tried for treating autism. But recent studies and reviews of published studies show that cannabis and cannabinoids do have potential and have been used in the treatment of not only core symptoms of ASD but also irritability and behavioral problems of autism.[88] Current research, although limited, shows that CBD-rich CUAT seems to be safe[89] and an effective, tolerable, option for many symptoms associated with ASD. Data from a recent cross-sectional survey of 269 autistic individuals of under 16 years of age in U.K. showed that among them there was a higher prevalence and frequency of CBD use, but not cannabis use. Further, they trusted the news and doctors less as sources of cannabinoid-related information than nonautistic controls.[90] Bilge and Ekici[91] also reported that treatment with CBD (containing <3%THC) at an average daily dose of 0.7 mg/kg/d (0.3-2 mg/kg/d) for a period of 6.5 months improved the behavioral problems, cognition, expressive language, and social interaction in 33 (27 males and 6 females; mean age of 7.7+5.5 years) autistic individuals. The authors also reported that according to recent studies, the average dose of CBD tested in individuals with autism was 3.8±2.6 mg/kg/d, with a 20:1 ratio of CBD to THC in the used preparations.

In fact, the following study is an excellent illustration of positive effects of CBD in autism. In an observational study of autistic patients, CBD-enriched cannabis extract was effective in improving autistic symptoms.[92] Of the 18 autistic patients undergoing treatment with compassionate use of standardized CBD-enriched cannabis sativa extract (CE; with a CBD to THC ratio of 75/1), among 15 patients who adhered to the treatment (10 with and 5 without epilepsy), only one patient showed lack of improvement in autistic symptoms. Due to adverse effects, three patients discontinued CE use before 1 month. After 6 to 9 months of treatment, most patients showed some level of improvement in more than one of the several symptom categories. It is important to note that the strongest improvements were reported for seizures, attention deficit/hyperactivity and social interaction deficits, especially seen in the 10 patients without epilepsy, nine of whom presented improvement equal to or above 30% in at least one of the eight categories; six presented improvements of 30% or more in at least two categories, and four presented improvements equal to or above 30% in at least four symptom categories. Ten out of the 15 patients were using other medicines, and nine of these were able to keep the improvements even after reducing or withdrawing other medications. These reported results are certainly promising to indicate that CBD-enriched CE may ameliorate multiple ASD symptoms even in patients without epilepsy, with substantial increase in life quality for both ASD patients and caretakers.

In a retrospective study of 60 children (age = 11.8 + 3.5, range 5.0 to 17.5 years) with ASD and severe behavioral problems, CBD-rich cannabis treatment was also safe and improved the behavioral outbreaks in 61% of patients, suggesting feasibility of CBD-based cannabis trials in children with ASD.[93]

To test a hypothesis, that there would be a different fMRI response to CBD in people with autism, in a placebo-controlled, randomized, double-blind, repeated-measure, cross-over study, Pretzsch and colleagues[94] acquired task-free fMRIs in 34 healthy men (half with ASD and no other identified problems) following oral administration of 600 mg CBD or matched placebo. Results showed that CBD significantly increased low frequency fluctuations (fALFF) in the cerebellar vermis and the right fusiform gyrus. However, posthoc within-group analyses revealed that this effect was primarily driven by the ASD group, with no significant change in controls. Within the ASD group only, CBD also significantly altered vermal functional connectivity (FC) with several of its subcortical (striatal) and cortical targets but did not affect fusiform FC with other regions in either group. These data suggest, especially in ASD, that CBD alters regional fALFF and FC in/between regions consistently implicated in ASD. The investigators suggested that future studies should examine if this alteration affects the complex behaviors these regions modulate.

Besides CBD, another nonpsychoactive cannabinoid, a propyl derivative of CBD, cannabidivarin (CBDV), seems to show potential for treating autism spectrum.[95-97] Like the effects of CBD on brain excitatory-inhibitory systems in autism,[98] and based on preclinical evidence, it was suggested that CBDV may also modulate brain excitatory–inhibitory systems, which are implicated in ASD. Thus, Pretzsch and colleagues[99] determined if, within ASD, brain responsivity to CBDV challenge is related to baseline biological phenotype. In a double-blind, randomized-order, cross-over design, they used magnetic resonance spectroscopy (MRS) to compare glutamate (Glx = glutamate + glutamine) and GABA+ (GABA + macromolecules) levels following placebo (baseline) and 600 mg CBDV in 34 healthy (without other identified problems) men with ($N = 17$) and without ($N = 17$) ASD. CBDV significantly increased Glx in the basal ganglia of both groups. However, this effect was not uniform across individuals. In the ASD group, and not in the typically developing controls, the "shift" in Glx correlated negatively with baseline Glx concentration. In contrast, CBDV had no significant impact on Glx in the dorsomedial prefrontal cortex, or on GABA+ in either voxel in either group. These findings suggest that, as measured by MRS, CBDV modulates the glutamate-GABA system in the basal ganglia but not in frontal regions. Moreover, there is individual variation in response depending on baseline biochemistry.

Parkinson Disease

Limited data are available from controlled clinical trials where patients with Parkinson disease (PD) were treated with cannabinoids. In one study of seven patients[100] and in another study of 19 patients,[101] oral nabilone (THC) showed no beneficial effects on the disease. In a more recent study, Lotan et al.[102] treated 22 patients with PD symptoms with smoked cannabis and showed significant improvement of sleep and pain scores without developing any adverse effects. In the case of CBD, in an exploratory double-blind trial, the investigators[103] treated seven PD patients each with either placebo, 75 mg/day CBD or 300 mg/day of CBD and found no significant effect on motor and general symptoms: however, quality of life improved. THCV has been shown to have antioxidant and neuroprotective effects via activation of CB_2 and not blocking CB_1 receptors in rats and mice and thus has potential to reduce motor problems of PD. But currently there is no clinical evidence that THCV could treat patients with PD.[104,105]

In a survey of patients with PD,[106] cannabis use was reported by 8.4% of patients and associated with younger age, living in large cities and better knowledge about the legal and clinical aspects of CUAT. Reduction of pain and muscle cramps was reported by more than 40% of cannabis users. The symptoms like stiffness/akinesia, freezing, tremor, depression, anxiety, and restless legs syndrome subjectively improved for more than 20%, and overall tolerability was good. Improvement of symptoms was reported by 54% of people using CUAT who applied oral CBD and 68% who inhaled THC-containing cannabis. Compared to CBD intake, inhalation of THC was more frequently reported to reduce akinesia and stiffness (50.0% versus 35.4%; $p < 0.05$). Importantly, this was not a clinical trial, but rather a self-report survey from which conclusions about cause and effect cannot be made. Interest in using CUAT was reported by 65% of those not using it. The authors concluded that CUAT is considered as a therapeutic option by many PD patients. However, in a most recent review of the published literature on cannabis or cannabis products for treating PD, Figura and colleagues[107] conclude that currently there is insufficient data to support the use of cannabinoids to treat patients with PD. Larger, randomized studies of cannabis use in PD should be conducted.

Spinal Cord Injuries

Limited data on the efficacy of cannabis or cannabis extract for the treatment of spinal cord injuries are available from three case reports involving a total of 10 patients. In one report of five patients,[108] in another of one patient,[109] and a third of four patients,[110] oral THC or *C. sativa* extract containing cannabidiol or a combination of the two (nabiximols) was associated with some improvement of spasticity muscle spasm, pain, vesical dysfunction and sleep quality.

Brain Injury/Stroke

There is no clinical evidence to suggest that cannabis or any other cannabinoid could treat neuronal injury or stroke in humans at this time. Much more preclinical and clinical research is needed to support the use of CBD or other cannabinoid as a therapeutic agent for treating stroke or brain injury in humans.

Dystonia

Dystonia involves overactivity of muscles required for normal movement, with extra force or activation of nearby but unnecessary muscles, including those that should be turned off to facilitate movement, and is often painful in addition to interfering with function. In an illustrative case, a 52-year-old woman dependent on cannabis and with multiple sclerosis, paroxysmal dystonia, and complex vocal tics, was started on an empirical trial of dronabinol. The patient reported a dramatic reduction of craving and illicit use without experiencing the "high" on dronabinol. She also reported an improvement in the quality of her sleep with diminished awakenings during the night, decreased vocalizations, and the tension associated with their emission, decreased anxiety, and a decreased frequency of *paroxysmal dystonia*.[111] However, in a randomized double-blind cross-over placebo-controlled study of 15 patients, oral THC (nabilone) showed no beneficial effects on generalized and segmental dystonia.[112] In the case of CBD, in a small pilot of 25 patients aged 1 to 17 years with complex motor disorder, two products of CBD enriched 5% oil formulation of cannabis were compared: one with 0.25% THC 20:1 group, the other with 0.83% THC 6:1 group for five months. Significant improvement in spasticity and dystonia, sleep difficulties, pain severity, and QOL was observed in the total study cohort, regardless of treatment assignment. Adverse effects included worsening of seizures in two patients, behavioral changes in two and somnolence in one.[113] Although the current evidence for CBD to treat movement disorders effectively is not strong, CBD does emerge as a compound deserving further study to treat and/or prevent movement disorders.[114]

Gilles de la Tourette Syndrome

A few clinical studies have been conducted by Muller-Vahl and colleagues on patients with Gilles de la Tourette syndrome (GTS).[115-120] In randomized, double-blind, placebo controlled studies involving 12 patients in one study (118) and 24 patients in another study,[117] oral THC (up to 10 mg/day for 6 weeks) significantly reduced the frequency of tics. There were no serious adverse effects; one patient dropped out due to anxiety and agitation. Currently there are no data from additional clinical studies to show if CBD, or any other cannabinoid, alone or a combination of more than one, can treat GTS in humans.

Posttraumatic Stress Disorder

There are a number of psychiatric conditions including PTSD, agitation in Alzheimer disease and Tourette disorder that qualify for state-authorized use of CUAT in many states in the U.S.[121] In a double-blind, randomized, placebo-controlled, cross-over study of patients with PTSD,[122] smoked cannabis was tested at three concentrations of THC (high THC, approximately 12% THC and < 0.05% CBD; high CBD = 11% CBD and 0.50% THC; THC+CBD = approximately 7.9% THC and 8.1% CBD, and placebo = < 0.03% THC and < 0.01% CBD). All treatment groups, including placebo, showed good tolerability and significant improvements in PTSD symptoms during 3 weeks of treatment, but no active treatment statistically outperformed placebo in this brief, preliminary trial. The investigators suggested that additional well-controlled and adequately powered studies with cannabis suitable for FDA drug development are needed to determine whether smoked cannabis improves symptoms of PTSD. On the other hand, a review by the Institute of Medicine[123] showed that there is no credible clinical evidence to support the use of cannabis for any of these conditions. On the contrary, among the 14.6% of 719 male veterans who reported using cannabis in the past 6 months,[124] cannabis use was associated with hazardous alcohol use, tobacco and other drug use, severity of PTSD, severe depression and suicidality.[121] Wilkinson and colleagues[125] and more recently, Bonn-Miller et al.[122] have observed that there is a need to conduct double-blind, randomized, placebo-or-active-controlled studies on the efficacy and safety of cannabis or its active constituent cannabinoids for psychiatric conditions. Thus, the use of cannabis or THC for treating PTSD should be considered carefully before being recommended or prescribed. Considerations should include the adverse physical and psychological adverse effects, hypotensive effects, and development of substance use disorder.

Glaucoma

Cannabinoids, have been investigated as possible anti-glaucoma drugs since the early 1970s.[123,126] In addition, there are several anecdotal reports of treatment of glaucoma with cannabinoids. In earlier studies, Crawford and Merritt[127] showed that 2.8% THC inhaled reduced intra-ocular pressure (IOP), but also increased systolic and diastolic blood pressure in people with glaucoma. The intensity and duration (3-4 hours) of the arterial and ocular pressure responses to THC inhalation were greater in hypertensives (N = 8) than in normotensive patients (N = 8). In a later randomized, balanced, double-blind study, Merritt et al.[128] found that 0.05 and 0.1% THC topically applied was not effective in reducing IOP in patients with open-angle glaucoma. In fact, the smoking of cannabis with higher concentrations of THC (2.5%) resulted in significant hypotension within 5 to 10 minutes of smoking in three patients.[128] The orthostatic episodes that clinically simulated the typical "faint" were characterized by the absence of tachycardia and their relief by assuming a reclining position. Postural hypotension occurred despite differences in inhalation technique, level of delta (9)-THC present in plasma, previous cannabis experience of body habitus. Another study[129] showed that eye drops containing 0.05, and 0.1%, but not the lower 0.01% THC, significantly reduced the IOP. However, there were significant adverse effects such as tachycardia, palpitations, postural hypotension, and alterations in mental status.[130] In fact, the IOP-lowering effects are well correlated with plasma levels of THC after smoking cannabis cigarettes.[131] In another study, Tomida and colleagues[132] showed that a single 5 mg sublingual dose of THC reduced the IOP temporarily and was well tolerated by most patients. Sublingual administration of 20 mg CBD did not reduce IOP, whereas 40 mg CBD produced a transient increase IOP rise. Recently, in an review of the published literature, Passani and colleagues[133] suggest that either orally administered, inhaled, topical or intravenous cannabinoids, particularly THC, do significantly reduce IOP in patients with glaucoma. However, THC lowered the IOP in some patients and was short-lived while in others it failed to lower IOP. In the case of CBD, a sublingual dose of 20 mg CBD did not reduce IOP, whereas 40 mg CBD produced a transient increase in IOP in humans.[132] Colasanti and colleagues[134] tested THC, CBD, cannabigerol, and cannabichromene in rats and cats to determine if one of these would reduce ocular tension. In one study, cannabigerol reduced the ocular tension, but cannabichromene did not,[135] while CBD reduced IOP by about 3 to 4 mm in cats.[136] However, during chronic treatment, the ocular toxicity consisting of conjunctival chemosis, erythema, and hyperemia were sustained, and corneal opacities approximating the site of drug delivery became evident within three to five days. Interestingly, CBD and THC seem to show differential effects on intraocular pressure in mice. Miller and colleagues[137] report on differential effects of THC and CBD on IOP in mice. A single topical application of THC lowered IOP by about 28% in male mice but not in female mice, and via activation of CB_1 and g-protein couple receptors (GPR18) receptors, while CBD prevented THC from lowering IOP. In addition, significant corneal endothelial cell density has been observed in people who chronically used cannabis.[138] More clinical research with other cannabinoids is needed before any can be used to treat glaucoma in humans. But as Sun and colleagues[139] point out, even if THC is developed to treat glaucoma, the frequent use of THC or cannabis for glaucoma might lead to significant adverse effects including development of CUD and/or withdrawal symptoms. The latter outweigh the benefits of its IOP-lowering capacity in glaucoma patients. Thus, the use of cannabis or THC for treating glaucoma should be considered carefully before being recommended or prescribed. Considerations should include the adverse physical and psychological adverse effects, hypotensive effects, and development of substance use disorder. More clinical research, including alternate routes of delivery of THC, CBD, and other cannabinoids, is needed before any can be used to treat glaucoma in humans.

Infections Co-Occurring in Persons With Substance Use Disorders

Cannabis use has a dichotomous relationship with viral infections.[140] On the one hand, people living with chronic viral infections such as HIV, Hepatitis C, and HTLV-1 have increased recreational use of cannabis; on the other hand, cannabis use can predispose one to develop higher risk in acquiring and/or transmitting infections such as HIV. Several investigators have suggested that cannabis use can have undesirable effects on the immune system and exacerbate the frequency of acquisition of bacterial and viral infections, including opportunistic infections.[141-144]

A significant amount of research has been performed in evaluating whether cannabis use is beneficial for patients with viral diseases. Most studies have demonstrated that cannabis use may not influence progression of chronic viral infections, such as HIV infection.[145] Other benefits of using cannabinoid drugs for improving morbidity of people with HIV (PWH) is not supported by clinical trials. Neither have studies shown a benefit for cannabinoids in improving adherence to antiretroviral therapy (ART).[146] In fact, people with cannabis use dependence (DSM-IV) report lower adherence to HIV therapy and greater HIV symptoms/anti-retroviral therapy (ART) side effects than cannabis users and cannabis use-nondependents with HIV[146] suggesting that cannabis use should be discouraged when patients are on anti-retroviral therapy.

There are fewer studies that have shown other beneficial effects of cannabinoid use in PWH. Some studies have also suggested that cannabis use is associated with anti-inflammatory effects and thus, may have a secondary benefit in preventing or hastening end organ damage in chronic HIV infection.[147] This has been best studied with neurocognitive impairment in PWH, where there was a significant improvement in neurocognitive function with cannabis use in PWH.[147] It has been suggested that the antioxidant and anti-inflammatory properties of cannabinoid drugs may justify its use as an adjunct therapy in PWH. It should be noted that there are no major clinical trial data that support this point of view now.

Other chronic viral infections such as hepatitis C are also influenced by cannabinoid use. Recent studies have shown cannabinoid use in chronic hepatitis C patients is associated with progression of liver fibrosis.[148] However, studies have also demonstrated that use of cannabinoids is associated with lower degree of hepatic steatosis among patients with both HIV and HCV infections.[149] This study warrants the need for a larger clinical trial to demonstrate beneficial effects of cannabis on hepatic steatosis.

People who use cannabis acquire viral and bacterial infections.[150] Hence, the impact of cannabinoid use in patients with SARS-CoV-2 or HTLV-I infections, which are associated with significant neurological disability, cannot be ruled out.[151] People who use cannabis may be vulnerable to SARS-CoV-2 infection and worsening of their clinical condition due to COVID-19 and associated morbidity and thus deserve more clinical attention by clinicians worldwide.[152] Ongoing studies will answer the questions of possible adverse effects of cannabinoid use in patients with these diseases.

Substance Use Disorders

Can cannabinoids, especially CBD, be used to treat substance use disorders? Limited research suggests that CBD has potential to treat disorders of substance use including tobacco, cannabis, and opioids. In a study of people who smoke tobacco, a CBD inhaler used over a week reduced the number of tobacco cigarettes by 40% while the placebo did not.[153] In a randomized, double-blind, placebo-controlled cross-over study, a single dose of 800 mg oral dose of CBD, reduced the salience and pleasantness of tobacco cigarette cues, compared with placebo, after overnight tobacco cigarette abstinence in individuals with tobacco use disorder. But CBD did not influence tobacco craving or withdrawal or any subjectively rated side effects.[154,155] On the other hand, CBD at doses of 7.5, 15, or 30 mg/kg/d, without dose-response, did prevent nicotine withdrawal in rats.[156] Additional trials are needed to determine if CBD would reduce the number of cigarettes used and/or reduce the adverse health consequences of tobacco use in people with tobacco use disorder.

In the case of CUD, in an open-label pragmatic trial, Beale and colleagues[157] treated people who regularly used cannabis with 200 mg/day of CBD over a 10-week period. CBD treatment reduced the neuroanatomical damage in the hippocampus without causing any significant adverse side effects thereby suggesting the need for more study of a potential neuroprotective role of CBD against brain structural harm conferred by chronic cannabis use. In a phase 2a, double-blind, placebo-controlled, randomized, adaptive Bayesian trial, Freeman and colleagues[158] also report that synthetic CBD at doses of 400 mg (2 capsules of 100 mg each twice daily) or 800 mg (2 capsules of 200 mg each twice daily) for 4 weeks, compared to placebo, was safe and effective in reducing cannabis use in patients with CUD. The dose of 200 mg was ineffective. In another randomized, double-blind, placebo-controlled trial, nabiximols combined with Motivational Enhancement Therapy and Cognitive-Behavioral Therapy (MET/CBT), was well tolerated and reduced cannabis use and craving but not withdrawal symptoms in people who chronically used cannabis.[159] Future trials with higher doses of CBD were recommended for patients with CUD. In another study of 128 patients with CUD (98 men and 30 women), treatment with placebo or nabiximols (47.5 mg THC+44 mg CBD), combined with psychosocial interventions was found to be a safe approach for reducing cannabis use among individuals with cannabis dependence who are seeking treatment.[160] In a later study, Lintzeris et al.[161] also reported that the benefit of treatment incorporating nabiximols with psychosocial interventions in reducing cannabis use appears to persist for up to three months after the cessation of treatment, proposing a stepped care model of treatment. In yet another double-blind randomized clinical inpatient trial with a 28-day follow-up study,[162] a group of 51 people with DSM-IV-TR cannabis-dependence who were treatment seeking in New South Wales, Australia, a 6-day regimen of nabiximols (maximum daily dose, 86.4 mg of Δ9-THC and 80 mg of CBD) or placebo with standardized psychosocial interventions during a 9-day admission, showed that nabiximols attenuated cannabis withdrawal symptoms and improved patient retention in treatment. However, placebo was as effective as nabiximols in promoting long-term reductions in cannabis use following medication cessation. Nevertheless, the data do support further evaluation of nabiximols for management of CUD and withdrawal in treatment-seeking populations. Solowij and colleagues[163] also reported that CBD was well tolerated by people who chronically used cannabis for at least 6 months without affecting their cognitive or psychological function. The participants reported reduced euphoria when smoking cannabis, significantly fewer depressive and psychoticlike symptoms at posttreatment relative to baseline, and exhibited improvements in attentional switching, verbal learning, and memory. Increased plasma CBD concentrations were associated with improvements in attentional control and beneficial changes in psychological symptoms. Greater benefits were observed in dependent than in nondependent people who used cannabis; however, the authors did not clarify if this was DSM-defined cannabis dependence or simply physiologically dependent. The investigators concluded that prolonged treatment with CBD appeared to have promising therapeutic effects for improving psychological symptoms and cognition in people who regularly used cannabis and that CBD might be a useful adjunct treatment for CUD. CBD also was effective in the treatment of cannabis withdrawal in a 19-year-old woman with cannabis dependence and cannabis withdrawal syndrome.[164] In another case report, since CBD is known to reduce the toxic effects of THC, Shannon and Opilla-Lehman[165] also reported a case of a 27-year-old male with bipolar disorder and addiction to cannabis use where CBD oil decreased the addictive use of cannabis and provide anxiolytic and sleep benefits.[165] Furthermore, research also shows that dronabinol, nabilone, or nabiximols, either alone or in combination with other medications, may have promise in reducing cannabis withdrawal symptoms, probably with a dose-dependent effect.[166]

For opioid use disorder (OUD), Hurd and colleagues[167] reported that CBD reduced the cue-induced craving and anxiety in people with OUD but suggested large clinical trials are needed to confirm its efficacy as a treatment. At the time of this writing, a larger study is in progress.

THE PHYSICIAN'S ROLE IN PRESCRIBING CANNABIS OR CANNABINOIDS USED AS TREATMENT

Physicians in addiction medicine today are confronted with questions from individuals, families, medical colleagues, addiction counselors, community leaders, schoolteachers, and policymakers about the potential therapeutic effects of and controversies about cannabis, CBD, THC, and other cannabinoids. Questions about the source, THC content, efficacy, tolerability, and safety related to varying doses of CBD, THC and other cannabinoids also are of critical importance. Additionally, concerns about unproven and exaggerated medical claims about cannabis products must be understood by addiction physicians, their patients, and the public alike. The impact of the commercial promotion of so-called "medicinal" cannabis on perceptions of cannabis among youth should be of concern to both addiction physicians and the public. In addition to the discussion below, please also see sidebar to Chapter 126, "Legal and Ethical Considerations When Choosing Whether to Recommend Dispensation of "Medical" Marijuana four Your Patient."

As discussed above, both nabilone and dronabinol (synthetic THC) are approved medications for treatment of nausea and vomiting associated with cancer chemotherapy, and for treating appetite stimulant in AIDS-related wasting. CBD is approved for treatment of rare forms of seizures—Lennox-Gastaut Dravet syndromes in young children and seizures from a rare brain tumor. In addition, nabiximols, indicated for chemotherapy induced nausea, intractable cancer pain, and multiple sclerosis, is available in 28 countries including Europe and Canada but not in the U.S. Currently, it is undergoing Phase III clinical trials in the United States. Nabiximols may have an indication for neuropathic pain, however, it is not clear whether its analgesic effect is related to CBD or the combination of CBD and THC. Given the intoxicating and addictive properties of THC, as well as its potential adverse effects on mental health, particularly at high doses with longer durations and earlier onset of initiation, this influence on youth also should be of great concern to addiction physicians. In the case of CBD, although it is not addictive[168] and relatively safe, it is associated with adverse effects including drug-drug interactions, hepatic abnormalities, diarrhea, fatigue, vomiting, and somnolence even at therapeutic doses.[167,169] Also, validity of concentrations of CBD versus THC on product labels are often not regulated by any entity, and thus may be unreliable and invite unwanted exposures to THC. In addition, a case of a 56-year-old man, who suffered profound neurologic, cardiac, and respiratory depression resulting in ICU admission after ingesting 350 mg CBD from seven CBD gummies each containing 50 mg CBD, has been reported.[170] Thus, addiction physicians must be cognizant and wary that the risks and adverse effects of THC and CBD use or recommendation of products containing THC must be weighed against the benefits for any disorder at any dose.

In 2016, the Federation of State Medical Boards, which include 70 state and territorial medical licensing boards in the United States, examined the issue of physicians and CUAT[171] and made recommendations that might be called responsible prescribing. The Board issued ten expectations of licensed physicians who recommend or prescribe cannabis. These are:

1. Patient-physician relationship.
2. Patient evaluation.
3. Informed and shared decision making.
4. Treatment agreement that should review other measures intended to relieve the symptoms.
5. Qualifying conditions.
6. Ongoing monitoring.
7. Consultation and referral of those with a known or suspected history of a substance use disorder or co-occurring mental health disorder with psychiatric, addiction or mental health specialists.
8. Detailed medical records.
9. Lack of any physician conflict of interest.
10. Physician use of cannabis such that the physician does not use cannabis themselves.

The Board recommended that the prescribing physicians should be familiar with the document and its recommendations.

Addiction physicians should also be familiar with the current American Society of Addiction Medicine (ASAM), American Psychiatric Association (APA), American Medical Association (AMA) and World Anti-Doping Agency (WADA) policy statements regarding recreational cannabis, CUAT, CBD, or other cannabinoids. ASAM (https://www.asam.org/advocacy/public-policy-statements/details/public-policy-statements/2020/10/10/cannabis) recommends the following:

1. Cannabis and cannabis-derived products recommended for medical indications should be subject to FDA review and approval to ensure their safety and effectiveness.
2. Healthcare professionals should avoid recommending cannabis to pregnant women, and should recommend cannabis with great caution, if at all, to those with substance use disorders or psychiatric disorders, or to children and adolescents. In fact, CDC also notes that cannabis use by pregnant woman can have teratogenic effects causing birth defects (https://www.cdc.gov/marijuana/factsheets/pregnancy.htm).
3. Healthcare professionals should not recommend cannabis use for the treatment of OUD.
4. Potency of non-FDA approved cannabis should be determined and clearly displayed on the label.
5. Healthcare professionals should consider the ratio of CBD to THC with respect to the indication and minimize potential adverse effects.

On the other hand, the American Psychiatric Association[172] does not find cannabis as beneficial for the treatment of any psychiatric disorder and thus does not endorse CUAT. In fact, APA finds a strong association of cannabis use with the onset of psychiatric disorders, and that adolescents are particularly vulnerable to harm, given the effects of cannabis on neurological development. It recommends additional research on adverse health effects in adolescents. The content and potency of various cannabinoids contained in cannabis can also vary, making dose standardization a challenging task. It recommends that prescribers and patients should be aware that the dosage administered by smoking is related to the depth and duration of the inhalation and therefore difficult to standardize, and that physicians who recommend use of cannabis for "medicinal" purposes should be fully aware of the risks and liabilities inherent in doing so In addition, physicians recommending cannabis to patients should do so within the context of a patient-physician relationship that includes the creation of a medical record and follow-up visits to assess the results of physician-recommended clinical interventions so that treatment plans can be amended, as indicated. ASAM, APA and AMA reject smoking as a means of drug delivery.[173,174] The World Anti-Doping Agency (WADA) has not included CBD on the WADA Prohibited List for athletic competitions (https://www.wada-ama.org/en/prohibited-list). However, The U.S. Food and Drug Administration and Federal Trade Commission have sent letters to cannabis companies warning them against making exaggerated medical claims about CBD.[175,176] The FDA also took issue with the businesses marketing CBD products as dietary supplements. False claims include using CBD to treat the following conditions: alcohol use disorder, Alzheimer disease, arthritis, autism, blood pressure and heart rate, cancer, chronic traumatic encephalopathy, cardiovascular disease, chemotherapy-induced hearing loss, colitis, concussions, depression, diabetes, leukemia, liver inflammation, lupus, Lyme disease, neurological damage, Parkinson disease, stroke, schizophrenia, traumatic brain injury (TBI), and tumors. A physician may prescribe any of these medications for an FDA-approved indication or for an off-label indication. However, based on the evidence reviewed above and as recommended by the Institute of Medicine (IOM), more research is needed from well-designed randomized placebo-controlled clinical trials before physicians prescribe either cannabis, cannabis extract, CBD, or any of the 125 cannabinoids that have not gone through rigorous FDA-required good manufacturing practices (GMP) good clinical practices (GCP), and good laboratory practices (GLP) guidelines, for any clinical condition.

Thus, it behooves addiction physicians to be knowledgeable about the fundamentals of research and clinical practice of prescribing or recommending cannabis and related products including the FDA approved medications, and other cannabis products available at cannabis dispensaries and through the internet. Given the legalization of CUAT in many states, addiction physicians should familiarize themselves about the content of THC, CBD, other cannabinoids in the cannabis plant, and other substances/adulterants that influence the efficacy and safety of the cannabis product that the patient wants prescribed. For example, in the DEA-seized cannabis samples, the concentration of THC significantly changed from 3.96% in 1995 to 14.35%, while that of CBD remained unchanged from 0.28% in 1995 to 0.24% in 2019 (https://nida.nih.gov/research-topics/marijuana/cannabis-marijuana-potency), suggesting that the use of currently available cannabis in dispensaries may be much more potent and may cause serious adverse health consequences. Finally, addiction physician should be familiar with the policy statements and recommendations made by the ASAM and APA, and AMA regarding CUAT and cannabinoids including CBD.

Regarding the impact of CUAT or cannabinoids in the workplace, since cannabis use is associated with cognitive deficits, motivation problems, and perceptual distortions, there should be an effective workplace cannabis policy constructed with a collaborative effort of addiction professionals, labor attorneys, and human resource professionals. Only then can the ultimate workplace cannabis policy comply with relevant laws, protect workplace safety and productivity, and support employees while remaining flexible enough to adapt to changes in the legal environment.[177] Currently, because the evidence to support therapeutic use of cannabinoids for treatment of psychiatric disorders is insufficient, the FDA has not approved cannabis or any of its products for treating any psychiatric indication. However, the evidence supporting cannabinoid prescription beyond the FDA indications is strongest for the management of pain and spasticity. But it must be noted that cannabinoids do have a potential for harm in vulnerable populations such as adolescents and those with psychotic disorders.[178]

We are faced with three important issues. Firstly, since synthetic CBD is now available, and both natural, plant-extracted CBD are pharmacologically similar,[179] it remains to be seen whether synthetic CBD would become the standard chemical in research and/or clinical practice. Secondly, and interestingly, recent genomic research shows that the NIDA-supplied cannabis varieties, used in basic and clinical research, are divergent from the private legal commercial varieties in terms of cannabinoid profile. The NIDA supplied cannabis varieties lack diversity in the single-copy portion of the genome, the maternally inherited genomes, the cannabinoid genes, and in the repetitive content of the genome. Therefore, the investigators[180] conclude that results based on NIDA's varieties are not generalizable regarding the effects of cannabis after consumption. Finally, it is important to note that in its 92-year history, the U.S. FDA has approved only two botanical drugs (whole plant-products—such as sinecatechins, and crofelemer) as medicine, mainly because of immense technical/chemical and other problems in obtaining well-characterized product from chemically complex nature of a plant. Therefore, it seems highly unlikely that the FDA will approve whole cannabis plant or its extract as medicine, since its purified individual chemical components like THC, CBD or other cannabinoids can be more readily obtained and used in research as well as in treatment.

CONCLUSION

Generally, of the hundreds of chemical constituents found in a plant, there is one main pharmacologically active chemical constituent like nicotine (Tobacco plant), cocaine (*Erythroxylon coca*), morphine (*Papaver somniferum*), and so on. But the *C. sativa*, plant appears to be unique in the plant kingdom in that it has not one but several pharmacologically active chemical constituents. There is understandable interest in the *potential* of cannabis or its cannabinoid constituents such as CBD and others discussed above to be utilized as CUAT to treat a wide range of clinical conditions briefly summarized in **Table 126-1**. Based upon this interest, as well as a powerful and growing cannabis industry/financial influence (see Chapter 9, "Impact of the Cannabis Industry on Cannabis Use Disorders"), there has been a strong movement in the U.S. and elsewhere to use or promote CUAT and to legalize it outside of regular channels and laws. This effort has been very successful so that in many states one can go to a pharmacy to fill a

TABLE 126-1 Therapeutic Potential of Cannabinoids Based on Research Reviewed

Cannabinoid	Pharmacologic activity	Potential indication
Cannabidiol	Anti-inflammatory, neuroprotective, antioxidant, cardioprotective, anti-angiogenesis	Anxiety (94[a]), Alzheimer's, autism, depression (61[a]), epilepsy/seizures (44[a]), inflammation, multiple sclerosis (7[a]), pain (64[a]), Parkinson disease (4[a]), trauma, colitis, skin disorders, substance use disorders (15[a])
Cannabichromene	Anti-inflammatory, neuroprotective	Epilepsy, skin disorders
Cannabidivarin	Anti-inflammatory, neuroprotective	Autism, epilepsy, skin disorders,
Tetrahydrocannabivarin	Anti-inflammatory, neuromodulatory, antioxidant, cardioprotective	Cancer, cardiovascular dysfunction, diabetes, neuropathy, nephropathy, pain, retinopathy
Cannabigerol	Anti-inflammatory, neuroprotective, anti-proliferative	Inflammation, pain, multiple sclerosis, colitis, skin disorders, cancer

[a]Number of clinical trials investigating clinical conditions registered at https://clinicaltrials.gov

prescription or go to a dispensary to purchase it for treatment. However, the IOM[181] and the ASAM recommended that additional research be conducted before cannabis is recommended by a physician for an unapproved clinical indication.

As discussed above, data from preclinical, case reports, clinical studies and/or trials showed that oral THC (FDA-approved nabilone or dronabinol) is effective for treating chemotherapy-associated nausea/vomiting. Oral THC is also approved as appetite stimulant in HIV-infected patients. Based on clinical evidence, although Health Canada approved nabiximols for the treatment of neuropathic pain, the U.S. FDA has not approved nabiximols for neuropathic pain yet. Currently, 289 clinical trials are in progress investigating the efficacy of CBD for treating one or more clinical conditions (see **Table 126-1**). But additional well-designed clinical studies and trials, *specific for each clinical indication*, are needed to obtain the FDA approval for CBD and other cannabinoids as CUAT for treating a wide range of clinical indications.

Despite the widespread publicity and many reviews on CUAT, objective review of all the available data suggests that it is premature to draw any definitive conclusions regarding the efficacy of cannabis or cannabinoids as treatment for all the potential clinical indications. Adoption of cannabis in practice by some clinicians may therefore take place in the absence of indications based on well-constructed studies. This can potentially lead to unhealthy use of the drug. Further clinical research to better characterize the pharmacological, physiological, and therapeutic effects of this class of drugs in clinical practice is needed. In addition, a recent review and meta-analysis of 20 published studies[58] showed that a strong placebo response contributed significantly to the perception of pain reduction observed in clinical trials of cannabis-based therapies. The study also suggests that media coverage of cannabis trials may promote high expectations of pain relief in clinical trial participants, thus increasing the placebo effect. Most importantly, the clinical trials for each clinical indication must be carried out in compliance with the FDA's strict guidelines such GLPs, GMPs, and GLPs before any cannabinoid including CBD, but not uncharacterized cannabis plant of unproven clinical efficacy, as therapeutic in clinical practice.

SUMMARY

Overall, synthetic THC (dronabinol) is approved by the U.S. FDA and other regulatory bodies as medication for treating chemotherapy-induced nausea and vomiting, and weight loss in HIV/AIDS-related wasting. A cannabis-derived product, nabiximols (combination of CBD and THC in 1:1 ratio), also has been approved by Health Canada and other health regulatory bodies in the world for treating neuropathic pain. However, for the treatment of other potential clinical conditions such as multiple sclerosis (MS), dystonia, Tourette syndrome, Parkinson disease, or glaucoma, no other cannabis-derived product is approved for lack of sufficient data from clinical trials. Though CB_2 pharmacology is suggestive that the endocannabinoid system may offer targets for PTSD intervention, clinical evidence from randomized clinical trials is lacking. Currently, the "medical product" that is available in the market, has not undergone the required testing complying with the FDA's GMP, GLP and GCP guidelines, and other clinical testing and prescribing requirements of any health regulatory body prior to use in clinical practice. In addition, medical organizations such as the IOM and ASAM recommend that additional research is needed to allow CUAT. Despite the widespread publicity and many reviews on cannabis or CUAT, objective review of the available data suggests that it is premature to draw any definitive conclusions regarding the efficacy of cannabis or CUAT for many of the potential clinical conditions. Adoption of cannabis in practice by some clinicians may therefore take place in the absence of indications based on well-constructed studies. This can potentially lead to unhealthy use of the drug by patients. Before any of these products are used in clinical practice, further clinical research from pivotal well-designed, randomized, double-blind, placebo-controlled trials in compliance with the GLP, GMP and GCP guidelines, with large enough sample size is needed to better characterize the pharmacological, physiological, and therapeutic effects and that have received approval from a health regulatory agency like the U.S. FDA.

KEY POINTS

Synthetic THC (dronabinol) is approved for treating chemotherapy-associated nausea and vomiting.

- Synthetic THC (nabilone) is approved for treating chemotherapy-associated nausea and vomiting; and for stimulating appetite in HIV-infected patients.
- CBD is approved for treating two rare forms of seizures: (1) Lennox-Gastaut and Dravet syndromes in young children, and (2) tuberous sclerosis from a benign brain tumor.
- CBD plus THC in 1:1 ratio (nabiximols) is approved in 28 countries (but not by the United States) for treating MS-associated spasticity/neuropathic pain.
- Although CBD and other cannabinoids may have potential as therapeutics, *none is approved as medicine by the FDA or any other regulatory authority* for any of the several clinical indications that are being promoted. Further, the FDA also has *not approved* cannabis or cannabis extract for any clinical condition.

REFERENCES

1. Watts G. Cannabis confusions. *BMJ Open*. 2006;332:175-176.
2. United Nations. *Single Convention on Narcotic Drugs*. United Nations; 1961.
3. United Nations Office on Drugs and Crime. *World Drug Report*. United Nations; 2021.
4. Substance Abuse and Mental Health Services Administration. *Key Substance Use and Mental Health Indications in the United States: Results from the 2019 National Survey on Drug Use and Health*. Accessed August 7, 2023. https://www.samhsa.gov/data/sites/default/files/reports/rpt29393/2019NSDUHFFRPDFWHTML/2019NSDUHFFR1PDFW090120.pdf

5. Hasin DS, Saha TD, Kerridge BT, et al. Prevalence of marijuana use disorders in the United States Between 2001-2002 and 2012-2013. *JAMA Psychiatry.* 2015;72(12):1235-1242.
6. Lopez-Quintero C, Pérez de los Cobos J, Hasin DS, et al. Probability and predictors of transition from first use to dependence on nicotine, alcohol, cannabis, and cocaine: results of the National Epidemiologic Survey on Alcohol and Related Conditions (NESARC). *Drug Alcohol Depend.* 2011;115(1-2):120-130.
7. Chen CY, O'Brien MS, Anthony JC. Who becomes cannabis dependent soon after onset of use? Epidemiological evidence from the United States: 2000-2001. *Drug Alcohol Depend.* 2005;79(1):11-22.
8. National Institute on Drug Abuse. *Marijuana, Research Report.* 2021. Accessed August 7, 2023. https://nida.nih.gov/publications/research-reports/marijuana/letter-director
9. ElSohly MA, Mehmedic Z, Foster S, Gon C, Chandra S, Church JC. Changes in cannabis potency over the last 2 decades (1995-2014): analysis of current data in the United States. *Biol Psychiatry.* 2016;79(7):613-619.
10. Stuyt E. The problem with the current high potency THC marijuana from the perspective of an addiction psychiatrist. *Mo Med.* 2018;115(6):482-486.
11. Bachman JG, Johnson LD, O'Malley PM. Explaining recent increases in students' marijuana use: impacts of perceived risks and disapproval, 1976 through 1996. *Am J Public Health.* 1998;88(6):887-892.
12. Compton WM, Han B, Jones CM, Blanco C. Cannabis use disorders among adults in the United States during a time of increasing use of cannabis. *Drug Alcohol Depend.* 2019;204:107468.
13. Han B, Compton WM, Jones CM, Blanco C. Cannabis use and cannabis use disorders among youth in the United States, 2002-2014. *J Clin Psychiatry.* 2017;78(9):1404-1413.
14. Radwan MM, Chandra S, Gul S, ElSohly MA. Cannabinoids, phenolics, terpenes and alkaloids of cannabis. *Molecules.* 2021;26(9).
15. Smith DE. Review of the American Medical Association Council on Scientific Affairs report on medical marijuana. *J Psychoactive Drugs.* 1998;30(2):127-136.
16. Kendall DA, Yudowski GA. Cannabinoid receptors in the central nervous system: their signaling and roles in disease. *Front Cell Neurosci.* 2016;10:294.
17. Wei D, Piomelli D. Cannabinoid-based drugs: potential application in addiction and other mental disorders. *Focus.* 2015;13(3):307-316.
18. Izzo AA, Borrelli F, Capasso R, Di Marzo V, Mechoulam R. Non-psychotropic plant cannabinoids: new therapeutic opportunities from an ancient herb. *Trends Pharmacol Sci.* 2009;30(10):515-527.
19. Sholler DJ, Schoene L, Spindle TR. Therapeutic efficacy of cannabidiol (CBD): a review of the evidence from clinical trials and human laboratory studies. *Curr Addict Rep.* 2020;7(3):405-412.
20. Li H. An archaeological and botanical account of cannabis in China. *Econ Bot.* 1974;28:437-448.
21. Gaoni Y, Mechoulam R. The isolation and structure of delta-1-tetrahydrocannabinol and other neutral cannabinoids from hashish. *J Am Chem Soc.* 1971;93(1):217-224.
22. Mechoulam R, Gaoni Y. Recent advances in the chemistry of hashish. *Fortschr Chem Org Naturst.* 1967;25:175-213.
23. Kumar RN, Chambers WA, Pertwee RG. Pharmacological actions and therapeutic uses of cannabis and cannabinoids. *Anaesthesia.* 2001;56(11):1059-1068.
24. Millar SA, Stone NL, Bellman ZD, Yates AS, England TJ, O'Sullivan SE. A systematic review of cannabidiol dosing in clinical populations. *Br J Clin Pharmacol.* 2019;85(9):1888-1900.
25. Millar SA, Stone NL, Yates AS, O'Sullivan SE. A systematic review on the pharmacokinetics of cannabidiol in humans. *Front Pharmacol.* 2018;9:1365.
26. Batalla A, Bos J, Postma A, Bossong MG. The impact of cannabidiol on human brain function: a systematic review. *Front Pharmacol.* 2020;11:618184.
27. Khan R, Naveed S, Mian N, Fida A, Raafey MA, Aedma KK. The therapeutic role of cannabidiol in mental health: a systematic review. *J Cannabis Res.* 2020;2(1):2.
28. Ben AM. Cannabinoids in medicine: a review of their therapeutic potential. *J Ethnopharmacol.* 2006;105(1-2):1-25.
29. Russo EB, Jiang HE, Li X, Sutton A, et al. Phytochemical and genetic analyses of ancient cannabis from Central Asia. *J Exp Bot.* 2008;59(15):4171-4182.
30. Bitencourt RM, Takahashi RN, Carlini EA. From an alternative medicine to a new treatment for refractory epilepsies: can cannabidiol follow the same path to treat neuropsychiatric disorders? *Front Psychiatry.* 2021;12:638032.
31. Food and Drug Administration. *FDA approves Valeant's Cesamet.* Accessed October 30, 2023. https://www.fdanews.com/articles/87057-fda-approves-valeant-s-cesamet
32. Levitt M. Nabilone vs. placebo in the treatment of chemotherapy-induced nausea and vomiting in cancer patients. *Cancer Treat Rev.* 1982;9(Suppl B):49-53.
33. Stuart-Harris RC, Mooney CA, Smith IE. Levonantradol: a synthetic cannabinoid in the treatment of severe chemotherapy-induced nausea and vomiting resistant to conventional anti-emetic therapy. *Clin Oncol.* 1983;9(2):143-146.
34. Chang AE, Shiling DJ, Stillman RC, et al. Delata-9-tetrahydrocannabinol as an antiemetic in cancer patients receiving high-dose methotrexate. A prospective, randomized evaluation. *Ann Intern Med.* 1979;91(6):819-824.
35. Chang AE, Shiling DJ, Stillman RC, et al. A prospective evaluation of delta-9-tetrahydrocannabinol as an antiemetic in patients receiving adriamycin and cytoxan chemotherapy. *Cancer.* 1981;47(7):1746-1751.
36. Levitt MFC, Hawks R, Wilson A. Randomized double-blind comparison of delta-9-tetrahydrocannabinol (THC) and marijuana as chemotherapy antiemetics. *Proceedings of the American Society for Clinical Oncology.* 1984;3:91.
37. Davis MP. Cannabinoids for symptom management and cancer therapy: the evidence. *J Natl Compr Canc Netw.* 2016;14(7):915-922.
38. Walsh KB, McKinney AE, Holmes AE. Minor cannabinoids: biosynthesis, molecular pharmacology and potential therapeutic uses. *Front Pharmacol.* 2021;12:777804.
39. Rock EM, Limebeer CL, Pertwee RG, Mechoulam R, Parker LA. Therapeutic potential of cannabidiol, cannabidiolic acid, and cannabidiolic acid methyl ester as treatments for nausea and vomiting. *Cannabis Cannabinoid Res.* 2021;6(4):266-274.
40. Beal JE, Olson R, Laubenstein L, et al. Dronabinol as a treatment for anorexia associated with weight loss in patients with AIDS. *J Pain Symptom Manage.* 1995;10(2):89-97.
41. Beal JE, Olson R, Lefkowitz L, et al. Long-term efficacy and safety of dronabinol for acquired immunodeficiency syndrome-associated anorexia. *J Pain Symptom Manage.* 1997;14(1):7-14.
42. Jatoi A, Windschitl HE, Loprinzi CL, et al. Dronabinol versus megestrol acetate versus combination therapy for cancer-associated anorexia: a North Central Cancer Treatment Group study. *J Clin Oncol.* 2002;20(2):567-573.
43. Abrams DI, Hilton JF, Leiser RJ, et al. Short-term effects of cannabinoids in patients with HIV-1 infection: a randomized, placebo-controlled clinical trial. *Ann Intern Med.* 2003;139(4):258-266.
44. Spanagel R, Bilbao A. Approved cannabinoids for medical purposes - Comparative systematic review and meta-analysis for sleep and appetite. *Neuropharmacology.* 2021;196:108680.
45. Holdcroft A, Smith M, Jacklin A, et al. Pain relief with oral cannabinoids in familial Mediterranean fever. *Anaesthesia.* 1997;52(5):483-486.
46. Notcutt W, Price M, Miller R, et al. Initial experiences with medicinal extracts of cannabis for chronic pain: results from 34 'N of 1' studies. *Anaesthesia.* 2004;59(5):440-452.
47. Raft D, Gregg J, Ghia J, Harris L. Effects of intravenous tetrahydrocannabinol on experimental and surgical pain. Psychological correlates of the analgesic response. *Clin Pharmacol Ther.* 1977;21(1):26-33.
48. Noyes R Jr, Brunk SF, Avery DA, Canter AC. The analgesic properties of delta-9-tetrahydrocannabinol and codeine. *Clin Pharmacol Ther.* 1975;18(1):84-89.

49. Noyes R Jr, Brunk SF, Baram DA, Canter A. Analgesic effect of delta-9-tetrahydrocannabinol. *J Clin Pharmacol.* 1975;15(2-3):139-143.
50. Staquet M, Gantt C, Machin D. Effect of a nitrogen analog of tetrahydrocannabinol on cancer pain. *Clin Pharmacol Ther.* 1978; 23(4):397-401.
51. Jochimsen PR, Lawton RL, VerSteeg K, Noyes R Jr. Effect of benzopyranoperidine, a delta-9-THC congener, on pain. *Clin Pharmacol Ther.* 1978;24(2):223-227.
52. Jain AK, Ryan JR, McMahon FG, Smith G. Evaluation of intramuscular levonantradol and placebo in acute postoperative pain. *J Clin Pharmacol.* 1981;21(S1):320s-326s.
53. Karst M, Salim K, Burstein S, Conrad I, Hoy L, Schneider U. Analgesic effect of the synthetic cannabinoid CT-3 on chronic neuropathic pain: a randomized controlled trial. *JAMA.* 2003;290(13):1757-1762.
54. Buggy DJ, Toogood L, Maric S, Sharpe P, Lambert DG, Rowbotham DJ. Lack of analgesic efficacy of oral delta-9-tetrahydrocannabinol in postoperative pain. *Pain.* 2003;106(1-2):169-172.
55. Naef M, Curatolo M, Petersen-Felix S, Arendt-Nielsen L, Zbinden A, Brenneisen R. The analgesic effect of oral delta-9-tetrahydrocannabinol (THC), morphine, and a THC-morphine combination in healthy subjects under experimental pain conditions. *Pain.* 2003;105(1-2):79-88.
56. Berman JS, Symonds C, Birch R. Efficacy of two cannabis based medicinal extracts for relief of central neuropathic pain from brachial plexus avulsion: results of a randomised controlled trial. *Pain.* 2004;112(3):299-306.
57. Ware MA, Wang T, Shapiro S, et al. Smoked cannabis for chronic neuropathic pain: a randomized controlled trial. *CMAJ.* 2010;182(14): E694-E701.
58. Gedin F, Blome S, Ponten M, et al. Placebo response and media attention in randomized clinical trials assessing cannabis-based therapies for pain: a systematic review and meta-analysis. *JAMA Netw Open.* 2022;5(11):e2243848.
59. Darkovska-Serafimovska M, Serafimovska T, Arsova-Sarafinovska Z, Stefanoski S, Keskovski Z, Balkanov T. Pharmacotherapeutic considerations for use of cannabinoids to relieve pain in patients with malignant diseases. *J Pain Res.* 2018;11:837-842.
60. Mücke M, Phillips T, Radbruch L, Petzke F, Häuser W. Cannabis-based medicines for chronic neuropathic pain in adults. *Cochrane Database Syst Rev.* 2018;3(3):CD012182.
61. Häuser W, Fitzcharles MA, Radbruch L, Petzke F. Cannabinoids in pain management and palliative medicine. *Dtsch Arztebl Int.* 2017;114(38):627-634.
62. Genaro K, Fabris D, Arantes ALF, Zuardi AW, Crippa JAS, Prado WA. Cannabidiol is a potential therapeutic for the affective-motivational dimension of incision pain in rats. *Front Pharmacol.* 2017;8:391.
63. Gray RA, Whalley BJ. The proposed mechanisms of action of CBD in epilepsy. *Epileptic Disord.* 2020;22(S1):10-15.
64. Carlini EA, Cunha JM. Hypnotic and antiepileptic effects of cannabidiol. *J Clin Pharmacol.* 1981;21(S1):417s-427s.
65. Caraballo R, Reyes G, Demirdjian G, Huaman M, Gutierrez R. Long-term use of cannabidiol-enriched medical cannabis in a prospective cohort of children with drug-resistant developmental and epileptic encephalopathy. *Seizure.* 2022;95:56-63.
66. Tzadok M, Uliel-Siboni S, Linder I, et al. CBD-enriched medical cannabis for intractable pediatric epilepsy: the current Israeli experience. *Seizure.* 2016;35:41-44.
67. Cunha JM, Carlini EA, Pereira AE, et al. Chronic administration of cannabidiol to healthy volunteers and epileptic patients. *Pharmacology.* 1980;21(3):175-185.
68. Devinsky O, Marsh E, Friedman D, et al. Cannabidiol in patients with treatment-resistant epilepsy: an open-label interventional trial. *Lancet Neurol.* 2016;15(3):270-278.
69. Anderson CL, Evans V, Gorham L, Liu Z, Johnson CR, Carney PR. Seizure frequency, quality of life, behavior, cognition, and sleep in pediatric patients enrolled in a prospective, open-label clinical study with cannabidiol. *Epilepsy Behav.* 2021;124:108325.
70. Bialer M, Johannessen SI, Levy RH, Perucca E, Tomson T, White HS. Progress report on new antiepileptic drugs: a summary of the Twelfth Eilat Conference (EILAT XII). *Epilepsy Res.* 2015;111:85-141.
71. Hill AJ, Mercier MS, Hill TD, et al. Cannabidivarin is anticonvulsant in mouse and rat. *Br J Pharmacol.* 2012;167(8):1629-1642.
72. Hill TD, Cascio MG, Romano B, et al. Cannabidivarin-rich cannabis extracts are anticonvulsant in mouse and rat via a CB1 receptor-independent mechanism. *Br J Pharmacol.* 2013;170(3):679-692.
73. Morano A, Cifelli P, Nencini P, et al. Cannabis in epilepsy: from clinical practice to basic research focusing on the possible role of cannabidivarin. *Epilepsia Open.* 2016;1(3-4):145-151.
74. Amada N, Yamasaki Y, Williams CM, Whalley BJ. Cannabidivarin (CBDV) suppresses pentylenetetrazole (PTZ)-induced increases in epilepsy-related gene expression. *PeerJ.* 2013;1:e214.
75. Hill AJ, Weston SE, Jones NA, et al. Δ^9-Tetrahydrocannabivarin suppresses in vitro epileptiform and in vivo seizure activity in adult rats. *Epilepsia.* 2010;51(8):1522-1532.
76. Gaston TE, Friedman D. Pharmacology of cannabinoids in the treatment of epilepsy. *Epilepsy Behav.* 2017;70(Pt B):313-318.
77. Zajicek J, Fox P, Sanders H, et al. Cannabinoids for treatment of spasticity and other symptoms related to multiple sclerosis (CAMS study): multicentre randomised placebo-controlled trial. *Lancet.* 2003;362(9395):1517-1526.
78. Zajicek JP, Sanders HP, Wright DE, et al. Cannabinoids in multiple sclerosis (CAMS) study: safety and efficacy data for 12 months follow up. *J Neurol Neurosurg Psychiatry.* 2005;76(12):1664-1669.
79. Wade DT, Makela P, Robson P, House H, Bateman C. Do cannabis-based medicinal extracts have general or specific effects on symptoms in multiple sclerosis? A double-blind, randomized, placebo-controlled study on 160 patients. *Mult Scler.* 2004;10(4):434-441.
80. Rog DJ, Nurmikko TJ, Friede T, Young CA. Randomized, controlled trial of cannabis-based medicine in central pain in multiple sclerosis. *Neurology.* 2005;65(6):812-819.
81. Lus G, Cantello R, Danni MC, et al. Palatability and oral cavity tolerability of THC:CBD oromucosal spray and possible improvement measures in multiple sclerosis patients with resistant spasticity: a pilot study. *Neurodegener Dis Manag.* 2018;8(2):105-113.
82. Markovà J, Essner U, Akmaz B, et al. Sativex(®) as add-on therapy vs. further optimized first-line ANTispastics (SAVANT) in resistant multiple sclerosis spasticity: a double-blind, placebo-controlled randomised clinical trial. *Int J Neurosci.* 2019;129(2):119-128.
83. Celius EG, Vila C. The influence of THC:CBD oromucosal spray on driving ability in patients with multiple sclerosis-related spasticity. *Brain Behav.* 2018;8(5):e00962.
84. Vermersch P, Trojano M. Tetrahydrocannabinol:cannabidiol oromucosal spray for multiple sclerosis-related resistant spasticity in daily practice. *Eur Neurol.* 2016;76(5-6):216-226.
85. Rudroff T, Sosnoff J. Cannabidiol to improve mobility in people with multiple sclerosis. *Front Neurol.* 2018;9:183.
86. Granja AG, Carrillo-Salinas F, Pagani A, et al. A cannabigerol quinone alleviates neuroinflammation in a chronic model of multiple sclerosis. *J Neuroimmune Pharmacol.* 2012;7(4):1002-1016.
87. Holdman R, Vigil D, Robinson K, Shah P, Contreras AE. Safety and efficacy of medical cannabis in autism spectrum disorder compared with commonly used medications. *Cannabis Cannabinoid Res.* 2022;7(4):451-463.
88. Fusar-Poli L, Cavone V, Tinacci S, et al. Cannabinoids for people with ASD: a systematic review of published and ongoing studies. *Brain Sci.* 2020;10(9):572.
89. Ganesh A, Shareef S. Safety and efficacy of cannabis in autism spectrum disorder. *Pediatr Neurol Briefs.* 2020;34:25.
90. Hua DY, Lees R, Brosnan M, Freeman TP. Cannabis and cannabidiol use among autistic and non-autistic adults in the UK: a propensity score-matched analysis. *BMJ Open.* 2021;11(12):e053814.
91. Bilge S, Ekici B. CBD-enriched cannabis for autism spectrum disorder: an experience of a single center in Turkey and reviews of the literature. *J Cannabis Res.* 2021;3(1):53.

92. Fleury-Teixeira P, Caixeta FV, Ramires da Silva LC, Brasil-Neto JP, Malcher-Lopes R. Effects of CBD-enriched *Cannabis sativa* extract on autism spectrum disorder symptoms: an observational study of 18 participants undergoing compassionate use. *Front Neurol.* 2019;10:1145.
93. Aran A, Cassuto H, Lubotzky A, Wattad N, Hazan E. Brief report: cannabidiol-rich cannabis in children with autism spectrum disorder and severe behavioral problems-a retrospective feasibility study. *J Autism Dev Disord.* 2019;49(3):1284-1288.
94. Pretzsch CM, Voinescu B, Mendez MA, et al. The effect of cannabidiol (CBD) on low-frequency activity and functional connectivity in the brain of adults with and without autism spectrum disorder (ASD). *J Psychopharmacol.* 2019;33(9):1141-1148.
95. Zamberletti E, Rubino T, Parolaro D. Therapeutic potential of cannabidivarin for epilepsy and autism spectrum disorder. *Pharmacol Ther.* 2021;226:107878.
96. Loss CM, Teodoro L, Rodrigues GD, et al. Is cannabidiol during neurodevelopment a promising therapy for schizophrenia and autism spectrum disorders? *Front Pharmacol.* 2020;11:635763.
97. Alves P, Amaral C, Teixeira N, Correia-da-Silva G. *Cannabis sativa*: much more beyond Δ(9)-tetrahydrocannabinol. *Pharmacol Res.* 2020;157:104822.
98. Pretzsch CM, Freyberg J, Voinescu B, et al. Effects of cannabidiol on brain excitation and inhibition systems; a randomised placebo-controlled single dose trial during magnetic resonance spectroscopy in adults with and without autism spectrum disorder. *Neuropsychopharmacology.* 2019;44(8):1398-1405.
99. Pretzsch CM, Voinescu B, Lythgoe D, et al. Effects of cannabidivarin (CBDV) on brain excitation and inhibition systems in adults with and without Autism Spectrum Disorder (ASD): a single dose trial during magnetic resonance spectroscopy. *Transl Psychiatry.* 2019;9(1):313.
100. Sieradzan KA, Fox SH, Hill M, Dick JP, Crossman AR, Brotchie JM. Cannabinoids reduce levodopa-induced dyskinesia in Parkinson's disease: a pilot study. *Neurology.* 2001;57(11):2108-2111.
101. Carroll CB, Bain PG, Teare L, et al. Cannabis for dyskinesia in Parkinson disease: a randomized double-blind crossover study. *Neurology.* 2004;63(7):1245-1250.
102. Lotan I, Treves TA, Roditi Y, Djaldetti R. Cannabis (medical marijuana) treatment for motor and non-motor symptoms of Parkinson disease: an open-label observational study. *Clin Neuropharmacol.* 2014;37(2):41-44.
103. Chagas MH, Zuardi AW, Tumas V, et al. Effects of cannabidiol in the treatment of patients with Parkinson's disease: an exploratory double-blind trial. *J Psychopharmacol.* 2014;28(11):1088-1098.
104. García C, Palomo-Garo C, García-Arencibia M, Ramos J, Pertwee R, Fernández-Ruiz J. Symptom-relieving and neuroprotective effects of the phytocannabinoid Δ^9-THCV in animal models of Parkinson's disease. *Br J Pharmacol.* 2011;163(7):1495-1506.
105. Espadas I, Keifman E, Palomo-Garo C, et al. Beneficial effects of the phytocannabinoid Δ(9)-THCV in L-DOPA-induced dyskinesia in Parkinson's disease. *Neurobiol Dis.* 2020;141:104892.
106. Yenilmez F, Fründt O, Hidding U, Buhmann C. Cannabis in Parkinson's disease: the patients' view. *J Parkinsons Dis.* 2021;11(1):309-321.
107. Figura M, Koziorowski D, Sławek J. Cannabis in Parkinson's Disease - the patient's perspective versus clinical trials: a systematic literature review. *Neurol Neurochir Pol.* 2022;56(1):21-27.
108. Hanigan WCDR, Truong XT. The effects of delta-9-THC on human spasticity. *Clinic Pharmacol Ther.* 1986;39:198.
109. Maurer M, Henn V, Dittrich A, Hofmann A. Delta-9-tetrahydrocannabinol shows antispastic and analgesic effects in a single case double-blind trial. *Eur Arch Psychiatry Clin Neurosci.* 1990;240(1):1-4.
110. Wade DT, Robson P, House H, Makela P, Aram J. A preliminary controlled study to determine whether whole-plant cannabis extracts can improve intractable neurogenic symptoms. *Clin Rehabil.* 2003;17(1):21-29.
111. Deutsch SI, Rosse RB, Connor JM, Burket JA, Murphy ME, Fox FJ. Current status of cannabis treatment of multiple sclerosis with an illustrative case presentation of a patient with MS, complex vocal tics, paroxysmal dystonia, and marijuana dependence treated with dronabinol. *CNS Spectr.* 2008;13(5):393-403.
112. Fox SH, Kellett M, Moore AP, Crossman AR, Brotchie JM. Randomised, double-blind, placebo-controlled trial to assess the potential of cannabinoid receptor stimulation in the treatment of dystonia. *Mov Disord.* 2002;17(1):145-149.
113. Libzon S, Schleider LB, Saban N, et al. Medical cannabis for pediatric moderate to severe complex motor disorders. *J Child Neurol.* 2018;33(9):565-571.
114. Peres FF, Lima AC, Hallak JEC, Crippa JA, Silva RH, Abílio VC. Cannabidiol as a promising strategy to treat and prevent movement disorders? *Front Pharmacol.* 2018;9:482.
115. Müller-Vahl KR, Koblenz A, Jöbges M, Kolbe H, Emrich HM, Schneider U. Influence of treatment of Tourette syndrome with delta9-tetrahydrocannabinol (delta9-THC) on neuropsychological performance. *Pharmacopsychiatry.* 2001;34(1):19-24.
116. Müller-Vahl KR, Kolbe H, Schneider U, Emrich HM. Cannabinoids: possible role in patho-physiology and therapy of Gilles de la Tourette syndrome. *Acta Psychiatr Scand.* 1998;98(6):502-506.
117. Müller-Vahl KR, Prevedel H, Theloe K, Kolbe H, Emrich HM, Schneider U. Treatment of Tourette syndrome with delta-9-tetrahydrocannabinol (delta 9-THC): no influence on neuropsychological performance. *Neuropsychopharmacology.* 2003;28(2):384-388.
118. Müller-Vahl KR, Schneider U, Koblenz A, et al. Treatment of Tourette's syndrome with delta 9-tetrahydrocannabinol (THC): a randomized crossover trial. *Pharmacopsychiatry.* 2002;35(2):57-61.
119. Müller-Vahl KR, Schneider U, Kolbe H, Emrich HM. Treatment of Tourette's syndrome with delta-9-tetrahydrocannabinol. *Am J Psychiatry.* 1999;156(3):495.
120. Müller-Vahl KR, Schneider U, Prevedel H, et al. Delta 9-tetrahydrocannabinol (THC) is effective in the treatment of tics in Tourette syndrome: a 6-week randomized trial. *J Clin Psychiatry.* 2003;64(4):459-465.
121. Gentes EL, Schry AR, Hicks TA, et al. Prevalence and correlates of cannabis use in an outpatient VA posttraumatic stress disorder clinic. *Psychol Addict Behav.* 2016;30(3):415-421.
122. Bonn-Miller MO, Sisley S, Riggs P, et al. The short-term impact of 3 smoked cannabis preparations versus placebo on PTSD symptoms: a randomized cross-over clinical trial. *PLoS One.* 2021;16(3):e0246990.
123. Watson SJ, Benson JA Jr, Joy JE. Marijuana and medicine: assessing the science base: a summary of the 1999 Institute of Medicine report. *Arch Gen Psychiatry.* 2000;57(6):547-552.
124. Krumm BA. Cannabis for posttraumatic stress disorder: A neurobiological approach to treatment. *Nurse Pract.* 2016;41(1):50-54.
125. Wilkinson ST, Radhakrishnan R, D'Souza DC. A systematic review of the evidence for medical marijuana in psychiatric indications. *J Clin Psychiatry.* 2016;77(8):1050-1064.
126. Tomida I, Pertwee RG, Azuara-Blanco A. Cannabinoids and glaucoma. *Br J Ophthalmol.* 2004;88(5):708-713.
127. Crawford WJ, Merritt JC. Effects of tetrahydrocannabinol on arterial and intraocular hypertension. *Int J Clin Pharmacol Biopharm.* 1979;17(5):191-196.
128. Merritt JC, Cook CE, Davis KH. Orthostatic hypotension after delta 9-tetrahydrocannabinol marihuana inhalation. *Ophthalmic Res.* 1982;14(2):124-128.
129. Merritt JC, Crawford WJ, Alexander PC, Anduze AL, Gelbart SS. Effect of marihuana on intraocular and blood pressure in glaucoma. *Ophthalmology.* 1980;87(3):222-228.
130. Merritt JC, Olsen JL, Armstrong JR, McKinnon SM. Topical delta 9-tetrahydrocannabinol in hypertensive glaucomas. *J Pharm Pharmacol.* 1981;33(1):40-41.
131. Mosaed S, Smith AK, Liu JHK, et al. The relationship between plasma tetrahydrocannabinol levels and intraocular pressure in healthy adult subjects. *Front Med (Lausanne).* 2021;8:736792.
132. Tomida I, Azuara-Blanco A, House H, Flint M, Pertwee RG, Robson PJ. Effect of sublingual application of cannabinoids on intraocular pressure: a pilot study. *J Glaucoma.* 2006;15(5):349-353.

133. Passani A, Posarelli C, Sframeli AT, et al. Cannabinoids in glaucoma patients: the never-ending story. *J Clin Med.* 2020;9(12):3978.
134. Colasanti BK, Craig CR, Allara RD. Intraocular pressure, ocular toxicity and neurotoxicity after administration of cannabinol or cannabigerol. *Exp Eye Res.* 1984;39(3):251-259.
135. Colasanti BK, Powell SR, Craig CR. Intraocular pressure, ocular toxicity and neurotoxicity after administration of delta 9-tetrahydrocannabinol or cannabichromene. *Exp Eye Res.* 1984;38(1):63-71.
136. Colasanti BK, Brown RE, Craig CR. Ocular hypotension, ocular toxicity, and neurotoxicity in response to marihuana extract and cannabidiol. *Gen Pharmacol.* 1984;15(6):479-484.
137. Miller S, Daily L, Leishman E, Bradshaw H, Straiker A. Δ9-Tetrahydrocannabinol and cannabidiol differentially regulate intraocular pressure. *Invest Ophthalmol Vis Sci.* 2018;59(15):5904-5911.
138. Polat N, Cumurcu B, Cumurcu T, Tuncer İ. Corneal endothelial changes in long-term cannabinoid users. *Cutan Ocul Toxicol.* 2018;37(1):19-23.
139. Sun X, Xu CS, Chadha N, Chen A, Liu J. Marijuana for glaucoma: a recipe for disaster or treatment? *Yale J Biol Med.* 2015;88(3):265-269.
140. Maggirwar SB, Khalsa JH. The link between cannabis use, immune system, and viral infections. *Viruses.* 2021;13(6):1099.
141. Rom S, Persidsky Y. Cannabinoid receptor 2: potential role in immunomodulation and neuroinflammation. *J Neuroimmune Pharmacol.* 2013;8(3):608-620.
142. Henriquez JE, Rizzo MD, Crawford RB, Gulick P, Kaminski NE. Interferon-α-mediated activation of T cells from healthy and HIV-infected individuals is suppressed by δ(9)-tetrahydrocannabinol. *J Pharmacol Exp Ther.* 2018;367(1):49-58.
143. Rizzo MD, Henriquez JE, Blevins LK, Bach A, Crawford RB, Kaminski NE. Targeting cannabinoid receptor 2 on peripheral leukocytes to attenuate inflammatory mechanisms implicated in HIV-associated neurocognitive disorder. *J Neuroimmune Pharmacol.* 2020;15(4):780-793.
144. Abrams DI, Guzman M. Cannabis in cancer care. *Clin Pharmacol Ther.* 2015;97(6):575-586.
145. Kaslow RA, Blackwelder WC, Ostrow DG, et al. No evidence for a role of alcohol or other psychoactive drugs in accelerating immunodeficiency in HIV-1-positive individuals. A report from the Multicenter AIDS Cohort Study. *JAMA.* 1989;261(23):3424-3429.
146. Bonn-Miller MO, Oser ML, Bucossi MM, Trafton JA. Cannabis use and HIV antiretroviral therapy adherence and HIV-related symptoms. *J Behav Med.* 2014;37(1):1-10.
147. Watson CW, Paolillo EW, Morgan EE, et al. Cannabis exposure is associated with a lower likelihood of neurocognitive impairment in people living with HIV. *J Acquir Immune Defic Syndr.* 2020;83(1):56-64.
148. Hézode C, Roudot-Thoraval F, Nguyen S, et al. Daily cannabis smoking as a risk factor for progression of fibrosis in chronic hepatitis C. *Hepatology.* 2005;42(1):63-71.
149. Nordmann S, Vilotitch A, Roux P, et al. Daily cannabis and reduced risk of steatosis in human immunodeficiency virus and hepatitis C virus-co-infected patients (ANRS CO13-HEPAVIH). *J Viral Hepat.* 2018;25(2):171-179.
150. Reiss CS. Cannabinoids and viral infections. *Pharmaceuticals (Basel).* 2010;3(6):1873-1886.
151. Khalsa JH, Bunt G, Maggirwar SB, Kottilil S. COVID-19 and cannabidiol (CBD). *J Addict Med.* 2021;15(5):355-356.
152. Borgonhi EM, Volpatto VL, Ornell F, Rabelo-da-Ponte FD, Kessler FHP. Multiple clinical risks for cannabis users during the COVID-19 pandemic. *Addict Sci Clin Pract.* 2021;16(1):5.
153. Morgan CJ, Das RK, Joye A, Curran HV, Kamboj SK. Cannabidiol reduces cigarette consumption in tobacco smokers: preliminary findings. *Addict Behav.* 2013;38(9):2433-2436.
154. Hindocha C, Freeman TP, Grabski M, et al. The effects of cannabidiol on impulsivity and memory during abstinence in cigarette dependent smokers. *Sci Rep.* 2018;8(1):7568.
155. Hindocha C, Freeman TP, Grabski M, et al. Cannabidiol reverses attentional bias to cigarette cues in a human experimental model of tobacco withdrawal. *Addiction.* 2018;113(9):1696-1705.
156. Smith LC, Tieu L, Suhandynata RT, et al. Cannabidiol reduces withdrawal symptoms in nicotine-dependent rats. *Psychopharmacology (Berl).* 2021;238(8):2201-2211.
157. Beale C, Broyd SJ, Chye Y, et al. Prolonged cannabidiol treatment effects on hippocampal subfield volumes in current cannabis users. *Cannabis Cannabinoid Res.* 2018;3(1):94-107.
158. Freeman TP, Hindocha C, Baio G, et al. Cannabidiol for the treatment of cannabis use disorder: a phase 2a, double-blind, placebo-controlled, randomised, adaptive Bayesian trial. *Lancet Psychiatry.* 2020;7(10):865-874.
159. Trigo JM, Soliman A, Quilty LC, et al. Nabiximols combined with motivational enhancement/cognitive behavioral therapy for the treatment of cannabis dependence: a pilot randomized clinical trial. *PLoS One.* 2018;13(1):e0190768.
160. Lintzeris N, Bhardwaj A, Mills L, et al. Nabiximols for the treatment of cannabis dependence: a randomized clinical trial. *JAMA Intern Med.* 2019;179(9):1242-1253.
161. Lintzeris N, Mills L, Dunlop A, et al. Cannabis use in patients 3 months after ceasing nabiximols for the treatment of cannabis dependence: results from a placebo-controlled randomised trial. *Drug Alcohol Depend.* 2020;215:108220.
162. Allsop DJ, Copeland J, Lintzeris N, et al. Nabiximols as an agonist replacement therapy during cannabis withdrawal: a randomized clinical trial. *JAMA Psychiatry.* 2014;71(3):281-291.
163. Solowij N, Broyd SJ, Beale C, et al. Therapeutic effects of prolonged cannabidiol treatment on psychological symptoms and cognitive function in regular cannabis users: a pragmatic open-label clinical trial. *Cannabis Cannabinoid Res.* 2018;3(1):21-34.
164. Crippa JA, Hallak JE, Machado-de-Sousa JP, et al. Cannabidiol for the treatment of cannabis withdrawal syndrome: a case report. *J Clin Pharm Ther.* 2013;38(2):162-164.
165. Shannon S, Opila-Lehman J. Cannabidiol oil for decreasing addictive use of marijuana: a case report. *Integr Med (Encinitas).* 2015;14(6):31-35.
166. Werneck MA, Kortas GT, de Andrade AG, Castaldelli-Maia JM. A systematic review of the efficacy of cannabinoid agonist replacement therapy for cannabis withdrawal symptoms. *CNS Drugs.* 2018;32(12):1113-1129.
167. Hurd YL, Spriggs S, Alishayev J, et al. Cannabidiol for the reduction of cue-induced craving and anxiety in drug-abstinent individuals with heroin use disorder: a double-blind randomized placebo-controlled trial. *Am J Psychiatry.* 2019;176(11):911-922.
168. WHO. *Cannabidiol Critical Review Report WHO Expert Committee on Drug Dependence Fortieth Meeting Geneva*, June 4-7, 2018.
169. Huestis MA, Solimini R, Pichini S, Pacifici R, Carlier J, Busardò FP. Cannabidiol adverse effects and toxicity. *Curr Neuropharmacol.* 2019;17(10):974-989.
170. Bass J, Linz DR. A case of toxicity from cannabidiol gummy ingestion. *Cureus.* 2020;12(4):e7688.
171. Chaudhry HJ, Hengerer AS, Snyder GB. Medical board expectations for physicians recommending marijuana. *JAMA.* 2016;316(6):577-578.
172. American Psychiatric Association. *Position Statement in Opposition to Cannabis as Medicine.* APA; 2019.
173. Anonymous. Cannabis and Cannabinoids. *JAMA.* 2016;316(22):2424-2425.
174. Marlowe DB. Malpractice liability and medical marijuana. *The Health Lawyer.* 2016;29:1-3.
175. Food and Drug Administration. *Warning Letters and Test Results for Cannabidiol-Related Products.* FDA; 2022.
176. Federal Trade Commission. *FTC Sends Warning Letters to Companies Advertising their CBD-Infused Products as Treatments for Serious Conditions Including Cancer, Alzheimer's and Multiple Sclerosis.* Accessed August 7, 2023. https://www.ftc.gov/news-events/news/press-releases/2019/09/ftc-sends-warning-letters-companies-advertising-their-cbd-infused-products-treatments-serious
177. Hazle MC, Hill KP, Westreich LM. Workplace cannabis policies: a moving target. *Cannabis Cannabinoid Res.* 2022;7(1):16-23.

178. Hill KP, Gold MS, Nemeroff CB, et al. Risks and benefits of cannabis and cannabinoids in psychiatry. *Am J Psychiatry*. 2022;179(2):98-109.
179. Maguire RF, Wilkinson DJ, England TJ, O'Sullivan SE. The pharmacological effects of plant-derived versus synthetic cannabidiol in human cell lines. *Med Cannabis Cannabinoids*. 2021;4(2):86-96.
180. Vergara D, Huscher EL, Keepers KG, et al. Genomic evidence that governmentally produced cannabis sativa poorly represents genetic variation available in state markets. *Front Plant Sci*. 2021;12:668315.
181. National Academies of Sciences Engineering, and Medicine; Health and Medicine Division; Board on Population Health and Public Health Practice; Committee on the Health Effects of Marijuana: An Evidence Review and Research Agenda. *The Health Effects of Cannabis and Cannabinoids: The Current State of Evidence and Recommendations for Research*. Accessed August 7, 2023. https://www.ncbi.nlm.nih.gov/books/NBK423845/

Sidebar

Legal and Ethical Considerations for Clinicians Recommending Cannabis Used as Treatment

Nassima Ait-Daoud Tiouririne and Jeffrey Katra

Most states that allow cannabis used as treatment (CUAT) usually permit it for conditions like chronic pain, anxiety, posttraumatic stress disorder (PTSD), dementia, seizures, neuromuscular disorders, cancer, glaucoma, inflammatory bowel disease, opioid use disorder, HIV, and autism spectrum disorder.[1] The decision for physicians to recommend or not recommend CUAT is a tricky one. It is illegal for providers to "prescribe" or authorize the use of cannabis as treatment, but is it ethical to withhold a cannabis authorization from a suffering patient when other treatment modalities have failed, and data indicate some level of cannabis efficacy? Is it ethical to offer a treatment when the evidence supporting effectiveness is limited, poor, or clearly shows no benefit, and assessment for risks is either not well-studied, not well-discussed, or both? The therapeutic effectiveness of cannabis and cannabinoids is fairly limited in scope and impact (more so than what some states have approved, as outlined above. See Chapter 126, "Therapeutic Effectiveness of Cannabis and Cannabinoids," for a review).

LEGALITY OF A CANNABIS RECOMMENDATION FROM A MEDICAL CLINICIAN

For most states, once a licensed clinician with prescriptive authority writes a patient a recommendation for CUAT, the patient must register with their state's database to obtain a "marijuana ID card," that allows them to purchase various forms of cannabis from a dispensary of their choice. The card allows a patient to obtain or possibly even grow cannabis without violating state law but provides no protection against violations of federal law.[2]

Currently, it is illegal for medical clinicians to "*prescribe*" cannabis even in states where it is legal because of its DEA Schedule I status. However, in states where CUAT is legal, "recommending" providers are making a recommendation and are attesting that they determined the patient suffers from one of the conditions cannabis is approved for; and ideally that certain contraindications are not problematic, that the benefits outweigh the risks of CUAT, and that an informed consent has been given to the patient about the risks, benefits, and side effects. However, whether these latter actions are being completed is largely unknown.

A federal court decision examined the differences between a "prescription" for CUAT and a "recommendation" and determined that while a cannabis prescription is illegal, a recommendation is different and is allowed. This "loophole" was upheld by the U.S. Court of Appeals for the Ninth Circuit in *Conant v. Walters 2002*, which affirmed the right of physicians to recommend CUAT (referred to in the case as "medical marijuana"). A physician discussing the potential benefits of "medicinal marijuana" and making such recommendations constitute protected speech under the First Amendment.[3] The U.S. (2002) Supreme Court refused to hear an appeal of the case.[3]

Accordingly, any state requiring that providers "prescribe" cannabis would expose them to criminal liability. Requiring a "prescription" or requiring physicians to specify dosage likely crosses the line from recommending to prescribing, which is illegal. By contrast, a "recommendation" that a patient has a state qualifying condition and could benefit from medical cannabis is permissible.[4]

These rulings however bypass the Food and Drug Administration's (FDA) processes that are meant to ensure both efficacy and safety. Physicians may discuss merits and risks of over the counter medications and dietary supplements with their patients based upon the known research and evidence base for the respective clinical condition.[5] However, even aspirin may be more regulated than CUAT as evidenced by the Code of Federal Regulations for its human use.[6]

ETHICAL CONSIDERATIONS

The ethical principles guiding patient care and treatment with cannabis should be akin to those of drugs for medical use, including ensuring a favorable benefit-to-risk ratio, fully informed consent, and careful monitoring for safety and side effects. The term "medical" infers[1] that the ingredients are well-defined and measurable (yet, cannabis has over 125 ingredients which vary),[7] ingredients should be consistent from one dose to the next,[8] indications for use should be reasonably evidence-based,[9] with well-established safe dosing ranges, and have clinical warnings and precautions within the product labeling[10]; and are prescribed and clinically supervised throughout care by a medically trained professional with expertise in the condition for which the patient is seeking treatment.[11] As well, clinicians recommending CUAT may still be held to medical malpractice risks and standards.

A primary ethical concern is whether the benefits of medical use of cannabis exceed its known risks. CUAT has not undergone any FDA or health regulatory body review before making claims about its benefits, assessment for risks, and monitoring of marketing practices. There is also concern that, without clinical trials or postmarketing surveillance as well as clinical reporting, adverse effects of cannabis may still be unreported and unknown. Many of the published trials are compromised by their small sample sizes, heterogeneous populations, and importantly, differing delivery vehicles and concentrations of the major cannabis compounds.[5] While there is some data supporting that cannabis may have some therapeutic benefits for patients with chronic neuropathic pain, chemotherapy-induced nausea and vomiting, and severe multiple sclerosis symptoms,[12] there remains some debate. Again, the reader is referred to Chapter 126 for a review of each of the possible uses of cannabis. A recent review and meta-analysis of 20 published studies showed that a strong placebo response contributed significantly to the perception of pain reduction observed in clinical trials of cannabis-based therapies. The study also suggests that media coverage of cannabis trials may promote high expectations of pain relief in clinical trial participants, thus increasing the placebo effect.[13]

Another ethical concern is how cannabis is governed by state laws. The laws of some states have been very noncommittal in their specification on what and how to "*prescribe*," to avoid the trap of prescription illegality, leaving it up to the consumer to decide on how much and what type of cannabis to use. Often the type of cannabis and mode of delivery is determined by the recommendations of dispensary employees. There are often no significant standards, qualifications, or regulations around the hiring, training, or expertise of dispensary staff. The goal of dispensaries is to increase sales as the market is becoming increasingly competitive, leaving vulnerable individuals in the hands of determined salespeople. There may be a lack of regulations on how much cannabis can be sold per day, per consumer, or per episode. On the other hand, state medical cannabis laws that require doctors to specify dosage, routes of administration, or strains, force physicians to "prescribe" instead of recommend.

Finally, FDA-approved drugs are carefully evaluated for safety, efficacy, and quality. Cannabis and its growing and cultivation are largely unregulated and unstandardized. There have been reports of pesticides, molds, and other contaminants in cannabis products, the consumption of which could lead to serious health problems.[14] Cannabis "recommenders" are recommending a compound, but what the patient gets at the dispensary may be a totally different compound. There is no clear optimal dose of CUAT for any of its state-approved conditions even if one could legally specify the dose. Some state-approved qualifying conditions lack evidence for benefit from CUAT, and in some cases have evidence for harm from CUAT with little to no evidence for benefit for the qualifying condition. The concentration of the different cannabinoids varies from one product to another and from one dispensary to another rendering any recommendations challenging.[2,15]

The field of CUAT is riddled with ideological conflicts. Research stakeholders, motivated by their faith in the utility of cannabis, can be resistant to disconfirming evidence. Certain political stakeholders, motivated perhaps by anti-drug sentiment, are resistant to drug policy change. This atmosphere creates a difficult environment for physicians who seek to treat their patients with compassion.

GUIDELINES FOR CANNABIS RECOMMENDATIONS

Unlike a prescription, a recommendation is a discussion about the pros and cons of consuming a substance. It is important to avoid prescribing "cannabis" by writing down the dose or strength of the product to be taken. One should simply affirm when they believe the patient may benefit from cannabis for an approved condition after careful assessment. The California Medical Association has issued a list of guidelines to physicians interested in recommending CUAT and advised against specifying dosage or the mode of administration.[16]

Physicians should carefully evaluate and document the risks involved before recommending cannabis use. They should keep in mind that cannabis remains a DEA Schedule I drug that it is not approved nor regulated by the FDA, and that the use of cannabis by individuals carries inherent risks.[12,14,17] Physicians should have sufficient knowledge and training in the field of cannabis. More states are mandating that physicians complete continuing medical education credit on medical cannabis before they are allowed to certify a patient for medical cannabis. It is notable that such states may have a very broad range of disorders qualifying for CUAT, extending into most every medical specialty; and yet the state required trainings of physician recommenders, if any, may only be two hours to cover not only cannabis but to also learn about the diagnosis and management of those qualifying disorders, which may lie outside the recommenders' typical practice, expertise, or training. This may place the recommending physician in a risky medicolegal position.

It is important for physicians to document a failure of other conventional, more evidence-based or safer approaches to treat the patient before recommending CUAT. It is also advisable to not only counsel the patient on the benefits and risks of medical cannabis but also to have them sign some type of consent form to document their understanding.[16]

With any recommendation, physicians should monitor their patients regularly and assess for the development of signs and symptoms of cannabis adverse effects such as increased heart rate, sleepiness, dizziness, dry mouth/dry eyes, paranoia, worsening anxiety, impaired attention, impaired memory, psychosis, cardiovascular sequelae, hyperemesis syndrome as well as respiratory symptoms if cannabis is smoked.[12] Physicians should also monitor for the development of unhealthy use, a cannabis use disorder, other substance use disorder, diversion, and or worsening of the underlying condition that qualified them for a cannabis card.[17] This is particularly challenging as many of these cannabis recommenders are not trained to diagnose or treat that particular underlying condition, for example a podiatrist recommending CUAT for dementia, or a clinician lacking experience or training in PTSD recommending CUAT for a veteran struggling with PTSD for whom no FDA-approved medications or evidence-based medications or psychotherapies have been recommended first. Useful strategies include enlisting patients in tracking dose, symptoms, relief, and adverse effects in a journal that they bring to their visit.[18]

CONCLUSION

In a field characterized by both pro- and anti-drug agendas, and federal drug laws increasingly in conflict with state-based legalization of cannabis, health care providers interested in CUAT struggle with the dilemma to recommend or not. Per the preceding chapter on therapeutic effectiveness of cannabis in this section of the textbook, cannabis has some efficacy, but for a very few and narrowly defined conditions; far fewer than those typically listed as qualifying disorders by state authorities. Further, cannabis-based products largely lack FDA evaluation and approval. To date, the FDA also has not approved cannabis or cannabis extract for any clinical condition with the exception of Epidolex®, a cannabidiol containing product that is approved for treatment of two rare childhood seizure disorders, and tuberous sclerosis from a benign brain tumor. Physicians can only make a recommendation for the use of cannabis for a state approved condition and should do so only if fully trained and knowledgeable, and only after careful assessment and documentation, and ongoing condition monitoring.

While scientific advances influence policy decisions about drugs such as DEA scheduling, social beliefs about drugs and the criminalization of their use have a strong impact as well. Policymakers should adopt an approach to cannabis scheduling that addresses safety and efficacy data deficiencies, allows cannabis-related medical research, improves the monitoring of the cannabis supply, and provides for FDA and other oversights in line with the standard of care for medications and medical practice. Physicians should be transparent and objective in their recommendations and practice according to ethical guidance set by the American Medical Association.

REFERENCES

1. ProCon.org. *State-by-State Medical Marijuana Laws*. Accessed September 1, 2022. https://medicalmarijuana.procon.org/legal-medical-marijuana-states-and-dc/#:~:text=to%2012%20plants-,Approved%20Conditions,spasms%20(including%20multiple%20sclerosis
2. Gregorio J. Physicians, medical marijuana, and the law. *Virtual Mentor*. 2014;16(9):732-738. doi:10.1001/virtualmentor.2014.16.9.hlaw1-1409
3. Conant v. Walters, 309 F.3d 629, (9th Cir 2002). Accessed August 7, 2023. https://www.justice.gov/osg/brief/walters-v-conant-petition
4. Thompson JW Jr, Koenen MA. Physicians as gatekeepers in the use of medical marijuana. *J Am Acad Psychiatry Law*. 2011;39(4):460-464. PMID: 22159973. https://jaapl.org/content/39/4/460
5. Mack A, Joy J. *Marijuana as Medicine? The Science Beyond the Controversy*. National Academies Press (US); 2000. 11, LEGAL ISSUES: https://www.ncbi.nlm.nih.gov/books/NBK224398/
6. National Archives, Code of Federal Regulations. *Part 343 – Internal analgesic, antipyretic, and antirheumatic drug products for over-the-counter human use*. Accessed March 1, 2023. https://www.ecfr.gov/current/title-21/chapter-I/subchapter-D/part-343
7. Fish JM. *Drugs and Society: U.S. Public Policy*. Rowman & Littlefield Publishers; 2006:149-162.
8. Balkansky A. *The Founding Fathers: Life, Liberty and…Beer!* Accessed September 1, 2022. https://blogs.loc.gov/headlinesandheroes/2018/05/founding-fathers-beer/
9. Drug Policy Alliance. *A History of the Drug War*. Accessed September 1, 2022. https://drugpolicy.org/issues/brief-history-drug-war
10. Global Commission on Drug Policy. *The War on Drugs*. Accessed September 1, 2022. https://www.globalcommissionondrugs.org/reports/the-war-on-drugs
11. Belouin SJ, Henningfield JE. Psychedelics: where we are now, why we got here, what we must do. *Neuropharmacology*. 2018;142:7-19.
12. National Academies of Sciences, Engineering, and Medicine. *The Health Effects of Cannabis and Cannabinoids: The Current State of Evidence and Recommendations for Research*. The National Academies Press; 2017. doi:10.17226/24625
13. Gedin F, Blome S, Ponten M, et al. Placebo response and media attention in randomized clinical trials assessing cannabis-based therapies for pain: a systematic review and meta-analysis. *JAMA Netw Open*. 2022;5(11):e2243848.1.
14. Seltenrich N. Into the weeds: regulating pesticides in cannabis. *Env Health Pers*. 2019;127:4. doi:10.1289/EHP5265
15. Wilkinson ST, D'Souza DC. Problems with the medicalization of marijuana. *JAMA*. 2014;311(23):2377-2378.
16. Marijuana Policy Project "Prescribing versus "recommending" medical cannabis. Accessed September 1, 2022. https://www.mpp.org/files/uploads/2016/09/Prescribing-vs.-Recommending.pdf
17. Volkow ND, Baler RD, Compton WM, Weiss SR. Adverse health effects of marijuana use. *N Engl J Med*. 2014;370(23):2219-2227. doi:10.1056/NEJMra1402309
18. Voth EA. Guidelines for prescribing medical marijuana. *West J Med*. 2001;175(5):305-306. doi:10.1136/ewjm.175.5.305

CHAPTER

127 Practical Considerations in Drug Testing

Jennifer A. Collins

CHAPTER OUTLINE

- Introduction
- The evolution of drug testing
- The science of drug testing
- Choice of testing matrix
- Limitations of drug testing
- Biomarkers of alcohol consumption
- Ethical issues in alcohol and drug testing

INTRODUCTION

Drug testing is the technology of addiction medicine and, increasingly, of other branches of medicine that involve evaluation and management of substance use disorders, the prescription of controlled substances, or both. It brings a critical measure of objectivity to patients' self-reports regarding their use of alcohol, prescribed medications, and other drugs.

Patients are not always fully disclosing with their physicians,[1,2] and physicians sometimes cannot reliably determine whether their patients are prevaricating.[3] This is particularly true in therapeutic relationships that involve the prescribing of controlled substances. For example, a study of 470 patients in a tertiary care pain program who were prescribed long-term opioid therapy, and who underwent random urine drug testing, found that 45% of the test results did not comport with information provided by the patient. Specifically, 20.2% of the test results were positive for an illicit substance, 14.5% were positive for an unreported prescription controlled substance, and 10.2% were negative for the prescribed opioid, while 2.6% of patients attempted to subvert the test.[4] These results are generally consistent with the findings of other studies involving long-term opioid therapy in specialty pain practices[5-7] and in primary care practices,[8,9] as well as in specialized addiction treatment programs.[10]

Drug testing serves at least two important purposes: to verify adherence to controlled substance-based pharmacotherapies and to detect the unauthorized use of prescription and illicit drugs. Another purpose of drug testing is to deter unauthorized drug use, but the literature on its effectiveness for this purpose is conflicting and may be dependent on the environment and circumstances under which it is applied.[11-14]

Drug testing in a clinical environment can inform medical diagnosis and treatment. However, it is not a stand-alone technique for monitoring recovery from a substance use disorder or the safety of pharmacotherapies involving controlled substances. It should be integrated, as necessary, with patient conversations and physical examinations, information from collaterals, queries of prescription drug monitoring program databases, and medication reconciliation.

This chapter provides a practical overview of the uses of drug testing in clinical settings, with a focus on optimizing the application of these technologies to enhance efforts to prevent substance use disorders, as well as the identification, treatment, and long-term management of individuals who have such disorders.

THE EVOLUTION OF DRUG TESTING

Alexander Gettler (1883–1968), who was the chief toxicologist in the New York City Office of the Chief Medical Examiner from 1918 to 1959, has been called "the father of forensic toxicology." Gettler revolutionized the application of chemical analysis to forensic investigations, and his work laid the foundation for more sophisticated techniques to detect and measure toxins in body tissues and fluids that remain in use today.[15]

One of the methods used in biochemical analysis of drugs is chromatography, which has many variations but which was initially described in 1900. In the mid-20th century, chromatographic techniques were refined, and gas and liquid chromatography applications for drug analyses became widely available. In 1960, Yalow and Berson described the first immunoassay,[16] a technique that would soon be applied to drug testing and would grow to dominate the drug testing market for decades.

The roots of mass spectrometry extend back to the 19th century, but modern mass spectrometric methods were first described by Dempster[17] and Aston[18] early in the 20th century. In 1952, James and Martin described the adaptation of a mass spectrometer (MS) to function as a detector for a gas chromatograph, leading to the first GC-MS instrument.[19] A few years later, quadrupole mass spectrometers, which offer compactness and rapid scanning, were invented by Wolfgang Paul.[20] For decades, GC-MS using a quadrupole mass filter was considered the gold standard for drug testing.

The combination of liquid chromatography with mass spectrometric detection (LC-MS) was more technically complex and followed GC-MS about two decades later. In 1968, Jennings and McLafferty introduced collision-induced dissociation, the principle on which tandem mass spectrometry is based.[21] Today, most drug testing is performed using immunoassay, GC-MS, or liquid chromatography-tandem mass spectrometry (LC-MS/MS) and sometimes a combination of those analytical techniques (eg, screening by immunoassay and confirmation by GC-MS or LC-MS/MS).

Urine drug testing was first used systematically in the methadone maintenance pilot programs of the 1960s.[22] A vital part of those programs was monitoring for continued heroin use and, as the technology became available, monitoring other drug use—thus supporting the therapeutic goal of abstinence from all potentially addictive substances.

Models for broader application of drug screening have roots in military drug testing programs. In 1971, President Nixon ordered the Department of Defense to test military personal prior to their return from Vietnam, using a newly developed immunoassay technique.[23] In the early 1980s, a confluence of events, including a Marine Prowler aircraft crash on the deck of the USS *Nimitz*, prompted wider use of drug testing in the military and the development of a forensically credible testing program.[24]

The military testing program served as a template, with some modifications, for President Reagan's Executive Order 12564 issued in 1986, which established a drug-free federal workplace. Subsequently, many private employers implemented drug-free workplace policies, which usually included pre-employment and for-cause testing. Random testing was not typically a feature of these programs unless public safety was an issue, as with truck and bus drivers, railroad engineers, and airline pilots.

Technical specifications for the federal workplace drug testing program were developed by the Research Triangle Institute in North Carolina and implemented by the National Institute on Drug Abuse (NIDA) as the National Laboratory Certification Program (NLCP), which certified laboratories to perform drug tests on federal employees. The Mandatory Guidelines for Federal Workplace Drug Testing Programs were implemented January 1, 1990. Administration of the program was later transferred from NIDA to the Substance Abuse and Mental Health Services Administration (SAMHSA), where it resides today. In 1991, the U.S. Congress enacted the Omnibus Transportation Employee Testing Act, which required industries regulated by the Department of Transportation to implement drug and alcohol testing procedures for all of their safety-sensitive employees, using laboratories certified by the NLCP.[25]

Other applications of drug screening programs include monitoring physicians and medical professionals in state Physician Health Programs[26] and detecting use of performance-enhancing drugs in sport.[27]

Drug testing has expanded in recent years to include a wide range of clinical settings, especially where controlled substances are prescribed on a regular basis. In clinical applications, drug test menus may be more extensive and include prescription medications (eg, opioids and benzodiazepines) as well as illicit drugs (including amphetamines, cannabinoids, and cocaine). These analyses are used to monitor patients' use of prescribed medications and to detect the use of both non-prescribed medications and illicit drugs.

In several important respects, drug testing in clinical settings differs from drug testing in forensic (workplace) and other programs focused on deterrence rather than diagnostic or medication compliance.

- Unlike drug testing in many other settings, the tests are ordered by healthcare professionals, as opposed to administrative personnel. In this regard, they are considered a component of medical care, much like any other medical laboratory test. Forensic urine drug test results are considered evidentiary and potentially subject to litigation.
- Whereas forensic urine drug testing results require review by a certified Medical Review Officer (MRO), this requirement does not exist for drug testing in clinical settings. Interpretation of drug test results in clinical settings falls to the healthcare professional, perhaps in consultation with a clinical chemist and/or toxicologist.
- Forensic urine drug testing focuses on minimizing the risk of false-positive test results by maximizing the specificity of the analytical method, in contrast to clinical settings, where unexpected negative and positive test results both are important, so the focus is on both the sensitivity and specificity of the tests.
- Forensic urine drug testing is almost exclusively intended to detect illicit drug use, whereas testing in clinical settings is intended not only to detect illicit drug use but also to verify legitimate use of prescribed medications. As a result, the breadth of the testing panel, as well as detection thresholds used, can differ significantly.

The additional demands of drug testing in clinical settings, along with the mostly unregulated environment in which it occurs, have led to a spectrum of laboratory strategies to meet specific needs, from the use of point-of-care screening devices with no confirmatory testing to sophisticated LC-MS applications that detect and quantify dozens of drugs in a single analytical cycle.

THE SCIENCE OF DRUG TESTING

Assessment of Laboratory Test Results

Laboratory tests typically are intended to inform the clinician of pathological conditions. Toward that objective, the performance of a test can be characterized by its clinical sensitivity and specificity with respect to the disease the test is intended to detect (the suspected disease). *Clinical* sensitivity and specificity are distinct from *analytical* sensitivity and specificity, which refer to the lowest concentration of drug detectable and the degree to which the method is free from interferences, respectively. For the purpose of this discussion, the following definitions apply:

- True positive (TP) = An abnormal laboratory result in a patient who has the suspected disease
- True negative (TN) = A normal laboratory result in a patient who does *not* have the suspected disease

- False positive (FP) = An abnormal laboratory result in a patient who does *not* have the suspected disease
- False negative (FN) = A normal laboratory result in a patient who does have the suspected disease

Given these parameters, the *sensitivity* of a laboratory test is defined as:

$$\text{Sensitivity} = \frac{\text{TP}}{\text{TP} + \text{FN}}$$

The denominator in this equation, TP + FN, corresponds to all of the patients who have the suspected disease; thus, the sensitivity is the fraction of patients with the suspected disease who produce a positive test result. Sensitivity is sometimes called "positivity in the presence of disease."

The *specificity* of a laboratory test is defined as:

$$\text{Specificity} = \frac{\text{TN}}{\text{TN} + \text{FP}}$$

In this case, the denominator of the equation, TN + FP, corresponds to all of the patients who do *not* have the suspected disease. The specificity is the fraction of patients without the suspected disease who produce a negative test. Specificity is sometimes called "negativity in the absence of disease."

The sensitivity and specificity of urine drug screening immunoassays must meet the requirements of the Food and Drug Administration (FDA) if the test is to be approved for in vitro diagnostic use, as published in the product insert. However, these data can be misleading.

To determine sensitivity, the test is applied to specimens confirmed to contain the drug at a concentration above the positive threshold. This is equivalent to testing patients who are already known to be positive for the drug. While the assessment provides a measure of the ability of the assay to reliably detect the drug when present, it does not necessarily provide a reliable estimate of the likelihood that a patient taking the drug will test positive, because the latter may be affected by multiple factors, including absorption, metabolism, and clearance of the drug, drug dose and pattern of administration, and hydration status.

The specificity of a urine drug screening test also is difficult to evaluate, because potential cross-reactivity is exceedingly difficult to predict, and there is a practical limit to the number of compounds that can be tested for interference. Therefore, estimates of specificity are inevitably inflated because there always are compounds that might interfere but were not tested. Experience in drug testing teaches that screening methods occasionally produce positive test results that are not confirmed by more specific analytical methods. The reason for the positive test result often cannot be determined.

A more useful measure of the clinical performance of a laboratory test is its *predictive value*. The predictive value of a positive test (PV_+) is defined as:

$$\text{Predictive value}(+) = \frac{\text{TP}}{\text{TP} + \text{FP}}$$

The denominator in this equation is the total number of positive results, so the PV_+ represents the likelihood that a positive test result is a true positive (ie, correctly identifies a patient with the suspected disease). Unlike sensitivity and specificity, which characterize the performance of a test when the patient already has been classified as positive or negative, the predictive value is an estimate of the probability that a patient who tests positive has the suspected disease. For a laboratory test with established specificity, the number of false-positive results it produces depends on the frequency of negative specimens. If all specimens are negative, then all positive results will be false positives.

However, if all specimens are positive, then all positive results will be true positives. Therefore, the FP in the equation, and consequently the predictive value of the test, depends on the frequency of positive patients among the population being tested. As a result, the predictive value of drug screening tests will vary from one practice to another, depending on the frequency with which patients meet the expectations that prompted use of the drug test. Studies that have assessed the predictive value of positive urine drug test results have produced estimates ranging from 10% to 100%, depending on the drug being screened.[28]

Methods of Detecting Drugs

Drug tests in this context are chemical analyses performed to detect the presence or absence of specific drugs and/or metabolites in a biological sample. Tests can be targeted to a specific drug or metabolite, to multiple compounds within a drug class (eg, opiates, amphetamines) or designed to monitor a comprehensive panel of analytes.

Common nomenclature in drug testing has evolved over the last decade and can be confusing. Traditionally, drug testing has been defined in terms of screening and confirmation testing. Screening tests are typically performed by immunoassay or enzymatic methods and confirmatory testing is performed by methods employing chromatography coupled to mass spectrometry. As testing expanded to include components for which there were no immunoassay methods, methodology became less related to these terms. When Current Procedural Terminology (CPT) codes were updated by the American Medical Association (AMA) in 2015, the terms presumptive and definitive were introduced and have now become commonplace. This terminology is maintained in the 2022 CPT code set. In general, the term "presumptive" can be used interchangeably with "screen" and "definitive" with "confirmation." This replaces the previous terminology of "qualitative" and "quantitative," which did not adequately reflect the underlying laboratory methodology applied to the testing. While presumptive drug tests are usually reported qualitatively (ie, as negative or positive), that is not always the case. Definitive tests may be reported either qualitatively or quantitatively with a numeric result for the target drugs/metabolites.

Immunoassay

Immunoassay methods are based on the ability of an antibody to selectively bind to specific antigens. Yalow and Berson used this principle to develop a method to measure insulin, creating the first immunoassay.[16] Now commonplace in medical diagnostic testing, immunoassays are available in a wide variety of formats and applications. For drug testing purposes, the assays are generally based on the interaction between a drug or drug metabolite (antigen) in a patient/donor sample and an antibody to the drug in a specialized reagent system. The most commonly used methods in clinical and forensic drug testing are competitive immunoassays in which a labeled antigen (drug derivative) in the reagent competes with antigen (drug) in the donor sample for binding sites on antibodies targeted to the drug. These assays may be considered *heterogeneous,* in which bound and unbound drug is separated prior to completion of the analysis, or *homogeneous,* in which the test is performed and results measured "in place." Homogeneous immunoassays are amenable to automation and are often performed on standard automated chemistry analyzers in the laboratory (**Fig. 127-1**).

Point-of-care or point-of-collection (POC) technology involves single test devices used to screen for drugs outside of a traditional laboratory setting. These tests follow the general design of a competitive heterogeneous immunoassay but involve lateral flow of the specimen across a solid support to which antibodies have been attached. Endogenous drugs compete with labeled analogues for binding to

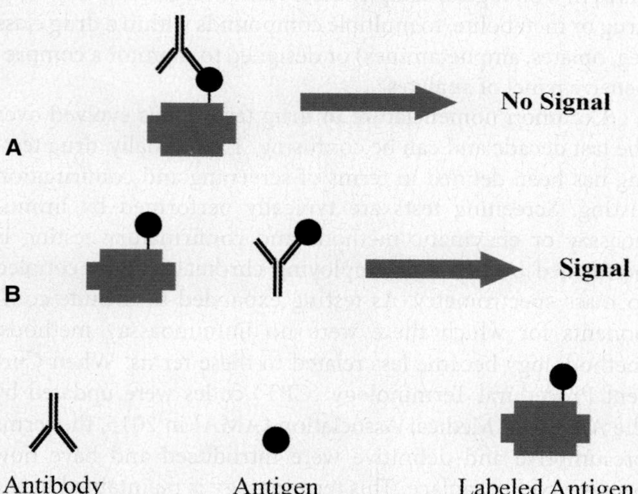

Figure 127-1. General design of a homogeneous immunoassay. A marker—such as an enzyme, fluorescent probe, or microparticle—is labeled with the drug to be detected. When an antibody binds to the drug attached to the marker, the activity of the marker (enzymatic activity, fluorescence, turbidity) is affected and can be detected as a negative test result **(A)**. However, in the presence of free drug in the urine specimen, the antibodies are saturated and do not react with the marker-labeled drugs; the signal detected therefore indicates a positive test result **(B)**. Positive test results may correspond to either the presence or absence of signal, depending on the properties of the specific marker. Enzymes are typically inhibited by the bound antibody, whereas markers involving fluorescence or turbidity may be activated by the antibody.

the immobilized antibodies. The method is called *lateral flow immunochromatography* or *lateral flow immunoassay* (**Fig. 127-2**).

Use of immunoassays in compliance drug testing programs can be an effective and economical approach provided practitioners and those interpreting the results understand the technology and associated strengths and limitations.

Assays may be designed to detect specific drugs or metabolites such as those for cocaine metabolite or may be designed to detect multiple drugs within a class, such as opiate assays that detect codeine, morphine, and the semisynthetic opiate hydrocodone. This characteristic of immunoassay methodology is referred to as cross-reactivity. The term cross-reactivity refers to the degree to which a drug or metabolite binds to the antibody and generates a signal in the detection system. Antibodies do not have absolute specificity, only relative selectivity, for the antigen (drug) against which they were produced. Thus, antibodies have the potential for cross-reactivity both with compounds that are structurally similar to the target compound and with unrelated compounds. This can be beneficial in that a single test reagent can be used to detect the presence of multiple compounds within a class such as opiates and barbiturates, obviating the need to perform tests for each individual drug. Tests that are more prone to nonspecific cross-reactivity (ie, detection of unrelated compounds) have diminished utility unless definitive testing is performed eliminate false-positive results.

In drug screening immunoassays, the extent of cross-reactivity with other compounds varies by target compound and by manufacturer. Amphetamine screening immunoassays, for example, are often susceptible to cross-reacting analytes because there are many drugs, both prescription and nonprescription, with the same or similar phenethylamine structure. Other screening immunoassays—for example, cocaine metabolite (benzoylecgonine)—are highly specific, so false-positive test results are uncommon. Cannabinoid immunoassays, while fairly specific for the delta-9-THC metabolite most commonly used to indicate cannabis use, also show cross-reactivity to other cannabinoid analogs such as delta-8-THC. Derived from hemp, delta-8-THC products have recently become widely available in some markets and are commonly detected in urine following use. Unlike cannabidiol (CBD), which has little or no cross-reactivity in standard immunoassays, delta-8-THC will generate a presumptive positive result. Definitive testing must be performed to distinguish the specific THC isomer.

While much of the discussion surrounding limitations of immunoassays centers on cross-reactivity to nontargeted compounds leading to false-positive results, it is equally important to understand what compounds of interest are not detected well, leading to false-negative results. Cross-reactivity of immunoassays to multiple drugs within a drug class may not be equivalent. For example, opiate class immunoassays are typically optimized to detect morphine and codeine, and have some cross-reactivity to hydrocodone and hydromorphone, but have limited, if any, cross-reactivity to oxycodone and oxymorphone. To effectively test for the presence of oxycodone and

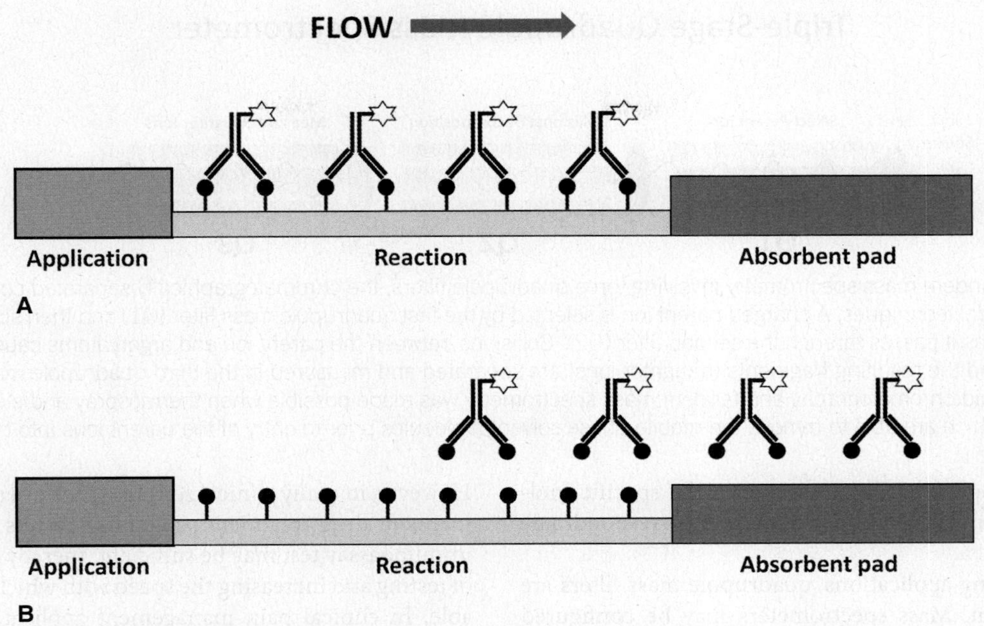

Figure 127-2. Design of immunochromatographic assay, often used for point-of-care drug testing devices. The drugs to be detected are immobilized on a reaction bed. The urine specimen and labeled antibodies to the drugs are applied to the device and are carried across the reaction bed by capillary action. When a drug is absent in the urine, antibodies bind to the immobilized drug on the reaction pad and a signal is detected **(A)**. When a drug is present in the urine specimen, the labeled antibodies are saturated and cannot bind to the immobilized drugs on the reaction pad **(B)**. Hence, in these devices, color development on the reaction pad is a negative test result, whereas lack of color development is a positive test result. The devices are typically configured to detect multiple drugs or metabolites by dividing the reaction pad into drug/metabolite-specific regions.

metabolites, a specific targeted oxycodone test is available and should be used. Similarly, while most benzodiazepine class assays provide good detection of oxazepam, temazepam, and alprazolam, cross-reactivity to lorazepam and clonazepam metabolites is often limited.[29,30] Therefore, when using a drug screening immunoassay to determine whether a patient has taken a drug, the reactivity of the immunoassay toward that particular drug and/or its metabolite(s) must be considered. The performance specifications of immunoassays, including cross-reactivity data, are included in the manufacturer's product insert. Laboratories performing drug screens can also provide this information on request. It should be noted, however, that standard cross-reactivity studies performed by reagent manufacturers may not be comprehensive and the presence of metabolites and untested compounds in patient urines can lead to unexpected results.

Chromatography/Mass Spectrometry

Definitive, or confirmation testing, is typically performed by chromatography with mass spectrometry. This coupled technology incorporates a method to separate components of a sample such as gas or liquid chromatography with a detection system based on identification of molecular mass fragments—mass spectrometry—to identify specific compounds.

Chromatographic methods utilize the chemical characteristics of individual compounds to separate components of a mixture by partitioning between a mobile phase and a stationary phase in the chromatographic system. In gas chromatography (GC), the mobile phase is a gas such as helium or hydrogen, while the mobile phase in liquid chromatography (LC, HPLC) is a liquid, usually an aqueous/solvent mixture. GC methods have exquisite resolution (ie, the ability to separate, or "resolve," similar compounds) but require analyte molecules that are thermally stable enough to be vaporized, since the mobile phase is gaseous. Many organic compounds do not chromatograph well or decompose at temperatures below their vapor point, so for GC analysis, they must be chemically modified to make them more volatile, a process known as "derivatization." LC methods do not require volatile analytes and, as a consequence, are more versatile. However, LC methods do not have the resolution of GC and may be more susceptible to chromatographic interference from comigrating compounds.

Chromatography alone does not detect or measure the components it separates; instead, a detector is required. The most commonly used detector for drug testing methodologies is the mass spectrometer, which has been adapted for use with both GC and LC systems.

Mass spectrometers use an energy source to ionize and break molecules into charged molecular weight fragments or ions that can be separated and measured through use of a mass filter. A plot of the ion abundance versus the mass to charge ratio of the fragments represents the mass spectrum of a given compound. The fragmentation pattern of a molecule is determined by the stability of the individual chemical bonds that

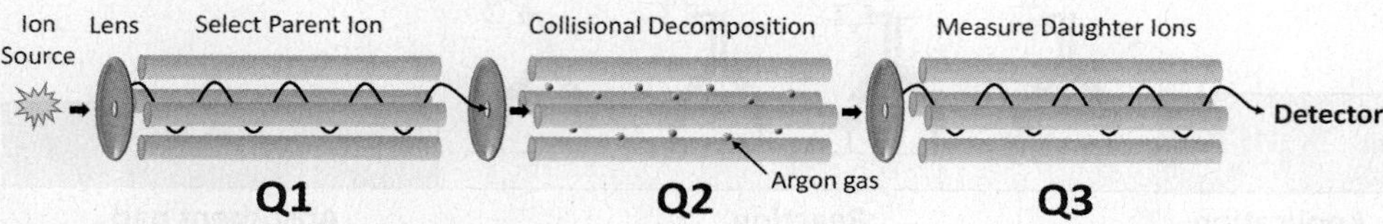

Figure 127-3. In tandem mass spectrometry involving three quadrupole filters, the chromatographically separated components are ionized by one of several techniques. A charged parent ion is selected by the first quadrupole mass filter (Q1) and then subjected to an inert gas such as argon as it passes through the second filter (Q2). Collisions between the parent ion and argon atoms causes decomposition of the molecule, and the resulting fragments (daughter ions) are separated and measured in the third quadrupole mass filter (Q3). The combination of liquid chromatography and tandem mass spectrometry was made possible when thermospray and electrospray ionizers were developed, which are able to remove the mobile phase solvent molecules prior to entry of the parent ions into the mass analyzer.

hold it together and typically is unique to the specific molecule, although similar molecules may have correspondingly similar mass spectra.

For drug testing applications, quadrupole mass filters are the most common. Mass spectrometers may be configured with an individual quadrupole system (ie, single-stage mass spectrometer, MS), or with two or more mass analyzers coupled together as a tandem mass spectrometer (ie, MS/MS or MS^x) to provide enhanced sensitivity and selectivity. In a tandem MS, the molecule is fragmented in an ionization chamber and a specific fragment ("parent ion") is selected by the first quadrupole. In the second quadrupole, the parent ion is exposed to an inert gas such as argon. Collisions with the gas atoms cause further decomposition of the parent ion into "daughter" ions. The third quadrupole separates and measures the daughter ions to identify the original molecule (**Fig. 127-3**).

Chromatography combined with mass spectrometry is considered a confirmatory method for drugs because no other analytical method has greater specificity. Identification of compounds incorporates both the retention time from the chromatographic system and the molecular fragmentation profile from the mass spectrometer to generate a result. When properly configured, drug analyses by GC-MS, LC-MS, or LC-MS/MS have a vanishingly small chance of producing a false-positive test result.

While GC-MS was once the more prevalent technique, LC-MS/MS has grown rapidly in recent years as a versatile and sensitive method for identification and quantification of drugs and drug metabolites in various body fluids, including blood, urine, and oral fluid.

Selection of Methodology in Testing Programs

The type of methodology and paradigm used in drug testing programs should be appropriate for the intended application.

In workplace forensic testing, immunoassay screening tests are commonly used to eliminate specimens with no detectable drug, and positive test results are followed by confirmation with GC-MS or LC-MS/MS. Confirmation of presumptive test results is compulsory in workplace and other settings, especially when there are serious consequences for a positive test. However, in many clinical settings (such as emergency departments or drug treatment programs), results of a presumptive immunoassay test may be sufficient, thereby reducing the cost of testing and increasing the speed with which results are available. In clinical pain management applications, particularly when a more comprehensive test menu is desired, LC-MS/MS testing without an immunoassay screen may be preferred.

A frequently asked question is "How accurate is the drug test?" When the two-step process (including the immunoassay screen and the mass spectrometry confirmation) is employed, the drug identification process is highly accurate. If a specific drug or metabolite is identified by a confirmatory test in a specimen from a donor, that drug or metabolite was present in the donor's body. A toxicologist or medical review officer (MRO) can determine whether the positive test result may be due to food products, nonregulated health aids, or over-the-counter medications.

Screening tests alone can be useful, but positive screening test results should never be considered proof that a drug or drug metabolite is present in the specimen. Likewise, negative screening results do not rule out the presence of a drug, since the drug may be present at a concentration below the detection threshold of the screening test.

There are often significant differences in cost between presumptive and definitive testing approaches and testing may be defined or limited by payer policies. From a practical perspective, the testing ordered should provide relevant and useful information consistent with regulatory requirements, individual patient needs, as well as the benefits and limitations of individual testing methodologies.

In the context of clinical addiction medicine, current guidance for the effective use of drug testing to support diagnosis, treatment, and promote recovery includes both presumptive and definitive testing paradigms.[31]

CHOICE OF TESTING MATRIX

There is no universal "best" matrix for drug testing. The choice of testing matrix should be based on situational considerations, including the particular drugs of interest, the desired window of detection, the probability of drug test subversion by the patient, and available clinical resources.

Urine

Urine is the oldest and most commonly used matrix for clinical drug testing, dating back at least to the methadone maintenance pilot programs of the mid-1960s.[32] Its advantages include its abundance and rapid, continual production; simple, noninvasive collection; high concentration of analytes relative to blood, thus providing a wider window of detection of up to several days for many drugs (or weeks, in the case of long-term use of lipid-soluble drugs); relatively rapid and simple preparation of samples for analysis; and decades of accumulated knowledge about the disposition of a large number of drugs and their metabolites.

The single most important limitation to urine as a testing matrix is that its collection is generally unobserved, thus providing the opportunity for test subversion through such means as sample dilution (with water or another fluid), adulteration (with an oxidizing agent, bleach, or another chemical additive), and substitution (with another specimen). Subversion can be minimized through observed collections, but this is widely considered intrusive and uncomfortable for both donor and staff and is not commonly used in clinical testing situations. Subversion often can be detected by assessing specimen integrity—including its color, pH, odor, temperature, specific gravity, creatinine, and presence of oxidants—at the point of collection or by laboratory testing. However synthetic urine products readily available for purchase have made detection more challenging.[33] Indicators of an invalid specimen should prompt an immediate observed recollection conducted by a same-gender collector.

A limitation of urine, compared to blood, is the inability to correlate the concentration of drug and drug metabolite with drug dose and schedule of administration. Determinants of drug and metabolite concentrations include the specific drug of interest, drug dose and route of administration, chronicity of use, time between last drug administration and collection of urine sample, the donor's pharmacogenetic and (often dynamic) pharmacokinetic profiles, urinary pH, and the donor's hydration status. In addition, with the exception of blood alcohol concentrations, which have an established relationship to impairment, drug concentrations in urine and other matrices do not correlate to impairment. This is due to multiple factors, including the phenomenon of tolerance as well as interindividual pharmacokinetic variability. In the case of cannabis, for example, the THC is rapidly removed from the blood but retained in the brain, so that following administration, the blood concentration falls rapidly even as impairment is increasing.

Oral Fluid

Oral fluid has the potential to address the most important limitation of urine as a testing matrix: privacy concerns. With oral fluid, the donor can be observed throughout the collection process, minimizing opportunities for test subversion. The matrix, however, may be vulnerable to "spiking" with drugs that are prescribed but not administered, by placing a small amount of drug in the oral cavity in the minutes to hours prior to the test. In such a case, residual drug may be detected, thereby creating an illusion of adherence. This concern can be obviated with the measurement of drug metabolites.

Oral fluid shares some of urine's other advantages, such as simple collection and relatively easy preparation for analysis. While oral fluid can be collected by direct expectoration, most commercially available oral fluid collection devices include an absorbent collection pad with a transport tube containing a buffer that stabilizes the oral fluid specimen and facilitates recovery of drugs from the pad. Both Point of Collection (POC) devices and laboratory-based testing is available using methodologies similar to those employed in urine testing.

Drugs enter the oral fluid primarily by passive diffusion from the blood.[34,35] Drugs are also deposited in the oral cavity during active drug use by oral, transmucosal, smoked, and inhaled or intranasal routes of administration. The transfer of drugs from blood into oral fluid depends on the physiochemical properties of the drug such as lipid solubility, degree of ionization, and binding with plasma proteins.[36] Parent drugs tend to be more lipid soluble than their respective metabolites, so the unmetabolized drug is more frequently detected in oral fluid as compared to urine. In addition, because the pH of oral fluid is slightly lower than plasma pH, weakly basic drugs such as cocaine and amphetamines tend to concentrate in oral fluid due to "ion trapping" and have higher oral fluid concentrations relative to plasma as a result.[37] 6-Acetylmorphine has also been shown to accumulate in oral fluid following heroin administration, making it advantageous in detecting heroin use. Weak acids such as barbiturates, and highly protein-bound drugs such as benzodiazepines, are present in oral fluid in lower concentrations. This partitioning of a drug between oral fluid and plasma is expressed as the saliva/plasma ratio (S/P ratio). Average saliva/plasma ratios of some commonly measured drugs are shown in **Table 127-1**.

Compared to urine, oral fluid has a narrower temporal window of detection. Some drugs may be detected earlier in oral fluid—for example, within minutes to hours of administration—but at the expense of diminished later detection. In clinical practice, however, where more chronic drug use is common, a more extended window of detection may be observed.[38] Studies performed in patients subject to drug testing in chronic pain and opioid treatment programs have demonstrated reasonable concordance between oral fluid and urine in compliance monitoring, with some differences in detection rates for certain drug classes.[39,40]

Hair

Because drugs and their metabolites are incorporated, in varying degrees, into the developing hair follicle, hair offers the longest window of detection of the commonly used matrices. Hair is unaffected by short-term drug or alcohol abstinence.

TABLE 127-1 Average Saliva/Plasma Ratios

Drug	Average S/P ratio
Ethyl alcohol	1.07
Barbiturates	0.3
Buprenorphine	1.0
Codeine	4.0
Methamphetamine	2.0
MDMA	7.0
Cocaine	3.0
Diazepam	0.02
Methadone	1.6
Morphine	0.8
THC	1.2
Tramadol	9.0

Data from Drummer OH. Drug testing in oral fluid. *Clin Biochem Rev.* 2006;27:147-159.

Additional advantages include simple, noninvasive collection, stability at room temperature (in dry, dark conditions), and relative invulnerability to adulterants.

Hair typically is collected from the vertex posterior section of the scalp, where growth is rapid and uniform. Because it takes approximately 7 to 10 days for hair from the follicle to emerge from the scalp, it is unsuitable for assessment of recent drug use, although hair also incorporates drug from sweat and sebum as well as from environmental exposure. A sample of hair is collected and its proximal portion is identified. Laboratories typically test the proximal 3 cm—corresponding roughly to the most recent 3 months of growth—because with longer samples, the natural washout of drug over time could dilute analytes of interest to below the cutoff concentration of the assay.

There are limitations to the use of hair as a testing matrix. Most studies have reported the lack of a linear relationship between drug dose and drug concentration in hair.[41] Drug concentration in hair depends on several factors, including dose and frequency of administration, metabolic factors, basicity of the drug, hair color, and percentage of collected hairs in the anagen (growth) and telogen (dormant) phases, as well as prolonged exposure to sunlight or other sources of ultraviolet radiation[42] and cosmetic treatments.[43,44] Hair testing can be subverted by shaving the head; in these instances, hair may be collected from other sites, including underarm, beard, or pubic locations; however, differing growth patterns in nonhead hair impact detection windows and thus interpretation of results. Costs of hair tests are higher than for urine or oral fluid, primarily due to increased cost and complexity of sample preparation required prior to analysis.

Melanin is thought to play an important role in the incorporation of basic drugs (such as amphetamines, cocaine, ketamine, opiates, and their metabolites) into hair.[45-47] Nevertheless, Mieczkowski found only minor effects of hair color on the incorporation of cocaine and benzoylecgonine into hair.[48] There is little interaction between melanin and acidic drugs and drug metabolites (eg, benzodiazepines, ethyl glucuronide, and THC-COOH). Thus, for some basic drugs, concentrations may be greater in pigmented than in nonpigmented hair,[49] while the concentrations of acidic drugs such as ethyl glucuronide[50,51] are not influenced by pigmentation.

Notwithstanding the relationship between the melanin content of hair and drug incorporation, the significance and impact of hair color on positive rates in populations subject to testing continues to be a topic of discussion.[52-54]

Analysis of hair has limitations in detecting moderate-risk drug use. In one study of a primary care patient population, study subjects were selected for moderate-risk drug use over the preceding 3 months. Of 243 participants who reported cannabis use over the preceding 3 months, 127 (52%) were confirmed positive for the cannabis metabolite in hair. Of 46 participants who reported cocaine use, 30 (65%) were confirmed positive for cocaine, its metabolites, or both. Of 33 participants who reported amphetamine use, only 8 (24%) were confirmed positive for amphetamine, methamphetamine, or MDMA. The authors suggest that using hair as the drug test matrix may under-identify people who use substances at a low frequency.[55]

LIMITATIONS OF DRUG TESTING

A drug test that measures all drug use or exposure does not exist and never will. It is impossible for any laboratory to develop a validated method for the detection of each and every drug with a potential for unhealthy use or addiction, the list of which is vast and continually growing. However, the ability to detect use of every drug is not usually necessary for the purposes of assessing recovery status and/or the need to modify the treatment plan. Some laboratories offer tests for extensive arrays of analytes, while other laboratories have relatively limited menus, so the clinician should be acquainted with the capabilities of the specific laboratory being used and ensure that the testing performed is relevant to patient care.

As noted earlier, drug testing typically begins with a screening immunoassay, the results of which sometimes require confirmation with a definitive technique. Screening immunoassays have inherent limitations based on the imperfect specificity of antigen-antibody reactions. Thus, all nonnegative immunoassay screening test results are labeled "presumptive" and require mass spectrometry-based testing if definitive identification of an analyte is necessary.

In addition, screening immunoassays may have clinically important sensitivity limitations, particularly with regard to the class-specific assays (such as those for amphetamines, barbiturates, benzodiazepines, and opiates) in which an antibody directed against a specific member of the drug class will have varying, but usually lesser, degrees of cross-reactivity with other class members. Thus, a negative result may indicate the absence of the drug, the presence of the drug below the assay cutoff, or inadequate sensitivity of the assay for the drug. Negative immunoassay results, particularly when the results are unexpected, may be more properly regarded as "presumptive negative" results.

Mass spectrometry-based definitive techniques are highly specific. Their sensitivity, however, is defined by the validated administrative cutoff concentration, which depends on the lower limit of quantification. These limits vary by analyte, by matrix, and by laboratory.

For drugs that are represented on a laboratory's menu of assays, the detection windows are determined by several factors, including (but not limited to) quantity, frequency, and recency of drug administration, the testing matrix, and the analytical capabilities of the specific assay. With regard to testing matrix, oral fluid and urine typically have windows of detection of up to several days. Head hair, which grows, on average, 1 cm per month and which by convention involves the testing of a proximal 3-cm segment of hair, provides a window of detection of approximately 3 months.

Drug test results do not permit the clinician to determine the drug dose, quantity or frequency of administration, the specific time of last use, or the route of administration. Despite claims to the contrary by some commercial laboratories, there is no peer-reviewed scientific basis for the use of propriety algorithms to determine adherence with prescription medication instructions based on the concentration of a drug or metabolite in urine.

Quantitative drug levels in urine are highly variable and are dependent on urinary water content, which can vary significantly in a 24-hour period. Normalizing quantitative values to urinary creatinine concentration removes some variability due to hydration status of the donor. This may be relevant when tracking values of a consistently-taken prescribed medication in a patient over time, however it does not remove inter-individual variability. Evaluation of serial creatinine-corrected concentrations of carboxy-THC has been used to differentiate new use from residual,[56,57] and using quantitative values to calculate a norbuprenorphine/buprenorphine ratio may prove helpful in identifying poor adherence in patients receiving buprenorphine for opioid use disorder.[58,59]

A positive drug test result is not diagnostic of a substance use disorder in an individual who has no history of such a disorder. A confirmed positive drug test result verifies the presence of a drug or drug metabolite at or above a cutoff concentration or detection limit, but a diagnosis of substance use disorder is made on the basis of a constellation of clinical signs and symptoms.[60] Hence, an unexpected drug test result should prompt a conversation with the patient about the meaning of the result. In the case of an individual who has a history of substance use disorder, an inappropriate drug test result may signal recurrence of use that may be brief or more prolonged. Again, accurate diagnosis and appropriate response require a conversation with the patient about the meaning of the test result.

Similarly, a negative drug test result does not prove that a drug or metabolite of interest was absent from the testing matrix. Rather, it means that, *if* the drug or metabolite is present, it is present below the cutoff concentration for the test that was used. An *unexpected*, confirmed negative drug test requires a behavioral explanation for the test result. For example, the differential diagnosis includes running out of the medication several days or more prior to the test because of a substance use disorder; as-needed medication use, with little or no use in the days preceding the drug test; sample adulteration; and medication diversion.

Mass spectrometry-based drug testing techniques are capable of providing results of exquisite sensitivity and specificity, but they have the aforementioned limitations. Thus, while drug testing is an essential component of the care of individuals with substance use disorders and individuals who are prescribed long-term controlled substance therapies, it is not a sufficient stand-alone monitoring technique and does not obviate the need for spending time talking with patients about how they are doing in life, speaking with the patients' loved ones (with the patient's permission), checking state prescription drug monitoring databases, and performing medication reconciliations.

BIOMARKERS OF ALCOHOL CONSUMPTION

Alcohol enjoys a special status in the United States and in many other countries. It can be used legally in the United States by persons over the age of 21, although its use and sometimes hazardous use by younger persons—college students, in particular—is pervasive.[61] It is ubiquitous. No prescription is necessary. And its unhealthy use does far more harm than any other drug or drug class, with the exception of tobacco.[62]

At one time, alcohol testing was limited almost entirely to the measurement of blood and breath in cases of acute intoxication and suspected impairment. This was true, in part, because of alcohol's pharmacokinetics: it is rapidly metabolized by first-order kinetics, so that even in the setting of chronic, heavy use, it generally cannot be detected in blood, breath, and urine more than several hours after use.[63]

Knowledge of an individual's alcohol consumption beyond acute use or intoxication is important in several clinical contexts, including substance use disorder treatment programs and posttreatment monitoring programs. It is vitally important in the impaired professionals' health programs, in which there is zero tolerance for alcohol consumption. Finally, it should be regarded as important in patients receiving long-term treatment with opioids or benzodiazepines because the co-consumption of alcohol plays an important role in the morbidity and mortality associated with those medications. None of the traditional, indirect biomarkers of heavy alcohol use—carbohydrate-deficient transferrin (CDT), gamma-glutamyl transferase (GGT), or mean corpuscular volume (MCV)—have the necessary sensitivity and specificity[64] for these purposes. To that end, ethyl glucuronide and ethyl sulfate, and more recently phosphatidyl ethanol, have been identified as widely available, longer-lasting, direct biomarkers of alcohol consumption.

Ethyl Glucuronide and Ethyl Sulfate

Ethyl glucuronide (EtG) and ethyl sulfate (EtS) are minor ethanol metabolites, which are formed by the conjugation of ethanol with glucuronic acid (via UDP-glucuronosyltransferases) and sulfate (via sulfotransferase), respectively. They can be detected in a variety of biological matrices. EtG and EtS are commonly measured in urine; EtG can also be measured in hair. They are the most appropriate biomarkers for assessment of alcohol abstinence. They appear in the urine within 1 hour of alcohol consumption and, depending on the drinking pattern and the cutoff concentration of the assay, may be detected for 72 hours or more after the last drink.[65]

It has been demonstrated that EtG can be synthesized in vitro in the presence of alcohol; as a result, in patients with glycosuria and *Escherichia coli* urinary tract infection, clinical false-positive EtG test results can be produced.[66] Conversely, *E. coli* also can hydrolyze EtG in vitro leading to false-negative results.[66] Genetic polymorphisms of the UGT 1A1 gene, which encodes several UDP-glucuronosyltransferases, have the potential to interfere with EtG production.[65] In contrast, EtS appears to be stable under these conditions and is not vulnerable to known genetic polymorphisms, making it a useful complementary biomarker of alcohol consumption.

Commercial immunoassays and laboratory-developed tests by mass spectrometry are used to identify EtG and EtS in urine and other matrices. It has been suggested that verifying alcohol abstinence requires urinary EtG and EtS cutoffs of 100 and 25 ng/mL, respectively. Some laboratories, however, offer higher EtG and EtS cutoff concentrations (500 and 250 ng/mL are common) in an effort to minimize the potential for a positive test resulting from incidental alcohol exposure. Unfortunately, there is no known cutoff that distinguishes incidental exposure to alcohol from consumption of alcohol beverages. The lower cutoffs reduce the specificity of the source of alcohol, because EtG, EtS, or both are detectable following consumption of nonalcoholic beer and wine, fruit juices, and ripe bananas, as well as ethanol-containing mouthwashes and hand sanitizers. Patients for whom there is a zero tolerance for alcohol consumption should be counseled to avoid such exposures.

In head hair, it has been proposed that EtG concentrations of less than 7 pg/mg indicate either abstinence or low intake of alcohol during the preceding 3 months. It also proposed that EtG concentrations of 7 to 30 pg/mg suggest repeated alcohol consumption and that concentrations greater than 30 pg/mg suggest chronic heavy use.[67] The incorporation of EtG into hair can be influenced by cosmetic and thermal treatments. It has also been reported that EtG and, less frequently, EtS were detected in several commercially available hair tonics, using cutoff concentrations of 50 and 10 ng/mL, respectively.[68]

Phosphatidyl Ethanol

Phosphatidyl ethanol (PEth) constitutes a group of phospholipids, each consisting of a glycerol backbone, a phosphoethanol headgroup, and two fatty acid chains, which are produced in red blood cell membranes by the action of enzyme phospholipase D on phosphatidylcholine in the presence of ethanol.[69] Forty-eight PEth homologues have been identified in humans; generally only the predominant 16:0/18:1 species is analyzed and reported by laboratories. PEth becomes detectable in blood within hours of a heavy drinking episode and has an elimination half-life of 4.5 to 12 days,[69] although elimination rates between individuals and between different PEth forms have been reported.[70] It can be measured in whole blood, including capillary blood collected on filter paper ("dried blood spot"), which simplifies collection, transport, and storage.

For these reasons, PEth has been promoted as a biomarker for binge and chronic alcohol consumption.[71] However, clinical studies have reported considerable interindividual variability in PEth levels, which may limit its use in identifying high-risk versus moderate alcohol consumption.[72] In addition, differences in analytical technique, source of PEth (ie, whole blood versus dried blood spot), and the specific PEth homologue(s) measured make laboratory-to-laboratory comparison of PEth values potentially problematic.

ETHICAL ISSUES IN ALCOHOL AND DRUG TESTING

Beauchamp and Childress have developed a widely used approach to bioethical reasoning. Their four principles—beneficence, nonmaleficence, justice, and respect for autonomy—provide a lens through which to examine the ethical aspects of clinical drug testing.[73]

Beneficence refers to the ethical principle that clinicians are obliged to act for the benefit of their patients. Drug testing is a diagnostic tool that, when integrated with other information, can be helpful in diagnosing, or monitoring the status of, substance use disorders. As with every diagnostic test, the result should be used to inform medical care and not to punish patients for displaying signs of a medical disorder. Additionally—and especially for patients in the early stages of substance use disorder treatment—appropriate drug test results can provide positive reinforcement, thereby supporting their recovery efforts.[74]

Nonmaleficence refers to the ethical principle that clinicians should refrain from acts that may harm their patients. Drug testing poses a number of potential harms, the most important of which accrue from errors in the ordering of tests and interpretation of test results, and from inappropriate responses to test results.[74] Errors of ordering and interpretation are commonplace and generally result from inadequate education.[75-77] With regard to the ordering of drug tests, the clinician should be knowledgeable about the composition of the drug test panel and the analytical limitations of the test.

Drug tests are never "general" tests for ruling out the presence of one or more of the ever-increasing number of drugs with a potential for hazardous use. Rather, drug tests, regardless of the analytical technique, are directed toward a panel—and often a very limited panel—of drugs. Thus, the clinician must be certain that the drugs of interest are represented on the panel and understand what may not be detected due to limitations of the analytical methodology.

Inappropriate, punitive clinical responses to drug test results can have important and enduring consequences for patients. Such responses may diminish the patient's trust in the clinician and may harm the therapeutic relationship. The most draconian response to an inappropriate drug test result—discharging the patient from a practice—is only rarely an acceptable option. Such acts foreclose opportunities to discuss the reason for the test results, to determine whether there might be a substance use disorder (or recurrence of this disease), and, if so, to initiate treatment or referral. Furthermore, it may precipitate uncomfortable and sometimes dangerous withdrawal syndromes or drive the patient to seek controlled substances from emergency rooms or nonmedical sources.[74]

Finally, as medical records are increasingly likely to follow patients through the healthcare system, misinformation (such as an incorrect interpretation of test results, characterizing patients as nonadherent with prescription instructions, or misdiagnosing patients as having substance use disorders on the basis of drug test results) has the potential to negatively affect the care patients receive from future clinicians and may have consequences for insurance coverage.[74]

The ethical principle of *justice* dictates that patients be treated fairly and equitably. This means that drug testing must be driven by patient-specific considerations, such as the risk of development or recurrence of a substance use disorder. There is no empirical or ethical justification for drug testing on the basis of patient ethnicity, race, religion, sexual orientation, or likeability.[76]

The fourth ethical principle, *respect for autonomy*, refers to the patient's right to self-rule, free from interference from others or from inadequate understanding of clinical choices. In the context of this chapter, respect for autonomy pertains chiefly to treatment involving prescribed and nonprescribed controlled substances.

With regard to the former, it involves discussions about the risks, benefits, costs, and alternatives associated with the use of medications and the rationale for the use of drug testing as one component of monitoring the safety and effectiveness of their administration. Such discussions typically are codified in the form of an informed consent document, a medication treatment agreement, or both. These documents should memorialize, but not substitute for, a conversation between the clinician and the patient.

With regard to drug testing, the conversation should include the details of testing protocols, including the testing schedule (random, scheduled, or for-cause) and testing matrices (urine, oral fluid, or hair), but should not include disclosure of the composition of the test panel, as this would undermine the deterrent effects of drug testing. In the case of urine, the discussion should include methods of collection (unmonitored, monitored, directly observed) and behaviors that would trigger monitored or observed collections, consequences of refusal to test, and clinical actions that may be taken in response to inappropriate test results. Reasonable actions might include instituting closer follow-up and otherwise enhancing treatment boundaries, involving family in the care plan, modifying the treatment plan, or referring the patient to an addiction specialist for evaluation and management. Provisions stipulating that failed drug test results will result in patient dismissal will effectively foreclose patient disclosures about their substance use and have no legitimate medical or ethical basis.[74]

Ultimately, some patients will not agree to such informed consent or treatment agreements or, if they do agree, will subsequently refuse a test. Again, this should prompt discussion, but if the issue cannot be resolved, further controlled substance prescribing generally will be contraindicated. In its place, the clinician should design a therapeutic plan without controlled substances or refer the patient elsewhere for care.[74]

ACKNOWLEDGMENT

The author would like to acknowledge Gary M. Reisfield, Roger L. Bertholf, Bruce A. Goldberger, and Robert L. DuPont for their original version of this chapter published in the previous edition.

REFERENCES

1. Reddy S. "I don't smoke, Doc," and other patient lies. *Wall St J.* February 18, 2013. Accessed July 12, 2023. https://www.wsj.com/articles/SB10001424127887323478004578306510461212692
2. Raymond J. What we lie to doctors about and why it matters. *Newsweek.* January 7, 2009. Accessed July 12, 2023. https://www.newsweek.com/what-we-lie-doctors-about-and-why-it-matters-78235
3. Ekman P, O'Sullivan M. Who can catch a liar? *Am Psychol.* 1991;46:913-920.
4. Michna E, Jamison RN, Pham LD, et al. Urine toxicology screening among chronic pain patients on opioid therapy: frequency and predictability of abnormal findings. *Clin J Pain.* 2007;23:173-179.
5. Manchikanti L, Cash KA, Damron KS, Manchukonda R, Pampati V, McManus CD. Controlled substance abuse and illicit drug use in chronic pain patients: an evaluation of multiple variables. *Pain Physician.* 2006;9:215-225.
6. Katz NP, Sherburne S, Beach M, et al. Behavioral monitoring and urine toxicology testing in patients receiving long-term opioid therapy. *Anesth Analg.* 2003;97:1097-1102.
7. Fishbain DA, Cutler RB, Rosomoff HL, Rosomoff RS. Validity of self-reported drug use in chronic pain patients. *Clin J Pain.* 1999;15:184-191.
8. Turner JA, Saunders K, Shortreed SM, et al. Chronic opioid therapy urine drug testing in primary care: prevalence and predictors of aberrant results. *J Gen Intern Med.* 2014;29:1663-1671.
9. Fleming MF, Balousek SL, Klessig CL, Mundt MP, Brown DD. Substance use disorders in a primary care sample receiving daily opioid therapy. *J Pain.* 2007;8:573-582.
10. Kirsh KL, Heit HA, Huskey A, Strickland J, Egan K, Passik SD. Trends in drug use from urine drug testing of addiction treatment clients. *J Opioid Manag.* 2015;11:61-68.

11. Dunn M, Thomas JO, Swift W, Burns L, Mattick RP. Drug testing in sport: the attitudes and experiences of elite athletes. *Int J Drug Policy.* 2010; 21:330-332.
12. Goldberg L, Elliot DL, MacKinnon DP, et al. Outcomes of a prospective trial of student-athlete drug testing: the Student Athlete Testing Using Random Notification (SATURN) study. *J Adolesc Health.* 2007; 41:421-429.
13. Carpenter CS. Workplace drug testing and worker drug use. *Health Serv Res.* 2007;42:795-810.
14. Manchikanti L, Manchukonda R, Pampati V, et al. Does random urine drug testing reduce illicit drug use in chronic pain patients receiving opioids? *Pain Physician.* 2006;9:123-129.
15. Freimuth HC, Alexander O. Gettler (1883–1968): a reflection. *Am J Forensic Med Pathol.* 1983;4:303-305.
16. Yalow RS, Berson SA. Immunoassay of endogenous plasma insulin in man. *J Clin Invest.* 1960;39:1157-1175.
17. Dempster AJ. Thirty years of mass spectroscopy. *Sci Mon.* 1948; 67:145-153.
18. Downard KM. Historical account: Francis William Aston—the man behind the mass spectrograph. *Eur J Mass Spectrom.* 2007;13:177-190.
19. James AT, Martin AJ. Gas–liquid partition chromatography: the separation and micro-estimation of volatile fatty acids from formic acid to dodecanoic acid. *Biochem J.* 1952;50:679-690.
20. Paul W. Electromagnetic traps for charged and neutral particles. *Rev Mod Phys.* 1990;62:531-540.
21. McLafferty FW, ed. *Tandem Mass Spectrometry*. John Wiley & Sons; 1983.
22. Dole VP, Kim WK, Eglitis I. Detection of narcotic drugs, tranquilizers, amphetamines, and barbiturates in urine. *JAMA.* 1966;198:349-352.
23. Baker SL Jr. U.S. Army heroin abuse identification program in Vietnam: implications for a methadone program. *Am J Public Health.* 1972;62:857-860.
24. Irving J. Drug testing in the military: technical and legal problems. *Clin Chem.* 1988;34:637-640.
25. *Omnibus Transportation Employee Testing Act of 1991, Pub.L. 102-143, Title V, 105 Stat. 952.* Accessed May 8, 2022. https://www.transportation.gov/sites/dot.gov/files/docs/199111028_Omnibus_Act.pdf
26. Altchuler SI. The use of drug testing in monitoring the impaired medical professional. *J Medical Licens Discip.* 2005;91(4):13-16.
27. Trout GJ, Kazlauskas R. Sports drug testing: an analyst's perspective. *Chem Soc Rev.* 2004;33:1-13.
28. Bertholf RL, Sharma R, Reisfield GM. Predictive value of positive drug screening results in an urban outpatient population. *J Anal Toxicol.* 2016;40:726-731.
29. West R, Pesce A, West C, et al. Comparison of clonazepam compliance by measurement of urinary concentration by immunoassay and LC-MS/MS in pain management population. *Pain Physician.* 2010;13(1):71-78.
30. Moeller KE, Lee KC, Kissack JC. Urine drug screening: practical guide for clinicians. *Mayo Clin Proc.* 2008;83(1):66-76.
31. Jarvis M, Williams J, Hurford M, et al. Appropriate use of drug testing in clinical addiction medicine. *J Addict Med.* 2017;11(3):163-173.
32. Goldstein A, Brown BW Jr. Urine testing schedules in methadone maintenance treatment of heroin addiction. *JAMA.* 1970;214:311-315.
33. Goggin M, Tann CM, Miller A, et al. Catching fakes: new markers of urine sample validity and invalidity. *J Anal Toxicol.* 2017;41(2):121-126.
34. Cone EJ, Huestis MA. Interpretation of oral fluid tests for drugs of abuse. *Ann NY Acad Sci.* 2007;1098:51-103.
35. Drummer OH. Drug testing in oral fluid. *Clin Biochem Rev.* 2006; 27:147-159.
36. Jusko WJ, Milsap RL. Pharmacokinetic principles of drug distribution in saliva. *Ann NY Acad Sci.* 1993;694:36-47.
37. Cone EJ. Saliva testing for drugs of abuse. *Ann NY Acad Sci.* 1993; 694:91-127.
38. Allen KR. Screening for drugs of abuse: which matrix, oral fluid or urine? *Ann Clin Biochem.* 2011;48(6):531-541.
39. Heltsley R, DePriest A, Black DL, et al. Oral fluid drug testing of chronic pain patients. II. Comparison of paired oral fluid and urine specimens. *J Anal Toxicol.* 2012;36:75-80.
40. Vindenes V, Yttredal B, Oiestad EL, et al. Oral fluid is a viable alternative for monitoring drug abuse: detection of drugs in oral fluid by liquid chromatography-tandem mass spectrometry and comparison to the results from urine samples from patients treated with methadone or buprenorphine. *J Anal Toxicol.* 2011;35:32-39.
41. Cooper GA, Kronstrand R, Kintz P. Society of hair testing guidelines for drug testing in hair. *Forensic Sci Int.* 2012;218:20-24.
42. Salomone A, Tsanaclis L, Agius R, Kintz P, Baumgartner MR. European guidelines for workplace drug and alcohol testing in hair. *Drug Test Anal.* 2016;8:996-1004.
43. Tanaka S, Iio R, Chinaka S, Takayama N, Hayakawa K. Identification of reaction products of methamphetamine and hydrogen peroxide in hair dye and decolorant treatments by high-performance liquid chromatography/mass spectrometry. *Biomed Chromatogr.* 2001;15:45-49.
44. Pritchett JS, Phinney KW. Influence of chemical straightening on the stability of drugs of abuse in hair. *J Anal Toxicol.* 2015;39:13-16.
45. Borges CR, Wilkins DG, Rollins DE. Amphetamine and N-acetylamphetamine incorporation into hair: an investigation of the potential role of drug basicity in hair color bias. *J Anal Toxicol.* 2001; 25:221-227.
46. Xiang P, Shen M, Zhuo X. Hair analysis for ketamine and its metabolites. *Forensic Sci Int.* 2006;162:131-134.
47. Rollins DE, Wilkins DG, Krueger GG, et al. The effect of hair color on the incorporation of codeine into human hair. *J Anal Toxicol.* 2003;27:545-551.
48. Mieczkowski T, Kruger M. Interpreting the color effect of melanin on cocaine and benzoylecgonine assays for hair analysis: brown and black samples compared. *J Forensic Leg Med.* 2007;14:7-15.
49. Lee S, Han E, Kim E, et al. Simultaneous quantification of opiates and effect of pigmentation on its deposition in hair. *Arch Pharm Res.* 2010;33:1805-1811.
50. Appenzeller BM, Schuman M, Yegles M, Wennig R. Ethyl glucuronide concentration in hair is not influenced by pigmentation. *Alcohol Alcoholism.* 2007;42:326-327.
51. Musshoff F, Madea B. Review of biologic matrices (urine, blood, hair) as indicators of recent or ongoing cannabis use. *Ther Drug Monit.* 2006;28:155-163.
52. Mieczkowski T. Assessing the potential for racial bias in hair analysis for cocaine: examining the relative risk of positive outcomes when comparing urine samples to hair samples. *Forensic Sci Int.* 2011;206:29-34.
53. Kelly RC, Mieczkowski T, Sweeney SA, Bourland JA. Hair analysis for drugs of abuse. Hair color and race differentials or systematic differences in drug preferences? *Forensic Sci Int.* 2000;107:63-86.
54. Kidwell DA, Lee EH, DeLauder SF. Evidence for bias in hair testing and procedures to correct bias. *Forensic Sci Int.* 2000;107(1-3):39-61.
55. Gryczynski J, Schwartz RP, Mitchell SG, O'Grady KE, Ondersma SJ. Hair drug testing results and self-reported drug use among primary care patients with moderate-risk illicit drug use. *Drug Alcohol Depend.* 2014;141:44-50.
56. Huestis MA, Cone EJ. Differentiating new marijuana use from residual drug excretion in occasional marijuana users. *J Anal Toxicol.* 1998;22(6):445-454.
57. Schwilke EW, Gullberg RG, Darwin WD, et al. Differentiating new cannabis use from residual urinary cannabinoid excretion in chronic, daily cannabis users. *Addiction.* 2011;106(3):499-506.
58. McMillin G, Davis R, Carlisle H, Clark C, Marin SJ, Moody DE. Patterns of free (unconjugated) buprenorphine, norbuprenorphine, and their glucuronides in urine using liquid chromatography-tandem mass spectrometry. *J Anal Toxicol.* 2012;36(2):81-87.
59. Donroe JH, Holt SR, O'Connor PG, Sukumar N, Tetrault JM. Interpreting quantitative urine buprenorphine and norbuprenorphine levels in office-based clinical practice. *Drug Alcohol Depend.* 2017;180:46-51.
60. American Psychiatric Association (APA). *Diagnostic and Statistical Manual of Mental Disorders.* 5th ed. American Psychiatric Association; 2013.
61. Skidmore CR, Kaufman EA, Crowell SE. Substance use among college students. *Child Adolesc Psychiatr Clin N Am.* 2016;25:735-753.

62. Nutt DJ, King LA, Phillips LD. Drug harms in the UK: a multicriteria decision analysis. *Lancet.* 2010;376:1558-1565.
63. Helander A, Beck O, Jones AW. Laboratory testing for recent alcohol consumption: comparison of ethanol, methanol, and 5-hydroxytryptophol. *Clin Chem.* 1996;42:618-624.
64. Cabarcos P, Alvarez I, Tabernero MJ, Bermejo AM. Determination of direct alcohol markers: a review. *Anal Bioanal Chem.* 2015;407:4907-4925.
65. Jatlow PI, Agro A, Wu R, et al. Ethyl glucuronide and ethyl sulfate assays in clinical trials, interpretation, and limitations: results of a dose ranging alcohol challenge study and 2 clinical trials. *Alcohol Clin Exp Res.* 2014;38:2056-2065.
66. Helander A, Olsson I, Dahl H. Postcollection synthesis of ethyl glucuronide by bacteria in urine may cause false identification of alcohol consumption. *Clin Chem.* 2007;53:1855-1857.
67. Kintz P. 2014 Consensus for the use of alcohol markers in hair for assessment of both abstinence and chronic excessive alcohol consumption. *Forensic Sci.* 2015;249:A1-A2.
68. Arndt T, Schrofel S, Stemmerich K. Ethyl glucuronide identified in commercial hair tonics. *Forensic Sci Int.* 2013;231:195-198.
69. Gnann H, Weinmann W, Thierauf A. Formation of phosphatidylethanol and its subsequent elimination during an extensive drinking experiment over 5 days. *Alcohol Clin Exp Res.* 2012;36:1507-1511.
70. Helander A, Böttcher M, Dahmen N, Beck O. Elimination characteristics of the alcohol biomarker phosphatidylethanol (PEth) in blood during alcohol detoxification. *Alcohol and Alcoholism.* 2019;54(3):251-257.
71. Dasgupta A. Alcohol biomarkers: an overview. In: Dasgupta A, ed. *Alcohol and Its Biomarkers.* Elsevier; 2015.
72. Helander A, et al. Monitoring of the alcohol biomarkers PEth, CDT and EtG/EtS in an outpatient treatment setting. *Alcohol and Alcoholism.* 2012;47(5):552-557.
73. Beauchamp TL, Childress JF. *Principles of Biomedical Ethics.* 6th ed. Oxford University Press; 2009.
74. Reisfield GM, Maschke KJ. Urine drug testing in long-term opioid therapy: ethical considerations. *Clin J Pain.* 2014;30:679-684.
75. Starrels JL, Fox AD, Kunins HV, Cunningham CO. They don't know what they don't know: internal medicine residents' knowledge and confidence in urine drug test interpretation for patients with chronic pain. *J Gen Intern Med.* 2012;27:1521-1527.
76. Reisfield GM, Bertholf R, Barkin RL, Webb F, Wilson G. Urine drug test interpretation: what do physicians know? *J Opioid Manag.* 2007;3:80-86.
77. Reisfield GM, Webb FJ, Bertholf RL, Sloan PA, Wilson GR. Family physicians' proficiency in urine drug test interpretation. *J Opioid Manag.* 2007;3:333-337.

Sidebar

Workplace Drug Testing and the Role of the Medical Review Officer

James L. Ferguson and Robert L. DuPont

A Medical Review Officer (MRO) is a physician, MD or DO, who is licensed in at least one state, Canada, or Mexico, and whose duty it is to act as an impartial gatekeeper and to advocate for the accuracy and integrity of a drug testing program. MROs are commonly used for workplace drug testing programs, but recently the need for MRO impartiality and objectivity has been recognized by many programs other than in the workplace. Examples include addiction treatment programs, recovery monitoring programs, and pain medicine clinics.

DUTIES OF THE MRO

MROs perform their duties by verifying chain-of-custody documentation, as well as interpreting and verifying laboratory-non negative and other problematic drug test results. The MRO receives all positive, adulterated, substituted, or invalid drug test results before those results go to the individual or organization that requested the drug test. In all federally regulated drug testing programs and many monitoring programs, the MRO also receives and reviews all negative test results. The MRO's task is to verify that the required drugs were included in the tests, that proper procedures were maintained in conducting the test, and that the results are forensically defensible.

In addition, the MRO establishes whether there is an acceptable, legitimate medical explanation for nonnegative laboratory results. An example of this process is the verification by the MRO of a prescription for mixed amphetamine salts in the name of a donor who had a confirmed positive test result for amphetamine. In this case, after speaking with the donor and verifying that the prescription for the amphetamine was valid for that individual at the time of the drug test, the MRO reported the drug test result as negative. In such a case, the employer is not informed by the laboratory of the positive test result, the fact that the employee had been diagnosed with attention deficit hyperactivity disorder, or that the employee had been prescribed for mixed amphetamine salts for that condition.

However, if in the reasonable medical judgment of the MRO, the prescription for mixed amphetamine salts is likely to pose a risk to safety or to be a violation of an applicable regulation, then the MRO is responsible for reporting a safety concern to the employer at the time the negative drug test result is presented. It is then the employer's obligation to conduct appropriate follow-up to determine if that employee is fit for duty. The MRO may assist in the follow-up process to the extent that it is feasible to do so but should not remove the safety warning unless verification is received that the safety risk no longer exists. MROs by themselves do not make fitness for duty decisions. An MRO practice is forensic and administrative in nature, and not clinical.

REGULATORY FRAMEWORK FOR MRO PRACTICE

MROs are required to be knowledgeable about the often complex and frequently changing regulations and practices that govern workplace drug testing. A 1986 Presidential Executive Order directed the U.S. Department of Health and Human Services (DHHS) to develop and publish scientific and technical guidelines for workplace drug testing of federal employees. Those guidelines[1], which are overseen by the Substance Abuse and Mental Health Services Administration (SAMHSA) within DHHS, significantly increased public acceptance of drug testing by establishing certification procedures for laboratories and placing final responsibility for the review of drug tests with a physician—designated, for the first time, as an MRO.

The medical review field grew dramatically when the U.S. Department of Transportation (DOT) mandated testing of transportation workers in safety-sensitive positions as part of the Drug-Free Workplace Act of 1988[2], which included a requirement for medical review. Further growth in the role of the MRO occurred as the courts, government agencies, and private employers acknowledged the protection offered by the expertise of a physician and added MROs to their testing programs, even when not required to do so.

The DOT regulations have been updated several times to reflect evolving research data and almost three decades of experience with workplace alcohol and drug testing. Such changes include issues of specimen validity to reduce the risk of cheating, as well as identifying new drugs to be added to the federal drug testing panel. The May 2012 update reflects the latest testing technology as it focused on the detection of 6-acetylmorphine (6-AM), a unique metabolite of heroin.[3,4] Effective July 3, 2012, laboratories and MROs "will no longer be required to consult with one another regarding the testing for the presence of morphine when the laboratory confirms the presence of 6-AM. This rule is intended to streamline the laboratory process for analyzing and reporting 6-AM positive results and will facilitate MRO verification of 6-AM positive results."

On January 23, 2017, SAMHSA authorized testing for Schedule II opioids, hydrocodone, hydromorphone, oxycodone and oxymorphone in the testing of federal employees. DOT issued a final order dated January 1, 2018 including these opioids in the DOT testing panel as well.

On September 10, 2020, SAMHSA published proposed Mandatory Guidelines for the testing of hair specimens in the federal workforce. At this writing, this proposal is under review at the Office of Management and Budget, which will have to be completed before the Guidelines become final.

A Notice of Proposed Rulemaking (NPRM) was published by DOT on February 28, 2022, to include oral fluid testing in the DOT testing protocols.[5] A Final Rule was issued by DOT on May 2, 2023 authorizing oral fluid testing beginning June 1, 2023. SAMHSA previously authorized oral fluid testing in its Mandatory Guideline that became effective on January 1, 2020. These authorizations are both contingent on laboratories becoming certified by the National Laboratory Certification Program to do the testing and, as of this writing, none have done so.

On April 7, 2022, SAMHSA published proposed updates to the Oral Fluid Mandatory Guidelines (OFMG) and the Urine Mandatory Guidelines (URMG) that will alter MRO practice in reviewing results using those specimen matrices if adopted.[6,7]

The SAMHSA guidelines and DOT drug testing regulations together are considered the "gold standard" of drug testing. Many non-DOT testing programs are modeled after the DOT program because they are the most widely used standards and because they have successfully withstood legal challenges. In addition to the DOT regulations—which cover testing of commercial drivers, pilots, mariners, railroad and other transit workers, among others—separate regulations govern testing of federal employees and employees regulated by the Nuclear Regulatory Commission (NRC). When such testing is done, it is essential that the MRO understand the applicable regulations.

This chapter sidebar focuses on SAMHSA Mandatory Guidelines and the DOT regulations because they cover the largest number of workers and because they are considered the standard against which other forensically defensible drug tests are judged. Although most workplace testing is not regulated by DOT, these regulations and Guidelines provide useful guidance for all workplace settings.

MRO Qualifications

The guidelines initially promulgated by DHHS specified only that an MRO had to be a licensed physician with knowledge of substance use disorders. Later, it became apparent that additional, more specific qualifications were needed. The 2001 regulations required (under Subpart G: Medical Review Officers and Verification Process) that MROs be licensed physicians and have "clinical experience in controlled substance abuse disorders[8]." The updated regulations require that prospective MROs obtain certification from a nationally recognized certifying board (the Medical Review Officer Certification Council or the American Association of Medical Review Officers) and recertify every 5 years. Initial and refresher training is required by each of the certifying organizations.

It is important for physicians performing as MROs to recognize that MRO practice, and all of workplace drug testing, constitutes forensic practice rather than clinical or diagnostic practice. No doctor–patient relationship exists, nor is it desired, between the MRO and the donor of the specimen. For clinicians, especially addiction medicine clinicians, this distinction may be challenging. MROs are involved as the final step to ensure the accuracy and objectivity of a process that is essentially a search-and-seizure governed by the Fourth Amendment of the Constitution and upheld by several Supreme Court decisions. While workplace drug testing is intended to deter drug use in the workplace, it cannot detect every incidence of drug use in the workplace. Multiple forensic layers of protection are established so that no specimen donor may be wrongly accused of being a drug user. Because of all of these protections some authors have assumed a high likelihood that those who test positive in workplace testing, without a documented, valid prescription as described above, may indeed have a substance use disorder.[9]

As the laws and regulations governing workplace drug testing change and as individuals who use drugs devise ever more challenging ways to evade detection by workplace testing systems, MROs must keep their knowledge up-to-date. A list of recommended online resources is presented in **Table 127-2**.

Contractual Issues

Before beginning the medical review process, the MRO should have a written contract with the employer, spelling out in detail the services to be provided. Medical review is only one of many components of a drug-free workplace program. The successful MRO will either provide the other components or be able to direct the employer to them.

Organizations called "consortia" or "third-party administrators" (C/TPAs) provide overall testing program management, policy review, educational materials, training programs, and random sampling of employees, while contracting out for laboratory, MRO, and collection services. MROs may function as C/TPAs, but must be careful to follow the regulations that prohibit them from having a financial relationship with laboratories whose tests they review.

TABLE 127-2 Useful Websites

Organization	Web Address
American Association of Medical Review Officers (AAMRO)	www.aamro.com
Drug and Alcohol Testing Industry Association (DATIA)	www.datia.org
Medical Review Officer Certification Council (MROCC)	www.mrocc.org
Substance Abuse and Mental Health Services Administration (SAMHSA), Division of Workplace Programs	www.samhsa.gov/workforce
Substance Abuse Program Administrators Association (SAPAA)	www.sapaa.com
U.S. Department of Transportation (DOT), Office of Drug & Alcohol Policy & Compliance	www.transportation.gov/odapc

THE MEDICAL REVIEW PROCESS

The medical review process begins when an MRO receives a drug test result from a laboratory and ends when the results are reported. When dealing with urine testing for the drugs specified by the DHHS for federally mandated workplace testing programs, it is required that the MRO work with a laboratory that has been certified under the DHHS rules regarding academic credentials, regular inspections, and satisfactory performance in testing regularly submitted blind proficiency specimens.[10,11]

When testing materials other than urine are used, laboratory selection involves careful review of laboratory credentials and quality control procedures. Consultation with a forensic toxicologist may be desirable in evaluating the competence of a particular laboratory.

Collection of Specimens

Although federal guidelines minimize the MRO's responsibility for collection of laboratory specimens, the MRO is required to check each custody and control form for signatures and collector remarks. In addition to this administrative function, the MRO should confirm that, in cases involving nonnegative test results, the chain of custody was not broken. The MRO also should be prepared to evaluate problems that arise when donors are unable to provide adequate amounts of urine for test purposes, otherwise known as "shy bladder" cases. Some of the most challenging MRO cases involve questions of urine specimen dilution, substitution, adulteration, and other issues involving interference with laboratory-testing techniques.

Choice of Specimen

The choice of specimen (eg, urine, hair, oral fluid) affects both the detectability of drug use and the interpretation of test results. The SAMHSA Drug Testing Advisory Board is developing standards for the inclusion of hair testing in the federal testing program.

Negative Test Results

When a test result is negative, the MRO's role is twofold. First, the MRO (or an MRO team member who is under the direct personal supervision of the MRO) reviews the custody and control form (CCF) and the laboratory result to determine whether the specimen was diluted, whether it was within the acceptable temperature range, and whether there were any other issues that may have had an adverse effect on the testing process.

If identified, such conditions would be reported to the employer, possibly with a recommendation for appropriate action to be taken in response. As the gatekeepers of the drug testing process, MROs are responsible for verifying that correctable errors are, in fact, corrected if it is possible to do so.

Nonnegative Test Results (Including Positive, Adulterated, Substituted, and Invalid Test Results)

Before reporting a nonnegative result, the MRO should be satisfied that (1) the correct specimen was tested (and not inadvertently confused with someone else's sample), (2) the laboratory accurately performed the necessary analyses, and (3) there was no acceptable, legitimate medical explanation for the nonnegative test result.

To resolve these questions, an MRO must understand forensic collection and chain-of-custody procedures, understand the role of the toxicology laboratory, and be familiar with the relevant laws and regulations.

Before a laboratory can report a result as a confirmed positive, its designated analyte must test positive by an approved screening method that includes, but is not limited to, immunoassay, as well as by a confirmatory test, typically performed with gas chromatography–mass spectrometry (GC–MS), liquid chromatography–mass spectrometry (LC–MS), or either of those two in tandem with mass spectrometry (GC–MS–MS, LC–MS–MS). The confirmatory test is so specific that it often is referred to as a "chemical fingerprint." Screening tests are less specific than the confirmation procedures and may be positive on the basis of compounds that are in some way chemically similar to the sought-after analytes.

Workplace drug testing is a forensic program designed to deter the use of drugs by a workforce. The majority of those being tested do not engage in unhealthy drug use. Therefore to discount the possibility of confirmed positive results being caused only by passive or incidental exposure to a drug, DHHS has established testing cutoff levels below which an analyte may be present but is not reportable. The DHHS certification program only addresses the DHHS-5 drugs. The panel is still referred to as DHHS-5, even though the number of analytes being tested for is now 14: benzoylecgonine (the cocaine metabolite), carboxy THC (the marijuana metabolite), phencyclidine (PCP), amphetamines [including methamphetamine, amphetamine, methylenedioxymethamphetamine (MDMA), methylenedioxyamphetamine (MDA)], the opiates morphine, codeine, 6-acetylmorphine, and the opioids hydrocodone, hydromorphone, oxycodone, and oxymorphone. It includes only certification for the testing of controlled substances that are listed in Schedule I or II of the federal Controlled Substance Act (CSA) and does *not* include benzodiazepines or barbiturates, which often are included in non–federally mandated testing panels. The inclusion of fentanyl and its metabolite are currently under discussion by SAMHSA.

Each employee who has a laboratory-confirmed nonnegative test must be offered an opportunity to be interviewed and the relevant paperwork from the laboratory and collection sites reviewed by the MRO. During this review, the MRO may find it necessary to speak with the designated employer representative (DER), with the individual who collected the urine, with laboratory personnel, and/or with the employee's physician or pharmacy. On occasion, the MRO may wish to have the worker examined by an independent physician. Additional laboratory testing may be required, possibly including reanalysis of the specimen.

Invalid Tests

Some specimens cannot be tested because of an interfering substance, because they are too diluted or too concentrated or because their pH is out of range. Some medications interfere with the screening process, and occasionally, adulterating substances may be added to the specimen. When a certified laboratory cannot complete testing of a specimen because of one of these unusual characteristics, the results are reported to the MRO as "invalid." MROs must remember that an invalid specimen is not synonymous with an adulterated specimen nor is it necessarily an attempt by a donor to subvert the testing process.

The MRO must review such results, interview the donor, and report the results to the employer as "test cancelled." If there is no acceptable medical explanation for the laboratory finding, the MRO will direct the DER to obtain an immediate observed re-collection of urine from that donor; however, if it appears that there may have been a legitimate explanation for the problem (rather than an attempt to subvert), a repeat of the test may not be necessary unless a negative result is required.

Adulterated or Substituted Tests

If the laboratory confirms an adulterant, the result is reported to the MRO as "adulterated." In cases of extreme dilution that are not consistent with normal human urine, the results are reported to the MRO as "substituted." Adulterated and substituted test results also must be reviewed by the MRO. Unless the donor offers a valid medical basis for the result, it is reported to the employer as "refusal to test," along with the reason (eg, "refusal to test because of adulteration with glutaraldehyde").

Record Keeping

When a test result is reported as nonnegative, a file should be created for all the relevant paperwork, including notes of the MRO's interactions with the test donor and others. Because the information in such a file may be subpoenaed, the MRO should treat it with at least as much care as is used in a clinical chart. Under federal testing programs, the MRO is required to keep records of all nonnegative tests for 5 years. In practice, this is a good rule for unregulated programs as well. Many MROs retain such records even longer.

The MRO Interview

When an interview is required, the MRO should make at least three attempts to contact the donor at the telephone number provided by the CCF during the 24 hours after the information is received. If the MRO is unable to contact the donor during that time, they should ask the DER to contact the donor and direct them to call the MRO within 72 hours. The DER also should warn the donor that if they do not contact the MRO, the MRO will report the results to the employer after 72 hours.

If contact is made, the MRO should identify the donor by asking them to provide the identification number used during the drug test collection. This number may be the donor's Social Security number (SSN) or any other number that is chosen by the employer and the donor. In cases where the SSN is used, to help preserve confidentiality the MRO may ask for only the last 4 digits. The MRO should explain the review process and the MRO's role in that process. Most importantly, the MRO must warn the donor that the MRO is required to provide to the employer and/or appropriate government agencies any information disclosed to the MRO during the review process if it might affect the performance of safety-sensitive duties. Some have called this a drug testing "Miranda warning."

The MRO should inform the donor of the drug detected and ask them about any medication use that might explain the result. (It is not appropriate for the MRO to ask about other medications being taken or about medical treatments other than those that could explain the drug test result.)

When the donor claims the confirmed positive result is caused by their own prescription medicine, the MRO must verify that prescription. There are many ways to do that and to help minimize the issue of prescription forgery, and it is currently recommended that MROs do a dual verification procedure. One example of this type of procedure is to ask the donor to provide a photo of the bottle label, after which the MRO calls the pharmacy and verifies the RX using the RX identification number.

Reporting Test Results

At the conclusion of the review process, the MRO notifies the donor and employer of the findings, which may be:

- *Negative* (including reversals on the basis of MRO verified legitimate medical explanations) and *negative, dilute*
- *Positive* (including positives confirmed on reanalysis) and *positive, dilute*. Positive reports must include the name of the verified positive drug
- *Cancelled* because of:
  - Fatal flaws or uncorrected correctable flaws
  - Failure to reconfirm on reanalysis
  - Invalid specimens, with or without medical justification
  - Shy bladder in a current employee who has an acceptable medical explanation
- *Refusal to test* because of:
  - Specimen adulterated, with a report that must include the name of the confirmed adulterating substance
  - Specimen substituted
  - Insufficient amount of urine provided, without a legitimate explanation
  - Donor late for test or left the collection site before the test could be completed
  - Donor refused to permit direct observation of the test, as required
  - Donor refused to cooperate with the testing process or refused to take a second test when asked to do so

THE FUTURE OF MRO PRACTICE

The contemporary perspective on alcohol and drug use in the workplace is rooted in the current understanding of addiction as a biopsychosocial disorder, with a renewed emphasis on brain biology.[12,13] As a consequence, MRO practice is challenging and constantly changing, providing physicians who specialize in addiction medicine with an additional arena in which to exercise their expertise and professional interest. This is especially important now, in view of the ongoing nationwide epidemic of unhealthy substance use including addiction.

In addition to the rapidly evolving science of addiction, the regulations governing drug testing also continue to evolve. Nonfederal testing programs have long included the Schedule II opioids and alternative specimen testing, as well as expanded drug panels including benzodiazepines, synthetics, and many opioids not in the federal program. This makes MRO practice even more challenging and necessary, especially now that the federal program is "catching up" with the Schedule II opioids and alternative specimens. Advances in drug testing technology benefit not only the federal testing program but also nonfederal workplace testing, addiction treatment and monitoring settings, pain medicine clinics, and beyond. Knowledgeable MROs are useful in all of these settings.

The MRO provides useful oversight of the drug testing process and sophisticated interpretation of drug test results to help ensure program fairness, accuracy, and testing that achieves the highest level of modern science. Many drug test results are relatively simple to interpret, while others benefit from the sophistication of the MRO.

In a free and open society, the hurdles faced by workplace alcohol and drug testing programs are complex and will not be dealt with easily. Workplace drug testing programs are important both in preventing unhealthy substance use and in providing a useful path to recovery for many employees who have substance use disorders. In addition, workplace testing programs promote safety and productivity.

The major challenge for the future of workplace programs is to develop and maintain comprehensive programs that are fair and reasonable, as well as strong. Such programs must operate in the public interest in ways that respect not only the interests of all parties involved, but also the dignity of workers and their families, including the dignity of persons who have substance use disorders.

REFERENCES

1. U.S. Department of Health and Human Services (DHHS). Mandatory guidelines for federal workplace drug testing programs. *Federal Register.* 1988;53:11970.
2. U.S. Department of Labor (DOL). Drug-Free Workplace Advisor: Drug-Free Workplace Act of 1988 Requirements. http://www.dol.gov/elaws/asp/drugfree/screenr.htm
3. U.S. Department of Transportation (DOT). Procedures for transportation workplace drug and alcohol testing programs. Overview of 49 CFR Part 40. 2013. Accessed 7 May, 2023. http://www.dot.gov/odapc/part40.html
4. U.S. Department Transportation (DOT). Procedures for transportation workplace drug and alcohol testing programs: 6-acetylmorphine (6-AM) testing. *Federal Register.* 2012;77(87):26471-26473. Accessed 7 May, 2023. http://www.gpo.gov/fdsys/pkg/FR-2012-05-04/pdf/2012-10665.pdf
5. *Federal Register* / Vol. 87, No. 39 / Monday, February 28, 2022 / Proposed Rules, pp 11156-11186.
6. *Federal Register* / Vol. 87, No. 67 / Thursday, April 7, 2022 / Proposed Rules, pp 20555-20557.
7. *Federal Register* / Vol. 87, No. 66 / Wednesday, April 6, 2022 / Notices, pp 19923-19924.
8. U.S. Department Transportation (DOT). Procedures for transportation workplace drug and alcohol testing programs. *Federal Register.* 2001;66:41951. Accessed 7 May, 2023. http://www.gpo.gov/fdsys/pkg/FR-2000-12-19/pdf/00-31251.pdf
9. DuPont RL, Griffin DW, Siskin BR, Shiraki S, Katze E. Random drug tests at work: the probability of identifying frequent and infrequent users of illicit drugs. *J Add Dis.* 1995;14:1-17.
10. DuPont RL. Drugs in the American workplace: Conflict and opportunity, Part II. Controversies in workplace drug use prevention. *Soc Pharmacol.* 1989;3:147-164.
11. DuPont RL. Medicines and drug testing in the workplace. *J Psychoactive Drugs.* 1990;22:451-459.
12. Nahas GG, Burks TF. *Drug Abuse in the Decade of the Brain.* IOS Press; 1997.
13. DuPont RL. *The Selfish Brain: Learning from Addiction.* Hazelden; 2000.

CHAPTER

128 Reducing Substance Use in Court-Leveraged Treatment

Douglas B. Marlowe

CHAPTER OUTLINE

- Scope of the problem
- Court-leveraged treatment
- Dimensions of court-leveraged treatment
- Matching participants to court-leveraged programs
- Cultural equity
- Medication for opioid use disorder
- Conclusion

SCOPE OF THE PROBLEM

More than half of U.S. persons incarcerated in state jails and prisons or sentenced to community probation have a moderate to severe substance use disorder.[1,2] Between 65% and 85% of individuals arrested for property, financial, and violent crimes test positive for illegal drugs or report recent use at the time of their arrest.[3] Among persons with substance use disorders involved in the criminal justice or criminal legal system, resuming substance use is one of the most potent predictors of criminal recidivism, increasing the odds of a new offense by two to four times.[4] Providing substance use treatment can reduce crime and substance use if participants receive an adequate dose of evidence-based services.[5] Unfortunately, the more persons need treatment and the greater their likelihood of recidivism, the less likely they will enter or complete treatment.[6] Note: some scholars and commentators use the term *criminal legal system* rather than *criminal justice system* because the system has often fallen short in providing equity and fairness for all persons. Other commentators take a contrary view that removing justice from the name suggests that equity is unachievable or might be misinterpreted as absolving system actors from its pursuit. Both terms are used in this chapter to recognize both perspectives.

Persons referred to treatment by the criminal justice or criminal legal system often lack intrinsic motivation for change and require external pressure and accountability to ensure they stay in treatment long enough to receive therapeutic benefits.[7,8] Compared with self-initiated treatment, outcomes are as, or more, effective for persons who choose to enter and remain in treatment primarily or exclusively to avoid serious negative legal repercussions from their substance use, such as impending incarceration.[9,10] Referred to as *leveraged* treatment, this arrangement differs from *compulsory* or *mandated* treatment in which persons have no choice but to attend treatment, as in cases of involuntary civil commitment or detainment in compulsory penal treatment centers. Compulsory treatment offers questionable therapeutic benefits[11] and raises serious concerns about potential due process and human rights violations.[12] Leveraged treatment is more effective and poses fewer due process concerns because persons are given the choice, often with the assistance of counsel, whether to choose treatment or to proceed as usual with adjudication.

COURT-LEVERAGED TREATMENT

In court-leveraged treatment, persons who are charged with or convicted of a crime receive a court-monitored rehabilitative disposition in lieu of traditional prosecution or sentencing. Eligibility criteria for most programs require candidates to (1) have a moderate to severe substance use disorder pursuant to DSM-5-TR diagnostic criteria or substance dependence pursuant to earlier DSM-IV-TR criteria, and (2) be charged with a drug- or alcohol-related offense such as possession or sale of a controlled substance, driving under the influence (DUI) of drugs or alcohol, or theft or forgery to support a substance use disorder. Although many programs exclude persons with violence charges or histories, some programs serve persons charged with certain types of violent offenses such as domestic violence.

Most court-leveraged programs require defendants to plead guilty or no contest to the arrest charge(s). Requiring a guilty plea is intended to keep participants engaged in treatment because the case ordinarily proceeds to sentencing in the event of treatment attrition or other repetitive rule violations. The plea is held in abeyance (suspended temporarily) while participants attend treatment and is reduced or withdrawn upon completion. Some programs expunge the arrest or guilty plea from participants' record if they remain arrest-free for an additional waiting period (typically 1 to 2 years) after completing treatment, which avoids some of the negative collateral consequences of a criminal conviction, such as barriers to employment, subsidized housing, or voting.

Some individuals are not eligible by statute or prosecutorial policy to avoid prosecution because of the seriousness of their crime or their criminal history. Such individuals may be sentenced to a court-monitored rehabilitative program in lieu of incarceration as a condition of probation. Failing to abide by the conditions of the program may result in a return to court, revocation of probation, and placement in custody.

DIMENSIONS OF COURT-LEVERAGED TREATMENT

Court-leveraged programs differ along several dimensions, making them differentially effective and sometimes counterproductive for persons with varying levels of treatment needs and risk factors for criminal recidivism or treatment attrition. As will be discussed, assigning persons to programs that are too intensive or not intensive enough to meet their needs is often ineffective and may increase the recurrence of substance use, criminal recidivism, or other undesirable outcomes like unstable housing or underemployment.

Court Calendar

Most court-leveraged programs have specialized calendars or dockets requiring participants to appear before the same judge until final resolution of the case to ensure consistency and continuity in case processing.

- ***Status Calendar.*** The most intensive programs employ status calendars, in which participants appear routinely in court for the judge to review their progress in treatment, offer advice and encouragement, and administer incentives for their accomplishments and sanctions for infractions. Examples of incentives include verbal praise, reduced supervision requirements, or small gifts (eg, coffee mugs, healthy snacks). Examples of sanctions include verbal reprimands, increased supervision requirements, home detention, or brief jail detention usually ranging from a few days to a few weeks. Status hearings typically begin on a weekly or biweekly (every 2 weeks) basis and may be tapered to monthly as participants settle into a treatment routine and achieve clinical stability.
- ***Compliance Calendar.*** Less intensive programs employ compliance calendars, in which participants return to court when they have completed treatment or if they are alleged to have committed a serious rule infraction, such as absconding from treatment. Compliance calendars have dedicated time slots, allowing hearings to be scheduled rapidly in response to alleged infractions. Probation officers or case managers from treatment agencies deliver progress reports to the court and may be present during compliance hearings to answer questions from the judge or offer recommendations about suitable consequences to impose.

Multidisciplinary Team

In the traditional court system, judges function as neutral arbiters and may not discuss defendants' progress with treatment providers or other practitioners outside of court or without all counsel (prosecutor and defense) present. To do so would violate defendants' constitutional due process rights to be treated impartially and to dispute any evidence that is offered. In court-leveraged programs, however, defendants commonly waive these rights and permit judges to work collaboratively with other professionals.

- ***Team Staffings.*** In the most intensive programs, judges function essentially as the leader of a multidisciplinary team, which often includes clinical case managers, probation officers, defense counsel, the prosecutor, and social service professionals. Team members meet routinely in staff meetings outside of court to review participant progress, contribute expertise, and offer recommendations to the judge for suitable consequences to impose.
- ***Compliance Reviews.*** In programs employing compliance calendars, judges usually do not meet routinely with other team members to review participant progress; however, they receive progress reports and schedule rapid compliance hearings for alleged infractions. In advance of the compliance hearings, judges may meet collaboratively with other team members in compliance reviews to prepare for their interactions with participants in court.

Consequences for Substance Use

Court-leveraged programs vary considerably in their responses to new incidences of substance use. Some programs view illegal drug or alcohol use as a serious rule violation and potential public safety threat. Staff in these programs may consider punitive sanctions to be essential for holding participants accountable for their actions and deterring other participants from similar misconduct. After delivering stern warnings and low-magnitude sanctions for the first few instances of substance use, they may deliver high-magnitude sanctions including home detention or jail detention, which escalate progressively in length or severity in response to successive instances of substance use or other infractions. Other programs, in contrast, view substance use as a symptom of a chronic and compulsive illness requiring treatment, not punishment. Punishing individuals for symptoms that are beyond their control interferes with the treatment process and can cause learned helplessness, in which persons become despondent and resentful because they are unable to avoid punishment, leading to higher rates of substance use, emotional distress, and crime.[13] Evidence supports both perspectives—but for different individuals. Reconciling these divergent strategies requires careful consideration of participants' diagnostic status and treatment needs.

Compulsive Substance Use ("High Need Persons")

In court-leveraged treatment programs, the term *high need* refers to a substance use disorder that includes compulsive features (described below) or other serious treatment or social service needs, such as mental health disorders or homelessness, and is distinguished from *high risk*, which refers to a high likelihood of treatment attrition or criminal recidivism. Common examples of high risk-factors include extensive criminal records, antisocial personality traits, antisocial peer groups, or impulsivity. This terminology may differ from that of the treatment field, which often uses *high risk* to refer to a high likelihood of continued substance use.

Some individuals charged with substance-related crimes have a substance use disorder that includes one or more of the following compulsive symptoms:

- persistent cravings for the substance,
- withdrawal symptoms,

- persistent but unsuccessful efforts to stop using the substance, and/or
- loss of control over usage leading to recurrent binge episodes (ie, use often substantially exceeds the person's intentions or expectations).

These symptoms are often indicative of severe and enduring neurochemical changes in the brain and reflect physiologic dependence or a substantial inability to avoid or control use.[14] For such high need individuals, abstinence is often an arduous goal to achieve. Delivering high-magnitude sanctions for failing to meet arduous goals interferes with treatment, is a sure recipe for learned helplessness, and can cause criminal justice or criminal legal professionals to exhaust their quiver of sanctions too quickly before treatment has had a chance to work. Instead, treatment adjustments or low-magnitude sanctions like verbal admonitions, writing assignments, or journaling exercises are ordinarily indicated for new instances of substance use until, at a minimum, participants are clinically stable and no longer experiencing debilitating symptoms like substance cravings or withdrawal.[15,16] High magnitude sanctions like jail detention are indicated only, if at all, for willful infractions such as delivering tampered drug test specimens or neglectful infractions such as overlooking treatment obligations.[17]

Noncompulsive Substance Use ("Low Need Persons")

Not all persons arrested for substance-related offenses have compulsive symptoms. Some individuals engage repeatedly in problematic substance use that gets them into frequent trouble with the law and may interfere with other critical responsibilities like childcare; however, their use is largely under volitional control. Delivering weak or no sanctions for noncompulsive substance use may encourage these low need participants to test the limits of the program's tolerance, leading to more of the same or increased substance use. Delivering weak sanctions for willful or neglectful infractions can cause habituation, in which persons become accustomed and thus less responsive to the threat of punishment, leading to higher rates of substance use and other infractions.[18] Deciding whether to deliver sanctions or treatment adjustments requires a careful consideration of participants' treatment needs and capacity to avoid substance use.

MATCHING PARTICIPANTS TO COURT-LEVERAGED PROGRAMS

No program works for everyone. Providing too much, too little, or the wrong kind of services does not improve outcomes, and in fact can worsen outcomes by allowing problems to fester for needy persons or by overburdening less impaired individuals and interfering with their ability to engage in productive activities like work or school. This is the foundation for a body of evidence-based principles referred to as *risk, needs, responsivity* or RNR.[19] RNR is derived from decades of research finding that the best outcomes are achieved when the intensity of criminal justice or criminal legal supervision is matched to participants' risk for recidivism or likelihood of attrition from treatment, and services focus primarily on the specific disorders or conditions that are responsible for participants' crimes. Most important, mixing participants with different levels of risk or need in the same treatment groups or residential programs has been shown to increase crime, substance use, and other undesirable outcomes because it exposes low-risk individuals to antisocial peers and values.[20,21]

Consistent with RNR principles, court-leveraged programs are most effective when they match services to participants' treatment needs and risk factors for treatment attrition or criminal recidivism. **Table 128-1** depicts a quadrant model

TABLE 128-1 Examples of Effective Court-Leveraged Programs for Persons With Different Risk and Need Profile

		Risk for criminal recidivism or treatment attrition	
		High	**Low**
Need for treatment for compulsive substance use disorder	*High*	**Drug court or DUI court** • Status calendar • Multidisciplinary team staffing • Intensive treatment and probation counseling • Treatment adjustments or low magnitude sanctions for substance use until clinically stable • Higher magnitude sanctions for willful or neglected infractions	**Court-monitored treatment diversion** • Compliance calendar • Progress reports and compliance reviews • Intensive treatment • Treatment adjustments or low magnitude sanctions for substance use until clinically stable • Higher magnitude sanctions for willful or neglected infractions
	Low	**HOPE court** • Compliance calendar • Progress reports and compliance reviews • Intensive probation counseling • Escalating higher magnitude sanctions for substance use and willful or neglectful infractions	**Minimal court involvement** • Traditional calendar • Remote check-ins with supervision officer or case manager

HOPE, Honest Opportunity Probation with Enforcement.

Adapted with permission from Marlowe DB. Evidence-based sentencing for drug offenders: an analysis of prognostic risks and criminogenic needs. *Chapman J Crim Justice.* 2009;1:167-201.

of RNR that crosses two levels of risk (high or low) with two levels of need, yielding four generic profiles of persons charged with drug or alcohol-related offenses.[22] Services that are required to rehabilitate persons in the high risk or need quadrants will often be unnecessary or counterproductive for those in the low risk or need quadrants. Studies have found that matching participants to court-leveraged services pursuant to the quadrant model led to significant improvements in treatment attendance, substance use, criminal recidivism and cost-effectiveness compared with programming as usual.[23,24]

High Risk and High Need Persons

Persons in the upper left quadrant have a compulsive substance use disorder as defined earlier and a high need for substance use treatment, and they often require mental health treatment and other social services as well, such as job training or remedial education. They also have substantial risk factors for criminal recidivism or premature attrition from treatment, such as extensive criminal histories, antisocial personality traits, antisocial peer groups, or impulsivity. Outcomes are significantly better when high risk and high need individuals appear every two weeks or more often in court for status hearings,[25-27] a multidisciplinary team meets frequently to review their progress and coordinate services,[25] participants receive intensive substance use treatment and probation counseling,[22-27] high-magnitude sanctions like jail detention are reserved for willful infractions such as absconding from treatment,[16] and treatment adjustments are applied for new instances of substance use.[15]

Drug Courts and DUI Courts

Rigorously evaluated programs that contain each of the above elements and are proven to enhance outcomes for high risk and high need persons charged with substance-related offenses include, but are not limited to, drug courts for persons charged with drug-related offenses and DUI courts for persons charged with repeated DUI offenses. The defining ingredients of these programs include frequent status hearings, service coordination by a multidisciplinary team, intensive substance use treatment, probation supervision, and distinguishing carefully between willful or neglectful infractions meriting higher-magnitude sanctions and compulsive substance use meriting low-magnitude sanctions or treatment adjustments.[28,29]

Meta-analyses and multisite studies have determined that drug courts and DUI courts significantly reduced criminal recidivism by an average of approximately 12%, with the most effective programs reducing recidivism by 50% to 85%,[25,27,30,31] and they generated net cost-benefits of approximately $9,000 per participant compared with incarceration or community supervision as usual.[32] Reductions in recidivism were found to last for at least three years after program entry,[27] and in two studies the effects lasted at least 15 years.[33,34] A national study of 23 adult drug courts found that drug courts also significantly reduced illegal drug use, improved participants' family relationships, reduced family conflicts, and increased participants' access to needed financial and social services.[30]

Importantly, the effects of drug courts and DUI courts are substantially moderated by the risk and need levels of participants. Programs are approximately twice as effective at reducing crime and 50% more cost-effective when they serve high risk and high need participants[25,35,36]; however, they can increase treatment attrition and recidivism when they imprudently serve persons with low levels of risk or need.[35,37] Harmful outcomes for low risk and need individuals may result from increased interactions with high-risk peers, or excessive treatment or supervision requirements may interfere with productive activities like work or childcare.

High Risk and Low Need Persons

Persons in the lower left quadrant do not have a compulsive substance use disorder as defined previously or other pressing treatment needs, but they have serious risk factors for criminal recidivism or attrition from traditional rehabilitation programs, such as extensive criminal records and antisocial peers. Delivering high-magnitude sanctions for substance use can be effective for such individuals, but only if they also receive counseling and social services addressing their risk factors for recidivism, a dedicated judge reviews noncompliance allegations expeditiously, and a multidisciplinary team coordinates services and keeps the judge apprised of participant progress.

HOPE Court

Honest Opportunity Probation with Enforcement (HOPE) is one example of a court-leveraged program showing promise for high risk and low need individuals. Participants are drug tested frequently and receive swift, certain, and brief jail sanctions (typically ranging from 2 to 15 days) for positive or missed drug tests or other infractions such as missed probation appointments. Participants are assigned to a compliance review calendar with a specially trained judge who orients them to the program, schedules prompt hearings in response to alleged infractions, ensures they are treated in an encouraging and procedurally fair manner, and imposes expeditious jail sanctions for proven violations. Participants are supervised by probation officers who deliver progress reports to the court and are well trained in evidence-based counseling strategies addressing participants' risk factors for recidivism, such as antisocial peer interactions, impulsivity, and antisocial thinking. Participants are also triaged to substance use treatment and other indicated services if they request them or are unable to refrain from illegal drug or alcohol use despite the sanctioning protocol. A randomized trial of the original HOPE program in Hawaii found that participants were 55% less likely than control participants to be arrested for a new crime, 72% less likely to test positive for illegal drugs, 61% less likely to miss probation appointments, and 53% less likely to have their probation revoked.[38] Many of these positive effects lasted for at least 10 years.[39]

Efforts to replicate the impressive results from the original HOPE program have had mixed success, with some studies reporting comparably favorable outcomes[40] and others finding no improvements or increases in probation violations.[41] Discrepant findings appear to be attributable to inconsistent implementation of the model. Although most programs rigorously apply the sanctioning elements, many fall short in delivering counseling or social services addressing participants' risk factors for recidivism or attrition from rehabilitation.[42] Sanctioning drug use without providing indicated services is unlikely to improve outcomes for high-risk individuals.[43] More important, HOPE is not suited for persons with compulsive substance use disorders for whom punitive sanctions for substance use are contraindicated.[15,16,18] Such persons should be referred to a treatment-oriented program like a drug court.[44]

Low Risk and High Need Persons

Persons in the upper right quadrant have a compulsive substance use disorder and high need for substance use treatment and other indicated services, but they do not have serious risk factors for criminal recidivism or treatment attrition. These individuals have a favorable prognosis if they are given reasonable access to an adequate dosage of evidence-based treatment and social services, and the court limits its role to monitoring treatment adherence and addressing attrition from treatment or other serious infractions.

Court-Monitored Treatment Diversion

A 2000 voter initiative in California referred to as Proposition 36 provides an instructive example of court-monitored diversion to treatment for low risk and high need persons.[45] Extensive research on Proposition 36 offers cautionary insights to avoid negative effects from treatment diversion programs and ensure adequate court oversight. Proposition 36 entitles persons charged with drug possession who do not have a violent or other serious exclusionary offense in their record to plead guilty in exchange for probation with conditions for substance use treatment and other indicated services. If participants are charged subsequently with a new drug possession offense or drug-related probation violation, they are again entitled to probation with increased conditions for treatment or other indicated services. The court may only impose a jail sanction or sentence if a participant is convicted of three drug possession offenses or determined by the judge to be a threat to public safety or unamenable to the treatments that are reasonably available in the community. Upon successful completion of treatment and probation, the guilty plea is vacated, and the case is expunged from the participant's record.

Results from Proposition 36 were largely disappointing; however, promising findings emerged for a subset of low risk and high need individuals. In the aggregate, large percentages of Proposition 36 participants did not enter treatment or left prematurely, and new arrests for drug and property crimes were significantly higher than in preimplementation years.[46] Importantly, however, roughly 25% of the participants were determined to be high risk due to serious criminal records or a history of premature attrition from treatment, and this subset of participants accounted for more than 80% of the criminal recidivism and criminal system costs.[47] Because Proposition 36 removed nearly all leverage from criminal justice or criminal legal authorities, it prevented the courts from managing these high-risk individuals safely or effectively. Superior outcomes for high-risk individuals are achieved in programs delivering greater supervision and accountability, like drug courts.[48]

When high risk persons were excluded from the analyses, Proposition 36 showed significant improvement for high need persons who were suffering from severe substance use disorders, including heroin and methamphetamine use disorders, when they received residential treatment or medication for addiction treatment commensurate with their treatment needs.[49] These findings suggest that diverting high need persons out of the aegis of the criminal justice or criminal legal system and into community treatment can be effective, but only if participants do not require concomitant monitoring and behavioral management from the court to ensure they attend treatment, desist from crime, and comply with other probation conditions. Courts should retain authority to confer with other professionals, schedule rapid compliance hearings where indicated, and administer substantial sanctions for repeated willful or neglectful infractions including illegal drug or alcohol use by persons who do not have a compulsive substance use disorder.

Low Risk and Low Need Persons

Finally, persons in the lower right quadrant do not have significant treatment needs or risk factors for recidivism and are likely to refrain on their own from further involvement with the criminal justice or criminal legal system. Such individuals require minimal, if any, court supervision. Low risk and low need persons can often be managed safely and effectively by having them check-in remotely with a supervision officer or case manager, such as through periodic phone conferences.[50] In the unlikely event of a serious rule infraction or new offense, the individual can appear in a traditional court hearing and be considered for a more intensive program.

CULTURAL EQUITY

Court-leveraged treatment programs were created to improve a troubled criminal justice or criminal legal system, not to mirror its worst attributes, yet racial and ethnic disparities exist in many programs, reflecting and possibly exacerbating systemic injustices. A study of more than 14,000 participants in 105 drug courts reported an average graduation rate of 36% for Black or African American participants and 46% for Latinx or Hispanic participants compared with 53% for non-Hispanic White participants.[51] Another study in ten geographically diverse communities in the U.S. found that Black persons arrested for drug offenses were roughly half as likely as White persons to be referred to drug court; of those referred, Black persons were less likely to be admitted in seven of the eight jurisdictions for which admission data were available; and of those admitted, Black persons were less likely to graduate in six of the ten jurisdictions.[52] Studies of Proposition 36 reported that Black and Hispanic participants were less likely than non-Hispanic White participants to receive services commensurate with their treatment needs, although legal outcomes were roughly equivalent.[53] These findings suggest that cascading inequities at successive stages in the criminal justice or criminal legal process may contribute additively or multiplicatively to higher legal system involvement for Black and Hispanic persons, lesser access to needed treatment and social services, and poorer legal and health outcomes.

Best practice standards promulgated by the National Association of Drug Court Professionals (NADCP) provide that drug courts should monitor their operations at least annually for evidence of racial, ethnic, and other cultural disparities and adjust their eligibility criteria, assessment procedures and treatment services to eliminate disparities that are detected.[54] To help drug courts meet these obligations, NADCP developed a suite of resources to measure disparities, increase entry and engagement of various racial, ethnic, and other groups, and apply culturally proficient practices to improve outcomes.[55] Technical assistance is required to help drug courts and other court-leveraged programs apply these tools to diagnose disparities, implement remedial measures and evaluate the success of their efforts.

MEDICATION FOR OPIOID USE DISORDER

Medication for opioid use disorder (MOUD) is a critical component of the evidence-based standard of care for treating persons with opioid use disorder.[56] Buprenorphine or methadone maintenance instituted in jail or prison and continued after release has been shown to increase retention in treatment and reduce nonprescribed opioid use, opioid overdose and mortality rates, and transmission of HIV and hepatitis C infections among individuals with opioid use disorder.[57] Improved outcomes are also reported for a different class of medication, naltrexone, which unlike methadone and buprenorphine, does not produce or sustain physiologic dependence.[57]

Despite compelling evidence of safety and effectiveness, only about 5% of persons with opioid use disorders receive these medications in court-referred programs.[58] Studies in drug courts have observed unwarranted hindrances in MOUD provision, including substantial delays in starting the medication regimens, stigmatizing attitudes held by some staff members or fellow clients, and greater use of naltrexone over methadone or buprenorphine in some programs, which might not have been medically indicated.[59-61] NADCP standards provide that drug courts should learn the scientific facts about MOUD, obtain expert medical consultation, and allow the use of all FDA-approved medications when prescribed by a qualified medical professional.[54] NADCP tool kits are available that provide sample letter templates to educate legal officials about the proven benefits of MOUD, alert them to practice standards governing its use, and include model agreements delineating the appropriate roles and responsibilities of drug court team members, partnering agencies, medical practitioners, and clients receiving MOUD.[62]

CONCLUSION

More than 30 years of research on court-leveraged treatment has identified the requisite ingredients for safe, effective, equitable, and cost-efficient interventions for substance-related crime. Studies have determined how persons should be matched to programs and identified best practices to enhance outcomes. This work is not finished, however, until the lessons are communicated effectively to practitioners and implemented in daily operations. Efforts are needed to educate legal officials, policy makers, and the public about evidence-based practices and ensure those practices are administered correctly in the court system.

REFERENCES

1. Bronson J, Stroop J, Zimmer S, Berzofsky M. *Drug Use, Dependence, and Abuse Among State Prisoners and Jail Inmates, 2007-2009*. Bureau of Justice Statistics; 2017. NCJ 250546. Accessed June 8, 2022. https://www.bjs.gov/content/pub/pdf/dudaspji0709.pdf
2. Fearn NE, Vaughn MG, Nelson EJ, Salas-Wright CP, DeLisi M, Qian Z. Trends and correlates of substance use disorders among probationers and parolees in the United States, 2002-2014. *Drug Alcohol Depend*. 2016;167:128-139.
3. Office of National Drug Control Policy. *2013 Annual Report, Arrestee Drug Abuse Monitoring Program II*. Accessed June 8, 2022. https://obamawhitehouse.archives.gov/sites/default/files/ondcp/policy-and-research/adam_ii_2013_annual_report.pdf
4. Kopak AM, Hoffman NG, Proctor SL. Key risk factors for relapse and rearrest among substance use treatment patients involved in the criminal justice system. *Am J Crim Justice*. 2016;41:14-30.
5. Holloway KR, Bennett TH, Farrington DP. The effectiveness of drug treatment programs in reducing criminal behavior: a meta-analysis. *Psicothema*. 2006;18(3):620-629.
6. Ternes M, Richer I, MacDonald SF. Distinguishing the features of offenders who do and do not complete substance use treatment in corrections: extending the reach of psychological services. *Psychol Serv*. 2020;17(4):422-432.
7. Gregoire TK, Burke AC. The relationship of legal coercion to readiness to change among adults with alcohol and other drug problems. *J Subst Abuse Treat*. 2004;26(1):337-343.
8. Lilach S, Blankers M, Koeter MWJ, Schippers GM, Goudriaan AE. The role of motivation in predicting addiction treatment entry among offenders with substance use disorders under probation supervision. *Int J Offender Ther Comp Criminol*. 2019;63(14):2453-2464.
9. Perron BE, Bright CL. The influence of legal coercion on dropout from substance abuse treatment: results from a national survey. *Drug Alcohol Depend*. 2008;92(1-3):123-131.
10. Kelly JF, Finney JW, Moos M. Substance use disorder patients who are mandated to treatment: characteristics, treatment process, and 1- and 5-year outcomes. *J Subst Abuse Treat*. 2005;28(3):213-223.

11. Werb D, Kamarulzaman A, Meacham MC, et al. The effectiveness of compulsory drug treatment: a systematic review. *Int J Drug Policy.* 2016;28:1-9.
12. United Nations Office of Drugs and Crime. *From coercion to cohesion: treating drug dependence through health care, not punishment.* Accessed June 8, 2022. https://www.unodc.org/docs/treatment/Coercion/From_coercion_to_cohesion.pdf
13. Seligman MEP. *Helplessness: on depression, development, and death.* W.H. Freeman; 1975.
14. Volkow ND, Warren KR. Drug addiction: the neurobiology of behavior gone awry. In: Ries RK, Fiellin DA, Miller SC, Saitz R, eds. *The ASAM Principles of Addiction Medicine.* 5th ed. Wolters Kluwer; 2014:3-18.
15. Boman JH, Mowen TJ, Wodahl EJ, Miller BL, Miller JM. Responding to substance-use-related probation and parole violations: are enhanced treatment sanctions preferable to jail sanctions? *Crim Justice Stud.* 2019;32(4):356-370.
16. Brown RT, Allison PA, Nieto J. Impact of jail sanctions during drug court participation upon substance abuse treatment completion. *Addict.* 2010;106(1):135-142.
17. Matejkowski J, Festinger DS, Benishek LA, Dugosh KL. Matching consequences to behavior: implications of failing to distinguish between noncompliance and nonresponsivity. *Int J Law Psychiatry.* 2011;34(4):269-274.
18. Marlowe DB, Kirby KC. Effective use of sanctions in drug courts: lessons from behavioral research. *Natl Drug Court Inst Rev.* 1999;2(1):1-31.
19. Bonta J, Andrews DA. *The Psychology of Criminal Conduct.* 6th ed. Routledge; 2017.
20. Lloyd CD, Hanby LJ, Serin RC. Rehabilitation group coparticipants' risk levels are associated with offenders' treatment performance, treatment change, and recidivism. *J Consult Clin Psychol.* 2014;82(2):298-311.
21. Lowenkamp CT, Latessa EJ. Increasing the effectiveness of correctional programming through the risk principle: identifying offenders for residential placement. *Criminol Public Policy.* 2005;4(1):501-528.
22. Marlowe DB. Evidence-based sentencing for drug offenders: an analysis of prognostic risks and criminogenic needs. *Chapman J Crim Justice.* 2009;1:167-201.
23. Carey SM, Ho T, Johnson AJ, Rodi M, Waller MS, Zil CE. *Missouri treatment courts: implementing RNR in a drug court setting — The 4-track model in practice outcome and cost study.* Accessed June 8, 2022. https://npcresearch.com/wp-content/uploads/MO-4-Track-Outcome-and-Cost-Summary.pdf
24. Zilius C, Nuzzo W, Rivera M, Carey S. *Longitudinal outcomes of the San Joaquin DUI monitoring court.* Accessed June 9, 2022. https://npcresearch.com/wp-content/uploads/SJDMC_Longitudinal-Evaluation-Report.pdf
25. Carey SM, Mackin JR, Finigan MW. What works? the ten key components of drug court: research-based best practices. *Drug Court Rev.* 2012;7(1):6-42.
26. Marlowe DB, Festinger DS, Dugosh KL, Lee PA, Benasutti KM. Adapting judicial supervision to the risk level of drug offenders: discharge and six-month outcomes from a prospective matching study. *Drug Alcohol Depend.* 2007;88S:4-13.
27. Mitchell O, Wilson DB, Eggers A, MacKenzie DL. Assessing the effectiveness of drug courts on recidivism: a meta-analytic review of traditional and nontraditional drug courts. *J Criminal Justice.* 2012;40(1):60-71.
28. National Association of Drug Court Professionals. *Defining drug courts: the key components.* Accessed June 8, 2022. https://www.ncjrs.gov/pdffiles1/bja/205621.pdf
29. National Center for DWI Courts. *The ten guiding principles of DWI courts.* Accessed June 8, 2022. http://www.dwicourts.org/sites/default/files/ncdc/Guiding_Principles_of_DWI_Court_0.pdf
30. Rossman SB, Rempel M, Roman JK, et al. *The multisite adult drug court evaluation: the impact of drug courts.* Vol. 4. Accessed June 8, 2022. http://www.courtinnovation.org/sites/default/files/documents/MADCE_4.pdf
31. Trood MD, Spivak BL, Ogloff JRP. A systematic review and meta-analysis of the effects of judicial supervision on recidivism and well-being factors of criminal offenders. *J Crim Justice.* 2021;74:101796.
32. Washington State Institute of Public Policy. *Benefit-cost results.* Accessed June 8, 2022. https://www.wsipp.wa.gov/BenefitCost
33. Finigan M, Carey SM, Cox A. *The impact of a mature drug court over 10 years of operation: recidivism and costs.* Accessed June 8, 2022. https://www.ncjrs.gov/pdffiles1/nij/grants/219224.pdf
34. Kearley BW, Gottfredson D. Long term effects of drug court participation: evidence from a 15-year follow-up of a randomized controlled trial. *J Exp Criminol.* 2019;16(3):27-47.
35. Cissner AB, Rempel M, Franklin AW, et al. *A statewide evaluation of New York's adult drug courts: identifying which policies work best.* Accessed June 8, 2022. https://www.bja.gov/Publications/CCI-UI-NYS_Adult_DC_Evaluation.pdf
36. *Minnesota DWI courts: a summary of evaluation findings in nine DWI court programs.* Accessed June 8, 2022. https://dps.mn.gov/divisions/ots/reports-statistics/Documents/mn-dwi-summary.pdf
37. Reich WA, Picard-Fritsche S, Rempel M, Farley EJ. Treatment modality, failure, and re-arrest: a test of the risk principle with substance-abusing criminal defendants. *J Drug Issues.* 2016;46(3):234-246.
38. Hawken A, Kleiman M. *Managing drug involved probationers with swift and certain sanctions: evaluating Hawaii's HOPE.* Accessed June 8, 2022. http://www.ncjrs.gov/pdffiles1/nij/grants/229023.pdf
39. Hawken A, Kulick J, Smith K. *HOPE II: A follow-up to Hawaii's HOPE evaluation.* Accessed June 8, 2022. https://www.ncjrs.gov/pdffiles1/nij/grants/249912.pdf
40. Hamilton Z, Campbell CM, van Wormer J, Kigerl A, Posey B. Impact of swift and certain sanctions: evaluation of Washington State's policy for offenders on community supervision. *Criminol Public Policy.* 2016;15(4):1009-1072.
41. Lattimore PK, MacKenzie DL, Zajac G, Dawes D, Arsenault E, Tueller S. Outcome findings from the HOPE demonstration field experiment: is swift, certain, and fair an effective supervision strategy? *Criminol Public Policy.* 2016;15(4):1103-1141.
42. Frailing K, Kennedy J, Taylor R, Rapp V. Swift and certain probation: assessing fidelity to the HOPE model. *Eur J Probation.* 2021;12(3):doi:10.1177/2066220320976111
43. Cullen FT, Pratt TC, Turanovic J. It's hopeless: beyond zero-tolerance supervision. *Criminol Public Policy.* 2016;15(4):1215-1227.
44. Alm SS. HOPE probation and the new drug court: a powerful combination. *Minnesota Law Rev.* 2015;99:1665-1695.
45. California Substance Abuse and Crime Prevention Act, 2000 Cal. Legis. Serv. Prop 36 (West), amending Cal. Penal Code §§ 1210, 3062, 3063; Cal. Health & Safety Code § 11999 (Deering).
46. Urada D, Evans E, Yang J, et al. *Evaluation of Proposition 36: the Substance Abuse and Crime Prevention Act of 2000: 2008 report.* Accessed June 8, 2022.
47. Urada D, Hawkins A, Connor BT, et al., *Evaluation of Proposition 36: the Substance Abuse and Crime Prevention Act of 2000: 2008 report.* Accessed June 8, 2022. https://www.uclaisap.org/prop36/documents/2008%20Final%20Report.pdf
48. Evans E, Li L, Urada D, Anglin MD. Comparative effectiveness of California's Proposition 36 and drug court programs before and after propensity score matching. *Crime Delinq.* 2014;60(6):909-938.
49. *Evaluation of the Substance Abuse and Crime Prevention Act: Final report.* Accessed June 8, 2022. https://www.uclaisap.org/prop36/documents/SACPAEvaluationReport.pdf
50. Barnes GC, Hyatt JM, Ahlman LC, Kent DTL. The effects of low-intensity supervision for lower-risk probationers: updated results from a randomized controlled trial. *J Crime Justice.* 2012;35:200-220.
51. Ho T, Carey SM, Malsch AM. Racial and gender disparities in treatment courts: do they exist and is there anything we can do to change them? *J Advancing Justice.* 2018;1:5-34.
52. Cheesman F, Genthon K, LaFountain N, Allred A, Kelliher C. *Results from the pilot testing of the Equity and Inclusion Assessment Tool.* National Center for State Courts; 2019.

53. Fosado R, Evans E, Hser Y. Ethnic differences in utilization of drug treatment services and outcomes among Proposition 36 offenders in California. *J Subst Abuse Treat.* 2007;33:391-399.
54. National Association of Drug Court Professionals. *Adult drug court best practice standards, vol. I text revision.* Accessed June 8, 2022. https://allrise.org/wp-content/uploads/2023/06/Adult-Drug-Court-Best-Practice-Standards-Volume-I-Text-Revision-December-2018.pdf
55. National Association of Drug Court Professionals. *Equity and inclusion toolkit.* Accessed June 8, 2022. https://allrise.org/wp-content/uploads/2023/05/Equity-and-Inclusion-Toolkit.pdf
56. National Academies of Sciences, Engineering, and Medicine. *Medications for opioid use disorder save lives.* 2019. Accessed June 8, 2022. https://www.nap.edu/catalog/25310/medicationsfor-opioid-use-disorder-save-lives
57. Substance Abuse and Mental Health Services Administration. *Use of medication-assisted treatment for opioid use disorder in criminal justice settings.* 2019. HHS Pub. No. PEP19-MATUSECJS. Accessed June 8, 2022. https://store.samhsa.gov/product/Use-of-Medication-Assisted-Treatment-for-Opioid-Use-Disorder-in-Criminal-Justice-Settings/PEP19-MATUSECJS
58. Krawczyk N, Picher CE, Feder KA, Saloner B. Only one in twenty justice-referred adults in specialty treatment for opioid use receive methadone or buprenorphine. *Health Aff (Project Hope).* 2017;36(12):2046-2053.
59. Baughman M, Tossone K, Singer MI, Flannery DJ. Evaluation of treatment and other factors that lead to drug court success, substance use reduction, and mental health symptomatology reduction over time. *Int J Offender Ther Comp Criminol.* 2019;63(2):257-275.
60. Dugosh KL, Festinger DS. *Ohio addiction treatment program evaluation and final report.* Treatment Research Institute; 2017. Accessed June 9, 2022. https://mha.ohio.gov/static/CommunityPartners/criminal-justice/atp/ATP-Evaluation-Final-Report-FY2016-2017977f.pdf
61. Fendrich M, LeBel T. Implementing access to medication assisted treatment in a drug treatment court: correlates, consequences, and obstacles. *J Offender Rehabil.* 2019;58(3):178-198.
62. Marlowe DB. *Treatment court practitioner tool kit: model agreements and related resources to support the use of medications for opioid use disorder.* Accessed June 8, 2022. https://allrise.org/wp-content/uploads/2022/07/NADCP_MOUD_toolkit_.pdf

Sidebar

Reducing Disparities in Substance Use Services in Legal System Settings Among BIPOC and Minority Groups

Fred Rottnek

INTRODUCTION

Black, Indigenous, People of Color (BIPOC) and other minority groups do not have the same access to prevention services, treatment, and recovery support in the U.S. as White people do. BIPOC and other minority groups have worse outcomes with every interaction with the legal system than White people do in the U.S. Imposition of one system over the other only amplifies these disparities.

This sidebar explores the histories of these disparities, the current state of substance use disorder (SUD) treatment among BIPOC and other minority groups in the legal system and opportunities for improvement of services while mitigating involvement of individuals in the legal system.

HISTORY OF SUBSTANCE USE-RELATED STIGMA AMONG BIPOC AND OTHER MINORITY GROUPS

The U.S. has a long history of both demonizing and racializing substance use. Examples include "Chinese opioid dens"[1] in the mid-1800s, the drunken American Indian stereotype,[2] "Reefer Madness" in 1936,[3] and blaming the current rise in U.S. overdose deaths on illegal immigration from Central and South America.[4,5] Media hyperbole and sensationalism amplify addiction as the morally fragile succumbing to the temptations of substance use. This negative messaging perpetuates stigma against those who use or have used drugs. This stigma includes stigma consciously or unconsciously held by the public, stigma that affects the practice of professionals, and internalized stigma held by those who use drugs.[6-8]

HISTORY OF HYPER-INCARCERATION AMONG BIPOC AND OTHER MINORITY GROUPS

Drug policies have seldom followed evidence-based practices or practice-informed research. Instead, policies typically respond to social practices and perceptions of blame among those using and selling drugs. Traditional approaches have focused on interdiction of drug supply and punishment of those who distribute and use substances. Proactive approaches to prevent drug use and mitigate the effects of risky use have typically been underfunded and under-messaged. Other public and professional education, such as responsible prescribing practices and safe drug disposal, are also part of the puzzle. But these practices are not enough to address the pressures that drive people toward unhealthy substance use and disorders.[9]

These suboptimal policies are perhaps most dramatically illustrated in the increased rate of incarceration at the beginning of the 1980s. A bundle of once-considered "common sense" policies and programs included the War on Drugs,[10] with state and federally legislated mandatory minimums on certain drug offenses,[11] which spurred hyper-incarceration rates for the next three decades. The impact of such drug policies has paralleled and fomented a system of criminal justice in the U.S. that disproportionately incarcerates people of color. In the U.S., BIPOC and minority populations tend to have lower income, fewer resources, less access to legal services, and experience more negative outcomes at every step throughout the legal system. As an example, even though Hispanic and non-Hispanic Blacks make up about 30% of the U.S. population, they make up more than 60% of the U.S. prison population.[12]

THE OPIOID OVERDOSE EPIDEMIC, COVID-19, AND OTHER UNEXPECTED SOCIAL EXPERIMENTS

While incarceration rates have been falling since 2009, Whites have almost exclusively benefitted from sentencing reforms and other practices, such as treatment courts, home arrest, home monitoring, and utilization of practices of smart incarceration. Smart decarceration is a model that begins with a holistic view of policy, safety, and desired outcomes of criminal justice involvement. It requires revisiting the status quo that U.S. practices have created for those incarcerated, those impacted by familial loss in the community, and the communities that have lost generations of parents, citizens, and wage earners.[13] Meanwhile, imprisonment of Blacks has continued to increase. Black women are twice as likely to be incarcerated than are White women; Black men are incarcerated at six times the rate of White men.[14]

The COVID-19 pandemic has pushed overdose deaths to new highs; however, it also forced many U.S. jails, prisons, and detention facilities to reduce the census in their facilities to decrease population density and allow some degree of social distancing.[15] Many cities suspended or eliminated cash bonds so that people could remain at home prior to court appearances, and many states released prisoners early to community corrections.[16] However, as the public health emergency eased, incarceration rates are largely returning to prepandemic levels.[16a]

On the policy front, the opioid overdose epidemic has changed not only the amount the U.S. is spending for SUD treatment, it has also prompted changes in services being supported. In fact, the 21st Century Cures Act, passed in 2016, was the first wide-spread legislation to address a large-scale prevention, treatment, and recovery support model to reduce the demand for substances in the U.S. However, many advocates, particularly among BIPOC and other minority communities, point out that it took an epidemic that primarily involved Whites to reframe issues of spending on research and treatment and prompt a meaningful fiscal investment in mitigating the current epidemic.[17]

A ROADMAP FOR IMPROVEMENT

These multiple, complex system changes provide opportunities to create significant and lasting change in the legal system. One useful framework to explore these opportunities is the Sequential Intercept Model (SIM) developed by the Substance Abuse and Mental Health Service Administration's (SAMHSA) GAINS Center[18] (**Fig. 128-1**). Originally developed to identity opportunities—or intercepts—for interventions to mitigate exposure of a person with mental illness to the legal system, SIM offers a model to explore current opportunities to improve the health and well-being of BIPOC and minority population, who are disproportionately represented at each intercept, through provision of SUD treatment services.[19,20]

This section explores opportunities to reform current practices to decrease disparities in legal system policies and substance use services at each intercept of SIM.

Intercept 0: Community Services involves getting a person into services prior to accessing police—particularly during a mental health or substance use crisis.

Substance use is commonly associated with behaviors prompting police involvement,[21] with alcohol and other drug use more likely to be associated with a drug-related crime or property crime rather than a violent crime. Thirty-one percent of state prisoners and 25% of federal prisoners reported drinking alcohol at the time of the offense. Nearly 4 in 10 state prisoners (39%) and 3 in 10 federal prisoners (31%) reported using drugs at the time of the offense. State prisoners serving time for a drug (55%) or a property (49%) offense were more likely than those serving time for a violent offense (35%) to report using drugs at the time of the offense. State prisoners serving time for a violent (35%) offense were less likely than those serving time for a drug (55%) or a property (49%) offense to report using drugs at the time of the offense.[21] Additionally, a significant percentage of the prison population met criteria for a SUD in the 12 months prior to imprisonment.[21]

Effective prevention and treatment services decrease behaviors associated with police involvement.[22]

Opportunities for improvement include expanding Medicaid coverage and services to maximize eligibility for SUD treatment services; public health education about treatment for SUDs; providing adequate, accessible SUD and mental health services[22]; combining in-person and telehealth services to reach people and families facing barriers to access; evaluating and, if appropriate, implementing mental health and SUD urgent care and/or sobering centers.[23]

Intercept 1: Law Enforcement involves law enforcement or other service providers diverting a person into services rather than arresting them—particularly during a mental

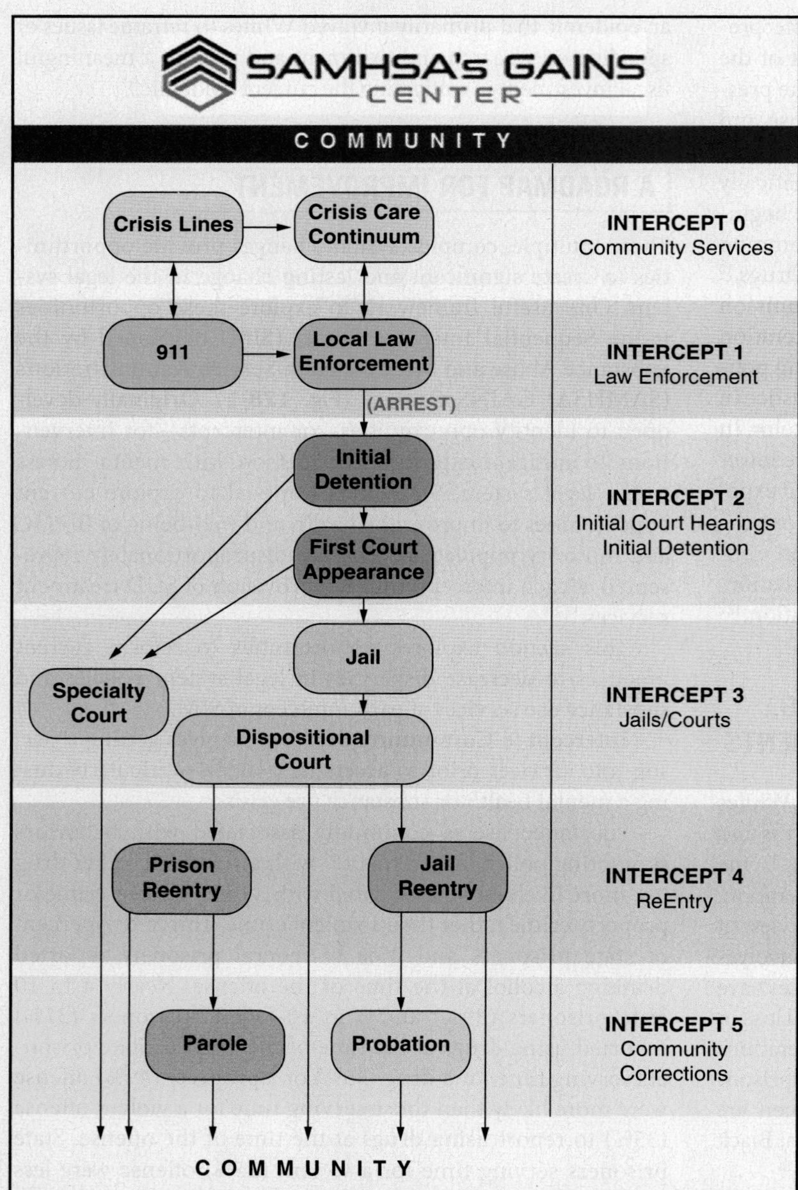

Figure 128-1. The Sequential Intercept Model. (From Substance Abuse and Mental Health Services Administration. *The Sequential Intercept Model (SIM).* https://www.samhsa.gov/criminal-juvenile-justice/sim-overview)

health or substance use crisis. These diversion services would mitigate exposure to the legal system while providing prevention and treatment services to decrease the likelihood of future police interactions.

BIPOC populations are more likely than Whites to be arrested for drug-related crimes, and they are more likely to serve time for offenses.[24,25]

Opportunities for improvement include expanding CIT (Crisis Intervention Team) services in neighborhoods with high crisis rates; public health education about the role of CIT in providing services while diverting people away from jails and minimizing contact with criminal justice systems.[26]

Intercept 2: Initial Court Hearings/Initial Detention occurs after someone has been brought into the jail and is engaged in the initial intake process, booking, medical assessment, or other evaluation, and the person is diverted to a treatment program rather than further time in the jail.

Opportunities for improvement include bolstering evidence-based screening tools to assess an arrestee for SUD and/or mental health diagnosis or crisis, partnering with local health care providers to co-locate a certified peer specialist, community health worker, or other professional in the intake process at the local jail or detention center, and adequately funding public defenders' and prosecuting attorneys' offices so that persons can move through a jail or detention center as quickly as possible in order to minimize deleterious effects of incarceration.[27,28]

Intercept 3: Jails/Courts involves getting a person into services through established jail or court processes after booking. This intercept includes services to the person while in the jail so that health conditions do not worsen.

Opportunities include providing adequate health care so that a person can be screened, diagnosed, and treated for serious/life-threatening acute and chronic diseases.[27]

Intercept 3: Specialty Courts involves a court-based diversion program so that a participant can be successful in achieving and sustaining recovery in the community while meeting the court-mandated elements of SUD programming.

BIPOC populations are less likely to be referred to specialty courts/diversion courts/treatment courts.[29-31] and those who are referred face greater barriers in successfully completing programs.[32]

Opportunities for improvement include following evidence-based and practice-informed programming and connecting the participant to treatment services, transitional and other affordable housing, occupational training, financial trainings, and other services as needed.[33,34]

Intercept 3.5: Jail/Prison SUD Treatment involves medically supervised withdrawal from substances and access to medications to treat SUDs (including opioid agonist therapies) and prevent relapse while a person is incarcerated. (Note: Intercept 3.5: Jail/Prison SUD Treatment is not part of the Sequential Intercept Model. It has been added here to illustrate opportunities for treatment for a person during incarceration).

Currently a minority of state and federal incarcerated persons who meet diagnostic criteria for an SUD receive treatment. An estimated 33% of state and 46% of federal prisoners who met the criteria for having a SUD in the 12 months prior to admission to prison participated in any alcohol or drug treatment program since admission to prison. About 12% of state and 15% of federal prisoners who met the criteria for having a SUD in the 12 months prior to admission to prison received alcohol or drug treatment in a residential facility or unit since admission. Among those who met the criteria for having a SUD, an estimated 27% of state and 25% of federal prisoners had participated in a self-help group or in peer counseling for drug or alcohol use since admission.[21]

Racial differences in perception of self and trust in treatment services further exacerbate treatment disparities in BIPOC and other minorities.[35,36]

Opportunities for improvement include provision of a medically-supervised withdrawal process, including medications and hydration to prevent potentially life-threatening withdrawal conditions, establishing relationships with outside healthcare facilities when a higher acuity of care is required, and provision of free-of-cost SUD medication treatment on-demand for those interested in treatment.[37,38]

Intercept 4: ReEntry involves a coordinated, support effort to help a person prepare for reentry back into the community with a "warm handoff" to a community provider so that a person can continue SUD or mental health services.

Opportunities include pre-arranging an appointment in the community for a person to continue SUD and/or mental health services, providing naloxone along with opioid overdose education and crisis information numbers upon discharge, assuring that medication started during incarceration will be continued during reentry, and engaging a certified peer specialist for follow-up following discharge from the facility.[39,40]

Intercept 5: Community Corrections involves additional services a person may receive under legal system supervision (eg, probation or parole) to stay connected to community services and reduce risk of violations and re-entering an institution.[20,41,42]

Opportunities include optimizing support for people on probation and parole to continue or initiate treatment for SUD and other health conditions, offering referrals to health and other social services as needed, facilitating transportation to treatment and services, and promoting interventions that will assist a person to avoid returning to use and to thrive in the community.[43,44]

CONCLUSION: IN THE MIDST OF CHAOS, THERE IS ALSO OPPORTUNITY TO ADDRESS BOTH INSULT AND INJURY

While U.S. policymakers work to reform the legal system,[45,46] health professionals can seize the opportunity to optimize services for those involved in the current system.

Addiction Medicine has a unique skillset to contribute to healthier communities by engaging with agencies and institutions at these SIM intercepts. By addressing underlying substance use and mental health issues, particularly among BIPOC and other minority populations, addiction specialists can promote health equity in historically underrecognized and exploited communities.[47,48] And by promoting health equity, we can also decrease the longstanding disparities within the legal system.

After all, these unexpected social experiments have again taught us that the well-being of all of us depends on the well-being of those of us who have the least. And, as Maya Angelou has encouraged us: *Do the best until you know better. Then, when you know better, do better.* Now is our time to do better.

REFERENCES

1. Hickman TA. Drugs and race in american culture: orientalism in the turn-of-the-century discourse of narcotic addiction. *Am Stud.* 2000;41(1):71-91.
2. Halpern LW. Study challenges views on alcohol consumption in Native Americans. *Am J Nurs.* 2016;116(5):17. doi: 10.1097/01.naj.0000482951.11479.62
3. *Reefer Madness*. Accessed August 23, 2023. https://www.imdb.com/title/tt0028346/
4. Holpuch A. Six key things to know about Trump's border wall speech. *The Guardian*. January 20, 2019; Accessed August 23, 2023. https://www.theguardian.com/us-news/2019/jan/08/trump-fact-check-speech-immigration-border-security
5. Grillo I. Opinion—Trump Can't Blame Mexico for U.S. Drug Problems. *The New York Times*. April 15, 2019; Accessed April 20, 2022. https://www.nytimes.com/2019/04/15/opinion/trump-mexico-drugs.html?auth=login-google1tap&login=google1tap
6. Legislative Analysis and Public Policy Association, Rulo Strategies LLC. *The Stigmatization of Justice-involved Individuals with Substance Use Disorders. Perspectives from Criminal Justice Practitioners and those with Lived Experience*. Accessed April 20, 2022. https://legislativeanalysis.org/

wp-content/uploads/2022/03/The-Stigmatization-of-Justice-involved-Individuals-with-Substance-Use-Disorders.pdf

7. Tipps RT, Buzzard GT, McDougall JA. The opioid epidemic in Indian Country. *J Law Med Ethics.* 2018;46(2):422-436. doi: 10.1177/1073110518782950
8. Skewes MC, Blume AW. Understanding the link between racial trauma and substance use among American Indians. *Am Psychol.* 2019;74(1):88-100. doi: 10.1037/amp0000331
9. The White House. *A Drug Policy for the 21st Century.* Accessed August 23, 2023. https://obamawhitehouse.archives.gov/ondcp/drugpolicyreform
10. Netherland J, Hansen HB. The war on drugs that wasn't: wasted whiteness, "dirty doctors," and race in media coverage of prescription opioid misuse. *Cult Med Psychiatry.* 2016;40(4):664-686. doi: 10.1007/s11013-016-9496-5
11. Mullen S, Kruse LR, Goudsward AJ, Bogues A. *Crack vs. Heroin. An unfair system arrested millions of blacks, urged compassion for whites.* Accessed August 23, 2023. https://www.app.com/in-depth/news/local/public-safety/2019/12/02/crack-heroin-race-arrests-blacks-whites/2524961002/
12. Acevedo A, Garnick DW, Dunigan R, et al. Performance measures and racial/ethnic disparities in the treatment of substance use disorders. *J Stud Alcohol Drugs.* 2015;76(1):57-67. doi: 10.15288/jsad.2015.76.57
13. Pettus-Davis C, Epperson M. *From mass incarceration to smart decarceration.* American Academy of Social Work and Social Welfare Grand Challenges Initiative Concept Paper. Accessed August 23, 2023. https://openscholarship.wustl.edu/cgi/viewcontent.cgi?article=1575&context=csd_research
14. Berman M. Prison populations decline again, Justice Department report shows. *Washington Post.* Accessed April 20, 2022. https://www.washingtonpost.com/national/prison-and-jail-populations-declined-again-justice-dept-report-shows/2019/04/25/7a678c7a-6779-11e9-8985-4cf30147bdca_story.html
15. Vera Institute of Justice. *COVID-19 - Data.* Accessed April 20, 2022. https://www.vera.org/publications/covid19-jail-population-decline
16. Minton T, Zeng Z, Maruschak L; BJS Statisticians. *Impact of COVID-19 on the Local Jail Population, January-June 2020.* Accessed August 23, 2023. https://bjs.ojp.gov/content/pub/pdf/icljpjj20.pdf

16a. Prison Policy Initiative. *New Data: The Changes in Prisons, Jails, Probation, and Parole in the First Year of the Pandemic.* Prison Policy Initiative. Published January 11, 2022. https://www.prisonpolicy.org/blog/2022/01/11/bjs_update/

17. Cole DM, Thomas DM, Field K, et al. the 21st century cures act implications for the reduction of racial health disparities in the U.S. criminal justice system: a public health approach. *J Racial Ethn Health Disparities.* 2017;5(4):885-893. doi: 10.1007/s40615-017-0435-0
18. Munetz MR, Griffin PA. Use of the sequential intercept model as an approach to decriminalization of people with serious mental illness. *Psychiatr Serv.* 2006;57(4):544-549. doi: 10.1176/ps.2006.57.4.544
19. American Society of Addiction Medicine. *Advancing Racial Justice in Addiction Medicine.* Accessed April 20, 2022. https://www.asam.org/advocacy/public-policy-statements/details/public-policy-statements/2021/02/25/public-policy-statement-on-advancing-racial-justice-in-addiction-medicine
20. Brinkley-Rubinstein L, Zaller N, Martino S, et al. Criminal justice continuum for opioid users at risk of overdose. *Addict Behav.* 2018;86:104-110. doi: 10.1016/j.addbeh.2018.02.024
21. Maruschak LM, Bronson J, Alper M. *Survey of Prison Inmates, 2016, Alcohol and Drug Use and Treatment Reported by Prisoners.* Accessed August 23, 2023. https://legislativeanalysis.org/wp-content/uploads/2021/07/Alcohol-and-Drug-Use-and-Treatment-Reported-by-Prisioners-July-2021.pdf
22. Substance Abuse and Mental Health Services Administration. *Executive Order Safe Policing for Safe Communities: Addressing Mental Health, Homelessness, and Addiction Report.* Accessed August 23, 2023. https://www.samhsa.gov/sites/default/files/safe-policing-safe-communities-report.pdf
23. Jarvis SV, Kincaid L, Weltge AF, Lee M, Basinger SF. Public intoxication: sobering centers as an alternative to incarceration, Houston, 2010-2017. *Am J Pub Health.* 2019;109(4):597-599. doi: 10.2105/ajph.2018.304907
24. Lilley DR, DeVall K, Tucker-Gail K. Drug courts and arrest for substance possession: was the African American community differentially impacted? *Crime Delinq.* 2019;65(3):352-374. doi: 10.1177/001112871878985
25. Acevedo A, Miles J, Panas L, Ritter G, Campbell K, Garnick D. Disparities in criminal justice outcomes after beginning treatment for substance use disorders: the influence of race/ethnicity and place. *J Stud Alcohol Drugs.* 2019;80(2):220-229. doi: 10.15288/jsad.2019.80.220
26. Substance Abuse and Mental Health Services Administration. *Crisis Intervention Team (CIT) Methods for Using Data to Inform Practice: A Step-By-Step Guide.* Accessed August 23, 2023. https://store.samhsa.gov/sites/default/files/d7/priv/sma18-5065.pdf
27. Substance Abuse and Mental Health Services Administration. *Screening and Assessment of Co-Occurring Disorders in the Justice System.* Accessed August 23, 2023. https://store.samhsa.gov/sites/default/files/d7/priv/pep19-screen-codjs.pdf
28. Daniels AE. *Suicide in Jails and Prisons Preventive and Legal Perspectives: A Guide for Correctional and Mental Health Staff, Experts, and Attorneys.* AE Daniels; 2022.
29. Nicosia N, MacDonald JM, Arkes J. Disparities in criminal court referrals to drug treatment and prison for minority men. *Am J Public Health.* 2013;103(6):e77-e84. doi: 10.2105/ajph.2013.301222
30. Bureau of Justice Assistance. *Journal for Advancing Justice Volume I: Identifying and Rectifying Racial, Ethnic, and Gender Disparities in Treatment Courts.* Accessed April 20, 2022. https://bja.ojp.gov/library/publications/journal-advancing-justice-volume-i-identifying-and-rectifying-racial-ethnic
31. Chen E, Nomura K. And justice for all? racial and ethnic disparities in federal drug courts in California and the US. *Cal J Politics Policy.* 2015;7(2). doi: 10.5070/p2cjpp7227275
32. Gallagher JR, Wahler EA. Racial disparities in drug court graduation rates: the role of recovery support groups and environments. *J Soc Work Pract Addict.* 2018;18(2):113-127. doi: 10.1080/1533256x.2018.1448277
33. U.S. Department of Health and Human Services. *What Are Drug Courts?* Accessed August 23, 2023. https://www.hhs.gov/opioids/treatment/drug-courts/index.html#:~:text=As%20an%20alternative%20to%20incarceration
34. Randall-Kosich O, Whitaker DJ, Guastaferro WP, Rivers D. Predicting drug court graduation: examining the role of individual and programmatic characteristics. *J Subst Abuse Treat.* 2022;135:108654. doi: 10.1016/j.jsat.2021.108654
35. Kerrison EM. Exploring how prison-based drug rehabilitation programming shapes racial disparities in substance use disorder recovery. *Soc Sci Med.* 2018;199:140-147. doi: 10.1016/j.socscimed.2017.08.002
36. Zgoba KM, Reeves R, Tamburello A, Debilio L. Criminal recidivism in inmates with mental illness and substance use disorders. *J Am Acad Psychiatry Law.* 2020;48(2):209-215. doi: 10.29158/JAAPL.003913-20
37. Hollander MAG, Chang CCH, Douaihy AB, Hulsey E, Donohue JM. Racial inequity in medication treatment for opioid use disorder: exploring potential facilitators and barriers to use. *Drug Alcohol Depend.* 2021;227:108927. doi: 10.1016/j.drugalcdep.2021.108927
38. Godette DC, Mulatu MS, Leonard KJ, Randolph SM, Williams ND. Racial/ethnic disparities in patterns and determinants of criminal justice involvement among youth in substance abuse treatment programs. *J Correct Health Care.* 2011;17(294):308.
39. Rosenberg A, Groves AK, Blankenship KM. Comparing Black and White drug offenders. *J Drug Issues.* 2016;47(1):132-142. doi: 10.1177/0022042616678614
40. Tyler ET, Brockmann B. Returning home: incarceration, reentry, stigma and the perpetuation of racial and socioeconomic health inequity. *J Law Med Ethics.* 2017;45(4):545-557. doi: 10.1177/1073110517750595

41. Evans EA, Wilson D, Friedmann PD. Recidivism and mortality after in-jail buprenorphine treatment for opioid use disorder. *Drug Alcohol Depend.* 2022;231:109254. doi: 10.1016/j.drugalcdep.2021.109254
42. Jannetta J, Breaux J, Ho H, Porter J. *Examining Racial and Ethnic Disparities in Probation Revocation. Summary Findings and Implications from a Multisite Study*. Accessed August 23, 2023. https://www.urban.org/sites/default/files/publication/22746/413174-Examining-Racial-and-Ethnic-Disparities-in-Probation-Revocation.PDF
43. Pew.org. *Comprehensive Policies Can Improve Probation and Parole.* Accessed August 23, 2023. https://www.pewtrusts.org/en/research-and-analysis/fact-sheets/2020/04/comprehensive-policies-can-improve-probation-and-parole
44. Goger A, Harding DJ, Henderson H. *A Better Path Forward for Criminal Justice: Prisoner Reentry*. Accessed August 23, 2023. https://www.brookings.edu/research/a-better-path-forward-for-criminal-justice-prisoner-reentry/
45. Hopwood S. *The Effort to Reform the Federal Criminal Justice System*. Accessed August 23, 2023. https://www.yalelawjournal.org/pdf/Hopwood_evjni3rp.pdf
46. Brennan Center for Justice. *Criminal Legal Reform One Year into the Biden Administration*. Accessed April 20, 2022. https://www.brennancenter.org/our-work/research-reports/criminal-legal-reform-one-year-biden-administration
47. Toro JD, Fine A, Wang MT, et al. The longitudinal associations between paternal incarceration and family well-being: implications for ethnic/racial disparities in health. *J Am Acad Child Adolesc Psychiatry.* 2022;61(3):423-433. doi: 10.1016/j.jaac.2021.08.005
48. National Sheriffs Association. *Jail-Based Medication-Assisted Treatment: Promising Practices, Guidelines, and Resources for the Field.* Accessed August 23, 2023. https://www.sheriffs.org/publications/Jail-Based-MAT-PPG.pdf

Index

Note: Page numbers followed by *f* denote figures; those followed by *t* denote tables; and page numbers followed by *b* denote boxes.

A

AA. *See* Alcoholics anonymous
AAAP. *See* American Academy of Addiction Psychiatry
AAS. *See* Anabolic–androgenic steroids
ABCT. *See* Alcohol behavioral couples therapy
Abdomen, medical care of patients, with unhealthy substance use, 1315
Abdominal pain, 1391
Abdominal tenderness, 1325
Ability for Self-Care subdomain, ASAM, 1842, 1842*t*
Abnormal eye movements, 1424
Abscess, IDUs and, soft-tissue infections, 1445
Absorption
  alcohol, 150
  anabolic androgenic steroids, 329–330
  bioavailability, 130
  gastric emptying, 130
  inhaled (smoked or vaporized) substances, 129
  nicotine, 232–234, 1033
  orally administered, 129
  psychoactive drugs and, 129
  rate hypothesis, 129
  venous drug concentrations, 129
Abstinence. *See also* Abstinent patients
  alcohol, 1427
  alcoholics anonymous and, 1298
  chemical aversion therapy, 1191–1192
  DSM-5, 1563
  methadone community clinics, 1133
  office-based opioid treatment, 1003, 1006
  pregnant women, 1207
  rates, reinforcements and follow-up support, 1194*t*
  substance-induced mental disorders, 1550
  violation effect, 1220
  voucher-based contingency management, 1135
  withdrawal and, 865–866
Abstinence stage interventions, social support, 1151–1152
Abstinence syndrome
  alprazolam and, 893
  for intrauterine cocaine, 1519
  lorazepam and, 893
  opioid withdrawal, 913
Abstinence-based treatment, opioid use disorder, 1797
Abstinence-oriented care, 1271–1272
Abstinence-oriented groups, 957
Abstinence-oriented Protestantism, 630
Abstinent patients, 1470
"Abuse-deterrent" formulations ("ADF"), 1931
Acamprosate, 949–950, 1119, 1230, 1359
  alcohol, adolescent SUDs, 1874
  alcohol dependence, 949–950
  clinical considerations, 950
  naltrexone *vs.*, 950
Acamprosate/naltrexone combination therapy, 950
Acceptance and commitment therapies (ACT), 1120, 1156, 1713, 1719, 1731, 1864
Acceptance, chronic pain, 1719
Accreditation Council for Graduate Medical Education (ACGME), 65–66, 588–590
Accreditation of treatment programs, 771
Accredited Addiction Medicine Fellowships, 589
Acculturation, 631
Acetaldehyde, 1335–1336
Acetaminophen, 1747–1748
  hepatotoxicity of, after ethanol ingestion, 1357
Acetazolamide, 318
Acetylcholine (ACh)
  nicotine, 238, 1034
  stimulants and, 209
Acetylcholine nicotinic receptors, alcohol and, 155
ACh. *See* Acetylcholine
Acid-base disturbances, 1377
Acquired immunodeficiency syndrome (AIDS)/ human immunodeficiency virus (HIV), 1453–1456
  classification, 1453–1454
  diagnosis, 1454
    acute infection, 1454
    testing, types of, 1454
  epidemiology and pathogenesis, 1453
  interactions of opioid agonist treatment, 981–982
  prevention, 1456
  treatment, 1454–1456
    drug interactions, 1456
    health maintenance and substance use disorders, 1455
    initiation and ART basics, 1454–1455
    response to, 1455
Acrolein, electronic drug delivery devices, 340–341
ACT. *See* Acceptance and commitment therapy
ACTH. *See* Adrenocorticotropin
Action stage, 1075, 1078
Activated charcoal
  alcohol intoxication, 869, 889
  benzodiazepines, 889
Active addiction, 1101
Active metabolites, cytochrome P450 enzymes, 166*t*
Active participation, 1256
Activity-contingent dosing, 1774
Acupuncture
  AWS, 876
  and unhealthy alcohol use, 1060
Acute alcohol poisoning, 1841
Acute alcohol-associated hepatitis, 1359–1360
Acute cardiovascular toxicity from MDMA, 936
Acute care, 64–65
Acute coronary syndrome, 1342
Acute hepatic toxicity from MDMA, 936
Acute hepatitis B, 1361–1362
Acute ingestion and withdrawal
  alcohol, adolescent SUDs, 1873–1874
  cannabis, adolescent SUDs, 1874–1875
  cocaine and methamphetamine, adolescent SUDs, 1877
  opioids, adolescent SUDs, 1876
Acute intoxication and withdrawal potential, 726
Acute kidney injury (AKI), 1376, 1377*t*, 1383
Acute metabolic acidosis, 1409
Acute myocardial infarction, cocaine, 202
Acute necrotizing ulcerative gingivitis (ANUG), 1446
Acute opioid withdrawal, 913
Acute pain management, 1763
Acute pancreatitis, management of, 1392
Acute renal injury, misdiagnosis of, 1379
Acute respiratory distress syndrome (ARDS), 1406–1407, 1409–1410
Acute stimulant administration, 202
Acute Stress Disorder (ASD), 1664
Acute tubular necrosis, 1376
Adapted cocaine dependency self-test, 1130*t*
Addiction, 111, 1052. *See also* Addictive disease; Co-occurring addiction disorder; Nonaddicted populations; Physician addiction
  American Academy of Pain Medicine, 1806
  anatomy of, 34–47
  biopsychosocial model, 1198–1200
    biological factors, 1199
    cultural factors, 1200
    psychological factors, 1199
    social factors, 1199–1200
  brain regions, 1064–1066, 1065*f*
    cortical projections, modulating striatum via, 1065
    frontal-striatal circuitry as neuromodulation therapeutics, 1066
    prefrontal cortex, 1065–1066
    striatum, 1064–1065
  comorbidity, physician addiction, 557
  cultural integration, 623–624, 624*f*
  as developmental disorder, 4–5, 5*f*
  disease, 581
  drug metabolism and, 131
  gender biases in, 622–623
  labelling smoking, 92
  liability, 157–159
  mindfulness-based interventions for, 1236–1245
    clinical strategies for, 1242–1243
    decreasing craving and drug cue-reactivity, 1242
    dissemination and implementation challenges, 1245
    diverse clinical populations, 1243–1244
    dose-response relationships, 1244–1245
    efficacy of, 1237
    implementation, directions for, 1243–1245
    operationalizing construct of mindfulness, 1236–1237
    restructuring reward processes, 1239–1240, 1240*f*, 1241*f*
    strengthening cognitive control, 1238, 1239*f*

Addiction (*Continued*)
stress and negative emotions, 1240–1242
therapeutic mechanisms of, 1238–1242, 1238*f*–1239*f*
treatment combinations and sequencing, 1244
multidisciplinary teamwork, 526–527, 559, 746–749, 751, 1734–1735
neuromodulation techniques for, 1069–1070
deep brain stimulation, 1070
focused ultrasound, 1069–1070
transcranial direct current stimulation, 1069
neuroscience of, 1236
pain
vs. clinical interface between, 1697–1703
DSM-IV criteria, limitations of, 1589
pathophysiology of, 1691–1707
physical dependence *vs.*, 1802*t*
"process" or "behavioral", 64
professionals, 1101, 1290, 1762
smoking tobacco, 95
specialist assessment needs and tools, 529–530
structural competency, 623–624, 624*f*
therapy with, specialized knowledge, 1270
transcranial magnetic stimulation for, 1066–1069
with cognitive therapy, 1068–1069
to DLPFC, 1067
dopamine, effects of, 1066–1067
as intervention, 1069
to MPFC, 1067–1068, 1068*f*
and pharmacotherapy, 1069
repetitive TMS, 1066
SUDs, application of, 1067
treatment
with pain, 1797
and research, 623–624
in United States, 701–702
vulnerability to, 11–13
Addiction behaviors checklist, 1768
Addiction clinical practice
consent and confidentiality in, 1904–1910
ethical issues in, 1896–1903
Addiction Consult Services, 748–749
Addiction continuum of care. *See* Continuum of addiction care
Addiction disorders (ADs)
cultural issues in, 627–634
cultural recovery in, 631–633
individual dynamic therapy *vs.*, 1113
Addiction medicine, 64–65
1970–2023, 586–587
in America, history of, 580–593
birth of, 580–593
collaborative care clinicians, 65–66
concepts and terminology, 27–30
cultural issues in, 627–634
definition, 27
disease, 29–30
future research, 592
implications for, 113–114
nonstigmatizing, recommendations for, 31*t*–32*t*
physician, 65–66
transformational change, 66–67
professionalism and medical advancements, 582–584
spectrum of use, 28–29, 28*f*
treatment, 30
Addiction Medicine and Cardiovascular Medicine, 1336
Addiction medicine clinicians, climate change, 85–86, 86*f*
Addiction Medicine Practice-based Research Network (AMNet), 774
Addiction Severity Index (ASI), 55, 530, 745, 1130*t*
Addiction Technology Transfer Centers (ATTCs), 646–647, 1124
Addiction treatment, 1164
building system capacity, effective care, 771–773
outcomes for, defining and measuring, 768–771
programs
accreditation for, 771
demedicalization and collapse of, 584–585
rebirth of, 586
psychiatric services, 740–757
psychotherapy *vs.*, 1271
quality improvement, 768–786
principles, 773–774
research on quality improvement, 773
services, outcomes for, 768
treatment provider organizations, performance measurement, 770
work force, diversity, 742
Addiction-focused scales, 57
Addiction-related disorders
case study, 1867*b*
family therapies, 1864–1865
multidimensional family therapy, 1864
multisystemic therapy, 1865
gender-responsive approaches, 1867
individual behavioral treatments, 1862–1864
adolescent community reinforcement approach, 1863
cognitive-behavioral therapy, 1862–1863
contingency management, 1863–1864
mindfulness-based approaches, 1864
motivational treatment, 1863
multiple approaches, 1866
opioid use disorder, 1866
race and cultural factors, 1867
return to use and continuing care, 1866–1867
treatment modalities, 1862
twelve-step approaches, 1865–1866
Addictive disorders, 788
Addicts Anonymous, 1107–1108
Adenosine
alcohol and, 155
caffeine and, 220
ADH. *See* Alcohol dehydrogenase
ADHD. *See* Attention deficit hyperactivity disorder
Adherence
monitoring, 1778
Opioid treatment program model, 461, 462*f*
treatment and medications, RP and, 1231
ADI. *See* Adolescent Drinking Inventory
Adjunctive gabapentin, 916
Adolescent(s). *See also specific substance abuse i.e. marijuana*
addiction-related disorders
case study, 1867*b*
family therapies, 1864–1865
gender-responsive approaches, 1867
individual behavioral treatments, 1862–1864
multiple approaches, 1866
opioid use disorder, 1866
race and cultural factors, 1867
return to use and continuing care, 1866–1867
treatment modalities, 1862
twelve-step approaches, 1865–1866, 1865*t*
alcohol drinking, 112–113
assessment, 1833–1837
athletes, nutritional supplements, 321–322
cigarette smoking
illicit drugs, 368
prevention, 13–14
treatment, 14–15
comprehensive assessment instruments, 1835–1836
co-occurring mental or behavioral disorders, 1834–1835
CRA, 1137
definition, 1838
detoxification and, 866
developmental considerations, 1833
drug testing, 1814–1816
drug-involved, cognitive/behavioral/ emotional conditions, 1841
early intervention, 1844
eating disorders, 1679–1680
efficacy of alcohol SBI, 484–485
factors, psychosocial, 1834–1835
family, 1818
family approaches with, 1204–1205
behavioral exchange systems training, 1204
brief strategic family therapy, 1204
multidimensional family therapy, 1204
multisystemic therapy, 1204–1205
follow-up, 1818–1819
illicit drug use, 941
informed consent and, 1904–1906
interviewing style, 1811–1812
placement, 1838–1839
placement, developmental considerations, 1838–1839
prevalence rates, 390–391
prevention, 390–398
etiology and implication, 391–392
interventions, 392–396
meta-analyses of, 393–395
psychological benefits, 1834–1835
referral to treatment, 1818
SBI in, 482
SBI in, alcohol use, 484–485
substance abuse
assessment instruments, 1833
comprehensive assessment instruments, 1833
developmental considerations, 1833
early intervention, 1844
prevalence rates, 390–391

protective factors, 392
psychologic benefits, 1834
risk factors, 392
transitional age youth, 1839
treatment` matching, placement criteria and strategies, 1844
Adolescent community reinforcement approach (A-CRA), 1139, 1863
Adolescent psychosocial smoking prevention programs, 393
Adolescent self-assessment profile, 1836
Adolescent SUDs
pharmacotherapy
alcohol, 1873–1874
cannabis, 1874–1875
clinical considerations, 1878–1879
cocaine and methamphetamine, 1877–1878
opioids, 1875–1877
tobacco/nicotine, 1871–1873
Adrenergic receptor antagonists, stimulant use disorders, 1019
Adrenocorticotropic hormone, 221
Adrenocorticotropin (ACTH), pharmacodynamics, 186
ADs. *See* Addiction disorders
Adult Alcohol Expectancy Questionnaire, 533
Adult hippocampal neurogenesis (AHN), 1695
Adults
alcohol screening, SBI for, 476–478
couple and family modalities for, 1203–1204
alcohol behavioral couple therapy, 1203
behavioral couples therapy, 1203–1204
brief family-involved treatment, 1203
SBI, alcohol screening, 476–477, 477*t*
use, cannabinoids, 249
Advanced personal vaporizers (APVs), 337–338, 338*f*
Adverse childhood experiences (ACES), 668
Adverse drug reactions, 142–143
Adverse effects, physical health, effects of, 224
Advertising, of cannabis, 121–122
AEA. *See* Anandamide
AEDs. *See* Anticonvulsant/antiepileptic drugs
Aerosol, 1340–1341
Aesthetes, AAS, 324
Affective and cognitive reactivity, 846
Affinity, 140
Affirmations, 1086
Affordable Care Act (ACA), 617, 702
African Americans, 1293
Aftercare, 1847–1848
programs, 599
therapeutic communities (TCs), 1180
2-AG, of endocannabinoids, 254–255
Against medical advice, 537
Age
AA/NA, 1293–1294
alcohol use disorders, 372–373
benzodiazepine withdrawal and, 896
drug/alcohol use disorders, 372–373
effects, 368
stimulant use disorders, 1023
Agency for Healthcare Research and Quality (AHRQ), 1806
Agitated delirium, 1485–1486
Agitation, and transient psychotic symptoms, 1613
Agonist binding sites, drugs targeting, 140
Agonist-antagonist opioids, pain treatment, limitations, 1770
Agoraphobia, 1590*t*, 1594
AHEAD (Alcohol Health Evaluation and Disease management) study, 746–747
AIDS. *See* Acquired immunodeficiency syndrome; Human immunodeficiency virus (HIV)
Air fresheners, 357
Air pollution, climate change and, 78
Airway, pathophysiology, 1403–1404
Alanine aminotransferase (ALT), 613, 1323, 1358
Al-Anon, 1202
facilitation therapy, 1167
literature, 1284
members, 1284
membership and meetings, 1284
TSF and, physician role and, 1284
Alateen, 1284
Albumin, 131
Alcohol, 4–5, 308, 610, 1320, 1322. *See also* College student drinking; Drinkers; Drinking
abuse
adolescents, brief intervention, 1811
altered mentation, 1420–1421
brief intervention, pregnant women, 498–501
action, molecular sites of, 152
addiction, 584
aversion therapy for, 1190
adolescents, prevalence rates and progression, 390–391
amount consumed, alcohol-related liver disease, 1355
and anxiety, 1592–1594
benzodiazepine withdrawal and, 889
biomarkers, 519
bone health consequences, 1493
brain and, P450 cytochromes, 136
brief interventions, 114*b*
caffeine and, 225
cardiovascular disorders, substance use, 1335–1339
alcohol-related cardiomyopathy, 1336–1337
atrial fibrillation and arrhythmias, 1338
coronary artery disease and stroke, 1339
direct effects, 1335–1336
heart failure, 1337–1338
hypertension, 1338
CBT plus naltrexone, RP and, 1222–1223
clinical effects, 869*t*
clinical uses for, 148–149
cocaine, 197
common liver diseases associated with, 1356*t*
detoxification, inpatient, 863
drug testing and ethical issues in, 1966–1967
drug–drug interactions, 151
endocrinological consequences, 1493–1494
epidemiology, 149–150
estimated blood levels, 150, 150*t*
family history of, benzodiazepine withdrawal, 895
future research, 159–160
gastrointestinal cancer, 1393
headache, 1422
hepatitis C virus, 1367
historical features, 149
human clinical studies, 152
hyperglycemia, 1492
hypoglycemia, 1490–1492
and interpersonal violence, 1483
intoxication (*see* Intoxication)
laboratory testing, 1814–1816
LGBTQ, 669–670
liver disorders, 1355–1370
low-risk use (or lower risk), 28
managed alcohol programs, 431–432
medical complications, 158–159
metabolic disorders, 1377–1379
movement disorders, 1434
neurobehavioral and cognitive disorders, 1424–1425
acute effects, 1424–1425
chronic effects, 1425
neurobiology of, 151–157
neuromuscular (nerve, muscle, and spinal cord) disorders, 1433
in older adults, 653
and opioids, 1047
pharmacodynamics, 150–151
pharmacokinetics of, 150
pharmacology of, 148–164
pharmacotherapy, adolescent SUDs
acamprosate, 1874
acute ingestion and withdrawal, 1873–1874
baclofen, 1874
disulfiram, 1874
5-HT_3 receptor antagonist ondansetron, 1874
naltrexone, 1874
topiramate, 1874
physician addiction, 555
PLMS and, 1470
psychotherapy, 1167
recovery, sleep during, 1469–1470
rehabilitation, medications for, 946–960
relapse rates, 1220–1221
renal and metabolic complications, 1377*t*
reproductive consequences, 1492–1493
screening for, 472–473, 564
and sedatives, pregnancy, substance use during, 1514–1516
prenatal alcohol exposure, 1514–1516
sedative use in, 1514
seizures, 1427
and self-harm, 1483
sleep disorders, 1468–1470
sleep-related breathing disorders, 1470
"standard drink", 610, 610*t*
stroke, 1430
and substance-induced depressive disorder, 1546
substance-induced mental disorders, 1549
targeted nalmefene for, 429
TBI, 1420
testing for, 861
and tobacco, 1047
traumatic injuries, 1482–1486
withdrawal
clinical presentation, 870–872
delirium, 871–872, 881–883

Alcohol (*Continued*)
- diagnostic classification, 875–876
- dosing schedule, 877–878
- DSM-IV diagnostic criteria, 872
- genetics, 875
- hallucinations, 871
- magnesium, 880
- management, 868–887
- pathophysiology, 875
- pharmacologic treatment regimens, 879*t*
- seizure management, 871
- severity scales, 872–875
- treatment issues, 883–884
- in U.S. Jails, 883–884
- in women, 636–637

Alcohol and other drug use (AOD), 1289
- epidemiology of, 1482–1484
  - alcohol- and motor vehicle-related injuries and fatalities, 1482–1483
  - alcohol- and non-motor vehicle-related injuries and fatalities, 1483
  - alcohol use and interpersonal violence, 1483
  - alcohol use and self-harm, 1483
  - other drug use and motor vehicle injuries and fatalities, 1483–1484
  - other drug use and self-harm, 1484
  - other drug use and violent injuries, 1484
  - overall risks, 1482
  - unintentional injury, 1482–1483
- perioperative management
  - benzodiazepine use disorder, 1538
  - cannabis, 1539
  - nicotine, 1538–1539
  - opioid use disorder, 1535–1538
  - stimulant use disorder, 1539
  - substance use disorders, 1539–1540
  - unhealthy alcohol use, 1530–1535
- traumatic injuries, 1485–1486
  - alcohol and other drug use, 1482–1486
  - alcohol, other drugs and, 1484–1485
  - COVID-19-related alcohol, other drug use and injury issues, 1485
  - electronic cigarette use and injuries, 1485
  - excited delirium, 1485–1486

Alcohol behavioral couples therapy (ABCT), 1203, 1223

Alcohol consumption
- ethyl glucuronide and ethyl sulfate, 1966
- phosphatidyl ethanol, 1966
- of *Pueraria lobata* extract, 1054–1055

Alcohol dehydrogenase (ADH), 149–150

Alcohol dependence
- CRA plus vouchers treatment, 1139–1140
- Wernicke disease, 881

Alcohol industry
- adult population groups, 112–113
- corporate activities, 108–111, 110*b*
- corporate commercial strategies and tactics, 108, 108*t*
- corporate political strategies and tactics, 109, 109*t*
- legal action, 109, 110*b*

Alcohol intoxication
- clinical picture, 868
- management, 868–869

Alcohol myopathy, 1433

Alcohol problems, spouses, RP intervention studies, 1225

Alcohol research, public health policy, 113

Alcohol screening, 564
- adult, 476–477, 477*t*
- in adults, 476–477
- youth, 479

Alcohol, Smoking, and Substance Involvement Screening Test (ASSIST), 486–487, 504, 657

Alcohol urges, support group attendance *vs.*, abstinence *vs.*, 1194*t*

Alcohol use. *See also* Alcohol use disorders
- acute, 1408–1409
- complements or substitutes for, 119
- laboratory testing, 519
- medical care costs, 400
- medical complications related to, 1323–1327
  - cardiovascular, 1323
  - endocrinologic, 1326
  - fetal, neonatal, and infant, 1326
  - gastrointestinal, 1324–1325
  - hematologic, 1326
  - infectious diseases, 1325
  - injury/trauma, 1326
  - liver, 1323–1324
  - musculoskeletal, 1326–1327
  - neurologic, 1325
  - oncologic, 1326
  - perioperative, 1327
  - renal and metabolic, 1324
  - respiratory, 1325
  - sleep, 1325
  - vitamin deficiencies, 1327
- in military, 456–457
- military occupational stressors and sexual trauma, 1206
- prevention, meta-analyses of, 394
- risk factor, 112
- and surgical risk, 1532
- systemic reviews for, SBI for, 482–484
- unhealthy, severity in, 610
- unintentional injury, 1483
- violence and crime, 400
- by women, 112

Alcohol use disorder (AUD), 13, 1357, 1409
- alcohol industry contributions to, 105–114
- MPFC, TMS to, 1068
- in older adults, 655
- pharmacotherapy of, 694–695
- primary psychotic disorder with co-occurring substance use disorder, 1602
- treatment situations, 1021–1022

Alcohol use disorder identification test (AUDIT), 477, 504, 528, 531, 657, 1205
- pharmacy-based SBI, 489
- primary care assessment needs and tools, 528

Alcohol Use Disorder Identification Test-Consumption (AUDIT-C), 528, 531, 657

Alcohol use disorders (AUDs), 49–50, 170, 472, 1335–1337, 1589
- abstainers and lower-risk drinkers, 614
- acamprosate, 949–950
- and antidepressant treatment of unipolar depression, 955–956
- approved medications, U.S. Food and Drug Administration, 946
- at-risk/hazardous alcohol use, 614
- bipolar disorder and, mood-stabilizer treatment, 956
- CID heuristic model, 106
- continuum of severity, 614–616
- co-occurring psychiatric symptoms and, medications treating, 954–956
- direct and indirect impact on, 111–113
- dream content in, 1469
- drug use, comorbidity of, 373–374
- FDA, approved medications for, 946, 947*t*
- incidence, 370
- lower risk use, 614
- in military, 456–457
- people with, 614–616
- pharmacotherapies, 956
- pharmacotherapy, 661
- prevalence, 370–372, 609
- risk factors, 370
- sleep, 1468–1469
- substance-associated suicidal behavior, 1548–1549
- substance-induced psychosis, 1605–1606
- subtypes, 953
- systems of care, 617
- treatment
  - and behavior change, 616–617
  - continuum of severity, 614–616
  - evidence-based medicine, 609
  - group therapy and therapeutic community, 611
  - measuring drinking behavior, 613–614
  - Minnesota Model, 610–611
  - modern approaches to, 610–611
  - outcomes, 611–613
  - personalizing practice, 617–618
  - pharmacotherapy, 609, 611
  - spectrum of severity, 610
  - systems of care, 617

Alcohol use outcomes, twelve-step facilitation group, integrated therapy approach *vs.*, 1101

Alcohol withdrawal
- clinical presentation, 870–872
- delirium, 871–872, 1325
- diagnostic classification, 875–876
- dosing schedule, 877–878
- DSM-IV diagnostic criteria, 872
- magnesium, 880
- management, 868–887, 1531–1532
- pharmacologic treatment regimens, 879*t*
- seizures, 871, 1427
- severity scales, 872–875
- sleep in, 1469
- treatment issues, 883–884
- in U.S. Jails, 883–884

Alcohol withdrawal syndrome (AWS), 659, 870
- management of
  - laboratory test, 876
  - medical and psychiatric problem assessment, 876
  - nonpharmacologic care, 876
  - pharmacologic management, 876–881, 879*t*
  - principles, 876
  - supportive measure, 876
  - supportive nonpharmacologic care, 876

pharmacologic management of
anticonvulsants, 878–880
benzodiazepines, 876–877
beta-adrenergic-blocking agents, 880
dosing schedule determination, 877–878
intravenous alcohol infusions, 880–881
magnesium levels, 880
neuroleptic agents, 880
thiamine, 881
Alcohol-associated cirrhosis, 1358
Alcohol-associated fatty liver/steatosis, 1357
Alcohol-associated hepatitis, 1357–1358, 1358*t*, 1360
Alcohol-associated liver disease (AALD), 1355–1360, 1532–1534
clinical features of, 1357–1358
diagnosis and assessment of severity of, 1358–1359
epidemiology, 1355
pathogenesis of, 1357
risk factors for, 1355–1357
amount of alcohol consumed, 1355
chronic viral hepatitis, 1357
genetic factors, 1356
ingestion of hepatotoxins, 1357
obesity and metabolic-associated fatty liver disease, 1356–1357
sex, 1355–1356
treatment of, 1358–1359
acute alcohol-associated hepatitis, 1359–1360
alcohol-associated cirrhosis, 1360
causative factors, 1359
liver transplantation, 1360
Alcohol-fed rats, 1356–1357
Alcohol-focused behavioral couples therapy (ABCT), 1296–1297
Alcoholic beverages
classes of, substances in, 148
formulations, methods of use, 148, 149*t*
Alcoholic cardiomyopathy, 1336
Alcoholic cirrhosis, 1532–1533
Alcoholic coma, 868
Alcoholic fatty liver, 1532
Alcoholic hallucinosis, 1606
Alcoholic heart disease, 1335
Alcoholic hepatitis, 1532
obesity, 1356–1357
Alcoholic inebriety, 583
Alcoholic liver disease (ALD), 1532–1534
chronic viral hepatitis, 1357
epidemiology of, 1355
ingestion of hepatotoxins, 1357
level of alcohol consumption, 1355
prevalence of, 1355
risk factors for, 1355–1357
sex, 1355–1356
viral hepatitis (*see* Hepatitis A virus (HAV); Hepatitis B virus (HBV); Hepatitis C virus (HCV))
Alcoholic pancreatitis, 1491
Alcoholics anonymous (AA), 30, 456, 472, 552, 586, 609, 957, 1095, 1097, 1103, 1107–1108, 1167, 1213, 1302, 1865
12 promises of, 1279, 1280*t*
active ingredients, influence of, 1298–1299
age-specific groups, 1293–1294
birth of, 1282–1283
clinician role and, 1285–1286
co-occurring disorder patients, 1101
effectiveness of, 1295–1298, 1303
engaging patients with, 1298
fellowship, 1279
group types, 1280
growth of, 1283
history of, 1279
involvement and prediction of treatment outcomes, 1297–1298
mechanisms of change in, 1298–1302
meetings, 1279
membership, 1279
outcome, 1286
patterns of utilization of, 1290–1291
peer support, 1256
population subgroups, 1292–1295, 1303
predecessors to, 1281–1282
in professional context, 1311
promises, 1279, 1280*t*
psychological variables, 1301–1302
purpose, 1279
recovery in, spiritually grounded, 1309–1310
SAD, 1593
slogans, 1286
sobriety anniversaries, 1281
as spiritual recovery movement, 1308
sponsorship, 1281
successful affiliation with, factors associated, 1291–1292
treatments based on, effectiveness of, 1297
twelve steps of, 1279, 1280*t*
twelve traditions of, 1279, 1280*t*
utilization of, 1290–1291
help-seeking populations, 1290
mandated populations, 1290
patterns of, 1290–1291
population studies, 1290
Alcohol-induced ciliary dysfunction (AICD), 1403–1404
Alcohol-induced fasting hypoglycemia, 1490
Alcohol-induced psychotic disorder (AIPD), 1606
Alcohol-interactive (AI) medications, 656–657
Alcoholism, 582, 1214. *See also* Alcohol dependence; Alcohol use; Alcohol use disorders; Heavy drinking
Alcohol-related birth defects (ARBD), 1515
Alcohol-related cardiomyopathy, 1336–1337
Alcohol-related dementia, 1425
Alcohol-related gastritis, 1390
Alcohol-related liver disease (ALD), 637
respiratory complications from, 1410
Alcohol-related neurodevelopmental disorder (ARND), 1515
Alcohol-related pancreatitis, 1390
susceptibility to, 1391
Alcohol-related peripheral neuropathy, 1325
Alcohol-related seizures, 1427
Alcohol-sensitizing agents, 950–951
Alcohol-vehicle-related injuries, 1482–1483
unintentional injury, 1483
ALD. *See* Alcoholic liver disease
Alexithymia, 560
Alfentanil
physician addiction, 555
screens, 563–564
Alkanes, 308
Alkyl nitrites, 308
17-Alkylated androgens, HDL cholesterol, 325
Alleles. *See* Polymorphisms
Allodynia, 1694, 1699–1700
Allosteric partial positive modulators, 140
Alpha-2 adrenergic agents
buprenorphine, withdrawal management, 915–916
clonidine, 916
combined clonidine and naltrexone treatment, 914
lofexidine, 916
methadone-to-buprenorphine transfer, studies assessing, 916
pain syndromes and, 1754
Alpha adrenergic antagonists, 953–954
Alpha-adrenergic agonists
alcohol withdrawal, 880
withdrawal seizures and, 880
Alpha-1-antitrypsin deficiency, 1405
Alpha-fetoprotein (AFP), 1368
α-adrenergic agents
opioid use disorder, 971
Alprazolam, 962, 962*t*, 964*t*, 965
abstinence syndromes, 893
addiction liability, 170–171
disorders related to, 1499
medical complications, 173
uncomplicated withdrawal syndrome, 877
ALT, 519
Altered biotransformation, 168
Altered mentation, 1420–1421
Alternative treatment options, 1904
Alveolar macrophage, 1404
Alzheimer's disease, 159
AMA (American Medical Association)
physician health programs, 561
Ambivalence, relapse and, 1224–1225
American Academy of Addiction Psychiatry (AAAP), 587–588
American Academy of Pediatrics (AAP)'s Committee, 750
American Association for the Cure of Inebriety (AACI), 583
American Association for the Study of Liver Diseases (AASLD), 1360
American Board of Addiction Medicine (ABAM), 588, 775
American Board of Medical Specialties (ABMS), 65–66
American Board of Preventive Medicine (ABPM), 589–590
American College of Academic Addiction Medicine (ACAAM), 591–592
American College of Rehabilitation Medicine (ACRM), 686
American Medical Association (AMA), physician health programs, 561
American Medical Temperance Association (AMTA), 584
American medicine, 64–65
American Osteopathic Association (AOA), 590
American Psychiatric Association (APA), 29, 95, 774, 788, 1255

American Public Health Association (APHA), 124–125
American Society of Addiction Medicine (ASAM) Criteria, 27, 588, 591–592, 597, 615, 647, 774, 861, 864, 1256, 1601, 1839–1849, 1947
 adolescent criteria
  behavioral conditions, 1840*t*
  emotional conditions, 1840*t*
 application, 731*t*–732*t*
 appropriate services, 726
 assessment dimensions, 728–729, 728*t*
 assessment-based treatment matching and clinical appropriateness, 1839–1840, 1840*t*
 clinical *vs.* reimbursement considerations, 727–728
 CONTINUUM, 734–735
 Continuum of Care for adults, 659
 co-occurring disorders, 729–730, 731*t*
 criteria
  assessment, 725
  publications, 725
 data gathering, systems of care, 732–733, 733*t*
 evolution of standardized toolkit, 736
 fidelity to, 734
 individualized treatment plan, 727
 levels of care, 729–733, 730*t*, 1848
 logistical impediments, 732
 mandated level of care or length of service, 732
 matching calculations, 734
 missions, 732
 objectivity, 729
 placement and treatment considerations by assessment dimension, 1840–1844
 research on, 733–734
 safe recovery environment, 732
 social impact, 735–736
 software, 734–735
 standard implementation, 734–735
 treatment failure, 728
American Society of Addiction Medicine Patient Placement Criteria (ASAM PPC), 1838
 assessment dimension, placement and treatment considerations, 1840–1844, 1840*t*
 assessment-based treatment matching and clinical appropriateness, 1839–1840, 1840*t*
 fidelity to, 734
 placement and treatment considerations by assessment dimension, 1840–1844
 treatment dose and utilization management, 1847–1848
 validation of placement criteria, 1848–1849
American Society of the Interventional Pain Physicians, 1806, 1807*t*
American Standard Classified Nomenclature of Disease, 585
Americans with Disabilities Act (ADA), 544–545
AMERSA (Association for Medical Education and Research in Substance Abuse), 590
Amitriptyline, 1395, 1749–1750
AMPA/kainate receptors, 154
Amphetamine(s), 5, 37, 1003, 1369, 1383
 ADHD, 1630–1631
 biogenic amines, 139*t*
 cardiovascular disorders, substance use, 1343–1344
  cardiomyopathy, 1344
  coronary artery disease, stroke, valvular heart disease, 1344
  hemodynamic effects, 1343–1344
 cocaine, 37, 1431
 dopamine and, 206
 endocrine and reproductive disorders, 1498
 glutamate and, 208
 headache, 1423
 mechanisms of action, 204–210
 metabolism of, 199
 movement disorders, 1434–1435
 neurobehavioral and cognitive disorders, 1425–1426
 norepinephrine, 207
 phase I oxidation, 131
 physician addiction, 556
 and psychosis, 1608
 renal and metabolic complications, 1377*t*
 screening tests for, 520
 seizures, 1427–1428
 serotonin, 208
 stimulant use, 1412
 stroke, 1430–1432
 substance-induced mental disorders, 1550
Amphetamine-induced obsessive-compulsive disorder (AIOCD), 1548
Amphetamine-type stimulants, 1404
 LGBTQ, 671
Amphetamine-type stimulants use disorder, 1020–1021
AMTA. *See* American Medical Temperance Association
Amygdala (AMY), 1660–1661
Amyl nitrite (poppers), LGBTQ, 670–671
Amyloid A (AA) amyloidosis, 1380
AN. *See* Anorexia nervosa
Anabolic androgenic steroids (AAS), 1045, 1432
Anabolic steroids, 1415
 endocrine and reproductive disorders, 1499–1500
 viral hepatitis, 1370
Anabolic Steroids Control Act, 318
Anabolic–androgenic steroids (AAS), 317–336
 absorption and metabolism, 329–330
 addiction liability, 327–329
 adverse effects, 325–327
 aesthetics, 324
 athletes, 323–324
 at-risk populations, 318–323
 diagnostic classifications, 329
 drugs in class, 317–323
 future vistas, 331
 history, 317
 for human use, 319*t*–320*t*
 mechanisms of action, 330–331
 pharmacology of, 317–336
 side effects of, 322–323, 322*f*
 supplements, minerals and other products, 319*t*–320*t*
 therapeutic use, 323
 unhealthy use, 323–324
 veterinary products, 319*t*–320*t*
Analgesic tolerance, opioid-induced hyperalgesia, 1700
Analytical sensitivity, 515
Analytical specificity, 515
Anandamide (AEA), 250, 254
Ancillary service model, 1183
Androgen, AAS, 330
Androgen supplementation, LGBTQ, 672
Androgenic steroids, viral hepatitis, 1370
Anemia, alcohol-dependent patients, 1531
Anesthesiologists
 physician addiction, 552, 553*t*
 remifentanil, 555
Anesthetics, 1752–1753
Anger, 1712
Animal addiction liability, cannabinoids, 255–256
Animal experiments, quantal dose-response graph, 138
Animal models
 drug reinforcement, 38
 inhalants, 314
 opioid reward, 40
 pain threshold, 1701–1702
Animal self-administration studies, 41
Animal studies
 drug interactions, caffeine and, 225
 electronic drug delivery devices, 345–346
 neurotoxicity, 313
 self-administration heroin, 41
Anion gap metabolic acidosis, 1378
Annis's cognitive-behavioral approach, RP and, 1226
Anorexia nervosa (AN)
 acute psychological management, 1684–1685
 adolescent substance abuse and, 1891
 biologic management of
  acute, 1682
  long-term, 1683
  subacute, 1682–1683
 definition, 1678
 prevalence, 1679–1680
 recovery rates, 1685
 subacute psychological management, 1685
Antagonists, 141, 1370
 therapies, using naltrexone, 604–605
Anterior cingulate cortex (ACC), 1066–1067
Anterior cortex, 36
Anterograde amnesia, 172
Antibiotics
 acute pancreatitis, 1392
 infective endocarditis, 1445
 osteomyelitis, 1451
Anticholinergics, 1395
Anti-convulsants, 1750–1752
 alcohol use disorder, 948
 amphetamine-type stimulants use disorder, 1020
 benzodiazepines and, 167–168, 901
 bipolar disorder
  adolescents, 1886–1887
 hypnotic sedative withdrawal, 901–903
 nonbenzodiazepines and, 168
 for pain, 1752
 sedative–hypnotics withdrawal, 964
 stimulant use disorders, 1019

SUDs, 1579
uncomplicated withdrawal syndrome, 878–880
Antidepressants, 195–196, 1749–1750
amphetamine-type stimulants use disorder, 1021
anxiety, 1698
compulsive sexual behavior disorder, 837
co-occurring substance use disorders, 1592
medication, 1572–1575
placebo-controlled trials, 1573–1574
stimulant use disorders, 1015–1016
unipolar depression, alcohol use disorder and, 955–956
Antidiuretic hormone release, 1495
Anti-Drug Abuse Act, 591
Antiepileptic drugs (AEDs), 1750–1752
Antihistamines, 455
Antimicrobial therapy, 1447
Antiparkinson agents, stimulant use disorders, 1017
Antipsychotics
amphetamine-type stimulants use disorder, 1021
co-occurring psychiatric symptoms and, 955
medications, co-occurring psychosis, 1603
stimulant use disorders, 1018
substance use disorder with co-occurring psychosis, 1613–1614
Antiretroviral therapy (ART), 1453–1455
Antisocial P, 1652
Antisocial PD (ASPD), 1650
Antisocial personality disorder (ASPD), 1626, 1629
adolescent substance abuse and, 1890
Anti-spasmodic agents, 1755
Antiviral treatment
hepatitis C virus, 1367
ANUG (acute necrotizing ulcerative gingivitis), 1446
Anxiety
alcohol, 1549
effects of cannabis, 259
high-volume sexual behaviors, 830
Anxiety disorders, 962
adolescent drug use, 1887
alcohol and, 1592–1594
benzodiazepines, prescribing for, 1912
caffeine and, 221
cannabis (marijuana) and, 1596
chronic pain and, 1695–1697
nicotine and, 1594
opioids and, 1595–1596
pain and, 1697
stimulants and, 1597
in women, 639
Anxiety management therapy, 1665–1666
Anxiety sensitivity (AS), 1711
Anxiety/stress management therapy, 1664
Anxiolytics
co-occurring anxiety disorders, alcohol use disorder, 956
co-occurring psychiatric symptoms and, 955
substance-induced mental disorders, 1549
AOD. *See* Alcohol and other drug use
Aortic dissection, cocaine, cardiovascular disorders, 1343
Approach bias, 845–846
Apps, substance use disorders, digital health interventions for, 1252–1255
Aquatic therapy, 1737
Arginine vasopressin (AVP), 1383
Aromatization, 325
Arrhythmias
alcohol, cardiovascular disorders, 1338
tobacco/nicotine, 1339
Arterial vasoconstriction, 1342
Arthrocentesis, 1451–1452
Articaine, 1192–1193
Arylcyclohexylamines
chemical structures of, 293, 294*f*
illicit, 295
intoxication, 303
neurobiology, 300
overdose, 303
pharmacodynamics, 296–297
ASAM PPC. *See* American Society of Addiction Medicine Patient Placement Criteria
ASAM standard workgroup, 774
Ascites, 1410
ASI. *See* Addiction Severity Index
Asian Americans, 373
drug/alcohol use disorders, 373
Ask-Counsel- Treat model, 1872
Aspartate aminotransferase (AST), 519, 613, 1323, 1358
ASPD. *See* Antisocial personality disorder
Aspiration syndromes, 1408–1409
Aspirin, 1748
Assertive Community Treatment (ACT), 1582
Assertive Continuing Care (ACC), 1866–1867
Assertiveness training, chronic pain, 1719
Assessment, 526–550, 725
adolescent drug abuse, 1833–1837
dimensions, ASAM Criteria, 728–729, 728*t*
of imminent danger, 730–732
information, sources of, 530
instruments, adolescent drug abuse, 1833
integrating, 533–534
patients with substance use, 526
physician addiction, 559
principles of, adolescent drug use, 1833
process, tasks of, 527
results, assessment information, 530
tools, 530–533
co-occurring conditions and functioning, 532–533
diagnostic assessment tools, 532
intoxication, 532
right, selection of, 528
withdrawal, 532
Assessment-based treatment matching, 1839–1840, 1840*t*
Assessors, needs of, 528–530
ASSIST (Alcohol, Smoking and Substance Involvement Screening Test), 1812
Association for Medical Education and Research in Substance Abuse (AMERSA), 590
Association for Multidisciplinary Education and Research in Substance use and Addictions (AMERSA) nursing competencies, 713
AST. *See* Aspartate aminotransferase (AST)
AST to Platelet Ratio Index (APRI), 1362–1363
Asthma, 1409
Asymptomatic LV dysfunction, 1337
Atenolol
alcohol withdrawal, 880
withdrawal seizures and, 880
Athletes. *See also* Adolescent(s)
anabolic androgenic steroids, 323–324
anabolic steroids, 1499
female, eating disorders, 1680–1681
Atomoxetine, attention deficit hyperactivity disorder, 1632
ATP-gated ion channels, alcohol and, 155
Atrial fibrillation, alcohol, cardiovascular disorders, 1338
At-risk drinking, 477
Attention and pain perception, 1712
Attention bias, 845–846
Attention deficit hyperactivity disorder (ADHD), 1912–1913
adolescent substance abuse and, 1889–1890
child and adolescent treatment considerations, 1637
cigarette smoking, 235
comorbid with SUDs, 1889–1890
diagnosis of, 1622–1625
co-occurring psychiatric disorders, 1624–1625
difficulties in, 1623–1624
neuropsychological testing, 1623
screening instruments, utility of, 1622–1623
epidemiology of, 1625–1626
genetic, 1627–1628
high-volume sexual behaviors, 830
impact of, 1629
neuroimaging, 1628–1629
possible reasons for linkage of, 1626–1627
prevalence and prognostic effects, 1565–1567
psychiatric comorbidity, 1022
treatment of, 1629–1636
nonstimulant medications, 1632
pharmacotherapeutic options for, 1630–1632
pharmacotherapy selection for, 1632–1636, 1633*t*
prescription stimulants, short *versus* long-acting formulations of, 1631–1632
psychostimulants, nonmedical use potential of, 1631
psychotherapeutic interventions for, 1636
stimulant medications, 1630–1631
stratification, 1635*t*
Attention Process Training (APS), 693
Attention training, 692
Attention-Deficit Scales for Adults (ADSA), 1623
AUD. *See* Alcohol use disorders
AUDIT. *See* Alcohol use disorder identification test
AUDIT-C. *See* Alcohol Use Disorder Identification Test-Consumption
Auditory hallucinations, 1607–1608
Autism spectrum disorder (ASD), cannabis treatment, 1942–1943
Autodigestion, 1391, 1391*f*
Autonomy
dysfunction, 1433
SUDs treatment, 1896–1898

Aversion effects
on cocaine craving, 1195–1196
craving for alcohol, 1194
Aversion therapies, 1189–1196
alcohol addiction, 1190
cannabis use disorder, 1192
cocaine, 1192–1193
conditioning, principles of, 1190
further research, need for, 1195*f*, 1196
heroin, 1193–1194
methamphetamine, 1192–1193
multimodality treatment programs and, 1189–1190
opioid use disorder, 1193–1194
prescription opioids, 1193–1194
stimulant use disorder, 1192–1193
taste aversion, principles of, 1190
tobacco/nicotine use disorder, 1192
uses of, 1190–1194
AWS. *See* Alcohol withdrawal syndrome

B

B vitamins, 881
Back pain, 1709
Baclofen, 1359
alcohol, adolescent SUDs, 1874
alcohol dependence, 952–953
neural injury, 1755
Bacteremia, 1452
Band-Aid approach, 66
Barb blisters, 889
Barbiturates, 1414
albumin, 131
endocrine and reproductive disorders, 1499
GABA receptor, 141
headache, 1422
historical features, 165–166
neurobehavioral and cognitive disorders, 1425
sedative use in pregnant people, 1514
sedative–hypnotic addiction/withdrawal, 889
sedative–hypnotic use disorder/withdrawal, 961, 962*t*
seizures, 1427
Bariatric surgery, 1680
benzodiazepine withdrawal and, 896
Barriers, receiving psychological care, 1720–1721
Basal ganglia
addiction and, 34
limbic system and, 35–36, 35*f*
Basic science, 2–26
Bath salts, 357, 1551
BATL (Boston Assessment of Traumatic Brain Injury-Lifetime), 687
BCT. *See* Behavioral couples therapy
military occupational stressors and sexual trauma, 1207
BDD. *See* Body dysmorphic disorder
Beck Depression Inventory (BDI), 1130*t*, 1728
BED. *See* Binge eating disorder
Beecher, L., 581–582
Beer, 148, 149*t*
Behavior
aggressive, ASS, 326–327
management, ASAM adolescent criteria, 1841–1842
modification, 1846
neurobiology of, drug addiction and, 2–26
stereotyping, drug and, 39–40
Behavior change techniques (BCTs), 1250
technology model and science of, 1108–1111
Behavioral addictions, 789
Behavioral approaches, problematic sexual behaviors, 836
Behavioral conditions, ASAM adolescent criteria, 1841–1842
Behavioral contingencies, 1715
Behavioral counseling, 1034–1035
Behavioral couples therapy (BCT), 1203–1204, 1268
Behavioral disinhibition pathway, 1645
Behavioral exchange systems training (BEST), 1204
Behavioral Family Therapy (BFT), 1864
Behavioral Health System of Care (BHSOC), 453
Behavioral interventions
eating disorders, 1682
smoking cessation, 1143–1157
Behavioral naltrexone therapy (BNT), 1265
Behavioral neuropharmacology, 20
Behavioral norms, 630
Behavioral procrastination, 1074–1075
Behavioral sensitization, 209
Behavioral therapies, 58, 601, 1575
common elements of, 1111–1114, 1112*t*
development of, 1108–1111, 1110*t*
effectiveness in real world treatment settings, 1109
efficacy, 1109
initial therapy development and pilot testing, 1108–1109
innovative, development of, 1124
LGBTQ, 674–675
rationales for combining medications with, 1122*t*
stage model, 1110*t*
Beneficence, 1966
ethical issues in, 1898
Benezet, A., 581
Benzodiazepine(s), 653–654, 915–916, 936, 956, 1205, 1555. *See also* Nonbenzodiazepine compounds
addiction liability, 170–171
albumin, 131
alcohol withdrawal seizures, 871
anticonvulsants and, 901
benefits and risks for, 1912
biotransformation of, 168
breastfeeding, 1522
cessation/detoxification
evaluation, 896–898
management, 898–901
co-occurring anxiety disorders, alcohol use disorder, 956
co-occurring psychiatric symptoms and, 955
co-occurring psychosis, 1603
co-occurring substance use disorders, 1592
cytochrome P450 enzymes, 166*t*
discontinuation, 891–894
drug–drug interactions, 169, 300
DTs, 878–879
endocrine and reproductive disorders, 1499
equivalency, 964*t*
formulations/chemical structure, 165, 165*f*, 166*t*
GABA receptor, 141
headache, 1422
historical features, 165–167
immunoassays for, 520
intoxication syndrome, 872
ionotropic receptors and, 139*t*
LGBTQ, 671
medical complications, 172–173
neural injury, 1755
neurobehavioral and cognitive disorders, 1425
OBOT, 1003
and opioids, 169–170
overdose, opioid overdose and, 909
panic disorder, 1592
pharmacodynamics, 167–168
pharmacogenomics, 168–169
pharmacokinetics, 168
pharmacologic characteristics affecting, 894
physician addiction, 554–556
prenatal alcohol exposure, 1515
prolonged/post-acute withdrawal syndrome, 892
for PTSD, 1669
respiratory depression, 961–963
schedule IV and, 1801
sedative use in pregnant people, 1514
sedative-hypnotics, 1414
sedative–hypnotics withdrawal, 963–966
seizures, 1427
sleep, 1473–1474
sleep-disordered breathing, 1414
tolerance and withdrawal mechanism, 170
toxicities, 172
treatment for, 661–662
treatment issues, 904
uncomplicated withdrawal syndrome, 876–877
use and unhealthy use of, 171
use disorder, perioperative care, 1538
withdrawal
concurrent medical conditions, 896
concurrent use of other substances, 895
dose and duration of use, 894
drug potency and, 894
host factors affecting, 894–896
other substances and, concurrent use of, 895
pharmacokinetics, 894
prolonged, 903–904
psychiatric comorbidity, 894–895
seizures and, 876–877
Benzoylecgonine, 1427–1428
Bernstein, SBI, 490
BES. *See* Binge Eating Scale
Beta blockers, 1342
alcohol withdrawal, 880
GAD, 1593
withdrawal seizures and, 871
Beta-adrenergic blocking agents, alcohol withdrawal, 880
Beta-adrenergic receptor blockers, 1342
Beta-carbolines, 141
Beta-endorphin, 182, 186–187
Beta-FNA, 41
β-Endorphin, 156

BI. *See* Brief intervention
Bias, 624
  ethical considerations, prescribing medications with, 1921
Biased agonism, 140–141, 141*f*
Biased research design, 110–111
Bibliotherapy, 1149, 1202
BIDI Stick, electronic drug delivery devices, 339–340
Biennial mammography, 1317
Binge drinking, 373, 472
Binge eating disorder (BED)
  conceptualization, 801
  definition, 801, 1679
  epidemiology, 803–804
  evaluation for, eating disorders with SUD comorbidity, 1681
  management of, 1683
  neurobiology
    neurochemistry, 801–803
    neurocircuitry and structure, 803
    neurocognition, 803
  patients, SUDs, 1680
  prevalence, 1680–1681
  recovery issues, 1685
  treatment, 804
Binge Eating Scale (BES), 1681–1682
Binge use, of stimulants, 196
Binge–intoxication stage, neurobiology of, 5–6, 6*f*–7*f*
Bioavailability, 130
Biochemical markers, 234
Biofeedback, 1697
Biogenic amines, 139*t*
Biogenic volatile organic compounds (BVOCs), 84
Biologic membranes, 130
Biological factors, biopsychosocial model, 1199
Biomarkers
  alcohol consumption, 519
    ethyl glucuronide and ethyl sulfate, 1966
    phosphatidyl ethanol, 1966
Biomedical conditions, 726
  ASAM adolescent criteria, 1841
Biopsychosocial model
  addiction and recovery, family member role in, 1198–1200
    biological factors, 1199
    cultural factors, 1200
    psychological factors, 1199
    social factors, 1199–1200
Bipolar disorders
  alcohol use disorder and, mood-stabilizer treatment, 956
  behavioral treatments, 1581–1582
  comorbid with SUDs, adolescents, 1886–1887
  diagnosing, 1570–1571
  DSM-5, 1560, 1562*t*
  medication treatment, 1579–1580
  pharmacological treatments, 1579–1581
  psychiatric comorbidity, 1022
Birthweight, tobacco and, 244
Bisexual individuals, AA, 1294–1295
Black, Indigenous and People of Color (BIPOC), 758
Black, Indigenous, People of Color (BIPOC)
  hyper-incarceration, 1982–1983
  substance use-related stigma, 1982
Blood
  alcohol concentration, 151–152
  cultures, infective endocarditis, 1447
  flow, 131
  testing, 515–516
Blood alcohol concentration (BAC), 613
Blood pressure
  alcohol and, 1494
Bloodstream, nicotine and, 232
BMI (brief motivational intervention), 1123
  clinical monitoring/management stage, 705
  college student drinking, 442–444
BMI score. *See* Body mass index score
BN. *See* Bulimia nervosa
BNI (brief negotiated interview), 488
BNT (behavioral naltrexone therapy), 1265
Body dysmorphic disorder (BDD), AAS, 329
Body mass index (BMI) score, 1378, 1684
Body packing, 1397
Bodybuilders, 323–326, 328–329
  LGBTQ, 672
Bone
  density
    caffeine and, 1498
    opioids, 1496
  health
    alcohol and, 1493
    consequences, alcohol, 1493
    tobacco, 1494–1495
  and joint infections, 1451–1452
    osteomyelitis, 1451
    septic arthritis, 1451–1452
  pain, NSAIDs, 1764–1765
Bone mineral density (BMD), 1318
Bong, 251–252
Booster aversion treatments, 1194, 1194*t*
Borderline personality disorder, 1649–1650, 1652
  in women, 641–642
Boston Assessment of Traumatic Brain Injury-Lifetime (BATL), 687
Botanical remedies with antiaddictive potential, 1052–1055
Botulinum toxin, 1754
BPD. *See* Borderline personality disorder
BPN. *See* Buprenorphine
Brain
  abscess, 1446, 1452
  addiction, 17
  adolescent substance abuse, 392
  alcohol and, P450 cytochromes, 136
  circuits, multiple, addiction and, 15
  drugs and, 136
  imaging
    during cocaine withdrawal, 201
    dopamine, 207
  limbic system, 35–36, 35*f*
  metabolism, psychoactive drugs and, 129
  nicotine and, 232, 242
  stem, 37–38, 38*f*
  structure and function, effects of cannabis, 259
  structures, addiction and, 34–35
  tissue, addiction and, 3, 4*f*
Brain disease, 1085–1086
Brain injury/stroke
  cannabis treatment, 1943
Brain regions
  addiction, 1064–1066, 1065*f*
    cortical projections, modulating striatum via, 1065
    frontal-striatal circuitry as neuromodulation therapeutics, 1066
    prefrontal cortex, 1065–1066
    striatum, 1064–1065
Breast, medical care of patients, with unhealthy substance use, 1315
Breastfeeding, pregnancy, substance use during, 1522
Bremazocine, 40
BRENDA, 1119
Brief Addiction Monitor (BAM), 657
Brief Assessment of Recovery Capital (BARC), 533
Brief demographics questionnaire, 1130*t*
Brief family-involved treatment, 1203
Brief intervention (BI), 1510. *See also* Screening and Brief intervention
  adolescent substance use, 1811
  adolescents, 1811–1821
  older adults, 1205–1206
  smoking cessation, 1148–1149
  substance use disorders, 599–600
Brief motivational intervention (BMI), 1123
  clinical monitoring/management stage, 705
  college student drinking, 442–444
Brief negotiated interview (BNI), 488
Brief psychotherapies, 1107–1108
Brief strategic family therapy (BSFT), 1204
Brief Strategic Family Therapy (BSFT), 1120–1121, 1864
British American Tobacco (BAT), 98
Bronchiolitis obliterans-organizing pneumonia, 203
Bronchoalveolar lavage, 1411
Bronchospasm, 1413
BSFT. *See* Brief strategic family therapy
Buddy system, CRA, 1137–1138
Bulimia nervosa (BN)
  biologic management of
    acute, 1683
    long-term, 1683
    subacute, 1683
  definition, 1678
  prevalence, 1679–1680
  recovery rates, 1685
  SUDs, 1891
Bulimia Test—Revised (BULIT-R), 1681
Bullous emphysema, 1412
Buprenorphine (BPN), 180, 647, 742, 745–746, 915–916, 971–972, 1370, 1513, 1516, 1765
  in agonist-to-antagonist treatment, 982–984
  clonidine *vs.*, 915
  glucuronide conjugates, 980
  versus methadone, comparative efficacy, 979–985
  methadone *vs.*
    maintenance therapy, 1496
  network therapy, 1171
  norbuprenorphine, 980
  OBOT, 1001
  opioid use disorder, 970

Buprenorphine (BPN) (*Continued*)
opioid use disorder, treatment
buccal/sublingual, pharmacology of, 977
buprenorphine-medication interactions, 978
diversion and nonmedical use, 979
dose adjustment, 978
extended-release (XR) injectable, 977–978
federal regulations, 978–979
initiation and precipitated withdrawal, 978
low-dose initiation, 978
Patient Selection, 979
setting, 978
sublingual, 978–979
opioids
adolescent SUDs, 1876
withdrawal, 915–916
partial agonist properties, 140
pharmacodynamics, 186
pharmacokinetics, 185–186
as schedule III medication, 1802*t*
stimulant use disorders, 1018
Buprenorphine/naloxone combination, 746
OBOT, 1001
Bupropion, 1033–1034
contingency management and, 1268
stimulant use disorders, 1016
tobacco/nicotine, adolescent SUDs, 1872–1873
Bupropion and extended-release naltrexone, cocaine and methamphetamine, adolescent SUDs, 1878
Bupropion SR, 1149
Burnout
physician addiction, 554
Buspirone
benzodiazepine withdrawal, 903
co-occurring anxiety disorders, alcohol use disorder, 956
GAD, 1593
stimulant use disorders, 1017
Butorphanol, 318, 1772
Butyrophenone antipsychotics, 1614
Butyrophenones haloperidol, 880

C

CA. *See* Cocaine Anonymous
Ca^{2+} phosphoinositide signaling pathway, 139–140
Cadaver pituitary growth hormone, 318
Caffeine, 191
A_1 receptor–mediated inhibition, 220
abstinence, 223*t*
A_{2A}-D_2 receptor heteromers, 220
adenosine–dopamine receptor heteromers, 220
analgesic properties, 1698
anxiety and, 221
arousal effects of, 220
cognitive performance, 221
dependence, 223
dietary guidelines, 224
discriminative stimulus effect, 225
drugs in class, 217, 218*f*
elimination, 221
endocrine and reproductive disorders, 1498–1499
epidemiology for, 218
genetics, 224
headache, 1422–1423
health effects, adverse, 224
history, 217
human performance and, 221–222
intoxication, 222
neurobiology, 220
pharmacokinetics of, 220–221
absorption and distribution, 220–221
metabolism, 221
pharmacology and clinical effects, 217–229
physical health and, 224–225
physical performance, 221
physiologic effects of, 221
psychomotor activating effect, 220
psychosis, 1612
psychostimulant pharmacologic profile, 220
reinforcing effects, 222
reversal of withdrawal effect, 221–222
sleep and performance effects, 1472
sources of, 218, 219*t*
subjective effects, 221
substance use disorder, 223
substance-induced mental disorders, 1549
therapeutic uses, 218–220
tolerance, 222
use, heritability of, 224
withdrawal, 222–223
Caffeine-induced anxiety disorder, 221, 224
CAGE questionnaire, 531
for adolescents, 1812
CAGE-AID (Cut down, Annoyed, Guilty, Eye-opener Tool), 1728–1729
Calcium acetyl homotaurinate, 949
California 24 cities project, 403
California Narcotics Hospital, 585
Callback schedule, OBOT, 1008–1009
Cambridge Filter Method, 94
cAMP (cyclic adenosine monophosphate pathway), 139
Campral. *See* Acamprosate
Cancer
caffeine and, 224
cannabinoids and, 260
electronic drug delivery devices, 345–346
pain, 1761–1762
screening, medical care of patients, with unhealthy substance use, 1317–1318
therapeutic ladder, opioids and, 1763–1764
Cancer-related pain, 1761, 1765
Candida, 1410, 1436
Cannabichromene (CBC), 1937–1938
Cannabicyclol (CBL), 1937–1938
Cannabidiol (CBD), 251, 1396, 1937–1938
stimulant use disorders, 1019
Cannabinoid(s), 41–42
addiction liability
animal, 255–256
human, 256
adverse effects, 258–261
antagonist, 248
binge eating disorder, 803
cannabis withdrawal, 257
cardiovascular disorders, substance use, 1345–1346
clinical uses, 255
complications, 1330–1331
cardiovascular, 1330–1331
endocrinologic, 1331
fetal, neonatal, and infant, 1331
gastrointestinal, 1331
hematologic, 1331
injury, 1331
neurologic, 1331
renal and metabolic, 1331
respiratory, 1330
vitamin deficiencies, 1331
endocannabinoid system, 253–255
endogenous, 248
epidemiology, 249–250
exogenous, 248
formulations, 251–252
headache, 1423–1424
historical features, 251–252
history, 248
immune system, 254
legal status, 248
movement disorders, 1435
neurobehavioral and cognitive disorders, 1426
pain perception and, 1698
pharmacokinetics, 252–253
absorption, 252
distribution, 252–253
elimination, 253
metabolism, 253
pharmacology of, 248–268
pregnant women, 261–262
preparations, 252
psychiatric effects, 258–259
receptors, drugs of abuse, 139*t*
renal and metabolic complications, 1377*t*
renal and metabolic effects of, 1384
seizures, 1428
self-administration, 42
sexual and reproductive function, 261
spice, 251
stroke, 1432
substances, 250–252
synthetic, 250–251
THC concentrations in, 251
therapeutic potential of, 1948–1949, 1948*t*
tolerance, 257–258
Cannabinoid hyperemesis syndrome (CHS), 1384
Cannabinoid type 1 receptor (CB1), 1384
of endocannabinoids, 253
Cannabinoid type 2 (CB2) receptor, 1384
of endocannabinoids, 253
Cannabis (marijuana), 1368, 1396–1397, 1602–1603, 1753–1754
for adult non-medical use, 116
and anxiety disorders, 1596
behavioral effects, 258
and cannabinoids as medicine
analgesic effect, 1940
antiemetic effects, 1939
appetite stimulant effect, 1939–1940
brain injury/stroke, 1943
CB_1 receptor, 1939

CB$_2$ receptors, 1939
dystonia, 1943–1944
epilepsy, 1940–1941
Food and Drug Administration, 1939
Gilles de la Tourette syndrome, 1944
glaucoma, 1944–1945
HIV, Hepatitis C, and HTLV-1 infections, 1945
multiple sclerosis, 1941–1942
nabiximol, 1949
Parkinson disease, 1943
physician's role in, 1946–1948
posttraumatic stress disorder, 1944
spinal cord injuries, 1943
substance use disorders, 1945–1946
Cannabis sativa, 1937
cannabis-related perceptions and behaviors, 1829
chemistry of, 1937–1938
climate change and, 82–84, 83*f*, 84*f*
clinical trials, 255
cognitive effect, 258
cultivation, 84, 1937
definition, 1937
electronic drug delivery devices, 349–350
environmental impacts, 84*f*
epidemiology, 1937
ethical considerations, 1955
future developments, 262
glaucoma, 261
governmental policy on, 1827*b*
guidelines for, 1955–1956
high potency cannabis use, 1829
impact of advertising and marketing, 121–122
impact of exposure to outlets/dispensaries, 122–123
intoxication, 256–257, 930–931
management, 930–931
physical effects, 930
psychological and behavioral effects, 930
legal considerations, 1954–1955
legalization, 124–125, 1827*b*
legalization impacts on youth, 1828–1829
liberalization, 1830
market, size and structure of, 120–121, 120*t*–121*t*
and mental illness, 119
in Navy personnel, 455
in older adults, 654
overdose, 253–254
perioperative care, 1539
pharmacotherapy, adolescent SUDs, 1874–1875
acute ingestion and withdrawal, 1874–1875
emerging therapies, 1875
N-acetyl cysteine, 1875
topiramate, 1875
phencyclidine, combination, 1046
physician addiction, 556, 569–570
during pregnancy effects, 261–262
pregnancy, substance use during, 1518
pricing, 123
psychomotor effects, 257–258
smoking, respiratory system, 260
stakeholder marketing (lobbying), 123–124
state-and country-level regulation, 248–249
substance use and harms, 1829
substance-induced mental disorders, 1550
substance-induced psychosis, 1606–1607
synthetic, 250
terminology, 1937
tetrahydrocannabinol, 455
tolerance, 257–258
urine screening tests, 523
use, 249–250
viral hepatitis, 1370
withdrawal, 257, 931
in women, 638
Cannabis and cannabis used as treatment (CUAT), 1518
Cannabis (or cannabinoid) hyperemesis syndrome (CHS)
cannabinoids and, 260–261
Cannabis indica, 250
Cannabis potency, 251
Cannabis Production Companies, by market capitalization, 120, 120*t*
Cannabis ruderalis, 250
Cannabis sativa, 248
complexity of, 250
Cannabis use disorder (CUD), 250
age, distribution of, 116, 117*f*
aversion therapies, 1192
cannabis industry contributions to, 116–125
incidence, 371
prevalence, 370–371
risk factors, 256
substance-induced psychosis, 1607
in United states
additional groups, 117
cannabis consumption, 118
complement or substitution, 119
COVID-era developments, 118
gender, 117
national, 116
prevalence of, 118
product development and vulnerability, 118–119
racial differences, 117
young people, 116–117
Cannabis use rates, mobile applications, 1254
Cannabis used as treatment (CUAT), 120, 249, 1423–1424, 1796
clinical trials and reviews, 255
Cannabis Youth Treatment (CYT) study, 1863
Capsaicin, 1396–1397
neuropathic pain, 1754
Carbamazepine, 878–879, 964–965, 1750–1751
benzodiazepine withdrawal, 901–902
bipolar disorder
adolescents, 1886–1887
CYP3A4 inducers, 169
CYP3A4 inducers and, 135
pain, 1750–1751
Carbon footprint, 84
Carbon monoxide (CO) monitoring, 1254–1255
Carceral-involved youth
substance use disorders in
challenges, 1858
interventions for, 1857–1858
screening and assessment, 1856
screening tools, 1856–1857
shared risk factors, 1856
transitional age youth, 1859
youth with, 1856
Carcinogenic carbonyls, 1408
Cardiac magnetic resonance imaging (MRI), alcohol-related cardiomyopathy, 1337
Cardiac output, 1335
Cardinal rules, 1179
Cardiomyopathy
amphetamines, cardiovascular disorders, 1344
cocaine, cardiovascular disorders, 1343
Cardiopulmonary functions, alcohol and, sleep and, 1469
Cardiotoxicity, inhalants, 312
Cardiovascular
cannabinoids, complications, 1330–1331
medical care of patients, with unhealthy substance use, 1315
opioids, stimulants, 1329–1330
tobacco use, complications related to, 1327
Cardiovascular diseases, 1320–1322
electronic drug delivery devices, 345–346
Cardiovascular disorders
detoxification and, 865
substance use, 1335–1346
alcohol, 1335–1339
alcohol and drugs, 1336*t*
amphetamines, 1343–1344
cannabinoids, 1345–1346
cocaine, 1341–1343
opioids, 1344–1345
tobacco/nicotine, 1339–1341
Cardiovascular system, 224
cannabinoids and, 260
stimulants, 202
tobacco smoke, 243
CARF (Commission on Accreditation of Rehabilitation Facilities), 771
Carfentanil, 911
Carisoprodol, 1754–1755
Case management, 599
Catecholamine systems, anatomic projections of, 37–38
Catecholamines, 1343
Catha edulis, 1551, 1610
Catha edulis plant, 193
Cathinones, 1383
clinical implications, 362
epidemiology, 361–362
history, 361
legal status, 362
pharmacology, 362
CATI. *See* Coolidge Axis II Inventory
Causative factors, alcohol-associated liver disease, treatment of, 1359
CB$_1$ antagonists, 251
CB$_2$ receptors, cannabinoids, 254
CBD. *See* Compulsive buying disorder
CBT. *See* Cognitive behavioral therapy
CBT for Internet addiction (CBT-IA), 853–854
CCM. *See* Chronic care management model
CD4 lymphocytes, 1454
CDC. *See* Centers for Disease Control and Prevention
CDM. *See* Chronic disease management
CDs (conduct disorders)
adolescent drug abuse, 1834
adolescent substance abuse and, 1889–1890

Cellulitis, soft-tissue infections, IDUs and, 1445
Center for Medicare and Medicaid Innovation (CMMI), 1075
Center for Substance Abuse Treatment (CSAT), 646–647, 653, 1862
Centers for Disease Control and Prevention (CDC), 655, 1340, 1453, 1804–1806, 1935
Central nervous system (CNS), 1402
  alcohol, 150–151
  benzodiazepines, CNS
  intoxication, stimulants in, 200–201
  nicotine, 235, 1030
  nicotinic mechanisms in, 239
  NSAIDs, 1747
  opioids
    medical management, 183
    withdrawal, 908
  sedative hypnotic agents, 961
  substance use, pulmonary pathophysiology and immunology of, 1402
Central pontine myelinolysis, 1437
Central sensitization, 1694–1695, 1694*f*
Central sleep apnea (CSA), 1466
Centralization of addiction services within existing primary care systems, 750
Centralized models, of linked service, 744–746, 744*t*
Cerebellar degeneration, 1437
Cerebral ischemia, 1431
Cerebral vasculitis, 1431
Certificate of Confidentiality (CoC), 59
Certification of Office-Based Opioid Treatment Clinicians, 770–771
Chain-of-custody procedures, 518
Change model, stages of, 1087
Change process
  motivation to, enhancing, 1074–1083
  principles in, 1079–1082
  stages of, 1074–1075
Change stages, 1086–1088
  conceptualizing patient change, 1087–1088, 1087*f*
  four processes, 1086–1087, 1086*t*
Change talk, 1086, 1086*t*
Chatbots, 1256
Chemoprophylaxis, 1319
Chest, medical care of patients, with unhealthy substance use, 1315
Chest pain
  cocaine-related, 1342
  endocarditis, 1446–1447
Child abuse and neglect, confidentiality requirements, 1908
Child Abuse Prevention and Treatment Act, 1523
Child and Turcotte classification, 1533, 1534*t*
Child Protective Services (CPS), 1522–1523
Child Reunification, 644
Childhood trauma
  aggression, adolescent drug abuse, 1835
  physician addiction, 557
Children
  alcohol drinking, 112
  prevention, substance use, 390–398
Children's Health Act of 2000, 1001
Chlordiazepoxide, 962*t*
  alcohol withdrawal, 896
  medical complications, 173
  respiratory compromise and, 889
  Substitution Dose Conversion, 899, 899*t*
  uncomplicated withdrawal syndrome, 877
Chlorpromazine, 1128
Choices, 1081
Cholecystectomy, 1533
Cholinergic agents, stimulant use disorders, 1017
Cholinergic systems, 238–239
Chromatography, drug detecting method, 1961–1962
Chronic airflow obstruction, 1405
Chronic alcohol, 1391, 1391*f*
  consumption, 1357
  intake, neural effects, 875
Chronic care, ASAM criteria, 1847–1848
Chronic care management (CCM) model, 703–704, 746–747
  clinical monitoring/management stage
    clinical practices, 707–708
    goal, 707
    indications for transition, 708–709
    self-disclosed or positive biologic tests, 708
    social determinants of health, 708
  early identification/intervention stage
    brief motivational interventions, 705
    clinical practices, 705
    goal of, 704–705
    indication for transition, 705–706
    screening, 705
  personal self-management stage, 709–710
  stabilization
    clinical practice, 706–707
    continuum of care, 706
    goal in, 706
    stage of care, 707
Chronic care model (CCM), 716–717
Chronic contemplation, 1074–1075
Chronic disease management (CDM) model, 746–747
Chronic heavy alcohol, 1433
Chronic hepatitis B, 1362–1363, 1362*f*
  treatment of, 1362–1363
Chronic nociceptive pain, 1691, 1697
Chronic noncancer pain (CNCP), 1710–1711, 1717, 1726
  ACT, 1719
  assertiveness training, 1719
  cognitive therapy, 1718
  cognitive-behavioral therapy for, 1718–1720
  family therapy, 1719
  guideline, 1806
  messages for families, 1719–1720
  mindfulness meditation, 1718–1719
Chronic nonmalignant pain (CNMP), 1720
Chronic obstructive pulmonary disease (COPD), 1327–1328
  nicotine-dependent patient, of tobacco smoke, 243
Chronic opioid therapy (COT), 1806
Chronic opioid use, 1404
Chronic pain, 691, 1596, 1691–1697
  from acute pain, progression of, 1711
  anger, forgiveness, empathy, 1712
  attention and pain perception, 1712
  cognitions and coping, 1713
  cycle, acute to chronic, 1695*f*
  emotional distress, 1710
  expectations and goal setting, 1712
  fear-avoidance model, 1712–1713
  kinesiophobia, 1712–1713
  pathophysiology of, 1691–1707
  patient, detoxification and, 865
  patients with, 1702–1703
  psychological issues in, 1708–1725
  and suicide, 1726
    coping, 1728
    opioid dosing, 1728
    pain intensity, 1727–1728
    pain type, 1727
    risk factors, 1727–1728
    sleep disturbance, 1727
  treatment, 1717–1721
  WHO model, 1693*f*
Chronic pain syndrome (CPS), 1714
Chronic pancreatitis, 1393–1394
  management of, 1392–1393
Chronic postsurgical pain (CPSP), 1709
Chronic toxicity, inhalants, 312–313
Chronic viral hepatitis, 1370
  alcohol-associated liver disease, 1357
Cig-a-likes cigarettes, 337
Cigarette business, economic realities of, 100–101
Cigarette company business records, nicotine, role of, 90, 91*t*
Cigarette smoking, 1339–1340, 1384. *See also* Electronic cigarettes (e-cigarettes)
  addictions treatment, relevance for, 236–237
  adolescent(s)
    monoamine oxidase B, 13
    prevention, 223
    treatment, 14–15
  caffeine and, 225
  causes, 1037–1038
  cellular results to, hypothesis, 240–242, 242*f*
  discrimination and self-administration, 236
  dyslipidemia, 1494
  environmental footprint of, 79
  epidemiology, 197
  genetic predisposition for, 236
  measures of, 234
  neurobiology, 1030–1031
  persistent cultural attitudes, 1031
  pharmacologic actions, 1030–1044
  pharmacotherapies, 1032–1034
    metabolism rate, 1035–1036
    optimizing methods, 1036
  physiologic effects, 243
  prevalence, 1031
  psychiatric comorbidity to, 237–238
  receptor changes, 241
  second hand and third hand exposure, 342–343
  toxicities, 243
  treating, schematic for, 1146, 1147*f*
  treatments, 1037–1038
  withdrawal, 237, 1037–1038
Ciliated cells, 1403–1404
Circadian rhythm disorders, 1467
Cirrhosis, 158–159, 373, 1323–1324, 1410, 1532–1533
  alcohol related, 1355
  effect on surgical risk, 1533

Cirrhosis associated diseases, 1378
Cirrhotic cardiomyopathy, 1336–1337
Citalopram
  alcohol use disorder, 955–956
  BED with comorbid SUD, 1683
Classic alcohol-related hepatitis, 1323
Classic family therapy, 1864
Classical conditioning, 1190
Classical hallucinogens, 269
  structures of, 269, 272*f*
  substance-induced mental disorders, 1550
Clearance (CI)
  calculation of, 132
  defining, 132
Clenbuterol, 318, 319*t*–320*t*
Climate change (CC)
  addiction medicine clinicians, 85–86, 86*f*
  definition, 76–88
  direct and indirect impacts, 76
  drivers, 76
  greater identification with environment, 77
  patient approach, 84–85
  substance use and environmental degradation
    cannabis, 82–84, 83*f*, 84*f*
    nicotine and tobacco, 79–82, 82*f*–83*f*
  and substance use, interactions
    air pollution and wildfires, 78
    drought, 79
    extreme weather events, 78–79
    heat waves, 77–78, 78*f*
  vulnerable populations, 77
Climate drivers. *See* Climate change drivers
Climate forcings. *See* Climate change drivers
Climax, 308
Clinical Antipsychotic Trial of Intervention Effectiveness (CATIE), 1602
Clinical assessment, cultural aspects of, 631
Clinical cultural competence, 627
Clinical dependence, alcohol, 225
Clinical Institute Withdrawal Assessment of Alcohol Scale, Revised (CIWA-Ar), 872, 873*t*–874*t*
Clinical management elements, 1178–1179
Clinical observation, 1834
Clinical Opiate Withdrawal Scale (COWS), 774, 913, 914*t*
Clinical populations, mindfulness-based treatment of addiction, 1243–1244
Clinical presentations, ASAM criteria and, 727–728
Clinical significance, identification of, adolescent drug abuse, 1833
Clinical studies. *See also* Animal experiments; Animal models; Clinical trials
  acamprosate, 950
  back pain, psychologic response, 1709
  cold-pressor pain, addict *vs.* nonaddict, 1701–1702
  COMBINE (Combining Medications and Behavioral Interventions for Alcoholism), 950
  pain rehabilitation program, comorbid addictions and, 1712
  SBI in, drug use, 487–488
Clinical trials, 1116
  blinding, 51
  comparative effectiveness studies, 51
  effect size, 51–52
  effectiveness trials, 50–51
  efficacy trials, 49–50
  male violence, co-occurring disorders and, group therapies for, 1101
  monitoring and quality control, 58–59
  outcome metrics
    addiction-focused scales, 57
    cognitive function, 56
    cost analysis–related measures, 57–58
    drug craving, 56
    healthcare service utilization measures, 57
    patient-reported outcome measures, 57
    pharmacokinetic measures, 57
    psychiatric scales, 56–57
    quantification of substance use, 55–56
    treatment adherence measures, 58
    withdrawal syndromes, 56
  phase IV trials, 50
  phases, 60*b*
  power, 51–52
  randomization, 51
  sample size, 51–52
  statistical analysis plans, 52
  statistical significance and effect sizes, 52–53
  substance-using populations
    elements, 48–49
    features, 51–53
    types, 49–51
  trial design aspects
    adaptive designs, 54–55
    non inferiority designs, 54
    superiority designs, 53–54
  uncomplicated withdrawal syndrome, 880
Clinical trials network (CTN), 50, 1109, 1258, 1634
Clinically preventable burden (CPB), SBI for, 483
Clinically significant portal hypertension (CSPH), 1358–1359
Clinic-based and institutional strategies
  inequities of care reduction, 762–763
Clinician(s), role of, patients with addiction, 1285–1286
Clinician-Administered PTSD Scale for DSM-5 (CAPS-5), 1662
Clomipramine, OCD, 1594
Clonazepam, 962*t*, 963–964, 1752
  addiction liability, 170–171
  benzodiazepines and, 171
  sedative-hypnotics withdrawal, 962*t*, 963–964
Clonidine, 1395, 1517–1518. *See also* Transdermal clonidine
  alcohol withdrawal, 862–863
  benzodiazepine withdrawal, 903
  drug–drug interactions, 300
  euphoria, 912
  and naltrexone treatment, 915
  nonopioid medication treatments, 972
  opioid use disorder, 971
  opioid withdrawal, 913–914
  opioid-dependent patient, 864–865
  sleep difficulties, 1474
  withdrawal management, 913–914
Clorazepate (Tranxene), 962*t*
"Closed distribution system," controlled substances and, 1000
Clostridium botulinum, 1436, 1452
Clostridium tetani, 1452–1453
Clostridium tetanus, 1436
Clozapine, psychosis, 1611
Club drugs, 827, 935
Club drugs/empathogens
  LGBTQ, 671
Cluster A disorders, 1648
Cluster B disorders, 1648–1651
Cluster C disorders, 1651
CM. *See* Contingency management
CMCA (Communities Mobilizing for Change on Alcohol Project), 403
CMCP (Communities Mobilizing for Change Project), 401–402
CNMP (chronic nonmalignant pain), 1720
CNS. *See* Central nervous system
CNS depressants, LGBTQ, 671
CNS stimulants, analgesic properties, 1698
Coagulopathy, 1326
Coated pits, 142
Coca leaves, 191, 196
Coca tea, 191, 196, 198
Coca-Cola, 197
Cocaethylene, 200, 1413
Cocaine, 5, 909, 1053–1054, 1368–1369, 1404
  abstinence, 1129
    duration of, 1134*f*
    mean durations of, 1133, 1134*f*
  abusers, CBT, 13
  acetylcholine, 209
  addiction
    prescription medications for, 13
    Twelve-Step programs, 1293
  alcohol drinkers, 197
  analgesic properties, 1698
  aversion therapies, 1192–1193
  biogenic amines, 139*t*
  breastfeeding, 1522
  cardiovascular disorders, substance use, 1341–1343
    aortic dissection, 1343
    cardiomyopathy, 1343
    coronary artery disease, 1341–1343
    hemodynamic effects, 1341
    stroke, 1343
  chemical structures, 191, 192*f*–193*f*
  clinical uses, 195
  craving, aversion therapy and, 1194
  dopamine and, 206
  drug–drug interactions, 5
  endocrine and reproductive disorders, 1497–1498
  epidemiology, 197
  formulations and methods, 191–196
  glutamate and, 208
  headache, 1423
  LGBTQ, 671
  mechanisms of action, 204–205
  movement disorders, 1434–1435
  neurobehavioral and cognitive disorders, 1425–1426
  neurotoxicity, 210
  norepinephrine, 207
  pharmacokinetics, absorption and distribution, 198
  phencyclidine, combination, 1046

Cocaine (*Continued*)
physician addiction, 556
and psychosis, 1607–1608
receptors, drugs of abuse, 139*t*
renal and metabolic complications, 1377*t*
seizures, 1427–1428
self-administration, 38–39
serotonin, 207
sleep difficulties, 1471
smoking
adverse effects, 203
stimulants, renal and metabolic effects of, 1381–1383
cocaine-associated thrombotic microangiopathy-hemolytic uremic syndrome, 1383
cocaine-associated vasculitis, 1382
hypertension and renal disease, 1382
rhabdomyolysis, 1382
street forms of, 202–203
stroke, 1430–1432
substance-induced mental disorders, 1550
urine testing, 520–521
in vitro experiments, 37
withdrawal, brain imaging during, 201
Cocaine and methamphetamine
adolescent SUDs, 1877–1878
pharmacotherapy, adolescent SUDs, 1877–1878
acute ingestion and withdrawal management, 1877
bupropion and extended-release naltrexone, 1878
cocaine use disorder, 1877–1878
mirtazapine, 1878
psychostimulants, 1878
Cocaine anonymous (CA), 1216, 1283, 1865
population subgroups, 1292–1295
Cocaine Collaborative Study
counsellors in, 1102–1103
FPW and, 1099
Cocaine Dependency Self-Test, 1130*t*
Cocaine hydrochloride, 520
Cocaine inebriety, 583
Cocaine use disorder (CUD), 371, 1014–1015
cocaine and methamphetamine, adolescent SUDs, 1877–1878
contingency management for, individual psychotherapy in, 1117–1118
CRA plus vouchers treatment, 1128
individual psychotherapy for, 1116
intake assessment, instruments used in, 1130*t*
voucher-based contingency management, 1133–1134
Cocaine users
CBT *vs.* TSF, 1222
limbic activation in, 43–44
Cocaine-associated hepatitis, 1368–1369
Cocaine-associated thrombotic microangiopathy-hemolytic uremic syndrome, 1383
Cocaine-associated vasculitis, 1382
Cochrane Group
alcohol abuse and, 483
drug use, SBI for, 483
Cochrane Review
CM, 1135
community-based prevention, effectiveness/meta analysis of, 396
smoking prevention, meta-analyses of, 393
substance use prevention, meta-analyses of, 394
Codeine, 178
pharmacodynamics, 186
pharmacokinetics, 184
phase I oxidation, 131
Schedule IV and, 1801
Coerced treatment, voluntary *vs.*, addiction treatments and, 1897–1898
Coffee, gastroesophageal reflux and, 224
Cognition, effects of cannabis, 258
Cognitive behavioral techniques, 1764
Cognitive behavioral therapy (CBT), 51, 1296
AA, 1295–1296
ACT, 1719
AN, 803
assertiveness training, 1719
benzodiazepine withdrawal, 903
BN, 803
with comorbid addiction disorder, 795
chronic pain, 1719
CM *vs.*, CBT/CM combination *vs.*, 1223
CNMP, 1720
cognitive therapy, 1718
co-occurring disorders and, group therapies, 1101
family therapy, 1719
messages for families, 1719–1720
mindfulness meditation, 1718–1719
naltrexone, 947
alcohol, RP and, 1222–1223
network therapy, 1165
problematic sexual behaviors, 836–837
psychotherapy, 1116
RP and, 1222
SUD, 1591
TSF *vs.*, 1215
Cognitive bias modification (CBM) studies, 693
Cognitive conditions, ASAM adolescent criteria, 1841–1842
Cognitive control, 1238, 1239*f*
Cognitive defects, adolescents, 1885
Cognitive disorders, 1424–1427
alcohol, 1424–1425
barbiturates, benzodiazepines, 1425
cannabinoids, 1426
cocaine, amphetamines and MDMA, 1425–1426
dissociative anesthetics, 1426
hallucinogens, 1426
inhalants, 1426–1427
opioids, 1426
Cognitive distortions, RP and, 1229–1230
Cognitive enhancement, addiction science, 1121–1122
Cognitive function, 56
Cognitive impairment, 1325
Cognitive interventions, RP and, 1229
Cognitive processing models, 1243
Cognitive processing therapy (CPT), 1665
Cognitive rehabilitation
for substance use disorder, 693
for traumatic brain injury, 692–693
Cognitive self-control strategies, 1227
Cognitive shifts, AA ingredients and, 1301
Cognitive therapy
TMS with, 1068–1069
Cognitive-behavioral approaches, 1116
Cognitive-behavioral group therapy (CBGT), 1094
Cognitive-behavioral model of relapse, 1226–1227, 1226*f*
Cognitive-behavioral reuse prevention (RP), 1866
Cognitive-behavioral therapies (CBTs), 601, 1591, 1862–1863
ADHD, 1636
LGBTQ, 674
mindfulness-based treatment of addiction, 1245
mobile applications/apps/stand-alone websites, 1253–1254
for PTSD, 1664
anxiety management therapy, 1665–1666
cognitive-focused therapy, 1665
for co-occurring PTSD-SUD, 1666–1668
effectiveness of, 1666
exposure-based therapy, 1664–1665
integrated treatment models, 1667
for strengthening recognition of maladaptive cognition, 845–846
TMS with cognitive therapy, 1068–1069
Cognitive–behavioral-based interventions, 854
Cognitive-focused therapy, 1664–1665
Cognitive-perceptual abnormalities, 1652
Cohort effects, 368
Cold-pressor pain, 1698–1699, 1701–1702
clinical studies, 1702–1703
tolerance, 1701–1702
Collaboration, 1085
ethical considerations, prescribing medications with, 1921
Collaboration on FASD Prevalence (CoFASP), 1515
Collaborative systems approach, 70–71
Collateral information, pain, 559
College on Problems of Drug Dependence, 586
College student drinking
athletics, 439
consequences, 437–441
damage
institution, 438
to others, 437–438
self, 437
drinking rates and disorders, 437
fraternity and sorority organizations, 439
individual and environmental risk factors, 440–441
individually focused interventions, 442–444
interventions, 441–446
misperceptions, 440–441
prevalence, 437–441
prevention strategies, 441–446
risk factors, 438–439
sex and ethnicity, 438
sexual minority status, 439
social norms, 440–441
College students, SBI in, alcohol use, 485–486
Colon, gastrointestinal disorders, 1393
Colorectal cancer screening, 1318

Columbia Suicide Severity Rating Scale (C-SSRS), 1549, 1729
Coma, 1381
cocktail, 890
Combination strategies, medication treatment and behavioral interventions, 1269
COMBINE (Combining Medications and Behavioral Interventions for Alcoholism), 950
Combined antiretroviral therapy (cART), 418
Combusted substance use, 1405–1407
Combustible tobacco use, pulmonary complications of, 1320
Commercial Determinant of Health (CDoH), 106
Commission on Accreditation of Rehabilitation Facilities (CARF), 771
Communication skills, RP and, 1228–1229
Communities Mobilizing for Change on Alcohol Project (CMCA), 403
Communities Mobilizing for Change Project (CMCP), 401–402
Community and clinical management, 1184
Community Care in Reach program, 749–750
Community enhancement activities, 1175, 1184
Community reinforcement and family training (CRAFT), 1140, 1202
individual psychotherapy, 1120
Community reinforcement approach (CRA), 602, 1132–1133, 1251–1252
control groups *vs.*, dependent measures and, 1138*f*
developing, 1138
empirical support, 1133–1140
individual psychotherapy, 1116–1117
initial study, 1139
multidimensional family therapy, 1139
plus disulfiram, unmarried subjects, abstinence and, 1138
plus vouchers treatment
contingency management, 1131–1132
elements of, 1131
therapist characteristics, 1131
treatment and technique, 1131–1133
special populations, 1138–1139
standard treatment *vs.*, 1139*f*
Community residential rehabilitation, 598
Community trials (CT) project, 402
Community-acquired pneumonia, 1410
Community-as-method, therapeutic communities (TCs), 1176
Community-based family involvement, 1172
Community-based prevention programs, 396
adolescents, 396
effectiveness/meta-analyses of, 396
environmental approaches, 399–407
Community-based treatment for criminal legal populations, 600
Community-based treatment programs (CTPs), 1108–1109
Comorbid chronic pain, SUDs, opioid use disorder. *see* Opioid use disorders (OUDs)
Comparative effectiveness studies, 51
Competencies, 1897
enhancement, adolescents, substance abuse, 393
for healthcare clinicians, 713–714
Complementary strategies, medication treatment and behavioral interventions, 1268–1269
Complementary techniques, substance use disorders, 1052–1063
Complex regional pain syndrome (CRPS), 1694–1695, 1697
Compliance calendar, court-leveraged treatment, 1976
Compliance enhancement therapy, 1119
Compliance, medication regimens, 1267
Composite International Diagnostic Interview (CIDI), 1663
Composite International Diagnostic Interview Substance Abuse Module (CIDI-SAM), 530
Comprehensive Assessment and Treatment Outcome Research (CATOR), 1865–1866
Comprehensive assessment instruments, 1835–1836
Compulsive buying disorder (CBD), 798–799
definition and conceptualization, 798
epidemiology, 798
neurobiology, 798
neurocircuitry, 798
treatment, 798–799
Compulsive sex in combination with substance use, 832–834
special populations, 833–834
Compulsive sexual behavior disorder (CSBD). *See also* Problematic sexual behaviors (PSB)
biopsychosocial assessment, 826
conceptualization, 799
definition, 799
epidemiology, 800
equity and diversity, 827–828
high-volume sexual behaviors, 828–830
historical and cultural contexts, 827–828
neurobiology
neurochemistry, 799
neurocircuitry and structure, 800
pharmacotherapy strategies
antidepressants, 837
hormonal therapies, 838
opioid antagonists, 838
selective serotonin reuptake inhibitors, 837–838
problematic, 826
treatment, 800–801
Compulsive substance use ("high need persons"), 1976–1977
Computed tomography (CT) scan
co-occurring psychosis and substance use disorders, 1604
osteomyelitis, 1451
Computer-assisted therapies (CAT), 603–604
Computerized brief intervention, 487
Concentric hypertrophy, 1344
Concerned significant others (CSOs), 1140, 1202
Concomitant use of alcohol, 1342
Concurrent opioid use disorder, treatment situations, 1021
Concurrent substance use disorders, treatment situations, 1021–1022
Concurrent Treatment of PTSD and Cocaine Dependence (CTPCD), 1667–1668
Concurrent Treatment of PTSD and Substance Use Disorders using Prolonged Exposure (COPE), 1667–1668
Conditioned nausea responses, covertsensitization and, 1191
Conditioned place preference (CPP)
animal drug addiction liability, cannabinoids, 255–256
Conditioned Place Preference (CPP), 1058–1059
Conditioned tolerance, 142
Conduct disorders (CDs), 1626
adolescent substance abuse and, 1889–1890
Confidentiality, 1904–1910
in addiction practice, 1904–1910
basis of, 1907
Federal laws, 1907–1908
linked services, 742–743
principles, 1908–1909
requirements, 1908
state laws, 1908
Conflict, 630
Congestive heart failure, 1321–1322
Conners' Adult ADHD Diagnostic Interview for the DSM-IV (CAADID), 1623
Consciousness raising, pre-contemplation stage and, 1080
Consent
in addiction practice, 1904–1910
confidentiality requirements, 1908
to treatment, 1905
Console, infant assessment, parameters for, 1517*t*
Constipation, 1775
Consultation, ethical issues in, 1902
Contaminants, 340
Contemplation, 1074–1075
Contingency management (CM), 51, 1131–1132, 1863–1864
bupropion and, 1268
cocaine use disorder, individual, 1117–1118
into community clinics, 1135
community reinforcement approach and, 1128–1140
conclusions on, 1137
initial study, 1133–1135
LGBTQ, 675
literature, growth of, 1135
longer-term outcomes of, 1136
opioid use, individual psychotherapy, 1116
pre-contemplation stage and, 1081
problematic sexual behaviors, 836
special populations, 1135–1136
therapist characteristics, 1131
tobacco use disorder, intensive interventions for, 1152
Continued problem potential, dimension 5, ASAM, 1843
Continued service, ASAM, 729
Continued use, dimension 5, ASAM, 1843
Continuing education (CE) programs, 714
Continuous learning and introspection, 762
Continuous pain, topical agents, 1754
Continuum of addiction care, 727
circa, 870

Contraceptives, oral, benzodiazepines, 169
Contract for life, adolescent smoking, 1817
Control groups, 1253
  CRA *vs.*, dependent measures and, 1138
Control issues, BPD, 1274
Controlled substances
  analogues, 318
  informed consent and, 1761–1762
Controlled Substances Act (CSA), 248, 318, 358–359, 409, 1801, 1802*t*, 1925, 1929–1930
  drug schedules, 293–294
  opioids, 1761–1762
Conventional cigarette. *See also* Electronic cigarettes (e-cigarettes)
  vs. pen-style tank EDDDs, 337
Convergent strategies, medication treatment and behavioral interventions, 1267–1268
Co-occurring addiction disorders. *See also specific i.e. Co-occurring substance use* disorders
  and anxiety disorders, 1589–1600
Co-occurring anxiety disorders, alcohol use disorder, treatment of, 956
Co-occurring disorders, 1183–1187, 1883
  ASAM criteria and, 729–730, 731*t*
  group therapies for, 1100–1102
  modified TC, 1184
  RP and, 1231
  services and, 726
Co-occurring mental or behavioral disorders, 1834–1835
Co-occurring mood disorders, substance use disorders
  bipolar disorders, DSM-5, 1560–1563, 1562*t*
  comorbidity, 1565–1566, 1565*t*
  depression, 1566
  depressive disorders, DSM-5, 1560, 1561*t*
  diagnostic criteria, 1559–1565
  diagnostic methods, 1569–1570, 1569*t*
  differential diagnosis, 1567–1572
  distinguishing mood symptoms, 1563–1565, 1564*t*
  DSM-IV and DSM-5, 1560
  etiological relationships, 1567, 1568*t*
  management, 1572–1583
  predictive validity, 1569–1570, 1569*t*
  prevalence, 1565–1567
  primary care, 1567
  prognostic effects, 1566–1567
  psychiatric populations, 1567
  significance, 1559–1560
  treatment, 1563
Co-occurring pain
  and substance use disorders, 1791–1799
    diagnostic confounds, 1792
    reciprocal vulnerability, 1791–1792
    treatment impediments, 1792
Co-occurring psychiatric disorders, 814–815, 966, 1624–1625
  in adolescents, 1883–1894
    diagnosis and management, 1884–1885
    incidence and prevalence, 1883–1884
    pharmacotherapy, 1885
    psychosocial treatment, 1885
  detoxification and, 865–866
  opioid use disorder, 985
    major depression, 985
    persistent depressive disorder, 985
    sleep disorders, 985
  prevalence of, 372
Co-occurring psychiatric symptoms, alcohol use disorder patients and, medications treating, 954–956
Co-occurring psychosis, 1601–1602, 1613–1615
  additional medication decisions, 1612
  alcohol use disorders and psychosis, 1605–1606
  amphetamines and psychosis, 1608
  cannabis and psychosis, 1606–1607
  clinical presentation of, 1605–1611
  cocaine and psychosis, 1607–1608
  definition of, 1601, 1602*t*
  diagnostic assessment, 1603–1604
  differential diagnosis, 1604–1605, 1604*t*
  dissociatives and psychosis, 1609
  hallucinogens and psychosis, 1608–1609
  longer-term management, 1616–1617
  management of, 1611–1615
  MDMA ("Ecstasy") and psychosis, 1609–1610
  multiple substance use and psychosis, 1611
  new psychoactive substances and psychosis, 1610–1611
  other outpatient treatment approaches, 1615–1616
  pharmacological treatment, 1611, 1613–1615
  prevalence of, 1601–1603
    primary psychotic disorder with co-occurring substance use disorder, 1602–1603
    substance-induced psychosis, 1601–1602
  primary psychotic disorder with, 1602–1603
  psychosocial interventions, 1612–1615
  substances and antipsychotic medications, 1612
Co-occurring substance use disorders
  longer-term management, 1616–1617
    recovery, 1616–1617
  management of, 1611–1615
    additional medication decisions, 1612
    pharmacological treatment, 1611
    psychosocial interventions, 1612–1613
    substances and antipsychotic medications, 1612
  other outpatient treatment approaches, 1615–1616
  prevalence, 1589–1590
  primary psychotic disorder with, 1602–1603
  screening and differential diagnosis, 1590–1591
  treatment considerations, 1591–1592
Coolidge Axis II Inventory (CATI), 1645–1646
Coombs test, 1381
Coordination of care, 1320–1321
Co-oximetry, 1415
COPD. *See* Chronic obstructive pulmonary disease
Coping skills
  adolescent substance abuse, ASAM, 1846
  cognitive-behavioral model
    of relapse, revised, 1227
    RP and, 1227
  individual psychotherapy, 1113
  relapse and, 1224–1225
  teaching, individual psychotherapy, 1102
  therapies, 1116
Coping/social skills training model, RP and, 1226
Cor pulmonale, 1406
Coronary artery bypass graft (CABG), 621–622
Coronary artery disease (CAD), 1320
  alcohol, cardiovascular disorders, 1339
  amphetamines, cardiovascular disorders, 1344
  cocaine, cardiovascular disorders, 1341–1343
  tobacco/nicotine, cardiovascular disorders, 1339–1340
Coronary atherosclerosis, 1339
Coronary calcification, 1339
Corporate social responsibility (CSR), 110
Corporate-induced Disorder (CID) heuristic model, 106, 107*t*, 107*f*
Corporate-induced disorders, 113
Cortical involvement, 36
Cortical projections, modulating striatum, 1065
Corticosteroids, 1323
Corticostriatal and forebrain neuromodulatory systems
  in gambling disorder, 792
Corticotropin-releasing hormone (CRH), 1661
Cortisol
  benzodiazepine(s), 1499
  caffeine and, 221
  marijuana and, 1497
Cost analysis–related measures, 57–58
Cough-inducing procedures, 1450
Counseling
  groups, 1095
  medication-assisted treatment, 53–54
  tobacco use, treatment planning, 1146, 1147*f*
Counselor
  addiction treatment
    network therapy, 1171, 1270
  collaborative care with, 1269–1274
  psychotherapists and, 1270
  satisfaction, 1103
  supervision, 1102–1103
  training, 1102
Counter conditioning, pre-contemplation stage and, 1081
Couples therapy, network therapy with, 557–558
Course of illness subdomain, ASAM, 1842, 1842*t*
Court calendar, court-leveraged treatment, 1976
Court-leveraged treatment
  cultural equity, 1979–1980
  dimensions of, 1976–1977
  effective court-leveraged programs, 1977*t*
  eligibility criteria, 1975
  high risk and high need persons, 1978
  high risk and low need persons, 1978–1979
  low risk and high need persons, 1979
  low risk and low need persons, 1979
  medication for opioid use disorder, 1980
  reducing substance use, 1975–1987
Courts. *See* Drug courts; Drug treatment courts
Covert sensitization, conditioned nausea responses and, 1191–1192
COVID-19 pandemic, 181–182, 544, 1250–1251, 1666–1667, 1983
  alcohol, traumatic injuries, 1485
  cannabis treatment, 1945

cannabis use disorder, 118
effects of, 1284–1285
quality care, 774
respiratory infections, 1449
telehealth, 1255
COX (Cyclooxygenase inhibition), 1748
COX-2 selective inhibitors, 1748
CPS. *See* Chronic pain syndrome
CRA. *See* Community reinforcement approach
"Crack" cocaine, 198*t*, 203–204
Crack lung, 1413
CRAFFT (Car, Relax, Alone, Family, Forget, Trouble), 1812, 1835
interview, 1862
CRAFT model, 1165
Craving, 1242, 1310, 1611
alcohol and, 152
cognitive processing models, 1243
relapse and, 1224
RP and, 1229
Craving behavioral intervention (CBI), 854
Creatine kinase (CK), 1433
Criminal justice system, 1855
persons referral, 1975
populations
detoxification, 866
Criminal legal system, women and, 647–648
Criminal recidivism, 1975
Crohn disease (CD), 1395–1396
Cross-reactivity, 515, 517*t*
Cross-tolerance, 142
Crothers, T.D., 583
CRPS (complex regional pain syndrome), 1694–1695, 1697
Cryoglobulinemia, 1380
CSA. *See* Controlled Substances Act
CSAT. *See* Center for Substance Abuse Treatment
CSAT's Addiction Technology Transfer Centers (ATTCs), 646–647
CSAT/SAMHSA (Center for Substance Abuse Treatment/Substance Abuse and Mental Health Services Administration), 1796
CSB. *See* Compulsive sexual behavior
CTI. *See* Computerized tailored intervention
CTN. *See* Clinical Trials Network
Cue exposure therapy (CE), 1670
Cue extinction model (CE), RP and, 1226, 1229
Cues, RP and, 1229
Cultural aspects of clinical assessment, 631
Cultural competence, LGBTQ, 669
Cultural factors, biopsychosocial model, 1200
Cultural identity, 630
Cultural issues, in addiction medicine, 627–634
Cultural resilience, LGBTQ, 669
Cultural subgroups, alcoholics anonymous, 1293
Cultural values in military, 681
Culturally adapted MI interventions (CAMIs), 1089
Culture(s), 627
patterns of substance use, 630–631
recovery, 631–633
Culture-specific treatment, 633
Cumulative incidence proportion, 385
Cumulative mass balance model, 79
Current Opioid Misuse Measure (COMM), 1729
Cut down, Annoyed, Guilty, Eye-opener Tool (CAGE-AID), 1728–1729
Cutaneous opioids, 1330
Cyclic adenosine monophosphate (cAMP), 139
"Cycling," AAS, 323–324
CYP3A4, 132
benzodiazepines, 168–169
drug metabolism, 132
CYP1A2, drug metabolism, 169, 185, 221, 224, 1472
CYP2B6 family, 132
CYP2C19
benzodiazepines metabolism, 169
polymorphisms of, 169
CYP2C9, drug metabolism, 168–169
CYP2D6, drug metabolism, 132
CYP2E1, drug metabolism, 136
Cysts, 148
Cytochrome (CYP) 450 activity, 131–132
barbiturates, 1499
benzodiazepines, 169
caffeine and, 221
elimination half-life, 166*t*
isoenzymes, 1369
isozymes, 133*t*–134*t*
Cytochrome P-450 2A6 (CYP2A6)
drug metabolism, 233–234
Cytochrome P-450 1A2 isoenzyme (CYP1A2)
psychosis, 1612
Cytochrome P-450 2E1 (CYP2E1) oxidizes ethanol, 1357
Cytomegalovirus retinitis, 1453

D

Dabbing wax, 349
Daley's psychoeducational approach, RP and, 1226
Dangerousness/lethality subdomain, ASAM, 1842, 1842*t*
DAST. *See* Drug Abuse Screening Test
DAST (Drug Abuse Screening Test), 1728–1729
DATA 2000. *See* Drug Addiction Treatment Act of 2000 (DATA 2000)
Data and Safety Monitoring Board (DSMB), 59
Date rape pill. *See* Flunitrazepam
Davidson Brief Social Phobia questionnaire, 1103
DAWN. *See* Drug Abuse Warning Network
DBT. *See* Dialectical behavioral therapy
DBT Substance Abuse (DBT-S), 1649, 1651
D-cycloserine (DCS), co-occurring PTSD-SUD, 1670
D4 dopamine receptor (DRD4), 1627–1628
DEA. *See* Drug Enforcement Administration
Death, 280
alcohol-related, 399
benzodiazepine(s), 169–170, 889
inhalants, 312
opioids, 169–170
smoking and, 1143
Decision making, ethical issues, 1902
Deep brain stimulation (DBS), 1070, 1660–1661
Default Mode Network (DMN), 1628
Degree of ambivalence, 1088–1089
Delaying tactics, climate change and, 85
Delirium tremens (DTs), 881–883, 1485–1486
Delivery, pregnancy, substance use during, 1521
Delta infection, 1368
Δ⁹-Tetrahydrocannabinol (THC), 248, 1396, 1518, 1937
analgesic effect, 1940
intravenous self-administration (IVSA), 256
in marijuana, 455
oral, 1939–1940
physical dependence/withdrawal, 257
sleep and, 1472–1473
substance-induced psychosis, 1606
Demographics, college student drinking, 438–439
Denial. *See* Patient(s)
Department of Children Youth Services (DCYS) system, 625
Department of Defense (DoD), 680
cross-sectional surveys of health-related behaviors among military personnel, 453–455
Population Health Improvement, 458–459, 458*f*
task force, 453–454
TRICARE role, 460
zero-tolerance policy, 455
Department of Health, Education, and Welfare ("HEW"), 1930
Department of Transportation (DOT), 518, 1958
Department of Veterans Affairs (VA), 1289–1290
Dependence. *See also specific substance i.e. alcohol dependence*
addiction liability and, 158
hallucinogen(s), 275–276
inhalants, 312
nicotine and, 237
Depolarization-induced suppression of excitation (DSE), 254–255
Depolarization-induced suppression of inhibition (DSI), 254–255
Depression, 1752. *See also* Depressive disorders
bodybuilders and, AAS, 329
fibromyalgia, 1696
high-volume sexual behaviors, 830
pain and, 1696
psychiatric comorbidity, 1022
Seligman's model of learned helplessness, 1713
sleep disorders, 1467, 1471
substance-induced mental disorders, 1885
Depressive disorders, 1547
antidepressant medication, 1572–1575
chronic pain and, 1696
comorbid with SUDs, adolescents, 1885–1886
DSM-5, 1560, 1561*t*
nicotine, 1577–1578
placebo response rate, 1573–1574
prevalence and prognostic effects, 1565–1567
primary care, 1577
suicidal behavior, 1577
tobacco, 1577–1578
treatment
adolescents, 1576
late life, 1576–1577
Depressive disorders, with SUDs, adolescents, 1885–1886
DER. *See* Designated employer representative
Desensitization
cigarette smokers, 239–240
receptor(s), 142

Designated employer representative (DER), 1972
Designer drugs, 861, 1551
Desipramine, BN with comorbid addiction disorder, 1683
Desomorphine. *See* Krokodil
Desyrel. *See* Trazodone
Detoxification, 538
  goals of, 861–862
  inpatient, 863
  management principles, 862
  outpatient, 863
  pharmacologic management, 862–863
  settings, selection considerations, 863–864
  substance abuse treatment *vs.*, 861–862
Developmental disabilities, adolescents, SUDs, 1888
Developmental stages, events, 1074
Dextroamphetamine, opioid induced sedation, 1775–1776
Dextromethorphan (DXM), 293, 910, 931–932, 1046, 1424, 1550, 1609
  abuse, epidemiology, 295–296
  drug–drug interactions, 300
  historical features, 294–295
  medical preparation, 294
  neurobehavioral and cognitive disorders, 1426
  pharmacodynamics, 299
  pharmacokinetics, 296–297
  seizures, 1428
  serotonin syndrome and, 299–300
  stroke, 1432
Dextrorphan, 1550
DFST. *See* Dual-focus schema therapy
Diabetes mellitus, 1320
  chronic pancreatitis, 1392–1393
  opioids, endocrine effects, 1496–1497
Diabetic ketoacidosis, 1490, 1497–1498
Diacetyl, 1408
Diacetylmorphine. *See* Heroin
Diagnosis, Intractable Risk and Efficacy Score (DIRE), 1729
Diagnosis-program-driven treatment, 727
Diagnostic and Statistical Manual of Mental Disorders (DSM), 2, 29, 105
Diagnostic and Statistical Manual of Mental Disorders-5 (DSM-5), 30, 1713–1714
  addiction, 30
  for ADHD, 1624
  bipolar disorders, 1560, 1562*t*
  caffeine intoxication, 222
  caffeine withdrawal, 222–223, 223*t*
  cannabis use disorder, 118
  depressive disorders, 1560, 1561*t*
  diagnostic criteria, AUD, 610
  primary *vs.* substance-induced mood disorders, 1567
  PTSD, 1658
  substance use disorders, 368–369
Diagnostic and Statistical Manual of Mental Disorders, Third Edition (DSM-III), 1658
Diagnostic and Statistical Manual of Mental Disorders-IV (DSM-IV), 30, 1713–1714
  AAS, 329
  addiction, group therapy, 1094, 1101
  alcohol use disorders, 370
  diagnostic criteria, AUD, 610
  drug use disorders, 371
  food addiction, 1679, 1679*t*
  inhalant abuse, 313
  nicotine dependent adults, 370
  opioid dependence, 1001
  psychiatric disorders, 1680
  sedative-hypnotics, 962
  sleep disorders, 1470
  substance-induced mental disorders, 1545
  SUDs, 1560, 1835
Diagnostic Interview for Children and Adolescents, 1835
Diagnostic Interview Schedule for Children, 1835
Diagnostic interviews, SUDs, 1835
Dialectical behavioral therapy (DBT), 1113–1114, 1649, 1668, 1864
Dialectical techniques, climate change and, 85
Diarrhea, 1393
Diazepam, 166*t*, 962, 962*t*
  addiction liability, 170–171
  benzodiazepines and, 167
  breastfeeding, 1522
  co-occurring anxiety disorders, alcohol dependence, 956
  disorders related to, 1499
  DTs, 881
  ketamine, 293
  medical complications, 173
  uncomplicated withdrawal syndrome, 876–877
  withdrawal and, 862–863
  withdrawal seizures and, 881
Dieting and purging, 1680
Diffuse alveolar hemorrhage, 1413
Diffusion tensor imaging (DTI)
  in gambling disorder, 792
Digital health
  definition, 1250–1251
  for substance use disorders, 1250–1259
Digital health interventions
  for substance use disorders, 1250–1259
    digital therapeutics for, 1251–1252
    evolution of, 1250–1251
    future opportunities and responsible digital health, 1257–1259
    integration into practice, 1257
    mobile applications or websites reviews with guided components, 1254–1255
    mobile applications/apps/stand-alone websites, 1252–1255
    newer digital technologies, 1255–1257
    telehealth, 1255
Digital mental health, 1258–1259
Digital technologies
  substance use disorders, digital health interventions for, 1255–1257
    chatbots, 1256
    peer support, 1256
    social media, 1256
    virtual reality, 1257
    wearables and tracking, 1256–1257
Digital therapeutics, 1251–1252
  substance use disorders, digital health interventions for, 1251–1252
Dilated cardiomyopathy, 1336
Dilaudid. *See* Hydromorphone
Diltiazem, CYP3A4 inhibitors and, 135
Dipeptidyl peptidase-4 (DPP-4) inhibitors, 1392–1393
Direct cerebral vasoconstriction, 1431
Direct-acting agents (DAAs), 745–746
Direct-acting antivirals (DAAs), 1363–1364, 1380
  hepatitis C virus, 1367
Disability
  interdisciplinary pain programs, 1720
  secondary and tertiary gains, 1715–1716
Disabled social network, 632*t*
Disagreements, ethical considerations, prescribing medications with, 1921–1922
Discharge criteria, ASAM, 729
Disciplinary actions, physician and, controlled substances, 1908
Diseases, drug addiction, 14–15
Disruptive mood dysregulation disorder (DMDD), 1559–1560
Disseminated candidiasis, 1436
Dissociative anesthetics, 293, 931–934
  Dizocilpine (MK-801), 295
  drugs in class, 293
  formulation, methods of use, 293–294
  headache, 1424
  historical features, 294–295
  intoxication
    physical effects, 932
    psychological and behavioral effects, 931–932, 932*t*
  neurobehavioral and cognitive disorders, 1426
  neurobiology, 300
  seizures, 1428
  stroke, 1432
  substances in class, 293
  withdrawal syndrome, 932
Dissociatives, 1046
  LGBTQ, 671
  and psychosis, 1609
Distraction, pain and, 1712
Distribution, 130–131
  drug, 130
  protein binding, 131
  rate of blood flow, 131
  volume of distribution, 130
Distributive integrated service models, 744*t*
Distributive models, SUDs, 747–749
Disulfiram, 951, 1273*t*, 1359, 1670
  alcohol, adolescent SUDs, 1874
  aversion therapy *vs.*, 1189–1190
  clinical use of, 951
  co-occurring substance use disorders, 1591
  medication adherence and, BPD, 1272
  pharmacology of, 951
  RP and, 1222–1223
  stimulant use disorders, 1017
Disulfiram-ethanol reaction (DER), 950
Divalproex, 956
D-lysergic acid diethylamide (LSD), 1423
DoD
  Forensic Drug Testing Labs, 455
DOM. *See* 3,5-Dimethoxy-4-methylamphetamine (DOM)

Domestic violence, women, 645–646
Dopamine (DA), 191, 1064
addiction, transcranial magnetic stimulation for, 1066–1067
alcohol, 155–156
antagonists, cocaine action, 39
binge–intoxication stage, 5–6
cocaine and, 1497–1498
cocaine binding, 37
disulfiram, 951
drug metabolism, 131
in gambling disorder, 791
psychostimulants and, 41
receptors, drugs of abuse, 139*t*
reward systems, 151
stimulants and, 205*t*, 206–207, 207*t*
in VTA, 41
Dopamine agonists (antiparkinson agents), stimulant use disorders, 1017
Dopamine receptors, and pharmacological actions, $_L$-THP, 1053–1054, 1053*f*
Dopamine transporter (DAT), 1627–1628
ADHD, 1630
Dopamine-regulated circuits, neurons and, 11
Dopaminergic neurons, nicotine and, 239
Dorsal striatum, ventral striatum and, 36–37, 36*f*
Dorsolateral prefrontal cortex (DLPFC), 1065–1066
TMS to, 1067
TMS with cognitive therapy, 1068–1069
Dose–receptor bound graphs, 137, 137*f*
Dose-response curves, 137*f*
Dose-response relationships, 1244–1245
ASAM, 1847
Dose–response studies, 53
Dosing, DXM intoxication syndrome, 303
DOT. *See* Department of Transportation
Drake, Daniel, 581
Dramatic relief, precontemplation stage and, 1080
Dravet syndrome, 1938
D_2 receptor agonists, 12
Drinkers. *See also* College student drinking; Drivers; Underage drinking
heavy, 1153
motives, college student drinking, 440
Drinking
and drug use, alcohol environment, effects of, 400
reduction/stopping, medications for, 946–954
Drinking partnership, 1199
Drinking patterns, 111
Drivers
designated, 424*t*, 432
DXM-positive, 295–296
intoxicated, 400–401, 485, 1817
Dronabinol, 1938
Droughts, climate change and, 79
Drug(s). *See also* Addiction; Adolescent(s); Controlled substances; Dose-response curves; Dose-response relationship; Dosing; Drug addiction(s); Drug testing; Drug use; Drug use disorder; Drug withdrawal; Drug-drug interactions; Drugs of abuse; Illicit drug; Medications; Multiple drugs; Prescription medications; specific i.e. psychostimulant drugs
access, 554–555
activity, drug concentrations and, 131
adults, 476–477, 477*t*
animal self-administration studies, 42
changing trends, in, 861
of choice, biologic effect of, physician addiction, 555
concentrations, drug activity and, 131
craving, 42–43
dependence, 2
designer, 861
discontinuation, written agreement, 1906–1907
disorders related to, 1355, 1463–1464, 1468–1477, 1497–1500
elimination, 132–135
inhaled, 129
interactions
alcohol, 225
altered biotransformation and, 168
caffeine and, 225
cigarette smoking, 225
cytochromes and, 135
energy drinks, 225
nicotine, 225
TSF, 1216
metabolism, 11, 131–132, 185
misuse of, 491
molecular-cellular level, 11
oral, absorption of, 129
physician addiction, 556
pregnant women
illicit drugs, 500–501
reinforcement, preclinical studies, 37–42
screening, differential diagnosis with, 860
selection, prescriptions and, 866
sleep and, 1470–1474
treatment, adolescents, 1835
withdrawal, drug addiction, 7
in women, 638
youth, 478–480, 479*t*–480*t*
Drug abuse, 1522–1523
Drug Abuse Screening Test (DAST), 504, 531, 1728–1729
for Adolescents, 1835
Drug Abuse Warning Network (DAWN), 260
Drug addiction(s)
behavior and, neurobiology of, 2–26
combative strategies, 13–19
disease of brain, 4*f*
environmental factors, 12
genetic factors, 11
neuroanatomy of, 42–44
neurobiology of, 5–6
pharmacologic intervention, 15–17, 15*t*, 16*f*
preventing, 13–14
treatment, 14–15
medications for, 14–15
Drug Addiction Treatment Act of 2000 (DATA 2000), 180, 745, 770–771, 1001
Drug binding, alpha$_1$-acid glycoprotein, 131
Drug Consumption Venues (DCVs), 428
Drug control policy, 1927–1933
Drug craving, 56
Drug criminalization, 761
Drug cue-reactivity, 1242
Drug discrimination studies
animal drug addiction liability, cannabinoids, 255–256
Drug Enforcement Administration (DEA), 409–410, 775, 1800–1803, 1911, 1924, 1930
Drug Enforcement Agency (DEA), 1255
Drug half-life, 184
Drug interactions, 135–136
human immunodeficiency virus, 1456
Drug metabolism, 131
Drug monitoring programs, 1806–1807
Drug potency, 137–138
Drug screening, patient permission and, 884, 1901
Drug testing
alcohol consumption, biomarkers of ethyl glucuronide and ethyl sulfate, 1966
phosphatidyl ethanol, 1966
clinical, 1957
at dance parties, contaminants ingestion reduction, 430
ethical issues in alcohol and, 1966–1967
evolution of
chromatography, 1957
federal workplace drug testing program, 1958
immunoassay technique, 1957–1958
LC-MS and GC-MS, 1957–1958
liquid chromatography-tandem mass spectrometry, 1957–1958
mass spectrometry, 1957
military testing program, 1958
urine drug testing, 1958
laboratory tests, 1958–1959
limitations of, 1964–1965
matrix for, 1962–1964
hair, 1963–1964
oral fluid, 1963, 1964*t*
urine, 1963
Medical Review Officer role and workplace duties of, 1969–1970
practice, 1973
process, 1971–1973
regulatory framework, 1970–1971
useful web sites, 1971*t*
methods, 1959–1962
chromatography, 1961–1962
immunoassay, 1959–1961, 1960*f*, 1961*f*
mass spectrometry, 1961–1962, 1962*f*
in military personnel, 455–456
selection of methodology, 1962
Drug use
infectious diseases, 1444–1457
liver disorders, 1355–1370
sleep disorders, 1463–1464, 1468–1477
Drug use disorder (DUD)
incidence, 371
incidence of, 371
prevalence, 371
risk factors, 371
Drug–drug interactions
alcohol, 151
benzodiazepines, 169
NSAIDs, 1755
stimulants, 199–200
Drug-Free Workplace Act (DFWP), 546–547

Drugs of abuse, 138, 139*t*. *See also* Illicit drug; Substance abuse
analgesic effects, 1698
mechanistic classification of, 138, 139*t*
renal problems, 1376
DSM-III. *See* Diagnostic and Statistical Manual of Mental Disorders-III
DSM-IV. *See* Diagnostic and Statistical Manual of Mental Disorders-IV
DSM-5-TR, 1250
DTx, 1251
Dual Assessment & Recovery Track (DART), 1186–1187
Dual diagnosis, 1183, 1889
AA/NA, 1292
Dual disorders. *See* Dual diagnosis
Dual Recovery Therapy (DRT), 1615
Dual-focus schema therapy (DFST), 1651
DUD. *See* Drug use disorder
Duloxetine
depression with comorbid pain syndromes, 1750
peripheral neuropathy, 1750
Duration, sedative–hypnotic, 894
Duty to warn, confidentiality requirements, 1908
DXM. *See* Dextromethorphan (DXM)
Dynamic model of relapse, 1227*f*
Dysesthetic pain, gabapentin, 1751
Dyslipidemia, 1494
Dysphoric effects, management, 200
Dyspnea, 1411
Dysregulated serotonin metabolism, pulmonary vasculature, 1405
Dysthymia, 1566–1567
Dystonia, cannabis, 1943–1944
Dystonic reactions, 1434

E

EA. *See* Electroacupuncture
Early intervention, adolescent substance abuse, 1844
Early- *versus* late-onset substance use, in older adults, 655
Ears, medical care of patients, with unhealthy substance use, 1315
Eat, infant assessment, parameters for, 1517*t*
Eating Disorder Diagnostic Scale (EDDS), 1681
Eating Disorder Examination Questionnaire (EDE-Q), 1681
Eating disorders
acute treatment, 1682
in adolescents, SUDs, 1891
BES, 1681–1682
BULIT-R, 1681
co-occurrence SUDs, 1685
co-occurring substance, 1685
definition, 1678
differential diagnosis, 1681
EDDS, 1681
EDE-Q, 1681
EDI-3, 1681
identification, 1681
long-term treatment, 1682
management of
acute psychological management, 1684–1685
biologic, 1682–1684
long-term psychological management, 1685
subacute psychological management, 1685
NESS, 1682
prevalence, 1679*t*
general population, 1679–1680
primary care population, 1680–1681
psychiatric disorder patients, 1680
SUDs patients, 1680
screening instruments, 1681–1682
subacute treatment, 1682
substance use with, 1681
in women, 641
YFAS, 1682
Eating Disorders Anonymous (EDA), 1685
Eating Disorders Inventory, Third Edition (EDI-3), 1681
EBQ. *See* Eating Behaviors Questionnaire
Echocardiography, 1346
alcohol-related cardiomyopathy, 1337
E-cigarette or vaping product use-associated lung injury (EVALI), 1408, 1871–1872
e-cigarettes. *See* Electronic Drug Delivery Devices (EDDD)
Ecoanxiety, 76–77
Ecological grid, 76–77
Ecological momentary assessment, 1123
Economic availability, 109–110
Economic informed consent, managed care, 1902
Ecoparalysis, 76–77
Ecstasy/MDMA, 935–936, 1383, 1550
pulmonary vasculature, 1405
sleep difficulties, 1471
ED. *See* Emergency department
ED50. *See* Median effective doses
EDA. *See* Eating Disorders Anonymous
EDDS. *See* Eating Disorder Diagnostic Scale
EDE-Q. *See* Eating Disorder Examination Questionnaire
EDI-3. *See* Eating Disorders Inventory-Third Edition (EDI-3)
Education
drug/alcohol use disorders, 375–376
EEG. *See* Electroencephalogram
Efavirenz (EFV)
CYP3A4 inducers, 135
CYP3A4 inducers and, 135
Effectiveness
clinical trials, 50–51, 53
court-leveraged programs, 1977*t*
of traditional therapeutic communities, 1181–1182
Efficacy
clinical trials, 49–50
pharmacodynamics, 137–142
research, individual psychotherapy, 1109
EFV. *See* Efavirenz
"E-juice," electronic drug delivery devices, 338
Elderly
alcohol use disorders, 372
benzodiazepines, 172
Elective surgery, 1327
Electrical stimulation therapy, 1742–1744
Electroencephalogram (EEG)
alcohol withdrawal seizures, 871
withdrawal seizure, 871
Electrolytes
alcohol and, 1494
DTs, 875
Electronic cigarettes, 1407–1408
aerosol, 1404
traumatic injuries, 1485
Electronic drug delivery devices (EDDDs), 370, 1036, 1340–1341, 1395, 1429–1430, 1513–1514, 1549, 1603
battery-powered devices, 337
cannabis, 349–350
cell and animal studies, 339
combustible cigarette, 338*f*
fine particles, 341
flavorants (flavorings), 339–340
health effects of, 344–346
history, 337
humectant, 338
marketing, 122
nicotine, 338–339
containing e-liquids, 338–339
delivery level, 341–342
pharmacokinetic studies, 341
nonnicotine substance use, 349
policy approach to, 350
prevalence of use, 343
propylene glycol and vegetable glycerin, 338
regulation of, 350–351
second-hand and third hand exposure, 342–343
toxicant exposures, 344–346
types, 337, 338*f*
use and stopping smoking
as clinical tool, 346–347
at population level, 347–348
vaporizers, 349–350
variation, 348–349
volatile organic compounds, 340–341
Electronic nicotine delivery systems (ENDS), 338*f*
Elimination, 132–135
caffeine and, 221
nicotine, 232–234
"E-liquid," electronic drug delivery devices, 338
Emergency department (ED)
alcohol use, 480
settings, SBI in, 480–481
Emergency personnel/police, 1603–1604
Emerging therapies, cannabis, adolescent SUDs, 1875
Emetine, 1190–1191
aversion therapy, 1192–1193
Emetric therapy data, aversion therapy and, 1195–1196
Emotion(s)
pain and, 1695–1697, 1709–1710
regulation, 1222
Emotional conditions, ASAM adolescent criteria, 1841–1842
Emotional distress, chronic pain and, 1710
Emotional states
relapse and, 1227
RP and, 1229
Emotional vulnerability factors, 1155
Empathogens, LGBTQ, 671
Emphysema, 1412
Empiric therapy, osteomyelitis, 1451
Employee assistance program (EAP), 544, 546–547, 702
Employer resources
employee assistance program, 546–547

labor union resources, 548
peer support groups, 547–548
screening and brief intervention, 548
Employment drug testing, 546
Employment, drug/alcohol use disorders, 628
Employment status, drug/alcohol use disorders, 375
EMR. *See* Electronic medical record
Encephalopathy, 1377
Endocannabinoid system (ECS), 253–255
Endocannabinoids (ECs), 7–8, 250
adverse effects, 258–259
alcohol and, 157
neurobiology of, 6
schizophrenia and, 258–259
Endocarditis, 1452
clinical presentation, 1446–1447
diagnosis, 1447
epidemiology, 1446
opioids, cardiovascular disorders, 1344–1345
outcome and prevention, 1448
pathogenesis, 1446
treatment, 1447–1448
valve surgery for, 1540
Endocrine disorders, substance use, 1490–1500
Endocrine syndromes, 1491*t*
Endocrine system, 203
stimulants, 203, 1776
Endocrinological consequences
alcohol, 1493–1494
alcohol use, medical complications related to, 1326
cannabinoids, 1331
opioids, 1330
tobacco use, complications related to, 1328
Endocytosis, 142
Endogenous catecholamine neurotransmitters
chemical structures of, 193*f*
Endogenous opiates, 208
Endophthalmitis, 1453
Endoscopic retrograde cholangio-pancreatography (ERCP), chronic pancreatitis, 1392
Endoscopic therapy, chronic pancreatitis, 1392
Endotoxin, 1357
End-stage liver disease, 1323–1324
Engagement, ASAM, 1843
Enkephalin, 182
Entecavir (ETV), 1363
Environment
addiction and, 12
community-based prevention programs, 399–407
events, 1074
pain, 1714–1715
role of, 1714–1716
safe, ASAM criteria and, 727
Environmental re-evaluation, pre-contemplation stage and, 1080
Enzymatic receptors, activated, 138
Enzymes, drug metabolism, 131
Ephedra, 192, 193*f*, 1431
Ephedrine
norepinephrine, 207
Epidemiologic Catchment Area (ECA) study, 368, 370, 1290–1291
Epidemiology
primary, secondary, and tertiary prevention, 385*t*, 385*b*
principles, 367–370
Epigenetics, 144
Epilepsy, cannabis treatment for, 1940–1941
Epinephrine, caffeine and, 1498
Equitable care, 1258
Erectile dysfunction, 243
Erythromycin, CYP3A4 inhibitors and, 135
Escitalopram (Lexapro), 1593
Esophagus, 1389–1390
gastrointestinal disorders, 1389–1390
Esquirol, Jean-Étienne Dominique, 582
Estimated glomerular filtration rates (eGRF), 621–622
Estrogen, 243, 1328
Eszopiclone
addiction liability, 171
nonbenzodiazepines and, 165, 166*t*, 167–168
Ethanol, 154–155, 308, 880–881, 1335, 1357, 1391, 1391*f*, 1393
laboratory testing, 519–520
Ethanol-induced neurotoxicity, 159
alcohol and, 159
Ethical dilemmas, resources for, 1902
Ethics
issues, addiction practice, 1896–1903
principle, 1896–1900
Ethnic groups, physician addiction, 552, 627
Ethnicity
definitions and concepts, 622
drug/alcohol use disorders, 373–374
Ethnic/racial subgroups, 1293
Ethyl alcohol, 148
Ethyl glucuronide (EtG), 519, 1512, 1966
Ethyl sulfate (EtS), 519, 1512, 1966
Ethylcocaine, 1369
Ethylene glycol, 1378–1379
toxicity, 1379
Euphoria, clonidine, 912
Euphorigenic cannabinoid delta-9 tetrahydrocannabinol (Δ9-THC), 1045
Eutectic mixture of local anesthetics (EMLA), 1752
EVALI syndrome, 386–387
"Eve", 520
Evidence-based approach, for substance use disorders, 1088
Evidence-based behavioral therapies, LGBTQ, 674–675
Evidence-based couple
substance use disorders, 1201–1202
community reinforcement and family training, 1202
inpatient treatment, engaging family members during, 1201–1202
motivational interviewing, 1201
Evoking
motivational interviewing processes, 1086
Excited delirium, 1485–1486
Exclusive/stand-alone model, 1183
Excretion, 135
Executive function, 37, 693
Exercise
AAS, 326
pain management, 1737
Exocrine insufficiency, chronic pancreatitis, 1392
Expectancy challenge interventions, college student drinking, 442
Experimental studies, 367–368. *See also* Animal experiments; Clinical studies
Explicit memory, 1425
Exposure-based therapy, 1664
Extended amygdala, 157–158
Extended-release formulation of naltrexone (XR-NTX), 983
Extension for Community Healthcare Outcomes (ECHO), 749
Extra-hypothalamic corticotropin- releasing factor system (CRF) system, 237
Extrapulmonary tuberculosis, 1450
Extreme weather events, climate change and, 78–79
Eye movement desensitization reprocessing (EMDR), 1664–1666
Eyes
infections, 1453
medical care of patients, with unhealthy substance use, 1315

F

Facebook, 1256
Facial pain, 1696
Family. *See also* Addicted families; Spouses with addiction (*See also* Recovered family)
adolescent substance abuse, 1834
ASAM, 1842
chaotic, adolescent assessment, 1843
interventions, 1120–1121
therapies
AN, 801
Family and Medical Leave Act (FMLA), 545
Family history
benzodiazepine withdrawal, 895
drug/alcohol use disorder, 376
gambling disorder, 815
Family history density (FHD), 1201
Family involvement
in addiction, treatment, and recovery, 1198–1208
biological factors, 1199
cultural factors, 1200
psychological factors, 1199
social factors, 1199–1200
couple and family modalities for adults, 1203–1204
alcohol behavioral couple therapy, 1203
behavioral couples therapy, 1203–1204
brief family-involved treatment, 1203
family approaches with adolescents, 1204–1205
behavioral exchange systems training, 1204
brief strategic family therapy, 1204
multidimensional family therapy, 1204
multisystemic therapy, 1204–1205
family psychoeducation and 12-step program engagement, 1202–1203
bibliotherapy, 1202
mutual support groups, 1202–1203
psychoeducation, 1202
population-specific considerations, 1205–1208
for military members and veterans, 1206–1207
for older adults, 1205–1206
for pregnant women, 1207–1208

Family members
  biopsychosocial model of, 1198–1200
  during inpatient treatment, 1201–1202
Family programs, 395–396
Family psychoeducation
  and 12-step program engagement, 1202–1203
    bibliotherapy, 1202
    mutual support groups, 1202–1203
    psychoeducation, 1202
Family recovery, 1099
Family regulation system, structural determinant of care, 760*b*
Family Smoking Prevention and Tobacco Control Act, 98, 350
Family studies of addiction, 789
Family Support Network, 1863
Family therapies, 1864–1865
  individual psychotherapy, 1120–1121
Family treatments
  substance use disorders, 1201–1202
    community reinforcement and family training, 1202
    inpatient treatment, engaging family members during, 1201–1202
    motivational interviewing, 1201
Family-based prevention
  approaches, 395–396
  effectiveness of, 395–396
  family programs, 395–396
  parenting programs, 395
Family-focused therapy, 1581–1582
Faradic aversion therapy, alcohol, 1191
FASD. *See* Fetal alcohol spectrum disorder (FASD)
Fatty acid ethyl esters (FAEE), 1512
Fatty liver, 1532
FDA. *See* Food and Drug Administration
Fear
  avoidance model, 1712–1713
  circuitry of, 1697
Fear of injury, impairment and, 1712–1713
Federal Aviation Administration (FAA), 545
Federal Bureau of Narcotics (FBN), 1929
Federal collaboration, 590
Federal confidentiality laws, 1907–1908
Federal Food, Drug and Cosmetic Act, 92, 98
Federal legislative changes, 617
Federal methadone regulations, 1000
Federal Motor Carrier and Safety Administration (FMCSA), 545
Federation of State Medical Board (FSMB) guidelines, 1806
Federation of State Physician Health Programs, pain treatment, guidelines, 561
Feedback, counsellor supervision, 1102–1103
Feedback-only interventions, college student drinking, 444
Female gonadal function, 1496
Fenfluramine, 1412
Fentanyl, 908, 1611, 1770. *See also* Transdermal fentanyl
  anesthesiologists, 552
  clinical implications, 359
  epidemiology, 359
  history, 358–359
  legal status, 359
  OIH, 1702
  pharmacology, 359
  physician addiction, 555, 563–564
  screens, 563–564
  substance-induced psychosis, 1602
Fentanyl overdose
  deaths, 409*f*, 411
  naloxone and, 911
Fetal
  alcohol use, medical complications related to, 1326
  cannabinoids, 1331
  opioids, 1330
  tobacco use, complications related to, 1328
Fetal alcohol spectrum disorder (FASD), 112, 159, 637, 1378, 1514, 1515*t*
Fetal alcohol syndrome (FAS), 1514
Fetal distress, 864–865
Fetal solvent syndrome, inhalants, 313
FIB-4, 1362–1363
Fibromyalgia
  depression and, 1696
  duloxetine, 1750
  risk of suicide, 1727
Fidelity, ethical issues in, 1900
Field of addiction medicine, 584, 589
  definition of, 589
  "time in practice" in, 590
Fighting elite, AAS, 324
Filtered cigarettes, 94, 94*f*
Finnegan Neonatal Abstinence Scoring System (FNASS), 1513
First-order elimination kinetics, 132
First-pass metabolism, 130
Flavorants (flavorings), electronic drug delivery devices, 339–340
Floppy baby syndrome, 172
Flualprazolam/etizolam
  clinical implications, 361
  history, 360–361
  legal status, 361
  pharmacology, 361
Flumazenil, 963
  beta-carboline activity, 141
  midazolam and, 902
  sedative-hypnotics withdrawal, 963
Flunitrazepam, 940
  addiction liability, 170–171
Flurazepam, 166*t*, 169
Fluvoxamine
  BED with comorbid addiction, 1683
  BN with comorbid addiction disorder, 1683
  OCD, 1593
fMRI. *See* Functional magnetic resonance imaging
Focal and segmental glomerulosclerosis (FSGS), 1379
Focused attention, 1236
Focusing, motivational interviewing processes, 1086
Folate deficiency, 1326, 1393
Follicle-stimulating hormone (FSH), 1494
Follow-up sessions, 1150
Food addiction, 1679
Food and Drug Administration (FDA)
  alcoholic dependence, approved medications for, 946, 947*t*
  cannabinoids, 1939
  OBOT, 1001
  opioids, 180
Food and Drug Agency (FDA), 1803–1804
Foods, caffeine content of, 219*t*
Forced nicotine abstinence, 1031
Foreign body granulomatosis, 1411
Forgiveness, 1712
Four-chamber enlargement
  alcohol-related cardiomyopathy, 1337
Four-Dimensional Symptom Questionnaire (4DSQ), 1590–1591
FPWs. *See* Family psychoeducational workshops
Fractional anisotropy (FA), 797
Fraternity and sorority organizations, 439
Freebase nicotine, electronic drug delivery devices, 339
Freebasing cocaine, 191–192
Freud, S., 197
Frontal-striatal circuitry
  as primary for neuromodulation therapeutics, 1066
Frontier drinking, 581
FSH. *See* Follicle-stimulating hormone
FTC method, 94
Fuels, 308–309, 309*t*
Fuels, volatile, 308–309
Full agonists, 140
Full CB_1 agonists, 251
Full opioid agonists, 912
Functional brain chemistry research, 1697
Functional family therapy (FFT), 1858
Functional impairment
  gambling disorder, 814
  pain, 1712–1713
Functional magnetic resonance imaging (fMRI)
  ADHD, 1628
  drug addiction, 42–43
Fungal endocarditis, 1344–1345
Furosemide, 318, 319*t*–320*t*

G

G protein receptors
  cyclic adenosine monophosphate, 139
  pharmacodynamic tolerance, 142
  serotonin, 139
  serpentine receptors, 139
G protein–coupled receptor (GPCR), 251
GABA. *See* Gamma-aminobutyric acid
GABAA. *See* Gamma-aminobutyric acid A
$GABA_A$-gated chloride ion channels, drug agents and, 141
GABA-benzodiazepine receptor complex, 892–894, 893*f*
GABAergic agents, 951–953
Gabapentin, 952
  benzodiazepine withdrawal, 902
  dysesthetic pain, 1750–1751
  pain, 1750–1751
  sleep difficulties, 1474
GAD. *See* Generalized anxiety disorder (GAD)
Gallstones, 1391
Gamblers anonymous, 1284
Gambling disorder
  assessment, 813–815, 818–820
  clinical characteristics, 813–814
  conceptualization, 789
  cultures, 628*t*–629*t*
  definition, 789
  epidemiological studies, 792–793

epidemiology, 812–813
family history, 815
functional impairment, 814
legal difficulties, 814
neurobiology, 789–792
genetic and environmental factors, 789–790
neurochemistry, 790–792
neurocognition, 790
pharmacotherapy, 818–820
psychiatric comorbidity, 814–815
psychologically based treatments, 815, 816*t*–820*t*
psychopharmacological interventions, 793–794
psychotherapeutic interventions, 793–794
quality of life, 814
treatment, 815–821
Gamma hydroxybutyrate (GHB), 1413–1414
Gamma-aminobutyric acid A ($GABA_A$) receptors, 167–168, 961
Gamma-aminobutyric acid ($GABA_A$) receptors, 1697
alcohol and, 152–154, 152*t*, 159–160
drugs acting on, 141
sedative–hypnotic, 888, 961
Gamma-glutamyl transferase (GGT), 519, 744, 861, 1965–1966
Gamma-glutaryl transferase (GGT), 613
Gamma-hydroxybutyrate (GHB)
intoxication, 937
withdrawal, 937
γ-Amino-butyric acid (GABA), 208
γ-glutamyl transpeptidase (γGT), 1358, 1370
Gas chromatography, 518
Gas chromatography/mass spectrometry (GC/MS), 519
Gastric emptying time, 130
Gastric lavage, 869
Gastric mucosa, 1389
Gastric secretions, 150–151
Gastritis, alcohol, 1390
Gastro-esophageal reflux disease (GERD), 224, 1395
Gastrointestinal
alcohol use, medical complications related to, 1324–1325
cannabinoids, complications, 1331
opioids, stimulants, 1330
tobacco use, complications related to, 1327
Gastrointestinal cancer, 1393–1394
Gastrointestinal disorders
colon, 1393
esophagus, 1389–1390
gastrointestinal cancer, 1393–1394
gastrointestinal symptoms associated with other drugs, 1394–1397
anticholinergics, 1395
body packing, 1397
cannabis, 1396–1397
laxatives, 1395
opioids, 1394–1395
psychostimulants, 1396
tobacco, 1395–1396
oral cavity, 1389
pancreas, 1390–1393
parotid glands, 1389
small intestine, 1393
stomach, 1390
Gastrointestinal infections, 1451
Gastrointestinal malignancy, 1396
Gastrointestinal system, caffeine and, 222
Gastrointestinal tract, problems, alcohol and, 1389
Gate theory, of pain transmission, 1692, 1694
Gated protocols, alcohol use disorders, 369–370
Gatekeepers, prevention programs, 400–401
Gating system, pain and, 1692–1693
Gay men, AA, 1294–1295
GBD. *See* Global Burden of Disease
GC-MS. *See* Gas chromatography/mass spectrometry (GC/MS)
GDC. *See* Group drug counseling
Gender
alcohol and other drug use, 374
nicotine and, 235–236
physician addiction, 552
reproductive consequences and, alcohol and, 1492
Gender biases in addiction, 622–623
Gender-specific issues, stimulant use disorders, 1022–1023
Gene expression, 209
General anesthetic, ketamine, 298
General meetings, 1178
General population, eating disorders, 1679–1680
General psychiatric management (GPM), 1649
General recovery rates, eating disorders, 1685
Generalized anxiety disorder (GAD), 1590*t*, 1592
differential diagnosis, 1592–1593
GAD-7, 774
smoking and, 1595
stimulants and, anxiety disorders and, 1597
treatment, 1593
Generalized tetanus, 1436
Genes, addiction and, 4
Genetic factors
addiction and, 11
alcohol-related liver disease, 1356
cigarette smoking, 236
Genetic polymorphisms, 144
Genetics
alcohol withdrawal, 875
OIH and, 1703
physician addiction, 553
Genitalia, medical care of patients, with unhealthy substance use, 1315–1316
Genome-wide association studies (GWASs), 11, 789–790, 1356
Gepirone, stimulant use disorders, 1017
GERD. *See* Gastroesophageal reflux disease
Geriatric Addictions Program (GAP), 659
GFR. *See* Glomerular filtration rate, renal function and
GGT. *See* Gamma-glutamyltransferase (GGT)
Ghrelin, binge eating disorder, 802
Gingivitis, IDUs and, 1446
Glasgow Coma Scale (GCS), 686, 910–911
Glaucoma
cannabinoids, 1944–1945
cannabis, 261
Global Appraisal of Individual Needs, Chestnut Health Systems group, 1848
Global Center for Credentialing and Certification (GCCC), 776
Global Initiative for Chronic Obstructive Lung Disease (GOLD), 1405
Global Severity Index (GSI) scores, 746
Global tobacco supply chain, environmental impacts and contribution, 83*f*
Glomerular filtration rate (GFR), 1376
renal function and, 1376
Glomerulonephritis, hepatitis C virus, 1380
Glucagon-like peptide-1 (GLP-1) agonists, 1392–1393
Glucose metabolism
caffeine and, 1498
cocaine and, 1497–1498
Glucose solutions, B vitamins, 881
Glucuronide, benzodiazepines, 168
Glutamate
activated ion channels, 154
receptors, 893
Glutamatergic agents, stimulant use disorders, 1019
Glutamatergic pathway, 10–11
Glutamatergic (Glu) system, 170
Glutethimide, 1429
Glycine receptors, alcohol and, 152–154, 152*t*
Goal Management Training (GMT), 693
Goal-oriented attentional self-regulation (GOALS), 693
Gonadotropins, 1495
Good Grief Network, climate change and, 85
Good Samaritan laws, 426
Google's Recover Together, 1256
Gooseflesh, 912
Gorski's neurologic impairment model, RP and, 1226
Gout, 1326–1327
G-protein-coupled receptors
allosteric modulation of, 140
signaling, 139
G-protein-independent pathway, endocannabinoids, 254
Graduation, therapeutic communities (TCs), 1180
Grapefruit juice, drugs and, 130
Graves disease, 1328
Gray death, 911
Grayken Center for Addiction at the Boston Medical Center, 1256
Greek system, fraternity/sorority, college student drinking, 439
Grindrod, R.B., 582
GRKs. *See* G protein-coupled receptor kinases
Group drug counseling (GDC), 1101, 1121
Group leaders, interventions of
behavioral assignments, 1097
brief stories, 1097
creative media, 1097
educational presentations, 1097
guest presenters with expertise, 1097
health lifestyle strategies, 1097
PowerPoint slides, 1097
problem, conflict/recovery issue, 1097
readings, 1097
video or audio, 1097
visual handouts, 1097
in vivo role-plays, 1097
workbooks, journals/worksheets, 1097
Group motivational interviewing (GMI), 1099

Group process, issues, 1098
Group sessions, adherence to, treatment dropout and, 1100
Group therapy, 1006
  for co-occurring disorders, 1100–1102
  dropping out, reasons, 1101–1102
  empirical validation of, 1099–1100
  family psychoeducational workshops, 1098–1099
  format of, 1095–1097
  goals of, 1094
  individual psychotherapy, 1121
  leaders, interventions of, 1097–1099
  limitations of, 1103
  obstacles to, 1098
  organization of, 1094–1099
  patients to groups, organization of, 1094–1099
  phase 1, 1097–1098
  phase 2, problem-solving, 1098
  physician input and support, need for, 1101–1102
  sessions, 1097–1098
  survey of group therapists, 1102–1103
  treatment discontinuation, reasons for, 1100
  types of, 1095, 1096*t*
    coping skill groups, 1095
    Milieu groups, 1095
    psychoeducational recovery groups, 1095
    specialized groups, 1095
    therapy or counseling, 1095
Group treatment research, limitations for, 1100
Groups-counselling, 1177–1178
Growth hormone, 1496
  anabolic steroids, 1499
  benzodiazepines, 1499
  naloxone, 1496
  opioids, 1496
Guanfacine, attention deficit hyperactivity disorder, 1632
Gut-liver-lung axis, 1404–1405

H

HAART. *See* Highly active antiretroviral therapy
Habitual drinking, 581
Hair
  adolescent drug use, 1834
  of dog, 1189
  drug testing matrix, 1963–1964
  gas chromatographic test, AAS and, 317–318
  testing, 517
Halazepam, addiction liability, 170–171
Hallucinations, 1601
  in AIPD, 1606
  alcohol withdrawal and, 871
    delirium, 881–883
    predictors of, 875
    seizures, 871
    severity scales, 873*t*–874*t*, 875
Hallucinogen(s), 1048
  addiction liability, 279
  brain functional activity, 278–279
  clinical implications, 362
  clinical uses, 272–273
  definition, 269
  drug–drug interactions, 284–285
  drugs in class, 269
  epidemiology, 274–276, 362
  flashbacks and, 1840
  glutamate, 277–278
  headache, 1423
  historical features, 273–274
  history, 362
  intoxication, 927–930
    management, 928–930
    physical effects, 928
    psychological and behavioral effects, 927–928, 928*t*
  legal status, 362
  mechanisms of action, 276–279
  neurobehavioral and cognitive disorders, 1426
  neurobiology, 276–279
  nonmedical use, 273
  pharmacology, 362
  prevalence, 275*t*
  and psychosis, 1608–1609
  representative, 270*t*–271*t*
  serotonergic, 284
  substances, 269
  use disorders, 279
  withdrawal, 930
Hallucinogen persisting perception disorder (HPPD), 1608–1609
Haloperidol, 1396–1397
Halothane, 308
Hamilton Depression Rating Scale, 955, 1547
Hangover, 870
  non-addicted populations, 1189
  pathophysiology, 870
  symptoms, interventions, 870
Han's Acupoint Nerve Stimulator (HANS), 1056
Hardware, 308
Harm, mechanisms of, 111
Harm reduction
  alcohol-impaired driving, 432
  definition, 423
  history of, 423–424
  integration of, addiction treatment programs, 424–425
  principles, 425
  strategies and mechanisms, 423, 424*t*
  substance use, overdose prevention of
    drug testing at dance parties, 430
    fentanyl test strips, 430
    Housing First programs, 432
    injectable opioid agonist treatment programs, 431
    managed alcohol programs, 431–432
    medications, 429
    opioid antagonists, 429
    overdose prevention online resources, 425*b*
    overdose prevention sites, 428–429
    overdose risk education and naloxone, 425–426
    portable high specificity drug-checking, 431
    post-substance use observation sites, 429
    pre- and post-HIV exposure prophylaxis, 429–430
    safer smoking and sniffing supply programs, 428
  supervised drug consumption venues, 423–424
Harm reduction policies, 417
Harm reduction services, 748
Harm reduction-informed support services, 762
Harmful substance use, 29
Harms
  associated with SUD, 690–691
  associated with TBI, 690–691
    chronic pain, 691
    life satisfaction and vocation, 691
    mood/affect impairment, 691
    mortality, 690
    neurocognitive performance, 690–691
    violent behavior, 690
Harrison Anti-Narcotic Act of 1914, 584–585
Harrison Narcotic Act, 1000
Harrison Narcotics Tax Act of 1914, 599, 1928
Hashish, 248–249
Hashish/hash oil, substance-induced mental disorders, 1550
Hazelden Foundation treatment program, 1297
HCV. *See* Hepatitis C virus
HDACs. *See* Histone deacetylases
HDL cholesterol, -alkylated androgens, 325
Head
  medical care of patients, with unhealthy substance use, 1315
  and neck, 203–204, 221, 556, 883
Head mounted displaces (HMD), 1257
Headache
  alcohol, 1422
  barbiturates, 1422
  benzodiazepines, 1422
  caffeine, 1422–1423
  cannabinoids, 1423–1424
  cocaine, amphetamines, and MDMA, 1423
  dissociative anesthetics, 1424
  hallucinogens, 1423
  opioids, 1423
  tobacco and nicotine, 1423
HEADSS psychosocial interview, for adolescents, 1812
Healing, persistent pain and, 1763
Health care approach, 67–73
Health care populations, eating disorders, 1680–1681
Health care professionals
  after patient overdose death, 575*b*
  duty to report, 1910
  engagement and enrollment, 1909–1910
  federal laws, 1910
  issues with, 1909
  protections for patient records, 1910
  quarterly and monthly reports, 1910
  treatment records, 1910
Health care providers, HIPAA, 1908
Health inequality, 621–622
Health Insurance Portability and Accountability Act (HIPAA), 1907
Health Resources and Services Administration, 774–775
Healthcare service utilization, 57
Healthy controls, 1702
Healthy immigrant, 1200
Heart disease
  caffeine and, 224
  opioids, cardiovascular disorders, 1345

Heart failure, alcohol, cardiovascular disorders, 1337–1338
Heart failure with reduced ejection fraction (HFrEF), 1343
alcohol-related cardiomyopathy, 1337
Heart rate variability (HRV), 1238, 1241
Heat, pain management, 1740–1742
Heat waves, climate change and, 77–78
Heat-not-burn (HNB) tobacco products, 348–349, 1340
Heavy alcohol use, 1153
Heavy drinking, 459
relapse to, 952, 1268
Helping relationships, pre-contemplation stage and, 1081
Helplessness, pain, 1713
Help-seeking populations, AA, 1290
Hematemesis, 1324
Hematologic
alcohol use, medical complications related to, 1326
cannabinoids, 1331
Hematuria, 1376
Hemodynamic effects, 1339
Amphetamines, cardiovascular disorders, 1343–1344
cocaine, cardiovascular disorders, 1341
Hemoptysis
cocaine, 203
smokers and, 203
Hemorrhage, 1343
Hemorrhagic stroke, 1430, 1432
Hepatic cirrhosis, 1451
Hepatic clearance, 132
Hepatic disorders, detoxification and, 865
Hepatic infections, 1451
Hepatic injury, 1369
Hepatic ischemia, 1369
Hepatic P450, opioid use disorder, 1699
Hepatic steatosis, 1323
Hepatic toxicity, 1368–1370
agents, 1369–1370
androgenic/anabolic steroids, 1370
cannabis, 1370
cocaine and stimulants, 1368–1369
coinjected materials, toxicity from, 1370
opioids, 1370
Hepatitis, 1532
Hepatitis A virus (HAV), 1360–1361
Hepatitis B E antigen (HBeAg), 1379
Hepatitis B vaccination, 1319
Hepatitis B virus (HBV), 1361–1363
acute hepatitis B, 1361–1362
chronic hepatitis B, 1362–1363, 1362*f*
CRA plus vouchers treatment, 1132
diagnosis, 1361, 1361*t*
epidemiology, 1361
outcome of infection with, 1361
transmission, 1361
treatment-naive hepatitis B, current first-line therapies for, 1363
virology, 1361
Hepatitis C virus (HCV), 745, 748–749, 751, 1317, 1329, 1363–1364. *See also* Advanced hepatitis C
clinical manifestations, 1365
chronic infection, 1365
primary infection, 1365
CRA plus vouchers treatment, 1132
diagnosis, 1365, 1366*t*
drug addiction, 17–18
epidemiology, 1363, 1364*f*
management issues, 1365–1368
access to health care and, 1365–1366
alcohol, 1367
antiviral treatment, 1367
assessing severity of the disease, 1367
dietary guidelines, 1367
direct-acting antivirals, 1367
hepatitis A and B vaccination, 1367
hepatocellular carcinoma, 1368
liver transplantation, 1368
management of risk factors, 1367
pre- and posttest counseling issues, 1366–1367
standard of care treatment regimens, 1368
treatment during pregnancy, 1368
opioid withdrawal, 913
outcome of infection with, 1365
prescription medication misuse, 413
in special populations, 1364–1365
carceral systems, individuals in, 1364–1365
prevalence, people born in countries, 1365
transmission, 1363–1364
injecting drug use, 1363–1364, 1364*t*
virology, 1363
Hepatitis C virus–related glomerulonephritis, 1380
Hepatitis D, 1368
Hepatitis virus–associated nephrotic syndrome, 1379
Hepatocellular carcinoma
hepatitis C virus, 1368
Hepatocellular carcinoma (HCC), 1323–1324, 1394
Hepatorenal syndrome (HRS), 1324, 1378
Hepatotoxic effects, 951
Hepatotoxicity, 1369
Herbal and plant-derived products, stimulant use disorders, 1019
Herbal highs, 357
Herbs, psychoactive, 937–940, 938*t*–939*t*
Heroin (diacetylmorphine), 178, 1411
aversion therapies, 1193–1194
diagnosis, 909–910
methadone and, 911
nephropathy, 1377*t*
opioid use disorder, 970
opioid withdrawal, 913
overdose deaths, 409*f*
pharmacokinetics, 184
withdrawal, 860
Heroin pyrolysate, vapors of, 1435
Heroin-associated nephropathy (HAN), 1379–1380
Heroin-related emergency department visits, 999
High-dose opioid therapy, OIH, 1702
Highest scoring drug (HSD), 487
High-risk behaviors, monitoring, 1918–1921
High-volume sexual behaviors (HVSB), 826–830
neurobiology, 829
psychiatric comorbidity, 829–830
HIPAA. *See* Health Insurance Portability and Accountability Act
Hispanic groups, 373
Historical pattern of use subdomain, ASAM, 1843
Histrionic personality disorder (HPD), 1650–1651
HIV-associated nephropathy (HIVAN), 1379
HIV-related infection, opioid overdose, 910
Holiday heart, 1338. *See also* Atrial fibrillation
Home, Education, Activities, Drugs, Sex, Suicidality (HEADSS) psychosocial interview, 1812
Home environments, chaotic, ASAM, 1843
Homeless population, 749–750, 1139
Hormonal therapies, compulsive sexual behavior disorder, 838
Hormone helpers, 318
Hormone releasing factors, 1490
Hormone replacement therapy, AN, 1683
Hormone supplementation
nonprescription use, 673
in transgender persons, 672–673
Hospital(s). *See also* Partial hospital programs
admission, alcohol withdrawal, 877, 883
program, adolescent substance abuse, ASAM, 1844–1845
Hospital Anxiety and Depression Scale (HADS), 1590–1591
Hospital-based addiction care, 535–542
clinical best practices, 536–537
evidence base, 536
harm reduction, 538
hospital care standards, 536*b*
hospital policies, 538–539
opioid use disorder, 537–538
posthospital transitions and care linkages, 539
workforce education, 539
Hospital-based clinicians, 597
Hospitalization, 597
care during, 1320–1321
Hospitalized patients, SBI, 491
Host defenses, IDUs and, 1444–1445
Hostility, 1554
House meetings, 1178
House rules, 1179
HPA axis. *See* Hypothalamic-pituitary-adrenal (HPA) axis
HPD. *See* Histrionic PD
5-HT. *See* Serotonin (5-HT)
5-HT_3 receptor antagonist ondansetron, alcohol, adolescent SUDs, 1874
5-HT_3 receptors, alcohol and, 139*t*, 154–155
Human addiction liability, cannabinoids, 256
Human growth hormone, 318
Human immunodeficiency virus (HIV), 745–748, 1000, 1132, 1453–1456. *See also* Neonatal abstinence syndrome
classification, 1453–1454
co-occurring disorders and, group therapies for, 1100–1101
CRA plus vouchers treatment, 1132
detoxification and, 862, 865
diagnosis, 1454
acute infection, 1454
testing, types of, 1454
drug addiction, 17–18

Human immunodeficiency virus (HIV) (*Continued*)
epidemiology and pathogenesis, 1453
interactions of opioid agonist treatment, 981–982
LGBTQ, 675
linked services and, 741, 744*t*
oral THC treatment, 1939–1940
prevention, 1456
prevention and treatment, 418
and sexually-transmitted infections in women, 642–643
TCAs, 1749–1750
treatment, 1454–1456
drug interactions, 1456
health maintenance and substance use disorders, 1455
initiation and ART basics, 1454–1455
response to, 1455
Human monkeypox virus (hMPXV), 666–667
Human services, therapeutic communities (TCs), 1182–1183
Human T-cell lymphotropic virus type I/II (HTLV-I/II), 1437
Humanity, classification of, 622
Humectant, electronic drug delivery devices, 338
Huss, M., 582
Hydrocodone, 179
pharmacokinetics, 185
rescheduling of, 1801
reward effects, 1766–1767
Hydrocollator therapy, 1740–1741
Hydromorphone, 179
opioid use disorder, 970
pharmacokinetics, 184
reward effects, 1766–1767
Hydroxyzine, 1592
Hyoscine, 1395
Hyperalgesia, 1694, 1700, 1765–1766
Hypercapnia, 1402
Hyperglycemia, 1324
alcohol, 1492
Hyperpathia, 1695
Hyperpyrexia, 1369
Hypersexual disorder, 828–830
Hypersexuality, 826–827
Hypertension, 1320, 1377*t*
alcohol, cardiovascular disorders, 1338
postinfectious glomerulonephritis, 1381
stimulants, renal and metabolic effects of, 1382
Hyperuricemia, 1326–1327
Hypnosis, 1060–1061
Hypnotic sedative withdrawal, anticonvulsants and, 889
Hypoadrenalism, marijuana and, 1497
Hypoglycemia, alcohol, 1490–1492
Hypogonadism, LGBTQ, 672
Hypokalemia, 1324, 1377–1378
Hypomagnesemia, 1324, 1378
Hypomania, 1570, 1579
Hyponatremia, 1750–1751
Hypophosphatemia, 1378
Hypothalamic-pituitary-adrenal (HPA) axis, 7, 156–157, 203
and PTSD, 1661, 1661*f*
Hypoventilation, 1402
Hypoxemia-related pulmonary hypertension, 1406
Hypoxia, opioid overdose, 911

I

IAT. *See* Internet Addiction Test
ICD-defined dependence, 111
ICDs. *See* Impulse control disorders
Ideal norm, 630
Identified Patients (IPs), 1202
Identity and internet, 845
Idiopathic nodular glomerulosclerosis, 1384
IDUs. *See* Injection drug users
IED. *See* Intermittent explosive disorder
IGT. *See* Integrated group therapy
Illegal behaviors, adolescent substance abuse, ASAM, 1846
Illegal drugs. *See also* Illicit drug
community reinforcement approach as, 1138
use of, SBI for, individual studies, 487
Illicit drug overdose, deaths, 64–65, 65*f*
Illicit drug use, 394–395
clinical testing and limited use, 456
deterrence testing, 455–456
factor in aircraft crash, 455
forensic testing, 455–456
prevalence of, 459
Vietnam war, 453
zero tolerance, 453
Illness behaviors, conditioning, 1715
Imaging studies
alcohol and, 152
drug addiction, 42, 43*f*
environmental factors and, addiction an, 12
Imipramine, 1749–1750
BN with comorbid addiction disorder, 1683
Immigrants, substance use, 636
Immigration paradox, 1200
Immigration, substance use and, 630
Imminent danger, assessing for, ASAM criteria and, 730–732
Immune system
cannabinoids and, 254
stimulants, 204
Immunizations, medical care of patients, with unhealthy substance use, 1318–1319, 1318*t*
Immunoassays, 517–518, 517*t*
for benzoylecgonine, 520–521
Immunoassays, drug detecting method, 1959–1961, 1960*f*, 1961*f*, 1964
Immunoglobulin A (IgA), 1378
Immunosuppressive drugs, 1363
Immunosuppressive therapy, 1380
Impaired Healthcare Personnel Program (IHCPP), 453
Implementation science, of SBI, 488
Implicit bias and discrimination, 762
Impulse control disorders (ICDs), 788
Impulse Control Disorders Not Elsewhere Classified, 788
Impulse-control disorder, 826–827
Impulsivity, 790, 1626
In utero opioid-exposed newborn, identification and treatment of, 1517
INCB. *See* International Narcotics Control Board
Inclusive model, 1183
Income, drug/alcohol use disorders, 375
Independent mood disorder, 1567, 1569*t*
Indian hemp, 248–249
"Indicated" prevention tactics, 388
Indigenous American Church, 630
Indigenous American healers, 581
Indinavir, CYP3A4 inhibitors, 133*t*–134*t*
Individual and interpersonal strategies, 762
Individual drug counseling (IDC), 1113
Individual patient data meta-analysis (IPDMA), 1254
Individual psychotherapy
acceptance and commitment therapy, 1120
behavior change, technology model and science of, 1108–1111
brief advice, clinician, 1115
CM, 1117–1118
cognitive-behavioral relapse prevention, 1120
computer-delivered technology-based interventions, 1123
CRA, 1116–1117
CRAFT model, 1120
development of, 1108–1111
differential therapeutics, 1122–1123
drug counselling, 1118
efficacy research, 1109
elements of
coping skills, 1113
interpersonal functioning, 1114
managing painful effects, 1113–1114
reinforcement contingencies, 1113
social support, 1114
substance use, 1111–1113
treatment alliance, 1114
treatment plan, 1113
family therapies, 1120–1121
group therapy, 1121
history of, 1107–1108
medical management, 1119
medications for addictive disorders, 1121–1122
mental health therapeutics, 1122
mindfulness based therapies, 1119
motivational enhancement therapy, 1114–1115
motivational interviewing, 1114–1115
network therapy, 1120
supportive-expressive therapy, 1115–1116
technology transfer, 1123–1124
twelve-step facilitation, 1118–1119
virtual therapy, 1123
Individual therapy
ASAM criteria and, 727
network therapy complementing, 1168–1169
plan, ASAM, 727
Individualized counseling, substance use disorders, 602–603
Indoleamine 2,3-dioxygenase 1 (IDO1), 1710–1711
Indoor cannabis (marijuana) grow operations (IMGOs), 84
InDUC. *See* Inventory of Drug Use Consequences
Industry-sponsored social aspects and public relations organizations (SAPROs), 106

Inebriate asylums, 582–583
Inebriety, 583
Inequality in health outcomes, 621
Inequities of care reduction
  changes in practice, 758–767
  clinic-based and institutional strategies, 762–763
  individual and interpersonal strategies, 762
  institutional determinants of care, 758–759, 759*b*
  interpersonal determinants of care, 760
  intersecting racial inequities, 763, 764*t*
  limitations to change in practice, 761–765
  policy and regulations, 761–765
  structural determinants of care, 758
  structural strategies
    advocate for primary prevention, 764
    family regulation policies, 764
    programmatic, clinical, policy, and research priorities, 764–765
    punitive policies, removal of, 763–764
  theoretical frameworks, 758–760
  toxicology, 763
  unnecessary barriers to treatment, 763
Infants
  alcohol use, medical complications related to, 1326
  benzodiazepines, 172
  cannabinoids, 1331
  opioids, 1330
  tobacco use, complications related to, 1328
Infection
  DTs, 875
  respiratory infections, 1450
  tobacco use, complications related to, 1328
Infectious diseases
  alcohol use, medical complications related to, 1325
  confidentiality requirements, 1908
  medical care of patients, with unhealthy substance use, 1317
  substance use, 1444–1457
Infective endocarditis (IE), 1446
Inflammation, 1362
  pain and, 1696
Inflammatory bowel disease, 1395–1396
Influenza, respiratory infections, 1450
Informed consent
  adolescents treatment
    adolescent's parent, 1905
    parental consent, 1905
    refusal of, 1905
    without parental consent, 1905
  agreement for treatment and, 1906–1907
  benzodiazepine cessation, 898
  competency (decisional capacity), 1904
  information, 1904
  legal requirements, prescribing drugs, 1925
  older adults treatment, 1906
  treatment
    agreement and, 1915
    proposed plan, 1916–1917
Inhalant
  intoxication, 934
  withdrawal, 934
Inhalant death syndrome, adolescents and, 1841
Inhalants, 1046
  addiction liability, 312
  case study, 315*b*
  endocrine and reproductive disorders, 1499
  future research, 314
  mechanisms of action, 311–312
  neurobehavioral and cognitive disorders, 1426–1427
  neuromuscular (nerve, muscle, and spinal cord) disorders, 1433
  pharmacodynamics, 311–312
  pharmacokinetics, 311
  pharmacologic classification of, 309*t*
  prevalence estimates, 310–311, 310*f*
  renal and metabolic effects of, 1384
  seizures, 1428–1429
  toxicity/adverse effects, 312
    acute effects, 312
    chronic toxicity, 312–313
    intoxication management, 314, 314*t*
    neurotoxicity, 313
  unhealthy use, 308–316
    annual prevalence, trends in, 310*f*
    definition, 308
    epidemiology, 310–311
    history, 309–310
    substances in class, 308–309
Inhibitory ion channels, properties of, 152, 152*t*, 153*f*
Initiative on Methods, Measurements and Pain Assessment in Clinical Trials (IMMPACT), 1728
Injecting drug use
  hepatitis C virus, 1363–1364, 1364*t*
Injection drug use, 1436–1437
  complications, 1328–1330
  endocarditis, 1344–1345
  immunizations, 1319
  nephrotic syndromes with, 1379–1380
    hepatitis virus–associated nephrotic syndrome, 1379
    heroin-associated nephropathy, 1379–1380
    HIV-associated nephropathy, 1379
    subcutaneous drug use–associated amyloidosis, 1380
  renal and metabolic complications, 1377*t*
  renal diseases
    nephritic syndromes associated with, 1380–1381
    nephritic-nephrotic syndromes associated with, 1380
    nephrotic syndromes associated with, 1379–1380
  unhealthy opioid use and, 1410–1412
Injection drug use–related renal disease, 1379–1381
  nephrotic syndromes associated with injection drug use, 1379–1380
Injection drug users (IDUs)
  adolescents and, 1841
  host defenses, 1444–1445
Injury
  cannabinoids, 1331
  tobacco use, complications related to, 1328
Injury/trauma
  alcohol use, medical complications related to, 1326
Inoculation method, 1665–1666
Inpatient settings, SBI in, 481
Insect repellent, 357
Insomnia, 1325, 1467
  pharmacotherapy, 1465*t*, 1475–1477
  sedative–hypnotics withdrawal, 963*t*, 964
Institutes of Medicine (IOM), 454, 621–622, 768–769, 1947
Institutional determinants of care
  drug user health hubs, 759*b*
  inequities of care reduction, 758–759, 759*b*
Institutional review board (IRB), 48, 59
Institutionalize health equity, inequities of care reduction, 763
Insulin
  alcohol abuse, 1491
  AOD, 1491
  caffeine and, 221
  resistance, 1490, 1492, 1494
Insulin therapy, cocaine and, 1497–1498
Integrase inhibitors, 1456
Integrase strand transfer inhibitors (INSTIs), 1455
Integrated care, substance use disorders, 701–712
Integrated cognitive–behavioral group treatment (IGT), 1101
Integrated group therapy (IGT), 1582. *See also* Network therapy
Integrated models, at-risk populations, 749–750
Integrative Behavioral Couple Therapy (IBCT), 1206
Integrative techniques, substance use disorders, 1052–1063
Intensive clinical interventions, smoking cessation, 1150
Intensive outpatient treatment
  adolescent substance abuse, 1844–1845
  outpatient settings, 597–598
Interdisciplinary pain programs, 1720
  CNMP, 1720
  services in, 1720
Interference with Addiction Recovery Efforts, ASAM, 1842, 1842*t*
Interferential current therapy (IFC) therapy, 1743
Interferon gamma release assays (IGRAs), 1450
Interferon (IFN) monotherapy, hepatitis C virus, 1367
International Center for Credentialing and Education of Addiction Professionals (ICCE), 776
International classification of diseases (ICD-11), 105, 788
International Classification of Diseases, 10th Edition (ICD-10)
  PTSD diagnostic criteria, 1663
International Consortium of Universities for Drug Demand Reduction (ICUDDR), 776
International Narcotics and Law Enforcement Affairs (INL), 776
International Network on Brief Interventions for Alcohol and Other Drugs (INEBRIA), 113, 114*b*
International Telecommunications Union (ITU), 1250
Internet, 842
  and identity, 845
  network therapy and, 1171

Internet addiction (IA), 796–798, 842–843, 845, 847. *See also* Problematic internet use (PIU)
Internet addiction disorder (IAD), 843–844
  conflict, 847
  construct, 847–849
  neuroimaging and neuropsychological correlates, 846–847
  polythetic approach, 847–848
  recurrence ("relapse"), 847
  salience, 847
  tolerance, 847
  withdrawal symptoms, 847
Internet characteristics, 850
Internet gaming disorder (IGD), 788, 842–843
  definition and conceptualization, 794
  diagnostic characteristics, 794
  epidemiology, 795–796
  neurobiology
    genetics, 794
    neurochemistry, 794
    neurocircuitry and Structure, 795
    neurocognition, 794–795
  neuroimaging and neuropsychological correlates, 847
  psychiatric diagnosis, 794
  treatment, 796
Internetbased CBT (iCBT), 1721
Interoceptive exposure therapy, tobacco dependence, anxiety disorder, 1595
Interpersonal determinants of care, inequities of care reduction, 760
Interpersonal determinants, relapse and, 1225–1226
Interpersonal functioning, improving, substance dependence and, 1114
Interpersonal relationships, RP and, 1228–1229
Interpersonal social rhythm therapy, 1581–1582
Interpersonal violence
  alcohol and, 1483
  unintentional injury, 1483
  in women, 643
Interprofessional addiction consult services (ACS), 536
Interprofessional collaborative practice (IPCP) research, 718, 719*t*–721*t*
Interprofessional education (IPE), 714, 715*t*
Interprofessional practice models
  chronic care model, 716–717
  Massachusetts collaborative care model, 717–718
  recommendations, substance use continuum, 722, 722*b*
  screening, brief intervention, treatment and referral to treatment, 716
Interprofessional substance use-related education
  continuing education (CE) programs, 714
  higher education, 714
Interstitial lung disease (ILD), 1406
Interstitial nephritis, 1384
Intervention acceptability, 1245
Intervention delivery, novel methods of, 1156
Interventions
  modes of, physician addiction, 558–559
  network therapy *vs.*, 1165, 1169
Interviewer-rated assessment of PTSD, 1662–1663
  Clinician-Administered PTSD Scale for DSM-5 (CAPS-5), 1662
  Composite International Diagnostic Interview (CIDI), 1663
  MINI, 1662
  Posttraumatic Diagnostic Scale for DSM-5, 1663
  PTSD Checklist for DSM-5, 1663
  PTSD Symptom Scale—Interview for DSM-5 (PSSI-5), 1662
  Structured Clinical Interview for DSM-5 Disorders (SCID), 1662
Intimate social network. *See* Social network
IntNSA. *See* International Nurses Society on Addictions
Intoxication, 111, 1199, 1326. *See also* Acute intoxication
  ASAM, 1840–1841
  assessment tools, 532
  cannabis, 256–257
  clinical effects of, 868, 869*t*
  with cocaine, 1570
  hangover, 870
  identification of, 860–861
  with inhalants, 312–314, 314*t*
  management, 860–861, 868–869
  syndrome, 870
Intoxication management, substance use disorders, 600–601
Intracerebral hemorrhages (ICHs), 1429
Intra-cranial self-stimulation procedures, animal drug addiction liability, cannabinoids, 255–256
Intractable pain, 1714
Intrapersonal determinants, relapse and, 1224–1225
Intrathecal analgesia, 1720, 1772–1773
Intrauterine abstinence syndrome (IAS), 981
Intravenous drug self-administration procedures animal drug addiction liability, cannabinoids, 255–256
Intravenous thiamine, alcohol intoxication, 881
Intrinsic clearance, 132
Intrinsic sleep disorders, 1475
Inventory of Drug Use Consequences (InDUC), 532
Inverse agonists, 141
Investigational new drug (IND), 48, 59
IOM. *See* Institute of Medicine
Ionotropic receptors, drugs and, 139*t*
Iontophoresis, 1743–1744
Iowa gambling task (IGT), 790
IQOS (I-Quit-Ordinary-Smoking), 348–349
I-Quit-Ordinary-Smoking (IQOS), 348–349
ISAM. *See* International Society of Addiction Medicine
Ischemic strokes, 1432
Isoflurane, 308
Isoniazid, 1450
Isopropyl alcohol (IPA), 1378–1379
Isorhynchophylline, structure of, 1054, 1054*f*

J

Jails, U.S., alcohol withdrawal, 883–884
JCAHO. *See* Joint Commission on Accreditation of Health Care Organizations
Job Club, 1132
Johnson Model Intervention, physician addiction, 553–554
Joint Commission on Accreditation of Health Care Organizations (JCAHO), 412
Jones, J., 582
Journal of Inebriety, 583
J-shaped curve, 1339, 1425
Justice, ethical issues in, 1899–1900

K

KAP (Knowledge Application Program), 775
Kava, 1369
Ketamine, 298–299, 931–932, 1046, 1424
  abuse, epidemiology, 295
  dissociatives and psychosis, 1609
  drug–drug interactions, 300
  ionotropic receptors, 139*t*
  LGBTQ, 671
  neurobehavioral and cognitive disorders, 1426
  neurobiology, 300
  new psychoactive substances, 1610
  pharmacodynamics, 298
  pharmacokinetics, 296
  physician addiction, 556
  renal and metabolic effects of, 1384
  seizures, 1428
  stroke, 1432
  substance-induced mental disorders, 1550
Ketamine hydrochloride, unhealthy use of, 293–294
Ketoacidosis, 1324, 1377, 1490, 1497–1498
Ketoconazole, CYP3A4 inhibitors and, 135, 169
Ketones, 1324
Khat, 193–194, 193*f*, 1610
Khat ingestion, 1369
Kidney functions, 1376
Kindling effect, alcohol withdrawal and, 871
Kinesiophobia, 1712–1713
Knowledge Application Program (KAP) Key, 775
Knowledge, skills, and attitudes (KSA), 713
Kolb, L., 585
Korsakoff syndrome, 1425
Kraeplin, E., model of psychopathology, 1308–1309
Kratom, 934–935, 1048, 1369–1370
  clinical implications, 360
  epidemiology, 359
  history, 359
  legal status, 360
  Mitragyna speciosa, 359
  pharmacology, 360
Kryger's Subjective Measurements, 1728

L

LAAM. *See* Levo-alpha-acetylmethadol
Labor, pregnancy, substance use during, 1521
Laboratory drug screens
  ordering, patient autonomy and, 1901
  patient permission and, 1901
Laboratory studies, sedative–hypnotics, 962
Laboratory tests
  adolescent substance use, 1814–1816
  clinical laboratories, 518
  confirmatory tests, 515
  duration of detection time, 515–516, 516*t*

federal regulations, 518
mass spectrometry, 518
measuring drinking behavior, 613
on-site testing, 518
ordering, patient autonomy and, 1901
pregnancy, substance use during, 1511–1512
regulation of, 518–519
screening immunoassay tests, 517–518, 517*t*
specimen types, 515–517
blood, 516
hair, 517
meconium and umbilical cord tissue, 516
oral fluid, 516
sweat, 517
urine, 515–516, 516*t*
substance-specific tests
amphetamines, 520
benzodiazepines, 520
cocaine, 520–521
ethanol, 519–520
fentanyl, 521
opiates, 521–522
opioids, 521–522
Laboratory-induced nociception, in animals, 1692
Lamotrigine, neuropathy, 1751–1752
Lancinating pain, valproic acid, 1751
Lapse risk, clinical RP interventions, 1227
Large sample, simple trials (LSSTs), 50
Lateral flow immunochromatography, 1960, 1961*f*
Laughing gas, 308–309, 1415
Law enforcement, 1486
Laxatives, 1395
Lazarus and Folkman's model, 1665–1666
LD50, 1369
LDL cholesterol, -alkylated androgens, 325
Learned tolerance, 142
Learning About Healthy Living (LAHL), 1603
Learning disorders (LDs)
ASAM adolescent criteria, 1840
substance abuse and, 1888
Legal considerations, 1808, 1911–1936
Legal consultation, ethical issues in, 1902
Legal difficulties, gambling disorder, 814
Legal highs, 357
Legal issues, pregnancy, substance use during, 1522–1523
Legal requirements, prescribing medication
adequate medical records, 1925
medical records, 1925
prescription order, 1925
Legalization, of cannabis, 124–125
LEK-8829, 1054
Length of coma (LOC), 686
Length of service, mandated, 732
Length of stay, 725
Lennox-Gastaut syndrome, 1938
Leptin, binge eating disorder, 801–802
Lesbian, AA, 1294–1295
Lesbian, Gay, Bisexual, Transexual, Questioning, Queer, Intersex, Asexual, Pansexual, and Allies (LGBTIA+)
substance use, 635–636
Lesbian, gay, bisexual, transgender, queer, and/or questioning (LGBTQ+) individuals, 1867
cannabis use disorder, 117
clinic templates, 667
patients, treatment considerations, 666–679
substance use
alcohol, 669–670
amphetamine-type stimulants, 671
amyl nitrite (poppers), 670–671
benzodiazepines, 671
club drugs/empathogens, 671
CNS depressants, 671
cocaine, 671
cultural competence, 669
cultural resilience, 669
dissociatives, 671
epidemiology, 669–673, 670*t*
evidence-supported recommendations for clinicians, 673–675
GHB receptors, 671
history and context of, 668–669
mitigating risk of HIV AND STIs, 675
personal resilience, 668
pro-erectile drugs, 672
sex hormones, 672–673
tobacco and nicotine products, 672
terminology and recommended best practices, 667
Levamisole, 1382, 1412–1413
Levamisole-induced syndrome, 1382
Levels of care
ASAM criteria, 729–733, 730*t*
assessing for, 728–729, 728*t*
placement and treatment considerations, 1848
mandated, 732
progress through, 727
transition between, RP and, 1230–1231
Levo-alpha-acetylmethadol (LAAM), 180
opioid use disorder, 970
pharmacokinetics, 185
Levorphanol, 1766–1767
pain treatment, limitations, 1766–1767
respiratory depression and, 1774–1775
Lexapro. *See* Escitalopram
Licensed health care workers, 545
Licensed providers, psychosocial interventions, 1270–1271
Lidocaine, 910
Lidocaine patch, neuropathic pain, 1752
Life Events Questionnaire, 1915
Life in Recovery Surveys, 1199
Life satisfaction, 1285
Life satisfaction and vocation, 691
Lifestyle
RP and, 1230
smoking cessation, 1152
Ligand-gated ion channels, 159–160
Ligand-gated ion channels, alcohol, 155
Light, A., research studies, addiction- related, 585
"Light" and "ultra-light" cigarettes, 94
Limbic system, addiction and, 35–36, 35*f*
Linked services
barriers to, 741–743
benefits of, 740–741, 741*t*
improved, prospects for, 751
models of, 743–751, 744*t*
payment systems, 743
Lipid solubility, absorption, 130
Liquid chromatography, 515
Liquid chromatography/mass spectrometry (LC/MS) method, 515
Lisdexamfetamine, 1630–1631
Literature
Al-Anon, 1284
NA, 1283
Lithium
bipolar disorder, adolescents, 1886–1887
co-occurring psychiatric symptoms and, 955
Liver
alcohol use, 1323–1324
caffeine and, 221
nicotine and, 233
stimulants, 203
Liver biopsy, 1358–1359
Liver cirrhosis, 373
women *vs.* men, 112
Liver disease , alcohol use, modes of transmission, 1355–1357, 1364–1370
Liver enzymes, 325, 1380
Liver injury, 1362
Liver stiffness, 1358
Liver transplantation, 1323–1324, 1360
hepatitis C virus, 1368
Loading dose (D1), 878–879, 901
Loading dose therapy, 878
LOC. *See* Internal locus of control
Locker room, 308
Locus coeruleus (LC), 37–38
Lofexidine, 916
opioid detoxification and, 915
opioid use disorder, 971
Logistical impediments, ASAM criteria and, 732
Long-acting medications, pain treatment, limitations, 1773
Long-acting naltrexone (Vivitrol), 947*t*
Long-acting opioids, short-acting opioids *vs.*, 1773
Long-term depression (LTD), 254–255
Long-term opioid use
side effects, 1773
toxicology studies, 1773
Long-term residential care, eating disorders, 1686
Lorazepam, 962*t*, 963–964
abstinence syndromes, 893
addiction liability, 170–171
alcohol withdrawal, 876–877
benzodiazepines and, 168–169
epidemiology, 171
intoxication syndrome, 869
medical complications, 173
uncomplicated withdrawal syndrome, 876–877
withdrawal seizures and, 881
Lorcaserin, stimulant use disorders, 1017
Low intensity focused ultrasound (LIFU), 1069–1070
Low nicotine research program, 99*f*
Low threshold treatment models, 747–749
Low-dose computed tomography (LDCT), 1317
Lower yield product, 94
LPV/R. *See* Lopinavir/ritonavir
Lungs
cancer, 234, 1406
function, 1413

Luvox. *See* Fluvoxamine
Lymph nodes, medical care of patients, with unhealthy substance use, 1316
Lymphatics, 1453
Lysergic acid diethylamide (LSD), 1608
neurobehavioral and cognitive disorders, 1426
pharmacodynamics, 279–280
pharmacokinetics, 279
seizures, 1428
stroke, 1432

M

MacLean, limbic system, addiction and, 35, 35*f*
Maddrey Discriminant Function (MDF), 1357–1358
Magnesium silicate, 1411
Magnetic resonance imaging, osteomyelitis, 1451
Main pancreatic duct (MPD)
chronic pancreatitis, 1392
Maintenance
smoking behavior, 1151
stage of change, 1075
Major anxiety disorders, 1589–1590, 1590*t*
Major depressive disorder (MDD), 1155, 1696
Major rules, disciplinary sanctions, 1179
Making Alcoholics Anonymous Easier (MAAEZ), 1296
Male gonadal function, 1495–1496
methadone maintenance therapy, 1495–1496
Malignant hyperthermia syndrome, 1369
Malingering, 1714
Mallory-Weiss syndrome, 1390
Mallory-Weiss tears, 1324
Malnutrition, alcohol abuse, 1490, 1493
Managed care, physician–patient relationship, 1903
Mandated populations, alcoholics anonymous, 1290
Mandatory smoking prohibition programs, 1340
Mania, 1579
Marchiafava-Bignami disease, 1424–1425
Marihuana Tax Act, 248, 1929
Marijuana (Cannabis), 5, 556, 569–570. *See also* Cannabinoid(s)
adolescents, 1813*t*–1814*t*
age and, 4–5, 5*f*
anonymous, 1283
Cannabis sativa, 1937
chemistry of, 1937–1938
cultivation, 1937
definition, 1937
endocrine and reproductive disorders, 1497
epidemiology, 1937
ethical considerations, 1955
guidelines for, 1955–1956
legal considerations, 1954–1955
as medicine
analgesic effects, 1940
antiemetic effects, 1939
appetite stimulant effects, 1939–1940
autism, 1942–1943
brain injury/stroke, 1943
CB_1 receptors, 1939
CB_2 receptors, 1939
dystonia, 1943–1944
epilepsy, 1940–1941
Food and Drug Administration, 1939
Gilles de la Tourette syndrome, 1944
glaucoma, 1944–1945
HIV, Hepatitis C, and HTLV-1 infections, 1945
multiple sclerosis, 1941–1942
nabiximol, 1949
Parkinson disease, 1943
physician's role in, 1946–1948
posttraumatic stress disorder, 1944
spinal cord injuries, 1943
substance use disorders, 1945–1946
in Navy personnel, 455
schedule I substance, 1802
sleep and, 1472–1473
terminology, 1937
tetrahydrocannabinol, 455
Marital status, 376
drug/alcohol use disorders, 376
Marketing spending, of cannabis, 121–122
Marlatt and Gordon's cognitive-behavioral approach, 1226
Marlatt-based relapse prevention, 1222
Mass spectrometry, 518
Mass spectrometry, drug detecting method, 1961–1962, 1962*f*
Massachusetts collaborative care model, 717–718
Massachusetts Youth Screening Instrument—Second Version (MAYSI-2), 1856–1857
Massage therapy, 1744, 1744*t*
Master Settlement Agreement (MSA), 98
MAST-G. *See* Michigan Alcoholism Screening Test-Geriatric version
Maternal Opioid Treatment:Human Experimental Research (MOTHER) study, 980
Matrix approach
methamphetamine and, 1223
relapse prevention and, 1226
Matrix Model, 1095
Mazindol, chemical structures, 191, 192*f*–193*f*
MBRP. *See* Mindfulness-Based Relapse Prevention
MBT. *See* Mentalization-based therapy
McGill Pain Questionnaire, 1751
McKenzie therapy, 1738
MDD. *See* Major depressive disorder
MDF. *See* Maddrey discriminant function
MDFT. *See* Multidimensional family therapy
Mean corpuscular volume (MCV), 613
Measurement Based Care (MBC), 774
Meconium, 1511
and umbilical cord tissue testing, 516
Medial prefrontal cortex (MPFC), 1066–1067
TMS to, 1067–1068, 1068*f*
Median effective doses, 138
Median toxic doses, 138
Medicaid, 1245
Medical care of patients, with unhealthy substance use, 1314–1332
cancer screening, 1317–1318
care during hospitalization, 1320–1321
co-occurring medical issues, 1321
pain, 1321
perioperative care, 1321
withdrawal, 1320–1321
chemoprophylaxis, 1319
immunizations, 1318–1319, 1318*t*
medical history, 1314–1315
older adults, 1321–1322
other infectious diseases, 1317
physical examination, 1315–1316
abdomen, 1315
breast, 1315
chest/cardiovascular, 1315
genitalia, 1315–1316
head, eyes, ears, nose, and throat, 1315
lymph nodes, 1316
neurologic, 1316
skin, 1315
vital signs and measurements, 1315
preventive counseling, 1318
primary and preventive care, 1314–1319
screening tests, 1316–1318, 1316*t*
sexually transmitted infections, 1317
substance use and treatment of medical conditions, 1319–1320
substance use, medical complications related to, 1322–1331, 1322*t*
alcohol use, 1323–1327
cannabinoids, 1330–1331
opioids, stimulants and injection drug use, 1328–1330
tobacco use, 1327–1328
testing for other conditions, 1318
Medical care settings, substance abuse treatment, national recommendations on, 473
Medical comorbidities
endocrine effects, 1776
interdisciplinary pain programs, 1720
stimulant use disorders, 1022
surgical setting, 1531
Medical management (MM), 57–58
collaborative care
to achieve patients treatment adherence, 1272–1274
counsellors, 1270
licensed providers, 1270–1271
pharmacotherapy support from nonphysicians, 1272
psychotherapists, 1271–1272
control issues, 1274
engagement, 1261–1274
intrinsic themes, 1265
medication adherence, 1264–1265
medication compliance plan, 1265–1266
motivational interviewing, 1263
nonphysicians, pharmacotherapy support from, 1272
Project COMBINE, 1265
strategies
combination strategies, 1269
complementary strategies, 1268–1269
convergent strategies, 1267–1268
principles for care integration, 1269
Project MATCH, 1267
therapies in withdrawal management, 1263–1264
withdrawal management, 1263–1264
Medical necessity, 1839
Medical outcome study (MOS), 57
Medical problems, military sexual trauma, 682

Medical Review Officer (MRO)
  duties of, 1969–1970
  practice, 1973
  process, 1971–1973
  regulatory framework, 1970–1971
  useful web sites, 1971*t*
Medical systems, inequities of care reduction, 763
Medical training, 741–742
Medical treatment systems, addiction treatment and, 740–757
Medicalized addiction, 1928
Medical-legal issues, opioid use disorder and, physician addiction, 568
Medically integrated therapeutic community, 1187
Medically managed intensive inpatient (hospital) treatment, 1847
Medication call-backs, OBOT, 1008–1009
Medication event monitoring systems (MEMS), 58
Medication for opioid use disorder (MOUD), 536–537, 999, 1980
Medication therapy
  discontinue, 1920–1921
  in prescribing medication, 1917–1918
Medication-induced obsessive-compulsive disorders, 1548
Medications. *See also* Nonstimulant medications; specific i.e. quazepam
  alcohol consumption and reduction of, 946–949
  alcohol rehabilitation, 956
  alcoholic dependence, U.S. Food and Drug Administration, 946, 947*t*
  alcohol-sensitizing agents, 950–951
  co-occurring psychiatric symptoms in patient, 954–956
  with psychosocial treatments, RP and, 1230
  sedative hypnotic use disorder, 962–963
Medications for opioid use disorder (MOUD), 600, 604, 1516
  breastfeeding, 1522
Medicine, patient autonomy, 1896–1897
Medium-intensity residential treatment, adolescent substance abuse, ASAM, 1845
Meeting attendance, alcoholics anonymous and, 1301
MEG. *See* Magnetoencephalography
Melanin, hair and drug incorporation, 1964
MELD. *See* Model for end-stage liver disease
Mellanby effect, 158
Memantine, 916
Membrane trafficking of endocannabinoids, 254
Memory training, 692–693
MEMS. *See* Medication event monitoring systems
Mendelian randomization, 1323
Meningovascular syphilis, 1452
Mental disorders
  primary, secondary, and tertiary prevention, 388, 388*f*
  in women, 639–642
Mental Health Parity and Addiction Equity Act (MHPAEA), 617, 702, 1899
Mental health screening, 1728
Mental illness, and cannabis, 119
Mental illness, comorbidity with, addiction and, 12–13
Mental status examination, adolescents, 1884–1885
Mentalization based therapy (MBT), 1649
Meperidine, 179, 1428
  abstinence syndrome, 910
  pharmacokinetics, 184
  physician addiction, 554–555
Mephedrone, 1551
Mescaline, 1423
  neurobehavioral and cognitive disorders, 1426
  pharmacodynamics, 282
  pharmacokinetics, 282
  seizures, 1428
  stroke, 1432
Mesocorticolimbic neurons, nicotine and, 239–240
MET. *See* Motivational enhancement therapy
Metabolic
  cannabinoids, 1331
  opioids, 1330
Metabolic acidosis, 1324
Metabolic disorders
  alcohol, 1377–1379
    hepatorenal syndrome and cirrhosis associated diseases, 1378
    toxic alcohols, 1378–1379
  cannabinoids, 1384
  inhalants, 1384
  ketamine, 1384
  opioids, 1377*t*, 1381
    prescription opioids, injection use of, 1381
    rhabdomyolysis, 1381
    urologic effects of, 1381
  stimulants, 1381–1383
    amphetamines, 1383
    cathinones, 1383
    cocaine, 1381–1383
    MDMA, 1383
  substance use, 1376–1385
  tobacco use, 1384
Metabolic-associated fatty liver disease (MAFLD), 1355
  obesity and, 1356–1357
Metabolism
  alcohol, 150, 158–159
  amphetamines, 199
  anabolic–androgenic steroids, 329–330
  caffeine, 221
  nicotine, 232–234
  phase I oxidation, drugs, 131–132, 133*t*–134*t*
  phase II reactions, drugs, 132
  stimulant, 199
Metabotropic glutamate receptors (mGluR), alcohol and, 157
Metabotropic-induced suppression of excitation (MSE), 254–255
Metabotropic-induced suppression of inhibition (MSI), 254–255
Methadone, 180, 647, 745, 914–915, 1320–1321, 1345, 1368, 1370, 1456
  benzodiazepine, 169
  community clinics, abstinence and, 1133
  detoxification, 865
    adolescents, 866
  directly observed treatment, 461
  drug–drug interactions, 188
  heroin and, overdose, naloxone and, 909–910
  office-based opioid therapy
    agonist therapy, 1000–1001
    pharmacotherapy, 1003
  opioid agonist treatment with, 1701–1702
  opioid use disorder, treatment
    adequacy of dose, 975
    benzodiazepines and, 977
    blood levels, 975
    continued illicit opioid use *versus*, 973–974
    duration and dose, 974–975
    heroin-simulated 24-hour dose-response, 973, 973*f*–974*f*
    induction, 974
    initial dose, 974
    medical monitoring, 977
    methadone medical maintenance, 976
    methadone-medication interactions, 976
    observed doses and take-home medication, 976
    patient stability, 976
    and QT interval, 976–977
    stabilization and steady state, 974
    at steady state, 973, 974*f*
    therapeutic window, 974
  opioids, adolescent SUDs, 1876–1877
  pharmacodynamics, 186
  pharmacokinetics, 185
  respiratory depression and, 1774–1775
  tolerance, 187
  treatment methods, 186
Methadone dosing in pregnancy, 980
Methadone maintenance (MM)
  community reinforcement approach, 1138
  CRA, 1138
Methadone maintenance therapy (MMT)
  buprenorphine therapy, 1496
  male gonadal function, 1495–1496
  opioid addiction, 1767
Methadone maintenance treatment programs (MMTP), 181–182
Methadone treatment, voucher-based reinforcement therapy in, 602
Methadone-metabolite ratios (MMR), 975
Methadone-to-Buprenorphine Transfer, 982
Methamphetamine(s), 5, 1053–1054, 1369, 1396, 1456–1457, 1554, 1630–1631
  aversion therapies, 1192–1193
  cardiovascular disease, 1344
  dependence, relapse rates and, 1220–1221
  epidemiology, 197
  matrix approach and, 1223
  neurobehavioral and cognitive disorders, 1425
  and psychosis, 1608
  substance-induced mental disorders, 1550
  use disorders, 51–52
    contingency-management, 1136–1137
Methamphetamine use disorder, 371
  stimulants and substance-induced depressive disorder, 1546
Methamphetamine-induced depressive symptoms, 1546

Methanol, 1378
Methaqualone, 1429
Methocarbamol, 1754–1755
Methoxetamine, 1551
Methyl ethyl ketone, 313–314
3,4-Methylenedioxymethamphetamine (MDMA), 191, 269–272, 520, 935–936, 1369, 1383
- addiction liability, 279
- eating disorders *vs.*, 1681
- headache, 1423
- intoxication, 935–936
  - physical effects, 936
  - psychological and behavioral effects, 935–936
- movement disorders, 1434–1435
- neurobehavioral and cognitive disorders, 1425–1426
- pharmacodynamics, 283–284
- pharmacokinetics, 283
- renal and metabolic complications, 1377*t*
- seizures, 1427–1428
- sleep difficulties, 1471
- stroke, 1430–1432
- substance-induced mental disorders, 1550
- substance-induced psychosis, 1609–1610
- withdrawal, 936
  - physical effects, 936

3,4-Methylenedioxypyrovalerone (MDPV), 1551
Methylone, 1551
Methylphenidate, 191, 192*f*–193*f*, 1634
- ADHD, 1630–1631
- chemical structures, 191, 192*f*–193*f*
- opioid induced sedation, 1775–1776

Mexiletine, neuropathic pain, 1752
MHPAEA. *See* Mental Health Parity and Addiction quity Act (MHPAEA)
Michigan Alcoholism Screening Test (MAST), 1130*t*, 1205
Microprocessors, 842
Midazolam, flumazenil and, 890
Midbrain ventral tegmental area (VTA), 151
Migration, substance use and, 631
Mild substance use disorders, 30
Mild to borderline intellectual disability (MBID), 1888
Milieu groups, 1095
Military culture, 681
Military members and veterans, population-specific considerations, 1206–1207
- military occupational stressors and sexual trauma, 1206–1207
- for pregnant women, 1207–1208
- VA, support for family treatment at, 1206

Military occupational stressors, 1206–1207
Military Personnel Drug Abuse Testing Program, 455
Military personnel, substance use disorders
- alcohol use and alcohol use disorder, 456–457
- Department of Defense Task Force, 453–454
- drug amnesty and rehabilitation, 454–455
- drug testing, 455–456
- policy and leadership, historical perspectives on, 453–455
- potential legal issues, 457
- Presidential directive, 455
- prevalence
  - sociodemographic characteristics of active duty personnel, 459
  - surveys, 459
  - trends in alcohol and substance use, 459
- tobacco, 457–459
- treatment, 459–460
  - Institute of Medicine review, 454
  - privacy and confidentiality, 459
- Vietnam experience, 454

Military sexual trauma (MST), 468
- assessment, 681–682
- barriers, 681
- clinical issues, 681–682
- military culture, 681
- physical and mental health, 680
- physical examination, 682
- psychosocial treatment, 682
- risk of, 680
- screening, 681

Millon Clinical Multiaxial Inventory-III (MCMIIII), 1645–1646
Mind–body connection, 1708–1709
Mind-body therapies, 1156
Mindfulness Based Cognitive Therapy (MBCT), 1237
Mindfulness based therapies, 1119
Mindfulness treatments, chronic pain, 1718–1719
Mindfulness-based approaches, 1864
Mindfulness-based cognitive therapy, 1864
Mindfulness-based interventions (MBIs), 1236–1237
- for addiction, 1237

Mindfulness-based relapse prevention (MBRP), 1229, 1237, 1616, 1864
Mindfulness-based reuse prevention (MBRP), 1866
Mindfulness-based therapeutic community (MBTC), 1864
Mindfulness-based treatment of addiction, 1236–1245
- clinical strategies for, 1242–1243
- implementation, directions for, 1243–1245
  - dissemination and implementation challenges, 1245
  - diverse clinical populations, 1243–1244
  - dose-response relationships, 1244–1245
  - treatment combinations and sequencing, 1244
- operationalizing construct of mindfulness, 1236–1237
- therapeutic mechanisms of, 1238–1242, 1238*f*–1239*f*
  - decreasing craving and drug cue-reactivity, 1242
  - restructuring reward processes, 1239–1240, 1240*f*, 1241*f*
  - strengthening cognitive control, 1238, 1239*f*
  - stress and negative emotions, 1240–1242

Mindfulness-Oriented Recovery Enhancement (MORE), 1237–1238
Mindfulness-to-Meaning Theory, 1241–1242
Mini International Neuropsychiatric Interview, 1662
- co-occurring substance use disorders, 1590–1591, 1591*t*

Mini-International Neuropsychiatric Interview (MINI), 530
Minnesota Multiphasic Personality Inventory (MMPI), 897
- Personality Disorder Scales, 1645–1646

Mirtazapine
- benzodiazepine withdrawal, 903
- cocaine and methamphetamine, adolescent SUDs, 1878
- generalized anxiety disorder, 1592

Missing at random (MAR), 52
Missing completely at random (MCAR), 52
Missing not at random (MNAR), 52
Misuse
- opioids
  - differential diagnosis of, 1768
  - risk factors for, 1768
- prescription medication, prevention of
  - age-adjusted death rates, 409*f*
  - CDC guidelines, 416*t*
  - classes, 411–414
  - co-occurrence with other substance and psychiatric disorders, 411
  - deterrent formulations, 417
  - drug monitoring programs, 417
  - emergency department visits, 410
  - epidemiology, 410–411
  - evidence-based treatment, 418–419
  - harm reduction policies, 417
  - healthcare utilization, 410
  - historical perspective, 409–410
  - HIV prevention and treatment, 418
  - naloxone, 417–418
  - prescriber education, 415–417
  - prevalence of, 410
  - prevention programs, 414
  - research, 419
  - syringe service programs, 418
  - take-back programs, 414–415

Mitragynine, 360
Mixed overdoses, 890
MK-801 (dizocilpine), 295
MM. *See* Medical management
MMM. *See* Methadone medical maintenance
MMPI. *See* Minnesota Multiphasic Personality inventory
MMT. *See* Methadone maintenance therapy
Mobile applications
- substance use disorders, 1254–1255
- substance use disorders, digital health interventions for, 1252–1255

Mobile medical applications (MMAs), 1251
Mobile TUD applications, 1156
Modafinil, 1631
- chemical structures, 191, 192*f*–193*f*

Model for End-Stage Liver Disease (MELD), 1357–1358, 1533
Model of spirituality, 1308–1309
Moderate mild substance use disorders, 30
Modern alcoholism movement, 586
Modified therapeutic communities (MTCs)
- continuity of care, 1186–1187
- co-occurring disorders, 1183–1187
- interventions, 1184
- medically integrated therapeutic community, 1187

mental and substance use disorders, 1183–1187
meta-analysis, 1186*f*
other modifications, 1183–1184
outcomes, 1184
outpatient models, 1186–1187
principles and methods, 1183
residential aftercare models, 1186
Modulation, chronic nociceptive pain and, 1692
Molecular genetic research, 789–790
Monitored recovery, physician addiction, 563–564
Monitoring, for high-risk behaviors
continued, revised, or terminate medication, 1919
tapering/discontinuing medication therapy, 1919–1921
Monitoring plan, office-based opioid therapy, 1009
Monitoring the Future (MTF) study, substance use disorders, 369
Monoamine neurotransmitters, 37
Monoamine oxidase (MOA), 242
Monoamine oxidase inhibitors (MAOIs), 179
drug–drug interactions, 199–200
for PTSD, 1669
stimulant use disorders, 1016
Monozygotic twins, alcohol-related liver disease, 1356
Mood disorders
substance use disorders and, 1695, 1698
in women, 640–641
Mood effects of cannabis, 259
Mood modification, 847
Mood stabilizers, 1579
bipolar disorder, adolescents, 1891
treatment, bipolar disorder and, 956
Mood/affect impairment, traumatic brain injury, 691
Morbidity, tobacco and, 244
Morphine, 178, 908, 1410
opioid-induced hyperalgesia, 1700–1703
pharmacokinetics, 183–184
Mortality
anorexia nervosa, 1685
tobacco and, 244
traumatic brain injury, 690
MOS. *See* Medical Outcome Study
Motivation, 850, 1176, 1615
behavioral interventions, 1145
contingency management, 1130
enhancing motivation to change, 1076–1082
interventions and, 1130
relapse prevention, 1224–1225
substance use, reduction, 1113
Motivation enhancement (ME)
mobile applications/apps/stand-alone websites, 1253
Motivational enhancement therapy (MET), 601, 854, 1216, 1857–1858, 1863
relapse prevention and, 1222, 1224–1225
Motivational enhancement therapy plus CBT (MET/CBT), 1139
Motivational interviewing (MI), 898, 1078, 1085–1089, 1091, 1857–1858, 1863
American Society of Addiction Medicine, 1843
behavioral interventions, 1263
brief interventions, 1811–1812
climate change and, 85–86
combining with other therapeutic modalities, 1088
as evidence-based approach, for substance use disorders, 1088
LGBTQ, 674–675
mindfulness-based treatment of addiction, 1245
mobile applications/apps/stand-alone websites, 1253
processes and stages of change, 1086–1088
conceptualizing patient change, 1087–1088, 1087*f*
four processes, 1086–1087, 1086*t*
skills, 1086, 1086*t*
and social justice, 1089
spirit, 1085–1086
in substance use disorder treatment, patient profiles and response, 1088–1089
degree of ambivalence, 1088–1089
marginalized racial and ethnic backgrounds, patients from, 1089
severity of, 1088
substance use disorders, 1201
TUD, 1148
unhealthy drug use, 487
Motivational treatment, 1863
Motivation-based dual diagnosis treatment model, 1614–1615
Motor vehicle crashes (MVCs), 1482, 1484, 1486
Motor vehicle injuries, 1482–1484
Movement disorders, 1434–1435
alcohol, 1434
cannabinoids, 1435
cocaine, amphetamines, and MDMA, 1434–1435
opioids, 1435
tobacco and nicotine, 1435
MRI. *See* Magnetic resonance imaging
MRO. *See* Medical review officer
MST. *See* Multisystemic therapy
MTCs. *See* Modified therapeutic communities
Mu opioid agonists, 1770
Mu opioid receptors, 908
expression, 1770
polymorphism, 1766
Multicomponent skills-based interventions, college student drinking, 442
Multidimensional family therapy (MDFT), 603, 1204, 1864
community reinforcement approach, 1139
Multidisciplinary team, court-leveraged treatment, 1976
Multifamily group therapy (MFGT), 853–854
Multimodal Study of ADHD (MTA), 1625
Multiple behaviors, 1082–1083
Multiple domains, of well-being, 1082–1083
Multiple marginalization, 1089
Multiple sclerosis (MS), cannabis, 1941–1942
Multiple sedative-hypnotics, 940
withdrawal from, 940
Multiple sleep latency test, 1463, 1468, 1472, 1475
Multiple substance use disorders, 1045–1051
Multiple substance use, substance-induced psychosis, 1611
Multiscale questionnaires, adolescent drug use, 1836
Multi-substance, 1512
Multisystemic therapy (MST), 603, 1204–1205, 1858, 1864–1865
Mu-opioid gene receptor (OPRM), 1699
Muscle ischemia, 1382
Muscle relaxants, pain and, 1754–1755
Musculoskeletal, alcohol use, medical complications related to, 1326–1327
Musculoskeletal system, stimulants, 203
Mutual help groups, 662
Mutual support groups, 1202–1203
Mutual support programs, 1099
μ-Opioid receptor (mOR) antagonists
stimulant use disorders, 1018
Mycotic aneurysm, 1448
Myocardial infarction (MI)
alcohol-related cardiomyopathy, 1337
electronic drug delivery devices, 345

N

NA. *See* Narcotics Anonymous
Nabilone, 1938
Nabiximols, 1949
N-acetylcysteine (NAC), 954, 1360, 1670
cannabis, adolescent SUDs, 1875
nACHRs. *See* Nicotinic acetylcholine receptors
NAc/NAcc. *See* Nucleus accumbens
NAFLD. *See* Non-alcoholic fatty liver disease
Najavits' Seeking Safety (SS), 1100
Nalbuphine, 318, 319*t*–320*t*
pain treatment, limitations, 1766
Nalmefene, 429
alcohol consumption and, 949
Nalmefene (Revex), 179
Naloxone, 179, 915, 1345
alcohol and, 156
nonmedical use, 417–418
opioid use disorder, 970
opioids
overdose, follow-up care, 912
withdrawal, clonidine and, 910
Naltrexone, 429, 838, 912, 914, 946–949, 1119, 1359, 1670
with acamprosate, 950
alcohol, adolescent SUDs, 1874
alcohol and, 156
alcohol consumption, reduction of, 946–949
antagonist therapies using, 604–605
for behavioral interventions, 1267
clinical considerations, 948–949
co-occurring substance use disorders, 1591
extended-release formulations, 983
management of patients, 1535
opioid use disorder, 970
opioid use disorder, treatment, 982–984
opioids
dependence with psychosocial treatments, 1230
withdrawal, 915
opioids, adolescent SUDs, 1876
physician addiction, 568
relapse prevention and, 1230
substance use disorder with co-occurring psychosis, 1613

N-arachidonoyl-PE by a unique phospholipase D *(NAPEPLD)*, 254
Narcissistic personality disorder (NPD), 1650–1651
Narcolepsy, clinical approaches to, 1470–1471, 1475
Narcotic Addict Treatment Act, 770–771, 1001
Narcotics Anonymous (NA), 1095, 1107–1108, 1283, 1865
  COVID-19 pandemic, 1285
  groups, 1107–1108
  history, 1283
  literature, 1283
  population subgroups, 1293
NAS. *See* Neonatal abstinence syndrome
Nasal insufflation of cocaine, 1412
National Academy of Medicine (NAM), 768–769. *See* Institute of Medicine (IOM)
National Addiction Technology Transfer Center, 1271
National Association of State Alcohol and Drug Abuse Directors (NASADAD), 725
National Birth Defect Prevention Study, 1515
National Center for Health Statistics *(NCHS)*, 181–182
National Comorbidity Survey (NCS), substance use disorders, 368
National Epidemiologic Survey on Alcohol and Related Conditions (NESARC), 370–371, 812–813, 1595–1596, 1602, 1625
  alcohol use disorder, 376
  drug use disorders, 371
  ethnicity, 373–374
  generalized anxiety disorder, 1592, 1595
  opioid use disorders, 1595–1596
  social anxiety disorder and, 1593, 1595
  substance use disorders, 368
National Forensic Laboratory Information System (NFLIS), 181–182
National Institute of Alcohol Abuse and Alcoholism (NIAAA), 30, 49–50, 586
  Epidemiological Study on Alcohol and Related Conditions (NESARC-III), 610
  outcomes and, 1222
  "standard drink", 610, 610*t*
National Institute on Alcohol Abuse and Alcoholism (NIAAA), 636, 653, 1862
National Institute on Drug Abuse (NIDA), 30, 50, 586, 646–647, 1256, 1812–1814, 1862
National Institutes of Health (NIH), 691, 1075, 1289–1290
National Laboratory Certification Program, 518
National Quality Forum (NQF), 770, 770*t*
National Standards for Culturally and Linguistically Appropriate Services, 627
National Summit for Opioid Safety, 1806, 1807*t*
National Survey of Sexual Health and Behavior, 828–829
National Survey of Substance Abuse Treatment Services (N-SSATS), 771
National Survey on Drug Use and Health (NSDUH), 116, 370–371
  employment status, 375
  gender, 374
  occupation, 375
  race and ethnicity, 373
  substance use disorders, 368–369
National Youth Tobacco Survey (NYTS), 370
Natural CC drivers, 76
Nausea aversion therapy, conditioned nausea responses, 1190–1191
N-benzylpiperazine, 1610
NCPE. *See* Noncardiogenic pulmonary edema
NCS. *See* National Comorbidity Survey
NCS-R, 793
NE. *See* Norepinephrine
Necrotizing fasciitis, injection drug use and, 1445
Nefazodone, for PTSD, 1668–1669
Negative allosteric modulators or inverse agonists, 141
Negative emotions
  mindfulness-based treatment of addiction, 1240–1242
Negative myoclonus, 1434
Negative Quick Screen, 475, 475*t*
Neonatal abstinence syndrome (NAS), 1512–1513, 1517–1518
Neonatal drug exposure, 940–941
Neonatal opioid withdrawal (NOW), 1513, 1517–1518
Neonatal opioid withdrawal syndrome (NOWS), 980–981
Neonatal opioid withdrawal/neonatal abstinence syndrome, 1517–1518
  pharmacologic treatment of, 1517–1518
  pharmacotherapy for, 1518*t*
  in utero opioid-exposed newborn, identification and treatment of, 1517
Neonatal withdrawal syndromes, 172
Neonate(s). *See also* Neonatal abstinence syndrome (NAS); Neonatal intoxication
  alcohol use, medical complications related to, 1326
  benzodiazepines, 172
  cannabinoids, 1331
  opioids, 1330
  tobacco use, complications related to, 1328
Nephritic syndrome, 1376, 1377*t*
  with injection drug use, 1380–1381
    postinfectious glomerulonephritis, 1380–1381
Nephritic-nephrotic syndrome, 1377*t*
  with injection drug use, 1380
    hepatitis C virus–related glomerulonephritis, 1380
Nephrology, 1376–1377
Nephrotic syndrome, 1376, 1377*t*
  with injection drug use, 1379–1380
    hepatitis virus–associated nephrotic syndrome, 1379
    heroin-associated nephropathy, 1379–1380
    HIV-associated nephropathy, 1379
    subcutaneous drug use–associated amyloidosis, 1380
Nerve damage, pain, 1695
Nervous system infections, drug users, 1452–1453
NESARC. *See* National Epidemiologic Study on Alcoholism and Related Conditions
NESS. *See* Night Eating Symptom Scale
Network therapy, 1164–1173
  adaptations of, 1171–1172
  addictive problem, 1169
  agenda, focusing on, 1173
  alcoholics anonymous, 1167
  cognitive-behavioral therapy, 1165
  community reinforcement, 1165
  community-based family involvement, 1172
  ending, 1171
  individual psychotherapy, 1120
  key elements, 1164–1165
  medication observation, 1168
  meeting arrangements, 1168
  membership in, 1166–1167
  network's membership, 1166–1167
  network's task, 1167
  patient selection, 1166
  pharmacotherapy, 1167–1168
  principles of, 1172–1173
  relevant research, 1170–1171
  research on, 1170–1171
  social network, 1165
  task of, 1167
  technique, 1164–1165, 1170
  treatment, principles of, 1172–1173
  typical, 1170
Neural axis, catecholamine systems and, 37–38
Neural patterns, 1310–1311
Neuroadaptation, 209–210
Neuroanatomy, limbic system, 35–36, 35*f*
Neurobehavioral and cognitive disorders, alcohol, 1424–1425
Neurobehavioral Cognitive Status Examination (NCSE), 690–691
Neurobehavioral Disorder with Prenatal Alcohol Exposure (ND-PAE), 1515
Neurobehavioral disorders, 1424–1427
  alcohol, 1424–1425
  barbiturates, benzodiazepines, 1425
  cannabinoids, 1426
  cocaine, amphetamines and MDMA, 1425–1426
  dissociative anesthetics, 1426
  hallucinogens, 1426
  inhalants, 1426–1427
  opioids, 1426
Neurobiology, 1310–1311
  binge–intoxication stage, 5–6, 6*f*–7*f*
  brain functional activity effects, 278–279
  conceptual framework for, 3*f*
  GABA, 278
  glutamate, 277–278
  mechanisms of action, 276–279
  preoccupation–anticipation stage, 9–11, 9*f*, 10*f*
  withdrawal-negative affect stage, 7–9, 8*f*
Neurocircuitry, in gambling disorder, 792
Neurocognition, traumatic brain injury, 690–691
Neurocognitive deficits, 1548
Neurocognitive disorder (NCD), 1548
Neuroimaging, attention deficit hyperactivity disorder, 1628–1629
Neuroimmune modulators, alcohol and, 157
Neuroleptics, 1614

Neurological disorders
  alcohol use, medical complications related to, 1325
  cannabinoids, 1331
  complications, 1437
  detoxification and, 865
  medical care of patients, with unhealthy substance use, 1316
  movement disorders, 1434–1435
    alcohol, 1434
    cannabinoids, 1435
    cocaine, amphetamines, and MDMA, 1434–1435
    opioids, 1435
    tobacco and nicotine, 1435
  neurobehavioral and cognitive disorders, 1424–1427
    alcohol, 1424–1425
    barbiturates, benzodiazepines, 1425
    cannabinoids, 1426
    cocaine, amphetamines and MDMA, 1425–1426
    dissociative anesthetics, 1426
    hallucinogens, 1426
    inhalants, 1426–1427
    opioids, 1426
  neurological complications, substance use resulting from infections, 1435–1437
  neuromuscular (nerve, muscle, and spinal cord) disorders, 1432–1433
    alcohol, 1433
    inhalants, 1433
    opioids, 1433
  seizures, 1427–1429
    alcohol, 1427
    barbiturates, benzodiazepines, 1427
    cannabinoids, 1428
    cocaine, amphetamines and MDMA, 1427–1428
    dissociative anesthetics, 1428
    inhalants, 1428–1429
    opioids, 1428
    psychedelics, 1428
  stroke, 1429–1432
    alcohol, 1430
    cannabinoids, 1432
    cocaine, amphetamines, and MDMA, 1430–1432
    dissociative anesthetics, 1432
    opioids, 1432
    psychedelics, 1432
    tobacco and nicotine, 1429–1430
  tobacco use, complications related to, 1328
  trauma, 1420–1422
  traumatic brain injury, 1420–1422
Neuromodulation techniques
  for addiction, 1069–1070
    deep brain stimulation, 1070
    focused ultrasound, 1069–1070
    transcranial direct current stimulation, 1069
  for substance use disorders, 1064–1070
    for addiction, 1066–1070
    addiction, brain regions, 1064–1066
    focused ultrasound, 1069–1070
    transcranial direct current stimulation, 1069
    transcranial magnetic stimulation for, 1066–1069
Neuromodulation therapeutics
  frontal-striatal circuitry, 1066
  substance use disorder, 694
  traumatic brain injury, 694
Neuromuscular (nerve, muscle, and spinal cord) disorders, 1432–1433
  alcohol, 1433
  inhalants, 1433
  opioids, 1433
Neurons
  dopamine-regulated circuits, 11
  drugs and, 11
Neuropathic pain, 1692
  capsaicin, 1754
  pregabalin, 1751
  tricyclic antidepressants, 1749–1750
Neuropathy, 1433
  lamotrigine, 1751–1752
Neuropeptide(s), 156–157
Neuropsychiatric opioids, 1330
Neurosyphilis, 1436–1437
Neurotoxicity, 210
  inhalants, 313
  MDMA, 283
Neurotoxin 6-hydroxydopamine (6-OH-DA), 41
Neurotoxins, psychostimulants and, 39
Neurotransmitter systems
  alcohol, 155–157, 156*t*
  severe alcohol withdrawal, 875
  stimulants, 204
Neutral allosteric modulators or antagonists, 141
Neutrophilia, 1357–1358
New Drug Application (NDA), 59
New psychoactive substances (NPS), 1931
  substance-induced psychosis, 1610–1611
N-hydroxynorcocaine, 1369
NIAAA Single Alcohol Screening Question (SASQ), 657
NIAAA (National Institute on Alcoholism and Alcohol Abuse) Youth Alcohol Screening Tool, 1812
NIATx model, 771–773, 776
Nicotine (tobacco), 5, 89, 1046–1047, 1328, 1514. *See also* Cigarette smoking; Smoking cessation; Tobacco; Tobacco addiction; Tobacco smoke; Tobacco use disorder; Transdermal nicotine patch (TNP)
  anxiety disorders and, 1594
  caffeine and, 225
  chemical structure of, 231*f*
  depression, 1577–1578
  drug interactions with, 230, 234–235
  electronic drug delivery devices, 338–339
    containing e-liquids, 338–339
    delivery level, 341–342
    pharmacokinetic studies, 341
  epidemiology, 231–232
  exposure
    biochemical assessment of, 234
  gum, 237
  headache, 1423
  historical features, 231–232
  ionotropic receptors and, 139*t*
  levels, 99–100
  LGBTQ, 672
  mechanisms of action, neurobiologic, 238–242
  methods of use, 230–231
  movement disorders, 1435
  perioperative care, 1538–1539
  pharmacokinetics of, 232–235
  pharmacologic actions, 235–236
  physician addiction, 555
  primary psychotic disorder with co-occurring substance use disorder, 1603
  psychoactive effects, 235–236
  public awareness, 96
  sleep and, 1472
  stroke, 1429–1430
  substance-induced mental disorders, 1549
  treatment history, 1144
  withdrawal, anxiety and arousal association, differential diagnosis, 1594
Nicotine addiction, in smoking behavior, 95–96, 97*f*
Nicotine anonymous, 1149, 1283
Nicotine dependence, 370
Nicotine Dependence Scale, 369
Nicotine gum, 95–96, 1032–1033
Nicotine inhaler, 1033
Nicotine lozenge, 1033
Nicotine nasal spray, 1033
Nicotine replacement therapies (NRT), 89, 1032–1033, 1513–1514, 1872
  tobacco and nicotine, 1429–1430
  tobacco/nicotine, adolescent SUDs, 1872
Nicotine/tobacco control policy
  climate change and, 85
Nicotine/tobacco use disorder (NTUD)
  causes, 1037–1038
  development, novel treatment approach, 1144
  neurobiology, 1030–1031
  in older adults, 655
  persistent cultural attitudes, 1031
  pharmacologic actions, 1030–1044
  pharmacotherapies, 1032–1034
    metabolism rate, 1035–1036
    optimizing methods, 1036
  prevalence, 1031
  treatments, 1037–1038
    behavioral treatments, 1148–1149
    brief clinical intervention, 1149–1150
    history of, 1144
    motivating smokers to quit, 1148
    motivation, 1145
    planning, 1146–1148
    skills-based behavioral treatments, 1145–1146
  withdrawal, 1037–1038
Nicotinic acetylcholine receptors (nAChRs), 238, 1030
Night Eating Symptom Scale (NESS), 1682
NIH (U.S. National Institutes of Health), 48
NIH HEAL Initiative (Helping to End Addiction Long Term Initiative), 986
Nitrates, 1415
Nitrous oxide, 308, 1415
  action of, 301
  classification, 293
  clinical use, 293
  as "laughing gas", 295

NMDA-antagonist action, tolerance, 185
N-methyl-D-aspartate (NMDA), 293, 893–894, 1394–1395
neurobiology, 300
receptors
alcohol, 159
antagonist activity, 303
substance-induced mental disorders, 1550
toxicity/adverse effects, 301–302
N,N-Dimethyltryptamine (DMT), 269, 281–282
pharmacodynamics, 281–282
pharmacokinetics, 281
Nociception, 7–8, 1692–1693
Nociceptive amygdala, 1697
Nocturnal polysomnogram (PSG), 1463
Node-link mapping, 1636
Nonadrenaline cells (NA cells), 37
Nonalcohol sedative hypnotics, 165–177
Nonalcohol SUDs, pharmacotherapy of, 695
Nonalcoholic fatty liver disease (NAFLD), 1356
Nonbenzodiazepine compounds, sedative–hypnotic withdrawal and, 889, 891
Nonbenzodiazepine hypnotics
biotransformation of, 168
formulations/chemical structure, 165, 166*t*
historical features, 165–167
pharmacodynamics, 167–168
Noncardiac vascular infections, 1448
clinical presentation, 1448
diagnosis, 1448
epidemiology and pathogenesis, 1448
treatment, 1448
Noncardiogenic acute pulmonary edema, pulmonary vasculature, 1405
Noncompetitive agonists, 141
Noncompliance, non-opioid analgesics, opioid use and, 1769
Noncompulsive substance use ("low need persons"), 1977
Nonfatal opioid overdose, 912
Nonjudgmental care, 1524
Nonmaleficence, 1966
ethical issues in, 1898–1899
Nonmedical use, of hallucinogen(s), 273
Nonmedical Use of Prescription Medications (NUPM), 181
Non-motor vehicle-related injuries and fatalities, unintentional injury, 1483
Non-NMDA (N-methyl-d-aspartate) AMPA and kainate, 893–894
Nonopioid analgesics, 1747–1749
Nonopioid medication(s), 1747–1760
pain management, 1747–1760
Nonpharmaceutical synthetic opioids, 357
Nonphysicians, pharmacotherapy support from, 1272
Non-rapid eye movement (NREM) sleep, 1463
sleep architecture, 1464
Nonsmoking skills, 1145
Non–12-step recovery groups, SMART recovery, 1284
Nonsteroidal antiinflammatory drugs (NSAIDs), 1748–1749
chronic pancreatitis, 1392
Nontraumatic chest pain, 926
Noradrenaline, 37
Norepinephrine (NE), 204, 205*t*, 205*f*
and arousal, in gambling disorder, 791
Norepinephrine reuptake inhibitor atomoxetine, stimulant use disorders, 1016
Norm gap, 630
Normative education, adolescents, substance use, 393
Nose, medical care of patients, with unhealthy substance use, 1315
Nosocomial transmission, of hepatitis C, 1364
Novel psychoactive substances (NPS)
cathinones
clinical implications, 362
epidemiology, 361–362
history, 361
legal status, 362
pharmacology, 362
designation of, 357
for drug screening, 357
flualprazolam/etizolam
clinical implications, 361
history, 360–361
legal status, 361
pharmacology, 361
hallucinogens
clinical implications, 362
epidemiology, 362
history, 362
legal status, 362
pharmacology, 362
history, 357
identifying and accessing information on, 363
Kratom
clinical implications, 360
epidemiology, 359
history, 359
legal status, 360
Mitragyna speciosa, 359
pharmacology, 360
nonpharmaceutical fentanyl analogues
clinical implications, 359
epidemiology, 359
history, 358–359
legal status, 359
pharmacology, 359
phenibut
clinical implications, 360
history, 360
legal status, 360
pharmacology, 360
specific examples, 358–362
substance-induced mental disorders, 1551
treatment, 358
types, 357
xylazine
clinical implications, 361
history, 361
legal status, 361
pharmacology, 361
NPD. *See* Narcissistic personality disorder
NPI-025, 1053
NPS. *See* Novel psychoactive substances
NS5A inhibitors, 1367
NS3/4A protease inhibitors, 1367
NSAIDs. *See* Nonsteroidal antiinflammatory drugs
NS5B inhibitors, 1367
NSDUH. *See* National Survey on Drug Use and Health
NTUD. *See* Nicotine/tobacco use disorder
Nubain. *See* Nalbuphine
Nuclear transcription, 140
Nucleoside reverse transcriptase inhibitors (NRTIs), 1455
Nucleus accumbens (NAc/NAcc), 36, 1064
binge–intoxication stages, 5–6
Nursing mothers
benzodiazepines, 172
detoxification and, 864–865
Nutritional supplements
adolescent athletes, 321–322
alcohol-related cirrhosis, 1357
stimulant use disorders, 1019

O

OAT. *See* Opioid agonist therapy
Obesity
alcohol-related liver disease, definition, 1679
biological management of
acute, 1683–1684
long-term, 1684
subacute, 1682–1683
and metabolic-associated fatty liver disease, 1356–1357
obstructive sleep apnea, 1466
substance use disorders, 1680
Objective Opioid Withdrawal Scale, 913
OBOT. *See* Office-based opioid treatment
Observational studies, epidemiologic principles, 367–368
Obsessive–compulsive disorder (OCD), 1590*t*, 1596–1597
differential diagnosis, 1594
smoking and, 1595
treatment, 1594
Obsessive-Compulsive-Inventory-4, 1590–1591
Obstructive airway disease, 1405–1406
Obstructive sleep apnea (OSA), 1465*t*, 1466, 1475
Occupation, drug/alcohol use disorders, 375
Occupational Alcohol Programs (OAPs), 547
Occupational exposures, 1408
Occupational therapy (OT)
occupational work rehabilitation, 1739, 1740*t*
posture and body mechanics, 1739
OCD. *See* Obsessive-compulsive disorder (OCD)
Odds ratio, 367
Office of National Drug Control Policy (ONDCP), 590
Office-based clinical trials, network therapy, 1170
Office-based opioid treatment (OBOT), 718, 999
clinical issues, 1008–1010
epidemiologic and regulatory issues, 999–1001
research issues, 1001–1008
office-based practice, patients entering directly into, 1001–1008, 1004*t*–1005*t*
stable, long-term patients in office-based practice, 1001, 1002*t*
setting, 596
special issues in, 999–1013
OIH. *See* Opioid-induced hyperalgesia
Olanzapine, psychosis, 1611

Older adults. *See also* Elderly
detoxification, 866
illicit drug use, 941
medical care of patients, with unhealthy substance use, 1321–1322
misusing alcohol/drugs, 1901
population-specific considerations for, 1205–1206
brief intervention, 1205–1206
family treatment modalities, 1205
screening and assessment, 1205
SBI in, alcohol use, 486–487
screening, unhealthy alcohol and drug use in
brief interventions, 512
diagnosis, 511–512
epidemiology, 510, 510*t*
screening tools, 511
self-administered screening approaches, 511
unique vulnerabilities, 510–511
substance use disorders in, 653–665
alcohol and prescription medications, 656–657
alcohol in social settings, 657
chronic pain, 656
cognitive impairment, 656
comorbidity, 656
co-occurring disorders, 656
issues, 655–657
metabolic changes, 655
pharmacotherapy, 660–662
prevention of return to use, 662
recovery support, 662
sleep problems, 656
suicidality, 656
treatment outcome research, limitations of, 660
OMT. *See* Opioid maintenance treatment
Onanism, 827
Oncologic
alcohol use, medical complications related to, 1326
tobacco use, complications related to, 1328
Oncologic toxicity, 243
Ondansetron, stimulant use disorders, 1017
Ondansetron study, 953
ONDCP. *See* White House Office of National Drug Control Policy
One-size-fits-all approach, 1122–1123
"Onion skin" hypertrophy, 1383
On-site testing, 518
Open-ended questions, 1086
Operant conditioning, 1190
Operation Enduring Freedom (OEF), 681
Operational Iraqi Freedom (OIF), 681
Opioid(s), 40–41, 521–522
abrupt cessation, 1764
abstinence syndrome, 913
abuse-deterrent formulations, 180, 180*t*
acute use, side effects, 1774–1776
addiction, 999–1000
alcohol and, 156–157
alcohol-related consumption, reduction of, 946–947
anesthesiologists, 552
antagonists, 429
anxiety disorders and, 1595–1596
benzodiazepines and, 169–170
blood level, reward and, 1767
buprenorphine, partial agonist properties, 140
central nervous system, medical management, 183
challenge, long-term opioid use, 1767–1768
chronic pain, 1933
classification, 908
clinical management variables, 1770–1779
CNS side effects, 1766*f*, 1767*f*
confirmatory testing for, 522, 522*t*
craving, 912
definition of, 178–181
dose requirements, 1773
dose-response curves, 137–138, 137*f*
dosing, 1773–1774
drug selection, 1770–1772
drug–drug interactions, 188
efficacy, 1773
endocrine effects, 1776
epidemiology of, use disorder, 181–183
equianalgesic doses, 1770–1772
federal agencies
Drug Enforcement Administration, 1803
FDA and REMS, 1803–1804
federal regulations
controlled substances, 1800
legitimate medical purposes, 1801–1802
schedule determination, 1801, 1802*t*
state and, 1802
three-day rule, 1801–1802
unhealthy use, 1800
harm reduction-oriented approach, 429
historical perspectives, 1761–1763
hydrocodone, rescheduling of, 1801
immune effects, 1776
intoxication and overdose
assessment, 909–910
clinical presentation, 908–912
diagnosis, 909–910, 909*t*
follow-up care, 912
management, 910–911, 911*t*
pharmacologic therapies, 911
legal and regulatory considerations in, 1800
long *vs.* short-acting, 1773
mechanisms of action, 182–183
medical complications of, 187–188
medications, pain management, 1762
mental health issues, 1768
metabolites, 522
MOP-r signaling properties, 183
naltrexone (ReVia), 1230
dependence with psychosocial treatments, 1230
overdose, follow-up care, 912
withdrawal, clonidine and, 910
neurobiology, 182–183
overdose deaths, 187, 409*f*, 411
patient-controlled analgesia, 1774
pharmacodynamics, 186–187
pharmacokinetics, 183–186
physician addiction, 554–556
position of, pain treatment, 1763–1764
prescribing guidelines
American Society of the Interventional Pain Physicians, 1806, . 1807*t*
Centers for Disease Control and Prevention, 1804–1806, 1805*t*
Chronic Non-Cancer Pain, 1806
Federation of State Medical Board, 1806
National Summit for Opioid Safety, 1806, 1807*t*
Prescription Drug Monitoring Programs, 1806–1807
prescription medication misuse, 412–413
receptors types of, 178
respiratory depression, 1774–1775
reward, animal models, 40
risk mitigation, 1779–1782
risk of suicide, dosing, 1728
rotation, 1776–1777
rotation of, 1776–1777
routes of administration, 1772–1773
schedule of administration, 1767*f*
scheduled *vs.* as-needed, 1774
screening immunoassay, 521–522
screens, 563–564
severe pain, 1747
side effects, management, 1774–1776
sleep and, 1471–1472
special issues, 1764–1770
state-controlled substance regulations, 1802
substance use disorders, 1761, 1769*t*
substance-induced mental disorders, 1550
substances included, 178–181
symptoms, 1763
tapering, 1777–1779
tolerance, 187
toxicity states medical management of, 187–188
treatment, 429
unhealthy use, differential diagnosis, 1767–1768, 1767*t*
withdrawal, 912–918, 1535–1536
acute, 917
alpha-2 adrenergic agents, 916
assessment, 913
chronic, 917
clinical presentation, 912–913, 914*t*
co-occurring conditions, 917–918
diagnosis, 913
follow-up care, 918
full opioid agonists, 913–914
management, 913
medical and psychiatric conditions, 917
other opioid agonists, 916
pharmacological therapies for, 913–917
protracted abstinence, 913
withdrawal, management, 1779
Opioid addiction
anesthesiologists, profession return, 552
methadone maintenance therapy, 1767
Opioid agonist(s)
and partial agonists, 971–972
treatment with methadone, 1701–1702
withdrawal of, 914–916
Opioid agonist therapy (OAT), 1000
climate change and, 84–85
opioid dependence, with psychosocial treatments, 1230
perioperative care, 1536
psychoactive medications, incarceration and, 864–865

Opioid agonist treatment (OAT)
history and context, 969
pain management
acute, buprenorphine, 984
acute, methadone and, 984
chronic, 984
treatment access through emergency departments, 984–985
Opioid alternative analgesics, 1749–1755
Opioid antagonists
amphetamine-type stimulants use disorder, 1020
compulsive sexual behavior disorder, 838
Opioid dependence, 745
network therapy and, 1265
randomized controlled trial and, 1264
Opioid overdose epidemic, 1983
Opioid receptor ligands, stimulant use disorders, 1018
Opioid Risk Tool (ORT), 1729
Opioid systems, in gambling disorder, 791–792
Opioid treatment agreement (OTA), 1779
Opioid Treatment Program (OTP) setting, 596
Opioid treatment system, 985–986
Opioid use disorder (OUD), 72, 371, 425, 596, 1154, 1251, 1509–1510, 1866
aversion therapies, 1193–1194
buprenorphine treatment
buprenorphine-medication interactions, 978
diversion and nonmedical use, 979
dose adjustment, 978
extended-release (XR) injectable, 977–978
federal regulations and sublingual buprenorphine, 978–979
initiation and precipitated withdrawal, 978
low-dose initiation, 978
patient selection, 979
setting, 978
sublingual/buccal, pharmacology of, 977
chronic pain, diagnosis, 1793–1794
clinical issues, pharmacotherapy, 972–973
goals, 972–973
medications, profile of, 973
opioid physical dependence, 973
protracted withdrawal syndrome, 973
diagnosis, 1596
genetics of, 1699–1700
methadone, treatment using
adequacy of dose, 975
benzodiazepines and, 977
blood levels, 975
continued illicit opioid use *versus*, 973–974
duration and dose, 974–975
heroin-simulated 24-hour dose-response, 973, 973*f*–974*f*
induction, 974
initial dose, 974
medical monitoring, 977
methadone medical maintenance, 976
methadone-medication interactions, 976
observed doses and take-home medication, 976
patient stability, 976
and QT interval, 976–977
stabilization and steady state, 974
at steady state, 973, 974*f*
therapeutic window, 974
monitoring for unhealthy use, 1793
NESARC, 1595–1596
pain and, 1699–1703
perioperative care, 1535–1538
acute pain, 1536–1538
medications, 1536
opioid agonist therapy, 1536–1538, 1536*t*
opioid withdrawal, 1535–1536
preoperative evaluation, 1535
pharmacological treatment
medication combinations, 972
nonopioids, 971
opioid antagonists, 970
opioid full and partial agonists, 970
pharmacotherapy, 661
physicians, re-entry of, 569
positron emission tomography of cerebral metabolism, 970
pregnancy
nonprescribed opioids during, 979–980
opioid agonist treatment, 979–981
special issues, medication treatment, 979–985
substance-induced psychosis, 1602
treatments, 537–538, 1596
unique effects of, 1699–1703
withdrawal management, 1263
in women, 638
Opioid withdrawal management
with transcutaneous electrical acupuncture, 1056–1058
animal studies, 1056
human studies, 1056
multiple daily treatment, 1057–1058
single treatment, 1056–1057
Opioid withdrawal syndrome (OWS)
α_2-adrenergic agonists, 972
lofexidine, 972
and medically supervised withdrawal, 971–972
medication combinations, 972
nonopioid medication treatments, 972
opioid agonists, 971–972
partial agonists, 971–972
Opioid-based medically supervised withdrawal, 971
Opioidergic agents, 946–949
Opioid-induced bowel dysfunction (OIBD), 1394
Opioid-induced constipation (OIC), 1394
Opioid-induced GI hyperalgesia (OIH), 1394–1395
Opioid-induced hyperalgesia (OIH), 1700
clinical evidence of, 1701, 1701*t*
genetics of, 1703
mechanisms of, 1700–1701
response, genetic factors, 1699
surgical patients, 1702
and tolerance, 1700
Opioid-induced noncardiogenic pulmonary edema, 1410–1411
Opioid-induced pulmonary edema, 1410
Opioid-induced respiratory depression, 1774–1775
Opioid-induced sedation, 1775–1776
Opioid-related myoclonus, 1435
Opioids, 1052–1053
and alcohol, 1047
binge eating disorder, 802–803
cardiovascular, 1329–1330
cardiovascular disorders, substance use, 1344–1345
endocarditis, 1344–1345
heart disease and stroke, 1345
prolonged QT, 1345
central nervous system and respiratory drive, 1402
chronic pain, treatment of, 1792–1793
chronic pancreatitis, 1392
complications, 1328–1330
craving, prevention, 1058–1060
animal procedures, 1058–1059
human study, 1059–1060
cutaneous, 1330
endocrine and reproductive disorders, 1495–1497
endocrinologic, 1330
fetal, neonatal, and infant, 1330
gastrointestinal, 1330
gastrointestinal symptoms associated with other drugs, 1394–1395
headache, 1423
movement disorders, 1435
neurobehavioral and cognitive disorders, 1426
neuromuscular (nerve, muscle, and spinal cord) disorders, 1433
neuropsychiatric, 1330
with other substances, 1047–1048
pharmacotherapy, adolescent SUDs, 1875–1877
acute ingestion and withdrawal management, 1876
buprenorphine, 1876
methadone, 1876–1877
naltrexone, 1876
pregnancy, substance use during, 1516–1518
neonatal opioid withdrawal/neonatal abstinence syndrome, 1517–1518
pharmacotherapy in, 1516–1517
pulmonary vasculature, 1405
renal and metabolic, 1330
renal and metabolic complications, 1377*t*, 1381
prescription opioids, injection use of, 1381
rhabdomyolysis, 1381
urologic effects of, 1381
respiratory, 1329
resumed use, 1058–1060
seizures, 1428
and stimulants, 1047–1048
stroke, 1432
and substance-induced depressive disorder, 1547
and tobacco, 1047
viral hepatitis, 1370
in women, 638
Opioids, adolescent SUDs, 1875–1877
Opium, 178
Opium Advisory Committee ("OAC"), 1928
Opium inebriety, 583

Oppositional defiant disorder (ODD), 1889–1890
  adolescent drug abuse, 1835
Oral antiviral agents, 1363
Oral cavity, gastrointestinal disorders, 1389
Oral fluid testing, 516
Orbital frontal cortex (OFC), 689–690, 790, 1066–1067
Orbitofrontal PFC, 37
Oregon Reducing Youth Access to Alcohol Project, 402–403
Orexins, binge eating disorder, 802
Organ systems
  alcohol, 158–159
  drug addiction, 17–18
  drug distribution, 131
  inhalants, 313
  transplantation, substance use disorders, 1539–1540
Organization of American States (OAS), 776
Oropharyngeal lesions, 1446
Osmitrol. *See* Mannitol
Osmolar gap, 1378–1379
Osmotic release oral system (OROS), 1634
Osteomyelitis, 1451
Outcome(s), 1081–1082
  addiction treatment services, 768
  aversion therapy, cocaine-amphetamine dependence, 1192
  expectancy, relapse and, 1224
Outcomes-driven treatments, 727, 729
Outpatient treatments, 597
  adolescent substance abuse, 1844
Overdose
  marijuana (Cannabis), 253–254
  mixed, 890
  naloxone and, 912
  nonfatal opioid, 912
  propoxyphene, 187
  sedative–hypnotic intoxication, 889–890
  sedative-hypnotics, 1414
Overdose education and naloxone distribution (OEND, 985
Overdose prevention centers, 748
Overdose Prevention Sites (OPS), 428–429
Oversees drug testing, 518
Oxazepam (Serax), 962*t*, 963–964, 964*t*
  benzodiazepines and, 166*t*, 168
Oxcarbazepine, 1750–1751
Oxford House (OH) model, 460–461
Oxycodone (OxyContin), 179
  dependence, treatment for, 1193
  pharmacokinetics, 184
  reward effects, 1766–1767

P

Pain, 1321
  addiction *vs.* clinical interface, 1697–1703
  anatomy of, 1692–1695, 1693*f*
  anticonvulsants, 1752
  anxiety sensitivity, 1711
  attention, 1712
  bedside examination, findings and meanings, 1693*t*
  behavioral contingencies, 1715
  biopsychosocial approach
    barriers to receiving psychological care, 1720–1721
    cognitive–behavioral therapy, 1718–1720
    exercises, 1717
    interdisciplinary pain programs, 1720
  cannabinoids and, 1698
  catastrophizing, 1713
  chronic pancreatitis, 1392
  cognitions and coping, 1713
  developmental issues, 1716
  disorders, comorbid psychologic factors, 1698
  emotional distress, 1710
  vs. emotions, 1695–1697, 1709–1710
  expectations and goal setting, 1712
  fear-avoidance model, 1712–1713
  genetics of, 1699–1700
  helplessness *vs.* self-efficacy, 1713
  kinesiophobia, 1712–1713
  management
    non-opioid treatments, 1747–1760
    rehabilitation approaches, 1734
  management, benzodiazepines and opioids, 170
  memory, 1697
  mind–body connection, 1708–1709
  opioid use disorders, 1596
  pathophysiology of, addiction interfaces and, 1691–1707
  perception, 1712
  physician addiction, 557
  physiology, 1692–1695
  prevalence of, 1763
  psychogenic components, 1714
  substance use disorder, 1697–1703, 1716–1717, 1717*t*
  syndromes classification
    alpha2-adrenergic agonists, 1755
    chronic pain syndrome, 1714
    DSM-IV and DSM-5, 1713–1714
    malingering, 1714
Pain management, opioid agonist treatment
  acute, buprenorphine, 984
  acute, methadone and, 984
  chronic, 984
Pain Medication Questionnaire (PMQ), 1729
Pain medicine, universal precautions, 1793, 1793*t*
Pain neuroscience education (PNE), 1738–1739
Pain-related fear, 1711
Palatine-like phospholipase domain-containing protein 3 (PNPLA3), 1356
Pancreas
  gastrointestinal disorders, 1390–1393
    acute pancreatitis, management of, 1392
    alcohol-related pancreatitis, 1390
    chronic pancreatitis, management of, 1392–1393
    definitions, 1391
    diagnosis, 1391–1392
    etiology, 1390–1391
    pathogenesis, 1391, 1391*f*
    susceptibility to alcohol-related pancreatitis, 1391
Pancreatic disease, 1395
Pancreatic fibrosis, 1391
Pancreatitis, chronic, 1393–1394
Panic disorder(s), 1590*t*
  differential diagnosis, 1594
  Mini-International Neuropsychiatric Interview, 1591*t*
  selective serotonin reuptake inhibitors, 1594
  smoking and, 1595
  treatment, 1594
  with/without agoraphobia, 1594
Paraphilias, 827, 830–831
  definitions and diagnosis, 830–831
  development, 831
  etiology, 831
  prevalence, 831
  and sex with minors, 831–832
Paraphilic disorders, 830–831
  definitions and diagnosis, 830–831
  development, 831
  etiology, 831
  prevalence, 831
  and sex with minors, 831–832
Parenchymal destruction, 1405
Parenchymal lung disease, 1413
Parenting and attachment, 645–646
Parents, adolescent substance abuse, 1835
Parkinson's disease, 1435
  caffeine and, 224–225
  cannabis treatment for, 1943
Parotid glands, gastrointestinal disorders, 1389
Paroxetine, for PTSD, 1668–1669
Paroxetine (Paxil), social anxiety disorder, 1593
Parrish, J., 583
Partial agonists, 140
Partial CB_1 agonists, 250–251
Partial hospital programs, adolescent substance abuse, 1844–1845
Partial hospitalization programs (PHP), 597–598
Partial mu agonists, pain treatment, limitations, 1770
Particles, electronic drug delivery devices, 341
Particulate matter (PM), 78
Partnership, 1085
Partnership, acceptance, compassion, and evocation (PACE), 1085
Passive-reactive paradigm, 1076
Pathologic(al) gambling. *See* Gambling disorder
Pathological computer use, 845
Pathological gambling (PG), 788
Pathological Internet use (PIU), 845, 848
Patient(s)
  assessment, risk stratification, 1912–1913
  autonomy, addiction practice, 1896–1903
  denial, dealing with, 1900–1901
  eating disorders, 1681
  perspective, linked services and, 740–741, 741*t*
  placement criteria, 733
  preparation and selection, 1130
  psychiatric disorders, 1680
  self-report, 530
  with substance use disorders, 1680
  tools, 528, 529*t*
Patient change, conceptualizing, 1087–1088, 1087*f*
Patient Health Questionnaire (PHQ-2), 774
Patient Health Questionnaire-9 (PHQ-9), 1549, 1553, 1728
Patient Placement Criteria for the Treatment of Psychoactive Substance Use Disorders, 725
Patient safety, 1603
Patient self-management stage, 709–710

Patient Stress Questionnaire, 1915
Patient-centered counseling, 1088
Patient-controlled analgesia (PCA), acute pain and, 1767, 1774
Patient-Reported Outcome Measures, 57
Patient-Reported Outcome Measures Information System (PROMIS), 57
Patient-reported outcomes (PROs), 774
Patients with chronic pain, 1702–1703
Paxil. *See* Paroxetine
P-4 Brief Assessment, 1729
PDAs. *See* Personal digital assistants
PDMP. *See* Prescription Drug Monitoring Program (PDMP)
PDs. *See* Personality disorders
PE therapy. *See* Prolonged exposure therapy
Peak drug concentration, drug exposure, 129
Peer recovery specialists, 599
Peer recovery support group participation, 709–710
Peer support, 1256
Peer-based recovery support services, 713–714
Peers
  adolescent drug abuse, 1834
  adolescent substance abuse, 1834
  confrontation, therapeutic communities, 1179
Pegylated interferon-alpha (PEG-IFN-α), 1363
Peliosis hepatitis, 17-alkylated androgens, 325
Pellagra, 1424
Pen-style tank EDDDs, 337
Pentazocine, 179–180
  pain treatment, limitations, 1766, 1772
  pharmacodynamics, 186
  pharmacokinetics, 184
Pentobarbital, 131, 899*t*, 965
Penylethylamines, hallucinogens, 269
People who inject drugs (PWID), 427, 427*b*, 1317, 1328–1329
  HAV, 1361
  HCV, 1365–1366
  hepatitis virus–associated nephrotic syndrome, 1379
  pneumonia, 1410, 1449
  pulmonary hypertension, 1411
  septic pulmonary emboli, 1411
People who use drugs (PWUD), 758
  sexually transmitted diseases, 1456–1457
People who use substances during pregnancy (PSP), 1509–1510
Peptic ulcer disease, 1390
Peptic ulceration, 1395
Perception, chronic nociceptive pain and, 1692
Performance enhancers, new-generation, 318
Performance-in-Practice (PIP) activity, 775
Perinatal SUD, 1509
Period effects, 368
Periodic limb movements of sleep (PLMS)
  alcohol and, 1470
  clinical approaches, 1465
Perioperative care, alcohol and other drug use
  benzodiazepine use disorder, 1538
  cannabis, 1539
  encephalopathy grade, 1534*t*
  nicotine, 1538–1539
  opioid use disorders, 1535–1536
  stimulant use disorders, 1539
  substance use disorders, 1539–1540
  unhealthy alcohol use, 1530–1535
Peripheral edema, 1737
Peripheral insulin resistance, ethanol, 1490, 1492
Peripheral nerve lesions, EMLA, 1752
Peripheral neuropathy, 1753
Peripheral sensitization, 1693–1694, 1693*t*, 1694*f*
Peripherally acting μ-opioid receptor agonists (PAMORAs), 1394
Permanent Central Opium Board, 1928–1929
Personal Experience Inventory, 1836
Personal Experience Screening Questionnaire, 1835
Personal problems, group therapies and, 1103
Personal resilience, LGBTQ, 668
Personality disorders (PDs)
  classification system, 1643
  co-occurring models, 1644
  definition, 1643
  diagnosis, 1644–1648
  diagnostic challenges, 1646, 1647*t*
  epidemiology, 1643–1644
  etiologic diagnoses, 1644–1645
  etiology, 1644
  high-volume sexual behaviors, 830
  integrated, 1651
  medical illness, 1647–1648
  pharmacologic treatments, 1651–1652
  practical issues, 1645–1648
  psychiatric illness, 1646
  substance use, 1646–1647
  theoretical issues, 1644–1645
  treatment
    evidence-based psychosocial and pharmacologic, 1648
    outcomes, 1648
    psychosocial treatments, 1648–1651
Personality profiles
  anabolic androgenic steroid, 324–325
  physician addiction, 553–554
Personalized medicine, 1023
Person-centered care, 630
Person-centered language, 762
Person-centered treatment planning, 659
Perspective, linked services and, 740–741, 741*t*
PET. *See* Positron emission tomography
Peyote, 274
Peyotism, 630
PFC. *See* Prefrontal cortex
pH, nicotine, 232
Pharmacodynamics, 137–142, 186–187
  dose-response and dose-receptor-bound graphs, 137, 137*f*
  drug potency, 137–138
  efficacy, 137–138
  graded dose-response graph, 137–138, 137*f*
  log drug concentration, 137, 137*f*
  lysergic acid diethylamide, 279–280
  median effective dose, 138
  median toxic dose, 138
  mescaline, 282
  3,4-methylenedioxy-N-methylamphetamine, 283–284
  N,N-dimethyltryptamine, 281–282
  principles, 137–142
  psilocin, 281
  psilocybin, 281
  salvinorin A, 284
  spare receptors, 137–138, 137*f*
Pharmacogenetics, 142–143
Pharmacogenomics, 142–144
Pharmacokinetic(s), 183–186, 952
  and brain, 136
  lysergic acid diethylamide, 279
  measures, 57
  mescaline, 282
  3,4-methylenedioxy-N-methylamphetamine, 283
  N,N-dimethyltryptamine, 281
  and pregnancy, 136–137
  principles, 129–147
  psilocin, 280–281
  psilocybin, 280–281
  Salvinorin A, 284
  tolerance, 142
Pharmacologic interventions
  drug addiction, 15–17, 15*t*
  for SUD and TBI, 694–695
Pharmacologic therapies, substance use disorders, 604–605
Pharmacology, 961–962
Pharmacotherapy
  AaLD, 1360
  for alcohol use disorder, 946–960
  college student drinking, 444
  compulsive sexual behavior disorder
    antidepressants, 837
    hormonal therapies, 838
    opioid antagonists, 838
    selective serotonin reuptake inhibitors, 837–838
  of co-occurring PTSD-SUD, 1669–1670
  gambling disorder, 818–820
  insomnia, 1465*t*, 1475–1477
  office-based opioid therapy, 999–1000, 1003, 1006
  in pregnancy, 1516–1517
  pregnant and postpartum individual, substance use disorder treatment in, 1519–1521
  for PTSD, 1668–1670
  restless legs syndrome, 1465*t*, 1477
  TMS and, 1069
Pharmacotherapy, adolescent SUDs
  alcohol
    acamprosate, 1874
    acute ingestion and withdrawal, 1873–1874
    baclofen, 1874
    disulfiram, 1874
    5-HT_3 receptor antagonist ondansetron, 1874
    naltrexone, 1874
    topiramate, 1874
  cannabis, 1874–1875
    acute ingestion and withdrawal, 1874–1875
    emerging therapies, 1875
    N-acetyl cysteine, 1875
    topiramate, 1875
  clinical considerations, 1878–1879
  cocaine and methamphetamine, 1877–1878
    acute ingestion and withdrawal management, 1877

bupropion and extended-release naltrexone, 1878
cocaine use disorder, 1877–1878
mirtazapine, 1878
psychostimulants, 1878
future directions, 1879
opioids, 1875–1877
acute ingestion and withdrawal management, 1876
buprenorphine, 1876
methadone, 1876–1877
naltrexone, 1876
psychosocial treatments, 1878
tobacco/nicotine, 1871–1873
bupropion, 1872–1873
nicotine replacement therapy, 1872
varenicline, 1873
Phase IV clinical trials, 50
Phencyclidine (PCP), 293, 931–932, 1046, 1424, 1428
with cocaine or cannabis, combination, 1046
dissociatives and psychosis, 1609
epidemiology, 295
historical features, 294–295
medical commercial preparation, 294
neurobehavioral and cognitive disorders, 1426
neurobiology, 300
pharmacodynamics, 297–298, 299*t*, 299*f*
pharmacokinetics, 296–297
seizures, 1428
stroke, 1432
substance-induced mental disorders, 1550
Phenethylamine stimulant drugs, chemical structures of, 193*f*
Phenethylamines, 1610
Phenibut
clinical implications, 360
history, 360
legal status, 360
pharmacology, 360
Phenobarbital, 1517–1518
CYP3A4 inducers and, 135
induction and taper protocol, 900–901
sedative–hypnotics withdrawal, 965
urine alkalization, 901
Phenothiazine, 1614
Phentermine, norepinephrine, 207
Phenylephrine, 195–196
Phenylpropanolamine, 196, 201–202, 205
Phenytoin, 879–880
pain, 1750–1751
Phosphate, 1378
Phosphatidyl ethanol (PEth), 519–520, 1966
Phosphatidylinositol 3-kinase (PI3K), 254
PHPs. *See* Physician health programs
Physical availability, 109–110
Physical dependence, 142
definition of, 962
drug dependence *vs.* drug addiction, 2
opioids, 1764–1765
substance use disorders, 1697
Physical health, effects of
adverse health effects, 224
health protective effects, 224–225
Physical restraints, 1603
substance use disorder with co-occurring psychosis, 1613
Physical therapy (PT)
aquatic therapy, 1737
cold therapy, 1742
heat therapy, 1740–1742
hot packs, 1740–1741
ultrasound, 1741–1742
lumbar and cervical stabilization, 1737–1738
mechanical diagnosis and therapy, 1738
passive, 1740–1742
stretching techniques, 1736–1737
Physical violence, in women, 645–646
Physician(s)
for addiction, 529–530
brief advice, adolescents, 1811
diversion programs, 561
smokers and, 1146
support, group therapies and, 1101–1102
Physician addiction, 552, 553*t*
age distribution, 552
anesthesiologists, 552, 553*t*
assessment, components of, 559
comorbidity, 557
co-occurring conditions, 557
drug access, 554–555
identification of, 557–558, 558*t*
as patients, clinical considerations with, 559–560
personality profiles, 553–554
physician health programs, 551–578
prevalence, 551
risk factors, 553–555
theories of, 553
treatment, 559–561
characteristics of, 560–561
Physician health programs (PHPs)
education and outreach, 566
function, 562–563, 563*t*
history, 561–562
outcome data, 565–566
physician addiction and, 551–578
pre-monitoring activities, 563
recovery monitoring, 563–564
recovery support, 564
return to use, 564–565
return to work, 565
structure, 562
Physician–patient relationship
alexithymia, 560
beneficence, 1898
Phytocannabinoids, 250
Piperazines, 1610
Pittsburgh Sleep Quality Index, 1728
Placement criteria
uses of, 733
validation of, ASAM criteria, 1848–1849
Plan-Do-Study-Act cycle, 67
Planned interventions, 1074, 1076
Planning, motivational interviewing processes, 1086–1087
Plant alkaloids, 191
Plant food, 357
Plant-based psychedelic compounds, 1055
Plant-derived stimulants, 191–194
Plasma pharmacokinetics, 57
Plasma pseudocholinesterase, 1369
PLMS. *See* Periodic limb movements of sleep
Pneumococcal vaccination, 1319
Pneumonia, 1409–1410
Pneumothorax, 1405–1406
Pocket vaporizers, 349–350
Pod e-cigarettes, 337–338
Point Subtraction Aggression Paradigm, ASS, 326–327
Point-prevalence abstinence rates, posttreatment follow-up, 1135, 1136*f*
Policy and leadership, 453–470
alcohol use, 456–457
COVID-19 pandemic, 461
global health, 461
historical perspectives, 453–455
Oxford House (OH) model, 460–461
potential legal issues, 457
tobacco use, 457–459
Policy studies, efficacy trials and, 401–403
Polyarteritis, 1383
Polyethylene oxide (PEO) coating, 1381
Polymicrobial endocarditis, 1344–1345
Polymicrobial infections, 1344–1345
Polymorphisms (alleles), addiction and, 11
Polysubstance, sedative–hypnotic use, 900
Polysubstance use, 1402
Poppers, 308
LGBTQ, 670–671
Population(s). *See also* Special populations; Substance using populations
alcoholics anonymous subgroups, 1292–1295
alcoholics anonymous studies, 1290
Population Assessment of Tobacco and Health (PATH) dataset, 369–370
Population-based simulation modeling, 99–100
Portopulmonary hypertension, 1410
Positive allosteric modulator, 140
Positive Quick Screen, 475, 475*t*
Positive screen, 477
Positron emission tomography (PET)
ADHD, 1628
dopamine, TMS on, 1066–1067
drug addiction, 42
Post-acute withdrawal syndrome, 892
Postconcussion syndrome (PCS), 686
Postdeployment alcohol, 1206–1207
Postinfectious glomerulonephritis, 1380–1381
Postpartum care, pregnancy, substance use during, 1523–1524
Post-substance use observation programs, 429
Post-synaptic Gq/11-coupled receptors, 254–255
Posttraumatic amnesia (PTA), 686
Posttraumatic Diagnostic Scale for DSM-5, 1663
Post-traumatic stress disorder (PTSD), 625, 1708, 1711
cannabis, 1944
cognitive-behavioral therapies for, 1664
anxiety management therapy, 1665–1666
cognitive-focused therapy, 1665
for co-occurring PTSD-SUD, 1666–1668
effectiveness of, 1666
exposure-based therapy, 1664–1665
integrated treatment models, 1667
comorbid SUDs, adolescents, 1887–1888
epidemiology, 1659–1660
fibromyalgia, 1696

Post-traumatic stress disorder (PTSD) (*Continued*)
  interviewer-rated assessment of, 1662–1663
    Clinician-Administered PTSD Scale for DSM-5 (CAPS-5), 1662
    Composite International Diagnostic Interview (CIDI), 1663
    MINI, 1662
    Posttraumatic Diagnostic Scale for DSM-5, 1663
    PTSD Checklist for DSM-5, 1663
    PTSD Symptom Scale—Interview for DSM-5 (PSSI-5), 1662
    Structured Clinical Interview for DSM-5 Disorders (SCID), 1662
  limbic system and, 1697
  military occupational stressors and sexual trauma, 1206–1207
  military sexual trauma, 681–682
  pharmacotherapy for, 1668–1670
  phenomenology, 1658–1659
  physician addiction, 557
  prevalence and prognostic effects, 1566
  prevalence, co-occurring, 1660
  relapse prevention and, 1231
  self-report assessment of, 1663
  substance use disorders (SUD)
    assessment of, 1661–1663
    etiological relationship, 1660
    neurobiological factors, 1660–1661
  substance-induced anxiety disorder, 1547, 1555
  treatment of, 1663–1670
  in women, 639–640
Post-treatment abstinence, aversion therapy and, 1192–1193
Postural tremor, 1434
Potassium and calcium selective ion channels, alcohol and, 155
Practical needs assessment questionnaire, 1130*t*. *See also* Beck Depression Inventory
Pragmatism, TSF and, 1214
Prazepam, addiction liability, 170–171
Precontemplation stage, processes in, 1074, 1076
Preexposure prophylaxis (PrEP), 1456
Prefrontal cortex (PFC), 1065–1066, 1627–1628
  regions of, 37
Pregabalin, 952
  generalized anxiety disorder, 1592–1593
  McGill Pain Questionnaire, 1751
  neuropathic pain, 1751
Pregnancy
  alcohol abuse
    brief intervention, 498–501
    conclusions and recommendations, 501–502
    screening for, 496–498
  alcohol and other drug use, 159
  benzodiazepines, 172
    withdrawal and, 896
  detoxification and, 864–865
  hepatitis C virus, 1368
  opioid use disorder
    nonprescribed opioids during, 979–980
    opioid agonist treatment, 979–981
  with opioid use disorder, 647
  population-specific considerations for, 1207–1208
  screening and brief intervention for, 496*b*
  substance use during, 1509–1524
    alcohol and sedatives, 1514–1516
    breastfeeding, 1522
    cannabis, 1518
    labor and delivery, 1521
    legal issues, 1522–1523
    neonatal abstinence syndromes, 1512–1513
    opioids, 1516–1518
    postpartum care, 1523–1524
    pregnant people, approach to, 1509–1510
    screening, 1510–1512
    stimulants, 1518–1519
    teratogenicity, 1512
    tobacco, 1513–1514
    treatment and postpartum individual, 1519–1521, 1520*t*, 1521*f*
  substance-abusing teenagers, 1841
  T-ACE questionnaire, drinking and, 497
  testing, opioid withdrawal, 917–918
  tobacco and, 243–244
Premarket tobacco product application (PMTA), 350
Premature termination, 1077, 1077*f*
Prenatal alcohol exposure (PAE), 1514
  pregnancy, substance use during, 1514–1516
  in women, 637
Prenatal care, routine office visits for, 1511
Prenatal education, 1511
Preparation stage, 1075, 1078
  smokers and, 1148
Prescription drug monitoring programs (PDMPs), 415–417, 775–776, 1806, 1913, 1930, 1935
Prescription drug use disorders, prevalence of, 410
Prescription Drug Use Questionnaire (PDUQ), 1729
Prescription drugs, in older adults, 653–654
Prescription medications
  challenges, 1914–1915
  ethical considerations, 1921–1924
    aberrant medication-taking behaviors, 1922–1923
    cognitive impairment and disordered impulse control, 1923
    disagreements, 1921–1922
    discontinuing prescribing or "firing", 1923
    illegal medication-related behavior, 1923–1924
    professionalism, collaboration, bias, 1921
    treatment agreements, 1922
  factors contributing, 1911–1915
  guidelines, regulations and other resources, 1915, 1916*t*
  misuse, prevention of
    classes, 411–414
    co-occurrence with other substance and psychiatric disorders, 411
    deterrent formulations, 417
    drug monitoring programs, 417
    epidemiology, 410–411
    evidence-based treatment, 418–419
    harm reduction policies, 417
    healthcare utilization, 410
    historical perspective, 409–410
    HIV prevention and treatment, 418
    naloxone, 417–418
    prescriber education, 415–417
    prevalence of, 410
    prevention programs, 414
    research, 419
    syringe services programs, 418
    take-back programs, 414–415
  opioids, 999
    misuse, SBI for, 481–482
  special precautions with, 1918
  vs. SUDs, 1913–1914
  universal precautions, 1915–1921
Prescription opioids, aversion therapies, 1193–1194
Prescription order, executing, 1925
President's Emergency Plan for AIDS Relief (PEPFAR), 461
Pretherapy stage, 1077*f*
Pretreatment issues, 1130–1131, 1215–1216
Prevention of HIV infection (PrEP), 1319
Prevention programs
  adolescents, 390
  benzodiazepines dependence, 904
  environmental strategies
    California 24 cities project, 403
    CMCA project, 403
    Community Trials (CT) project, 402
    domains of, 401
    educational programs, 401–402
    implementation science, 405
    versus individual approaches, 400–401
    medical professionals, 405
    Oregon Reducing Youth Access to Alcohol Project, 402–403
    Safer California Universities Project, 402
    SNAPP, 402
    social ecology, of alcohol use, 403–404, 404*f*
    Southwest California Indians Project, 403
    Stockholm Prevents Alcohol and Drug problems, 402
    Study to Prevent Alcohol-Related Consequences, 403
    substance addiction, environmental approaches, 399–407
  substance use, children and adolescents, 390–398
Preventive counseling, medical care of patients, with unhealthy substance use, 1318
Pricing, of cannabis, 123
Prilocaine and lidocaine. *See* Eutectic mixture of local anesthetics (EMLA)
Primary analgesics, 1747
Primary angioplasty, 1342–1343
Primary care, 740
  assessment needs and tools, 528, 529*t*
  clinicians, 774–776
  depression, 1577–1578
  disease management and, 744
  linked services and, 740–741, 741*t*
  populations
    addiction and, 1589–1590
    eating disorders, 1680–1681
  and psychiatric populations, 1567
  screening and brief intervention in
    alcohol use, 484
    Project Health, 484
  therapists, 1165

Primary care physicians (PCPs), 759
Primary care providers (PCPs), 1811
Primary mood disorder, 1567, 1569*t*
Primary psychotic disorder (PPD), 1547
  with co-occurring substance use disorder, 1602–1603
Principles, confidentiality *vs.*
  employer *vs.* employee, 1908–1909
  society *vs.* patient, 1909
PRISM. *See* Psychiatric Research Interview for Substance and Mental Disorders (PRISM)
Prison system, 750
  therapeutic communities, 1178
Prison-based treatment
  programs, 600
  women and, 648
Privacy, safety *vs.* physician addiction, 566–567
Problem gambling, 812, 815
Problem Oriented Screening Instrument for Teenagers, 1835
Problematic internet use (PIU), 796–798
  definition and conceptualization, 796
  epidemiology, 797
  neurobiology
    genetics, 796
    neurochemistry, 797
    neurocircuitry and structure, 797
    neurocognition, 797
  treatment, 798
Problematic sexual behaviors (PSB). *See also* Compulsive sexual behavior disorder (CSBD)
  assessment, 834, 835*t*
  behavioral approaches, 836
  cognitive behavioral therapy, 836–837
  contingency management, 836
  psychoanalysis, 837
  12-step and self-help groups, 837
  treatment approaches, 834
Problem-focused interviews, adolescents, 1836
Problem-solving groups, group therapy, 1095
Process groups, 1095
Process improvement, NIATx model, 771–773
  Agency change, 772
  change leader, 772
  customer understanding, 772
  PDSA cycles, 773
  seek outside ideas and encouragement, 772–773
"Process" or "behavioral" addictions, 64
Process, principles in, 1079–1081
Pro-erectile drugs, LGBTQ, 672
Professional health monitoring programs (PHPs), 545
Professional Standards or Codes of Ethics, ethical issues in, 1902
Professionalism, ethical considerations, prescribing medications with, 1921
Progress, in therapy, 1078
Progressive liver fibrosis, 1357
Project COMBINE, 1265
Project Health, primary care and, SBI in, 484
Project MATCH, 1122, 1215, 1222, 1293, 1615
  alcoholics anonymous, 1296–1297, 1301
  population subgroups and, 1293
Project TrEAT
  older adults, 486–487
  primary care and, SBI in, 484
Prolapse, 1219–1220
Prolonged Exposure therapy (PE), 1664
Prolonged psychiatric sequelae, 932–934, 933*t*
Prolonged QT, opioids, cardiovascular disorders, 1345
PROMIS Pain Interference, 774
Propofol
  anesthesiologists, 556
  physician addiction, 556
Propoxyphene, overdose, 187
Propranolol
  anxiety and tremors, 903–904
  benzodiazepine withdrawal, 902–903
  for PTSD, 1669
Propylene glycol, electronic drug delivery devices, 338
Propylene oxide, 1340–1341
Prostate cancer screening, 1317–1318
Protein(s), 152
Protein restriction, 1360
Proteinuria, 1377
Protracted abstinence syndrome, 913, 965–966
Protracted withdrawal symptoms, sedative–hypnotics withdrawal, 965–966
Provider Clinical Support System (PCSS) guidance, 982
Provider's Clinical Support System for Medication Assisted Treatment (PCSS-MAT), 775
Pseudoaddiction, 1768
Pseudoephedrine, 192
Pseudowithdrawal, benzodiazepines and, 892
Psilocin
  pharmacodynamics, 281
  pharmacokinetics, 280–281
Psilocybin, 1423
  neurobehavioral and cognitive disorders, 1426
  pharmacodynamics, 281
  pharmacokinetics, 280–281
  seizures, 1428
  stroke, 1432
PSTD. *See* Posttraumatic stress disorder
Psychedelic drugs, 1330–1331
Psychedelics, 953, 1608. *See also* Hallucinogens
  anesthesiologists, 552
  seizures, 1428
  stroke, 1432
Psychiatric and cognitive conditions, 726
Psychiatric comorbidity
  co-occurring disorders and, group therapies for, 1096*t*
  detoxification and, 862
  gambling disorder, 814–815
Psychiatric disorders. *See also specific i.e. mood disorders*
  coexisting, 1285
  co-occurring disorders, 1103
  eating disorders, 1680
  inhalants, 313
Psychiatric populations
  tobacco use disorder, 1154–1155
    addressing and co-occurring tobacco and psychiatric problems, 1155
Psychiatric problems, addressing and co-occurring, 1155
Psychiatric Research Interview for Substance and Mental Disorders (PRISM), 1560, 1569–1570, 1569*t*
Psychiatric scales, 56–57
Psychiatric treatment populations, primary care and, 1567
Psychiatric treatment systems, addiction treatment and, linking, 740–757
Psychiatry, 585
Psychiatry consult liaison services, 536
Psychoactive drugs
  absorption, 129–130
  distribution, 130–131
Psychoactive herbs, 937–940, 938*t*–939*t*
Psychoactive substance abuse, socialization into, 633
Psychoanalysis, problematic sexual behaviors, 837
Psychoeducation, 1202, 1664, 1718
Psychoeducational recovery groups, 1095
Psychogenic pain, 1714, 1716
Psychological dysfunction, 1175
Psychological factors, biopsychosocial model, 1199
Psychological modulation, 1709–1710
  developmental issues, 1716
  stages of, 1692–1693
  threshold, OIH, 1701–1702
  tolerance, OIH, 1701–1702
Psychological support, benzodiazepine cessation, 898
Psychological variables, alcoholics anonymous, 1301–1302
Psychomotor effects, 257–258
Psychopathology, model of, 1308–1309
Psychosis, 1601
  effects of cannabis, 258–259
  substance-induced psychosis, 1605–1606
Psychosocial evaluation, 1360
Psychosocial interventions, stimulants and, anxiety disorders and, 1597
Psychosocial therapies, 709
Psychosomatic concepts, evaluation of, 1696
Psychostimulants, 38–40, 1396
  attention deficit hyperactivity disorder, 1631
  cocaine and methamphetamine, adolescent SUDs, 1878
  cognition, 1425
  sites of action, 38–39
Psychoterratic syndromes, 76–77
  climate change and, 84
Psychotherapeutic support, benzodiazepine cessation, 898
Psychotherapy, 1682
  binge eating disorder, 1684–1685
  substance use disorders, 602–603
PTSD Checklist for DSM-5 (PCL-5), 1663
PTSD Symptom Scale—Interview for DSM-5 (PSSI-5), 1662
Public health approach, 66
  alcohol and, 399
  tobacco use and, 1143
Public Health Emergency, 1258
Public health policy, alcohol research, 113
Public policy intervention, climate change and, 85
Pueraria lobata, 1054–1055
Pugh classifications, 1533, 1533*t*

Pulmonary disease complications, electronic drug delivery devices, 346
Pulmonary disorders
  substance use, 1402–1415
    airway pathophysiology, 1403–1404
    central nervous system and respiratory drive, 1402
    pulmonary immune function, 1404–1405, 1404*f*
    pulmonary pathophysiology and immunology of, 1402–1405
    pulmonary vasculature, 1405
    respiratory system complications and diseases associated with, 1403*t*
Pulmonary edema, 1410–1411
  stimulant use, 1413
Pulmonary effects
  substance use, 1405–1415
    acute and chronic unhealthy alcohol use, 1408–1410
    sedative-hypnotics, 1413–1414
    smoked (combusted) substance use, 1405–1407
    stimulant use, 1412–1413
    unhealthy opioid use and injection drug use, 1410–1412
    "vaping" and electronic cigarettes, 1407–1408
Pulmonary emphysema, 1405
Pulmonary function tests, 1411
Pulmonary hypertension, 1406
  stimulant use, 1412–1413
  unhealthy opioid use, 1411–1412
Pulmonary immune function, substance use, pulmonary pathophysiology and immunology of, 1404–1405
Pulmonary Langerhans cell histiocytosis, 1406
Pulmonary microvascular vasodilation, 1410
Pulmonary system
  adverse effects, stimulants, 203
  cannabinoids and, 260
  tobacco smoke, 243
Pulmonary vasculature, 1405
Punishment, aversion therapy *vs.*, 1189
Punitive policies, 761
Pure Food and Drug Act, 92
Purkinje cells, 1434
P2Y12 receptor, 1342
Pyramiding, AAS, 323–324

Q

QALYs. *See* Quality-adjusted life-year (QALY)
Quality chasm series, 751
Quality of life, 1658
  gambling disorder, 814
  measurement, 57
  opioid therapy, 1770
Quality-adjusted life-year (QALY), 483, 1252
Quantification of substance use, 55–56
Quasi-medical use of opium, 1928
Quasi–office-based approach, 1006
Quazepam, addiction liability, 170–171
Quick Screen, NIDA, SBI, 475, 475*t*
Quitting smoking, 1146, 1150

R

Race/racism
  in addiction, 622
  definitions and concepts, 622
  drug/alcohol use disorders, 373–374
  levels of, 622
  nicotine metabolism and, 230
  physician addiction, 552
  as social determinant of health, 621–622
  systemic, 622
Racial and ethnic minorities
  Black and African Americans, 1152–1153
  Hispanics/Latinos, 1153
  Indigenous American, 1153
Racial inequities of care reduction, 763, 764*t*
Racial subgroups, AA, 1293
RAFFT (Relax, Along, Friends, Family, Trouble), 1728–1729
Randomized controlled trials (RCTs), 51
  alcoholics anonymous, 1295–1297
Rapid eye movement (REM)
  alcohol recovery, sleep during, 1470
  sleep architecture, 1464
Rapid-cycling bipolar disorders, 1570–1571
Rate hypothesis, 129
Rate of increase, opioids, 1766–1767, 1766*f*
RCTs. *See* Randomized controlled trials
Reactive hypoglycemia, 1490
Readiness and resources, 726
Readiness to Change, dimension 4, ASAM, 1842–1843
Rebound, benzodiazepines and, 892
Receptor(s), 138–140
  drugs of abuse, 138, 139*t*
  historical perspective, 138
  physical dependence, 142
  receptor-effector linkage, 138*f*
    desensitization, 142
    G proteins and second messenger, 139–140
    with intrinsic enzyme activity, 140
    ligand-gated ion channels, 138–139
    nuclear transcription, 140
  regulating nuclear transcription, 140
  tolerance and sensitization, 142
Receptor-effector linkage, types, 138, 138*f*
Receptor-effector system, 138–140, 138*f*
Recombinant human growth hormone, 318
Recovery, 1097–1098, 1220, 1616–1617
  biopsychosocial model, 1198–1208
    biological factors, 1199
    cultural factors, 1200
    psychological factors, 1199
    social factors, 1199–1200
  capital, 1309
  conceptualizing addiction, 1308–1309
  eating disorders, 1685
  family recovery, 1099
  groups, issues addressed, 1094, 1096*t*
  issues in, BPD/SUD, 1685–1686
  living environment, dimension 6, ASAM, 1843–1844
  neurobiology, 1310–1311
  nicotine anonymous, 1283
  pain and, 1765
  physician addiction, 567–568
  process, spirituality and, 1308–1311
  rates, eating disorders, 1685
  rehabilitation and, 1308–1309
  social network, RP and, 1228–1229
  supports for, physician addiction, 564
  twelve step programs, 1279–1287
Recovery Attitude and Treatment Evaluator (RAATE), 533
Recovery capital (RC), 774, 1309
Recovery coaches, 599
Recovery environment, 453, 726
Recovery Research, 1256
Recreational cannabis, legalization of, 119
Recruitment, 1076–1077
Re-entry modified TC (RMTC), 1184
Refeeding treatment, anorexia nervosa, 1682
Reference method, 515
Referral management and care coordination for older adult with unhealthy substance use, 660*t*
Reflections, 1086
Reflex sympathetic dystrophy (RSD), 1697
Regulation, 1800
Regulatory considerations, pain management, 1800
Rehabilitation
  addiction treatment, 1166
  pain management, 1734
    active physical therapy, 1736–1739
    acute and chronic pain conditions, 1740–1744
    occupational therapy, 1739
    psychological interventions, 1739–1740, 1740*t*
  recovery and, 1308–1309
  substance abuse, 861–862
Reinforcement aversion treatments, 1194
Reinforcement contingencies, substance dependence and, 1113
Relapse, 1006, 1219–1220
  alcoholics anonymous, 1302
  alcohol-sensitizing agents, 950–951
  aversion therapy, 1192
  determinants of, 1223–1226
  dimension 5, ASAM, 1843
  early, reasons, 1081
  expectancy and, 1224
  rates, treatment outcomes and, 1220–1221
  risk, clinical RP interventions, 1227–1231
  smoking and, 1151
Relapse prevention (RP)
  clinical models, intervention strategies, 1219–1231
  comorbid psychiatric disorders, 1231
  co-occurring disorders and, 1231
  effectiveness and efficacy of, 1221–1223
  models of, 1226–1231
  strategies, 1219–1231
  substance use disorders, 1219
Relapse Replication Extension Project (RREP), 1223
Relative risk (RR), 367
  of stroke, 1430
Relatives, treatment-resistant persons and, 1139–1140

Relax, Along, Friends, Family, Trouble (RAFFT), 1728–1729
Releasers, 204
REM. *See* Rapid eye movement
Remifentanil
anaesthesiologists, 555
opioid-induced hyperalgesia, 1702
Renal
cannabinoids, 1331
opioids, 1330
tobacco use, complications related to, 1327
Renal clinical syndromes, 1376–1377
Renal diseases
alcohol, 1377–1379
hepatorenal syndrome and cirrhosis associated diseases, 1378
toxic alcohols, 1378–1379
alcohol use and, 203
cannabinoids, 1384
inhalants, 1384
injection drug use-related renal disease
nephritic syndromes associated with injection drug use, 1380–1381
nephritic-nephrotic syndromes associated with injection drug use, 1380
nephrotic syndromes associated with injection drug use, 1379–1380
ketamine, 1384
opioids, 1377*t*, 1381
prescription opioids, injection use of, 1381
rhabdomyolysis, 1381
urologic effects of, 1381
stimulants, 1381–1383
amphetamines, 1383
cathinones, 1383
cocaine, 1381–1383
MDMA, 1383
stimulants, renal and metabolic effects of, 1382
substance use, 1376–1385
tobacco use, 1384
Renal diseases, detoxification and, 865
Renal function, measurement of, 1376–1377
Renal syndromes, 1377*t*
drugs and alcohol, 1377*t*
Reperfusion therapy, 1342–1343
Repetitive TMS (rTMS), 1066
Reporting results, in journal article, 59
Reproductive consequences
alcohol, 1492–1493
tobacco, 1494
Research. *See also specific i.e. association of medical education and research in substance abuse*
alcohol treatment, 499
alcoholics anonymous, 1290–1291
ASAM, 733–734
aversion therapies, 1192–1193
chemicals, 357
office-based opioid treatment, 1001–1008, 1002*t*
studies, addiction-related, 1297
twelve step programs, 1289–1303
reSET-O, 1252
Residential aftercare models, modified therapeutic communities, 1186
Residential interventions, 1185*t*
Residential programs, 598–600
Residential treatment programs, adolescent substance abuse, ASAM, 1845–1847
Resource-intensive intervention models, 745
Respiratory
alcohol use, medical complications related to, 1325
cannabinoids, complications, 1330
opioids, stimulants, 1329
tobacco use, complications related to, 1327–1328
Respiratory alkalosis, 1409
Respiratory automaticity, 1402
Respiratory bronchiolitis-associated ILD (RB-ILD), 1406
Respiratory depression
alcohol intoxication, 869
opioids medical complications, 1774–1775
sedative–hypnotics intoxication, 961–963
Respiratory drive
substance use, pulmonary pathophysiology and immunology of, 1402
Respiratory impairment, 1402
Respiratory infections, 1448–1450
COVID, 1449
epidemiology and pathogenesis, 1449
influenza, 1450
pneumonia, 1449
tuberculosis, 1449–1450
Respiratory tract, 1402
cannabis smoking, 260
Response elements, 140
Responsible beverage service (RBS) programs, 400–401
Restless legs syndrome (RLS), 1465–1466, 1465*t*, 1477
Restructuring reward processes, mindfulness-based treatment of addiction, 1239–1240, 1240*f*, 1241*f*
Retention, substance abuse in women, 1077–1078, 1077*f*
Retrograde endocannabinoid-mediated synaptic plasticity, 254–255
Reverse anorexia, anabolic androgenic steroids, 324–325, 329
Reversible cerebral vasoconstriction syndrome (RCVS), 1431
Revix. *See* Nalmefene
Reward(s)
interference of pain, 1767
opioids
factors affecting, 1766–1767
mechanisms of, 1766
oxycodone effects, 1766–1767
Reward Cycle, 1766–1767
Reward pathways
anabolic–androgenic steroids, 327–328
dopamine depletion and, 1698
Reward sensitivity pathway, 1645
Rhabdomyolysis, 926, 1368–1369, 1381–1383
Rhynchophylline, structure of, 1054, 1054*f*
Rifampin, 1450
Rifapentine, 1450
Righting reflex, 1085–1086
Riluzole, amphetamine-type stimulants use disorder, 1021
Risk assessment
suicide, 1728–1729
mental health screening, 1728
screening tools for, 1729
sleep disturbance, 1728
Risk Evaluation and Mitigation Strategies (REMS), 1803, 1930
Risperidone, psychosis, 1611
Ritanserin, stimulant use disorders, 1017
RLS. *See* Restless legs syndrome
Roid rage, 326
Roman Catholicism, substance use and, 630
Roofies. *See* Flunitrazepam
Routine office visits, for prenatal care, 1511
Roux-en-Y gastric bypass, 1683–1684
RREP. *See* Relapse Replication Extension Project
RSD. *See* Reflex sympathetic dystrophy
RTV. *See* Ritonavir
Rush, B., 580–581
Rush feeling, 42–43, 308
Ryan Haight Online Pharmacy Consumer Protection Act of 2008, 1258

S

SAD. *See* Social anxiety disorder (SAD)
SADD (Students Against Destructive Decisions), 1817
SAEs (serious adverse events), 58
Safer California Universities Project, 402
Safety, privacy *vs.* physician addiction, 566–567
Saint John's wort, methadone and, 135
Salience, 9–10
Saliva testing, adolescent drug use, 1834
Salvia divinorum, 284, 1551, 1610–1611
Salvinorin A, 284
pharmacodynamics, 284
pharmacokinetics, 284
SAM. *See* American Society of Addiction Medicine
SAMHSA (Substance Abuse and Mental Health Services Administration), 518, 691, 769, 771, 781, 1114
SAMHSA Treatment Improvement Protocol (TIP), 658
SAMHSA's Drug Abuse Warning Network, 119
Saquinavir, CYP3A4, 135
Sativex® (nabiximols), 251
Savoring technique, 1240
SBI. *See* Screening and brief intervention (SBI)
S2BI (Screening to Brief Intervention), 1812–1814
SBIRT (Screening, brief intervention, and referral to treatment), 72, 482, 617, 657–658, 691, 1811
brief intervention, 658
screening, 657–658
treatment programs, 658–660
SCAT-3 (Sports Concussion Assessment Tool-V3), 687
Schedule II opioids, prescribing, 1802–1803
Schedule IV, drugs in, 1801
Schedule I-V prescriptions, 1800, 1801*t*
Schema-focused therapy (SFT), 1649–1650
Schizoaffective disorder, psychosis, 1611

Schizophrenia, 1554, 1608–1609, 1616
endocannabinoids and, 258–259
psychiatric comorbidity, 1022
psychosis, 1611
substance abuse and, 1888–1889
substance-induced psychosis, 1602
tobacco addiction, 258–259
Schizotypal PD, 1652
School, adolescents, substance abuse, 369
School-based prevention
adolescents, substance abuse, 392–393
effectiveness of, 393–395
literature, meta-analyses of, adolescents, 393–394
meta-analyses of, adolescents, 393–395
School-based smoking prevention program, 393
SCID-5 (structured clinical interview for DSM-5), 56–57
Science of Behavior Change (SOBC), 1108–1109
Screener and Opioid Assessment for Patients in Pain-Revised (SOAPP-R), 482, 1768
Screener and Opioid Assessment for Patients with Pain (SOAPP), 1717*t*, 1729
Screener and Opioid Assessment for Patients with Pain-Revised (SOAPP-R), 504
Screening
adolescents, 1812–1816
annual visits, 1812
comprehensive assessment, adolescent drug abuse, 1835–1836
comprehensive screens, 1835
co-occurring SUDs, 1590–1591
drugs, differential diagnosis with, 860
goals with in, 496–498
high-risk substance use features, 1818*t*
instrumentation, adolescent drug use, 1835–1836
mild to moderate SUD, 1817
multi-problem screens, 1835
non-alcohol drugs, 1835
positive reinforcement, 1816
pregnancy, substance use during
laboratory testing, 1511–1512
pregnant women, 483
riding/driving risk counseling, 1817
severe SUD, 1817–1818
substance abuse, 473
substance use screens, 1835
unhealthy alcohol and drug use, in older adults
brief interventions, 512
diagnosis, 511–512
epidemiology, 510, 510*t*
screening tools, 511
self-administered screening approaches, 511
unique vulnerabilities, 510–511
validated screen options, 1812–1814
without SUD, 1816–1817
Screening and brief intervention (SBI)
adults
adult alcohol screening, 476–477, 477*t*
brief intervention, alcohol, 477–478
severity, assessment of, 477
alcohol use, individual studies, 487–488
clinical guidelines, 473–480
in clinical settings using quality improvement principles, 506–507
current evidence on, 480–482
employer resources, 548
five A's (Ask, Advise, Assess, Assist, Arrange), 473
illicit drug use, 472
individual studies, 484–487
national recommendations on, 473
in pregnancy, 496*b*
primary care settings, 473–475
severity, assessment of, 477
substance abuse, 472–495
system at reviews of, alcohol use, 482–484
in trauma centers, hospitals, and emergency departments, 504*b*
unhealthy alcohol use, 472–473
unhealthy substance use screening, 475, 475*t*
youth
alcohol screening, 479, 479*t*
assessment questionnaires, 479–480
brief intervention, 480
confidentiality and parental involvement, 478
severity, assessment of, 479, 480*t*
substance use, 478
Screening, brief intervention, and referral to treatment (SBIRT), 774–775
interprofessional practice models, 716
LGBTQ, 673
Screening immunoassay tests, 517–518, 517*t*
Screening methods for adolescents, 1812
Screening Test for At-risk Drinking (STAD), 504
Screening tests, medical care of patients, with unhealthy substance use, 1316–1318, 1316*t*
Screening to Brief Intervention (S2BI), 1862
Screening tools
for adolescent substance use, 1813*t*–1814*t*
to patient assessment, 528, 529*t*
SCS. *See* Sexual Compulsivity Scale; Spinal cord stimulation
SDMs (syringe-dispensing vending machines), 427
Second messenger systems, 139–140
Secondary depression, adolescents, 1886
Secondary gain, as pain, 1715–1716
Secondary hyperalgesia, 1694
Secondary psychopathology model, 1645
Sedative, pregnancy, substance use during, 1514
Sedative–hypnotic agents, 961, 1425. *See also* Sedative-hypnotic withdrawal
addiction liability, 170–171
CNS and, 961
delirium, 872
discontinuation of, signs and symptoms, 890–891, 891*t*
interventions for, 963–966
intoxication syndrome, 869
medical complications, 172–173
pharmacology of, 961–962
uncomplicated withdrawal syndrome, 877
withdrawal
overview, 890
signs and symptoms, 890–891, 891*t*
Sedative–hypnotic intoxication
management, 963
overdose, 889–890
clinical presentation, 889
management, 889–890
and withdrawal, management of, 890–896
Sedative–hypnotic tolerance testing, 891
Sedative–hypnotic use disorder
classes, 962*t*
co-occurring disorders, treatment of, 966
definitions, 962
intoxication and overdose, management of, 963
medications, use of, 962–963
pharmacological interventions for, 961–968
pharmacology, 961–962
withdrawal, 963–966, 963*t*
anticonvulsants, 965
benzodiazepine taper, 964–965
flumazenil, 965
management, 964–965
phenobarbital, 965
protracted withdrawal symptoms, 965–966
treatment setting, 966
Sedative–hypnotic withdrawal
clinical manifestations of, 889, 891*t*
management, 963–966, 963*t*
anticonvulsants, 965
benzodiazepine taper, 964–965
flumazenil, 965
phenobarbital, 965
protracted withdrawal symptoms, 965–966
management of, 890–896
seizures, treatment, 862
syndrome, 890
time-course of, 890, 890*f*
treatment setting, 966
Sedative-hypnotics
multiple, 940
with other drugs, 940
Sedative–hypnotics, 1413–1414
overdose, 889–890, 1414
sleep-disordered breathing, 1414
substance-induced mental disorders, 1549
withdrawal syndromes, 1414
Sedatives, 1370, 1425
Sedatives–tranquilizers, prescription medication misuse, 414
Seeking Safety (SS), 1667, 1669
Seeking Safety, in women, 645
Seizures, 1424–1425, 1427–1429
alcohol, 1427
barbiturates, benzodiazepines, 1427
cannabinoids, 1428
cocaine, amphetamines and MDMA, 1427–1428
dissociative anesthetics, 1428
inhalants, 1428–1429
opioids, 1428
psychedelics, 1428
Selective serotonin reuptake inhibitors (SSRIs), 1750
compulsive sexual behavior disorder, 837–838
panic disorder, 1594

for PTSD, 1668–1669
social anxiety disorder, 1593
stimulant use disorders, 1016
Self-administration heroin, 41
Self-administration studies
drug reinforcement, 38
opioids, 40
Self-awareness, TSF, 1286
Self-deflation, TSF, 1286
Self-efficacy
for alcohol-related situations, 533
helplessness, pain, 1713
relapse and, 1224
Self-examination, physician-patient, 560
Self-governance, 1286
Self-guided recovery, physician addiction, 567–568
Self-harm
alcohol and, 1483
other drug use and, 1484
Self-help and mutual self-help, 1176
Self-help groups, 1222
smoking cessation, 1149
Self-help RP interventions, 1222
Self-induced disease, 1360
Self-liberation, pre-contemplation stage and, 1081
Self-management approaches, 1220
Self-medication, psychosis, 1612
Self-monitoring, smoking behavior, 1150–1151
Self-re-evaluation, pre-contemplation stage and, 1080–1081
Self-report assessment
adolescent drug use, 1834
posttraumatic stress disorder (PTSD), 1663
validity and alternatives, adolescent drug use, 1834
Self-report instruments, 532
Semistructured drug history interview, 1130*t*
Sensitization, 1607–1608
addiction liability and, 158
drug and, 142
stimulants and, 209
Sensory axons, pain and, 1693
Separate from hardware (SaMD), 1251
Septic arthritis, 1451–1452
Septic pulmonary emboli, 1411
Sequential Intercept Model (SIM), 1983, 1984*f*
community corrections, 1985
initial court hearings/initial detention, 1984
jail/prison SUD treatment, 1985
jails/courts, 1984
law enforcement, 1983–1984
ReEntry, 1985
specialty courts, 1985
Serenity prayer, AA, 1098
Serotonergic agents
alcohol use disorder, 953
stimulant use disorders, 1017
Serotonergic hallucinogens, 284
Serotonin (5-hydroxytryptamine), 269
alcohol and, 157
binge eating disorder, 802
G proteins receptors, 139
in gambling disorder, 790–791
psychostimulants, 38–39
stimulants, 205*t*, 207–208
Serotonin reuptake inhibitors (SRIs), 954–956
Serotonin syndrome, DXM, 299–300
Serotonin transporter (SERT), 1426
Serotonin-norepinephrine reuptake inhibitors (SNRIs), 1592
for PTSD, 1668–1669
stimulant use disorders, 1016
Sertraline (Zoloft), 955
multicenter trial of, 955
social anxiety disorder, 1593
Sertraline, for PTSD, 1668–1669
Sevoflurane, 308
Sex
alcohol-related liver disease, 1355–1356
benzodiazepine withdrawal and, 896
Sex addiction, 826–827
Sex hormones, LGBTQ, 672–673
Sexual abuse, in women, 645–646
Sexual addiction, 828–830
Sexual and reproductive function, cannabinoids and, 261
Sexual assault, barriers, 681
Sexual behavior, high-risk, ASAM adolescent criteria, 1842
Sexual desires or orientations, 827
Sexual function, stimulants and, 204
Sexual harassment and assaults, 1206
Sexual health/behaviors, military sexual trauma (MST), 682
Sexual orientation
and gender identity minorities, 827–828
and identity, drug/alcohol use disorders, 374–375
racial and cultural backgrounds, 827–828
Sexual performance, 158–159
Sexual transmission, 1364
Sexual trauma, 1206–1207
Sexual violence, 1658–1659
Sexual violence victimization, 1199
Sexually transmitted diseases (STD), 1456–1457
Sexually transmitted infections
alcohol use, medical complications related to, 1325
medical care of patients, with unhealthy substance use, 1317
Short half-life agents, medical complications, 173
Short Michigan Alcoholism Screening Test-Geriatric Version (SMAST-G), 657
Short Opiate Withdrawal Scale, 774
Short Opioid Withdrawal Scale, 913
Short self-report instruments, 532
Short-acting opioids, long-acting opioids *vs.*, 173, 1773
SHS (second hand smoke), 244
Sialosis, 1389
SIFs (supervised injection facilities), 428
Signal transduction, 209
Simple Screening Instrument for Alcohol and Other Drug Abuse, adolescent drug use, 1834
Single Alcohol Screening Question (SASQ), 657
Single Convention on Narcotics Drugs, 1929
Single entity, AA as, 1302–1303
Single-group evaluations, Twelve Step principles, 1297
Situational Confidence Questionnaire (SCQ), 533
Skill groups, 1095
Skills, smoking cessation, 1145–1146
Skin and soft tissue infections (SSTI), 1328–1329
Skin infections, IDUs and, 1445–1446
Skin medical care of patients, with unhealthy substance use, 1315
Skin ulcers
contamination of, 1452
drug users, 1445
IDUs and, 1445
Sleep
alcohol use, 1468–1470
alcohol use, medical complications related to, 1325
architecture, alcohol effects on, 1463–1464
deprivation, 1463
disorders
addiction and, 1698
circadian rhythm disorders, 1467
clinical approaches to, 1474–1475
insomnia, 1466–1467
medical and psychiatric factors, 1467
obstructive sleep apnea, 1466
restless legs syndrome, 1465–1466
understanding, drive/sleep need, 1463
disturbance, 1727–1728
extrinsic factors affecting, 1467
infant assessment, parameters for, 1517*t*
rhythms, 1464
stimulants, 1330
tobacco use, complications related to, 1328
Sleep need, 1463
Sleep-disordered breathing, 1409, 1414
Sleep-related breathing disorders, alcohol and, 1470
Slow release oral morphine, opioid use disorder, 970
Small intestine, gastrointestinal disorders, 1393
SMART (Sequential Multiple Assignment Randomized trial) design, 54–55
peer support, 1256
SMART recovery, 1284, 1865
SMI (severe mental illness), 1075–1077
SMM (standard medical management), 53–54
Smoked cannabis, 1407
Smoked "crack" cocaine and "crystal" methamphetamine, 1407
Smoked opioids, 1407
Smoked (combusted) substance use, 1405–1407
smoked cannabis, 1407
smoked "crack" cocaine and "crystal" methamphetamine, 1407
smoked opioids, 1407
smoked tobacco, 1405–1407
Smoked tobacco, 1405–1407
acute respiratory distress syndrome, 1406–1407
interstitial lung disease, 1406
lung cancer, 1406
obstructive airway disease, 1405–1406
pneumothorax, 1406
pulmonary hypertension and cor pulmonale, 1406
Smokers
abstinence, 1079*f*
host defenses, 1444

Smoking. *See also* Smoking cessation
  behavior, self-monitoring of, 1150–1151
  cardiovascular, 1327
  cardiovascular toxicity, 345
  depression and, 13
  generalized anxiety disorder and, 1595
  immunizations, 1319
  machine tests, 341
  myocardial infarction, 345
  obsessive–compulsive disorder and, 1595
  panic disorder and, 1595
  passive, dyslipidemia, 1494
  physician addiction, 555
  prevention, 393–394
  RP, randomized trials for, 1222
Smoking cannabis, 1449
Smoking cessation
  behavioral interventions in, 1143–1157
  behavioral treatments, choice of, 1148–1149
  benefits, 245, 1033–1034
  follow-up sessions, 1150
  initiating, timing of, 1144
  lifestyle change, 1152
  managing slips, 1152
  motivation, 1150
  preparation for, 1150
  racial and ethnic minorities, 1152–1153
SNAP-25, 1627–1628
SNAPP (Sacramento Neighborhood Alcohol Prevention Project), 402
Snoring, OSA, 1466
SO (significant other), CRA plus vouchers treatment, 1120–1121, 1132, 1138
SOAPP. *See* Screener and Opioid Assessment for Patients with Pain (SOAPP)
SOAPP-R. *See* Screener and Opioid Assessment for Patients in Pain-Revised (SOAPP-R)
Sobriety
  secular organizations for, 1284
  women for, 1284
Social adaptation to technological change, 844–845
Social anxiety disorder (SAD), 1590*t*
  differential diagnosis, 1593
  Mini-International Neuropsychiatric Interview, 1591*t*
  smoking, 1595
  stimulants and, anxiety disorders and, 1597
  treatment, 1593
Social availability, 109–110
Social determinants of health, 66
Social factors
  biopsychosocial model, 1199–1200
  drug/alcohol use disorders, 375–376
Social functioning subdomain, ASAM, 1842
Social justice, 66
  motivational interviewing and, 1089
Social learning, 1176
Social liberation, 1081
Social media, 842–858, 1256
  assessment, 849–850
  epidemiology and comorbidity, 843–845
  historical perspective, 843
  indications for treatment
    morbidity, 852
    mortality, 851–852
  pretreatment issues
    general and stage-specific interventions, 852–853
    interventions, choice and timing, 852
    motivation, 852
    patients/suitability, selection and preparation, 852
    therapist characteristics, 852
  relevant treatment research
    pharmacotherapy and psychologically based treatments, 854–855
    psychologically based treatments, 853–854
  treatment planning, 850–851
    diagnosis, 850–851
    rating scales, 851
Social medicine, 66
Social network, 631–632, 632*t*
  AA and, 1300
  CRA plus vouchers treatment, 1132
  network therapy, 1166
Social organization, therapeutic communities (TC), 1177
Social phobias, comorbid SUDs, adolescents, 1887
Social prescriptions, climate change and, 85
Social resistance skills, adolescents, substance abuse, 393
Social supports
  cessation stage interventions, 1151
  network therapy, 1165
Social-ecological framework of opioid misuse, 68, 69*f*
Society, challenges for, 19–20
Sociocultural interventions, 633
SOCRATES (Stages of Change Readiness and Treatment Eagerness Scale), 532–533, 1130*t*
Sodium valproate, 902
  benzodiazepine withdrawal, 902
Soft-tissue infections, IDUs and, 1445–1446
SOGS. *See* South Oaks Gambling Screen (SOGS)
Solastalgia, definition, 76–77
Soldier's disease, 409
Solvents, 308–309
Some over-the-counter (OTC), 195
South Oaks Gambling Screen, 812–813
Southwest California Indians Project, 403
SPARC (Study to Prevent Alcohol-Related Consequences), 403
Special populations
  CM, 1135–1136
  CRA, 1138–1139, 1139*f*
  detoxification and, 864–866
Specialized Addiction Treatment in Older Adulthood, 659–660
Specialty, physician addiction, 552, 553*t*
Spinal cord injury, 1421
  cannabis treatment, 1943
Spinal cord stimulation, 1720
Spiritual awakening, 1299, 1301, 1309
Spirituality
  AA ingredients and, 1300–1301
  defined, 1308
  neurobiology, 1310–1311
  phenomenon, 1308–1309
  principle, TSF, 1287
  recovery capital, 1309
  recovery process and, 1308–1311
  religious experience and, 1310
  TSF and, 1214
  Twelve-step programs, 1308
  without theism, 1310
Spirometry, 1405
Spironolactone, 318
Spontaneous abortion, 1378
Spontaneous aversions, 1190
Spontaneous bacterial peritonitis (SBP), 1451
Sports Concussion Assessment Tool-V3 (SCAT-3), 687
Spouses, alcohol problems, RP intervention studies and, 1223
Squamous cell carcinoma (SCC), 1393
SRIs. *See* Serotonin reuptake inhibitors (SRIs)
SSPs (syringe service programs), 426–428
SSRIs. *See* Selective serotonin reuptake inhibitors (SSRIs)
Stacking, 323–324
STAD (Stockholm Prevents Alcohol and Drug Problems), 402
Staff facilitates community-as-method, 1177
Stage effect, 1078
Stage 3 pain states, 1695
Stages of change, 1086–1088
  conceptualizing patient change, 1087–1088, 1087*f*
  four processes, 1086–1087, 1086*t*
  model, 1076–1082, 1087
Stages of Change Readiness and Treatment Eagerness Scale (SOCRATES), 1130*t*
Stakeholder marketing (lobbying), cannabis consumption, 123–124
Stand-alone websites, substance use disorders, digital health interventions for, 1252–1255
Standardized questionnaires, intoxication states, 860
Staphylococcus aureus, 1380–1381
State certification, ASAM criteria, 729
State laws, medical information and, 1908
State licensure, ASAM criteria, 729
State-by-trait interaction, 1236–1237
State-controlled substance regulations, 1802
State-level drug use policies, drug/alcohol use disorders, 376
Statistical analysis plans, 52
Status calendar, court-leveraged treatment, 1976
Status epilepticus, 1427
12-step and self-help groups, problematic sexual behaviors, 837
12-step program engagement
  family psychoeducation and, 1202–1203
    bibliotherapy, 1202
    mutual support groups, 1202–1203
    psychoeducation, 1202
12-Step recovery support groups, 662
Stereotypic behavior, 1607–1608
Steroids, 317
Stevens-Johnson syndrome, 204, 1750–1751
Stigma, 537, 624, 1250–1251
  linked services, 742–743
Stimulant(s). *See also* Prescription stimulants
  addiction, RP studies, 1223
  anxiety disorders and, 1597

class of, substances in, 191
clinical uses, 194*t*, 195–196
drug-drug interactions, 199–200
epidemiology, 197–198
history of, 196–197
neurobiology of, mechanisms of action, 204–210, 205*t*, 205*f*
nonmedical use and addiction, 196
pharmacodynamic actions, 200–204
acute stimulant administration, 202
adverse health effects, 200
behavioral pharmacology, 201
cardiovascular system, 202
chronic effects, 201
CNS intoxication, 200–201
endocrine, 203
gastrointestinal system, 203
head and neck, 203–204
immune system, 204
liver, 203
musculoskeletal system, 203
pulmonary, 203
renal system, 203
reproductive, fetal, and neonatal health, 204
sexual function, 204
withdrawal, 201
pharmacokinetics
absorption and distribution, 198
elimination, 199
metabolism of, 199
parameters of oral stimulants, 199*t*
pharmacology of, 191–216
plant-derived, 191–194
prescription medication misuse, 413–414
sleep and, 1470–1471
synthetic, 193*f*, 194–195, 194*t*
Stimulant psychosis, 200
Stimulant tolerance, 210
Stimulant use disorders, 371
acupuncture, 1020
aversion therapies, 1192–1193
concurrent substance use disorders, 1021–1022
medication combinations, 1020
parenteral treatment, 1023
perioperative care, 1539
pharmacodynamic approach, 1023
pharmacological treatment, 1014–1029
behavioral mechanisms, 1015*t*
goals of, 1014
mechanisms, 1015
psychiatric comorbidity, 1022
treatment situations, 1021–1023
Stimulant use, substance use, pulmonary effects of, 1412–1413
administration, consequences of, 1412
diffuse alveolar hemorrhage, 1413
lung function, 1413
parenchymal lung disease, 1413
pulmonary edema, 1413
pulmonary hypertension, 1412–1413
Stimulant-associated acute coronary syndrome, 926
Stimulants, 923–927
amphetamine-type stimulants use disorder, 1020
benefits and risks for, 1912–1913
complications, 1328–1330
intoxication, 923–927, 925*t*
management of medical effects, 926–927
physical effects, 925–926
psychological and behavioral effects, 924–925
and opioids, 1047–1048
pharmacological treatment, 1014–1029
postsynaptic receptors, 924
pregnancy, substance use during, 1518–1519
presynaptic catecholamine reuptake sites, 924
renal and metabolic effects of, 1381–1383
amphetamines, 1383
cathinones, 1383
cocaine, 1381–1383
MDMA, 1383
seizures, 1428
sleep, 1330
and substance-induced depressive disorder, 1546
substance-induced mental disorders, 1550
and tobacco, 1047
withdrawal, 927
management, 927
physical effects, 927
in women, 638
Stimulus conditioning, in rats, 1191
Stimulus control, pre-contemplation stage and, 1081
Stockholm Prevents Alcohol and Drug Problems (STAD), 402
Stomach
gastrointestinal disorders, 1390
alcohol-related gastritis, 1390
peptic ulcer disease, 1390
nicotine and, 232, 1034
Stopping smoking, 1340
Strengths model, 68
for case management, 69, 70*f*
Streptococci, soft-tissue infections, 1445
Stress, 1113–1114
addiction and, 1699
alcohol use disorders, 375
fibromyalgia, 1696
mindfulness-based treatment of addiction, 1240–1242
pain, 1715
physician addiction, 554
Stress Inoculation Training (SIT), 1665–1666
Stress reduction pathway, 1645
Striatal dopamine D_2 receptor binding, 42
Striatum, 1064–1065
Stroke, 1429–1432
alcohol, 1430
alcohol, cardiovascular disorders, 1339
amphetamines, cardiovascular disorders, 1344
cannabinoids, 1432
cocaine, amphetamines, and MDMA, 1430–1432
cocaine, cardiovascular disorders, 1343
dissociative anesthetics, 1432
opioids, 1432
opioids, cardiovascular disorders, 1345
psychedelics, 1432
tobacco and nicotine, 1429–1430
Structural competency in training, inequities of care reduction, 762–763
Structural determinants of care, inequities of care reduction, 758
Structural factors, drug/alcohol use disorders, 376
Structural interventions, college student drinking, 444–446
Structural racism, 622
Structural strategies, inequities of care reduction
advocate for primary prevention, 764
family regulation policies, 764
programmatic, clinical, policy, and research priorities, 764–765
punitive policies, removal of, 763–764
Structural–strategic family therapy, 1864
Structured Assessment and Screening Instrument (SAVRY), 1857
Structured Clinical Interview for DSM-5 Disorders (SCID), 1662
Structured Clinical Interview for DSM-5 Personality Disorders (SCID-5-PD), 1645–1646
Structured Interview of Personality Organization (STIPO), 1645–1646
STTR (seek, test, treat, and retain model of care), 418
Subacute withdrawal, 954–955
Subcultures, 628–629
Subcutaneous drug use–associated amyloidosis, 1380
Subjective Opioid Withdrawal Scale, 913
Subjective/psychological availability, 109–110
Sublingual buprenorphine, 1516, 1796
Substance abuse. *See also* Substance use disorders
eating disorders *vs.*, 1680
screening
and brief intervention, 472–495
national recommendation, 473
treatment, 1143
Substance Abuse and Mental Health Services Administration (SAMHSA), 653, 691, 713–714, 1075, 1205, 1548–1549, 1616, 1729
Facility Locator, 635
telehealth, 1255
treatment services, 1817–1818
Substance Dependence Posttraumatic Stress Disorder Therapy (SDPT), 1667
Substance intoxication, 1569–1571
Substance use. *See also* Substance use disorders
adolescents
prevalence rates and progression, 390–391
prevention, 390–398
BIPOC and minority groups, 1982
cardiovascular disorders, 1335–1346
alcohol, 1335–1339
alcohol and drugs, 1336*t*
amphetamines, 1343–1344
cannabinoids, 1345–1346
cocaine, 1341–1343
opioids, 1344–1345
tobacco/nicotine, 1339–1341
consequences for, 1976–1977
and co-occurring conditions in women, 635–652

Substance use. *See also* Substance use disorders (*Continued*)
epidemiology, 635
interprofessional coordination, 644
management and retention issues, 643–644
preliminary assessment, 645
problem severity, 644
treatment, 643–648
treatment culture, 646–647
treatment manuals, 644–645
cultures, 628–631, 628*t*–629*t*
developmental perspective on etiology, 391
endocrine disorders, 1490–1500
gastrointestinal disorders, 1394–1397
anticholinergics, 1395
body packing, 1397
cannabis, 1396–1397
colon, 1393
esophagus, 1389–1390
gastrointestinal cancer, 1393–1394
laxatives, 1395
opioids, 1394–1395
oral cavity, 1389
pancreas, 1390–1393
parotid glands, 1389
psychostimulants, 1396
small intestine, 1393
stomach, 1390
tobacco, 1395–1396
harm reduction of
drug testing at dance parties, 430
fentanyl test strips, 430
Housing First programs, 432
injectable opioid agonist treatment programs, 431
managed alcohol programs, 431–432
medications, 429
opioid antagonists, 429
overdose prevention online resources, 425*b*
overdose prevention sites, 428–429
overdose risk education and naloxone, 425–426
portable high specificity drug-checking, 431
post-substance use observation sites, 429
pre- and post-HIV exposure prophylaxis, 429–430
safer smoking and sniffing supply programs, 428
virtual spotting, 429
in legal system settings, 1982
military occupational stressors and sexual trauma, 1206–1207
military sexual trauma (MST), 681
patterns of, 630–631
perioperative care
benzodiazepine use disorder, 1538
cannabis, 1539
encephalopathy grade, 1534*t*
nicotine, 1538–1539
opioid use disorders, 1535–1536
stimulant use disorders, 1539
substance use disorders, 1539–1540
unhealthy alcohol use, 1530–1535
during pregnancy, 1509–1524
alcohol and sedatives, 1514–1516
breastfeeding, 1522
cannabis, 1518
labor and delivery, 1521
legal issues, 1522–1523
neonatal abstinence syndromes, 1512–1513
opioids, 1516–1518
postpartum care, 1523–1524
pregnant people, approach to, 1509–1510
screening, 1510–1512
stimulants, 1518–1519
teratogenicity, 1512
tobacco, 1513–1514
treatment and postpartum individual, 1519–1521, 1520*t*, 1521*f*
prevention, 391–392
on family level, 392
on individual level, 392
interventions, 392–396
risk and protective factors, 392
school/community level, 392
pulmonary effects of, 1405–1415
acute and chronic unhealthy alcohol use, 1408–1410
sedative-hypnotics, 1413–1414
smoked (combusted) substance use, 1405–1407
stimulant use, 1412–1413
unhealthy opioid use and injection drug use, 1410–1412
"vaping" and electronic cigarettes, 1407–1408
pulmonary pathophysiology and immunology of, 1402–1405
airway pathophysiology, 1403–1404
central nervous system and respiratory drive, 1402
pulmonary immune function, 1404–1405, 1404*f*
pulmonary vasculature, 1405
quantification of, 55–56
renal and metabolic disorders, 1376–1385
alcohol, 1377–1379
cannabinoids, 1384
inhalants, 1384
injection drug use–related renal disease, 1379–1381
ketamine, 1384
opioids, 1377*t*, 1381
stimulants, 1381–1383
stimulants, renal and metabolic effects of, 1382
substance use, 1376–1385
tobacco use, 1384
social influences among young, 391
special populations, 635–636
traumatic injuries, 1490–1500
trends in, 459
Substance Use
gastrointestinal problems and, 1389–1397
Substance Use Brief Screen (SUBS), 657
Substance use disorder
course, 1834–1835
criteria, 1833
Substance use disorder (SUD), 29–30, 48–49, 64, 256–257, 1085–1086, 1175, 1768–1770
age, 372–373
assessment, 691–692
behavioral, cognitive, and emotional characteristics, 1176*t*
behavioral interventions, 17
chronic care management model
clinical monitoring/management stage, 707–709
clinical stages, 703–704, 703*t*
early identification/intervention stage, 704–706
personal self-management stage, 709–710
stabilization, 706–707
cognitive rehabilitation for, 693–694
community reinforcement approach, 1139–1140
comorbidity of, 1883–1884
continuum of care, 527, 527*t*
co-occurring mood disorders and
behavioral treatments, 1575
bipolar disorders, DSM-5, 1560, 1562*t*
depressive disorders, DSM-5, 1560, 1561*t*
diagnostic criteria, 1559–1565
diagnostic methods, 1569–1570, 1569*t*
differential diagnosis, 1567–1572
DSM-IV and DSM-5, 1560
etiological relationships, 1567, 1568*t*
management, 1572–1583
medication treatments, 1575
predictive validity, 1569–1570, 1569*t*
prevalence, 1565–1567
primary care, 1567
prognostic effects, 1566–1567
psychiatric populations, 1567
significance, 1559–1560
symptoms, 1563–1565, 1564*t*
treatment, 1563
co-occurring mood disorders and group therapies for, 1100–1102
cultural recovery in, 632–633
disordered eating after, 1685–1686
effects of, 1098
epidemiology of, 367–385
functional MRI studies, 1195
harm reduction, 18–19
harms associated with, 690–691
historical perspective, 1128–1129
inhalants, 311
integrated care for, 701–712
medications for, 1580–1581
in military personnel
alcohol use and alcohol use disorder, 456–457
Department of Defense Task Force, 453–454
drug amnesty and rehabilitation, 454–455
drug testing, 455–456
IOM recommendations, 457
policy and leadership, historical perspectives on, 453–455
potential legal issues, 457
Presidential directive, 455
prevalence, 459
tobacco, 457–459
treatment, 459–460
Vietnam experience, 454
motivational interviewing, 1088–1089

degree of ambivalence, 1088–1089
marginalized racial and ethnic backgrounds, patients from, 1089
severity of, 1088
motivational interviewing, as evidence-based approach for, 1088
neurobiological basis for overlap of allostatic states of, 1699
neuromodulation, 17
neuromodulation treatments, 694
opioids and, 1768–1770
organ transplantation, 1539–1540
overview of evidence-based psychotherapies, 1114–1120
pain treatment, 1717, 1717*t*
general effects, 1698–1699
neurobiological interface, 1698
patients with, eating disorders, 1680
pharmacologic interventions for, 694–695
pharmacological interventions, 15–17, 15*t*, 16*f*
prevalence, 687–688
prevalence of, 1883–1884
prevention, 13–14, 14*f*
primary care clinicians, 774–776
psychotherapy, history of, 1107–1108
remission and treatment, 376–377
risk for, 12–13
sedative–hypnotics, 962
technology model, 1108–1111, 1110*t*
therapeutic communities, 1175–1183
motivation, 1176
perspectives, 1175–1176
self-help and mutual self-help, 1176
social learning, 1176
view of disorder, 1175
view of person, 1175–1176
view of recovery, 1176
view of right living, 1176
traumatic brain injury and, 689
treating comorbidities, 17–18, 18*f*
treatment, 14–15, 701–702
treatment approaches, 692–695
treatment programs, 530
women with, 1099–1100, 1891
Substance Use Disorder Clinical Care (SUDCC), 453
Substance use disorder treatment/rehabilitation, 861–862
Substance use disorders (SUDs)
aging process, 653, 655
alcohol–medication interactions, 655
application of, 1067
attention deficit hyperactivity disorder
child and adolescent treatment considerations, 1637
co-occurring psychiatric disorders, 1624–1625
diagnosis of, 1622–1625
difficulties in, 1623–1624
epidemiology of, 1625–1626
genetic, 1627–1628
impact of, 1629
neuroimaging, 1628–1629
neuropsychological testing, 1623
nonstimulant medications, 1632
pharmacotherapeutic options for, 1630–1632
pharmacotherapy selection for, 1632–1636, 1633*t*
possible reasons for linkage of, 1626–1627
prescription stimulants, short *versus* long-acting formulations of, 1631–1632
psychostimulants, nonmedical use potential of, 1631
psychotherapeutic interventions for, 1636
screening instruments, utility of, 1622–1623
stimulant medications, 1630–1631
stratification, 1635*t*
treatment of, 1629–1636
behavioral therapy, 601
cannabis treatment, 1945–1946
in carceral-involved youth
challenges, 1858
interventions for, 1857–1858
screening and assessment, 1856
screening tools, 1856–1857
shared risk factors, 1856
transitional age youth, 1859
youth with, 1856
cognitive-behavioral therapy, 601
community reinforcement approach, 602
community-based treatment for criminal legal populations, 600
comorbid psychiatric disorders, RP and, 1230–1231
complementary interventions, 1052–1063
computer-assisted therapies, 603–604
co-occurring, 1153–1154, 1791–1799
and co-occurring personality disorders, 1643–1657
co-occurring psychosis, 1601–1602, 1613–1615
additional medication decisions, 1612
alcohol use disorders and psychosis, 1605–1606
amphetamines and psychosis, 1608
cannabis and psychosis, 1606–1607
clinical presentation of, 1605–1611
cocaine and psychosis, 1607–1608
differential diagnosis, 1604–1605, 1604*t*
dissociatives and psychosis, 1609
hallucinogens and psychosis, 1608–1609
longer-term management, 1616–1617
management of, 1611–1615
MDMA ("Ecstasy") and psychosis, 1609–1610
multiple substance use and psychosis, 1611
new psychoactive substances and psychosis, 1610–1611
other outpatient treatment approaches, 1615–1616
pharmacological treatment, 1611, 1613–1615
prevalence of, 1601–1603
primary psychotic disorder with, 1602–1603
psychosocial interventions, 1612–1615
substances and antipsychotic medications, 1612
criminal legal settings, 600
digital health interventions for, 1250–1259
digital therapeutics for, 1251–1252
evolution of, 1250–1251
future opportunities and responsible digital health, 1257–1259
integration into practice, 1257
mobile applications or websites reviews with guided components, 1254–1255
mobile applications/apps/stand-alone websites, 1252–1255
newer digital technologies, 1255–1257
telehealth, 1255
effective screening and identification of, 1201
family history density, 1201
evidence-based couple and family treatments for, 1201–1202
community reinforcement and family training, 1202
inpatient treatment, engaging family members during, 1201–1202
motivational interviewing, 1201
individualized counseling, 602–603
integrative interventions, 1052–1063
longitudinal studies, 1219
motivational enhancement therapy, 601
multidimensional family therapy, 603
multiple, pharmacological interventions, 1045–1051
multisystemic therapy, 603
neuromodulation for, 1064–1070
for addiction, 1066–1070
addiction, brain regions, 1064–1066
focused ultrasound, 1069–1070
transcranial direct current stimulation, 1069
transcranial magnetic stimulation for, 1066–1069
in older adults, 653–665
alcohol and prescription medications, 656–657
alcohol in social settings, 657
chronic pain, 656
cognitive impairment, 656
comorbidity, 656
co-occurring disorders, 656
issues, 655–657
metabolic changes, 655
pharmacotherapy, 660–662
prevention of return to use, 662
recovery support, 662
sleep problems, 656
suicidality, 656
treatment outcome research, limitations of, 660
pharmacologic therapies, 604–605
posttraumatic stress disorder (PTSD), 1660
assessment of, 1661–1663
etiological relationship, 1660
neurobiological factors in co-occurring, 1660–1661
prison-based treatment programs, 600
psychotherapies, 602–603
and suicide, 1726
risk assessment, 1728–1729
treatment, 512, 594–608
acute pain, 1794
acute-on-chronic pain, 1794
chronic pain, 1795–1796
clinical monitoring, 600
delivery system, 594–598

Substance use disorders (SUDs) (*Continued*)
- frequent emergency department visits, 1795
- goals of, 594, 595*t*–596*t*
- intoxication management, 600–601
- opioid agonist therapy, patients, 1794–1796
- in outpatient office, 599–600
- pain, 1794–1797
- pharmacologic and psychosocial, 594
- rewarding medications, 1796–1797
- screening and brief intervention, 599–600
- services, 600–604
- withdrawal management, 600–601

trends in, 459
voucher-based reinforcement therapy, 602
- day treatment with abstinence contingencies, 602
- in methadone treatment, 602

Substance use during pregnancy, 750
Substance use. *See also* Substance use disorders
- adolescents, 1811
- history of alcohol use, 1817

Substance use services, reducing disparities, 1982–1987
Substance use-related care, interprofessional collaborative practice, 713–724
Substance use-related consequences, in women, 636–638
Substance use–related risks, 726
Substance withdrawal, 1513
Substance-associated suicidal behavior (SASB), 1548–1549
Substance-induced anxiety disorder (SIAD), 1547
Substance-induced bipolar disorder (SIBD), 1545, 1547
Substance-induced depressive disorder (SIDD), 1545–1547
- alcohol and, 1546
- opioids and, 1547
- stimulants and, 1546

Substance-induced mental disorders (SIMD), 1545
- diagnosis, 1545–1546, 1551
- prevalence and course of, 1546–1549
  - substance-associated suicidal behavior, 1548–1549
  - substance-induced anxiety disorder, 1547
  - substance-induced bipolar and related disorder, 1547
  - substance-induced depressive disorder, 1546–1547
  - substance-induced neurocognitive disorder, 1548
  - substance-induced psychotic disorders, 1547
  - substance/medication-induced obsessive-compulsive and related disorders, 1548
- substance-induced symptoms, 1549–1551
- treatment of, 1551–1556
  - diagnostic considerations, 1552–1555
  - treatment considerations, 1552–1556
  - treatment issues, 1554

Substance-induced neurocognitive disorder, 1885
Substance-induced neurocognitive disorder (SINCD), 1548
Substance-induced obsessive-compulsive disorders (SIOCD), 1545, 1548
Substance-induced psychosis, 1601–1602
- clinical presentation of, 1605–1611
  - alcohol use disorders and psychosis, 1605–1606
  - amphetamines and psychosis, 1608
  - cannabis and psychosis, 1606–1607
  - cocaine and psychosis, 1607–1608
  - dissociatives and psychosis, 1609
  - hallucinogens and psychosis, 1608–1609
  - MDMA ("Ecstasy") and psychosis, 1609–1610
  - multiple substance use and psychosis, 1611
  - new psychoactive substances and psychosis, 1610–1611

Substance-induced psychotic disorders (SIPD), 1547
Substance-induced seizures, 1427
Substance/medication-induced anxiety disorder (SIAD), 1590*t*
Substance/medication-induced obsessive-compulsive disorders (SIOCD), 1548
Substance-Related and Addictive Disorders module of the Structured Clinical Interview for DSM-5 (SCID-5), 530
Substances
- adolescent use, 1829
- interviewing adolescents, 1811–1812
- signs, 1815*t*

Substances, psychoactive, 1887
Substance-use-related pregnancy-associated deaths, 1523
Substance-using populations
- ADHD screening instruments in, 1622–1623
- difficulties, in diagnosing adult ADHD, 1623–1624
  - overdiagnosis, potential reasons for, 1624
  - underdiagnosis, potential reasons for, 1623–1624

Substitution and taper, benzodiazepine cessation, 899–900, 899*t*
Substitution Dose Conversion, 899, 899*t*
Subthreshold exposure, 1512
Sudden infant death syndrome (SIDS), 1514
SUDs. *See* Substance use disorders (SUDs)
Sufentanil
- OIH, 1702
- physician addiction, 555
- screens, 563–564

Suicidal behavior, depression, 1577
Suicidal ideation, 1730
- pain coping, 1728
- pain intensity, 1727–1728
- pain type for, 1727
- prevalence of, 1726
- risk factors for, 1726
- sleep disturbance, 1727
- substance use disorders, 1727

Suicide, 1483
- and chronic pain, 1726
  - coping, 1728
  - opioid dosing, 1728
  - pain intensity, 1727–1728
  - pain type, 1727
  - risk factors, 1727–1728
  - sleep disturbance, 1727
- mitigation strategies, 1729
  - risk stratification, 1729
  - treatment options, 1729
- risk assessment, 1728–1729
  - mental health screening, 1728
  - screening tools for, 1729
  - sleep disturbance, 1728
- and substance use disorders, 1726
  - risk assessment, 1728–1729
  - risk factors, 1727–1728

Suicide, alcohol use, 400
Suicide Assessment Five-Step Evaluation and Triage (SAFE-T) assessment tool, 1729
Sulfonylureas, AOD, 1491
Summaries, 1086
Supervised injection facilities (SIFs), 428
Support group attendance, abstinence *vs.*, alcohol urges, 1194*t*
Support programs, after aversion therapy, 1194
Supportive-expressive therapy, 1115–1116
Surreptitious laxative, 1395
Survival and ventricular enlargement (SAVE), 1337–1338
Sustained virologic response (SVR), 1367
Sweat testing, 517
Swedish Twin Registry, 1339
Sweep testing, Navy's program, 455
Sweetser, William, 581
Symptom Checklist-90-Revised (SCL-90-R), 1130*t*
Symptom recurrence, benzodiazepines and, 891
Symptom-triggered therapy, 878
Synaptic plasticity, drug addiction, 11
Syndemic, 668
Synesthesia, 1608
Synthetic cannabinoids, 250, 1346, 1384, 1426, 1938
- substance-induced mental disorders, 1551
- substance-induced psychosis, 1610

Synthetic cathinones, 357, 1551
- substance use disorder with co-occurring psychosis, 1614

Synthetic marijuana, substance-induced psychosis, 1610
Syphilis, 1436–1437
Syringe service programs (SSPs), 418, 426–428
Systematic discontinuation, benzodiazepine cessation, 898–899
Systems of care, gathering data, 732–733, 733*t*

T

$t_{1/2}$. *See* Drug half-life ($t_{1/2}$)
Tabes dorsalis, 1436–1437
Tabletop vaporizers, 349–350
T-ACE questionnaire, pregnant women, drinking and, 497
Tachypnea, 1325, 1414
Tactile hallucinations, 871
Take-back programs, 414–415
Talc, 1411
Talwin. *See* Pentazocine
Transmission, chronic nociceptive pain and, 1692
Tapering
- benzodiazepine cessation, 899
- opioid therapy, 1777–1779

Tapering/discontinuing medication therapy, 1919–1921
Taste aversion, principles of, aversion therapies, 1190
TAU (treatment-as-usual) group, 50–51
TBI. *See* Traumatic brain injury (TBI)
TCAs. *See* Tricyclic antidepressants
TCs. *See* Therapeutic communities (TCs)
TEAS. *See* Transcutaneous electrical acupuncture stimulation (TEAS)
Telehealth, 1255
 DATA-waived providers, 782*f*
 federal and state regulatory requirements and decisions, 784–785
 implementation, challenges and barriers, 784
 patient acceptability, satisfaction, and outcomes, 782–783
 provider receptivity and satisfaction, 783–784
 recovery support services access barriers, 780, 782*f*
 research on the effectiveness and benefits, 782–784, 783*t*
 SUD-related services
  during COVID-19 pandemic, 781
  prior to COVID-19 pandemic, 780–781
Telemedicine, 1123, 1255
Telephone counseling, 1156
Temazepam (Restoril), 962*t*, 963–964
 benzodiazepines, 166*t*, 169
 disorders related to, 1499
 medical complications, 173
Temperament
 ASAM, 1846
Tennessee Recovery Navigators, 599
Tenofovir alafenamide (TAF), 1363
Tenofovir disoproxil fumarate, 1456
Tenofovir disoproxil fumarate (TDF), 1363
TENS. *See* Transcutaneous electrical nerve stimulation (TENS)
Teratogen, 1512
Teratogenicity, pregnancy, substance use during, 1512
Termination stage, 1075
Terry, C., research studies, addiction-related, 585
Tertiary gain, as pain, 1715–1716
Testosterone, 317
 marijuana and, 1497
 mechanisms of action, 330
 testicular size and, 325
Testosterone and Pain (TAP), 1496
Tetanus, 1436, 1452–1453
Tetrahydrocannabinol (THC), 523, 1330–1331, 1345, 1408
 substance-induced mental disorders, 1550
Tetrahydroquinolines (TIQs), 156
Text messaging interventions, TUD, 1156
TGF-β1, 1357
THC. *See* Δ^9-tetrahydrocannabinol (THC)
THCV (tetrahydrocannabivarin), 1937–1938
The Addiction Medicine Foundation (TAMF), 589
The American Psychiatric Association's Climate Psychiatry Alliance, 86
The Drug Abuse Warning Network (DAWN), 181–182
The Drug Taking Confidence Questionnaire, 533
The Human Intervention Motivational Study (HIMS) program, 545
The International Classification of Sleep Disorders, Revised (ICSD-3), 1465
The Pain, Enjoyment of Life and General Activity (PEG) scale, 1918
The Population Assessment of Tobacco and Health (PATH) study
 substance use disorders, 369
Thebaine, 178–179
Theory of change, 850
Therapeutic alliance, 1245
Therapeutic communities (TCs), 598–600, 1270
 community-as-method, 1176
 modified
  continuity of care, 1186–1187
  co-occurring disorders, 1183–1187
  interventions, 1184
  medically integrated therapeutic community, 1187
  mental and substance use disorders, 1183–1187
  other modifications, 1183–1184
  outcomes, 1184
  outpatient models, 1186–1187
  principles and methods, 1183
  residential aftercare models, 1186
 research, 1184–1186, 1186*f*
 therapeutic–educative activities (*see* Groups-counseling)
 traditional
  applications, 1182–1183
  clinical management elements, 1178–1179
  community enhancement activities, 1178
  disciplinary sanctions, 1179
  effectiveness, 1181–1182
  evolution, 1182–1183
  in human services, 1182–1183
  methods, 1177–1179
  modifications, 1182–1183
  peers as role models, 1177
  program model, 1177
  program stages and phases, 1179–1180
  residential TC treatment, 1180–1181
  staff as rational authorities, 1177
  structure/social organization, 1177
  traditional, 1175–1183
 work as education and therapy, 1177
 worldwide, 1182
Therapeutic Education System (TES), 1251
Therapeutic index, 138
Therapeutic interventions, addiction practice, 1898
Therapeutic–educative activities, 1184. *See also* Groups-counseling
Therapist
 characteristics
  CRA and, 1131
  pretreatment issues and, 1215–1216
 therapeutic skills of, 1215–1216
 TSF and, 1214
Thiamine, 881
Thiamine deficiency, 1393
Thirdhand smoke, 244
Third-party payer, patient permission and, 1901
"Throat hit," electronic drug delivery devices, 338
Throat medical care of patients, with unhealthy substance use, 1315
Thrombocytopenia, 1326
Thromboembolic disorders, 17-alkylated androgens, 325
Thrombotic microangiopathic anemia (TMA), 1381
Thyroid disease, 1494
TikTok, 1256
Timing, sleep-wake circadian rhythm, 1475
TIP. *See* Treatment improvement protocol (TIP)
TIQs (tetrahydroquinolines), 156
Tizanidine, neural injury, 1755
TJC (The Joint Commission), 771
Tobacco, 230–247, 1047
 addiction, 236–237
 adherence to, 1035
 and alcohol, 1047
 depression, 1577–1578
 drug interactions with, 234–235
 exposure to, biochemical assessment of, 234
 gastrointestinal symptoms associated with drugs, 1395–1396
  gastro-esophageal reflux, 1395
  gastrointestinal malignancy, 1396
  inflammatory bowel disease, 1395–1396
  pancreatic disease, 1395
  peptic ulceration, 1395
 headache, 1423
 infants, 244
 LGBTQ, 672
 mortality, 244
 movement disorders, 1435
 and opioids, 1047
 other addictions and, 244–245
 physician addiction, 555
 pregnancy, 243–244
 pregnancy, substance use during, 1513–1514
 pregnant women, 472–473
 related disorders, 1494–1495
 and stimulants, 1047
 stroke, 1429–1430
 withdrawal, 237
Tobacco cessation, pharmacological intervention for, 476
Tobacco cessation, treatment and technique, 1148–1151
Tobacco Control Act, 98
Tobacco dependence
 monoamine oxidase, 242
 treatment, 1595
Tobacco problems, addressing and co-occurring, 1155
Tobacco products
 with anxiety disorder, treatment, 1594–1595
 design, 90–92
 history of, 92*f*
Tobacco smoke
 gaseous components of, 242–243
 lung and, 260
 particulate components of, 242–243
 pulmonary immune function, 1404
 systemic toxicity, 242–245
Tobacco smoking, climate change and, 79–82, 82*f*–83*f*

Tobacco use
  adolescents, prevalence rates and progression, 390–391
  behavioral treatment, 1145–1146
  complications related to, 1327–1328
    cardiovascular, 1327
    endocrinologic, 1328
    fetal, neonatal, and infant, 1328
    gastrointestinal, 1327
    infections, 1328
    injury, 1328
    neurologic, 1328
    oncologic, 1328
    perioperative, 1328
    renal, 1327
    respiratory, 1327–1328
    sleep, 1328
  renal and metabolic effects of, 1384
  treatment planning, 1146–1148, 1147*f*
Tobacco use disorder (TUD)
  acceptance and commitment and mind–body therapies, 1156
  aversion therapies, 1192
  causes, 1037–1038
  definition, 89
  development, novel treatment approach in, 1152, 1156
  diagnostic criteria, 89
  economic realities, 100–101
  intensive interventions for, 1152
    contingency management, 1152
  intervention delivery, novel methods of, 1156
  mass marketing, 93–94, 94*f*
  MBI, 1238
  mood altering effects, 89
  neurobiology, 1030–1031
  nicotine, 89
  persistent cultural attitudes, 1031
  pharmacologic actions, 1030–1044
  pharmacotherapies, 1032–1034
    metabolism rate, 1035–1036
    optimizing methods, 1036
  prevalence, 1031
  primary psychotic disorder with co-occurring substance use disorder, 1603
  systematically excluded populations, treatment considerations for, 1152–1155
    individuals with co-occurring substance use disorders, 1153–1154
    population subgroups, 1153
    psychiatric populations, 1154–1155
    racial and ethnic subgroups, 1152–1153
  tobacco cigarette industry contributions to, 89–101
  tobacco product design, 90–92
  treatments, 1037–1038, 1595
    access and utilization, 1038
  withdrawal, 1037–1038
Tobacco use disorders, 370
Tobaccoism, 1144
Tobacco/nicotine
  cardiovascular disorders, substance use, 1339–1341
    arrythmia, 1339
    coronary artery disease, 1339–1340
    Electronic Drug Delivery Devices, 1340–1341
    hemodynamic effects, 1339
  pharmacotherapy, adolescent SUDs, 1871–1873
    bupropion, 1872–1873
    nicotine replacement therapy, 1872
    varenicline, 1873
Tobacco-related disparities, 1038
Tolerance
  AAS, 328
  addiction liability and, 158
  American Academy of Pain Medicine, 1765
  caffeine, 222, 224
  cannabinoid, 257–258
  definition of, 962
  development, 187
  inhalants, 312
  opioid-induced hyperalgesia, 1700
  short-acting opioids, 187
  stimulants and, 210
  SUDs, 1703
Toluene, 308–309, 312, 1426–1427
Topical agents, continuous pain, 1754
Topical NSAID, neuropathic pain, 1749
Topiramate (Topamax), 951–952, 1359
  alcohol, adolescent SUDs, 1874
  alcohol use disorder, 951–952
  BED with comorbid addiction, 1683
  cannabis, adolescent SUDs, 1875
Torrance, E., research studies, addiction-related, 585
Torsades de Pointes, 1345
Torsades de pointes syndrome, levorphanol, 1770–1772
Toxic alcohols, 1378–1379
  metabolic disorders
    ethylene glycol, 1378–1379
    isopropyl alcohol, 1379
Toxic oxidative metabolites, 1369
Toxicity, 111
  from coinjected materials, 1370
Toxicity states, medical management of, 187–188
Toxicology
  long-term opioid use, 1768
  written agreement, 1906
Toxin, 1452
Tracking, digital technologies, 1256–1257
Traditional cigarettes (TCs), 337, 339, 344
Traditional therapeutic communities (TCs), 1175–1183
  applications, 1182–1183
    to special populations, 1182
  clinical management elements, privileges, 1179
  community enhancement activities, 1178–1179
  community-as-method, 1176–1177
  disciplinary sanctions, 1179
    peer confrontation/verbal affirmations and correctives, 1179
    surveillance, 1179
  effectiveness, 1181–1182
  evolution, 1182–1183
  in human services, 1182–1183
  methods, 1177–1179
  modifications, 1182–1183
  modified
    co-occurring disorders, 1183–1187
    mental and substance use disorders, 1183–1187
    principles and methods, 1183
  peers as role models, 1177
  perspectives, 1175–1176
  program model, 1177
  program stages and phases, 1179–1180
    aftercare, 1180
    graduation, 1180
    orientation–induction (0–60 days), 1180
    primary treatment (2–12 months), 1180
    reentry (13–24 months), 1180
  residential TC treatment, 1180–1181
  staff as rational authorities, 1177
  structure/social organization, 1177
  therapeutic–educative activities (*see* Groups-counseling)
  traditional, 1175–1176
Traffic crashes, alcohol-related, 399
Training drugs, animal models, 42
Trajectory analyses, drinking measuring method, 613
Tramadol, 916, 1428
  pain treatment, limitations, 1763
  physician addiction, 556
Transcranial direct current stimulation (tDCS), 1069
Transcranial magnetic stimulation (TMS), 694, 1660–1661
  for addiction, 1066–1069
    with cognitive therapy, 1068–1069
    to DLPFC, 1067
    dopamine, effects of, 1066–1067
    as intervention, 1069
    to MPFC, 1067–1068, 1068*f*
    and pharmacotherapy, 1069
    repetitive TMS, 1066
    SUDs, application of, 1067
Transcutaneous electrical acupoint stimulation (TEAS), 1056
Transcutaneous electrical acupuncture
  opioid withdrawal management with, 1056–1058
    animal studies, 1056
    human studies, 1056
    multiple daily treatment, 1057–1058
    single treatment, 1056–1057
  for unhealthy alcohol and substance use, 1055–1056
Transcutaneous electrical nerve stimulation (TENS), 1740, 1741*t*, 1743
  iontophoresis, 1743–1744
  pain management, 1743
  precautions and contraindications, 1743
Transdermal nicotine patch, 1033
Transduction, chronic nociceptive pain and, 1692
Transfer/Discharge Criteria, 729
Transference-focused psychotherapy (TFP), 1649–1650
Transient elastography (TE), 1358
Transient ischemic attacks (TIAs), 1431
Transient paranoia, 1607–1608

Transient receptor potential vanilloid-1 receptor (TRPV-1), 1396–1397
Transitional age youth, 1839
Transitional age youth (TAY), 1859
Transjugular intrahepatic portosystemic shunt (TIPS), 1410
7-transmembrane-domain G-protein coupled receptors (GPCRs), 253
Transporter blockers, 204, 205*f*
Transporter substrates, 204, 205*f*
Trauma
  adolescents, 1887
  alcohol use, medical complications related to, 1326
  fibromyalgia, 1696
  informed assessment, 526–527
  neurological disorders, 1420–1422
Trauma-Informed Guilt Reduction Therapy (TriGR), 1666
Trauma-informed systems and interventions, 646
Trauma-related difficulties, 645–646
Traumatic brain injury (TBI)
  animal models, 686–687
  assessment, 687, 691–692
  classification, 686, 686*t*
  cognitive rehabilitation for, 692–694
  definition, 685–687
  diagnosis, 686–687
  dopaminergic agonist treatment, 688–689
  epidemiology, 687
  factors, 689, 695
  harms associated with, 690–691
  high-impact sports, 687
  in military populations, 686–687
  neurocircuitry, 688
  neurological disorders, 1420–1422
  neuromodulation treatments, 694
  pharmacologic interventions for, 694–695
  prevalence, 687–688
  risk factors, 688–690
  and substance use disorders, 689
  treatment approaches, 692–695
Traumatic event, 1658–1659
Traumatic injuries
  alcohol and other drug use, 1482–1486
  alcohol, other drugs and, 1484–1485
  special considerations, 1485–1486
    COVID-19-related alcohol, other drug use and injury issues, 1485
    electronic cigarette use and injuries, 1485
    excited delirium, 1485–1486
  substance use, 1490–1500
Trazodone, 903
  benzodiazepine withdrawal, 903
Treatment, 1591–1592. *See also* Pretreatment
  AAS, 329
  ASAM, 1844
  choice of, 1130
  compliance, 1137–1138, 1292
  co-occurrence SUDs, 1682
  detoxification *vs.*, 862
  GAD, 1593
  groups of, 725, 1095
  individualized plan, 727
  levels, choice of, 727
  matching, evolving approaches, 734
  modalities, adolescent substance abuse, 1120–1121
  models, 1129, 1145, 1213–1214
  outcomes
    ASAM criteria, 1844
    prediction of, 1297–1298
    relapse rates and, 1220–1221
  physician addiction, 559–561
  plan, 1129–1130
    consent to, 1905
    SUDs and, 1129
  programs
    pregnant women, 472–473
    proposed plan, 1916–1917
  rehabilitation, withdrawal and, 861–862
  retention, OBOT, 1003–1006
  SAD, 1593
  settings, sedative–hypnotics withdrawal, 963–966
  tobacco/nicotine, 1595
  of unhealthy alcohol use, 610
Treatment adherence
  behavioral interventions and, 1272–1274
  measures, 58
Treatment as prevention (TasP), 666–667
Treatment Episode Data Set (TEDS), 181–182
Treatment improvement protocols (TIPs), 775, 884, 1170, 1205
Treatment-naive hepatitis B, current first-line therapies for, 1363
Treatment-resistant persons, CRA and, 1139–1140
Trental. *See* Pentoxifylline
Triamterene, 318
Triazolam (Halcion), 166*t*, 889, 899*t*, 962*t*, 964*t*, 965, 1499
Triazolobenzodiazepines
  sedative–hypnotics withdrawal, 965
  withdrawal, 965
Trichloroethane, 312
Tricyclic antidepressants (TCAs)
  attention deficit hyperactivity disorder, 1632
  neuropathic pain, 1749–1750
  for PTSD, 1669
  stimulant use disorders, 1016
Trigger point injections, 1737
Triggers, eating disorders, 1684
Triglyceride synthesis, 1493
Tropic spastic araparesis (TSP), 1437
Troponin, 1342
Trotter, Thomas, 581
Tryptophan hydroxylase 2 (TPH2), 1627–1628
TSF. *See* Twelve step facilitation (TSF)
TTM (transtheoretical model), 1075, 1081–1082
T-total pledge, 582
Tuberculosis, 1325
  alcohol/drug use, 1444
  host defenses, 1444–1445
  respiratory infections, 1449–1450
Tuberculous peritonitis, 1451. *See also* Spontaneous bacterial peritonitis
Tumors
  alcohol, 158–159
  morphine and, 40
Turner, J., 584
TWEAK questionnaire, pregnant women, 497
Tweaking, 1550
Twelve Promises, 1289
Twelve step facilitation (TSF), 1222
  AA, 1295–1296
  approaches, 1213–1217
  CBT *vs.*, 948, 1215, 1267, 1286
  features of, 1214
  historical perspective, 1213
  indications for treatment, 1215
  individual psychotherapy, 1118–1119
  integrated therapy approach *vs.*, alcohol use outcomes, 1101
  pretreatment issues
    motivation, 1215
    therapist characteristics, 1215–1216
  referral to, clinician role and, 1285–1286
  relevant research, 1216–1217
  RP and, 1222
  summary and conclusions, 1217
  theory of change, 1214
  treatment
    indications, 1215
    models, 1213–1214
    planning and evaluation, 1214–1215
Twelve step-oriented treatment, 1297
Twelve-step community support groups, 616–617
Twelve-step facilitation, 611
Twelve-step groups, recovery. *See* Twelve-step programs
Twelve-step programs, 1108, 1215, 1230–1231, 1279–1287, 1289
  adolescent substance abuse, 1293–1294
  benefits of, 1286
  clinician facilitation of, 1285–1286
  effective, 1286–1287
  integration of, 1287, 1311
  naturalistic studies of treatments based on, 1297
  practical information and advice on, 1285–1286
  principles, 1297
  research, 1279–1287, 1289–1303
Twin studies, 789
Twitter, 1256
Two-phase model, sleep rhythms, 1464

U

U-47700, 357, 911
Uber Coca, 197
UCSA (Uniform Controlled Substances Act), 1930
UDT (urine drug testing), 1780–1781
Ulcerative colitis (UC), 1395–1396
Ultrarapid opioids, anesthesia assisted, 916
Ultrasound-based transient elastography, 1362–1363
Unbundled treatment, 735
Unbundling, 735
Uncaria rhynchophylla, structure of, 1054, 1054*f*
Uncomplicated substitution and taper, benzodiazepine cessation, 900
Underage drinking, 400–403
Unemployed patients, CRA plus vouchers treatment, 1132
Ungated protocols, 369–370

Unhealthy alcohol and drug use
acute and chronic, 1408–1410
acute metabolic acidosis and respiratory alkalosis, 1409
acute respiratory distress syndrome, 1409–1410
alcohol-related liver disease, respiratory complications from, 1410
aspiration syndromes, 1408–1409
asthma, 1409
pneumonia, 1409
sleep-disordered breathing, 1409
in older adults, screening
brief interventions, 512
diagnosis, 511–512
epidemiology, 510, 510*t*
screening tools, 511
self-administered screening approaches, 511
unique vulnerabilities, 510–511
perioperative care, 1530–1535
alcohol withdrawal, 1531–1532
alcohol-associated liver disease, 1532–1534
naltrexone pharmacotherapy, 1535
preoperative evaluation, 1531
surgical risk, 1532
primary, secondary, and tertiary prevention, 387, 387*t*
spectrum of severity in, 610
Unhealthy opioid use
and injection drug use, 1410–1412
emphysema, 1412
foreign body granulomatosis, 1411
pneumonia, 1410
pulmonary edema, 1410–1411
pulmonary hypertension, 1411–1412
septic pulmonary emboli, 1411
Unhealthy prescription medication use and opioid treatment, 638
Unhealthy substance use, 64–66, 77–78
medical care of patients with, 1314–1332
Uniform Controlled Substances Act (“UCSA”), 1930
Unintentional injury, 1482–1483
alcohol- and motor vehicle–related injuries and fatalities, 1482–1483
alcohol- and non–motor vehicle-related injuries and fatalities, 1483
alcohol use and interpersonal violence, 1483
Unipolar depression, antidepressants, alcohol use disorder and, 955–956
United Nations Office on Drugs and Crime (UNODC), 776, 1551, 1610
United States Controlled Substances Act, 1551
United States Medical Licensing Examination (USMLE), 1710
United States Pharmacopeia (USP), 92
United States Preventative Task Force, 1872
United States Preventive Services Task Force, 1406
United States (US), standard drink in, 610, 610*t*
Universal alcohol prevention programs, metaanalyses of, adolescents, 394
“Universal” prevention tactics, 388
Unmarried subjects, CRA plus disulfiram, abstinence and, 1138
Urinalysis, adolescent drug use, 1834
Urinary calcium, 224
Urinary incontinence, caffeine and, 224
Urine
alkalization, phenobarbital, 889–890
drug screens, 897
drug testing, 1963
immunoassays, 517*t*
opioid overdose, 909
PHPs, 563–564
samples, detection times for drugs and alcohol, 56*t*
testing, 515–516, 516*t*, 1003, 1179
amphetamines, 520
cannabis, 523
cocaine, 520–521
patient permission and, 1901
Urine drug testing (UDT), 1780–1781
Urine toxicology, 910
U.S. addiction treatment system, 624
U.S. Controlled Substances Act, 1761–1762
U.S. Current Population Survey-Tobacco Use Supplement (CPS-TUS), 347–348
U.S. Department of Health and Human Services, 1872
U.S. Department of Veterans Affairs, 29
U.S. Drug Enforcement Administration, 1000
U.S. Drug-Free Workplace Act, 544
U.S. Food and Drug Administration (FDA), 1001, 1611
U.S. Harrison Narcotics Act, 409
U.S. National Certification Commission of Addiction Professionals (NCCAP), 776
U.S. National Institute on Alcohol Abuse and Alcoholism (NIAAA), 1321
US “war on drugs,” 1971, 591
USPSTF (U.S. Preventive Services Task Force), 472–473, 511
Utilization
AA, 1303
ASAM, 1847–1848

V

Vaccination
hepatitis A and B, 1367
influenza, 1450
Valproic acid, 1751
bipolar disorder, adolescents, 1886–1887
Valve surgery, for endocarditis, 1540
Valvular heart disease, amphetamines, cardiovascular disorders, 1344
Vaping, 1871–1872
"Vaping" cigarettes, 1407–1408
Vapor chemicals, 1404
Varenicline, 954, 1034, 1047, 1149
tobacco/nicotine, adolescent SUDs, 1873
Variable-centered analyses, drinking measuring method, 613
Varicella vaccine, immunizations, 1319
Vasculitis, 1431–1432
Vd (volume of distribution), drug distribution, 130
Vegetable glycerin, electronic drug delivery devices, 338
Venlafaxine
depression with comorbid pain syndromes, 1750
peripheral neuropathy, 1750
for PTSD, 1668–1669
Venlafaxine XR, GAD, 1592
Ventral cingulate cortex, 37
Ventral striatum, 36–37
beta-FNA, 41
dorsal striatum, 36–37, 36*f*
Ventral tegmental area (VTA), 1031
Ventromedial areas, 36
Ventromedial prefrontal cortex (vmPFC), 790
Vertebral osteomyelitis, 1451
Vertical transmission, 1364
Veterans Administration Cooperative Studies Group, disulfiram, 950–951
Veterans Affairs (VA), 680
health care system, 683
Medical Centers, 681
VHA (Veterans Health Administration), 769
Vibrio vulnificus, IDUs and, 1446
Vicodin. *See* Hydrocodone
Vietnam Twin Era Registry, 789
Vigabatrin, alcohol withdrawal, 880
Violence, traumatic brain injury, 690
Violent injuries, other drug use and, 1484
Viral hepatitis, 1000, 1360–1364, 1451
hepatic toxicity associated with other drug use, 1368–1370
agents, 1369–1370
androgenic/anabolic steroids, 1370
cannabis, 1370
cocaine and stimulants, 1368–1369
coinjected materials, toxicity from, 1370
opioids, 1370
hepatitis A, 1360–1361
hepatitis B, 1361–1363
hepatitis C virus, 1363–1364
hepatitis D, 1368
Virtual reality (VR), 1257
Virtual spotting, 429
Virtual therapy, 1123
Visual analogue scale (VAS), 854, 1059–1060
Visual Analogue Scale for Opioid Craving, 774
Visual hallucinations, 1607–1608
alcohol withdrawal and, 871
Vitamin deficiencies
alcohol use, medical complications related to, 1327
cannabinoids, 1331
Vitamins, 881
Vivitrol. *See* Naltrexone
VOCs (volatile organic compounds), electronic drug delivery devices, 340–341
Volatile alkyl nitrites, 308–309, 309*t*
Volatile anesthetics, 308–309, 309*t*
Volatile organic compounds (VOCs), 340–341
Volatile solvents, 308–309, 309*t*
Volatile substances, 1414–1415
Voltage-gated ion channels, 159–160
Volume repletion, AWS, 876
Volunteer treatment, coercion *vs.*, addiction treatments and, 1897–1898
Voucher-based contingency management
CBT *vs.*, CBT/CM combination *vs.*, 1223
illicit drug use disorders, 1138
Voucher-based reinforcement therapy, 602
day treatment with abstinence contingencies, 602
in methadone treatment, 602